# CONGRATULATIONS

## You now have access to Mosby's "Get Connected" Bonus Package!

### Here's what's included to help you "Get Connected"

**sign on at:**

http://www.mosby.com/MERLIN/Dictionary

A Website just for you with the new 6th edition of **Mosby's Medical, Nursing, & Allied Health Dictionary**

**what you will receive:**

Whether you're a student, an instructor, or a clinician, you'll find information just for you. Things like:
- Content Updates
- Links to Related Products
- Activities
- Consultant Information . . . and more

**plus:**

 WebLinks

An exciting new program that allows you to directly access hundreds of active websites keyed specifically to the content of this book. The WebLinks are continually updated, with new ones added as they develop.

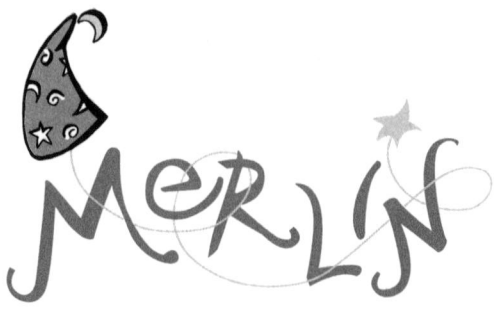

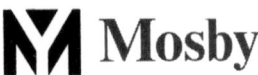 Mosby

Mosby's Electronic Resource Links & Information Network

# MOSBY'S
## MEDICAL, NURSING,
## & ALLIED HEALTH
# DICTIONARY

# MOSBY'S
## MEDICAL, NURSING, & ALLIED HEALTH
# DICTIONARY

**SIXTH EDITION**

Illustrated in full color throughout
With Over 2200 Illustrations

*Chief Lexicographer*
Douglas M. Anderson, MA

*Lexicographers*
Jeff Keith, MA
Patricia D. Novak, PhD

*Lexicographic Coordinator*
Michelle A. Elliot, BA

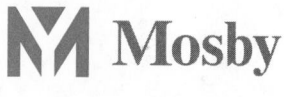

Mosby

*An Affiliate of Elsevier*

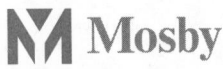

*An Affiliate of Elsevier*

*Vice President, Publishing Director:* Sally Schrefer
*Executive Editor, Nursing:* Darlene Como
*Developmental Editor:* Tamara A. Myers
*Project Manager:* Pat Joiner
*Manager, Intellectual Property Resources:* Tripp Narup
*Designer:* Mark A. Oberkrom
*Permission Assistant:* Allen K. Berry

*Cover illustrations:*
**Cardiac nuclear scanning** from Cannobio MM:
  *Cardiovascular disorders,* St. Louis, 1990, Mosby.
**Chromobacteriosis** from Baron EJ, Peterson LR, Finegold SM:
  *Bailey and Scott's diagnostic microbiology,* ed 9, St. Louis,
  1994, Mosby.
**Cryosurgery** from Jaffe ND: *Atlas of ophthalmic surgery,* ed 2,
  St. Louis, 1996, Mosby.
**Duodenal ulcer** from Seidel HM, Benedict GW, Ball JW, and
  Dains JE: *Mosby's guide to physical examination,* ed 4,
  St. Louis, 1999, Mosby.
**Fluorescent antibody test** from Baron EJ, Peterson LR,
  Finegold SM: *Bailey and Scott's diagnostic microbiology,*
  ed 9, St. Louis, 1994, Mosby.
**Single-photon emission computed tomography** from Chipps EM,
  Clanin NJ, Campbell VG: *Neurologic disorders,* St. Louis,
  1992, Mosby.

Mosby
*An Affiliate of Elsevier*
11830 Westline Industrial Drive
St. Louis, Missouri 63146

Printed in the United States of America

**International Standard Book Numbers**

0-323-03736-4 (professional)
0-723-43225-2 (UK)
Revised Reprint
05  06  07  08  09  CL/VER  9  8  7  6  5  4  3  2  1

# CONTENTS

# DEDICATION

*This edition is dedicated to Kenneth N. Anderson (1921-2001), a fine lexicographer and an extraordinary individual.*

# STAFF

**Chief Lexicographer:**
Douglas M. Anderson

**Lexicographers:**
Jeff Keith, Patricia D. Novak

**Lexicographic Coordinator:**
Michelle A. Elliot

**Editorial Consultants:**
Terry Eynon, Dana L. Knighten, Carolyn Kruse, Matt T. Lee,
Jeffrey M. Downing, Laurie Sparks

**Programing and Composition by:**
The Clarinda Company

**Artists and Photographers:**
Michael Abbey, Peter Arnold, Molly Babich, Ernest W. Beck,
Joan M. Beck, Scott Bodell, G. David Brown, Rob Callantine, Lisa Chuck,
Terry Cockerham, Barbara Cousins, John Daugherty, Marsha J. Dohrmann,
Ronald J. Ervin, Andrew P. Evan, Jody L. Fulks, H.M. Gilles,
Michael Godomski, Andrew Grivas, John V. Hagen, Marcia Hartsock,
Jon Henke, R.T. Hutchings, Carlyn Iverson, Lisa Shoeme Kerl,
Christy Krames, James M. Kron, David J. Mascaro, M. Moore,
William Ober, Laurie O'Keefe, Christine Oleksyk, Mary Osbourne,
Kevin Patton, David M. Phillips, Ed Reschke, F. Rinnerthaler,
Jeanne Robertson, David Scharf, Michael Schenk, J.V. Small,
Howard Sochurek, Nadine Sokol, Kevin A. Somerville, Tom Stack,
Trent Stephens, Karen Waldo, George J. Wassilchenko, Patrick Watson,
Klaus Weber, Nancy S. Wexler, Steve Young

# PUBLISHER'S FOREWORD

Medical and biological science and technology are advancing at a staggering rate. The language of health care and science evolves constantly to keep pace with these changes. To master the body of knowledge essential to their professional practice and to communicate effectively with their colleagues in various disciplines, health professionals must have access to the language of this vast and vital field.

*Mosby's Medical, Nursing, & Allied Health Dictionary* was developed to provide a single source of authoritative, up-to-date information concerning health and health care terminology. Now in its sixth edition, *Mosby's Dictionary* has been praised by educators, students, and practitioners for its clarity, comprehensiveness, reliability, currency, and acclaimed illustrations. The hallmarks of our dictionary include the use of a large, easy-to-read typeface; encyclopedic definitions for many key terms; comprehensive entries for numerous drugs; commonsense, strictly alphabetical organization; the detailed Color Atlas of Human Anatomy; and the wealth of useful reference information provided in the appendixes. To assist our readers in recognizing alternate spellings, selected British spellings are included where appropriate.

One of *Mosby's Dictionary's* most distinctive features is the inclusion of more than 2200 high-quality full-color illustrations and photographs throughout the dictionary to enhance and clarify definitions of terms that cannot be adequately explained by words alone. *Mosby's Dictionary* was the first English-language medical, nursing, or allied health dictionary to use full color to show anatomy, disorders, and essential equipment throughout the dictionary, giving new meaning to the adage "one picture is worth a thousand words." For the sixth edition over 1200 figures have been added or updated. A list of the illustrations appears on p. xi. In addition, the 43-page Color Atlas of Human Anatomy has been updated with numerous full-color illustrations and is placed in the front of the dictionary for easy access.

To reflect new developments in many different facets of health care, approximately 3000 entirely new entries have been added to the sixth edition. Furthermore, all new and existing entries were thoroughly reviewed by experts to reflect current knowledge and practice. More than 10,000 definitions have been revised based on our consultants' recommendations. Our consultant board of over 100 individuals represents not only diverse specialties and disciplines but also Canadian and international interests. We are indebted to our consultants for their invaluable advice and assistance in the selection of new entries, as well as for the revision and refinement of definitions.

A total of 70 new and updated tables appear throughout the dictionary to provide key reference information to supplement the definitions. A list of boxes and tables is included on p. xxii to facilitate quick reference.

The appendixes offer an extensive compendium of useful reference information. Appendixes include information on normal laboratory values for adults and children, units of measurement, complete anatomy tables, common drug interactions, assessment guides, nutrition guidelines, directories of key health organizations, Spanish and French translations for commonly used vocabulary, immunizations, infection control, diagnosis-related groups, and the latest NANDA-approved nursing diagnoses, including an extensive listing of nursing diagnoses related to numerous diseases, disorders, and procedures. All appendixes have been updated to include the latest information.

Appendixes new to this edition include contemporary and alternative medicine, herbs and natural supplements, herb–laboratory test interferences, American Sign Language guidelines, and key information for three important nursing taxonomies: the Nursing Interventions Classification, the Nursing Outcomes Classification, and the Omaha Classification System. The lists of resources and organizations have been extensively updated and expanded. The appendixes alone make *Mosby's Dictionary* an indispensable resource for students and professionals in the health sciences.

In addition to the many printed resources available in *Mosby's Dictionary,* we have provided a unique website on Mosby's Electronic Resource Links & Information Network (MERLIN). This website provides hundreds of links to key medical, nursing, and allied health organizations; answers to frequently asked questions; current contact information; and much more. The MERLIN website is updated regularly.

All the virtues of the first five editions of *Mosby's Dictionary* have been retained. Word roots and pronunciations are provided for principle entries to assist in learning and using vocabulary. Among the entries on diseases, drugs and procedures, over 1000 include practical information presented under separate headings such as Methods, Adverse Effects, Nursing Considerations, and Outcome Criteria. The rationales for all procedures is given due attention. Headings for Defining Characteristics, Risk Factors, and Related Factors have been added to the entries for nursing diagnoses to assist the reader to quickly locate this information. The inclusion of numerous prefixes and suffixes gives the reader additional access not only to the meanings of defined terms but also to terms that are not included in this dictionary and that, to a large extent, are not found in other reference works. The myriad cross-references from definition to definition are well chosen and contribute to the dictionary's encyclopedic dimensions. As with the prior editions, *Mosby's Dictionary* continues to serve nursing and allied health students and professionals as the most comprehensive, authoritative, and up-to-date dictionary available.

It is impossible to acknowledge specifically the many individuals who have contributed to the sixth edition of *Mosby's Dictionary.* However, we would like to thank our board of consultants who graciously gave of their time and expertise, helping ensure that the new edition of our dictionary would be a comprehensive, reliable, up-to-date resource for students and professionals in the health sciences. We are especially grateful to the many Mosby, WB Saunders, Churchill Livingstone, Wolfe, and Gower authors and artists whose photographs and line drawings appear in this new edition of our dictionary. We also gratefully acknowledge the extensive contributions made by Ken and Lois Anderson and Walter Glanze to the first five editions of *Mosby's Dictionary.* Their knowledge, dedication, professionalism, and commitment to quality were critical to the success of our dictionary. These people and many others played important roles in the development and publication of our new edition. We appreciate their contributions and trust that they will be proud to be associated with the sixth edition of *Mosby's Medical, Nursing, & Allied Health Dictionary.*

# CONSULTANTS

**Mary A. Allen, RN, MS**
Clinical Trials Specialist
National Institutes of Allergy and
    Infectious Diseases
National Institutes of Health
Bethesda, Maryland

**Aris J. Andrews, RN, BA, MS**
Assistant Professor
School of Nursing
Creighton University Hastings Campus
Hastings, Nebraska

**Linda L. Andrews, RN, EdD**
Associate Professor
Nursing Program–School of Health
    Science and Human Performance
Lynchburg College
Lynchburg, Virginia

**Jean Krajicek Bartek, PhD, ARNP**
Associate Professor
Colleges of Nursing and Medicine
University of Nebraska Medical
    Center
Omaha, Nebraska

**Patricia Bates, RN, BSN, CURN**
Clinical Urology Nurse
Kaiser Permanente
Portland, Oregon

**Jane J. Benedict, RN, BSN, MSN**
Associate Professor of Nursing
Pennsylvania College of Technology
Williamsport, Pennsylvania

**Barbara Billek-Sawhney, MS, PT**
Director, Associate Professor
School of Physical Therapy
Slippery Rock University
Slippery Rock, Pennsylvania

**Jacqueline J. Birmingham, RN, MS, CMAC**
Consultant, Educator, Writer
Suffield, Connecticut

**Christi A. Blair, RN, MSN**
Practical Nursing Instructor
Holmes Community College
Kosciusko, Mississippi

**Margie E. Brown, RNC, MS, ANP**
Clinical Associate, Surgery
St. Mary's Medical Center
Long Beach, California

**Susan Burkett, RN, MSN, CPNP, CPN**
VP Erlanger Health System,
    Administrator TCTCH
TC Thompson Children's Hospital
Chattanooga, Tennessee

**Jeanie Burt, MA, RN, MSN**
Assistant Professor of Nursing
School of Nursing
Harding University
Searcy, Arkansas

**Darlene Nebel Cantu, MSN, RNC**
Director
Baptist Health System
School of Professional Nursing
Adjunct Faculty
San Antonio College
San Antonio, Texas

**Kathlyn M. Carlson, BSN, MA, CPAN**
Clinical Nurse
Surgical Services, Pre- and
    Post-Anesthesia Care
Abbott-Northwestern Hospital
Minneapolis, Minnesota

**Paul W. Cascella, PhD, CCC-SLP**
Assistant Professor
Department of Communication
    Disorders
Southern Connecticut State University
New Haven, Connecticut

**Janice T. Chussil, MSN, RNC, DNC**
Adult Nurse Practitioner
Dermatology Associates
Portland, Oregon

**Michael S. Clement, MD**
Fellow
American Academy of Pediatrics
Clinical Lecturer
Department of Family and Community
    Medicine
University of Arizona
Mesa, Arizona

**Linda A. Copenhaver, MSN, RN, C**
Associate Professor, Nursing
Austin Community College
Austin, Texas

**Joan A. Daly, RT(R), MBA**
Faculty
Clinical Coordinator
Radiology Program
Portland Community College
Portland, Oregon

**James J. Dempsey, PhD**
Associate Professor/Coordinator of
    Audiology
Department of Communication
    Disorders
Southern Connecticut State University
New Haven, Connecticut

**Kathleen Dietz-Lovett, RN, MS, CANP, AOCN**
Adult Nurse Practitioner
Oncology CNS
Independent Consultant
Marstons Mills, Massachusetts

**Deborah Oldenburg Erickson, BSN, MSN**
Instructor
Methodist Medical Center
School of Nursing
Peoria, Illinois

**Carol Feingold, MS, RN**
Senior Lecturer
College of Nursing
University of Arizona
Tucson, Arizona

**Michael A. Fiedler, MS, CRNA**
Doctoral Student
University of Tennessee at Memphis
Memphis, Tennessee

**Donna G. Friedman, PhD**
Professor
Department of Chemistry
St. Louis Community College at
    Florissant Valley
St. Louis, Missouri

**John Fritz, RN, MN**

**Stephanie D. Garrison, RN, MSN, DSN**
Associate Professor
College of Nursing
University of South Alabama
Mobile, Alabama

**Florencetta Hayes Gibson, BSN, MEd, MSN, CNS**
Associate Professor
Adult Health Department
College of Nursing
University of Louisiana at Monroe
Monroe, Louisiana

**Kate Goldblum, MSN, RN, CS, CRNO, CFNP**
Nurse Practitioner
Goldblum Family Eye Care Center
Albuquerque, New Mexico

**Linda B. Haas, PhD, RN, CDE**
Endocrinology Clinical Nurse
    Specialist
VA Puget Sound Health Care System,
    Seattle Division
Primary and Specialty Care
Seattle, Washington

**Heidi Hahn, MHS, PT, CCS**
Physical Therapist
Barnes-Jewish Hospital
St. Louis, Missouri

**Patty Hale, PhD, RN, FNP-C**
Associate Professor
Lynchburg College
School of Health Science
Lynchburg, Virginia

**Mary Martha Hall, MSN, RN, FNP**
Nurse Practitioner, Clinical Nurse
    Specialist
Emergency Consultants, Inc.
Memorial Hermann Healthcare System
Houston, Texas

**Patricia C. Hart, PhD, RD**
Associate Professor
Department of Human Sciences and
    Design
Samford University
Birmingham, Alabama

**Monica M. Hentemann, RN, BSN**
Staff Nurse
Spectrum Health Oncology
Grand Rapids, Michigan

**Dorothy G. Herron, PhD, RN, CS**
Assistant Professor
Adult Health Department
School of Nursing
University of Maryland
Baltimore, Maryland

**Mary G. Hirsch, RN, MSN,
CWOCN**
Health Care Economics
Mallinckrodt, Inc.
St. Louis, Missouri

**Diana Hughes, PhD, CCC-SLP**
Professor
Department of Communication
    Disorders
Central Michigan University
Mount Pleasant, Michigan

**Trudi James-Parks, RT(R)**
Professor, Radiologic Technology
Lorain County Community College
Elyria, Ohio

**Gail I. Jones, PhD, MT(ASCP), SC**
Medical Technologist/Instructor
Biology Department
Texas Christian University
Fort Worth, Texas

**JaCinda L. Jones, PharmD**
Manager, Pharmaceutical Care and
    Disease Management
Medicine Shoppe International, Inc.
St. Louis, Missouri

**Josephine A. Kahler, EdD, RN, CS**
Associate Professor/Satellite Director
Medical University of South Carolina
Francis Marion University
Florence, South Carolina

**Judy Kaye, ARNP, PhDc, CNRN,
CCRN, GNP, CS**
Research Specialist, Adult and
    Gerontology Nurse Practitioner
University Hospital
Augusta, Georgia

**Judith Ann Kilpatrick, MSN, RNC**
Lecturer
School of Nursing
Widener University
Chester, Pennsylvania

**Carl A. Kirton, RN, MA, ACRN,
ANP-CS**
Clinical Assistant Professor of Nursing
Division of Nursing
New York University
New York, New York

**Larry H. Knipp, BA, MS, PhD**
Professor and Chair
Department of Biology
North Park University
Chicago, Illinois

**Barbara Krainovich-Miller, EdD, RN**
Visiting Professor
New York University
The Steinhardt School of Education
Division of Nursing, Graduate
    Program
New York, New York

**Anne R. Lewis, MA, RN**
Neuroscience Clinical Nurse Specialist
Genesis Medical Center
Davenport, Iowa

**David E. Lewis, PhD**
Professor of Chemistry
Department of Chemistry
University of Wisconsin–Eau Claire
Eau Claire, Wisconsin

**Kim Litwack, PhD, RN, FAAN,
CFNP**
Associate Professor
Grand Valley State University
Department of Nursing
Allendale, Michigan

**Janis Luft, RN, NP, MSN**
Women's Health Nurse Practitioner
University of California–San Francisco
San Francisco, California

**Melanie S. MacNeil, RN, BSCN, MN**
Professor
Advanced Anatomy and Wellness
    Chair
Nursing
Brock University
St. Catherine's, Ontario

**Lisa McClane, RNC, MSN, CNS**
Program Administrator
Women's & Infant's Services
Erlanger Health System
Chattanooga, Tennessee

**Jennifer L. McQuade, PharmD**
Medical Information Consultant
Douglasville, Georgia

**Mary Merchant, RN, MSN, FNP**
Continuum of Care Manager
Medical University of South Carolina
Charleston, South Carolina

**William R. Metcalf**
Division Chief
EMS and Special Services
North Lake Tahoe Fire Protection
    District
Incline Village, Nevada

**Claudia L. Mitchell, RN, BSN, MSN**
Professor of Nursing
Santa Barbara City College
Santa Barbara, California

**Kathleen Mulryan, RN, BSN, MSN**
Professor of Nursing
LaGuardia Community College
Department of Natural and Applied
    Sciences
Long Island City, New York

**Elaine K. Neel, BSN, MSN**
Nursing Instructor
Methodist Medical Center of Illinois
School of Nursing
Peoria, Illinois

**Patricia J. Nunn, RDH, MS**
Associate Professor and Chair
Department of Dental Hygiene
College of Dentistry
University of Oklahoma
Oklahoma City, Oklahoma

**Susan M. Caley Opsals, BS, MS**
Instructor, Anatomy and Physiology
Division of Natural Sciences and
    Mathematics
Illinois Valley Community College
Oglesby, Illinois

**Jeffrey Papp, PhD, RT(R) (QM)**
Professor
Physics and Diagnostic Imaging
College of DuPage
Department of Health Sciences
Glen Ellyn, Illinois

**Kevin T. Patton, PhD**
Professor of Life Sciences
St. Charles Community College
St. Peters, Missouri;
Adjunct Assistant Professor of
    Physiology
St. Louis University Medical School
St. Louis, Missouri

**Lorraine Williams Pedretti, MS, OTR**
Professor Emeritus
San Jose State University
Department of Occupational Therapy
San Jose, California

**Leonard A. Piché, PhD, RD**
Associate Professor
Nutrition Program
University of Western Ontario
Brescia College
London, Ontario

**Melissa Powell, RN, MSN**
Assistant Professor
Associate Degree Nursing
Eastern Kentucky University
Richmond, Kentucky

**Elaine T. Princevalli, RN, BSN, MS**
Instructor
Practical Nurse Education Program
Eli Whitney Reg. Vo-Tech School
Hamden, Connecticut

**Jean A. Proehl, RN, MN, CEN,
CCRN**
Emergency Clinical Nurse Specialist
Dartmouth-Hitchcock Medical Center
Lebanon, New Hampshire

**Patti D. Quenzer, RN, RT, BSN, MSN**
Associate Professor
Southern West Virginia Community
    and Technical College
Williamson, West Virginia

**Patricia Reese, MSN, CNS**
Skills Lab Supervisor
Penn Valley Community College
Kansas City, Missouri

**Karen D. Robinson, RN, MN, MPM**
Administrative Director, Radiation
    Oncology
University of Pittsburgh Cancer
    Institute
Pittsburgh, Pennsylvania

**Susan C. Ruda, MS, RN, ONC**
Clinical Nurse Specialist
Parkview Musculoskeletal Institute
Palos Heights, Illinois

**Darlene T. Schelper, RN, MSN,
CEN, RNC**
Clinical Nurse Educator–Emergency
    Services
The Milton S. Hershey Medical
    Center
Nursing Education and Professional
    Development
Hershey, Pennsylvania

**Roberta J. Secrest, PhD, PharmD**
Scientist
Manager
US Medical Research
Aventis Pharmaceuticals, Inc.
Kansas City, Missouri

**Sarah C. Smith, RN, MA, CRNO**
Educational Associate
University of Iowa Health Care
Department of Ophthalmology
Iowa City, Iowa

**Jean Sparks, PhD, MT(ASCP)**
Assistant Professor
Department of Medical Laboratory
    Sciences
University of Texas Southwestern
Allied Health Sciences School
Dallas, Texas

**A. Christy Tamisiea, RN, MSN**
Instructor
Medical-Surgical Nursing
Nursing Department
Clarkson College
Omaha, Nebraska

**Rowena Tessmann, DCur, RN-CS**
Associate Professor
University of Maine at Fort Kent
Division of Nursing
Fort Kent, Maine

**Gary A. Thibodeau, PhD**
Chancellor Emeritus and Professor
    Emeritus, Biology
University of Wisconsin—River Falls
River Falls, Wisconsin

**Kathleen K. Tyser, BSN, MS**
Assistant Professor, Nursing
Clarkson College
Omaha, Nebraska

**Peggy Vernon, RN, MA, C-PNP**
Pediatric Nurse Practitioner
Dermatology Nurse Practitioner
Aurora/Parker Skin Care Center
Cara Mia Medical Day Spa
Parker, Colorado

**Lois L. VonCannon, RN, MSN**
Clinical Assistant Professor
University of North Carolina at
    Greensboro
Greensboro, North Carolina

**Terri A. Watson, CDA**
Program Director, Dental Assistant
    Program
Omaha College of Health Careers
Dental Assistant Program
Omaha, Nebraska

**Mary E. Wilbur, MSN, RN**
Continuum of Care Manager
Department of Outcomes Management
Medical University of South Carolina
Charleston, South Carolina

**Thomas J. Zwemer, DDS, MSD**
Vice President of Academic Affairs
    Emeritus
Medical College of Georgia
Augusta, Georgia

# LIST OF BOXES AND TABLES

## A. ALPHABETIC ORDER

The entries are alphabetized in dictionary style, that is, letter by letter, disregarding spaces or hyphens between words:

| | |
|---|---|
| **analgesic** | **artificial lung** |
| **anal membrane** | **artificially acquired immunity** |
| **analog** | **artificial pacemaker** |

(Alphabetized in telephone-book style, that is, word by word, the order would be different: **anal membrane / analgesic / analog; artificial lung / artificial pacemaker / artificially acquired immunity.**)

The alphabetization is alphanumeric; that is, words and numbers form a single list, numbers being positioned as though they were spelled-out numerals: **Nilstat/90-90 traction/ninth nerve.** (An example of the few exceptions to this rule is the sequence **17-hydroxycorticosteroid / 11-hydroxyetiocholanolone / 5-hydroxyindoleacetic acid,** which can be found between the entries **hydroxochloroquine sulfate** and **hydroxyl,** not, as may be expected, **17-.** . . in letter "S," **11-.** . . in letter "E," and **5-.** . . in letter "F.")

Small subscript and superscript numbers are disregarded in alphabetizing: **No / N₂O / nobelium**

For the alphabetization of prefixes and suffixes, see F.

## B. COMPOUND HEADWORDS

Compound headwords are given in their natural word order: **abdominal surgery,** not **surgery, abdominal; achondroplastic dwarf,** not **dwarf, achondroplastic.**

When appropriate, a reference is made elsewhere to the nonalphabetized element; the entry **dwarf,** for example, shows this indirect cross-reference: ". . . Kinds of dwarfs include **achondroplastic dwarf,** . . ." (followed by additional terms ending in "dwarf").

There are few exceptions to this natural word order; nearly all of these concern formal classifications, for example: "**coping, commonity, ineffective,** a nursing diagnosis accepted by the Eleventh National Conference on the Classification of Nursing Diagnoses . . ."

(NOTE: In this guide, the term "headword" is used to refer to any alphabetized and nonindented definiendum, be it a single-word term or a compound term.)

## C. MULTIPLE DEFINITIONS

If a headword has more than one meaning, the meanings are numbered and are often accompanied by an indication of the field in which a sense applies: "**fractionation, 1.** (in neurology) . . . **2.** (in chemistry) . . . **3.** (in bacteriology) . . . **4.** (in histology) . . . **5.** (in radiology) . . ."

Smaller differences in meaning are occasionally separated by semicolons: "**enervation, 1.** the reduction or lack of nervous energy; weakness; lassitude, languor. **2.** removal of a complete nerve or of a section of nerve."

Words that are spelled alike but have entirely different meanings and origins are usually given as separate entries, with superscript numbers: "**aural**[1], of or pertaining to the ear or hearing . . ." followed by "**aural**[2], of or pertaining to an aura."

For reference entries that appear in the form of numbered senses, see the example of **hyperalimentation** at E.

## D. THE BOLDFACE ELEMENTS OF AN ENTRY

After the entry headword, which has large boldface type, the following elements may occur in boldface, in this order:

In boldface:

■ HEADWORD ABBREVIATIONS: **central nervous system (CNS)**

A corresponding abbreviation entry is listed: "**CNS,** abbreviation for **central nervous system.**" (For abbreviation entries, see F.)

Occasionally the order is reversed: "**DDT (dichlordiphenyltrichloroethane),**" with a corresponding reference entry: "**dichlordiphenyltrichloroethane. See DDT.**" (For reference entries, see E below.)

■ PLURAL OR SINGULAR FORMS that are not obvious. The first form shown is the more common except when plurals are of more or less equal frequency: "**carcinoma,** *pl.* **carcinomas, carcinomata**"; "**cortex,** *pl.* **cortices**"; "**data,** *sing.* **datum**"

A reference entry is listed only when the terms are alphabetically separated; for example, there are several entries between **data** and "**datum. See data.**"

■ HIDDEN ENTRIES, that is, terms that can best be defined in the context of a more general entry. For example, the definition of the entry **equine encephalitis** continues as follows: ". . . **Eastern equine encephalitis (EEE)** is a severe form of the infection . . . **western equine encephalitis (WEE),** which occurs . . . **Venezuelan equine encephalitis (VEE),** which is common in . . ."

The corresponding reference entries are "**eastern equine encephalitis. See equine encephalitis.**"; "**western equine encephalitis. See equine . . .**"; and so forth. For further reference, from the abbreviations **EEE, WEE,** and **VEE,** see F.

■ INDIRECT CROSS-REFERENCES to other defined entries, shown as part of the definition and usually introduced by "Kinds of": "**dwarf,** . . . Kinds of dwarfs include **achondroplastic dwarf, asexual dwarf,** . . . , and **thanatophoric dwarf.**"

The entry referred to may or may not show a reciprocal reference, depending on the information value.

■ SYNONYMOUS TERMS, preceded by "Also called," "Also spelled," or, for verbs and adjectives, "Also": "**abducens nerve,** . . . Also called **sixth nerve.**"

A corresponding reference entry is usually given: "**sixth nerve. See abducens nerve.**"

Occasionally the synonymous term is accompanied by a usage label: "**abdomen,** . . . Also called *(informal)* **belly.**"

If a synonymous term applies to only one numbered sense, it precedes rather than follows the definition, to avoid ambiguity: "**algology, 1.** the branch of medicine that is concerned with the study of pain. **2.** also called **phycology.** the branch of science that is concerned with algae." (Whenever a synonymous term *follows* the last numbered sense, it applies to all senses of the entry.)

■ (DIRECT) CROSS-REFERENCES, preceded by "See also" or "Compare," referring to another defined entry for additional information: "**abdominal aorta,** . . . See also **descending aorta.**"

The cross-reference may or may not be reciprocal.

Cross-references are also made to illustrations, to tables, to the color atlas, and to the appendixes.

For cross-references from an abbreviation entry (with "See"), see F.

■ PARTS OF SPEECH related to the entry headword, shown as run-on entries that do not require a separate definition: "**abalienation,** . . . —**abalienate,** *v.,* **abalienated,** *adj.*"

## E. REFERENCE ENTRIES

Reference entries are undefined entries referring to a defined entry. There, they usually correspond to the boldface terms for which reference entries are mentioned at D above.

However, many of the less frequently used synonymous terms are listed as a reference only; at the entry referred to, the reader's attention is not drawn to them with "Also called."

A reference entry may also refer to a defined entry for other reasons: A particular lightface term in the definition is occasionally referred to: "**motion sickness,** . . . air sickness . . ."—with the reference entry "**air sickness: See motion sickness.**"

Some reference entries appear in the form of a numbered sense of a defined entry: "**hyperalimentation, 1.** overfeeding or the . . . in excess of the demands of the appetite. **2.** See **total parenteral nutrition.**" The latter entry says "Also called **hyperalimentation.**"

If two or more alphabetically adjacent terms refer to the same entry or entries, they are styled as one reference entry: "**coxa adducta, coxa flexa.** See **coxa vara.**"

A reference entry that would be derived from a boldface term in an immediately adjacent entry is not listed again as a headword; it becomes a "hidden reference entry": "**acardius amorphus,** . . . Also called **acardius anceps.**" But **acardius anceps** is not listed again as a reference entry because it would immediately *follow* the entry, the next entry being **acariasis.** Likewise: "**acoustic neuroma,** . . . Also called **acoustic neurilemmoma, acoustic neurinoma, acoustic neurofibroma.**" But the three synonymous terms are not listed again as reference entries because they would immediately *precede* the entry, the entry ahead being **acoustic nerve.** Therefore:

> If a term is not listed at the expected place, the reader might find it among the boldface terms of the immediately preceding or the immediately following entry.

Selected British spellings are included where appropriate. These are included as reference entries which refer the reader to the American spelling containing the definition. After the definition, the British spelling is given as an alternate spelling. For example: "**haematology.** See **hematology.**" The end of the definition for **hematology** says "Also spelled **haematology.**" As with other reference entries, when the reference entry would immediately precede or follow the main entry, it is not included as a separate entry, such as "**hyperkalemia** . . . Also spelled **hyperkalaemia.**"

## F. OTHER KINDS OF ENTRIES

■ ABBREVIATION ENTRIES: Most abbreviation entries, including symbol entries, show the full form of the term in boldface: "**ABC,** abbreviation for **aspiration biopsy cytology.**" "**H,** symbol for the element **hydrogen.**" Implied reference is made to the entries **aspiration biopsy cytology** and **hydrogen** respectively.

Abbreviation entries for which there is no corresponding entry show the full form in italics: "**CBF,** abbreviation for *cerebral blood flow.*" "**f,** symbol for *respiratory frequency.*"

A combination of abbreviation entry and reference entry occurs when the abbreviation is that of a boldface or lightface term appearing under another headword. For example, the hidden entries at D (in addition to the reference entries shown there) are also referred to in the following manner: "**EEE,** abbreviation for **eastern equine encephalitis.** See **equine encephalitis.**" An example with a lightface term: "**HLA-A,** abbreviation for *human leukocyte antigen A.* See **human leukocyte antigen.**" The latter entry says ". . They are HLA-A, HLA-B, HLA-C . . ."

■ PREFIXES AND SUFFIXES: The large amount and the nature of prefix and suffix entries are an important feature of this dictionary. Through these entries the reader has additional access to the meanings of headwords and the words used in defining them. But such entries also give access to thousands of terms that are not included in this dictionary (and, to a large extent, are not found in any other reference work). For example, the entries **xylo-** and **-phage** (plus **-phagia, phago-,** and **-phagy**) may lead to the meaning of "xylophagous," namely, "wood-eating."

Prefix and suffix headwords consisting of variants are alphabetized by the first variant only. For example, "**epi-, ep-,** a prefix meaning 'on, upon' . . ." is followed by **epiblast** (notwithstanding "**ep-**"). The other variant or variants are listed in their own alphabetical place as reference entries referring to the first variant: "**ep-.** See **epi-.**"

■ ENTRIES WITH SPECIAL PARAGRAPHS: Among the entries on diseases, drugs, and procedures, at least 1000 feature special paragraphs, with headings such as:

*observations, intervention,* and *nursing considerations.* (for disease entries),

*indications, contraindications,* and "*adverse effects.*" (for drug entries),

"*method,*" "*nursing interventions,*" and "*outcome criteria.*" (for procedure entries).

## G. FURTHER COMMENTS

■ EPONYMOUS TERMS THAT END IN "SYNDROME" OR "DISEASE" are given with an apostrophe (and "s" where appropriate) if they are based on the name of one person: **Adie's syndrome; Symmers' disease; Treacher Collins' syndrome** (the ophthalmologist Edward Treacher Collins). If they are based on the names of several people, they are without apostrophe: **Bernard-Soulier syndrome; Brill-Symmers disease.**

■ ABBREVIATIONS AND LABELS IN ITALIC TYPE: The abbreviations are *pl.* (plural), *npl.* (noun plural), *sing.* (singular); *n.* (noun), *adj.* (adjective), *v.* (verb). The recurring labels are *slang, informal, nontechnical, obsolete, archaic; chiefly British, Canada, U.S.*

■ DICTIONARY OF FIRST REFERENCE for general spelling preferences is *Webster's New Collegiate Dictionary;* thereafter: *Webster's Third New International Dictionary.*

## H. PRONUNCIATION

■ SYSTEM: See the Pronunciation Key on p. xxvi. The pronunciation system of this dictionary is basically a system that most readers know from their use of popular English dictionaries, especially the major college or desk dictionaries. All symbols for English sounds are ordinary letters of the alphabet with few adaptations, and with the exception of the schwa, /ə/ (the neutral vowel).

■ ACCENTS: Pronunciation, given between slants, is shown with primary and secondary accents, and a raised dot shows that two vowels or, occasionally, two consonants, between the slants are pronounced separately:

> **anoopsia** /an′ō·op′sē·ə/
> **cecoileostomy** /sē′kō·il′ē·os′təmē/
> **methemoglobin** /met′hēməglō′bin, met·hē′məglōbin/

Without the raised dot, the second /th/ in the last example would be pronounced as in "thin." (The pronunciation key lists the following paired consonant symbols as representing a single sound: /ch/, /ng/, /sh/, /th/, /t͟h/, /zh/, and the foreign sounds /kh/ and /ᴋh/—if no raised dot intervenes.)

■ TRUNCATION: Pronunciation may be given in truncated form, especially for alternative or derived words:

> **defibrillate** /difī′brilāt, difib′-/
> **bacteriophage** /baktir′ē·əfāj′, . . .—**bacteriophagy** /-of′əjē/, *n.*

In the last example, the reader is asked to make the commonsense assumption that the primary accent of the headword becomes a secondary accent in the run-on term: /baktir′ē·of′əjē/.

■ LOCATION: Pronunciation may be given for any boldface term and may occur anywhere in an entry:

> **aura** /ôr′ə/, **1.** *pl.* **aurae** /ôr′ē/, a sensation . . . **2.** *pl.* **auras,** an emanation of light . . .
> **micrometer, 1.** /mīkrom′ətər/, an instrument used for . . . **2.** /mī′krōmē′tər/, a unit of measurement . . .

Occasionally it is given for a lightface term:

> **b.i.d.,** (in prescriptions) abbreviation for *bis in die* /dē′ā/, a Latin phrase meaning . . .
> **boutonneuse fever.** . . ., an infectious disease . . . a tache noire /täshnô·är′/ or black spot . . .

■ LETTERWORD VERSUS ACRONYM: Letterwords are abbreviations that are pronounced by sounding the names of each letter, whereas acronyms are pronounced as words. If the pronunciation of an abbreviation is not given, the abbreviation is usually a letterword:

**ABO blood groups** [read /ā′bē′ō′/, not /ā′bō/]

If the pronunciation is an acronym, this is indicated by pronunciation:

**AWOL** /ā′wôl/

Some abbreviations are used as both:

*JAMA* /jä′mä, jam′ə, jā′ā′em′ā′/

■ FOREIGN SOUNDS: Non-English sounds do not occur often in this dictionary. They are represented by the following symbols:

| | |
|---|---|
| /œ/ | as in (French) **feu** /fœ/, **Europe** /œrôp′/; (German) **schön** /shœn/, **Goethe** /gœ′tə/ |
| /Y/ | as in (French) **tu** /tY/, **déjà vu** /dāzhävY′/; (German) **grün** /grYn/, **Walküre** /vulkY′rə/ |
| /kh/ | as in (Scottish) **loch** /lokh/; (German) **Rorschach** /rôr′shokh/, **Bach** /bokh, bäkh/ |
| /kh/ | as in (German) **ich** /ikh/, **Reich** /rīkh/ (or, approximated, as in English **fish:** /ish/, /rīsh/) |
| /N/ | This symbol does not represent a sound but indicates that the preceding vowel is a nasal, as in French **bon** /bôN/, **en face** /äNfäs′/, or **international** /aNternäsyōnäl′/. |
| /nyə/ | Occurring at the end of French words, this symbol is not truly a separate syllable but an /n/ with a slight /y/ (similar to the sound in "onion") plus a near-silent /ə/, as in **Bois de Boulogne** /boolō′nyə/, **Malgaigne** /mälgā′nyə/. |

Because this work is a subject dictionary rather than a language dictionary, certain foreign words and proper names are rendered by English approximations. Examples are **Müller** /mil′ər/ (which is closer to German than /mY′lər/), **Niemann** /nē′mon/ (which is closer than /nē′män/), **Friedreich** /frēd′rīsh/ (which is close enough for anyone not used to pronouncing /kh/), or **jamais vu,** for which three acceptable pronunciations are given: /zhämävY′/ (near-French) and the approximations /zhämävē′/ and /zhämävoo′/ (/-vē′/ being much closer to French than /-voo′/). Depending on usage, a foreign word or name may be given with near-native pronunciation, with entirely assimilated English pronunciation (as **de Quervain's fracture** /də kärvānz′/), or with both (as **Dupuytren's contracture** /dYpYi-traNs′, dēpē·itranz′/ or **Klippel-Feil syndrome** /klipel′fel′, klip′-əlfil′/).

At any rate, the English speaker should not hesitate to follow whatever is usage in his or her working or social environment.

Many of the numerous *Latin* terms in this dictionary are not given with pronunciation, mainly because there are different ways (all of them understood) in which Latin is pronounced by the English speaker and may be pronounced by speakers elsewhere. However, guidance is given in many cases, often to reflect common usage.

■ LATIN AND GREEK PLURALS: The spelling of Latin and Greek plurals is shown in most instances. However, when the plural formation is regular according to Latin and Greek rules, the pronunciation is usually not included. Therefore, the following list shows the suggested pronunciation of selected plural endings that are frequently encountered in the field of medicine:

| PLURAL ENDINGS | EXAMPLES |
|---|---|
| **-a** /-ə/ | **inoculum,** *pl.* **inocula** /inok′yoolə/ |
| **-ae** /-ē/ | **vertebra,** *pl.* **vertebrae** /vur′təbrē/ |
| **-ces** /-sēz/ | **thorax,** *pl.* **thoraces** /thôr′əsēz/ |
| | **apex,** *pl.* **apices** /ā′pisēz/ |
| **-era** /-ərə/ | **genus,** *pl.* **genera** /jen′ərə/ |
| **-ges** /-jēz/ | **meninx,** *pl.* **meninges** /minin′jēz/ |
| **-i** /-ī/ | **calculus,** *pl.* **calculi** /kal′kyəlī/ |
| | **coccus,** *pl.* **cocci** /kok′sī/ |

| PLURAL ENDINGS | EXAMPLES |
|---|---|
| **-ia** /-ē·ə/ | **criterion,** *pl.* **criteria** /krītir′ē·ə/ |
| **-ides** /-idēz/ | **epulis,** *pl.* **epulides** /ipyoo′lidēz/ |
| **-ina** /-ənə/ | **foramen,** *pl.* **foramina** /fəram′ənə/ |
| **-ines** /-ənēz/ | **lentigo,** *pl.* **lentigines** /lentij′ənēz/ |
| **-omata** /-ō′mətə/ | **hemotoma,** *pl.* **hematomata** /hē′mətō′mətə/ |
| **-ones** /-ō′nēz/ | **comedo,** *pl.* **comedones** /kom′ədō′nēz/ |
| **-ora** /-ərə/ | **corpus,** *pl.* **corpora** /kôr′pərə/ |
| | **femur,** *pl.* **femora** /fem′ərə/ |
| **-ses** /-sēz/ | **analysis,** *pl.* **analyses** /ənal′əsēz/ |
| **-udes** /-oo′dēz/ | **incus,** *pl.* **incudes** /inkoo′dēz/ |
| **-us** /-oos/ | **ductus** (/duk′təs/), *pl.* **ductus** /duk′toos/ |

NOTE: Notwithstanding the listing of Latin and Greek plurals in this dictionary, and notwithstanding the foregoing examples, in most instances it is acceptable or even preferable to pluralize Latin and Greek words according to the rules of English words. (For certain kinds of entries, both the English and the foreign plurals are given in this dictionary, usually showing the English form first, as, for example, in nearly all **-oma** nouns: **hematoma,** *pl.* **hematomas, hematomata.**)

W.D.G.

## I. ETYMOLOGIES AND EPONYMS

The word roots, or etymologies, of the headwords in this dictionary are shown in square brackets following the pronunciations of the headwords. Meanings are given in roman typeface and represent the original connotation of the word from which the medical term is derived. In compound medical terms formed from two or more elements, a plus sign (+) is used to indicate an element has been translated in a previous headword, as in [L *acidus* + Gk *philein* to love]. A semicolon (;) is used to separate word elements having more than one origin, as in [L *abdomen;* Gk *skopein* to view]. Word fragments representing etymologic elements, such as prefixes, are separated from the rest of the word root by a comma (,), as in [Gk *a, basis* not step]. A comma is also used to separate the abbreviation for the language of origin and its translation when the English-language equivalent for the word is the same, as in the term **ala** [L, wing].

The following abbreviations are used to identify language sources:

| | | | |
|---|---|---|---|
| Afr | African | Jpn | Japanese |
| Ar | Arabic | L | Latin |
| AS | Anglo-Saxon | ME | Middle English |
| Dan | Danish | OFr | Old French |
| D | Dutch | ONorse | Old Norse |
| Fr | French | Port | Portuguese |
| Ger | German | Scand | Scandinavian |
| Gk | Greek | Sp | Spanish |
| Heb | Hebrew | Swe | Swedish |
| It | Italian | Turk | Turkish |

Some other languages sources, such as Singhalese or Welsh, may be indicated without abbreviations.

Eponymous entries, in which the surname of an individual is incorporated in the headword, are also treated in square brackets with brief biographic details, as in **Alcock's canal** [Benjamin Irish anatomist, b. 1801]. When an eponym contains two or more surnames, a semicolon (;) is used to separate the identities of the individuals. Medical terms derived from other proper nouns, such as geographic sites, are presented in a similar manner, as **calabar swelling** [Calabar, a Nigerian seaport], or **ytterbium (Yb)** [Ytterby, Sweden].

K.N.A.

# PRONUNCIATION KEY

## Vowels

| SYMBOLS | KEY WORDS |
|---|---|
| /a/ | hat |
| /ä/ | father |
| /ā/ | fate |
| /e/ | flesh |
| /ē/ | she |
| /er/ | **air, ferry** |
| /i/ | sit |
| /ī/ | **eye** |
| /ir/ | **ear** |
| /o/ | proper |
| /ō/ | nose |
| /ô/ | saw |
| /oi/ | boy |
| /o͞o/ | move |
| /o͝o/ | book |
| /ou/ | **ou**t |
| /u/ | cup, love |
| /ur/ | **fur, first** |
| /ə/ | (the neutral vowel, always unstressed, as in) **ago**, focus |
| /ər/ | teach**er**, doct**or** |

## Consonants

| SYMBOLS | KEY WORDS |
|---|---|
| /b/ | **b**ook |
| /ch/ | **ch**ew |
| /d/ | **d**ay |
| /f/ | **f**ast |
| /g/ | **g**ood |
| /h/ | **h**appy |
| /j/ | **g**em |
| /k/ | **k**eep |
| /l/ | **l**ate |
| /m/ | **m**ake |
| /n/ | **n**o |
| /ng/ | si**ng**, dri**nk** |
| /ng·g/ | fi**ng**er |
| /p/ | **p**air |
| /r/ | **r**ing |
| /s/ | **s**et |
| /sh/ | **sh**oe, lo**ti**on |
| /t/ | **t**one |
| /th/ | **th**in |
| /*th*/ | **th**an |
| /v/ | **v**ery |
| /w/ | **w**ork |
| /y/ | **y**es |
| /z/ | **z**eal |
| /zh/ | a**z**ure, vi**si**on |

For /œ/, /Y/, /kh/, /*kh*/, /N/, and /nyə/,
see FOREIGN SOUNDS, p. xxv.

# COLOR ATLAS
# OF HUMAN ANATOMY

# SKELETAL SYSTEM

**ANTERIOR VIEW OF SKELETON**

**POSTERIOR VIEW OF SKELETON**

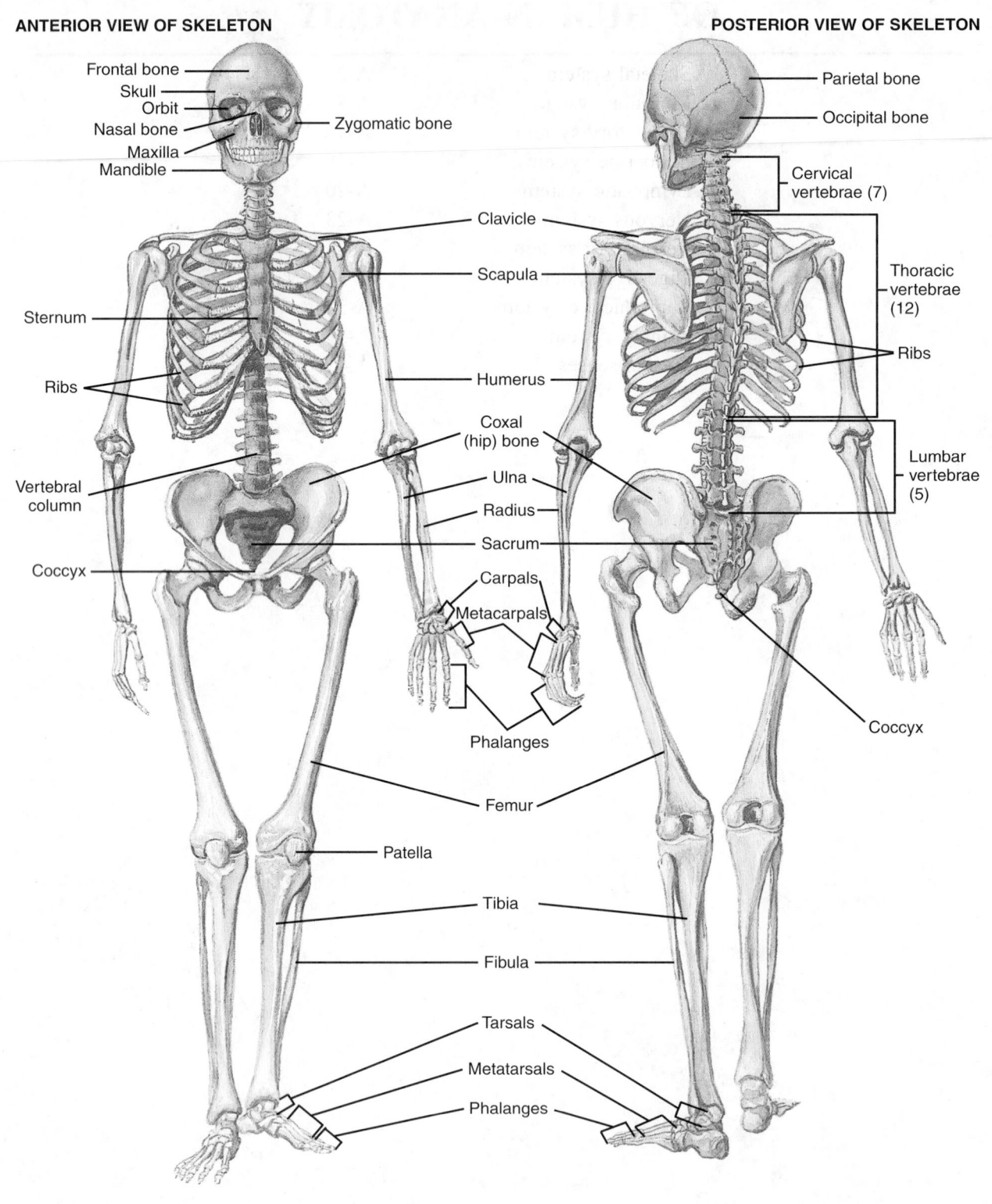

Frontal bone
Skull
Orbit
Nasal bone
Maxilla
Mandible
Zygomatic bone
Sternum
Ribs
Vertebral column
Coccyx
Clavicle
Scapula
Humerus
Coxal (hip) bone
Ulna
Radius
Sacrum
Carpals
Metacarpals
Phalanges
Femur
Patella
Tibia
Fibula
Tarsals
Metatarsals
Phalanges
Parietal bone
Occipital bone
Cervical vertebrae (7)
Thoracic vertebrae (12)
Ribs
Lumbar vertebrae (5)
Coccyx

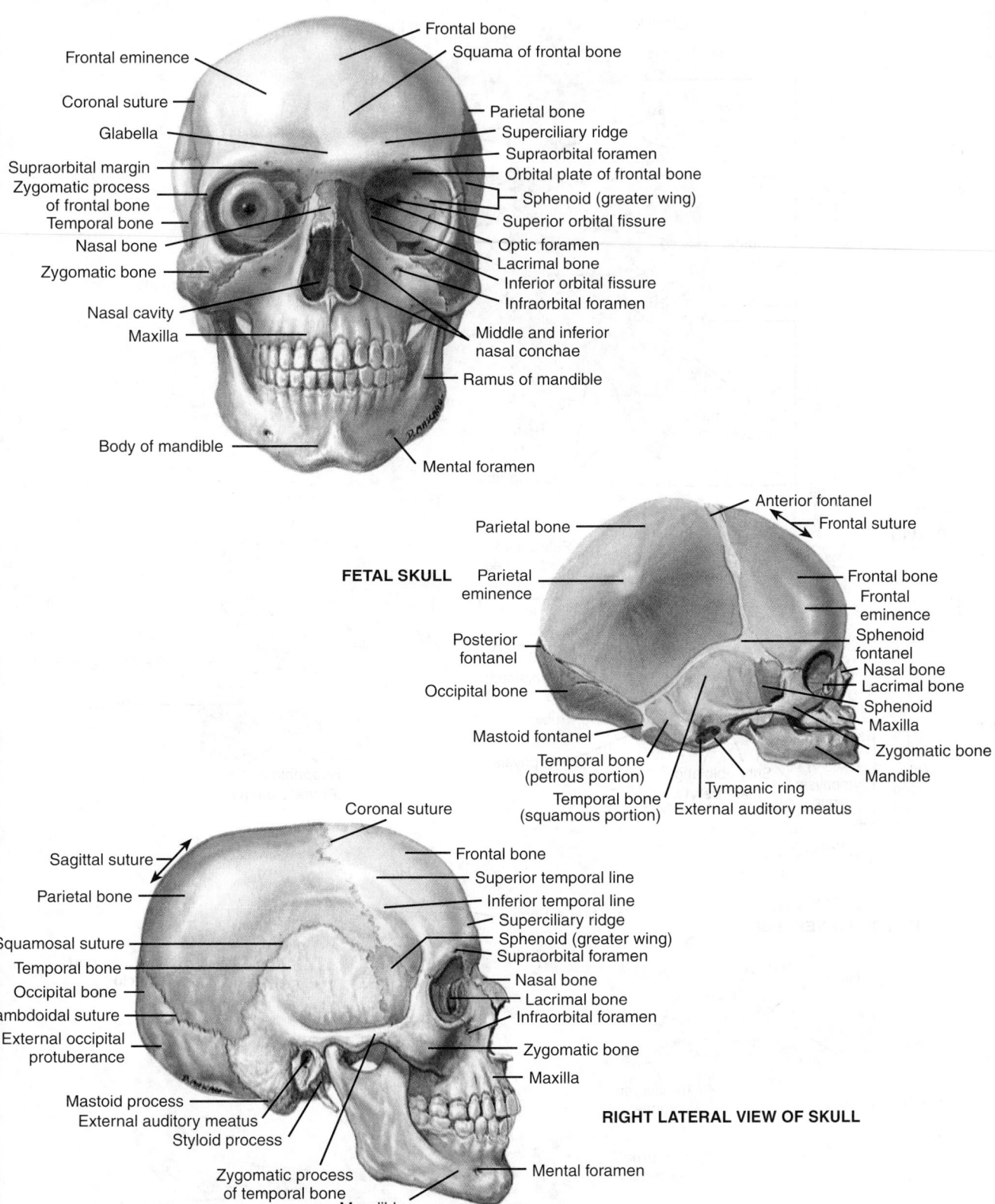

**ANTERIOR VIEW OF SKULL**

Frontal bone
Squama of frontal bone
Frontal eminence
Coronal suture
Parietal bone
Glabella
Superciliary ridge
Supraorbital margin
Supraorbital foramen
Zygomatic process
of frontal bone
Orbital plate of frontal bone
Temporal bone
Sphenoid (greater wing)
Superior orbital fissure
Nasal bone
Optic foramen
Zygomatic bone
Lacrimal bone
Inferior orbital fissure
Nasal cavity
Infraorbital foramen
Maxilla
Middle and inferior
nasal conchae
Ramus of mandible
Body of mandible
Mental foramen

**FETAL SKULL**

Anterior fontanel
Frontal suture
Parietal bone
Frontal bone
Parietal
eminence
Frontal
eminence
Sphenoid
fontanel
Posterior
fontanel
Nasal bone
Lacrimal bone
Occipital bone
Sphenoid
Maxilla
Mastoid fontanel
Zygomatic bone
Temporal bone
(petrous portion)
Mandible
Tympanic ring
Temporal bone
(squamous portion)
External auditory meatus

Coronal suture
Sagittal suture
Frontal bone
Superior temporal line
Parietal bone
Inferior temporal line
Superciliary ridge
Squamosal suture
Sphenoid (greater wing)
Temporal bone
Supraorbital foramen
Occipital bone
Nasal bone
Lacrimal bone
Lambdoidal suture
Infraorbital foramen
External occipital
protuberance
Zygomatic bone
Maxilla
Mastoid process
External auditory meatus
**RIGHT LATERAL VIEW OF SKULL**
Styloid process
Zygomatic process
of temporal bone
Mental foramen
Mandible

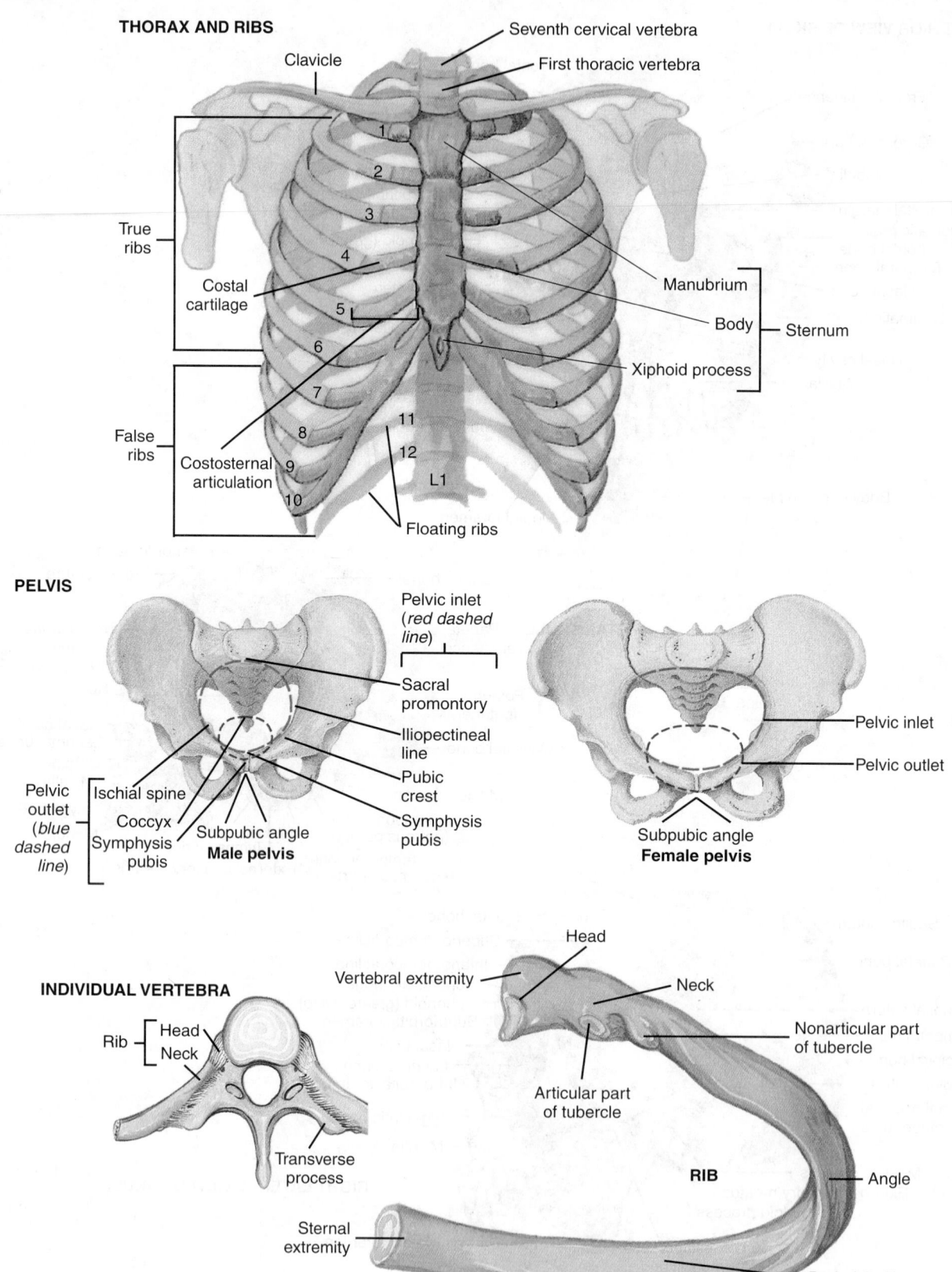

**THORAX AND RIBS**

Seventh cervical vertebra

First thoracic vertebra

Clavicle

1
2
3
4
5
6
7
8
9
10
11
12
L1

True ribs

Costal cartilage

False ribs

Costosternal articulation

Floating ribs

Manubrium

Body

Xiphoid process

Sternum

**PELVIS**

Pelvic inlet (*red dashed line*)

Sacral promontory

Iliopectineal line

Pubic crest

Symphysis pubis

Ischial spine

Coccyx

Symphysis pubis

Subpubic angle

**Male pelvis**

Pelvic outlet (*blue dashed line*)

Pelvic inlet

Pelvic outlet

Subpubic angle

**Female pelvis**

**INDIVIDUAL VERTEBRA**

Rib

Head

Neck

Transverse process

Vertebral extremity

Head

Neck

Articular part of tubercle

Nonarticular part of tubercle

**RIB**

Angle

Sternal extremity

Body (shaft)

**VERTEBRAL COLUMN**

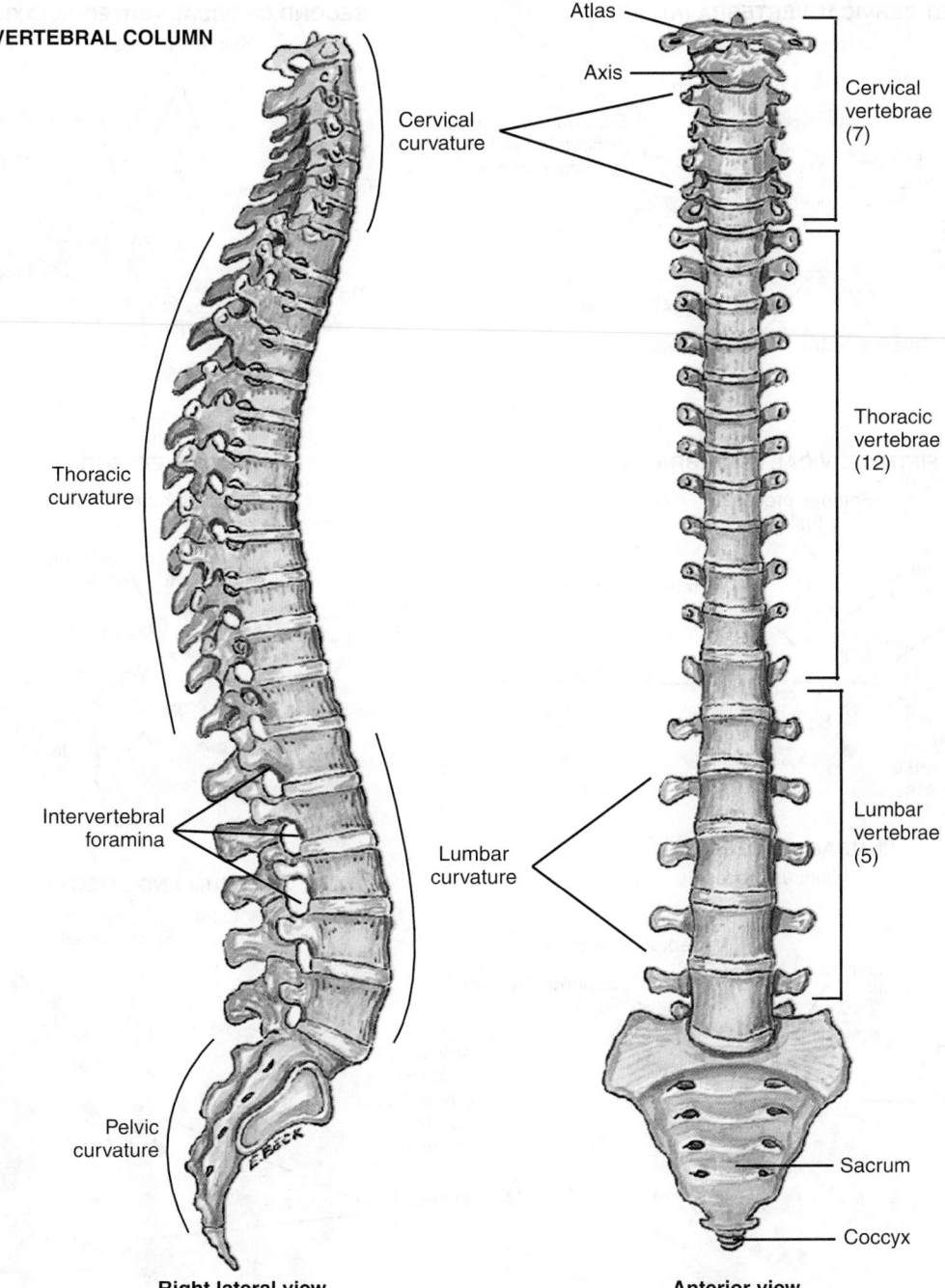

Cervical curvature

Thoracic curvature

Intervertebral foramina

Pelvic curvature

**Right lateral view**

Atlas

Axis

Cervical vertebrae (7)

Thoracic vertebrae (12)

Lumbar curvature

Lumbar vertebrae (5)

Sacrum

Coccyx

**Anterior view**

### FIRST CERVICAL VERTEBRA (ATLAS)

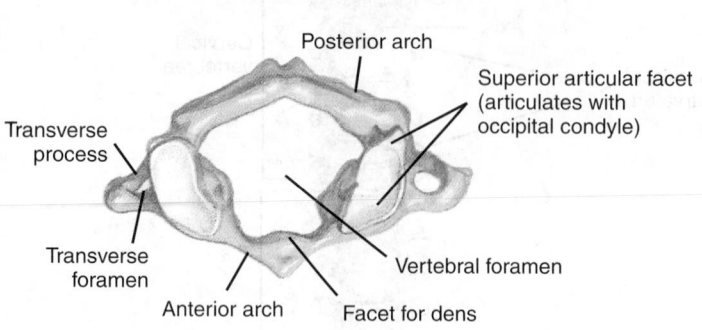

- Posterior arch
- Superior articular facet (articulates with occipital condyle)
- Transverse process
- Transverse foramen
- Anterior arch
- Facet for dens
- Vertebral foramen

### SECOND CERVICAL VERTEBRA (AXIS)

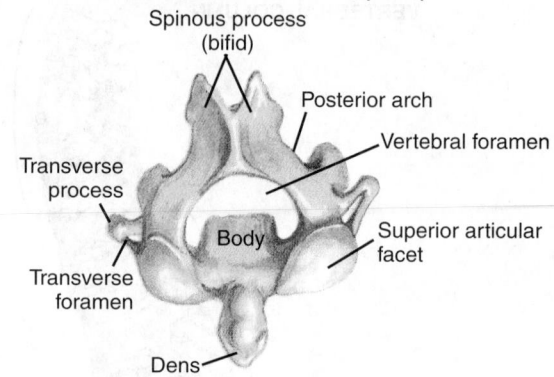

- Spinous process (bifid)
- Posterior arch
- Vertebral foramen
- Transverse process
- Superior articular facet
- Transverse foramen
- Body
- Dens

### FIFTH CERVICAL VERTEBRA

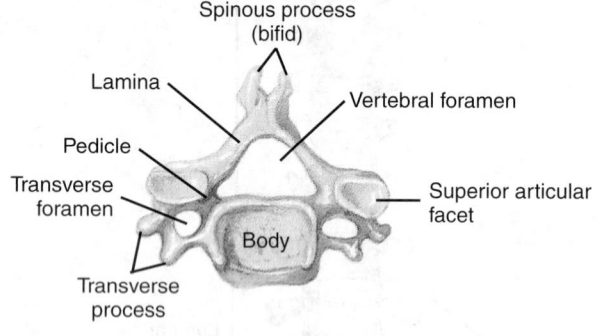

- Spinous process (bifid)
- Lamina
- Vertebral foramen
- Pedicle
- Transverse foramen
- Superior articular facet
- Body
- Transverse process

### THORACIC VERTEBRA

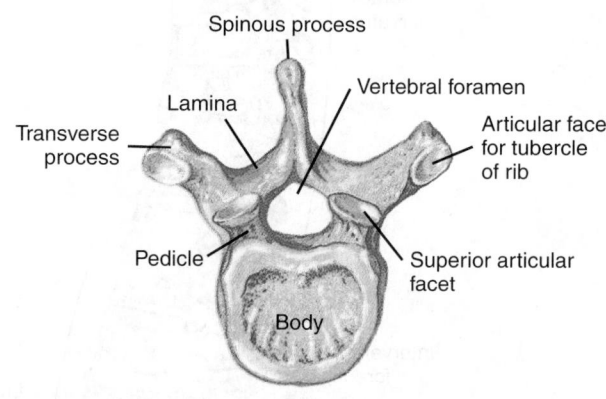

- Spinous process
- Vertebral foramen
- Lamina
- Articular facet for tubercle of rib
- Transverse process
- Pedicle
- Superior articular facet
- Body

### LUMBAR VERTEBRA

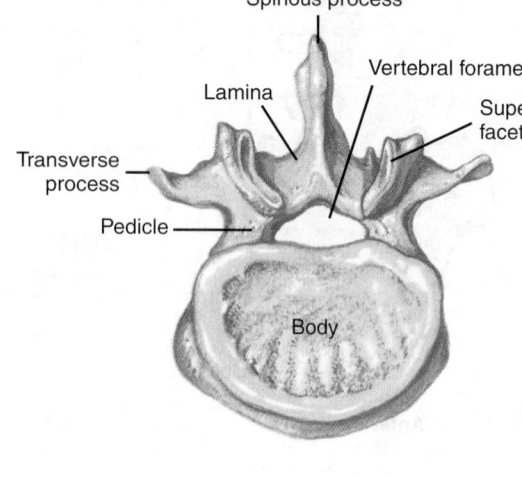

- Spinous process
- Vertebral foramen
- Lamina
- Superior articular facet
- Transverse process
- Pedicle
- Body

### SACRUM AND COCCYX

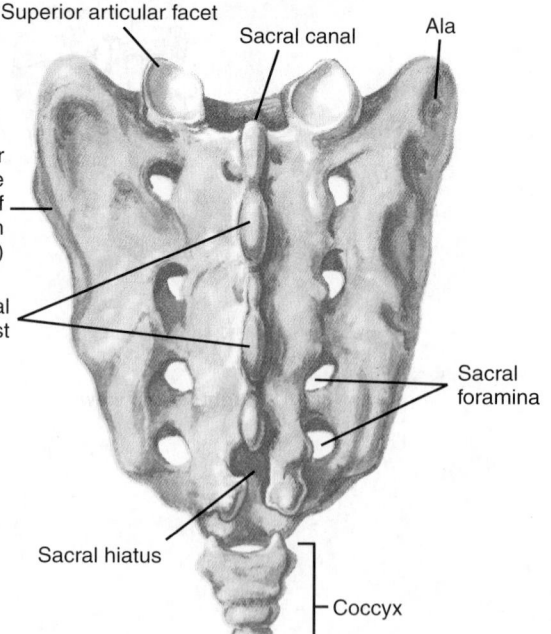

- Superior articular facet
- Sacral canal
- Ala
- Articular surface (point of articulation with coxa)
- Median sacral crest
- Sacral foramina
- Sacral hiatus
- Coccyx

# MICROSCOPIC STRUCTURE OF BONE

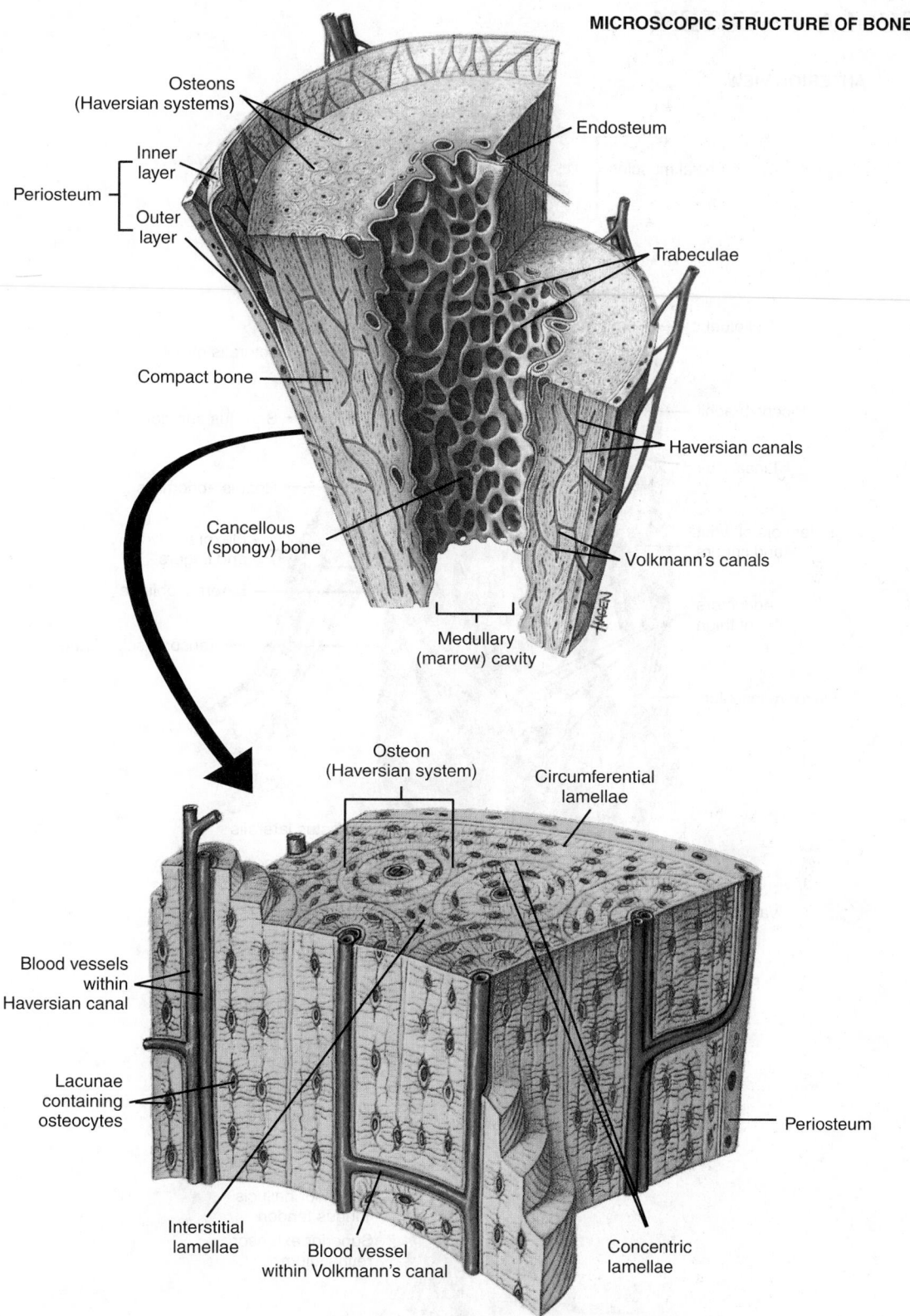

Osteons (Haversian systems)

Periosteum
- Inner layer
- Outer layer

Endosteum

Trabeculae

Compact bone

Haversian canals

Cancellous (spongy) bone

Volkmann's canals

Medullary (marrow) cavity

Osteon (Haversian system)

Circumferential lamellae

Blood vessels within Haversian canal

Lacunae containing osteocytes

Periosteum

Interstitial lamellae

Blood vessel within Volkmann's canal

Concentric lamellae

# MUSCULAR SYSTEM

**ANTERIOR VIEW**

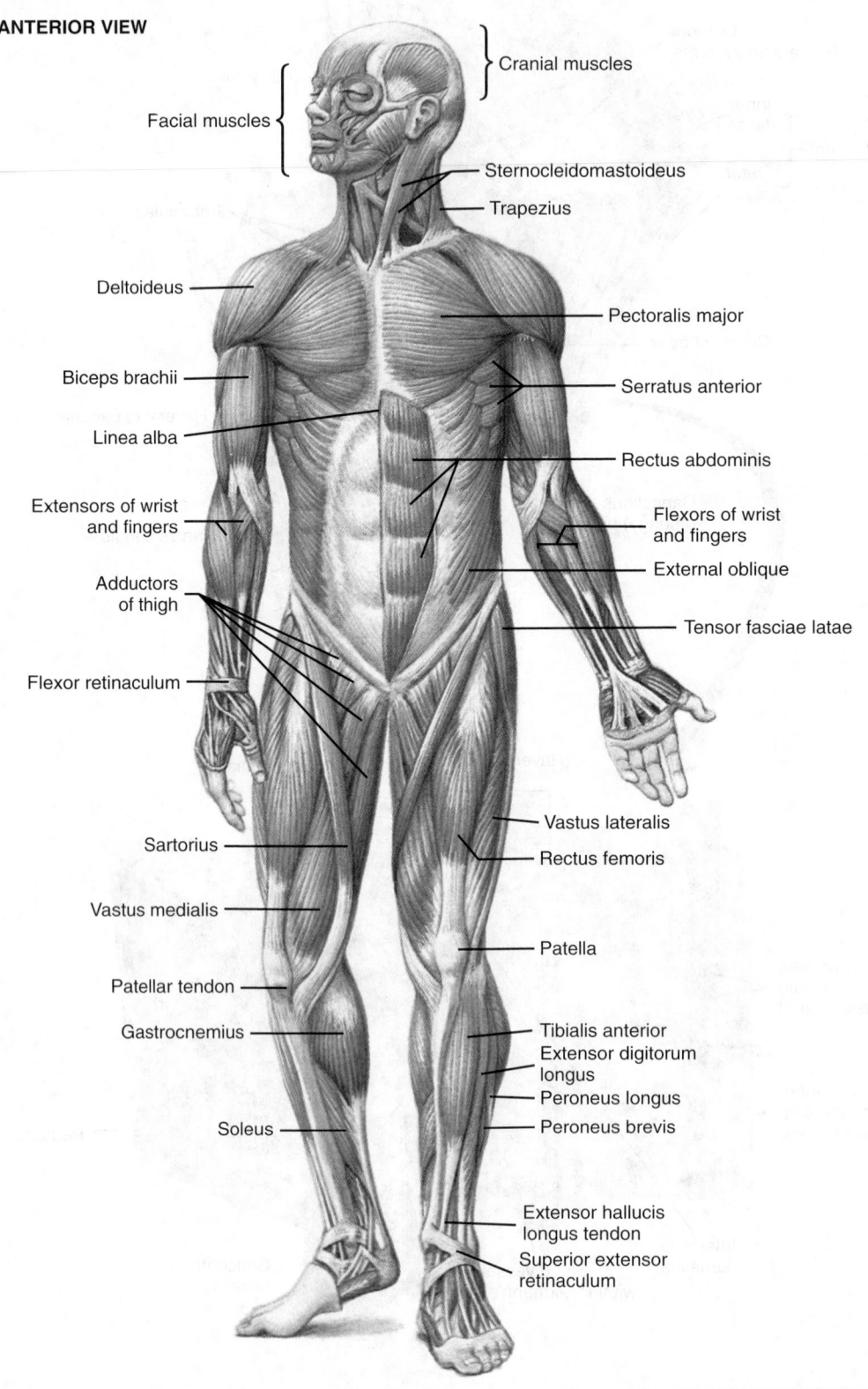

Cranial muscles

Facial muscles

Sternocleidomastoideus

Trapezius

Deltoideus

Pectoralis major

Biceps brachii

Serratus anterior

Linea alba

Rectus abdominis

Extensors of wrist
and fingers

Flexors of wrist
and fingers

External oblique

Adductors
of thigh

Tensor fasciae latae

Flexor retinaculum

Vastus lateralis

Sartorius

Rectus femoris

Vastus medialis

Patella

Patellar tendon

Tibialis anterior

Gastrocnemius

Extensor digitorum
longus

Peroneus longus

Peroneus brevis

Soleus

Extensor hallucis
longus tendon

Superior extensor
retinaculum

**POSTERIOR VIEW**

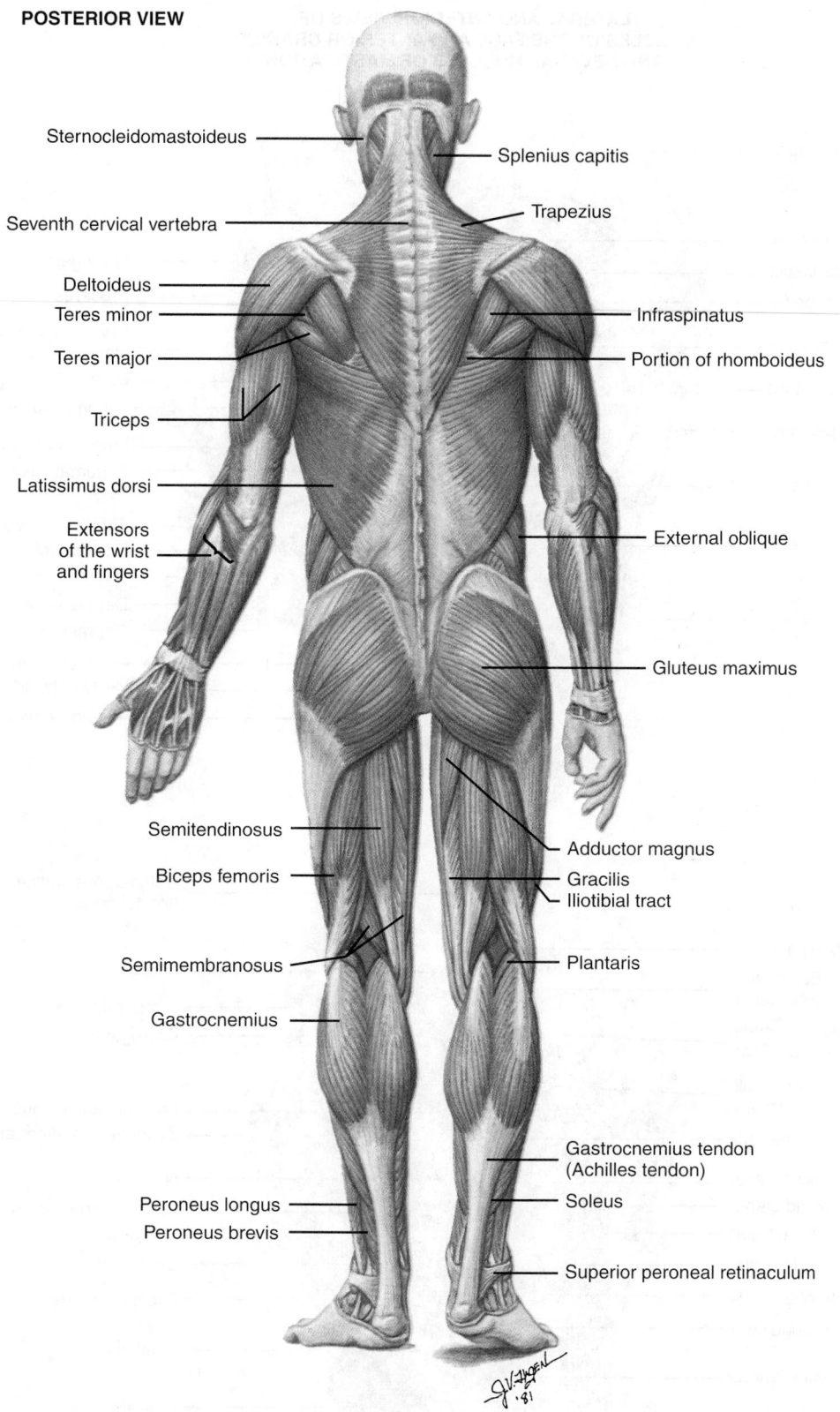

Sternocleidomastoideus

Seventh cervical vertebra

Deltoideus

Teres minor

Teres major

Triceps

Latissimus dorsi

Extensors
of the wrist
and fingers

Splenius capitis

Trapezius

Infraspinatus

Portion of rhomboideus

External oblique

Gluteus maximus

Semitendinosus

Biceps femoris

Semimembranosus

Gastrocnemius

Adductor magnus

Gracilis
Iliotibial tract

Plantaris

Gastrocnemius tendon
(Achilles tendon)

Peroneus longus

Peroneus brevis

Soleus

Superior peroneal retinaculum

**LATERAL AND ANTERIOR VIEWS OF
MUSCLES OF THE FACE AND ANTERIOR CRANIUM
AND SEVERAL MUSCLES OF MASTICATION**

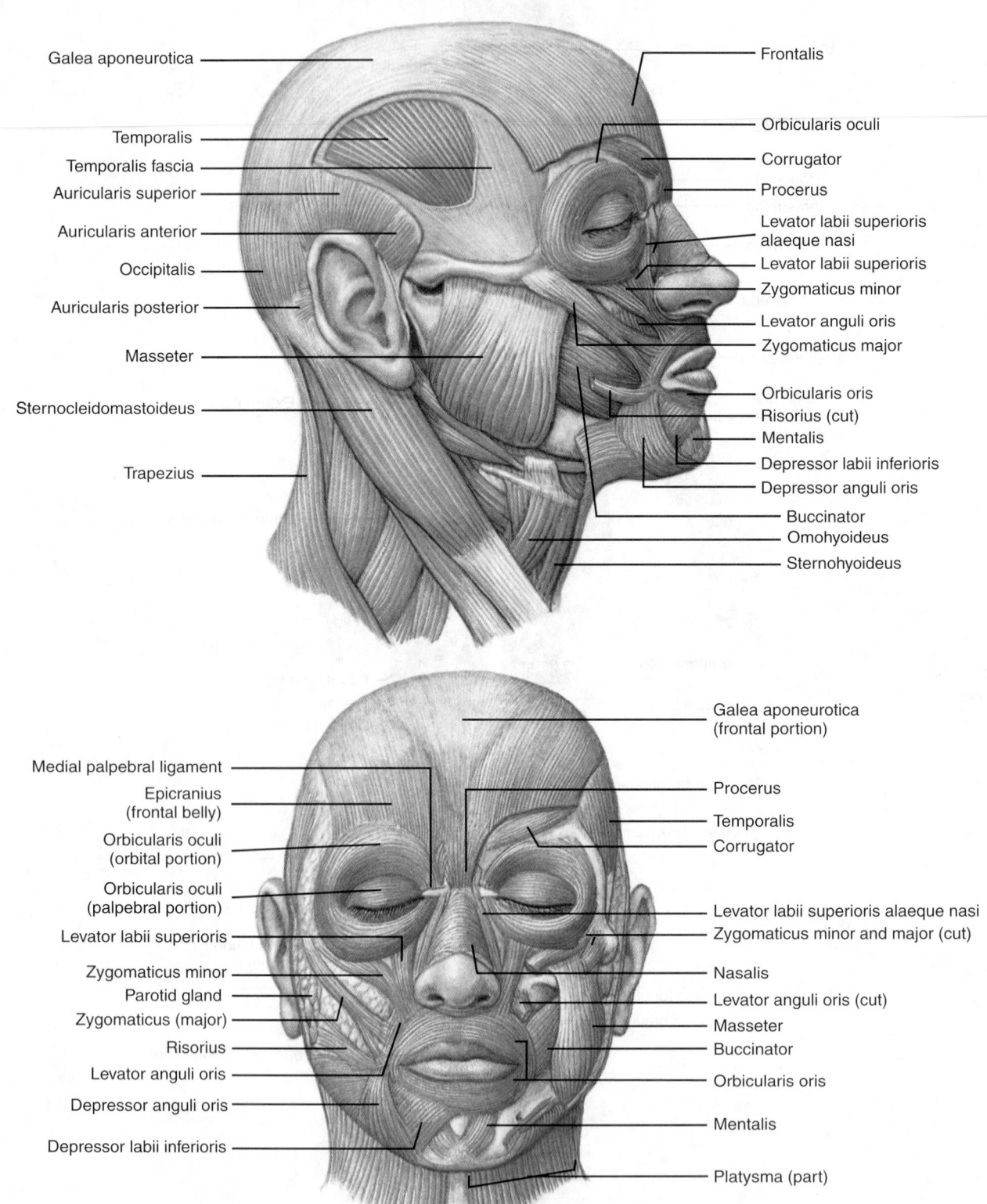

Galea aponeurotica

Temporalis

Temporalis fascia

Auricularis superior

Auricularis anterior

Occipitalis

Auricularis posterior

Masseter

Sternocleidomastoideus

Trapezius

Frontalis

Orbicularis oculi

Corrugator

Procerus

Levator labii superioris alaeque nasi

Levator labii superioris

Zygomaticus minor

Levator anguli oris

Zygomaticus major

Orbicularis oris

Risorius (cut)

Mentalis

Depressor labii inferioris

Depressor anguli oris

Buccinator

Omohyoideus

Sternohyoideus

Medial palpebral ligament

Epicranius (frontal belly)

Orbicularis oculi (orbital portion)

Orbicularis oculi (palpebral portion)

Levator labii superioris

Zygomaticus minor

Parotid gland

Zygomaticus (major)

Risorius

Levator anguli oris

Depressor anguli oris

Depressor labii inferioris

Galea aponeurotica (frontal portion)

Procerus

Temporalis

Corrugator

Levator labii superioris alaeque nasi

Zygomaticus minor and major (cut)

Nasalis

Levator anguli oris (cut)

Masseter

Buccinator

Orbicularis oris

Mentalis

Platysma (part)

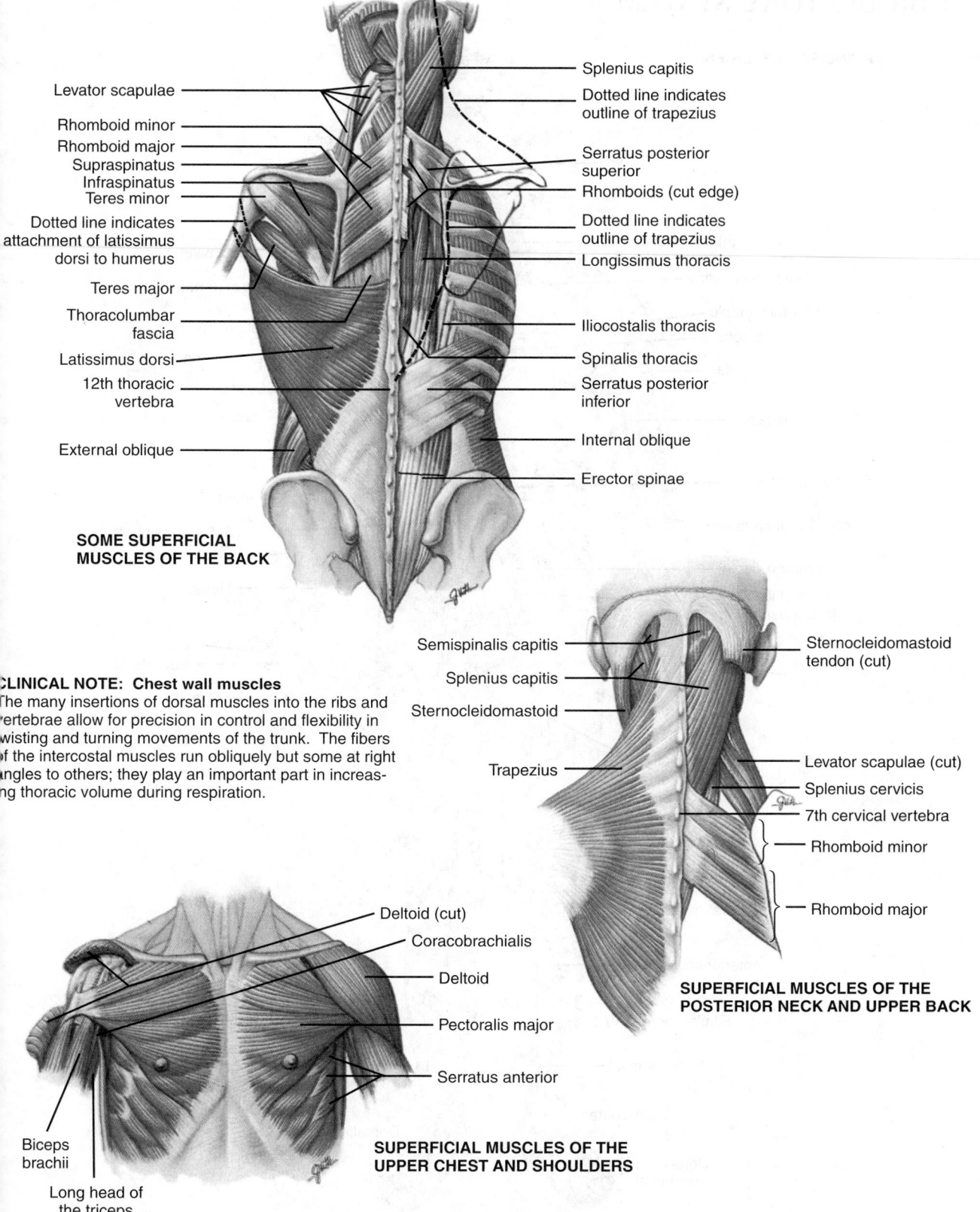

Splenius capitis

Dotted line indicates outline of trapezius

Levator scapulae

Rhomboid minor

Rhomboid major

Supraspinatus

Infraspinatus

Teres minor

Serratus posterior superior

Rhomboids (cut edge)

Dotted line indicates attachment of latissimus dorsi to humerus

Dotted line indicates outline of trapezius

Longissimus thoracis

Teres major

Thoracolumbar fascia

Iliocostalis thoracis

Latissimus dorsi

Spinalis thoracis

12th thoracic vertebra

Serratus posterior inferior

External oblique

Internal oblique

Erector spinae

**SOME SUPERFICIAL MUSCLES OF THE BACK**

**CLINICAL NOTE: Chest wall muscles**

The many insertions of dorsal muscles into the ribs and vertebrae allow for precision in control and flexibility in twisting and turning movements of the trunk. The fibers of the intercostal muscles run obliquely but some at right angles to others; they play an important part in increasing thoracic volume during respiration.

Semispinalis capitis

Sternocleidomastoid tendon (cut)

Splenius capitis

Sternocleidomastoid

Trapezius

Levator scapulae (cut)

Splenius cervicis

7th cervical vertebra

Rhomboid minor

Rhomboid major

**SUPERFICIAL MUSCLES OF THE POSTERIOR NECK AND UPPER BACK**

Deltoid (cut)

Coracobrachialis

Deltoid

Pectoralis major

Serratus anterior

Biceps brachii

Long head of the triceps

**SUPERFICIAL MUSCLES OF THE UPPER CHEST AND SHOULDERS**

# CIRCULATORY SYSTEM

**PRINCIPAL ARTERIES**

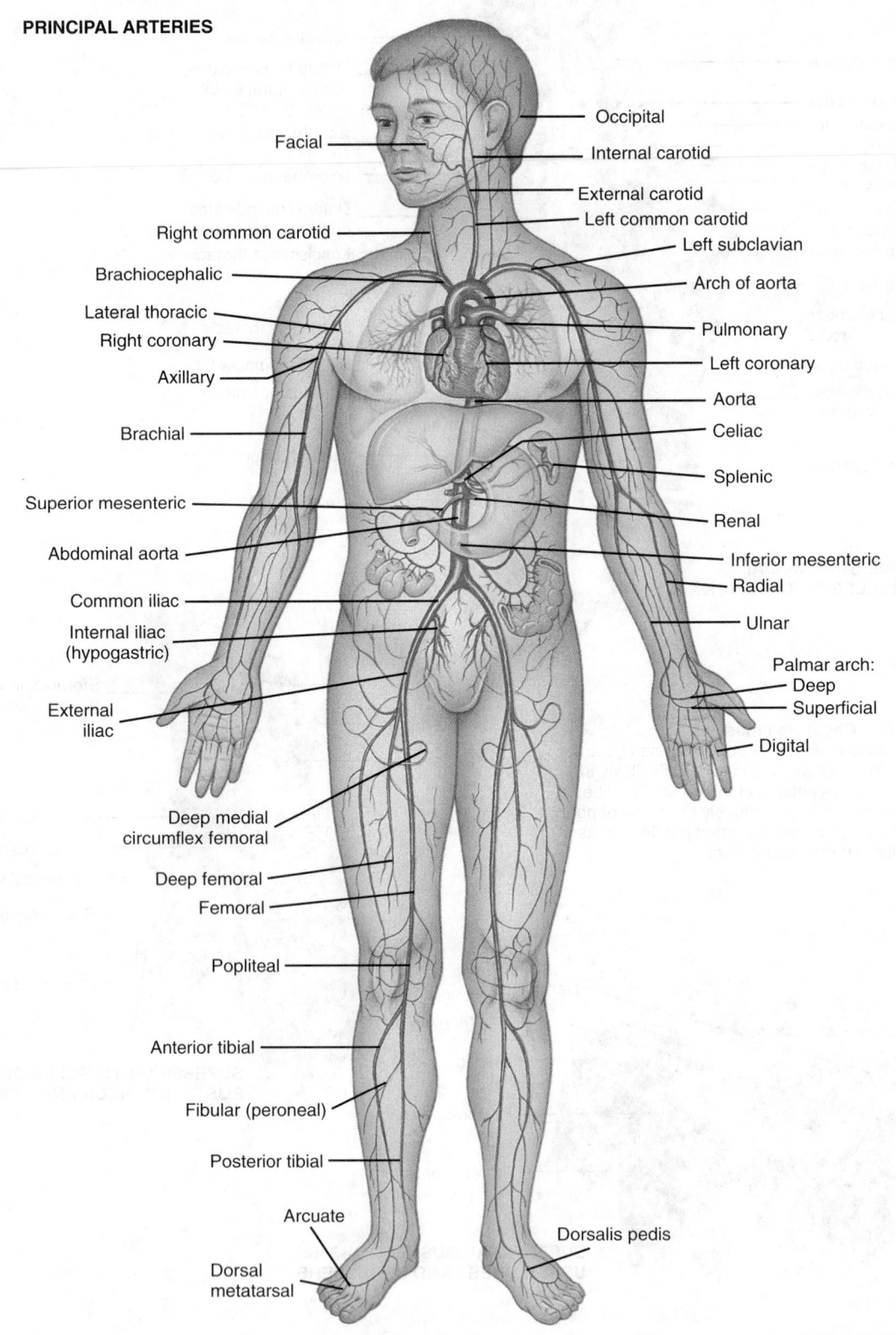

Occipital

Facial

Internal carotid

External carotid

Right common carotid

Left common carotid

Left subclavian

Brachiocephalic

Arch of aorta

Lateral thoracic

Pulmonary

Right coronary

Left coronary

Axillary

Aorta

Brachial

Celiac

Splenic

Superior mesenteric

Renal

Abdominal aorta

Inferior mesenteric

Radial

Common iliac

Ulnar

Internal iliac
(hypogastric)

Palmar arch:
Deep
Superficial

External
iliac

Digital

Deep medial
circumflex femoral

Deep femoral

Femoral

Popliteal

Anterior tibial

Fibular (peroneal)

Posterior tibial

Arcuate

Dorsalis pedis

Dorsal
metatarsal

**PRINCIPAL VEINS**

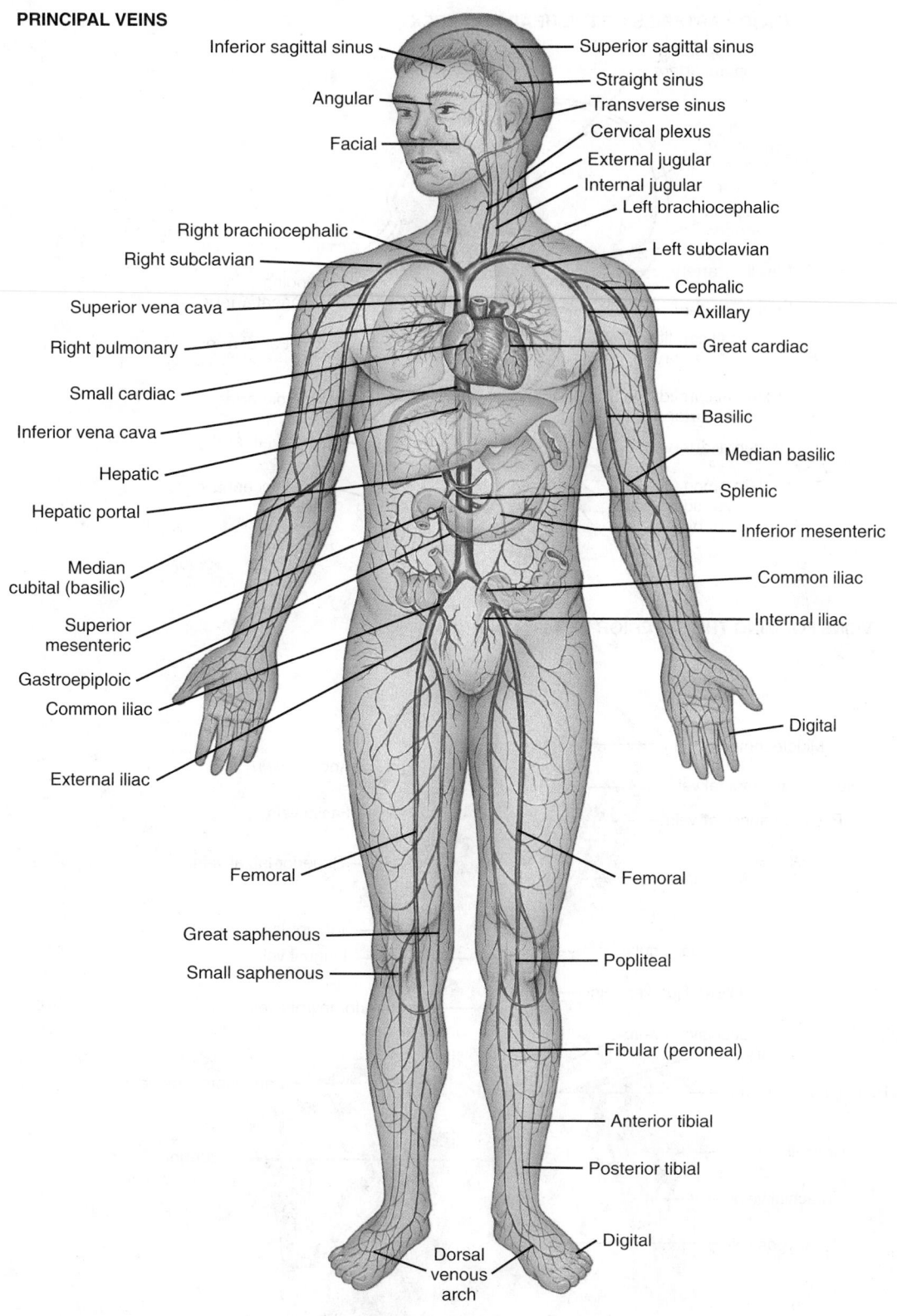

Inferior sagittal sinus

Angular

Facial

Right brachiocephalic

Right subclavian

Superior vena cava

Right pulmonary

Small cardiac

Inferior vena cava

Hepatic

Hepatic portal

Median
cubital (basilic)

Superior
mesenteric

Gastroepiploic

Common iliac

External iliac

Femoral

Great saphenous

Small saphenous

Superior sagittal sinus

Straight sinus

Transverse sinus

Cervical plexus

External jugular

Internal jugular

Left brachiocephalic

Left subclavian

Cephalic

Axillary

Great cardiac

Basilic

Median basilic

Splenic

Inferior mesenteric

Common iliac

Internal iliac

Digital

Femoral

Popliteal

Fibular (peroneal)

Anterior tibial

Posterior tibial

Digital

Dorsal
venous
arch

A-13

## MAJOR ARTERIES OF THE HEAD AND NECK

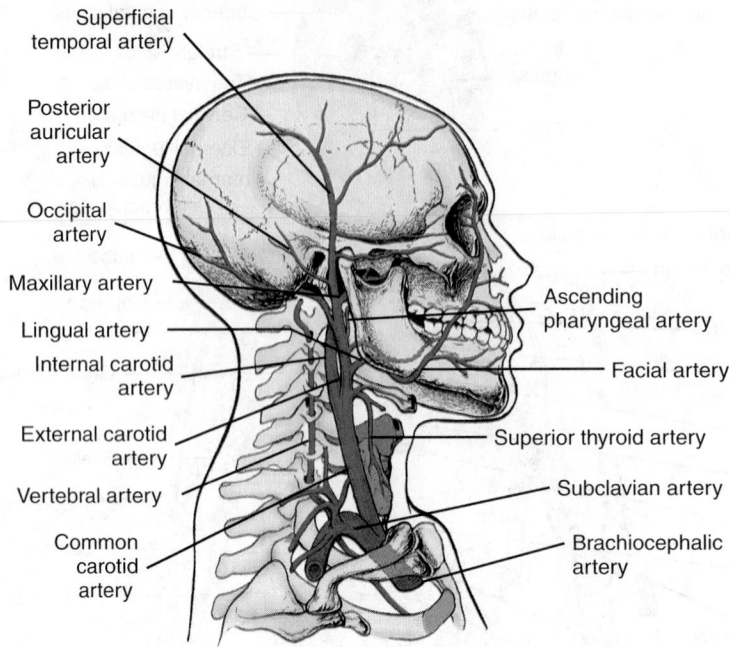

Superficial temporal artery

Posterior auricular artery

Occipital artery

Maxillary artery

Lingual artery

Internal carotid artery

External carotid artery

Vertebral artery

Common carotid artery

Ascending pharyngeal artery

Facial artery

Superior thyroid artery

Subclavian artery

Brachiocephalic artery

## VEINS FORMING THE SUPERIOR VENA CAVA

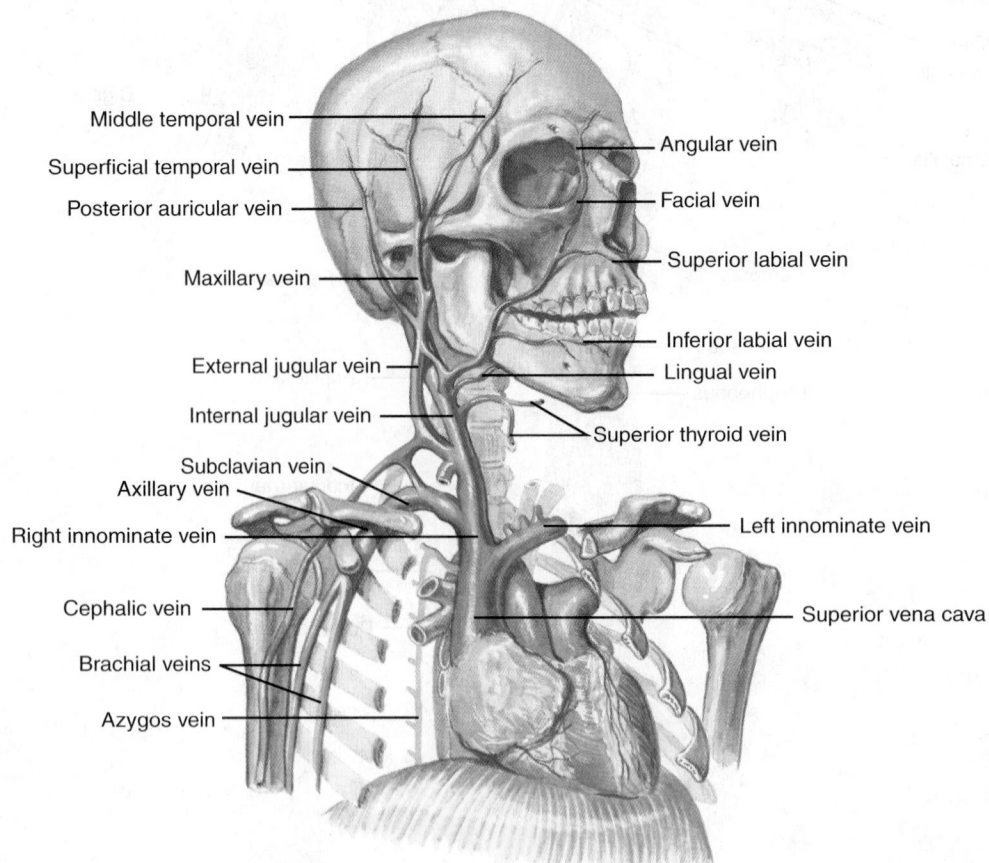

Middle temporal vein

Superficial temporal vein

Posterior auricular vein

Maxillary vein

External jugular vein

Internal jugular vein

Subclavian vein

Axillary vein

Right innominate vein

Cephalic vein

Brachial veins

Azygos vein

Angular vein

Facial vein

Superior labial vein

Inferior labial vein

Lingual vein

Superior thyroid vein

Left innominate vein

Superior vena cava

## ANTERIOR VIEW OF THE HEART

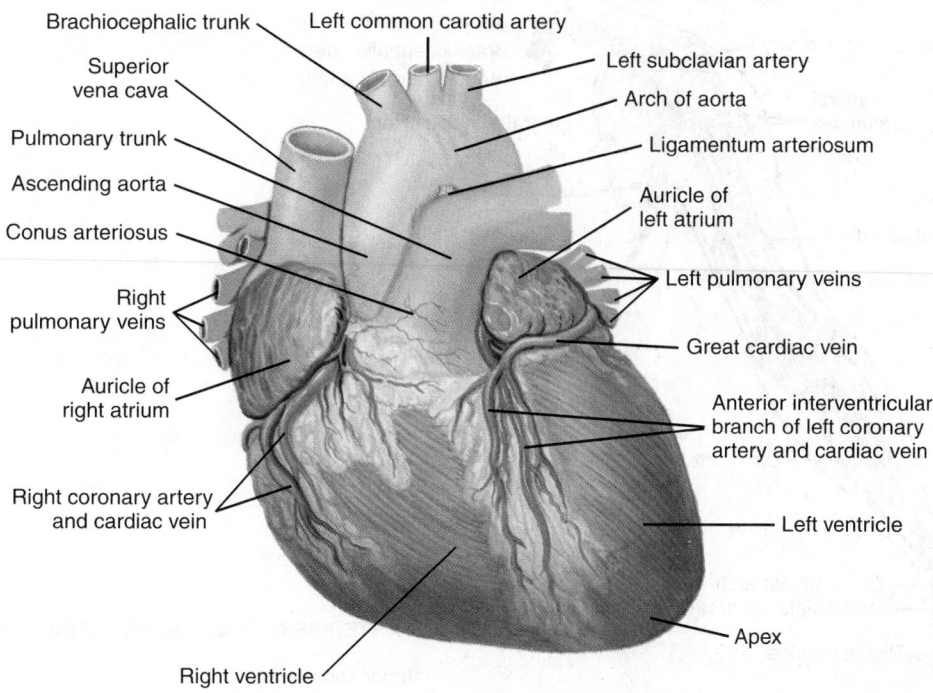

Brachiocephalic trunk

Left common carotid artery

Superior vena cava

Left subclavian artery

Pulmonary trunk

Arch of aorta

Ascending aorta

Ligamentum arteriosum

Conus arteriosus

Auricle of left atrium

Right pulmonary veins

Left pulmonary veins

Great cardiac vein

Auricle of right atrium

Anterior interventricular branch of left coronary artery and cardiac vein

Right coronary artery and cardiac vein

Left ventricle

Apex

Right ventricle

## POSTERIOR VIEW OF THE HEART

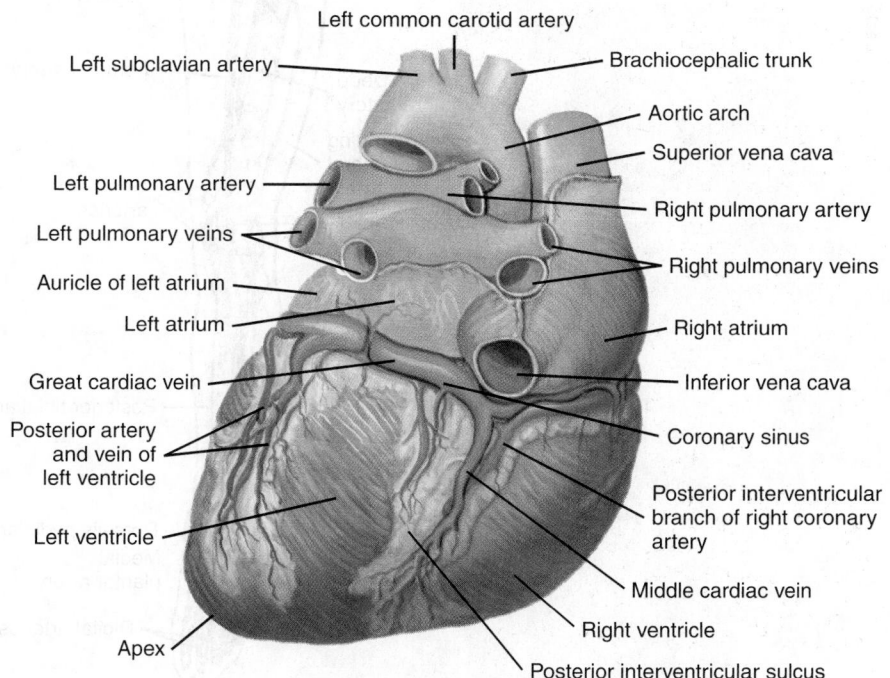

Left common carotid artery

Left subclavian artery

Brachiocephalic trunk

Aortic arch

Superior vena cava

Left pulmonary artery

Right pulmonary artery

Left pulmonary veins

Right pulmonary veins

Auricle of left atrium

Left atrium

Right atrium

Great cardiac vein

Inferior vena cava

Posterior artery and vein of left ventricle

Coronary sinus

Posterior interventricular branch of right coronary artery

Left ventricle

Middle cardiac vein

Apex

Right ventricle

Posterior interventricular sulcus

## MAJOR ARTERIES OF THE UPPER EXTREMITY

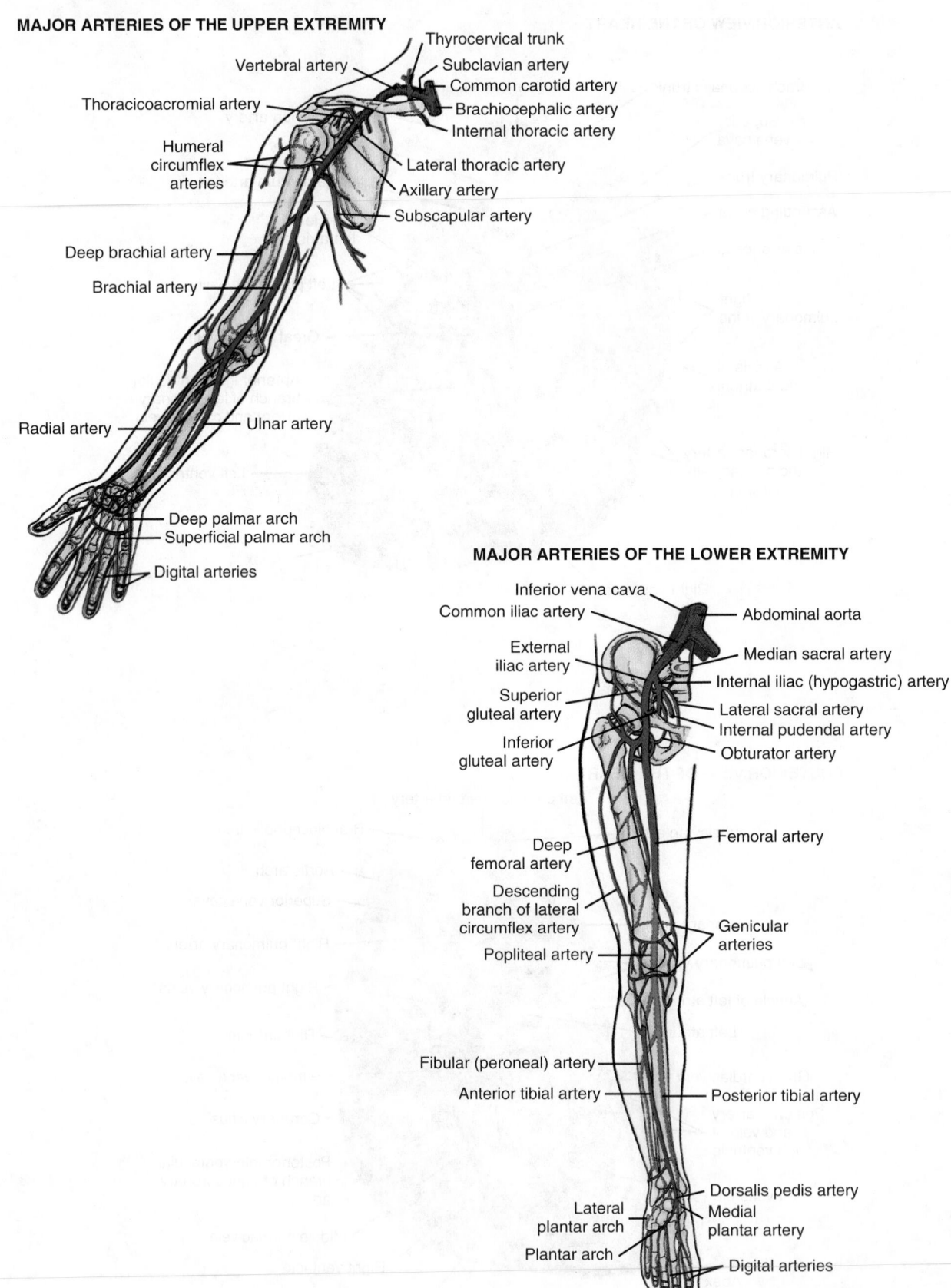

Thyrocervical trunk
Vertebral artery
Subclavian artery
Common carotid artery
Thoracicoacromial artery
Brachiocephalic artery
Internal thoracic artery
Humeral circumflex arteries
Lateral thoracic artery
Axillary artery
Subscapular artery
Deep brachial artery
Brachial artery
Radial artery
Ulnar artery
Deep palmar arch
Superficial palmar arch
Digital arteries

## MAJOR ARTERIES OF THE LOWER EXTREMITY

Inferior vena cava
Common iliac artery
Abdominal aorta
External iliac artery
Median sacral artery
Internal iliac (hypogastric) artery
Superior gluteal artery
Lateral sacral artery
Internal pudendal artery
Inferior gluteal artery
Obturator artery
Deep femoral artery
Femoral artery
Descending branch of lateral circumflex artery
Genicular arteries
Popliteal artery
Fibular (peroneal) artery
Anterior tibial artery
Posterior tibial artery
Dorsalis pedis artery
Lateral plantar arch
Medial plantar artery
Plantar arch
Digital arteries

**MAJOR VEINS OF THE UPPER EXTREMITY**

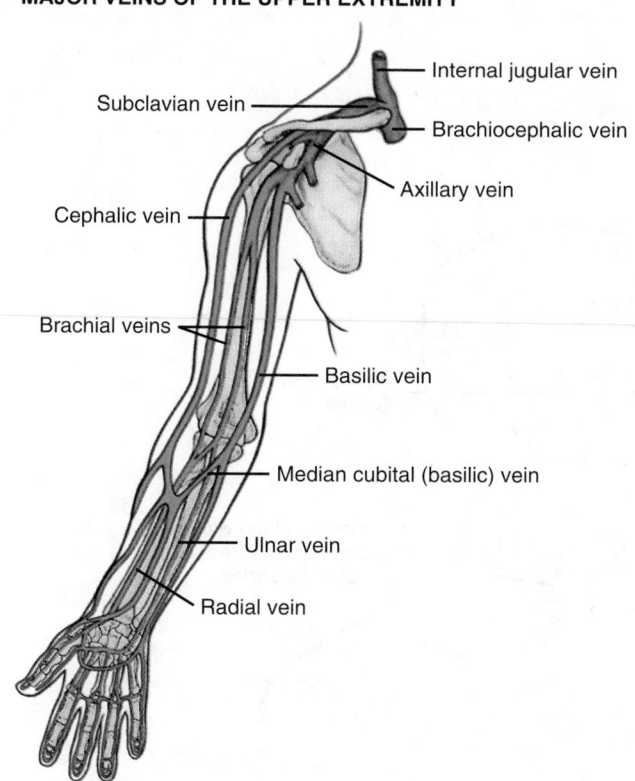

Internal jugular vein

Subclavian vein

Brachiocephalic vein

Axillary vein

Cephalic vein

Brachial veins

Basilic vein

Median cubital (basilic) vein

Ulnar vein

Radial vein

**MAJOR VEINS OF THE LOWER EXTREMITY**

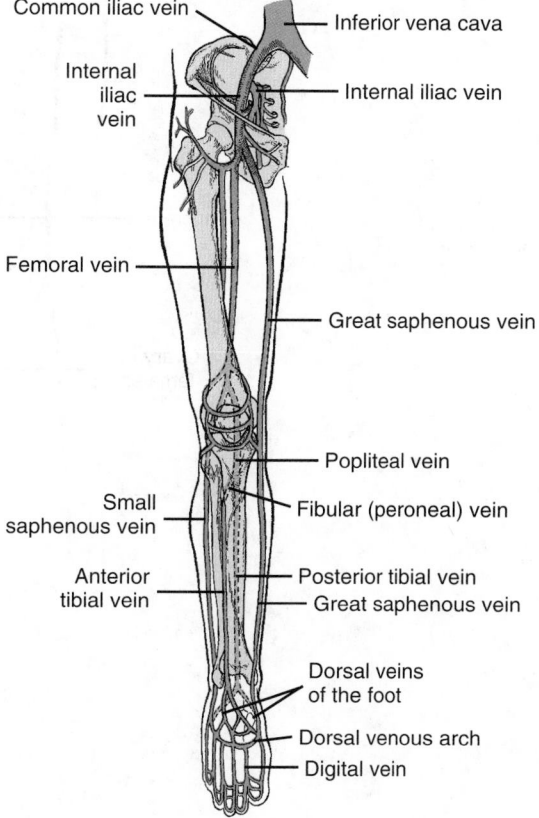

Common iliac vein

Inferior vena cava

Internal iliac vein

Internal iliac vein

Femoral vein

Great saphenous vein

Popliteal vein

Small saphenous vein

Fibular (peroneal) vein

Anterior tibial vein

Posterior tibial vein

Great saphenous vein

Dorsal veins of the foot

Dorsal venous arch

Digital vein

# ENDOCRINE SYSTEM

**GLANDS OF THE ENDOCRINE SYSTEM**

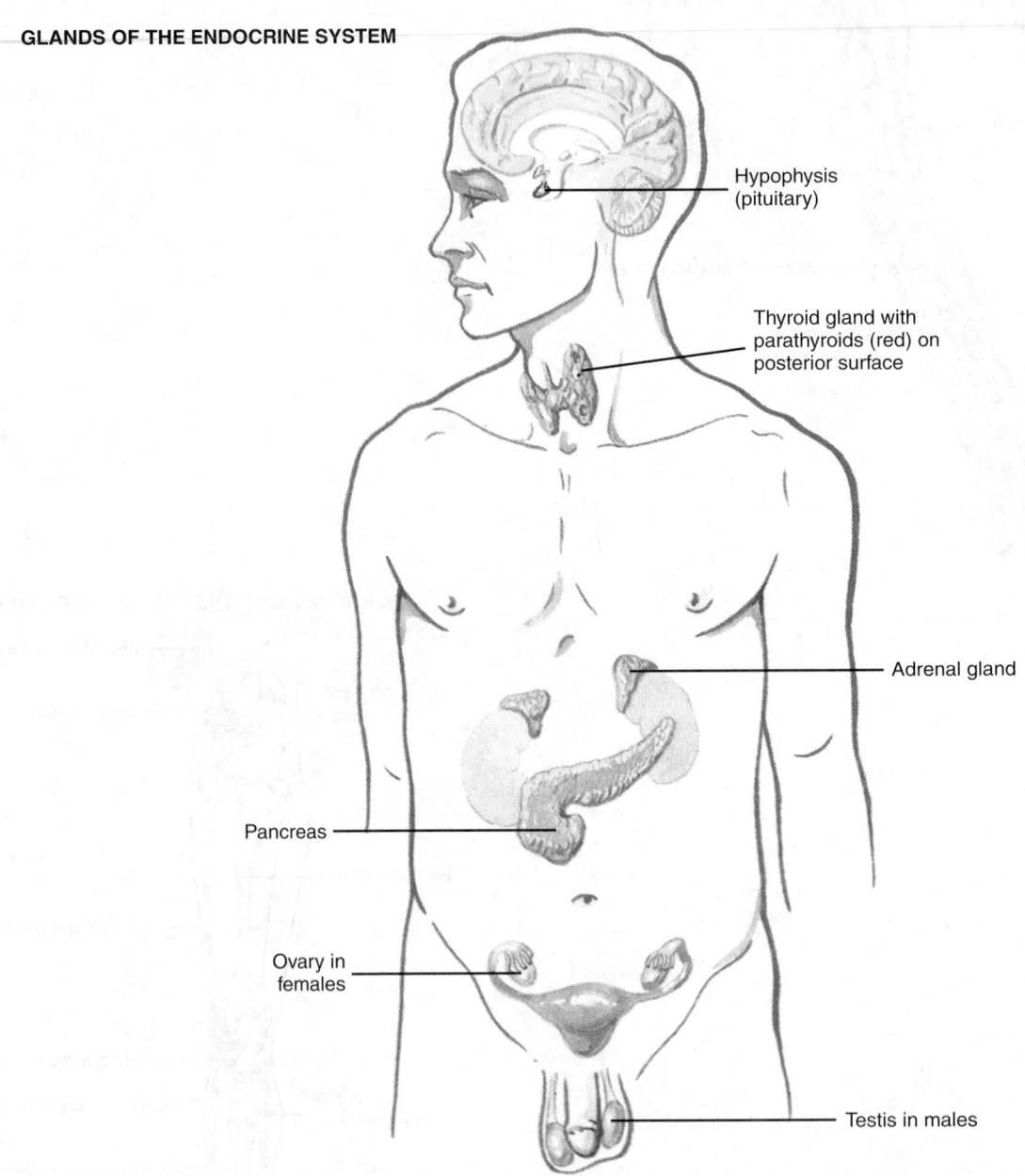

Hypophysis (pituitary)

Thyroid gland with parathyroids (red) on posterior surface

Adrenal gland

Pancreas

Ovary in females

Testis in males

**LOCATION OF THE PITUITARY AND PINEAL GLANDS**

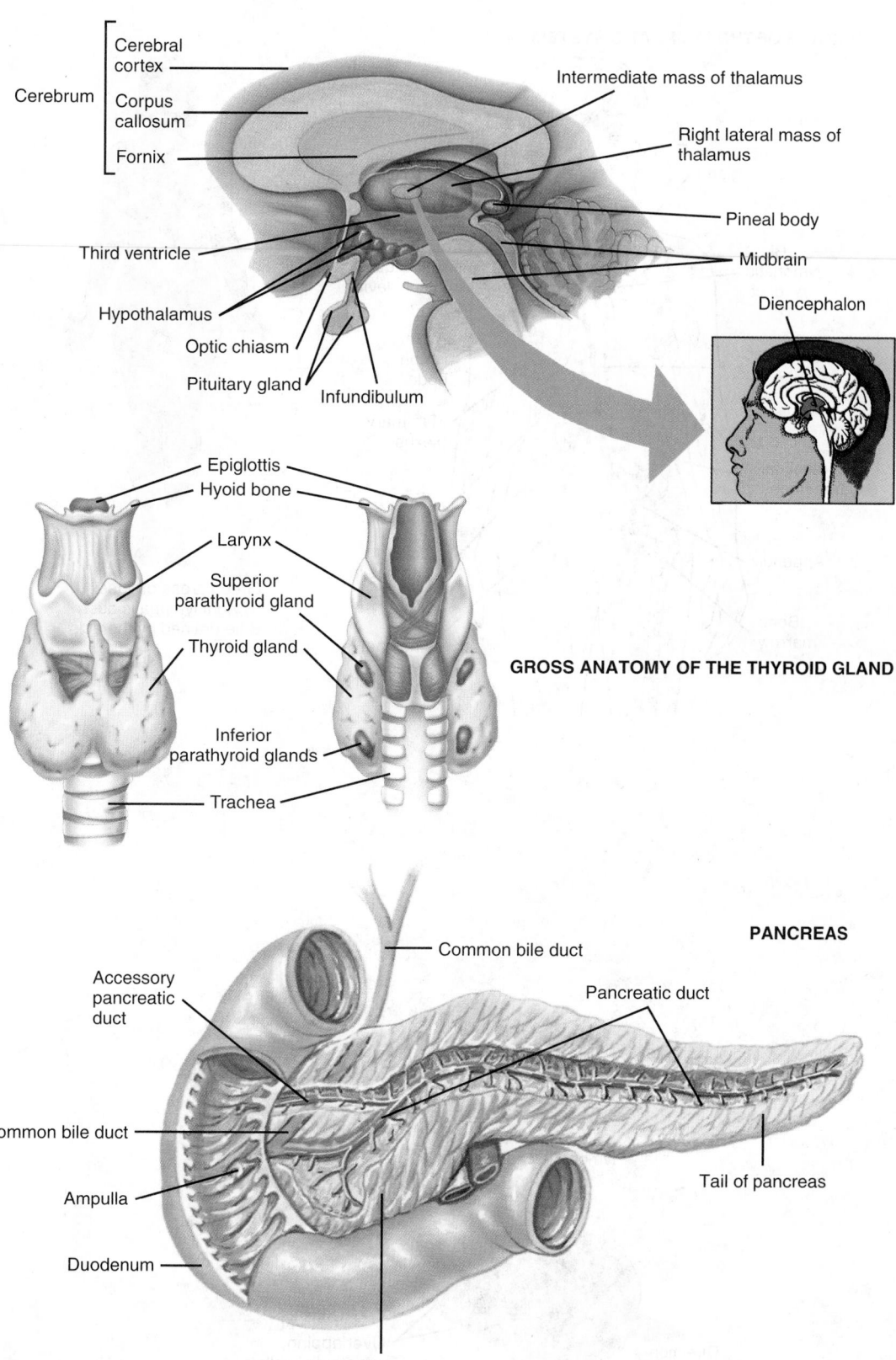

Cerebrum
- Cerebral cortex
- Corpus callosum
- Fornix

Intermediate mass of thalamus

Right lateral mass of thalamus

Pineal body

Midbrain

Third ventricle

Hypothalamus

Optic chiasm

Pituitary gland

Infundibulum

Diencephalon

Epiglottis

Hyoid bone

Larynx

Superior parathyroid gland

Thyroid gland

Inferior parathyroid glands

Trachea

**GROSS ANATOMY OF THE THYROID GLAND**

**PANCREAS**

Common bile duct

Pancreatic duct

Accessory pancreatic duct

Common bile duct

Ampulla

Duodenum

Tail of pancreas

Head of pancreas

# LYMPHATIC SYSTEM

## ORGANS OF THE LYMPHATIC SYSTEM

Thymus gland

Tonsils

Cervical lymph node

Right lymphatic duct

Entrance of thoracic duct into subclavian vein

Thoracic duct

Axillary lymph node

Mammary plexus

Intestinal lymph nodes

Appendix

Spleen

Peyer's patches in intestinal wall

Bone marrow

Inguinal lymph nodes

Green areas drained by right lymphatic duct. Blue drained by thoracic duct.

## STRUCTURE OF A LYMPHATIC CAPILLARY

Fluid entering lymphatic capillary

Valve closed

Valve open

Direction of flow

Overlapping endothelial cells

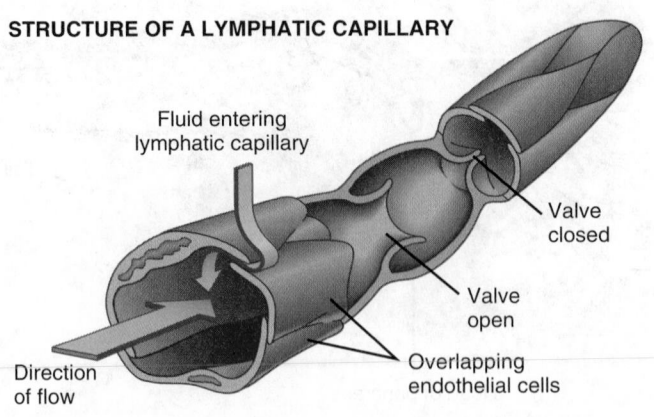

## STRUCTURE OF THE SPLEEN

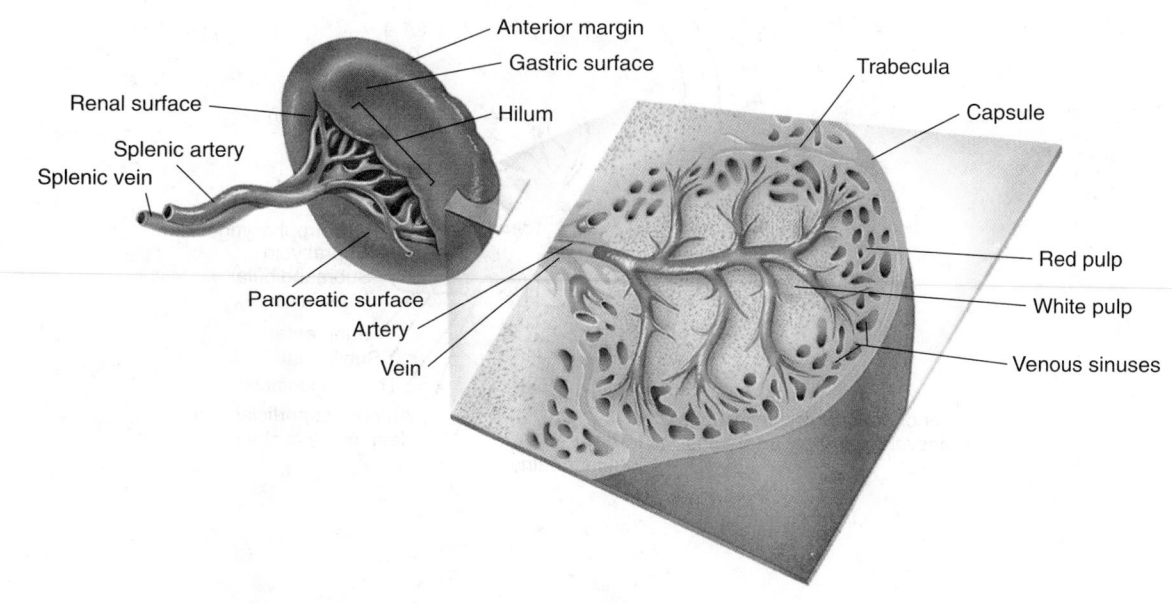

## LOCATION AND GROSS ANATOMY OF THE THYMUS

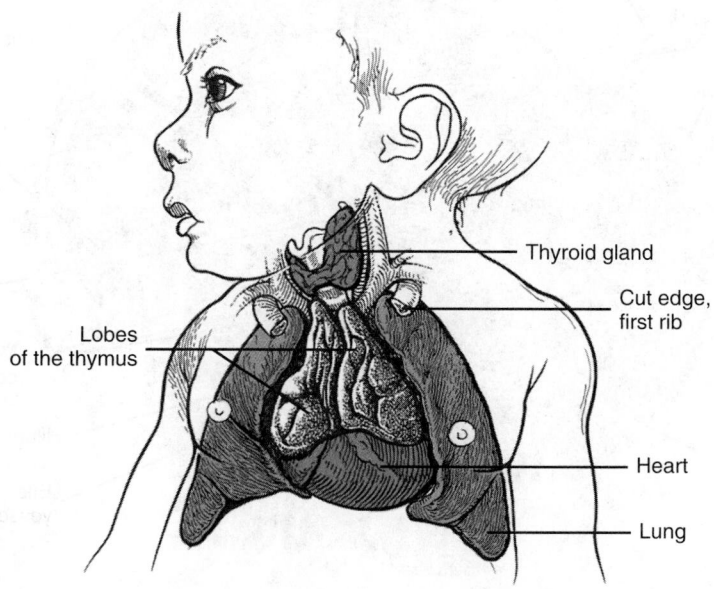

## LYMPHATIC DRAINAGE SYSTEM OF THE HEAD AND NECK

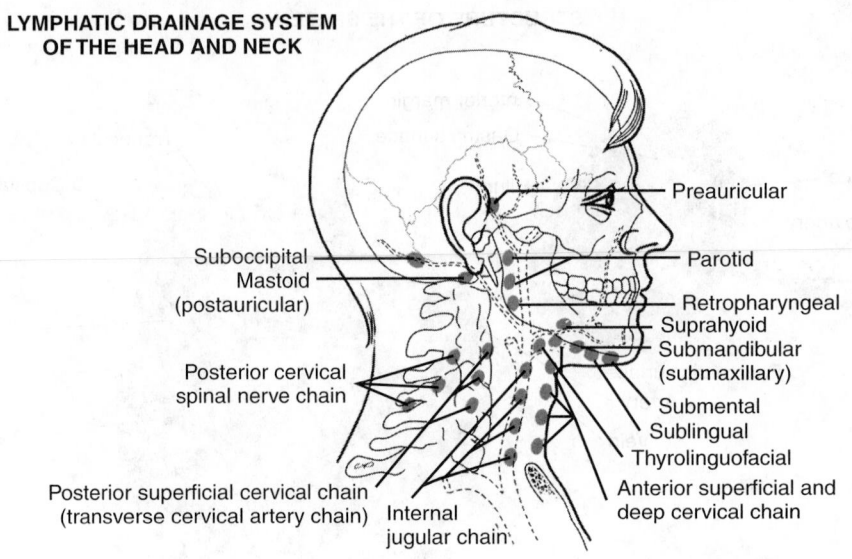

Preauricular

Suboccipital

Mastoid (postauricular)

Parotid

Retropharyngeal

Suprahyoid

Submandibular (submaxillary)

Posterior cervical spinal nerve chain

Submental

Sublingual

Thyrolinguofacial

Posterior superficial cervical chain (transverse cervical artery chain)

Internal jugular chain

Anterior superficial and deep cervical chain

## SCHEMATIC SECTION OF A LYMPH NODE

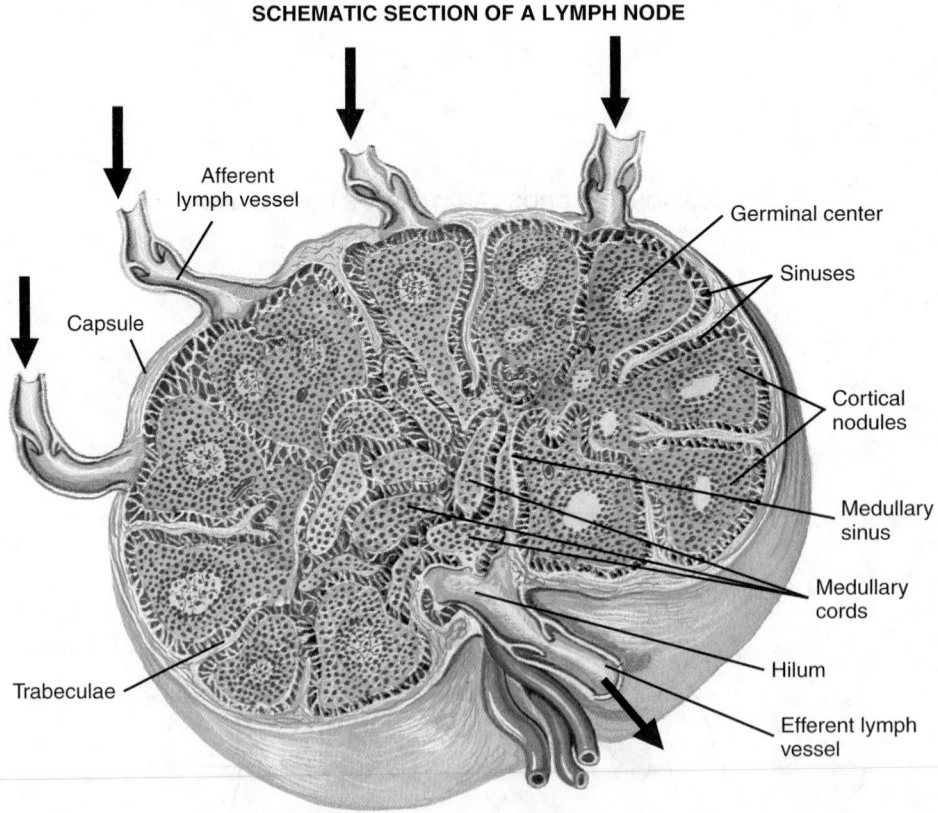

Afferent lymph vessel

Germinal center

Sinuses

Capsule

Cortical nodules

Medullary sinus

Medullary cords

Hilum

Trabeculae

Efferent lymph vessel

# NERVOUS SYSTEM

**SIMPLIFIED VIEW OF THE NERVOUS SYSTEM**

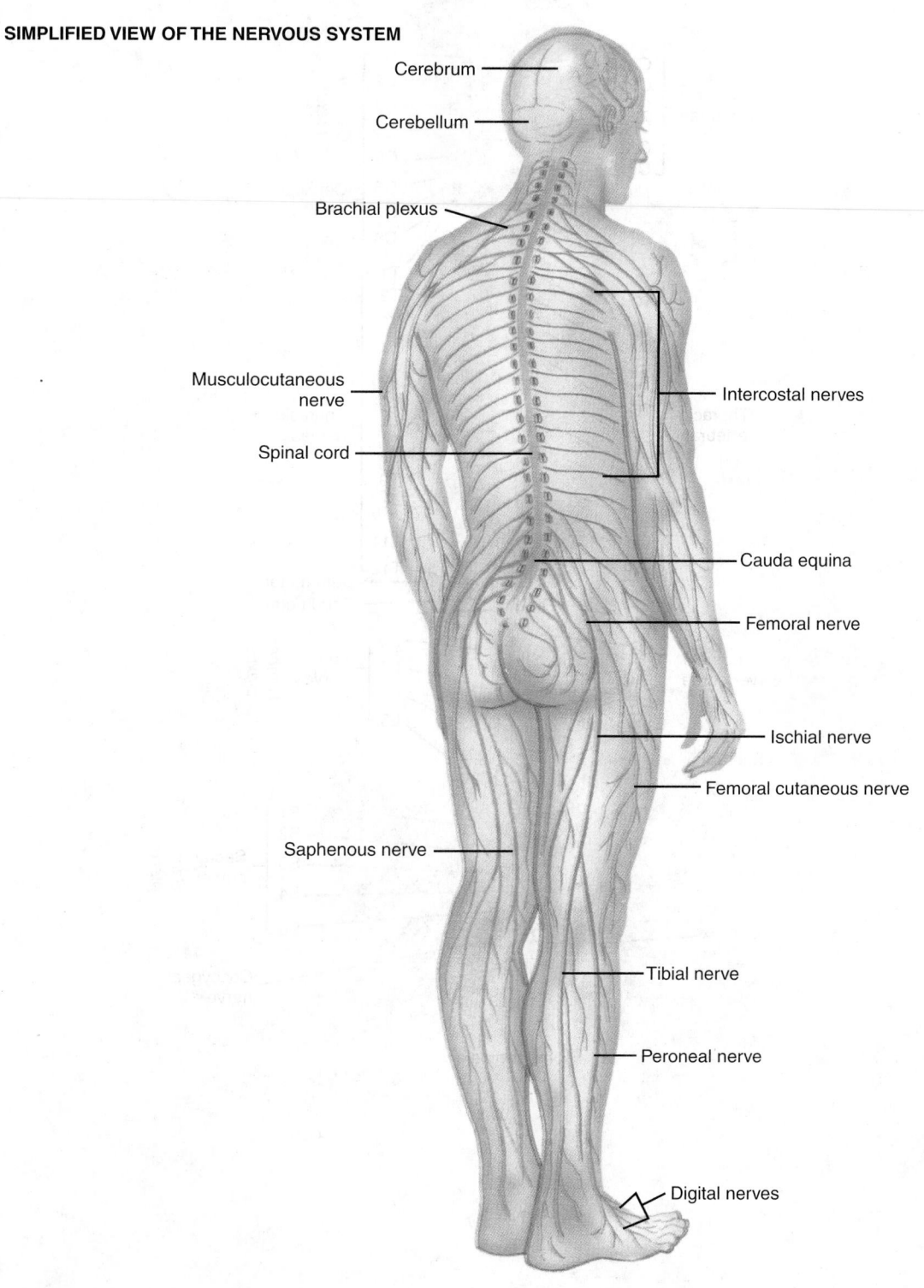

Cerebrum

Cerebellum

Brachial plexus

Musculocutaneous nerve

Spinal cord

Intercostal nerves

Cauda equina

Femoral nerve

Ischial nerve

Femoral cutaneous nerve

Saphenous nerve

Tibial nerve

Peroneal nerve

Digital nerves

## GROSS ANATOMY OF THE SPINAL CORD

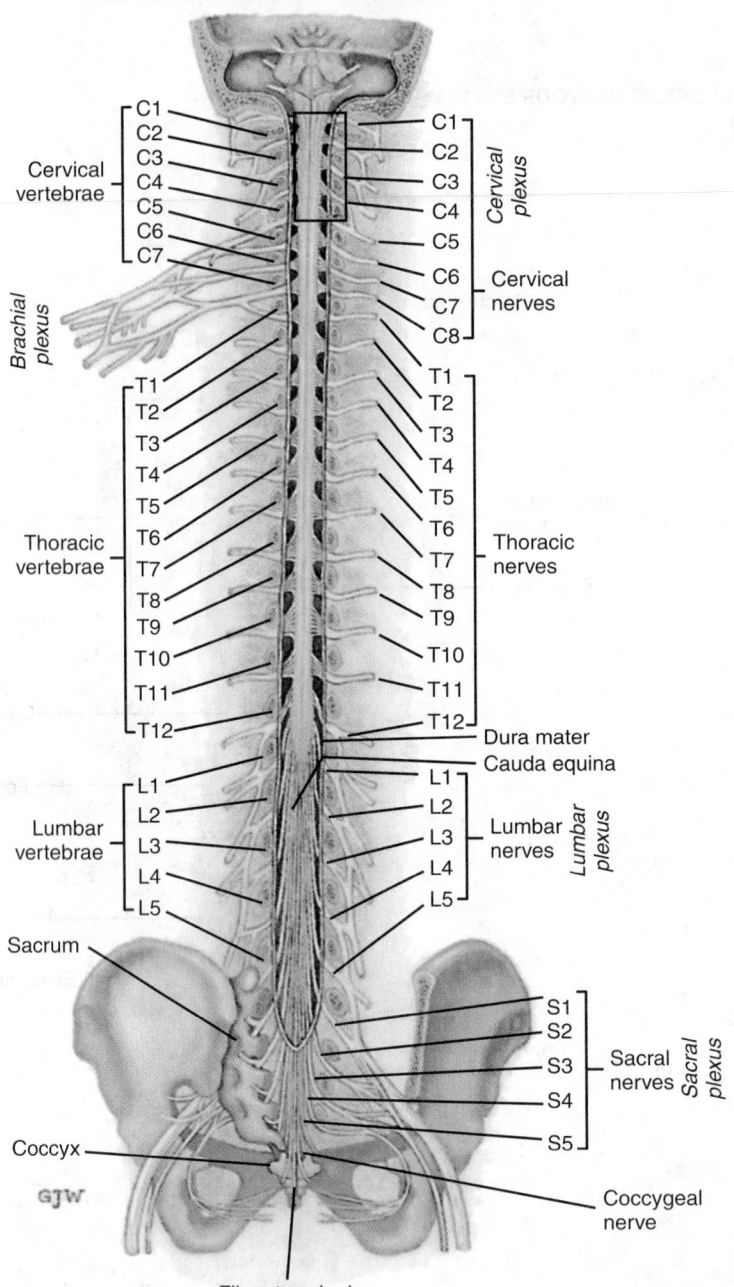

Cervical vertebrae

C1
C2
C3
C4
C5
C6
C7

*Brachial plexus*

T1
T2
T3
T4
T5
T6
T7
T8
T9
T10
T11
T12

Thoracic vertebrae

Lumbar vertebrae

L1
L2
L3
L4
L5

Sacrum

Coccyx

GJW

Filum terminale

C1
C2
C3
C4
C5
C6
C7
C8

*Cervical plexus*

Cervical nerves

T1
T2
T3
T4
T5
T6
T7
T8
T9
T10
T11
T12

Thoracic nerves

Dura mater
Cauda equina

L1
L2
L3
L4
L5

Lumbar nerves

*Lumbar plexus*

S1
S2
S3
S4
S5

Sacral nerves

*Sacral plexus*

Coccygeal nerve

## CEREBRAL NUCLEI

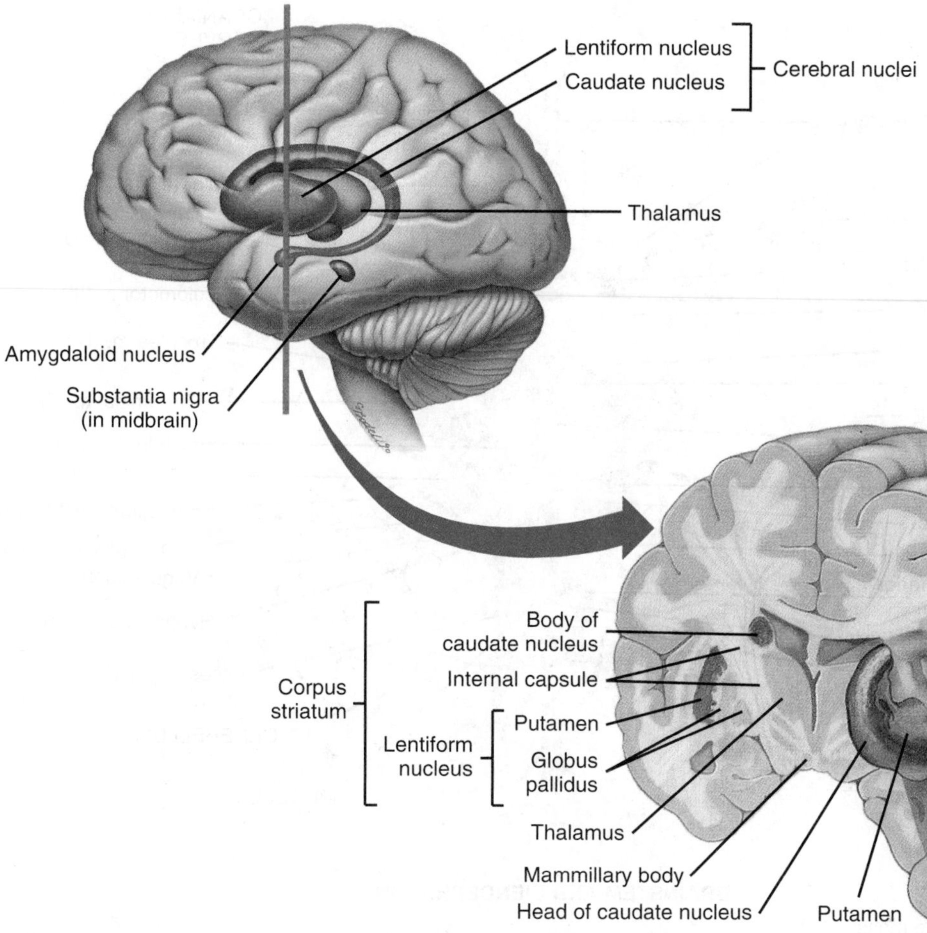

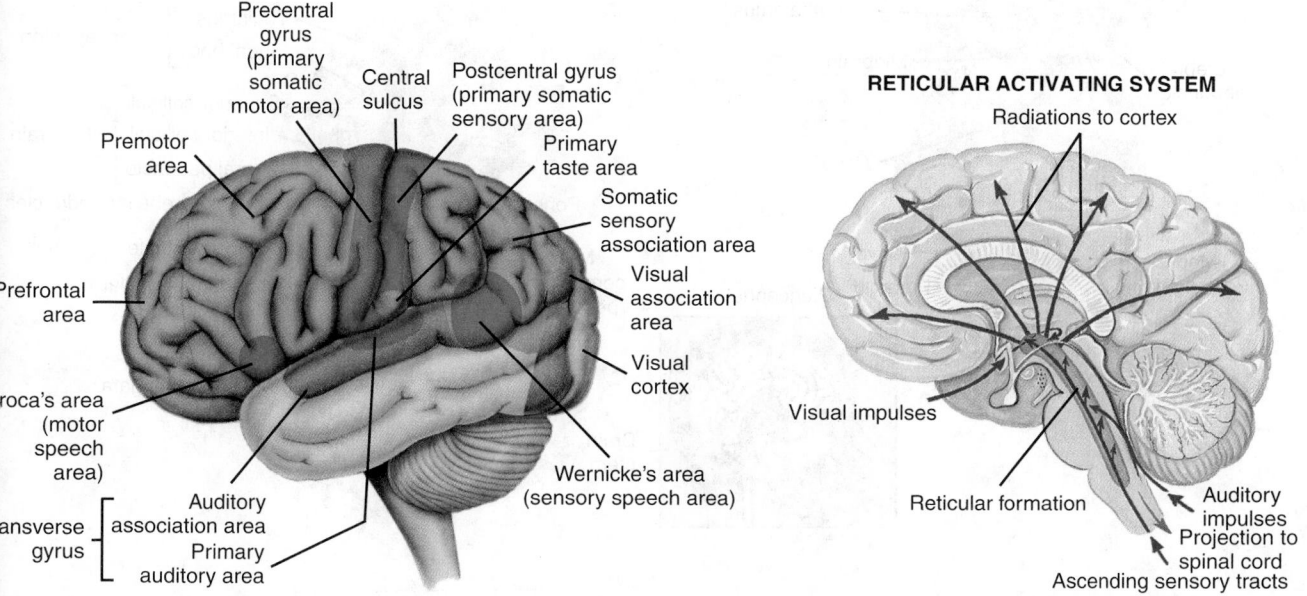

Lentiform nucleus
Caudate nucleus
Cerebral nuclei
Thalamus

Amygdaloid nucleus
Substantia nigra
(in midbrain)

Corpus
striatum

Body of
caudate nucleus
Internal capsule

Lentiform
nucleus
Putamen
Globus
pallidus

Thalamus
Mammillary body
Head of caudate nucleus
Putamen

## FUNCTIONAL AREAS OF THE CEREBRAL CORTEX

Precentral
gyrus
(primary
somatic
motor area)

Central
sulcus

Postcentral gyrus
(primary somatic
sensory area)

Primary
taste area

Premotor
area

Somatic
sensory
association area

Prefrontal
area

Visual
association
area

Visual
cortex

Broca's area
(motor
speech
area)

Wernicke's area
(sensory speech area)

Transverse
gyrus

Auditory
association area
Primary
auditory area

## RETICULAR ACTIVATING SYSTEM

Radiations to cortex

Visual impulses

Reticular formation

Auditory
impulses
Projection to
spinal cord
Ascending sensory tracts

## BASE OF THE BRAIN

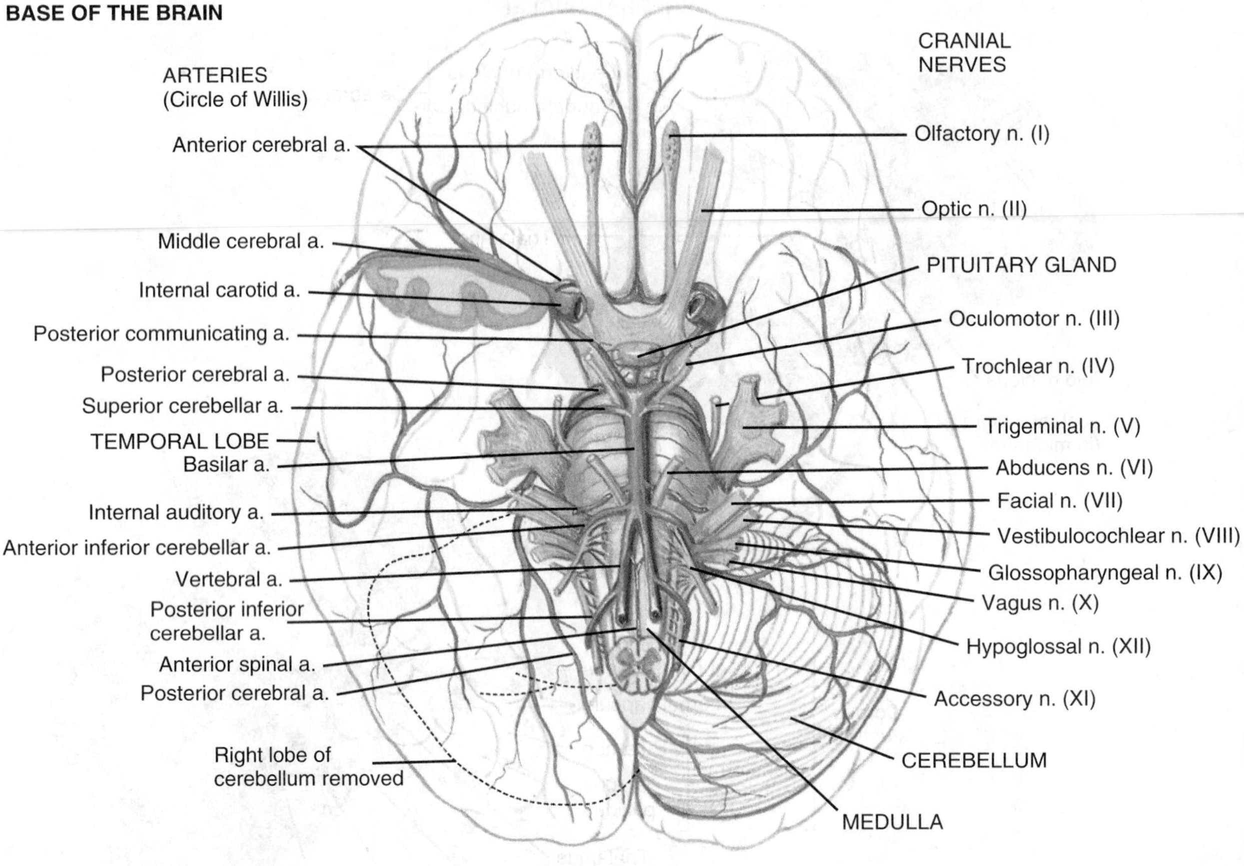

ARTERIES
(Circle of Willis)

Anterior cerebral a.

Middle cerebral a.

Internal carotid a.

Posterior communicating a.

Posterior cerebral a.

Superior cerebellar a.

TEMPORAL LOBE

Basilar a.

Internal auditory a.

Anterior inferior cerebellar a.

Vertebral a.

Posterior inferior cerebellar a.

Anterior spinal a.

Posterior cerebral a.

Right lobe of cerebellum removed

CRANIAL NERVES

Olfactory n. (I)

Optic n. (II)

PITUITARY GLAND

Oculomotor n. (III)

Trochlear n. (IV)

Trigeminal n. (V)

Abducens n. (VI)

Facial n. (VII)

Vestibulocochlear n. (VIII)

Glossopharyngeal n. (IX)

Vagus n. (X)

Hypoglossal n. (XII)

Accessory n. (XI)

CEREBELLUM

MEDULLA

## BRAINSTEM AND DIENCEPHALON

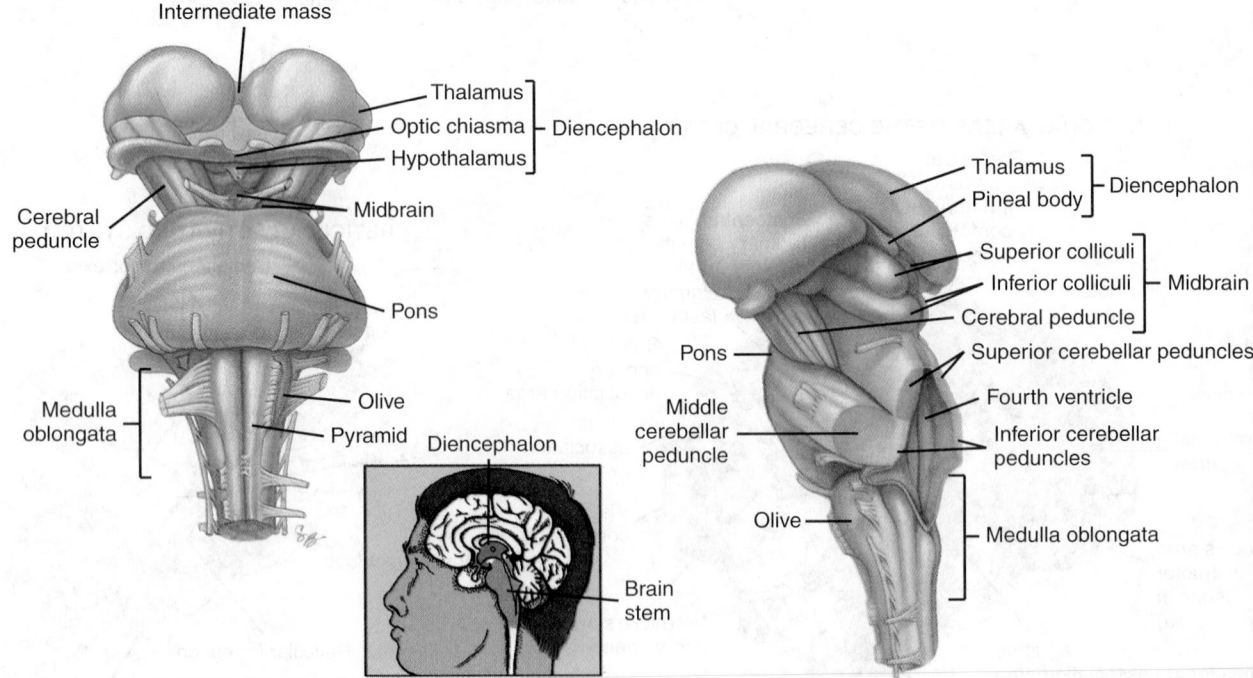

Intermediate mass

Thalamus
Optic chiasma — Diencephalon
Hypothalamus

Cerebral peduncle

Midbrain

Pons

Medulla oblongata

Olive
Pyramid

Diencephalon

Brain stem

Thalamus
Pineal body — Diencephalon

Superior colliculi
Inferior colliculi — Midbrain
Cerebral peduncle

Superior cerebellar peduncles

Fourth ventricle

Inferior cerebellar peduncles

Medulla oblongata

Pons

Middle cerebellar peduncle

Olive

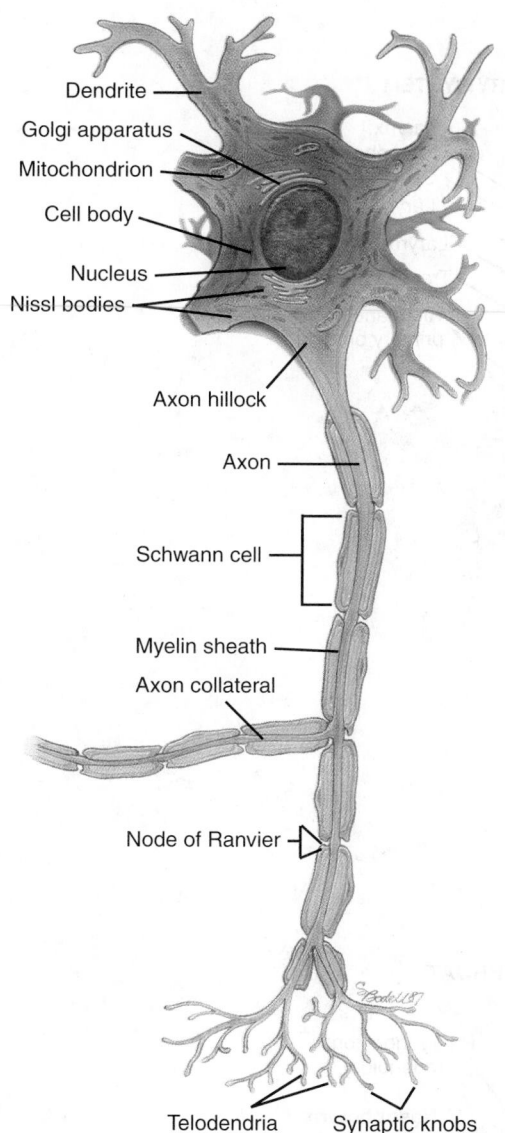

**BASIC STRUCTURE OF THE NEURON**

Dendrite

Golgi apparatus

Mitochondrion

Cell body

Nucleus

Nissl bodies

Axon hillock

Axon

Schwann cell

Myelin sheath

Axon collateral

Node of Ranvier

Telodendria   Synaptic knobs

**MYELINATED AXON**

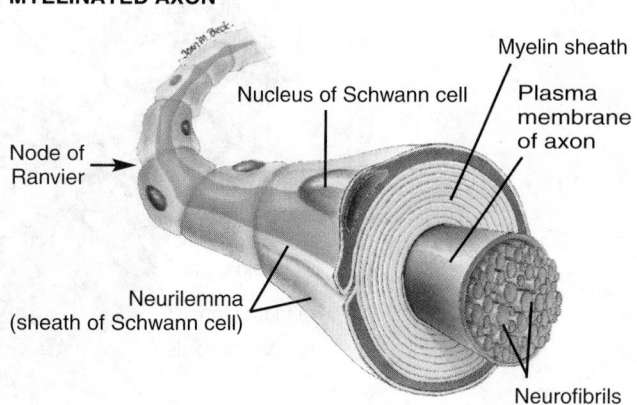

Node of Ranvier

Nucleus of Schwann cell

Myelin sheath

Plasma membrane of axon

Neurilemma (sheath of Schwann cell)

Neurofibrils

# RESPIRATORY SYSTEM

## ORGANS OF THE RESPIRATORY SYSTEM

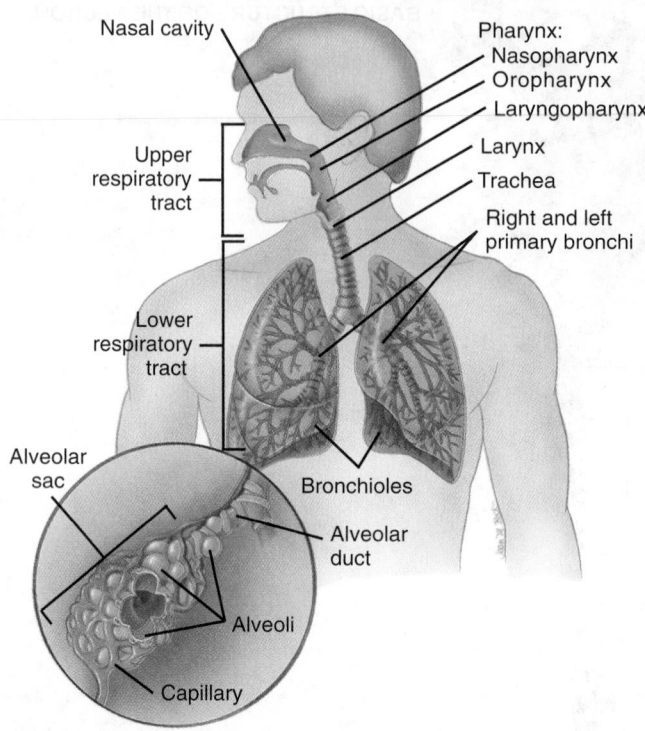

Nasal cavity

Pharynx:
Nasopharynx
Oropharynx
Laryngopharynx

Larynx

Trachea

Right and left
primary bronchi

Upper
respiratory
tract

Lower
respiratory
tract

Alveolar
sac

Bronchioles

Alveolar
duct

Alveoli

Capillary

## NASAL PASSAGES AND THROAT

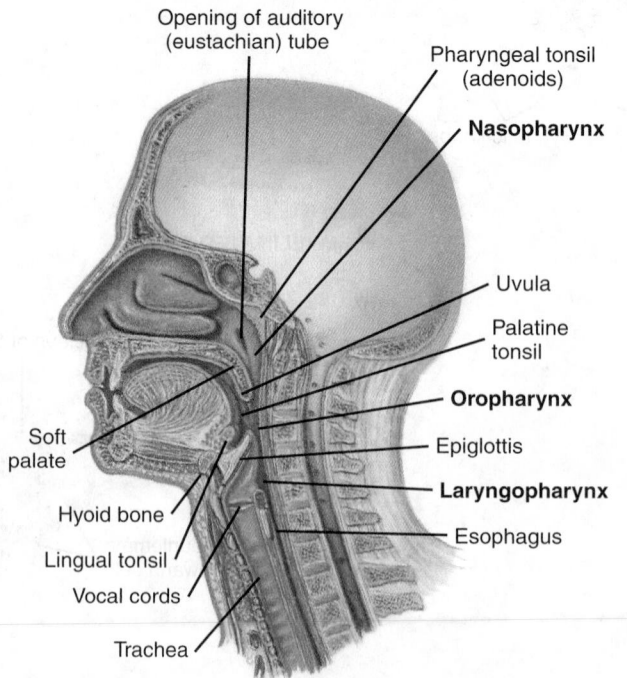

Opening of auditory
(eustachian) tube

Pharyngeal tonsil
(adenoids)

**Nasopharynx**

Uvula

Palatine
tonsil

**Oropharynx**

Epiglottis

**Laryngopharynx**

Esophagus

Soft
palate

Hyoid bone

Lingual tonsil

Vocal cords

Trachea

## NASAL SEPTUM

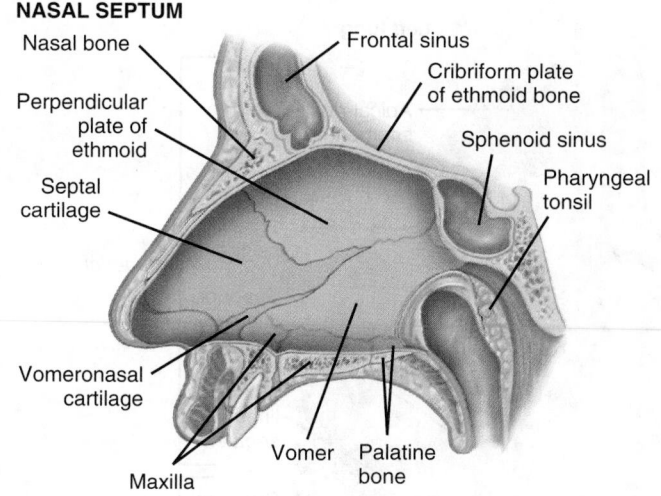

Nasal bone
Frontal sinus
Cribriform plate of ethmoid bone
Perpendicular plate of ethmoid
Sphenoid sinus
Septal cartilage
Pharyngeal tonsil
Vomeronasal cartilage
Maxilla
Vomer
Palatine bone

## NASAL CAVITY

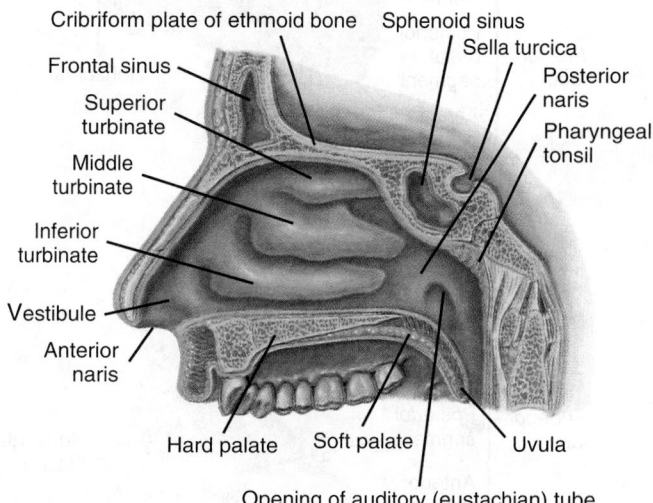

Cribriform plate of ethmoid bone
Sphenoid sinus
Sella turcica
Frontal sinus
Posterior naris
Superior turbinate
Pharyngeal tonsil
Middle turbinate
Inferior turbinate
Vestibule
Anterior naris
Hard palate
Soft palate
Uvula
Opening of auditory (eustachian) tube

## BONES OF THE NASAL CAVITY

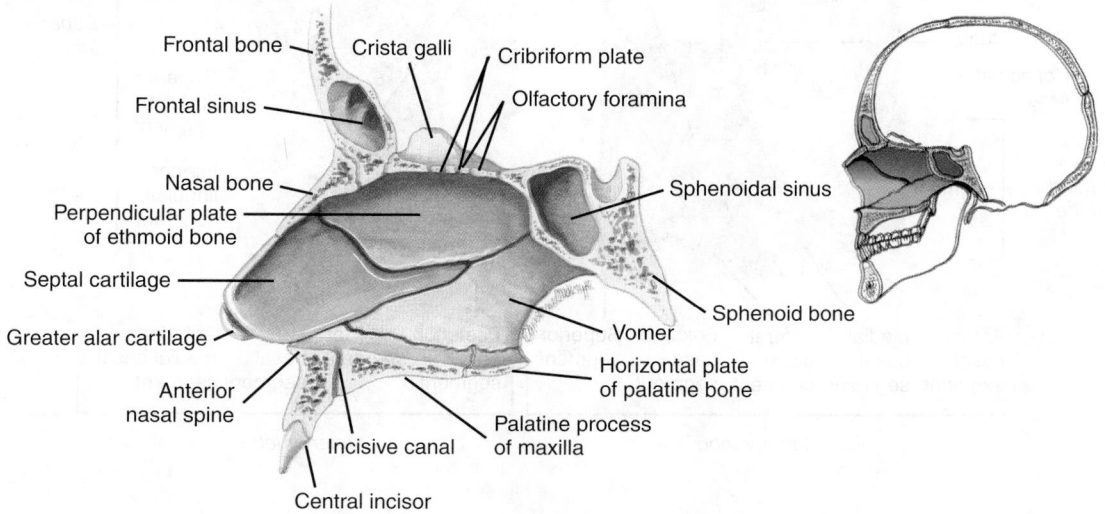

Frontal bone
Crista galli
Cribriform plate
Frontal sinus
Olfactory foramina
Nasal bone
Perpendicular plate of ethmoid bone
Sphenoidal sinus
Septal cartilage
Greater alar cartilage
Sphenoid bone
Anterior nasal spine
Vomer
Horizontal plate of palatine bone
Incisive canal
Palatine process of maxilla
Central incisor

**LUNGS**

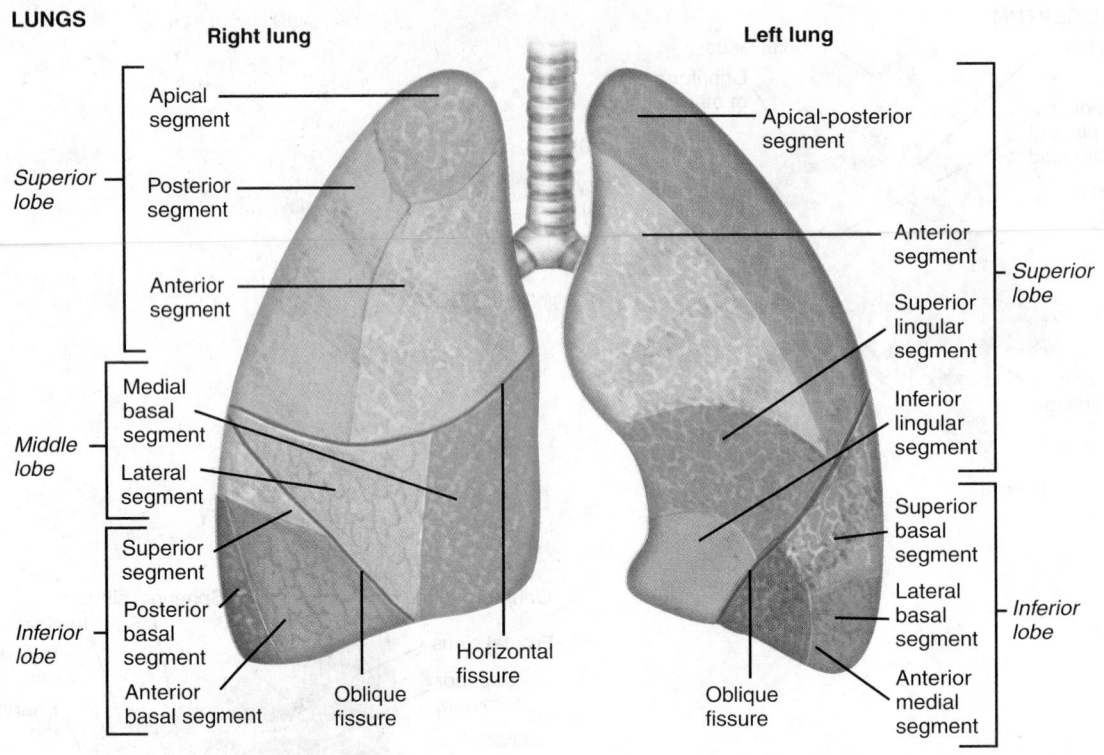

**Right lung**

Apical segment
Posterior segment
Anterior segment

*Superior lobe*

*Middle lobe*

Medial basal segment
Lateral segment

*Inferior lobe*

Superior segment
Posterior basal segment
Anterior basal segment

Oblique fissure

Horizontal fissure

**Left lung**

Apical-posterior segment
Anterior segment
Superior lingular segment
Inferior lingular segment

*Superior lobe*

Superior basal segment
Lateral basal segment
Anterior medial segment

Oblique fissure

*Inferior lobe*

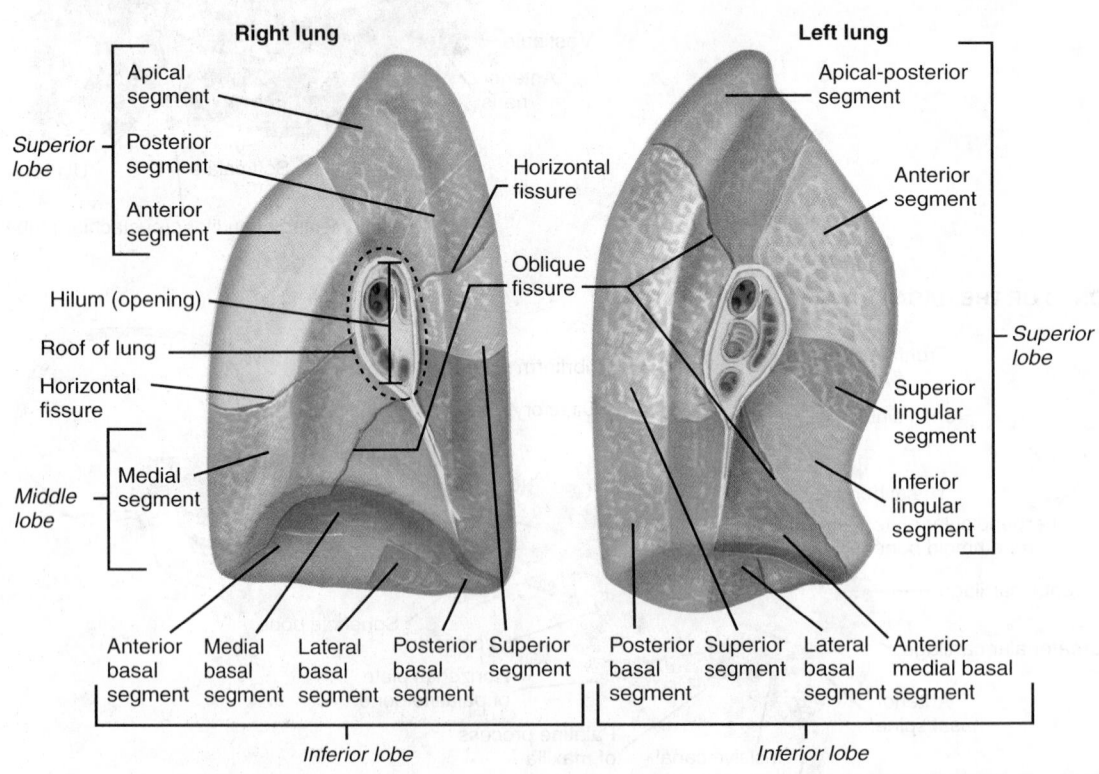

**Right lung**

Apical segment
Posterior segment
Anterior segment

*Superior lobe*

Hilum (opening)
Roof of lung
Horizontal fissure

*Middle lobe*

Medial segment

Horizontal fissure
Oblique fissure

Anterior basal segment
Medial basal segment
Lateral basal segment
Posterior basal segment
Superior segment

**Left lung**

Apical-posterior segment
Anterior segment

*Superior lobe*

Superior lingular segment
Inferior lingular segment

Posterior basal segment
Superior segment
Lateral basal segment
Anterior medial basal segment

*Inferior lobe*

*Inferior lobe*

## LARYNX AND UPPER TRACHEA

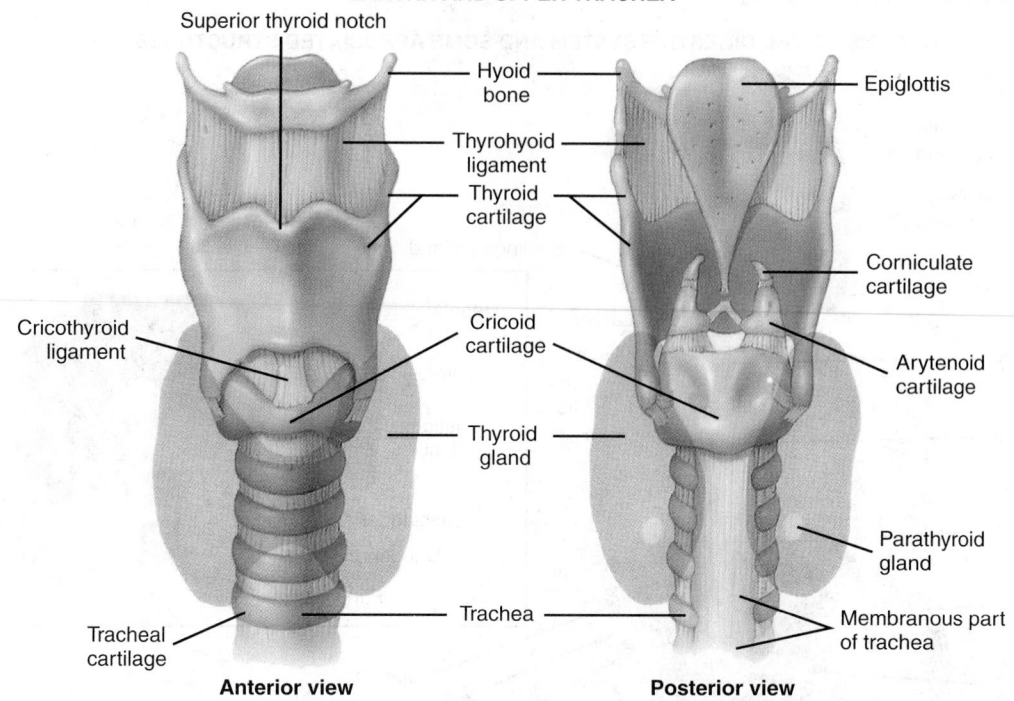

Superior thyroid notch

Hyoid bone

Epiglottis

Thyrohyoid ligament

Thyroid cartilage

Corniculate cartilage

Cricothyroid ligament

Cricoid cartilage

Arytenoid cartilage

Thyroid gland

Parathyroid gland

Tracheal cartilage

Trachea

Membranous part of trachea

**Anterior view**

**Posterior view**

## GAS-EXCHANGE STRUCTURES OF THE LUNG

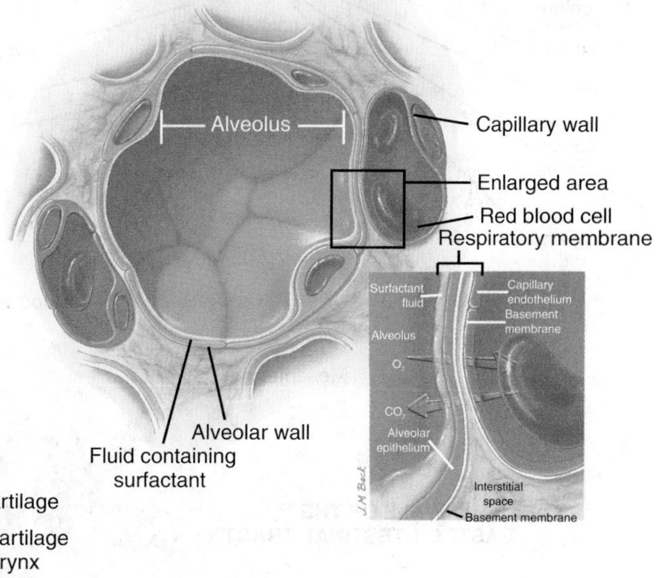

Alveolus

Capillary wall

Enlarged area

Red blood cell
Respiratory membrane

Surfactant fluid

Capillary endothelium

Basement membrane

Alveolus

$O_2$

$CO_2$

Alveolar epithelium

Interstitial space

Basement membrane

Alveolar wall

Fluid containing surfactant

## LARYNX

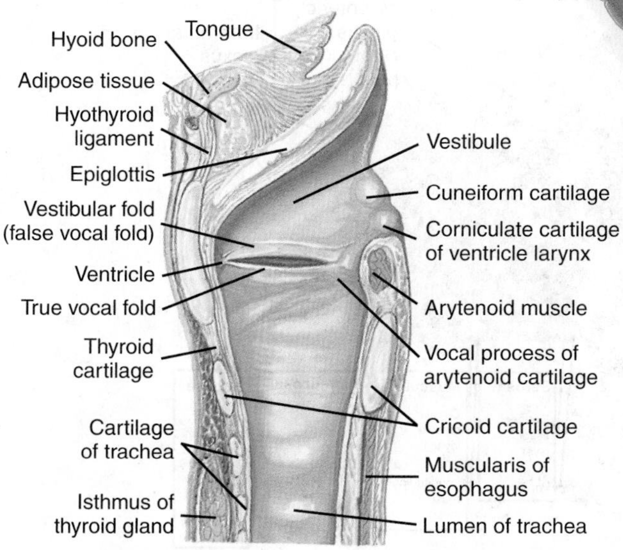

Tongue

Hyoid bone

Adipose tissue

Hyothyroid ligament

Epiglottis

Vestibular fold (false vocal fold)

Ventricle

True vocal fold

Thyroid cartilage

Cartilage of trachea

Isthmus of thyroid gland

Vestibule

Cuneiform cartilage

Corniculate cartilage of ventricle larynx

Arytenoid muscle

Vocal process of arytenoid cartilage

Cricoid cartilage

Muscularis of esophagus

Lumen of trachea

# DIGESTIVE SYSTEM

## ORGANS OF THE DIGESTIVE SYSTEM AND SOME ASSOCIATED STRUCTURES

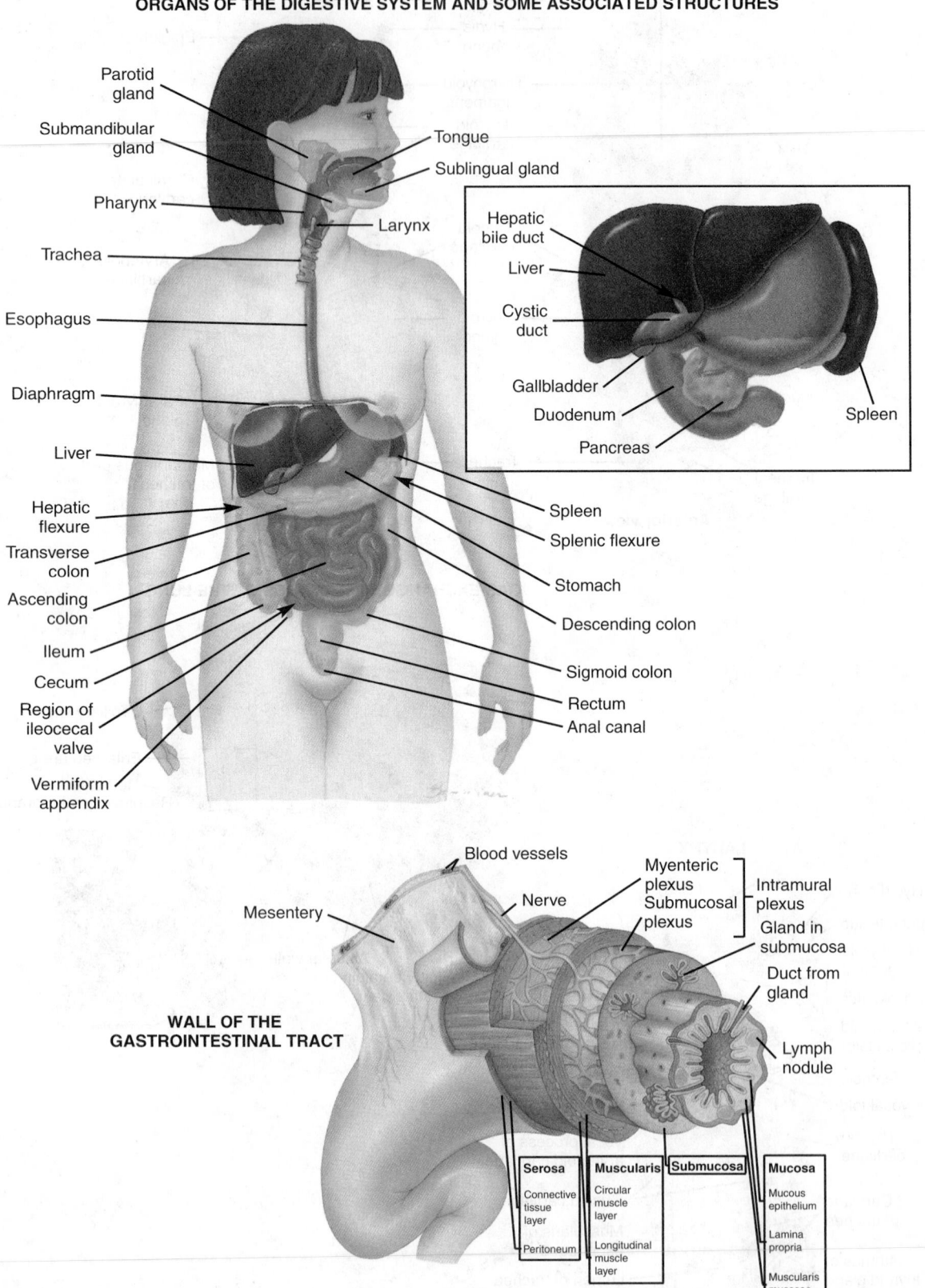

**WALL OF THE GASTROINTESTINAL TRACT**

# LOCATION OF THE SALIVARY GLANDS

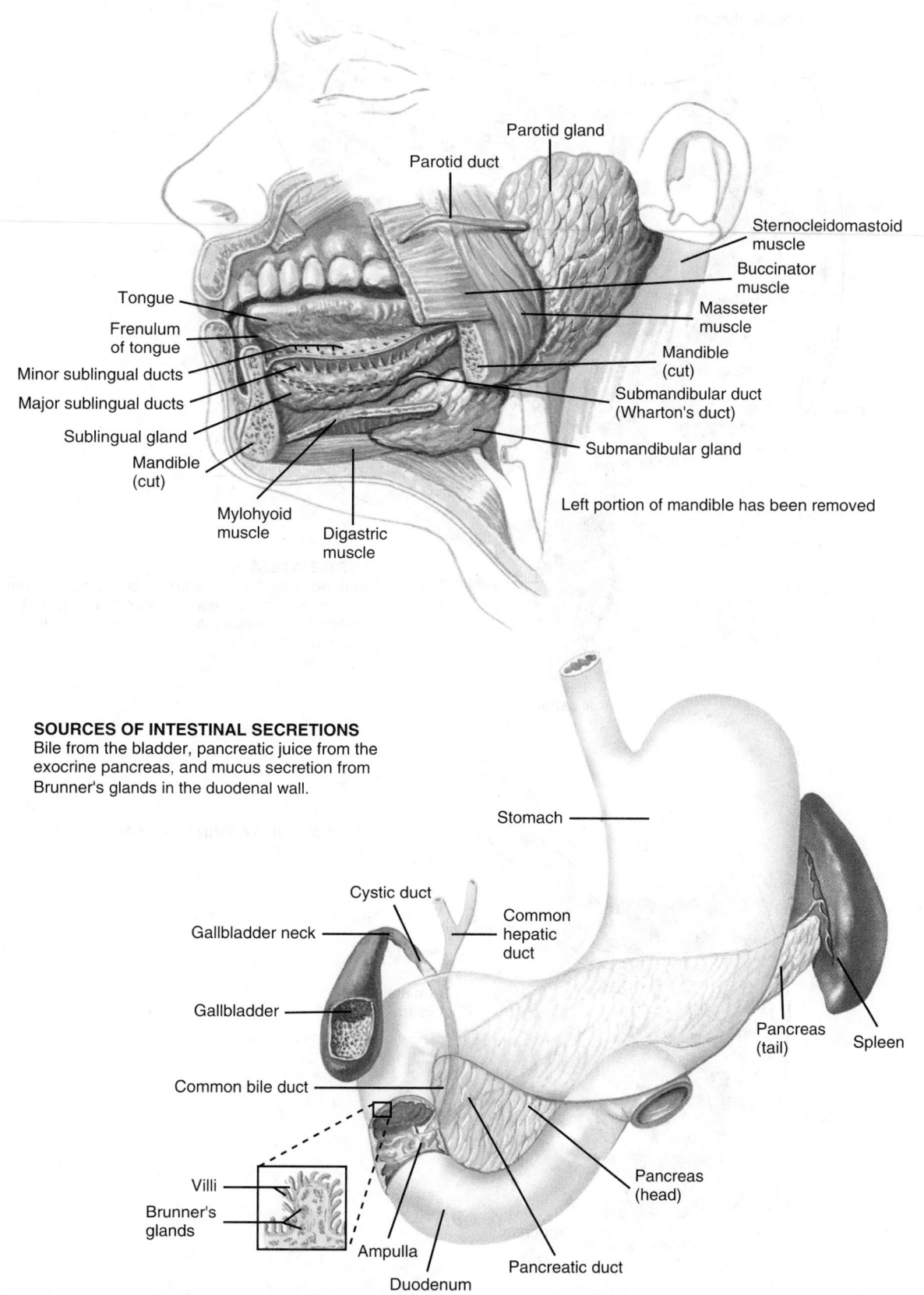

Parotid gland

Parotid duct

Sternocleidomastoid muscle

Buccinator muscle

Masseter muscle

Tongue

Frenulum of tongue

Minor sublingual ducts

Major sublingual ducts

Sublingual gland

Mandible (cut)

Mandible (cut)

Submandibular duct (Wharton's duct)

Submandibular gland

Mylohyoid muscle

Digastric muscle

Left portion of mandible has been removed

## SOURCES OF INTESTINAL SECRETIONS
Bile from the bladder, pancreatic juice from the exocrine pancreas, and mucus secretion from Brunner's glands in the duodenal wall.

Stomach

Cystic duct

Gallbladder neck

Common hepatic duct

Gallbladder

Common bile duct

Pancreas (tail)

Spleen

Villi

Brunner's glands

Ampulla

Duodenum

Pancreatic duct

Pancreas (head)

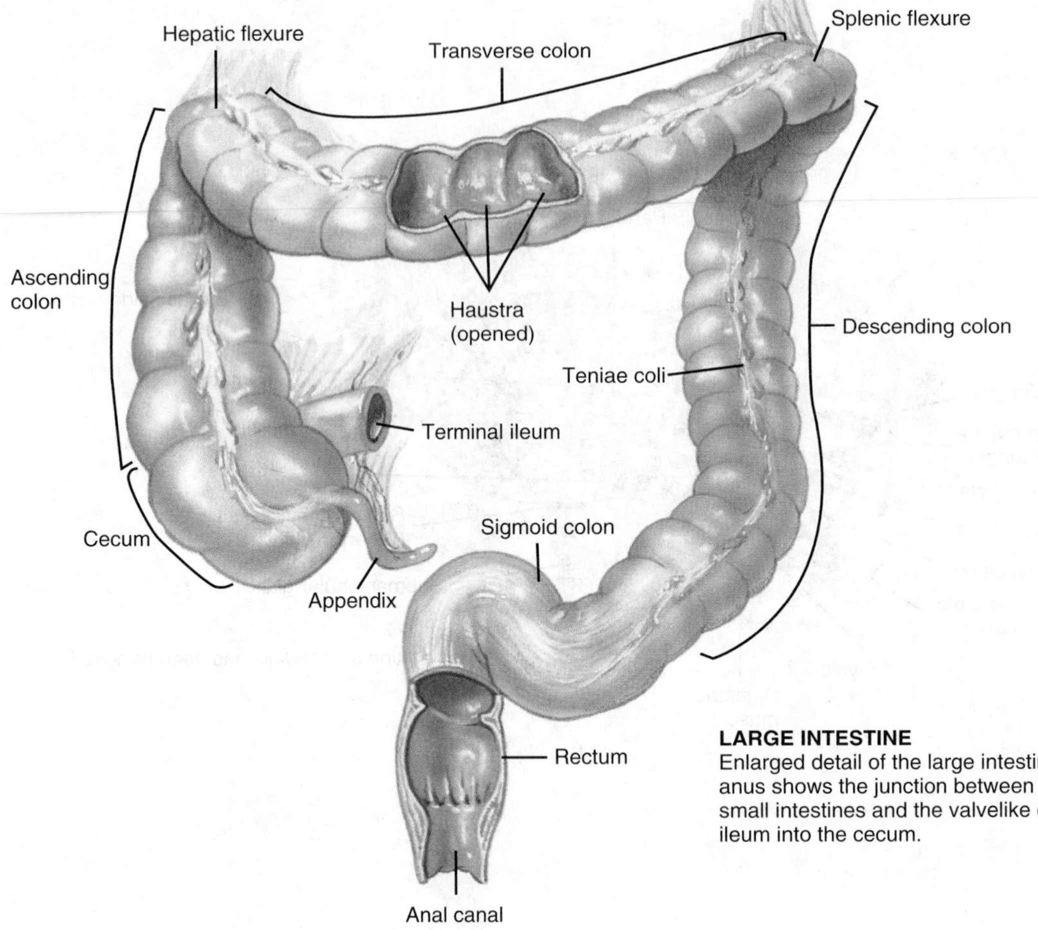

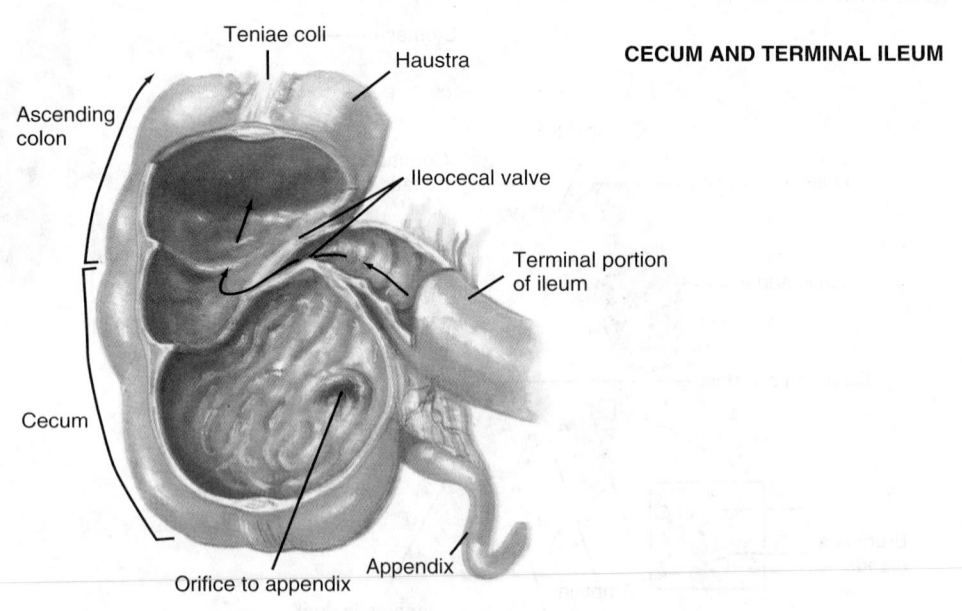

Hepatic flexure

Transverse colon

Splenic flexure

Ascending colon

Haustra (opened)

Descending colon

Teniae coli

Terminal ileum

Cecum

Sigmoid colon

Appendix

Rectum

**LARGE INTESTINE**
Enlarged detail of the large intestine, rectum, and anus shows the junction between the large and small intestines and the valvelike entry of the ileum into the cecum.

Anal canal

Teniae coli

Haustra

**CECUM AND TERMINAL ILEUM**

Ascending colon

Ileocecal valve

Terminal portion of ileum

Cecum

Orifice to appendix

Appendix

# REPRODUCTIVE SYSTEM

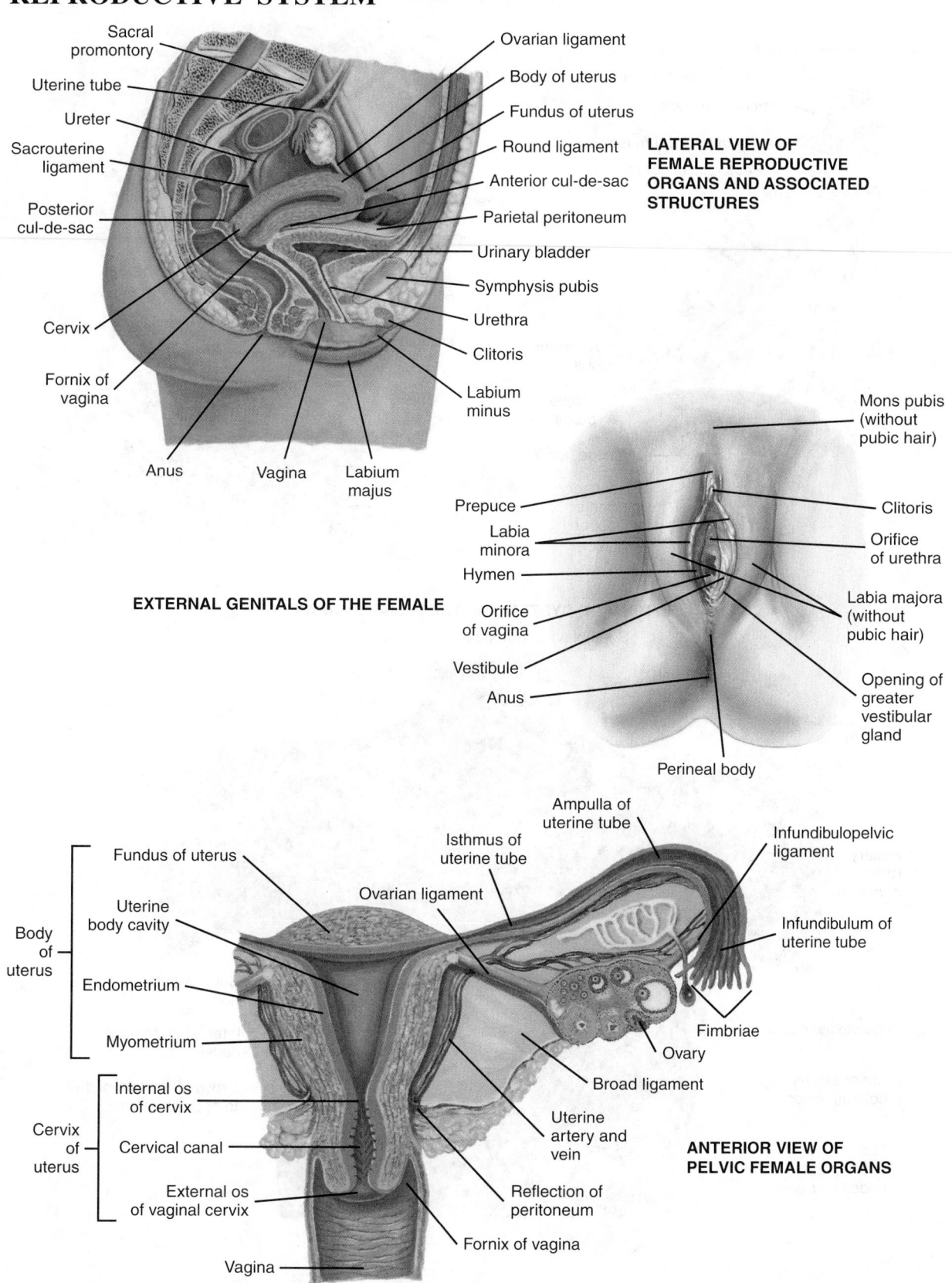

Sacral promontory
Uterine tube
Ureter
Sacrouterine ligament
Posterior cul-de-sac
Cervix
Fornix of vagina
Anus
Vagina
Labium majus

Ovarian ligament
Body of uterus
Fundus of uterus
Round ligament
Anterior cul-de-sac
Parietal peritoneum
Urinary bladder
Symphysis pubis
Urethra
Clitoris
Labium minus

**LATERAL VIEW OF FEMALE REPRODUCTIVE ORGANS AND ASSOCIATED STRUCTURES**

**EXTERNAL GENITALS OF THE FEMALE**

Prepuce
Labia minora
Hymen
Orifice of vagina
Vestibule
Anus

Mons pubis (without pubic hair)
Clitoris
Orifice of urethra
Labia majora (without pubic hair)
Opening of greater vestibular gland

Perineal body

Fundus of uterus
Uterine body cavity
Body of uterus
Endometrium
Myometrium
Internal os of cervix
Cervix of uterus
Cervical canal
External os of vaginal cervix
Vagina

Ampulla of uterine tube
Isthmus of uterine tube
Ovarian ligament
Infundibulopelvic ligament
Infundibulum of uterine tube
Fimbriae
Ovary
Broad ligament
Uterine artery and vein
Reflection of peritoneum
Fornix of vagina

**ANTERIOR VIEW OF PELVIC FEMALE ORGANS**

## FEMALE BREAST

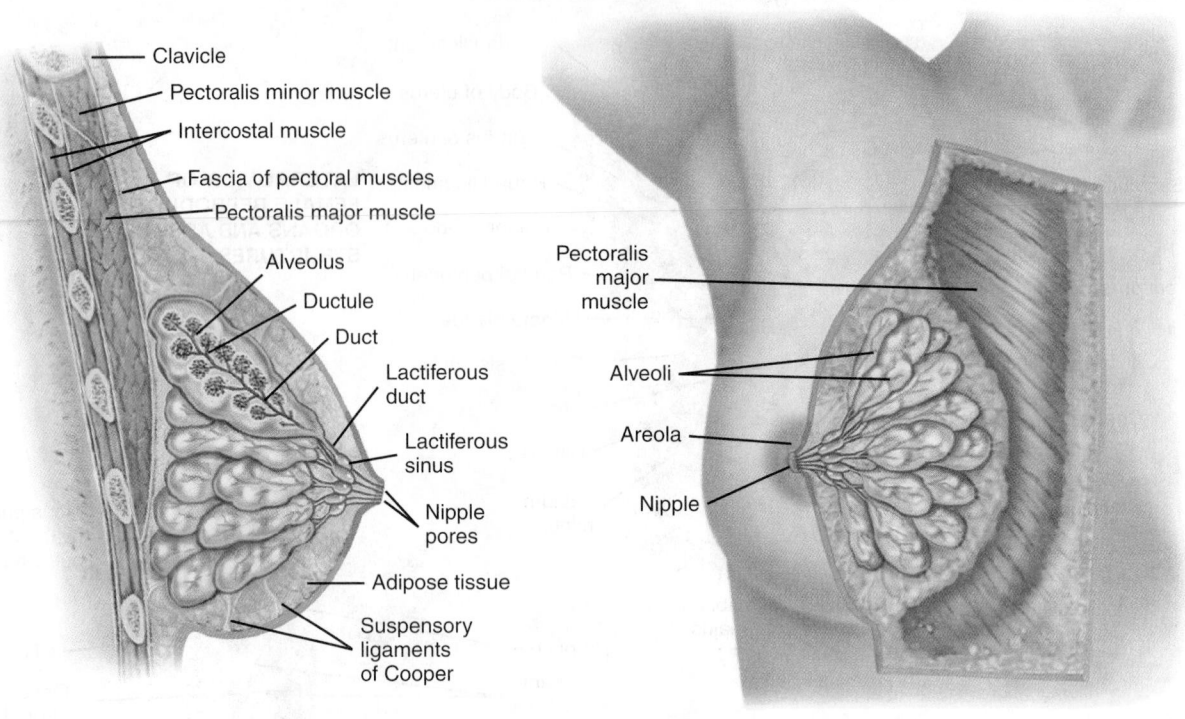

Clavicle
Pectoralis minor muscle
Intercostal muscle
Fascia of pectoral muscles
Pectoralis major muscle
Alveolus
Ductule
Duct
Lactiferous duct
Lactiferous sinus
Nipple pores
Adipose tissue
Suspensory ligaments of Cooper

Pectoralis major muscle
Alveoli
Areola
Nipple

## LYMPHATIC SYSTEM AND THE FEMALE BREAST

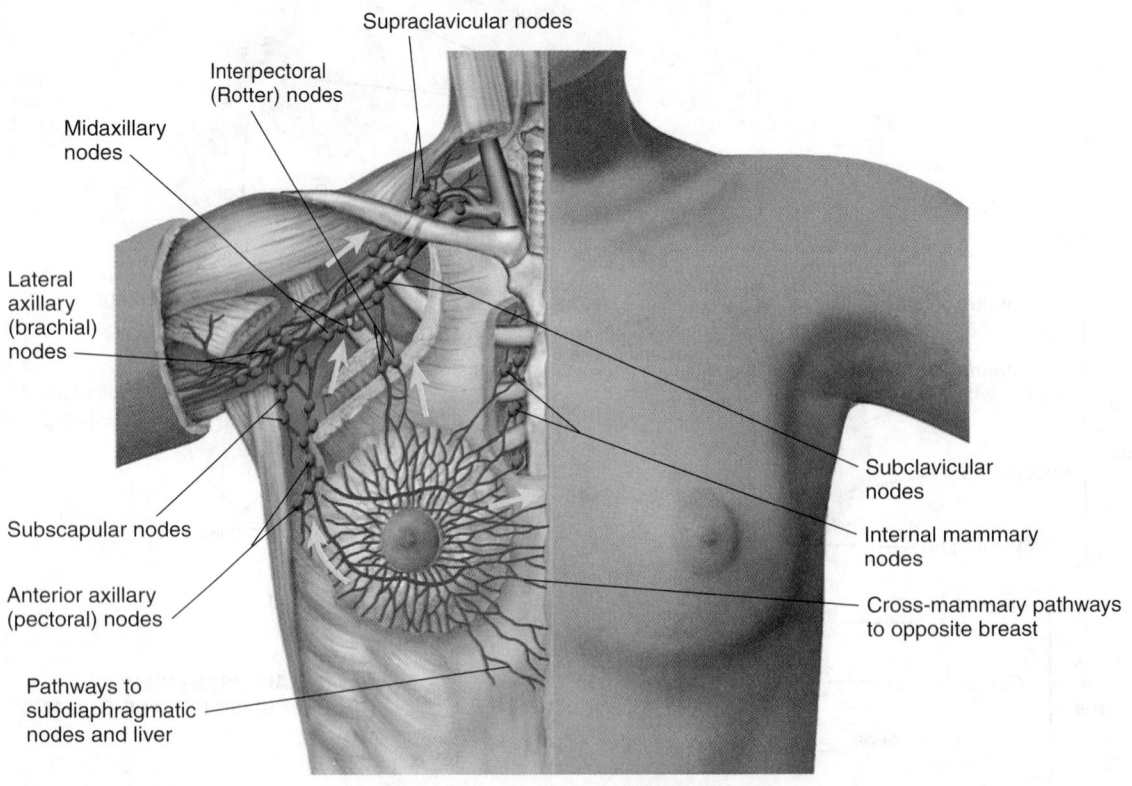

Supraclavicular nodes
Interpectoral (Rotter) nodes
Midaxillary nodes
Lateral axillary (brachial) nodes
Subscapular nodes
Anterior axillary (pectoral) nodes
Pathways to subdiaphragmatic nodes and liver

Subclavicular nodes
Internal mammary nodes
Cross-mammary pathways to opposite breast

## MALE REPRODUCTIVE ORGANS AND
## ASSOCIATED STRUCTURES

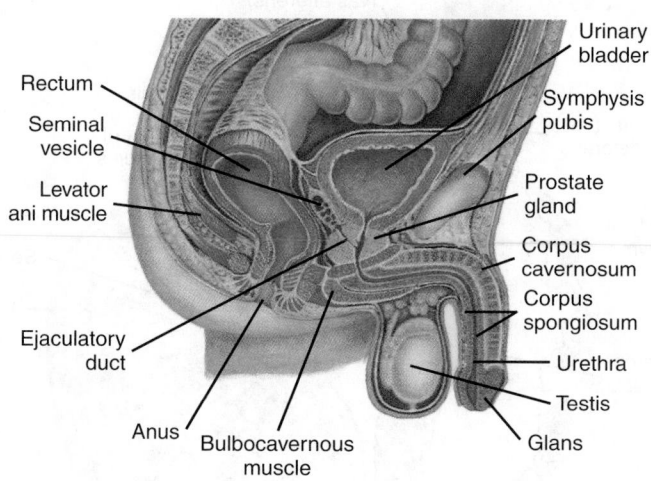

Rectum

Seminal
vesicle

Levator
ani muscle

Ejaculatory
duct

Anus

Bulbocavernous
muscle

Urinary
bladder

Symphysis
pubis

Prostate
gland

Corpus
cavernosum

Corpus
spongiosum

Urethra

Testis

Glans

## EXTERNAL GENITALS OF
## THE MALE

Location of
symphysis pubis

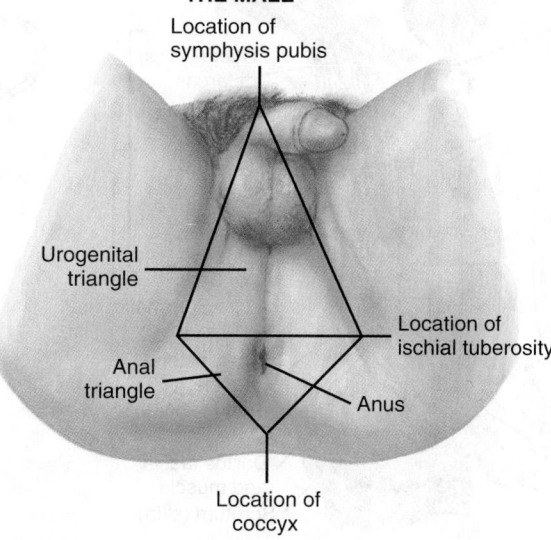

Urogenital
triangle

Anal
triangle

Location of
ischial tuberosity

Anus

Location of
coccyx

A-37

## TUBULES OF THE TESTIS AND EPIDIDYMUS

Spermatic cord

Nerves and blood vessels (vas afferens)

Head of epididymis

Ductus (vas) deferens

Efferent ductules

Rete testis

Body of epididymis

Septum

Lobule

Afferent blood vessels

Tail of epididymis

Tunica albuginea

Seminiferous tubules

## ANTERIOR VIEW OF MALE REPRODUCTIVE STRUCTURES

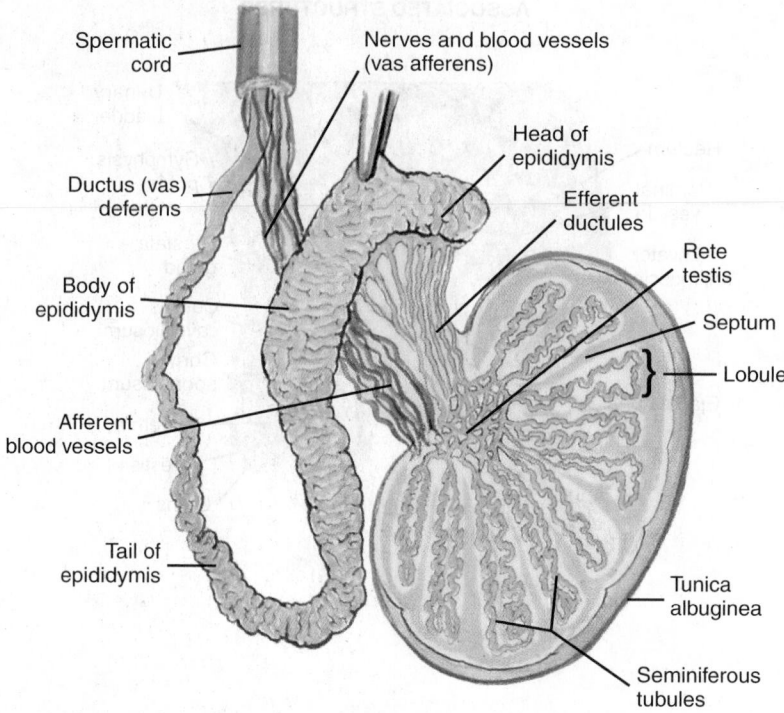

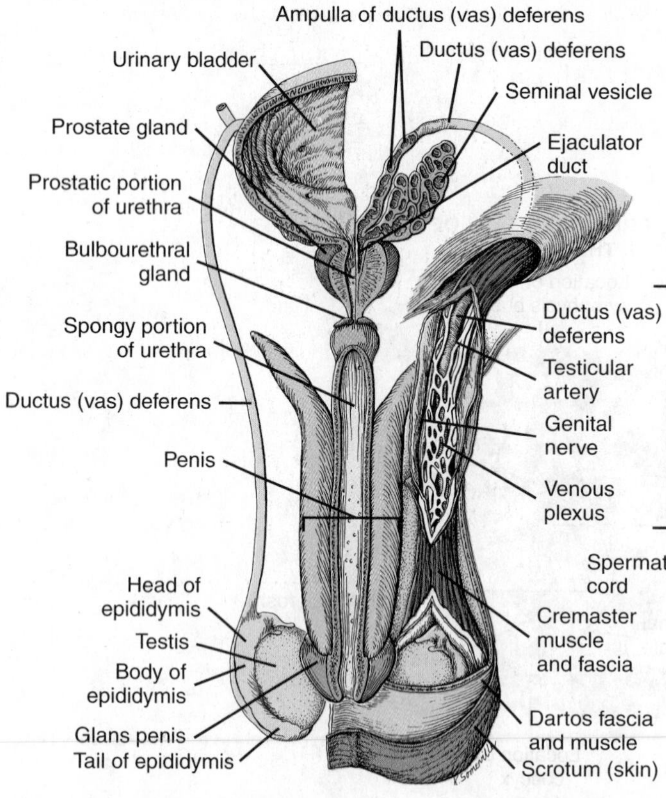

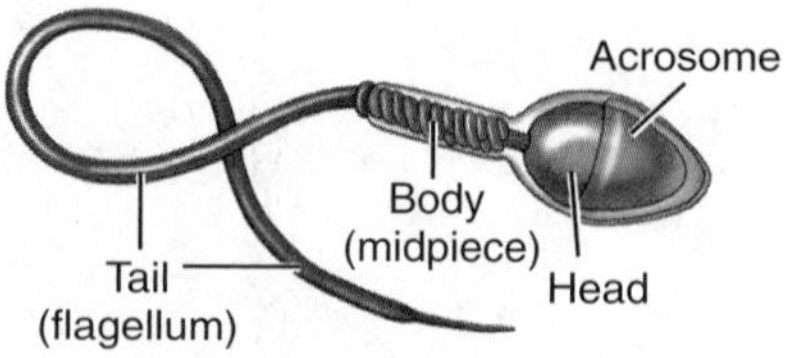

Ampulla of ductus (vas) deferens

Urinary bladder

Ductus (vas) deferens

Prostate gland

Seminal vesicle

Prostatic portion of urethra

Ejaculator duct

Bulbourethral gland

Ductus (vas) deferens

Spongy portion of urethra

Testicular artery

Ductus (vas) deferens

Genital nerve

Penis

Venous plexus

Spermatic cord

Head of epididymis

Cremaster muscle and fascia

Testis

Body of epididymis

Glans penis

Dartos fascia and muscle

Tail of epididymis

Scrotum (skin)

Acrosome

Body (midpiece)

Tail (flagellum)

Head

# URINARY SYSTEM

**URINARY SYSTEM AND SOME ASSOCIATED STRUCTURES**

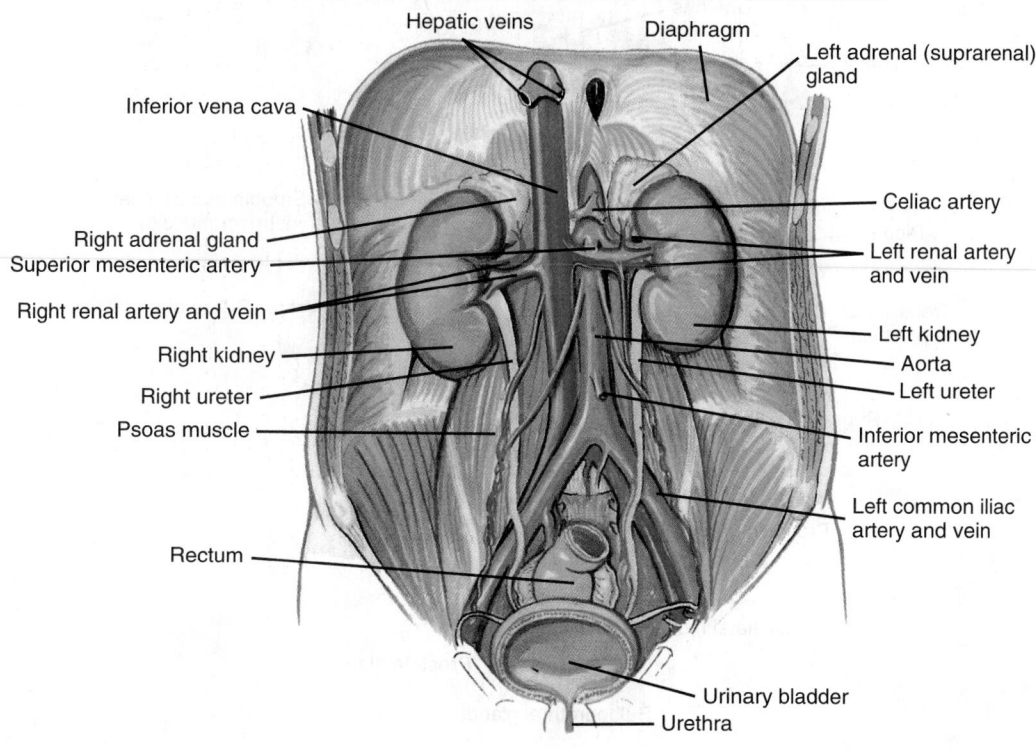

Hepatic veins

Diaphragm

Left adrenal (suprarenal) gland

Inferior vena cava

Celiac artery

Right adrenal gland

Left renal artery and vein

Superior mesenteric artery

Right renal artery and vein

Left kidney

Right kidney

Aorta

Right ureter

Left ureter

Psoas muscle

Inferior mesenteric artery

Left common iliac artery and vein

Rectum

Urinary bladder

Urethra

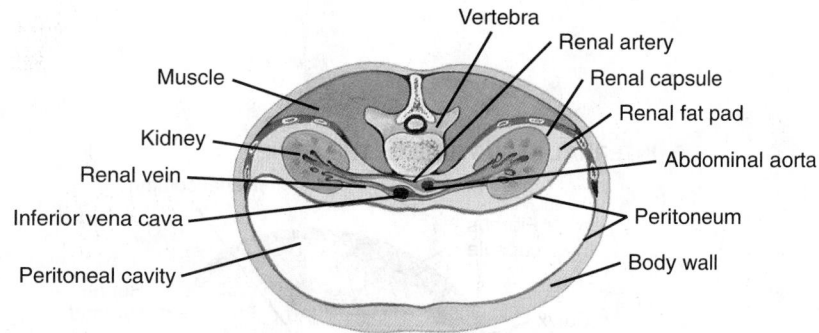

Vertebra

Renal artery

Muscle

Renal capsule

Renal fat pad

Kidney

Renal vein

Abdominal aorta

Inferior vena cava

Peritoneum

Peritoneal cavity

Body wall

**BLADDER**

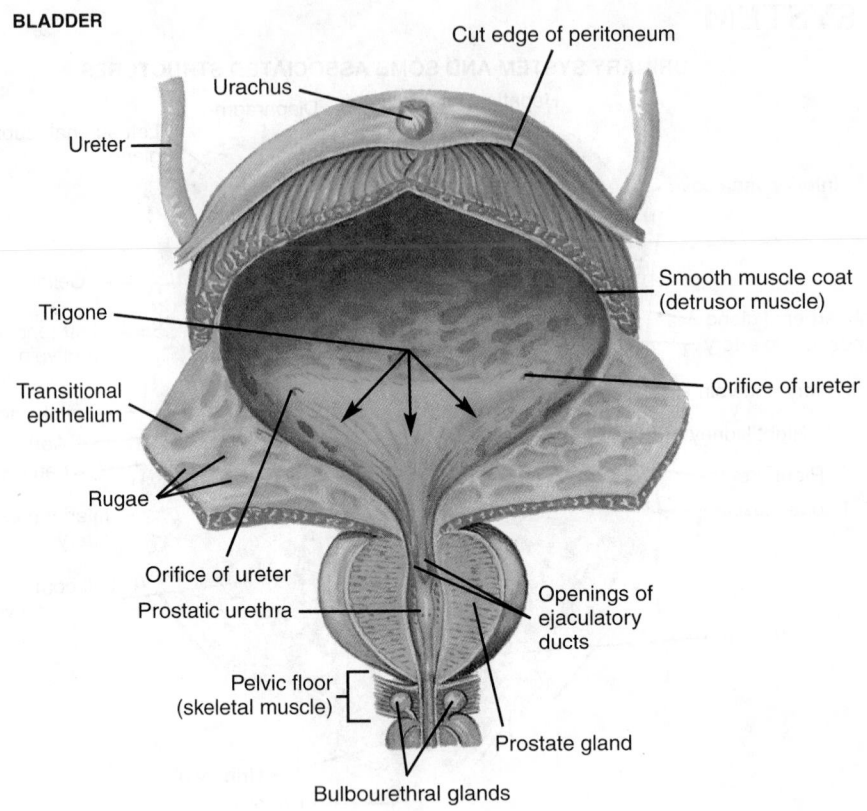

Urachus

Cut edge of peritoneum

Ureter

Smooth muscle coat
(detrusor muscle)

Trigone

Orifice of ureter

Transitional
epithelium

Rugae

Orifice of ureter

Prostatic urethra

Openings of
ejaculatory
ducts

Pelvic floor
(skeletal muscle)

Prostate gland

Bulbourethral glands

**INTERNAL STRUCTURE OF THE KIDNEY**

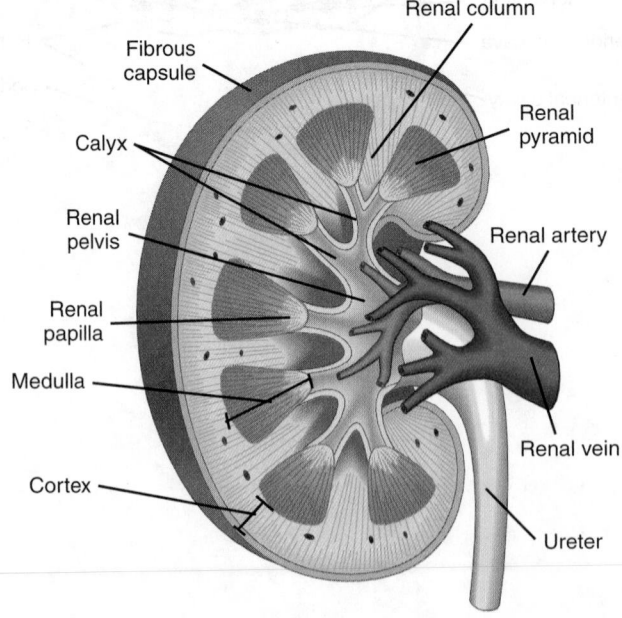

Renal column

Fibrous
capsule

Renal
pyramid

Calyx

Renal artery

Renal
pelvis

Renal
papilla

Renal vein

Medulla

Cortex

Ureter

**NEPHRON**

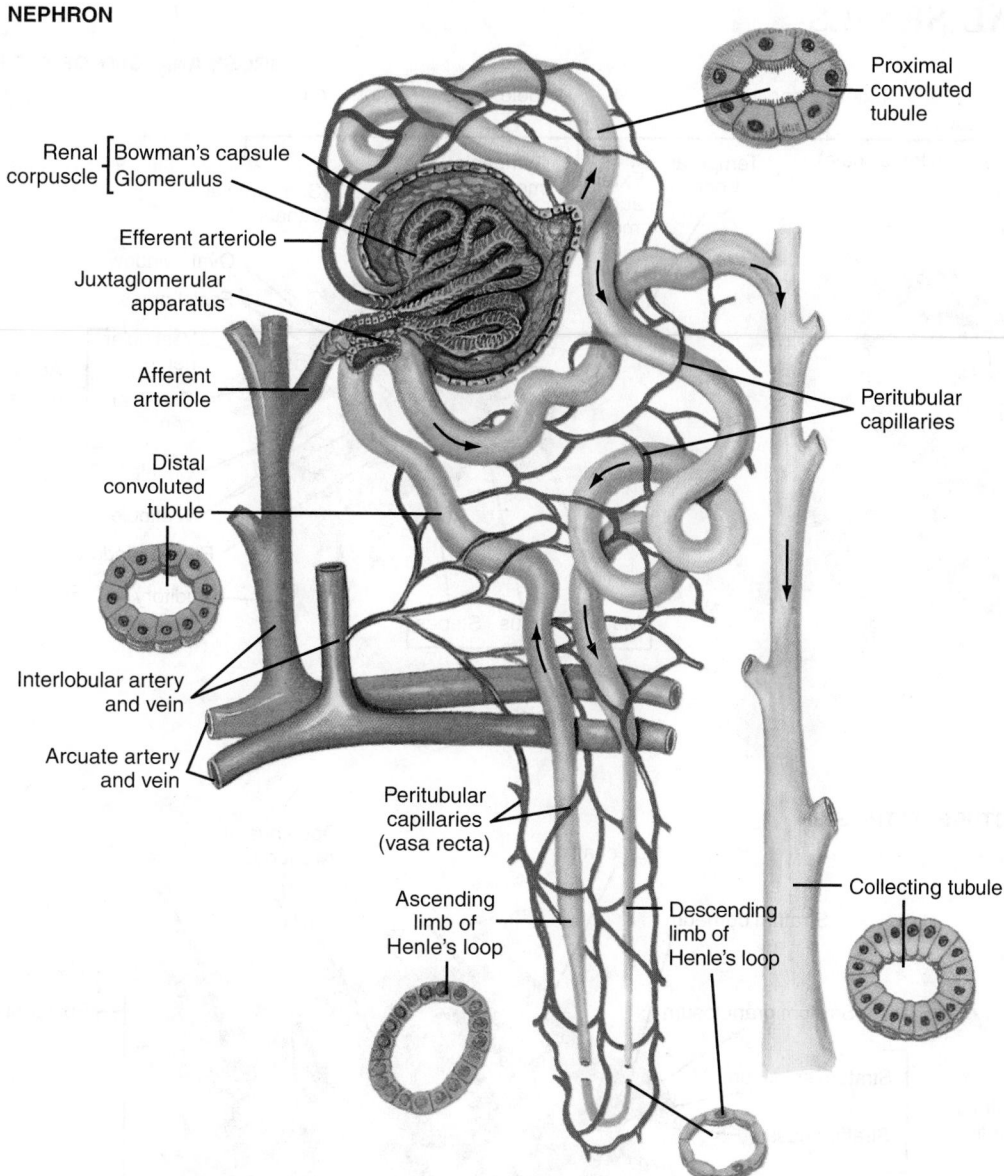

Proximal
convoluted
tubule

Renal { Bowman's capsule
corpuscle { Glomerulus

Efferent arteriole

Juxtaglomerular
apparatus

Afferent
arteriole

Peritubular
capillaries

Distal
convoluted
tubule

Interlobular artery
and vein

Arcuate artery
and vein

Peritubular
capillaries
(vasa recta)

Collecting tubule

Ascending
limb of
Henle's loop

Descending
limb of
Henle's loop

# SPECIAL SENSES

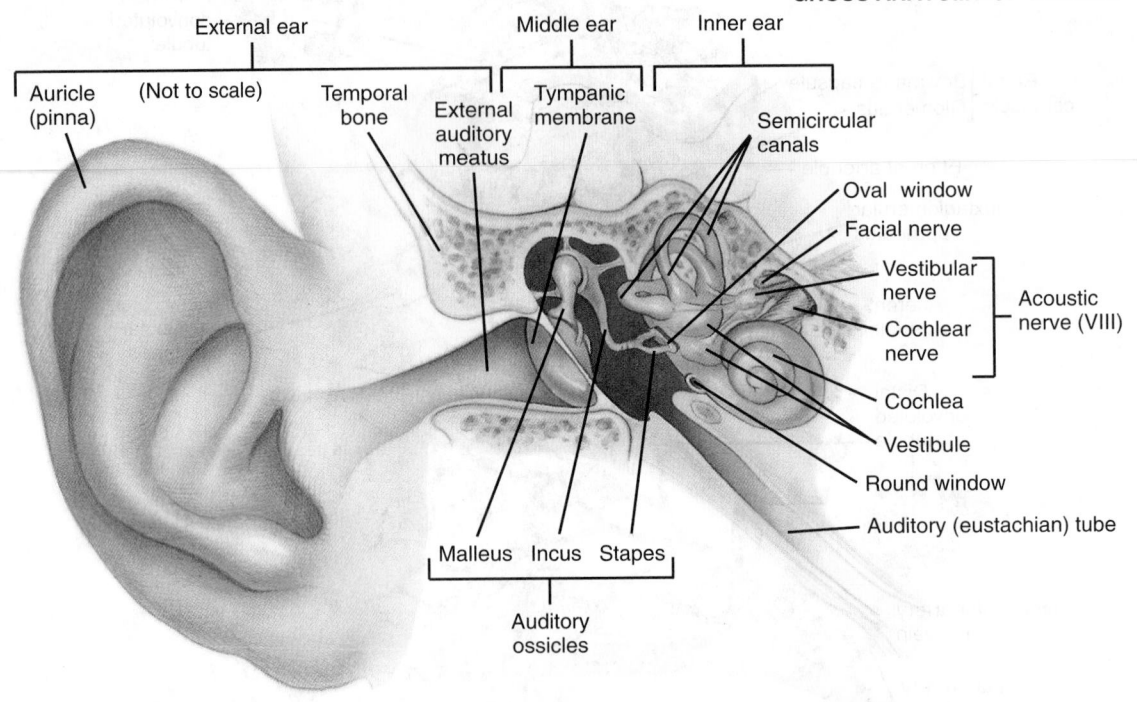

**GROSS ANATOMY OF THE EAR**

External ear

Middle ear

Inner ear

Auricle (pinna)

(Not to scale)

Temporal bone

External auditory meatus

Tympanic membrane

Semicircular canals

Oval window

Facial nerve

Vestibular nerve

Cochlear nerve

Acoustic nerve (VIII)

Cochlea

Vestibule

Round window

Auditory (eustachian) tube

Malleus   Incus   Stapes

Auditory ossicles

## STRUCTURE OF THE SKIN

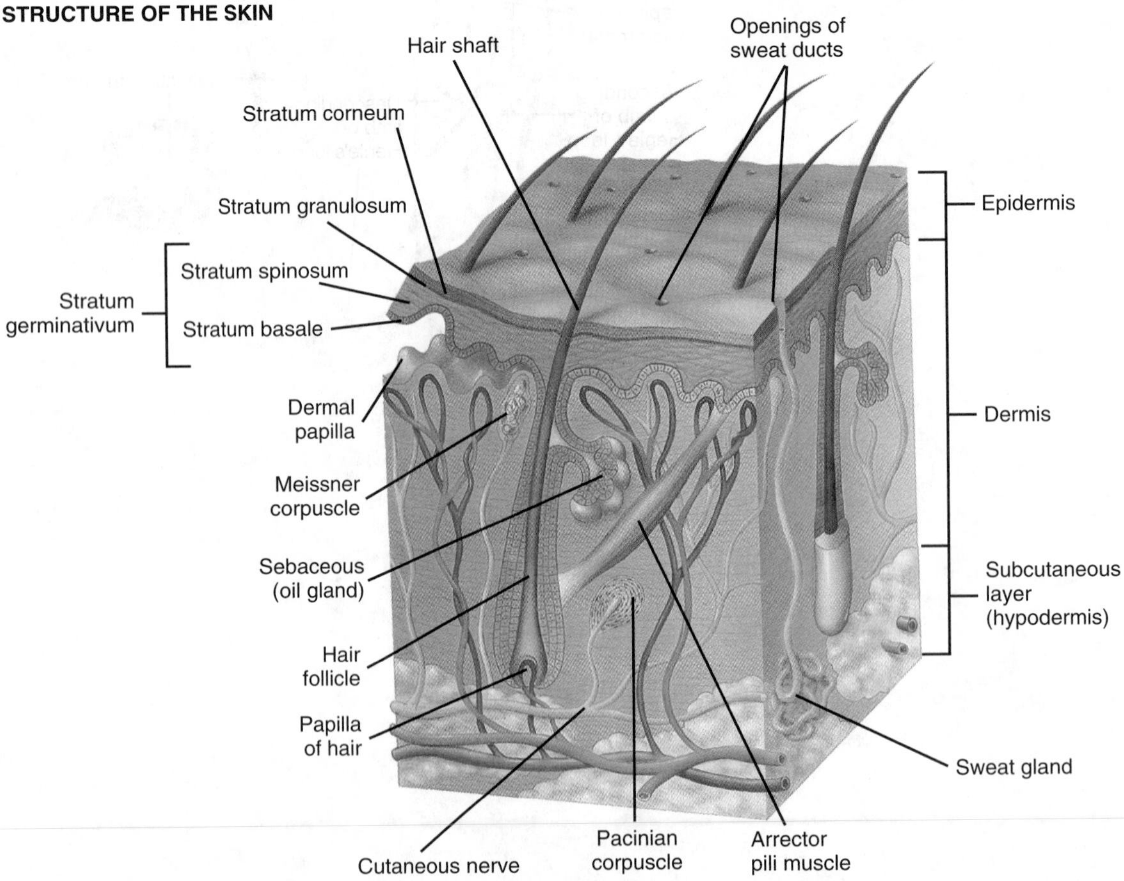

Hair shaft

Openings of sweat ducts

Stratum corneum

Stratum granulosum

Stratum spinosum

Stratum basale

Stratum germinativum

Epidermis

Dermal papilla

Dermis

Meissner corpuscle

Sebaceous (oil gland)

Hair follicle

Papilla of hair

Subcutaneous layer (hypodermis)

Sweat gland

Cutaneous nerve

Pacinian corpuscle

Arrector pili muscle

**A-42**

# CROSS-SECTIONAL VIEW OF THE EYE

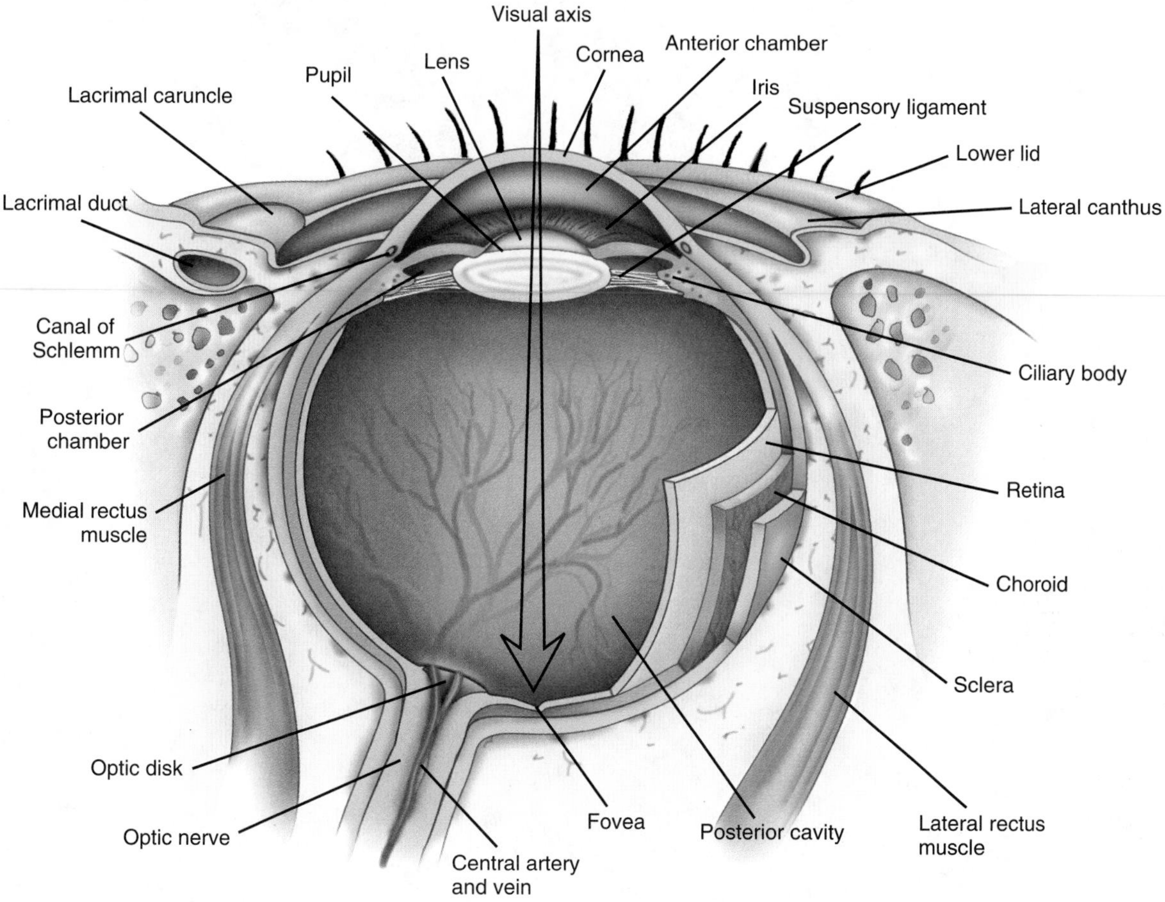

Visual axis

Pupil

Lens

Cornea

Anterior chamber

Iris

Suspensory ligament

Lower lid

Lacrimal caruncle

Lateral canthus

Lacrimal duct

Ciliary body

Canal of Schlemm

Posterior chamber

Retina

Medial rectus muscle

Choroid

Sclera

Optic disk

Optic nerve

Fovea

Posterior cavity

Lateral rectus muscle

Central artery and vein

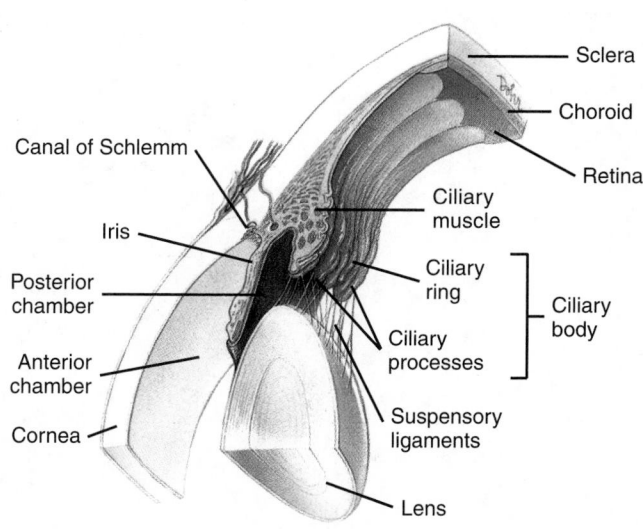

Sclera

Canal of Schlemm

Choroid

Retina

Iris

Ciliary muscle

Posterior chamber

Ciliary ring

Ciliary body

Anterior chamber

Ciliary processes

Cornea

Suspensory ligaments

Lens

**a,** **1.** symbol for **arterial blood,** as in PaO$_2$.

**A,** **1.** abbreviation for **accommodation. 2.** symbol for alveolar gas. **3.** abbreviation for **ampere. 4.** abbreviation for **anterior. 5.** abbreviation for **atomic weight (mass). 6.** abbreviation for **axial. 7.** symbol for **mass number.**

**Å, α.** See **alpha.**

**Å,** symbol for **angstrom,** a unit for distance. 1Å = 10$^{-10}$ m.

**a-,** **1.** a prefix meaning 'before' from Latin, *ante.* **2.** a prefix meaning 'without,' 'away from,' 'not,' from Greek *a.*

**A68,** symbol for a protein found in the brain tissue of Alzheimer's disease patients. It is also found in the developing normal brains of fetuses and infants but begins to disappear by the age of 2 years.

**AA,** **1.** abbreviation for **achievement age. 2.** abbreviation for **Alcoholics Anonymous. 3.** abbreviation for **amplitude of accommodation. 4.** abbreviation for **anesthesiologist's assistant. 5.** abbreviation for **amino acid.**

**a̅a̅, AA,** (in prescriptions) abbreviation for *ana,* indicating an equal amount of each ingredient to be compounded.

**AAA,** abbreviation for *American Association of Anatomists.*

**AAAI,** abbreviation for **American Academy of Allergy and Immunology.**

**AACN,** **1.** abbreviation for **American Association of Colleges of Nursing. 2.** abbreviation for **American Association of Critical Care Nurses.**

**AAFP,** abbreviation for *American Academy of Family Physicians.*

**AAI,** abbreviation for **ankle-arm index.** See **anklebrachial index.**

**AAIN,** abbreviation for **American Association of Industrial Nurses.**

**AAL,** abbreviation for **anterior axillary line.**

**AAMC,** abbreviation for **American Association of Medical Colleges.**

**AAMI,** abbreviation for **Association for the Advancement of Medical Instrumentation.**

**AAN,** abbreviation for **American Academy of Nursing.**

**AANA,** abbreviation for **American Association of Nurse Anesthetists.**

**AANN,** **1.** abbreviation for **American Association of Neuroscience Nurses. 2.** abbreviation for **American Association of Neurological Nurses.**

**AAOHN,** abbreviation for *American Association of Occupational Health Nurses.*

**AAOMS,** abbreviation for *American Association of Oral and Maxillofacial Surgeons.*

**AAPA,** abbreviation for **American Academy of Physicians' Assistants.**

**AAPB,** abbreviation for **American Association of Pathologists and Bacteriologists.**

**AAPMR,** abbreviation for **American Academy of Physical Medicine and Rehabilitation.**

**Aaron's sign** [Charles D. Aaron, American physician, 1866–1951], a diagnostic sign in appendicitis indicated by pain or distress when pressure is applied over McBurney's point in the epigastric region. See also **McBurney's point.**

**AARP,** abbreviation for **American Association of Retired Persons.**

**Aarskog syndrome** /ärs′kog/ [Dagfinn Charles Aarskog, Norwegian pediatrician, b. 1928], an X-linked syndrome characterized by ocular hypertelorism, anteverted nostrils, broad upper lip, peculiar scrotal "shawl" above the penis, and small hands. Also called **faciodigitogenital syndrome, faciogenital dysplasia.**

**AART,** abbreviation for **American Association for Respiratory Therapy.**

**Aase syndrome** /äz/ [Jon Morton Aase, American pediatrician, b. 1936], a familial syndrome characterized by mild growth retardation, hypoplastic anemia, variable leukocytopenia, triphalangeal thumbs, narrow shoulders, and late closure of fontanels, and occasionally by cleft lip, cleft palate, retinopathy, and web neck. A recessive mode of inheritance has been suggested.

**AAUP,** abbreviation for **American Association of University Professors.**

**AAV,** abbreviation for **adenoassociated virus.**

**Ab,** abbreviation for **antibody.**

**ab-, abs-,** a prefix meaning 'from, off, away from': *abstract, abnormal.*

**abacavir,** an antiviral.

▪ INDICATIONS: It is prescribed in combination with other antiretroviral agents for HIV-1 infection.

▪ CONTRAINDICATIONS: Known hypersensitivity to this drug prohibits its use.

▪ ADVERSE EFFECTS: Life-threatening adverse effects include granulocytopenia, anemia, fatal hypersensitivity reactions, and lactic acidosis. Common side effects include fever, headache, malaise, insomnia, nausea, vomiting, diarrhea, anorexia, and rash.

**abacterial** /ab′aktir′ē·əl/, any atmosphere or condition free of bacteria; literally, without bacteria.

**abaissement** /ä′bāsmäN′/ [Fr, a lowering], **1.** a falling or depressing. **2.** (in ophthalmology) the displacement of a lens.

**abalienation** /abāl′yənā′shən/, a state of physical deterioration or mental decay.—**abalienate,** *v.,* **abalienated,** *adj.*

**A band,** the area between two I bands of a sarcomere, marked by partial overlapping of actin and myosin filaments and appearing dark.

**abandonment of care** /əban′dənment/, (in law) wrongful cessation of the provision of care to a patient, usually by a physician or a nurse.

**abapical** /abap′əkəl/, opposite the apex.

**abarognosis** /aber′agnō′sis/ [Gk, *a,* not, *baros,* weight, *gnosis,* knowledge], an inability to judge or compare the weight of objects, particularly those held in the hand.

**abarthrosis.** See **synovial joint.**

**abarticular** /ab′ärtik′yŏŏlər/, **1.** pertaining to a condition that does not affect a joint. **2.** pertaining to a site or structure remote from a joint.

**abarticular gout** [L, *ab,* away from, *articulus,* joint], gout that affects structures other than joints, such as ligaments.

**abarticulation** /ab′ärtik′yəlā′shən/, **1.** dislocation of a joint. **2.** a synovial joint.

**abasia** /əbā′zhə/ [Gk, *a, basis,* not step], the inability to walk, caused by lack of motor coordination. —**abasic, abatic,** *adj.*

**abasia-astasia.** See **astasia-abasia.**

**abate** /əbāt′/ [ME, *abaten,* to beat down], to decrease or reduce in severity or degree.

**abatement** /əbāt′mənt/, a decrease in severity of symptoms.

**abatic,** pertaining to an inability to walk.

**abaxial** /abak′sē·əl/ [L, *ab, axis* from axle], **1.** pertaining to a position outside the axis of a body or structure. **2.** pertaining to a position at the opposite extremity of a structure.

**Abbe-Estlander operation** /ab′ē·est′-/ [Robert Abbé, American surgeon, 1851–1928; Jakob A. Estlander, Finnish surgeon, 1831–1881], a surgical procedure that transfers a full-thickness section of one oral lip to the other lip, using an arterial pedicle for ensuring survival of a graft.

**Abbé-Zeiss apparatus** /äbā′tsīs′/ [Ernst K. Abbe, German physicist, 1840–1905; Carl Zeiss, German optician, 1816–1885], an apparatus for calculating the number of blood cells in a measured amount of blood. See also **hemacytometer.**

**Abbokinase,** a trademark for a plasminogen activator (urokinase).

**Abbott-Miller tube.** See **Miller-Abbott tube**

**Abbott pump,** a trademark for a small portable pump that can be adjusted and finely calibrated to deliver precise amounts of medication in solution through an IV infusion set. It is similar to a Harvard pump, but the flow rate may be increased or decreased by smaller increments. See also **Harvard pump.**

**ABC,** abbreviation for **aspiration biopsy cytology.**

**abciximab,** a platelet aggregation inhibitor.

■ INDICATIONS: It is prescribed as an adjunct to percutaneous transluminal coronary angioplasty or atherectomy.

■ CONTRAINDICATIONS: The drug should not be given to patients with active internal bleeding, recent GI or urinary bleeding of significance, history of stroke, thrombocytopenia, or recent major surgery.

■ ADVERSE EFFECTS: The side effects most often reported include bleeding, thrombocytopenia, pulmonary edema, atrioventricular block, and atrial fibrillation.

**Abdellah, Faye Glenn,** (b. 1919–), a nursing theorist who introduced a typology of 21 nursing problems in 1960 in *Patient-Centered Approaches to Nursing.* The concepts of nursing, nursing problems, and the problem-solving process are central to Abdellah's work. The typology is divided into three areas: (1) the physical, sociological, and emotional needs of the patient; (2) the types of interpersonal relationships between the nurse and the patient; and (3) the common elements of patient care. It was formulated in terms of nursing-centered services that can be used to determine the patient's needs and to teach and evaluate nursing students. It was based on systematic research studies. The typology provided a scientific body of knowledge unique to nursing, making it possible to move away from the medical model of educating nurses. The nursing diagnosis classification system may be considered an outgrowth of Abdellah's typology.

**abdomen** /ab′dəmən, abdō′mən/ [L, belly], the portion of the body between the thorax and the pelvis. The abdominal cavity is lined by the peritoneum; contains the inferior portion of the esophagus, the stomach, the intestines, the liver, the spleen, the pancreas, and other organs; and is bounded by the diaphragm and the pelvis. Also called *(informal)* **belly.** See also **abdominal regions.** —**abdominal** /abdom′-/, *adj.*

**abdominal actinomycosis.** See **actinomycosis.**

**abdominal adhesion** /abdom′inəl/, the binding together of tissue surfaces of abdominal organs, usually involving the intestines and causing obstruction. The condition may result from trauma or inflammation and may form after abdominal surgery. The patient experiences abdominal distension, pain, nausea, vomiting, and increased pulse rate. Surgery may be required.

**abdominal aorta,** the portion of the descending aorta that passes from the aortic hiatus of the diaphragm into the abdomen, descending ventral to the vertebral column, and ending at the fourth lumbar vertebra, where it divides into the two common iliac arteries. It supplies blood to abdominal structures, such as the testes, ovaries, kidneys, and stomach. Its branches are the celiac, superior mesenteric, inferior mesenteric, middle suprarenal, renal, testicular, ovarian, inferior phrenic, lumbar, middle sacral, and common iliac arteries. See also **descending aorta.** Compare **thoracic aorta.**

**abdominal aortic aneurysm,** a common type of aneurysm, found in the abdominal aorta, usually in an area of severe atherosclerosis.

**abdominal aortography,** a radiographic study of the abdominal aorta after the introduction of a contrast medium through a catheter in the femoral artery.

**abdominal aponeurosis,** the conjoined sheetlike tendons of the oblique and transverse skeletal muscles of the abdomen.

**abdominal bandage,** a broad absorbent gauze or other material commonly used after abdominal surgery.

**abdominal binder,** a bandage or elasticized wrap that is applied around the lower part of the torso to support the abdomen. It is sometimes applied after abdominal surgery to decrease discomfort, thereby increasing a patient's ability to begin ambulatory activities and accelerating convalescence.

**abdominal breathing,** a pattern of inhalation and exhalation in which most of the ventilatory work is done with the abdominal muscles. The contractile force of the abdomen is used to elevate the diaphragm. See also **diaphragmatic breathing.**

**abdominal cavity,** the space within the abdominal walls between the diaphragm and the pelvic area, containing the liver, stomach, intestines, spleen, gallbladder, kidneys, and associated tissues and blood and lymph vessels.

**abdominal decompression,** an obstetric technique to reduce pressure on the abdomen during the first stage of labor. The abdomen is enclosed in a chamber that permits surrounding pressure to be controlled. The technique is no longer used.

**abdominal delivery,** the delivery of a child through a surgical incision in the abdomen. See **cesarean section.**

**abdominal examination,** the physical assessment of a patient's abdomen by visual inspection and the use of auscultation, percussion, and palpation. Visual inspection of the normally oval shape of the abdominal surface while the patient is supine may reveal abnormal surface features indicating effects of disease, surgery, or injury. Subsurface tumors, fluid accumulation, or hypertrophy of the liver or spleen may be observed as an abnormal surface feature. Auscultation may reveal vascular sounds that provide information about arterial disorders such as aortic aneurysms as well as bowel sounds that are indicative of intestinal function. In the pregnant patient, auscultation can detect fetal heartbeat and blood circulation in the placenta. Percussion involves gently striking the abdominal wall at various points to produce

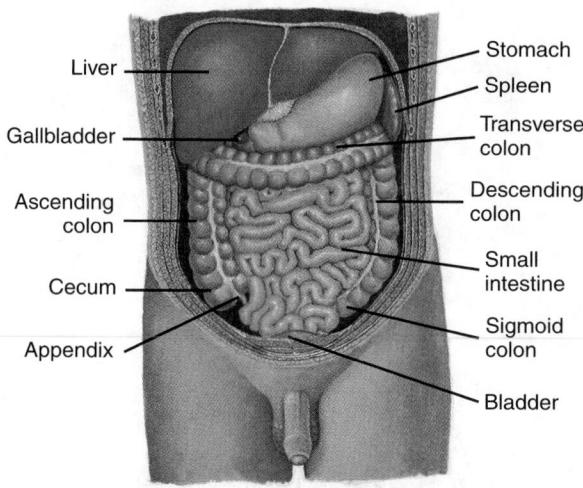

**Abdominal cavity** *(Seidel et al, 1995)*

*abdominis* is a long, flat muscle that runs the entire length of the front of the abdomen. The *pyramidalis* is a small triangular muscle at the bottom front of the abdomen. The abdominal muscles compress the abdominal contents during urination, defecation, vomiting, parturition, and forced expiration.

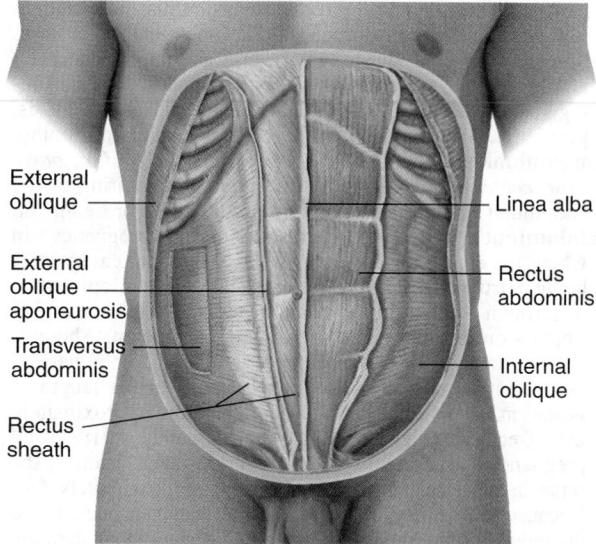

**Abdominal muscles** *(Seidel et al, 1999)*

sounds. The sounds help detect the condition of internal organs. In palpation, indirect exploration of the abdomen is performed by using the examiner's sense of touch to detect areas of tenderness or rigidity, muscle tone and skin condition, and shapes and sizes of subsurface organs or masses.

**abdominal fistula,** an abnormal passage from an abdominal organ to the surface of the abdomen. In a colostomy, a passage from the bowel to an opening on the surface of the abdomen is created surgically.

**abdominal gestation,** the implantation of a fertilized ovum outside the uterus but within the peritoneal cavity. See also **ectopic pregnancy.**

**abdominalgia** /abdom′ənal′jə/ [L, *abdomen,* belly; Gk, *algos,* pain], a pain in the abdomen.

**abdominal girth,** the circumference of the abdomen, usually measured at the umbilicus.

**abdominal hernia,** a hernia in which a loop of bowel protrudes through the abdominal musculature, often through the site of an old surgical scar that has stretched and thinned. Also called **ventral hernia.** See also **hernia.**

**abdominal hysterectomy,** the excision of the uterus through the abdominal wall. Also called **abdominohysterectomy.**

**abdominal inguinal ring,** an opening of the inguinal canal on the abdominal wall, through which the male spermatic cord and the female round ligament pass. The deep abdominal inguinal ring is marked by an oval depression on the deep aspect of the anterior abdominal wall, just above the inguinal ligament. The superficial abdominal inguinal ring is a triangle-shaped opening in the aponeurosis of the external oblique muscle.

**abdominal muscles,** the set of muscles that make up the ventral abdominal wall, including the external oblique *(obliquus externus abdominis),* internal oblique *(obliquus internus abdominis),* transversalis *(transversus abdominis),* rectus abdominis, and pyramidalis. Broad and thin, the external oblique muscle is the largest and most superficial of the abdominal muscles; it is situated in the lateral and ventral walls of the abdomen. The internal oblique muscle is also situated in the lateral and ventral walls of the abdomen, but is smaller and thinner. The *transversus abdominis* is the most internal of the flat muscles of the abdomen. The *rectus*

**abdominal nephrectomy** [L, *abdominis,* belly; Gk, *nephr,* kidney, *ektomē,* cutting out], the surgical removal of a kidney through an abdominal incision.

**abdominal pain,** acute or chronic, localized or diffuse pain in the abdominal cavity. Abdominal pain is a significant symptom because its cause may require immediate surgical or medical intervention. The most common causes of severe abdominal pain are inflammation, perforation of an intraabdominal structure, circulatory obstruction, intestinal or ureteral obstruction, intestinal cramping, or rupture of an organ located within the abdomen. Specific conditions include appendicitis, perforated gastric ulcer, strangulated hernia, superior mesenteric arterial thrombosis, diverticulitis, and small and large bowel obstruction. Differential diagnosis of the cause of acute abdominal pain requires its localization and characterization by means of light and deep palpation, auscultation, percussion, and abdominal, rectal, or pelvic examination. Direct physical examination may be supplemented by various laboratory and radiologic examinations. Aspiration of peritoneal fluid (paracentesis) for bacteriologic and chemical evaluation is sometimes indicated. Conditions producing acute abdominal pain that may require surgery include appendicitis, acute or severe and chronic diverticulitis, acute and chronic cholecystitis, cholelithiasis, acute pancreatitis, perforation of a peptic ulcer, various intestinal obstructions, abdominal aortic aneurysms, and trauma affecting any of the abdominal organs. Gynecologic causes of acute abdominal pain that may require surgery include acute pelvic inflammatory disease, ruptured ovarian cyst, and ectopic pregnancy. Abdominal pain associated with pregnancy may be caused by the weight of the enlarged uterus; rotation, stretching, or compression of the round ligament; or squeezing or displacement of the bowel. In addition, uterine contractions associated with premature labor may produce severe abdominal pain. Chronic abdominal pain may be functional or may result from overeating or excessive air swallowing (aerophagia). When symptoms are recurrent, an organic cause is considered. Organic sources of abdominal pain include peptic ulcer, hiatal hernia, gastritis, chronic cholecystitis and cholelithiasis, chronic pancreatitis, pancreatic carcinoma, chronic diverticulitis, intermittent low-grade intestinal obstruction, and functional indigestion. Some systemic conditions may cause abdominal pain. Examples include systemic lupus erythematosus, lead poisoning, hypercalcemia, sickle cell anemia, diabetic acidosis, porphyria, tabes dorsalis, and black widow spider poisoning.

**abdominal paracentesis** [L, *abdominis,* belly; Gk, *para,* near, *kentesis,* puncturing], the surgical puncturing of the abdominal cavity to remove fluid for diagnosis or treatment.

**abdominal pregnancy,** an extrauterine pregnancy in which the conceptus develops in the abdominal cavity after being extruded from the fimbriated end of the fallopian tube or through a defect in the tube or uterus. The placenta may implant on the abdominal or visceral peritoneum. Abdominal pregnancy may be suspected when the abdomen has enlarged but the uterus has remained small for the length of gestation. Abdominal pregnancies constitute approximately 2% of ectopic pregnancies and approximately 0.01% of all pregnancies. The condition results in perinatal death of the fetus in most cases, maternal death in approximately 6%. Because of its rarity, the condition may be unsuspected, and diagnosis is often delayed. Ultrasound or x-ray visualization showing gas in the maternal bowel below the fetus is diagnostic of the condition. Surgical removal of the placenta, sac, and embryo or fetus is necessary if attached to the posterior part of the tube, ovary, broad ligament and uterus. The procedure is often complicated by massive bleeding, and, because the placenta tends to adhere firmly to the peritoneum and to the bowel, complete removal is seldom possible. Allowing it to be absorbed presents fewer problems. Postoperative sequelae may include retained placental tissue, infection, continued bleeding, and sterility.

**abdominal pulse,** the pulse of the abdominal aorta.

**abdominal quadrant,** any of four topographic areas of the abdomen divided by two imaginary lines, one vertical and one horizontal, intersecting at the umbilicus. The divisions are the left upper quadrant (LUQ), the left lower quadrant (LLQ), the right upper quadrant (RUQ), and the right lower quadrant (RLQ).

**abdominal reflex,** a superficial neurologic reflex obtained by firmly stroking the skin of the abdomen. It normally results in a brisk contraction of abdominal muscles in which the umbilicus moves toward the site of the stimulus. This reflex is lost in diseases of the pyramidal tract. See also **superficial reflex.**

**abdominal regions,** the nine topographic subdivisions of the abdomen, determined by four imaginary lines, in a tic-tac-toe pattern, imposed over the anterior surface. The upper horizontal line passes along the level of the cartilages of the ninth rib; the lower along the iliac crests. The two vertical lines extend on each side of the body from the cartilage of the eighth rib to the center of the inguinal ligament. The lines divide the abdomen into three upper, three middle, and three lower zones: right hypochondriac, epigastric, and left hypochondriac regions (upper zones); right lateral (lumbar), umbilical, and left lateral (lumbar) regions (middle zones); right inguinal (iliac), pubic (hypogastric), and left inguinal (iliac) regions (lower zones).

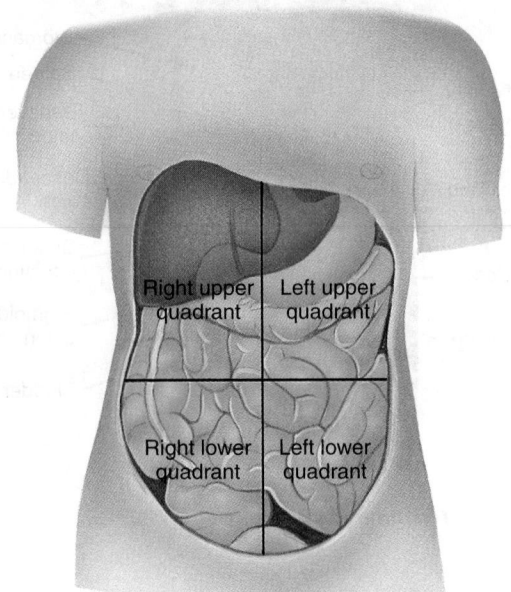

**Abdominal quadrants**
*(Thibodeau and Patton, 1999/Nadine Sokol)*

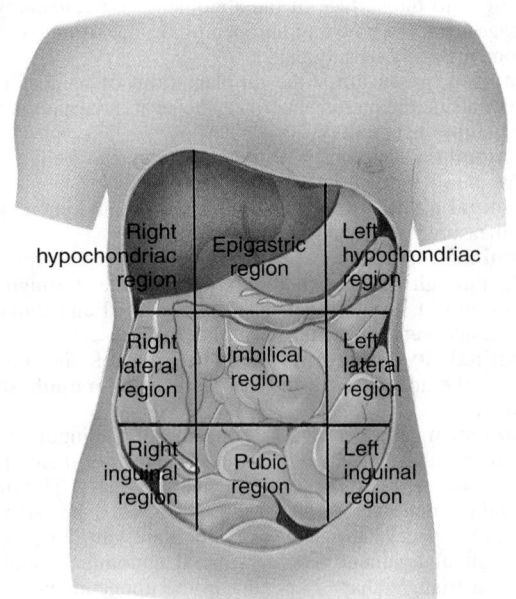

**Abdominal regions** *(Thibodeau and Patton, 1999/Nadine Sokol)*

**abdominal splinting,** a rigid contraction of the abdominal wall muscles. It usually occurs as an involuntary reaction to the pain of a visceral disease or disorder or postoperative discomfort. Abdominal splinting, in turn, may result in hypoventilation and respiratory complications. Also called **guarding.**

**abdominal sponge** [L, *abdominis,* belly; Gk, *spongia,* sponge], a special type of gauze pad used as an absorbent and covering for the viscera. See also **sponge.**

**abdominal surgery,** any operation that involves an incision into the abdomen. To prepare for surgery, laboratory, radiographic, and cardiac tests and consultations may be done. Immediately before surgery, body hair is clipped and skin is cleansed from the nipple line to the pubis. Food and fluids by mouth are withheld for up to 6 hours or more before surgery. After surgery the nurse ensures that the airway is patent and vital signs are stable, checks tubes and catheters, connects drainage tubes to collection containers, and checks the dressing for excessive bleeding or drainage, and records fluid intake and output. The patient is turned and is helped to breathe deeply every hour and, if secretions are present, to cough. Medication is given as needed for pain relief. Some kinds of abdominal surgery are **appendectomy, cholecystectomy, colostomy, gastrectomy, herniorrhaphy,** and **laparotomy.** See also **acute abdomen, laparotomy.**

**abdominal tenaculum.** See **tenaculum.**

**abdominal ultrasound test,** an ultrasound test that provides accurate visualization of the abdominal aorta, liver, gallbladder, pancreas, bile ducts, kidneys, ureters, and bladder. This test is used to diagnose and locate cysts, tumors, calculi, and malformations; to document the progression of various diseases; and to guide the insertion of instruments during surgical procedures.

**abdominal wound,** a break in the continuity of the abdominal wall. A wound that exposes or penetrates the viscera raises the danger of infection or peritonitis.

**abdomino-** /abdom′inō-/, a combining form meaning 'abdomen': *abdominoscopy, abdominovesical.*

**abdominocardiac reflex** /-kär′dē·ək/, an immediate, involuntary response of the heart to stimulation of the abdominal viscera. The reflex is mediated through the vagus nerve.

**abdominocentesis.** See **paracentesis.**

**abdominocyesis** /abdom′inōsī·ē′sis/, an abdominal pregnancy.

**abdominocystic.** See **abdominovesical.**

**abdominogenital** /-jen′itəl/, pertaining to the abdomen and reproductive system.

**abdominohysterectomy.** See **abdominal hysterectomy.**

**abdominohysterotomy** /-his′tərot′əmē/, hysterotomy through an abdominal incision. See **hysterotomy.**

**abdominopelvic cavity** /-pel′vik/, the space between the diaphragm and the groin. There is no structurally distinct separation between the abdomen and pelvic regions.

**abdominoperineal** /-per′inē′əl/, pertaining to the abdomen and the perineum, including the pelvic area, female vulva and anus, and male anus and scrotum.

**abdominoplasty,** a surgical procedure to tighten the abdominal muscles. Also called **tummy tuck.**

**abdominoscopy** /abdom′inos′kəpē/ [L, *abdomen;* Gk, *skopein,* to view], a procedure for examining the contents of the peritoneum in which an electrically illuminated tubular device is passed through a trocar into the abdominal cavity. Also called **peritoneoscopy.** See also **endoscopy, laparoscopy.**

**abdominoscrotal** /-skrō′təl/, pertaining to the abdomen and scrotum.

**abdominothoracic arch** /-thôras′ik/, the boundary between the thorax and the abdomen.

**abdominovaginal** /-vaj′inəl/, pertaining to the abdomen and vagina.

**abdominovesical** /-ves′ikəl/, pertaining to the abdomen and bladder. Also **abdominocystic.**

**abducens** /abdōō′sənz/ [L, drawing away], pertaining to a movement away from the median line of the body.

**abducens muscle,** the extraocular lateral rectus muscle that moves the eyeball outward.

**abducens nerve** [L, *abducere,* to take away], either of the paired sixth cranial nerves. It arises in the pons near the fourth ventricle, leaves the brainstem between the medulla oblongata and pons, and passes through the cavernous sinus and the superior orbital fissure. It controls the lateral rectus muscle, turning the eye outward. Also called **abducent nerve, nervus abducens, sixth cranial nerve.**

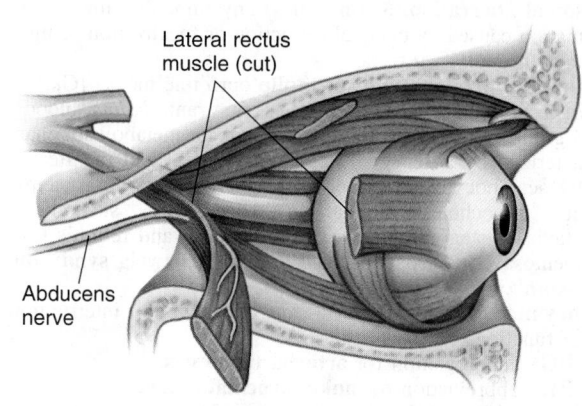

**Abducens nerve**

**abduct** /abdukt′/, to move away from an axis of the body.

**abduction** [L, *abducere,* to take away], movement of a limb away from the body. Compare **adduction.**

**abduction boots,** a pair of orthopedic casts for the lower extremities, available in both short-leg and long-leg configurations, with a bar incorporated at ankle level to provide hip abduction. Abduction boots are used for postoperative positioning and immobilization after hip adductor releases with total hip arthroplasty or hip prosthesis implantation. They also promote proper positioning during healing after surgical repair of the lower extremities.

**abductor** /abduk′tər/ [L, *abducere*], a muscle that draws a body part away from the midline or axis, or one part from another. Compare **adductor.**

**abembryonic** /ab′embrē·on′ik/, opposite the position of the embryo.

**Abernethy's sarcoma** /ab′ərnē′thēz/ [John Abernethy, British surgeon, 1764–1831], a malignant neoplasm of fat cells, usually occurring on the trunk.

**aberrancy.** See **aberrant ventricular conduction.**

**aberrant** /aber′ənt/ [L, *aberrare,* to wander], **1.** pertaining to a wandering from the usual or expected course, such as various ducts, nerves, vessels in the body, or cardiac conduction. **2.** (in botany and zoology) pertaining to an abnormal individual, such as certain atypical members of a species.

**aberrant conduction.** See **aberrant ventricular conduction.**

**aberrant goiter,** an enlargement of a supernumerary or ectopic thyroid gland.

**aberrant ventricular conduction (AVC),** the temporary abnormal intraventricular conduction of a supraventricular impulse. It is usually associated with an increase in the duration of the QRS complex to more than 120 msec. This conduction pattern is fairly common after a very premature atrial beat and during the paroxysmal supraventricular tachycardia that is caused by orthodromic circus movement tachycardia (using the atrioventricular node intergradely and an accessory pathway retrogradely). Also called **aberrancy, aberrant conduction, ventricular aberration.**

**aberration** /ab′ərā′shən/ [L, *aberrare,* to wander],   **1.** any departure from the usual course or normal condition. **2.** abnormal growth or development. **3.** (in psychology) an illogical and unreasonable thought or belief, often leading to an unsound mental state. **4.** (in genetics) any change in the number or structure of the chromosomes. See also **chromosomal aberration. 5.** (in optics) any imperfect image formation caused by unequal refraction or focalization of light rays through a lens.

**abetalipoproteinemia** /əbā′təlip′ōprō′tinē′mē·ə/ [Gk, *a, beta,* not beta, *lipos,* fat, *proteios,* first rank, *haima,* blood], a group of rare inherited disorders of fat metabolism, characterized by absence of apoprotein B-100 and manifested by acanthocytosis, low or absent serum beta-lipoproteins, and hypocholesterolemia. In severe cases steatorrhea, ataxia, nystagmus, motor incoordination, and retinitis pigmentosa occur. Also called **Bassen-Kornzweig syndrome** /-kôrn′zwīg/.

**abeyance** /əbā′əns/ [Fr],   a state of inaction or interruption of function.

**ABG,**   abbreviation for **arterial blood gas.**

**ABI,**   abbreviation for **ankle-brachial index.**

**abient** /ab′ē·ənt/ [L, *abire,* to go away],   characterized by a tendency to move away from stimuli. Compare **adient.** —**abience,** *n.*

**ability** /əbil′itē/,   the capacity to act in a specified way because of the possession of appropriate skills and mental or physical fitness.

**abiogenesis** /ab′ē·ōjen′əsis/ [Gk, *a + bios,* not life, *genein,* to produce],   spontaneous generation; the idea that life can originate from inorganic, inanimate matter. Compare **biogenesis.** —**abiogenetic,** *adj.*

**abiosis** /ab′ē·ō′sis/ [Gk, *a + bios* not life],   a nonviable condition or a situation that is incompatible with life. —**abiotic,** *adj.*

**abiotrophy** /ab′ē·ot′rəfē/ [Gk, *a + bios + trophe* nutrition],   a premature depletion of vitality or the deterioration of certain cells and tissues, especially those involved in genetic degenerative diseases. See also **atrophy.** —**abiotrophic** /ab′ē·ətrō′fik/, *adj.*

**ablastemic** /ab′lastem′ik/,   nongerminal or not germinating.

**ablate** /ablāt′/ [L, *ab + latus,* carried away],   to cut away or remove, as in ablation.

**ablation** /ablā′shən/ [L, *ab + latus,* carried away],   an amputation, an excision of any part of the body, or a removal of a growth or harmful substance.

**ablatio placentae.**   See **abruptio placentae.**

**ABLB test,**   abbreviation for **alternate binaural loudness balance test.**

**-able, -ible,**   a suffix indicating 'ability or capacity': *intractable, flexible.*

**ablepharia** /ab′ləfer′ē·ə/,   a defect characterized by partial or total absence of the eyelids.

**ablepsia** /əblep′sē·ə/ [Gk, *a + blepein,* not to see],   the condition of being blind. Also called **ablepsy.**

**abluent,**   pertaining to the ability of a substance to cleanse or wash away.

**ablution** /ablōō′shən/,   the act of washing or bathing.

**ABMS,**   abbreviation for *American Board of Medical Specialties.*

**abnerval current** /abnur′vəl/ [L, *ab,* from; Gk, *neuron,* nerve],   an electrical current that passes from a nerve to and through muscle.

**abneural** /abnŏŏr′əl/,   away from the central nervous system or the neural axis.

**abnormal behavior** /abnôr′məl/ [L, *ab + norma,* away from rule],   behavior that deviates from the norms of the group or society. See also **behavior disorder.**

**abnormality** /ab′nôrmal′itē/ [L, *ab,* away from, *norma,* the rule],   a condition that differs from the usual cultural or scientifically accepted norms.

**abnormal psychology,**   the study of any behavior that deviates from culturally accepted norms.

**abnormal tooth mobility,**   excessive movement of a tooth within its socket as a result of injury or disease in the supporting tissues.

**ABO blood group,**   a system for classifying human blood based on the antigenic components of red blood cells and their corresponding antibodies. The ABO blood group is identified by the presence or absence of two different antigens, A and B, on the surface of the red blood cell. The four blood types in this grouping, A, B, AB, and O, are determined by and named for these antigens. Type AB indicates the presence of both antigens; type O the absence of both. Corresponding antibodies, anti-A and anti-B agglutinins, can be found in the plasma of type O blood. The plasma components of type A and type B blood are, respectively, devoid of anti-A and anti-B agglutinins; both agglutinins are absent from type AB blood plasma. In addition to its significant role in transfusion therapy and transplantation, the ABO blood grouping contributes to forensic medicine, to genetics, and, together with the less important blood groups, to anthropology and legal medicine. See also **blood group, Rh factor, transfusion.**

**aboiement** /ä′bô·ämäN′/,   an involuntary making of abnormal, animal-like sounds, such as barking. Aboiement may be a clinical sign of Gilles de la Tourette's syndrome.

**abort** /əbôrt′/ [L, *ab,* away from, *oriri,* to be born],   **1.** to deliver a nonviable fetus; to miscarry. See also **spontaneous abortion. 2.** to terminate a pregnancy before the fetus has developed enough to live outside the uterus. See also **induced abortion. 3.** to terminate in the early stages or to discontinue before completion, as to arrest the usual course of a disease, to stop growth and development, or to halt a project.

**aborted systole,**   a contraction of the heart that is usually weak and is not associated with a radial pulse.

**abortifacient** /əbôr′tifā′shənt/,   **1.** producing abortion. **2.** any agent that causes abortion.

**abortion** /əbor′shən/ [L, *ab + oriri*],   the spontaneous or induced termination of pregnancy before the fetus has developed to the stage of viability. Kinds of abortion include **habitual abortion, infected abortion, septic abortion, threatened abortion,** and **voluntary abortion.** See also **complete abortion, elective abortion, incomplete abortion, induced abortion, medical abortion, missed abortion, spontaneous abortion, therapeutic abortion.**

**abortionist,**   a person who performs abortions.

**abortion on demand,**   a concept promoted by prochoice health advocates that it is the right of a pregnant woman to have an abortion performed at her request. That right may be limited by time of gestation, or it may pertain to any period of gestation.

**abortion pill.**   See **mifepristone.**

**abortive infection** /əbôr′tiv/, an infection in which some or all viral components have been synthesized, but no infective virus is produced. The situation may result from an infection with defective viruses or because the host cell is non-permissive and prohibits replication of the particular virus.

**abortus** /əbôr′təs/, any incompletely developed fetus that results from an abortion, particularly one weighing less than 500 g.

**abortus fever,** a form of brucellosis, the only one endemic to North America. It is caused by *Brucella abortus,* an organism so named because it causes abortion in cows. Infection in humans results from the ingesting contaminated milk or milk products from cows infected with *B. abortus,* from handling infected meat, or from skin contact with the excreta of living infected animals. A prolonged course of combination antibiotic therapy is required: doxycycline and a parenteral aminoglycoside followed by oral therapy with doxycycline and rifampin. Also called **Rio Grande fever.** See also **brucellosis.**

**abouchement** /ä′bo͞oshmäN′/ [Fr, a tube connection], the junction of a small blood vessel with a large blood vessel.

**aboulia.** See **abulia.**

**ABP,** abbreviation for **arterial blood pressure.**

**ABPM,** abbreviation for **ambulatory blood pressure monitoring.**

**ABR,** abbreviation for **auditory brainstem response.**

**abrachia** /əbrā′kē·ə/ [Gk, *a + brachion,* without arm], the absence of arms. —**abrachial,** *adj.*

**abrachiocephalia.** See **acephalobrachia.**

**abrade** /əbrād′/, to remove the epidermis, usually by scraping or rubbing.

**abrasion** /əbrā′zhən/ [L, *abradere,* to scrape off], a scraping, or rubbing away of a surface, such as skin or teeth, by friction. Abrasion may be the result of trauma, such as a skinned knee; of therapy, as in dermabrasion of the skin for removal of scar tissue; or of normal function, such as the wearing down of a tooth by mastication. Compare **laceration.** See also **bruxism, friction burn.** —**abrade,** *v.,* **abrasive,** *adj.*

**abrasive,** **1.** pertaining to a substance that can grind or wear down another substance. **2.** an object or surface that can cause an abrasion.

**abreact** /ab′rē·akt′/, **1.** to release a repressed emotion. **2.** to work off by catharsis effects of a repressed disagree-

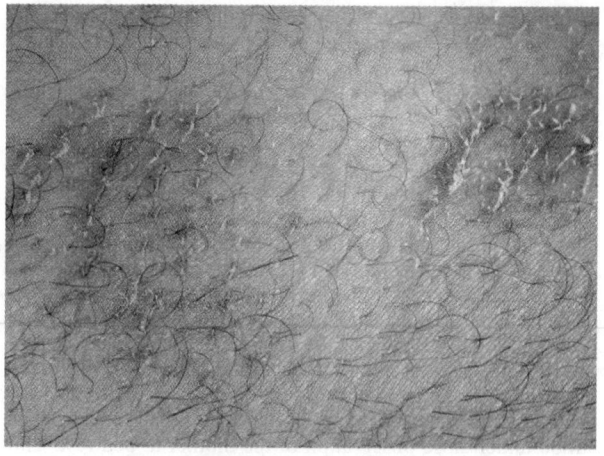

**Abrasion of the skin**
*(Cotran, Kumar, and Collins, 1999/from the teaching collection of the Department of Dermatology, Southwestern Medical School, Dallas)*

able experience. **3.** to mentally relive or bring into consciousness repressed experiences.

**abreaction** /ab′rē·ak′shən/ [L, *ab,* from, *re,* again, *agere,* to act], an emotional release resulting from mentally reliving or bringing into consciousness, through the process of catharsis, a long-repressed, painful experience. See also **catharsis.**

**abrosia** /əbrō′zhə/ [Gk, fasting], a condition caused by fasting or abstaining from food. See also **anorexia.**

**abruption** [L, *ab,* away from, *rumpere,* rupture], a sudden breaking off or tearing apart.

**abruptio placentae** [L, *ab,* away from, *rumpere,* to rupture], separation of the placenta implanted in normal position in a pregnancy of 20 weeks or more or during labor before delivery of the fetus. It occurs in approximately 1 in 200 births, and, because it often results in severe hemorrhage, it is a significant cause of maternal and fetal mortality. Hypertension and preeclampsia are associated with increased rates of occurrence; in many cases, however, there is

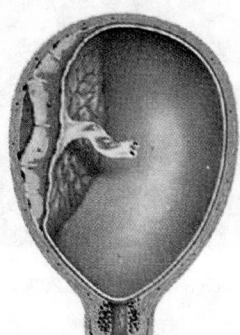
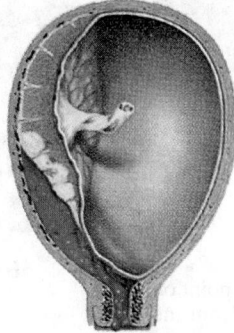
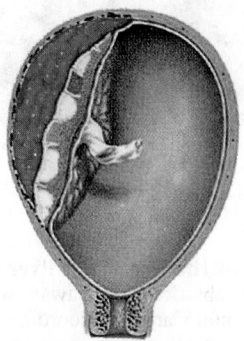

Partial separation (concealed hemorrhage)

Partial separation (apparent hemorrhage)

Complete separation (concealed hemorrhage)

**Abruptio placentae** *(Lowdermilk, Perry, and Bobak, 2000)*

no explanation. Complete separation causes immediate death of the fetus. Bleeding from the site of separation causes abdominal pain, uterine tenderness, and tetanic uterine contraction. Bleeding may be concealed within the uterus or may be evident externally, sometimes as sudden massive hemorrhage. In severe cases, shock and death can result in minutes. Cesarean section must be performed immediately and rapidly. Extensive extravasation of blood within the uterine wall may deplete fibrinogen, prolong clotting time, bring about intractable bleeding, lead to disseminated intravascular coagulation, and, by damaging the uterine musculature, prevent the uterus from contracting well after delivery. Hysterectomy may be necessary to prevent exsanguination. Partial separation may cause little bleeding and may not interfere with fetal oxygenation. If the pregnancy is near term, labor may be permitted or induced by amniotomy. A premature pregnancy may be allowed to continue under close observation of the mother at bed rest. The nurse must be alert to the possibility that bleeding is present but concealed internally and that if all the blood can escape, there may be little pain. Also called **ablatio placentae, accidental hemorrhage, placental abruption.** Compare **placenta previa.** See also **Couvelaire uterus.**

**abscess** /ab′səs/ [L, *abscedere,* to go away], **1.** a cavity containing pus and surrounded by inflamed tissue, formed as a result of suppuration in a localized infection (characteristically, a staphylococcal infection). Healing usually occurs when an abscess drains or is incised. If an abscess is deep in tissue, drainage is done by means of a sinus tract that connects it to the surface. In a sterile abscess, the contents are not the result of pyogenic bacteria. **2. dental abscess,** an abscess that develops anywhere along the root length of a tooth. It is usually characterized by pain caused by the pressure of pus against the nerve tissue, redness caused by blood accumulation, and swelling caused by the suppuration.

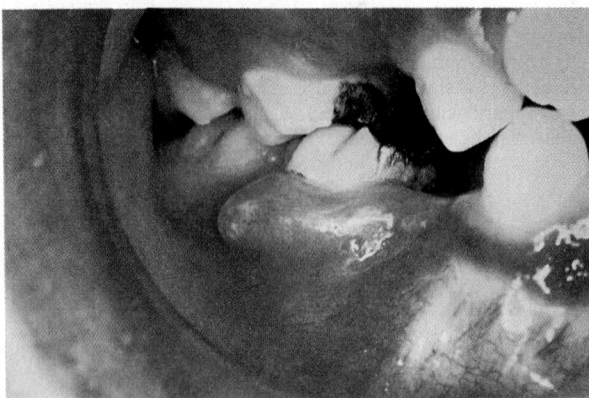

**Dental abscess** *(Stone and Gorbach, 2000)*

**abscess of the liver** See **liver abscess.**
**abscissa** /absis′ə/ [L, *ab,* away; *scindere,* to cut], a point on a horizontal Cartesian coordinate plane measured from the *y*- (or vertical) axis running perpendicular to the plane, or *x*-axis.
**abscission** /absish′ən/ [L, *abscinere,* to cut away], the process of cutting away, as in corneal abscission, removal of the prominence of the cornea.

**absconsio** /abskon′shō/ [L, *ab,* away from, *condo,* hidden], a cavity or fossa.
**abscopal** /abskō′pəl/, pertaining to the effect of irradiated tissue on remote tissue not exposed to radiation.
**absence seizure,** an epileptic seizure characterized by a sudden, momentary loss of consciousness. Occasionally it is accompanied by minor myoclonus of the neck or upper extremities, slight symmetric twitching of the face, or loss of muscle tone. The seizures usually occur many times a day without a warning aura and are most frequent in children and adolescents, especially at puberty. The patient experiencing a typical seizure has a vacant facial expression and ceases all voluntary motor activity; with the rapid return of consciousness, the patient may resume conversation at the point of interruption without realizing what occurred. During and between seizures, the patient's electroencephalogram shows 3-Hz spike-and-wave discharges. Anticonvulsant drugs used to prevent absence seizures include ethosuximide, trimethadione, and valproic acid. Also called **absentia epileptica, petit mal seizure.** See also **epilepsy.**
**absenteeism** /ab′səntē′izəm/, (for health or related reasons) absence from work. Absenteeism varies according to job assignments, with professional and managerial personnel taking average annual sick leave of 4 days, whereas unskilled workers claim an average of 18 days sick leave during the year. Surveys also indicate that fewer than 10% of workers account for nearly 50% of all absenteeism. The most common causes of absenteeism include influenza and occupationally related skin diseases.
**absentia epileptica.** See **absence seizure.**
**absent without leave (AWOL)** /ā′wôl/ [L, *absentia*], a term used to describe a patient who departs from a psychiatric facility without authorization.
**abs feb,** abbreviation for *absente febre,* a Latin phrase meaning in the absence of fever.
*Absidia* /absid′ē·ə/, a genus of fungus belonging to the class Phycomycetes. Several species have been found to cause infections of otosclerosis and pulmonary and general mycosis in humans. Other pathogenic species cause diseases in livestock.

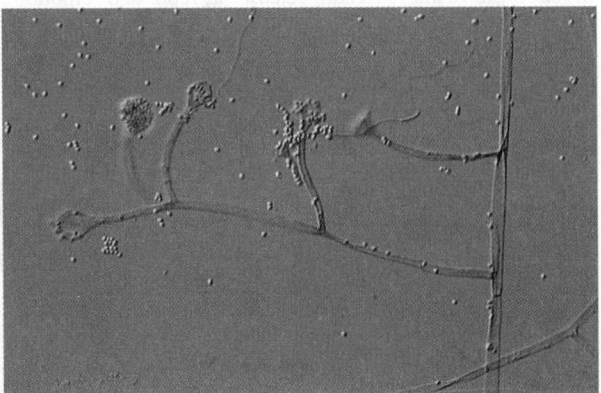

***Absidia* species** *(Mahon and Manuselis, 2000)*

**absolute,** unconditional, unrestricted, or independent of arbitrary standards.
**absolute agraphia** [L, *absolutus,* set loose; Gk, *a,* not, *graphein,* to write], a complete inability to write caused by

a central nervous system lesion. The person is unable to write even the letters of the alphabet. See also **agraphia.**

**absolute alcohol.**   See **dehydrated alcohol.**

**absolute cephalopelvic disproportion.**   See **cephalopelvic disproportion.**

**absolute discharge** /ab′səlo͞ot/ [L, *absolutus,* set free], a final and complete termination of the patient's relationship with a care-giving agency.

**absolute glaucoma** /ab′səlo͞o′t/ [L, *abolutus* + Gk, *cataract*], complete blindness in which a glaucoma-induced increase in intraocular pressure results in permanent vision loss. The optic disc is white and deeply excavated, and the pupil is usually widely dilated and immobile. Also called absolutum glaucoma, **glaucoma consummatum.**

**absolute growth,** the total increase in size of an organism or a particular organ or part, such as the limbs, head, or trunk.

**absolute humidity,** the actual mass or content of water in a measured volume of air. It is usually expressed in grams per cubic meter or pounds per cubic foot or cubic yard.

**absolute neutrophil count (ANC),** the number of neutrophils in a milliliter of blood, having a reference value of approximately 1500–7700 per μL. The ANC is a measure of a person's immune status. Generally, if the count is above 1000 the person may safely mingle with other people or undergo chemotherapy, while a count below 500 indicates that a person is at high risk for infection and should be kept away from those with infectious diseases.

**absolute refractory period.**   See **refractory period.**

**absolute temperature,** temperature that is measured from a base of absolute zero on the Kelvin scale or the Rankine scale.

**absolute threshold** [L, *absolutus,* set loose; AS, *therscold*], **1.** the lowest point at which a stimulus can be perceived. **2.** pertaining to millivolts of electrical charge determined by ion fluctuations or movement across cell membranes that result in nerve stimulation.

**absolute zero,** the temperature at which all molecular activity except vibration ceases. It is a theoretical value derived by calculations and projections from experiments with the behavior of gases at extremely low temperatures. On the Celcius scale, absolute zero is estimated to be equal to −273° C. On the Fahrenheit scale, the equivalent temperature is calculated at −460° F.

**absorb** /absôrb′, əbzôrb′/ [L, *absorbere,* to swallow], **1.** the act of drinking in, wholly engulfing, assimilating, or taking up various substances; for example, the tissues of the intestines absorb fluids. **2.** the energy transferred to tissues by radiation, such as an absorbed dose of radioactivity.

**absorbable gauze** /əbsôr′bəbəl/, a material, produced from oxidized cellulose, that can be absorbed. It is applied directly to tissue to stop bleeding.

**absorbable surgical suture** [L, *absorbere,* to suck up; Gk, *cheirourgos,* surgery; L, *sutura*], a suture made from material that can be completely removed by the body's phagocytes.

**absorbance** /əbsôr′bəns/, the degree of absorption of light or other radiant energy by a medium that is exposed to the energy. It is expressed as the logarithm of the ratio of energy transmitted through a pure solvent to the energy transmitted through the medium. Absorbance varies with factors such as wavelength, solution concentration, and path length.

**absorbed dose,** the energy imparted by ionizing radiation per unit mass of irradiated material at the place of interest. The SI unit of absorbed dose is the gray, which is 1 J/kg and equals 100 rad.

**absorbent** /absôr′bənt/ [L, *absorbere,* to suck up], **1.** capable of attracting and absorbing substances into itself. **2.** a product or substance that can absorb liquids or gases.

**absorbent dressing,** a dressing of any material applied to a wound or incision to absorb secretions.

**absorbent gauze,** a fabric or pad with various forms, weights, and uses. It may be a rolled, single-layered fine fabric for spiral bandages, or it may be a thick, multilayered pad for a sterile pressure dressing. There may also be an adhesive backing.

**absorbent point.**   See **paper point.**

**absorbefacient** /absôr′bifā′shənt/ [L, *absorbere* + *facere,* to make], **1.** any agent that promotes or enhances absorption. **2.** causing or enhancing absorption.

**absorption** /absôrp′shən/ [L, *absorptio*], **1.** the incorporation of matter by other matter through chemical, molecular, or physical action, such as the dissolving of a gas in a liquid or the taking up of a liquid by a porous solid. **2.** (in physiology) the passage of substances across and into tissues, such as the passage of digested food molecules into intestinal cells or the passage of liquids into kidney tubules. Kinds of absorption are **agglutinin absorption, cutaneous absorption, external absorption, intestinal absorption, parenteral absorption,** and **pathologic absorption. 3.** (in radiology) the process of absorbing radiant energy by living or nonliving matter with which the radiation interacts.

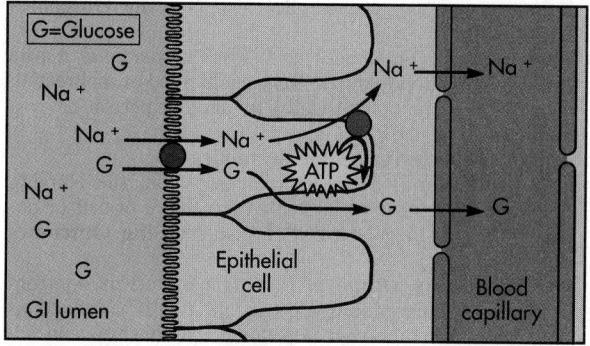

**Absorption of sodium, glucose, and amino acids**
*(Thibodeau and Patton, 1999/Rolin Graphics)*

**absorption coefficient,** the fractional loss in intensity of electromagnetic energy as it interacts with an absorbing material. It is usually expressed per unit thickness or per unit mass.

**absorption rate constant,** a value describing how much drug is absorbed per unit of time.

**absorption spectrum,** a plot of percent transmittance, absorbance, logarithm of absorbance, or absorptivity of a compound as a function of wavelength, wave number, or frequency of radiation.

**absorptivity** /ab′sôrptiv′itē/, absorbance at a particular wavelength divided by the product of the concentration of a substance and the sample path length.

**abstinence** /ab′stinəns/, voluntarily avoiding a substance, such as food or alcohol, or refraining from the performance of an act, such as sexual intercourse.

**abstinence syndrome** [L, *abstinere,* to hold back; Gk, *syn,* together, *dromos,* course], the withdrawal symptoms experienced by a chemically dependent person who is suddenly deprived of a regular intake of alcohol or other addictive substance.

**abstract** /ab′strakt, abstrakt′/, **1.** a condensed summary of a scientific article, literary piece, or address. **2.** to collect data such as from a medical record.

**abstraction** /abstrak′shən/ [L, *abstrahere,* to drag away], a condition in which all or part of the dental arch is farther from the Frankfurt horizontal plane than normal.

**abstract thinking,** the final, most complex stage in the development of cognitive thinking, in which thought is characterized by adaptability, flexibility, and the use of concepts and generalizations. Problem solving is accomplished by drawing logical conclusions from a set of observations, such as making hypotheses and testing them. This type of thinking appears from about 12 to 15 years of age, usually after some degree of education. In psychiatry, many disorders are characterized by the inability to think abstractly. Compare **concrete thinking, syncretic thinking.**

**abulia** /əboo′lyə/ [Gk, *a + boule,* without will], a loss of the ability or reduced capacity to exhibit initiative or to make decisions. Also spelled **aboulia.**

**abuse** /abyoos′/ [L, *abuti,* to waste], **1.** improper use of equipment, a substance, or a service, such as a drug or program, either intentionally or unintentionally. See also **substance abuse. 2.** to physically or verbally attack or injure. An example is **child abuse.**

**abuse cessation,** a nursing outcome from the Nursing Outcomes Classification (NOC) defined as evidence that the victim is no longer abused. See also **Nursing Outcomes Classification.**

**abused person** [Fr, *abuser,* to disuse, L, *persona,* a role played], an individual who has been harmed or maltreated, verbally, sexually, or physically, by another person or by a situation.

**abuse of the elderly.** See **elder abuse.**

**abuse protection,** a nursing outcome from the Nursing Outcomes Classification (NOC) as protection of self or dependent others from abuse. See also **Nursing Outcomes Classification.**

**abuse protection support,** a nursing intervention from the Nursing Interventions Classification (NIC) defined as identification of high-risk, dependent relationships and actions to prevent further infliction of physical or emotional harm. See also **Nursing Interventions Classification.**

**abuse protection support: child,** a nursing intervention from the Nursing Interventions Classification (NIC) defined as identification of high-risk, dependent child relationships and actions to prevent possible or further infliction of physical, sexual, or emotional harm or neglect of basic necessities of life. See also **Nursing Interventions Classification.**

**abuse protection support: domestic partner,** a nursing intervention from the Nursing Interventions Classification (NIC) defined as identification of high-risk, dependent domestic relationships and actions to prevent possible or further infliction of physical, sexual, or emotional harm, or exploitation of a domestic partner. See also **Nursing Interventions Classification.**

**abuse protection support: elder,** a nursing intervention from the Nursing Interventions Classification (NIC) defined as identification of high-risk, dependent elder relationships and actions to prevent possible or further infliction of physical, sexual, or emotional harm; neglect of basic necessities of life; or exploitation. See also **Nursing Interventions Classification.**

**abuse protection support: religious,** a nursing intervention from the Nursing Interventions Classification (NIC) defined as identification of high-risk, controlling, religious re-

lationships and actions to prevent infliction of physical, sexual, or emotional harm and/or exploitation. See also **Nursing Interventions Classification.**

**abuse recovery: emotional,** a nursing outcome from the Nursing Outcomes Classification (NOC) defined as healing of psychologic injuries due to abuse. See also **Nursing Outcomes Classification.**

**abuse recovery: financial,** a nursing outcome from the Nursing Outcomes Classification (NOC) defined as regaining monetary and legal control or benefits following financial exploitation. See also **Nursing Outcomes Classification.**

**abuse recovery: physical,** a nursing outcome from the Nursing Outcomes Classification (NOC) defined as healing of physical injuries due to abuse. See also **Nursing Outcomes Classification.**

**abuse recovery: sexual,** a nursing outcome from the Nursing Outcomes Classification (NOC) defined as healing following sexual abuse or exploitation. See also **Nursing Outcomes Classification.**

**abusive behavior self-control,** a nursing outcome from the Nursing Outcomes Classification (NOC) defined as self-restraint of own behaviors to avoid abuse and neglect of dependents or significant others. See also **Nursing Outcomes Classification.**

**abutment** /əbut′mənt/ [Fr, *abouter* to place end to end], a tooth, root, or implant that supports and provides retention for a fixed or movable prosthesis.

**abutment tooth,** a tooth selected to support a prosthesis.

**ABVD,** an anticancer drug combination of doxorubicin, bleomycin, vinblastine, and dacarbazine.

**Ac,** symbol for the element **actinium.**

**AC, 1.** abbreviation for **alternating current. 2.** abbreviation for *accommodative convergence.* See **AC/A ratio.**

**ac-.** See **ad-.**

**a.c.,** (in prescriptions) abbreviation for *ante cibum,* a Latin phrase meaning 'before meals.'

**A-C,** abbreviation for *alveolar-capillary.*

**acacia gum,** a dried, gummy exudate of the acacia tree (*Acacia senegal*) used as a suspending or emulsifying agent in medicines.

**academic ladder** /ak′ədem′ik/ [Gk, *akademeia,* school], the hierarchy of faculty appointments in a university through which a faculty member advances from the rank of instructor to assistant professor to associate professor to professor.

**acalculia** /a′kalkoo′lyə/ [Gk, *a,* not; L, *calculare,* to reckon], a type of aphasia characterized by the inability to perform simple mathematic calculations previously known. It is commonly seen in neurological disorders.

**acampsia** /əkamp′sē·ə/ [Gk, *a + kampsein,* not to bend], a condition in which a joint is rigid. See also **ankylosis.**

**acanth-, acantho-,** /əkan′thə/ [Gk, *akantha,* thorn], a combining form meaning 'thorny or spiny': *acanthesia, acanthocytosis.*

**acanthamebiasis** /əkan′thəmēbī′əsis/, a potentially fatal meningoencephalitis infection caused by strains of *Acanthamoeba.* It is commonly acquired by swimming in water contaminated by the microorganism, but cleaning contact lenses in contaminated solution also has caused keratins.

*Acanthamoeba* /əkan′thəmē′bə/, a genus of free-living amebas typically found in soil and water. The organisms may enter the body through a break in the skin, causing a localized infection, or even though the nose, causing systemic infections of the lung, genitourinary system, brain, and central nervous system. Although an infection may be fatal, cases are more commonly chronic.

**acanthesia** /ak′anthē′zhə/, pin prick paresthesia; an abnormality of cutaneous sensory perception that causes a simple touch to be felt as a painful pin prick.

**acanthiomeatal line** /əkan'thē-ō'mē-ā'təl/, a hypothetical line extending from the external auditory meatus to the acanthion. In dentistry a full maxillary denture is constructed so that its occlusal plane is parallel with this line.

**acanthion,** a point at the center of the base of the anterior nasal spine.

*Acanthocheilonema perstans* /akan'thōkī'lənē'mə/, a threadworm usually found in Africa. It commonly infects wild and domestic animals and occasionally invades the bloodstream of humans, causing a skin rash, muscle and joint pains, various neurologic disorders, and nodules in the subcutaneous tissues. The larvae are also found in the cerebrospinal fluid of affected patients.

**acanthocheilonemiasis.** See **mansonellosis.**

**acanthocyte** /əkan'thəsīt'/ [Gk, *akantha* + *kytos,* cell], an abnormal red blood cell with spurlike projections. Large numbers are present in abetalipoproteinemia; fewer occur in cirrhosis and in certain malabsorption syndromes. Compare **burr cell.** See also **abetalipoproteinemia, acanthocytosis.**

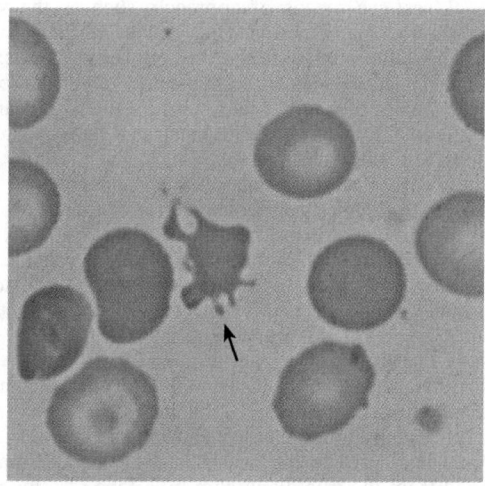

**Acanthocyte** *(Carr and Rodak, 1999)*

**acanthocytosis** /akan'thōsītō'sis/ [Gk, *akantha* + *kytos* + *osis,* condition], the presence of acanthocytes in the circulating blood, most commonly associated with abetalipoproteinemia, in which as many as 80% of the erythrocytes are acanthocytes. See also **abetalipoproteinemia, elliptocytosis.**

**acanthoid,** resembling a spinous process.

**acanthoma** /ak'anthō'mə/ [Gk, *akantha* + *oma,* tumor], hypertrophy arising from the prickle-cell layer of the epidermis which is localized rather than diffuse. It may be benign or malignant.

**acanthoma adenoides cysticum.** See **trichoepithelioma.**

**acanthoma fissuration,** development of a fissure bordered by increased thickening at sites of friction of the prickle-cell level of epidermis.

**acanthoma verrucosa seborrheica.** See **seborrheic keratosis.**

**acanthorrhexis** /əkan'thôrek'sis/, the rupture of intercel-

lular bridges of the prickle-cell layer of epidermis, as in eczema or allergic contact dermatitis.

**acanthosis** /ak'ənthō'sis/ [Gk, *akantha* + *osis,* condition], an abnormal, diffuse hypertrophy of the prickle-cell layer of the skin, as in eczema and psoriasis. See also **acanthosis nigricans, epidermis. —acanthotic,** *adj.*

**acanthosis nigricans** /nē'grikanz'/, a skin disease characterized by hyperpigmented, velvety thickening of the skin, common in the neck, axilla, and groin. There are benign and malignant forms; the latter is most often associated with cancers of the GI tract. See also **acanthosis.**

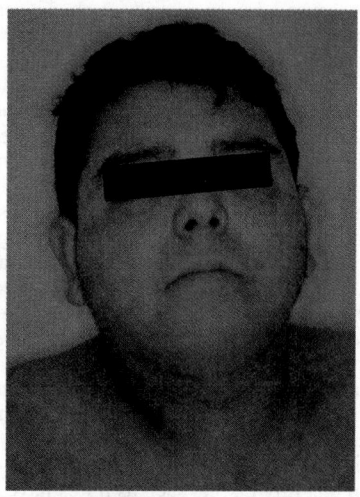

**Acanthosis nigricans on the neck** *(Lemmi and Lemmi, 2000)*

**acanthotic.** See **acanthosis.**

**acapnia** /akap'nē-ə/, a deficiency of carbon dioxide in the blood. The condition is usually the result of hyperventilation.

**AC/A ratio,** (in ophthalmology) the proportion between accommodative convergence (AC) and accommodation (A), or the amount of convergence automatically resulting from the dioptric focusing of the eyes at a specified distance. The ratio of accommodative convergence to accommodation is usually expressed as the quotient of accommodative convergence in prism diopters divided by the accommodative response in diopters.

**acarbia** /akär'bē-ə/ [Gk, *a,* not; L, *carbo,* coal], **1.** a decrease in the bicarbonate level in the blood. **2.** any condition that lowers the bicarbonate level in the blood.

**acarbose,** an insulin-control drug.

■ INDICATIONS: It is prescribed in the treatment of type 2 diabetes mellitus; it slows the digestion of complex carbohydrates and reduces the demand for insulin. The drug is indicated for use with dietary modifications or other medications that treat diabetes in patients whose hyperglycemia is not sufficiently controlled by diet alone.

■ CONTRAINDICATIONS: It should not be used by patients with diabetic ketoacidosis or intestinal diseases that may impair digestion or absorption. Caution is advised for use in patients with renal dysfunction.

■ ADVERSE EFFECTS: The side effects most often reported include flatulence, diarrhea, and abdominal pain. Increased transaminase levels have been reported in patients taking high doses.

**acardia** /äkär′dē·ə/ [Gk, *a* + *kardia,* without heart], a rare congenital anomaly in which the heart is absent. It is sometimes seen in a conjoined twin whose survival depends on the circulatory system of its twin. —**acardiac,** *adj.*

**acardius acephalus,** an acardiac fetus that lacks a head and most of the upper part of the body.

**acardius acormus,** an acardiac fetus that has a grossly defective trunk.

**acardius amorphus,** an acardiac fetus with a rudimentary body that does not resemble the normal form. Also called **acardius anceps.**

**acariasis** /ak′ərī′əsis/ [Gk, *akari,* mite, *osis,* condition], any disease caused by an acarid, such as scrub typhus, which is transmitted by trombiculid mites.

**acarid** /ak′ərid/, one of the many mites that are members of the order Acarina, which includes a great number of parasitic and free-living organisms. Most are yet not described, but several types are of medical interest because they infect humans. Those associated with disease act as intermediate hosts of pathogenic agents, directly cause skin or tissue damage, and cause loss of blood or tissue fluids. Important as vectors of scrub typhus and other rickettsial agents are the six-legged larvae of trombiculid mites, which are parasitic of humans, many other mammals, and birds. See also **chigger, scabies.**

**acaro-,** a combining form meaning 'mites': *acarodermatitis, acariasis.*

**acarodermatitis** /ak′ərōdur′mətī′tis/ [Gk, *akari,* mite, *derma,* skin, *itis,* inflammation], a skin inflammation caused by mites or ticks.

**acarophobia** /-fō′bē·ə/, a morbid dread of tiny parasites or the delusion that tiny insects such as mites have invaded the skin.

**acaudal** /ākô′dəl/ [Gk, *a,* without; L, *cauda,* tail], without a tail.

**acc, Acc,** abbreviation for **accommodation.**

**ACC,** abbreviation for *American College of Cardiology.*

**accelerated hypertension.** See **malignant hypertension.**

**accelerated idiojunctional rhythm,** an automatic junctional rhythm whose rate is greater than 59 beats/min but less than 100 beats/min.

**accelerated idioventricular rhythm (AIVR),** an automatic ectopic ventricular rhythm, whose rate is greater than 49 beats/min but less than 100 beats/min, without retrograde conduction to the atria. In acute myocardial infarction an AIVR can be a sign of spontaneous reperfusion or a result of thrombolytic therapy.

**accelerated junctional rhythm,** an ectopic junctional heart rhythm whose rate exceeds the normal firing rate of junctional tissue, with or without retrograde atrial conduction.

**accelerated respiration,** an abnormally rapid rate of breathing, usually more than 25 breaths per minute. See also **tachypnea.**

**acceleration** /aksel′ərā′shən/ [L, *accelerare,* to quicken], an increase in the speed or velocity of an object or reaction. Compare **deceleration.** —**accelerator,** *n.*

**acceleration-deceleration injury,** injury resulting from a collision between a body part and another object or body part while both are in motion.

**acceleration phase,** (in obstetrics) the first period of active labor, stage I, characterized by an increased rate of dilation of the cervical canal as charted on a Friedman curve.

**accelerator** /aksel′ərā′tər/ [L, *accelerare,* to quicken], **1.** a nerve or muscle that increases the rate of performance

of some function. **2.** an agent or apparatus that is used to increase the rate at which a substance acts or a function proceeds.

**accelerator urinae.** See **bulbocavernosus.**

**accentuation** /aksen′chōō·ā′shən/ [L, *accentus,* accent], an increase in distinctness or loudness, as in heart sounds.

**acceptable daily intake (ADI)** the maximum amount of any substance that can be safely ingested by a human. Ingestion that exceeds this amount may cause toxic effects.

**acceptance: health status,** a nursing outcome from the Nursing Outcomes Classification (NOC) defined as reconciliation to health circumstances. See also **Nursing Outcomes Classification.**

**acceptance of individuality** /aksep′təns/, (in psychiatry) an index of family health in which differentiation or individuation is a valued goal.

**acceptance of separation,** an indicator of mental well-being in which a loss is mourned in a healthy manner. It indicates higher level of adaptability.

**acceptor** /aksep′tər/ [L, *accipere,* to receive], **1.** an organism that receives from another person or organism living tissue, such as transfused blood or a transplanted organ. **2.** a substance or compound that combines with a part of another substance or compound. Compare **donor.**

**access** /ak′ses/, a means of approach, such as the space needed for the manipulation of dental or surgical instruments. An example is vascular access in hemodialysis.

**access cavity** [L, *accedere,* to approach], a coronal opening to the center of a tooth, required for effective cleaning, shaping, and filling of the pulp canal and chamber during endodontic or root canal therapy.

**accessory** /akses′ərē/ [L, *accessonis,* appendage], **1.** a supplement used chiefly for convenience or for safety, such as the electric elevator mechanisms for hospital beds. **2.** a structure that serves one of the main anatomic systems, such as the accessory sex organs in men and women; the accessory organs of the skin; the hair; the nails; and the skin glands. **3.** one who aids in perpetrating a crime.

**accessory chromosome.** See **monosome.**

**accessory diaphragm,** a congenital defect in which a second diaphragm or portion of a diaphragm develops in the chest. It is usually found on the right side and is oriented upward and backward to the posterior chest wall. It may be separated from the true diaphragm by a lobe of a lung.

**accessory gland,** glandular tissue that contributes in a secondary way to the function of a similar gland, which may be nearby or some distance away.

**accessory ligament** [L, *accessus,* extra, *ligare,* to bind], a ligament that helps strengthen a union between two bones, even though it is not part of a joint capsule.

**accessory movement,** a joint movement that is necessary for a full range of motion but is not under direct voluntary control. Examples include rotation and gliding motions.

**accessory muscle,** a relatively rare anatomic duplication of a muscle that may appear anywhere in the muscular system. The most common sign associated with an accessory muscle is the appearance of a soft-tissue mass. Differential diagnosis without surgical intervention and exploration is difficult because of the similar appearance of some tumors or soft-tissue masses, such as ganglia. The appearance of the soft-tissue mass associated with an accessory muscle may be transient, or it may be constant, depending on the location of the accessory muscle in relation to motion. In many individuals with accessory muscles, specific treatment is not indicated unless the accessory muscle interferes with normal function.

**accessory muscles of respiration,** muscles of the neck,

back, and abdomen that may assist the diaphragm and the internal and external intercostal muscles in respiration, especially in some breathing disorders or during exercise.

**accessory nasal sinuses** [L, *accessus,* extra, *nasus,* nose, *sinus,* hollow], the paranasal sinuses that occur as hollows within the skull but open into the nasal cavity and are lined with a mucous membrane that is continuous with the nasal mucous membrane.

**accessory nerve,** either of a pair of cranial nerves essential for speech, swallowing, and certain movements of the head and shoulders. Each nerve has a cranial and a spinal portion, communicates with certain cervical nerves, and connects to the nucleus ambiguus of the brain. Also called **eleventh nerve, nervus accessorius, spinal accessory nerve.**

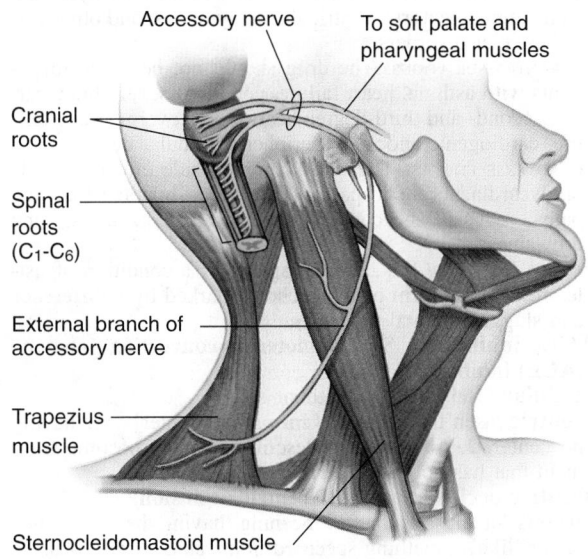

Accessory nerve

Accessory nerve

To soft palate and pharyngeal muscles

Cranial roots

Spinal roots (C₁-C₆)

External branch of accessory nerve

Trapezius muscle

Sternocleidomastoid muscle

**accessory organ,** an organ or other distinct collection of tissues that contributes to the function of another similar organ, such as the ocular muscles and eyelids, which contribute to the function of the eye.

**accessory pancreas** [L, *accessus,* extrig; Gk, *pan,* all, *kreas,* flesh], small clusters of pancreas cells detached from the pancreas and sometimes found in the wall of the stomach or intestines.

**accessory pancreatic duct,** a small duct opening into the pancreatic duct or duodenum near the mouth of the common bile duct.

**accessory pathway,** an abnormal conduction path between an atrium and a ventricle. Ventricular activation via an accessory pathway slows initial ventricular contraction, producing preexcitation and the delta wave of Wolff-Parkinson-White syndrome. The delta wave shortens the P-R interval, and broadens the QRS complex. The most common associated arrhythmias are paroxysmal supraventricular tachycardia and atrial fibrillation. Patients may be cured by transvenous radiofrequency ablation of the accessory pathway or treated medically.

**accessory phrenic nerve,** the nerve that joins the phrenic nerve at the root of the neck or in the thorax, forming a loop around the subclavian vein. It may arise from the nerve to the subclavius or from the fifth cervical nerve. Compare **phrenic nerve.**

**accessory placenta** [L, *accessionis,* a thing added, *placenta,* flat cake], a small placenta that may develop attached to the main placenta by umbilical blood vessels. Also called **succenturiate placenta.**

**accessory root canal,** a lateral branching of the pulp canal in a tooth, usually occurring in the apical third of the root.

**accessory sign,** a sign that is not typical or characteristic of a particular disease.

**accessory sinus of the nose.** See **paranasal sinus.**

**accessory spleen** [L, *accessus,* extra; Gk, *splen*], small nodules of spleen tissue that may occur in the gastrosplenic ligament, greater omentum, or other visceral sites.

**accessory thymus** [L, *accessus,* extra; Gk, *thymos,* thymelike], a nodule of thymus tissue that is isolated from the gland.

**accessory tooth,** a supernumerary tooth that does not resemble a normal tooth in size, shape, or position.

**access time,** the amount of time required for a computer to retrieve data from its disk drive.

**ACCH,** abbreviation for **Association for the Care of Children's Health.**

**accident** /ak′sidənt/ [L, *accidere,* to happen], any unexpected or unplanned event that may result in death, injury, property damage, or a combination of serious effects. The victim may or may not be directly involved in the cause of the accident. Accidents frequently are the result of both physical and mental factors that can result in unsafe operating systems at work, home, or other sites.

**accidental hemorrhage.** See **abruptio placentae.**

**accident-prone,** describing a person who experiences accidents and accompanying injuries at a much greater than average rate.

**acclimate** /əklī′mit, ak′limāt/ [L, *ad,* toward; Gk, *klima,* region], to adjust physiologically to a different climate or environment, or to changes in altitude or temperature. Also **acclimatize** /əklī′mətīz′/. —**acclimation, acclimatization,** *n.*

**acclimatization to heat** [L, *ad,* toward; Gk, *klima,* region], a process whereby the body adapts to warmer environmental temperatures.

**accommodation (A, acc, Acc)** /əkom′ədā′shən/ [L, *accommodatio,* adjustment], **1.** the state or process of adapting or adjusting one thing or set of things to another. **2.** the continuous process or effort of the individual to adapt or adjust to surroundings to maintain a state of homeostasis, both physiologically and psychologically. **3.** the adjustment of the eye to variations in distance. See also **accommodation reflex. 4.** (in sociology) the reciprocal reconciliation of conflicts between individuals or groups concerning habits and customs, usually through a process of compromise, arbitration, or negotiation. Also called **adjustment.** Compare **adaptation.**

**accommodation reflex,** an adjustment of the eyes for near vision, consisting of pupillary constriction, convergence of the eyes, and increased convexity of the lens. Also called **ciliary reflex.** See also **light reflex.**

**accommodative strabismus** /əkom′ədā′tiv/ [L, *accommodatio,* adjustment; Gk, *strabismos,* squint], **1.** strabismus resulting from abnormal demand on accommodation, such as convergent strabismus due to uncorrected hyperopia or divergent strabismus due to uncorrected myopia. **2.** strabismus resulting from the act of accommodation in association with a high AC/A ratio.

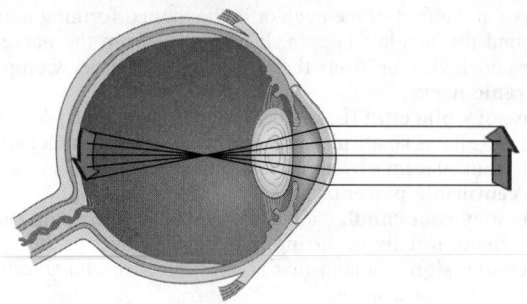

Distant image: lens is flattened

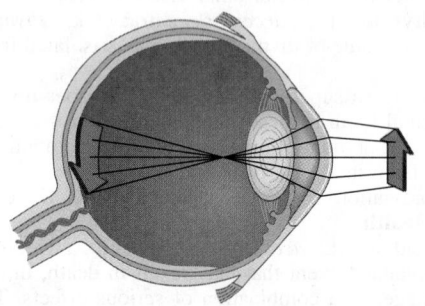

Close image: lens is rounded

**Accommodation reflex**
*(Thibodeau and Patton, 1999/Network Graphics)*

**accomplishment quotient** /əkom′plishmənt/, a numeric evaluation of a person's achievement age compared with mental age, expressed as a ratio multiplied by 100. See also **achievement quotient, intelligence quotient.**

**accountability** /əkoun′təbil′itē/, being accountable or responsible for the moral and legal requirements of proper patient care.

**accreditation** /əkred′itā′shən/, a process whereby a professional association or nongovernmental agency grants recognition to a school or institution for demonstrated ability to meet predetermined criteria, such as the accreditation of hospitals by the Joint Commission on Accreditation of Healthcare Organizations or of nursing schools by the National League for Nursing. Compare **certification, licensure.**

**accrementition** /ak′rəmentish′ən/, growth or increase in size by the addition of similar tissue or material, as in cellular division, simple fission, budding, or gemmation.

**accrete.** See **accretion.**

**accretio cordis** /əkrē′shē·ō/ [L, *accrescere,* to increase, *cordis,* heart], an abnormal condition in which the pericardium adheres to a structure around the heart.

**accretion** /əkrē′shən/ [L, *accrescere,* to increase], **1.** growth by the addition of material similar to that already present. **2.** the adherence or growing together of parts that are normally separated. **3.** an accumulation of foreign material, especially within a cavity. —**accrete,** *v.,* **accretive,** *adj.*

**acculturation** /əkul′chərā′shən/, the process of adopting the cultural traits or social patterns of a different population group.

**accumulated dose equivalent** /əkyōō′myəlā′tid/, an estimate of an individual's absorbed dose of radiation over a lifetime, expressed in rem. Occupationally exposed persons are allowed no more than 5 rem per year, or 1 rem times age at any time during the person's lifetime. See also **rem.**

**accuracy** /ak′yərəsē′/, the extent to which a measurement is close to the true value.

**accurate empathy** /ak′yərit/, a communication technique used by a nurse to convey an understanding of the patient's feelings and experiences.

**Accurbron,** a trademark for a bronchodilator (theophylline).

**Accutane,** a trademark for an antiacne agent (isotretinoin).

**AC/DC,** slang term for a person who is both heterosexual and homosexual. See also **bisexual.**

**ACE,** abbreviation for **angiotensin-converting enzyme.**

**Ace bandage,** a trademark for a woven elastic bandage.

**acebutolol** /as′əbōō′təlol/, a beta-adrenergic blocking agent.

■ INDICATIONS: It is prescribed in the treatment of hypertension, angina pectoris, ventricular arrhythmias, and other cardiovascular disorders.

■ CONTRAINDICATIONS: The drug should not be given to patients with asthma, heart failure, persistent severe bradycardia, second- and third-degree heart block, overt cardiac failure, cardiogenic shock, or peripheral vascular disease.

■ ADVERSE EFFECTS: The most common side effects include bradycardia, bronchospasm, flatulence, hypotension, leg pains, nausea, headache, skin rashes, dizziness, and drowsiness.

**acedia** /əsē′dē·ə/ [Gk, *akedia,* apathy], a condition of listlessness and a form of melancholy, marked by indifference and sluggish mental processes.

**ACE inhibitor.** See **angiotensin-converting enzyme (ACE) inhibitor.**

**acellular** /āsel′yə lər/, without cells.

**acentric** /āsen′trik/ [Gk, *a, kentron,* not center], **1.** having no center. **2.** (in genetics) describing a chromosome fragment that has no centromere.

**acentric occlusion.** See **eccentric occlusion.**

**-aceous** /-ā′shəs/, a suffix meaning 'having the appearance of' or 'like' something specified: *foliaceous, testaceous.*

**ACEP,** abbreviation for **American College of Emergency Physicians.**

**acephal-, acephalo-,** a combining form meaning 'having no head': *acephalobrachia, acephaly.*

**acephalia,** congenital absence of the head.

**acephalism.** See **acephalia.**

**acephalobrachia** /asef′əlōbrā′kē·ə/ [Gk, *a + kephale,* without head, *brachion,* arm], a congenital anomaly in which a fetus lacks both arms and a head. Also called **abrachiocephalia.**

**acephalocardia** /-kär′dē·ə/ [Gk, *a,* not, *kephale,* head, *cardia,* heart], congenital absence of both head and heart.

**acephalus** /əsef′ələs/ [Gk, *a,* not, *kephale,* head], a headless fetus.

**acephaly** /əsef′əlē/ [Gk, *a, kephale,* without head], a congenital defect in which the head is absent or not properly developed. Also called **acephalia** /as′əfā′lē·ə/, **acephalism** /əsef′əliz′əm/. —**acephalic,** *adj.*

**acerola** /as′ərō′lə/, a small, cherrylike fruit of the genus *Malpighia* that grows in tropical climates. It is a richer source of vitamin C than any other known fruit. Also called **Barbados cherry.**

**acesulfame-K** /as′əsul′fām/, a synthetic noncaloric sweetener marketed under the trademark Sunnette. It is approximately 200 times sweeter than sucrose. Heat does not affect its sweetening ability, an advantage over aspartame. Also called **acesulfame potassium.**

**acet,** abbreviation for an acetate carboxylate anion.

**acet-,** a combining form meaning 'vinegar': *acetoin, acetyl.*

**acetabula.** See **acetabulum.**

**acetabular** /as′ətab′yələr/ [L, *acetabulum,* little saucer], pertaining to the acetabulum, the cup-shaped hip socket into which the head of the femur is set.

**acetabular notch,** an indentation in the margin of the acetabulum, the cup-shaped socket of the hip bone.

**acetabuloplasty** /as′ətab′yəlōplas′tē/, plastic surgery performed on the acetabulum.

**acetabulum** /as′ətab′yələm/, *pl.* **acetabula** [L, vinegar cup], the large, cup-shaped cavity at the juncture and lateral surface of the ilium, the ischium, and the pubis, in which the ball-shaped head of the femur articulates.

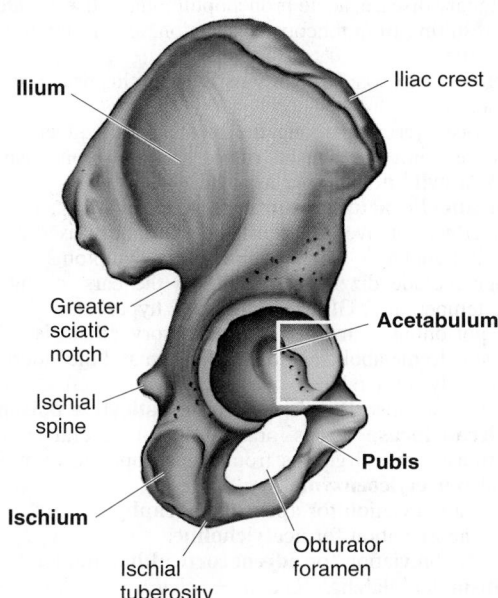

Ilium

Iliac crest

Greater
sciatic
notch

**Acetabulum**

Ischial
spine

**Pubis**

**Ischium**

Obturator
foramen

Ischial
tuberosity

**Acetabulum at the junction of the ilium,
ischium, and pubis**
*(Herlihy and Maebius, 2000)*

**acetal,** **1.** a colorless liquid, $C_2H_4$ $(OC_2H_5)_2$, sometimes used as a hypnotic. Also called **diethyl acetal. 2.** any compound with the general formula $R_2C(OR)_2$ or $RCH(OR)_2$, in which R indicates an alkyl or aryl group.

**acetaldehyde ($CH_3CHO$)** /as′ətəldē′hīd/, a colorless, volatile liquid aldehyde with a pungent odor produced by the oxidation of ethyl alcohol. Its systematic (IUPAC) name is ethanol. In the human body, acetaldehyde is produced in the liver by the action of alcohol dehydrogenase and other enzymes. It is used commercially in the manufacture of acetic acid and various aromas and flavors. Exposure to high levels of acetaldehyde can result in headache, corneal injury, rhinitis, and respiratory disorders.

**acetaminophen** /əset′əmin′əfin/, an analgesic and antipyretic drug used in many nonprescription pain relievers. It has no antiinflammatory properties. It may be used in combination with other products.

■ INDICATIONS: It is often recommended for treatment of mild to moderate pain and fever.

■ CONTRAINDICATION: Known hypersensitivity to acetaminophen prohibits its use. It should not be used in the presence of liver disease.

■ ADVERSE EFFECTS: Among the most serious adverse reactions are anaphylaxis, hepatotoxicity, and hemolytic anemia. Overdosage can result in fatal cyanosis and hepatic necrosis.

**acetaminophen poisoning,** a toxic reaction to the ingestion of excessive doses of acetaminophen. Dosages exceeding 140 mg/kg can produce liver failure, and larger doses can be fatal. Large amounts of acetaminophen metabolites can overwhelm the glutathione-detoxifying mechanism of the liver, resulting in progressive necrosis of the liver within 5 days. The onset of symptoms may be marked by nausea and vomiting, profuse sweating, pallor, and oliguria. The nausea and vomiting increase, accompanied by jaundice and pain in the upper abdomen, hypoglycemia, encephalopathy, and kidney failure. Treatment requires emesis or gastric lavage, depending on the length of time since the ingestion. Acetylcysteine may prevent extensive liver damage if given soon after ingestion (via nasogastric tube).

**acetate** /as′itāt/, an anion of formula $C_2H_3O_2$, conjugate base of acetic acid.

**acetate kinase,** an enzyme that catalyzes the transfer of a phosphate group from adenosine triphosphate to acetate. Also called **acetokinase.** /as′ətōkī′nās, əsē′tō-/.

**acetazolamide** /as′ətəzō′ləmīd/, a carbonic anhydrase inhibitor diuretic agent.

■ INDICATIONS: It is prescribed for adjunctive treatment for edema, glaucoma, epilepsy (primarily petit mal), and prevention of symptoms associated with acute mountain sickness.

■ CONTRAINDICATIONS: Hyponatremia, hypocalcemia, severe liver or kidney disease or dysfunction, Addison's disease, or known hypersensitivity to this drug prohibits its use.

■ ADVERSE EFFECTS: Among the most serious adverse reactions are anorexia and depression, particularly in the elderly; acidosis; hyperuricemia; and crystalluria. Paresthesias, GI disturbances, and lethargy are common.

**Acetest,** a trademark for a product used to test for the presence of abnormal quantities of acetone in the urine of patients with diabetes mellitus or other metabolic disorders. A large quantity of acetone causes a rapid change in the color of the Acetest tablet. See also **acidosis, ketone bodies.**

**acetic** /əsē′tik, əset′ik/ [L, *acetum,* vinegar], pertaining to substances having the sour properties of vinegar or acetic acid; also, to chemical compounds possessing the radical, $CH_3CO$—.

**acetic acid ($HC_2H_3O_2$),** a clear, colorless, pungent liquid that is miscible with water, alcohol, glycerin, and ether and that constitutes 3% to 5% of vinegar. Acetic acid is produced commercially by the reaction of methyl alcohol with carbon monoxide in the presence of a catalyst, or it may be converted from ethyl alcohol by the action of many aerobic bacteria. Various concentrations are used in the manufacture of plastics, dyes, insecticides, cellulose acetate, photographic chemicals, and pharmaceutic preparations, including vaginal jellies and antimicrobial solutions for the treatment of superficial infections of the external auditory canal. Also called **ethanoic acid.**

**acetic fermentation,** the production of acetic acid or vinegar from a weak alcoholic solution.

**acetoacetic acid** /as′ətō·əsē′tik, əsē′tō-/, a colorless, oily keto acid produced by the metabolism of lipids and pyruvates. It is excreted in trace amounts in normal urine and in elevated levels in diabetes mellitus, especially in ketoacidosis. Acetoacetic acid is also increased during starvation as a result of incomplete oxidation of fatty acids. Soluble in water, alcohol, and ether, acetoacetic acid decomposes at temperatures below 100° C to acetone and carbon dioxide. Also called **acetone carboxylic acid** /kär'boksil'ik/, **acetylacetic acid** /əsē'tiləsē'tik, as'ətil-/, **beta-ketobutyric acid** /bet'əkē'tōbyōōtir'ik/, **diacetic acid** /dī·əsē'tik/.

**acetohexamide** /-hek'səmīd/, a sulfonylurea oral antidiabetic.

■ INDICATION: It may be prescribed in the treatment of type 2 diabetes mellitus.

■ CONTRAINDICATIONS: Its use is prohibited as sole therapy in type 1 diabetes, diabetic ketoacidosis, severe liver or kidney dysfunction, or known hypersensitivity to this drug or to other sulfonylureas.

■ ADVERSE EFFECTS: Among the most serious adverse reactions are blood dyscrasias, hypoglycemia, and allergic reactions. GI disturbances are common.

**acetokinase.** See **acetate kinase.**

**acetol kinase,** an enzyme that catalyzes the transfer of a phosphate group from adenosine triphosphate to hydroxyacetone.

**acetonaemia.** See **ketonemia.**

**acetone** /as'ətōn/, a colorless, aromatic, volatile liquid ketone body found in small amounts in normal urine and in larger quantities in the urine of diabetics experiencing ketoacidosis or starvation's also called 2-propanone. It is one of the group of compounds called ketones. Commercially prepared acetone is used to clean the skin before injections, but prolonged exposure to the compound can be irritating. It also has many varied industrial uses.

**acetone bodies.** See **ketone bodies.**

**acetone carboxylic acid.** See **acetoacetic acid.**

**acetone in urine test,** a test for the presence of dimethylketone in the urine of patients, used as a laboratory indication of ketosis and the severity of diabetes mellitus. Chemically treated test paper strips or sticks are exposed to urine. If acetone is present in the urine as the result of incomplete breakdown of fatty and amino acids in the body, the test strips change color. A similar test uses a compound added directly to a urine sample.

**acetonide grouping,** an acetone-based ketal, or ketone-alcohol derivative, present in some corticosteroid drugs, such as fluocinolone acetonide.

**acetonuria** /as'ətōnŏŏr'ē·ə/, the presence of acetone and diacetic bodies in the urine. See also **ketoaciduria.**

**acetophenetidin.** See **phenacetin.**

**acetpyrogall** /as'ətpī'rəgal/, a topical irritant used as a caustic and keratolytic agent. Also called **pyrogallol triacetate.**

**acetyl (CH₃CO),** a monovalent radical associated with derivatives of acetic acid, sometimes indicated by the symbol Ac.

**acetylacetic acid.** See **acetoacetic acid.**

**acetylcholine (ACh)** /as'ətilkō'lēn, əsē'til-/, a direct-acting cholinergic neurotransmitter agent widely distributed in body tissues, with a primary function of mediating synaptic activity of the nervous system and skeletal muscles. Its half-life and duration of activity are short because it is rapidly destroyed by acetylcholinesterase. Its activity also can be blocked by atropine at junctions of nerve fibers with glands and smooth muscle tissue. It is a stimulant of the vagus and parasympathetic nervous system and functions as a vasodilator and cardiac depressant. Acetylcholine is used therapeutically as an adjunct to eye surgery and has limited benefits in certain circulatory disorders because of its short half-life.

**acetylcholinesterase (AChE)** /-kō'lines'tərās/, an enzyme present at endings of voluntary nerves and parasympathetic involuntary nerves. It inactivates and prevents accumulation of the neurotransmitter acetylcholine released during nerve impulse transmission by hydrolyzing the substance to choline and acetate. The action reduces or prevents excessive firing of neurons at neuromuscular junctions.

**acetylcoenzyme A** /əsē'til·kō·en'zīm, as'ətil-/, a biomolecule that carries an activated form of the 2-carbon acetyl unit that is found in the course of several important metabolic processes. The formation of acetylcoenzyme A is the critical intermediate step between anaerobic glycolysis and the citric acid cycle. Also called **acetyl-CoA.** See also **citric acid cycle, tricarboxylic acid cycle.**

**acetylcysteine** /-sis'tēn/, a mucolytic and acetaminophen antidote.

■ INDICATIONS: It is prescribed in the treatment of chronic pulmonary disease, acute bronchopulmonary disease, atelectasis resulting from mucous obstruction, and acetaminophen poisoning.

■ CONTRAINDICATION: Known sensitivity to this drug prohibits its use.

■ ADVERSE EFFECTS: Among the most serious adverse reactions are stomatitis, nausea, rhinorrhea, and bronchospasm.

**acetylsalicylic acid.** See **aspirin.**

**acetylsalicylic acid poisoning** /əsē'təlsal'isil'ik, as'itəl-/, toxic effects of overdosage of the commonly used antipyretic and analgesic drug, aspirin. Early symptoms of overdosage include dizziness, ringing in the ears, changes in body temperature, GI discomfort, and hyperventilation. Severe poisoning is marked by respiratory alkalosis, which may lead to metabolic acidosis. Children and the elderly are particularly vulnerable to the potential toxic effects of salicylates. See also **Reye's syndrome, salicylate poisoning.**

**acetyltransferase** /-trans'fərās/, any of several enzymes that transfer acetyl groups from one compound to another. See also **acetylcoenzyme A.**

**ACG,** abbreviation for **apexcardiography.**

**ACh,** abbreviation for **acetylcholine.**

**ACH,** abbreviation for **adrenocortical hormone.**

**achalasia** /ak'əlā'zhə/ [Gk, *a* + *chalasis*, without relaxation], an abnormal condition characterized by inability of a muscle to relax (cardiospasm), particularly the lower esophageal sphincter. Compare **corkscrew esophagus.** See also **dysphagia.**

**Achard-Thiers syndrome** /äsh'ärtērz'/ [Emile C. Achard, French physician, 1860–1941; Joseph Thiers, French physician, b. 1885], a hormonal disorder seen in postmenopausal women with diabetes, characterized by growth of body hair in a masculine distribution. Treatment includes mechanical removal or bleaching of excess hair and hormonal therapy to correct endocrine imbalances related to systemic disease. See also **hirsutism.**

**ache** /āk/ [OE, *acan*, to hurt], **1.** a pain characterized by persistence, dullness, and, usually, moderate intensity. An ache may be localized, as a stomach ache, headache, bone ache; or a general ache, as in the myalgia that accompanies a viral infection or a persistent fever. **2.** to suffer from a dull, persistent pain of moderate intensity.

**AChE,** abbreviation for **acetylcholinesterase.**

**acheiria** /əkī'rē·ə/ [Gk, *a*, not, *cheir*, hand], congenital absence of one or both hands.

**acheiropody** /ak'īrop'ədē/ [Gk, *a*, not, *cheir*, hand, *pous*, foot], absence of hands and feet.

**achievement age** /əchēv'mənt/, the level of a person's educational development as measured by an achievement

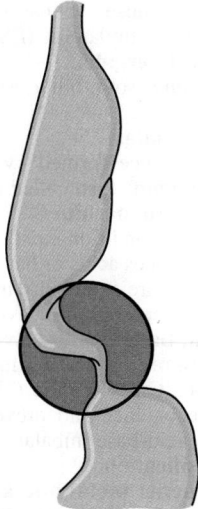

**Esophageal achalasia: advanced stage**
*(Phipps, Sands, and Marek, 1999)*

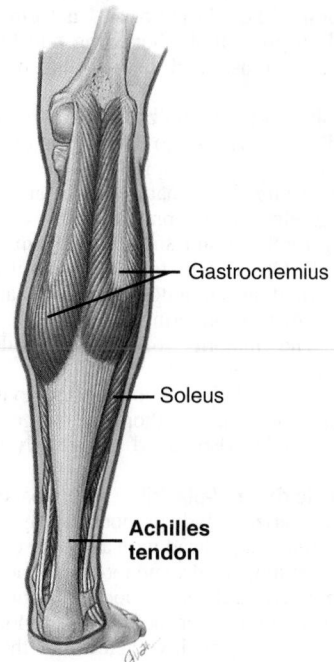

test and compared with the normal score for chronologic age. Compare **mental age.** See also **developmental age.**

**achievement quotient (AQ),** a numeric expression of a person's achievement age, determined by various achievement tests, divided by the chronologic age and expressed as a multiple of 100. Compare **intelligence quotient.** See also **accomplishment quotient.**

**achievement test,** a standardized test for the measurement and comparison of knowledge or proficiency in various fields of vocational or academic study. Compare **aptitude test, intelligence test, personality test, psychologic test.**

**Achilles jerk.** See **Achilles tendon reflex.**

**Achilles tendon** /əkil′ēz/ [*Achilles,* Greek mythologic hero], the common distal tendon of the soleus and gastrocnemius muscles of the leg. It is the thickest and strongest tendon in the body and connects triceps surae muscle to the heel bone. In an adult it is about 15 cm long. The tendon becomes contracted about 4 cm above the heel and flares out again to insert into the calcaneus. Also called **tendo calcaneus.**

**Achilles tendon reflex,** a deep tendon reflex consisting of plantar flexion of the foot when a sharp tap is given directly to the tendon of the gastrocnemius muscle at the back of the ankle. This reflex is often absent in people with peripheral neuropathies or diabetes. A sluggish return of the flexed foot may occur in patients with hypothyroidism. A hyperactive reflex may be caused by hyperthyroidism or by pyramidal tract disease. Also called **Achilles jerk, ankle reflex.** See also **deep tendon reflex.**

**achiral,** pertaining to the absence of chirality in a compound, as in stereochemical isomers.

**achlorhydria** /ā′klôrhī′drē·ə/ [Gk, *a + chloros,* not green, *hydor,* water], an abnormal condition characterized by the absence of hydrochloric acid in gastric secretions. Achlorhydria occurs most commonly in atrophy of the gastric mucosa, gastric carcinoma, and pernicious anemia. It is also found in severe iron deficiency anemia. Malignancy is expected when achlorhydria is seen in combination with gastric ulceration. Protein digestion is severely impaired in patients with achlorhydria, but overall digestion in the alimentary tract is relatively normal, because trypsin and

**Achilles tendon** *(Thibodeau and Patton, 1999/John V. Hagen)*

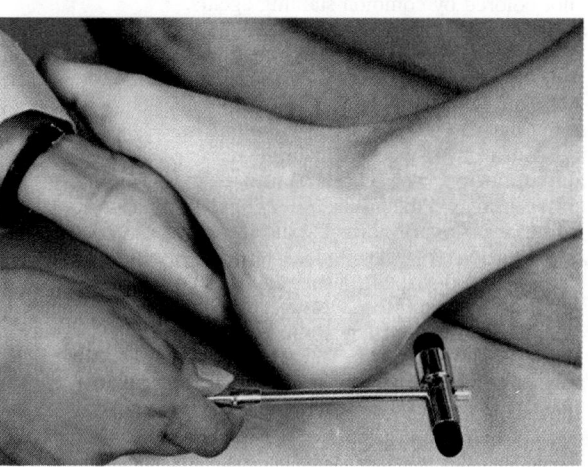

**Elicitation of the Achilles tendon reflex**
*(Barkauskas et al, 1998)*

other enzymes of the pancreas and small intestine are not affected. See also **achylia, pernicious anemia. —achlorhydric,** *adj.*

**achloropsia** /ā′klôrop′sē·ə/ [Gk, *a,* not, *chloros,* green, *opsis,* vision], an inability to see green; green blindness.

**acholia** /akō′lē·ə/ [Gk, *a + chole,* without bile], **1.** the absence or decrease of bile secretion. **2.** any condition that suppresses the flow of bile into the small intestine. **—acholic,** *adj.*

**acholuria** /ak′əlŏŏr′ē·ə/ [Gk, *a + chole,* without bile, *ouron,* urine], the absence or lack of bile pigments in the urine.

**achondrogenesis** /ākon'drōjen'əsis/, a form of dwarfism characterized by gross limb shortening and hydropic head and trunk. It is transmitted by an autosomal recessive gene.

**achondroplasia** /ākon'drōplā'zhə/ [Gk, *a* + *chondros,* without cartilage, *plassein,* to form], a disorder of the growth of cartilage in the epiphyses of the long bones and skull. It results in premature ossification, permanent limitation of skeletal development, and dwarfism typified by protruding forehead and short, thick arms and legs on a normal trunk. Onset is in fetal life. Familial achondroplasia is inherited as an autosomal dominant gene; the chance is 50% that an offspring of an affected parent will be affected. The majority of affected individuals die during gestation or the first year of life. The minority that survive have relatively normal longevity. There is no treatment other than orthopedic surgery. Antenatal diagnosis is possible. Also called **chondrodystrophy, fetal rickets.**

**achondroplastic dwarf** /-plas'tik/, the most common type of dwarf, characterized by disproportionately short limbs, a normal-sized trunk, large head with a depressed nasal bridge and small face, stubby hands, and lordosis. The condition results from an inherited defect in bone-forming tissue and is often associated with other defects or abnormalities, although there is usually no involvement of the central nervous system and intelligence is normal. See also **achondroplasia.**

**achroma** akrō'mə/ [Gk, *a,* without, *chroma,* color], lack of color.

**achromatic,** **1.** free of color. **2.** color blind. **3.** a substance not colored by common staining agents.

**achromatic lens** /ak'rəmat'ik/, [Gk, *a,* without, *chroma,* color; L, *lens*], a lens in which the focal lengths for red and blue colors of the spectrum are the same, refracting light without decomposing it into its component colors.

**achromatic vision.** See **color blindness.**

**achromatocyte.** See **achromocyte.**

**achromatopsia.** See **color blindness.**

**achromia** /akrō'mēə/ [Gk, *a* + *chroma,* without color], the absence or loss of normal skin pigment.

*Achromobacter* /akrō'mōbak'tər/, a genus of gramnegative, rod-shaped, flagellated bacteria that do not form pigment on agar. Most species in the genus are saprophytic, nonpathogenic organisms found in water, soil, or the human digestive tract.

**achromocyte** /ākrō'məsīt/, a sickle-shaped, abnormally pale erythrocyte. Also called **achromatocyte.**

**Achromycin V,** a trademark for an antibiotic (tetracycline hydrochloride).

**achylia** /ākī'lē·ə/ [Gk, *a, chylos,* not juice], an absence or severe deficiency of hydrochloric acid and pepsinogen (pepsin) in the stomach. This condition may also occur in the pancreas when the exocrine portion of that gland fails to produce digestive enzymes. Also called **achylosis.** See also **achlorhydria.**

**achylous** /əkī'ləs/, **1.** pertaining to a lack of gastric juice or other digestive secretions. **2.** pertaining to a lack of chyle.

**acicular** /əsik'yələr/ [L, *aciculus,* little needle], needle-shaped, such as certain leaves and crystals.

**acid** /as'id/ [L *acidus* sour], **1.** a compound that yields hydrogen ions when dissociated in aqueous solution (Arrhenius definition) or acts as a hydrogen ion donor (Brönsted definition) or acts as an electron pair acceptor (Lewis definition). Acids turn blue litmus red, have a sour taste, and react with bases to form salts. Acids have chemical properties essentially opposite to those of bases. See also **alkali.** **2.** *slang.* lysergic acid diethylamide (LSD). **3.** sour or bitter to the taste. See also **lysergide.**

**acid-,** a prefix meaning 'sour, bitter, acid': *acidemia, acidophil.*

**acidaemia.** See **acidemia.**

**acidalbumin,** a substance formed by the action of mild acid solutions on albumin. Also called **metaprotein.**

**acidaminuria.** See **aminoaciduria.**

**acid-base balance,** a condition existing when the net rate at which the body produces acids or bases equals the net rate at which acids or bases are excreted. The result of acid-base balance is a stable concentration of hydrogen ions in body fluids. See also **acid, base.**

**acid-base management,** a nursing intervention from the Nursing Interventions Classification (NIC) defined as promotion of acid-base balance and prevention of complications resulting from acid-base imbalance. See also **Nursing Interventions Classification.**

**acid-base management: metabolic acidosis,** a nursing intervention from the Nursing Interventions Classification (NIC) defined as promotion of acid-base balance and prevention of complications resulting from serum $HCO_3$ levels lower than desired. See also **Nursing Interventions Classification.**

**acid-base management: metabolic alkalosis,** a nursing intervention from the Nursing Interventions Classification (NIC) defined as promotion of acid-base balance and prevention of complications resulting from serum $HCO_3$ levels higher than desired. See also **Nursing Interventions Classification.**

**acid-base management: respiratory acidosis,** a nursing intervention from the Nursing Interventions Classification (NIC) defined as promotion of acid-base balance and prevention of complications resulting from serum $pCO_2$ levels higher than desired. See also **Nursing Interventions Classification.**

**acid-base management: respiratory alkalosis,** a nursing intervention from the Nursing Interventions Classification (NIC) defined as promotion of acid-base balance and prevention of complications resulting from serum $pCO_2$ levels lower than desired. See also **Nursing Interventions Classification.**

**acid-base metabolism,** the metabolic processes that maintain the balance of acids and bases essential in regulating the composition of body fluids. Acids release hydrogen ions, and bases accept them; the concentration of hydrogen ions present in a solution governs whether it is acid, alkali, or neutral. Hydrogen ions in water are measured on a pH scale of 0.0 to 14.0, with a reading of 7.0 indicating neutral at 25° C. Above 7.0, the solution is alkaline; below 7.0, it is acid. Blood is slightly alkaline, ranging from 7.35 to 7.45. Metabolic buffer systems within the body maintain this ratio, and, when the ratio is upset, either acidosis or alkalosis results. Acidosis may be caused by diarrhea, vomiting, uremia, diabetes mellitus, and the action of certain drugs. Alkalosis may be caused by overingestion of alkaline drugs, loss of chloride in gastric vomitus, and the action of certain diuretic drugs. See also **acid-base balance, acidosis, alkalosis, pH.**

**acid-base monitoring,** a nursing intervention from the Nursing Interventions Classification (NIC) defined as collection and analysis of patient data to regulate acid-base balance. See also **Nursing Interventions Classification.**

**acid bath,** a bath taken in water containing a mineral acid to help reduce excessive sweating.

**acid burn,** damage to tissue caused by exposure to an acid. The severity of the burn is determined by the strength of the acid and the duration and extent of exposure. Emergency treatment includes irrigating the affected area with large amounts of water. Compare **alkali burn.**

**acid dust,** an accumulation of highly acidic particles of dust. Such substances accumulate in the atmosphere and account for much of the smog hanging over large metropolitan areas. Many respiratory illnesses, such as lung cancer and asthma, may be aggravated or caused by such dust. See also **acid rain.**

**acid dyspepsia,** a digestive disorder associated with excessive stomach acidity. It occurs in peptic ulcer disease and gallbladder disease.

**acidemia** /as'idē'mē·ə/, decreased pH status of the blood or abnormal acidity in the blood. Specific types are denoted by prefixes: *lactacidemia, lipacidemia.* Also spelled **acidaemia.**

**acid etching,** cutting of the surface of dental enamel with an acid in order to roughen it, increase retention of resin sealant, and promote mechanical retention.

**acid-fast bacillus (AFB),** a type of bacillus that resists decolorizing by acid after accepting a stain. Examples include *Mycobacterium tuberculosis* and *M. leprae.*

**acid-fast stain,** a method of staining used in bacteriology in which a smear on a slide is treated with carbol-fuchsin stain, decolorized with acid alcohol, and counterstained with methylene blue to identify acid-fast bacteria. Acid-fast organisms resist decolorization and appear red or yellow against a dark background when viewed under a microscope. The stain may be performed on any clinical specimen but is most commonly used in examining sputum for *Mycobacterium tuberculosis,* an acid-fast bacillus. See also **Ziehl-Neelsen test.**

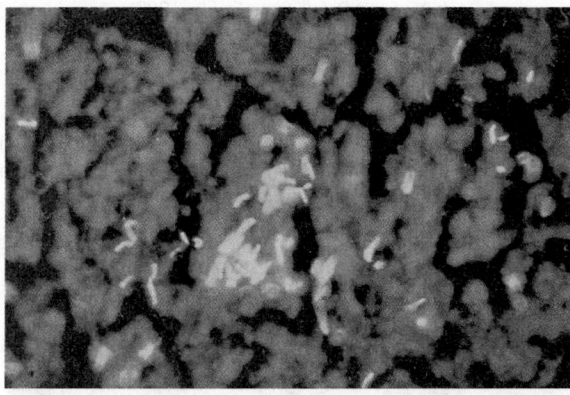

**Acid-fast stain of *Mycobacterium tuberculosis***
(Murray et al, 1998)

**acid flush,** a runoff of precipitation with a high acid content, as may occur during thaws in various parts of the world. Acid flushes may pollute rivers and reservoirs, killing fish and endangering the natural balance of the ecosystem. See also **acid rain.**

**acidify** /asid'əfī/, 1. to make a substance acidic, as through the addition of an acid. 2. to become acidic. Compare **alkalinize.**

**acidity** /asid'itē/ [L, *acidus,* sour], the degree of sourness, sharpness of taste, or ability of a chemical to yield hydrogen ions in an aqueous solution.

**acidity of the stomach,** the degree of gastric acid in the stomach. The acidity varies during any 24-hour period but averages from of pH 0.9 to 1.5. The main source of stomach acidity is hydrochloric acid secreted by gastric glands of the stomach.

**acid mist,** mist containing a high concentration of acid or particles of any toxic chemical, such as carbon tetrachloride or silicon tetrachloride. Such chemicals are often used by industry and stored in tanks that may leak their contents into residential areas, becoming especially dangerous if the toxic substance mixes with fog. Inhalation of acid mists may irritate the mucous membranes, the eyes, and the respiratory tract and seriously upset the chemical balances of the body. See also **acid rain.**

**acid mucopolysaccharide,** a major chemical constituent of ground substance in the dermis.

**acidophil** /as'idōfil, əsid'əfil/ [L, *acidus* + Gk, *philein,* to love], 1. a cell or cell constituent with an affinity for acid dyes. 2. an organism that thrives in an acid medium. —**acidophilic,** *adj.*

**acidophilic adenoma,** a tumor of the pituitary gland characterized by cells that can be stained red with an acid dye. Gigantism and acromegaly can be caused by an acidophilic adenoma. Also called **eosinophilic adenoma.**

**acidophilus milk** /as'idof'ələs/, milk inoculated with cultures of *Lactobacillus acidophilus,* used in various enteric disorders to change the bacterial flora of the GI tract.

**acidosis** /as'idō'sis/ [L, *acidus* + Gk, *osis,* condition], an abnormal increase in hydrogen ion concentration in the body, resulting from an accumulation of an acid or the loss of a base. It is indicated by a blood pH below the normal range (7.35 to 7.45). The various forms of acidosis are named for their cause; for example, renal tubular acidosis results from failure of the kidney to secrete hydrogen ions or reabsorb bicarbonate ions, respiratory acidosis results from respiratory retention of $CO_2$, and diabetic acidosis results from an accumulation of ketones associated with lack of insulin. Treatment depends on diagnosis of the underlying abnormality and concurrent correction of the acid-base imbalance. Compare **alkalosis.** —**acidotic,** *adj.*

**acidosis dialysis,** a type of metabolic acidosis that may develop when contaminating bacteria alter the pH of the dialysis bath.

**acidotic,** pertaining to acidosis, either depletion of base or accumulation of acid.

**acid phosphatase,** an enzyme found in the kidneys, serum, semen, and prostate gland. It is elevated in serum in cancers of the prostate and in trauma. Normal concentrations in serum are 0 to 1.1 Bodansky U/ml. See also **alkaline phosphatase.**

**acid phosphatase test,** a blood test used primarily to diagnose end stage prostatic carcinoma and to monitor the efficacy of treatment.

**acid poisoning,** a toxic condition caused by the ingestion of a toxic acid agent such as hydrochloric, nitric, phosphoric, or sulfuric acid, some of which are ingredients in common household cleaning compounds. Compare **alkali poisoning.**

**acid rain,** the precipitation of moisture, as rain, with high acidity caused by release into the atmosphere of pollutants from industry, motor vehicle exhaust, and other sources. Acid precipitation with a pH of 5.6 or lower is blamed by various authorities for numerous human health problems, fish kills, and the destruction of timber. Also called **acid precipitation, acid snow.**

**acid rebound,** a condition of hypersecretion of gastric acid that may occur after the initial buffering effect of an antacid. It occurs most noticeably when antacids containing calcium carbonate are used.

**acid salt,** a salt that is formed from only partial replacement of hydrogen ions from the related acid, leaving some degree of acidity. An example is sodium bicarbonate, which is also identified as sodium acid carbonate or sodium hydrogen carbonate.

**acid snow.** See **acid rain.**

**acid therapy,** a method for removing warts that uses plaster patches impregnated with acid, such as 40% salicylic acid, or with acid drops, such as 5% to 16.7% salicylic and lactic acids in flexible collodion. The application is made every 12 to 24 hours for 2 to 4 weeks. Acid therapy is not usually recommended for body areas that perspire heavily or that are likely to become wet or for exposed body parts where the patches would detract from the patient's appearance.

**acidulous** /əsid′yələs/, slightly acidic or sour.

**aciduria** [L, *acidus* + Gk, *ouron*, urine], the presence of acid in the urine. The condition may be caused by a diet rich in meat proteins or certain fruits, a medication used to treat a urinary tract disorder, an inborn error of metabolism, or ketoacidosis.

**acinar adenocarcinoma.** See **acinic cell adenocarcinoma.**

**acinar cell** /as′inər/ [L, *acinus,* grape], a cell of the tiny lobules of a compound gland or similar saclike structure such as an alveolus.

*Acinetobacter* /as′inē′təbak′tər/, a genus of nonmotile, aerobic bacteria of the family Neisseriaceae that often occurs in clinical specimens. The *Acinetobacter* contains gram-negative or gram-variable cocci and does not produce spores. This bacterium grows on regular medium without serum and is oxidase negative and catalase positive.

**acini.** See **acinus.**

**acinic cell adenocarcinoma** /asin′ik/ [L, *acinus,* grape], an uncommon low-grade malignant neoplasm that develops in the secreting cells of racemose glands, especially the salivary glands. The tumor consists of cells with clear or slightly granular cytoplasm and small eccentric dark nuclei. Also called **acinar adenocarcinoma, acinous adenocarcinoma.**

**aciniform** /asin′ifôrm/ [L, *acinus,* grape; *forma,* shape], shaped like a cluster of grapes. The term refers particularly to glandular tissue.

**acinitis** /as′inī′tis/, any inflammation of the tiny, grape-shaped portions of certain glands.

**acinotubular gland** /as′inōt(y)o͞ob′yələr/ [grape-shaped], a gland in which the acini are tube-shaped.

**acinous adenocarcinoma.** See **acinic cell adenocarcinoma.**

**acinus** /as′inəs/, *pl.* **acini** [L, grape], **1.** any small saclike structure, particularly one found in a gland. **2.** a subdivision of the lung consisting of the tissue distal to a terminal bronchiole. Also called **alveolus.**

**A.C. joint,** abbreviation for *acromioclavicular joint.* See **acromioclavicular articulation.**

**Aclovate,** a trademark for a topical corticosteroid (alclometasone dipropionate).

**ACLS,** abbreviation for **advanced cardiac life support.**

**ACMC,** abbreviation for **Association of Canadian Medical Colleges.**

**acme** /ak′mē/ [Gk, *akme,* point], the peak or highest point, such as the peak of intensity of a uterine contraction during labor.

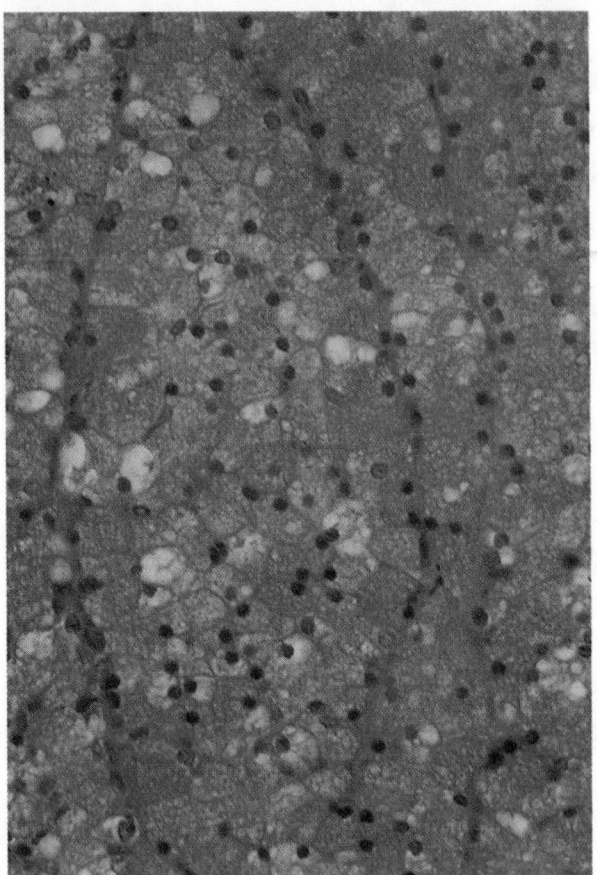

**Acinic cell adenocarcinoma**
*(Silverberg, DeLellis, and Frable, 1997)*

**acne** /ak′nē/ /ak′nē/, a disease of the skin common where sebaceous glands are numerous (face, upper back, and chest). Characteristic lesions include open (blackhead) and closed (whitehead) comedo, inflammatory papules, pustules, nodules and cysts. It seems to result from thickening of the follicular opening, increased sebum production, the presence of bacteria, and the host's inflammatory response.

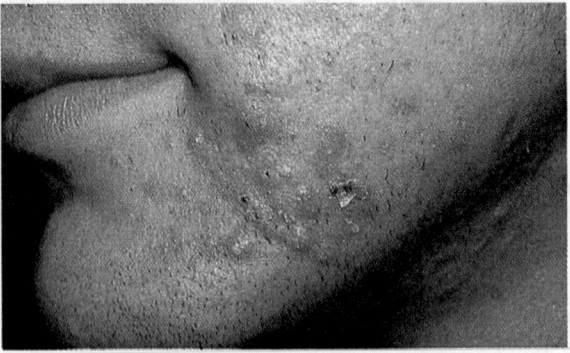

**Moderate acne** *(White, 1994)*

Treatment includes the use of topical and oral antibiotics, topical and oral retinoids, benzoyl peroxide, sala, and azelaic acid. Kinds of acne include **acne conglobata, chloracne,** and **acne fulminas.** Also called **acne vulgaris.** See also **comedo.**

**acne atrophica** /atrof′ikə/, a skin disorder characterized by small scars or pits left by an earlier occurrence of acne vulgaris.

**acne cachecticorum,** an eruption or irritation of the skin that may occur in patients who are very weak and debilitated. It is characterized by soft, mildly infiltrated pustular lesions.

**acne conglobata** /kong′glōbā′tə/, a severe form of acne with abscess, cyst, scar, and keloid formation. It may affect the lower back, buttocks, and thighs, as well as the face and chest. It affects more males than females. Also called **cystic acne.**

**acneform** /ak′nifôrm/, resembling acne. Also **acneiform** /aknē′əfôrm/.

**acneform drug eruption,** any of various skin reactions to a drug characterized by papules and pustules resembling acne.

**acne fulminans,** a form of severe nodular acne characterized by inflamed nodules and plaques that can result in skin ulcers and severe scarring. The condition mainly affects teenage boys and may be accompanied by fever, arthritis, and blood disorders.

**acnegenic** /ak′nijen′ik/ [Gk, *akme + genein,* to produce], causing or producing acne.

**acneiform.** See **acneform.**

**acne keloid** [Gk, *akme,* point, *kelis,* spot, *eidos,* form], excessive scar tissue that has developed at the site of an acne lesion.

**acne necrotica miliaris,** a rare, chronic type of pruritic, pustular folliculitis of the scalp, occurring mostly in adults and characterized by tiny pustules, probably a pyoderma or tuberculid. Also called **acne varioliformis.**

**acne neonatorum,** a skin condition of newborns caused by sebaceous gland hyperplasia and characterized by the localized formation of grouped comedones on the nose, cheeks, and forehead.

**acne papulosa,** a common skin condition in which comedones develop moderately inflamed papules. It is considered a papular form of acne vulgaris.

**acne pustulosa,** a form of acne in which the predominant lesions are pustular and may result in scarring.

**acne rosacea.** See **rosacea.**

**acne urticaria** /ur′tiker′ē·ə/, a form of acne marked by papules that are predominantly edematous and wheallike and that have been aggravated by scratching.

**acne varioliformis.** See **acne necrotica miliaris.**

**acne vulgaris.** See **acne.**

**ACNM,** abbreviation for *American College of Nurse-Midwives.*

**ACOG,** abbreviation for **American College of Obstetricians and Gynecologists.**

**acognosia** /ak′og·nō′zhə/, a knowledge of remedies.

**acorea** /ā′kôrē′ə/ [Gk, *a,* without, *kore,* pupil], an absence of the pupil of the eye.

**acoria** /akôr′ē·ə/ [Gk, *a,* without, *koros,* satiety], a condition characterized by constant hunger and eating, even when the appetite is small.

**acorn-tipped catheter,** a flexible catheter with an acorn-shaped tip used in various diagnostic procedures, especially in urology.

**acous-, acus-, acust-, acousto-,** combining form meaning 'hearing': *acoustic, acousma.*

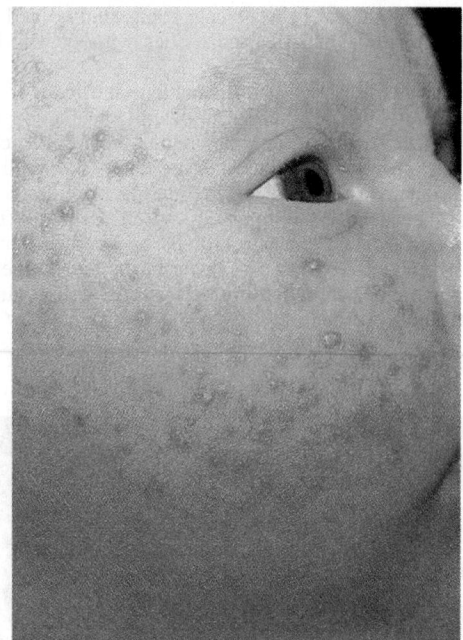

**Acne neonatorum** *(Zitelli and Davis, 1997)*

**-acousia, -acusia, -acusis, -akusis,** suffix meaning a '(specified) condition of the hearing.'

**acousma** /əkooz′mə/, *pl.* **acousmas, acousmata** [Gk, *akousma,* something heard], a hallucinatory impression of strange sounds.

**acoustic** /əkoos′tik/ [Gk, *akouein,* to hear], pertaining to sound or hearing. Also **acoustical.**

**-acoustic, -acoustical, 1.** a suffix meaning 'the hearing organs': *entacoustic, otacoustic.* **2.** a suffix meaning 'amplified sound waves': *microcoustic, stethacoustic.*

**acoustic apparatus,** the various components of the sense of hearing. See also **internal ear, cochlea, organ of Corti.**

**acoustic cavitation,** a potential biologic effect of ultrasonography, marked by large-amplitude oscillations of microscopic gas bubbles. As normally used, ultrasound pulses are too short to cause acoustic cavitation in human tissues.

**acoustic center,** the portion of the brain, in the temporal lobe of the cerebrum, in which the sense of hearing is located. Also called **auditory cortex.**

**acoustic hair cell.** See **auditory hair.**

**acoustic-immittance audiometry,** an audiologic testing used to evaluate the status of the outer and middle ears and of the acoustic reflex arc. It includes tympanometry, static-compliance testing, and acoustic reflex measures.

**acoustic impedance,** interference with the passage of sound waves by objects in the path of those waves. It equals the velocity of sound in a medium times the density of the medium. The acoustic impedance of bone may be nearly five times as great as that of blood. Testing of middle ear acoustic impedance is part of audiologic evaluation batteries used to detect middle ear problems.

**acoustic meatus** [Gk, *akoustikos,* hearing; L, *meatus,* a passage], the external or internal canal of the ear.

**acoustic microscope,** a microscope in which the object being viewed is scanned with sound waves and its image reconstructed with light waves. Acoustic microscopes produce excellent resolution of the objects being studied and allow close examination of cells and tissues without staining or damaging the specimen.

**acoustic nerve.** See **vestibulocochlear nerve.**

**acoustic neuroma,** a benign unilateral or bilateral tumor that develops from the eighth cranial (vestibulocochlear) nerve and grows within the auditory canal. Depending on the location and size of the lesion, tinnitus, progressive hearing loss, headache, facial numbness, papilledema, dizziness, and an unsteady gait may result. Paresis and difficulty in speaking and swallowing may occur in the later stage. Also called **acoustic neurilemmoma, acoustic neurinoma, acoustic neurofibroma.**

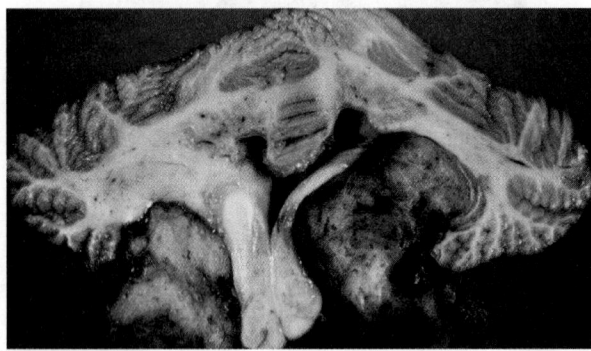

**Acoustic neuroma**
(Cotran, Kumar, and Collins, 1999/courtesy Dr. K.M. Earle)

**acoustic reflex,** contraction of the stapedius and tensor tympani muscles in the middle ear in response to a loud sound. The muscle contractions pull the stapes out of the oval window and thus protects the inner ear from damage caused by loud noise. The **acoustic reflex threshold** is the lowest level of sound that will elicit an acoustic reflex and is in the range of 85 to 90 dB hearing level in individuals with normal hearing. Acoustic reflexes are usually elevated or absent in cases of conductive or neural hearing loss and present at normal or lower levels in the case of cochlear (inner ear) hearing loss.

**acoustics** /əkōōs′tiks/ [Gk, akoustikos, hearing], the science of sound.

**acoustic shadow,** in an ultrasound image, the absence of echoes produced by the presence of dense material, such as calculi, which impede the transmission of sound waves. It is often used to detect gallstones.

**acoustic trauma,** a sudden loss of hearing, partial or complete, caused by an extremely loud noise, a severe blow to the head, or other trauma. The greatest loss of hearing occurs at 4000 Hz. It may be temporary or permanent. Compare **noise-induced hearing loss.**

**acoustooptics** /əkōōs′tō·op′tiks/, a field of physics that studies the generation of light waves by ultra-high-frequency sound waves. Knowledge gained by such study is applied chiefly in the transmission of information by acoustooptic devices.

**ACP, 1.** abbreviation for *American College of Pathologists.* **2.** abbreviation for **American College of Physicians. 3.** abbreviation for **American College of Prosthodontists.**

**acquired** /əkwī′ərd/ [L, acquirere, to obtain], pertaining to

a characteristic, condition, or disease originating after birth, not caused by hereditary or developmental factors but by a reaction to environmental influences outside of the organism. An example is acquired immunity. Compare **congenital, familial, hereditary.**

**acquired epileptic aphasia.** See **Landau-Kleffner syndrome.**

**acquired hypogammaglobulinemia** [L, *acquirere,* to obtain; Gk, *hypo,* a deficiency, *gamma,* third letter of Greek alphabet; L, *globulus,* small globe; Gk, *haima,* blood], an acquired deficiency of the gamma globulin blood fraction. See also **hypogammaglobulinemia.**

**acquired immunity,** any form of immunity that is not innate and is obtained during life. It may be naturally or artificially acquired and actively or passively induced. **Naturally acquired immunity** is obtained by the development of antibodies resulting from an attack of infectious disease or by the transmission of antibodies from the mother through the placenta to the fetus or to the infant through colostrum and breast milk. **Artificially acquired immunity** is obtained by vaccination or by the injection of immune globulin. Compare **natural immunity.** See also **active immunity, passive immunity.**

**acquired immunodeficiency syndrome (AIDS),** a syndrome involving a defect in cell-mediated immunity that has a long incubation period, follows a protracted and debilitating course, is manifested by various opportunistic infections, and without treatment has a poor prognosis. The disorder originally was found in homosexual men and IV drug users but now occurs increasingly among heterosexual men and women and children of those with the disease. More than 1 million cases of AIDS have appeared in the United States, where in the 1990s it was the leading cause of death among men between 25 and 44 years of age and the fourth leading cause of death among women of the same age group. A total of 36.1 million cases of AIDS, including 16.5 million women and 1.4 million children younger than 15 years of age, are estimated worldwide by 2001. An estimated 21.5 million had died from the epidemic by the end of 2000. The disease is particularly prevalent in sub-Saharan Africa, where the estimated number of cases in 2001 exceed 24 million, including 12.9 million women and 1 million children under 15 years of age.

■ OBSERVATIONS: AIDS is caused by either of two varieties of the human immunodeficiency virus, designated HIV-1 and HIV-2. HIV is a retrovirus that attracts and kills CD4+ lymphocytes (T helper cells), weakening the immune system's ability to prevent infection. The virus may also invade macrophages, in which it replicates freely, undetected by the immune system. HIV is not spread by casual contact but rather by sexual intercourse or exposure to contaminated blood, semen, breast milk, or other body fluids of infected persons. A patient may be diagnosed as having AIDS if he or she is infected with HIV, has a CD4+ count below 200 to 500/ml, and exhibits one or more of the following signs and symptoms: extreme fatigue, intermittent fever, night sweats, chills, lymphadenopathy, enlarged spleen, anorexia and consequent weight loss, severe diarrhea, apathy, and depression. As the disease progresses, characteristics are a general failure to thrive, anergy, and any of a variety of recurring infections, most commonly *Pneumocystis carinii* pneumonia, tuberculosis, meningitis, and encephalitis caused by aspergillosis, candidiasis, cryptococcosis, cytomegalovirus, toxoplasmosis, or herpes simplex. Some patients with AIDS are susceptible to malignant neoplasms, especially Kaposi's sarcoma, Burkitt's lymphoma, and non-Hodgkin's lymphoma, that both cause and result from immunodeficiency.

Psychological complications of AIDS may include chronic anxiety, depression, substance dependence, organic mental disorders, and suicidal ideation.

■ INTERVENTIONS: Treatment consists primarily of chronic symptom management and combined chemotherapy to counteract the opportunistic infections. There is no known cure for AIDS. Drugs used in the treatment of AIDS include reverse transcriptase inhibitors, such as zidovudine and didanosine, which interfere with the virus' ability to synthesize DNA within host cells, and protease inhibitors, such as ritonavir and indinavir, which cause the production of non-infectious HIV particles. These drugs are given in combinations (often called *cocktails*); one commonly used combination is made up of two reverse transcriptase inhibitors and a potent protease inhibitor. Vaccines routinely recommended for AIDS include those directed against pneumococcal influenza, hepatitis B, and general childhood infections, as well as infections that may be endemic in countries where the patient may travel, such as typhoid and yellow fever.

■ NURSING CONSIDERATIONS: Nursing care of the patient with AIDS varies with the patient's symptoms. These may include dyspnea, nutritional wasting, fatigue, pain and incontinence. Intervention is directed at providing education to prevent the spread of disease and infection, promoting self-care and optimal nutrition, and providing emotional support for patients and their families. Patients with tumors, hematologic abnormalities, and infections require routine treatment for those disorders concurrently with care for their HIV-related complaints. See also **AIDS-dementia complex, AIDS-wasting syndrome, CD4, CD8, gp160, human immunodeficiency virus, retrovirus.**

**acquired pellicle,** an acellular film composed of salivary glycoproteins that closely and firmly adheres to the oral cavity. It is distinct from plaque, which is cellular and loosely adhered to the teeth until calcified into calculus. Acquired pellicle that has become discolored as a result of poor oral hygiene is called brown pellicle. Compare **bacterial plaque.**

**acquired reflex.** See **conditioned reflex.**

**acquired sterility** [L, *acquirere,* to obtain, *sterilis,* barren], the failure to conceive after once bearing a child. Also called **one-child sterility, secondary infertility.**

**acquired trait** [L, *acquirere,* to obtain + *trahere,* to draw], a physical characteristic that is not inherited but may be an effect of the environment or of a somatic mutation.

**ACR,** abbreviation for **American College of Radiology.**

**acral** /ak′rəl/ [Gk, *akron,* extremity], pertaining to an extremity or apex.

**acrid** /ak′rid/ [L, *acris,* sharp], sharp or pungent, bitter and unpleasant to the smell or taste.

**acridine** /ak′ridēn/, a dibenzopyridine compound used in the synthesis of dyes and drugs. Its derivatives include fluorescent yellow dyes and the antiseptic agents acriflavine hydrochloride, acriflavine base, and proflavine.

**acrimony** /ak′rəmō′nē/ [L, *acrimonia,* pungency], a quality of bitterness, harshness, or sharpness.

**acrivistane,** an antihistamine and decongestant.

■ INDICATIONS: When combined with pseudoephedrine hydrochloride, it is prescribed in the treatment of allergic rhinitis.

■ CONTRAINDICATIONS: The drug should not be given to patients with known sensitivity to acrivistane or other alkylamine antihistamines or any components of the formulation. Its use is contraindicated in patients using monoamine oxidase inhibitors or in those with severe coronary artery disease or severe hypertension.

■ ADVERSE EFFECTS: The side effects most often reported include somnolence, headache, dizziness, nervousness, insomnia, dry mouth, and asthenia.

**acro-,** a prefix meaning 'extremities': *acrocentric, acrocyanosis.*

**acrocentric** /ak′rōsen′trik/ [Gk, *akron,* extremity, *kentron,* center], pertaining to a chromosome in which the centromere is located near one of the ends so that the arms of the chromosome are extremely uneven in length. Compare **metacentric, submetacentric, telocentric.**

**acrocephalopolysyndactyly** [*acrocephaly* + *polysyndactyly*], acrocephaly (see **oxycephaly**) and syndactyly with polydactyly as an additional feature. Four types are distinguished: *type I* is Noack's syndrome, *type II* is Carpenter's syndrome, *type III* is Sakati-Nyhan syndrome, and *type IV* is Goodman syndrome.

**acrocephalosyndactylism.** See **acrocephalosyndactyly.**

**acrocephalosyndactyly** /ak′rō·sef′ə·lō·sin·dak′ti·lē/ [*acrocephaly* + *syndactyly*], craniostenosis characterized by acrocephaly and syndactyly; the term is often used alone to denote **Apert's syndrome.** Sometimes, however, Apert's syndrome is designated *acrocephalosyndactyly, type I,* and acrocephalosyndactyly occurring with other anomalies is split into *acrocephalosyndactyly, type III* (**Saethre-Chotzen syndrome),** *acrocephalosyndactyly, type IV* (**Waardenburg's syndrome),** and *acrocephalosyndactyly, type V)* (**Pfeiffer type acrocephalosyndactyly,** which is the same as **Noack's syndrome).**

**acrocephaly.** See **oxycephaly.**

**acrochordon** /ak′rōkôr′don/, a benign, pedunculated growth commonly occurring on the eyelids, neck, axilla, or groin. Also called **skin tag.**

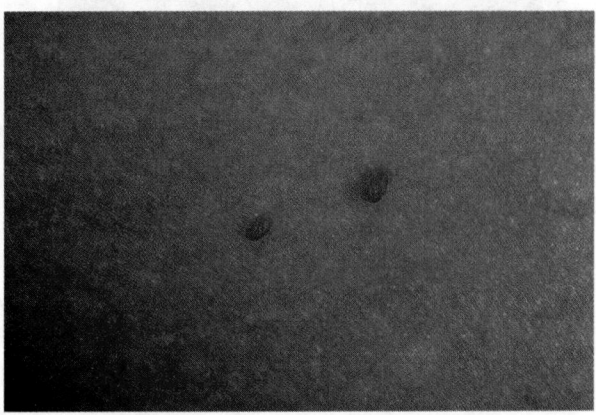

**Acrochordon** *(Lemmi and Lemmi, 2000)*

**acrocyanosis.** See **Raynaud's phenomenon.**

**acrodermatitis** /-dur′mətī′tis/ [Gk, *akron* + *derma,* skin, *itis,* inflammation], any eruption of the skin of the hands and feet caused by a parasitic mite belonging to the order Acarina.

**acrodermatitis enteropathica** /en′tərōpath′ikə/, a rare, chronic disease of infants characterized by vesicles and bullae of the skin and mucous membranes, alopecia, diarrhea, and failure to thrive. An autosomal recessive disorder of zinc malabsorption, the disease may be lethal if not treated. Zinc sulfate is usually prescribed.

**acrodermatitis papulosa infantum.** See **Gianotti-Crosti syndrome.**

**acrodynia** /ak'rō·din'ē·ə/ [Gk, *akron* + *odyne,* pain], a disease that occurs in infants and young children. Symptoms include edema, pruritus, generalized skin rash, pink coloration of the extremities and scarlet coloration of the cheeks and nose, swollen, painful extremities, cold and clammy skin, profuse sweating, digestive disturbances, photophobia, polyneuritis, extreme irritability alternating with periods of listlessness and apathy, and failure to thrive. Mercury poisoning is strongly implicated. Also called **erythredema polyneuropathy, Feer's disease, pink disease, Swift's disease.**

**acroesthesia** /ak'rō·esthē'zhə/ [Gk, *akron,* extremity, *aisthesis,* sensation], a condition of increased sensitivities or pain in the hands or feet.

**acrokeratosis verruciformis** /ak'rōker'ətō'sis/, a skin disorder characterized by the appearance of flat wartlike lesions on the dorsum of the hands and feet and occasionally on the wrists, forearms, and knees. It is an inherited disease, transmitted as a dominant trait.

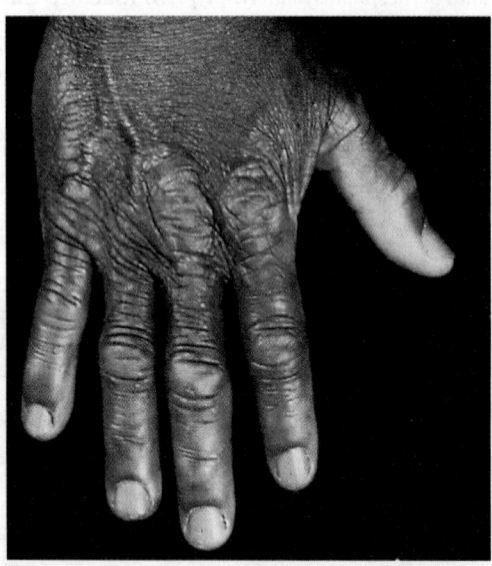

**Acrokeratosis verruciformis** (du Vivier, 1993)

**acrokinesis** /-kīnē'sis/ [Gk, *akron,* extremity, *kinesis,* motion], a state in which the limbs possess an abnormally wide range of motion.

**acromegalia.** See **acromegaly.**

**acromegalic eunuchoidism** /-məgal'ik/, a rare disorder characterized by genital atrophy and development of female secondary sex characteristics occurring in men with advanced acromegaly caused by a tumor in the anterior pituitary gland. Initially the gonadal function of the anterior lobe may be stimulated, but with the growth of the tumor the patient may become impotent; lose facial, axillary, and pubic hair; and acquire soft skin and a feminine distribution of fat. Also called **retrograde infantilism.**

**acromegaly** /ak'rəmeg'əlē/ [Gk, *akron* + *megas,* great], a chronic metabolic condition characterized by a gradual, marked enlargement and thickening of the bones of the face

and jaw. The condition, which afflicts middle-aged and older persons, is caused by the overproduction of growth hormone and is treated by radiation, pharmacologic agents, or surgery, often involving partial resection of the pituitary gland. Also called **acromegalia.** Compare **gigantism.** See also **adenohypophysis, growth hormone.** —**acromegalic,** *adj.*

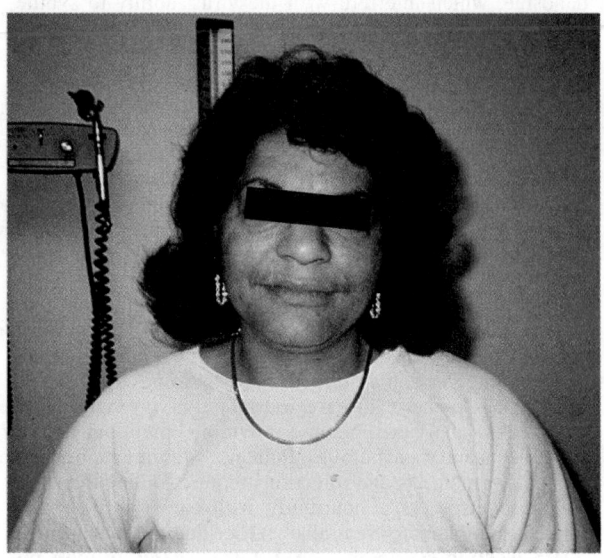

**Acromegaly**
(Seidel et al, 1999/courtesy Gary Wand, MD, The Johns Hopkins University and Hospital, Baltimore)

**acromial.** See **acromion.**

**acromial process** /əkrō'mē·əl/ [Gk, *akron,* extremity, *omos,* shoulder], a flat, triangular lateral extension of the scapula.

**acromicria** /ak'rəmik'rē·ə/, an anomaly characterized by abnormally small hands and feet. The person may also possess unusually small facial features, such as nose and ears.

**acromioclavicular articulation** /-mī'ōklavik'yələr/, the gliding joint between the acromial end of the clavicle and the medial margin of the acromion process of the scapula. It forms the highest part of the shoulder. The joint has six ligaments.

**acromiocoracoid** /-kôr'əkoid/, pertaining to the acromion and coracoid process.

**acromiohumeral** /-hyōō'mərəl/, pertaining to the acromion and the humerus.

**acromion** /əkrō'mē·ən/ [Gk, *akron* + *omos,* shoulder], the lateral extension of the spine of the scapula, forming the highest point of the shoulder and connecting with the clavicle at a small oval surface in the middle of the spine. It gives attachment to the deltoideus and trapezius muscles. Also called **acromion process.** Compare **coracoid process.** —**acromial,** *adj.*

**acromioscapular** /-skap'yələr/, pertaining to the acromion and the scapula.

**acroosteolysis** /ak'rō·os'tē·ol'isis/, an occupational disease that mainly affects people who work with polyvinylchloride (PVC) plastic materials. It is characterized by Raynaud's phenomenon, loss of bone tissue in the hands, and sensitivity to cold temperatures. A nonoccupational form of the disease is believed to be inherited.

**acroparesthesia** /ak′rōpar′isthē′zhə/ [Gk, *akron* + *para,* near, *aisthesis,* feeling], **1.** an extreme sensitivity at the tips of the extremities of the body, caused by nerve compression in the affected area or by polyneuritis. **2.** a disease characterized by tingling, numbness, and stiffness in the extremities, especially in the fingers, the hands, and the forearms. It sometimes produces pain, skin pallor, or mild cyanosis. The disease occurs in a simple form, which may produce acrocyanosis, and in an angiospastic form, which may produce gangrene.

**acrophobia** [Gk, *akron* + *phobos,* fear], a pathologic fear or dread of high places that results in extreme anxiety. Therapy attempts to overcome or eliminate the phobic response. See also **obsession, phobia.**

**acrosomal.** See **acrosome.**

**acrosomal cap, acrosomal head cap.** See **acrosome.**

**acrosomal reaction** /ak′rəsō′məl/, the pattern of various chemical changes that occur in the anterior of the head of the spermatozoon in response to contact with the ovum and that lead to the sperm's penetration and fertilization of the ovum.

**acrosome** /ak′rəsōm′/ [Gk, *akron* + *soma,* body], the cap-like structure surrounding the anterior end of the head of a spermatozoon. It is derived from the Golgi apparatus within the cytoplasm and contains degradative enzymes that function in the penetration of the ovum during fertilization. Also called **acrosomal cap, acrosomal head cap.** See also **acrosomal reaction.** —**acrosomal,** *adj.*

**acrotic** /əkrot′ik/ [Gk, *a* + *krotos,* not beating], **1.** pertaining to the surface of the body or to the skin glands. **2.** pertaining to an absent or weak pulse.

**acryl-, acrylo-,** a prefix for terms meaning 'acrylic compound.'

**acrylate,** an anion, salt, ester, or conjugate base of acrylic acid. Also called **2-propenoate.**

**acrylic acid (CH₂CHCOOH)** /əkril′ik/, a corrosive liquid used in the production of plastic materials used in medical and dental procedures. Also called **2-propenoic acid.**

**acrylic resin base,** a denture base made of acrylic resin.

**acrylic resin dental cement,** a cement for restoring or repairing damaged teeth. In powder form it contains polymethyl methacrylate, which acts as a filler, plasticizer, and polymerization initiator. In liquid form it contains methyl methacrylate with an inhibitor and an activator.

**ACS, 1.** abbreviation for *American Cancer Society.* **2.** abbreviation for *American Chemical Society.* **3.** abbreviation for **American College of Surgeons. 4.** abbreviation for *anodal closing sound.* **5.** abbreviation for **acute confusional state.**

**ACSM,** abbreviation for *American College of Sports Medicine.*

**act-,** prefix meaning 'to do, drive, act': *action, activate.*

**ACTH,** abbreviation for **adrenocorticotropic hormone.**

**Acthar,** a trademark for adrenocorticotropic hormone injection (corticotropin).

**-actide,** combining form designating a synthetic corticotropin.

**Actidil,** trademark for an antihistamine (triprolidine hydrochloride).

**Actifed,** trademark for a fixed-combination drug containing an adrenergic vasoconstrictor (pseudoephedrine hydrochloride) and an antihistamine (triprolidine hydrochloride).

**actigraph** /ak′tigraf′/, any instrument that records changes in the activity of a substance or an organism and produces a graphic record of the process, such as an electrocardiograph machine, which produces a record of electrical cardiac activity.

**actin,** a protein forming the thin filaments in muscle fibers that are pulled on by myosin cross-bridges to cause a muscle contraction. See also **myosin.**

**actin-.** See **actino-.**

**acting out,** the expression of intrapsychic conflict or painful emotion through overt behavior that is usually pathologic, defensive, and subconscious and that may be destructive or dangerous. In controlled situations such as psychodrama, Gestalt therapy, or play therapy, such behavior may be therapeutic in that it may serve to reveal to the patient the underlying conflict governing the behavior. See also **transference.**

**actinic** /aktin′ik/ [Gk, *aktis,* ray], pertaining to radiation, such as sunlight or x-rays.

**actinic burn,** a burn caused by exposure to sunlight or other source of ultraviolet radiation.

**actinic conjunctivitis** [Gk, *actis,* ray, + L, *conjunctivus,* connecting; Gk, *itis,* inflammation], an inflammation of the conjunctiva caused by exposure to the ultraviolet radiation (UV) of sunlight or other UV sources, such as acetylene torches, therapeutic lamps (sun lamps), and klieg lights. Also called **actinic ophthalmia.**

**actinic dermatitis,** a skin inflammation or rash resulting from exposure to sunlight, x-ray, or atomic particle radiation. Chronic or recurrent actinic dermatitis can predispose to skin cancer. See also **actinic keratosis.**

**actinic keratosis,** a slowly developing, localized thickening and scaling of the outer layers of the skin as a result of chronic, prolonged exposure to the sun. Treatment of this premalignant lesion includes surgical excision, cryotherapy, and topical chemotherapy. Also called **senile keratosis, senile wart, solar keratosis.**

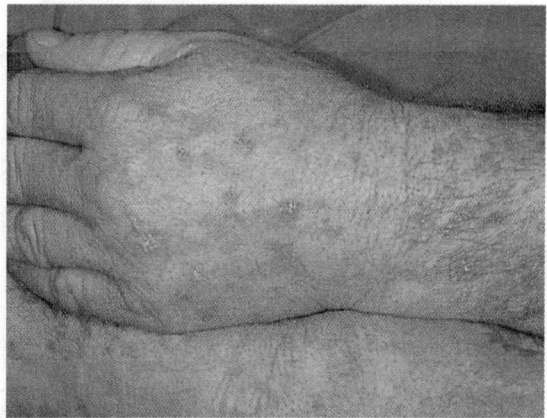

**Actinic keratosis**
*(Greenberger and Hinthorn, 1993/courtesy Dr. Loren H. Amundson, University of South Dakota, Sioux Falls)*

**actinic ophthalmia.** See **actinic conjunctivitis.**

**actinism,** the ability of sunlight or similar forms of radiation to produce chemical changes.

**actinium (Ac),** a rare, radioactive metallic element. Its atomic number is 89; its atomic mass is 227. It occurs in some ores of uranium.

**actino-, actin-,**   prefix meaning 'ray or radiation': *actino-cardiogram, actiniform.*

*Actinobacillus* /ak'tinōbasil'əs/,   a genus of small, gram-negative bacillus, with members that are pathogenic for humans and other animals. The species *Actinobacillus actinomycetemcomitans* is the cause of actinomycosis in humans.

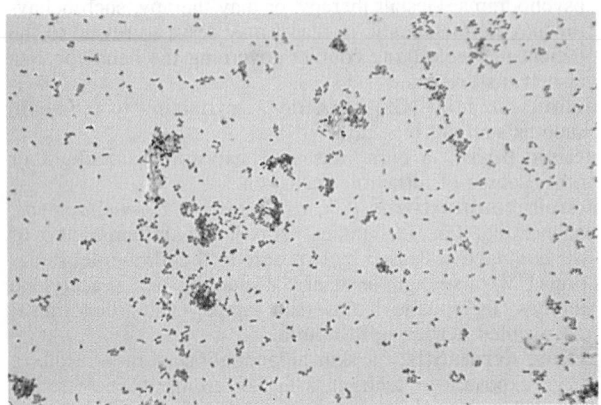

***Actinobacillus actinomycetemcomitans***
*(Mahon and Manuselis, 2000)*

*Actinomyces* /ak'tinōmī'sēz/ [Gk, *aktis,* ray, *mykes,* fungus], a genus of anaerobic or facultative anaerobic, gram-positive bacteria. Species that may cause disease in humans, such as *Actinomyces israelii,* are normally present in the mouth and throat. See also **actinomycosis.**

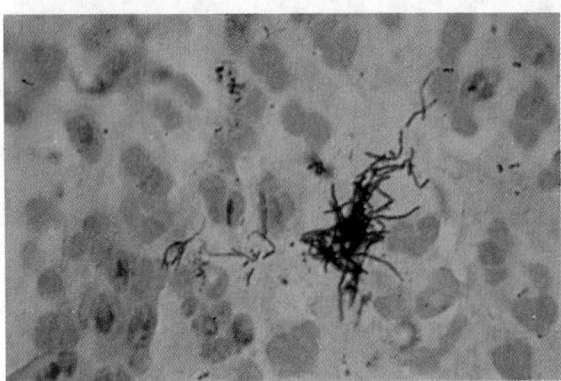

***Actinomyces israelii*** *(Baron, Peterson, and Finegold, 1994)*

**actinomycin A**   the first of a group of chromopeptide antibiotic agents derived from soil bacteria. Most are derivatives of phenoxazine and contain actinocin. They are generally active against gram-positive and gram-negative bacteria and some fungi. Because of their cytotoxic properties, they are effective for certain types of neoplasms. See **dactinomycin.**
**actinomycin B,**   an antibiotic antineoplastic agent derived from *Actinomyces antibioticus.*
**actinomycin D.**   See **dactinomycin.**

**actinomycosis** /ak'tinōmīkō'sis/,   a chronic, systemic disease characterized by deep, lumpy abscesses that extrude a thin, granular pus through multiple sinuses. The disease occurs worldwide but is seen most frequently in those who live in rural areas. It is not spread from person to person or from animals to humans. The most common causative organism in humans is *Actinomyces israelii,* a normal inhabitant of the bowel and mouth. Disease occurs after tissue damage, usually in the presence of another infectious organism. It can be diagnosed by microscopic identification of sulfur granules, pathognomonic of *Actinomyces,* in the exudate. There are several forms of actinomycosis. **Orocervicofacial actinomycosis** occurs with the spread of the bacterium into the subcutaneous tissues of the mouth, throat, and neck as a result of dental or tonsillar infection. **Thoracic actinomycosis** may represent proliferation of the organism from cervicofacial abscesses into the esophagus, or it may result from inhalation of the bacterium into the bronchi. **Abdominal actinomycosis** usually follows an acute inflammatory process in the stomach or intestines, such as appendicitis, diverticulum of the large bowel, or a perforation found in the groin or another area that drains exudate into the stomach. A large mass may be palpated, and sinus tracts from abscesses deep in the abdomen may form. **Pelvic actinomycosis** is most commonly associated with intrauterine devices. Central nervous system actinomycosis is a rare cause of brain abscess. **Musculoskeletal actinomycosis** involves subcutaneous tissue, muscle, and bone. **Disseminated actinomycosis** follows hematogenous spread of the infection and may involve the skin, brain, liver, and urogenital system. All forms of actinomycosis are treated with at least 6 weeks of daily injections of penicillin in large doses. Abdominal actinomycosis can be cured in 40% of cases, thoracic actinomycosis in 80%, and orocervicofacial actinomycosis in 90%.

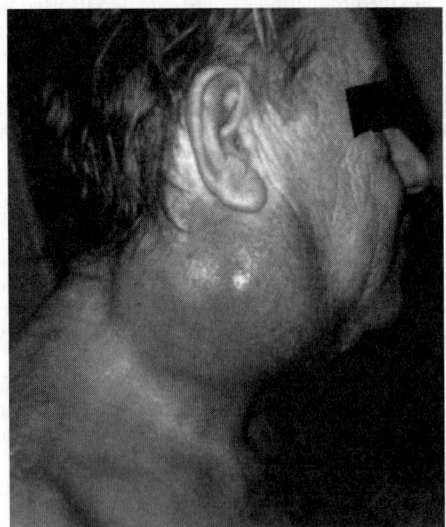

**Cervical actinomycosis** *(Stone and Gorbach, 2000)*

**actinotherapy,**   the use of ultraviolet, other parts of the spectrum of the sun's rays, or x-rays to treat various disorders, particularly skin diseases.
**action,**   activity used to carry out a function or produce an effect.

**action current.** See **action potential.**

**action level,** the level of concentration at which an undesirable or toxic component of a food is considered dangerous enough to public health to warrant government prohibition of the sale of that food. The U.S. Food and Drug Administration tests foods for action levels.

**action potential,** an electrical impulse consisting of a self-propagating series of polarizations and depolarizations, transmitted across the plasma membranes of a nerve fiber during the transmission of a nerve impulse and across the plasma membranes of a muscle cell during contraction or other activity. In the absence of an impulse, the inside is electrically negative and the outside is positive (the resting potential). During the passage of an impulse at any point on the nerve fiber, the inside becomes positive and the outside, negative. Also called **action current.**

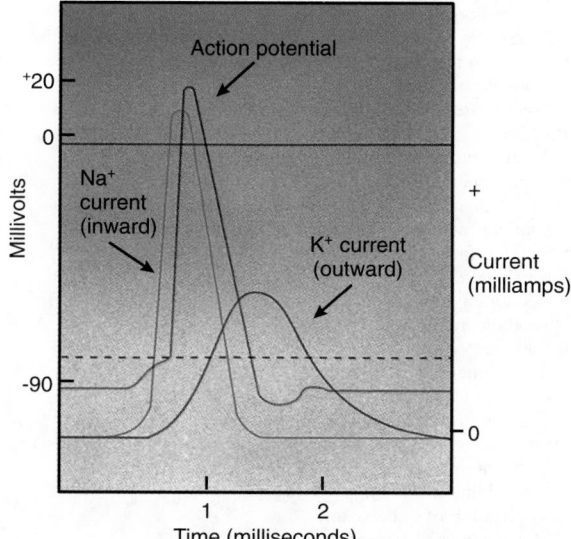

**Action potential** *(Potter and Perry, 1993)*

**action tremor** [L, *agere,* to do, *tremor,* shaking], a slight shaking that occurs or is evident during voluntary movements of the upper extremities. Also called **intention tremor.**

**Activase,** a trademark for a commercial form of tissue plasminogen activator (alteplase recombinant).

**activate** /ak'təvāt/ [L, *activus,* active], to induce or prolong an activity or render optimal action.

**activated charcoal,** a general-purpose emergency antidote and a powerful pharmaceutic adsorbent.

■ INDICATIONS: It is prescribed in the treatment of acute poisoning and the control of flatulence.

■ CONTRAINDICATIONS: There are no known contraindications, but activated charcoal is ineffective in poisoning caused by a strong acid or alkali or by cyanide. It should not be administered to unconscious persons.

■ ADVERSE EFFECTS: There are no known adverse effects.

**activated clotting time test (ACT),** a blood test primarily used to measure the effect of heparin as an anticoagulant during cardiac angioplasty, hemodialysis, and cardiopulmonary bypass surgery (CPB). It can also be used to monitor

the dose of protamine sulfate required to reverse the effect of heparin. The test measures the time required for whole blood to clot after the addition of particulate activators.

**activated 7-dehydrocholesterol.** See **vitamin D₃.**

**activated partial thromboplastin time (APTT),** See **partial thromboplastin time.**

**activated resin.** See **self-curing resin.**

**activating enzyme,** an enzyme that promotes or sustains an activity, such as catalyzing the combining of amino acids to form peptides or proteins.

**activation** /ak'tivā'shən/, the promotion or production of an activity, such as the generation of a catalyst, protein synthesis, or enzymatic function.

**activation energy** [L, *activus,* active], the energy required to convert reactants to transition-state species that will spontaneously proceed to products.

**activation factor.** See **factor XII.**

**activator** /ak'tivā'tər/, **1.** a substance, force, or device that stimulates activity in another substance or structure, especially a substance that activates an enzyme. **2.** a substance that stimulates the development of an anatomic structure in the embryo. **3.** an internal secretion of the pancreas. **4.** an apparatus for making substances radioactive, such as a cyclotron or neutron generator. **5.** (in dentistry) a removable orthodontic appliance that functions as a passive transmitter and stimulator of the perioral muscles.

**active algolagnia.** See **sadism.**

**active anaphylaxis** [Gk, *ana,* up, *phylaxis,* protection], a condition of hypersensitivity caused by the reaction of the immune system to the injection of a foreign protein. See also **anaphylaxis.**

**active assisted exercise** [L, *activus*], the movement of the body or any of its parts primarily through the individual's own efforts but accompanied by the aid of a member of the health care team or some device, such as an exercise machine. See also **exercise, passive exercise, range of motion.**

**active carrier** [OFr, *carier*], a person without signs or symptoms of an infectious disease who carries the causal microorganisms and can transmit the disease to others.

**active electrode** [Gk, *elektron,* amber, *hodos,* way], an electrode that is applied at a specific point to produce stimulation in a concentrated area in electrotherapy.

**active euthanasia.** See **euthanasia.**

**active exercise,** repetitive movement of a part of the body as a result of voluntary contraction and relaxation of the controlling muscles. Compare **passive exercise.** See also **aerobic exercise, anaerobic exercise.**

**active expiration** [L, *expirare,* to breathe out], forced exhalation, using the abdominal wall, internal intercostal muscles, and diaphragm.

**active hyperemia** [L, *activus* + Gk, *hyper,* excessive, *haima,* blood], the increased flow of blood into a particular body part.

**active immunity,** a form of long-term, acquired immunity; it protects the body against a new infection as the result of antibodies that develop naturally after an initial infection or artificially after a vaccination. Compare **passive immunity.** See also **immune response.**

**active labor** [L, *activus,* active, *labor,* work], the normal progress of the birth process, including uterine contractions, dilation of the cervix, and descent of the fetus into the birth canal.

**active listening**[1], the act of alert intentional hearing and demonstration of an interest in what a person has to say through verbal signal, nonverbal gestures, and body language.

**active listening**[2], a nursing intervention from the Nursing Interventions Classification (NIC) defined as attending closely to and attaching significance to a patient's verbal and nonverbal messages. See also **Nursing Interventions Classification.**

**active movement,** muscular action at a joint as a result of voluntary effort. Compare **passive movement.**

**active-passive,** (in psychiatry) a concept that characterizes persons as either actively involved in shaping events, such as being proactive, or passively reacting to them, such as being reactive.

**active play,** any activity from which one derives amusement, entertainment, enjoyment, or satisfaction by taking a participatory rather than a passive role. Children of all age groups engage in various forms of active play, from the exploration of objects and toys by the infant and toddler to the formal games, sports, and hobbies of the older child. Compare **passive play.**

**active range of motion (AROM),** the range of movement through which a patient can actively (without assistance) move a joint by the adjacent muscles.

**active resistance exercise,** the movement or exertion of the body or any of its parts performed totally through the individual's own efforts against a resisting force. See also **progressive resistance exercise.**

**active resistance training (ART),** a conditioning or rehabilitation program designed to enhance a patient's muscular strength, power, and endurance through progressive active resistance exercises and muscle overloading.

**active sensitization** [L, *agere,* to do, *sentire,* to feel], the condition that results when a specific antigen is injected into a person known to be susceptible. See also **sensitization.**

**active site,** the place on the surface of an enzyme where its catalytic action occurs.

**active specific immunotherapy,** a therapy in which a cancer patient is exposed to irradiated tumor cells. The injected cells stimulate the production of antibodies that destroy the tumor cells.

**active transport,** the movement of materials across the membranes and epithelial layers of a cell by means of chemical activity that allows the cell to admit otherwise impermeable molecules against a concentration gradient. Expediting active transport are carrier molecules within the cell that bind and enclose themselves to incoming molecules. Active transport is the means by which the cell absorbs glucose and other substances needed to sustain life and health. Certain enzymes play a role in active transport, providing a chemical "pump" that typically uses adenosine triphosphate to help move substances through the plasma membrane. Compare **osmosis, passive transport.**

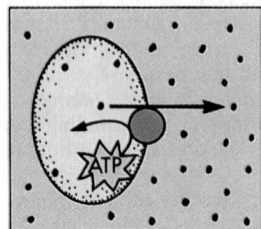

**Active transport** *(Potter and Perry, 1993)*

**activities of daily living (ADL)** /aktiv'itēz/, the activities usually performed in the course of a normal day in the person's life, such as eating, toileting, dressing, bathing, or brushing the teeth. The ability to perform ADL may be compromised by a variety of causes, including chronic illnesses and accidents. The limitation may be temporary or permanent; rehabilitation may involve relearning the skills or learning new ways to accomplish ADL. The goal of health care professionals is to promote the greatest degree of independence for the patient. An ADL checklist is often used before discharge from a hospital. If any activities cannot be ad-

### Specific elements to consider in activities of daily living training

**Feeding:**
- Utensil, cup, plate management, and napkin use.
- Tidiness/organization.
- Awareness of swallowing, chewing, or pocketing problems.
- Ability to handle different food consistencies (e.g., finger foods versus soups).
- Mouth care after eating.

**Bathing:**
- Assembling of items and appropriate equipment.
- Management of caps, lids, sprays, etc.
- Facial cleansers and cosmetic application.
- Shaving foam or soap application versus electric razor.
- Shaving face, underarms, and/or legs.
- Hair care.
- Deodorant application.
- Tooth/denture care.
- Nail care.
- Replacement of care items.
- Location of bath facilities in hospital and home.
- Transfer ability to bathtub or shower.

**Dressing:**
- Selection of clothing.
- Assembling of clothing.
- Application of underwear.
- Management of fasteners.
- Application of trousers/slacks, belt, or suspenders.
- Management of pullover tops.
- Application of shirt, jacket, dress (front opening), or tie.
- Management of buttons.
- Application of socks or stockings.
- Application of shoes and tying laces.
- Location of dressing activities: bed, sitting or standing.
- Ability to care for and apply glasses, contact lenses, or hearing aid.

**Toileting and elimination management:**
- Transfer ability.
- Clothing management.
- Cognitive function.
- Bowel and bladder control.
- External devices: assembly, application, removal, and care of equipment.
- Suppository insertion (include preparation of suppository and cleaning of insertion device if used).
- Post toileting hygiene.
- Timing of bowel program (morning or evening).
- Employment/school/home/environment considerations.
- Colostomy or ileal conduit care.
- Performance of bladder management programs.
- Accident management.

Adapted from Mumma CM, editor: *Rehabilitation nursing concepts and practice: a core curriculum,* ed 2, Skokie, Ill, 1987, Rehabilitation Nursing Foundation.

equately performed, arrangements are made with an outside agency, health care professionals, or family members to provide the necessary assistance. See also **Barthel Index.**

**activity,** the action of an enzyme on an amount of substrate that is converted to product per unit time under defined conditions.

**activity coefficient,** a proportionality constant, $\gamma$, relating activity, $\alpha$, to concentration, $c$, expressed in the equation, $\alpha = \gamma c$.

**activity intolerance,** a nursing diagnosis accepted by the Fifth National Conference on the Classification of Nursing Diagnoses. Activity intolerance is a state in which an individual has insufficient physiologic or psychologic energy to endure or complete required or desired daily activities. The cause of the condition may be generalized weakness, a sedentary life-style, imbalance between oxygen supply and demand, or bed rest or immobility.

■ DEFINING CHARACTERISTICS: The defining characteristics include verbal report of fatigue or weakness, abnormal heart rate or blood pressure response to activity, exertional discomfort or dyspnea, electrocardiographic changes reflecting arrhythmias or ischemia, and changes in skin color or moisture.

■ RELATED FACTORS: The related factors include generalized weakness, sedentary life-style, imbalance between oxygen supply and demand, bed rest or immobility. See also **nursing diagnosis.**

**activity intolerance, risk for,** a nursing diagnosis accepted by the Seventh National Conference on the Classification of Nursing Diagnoses. Risk for activity intolerance is a state in which an individual is at risk of experiencing insufficient physiologic or psychologic energy to endure or complete required or desired daily activities.

■ RISK FACTORS: Risk factors are a history of previous intolerance, deconditioned status, presence of circulatory or respiratory problems, and inexperience with activity. See also **nursing diagnosis.**

**activity theory,** a concept proposed by Robert J. Havighurst, an American educator and gerontologist, that continuing activities from middle age promotes well-being and satisfaction in aging. Thus older adults who are actively involved in a variety of situations and who establish new roles and relationships are more likely to age with a sense of satisfaction.

**activity therapy,** a nursing intervention from the Nursing Interventions Classification (NIC) defined as prescription of and assistance with specific physical, cognitive, social, and spiritual activities to increase the range, frequency, or duration of an individual's (or group's) activity. See also **Nursing Interventions Classification.**

**activity tolerance**[1], the type and amount of exercise a patient may be able to perform without undue exertion or possible injury.

**activity tolerance**[2], a nursing outcome from the Nursing Outcomes Classification (NOC) defined as responses to energy-consuming body movements involved in required or desired daily activities. See also **Nursing Outcomes Classification.**

**actomyosin** /ak'təmī'əsin/, the complex consisting of parallel threads of actin and myosin proteins that constitutes muscle fibers. It is responsible for contraction and relaxation of muscle. When a muscle fiber contracts, the two proteins slide past each other, shortening the fiber while increasing its apparent thickness. See also **sliding filaments.**

**actual cautery** /ak'chōō·əl/ [L, *actus,* act], the application of heat, rather than a chemical substance, in the destruction of tissue.

**actual charge,** the amount actually charged or billed by a practitioner for a service. The actual charge usually is not the same as that paid for the service by an insurance plan.

**actual damages.** See **damages.**

**actual focal spot.** See **focal spot.**

**actualize** /ak'chōō·əlīz'/, the act of fulfilling a potential, as by a person who may develop capabilities through experience and education.

**acu-,** combining form meaning 'sharp, clear, needle': *acuity, acupuncture.*

**acuity** /əkyōō'itē/ [L, *acuere,* to sharpen], the clearness or sharpness of perception, such as visual acuity.

**acuminate** /ə·kyōō'mi·nāt/ [L, *acuminatus*], sharp-pointed.

**acuminate wart.** See **genital wart.**

**acupressure**[1] /ak'yəpresh'ər/ [L, *acus,* needle, *pressura,* pressure], a therapeutic technique of applying digital pressure in a specified way on designated points on the body to relieve pain, produce anesthesia, or regulate a body function.

**acupressure**[2], a nursing intervention from the Nursing Interventions Classification (NIC) defined as the application of firm, sustained pressure to special points on the body to decrease pain, produce relaxation, and prevent or reduce nausea. See also **Nursing Interventions Classification.**

**acupressure needles,** needles inserted near a source of bleeding to help control blood loss. The needles exert pressure on tissues adjacent to the damaged vessel.

**acupuncture** /ak'yəpunk'chər/ [L, *acus* + *punctura,* puncture], a traditional Chinese method of producing analgesia or altering the function of a body system by inserting fine, wire-thin or hollow needles into the skin at specific sites on the body along a series of lines, or channels, called meridians. See also **moxibustion. —acupuncturist,** *n.*

**acupuncture point,** one of many discrete points on the skin along the several meridians, or chains of points of the body. Stimulation of any of the various points may induce an increase or decrease in function or sensation in an area or system of the body.

**acus** /ā'kəs/ [L], any needlelike structure.

**-acusis.** See **-acousia.**

**acute** /əkyōōt'/ [L, *acutus,* sharp], **1.** (of a disease or disease symptoms) beginning abruptly with marked intensity or sharpness, then subsiding after a relatively short period. **2.** sharp or severe. Compare **chronic.**

**acute abdomen,** an abnormal condition characterized by the acute onset of severe pain within the abdominal cavity. An acute abdomen requires immediate evaluation and diagnosis because it may indicate a condition that calls for surgical intervention. Information about the onset, duration, character, location, and symptoms associated with the pain is critical in making an accurate diagnosis. The patient is asked what decreases or increases the pain; constant, increasing pain is generally associated with appendicitis and diverticulitis, whereas intermittent pain is more likely indicative of a bowel obstruction, ureteral calculi, or gallstones. Appendicitis may often be differentiated from a perforated ulcer by the slower onset or development of pain. Although the patient's report of the location of the pain is sometimes misleading because of referral, radiation, or reflection of pain, it may serve to identify a specific organ or system. Factors in the patient's history that are useful in the diagnosis and management of an acute abdomen include changes in bowel habits, weight loss, bloody stool, diarrhea, menses, vomiting, clay-colored stool, and previous abdominal surgery. Also called **surgical abdomen.** See also **abdominal pain.**

**acute abscess** [L, *acutus,* sharp, *abscedere,* to go away], a collection of pus in a body cavity accompanied by localized inflammation, pain, pyrexia, and swelling.

**acute air trapping,** a condition of bronchiolar obstruction that results in early airway closure and trapping of air distal to the affected bronchiole. Air trapping can occur in persons with chronic obstructive pulmonary disease or asthma. Persons prone to episodes of acute air trapping learn to control exhalations through pursed-lip breathing.

**acute alcoholism,** drunkenness or intoxication resulting from excessive consumption of alcoholic beverages. The syndrome is temporary and is characterized by depression of the higher nerve centers, causing impaired motor control, stupor, lack of coordination, and often nausea, dehydration, headache, and other physical symptoms. Compare **chronic alcoholism.** See also **alcoholism.**

**acute angle** [L, *acutus* + *angulus*], any angle of less than 90 degrees.

**acute anicteric hepatitis** [Gk, *a,* without, *ikteros,* jaundice, *hēpar,* liver, *itis,* inflammation], an acute hepatitis that is not accompanied by jaundice.

**acute articular rheumatism** [L, *articulare,* to divide into joints; Gk, *rheumatismos,* that which flows], a common form of adult rheumatism, possibly associated with a pyogenic infection in the joints. Symptoms include fever and arthritis.

**acute ascending myelitis** [L, *ascendere,* to go up; Gk, *myelos,* marrow, *itis,* inflammation], a severe inflammation of the spinal cord that extends progressively upward with corresponding interference in nerve functions. See also **myelitis.**

**acute ascending spinal paralysis,** a severe progressive spinal paralysis that spreads upward toward the brain.

**acute atrophic paralysis** [Gk, *a, trophe,* without nourishment, *paralyein,* to be palsied], a severe poliomyelitis involving the anterior horns of the spinal cord. It results first in flaccid paralysis of involved muscle groups and later by atrophy of those muscles.

**acute bacterial arthritis.** See **septic arthritis.**

**acute bronchitis.** See **bronchitis.**

**acute care,** a pattern of health care in which a patient is treated for a brief but severe episode of illness, for the sequelae of an accident or other trauma, or during recovery from surgery. Acute care is usually given in a hospital by specialized personnel using complex and sophisticated technical equipment and materials, and it may involve intensive care or emergency care. This pattern of care is often necessary for only a short time, unlike chronic care.

**acute catarrhal sinusitis** [Gk, *kata* + *rhoia,* flow; L, *sinus,* hollow], an inflammation that involves the nose and sinuses.

**acute cervicitis.** See **cervicitis.**

**acute childhood leukemia,** a progressive, malignant disease of the blood-forming tissues. It is characterized by the uncontrolled proliferation of immature leukocytes and their precursors, particularly in the bone marrow, spleen, and lymph nodes. It is the most frequent cancer in children, with a peak onset occurring between 2 and 5 years of age.

■ OBSERVATIONS: Acute leukemia is classified according to cell type: **acute lymphoid leukemia (ALL)** includes lymphatic, lymphocytic, lymphoblastic, and lymphoblastoid types; **acute nonlymphoid leukemia (ANLL)** includes granulocytic, myelocytic, monocytic, myelogenous, monoblastic, and monomyeloblastic types (the myelocytic and monocytic series are abbreviated **AML**). ALL is predominantly a disease of childhood, whereas AML and ANLL occur in all age groups. The traditional classification of leuke-

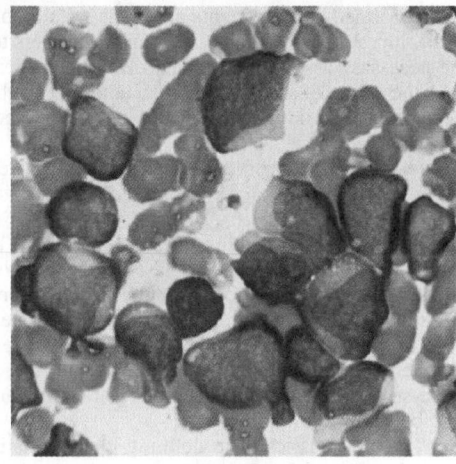

**Acute childhood leukemia** *(Carr and Rodak, 1999)*

mia into chronic and acute types is based on duration or expected course of the illness and the relative maturity of the leukemic cells. The exact cause of the disease is unknown, although various factors are implicated, including genetic defects, immune deficiency, viruses, and carcinogenic environmental factors, primarily ionizing radiation. In acute leukemia, large immature leukocytes accumulate rapidly and infiltrate other body tissues, especially the reticuloendothelial system, causing decreased production of erythrocytes and platelets. Neutropenia, anemia, increased susceptibility to infection and hemorrhage, and weakening of the bones with a tendency to fracture also occur. Initial symptoms of the disease include fever; pallor; fatigue; anorexia; secondary infections (usually of the mouth, throat, or lungs); bone, joint, and abdominal pain; subdermal or submucosal hemorrhage; and enlargement of the spleen, liver, and lymph nodes. Onset may be abrupt or may follow a gradual, progressive course. Involvement of the central nervous system may lead to leukemic meningitis. Characteristically, a peripheral blood smear reveals many immature leukocytes. The diagnosis is confirmed by bone marrow aspiration or biopsy and examination, which in ALL reveal a highly elevated number of lymphoblasts with almost complete absence of erythrocytes, granulocytes, and megakaryocytes. The prognosis is poor in untreated cases, and death occurs usually within 6 months after onset of symptoms. Survival rates have dramatically increased in recent years with the use of antileukemic agents in combination regimens. Remission of 5 years or longer occurs in 50% to 70% of children with ALL, with 20% to 30% achieving complete remission. Children with AML have a poorer prognosis, and the remission rate is far less than for ALL.

■ INTERVENTIONS: Treatment of acute leukemia consists of a three-stage process involving the use of chemotherapeutic agents and irradiation. In the first phase (remission induction), complete destruction of all leukemic cells is achieved within a 4- to 6-week period with the use of a combination drug-therapy regimen. The main drugs used in ALL are the corticosteroids, usually three daily oral doses of prednisone; vincristine, administered intravenously once a week; and L-asparaginase, given intramuscularly three times a week for a total of nine doses. Allopurinol, a xanthine-oxidase inhibitor, is usually administered to inhibit uric acid production. Other drugs used in various combination regimens in sequential cycles include methotrexate, 6-mercaptopurine, cyclophosphamide, cytosine arabinoside, hydroxyurea, daunorubicin, and doxorubicin. In children with AML the primary drugs for induction remission are 6-thioguanine, daunomycin, cytosine arabinoside, 5-azacytidine, vincristine, and prednisone. The child is usually hospitalized for part or all of the treatment because of the many side effects of the drugs and the high risk of complications, especially infection and hemorrhage. If severe hemorrhaging occurs and does not respond to local treatment, platelet transfusions may be necessary, and in cases of severe anemia, especially during induction therapy, whole blood or packed red cells may be needed to raise hemoglobin levels. The second stage of treatment involves prophylactic maintenance to prevent leukemic infiltration of the central nervous system. Because chemotherapy drugs do not cross the blood-brain barrier, therapy usually consists of daily high-dose cranial irradiation for about 2 weeks after induction remission and weekly or twice-weekly doses of intrathecal methotrexate, for a total of five or six injections; in some cases only the drug is given. In small children the irradiation is limited to the cranium to prevent retardation of linear growth, but older children may receive craniospinal radiation. Therapy to maintain remission usually begins after the child is discharged from the hospital and consists of various regimens of drugs in combination. A common schedule includes daily oral doses of 6-mercaptopurine and weekly doses of oral methotrexate, intermittent short-term therapy with prednisone and vincristine, and periodic doses of intrathecal methotrexate for prophylaxis against spread to the central nervous system. Complete blood counts are done weekly or monthly, and bone marrow examinations are performed every 3 to 4 months to detect myelosuppression and drug toxicity. Maintenance therapy is discontinued after a period of 2 to 3 years if initial remission is maintained. Continuous treatment beyond 3 years is not advised, as the adverse affects of the medications increase with prolonged use. Relapse occurs in as many as 20% of treated children. If relapse occurs, the child begins the treatment cycle again, usually with prednisone, vincristine, and a combination of other drugs not previously tried. With each relapse the prognosis becomes poorer. Other treatments for prolonging remission include immunotherapy using periodic inoculation with bacille Calmette-Guérin vaccine or bone marrow transplantation, which has been successful in inducing long-term remissions in about 10% to 20% of the cases, especially those with AML or severe, terminal ALL.

■ NURSING CONSIDERATIONS: Nursing care for the child with acute leukemia involves intensive physical and emotional support during all phases of the disease, its diagnosis, and treatment. Foremost is the preparation of the child and parents for the various diagnostic and therapeutic procedures, including venipuncture, bone-marrow aspiration or biopsy, lumbar puncture, and x-ray treatment. Specific medical and nursing management depends on the particular regimen of drug therapy, although most of the chemotherapeutic agents used in treatment cause myelosuppression that may lead to secondary complications of infection, hemorrhage, and anemia. Overwhelming infection is a major problem and one of the most frequent causes of death. Severe neutropenia indicates increased risk of infection. It may occur during immunosuppressive therapy or after prolonged antibiotic therapy. The most common infectious organisms are viruses, especially varicella, herpes zoster, herpes simplex, measles, mumps, rubella, and poliomyelitis; both gram-positive and gram-negative bacteria, including *Staphylococcus aureus, S. epidermidis,* group-A beta-hemolytic *Streptococcus,*

*Pseudomonas aeruginosa, Escherichia coli, Proteus,* and *Klebsiella;* and various parasites and fungi, especially *Pneumocystis carinii* and *Candida albicans.* To prevent infection, the nurse isolates the child as much as possible, screens visitors for active infection, institutes strict aseptic procedures, monitors temperature closely, evaluates possible infection sites (such as needle punctures), encourages adequate nutrition, helps the child to avoid exertion or fatigue, and, at discharge, teaches the child and parents the necessity for avoiding all known sources of infection, primarily the common childhood communicable diseases. Preventive measures to control infection also help decrease the tendency toward hemorrhage. Special attention is given to skin care, oral hygiene, cleanliness of the perineal area, and restriction of activities that could result in accidental injury. A major nursing consideration is the management of the many side effects resulting from drug toxicity and irradiation, including nausea and vomiting, anorexia, oral and rectal ulceration, alopecia, hemorrhagic cystitis, and peripheral neuropathy, including weakness and numbing of the extremities and severe jaw pain. Although corticosteroid treatment usually increases the appetite and produces a euphoric sense of well-being in the child, it also causes moon face, which is reversed with cessation of the steroid therapy. During maintenance therapy, the nurse continues to provide emotional support and guidance, specifically teaching parents which side effects are normal reactions to drugs and which indicate toxicity and require medical attention. In terminal stages of the disease, relief of discomfort and pain becomes the primary focus. Effective measures include careful physical handling of the child, frequent position changes, prevention of pressure on painful areas, and control of annoying environmental factors, such as excessive light and noise. Nonsalicylate analgesics are used as needed, depending on the severity of pain. See also **acute lymphocytic leukemia, acute myelocytic leukemia, leukemia.**

**acute cholecystitis.** See **cholecystitis.**

**acute circulatory failure** /sur′kyələtôr′ē/, a drop in cardiac output resulting from cardiac or noncardiac causes and leading to tissue hypoxia. Acute circulatory failure usually happens so rapidly that the body does not have time to adjust to the changes. If not controlled immediately, the condition usually progresses to shock.

**acute circumscribed edema** [L, *circum,* around, *scribere,* to draw; Gk, *oidema,* swelling], a localized edema, often associated with an inflammatory lesion or process.

**acute confusional state,** a form of delirium caused by interference with the metabolic or other biochemical processes essential for normal brain functioning. Symptoms may include disturbances in cognition, levels of awareness, short-term memory deficit, retrograde and enterograde amnesia, and orientation, accompanied by restlessness, apprehension, irritability, and apathy. The condition may be associated with an acute physiologic state, delirium, toxic psychosis, or acute brain syndrome. An acute stress reaction to new surroundings or new demands is common in adolescence; it generally subsides as person adjusts.

**acute delirium,** an episode of acute organic reaction that is sudden, severe, and transient. See also **delirium.**

**acute diarrhea** [Gk, *dia + rhein,* to flow], a sudden severe attack of diarrhea.

**acute diffuse peritonitis** [L, *diffundere,* to pour out; Gk, *peri,* near, *tenein,* to stretch, *itis,* inflammation], an acute widespread attack of peritonitis affecting most of the peritoneum and usually caused by a perforation of an abdominal organ (e.g., stomach or appendix). It is also a complication of peritoneal dialysis. Also called **generalized peritonitis.**

**acute disease,** a disease characterized by a relatively sudden onset of symptoms that are usually severe. An episode of acute disease results in recovery to a state comparable to the patient's condition of health and activity before the disease, in passage into a chronic phase, or in death. Examples are pneumonia and appendicitis. See also **chronic disease.**

**acute disseminated encephalitis.** See **acute disseminated encephalomyelitis.**

**acute disseminated encephalomyelitis,** a form of encephalitis that commonly develops after an acute viral infection, such as measles, apparently as an immune attack on the myelin tissue of the nervous system. Early symptoms may include fever, headache, vomiting, and drowsiness and progress to seizures, coma, and paralysis. Frequently patients who recover experience neurologic disorders. Also called **acute disseminated encephalitis.**

**acute diverticulitis,** a sudden severe, painful disorder of the intestinal tract, resulting from inflammation of one or more diverticula, or pouches, in the wall of the bowel. The condition is typically diagnosed through x-rays and treated surgically. If left untreated, the inflamed pouches may rupture, spilling fecal matter into the abdominal cavity and causing peritonitis.

**acute endarteritis** [Gk, *endon,* within, *arteria,* windpipe, *itis,* inflammation], inflammation of the cells lining an artery. It may be caused by an infection or the proliferation of fibrous tissue inside the arterial wall.

**acute epiglottitis,** a severe, rapidly progressing bacterial infection of the upper respiratory tract that occurs in young children, primarily between 2 and 7 years of age. It is characterized by sore throat, croupy stridor, and inflamed epiglottis, which may cause sudden respiratory obstruction and possibly death. The infection is generally caused by *Haemophilus influenzae,* type B, although streptococci may occasionally be the causative agent. Transmission occurs by infection with airborne particles or contact with infected secretions. The diagnosis is made by bacteriologic identification of *H. influenzae,* type B, in a specimen taken from the upper respiratory tract or in the blood. A lateral x-ray film of the neck shows an enlarged epiglottis and distension of the hypopharynx, which distinguishes the condition from croup. Direct visualization of the inflamed, cherry-red epiglottis by depression of the tongue or indirect laryngoscopy is also diagnostic but may produce total acute obstruction and should be attempted only by trained personnel with equipment to establish an airway or to provide respiratory resuscitation, if necessary. Compare **croup.**

■ OBSERVATIONS: The onset of the infection is abrupt, and it progresses rapidly. The first signs—sore throat, hoarseness, fever, and dysphagia—may be followed by an inability to swallow, drooling, varying degrees of dyspnea, inspiratory stridor, marked irritability and apprehension, and a tendency to sit upright and hyperextend the neck to breathe. Difficulty in breathing may progress to severe respiratory distress in minutes or hours. Suprasternal, supraclavicular, intercostal, and subcostal inspiratory retractions may be visible. The hypoxic child appears frightened and anxious; the skin color ranges from pallor to cyanosis.

■ INTERVENTIONS: Establishment of an airway is urgent, either by endotracheal intubation or by tracheostomy. Humidity and oxygen are provided, and airway secretions are drained or suctioned. IV fluids are usually required, and antibiotic therapy is initiated immediately, usually with ceftriaxone, cefuroxime, or ampicillin/sulbactam. Sedatives are contraindicated because of their depressant effect on the respiratory system, and antihistamines and adrenergic drugs are not usually of any therapeutic value. Steroids are useful.

■ NURSING CONSIDERATIONS: The nurse may assist with intubation or tracheostomy once the diagnosis is confirmed. Intensive nursing care is required for a child with acute epiglottitis. The most acute phase of the condition passes within 24 to 48 hours, and intubation is rarely needed beyond 3 to 4 days. As the child responds to therapy, breathing becomes easier; rapid recovery usually occurs so that bed rest and quiet activity to relieve boredom become primary nursing concerns. The infection may spread, causing such complications as otitis media, pneumonia, and bronchiolitis. Complications of the tracheostomy may also develop, including infection, atelectasis, cannula occlusion, tracheal bleeding, granulation, stenosis, and delayed healing of the stoma. Also called **acute epiglottiditis.**

**acute fatigue,** a sudden onset of physical and mental exhaustion or weariness, particularly after a period of mental or physical stress. Physical factors usually include an accumulation of waste products of muscle contractions. Boredom is a common mental factor. Recovery follows a period of rest and restoration of energy sources.

**acute febrile neutrophilic dermatosis.** See **Sweet's syndrome.**

**acute febrile polyneuritis.** See **Guillain-Barré syndrome.**

**acute fibrinous pericarditis** [L, *fibra,* fibrous; Gk, *peri,* near, *kardia,* heart, *itis,* inflammation], acute inflammation of the endothelial cells of the pericardium with fibers extending into the pericardial sac.

**acute gastritis.** See **gastritis.**

**acute glaucoma.** See **glaucoma.**

**acute glomerulonephritis.** See **postinfectious glomerulonephritis.**

**acute goiter** [L, *guttur,* throat], a condition of sudden enlargement of the thyroid gland. Clinical manifestations are those of hyperthyroidism.

**acute granulocytic leukemia (AGL).** See **acute myelocytic leukemia.**

**acute hallucinatory paranoia,** a form of psychosis in which hallucinations are combined with delusions of paranoia.

**acute hallucinosis.** See **alcoholic hallucinosis.**

**acute hemorrhagic conjunctivitis,** a highly contagious eye disease usually caused by enterovirus type 70 but also by coxsackie AZA. The disease is found primarily in densely populated humid areas, particularly the developing

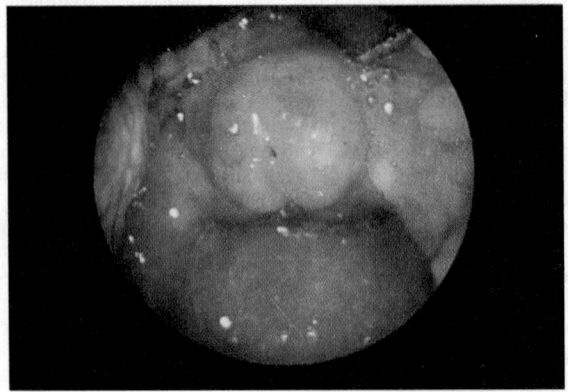

**Acute epiglottis: endoscopic view**
(Bingham, Hawke, and Kwok, 1992/courtesy Dr. Bruce Benjamin)

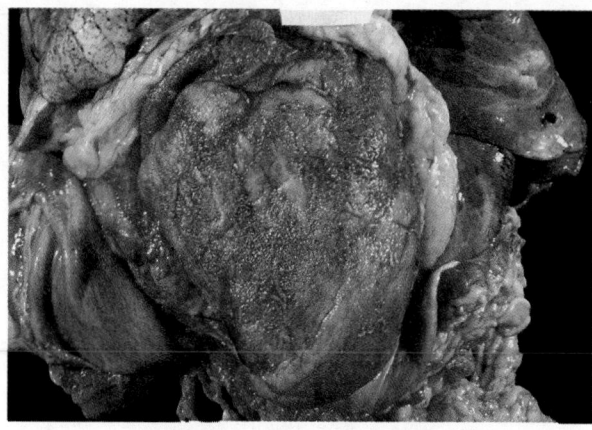

**Acute fibrinous pericarditis**
*(Kumar, Cotran, and Robbins, 1997)*

countries or places with a large immigrant population. Clinical features include sudden onset of severe ocular pain, blurred vision, photophobia, subconjunctival hemorrhage, chemosis, and profuse watery discharge from the eye. Spontaneous improvement occurs within 2 to 4 days and is complete by 7 to 10 days. Treatment consists of hygienic measures and ophthalmic preparations.

**acute hemorrhagic leukoencephalitis.** See **acute necrotizing hemorrhagic encephalopathy.**

**acute hemorrhagic pancreatitis** [Gk, *haima,* blood, *rhegnynei,* to gush, *pan,* all, *kreas,* flesh], a potentially fatal inflammation of the pancreas characterized by bleeding, tissue necrosis, and digestive tract paralysis.

**acute hypoxia,** a sudden or rapid depletion in available oxygen at the tissue level. The condition may result from asphyxia, airway obstruction, acute hemorrhage, blockage of the alveoli by edema or infectious exudate, or abrupt cardiorespiratory failure. Clinical signs may include hypoventilation or hyperventilation to the point of air hunger and neurologic deficits ranging from headache and confusion to loss of consciousness.

**acute idiopathic polyneuritis.** See **Guillain-Barré syndrome.**

**acute idiopathic thrombocytopenic purpura.** See **idiopathic thrombocytopenic purpura.**

**acute illness,** any illness characterized by signs and symptoms that are of rapid onset and short duration; it may be severe and impair normal functioning.

**acute immune disease.** See **autoimmunity.**

**acute infectious paralysis** [L, *inficere,* to stain; Gk, *paralyein,* to be palsied], **1.** an alternative term for acute anterior poliomyelitis. **2.** infectious polyneuritis.

**acute infective hepatitis.** See **hepatitis A.**

**acute intermittent porphyria (AIP),** an autosomal dominant, genetically transmitted metabolic hepatic disorder characterized by acute attacks of neurologic dysfunction that can be started by environmental or endogenous factors. Women are affected more frequently than men, and attacks often are precipitated by starvation or severe dieting, alcohol ingestion, bacterial or viral infections, and a wide range of pharmaceutic products. Any part of the nervous system can be affected, and an initial common effect is mild to severe abdominal pain. Other effects can include tachycardia, hypertension, hyponatremia, peripheral neuropathy, and organic brain dysfunction marked by seizures, coma, hallucinations, and respiratory paralysis. A frequent diagnostic factor is a high level of porphyrin precursors in the urine, which usually increases during periods of acute attacks. Treatment is generally symptomatic, with emphasis on respiratory support, beta blockers, pain control and education of the patient about environmental factors, particularly medications such as barbiturates, that are known to cause an onset of symptoms. A high-carbohydrate diet is reported to reduce the risk of acute attacks because glucose tends to block the induction of hepatic gamma-aminolevulinic acid (ALA) synthetase, an enzyme involved in the porphyrias. See also **porphyria.**

**acute interstitial nephritis.** See **interstitial nephritis.**

**acute laryngotracheobronchitis.** See **croup.**

**acute lichenoid pityriasis.** See **Mucha-Habermann disease.**

**acute lobar pneumonia,** a form of pneumonia characterized by lobar distribution of the consolidation of the serofibrous fluid exuded by the alveoli. The condition results from an infection by a virulent type of *Streptococcus pneumoniae.* Onset is sudden. Symptoms include a pleuritic chest pain, dry cough, and rust-colored sputum.

**acute lymphoblastic leukemia.** See **acute lymphocytic leukemia.**

**acute lymphocytic leukemia (ALL),** a hematologic, malignant disease characterized by large numbers of immature cells, lymphoblasts in the bone marrow, circulating blood, lymph nodes, spleen, liver, and other organs. The number of normal blood cells is usually reduced. More than three-fourths of the cases in the United States occur in children, with the greatest number diagnosed between 2 and 5 years of age. The risk of the disease is increased for people with Down syndrome and for siblings of leukemia patients. The disease has a sudden onset and rapid progression marked by fever, pallor, anorexia, fatigue, anemia, hemorrhage, bone pain, splenomegaly, and recurrent infection. Blood and bone marrow studies are used for diagnosis and for determination of the type of proliferating lymphocyte, which may be B cells, T cells (which usually respond poorly to therapy), or null cells that lack T- or B-cell characteristics. Treatment includes intensive combination chemotherapy, therapy for secondary infections and hyperuricemia, irradiation, and intrathecal methotrexate.

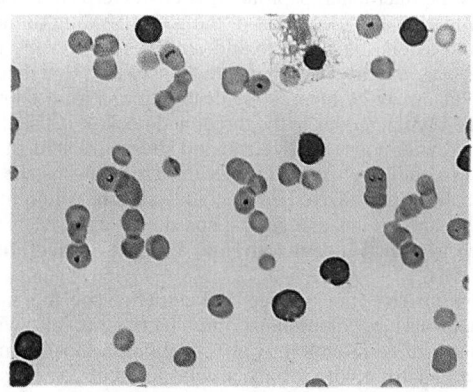

**Peripheral blood smear of acute lymphocytic leukemia**
*(Zitelli and Davis, 1997)*

**acute lymphoid leukemia (ALL).** See **acute childhood leukemia.**

**acute mastitis.** See **mastitis.**

**acute mountain sickness.** See **altitude sickness.**

**acute myelitis,** a sudden, severe inflammation of the spinal cord. See also **acute transverse myelitis, myelitis.**

**acute myelocytic leukemia (AML),** a malignant neoplasm of blood-forming tissues characterized by the uncontrolled proliferation of immature granular leukocytes that usually have azurophilic Auer rods in their cytoplasm. Typical symptoms are spongy bleeding gums, anemia, fatigue, fever, dyspnea, moderate splenomegaly, joint and bone pains, and repeated infections. AML occurs most frequently in adolescents and young adults. The risk of the disease is increased among people who have been exposed to massive doses of radiation and who have certain blood dyscrasias, such as polycythemia vera, primary thrombocytopenia, and refractory anemia. Variants of AML, in which only one cell line proliferates, are erythroid, eosinophilic, basophilic, monocytic, and megakaryocytic leukemias. The diagnosis is based on blood counts and bone marrow biopsies. Radiotherapy, chemotherapy, biotherapy, and bone marrow transplantation are used, but long remissions resulting from any form of treatment are rare. Also called **acute granulocytic leukemia (AGL), acute myelogenous leukemia, acute nonlymphocytic leukemia (ANLL), myeloid leukemia, splenomedullary leukemia, splenomyelogenous leukemia.** See also **acute childhood leukemia, chronic myelocytic leukemia.**

**acute myocardial infarction (AMI)** [L, *acutus,* + Gk, *mys,* muscle, *kardia,* heart; L, *infarcire,* to stuff], the early critical stage of necrosis of heart muscle tissue caused by blockage of a coronary artery. It is characterized by elevated S-T segments in the reflecting leads and elevated levels of cardiac enzymes. See also **myocardial infarction.**

**acute necrotizing hemorrhagic encephalopathy,** a degenerative brain disease, characterized by marked edema, numerous minute hemorrhages, necrosis of blood vessel walls, demyelination of nerve fibers, and infiltration of the meninges with neutrophils, lymphocytes, and histiocytes. Typical signs are severe headache, fever, and vomiting; convulsions may occur, and the patient may rapidly lose consciousness. Treatment consists of decompression by withdrawing cerebrospinal fluids. Also called **acute hemorrhagic leukoencephalitis.**

**acute necrotizing ulcerative gingivitis (ANUG),** a recurrent periodontal disease of sudden onset that primarily affects the interdental papillae. It is characterized by painful inflammation and ulceration of the gums, leading to the formation of craterlike defects and ulcers. The necrotic tissue appears as a gray membrane that is easily sloughed off. There also may be fever, bone destruction, a fetid odor, and enlarged lymph nodes in the throat and neck. It is usually associated with poor oral hygiene and stress and is most common in conditions in which there is crowding of the teeth and malnutrition. Treatment includes chlorhexidine mouthwashes, antibiotics, analgesics, and dental care. Also called **trench mouth, Vincent's angina, Vincent's infection.** See **gingivitis.**

**acute nephritis,** a sudden inflammation of the kidney, characterized by albuminuria and hematuria, but without edema or urine retention. It affects children most commonly and usually involves only a few glomeruli. See also **nephritis.**

**acute nicotine poisoning** [L, *Nicotiana, potio,* drink], a toxic effect produced by nicotine. Characteristics include burning sensation in the mouth, nausea and vomiting, diar-

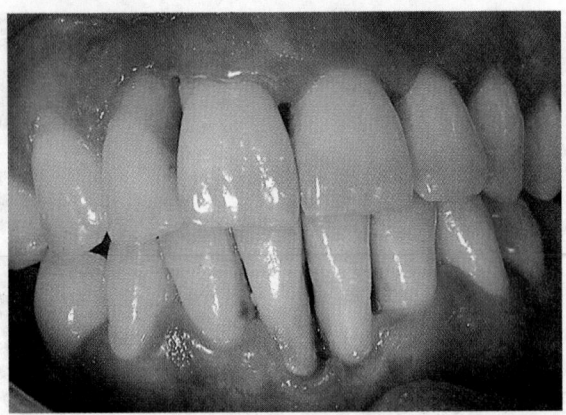

**Acute necrotizing ulcerative gingivitis** *(Murray et al, 1994)*

rhea, palpitations, salivation, agitation, respiratory, depression, and convulsions that may lead to death.

**acute nongonorrheal vulvitis** [L, *non,* not; Gk, *gone,* seed, *rhoia,* flow; L, *vulva,* wrapper; Gk, *itis,* inflammation], an inflammation of the vulva resulting from chafing, accumulation of sebaceous material, atopic reactions, local infections, or other causes that are nonvenereal.

**acute nonlymphocytic leukemia (ANLL).** See **acute myelocytic leukemia.**

**acute nonspecific pericarditis** [Gk, *peri,* around, *kardia,* heart, *itis,* inflammation], inflammation of the pericardium, with or without effusion. It often is associated with myocarditis but usually resolves without complications. See also **pericarditis.**

**acute pain,** severe pain, as may follow surgery or trauma or accompany myocardial infarction or other conditions and diseases. Acute pain occurring in the first 24 to 48 hours after surgery is often difficult to relieve, even with drugs. Some studies show that patients over 50 years of age need less analgesia to relieve acute pain than do younger patients. Another study indicates that 23% of surgical patients, except for orthopedic patients, do not require analgesia. Acute pain in individuals with orthopedic problems originates from the periosteum, the joint surfaces, and the arterial walls. Muscle pain associated with bone surgery results from muscle ischemia rather than muscle tension. Acute abdominal pain often causes the individual involved to lie on one side and draw up the legs in the fetal position. Compare **chronic pain.** See also **pain, pain intervention, pain pathway.**

**acute pancreatitis** [Gk, *pan,* all, *kreas,* flesh, *itis,* inflammation], a sudden inflammation of the pancreas caused by autodigestion and marked by symptoms of acute abdomen and escape of pancreatic enzymes into the pancreatic tissues. The condition is associated with biliary disease or alcoholism. The autodigestion is caused by premature activation of the digestive enzymes. The disorder can also be of unknown cause. See also **pancreatitis.**

**acute paranoid disorder,** a psychopathologic condition characterized by persecutory delusional thoughts of rapid onset, quick development, and short duration, usually lasting less than 6 months. The disorder, which rarely becomes chronic, is most commonly seen in persons who have experienced drastic changes in their environment, such as immigrants, refugees, prisoners, military inductees, and, in a less severe form, those leaving home for the first time.

**acute parapsoriasis.** See **Mucha-Habermann disease.**

**acute pharyngitis,** sudden, severe inflammation of the pharynx. See also **pharyngitis.**

**acute pleurisy,** inflammation of the pleura, often as a result of lung disease. It is characterized by irritation without recognizable effusion and is localized. See also **pleurisy.**

**acute primary myocarditis, 1.** inflammation of the heart muscle most commonly caused by a bacterial infection initiated locally or carried through the bloodstream. **2.** severe inflammation of the heart muscle associated with degeneration of the muscle fibers and release of leukocytes into the interstitial tissues. See also **myocarditis.**

**acute promyelocytic leukemia (AProL),** a malignancy of the blood-forming tissues, characterized by the proliferation of promyelocytes and blast cells with distinctive Auer rods. Symptoms include severe bleeding and bruises. The patient may also have low fibrinogen level and platelet count. Management of the disease typically requires replacement of coagulation factors and administration of cytotoxic drugs. See **leukemia.**

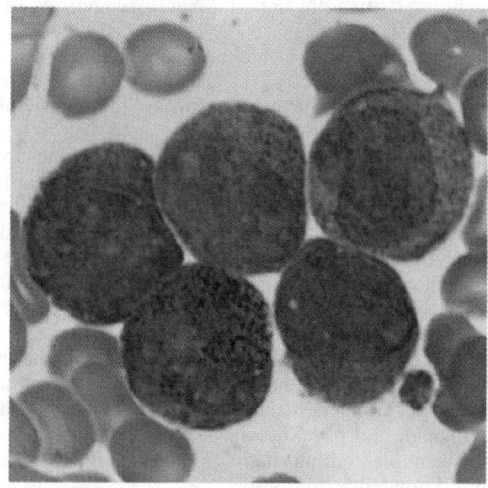

**Acute promyelocytic leukemia** *(Carr and Rodak, 1999)*

**acute prostatitis** [L, *acutus,* sharp; Gk, *prostates,* one standing before, *itis,* inflammation], a sudden, severe inflammation of the prostate. See also **prostate, prostatitis.**

**acute psychosis,** one of a group of disorders in which ego functioning is either impaired or inhibited. The ability to process reality-based information is diminished and disordered. The cause of the particular disorder may be a known physiologic abnormality. In situations where the physiologic abnormality is not recognized, the functional impairment is still clearly present.

**acute pyelonephritis.** See **pyelonephritis.**

**acute pyogenic arthritis,** an acute bacterial infection of one or more joints, caused by trauma or a penetrating wound and occurring most frequently in children. Typical signs are pain, redness, and swelling in the affected joint; muscular spasms in the area; chills; fever; sweating; and leukocytosis. Treatment consists of immobilization of the joint, analgesia, sedation, and IV administration of an antibiotic. If required, the joint may be irrigated with normal saline solution and an antibiotic. Hospitalization is usually required.

**acute radial nerve palsy.** See **radial nerve palsy.**

**acute radiation exposure.** See **radiation exposure.**

**acute rejection** [L, *rejicere,* to throw back], following organ transplantations, the rapid reaction against allograft or xenograph tissue that is incompatible. It often occurs after a week after treatment, during which the immune response increases in intensity.

**acute renal failure.** See **renal failure.**

**acute respiratory distress syndrome.** See **adult respiratory distress syndrome.**

**acute respiratory failure (ARF)** [L, *acutus + respirare,* respiratory, *fallere,* to deceive], a sudden inability of the lungs to maintain normal respiratory function. The condition may be caused by an obstruction in the airways or by failure of the lungs to exchange gases in the alveoli.

**acute rheumatic arthritis,** arthritis that occurs during the acute phase of rheumatic fever.

**acute rhinitis.** See **rhinitis.**

**acute schizophrenia,** a disorder consisting of various degrees of psychosis that is characterized by the sudden onset of personality disorganization. Symptoms include disturbances in thought, mood, and behavior. Positive symptoms include delusions, which may be bizarre in nature; hallucination, especially auditory; disorganized speech; inappropriate affect; and disorganized behavior. Negative symptoms include flat affect, avolition, alogia, and anhedonia. Episodes appear suddenly in persons whose previous behavior has been relatively normal and are usually of short duration. Recurrent episodes are common, and in some instances a more chronic type of the disorder may develop. See also **schizoaffective disorder, schizophrenia, schizophreniform disorder.**

**acute secondary myocarditis,** sudden, severe inflammation of the heart muscle, as a result of a disease of the endocardium or pericardium or to a generalized infection. See also **myocarditis.**

**acute septic myocarditis** [Gk, *septikos,* putrid, *mys,* muscle, *kardia,* heart, *itis,* inflammation], severe inflammation of the myocardium associated with pus formation, necrosis, and abscess formation. See also **myocarditis.**

**acute suppurative arthritis** [L, *suppurare,* to form pus], a form of arthritis characterized by an invasion of the joint space by pyogenic organisms and the formation of pus in the joint cavity.

**acute suppurative sinusitis** [L, *acutus,* sharp, *suppurare,* to form pus, *sinus,* hollow; Gk, *itis,* inflammation], a purulent infection of the sinuses. Symptoms are pain over the inflamed area, headache, chills, and fever.

**acute tonsillitis** [L, *acutus,* sharp, *tonsilla;* Gk, *itis,* inflammation], an inflammation of the tonsil(s) associated with a catarrhal exudate over the tonsil or the discharge of caseous or suppurative material from the tonsil crypts.

**acute toxicity,** the harmful effect of a toxic agent that manifests itself in seconds, minutes, hours, or days after entering the patient.

**acute transverse myelitis,** an inflammation of the entire thickness of the spinal cord, affecting both the sensory and motor nerves. It can develop rapidly, accompanied by necrosis and neurologic deficit that commonly persist after recovery. Patients in whom spastic reflexes develop soon after the onset of this disease are more likely to recover. This disorder may result from a variety of causes, such as multiple sclerosis, measles, pneumonia, and the ingestion of certain toxic agents such as carbon monoxide, lead, and arsenic. Such poisonous substances can destroy the entire circumference of the spinal cord, including the myelin sheaths, the axis cylinders, and the neurons, and can also cause hemorrhage and necrosis. There is no effective treatment, and the prognosis for complete recovery is poor. Nursing care includes frequent assessment of vital signs, vigilance for signs of spinal shock, maintenance of a urinary catheter, and proper skin care.

**acute tubular necrosis (ATN)** [L, *tubulus,* tubule; Gk, *nekros,* dead, *osis,* condition], sudden failure of the kidney tubules. The condition is commonly caused by an interruption of the blood supply to the tubules, resulting in ischemia. See also **renal failure.**

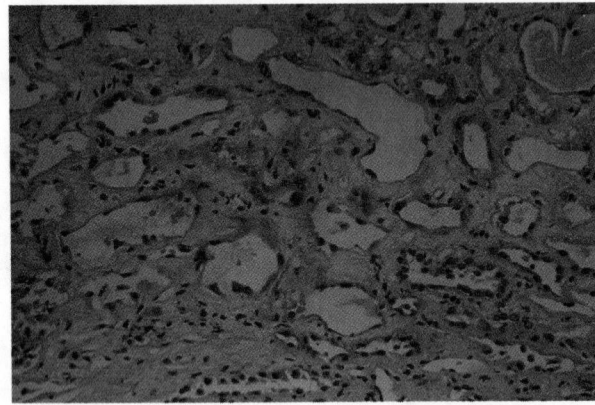

**Ischemic acute tubular necrosis**
*(Cotran, Kumar, and Collins, 1999)*

**acute urethral syndrome** [Gk, *ourethra,* urethra, *syn,* together, *dromos,* course], a group of pelvic symptoms experienced by women, including dysuria, urinary frequency, urinary tenesmus, lower back pain, and suprapubic aching and cramping. Clinical evidence of a pathogen or other factor to account for the symptoms may be absent, and further testing may be required.

**acyanotic** /ā′sī·ənot′ik/ [Gk, *a,* not, *kyanos,* blue], lacking a blue appearance of the skin and mucous membranes. See also **cyanosis.**

**acyanotic congenital defect** [Gk, *a, kyanos,* not blue], a heart defect present at birth that does not produce blue discoloration of the skin and mucous membranes under normal circumstances. However, the condition does increase the load on the pulmonary circulation and may lead to cyanosis, right ventricular failure, or other complications during physical exertion.

**acyclovir** /əsī′klōvir/, an antiviral agent with activity against herpesvirus types 1 and 2 and varicella zoster virus. Acyclovir inhibits the application of herpesvirus deoxyribonucleic acid (DNA) molecules.

■ INDICATIONS: It is prescribed topically in an ointment for the treatment of herpes simplex keratitis and both topically and systemically (oral and IV) in other types of herpes infections, including genital herpes.

■ CONTRAINDICATION: Known sensitivity to this drug prohibits its use.

■ ADVERSE EFFECTS: After topical use, irritation or pruritus may occur; after systemic use, diaphoresis, headache, and nausea may occur. When it is administered intravenously in the treatment of immunosuppressed patients, there may be pain at the site of the injection.

**acyesis** /ā′sī·ē′sis/, **1.** the absence of pregnancy. **2.** a condition of sterility in women.

**acyl** /ā′sil /, an organic radical derived from an organic acid by removal of the hydroxyl group from the carboxyl group.

**acylation** /as′ilā′shən/, the incorporation into a molecule of an organic compound of an acyl group, R—CO—.

**AD,** abbreviation for **Alzheimer's disease.**

**ad-,** prefix meaning 'to, toward, addition to, or intensification': *adneural, adrenal.*

**-ad,** suffix meaning 'toward (a specified terminus)': *cephalad.*

**a.d.,** abbreviation for **auris dextra,** or right ear.

**A/D,** abbreviation for **analog-to-digital, anodal duration; average deviation.**

**ADA,** **1.** abbreviation for **American Dental Association. 2.** abbreviation for **American Diabetes Association. 3.** abbreviation for **American Dietetic Association. 4.** abbreviation for **adenosine deaminase.**

**adactyly** /ādak′tilē/ [Gk, *a + daktylos,* not finger or toe], a congenital defect in which one or more digits of the hand or foot are missing.

**Adair-Dighton's syndrome** [Charles Adair-Dighton, twentieth century British physician]. See **osteogenesis imperfecta.**

**Adalat,** trademark for a calcium channel blocker (nifedipine).

**adamantinoma, adamantoblastoma.** See **ameloblastoma.**

**Adam, Evelyn,** a Canadian nursing theorist who applied the structure of a conceptual model for nursing in her book, *Être Infirmière* in 1979 (*To Be a Nurse,* 1980). A conceptual model consists of assumptions, beliefs and values, and major units. Adam believes that a theory is useful to more than one discipline, but that a conceptual model for a discipline is useful only to that discipline. Adam developed Virginia Henderson's concepts within Dorothy Johnson's structure of a conceptual model. She describes the goal of nursing as maintaining or restoring the client's independence in the satisfaction of 14 fundamental needs. Each need has biological, physiological, and psychosocial aspects. The nurse has the role of complementing and supplementing the client's strength, knowledge, and will.

**ADAMHA,** abbreviation for U.S. *Alcohol, Drug Abuse, and Mental Health Administration.*

**Adam's apple,** *informal,* the bulge at the front of the neck produced by the thyroid cartilage of the larynx. Also called **laryngeal prominence.**

**Adams-Stokes syndrome** [Robert Adams, Irish surgeon, 1791–1875; William Stokes, Irish physician, 1804–1878], a condition characterized by sudden, recurrent episodes of loss of consciousness caused by incomplete heart block. Seizures may accompany the episodes. Also called **Stokes-Adams syndrome.** See also **infranodal block.**

**adaptation** /ad′aptā′shən/ [L, *adaptatio,* act of adapting], a change or response to stress of any kind, such as inflammation of the nasal mucosa in infectious rhinitis or increased crying in a frightened child. Adaptation may be normal, self-protective, and developmental, as when a child learns to talk; it may be all-encompassing, creating further stress, as in polycythemia, which occurs naturally at high altitudes to provide more oxygen-carrying red blood cells but may also lead to thrombosis, venous congestion, or edema. The degree and nature of adaptation shown by a patient are evaluated regularly by the nurse. They constitute a measure of the effectiveness of nursing care, the course of the disease, and the ability of the patient to cope with stress. Compare **accommodation.**

**adaptation model,** (in nursing) a conceptual framework that focuses on the patient as an adaptive system, one in which nursing intervention is required when a deficit develops in the patient's ability to cope with the internal and external demands of the environment. These demands are classified into four groups: physiologic needs, the need for a positive self-concept, the need to perform social roles, and the need to balance dependence and independence. The nurse assesses the patient's maladaptive response and identifies the kind of demand that is causing the problem. Nursing care is planned to promote adaptive responses to cope successfully with the current stress on the patient's well-being. This model, first proposed by Sister Callista Roy, is frequently used as a conceptual framework for programs of nursing education.

**adaptation syndrome.** See **general adaptation syndrome.**

**adapted clothing,** clothing that has been modified, such as with taped hook and loop or Velcro fasteners, to permit disabled persons to dress themselves with minimal difficulty.

**adapter** [L, *adaptatio,* the process of adjusting], a device for joining or connecting two or more parts of a system to enable it to function properly, usually with tubing.

**adaptive capacity, decreased intracranial,** a nursing diagnosis accepted by the Eleventh National Conference on the Classification of Nursing Diagnoses. Adaptive capacity, decreased: intracranial is a clinical state in which intracranial fluid dynamic mechanisms that normally compensate for increases in intracranial volumes are compromised, resulting in repeated disproportionate increases in intracranial pressure (ICP) in response to a variety of noxious and nonnoxious stimuli.

■ DEFINING CHARACTERISTICS: Major defining characteristics include repeated increases in ICP of greater than 10 mm Hg for more than 5 minutes after any of a variety of external stimuli. Minor defining characteristics include disproportionate increases in ICP after a single environmental or nursing maneuver stimulus; elevated component of $P_2$ ICP waveform; volume pressure response test variation (volume pressure ratio $>2$, pressure-volume index $<10$); baseline ICP equal to or greater than 10 mm Hg; and wide-amplitude ICP elevation.

■ RELATED FACTORS: Factors include brain injuries; sustained increase in ICP $\geq 10$ to 15 mm Hg; decreased cerebral perfusion pressure $\leq 70$ mm Hg; and systemic hypotension with intracranial hypertension. See also **nursing diagnosis.**

**adaptive device** /adap'tiv/ [L, *adaptatio,* process of adapting; OFr, *devise*], any structure, design, instrument, contrivance, or equipment that enables a person with a disability to function independently. Examples include plate guards, grab bars, and transfer boards. Also called **self-help device** or **assistive device.**

**adaptive hypertrophy** [L, *adaptatio,* process of adapting; Gk, *hyper,* excessive, *trophe,* nourishment], a reactive increase in amount of tissue that compensates for a loss of the same or similar tissue so that function is not impaired.

**adaptive response,** an appropriate reaction to an environmental demand.

**adaptor RNA.** See **transfer RNA.**

**ADC,** abbreviation for **AIDS-dementia complex.**

**ADC Van Disal** /ā'dē'sē'vandī'səl/, a term used as a mnemonic device for recalling the protocol of hospital admission orders. The letters stand for **A**dmission authorization, **D**iagnosis, **C**ondition, **V**ital signs, **A**ctivity, **D**rugs, **I**nstructions, **S**pecial studies, **A**llergies, **L**aboratory tests.

**Addams, Jane** (1860–1935), an American social reformer. In Chicago in 1889 she founded Hull House, one of the first social settlements in the United States, where volunteers from many disciplines, including nursing, lived and worked in their professions. She played a central role in most of the social reforms of her time and provided an inspiration to those in the nursing profession who were striving to establish high educational standards and better working conditions. She was co-recipient of the Nobel peace prize in 1931.

**addict** /ad'ikt/ [L, *addicere,* to devote], a person who has become physiologically or psychologically dependent on a chemical such as alcohol or other drugs to the extent that normal social, occupational, and other responsible life functions are disrupted.

**addiction** /ədik'shən/ [L, *addicere,* to devote], compulsive, uncontrollable dependence on a chemical substance, habit, or practice to such a degree that cessation causes severe emotional, mental, or physiologic reactions. Compare **habituation.**

**addictive personality** /ədik'tiv/, a personality marked by traits of compulsive and habitual use of a substance or practice in an attempt to cope with psychic pain engendered by conflict and anxiety.

**addisonian anemia.** See **pernicious anemia.**

**addisonian crisis.** See **adrenal crisis.**

**addisonism,** [Thomas Addison, London physician, 1793–1860], a condition characterized by the physical signs of Addison's disease, although loss of adrenocortical functions is not involved. The signs include increase in bronze pigmentation of the skin and mucous membranes caused by increased melanocyte-stimulating hormone (MSH), as well as general debility.

**Addison's crisis.** See **adrenal crisis.**

**Addison's disease** [Thomas Addison], a life-threatening condition caused by partial or complete failure of adrenocortical function, often resulting from autoimmune processes, infection (especially tubercular or fungal), neoplasm, or hemorrhage in the gland. All three general functions of the adrenal cortex (glucocorticoid, mineralocorticoid, and androgenic) are lost. Also called **Addison's syndrome.** See also **adrenal crisis.**

■ OBSERVATIONS: The disease is characterized by increased bronze pigmentation of the skin and mucous membranes; weakness; decreased endurance; anorexia; dehydration; weight loss; GI disturbances; salt cravings; anxiety, depression, and other emotional distress; and decreased tolerance

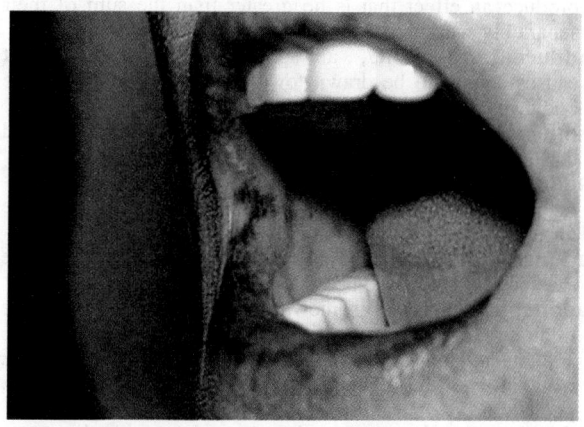

**Addison's disease: buccal pigmentation**
*(Lawrence and Cox, 1993)*

to physical and emotional stress. The person's requirements for glucocorticoid, mineralocorticoid, and salt are increased by stress, as in infection, trauma, and surgical procedures. The onset is usually gradual, over a period of weeks or months. Laboratory tests reveal abnormally low blood concentrations of sodium and glucose, a greater than normal level of serum potassium, and a decreased urinary output of certain steroids. The diagnosis is established if the amount of cortisol in the plasma and steroid in the urine does not increase after stimulation with ACTH.

■ INTERVENTIONS: Treatment includes replacement therapy with glucocorticoid, and mineralocorticoid drugs, an adequate fluid intake, control of sodium and potassium balance, and a diet high in complex carbohydrate and protein. Follow-up care includes continued administration of glucocorticoid drugs.

■ NURSING CONSIDERATIONS: The complications of Addison's disease include high fever, confused behavior, and adrenal crisis (addisonian crisis). With careful management, the patient's resistance to infection, capacity for work, and general well-being can be maintained. Nursing care includes administering corticosteroids and other drugs, observing the patient for signs of abnormal sodium and potassium levels, monitoring body weight and fluid intake and output, and encouraging adequate intake of nutrients. The patient also needs protection against stress while in the hospital and instruction in the importance of avoiding stress at home. The significance of emotional distress, the value of wearing a medical-alert bracelet or tag, the signs of impending crisis, the use of a prepared kit for emergencies, and the importance of scrupulous attention to drug and diet regimens are emphasized before discharge. Discharge teaching also emphasizes the need to take cortisone after meals or with milk to prevent gastric irritation and the development of ulcers.

**Addison's keloid.** See **morphea.**

**Addison's syndrome.** See **Addison's disease.**

**addition** [L, *additio,* something added], a chemical reaction in which two complete molecules combine to form a new product, usually by attachment to carbon atoms at a double or triple bond of one of the molecules.

**additive** /ad′itiv/, any substance added intentionally or indirectly that becomes a part of the food, pharmaceutical, or other product. Additives may be introduced in growing, processing, packaging, storage, or cooking or other final preparation for consumption.

**additive effect** [L, *additio,* something added, *effectus*], the combined effect of drugs that when used in combination produce an effect that is no greater than the sum of their separately measured individual effects.

**adducent** /ədo͞o′sənt/, an agent or other stimulus that causes a limb to be drawn toward the median axis of the body, or causes the fingers or toes to move together.

**adduct** /ədukt′/ [L, *adducere,* to bring to], to move toward the median axis of the body.

**adduction** /əduk′shən/ [L, *adducere,* to bring to], movement of a limb toward the median axis of the body. Compare **abduction.** —**adduct,** *v.*

**adductor** /əduk′tər/, a muscle that draws a part toward the axis or midline of the body. Compare **abductor, tensor.**

**adductor brevis,** a somewhat triangular muscle in the thigh and one of the five medial femoral muscles. It acts to adduct and rotate the thigh medially and to flex the leg. Compare **adductor longus, adductor magnus, gracilis, pectineus.**

**adductor canal,** a triangular channel beneath the sartorius muscle and between the adductor longus and vastus medialis through which the femoral vessels and the saphe-

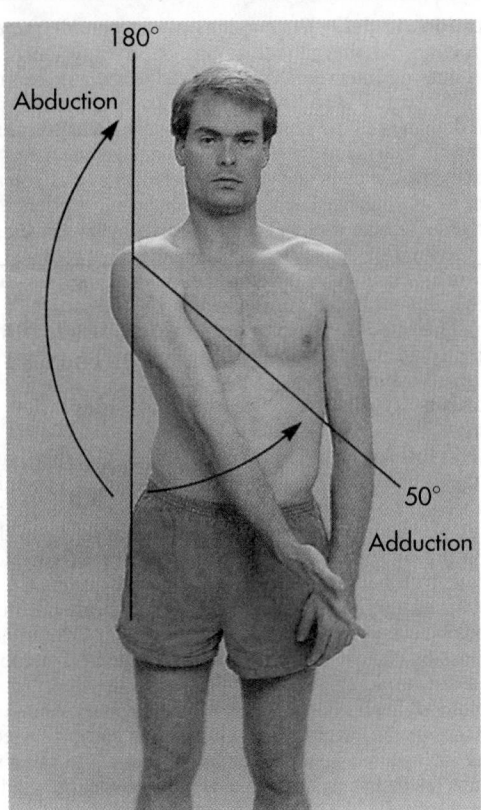

**Adduction and abduction of the shoulder**
(Seidel et al, 1995/Patrick Watson)

nous nerve pass. Also called **Hunter's canal, subsartorial canal.**

**adductor longus,** the most superficial of the three adductor muscles of the thigh and one of five medial femoral muscles. It functions to adduct and flex the thigh. Compare **adductor brevis, adductor magnus, gracilis, pectineus.**

**adductor magnus,** the long, heavy triangular muscle of the medial aspect of the thigh. The adductor magnus acts to adduct the thigh. The proximal portion acts to rotate the thigh medially and to flex it on the hip; the distal portion acts to extend the thigh and rotate it laterally.

**aden-.** See **adeno-.**

**adenalgia** /ad′ənal′jə/ [Gk, *aden,* gland, *algos,* pain], pain in any of the glands. Also called **adenodynia** /ad′ənōdin′ē-ə/.

**adenectomy** /ad′ənek′təmē/ [Gk, *aden + ektomē,* excision], the surgical removal of any gland.

**Aden fever.** See **dengue fever.**

**-adenia,** suffix meaning '(condition of the) glands': *anadenia, heteradenia.*

**adenine** /ad′ənin/, a purine base that is a component of DNA, RNA, adenosine monophosphate (AMP), cyclic AMP, adenosine diphosphate (ADP), and adenosine triphosphate (ATP). See **adenosine triphosphate, deoxyribonucleic acid, ribonucleic acid.**

**adenine arabinoside.** See **vidarabine.**

**adenine-D-ribose.** See **adenosine.**

**adenitis** /ad′ənī′tis/, an inflammatory condition of a lymph node. Acute adenitis of the cervical lymph nodes may ac-

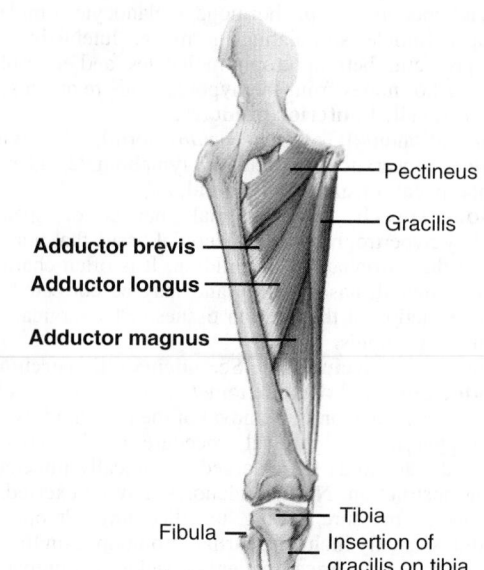

**Adductor brevis, adductor longus, and adductor magnus muscles of the anterior thigh**
*(Thibodeau and Patton, 1999/John V. Hagen)*

of the glands. Specific tumors are diagnosed and named by cytologic identification of the tissue affected; for example, an adenocarcinoma of the uterine cervix is characterized by tumor cells resembling the glandular epithelium of the cervix. **—adenocarcinomatous,** *adj.*

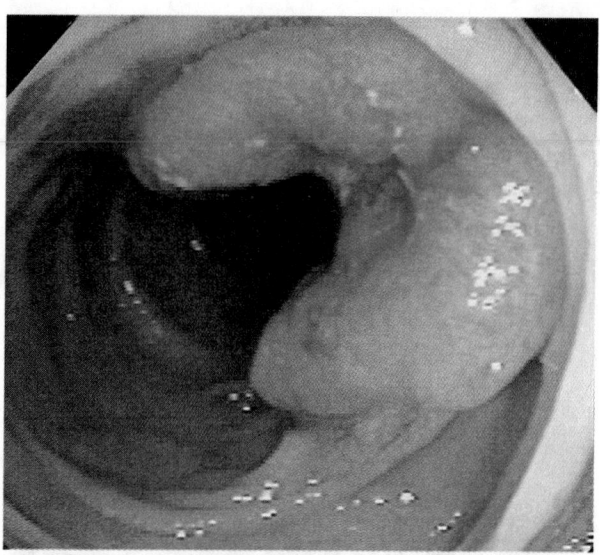

**Adenocarcinoma of the sigmoid colon** *(Wilcox, 1995)*

company a sore throat and stiff neck, simulating mumps if severe. It is most often related to an oral, pharyngeal, or ear infection. Scarlet fever may cause an acute suppurative cervical adenitis. Swelling of the lymph nodes in the back of the neck is often the result of a scalp infection, insect bite, or infestation by head lice. Inflammation of the lymph nodes of the mesenteric portion of the peritoneum often produces pain and other symptoms similar to those of appendicitis. Mesenteric adenitis may be mistaken for appendicitis, but characteristically mesenteric adenitis is preceded by a respiratory infection, the pain is less localized and less constant than in appendicitis, and it does not increase in severity. Generalized adenitis is a secondary symptom of syphilis. Therapy requires treatment of the primary infection by the administration of antimicrobial agents, application of warm compresses, and, in some cases, when fluctuation is present, incision and drainage. Also called **lymphadenitis.** Compare **acinitis.**

**adeno-, aden-,** prefix meaning 'gland': *adenocarcinoma, adenectomy.*

**adenoacanthoma** /ad'ənō·ak'anthō'mə/ [Gk, *aden* + *akantha,* thorn, *oma,* tumor], a neoplasm that may be malignant or benign, derived from glandular tissue with squamous differentiation shown by some of the cells.

**adenoameloblastoma** /ad'ənō-amel'ōblastō'mə/, *pl.* **adenoameloblastomas, adenoameloblastomat,** a benign tumor of the maxilla or mandible composed of ducts lined with columnar or cuboidal epithelial cells. It develops in tissue that normally gives rise to the teeth, and it most often occurs in young people.

**adenoassociated virus (AAV)** /ad'ənō-/, a defective virus that can reproduce only in the presence of adenoviruses. It is not yet known what role, if any, these organisms have in causing disease.

**adenocarcinoma** /ad'ənōkärsinō'mə/, *pl.* **adenocarcinomas, adenocarcinomata** [Gk, *aden* + *karkinos,* crab, *oma*], any one of a large group of malignant, epithelial cell tumors

**adenocarcinoma in situ,** a localized growth of abnormal glandular tissue that may become malignant. However, the abnormal cells do not extend beyond the basement membrane. It is most common in the endometrium and in the large intestine.

**adenocarcinoma of the kidney.** See **renal cell carcinoma.**

**adenocarcinoma of the lung,** a type of bronchogenic carcinoma made up of a discrete mass of cuboidal or columnar cells, generally at the lung periphery. Most of these tumors form glandular structures that contain mucin, although a few lack mucin and are solid. Growth is slow, but there may be early invasion of blood and lymph vessels, with metastases while the primary lesion is still asymptomatic. There are two types of lung adenocarcinomas, **bronchogenic adenocarcinoma** and **bronchioloalveolar carcinoma.**

**adenocarcinomatous.** See **adenocarcinoma.**

**adenocele** /ad'ənōsēl'/, a cystic, glandular tumor.

**adenochondroma** /ad'ənōkondrō'mə/, *pl.* **adenochondromas, adenochondromata** [Gk, *aden* + *chondros,* cartilage, *oma*], a neoplasm of cells derived from glandular and cartilaginous tissues, as a mixed tumor of the salivary glands. Also called **chondroadenoma.**

**adenocyst** /ad'ənōsist'/ [Gk, *aden* + *kytis,* bag], a benign tumor in which the cells form cysts. A kind of adenocyst is **papillary adenocystoma lymphomatosum.** Also called **adenocystoma.**

**adenocystic carcinoma,** a malignant neoplasm composed of cords of uniform small epithelial cells arranged in a sievelike pattern around cystic spaces that often contain mucus. The tumor occurs most frequently in the salivary glands, breast, mucous glands of the upper and lower respiratory tract, and, occasionally, in vestibular glands of the vulva. The malignant slow growth tends to spread along nerves, causing neurologic damage. Facial paralysis often results from adenocystic carcinoma of the salivary gland. Blood-borne metastases to bones and liver have been reported. Also called **adenoid cystic carcinoma, adenomyoepithelioma, cribriform carcinoma, cylindroma.**

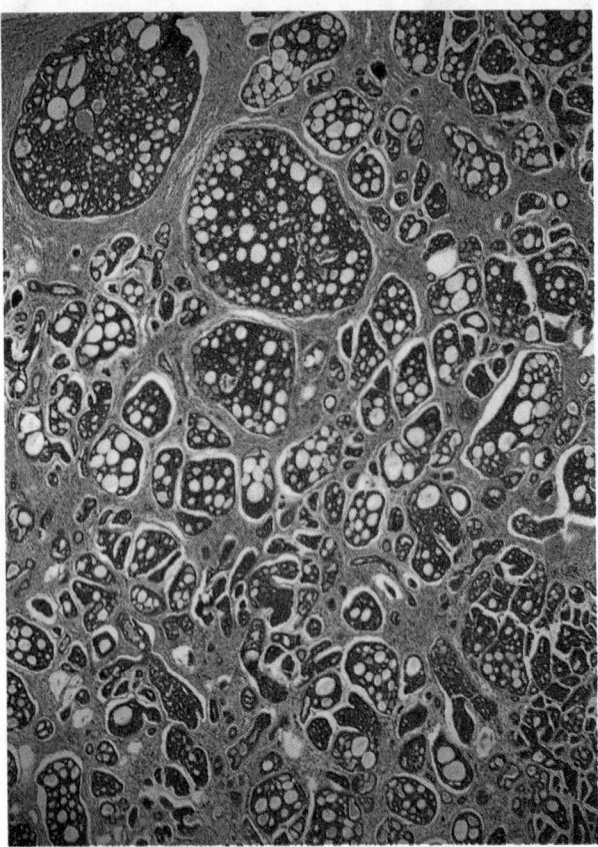

**Adenocystic carcinoma** *(Silverberg, DeLellis, and Frable, 1997)*

**adenocystoma.** See **adenocyst.**

**adenodynia.** See **adenalgia.**

**adenoepithelioma** /ad′ənō·ep′ithē′lē·ō′mə/, *pl.* **adenoepitheliomas, adenoepitheliomata** [Gk, *aden* + *epi,* on, *thele* nipple, *oma*], a neoplasm consisting of glandular and epithelial components.

**adenofibroma** /ad′ənōfībrō′mə/, *pl.* **adenofibromas, adenofibromata** [Gk, *aden* + L, *fibra,* fiber, *oma*], a tumor of the connective tissues that contains glandular elements.

**adenofibroma edematodes,** a neoplasm consisting of glandular elements and connective tissue in which marked edema is present.

**adenofibromata.** See **adenofibroma.**

**adenohypophysis** /ad′ənō′hīpof′isis/ [Gk, *aden* + *hypo,* beneath, *phyein,* to grow], the anterior lobe of the pituitary gland. It secretes growth hormone, thyroid stimulating hor-

mone, adrenocorticotropic hormone, melanocyte stimulating hormone, follicle stimulating hormone, luteinizing hormone, prolactin, beta lipotropin molecules, and endorphins. Releasing hormones from the hypothalamus regulate secretions. Also called **anterior pituitary.**

**adenoid** /ad′ənoid/ [Gk, *aden* + *eidos,* form], **1.** having a glandular appearance, particularly lymphoid. **2.** adenoids, the pharyngeal tonsils. —**adenoidal,** *adj.*

**adenoidal speech,** an abnormal manner of speaking caused by hypertrophy of the adenoidal tissue that normally exists in the nasopharynx of children. It is often characterized by a muted, nasal quality and may be corrected by a natural reduction of the swollen tissues or by surgical excision of the adenoids.

**adenoid cystic carcinoma.** See **adenocystic carcinoma.**

**adenoidectomy** /ad′ənoidek′təmē/ [Gk, *aden* + *eidos,* form, *ektomē,* excision], removal of the lymphoid tissue in the nasopharynx. The surgical procedure may be performed because the adenoids are enlarged, chronically infected, or causing obstruction. Normal adenoids may be excised as a prophylactic measure during tonsillectomy. Preoperative procedures usually include a partial thromboplastin time test and for African-American patients a sickle cell preparation test. The operation is performed with general anesthesia in children, but local anesthesia may be used in adults. After removal of the adenoids, bleeding is stemmed with pressure or vessels may be ligated with sutures or electrocoagulation current may be used. Postoperatively, the patient is observed for signs of hemorrhage, and the pulse, blood pressure, and respiration are checked every 15 minutes for the first hour and every 30 minutes for several hours thereafter. See also **tonsillectomy.**

**adenoid facies,** the dull expression, with open mouth, sometimes seen in children with hypertrophy of the pharyngeal tonsils ("adenoids").

**adenoid hyperplasia,** a condition of enlarged adenoid glands, especially in children. Enlarged adenoids, often in association with enlarged tonsils, are a frequent cause of recurrent otitis media, sinusitis, conduction hearing loss, and partial respiratory obstruction. Severe obstruction can result in alveolar hypoventilation and pulmonary hypertension with congestive heart failure. Treatment usually consists of surgical removal of the adenoids.

**adenoid hypertrophy** [Gk, *aden,* gland, *eidos,* form, *hyper,* excessive, *trophe,* nourishment], an enlargement of the pharyngeal tonsil.

**adenoiditis** /ad′ənoidī′tis/, inflammation of the adenoids or pharyngeal tonsils.

**adenoids,** small masses of lymphoid tissue forming the pharyngeal tonsils on the posterior wall of the nasopharynx. Also called **pharyngeal tonsils.**

**adenoid tissue,** the lymphoid tissue that forms the pharyngeal tonsils.

**adenoleiomyofibroma** /ad′ənōlī′ōmī′ōfībrō′mə/, *pl.* **adenoleiomyofibromas, adenoleiomyofibromata** [Gk, *aden* + *leios,* smooth, *mys,* muscle; L, *fibra,* fiber; Gk, *oma*], a glandular tumor with smooth muscle, connective tissue, and epithelial elements.

**adenolipoma** /ad′ənōlipō′mə/, *pl.* **adenolipomas, adenolipomata** [Gk, *aden* + *lipos,* fat, *oma*], a neoplasm consisting of elements of glandular and fatty tissue.

**adenolipomatosis** /ad′ənōlip′ōmətō′sis/, a condition characterized by the growth of adenolipomas in the groin, axilla, and neck.

**adenolymphoma.** See **papillary adenocystoma lymphomatosum.**

**adenoma** /ad'ənō'mə/, *pl.* adenomas, adenomata [Gk, *aden* + *oma*], a tumor of glandular epithelium in which the cells of the tumor are arranged in a recognizable glandular structure. An adenoma may cause excess secretion by the affected gland, such as acidophilic pituitary adenoma resulting in an excess of growth hormone. Kinds of adenomas include **acidophilic adenoma, basophilic adenoma, fibroadenoma,** and **insulinoma.** —**adenomatous,** *adj.*

**-adenoma,** suffix meaning a 'tumor composed of glandular tissue or glandlike in structure': *sarcoadenoma, splenadenoma.*

**adenoma sebaceum** /sebā'sē·əm/, an abnormal skin condition consisting of multiple wartlike, yellowish red, waxy papules on the face that are not sebaceous, composed chiefly of fibrovascular tissue. The lesions are usually benign. See also **tuberous sclerosis.**

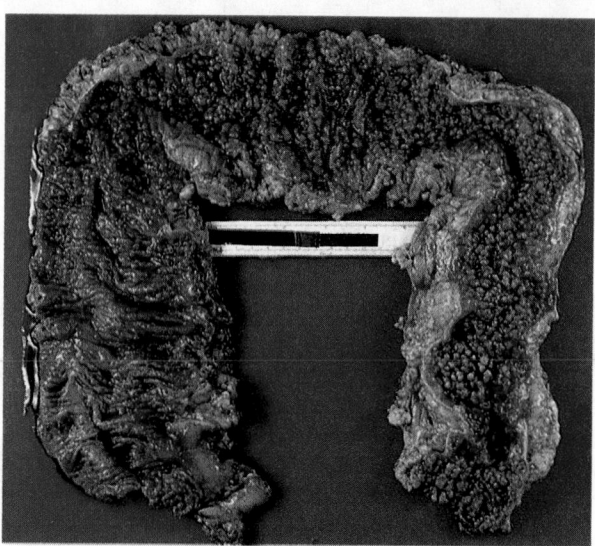

**Familial adenomatous polyposis**
*(Silverberg, DeLellis, and Frable, 1997)*

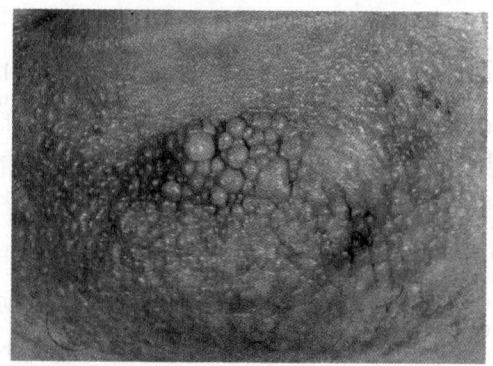

**Adenoma sebaceum** *(du Vivier, 1993)*

**adenomatoid** /ad'ənō'mətoid/ [Gk, *aden* + *oma* + *eidos,* form], resembling a glandular tumor.

**adenomatosis** /ad'ənōmətō'sis/, an abnormal condition in which hyperplasia or tumor development affects two or more glands, usually the thyroid, adrenals, or pituitary.

**adenomatous.** See **adenoma.**

**adenomatous goiter** /ad'ənō'mətəs/, an enlargement of the thyroid gland caused by an adenoma or numerous colloid nodules.

**adenomatous polyp** [Gk, *aden,* gland, *oma,* tumor, *polys,* many, *pous,* foot], a tumor that develops in glandular tissue. It is characterized by neoplastic changes in epithelium.

**adenomatous polyposis coli (APC),** a gene associated with **familial adenomatous polyposis (FAP),** an inherited disorder characterized by the development of myriad polyps in the colon, beginning in late adolescence or early adulthood. Untreated, the condition nearly always leads to colon cancer. The gene is located on chromosome 5.

**adenomyoepithelioma.** See **adenocystic carcinoma.**

**adenomyofibroma** /ad'ənōmī'ōfibrō'mə/, *pl.* **adenomyofibromas, adenomyofibromata** [Gk, *aden* + *mys,* muscle; L, *fibra,* fiber; Gk, *oma*], a fibrous tumor that contains glandular and muscular components.

**adenomyoma** /ad'ənōmī·ō'mə/, *pl.* **adenomyomas, adenomyomata,** a tumor of the endometrium of the uterus characterized by a mass of smooth muscle containing endometrial tissue and glands.

**adenomyomatosis** /ad'ənōmī'ōmətō'sis/, an abnormal condition characterized by the formation of benign nodules resembling adenomyomas, found in the uterus or in parauterine tissue.

**adenomyosarcoma** /ad'ənōmī'ōsärkō'mə/, *pl.* **adenomyosarcomas, adenomyosarcomata,** a malignant tumor of soft tissue containing glandular elements and striated muscle.

**adenomyosis** /ad'ənōmī·ō'sis/, **1.** an invasion of the muscular wall of the uterus by the endometrium.

**adenopathy** /ad'ənop'əthē/ [Gk, *aden* + *pathos,* suffering], an enlargement of any gland. —**adenopathic,** *adj.*

**adenopharyngitis** /ad'ənōfer'injī'tis/, an inflammation of the adenoid tonsils and the pharynx.

**adenosarcoma** /ad'ənōsärkō'mə/, *pl.* **adenosarcomas, adenosarcomata** [Gk, *aden* + *sarx,* flesh, *oma*], a malignant glandular tumor of the soft tissues of the body.

**adenosarcorhabdomyoma** /ad'ənōsär'kōrab'dōmīō'mə/, *pl.* **adenosarcorhabdomyomas, adenosarcorhabdomyomata,** a tumor composed of glandular and connective tissue, and striated muscle elements.

**adenosine** /əden'əsin, -sēn/, a compound derived from nucleic acid, composed of adenine and a sugar, D-ribose. Adenosine is the major molecular component of the nucleotides adenosine monophosphate, adenosine diphosphate, and adenosine triphosphate and of the nucleic acids deoxyribonucleic acid and ribonucleic acid. Also called **adenine-D-ribose.** See also **adenosine phosphate.**

**adenosine 3′,5′-cyclic monophosphate.** See **cyclic adenosine monophosphate.**

**adenosine deaminase (ADA)** /dē·am'inās/, an enzyme that catalyzes the conversion of adenosine to the nucleoside inosine through the removal of an amino group. A deficiency of ADA can lead to **severe combined immunodeficiency syndrome (SCIDS).** See also **adenosine.**

**adenosine diphosphate (ADP),** a product of the hydrolysis of adenosine triphosphate.

**adenosine hydrolase,** an enzyme that catalyzes the conversion of adenosine into adenine and ribose.

**adenosine kinase,** an enzyme in the liver and kidney that catalyzes the transfer of a phosphate group from adenosine triphosphate to produce adenosine diphosphate.

**adenosine monophosphate (AMP),** an ester, composed of adenine-D-ribose and phosphoric acid, that participates in energy released by working muscle. Also called **adenylic acid.**

**adenosine phosphate,** a compound consisting of the nucleotide adenosine attached through its ribose group to one, two, or three phosphate units, or phosphoric acid molecules. Kinds of adenosine phosphate, all of which are interconvertible, are **adenosine diphosphate, adenosine monophosphate,** and **adenosine triphosphate.**

**adenosine triphosphatase (ATPase),** an enzyme in skeletal muscle and other tissues that catalyzes the hydrolysis of adenosine triphosphate to adenosine diphosphate and inorganic phosphate. Among various enzymes in this group, mitochondrial ATPase is involved in obtaining energy for cellular metabolism, and myosin ATPase is involved in muscle contraction.

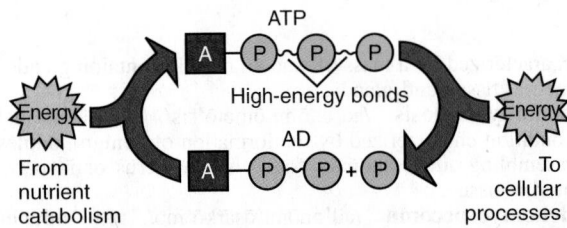

**Role of adenosine triphosphate (ATP) in metabolism**
*(Thibodeau and Patton, 1999/Rolin Graphics)*

**adenosine triphosphate (ATP),** a compound consisting of the nucleotide adenosine attached through its ribose group to three phosphoric acid molecules. It serves to store energy in muscles; energy is released when it is hydrolyzed to adenosine diphosphate.

**adenosis** /ad′ənō′sis/, **1.** any disease of the glands, especially a lymphatic gland. **2.** an abnormal development or enlargement of glandular tissue.

**adenotomy** /ad′ənot′əmē/ [Gk, *aden,* gland, *tome,* a cutting], dissection or incision of a gland.

**adenotonsillectomy** /ad′ənōton′silek′təmē/, surgical removal of the adenoids and tonsils. Compare **tonsillectomy.**

**adenovirus** /ad′ənōvī′rəs/ [Gk, *aden* + L, *virus,* poison], any one of the 49 medium-sized viruses of the Adenoviridae family, pathogenic to humans, that cause conjunctivitis, upper respiratory infection, cystitis, or GI infection. After the acute and symptomatic period of illness, the virus may persist in a latent stage in the tonsils, adenoids, and other lymphoid tissue. Compare **rhinovirus. —adenoviral,** *adj.*

**adenylate** /əden′ilāt/, a salt or ester of adenylic acid.

**adenylate cyclase,** an enzyme that initiates the conversion of adenosine triphosphate (ATP) to cyclic adenosine monophosphate (cAMP), a mediator of many physiologic activities.

**adenylate kinase,** an enzyme in skeletal muscle that makes possible the reaction ATP + AMP = 2ADP. Also called **myokinase.**

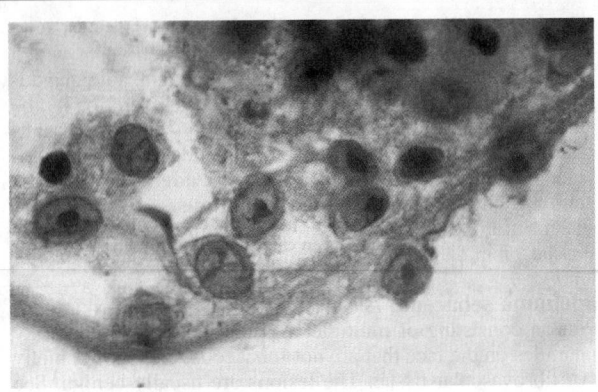

**Adenovirus infection within transitional cells**
*(Silverberg, DeLellis, and Frable, 1997)*

**adenylic acid.** See **adenosine monophosphate.**

**adequate and well-controlled studies,** clinical and laboratory studies that the sponsors of a new drug are required by law to conduct to demonstrate the truth of the claims made for its effectiveness.

**adermia** /ədur′mē·ə/ [Gk, *a* + *derma,* without skin], a congenital or acquired skin defect or the absence of skin.

**ADH,** abbreviation for **antidiuretic hormone.**

**ADHA,** abbreviation for the **American Dental Hygienists' Association.**

**adhere** /adhir′/, to stick together or become fastened together, as two surfaces.

**adherence** /adhir′əns/, **1.** the quality of clinging or being closely attached. **2.** the process in which a person follows rules, guidelines, or standards, especially as a patient follows a prescription and recommendations for a regimen of care.

**adherence behavior,** a nursing outcome from the Nursing Outcomes Classification (NOC) defined as self-initiated action taken to promote wellness, recovery, and rehabilitation. See also **Nursing Outcomes Classification.**

**adherent** /adhir′ənt/ [L, *adhaerens,* sticking to], having the tendency to cling, as one substance to the surface of another substance.

**adherent pericardium.** See **pericardial adhesion.**

**adherent placenta** [L, *adhaerens,* sticking to, *placenta,* flat cake], a placenta that remains attached to the uterine wall beyond the normal time after birth of the fetus. See also **placenta accreta.**

**adhesin** /adhē′sin/, a bacterial product that can split proteins. It combines with epithelial cell glycoproteins or glycolipid receptors.

**adhesion** /adhē′zhən/ [L, *adhaerens,* sticking to], a band of scar tissue that binds anatomic surfaces that normally are separate from each other. Adhesions most commonly form in the abdomen, after abdominal surgery, inflammation, or injury. A loop of intestine may adhere to unhealed areas. Scar tissue constricting the bowel's lumen causes obstruction, blocking the intestinal flow and causing abdominal pain, nausea and vomiting, and distension. Nasogastric intubation and suction may relieve the symptoms. If the blockage does not resolve spontaneously, surgery to lyse adhesions may be necessary. See also **adhesiotomy, intestinal obstruction.**

**adhesiotomy** /adhē′sē·ot′əmē/ [L, *adhaerens* + Gk, *temnein* to cut], the surgical dividing or separating of adhesions, usually performed to relieve an intestinal obstruction. Also called **lysis of adhesions.** See also **abdominal surgery.**

**adhesive** /adhē′siv/ [L, *adhaerens,* sticking to], a quality of a substance that enables it to become attached to another substance.

**adhesive capsulitis,** shoulder condition characterized by stiffness, pain, and limited range of motion. It most often occurs in midlife. Also called **frozen shoulder.** See also **capsulitis.**

**adhesive pericarditis,** a condition characterized by adhesions between the visceral and parietal layers of the pericardium or by adhesions between the pericardium and the mediastinum, diaphragm, or chest wall. Adhesions between the pericardial layers may completely obstruct the pericardial cavity. Adhesive pericarditis may seriously impair normal heart movements.

**adhesive peritonitis,** an inflammation of the peritoneum, characterized by adhesions between adjacent serous surfaces. This condition may be marked by an exudate of serum, fibrin, cells, and pus, accompanied by abdominal pain and tenderness, vomiting, constipation, and fever.

**adhesive phlebitis.** See **obliterative phlebitis.**

**adhesive plaster.** See **adhesive tape.**

**adhesive pleurisy,** inflammation of the pleura with exudation. It causes obliteration of the pleural space through the fusion of the visceral pleural layer covering the lungs and the parietal layer lining the walls of the thoracic cavity.

**adhesive skin traction,** one of two kinds of skin traction in which the therapeutic pull of traction weights is applied with adhesive straps that stick to the skin over the body structure involved, especially a fractured bone. Adhesive skin traction is a short-term treatment used only when continuous traction is desired and skin care for the affected area is easily maintained. It is not suitable for clients with fragile skin. Compare **nonadhesive skin traction.**

**adhesive tape,** a strong fabric material covered on one side with an adhesive. Often water-repellent, it may be used to hold bandages and dressings in place, to immobilize a part, or to exert pressure. Also called **adhesive plaster.**

**ADI,** abbreviation for **acceptable daily intake.**

**adiadochokinesia** /ā′dē·ad′əkō′kinē′zhə, ədī′ədō′kō-/, an inability to perform rapidly alternating movements, such as pronation and supination, or elbow flexion and extension. The activity is commonly included in a neurologic examination.

**adiaphoresis** /ā′dē·əfôrē′sis/, an absence or deficiency of sweat.

**adiastole** /ā′dī·as′təlē/ [Gk, *a,* not, *dia,* across, *stellein,* to set], the absence or imperceptibility of the diastolic stage of the cardiac cycle. See also **diastole.**

**adiathermance** /a′dī·əthur′məns/ [Gk, *a* + *dia,* not across, *therme,* heat], the quality of being unaffected by radiated heat.

**adient** /ad′ē·ənt/ [L, *adire,* moving toward], characterized by a tendency to move toward rather than away from stimuli. Compare **abient. —adience,** *n.*

**Adie's pupil** /ā′dēz/ [William J. Adie, English physician, 1886–1935], an abnormal condition of the eyes marked by one pupil that reacts much more slowly to light changes or to accommodation or convergence than the pupil of the other eye. It is considered a pupillary muscle problem. There is no specific treatment. Also called **tonic pupil.**

**Adie's syndrome** [William J. Adie], the condition of Adie's pupil accompanied by depressed or absent tendon reflexes, particularly the ankle and knee-jerk reflexes. See also **Adie's pupil.**

**adip-.** See **adipo-.**

**adipectomy.** See **lipectomy.**

**adiphenine hydrochloride** /ədif′ənin/, an anticholinergic agent with smooth muscle relaxant properties that has been used for spastic disorders of the GI and genitourinary tracts.

**adipic** /ədip′ik/ [L, *adeps,* fat], pertaining to fatty tissue.

**adipo-, adip-,** combining form meaning 'fat': *adipocele, adipogenesis.*

**adipocele** /ad′ipōsēl′/ [L, *adeps* + Gk, *kele,* hernia], a hernia containing fat or fatty tissue. Also called **lipocele.**

**adipocyte** /ad′ipōsīt′/, a fat (adipose) cell, potentially containing a large fat vacuole consisting mainly of triglycerides.

**adipofibroma** /ad′ipōfībrō′mə/, *pl.* **adipofibromas, adipofibromata** [L, *adeps* + *fibra,* fiber; Gk, *oma*], a fibrous neoplasm of the connective tissue with fatty components.

**adipokinesis** /ad′ipō′kinē′sis/, the mobilization of fat or fatty acids in lipid metabolism.

**adipokinin** /ad′ipokī′nin/, a hormone of the anterior pituitary that causes mobilization of fat from adipose tissues.

**adipometer** /ad′ipom′ətər/, an instrument for measuring the thickness of a skin area as a guide to calculating the amount of subcutaneous fat.

**adiponecrosis** /ad′ipōnikrō′sis/, [L, *adeps* + Gk, *nekros,* dead, *osis* condition], a necrosis of fatty tissue in the body. The condition may be associated with hemorrhagic pancreatitis. **—adiponecrotic,** *adj.*

**adiponecrosis subcutanea neonatorum,** an abnormal dermatologic condition of the newborn characterized by patchy areas of hardened subcutaneous fatty tissue and a bluish-red discoloration of the overlying skin. The lesions, often a result of manipulation during delivery, spontaneously resolve within a period of days to several weeks without scarring. Also called **pseudosclerema, subcutaneous fat necrosis.**

**adiponecrotic.** See **adiponecrosis.**

**adipose** /ad′ipōs/, fatty. Adipose tissue is composed of fat-containing cells arranged in lobules. See also **fat, fatty acid, lipoma.**

**adipose capsule** [L, *adeps,* fat, *capsula,* little box], a capsule of fatty tissue surrounding the kidney. Also called **renal fat.**

**adipose degeneration.** See **fatty degeneration.**

**adipose tissue** [L, *adeps,* fat; OFr, *tissu*], a collection of fat cells. See also **fatty tissue.**

**adipose tumor.** See **lipoma.**

**adiposis dolorosa.** See **Dercum's disease.**

**adiposogenital dystrophy** /ad′ipō′sōjen′itəl/ [L, *adeps* + *genitalis,* generation], a disorder occurring in males, characterized by genital hypoplasia and feminine secondary sex characteristics, including female distribution of fat. It is caused by hypothalamic malfunction or by a tumor in the anterior pituitary gland. Subnormal body temperature, low blood pressure, and reduced blood glucose level are frequently associated with the disorder. Diabetes insipidus also results from hyposecretion of antidiuretic hormone, which causes increased diluted urine output, electrolyte imbalances, and thirst. In addition, involvement of the hypothalamic satiety center may induce overeating and result in pronounced obesity. If a tumor is present, there may be drowsiness and symptoms of increased intracranial pressure (for example, subtle locus of control [LOC] changes and headache). Treatment may include the administration of testosterone and a weight reduction program, excision or radiologic ablation of a tumor, and replacement of hormones, as necessary. Also called **adiposogenital syndrome, Fröhlich's syndrome.**

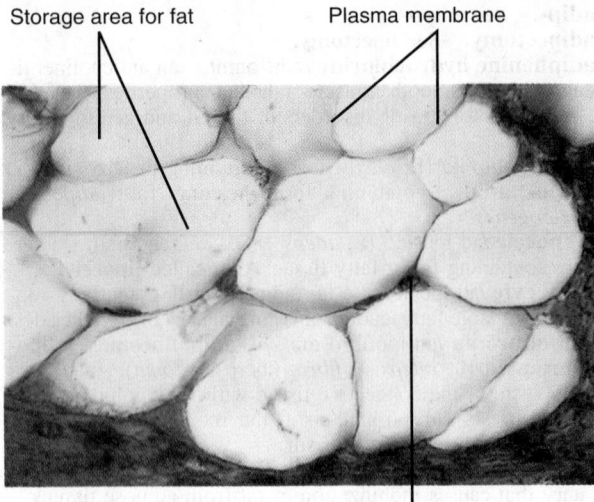

Storage area for fat     Plasma membrane

Nucleus of adipose cell

**Adipose tissue** (© Ed Reschke; used with permission)

**adipsia** /ādip'sē·ə/ [Gk, a + dipsa, not thirst], absence of thirst.

**aditus** /ad'itəs/ [L, going to], an approach or an entry.

**adjunct** /ad'jungkt/ [L, adjungere, to join], (in health care) an additional substance, treatment, or procedure used for increasing the efficacy or safety of the primary substance, treatment, or procedure or for facilitating its performance. —**adjunctive,** adj.

**adjunctive group** /adjungk'tiv/, a group with specific activities and focuses, such as socialization, perceptual stimulation, sensory stimulation, or reality orientation.

**adjunctive psychotherapy,** a form of psychotherapy that concentrates on improving a person's general mental and physical well-being without trying to resolve basic emotional problems. Some kinds of adjunctive psychotherapy are **music therapy, occupational therapy, physical therapy,** and **recreational therapy.**

**adjunct to anesthesia,** one of a number of drugs or techniques used to enhance anesthesia but that are not classified as anesthetics. They may include heat, ice, hypnosis healing touch, NSAIDs such as ketorolac, and antiemetics such as H₂ blockers. Each has a use in anesthetic procedures, as well as a therapeutic indication in other aspects of health care. Adjuncts to anesthesia are used before anesthetic as premedications and during anesthesia to intensify anesthetic effects or to reduce the amount of anesthetic needed. Premedications are given to reduce anxiety, sedate the patient, and reduce oral and respiratory secretions. Opioid analgesics, sedatives and hypnotics, phenothiazines, anticholinergics, and antianxiety agents are common premedications. Neuromuscular blocking agents are given to produce paralysis of the skeletal muscles during the surgical procedure. These agents are of two kinds: depolarizing and nondepolarizing. The only depolarizing agent, succinylcholine, acts by depolarizing the postsynaptic membranes at the neuromuscular junction, rendering them refractory to stimulation and producing muscle paralysis. Nondepolarizing agents such as vecuronium, rocuronium, atracurium, mivacurium, and pancuronium act by competing with acetylcholine for occupation of postsynaptic receptors at the neuromuscular junction,

thus producing skeletal muscle paralysis. The use of these agents requires controlled respiration and a careful evaluation of the recovery of neuromuscular transmission before emergence from anesthesia and in the postoperative period.

**adjustable axis face-bow.** See **kinematic face-bow.**

**adjustable orthodontic band** /adjus'təbəl/, a thin metal ring, usually made of stainless steel, equipped with an adjusting screw to allow alteration in size, that is fitted to a tooth and allows the attachment of orthodontic appliances. See also **orthodontic band.**

**adjusted death rate.** See **standardized death rate.**

**adjustment.** See **accommodation.**

**adjustment disorder** [L, adjuxtare, to bring together], a temporary disorder of varying severity that occurs as an acute reaction to overwhelming stress in persons of any age who have no apparent underlying mental disorders. Symptoms include anxiety, withdrawal, depression, brooding, impulsive outbursts, crying spells, attention-seeking behavior, enuresis, loss of appetite, aches, pains, and muscle spasms. It can be persistent if symptoms continue for six months or more. It can develop in response to an identifiable stressor and result from such situations as separation of an infant from its mother, the birth of a sibling, loss or change of job, death of a loved one, or forced retirement. Symptoms usually recede and eventually disappear as stress diminishes. See also **anxiety disorder.**

**adjustment, impaired,** a nursing diagnosis accepted by the Seventh National Conference on the Classification of Nursing Diagnoses (revised 1998). Impaired adjustment is a state in which the individual is unable to modify his or her life-style or behavior in a manner consistent with a change in health status.

■ DEFINING CHARACTERISTICS: The defining characteristics include a denial of health status change, a failure to achieve optimal sense of control, a failure to take actions that would prevent further health problems and a demonstration of nonacceptance of health status change.

■ RELATED FACTORS: Related factors include a disability requiring a change in life-style; lack of motivation to change; multiple stressors; absence of social support for changed beliefs and practices; intense emotional state; low state of optimism; negative attitudes towards health behavior; and failure to intend to change behavior. See also **nursing diagnosis.**

**adjuvant** /ad'jəvənt/ [L, ad + juvare, to help], 1. a substance, especially a drug, added to a prescription to assist in the action of the main ingredient. 2. (in immunology) a substance added to an antigen that enhances or modifies the antibody response to the antigen. 3. an additional treatment or therapy.

**adjuvant chemotherapy,** the use of anticancer drugs after or in combination with another form of cancer treatment, as after apparently complete surgical removal of a cancer. The method is used when there is a significant risk that undetected cancer cells may still be present. Adjuvant chemotherapy is most commonly used in treating breast cancer.

**adjuvant therapy,** the treatment of a disease with substances that enhance the action of drugs, especially drugs that promote the production of antibodies.

**ADL,** abbreviation for **activities of daily living.**

**adlerian psychology** [Alfred Adler, Viennese psychiatrist, 1870–1937], a branch of psychoanalysis that focuses on physical security, sexual satisfaction, and social integration. See also **individual psychology.**

**ad lib,** abbreviation of the Latin phrase ad libitum, meaning to be taken as desired.

**administration of parenteral fluids** /admin'istrā'shən/,

the IV infusion of various solutions to maintain adequate hydration, restore and/or maintain fluid volume, reestablish lost electrolytes, or provide partial nutrition. See **parenteral.**

■ METHOD: Fluid is administered parenterally through a closed system consisting of a bottle or bag of sterile solution and tubing which has been attached to an intracatheter or butterfly needle that is inserted into a peripheral vein and securely taped to the patient's arm, leg, or scalp. The fluid is infused at a rate appropriate to the client's clinical condition. Five percent dextrose in distilled water may be used to maintain volume and provide nutrients; ascorbic acid and B vitamins are often added to the solution. Five percent dextrose in saline solution plus potassium chloride may be infused to reestablish electrolyte balance, but potassium is contraindicated in renal failure and untreated adrenal insufficiency. A one-sixth molar lactate solution may be administered if sodium is deficient, and an ammonium chloride solution may be administered when chloride must be replaced. Distilled water containing 10% to 20% glucose or fructose may be used to supply carbohydrate, but, because these solutions are hypertonic, additional hydration is needed for proper excretion. Low-molecular-weight dextran is frequently used as a plasma volume expander in treating shock, but it increases bleeding time and is contraindicated in pregnancy and severe renal disease. During parenteral fluid administration, the venipuncture site is observed every 1 to 2 hours for signs of infiltration, which is evidenced by localized swelling, coolness, pallor, and discomfort at the site; for the patient's complaints of pain or discomfort; for the security and comfort of the tape; and for the position of the patient's extremity. The flow rate, level, color, and clarity of the fluid; the label; and the patency of the tubing and needle are checked, and the patient is monitored for signs of dehydration, fever, and signs of circulatory overload, such as headache, tachycardia, elevated blood pressure, weight gain, dyspnea, engorged neck veins, and pulmonary edema. The patient is also monitored for signs and symptoms of phlebitis: redness, warmth, and swelling at the IV site and burning pain along the vein.

■ INTERVENTIONS: Depending on the purpose and patient's specific condition, the nurse may select the necessary equipment, prepare the venipuncture site, check the labels of fluid bottles for content, and perform the venipuncture. During fluid administration, the nurse keeps the system closed, watches the flow rate, records the amount of solution given, and observes the venipuncture site and the patient's general condition. If there are any signs of increased blood volume, the nurse reduces the flow of the infusion until further orders are obtained. The nurse changes the dressing according to institutional protocol and ensures that the patient understands the importance of not disturbing the tubing, of reporting pain or swelling, of avoiding sudden twisting or turning movements of the extremity, and of reporting pain or swelling at the IV site or blood in the IV tubing.

■ OUTCOME CRITERIA: Parenteral fluid therapy is usually uneventful. Patients requiring special attention include infants, elderly patients with circulatory or renal impairment or confusion, and burn patients, whose plasma may shift suddenly from interstitial tissue, causing increased blood volume.

**Administration on Aging (AOA),** the principal U.S. agency designated to carry out the provisions of the Older Americans Act of 1965. The AOA advises the U.S. Secretary of the Department of Health and Human Services and other federal departments and agencies on the characteristics and needs of older people and develops programs designed to promote their welfare.

**admission,** **1.** the act of being received into a place or class of things. **2.** a patient accepted for inpatient service in a hospital. **3.** a concession or acknowledgment.

**admission care,** a nursing intervention from the Nursing Interventions Classification (NIC) defined as facilitating entry of a patient into a health care facility. See also **Nursing Interventions Classification.**

**ADN,** abbreviation for **Associate Degree in Nursing.**

**ad nauseam** [L, *ad,* to; Gk, *nausia,* seasickness], to the extent of inducing nausea and vomiting.

**adneural** /adnoo′əl/, **1.** located near or toward a nerve or nerve ending. **2.** pertaining to the stage of a nervous disorder in which the symptoms are apparent. Also **adnerval.**

**adnexa** /adnek′sa/, *sing.* **adnexus** [L, *adnectere,* to tie together], tissue or structures in the body that are adjacent to or near another, related structure. The ovaries and the uterine tubes are adnexa of the uterus. Also called **annexa.** —**adnexal,** *adj.*

**adnexal** [L, *adnectere,* to tie together], pertaining to accessory organs or tissues, as in the relationship of the fallopian tubes and uterus.

**adnexa oculi,** the accessory organs of the eye: the eyelids, lashes, eyebrows, conjunctival sac, lacrimal apparatus, and extrinsic muscles of the eye.

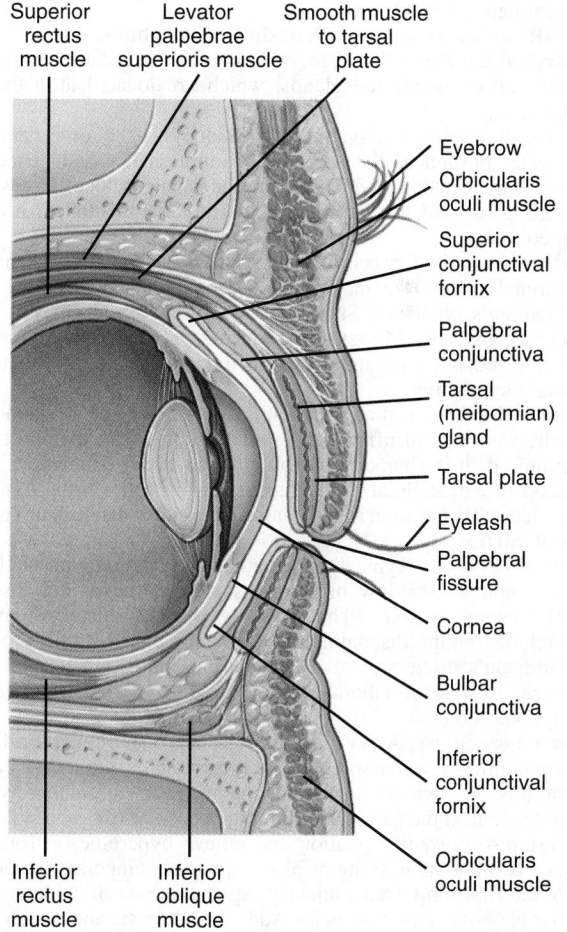

Superior rectus muscle — Levator palpebrae superioris muscle — Smooth muscle to tarsal plate — Eyebrow — Orbicularis oculi muscle — Superior conjunctival fornix — Palpebral conjunctiva — Tarsal (meibomian) gland — Tarsal plate — Eyelash — Palpebral fissure — Cornea — Bulbar conjunctiva — Inferior conjunctival fornix — Orbicularis oculi muscle — Inferior rectus muscle — Inferior oblique muscle

**Adnexa oculi** *(Thibodeau and Patton, 1999/Barbara Cousins)*

**adnexa uteri,** the uterine appendages: the ovaries, fallopian tubes, and associated ligaments.

**adnexectomy** /ad'neksek'təmē/ [Gk, *ektomē,* excision], surgical removal of accessory structures.

**adnexitis** /ad'neksī'tis/, an inflammation of the adnexal organs of the uterus, such as the ovaries or the fallopian tubes.

**adnexopexy** /adnek'sōpek'sē/, a surgical procedure in which the fallopian tubes and ovaries are elevated and sutured to the abdominal wall.

**adnexus.** See **adnexa.**

**-adol,** combining form designating an analgesic.

**adolescence** /ad'əles'əns/ [L, *adolescere,* to grow up], **1.** the period in development between the onset of puberty and adulthood. It usually begins between 11 and 13 years of age, with the appearance of secondary sex characteristics, and spans the teenage years, terminating at 18 to 20 years of age with the completion of the development of the adult form. During this period the individual undergoes extensive physical, psychologic, emotional, and personality changes. **2.** the state or quality of being adolescent or youthful. See also **postpuberty, prepuberty, psychosexual development, psychosocial development, pubarche.**

**adolescent,** **1.** pertaining to characteristic of adolescence. **2.** one in the state or process of adolescence; a teenager.

**adolescent vertebral epiphysitis.** See **Scheuermann's disease.**

**adoption** /ədop'shən/ [L, *adoptere,* to choose], a selection and inclusion in an established relationship or a choice of treatment protocol.

**ADP,** abbreviation for **adenosine diphosphate.**

**adrenal** /ədrē'nəl/ [L, *ad,* to, *ren,* kidney], pertaining to the adrenal, or suprarenal glands, which are located atop the kidneys.

**adrenal cortex** [L, *ad,* to, *ren,* kidney], the outer and greater portion of the adrenal, or suprarenal, gland, fused with the gland's medulla. It produces mineralocorticoids, androgens, and glucocorticoids, hormones essential to homeostasis.

**adrenal cortical carcinoma,** a malignant neoplasm of the adrenal cortex that may cause adrenogenital syndrome or Cushing's syndrome. Such tumors vary in size and may occur at any age. Metastases frequently occur in the lungs, liver, and other organs. See also **adrenal virilism, Cushing's syndrome.**

**adrenal crisis,** an acute, life-threatening state of profound adrenocortical insufficiency in which immediate therapy is required. It is characterized by glucocorticoid deficiency, a drop in extracellular fluid volume, and hyperkalemia. Also called **addisonian crisis.** See also **Addison's disease, adrenal cortex.**

■ OBSERVATIONS: Typically, the patient appears to be in shock or coma with a low blood pressure, weakness, and loss of vasomotor tone. The person's medical history may include abrupt discontinuation of exogenous steroids or Addison's disease or reveal symptoms indicating its presence. Results of laboratory tests show hyperkalemia and hyponatremia.

■ INTERVENTIONS: An IV isotonic solution of sodium chloride containing a water-soluble glucocorticoid is administered rapidly. Vasopressor agents may be necessary to combat hypotension. If the patient is vomiting, a nasogastric tube is inserted to prevent aspiration and relieve hyperemesis. Total bed rest and monitoring of blood pressure, temperature, and other vital signs are mandatory. After the first critical hours, the patient is followed as for Addison's disease, and corticosteroid dosage is tapered to maintenance levels. Infection and a failure to increase the maintenance glucocorticoid

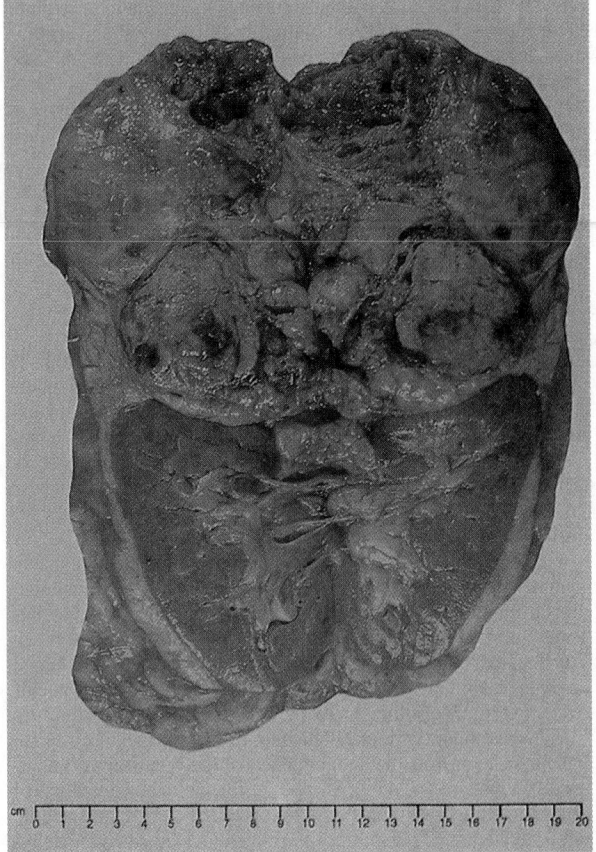

**Adrenal cortical carcinoma**
*(Silverberg, DeLellis, and Frable, 1997)*

(steroid) dose are common causes of crisis in people who have Addison's disease.

■ NURSING CONSIDERATIONS: Nursing care during adrenal crisis includes eliminating all forms of stimuli, especially loud noises or bright lights. The patient is not moved unless absolutely necessary and is not allowed to perform self-care activities. If the condition is identified and treated promptly, the prognosis is good. Discharge instructions include a reminder to the patient to seek medical attention in any stressful situation, whether physiologic or psychologic, to prevent a recurrence of the crisis.

**adrenalectomy** /ədrē'nəlek'təmē/ [L, *ad* + *ren* + Gk, *ektomē,* excision], the total or partial surgical resection of one or both adrenal glands. It is performed to reduce the excessive secretion of adrenal hormones caused by an adrenal tumor or a malignancy of the breast or prostate. The incision is made under the twelfth rib in the rear flank area with the patient under general anesthesia. Preoperative laboratory tests include electrolytes, fasting blood glucose, glucose tolerance, and fluid states and adrenergic and blockade if needed. Hemodynamic monitoring and preoperative steroid replacement are performed. Before surgery a nasogastric tube may be inserted. Careful intraoperative positioning is necessary for the patient with Cushing's syndrome because of osteoporosis, fragile bone, and muscle wasting. In patients with pheochromocytoma, intraoperative manipulation of an adrenal tumor can cause a surge of catecholemines, resulting in a blood pressure increase. Postoperative care focuses on maintaining blood pressure with vasopressors or vasodilators as needed, giving replacement doses of corticosteroids, and monitoring fluid and electrolyte status. When both glands are removed, the maintenance dosage of steroids continues for life. Stress and fatigue must be avoided. See also **Addison's disease, Cushing's syndrome, pheochromocytoma.**

**adrenal gland,** either of two secretory organs perched atop the kidneys and surrounded by the protective fat capsule of the kidneys. Each consists of two parts having independent functions: the cortex and the medulla. The adrenal cortex, in response to adrenocorticotropic hormone secreted by the anterior pituitary, secretes cortisol and androgens. Adrenal androgens serve as precursors that are converted by the liver to testosterone and estrogens. Renin from the kidney controls adrenal cortical production of aldosterone. The adrenal medulla manufactures the catecholamines epinephrine and norepinephrine. Also called **suprarenal gland.**

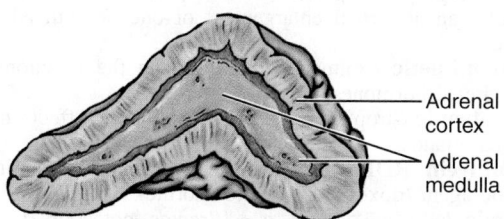

**Cross section of the adrenal gland**
(Herlihy and Maebius, 2000)

**Adrenalin,** trademark for an adrenergic (epinephrine).

**adrenaline.** See **epinephrine.**

**adrenal insufficiency** [L, *ad,* to, *ren,* kidney, *in,* not, *sufficere,* to suffice], a condition in which the adrenal gland is unable to produce adequate amounts of cortical hormones. See also **Addison's disease.**

**adrenalize** /ədrē′nəlīz/, to stimulate or excite.

**adrenal medulla,** the inner portion of the adrenal gland. Adrenal medulla cells secrete epinephrine and norepinephrine when stimulated by the sympathetic division of the autonomic nervous system. See also **adrenal cortex.**

**adrenal virilism,** a condition characterized by hypersecretion of adrenal androgens, resulting in somatic masculinization. Excessive production of the hormone may be caused by a virilizing adrenal tumor, congenital adrenal hyperplasia, or an inborn deficiency of enzymes required to transform endogenous androgenic steroids to glucocorticoids. Girls born with adrenogenitalism may be pseudohermaphroditic with clitoral enlargement and labial fusion in infancy and later have low vocal pitch, acne, amenorrhea, and masculine distribution of hair and muscle development. Boys with congenital adrenogenitalism show precocious development of the penis, the prostate, and pubic and axillary hair; but their testes remain small and immature because negative feedback from the high level of adrenal androgens prevents the normal pubertal increase in pituitary gonadotropin. Children with the disorder are unusually tall, but their epiphyses close prematurely, and as adults they are abnormally short.

Virilizing tumors are more common or more frequently diagnosed in women. They usually occur between 30 and 40 years of age but may arise later, after the menopause. Signs of the tumor in women include hirsutism, amenorrhea, oily skin, ovarian changes, muscular hypertrophy, and atrophy of the uterus and breasts. Treatment may involve tumor resection, cortisol administration, and cosmetic surgical procedures. Electrolytic hair removal may be indicated. Also called **adrenogenital syndrome.** See also **congenital adrenal hyperplasia, pseudohermaphroditism, virilization.**

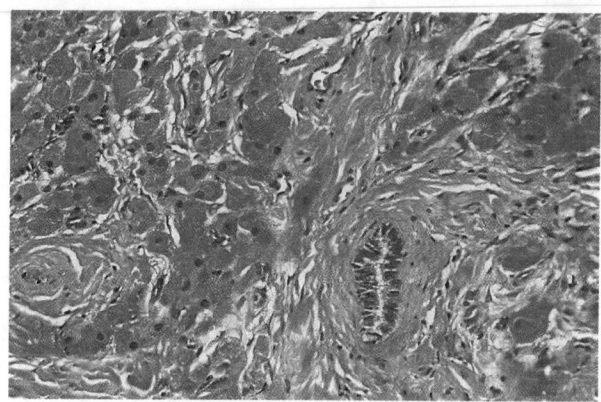

**Adrenal virilism** (Fletcher, 2000)

**adrenarche** /ad′rinär′kē/ [L, *ad* + *ren* + Gk, *arche,* beginning], the intensified activity in the adrenal cortex that occurs at about 8 years of age and increases the elaboration of various hormones, especially androgens.

**adrenergic** /ad′rinur′jik/ [L, *ad* + *ren;* Gk, *ergon,* work], pertaining to sympathetic nerve fibers of the autonomic nervous system that liberate norepinephrine at a synapse where a nerve impulse passes. Compare **cholinergic.** See also **sympathomimetic.**

**adrenergic blocking agent.** See **antiadrenergic.**

**adrenergic bronchodilator,** a drug that acts on the beta-2 sympathetic nervous system receptors to relax bronchial smooth muscle cells. Examples include drugs that contain epinephrine, ephedrine, isoproterenol, or albuterol.

**adrenergic drug.** See **sympathomimetic.**

**adrenergic fibers,** nerve fibers of the autonomic nervous system that release the neurotransmitter norepinephrine and, in some areas, dopamine. Most postganglionic sympathetic nerve fibers are of this type.

**adrenergic receptor** [L, *ad* + *ren,* kidney; Gk, *ergon,* work; L, *recipere,* to receive], a site in a sympathetic effector cell that reacts to adrenergic stimulation. Two types of adrenergic receptors are recognized: **alpha-adrenergic,** which act in response to sympathomimetic stimuli, and **beta-adrenergic,** which block sympathomimetic activity. In general, stimulation of alpha receptors is excitatory of the function of the host organ or tissue, and stimulation of the beta receptors is inhibitory.

**-adrenia,** combining form meaning '(degree or condition of) adrenal activity': *anadrenia, hypadrenia.*

**adrenocortical** /-kôr′tikəl/ [L, *ad* + *ren* + *cortex,* bark], pertaining to the outer or superficial portion of the adrenal gland.

**adrenocortical hormone (ACH)** [L, *ad,* to, *ren,* kidney, *cortex,* bark; Gk, *hormaein,* to set in motion], any of the hormones secreted by the cortex of the adrenal gland, including the glucocorticoids, mineralocorticoids, and androgens.

**adrenocorticotrophic hormone.** See **adrenocorticotropic hormone.**

**adrenocorticotropic** /ədrē′nōkôr′tikōtrop′ik/ [L, *ad* + *ren* + *cortex,* bark; Gk, *trope,* a turning], pertaining to stimulation of the adrenal cortex. Also **adrenocorticotrophic** /-trof′ik/.

**adrenocorticotropic hormone (ACTH),** a hormone of the anterior pituitary gland that stimulates the growth of the adrenal gland cortex and the secretion of corticosteroids. ACTH secretion, regulated by corticotropin releasing hormone (CRH) from the hypothalamus, increases in response to a low level of circulating cortisol and to stress, fever, acute hypoglycemia, and major surgery. Under normal conditions a diurnal rhythm occurs in ACTH secretion, with an increase beginning after the first few hours of sleep and reaching a peak at the time a person awakens and a low in the evening. A purified preparation of ACTH in capsules is widely used in the treatment of rheumatoid arthritis, acquired hemolytic anemia, intractable allergic states, various dermatologic diseases, and many other disorders. Normal of ranges are from 15 to 100 pg/ml or 10 to 80 ng/L in the AM to less than 50 pg/ml or 50 ng/L in the PM. Also called **adrenocorticotrophic hormone, corticotropin.**

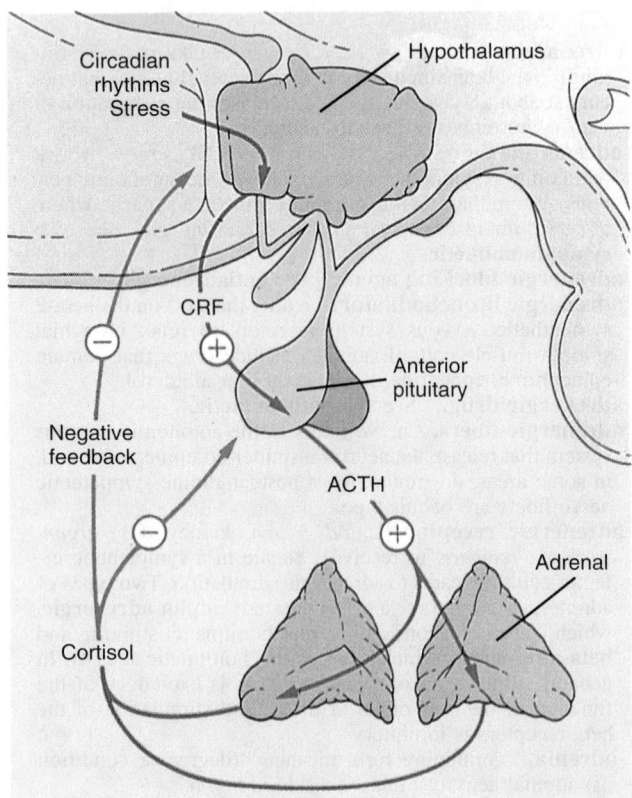

**Feedback regulation of ACTH** *(Zitelli and Davis, 1997)*

Circadian rhythms
Stress
Hypothalamus
CRF
Anterior pituitary
Negative feedback
ACTH
Adrenal
Cortisol

**adrenocorticotropic hormone test,** a blood test used to study the anterior pituitary gland's functioning by measuring cortisol levels. The test is used to diagnose Cushing's syndrome and Addison's disease, which are characterized by overproduction and underproduction of cortisol, respectively.

**adrenocorticotropin** /-trop′in/, the adrenocorticotropic hormone **(ACTH)** secreted by the anterior pituitary gland that stimulates secretion of other hormones by the adrenal cortex.

**adrenodoxin** /ədrē′nōdok′sin/, a nonheme iron protein, produced by the adrenal glands, that participates in the transfer of electrons within animal cells.

**adrenogenital syndrome.** See **adrenal virilism.**

**adrenoleukodystrophy (ALD),** a rare hereditary childhood metabolic disease that is transmitted as a recessive sex-linked trait and affects mainly males. It is characterized by adrenal atrophy and widespread cerebral demyelination, producing progressive mental deterioration, aphasia, apraxia, eventual blindness and quadriplegia. Prognosis is poor, with death occurring usually in 1 to 5 years. ALD was formerly classified under Schilder's disease.

**adrenomegaly** /-meg′əlē/ [L, *ad* + *ren* + Gk, *megaly,* large], an abnormal enlargement of one or both adrenal glands.

**adrenomimetic** /-mimet′ik/, mimicking the functions of the adrenal hormones.

**adrenotropic** /-trop′ik/, having a stimulating effect on the adrenal glands.

**Adriamycin RDF,** trademark for an antibiotic antineoplastic agent (doxorubicin hydrochloride).

**adromia** /ədrō′mē·ə/ [Gk, *a* + *dromos,* not course], the absence of the conductive capacity of any nerve that normally innervates a muscle.

**Adrucil,** trademark for an antineoplastic (fluorouracil).

**ADRV,** abbreviation for **adult rotavirus.**

**ADS,** abbreviation for **antidiuretic substance.**

**Adson's maneuver** [Alfred W. Adson, American surgeon, 1887–1951], a test for the thoracic outlet syndrome. It is performed with the patient sitting with hands on the thighs. The examiner palpates both radial pulses as the patient takes a deep breath and holds it while extending the neck and turning the head toward the affected side. If the radial pulse on the affected side is significantly diminished or there is numbness or tingling in the hand, the result is regarded as positive. Also called **Adson's test.**

**adsorb,** to attract and hold other material on the surface.

**adsorbent** /adsôr′bənt/, a substance that takes up another by the process of adsorption, as by the attachment of one substance to the surface of the other.

**adsorption** /adsôrp′shən/ [L, *ad* + *sorbere,* to suck in], a natural process whereby molecules of a gas or liquid adhere to the surface of a solid. The phenomenon depends on an assortment of factors such as surface tension and electrical charges. Many biologic reactions involve adsorption. In chemistry, adsorption is the principle on which chromatography is based and which allows for the separation of a mixture into component fractions for qualitative analysis. See also **chromatography.**

**ADT,** abbreviation for *Accepted Dental Therapeutics,* a journal published by the Council on Dental Therapeutics of the American Dental Association.

**adult** /ədult′, ad′ult/ [L, *adultus,* grown up], **1.** one who is fully developed and matured and who has attained the intellectual capacity and the emotional and psychologic stability characteristic of a mature person. **2.** a person who has reached full legal age. Compare **child. 3.** any fully grown and mature organism.

**adult celiac disease.** See **celiac disease.**

**adult ceroid-lipofuscinosis.** See **Kufs' disease.**

**adult day-care center,** a facility for the supervised care of older adults, providing such activities as meals and socialization one or more days a week during specified daytime hours. The participants, primarily persons with physical and/or mental problems who need socialization, physical assistance, and/or physical assistance, return to their homes each evening. The program is often used as respite by family members caring for an older person who cannot be left alone safely in the home.

**adult ego state,** (in psychiatry) a part of the self that analyzes and solves problems, using information received from the parent ego and child ego states. It is assumed to be fully developed in a normal individual at the age of 12. The term is used in transactional analysis.

**adulteration** /ədul′tərā′shən/ [L, *adulterare,* to defile], the debasement or dilution of the purity of any substance, process, or activity by the addition of extraneous material.

**adult hemoglobin.** See **hemoglobin A.**

**adulthood,** the phase of development characterized by physical and mental maturity.

**adult nurse practitioner,** a registered nurse who has received additional education in the primary health care of adults. The additional education may be obtained through a master's degree program or a nondegree-granting continuing education certificate program.

**adult-onset diabetes.** See **type 2 diabetes mellitus.**

**adult polycystic disease.** See **polycystic kidney disease.**

**adult respiratory distress syndrome (ARDS),** severe pulmonary congestion characterized by diffuse injury to alveolar-capillary membranes. Fulminating sepsis, especially when gram-negative bacteria are involved, is the most common cause. ARDS may occur after trauma; neardrowning; aspiration of gastric acid; paraquat ingestion; inhalation of corrosive chemicals, such as chlorine, ammonia, or phosgene; or use of certain drugs, including barbiturates, chlordiazepoxide, heroin, methadone, propoxyphene, and salicylates. Other causes include diabetic ketoacidosis, fungal infections, high altitude, pancreatitis, tuberculosis, and uremia. Also called **acute respiratory distress syndrome, congestive atelectasis, hemorrhagic lung, noncardiogenic pulmonary edema, pump lung, shock lung, stiff lung, wet lung.** See also **chronic obstructive pulmonary disease.**

■ OBSERVATIONS: Signs and symptoms of ARDS include breathlessness, dyspnea, tachypnea, hypoxemia, and decreased lung compliance. Changes occurring within the lung include damage to the alveolar-capillary membranes, leakage of plasma proteins into the alveoli, dilution of surfactant, cessation of surfactant production, hemorrhage, interstitial edema, impaired gas exchange, and ventilation-perfusion abnormalities.

■ INTERVENTIONS: Treatment includes establishing an airway, administering oxygen, improving the underlying condition, removing the cause of ARDS, suctioning the respiratory passages as necessary, and reducing oxygen consumption. When ventilation cannot be maintained and there is evidence of a rising $PaCO_2$, mechanical ventilation is necessary. PEEP is widely used in the treatment of ARDS. All interventions for ARDS are supportive; there is no cure.

■ NURSING CONSIDERATIONS: The patient with ARDS requires constant and meticulous care, reassurance, and observation for changes in respiratory function and adequacy, including signs of hypercapnia, hypoxemia, especially confusion, skin flushing, and behavior changes such as agitation and restlessness. Increasing hypoxia may be signaled by tachycardia, elevated blood pressure, increased peripheral resistance, and fulminant respiratory failure. If PEEP is being used, the patient is carefully observed for a sudden disappearance of breath sounds accompanied by signs of respiratory distress—an indication that pneumothorax may be present. Respiratory therapy, sterile suction techniques, and position changes are continued as necessary. The patient's weight is measured frequently, chest x-ray films are evaluated, and bacteriologic cultures of secretions are analyzed for the causative organism. Throughout treatment, ventilation is carefully monitored through analysis of arterial blood gases.

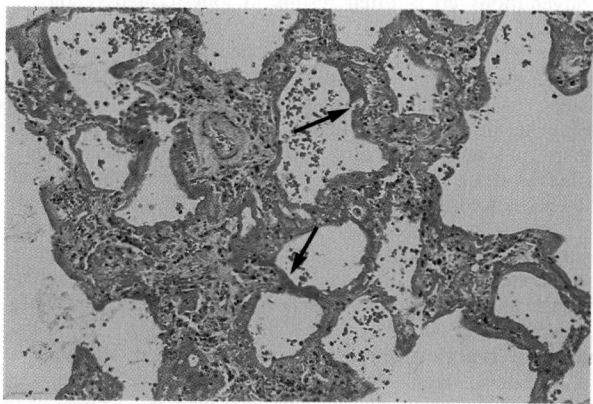

**Adult respiratory distress syndrome:
diffuse alveolar damage**
*(Kumar, Cotran, and Robbins, 1997)*

**adult rickets.** See **osteomalacia.**

**adult rotavirus (ADRV),** a form of rotavirus that causes severe diarrhea in adults. The virus resembles the usual rotavirus and its genome, but it is not antigenically related and does not react against rotavirus antibodies. ADRV antibodies have been found in adults in China and Australia. See also **rotavirus.**

**advanced cardiac life support (ACLS),** emergency medical procedures in which basic life support efforts of cardiopulmonary resuscitation are augmented by establishment of an IV fluid line, possible defibrillation, drug administration, control of cardiac arrhythmias, endotracheal intubation, and use of ventilation equipment.

**advance directive** [Fr, *avancer,* to move forward; L, *dirigere,* to direct], an advance declaration by a person of treatment preferences if he or she is unable to communicate his or her wishes. See **durable power of attorney for health care** and **living will.**

**advanced life support (ALS),** a higher level of emergency medical care, usually provided by EMT-intermediates or paramedics. Typically ALS includes invasive techniques such as IV therapy, intubation, and/or drug administration.

**advanced practice nurse (APN),** a nurse with a master's degree in nursing, advanced education in pharmacology and physical assessment, and certification and expertise in a specialized area of practice. An APN usually works in a critical, acute, restorative, or community health care agency.

**advancement** /advans′/ [Fr, *avancer,* to move forward], a surgical technique in which a muscle or tendon is drawn forward.

**adventitia** /ad'ventish'ə/ [L, *adventitius,* coming from abroad], the outermost layer, composed of connective tissue with elastic and collagenous fibers, of an artery or other structure.

**adventitious** [L, *adventitius,* from outside sources], **1.** pertaining to an accidental condition or an arbitrary action. **2.** not hereditary. **3.** occurring at an inappropriate place, such as a coating on an artery.

**adventitious bursa,** an abnormal bursa that develops as a response to friction or pressure.

**adventitious crisis,** a rare accidental and unexpected tragedy that may affect an entire community or population, such as an earthquake, flood, or airplane crash. In addition to injuries, loss of life, and property damage, an adventitious crisis often results in long-term psychologic effects.

**adventitious sound,** a breath sound that is not normally heard, such as a crackle, gurgle, or wheeze. It may be superimposed on normal breath sounds.

**adverse drug effect** /advurs', ad'vers/, an unintended harmful reaction to a drug administered at normal dosage.

**adverse drug reaction** any harmful effect on the body of therapeutic drugs, drugs of abuse, or the interaction of two or more pharmacologically active agents within a short time span. Drugs most likely to cause adverse reactions include hypnotics, central nervous system stimulants, antidepressants, tranquilizers, and muscle relaxants. Also called **drug reaction.**

**adverse reaction,** any harmful, unintended effect of a medication, diagnostic test, or therapeutic intervention.

**advocacy** /ad'vəkas'ē/, **1.** a process whereby a nurse provides a patient with the information to make certain decisions. **2.** a method by which patients, their families, attorneys, health professionals, and citizen groups can work together to develop programs that ensure the availability of high-quality health care for a community. **3.** pleading a cause on behalf of another, such as a nurse pleading for better care of a patient.

**adynamia** /ad'inā'mē-ə/ [Gk, *a* + *dynamis,* not strength], lack of physical strength resulting from a pathologic condition. See also **asthenia. —adynamic,** *adj.*

**adynamia episodica hereditaria,** a condition seen in infancy, characterized by periodic muscle weakness and episodes of flaccid paralysis. It is inherited as an autosomal dominant trait. Also called **hyperkalemic periodic paralysis.**

**adynamic.** See **adynamia.**

**adynamic fever,** an elevated temperature with a feeble pulse, and cool, moist skin. Also called **asthenic fever.**

**adynamic ileus.** See **ileus, paralytic ileus.**

**AE,** abbreviation for *above the elbow* amputation. A short AE amputation (near the shoulder) results in the loss of shoulder rotation. After a long AE amputation (just above the elbow) the patient should retain good shoulder function.

**AEC syndrome.** See **Hay-Wells syndrome.**

*Aedes* /ā·ē'dēz/ [Gk, *aedes,* unpleasant], a genus of mosquito, prevalent in tropical and subtropical regions. Several species are capable of transmitting pathogenic organisms to humans, including dengue, equine encephalitis, St. Louis encephalitis, tularemia, and yellow fever.

**-aemia.** See **-emia.**

**aequator.** See **equator.**

**aer-.** See **aero-.**

**aerate** /er'āt/ [Gk, *aer,* air], to charge a substance or a structure with air, carbon dioxide, or oxygen.

**aeration** [Gk, *aer,* air], **1.** exchange of carbon dioxide for oxygen by blood in the lungs. **2.** the process of exposing a tissue or fluid to air or artificially charging it with oxygen or another gas, such as carbon dioxide.

**aero-, aer-,** combining form meaning 'air or gas': *aerobe, aerate.*

*Aerobacter aerogenes.* See *Enterobacter cloacae.*

**aerobe** /er'ōb/ [Gk, *aer* + *bios,* life], a microorganism that lives and grows in the presence of free oxygen. An aerobe may be **facultative** or **obligate.** Compare **anaerobe, microaerophile.**

**aerobic** /erō'bik/, **1.** pertaining to the presence of air or oxygen. **2.** able to live and function in the presence of free oxygen. **3.** requiring oxygen for the maintenance of life.

**aerobic capacity.** See **maximum oxygen uptake.**

**aerobic exercise,** any physical exercise that requires additional effort by the heart and lungs to meet the skeletal muscles' increased demand for oxygen. Aerobic exercise increases the breathing rate and ultimately raises heart and lung efficiency. Prolonged aerobic exercises (at least 20 minutes three times per week) is recommended for the maintenance of a healthy cardiovascular system. Examples of aerobic exercise include running, jogging, swimming, and vigorous dancing or cycling. Also called **aerobics.** See also **active exercise, passive exercise.**

**aerobic glycolysis.** See **glycolysis.**

**aerobics.** See **aerobic exercise.**

**aerodermectasia.** See **subcutaneous emphysema.**

**aerodontalgia** /er'ōdontal'jə/ [Gk, *aer* + *odous,* tooth, *algos,* pain], a painful sensation in the teeth caused by a change in atmospheric pressure, as may occur at high altitudes.

**aerodynamics,** the study of air or other gases in motion or of bodies moving in air.

**aerodynamic size,** pertaining to the behavior of various aerosol particle sizes and densities.

**aeroembolism.** See **air embolism.**

*Aeromonas* /er'ōmō'nəs/, a genus of pathogenic rod-shaped gram-negative bacteria found in fresh and salt water and also soil and sewage. Various species affect fish and animals as well as humans, causing wound infections and gastroenteritis.

**aerophagy** /erof'əjē/ [Gk, *aer* + *phagein,* to eat], the swallowing of air, usually followed by belching, gastric distress, and flatulence. Also called **aerophagia** /er'ōfā'jē-ə/.

**aerosinusitis** /er'ōsī'nəsī'tis/ [Gk, *aer* + L, *sinus,* curve; Gk, *itis*], inflammation, edema, or hemorrhage of the frontal sinuses, caused by expansion of air within the sinuses when barometric pressure is decreased, as in aircraft at high altitudes. Also called **barosinusitis.**

**aerosol** /er'əsol'/ [Gk, *aer*; L, *solutus,* dissolved], **1.** nebulized particles suspended in a gas or air. **2.** a pressurized gas containing a finely nebulized medication for inhalation therapy. **3.** a pressurized gas containing a nebulized chemical agent for sterilizing the air of a room.

**aerosol bronchodilator therapy,** the use of drugs that relax the respiratory tract smooth muscle tissue when administered as tiny droplets or a mist to be inhaled.

**aerospace medicine** /er'ōspās/, a branch of medicine concerned with the physiologic and psychologic effects of living and working in an artificial environment beyond the atmospheric and gravitational forces of the earth. The stress of extraterrestrial travel requiring long periods of weightlessness is a major concern. See also **aviation medicine.**

**Aerosporin,** trademark for an antibiotic (polymyxin B sulfate).

**aerotherapy** /er'ōther'əpē/, the use of air in treating disease, as in hyperbaric oxygen treatments.

**aerotitis** /er'ətī'tis/ [Gk, *aer* + *otikos,* ear, *itis*], an inflammation of the ear caused by changes in atmospheric pressure. Also called **barotitis.**

**aerotitis media,** inflammation or bleeding in the middle ear caused by a difference between the air pressure in the middle ear and that of the atmosphere, as occurs in sudden changes in altitude, in scuba diving, and in hyperbaric chambers. Symptoms are pain, tinnitus, diminished hearing, and vertigo. Also called **barotitis media.**

**Æsculapius** /es'kyo͞olā'pē-əs/, the ancient Greek god of medicine. According to legend, Æsculapius, the son of Apollo, was trained by the centaur Chiron in the art of healing; he became so proficient that he not only cured sick patients but also restored the dead to life. Because Zeus feared that Æsculapius could help humans escape death altogether, he killed the healer with a bolt of lightning. Later, Æsculapius was raised to the stature of a god and was worshipped also by the Romans, who believed he could prevent pestilence. Serpents were regarded as sacred by Æsculapius, and he is symbolized in modern medicine by a staff with a serpent entwined about it. See **staff of Æsculapius.**

**aesthesia.** See **esthesia.**

**-aesthesia, -esthesia,** suffix meaning '(condition of) feeling, perception, or sensation': *allaesthesia, hypercrysaesthesia.*

**-aesthetic.** See **-esthetic.**

**aesthetics.** See **esthetics.**

**AF,** 1. abbreviation for **atrial fibrillation.** 2. abbreviation for **atrial flutter.**

**af-.** See **ad-.**

**AFB,** abbreviation for **acid-fast bacillus.**

**afebrile** /āfē'bril, āfeb'ril/ [Gk, *a* + *febris,* not fever], without fever.

**affect** /əfekt'/ [L, *affectus* influence], an outward, observable manifestation of a person's expressed feelings or emotions, such as bland or bright. —**affective,** *adj.*

**affection** /əfek'shən/ [L, *affectus,* influence], 1. an emotional state expressed as by a warm or caring feeling toward another individual. 2. a morbid process affecting all or a part of the human body.

**affective** /əfek'tiv/ [L, *affectus*], pertaining to emotion, mood, or feeling.

**affective disorder.** See **mood disorder.**

**affective intimacy,** a measure of well-being in a family group that focuses on whether members feel close to one another yet do not lose their individuality.

**affective learning,** the acquisition of behaviors involved in expressing feelings in attitudes, appreciations, and values.

**affective melancholia** [L, *affectus,* influence; Gk, *melas,* black, *chole,* bile], a form of severe depression characterized by a lack of interest in normally pleasant activities. The condition may occur in the depressed phase of a bipolar disorder.

**affective psychosis,** a psychologic reaction in which the ego's functioning is impaired and the primary clinical feature is a severe disorder of mood or emotions.

**affect memory,** a particular emotionally expressed feeling that recurs whenever a significant experience is recalled.

**afferent** /af'ərənt/ [L, *ad* + *ferre,* to carry], proceeding toward a center, as applied to arteries, veins, lymphatics, and nerves. Compare **efferent.**

**afferent glomerular arteriole.** See **vas afferens.**

**afferent nerves** [L, *ad* + *ferre,* to bear, *nervus*], nerve fibers that transmit impulses from the periphery toward the central nervous system.

**afferent pathway** [L, *ad* + *ferre,* to bear; AS, *paeth* + *weg*], the course or route taken, usually by a linkage of neurons, from the periphery of the body toward the center.

**afferent tract** [L, *ad* + *ferre,* to bear, *tractus*], a pathway for nerve impulses traveling inward or toward the brain, the center of an organ, or another body structure. Also called **ascending tract.**

**affidavit** /af'idā'vit/ [L, he has pledged], a written statement that is sworn to before a notary public or an officer of the court.

**affiliated hospital** /əfil'ē-ā'tid/ [L, *ad* + *filius,* to son], a hospital that is associated to some degree with a medical school, other health profession, a health program, or other health care institution.

**affinity** /əfin'itē/ [L, *affinis,* related], the measure of the binding strength of the antibody-antigen reaction.

**affirmation** [L, *affirmare,* to make firm], (in psychology) autosuggestion, the point at which a tendency toward positive reaction is observed by the therapist.

**affirmative defense** /əfur'mətiv/ [L, *affirmare,* to make firm], (in law) a denial of guilt or wrongdoing based on new evidence rather than on simple denial of a charge, as a plea of immunity according to a good Samaritan law. The defendant bears the burden of proof in an affirmative defense.

**afflux** /af'luks/ [L, *affluere,* to flow], the sudden flow of blood or other liquid to a part of the body.

**affusion** /afyo͞o'zhən/ [L, *affundere,* to pour out], a form of therapy in which water is sprinkled or poured over the body or a particular body part. It is used for pyrexia or other disease conditions.

**afibrinogenemia** /afī'brinō'jenē'mē-ə/ [Gk, *a,* not; L, *fibra,* fiber; Gk, *genein,* to produce, *haima,* blood], a relative lack or absence of fibrinogen in the blood. It may be the result of a primary, congenital blood dyscrasia or acquired, as in disseminated intravascular coagulation. Also spelled **afibrinogenaemia.**

**aflatoxins** /af'lātok'sins/ [Gk, *a,* not; L, *flavus,* yellow; Gk, *toxikon,* poison], a group of carcinogenic and toxic factors produced by *Aspergillus flavus* food molds. The mycotoxins cause liver necrosis and liver cancer in laboratory animals and are believed to be responsible for a high incidence of liver cancer among people in tropical regions of Africa and Asia who may consume moldy grains, peanuts, or other *Aspergillus*-contaminated foods. See *Aspergillus.*

**AFO,** abbreviation for **ankle-foot orthosis.**

**AFP,** abbreviation for **alpha-fetoprotein.**

**African lymphoma.** See **Burkitt's lymphoma.**

**African relapsing fever.** See **Dutton's relapsing fever.**

**African sleeping sickness.** See **African trypanosomiasis.**

**African tick fever.** See **relapsing fever.**

**African tick typhus,** a rickettsial infection transmitted by ixodid ticks and characterized by fever, chills, maculopapular rash, headache, myalgia, arthralgias, and swollen lymph nodes. At the onset of the infection, a local lesion called tache noire, a buttonlike ulcer with a black center, appears at the site of the tick bite. The rash usually begins on the forearms and spreads over the rest of the body. The fever may persist into the second week, but death or complications are rare.

**African trypanosomiasis,** a disease caused by the parasite *Trypanosoma brucei gambiense* (West African or Gambian trypanosomiasis) or *T. brucei rhodesiense* (East African or Rhodesian trypanosomiasis), transmitted to humans by the bite of the tsetse fly. African trypanosomiasis occurs only in the savannahs and woodlands of central and east Africa, where tsetse flies are found. The disease progresses through two phases: Stage 1 is marked by fever, lymphadenopathy, splenomegaly, and myocarditis. Stage 2 is marked by symptoms of central nervous system involvement, including lethargy, sleepiness, headache, convulsions, and coma. The disease is fatal unless treated, though it may be years before the patient reaches the neurologic phase. Antimicrobial medications specific for the treatment of trypanosomiasis (suramin, pentamidine, organic arsenicals difluoromethylorthinine and eflornithine) are available in the United States only from the Centers for Disease Control and Prevention. Kinds of African trypanosomiasis are **Gambian trypanosomiasis** and **Rhodesian trypanosomiasis.** Also called **African sleeping sickness, sleeping sickness.** See also **trypanosomiasis, tsetse fly.**

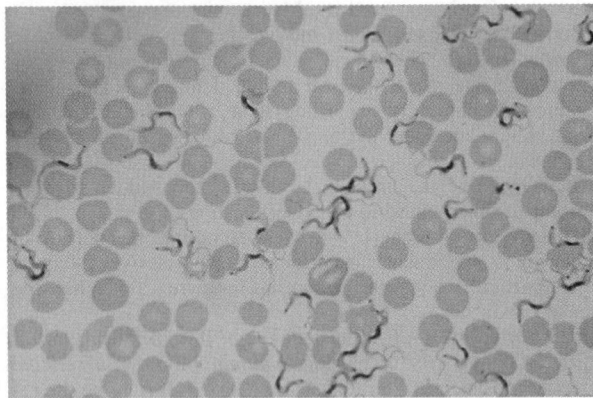

**African trypanosomiasis: bloodstream parasites**
*(Cotran, Kumar, and Collins, 1999)*

**Afrin,** trademark for an adrenergic vasoconstrictor (oxymetazoline hydrochloride).

**afterbirth** [AS, *aefter* + ME, *burth*], the placenta, the amnion, the chorion, and some amniotic fluid, blood, and blood clots expelled from the uterus after childbirth.

**aftercare** [AS, *aefter* + *caru*], health care offered a patient after discharge from a hospital or other health care facility. The patient may require a certain amount of medical or nursing attention for a health problem that no longer demands inpatient status.

**afterdepolarization** /-dēpō′lərizā′shən/, a membrane potential depolarization that follows an action potential. In cardiac muscles, it may be early (during phase 3 of the action potential) or delayed (during phase 4 ) and it is thought to cause atrial and ventricular tachycardia, especially in the setting of a long Q-T interval or digitalis toxicity. Also called **afterpotential.**

**aftereffect,** a physical or psychologic effect that continues after the stimulus is removed.

**afterimage,** a visual sensation that continues after the stimulus ends. The image may appear in colors complementary to those of the stimulus.

**afterload** [AS, *aefter* + ME, *lod*], the load, or resistance, against which the left ventricle must eject its volume of blood during contraction. The resistance is produced by the volume of blood already in the vascular system and by the constriction of the vessel walls.

**afterloading,** a technique in which an unloaded applicator or needle is placed within a patient at the time of an operative procedure and subsequently loaded with a radioactive source. The loading is done under controlled conditions in which health care personnel are protected against radiation exposure. See also **remote afterloading.**

**aftermovement,** an involuntary muscle contraction that causes a continued movement of a limb after a strong exertion against resistance has stopped. It is often demonstrated in abduction of the arm. Also called **Kohnstamm's phenomenon, rebound effect.**

**afterpains** [AS, *aefter* + Gk, *poine,* penalty], contractions of the uterus common during the first days after delivery. They tend to be strongest in nursing mothers during breastfeeding, in multiparas, after the birth of large babies, and when the uterus has been overdistended. They usually resolve spontaneously but may require analgesia. The nurse may reassure the mother that afterpains are normal and prove that the uterus is contracting as it should.

**afterperception,** the apparent perception of a stimulus that continues after the stimulus is removed.

**afterpotential.** See **afterdepolarization.**

**afterpotential wave** /-pəten′shəl/, either of two smaller waves, positive or negative, that follow the main spike potential wave of a nerve impulse, as recorded on an oscillograph tracing of an action potential that propagates along a nerve fiber.

**Ag,** symbol for the element **silver.**

**ag-.** See **ad-.**

**AGA,** abbreviation for **appropriate for gestational age.**

**against medical advice (ama),** a phrase pertaining to a client's decision to discontinue a therapy despite the advice of medical professionals.

**agalactia** /ā′gəlak′shə/ [Gk *a* + *gala,* not milk], the inability of the mother to secrete enough milk to breastfeed an infant after childbirth.

**agamete** /āgam′ēt/ [Gk *a* + *gamos* not marriage], **1.** any of the unicellular organisms, such as bacteria and protozoa, that reproduce asexually by multiple fission instead of producing gametes. **2.** any asexual reproductive cell, such as a spore or merozoite, that forms a new organism without fusion with another gamete. See also **fungus. —agametic, agamous,** *adj.*

**agametic** /āgəmē′tik/, asexual; without recognizable sex organs or gametes. Also called **agamous** /ag′əməs/.

**agamic** /āgam′ik/, reproducing asexually, without the union of gametes; asexual.

**agammaglobulinemia** /agam′əglob′yōōlinē′mē·ə/ [Gk *a* + *gamma,* not gamma (third letter of Greek alphabet); L, *globulus,* small sphere; Gk, *haima,* blood], the absence of the serum immunoglobulin gamma globulin, associated with an increased susceptibility to infection. The condition may be transient, congenital, or acquired. The transient form is common in infancy before 6 weeks of age, when the infant becomes able to synthesize the immunoglobulin. The congenital form is rare and sex-linked, affecting male children; it results in decreased production of antibodies. The acquired form usually occurs in malignant diseases such as leukemia, myeloma, or lymphoma. Also spelled **agammaglobulinaemia.** See also **Bruton's agammaglobulinemia, immune gamma globulin.**

**agamogenesis** /əgam′ōjen′əsis/ [Gk, *a* + *gamos,* not marriage, *genein,* to produce], asexual reproduction, as by budding, simple fission of cells, or parthenogenesis. **—agamocytogenic, agamogenetic, agamogenic, agamogonic,** *adj.*

**agamont.** See **schizont.**

**agamous.** See **agametic.**

**aganglionic megacolon.** See **Hirschsprung's disease.**

**aganglionosis** /əgang′lē·ənō′sis/ [Gk, *a,* not, *gagglion,* knot, *osis,* condition], absence of parasympathetic ganglion cells in the myenteric plexus, a diagnostic sign of congenital megacolon.

**agar-agar** /a′gärə′gär/ [Malay], a dried hydrophilic, colloidal product obtained from certain species of red algae. Because it is unaffected by bacterial enzymes, it is widely used as the basic ingredient in solid culture media in bacteriology. Agar-agar is also used as a suspending medium, as an emulsifying agent, and as a bulk laxative. Also called **agar.**

**agarose** /ag′ärōs/, an essentially neutral fraction of agar used as a medium in electrophoresis, particularly for separation of serum proteins, hemoglobin variants, and lipoprotein fractions.

**agastria** /əgas′trē·ə/ [Gk, *a + gaster,* without stomach], the absence of a stomach.

**agastric** /āgas′trik/ [Gk, *a + gaster,* without stomach], pertaining to lack of a stomach or digestive tract.

**AGC,** abbreviation for *absolute granulocyte count.*

**age** [L, *aetus*], **1.** a stage of development at which the body has arrived, as measured by physical and laboratory standards to what is normal for a male or female of the same chronologic span of life. See also **mental age. 2.** to grow old.

**age 30 transition,** (in psychiatry) a period between 28 and 33 years of age when an individual may reevaluate the choices made in his or her twenties.

**aged** /ājd/, a state of having grown older or more mature than others of the population group.

**ageism** /ā′jizəm/ [L, *aetas,* lifetime], an attitude that discriminates, separates, stigmatizes, or otherwise disadvantages older adults on the basis of chronologic age.

**agency** [L, *agere,* to do], **1.** (in law) a relationship between two parties in which one authorizes the other to act in his or her behalf as agent. It usually implies a contractual arrangement between two parties managed by a third party, the agent. **2.** the business of any power or firm empowered to act for another.

**Agency for Health Care Policy and Research (AHCPR),** an agency of the U.S. Public Health Service that supports and conducts scientific research, facilitates the development of clinical guidelines, and assesses health care technology.

**agenesia.** See **agenesis.**

**agenesia corticalis** /ā′jenē′zhə/ [Gk, *a + genein,* not to produce; L, *cortex*], the failure of the cortical cells of the brain, especially the pyramidal cells, to develop in the embryo, resulting in infantile cerebral paralysis and severe mental retardation.

**agenesis** /ājen′əsis/ [Gk, *a + genein,* not to produce], **1.** congenital absence of an organ or part, usually caused by a lack of primordial tissue and failure of development in the embryo. **2.** impotence or sterility. Also called **agenesia.** Compare **dysgenesis. —agenic,** *adj.*

**agenetic fracture** /ā′jenet′ik/, a spontaneous fracture caused by an imperfect bone development.

**agenic.** See **agenesis.**

**ageniocephaly** /ājen′ē·ōsef′əlē/ [Gk, *a + genein,* not to produce, *kephale,* head], a form of otocephaly in which the brain, cranial vault, and sense organs are intact but the lower jaw is malformed. Also called **ageniocephalia. —ageniocephalic, ageniocephalous,** *adj.*

**agenitalism** /ājen′itəliz′əm/, any condition caused by the lack of sex hormones and the absence or malfunction of the ovaries or testes.

**agenosomia** /əjen′əsō′mē·ə/, a congenital malformation characterized by the absence or defective formation of the

genitals and protrusion of the intestines through an incompletely developed abdominal wall.

**agenosomus** /əjen′əsō′məs/ [Gk, *a + genein,* not to produce, *soma,* body], a fetus with agenosomia.

**agent** [L, *agere,* to do], (in law) a party authorized to act on behalf of another and to give the other an account of such actions.

**Agent Orange,** a U.S. military code name for a mixture of two herbicides, 2,4-D and 2,4,5-T, used as a defoliant in Southeast Asia during the 1960s war in Vietnam. The herbicides were unintentionally contaminated with the highly toxic chemical dioxin, believed to be a cause of cancer and birth defects in animals and established as a cause of chloracne and porphyria cutanea tarda in humans. See **dioxin.**

**age of consent,** (in medical jurisprudence) the age at which an individual is legally free to act as an adult, without parental permission for such activities as marriage or sexual intercourse or giving permission for medical treatment or surgery. The specific age of consent varies from 13 to 21, according to local laws.

**age of majority,** the age at which a person is considered to be an adult in the eyes of the law.

**age-specific,** data in which the age of the individual is significant for epidemiologic or statistical purposes.

**ageusia** /əgyoo′sē·ə/ [Gk, *a + geusis,* without taste], a loss or impairment of the sense of taste. Also called **ageustia, gustatory anesthesia.**

**agger** /ag′ər, aj′ər/, a small mound or eminence of tissue, such as the curved elevation above the atrium of the nose.

**agglomerate** /əglom′ərāt/ [L, *glomus,* a ball], to collect or gather into a mass, ball, or cluster.

**agglomeration** [L, *agglomerare,* to gather into a ball], a mass or cluster of individual units.

**agglutinant** /əgloo′tənənt/ [L, *agglutinare,* to glue], something that causes adhesion, such as a circulating antibody that is stimulated by the presence of an antigen to adhere to it.

**agglutination** /əgloo′tinā′shən/ [L, *agglutinare,* to glue], the clumping together of cells as a result of interaction with specific antibodies called agglutinins. Agglutinins are used in blood typing and in identifying or estimating the strength of immunoglobulins or immune sera. See also **agglutinin, blood typing, precipitin.**

**agglutination-inhibition test,** a serologic technique useful in testing for certain unknown soluble antigens. The unknown antigen is mixed with a known agglutinin. If there is a reaction, the agglutinin can no longer adhere to the cells or particles that carry its corresponding antigen, and the unknown antigen is thus identified. One type of pregnancy test is based on agglutination inhibition.

**agglutination titer,** the highest dilution of a serum that will produce clumping of cells or particulate antigens. It is a measure of the concentration of specific antibodies in the serum.

**agglutinin** /əgloo′tinin/, an antibody that interacts with antigens, resulting in agglutination. Usually multivalent, agglutinins act on insoluble antigens in stable suspension to form a cross-linking lattice that may clump or precipitate. Compare **precipitin.** See also **agglutination, blood typing, hemagglutination.**

**agglutinin absorption,** the removal from immune serum of antibody by treatment with homologous antigen, followed by centrifugation and separation of the antigen-antibody complex.

**agglutinogen** /ag′lootin′əjin/ [L, *agglutinare + Gk, *genein,* to produce], any antigenic substance that causes agglutina-

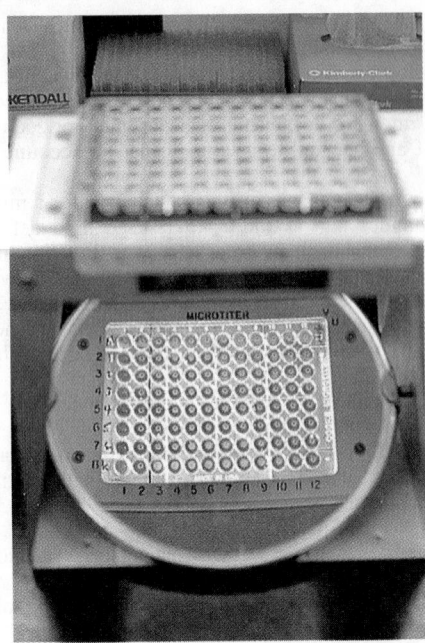

**Agglutination assay** (Mudge-Grout, 1992)

tion (clumping together of cells) by the production of agglutinin.

**aggregate** /ag′rəgāt/ [L, *ad* + *gregare,* to gather together], the total of a group of substances or components making up a mass or complex. Data on individual patients can be aggregated to allow conclusions about the patient population to be made.

**aggregate anaphylaxis,** an exaggerated immune reaction of immediate hypersensitivity induced by an antigen that forms a soluble antigen-antibody complex.

**aggregation** /ag′rəgā′shən [L, *ad* + *gregare,* to gather together], an accumulation of substances, objects, or individuals, as in the clumping of blood cells or the clustering of clients with the same disorder.

**aggression** /əgresh′ən/ [L, *aggressio,* to attack], a forceful behavior, action, or attitude that is expressed physically, verbally, or symbolically. It may arise from innate drives or occur as a defensive mechanism, often resulting from a threatened ego. It is manifested by either constructive or destructive acts directed toward oneself or against others. Kinds of aggression are **constructive aggression, destructive aggression,** and **inward aggression.**

**aggression control,** a nursing outcome from the Nursing Outcomes Classification (NOC) defined as self-restraint of assaultive, combative, or destructive behavior toward others. See also **Nursing Outcomes Classification.**

**aggressive personality** /əgres′iv/, a personality with behavior patterns characterized by irritability, impulsivity, destructiveness, or violence in response to frustration.

**aggressive-radical therapy,** (in psychiatry) a form of therapy that introduces the political and social viewpoints of the therapist into the therapeutic process. Proponents of this technique believe that making all values explicit, sometimes through actual didactic input, enables the patient to view the solution of an emotional conflict and the raising of political consciousness as one and the same.

**aging** [L, *aetas,* lifetime], the process of growing old, resulting in part from a failure of body cells to function normally or to produce new body cells to replace those that are dead or malfunctioning. Normal cell function may be lost through infectious disease, malnutrition, exposure to environmental hazards, or genetic influences. Among body cells that exhibit early signs of aging are those that normally cease dividing after reaching maturity. See also **assessment of the aging patient.**

**agitated** /aj′ətā′təd [L, *agitare,* to shake], describing a condition of psychomotor excitement characterized by purposeless, restless activity. Pacing, talking, crying, and laughing sometimes are characteristic and may serve to release nervous tension associated with anxiety, fear, or other mental stress. —**agitate,** *v.,* **agitation,** *n.*

**agitated depression,** a severe depressive disorder characterized by severe anxiety accompanied by continuous physical restlessness, and, frequently, somatic symptoms. Psychomotor agitation is prominenet. Delusions may also be present, as well as depression with psychotic features. See also **depression.**

**agitation,** a state of chronic restlessness and increased psychomotor activity that is generally observed as an expression of emotional tension.

**agitographia** /aj′itōgraf′ē·ə/ [L, *agitare* + Gk, *graphein,* to write], a condition characterized by abnormally rapid writing in which words or parts of words are unconsciously omitted. The condition is commonly associated with agitophasia.

**agitophasia** /aj′itōfā′zhə/ [L, *agitare* + Gk, *phasis,* speech], a condition characterized by abnormally rapid speech in which words, sounds, or syllables are unconsciously omitted, slurred, or distorted. The condition is commonly associated with agitographia. Also called **agitolalia.**

**aglossia** /əglos′ē·ə/ [Gk, *a* + *glossa,* without tongue], congenital absence of the tongue.

**aglycemia** /ā′glīsē′mē·ə/ [Gk, *a, glykis,* not sweet, *haima,* blood], an absence of blood glucose.

**agnathia** /ag·nath′ē·ə/ [Gk, *a, gnathos,* not jaw], a developmental defect characterized by total or partial absence of the lower jaw. Also called **agnathy** /ag′nəthē/. Compare **synotia.** See also **otocephaly.** —**agnathous,** *adj.*

**agnathocephalia, agnathocephalic, agnathocephalous.** See **agnathocephaly.**

**agnathocephalus** /ag·nath′əsef′ələs/, a fetus with agnathocephaly.

**agnathocephaly** /ag·nath′əsef′əlē/ [Gk, *a* + *gnathos* + *kephale,* head], a congenital malformation characterized by the absence of the lower jaw, defective formation of the mouth, and placement of the eyes low on the face with fusion or approximation of the zygomas and the ears. Also called **agnathocephalia.** See also **otocephaly.** —**agnathocephalic, agnathocephalous,** *adj.*

**agnathus** /ag·nath′əs/ [Gk, *a* + *gnathos,* without jaw], a fetus with agnathia.

**agnathy.** See **agnathia.**

**AgNO₃,** the chemical formula for silver nitrate.

**agnogenic myeloid metaplasia.** See **myeloid metaplasia.**

**agnosia** /ag·nō′zhə/ [Gk, *a* + *gnosis,* not knowledge], total or partial loss of the ability to recognize familiar objects or persons through sensory stimuli as a result of organic brain damage. The condition may affect any of the senses and is classified accordingly as auditory, visual, olfactory, gustatory, or tactile agnosia. Also called **agnosis.** See also **autotopagnosia.**

**-agnosia, -agnosis,** suffix meaning '(condition of the) loss of the faculty to perceive': *autotopagnosia, paragnosia.*

**-agogue, -agog,** suffix meaning an 'agent promoting the expulsion of a (specified) substance': *lymphagogue, uragogue.*

**agonal** /ag′ənəl/ [Gk, *agon,* struggle], pertaining to death and dying.

**agonal respiration.** See **Cheyne-Stokes respiration.**

**agonal thrombus,** a mass of blood platelets, fibrin, clotting factors, and cellular elements that forms in the heart of a dying patient.

**agonist** /ag′ənist/ [Gk, *agon,* struggle], **1.** a contracting muscle whose contraction is opposed by another muscle (an antagonist). **2.** a drug or other substance having a specific cellular affinity that produces a predictable response.

**agony** /ag′ənē/ [Gk, *agon*], severe physical or emotional anguish or distress, as in pain.

**agoraphobia** /ag′ərə-/ [Gk, *agora,* marketplace, *phobos,* fear], an anxiety disorder characterized by a fear of being in an open, crowded, or public place, such as a field, tunnel, bridge, congested street, or busy department store, where escape is perceived as difficult or help not available in case of sudden incapacitation.

**-agra,** suffix meaning a 'pain or painful seizure': *cardiagra, trachelagra.*

**agranular endoplasmic reticulum.** See **endoplasmic reticulum.**

**agranulocyte** /āgran′yoolōsīt′/ [Gk, *a,* not; L, *granulum,* small grain; Gk, *kytos,* cell], any leukocyte that does not contain predominant cytoplasmic granules, such as a monocyte or lymphocyte. Compare **granulocyte.** See also **leukocyte.**

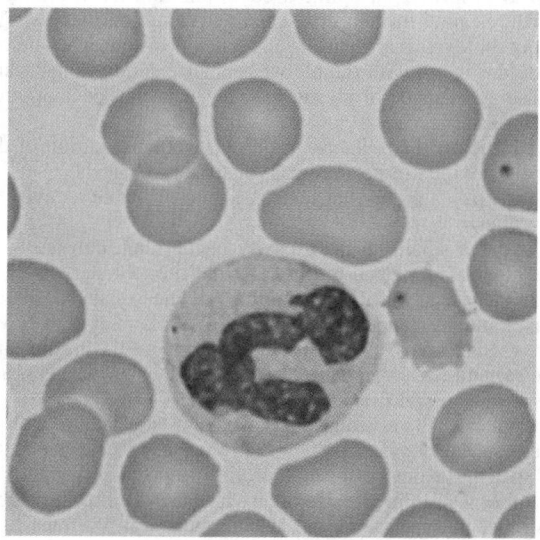

**Agranulocyte** *(Carr and Rodak, 1999)*

**agranulocytic** /-si′tik/ [Gk, *a,* not, *granule, kytos,* cell], pertaining to a white blood cell that, when stained, shows no granules in its cytoplasm.

**agranulocytosis** /āgran′yoolō′sītō′sis/, a severe reduction in the number of white blood cells (basophils, eosinophils, and neutrophils). Neutropenia results, whereby the body is severely depleted in its ability to defend itself. Fever, prostration, and bleeding ulcers of the rectum, mouth, and vagina may be present. The acute disease may be an adverse reaction to a medication or the result of radiation therapy or chemotherapy.

**agranulosis.** See **agranulocytosis.**

**agraphesthesia.** See **graphanesthesia.**

**agraphia** /āgraf′ē-ə/ [Gk, *a, graphein,* not to write], a loss of the ability to write, resulting from injury to the language center in the cerebral cortex. Compare **dysgraphia.** —**agraphic,** *adj.*

**A:G ratio,** the ratio of protein albumin to globulin in the blood serum. On the basis of differential solubility with neutral salt solution the normal values are 3.5 to 5 g/dl for albumin and 2.5 to 4 g/dl for globulin.

**agrimony,** an herb found in Asia, Europe, and the United States.

■ USES: This herb is used for mild diarrhea, gastroenteritis, intestinal mucus secretion, inflammation of the mouth and throat, cuts and scrapes, and amenorrhea.

■ CONTRAINDICATIONS: Agrimony is not recommended during pregnancy and lactation, in children, or in those with known hypersensitivity to this plant or roses.

**agrypnia.** See **insomnia.**

**agrypnocoma** /agrip′nōkō′mə/ [Gk, *agrypnos,* sleepless], a coma in which there is some degree of wakefulness. The condition may be manifested by extreme lethargy or drowsiness accompanied by delirium.

**agrypnotic** /ag′ripnot′ik/, **1.** insomniac. **2.** a drug or other substance that prevents sleep.

**AGS,** abbreviation for *American Geriatrics Society.*

**agyria** /əjī′rē-ə/, a cerebral cortex abnormality in which the gyri are poorly developed. The cortical tissue is reduced, leading to severe mental retardation. Also called **lissencephaly.**

**AHA,** abbreviation for **American Hospital Association.**

**"aha" reaction** /ähä′/, (in psychology) a sudden realization or inspiration, experienced especially during creative thinking. Some psychologists associate great scientific discoveries and artistic inspirations with this reaction, which is not necessarily related to intelligence. The term has apparently replaced **"aha" experience,** formerly used by psychologists, especially those of the Gestalt school, to label experiences in which an individual utters "Aha!" during a moment of revelation.

**AHCPR,** abbreviation for **Agency for Health Care Policy and Research.**

**AHF,** abbreviation for **antihemophilic factor.**

**AHH,** abbreviation for **aryl hydrocarbon hydroxylase.**

**Ahumada-del Castillo syndrome** /ä′hōōmä′dädel′kästē′-yō/, [Juan Carlos Ahumada; E.B. del Castillo; twentieth-century Argentine physicians], a form of secondary amenorrhea that may be associated with a pituitary gland tumor. It is characterized by both galactorrhea and amenorrhea in the absence of a pregnancy.

**AI, 1.** abbreviation for **artificial intelligence. 2.** abbreviation for **artificial insemination.**

**AICD,** abbreviation for **automatic implanted cardioverter defibrillator.**

**aid,** assistance given a person who is ill, injured, or otherwise unable to cope with normal demands of life.

**AID,** abbreviation for **artificial insemination donor.**

**AIDS** /ādz/, abbreviation for **acquired immunodeficiency syndrome.**

**AIDS-associated retinopathy.** See **HIV-associated retinopathy.**

**AIDS-dementia complex (ADC),** a neurologic effect of encephalitis or brain inflammation experienced by nearly one-third of all patients with acquired immunodeficiency syndrome (AIDS). The condition is characterized by memory loss and by varying levels and forms of dementia. It may be caused by the destruction of brain neurons by the AIDS virus, as autopsies indicate that the density of the neurons may be 40% lower in AIDS patients than in persons who have not had AIDS. Also called **AIDS-related dementia.**

**AIDS-related complex** See **AIDS-wasting syndrome.**

**AIDS serology test (AIDS screen, HIV antibody test, Western blot test, ELISA),** a blood, oral, or urine test used to detect the antibody to the human immunodeficiency virus (HIV), which causes AIDS. Home testing kits are now available in addition to the tests performed by health care providers.

**AIDS-wasting syndrome,** a syndrome associated with progressed acquired immunodeficiency syndrome (AIDS). Signs and symptoms may include weight loss, fever, malaise, lethargy, oral thrush, and immunologic abnormalities characteristic of AIDS. Formerly called **AIDS-related complex (ARC).**

**AIH,** abbreviation for **artificial insemination husband.**

**AILD,** abbreviation for **angioimmunoblastic lymphadenopathy with dysproteinemia.**

**ailment** [OE, *eglan*], any disease or physical disorder or complaint, generally of a chronic, acute, or mild nature.

**ainhum.** See **autoamputation.**

**air** [Gk, *aer*], the colorless, odorless gaseous mixture constituting the earth's atmosphere. It consists of 78% nitrogen; 20% oxygen; almost 1% argon; small amounts of carbon dioxide, hydrogen, and ozone; traces of helium, krypton, neon, and xenon; and varying amounts of water vapor.

**air bath,** the exposure of the naked body to warm air for therapeutic purposes. Also called **balneum pneumaticum.**

**airborne contaminants,** materials in the atmosphere that can affect the health of persons in the same or nearby environments. Particularly vulnerable are tissues of the upper respiratory tract and lungs, including the terminal bronchioles and alveoli. The effects depend in part on the solubility of the inhaled matter. Inhaled contaminants may cause tissue damage, tissue reaction, disease, or physical obstruction. Some airborne contaminants, such as carbon monoxide gas, may have little or no direct effect on the lungs but can be absorbed into the bloodstream and carried to other organs or damage the blood itself. Biologically inert gases may dilute the atmospheric oxygen below the normal blood saturation value, thereby disturbing cellular respiration.

**airborne precautions,** safeguards designed to reduce the risk of airborne transmission of infectious agents. Airborne droplet nuclei consist of small-particle residue (5 μm or smaller in size) of evaporated droplets that may remain suspended in the air for long periods of time. Airborne transmission occurs by dissemination of either airborne droplet nuclei or dust particles containing the infectious agent. Microorganisms carried in this manner can be widely dispersed by air currents and may become inhaled or deposited on a susceptible host from the source patient. Special air handling and ventilation are required to prevent airborne transmission. Airborne precautions apply to patients known or suspected to have serious illnesses that are transmitted by airborne droplet nuclei. Examples include measles, varicella-zoster virus infections, legionella, disseminated zoster, and tuberculosis. See also **standard precautions, transmission-based precautions.**

**aircast splint.** See **air splint.**

**air compressor,** a mechanical device that compresses air for storage and is used in handpieces and other air-driven medical and dental tools.

**air embolism** the abnormal presence of air in the cardiovascular system, resulting in obstruction of blood flow. Air embolism may occur if a large quantity of air is inadvertently introduced by injection, as during IV therapy or surgery, or by trauma, as a puncture wound. Also called **aeroembolism.** See also **decompression sickness, embolus, gas embolism.**

**air encephalography.** See **encephalography.**

**air entrainment,** the movement of room air into the chamber of a jet nebulizer used to treat respiratory diseases. Air entrainment increases the rate of nebulization and the amount of liquid administered per unit of time.

**airflow pattern,** the pattern of movement of respiratory gases through the respiratory tract. The pattern is affected by such factors as gas density and viscosity.

**air fluidization,** the process of blowing temperature-controlled air through a collection of microspheres to create a fluidlike movement. The technique is used in special mattresses designed to reduce pressure against a patient's skin. See also **air-fluidized bed.**

**air-fluidized bed,** a bed with body support provided by thousands of tiny soda-lime glass beads suspended by pressurized temperature-controlled air. The patient rests on a polyester filter sheet that covers the beads. The special bed is designed for use by patients with posterior pressure ulcers or at risk for pressure ulcers or posterior grafts, burns, or donor areas. Pressure against the skin surface of the patient is less than capillary filling pressure. The improved capillary blood flow to the skin speeds the growth of granulation tissue.

**air hunger,** a form of respiratory distress characterized by gasping, labored breathing, or dyspnea.

**airplane splint,** a splint used to immobilize a shoulder during healing from injury, such as a fractured humerus. The splint holds the arm in an abducted position at or below shoulder level, with the elbow bent. It extends to the waist and may be made of plastic or wire, or it may be supported by a plaster body.

**air pollution** [L, *polluere,* to defile], contamination of the air by noxious fumes, aromas, or toxic chemicals.

**air pump,** a pump that forces air into or out of a cavity or chamber.

**air sac,** a small, terminal cavity in the lung, consisting of the alveoli connected to one terminal bronchiole.

**air sickness,** a form of motion sickness caused by air travel and, in some cases, by traveling on land at high elevations. Symptoms usually include nausea and vomiting and are sometimes accompanied by headache or drowsiness. See also **motion sickness.**

**air spaces,** the alveolar ducts, alveolar sacs, and alveoli of the respiratory system.

**air splint,** a device for temporarily immobilizing fractured or otherwise injured extremities. It consists of an inflatable cylinder that can be closed at both ends and becomes rigid when filled with air under pressure. Also called **aircast splint.**

**air swallowing,** the intake of air into the digestive system, usually involuntary and during eating, drinking, or chewing gum. Air swallowing may also be an effect of anxious behavior. The problem occurs commonly in infants as a result of faulty feeding methods.

**air thermometer,** a thermometer using air as its expansible medium. See also **thermometer.**

**airway** [Gk, *aer* + AS, *weg,* way], **1.** a tubular passage for movement of air into and out of the lung. An airway with a diameter greater than 2 mm is defined as a large, or central, airway; one smaller than 2 mm is called a small, or periph-

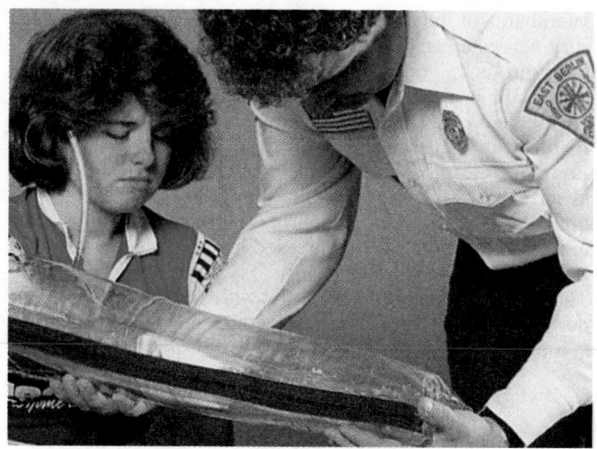

**Air splint** *(Judd and Ponsell, 1988)*

eral, airway. **2.** a respiratory anesthesia device. **3.** an oropharyngeal tube used for mouth-to-mouth resuscitation.

**airway clearance, ineffective,** a nursing diagnosis accepted by the Fourth National Conference on the Classification of Nursing Diagnoses (revised 1998). Ineffective airway clearance is a state in which an individual is unable to clear secretions or obstructions from the respiratory tract to maintain a clear airway.

■ DEFINING CHARACTERISTICS: The defining characteristics are abnormal breath sounds (crackles, gurgles, wheezes); cough, ineffective or absent; sputum; report of chest congestion; dyspnea; diminished breath sounds; orthopnea; cyanosis; difficulty vocalizing; wide-eyed changes in respiratory rate and rhythm; and restlessness.

■ RELATED FACTORS: Related factors include environmental elements, such as smoking, smoke inhalation, and secondhand smoke. Other related factors include airway spasm, retained secretions, excessive mucus, presence of an artificial airway, a foreign body in the airway, secretions in the bronchi, exudate in the alveoli, neuromuscular dysfunction, hyperplasia of the bronchial walls, chronic obstructive pulmonary disease, infection, asthma, and allergic airways. See also **nursing diagnosis.**

**airway conductance,** the instantaneous rate of gas flow in the airway per unit of pressure difference between the mouth, nose, or other airway opening and the alveoli. It is the reciprocal of airway resistance and is indicated by the symbol $G_{aw}$.

**airway division,** one of the 18 segments of the bronchopulmonary system. The segments are usually numbered from 1 to 10 for the right lung, which has three lobes, and from 1 to 8 for the left lung, which has two lobes.

**airway insertion and stabilization,** a nursing intervention from the Nursing Interventions Classification (NIC) defined as insertion or assisting with insertion and stabilization of an artificial airway. See also **Nursing Interventions Classification.**

**airway management,** a nursing intervention from the Nursing Interventions Classification (NIC) defined as facilitation of patency of air passages. See also **Nursing Interventions Classification.**

**airway obstruction,** a mechanical impediment to the delivery of air to the lungs or to the absorption of oxygen in the lungs.

■ OBSERVATIONS: If the obstruction is minor, as in sinusitis or pharyngitis, the person is able to breathe, but not normally. If the obstruction is acute, the person may grasp the neck, gasp, become cyanotic, and lose consciousness.

■ INTERVENTIONS: Acute airway obstruction requires rapid intervention to save the person's life. In cases of obstruction caused by a bolus of food, a collection of mucus, or a foreign body, the object may be removed manually, by suction, or with the Heimlich maneuver. Obstruction caused by an inflammatory or allergic reaction may be treated with bronchodilating drugs, corticosteroids, intubation, and administration of oxygen. An emergency tracheotomy may be required if the obstruction cannot be mechanically or pharmacologically relieved within a few minutes.

■ NURSING CONSIDERATIONS: The patient is usually very apprehensive and may physically resist assistance. Medical help is summoned, and emergency care is begun and includes removing the obstruction, administering oxygen, and performing cardiopulmonary resuscitation, if necessary. See also **aspiration, cardiopulmonary resuscitation, Heimlich maneuver.**

**airway resistance,** a measure of the impedance to airflow through the bronchopulmonary system. It is the reciprocal of airway conductance and is indicated by the symbol $R_{aw}$.

**airway suctioning,** a nursing intervention from the Nursing Interventions Classification (NIC) defined as removal of airway secretions by inserting a suction catheter into the patient's oral airway and/or trachea. See also **Nursing Interventions Classification.**

**AIUM,** abbreviation for *American Institute of Ultrasound in Medicine.*

**AKA,** abbreviation for *above the knee amputation.*

**akaryocyte** /āker′ē·əsīt′/ [Gk, *a,* not, *karyon,* kernel], a cell without a nucleus, such as an erythrocyte.

**akathisia** /ak′əthē′zhə/ [Gk, *a* + *kathizein,* not to sit], a pathologic condition characterized by restlessness and agitation, such as an inability to sit still. —**akathisiac,** *adj.*

**akeratosis** /āker′ətō′sis/, a skin condition in which there is a lack of horny tissue in the epidermis.

**akinesia** /ā′kinē′zhə, ā′kīnē′zhə/ [Gk, *a, kinesis,* without movement], an abnormal state of motor and psychic hypoactivity or muscular paralysis. Also called **akinesis.** —**akinetic,** *adj.*

**akinesthesia** /ākin′esthē′zhə/, a loss of the sense of movement.

**akinetic** /ā′kinet′ik/ [Gk, *a, kinesis*], without movement, pertaining to a loss of ability to move a part or all of the body.

**akinetic apraxia,** the inability to perform a spontaneous movement. See also **apraxia.**

**akinetic mutism,** a state of apparent alertness in which a person is unable or refuses to move or to make sounds, resulting from neurologic or psychologic disturbance.

**akinetic seizure,** a type of seizure disorder observed in children. It is a brief, generalized seizure in which the child suddenly falls to the ground.

**Akineton,** trademark for a peripheral anticholinergic (biperiden hydrochloride).

**-akusis.** See **-acousia.**

**Al,** symbol for the element **aluminum.**

**-al,** suffix designating a compound containing a member of the aldehyde group: *chloral, ethanal.*

**-al, -ale,** suffix meaning 'characterized by' or "pertaining to": *appendiceal, meningeal.*

**ala** /ā′lə/, *pl.* **alae** [L, wing], **1.** any winglike structure. **2.** the axilla.

**Ala,** abbreviation for the amino acid **alanine.**

**ALA,** abbreviation for **aminolevulinic acid.**

**ala auris,** the auricle of the ear.

**ala cerebelli** /ser′əbel′ī/, the ala of the central lobule of the cerebellum.

**ala cinerea** /sinir′ē·ə/, the triangular area on the floor of the fourth ventricle of the brain from which the autonomic fibers of the vagus nerve arise.

**alactasia.** See **lactase deficiency.**

**Alagille syndrome** /ä·lä·zhēl′/ [Daniel Alagille, French pediatrician, b. 1925], an autosomal dominant syndrome of neonatal jaundice, cholestasis with peripheral pulmonic stenosis, and occasionally septal defects or patent ductus arteriosus, resulting from low numbers or absence of intrahepatic bile ducts; it is characterized by unusual facies and ocular, vertebral, and nervous system abnormalities.

**ala nasi** /nā′sī/, the outer flaring cartilaginous wall of each nostril.

**alanine (Ala)** /al′ənin/, a nonessential amino acid found in many food protein sources as well as in the body. It is degraded in the liver to produce important biomolecules such as pyruvate and glutamate. Its carbon skeleton also can be used as an energy source. See also **amino acid, protein.**

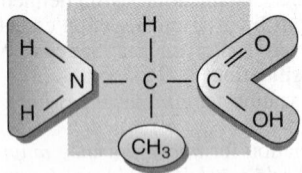

**Chemical structure of alanine**

**alanine aminotransferase (ALT),** an enzyme normally present in the serum and tissues of the body, especially the tissues of the liver. This enzyme catalyzes the transfer of an amino group from *l*-alanine to alpha-ketoglutarate, forming pyruvate and 1-glutamate. The reaction is reversible. The enzyme is released into the serum as a result of tissue injury and increases in persons with acute liver damage. Normal findings are 5-35 IU/L. Also called **alanine transferase.** Previously called **serum glutamic pyruvic transaminase.** Compare **aspartate aminotransferase.**

**alanine aminotransferase test (ALT or SGPT),** a blood test that measures levels of ALT, an enzyme found predominantly in the liver. Elevated levels of ALT are highly specific in indicating hepatocellular disease.

**alanine transferase.** See **alanine aminotransferase (ALT).**

**Al-Anon,** an international organization that offers guidance, counseling, and support for the relatives, friends, and associates of alcoholics. See also **Alcoholics Anonymous.**

**ala of the ethmoid,** a small projection on each side of the crista galli of the ethmoid bone. Each ala fits into a corresponding depression of the frontal bone.

**ala of the ilium,** the upper flaring portion of the iliac bone.

**ala of the sacrum,** the flat extension of bone on each side of the sacrum.

**alar** /ā′lär/ [L, *ala*, wing], pertaining to a winglike structure, such as the shoulder.

**ALARA,** an abbreviation for *as low as reasonably achievable.*

**alar lamina** [L, *ala*, wing, *lamina*, thin plate], the postero-

lateral area of the embryonic neural tube through which sensory nerves enter.

**alar ligament,** one of a pair of ligaments that connect the axis to the occipital bone and limit rotation of the cranium. Also called **check ligament, odontoid ligament.** Compare **membrana tectoria.**

**alarm reaction,** the first stage of the general adaptation syndrome. It is characterized by the release of ACTH by the pituitary gland and of epinephrine by the medulla of the adrenal gland, which cause increased blood glucose levels and faster respirations, increasing the oxygen level of the blood. These actions provide the body with increased energy to deal with a stressful situation. See also **general adaptation syndrome, stress.**

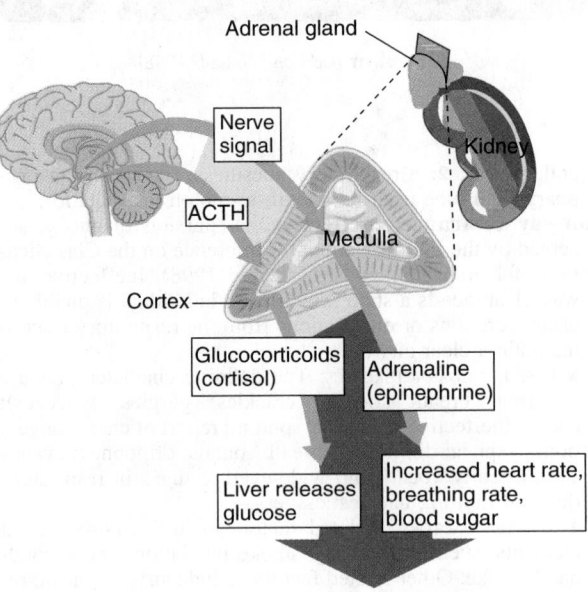

**Alarm reaction** *(Thibodeau and Patton, 1999/Precision Graphics)*

**alar process** [L, *ala*, wing, *processus*], a projection of the cribriform plate of the ethmoid bone articulating with the frontal bone.

**alaryngeal speech** /ā′lä·rin′je·əl spēch/ [Gk, *a*, without + *larynx*; ME, *speche*], a method of speech used after laryngectomy, with sound produced by vibration of the column of air in the esophagus against the sphincter between the esophagus and pharynx. Also called **esophageal speech.**

**alastrim** /al′əstrim/ [Port, *alastrar*, to spread], a mild form of smallpox, with little rash. It is thought to be caused by a weak strain of *Poxvirus variolae.* Unlike smallpox, alastrim is rarely fatal. Also called **Cuban itch, milkpox, variola minor.** See also **smallpox.**

**Alateen,** an international organization that offers guidance, counseling, and support for the children of alcoholics. See also **Alcoholics Anonymous.**

**alatrofloxacin/trovafloxacin,** an antiinfective.

■ INDICATIONS: This drug is used to treat nosocomial pneumonia, chronic bronchitis, acute sinusitis, complicated intraabdominal infections, pelvic infection, skin and skin structure infections, urinary tract infections, chronic bacterial prostatitis, urethral gonorrhea in males, pelvic inflammatory disease, and cervicitis caused by susceptible organisms.

■ CONTRAINDICATIONS: Known hypersensitivity to quinolones, seizure disorders, cerebral atherosclerosis, and photosensitivity prohibit the use of this drug.

■ ADVERSE EFFECTS: Life-threatening side effects include pseudomembranous colitis. Other adverse effects include headache, dizziness, insomnia, anxiety, nausea, flatulence, vomiting, diarrhea, abdominal pain, vaginitis, crystalluria, rash, pruritus, and photosensitivity.

**ala vomeris** /vō′məris/,   an extension of bone on each side of the upper border of the vomer.

**alb-,**  prefix meaning 'white': *albumin.*

**alba** /al′bə/,   literally, 'white,' as in *linea alba.*

**albedo** /albē′dō/ [L, *albus,* white],   a whiteness, particularly as a surface reflection.

**Albers-Schönberg disease** /-shœn′burg, -shōn′-/ [Heinrich E. Albers-Schönberg, Hamburg radiologist, 1865–1921],   a form of osteopetrosis characterized by marblelike calcification of bones. The condition, often discovered by chance during x-ray examination, is transmitted as an autosomal dominant trait. See also **osteopetrosis.**

**Albert's disease** [Eduard Albert, Austrian surgeon, 1841–1900],   an inflammation of the bursa that lies between the Achilles tendon and the calcaneus. It is most frequently caused by injury but may also result from the wearing of poorly fitted shoes, increased strain on the tendon, or rheumatoid arthritis. Treatment includes intrabursal injection of corticosteroid with lidocaine and warm compresses. If treatment is delayed, the inflammation may cause erosion of the calcaneus. Also called **anterior Achilles bursitis.**

**albicans** /al′bikənz/ [L, *albus,* white],   white or whitish. See also **corpus albicans.**

**albinism** /al′biniz′əm/,   a congenital hereditary condition characterized by partial or total lack of melanin pigment in the body. Total albinos have pale skin that does not tan, white hair, pink eyes, nystagmus, astigmatism, and photophobia. Albinos are prone to severe sunburn, actinic dermatitis, and skin cancer. Compare **piebald, vitiligo.**

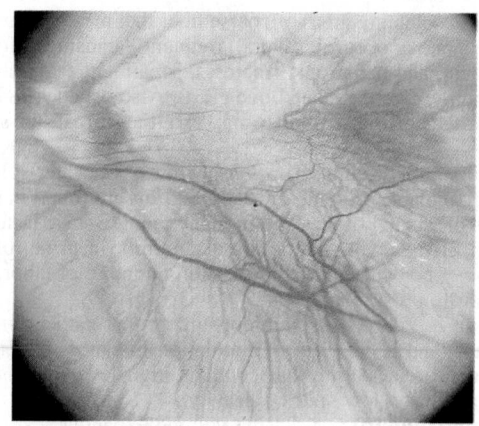

**Pale fundus of albinism** *(Zitelli and Davis, 1997)*

cause of a lack of eye pigment, the choroid is vulnerable to adverse effects of sunlight frequently resulting in photophobia, astigmatism, and other visual disorders. Lack of skin pigment predisposes the individual to skin cancer.

**albinuria** /al′binŏŏr′ē·ə/,   white or colorless urine.

**Albl's ring,**   a calcified ring-shaped shadow visible on a radiograph of an aneurysm of a cerebral artery.

**Albright's hereditary osteodystrophy** /awl′brīts/ [Fuller Albright, American physician and endocrinologist, 1900−1969],   See **pseudohypoparathyroidism.**

**Albright's syndrome** /ôl′brīts/ [Fuller Albright, Boston physician, 1900–1969],   a disorder characterized by fibrous dysplasia of bone, isolated brown macules on the skin, and endocrine dysfunction. It causes precocious puberty in girls but not in boys. The bone lesions are reddish gray, gritty fi-

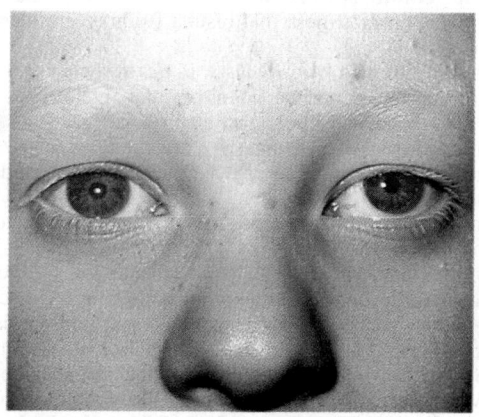

**White hair and pale skin of albinism**
*(Zitelli and Davis, 1997)*

**Albini's nodules** /äl·be′nēz/ [Giuseppe Albini, Italian physiologist, 1827−1911],   gray nodules the size of small grains, sometimes seen on the free edges of the atrioventricular valves of infants; they are remains of fetal structures.

**albino** /albī′nō/ [L, *albus,* white],   an individual with a marked deficiency of pigment in the eyes, hair, and skin. Be-

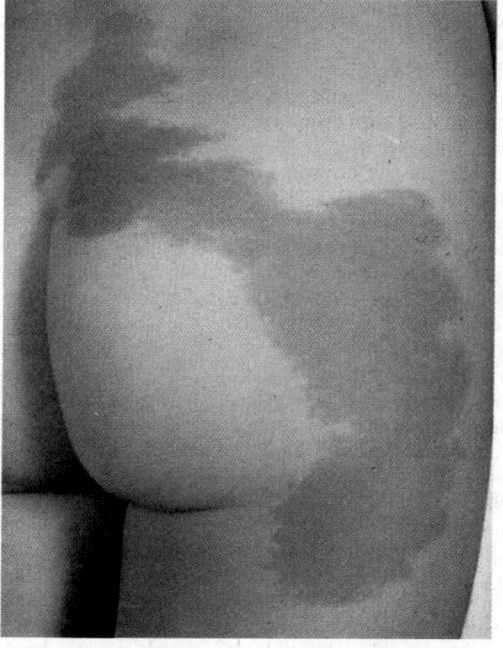

**Albright's syndrome**
*(du Vivier, 1997/courtesy Dr. David Atherton)*

bromas containing areas of coarse fiber that may be confined to one bone or occur in several, frequently causing deformities, pain, and pathologic fractures. Treatment may involve osteotomy, curettage, and bone grafts. Also called **Albright-McCune-Sternberg syndrome, osteitis fibrosa disseminata.**

**albumin** /alby$\overline{oo}$′min/ [L, *albus,* white], a water-soluble, heat-coagulable protein. Various albumins are found in practically all animal tissues and in many plant tissues. Determination of the levels and kinds of albumin in urine, blood, and other body tissues is the basis of a number of laboratory diagnostic tests.

**albumin A,** a blood serum constituent that gathers in cancer cells and is deficient in circulation in cancer patients.

**albuminaturia** urine that contains high level of albumin salts and has a low specific gravity.

**albumin (human),** a plasma-volume expander.
■ INDICATIONS: It is prescribed in the treatment of hypoproteinemia, hyperbilirubinemia, and hypovolemic shock.
■ CONTRAINDICATIONS: Severe anemia, cardiac failure, or allergic reaction to albumin prohibits its use.
■ ADVERSE EFFECTS: Among the most serious adverse reactions are chills, hypertension, fever, and urticaria.

**albuminous liver.** See **amyloid liver.**

**albumin test** [L, *albus,* white], any of several tests for the presence of albumin, a class of simple proteins, in the urine, a common sign of renal or chronic disease. One type of albumin test depends on the change in color of a chemically treated strip of paper in the presence of albumin.

**albuminuria.** See **proteinuria.**

**-albuminuria,** suffix meaning a '(specified) condition characterized by excess serum proteins in the urine': *noctalbuminuria, pseudalbuminuria.*

**albuterol,** a beta-2 receptor adrenergic agent.
■ INDICATION: It is prescribed in the treatment of bronchospasm in patients with reversible obstructive airway disease, including asthma.
■ CONTRAINDICATION: Known sensitivity to this drug prohibits its use.
■ ADVERSE EFFECTS: Among the most serious adverse reactions are tachycardia, insomnia, dizziness, and hypertension.

**alcalase,** an enzyme found in certain laundry detergents. It is a cause of enzymatic detergent asthma.

**alclometasone dipropionate,** a topical corticosteroid.
■ INDICATIONS: It is prescribed for the relief of symptoms of inflammation and pruritus of corticosteroid-responsive dermatoses.
■ CONTRAINDICATIONS: It is contraindicated in patients with hypersensitivity to the drug. Children may absorb proportionally greater amounts of the drug per area of skin surface and should be treated with the smallest amount of the drug needed.
■ ADVERSE EFFECTS: Among adverse reactions are burning, stinging, and itching.

**Alcock's canal** [Benjamin Alcock, Irish anatomist, b. 1801], a canal formed by the obturator internus muscle and the obturator fascia through which the pudendal nerve and vessels pass. Also called **pudendal canal.**

**alcohol** /al′kəhôl/ [Ar *alkohl* subtle essence], **1.** a preparation containing at least 92.3% and not more than 93.8% by weight of ethyl alcohol, used as a topical antiseptic and solvent. **2.** a clear, colorless, volatile liquid that is miscible with water, chloroform, or ether, obtained by the fermentation of carbohydrates with yeast. **3.** a compound derived from a hydrocarbon by replacing one or more hydrogen atoms with an equal number of hydroxyl (OH) groups. De-

pending on the number of hydroxyl groups, alcohols are classified as monohydric, dihydric, trihydric.

**alcohol bath,** a procedure for decreasing an elevated body temperature. It is not widely used because of the drying effect of alcohol. A tepid solution of 25% to 50% alcohol in water is sponged lightly on each limb, then on the trunk; the person is turned only once from supine to prone position if possible and then back again. Some sources recommend placing a hot-water bottle at the feet and a cold compress on the head to accelerate heat loss through vasodilation, to promote the comfort of the patient during the procedure, and to reduce the temperature of the circulation to the brain.

**Alcohol, Drug Abuse, and Mental Health Administration (ADAMHA),** an agency of the U.S. Department of Health and Human Services with three components—the National Institute on Alcohol Abuse and Alcoholism, the National Institute on Drug Abuse, and the National Institute of Mental Health. It conducts and supports research on the biologic, psychologic, epidemiologic, and behavioral aspects of alcoholism, drug abuse, and mental health and illness.

**alcoholic,** **1.** pertaining to alcohol or its effects on other substances. **2.** a person who has developed a dependency on alcohol through abuse of the substance.

**alcoholic ataxia** [Ar, *alkohl,* essence; Gk, *ataxia,* disorder], a loss of coordination in performing voluntary movements associated with peripheral neuritis as a result of alcoholism. A similar form of ataxia may occur with neuritis resulting from other toxic agents.

**alcoholic blackout,** a form of amnesia in which a person has no memory of what occurred during a period of alcohol abuse.

**alcoholic cardiomyopathy** [Ar, *alkohl,* essence; Gk, *kardia,* heart, *mys,* muscle, *pathos,* disease], a cardiac disease associated with alcohol abuse and characterized by an enlarged heart and low cardiac output. Treatment consists of abstinence from alcohol and results in marked reduction in heart size in over 50% of patients.

**alcoholic cirrhosis.** See **Laënnec's cirrhosis.**

**alcoholic coma** [Ar, *alkohl* + Gk, *koma,* deep sleep], a state of unconsciousness that results from severe alcoholic intoxication.

**alcoholic dementia** [Ar, *alkohl* + L, *de,* away, *mens,* mind], a deterioration of normal cognitive and intellectual functions associated with long-term alcohol abuse.

**alcoholic dyspepsia,** a digestive disorder characterized by abdominal discomfort and provoked by the consumption of alcohol.

**alcoholic fermentation,** the conversion of carbohydrates to ethyl alcohol.

**alcoholic hallucinosis,** a form of alcoholic psychosis characterized primarily by auditory hallucinations occuring in a clear sensorium, abject fear, and persecutory delusions. The condition develops in acute alcoholism as withdrawal symptoms shortly after stopping or reducing prolonged and heavy alcohol intake, usually within 48 hours. Also called **acute hallucinosis.** See also **alcoholic psychosis, hallucinosis.**

**alcoholic hepatitis,** acute toxic liver injury associated with excess ethanol consumption. It is characterized by necrosis, polymorphonuclear inflammation, and in many instances Mallory bodies.

**alcoholic ketoacidosis,** the fall in blood pH (acidosis) sometimes seen in alcoholics and associated with a rise in serum ketone bodies (acetone, beta-hydroxybutyric acid, and acetoacetic acid).

**alcoholic neuropathy.** See **alcoholic paralysis.**

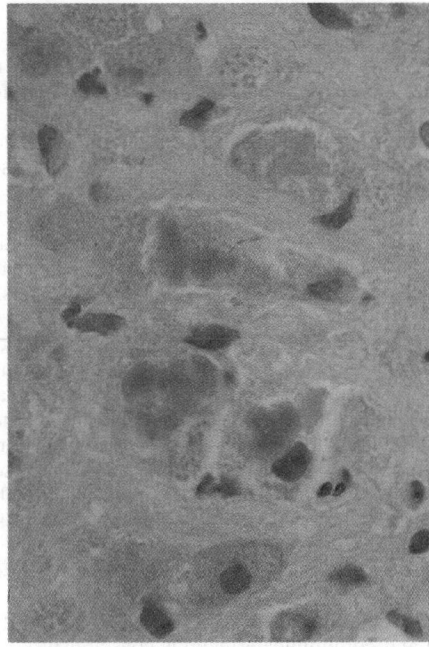

**Alcoholic hepatitis** *(Kumar, Cotran, and Robbins, 1997)*

**alcoholic-nutritional cerebellar degeneration,** a sudden, severe incoordination in the lower extremity characteristic of poorly nourished alcoholics. The patient walks, if at all, with an ataxic or wide-based gait. Cerebellar tumors, multiple sclerosis, and other neurologic disorders are characterized by similar motor impairments. Treatment consists of improved nutrition, abstinence from alcohol, and physical therapy. See also **alcoholism.**

**alcoholic paralysis** [Ar, *alkohl,* essence; Gk, *paralyein,* to be palsied], a paralysis affecting the peripheral nerves as a result of alcohol consumption. Also called **alcoholic neuropathy.**

**alcoholic psychosis,** any of a group of severe mental disorders in which the ego's functioning is impaired, such as pathologic intoxication, delirium tremens, Korsakoff's psychosis, and acute hallucinosis. It is characterized by brain damage or dysfunction that results from excessive alcohol use.

**Alcoholics Anonymous (AA),** an international nonprofit organization, founded in 1935, consisting of abstinent alcoholics whose purpose is to stay sober and help others recover from the disease of alcoholism through a 12-step program, including group support, shared experiences, and faith in a higher power. The AA program, which emphasizes both medical and religious resources for help in overcoming alcoholism, consists of attending meetings and coping with abstinence "one day at a time." Meetings are held at convenient times in factories, schools, churches, hospitals, and other community buildings. Similar groups who work with the children, relatives, friends, and associates of alcoholics are **Al-Anon** and **Alateen.**

**alcoholic trance,** a state of automatism resulting from ethanol intoxication.

**alcoholism** /al′kəhôliz′əm/, the extreme dependence on excessive amounts of alcohol, associated with a cumulative pattern of deviant behaviors. Alcoholism is a chronic illness with a slow, insidious onset, which may occur at any age. The cause is unknown, but cultural and psychosocial factors are suspect, and families of alcoholics have a higher incidence of alcoholism. ■ OBSERVATIONS: The most frequent medical consequences of alcoholism are central nervous system depression and cirrhosis of the liver. The severity of each may be greater in the absence of food intake. Alcoholic patients also may suffer from alcoholic gastritis, peripheral neuropathies, auditory hallucinations, and cardiac problems. Abrupt withdrawal of alcohol in addiction causes weakness, sweating, and hyperreflexia. The severe form of alcohol withdrawal is called delirium tremens. ■ INTERVENTIONS: Extreme caution should be used in administering drugs to the alcoholic patient because of the possibility of additive central nervous system depression and toxicity caused by inability of the liver to metabolize the drugs. Treatment of alcoholism consists of psychotherapy (especially group therapy, by organizations like Alcoholics Anonymous), or administration of drugs such as disulfiram that cause an aversion to alcohol. See also **acute alcoholism, chronic alcoholism, delirium tremens.**

**alcohol poisoning,** poisoning caused by the ingestion of any of several alcohols, of which ethyl, isopropyl, and methyl are the most common. Ethyl alcohol (ethanol) is found in beverages, hairspray, and mouthwashes. Ordinarily, it is lethal only if large quantities are ingested in a brief period. Isopropyl (rubbing) alcohol is more toxic. Methyl alcohol (methanol) is extremely poisonous: in addition to nausea, vomiting, and abdominal pain, it may cause blindness; death may follow the consumption of only 2 ounces. Treatment for alcohol poisoning may include gastric lavage and other supportive interventions.

**alcohol withdrawal syndrome,** the clinical symptoms associated with cessation of alcohol consumption. These may include tremor, hallucinations, autonomic nervous system dysfunction, and seizures.

**ALD,** abbreviation for **adrenoleukodystrophy.**

**Aldactazide,** trademark for a fixed-combination drug containing a potassium-wasting diuretic (hydrochlorothiazide) and a potassium-sparing diuretic (spironolactone).

**Aldactone,** trademark for a potassium-sparing diuretic (spironolactone).

**aldehyde** /al′dəhīd′/ [Ar, *alkohl* + L, *dehydrogenatum,* dehydrogenated], any of a large category of organic compounds derived from oxidation of a corresponding primary alcohol, as in the conversion of ethyl alcohol to acetaldehyde, also known as ethanal. Each aldehyde is characterized by a carbonyl group (—CO—) attached directly to a hydrogen (—CHO) in its formula, and can be converted into a corresponding acid by oxidation, as in the conversion of acetaldehyde to acetic acid.

**Aldoclor,** trademark for a fixed-combination antihypertensive drug containing chlorothiazide, a diuretic, and methyldopa, an antihypertensive.

**aldolase** /al′dəlās/, enzymes found in muscle tissue that catalyze the step in anaerobic glycolysis involving the breakdown of fructose 1,6-biphosphate to glyceraldehyde 3-phosphate (GAP). The enzyme can also catalyze the reverse reaction. Normal adult findings are 3 to 8.2 Sibley-Lehninger U/dl or 22 to 59 mU at 37° C. See also **glycolysis.**

**aldolase test,** a blood test that is most useful in indicating muscular or hepatic cellular injury or disease. It measures levels of aldolase, an enzyme that exists throughout most body tissues and that is used in the breakdown of glucose.

**Aldomet,** trademark for an antihypertensive (methyldopa).

**Aldoril,** trademark for a fixed-combination drug containing a potassium-wasting diuretic (hydrochlorothiazide) and an antihypertensive (methyldopa).

**aldose** /al'dōs/, the chemical form of monosaccharides in which the carbonyl group is an aldehyde.

**aldosterone** /al'dōstərōn', aldos'tərōn/, a mineralocorticoid steroid hormone produced by the adrenal cortex with action in the renal tubule to retain sodium, conserve water by reabsorption, and increase potassium excretion or increase of urinary excretion of potassium.

**aldosterone test,** a blood or 24-hour urine test used to diagnose hyperaldosteronism, which is associated with primary or secondary aldosteronism. Primary aldosteronism involves a tumor of the adrenal cortex or bilateral adrenal nodular hyperplasia, while secondary aldosteronism is associated with a variety of nonadrenal conditions.

**aldosteronism** /al'dōstərō'nizəm, aldos'-/, a condition characterized by hypersecretion of aldosterone, occurring as a primary disease of the adrenal cortex or, more often, as a secondary disorder in response to various extraadrenal pathologic processes. Primary aldosteronism, also called **Conn's syndrome,** may be caused by adrenal hyperplasia or by an aldosterone-secreting adenoma. Secondary aldosteronism is associated with increased plasma renin activity and may be induced by the nephrotic syndrome, hepatic cirrhosis, idiopathic edema, congestive heart failure, trauma, burns, or other kinds of stress. Hypersecretion of aldosterone promotes sodium retention and potassium excretion, leading to increased blood volume and blood pressure. The electrolyte imbalance in aldosteronism usually causes increased thirst and urination, treatment of primary aldosteronism caused by a tumor may include surgical resection and chemotherapy with the adrenal cytotoxic agent mitotane. Spironolactone, an aldosterone antagonist, or amiloride, a diuretic that blocks potassium excretion and sodium resorption, are frequently used to treat symptoms of aldosteronism. Also called **hyperaldosteronism.**

**aldosteronoma** /al'dōstir'ənō'mə/, *pl.* **aldosteronomas, aldosteronomata,** an aldosterone-secreting adenoma of the adrenal cortex that is usually small and occurs more frequently in the left than the right adrenal gland. Hyperaldosteronism with salt retention, expansion of the extracellular fluid volume, and increased blood pressure may occur.

**-aldrate,** suffix designating an antacid aluminum salt.

**alendronate,** a bone-resorption inhibitor.
■ INDICATIONS: This drug is used to treat osteoporosis in postmenopausal women and Paget's disease.
■ CONTRAINDICATIONS: Known hypersensitivity to biphosphonates prohibits the use of this drug.
■ ADVERSE EFFECTS: Side effects of this drug include anemia, hypokalemia, hypomagnesemia, hypophosphatemia, abdominal pain, anorexia, constipation, nausea, vomiting, bone pain, hypertension, urinary tract infection, and fluid overload.

**Aleppo boil.** See **oriental sore.**

**alertness** [Fr, *alerte*], a condition of being mentally quick, active, and keenly aware of the environment.

**aleukemia,** an acute form of leukemia characterized by a diminished total white cell content in the peripheral blood supply, accompanied by a loss of normal bone marrow function. Also spelled **aleukaemia.**

**aleukemic leukemia** /ā'lookē'mik/, a type of leukemia in which the total leukocyte count remains within normal limits and few abnormal forms appear in the peripheral blood. Diagnosis requires bone marrow biopsy. Also called **aleukocythemic leukemia, subleukemic leukemia.** See also **leukemia.**

**aleukemic myelosis.** See **myeloid metaplasia.**

**aleukia** /āloo'kē·ə/ [Gk, *a* + *leukos,* not white], a marked reduction in or complete absence of white blood cells or blood platelets. Compare **leukopenia, thrombocytopenia.** See also **aplastic anemia.**

**aleukocythemic leukemia.** See **aleukemic leukemia.**

**aleukocytosis** /āloo'kōsītō'sis/, an extreme decrease or absence of leukocytes in the blood.

**Alexander's disease** /al'eg·zan'dərz/ [W. Stewart Alexander, English pathologist, 20th century], an infantile form of leukodystrophy, characterized by eosinophilic material at the surface of the brain and around its blood vessels, resulting in brain enlargement.

**Alexander technique** [Frederick Matthias Alexander, Australian actor, 1869–1955, who developed and taught the technique], a body-focused alternative health therapy that focuses on individual variations in body musculature, posture, and the breathing process and on the correction of defects to avoid stress, tension, and possible dysfunction.

**alexia** /əlek'sē·ə/ [Gk, *a, lexis,* not speech], an inability to comprehend written words. See also **word blindness.** Compare **dyslexia.** —**alexic,** *adj.*

**alexic** /əlek'sik/ [Gk, *a,* without, *lexis,* speech], pertaining to alexia.

**alexithymia** /əlek'sithī'mē·ə, -thim'ē·ə/, an inability to experience and communicate feelings consciously.

**alfa.** See **alpha.**

**alfalfa,** an herb that is grown throughout the world.
■ USES: This herb is used for poor appetite, hay fever and asthma, and high cholesterol. It may also be used as a nutrient source.
■ CONTRAINDICATIONS: Alfalfa is not recommended during pregnancy and lactation, in children, or in those with known hypersensitivity to this product.

**ALG,** abbreviation for **antilymphocyte globulin.** See **antilymphocyte serum.**

**alg-.** See **algesi-.**

**alga** /al'gə/, *pl.* **algae** /al'jī, al'jē/ [L, seaweed], any of a large group of mostly photosynthetic protists. Many species of algae are found worldwide in fresh water, in salt water, and on land. —**algal,** *adj.*

**algesi-, alg-, alge-, algo-,** prefix meaning 'pain': *algesia, algophobia.*

**-algesia,** suffix meaning '(condition of) sensitivity to pain': *asphalgesia, hyperthermalgesia.*

**-algesic,** suffix meaning 'sensitivity to pain': *analgesic, paralgesic.*

**-algia, -algy,** suffix meaning 'pain, painful condition': *epigastralgia, uteralgia.*

**-algic,** suffix meaning 'pain': *cardialgic, tibialgic.*

**algid** /al'jid/ [L, *algere,* to be cold], chilly or cold.

**algid malaria** [L, *algere,* to be cold], a stage of malaria caused by the protozoan *Plasmodium falciparum.* It is characterized by coldness of the skin, profound weakness, and severe diarrhea. See also **falciparum malaria, malaria.**

**alginate** /al'ji·nāt /, a salt of alginic acid, extracted from marine kelp. The calcium, sodium, and ammonium alginates have been used as foam, clot, or gauze for absorbable surgical dressings. Soluble alginates, such as those of sodium, potassium, or magnesium, form a viscous sol that can be changed into a gel by a chemical reaction with compounds such as calcium sulfate; this makes them useful as materials for taking dental impressions.

**algo-.** See **algesi-.**

**algodystrophy** /al'gōdis'trəfē/, a painful wasting of the muscles of the hands, often accompanied by tenderness and a loss of bone calcium. The condition may begin in the hand or in the shoulder and spread over the entire limb, causing contractures, edema, and cyanosis of the skin. It may be associated with injury, heart disease, stroke, or a viral infection.

**algolagnia** /al'gōlag'nē·ə/ [Gk, *algos,* pain, *lagneia,* lust], a form of sexual perversion characterized by sadism or masochism. See also **sadism, sadomasochism.**

**algologist** /algol'əjist/, **1.** a person who specializes in the study of or the treatment of pain. **2.** also called **phycologist.** a person who specializes in the study of algae.

**algology, 1.** the branch of medicine that is concerned with the study of pain. **2.** the branch of science that is concerned with algae. Also called **phycology.**

**algophobia** [Gk, *algos,* pain, *phobos,* fear], an anxiety disorder characterized by an abnormal, pervasive fear of experiencing pain or of witnessing pain in others.

**algor** [L, cold], the sensation of cold or a chill, particularly in the first stage of a fever.

**algorithm** /al'gərith'əm/, **1.** a step-by-step procedure for the solution of a problem by a computer, using specific mathematic or logical operations. Compare **heuristic. 2.** an explicit protocol with well-defined rules to be followed in solving a health care problem.

**algor mortis,** the reduction in body temperature and accompanying loss of skin elasticity that occur after death. Also called **death chill.**

**algospasm** /al'gōspaz'əm/, an acute, painful spasm of the muscles.

**Alice in Wonderland syndrome,** perceptual distortions of space and size, as experienced by the character Alice in the Lewis Carroll story. Similar hallucinogenic experiences have been reported by individuals using drugs of abuse and by patients with certain neurologic diseases.

**alien** /āl'yən/ [L, *alienare,* to estrange], strange, unusual, or foreign.

**alienate** /āl'yənāt/ [L, *alienare,* to cause a withdrawal or transference of affection, or detachment.

**alienation** /āl'yənā'shən/ [L, *alienare,* to estrange], the act or state of being estranged or isolated. See also **depersonalization.**

**alignment** /əlīn'mənt/ [Fr, *aligner,* to put in a straight line], **1.** the arrangement of a group of points or objects along a line. **2.** the placing or maintaining of body structures in their proper anatomic positions, such as straightening the teeth or repairing a fractured bone. Also spelled **alinement.**

**aliment** [L, *alimentum,* to nourish], nutrition.

**alimentary** /al'əmen'tərē/ [L, *alimentum,* nourishment], pertaining to food or nourishment and to the digestive organs.

**alimentary bolus.** See **bolus,** def. 1.

**alimentary canal.** See **digestive tract.**

**alimentary duct,** the thoracic duct of the lymphatic system.

**alimentary system** [L, *alimentum,* nourishment; Gk, *systema*], the digestive system.

**alimentary tract.** See **digestive tract.**

**alimentation,** nourishment. See also **feeding.**

**alinement.** See **alignment.**

**aliphatic** /al'ifat'ik/ [Gk, *aleiphar,* oil], pertaining to fat or oil, specifically to those hydrocarbon compounds that are open chains of carbon atoms, such as the fatty acids, rather than aromatic ring structures. Aliphatic compounds do not have unsaturated cyclic structures as are found in the aromatic compounds benzene or nephthalene, etc.

**aliphatic acid,** an acid of a nonaromatic hydrocarbon.

**aliphatic alcohol,** an alcohol that contains an open chain or fatty series of hydrocarbons. Examples include ethyl alcohol and isopropyl alcohol, both of which have fat-solvent properties as well as bactericidal effects.

**-alis,** suffix meaning 'pertaining to' something specified.

**alitretinoin,** a second-generation retinoid.

■ INDICATIONS: It is used to treat the cutaneous lesions seen in Kaposi's sarcoma.

■ CONTRAINDICATIONS: Known hypersensitivity and pregnancy prohibit this drug's use.

■ ADVERSE EFFECTS: Side effects include rash, stinging, warmth, redness, erythema, blistering, crusting, peeling, contact dermatitis, and pain at the site of application.

**alkalemia** [Ar, *al* + *galiy,* wood ash; Gk, *haima,* blood], a condition of increased pH of the blood, above the normal range of 7.35 to 7.45. Also spelled **alkalaemia.**

**alkali** /al'kəlī/ [Ar, *al* + *galiy,* wood ash], a compound with the chemical characteristics of a base. Alkalis combine with fatty acids to form soaps, turn red litmus blue, and enter into reactions that form water-soluble carbonates. See also **acid, base. alkaline,** *adj.* **alkalinity,** *n.*

**alkali burn,** damage to tissue caused by exposure to an alkaline compound like lye. Treatment includes washing the area with copious amounts of water to remove the chemical. It takes much more water to irrigate an alkali burn than to irrigate an acid burn. The victim is immediately taken to a medical facility for assessment of tissue damage. Compare **acid burn.**

**-alkaline,** suffix meaning 'alkali': *subalkaline.*

**alkaline ash** /al'kəlīn/, residue in the urine having a pH higher than 7.0.

**alkaline ash–producing foods,** foods that may be ingested to produce an alkaline pH in the urine, thereby reducing the incidence of acidic urinary calculi, or that may be avoided to reduce the incidence of alkaline calculi. Some foods that result in alkaline ash are milk, cream, buttermilk, fruit (except prunes, plums, and cranberries), vegetables (except corn and lentils), almonds, chestnuts, coconuts, and olives.

**alkaline bath,** a bath taken in water containing sodium bicarbonate, used especially for skin disorders.

**alkaline phosphatase,** an enzyme present in bone, the kidneys, the intestine, plasma, and teeth. It may be elevated in the serum in some diseases of the bone and liver and in some other illnesses. The normal concentrations of this enzyme in the serum of adults are 1.5 to 4.5 Bodansky units; in children, 5 to 14 Bodansky units. See also **Bodansky unit.**

**alkaline phosphatase test (ALP),** a blood test used to determine a variety of liver and bone disorders such as extrahepatic and intrahepatic obstructive biliary disease, cirrhosis, hepatic tumors, hepatotoxic drugs, hepatitis, osteoblastic metastatic tumors, Paget's disease, rheumatoid arthritis, and hyperparathyroidism.

**alkaline reserve,** an additional amount of sodium bicarbonate the body produces to maintain a normal arterial blood pH (7.35 to 7.45) when the carbon dioxide level increases as a result of hypoventilation. The alkaline reserve is maintained by the kidneys, which control excretion of bicarbonate ions in the urine.

**alkalinity** /al'kəlin'itē/, pertaining to the acid-base relationship of any solution that has a lower concentration of hydrogen ions or a higher concentration of hydroxide ions than pure water, which is an arbitrarily neutral standard with a pH of 7.0 at 25° C.

**alkalinize** /al'kəlinīz/, **1.** to make a substance alkaline, as through the addition of a base. **2.** to become alkaline. Also **alkalize** /al'kəlīz/. Compare **acidify.**

**alkali poisoning,** a toxic condition caused by the ingestion of an alkaline agent like liquid ammonia, lye, and some detergent powders. Compare **acid poisoning.**

**alkali reserves** [Ar, *al + galiy,* the wood ashes,+ L, *reservare,* to save], the volume of carbon dioxide or carbonates at standard temperature and pressure in 100 mL of blood plasma. The principal buffer in blood is bicarbonate, which represents most of the alkali reserve. Hemoglobin phosphates and additional bases also act as buffers. If the alkali reserve is low, acidosis exists. If the alkali reserve is high, alkalosis exists.

**alkalize.** See **alkalinize.**

**alkaloid** /al′kəloid/ [Ar, *al + galiy* + Gk, *eidos,* form], any of a large group of nitrogen-containing organic compounds produced by plants, including many pharmacologically active substances, such as atropine, caffeine, cocaine, morphine, nicotine, and quinine.

**alkalosis** /al′kəlō′sis/ [Ar, *al + galiy* + Gk, *osis,* condition], an abnormal condition of body fluids, characterized by a tendency toward a blood pH level greater than 7.45, as from an excess of alkaline bicarbonate or a deficiency of acid. Respiratory alkalosis may be caused by hyperventilation, resulting from an excess loss of carbon dioxide and a carbonic acid deficit. Metabolic alkalosis may result from an excess intake or retention of bicarbonate, loss of gastric acid in vomiting, potassium depletion, or any stimulus that increases the rate of sodium-hydrogen exchange. When a buffer system, such as carbon dioxide retention or bicarbonate excretion, prevents a shift in pH, it is labeled compensating alkalosis. Treatment of uncompensated alkalosis involves correction of dehydration and various ionic deficits to restore the normal acid-base balance in which the ratio of carbonic acid to bicarbonate is 20:1. Compare **acidosis.**

**alkaptonuria** /alkap′tōnŏŏr′ē·ə/ [Ar, *al + galiy* + Gk, *haptein* to possess, *ouron* urine], a rare inherited disorder resulting from the incomplete metabolism of tyrosine, an amino acid, in which abnormal amounts of homogentisic acid are excreted as a result of incomplete metabolism of tyrosine, staining the urine dark. In this disorder, which is transmitted by an autosomal recessive gene, a key metabolic enzyme is absent from the body. Usually the condition does not cause symptoms until middle age, at which point ochronosis, a type of arthritis, may develop. The condition also can be caused by chronic phenol poisoning. See also **ochronosis. —alkaptonuric,** *adj.*

**alkene** /al′kēn/, an unsaturated aliphatic hydrocarbon containing one double bond in the carbon chain, such as ethylene (ethene). Also called **olefin.**

**Alkeran,** trademark for an alkylating antineoplastic agent (melphalan).

**alkyl** /al′kil/, a hydrocarbon fragment derived from alkane by the removal of one of the hydrogen atoms.

**alkylamine** /al′kiləmīn′/, an amine in which an alkyl group replaces one to three of the hydrogen atoms that are attached to the nitrogen atom, such as methylamine (aminomethane).

**alkylating agent** /al′kilā′ting/, any substance that contains an alkyl radical and is capable of replacing a free hydrogen atom in an organic compound, or one that acts by a similar mechanism. This type of chemical reaction results in interference with mitosis and cell division, especially in rapidly proliferating tissue. They are radiometric in that their action is similar to that of irradiation. The agents are useful in the treatment of cancer. Agents include cyclophosphamide. Adverse effects include nausea, vomiting, alopecia, and anemia.

**alkylation,** a chemical reaction in which an alkyl group is transferred from an alkylating agent. When such organic re-

actions occur with a biologically significant cellular constituent such as deoxyribonucleic acid (DNA), they result in interference with mitosis and cell division.

**ALL,** abbreviation for **acute lymphocytic leukemia.** See also **acute childhood leukemia.**

**all-.** See **allo-.**

**allachesthesia** /al′əkesthē′zhə/ [Gk, *allache,* elsewhere], a defect of touch sensation in which a stimulus is perceived to be at a point distant from where it is actually applied.

**allanto-,** combining form meaning 'allantois': *allantotoxicon.*

**allantoic.** See **allantois.**

**allantoidoangiopagus** /al′əntoi′dō·an′jē·op′əgəs/ [Gk, *allantoeides,* sausagelike, *angeion,* vessel, *pagos,* fixed], conjoined monozygotic twin fetuses of unequal size that are united by the vessels of the umbilical cord. Also called **omphaloangiopagus.** See also **omphalosite. —allantoidoangiopagous,** *adj.*

**allantoin** /əlan′tō·in/, a chemical compound (5-ureidohydantoin), $C_4H_6N_4O_3$, that occurs as a white crystallizable substance found in many plants and in the allantoic and amniotic fluids and fetal urine of primates. It is also present in the urine of mammals other than primates as a product of purine metabolism. The substance, which can be produced synthetically by the oxidation of uric acid, was once used to promote tissue growth in the treatment of suppurating wounds and ulcers.

**allantois** /əlan′tois/ [Gk, *allas,* sausage, *eidos,* form], a tubular extension of the endoderm of the yolk sac that extends with the allantoic vessels into the body stalk of the embryo. In human embryos, allantoic vessels become the umbilical vessels and the chorionic villi. See also **body stalk, umbilical cord. —allantoic** /al′əntō′ik/, *adj.*

**allele** /əlēl′/, **1.** one of two or more alternative forms of a gene that occupy corresponding loci on homologous chromosomes. Each allele encodes a phenotypic feature or a certain inherited characteristic. An individual normally has two alleles for each gene, one contributed by the mother and one by the father. If both alleles are the same, the individual is homozygous. If the alleles are different, the individual is heterozygous. In heterozygous individuals, one of the alleles is usually dominant, and the other is recessive. In humans, for example, the allele for brown eyes is dominant, and the allele for blue eyes is recessive. **2.** also called **allelomorph** /əlēl′əmôrf′/. One of two or more contrasting characteristics transmitted by alternative forms of a gene. **—allelic,** *adj.*

**allelo-,** combining form meaning 'another': *allelocatalysis, allelomorph.*

**allelomorph.** See **allele.**

**Allen-Doisy test** [Edgar Allen, U.S. endocrinologist, 1892–1943; Edward Doisy, U.S. biochemist and Nobel laureate, 1893–1986], a bioassay test for estrogen and gonadotropins in which ovariectomized mice are injected with an estrogenic substance. The appearance of cornified cells on vaginal smears is regarded as a positive finding.

**Allen test,** a test for the patency of the radial artery after insertion of an indwelling monitoring catheter. The patient's hand is formed into a fist while the nurse compresses the ulnar artery. Compression continues while the fist is opened. If blood perfusion through the radial artery is adequate, the hand should flush and resume normal pinkish coloration.

**allergen** /al′ərjin/ [Gk, *allos,* other, *ergein,* to work, *genein,* to produce], an environmental substance that can produce a hypersensitive allergic reaction in the body but may not be intrinsically harmful. Common allergens include pollen, animal dander, house dust, feathers, and various foods. Studies indicate that one of six Americans is hypersensitive to one or more allergens. Methods to identify specific allergens affecting individuals include the patch test, the scratch test, the radioallergosorbent (RAST) test, and the Prausnitz-Küstner (PK) test. —**allergenic,** *adj.* See also **allergic reaction, allergy.**

**allergenic** /al'ərjen'ik/, provoking allergic reactions.

**allergenic extract,** a protein-containing extract purified from a substance to which a person may be sensitive. The extract, may be used for diagnosis or for desensitization therapy.

**allergic** /əlur'jik/, **1.** pertaining to allergy. **2.** having an allergy.

**allergic alveolitis.** See **diffuse hypersensitivity pneumonia.**

**allergic arthritis,** appearance of symptoms of arthritis such as swollen joints after the ingestion of allergenic foods or medications.

**allergic asthma,** a form of asthma caused by exposure of the bronchial mucosa to an inhaled airborne antigen. The antigen causes the production of antibodies that bind to mast cells in the bronchial tree. The mast cells then release histamine, which stimulates contraction of bronchial smooth muscle and causes mucosal edema. Hyposensitization treatments are more effective for pollen sensitivity than for allergies to house dust, animal dander, mold, and insects. Psychologic factors may provoke asthma attacks in bronchi already sensitized by antigens. Medication, including immunotherapy, can help relieve allergy symptoms. Often a diurnal pattern of histamine release occurs, causing variable degrees of bronchospasm at different times of the day. Also called **atopic asthma, extrinsic asthma.** See also **asthma, asthma in children, asthmatic eosinophilia, status asthmaticus.**

**allergic bronchopulmonary aspergillosis,** a form of aspergillosis that occurs in asthmatics when the fungus *Aspergillus fumigatus,* growing within the bronchial lumen, causes a type I or type III hypersensitivity reaction. The characteristics of the condition are similar to those of asthma, including dyspnea and wheezing. Chest examination and pulmonary function tests may reveal airway obstruction. Serologic tests usually reveal precipitating antibodies to *A. fumigatus.* Bacteriologic and microscopic examination of sputum may reveal *A. fumigatus* in addition to Charcot-Leyden crystals. Eosinophilia is usually also present. Compare **aspergillosis.**

**allergic conjunctivitis,** inflammation of the conjunctiva caused by an allergy. Common allergens that cause this condition are pollen, grass, topical medications, air pollutants, occupational irritants, and smoke. It is bilateral, usually starts before puberty, and commonly recurs in a seasonal pattern for about 10 years.

■ OBSERVATIONS: The common signs include itching, burning and swelling around the eyes and excessive tearing. Eosinophils predominate in stained blood smears. Diagnosis is usually based on the results of cultures and sensitivity tests to identify the causative allergen.

■ INTERVENTIONS: Oral antihistamines and vasoconstrictor and corticosteroid eyedrops, such as prednisone acetate are typically prescribed. .

■ NURSING CONSIDERATIONS: Cold compresses may be administered. Also called **redeye.** See also **conjunctivitis.**

**allergic contact dermatitis.** See **allergic dermatitis.**

**allergic coryza,** acute rhinitis caused by exposure to any allergen to which the person is hypersensitive.

**allergic dermatitis** [Ger, *allergie,* reaction; Gk, *derma,* skin, *itis,* inflammation], an acute, cell-mediated inflammatory response of an area of skin after exposure of that area to a contact allergen to which the patient is hypersensitive. Such allergens include dyes, perfumes, poison ivy, certain chemicals, and metals. Also called **allergic contact dermatitis.**

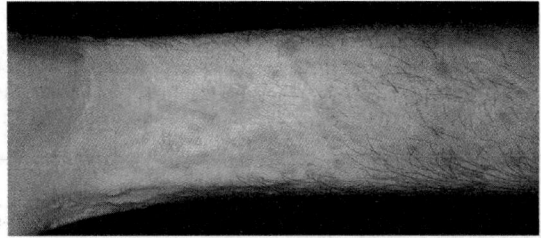

**Allergic dermatitis resulting from contact with poison ivy**
*(Goldstein and Goldstein, 1997)*

**allergic interstitial pneumonitis.** See **diffuse hypersensitivity pneumonia.**

**allergic purpura** [Gk, *allos,* other, *ergein,* to work; L, *purpura,* purple], a chronic disorder of the skin associated with urticaria, erythema, asthma, and rheumatic joint swellings. Unlike in other forms of purpura, platelet count, bleeding time, and blood coagulation are normal.

**allergic reaction,** an unfavorable physiologic response to an allergen to which a person has previously been exposed and to which the person has developed antibodies. The response may be characterized by a variety of symptoms including urticaria, eczema, dyspnea, bronchospasm, diarrhea, rhinitis, sinusitis, laryngospasm, and anaphylaxis. Allergic reactions may be immediate or delayed. Eosinophilia is usually present and is revealed in the differential white blood cell count.

**allergic rhinitis,** inflammation of the nasal passages, usually associated with watery nasal discharge and itching of the nose and eyes, caused by a localized sensitivity reaction

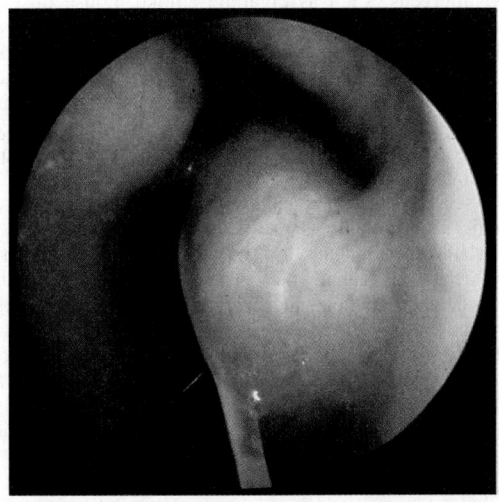

**Allergic rhinitis: view through fiberoptic rhinoscope**
*(Zitelli and Davis, 1997)*

to an allergen, such as house dust, animal dander, or pollen. The condition may be seasonal, as in hay fever, or perennial, as in allergy to dust or animals. Treatment may include the local, systemic, or topical administration of antihistamines or steroids, avoidance of the antigen, and hyposensitization by injections of diluted antigen in gradually increasing amounts.

**allergic vasculitis,** an inflammatory condition of the blood vessels that is induced by allergens, such as iodides, penicillin, sulfonamides, and thioureas. It is characterized by itching, malaise, and a slight fever and by the presence of papules, vesicles, urticarial wheals, or small ulcers on the skin.

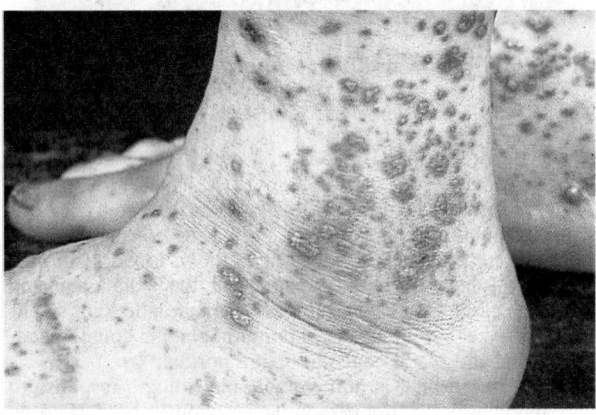

**Allergic vasculitis in the foot**
*(du Vivier, 1993/courtesy St. Mary's Hospital)*

**allergist** /al'ərjist/, a physician who specializes in the diagnosis and treatment of allergic disorders.

**allergy** /al'ərjē/ [Gk, *allos*, other, *ergein*, to work], a hypersensitive reaction to common, often intrinsically harmless, substances most of which are environmental. More than 20 million Americans have allergic reactions to airborne or inhaled allergens, such as cigarette smoke, house dust, and pollens. Symptoms of mild allergies, such as those associated with rhinitis, conjunctivitis, and urticaria, can be suppressed by antihistamines with glucocorticoids administered as supplements to primary therapy. Severe allergic reactions, such as anaphylaxis and angioneurotic edema of the glottis, can cause systemic shock and death and commonly require immediate therapy with subcutaneous epinephrine or IV steroids, such as dexamethasone sodium phosphate. See also **allergic reaction, allergy testing.**

**allergy blood test,** a blood test used to measure serum immunoglobulin E (IgE), which is an effective method of diagnosing allergy and of specifically identifying the allergen. This test can be helpful when results of an allergy skin test are questionable, when the allergen is not available in a form for dermal injection, when the allergen may incite an anaphylactic reaction if injected into the patient, or when skin testing is particularly difficult (i.e., in infants, or patients with dermographia or widespread skin disease).

**allergy management,** a nursing intervention from the Nursing Interventions Classification (NIC) defined as identification, treatment, and prevention of allergic responses to food, medications, insect bites, contrast material, blood, or other substances. See also **Nursing Interventions Classification.**

**allergy skin test,** a skin test used to detect allergic reactions. Properly performed, it is considered the most convenient and least expensive test for detecting such reactions. The test involves injecting an allergen into the skin and then evaluating the wheal (swelling) and flare (redness) responses that follow.

**allergy testing,** any one of the various procedures used in identifying the specific allergens that afflict a patient. Such tests are helpful in prescribing treatment to prevent allergic reactions or to reduce their severity. The most common is skin testing, which exposes the patient to small quantities of the suspected allergens. Positive reactions usually occur within 20 minutes as varying degrees of erythema. Factors considered in performing allergy tests include the medical history of the patient, the allergy history, the environment, and the diet. Individuals to be tested are usually instructed to discontinue the use of any antihistamines at least 24 hours before the test, because these drugs can interfere with normal test responses. The most common kinds of allergy testing are the **intradermal, scratch, patch, conjunctival, Prausnitz-Küstner (PK), radioallergosorbent (RAST),** and **use** tests.

**allesthesia** /al'esthē'zha/, a referred pain or other sensation that is perceived at a remote site on the same or opposite side of the body stimulated. Also called **alloesthesia.**

**all fours position,** the sixth stage in the Rood system of ontogenetic motor patterns. In this stage, the lower trunk and lower extremities are brought into a co-contraction pattern while stretching of the trunk and limb girdles develops co-contractions of the trunk flexors and extensors.

**allicin** /al'i·sin/ [*Allium*, the genus of garlic], an oily substance extracted from garlic, having antibacterial activity.

**allied health personnel.** See **paramedical personnel.**

**alligator forceps,** 1. a forceps with heavy teeth and a double clamp, used in orthopedic surgery. 2. a forceps with long, thin, angular handles and interlocking teeth. Also called **alligator clamp.**

**Allis forceps,** curved forceps with serrated edges, used for grasping tissues. Also called **Allis clamps.**

**allo-, all-,** combining form meaning 'differing from the normal, reversal, or referring to another': *allopathy, allergic.*

**alloantigen** /al'ō·an'tijen/ [Gk, *allos*, other], an isoantigen; a substance present in some members of a species which stimulates production of antibodies in other members of the species. An example is blood group antigens.

**allodiploid** /al'ōdip'loid/ [Gk, *allos*, other, *diploos*, double, *eidos*, form], 1. an individual, organism, strain, or cell that has two genetically distinct sets of chromosomes derived from different ancestral species, as occurs in hybridization. 2. pertaining to such an individual, organism, strain, or cell. Also called **allodiploidic.** Compare **autopolyploid.**

**allodiploidy** /al'ōdip'loidē/, the state or condition of having two genetically distinct sets of chromosomes derived from different ancestral species.

**alloeroticism, alloerotism.** See **heteroeroticism.**

**alloesthesia** See **allesthesia.**

**allogamy.** See **cross fertilization.**

**allogeneic.** See **allogenic.**

**allogenic** /al'ōjen'ik/ [Gk, *allos* + *genein*, to produce], 1. (in genetics) denoting an individual or cell type that is from the same species but genetically distinct. 2. (in transplantation biology) denoting tissues, particularly stem cells from either bone marrow or peripheral blood, that are from the same species but antigenically distinct; homologous. Compare **syngeneic, xenogeneic.**

**allograft** /al′əgraft/ [Gk, *allos,* other + *graphion,* stylus], a graft of tissue between two genetically dissimilar individuals of the same species, such as a tissue transplant between two humans who are not identical twins. Tissues commonly used for allografts include cornea, cartilage, bone, artery, and cadaver skin stored in a skin-tissue bank. Also called homogenous graft, **homograft, homologous graft.** Compare **autograft, isograft, xenograft.** See also **graft.**

**allohexaploid, allohexaploidic.** See **allopolyploid.**

**allokeratoplasty** /al′ōker′ətoplas′tē/, the repair of a cornea with synthetic transparent material.

**allometric.** See **allometry.**

**allometric growth,** the increase in size of different organs or parts of an organism at various rates. Also called **heterauxesis.** Compare **isometric growth.** See also **allometry.**

**allometron** /əlom′itron/, a quantitative change in the proportional relationship of the parts of an organism as a result of evolution.

**allometry** /əlom′itrē/ [Gk, *allos* + *metron,* measure], the measurement and study of the changes in proportions of the various parts of an organism in relation to the growth of the whole or of such changes in within a series of related organisms. See also **allometric growth. —allometric,** *adj.*

**allomorphism** /al′ōmôr′fizəm/ [Gk, *allos,* other, *morphe,* form], **1.** a change in crystalline form without a change in chemical composition. **2.** a change in the shape of a group of cells caused by pressure or other physical factors.

**allopathic physician** /al′ōpath′ik/, a physician who treats disease and injury with active interventions, such as medical and surgical treatment, intended to bring about effects opposite of those produced by the disease or injury. Almost all practicing physicians in the United States are allopathic. Compare **chiropractic, homeopathy, osteopathy.**

**allopathy** /əlop′əthē/ [Gk, *allos* + *pathos,* suffering], a system of medical therapy in which a disease or an abnormal condition is treated by creating an environment that is antagonistic to the disease or condition; for example, an antibiotic toxic to a pathogenic organism is given in an infection.

**allopentaploid, allopentaploidic.** See **allopolyploid.**

**alloplast** /al′ōplast/ [Gk, *allos,* other, *plassein,* to mold], a graft made of plastic, metal, or other material foreign to the human body.

**alloplastic** /al′ō·plas′tik /, **1.** pertaining to or characterized by alloplasty. **2.** pertaining to an alloplast.

**alloplastic maneuver** [Gk, *allos* + *plassein,* to mold], (in psychology) a process that is part of adaptation, involving an adjustment or change in the external environment. Compare **autoplastic maneuver.**

**alloplasty** /al′ōplas′tē/ [Gk, *allos,* other, *plassein,* to mold], plastic surgery in which materials foreign to the human body are implanted.

**alloploid, alloploidic.** See **allodiploid, allopolyploid.**

**alloploidy.** See **allodiploidy, allopolyploidy.**

**allopolyploid** /al′əpol′iploid/ [Gk, *allos* + *polyplous,* many times, *eidos* form], **1.** an individual, organism, strain, or cell that has more than two genetically distinct sets of chromosomes derived from two or more different ancestral species, as occurs in hybridization. Such individuals are referred to as allotriploid, allotetraploid, allopentaploid, allohexaploid, and so on, depending on the number of haploid sets of chromosomes they contain. **2.** pertaining to such an individual, organism, strain, or cell. Also **allopolyploidic.** See also **mosaic.** Compare **autopolyploid.**

**allopolyploidy** /al′əpol′iploi′dē/, the state or condition of having more than two genetically distinct sets of chromosomes derived from two or more different ancestral species. See also **mosaic.** Compare **autopolyploidy.**

**allopurinol** /al′əpyōōr′ənôl/, a xanthine oxidase inhibitor uricosuric agent.

■ INDICATIONS: It is prescribed in the treatment of gout and other hyperuricemic conditions.

■ CONTRAINDICATIONS: It is not prescribed for children (except those with hyperuricemia resulting from malignancy), lactating mothers, or people suffering an acute attack of gout. Known hypersensitivity to this drug prohibits its use.

■ ADVERSE EFFECTS: Among the most serious adverse reactions are blood dyscrasias and severe rashes and other allergic reactions. GI and ophthalmologic disturbances also may occur.

**allorhythmia** /al′ōrith′mē′ə/, an irregular heart rhythm that occurs repeatedly.

**all-or-none law,** **1.** the principle in neurophysiology stating that a stimulus must be strong enough to reach threshold to trigger a nerve impulse. Once theshold is achieved, the entire impulse is discharged. A weak stimulus will not produce a weak reaction. **2.** the principle that the heart muscle, under any stimulus above a threshold level, will respond either with a maximal strength contraction or not at all. Also called **Bowditch's law.**

**allosteric sites** /al′ōster′ik/ [Gk, *allos* + *stereos,* solid], the sites, other than the active site or sites, of an enzyme that bind regulatory molecules.

**allotetraploid, allotetraploidic.** See **allopolyploid.**

**allotransplantation,** transplantation of an allograft.

**allotrio-,** prefix meaning 'strange or foreign': *allotriodontia.*

**allotriodontia** /əlot′rē·ōdon′shə/, **1.** the development of a tooth in an abnormal location, such as in a dermoid tumor. **2.** the transplantation of teeth from one individual to another.

**allotriploid, allotriploidic.** See **allopolyploid.**

**allotropic,** **1.** pertaining to a substance that is changed by digestion to retain some of its nutritive value. **2.** pertaining to an element that may exist in two or more molecular forms, such as carbon in the diamond and graphite forms.

**allowable charge** /əlou′əbəl/, the maximum amount that a third party, usually an insurance company, will reimburse a provider for a specific service.

**allowable costs,** components of an institution's costs that are reimbursable as determined by a payment formula. In general, costs of services not considered to be reasonable or necessary to the proper provision of health services are excluded from allowable costs.

**allowable dose.** See **accumulated dose equivalent.**

**allowable error,** the amount of error that can be tolerated without invalidating the medical usefulness of the analytic result. Allowable error is defined as having a 95% limit of analytic error; only 1 sample in 20 can have an error greater than this limit.

**alloxan** /əlok′san/, an oxidation product of uric acid that is found in the human intestine in diarrhea. Alloxan has been used to produce diabetes in experimental animals by destroying the insulin-secreting islet cells of the pancreas.

**alloy** /al′oi/ [Fr, *aloyer,* to combine metals], a mixture of two or more metals or of substances with metallic properties. Most alloys are formed by mixing molten metals that dissolve in each other. A number of alloys have medical applications, such as those used for prostheses and in dental amalgams. See **amalgam.**

**almond oil,** an oil expressed from the kernels of the fruit of the sweet almond tree, *Prunus amygdalus,* which is native to the Mediterranean region. The fixed oil is a demulcent and mildly laxative. Bitter almond oil is a volatile oil that contains lethal prussic acid.

**aloe,** a succulent found throughout the world.

- ■ USES: Aloe vera gel is used externally for minor burns, skin irritations, minor wounds, frostbite, and radiation-caused injuries. Internally, it is used to heal intestinal inflammation and ulcers, and as a digestive aid to stimulate bile secretion.
- ■ CONTRAINDICATIONS: *Topically:* Hypersensitivity to this plant, garlic, onions, or tulips prohibits the use of aloe. Aloe also should not be used on deep wounds. *Internally:* The dried juice is contraindicated during pregnancy and lactation, in children less than 12 years of age, and in those with kidney or cardiac disease or bowel obstruction. This product should not be used long-term.

**alopecia** /al′əpē′shə/ [Gk, *alopex,* fox mange], partial or complete lack of hair resulting from normal aging, endocrine disorder, drug reaction, anticancer medication, or skin disease. Kinds of alopecia include **alopecia areata, alopecia totalis, alopecia universalis, androgenic female pattern, male pattern, premature alopecia and scarring.**

**alopecia areata** /er′ē·ā′tə/, a disease of unknown cause in which sudden well-defined bald patches occur. The bald areas are usually round or oval and located on the head and other hairy parts of the body with characteristic "exclamation point" formation by the hair at the end that leaves the scalp not clear. The condition is usually self-limited and often clears completely within 6 to 12 months without treatment. Recurrences are common. Compare **alopecia totalis, alopecia universalis.**

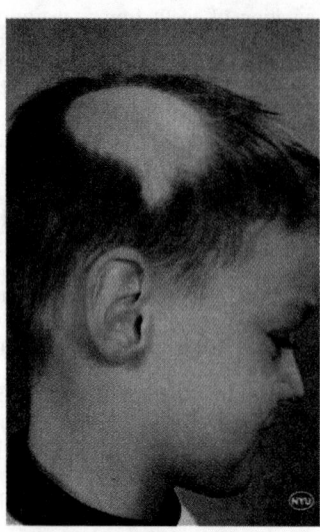

**Alopecia areata**
*(Barkauskas et al, 1998/courtesy American Academy of Dermatology and Institute for Dermatologic Communication and Education, Schaumburg, Illinois)*

**alopecia congenitalis,** congenital baldness in which there may be partial or complete absence of hair at birth.

**alopecia neurotica,** loss of hair, usually occurring at one site, after a disease or injury involving the nervous system.

**alopecia prematura,** baldness that occurs early in life, beginning as early as late adolescence.

**alopecia senilis,** a form of natural hair loss that affects older persons.

**alopecia totalis,** an uncommon condition characterized by the loss of all the hair on the scalp. The cause is unknown, and the baldness is usually permanent. No treatment is known. Compare **alopecia areata, alopecia universalis.**

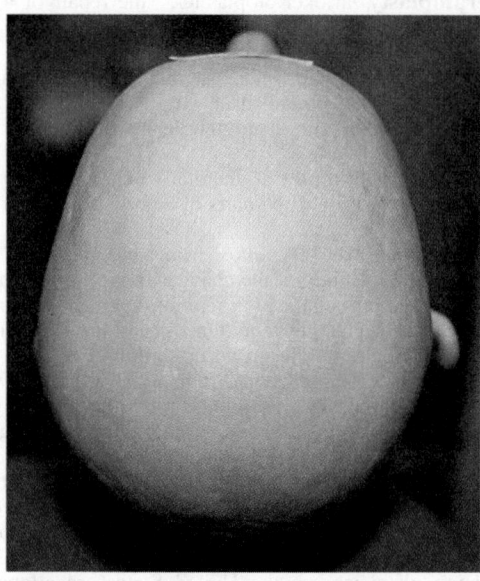

**Alopecia totalis** *(Hordinsky, Sawaya, and Scher, 2000)*

**alopecia toxica,** a form of hair loss attributed to a febrile illness.

**alopecia universalis,** a total loss of hair on all parts of the body. The condition is occasionally an extension of alopecia areata. Compare **alopecia areata, alopecia totalis.**

**alpha** /al′fə/, A, α, the first letter of the Greek alphabet. It is commonly used as a scientific notation, as in denoting the position of an atom in a molecule, identifying a nuclear particle, or designating a particular physiologic rhythm. For example, it is used in chemical nomenclature to distinguish one variation in a chemical compound from others.

**alpha-adrenergic.** See **adrenergic receptor.**

**alpha-adrenergic blocking agent.** See **antiadrenergic.**

**alpha-adrenergic receptor.** See **alpha receptor.**

**alpha alcoholism,** a mild form of alcoholism in which the dependence is psychologic rather than physical. The person may consume alcohol in excessive amounts to relieve physical pain or psychologic distress but is usually able to retain control when the distress subsides and can cease use of alcohol voluntarily.

**alpha-aminoisovalerianic acid.** See **valine.**

**alpha₁-antitrypsin** [Gk, *anti,* against, trypsin], a plasma protein produced in the liver that inhibits the action of proteolytic enzymes such as trypsin. Deficiencies are associated with hepatitis in children and panacinar emphysema in adults. The latter is an inherited condition.

**alpha₁-antitrypsin test,** a blood test administered to individuals with a family history of emphysema, since a familial tendency to have a deficiency of this antienzyme exists. A

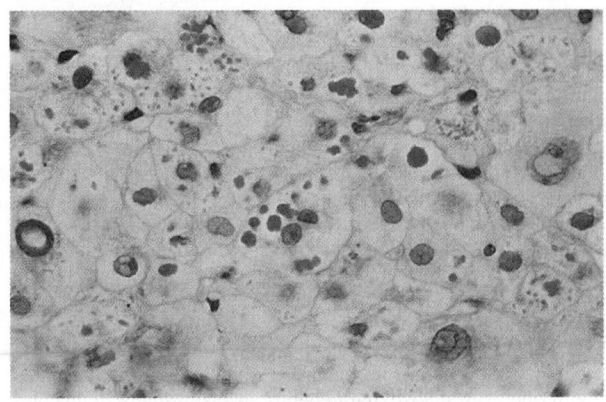

**Alpha₁-antitrypsin deficiency**
*(Cotran, Kumar, and Collins, 1999/courtesy Dr. I. Wanless, Toronto Hospital, Toronto, Ontario, Canada)*

similar deficiency also exists in children with cirrhosis and other liver diseases.

**alpha cell** [Gk, *alpha,* first letter of the Greek alphabet; L, *cella,* storeroom], one of a class of cells located in the anterior lobe of the pituitary gland or in the pancreatic islets. Alpha cells in the pancreas produce glucagon, which raises the level of glucose in the blood.

**alpha chain disease.** See **immunoproliferative small intestine disease.**

**alpha error.** See **type I error.**

**alpha-fetoprotein (AFP),** a protein normally synthesized by the liver, yolk sac, and GI tract of a human fetus, but it may be found at an elevated level in the sera of adults having certain malignancies. AFP measurements in amniotic fluid are used for early diagnosis of fetal neural tube defects, such as spina bifida and anencephaly. Elevated serum levels may be present in ataxia-telangiectasia, hereditary tyrosinemia, cirrhosis, alcoholic hepatitis, hepatocellular carcinoma, and viral hepatitis. Although not a specific marker for malignancies, AFP may be used to monitor effectiveness of surgical and chemotherapeutic management of hepatomas and germ cell neoplasms.

**alpha-fetoprotein test (AFP),** a blood test used to assist in diagnosing certain neoplastic conditions, such as hepatoma, some tumors and teratomas, Hodgkin's disease, lymphoma, and renal cell carcinoma. Elevated AFP levels also may indicate cirrhosis, chronic active hepatitis, and neural tube defects in the fetus.

**alpha-fucosidase,** a lysosomal enzyme that catalyzes the hydrolysis of fucosides. A deficiency of this enzyme is a cause of fucosidosis.

**alpha-galactosidase,** an enzyme that catalyzes the conversion of alpha-D-galactoside to D-galactose.

**alpha-globulins,** one of a group of serum proteins classified as alpha, beta, or gamma on the basis of their electrophoretic mobility. Alpha-globulins have the greatest negative charge.

**alpha hemolysis,** the development of a greenish zone around a bacterial colony growing on blood-agar medium, characteristic of pneumococci and certain streptococci and caused by the partial decomposition of hemoglobin. Compare **beta hemolysis.**

**alpha-hydroxypropionic acid.** See **lactic acid.**

**alpha₂-interferon** /in'tərfir'on/, a protein molecule effec-

tive in controlling the spread of common colds caused by rhinoviruses. It is administered as a nasal spray.

**alpha-methyldopa.** See **methyldopa.**

**alphanumeric,** data in the form of letters A-Z and numerals 0-9. The characters, which also may include punctuation marks, are used commonly in computer programming to code applications.

**alpha particle,** a particle emitted from an atom during one kind of radioactive decay. It consists of two protons and two neutrons, the equivalent of a helium nucleus. Ordinarily, alpha particles are a weak form of radiation with a short range and are not considered hazardous unless inhaled or ingested.

**alpha receptor,** any of the postulated adrenergic components of receptor tissues that respond to norepinephrine and to various blocking agents. The activation of the alpha receptors causes such physiologic responses as increased peripheral vascular resistance, dilation of the pupils, and contraction of pilomotor muscles. Also called **alpha-adrenergic receptor.** Compare **beta receptor.**

**alpha redistribution phase,** a period after IV administration of a drug when the blood level begins to fall from its peak. It is caused primarily by redistribution of the drug throughout the body.

**alpha rhythm.** See **alpha wave.**

**alpha state,** a condition of relaxed, peaceful wakefulness devoid of concentration and sensory stimulation. It is characterized by the alpha rhythm of brain wave activity, as recorded by an electroencephalograph, and is accompanied by feelings of tranquillity and a lack of tension and anxiety. Biofeedback training and meditation techniques are used to achieve this state.

**Alpha Tau Delta** /al'fə tou' del'tə/, a national fraternity of professional nurses.

**alpha-thalassemia** [Gk, *thalassa,* sea + *haema,* blood], thalassemia caused by decreased rate of synthesis of the alpha chains of hemoglobin. The homozygous form is incompatible with life, the stillborn infant displaying severe hydrops fetalis; the heterozygous form may be asymptomatic or marked by mild anemia.

**alpha-tocopherol.** See **vitamin E.**

**alphavirus** /al'favī'rəs/, any of a group of very small togaviruses consisting of a single molecule of single-stranded deoxyribonucleic acid (DNA) within a lipoprotein capsule. Many alphaviruses multiply in the cytoplasm of cells of arthropods and are transmitted to humans through insect bites, such as that causing equine encephalitis. See also **encephalitis, togaviruses.**

**alpha wave,** one of the four types of brain waves, characterized by a relatively high voltage or amplitude and a frequency of 8 to 13 Hz. Alpha waves are the "relaxed waves" of the brain and constitute the majority of waves recorded by electroencephalograms registering the activity of the parietal and the occipital lobes and the posterior parts of the temporal lobes when the individual is awake but nonattentive and relaxed, with the eyes closed. Opening and closing the eyes affect the patterns of the alpha waves and the beta waves. Also called **alpha rhythm, Berger wave.** Compare **beta wave, delta wave, theta wave.**

**Alport's syndrome** [A.C. Alport, South African physician, 1880–1959], a form of hereditary nephritis with symptoms of glomerulonephritis, hematuria, progressive sensorineural hearing loss, and occasional ocular disorders such as cataracts, drusen, and lenticonus. The trait is transmitted most often through females, who are often asymptomatic. In males kidney impairment tends to develop in the third decade; death from renal complications occurs in middle age. Treatment is directed toward relief of uremia or other kidney disorders. Kidney transplantation and dialysis are sometimes successful.

**alprazolam** /alpraz′ələm/, a benzodiazepine antianxiety agent.

■ INDICATIONS: It is prescribed in the treatment of anxiety disorders or the short-term relief of the symptoms of anxiety.

■ CONTRAINDICATIONS: Acute narrow-angle glaucoma or known sensitivity to this drug or other benzodiazepines prohibits its use. It is contraindicated with ketoconazole and itraconazole. Pregnancy is also a contraindication.

■ ADVERSE EFFECTS: Among the most serious adverse reactions are drowsiness and lightheadedness.

**alprostadil,** a proprietary form of prostaglandin E₁ used to maintain the patency of the ductus arteriosus in certain neonates.

■ INDICATIONS: It is recommended as palliative therapy for neonates awaiting surgery to correct congenital heart defects, such as tetralogy of Fallot and tricuspid atresia.

■ CONTRAINDICATIONS: There are no contraindications.

■ ADVERSE EFFECTS: The most common adverse effects are apnea, fever, seizures, cerebral bleeding, flushing, bradycardia, and hypertension.

**ALS,** **1.** abbreviation for **advanced life support.** See **Emergency Medical Technician-Advanced Life Support (EMT-ALS). 2.** abbreviation for **amyotrophic lateral sclerosis. 3.** abbreviation for **antilymphocyte serum.**

**Alström's syndrome** [Carl A. Alström, twentieth century geneticist], an inherited disease characterized by multiple system resistance to hormones. Clinical features include retinal degeneration leading to childhood blindness, insulin-resistant diabetes mellitus, infantile obesity, nerve deafness, baldness, hyperuricemia, and hypertriglyceridemia. Males may also have high plasma gonadotropin levels and hypogonadism. The condition is transmitted through an autosomal recessive gene.

**ALT,** abbreviation for **alanine aminotransferase.**

**altered mucous membrane, impaired,** a nursing diagnosis accepted by the Fifth National Conference on the Classification of Nursing Diagnoses. The condition is defined as a state in which an individual experiences disruptions in the tissue layers of the oral cavity.

■ DEFINING CHARACTERISTICS: Defining characteristics include oral pain or discomfort, coated tongue, xerostomia (dry mouth), stomatitis, oral lesions or ulcers, lack of or decreased salivation, leukoplakia, edema, hyperemia, oral plaque, desquamation, vesicles, hemorrhagic gingivitis, carious teeth, and halitosis.

■ RELATED FACTORS: Related factors include pathologic condition of the oral cavity caused by radiation to head or neck, dehydration, chemical trauma (including acidic foods, drugs, noxious agents, and alcohol), mechanical trauma (such as ill-fitting dentures, braces, endotracheal or nasogastric tubes, and surgery in the oral cavity), taking nothing by mouth for more than 24 hours, ineffective oral hygiene, mouth breathing, malnutrition, infection, lack of or decreased salivation, and medication. See also **nursing diagnosis.**

**altered state of consciousness (ASC)** [L, *alter,* other], any state of awareness that differs from the normal awareness of a conscious person. Altered states of consciousness have been achieved, especially in Eastern cultures, by many individuals using various techniques, such as prolonged fasting, deep breathing, whirling, and chanting. Researchers now recognize that such practices can affect body chemistry and help induce the desired state. Experiments suggest that telepathy, mystical experiences, clairvoyance, and other altered states of consciousness may be subconscious capabilities in most individuals and can be used to improve health and help fight disease.

**alteregoism** /ôl′tərē′gō·iz′əm/, an altruistic feeling for an individual who is similar to or in a similar situation as oneself.

**alternans** /ôl′tərnənz/ [L, *alternare,* to alternate], a regular heart rhythm that causes the pulse to alternate between strong beats and weak beats (pulsus alternans).

**alternate binaural loudness balance (ABLB) test,** comparison of the intensity levels at which a given pure tone sounds equally loud to the normal ear and the ear with hearing loss; done to determine recruitment with unilateral sensorineural loss.

**alternate generation** /ôl′tərnit/ [L, *alter,* other of two], a type of reproduction in which a sexual generation alternates with one or more asexual generations, as in many plants and simple animals. Also called **alternation of generations.**

**alternating current (AC)** /ôl′tərnā′ting/, an electric current that reverses direction, according to a consistent sinusoidal pattern. Compare **direct current.** See also **current.**

**alternating mydriasis,** a visual disorder in which there is abnormal dilation of the pupils that affects the left and right eyes alternately. See also **mydriasis.**

**alternating pulse.** See **pulsus alternans.**

**alternation,** the recurrent, successive occurrence of two functions or phases, as when a nerve fiber responds to every other stimulus, or when a heart produces an irregular beat with every other cardiac cycle.

**alternation of generations.** See **alternate generation.**

**alternation rules,** (in psychology) the sociolinguistic rules that establish options available to a person when he or she is speaking to someone else. The rules are influenced by social categories, such as kinship, sex, status, age, and type of interpersonal relationship.

**alternative inheritance** /ôltur′nətiv/, the acquisition of all genetic traits and conditions from one parent, as in self-pollinating plants and self-fertilizing animals.

**alternative medicine,** any of the systems of medical diagnosis and treatment differing in technique from that of the allopathic practitioner's use of drugs and surgery to treat disease and injury. Examples include faith healing, homeopathy, Indian Ayurvedic medicine, acupuncture, aroma therapy, and therapeutic touch.

**alternative pathway of complement activation,** a process of antigen-antibody interaction in which activation of the C3 step occurs without prior activation of C1, C4, and C2. The initiating substance may be endotoxin, yeast cell wall, bacterial capsule, or immunoglobulin A. Also called **properdin system.**

**alternator,** a device for generating an electric current that changes polarity a specified number of times per second.

**alternobaric vertigo,** a condition of dysequilibrium caused by unequalized pressure differences in the middle ear, as may be experienced by divers during ascent. The pressure difference exerts its effect on the oval window of the inner ear.

**alt hor,** (in prescriptions) abbreviation for the Latin phrase *alternis horis,* meaning 'every other hour.'

**altitude** /al′tityōod/ [L, *altitudo,* height], any location on earth with reference to a fixed surface point, which is usually sea level. Several types of health effects are associated with altitude extremes, including a greater intensity of ultraviolet radiation that results from a thinner atmosphere. There are fewer molecules per liter of atmosphere and lower oxygen partial pressure. At an altitude of 5500 m, inspired oxygen pressure is only 50% of that at sea level, although demands of physical effort and cellular respiration are the same at both altitudes. High-altitude intolerance is usually associated with a blood or pulmonary disorder. See also **altitude sickness.**

**altitude anoxia** [L, *altus,* high; Gk, *a,* without, *oxys,* sharp, *genein,* to produce], oxygen deprivation in a high-altitude atmosphere.

**altitude sickness,** a syndrome associated with the relatively low partial pressure (reduced barometric pressure) of oxygen in the atmosphere at altitudes encountered during mountain climbing or travel in unpressurized aircraft. The acute symptoms may include dizziness, headache, irritability, breathlessness, and euphoria. Older people and those affected by pulmonary or cardiac disorders may suffer pulmonary edema, heart failure, or prostration, requiring emergency treatment and removal to lower altitudes. A chronic form of altitude sickness is characterized by an increased production of red blood cells, resulting in blood that is thick and difficult to move through the circulatory system. Also called **acute mountain sickness, Monge's disease, "the bends."** See also **polycythemia.**

**altruism** /al′trōō·iz′əm/, a sense of unconditional concern for the welfare of others. It may be expressed at the level of the individual, group, or the larger social system.

**alum** /al′əm/ [L, *alumen*], a topical astringent, used primarily in lotions and douches.

**alum bath,** a bath taken in water containing the mineral salt alum, used primarily for skin disorders.

**aluminum (Al)** /əlōō′minəm/ [L, *alumen* alum], a widely used metallic element and the third most abundant of all the elements. Its atomic number is 13; its atomic weight (mass) is 26.97. It occurs in the ores feldspar, mica, and kaolin but most abundantly in bauxite. Aluminum is commonly obtained by purifying bauxite to produce alumina, which is reduced to aluminum. It is light and durable and used extensively in the manufacture of aircraft components, prosthetic devices, and dental appliances. Its compounds are components of many antacids, antiseptics, and astringents. Aluminum salts, such as aluminum hydroxychloride, can cause allergic reactions in susceptible individuals. Aluminum hydroxychloride is the most commonly used agent in antiperspirants and is also effective as a deodorant.

**aluminum acetate solution.** See **Burow's solution.**

**aluminum attenuator,** an aluminum filter used to control the hardness of an x-ray beam. The attenuator removes low-energy x-ray photons before they can reach the patient and be absorbed.

**aluminum hydroxide gel** [L, *alumen,* alum; Gk, *hydor,* water, *oxys,* sharp; L, *gelare,* to congeal], an antacid that works by chemical neutralization and also by adsorption of hydrochloric acid, gases, and toxins.

**Alupent,** trademark for a beta-adrenergic bronchodilator (metaproterenol sulfate).

**Alurate Elixir,** trademark for a sedative-hypnotic (aprobarbital).

**Alu sequences,** a family of repeated sequences found in large numbers in the human genome.

**alve-, alveolo-,** prefix meaning 'trough, channel, cavity': *alveolate, alveolus.*

**alveobronchitis** [L, *alveolus,* little hollow; Gk, *brongchos,* windpipe, *itis,* inflammation], inflammation of the alveoli and bronchioles. Also called **alveobronchiolitis.** See also **bronchopneumonia.**

**alveolar** /alvē′ələr/ [L, *alveolus,* little hollow], pertaining to an alveolus.

**alveolar adenocarcinoma** [L, *alveolus,* little hollow], a neoplasm in which the tumor cells form alveoli.

**alveolar air,** the respiratory gases in an alveolus of the lung. Alveolar air can be analyzed for its content of oxygen, carbon dioxide, or other gases by collecting the last portion of air expelled by maximum exhalation. Also called **alveolar gas.**

**alveolar air equation,** a mathematical expression relating the approximate alveolar oxygen tension to the arterial partial pressure of carbon dioxide, the fractional inspired oxygen, and the ratio of carbon dioxide production to oxygen consumption.

**alveolar-arterial end-capillary gas pressure difference,** the gas pressure difference between the partial pressure of a gas, such as $CO_2$, in alveolar air and that in pulmonary capillary blood as the blood leaves the alveoli. It is measured in torr or mm Hg.

**alveolar-arterial gas pressure difference,** the difference between the partial pressure of a gas, such as $CO_2$, in the alveoli and that in systemic arterial blood. The difference may indicate ventilation-perfusion mismatching. A negative difference indicates that the partial pressure of the gas is higher in systemic arterial blood than it is in alveolar air. It is measured in torr or mm Hg.

**alveolar bone.** See **alveolar process.**

**alveolar canal,** any of the canals of the maxilla through which the posterior superior alveolar blood vessels and the nerves to the upper teeth pass. Also called **dental canal.**

**alveolar-capillary membrane,** a lung tissue structure, varying in thickness from 0.4 to 2 μm, through which diffusion of oxygen and carbon dioxide molecules occurs during the respiration process. It consists of an alveolar cell separated from a capillary cell by an interstitial space and is essentially a fluid barrier.

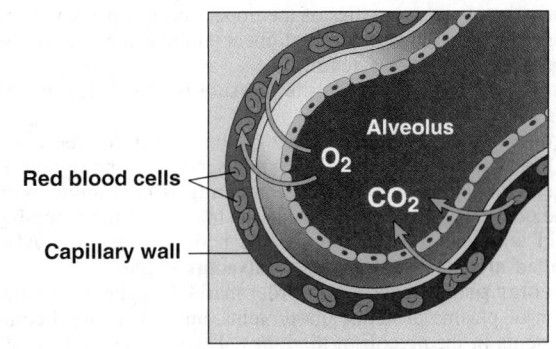

Exchange of gases between an alveolus and a lung capillary

**Alveolar-capillary membrane** *(Chabner, 2001)*

**alveolar carcinoma.** See **bronchioloalveolar carcinoma.**

**alveolar cell carcinoma,** a malignant pulmonary neoplasm that arises in a bronchiole and spreads along alveolar surfaces. The tumor consists of cuboidal or nonciliated columnar epithelial cells with abundant eosinophilic cytoplasm that may contain droplets of mucus. This form of lung cancer is often characterized by a severe cough and copious sputum. Also called **bronchiolar carcinoma, bronchioloalveolar carcinoma.**

**alveolar cleft,** a break in the continuity of the alveolar process, usually congenital. It typically occurs with a cleft lip and/or a cleft palate. See also **cleft lip, cleft palate.**

**alveolar cyst,** an air-filled cavity in a lung or visceral tissues caused by rupture of an alveolus.

**alveolar dead space.** See **dead space.**

**alveolar distending pressure,** the pressure difference between the alveoli and the intrapleural space.

**alveolar duct,** any of the air passages in the lung that branch out from the respiratory bronchioles. From the ducts arise the alveolar sacs.

**alveolar edema,** an accumulation of fluid within the alveoli. The cause is usually the movement of blood components through the pulmonary capillary walls as a result of a change in osmotic pressure, an increased permeability of the walls, or related factors.

**alveolar fiber,** any of the many white, collagenous fibers of the periodontal ligament that extend from the alveolar process to the intermediate plexus, where their terminations mix with those of the cemental fibers. Alveolar fibers surround the tooth and assist in resisting horizontal movements.

**alveolar fistula.** See **dental fistula.**

**alveolar gas.** See **alveolar air.**

**alveolar gas volume,** the aggregate volume of gas in the alveoli of the lungs. It is indicated by the symbol $V_A$.

**alveolar gingiva.** See **attached gingiva.**

**alveolar macrophage,** a cell of the reticuloendothelial system in the lungs that engulfs and digests foreign substances inhaled into the alveoli.

**alveolar microlithiasis,** a disease characterized by the presence of calcium phosphate deposits in the alveoli and other parts of the bronchopulmonary system. The fine, sandlike deposits may cause the entire lung to appear radiopaque. The disease is familial in about half of cases.

**alveolar periosteum** [L, *alveolus,* little hollow; Gk, *peri,* near, *osteon,* bone], a dense layer of connective tissue that lines the alveolar cavities of the upper and lower jaws, joining the bones to the horizontal fibers on the cementum of the teeth. See also **periosteum.**

**alveolar pressure ($P_A$),** the pressure in the alveoli of the lungs.

**alveolar process,** the portion of the maxilla or the mandible that forms the dental arch and serves as a bony investment for the teeth. Its cortical covering is continuous with the compact bone of the body of the maxilla or the mandible and with the spongy bone of the body of the jaws. Also called **alveolar bone.** See also **alveolar ridge.**

**alveolar proteinosis,** a disorder marked by the accumulation of plasma proteins, lipoproteins, and other blood components in the alveoli of the lungs. The disease tends to affect previously healthy young adults, with a higher incidence among males than females. The cause is unknown, and clinical signs vary, although only the lungs are affected. Some patients are asymptomatic, whereas others experience dyspnea and an unproductive cough. The condition may be treated with bronchopulmonary lavage. There is a risk of secondary infections.

**alveolar ridge,** the bony ridge of the maxilla or the mandible that contains the alveoli of the teeth. See also **alveolar process.**

**alveolar sac** [L, *alveolus,* little hollow; Gk, *sakkos*], an air sac at one of the terminal cavities of lung tissue.

**alveolar sinus.** See **dental fistula.**

**alveolar socket** [L, *alveolus,* little hollow; OFr, *soket*], a cavity in the alveolar process of the maxilla and mandible that accommodates a tooth.

**alveolar soft part sarcoma,** a tumor in subcutaneous or fibromuscular tissue, consisting of numerous large round or polygonal cells in a netlike matrix of connective tissue.

**alveolar ventilation,** the volume of air that ventilates all the perfused alveoli, equal to total ventilation minus dead space ventilation. The normal average is between 4 and 5 liters per minute.

**alveolectomy** /al′vē-əlek′təmē/ [L, *alveolus* + Gk, *ektomē,* excision], the excision of a portion of the alveolar process performed to aid the extraction of a tooth or teeth, modify the alveolar contour after tooth extraction, or prepare the mouth for dentures.

**alveoli** /al·vē′ō·lī /, See **alveolus.**

**alveolitis** /al′vē·əlī′tis/, inflammation of the alveoli caused by the inhalation of an allergen. It is characterized by acute episodes of dyspnea, cough, sweating, fever, weakness, and pain in the joints and muscles lasting from 12 to 18 hours. Recurrent episodes may lead to chronic obstructive pulmonary disease with weight loss, increasing exertional dyspnea, and interstitial fibrosis. X-ray films of the lungs may show cellular thickening of alveolar septa and ill-defined generalized infiltrates. Kinds of alveolitis include **bagassosis, farmer's lung,** and **pigeon breeder's lung.**

**alveoloplasty** /alvē′əlōplas′tē/, reconstruction by plastic surgery of a dental alveolus.

**alveolotomy** /al′vē·əlot′əmē/, incision of a dental alveolus performed to drain pus from a dental infection.

**alveolus** /alvē′ələs/, *pl.* **alveoli** [L, little hollow], **1.** a small outpouching of walls of alveolar space through which gas exchange between alveolar air and pulmonary capillary blood takes place. The term is often used interchangeably with acinus. See also **alveolar sac, dental alveolus, pulmonary alveolus. —alveolar,** *adj.* **2.** a tooth socket.

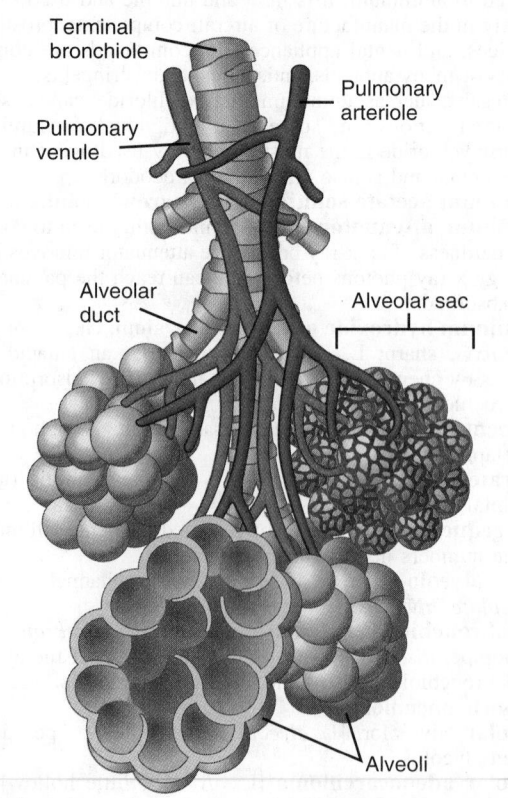

**Alveoli** *(Thibodeau and Patton, 1999/Network Graphics)*

Terminal bronchiole

Pulmonary arteriole

Pulmonary venule

Alveolar duct

Alveolar sac

Alveoli

**alvine constipation.** See **obstructive constipation.**

**alymphocytosis** /alim′fōsītō′sis/ [Gk, *a,* not; L, *lympha,* water; Gk, *kytos,* cell, *osis,* condition], a severe reduction in the total number of circulating lymphocytes in the blood. Compare **aplastic anemia, lymphocytopenia.** See also **leukocyte, lymphocyte.**

**Alzheimer's disease (AD)** /ôl′zīmərz/ [Alois Alzheimer, German neurologist, 1864–1915], progressive mental deterioration characterized by confusion, memory failure, disorientation, restlessness, agnosia, speech disturbances, inability to carry out purposeful movement, and hallucinosis. The patient may become hypomanic, refuse food, and lose sphincter control without focal impairment. The disease sometimes begins in middle life with slight defects in memory and behavior, but the symptoms worsen dramatically after the age of 70. Although it occurs with equal frequency in men and women, the familial risk is four times

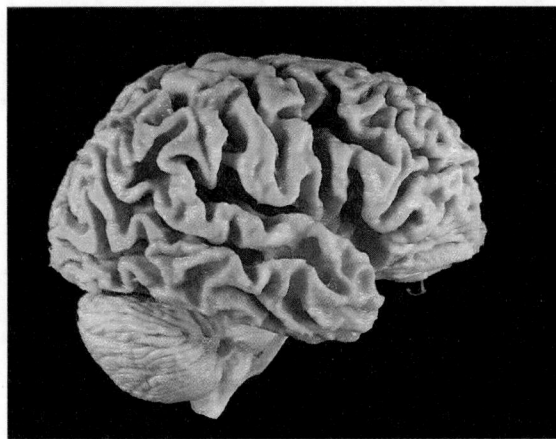

**Alzheimer's disease: narrowing of cerebral cortical gyri**
*(Kumar, Cotran, and Robbins, 1997)*

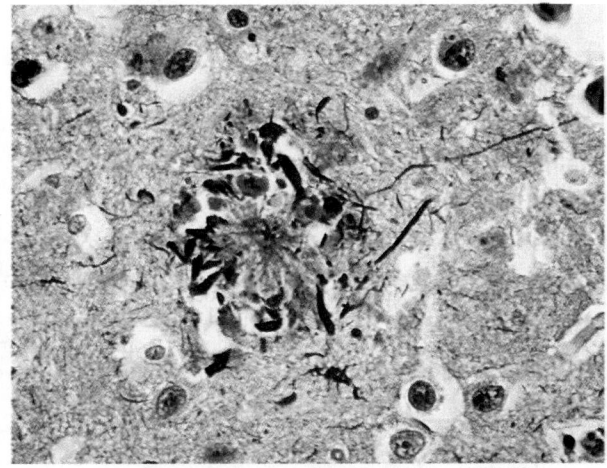

**Alzheimer's disease: senile plaque**
*(Kumar, Cotran, and Robbins, 1997/courtesy Eileen Bigio, MD, Department of Pathology, University of Texas Southwestern Medical Center, Dallas)*

that of the general population. Typical pathologic features are miliary plaques in the cortex and fibrillary degeneration in layers containing pyramidal ganglion cells. The cerebral cortex atrophies with widening of the cerebral sulci, especially in the frontal and temporal regions. Diagnostic criteria consist of a failure in at least three cognitive functions, including memory, use of language, visuospatial skills, personality, and calculating skills. The symptoms frequently begin with an inability to incorporate new knowledge despite the retention of old information, an inability to recall words, and an inability to orient to one's surroundings. Only palliative treatment is available. ■ NURSING CONSIDERATIONS: Nursing care is concerned primarily with promoting activity and sleep and preventing agitation, violence, and injury. Death usually occurs 8 to 12 years after the first symptoms appear. Also called **senile dementia-Alzheimer type (SDAT).**

**Alzheimer's sclerosis** [Alois Alzheimer; Gk, *sclerosis,* hardening], the degeneration of small cerebral blood vessels resulting in mental changes.

**Am,** symbol for the element **americium.**

**ama,** abbreviation for **against medical advice.**

**AMA,** 1. abbreviation for **American Medical Association.** 2. abbreviation for **antimitochondrial antibody.**

**amalgam** /əmal′gəm/ [Gk, *malagma,* soft mass], 1. a mixture or combination. 2. an alloy of mercury, silver, and other metals commonly used as a dental filling. 3. an alloy, usually made with mercury and another metal, in which the proportions of the metal components may be varied according to the desired hardness of the amalgam. Hardness can vary from that of a hard metal to that of a pliable plastic.

**amalgam carrier,** (in dentistry) an instrument used to pick up a quantity of amalgam and transfer it into a prepared tooth cavity (cavity prep) or mold.

**amalgam carver,** a dental instrument for shaping soft amalgam used in some tooth cavity fillings or restorations.

**amalgam condenser,** (in dentistry) an instrument used for compacting soft amalgam in filling teeth.

**amalgam core,** a rigid base for retaining a cast crown restoration, used in the replacement of a damaged tooth crown. The core may be held in place by undercuts, slots, pins, or the pulp chamber of an endodontically treated tooth. Compare **cast core, composite core.** See also **core.**

**amalgam tattoo,** a discoloration of the gingiva or buccal membrane caused by particles of silver that migrate from an amalgam filling and become embedded under the tissue surface. The condition causes no symptoms and is left untreated.

*Amanita* [Gk, *amanitai,* fungus], a genus of mushrooms. Some species, such as *Amanita phalloides,* are poisonous, causing hallucinations, GI upset, and pain that may be followed by liver, kidney, and central nervous system damage.

**amantadine hydrochloride** /əman′tədēn/, an antiviral and antiparkinsonian agent. ■ INDICATIONS: It is prescribed in the prophylaxis and early treatment of influenza virus A and in the treatment of parkinsonian symptoms and drug-induced extrapyramidal reactions. ■ CONTRAINDICATIONS: It is used with caution in patients with congestive heart failure and during pregnancy and lactation. Known hypersensitivity to this drug prohibits its use. ■ ADVERSE EFFECTS: Among the most serious adverse reactions are central nervous system effects and livedo reticularis. Nausea, dizziness, insomnia, nervousness, blurred vision, and slurred speech also may occur.

**amastia** /əmas′tē·ə/ [Gk, *a, mastos,* not breast], absence of the breasts in women caused by a congenital defect, an en-

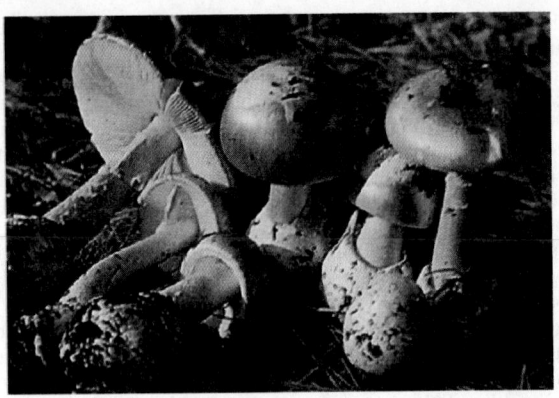

***Amanita phalloides*** *(Auerbach, 1995)*

tion of any air pollutant, such as lead, nitrogen dioxide, sodium hydroxide, or sulfur dioxide. Research and medical evidence show the strong correlation between many diseases and toxic chemicals, but little is known about the precise effects and movement of airborne pollutants.

**ambient noise** [L, *ambiens,* around; ME, clamor], the total noise in a given environment.

**ambient pressure,** the atmospheric pressure, or pressure in the environment or surrounding area. It is given a reference value of zero (0) cm $H_2O$.

**ambient temperature** [L, *ambi,* around, *temperatura*], the temperature of the environment.

**ambiguous** /ambig'yo͞o·əs/ [L, *ambiguus,* to wander], having more than one direction, development, or interpretation or meaning.

**ambiguous genitalia** [L, *ambigere,* to go around], external genitalia that are not normal and morphologically typical of either sex, as occurs in pseudohermaphroditism.

docrine disorder resulting in faulty development, lack of development of secondary sex characteristics, or a bilateral mastectomy. Also called **amazia.**

**amaurosis** /am'ôrō'sis/ [Gk, *amauroein,* to darken], blindness, especially lack of vision resulting from a systemic cause such as disease of the optic nerve or brain, diabetes, renal disease, after acute gastritis or systemic poisoning produced by excessive use of alcohol or tobacco, rather than from damage to the eye itself. Unilateral or, more rarely, bilateral amaurosis may follow an emotional shock and may continue for days or months. One kind of congenital amaurosis is transmitted as an autosomal recessive trait. —**amaurotic,** *adj.*

**amaurosis fugax** /fo͞o'gaks/, transient episodic blindness caused by decreased blood flow to the retina. Compare **amaurosis.**

**amaurosis partialis fugax,** transitory partial blindness, usually caused by vascular insufficiency of the retina or optic nerve as a result of carotid artery disease. Other related symptoms include dizziness, nausea, and vomiting.

**amaurotic.** See **amaurosis.**

**amaurotic familial idiocy.** See **Tay-Sachs disease.**

**amazia.** See **amastia.**

**amb-.** See **ambi-.**

**Ambenyl Cough Syrup,** trademark for a fixed-combination drug containing a opioid analgesic-antitussive (codeine phosphate), an antihistamine (bromodiphenhydramine hydrochloride), and alcohol.

**amber** [Ar, *anbar*], a hard fossilized resin derived from pine trees. An oil of amber, *Oleum succini,* has been used in some pharmaceutical preparations.

**amber mutation** [Ar, *anbar,* ambergris], a genetic alteration that causes the synthesis of a polypeptide chain to terminate prematurely because the triplet of nucleotides that normally codes for the next amino acid in the chain becomes uracil-adenine-guanine, the sequence that signals the end of the chain. Also called **nonsense mutation, ochre mutation.**

**ambi-, ambo-, amb-,** prefix meaning 'on both sides' or 'both': *ambidexterity, ambomalleal.*

**ambidextrous** /am'bēdek'strəs/ [L, *ambo,* both, *dexter,* right], able to use either the left or right hand to perform a task.

**ambient** /am'bē·ənt/ [L, *ambire,* on both sides], pertaining to the surrounding area or atmosphere, usually a defined area such as a room or other large enclosed space.

**ambient air standard,** the maximum tolerable concentra-

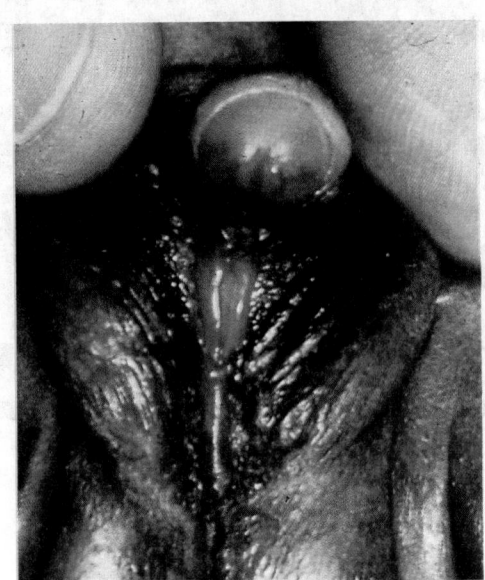

**Ambiguous genitalia** *(Zitelli and Davis, 1997)*

**ambilateral.** See **ambi-.**

**ambilhar.** See **niridazole.**

**ambiopia.** See **diplopia.**

**ambivalence** /ambiv'ələns/ [L, *ambo,* both, *valentia,* strength], **1.** a state in which a person concomitantly experiences conflicting feelings, attitudes, drives, desires, or emotions, such as love and hate, tenderness and cruelty, pleasure and pain toward the same person, place, object, or situation. To some degree, ambivalence is normal. Treatment in severe, debilitating cases consists of psychotherapy appropriate to the underlying cause. **2.** uncertainty and fluctuation caused by an inability to make a choice between opposites. **3.** a continuous oscillation or fluctuation. —**ambivalent,** *adj.*

**ambivalent** [L, *ambo,* both, *valentia,* strength], **1.** having equal power on both sides. **2.** (in psychology) having equally strong but opposing emotions, as love and hate for the same person.

**ambivert** /am'bivurt'/ [L, *ambo*, both, *vertere*, to turn], a person who possesses characteristics of both introversion and extroversion.

**amblyopia** /am'blē·ō'pē·ə/ [Gk, *amblys*, dull, *ops*, eye], reduced vision in an eye not correctable by a manifest refraction and with no obvious pathologic or structural cause. Typically, the vision in an amblyopic eye is 2 lines or more worse than in the fellow eye. See also **toxic amblyopia.**

**amblyopia cruciata.** See **crossed amblyopia.**

**ambo-.** See **ambi-.**

**ambon** [Gk, raised stage], a fibrocartilaginous ring that surrounds the cavity of a long bone socket.

**Ambu bag,** trademark for a resuscitator bag used to assist respiratory ventilation. See also **bag-valve-mask resuscitator.**

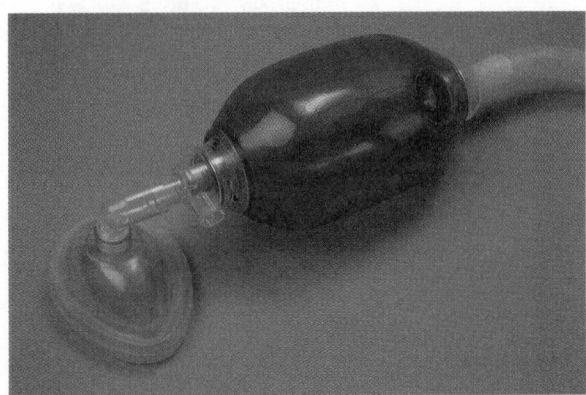

**Ambu bag** *(Zakus, 1995)*

**ambulance** /am'byələns/ a vehicle designed to transport patients who are not able to be transported in a normal manner. It may be used under emergency or nonemergency conditions and is equipped with supplies and personnel to provide patient care en route.

**ambulation: walking,** a nursing outcome from the Nursing Outcomes Classification (NOC) defined as ability to walk from place to place. See also **Nursing Outcomes Classification.**

**ambulation: wheelchair,** a nursing outcome from the Nursing Outcomes Classification (NOC) defined as ability to move from place to place in a wheelchair. See also **Nursing Outcomes Classification.**

**ambulatory** /am'byələtôr'ē/ [L, *ambulare*, to walk about], able to walk, hence describing a patient who is not confined to bed or designating a health service for people who are not hospitalized.

**ambulatory anesthesia,** anesthesia done on an outpatient basis for ambulatory surgery.

**ambulatory automatism,** aimless wandering or moving about or performance of mechanical acts without conscious awareness of the behavior. See also **fugue, poriomania.**

**ambulatory blood pressure monitoring (ABPM),** the recording a patient's blood pressure at regular intervals under normal living and working conditions.

**ambulatory care,** health services provided on an outpatient basis to those who visit a hospital or other health care facility and depart after treatment on the same day.

**ambulatory electrocardiograph.** See **Holter monitor.**

**ambulatory schizophrenia,** a mild form of psychosis, characterized mainly by a tendency to respond to questions with vague and irrelevant answers. The person also may seem somewhat eccentric and wander aimlessly.

**ambulatory splint.** See **functional splint.**

**ambulatory surgery center,** a medical facility designed and equipped to handle surgery cases, such as cataracts, herniorrhaphy, and meniscectomy, that do not require overnight hospitalization. Most patients who are in relatively good health may receive treatment at ambulatory surgery centers. The centers may be part of a community general hospital, a specialty hospital, or an independent medical facility with prearranged hospital backup. The centers are staffed with health professionals as in conventional surgery departments.

**Ambu simulator,** trademark for a manikin used in teaching cardiopulmonary resuscitation.

**am care** /ā·em'/, routine hygienic care that is given patients before breakfast or early in the morning.

**amcinonide** /amsin'ōnīd/, a topical corticosteroid.
- ■ INDICATION: It is used to treat inflammatory skin conditions.
- ■ CONTRAINDICATIONS: Circulation impairment or known hypersensitivity to steroids prohibits its use.
- ■ ADVERSE EFFECTS: Among the most common adverse reactions are itching, stinging, burning, and less frequently, various skin eruptions. Systemic side effects may result from prolonged or excessive application.

**amdinocillin** /am'dinōsil'in/, a penicillin derivative that is used as a parenteral antibiotic.
- ■ INDICATIONS: It is prescribed for the treatment of urinary infections caused by susceptible strains of *Escherichia coli* and various species of *Klebsiella* and *Enterobacter.*
- ■ CONTRAINDICATIONS: It is contraindicated in patients allergic to penicillin.
- ■ ADVERSE EFFECTS: Among the most serious adverse effects reported are eosinophilia, thrombocytosis, elevated serum aspartate aminotransferase and serum alkaline phosphatase, skin rash, thrombophlebitis, diarrhea, nausea, dizziness, and various blood disorders.

**ameba** /əmē'bə/ [Gk, *amoibe*, change], a microscopic, single-celled, parasitic organism. Several species may be parasitic in humans, including *Entamoeba coli* and *E. histolytica.* Also spelled **amoeba.** See also **amebiasis.** —**amebic,** *adj.*

**-ameba, -amoeba,** suffix meaning a '(specified) protozoan': *caudameba, Entamoeba.*

**amebiasis** /am'ēbī'əsis/, an infection of the intestine or liver by species of pathogenic amebas, particularly *Entamoeba histolytica,* acquired by ingesting fecally contaminated food or water. Infected carriers can be asymptomatic (luminal ambiasis); they may develop invasive intestinal disease with dysentery, colitis, or appendicitis or invasive extraintestinal disease with peritonitis and liver or lung abscess. Infection is most serious in infants, the elderly, and debilitated people. Amebiasis may require treatment with luminal amebicides (iodoquinole, paromycin) to eradicate cysts and/or systemic treatment with metronidazole. Also spelled **amoebiasis.** See also **ameba, amebic abscess, amebic dysentery, hepatic amebiasis.**

**amebic.** See **ameba.**

**amebic abscess** /əmē'bik/, a collection of pus formed by disintegrated tissue in a cavity, usually in the liver, caused by the protozoan parasite *Entamoeba histolytica.* Cysts of the organism, ingested in fecally contaminated food or water, pass into the intestine, where active trophozoites of the

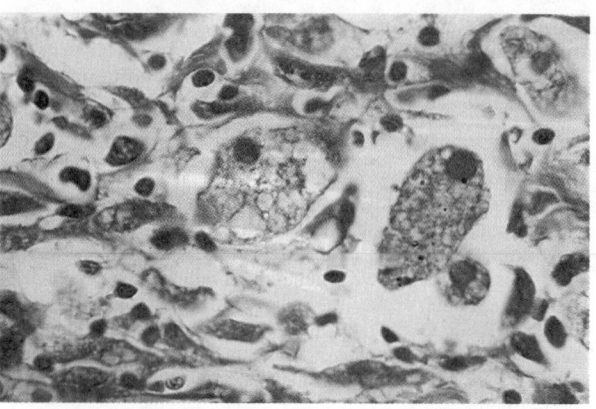

**Amebiasis of the colon** *(Cotran, Kumar, and Collins, 1999)*

parasite are released. The trophozoites enter the intestinal mucosa, causing ulceration, nausea, vomiting, abdominal pain, and severe diarrhea, and they may invade the liver and produce an abscess. Oral metronidazole and chloroquine hydrochloride administered orally or intramuscularly are used in treating hepatic amebic abscesses. See also **amebiasis.**

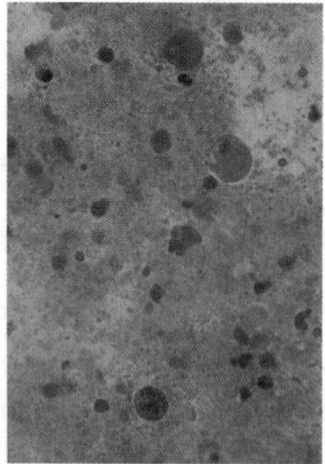

**Aspirate of hepatic amebic abscess**
*(Silverberg, DeLellis, and Frable, 1997)*

**amebic carrier state,** a condition in which a patient may be a carrier of amebic organisms without showing signs or symptoms of an amebic infection. A **precocious carrier** may appear healthy but may subsequently develop the amebic infection.

**amebic dysentery,** an inflammation of the intestine caused by infestation with *Entamoeba histolytica*. It is characterized by frequent, loose stools flecked with blood and mucus. Intestinal amebiasis may be accompanied by symptoms of liver involvement. Also called **intestinal amebiasis.** See also **amebiasis, hepatic amebiasis.**

**amebic hepatitis,** an inflammation of the liver caused by

an amebic infection, usually after an attack of amebic dysentery.

**amebicide** /əmē′bəsīd/, a drug or other agent that is destructive to amebae.

**ameboid movement** /əmē′boid/ [Gk, *amoibe,* ameba, *eidos,* form; L, *movere,* to move], the ameba-like movement of certain types of body cells that can migrate through tissues, such as white blood cells. The movement generally consists of extension of a portion of the cell membrane probably caused by internal rearrangement/movement of the cytoskeleton. See also **diapedesis.**

**amelanotic** /am′ilənot′ik/ [Gk, *a, melas,* not black], pertaining to tissue that is unpigmented because it lacks melanin.

**amelanotic melanoma,** a melanoma that lacks melanin. See also **melanoma.**

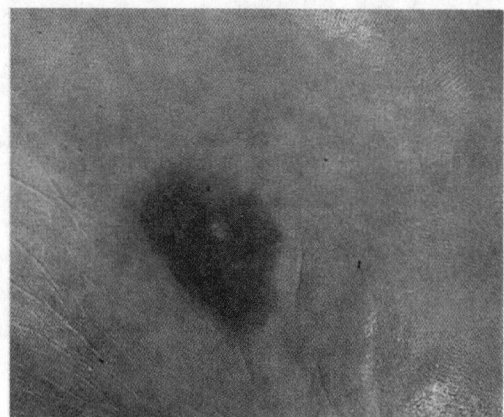

**Amelanotic malignant melanoma** *(du Vivier, 1993)*

**amelia** /əmē′lyə/ [Gk, *a, melos,* not limb], **1.** a birth defect, marked by the absence of one or more limbs. The term may be modified to indicate the number of legs or arms missing at birth, such as **tetramelia** for the absence of all four limbs. **2.** a psychologic trait of apathy or indifference associated with certain forms of psychosis.

**amelification** /əmel′ifikā′shən/ [OFr, *amel,* enamel; L, *facere,* to make], the differentiation of ameloblasts, or enamel cells, into the enamel of the teeth.

**amelioration** [L, *ad,* to, *melior,* better], an improvement in conditions.

**ameloblast** /am′ilōblast′/ [OFr, *amel* + Gk, *blastos,* germ], an epithelial cell from which tooth enamel is formed. **ameloblastic,** *adj.*

**ameloblastic fibroma,** an odontogenic neoplasm in which simultaneous proliferation of mesenchymal and epithelial tissues occurs without the formation of dentin or enamel.

**ameloblastic hemangioma,** a highly vascular tumor of cells covering the dental papilla. See also **hemangioma.**

**ameloblastic odontoma,** a malignant tumor of the jaw that forms cementum, dentin, enamel, and pulp tissue. See also **composite odontoma.**

**ameloblastic sarcoma,** a malignant odontogenic tumor, characterized by the proliferation of epithelial and mesenchymal tissue without the formation of dentin or enamel.

**ameloblastoma** /am′əlōblastō′mə/ [OFr, *amel* + Gk, *blastos,* germ, *oma*], a highly destructive, malignant, rapidly growing tumor of the jaw. Also called **adamantinoma, adamantoblastoma, epithelioma adamantinum.**

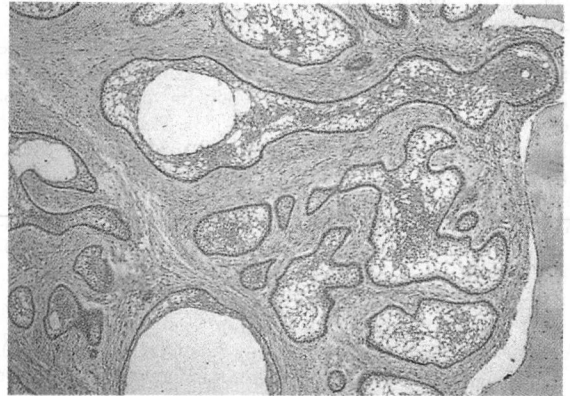

**Follicular ameloblastoma** *(Eveson and Skully, 1995)*

**amelodentinal** /am′əlōden′tinəl/ [OFr, *amel* + L, *dens,* tooth], pertaining to both the enamel and the dentin of the teeth.

**amelogenesis** /am′əlōjen′əsis/ [OFr, *amel* + Gk, *genein,* to produce], the formation of the enamel of the teeth. **—amelogenic,** *adj.*

**amelogenesis imperfecta,** a condition characterized by a brown coloration of the teeth and resulting from either severe hypocalcification or hypoplasia of the enamel. The condition, which is inherited as an autosomal dominant trait, is classified according to severity: in agenesis, there is a complete lack of enamel; in enamel hypoplasia, defective matrix formation causes the enamel to be normal in hardness but deficient in quantity; and in enamel hypocalcification, defective maturation of ameloblasts results in enamel that is normal in quantity but soft and undercalcified. Also called **hereditary brown enamel, hereditary enamel hypoplasia.** Compare **dentinogenesis imperfecta.** See also **enamel hypocalcification, enamel hypoplasia.**

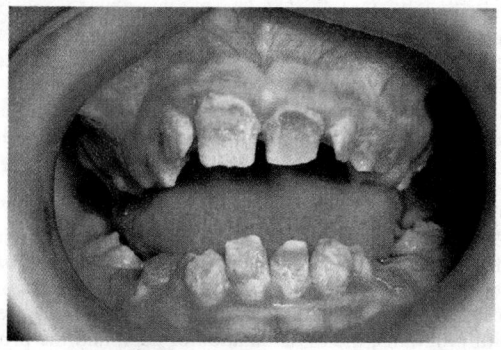

**Amelogenesis imperfecta** *(Christensen, 1994)*

**amenorrhea** /ā′menərē′ə/ [Gk, *a, men,* not month, *rhoia,* to flow], the absence of menstruation. Amenorrhea is normal before sexual maturity, during pregnancy, after menopause, and during the intermenstrual phase of the monthly hormonal cycle; it is otherwise caused by dysfunction of the hypothalamus, pituitary gland, ovary, or uterus, by the congenital absence or surgical removal of both ovaries or the uterus, or by medication. **Primary amenorrhea** is the failure of menstrual cycles to begin. **Secondary amenorrhea** is the cessation of menstrual cycles once established. Also spelled **amenorrhoea.** See also **dietary amenorrhea, hypothalamic amenorrhea, postpill amenorrhea. —amenorrheic.** *adj.*

**amentia** /āmen′shə/ [Gk, *a,* not; L, *mens,* mind], **1.** former term for mental retardation. **2.** dementia.

**American Academy of Allergy and Immunology (AAAI),** a national organization of physicians specializing in the diagnosis and treatment of allergies and immune system disorders.

**American Academy of Audiology,** a professional association for audiologists.

**American Academy of Nursing (AAN),** the honorary organization of the American Nurses Association, created to recognize superior achievement in nursing in order to promote advances and excellence in nursing practice, education, and research. A person elected to membership is given the title of Fellow of the American Academy of Nursing and may use the abbreviation FAAN as an honorific.

**American Academy of Physical Medicine and Rehabilitation (AAPMR),** a national association of professional health care workers concerned with the diagnosis of physical impairment and the development of therapies and devices to improve physical function.

**American Academy of Physicians Assistants (AAPA),** a national organization of physicians' assistants or associates.

**American Association for Respiratory Therapy (AART),** a national organization of respiratory therapists and other health workers involved in improving the ventilatory function of the respiratory tract.

**American Association of Colleges of Nursing (AACN),** a national organization of baccalaureate and higher degree programs in nursing that was established to address issues in nursing education.

**American Association of Critical Care Nurses (AACN),** a national organization of nurses working in critical care units.

**American Association of Industrial Nurses (AAIN),** a national professional association of nurses working in industry and concerned with issues in occupational health.

**American Association of Medical Colleges (AAMC),** a national organization of faculty members and deans of medical schools and colleges that was established to address issues in medical education.

**American Association of Neurological Nurses (AANN),** a national organization of nurses working in the field of neurology.

**American Association of Neuroscience Nurses (AANN),** a national organization of nurses working with neurologically impaired patients. The organization is affiliated with the American Association of Neurological Surgeons.

**American Association of Nurse Anesthetists (AANA),** a professional association of certified registered nurse anesthetists. See also **nurse anesthetist.**

**American Association of Pathologists and Bacteriologists (AAPB),** a national professional organization of specialists in pathology and bacteriology.

**American Association of Retired Persons (AARP),** a voluntary U.S. organization of older persons, who may or may not be retired, with the goal of improving the welfare of persons over 50 years of age. The AARP advises members of Congress and state legislatures about legislation affecting older individuals.

**American Association of University Professors (AAUP),** a national organization of faculty members of institutions of higher learning. The AAUP represents faculty in matters of academic freedom, appointment policies, and procedures and serves as the bargaining agent for the faculties of some universities.

**American College of Emergency Physicians (ACEP),** a national professional organization of physicians specializing in emergency medicine.

**American College of Obstetricians and Gynecologists (ACOG),** the national organization of obstetricians and gynecologists. It is concerned with the education of physicians in the specialty standards of practice, the continued education and well-being of its members, and the board certification of eligible members as fellows of the organization.

**American College of Physicians (ACP),** a national professional organization of physicians.

**American College of Prosthodontists,** an organization of dentists who specialize in the restoration of dental or oral prostheses, such as dentures, artificial crowns, and bridges, and in the diagnosis and treatment of temporomandibular joint and maxillofacial disorders.

**American College of Radiology (ACR),** a national professional organization of physicians who specialize in radiology.

**American College of Surgeons (ACS),** a national professional organization of physicians who specialize in surgery.

**American Dental Hygienists' Association (ADHA),** the largest organization of dental hygienists in the United States. Its mission is to advance the art and science of dental hygiene by increasing the awareness of and ensuring access to quality oral health care; by promoting the highest standards of dental hygiene education, licensure, practice, and research; and by representing the interests of dental hygienists. The ADHA is structured on local, state, and national levels and has its national headquarters in Chicago.

**American Hospital Association (AHA),** a national organization of individuals, institutions, and organizations that works to improve health services for all people. The AHA publishes several journals and newsletters.

*American Journal of Nursing,* the professional journal of the American Nurses Association (ANA). It contains articles of general and specialized clinical interest to nurses and is an important resource regarding the profession in the United States.

**American leishmaniasis,** a group of infections caused by various species of *Leishmania* of Central and South America, characterized by cutaneous lesions at the site of the sandfly bite and transmitting infection and causing disfiguring ulcerative lesions of the nose, mouth, and throat or visceral disease. Illness may be prolonged, rendering patients susceptible to serious secondary infections. Kinds of American leishmaniasis are **chiclero's ulcer, espundia, forest yaws,** and **uta.** Also called **mucocutaneous leishmaniasis, New World leishmaniasis.** See also **leishmaniasis.**

**American Medical Association (AMA),** a professional association whose membership is made up of approximately half of the total licensed physicians in the United States, including practitioners in all recognized medical specialties, as well as general primary care physicians. The AMA is governed by a board of trustees and house of delegates who represent various state and local medical associations and U.S. government agencies such as the Public Health Service and medical departments of the army, navy, and air force. The AMA maintains directories of all qualified physicians (including nonmembers) in the United States, including graduates of foreign medical colleges; evaluates prescription and nonprescription drugs; advises congressional and state legislators regarding proposed health care laws; and publishes a variety of journals that report on scientific and socioeconomic developments in the field of medicine. See also **British Medical Association, Canadian Medical Association.**

**American mountain fever.** See **Colorado tick fever.**

**American National Standards Institute (ANSI),** a private nonprofit organization that coordinates voluntary developments of standards for medical and other devices in the United States and represents the United States in matters related to international standardization.

**American Nephrology Nurses' Association (ANNA),** an organization of nurses and technicians working in the fields of dialysis and renal diseases.

**American Nurses Association (ANA),** the national professional association of registered nurses in the United States. It was founded in 1896 to improve standards of health and the availability of health care given in order to foster high standards for nursing, to promote the professional development of nurses, to advance the economic and general welfare of nurses, and to project a positive and realistic view of nursing. The ANA is made up of 54 constituent associations, from the 50 states, the District of Columbia, Guam, and the Virgin Islands, and the Federal Nurses Association (FedNA), representing more than 900 district associations. National conventions are held biennially in even-numbered years. Members may join one or more of the five divisions on nursing practice: Community Health, Gerontological, Maternal and Child Health, Medical-Surgical, and Psychiatric and Mental Health Nursing. These divisions are coordinated by the Congress for Nursing Practice. The Congress evaluates changes in the scope of practice, monitors scientific and educational developments, encourages research, and develops statements that describe ANA policies regarding legislation affecting nursing practice. In addition, the ANA is politically active on the federal level in all issues relevant to nursing and the public. Statistical services enable the association to fulfill its role as the most authoritative source of data on nursing in the United States. ANA publications include *American Nurse, Publications List,* and *The American Journal of Nursing.*

**American Nurses Association—Political Action Committee (ANA-PAC),** an organization that raises funds for political contributions to candidates for public office at the state and national levels. Formerly called **Nurses' Coalition for Action in Politics (N-CAP).**

**American Occupational Therapy Association.** See **AOTA.**

**American Psychiatric Association (APA),** a national professional association for physicians who specialize in psychiatry. It is concerned with the development of standards for psychiatric facilities, the formulation of mental health programs, the dissemination of data, and the promotion of psychiatric education and research. It publishes the *Diagnostic and Statistical Manual of Mental Disorders (DSM).*

**American Red Cross,** one of more than 120 national organizations that seek to reduce human suffering through various health, safety, and disaster relief programs in affiliation with the International Committee of the Red Cross.

The committee and all Red Cross organizations evolved from the Geneva Convention of 1864, following the example and urging of Swiss humanitarian Jean Henri Dunant, who aided wounded French and Austrian soldiers at the Battle of Solferino in 1859. The American Red Cross has more than 1.3 million members in about 1300 chapters throughout the United States. Some 97% of Red Cross staff is volunteer. Chapters maintain small paid staffs and employ some professionals but depend largely on the volunteers. The American Red Cross blood program collects and distributes more blood than any other single U.S. agency and coordinates distribution of blood and blood products to the U.S. Defense Department on request or during national emergencies. The organization annually collects about 4 million blood donations and gives blood to more than 4000 hospitals. American Red Cross nursing and health programs include courses in the home on parenthood, prenatal and postnatal care, hygiene, and venereal disease. Nursing students are enrolled for service in American Red Cross community programs and during disasters. Four area offices at Alexandria, Virginia; Atlanta, Georgia; St. Louis, Missouri; and San Francisco, California, supervise and assist 70 divisions of the American Red Cross and direct field staff members assigned to military installations. National headquarters of the organization is at 17th and D Streets, NW, Washington, DC 20006. The President of the United States is honorary chairman of the organization, for which a 50-member board of governors, all volunteers, develops policy. The symbol of the American Red Cross, like that of most other Red Cross societies throughout the world, is a red cross on a field of white; in Switzerland it is a white cross on a red field, in Muslim countries a red crescent, and in Israel a red star of David.

**American Registry of Radiologic Technologists (ARRT),** a national certifying body for radiologic technologists in the disciplines of radiography, nuclear medicine, radiation therapy, mammography, computed tomography, magnetic resonance imaging, quality management and cardiovascular-interventional technology. Certification is awarded following passage of an examination in each of these areas.

**American Sign Language (Ameslan, ASL),** a method of manual communication used by some deaf persons. Messages are conveyed by manipulation of the hands and fingers. ASL is a distinct language, with its own grammar and syntax. See also **sign language.**

**American Society of Parenteral and Enteral Nutrition (ASPEN),** an organization that provides education, support, and accreditation to persons who specialize in nutrition that is provided through IV, enteral, or related types of feeding.

**American Speech, Language, and Hearing Association (ASHA),** a professional association that certifies audiologists and speech-language pathologists.

**Americans With Disabilities Act,** legislation approved by the U.S. Congress in July 1990, that would bar discrimination against persons with physical or mental disabilities. The Act defines disability as a condition that "substantially limits" such activities as walking or seeing, and it applies to persons with acquired immunodeficiency syndrome (AIDS), as well as to alcoholics and drug users undergoing treatment. The law requires employers to make "reasonable accommodations" for workers who are otherwise qualified to carry out their job duties.

**American Type Culture Collection (ATCC),** a U.S. nonprofit, nongovernmental organization that is concerned with the preservation of specimens of cellular and microbiologic cultures and with the distribution of the cultures to research centers and laboratories in the academic, scientific, and medical communities.

**americium (Am)** /am′ərish′ē·əm/, a synthetic radioactive element of the actinide group. Its atomic number is 95; its atomic mass is 243.

**Ameslan** /am′islan/, abbreviation for **American Sign Language.**

**Ames test** /āmz/, a method of testing substances for possible carcinogenicity by exposing a strain of *Salmonella* bacteria to a sample of the substance. The rate of mutations observed is interpreted as an indication of the carcinogenic potential of the substance tested. Also called **mutagenicity test.**

**amethopterin.** See **methotrexate.**

**ametropia** /am′itrō′pē·ə/ [Gk, *ametros*, irregular, *opsis*, sight], a condition characterized by an optic defect involving an error of refraction, such as astigmatism, hyperopia, or myopia. **—ametropic,** *adj.*

**AMI,** abbreviation for **acute myocardial infarction.**

**Amicar,** trademark for a hemostatic (aminocaproic acid).

**amicrobic** /am′īkrob′ik/, not caused by or related to microbes.

**amidase** /am′i·dās /, 1. an enzyme that catalyzes the formation of a monocarboxylic acid and ammonia by hydrolytic cleavage of the C—N bond of a monocarboxylic acid amide. 2. more generally, a term used in the recommended and trivial names of some hydrolases acting on amides, particularly those acting on linear amides.

**amide,** 1. a chemical compound formed from an organic acid by the substitution of an amino ($NR_2$) group for the hydroxyl of a carboxyl (COOH) group. 2. a chemical compound formed by the deprotonation of an amine, $HNR_2$.

**amide local anesthetic,** any of more than two dozen compounds containing an amide group that are safe, versatile, and effective local anesthetics. If hypersensitivity to a drug in this group precludes its use, one of the ester-compound local anesthetics may provide analgesia without adverse effect. Examples of amide local anesthetics are **bupivacaine, lidocaine, mepivacaine,** and **prilocaine.**

**amido-,** prefix meaning 'the presence of the radical $NH_2$ along with the radical CO': *amidoacetal, amidobenzene.*

**amifostine,** a cytoprotective agent for cisplatin.

■ INDICATIONS: This drug is used to reduce renal toxicity when cisplatin is given to treat ovarian cancer.

■ CONTRAINDICATIONS: Known hypersensitivity to mannitol or aminothiol, hypotension, dehydration, and lactation prohibit the use of this drug.

■ ADVERSE EFFECTS: Dizziness, somnolence, sneezing, flushing, hiccups, hypocalcemia, rash, and chills are among this drug's side effects. Common side effects include hypotension, nausea, and vomiting.

**Amigo,** trademark for a battery-operated scooterlike vehicle that gives mobility to some patients who cannot walk.

**amikacin sulfate** /am′ikā′sin/, an aminoglycoside antibiotic.

■ INDICATIONS: It is prescribed in the treatment of various severe infections caused by susceptible strains of gram-negative bacteria.

■ CONTRAINDICATIONS: Concurrent use of certain diuretics or known hypersensitivity to this or other aminoglycosides prohibits its use. The drug is used with caution in patients who have impaired renal function or myasthenia gravis and those under the influence of neuromuscular blockers or other nephrotoxins.

■ ADVERSE EFFECTS: Among the most serious adverse reactions are nephrotoxicity, auditory and vestibular ototoxicity, and neuromuscular blockade. GI disturbances, pain at the site of injection, and hypersensitivity reactions may occur.

**Amikin,**  trademark for an aminoglycoside antibiotic (amikacin sulfate).

**amiloride hydrochloride** /am′ilôr′id/,  a potassium-sparing diuretic with antihypertensive activity.
■ INDICATIONS: It is prescribed as adjunctive therapy in the treatment of congestive heart failure or hypertension. It is often given with a thiazide medication.
■ CONTRAINDICATIONS: Concurrent use of potassium-conserving agents, hyperkalemia, impaired renal function, or known hypersensitivity to this drug prohibits its use.
■ ADVERSE EFFECTS: Among the most serious adverse reactions are headache, diarrhea, nausea and vomiting, anorexia, hyperkalemia, dizziness, encephalopathy, impotence, muscle cramps, photosensitivity, irregular heart rhythm, mental confusion, and paresthesia.

**amine** /am′in, əmēn′/ [L, *ammonia*],  (in chemistry) an organic derivative of ammonia in which one or more hydrogen atoms are replaced by alkyl or aryl groups.

**amine pump,**  *informal.* an active transport system in the presynaptic nerve endings that takes up released amine neurotransmitters. Adverse reactions to some drugs, notably tricyclic antidepressants, block this function, resulting in a high concentration of norepinephrine in cardiac tissue and resultant tachycardia and arrhythmia. See also **monoamine oxidase inhibitor.**

**amino-,**  prefix for a chemical name indicated by the monovalent radical $NH_2$.

**aminoacetic acid.**  See **glycine.**

**amino acid** /əmē′nō/,  an organic chemical compound composed of one or more basic amino groups and one or more acidic carboxyl groups. Twenty of the more than 100 amino acids that occur in nature are the building blocks of proteins. Peptide linkages between them form polypeptides or proteins (for example the structural components of muscle). The eight **essential amino acids** are isoleucine (Ile), leucine (Leu), lysine (Lys), methionine (Met), phenylalanine (Phe), threonine (Thr), tryptophan (Trp), and valine (Val). Arginine (Arg) and histidine (His) are essential in infants. Cysteine (Cys) and tyrosine (Tyr) are semiessential because they may be synthesized from methionine (Met) and phenylalanine (Phe), respectively. The main nonessential amino acids are alanine (Ala), asparagine (Asn), aspartic acid (Asp), glutamine (Glm), glutamic acid (Glu), glycine (Gly), proline (Pro), and serine (Ser). From their structures, the amino acids can be classified as basic (arginine, histidine, lysine), acidic (aspartic acid, glumatic acid), or neutral (the remainder); each group is transported across cell membranes by different carrier methods.

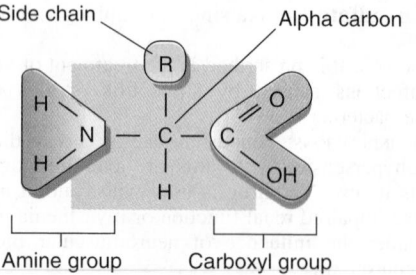

**Amino acid: basic chemical structure**

**amino acid group,**  a category of organic chemicals containing the monovalent amine radical $NH_2$, an acid or COOH, and a group idiosyncratic to that particular amino acid group.

**aminoacidopathy** /ə·mē′nō·as′id·op′ə·thē /,  any of various disorders caused by a defect in an enzymatic step in the metabolic pathway of one or more amino acids or in a protein mediator necessary for transport of an amino acid into or out of a cell.

**aminoaciduria** /amē′nō·as′idöōr′ē·ə/,  the abnormal presence of amino acids in the urine that usually indicates an inborn metabolic defect, as in cystinuria. Also called **acidaminuria.**

**aminobenzene.**  See **aniline.**

**aminobenzoic acid** /-benzō′ik/,  a metabolic product of the catabolism of the amino acid tryptophan. Also called **anthranilic acid.** See also **paraaminobenzoic acid (PABA).**

**aminocaproic acid** /əmē′nōkəprō′ik, am′inō-/,  a hemostatic.
■ INDICATION: It is prescribed to stop excessive bleeding that results from hyperfibrinolysis.
■ CONTRAINDICATION: Active intravascular coagulation prohibits its use.
■ ADVERSE EFFECTS: Among the most serious adverse reactions are thrombosis and hypotension. Inhibition of ejaculation, nasal congestion, diarrhea, and allergic reactions also may occur.

**aminoglycoside antibiotic.**  See **antibiotic.**

**aminohydrolase.**  See **deaminase.**

**aminolevulinic acid (ALA)**[1] /am′inōlev′ōōlin′ik/,  the aliphatic precursor of heme. It is formed in the body from the condensation of glycine and succinyl coenzyme A and undergoes further condensation to form porphobilinogen. Aminolevulinic acid may be detected in the urine of some patients with porphyria, liver disease, and lead poisoning.

**aminolevulinic acid**[2],  a photochemotherapeutic agent.
■ INDICATIONS: It is used to treat nonhyperkeratotic actinic keratoses of the face and scalp.
■ CONTRAINDICATIONS: Known hypersensitivity to porphyrins contraindicates this drug's use.
■ ADVERSE EFFECTS: Side effects include crusting, hypopigmentation or hyperpigmentation, ulceration, pain, itching, bleeding, and pustules at the site of application.

**aminophylline** /am′ənōfil′in, əmē′nō-/,  a bronchodilator.
■ INDICATIONS: It is prescribed in the treatment of bronchospasm associated with asthma, emphysema, and bronchitis.
■ CONTRAINDICATIONS: Known hypersensitivity to this drug or other xanthine medication prohibits its use. It is used with caution in patients who have peptic ulcer and those in whom cardiac stimulation would be harmful.
■ ADVERSE EFFECTS: Among the more serious adverse reactions are GI disturbances, central nervous system stimulation, palpitations, tachycardia, nervousness, and seizures.

**aminophylline poisoning,**  an adverse reaction to an excessive intake of a methylxanthine drug such as caffeine or theophylline. The patient appears alternately restless, excited, and lethargic. Symptoms may include nausea, diarrhea, vomiting, abdominal pain, and GI bleeding; headache, tinnitus, thirst, delirium, and seizures; tachycardia, cardiac arrhythmias, and blood pressure changes.

**aminopyrine** /-pī′rin/,  a white chemical compound with analgesic and antipyretic effects. Its continued or excessive use may lead to agranulocytosis.

**aminosalicylic acid.**  See **paraaminosalicylic acid (PAS, PASA).**

**aminosuccinic acid.**  See **aspartic acid.**

**aminotransferases** /-trans′fərās/,  enzymes that catalyze the transfer of an amino group from an amino acid to an alpha-keto acid, with pyridoxal phosphate and pyridoxamine phosphate acting as coenzymes. Aspartate amino transferase (AST), normally present in serum and various tissues, especially in the heart and liver, is released by damaged cells, and, as a result, a high serum level of AST may be diagnostic in myocardial infarction or hepatic disease. Alanine aminotransferase (ALT), a normal constituent of serum and especially in the liver, is released by injured tissue and may be present in high concentrations in the sera of patients with acute liver disease. Also called **transaminase** /transam'inās/.

**amiodarone hydrochloride,** an oral antiarrhythmic drug.
- INDICATIONS: It is prescribed for the treatment of life-threatening recurrent ventricular fibrillation and recurrent, hemodynamically unstable ventricular tachycardia refractory to other drugs.
- CONTRAINDICATIONS: This drug should not be given to patients with severe sinus-node dysfunction or second- and third-degree atrioventricular block or when episodes of bradycardia have resulted in syncope, except when used in conjunction with a pacemaker.
- ADVERSE EFFECTS: Among the most serious adverse effects are pulmonary toxicity, liver dysfunction, nausea, vomiting, constipation, anorexia, malaise, fatigue, tremor, involuntary movements, visual disorders, bradycardia, cyanosis, and congestive heart failure.

**Amipaque,** trademark for an intrathecal and intravascular diagnostic drug (metrizamide).

**amitosis** /am'ətō'sis/ [Gr, *a, mitos,* not thread], cell division in which there is simple fission of the nucleus and cytoplasm (as in bacteria) without the complex stages of chromosome separation that occur in mitosis. —**amitotic,** *adj.*

**amitriptyline** /am'itrip'tilin/, a tricyclic antidepressant.
- INDICATION: It is prescribed in the treatment of depression.
- CONTRAINDICATIONS: Concomitant administration of monoamine oxidase inhibitors, recent myocardial infarction, or known hypersensitivity to this drug or to other tricyclic medication prohibits its use. It is used with caution in patients having a seizure disorder or cardiovascular disease.
- ADVERSE EFFECTS: Among the more common adverse reactions are sedation and anticholinergic effects. A variety of cardiovascular and central nervous system effects may occur. This agent interacts with many other drugs.

**AML,** abbreviation for **acute myelocytic leukemia.**

**ammoni-, ammono-,** prefix meaning 'ammonium': *ammoniemia, ammonolysis.*

**ammonia (NH₃)** /amō'nē·a/ [Gk, *ammoniakos,* salt of Ammon, Egyptian god], a colorless pungent gas produced by the decomposition of nitrogenous organic matter. Some of its many uses are as an aromatic stimulant, a detergent, and an emulsifier.

**ammoniacal fermentation** /am'ənī'əkəl/, the production of ammonia and carbon dioxide from urea by the enzyme urease.

**ammonia exposure,** an adverse reaction to ammonia, which is formed as a product of amino acid and nucleic acid catabolism. Ammonia is converted to urea in the liver and excreted by the kidneys. In liver diseases such as cirrhosis, ammonia may accumulate in the blood, resulting in neurologic damage. Preventive measures include administering antibiotics that restrict the growth of ammonia-producing bacteria and limiting the amount of protein in the diet.

**ammonia level test,** a blood test used to help diagnose severe liver diseases such as fulminant hepatitis, cirrhosis, and hepatic encephalopathy.

**ammonium ion,** an $NH_4^+$ ion formed by the reaction of ammonia ($NH_3$) with a hydrogen ion ($H^+$). The ammonium ion is highly soluble in water but does not pass easily through cell membranes, as does the ammonia molecule, and its rate of excretion is influenced in part by the acidity of urine. The lower the pH, the greater the proportion of ammonium ions present, assuming a constant level of ammonia production from amino acid metabolism.

**Ammon's horn.** See **hippocampus.**

**ammonuria** /am'ōnŏŏr'ē·ə/, urine that contains an excessive amount of ammonia.

**amnesia** /amnē'zhə/ [Gk, *a, mnasthai,* to forget], a loss of memory caused by brain damage or by severe emotional trauma. Kinds of amnesia include **anterograde amnesia, posttraumatic amnesia,** and **retrograde amnesia.**

**amnesiac** /amnē'sē·ək/, a person with a loss of memory caused by brain damage or severe emotional trauma.

**amnesic** /amnē'sik/ [Gk, *a, mnasthai,* to forget], in a state of forgetfulness or showing signs of memory loss or impairment.

**amnesic aphasia** [Gk, *a, mnasthai + a, phasis,* without speech], an inability to remember spoken words or to use words for names of objects, circumstances, or characteristics.

**amnestic apraxia** /amnes'tik/, the inability to carry out a movement in response to a request because of a lack of ability to remember the request. See also **apraxia.**

**amnio-,** prefix meaning 'amnion': *amniogenesis, amniorrhexis.*

**amniocentesis** /am'nē·ōsentē'sis/ [Gk, *amnos,* lamb's caul, *kentesis,* pricking], an obstetric procedure in which a small amount of amniotic fluid is removed for laboratory analysis. It is usually performed between the sixteenth and twentieth weeks of gestation to aid in the diagnosis of fetal abnormalities.
- METHOD: With the use of ultrasound scanning techniques the position of the fetus and the location of the placenta are determined. The skin on the mother's abdomen is aseptically prepared, and a local anesthetic is usually injected. A needle attached to a syringe is introduced into a part of the uterus where there is the least chance of perforating the placenta or scratching the fetus. Between 20 and 25 ml of amniotic fluid is aspirated. Amniocentesis is performed to diagnose various genetic defects, including chromosomal abnormalities, neural tube defects, and Tay-Sachs disease. It is also performed to discover the sex of the fetus if certain sex-linked genetic defects are suspected. Later in pregnancy,

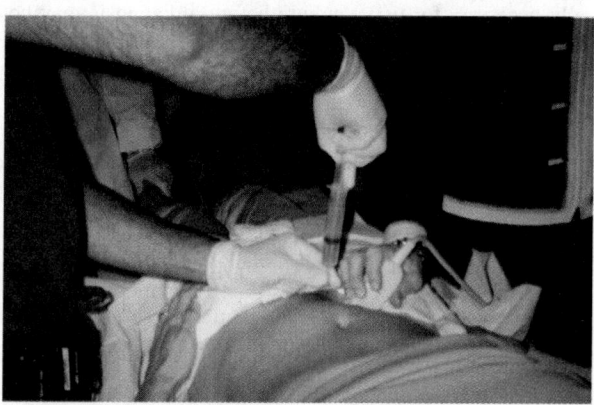

**Amniocentesis: placement of needle** *(Chabner, 2001)*

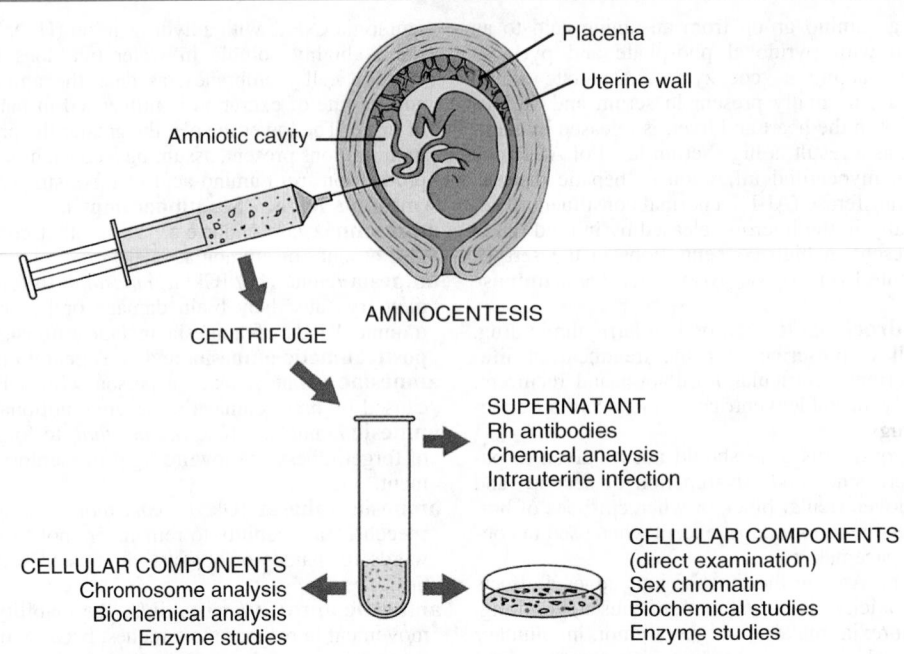

**Amniocentesis: laboratory use of amniotic fluid aspirant** *(Lowdermilk, Perry, Bobak, 2000)*

amniocentesis may be performed to assess fetal lung maturity by testing the lecithin-sphingomyelin (L/S) ratio and the presence of phosphatidyl-glycerol (PG) in the laboratory before elective delivery. The fluid may be tested for the concentration of creatinine, another indicator of fetal maturity. When postmaturity is suspected, amniocentesis is performed to examine the amniotic fluid for meconium.

■ NURSING CONSIDERATIONS: Proof of informed consent must be signed by the woman before amniocentesis. Specifically stated in the consent form are the reasons for performing the procedure and the facts that fluid is to be removed after needle puncture of the uterus, that ultrasound imaging techniques are usual adjuncts, that the procedure may fail to give the results intended, and that spontaneous abortion, nausea, abdominal pain, or fetal injury may occur. The woman is reassured that complications and failure are rare; she is given emotional support before, during, and after the procedure. In testing for genetic abnormalities 10 days to 2 weeks is usually necessary for tissue culture before a diagnosis may be made; this waiting period may be extremely stressful for the mother. The woman is warned to report any signs of infection or of the onset of labor. Rh immune globulin should be given to pregnant women who are Rh negative.

■ OUTCOME CRITERIA: Spontaneous abortion occurs in approximately 1% of women undergoing amniocentesis. Perforation of the placenta or a blood vessel in the umbilical cord or placenta may cause hemorrhage or isoimmunization and hemolytic disease of the fetus, possibly leading to fetal death. Maternal and fetal infection with attendant morbidity or mortality may occur, but it is rare. Premature rupture of the membranes, premature labor, or trauma to the fetus or umbilical cord may occur. Compare **chorionic villi sampling.**

**amniography** /am′nē·og′rəfē/, a procedure used to detect placement of the placenta by x-ray examination with injection of a radiopaque contrast medium into the amniotic fluid. It is seldom used, having been largely supplanted by ultrasonography.

**amnioinfusion,** a nursing intervention from the Nursing Interventions Classification (NIC) defined as infusion of fluid into the uterus during labor to relieve umbilical cord compression or to dilute meconium-stained fluid. See also **Nursing Interventions Classification.**

**amnion** /am′nē·on/ [Gk, *amnos,* lamb's caul], a membrane, continuous with and covering the fetal side of the placenta, that forms the outer surface of the umbilical cord. Compare **chorion.**

**amnionitis** /am′nē·ōnī′tis/, an inflammation of the amnion. The condition may develop after early rupture of the fetal membranes.

**amnioscopy** /am′nē·os′kəpē/, direct visual examination of the fetus and amniotic fluid with an endoscope that is inserted into the amniotic cavity through the uterine cervix or an incision in the abdominal wall.

**amniotic** /am′nē·ot′ik/, pertaining to the amnion.

**amniotic band disruption sequence syndrome,** an abnormal condition of fetal development characterized by the development of fibrous bands within the uterus that entangle the fetus, leading to deformities in structure and function. The syndrome is associated with a variety of congenital defects, including clubbed feet, missing limbs, simian creases, and skull and visceral defects. It can be detected in the womb. Interventions are specific to the varied symptoms, and genetic counseling is applied.

**amniotic cavity** [Gk, *amnion,* fetal membrane; L, *cavum*], the fluid-filled cavity of the amniotic sac surrounding the fetus.

**amniotic fluid,** a liquid produced by the fetal membranes and the fetus. It surrounds the fetus throughout pregnancy, protecting it from trauma and temperature variations, providing freedom of fetal movements, and helping to maintain the fetal oxygen supply. The volume totals about 1000 ml at

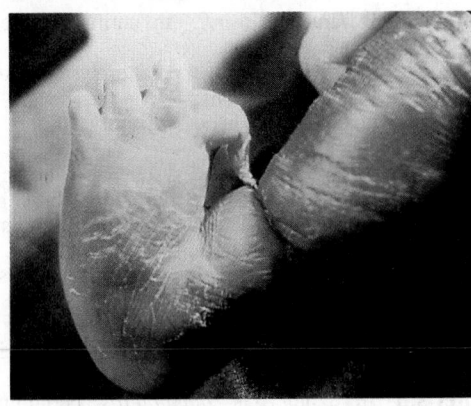

**Amniotic bands** *(Zitelli and Davis, 1997)*

term. In addition to providing the fetus with physical protection, the amniotic fluid is a medium of active chemical exchange. It is secreted and resorbed by cells lining the amniotic sac at a rate of 500 ml/hr at term and is swallowed, metabolized, and excreted as fetal urine at a rate of 50 ml/hr. Its chemical constituents are those of maternal and fetal plasma in different concentrations. Its pH is close to neutral. Amniotic fluid itself is clear, though desquamated fetal cells and lipids give it a cloudy appearance.

**amniotic fluid embolism** [Gk, *amnion;* L, *fluere,* to flow; Gk, *embolos,* plug], a quantity of amniotic fluid that enters the maternal blood system during labor and/or delivery and becomes lodged in a vessel. It is usually fatal to the mother if it is a pulmonary embolism.

**amniotic fold,** an embryonic growth feature observed in many vertebrates, particularly birds and reptiles. It consists of flaps of ectoderm and mesoderm that grow over the back of an embryo to form the amnion.

**amniotic sac,** a thin-walled bag that contains the fetus and amniotic fluid during pregnancy. It has a capacity of 4 to 5 L at term. The wall of the sac extends from the margin of the placenta. The amnion, chorion, and decidua that make up the wall are each a few cell layers thick. They are closely applied—though not fused—to each other and to the wall of the uterus. The intact sac and its fluid provide for the equilibration of hydrostatic pressure within the uterus. During labor, the sac effects the uniform transmission of the force of uterine contractions to the cervix for dilation. See also **amnion, chorion, decidua.**

**amniotomy** /am′nē·ot′əmē/, the artificial rupture of the fetal membranes (ARM). It is usually performed to stimulate or accelerate the onset of labor. The procedure is painless.

**amobarbital** /am′ōbär′bətal/, a barbiturate sedative-hypnotic.

■ INDICATIONS: It is prescribed as an anticonvulsant and a preanesthetic.

■ CONTRAINDICATIONS: Porphyria or known hypersensitivity to barbiturates prohibits its use. It is also contraindicated in patients with marked liver impairment or respiratory disease.

■ ADVERSE EFFECTS: Among the most serious adverse reactions are respiratory and circulatory depression, drug hangover, and various allergic reactions. It also interacts with many other drugs.

**A-mode,** amplitude modulation in diagnostic ultrasonography. It represents the time required for the ultrasound beam to strike a tissue interface and return its signal to the transducer. The greater the reflection at the interface, the larger the signal amplitude on the A-mode screen. See also **B-mode, M-mode.**

**A-mode ultrasound** [L, *ultra,* beyond, *sonus,* sound], a display of ultrasonic echoes in which the horizontal axis of the cathode ray tube display represents the time required for the return of the echo and the vertical axis represents the strength of the echo. The mode is used in echoencephalography. See also **A-mode.**

**amoeba.** See ameba.

**amoebiasis.** See amebiasis.

**amoebic dysentery.** See amebic dysentery.

**amok** [Malay, *amoq,* furious], a psychotic frenzy with a desire to kill anybody encountered. The murderous episodes may follow periods of severe depression.

**amorph** /ā′môrf, əmôrf′/ [Gk, *a, morphef,* not shape], **1.** a mutant allele that has little or no effect on the expression of a trait. Compare **antimorph, hypermorph, hypomorph.** —**amorphic,** *adj.* **2.** abbreviation for *amorphous,* as in amorph IZS (amorphous insulin zinc suspension).

**amorphic,** (in genetics) pertaining to a gene that is inactive or nearly inactive so that it has no determinable effect.

**amorphous** /əmôr′fəs/ [Gk, *a,* not, *morphe,* form], **1.** describing an object that lacks definite visible shape or form. **2.** (in chemistry) a substance that is not crystalline.

**amorphous crystals,** shapeless, ill-defined crystals, usually phosphates.

**amoxapine** /əmok′sepin/, an antidepressant similar to the tricyclics.

■ INDICATION: It is prescribed in the treatment of mental depression.

■ CONTRAINDICATIONS: It is used with caution in conditions in which anticholinergics are contraindicated, in seizure disorders, and in cardiovascular disorders. Concomitant administration of monoamine oxidase inhibitors, recent myocardial infarction, or known hypersensitivity to this drug prohibits its use.

■ ADVERSE EFFECTS: Among the most serious adverse reactions are sedation and anticholinergic side effects. A variety of GI, cardiovascular, and neurologic reactions may also occur. It is involved in many drug interactions.

**amoxicillin** /əmok′səsil′in/, a beta-lactam semisynthetic oral penicillin antibiotic.

■ INDICATIONS: It is prescribed in the treatment of infections caused by a susceptible gram-negative or gram-positive organism.

■ CONTRAINDICATION: Known hypersensitivity to any penicillin prohibits its use.

■ ADVERSE EFFECTS: Among the most serious adverse reactions are anaphylaxis, nausea, and diarrhea. Allergic reactions and rashes are common.

**Amoxil,** trademark for a beta-lactam antibiotic (amoxicillin).

**AMP,** abbreviation for **adenosine monophosphate.**

**ampere (A)** /am′pēr/ [André M. Ampere, French physicist, 1775–1836], a unit of measurement of the amount of electric current. An ampere, according to the meter-kilogram-second (MKS) system, is the amount of current passed through a resistance of 1 ohm by an electric potential of 1 volt; in the International System (SI), an ampere is a unit of electric current that carries a charge of 1 coulomb through a conductor in 1 second. The standard international ampere is the amount of current that deposits 0.001118 g of silver per second when passed, according to certain specifications, through a silver nitrate solution. See also **ohm, volt, watt.**

**amperometry** /am′parom′ətrē/, the measurement of current at a single applied potential.

**amph-.** See **amphi-**.

**amphetamine poisoning,** toxic effects of overdosage of amphetamines. Symptoms usually include excitement, tremors, tachycardia, hallucinations, delirium, convulsions, and circulatory collapse.

**amphetamines** /amfet′əmēnz/, a group of nervous system stimulants, including amphetamine and its chemical congeners dextroamphetamine and methamphetamine, that are subject to abuse because of their ability to produce wakefulness and euphoria. Abuse leads to compulsive behavior, paranoia, hallucinations, and suicidal tendencies. Amphetamines have many street names, such as **black beauties, lid poppers, pep pills, speed** (an injectable form), and **ice** (a crystalline form of methamphetamine that is smoked). See also **crank, dextroamphetamine sulfate, methamphetamine hydrochloride.**

**amphetamine sulfate,** a colorless water-soluble salt of amphetamine that stimulates the central nervous system. It has been used to treat certain respiratory complaints, to reduce fatigue, and to treat narcolepsy. It formerly was used to treat obesity.

**amphi-, amph-, ampho-,** prefix meaning 'on both sides, around, double': *amphiarthrosis, amphodiplopia.*

**amphiarthrosis.** See **cartilaginous joint.**

**amphidiarthrodial joint** /am′fēdī′ärthrō′dē·əl/ [Gk, *amphi,* both kinds], a type of joint that combines amphiarthrosis with diarthrosis, permitting movement in more than one direction, such as that of the lower jaw.

**amphigenesis.** See **amphigony.**

**amphigenetic** /am′fijənet′ik/ [Gk, *amphi,* both sides, *genein,* to produce], **1.** produced by the union of gametes from both sexes. **2.** bisexual; having both testicular and ovarian tissue. Compare **hermaphroditism, pseudohermaphroditism.**

**amphigenous inheritance** /amfij′ənəs/, the acquisition of genetic traits and conditions from both parents. Also called **biparental inheritance, duplex inheritance.**

**amphigonadism** /am′figō′nədiz′əm/, true hermaphroditism; the presence of both testicular and ovarian tissue. —**amphigonadic,** *adj.*

**amphigony** /amfig′ənē/ [Gk, *amphi* + *gonos,* generation], sexual reproduction. Also called **amphigenesis.** —**amphigonic** /am′figon′ik/, *adj.*

**amphikaryon** /am′fiker′ē·on/ [Gk, *amphi* + *karyon,* nucleus], a nucleus containing the diploid number of chromosomes. —**amphikaryotic,** *adj.*

**amphimixis** /am′fimik′sis/ [Gk, *amphi* + *mixis,* mingling], **1.** the union of germ cells in reproduction so that both maternal and paternal hereditary characteristics are derived; interbreeding. **2.** the union and integration of oral, anal, and genital libidinal impulses in the development of heterosexuality.

**amphipathic** /-path′ik/ [Gk, *amphi* both + *pathos* suffering], pertaining to a molecule having two sides with characteristically different properties, such as a detergent, which has both a polar (hydrophilic) end and a nonpolar (hydrophobic) end but is long enough so that each end demonstrates its own solubility characteristics.

**ampho-.** See **amphi-**.

**Amphojel,** trademark for aluminum hydroxide gel.

**amphoric breath sound** /amfôr′ik/ [Gk, *amphoreus,* jug], an abnormal, resonant, hollow, blowing sound heard with a stethoscope over the thorax. It indicates a cavity opening into a bronchus or a pneumothorax.

**amphoteric** /am′fōter′ik/ [Gk, *amphoteros,* pertaining to both], a substance that can act as an acid or base, depending on conditions.

**amphotericin B** /am′fəter′əsin/, an antifungal medication.

■ INDICATIONS: It is prescribed for topical or systemic use in the treatment of fungal infections.

■ CONTRAINDICATION: Known hypersensitivity to this drug prohibits its use.

■ ADVERSE EFFECTS: When it is used systemically, among the most serious adverse reactions are thrombophlebitis, blood dyscrasias, nephrotoxicity, nausea, and fever; chills and shaking may occur on administration. With topical use, local hypersensitivity reactions are the most common adverse reactions.

**amphotericin methyl ester (AME),** an antiviral drug used in experimental treatment of human immunodeficiency virus infections.

**amphoterism** /-ter′izəm/ [Gk, *amphoteros,* pertaining to both], a quality of a chemical compound that permits it to act as an acid or a base.

**ampicillin** /am′pəsil′in/, a semisynthetic aminopenicillin.

■ INDICATIONS: It is prescribed in the treatment of infections caused by a broad spectrum of sensitive gram-negative and gram-positive organisms.

■ CONTRAINDICATION: Known hypersensitivity to any penicillin prohibits its use.

■ ADVERSE EFFECTS: Among the most serious adverse reactions are anaphylaxis, nausea, and diarrhea. Fever, rashes, allergic reactions, and suprainfection also may occur.

**ampicillin sodium,** the sodium salt of ampicillin, prescribed as an antibiotic to treat gram-positive organisms and some gram-negative organisms.

**amplification** /am′plifikā′shən/ [L, *amplificare,* to make wider], **1.** a genetic engineering process in which the amount of plasmid DNA increased in proportion to the amount of bacterial DNA by treatment with certain substances, including chloramphenicol. **2.** the replication in bulk of an entire gene library. See also **polymerase chain reaction. —amplify,** *v.*

**amplifier,** a device that controls power from a mechanical, electrical, hydraulic, or other source so that the output is greater than the input.

**amplitude** /am′plityōod/ [L, *amplus,* wide], width or breadth of range or extent, such as amplitude of accommodation or amplitude of convergence.

**amplitude of accommodation (AA),** the total accommodative power of the eye, determined by the difference between the refractive power for farthest vision and that for nearest vision.

**amplitude of convergence,** the difference in the power needed to turn the eyes from their far point to their near point of convergence. Also called **fusional amplitude, vergence ability.**

**amprenavir,** an antiviral.

■ INDICATIONS: It is used to treat HIV in combination with other antiretroviral agents.

■ CONTRAINDICATIONS: Known hypersensitivity to this drug prohibits its use.

■ ADVERSE EFFECTS: Life-threatening side effects include Stevens-Johnson syndrome and acute hemolytic anemia. Other serious adverse effects include new-onset diabetes, hyperglycemia, and exacerbation of preexisting diabetes mellitus. Common side effects include diarrhea, abdominal pain, nausea, paresthesia, and rash.

**ampule** /am′pyōol/ [Fr, *ampoule,* phial], a small, sterile glass or plastic container that usually contains a single dose of a solution. Also spelled **ampoule.**

**ampulla** /ampōol′ə/ [L, flasklike bottle], a rounded, saclike dilation of a duct, canal, or any tubular structure, such

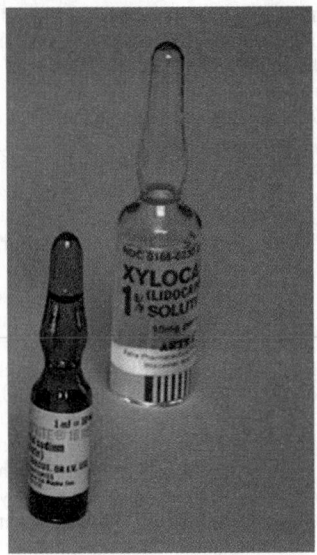

**Ampule** *(Potter and Perry, 2001)*

as the lacrimal duct, semicircular canal, uterine tube, rectum, or vas deferens.

**ampulla of the bile duct.** See **hepatopancreatic ampulla.**

**ampulla of the rectum,** a flask-shaped dilation near the end of the rectum.

**ampulla of Vater.** See **hepatopancreatic ampulla.**

**ampullary aneurysm.** See **saccular aneurysm.**

**ampullary tubal pregnancy** /ampo͞o'lərē, am'pəler'ē/, a kind of tubal pregnancy in which implantation occurs in the ampulla of one of the fallopian tubes. See also **tubal pregnancy.**

**ampullula** /ampo͞ol'yələ/, a spherical dilation of a minute lymph or blood vessel or duct. Compare **ampulla.**

**amputation** /am'pyo͞otā'shən/ [L, *amputare,* to excise], the surgical removal of a part of the body or a limb or part of a limb. It is performed to treat recurrent infections or gangrene in peripheral vascular disease, to remove malignant tumors, and to treat severe trauma. With the patient under anesthesia, the part is removed and a shaped flap is cut from muscular and cutaneous tissue to cover the end of the bone. A section may be left open for drainage if infection is present. Preoperative care can include an assessment of circulation in the affected part. After surgery a lower leg amputation is elevated on a pillow for no more than 24 to 48 hours, and, if necessary, protected with plastic from urinary and fecal contamination. Vital signs are monitored carefully. If a soft dressing is used, it is watched for excessive bleeding. The stump is moved frequently to prevent circulatory complications, contractures, and tissue necrosis. If the dressing is rigid (a cast), it must remain in place for 8 to 14 days. Should the cast come off accidentally, the stump must be wrapped tightly at once with an elastic compression bandage and plans must be made to replace the cast. The patient is fit for a prosthesis, either delayed or immediately. Medication may relieve incisional and phantom limb pain. Kinds of amputation include **closed amputation, congenital amputation, open amputation, primary amputation,** and **secondary amputation.**

**amputation care,** a nursing intervention from the Nursing Interventions Classification (NIC) defined as promotion of physical and psychological healing after amputation of a body part. See also **Nursing Interventions Classification.**

**amputation flap,** a flap of skin used to cover the end of an amputation stump.

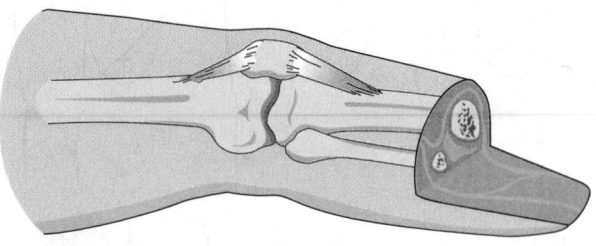

Flap amputation

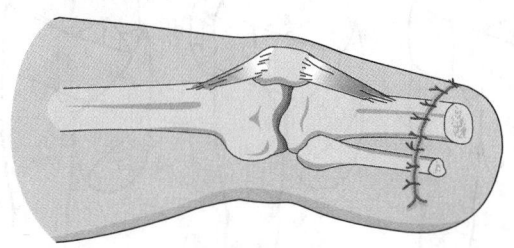

Secured flap amputation

**Amputation flaps** *(Beare and Myers, 1998)*

**amputation neuroma,** a form of traumatic neuroma that may develop near the stump after the amputation of an extremity.

**amputation-stump bandage,** an elastic figure-eight bandage applied to cover the stump after an amputation. It helps control edema and shape the remaining portion of the limb. (See figure, p. 86.)

**amputee** /am'pyətē'/, a person who has had one or more extremities traumatically or surgically removed. See also **congenital amputation.**

**AMRA,** abbreviation for *American Medical Records Association.*

**amrinone lactate** /am'rinōn/, an IV cardiac inotropic drug.

■ INDICATIONS: It is prescribed in the short-term management of congestive heart failure in patients who do not respond to therapy with digitalis, diuretics, and vasodilators.

■ CONTRAINDICATIONS: Concomitant use with disopyramide and any combination therapy should be closely monitored for potential interactions.

■ ADVERSE EFFECTS: Among the more serious adverse reactions are thrombocytopenia, arrhythmias, hypotension, nausea, vomiting, liver impairment, and hypersensitivity effects.

**Amsler grid** [Marc Amsler, Swiss ophthalmologist, 1891–1968], a checkerboard grid of intersecting dark horizontal and vertical lines with one dark spot in the middle. To discover a visual field defect, the person simply covers or closes one eye and looks at the spot with the other. A visual field defect is perceived as a defect, distortion, blank, or

Start of second bandage

**Amputation-stump bandaging for
above-the-knee stump**
*(Lewis, Heitkemper, and Dirksen, 2000)*

other fault in the grid. The person may record the defects directly on a paper copy of the grid that may be kept as a permanent record.

**AMT,** abbreviation for *American Medical Technologists.*

**amu,** abbreviation for **atomic mass unit.**

**amusia** /ə·myo͞o′zē·ə/ [Gk, *amousia*, want of harmony], inability to recognize the significance of sounds manifest as loss of the ability to recognize or produce music.

**amyelia** /am′ī·ēl′yə/ [Gk, *myelos*, marrow], the absence of a spinal cord.

**amyelinic neuroma** /amī′əlin′ik/ [Gk, *a, myelos*, without marrow, *neuron*, nerve, *oma*], a tumor that contains only nonmyelinated nerve fibers.

**amygdala** /amig′dələ/ [Gk, *amygdale*, almond], an almond-shaped mass of gray matter in the front portion of the temporal lobe of the brain that may play a major role in memory processing and "learned fear."

**amygdalin** /əmig′dəlin/ [Gk, *amygdale*, almond], a naturally occurring cyanogenic glycoside obtained from bitter almonds and apricot pits. It has been promoted as a potential cancer remedy under the trademark of Laetrile. Also called **vitamin B₁₇.**

**amygdaloid** /-dəloid/, resembling a tonsil.

**amygdaloid fossa** [Gk, *amylon, eidos*, starchlike; L, *fossa*, ditch], a space in the wall of the oropharynx, between the pillars of the fauces, that is occupied by the palatine tonsil. Also called **tonsillar fossa.**

**amygdaloid nucleus** [Gk, *amygdale*, almond, *eidos*, form; L, *nucleus*, nut], one of the basal nuclei, found in the inferior horn of the lateral ventricle.

**amyl-.** See **amylo-.**

**amyl alcohol** /am′il/ [Gk, *amylon*, starch], a colorless, oily liquid that is only slightly soluble in water but can be mixed with ethyl alcohol, chloroform, or ether.

**amyl alcohol, tertiary.** See **amylene hydrate.**

**amylase** /am′ilās/ [Gk, *amylon*, starch], an enzyme that catalyzes the hydrolysis of starch into smaller carbohydrate molecules. Alpha-amylase, found in saliva, pancreatic juice, malt, certain bacteria, and molds, catalyzes the hydrolysis of starches to dextrins, maltose, and maltotriose. Beta-amylase, found in grains, vegetables, malt, and bacteria, is involved in the hydrolysis of starch to maltose. Normal blood findings are 56 to 190 IU/L. See also **enzyme.**

**amylase test,** an easily and rapidly performed blood or urine test that is most specific for pancreatitis and other pancreatic disorders. Elevated amylase levels may also indicate nonpancreatic disorders such as bowel perforation, penetrating peptic ulcer, duodenal obstruction, and others.

**amylene hydrate** /am′əlēn/, a clear, colorless liquid with a camphorlike odor, miscible with alcohol, chloroform, ether, or glycerin and used as a solvent and a hypnotic.

**amylic fermentation** /əmil′ik/, the formation of amyl alcohol from sugar.

**amyl nitrite,** a vasodilator.

■ INDICATION: It is prescribed to relieve the vasospasm of angina pectoris and cyanide poisoning.

■ CONTRAINDICATION: Known hypersensitivity to this drug or to other nitrites prohibits its use.

■ ADVERSE EFFECTS: Among the serious adverse reactions are hypotension, allergic reactions, nausea, headache, and dizziness.

**amylo-, amyl-,** combining form meaning 'starch': *amylodextrin, amylase.*

**amylobarbitone.** See **amobarbital.**

**amyloid** /am′iloid/ [Gk, *amylon*, starch, *eidos*, form], **1.** pertaining to or resembling starch. **2.** a starchlike protein-carbohydrate complex that is deposited abnormally in some tissues during certain chronic disease states, such as amyloidosis, rheumatoid arthritis, tuberculosis, and Alzheimer's disease.

**amyloid disease.** See **amyloidosis.**

**amyloid liver** [Gk, *amylon*, starch, *eidos*, form; AS, *lifer*], liver in which the cells have been infiltrated with amyloid deposits. Also called **albuminous liver.**

**amyloidosis** /am′iloidō′sis/ [Gk, *amylon* + *eidos*, form, *osis*, condition], a disease in which a waxy, starchlike glycoprotein (amyloid) accumulates in tissues and organs, impairing their function. There are two major forms of the condition. **Primary amyloidosis** usually occurs with multiple myeloma. Patients with **secondary amyloidosis** usually suffer from another chronic infectious or inflammatory disease, such as tuberculosis, osteomyelitis, rheumatoid arthritis, or Crohn's disease. The cause of both types of amyloidosis is unknown. Almost all organs are affected, most often the heart, lungs, tongue, and intestines in primary amyloidosis, and the kidneys, liver, and spleen in the secondary type. Elderly patients tend to experience cardiac effects of the disease. Diagnosis is made through biopsy of the suspected organ. There is no known cure for amyloidosis, and treatment in the secondary type is aimed at alleviating the underlying chronic disease. Patients with renal amyloidosis are frequently candidates for kidney dialysis and transplantation.

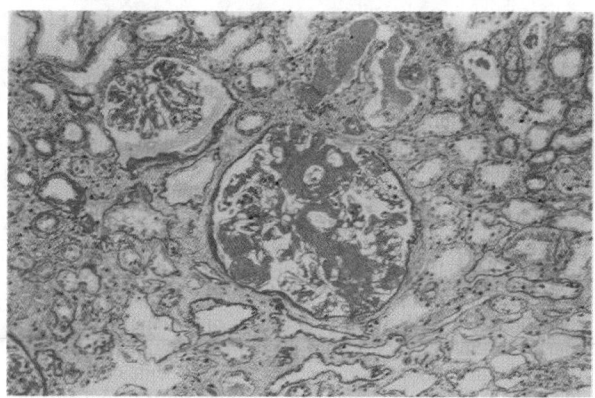

**Amyloidosis of the kidney**
*(Kumar, Cotran, and Robbins, 1997)*

**amylolysis** /am′ēlol′isis/, [Gk, *amylon,* starch, *lysis,* loosening], the digestive process whereby starch is converted into sugars and dextrins by hydrolysis or by enzymatic activity.

**amylopectinosis.** See **Andersen's disease.**

**amylose** /am′ə·lōs/ [Gk, *amylon,* starch + -*ose,* carbohydrate suffix], a lesser constituent of starch consisting of a chain of glucose residues; it stains blue with iodine.

**amyoplasia congenita.** See **arthrogryposis multiplex congenita.**

**amyotonia** /ā′mī·ōtō′nē·ə/ [Gk, *a, mys,* not muscle, *tonos,* tone], an abnormal condition of skeletal muscle, characterized by a lack of tone, weakness, and wasting, usually the result of motor neuron disease. See also **myotonia.** —**amyotonic,** *adj.*

**amyotrophic lateral sclerosis (ALS)** /ā′mī·ōtrof′ik/ [Gk, *a, mys* + *trophe,* nourishment], a degenerative disease of the motor neurons, characterized by weakness and atrophy of the muscles of the hands, forearms, and legs, spreading to involve most of the body and face. It results from degeneration of the motor neurons of the anterior horns and corticospinal tracts, beginning in middle age and progressing rapidly, causing death within 2 to 5 years. There is no known treatment. Also called **Lou Gehrig's disease, wasting palsy.** See also **Aran-Duchenne muscular atrophy.**

**Amytal Sodium,** trademark for a barbiturate (sodium amobarbital).

**an-, ana-,** prefix meaning 'not, without': *anoxia, analgesia.*

**-an, -ian,** suffix meaning 'belonging to, characteristic of, similar to': *protozoan, salpingian.*

**ANA,** 1. abbreviation for **American Nurses Association.** 2. abbreviation for **antinuclear antibody.**

**ana.** See **a̅a̅, A̅A̅**

**anabolic steroid** /an′əbol′ik/ [Gk, *anaballein,* to build up], any one of several compounds derived from testosterone or prepared synthetically to promote general body growth, to oppose the effects of endogenous estrogen, or to promote masculinizing effects. All such compounds cause a mixed androgenic-anabolic effect.

■ INDICATIONS: Anabolic steroids are prescribed in the treatment of aplastic anemia, red-cell aplasia, and hemolytic anemia and in anemias associated with renal failure, myeloid metaplasia, and leukemia.

■ CONTRAINDICATIONS: They are contraindicated in palliation of carcinoma of the breast; in pregnancy and serious cardiac, renal, and hepatic diseases; and with known hypersensitivity.

■ ADVERSE EFFECTS: Among the most serious adverse effects are acne, growth of facial hair, and hoarsening or deepening of the voice; other masculinizing features are common. Continued use of these compounds in women may also produce prominent musculature, excessive body hair, and hypertrophy of the clitoris.

**anabolism** /ənab′əliz′əm/ [Gk, *anaballein,* to build up], constructive metabolism characterized by the conversion of simple substances into the more complex compounds of living matter. Compare **catabolism.** —**anabolic** /an′əbol′ik/, *adj.*

**anabolite** /ənab′ōlīt/ [Gk, *anaballein,* to build up], a product of the process of anabolism.

**anacatadidymus** /an′əkat′ədid′iməs/ [Gk, *ana,* up, *kata,* down, *didymos,* twin], conjoined twins that are fused in the middle but separated above and below.

**anaclisis** /an′əklī′sis/ [Gk, *ana* + *klisis,* leaning], 1. a condition, normal in childhood but pathologic in adulthood, in which a person is emotionally dependent on other people. 2. a condition in which a person consciously or unconsciously chooses a love object because of a resemblance to the mother, father, or other person who was an important source of comfort and protection in infancy. —**anaclitic** /an′əklit′ik/, *adj.*

**anaclitic depression** /an′əklit′ik/, a syndrome occurring in infants, usually after sudden separation from the mothering person. Symptoms include apprehension, withdrawal, detachment, incessant crying, refusal to eat, sleep disturbances, and, eventually, stupor leading to severe impairment of the infant's physical, social, and intellectual development. If the mothering figure or a substitute is made available within 1 to 3 months, the infant recovers quickly with no long-term effects. See also **hospitalism.**

**anacrotic** /an′əkrot′ik/, pertaining to anacrotism, or a pulse with more than one expansion of the artery and observed as a double heartbeat.

**anacrotic pulse** [Gk, *ana* + *krotos,* stroke], a pulse characterized by a transient drop in amplitude of the primary elevation on a sphygmographic tracing. It is seen in valvular aortic stenosis.

**anacrotism** /ənak′rətiz′əm/ [Gk, *ana, krotos,* stroke], a condition characterized by two arterial expansions per heartbeat and observed as a notch on the ascending limb of an arterial pulse pressure tracing. —**anacrotic,** *adj.*

**anacusis** /an′əko͞o′sis/ [Gk, *a, akouein,* not to hear], a total loss of hearing.

**anadicrotic pulse** /an′ədīkrot′ik/ [Gk, *ana* + *dis,* twice, *krotos,* stroke], (on a sphygmographic tracing) a pulse characterized by two transient drops in amplitude on the curve of primary elevation.

**anadidymus** /an′ədid′iməs/ [Gk, *ana* + *didymos,* twin], conjoined twins that are united at the pelvis and lower extremities but are separated in the upper half. Also called **duplicatus anterior.**

**anadipsia** /an′ədip′sē·ə/ [Gk, *ana* + *dipsa,* thirst], extreme thirst, often occurring in the manic phase of bipolar mood disorder. The condition is the result of dehydration caused by the excessive perspiration, electrolyte imbalance, continuous urination, and relentless physical activity produced by the intense excitement characteristic of the manic phase. See also **polydipsia.**

**Anadrol-50,** trademark for an androgen (oxymetholone).

**anaemia.** See **anemia.**

**anaerobe** /aner′ōb/ [Gk, *a* + *aer,* not air, *bios,* life],   a microorganism that grows and lives in the complete or almost complete absence of oxygen. An example is *Clostridium botulinum.* Anaerobes are widely distributed in nature and in the body. Types include the **facultative anaerobe** and the **obligate anaerobe.** Compare **aerobe, microaerophile.** See also **anaerobic infection.**

**anaerobic** /an′ərō′bik/,   **1.** pertaining to the absence of air or oxygen. **2.** able to grow and function without air or oxygen.

**anaerobic catabolism,**   the breakdown of complex chemical substances into simpler compounds, with the release of energy, in the absence of oxygen.

**anaerobic exercise,**   any short-duration exercise that is powered primarily by metabolic pathways that do not use oxygen. Such pathways produce lactic acid, resulting in metabolic acidosis. Examples of anaerobic exercise include sprinting and weight lifting. Compare **aerobic exercise.** See also **active exercise, passive exercise.**

**anaerobic glycolysis.**   See **glycolysis.**

**anaerobic infection,**   an infection caused by an anaerobic organism, usually occurring in deep puncture wounds that exclude air or in tissue that has diminished oxygen-reduction potential as a result of trauma, necrosis, or overgrowth of bacteria. Kinds of anaerobic infection are **gangrene** and **tetanus.** See also *Clostridium.*

**anaerobic myositis.**   See **gas gangrene.**

**anaesthesia.**   See **anesthesia.**

**anaesthetic.**   See **anesthetic.**

**anaesthetist.**   See **anesthetist.**

**anagen.**   See **hair.**

**anagrelide,**   an antiplatelet agent.

■ INDICATIONS: This drug is prescribed for essential thrombocythemia.

■ CONTRAINDICATIONS: Known hypersensitivity to this drug and hypotension prohibit its use.

■ ADVERSE EFFECTS: Life-threatening effects include congestive heart failure, myocardial infarction, cardiomyopathy, cardiomegaly, complete heart block, atrial fibrillation, anemia, thrombocytopenia, ecchymosis, and lymphadenoma. Other serious effects include tachycardia, palpitations, arrhythmia, and seizures. Common side effects include postural hypotension and rash.

**Ana-Kit,**   trademark for an insect sting treatment emergency kit containing epinephrine in a sterile 1-ml syringe.

**anal** /ā′nəl/ [L, *anus*],   pertaining to the anus.

**anal agenesis.**   See **imperforate anus.**

**anal canal,**   the final portion of the alimentary tract, about 4 cm long, between the rectum and the anus.

**anal character,**   (in psychoanalysis) type of personality exhibiting patterns of behavior originating in the anal phase of childhood. It is characterized by extreme orderliness, obstinacy, perfectionism, cleanliness, punctuality, and miserliness, or their extreme opposites. Also called **anal personality.** See also **anal stage, psychosexual development.**

**anal column,**   the highly vascular longitudinal folds of the anal canal, in which are found the hemorrhoidal blood vessels.

**anal crypt,**   the depression between rectal columns that encloses networks of veins that, when inflamed and swollen, are called hemorrhoids.

**analeptic.**   See **central nervous system stimulant.**

**anal eroticism,**   (in psychoanalysis) libidinal fixation at or regression to the anal stage of psychosexual development, often reflected in such personality traits as miserliness, stubbornness, and overscrupulousness. Also called **anal erotism.** Compare **oral eroticism.** See also **anal character.**

**anal fissure,**   a painful linear ulceration or laceration of the skin at the margin of the anus. Also called **fissure-in-ano.**

**anal fistula,**   an abnormal opening on the cutaneous surface near the anus, usually resulting from a local crypt abscess and also common in Crohn's disease. A perianal fistula may or may not communicate with the rectum. Also called **fistula-in-ano.**

**analgesia** /an′əljē′zē·ə/ [Gk, *a, algos,* without pain],   a decreased or absent sensation of pain.

**analgesic** /an′əljē′zik/,   **1.** relieving pain. **2.** a drug that relieves pain. The opioid analgesics act on the central nervous system and alter the patient's perception; they are more often used for severe pain. The nonopioid analgesics act primarily at the periphery, do not produce tolerance or dependence, and do not alter the patient's perception; they are used for mild to moderate pain. See also **pain intervention.**

**analgesic administration,**   a nursing intervention from the Nursing Interventions Classification (NIC) defined as use of pharmacologic agents to reduce or eliminate pain. See also **Nursing Interventions Classification.**

**analgesic administration: intraspinal,**   a nursing intervention from the Nursing Interventions Classification (NIC) defined as administration of pharmacologic agents into the epidural or intrathecal space to reduce or eliminate pain. See also **Nursing Interventions Classification.**

**analgesic nephropathy** [Gk, *a, algos,* without pain, *nephros,* kidney, *pathos,* disease],   kidney damage resulting from the consumption of excessive amounts of nonsteroidal antiinflammatory drugs (NSAIDs) or similar analgesic medications.

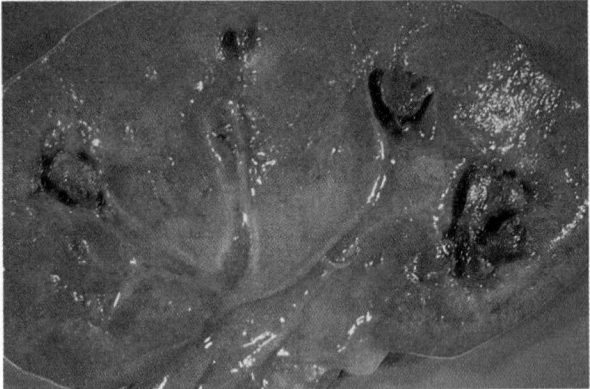

**Analgesic nephropathy** *(Cotran, Kumar, and Collins, 1999)*

**analgia** [Gk, *ana,* without, *algos,* pain],   an absence of pain.

**anal incontinence** [L, *anus, incontinentia,* an inability to retain],   the lack of voluntary control over fecal discharge.

**anal membrane.**   See **cloacal membrane.**

**anal membrane atresia.**   See **imperforate anus.**

**analog** /an′əlog/ [Gk, *analogos,* proportionate],   **1.** a substance, tissue, or organ that is similar in appearance or function to another but differs in origin or development, such as the eye of a fly and the eye of a human. **2.** a drug or other chemical compound that resembles another in structure or constituents but has different effects. Also spelled **analogue.** Compare **homolog.**

**analog computer,**   a computer that processes information as a physical quantity, such as voltage, amperage, weight, or length and presents results of calculations that can be continuously varied and measured. Compare **hybrid computer.**

**analogous** /ənal'əgəs/ [Gk, *analogos,* proportionate], similar in function but different in origin or structure, such as wings of birds and flies.

**analog signal,** a continuous electrical signal representing a specific condition, such as temperature, electrocardiogram waveforms, telephones, or computer modems.

**analog-to-digital converter,** a device for converting analog information, such as temperature or electrocardiographic waveforms, into digital form for processing by a digital computer. Also called **A/D converter.**

**analogue.** See **analog.**

**analogy** /ənal'əjē/ [Gk, *analogos*], similar to a degree in function or form but different in structure or origin.

**anal orifice** [L, *orificium,* an opening], **1.** the external opening at the end of the anal canal. **2.** the anus, surrounded by the anal sphincter muscle.

**anal personality.** See **anal character.**

**anal phase.** See **anal stage.**

**anal reflex,** a superficial neurologic reflex obtained by stroking the skin or mucosa of the region around the anus, which normally results in a contraction of the external anal sphincter. This reflex may be lost in disease of the pyramidal tract above the upper lumbar spine level (S3-S4). See also **superficial reflex.**

**anal sadism,** (in psychoanalysis) a sadistic form of anal eroticism, manifested by such behavior as aggressiveness and selfishness. Compare **oral sadism.**

**anal stage,** (in psychoanalysis) the pregenital period in psychosexual development, occurring between 1 and 3 years of age, when preoccupation with the function of the bowel and the sensations associated with the anus are the predominant source of pleasurable stimulation. It is regarded as an important determinant of ultimate personality type. Adult patterns of behavior associated with fixation on this stage include extreme neatness, orderliness, cleanliness, perfectionism, and punctuality or their extreme opposites. Also called **anal phase.** See also **anal character, psychosexual development.**

**anal stenosis.** See **imperforate anus.**

**anal verge** [L, *anus + vergere,* to bend], the area between the anal canal and the perianal skin.

**analysand** /ənal'isand'/, a person undergoing psychoanalysis.

**analysis** /ənal'əsis/ [Gk, *ana + lyein,* to loosen], **1.** the separation of substances into their constituent parts and the determination of the nature, properties, and composition of compounds. In chemistry, **qualitative analysis** is the determination of the elements present in a substance; **quantitative analysis** is the determination of how much of each element is present in a substance. **2.** an informal term for **psychoanalysis.** —**analytic,** *adj.,* **analyze,** *v.*

**analysis of variance (ANOVA),** a series of statistical procedures for comparing differences among two or more groups to determine if differences are due to chance. It is accomplished by examining the differences within the groups as well.

**analyst** /an'əlist/, **1.** a psychoanalyst. **2.** a person who analyzes the chemical, physical, or other properties of a substance or product.

**analyte** /an'əlīt/, any substance that is measured. The term is usually applied to a component of blood or other body fluid.

**analytic.** See **analysis.**

**analytical chemistry,** a branch of chemistry that deals with identification (qualitative) and measurement (quantitative) of the components of chemical compounds or mixtures of compounds.

**analytic psychology** /an'əlit'ik/, **1.** the system in which phenomena such as sensations and feelings are analyzed and classified by introspection rather than by experimental methods. Compare **experimental psychology. 2.** also called **Jungian psychology,** a system of analyzing the psyche according to the concepts developed by Carl Gustav Jung. It differs from the psychoanalysis of Sigmund Freud in stressing a "collective unconscious" and a mystic, religious factor in the development of the personal unconscious while minimizing the role of sexual influence on early emotional and psychologic development.

**analyze.** See **analysis.**

**analyzing** /an'əlī'zing/, (in five-step nursing process) a category of nursing behavior in which the health care needs of the client are identified and the goals of care are defined. The nurse interprets data; identifies problems (nursing diagnoses) involving the patient, the patient's family, and significant others; defines goals and establishes priorities; integrates the information; and projects the expected outcomes of nursing activities. Although analyzing follows assessing and precedes planning in the five steps of the nursing process, in practice, analyzing is integral to effective nursing practice at all steps of the process. See also **assessing, evaluating, implementing, nursing process, planning.**

**anamnesis** /an'amnē'sis/ [Gk, *anamimneskein,* to recall], **1.** remembrance of the past. **2.** the accumulated data concerning a medical or psychiatric patient and the patient's background, including family, previous environment, experiences, and, particularly, recollections, for use in analyzing his or her condition. Compare **catamnesis.**

**anamnestic** /an'amnes'tik/, **1.** pertaining to amnesia or memory. **2.** pertaining to the immunologic memory and the immune response to an antigen to which immunocompetent cells have been exposed.

**ANA-PAC,** abbreviation for **American Nurses Association-Political Action Committee.**

**anaphase** /an'əfāz/ [Gk, *ana + phainein,* to appear], the third of four stages of nuclear division in mitosis and in each of the two divisions of meiosis. In anaphase of mitosis and of the second meiotic division, the centromeres divide, and the two chromatids, which are arranged along the equatorial plane of the spindle, separate and move to the opposite poles of the cell, forming daughter chromosomes. In anaphase of the first meiotic division, the pairs of homologous chromosomes separate from each other and move intact to the opposite poles of the cell. See also **cytokinesis, interphase, meiosis, metaphase, mitosis, prophase, telophase.**

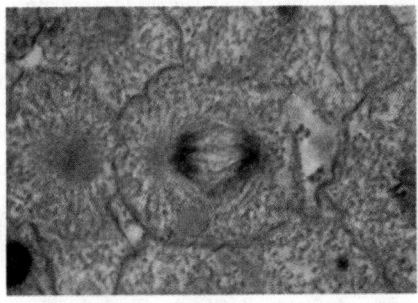

**Anaphase** *(© Ed Reschke; used with permission)*

**anaphia** /ənā′fē·ə/,   an inability to perceive tactile stimuli.

**anaphoresis,**   (in electrophoresis) the movement of anions in a solution or suspension toward the anode.

**anaphylactic** /an′əfilak′tik/ [Gk, *ana,* up, *phylaxis,* protection],   pertaining to anaphylaxis.

**anaphylactic hypersensitivity,**   an immediate, systemic hypersensitivity response to an exogenous antigen mediated by immunoglobulin E or G. It can be triggered by many substances, including drugs, especially penicillin and other antibiotics; foreign proteins used as therapeutic agents, such as insulin, vaccines, allergen extracts, and muscle relaxants; insect venom, especially from bees, wasps, hornets, and fire ants; and certain foods such as shellfish, berries, chocolate, eggs, and nuts. Also called **type I hypersensitivity.** Compare **cell-mediated immune response, cytotoxic anaphylaxis, immune complex hypersensitivity.** See also **anaphylactic shock, immunoglobulin.**

**anaphylactic reactions** [Gk, *ana, phylaxis,* protection; L, *re, agere,* to act],   acute allergic responses involving IgE-mediated antigen-stimulated mast cell activation resulting in histamine release. Exposure to the antigen may result in dyspnea, airway obstruction, shock, urticaria, and, in some cases, death. Anaphylactic reactions may be caused by Hymenoptera (bee) stings, foods, allergen extract; medications, or exercise. Rapid administration of subcutaneous epinephrine is the treatment of choice for severe reactions.

**anaphylactic shock,**   a severe and sometimes fatal systemic allergic reaction to a sensitizing substance, such as a drug, vaccine, specific food, serum, allergen extract, insect venom, or chemical. This condition may occur within seconds to minutes from the time of exposure to the sensitizing factor (allergen) and is commonly marked by respiratory distress and vascular collapse. The quicker the systemic atopic reaction occurs in the individual after exposure, the more severe the associated shock is likely to be.

■ OBSERVATIONS: The first symptoms are intense anxiety, weakness, and a feeling of impending doom. Sweating and shortness of breath may occur. These are often followed, often quickly, by pruritus and urticaria. Other symptoms include hypotension, shock, arrhythmia, respiratory congestion, laryngeal edema, nausea, and diarrhea.

■ INTERVENTIONS: Treatment requires the immediate injection of intramuscular or subcutaneous epinephrine with vigorous massage of the injection site to ensure faster distribution of the drug. The airway is maintained, and the patient is carefully monitored for signs of laryngeal edema, which may require the insertion of an endotracheal tube or a cricothyrotomy and oxygen therapy. The signs of laryngeal edema include stridor, hoarseness, and dyspnea. Cardiopulmonary resuscitation may be required for cardiac arrest.

■ NURSING CONSIDERATIONS: Nursing care of patients experiencing anaphylactic shock requires appropriate emergency treatment and the close monitoring of the patient for respiratory distress, hypotension and decreased circulatory volume. Patients with a history of severe allergic reactions are instructed to avoid offending allergens; some patients must carry emergency anaphylaxis kits. Such kits contain injectable epinephrine, such as an Epi-Pen Auto-Injector.

**anaphylactoid purpura.** See **Henoch-Schönlein purpura.**

**anaphylatoxin** /an′əfī′lətok′sin/,   a polypeptide derived from complement. Along with other mechanisms, it mediates changes in mast cells leading to the release of histamine and other immunoreactive or inflammatory reactive substances.

**anaphylaxis** /an′əfilak′sis/ [Gk, *ana + phylaxis,* protection],   an exaggerated, life-threatening hypersensitivity reaction to a previously encountered antigen. It is mediated by antibodies of the E or G class of immunoglobulins and results in the release of chemical mediators from mast cells. The reaction may consist of a localized wheal and flare of generalized itching, hyperemia, angioedema, and in severe cases vascular collapse, bronchospasm, and shock. The severity of symptoms depends on the original sensitizing dose of the antigen, the number and distribution of antibodies, and the route of entry and dose of subsequently encountered antigen. Penicillin injection is the most common cause of anaphylactic shock. Insect stings, radiopaque contrast media containing iodide, aspirin, antitoxins prepared with animal serum, and allergens used in testing and desensitizing patients who are hypersensitive also produce anaphylaxis in some individuals. Kinds of anaphylaxis are **aggregate anaphylaxis, antiserum anaphylaxis, cutaneous anaphylaxis, cytotoxic anaphylaxis, indirect anaphylaxis,** and **inverse anaphylaxis.** —**anaphylactic,** *adj.*

**anaphylaxis management,**   a nursing intervention from the Nursing Interventions Classification (NIC) defined as promotion of adequate ventilation and tissue perfusion for a patient with a severe allergic (antigen-antibody) reaction. See also **Nursing Interventions Classification.**

**anaplasia** /an′əplā′zhə/ [Gk, *ana + plassein,* to shape],   a change in the structure and orientation of cells, characterized by a loss of differentiation and reversion to a more primitive form. Anaplasia is characteristic of malignancy. Compare **aplasia.** —**anaplastic** /an′əplas′tik/, *adj.*

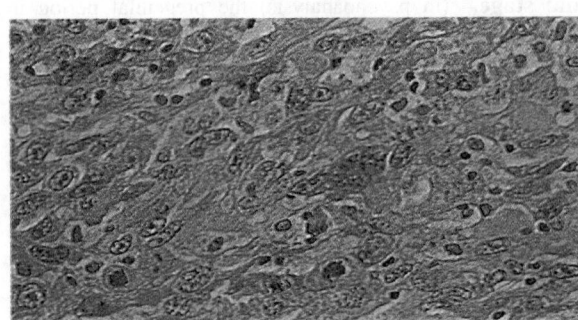

**Anaplasia** *(Besser and Thorner, 1994)*

**anaplastic** [Gk, *ana,* backward, *plassein,* to mold],   pertaining to anaplasia.

**anaplastic astrocytoma.** See **glioblastoma multiforme.**

**anapnea** /anap′nē·ə/ [Gk, *ana, pnoia,* breath],   respiration or restoration of breathing after a period of halted respiration.

**anapophysis** /an′ə·pof′i·sis/ [Gk, *an-,* not, without + *apophysis,* a growing away],   an accessory vertebral process, especially one on a thoracic or lumbar vertebra.

**Anaprox,**   trademark for a nonsteroidal antiinflammatory drug (naproxen sodium).

**anarthria** /anär′thrē·ə/ [Gk, *a, arthron,* not joint],   a loss of control of the muscles of speech, resulting in the inability to articulate words. The condition is usually caused by damage to a central or peripheral motor nerve.

**anasarca** /an′əsär′kə/ [Gk, *ana + sarx,* flesh],   severe generalized, massive edema. Anasarca often occurs in severe cardiovascular renal disease. See also **edema.** —**anasarcous,** *adj.*

**anastomose** /ənas′təmōs/ [Gk, *anastomoien,* to provide a mouth], to open a channel or passage between two vessels or cavities that are normally separate.

**anastomosis** /ənas′tōmō′sis/ *pl.* **anastomoses** [Gk, *anastomoien,* to provide a mouth], **1.** a connection between two vessels. **2.** a surgical joining of two ducts, blood vessels, or bowel segments to allow flow from one to the other. A vascular anastomosis may be performed to bypass an aneurysm or a vascular or arterial occlusion. With the patient under anesthesia, a section of the saphenous vein or a synthetic prosthesis is grafted to the prepared vessels. Postoperative nursing care includes preventing tissue injury and wound infection. An adequate airway is maintained, oxygen is given if necessary, and vital signs are closely monitored. Lack of blood flow may allow the graft to close. Pulses distal to the anastomosis are evaluated and their locations marked. Capillary filling time and the color and temperature of the skin are checked. Prophylactic antibiotic therapy may be started within hours. Urinary output is monitored. The patient is turned and frequently encouraged to breathe deeply to cough. Kinds of anastomoses are **end-to-end anastomosis, side-to-side anastomosis.** See also **aneurysm, bypass.**

**anastomosis at elbow joint,** a convergence of blood vessels at the elbow joint, consisting of various veins and portions of the brachial and deep brachial arteries and their branches.

**anastomotic** /ənas′təmot′ik/, pertaining to or resembling an anastomosis.

**anastrozole,** a nonsteroidal aromatase inhibitor.

■ INDICATIONS: It is prescribed in the treatment of advanced breast cancer for postmenopausal women whose disease has not responded to treatment with tamoxifen.

■ CONTRAINDICATIONS: The drug is usually effective only in patients with estrogen-dependent tumors.

■ ADVERSE EFFECTS: The side effects most often reported include diarrhea, fatigue, nausea, headache, hot flashes, and back pain.

**anatomic** [Gk, *ana* + *temnein,* to cut], pertaining to the structure of the body.

**anatomic age,** the estimated age of an individual based on the stage of development or deterioration of the body as compared to that of other persons of the same chronologic age.

**anatomic crown,** the portion of the dentin of a tooth that is covered by enamel. See also **artificial crown, clinical crown, partial crown.**

**anatomic curve,** the curvature of the different segments of the vertebral column. In the lateral contour of the back, the cervical and lumbar curves appear concave, the thoracic and sacral curves appear convex.

**anatomic dead space.** See **dead space.**

**anatomic height of contour,** an imaginary line that encircles a tooth at the level of greatest circumference. Also called **surveyed height of contour.** See also **height of contour.**

**anatomic impotence.** See **impotence.**

**anatomic neck of the humerus** [Gk, *ana,* up, *temnein,* to cut; AS, *hnecca;* L, *humerus,* shoulder], the portion of the humerus where there is a slight constriction adjoining the head.

**anatomic pathology** [Gk, *ana,* up, *temnein,* to cut, *pathos,* disease, *logos,* science], the study of the effects of disease on the structure of the body.

**anatomic position,** a standard position of the body: standing erect, facing directly forward, feet pointed forward and slightly apart, and arms hanging down at the sides with

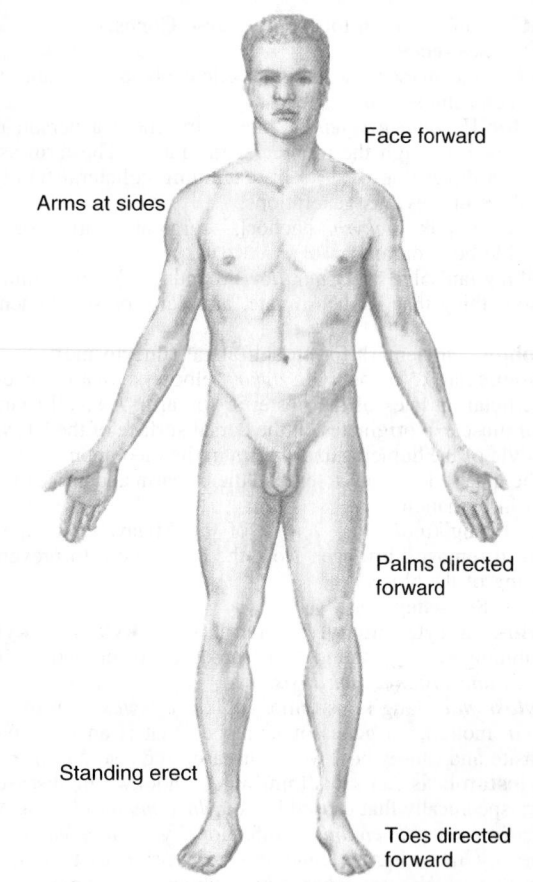

Face forward

Arms at sides

Palms directed forward

Standing erect

Toes directed forward

**Anatomic position** *(Applegate, 2000)*

palms facing forward. This position is used as a reference to describe sites or motions of various parts of the body.

**anatomic snuffbox,** a small, cuplike depression on the back of the hand near the wrist formed by the tendons reaching toward the thumb and index finger as the thumb is abducted, the wrist flexed, and the digits extended.

**anatomic topography** [Gk, *ana* + *temnein,* to cut, *topos,* place, *graphein,* to write], a system of identification of a body part in terms of the region in which it is located and its nearby structures.

**anatomic zero joint position,** the beginning point of a joint range of motion.

**anatomy** /ənat′əmē/ [Gk, *ana* + *temnein,* to cut], **1.** the study, classification, and description of structures and organs of the body. **2.** the structure of an organism. See also **applied anatomy, comparative anatomy, gross anatomy, microscopic anatomy, surface anatomy.** Compare **physiology.**

**anatripsis** /an′ətrip′sis/, a therapy that involves rubbing or friction with or without a simultaneous application of a medicine.

**Anavar,** trademark for an androgen (oxandrolone).

**ANC,** abbreviation for *absolute neutrophil count,* calculated by adding the number of segmented neutrophils and the number of basal neutrophis and multiplying the sum by the total white blood cell count. The formula is ANC = Total WBC count $\times$ (% neutrophils + % bands)/100.

**A.N.C.,** abbreviation for **Army Nurse Corps.**

**-ance.** See **-ency.**

**Ancef,** trademark for a semisynthetic cephalosporin antibiotic (cefazolin sodium).

**ancestor** [L, *antecessorem*], one from whom a person is descended, through the mother or the father. The term assumes a direct line of descent, excluding collateral family members of previous generations.

**anchorage** [Gk, *agkyra*, anchor], surgical fixation of a movable body organ.

**ancillary** /an'səler'ē/ [L, *ancillaris*, handmaid], pertaining to something that is subordinate, auxiliary, or supplementary.

**Ancobon,** trademark for an antifungal (flucytosine).

**anconeus** /angkō'nē·əs/ [Gk, *agkon*, elbow], one of seven superficial muscles of the posterior forearm. A small triangular muscle, it originates on the dorsal surface of the lateral condyle of the humerus and inserts in the olecranon process of the ulna. It functions to extend the forearm and abduct the ulna in pronation.

**ancrod** /ang'krod/, the venom of the Malayan pit viper, used to remove fibrinogen from the circulation, to prevent clotting of the blood.

**-ancy.** See **-ency.**

**ancylo-, ancyl, anchyl-, anchylo-, ankylo-, ankyl,** combining form meaning 'bent or crooked, curved, stiff, fixed': *ancylostoma, ankylosis.*

**Ancylostoma** /ang'kilos'təmə/ [Gk, *agkylos*, crooked, *stoma*, mouth], a genus of nematode that is an intestinal parasite and causes hookworm disease. See also *Necator.*

**ancylostomiasis** /an'səlos'təmī'əsis/, hookworm disease, more specifically that caused by *Ancylostoma duodenale, A. braziliense,* or *A. caninum.* Infection by *A. duodenale* is generally more harmful and less responsive to treatment than that by *Necator americanus,* which is the hookworm most often found in the southern United States. Clinical manifestations and treatment are similar for all types of hookworms. Infection may be prevented by eliminating fecal pollution of soil and by wearing shoes. See also **hookworm.**

**Andersen's disease** [Dorothy H. Andersen, American pathologist, 1901–1963], a rare glycogen storage disease characterized by a genetic deficiency of branching enzyme (alpha-1:4, alpha 1:6 transglucosidase), causing the deposition in tissues of abnormal glycogen with long inner and outer chains. Infants with the disease are normal at birth but fail to thrive and soon show hepatomegaly, splenomegaly, and hypotonia of muscle associated with the progressive development of liver cirrhosis or heart failure of unknown mechanisms. Diagnosis is by enzyme assays of white blood cells and fibroblasts. There is no specific therapy for the disease, which is usually fatal in the first few years of life. Also called **amylopectinosis, brancher glycogen storage disease, glycogen storage disease type IV.**

**-andr-,** combining form designating an androgen (steroid hormone).

**andreioma, androblastoma.** See **arrhenoblastoma.**

**andro-, andr-,** prefix meaning 'man or male': *androcyte, androgen.*

**androgamone** /an'drōgam'ōn/ [Gk, *andros*, man, *gamos*, marriage], a chemical secreted by male gametes that is believed to attract female gametes.

**androgen** /an'drəjin/ [Gk, *andros* + *genein*, to produce], any steroid hormone that increases male characteristics. Natural hormones, such as testosterone and its esters and analogs, are primarily used as substitutional therapy during the male climacteric. **—androgenic** /an'drōjen'ik/, *adj.*

**androgenic** [Gk, *andros*, man, *genein*, to produce], pertaining to the production or development of masculine characteristics.

**androgynous** /androj'inəs/, **1.** (of a man or woman) having some characteristics of both sexes. Social role, behavior, personality, and appearance are reflections of individuality and are not determined by gender. **2.** hermaphroditic. Compare **gynandrous. —androgyny** /-droj'ənē/, *n.*

**android** [Gk, *andros* + *eidos,* form], pertaining to something that is typically masculine, or manlike, such as an android pelvis.

**android pelvis,** a type of pelvis with a structure characteristic of the male. It is not uncommon in women. The bones are thick and heavy, and the inlet is heart-shaped. The sacrum inclines anteriorly, the side walls are convergent, and the pubic arch is small. The diameters of the midplane and the outlet are smaller than in the normal gynecoid pelvis. Vaginal delivery is likely to be difficult unless the overall pelvis is large and the fetus small. See also **pelvis.**

**andrology** /androl'əjē/ [Gk, *andros*, man, *logos*, science], the study of the health of males.

**androma.** See **arrhenoblastoma.**

**andropause** /an'drəpôs/, a change of life for males that may be expressed in terms of a career change, divorce, or reordering of life. It is associated with a decline in androgen levels that occurs in men during their late forties or early fifties. See also **menopause.**

**androstenedione test,** a blood test used to help diagnose the presence of virilizing hormones, especially in females, and polycystic ovary syndrome (Stein-Leventhal syndrome).

**androsterone** /andros'tərōn/ [Gk, *andros* + *stereos,* solid], originally believed to be the principal male sex hormone, it is used less frequently in therapy since the discovery of testosterone. The greater potency of several other male sex hormones has relegated androsterone largely to historic biochemical interest. See also **anabolic steroid, testosterone.**

**-ane,** suffix designating a saturated hydrocarbon of the methane series: *butane, propane.*

**anecdotal** /an'əkdot'əl/ [Gk, *anekdotos,* unpublished], pertaining to knowledge based on isolated observations and not yet verified by controlled scientific studies.

**anecdotal records,** medical findings usually based on one or a few observed episodes of patient care, as distinguished from results compiled in a large-scale scientific or systematic study.

**anechoic** /an'ekō'ik/, (in ultrasonography) free of echoes.

**Anectine,** trademark for a depolarizing neuromuscular blocker (succinylcholine chloride), used as an adjunct to anesthesia.

**anemia** /ənē'mē·ə/ [Gk, *a* + *haima,* without blood], a decrease in hemoglobin in the blood to levels below the normal range of 12-16 g/dL for women and 13.5-18 g/dL for men. Anemia may be caused by a decrease in red cell production, an increase in red cell destruction, or a loss of blood. A morphologic classification system describes anemia by the hemoglobin content of the red cells (normochromic or hypochromic) and by differences in red cell size (macrocytic, normocytic, or microcytic). Also spelled **anaemia.** See also **hemolytic anemia, hypoplastic anemia, iron deficiency anemia, iron metabolism.**

■ OBSERVATIONS: Depending on severity, anemia may be accompanied by clinical findings that stem from the diminished oxygen-carrying capacity of the blood. Signs and symptoms include fatigue, exertional dyspnea, dizziness, headache, insomnia, and pallor. Signs may also include confusion or disorientation. Anorexia, dyspepsia, palpitations, tachycardia, cardiac dilation, and systolic murmurs also may occur. Iron deficiency is the most common causative factor. Additional laboratory studies may be required to establish the less common forms of anemia.

■ INTERVENTIONS: The therapeutic response to anemia is variable and depends on the causative factors. Moderate to severe anemia, with hemoglobin levels that are below 7 to 8 g/dL, may require transfusion of one or more units of blood (packed red blood cells), especially if the condition is acute and specific clinical signs are present. Depending on the kind of anemia, treatment includes providing supplements of the deficient component, eliminating the cause of the blood loss, or alleviating the hemolytic component. The latter may involve administration of adrenal corticosteroids or splenectomy. Appropriate laboratory tests are repeated at intervals to monitor the response and need for continued therapy. Erythropoietin injections may be used to stimulate red cell production when anemia is secondary to chronic renal failure, the anemia of chronic disease, or in chemotherapy.

**-anemia, -anaemia, -nemia** suffix meaning (condition of) red blood cell deficiency: *achylanemia, melanemia, sulfanemia.*

**anemia of chronic disease,** a decrease in the number of circulating erythrocytes as a result of a chronic inflammatory state.

**anemia of pregnancy,** a condition of pregnancy characterized by a reduction in the concentration of hemoglobin in the blood. It may be physiologic or pathologic. In physiologic anemia of pregnancy, the reduction in concentration results from dilution because the plasma volume expands more than the red blood cell volume. The hematocrit in pregnancy normally drops several points below its pregnancy level. In pathologic anemia of pregnancy, the oxygen-carrying capacity of the blood is deficient because of disordered erythrocyte production or excessive loss of erythrocytes through destruction or bleeding. Pathologic anemia is a common complication of pregnancy occurring in approximately half of all pregnancies. Disordered production of erythrocytes may result from nutritional deficiency of iron, folic acid, or vitamin $B_{12}$, or from sickle cell or other chronic disease, malignancy, chronic malnutrition, or exposure to toxins. Destruction of erythrocytes may result from inflammation, chronic infection, sepsis, autoimmune disorders, microangiopathy, or a hematologic disease in which the red cells are abnormal. Excessive loss of erythrocytes through bleeding may result from abortion, bleeding hemorrhoids, intestinal parasites such as hookworm, placental abnormalities such as placenta previa and premature separation, or postpartum uterine atony.

**anemic** /ənē′mik/ [Gk, *a,* without, *haima,* blood], pertaining to anemia. See also **Cabot rings.**

**anemic anoxia,** a condition characterized by an oxygen deficiency in body tissues, resulting from a decrease in the number of erythrocytes or in the amount of hemoglobin in the blood.

**anemic infarct.** See **pale infarct.**

**anemo-,** prefix meaning 'wind': *anemophobia.*

**anencephalus** /an′ən·sef′ə·ləs/, an infant with anencephaly.

**anencephaly** /an′ensef′əlē/ [Gk, *a + encephalos,* without brain], congenital absence of major portions of the brain and malformation of the brainstem. The cranium does not close and the vertebral canal remains a groove. Transmitted genetically, anencephaly is not compatible with life. It can be detected early in gestation by amniocentesis and analysis or by ultrasonography. See also **neural tube defect.** —**anencephalous,** *adj.*

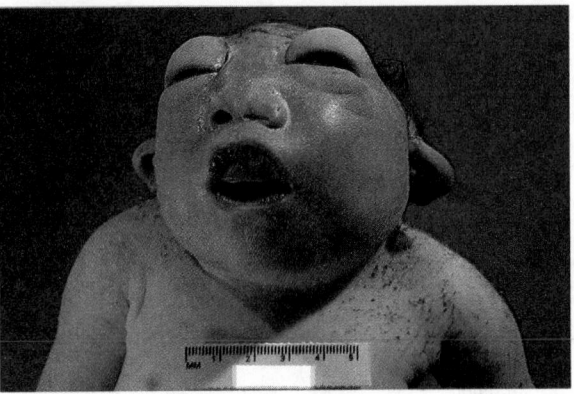

**Anencephaly** *(Kumar, Cotran, and Robbins, 1997)*

**anephric** /ā·nef′rik/ [Gk, *a, nephros* without kidney], without kidneys.

**anephrogenesis** /anef′rōjen′əsis/ [Gk, *a,* without, *nephros,* kidney, *genein,* to produce], the condition of being born without kidneys.

**anergia** /ənur′jə/, **1.** a condition of lethargy or lack of physical activity. **2.** a diminished or absent sensitivity to commonly used test antigens.

**anergic** /ənur′jik/, pertaining to a lack of energy or activity.

**anergic stupor,** a kind of dementia characterized by quietness, listlessness, and nonresistance.

**anergy** /an′ərjē/ [Gk, *a, ergon,* not work], **1.** lack of activity. **2.** an immunodeficient condition characterized by a lack of or diminished reaction to an antigen or group of antigens. This state may be seen in advanced tuberculosis and other serious infections, acquired immunodeficiency syndrome, and some malignancies. —**anergic,** *adj.*

**aneroid** /an′əroid/, not containing a liquid; used especially to describe a device in contrast to one that performs a similar function that does contain liquid, such as an aneroid sphygmomanometer, which does not contain a column of liquid mercury.

**aneroid barometer,** a device consisting of a flexible spring in a sealed, evacuated metal box that is used to measure atmospheric pressure. It is less accurate than a mercury barometer and is generally used for nonscientific work.

**Anestacon,** trademark for an endourethral local anesthetic solution (2% lidocaine hydrochloride).

**anesthesia** /an′esthē′zhə/ [Gk, *anaisthesia,* lack of feeling], the absence of all sensation, especially sensitivity to pain, as induced by an anesthetic substance or by hypnosis or as occurs with traumatic or pathophysiologic damage to nerve tissue. Anesthesia induced for medical or surgical purposes may be topical, local, regional, or general and is named for the anesthetic agent used, the method or procedure followed, or the area or organ anesthetized. Also spelled **anaesthesia.** See also **general anesthesia, local anesthesia, regional anesthesia, topical anesthesia,** and specific anesthetic agents.

**anesthesia administration,** a nursing intervention from the Nursing Interventions Classification (NIC) defined as preparation for and administration of anesthetic agents and monitoring of patient responsiveness during administration. See also **Nursing Interventions Classification.**

## Common postanesthesia problems

**Apnea, hypoventilation, and hypoxia**
Contributing factors
  Airway obstruction
  Respiratory depressant drugs
  Residual effects of muscle relaxants
  Pain
  Constrictive abdominal or thoracic dressings
Treatment
  Airway maintenance
  Oxygen administration
  Reversal of anesthetic agents by narcotic antagonists and
    anticholinesterases
  Respiratory stimulants
  Wake-up regimen
  Pain relief

**Hypotension**
Contributing factors
  Hypovolemia (blood loss; fluid deficit)
  Cutaneous vasodilation with rewarming
  Loss of sympathetic tone
  Myocardial dysfunction
  Drugs
  Technical problems
Treatment
  Determine cause
  Replace volume deficits
  Place patient in Trendelenburg position
  Administer vasopressors

**Hypertension**
Contributing factors
  Pain
  Delirium and agitation
  Hypoxia
  Hypercarbia
  Excess fluid administration
  Moderate hypothermia
  Gastric or bladder distension
  Preoperative hypertension
Treatment
  Determine cause
  Drug therapy (analgesics; sedation)

From Beare PG, Myers JL: *Principles and practice of adult health nursing,* ed 3, St Louis, 1998, Mosby.

**anesthesia machine,** an apparatus for administering inhalation anesthetic gases and vapors that is capable of controlling ventilation. Although there are many different models, all have the following features: a delivery system for gas; a flowmeter to measure gas flow; vaporizers for volatilizing and combining the anesthetic agents with oxygen and carrier gases; a circuit for delivering the gas to the patient; monitoring equipment or gauges; and a ventilator and a scavenging system to contain and discharge excess gas.

**anesthesia patients, classification of,** the system by which the American Society of Anesthesiologists classifies patients in five categories by physical status. Class I includes patients who are healthy and who are without organic, physiologic, biochemical, or psychiatric problems. Class II includes patients who have mild to moderate systemic disease, whether involving or extraneous to the condition requiring anesthesia, such as anemia, mild diabetes, moderate hypertension, obesity, or chronic bronchitis. Class III includes patients who have severe systemic disturbances or disease, whether or not related to the procedure requiring surgical anesthesia. Class IV includes patients who have severe systemic disease that is a constant threat to life that may or may not be related to the intended surgical procedure. Class V includes the moribund patient who is not expected to survive more than 24 hours with or without surgical intervention, such as a person in shock with a ruptured abdominal aneurysm or a massive pulmonary embolus. The letter *E* is added to the roman numeral to indicate an emergency procedure, as when the condition of a patient scheduled for an elective herniorrhaphy requires emergency treatment when the hernia strangulates.

**anesthesia screen,** a metal, inverted U-shaped frame that attaches to the sides of an operating table, 12 to 18 inches above a patient's upper chest. It is covered with a sheet to prevent contamination of an operative site on the chest or abdomen by airborne infection from the patient or the anesthetist and to provide a wide sterile field for the surgeon.

**anesthesiologist** /an'əsthē'zē·ol'əjist/, a physician who completes an accredited of residency in anesthesia. Although anesthesiologists do administer anesthesia directly, they more often supervise nurse anesthetists in the delivery of anesthesia, act as consultants, head anesthesia departments or divisions, or direct intensive care units or pain management clinics. Compare **nurse anesthetist.**

**anesthesiologist assistant (AA),** an allied health professional who, under the supervision of a licensed anesthesiologist, assists in developing and implementing the anesthesia care plan. Duties may include collecting preoperative data, such as taking an accurate health history and performing an appropriate physical examination; performing various preoperative tasks, such as the insertion of IV and arterial lines, central venous pressure monitors, and special catheters; managing the airway and administering drugs for induction and maintenance of anesthesia; administering supportive therapy, such as IV fluids and vasodilators; providing recovery room care and performing other functions and tasks relating to care in an intensive care unit or pain clinic; providing anesthesia monitoring services; and performing administrative and educational functions and tasks.

**anesthesiologist's assistant (AA),** an allied health professional who assists the anesthesiologist in collecting preoperative data, such as taking the health history and performing an appropriate physical examination; in performing various preoperative tasks, such as the insertion of IV and arterial lines, central venous pressure monitors, and special catheters; in managing the airway and administering medications for induction and maintenance of anesthesia; in administering supportive therapy, such as IV fluids and vasodilators; in providing postanesthesia care unit (PACU) care under the care of a registered nurse with expertise in preanesthesia care and in performing other functions and tasks relating to care in an intensive care unit or pain clinic; in providing anesthesia monitoring services; and in performing administrative functions and tasks, such as staff education.

**anesthesiology** /-ol'əjē/, the branch of medicine that is concerned with the relief of pain and with the administration of medication to relax muscles and obliterate consciousness during surgery. It is a specialty requiring competency in general medicine, a broad understanding of surgical procedures, and a comprehensive knowledge of clinical obstetrics, chest medicine, neurology, pediatrics, pharmacology, biochemistry, cardiology, and cardiac and respiratory physiology. See also **anesthesiologist, nurse anesthetist.**

**anesthetic** /an'esthet'ik/, a drug or agent that is capable of producing a complete or partial loss of feeling (anesthesia). Also spelled **anaesthetic.**

**anesthetist** /ənes'thətist/, a person who administers anesthesia. Also spelled **anaesthetist.** See also **nurse anesthetist,** also called anesthesia technician.

**anesthetize** /ənes'thətīz/ [Gk, *anaisthesia,* lack of feeling], to induce a state of anesthesia.

**anetoderma** /an'ətōdur'mə/ [Gk, *anetos,* relaxed, *derma,* skin], an idiopathic clinical change produced by focal damage to elastin fibers that results in looseness of skin. There is no known effective treatment.

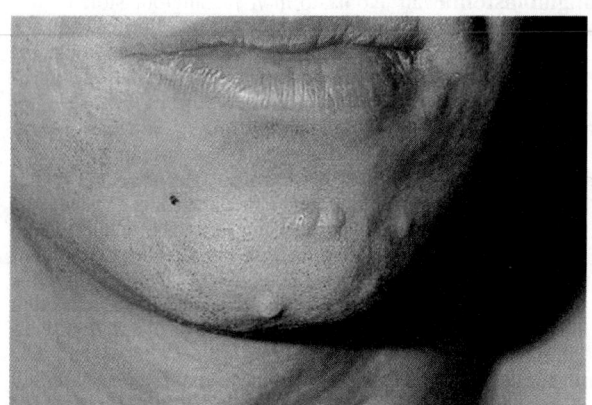

**Anetoderma** *(Lawrence and Cox, 1993)*

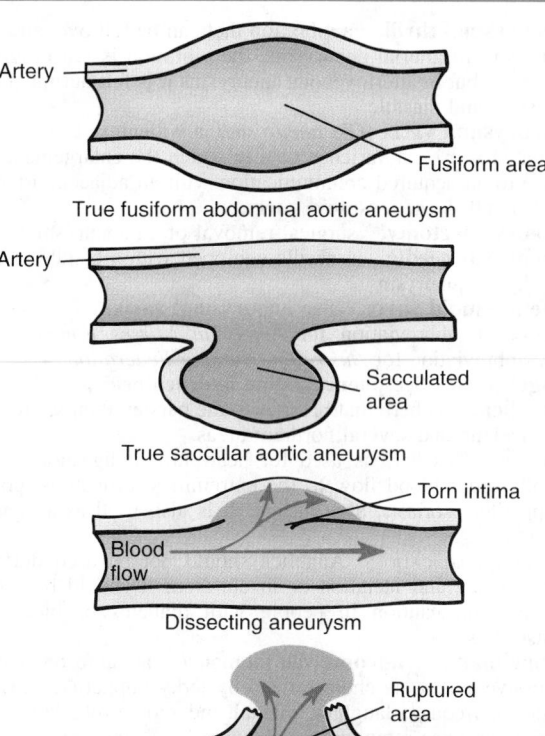

Artery — Fusiform area

True fusiform abdominal aortic aneurysm

Artery — Sacculated area

True saccular aortic aneurysm

Torn intima — Blood flow

Dissecting aneurysm

Ruptured area — Blood flow

Pseudoaneurysm

**Aneurysms** *(Lewis, Heitkemper, and Dirksen, 2000)*

**aneuploid** /an'yŏŏploid/ [Gk, *a, eu,* not good, *ploos,* fold, *eidos,* form], **1.** an individual, organism, strain, or cell that has a chromosome number that is not an exact multiple of the haploid number characteristic of the species. **2.** pertaining to such an individual, organism, strain, or cell. Also called **aneuploidic** /-ploi'dik/. Compare **euploid.** See also **monosomy, trisomy.**

**aneuploidy** /an'yŏŏploi'dē/, any variation in chromosome number that involves individual chromosomes rather than entire sets of chromosomes. There may be fewer chromosomes, as in Turner's syndrome (one X chromosome in females), or more chromosomes, as in Down syndrome (three copies of chromosome 21). Such individuals have various abnormal physiologic and morphologic traits. See also **chromosomal aberration.** Compare **euploidy.** See also **monosomy, trisomy.**

**aneurysm** /an'yŏŏriz'əm/ [Gk, *aneurysma,* widening], a localized dilation of the wall of a blood vessel. It may be caused by atherosclerosis and hypertension, or, less frequently, by trauma, infection, or a congenital weakness in the vessel wall. Aneurysms are common in the aorta but also occur in peripheral vessels, especially in the popliteal arteries of older people. A sign of large arterial aneurysm is a pulsating swelling that produces a blowing murmur on auscultation. Small aneurysms may produce no sound at all. An aneurysm may rupture, causing hemorrhage, or thrombi may form in the dilation and give rise to emboli that may obstruct smaller vessels. Also called **vascular tumor.** Kinds of aneurysms include **aortic, bacterial, berry, cerebral, compound, dissecting, fusiform, mycotic, racemose, Rasmussen's, saccular, varicose,** and **ventricular aneurysm.** —**aneurysmal** /an'yooriz'məl/, *adj.*

**aneurysmal bone cyst,** a cystic lesion that tends to develop in the metaphyseal region of long bones but may occur in any bone, including the vertebrae. It may produce pain and swelling and generally increases in size gradually. It is usually removed surgically, but radiation may be used in cases when the tumor is not readily accessible.

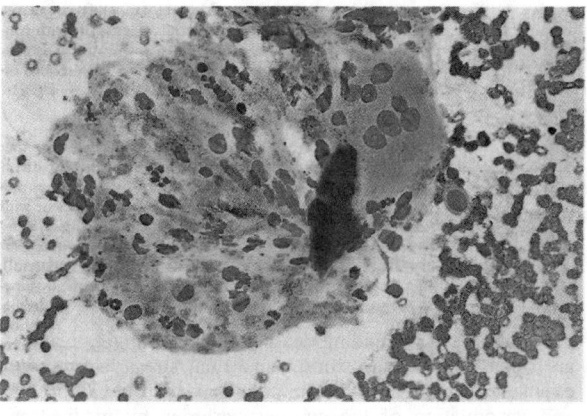

**Aneurysmal bone cyst** *(Silverberg, DeLellis, and Frable, 1997)*

**aneurysmal thrill,** a vibration that can be felt over an aneurysm. In arterial aneurysms, the vibration is felt only in systole, but in arteriovenous aneurysms it is felt during both systole and diastole.

**aneurysmal varix** [Gk, *aneurysma,* a widening; L, *varix,* a dilated vein], a varicose vein in which the enlargement is due to an acquired communication with an adjacent artery. Also called **aneurysmoid varix.**

**aneurysmectomy,** surgical removal of an aneurysm.

**aneurysm needle,** a needle equipped with a handle, used to ligate aneurysms.

**aneurysmoid varix.** See **aneurysmal varix.**

**ANF,** **1.** abbreviation for *American Nurses Foundation.* **2.** abbreviation for *Australian Nursing Federation.*

**angel dust.** See **phencyclidine hydrochloride.**

**angelica,** an herb that belongs to the parsley family, grown in Iceland and several northern areas.

■ USES: This herb is used for heartburn, indigestion, gas, colic, poor blood flow to the extremities, bronchitis, poor appetite, psoriasis, and vitiligo. It is also used as an antiseptic.

■ CONTRAINDICATIONS: Angelica should not be used during pregnancy and lactation or in children; it should be used only with caution in people with diabetes or bleeding disorders.

**Angelman's syndrome** /ān′jəl·mənz/, an autosomal recessive syndrome characterized by jerky puppetlike movements, frequent laughter, mental and motor retardation, a peculiar open-mouthed facial expression, and seizures. It can be caused by a deletion on chromosome 15 inherited from the mother; the same deletion inherited from the father causes **Prader-Willi syndrome.**

**anger** [L, *angere,* to hurt], an emotional reaction characterized by extreme displeasure, rage, indignation, or hostility. It is considered to be of pathologic origin when such a response does not realistically reflect a person's actual circumstances. However, expressions of anger vary widely in different individuals cultures and may be considered functional under certain controlled circumstances.

**anger control assistance,** a nursing intervention from the Nursing Interventions Classification (NIC) defined as facilitation of the expression of anger in an adaptive nonviolent manner. See also **Nursing Interventions Classification.**

**angi-.** See **angio-.**

**angiitis** /anjē·ī′tis/ [Gk, *angeion,* vessel, *itis*], inflammation of a vessel, chiefly a blood or lymph vessel. See also **vasculitis.**

**angina** /anjī′nə, an′jinə/ [L, *angor,* quinsy (strangling)], **1.** a spasmodic, cramplike choking feeling. **2. angina pectoris. 3.** characterized by a feeling of choking, suffocation, or crushing pressure and pain. Kinds of angina are **decubitus, intestinal, Ludwig's, stable, preinfarction, Prinzmetal's, streptococcal** and **unstable,** and **angina. —anginal,** *adj.*

**-angina,** suffix meaning 'severe ulceration, usually of the mouth or throat.'

**anginal** /anji′nal/, pertaining to angina.

**angina pectoris,** a paroxysmal thoracic pain caused most often by myocardial anoxia as a result of atherosclerosis or spasm of the coronary arteries. The pain usually radiates along the neck, jaw, and shoulder and down the inner aspect of the left arm. It is frequently accompanied by a feeling of suffocation and impending death. Attacks of angina pectoris are often related to exertion, emotional stress, eating, and exposure to intense cold. The pain may be relieved by rest and vasodilation of the coronary arteries by medication, such as nitroglycerin. Also called **cardiac pain.**

**angina sine dolore** /sē′nə dolôr′ə, sī′nē/, a painless episode of coronary insufficiency. See also **silent ischemia.**

**angina trachealis.** See **croup.**

**angio-, angei-, angi-,** combining form meaning 'a vessel, usually a blood vessel': *angioblastic, angiitis.*

**angioblast** /an′jēō·blast′/ [Gk, *angeion,* vessel + *blastos,* germ], **1.** the mesenchymal tissue of the embryo from which the blood cells and blood vessels differentiate. **2.** an individual vessel-forming cell.

**angioblastic meningioma** /an′jē·ōblas′tik/, a tumor of the blood vessels of the meninges covering the spinal cord or the brain.

**angioblastoma** /an′jē·ōblastō′mə/, *pl.* angioblastomas, angioblastomata [Gk, *angeion,* vessel, *blastos,* germ, *oma*], a tumor of blood vessels in the brain. Kinds of angioblastomas are **angioblastic meningioma** and **cerebellar angioblastoma.**

**angiocardiogram** /an′jē·ōkär′dē·ōgram′/, a series of radiographic images produced by angiocardiography.

**angiocardiography** /-kär′dē·og′rəfē/ [Gk, *angeion* + *kardia,* heart, *graphein,* to record], the process of producing a radiograph of the heart and its great vessels. A radiopaque contrast medium is injected directly into the heart by a catheter introduced through the antecubital or femoral veins. X-ray films are taken as the contrast medium passes through the heart and great vessels. Also called **cardiac angiography.** See also **angiography.**

**angiocardiopathy** /-kär′dē·op′əthē/ [Gk, *angeion,* vessel, *kardia,* heart, *pathos,* disease], a disease of the blood vessels of the heart.

**angiocarditis** /-kärdī′tis/, inflammation of the heart and large blood vessels.

**angiocatheter** /an′jē·ōkath′ətər/, a hollow, flexible tube inserted into a blood vessel to withdraw or instill fluids.

**angiochondroma** /an′jē·ōkondrō′mə/, *pl.* **angiochondromas, angiochondromata** [Gk, *angeion* + *chondros,* cartilage, *oma*], a cartilaginous tumor characterized by an excessive formation of blood vessels.

**angioedema** /an′jē·ō′ide′mə/, a dermal, subcutaneous, or submucosal swelling that is acute, painless, and of short duration. It may involve the face, neck, lips, larynx, hands, feet, genitalia, or viscera. Angioedema may be hereditary or the result of food or drug allergy, infection, emotional stress, or a reaction to blood products. Treatment depends on the

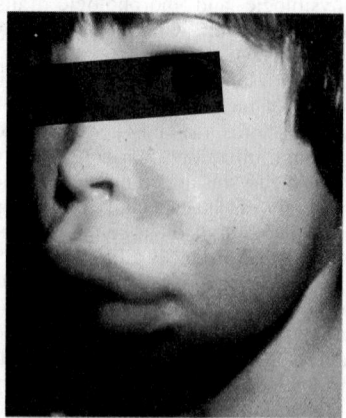

**Angioedema** *(Zitelli and Davis, 1997)*

cause. Severe angioedema may require subcutaneous injections of epinephrine, intubation, or tracheotomy to prevent respiratory obstruction. Prevention depends on the identification and avoidance of causative factors. Also called **angioneurotic edema.** See also **anaphylaxis, serum sickness, urticaria.**

**angioendothelioma.** See **hemangioendothelioma.**

**angiofibroma** /an'jē·ōfĭbrō'mə/, *pl.* **angiofibromas, angiofibromata** [Gk, *angeion* + L, *fibra,* fiber; Gk, *oma*], an angioma containing fibrous tissue. Also called **fibroangioma, telangiectatic fibroma.**

**angiogenesis** /an'jē·ōjen'əsis/ [Gk, *angeion* + *genesis,* origin], the ability to evoke blood vessel formation, a common property of malignant tissue. The presence of angiogenesis in breast tissue is regarded as a precursor of histologic evidence of breast cancer.

**angiogenin** /an'jē·ōjen'in/, a protein that mediates the formation of blood vessels. A single-chain basic protein cloned from molecules of the tumor angiogenesis factor (TAF) in human colon cancer cells. Angiogenin is used experimentally to stimulate the development of new blood vessels in wound healing, stroke, or coronary heart disease. See also **tumor angiogenesis factor.**

**angioglioma** /an'jē·ōglē·ō'mə/, *pl.* **angiogliomas, angiogliomata** [Gk, *angeion* + *glia,* glue, *oma*], a highly vascular tumor composed of neuroglia.

**angiogram** /an'jē·əgram/ [Gk, *angeion,* vessel, *gramma,* writing], a radiographic image of a blood vessel following injection of a radiopaque contrast medium. Also called **arteriogram.**

**angiograph** /an'jē·əgraf/ [Gk, *angeion,* vessel, *graphein,* to record], an instrument that records the patterns of pulse waves. See also **sphygmograph.**

**angiography** /an'jē·og'rəfē/ [Gk, *angeion* + *graphein,* to record], the x-ray visualization of the internal anatomy of the heart and blood vessels after the intravascular introduction of radiopaque contrast medium. The procedure is used as a diagnostic aid in myocardial infarction, vascular occlusion, calcified atherosclerotic plaques, cerebrovascular accident, portal hypertension, renal neoplasms, renal artery stenosis as a causative factor in hypertension, pulmonary emboli, and congenital and acquired lesions of pulmonary vessels. The contrast medium may be injected into an artery or vein or introduced into a catheter inserted in a peripheral artery and threaded through the vessel to a visceral site. Because the iodine in the contrast medium may cause a marked allergic reaction in some patients and may lead to death in severe cases, testing for hypersensitivity is indicated before the radiopaque substance is used. After the procedure the patient is monitored for signs of bleeding at the puncture site, and bed rest for a number of hours is indicated. —**angiographic,** *adj.*

**angiohemophilia.** See **von Willebrand's disease.**

**angioimmunoblastic lymphadenopathy with dysproteinemia (AILD),** a systemic disorder resembling lymphoma, characterized by fever, night sweats, weight loss, and generalized lymphadenopathy; there is a cellular infiltrate of lymphocytes, immunoblasts, and plasma cells, change or effacement of lymph node architecture, hepatosplenomegaly, maculopapular rash, polyclonal hypergammaglobulinemia, and Coombs-positive hemolytic anemia. It is considered to be a nonmalignant hyperimmune reaction to chronic antigenic stimulation; there is proliferation of B cells and profound deficiency of T cells. The disease follows a progressive but variable course; some patients have long survival without chemotherapy, whereas others have a rapid course with death from overwhelming infection.

**angiokeratoma** /an'jē·ōker'ətō'mə/, *pl.* **angiokeratomas, angiokeratomata** [Gk, *angeion* + *keras,* horn, *oma*], a vascular, horny neoplasm on the skin, characterized by clumps of dilated blood vessels, clusters of warts, and thickening of the epidermis, especially the scrotum and the dorsal aspect of the fingers and toes.

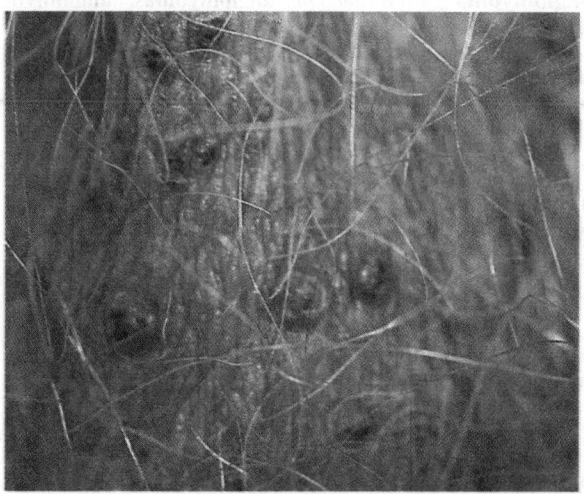

**Angiokeratoma** *(du Vivier, 1993)*

**angiokeratoma circumscriptum,** a rare skin disorder characterized by discrete papules and nodules in small patches on the legs or on the trunk.

**angiokeratoma corporis diffusum,** an uncommon familial disease in which phospholipids are stored in many parts of the body, especially in the venal and cardiovascular systems, causing vasomotor, urinary, and cutaneous disorders and, in some cases, muscular abnormalities. Characteristic signs of the disease are dilation of blood vessels in the "bathing suit areas," edema, hypertension, and cardiomegaly, especially enlargement of the left ventricle; diffuse nodularity of the skin; albumin, erythrocytes, leukocytes, and casts in the urine; and vacuoles in muscle bundles. Also called **Fabry's disease.**

**angiokeratomata.** See **angiokeratoma.**

**angiolipoma** /an'jē·ōlipō'mə/, *pl.* **angiolipomas, angiolipomata** [Gk, *angeion* + *lipos,* fat, *oma*], a benign neoplasm containing blood vessels and tissue. Also called **lipoma cavernosum, telangiectatic lipoma.**

**angioma** /an'jē·ō'mə/, *pl.* **angiomas, angiomata** [Gk, *angeion,* vessel, *oma* tumor], any benign tumor with blood vessels (hemangioma) or lymph vessels (lymphangioma). Most angiomas are congenital; some, such as cavernous hemangiomas, may disappear spontaneously.

**-angioma,** suffix meaning a 'tumor composed chiefly of blood and lymph vessels': *fibroangioma, glomangioma.*

**angioma arteriale racemosum** /ärtir'ē·ā'lē ras'əmō'səm/ [Gk, *angeion* + *oma* + L, *arteria,* airpipe, *racemus,* grape], a vascular neoplasm characterized by the intertwining of many small, newly formed dilated blood vessels. Normal blood vessels become affected.

**angioma cavernosum.** See **cavernous hemangioma.**

**angioma cutis,** a nevus composed of a network of dilated blood vessels.

**angioma lymphaticum.** See **lymphangioma.**

**angioma serpiginosum** /sərpij′inō′səm/ [Gk, *angeion* + *oma* + L, *serpere,* to creep], a cutaneous disease characterized by rings of tiny vascular points appearing as red dots.

**angiomatosis** /an′jē·ōmətō′sis/, a condition characterized by numerous vascular tumors.

**angiomyoma** /-mī·ō′mə/, *pl.* **angiomyomas, angiomyomata** [Gk, *angeion* + *mys,* muscle, *oma*], a tumor composed of vascular and muscular tissue elements.

**angiomyoneuroma.** See **glomangioma.**

**angiomyosarcoma** /-mī′ōsärkō′mə/, *pl.* **angiomyosarcomas, angiomyosarcomata** [Gk, *angeion* + *mys* muscle, *sarx,* flesh, *oma*], a tumor containing vascular, muscular, and connective tissue elements.

**angioneuroma.** See **glomangioma.**

**angioneurotic anuria** /-nŏŏrot′ik ənyŏŏr′ē·ə/ [Gk, *angeion* + *neuron,* nerve, *a* + *ouron,* not urine], an abnormal condition characterized by an almost complete absence of urination caused by destruction of tissue in the renal cortex.

**angioneurotic edema.** See **angioedema.**

**angioneurotic gangrene** [Gk, *angeion* + *neuron,* nerve, *gaggraina*], the death and putrefaction of tissue caused by an interruption of the blood supply resulting from thrombotic arteries or veins.

**angiopathy** /an′jē·op′əthē/ [Gk, *angeion,* vessel, *pathos,* disease], a disease of the blood vessels.

**angioplasty** /an′jēōplas′tē/ [Gk, *angeion,* vessel, *plassein,* to mold], the reconstruction of blood vessels damaged by disease or injury.

**angiopoiesis** /-poi·ē′sis/ [Gk, *angeion,* vessel, *poien,* to make], the process of blood vessel formation.

**angiorrhaphy** /an′jē·ôr′əfē/ [Gk, *angeion,* vessel, *rhaphe,* suture], the repair by suture of any blood vessel.

**angiosarcoma** /-särkō′mə/, a rare, malignant tumor consisting of endothelial and fibroblastic tissue that proliferates and eventually surrounds vascular channels. The condition usually occurs in older persons. Angiosarcoma has been associated with exposure to vinyl chloride and arsenic. Also

called **hemangiosarcoma, malignant hemangioendothelioma.** Compare **angioma.**

**angiosclerosis** /-sklerō′sis/ [Gk, *angeion,* vessel, *skleros,* hard, *osis,* condition], a thickening and hardening of the walls of the blood vessels. See also **atherosclerosis.**

**angioscope** /an′jē·əskōp′/, a type of microscope that permits inspection of the capillary vessels.

**angiospasm** /an′jē·ōspaz′əm/, a sudden, transient constriction of a blood vessel. Also called **vasomotor spasm, vasospasm.** See also **vasoconstriction.**

**angiostrongyliasis** /an′jē·ō·stron′ji·lī′ə·sis/, infection by a species of *Angiostrongylus,* usually *A. cantonensis* in humans; infection comes after eating contaminated raw hosts such as snails, slugs, prawns, or crabs. The larval worms migrate to the central nervous system and cause eosinophilic meningitis.

*Angiostrongylus* [Gk, *angeion,* vessel + *strongylos,* round], a genus of parasitic nematodes; species *A. cantonensis* and *A. costaricensis* normally infect other animals but can cause angiostrongyliasis in humans.

**angiotensin** /-ten′sin/ [Gk, *angeion* + L, *tendere,* to stretch], a polypeptide in the blood that causes vasoconstriction, increased blood pressure, and the release of aldosterone from the adrenal cortex. Angiotensin is formed by the action of renin on angiotensinogen, an alpha-2-glycoprotein that is produced in the liver and constantly circulates in the blood. Renin, stimulated by juxtaglomerular cells in the kidney in response to decreased blood volume and serum sodium, acts as an enzyme in the conversion of angiotensinogen to angiotensin I, which is rapidly hydrolyzed to form the active compound, angiotensin II. The vasoconstrictive action of angiotensin II decreases the glomerular filtration rate, and the concomitant action of aldosterone promotes sodium retention, with the result that blood volume and sodium reabsorption increase. Plasma angiotensin II increases during the luteal phase of the menstrual cycle and is probably responsible for an elevated level of aldosterone during that period. Angiotensin is inactivated by peptidases, called angiotensinases, in plasma and tissues.

**angiotensin-converting enzyme (ACE),** a glycoprotein (dipeptidyl carboxypeptidase) that catalyzes the conversion of angiotensin I to angiotensin II by splitting two terminal amino acids. ACE-inhibiting agents are used in hypertension control and for protection of the kidneys in type 1 diabetes mellitus.

**angiotensin-converting enzyme (ACE) inhibitor,** a protease inhibitor found in serum that promotes vasodilation by blocking the formation of angiotensin II and slowing the degradation of bradykinin and other kinins. It decreases sodium retention, water retention, blood pressure, and heart size and increase cardiac output.

**angiotensin-converting enzyme test (ACE),** a blood test used to detect and monitor the clinical course of sarcoidosis, to differentiate sarcoidosis from other granulomatous diseases, and to differentiate between active and dormant sarcoid disease.

**angiotensinogen** /-tensin′əjən/, a serum glycoprotein produced in the liver that is the precursor of angiotensin.

**angiotensin sensitivity test (AST),** a test for sensitivity to angiotensin II by infusion of angiotensin II amide into the right cubital vein. Angiotensin is metered in doses that increase by 1 ng/kg/min at 5-minute intervals. A positive AST result is an effective pressor dose, or one that causes a 20 mm Hg rise in diastolic blood pressure at an infusion rate of less than 10 ng/kg/min.

**angle** /ang′gəl/ [L, *angulus*], **1.** the space or the shape formed at the intersection of two lines, planes, or borders.

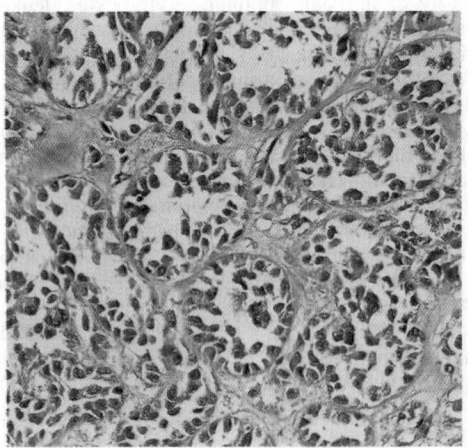

**Epithelial angiosarcoma**
*(Silverberg, DeLellis, and Frable, 1997)*

The divergence of the lines, planes, or borders may be measured in degrees of a circle. **2.** (in anatomy and physiology) the geometric relationships between the surfaces of body structures and the positions affected by movement.

**angle board,** a device used in denistry to establish reproducible angular relationships between a patient's head, the x-ray beam, and the x-ray film during radiography.

**angle-closure glaucoma.** See **glaucoma.**

**angle former,** a hoe-shaped, paired dental instrument whose cutting edges are at an oblique angle to the axis of the blade. It is used to accent angles in class III dental caries. Also called **bayonet angle former.**

**angle of convergence,** an angle formed between the visual axis of an eye focused on an object and a median line.

**angle of incidence,** the angle at which an ultrasound beam hits the interface between two different types of tissues, such as the facing surfaces of bone and muscle. The angle is also affected by the difference in acoustic impedance of the different tissues.

**angle of iris,** the angle formed between the cornea and the iris at the periphery of the anterior chamber of the eye. The aqueous fluid normally drains through this angle, which may be blocked in glaucoma. Also called **filtration angle.**

**angle of Louis** [Pierre C. A. Louis, French physician, 1787–1872], the sternal angle between the manubrium and the body of the sternum.

**angle of mandible,** the measure in degrees of the relationship between the body and the ramus of the mandible. It is used in cephalometric measurements of skull radiographs. Also called **gonial angle.**

**angle of refraction** [L, *angulus* + *refringere,* to break apart], the angle that a refracted ray of light makes with a line perpendicular to the refracting surface at the point of refraction. Also called **refracting angle.**

**angle of Treitz** /trīts/ [Wenzel Treitz, Czech physician, 1819–1872], a sharp curve or flexure at the junction of the duodenum and jejunum.

**Angle's Classification of Malocclusion (modified)** [Edward Hartley Angle, American orthodontist, 1855–1930], a classification of the various types of malocclusion, or abnormal contact between the teeth of the maxilla and those of the mandible. The classification is based on where the buccal groove of the mandibular first molar contacts the mesiobuccal cusp of the maxillary first molar: on the cusp (Class I, neutroclusion, or normal occlusion); distal to the cusp by at least the width of a premolar (Class II, distocclusion); or mesial to the cusp (Class III, mesiocclusion). Each class contains two or more types or divisions. See also **classification of malocclusion.**

**angor** /ang′gôr/, a condition of extreme distress, usually occurring in abdominal or pectoral angina or during a sudden attack of blindness.

**angstrom (Å)** /ang′strəm/ [Anders J. Angström, Swedish physicist, 1814–1874], a unit of measure of length equal to 0.1 nanometer (1/10,000,000,000 meter), or $10^{-10}$ meter. Also called **angstrom unit, a.u.**

**angular artery** /ang′gu·lər är′tə·re /, a branch of the facial artery that supplies the lacrimal sac, lower eyelid, and nose.

**angular gyrus** /ang′gyələr/ [L, *angulus* + Gk, *gyros*], a folded convolution in the inferior parietal lobe where it unites with the temporal lobe of the cerebral cortex.

**angular movement** [L, *angularis,* sharply bent], one of the four basic movements allowed by the various joints of the skeleton. It is a movement in which the angle between two adjoining bones is decreased, as in flexion, or increased, as in extension. Compare **circumduction, gliding, rotation.**

**angular spinal curvature** [L, *angulus* + *spina,* backbone,

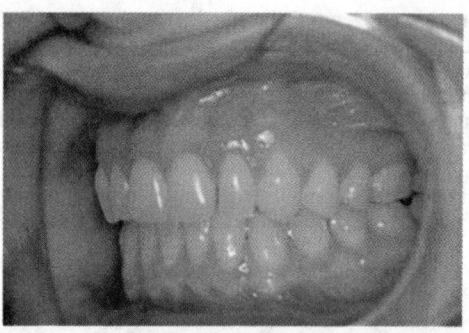

Class I malocclusion

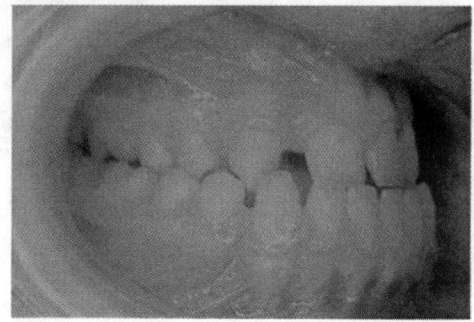

Class III malocclusion

**Angle's classification of malocclusion**
(Seidel et al, 1999/courtesy Drs. Abelson and Cameron, Lutherville, MD)

*curvatura,* bend], a sharp bending or sloping of the vertebral column. See also **gibbus.**

**angular stomatitis,** inflammation at the corner of the mouth.

**angular vein,** one of a pair of veins of the face, formed by the junction of the frontal and the supraorbital veins. At the root of the nose each angular vein receives the flow of venous blood from the infraorbital, the superior palpebral, the inferior palpebral, and the external nasal veins, becoming the first part of one of the two facial veins.

**angulated fracture** /ang′gyəlā′tid/, a fracture in which the fragments of bone are at angles to one another.

**angulation** [L, *angulatus,* bent], **1.** an angular shape or formation. **2.** the discipline of precisely measuring angles, as in mechanical drafting and surveying. **3.** (in radiography) the direction of the primary beam of radiation in relation to the object being radiographed and the film used to record its image. See also **horizontal angulation, vertical angulation.**

**anhedonia** /an′hēdō′nē·ə/ [Gk, *a* + *hedone,* not pleasure], the inability to feel pleasure or happiness in response to experiences that are ordinarily pleasurable. It is often a characteristic of major depression and schizophrenia. —**anhedonic,** *adj.*

**anhidrosis** /an′hidrō′sis, an′hī-/ [Gk, *a* + *hidros,* without sweat], an abnormal condition characterized by inadequate perspiration.

**anhidrotic** /an′hidrot′ik, an′hī-/, **1.** pertaining to anhidrosis. **2.** an agent that reduces or suppresses sweating.

**anhidrotic ectodermal dysplasia,** a congenital X-linked disorder fully expressed in males, or rarely an autosomal recessive trait with full expression in both sexes, characterized by ectodermal dysplasia associated with aplasia or hypoplasia of the sweat glands, hypothermia, alopecia, anodontia, conical teeth, and typical facies with frontal bossing, midfacial hypoplasia, saddle nose, large chin, and thick lips. Also called **Christ-Siemens-Touraine syndrome, congenital ectodermal defect, hypohidrotic ectodermal dysplasia.**

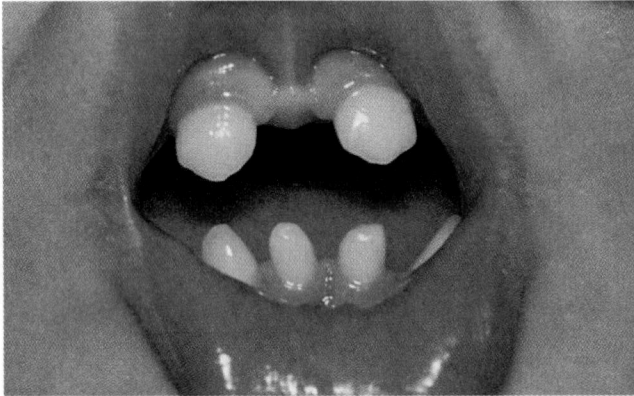

**Anhidrotic ectodermal dysplasia**
*(Hordinsky, Sawaya, and Scher, 2000)*

**anhydrase** /anhī′drās/ [Gk, *a,* not, *hydor,* water], an enzyme that catalyzes the elimination of water molecules from certain compounds, as carbonic anhydrase dehydrates carbonic acid, thereby controlling the amount of carbon dioxide in the blood and lungs.

**anhydration.** See **dehydration.**

**anhydride** /anhī′drīd/ [Gk, *a* + *hydor,* without water], a chemical compound derived by the removal of water from one or more substances, especially an acid.

**anhydrous** /anhī′drəs/ [Gk, *a,* without, *hydor,* water], an absence of water.

**anicteric** /an′ikter′ik/ [Gk, *a* + *icterus,* not jaundice], pertaining to the absence of jaundice.

**anicteric hepatitis,** a mild form of hepatitis in which there is no jaundice (icterus). Symptoms include anorexia, GI disturbances, and slight fever. Aspartate aminotransferase and alanine aminotransferase are elevated. The infection may be mistaken for influenza or be undetected. Compare **hepatitis.** See also **acute anicteric hepatitis, jaundice.**

**anidean** /anid′ē-ən/ [Gk, *a* + *eidos,* not form], formless; shapeless; denoting an undifferentiated mass, such as an anideus. Also **anidian, anidous** /an′idəs/.

**anideus** /anid′ē-əs/, an anomalous, rudimentary embryo consisting of a simple rounded mass with little indication of the body parts. A kind of anideus is **embryonic anideus.** Also called **fetus anideus.**

**anidian, anidous.** See **anidean.**

**aniline (C₆H₅NH₂)** /an′ilēn/ [Ar, *alnil,* indigo], an oily, colorless poisonous liquid with a strong odor and burning taste, formerly extracted from the indigo plant and now made synthetically by using nitrobenzene in the manufacture of aniline dyes. Industrial workers exposed to aniline are at risk of developing methemoglobinemia and bone mar-

row depression. Also called **amidobenzene, aminobenzene.**

**anilingus** /ā′niling′gəs/, sexual stimulation of the anus by the tongue or lips.

**anilism** [Ar, *alnil,* indigo; Gk, *ismos,* state], a condition of poisoning resulting from exposure to aniline compounds. Symptoms generally include cyanosis, weakness, cold sweats, irregular pulse, breathing difficulty, coma, convulsions, and possible sudden heart failure. Also called **anilinism.** See also **aniline.**

**anima** /an′imə/ [L, soul], **1.** the soul or life. **2.** the active ingredient in a drug. **3.** (in Jungian psychology) a person's true inner unconscious being or personality, as distinguished from overt personality, or persona. **4.** (in analytic psychology) the female component of the male personality. Compare **animus.**

**animal,** a multicellular organism that subsists on the breakdown of organic substances taken into the body, usually by ingestion. Most animals are capable of movement as a result of the actions of nervous tissue and muscle tissue, which are unique to animals.

**animal-assisted therapy,** a nursing intervention from the Nursing Interventions Classification (NIC) defined as purposeful use of animals to provide affection, attention, diversion, and relaxation. See also **Nursing Interventions Classification.**

**animal pole** [L, *anima*], the active, formative part of an ovum. It contains the nucleus and the bulk of the cytoplasm and is the site where the polar bodies form. In mammals, the animal pole is also the site where the inner cell mass develops and gives rise to germ layers, such as the ectoderm. Also called **germinal pole.** Compare **vegetal pole.**

**animal starch.** See **glycogen.**

**animation,** **1.** the state of being alive. **2.** an ability to put into action a vivid appearance of life.

**animus** /an′iməs/ [L, spirit], **1.** the active or rational soul; the animating principle of life. **2.** (in analytic psychology) the male component of the female personality. **3.** (in psychiatry) a deep-seated antagonism that is usually controlled but may erupt with virulence under stress. Compare **anima.**

**anion** /an′ī-ən/ [Gk, *ana* + *ion,* backward going], **1.** a negatively charged ion that is attracted to the positive electrode (anode) in electrolysis. Compare **cation.**

**anion-exchange resin,** any one of the simple organic polymers with high molecular weights that exchange anions with other ions in solution. Anion exchange resins are used as antacids in treating ulcers. Compare **cation-exchange resin.**

**anion gap,** the difference between the concentrations of serum cations and anions, determined by measuring the concentrations of sodium cations and chloride and bicarbonate anions. It is helpful in the diagnosis and treatment of acidosis, and it is estimated by subtracting the sum of sodium and bicarbonate concentrations in the plasma from that of sodium. It is normally about 8 to 14 mEq/L and represents the negative charges contributed to plasma by unmeasured ions or ions other than those of chloride and bicarbonate, mainly phosphate, sulfate, organic acids, and plasma proteins. Anions other than chloride and bicarbonate normally constitute about 12 mEq/L of the total anion concentration in plasma. Acidosis can develop with or without an associated anion increase. An increase in the anion gap often suggests diabetic ketoacidosis, drug poisoning, renal failure, or lactic acidosis and usually warrants further laboratory tests.

**anion gap test,** a blood test used to help identify the causes of metabolic acidosis, most of which are associated with an increased anion gap.

**anionic** /an'ī·on'ik/ [Gk, *ana*, not, *ion*, going], pertaining to an anion.

**aniridia** /an'i·rid'ē·ə/ [Gk, *a*, without + *iris*], absence of the iris, a usually bilateral, hereditary anomaly; often a rudimentary stump is visible through a gonioscope.

**anisakiasis** /an'i·sə·kī'ə·sis/, infection of humans or other animals with a nematode of the family Anisakidae, usually *Anisakis marina*. Human infection is usually caused by third-stage larvae eaten in undercooked infected marine fish such as herring; the larvae then burrow into the stomach wall, producing an eosinophilic granulomatous mass. Also called **eosinophilic granuloma.**

*Anisakis* /an'i·sa'kis/ [Gk, *an-*, not, without + Gk, *isos*, equal + Gk, *akis*, point], a genus of nematodes of the family Anisakidae; species *A. marina* is the usual cause of human anisakiasis.

**anise** /an'is/, the fruit of the *Pimpinella anisum* plant. Extract of anise is used in the preparation of carminatives and expectorants.

**aniseikonia** /an'īsīkō'nē·ə/ [Gk, *anisos*, unequal, *eikon*, image], an abnormal ocular condition in which each eye perceives the same image as being of a different form and size.

**anismus** /ānis'məs/, extreme contraction of the external sphincter of the anus.

**aniso-, anis-** /anī'sō-/, prefix meaning 'unequal, asymmetric, or dissimilar': *aniseikonia, anisognathous.*

**anisocoria** /-kôr'ē·ə/ [Gk, *anisos*, unequal, *kore*, pupil], an inequality of the diameter of the pupils of the two eyes.

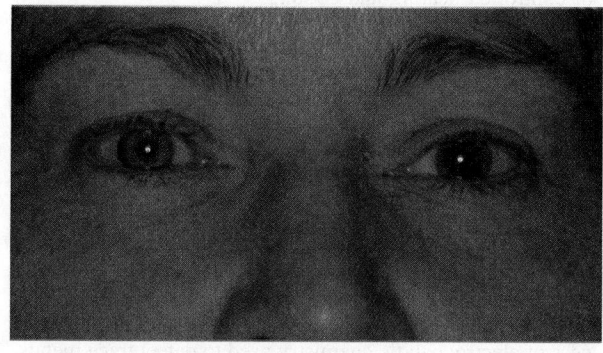

**Anisocoria** *(Lemmi and Lemmi, 2000)*

**anisocytosis** /anī'sōsīto'sis/ [Gk, *anisos* + *kytos*, cell], an abnormal condition of the blood characterized by excessive red blood cells of variable and abnormal size. Compare **poikilocytosis.** See also **macrocytosis, microcytosis.**

**anisogamete** /-gam'ēt/ [Gk, *anisos* + *gamos*, marriage], a gamete that differs considerably in size and structure from the one with which it unites, as the macrogamete and microgamete of certain sporozoa. Compare **heterogamete, isogamete.** —**anisogametic,** *adj.*

**anisogamy** /an'īsog'əmē/, sexual conjugation of gametes that are of unequal size and structure, as in certain thallophytes and sporozoa. Compare **heterogamy, isogamy.** —**anisogamous,** *adj.*

**anisognathy** /an'īsōnath'ik/ [Gk, *anisos* + *gnathos*, jaw], an abnormal condition in which the maxillary and mandibular arches or jaws are of significantly different sizes. —**anisognathic,** *adj.*

**anisokaryosis** /anī'sōker'ē·ō'sis/, a significant variation in nuclear size among cells of the same general type. —**anisokaryotic,** *adj.*

**anisomastia** /anī'sōmas'tē·ə/, a condition in which one female breast is much larger than the other.

**anisometropia** /anī'sōmetrō'pē·ə/ [Gk, *anisos* + *metron*, measure, *ops*, eye], an abnormal ocular condition characterized by a difference in the refractive powers of the eyes.

**anisopia** /an'īsō'pē·ə/, a condition in which the visual power of one eye is greater than that of the other.

**anisopiesis** /an'īsōpī·ē'sis/ [Gk, *anisos*, unequal, *piesis*, pressure], a condition of unequal arterial blood pressure on the left and right sides of the body.

**anisotropine methylbromide,** an anticholinergic.

■ INDICATION: It is prescribed as adjunctive therapy in the treatment of peptic ulcer.

■ CONTRAINDICATIONS: Glaucoma, obstructive uropathy, obstructive conditions of the GI tract, paralytic ileus, intestinal atony, unstable cardiovascular status in acute hemorrhage, severe ulcerative colitis or toxic megacolon complicating ulcerative colitis, or myasthenia gravis prohibits its use.

■ ADVERSE EFFECTS: Among the most serious adverse reactions are blurred vision, tachycardia, mydriasis, cycloplegia, impotence, mental confusion, urinary retention, constipation, allergic reactions, and urticaria.

**ankh** /ängk/, an ancient Egyptian symbol of life. It resembles a cross with a loop instead of the top beam.

**ankle** [AS, *ancleow*], **1.** the joint of the tibia and fibula of the leg with the talus of the foot. **2.** the part of the leg where this joint is located.

**ankle-arm index (AAI).** See **ankle-brachial index.**

**ankle bandage,** a figure-eight bandage looped under the sole of the foot and around the ankle. The heel may be covered or left exposed, although covering is preferable because it prevents "window edema."

**ankle bone.** See **talus.**

**ankle-brachial index (ABI),** the ratio of ankle systolic blood pressure to arm systolic blood pressure. It is calculated by dividing the higher of the left and right ankle pressures by the higher of the two brachial artery pressures. Also called **ankle-arm index (AAI).**

**ankle clonus,** an involuntary tendon reflex that causes repeated flexion and extension of the foot. It may be caused by pressure on the foot or corticospinal disease.

**ankle-foot orthosis (AFO),** any of a variety of protective external devices that can be applied to the ankle area to prevent injury in a high-risk athletic activity, to protect a previous injury such as a sprain, or to assist patients with chronic joint instability with walking. An AFO is often used by patients who are unable to dorsiflex the ankle during gait.

**ankle joint** [AS, *ancleow* + L, *jungere*, to join], a synovial hinge joint between the leg and the foot. The rounded malleolar prominences on each side of the joint form a mortise for the upper surface of the talus.

**ankle reflex.** See **Achilles tendon reflex.**

**ankylo-.** See **ancylo-.**

**ankyloblepharon** /ang'kə·lō·blef'ə·ron/ [Gk, *agkylos*, crooked + *blepharon*, eyelid], the adhesion of the ciliary edges of the eyelid to each other.

**ankyloblepharon−ectodermal dysplasia−clefting syndrome.** See **Hay-Wells syndrome.**

**ankyloglossia** /ang'kilōglos'ē·ə/ [Gk, *agkylos*, crooked, *glossa* tongue], a severe restriction of tongue movement as a result of fusion or adherence of the tongue to the floor of the mouth. Partial ankyloglossia (also called **tongue-tie**) is caused by a lingual frenum that is abnormally short or is attached too close to the tip of the tongue; this condition may

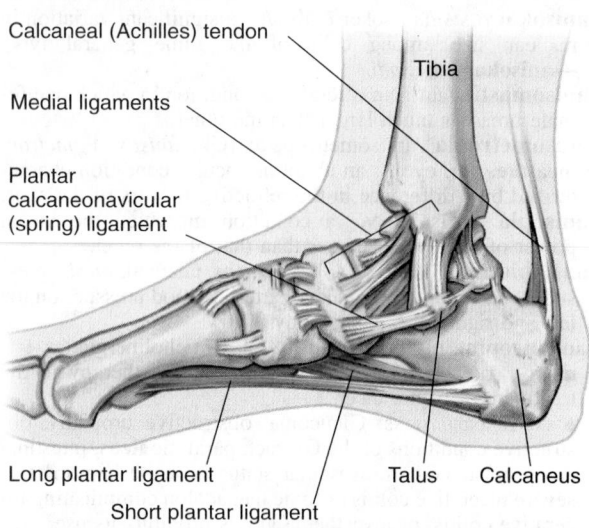

Calcaneal (Achilles) tendon

Tibia

Medial ligaments

Plantar calcaneonavicular (spring) ligament

Long plantar ligament

Short plantar ligament

Talus      Calcaneus

**Ankle joint of the right foot: medial view**

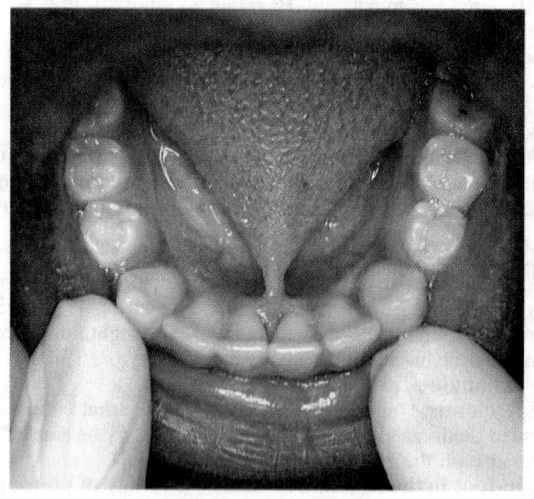

**Ankyloglossia** *(Zitelli and Davis, 1997)*

be surgically corrected by a simple excision. Complete ankyloglossia requires extensive surgical reconstruction of the tongue and the floor of the mouth.

**ankylosed** /ang'kilōst/, pertaining to the immobility of a joint resulting from pathologic changes in it or in adjacent tissues.

**ankylosing spondylitis** /ang'kilō'sing/, a chronic inflammatory disease of unknown origin, first affecting the spine and adjacent structures and commonly progressing to eventual fusion (ankylosis) of the involved joints. In extreme cases a forward flexion of the spine, called a "poker spine" or "bamboo spine," develops. The disease primarily affects males under 30 years of age and generally follows a course of 20 years. There is a strong hereditary tendency. In addition to the spine, the joints of the hip, shoulder, neck, ribs, and jaw are often involved. When the costovertebral joints are involved, the patient may have difficulty in expanding

the rib cage while breathing. Ankylosing spondylitis is a systemic disease, often affecting the eyes and heart. Many patients also have inflammatory bowel disease. The aim of treatment is to reduce pain and inflammation in the involved joints, usually with nonsteroidal antiinflammatory drugs. Physical therapy helps keep the spine as erect as possible to prevent flexion contractures. In advanced cases, surgery may be performed to straighten a badly deformed spine. Compare **rheumatoid arthritis.** See also **ankylosis.** Also called **Marie-Strümpell disease.**

**ankylosis** /ang'kilō'sis/ [Gk, *ankylosis,* bent condition], **1.** fixation of a joint, often in an abnormal position, usually resulting from destruction of articular cartilage and subchondral bone, as occurs in rheumatoid arthritis. It may also occur in immobilized patients when active or passive range of motion is not provided. Also called **true ankylosis. 2.** Surgically induced fixation of a joint to relieve pain or provide support. Also called **arthrodesis, fusion.**

**anlage** /on'lägə/ [Ger, *Anlage,* disposition, aptitude], (in embryology) the undifferentiated layer of cells from which a particular organ, tissue, or structure develops; primordium rudiment. See also **blastema.**

**ANLL,** abbreviation for **acute nonlymphocytic leukemia.** See **acute myelocytic leukemia.**

**ANNA.** abbreviation for **American Nephrology Nurses' Association.**

**anneal** [AS, *aelan,* to burn], **1.** a method of tempering metals, glass, or other materials by controlled heating and cooling to make them more malleable and ductile. **2.** a process whereby two separate strands of nucleic acid interact to form a duplex molecule, often by using a related technique of controlled heating and cooling.

**annexa.** See **adnexa.**

**annihilation** /ənī'əlā'shən/, the total transformation of matter into energy, as when an antimatter positron collides with an electron. Two photons are created, each equaling the mass of the individual particles at rest.

**annular.** See **anular.**

**annular ligament.** See **anular ligament.**

**annulus** /an'yələs/ [L, a ring], any ring-shaped structure, such as the outer edge of an intervertebral disk.

**annulus conjunctivae.** See **conjunctival ring.**

**anodal** [Gk, *ana + hodas,* way], relating to an anode.

**anode,** the electrode at which oxidation occurs.

**anodic stripping voltammetry** /ənō'dik, anod'ik/, a process of electroanalytic chemistry used to detect trace metals. It involves the use of a metal-exchange reagent that releases lead or other metals from macromolecular binding sites.

**anodontia** /an'ōdon'tē·ə/ [Gk, *a,* not, *odous,* tooth], a congenital defect in which some or all of the teeth are missing. The term is generally applied to cases in which most teeth are missing and no tooth follicles are present.

**anodyne** /an'ədīn/ [Gk *a + odyne,* not pain], a drug that relieves or lessens pain. Compare **analgesic.**

**anomalo-, anomal-,** combining form meaning 'uneven, deviation from normal, or irregular': *anomalopia, anomalous.*

**anomalous** /ə·nom'ə·ləs/ [Gr. *anōmalos*], irregular; marked by deviation from the natural order. Applied particularly to congenital and hereditary defects.

**anomaly** /ənom'əlē/ [Gk, *anomalos,* irregular], **1.** deviation from what is regarded as normal. **2.** congenital malformation, such as the absence of a limb or the presence of an extra finger. **—anomalous,** *adj.*

**anomia** /ənō'mē·ə/ [Gk, *a + onoma,* without name], a form of aphasia characterized by the inability to name objects. Comprehension and repetition are unaffected.

**anomie** /an′əmē/, a state of apathy, alienation, anxiety, personal disorientation, and distress, resulting from the loss of social norms and goals previously valued. Also spelled **anomy.**

**anonychia** /an′ō·nik′e·ə/ [Gk, *a, onyx* without nail], absence of the nail(s).

**anoopsia** /an′ō·op′sē·ə/ [Gk, *ana,* up, *ops,* eye], a strabismus in which one or both eyes are deviated upward. Also called **hypertropia.**

*Anopheles* /ənof′əlēz/ [Gk, *anopheles,* harmful], a genus of mosquito, many species of which transmit malaria-causing parasites to humans. See also **malaria,** *Plasmodium.*

**anopia** /anō′pē·ə/ [Gk, *a + ops,* not eye], blindness resulting from a defect in or the absence of one or both eyes.

**-anopia, -anopsia,** 1. suffix meaning '(condition involving) nonuse or arrested development of the eye': *hemianopia, quadrantanopsia.* 2. suffix meaning '(condition of) defective color vision': *cyanopia, tritanopia.*

**anoplasty** /an′ōplas′tē/ [L, *anus* + Gk, *plassein,* to shape], a restorative operation on the anus.

**-anopsia.** See **-anopia.**

**anorchia** /anôr′kē·ə/ [Gk, *a + orchis,* not testis], congenital absence of one or both testes. Also called **anorchism.**

**anorchidism.** See **anorchia.**

**anorectal** /ān′ōrek′təl, ā′nō-/ [L, *anus + rectus,* straight], pertaining to the anal and rectal portions of the large intestine.

**anorectal abscess** [L, *anus + rectus,* straight, *abscedere,* to go away], an abscess in the area of the anus and rectum. See also **abscess.**

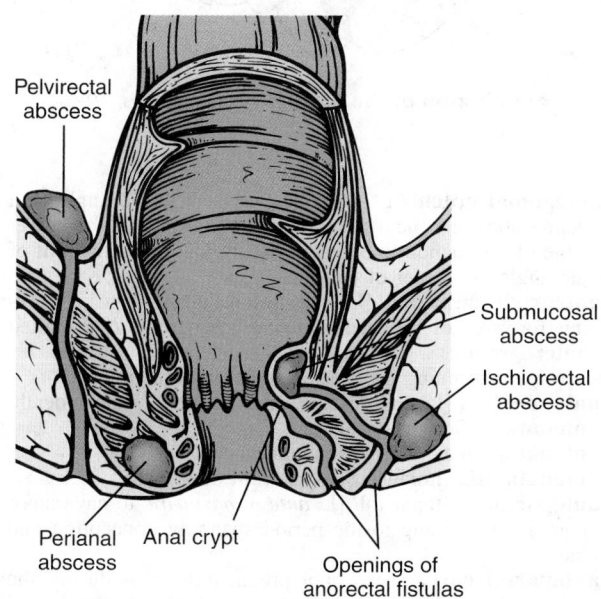

**Anorectal abscess: common sites**
*(Lewis, Heitkemper, and Dirksen, 2000)*

Pelvirectal abscess
Submucosal abscess
Ischiorectal abscess
Perianal abscess   Anal crypt
Openings of anorectal fistulas

**anorectal stricture** [L, *anus + rectus,* straight, *strictura,* compression], a narrowing of the anorectal canal. It is sometimes congenital but also may result from surgery to correct a fissure or to remove hemorrhoids.

**anorectic** /an′ōrek′tik/, 1. pertaining to anorexia. 2. lacking appetite. 3. causing a loss of appetite, as an anorexiant drug. Also **anorectous, anorexiant, anorexic.**

**anorexia** /an′ōrek′sē·ə/ [Gk, *a + orexis,* not appetite], lack or loss of appetite, resulting in the inability to eat. The condition may result from poorly prepared or unattractive food or surroundings, unfavorable company, or various physical and psychologic causes. Compare **pseudoanorexia.** See also **anorexia nervosa.**

**anorexia nervosa,** a disorder characterized by a prolonged refusal to eat, resulting in emaciation, amenorrhea, emotional disturbance concerning body image, and fear of becoming obese. The condition is seen primarily in adolescents, predominantly in girls, and is usually associated with emotional stress or conflict, such as anxiety, irritation, anger, and fear, which may accompany a major change in the person's life. Treatment consists of measures to improve nourishment, followed by therapy to overcome the underlying emotional conflicts.

**anorexiant** /an′ôrek′sē·ənt/, a drug or other agent that suppresses the appetite, such as amphetamine. See also **anorectic.**

**anorexic.** See **anorectic.**

**anorgasmy** /an′ôrgaz′mē/, failure to achieve orgasm.

**anorthopia** /an′ôrthō′pē·ə/, a visual disorder in which straight lines appear to be curved or angular. The person also may have a diminished perception of symmetry.

**anosigmoidoscopy** /an′ōsig′moidos′kəpē/, a procedure in which an endoscope is used for direct examination of the lining of the anus, rectum, and sigmoid colon.

**anosmia** /anoz′mē·ə/ [Gk, *a + osme,* without smell], loss or impairment of the sense of smell. It usually occurs as a temporary condition resulting from a head cold or respiratory infection or when intranasal swelling or other obstruction prevents odors from reaching the olfactory region. It becomes a permanent condition when the olfactory neuroepithelium or any part of the olfactory nerve is destroyed as a result of intracranial trauma, neoplasms, or disease, such as atrophic rhinitis or the chronic rhinitis associated with the granulomatous diseases. In some instances, the condition may be caused by psychologic factors, such as a phobia or fear associated with a particular smell. Kinds of anosmia include **anosmia gustatoria** and **preferential anosmia.** Also called **anosphresia, olfactory anesthesia.** —**anosmatic, anosmic,** *adj.*

**anosmia gustatoria,** the inability to smell foods.

**anosmic** [Gk, *a + osme,* without smell], pertaining to a loss of the sense of smell.

**anosognosia** /an′əsog·nō′zhə/ [Gk, *a + nosos,* not disease, *gnosis,* knowing], lack of awareness or denial of a neurologic defect, especially paralysis, on one side of the body. It may be attributable to a lesion in the right parietal lobe of the brain.

**anosphresia.** See **anosmia.**

**anotia** /anō′tē·ə/ [Gk, *a,* without, *ous,* ear], a congenital absence of one or both ears.

**ANOVA,** abbreviation for **analysis of variance.**

**anovaginal** /ā′nōvaj′inəl/ [L, *anus + vagina,* sheath], pertaining to the perineal region of the anus and vagina.

**anovarianism.** See **anovarism.**

**anovarism** /an·ō′vər·iz·əm/ [Gk, *a,* without; L, *ovum,* egg], absence of the ovaries. Also called **anovarianism.**

**anovesical** /-ves′ikəl/ [L, *anus + vesicula,* small bladder], pertaining to the anus and bladder.

**anovular** /anov′yələr/ [Gk, *a,* not, *ovulum*], pertaining to menstrual discharge not associated with the production or release of an ovum.

**anovular menstruation** [Gk, *a* + *ovulum,* not egg], menstrual bleeding that occurs although ovulation has not taken place. The ovum either remains within the follicle and undergoes degeneration or in rare cases becomes impregnated, resulting in an ovarian pregnancy.

**anovulation** /an′ovyəlā′shən/, failure of the ovaries to produce, mature, or release eggs. The condition may be a result of ovarian immaturity or postmaturity; of altered ovarian function, as in pregnancy and lactation; of primary ovarian dysfunction, as in ovarian dysgenesis; or of disturbance of the interaction of the hypothalamus, pituitary gland, and ovary, caused by stress or disease. Hormonal contraceptives prevent conception by suppressing ovulation. Anovulation may be an adverse side effect of medications prescribed in the treatment of other disorders. —**anovulatory** /anov′yəl ətôr′ē/, *adj.*

**anoxemia** /an′oksē′mē·ə/, a deficiency of oxygen in the blood. Also spelled **anoxaemia.** See also **hypoxia.**

**anoxia** /anok′sē·ə/ [Gk, *a* + *oxys,* not sharp], an abnormal condition characterized by a local or systemic lack of oxygen in body tissues. It may result from an inadequate supply of oxygen to the respiratory system, an inability of the blood to carry oxygen to the tissues, or a failure of the tissues to absorb the oxygen from the blood. Kinds of anoxia include **anemic anoxia** and **stagnant anoxia.** See also **hypoxemia, hypoxia.** —**anoxic,** *adj.*

**-ans,** suffix meaning '-ing': *penetrans, proliferans.*

**ansa** /an′sə/, *pl.* **ansae** [L, handle], (in anatomy) a looplike structure resembling a curved handle of a vase.

**ansa cervicalis,** one of three loops of nerves in the cervical plexus, branches of which innervate the infrahyoid muscles. Also called **ansa hypoglossi.**

**-anserin,** suffix designating a serotonin antagonist.

**ANSER system,** a pattern of questionnaires for studying developmental defects in children.

**ANSI,** abbreviation for **American National Standards Institute.**

**ant-.** See **anti-.**

**Antabuse,** trademark for a blocker of alcohol oxidation (disulfiram).

**antacid** /antas′id/ [Gk, *anti,* against, *acidus,* sour], **1.** opposing acidity. **2.** a drug or dietary substance that buffers, neutralizes, or absorbs hydrochloric acid in the stomach. Nonsystemic antacids containing aluminum and calcium are constipating; those containing magnesium have a laxative effect. Systemic antacids such as sodium bicarbonate are rarely used.

**antagonism** /antag′əniz′əm/ [Gk, *antagonisma,* struggle], **1.** an inhibiting action between physiologic processes, such as muscle actions. An example is the opposition between the biceps and the triceps of the arm. The biceps flexes the arm while the triceps extends it. **2.** opposing actions of drugs.

**antagonist** /antagə′nist/ [Gk, *antagonisma,* struggle], **1.** one who contends with or is opposed to another. **2.** (in physiology) any agent, such as a drug or muscle, that exerts an opposite action to that of another or competes for the same receptor sites. Kinds of antagonists include the **antimetabolite, associated antagonist, direct antagonist,** and **narcotic antagonist.** Compare **agonist. 3.** (in dentistry) a tooth in the upper jaw that articulates during mastication or occlusion with a tooth in the lower jaw. —**antagonistic,** *adj.,* **antagonize,** *v.*

**antagonistic reflexes** [Gk, *antagonisma* + L, *reflectere,* to bend back], two or more reflexes initiated at the same time that produce opposite effects. The most adaptive or persistent response occurs.

**antagonize.** See **antagonist.**

**ante-,** prefix meaning 'before in time or in place': *anteflexion, antepartal.*

**antebrachial region** /an′tə·brā′kē·əl/ [L, *ante,* before + *brachium,* arm], an anatomical term denoting the forearm, divided into the anterior or palmar antebrachial region and the posterior or dorsal antebrachial region.

**antebrachium.** See **forearm.**

**antecardium.** See **epigastric region.**

**antecedent** /an′ti·sē′dənt/ [L, *antecedentem*], a thing or period that precedes others in time or order.

**antecubital** /-kyo͞o′bitəl/ [L, *ante,* before, *cubitum,* elbow], in front of the elbow; at the bend of the elbow.

**antecubital fossa** [L, *ante,* before, *cubitum,* elbow, *fossa,* ditch], a depression at the bend of the elbow.

**antecurvature** /-kur′vəchər/, a slight degree of anteflexion or forward curvature.

**antefebrile.** See **antipyretic.**

**anteflexion** /-flek′shən/ [L, *ante* + *flectare,* bend], an abnormal position in which an organ is tilted acutely forward, folded over on itself.

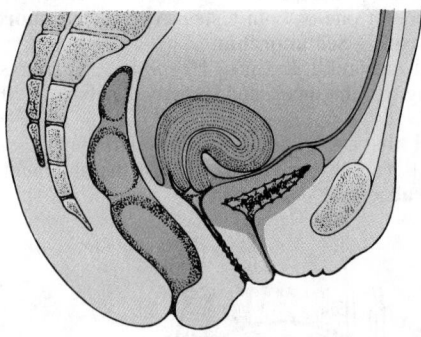

**Anteflexion of the uterus** *(Beare and Myers, 1998)*

**antegonial notch** /-gō′nē·əl/ [L, *ante* + *gonia,* angle], a depression or concavity commonly present on the lower edge of the mandible on each side, immediately in front of the angle, or corner of the jaw.

**antegrade** /an′təgrād/ [L, *ante,* before, *gredi,* to go], moving forward, or proceeding toward the front. Also called **anterograde.**

**-antel,** combining form designating an anthelmintic.

**ante mortem** [L, *ante,* before, *mors,* death], before death.

**antenatal.** See **prenatal.**

**antenatal care.** See **antepartal care.**

**antenatal diagnosis.** See **prenatal diagnosis.**

**antepartal** /an′təpär′təl/ [L, *ante* + *parturire,* to have labor pains], pertaining to the period spanning conception and labor.

**antepartal care,** care of a pregnant woman during the time in the maternity cycle that begins with conception and ends with the onset of labor. A medical, surgical, gynecologic, obstetric, social, and family history is taken, with particular emphasis on the discovery of familial or transmissible diseases. A physical examination is performed, including observation and evaluation of all body systems and pelvic organs. The vaginal part of the pelvic examination may include estimation of the size of the pelvis; a Papanicolaou (Pap) smear; and tests for *Neisseria gonorrhoeae, Candida albicans, Chlamydia* spp., *Trichomonas vaginalis,* syphilis, genital herpes, and other viral infections. Blood pressure, weight, urinalysis primarily for glucose and protein, measurement of the height of the fundus, and auscultation of the fetal heart are routinely performed at monthly intervals or even more frequently in the second and third trimesters. Laboratory tests are performed to determine blood type and Rh factor, rubella antibody titers, hematocrit, and hemoglobin or complete blood count. Ultrasound and/or amniocentesis may be performed if certain fetal abnormalities are suspected. Also called **antenatal care, prenatal care.** See also **intrapartal care, postpartal care.**

**antepartum hemorrhage** [Gk, *ante*, before; L, *parturire*, to have labor pains; Gk, *haima*, blood, *rhegnynai*, to burst forth], bleeding from the uterus during a pregnancy in which the placenta appears to be normally situated, particularly after the 28th week.

**antepyretic** /-pīret'ik/ [L, *ante*, before; Gk, *pyretos*, fever], before the onset of fever. Also called **antefebrile.**

**anterior (A)** /antir'ē·ər/ [L, *ante* + *prior*, foremost], **1.** the front of a structure. **2.** pertaining to a surface or part situated toward the front or facing forward. Compare **posterior.** See also **ventral.**

**anterior Achilles bursitis.** See **Albert's disease.**

**anterior asynclitism.** See **asynclitism.**

**anterior atlantoaxial ligament** /atlan'tō·ak'sē·əl/, one of five ligaments connecting the atlas to the axis. It is fixed to the inferior border of the anterior arch of the atlas and to the ventral surface of the body of the axis. Compare **posterior atlantoaxial ligament.**

**anterior atlantooccipital membrane,** one of two broad, densely woven fibrous sheets that form part of the atlantooccipital joint between the atlas and the occipital bone. Also called **anterior atlantooccipital ligament.** Compare **posterior atlantooccipital membrane.**

**anterior axillary line (AAL),** an imaginary vertical line on the body wall continuing the line of the anterior axillary fold with the upper arm.

**anterior cardiac vein,** one of several small vessels that return deoxygenated blood from the ventral portion of the myocardium of the right ventricle to the right atrium. See also **coronary sinus.**

**anterior central gyrus.** See **precentral gyrus.**

**anterior cerebral commissure** [L, *ante* + *prior*, foremost, *cerebrum*, brain, *commissura*, ajoining], a bundle of fibers in the anterior wall of the forebrain connecting the olfactory bulb and cortex on one side with the similar structures on the other side.

**anterior chamber** [L, *ante* + *prior*, foremost; Gk, *kamara*, an arched cover], the part of the anterior cavity of the eye in front of the iris. It contains the aqueous humor.

**anterior column.** See **anterior horn.**

**anterior common ligament.** See **anterior longitudinal ligament.**

**anterior corticospinal tract,** a group of nerve fibers in the anterior funiculus of the spinal cord, originating in the cerebral cortex.

**anterior cruciate ligament,** a strong band that arises from the posterior middle part of the lateral condyle of the femur, passes anteriorly and inferiorly between the condyles, and is attached to the depression in front of the intercondylar eminence of the tibia.

**anterior crural nerve.** See **femoral nerve.**

**anterior cutaneous nerve,** one of a pair of cutaneous branches of the cervical plexus. It arises from the second and the third cervical nerves and divides into the ascending and the descending branches. The ascending branches are distributed to the cranial, the ventral, and the lateral parts of the neck. The descending branches are distributed to the skin of the ventral and lateral parts of the neck as far down as the sternum.

**anterior determinants of cusp,** the characteristics of the anterior teeth that determine the cusp elevations and the fossa depressions in restoration of the postcanine teeth. Such determinants include occlusion, alignment overlaps, and the capacity to disocclude conjointly with condylar trajectories.

**anterior drawer sign or test,** a test for rupture of the anterior cruciate ligament. The result is positive if there is increased anterior glide of the tibia when the knee is flexed at a 90-degree angle. See also **drawer sign.**

**anterior elastic lamina.** See **Bowman's lamina.**

**anterior fontanel,** a diamond-shaped unossified area between the frontal and two parietal bones just above an infant's forehead at the junction of the coronal and sagittal sutures. Also called soft spot *(informal).* See also **fontanel.**

**anterior guide,** the portion of a dental articulator that is contacted by the incisal guide pin to maintain the selected separation of the upper and lower members of the articulator. The anterior guide influences the changing relationships of mounted casts in eccentric movements. Also called **incisal guide.** Compare **condylar guide.**

**anterior horn** [L, *ante* + *prior*, foremost, *cornu*, horn, *spina*, spine; Gk, *chorde*, string], one of the hornlike projections of gray matter into the white matter of the spinal cord. The anterior, or ventral, horn contains efferent fibers innervating skeletal muscle tissue. Also called **anterior column**

**anterior horn cell,** a large nerve cell, the body of a motor neuron, in the anterior column of the spinal cord.

**anterior longitudinal ligament,** the broad, strong ligament attached to the ventral surfaces of the vertebral bodies. It extends from the occipital bone and the anterior tubercle of the atlas to the sacrum. Also called **anterior common ligament.** Compare **posterior longitudinal ligament.**

**anterior mediastinal node,** a node in one of the three groups of thoracic visceral nodes of the lymphatic system that drains lymph from the nodes of the thymus, the pericardium, and the sternum. The nodes are located ventral to the brachiocephalic veins and to the arterial trunks from the aortic arch. Compare **posterior mediastinal node.** See also **lymph, lymphatic system, lymph node.**

**anterior mediastinum,** a caudal portion of the mediastinum in the middle of the thorax, bounded ventrally by the body of the sternum and parts of the fourth through the seventh ribs and dorsally by the parietal pericardium, extending downward as far as the diaphragm. Compare **middle mediastinum, posterior mediastinum, superior mediastinum.**

**anterior nares,** the ends of the nostrils that open anteriorly into the nasal cavity and allow the inhalation and the exhalation of air. Each is an oval opening that measures about 1.5 cm anteroposteriorly and about 1 cm in diameter. The anterior nares connect with the nasal fossae. Also called **nostrils.** Compare **posterior nares.**

**anterior nasal spine,** the sharp anterosuperior projection at the anterior extremity of the line of union of the two maxillae.

**anterior neuropore,** the opening of the embryonic neural tube in the anterior portion of the forebrain. Compare **posterior neuropore.** See also **horizon.**

**anterior pituitary.** See **adenohypophysis.**

**anterior-posterior diameter of the pelvic outlet,** the distance between the middle of the symphysis pubis and the upper border of the third sacral vertebra.

**anterior rhizotomy** [L, *anterior*, foremost; Gk, *rhiza*, root, *temnein*, to cut], the surgical cutting of the ventral root of a spinal nerve, usually to relieve persistent spasm, involuntary movement, or intractable pain.

**anterior tibial artery,** one of the two divisions of the popliteal artery, arising in back of the knee, dividing into six branches, and supplying various muscles of the leg and foot. Compare **posterior tibial artery.**

**anterior tibial node,** one of the small lymph glands of the lower limb, lying on the interosseous membrane near the proximal portion of the anterior tibial vessels. Compare **inguinal node, popliteal node.**

**anterior tooth,** any of the incisors or canines. Compare **posterior tooth.**

**anterior triangle of the neck,** a triangular area bounded by the median line of the neck in front, the lower border of the mandible, and a line extending back to the sternocleidomastoid muscle.

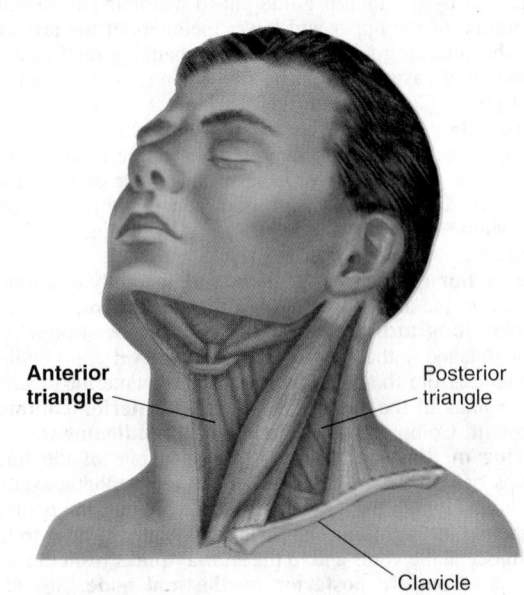

Anterior triangle — Posterior triangle

Clavicle

**Anterior triangle of the neck** *(Seidel et al, 1999)*

**antero-, anter-** /an'tərō-/, prefix denoting front: *anterolateral.*

**anterocclusion** /an'tərōklōo'shən/ [L, *ante* + *occludere,* to shut], a malocclusion in which the mandibular teeth are anterior to their normal position relative to the maxillary teeth. Compare **anteversion.**

**anteroexternal.** See **anterolateral.**

**anterograde.** See **antegrade.**

**anterograde amnesia** [L, *ante* + *prior,* foremost, *gredi,* to go], **1.** the inability to recall events that occur after the onset of amnesia. **2.** the inability to form new memories. Compare **anterograde memory, retrograde amnesia.**

**anterograde memory,** the ability to recall past events but not recent occurrences. Compare **anterograde amnesia.**

**anteroinferior** /an'tərō·infir'ē·ər/, situated in front of but at a lower level, such as the anteroinferior spine of the ilium.

**anterointernal.** See **anteromedial.**

**anterolateral** /-lat'ərəl/, in front and on each side of another structure or object.

**anterolateral thoracotomy,** a surgical technique in which entry to the chest is made with an incision below the breast but above the costal margins. The incision involves the pectoralis, serratus anterior, and intercostal muscles. Compare **median sternotomy, posterolateral thoracotomy.** See also **thoracotomy.**

**anteromedial** /an'tər·ō·mē'dē·əl/, located anteriorly and to the medial side; also called **anterointernal.**

**anteromedial central arteries of anterior communicating artery,** branches of the anterior communicating artery that supply the corpus callosum, septum pellucidum, lentiform nucleus, and caudate nucleus.

**anteroposterior (AP)** /an'tərōpostir'ē·ər/ [L, *ante* + *prior,* foremost, *posterus,* coming after], from the front to the back of the body.

**anteroposterior vaginal repair,** a surgical procedure in which the upper and lower walls of the vagina are reconstructed to correct relaxed tissue. Relaxed vaginal tissue may result from aging changes, childbirth, or surgical trauma or may be inherited.

**anterosuperior,** situated in front of but at a higher level, such as the anterosuperior spine of the ilium.

**anteversion** /-vur'shən/ [L, *ante* + *versio,* turning], **1.** an abnormal position of an organ in which it is tilted or bent forward on its axis, away from the midline. **2.** (in dentistry) the tipping or the tilting of teeth or other mandibular structures more anteriorly than normal. Compare **anterocclusion. 3.** the angulation created in the transverse plane between the neck and shaft of the femur. The normal angle is between 15 and 20 degrees.

**anteverted** /an'tivur'tid/, inclined or turned forward, as for example a uterus.

**anthelmintic** /ant'helmin'tik/ [Gk, *anti* + *helmins,* against worms], **1.** pertaining to a substance that destroys or prevents the development of parasitic worms, such as filariae, flukes, hookworms, pinworms, roundworms, schistosomes, tapeworms, trichinae, and whipworms. **2.** an anthelmintic drug. An anthelmintic may interfere with the parasites' carbohydrate metabolism, inhibit their respiratory enzymes, block their neuromuscular action, or render them susceptible to destruction by the host's macrophages. Drugs used in treating specific helmintic infections include piperazine, pyrantel pamoate, pyrvinium pamoate, mebendazole, niclosamide, hexylresorcinol, diethylcarbamazine, and thiabendazole.

**-anthema,** suffix meaning a '(specified) type of skin eruption or rash': *enanthema, exanthema.*

**anthraco-,** combining form meaning 'carbuncle or coal': *anthraconecrosis, anthracosis.*

**anthracosis** /an'thrəkō'sis/ [Gk, *anthrax,* coal, *osis,* condition], a chronic lung disease characterized by the deposit of coal dust in the lungs and by the formation of black nodules on the bronchioles, resulting in focal emphysema. The condition occurs in coal miners and is aggravated by cigarette smoking. There is no specific treatment; most cases are asymptomatic, and preventing further exposure to coal dust may halt progress of the condition. Also called **black lung disease, coal worker's pneumoconiosis, miner's pneumoconiosis.** See also **inorganic dust.**

**anthralin** /an'thrəlin/, a topical antipsoriatic.

■ INDICATIONS: It is prescribed in the treatment of psoriasis and chronic dermatitis.

■ CONTRAINDICATIONS: Renal dysfunction or known hypersensitivity to this drug prohibits its use. It is not applied to acute psoriatic eruptions or near the eyes.

■ ADVERSE EFFECTS: The most serious adverse reaction is nephrotoxicity resulting from systemic absorption.

**anthranilic acid.** See **aminobenzoic acid.**

**anthrax** /an′thraks/ [Gk, *anthrax,* coal, carbuncle], an acute infectious disease caused by spore-forming bacteria and occurring most frequently in herbivores (cattle, goats, sheep). It is caused by the bacterium *Bacillus anthracis.* Anthrax in animals is usually fatal. Inhalation causes the most serious form of anthrax in humans, but it is most often acquired when a break in the skin has direct contact with infected animals and their hides. The cutaneous form begins with a reddish brown lesion that ulcerates and then forms a dark scab surrounded by brawny edema. The signs and symptoms that follow include internal hemorrhage, muscle pain, headache, fever, nausea, and vomiting. The pulmonary form, called woolsorter's disease, is often fatal unless treated early. Treatment for both forms is ciprofloxacin or erythromycin. Contaminated surfaces should be cleaned with a 5% hypochlorite solution. A vaccine is available for veterinarians and for others for whom anthrax is an occupational hazard. The incubation period for anthrax is 2 to 60 days. Also called **malignant pustule.**

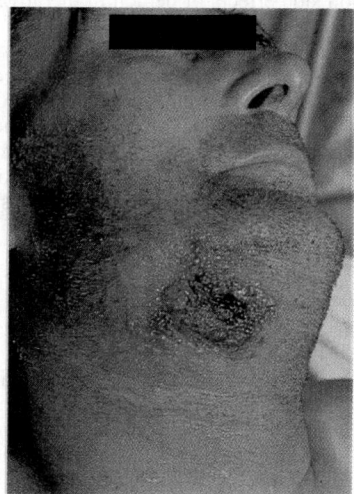

**Anthrax** *(Beeching and Nye, 1996)*

**anthropo-,** prefix meaning 'man or human': *anthropocentric, anthropoid.*

**anthropoid** /an′thrəpoid/ [Gk, *anthropos,* human, *eidos,* form], a noun or adjective generally applied to humanlike apes or other primates; also used to describe a certain kind of pelvis in gynecology and obstetrics. See also **pelvis.**

**anthropoid pelvis** [Gk, *anthropos,* human, *eidos,* form], a type of pelvis in which the inlet is oval; the anteroposterior diameter is much greater than the transverse. The posterior portion of the space in the true pelvis is much greater than the anterior portion. If the pelvis is large, vaginal delivery is not compromised, but the occiput posterior position of the fetus is favored. This type of pelvis is present in 40% of women who are not Caucasian and in more than 25% of Caucasian women. See also **pelvis.**

**anthropology** [Gk, *anthropos,* human, *logos,* science], the science of human beings, from animal-like characteristics to social and environmental aspects.

**anthropometry** /an′thrəpom′ətrē/ [Gk, *anthropos* + *metron,* measure], the science of measuring the human body

### Anthropometric measurements

| Test | Gender | Normal values | Values showing malnutrition |
|---|---|---|---|
| Triceps skinfold (TSF) | Male | 11-12.5 mm | 7.5-11 mm |
| | Female | 15-16.5 mm | 10-15 mm |
| Mid upper arm circumference (MUAC) | Male | 26-29 cm | 20-26 cm |
| | Female | 26-28.5 cm | 20-26 cm |
| Arm muscle circumference (AMC) | Male | 23-25 cm | 16-23 cm |
| | Female | 20-23 cm | 14-20 cm |
| AMC = MUAC − 0.314 = TSF | | | |

as to height, weight, and size of component parts, including skinfolds, to study and compare the relative proportions under normal and abnormal conditions. Also called **anthropometric measurement.** —**anthropometric,** *adj.*

**anthropomorphism** /an′thrəpōmôr′fizəm/ [Gk, *anthropos,* human, *morphe,* form], the assignment of human shapes and qualities to other animals.

**anti-, ant-,** prefix meaning 'against or over against': *antialexin, antacid.*

**antiadrenergic** /an′ti·ad′rənur′jik, an′tī-/ [Gk, *anti* + L, *ad* + *ren,* to kidney], **1.** pertaining to the blocking of the effects of impulses transmitted by the adrenergic postganglionic fibers of the sympathetic nervous system. **2.** an antiadrenergic agent. Drugs that block the response to norepinephrine bound to alpha-adrenergic receptors reduce the tone of smooth muscle in peripheral blood vessels, causing increased peripheral circulation and decreased blood pressure. Alpha$_1$-blocking agents include ergotamine derivatives, used in treating migraine; phenoxybenzamine and phentolamine, administered for Raynaud's disease, pheochromocytoma, and diabetic gangrene; and tolazoline hydrochloride, administered for spastic vascular disease. Agents that block beta$_1$-adrenergic receptors decrease the rate and force of heart contractions among other effects. Propranolol and its congeners are beta-blocking agents and are administered for hypertension, angina, and arrhythmias. Also called **sympatholytic.** Compare **adrenergic.**

**antiagglutinin** /-əgl$\overline{oo}$′tinin/ [Gk, *anti,* against; L, *agglutinare,* to glue], a specific antibody that counteracts the effects of an agglutinin.

**antiamebic** /an′ti·əmē′bik/, pertaining to a medication that treats amebic infections.

**antianabolic** /-an′əbol′ik/, pertaining to drugs or other agents that inhibit or retard anabolic processes, such as cell division and the creation of new tissue by protein synthesis.

**antianaphylaxis** /-an′əfilak′sis/ [Gk, *anti,* against, *ana,* back, *phylaxis,* protection], a procedure to prevent anaphylactic reactions by injecting a patient with small desensitizing doses of the antigen. Also called allergy immunotherapy.

**antianemic** /-ənē′mik/ [Gk, *anti* + *a* + *haima,* without blood], **1.** pertaining to a substance or procedure that counteracts or prevents a deficiency of erythrocytes. **2.** an agent used to treat or to prevent anemia. Whole blood is transfused in the treatment of anemia resulting from acute blood loss, and packed red cells are usually administered when the deficiency is caused by chronic blood loss. Transfusions of blood components are used in the treatment of aplastic anemia. Iron deficiency anemia, the most common form of anemia, is usually treated with oral preparations of ferrous sulfate, fumarate, or gluconate, but a parenteral preparation is indicated for people who are unable to absorb iron from the GI tract or for those who respond with nausea and diarrhea to oral administration of iron. Cyanocobalamin is administered parenterally in the treatment of pernicious anemia. Folic acid is prescribed to correct a deficiency of that vitamin in the anemias accompanying general malnutrition or alcoholic cirrhosis and to treat the common anemia of infants who are on an exclusive milk diet. A combination of folic acid and vitamin $B_{12}$ is prescribed for people who are anemic as a result of an inadequate dietary intake of both vitamins.

**antianginal drug** /-anjī′nəl/, any medication that reduces myocardial oxygen consumption or increases oxygen supply to the myocardium to prevent symptoms of angina pectoris.

**antiantibody** /an′ti·an′tibod′ē/ [Gk, *anti* + *anti* + AS, *bodig*], an immunoglobulin formed as the result of the administration of an antibody that acts as an immunogen. The antiantibody then interacts with the antibody. See also **antibody, immune gamma globulin.**

**antiantitoxin** /-tok′sin/ [Gk, *anti* + *anti* + *toxikon*, poison], an antiantibody that may form in the body during immunization, inhibiting or counteracting the effect of the antitoxin administered. See also **antiantibody.**

**antianxiety agent,** a drug that reduces anxiety. The group includes the benzodiazepine derivatives (diazepam and drugs related to it) and a few less widely used non-benzodiazepines such as meprobamate and hydroxyzine. Prolonged high dosage of benzodiazepine agents leads to tolerance and physical dependence, and sudden discontinuation of them may cause withdrawal symptoms. Also called **anxiolytic.**

**antiarrhythmic** /-ərith′mik/ [Gk, *anti* + *rhythmos*, rhythm], **1.** pertaining to a procedure or substance that prevents, alleviates, or corrects an abnormal cardiac rhythm. **2.** an agent used to treat a cardiac arrhythmia. A defibrillator that delivers a precordial electric shock is often used to restore a normal rhythm to rapid, irregular atrial or ventricular contractions. A pacemaker may be implanted in a patient with an extremely slow heart rate or other arrhythmia. The electrode catheter of an external pacemaker may be threaded through a vein to the heart in cases of ventricular standstill or complete heart block. Two of the major antiarrhythmic drugs are lidocaine, which increases the threshold of electrical stimulation in the ventricles during diastole, and a combination of disopyramide, procainamide, and quinidine, which decreases the excitability of the myocardium and prolongs the refractory period. The beta-adrenergic blocking agent propranolol may be used in treating arrhythmias. Isoproterenol is indicated for complete heart block and ventricular arrhythmias requiring an increased force of cardiac contractions to establish a normal rhythm. Atropine may be used in the treatment of bradycardia, a sedative in the treatment of tachycardia, and digitalis in the treatment of atrial fibrillation. Calcium blockers control arrhythmias by inhibiting calcium ion influx across the cell membrane of cardiac muscle, thus slowing atrioventricular (AV) conduction and prolonging the effective refractory period within the AV node. See also **arrhythmia.**

**antiarthritic** /-ärthrit′ik/ [Gk, *anti*, against, *arthron*, joint, *itis*, inflammation], pertaining to a therapy that relieves symptoms of arthritis.

**antibacterial** /-baktir′ē·əl/ [Gk, *anti* + *bakterion*, small staff], **1.** pertaining to a substance that kills bacteria or inhibits their growth or replication. **2.** an antibacterial agent. Antibiotics synthesized chemically or derived from various microorganisms exert their bactericidal or bacteriostatic effect by interfering with the production of the bacterial cell wall; by interfering with protein synthesis, nucleic acid synthesis, or cell membrane integrity; or by inhibiting critical biosynthetic pathways in the bacteria.

**antiberiberi factor.** See **thiamine.**

**antibiotic** /-bī·ot′ik/ [Gk, *anti* + *bios*, life], **1.** pertaining to the ability to destroy or interfere with the development of a living organism. **2.** an antimicrobial agent, derived from cultures of a microorganism or produced semisynthetically, used to treat infections. The penicillins, derived from species of the fungus *Penicillium* or manufactured semisynthetically, consist of a thiazolidine ring fused to a beta-lactam ring connected to side chains; these agents exert their action by inhibiting mucopeptide synthesis in bacterial cell walls during multiplication of the organisms. Penicillin G and V are widely used in treating many gram-positive coccal infections but are inactivated by the enzyme penicillinase produced by strains of staphylococci; cloxacillin, dicloxacillin, methicillin, nafcillin, and oxacillin are penicillinase-resistant penicillins. Broad-spectrum penicillins effective against gram-negative organisms are ampicillin, carbenicillin, and hetacillin. Hypersensitivity reactions, such as rash, fever, bronchospasm, vasculitis, and anaphylaxis, are relatively common side effects of penicillin therapy. Aminoglycoside antibiotics, composed of amino sugars in glycoside linkage, interfere with the synthesis of bacterial proteins and are used primarily for treating infections caused by gram-negative organisms. The aminoglycosides include gentamicin derived from *Micromonospora,* semisynthetic amikacin, kanamycin, neomycin, streptomycin, and tobramycin. These agents commonly cause nephrotoxic and ototoxic reactions as well as GI disturbances. Macrolide antibiotics, consisting of a large lactone ring and deoxamino sugar, interfere in protein synthesis of susceptible bacteria during multiplication without affecting nucleic acid synthesis. Oleandomycin, which is added to feed to improve the growth of poultry and swine, and broad-spectrum erythromycin, used to treat various gram-positive and gram-negative infections and intestinal amebiasis, are macrolides derived from species of *Streptomyces.* Erythromycin may cause mild allergic reactions and GI discomfort, but nausea, vomiting, and diarrhea occur infrequently with the usual oral dose. Polypeptide antibiotics derived from species of *Streptomyces* or certain soil bacilli vary in their spectra; most agents are nephrotoxic and ototoxic. Bacitracin and vancomycin are polypeptides used to treat severe staphylococcal infections; capreomycin and vancomycin are antituberculosis agents; and gramicidin is included in ointments for topical infections. Among polypeptide antibiotics effective against gram-negative organisms, colistin and neomycin are administered for diarrhea caused by enteropathogenic *Escherichia coli.* The tetracyclines, including the prototype derived from *Streptomyces,* chlortetracycline, demeclocycline, doxycycline, minocycline, and oxytetracycline, are active against a wide range of gram-positive and gram-negative organisms and some rickettsiae. Antibiotics in this group are primarily bacteriostatic and are thought to exert their effect by inhibiting protein synthesis in the organisms. Tetracycline therapy may cause GI irritation, photosensitivity, renal toxicity, and hepatic toxicity. Administering a drug of this group in patients during the last half of pregnancy or before 8 years of age may result in permanent discoloration of the teeth. The cephalosporins, derived from the soil fungus *Cephalosporium* or produced semisynthetically, inhibit bacterial cell wall synthesis and resist the action of penicillinase. They are used in treating infections of the respiratory tract, urinary tract, middle ear, and bones, as well as septicemia caused by a wide range of gram-positive and gram-negative organisms. The group includes cefadroxil, cefamandole, cefazolin, cephalexin, cephaloglycin, cephaloridine, cephalothin, cephapirin, and cephradine. Treatment with a cephalosporin may cause nausea, vomiting, diarrhea, enterocolitis, or an allergic reaction, such as a rash, angioneurotic edema, or exfoliative dermatitis; use of antibiotics in this group is contraindicated in patients who have shown hypersensitivity to a penicillin. Chloramphenicol, a broad-spectrum antibiotic initially derived from *Streptomyces venezuelae,* inhibits protein synthesis in bacteria. Because the drug may cause life-threatening blood dyscrasias, its use is reserved for the treatment of acute typhoid fever, serious gram-negative infections (including *Haemophilus influenzae* meningitis), and rickettsial diseases.

**antibiotic anticancer agents,** drugs that may have both antibiotic and anticancer activity. Examples include bleomycin, dactinomycin, daunorubicin, and mitomycin.

**antibiotic resistant,** pertaining to strains of microorganisms that either developed a resistance to antibiotic medications or were never sensitive to the drug.

**antibiotic sensitivity test,** a laboratory method for determining the susceptibility of organisms to therapy with antibiotics. After the infecting organism has been recovered from a clinical specimen, it is cultured and tested against several antibiotic drugs, often in two groups, gram-positive and gram-negative. If the growth of the organism is inhibited by the action of the drug, it is reported as sensitive to that antibiotic. If the organism is not susceptible to the antibiotic, it is reported as resistant to that drug. See also **Gram's stain, sensitivity test.**

**antibody (Ab)** /an'tibod'ē/ [Gk, *anti* + AS, *bodig*], an immunoglobulin produced by lymphocytes in response to bacteria, viruses, or other antigenic substances. An antibody is specific to an antigen. Each class of antibody is named for its action. Antibodies include agglutinins, bacteriolysins, opsonins, and precipitin. Also called **immune body.** See also **antiantibody, antigen determinant, plasma protein, T cell.**

**antibody absorption,** the process of removing or tying up undesired antibodies in an antiserum reagent by allowing them to react with undesired antigens.

**antibody-instructive model,** a hypothetical explanation for antibody formation. It postulates that each antigenic contact in the life of an individual causes a new antibody to develop, as when a B cell comes in contact with an antigen and subsequently produces plasma cells and memory cells. The model maintains that the random contact of B cells with antigens induces the reticuloendothelial system to instruct memory cells to produce antibodies against antigens at any time. This model is not supported by experimental evidence in favor of the **antibody-specific model.**

**antibody-specific model,** a proposed explanation for antibody formation which states that precommitted clones of lymphoid cells that are produced in the fetus are capable of interacting with a limited number of antigenic determinants with which they may have contact. Any such cells that encounter their specific antigenic determinant in utero are destroyed or suppressed. This action removes cells programmed to produce endogenous autoantibodies and prevents the development of autoimmune diseases, leaving intact those cells capable of reacting with exogenous antigens. The model holds that the body contains an enormous number of diverse clones of cells, each genetically programmed to synthesize a different antibody. Any antigen entering the body selects the specific clone programmed to synthesize the antibody for that antigen and stimulates the cells of the clone to proliferate and produce

more of the same antibody. Also called **clonal selection model.** Compare **antibody-instructive model.** See also **autoimmunity.**

**antibody therapy,** the administration of parenteral immunoglobulins as a treatment for patients with immunodeficiency diseases.

**antibody titer,** the concentration of antibodies circulating in the bloodstream of an individual. A rising titer usually indicates the body's response to antigens associated with a developing infection.

**antibromic.** See **deodorant.**

**anticancer diet** /-kan'sər/, a diet, based on recommendations of the American Cancer Society (ACS), National Cancer Institute (NCI), and National Academy of Sciences, to reduce cancer risk factors associated with eating habits.

**anticarcinogenic** /-kär'sinəjen'ik/ [Gk, *anti,* against, *karkinos,* crab, *oma,* tumor, *genein,* to produce], pertaining to a substance or device that neutralizes the effects of a cancer-causing substance.

**anticholinergic** /-kō'lənur'jik/ [Gk, *anti* + *chole,* bile, *ergein,* to work], **1.** pertaining to a blockade of acetylcholine receptors that results in the inhibition of the transmission of parasympathetic nerve impulses. **2.** an anticholinergic agent that functions by competing with the neurotransmitter acetylcholine for its receptor sites at synaptic junctions. Anticholinergic drugs are used to treat spastic disorders of the GI tract, to reduce salivary and bronchial secretions before surgery, or to dilate the pupil. Some anticholinergic agents reduce parkinsonian symptoms but are never considered primary agents for therapy. Atropine in large doses stimulates the central nervous system and in small doses acts as a depressant. Among numerous cholinergic blocking agents are atropine, belladonna, glycopyrrolate, hyoscyamine sulfate, methixene hydrochloride, trihexyphenidyl, and scopolamine. Also called **cholinergic-blocking, parasympatholytic.**

**anticholinergic agent.** See **anticholinergic.**

**anticholinergic poisoning,** poisoning caused by overdosage with an anticholinergic agent or by ingestion of plants such as jimsonweed that contain belladonna alkaloids. It is characterized by dry mouth, hot, dry, flushed skin, fixed and dilated pupils, sinus tachycardia, urinary retention, disorientation, agitation, impairment of short-term memory, slurred speech, hallucinations, respiratory depression, seizures, and coma; in rare cases death may occur. Treatment is by induced emesis and administration of activated charcoal; physostigmine may be used in severe cases to reverse the anticholinergic effects.

**anticholinesterase** /an'tikol'ənes'tərās/, a drug that inhibits or inactivates the action of acetylcholinesterase. Drugs of this class cause acetylcholine to accumulate at the junctions of various cholinergic nerve fibers and their effector sites or organs, allowing potentially continuous stimulation of cholinergic fibers throughout the central and peripheral nervous systems. Anticholinesterase drugs include physostigmine, neostigmine, edrophonium, and pyridostigmine. Neostigmine and pyridostigmine are prescribed in the treatment of myasthenia gravis; edrophonium in the diagnosis of myasthenia gravis and the treatment of overdosage of curariform drugs. Many agricultural insecticides have been developed from anticholinesterases; these are the highly toxic chemicals called organophosphates. Nerve gases developed as potential chemical warfare agents contain potent, irreversible forms of anticholinesterase.

**anticipation** /antis'ipā'shən/, an appearance before the expected time of a periodic sign or symptom, as a malarial paroxysm or a hereditary disorder.

**anticipatory adaptation** /antis'əpətôr'ē/ [L, *anticipare*, to receive before], the act of adapting to a potentially distressing situation before actually confronting the problem, as when a person tries to relax before learning the results of a medical examination.

**anticipatory grief,** feelings of grief that develop before, rather than after, a loss.

**anticipatory guidance[1],** the psychologic preparation of a person to help relieve fear and anxiety of an event expected to be stressful. An example is the preparation of a child for surgery by explaining what will happen and what it will feel like and showing equipment or the area of the hospital where the child will be. It is also used to prepare parents for normal growth and development.

**anticipatory guidance[2],** a nursing intervention from the Nursing Interventions Classification (NIC) defined as preparation of patient for an anticipated developmental and/or situational crisis. See also **Nursing Interventions Classification.**

**anticoagulant** /-kō·ag'yələnt/ [Gk, *anti* + *coagulare*, curdle], **1.** pertaining to a substance that prevents or delays coagulation of the blood. **2.** an anticoagulant drug. Heparin, obtained from the liver and lungs of domestic animals, is a potent anticoagulant that interferes with the formation of thromboplastin, with the conversion of prothrombin to thrombin, and with the formation of fibrin from fibrinogen. Phenindione derivatives administered orally or by injection are vitamin K antagonists that prevent coagulation by inhibiting the formation of vitamin K–dependent clotting factors. See also **antithrombotic.**

**anticoagulant therapy** [Gk, *anti* + L, *coagulare*, to curdle; Gk, *therapeia*], the administration of drugs such as heparin or warfarin that reduce the tendency of blood to coagulate, thereby reducing the risk of thrombosis.

**anticodon** /an'tikō'don/ [Gk, *anti* + *caudex*, book], a sequence of three nucleotides found in transfer RNA. Each anticodon pairs complementarily with a specific codon of messenger RNA during protein synthesis and specifies a particular amino acid in the protein. See also **genetic code, transcription, translation.**

**anticomplement,** a substance other than an antigen-antibody complex that activates serum complement, resulting in complement fixation.

**anticonvulsant** /-kənvul'sənt/ [Gk, *anti* + L, *convellere*, to shake], **1.** pertaining to a substance or procedure that prevents or reduces the severity of epileptic or other convulsive seizures. **2.** an anticonvulsant drug. Hydantoin derivatives, especially phenytoin, apparently exert their anticonvulsant effect by stabilizing the cell membrane and decreasing intracellular sodium, with the result that the excitability of the epileptogenic focus is reduced. Phenytoin prevents the spread of excessive discharges in cerebral motor areas and suppresses arrhythmias originating in the thalamus, frontal lobes, and other brain areas. Succinic acid derivatives, valproic acid, paramethadione, and various barbiturates are among the drugs prescribed to limit or prevent petit mal seizures. Some benzodiazepines also have been shown to be useful as anticonvulsants. Many of these agents have a potential for producing fetal malformations when administered to pregnant women.

**antideformity positioning and splinting** /-dəfôr'mitē/, the use of splints, braces, or similar devices to prevent or control contractures or other musculoskeletal deformities that may result from disuse, burns, or other injuries. Examples include the application of an axillary or airplane splint to prevent adduction contracture of the shoulder and a neck conformer splint to prevent flexion contractures of the neck.

**antidepressant** /-dəpres'ənt/, pertaining to a substance or a measure that prevents or relieves depression.

**antidiabetic** /-dī'əbet'ik/, pertaining to an agent that prevents or relieves symptoms of diabetes.

**antidiarrheal** /-dī'ərē'əl/, a drug or other agent that relieves the symptoms of diarrhea. Antidiarrheals absorb water from the digestive tract, alter intestinal motility, alter electrolyte transport, or adsorb toxins or microorganisms.

**antidiuretic** /-dī'əret'ik/ [Gk, *anti* + *dia*, through, *ourein*, to urinate], **1.** of or pertaining to the suppression of urine formation. **2.** an antidiuretic hormone (vasopressin), produced in hypothalamic nuclei and stored in the posterior lobe of the pituitary gland, that suppresses urine formation by stimulating the resorption of water in distal tubules and collecting ducts in the kidneys. —**antidiuresis,** *n.*

**antidiuretic hormone (ADH),** a hormone that decreases the production of urine by increasing the reabsorption of water by the renal tubules. ADH is secreted by cells of the hypothalamus and stored in the posterior lobe of the pituitary gland. ADH released in response to a decrease in blood volume or an increased concentration of sodium or other substances in plasma, or by pain, stress, or the action of certain drugs. ADH causes contraction of smooth muscle in the digestive tract and blood vessels, especially capillaries, arterioles, and venules. Acetylcholine, methacholine, nicotine, large doses of barbiturates, anesthetics, epinephrine, and norepinephrine stimulate ADH release; ethanol and phenytoin inhibit production of the hormone. Increased intracranial pressure promotes inappropriate increases and decreases in ADH. Synthetic ADH is used in the treatment of diabetes insipidus (caused by decreased ADH levels). Normal values are 1 to 5 pg/ml or less than 1.5 ng/L. Also called **vasopressin.**

**antidiuretic hormone (ADH) test,** a blood test that may be used to diagnose diabetes insipidus (both the neurogenic and nephrogenic forms) and the syndrome of inappropriate ADH secretion (SIADH), which is associated with tumors, pulmonary diseases, infection, trauma, Addison's disease, and myxedema.

**anti-DNA antibody test,** a blood test that is useful for the diagnosis and follow-up of systemic lupus erythematosus (SLE). High titers characterize SLE, while low to moderate levels may indicate other rheumatic diseases as well as chronic hepatitis, infectious mononucleosis, and biliary cirrhosis.

**antidotal** /-dō'təl/ [Gk, *anti*, against, *dotos*, that which is given], a substance that renders a poison or drug ineffective. See also **antidote.**

**antidote** /an'tidōt/ [Gk, *anti* + *dotos*, that which is given], a drug or other substance that opposes the action of a poison. An antidote may be mechanical, acting to coat the stomach and prevent absorption; chemical, acting to make the toxin inert; or physiologic, acting to oppose the action of the poison, as when a sedative is given to a person who has ingested a large amount of a stimulant, or when a receptor blocker is administered to a person who has taken a large dose of the receptor agonist.

**antidromic conduction** /an'tidrom'ik/ [Gk, *anti* + *dromos*, course], the conduction of a neural impulse backward from a receptor in the midportion of an axon. It is an unnatural phenomenon and may be produced experimentally. Because synaptic junctions allow conduction in one direction only, any backward, antidromic impulses that occur fail to pass the synapse, dying at that point. Compare **orthodromic conduction.**

**antiembolism hose** /-em'bəliz'əm/ [Gk, *anti* + *embolos*, plug], elasticized stockings worn to prevent the formation of emboli and thrombi, especially in patients who have had surgery or who have been restricted to bed. Return flow of the venous circulation is promoted, preventing venous stasis and dilation of the veins, conditions that predispose individuals to varicosities and thromboembolic disorders. Abbreviated **AE hose** or **TED (thromboembolic disorder) hose.**

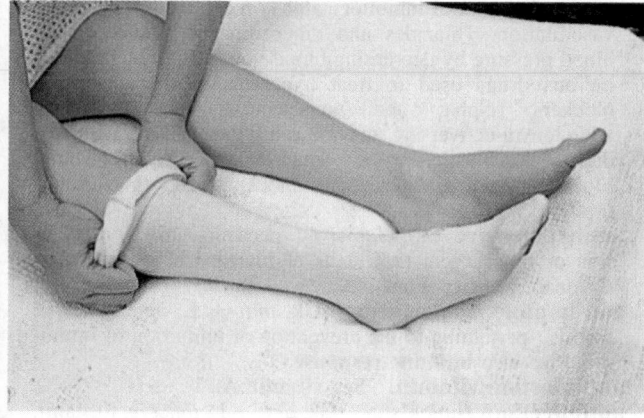

**Antiembolism hose** (Elkin, Perry, and Potter, 2000)

**antiemetic** /-imet′ik/ [Gk, *anti + emesis,* vomiting], **1.** pertaining to a substance or procedure that prevents or alleviates nausea and vomiting. **2.** an antiemetic drug or agent. Chlorpromazine and other phenothiazines are sometimes effective antiemetic agents. In motion sickness, scopolamine and antihistamines provide relief. Marijuana derivatives may alleviate the nausea induced by certain antineoplastic drugs in cancer patients. SHT₃-receptor antagonists may relieve chemotherapy-induced nausea.

**antiepileptic.** See **anticonvulsant.**

**antiestrogen drug** /-es′trəjən/, any of a group of hormone-based products used predominantly in cancer chemotherapy. The group includes tamoxifen. They are used mainly in treating estrogen-dependent tumors, such as breast cancer.

**antifebrile.** See **antipyretic.**

**antifibrillatory** /-fibril′ətôr′ē/, a medication or other agent that suppresses either atrial or ventricular fibrillation.

**antiflux** /an′ti·fluks/ [Gk, *anti,* against + L, *fluere,* to flow], a substance that prevents the attachment of solder.

**antifungal** /-fung′gəl/, **1.** pertaining to a substance that kills fungi or inhibits their growth or reproduction. **2.** an antifungal, antibiotic drug. Amphotericin B and ketoconazole, both effective against a broad spectrum of fungi, probably act by binding to sterols in the fungal cell membrane and changing the membrane's permeability. Griseofulvin, another broad-spectrum antifungal agent, binds to the host's new keratin and renders it resistant to further fungal invasion. Miconazole inhibits the growth of common dermatophytes, including yeastlike *Candida albicans;* nystatin is effective against yeast and yeastlike fungi. Also called **antimycotic.**

**antigalactic** /-gəlak′tik/, pertaining to a drug or other agent that prevents or reduces milk secretion in some mothers of newborns.

**anti-GBM disease,** a kidney disorder in which the glomerular basement membrane is damaged by an antigen-antibody reaction. The kidney itself may serve as the antigenic target in the reaction.

**antigen** /an′tijən/ [Gk, *anti + genein,* to produce], a substance, usually a protein, that the body recognizes as foreign and that can evoke an immune response.

**antigen-antibody reaction,** a process of the immune system in which immunoglobulin-coated B cells recognize a specific antigen and stimulate antibody production. T cells also play an essential role in the reaction. An antigen-antibody reaction begins with the binding of antigens to antibodies to form antigen-antibody complexes. These complexes may render toxic antigens harmless, agglutinize antigens on the surface of microorganisms, or activate the complement system by exposing the complement-binding sites on antibodies. Certain complement proteins immediately bind to these sites and trigger the activity of the other complement proteins, which cause antigen-bearing cells to lyse. Antigen-antibody reactions may start immediately with antigen contact or as much as 48 hours later. They normally produce immunity but may also be responsible for allergy, autoimmunity, and fetomaternal hematologic incompatibility. In the immediate allergic response, the antigen-antibody reaction activates certain enzymes and causes an imbalance between those enzymes and their inhibitors. Simultaneously released into the circulation are several pharmacologically active substances, including acetylcholine, bradykinin, histamine, immunoglobulin G, and leukotaxine. See also **allergen, allergic reaction, humoral immunity, serum sickness.**

**antigenic** /-jen′ik/, provoking an immune response or reacting with antibodies. Also called **immunogenic.**

**antigenic determinant,** a short sequence of amino acids in an antigen molecule that assume a particular shape and bind to a corresponding site of an antibody molecule or T cell receptor. Also called **epitope.** See also **antibody.**

**antigenic drift** [Gk, *anti,* against, *genein,* to produce; AS, *drifan,* drift], the tendency of a virus or other microorganism to alter its genetic makeup, periodically producing a mutant antigen requiring new antibodies and vaccines to combat its effects. See also **influenza.**

**antigenicity** /an′tijənis′ətē/, the ability to cause the production of antibodies. The degree of antigenicity of a substance depends on the kind and amount of that substance and on the degree to which the host is sensitive to it and able to produce antibodies. See also **antigen-antibody reaction.**

**antigenic shift,** a sudden, major change in the antigenicity of a virus, seen especially in influenza viruses, resulting from the recombination of the genomes of two virus strains; it is associated with pandemics because hosts do not have immunity to the new strain. Compare **antigenic drift.**

**antigen-presenting cell,** a cell that can break down protein antigens into peptides and present the peptides, in conjunction with major histocompatibility complex class II molecules, on the cell surface, where they can interact with T cell receptors. Macrophages are one type of antigen-presenting cell.

**antigen processing,** the steps that occur in an immune response after a protein is recognized as a foreign.

**antigen unit,** the smallest amount of antigen required to fix one unit of complement.

**antigerminal pole.** See **vegetal pole.**

**antiglobulin** /an′tiglob′yŏolin/ [Gk, *anti + L, globulus,* small globe], an antibody that occurs naturally or is prepared in laboratory animals to be used against human globulin. Specific antiglobulins are used in the detection of specific antibodies, as in blood typing. See also **antiglobulin test, Coombs' test, precipitin.**

**antiglobulin test,** a test for the presence of antibodies that coat and damage red blood cells as a result of any of several diseases or conditions. The test can detect Rh antibodies in maternal blood and is used to anticipate hemolytic disease of the newborn. It is also used to diagnose and screen for autoimmune hemolytic anemias and to determine the compatibility of blood types. When exposed to a sample of the patient's serum, the antiglobulin serum causes agglutination if human globulin antibody or its complement is present. Also called **Coombs' test.** See also **autoimmune disease, erythroblastosis fetalis.**

**antigravity muscles** /-grav′itē/, the muscle groups involved in stabilization of joints or other body parts by opposing the effects of gravity. Examples include the muscles of the jaw that automatically keep the mandible raised and the mouth closed.

**anti-G suit.** See **military antishock trousers.**

**antihemophilic C factor.** See **factor XI.**

**antihemophilic factor (AHF)** /-hē′mōfil′ik/, blood factor VIII, a systemic hemostatic.

■ INDICATION: It is prescribed in the treatment of hemophilia A, a deficiency of factor VIII.

■ CONTRAINDICATION: There are no known contraindications.

■ ADVERSE EFFECTS: The most serious adverse reaction is hepatitis, which occurs because the factor is obtained from pools of human plasma. Allergic reactions may also occur.

**antihemophilic factor plasma** [Gk, *anti*, against, *haima*, blood, *philein*, to love; L, *facere*, to make; Gk, *plassein*, to mold], blood plasma that contains the antihemophilic factor VIII.

**antihemorrhagic** /-hē′môraj′ik/, any drug or agent used to prevent or control bleeding, such as thromboplastin or thrombin, either of which mediates the blood clotting process.

**antihidrotic** /-hidrot′ik/ [Gk, *anti*, + *hidros*, sweat], an agent that inhibits or prevents the production of sweat.

**antihistamine** /-his′təmin/ [Gk, *anti* + *histos*, tissue, amine (ammonia compound)], any substance capable of reducing the physiologic and pharmacologic effects of histamine, including a wide variety of drugs that block histamine receptors. Many such drugs are readily available as nonprescription medicines for the management of allergies. Toxicity resulting from the overuse of antihistamines and their accidental ingestion by children is common and sometimes fatal. These substances do not completely stop the release of histamine, and the ways in which they act on the central nervous system are not completely understood. The antihistamines are divided into histamine $H_1$ and $H_2$ blockers, depending on the responses to histamine they prevent. The $H_1$ blocking drugs, such as the alkylamines, ethanolamines, ethylenediamines, and piperazines, are effective in the symptomatic treatment of acute allergies. Second-generation $H_1$ blockers, such as cetirizine (Zyrtec), fexofenadine (Allegra), and loratadine (Claritin), cause less sedation. The $H_2$ blocking drugs are effective in the control of gastric secretions and are often used in the treatment of gastroesophageal reflux disease. Antihistamines can both stimulate and depress the central nervous system.

**antihistamine poisoning,** an adverse reaction to an excessive intake of antihistamine medication. Symptoms include fatigue, lethargy, delirium, hallucinations, loss of voluntary muscle control, hyperreflexia, tachycardia, dilated pupils, and in severe cases coma.

**antihistaminic** [Gk, *anti* + *histos*, tissue, amine], pertaining to a substance that counteracts the effects of histamine.

**antihypercholesterolemic** /-hī′pərkō′les′tərōlē′mik/, a drug that prevents or controls an increase of cholesterol in the blood. See also **antilipidemic.**

**antihypertensive** /-hī·pərten′siv/, 1. pertaining to a substance or procedure that reduces high blood pressure. 2. an antihypertensive agent. Various drugs achieve their antihypertensive effect by depleting tissue stores of catecholamines in peripheral sites, by stimulating pressor receptors in the carotid sinus and heart, by blocking autonomic nerve impulses that constrict blood vessels, by stimulating central inhibitory alpha₂ receptors, or by direct vasodilation. Thiazides and other diuretic agents reduce blood pressure by decreasing blood volume. Among the numerous drugs used to treat hypertension are adrenergic blockers (alpha₁ and nonselective beta blockers), angiotensin-converting enzyme inhibitors, nonnitrate vasodilators (such as hydrazine), beta blockers, calcium channel blockers, angiotensin receptor blockers, and thiazide diuretics.

**antihypotensive** /-hī′pōten′siv/, pertaining to any medication or other agent that tends to increase blood pressure. Compare **antihypertensive.**

**antiimmune** /an′ti·imyo͞on′/ [Gk, *anti* + L, *immunis*, free from], pertaining to the prevention or inhibition of immunity. See also **immune response.**

**antiinfection vitamin.** See **vitamin A.**

**antiinfectious** /-infek′shəs/ [Gk, *anti* + L, *inficere*, to stain], pertaining to an agent that prevents or treats infection.

**antiinflammatory** /-inflam′ətor′ē/ [Gk, *anti* + L, *inflammare*, to set afire], pertaining to a substance or procedure that counteracts or reduces inflammation.

**antiinitiator** /-inish′ē·ātər/, a substance that is a potential cocarcinogen but that may protect cells against cancer development if given before exposure to an initiator. An example is the food additive butylated hydroxytoluene (BHT). An antiinitiator given after exposure to an initiator may also act as a promoter and encourage rather than block cancer development.

**antileprotic** /-leprot′ik/, a drug or other agent that is effective in treating leprosy.

**antilipidemic** /an′tilip′idē′mik/ [Gk, *anti* + *lipos*, fat, *haima*, blood], 1. pertaining to a regimen, diet, or agent that reduces the amount of lipids in the serum. Antilipidemic diets and drugs are prescribed to reduce the risk of atherosclerotic cardiovascular disease (ACVD) for two reasons: atheromatous plaques contain free cholesterol, and lower serum cholesterol levels and lower incidence of coronary heart disease are found in populations consuming a low-fat diet than in those on a high-fat diet. 2. a drug used to reduce the amount of lipids in the serum. A number of pharmacologic agents are used to reduce serum lipids. Among drugs used to reduce serum lipids are bile acid sequestrants and lovastatin. Cholestyramine and colestipol exert their antilipemic action by combining with bile acids in the intestine to form an insoluble complex that is excreted in the feces; they may reduce serum cholesterol but prevent the absorption of essential fat-soluble vitamins and may be associated with several serious side effects. Colestipol also binds and removes bile acids from the intestine. Lovastatin interferes with the biosynthesis of cholesterol. See also **hyperlipidemia.**

**Antilirium,** trademark for an acetylcholinesterase drug inhibitor (physostigmine salicylate).

**antilymphocyte serum (ALS)** /-lim′fəsīt/, a serum.

■ INDICATIONS: It is prescribed as an immunosuppressive agent for the reduction of rejection reactions in organ transplantation and as an adjunct in chemotherapy for malignant

neoplasms. Its effects have been promising in some cases of leukemia and in kidney transplantation.
- ADVERSE EFFECTS: It is associated with serious serum sickness, generalized infection, anaphylaxis, and antigen–antibody–induced glomerulonephritis. Also called **antilymphocyte globulin (ALG).**

**antimalarial** /-məler′ē·əl/, **1.** pertaining to a substance that destroys or suppresses the development of malaria plasmodia or to a procedure that exterminates the mosquito vectors of the disease, such as spraying insecticides or draining swamps. **2.** an antimalarial drug that destroys or prevents the development of plasmodia in human hosts. Chloroquine hydrochloride and hydroxychloroquine sulfate are effective against *Plasmodium vivax, P. malariae,* and certain strains of *P. falciparum.* Patients with drug-resistant *P. falciparum* are often treated with a combination of quinine, pyrimethamine, and sulfadoxine. See also **malaria.**

**antimessage,** a strand of viral RNA that cannot act as messenger RNA because of its negative coding sequence. It must be converted to a positive-strand sequence by a viral transcriptase before its message can be translated in a host cell.

**antimetabolite** /-mətab′əlīt/ [Gk, *anti* + *metabole,* change], a drug or other substance that is an antagonist to or resembles a normal human metabolite and interferes with its function in the body, usually by competing for its receptors or enzymes. Among the antimetabolites used as antineoplastic agents are the folic acid analog methotrexate and the pyrimidine analog fluorouracil. Antineoplastic mercaptopurine, an analog of the nucleotide adenine and the purine base hypoxanthine, is a metabolic antagonist of both compounds. Thioguanine, another member of a large series of purine analogs, interferes with nucleic acid synthesis. Cytarabine, used in the treatment of acute myelocytic leukemia, is a synthetic nucleoside that resembles cytidine and kills cells that actively synthesize deoxyribonucleic acid (DNA), apparently by inhibiting the enzyme DNA polymerase.

**antimicrobial** /-mīkrō′bē·əl/ [Gk, *anti* + *mikros,* small, *bios,* life], **1.** pertaining to a substance that kills microorganisms or inhibits their growth or replication. **2.** an agent that kills or inhibits the growth or replication of microorganisms. See also **antibiotic.**

**antimicrobial drugs** [Gk, *anti* + *mikros,* small, *bios,* life, Fr, *drogue*], drugs that destroy or inhibit the growth of microorganisms.

**antimicrobic** /-mīkrob′ik/, any agent that prevents or destroys microorganisms or inhibits their growth.

**Antiminth,** trademark for an anthelmintic (pyrantel pamoate).

**antimitochondrial antibody (AMA)** /-mī′tōkon′drē·əl/, an antibody that acts specifically against mitochondria. These antibodies are not normally present in the blood of healthy people. A laboratory test for the presence of antibodies in the blood is a valuable diagnostic aid in liver disease. Low titers may occur in chronic hepatitis, drug-induced hepatotoxicity, and various other diseases. High titers are virtually diagnostic of primary biliary cirrhosis.

**antimitochondrial antibody (AMA) test,** a blood test that is used primarily to help diagnose primary biliary cirrhosis. Patients with chronic active hepatitis, drug-induced cholestasis, autoimmune hepatitis, extrahepatic obstruction, or acute infection may also test positive for AMA.

**antimitotic** /-mītot′ik/, inhibiting cell division.

**antimony (Sb)** /an′təmō′nē/ [L *antimonium*], a bluish, crystalline metallic element occurring in nature. Various antimony compounds are used in the treatment of filariasis, leishmaniasis, lymphogranuloma, schistosomiasis, and trypanosomiasis and as emetics.

**antimony poisoning,** toxic effect caused by the ingestion or inhalation of antimony or antimony compounds, characterized by vomiting, sweating, diarrhea, and a metallic taste in the mouth. Irritation of the skin or mucous membrane may result from external exposure. Severe poisoning resembles arsenic poisoning. Antimony and antimony compounds are common ingredients of many substances used in medicine and industry.

**antimorph** /an′təmôrf/ [Gk, *anti* + *morphe,* form], a mutant allele that inhibits or antagonizes the influence of the normal allele in the expression of a trait. Compare **amorph, hypermorph, hypomorph.**

**antimuscarinic** /-mus′kərin′ik/ [Gk, *anti* + L, *musca,* fly], effective against the poisonous activity of muscarine. See also **muscarinic.**

**antimutagen** /-myōō′təjən/ [Gk, *anti* + L, *mutare,* to change; Gk, *genein,* to produce], **1.** any substance that reduces the rate of spontaneous mutations or counteracts or reverses the action of a mutagen. **2.** any technique that protects cells against the effects of mutagens. —**antimutagenic,** *adj.*

**antimycotic.** See **antifungal.**

**antimyocardial antibody test (AMA),** a blood test used to detect an autoimmune source of myocardial injury and disease, such as rheumatic heart disease, cardiomyopathy, postthoracotomy syndrome, and postmyocardial infarction. This test may also be used to monitor these conditions' response to treatment.

**antineoplastic** /-nē′ōplas′tik/ [Gk, *anti* + *neos,* new, *plasma,* something formed], **1.** pertaining to a substance, procedure, or measure that prevents the proliferation of malignant cells. **2.** a chemotherapeutic agent that controls or kills cancer cells. Drugs used in the treatment of cancer are cytotoxic but are generally more damaging to dividing cells than to resting cells. Cycle-specific antineoplastic agents are more effective in killing proliferating cells than in killing resting cells, and phase-specific agents are most active during a specific phase of the cell cycle. Most anticancer drugs prevent the proliferation of cells by inhibiting the synthesis of deoxyribonucleic acid (DNA) by various mechanisms. Alkylating agents, such as nitrogen mustard derivatives, ethylenimine derivatives, and alkyl sulfonates, interfere with DNA replication by causing cross-linking of DNA strands and abnormal pairing of nucleotides. Antimetabolites exert their action by interfering with the formation of compounds required for cell division. The folic acid analog and 5-fluorouracil, a pyrimidine analog, inhibit enzymes required for the formation of the essential DNA constituent thymidine. Hypoxanthine analog 6-mercaptopurine and 6-thioguanine, an analog of guanine, interfere with the biosynthesis of purine. Vinblastine and vincristine, alkaloids derived from the periwinkle plant, disrupt cell division by interfering with the formation of the mitotic spindle. Antineoplastic antibiotics, such as doxorubicin, daunomycin, and mitomycin, block or inhibit DNA synthesis; dactinomycin and mithramycin interfere with ribonucleic acid synthesis. Cytotoxic chemotherapeutic agents may be administered orally, intravenously, or by infusion. All have untoward and unpleasant side effects and are potentially immunosuppressive and dangerous. Estrogens and androgens, although not considered antineoplastic agents, frequently cause tumor regression when administered in high doses to patients with hormone-dependent cancers. See also **alkylating agent, antimetabolite.**

**antineoplastic antibiotic,** a chemical substance derived from a microorganism or a synthetic analog of the substance, used in cancer chemotherapy. Dactinomycin, used in the treatment of Wilms' tumor, testicular carcinoma, choriocarcinoma, rhabdomyosarcoma, and some other sarcomas, exerts its antineoplastic effect by interfering with ribonucleic acid (RNA) synthesis. Mithramycin, with a similar mechanism of action, is also administered for testicular cancer and for trophoblastic neoplasms. Doxorubicin, a broadspectrum agent that is especially useful in treating breast carcinoma, lymphomas, sarcomas, and acute leukemia, and closely related daunomycin, which is also effective in acute leukemias, block the biosynthesis of RNA. Mitomycin C, prescribed for gastric, breast, cervical, and head and neck carcinomas, cross-links strands of deoxyribonucleic acid (DNA). Bleomycin, used in the treatment of squamous cell carcinomas of the head and neck, testicular carcinoma, and lymphomas, damages DNA and prevents its repair. Antineoplastic antibiotics depress bone marrow and usually cause nausea and vomiting; several cause alopecia.

**antineoplastic hormone,** a chemical substance produced by an endocrine gland or a synthetic analog of the naturally occurring compound, used to control certain disseminated cancers. Hormonal therapy is designed to counteract the effect of an endogenous hormone required for tumor growth. The estrogens diethylstilbestrol (DES) and ethinyl estradiol may be used in palliative treatment of a prostatic carcinoma that is nonresectable or unresponsive to radiotherapy. An androgen, such as testosterone propionate, testolactone, or fluoxymesterone, may be administered postoperatively to control disseminated breast cancer in women whose tumor is estrogen-dependent. The antiestrogen tamoxifen produces responses in many patients with advanced estrogen-dependent breast cancer. Paradoxically, large doses of estrogen, frequently used to control disseminated breast cancer in postmenopausal women, apparently check the growth of tumors by inhibiting the secretion of estrogen by the adrenal gland. Some progestins produce a favorable response in women with disseminated endometrial carcinoma and, occasionally, in patients with prostatic or renal cancers. These progestins include megestrol acetate, medroxyprogesterone acetate, and 17-alphahydroxyprogesterone caproate.

**antineuritic vitamin.** See **thiamine.**

**antineutrophil cytoplasmic antibody test,** a blood test used to diagnose Wegener's granulomatosis (WG). It is also used to follow the course of the disease, monitor its response to therapy, and detect early relapse.

**antinuclear antibody (ANA)** /-nōō′klē·ər/, an autoantibody that reacts with nuclear material. Antinuclear antibodies are found in the blood serum of patients with rheumatoid arthritis, systemic lupus erythematosus, Sjögren's syndrome, polymyositis, and a number of nonrheumatic disorders ranging from lymphomas and leukemias to adverse drug reactions. The antibodies are often detected with an immunofluorescent assay technique.

**antinuclear antibody (ANA) test,** a blood test used primarily to help diagnose systemic lupus erythematosus (SLE), although a positive result may also indicate other autoimmune diseases such as Sjögren's syndrome, scleroderma, Raynaud's disease, mixed connective tissue disease, rheumatoid arthritis, primary biliary cirrhosis, thyroiditis, and chronic active hepatitis.

**antiodontalgia** /an′ti·ō′dontal′jə/, a toothache remedy.

**antioncogene** /an′ti·on′kəjēn/, a tumor-suppressing gene. It may act by controlling cellular growth. When an antioncogene is inactivated, tumor cellular proliferation begins and tumor activity accelerates.

**antioxidant** /-ok′sidənt/, a chemical or other agent that inhibits or retards oxidation of a substance to which it is added. Examples include butylated hydroxyanisole (BHA)

and butylated hydroxytoluene (BHT). These substances are added to foods containing fats or oils to prevent oxygen from combining with the fatty molecules, thereby causing them to become rancid.

**antioxidation** /-ok′sidā′shən/, the prevention of oxidation.

**antiparallel** /-per′ələl/ [Gk, *anti* + *parallelos,* side-by-side], pertaining to molecules, such as strands of DNA, that are parallel but are oriented in opposite directions.

**antiparasitic** /-per′əsit′ik/ [Gk, *anti* + *parasitos,* guest], **1.** pertaining to a substance or procedure that kills parasites or inhibits their growth or reproduction. **2.** an antiparasitic drug such as an amebicide, an anthelmintic, an antimalarial, a schistosomicide, a trichomonacide, or a trypanosomicide.

**antiparkinsonian** /-pär′kənsəniz′əm/, pertaining to a substance or procedure used to treat parkinsonism. Drugs for this neurologic disorder are of two kinds: those that compensate for the lack of dopamine in the corpus striatum of parkinsonism patients, and anticholinergic agents that counteract the activity of the abundant acetylcholine in the striatum. Synthetic levodopa, a dopamine precursor that crosses the blood-brain barrier, is administered to patients to reduce the rigidity, sluggishness, dysphagia, drooling, and instability characteristic of the disease, but the drug does not alter the relentless course of the disorder. Centrally active cholinergic blockers, notably benztropine, biperiden, procyclidine, and trihexyphenidyl, may relieve tremors and rigidity and improve mobility. The antiviral agent amantadine is often effective in the treatment of parkinsonism; its mechanism of action is not established, but it apparently increases release of dopamine in the brain. Therapeutic approaches to the relief of the symptoms of parkinsonism include alcohol injection, cautery, cryosurgery, and surgical excision performed to destroy the globus pallidus (reducing rigidity) and parts of the thalamus (reducing tremor). Extrapyramidal symptoms similar to those of idiopathic parkinsonism are frequently induced by antipsychotic drugs. See also **tardive dyskinesia.**

**antipathic** /-path′ik/, pertaining to a strong or excessive aversion or dislike.

**antipathy** /antip′əthē/ [Gk, *anti* + *pathos,* suffering], a strong feeling of aversion or antagonism to particular objects, situations, or individuals.

**antiperistalsis** /-per′əstal′sis/, a wave of contractions in the digestive tract that moves toward the oral end of the tract. In the duodenum, stomach, or esophagus it results in regurgitation. Also called **reverse peristalsis.**

**antiperistaltic** /-per′əstal′tik/ [Gk, *anti* + *peristellein,* to wrap around], **1.** pertaining to a substance that inhibits or diminishes peristalsis. **2.** an antiperistaltic agent. Opioids, such as paregoric, diphenoxylate, and loperamide hydrochloride, are antiperistaltic agents used to provide symptomatic relief in diarrhea. Anticholinergic (parasympatholytic) drugs reduce spasms of intestinal smooth muscle and are frequently prescribed to decrease excessive GI motility.

**antipernicious anemia factor.** See **cyanocobalamin.**

**antiplatelet** /-plat′lit/, any agent that destroys platelets or inhibits their function.

**antipode** /an′tipōd/, something that is diametrically opposite.

**antipraxia** /prak′sē·ə/, a condition in which functions or symptoms appear to oppose each other.

**antiprogestin** /-prōjes′tin/, a substance that interferes with the production, uptake, or effects of progesterone.

**antiprotease,** a substance that is capable of preventing the digestion of proteins.

**antiprothrombin** /prōthrom′bin/, a substance that inhibits the conversion of prothrombin to thrombin.

**antiprotoplasmatic** /-prō'təplasmat'ik/, pertaining to agents that damage the protoplasm of cells.

**antipruritic** /-prooŏrit'ik/ [Gk, *anti* + L, *prurire,* to itch], **1.** pertaining to a substance or procedure that tends to relieve or prevent itching. **2.** an antipruritic drug. Topical anesthetics, corticosteroids, and antihistamines are used as antipruritic agents.

**antipsoriatic** /an'tisôr'ē·at'ik/ [Gk, *anti* + *psora,* itch], pertaining to an agent that relieves the symptoms of psoriasis.

**antipsychotic** /-sīkot'ik/ [Gk, *anti* + *psyche,* mind, *osis,* condition], **1.** pertaining to a substance or procedure that counteracts or diminishes symptoms of a psychosis. **2.** an antipsychotic drug. Phenothiazine derivatives are the oldest antipsychotics for use in the treatment of schizophrenia and other major affective disorders. They apparently act by enhancing the filtering mechanisms of the reticular formation in the brainstem and by blocking central dopamine receptors. See also **neuroleptic, tranquilizer.**

**antipyresis** /-pīrē'sis/ [Gk, *anti* + *pyretos,* fever], treatment to reduce and ameliorate fever.

**antipyretic** /-pīret'ik/ [Gk, *anti* + *pyretos,* fever], **1.** pertaining to a substance or procedure that reduces fever. **2.** an antipyretic agent. Such drugs usually lower the thermodetection set point of the hypothalamic heat regulatory center, with resulting vasodilation and sweating. Widely used antipyretic agents are acetaminophen, aspirin, and NSAIDs. Also called **antifebrile, antithermic.**

**antipyretic bath,** a bath in which tepid water is used to reduce body temperature.

**antipyrotic** /-pīrot'ik/ [Gk, *anti* + *pyr,* fire], pertaining to the treatment of burns or scalds.

**antirachitic** /-rəkit'ik/, pertaining to an agent used to treat rickets.

**anti-Rh agglutinin,** an antibody to the Rh antigen present on Rh+ red blood cells that causes these cells to clump (agglutinate). This antibody is produced by Rh− persons after exposure to Rh+ red blood cells, as when an Rh− mother is pregnant with an Rh+ fetus.

**antirheumatic** /-rooŏmat'ik/ [Gk, *anti* + *rheumatismos,* that which flows], pertaining to the relief of symptoms of any painful or immobilizing disorder of the musculoskeletal system.

**antiscorbutic vitamin.** See **ascorbic acid.**

**antiseborrheic** /-seb'ərē'ik/, pertaining to a drug or agent that is applied to the skin to control seborrhea or seborrheic dermatitis.

**antisense** /an'tēsens/, pertaining to an RNA molecule that is complementary to the messenger RNA (mRNA) produced by transcription of a given gene. Antisense RNA synthesized in the laboratory will hybridize with the complementary mRNA molecules, thereby blocking the synthesis of specific proteins.

**antisense strand,** the strand of a double-stranded nucleic acid that is complementary to the sense strand, in DNA being thus the template strand on which the mRNA is synthesized. Compare **sense strand.**

**antisepsis** /-sep'sis/ [Gk, *anti* + *sepein,* putrefaction], destruction of microorganisms to prevent infection.

**antiseptic** /-sep'tik/, **1.** tending to inhibit the growth and reproduction of microorganisms. **2.** a substance that tends to inhibit the growth and reproduction of microorganisms.

**antiseptic dressing,** a fabric or pad treated with a solution and applied to a wound or an incision to prevent or treat infection. The solution may be an antiseptic, germicidal, or bacteriostatic.

**antiseptic gauze,** a dressing permeated with a solution to prevent infection.

**antiserum** /an'tisir'əm/, *pl.* **antisera, antiserums** [Gk, *anti* + L, whey], serum of an animal or human containing antibodies against a specific disease, used to confer passive immunity to that disease. Antisera do not provoke the production of antibodies. There are two types of antiserum: antitoxin is an antiserum that neutralizes the toxin produced by specific bacteria, but it does not kill the bacteria; antimicrobial serum acts to destroy bacteria by making them more susceptible to the leukocytic action. Polyvalent antiserum acts on more than one strain of bacteria; monovalent antiserum acts on only one strain. Antibiotic drugs have largely replaced antimicrobial antisera. Caution is always to be used in administration of antiserum of any kind, since hepatitis or hypersensitivity reactions can result. Also called **immune serum.** Compare **vaccine.**

**antiserum anaphylaxis,** an exaggerated hypersensitivity in a normal person after the injection of serum from a sensitized individual. Also called **passive anaphylaxis.** Compare **active anaphylaxis.**

**antishock garment,** trousers designed to apply pressure on circulation in the lower part of the body, thereby increasing the amount of blood in the upper part.

**antisialogog** /-sī·al'əgōg'/ [Gk, *anti* + *sialon,* saliva, *agogos,* leading], a drug that reduces saliva secretion.

**anti-smooth muscle antibody test,** a blood test used primarily to help diagnose autoimmune chronic active hepatitis, although a low-level positive result may also be associated with viral infections, malignancy, multiple sclerosis, primary biliary cirrhosis, and *Mycoplasma* infections.

**antisocial personality** /-sō'shəl/ [Gk, *anti* + L, *socius,* companion], a person who exhibits attitudes and overt behavior contrary to the customs, standards, and moral principles accepted by society. Also called **psychopathic personality, sociopathic personality.** See also **antisocial personality disorder.**

**antisocial personality disorder,** a condition characterized by repetitive behavioral patterns that are contrary to usual moral and ethical standards and cause a person to experience continuous conflict with society. Symptoms include aggressiveness, callousness, impulsiveness, irresponsibility, hostility, a low frustration level, a marked emotional immaturity, and poor judgment. A person who has this disorder overlooks the rights of others, is incapable of loyalty to others or to social values, is unable to experience guilt or to learn from past behaviors, is impervious to punishment, and tends to rationalize his or her behavior or to blame it on others. Also called **antisocial reaction.**

**antispasmodic** /-spazmod'ik/, a drug or other agent that prevents smooth muscle spasms, as in the uterus, digestive system, or urinary tract. Belladonna and dicyclomine hydrochloride are among drugs used in antispasmodic preparations. See also **anticholinergic, cholinergic blocking agent.**

**antispermatozoal antibody test,** a fluid analysis or blood test used as an infertility screening test. The test may be done on both men and women to detect the presence of sperm antibodies that may diminish fertility.

**antistreptolysin-O test (ASOT, ASO, ASLT)** /an'tistrep'təlī'sinō'/, a streptococcal antibody test for finding and measuring serum antibodies to streptolysin-O, an exotoxin produced by most group A and some group C and G streptococci. The test is often used as an aid in the diagnosis of rheumatic fever and glomerulonephritis. A low titer of antistreptolysin-O antibody is present in most people, since streptococcal infection is common. Elevated or increasing titers indicate a recent infection. The normal findings for adults are equal to or less than 160 Todd units/ml. See also **Lancefield's classification.**

**antithermic.** See **antipyretic.**

**antithrombin** /-throm'bin/, a substance that inhibits the action of thrombin.

**antithrombotic** /-thrombot'ik/, preventing or interfering with the formation of a thrombus or blood coagulation.

**antithymocyte globulin (ATG)** /an'tithī'məsīt/, a gamma globulin fraction rendered immune to T lymphocytes.

**antithyroglobulin antibody test,** a blood test used primarily in the differential diagnosis of thyroid diseases such as Hashimoto's thyroiditis or chronic lymphocytic thyroiditis in children. This test is usually performed in conjunction with the antithyroid microsomal antibody test.

**antithyroid drug** /-thī'roid/, a preparation that inhibits the synthesis of thyroid hormones and is commonly used in the treatment of hyperthyroidism. The major antithyroid drugs are thioamides, such as propylthiouracil, and methimazole. In the body such substances interfere with the incorporation of iodine into the tyrosyl residues of thyroglobulin required for the production of the hormones thyroxine and triiodothyronine. These drugs are often used to control hyperthyroidism during an anticipated remission and before a thyroidectomy.

**antithyroid microsomal antibody test,** a blood test used primarily in the differential diagnosis of thyroid diseases such as Hashimoto's thyroiditis or chronic lymphocytic thyroiditis in children. This test is usually performed in conjunction with the antithyroglobulin antibody test.

**antitoxin** /-tok'sin/ [Gk, *anti* + *toxikon,* poison], a subgroup of antisera usually prepared from the serum of horses immunized against a particular toxin-producing organism, such as botulism antitoxin given therapeutically in botulism and tetanus and diphtheria antitoxins given prophylactically to prevent those infections.

**antitrismus** /-tris'məs/, a tonic muscular spasm that forces the mouth to open.

**antitrust** /-trust'/, (in law) against the operation, establishment, or maintenance of a monopoly in the manufacture, production, or sale of a commodity, provision of a service, or practice of a profession.

**antitrypsin** /-trip'sin/, a protein, produced in the liver, that blocks the action of trypsin and other proteolytic enzymes. A deficiency of antitrypsin is associated with emphysema, in which the basic lesion is believed to result from effects of proteolytic enzymes on the walls of the alveoli. Also called **alpha-antitrypsin.**

**antitubercular** /-tŏŏbur'kyələr/, any agent or group of drugs used to treat tuberculosis. At least two drugs, and usually three, are required in various combinations in pulmonary tuberculosis therapy. These include isoniazid (INH), ethambutol (EMB), streptomycin (SM), and rifampin (RMP). Supplements of pyridoxine (vitamin $B_6$) also may be needed to relieve the symptoms of peripheral neuritis that can occur as an INH side effect.

**antitumor antibodies,** natural products that interfere with deoxyribonucleic acid (DNA) in such a way as to prevent its further replication and the transcription of ribonucleic acid.

**antitussive** /an'titus'iv/ [Gk, *anti* + L, *tussive,* cough], **1.** against a cough. **2.** any of a large group of opioid and nonopioid drugs that act on the central and peripheral nervous systems to suppress the cough reflex. Because the cough reflex is necessary for clearing the upper respiratory tract of obstructive secretions, antitussives should not be used with a productive cough. Codeine and hydrocodone are potent opioid antitussives. Dextromethorphan is an effective antitussive with no dependence liability. Antitussives are administered orally, usually in a syrup with a mucolytic or expectorant and alcohol, or, sometimes, in a capsule with an antihistaminic and a mild analgesic.

**antivenin** /an'tiven'in/ [Gk, *anti* + L, *venenum,* poison], a suspension of venom-neutralizing antibodies prepared from the serum of immunized horses. Antivenin confers passive immunity and is given as a part of emergency first aid for various snake and insect bites. Also called **antivenom.**

**Antivert,** trademark for an antihistaminic antivertigo agent (meclizine hydrochloride).

**antiviral,** destructive to viruses.

**antivitamin factor** [Gk, *anti* + L, *vita,* life, amine], a substance that inactivates a vitamin.

**antixerophthalmic vitamin.** See **vitamin A.**

**Anton's syndrome** [Gabriel Anton, German neuropsychiatrist, 1858–1933], a form of anosognosia in which a person with partial or total blindness denies being visually impaired, despite medical evidence to the contrary. The patient typically contrives excuses for the inability to see, such as suggesting that the light is inadequate.

**antr-.** See **antro-.**

**antra.** See **antrum.**

**antral gastritis** [Gk, *antron,* cave], an abnormal narrowing of the antrum, or distal portion of the stomach. The narrowing is not a true gastritis, but a radiographic finding that may represent gastric ulcer or tumor.

**antrectomy** /antrek'təmē/, the surgical excision of the pyloric part of the stomach.

**antro-, antr-,** prefix meaning 'antrum or sinus': *antrocele, antrodynia.*

**antrum,** *pl.* **antra** [Gk, *antron,* cave], a cavity or chamber that is nearly closed and usually surrounded by bone. The cardiac antrum is a dilation of the esophagus. The fluid-filled cavity in a mature graafian follicle is also termed an antrum.

**antrum cardiacum** /an'trəm/, a constricted passage from the esophagus to the stomach, lying just inside the opening formed by the cardiac sphincter.

**antrum of Highmore.** See **maxillary sinus.**

**Anturane,** trademark for a uricosuric (sulfinpyrazone).

**ANUG,** abbreviation for **acute necrotizing ulcerative gingivitis.**

**anular** /an'yələr/ [L, *annulus,* ring], describing a ring-shaped lesion surrounding a clear, normal, unaffected disk of skin.

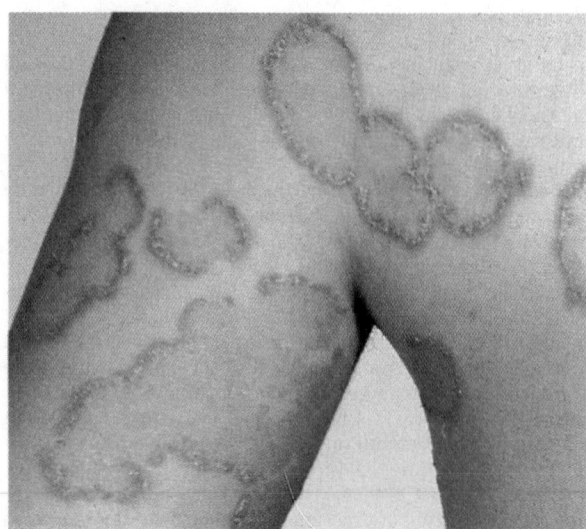

**Anular psoriasis** *(du Vivier, 1993)*

**anular ligament,** a ligament that encircles the head of the radius and holds it in the radial notch of the ulna. Distal to the notch, the anular ligament forms a complete fibrous ring.

**anulus** /an'yələs/, a ring of circular tissue, such as the whitish tympanic anulus around the perimeter of the tympanic membrane.

**anuresis.** See **anuria.**

**anuria** /ənŏŏr'ē·ə/ [Gk, *a, ouron,* not urine], the absence of urine production or a urinary output of less than 100 ml per day. Anuria may be caused by kidney failure or dysfunction, a decline in blood pressure below that required to maintain filtration pressure in the kidney, or an obstruction in the urinary passages. A rapid decline in urinary output, leading ultimately to anuria and uremia, occurs in acute renal failure. Kinds of anuria include **angioneurotic anuria, obstructive anuria, postrenal anuria, prerenal anuria,** and **renal anuria.** Also called **anuresis** /an'yŏŏrē'sis/. —**anuric, anuretic,** *adj.* Compare **oliguria.**

**anus** /ā'nəs/, the outlet at the terminal end of the anal canal lying in the fold between the buttocks.

**anxietas** /angzī'ətas/ [L, anxiety], a state of anxiety, nervous restlessness, or apprehension, often accompanied by a feeling of oppression in the epigastrium. Kinds of anxietas are **anxietas presenilis** and **restless legs syndrome.**

**anxietas presenilis** [L, *anxietas + prae,* before, *senex,* aged], a state of extreme anxiety associated with the climacteric period of life.

**anxietas tibiarum.** See **restless legs syndrome.**

**anxiety**[1] /angzī'ətē/ [L *anxietas*], anticipation of impending danger and dread accompanied by restlessness, tension, tachycardia, and breathing difficulty not associated with an apparent stimulus. Kinds of anxiety include **castration anxiety, generalized** or **"free-floating" anxiety, separation anxiety, panic anxiety,** and **situational anxiety.**

**anxiety**[2], a nursing diagnosis accepted by the Fifth National Conference on the Classification of Nursing Diagnoses. Anxiety is defined as a vague, uneasy feeling, the source of which is often nonspecific or unknown to the individual.

■ DEFINING CHARACTERISTICS: The defining characteristics of anxiety may be subjective or objective. Subjective characteristics include increased tension, apprehension, persistent increased helplessness, and feelings of uncertainty, inadequacy, fear, overexcitability, distress, worry, and impending doom. Objective characteristics include increased heart rate, dilated pupils, restlessness, insomnia, glancing about, poor eye contact, trembling, facial tension, quivering voice, self-focus, increased perspiration, and expressed concern regarding life events.

■ RELATED FACTORS: Related factors include an unconscious conflict regarding essential values or goals of life; threat to self-concept; threat of death; threat to or of change in health status, the environment, or interaction patterns; situational or maturational crises; interpersonal transmission of contagion, and unmet needs.

**anxiety attack,** an acute, psychobiologic reaction manifested by intense anxiety and panic. Symptoms include palpitations, shortness of breath, dizziness, faintness, profuse sweating, pallor of the face and extremities, GI discomfort, and a vague feeling of imminent doom or death. Attacks usually occur suddenly, last from a few seconds to an hour or longer, and vary in frequency from several times a day to once a month. Treatment consists of reassurance, separation of the individual from anxiety-producing situations, administration of a sedative if necessary, and appropriate psychotherapy to identify the stresses perceived as threatening. See also **anxiety.**

**anxiety complex.** See **castration anxiety.**

**Physiological, behavioral, cognitive, and affective responses to anxiety**

| Physiological | Physiological—cont'd | Behavioral | Cognitive | Affective |
|---|---|---|---|---|
| *Cardiovascular* | *Neuromuscular* | Restlessness | Impaired attention | Edginess |
| Palpitations | Increased reflexes | Physical tension | Poor concentration | Impatience |
| Heart racing | Startle reaction | Tremors | Forgetfulness | Uneasiness |
| Increased blood pressure | Eyelid twitching | Startle reaction | Errors in judgment | Tension |
| Faintness* | Insomnia | Rapid speech | Preoccupation | Nervousness |
| Actual fainting* | Tremors | Lack of coordination | Blocking of thoughts | Fear |
| Decreased blood pressure* | Rigidity | Accident proneness | Decreased perceptual field | Fright |
| Decreased pulse rate* | Fidgeting | Interpersonal withdrawal | Reduced creativity | Alarm |
| | Pacing | Inhibition | Diminished productivity | Terror |
| *Respiratory* | Strained face | Flight | Confusion | Jitteriness |
| Rapid breathing | Generalized weakness | Avoidance | Hypervigilance | Jumpiness |
| Shortness of breath | Wobbly legs | Hyperventilation | Self-consciousness | |
| Pressure on chest | Clumsy movement | | Loss of objectivity | |
| Shallow breathing | | | Fear of losing control | |
| Lump in throat | *Urinary Tract* | | Frightening visual images | |
| Choking sensation | Pressure to urinate* | | Fear of injury or death | |
| Gasping | Frequency to urination* | | | |
| *Gastrointestinal* | *Skin* | | | |
| Loss of appetite | Face flushed | | | |
| Revulsion toward food | Localized sweating (palms) | | | |
| Abdominal discomfort | Itching | | | |
| Abdominal pain* | Hot and cold spells | | | |
| Nausea* | Face pale | | | |
| Heartburn* | Generalized sweating | | | |
| Diarrhea* | | | | |

From Stuart GW, Sundeen: *Principles and practice of psychiatric nursing,* ed 5, St Louis, 1995, Mosby.
*Parasympathetic response.

**anxiety control,** a nursing outcome from the Nursing Outcomes Classification (NOC) defined as personal actions to eliminate or reduce feelings of apprehension and tension from an unidentifiable source. See also **Nursing Outcomes Classification.**

**anxiety, death,** a nursing diagnosis accepted by the Thirteenth National Conference on the Classification of Nursing Diagnoses. The condition is the apprehension, worry, or fear related to death or dying.

■ DEFINING CHARACTERISTICS: The condition is characterized by worrying about the impact of one's own death on significant others; feelings of powerlessness over issues related to dying; fear of loss of physical and/or mental abilities when dying; anticipated pain related to dying; deep sadness; fear of the process of dying; concerns of overworking the caregiver as terminal illness incapacitates self; concern about meeting one's creator or feeling doubtful about the existence of a higher being; total loss of control over any aspect of one's death; negative death images or unpleasant thoughts about any event related to death or dying; fear of delayed demise; fear of premature death because it prevents the accomplishment of important life goals; worry about being the cause of other's grief and suffering; fear of leaving family alone after death; fear of developing a terminal illness, and denial of one's own mortality or impending death.

■ RELATED FACTORS: Related factors are to be developed. See also **nursing diagnosis.**

**anxiety disorder,** a disorder in which anxiety is the most prominent feature. The symptoms range from mild, chronic tenseness, with feelings of timidity, fatigue, apprehension, and indecisiveness, to more intense states of restlessness and irritability that may lead to aggressive acts, persistent helplessness, or withdrawal. In extreme cases, the overwhelming emotional discomfort is accompanied by physical responses, including tremor, sustained muscle tension, tachycardia, dyspnea, hypertension, increased respiration, and profuse perspiration. Other physical signs include changes in skin color, nausea, vomiting, diarrhea, restlessness, immobilization, insomnia, and changes in appetite, all occurring without identification of a known underlying organic cause. See also **anxiety, anxiety attack, anxiety reaction, anxiety state, obsessive-compulsive disorder, phobia.**

**anxiety dream,** a dream that is accompanied by restlessness and a gradual increase in pulse rate. Anxiety dreams tend to occur in children, who usually recall the content clearly.

**anxiety reaction** [L, *anxietas + re, agere,* to act], a clinical characteristic in which anxiety is the predominant feature or is experienced by a person facing a dreaded situation to the extent that his or her functioning is impaired. The reaction may be expressed as a panic disorder, a phobia, or a compulsion.

**anxiety reduction,** a nursing intervention from the Nursing Interventions Classification (NIC) defined as minimizing apprehension, dread, foreboding, or uneasiness related to an unidentified source of anticipated danger. See also **Nursing Interventions Classification.**

**anxiety state** [L, *anxietas + state*], a mental or emotional reaction characterized by apprehension, uncertainty, and irrational fear. Anxiety states may be accompanied by physiologic changes such as sweating, tremors, rapid heartbeat, dilated pupils, and dry mouth.

**anxiolytic** /angk′sē-ōlit′ik/, a drug used primarily to treat episodes of anxiety. Common kinds of anxiolytics include barbiturates, benzodiazepines, and busperone.

**AOA,** abbreviation for **Administration on Aging.**

**AORN,** abbreviation for **Association of Operating Room Nurses.**

**aorta** /ā·ôr′tə/ [Gk, *aerein,* to raise], the main trunk of the systemic arterial circulation, comprising four parts: the ascending aorta, the arch of the aorta, the thoracic portion of the descending aorta, and the abdominal portion of the descending aorta. It starts at the aortic opening of the left ventricle, rises a short distance, bends over the root of the left lung, descends within the thorax on the left side of the vertebral column, and passes through the aortic hiatus of the diaphragm into the abdominal cavity. It branches into the two common iliac arteries.

**aortic** /ā·ôr′tik/ [Gk, *aerein,* to raise], pertaining to the aorta.

**aortic aneurysm,** a localized dilation of the wall of the aorta caused by atherosclerosis, hypertension, or, less frequently, syphilis. The lesion may be a saccular distension, a fusiform or cylindrical swelling of a length of the vessel, or a longitudinal dissection between the outer and middle layers of the vessel wall. Syphilitic aneurysms almost always occur in the thoracic aorta and usually involve the aortic arch. The more common atherosclerotic aneurysms are usually in the abdominal aorta below the renal arteries and above the bifurcation of the aorta. These lesions often contain atheromatous ulcers covered by thrombi that may discharge emboli, causing obstruction of smaller vessels. See also **dissecting aneurysm.**

**aortic angiogram.** See **aortogram.**

**aortic arch.** See **arch of the aorta.**

**aortic arch syndrome,** any of a group of occlusive conditions of the aortic arch producing a variety of symptoms related to obstruction of the large branch arteries, including the brachiocephalic, left common carotid, and left subclavian. It may be caused by atherosclerosis, Takayasu's arteritis, syphilis, and other conditions. Symptoms include syncope, temporary blindness, hemiplegia, aphasia, and memory loss.

**aortic atresia** [Gk, *aeirein + a, tresis,* a boring], a congenital anomaly in which the left side of the heart is defective and there is an imperforation of the aortic valve into the aorta.

**aortic balloon pump.** See **intraaortic balloon pump.**

**aortic body,** one of several small structures on the aortic arch that contain neural tissue sensitive to the chemical composition of arterial blood. The aortic bodies respond primarily to large reductions in blood oxygen content and trigger an increase in respiratory rate. See also **aortic-body reflex, carotid body.**

**aortic-body reflex,** a neural reflex in which a decrease in the oxygen content of arterial blood is sensed by the aortic bodies, which signal the medullary respiratory center to increase respiratory rate. See also **carotid-body reflex.**

**aortic insufficiency.** See **aortic regurgitation.**

**aortic notch** [Gk, *aeirein,* to raise; OFr, *enochier*], the dicrotic notch on the descending limb of an arterial pulse sphygmogram. It marks the closure of the aortic valve.

**aortic obstruction** [L, *obstruere,* to build against], a blockage or impediment that interrupts the flow of blood in the aorta.

**aortic regurgitant murmur** [Gk, *aeirein,* to raise; L, *re,* again, *gurgitare,* to flow, *murmur,* humming], a high-pitched, soft, blowing, decrescendo, early diastolic heart murmur that is a sign of aortic regurgitation.

**aortic regurgitation,** the flow of blood from the aorta back into the left ventricle during diastole, resulting from a failure of the aortic valve to close completely. Also called **aortic insufficiency.**

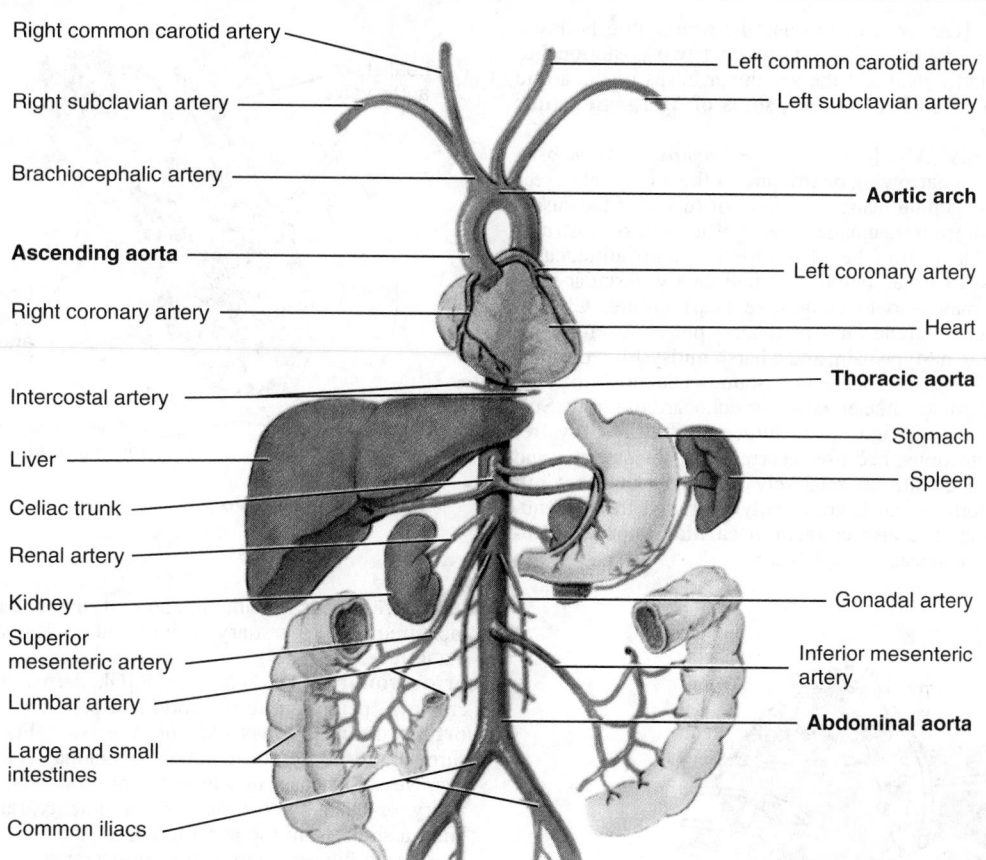

Right common carotid artery

Right subclavian artery

Brachiocephalic artery

**Ascending aorta**

Right coronary artery

Intercostal artery

Liver

Celiac trunk

Renal artery

Kidney

Superior mesenteric artery

Lumbar artery

Large and small intestines

Common iliacs

Left common carotid artery

Left subclavian artery

**Aortic arch**

Left coronary artery

Heart

**Thoracic aorta**

Stomach

Spleen

Gonadal artery

Inferior mesenteric artery

**Abdominal aorta**

**Branches of the aorta** *(Applegate, 2000)*

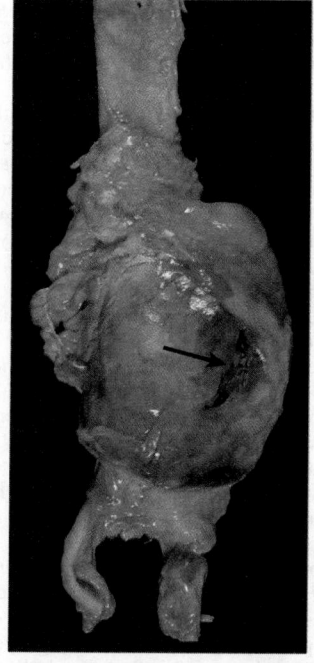

**Ruptured abdominal aortic aneurysm**
*(Cotran, Kumar, and Collins, 1999)*

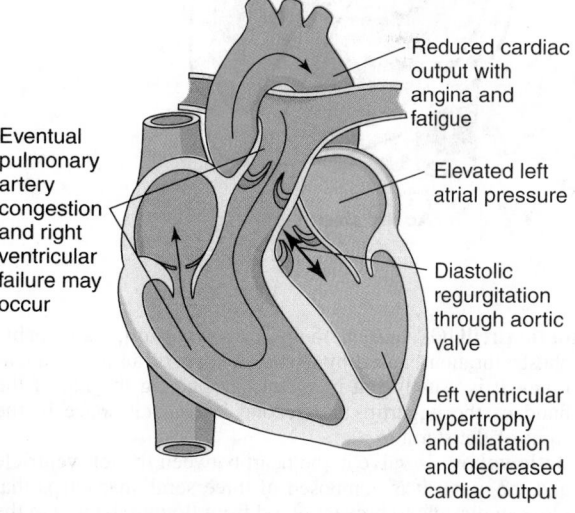

Eventual pulmonary artery congestion and right ventricular failure may occur

Reduced cardiac output with angina and fatigue

Elevated left atrial pressure

Diastolic regurgitation through aortic valve

Left ventricular hypertrophy and dilatation and decreased cardiac output

**Effects of aortic regurgitation** *(Beare and Myers, 1998)*

**aortic sinus** [Gk, *aeirein*, to raise; L, *sinus*, little hollow], any of three dilations, one anterior and two posterior, between the aortic wall and the semilunar cusps of the aortic valve. Also called **Petit's sinus, sinus of Morgagni, sinus of Valsalva.**

**aortic stenosis (AS)** [Gk, *aeirein* + *stenos*, narrow, *osis*, condition], a narrowing or stricture of the aortic valve secondary to congenital malformation or of fusion of the cusps, as may result from rheumatic fever. Aortic stenosis obstructs the flow of blood from the left ventricle into the aorta, causing decreased cardiac output and pulmonary vascular congestion. It may lead to congestive heart failure. Clinical manifestations include faint peripheral pulses, exercise intolerance, angina-type pain, and a harsh midsystolic murmur often introduced by an ejection sound. Diagnosis is confirmed by cardiac catheterization or echocardiography. Surgical repair may be indicated. Surgery is followed by frequent examinations, because recurrence of the stenosis and bacterial endocarditis are relatively common sequelae. Children with aortic stenosis are usually restricted from strenuous, activities. See also **congenital cardiac anomaly, valvular heart disease.**

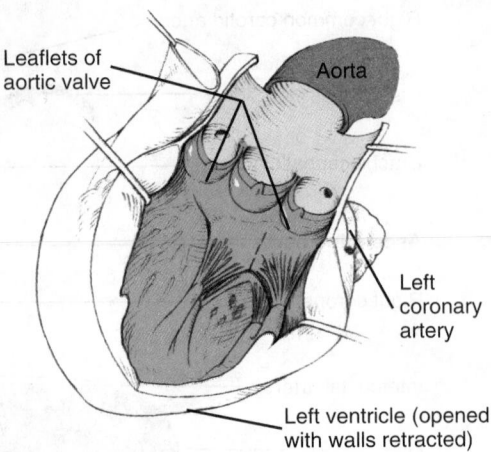

Leaflets of aortic valve

Aorta

Left coronary artery

Left ventricle (opened with walls retracted)

**Aortic valve** *(Stanford Project, 1996)*

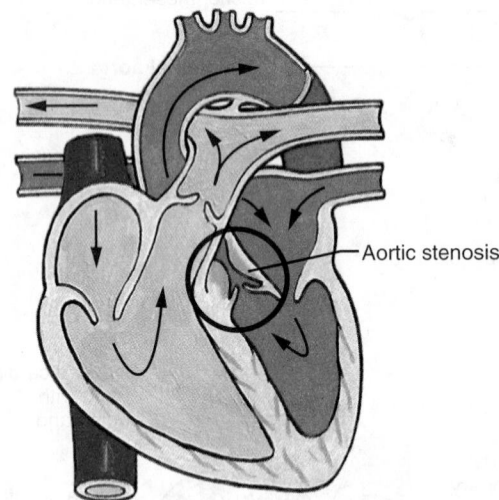

Aortic stenosis

**Aortic stenosis** *(Wong, 1999)*

**aortic thrill** [Gk, *aeirein*, to raise; AS, *thyrlian*], a palpable chest vibration caused by aortic stenosis or an aortic aneurysm. It is usually felt in systole by placing the flat of the hand or the fingertips the second intercostal space to the right of the sternum.

**aortic valve,** a valve in the heart between the left ventricle and the aorta. It is composed of three semilunar cusps that close in diastole to prevent blood from flowing back into the left ventricle from the aorta. The three cusps are separated by sinuses that resemble tiny buckets when they are filled with blood. These cup-shaped flaps grow from the lining of the aorta and, in systole, open to allow oxygenated blood to flow from the left ventricle into the aorta and on to the peripheral circulation. Compare **mitral valve, pulmonary valve, tricuspid valve.**

**aortic valvular stenosis.** See **subaortic stenosis.**

**aortitis** /ā′ôrtī′tis/, inflammation of the aorta. It occurs most frequently in tertiary syphilis and occasionally in rheumatic fever.

**aortocoronary** /ā·ôr′tōkôr′əner′ē/ [Gk, *aeirein* + L, *corona*, crown], pertaining to the aorta and coronary arteries.

**aortocoronary bypass** [AS, *bi*, alongside; Fr, *passer*], a surgical procedure, for treatment of angina pectoris or coronary vessel disease, in which a saphenous vein, mammary artery, or other blood vessel or a synthetic graft is used to build a shunt from the aorta to one of the coronary arteries in order to bypass a circulatory obstruction.

**aortogram** /ā·ôr′təgram/ [Gk, *aerein* + *gramma*, record], a radiographic image of the aorta made after the injection of a radiopaque contrast medium in the blood. Also called **aortogram.**

**aortography** /ā·ôrtog′rəfē/ [Gk, *aerein* + *graphein*, to record], a radiographic process in which the aorta and its branches are injected with any of various contrast media for visualization. —**aortographic,** *adj.*

**aortopulmonary fenestration** /ā·ôr′tōpul′məner′ē/ [Gk, *aerein* + L, *pulmoneus*, lung, *fenestra*, window], a congenital anomaly characterized by an abnormal fenestration in the ascending aorta and the pulmonary artery cephalad to the semilunar valve, allowing oxygenated and unoxygenated blood to mix, resulting in a decrease in the oxygen available in the peripheral circulation.

**aosmic.** See **anosmia.**

**AOTA,** abbreviation for **American Occupational Therapy Association.**

**AOTF,** abbreviation for *American Occupational Therapy Foundation.*

**ap-, apo-,** prefix meaning 'separation or derivation from; away from': *apeidosis, aponeurosis.*

**AP,** abbreviation for **anteroposterior.**

**APA,** 1. abbreviation for **American Psychiatric Association.** 2. abbreviation for *American Psychological Association.*

**APACHE** /əpach′ē/, abbreviation for *Acute Physiology and Chronic Health Evaluation,* a system of classifying severity of illnesses in intensive care patients.

**apareunia** /ā′pərōō′nē·ə/, an inability to perform sexual intercourse caused by a physical or psychologic sexual dysfunction.

**apathetic.** See **apathy.**

**apathetic hyperthyroidism** /ap'əthet'ik/, a form of thyrotoxicosis that tends to affect mainly older adults who have stereotyped "senile" physical features and whose behavior is apathetic and inactive rather than hyperkinetic. Medical treatment not only restores normal behavioral activity but also results in a loss of wrinkles and a more youthful physical appearance. Untreated, the patient is likely to succumb to the effects of stress or acute illness.

**apathy** /ap'əthē/ [Gk, *a, pathos,* not suffering], an absence or suppression of emotion, feeling, concern, or passion; an indifference to stimuli found generally to be exciting or moving. The condition is common in patients with neurasthenia, depressive disorders, and schizophrenia. —**apathetic,** *adj.*

**apatite** /ap'ətīt/ [Gk, *apate,* deceit], an inorganic mineral composed of calcium and phosphate that is found in the bones and teeth.

**APC,** **1.** abbreviation for **aspirin, phenacetin, caffeine.** **2.** abbreviation for *atrial premature contraction.* **3.** abbreviation for **adenomatous polyposis coli.**

**APD,** abbreviation for **adult polycystic disease.** See **polycystic kidney disease.**

**apepsia** /āpep'sē·ə/ [Gk, *a,* without, *pepsis,* digestion], a condition involving a failure of the digestive functions.

**aperient** /əpir'ē·ənt/ [L, *aperire,* to open], a mild laxative.

**aperistalsis** /āper'istal'sis/ [Gk, *a,* without, *peristellein,* to clasp], a failure of the normal waves of contraction and relaxation that move contents through the digestive tract.

**aperitive** /əper'itiv/ [L, *aperere,* to open], a stimulant of the appetite. Also called **aperitif** /əper'itif/.

**Apert's syndrome** /äperz'/ [Eugene Apert, French pediatrician, 1868–1940], a rare condition characterized by an abnormal craniofacial appearance in combination with partial or complete fusion of the fingers and toes. The specific cause of Apert's syndrome is unknown, but the condition appears to be the result of a primary germ plasm defect. A characteristic feature is the premature joining of cranial bones, with resultant growth disturbances. Signs of Apert's syndrome include a peaked and vertically elongated head, widespread and bulging eyes, and a high, arched posterior palate with bony defects of the maxilla and the mandible. The degree of fusion varies greatly and may be complete. Also called **acrocephalosyndactyly; acrocephalosyndactyly, type I.** See also **acrocephalosyndactyly.**

**aperture** /ap'ərchər/ [L, *apertura,* an opening], an opening or hole in an object or anatomic structure.

**aperture of frontal sinus,** an external opening of the frontal sinus into the nasal cavity.

**aperture of glottis,** an opening between the true vocal cords and the arytenoid cartilages.

**aperture of larynx,** an opening between the pharynx and larynx.

**aperture of sphenoid sinus,** a round opening between the sphenoid sinus and nasal cavity, situated just above the superior nasal concha.

**apex** /ā'peks/, *pl.* **apices** /ā'pisēz/ [L, tip], the top, the end, the summit, or the extremity of a structure, such as the apex of the heart or the apices of the teeth.

**apex beat,** a pulsation of the left ventricle of the heart, palpable and sometimes visible at the fifth intercostal space, approximately 9 cm to the left of the midline. Also called **apical beat.**

**apexcardiogram (ACG)** /-kär'dē·əgram'/, a graphic representation of the pulsations of the chest over the heart in the region of the cardiac apex. The purpose is to provide additional information regarding the diagnosis of ventricular abnormalities.

**apexcardiography (ACG)** /-kär'dē·og'rəfē/, the recording of heart pulsations obtained from the cardiac apex.

**apex cordis** [L, *apex + cordis,* of the heart], the pointed lower border of the heart. It is directed downward, forward, and to the left and is usually located at the level of the fifth intercostal space.

**apexification** /-if'ikā'shən/ [L, *apex + facere,* to make], a process of inducing tooth root development, usually by repeated treatments with calcium hydroxide, or of promoting apical closure of the root by the placement of hard material after an apicoectomy.

**apexigraph** /āpek'sigraf'/, a device used for determining the position of the apex of a tooth root.

**apex murmur** [L, *apex,* summit, *murmur,* humming], a heart sound heard best at the apex of the heart, which in most individuals is at the level of the fifth intercostal space. Also called **apical murmur.**

**apex of the lung,** the highest point of the lung as it extends to the level of the first rib at the base of the neck.

**apex pneumonia** [L, *apex,* summit; Gk, *pnemon,* lung], pneumonia in which consolidation is limited to the upper lobe of one lung. Also called **apical pneumonia.**

**apex pulmonis** /pəlmō'nis/ [L, *apex + pulmoneus,* lung], the rounded upper border of each lung, projecting above the clavicle.

**Apgar score** /ap'gär/ [Virginia Apgar, American anesthesiologist, 1909–1974], the evaluation of an infant's physical condition, usually performed 1 minute and again 5 minutes after birth, based on a rating of five factors that reflect the infant's ability to adjust to extrauterine life. Virginia Apgar, M.D., developed the system for the rapid identification of infants requiring immediate intervention or transfer to an intensive care nursery.

■ METHOD: The infant's heart rate, respiratory effort, muscle tone, reflex irritability, and color are scored from a low value of 0 to a normal value of 2. The five scores are combined, and the totals at 1 minute and 5 minutes are noted; for example, Apgar 9/10 is a score of 9 at 1 minute and 10 at 5 minutes.

■ NURSING CONSIDERATIONS: A low 1-minute score requires immediate intervention, including administration of oxygen, clearing of the nasopharynx, and usually transfer to an intensive care nursery. A baby with a low score that persists at 5 minutes requires expert care, which may include assisted ventilation, umbilical catheterization, cardiac massage, blood gas evaluation, correction of acid-base deficit, or medication to reverse the effects of maternal medication.

### Infant evaluation at birth: Apgar scoring system

| Sign | 0 | 1 | 2 |
| --- | --- | --- | --- |
| Heart rate | Absent | Slow, <100 | >100 |
| Respiratory effort | Absent | Irregular, slow, weak cry | Good, strong cry |
| Muscle tone | Limp | Some flexion of extremities | Well flexed |
| Reflex irritability | No response | Grimace | Cry, sneeze |
| Color | Blue, pale | Body pink, extremities blue | Completely pink |

From Wong DL: Whaley and Wong's *essentials of pediatric nursing,* ed 6, St Louis, 2001, Mosby.

■ OUTCOME CRITERIA: A score of 0 to 3 represents severe distress, a score of 4 to 7 indicates moderate distress, and a score of 7 to 10 indicates an absence of difficulty in adjusting to extrauterine life. The 5-minute total score is normally higher than the 1-minute score. Because a normal, vigorous, healthy newborn almost always has bluish hands and feet at 1 minute, the first score for color will include a 1 rather than a perfect 2; however, at 5 minutes the blueness may have passed, and a score of 2 may be given. A 5-minute overall score of 0 to 1 correlates with a 50% neonatal mortality rate; infants who survive exhibit three times as many neurologic abnormalities at 1 year of age as do children with a 5-minute score of 7 or more.

**APHA,** abbreviation for *American Public Health Association.*

**aphacia, aphacic.** See **aphakia.**

**aphagia** /əfā′jē·ə/ [Gk, *a* + *phagein*, not to eat], a condition characterized by the loss of the ability to swallow as a result of organic or psychologic causes. A kind of aphagia is **aphagia algera.** See also **dysphagia.**

**aphagia algera,** a condition characterized by the refusal to eat or swallow because doing so causes pain.

**aphakia** /əfā′kē·ə/ [Gk, *a, phakos*, not lens], (in ophthalmology) a condition in which the crystalline lens of the eye is absent, usually because it has been surgically removed, as in the treatment of cataracts. Also called **aphacia** /əfā′shə/. —**aphakic, aphacic,** *adj.*

**aphakic** /əfākik/ [Gk, *a*, without, *phakos*, lens], pertaining to the absence of the lens of the eye as a result of a congenital or surgical cause.

**aphasia** /əfā′zhə/ [Gk, *a* + *phasis*, not speech], an abnormal neurologic condition in which language function is disordered or absent because of an injury to certain areas of the cerebral cortex. The deficiency may be sensory or receptive, in which language is not understood, or expressive or motor, in which words cannot be formed or expressed. Aphasia may be complete or partial, affecting specific language functions. Most commonly, the condition is a mixture of incomplete expressive and receptive aphasia. It may occur after severe head trauma, prolonged hypoxia, or cardiovascular accident. It is sometimes transient, as when the swelling in the brain that follows a stroke or injury subsides and language returns. See also **Broca's area, Wernicke's aphasia**—**aphasic,** *adj.*

**aphemia** /əfē′mē·ə/, a loss of the ability to speak. The term is applied to emotional disorders as well as neurologic causes. A person may be **aphemic** because a fear of speaking or a refusal to participate in verbal communication.

**apheresis** /əfer′əsis, af′ərē′sis/ [Gk, *aphairesis*, removal], a procedure in which blood is temporarily withdrawn, one or more components are selectively removed, and the rest of the blood is reinfused into the donor. The process is used in treating various disease conditions in the donor and for obtaining blood elements for treatment of other patients or for research purposes. Also called **pheresis.** See also **leukapheresis, plasmapheresis, plateletpheresis.**

**-aphia, -haphia,** suffix meaning a 'condition of the sense of touch': *hyperaphia, paraphia.*

**aphonia** /āfō′nē·ə/ [Gk, *a, phone,* without voice], a condition characterized by loss of the ability to produce normal speech sounds that results from overuse of the vocal cords, organic disease, or psychologic causes, such as anxiety. Kinds of aphonia include **aphonia clericorum, aphonia paralytica, aphonia paranoica,** and **spastic aphonia.** See also **speech dysfunction.** —**aphonic, aphonous,** *adj.*

**aphonia paralytica** /par′əlit′ikə/, a condition characterized by a loss of the voice caused by paralysis or disease of the laryngeal nerves.

**aphonia paranoica,** an inability to speak that lacks an organic basis and that is characteristic of some forms of mental illness.

**aphonic.** See **aphonia.**

**aphonic pectoriloquy** /āfon′ik/, the abnormal transmission of voice sounds through a cavity or a serous pleural effusion, detected during auscultation of a lung.

**aphonic speech,** abnormal speech in which vocalizations are whispered.

**aphonous.** See **aphonia.**

**aphoria** /əfôr′ē·ə/, a condition in which physical weakness is not lessened as a result of exercise.

**aphrasia** /əfrā′zhə/, a form of aphasia in which a person may be able to speak single words or understand single words but is not able to communicate with words that are arranged in meaningful phrases or sentences.

**-aphrodisia,** suffix meaning a '(specified) condition of sexual arousal': *anaphrodisia, hypaphrodisia.*

**aphronia** /əfrō′nē·ə/ [Gk, *a, phronein,* not to understand], (in psychiatry) a condition characterized by an impaired ability to make commonsense decisions. —**aphronic,** *n., adj.*

**aphthae** /af′thē/ [Gk, *aphtha,* eruption], a common condition of shallow, painful ulcerations that usually affect the oral mucosa but not underlying bone. Aphthae occasionally may affect other body tissues, including those of the GI tract and the external genitalia. See also **aphthous stomatitis, foot-and-mouth disease.** —**aphthous,** *adj.*

**aphthous fever.** See **foot-and-mouth disease.**

**aphthous stomatitis** /af′thəs/ [Gk, *aptha,* eruption; *stoma,* mouth, *itis* inflammation], a recurring condition characterized by the eruption of painful ulcers (commonly called canker sores) on the mucous membranes of the mouth. Evidence suggests that the condition is an immune reaction. Heredity, some foods, emotional stress, cancer, and fever are also possible causes. See also **canker sore.**

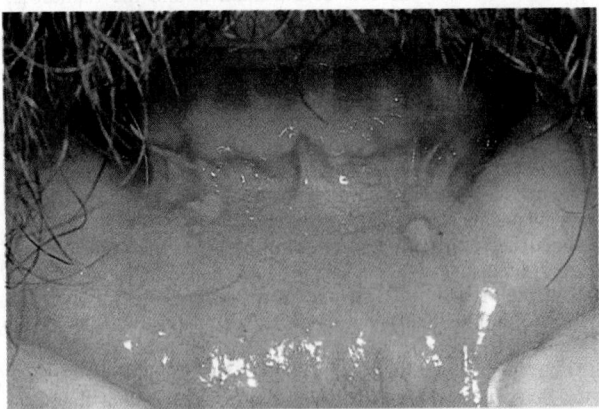

**Aphthous stomatitis** *(Michelson and Friedlaender, 1996)*

**APIC,** abbreviation for **Association for Professionals in Infection Control and Epidemiology.**

**apical** /ap′ikəl, ā′pi-/ [L, *apex,* tip], **1.** pertaining to the summit or apex. **2.** pertaining to the end of a tooth root or the lumenal surface of a cell.

**apical beat.**  See **apex beat.**

**apical curettage** [L, *apex;* Fr, scraping],  debridement of the apical surface of a tooth and removal of diseased soft tissues in the surrounding bony crypt. Compare **apicoectomy, root curettage, subgingival curettage.**

**apical fiber,**  one of the many fibers of the periodontal ligament. These fibers radiate around the apex of the tooth at approximately right angles to their cementum attachment, extending into the bone at the bottom of the alveolus. Apical fibers resist forces that tend to lift the tooth from the socket and, with the other fibers of the periodontal ligament, stabilize the tooth against tilting movements.

**apical impulse.**  See **precordial movement.**

**apical lordotic view** /lôrdot′ik/,  a radiograph made with the patient leaning backward at an angle of approximately 45 degrees, allowing visualization of the apices of the lung under the clavicle.

**apical murmur.**  See **apex murmur.**

**apical odontoid ligament** /ōdon′toid/,  a ligament connecting the axis to the occipital bone. It extends from the process of the axis to the anterior margin of the foramen magnum and lies between the two alar ligaments, blending with the anterior atlantooccipital membrane.

**apical periodontitis** [L, *apex,* summit; Gk, *peri,* near, *odous,* tooth, *itis,* inflammation],  an inflammation of the tissues around the apex of a tooth root.

**apical pneumonia.**  See **apex pneumonia.**

**apical pulse,**  the heartbeat as heard with a stethoscope placed on the chest wall adjacent to the cardiac apex.

**apicectomy.**  See **apicoectomy.**

**apices.**  See **apex.**

**apicitis** /ap′isī′tis/,  an inflammation of the apex of a body structure, such as the apex of a lung or root of a tooth.

**apicoectomy** /ap′isek′təmē/ [L, *apex* + Gk, *ektomē* excision],  the surgical removal of the apex or the apical portion of a tooth root, usually in conjunction with apical curettage or root canal therapy. Also called **apicectomy root amputation, root resection.**

**apicotomy** /ā′pikot′əmē/,  a surgical incision into the apex of a body structure.

**apituitarism** /ā′pityo͞o′itəriz′əm/ [Gk, *a,* without; L, *pituita,* phlegm; Gk, *ismos,* a state],  an absence or loss of function of the pituitary gland.

**APKD,**  abbreviation for *adult polycystic kidney disease.* See also **polycystic kidney disease.**

**aplasia** /əplā′zhə/ [Gk, *a, plassein,* not to form],  **1.** a developmental failure resulting in the absence of an organ or tissue. **2.** (in hematology) a failure of the normal process of cell generation and development. See also **aplastic anemia, hyperplasia.**

**aplasia cutis congenita** [Gk, *a, plassein;* L, *cutis,* skin, *congenitus* born with],  the congenital absence of a localized area of skin. The defect occurs predominantly on the scalp, less frequently on the limbs and trunk; it is usually covered by a thin, translucent membrane or scar tissue, or it may be raw and ulcerated. The condition is genetically transmitted, although the mode of inheritance is not known.

**aplastic** /āplas′tik/ [Gk, *a, plassein,* not to form],  **1.** pertaining to the absence or defective development of a tissue or organ. **2.** failure of a tissue to produce normal daughter cells by mitosis. See also **aplastic anemia.**

**aplastic anemia,**  a deficiency of all of the formed elements of blood (specifically red blood cells, white blood cells, and platelets), representing a failure of the cell-generating capacity of bone marrow. Neoplastic disease of bone marrow and destruction of bone marrow by exposure to toxic chemicals, ionizing radiation, or some antibiotics or other medications are common causes. Also spelled **anaemia.** Compare **alymphocytosis, hemolytic anemia, hypoplastic anemia.** See also **aleukia, leukopenia.**

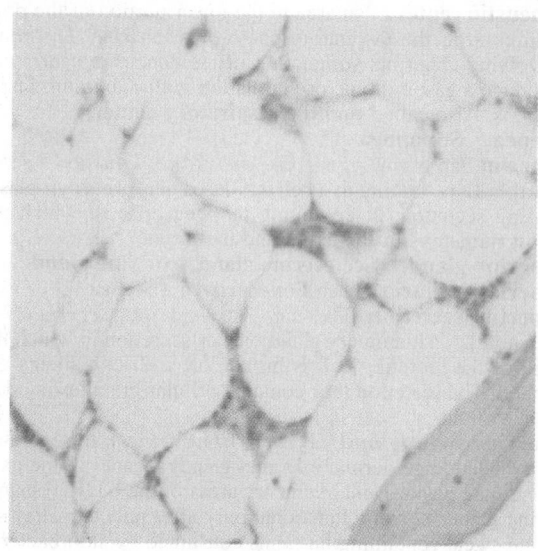

**Aplastic anemia: bone marrow smear**
*(Carr and Rodak, 1999)*

**Apley's scratch test,**  a method for assessing the range of motion of the shoulders. The patient is asked to scratch his or her back while reaching over the head with one hand and behind the back with the other hand. The test requires abduction and lateral rotation of one shoulder and adduction and medial rotation of the other shoulder.

**Aplisol,**  trademark for a tuberculin purified protein derivative.

**Aplitest,**  trademark for a tuberculin purified protein derivative.

**APMA,**  abbreviation for *American Podiatric Medical Society.*

**AP mobile projection.**  See **AP portable chest radiograph.**

**APN.**  Abbreviation for **advanced practice nurse.**

**apnea** /apnē′ə, ap′nē·ə/ [Gk, *a* + *pnein,* not to breath],  an absence of spontaneous respiration. Types of apnea include **cardiac apnea, deglutition apnea, periodic apnea of the newborn, primary apnea, reflex apnea, secondary apnea,** and **sleep apnea.** Also spelled **apnoea.** —**apneic,** *adj.*

**apnea monitor** [Gk, *a* + *pnein,* not to breathe],  a bed surface for infants, designed to sound an alarm if the child stops breathing for a given period of time. It may be a bed pad (alarm mattress) or a nasal flow sensor.

**apnea monitoring,**  the act of closely observing the respiration of individuals, particularly infants. The procedure may involve the use of electronic devices that detect changes in thoracic or abdominal movements and in heart rate. Such devices may include an alarm that sounds if breathing stops. See also **apnea monitor.**

**apneic.**  See **apnea.**

**apneumia** /ap·no͞o′mē·ə/ [Gk, *a, pneumon,* without lung],  congenital absence of the lungs.

**apneustic breathing** /apnōō′stik/ [Gk, *a, pneusis,* not breathing], a pattern of breathing characterized by a prolonged inspiratory phase followed by expiration apnea. The rate of apneustic breathing is usually around 1.5 breaths per minute. This breathing pattern is often associated with head injury.

**apneustic center,** an area in the lower portion of the pons that controls the inspiratory phase of respiration. Disorders involving abnormal stimulation of the apneustic center can produce a gasping type of ventilation with maximum inspirations. Also called **pontine respiratory center.**

**apnoea.** See **apnea.**

**apocrine** /ap′əkrīn, -krin/ [Gk, *apo,* from, *krinein,* to separate], **1.** pertaining to a cell that loses part of its cytoplasm during secretion. **2.** pertaining to sweat glands, which are most numerous in the axilla and the groin.

**apocrine gland.** See **eccrine gland, exocrine gland.**

**apocrine miliaria.** See **Fox-Fordyce disease.**

**apocrine secretion** [Gk, *apo* + *krinein;* L, *secernere,* to separate], a mammary gland type of secretion in which the end of the secreting cell is broken off and its contents expelled. The secretion thus contains cellular granules in addition to fluid.

**apocrine sweat gland** [Gk, *apo,* from, *krinein,* to separate], one of the large dermal exocrine glands located in the axillary, anal, genital, and mammary areas of the body. The apocrine glands become functional only after puberty. They secrete sweat containing nutrients consumed by skin bacteria. Bacterial waste products produce a characteristic odor. Compare **eccrine gland.** See also **exocrine gland.**

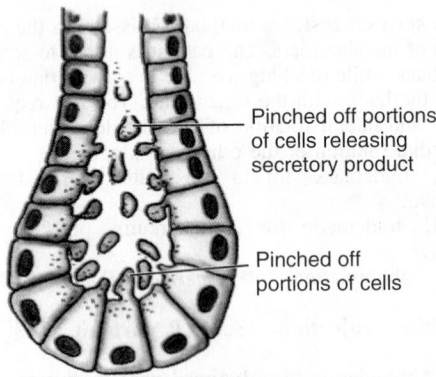

Pinched off portions of cells releasing secretory product

Pinched off portions of cells

**Apocrine sweat gland** *(Applegate, 2000)*

**apodal** /ə·pō′dəl/ [Gk, *a, pous,* without foot], having no feet. See also **symmelia.**

**apodial symmelia.** See **sirenomelia.**

**apoenzyme** /ap′ō·en′zīm/ [Gk, *apo* + *en,* into, *zyme,* ferment], the protein part of a holoenzyme. The nonprotein part is the prosthetic group, which is usually permanently attached to the apoenzyme.

**apogee** /ap′əjē/ [Gk, *apo* + *ge,* earth], the climax of a disease or the period of greatest severity of signs and symptoms, usually followed by a crisis.

**apolipoprotein** /ap′ōlip′ōprō′tēn/ [Gk, *apo* + *lipos,* fat, *protos,* first], the protein component of lipoprotein complexes.

**apolipoprotein A-I,** a protein component of lipoprotein complexes found in high-density lipoprotein (HDL) and chylomicrons. It is an activator of lecithin-cholesterol acyltransferase (LCAT), which forms cholesteryl esters in HDL. All apoproteins of plasma lipoproteins bind and transport lipid in the blood. A deficiency of apolipoprotein A-I is associated with low HDL levels and Tangier disease. See also **Tangier disease.**

**apolipoprotein A-II,** A protein component of lipoprotein complexes found in high-density lipoprotein (HDL) and chlyomicrons which activates hepatic lipase. See also **apolipoprotein A-I**

**apolipoprotein A-III,** one found in high-density lipoproteins; also called **apolipoprotein D.**

**apolipoprotein B, apoprotein B-48,** a protein component of lipoprotein involved in transport of chlyomicrons from the GI tract to the bloodstream.

**apolipoprotein B-100,** a protein component of lipoprotein involved in hepatic transport of lipid as very-low-density lipoprotein (VLDL) and low-density lipoprotein (LDL). Apoprotein B-100 links to cellulose LDL receptors. It is elevated in the plasma of patients with familial hyperlipoproteinemia. See also **hyperlipoproteinemia.**

**apolipoprotein C,** a class of apolipoproteins, apo C-I, C-II, and C-III, that occur in very-low-density lipoprotein (VLDL), high-density lipoprotein (HDL), and chylomicrons; apo C-II activates lipoprotein lipase, which hydrolyzes triglycerides for transfer from VLDL and chylomicrons to tissues.

**apolipoprotein C-I,** a protein component of lipid that activates lecithin-cholesterol acyltransferase (LCAT).

**apolipoprotein C-II,** a protein component of chylomicrons and very-low-density lipoprotein (VLDL) that activates lipoprotein lipase (LPL), an enzyme that hydrolyzes triglyceride to free fatty acids and monoglycerides.

**apolipoprotein D.** See **apolipoprotein A-III.**

**apolipoprotein E,** a protein component of lipoprotein complexes found in very low-density lipoprotein (VLDL), high-density lipoprotein (HDL), chylomicrons, and chylomicron remnants. It facilitates hepatic uptake of chylomicron and VLDL remnants and is elevated in patients with type III hyperlipoproteinemia. See also **hyperlipoproteinemia.**

**apolipoproteins test,** a blood test used to evaluate the risks of atherogenic disease of the heart and peripheral arteries. Specific levels of certain apolipoproteins are also associated with conditions such as Alzheimer's disease, familial hypercholesterolemia, some types of renal failure, nephrotic syndrome, and estrogen depletion in women over the age of 50.

**aponeurosis** /ap′ōnŏŏrō′sis/, *pl.* **aponeuroses** [Gk, *apo* + *neuron,* nerve, sinew], a strong flat sheet of fibrous connective tissue that serves as a tendon to attach muscles to bone or as fascia to bind muscles together or to other tissues at their origin or insertion.

**aponeurosis of the external abdominal oblique,** the strong membrane that covers the entire ventral surface of the abdomen and lies superficial to the rectus abdominis. Fibers from both sides of the aponeurosis interlace in the midline to form the linea alba. The upper part of the aponeurosis serves as the inferior origin of the pectoralis major; the lower part ends in the inguinal ligament.

**aponeurotic fascia** /-nŏŏrot′ik/ [Gk, *apo,* from, *neuron,* tendon], a thickened layer of connective tissue that provides attachment to a muscle.

**apophyseal** /ap′əfiz′ē·əl/, pertaining to an apophysis. Also **apophysial.**

**apophyseal fracture,** a fracture that separates a projection (apophysis) of a bone from the main osseous tissue at a point of strong tendinous attachment.

**apophysial.** See **apophyseal.**

**apophysis** /əpof′isis/ [Gk, a growing away], any small projection, process, or outgrowth, usually on a bone without an independent center of ossification. Examples include the zygomatic apophysis of the temporal bone and the basilar apophysis of the occipital bone.

**apophysitis** /əpof′əsī′tis/, inflammation of an outgrowth, projection, or swelling, especially a bony outgrowth that is still attached to the rest of the bone. Apophysitis occurs most frequently as a disorder of the foot caused by disease of the epiphysis of the quadrangular bone at the back of the tarsus.

**apoprotein** /ap′ōprō′tēn/, a polypeptide chain not yet complexed to its specific prosthetic group.

**apoptosis** /ā′pōtō′sis, ā′poptō′sis/ [Gk, apo, away, ptosis, falling], necrosis of keratinocytes in which the nuclei of the necrotic cells dissolve and the cytoplasm shrinks, rounds up, and is subsequently phagocytized. The term generally refers to "programmed" cell death.

**aposia** /āpō′shə/ [Gk, a, not, posis, thirst], a complete lack of thirst.

**apothecaries' measure** /əpoth′əker′ēz/ [Gk, apotheke, store], a system of graduated liquid volumes originally based on the minim, formerly equal to one drop of water but now standardized to 0.06 ml; 60 minims equals 1 fluid dram, 8 fluid drams equals 1 fluid ounce, 16 fluid ounces equals 1 pint, 2 pints equals 1 quart, 4 quarts equals 1 gallon. See also **apothecaries' weight, metric system.**

**apothecaries' weight,** a system of graduated amounts arranged in order of heaviness and based on the grain, formerly equal to the weight of a plump grain of wheat but now standardized to 65 mg; 20 grains equals 1 scruple, 3 scruples equals 1 dram, 8 drams equals 1 ounce, 12 ounces equals 1 pound. Compare **avoirdupois weight.** See also **apothecaries' measure, metric system.**

**apothecary** /əpoth′əker′ē/ [Gk, apotheke, store], a pharmacist. See also **apothecaries' measure, apothecaries' weight.**

**apparatus** /ap′ərat′əs/ [L, ad, toward, parare, to make ready], a device or a system composed of different parts that act together to perform some special function.

**apparent death.** See **death.**

**appendage.** See **appendix** (def. 1).

**appendectomy** /ap′əndek′təmē/ [L, appendere + Gk, ektomē, excision], the surgical removal of the vermiform appendix. The operation is performed in acute appendicitis to remove an inflamed appendix before it ruptures. Postoperative care and nursing considerations are the same as for any other abdominal operation. If the appendix has perforated and risk of peritonitis is high, a drain may be left in the incision, dressing changes are more frequent, and appropriate antibiotics are prescribed; ileus may develop within days, and pain may be acute. See also **abdominal surgery, peritonitis.**

**appendical.** See **appendiceal.**

**appendical reflex** /əpen′dikəl/, extreme tenderness at McBurney's point on the abdomen, a diagnostic finding in appendicitis.

**appendiceal** /ap′endish′əl/, pertaining to the vermiform appendix. Also **appendicial, appendical** /əpen′dikəl/.

**appendiceal abscess.** See **appendicular abscess.**

**appendicectomy** /əpen′disek′təmē/, **1.** surgical removal of the vermiform appendix. **2.** surgical removal of an appendage.

**appendices.** See **appendix.**

**appendices epiploicae.** See **appendix epiploica.**

**appendicial.** See **appendiceal.**

**appendicitis** /əpen′disī′tis/ [L, appendere + Gk, itis], inflammation of the vermiform appendix, usually acute, that, if undiagnosed, leads rapidly to perforation and peritonitis. The inflammation is caused by an obstruction such as a hard mass of feces or a foreign body in the lumen of the appendix, fibrous disease of the bowel wall, an adhesion, or a parasitic infestation. Appendicitis is most likely to occur in teenagers and young adults and is more prevalent in male patients.

■ OBSERVATIONS: The most common symptom is constant pain in the right lower quadrant of the abdomen around McBurney's point, which the patient describes as having begun as intermittent pain in midabdomen. Rebound pain occurs at McBurney's point as well. Pain may also occur on the left side. Extreme tenderness occurs over the right rectus muscle. To decrease the pain, the patient keeps knees bent to prevent tension of abdominal muscles. Appendicitis is characterized by vomiting, a low-grade fever of 99° to 102° F, an elevated white blood count, rebound tenderness, a rigid abdomen, and decreased or absent bowel sounds.

■ INTERVENTIONS: Treatment is appendectomy within 24 to 48 hours of the first symptoms because delay usually results in rupture and peritonitis as fecal matter is released into the peritoneal cavity. The fever rises sharply once peritonitis begins. The patient may have sudden relief from pain immediately after rupture, followed by increased, diffuse pain. The nurse is alert to the other indications of peritonitis: increasing abdominal distension, acute abdomen, rigid boardlike abdomen, tachycardia, rapid shallow breathing, and restlessness. If peritonitis is suspected, IV antibiotic therapy, fluids, and electrolytes are given. Kinds of appendicitis include **chronic appendicitis.** See also **McBurney's point, peritonitis.**

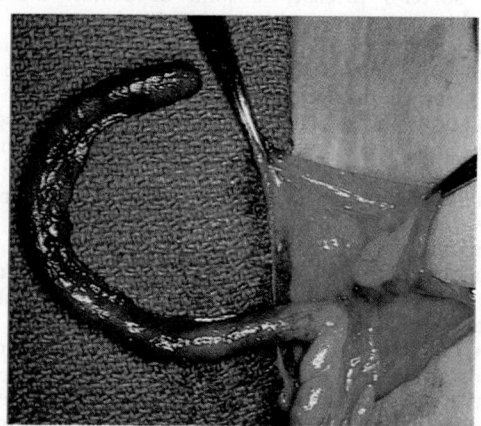

**Acute appendicitis** *(Zitelli and Davis, 1997)*

**appendicitis pain** [L, appendere, to hang upon, poena, penalty], severe general abdominal pain that develops rapidly and usually becomes localized in the lower right quadrant. It is accompanied by extreme tenderness over the right rectus muscle with rebound pain at McBurney's point. Occasionally, the pain is on the left side.

**appendicular** /ap'əndik'yələr/, **1.** pertaining to the vermiform appendix. **2.** pertaining to the limbs of the skeleton.

**appendicular abscess, 1.** an abscess on a limb. **2.** an abscess of the vermiform appendix. Also called **appendiceal abscess.**

**appendicular skeleton,** the bones of the limbs and their girdles, attached to the axial skeleton. See also **axial skeleton.**

**appendix** /əpen'diks/, *pl.* **appendixes, appendices, 1.** an accessory part attached to a main structure. Also called **appendage. 2.** See vermiform appendix.

**appendix dyspepsia** [L, *appendere* + Gk, *dys,* difficult, *peptein,* to digest], an abnormal condition characterized by impairment of the digestive function associated with chronic appendicitis. See also **dyspepsia.**

**appendix epididymidis** /ep'ididim'idis/, a cystic structure sometimes found on the head of the epididymis. It represents a remnant of the mesonephros.

**appendix epiploica** /əp'iplô'ikə/, *pl.* **appendices epiploicae** [L, *appendere* + Gk, *epiploon,* caul], one of the fat pads, 2 to 10 cm long, scattered through the peritoneum along the colon and the upper part of the rectum, especially along the transverse and the sigmoid parts of the colon.

**appendixes.** See **appendix.**

**appendix vermiformis.** See **vermiform appendix.**

**apperception** /ap'ərsep'shən/ [L, *ad,* toward, *percipere,* to perceive], **1.** mental perception or recognition. **2.** (in psychology) a conscious process of understanding or perceiving in terms of a person's previous knowledge, experiences, emotions, and memories. —**apperceptive,** *adj.*

**appestat** /ap'əstat/, a center in the hypothalamus of the brain that controls the appetite.

**appetite** /ap'ətīt/ [L, *appetere,* to long for], a natural or instinctive desire, such as for food.

**apple picker's disease,** an allergic reaction with respiratory complaints, associated with the handling of apples that have been treated with a fungicide.

**apple sorter's disease,** a form of contact dermatitis caused by chemicals used in washing apples.

**appliance** /əplī'əns/ [L, *applicare,* to apply], a device or instrument used to perform a specific medical function or to have a specific therapeutic effect.

**application** /ap'likā'shən/, a computer program used to process a particular type of data, such as payroll, inventory, data about patients, scheduling of procedures and activities, pharmacy requisition and control, recording of nursing notes, and care planning.

**applicator** /ap'likā'tər/, a rodlike instrument with a piece of cotton on the end, used for the local application of medication or probing of wound pockets/crevices. Also called a **cotton swab.**

**applied anatomy** /əplīd'/, the study of the structure of the organs of the body as it relates to the diagnosis and treatment of disease. Also called **practical anatomy.** See also **comparative anatomy, pathologic anatomy, radiologic anatomy, surgical anatomy.**

**applied chemistry,** the application of the study of chemical elements and compounds to industry and the arts.

**applied psychology, 1.** the interpretation of historical, literary, medical, or other data according to psychologic principles. **2.** any branch of psychology that emphasizes practical rather than theoretic approaches and objectives, such as clinical psychology, child psychology, industrial psychology, and educational psychology.

**applied science.** See **science.**

**AP portable chest radiograph,** a radiographic examination of the chest performed with a portable x-ray machine in the room of an immobilized patient. The film holder is placed behind the patient and the x-ray tube in front. The patient is positioned as upright as possible to allow for visualization of fluid levels in the lungs. Also called **AP mobile projection.**

**apposition** /ap'əsish'ən/ [L, *apponere,* to put to], the placing of objects in proximity, as in the layering of tissue cells or juxtapositioning of facing surfaces side-by-side.

**appositional growth,** an increase in size by the addition of new tissue or similar material at the periphery of a particular part or structure, as in the addition of new layers in bone and tooth formation. Compare **interstitial growth.**

**apposition suture,** a suture that holds the margins of an incision close together.

**approach,** the steps in a particular surgical procedure, from division of the most superficial parts of the anatomy through exposure of the operation site.

**approach-approach conflict** [L, *ad* + *propiare,* to draw near], a conflict resulting from the simultaneous presence of two or more incompatible impulses, desires, or goals, each of which is desirable. Also called **double-approach conflict.** See also **conflict.**

**approach-avoidance conflict,** a conflict resulting from the presence of a single goal or desire that is both desirable and undesirable. See also **conflict.**

**appropriate for gestational age (AGA) infant** /əprō'prē·it/ [L, *ad,* toward, *proprius,* ownership], a newborn whose size, growth, and maturation are normal for gestational age, whether delivered prematurely, at term, or later than term. Such infants, if born at term, fall within the average range of size and weight on intrauterine growth curves, measuring from 48 to 53 cm in length and weighing between 2700 and 4000 g.

**approximal** /əprok'siməl/ [L, *approximare,* to approach], close, or very near.

**approximate** /əprok'simāt/ [L, *ad* + *proximare,* to come near], to draw two tissue surfaces close together as in the repair of a wound or to draw the bones of a joint together as in physical therapy.

**approximator** /əprok'səmā'tər/, a medical instrument used to draw together the edges of divided tissues, as in closing a wound or in repairing a fractured rib.

**apraxia** /əprak'sē·ə/ [Gk, *a* + *pressein,* not to act], an impairment in the ability to perform purposeful acts or to manipulate objects in the absence or loss of motor power sensation or coordination. **Ideational apraxia** is characterized by impairment caused by a loss of the perception of the use of an object. **Motor apraxia** is characterized by an inability to use an object or perform a task although it is understood. **Amnestic apraxia** is characterized by an inability to perform the function because of an inability to remember the command to perform it. **Apraxia of speech** is an inability to program the position of speech muscles and the sequence of muscle movements necessary to produce understandable speech, although understanding of speech remains intact. —**apraxic,** *adj.*

**Apresoline Hydrochloride** trademark for a nonnitrate vasodilator antihypertensive (hydralazine hydrochloride).

**aprobarbital** /ap'rōbär'bital/, an intermediate-acting barbiturate.

■ INDICATIONS: It is prescribed as a sedative-hypnotic for sedation and induction of sleep on a short-term basis.

■ CONTRAINDICATIONS: The drug is contraindicated for patients with a known sensitivity to barbiturates or with a history of porphyria.

■ ADVERSE EFFECTS: The most common adverse effects include respiratory depression, nausea, vomiting, dizziness, nervousness, headache, skin rash, and purpura.

**aprosody** /āpros'odē/ [Gk, *a* + *prosodia,* not modulated voice], a speech disorder characterized by the absence of the normal variations in pitch, loudness, intonation, and rhythm of word formation.

**aprosopia** /ā'prəsō'pē·ə/ [Gk, *aprosopos,* faceless], a congenital absence of part or all of the facial structures. The condition is usually associated with other malformations.

**APTA,** abbreviation for *American Physical Therapy Association.*

**aptitude** /ap'tətyōōd/ [L, *aptitudo,* ability], a natural ability, tendency, talent, or capability to learn, understand, or acquire a particular skill; mental alertness.

**aptitude test,** any of a variety of standardized tests for measuring an individual's ability to learn certain skills. Compare **achievement test, intelligence test, personality test, psychologic test.**

**apyretic** /ā'pīret'ik/ [Gk, *a* + *pyretos,* without fever], an afebrile condition.

**apyrexia** /ā'pīrek'sē·ə/ [Gk, *a* + *pyrexis,* without fever], an absence or remission of fever.

**aq.** See **aqua.**

**AQ,** abbreviation for **achievement quotient.**

**aqua (aq)** /ä'kwə/, the Latin word for water.

**aqua amnii.** See **amniotic fluid.**

**AquaMEPHYTON,** trademark for a vitamin K compound (phytonadione).

**aquaphobia** /ä'kwəfō'bē·ə/ [L, *aqua,* water; Gk, *phobos,* fear], irrational fear of water.

**aquapuncture** /-pungk'chər/ [L, *aqua,* water, *punctura,* puncture], the injection of water under the skin or spraying of a fine jet of water onto the skin surface to relieve a mild irritation.

**aquatherapy.** See underwater exercise.

**aquathermia pad** /-thur'mē·ə/, a waterproof plastic or rubber pad that can be applied to areas of muscle sprain, edema, or mild inflammation. The pad contains channels through which heated or cooled water flows. The device is connected by hoses to a bedside control unit that contains a temperature regulator, a motor for circulating the water, and a reservoir of distilled water. Although generally safer than a conventional heating pad, the aquathermia pad should be checked periodically to avoid the risk of accidental burns. Also called **water flow pad.**

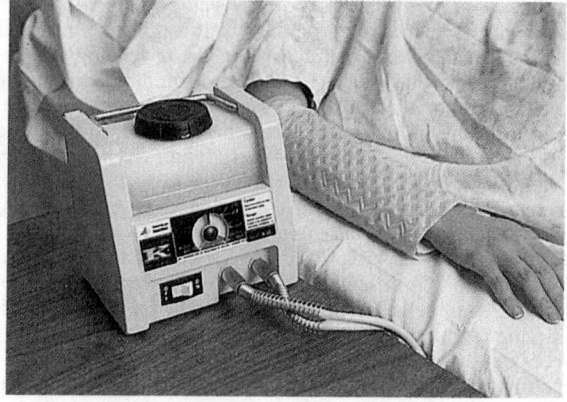

**Aquathermia pad** *(Potter and Perry, 2001)*

**aquatic exercise.** See underwater exercise.

**aqueduct** /-dukt/ [L, *aqua,* water, *ductus,* act of leading], any canal, channel, or passage through or between body parts, as the cerebral aqueduct in the brain.

**aqueduct of Sylvius.** See **cerebral aqueduct.**

**aqueductus** /ak'wəduk'təs/, the Latin word for canal.

**aqueous** /ā'kwē·əs, ak'wē·əs/ [L, *aqua*], **1.** watery or waterlike. **2.** a medication prepared with water. See also **aqueous humor.**

**aqueous chambers** [L, *aqua,* water; Gk, *kamara,* something with an arched cover], the anterior and posterior chambers of the eye, containing the aqueous humor.

**aqueous extract,** a water-based preparation of plant or animal substance containing the biologically active portion without the cellular residue.

**aqueous humor,** the clear, watery fluid circulating in the anterior chamber of the eye. It is produced by the ciliary body and is reabsorbed into the venous system at the iridocorneal angle by means of the sinus venosus, or canal of Schlemm.

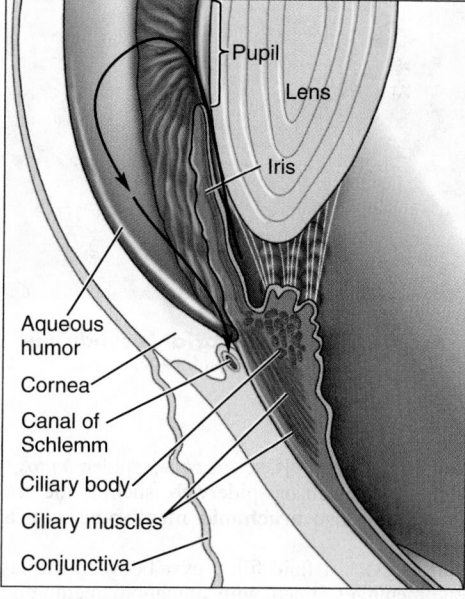

**Flow of aqueous humor** *(Herlihy and Maebius, 2000)*

**aqueous phase,** a fluid stage of a substance that may also exist in other forms during cycles of change, such as the occurrence of water in a liquid state and at other times as ice or water vapor.

**aqueous solution** [L, *aqua,* water + *solutus,* dissolved], a homogenous liquid preparation of any substance dissolved in water.

**Ar,** symbol for the element **argon.**

**AR,** abbreviation for *assisted respiration.*

**arabinofuranosylcytosine.** See **cytarabine.**

**arabinosylcytosine.** See **cytarabine**.

**arachidonic acid** /ar'əkidon'ik/ [L, *arachos,* a legume], a long-chain fatty acid that is a component of lecithin and a basic material in the biosynthesis of some prostaglandins. In mammals, arachidonic acid is synthesized from linoleic acid, which is an essential fatty acid.

**arachnid** [Gk, *arachne*, spider], an animal in the phylum Arthropoda, class Arachnida, which includes spiders, scorpions, mites, and ticks.

**arachnidism.** See **arachnoidism.**

**arachnitis** /ar′əknī′tis/, inflammation of the arachnoid membrane covering the brain. Also called **arachnoiditis.**

**arachno-, arachn-,** combining form meaning 'arachnoid membrane or spider': *arachnoidal, arachnoidea.*

**arachnodactyly** /ərak′nōdak′tilē/ [Gk, *arachne*, spider, *dactylos,* finger], a congenital condition of having long, thin, spiderlike fingers and toes. It is seen in Marfan's syndrome.

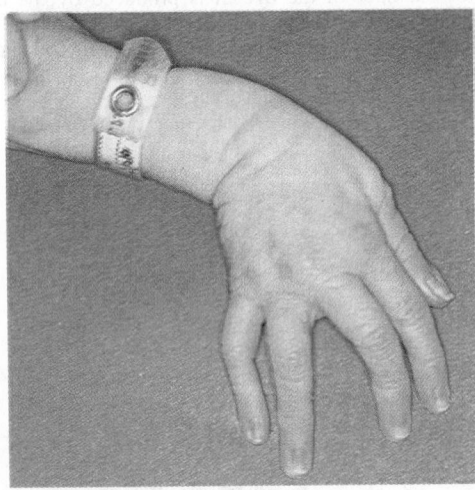

**Arachnodactyly in Marfan's syndrome**
*(Zitelli and Davis, 1997)*

**arachnoid** /ərak′noid/ [Gk, *arachne*, spider, *eidos,* form], resembling a cobweb or spiderweb, such as the arachnoid membrane. See also **arachnoid membrane. —arachnoidal,** *adj.*

**arachnoid cyst,** a fluid-filled cyst between the layers of the leptomeninges, lined with arachnoid membrane, most commonly occurring in the sylvian fissure. Also called **leptomeningeal cyst.**

**arachnoidism** /ərak′noidiz′əm/ [Gk, *arachne*, spider, *eidos,* form], the condition produced by the bite of a venomous spider. Also called **arachnidism** /ərak′nīdiz′əm/.

**arachnoiditis.** See **arachnitis.**

**arachnoid membrane,** a thin, delicate membrane enclosing the brain and the spinal cord, interposed between the pia mater and the dura mater. The subarachnoid space lies between the arachnoid membrane and the pia mater, and the subdural space lies between the arachnoid membrane and the dura mater. Also called **arachnoid sheath.**

**arachnoid sheath.** See **arachnoid membrane.**

**arachnoid villi** /vil′ī/ [Gk, *arachne*, spider, *villus,* shaggy hair], projections of fibrous tissue from the arachnoid membrane.

**arachnophobia** /ərak′nōfō′bē·ə/, a morbid fear of spiders.

**Aramine,** trademark for a beta-adrenergic agonist (metaraminol bitartrate).

**Aran-Duchenne muscular atrophy** /aran′dōōshen′/ [François A. Aran, French physician, 1817–1861; Guillaume B.A. Duchenne, French neurologist, 1806–1875], a form of amyotrophic lateral sclerosis affecting the hands, arms, shoulders, and legs at the onset before becoming more generalized. Also **progressive spinal muscular atrophy.**

**arbitrary inference** /är′bitrer′ē in′fərəns/, a form of cognitive distortion in which a judgment based on insufficient evidence leads to an erroneous conclusion.

**arbitrator** /är′bətrā′tər/ [L, *arbiter,* umpire], an impartial person appointed to resolve a dispute between parties. The arbitrator listens to the evidence presented by the parties in an informal hearing and attempts to arrive at a resolution acceptable to both parties. **—arbitration,** *n.*

**arborization test.** See **ferning test.**

**arbovirus** /är′bōvī′rəs/, any one of more than 300 insect-borne viruses that cause infections characterized by a combination of two or more of the following: fever, rash, encephalitis, and bleeding into the viscera or skin. Dengue, yellow fever, and equine encephalitis are three common arboviral infections. Treatment is symptomatic for all arbovirus infections. Vaccines have been developed to prevent infection from some arboviruses.

**arc** [L, *arcus,* bow], a part of the circumference of a circle.

**ARC.** See **AIDS-wasting syndrome.**

**arcade** [L, *arcus,* bow], an arch or series of arches.

**arch,** any anatomic structure that is curved or has a bow-like appearance. Also called **arcus.**

**arch-.** See **archi-.**

**arch bar,** any one of various types of wires, bars, or splints that conform to the arch of the teeth and are used in the treatment of fractures of the jaws and in the stabilization of injured teeth.

**arche-.** See **archi-.**

**-arche,** suffix meaning 'beginning': *menarche.*

**archentera, archenteric.** See **archenteron.**

**archenteric canal.** See **neurenteric canal.**

**archenteron** /arken′təron/, *pl.* **archentera** [Gk, *arche*, beginning, *enteron,* intestine], the primitive digestive cavity formed by the invagination into the gastrula which is lined with entoderm during the embryonic development of many animals. It corresponds to the tubular cavity in the vertebrates that connects the amniotic cavity with the yolk sac. Also called **archigaster, coelenteron, gastrocoele, primitive gut.** See also **gastrula. —archenteric,** *adj.*

**archeocortex.** See **olfactory cortex.**

**arches of the foot** [L, *arcus,* bow; AS, *fot*], the bony curves of the instep, including the longitudinal (anteroposterior) and the transverse arches.

**archetype** /är′kətīp′/ [Gk, *arche* + *typos,* type], **1.** an original model or pattern from which a thing or group of things is made or evolves. **2.** (in analytic psychology) an inherited primordial idea or mode of thought derived from the experiences of the human race and present in the subconscious of the individual in the form of drives, moods, and concepts. See also **anima. —archetypal, archetypic, archetypical,** *adj.*

**archi-, arch-, arche-,** prefix meaning 'first, beginning, or original': *archiblastoma, archetype.*

**archiblastoma** /är′kiblastō′mə/, *pl.* **archiblastomas, archiblastomata** [Gk, *arche* + *blastos,* germ, *oma*], a tumor composed of cells derived from the layer of tissue surrounding the germinal vesicle.

**archigaster.** See **archenteron.**

**archinephric canal, archinephric duct.** See **pronephric duct.**

**archinephron.** See **pronephros.**

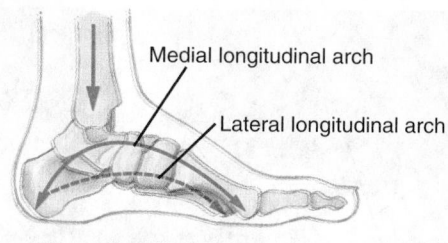

Normal longitudinal arch

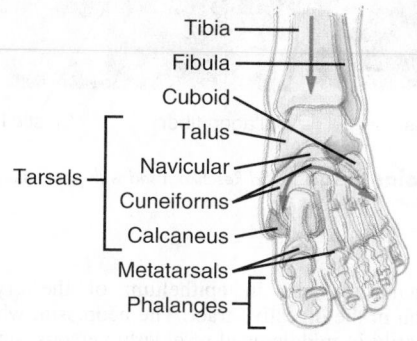

**Arches of the foot**
*(Thibodeau and Patton, 1999/Yvonne Wylie Watson)*

**archistome.** See **blastopore.**

**architectural barriers** /är′kətek′chərəl/, architectural features of homes and public buildings that limit access and mobility of disabled persons. Wheelchair access, for example, requires ramped entryways, a minimum of 32-inch-wide doorways, a space of at least 60 inches by 60 inches for wheelchair turns, and counters no more than 26.5 inches above floor level.

**architecture** /är′kitek′chər/ [Gk, *architekton,* master builder], the basic structure of a computer, including the memory, central processing unit, and input/output devices.

**architis** /ärkī′tis/ [Gk, *archos,* anus, *itis,* inflammation], an inflammation of the anus. Also called **proctitis.**

**arch length** /ärch/, the distance from the distal point of the most posterior tooth on one side of the upper or lower jaw to the same point on the other side, usually measured through the points of contact between adjoining teeth. See also **available arch length.**

**arch length deficiency,** the difference in any dental arch between the length required to accommodate all the natural teeth and the actual length.

**arch of the aorta,** the proximal one of the four portions of the aorta, giving rise to three arterial branches called the innominate (brachiocephalic), left common carotid, and left subclavian arteries. The arch rises at the level of the border of the second sternocostal articulation of the right side, passes to the left in front of the trachea, bends dorsally, and becomes the descending aorta. Also called **aortic arch.**

**arch width,** the distance between the left and right opposite in the upper or lower jaw. The intercanine, interpremolar, or intermolar distance may be cited as the arch width.

**arch wire,** an orthodontic wire fastened to two or more teeth through fixed attachments, used to cause or guide tooth movement. See also **full-arch wire, sectional arch wire.**

**arcing spring contraceptive diaphragm** /är′king/, a kind of contraceptive diaphragm in which the flexible metal spring that forms the rim is a combination of a flexible coil spring and a flat band spring made of stainless steel. The latex or silicone rubber dome is approximately 4 cm deep, and the diameter of the rubber-covered rim is between 55-100 mm. Seven sizes, in increments of 0.5 cm, allow the clinician to fit the diaphragm to a particular woman. The kind of spring and the size of the rim in millimeters are stamped on the rim, for example, 75 mm arcing spring. This kind of diaphragm is prescribed for a woman whose vaginal musculature is relaxed and does not afford strong support, as in first-degree cystocele, rectocele, or uterine prolapse. Compare **coil spring contraceptive diaphragm, flat spring contraceptive diaphragm.** See also **contraceptive diaphragm fitting.**

**arctation.** See **stenosis.**

**arcuate** /är′kyo͞o·at/ [L, *arcuatus,* bowed], an arch or bow shape.

**arcuate scotoma** [L, *arcuatus* bowed; Gk, *skotoma,* darkness], an arc-shaped blind area that may develop in the field of vision of a person with glaucoma. It is caused by damage to nerve fibers in the retina.

**arcus.** See **arch.**

**arcus senilis** /sene̅′lis/ [L, bow, aged], an opaque ring, gray to white in color, that surrounds the periphery of the cornea. It is caused by deposits of cholesterol in the cornea or hyaline degeneration and occurs primarily in older persons. Also called **gerontoxon.**

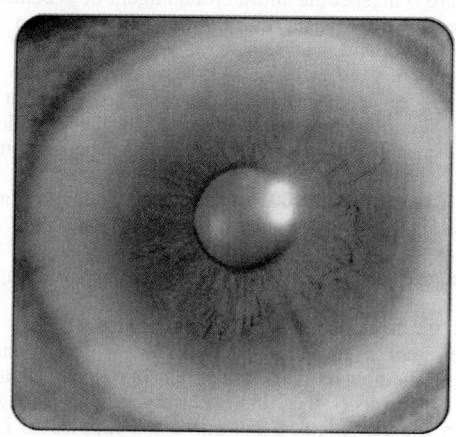

**Arcus senilis** *(Kanski and Nischal, 1999)*

**ardeparin,** an anticoagulant.
- INDICATIONS: This drug is used to prevent deep vein thrombosis after knee replacement surgery.
- CONTRAINDICATIONS: The following conditions prohibit the use of this drug: known hypersensitivity to this drug, pork products, heparin, or other anticoagulants; hemophilia, leukemia with bleeding, thrombocytopenic purpura, cerebrovascular hemorrhage, cerebral aneurysm, severe hypertension, and other severe cardiac disease.
- ADVERSE EFFECTS: Life-threatening consequences include intracranial bleeding, hemorrhage, anaphylaxis, and thrombocytopenia. Other adverse effects include fever, hypersensitivity, anemia, pruritus, superficial wound infection, ecchymosis, and rash.

**ARDS,** abbreviation for **adult respiratory distress syndrome.**

**area** /er′ē·ə/ [L, space], (in anatomy) a limited anatomic space that contains a specific structure of the body or within which certain physiologic functions predominate, such as the aortic area and the association areas of the cerebral cortex.

**area restriction,** a nursing intervention from the Nursing Interventions Classification (NIC) defined a limitation of patient mobility to a specified area for purposes of safety or behavior management. See also **Nursing Interventions Classification.**

**areata** /erē·ā′tə/, occurring in patches, such as hair loss in alopecia areata.

**area under the concentration curve (AUC),** a method of measurement of the bioavailability of a drug based on a plot of blood concentrations sampled at frequent intervals. It is directly proportional to the total amount of unaltered drug in the patient's blood.

**areflexia** /ā′rēflek′sē·ə/, the absence of the reflexes.

*Arenavirus* /er′inəvī′rəs/, a genus of viruses usually transmitted to humans by contact with or inhalation of aerosolized excreta of wild rodents. Individual arenaviruses are identified with specific geographic areas, such as **Bolivian hemorrhagic fever** in one river valley in Bolivia; **Lassa fever** in Nigeria, Liberia, and Sierra Leone; and **Argentine hemorrhagic fever** in two agricultural provinces in Argentina. Arenavirus infections are characterized by slow onset, fever, muscle pain, rash, petechiae, hemorrhage, delirium, hypotension, and ulcers of the mouth. Treatment is supportive; there is no specific antimicrobial agent or vaccine. Fluid and electrolyte balance, rest, and adequate nutrition are the goals of treatment.

**areola** /erē′ōlə/, *pl.* **areolae,** **1.** a small space or a cavity within a tissue. **2.** a circular area of a different color surrounding a central feature, such as the discoloration about a pustule or vesicle. **3.** the part of the iris around the pupil.

**areola mammae** /mam′ē/, the pigmented, circular area surrounding the nipple of each breast. Also called **areola papillaris.**

**areolar** /erē′ələr/ [L, *areola,* little space], pertaining to an areola.

**areolar gland,** one of the large modified sebaceous glands in the areolae encircling the nipples of the breasts of women. The areolar glands secrete a lipoid fluid that lubricates and protects the nipple during nursing and contain smooth muscle bundles that cause the nipples to become erect when stimulated. Also called **gland of Montgomery.**

**areolar tissue,** a kind of connective tissue having little tensile strength and consisting of loosely woven fibers and areolae. It occupies the interspaces of the body. Also called **fibroareolar tissue.** Compare **fibrous tissue.**

**areolitis** /er′ē·əlī′tis/, an inflammation of the areolas of the breasts.

**ARF,** abbreviation for **acute respiratory failure.**

**Arfonad,** trademark for a ganglion blocking agent antihypertensive (trimethaphan camsylate).

**Arg,** abbreviation for the amino acid **arginine.**

**argentaffin cell** /är′jentaf′in/ [L, *argentum,* gleaming, *affinitas,* affinity], a cell containing granules that stain readily with silver and chromium. Such cells occur in most regions of the GI tract and are especially abundant in the crypts of Lieberkühn. Also called **enterochromaffin cell, Kulchitsky's cell.** See also **carcinoid, carcinoid syndrome.**

**argentaffinoma** /är′jentaf′inō′mə/, *pl.* **argentaffinomas, argentaffinomata,** a carcinoid tumor arising most often

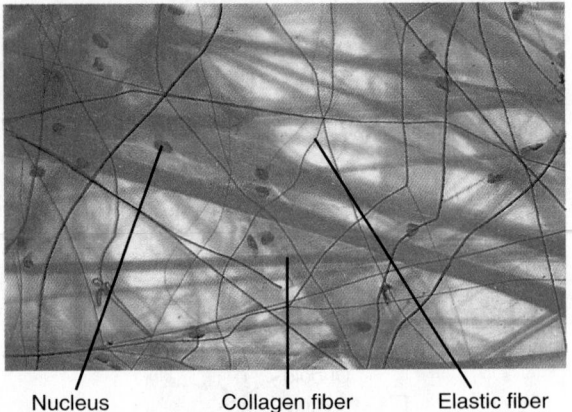

Nucleus    Collagen fiber    Elastic fiber

**Areolar tissue** (© Ed Reschke; used with permission)

from argentaffin cells in epithelium of the crypts of Lieberkühn in the digestive tract. The neoplasm, which occurs primarily in middle-aged or elderly persons, starts as a nodule or plaque and progresses to a growth encircling the bowel. Highly vascular tumors formed of silver-staining argentaffin cells may also develop in the bronchi.

**argentaffinoma syndrome.** See **carcinoid syndrome.**

**argentaffinomata.** See **argentaffinoma.**

**Argentine hemorrhagic fever,** an infectious disease caused by an arenavirus transmitted to humans by contact with or inhalation of aerosolized excreta of infected rodents. Initially, it is characterized by chills, fever, headache, myalgia, anorexia, nausea, vomiting, and a general feeling of malaise. As the disease progresses, the victim may develop a high fever, dehydration, hypotension, flushed skin, abnormally slow heartbeat, bleeding from the gums and internal tissues, hematuria, and hematemesis. There may be involvement of the central nervous system, shock, and pulmonary edema. There is no specific treatment for the disease other than hydration, rest, warmth, and adequate nutrition. Rarely, IV fluids and dialysis are necessary. Usually, the prognosis is complete recovery. See also *Arenavirus,* Bolivian hemorrhagic fever, Lassa fever.

**arginase** /är′jinās/, an enzyme that catalyzes the hydrolysis of arginine during the urea cycle, producing urea and ornithine. The enzyme is found primarily in the liver but also occurs in the mammary gland, testes, and kidney.

**arginase deficiency,** an autosomal recessive aminoacidopathy involving the biosynthesis of urea; arginine is elevated in blood and urine and may cause secondary cystinuria; orotic aciduria is common, but hyperammonemia is rare. Clinical signs include psychomotor retardation, hepatomegaly, and scalp discoloration. Also called **argininemia.**

**arginine (Arg)** /är′jinin/, an amino acid formed during the urea cycle by the transfer of a nitrogen atom from aspartate to citrulline. It can also be prepared synthetically. Certain compounds made from arginine, especially arginine glutamate and arginine hydrochloride, are used intravenously in the management of conditions in which there is an excess of ammonia in the blood caused by liver dysfunction. See also **urea cycle.**

**argininemia** /är′jininē′mē·ə/, arginase deficiency.

**argininosuccinic acidemia** /ärjin′inō′suksin′ik/, an inherited amino acid metabolism disorder in which the lack of an enzyme, argininosuccinase, results in an excess of argini-

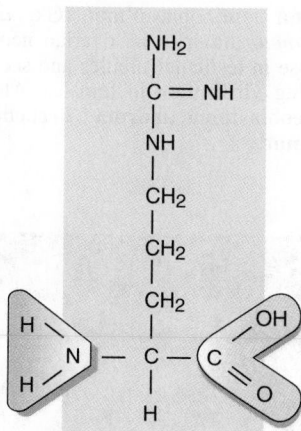

**Chemical structure of arginine**

nosuccinic acid in the blood. The condition is characterized by seizures and mental retardation. Treatment mainly involves a low-protein diet containing essential amino acids or amino acid analogs.

**argon (Ar)** /är′gon/ [Gk, *argos,* inactive], a colorless, odorless, chemically inactive gas and one of the six rare gases in the atmosphere. Its atomic mass is 39.95; its atomic number is 18. It forms no known compounds.

**Argyll Robertson pupil** [Douglas M.C.L. Argyll Robertson, Scottish ophthalmologist, 1837–1909], a pupil that constricts on accommodation but not in response to light. It is most often seen with miosis and in advanced neurosyphilis.

**argyria** /ärjī′rē·ə/ [Gk, *argyros,* silver], a dull blue or gray coloration of the skin, conjunctiva, and internal organs caused by prolonged exposure to silver salts.

**argyrophil** /ärjī′rəfil/ [Gk, *argyros,* silver, *philein,* to love], a cell or other object that is easily stained or impregnated with silver.

**arhythmia.** See **arrhythmia.**

**ariboflavinosis** /ārī′bōflā′vinō′sis/ [Gk, *a,* not, *ribose;* L, *flavus,* yellow; Gk, *osis*], a condition caused by deficiency of riboflavin (vitamin B$_2$) in the diet. It is characterized by bilateral lesions at the corners of the mouth, on the lips, and around the nose and eyes; by seborrheic dermatitis, and by various visual disorders. See also **riboflavin.**

**Arica therapy,** an alternative mental health treatment introduced by Oscar Ichazo that focuses on altered states of consciousness with a goal of increasing the powers of the mind. It requires a 40-day training program of physical exercise and meditation, climaxed by a mild form of sensory deprivation during which the patient practices self-observation.

**Arimidex,** trademark for an aromatase inhibitor (anastrozole).

**Aristocort,** trademark for a glucocorticoid (triamcinolone).

**-arit,** combining form designating an antirheumatic drug.

**arithmetic mean.** See **mean.**

**Arkansas stone** /är′kənsô/, a fine-grained stone of novaculite used to sharpen surgical instruments.

**Arlidin,** trademark for a beta-adrenergic agonist peripheral vasodilator (nylidrin hydrochloride).

**arm** [L, *armus*], **1.** the portion of the upper limb of the body between the shoulder and the elbow. The bone of the arm is the humerus. The muscles of the arm are the coracobrachialis, the biceps brachii, the brachialis, and the triceps brachii. **2.** *nontechnical.* the arm and the forearm. See also **shoulder joint.**

**ARM,** abbreviation for *artificial rupture of (fetal) membranes.* See also **amniotomy.**

**armamentarium** /är′məmenter′ē·əm/ [L, *armamentum,* implement], the total therapeutic assets of a physician or medical facility, including medicines and equipment.

**arm board, 1.** a board used to position the affected arm of a person with hemiplegia and of others with arm disabilities. It fastens to the arm rest of a wheelchair, supporting the flaccid arm in the correct position to prevent or decrease subluxation of the shoulder joint, and to prevent edema. **2.** a board used to keep the arm still to permit the drawing of blood or starting of an IV needle.

**arm bone.** See **humerus.**

**arm cylinder cast,** an orthopedic device of plaster of paris or fiberglass, used for immobilizing the upper limb from the wrist to the upper arm. It is most often applied to aid the healing of a dislocated elbow, for postoperative immobilization or positioning of the elbow, or in the correction of an elbow deformity.

**armpit.** See **axilla.**

**Army Nurse Corps (ANC),** a branch of the U.S. Army, founded February 2, 1901, with headquarters in Falls Church, Virginia.

**Arneth's classification of neutrophils** [Joseph Arneth, German physician, 1873–1953], a system expressed in chart form in which neutrophils are divided into five classes according to the number of segments of their nuclei and are further subdivided according to the shape of the nuclei. Immature neutrophils with a single lobed nucleus are placed on the far left side of the chart; those with multilobed nuclei are placed on the far right side.

**Arnold-Chiari malformation** /är′nəldkē·är′ē/ [Julius Arnold, German pathologist, 1835–1915; Hans Chiari, French pathologist, 1851–1916], a congenital herniation of the brainstem and lower cerebellum through the foramen magnum into the cervical vertebral canal. It is often associated with meningocele and spina bifida. See also **neural tube defect.**

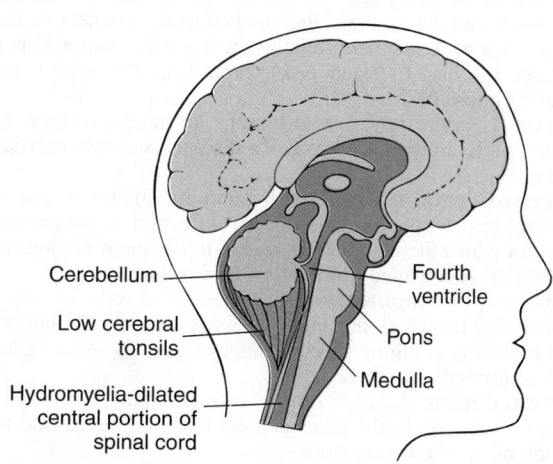

**Arnold-Chiari malformation** *(McCance and Huether, 1998)*

**Arnold, Friedrich** [German anatomist, 1803–1890], an investigator of structures and functions of the brain and nervous system, including the nerve center of the cough reflex.

**-arol,** combining form designating a dicoumarol-type anticoagulant.

**AROM,** **1.** abbreviation for **active range of motion.** **2.** abbreviation for *artificial rupture of (fetal) membranes.*

**aroma** [Gk, spice], any agreeable odor or pleasing fragrance, especially of food, drink, spices, or medication.

**aromatic** /er'ōmat'ik/ [Gk, *aroma*, spice], **1.** pertaining to a strong but agreeable odor such as a pleasant spicy odor. **2.** a stimulant or spicy medicine.

**aromatic alcohol,** a fatty alcohol in which part of the hydrogen of the alcohol radical is replaced by an aromatic ring.

**aromatic ammonia spirit** [Gk, *aroma*, Ammon temple, ancient source of ammonium chloride salt, *spiritus*, breath], a strongly fragrant solution of ammonium carbonate in dilute liquid ammonia, oils, alcohol, and water. It is used as a reflex stimulus, antacid, and a carminative to relieve flatulence. Also called **aromatic spirit of ammonia.**

**aromatic bath,** a medicated bath in which aromatic substances or essential oils are added to the water.

**aromatic compounds,** organic compounds that contain a benzene, naphthalene, or analogous ring. Many of these compounds have agreeable odors, which accounts for the use of this term for such compounds.

**aromatic elixir** [Gk, *aroma* + Ar, *al-iksir*, philosophers' stone], a pleasant smelling flavoring agent added to some medications.

**aromatic hydrocarbon** [Gk, *aroma*, spice; *hydor*, water; L, *carbo*, coal], an organic compound that has a benzene or other aromatic ring, as distinguished from an open-chain aliphatic compound.

**aromatic spirit of ammonia.** See **aromatic ammonia spirit.**

**arousal** [OE, to rise], a state of responsiveness to sensory stimulation.

**arousal level,** the state of sensory stimulation needed to induce active wakefulness in a sleeping infant. Arousal levels range from deep sleep to drowsy state.

**array** [ME, *aray*, preparation], an arrangement or order of components or other objects, usually according to a predetermined system or plan.

**arrector pili** /ä·rek'tor pī'lī/ *pl.* **arrectores pilorum** /ä·rek·tor'ez pī·lor'əm/ [L, raisers of the hair], minute smooth muscles of the skin, attached to the connective tissue sheath of the hair follicles; when they contract they cause the hair to stand erect, producing the appearance called goose flesh.

**arrest** [L, *ad, restare,* to withstand], to inhibit, restrain, or stop, as to arrest the course of a disease. See also **cardiac arrest.**

**arrested dental caries,** tooth decay in which the area of decay has stopped progressing and infection is not present but in which the demineralized area in the tooth remains as a cavity. Also called **eburnation of dentin.**

**arrested development,** the cessation of one or more phases of the developmental process in utero before normal completion, resulting in congenital anomalies. Also called **developmental arrest.**

**arrested labor** [L, *ad* + *restare,* to withstand, *labor,* work], an interruption in the labor process that may be caused by lack of uterine contractions.

**arrheno-,** prefix meaning 'male': *arrhenoblastoma, arrhenogenic.*

**arrhenoblastoma** /erē'nōblastō'mə/ [Gk, *arrhen,* male, *blastos,* germ, *oma,* tumor], an ovarian neoplasm whose cells mimic those in testicular tubules and secrete male sex hormone, causing virilization in females. Also called **andreioma, andreoblastoma, androma, arrhenoma, Sertoli-Leydig cell tumor.**

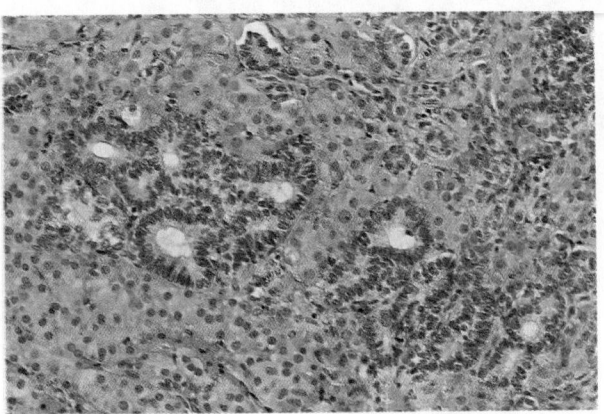

**Arrhenoblastoma** *(Fletcher, 2000)*

**arrhenogenic** /erē'nōjen'ik/, producing only male offspring.

**arrhenokaryon** /erē'nōker'ē·on/ [Gk, *arrhen,* male, *karyon,* nucleus], an organism that is produced from an egg that has only paternal chromosomes.

**arrhenoma.** See **arrhenoblastoma.**

**arrhythmia** /ərith'mē·ə, ərith'mē·ə/ [Gk, a + *rhythmos,* without rhythm], any deviation from the normal pattern of the heartbeat. Also spelled **arhythmia.** Compare **dysrhythmia.** —**arrhythmic, arrhythmical,** *adj.*

**arrhythmic** [Gk, *a, rhythmos,* without rhythm], pertaining to an absence or irregularity of normal rhythm in the heart's beating.

**ARRT,** abbreviation for **American Registry of Radiologic Technologists.**

**arsenic (As)** /är'sənik/ [Gk, *arsen,* strong], an element that occurs throughout the earth's crust in metal arsenides, arsenious sulfides, and arsenious oxides. Its atomic number is 33; its atomic mass is 74.92. The arsenic atom occurs in the elemental form and in trivalent and pentavalent oxidation states. This element has been used for centuries as a therapeutic agent and as a poison and continues to have limited use in some trypanosomicidal drugs such as melarsoprol and tryparsamide. The introduction of nonarsenic trypanosomicides with less dangerous side effects in the treatment of trypanosomiasis has greatly reduced its use. The average concentration in the human adult is about 20 mg, which is stored mainly in the liver, kidney, GI tract, and lungs. The mechanisms for the biotransformation of arsenics in humans are not well understood. Most arsenics are slowly excreted in the urine and feces, which accounts for the toxicity of the element. —**arsenic** /ärsen'ik/, *adj.*

**arsenic poisoning,** toxic effect caused by the ingestion or inhalation of arsenic or a substance containing arsenic, an ingredient in some pesticides, herbicides, dyes, and medicinal solutions. Small amounts absorbed over a period of time may result in chronic poisoning, producing nausea, headache, coloration and scaling of the skin, hyperkeratoses, anorexia, and white lines across the fingernails. Ingestion of large amounts of arsenic results in severe GI pain, diarrhea, vomiting, and swelling of the extremities. Renal failure and shock may occur, and death may result. Determination of the presence of arsenic in the urine, hair, or fingernails is diagnostic.

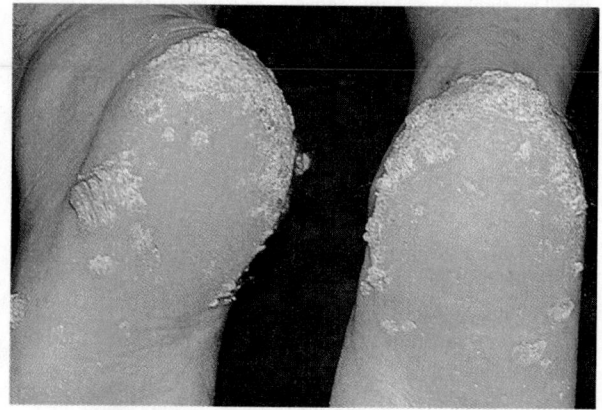

**Arsenic keratoses** (Lawrence and Cox, 1993)

**arsenic stomatitis** [Gk, *arsen,* strong; *stoma,* mouth, *itis,* inflammation],   an abnormal oral condition associated with arsenic poisoning, characterized by dry, red, painful oral mucosa; ulceration; bleeding beneath the mucosa; and mobility of teeth. Compare **Atabrine stomatitis, bismuth stomatitis.** See also **arsenic poisoning.**
**arsenic trihydride.**   See **arsine.**
**arsine (AsH$_3$),**   a colorless poisonous gas with an unpleasant odor. It occurs in various industries, particularly where scrap metal is used or produced. Also called **arsenic trihydride.**
**ART,**   abbreviation for **active resistance training.**
**Artane,**   trademark for an anticholinergic (trihexyphenidyl hydrochloride).
**artefact.**   See **artifact.**
**arterectomy** /är′tərek′təmē/,   the surgical removal of a segment of an artery.
**arteri-.**   See **arterio-.**
**arteria alveolaris inferior.**   See **inferior alveolar artery.**
**arterial** /ärtir′ē·əl/ [Gk, *arteria,* airpipe],   pertaining to an artery.
**arterial bleeding.**   See **arterial hemorrhage.**
**arterial blood gas (ABG),**   the oxygen and carbon dioxide content of arterial blood, measured by various methods to assess the adequacy of ventilation and oxygenation and the acid-base status of the body. Oxygen saturation of hemoglobin is normally 95% or higher. The partial pressure of arterial oxygen, normally 80 to 100 mm Hg, is increased in hyperventilation and decreased in cardiac decompensation, chronic obstructive pulmonary disease, and certain neuromuscular disorders. The partial pressure of carbon dioxide, normally 38 to 45 mm Hg, may be higher in emphysema, chronic obstructive pulmonary disease, and reduced respiratory center function; it may be lower in pregnancy and in the presence of pulmonary emboli and anxiety.

**Arterial blood gases**

| Respiratory function | Measurements | Normal value |
|---|---|---|
| Acid-base balance | pH-hydrogen ion concentration | 7.35-7.45 |
| Oxygenation | PaO$_2$: partial pressure of dissolved O$_2$ in blood | 80-100 mm Hg |
|  | SaO$_2$: percentage of O$_2$ bound to hemoglobin | 95%-98% |
| Ventilation | PaCO$_2$: partial pressure of CO$_2$ dissolved in blood | 38-45 mm Hg |

Modified from Phipps WF, Sands JK, and Marek JF: *Medical surgical nursing: concepts and clinical practice,* ed 6, St Louis, 1999, Mosby.

**arterial blood gases test (ABG),**   a blood test used to provide information that helps assess and manage a patient's respiratory (ventilation) and metabolic (renal) acid/base and electrolyte homeostasis, and to assess adequacy of oxygenation.
**arterial blood pressure (ABP),**   the pressure of the blood in the arterial system, which depends on the heart's pumping pressure, the resistance of the arterial walls, elasticity of vessels, the blood volume, and its viscosity.
**arterial capillaries,**   microscopic blood vessels (capillaries) extending beyond the terminal ends of arterioles.
**arterial catheter** [Gk, *arteria,* airpipe, *katheter,* a thing lowered into],   a tubular instrument that can be inserted into an artery either to draw blood or to measure blood pressure directly.
**arterial circle of Willis.**   See **circle of Willis.**
**arterial circulation** [Gk, *arteria* + L, *circulare,* to go around],   the movement of blood through the arteries directed away from the heart to the tissues, as opposed to venous circulation away from the tissues to the heart.
**arterial hemorrhage,**   the loss of blood from an artery, often associated with vessel trauma or the removal of a large-bore arterial catheter. Also called **arterial bleeding.**
**arterial insufficiency,**   inadequate blood flow in arteries. It may be caused by occlusive atherosclerotic plaques or emboli; damaged, diseased, or intrinsically weak vessels; arteriovenous fistulas; aneurysms; hypercoagulability states; or heavy use of tobacco. Signs of arterial insufficiency include

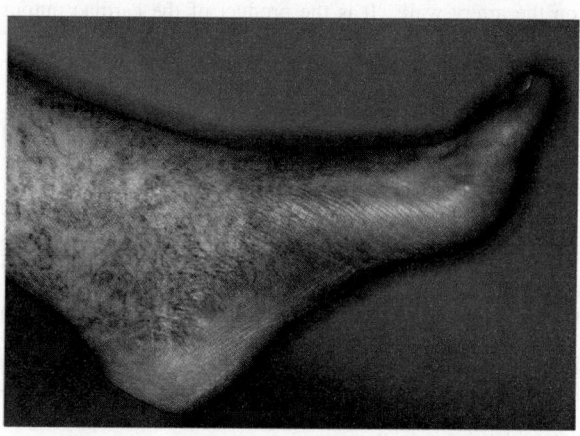

**Arterial insufficiency of the lower extremities**
(Lemmi and Lemmi, 2000)

pale, cyanotic, or mottled skin over the affected area, absent or decreased sensations, tingling, diminished sense of temperature, muscle pains, reduced or absent peripheral pulses, and, in advanced disease, arterial ulcers and atrophy of muscles in the involved extremity. Diagnosis includes checking and comparing peripheral pulses in contralateral extremities, angiography, ultrasound using a Doppler device, and skin temperature tests. Treatment may include a diet low in saturated fats, moderate exercise, sleeping on a firm mattress, use of a vasodilator, and, if indicated, surgical repair of an aneurysm or arteriovenous fistula. Use of tobacco products, prolonged standing, and sitting with the knees bent are discouraged.

**arterial insufficiency of lower extremities,** a condition characterized by hardening, thickening, and loss of elasticity of the walls of arteries in the legs. It causes decreased circulation, sensation, and function. Symptoms include sharp, cramping pain during exercise or rest at night; numbness; skin changes ranging from pallor to ulceration; thickened toenails; and loss of hair on the legs. Dorsalis pedis, posterior tibial, and popliteal pulses may be diminished or absent. Laboratory studies usually show elevated plasma lipid levels. See also **claudication.**

**arterial line (A-line, Art-line),** an arterial blood monitoring system consisting of a catheter inserted into an artery and connected to pressure tubing, a transducer, and a monitor. The device permits continuous direct blood pressure readings as well as access to the arterial blood supply when samples are needed for analysis.

**arterial murmur,** a sound produced by blood moving through narrowed artery.

**arterial nephrosclerosis** [Gk, *arteria,* airpipe, *nephros,* kidney, *sklera,* hard, *osis,* condition], arteriosclerosis of the renal arteries, leading to deprivation of oxygenated blood to the kidney tissues and their destruction.

**arterial network** [L, *rete,* net: Gk, *arteria*], an anastomotic network of small arteries at a point before they branch into arterioles and capillaries. Also called **rete arteriosum.**

**arterial palpitation** [Gk, *arteria,* airpipe; L, *palpitare,* to flutter], a pulsation felt in an artery.

**arterial pH,** the hydrogen ion concentration of arterial blood. Normal range is 7.35 to 7.45.

**arterial plethysmography,** a manometric test that is usually performed to rule out occlusive disease of the lower extremities. It can also be used to identify arteriosclerotic disease in the upper extremity.

**arterial pressure,** the stress exerted by circulating blood on the artery walls. It is the product of the cardiac output and the systemic vascular resistance. A number of extrinsic and intrinsic factors regulate and maintain a reasonably constant arterial pressure. Extrinsic factors include neurologic stimulation and hormones such as catecholamines and prostaglandins. Intrinsic factors include chemoreceptors and pressure-sensitive receptors in the arterial walls that cause vasoconstriction or vasodilation. Arterial pressure is commonly measured with a sphygmomanometer and a stethoscope. Stress, hypervolemia, hypovolemia, and various drugs may alter the arterial pressure. Also called **arterial tension.** See also **blood pressure.**

**arterial rete** /rē′tē/ [Gk, *arteria,* airpipe; L, *rete,* net], a network of arteries and arterioles.

**arterial sclerosis** [Gk, *arteria,* airpipe, *sklerosis,* hardening], a thickening of the arteries. See also **arteriosclerosis, atherosclerosis.**

**arterial tension.** See **arterial pressure.**

**arterial thrill,** a vibration that can be felt over an artery. It is unusually associated with turbulent blood flow within the artery.

**arterial wall,** the fibrous and muscular wall of vessels that carry oxygenated blood from the heart to structures throughout the body, and of the pulmonary arteries that carry deoxygenated blood from the heart to the lungs. The wall of an artery has three layers: the **tunica intima,** the inner coat; the **tunica media,** the middle coat; and the **tunica adventitia,** the outer coat. Nerves from the sympathetic system constrict the vessel and thus control the flow of blood into the areas served by the artery. The middle layer in smaller arteries is almost entirely muscular and in larger arteries is more elastic. The thickness of the outer layer varies with the location of the artery. In protected areas, such as the abdominal and cranial cavities, the outer layer of associated arteries is very thin, but in more exposed locations, as in the limbs, it is much thicker.

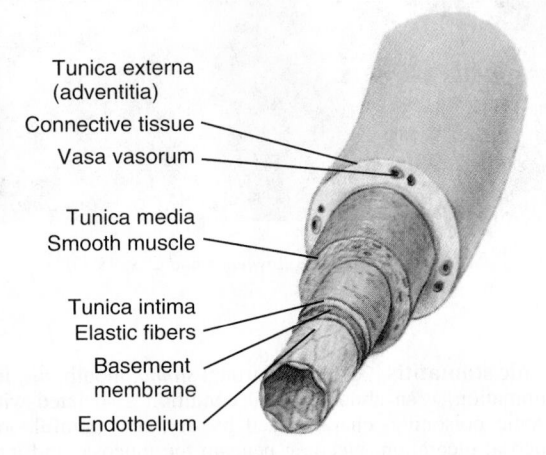

Tunica externa (adventitia)
Connective tissue
Vasa vasorum
Tunica media
Smooth muscle
Tunica intima
Elastic fibers
Basement membrane
Endothelium

**Arterial wall** *(Applegate, 2000)*

**arteriectomy** /ärtir′ē·ek′təmē/ [Gk, *arteria* + *ektomē,* excision], the surgical removal of a portion of an artery.

**arteries.** See **blood vessel.**

**arterio-, arteri-,** prefix meaning 'artery': *arteriosclerosis, arteritis.*

**arteriocapillary** /är·tēr′ē·ō·kap′i·lar′ē/ [Gk, *arteria* + L, *capillaris,* hairlike], pertaining to the arteries and the capillaries.

**arteriofibrosis** /ärtir′ē·ōfībrō′sis/, an inflammatory, fibrous thickening of the walls of the arteries and arterioles, resulting in a narrowing of the lumen of the vessels.

**arteriogram** /ärtir′ē·əgram′/, an x-ray film of an artery injected with a radiopaque medium. See also **arteriography.**

**arteriography** /ärtir′ē·og′rəfē/ [Gk, *arteria,* airpipe, *graphein,* to record], a method of radiologic visualization of arteries performed after a radiopaque contrast medium is introduced into the bloodstream or into a specific vessel by injection or through a catheter. See also **angiography.** —**arteriographic,** *adj.*

**arteriole** /ärtir′ē·ōl/ [L, *arteriola,* little artery], the smallest of the arteries. Blood flowing from the heart is pumped through the arteries, to the arterioles, to the capillaries, into the veins, and returned to the heart. The muscular walls of the arterioles constrict and dilate in response to both local factors and neurochemical stimuli; thus, arterioles play a significant role in peripheral vascular resistance and in regulation of blood pressure. Also called **arteriola.** See also **artery.**

**arteriolosclerosis** /ärtir′ē·ō′ləsklärō′sis/, pathologic thickening, hardening, and loss of elasticity of arteriolar walls.

**arteriopathy** /ärtir′ē·op′əthē/ [Gk, *arteria* + *pathos,* suffering], a disease of an artery.

**arterioplasty** /ärtir′ē·əplas′tē/ [Gk, *arteria* + *plassein,* to mold], plastic surgery of an artery. The procedure is often performed to correct an aneurysm.

**arteriosclerosis** /ärtir′ē·ō′sklärō′sis/ [Gk, *arteria* + *sklerosis,* hardening], a common disorder characterized by thickening, loss of elasticity, and calcification of arterial walls. It results in a decreased blood supply, especially to the cerebrum and lower extremities. The condition often develops with aging and in hypertension, nephrosclerosis, scleroderma, diabetes, and hyperlipidemia. Typical signs and symptoms include intermittent claudication, changes in skin temperature and color, altered peripheral pulses, bruits over an involved artery, headache, dizziness, and memory defects. Vasodilators and exercise may relieve symptoms, but there is no specific treatment. Preventive measures include therapy for predisposing diseases, adequate rest and exercise, avoidance of stress, and discontinuation of tobacco use. Kinds of arteriosclerosis include **atherosclerosis** and **Mönckeberg's arteriosclerosis.** Also called **arterial sclerosis, hardening of the arteries.—arteriosclerotic,** *adj.*

**arteriosclerosis obliterans** [Gk, *arteria* + *skleros* + L, *obliterare,* efface], a gradual narrowing of the arteries with thrombosis and degeneration of the intima. The condition may lead to complete occlusion of an artery and subsequent gangrene.

**arteriosclerotic** /-sklärot′ik/ [Gk, *arteria* + *skleros,* hard], pertaining to a thickening and hardening of the arterial wall.

**arteriosclerotic heart disease (ASHD),** a thickening and hardening of the walls of the coronary arteries.

**arteriosclerotic retinopathy** [Gk, *arteria,* airpipe, *sklerosis,* hardening; L, *rete,* net; Gk, *pathos,* disease], a disorder of the retina associated with hardening and thickening of the arteries supplying that part of the eye. It often accompanies hypertension.

**arteriospasm** /ärtir′ē·ōspaz′əm/ [Gk, *arteria* + *spasmos,* spasm], a spasm of an artery.

**arteriostenosis** /-stänō′sis/, a narrowing of an artery.

**arteriotomy** /ärtir′ē·ot′əmē/, a surgical incision in an artery.

**arteriovenous (AV)** /-vē′nəs/ [Gk, *arteria* + L, *vena,* vein], pertaining to arteries and veins.

**arteriovenous anastomosis** [Gk, *arteria* + L, *vena;* Gk, *anastomoein,* to form a mouth], a communication between an artery and a vein, either as a congenital anomaly or as a surgically produced link between vessels.

**arteriovenous aneurysm,** a dilation affecting both an artery and a vein, often as an abnormal linkage of the two.

**arteriovenous angioma of the brain,** a congenital tumor consisting of a tangle of coiled, usually dilated arteries and veins, islets of sclerosed brain tissue, and, occasionally, cartilaginous cells. The lesion, which may be distinguished by an intracranial bruit, generally arises in the vascular system of the pia mater and may grow to project deeply into the brain, causing seizures and progressive hemiparesis.

**arteriovenous fistula,** an abnormal communication between an artery and vein. It may occur congenitally or result from trauma, infection, arterial aneurysm, or a malignancy. A continuous murmur and palpable thrill may be detected over the fistula and may be obliterated by compressing the feeding artery; this maneuver may slow the heartbeat (Branham's sign). Chronic arteriovenous fistulas may cause varicosities, cutaneous ulcers, and cardiac enlargement. A congenital fistula may result in a cavernous hemangioma. If an

arteriovenous fistula is limited in size and is accessible, it can be treated by surgical excision. An arteriovenous fistula is often created surgically to provide vascular access for hemodialysis.

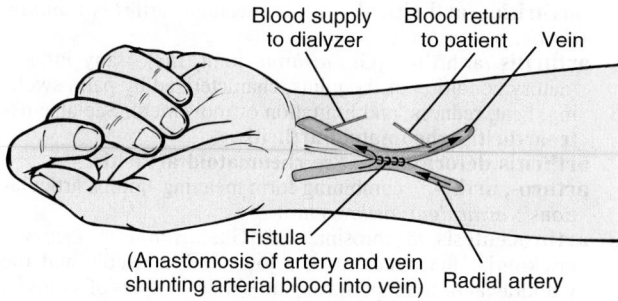

Blood supply to dialyzer   Blood return to patient   Vein

Fistula (Anastomosis of artery and vein shunting arterial blood into vein)   Radial artery

**Arteriovenous fistula** *(Lewis, Heitkemper, Dirksen, 2000)*

**arteriovenous oxygen (a-vo₂) difference,** the arterial oxygen content minus the central venous oxygen content.

**arteriovenous shunt (AV shunt),** a passageway, artificial or natural, that allows blood to flow from an artery to a vein without going through a capillary network.

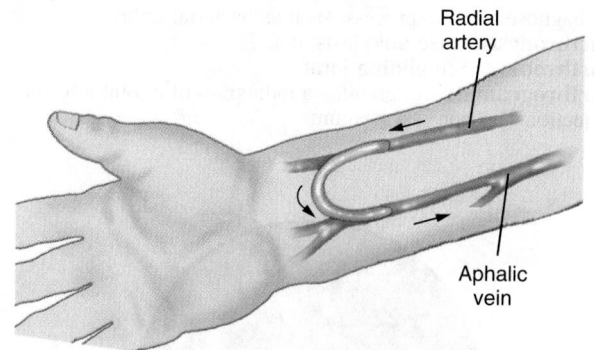

Radial artery

Aphalic vein

**Arteriovenous shunt** *(Sanders et al, 2000)*

**arteritis** /är′tərī′tis/ [Gk, *arteria* + *itis*], inflammation of the inner layers or the outer coat of one or more arteries. It may occur as a clinical entity or accompany another disorder, such as rheumatoid arthritis, rheumatic fever, polymyositis, or systemic lupus erythematosus. Kinds of arteritis include **infantile, rheumatic, Takayasu's,** and **temporal arteritis.** See also **endarteritis, periarteritis.**

**arteritis obliterans.** See **endarteritis obliterans.**

**arteritis umbilicalis,** septic inflammation of the umbilical artery in newborns, usually caused by the bacterium *Clostridium tetani.*

**artery** /är′tərē/ [Gk, *arteria,* airpipe], one of the large blood vessels carrying blood in a direction away from the heart to the tissues. See also **arterial wall, arteriole.** Compare **vein.**

**artery forceps,** any forceps used for grasping, compressing, and holding the end of an artery during ligation. Generally self-locking, its handles are scissorlike. Also called **hemostatic forceps.**

**arthral.** See **articular.**

**arthralgia** /ärthral'jə/ [Gk, *arthron,* joint, *algos,* pain], joint pain. —**arthralgic,** *adj.*

**-arthria,** suffix meaning a '(specified) condition involving the ability to articulate': *anarthria, dysarthria.*

**-arthritic, -arthritical,** suffix meaning 'arthritis': *antiarthritic, postarthritic.*

**arthritis** /ärthrī'tis/ [Gk, *arthron,* joint, *itis*], any inflammatory condition of the joints, characterized by pain, swelling, heat, redness, and limitation of movement. See also **osteoarthritis, rheumatoid arthritis.**

**arthritis deformans.** See **rheumatoid arthritis.**

**arthro-, arthr-,** combining form meaning 'joints, articulations': *arthralgia, arthrocentesis.*

**arthrocentesis** /är'thrōsintē'sis/ [Gk, *arthron + kentesis,* pricking], the puncture of a joint with a needle and the withdrawal of fluid, performed to obtain samples of synovial fluid for diagnostic purposes. It may also be used to instill medications and to remove fluid from joints to simply relieve pain. A local anesthetic is usually administered; surgical asepsis is observed in the procedure. Normal synovial fluid is a clear, straw-colored, slightly viscous liquid that forms a white, viscous clot when mixed with glacial acetic acid; if inflammation is present, as in rheumatoid arthritis, the fluid is watery and turbid, and its mixture with glacial acetic acid results in a flocculent, easily broken clot. The number of leukocytes, especially polymorphonuclear cells, and the protein content are increased, and the glucose level is decreased if inflammation is present. Synovial fluid samples are also cultured and examined microscopically to diagnose a septic process, such as bacterial arthritis.

**arthrodesis.** See **ankylosis,** def. 2.

**arthrodia.** See **gliding joint.**

**arthrogram** /är'thrəgram/, a radiogram of a joint after injection of a contrast medium.

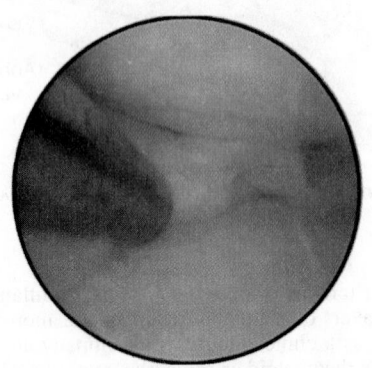

**Arthrogram of the knee** *(Johnson, 1981)*

**arthrography** [Gk, *arthron,* joint, *graphein,* to record], a method of radiographically visualizing the inside of a joint using a radiolucent or radiopaque contrast medium.

**arthrogryposis multiplex congenita** [Gk, *arthron + gryposis,* joint curve; L, *multus,* many, *plica,* fold, *congenitus,* born with], fibrous stiffness of one or more joints, present at birth. It is often associated with incomplete develop-

ment of the muscles that move the involved joints and degenerative changes of the motor neurons that innervate those muscles. The cause of the condition, which is uncommon, is unknown. Physiotherapy to loosen the joints is the only treatment. Also called **amyoplasia congenita** /əmī'ōplā'zhə/.

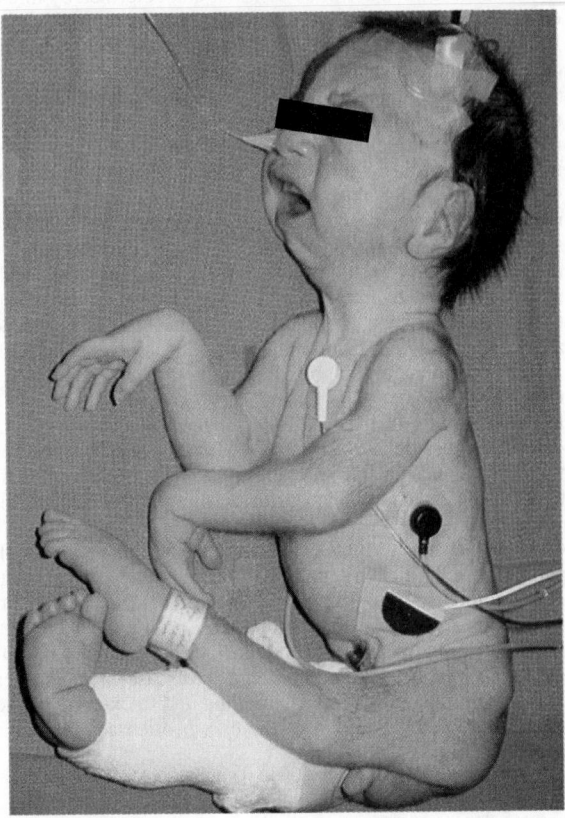

**Neonate with arthrogryposis multiplex congenita**
*(Moore, 1994/courtesy Dr. A.E. Chudley, Department of Pediatrics and Child Health, University of Manitoba, Children's Hospital, Winnipeg, Canada)*

**arthrokinematic** /är'thrəkin'əmat'ik/, pertaining to the movement of bone surfaces within a joint.

**arthron** /är'thron/ [Gk], a joint or articulation, including its various components of bones, cartilaginous inserts, all soft tissue structures intervening between the rigid skeletal parts, and the adjacent muscular elements.

**arthropathy** /ärthrop'əthē/ [Gk, *arthron + pathos,* suffering], any disease or abnormal condition affecting a joint. —**arthropathic,** *adj.*

**arthroplasty** /är'thrəplast'ē/ [Gk, *arthron + plassein,* to mold], the surgical reconstruction or replacement of a painful, degenerated joint, to restore mobility in osteoarthritis or rheumatoid arthritis or to correct a congenital deformity. Either the bones of the joint are reshaped and soft tissue or a metal disk is placed between the reshaped ends, or all or part of the joint is replaced with a metal or plastic prosthesis. Preoperative care may include the typing and crossmatching of blood. After surgery the patient may be placed in traction to immobilize the affected limb. Physical therapy to increase muscle strength and range of motion is allowed in a slow, progressive schedule. When a lower extremity is involved, weight-bearing may or may not be allowed. Frequent checks of distal circulation are made and the nurse watches for signs of surgical shock, thrombophlebitis, pulmonary embolism, or fat embolism. Antibiotics are usually given to prevent infection, which is the most common cause of failure of the surgery. See also **osteoarthritis.**

**arthropod** /är′thrəpod′/ [Gk, *arthron* + *pous,* foot], a member of the Arthropoda, a large phylum of animal life that includes crabs and lobsters as well as mites, ticks, spiders, and insects. Arthropods generally are distinguished by a jointed exoskeleton (shell) and paired, jointed legs; they bite, sting, cause allergic reactions, and may serve as vectors for viruses and other disease-causing agents.

**arthroscope** /-skōp′/ [Gk, *arthron* + *skopein,* to watch], a type of endoscope used to examine joints.

**arthroscopy** /ärthros′kəpē/ [Gk, *arthron* + *skopein,* to watch], the examination of the interior of a joint, performed by inserting a specially designed endoscope through a small incision. The procedure, used chiefly in knee problems, permits biopsy of cartilage or synovium, diagnosis of a torn meniscus, and, in some instances, removal of loose bodies in the joint space. —**arthroscopic,** *adj.*

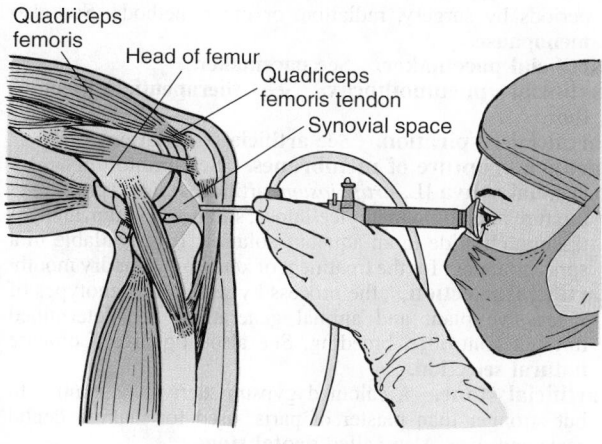

Quadriceps femoris
Head of femur
Quadriceps femoris tendon
Synovial space

**Arthroscopy** *(Beare and Myers, 1998)*

**arthrous** /är′thrəs/ [Gk, *arthron*], 1. pertaining to joints or the articulation of bones. 2. pertaining to a disease of a joint.

**Arthus reaction** /ärtoōs′/ [Nicholas M. Arthus, French physiologist, 1862–1945], a rare, severe, immediate nonatopic hypersensitivity reaction to the injection of a foreign substance, that usually is not irritating but in certain individuals is antigenic. The reaction is thought to involve the formation of an antigen-antibody complex that activates complement. Acute local inflammation, usually in the skin and marked by edema, hemorrhage, and necrosis, occurs at the site of injection. Also called **Arthus phenomenon.** See also **serum sickness.**

**articul-,** combining form meaning 'joint, structure and function': *articular, articulatio.*

**articular** /ärtik′yələr/ [L, *articulare,* to divide into joints], relating to a joint or the involvement of joints.

**articular capsule** [L, *articulare,* to divide into joints], an envelope of tissue that surrounds a freely moving joint, composed of an external layer of white fibrous tissue and an internal synovial membrane. See also **fibrous capsule.**

**articular cartilage** [L, *articulare* + *cartilago*], a type of hyaline connective tissue that covers the articulating surfaces of bones within synovial joints. See also **cartilage.**

**articular disk,** the platelike cartilaginous end of certain bones in movable joints, sometimes closely associated with surrounding muscles or with cartilage.

**articular fracture,** a fracture involving the articulating surfaces of a joint.

**articular head,** a projection on a bone that forms a joint with another bone.

**articular muscle,** a muscle that is attached to the capsule of a joint.

**articular process of vertebra,** a bony outgrowth on a vertebra that forms a joint with an adjoining vertebra.

**articulate** /ärtik′yəlāt/ [L, *articulare,* to divide into joints], 1. to form a joint. 2. to use speech that is distinct and connected.

**articulated** /ärtik′yəlā′tid/, 1. united by a movable joint. 2. expressed in clear speech.

**articulated partial denture.** See **partial denture.**

**articulatio cubiti.** See **elbow joint.**

**articulatio ellipsoidea.** See **condyloid joint.**

**articulatio genus.** See **knee joint.**

**articulation.** See **joint.**

**articulation of the pelvis** /ärtik′yəlā′shən/, any one of the connections between the bones of the pelvis, involving four groups of ligaments. The first group connects the sacrum and the ilium; the second, the sacrum and the ischium; the third, the sacrum and the coccyx; and the fourth, the two pubic bones.

**articulatio plana.** See **gliding joint.**

**articulatio sellaris.** See **saddle joint.**

**articulator** /ärtik′yəlā′tər/ [L, *articulare,* to divide into joints], a mechanical device used in the fabrication and testing of dental prostheses. It represents the temporomandibular joints and jaw members to which maxillary and mandibular casts may be attached. Some articulators are adjustable, allowing movement of attached casts into various eccentric relationships.

**articulus.** See **joint.**

**artifact** /är′təfakt/ [L, *ars,* skill, *facere,* to make], anything artificially made; may be extraneous, irrelevant, or unwanted, such as a substance, structure, or piece of data or information. In radiologic imaging, spurious electronic signals may appear as an artifact in an image with as much strength as the signals produced by the real objects, thereby confusing the radiologist and the results of any examination.

**artifactual modification** /är′təfak′choo·əl/, a change in protein structure caused by in vitro manipulation.

**artificial** /är′tifish′əl/ [L, *artificium,* not natural], 1. made by human work as a substitute for something that is natural. 2. simulated, resulting from art in imitation of nature.

**artificial abortion,** an abortion that is produced deliberately.

**artificial airway** [L, *artificiosum,* skillfully made], a plastic or rubber device that can be inserted into the upper or lower respiratory tract to facilitate ventilation or the removal of secretions.

**artificial airway management,** a nursing intervention from the Nursing Interventions Classification (NIC) defined as maintenance of endotracheal and tracheostomy tubes and preventing complications associated with their use. See also **Nursing Interventions Classification.**

**artificial ankylosis,** a surgical procedure in which two or more parts of a joint are fixed so that the joint becomes immovable.

**artificial anus,** a surgical opening into the bowel, as in a colostomy.

**artificial assists,** any prosthetic devices or contrivances that may enable a physically challenged person to function. Examples include heart pacemakers, crutches, and artificial limbs.

**artificial blood.** See **perfluorocarbons.**

**artificial classification of caries.** See **classification of caries.**

**artificial classification of cavities,** any cavity that may be classified in one of six groups, the first five of which are those proposed by G.V. Black. Class 1: cavities associated with structural tooth defects in the occlusal surfaces of posterior teeth, and lingual surfaces of anterior teeth, such as pits and fissures; class 2: cavities in the proximal surfaces of premolars and molars; class 3: cavities in the proximal surfaces of the canines and incisors that do not involve removal and restoration of the incisal angle; class 4: cavities in the proximal surfaces of canines and incisors that require the removal and restoration of the incisal angle; class 5: cavities, except pit cavities, in the gingival third of the labial, buccal, or lingual surfaces of the teeth; class 6: (not included in Black's classification) cavities on the incisal edges and cusp tips of the teeth. See also **cavity classification, simple cavity, smooth surface cavity.**

**artificial crown,** a dental prosthesis that restores part or all of the crown of a natural tooth. Compare **anatomic crown, clinical crown, partial crown.**

**artificial dentition.** See **dentition.**

**artificial eye,** a prosthetic device resembling the anterior surface of a normal eyeball. It is fitted under the upper and lower eyelid of an eye that has been removed.

**artificial fever,** an elevated body temperature produced by artificial means, such as the injection of malarial parasites or a vaccine known to produce fever symptoms or application of heat to the body. An artificial fever may be prescribed for a patient to arrest a disease that is sensitive to elevated body temperatures. Also called **fever therapy.**

**artificial heart,** a mechanical device of molded polyurethane, consisting of two ventricles implanted in the body and powered by an air compressor located outside the body. The first artificial heart for humans was implanted in December 1982 at the University of Utah Medical Center in Salt Lake City. It was attached to the atria and major blood vessels of the native heart with Dacron fittings and kept the patient alive for 112 days. See also **Jarvik-7.**

**artificial homologous insemination.** See **artificial insemination—husband (AIH).**

**artificial impregnation.** See **artificial insemination—husband.**

**artificial insemination (AI),** the introduction of semen into the vagina or uterus by mechanical or instrumental means rather than by sexual intercourse. The procedure is planned to coincide with the expected time of ovulation so that fertilization can occur. Kinds of artificial insemination are **artificial insemination—donor (AID)** and **artificial insemination—husband (AIH).** Also called **artificial impregnation.** See also **menstrual cycle.**

**artificial insemination—donor (AID),** artificial insemination in which the semen specimen is provided by an anonymous donor. The procedure is used primarily in cases where the husband is sterile. Also called **heterologous insemination.** Compare **artificial insemination—husband.**

**artificial insemination—husband (AIH),** artificial insemination in which the semen specimen is provided by the husband. The procedure is used primarily in cases of impotency, low sperm count, or a vaginal disorder or when the husband is incapable of sexual intercourse because of some physical disability. Also called **artificial homologous insemination.** Compare **artificial insemination—donor.**

**artificial intelligence (AI),** a system that makes it possible for a machine to perform functions similar to those performed by human intelligence, such as learning, reasoning, self-correcting, and adapting. Computer technology produces many instruments and systems that mimic and surpass some human capabilities, as speed of counting, correlating, sensing, and deducing.

**artificial kidney,** a device used to remove the body waste, commonly excreted in urine, from circulating blood. It usually consists of a set of tubes or catheters that pass the blood through a dialysate solution where wastes are removed by osmosis and diffusion. Also called **dialyzer, hemodialyzer, kidney machine.** See also **hemodialysis, peritoneal dialysis.**

**artificial labor** [L, *artificiosum,* artificial, *labor,* work], induced labor, as when started with drugs or mechanical devices.

**artificial limb.** See **prosthesis.**

**artificial lung.** See **Drinker respirator.**

**artificially acquired immunity.** See **acquired immunity.**

**artificial menopause** [L, *artificiosus,* artificial, *men,* month; Gk, *pauein,* to cease], the termination of menstrual periods by surgery, radiation, or other methods. See also **menopause.**

**artificial pacemaker.** See **pacemaker.**

**artificial pneumothorax.** See **therapeutic pneumothorax.**

**artificial respiration.** See **artificial ventilation.**

**artificial rupture of membranes.** See **amniotomy.**

**artificial saliva** [L, *artificiosum,* artifice, *saliva,* spittle], a mixture of carboxymethylcellulose, sorbitol, sodium, and potassium chloride in an aqueous solution. It is available in a spray container for the treatment of xerostomia, or dry mouth.

**artificial selection,** the process by which the genotypes of successive plant and animal generations are determined through controlled breeding. See also **eugenics.** Compare **natural selection.**

**artificial stone,** a calcined gypsum derivative similar to but stronger than plaster of paris, used for making dental casts and dies. Also called **dental stone.**

**artificial tears,** a pharmaceutical preparation of various polymers that can be instilled in the eyes of patients suffering from dry eye or keratoconjunctivitis sicca.

**artificial ventilation,** the process of supporting respiration by manual or mechanical means when normal breathing is inefficient or has stopped. If artificial ventilation is unsuccessful, the patient is repositioned and the airway is tested for the presence of an obstruction. Also called **artificial respiration.** See also **cardiopulmonary resuscitation, resuscitation, ventilator.**

**Art-line.** See **arterial line.**

**art therapist,** a human service professional who uses art media and images, the creative process, and client responses to artwork in order to assess, treat, and rehabilitate patients with mental, emotional, physical, or developmental disorders. Through art, the therapist attempts to help the client access and express memories, trauma, and psychic conflict often not easily reached with words.

**art therapy**[1], a type of adjunctive mental health treatment in which the patient is encouraged to express his or her feelings through various forms of artwork.

**art therapy²,** a nursing intervention from the Nursing Interventions Classification (NIC) defined as facilitation of communication through drawings or other art forms. See also **Nursing Interventions Classification.**

**aryepiglottic folds** /er′ē·ep′iglot′ik/, folds of mucous membrane that extend around the margins of the larynx from a junction with the epiglottis. They function as a sphincter during swallowing.

**aryl-,** prefix designating an alkyl monovalent radical derived from an aromatic hydrocarbon and used to denote aromatic groups.

**aryl hydrocarbon hydroxylase (AHH),** an enzyme that converts carcinogenic chemicals in tobacco smoke and in polluted air into active carcinogens within the lungs. Aryl hydrocarbon hydroxylase is the subject of numerous studies to determine why cancer develops in some smokers but not in others. Experimental blood tests indicate that the level of aryl hydrocarbon hydroxylase may be a factor in hereditary predisposition of a cigarette smoker to cancer.

**arytenoid cartilage** /ä·rit′ənoid kär′ti·ləj/ [Gk, *arytaina,* ladle + *eidos,* form; L, *cartilago*], one of the paired, pitcher-shaped cartilages of the back of the larynx at the upper border of the cricoid cartilage.

**As,** symbol for the element **arsenic.**

**AS,** abbreviation for **aortic stenosis.**

**as-.** See **ad-.**

**a.s.,** abbreviation for **auris sinistra.**

**ASA, 1.** abbreviation for *American Society of Anesthesiologists.* **2.** abbreviation for **aspirin** (acetylsalicylic acid).

**ASAHP,** abbreviation for *American Society of Allied Health Professionals; Association of Schools of Allied Health Professionals.*

**ASAP,** abbreviation for *as soon as possible.*

**asbestos** /asbes′təs/ [Gk, *asbestos,* unquenchable], a group of fibrous impure magnesium silicate minerals. Inhalation of the fibers can lead to pulmonary fibrosis if the fibers accumulate in terminal bronchioles. Continued exposure to asbestos fibers can result in lung cancer.

**asbestos body,** a structure found in the lungs of patients with asbestosis, consisting of an asbestos fiber engulfed by a macrophage or of a mass of asbestos spicules coated with calcium, iron salts, and other substances.

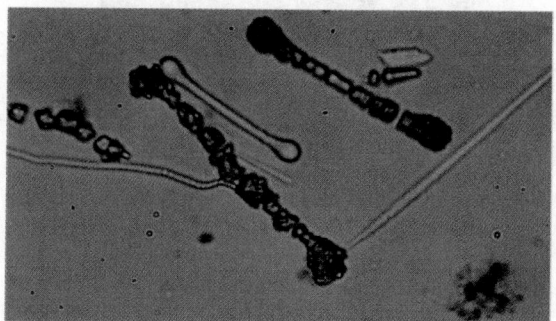

**Asbestos bodies** *(Silverberg, DeLellis, and Frable, 1997)*

**asbestosis** [Gk, *asbestos,* inextinguishable, *osis,* condition], a chronic lung disease caused by the inhalation of asbestos fibers that results in the development of alveolar, interstitial, and pleural fibrosis. Asbestos miners and workers are most frequently affected, but the disease sometimes occurs in other people who have been exposed to asbestos building materials. Chest x-ray films show the characteristic small linear opacities distributed throughout the lungs. The disease is progressive: Shortness of breath develops eventually into respiratory failure. Cigarette smoking and continuous exposure to asbestos aggravate the condition. Fatal mesothelial tumors sometimes occur. There is no treatment. See also **chronic obstructive pulmonary disease, inorganic dust.**

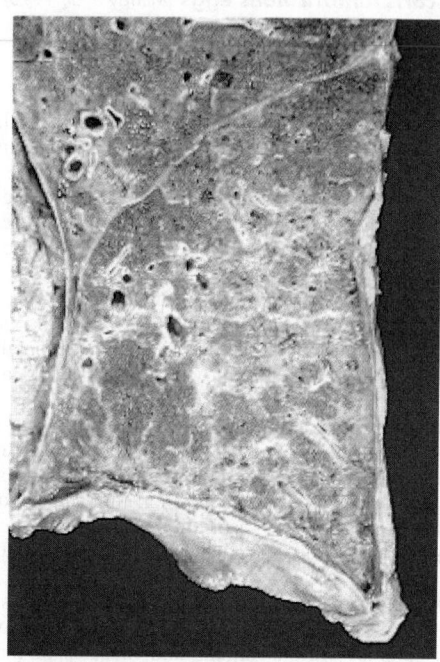

**Asbestosis** *(Kumar, Cotran, and Robbins, 1997)*

**ASC,** abbreviation for **altered state of consciousness.**

**ascariasis** /as′kərī′əsis/ [Gk, *askaris,* intestinal worm, *osis,* condition], an infection caused by a parasitic worm, *Ascaris lumbricoides,* that migrates through the lungs in its larval stage. The eggs are passed in human feces, contaminating the soil and allowing transmission to the mouths of others through hands, water, or food. After hatching in the small intestine, the larvae travel through the wall of the intestine and are carried by the lymphatics and blood to the lungs. Early respiratory symptoms of coughing, wheezing, hemoptysis, and fever are caused by the passage through the respiratory tract. The larvae are swallowed; they mature in the jejunum, where they release eggs; and the cycle is repeated. Intestinal infection may result in abdominal cramps and obstruction. In children migration of the adult worms into the liver, gallbladder, or peritoneal cavity may cause death. The infective eggs are readily identified in the feces. Piperazine citrate, pyrantel pamoate, mebendazole, and alberdazole are effective treatments. The disease can be prevented by educating people, especially children, about good hygiene such as handwashing.

*Ascaris* /as′kəris/, a genus of large parasitic intestinal roundworms, such as *Ascaris lumbricoides,* a cause of ascariasis, found throughout temperate and tropic regions.

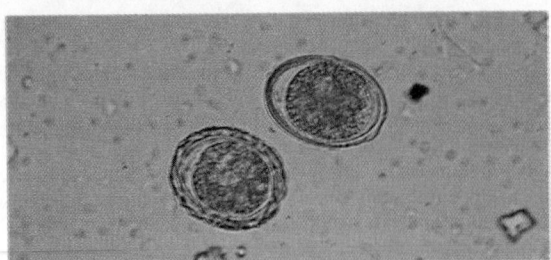

***Ascaris lumbricoides* eggs** *(Murray et al, 1990)*

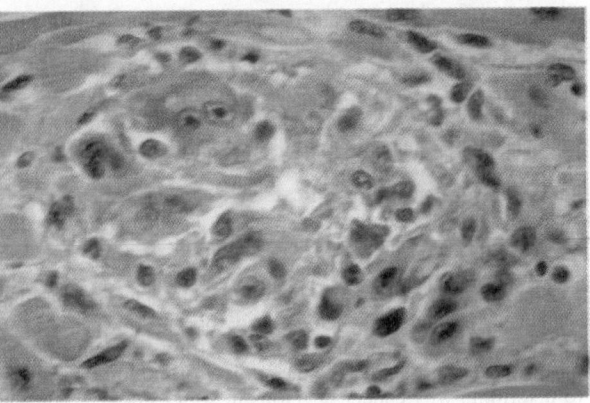

**Aschoff body**
*(Kumar, Cotran, and Robbins, 1997/courtesy Sid Murphree, MD, Department of Pathology, University of Texas Southwestern Medical School, Dallas)*

**ascending aorta** /asen'ding/ [L, *ascendere,* to climb], one of the four main sections of the aorta, branching into the right and left coronary arteries. See also **arch of the aorta.**

**ascending colon,** the segment of the colon that extends up the cecum in the lower right side of the colic fissure to the abdomen to the transverse colon at the hepatic flexure on the right side.

**ascending current.** See **centripetal current.**

**ascending neuritis** [L, *ascendere,* to rise; Gk, *neuron,* nerve, *itis,* inflammation], a nerve inflammation that begins on the periphery and moves upward along a nerve trunk.

**ascending neuropathy,** a disease of the nervous system that begins at a lower place in the body and spreads upward.

**ascending paralysis,** a condition in which there is successive flaccid paralysis of the legs, then the trunk and arms, and finally the muscles of respiration. Causes include poliomyelitis, Guillain-Barré syndrome, and exposure to toxic chemicals.

**ascending pharyngeal artery,** one of the smallest arteries that branch from the external carotid artery, deep in the neck. It supplies various organs and muscles of the head, such as the tympanic cavity, the longus capitis, and the longus colli. It divides into five branches: the pharyngeal, palatine, prevertebral, inferior tympanic, and posterior meningeal.

**ascending poliomyelitis** [L, *ascendere,* to rise; Gk, *polios,* gray, *myelos,* marrow, *itis,* inflammation], poliomyelitis that begins in the legs and spreads upward to involve the trunk and respiratory muscles. See also **ascending paralysis.**

**ascending tract** [L, *tractus*], a nervous system pathway found in the spinal cord that carries impulses toward the brain. Also called **afferent tract.**

**ascending urography.** See **urography.**

**asceticism** /aset'isiz'əm/ [Gk, *askein,* to exercise], (in psychiatry) a defense mechanism that involves repudiation of all instinctual impulses. The concept is derived from the religious doctrine that material things are evil and only spiritual things are good.

**Ascher's syndrome** /äsh'ərz/ [Karl Wolfgang Ascher, Czech-born American ophthalmologist, 1887–1971], relaxation of the skin of the eyelid and redundancy of the mucous membrane and submucous tissue of the upper lip in goiter.

**Aschoff bodies** [Karl A. L. Aschoff, German pathologist, 1866–1942; AS, *bodig*], tiny rounded or spindle-shaped nodules containing multinucleated giant cells, fibroblasts, and basophilic cells. They are found in joints, tendons, the pleura, and the cardiovascular system of rheumatic fever patients.

**ascites** /əsī'tēz/ [Gk, *askos,* bag], an abnormal intraperitoneal accumulation of a fluid containing large amounts of protein and electrolytes. Ascites may be detectable when more than 500 ml of fluid has accumulated. The condition may be accompanied by general abdominal swelling, hemodilution, edema, or a decrease in urinary output. Identification of ascites is made through palpation, percussion, and auscultation. Ascites is a complication, for example, of cirrhosis, congestive heart failure, nephrosis, malignant neoplastic disease, peritonitis, or various fungal and parasitic diseases. It is treated with dietary therapy and diuretic drugs; abdominal paracentesis may be performed to relieve pain and improve respiratory and visceral function by relieving the pressure of the accumulated fluid. A peritoneovenous shunt may be surgically inserted to drain the ascites via a tube from the peritoneal cavity to the superior vena cava. See also **paracentesis. —ascitic,** *adj.*

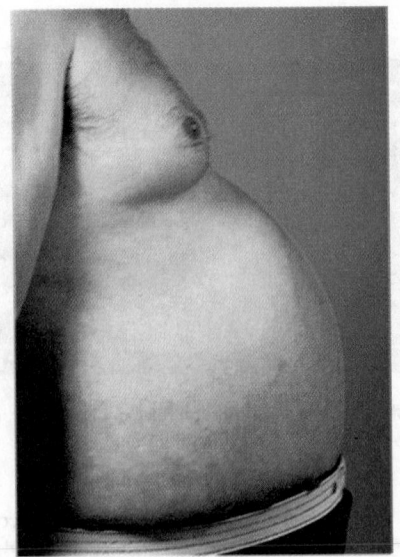

**Ascites** *(Lewis, Heitkemper, and Dirksen, 2000)*

**ascites adiposus.** See **chylous ascites.**

**ascites praecox** /prē′koks/ [Gk, *askos* + L, premature], an abnormal accumulation of fluid within the peritoneal cavity before the generalized edema associated with pericarditis. See also **ascites.**

**ascitic fluid** /əsit′ik/ [Gk, *askos,* bag], a watery fluid containing albumin, glucose, and electrolytes that accumulates in the peritoneal cavity in association with certain diseases, such as liver disease or congestive heart failure. The fluid occurs as leakage from the veins and lymphatics into extravascular spaces.

**ASCO,** abbreviation for *American Society of Clinical Oncology.*

**ascorbemia** /as′kôrbē′mē·ə/ [Gk, *a,* not; AS, *scurf,* scurvy; Gk, *haima,* blood], the presence of ascorbic acid in the blood in amounts greater than normal, usually reflecting only an excess of ascorbic acid intake. The condition is usually due to the use of ascorbic acid supplements.

**ascorbic acid** /əskôr′bik/ [Gk, *a,* not; AS, *scurf,* scurvy], a water-soluble, white crystalline vitamin present in citrus fruits, tomatoes, berries, potatoes, and fresh green and leafy vegetables, including broccoli, brussels sprouts, collards, turnip greens, parsley, sweet bell peppers, and cabbage. It is essential for the formation of collagen and fibrous tissue for normal intercellular matrices in teeth, bone, cartilage, connective tissue, and skin, and for the structural integrity of capillary walls. It also aids in fighting bacterial infections and interacts with other nutrients. Signs of deficiency are bleeding gums, tendency to bruise, swollen or painful joints, nosebleeds, anemia, lowered resistance to infections, and slow healing of wounds and fractures. Severe deficiency results in scurvy. A large excess of ascorbic acid may cause a burning sensation during urination, diarrhea, skin rash, and nausea and may disturb the absorption and metabolism of cyanocobalamin. Results of tests for glycosuria, uric acid, and iron may be inaccurate when the patient is receiving large amounts of the vitamin. Also called **antiscorbutic vitamin, vitamin C.** See also **ascorbemia, infantile scurvy, scurvy.**

**ascorburia** /as′kôrbyŏŏr′ē·ə/ [Gk, *a,* not; AS, *scurf,* scurvy; Gk, *ouron,* urine], the presence of ascorbic acid in the urine in amounts greater than normal. It usually reflects only an excess ascorbic acid intake, generally caused by the use of ascorbic acid supplements.

**ascribed role** /əskrībd′/, an assigned role in society, based on age, sex, or other factors about which the individual has no choice. See also **assumed role.**

**ASD,** abbreviation for **atrial septal defect.**

**-ase,** suffix used in naming enzymes; acts on the substance named in the word root (that precedes the suffix): *lipase, protease.*

**Asendin,** trademark for a tricyclic antidepressant (amoxapine).

**asepsis** /āsep′sis/ [Gk, *a, sepsis,* not decay], **1.** the absence of germs. **2. medical asepsis,** procedures used to reduce the number of microorganisms and prevent their spread. Examples include handwashing and "no touch" dressing technique. **3. surgical asepsis,** procedures used to eliminate any microorganisms; sterile technique. An example is sterilization of surgical instruments. —**aseptic,** *adj.*

**aseptic** /āsep′tik/ [Gk, *a,* without, *sepsis,* decay], pertaining to a condition free of living pathogenic organisms or infected material. See also **asepsis.**

**aseptic-antiseptic,** both aseptic and antiseptic.

**aseptic body image,** an awareness by operating room personnel of body, hair, makeup, clothing, jewelry, and placement with regard for maintenance of a sterile environment.

The body image also includes an awareness of changing proximities between sterile and contaminated areas as a field becomes progressively contaminated.

**aseptic bone necrosis,** a type of bone and joint damage that may occur in people who repeatedly breathe compressed air, as in diving or tunneling occupations. The condition apparently results from occlusion of small arteries in the bone by nitrogen bubbles, followed by infarction of bone tissue. It may also occur in total joint replacement and in patients taking corticosteroids. The condition may be asymptomatic or, if joint surfaces are involved, marked by severe pain and joint collapse.

**aseptic fever,** a fever not associated with infection. Mechanical trauma, as in a crushing injury, can cause fever even when no pathogenic microorganism is present. Although the exact mechanism is not understood, fever in such cases is believed to result from the breakdown of leukocytes or the absorption of avascular tissue.

**aseptic gauze,** any gauze that is free of microorganisms.

**aseptic meningitis,** an inflammation of the meninges that is caused by one of a number of viruses, including coxsackieviruses, nonparalytic polioviruses, echoviruses, and mumps, or may be drug induced, such as with high-dose IV immunoglobulin. Viral meningitis is especially common in children during the late summer and early fall. In about one third of the cases no pathogen can be demonstrated, but analysis of cerebrospinal fluid reveals increased numbers of white blood cells, usually lymphocytes; normal glucose concentration; slightly elevated protein levels; and no bacteria. Symptoms vary, depending on the causative agent and may include fever, headache, stiff neck and back, nausea, and skin rash. No specific treatment is available. Supportive therapy is directed to maintaining hydration and controlling fever. Complete recovery, without complication or residual effect, is usual. See also **viral meningitis.**

**aseptic necrosis** [Gk, *a, sepsis,* without decay, *nekros,* dead, *osis,* condition], cystic and sclerotic degenerative changes in tissues, as may follow an injury in the absence of infection.

**aseptic peritonitis** [Gk, *a, sepsis,* without decay, *peri,* near, *teinein,* to stretch, *itis,* inflammation], peritonitis in which inflammation of the peritoneum is caused by chemicals, radiation, or injury, rather than by an infectious agent.

**aseptic surgery** [Gk, *a, sepsis,* without decay, *cheirourgos,* surgeon], the prevention of contamination during surgical procedures.

**aseptic technique,** any health care procedure in which added precautions, such as use of sterile gloves and instruments, are used to prevent contamination of a person, object, or area by microorganisms.

**Asepto syringe,** trademark for a large bulb-fitted, blunt-tipped syringe used primarily for irrigating wounds.

**asexual** /āsek′shoo·əl/ [Gk, *a,* not; L, *sexus,* male or female]. **1.** not sexual. **2.** pertaining to an organism that has no sexual organs. **3.** pertaining to a process that is not sexual. —**asexuality,** *n.*

**asexual dwarf,** an adult dwarf whose genital organs are underdeveloped.

**asexual generation.** See **asexual reproduction.**

**asexuality.** See **asexual.**

**asexualization** /āsek′shoo·əlīzā′shən/, the process of making one incapable of reproduction; sterilization of an individual or animal by castration, vasectomy, removal of the ovaries, or use of chemicals.

**asexual reproduction,** any type of reproduction that occurs without the union of male and female gametes, such as fission, budding, sporulation, or parthenogenesis. Also called **asexual generation, direct generation, nonsexual generation.** Compare **sexual reproduction.**

**ASHA,** abbreviation for **American Speech, Language, and Hearing Association.**

**ASHD,** abbreviation for **arteriosclerotic heart disease.**

**Asherman syndrome,** secondary amenorrhea in a hormonally normal woman, caused by obliteration of the endometrial cavity by adhesions that form as a result of curettage or infection.

**asialorrhea.** See **hyposalivation.**

**Asian flu.** See **influenza.**

**asiderosis** /ā′sidərō′sis/, an iron deficiency and a cause of anemia.

**-asis,** suffix meaning an 'action, process, or result of': *metabasis, oxydasis.*

**ASL,** abbreviation for **American Sign Language.**

**ASLT,** abbreviation for **antistreptolysin-O test.**

**ASMT,** abbreviation for *American Society for Medical Technology.*

**Asn,** abbreviation for the amino acid **asparagine.**

**asocial** /āsō′shəl/ [Gk, *a*, without; L, *socius,* companion], withdrawn or disengaged from normal contacts with other individuals.

**asoma** /āsō′mə/ [Gk, *a*, not, *soma,* body], a fetus with an incomplete trunk and head.

**ASOT,** abbreviation for **antistreptolysin-O test.**

**asparaginase** /aspar′əjinās/ [Gk, *asparagos,* asparagus], an enzyme that catalyzes the hydrolysis of asparagine to asparaginic acid and ammonia. Asparaginase is used as a chemotherapeutic agent in the treatment of acute lymphoblastic leukemia and lymphosarcoma.

**asparagine (Asn)** /aspar′əjin/, a nonessential amino acid found in many food and body proteins. It is easily hydrolyzed to aspartic acid and has diuretic properties. See also **amino acid, protein.**

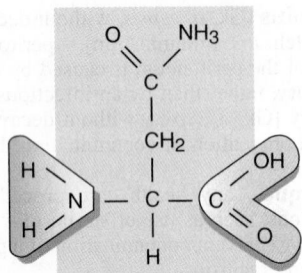

**Chemical structure of asparagine**

**aspartame** /aspär′tām, as′pərtām/, a white, almost odorless crystalline powder that is used as an artificial sweetener. It is formed by binding the amino acids of phenylalanine and aspartic acid. Approximately 180 times as sweet as the same amount of sucrose, it is used mostly to sweeten cold or uncooked foods. Unprotected aspartame tends to lose its sweetness in the presence of heat, moisture, and alkaline media. Excessive use of this nonnutritive sweetener should be avoided by patients with phenylketonuria (PKU) because the substance hydrolyzes to form aspartate and phenylalanine.

**aspartate aminotransferase (AST)** /aspär′tāt/, an enzyme normally present in body serum and in certain body tissues, especially those of the heart and liver. This enzyme affects the intermolecular transfer of an amino group from aspartic acid to alpha-ketoglutaric acid, forming glutamic acid and oxaloacetic acid. The reaction is reversible. The enzyme is released into the serum because of tissue injury and thus may increase as a result of myocardial infarction and liver damage. Normal findings for adults are 8 to 20 U/L or 5 to 40 IU/L. Previously called **glutamic-oxaloacetic transaminase, serum glutamic oxaloacetic transaminase (SGOT).** Compare **alanine aminotransferase.**

**aspartate aminotransferase test (AST, formerly called SGOT),** a blood test used in the evaluation of suspected coronary occlusive heart disease or hepatocellular diseases. AST is one of several enzymes tested in the cardiac enzyme series to help diagnose myocardial infarction.

**aspartate kinase,** an enzyme that catalyzes the transfer of a phosphate group from adenosine triphosphate to aspartate to produce phosphoaspartate.

**aspartate transaminase.** See **aspartate aminotransferase.**

**aspartic acid (Asp)** /aspär′tik/, a nonessential amino acid present in sugar cane, beet molasses, and breakdown products of many proteins. Pure aspartic acid is a water-soluble, colorless crystalline substance. In the citric acid cycle, aspartic acid and oxaloacetic acid are interconvertible. Aspartic acid is used in culture media, dietary supplements, detergents, fungicides, and germicides. Also called **aminosuccinic acid.** See also **amino acid, protein.**

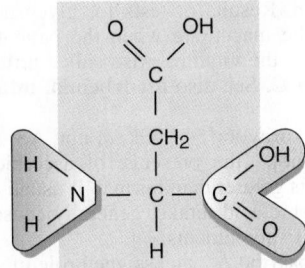

**Chemical structure of aspartic acid**

**aspastic** /āspas′tik/, not characterized by spasms.

**aspect** [L, *aspectus,* a look], the appearance, look, facing, or fronting of a person or object.

**Asperger's syndrome** /äs′pər·gərz/ [Hans Asperger, Austrian psychiatrist, 20th century], a pervasive developmental disorder similar to autistic disorder, characterized by severe impairment of social interactions and by restricted interests and behaviors, but lacking the delays in development of language, cognitive function, and self-help skills that additionally define autistic disorder. It may be equivalent to a high-functioning form of autistic disorder.

**aspergillic acid** /as′pərjil′ik/, an antibiotic substance derived from *Aspergillus flavus,* an aflatoxin-producing mold found on corn, grain, and peanuts. See **aflatoxins.**

**aspergillosis** /as′pərjilō′sis/ [L, *aspergere,* to sprinkle; Gk, *osis,* condition], an infection caused by inhalation of a fungus of the genus *Aspergillus* that can cause inflammatory, granulomatous lesions on or in any organ. The infection is relatively uncommon and typically occurs in an immunodeficient person already weakened by some other disorder. Topical fungicides can be used on the skin; amphotericin B is used to treat systemic aspergillosis, especially if it has spread to the lungs. Surgery may be required to remove a fungus ball. The prognosis, as for most systemic fungal infections, is poor. Compare **allergic bronchopulmonary aspergillosis.**

***Aspergillus*** /as'pərjil'əs/ [L, *aspergere,* to sprinkle], a genus of fungi that is a common contaminant in the laboratory and a cause of nosocomial infection. The fungus has hyphae and spores, lives in the soil, is ubiquitous, and proliferates rapidly. Inhalation of the spores of the two pathogenic species, *Aspergillus fumigatus* and *A. flavus,* is common, but infection is rare.

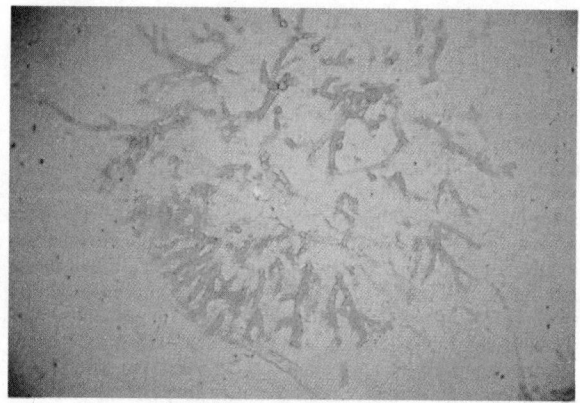

***Aspergillus fumigatus*** (Murray et al, 1998)

**aspermatic** /ā'spurmat'ik/, unable to secrete or ejaculate semen.

**aspermatogenesis** /āspur'mətōjen'əsis/, failure of the testes to produce spermatozoa.

**aspermia** /āspur'mē·ə/ [Gk, *a, sperma,* without seed], lack of formation or ejaculation of semen.

**asphyxia** /asfik'sē·ə/ [Gk, *a + sphyxis,* without pulse], severe hypoxia leading to hypoxemia and hypercapnia, loss of consciousness, and, if not corrected, death. Some of the more common causes of asphyxia are drowning, electrical shock, aspiration of vomitus, lodging of a foreign body in the respiratory tract, inhalation of toxic gas or smoke, and poisoning. Oxygen and artificial ventilation are promptly administered to prevent damage to the brain. The underlying cause is then treated. See also **artificial ventilation. —asphyxiate,** *v.,* **asphyxiated,** *adj.*

**asphyxia livida** /liv'ədə/, an abnormal condition in which a newborn's skin is cyanotic, the pulse is weak and slow, and the reflexes are slow or absent. Also called **blue asphyxia.**

**asphyxia neonatorum,** a condition in which a newborn does not breathe spontaneously. The asphyxia may develop before or during labor or immediately after delivery. The condition may involve placental or neonatal pulmonary dysfunction with underlying causes that can include abruptio placentae, umbilical compression, or uterine tetany. Other

factors include congenital defects, such as a diaphragmatic hernia, or adverse effects of anesthetics or analgesics administered to the mother. Immediate resuscitation is required to prevent death or brain damage. Also called **perinatal asphyxia.** See also **asphyxia livida, asphyxia pallida.**

**asphyxia pallida** /pal'ədə/, an abnormal condition in which a newborn appears pale and limp, shows signs of apnea, and suffers from bradycardia as marked by a heartbeat of 80 beats/min or less.

**asphyxiate** /asfik'sē·āt/ [Gk, *a + sphyxis,* without pulse], to induce an inability to breathe. Causes may include circulatory congestion, chemical poisoning, electrical shock, or physical suffocation.

**asphyxiated.** See **asphyxia.**

**asphyxiating thoracic dysplasia.** See **Jeune's syndrome.**

**asphyxiation** [Gk, *a + sphyxis,* without pulse], a state of asphyxia or inability to breathe.

**aspirant** /as'pirənt/, the fluid, gas, or solid particles that are withdrawn from the body by aspiration methods.

**aspirant maneuver,** a procedure used in making x-ray films of the laryngopharyngeal area. The patient exhales completely, then slowly inhales while making a harsh, high-pitched sound. The maneuver adducts the vocal cords so the ventricle of the larynx is clearly visible in the x-ray.

**aspirate** /-rāt/ [L, *aspirare,* to breathe upon], to withdraw fluid or air from a cavity. The process is usually aided by use of a syringe or a suction device. See **paracentesis, thoracentesis.**

**aspirating needle** /-rā'ting/, a long hollow needle used to remove fluid from a cavity, vessel, or structure of the body.

**aspirating syringe,** a hypodermic syringe used to inject local anesthetics, especially in dentistry. Checking for blood in the syringe after pulling back slightly on the plunger ensures that the anesthetic solution will not be deposited in a blood vessel.

**aspiration** /as'pirā'shən/, 1. drawing in or out by suction. 2. the act of withdrawing a fluid, such as mucus or serum, from the body by a suction device. See also **aspiration pneumonia. —aspirate,** *n.*

**aspiration biopsy,** the removal of living tissue, for microscopic examination, by suction through a fine needle attached to a syringe. The procedure is used primarily to obtain cells from a lesion containing fluid or when fluid is formed in a serous cavity. See also **cytology, needle biopsy.**

**aspiration biopsy cytology (ABC),** a microscopic examination of cells obtained directly from living body tissue by aspiration through a fine needle. It is used primarily as a diagnostic procedure, generally as a technique for detecting nuclear and cytoplasmic changes in cancerous tissue. Compare **exfoliative cytology.**

**aspiration control,** a nursing outcome from the Nursing Outcomes Classification (NOC) defined as personal actions to prevent the passage of fluid and solid particles into the lung. See also **Nursing Outcomes Classification.**

**aspiration drug abuse,** the inhalation of a liquid, solid, or gaseous chemical into the respiratory system for nontherapeutic purposes. Examples include glue and solvent sniffing and cocaine snorting.

**aspiration of vomitus,** the inhalation of regurgitated gastric contents into the pulmonary system. See also **aspiration pneumonia.**

**aspiration pneumonia,** an inflammatory condition of the lungs and bronchi caused by inhaling foreign material or acidic vomitus. Compare **bronchopneumonia.** See also **pneumonia.**

■ OBSERVATIONS: Aspiration pneumonia may occur during anesthesia or recovery from anesthesia or during a seizure of acute alcoholic intoxication or other condition characterized by vomiting and a decreased level of consciousness. Patients receiving enteral feeding therapies may also be at risk.

■ INTERVENTIONS: Treatment consists of prompt suctioning of the bronchi and administration of 100% oxygen. Continued artificial ventilation may be required. As long as oxygen is administered, frequent analyses of blood gas levels may be indicated. Corticosteroids may be given to diminish inflammation. The sputum is cultured regularly, and any bacterial infection thus diagnosed is treated with an appropriate antibiotic.

■ NURSING CONSIDERATIONS: The pulse rate and quality of respirations, level of consciousness, and skin color are carefully monitored. An oral airway is left in place until the patient's condition improves, and secretions are removed by suction as necessary. Infection and respiratory failure are frequent complications. Aspiration pneumonia may be prevented by positioning unconscious patients with the head elevated 15 to 30 degrees and turned to the side and by paying careful attention to the maintenance of enteral feeding therapy and an adequate airway.

**aspiration precautions,** a nursing intervention from the Nursing Interventions Classification (NIC) defined as prevention or minimization of risk factors in the patient at risk for aspiration. See also **Nursing Interventions Classification.**

**aspiration, risk for,** a nursing diagnosis accepted by the Eighth National Conference on the Classification of Nursing Diagnoses. Risk for aspiration is a state in which an individual is at risk for entry of gastric secretions, oropharyngeal secretions, or exogenous food or fluids into tracheobronchial passages caused by dysfunction or absence of normal protective mechanisms.

■ RISK FACTORS: Risk factors include reduced level of consciousness, depressed cough and gag reflexes, presence of a tracheostomy or endotracheal tube, overinflated tracheostomy or endotracheal tube cuff, inadequate inflation of a tracheostomy or endotracheal tube cuff, GI tubes, and bolus tube feedings or medication administration. Other risk factors are situations hindering elevation of the upper body, increased intragastric pressure, increased gastric residual, decreased GI motility, delay in gastric emptying, impaired swallowing, wired jaws, and facial, oral, or neck surgery or trauma. See also **nursing diagnosis.**

**aspirator** /as'pirā'tər/ [L, *aspirare*, to breathe upon], any instrument that removes a substance from a body cavity by suction, such as a bulb syringe, piston pump, or hypodermic syringe.

**aspirin (ASA)** /as'pirin/, an analgesic, antipyretic, and antiinflammatory. Also called **acetylsalicylic acid** /əsē'təlsal'isil'ik, as'itəl-/ **(ASA).**

■ INDICATIONS: It is prescribed to reduce fever and relieve pain and inflammation.

■ CONTRAINDICATIONS: Bleeding disorders, peptic ulcer, pregnancy, concomitant use of anticoagulants, or known hypersensitivity to salicylates prohibits its use.

■ ADVERSE EFFECTS: Among the most serious adverse reactions are ulcers, occult bleeding, clotting defects, renal toxicities, tinnitus, dyspepsia, and allergic reactions. Reye's syndrome has been associated with aspirin use in children.

**aspirin poisoning.** See **salicylate poisoning.**

**asplenia** /āsplē'nē·ə/ [Gk, *a*, without, *spleen*], absence of a spleen. The condition may be congenital or result from surgical removal.

**ASRT,** abbreviation for *American Society of Radiologic Technologists.*

**Assam fever.** See **kala-azar.**

**assault** /əsôlt'/ [L, *assilirere*, to leap upon], **1.** an unlawful act that places another person, without that person's consent, in fear of immediate bodily harm or battery. **2.** the act of committing an assault. **3.** to threaten a person with bodily harm or injury. See **battery.**

**assay** /asā', as'ā/ [Fr, *essayer*, to try], the analysis of the purity or effectiveness of drugs and other biologic substances, including laboratory and clinical observations.

**assertion training.** See **assertive training.**

**assertiveness** /əsur'tivnes/, behavior directed toward claiming one's rights without denying those of others.

**assertiveness training,** a nursing intervention from the Nursing Interventions Classification (NIC) defined as assistance with the effective expression of feelings, needs, and ideas while respecting the rights of others. See also **Nursing Interventions Classification.**

**assertive training** /əsur'tiv/ [L, *asserere*, to join to oneself], a therapeutic technique to help individuals become more self-assertive and self-confident in interpersonal relationships. It focuses on the direct, honest statement of feelings and beliefs, both positive and negative. The technique is learned by role playing in a therapeutic setting, usually in a group, followed by practice in actual situations. Also called **assertion training.**

**assess.** See **assessment.**

**assessing** /əses'ing/ [L, *assidere*, to sit beside], (in five-step nursing process) a category of nursing behavior that includes the gathering, verifying, and communicating of information related to the client. The nurse collects information from verbal interactions with the patient, the patient's family, and significant others; examines standard data sources for information; systematically checks for symptoms and signs; determines the patient's ability to perform self-care activities; assesses the patient's environment; and identifies reactions of the staff (including the nurse who is performing the assessment) to the patient and to the patient's family and significant others. To verify the data, the nurse confirms the observations and perceptions by gathering additional information; discusses the orders and decisions made by other members of the staff with them, when indicated; and personally evaluates and checks the patient's condition. The nurse reports the information that has been gathered and verified. Although assessing is the first of the five steps of the nursing process, preceding analyzing, in practice it is integral to effective nursing practice at all steps of the process. See also **analyzing, evaluating, implementing, nursing process, planning.**

**assessment** /əses'mənt/ [L, *assidere*, to sit beside], (in medicine and nursing) **1.** an evaluation or appraisal of a condition. **2.** the process of making such an evaluation. **3.** (in a problem oriented medical record) an examiner's evaluation of the disease or condition based on the patient's subjective report of the symptoms and course of the illness or condition and the examiner's objective findings, including data obtained through laboratory tests, physical examination, and medical history. See also **nursing assessment, problem-oriented medical record. —assess,** *v.*

**assessment of the aging patient,** an evaluation of the changes characteristic of advancing years exhibited by an elderly person.

■ METHOD: The patient is measured, weighed, examined, observed, and questioned about physical, functional, and behavioral changes; height normally diminishes 1 to 2 inches with aging, and weight steadily decreases in men over 65 years of age but increases in women. The skin is examined for dryness, wrinkles, sagging, thinning over the back of the hands, areas of vitiligo, keratoses, warts, changes in appearance of freckles and moles, skin tags, and senile telangiectases, and the hair for depigmentation, lack of luster, and thinning or loss on the scalp and in the axillary and pubic areas. Observations are made of enlargement of the nose and ears relative to face size, dryness of the eyes, opacity of the lens, discoloration of the sclera and iris, an opaque ring near the edge of the cornea (arcus senilis), decreased pupil size, and diminished peripheral vision. Tests are performed to determine whether there is hearing loss, especially of high-frequency tones; decreased tidal volume; diminished peripheral perfusion; exertional dyspnea; or deviation of the trachea, especially if scoliosis is present. Examination may reveal gum recession, loss of teeth and taste perception, and diminished salivation. It may also find decreased resting heart rate and cardiac output, increased diastolic and systolic blood pressure, and an easily palpable arterial pulse. The elderly patient may show decreased muscle mass, osteoarthritic joints, Heberden's or Bouchard's nodes at finger joints, contracture of lateral fingers, osteoporosis, a broad-based stance, and slow voluntary movements. The sense of position, of smell, and of touch and the sensitivity to heat and cold may be diminished, and deep tendon reflexes may be decreased. Signs of aging that may be found in women are pendulous, flaccid breasts; vaginal narrowing and shortening and diminished lubrication, causing painful coitus; and effects of long-term estrogen therapy. Signs of aging in men include decrease in the size and firmness of the testes and in the amount and viscosity of seminal fluid, increased diameter of the penis, and prostatic hypertrophy; libido and a sense of sexual satisfaction usually do not diminish. ■ NURSING CONSIDERATIONS: The nurse faces the patient during the evaluation, establishes eye contact, repeats questions if necessary, avoids shouting, and addresses the person by name. If the patient's visual perception and tactile sense are diminished, the nurse uses color contrasts and items of marked textural differences in the assessment. ■ OUTCOME CRITERIA: Aging does not progress at a uniform rate, and its effects may vary widely from one individual to the next, but, in many cases, changes once considered normal in elderly patients are disease processes that may respond to treatment. A thorough physical assessment distinguishes the effects of pathological disorders from those of aging and elucidates the care needed by the patient.

**assimilate** /əsim′əlāt/ [L, *assimilare,* to make alike],   to absorb nutritive substances from the digestive tract to the circulatory system and convert them into living tissues.

**assimilation** [L, *assimulare,* to make alike],   **1.** the process of incorporating nutritive material into living tissue; the end stage of the nutrition process, after digestion and absorption or simultaneous with absorption. **2.** (in psychology) the incorporation of new experiences into a person's pattern of consciousness. Compare **apperception. 3.** (in sociology) the process in which a person or a group of people of a different ethnic background become absorbed into a new culture. —**assimilate,** *v.*

**assist-control mode,**   a system of mechanical ventilation in which the patient is allowed to initiate breathing, although the ventilator delivers a set volume with each breath. The ventilator can also be programmed to initiate breathing if the patient's breathing slows beyond a certain point or stops altogether. Also called **continuous mandatory ventilation.**

**assisted breech** [L, *assistere,* to stand by],   an obstetric operation in which a baby being born feet or buttocks first is permitted to deliver spontaneously as far as its umbilicus and is then extracted. Also called **partial breech extraction.** Compare **breech extraction.**

**assisted circulation** [L, *assistere,* to stand, *circulare,* to go around],   a method of treating patients with severe circulatory deficiencies by introducing a mechanical pumping system to aid the blood flow.

**assisted death,**   a form of euthanasia in which an individual expressing a wish to die prematurely is helped to accomplish that goal by another person, either by counseling and/or by providing a poison or other lethal instrument. The assisted death may be regarded as a homicide or suicide by local authorities, and the person giving assistance may be held responsible for the death. See also **assisted suicide.**

**assisted reproductive technology,**   the manipulation of egg and sperm in treating infertility. The processes include the administration of drugs to induce ovulation, fertilization, gamete intrafallopian transfer, zygote intrafallopian transfer, and cryopreservation of gametes. See also **in vitro fertilization.**

**assisted suicide,**   a form of euthanasia in which a person wishes to commit suicide but feels unable to perform the act alone because of a physical disability or lack of knowledge about the most effective means. An individual who assists a suicide victim in accomplishing that goal may or may not be held responsible for the death, depending on local laws. The participation of health professionals, especially physicians, in assisted suicide is controversial. See also **euthanasia, suicide.**

**assisted ventilation,**   the use of mechanical or other devices to help maintain respiration, usually by delivering air or oxygen under positive pressure. See also **IPPB, respiration.**

**assistive listening device (ALD),**   a device other than a hearing aid that helps the deaf to hear. See also **hearing aid.**

**associated antagonist,**   one of a pair of muscles or group of muscles that pull in opposite directions but whose combined action results in moving a part in one direction.

**Associate Degree in Nursing (ADN)** /əsō′shē·āt/ [L, *associare,* to unite],   an academic degree awarded on satisfactory completion of a 2-year course of study, usually at a community or junior college. The recipient is eligible to take the national licensing examination to become a registered nurse. An associate degree in nursing is not available in Canada.

**associated movement,**   **1.** a movement of parts that act together, as of the eyes. **2.** see **contralateral reflexes, synkinesis.**

**associate nurse,**   **1.** (in primary nursing, United States) a nurse who is responsible for implementing a primary nurse's care plans. **2.** in some states, a registered nurse who holds a diploma from a hospital school of nursing or an associate degree.

**association** /əsō′shē·ā′shən/ [L, *associare,* to unite],   **1.** a connection, union, joining, or combination of things. **2.** (in psychology) the connection of remembered feelings, emotions, sensations, thoughts, or perceptions with particular persons, things, or ideas. Kinds of association are **association of ideas, clang association, controlled association, dream association,** and **free association.**

**association area,**   any part of the cerebral cortex involved in the integration of sensory information. Also called **association cortex.**

**Association for Professionals in Infection Control and Epidemiology (APIC),**   a national professional organization of nurses working in the field of infection control.

**Association for the Advancement of Medical Instrumentation (AAMI),** a nonprofit organization involved in education and standards relating to biomedical engineering.

**Association for the Care of Children's Health (ACCH),** an international, interdisciplinary organization concerned with the psychosocial needs of children and their families in health care settings. A quarterly journal and a bimonthly newsletter are available to members. There are affiliate organizations throughout the United States and Canada.

**associationist model of learning** /əsō'shē·ā'shənist/, a theory that defines learning as behavioral change that is a result of reinforced practice. If the response has not been reinforced repeatedly, an alternative behavior may be substituted.

**Association of Canadian Medical Colleges (ACMC),** a Canadian organization of the deans and faculty members of the nation's 16 medical schools. It is concerned with all aspects of the education of physicians and acts as the liaison between the member schools and other professional organizations and governmental agencies. The official languages of the ACMC are English and French.

**association of ideas,** a mental connection established between similar or simultaneously occurring ideas, feelings, or perceptions.

**Association of Operating Room Nurses (AORN),** a national organization of operating room nurses.

**Association of Women's Health, Obstetric, and Neonatal Nurses (AWHONN),** an organization of nurses working in obstetrics and gynecology in the United States. Formerly called **Nurses Association of the American College of Obstetrics and Gynecology (NAACOG).**

**association paralysis,** a motor neuron disease in which wasting, weakness, and fasciculation of the tongue, facial muscles, pharynx, and larynx occur. Also called **progressive bulbar paralysis.**

**association test,** a technique used in psychiatric diagnosis and in educational and psychologic evaluation in which a person is asked to respond to a stimulus word with the first word that comes to mind. The time taken to respond and the associations offered are compared with pretested responses and are classified and enumerated for diagnostic significance. Also called **word association test.** See also **free association.**

**associative looseness** /əsō'shətiv/, a form of thought disorder in which the patient is unable to maintain consistent thought for more than a few minutes and jumps from thought to thought in a conversation. Fragmentation of thoughts is generally noted in patients with schizophrenia.

**associative play,** a form of play in which a group of children participate in similar or identical activities without formal organization, group direction, group interaction, or a definite goal. The children may borrow or lend toys or pieces of play equipment, and they may imitate others in the group, but each child acts independently, as on a playground or among a group riding tricycles or bicycles. Compare **cooperative play.** See also **parallel play, solitary play.**

**assortive mating,** the matching of males and females for reproduction in a manner that avoids random selection.

**assumed role** /əsōomd'/, a role in life that an individual usually selects or achieves by choice, such as one's role in marriage or employment. See also **ascribed role.**

**AST,** 1. abbreviation for **aspartate aminotransferase.** 2. less frequently, abbreviation for **angiotensin sensitivity test.**

**-ast,** combining form designating an antiasthmatic or antiallergic drug not acting primarily as an antihistamine.

**astasia** /astā'zhə/, a lack of motor coordination marked by an inability to stand or sit without assistance.

**astasia-abasia** [Gk, *a, stasis,* not stand, *a, basis,* not step], a form of ataxia in which the patient is unable to stand or walk because of lack of motor coordination although able to carry out natural leg movements when sitting or lying down. Also called **abasia-astasia.**

**astatine (At)** [Gk, *astasis,* unsteady], a very unstable, radioactive element that occurs naturally in tiny amounts. Its atomic number is 85; the atomic mass of its longest lived isotope is 210.

**asteatosis** /as'tē·ətō'sis/ [Gk, *a, stear,* without tallow, *osis,* condition], a dry skin condition caused by a deficiency of sebaceous gland secretions. Scales and fissures may result from the dryness. The condition is treated with creams and ointments that replace the missing skin oils.

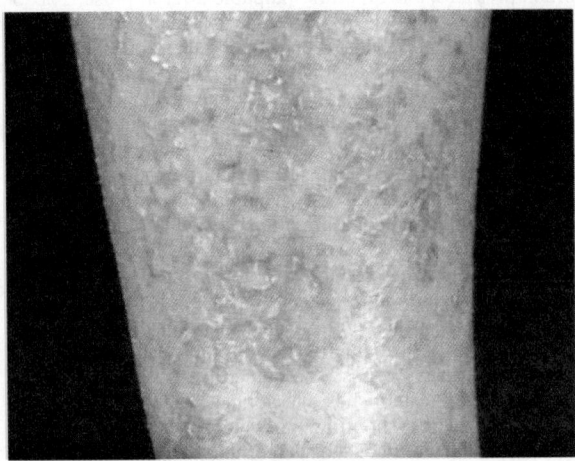

**Asteatotic eczema** *(du Vivier, 1993)*

**-aster,** suffix meaning 'star-shaped': *diaster, oleaster.*

**astereognosis** /əstir'ē·og·nō'sis/ [Gk, *a, stereos,* not solid, *gnosis,* knowledge], an inability to identify objects by touch.

**asterixis** /as'tərik'sis/ [Gk, *a, sterixis,* not fixed position], a hand-flapping tremor, often accompanying metabolic disorders. The tremor is usually induced by extending the arm and dorsiflexing the wrist. Asterixis is seen frequently in hepatic encephalopathy. Also called **flapping tremor, liver flap.**

**asteroid body** [Gk, *aster,* star, *eidos,* form], an irregular star-shaped structure that develops in the giant cells in certain diseases, including sarcoidosis, actinomycosis, and nocardiosis.

**asthenia** /asthē'nē·ə/ [Gk, *a + sthenos,* without strength], 1. the lack or loss of strength or energy; weakness; debility. 2. (in psychiatry) lack of dynamic force in the personality. Kinds of asthenia include **myalgic asthenia** and **neurocirculatory asthenia.** See also **adynamia. —asthenic,** *adj.*

**-asthenia,** suffix meaning '(condition of) debility, loss of strength and energy, depleted vitality': *neurasthenia, phlebasthenia.*

**asthenic** /asthen'ik/ [Gk, *a + sthenos,* without strength], pertaining to a condition of weakness, feebleness, or loss of vitality.

**asthenic fever.**   See **adynamic fever.**

**asthenic habitus** [Gk, *a + sthenos,* without strength; L, *habere,* to have],   a body structure characterized by a slender build with long limbs, an angular profile, and prominent muscles or bones. Compare **athletic habitus, pyknic.** See also **ectomorph.**

**asthenic personality,**   a personality characterized by low energy, lack of enthusiasm, depressed emotions, and oversensitivity to physical and emotional strain. A person who has this kind of personality may be easily fatigued and self-pitying and may place the burden of physical and emotional difficulties on others.

**asthenopia** /as′thənō′pē·ə/ [Gk, *a, sthenos + ops,* eye],   a condition in which the eyes tire easily because of weakness of the ocular or ciliary muscles. Symptoms include pain in or around the eyes, headache, dimness of vision, dizziness, and slight nausea.

**asthma** /az′mə/ [Gk, panting],   a respiratory disorder characterized by recurring episodes of paroxysmal dyspnea, wheezing on expiration and/or inspiration caused by constriction of the bronchi, coughing, and viscous mucoid bronchial secretions. The episodes may be precipitated by inhalation of allergens or pollutants, infection, cold air, vigorous exercise, or emotional stress. Treatment may include elimination of the causative agent, hyposensitization, aerosol or oral bronchodilators, beta-adrenergic drugs, methylxanthines, cromolyn, leukotriene inhibitors, and short-term use of corticosteroids. Sedatives and cough suppressants may be contraindicated. Also called **bronchial asthma.** See also **allergic asthma, asthma in children, exercise-induced asthma, intrinsic asthma, organic dust, status asthmaticus.**

reverse inflammatory condition resulting in bronchial constriction of the airways. See also **Nursing Outcomes Classification.**

**asthma crystal.**   See **Charcot-Leyden crystal.**

**asthma in children,**   a chronic inflammatory disorder of the airways in which many cells, including mast cells and eosinophils play a part. The inflammation causes symptoms associated with obstructive airflow and characterized by recurring attacks of paroxysmal dyspnea, wheezing, prolonged expiration, and an irritative cough that is a common, chronic illness in childhood. Onset usually occurs between 3 and 8 years of age. Asthmatic attacks are caused by constriction of the large and small airways, resulting from bronchial smooth muscle spasm, edema or inflammation of the bronchial wall, or excessive production of mucus. It is a complex disorder involving biochemical, immunologic, infectious, endocrinologic, and psychologic factors. Asthma attacks in the past were classified as either extrinsic or intrinsic. Most extrinsic attacks in children were associated with an allergenic hypersensitivity to a foreign substance, such as airborne pollen, mold, house dust, certain foods, animal hair and skin, feathers, insects, smoke, and various chemicals or drugs. In infants, especially those with a family history of allergic reactions, food allergy is a common precipitating factor. Intrinsic attacks were associated with physical stress resulting from fatigue or exercise, exposure to cold air, or psychologic stress; this system of classification has been abandoned because many of the triggering factors overlap.

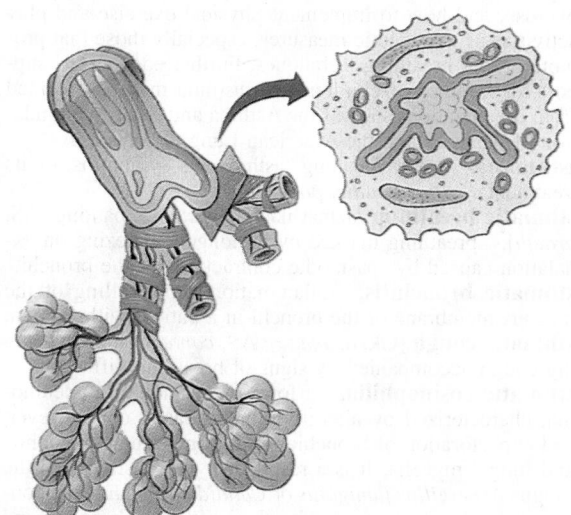

**Asthma: obstruction of airways by excessive mucous production and edema of respiratory mucosa**
*(Thibodeau and Patton, 1999/Rolin Graphics)*

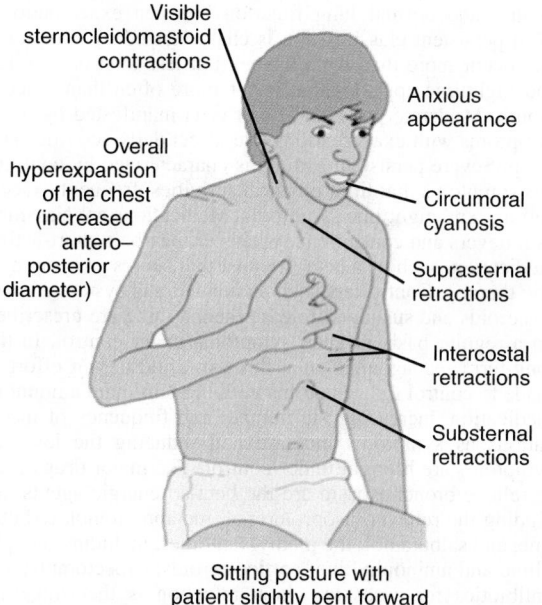

Visible sternocleidomastoid contractions

Anxious appearance

Overall hyperexpansion of the chest (increased antero-posterior diameter)

Circumoral cyanosis

Suprasternal retractions

Intercostal retractions

Substernal retractions

Sitting posture with patient slightly bent forward

**Asthma in children: physical findings**
*(Zitelli and Davis, 1997)*

**-asthma,**   suffix meaning '(condition of) labored breathing.'

**asthma control,**   a nursing outcome from the Nursing Outcomes Classification (NOC) defined as personal actions to

■ OBSERVATIONS: Asthma in children is often confused with acute middle and lower respiratory tract infections, congenital stridor, obstruction of the bronchi or trachea, bronchial or tracheal compression, and cystic fibrosis. The diagnosis is generally determined by observation during a physical examination, medical history, and familial allergic disease.

Laboratory tests and x-ray studies may eliminate identification of other diseases. A diagnostic feature is the presence of large numbers of eosinophils and Charcot-Leyden crystals in the sputum. Pulmonary function tests are valuable for assessing the degree of airway obstruction and the volume of gas exchange. Asthmatic episodes vary greatly in frequency, duration, and degree of symptoms. They may range from occasional periods of wheezing, mild coughing, and slight dyspnea to severe attacks that can lead to total airway obstruction and respiratory tract failure (status asthmaticus). An attack may begin gradually or abruptly and is often preceded by an upper respiratory infection. Typically an attack begins with signs of air hunger, yawning, sighing, shortness of breath, paroxysms of wheezing, and a hacking, nonproductive cough. As secretions increase, the expiratory phase becomes prolonged. A large quantity of thick, tenacious mucoid sputum is produced as the attack subsides. The child appears apprehensive, speaks in a panting manner, and may assume a bent-over position to facilitate breathing. The prolonged expiratory phase is not as noticeable in infants and young children. In severe spasm or obstruction the respirations become shallow and irregular. A sudden increase in the rate of respiration, repeated hacking, and nonproductive coughing are indicative of lack of air movement with impending ventilatory failure and asphyxia.

■ INTERVENTIONS: Management of asthma in children is based on four stages of severity: intermittent, mild persistent, moderate persistent, and severe persistent. Clinical features of intermittent asthma include symptoms that occur less than once a week, brief exacerbations of from a few hours to a few days, nighttime episodes that occur less than twice a month, and normal lung function between exacerbations. Mild persistent classification is characterized by symptoms that occur more than once a week but less than once a day and nighttime episodes that occur more often than twice a month. Moderate persistent severity is manifested by daily symptoms with exacerbations that affect daily activities and sleep. Severe persistent asthma is characterized by continuous symptoms that limit physical activities, frequent exacerbations, and nighttime symptoms. Medications are classified as relievers and controllers. A reliever may be a short-acting medication, such as a beta$_2$ agonist that serves as symptomatic therapy. Controllers such as inhaled and systemic corticosteroids and sustained-release theophylline are prescribed on a regular basis to keep symptoms under control. In the long-term management of asthma in children, an effort is made to control the symptoms with the minimum amount of medication, increasing the number and frequency of medications as symptoms increase and reducing the level as symptoms are brought under control. The major drugs used to relieve bronchospasm are the beta-adrenergic agents, including the relievers isoproterenol, metaproterenol, terbutaline, and salbutamol; the methylxanthines, including theophylline and aminophylline; corticosteroids; expectorants; and antibiotics for cases in which infection is the triggering mechanism. Rarely an acute attack does not respond to any of these measures, resulting in status asthmaticus. Hospitalization is required. The child is usually in a state of dehydration and acidosis with hypoxia and hypercapnia. Management consists of administration of IV fluids; humidified oxygen given by mask or cannula; administration of sodium bicarbonate or tromethamine to keep pH at acceptable levels; and use of bronchodilators to alleviate bronchospasm and of antibiotics to reduce risk of infection. Mild, intermittent episodes of asthma are treated with bronchodilators in aerosol sprays, which provide quick relief and are effective in controlling an attack; oral administration is preferred for younger children. Those with persistent chronic asthma receive daily oral doses of a bronchodilator, often theophylline, usually in combination with an expectorant and corticosteroids. Bronchospasm induced by exercise can be treated prophylactically with cromolyn sodium, a controller that inhibits the release of histamine in the lungs. Long-range management and treatment include physical training and exercises to induce physical and mental relaxation, improve posture, strengthen respiratory musculature, and develop better breathing patterns. Hyposensitization is recommended when an allergen is known and cannot be avoided. Prognosis varies considerably; many children lose their symptoms at puberty but the symptoms reappear in their 40s. The prognosis depends on the number and severity of symptoms, emotional factors, and the family history of allergy.

■ NURSING CONSIDERATIONS: The primary focus of nursing care for children with acute asthma is to relieve symptoms of respiratory distress by initiating IV infusion and oxygen therapy, correcting acidosis, and administering bronchodilators and corticosteroids. The nurse implements measures to promote physical comfort, induce rest, and reduce fatigue and anxiety. An especially important role is reassuring the child and parents about procedures, equipment, and prognosis. The nurse also plays a significant role in the long-term support of children with chronic asthma, primarily in teaching the child and parents about the disease and how to cope with the condition. Once an allergen is determined, the home environment must be modified to reduce or eliminate contact with possible causative agents, including presence of warm-blooded pets, tobacco smoke, cockroaches, dust mites, and fungi. The nurse teaches the child and parents how to use prescribed medications, especially nebulizers and aerosol devices, how to detect early signs of an attack so that it can be controlled with medication, how to determine any adverse effects of the drugs, especially the dangers of overuse, and how to implement physical exercise and play activities as therapeutic measures, especially those that promote proper breathing techniques. Further educational support for families of children with asthma may be obtained from organizations such as the Asthma and Allergy Foundation of America and the American Lung Association.

**-asthmatic,** suffix meaning 'asthma, its symptoms, or its treatment': *antiasthmatic, postasthmatic.*

**asthmatic breathing** /azmat'ik/ [Gk, *asthma*, panting; AS, *braeth*], breathing marked by prolonged wheezing on exhalation caused by spasmodic contractions of the bronchi.

**asthmatic bronchitis,** inflammation and swelling of the mucous membrane of the bronchi in a patient with asthma.

**asthmatic cough** [Gk, *asthma* + AS, *cohhetan*], a wheezing cough accompanied by signs of breathing difficulty.

**asthmatic eosinophilia,** a form of eosinophilic pneumonia, characterized by allergic bronchospasm, cough, fever, and expectoration of bronchial casts containing eosinophils and fungal mycelia. It is a result of hypersensitivity to the fungus *Aspergillus fumigatus* or *Candida albicans.* The condition usually occurs in the fourth or fifth decade of life and is twice as common in women as in men. Untreated, it may result in pleural effusion, pericarditis, ascites, encephalitis, hepatomegaly, and respiratory failure. Treatment is similar to that for asthma and includes administration of corticosteroids and antibiotics. Desensitization to the allergen is not usually effective. See also **allergic asthma, eosinophilic pneumonia.**

**Astiban,** trademark for a parasiticide (sodium stibocaptate).

**astigmatic** /as'tigmat'ik/ [Gk, *a, stigma,* without point], pertaining to astigmatism, or an error of refraction in which a ray of light is not sharply focused on the retinal tissue but is spread over a more diffuse area. Astigmatism is due to differences in curvature in the various meridians of the cornea and lens of the eye.

**astigmatism** /əstig′mətiz′əm/ [Gk, *a, stigma,* without point], an abnormal condition of the eye in which the light rays cannot be focused clearly in a point on the retina because the spheric curve of the cornea or lens is not equal in all meridians. Vision is typically blurred; if uncorrected, it often results in visual discomfort or asthenopia. The person cannot accommodate to correct the problem. The condition usually may be corrected with contact lenses or with eyeglasses ground to neutralize the condition.

**astro-,** prefix meaning 'star or star-shaped': *astroblastoma, astrocytoma.*

**astroblastoma** /as′trōblastō′mə/, *pl.* **astroblastomas, astroblastomata** [Gk, *aster,* star, *blastos,* germ, *oma,* tumor], a malignant neoplasm of the brain and spinal cord. Cells of an astroblastoma lie around blood vessels or around connective tissue septa.

**astrocyte** /as′trōsīt′/ [Gk, *aster* + *kytos,* cell], a large, star-shaped neuroglial cell with many branches, found in certain tissues of the nervous system.

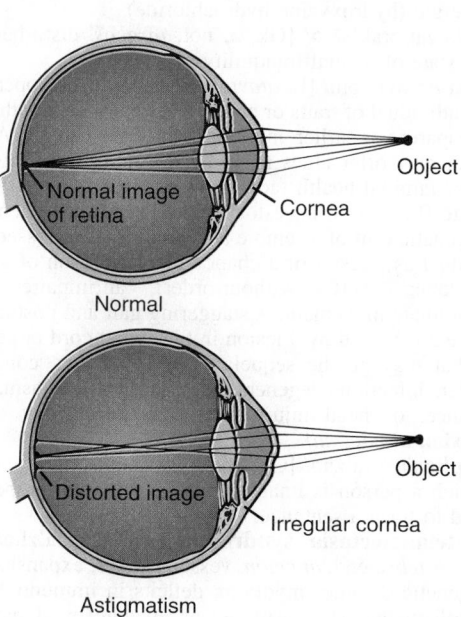

**Astigmatism**

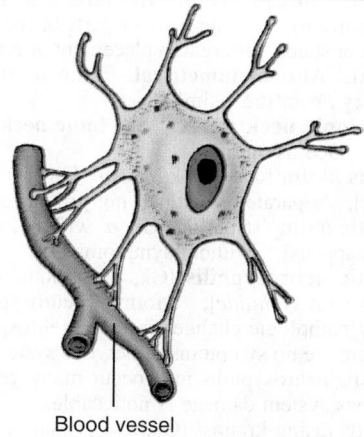

**Astrocyte** (Monahan and Neighbors, 1998)

**astrocytoma** /as′trōsītō′mə/, *pl.* **astrocytomas, astrocytomata** [Gk, *aster, kytos* + *oma*], a primary tumor of the brain composed of astrocytes and characterized by slow growth, cyst formation, invasion of surrounding structures, and often development of a highly malignant glioblastoma within the tumor mass. Complete surgical resection of an as-

**-astine,** combining form designating an antihistaminic.

**astragalus¹.** See **talus.**

**astragalus²,** an herb that is grown throughout the world, most commonly in China, Japan, and Korea.

■ USES: This herb is used as an immune stimulant; for viral infections, HIV/AIDS, cancer, and vascular disorders; to improve circulation; and to lower blood pressure. It may show efficacy in treating myasthenia gravis.

■ CONTRAINDICATIONS: Astragalus should not be used during pregnancy and lactation, in children, or during acute infections.

**astringent** /əstrin′jənt/ [Gk, *astringere,* to tighten], **1.** a substance that causes contraction of tissues on application, usually used locally. **2.** having the quality of an astringent. **—astringency,** *n.*

**astringent bath,** a bath in which alum, tannic acid, or another astringent is added to the water. An astringent contracts body tissue and therefore stops capillary bleeding or loosens secretions.

**astringent douche,** a cleansing stream containing substances such as alum that can contract the mucous membrane of the vagina.

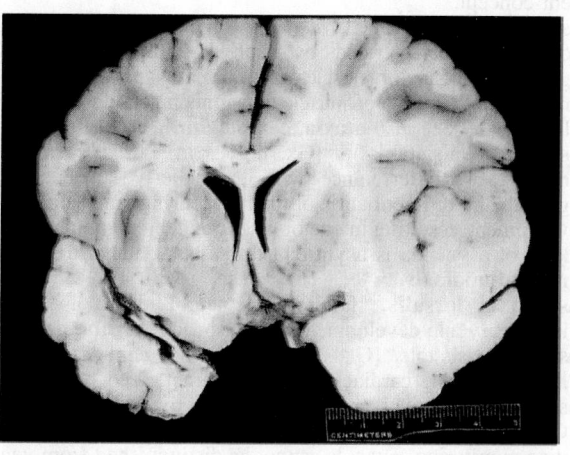

**Astrocytoma** (Kumar, Cotran, and Robbins, 1997)

trocytoma may be possible early in the development of the tumor. Also called **astrocytic glioma.**

**astrocytosis** /as'trōsītō'sis/ [Gk, *aster* + *kytos* + *osis,* condition], an increase in the number of neuroglial cells with fibrous or protoplasmic processes frequently observed in an irregular area adjacent to degenerative lesions, such as abscesses, certain brain neoplasms, and encephalomalacia. Astrocytosis represents a reparative process and in some cases may be diffuse in a large region.

**astrophobia.** See **tonitrophobia.**

**asylum** /əsī'ləm/ [Gk, *asylon,* inviolable], an institution for the care of physically or mentally handicapped persons judged incapable of caring for themselves.

**asymmetric** /ā'simet'rik, as'imet'rik/ [Gk, *a* + *symmetria,* without proportion], (of the body or parts of the body) unequal in size or shape; different in placement or arrangement about an axis. Also **asymmetrical.** Compare **symmetric.** —**asymmetry** /āsim'itrē, asim'-/, *n.*

**asymmetric tonic neck reflex.** See **tonic neck reflex.**

**asymmetry.** See **asymmetric.**

**asymphytous** /ə·sim'fə·təs/ [Gk, *a, symphysis,* not a growing together], separate or distinct; not grown together.

**asymptomatic** /āsimp'təmat'ik/ [Gk, *a,* without, *symptoma,* that which happens], without symptoms.

**asymptomatic neurosyphilis** [Gk, *a,* without, *symptoma, neuron,* nerve; Fr, *syphilide*], a form of neurosyphilis characterized by pathologic changes in the cerebrospinal fluid, although there are no symptoms of nervous system damage. Asymptomatic neurosyphilis may occur many years before actual nervous system damage is noticeable.

**asynchronous** /āsing'krənəs/ [Gk, *a* + *synchronos,* not simultaneous], (of an event or device) a computer operation in one command performed in response to a signal that the previous command has been completed. One operation is completed before the next is initiated.

**asynclitism** /āsing'klitiz'əm/ [Gk, *a* + *syn,* not together, *kleisis,* to lean], presentation of a parietal aspect of the fetal head to the maternal pelvic inlet in labor. The sagittal suture is parallel to the transverse diameter of the pelvis but anterior or posterior to it. In normal labor, the fetal head usually engages with some degree of asynclitism. **Anterior asynclitism,** in which the anterior part presents, is called Nägele obliquity. **Posterior asynclitism** is called Litzmann obliquity. See also **cardinal movements of labor, engagement.**

**asyndesis** /əsin'dəsis/, a mental disorder marked by an inability to assemble related ideas or thoughts into one coherent concept.

**asynergy** /āsin'ərjē/ [Gk, *a* + *syn* + *ergein,* to work], **1.** a condition characterized by faulty coordination among groups of organs or muscles that normally function harmoniously. **2.** the state of muscle antagonism found in cerebellar disease. See also **ataxia, cerebellum.**

**asyntaxia** /ā'sintak'sē·ə/ [Gk, *a* + *syn* + *taxis,* arrangement], any interference with the orderly sequence of growth and differentiation of the fetus during embryonic development, resulting in one or more congenital anomalies. A kind of asyntaxia is **asyntaxia dorsalis.** See also **developmental anomaly.**

**asyntaxia dorsalis,** failure of the neural tube to close during embryonic development. See also **neural tube defect.**

**asystole** /āsis'təlē/ [Gk, *a* + *systole,* not contraction], a life-threatening cardiac condition characterized by the absence of electrical and mechanical activity in the heart. Clinical signs include apnea and lack of pulse. Without cardiac monitoring, asystole cannot be distinguished from ventricular fibrillation. —**asystolic,** *adj.*

**asystolic cardiac rhythm** /ā'sistol'ik/, an electrocardiographic recording that appears as a flat line, indicating cardiac arrest.

**At,** symbol for the element **astatine.**

**at-.** See **ad-.**

**Atabrine Hydrochloride,** trademark for an antimalarial (quinacrine hydrochloride).

**Atabrine stomatitis,** an abnormal oral condition characterized by skin changes that resemble those of lichen planus. It may be associated with the use of Atabrine Hydrochloride. Compare **arsenic stomatitis, bismuth stomatitis.**

**ataractic** /at'ərak'tik/ [Gk, *ataraktos,* quiet], pertaining to a drug or other agent that has a tranquilizing or sedating effect.

**Atarax,** trademark for an antianxiety, antiemetic, and anticholinergic (hydroxyzine hydrochloride).

**ataraxia** /at'ərak'sē'ə/ [Gk, *a,* not, *tarakos,* disturbed], a vague state of mental tranquility.

**atavism** /at'əviz'əm/ [L, *atavus,* ancestor], the appearance in an individual of traits or characteristics more like those of a grandparent or earlier ancestor than of the parents. Atavistic data may offer clues to an examining physician of genetic or familial health factors. —**atavistic,** *adj.*

**atavistic** [L, *atavus,* ancestor], pertaining to the tendency for a genetic trait of a remote ancestor to be expressed in an individual as a result of a chance recombination of genes.

**ataxia** /ətak'sē·ə/ [Gk, without order], an impaired ability to coordinate movement. A staggering gait and postural imbalance are caused by a lesion in the spinal cord or cerebellum that may be the sequela of birth trauma, congenital disorder, infection, degenerative disorder, neoplasm, toxic substance, or head injury. See also **hereditary ataxia.** —**ataxial, ataxic,** *adj.*

**ataxiaphasia** /-fā'zhə/ [Gk, *ataxia,* without order], a state in which a person is unable to connect words properly as needed to form a sentence.

**ataxia-telangiectasia syndrome** /tələn'jē·ektā'zhə/ [Gk, *ataxia* + *telos,* end, *angeion,* vessel, *ektasis,* expansion], a rare genetic disorder involving deficits in immunoglobulin metabolism that is transmitted as an autosomal recessive trait. It usually begins in infancy with impaired motor control (ataxia) and progresses slowly with increasing cerebellar degeneration to severe disability. Permanent dilation of superficial blood vessels (telangiectasias) are most prominent on skin surfaces exposed to the sun: ears, face, and bulbar conjunctiva. Intellectual ability seems to stop at the level of 10 years of age in many cases. Affected individuals are susceptible to upper and lower respiratory infections and have an increased risk of malignancy, especially lymphoma. Also called **Louis-Bar syndrome.**

**ataxic.** See **ataxia.**

**ataxic aphasia.** See **motor aphasia.**

**ataxic breathing,** a type of breathing associated with a lesion in the medullary respiratory center and characterized by a series of inspirations and expirations. See also **Biot's respiration.**

**ataxic dysarthria,** abnormal speech characterized by faulty formation of sounds because of neuromuscular dysfunction of the cerebellum.

**ataxic gait.** See **cerebellar gait.**

**ataxic speech.** See **cerebellar speech.**

**ATCC,** abbreviation for **American Type Culture Collection.**

**-ate, 1.** suffix meaning 'acted upon or being in a (specified) state': *degenerate, enucleate.* **2.** suffix meaning 'possessing': *caudate, longipedate.* **3.** suffix meaning a 'chemical compound derived from a (specified) source': *silicate, opi-*

*ate.* **4.** suffix meaning an 'acid compound': *oxalate, phosphate.*

**atelectasis** /at′ilek′təsis/ [Gk, *ateles,* incomplete, *ektasis,* expansion], an abnormal condition characterized by the collapse of alveoli, preventing the respiratory exchange of carbon dioxide and oxygen in a part of the lungs. Symptoms may include diminished breath sounds, a mediastinal shift toward the side of the collapse, fever, and increasing dyspnea. As the remaining portions of the lungs eventually hyperinflate, oxygen saturation of the blood is often nearly normal. The condition may be caused by obstruction of the major airways and bronchioles, by compression of the lung as a result of fluid or air in the pleural space, or by pressure from a tumor outside the lung. Loss of functional lung tissue may secondarily cause increased heart rate, blood pressure, and respiratory rate. Secretions retained in the collapsed alveoli are rich in nutrients for bacterial growth, a condition often leading to stasis pneumonia in critically ill patients. See also **postoperative atelectasis, primary atelectasis.**

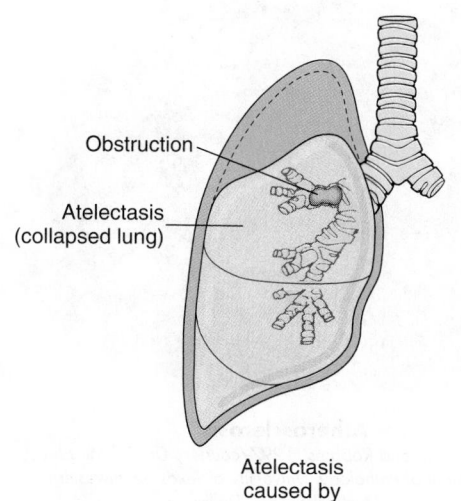

Obstruction
Atelectasis (collapsed lung)
Atelectasis caused by obstruction

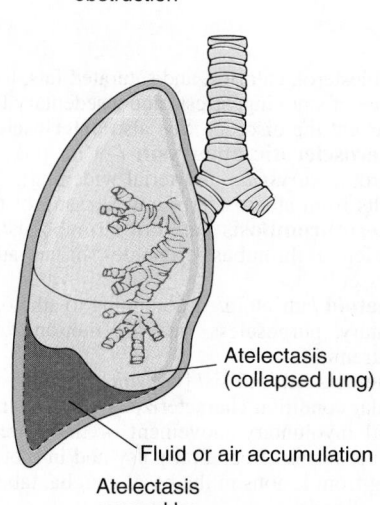

Atelectasis (collapsed lung)
Fluid or air accumulation
Atelectasis caused by accumulation

**Atelectasis** *(Chabner, 2001)*

**ateliosis** /ətē′lē·ō′sis/ [Gk, *ateles,* incomplete, *osis,* condition], a form of dwarfism caused by the absence or destruction of eosinophil cells of the adenohypophysis. The person may appear childlike and have poorly developed muscles.

**ateliotic dwarf** /at′əlē·ot′ik/, a dwarf whose skeleton is incompletely formed as a result of the nonunion of the epiphyses and diaphyses during bone development.

**atelo-,** prefix meaning 'imperfect or incomplete': *ateloglossia, atelopodia.*

**atelorachidia** /at′əlôr′əkid′ē·ə/ [Gk, *ateles,* incomplete, *rhachis,* spine], a defective, incomplete formation of the spinal column. Also spelled **atelorhachidia.**

**atenolol** /aten′əlôl/, a beta blocker.

■ INDICATION: It is prescribed for the treatment of hypertension.

■ CONTRAINDICATIONS: Sinus bradycardia, second- or third-degree atrioventricular block, cardiogenic shock, or cardiac failure prohibits its use.

■ ADVERSE EFFECTS: Among the more serious adverse reactions are bradycardia, dizziness, and nausea.

**ATG,** abbreviation for **antithymocyte globulin.**

**athelia** /āthē′lē·ə/ [Gk, *a,* not, *thele,* nipple], an absence of nipples.

**atherectomy** /ath′ərek′təmē/, surgical removal of an atheroma in a major artery.

**atherectomy catheter,** a specially designed catheter for cutting away atheromatous plaque from the lining of an artery. A tiny metal cone at the tip of the catheter has cutting edges for loosening the plaque and has openings through which the plaque fragments can be aspirated. The catheter is positioned and monitored by fluoroscopy.

**atheroembolic renal disease** /ath′ərō·embol′ik/, a condition of gradual or rapid kidney failure resulting from obstruction of the renal arteries by atheromas and emboli. It is associated with atherosclerosis and hypertension and occurs most frequently in persons over 60 years of age. The patient is usually azotemic and also experiences emboli in other body areas.

**atheroembolism** /ath′ərō·em′bəliz′əm/, obstruction of a blood vessel by a cholesterol-containing embolism originating from an atheroma in a major artery.

**atherogenesis** [Gk, *athere,* porridge, *oma,* tumor, *genein,* to produce], the formation of subintimal plaques in the lining of arteries.

**atheroma** /ath′ərō′mə/, *pl.* **atheromas, atheromata** [Gk, *athere,* meal, *oma,* tumor], an abnormal mass of fat or lipids, as in a sebaceous cyst or in deposits in an arterial wall. **—atheromatous,** *adj.*

**atheromatosis** /ath′ərōmətō′sis/, the development of many atheromas.

**atheromatous** [Gk, *athere,* meal, *oma,* tumor], pertaining to atheroma.

**atheromatous plaque,** a yellowish raised area on the lining of an artery formed by fatty deposits.

**atherosclerosis** /ath′ərō′sklərō′sis/ [Gk, *athere,* meal, *sklerosis,* hardening], a common disorder characterized by yellowish plaques of cholesterol, other lipids, and cellular debris in the inner layers of the walls of arteries. Atherosclerosis may be induced by injury to the arterial endothelium, proliferation of smooth muscle in vessel walls, or accumulation of lipids in hyperlipidemia. It usually occurs with aging and is often associated with tobacco use, obesity, hypertension, elevated low-density lipoprotein and depressed high-density lipoprotein levels, and diabetes mellitus. The condition begins as a fatty streak and gradually builds to a fibrous plaque or atheromatous lesion. The vessel walls become

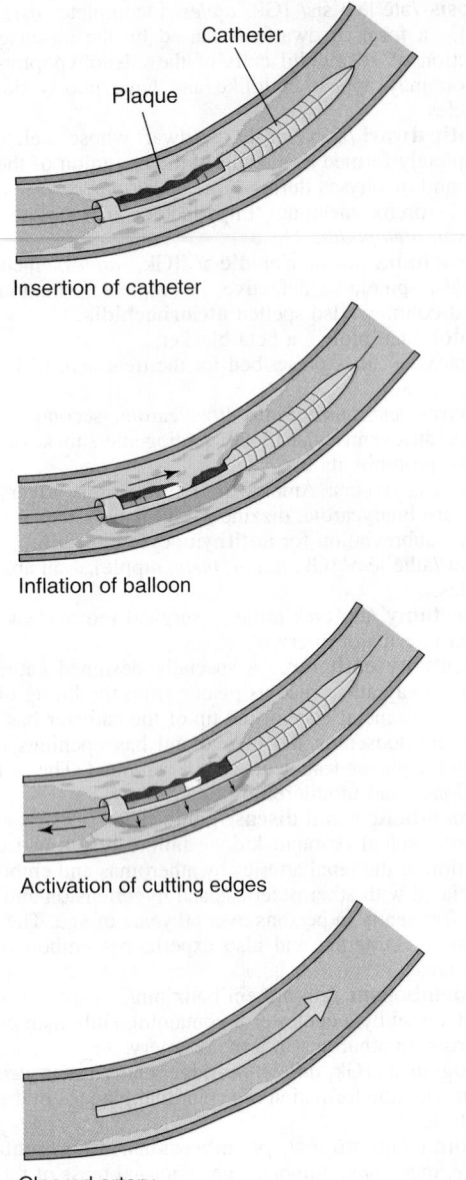

Insertion of catheter

Inflation of balloon

Activation of cutting edges

Cleared artery

**Atherectomy catheter** *(Beare and Myers, 1998)*

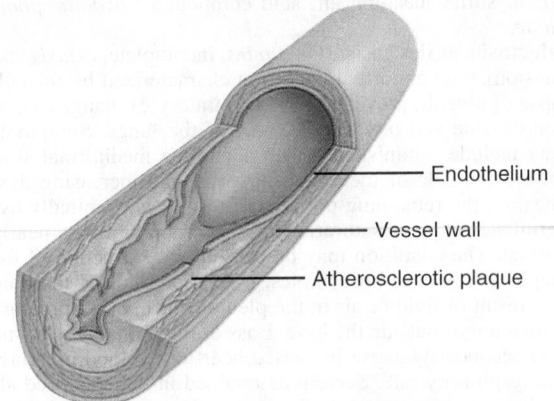

**Atherosclerosis: partial blockage of an artery by plaque** *(Thibodeau and Patton, 1999/Barbara Cousins)*

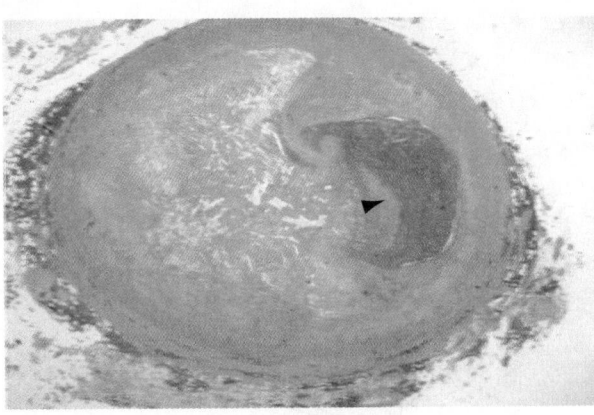

**Atherosclerosis**
*(Kumar, Cotran, and Robbins, 1997/courtesy Dr. Sid Murphree, Department of Pathology, University of Texas Southwestern Medical School, Dallas)*

thick, fibrotic, and calcified, and the lumen narrows, resulting in reduced blood flow to organs normally supplied by the artery. The plaque eventually creates a risk for thrombosis and is one of the major causes of coronary heart disease, angina pectoris, myocardial infarction, and other cardiac disorders. Plaque rupture is usually provoked by activation of the sympathetic nervous system, such as sudden awakening, heavy physical exertion, or anger. Antilipemic agents do not reverse atherosclerosis. Segments of arteries obstructed or severely damaged by atheromatous lesions may be replaced by patch grafts or bypassed, as in coronary bypass surgery; the lesion may be removed from the vessel via endarterectomy; or obstructed arteries may be opened by balloon angioplasty or by the insertion of stents. A diet low in cholesterol, calories, and saturated fats, together with avoidance of smoking, stress, and a sedentary life-style, may help prevent the disorder. See also **arteriosclerosis.**

**atherosclerotic aneurysm** /-ot'ik/ [Gk, *athere* + *skleros,* hard, *aneurysma,* an arterial widening], a dilation that results from atherosclerotic weakening of the arterial wall.

**atherothrombosis** /ath'ərō'thrombō'sis/, a condition in which a thrombus originates in an atheromatous blood vessel.

**athetoid** /ath'ətoid/, pertaining to athetosis, as in the involuntary, purposeless weaving motions of the body or its extremities.

**athetosis** /ath'ətō'sis/ [Gk, *athetos,* not fixed], a neuromuscular condition characterized by slow, writhing, continuous, and involuntary movement of the extremities, as seen in some forms of cerebral palsy and in motor disorders resulting from lesions in the basal ganglia, tabes dorsalis, or other conditions.

**athiaminosis** /əthī'əminō'sis/, a condition resulting from lack of thiamine in the diet. See also **beriberi, thiamin.**

**athlete's foot.** See **tinea pedis.**

**athlete's heart** /ath′lēts/,   an enlarged but otherwise normal heart of an athlete trained for endurance. It is characterized by a low heart rate, an increased pumping capacity, and a greater ability to deliver oxygen to skeletal muscles. Also called **athletic heart syndrome (AHS).**

**athletic habitus** /athlet′ik/,   a physique characterized by a well-proportioned, muscular body with broad shoulders, thick neck, deep chest, and flat abdomen. Compare **asthenic habitus, pyknic.** See also **mesomorph.**

**athletic heart syndrome.** See **athlete's heart.**

**athletic trainer,**   an allied health professional who, with the consultation and supervision of attending physicians, is an integral part of the health care system associated with sports. Through both academic preparation and practical experience, the athletic trainer provides a variety of services, including injury prevention and recognition and immediate care, treatment, and rehabilitation of athletic trauma.

**Athrombin-K,**   trademark for an anticoagulant (warfarin).

**Ativan,**   trademark for a benzodiazepine antianxiety agent (lorazepam).

**atlantal** /ətlan′təl/,   pertaining to the atlas, the first cervical vertebra.

**atlantoaxial** /ətlan′tō·ak′sē·əl/ [Gk, *atlas*, to bear, *axis*, pivot],   pertaining to the first two cervical vertebrae.

**atlantooccipital joint** /-oksip′itəl/ [Gk, *atlas*, to bear; L, *ob*, against, *caput*, head],   one of a pair of condyloid joints formed by the articulation of the atlas of the vertebral column with the occipital bone of the skull. It includes two articular capsules, two membranes, and two lateral ligaments. The atlantooccipital joint permits nodding and lateral movements of the head.

**atlas** [Gk, *atlas*, to bear, a mythical giant, compelled to uphold the world],   the first cervical vertebra, articulating with the occipital bone and the axis.

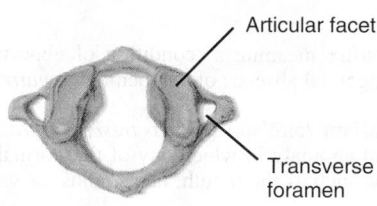

Articular facet

Transverse foramen

**Atlas** *(Applegate, 2000)*

**ATLS,**   abbreviation for *advanced trauma life support.*

**atm,   1.** abbreviation for **atmosphere. 2.** abbreviation for **atmospheric.**

**atman** /ät′män/,   (in psychiatry) a concept derived from Eastern Indian philosophy that the highest value is knowledge of one's true self. The atman represents the most inward reality, the innermost spirit, and the highest controlling power of a person.

**atmo-,**   prefix meaning 'steam or vapor': *atmolysis, atmotherapy.*

**atmosphere (atm)** /at′məsfir/ [Gk, *atmos*, vapor, *sphaira*, sphere],   **1.** the natural body of air, composed of approximately 21% oxygen, 78% nitrogen, and 1% argon and other gases, including trace levels of carbon dioxide and water vapor that covers the surface of the earth. **2.** an envelope of gas, which may or may not duplicate the natural atmosphere

in chemical components. **3.** a unit of gas pressure that is usually defined as being equivalent to the average pressure of the earth's atmosphere at sea level, or about 14.7 pounds per square inch or 760 mm Hg. —**atmospheric,** *adj.*

**atmospheric pressure** /-fer′ik/,   the pressure exerted by the weight of the atmosphere. The average atmospheric pressure at sea level is approximately 14.7 pounds per square inch. With increasing altitude the pressure decreases: at 30,000 feet, approximately the height of Mt. Everest, the air pressure is 4.3 pounds per square inch. Also called **barometric pressure.**

**ATN,**   abbreviation for **acute tubular necrosis.**

**atom** /at′əm/ [Gk, *atmos*, indivisible],   **1.** (in chemistry and physics) the smallest division of an element that exhibits all the properties and characteristics of the element. It comprises neutrons, electrons, and protons. The number of protons in the nucleus of every atom of any given element is the same and is called its atomic number. **2.** *nontechnical,* the amount of any substance that is so small that further division is not possible. —**atomic,** *adj.*

**atomic mass,**   the average mass, relative to an atom of carbon, of an atom of an element based on the natural isotopic mix of that element. Also called **atomic weight.** See also **atomic mass unit.**

**atomic mass unit (amu)** /atom′ik/,   the mass of a neutral atom of an element, expressed as 1/12 of the mass of the isotope carbon-12 which has a value of exactly 12. The energy equivalent of 1 amu is 931.2 MeV. The mass equivalent of 1 amu is $1.66(10^{-24}$ g).

**atomic number,**   the number of protons in the nucleus of an atom of a particular element. In a neutral atom, the atomic number equals the number of electrons. See also **atom, electron, proton.**

**atomic theory** [Gk, *atmos*, indivisible, *theoria*, speculation],   the concept that all matter is composed of submicroscopic atoms that are in turn composed of protons, electrons, and neutrons. A chemical element is identified by the number of protons in its atoms.

**atomic weight.**   See **atomic mass.**

**atomize.**   See **nebulize.**

**atomizer** /at′əmī′zər/,   a device used to reduce a liquid and eject it as a fine spray or vapor.

**atonia** /ātō′nē·ə/ [Gk, *a + tonos*, without tone],   decreased or absent muscle tone.

**atonic** /əton′ik/,   **1.** weak. **2.** lacking normal tone, as in the case of a muscle that is flaccid. **3.** lacking vigor, such as an atonic ulcer, which heals slowly. —**atony** /at′onē/, *n.*

**atonic bladder.**   See **flaccid bladder.**

**atonic constipation,**   constipation caused by failure of the colon to respond to the normal stimuli for evacuation, caused by loss of muscle tone. It may occur in elderly or bedridden patients or after prolonged dependence on laxatives. Also called **colon stasis, lazy colon.** See also **fecal impaction, fecalith, inactive colon, constipation.**

**atonic impotence.**   See **impotence.**

**atonicity**   See **atonia.**

**atony.**   See **atonic.**

**atopic** /ātop′ik/ [Gk, *a + topos*, not place],   pertaining to a hereditary tendency to experience immediate allergic reactions such as asthma or vasomotor rhinitis because of the presence of an antibody (atopic reagin) in the skin and sometimes the bloodstream. —**atopy** /at′opē/, *n.*

**atopic allergy** [Gk, *a*, not, *topos*, place],   a form of allergy that afflicts persons with a genetic predisposition to hypersensitivity to certain allergens. Examples include asthma, hay fever, and food allergies.

**atopic asthma.**   See **allergic asthma.**

**atopic dermatitis,** an intensely pruritic, often excoriated inflammation commonly found on the face and antecubital and popliteal areas of allergy-prone (atopic) individuals. In infancy and early childhood it is called infantile eczema and is characterized by erythema, oozing, crusting, and secondary bacterial infections. In adults the disease manifests itself with crusting, excoriation and lichenification. Treatment includes identification and avoidance of allergens and administration of topical corticosteroids, moisturizers and lubricants, antihistamines, and wet compresses. Also called **atopic eczema.** Compare **contact dermatitis.** See also **atopic.**

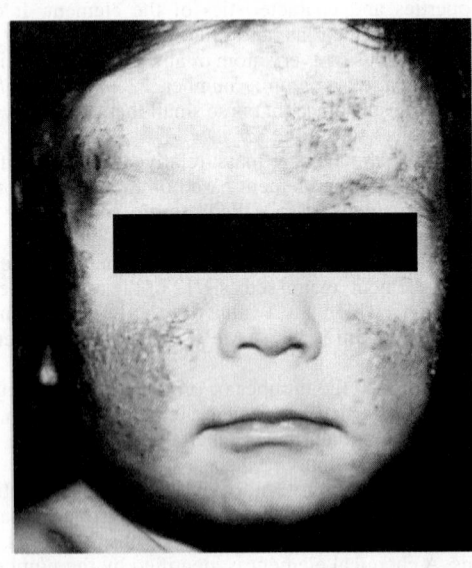

**Infantile atopic dermatitis** *(Zitelli and Davis, 1997)*

**atopic reagin.** See **reagin.**

**atopognosia** /ātop′əgnō′zhə/ [Gk, *a, topos,* not place, *gnosis,* knowledge], a form of agnosia in which a person is unable to locate a tactile sensation correctly.

**atopy.** See **atopic.**

**atorvastatin,** an antihyperlipidemic.

■ INDICATIONS: This drug is used as an adjunct in primary hypercholesterolemia, types Ia and Ib.

■ CONTRAINDICATIONS: Known hypersensitivity, pregnancy, lactation, and active liver disease prohibit the use of this drug.

■ ADVERSE EFFECTS: Liver dysfunction is a potentially life-threatening side effect of this drug. Other adverse effects include rash, pruritus, alopecia, dyspepsia, flatus, pancreatitis, lens opacities, myalgia, and headache.

**atoxic.** See **nontoxic.**

**ATP,** abbreviation for **adenosine triphosphate.**

**ATPase,** abbreviation for **adenosine triphosphatase.**

**ATPD,** abbreviation for *ambient temperature, ambient pressure, dry.*

**ATPS,** abbreviation for *ambient temperature, ambient pressure, saturated* (with water vapor). See also **volume ATPS.**

**atransferrinemic anemia** /ā′transfer′inē′mik/, an iron-transport deficiency disease characterized by a failure of iron to move from the liver or other storage sites to tissues in which erythrocytes develop. The condition may be caused by a molecular defect in transferrin, an iron-binding protein. In addition to anemia, the patient usually suffers from hemosiderosis.

**atraumatic** /ā′trômat′ik/ [Gk, *a,* without, *trauma*], pertaining to therapies or therapeutic instruments and devices that are unlikely to cause tissue damage.

**atresia** /ətrē′zhə/ [Gk, *a, tresis,* not perforation], the absence of a normal body opening, duct, or canal, such as of the anus, vagina, or external ear canal. —**atresic, atretic,** *adj.*

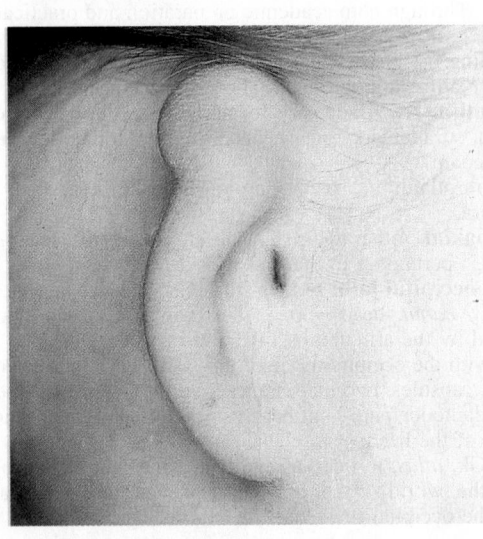

**Atresia of the right external ear** *(Zitelli and Davis, 1997)*

**-atresia,** suffix meaning a 'condition of abnormal occlusion' or congenital absence of an opening: *gynatresia, urethratresia.*

**atresic teratism** /ətrē′sik/ [Gk, *a, tresis* + *tera,* monster], a congenital anomaly in which any of the normal openings of the body, such as the mouth, nares, anus, or vagina, fails to form.

**atretic.** See **atresia.**

**atreto-,** prefix meaning 'closed, or lacking an opening': *atretoblepharia, atretorrhinia.*

**atria.** See **atrium.**

**atrial appendix.** See **auricle.**

**atrial extrasystole.** See **premature atrial complex.**

**atrial fibrillation** (AF) /ā′trē·əl/, a cardiac arrhythmia characterized by disorganized electrical activity in the atria accompanied by an irregular ventricular response that is usually rapid. The atria quiver instead of pumping in an organized fashion, resulting in compromised ventricular filling and reduced stroke volume. Stasis of left atrial flow increases the risk of stroke. AF is associated with rheumatic heart disease (left atrial dilation), mitral stenosis, acute myocardial infarction, and heart surgery, or it may be idiopathic (lone AF). Treatment goals are to control the ventricular rate creating atrioventricular block, to prevent stroke through the use of anticoagulants, and to convert to sinus rhythm. Treatment categories are acute, subacute, and chronic. AF is called uncontrolled and controlled if ventricular response is less than 100. If ventricular response is 100 or more, it is called uncontrolled atrial fibrillation; less than 100, controlled.

**atrial flutter (AF),** a type of atrial tachycardia characterized by contraction rates between 230/min and 380/min. Two kinds, typical and atypical, have been identified and are distinguished from each other by their rates and electrocardiographic (ECG) patterns. During typical atrial flutter the atrial rate is between 290/min and 310/min and produces "fence post" or "sawtooth" ECG waves. During atypical atrial flutter the artial rate is higher, and the ECG waves lack the sawtooth appearance, and are often sinusoidal. For both types, ventricular contractions usually follow atrial contractions in a 1:2, 1:3, 1:4, or variable ratio. Compare **atrial fibrillation.**

**atrial gallop.** See S$_4$.

**atrial myxoma,** a benign, pedunculated, gelatinous tumor that originates in the interatrial septum of the heart. The tumor is characterized by palpitations, disseminated neuritis, nausea, weight loss, fatigue, dyspnea, fever, and occasional sudden loss of consciousness. It is treated by surgical removal of the tumor.

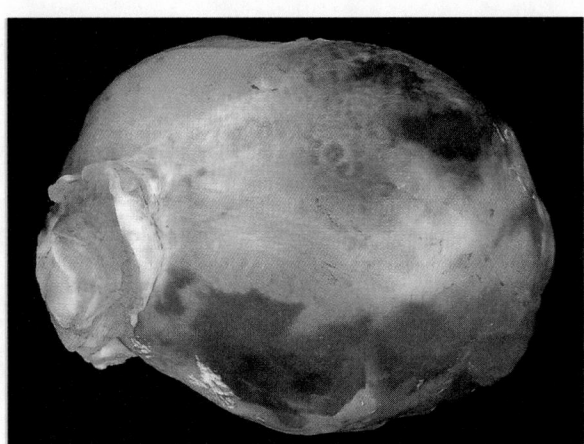

**Left atrial myxoma** (Fletcher, 2000)

**atrial natriuretic factor test (ANF),** a blood test used to detect levels of ANF, which have been shown to be a marker of congestive heart failure (CHF) severity in patients with known CHF. ANF is also used to predict which cardiac patients are likely to develop CHF and to predict the chance of developing CHF after acute myocardial infarction.

**atrial natriuretic peptide (ANP),** a hormone involved in natriuresis and the regulation of renal and cardiovascular homeostasis. It is generally 28 amino acids in length but varies somewhat; it is synthesized as a prohormone in the granules of the myocytes of the atrium and is released into the circulation in response to atrial dilation or increased intravascular fluid volume. It causes natriuresis, diuresis, and renal vasodilation; reduces circulating concentrations of renin, aldosterone, and antidiuretic hormone; and thereby normalizes circulating blood pressure and volume. Also called **atrial natriuretic factor.**

**atrial pacing.** See **pacing.**

**atrial premature beat, atrial premature complex (APC).** See **premature atrial complex.**

**atrial septal defect (ASD),** a congenital cardiac anomaly characterized by an abnormal opening between the atria.

The severity of the condition depends on the size and location of the opening, which are related to the stage at which embryonic development of the septum was arrested. ASDs are classified as **ostium primum defect,** in which there is inadequate development of the endocardial cushions of the first septum of the fetal heart; **ostium secundum defect,** in which the aperture in the second septum of the fetal heart fails to close; and **sinus venosus defect,** in which the superior portion of the atrium fails to develop. ASDs increase the flow of oxygenated blood into the right side of the heart, which is usually well tolerated, since the blood is delivered under much lower pressure than in ventricular septal defect. Clinical manifestations include a characteristic harsh, scratchy systolic murmur and a fixed splitting of the second heart sound, which does not vary with respiration. X-ray films and electrocardiograms generally show right atrial and right ventricular enlargement, although definitive diagnosis is made by cardiac catheterization or echocardiogram. Surgical closure is indicated in most cases but is usually postponed until later childhood, unless the defect is severe. See also **endocardial cushion defect.**

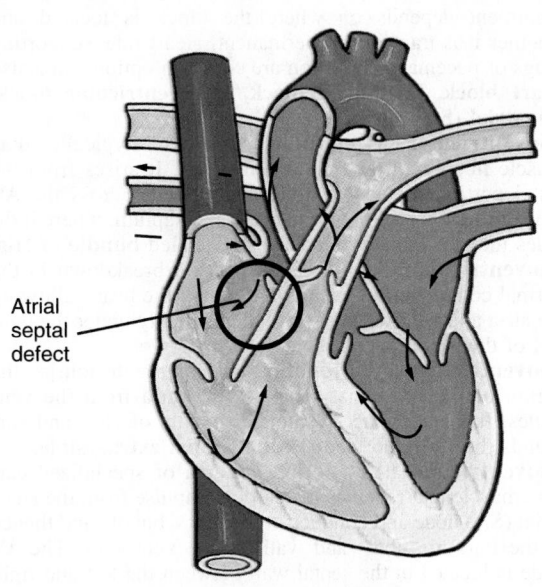

**Atrial septal defect** (Wong, 1999)

**atrial septum** [L, *atrium,* hall, *saeptum,* fence], a partition between the left and right atria of the heart.

**atrial standstill,** a condition of complete failure of the atria to contract. P waves are absent in all electrocardiogram surface leads, and A waves are absent in the jugular venous pulse and right atrial pressure tracings. Generally a junctional escape pacemaker maintains ventricular activity during atrial standstill.

**atrial systole,** the contraction of the atria of the heart, which precedes ventricular contraction by a fraction of a second.

**atrial tachycardia** [L, *atrium,* hall; Gk, *tachys,* quick, *kardia,* heart], rapid beating of the atria caused by abnormal automaticity, triggered activity, or intraatrial reentry. The atrial rate is usually less than 200/min; however, in cases of digitalis excess, the rate increases gradually to 130/min to

250/min as the digitalis is continued. When there is 2:1 conduction, the atrial rhythm is irregular in 50% of cases. The contour of the P′ waves is different from that of the sinus P wave except in cases of digitalis-induced atrial tachycardia, when the P′ wave is almost identical to the sinus P wave. Vagal maneuvers have no effect on atrial tachycardia, although they do cause atrioventricular block. Atrial tachycardia may be either nonparoxysmal (common) or paroxysmal (uncommon). Also called **auricular tachycardia.**

**atrichia** /ātrik′ē·ə/ [Gk, *a,* not, *thrix,* hair],   **1.** pertaining to a group of bacteria that lack flagella. **2.** the absence of hair.

**atrichosis** /ā′trikō′sis/ [Gk, *a* + *trichia* without hair, *osis,* condition],   a congenital absence of hair.

**atrio-,**   prefix meaning 'atrium of the heart' or entrance chamber: *atriocommissuropexy, atrionector.*

**atrioventricular (AV)** /ā′trē·ōventrik′yələr/ [L, *atrium,* hall, *ventriculus*],   pertaining to a connecting conduction event or anatomic structure between the atria and ventricles.

**atrioventricular block (AVB)** [L, *atrium* + *ventriculus,* little belly],   a disorder of cardiac impulse transmission that reflects prolonged, intermittent, or absent conduction of impulses between the atria and ventricles. It commonly occurs at the AV node or within the bundle branch system. Treatment depends on where the block is located and whether it is transient or permanent. Heart rate–supporting drugs or pacemaker insertion are common options. See also **heart block, intraatrial block, intraventricular block, sinoatrial (SA) block.**

**atrioventricular (AV) bundle,**   a band of atypical cardiac muscle fibers with few contractile units. It arises from the distal portion of the AV node and extends across the AV groove to the top of the intraventricular septum, where it divides into the bundle branches. Also called **bundle of His.**

**atrioventricular (AV) dissociation,**   a breakdown in the normal conduction of excitation through the heart, allowing the atria and ventricles to beat independently under the control of their own pacemakers.

**atrioventricular (AV) junction** [L, *jungere,* to join],   the region of the heart that separates the atria from the ventricles. It includes the AV bundle (bundle of His) and surrounds the AV node. See also **junctional extrasystole.**

**atrioventricular (AV) node,**   an area of specialized cardiac muscle that receives the cardiac impulse from the sinoatrial (SA) node and conducts it to the AV bundle and thence to the Purkinje fibers and walls of the ventricles. The AV node is located in the septal wall between the left and right atria.

**atrioventricular (AV) septum,**   a small portion of membrane that separates the atria from the ventricles of the heart.

**atrioventricular (AV) valve,**   a valve in the heart through which blood flows from the atria to the ventricles. The valve between the left atrium and left ventricle is the mitral (bicuspid) valve; the right AV valve is the tricuspid valve.

**at risk,**   the state of an individual's or population's being vulnerable to a particular disease or event. The factors determining risk may be environmental, psychosocial, psychologic, or physiologic. An example of an environmental factor is exposure to harmful substances or organisms. An example of a physiologic factor is genetic predisposition to a disease.

**atrium** /ā′trē·əm/, *pl.* **atria** [L, hall],   a chamber or cavity, such as the right and left atria of the heart or the nasal cavity.

**atrium of ear,**   the external part of the ear, including the auricle and the tubular portion of the external auditory meatus.

**atrium of the heart,**   one of the two upper chambers of the heart. The right atrium receives deoxygenated blood from

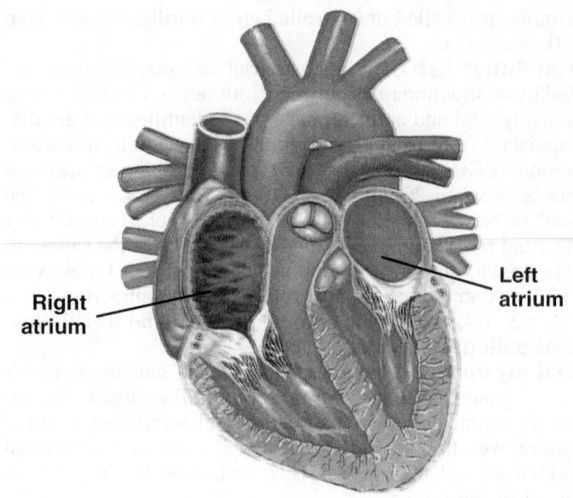

Right atrium

Left atrium

**Atria of the heart** *(Cannobio, 1990)*

the superior vena cava, the inferior vena cava, and the coronary sinus. The left atrium receives oxygenated blood from the pulmonary veins. Blood is emptied into the ventricles from the atria during diastole.

**Atromid-S,**   trademark for an antilipemic (clofibrate).

**-atrophia,**   **1.** suffix meaning a 'condition of nutrition and growth': *metatrophia, pantatrophia.* **2.** combining form meaning a 'progressive decline of a body part': *dermatrophia, neuratrophia.*

**atrophic** /ātrof′ik/ [Gk, *a,* without, *trophe,* nourishment],   characterized by a wasting of tissues, usually associated with general malnutrition or a specific disease state. See also **dystrophic.**

**atrophic arthritis.**   See **rheumatoid arthritis.**

**atrophic catarrh** [Gk, *a, trophe,* without nourishment, *kata,* down, *rhoia,* flow],   an abnormal condition characterized by inflammation and discharge from the mucous membranes of the nose, accompanied by the loss of mucosal and submucosal tissue. Compare **hypertrophic catarrh.** See also **catarrh.**

**atrophic cirrhosis** [Gk, *a* + *trophe,* without nourishment, *kirrhos,* yellow-orange],   a form of advanced portal cirrhosis with massive shrinking of the liver.

**atrophic fracture,**   a spontaneous fracture caused by bone atrophy, as in the bones of a person with osteoporosis.

**atrophic gastritis,**   a chronic inflammation of the stomach, associated with degeneration of the gastric mucosa. Seen in elderly patients and in persons with pernicious anemia, it rarely causes epigastric pain. See also **pernicious anemia.**

**atrophic glossitis,**   a pathologic condition in which the various papillae are lost from the dorsum of the tongue, resulting in a very sore and highly sensitive surface that makes eating difficult. See also **glossitis.**

**atrophic rhinitis** [Gk, *a* + *trophe,* without nourishment, *rhis,* nose, *itis,* inflammation],   a nasal condition in which there is atrophy of the mucous membrane of the nose, resulting in failure of the ciliary function and drying and crusting of the lining of the nasal passages. This may reduce the sense of smell.

**atrophic vaginitis** [Gk, *a* + *trophe*, without nourishment; L, *vagina*, sheath; Gk, *itis*, inflammation], degeneration of the vaginal mucous membrane after menopause. See also **vaginitis.**

**atrophied** /at′rōfīd/ [Gk, *a* + *trophe*, without nourishment], decreased in size because of disuse or disease, as an organ, tissue, or body part.

**atrophoderma** /at′rōfədur′mə/ [Gk, *a* + *trophe* + *derma*, skin], the wasting away or decrease in thickness of the skin. The atrophy may affect the entire body surface or only localized areas. The condition is often associated with aging and may occur as a primary or secondary symptom of various diseases.

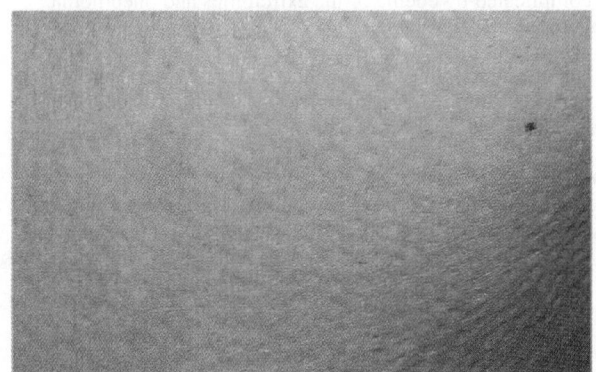

**Follicular atrophoderma** *(Lawrence and Cox, 1993)*

**atrophy** /at′rəfē/ [Gk, *a* + *trophe*, without nourishment], a wasting or decrease in size or physiologic activity of a part of the body because of disease or other influences. A skeletal muscle may undergo atrophy as a result of lack of physical exercise or neurologic or musculoskeletal disease. Cells of the brain and central nervous system may atrophy in old age because of restricted blood flow to those areas. See also **aging.** —**atrophic,** *adj.,* **atrophy,** *v.*

**atrophy of disuse** [Gk, *a, trophe* + L, *dis,* opposite of, *usus*], a shrinkage of tissues resulting from immobility or lack of exercise.

**atropine** /at′rōpin/ [Gk, *Atropos,* one of the three Fates], an alkaloid from *Atropa belladonna* and *Datura stramonium* plants. It is related to other drugs, such as scopolamine and hyoscyamine, and has a similar action of blocking parasympathetic stimuli by raising the threshold of response of effector cells to acetylcholine.

**atropine sulfate,** an antispasmodic and anticholinergic.
■ INDICATIONS: It may be prescribed in the treatment of GI hypermotility to decrease the tone of the detrusor muscle of the urinary bladder in urinary tract disorders, for cyclopegic refraction and dilation of the pupil in inflammation of the iris or the uvea, cardiac arrhythmias, and certain kinds of poisoning and as an adjunct to anesthesia.
■ CONTRAINDICATIONS: GI obstruction, glaucoma, hepatitis, liver or kidney dysfunction, porphyria, or known hypersensitivity to this drug or other anticholinergics prohibits its use.
■ ADVERSE EFFECTS: Among the more serious adverse reactions are tachycardia, angina, loss of taste, nausea, diarrhea, skin rash, blurred vision, and eye pain. Dry mouth and constipation are common effects.

**atropine sulfate poisoning** [Gk, *Atropos,* fate; L, *sulphur* + *potio,* drink], toxic effects of an overdose of a drug sometimes used as an adjunct to general anesthesia and to treat bradycardia. Symptoms include tachycardia, hot and dry flushed skin, dry mouth with thirst, restlessness and excitement, urinary retention, constipation, and a burning pain in the throat.

**attached epithelial cuff.** See **junctional epithelium.**

**attached gingiva,** gum tissue that covers and is firmly attached to the alveolar process in the maxilla and mandible. Also called **alveolar gingiva.**

**attachment** [Fr, *attachement*], **1.** the state or quality of being affixed or attached. **2.** (in psychiatry) a mode of behavior in which one individual relates in an affiliative or dependent manner to another; a feeling of affection or loyalty that binds one person to another. **3.** See **bonding. 4.** (in dentistry) any device, such as a retainer or artificial crown, used to secure a partial denture to a natural tooth in the mouth.

**attachment apparatus,** the various tissues that surround and support the teeth, including the cementum, the periodontal ligament, and the alveolar process. See also **masticatory system.**

**attachment promotion,** a nursing intervention from the Nursing Interventions Classification (NIC) defined as facilitation of the development of the parent-infant relationship. See also **Nursing Interventions Classification.**

**attack,** an episode in the course of an illness, usually characterized by acute and distressing symptoms.

**attending** [L, *attendo,* to notice], (in psychology) pertaining to an aroused readiness to perceive, with an adjustment of the brain and sense organs to focus on a situation.

**attending physician** [L, *attendere,* to stretch], the physician who is responsible for a particular patient. In a university hospital setting, an attending physician often also has teaching responsibilities, holds a faculty appointment, and supervises residents and medical students. Also called *(informal)* **attending.**

**attention** [L, *attendere,* to stretch], the element of cognitive functioning in which the mental focus is maintained on a specific issue, object, or activity.

**attention deficit disorder,** a syndrome affecting children, adolescents, and adults characterized by short attention span, hyperactivity, and poor concentration. The symptoms may be mild or severe and are associated with functional deviations of the central nervous system without signs of major neurologic or psychiatric disturbance. The people affected are usually of normal or above average intelligence. Other symptoms include impairment in perception, conceptualization, language, memory, and motor skills; decreased attention span; increased impulsivity; and emotional lability. The condition is 10 times more prevalent in boys than in girls and may result from genetic factors, biochemical irregularities, perinatal or postnatal injury, or disease. There is no known cure, and symptoms often subside or disappear with time. Medication with methylphenidate, pemoline, or the dextroamphetamines is frequently prescribed for children with hyperactive symptoms, and some form of psychotherapeutic counseling is often recommended. Some treatments include abstinence from certain foods and food additives. Also called **hyperactivity, hyperkinesis, minimal brain dysfunction.** See also **learning disability.**

**attention deficit hyperactivity disorder,** a childhood mental disorder with onset before 7 years of age and involving impaired or diminished attention, impulsivity, and hyperactivity. Also called **hyperactive child syndrome** in the twentieth century.

**attenuated** /əten′yōō·ā′tid/ [L, *attenuare,* to make thin], pertaining to the dilution of a solution or the reduction in virulence or toxicity of a microorganism or a drug by weakening it.

**attenuated virus** [L, *attenuare,* to make thin, *virus,* poison], a strain of virus whose virulence has been lowered by physical or chemical processes, or by repeated passage through the cells of another species. Vaccines made by attenuated strains are used to prevent tuberculosis, smallpox, measles, mumps, rubella, polio, and yellow fever.

**attenuation** /əten′yoo̅-ā′shən/ [L, *attenuare,* to make thin], the process of reduction, such as the attenuation of an x-ray beam by reducing its intensity, the weakening of the degree of virulence of a disease organism, or culturing under unfavorable conditions.

**attenuation coefficient,** in radiography or ultrasound, the difference between the energy that enters a body part and the energy that is not detected. The difference is caused by the absorption and scattering of energy within the body tissues.

**attenuator** /əten′yoo̅-ā′tər/ [L, *attenuare,* to make thin], an agent that weakens the toxicity of a poisonous substance or the virulence of a microorganism.

**Attenuvax,** trademark for an active immunizing agent (live measles virus vaccine).

**attic.** See **epitympanic recess.**

**attitude** /at′ətyoo̅d, -too̅d/ [L, *aptitude,* fitness], **1.** a body position or posture, particularly the fetal position in the uterus, as determined by the degree of flexion of the head and extremities. **2.** (in psychiatry) any of the major integrative forces in the development of personality that gives consistency to an individual's behavior. Attitudes are cognitive in nature, formed through interactions with the environment. They reflect the person's innermost convictions about situations good or bad, right or wrong, desirable or undesirable.

**attitudinal isolation** /at′ətyoo̅′dənəl/ [L, *attitudo,* posture], a type of social isolation that results from a person's own cultural or personal values.

**attitudinal reflex,** any reflex initiated by a change in position of the head or by a change in position of the head with respect to the position of the body. Kinds of attitudinal reflexes include **tonic neck reflex** and **tonic labyrinthine reflex.** Also called **statotonic reflex.**

**atto-,** a prefix in the metric system indicating a value of one quintillionth, or $10^{-18}$.

**attraction** [L, *attrahere,* to draw to], a tendency of the teeth or other maxillary or mandibular structures to become elevated above their normal position.

**attrition** /ətrish′ən/ [L, *atterere,* to wear away], the process of wearing away or wearing down by friction.

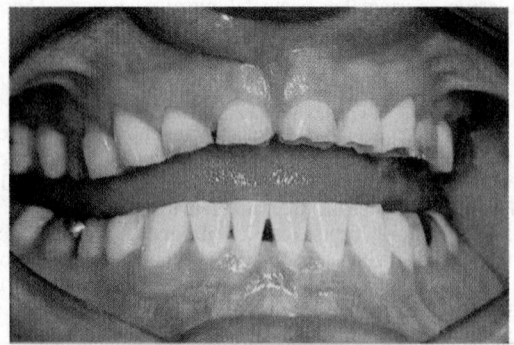

**Attrition of the teeth** *(Christensen, 1994)*

**-ature,** noun-forming combining form: *ligature, tubulature.*

**at. wt.,** abbreviation for **atomic weight.**

**atypia** /ātip′ē-ə/ [Gk, *a + typos,* without type], a condition of being irregular or nonstandard.

**atypical** /ātip′əkəl/ [Gk, *a + typos,* without type], a condition or object that is not of a usual or standard type.

**atypical measles syndrome (AMS),** a form of measles (rubeola) reported in persons immunized with a killed measles vaccine used in the United States from 1962 to 1967 and in Canada until 1970. Symptoms differ from those of typical measles, beginning with a sudden high fever, headache, abdominal pain, and coughing. The measles rash may appear only 1 or 2 days later, usually starting on the hands and feet rather than the head and neck. The infection may be complicated by edema of the extremities and pneumonia.

**atypical** *Mycobacterium* [Gk, *a + typos,* without type, *mykes,* fungus, *bakterion,* small staff], a group of mycobacteria, including pathogenic and nonpathogenic forms, that are classified according to their ability to produce pigments, growth characteristics, and reactions to chemical tests.

**atypical pneumonia** [Gk, *a + typos,* without type, *pneumon,* lung, *ia,* condition], a group of relatively mild symptoms of chills, headache, muscular pains, moderate fever, and coughing, but without evidence of a bacterial infection. Chest x-ray film may show mottling at the bases of the lungs. Eaton agent, or *Mycoplasma pneumoniae,* may be the cause of the symptoms.

**atypical somatoform disorder,** an abnormal condition marked by physical symptoms and complaints that appear related to a preoccupation with an imagined defect in one's personal appearance or ability.

**Au,** symbol for the element **gold.**

**audible** /ô′dəbəl/ [L, *audire,* to hear], capable of being heard. Some animals are able to hear sounds of higher or lower frequencies and different intensities than those audible to most humans.

**audio-,** combining form meaning 'hearing': *audiology.*

**audioanalgesia** /ô·dē·ō·an′əljē′sē·a/ [L, *audire,* to hear; Gk, *a, algos,* not pain], the use of music to enhance relaxation and to distract a patient's mind from pain, as during dentistry, during labor and childbirth, or during procedures with sedation or regional anesthetic techniques.

**audiogenic epilepsy.** See **auditory epilepsy.**

**audiogram** /ô′dē·əgram′/ [Gk, *audire + gramma,* record], a chart showing the faintest level at which an individual is able to detect sounds of various frequencies, usually in octaves from 125 Hz to 8000 Hz. See also **audiometry.**

**audiologic.** See **audiology.**

**audiologist,** a health professional with graduate education in normal hearing processes and hearing loss, who detects and evaluates hearing loss, and who determines how a client can best make use of remaining hearing. If a client can benefit from assistive learning devices such as hearing aids, the audiologist assists with the selection, fitting, and training in their use. See also **speech-language pathologist.**

**audiology** /-ol′əjē/ [L, *audire + Gk, logos,* science], a field of research and clinical practice devoted to the study of hearing disorders, assessment of hearing, hearing conservation, and aural rehabilitation. —**audiologic,** *adj.*

**audiometer** /ô′dē·om′ətər/ [L, *audire + Gk, metron,* measure], an electronic device for testing hearing. Earphones are placed over the ears (air-conduction testing), or a bone vibrator is placed on the mastoid (bone conduction testing). Hearing is tested by using tones from very low to very high frequencies at various decibels of intensity. The patient signals when a tone is heard, and the lowest level at which the patient hears is noted on an audiogram.

**audiometrist** /ô′dē·om′ətrist/, a technician who has received special training in the use of pure-tone audiometry equipment. An audiometrist conducts the hearing tests selected and interpreted by an audiologist, who supervises the process.

**audiometry** /ô′dē·om′ətrē/, the testing of the sensitivity of the sense of hearing. Various audiometric tests determine the lowest intensity of sound at which an individual can perceive auditory stimuli (hearing threshold) and distinguish different speech sounds. Pure tone audiometry assesses the person's ability to hear frequencies, usually ranging from 125 to 8000 hertz (Hz), and can indicate whether a hearing loss is caused by an outer ear, a middle ear, an inner ear, or an acoustic nerve problem. Speech audiometry tests the ability to understand selected words. Impedance audiometry is an objective method of assessing the resistance or compliance of the conducting mechanism of the middle ear with a probe inserted into the ear canal. —**audiometric,** *adj.*

**audiovisual** /ô′dē·ō·vizh′əl/, pertaining to communication that uses both sight and sound messages.

**audit** /ô′dit/, **1.** a final statement of account. **2.** a review and evaluation of health care procedures.

**auditory** /ô′dətôr′ē/ [L, *auditorius,* hearing], pertaining to the sense of hearing and the hearing organs involved.

**auditory amnesia** [L, *auditorius,* hearing; Gk, *amnesia,* forgetfulness], a loss of memory for the meaning of sounds. Also called **word deafness.**

**auditory area** [L, *auditorium,* hearing], the sound perception area of the cerebral cortex. It is located in the floor of the lateral fissure and on the dorsal surface of the superior temporal gyrus.

**auditory brainstem response (ABR),** an electrophysiologic test used to measure hearing sensitivity and evaluate the integrity of ear structures from the auditory nerve through the brainstem. It is also used to screen hearing of newborns.

**auditory canal.** See **auditory meatus.**

**auditory cortex.** See **acoustic center.**

**auditory epilepsy,** a reflex form of epilepsy provoked by sounds. Also called **audiogenic epilepsy.**

**auditory hair** [L, *audire,* to hear; AS, *haer*], one of the cells with hairlike processes in the spiral organ of Corti. The hairs, or cilia, function as sensory receptors. Also called **acoustic hair cell, cell of Corti.**

**auditory hallucination** [L, *audire,* to hear, *alucinari,* a wandering mind], a subjective experience of hearing voices or other sounds despite the absence of an actual reality based external stimulus to account for the phenomenon.

**auditory meatus** [L, *audire,* to hear, *meatus,* passage], **1.** the external auditory meatus, a tubelike channel of the external ear extending from the auricle to the tympanum of the middle ear. **2.** the internal auditory meatus, a short channel extending from the petrous part of the temporal bone to the fundus near the vestibule. It contains the eighth cranial nerve. Also called **auditory canal.**

**auditory nerve.** See **vestibulocochlear nerve.**

**auditory ossicles** [L, *audire* + *ossiculum,* little bone], the malleus, the incus, and the stapes, three small bones in the middle ear that articulate with each other. As the tympanic membrane vibrates, it transmits sound waves through the ossicles to the cochlea.

**auditory system assessment,** an evaluation of the patient's ears and hearing and an investigation of present and past diseases or conditions that may be responsible for an auditory impairment.

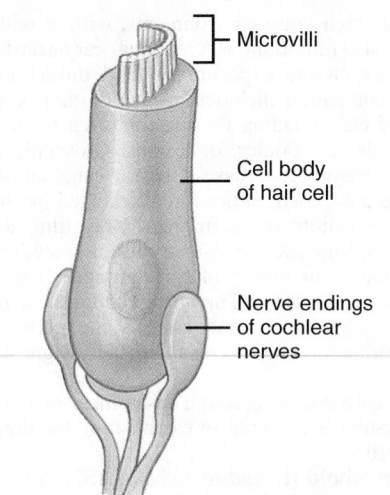

**Auditory hair cell**
*(Seeley, Stephens, and Tate, 1995/Barbara Cousins; used by permission of The McGraw-Hill Companies)*

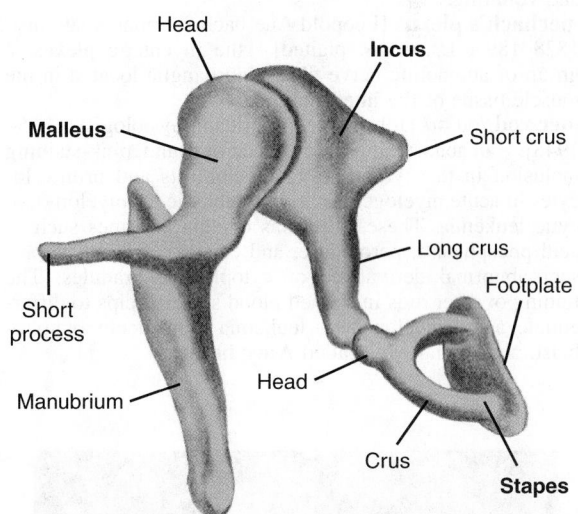

**Auditory ossicles** *(Thompson et al, 1993)*

■ METHOD: The client is questioned in verbal or written form regarding previous ear problems, especially childhood problems of otitis media, perforations of the eardrum, and drainage, and history of measles, mumps, or scarlet fever. Information is obtained about past or present ototoxic medications, such as aspirin, chemotherapeutic drugs, NSAIDS. streptomycin, aminoglycerides, or diuretics. Previous ear surgeries as well as tonsillectomy and adenoidectomy or head injury are also documented. Use of a hearing aid and problems with compacted cerumin are noted. Symptoms of dizziness, ringing in the ears, and hearing loss are recorded. Information regarding allergies, prematurity, and family members with hearing loss is documented. Chronic medical conditions such as diabetes or cancer as well as occupational exposures to high-noise environments, with or without protection, are also important. Recreational ear hazards, such as swimming or chronic exposure to loud music, are noted. Physical examination includes inspection and palpation of the external ear including the mastoid area for tenderness, swelling, redness, nodules, or lesions. Otoscopic examination is then performed to assess the ear canal and tympanic membrane. Diagnostic procedures indicated by the history may include audiometry, a mastoid x-ray film, Rinne and Weber tuning-fork tests, and microbiologic studies for potential pathogens in smears of ear drainage.

■ NURSING CONSIDERATIONS: The nurse conducts the interview, makes the observations, and collects the pertinent background information and the results of the diagnostic procedures.

■ OUTCOME CRITERIA: A thorough assessment of the patient's auditory system is essential in establishing the diagnosis of an ear disorder.

**auditory threshold** [L, *audire,* to hear; AS, *threscold*], the lowest intensity at which a sound may be heard. An audiologist typically determines a patient's threshold for pure tones and speech.

**auditory tube.** See **eustachian tube.**

**auditory vertigo** [L, *audire,* to hear, *vertigo,* dizziness], vertigo associated with ear disease. It is characterized by sensations of gyration and, when severe, with prostration and vomiting.

**Auerbach's plexus** [Leopold Auerbach, German anatomist, 1828–1897; L, *plexus,* plaited], the myenteric plexus, a group of autonomic nerve fibers and ganglia located in the muscle tissue of the intestinal tract.

**Auer rod** /ou′ər/ [John Auer, American physiologist, 1875–1948], an abnormal, needle-shaped or round, pink-staining inclusion in the cytoplasm of myeloblasts and promyelocytes in acute myelogenous, promyelocytic, or myelomonocytic leukemia. These inclusions contain enzymes such as acid phosphatase, peroxidase, and esterase and may represent abnormal derivatives of cytoplasmic granules. The finding of Auer rods in stained blood smears helps to differentiate acute myelogenous leukemia from acute lymphoblastic leukemia. Also called **Auer body.**

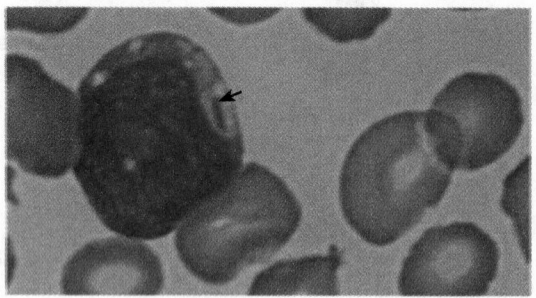

**Auer rod** *(Carr and Rodak, 1999)*

**augmentation** /ôg′məntā′shən/ [L, *augmentare,* to increase], **1.** stimulation of an increased rate of biologic activity, such as faster cell division or heartbeat. **2.** breast enlargement through mammoplasty.

**augmentation mammoplasty,** a surgical procedure to enlarge the breasts.

**aur-, auri-,** prefix meaning 'ear': *auricle, aural.*

**aura** /ôr′ə/ [L, breath], **1.** *pl.* **aurae** /ôr′ē/, a sensation, as of light or warmth, that may precede an attack of migraine or an epileptic seizure. **2.** *pl.* **auras,** an emanation of light or color surrounding a person as seen in Kirlian photography and studied in current nursing research in healing techniques.

**aural**[1] /ôr′əl/, pertaining to the ear or hearing. —**aurally,** *adv.*

**aural**[2], pertaining to an aura.

**aural forceps,** a dressing forceps with fine, bent tips used in surgery.

**aurally.** See **aural.**

**aural rehabilitation,** a form of therapy in which hearing-impaired individuals are taught to improve their ability to communicate. Methods taught include, but are not limited to, speech-reading, auditory training, use of hearing aids, and use of assistive listening devices such as telephone amplifiers.

**auramine** /ôr′əmēn/, a yellow aniline dye used in the manufacture of paints, textiles, and rubber products. The experimental carcinogen in animals has been identified as a cause of bladder cancer in humans. Also called **dimethyl aniline.**

**auramine O,** a fluorescent, yellow aniline dye used as a stain for the tubercle bacillus and for deoxyribonucleic acid (DNA).

**auranofin** /ôr′ənof′in/, an oral gold antiarthritic drug.

■ INDICATIONS: It is prescribed for the treatment of rheumatoid arthritis.

■ CONTRAINDICATIONS: Auranofin is contraindicated for patients who have disorders that are caused by or aggravated by medicines containing gold or who have impaired kidney function.

■ ADVERSE EFFECTS: Among the most severe adverse reactions are diarrhea, loose stools, abdominal pain, nausea, vomiting, rash, pruritus, stomatitis, anemia, leukopenia, granulocytopenia, thrombocytopenia, eosinophilia, proteinemia, hematuria, and elevated liver enzyme levels.

**aurantiasis cutis** /ôr′əntī′əsis/ [L, *aurantium,* orange; Gk, *osis,* condition; L, *cutis,* skin], a yellowish skin pigmentation that results from eating excessive amounts of foods containing carotene, such as carrots.

**auras.** See **aura.**

**Aureomycin,** trademark for a tetracycline antibiotic (chlortetracycline hydrochloride).

**auriasis.** See **chrysiasis.**

**auricle** /ôr′ikəl/ [L, *auricula,* little ear], **1.** the external ear. Also called **pinna. 2.** the left or right cardiac atrium, so named because of its earlike shape. Also called **atrial appendix.**

**auricular** /ôrik′yələr/, **1.** pertaining to the auricle of the ear. **2.** otic.

**auricular cervical nerve reflex.** See **Snellen's reflex.**

**auricularis anterior,** one of three extrinsic muscles of the ear. It functions to move the auricula forward and upward. Some people can voluntarily contract the auricularis anterior to move the ears. Compare **auricularis posterior, auricularis superior.**

**auricularis posterior,** one of three extrinsic muscles of the ear. It serves to draw the auricula backward. Compare **auricularis anterior, auricularis superior.**

**auricularis superior,** a thin, fan-shaped muscle that is one of three extrinsic muscles of the ear. It acts to draw the auricula upward. Compare **auricularis anterior, auricularis posterior.**

**auricular line,** a hypothetical line passing through the ex-

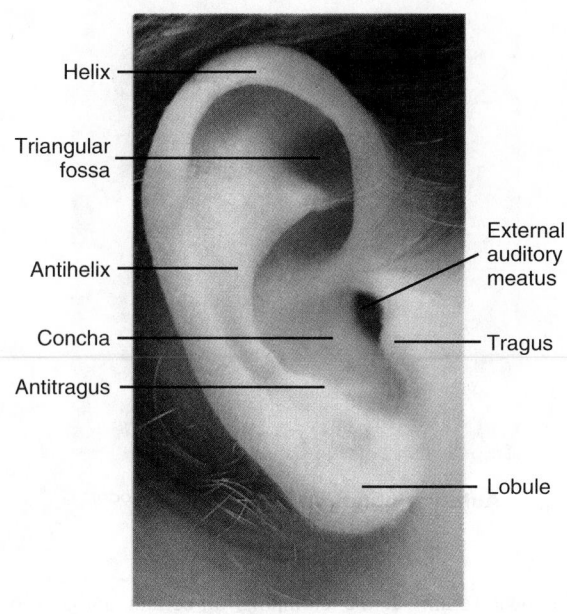

**Auricle** *(Seidel et al, 1999)*

Helix

Triangular fossa

Antihelix

Concha

Antitragus

External auditory meatus

Tragus

Lobule

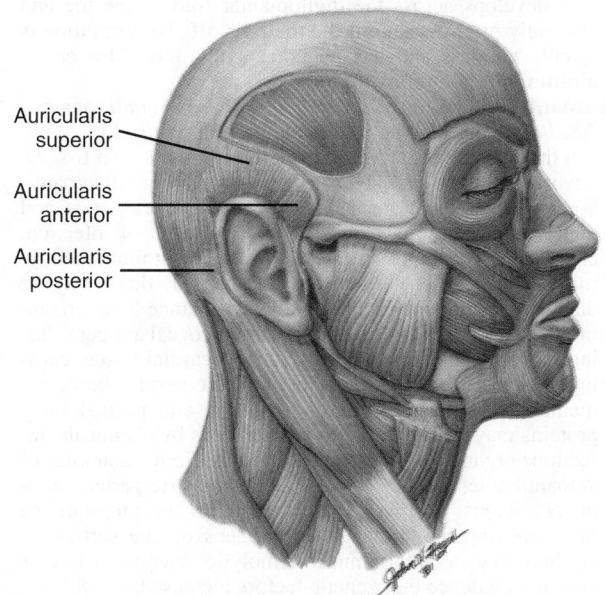

Auricularis superior

Auricularis anterior

Auricularis posterior

**Extrinsic muscles of the ear: auricularis anterior, auricularis posterior, and auricularis superior**
*(Thibodeau and Patton, 1999/John V. Hagen)*

ternal auditory meatuses and perpendicular to the Frankfort horizontal plane.

**auricular point,** the center of the external auditory meatus.

**auricular tachycardia.** See **atrial tachycardia.**

**auricular tubercle,** a small projection sometimes found on the edge of the helix of the ear, conjectured by some to be a relic of a simian ancestry. Also called **darwinian tubercle, Darwin's tubercle.**

**auriculin** /ôrik′yəlin/, a hormonelike substance with diuretic activity produced in the atria of the heart.

**auriculocranial** /-krā′nē-əl/, pertaining to the auricle of the ear and the cranium.

**auriculotemporal** /-tem′pərəl/, pertaining to the auricle of the ear and the temporal area of the skull.

**auriculoventriculostomy** /ôrik′yəlōventrik′yəlos′təmē/ [L, *auricula* + *ventriculus,* little belly; Gk, *stoma,* opening], a surgical procedure that directs cerebrospinal fluid into the general circulation in the treatment of hydrocephalus, usually in the newborn. In this procedure a polyethylene tube is passed from the lateral ventricle through a burr hole in the parietal skull area under the scalp and into the jugular vein or abdomen for the discharge of cerebrospinal fluid. The tube, which has valves, is inserted to prevent reflux of the blood into the ventricles and to maintain the draining of excess cerebrospinal fluid when ventricular pressure increases. This procedure is performed to correct the communicating and the obstructive forms of hydrocephalus. Also called **ventriculoatrial shunt, ventriculoatriostomy.**

**auris dextra (a.d.),** the Latin term for right ear.

**auris sinistra (a.s.),** the Latin term for left ear.

**aurothioglucose** /ôr′ōthī′ōgloo′kōs/, an organic gold antiarthritic used in chrysotherapy.

■ INDICATION: It is prescribed for adjunctive treatment of adult and juvenile rheumatoid arthritis.

■ CONTRAINDICATIONS: Severe uncontrolled diabetes, renal or hepatic dysfunction, a history of infectious hepatitis, hypertension, heart failure, systemic lupus erythematosus, agranulocytosis, hemorrhagic diathesis, pregnancy, urticaria, eczema, colitis, or known hypersensitivity to this drug prohibits its use.

■ ADVERSE EFFECTS: Among the most serious adverse effects are kidney and liver damage and allergic reactions. Dermatitis and lesions of mucous membranes are common.

**auscultate** /ôs′kəltāt/ [L, auscultare, to listen], to practice auscultation, or to listen and interpret sounds produced within the body.

**auscultation** /ôs′kəltā′shən/ [L, *auscultare,* to listen], the act of listening for sounds within the body to evaluate the condition of the heart, blood vessels, lungs, pleura, intestines, or other organs or to detect the fetal heart sound. Auscultation may be performed directly with the unaided ear, but most commonly a stethoscope is used to determine the frequency, intensity, duration, and quality of the sounds. —**auscultate,** *v.,* **auscultatory** /ôskul′tətôr′ē/, *adj.*

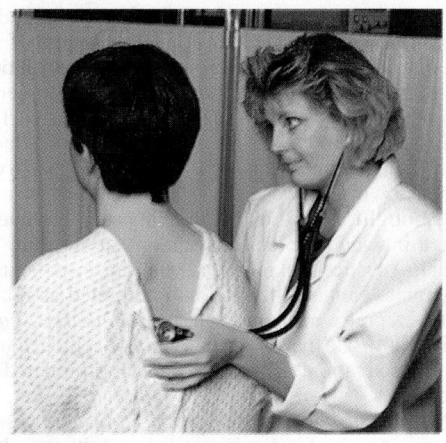

**Auscultation of the lungs** *(Belcher, 1992)*

**auscultatory gap,** time in which sound is not heard in the auscultatory method of measuring blood pressure with a sphygmomanometer, occurring particularly in hypertension and in aortic stenosis.

**auscultatory percussion.** See **auscultation, percussion.**

**Austin Flint murmur** [Austin Flint, American physiologist, 1812–1886], a low-pitched sound characteristic of severe aortic regurgitation without mitral valve disease. It is typically heard during ventricular middiastole at the mitral valve area. Amyl nitrate may help differentiate this murmur from that of mitral valve stenosis.

**Australia antigen,** hepatitis B surface antigen (HBsAg), found present in acute or chronic hepatitis B. See also **hepatitis.**

**Australian lift,** a type of shoulder lift used to move a patient who is unable to assume a sitting position on a bed or other surface. The lift is executed by two persons, one on each side of the patient, who place the shoulder near the patient under the patient's axillae. At the same time, the two lifters grasp each other's hands under the patient's thighs and make coordinated movements needed to lift the patient onto or from a bed or wheelchair.

**Australian Q fever.** See **Q fever.**

**autacoid** /ô′təkoid/, any of a group of substances, as hormones, that are produced in one organ and are transported via blood or lymph as a means to control a physiologic process in another part of the body.

**authenticity** /ô′thəntis′itē/, (in psychiatry) emotional and behavioral openness; a quality of being genuine and trustworthy.

**authoritarian personality,** a group of behavioral traits characteristic of one who advocates obedience and strict adherence to rules.

**authority** /ôthôr′ətē/, a relationship between two or more persons or groups characterized by the influence one may exercise over the other through ideas, commands, suggestions, or instructions.

**authority figure,** a person who by virtue of status, strength, knowledge, or other recognized superiority exerts influence over others.

**autism** [Gk, *autos,* self], a mental disorder characterized by extreme withdrawal and an abnormal absorption in fantasy, accompanied by delusion, hallucination, and inability to communicate verbally or otherwise relate to people. Schizophrenic children are often autistic. See also **infantile autism. —autistic,** *adj.*

**autistic disorder** /ôtis′tik/ [Gk, *autos,* self], a pervasive developmental disorder with onset in infancy or childhood, characterized by impaired social interaction, impaired communication, and a remarkably restricted repertoire of activities and interests. See also **infantile autism. —autistic,** *adj.*

**autistic phase,** a period of preoedipal development, according to Mahler's system of personality stages. It lasts from birth to around 1 month and is considered normal. Children then become aware that they cannot satisfy their body needs by themselves.

**autistic thought,** a form of thinking that is internally stimulated in which the ideas have a private meaning to the individual. Autistic thinking is a symptom in patients with schizophrenia. Fantasy life may be interpreted as reality.

**auto-, aut-,** prefix meaning 'self': *autocatharsis, autism.*

**autoactivation** /-ak′tivā′shən/ [Gk, *autos,* self, *activus,* active], self-activation, as when a gland is stimulated by its own secretions.

**autoagglutination** /-əglo̅o̅′tənā′shən/ [Gk, *autos,* self; L, *agglutinare,* to glue], **1.** also called **autohemagglutination.** The clumping of red blood cells caused by an individu-

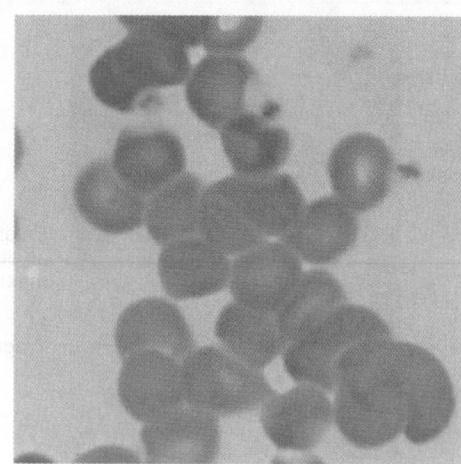

**Autoagglutination** *(Carr and Rodak, 1999)*

al's own serum. **2.** the clumping of certain antigens or antigen-bearing cells, such as bacteria.

**autoamputation** /-amp′yo̅o̅tā′shən/, the spontaneous detachment of a body part, usually the fourth or fifth toe, as occurs among the males of some African peoples. A depression develops across the digitoplantar fold of the toe and gradually progresses until the toe falls off. The condition is usually painless and has no other symptoms. Also called **ainhum** /ān′ho̅o̅m, īnyoon′/.

**autoantibody** /ô′tō-an′tibod′ē/ [Gk, *autos* + *anti,* against; AS, *bodig,* body], an immunoglobulin produced by a person that recognizes an antigen on that person's own tissues. Several mechanisms may trigger the production of autoantibodies: an antigen, formed during fetal development and then sequestered, may be released as a result of infection, chemical exposure, or trauma, as occurs in autoimmune thyroiditis, sympathetic uveitis, and aspermia; there may be disorders of immune regulatory or surveillance function; antibodies produced against certain streptococcal antigens during infection may cross-react with myocardial tissue, causing rheumatic heart disease, or with glomerular basement membrane, causing glomerulonephritis; and normal body proteins may be converted to autoantigens by chemicals, infectious organisms, or therapeutic drugs. Some examples of autoantibodies are those found against gastric parietal cells in pernicious anemia, against platelets in autoimmune thrombocytopenia, and against antigens on the surface of erythrocytes in autoimmune hemolytic anemia. There is growing evidence that genetic factors increase the incidence and severity of autoimmune diseases.

**autoantigen** /ô′tō-an′tijin/ [Gk, *autos* + *anti,* against, *genein,* to produce], an endogenous body constituent that stimulates the production of autoantibodies and an autoimmune reaction. An autoantigen associated with **Addison's disease** has been identified as the enzyme 17 α-hydroxylase. Also called **self-antigen.** See also **antibody-specific model, autoantibody, autoimmune disease.**

**autoantitoxin** /-an′titok′sin/, an antibody produced as protection against a toxin resulting from infection in the same individual, such as *Escherichia coli* endotoxin.

**autoaugmentation** /-ôg′məntā′shən/, a surgical procedure in which the detrusor muscle of the bladder is removed, leaving the bladder epithelium otherwise intact.

**autoblast** /ô′təblast/, an independent microorganism.

**autocatheterization** /-kath′ərizā′shən/,   the insertion of a catheter by the patient, usually referring to urinary catheterization. See also **self-catheterization.**

**autochthonous** /ôtok′thənəs/, [Gk, *autos,* self, *chthon,* earth],   **1.** relating to a disease or other condition that appears to have originated in the part of the body in which it was discovered. **2.** (in psychology) describing the sudden appearance of a system of delusions.

**autochthonous idea** [Gk, *autos + chthon,* earth],   an idea that originates in the unconscious and arises spontaneously in the mind, independent of the conscious train of thought.

**autoclassis** /ôtok′ləsis/ [Gk, *autos,* self, *klassis,* breaking],   the rupturing or breaking of a part of the body caused by a force or agent arising from within the body itself.

**autoclave** /ô′təklāv/,   an appliance used to sterilize medical instruments or other objects with steam under pressure.

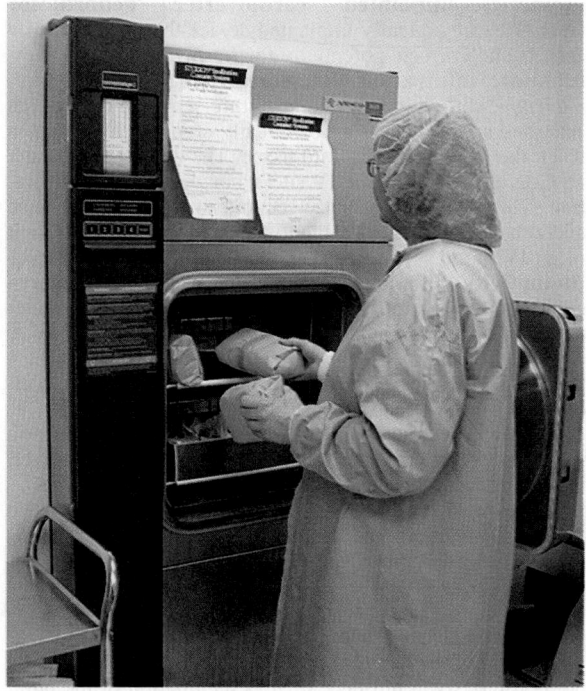

**Autoclave** *(Sorrentino, 2000)*

**autocrine** /ô′təkrin/,   denoting the effect of a hormone on cells that produce it.

**autodermic graft.**   See **autogenous graft.**

**autodigestion,**   a condition in which gastric juices in the pancreas or stomach digest the organ's own tissues.

**autodiploid** /ô′tōdip′loid/ [Gk, *autos + diploos,* double, *eidos,* form],   **1.** an individual, organism, strain, or cell containing two genetically identical or nearly identical chromosome sets that are derived from the same ancestral species and result from the duplication of the haploid set. **2.** pertaining to such an individual, organism, strain, or cell. Also **autodiploidic.** Compare **allodiploid.** See also **autopolyploid.**

**autodiploidy** /ô′tōdip′loidē/,   the state or condition of having two genetically identical or nearly identical chromo-

some sets from the same ancestral species. Such a state enables cell division to occur in a normal manner. Compare **allodiploidy.**

**autoeroticism** /-irot′əsiz′əm/ [Gk, *autos + eros,* love],   **1.** sensual, sexual gratification of the self, usually obtained through the stimulus of one's own body without the participation of another person. It is derived from such acts as stroking, masturbation, and fantasy, or from other oral, anal, or visual sources of stimulation. **2.** sexual feeling or desire occurring without any external stimulus. **3.** (in Freudian psychoanalytic theory) an early phase of psychosexual development, occurring in the oral and the anal stages. Also called **autoerotism.** Compare **heteroeroticism. —auto-erotic,** *adj.*

**autoerythrocyte sensitization** /ô′tō·ərith′rəsīt/ [Gk, *autos + erythros,* red, *kytos,* cell],   hypersensitivity to one's own red blood cells. It results in the spontaneous appearance of painful, hemorrhagic spots on the anterior aspects of the arms and legs. Autoimmune hemolytic anemia, an extreme example of the condition, may cause fulminant hemolysis, fever, abdominal pain, hyperbilirubinemia, thrombosis, and shock. Psychoneurotic disorders also may be associated with the condition.

**autoerythrocyte sensitization syndrome.**   See **Gardner-Diamond syndrome.**

**autogenesis** /ô′tōjen′əsis/ [Gk, *autos + genein,* to produce],   **1.** abiogenesis. **2.** a self-produced condition; a condition originating from within the organism. Also called **autogeny** /ôtoj′ənē/. Compare **heterogenesis, homogenesis. —autogenetic, autogenic,** *adj.*

**autogenic therapy** /-jen′ik/,   a mental health therapy introduced by Wolfgang Luthe. It is based on the concept that natural forces in the brain are able to remove disturbing influences so that functional harmony can be restored in the mind and body. It was developed from research on sleep and hypnosis and involves biofeedback exercises.

**autogenic training,**   a nursing intervention from the Nursing Interventions Classification (NIC) defined as assisting with self-suggestions about feelings of heaviness and warmth for the purpose of inducing relaxation. See also **Nursing Interventions Classification.**

**autogenous** /ôtoj′ənəs/,   **1.** self-generating. **2.** originating from within the organism, as a toxin or vaccine.

**autogenous graft** [Gk, *autos,* self, *genein,* to produce, *graphion,* stylus],   a skin graft transplanted from one site to another in the same individual.

**autogenous vaccine** [Gk, *autos,* self, *genein,* to produce; L, *vacca,* cow],   a vaccine prepared from cultures of an infectious agent taken from the patient to be treated.

**autogeny.**   See **autogenesis.**

**autograft** /ô′təgraft′/ [Gk, *autos + graphion,* stylus],   surgical transplantation of any tissue from one part of the body to another location in the same individual. Autografts are used in several kinds of plastic surgery, most commonly to replace skin lost in severe burns. Compare **allograft, isograft, xenograft.** See also **graft.**

**autographism.**   See **dermatographia.**

**autohemagglutination.**   See **autoagglutination.**

**autohemolysis** /-hēmol′isis/ [Gk, *autos,* self, *haima,* blood, *lysein,* to loosen],   the destruction of erythrocytes by hemolytic agents found in an individual's own blood.

**autohexaploid, autohexaploidic.**   See **autopolyploid.**

**autohypnosis** [Gk, *autos, hypnos,* sleep],   the self-induction of hypnosis by an individual who concentrates on one subject to attain an altered state of consciousness. It may also occur in a person who has become sensitized to the process by undergoing hypnosis a number of times.

**autoimmune** /-imyōōn′/ [Gk, *autos* + L, *immunus,* exempt], pertaining to an immune response to one's own tissues. See also **autoimmune disease.**

**autoimmune disease,** one of a large group of diseases characterized by altered function of the immune system of the body, resulting in the production of antibodies against the body's own cells. Antigens normally present on the body's cells stimulate the development of autoantibodies, which, unable to distinguish those antigens from external antigens, act against the body's cells to cause localized and systemic reactions. These reactions can affect almost any cell or tissue and cause a variety of diseases, including systemic lupus erythematosus (SLE) and autoimmune thyroiditis. Some autoimmune disorders, such as Hashimoto's disease, are tissue specific, whereas others, such as SLE, affect multiple organs and systems.
■ OBSERVATIONS: The manifestations and clinical characteristics depend on the specific disease and on the organ or organ systems affected. See specific diseases.
■ INTERVENTIONS: Therapy includes corticosteroid, antiinflammatory, and immunosuppressive drugs. Symptoms are treated specifically.
■ NURSING CONSIDERATIONS: Many autoimmune diseases are characterized by periods of crisis interrupted by periods of remission. During a crisis, the patient may be hospitalized and require extensive nursing care, with relief from pain, applications of heat or cold, range of motion exercises, or assistance in movement and ambulation. It is important also to teach the patient and the family the side effects of the drugs being prescribed and how the drugs are to be taken. See also **autoantibody, autoantigen.**

**autoimmune hypothesis,** a concept that defects occur in the body's immune system as one ages. As a result of the defects, a person's antibody-producing cells can no longer distinguish between "self" and "nonself" tissues. The body's own cells are then misidentified as foreign and are attacked by antibodies.

**autoimmune polyglandular syndromes.** See **polyglandular autoimmune syndromes.**

**autoimmune response.** See **indirect anaphylaxis.**

**autoimmunity** /-imyōō′nitē/, an abnormal condition in which the body reacts against constituents of its own tissues. Autoimmunity may result in hypersensitivity and autoimmune disease. Also called **acute immune disease.** See also **antibody-specific model, autoantibody, autoantigen, autoimmune disease.**

**autoimmunization** /-im′yəniza′shən/, the process whereby a person's immune system develops antibodies against one or more of the person's own tissues. See also **autoantibody, autoantigen, autoimmune disease.**

**autoinfection,** an infection by disease organisms already present in the body but developing in a different body part.

**autoinfusion** /-infyōō′zhən/, a technique for forcing blood from the extremities to the body core by applying bandages. It may be used to control bleeding and, in surgery, to create a relatively bloodless surgical field.

**autoinoculation** /-inok′yəlā′shən/ [Gk, *autos* + L, *inoculare,* to graft], the inoculation of a microorganism obtained by contact with a lesion on one's own body, producing a secondary infection.

**autointoxication** /-intok′sikā′shən/ [Gk, *autos* + L, *in;* Gk, *toxikon,* poison], a condition of poisoning by substances generated by one's own body, as by toxins resulting from a metabolic disorder.

**autokeratoplasty** /-ker′ətōplas′tē/, the surgical transfer of corneal tissue from one eye of a patient to repair the cornea of the other.

**autokinesia** /-kinē′zhə/, voluntary movement.

**autolesion** /-lē′zhən/, a self-inflicted injury.

**Autolet** /ô′tōlet/, trademark for a small, sharp instrument, as a lancet, that is used to obtain a capillary blood specimen.

**autologous** /ôtol′əgəs/ [Gk, *autos* + *logos,* ratio], pertaining to a tissue or structure occurring naturally and derived from the same individual such as blood donated by a patient before surgery to be returned to the patient during or after surgery.

**autologous graft** [Gk, *autos, logos, graphion,* stylus], the transfer of tissue from one site to another on the same body.

**autologous transfusion,** a procedure in which blood is removed from a donor and stored for a variable period before it is returned to the donor's circulation.

**autolysis** /ôtol′isis/, the spontaneous destruction of tissues by intracellular enzymes. It generally occurs in the body after death.

**automatic behavior.** See **automatism.**

**automatic bladder.** See **spastic bladder.**

**automatic implanted cardioverter defibrillator (AICD),** a surgically implanted device that automatically detects and corrects potentially fatal arrhythmias.

**automatic infiltration detector** /ô′təmat′ik/ [Gk, *automatismos,* self-action], a temperature-sensitive device that activates an alarm and automatically stops an IV infusion when the IV fluid passes into tissue. The device detects any cooling of the skin at the IV site, a common sign of infiltration. The detector is usually secured to the skin with tape and attaches by a small cable to the fluid-monitoring circuit of an IV pump.

**automaticity** /ô′tōmətis′itē/, a property of specialized excitable tissue that allows self-activation through spontaneous development of an action potential, as in the pacemaker cells of the heart.

**automatic mallet condenser.** See **mechanical condenser.**

**automatic speech,** speech composed of or containing words or phrases spoken without much conscious thought, often consisting of expletives, profanities, and greetings.

**automation** /ô′təmā′shən/, use of a machine designed to follow a predetermined sequence of individual operations repeatedly and automatically.

**automatism** /ôtom′ətiz′əm/ [Gk, *automatismos,* self-action], **1.** (in physiology) involuntary function of an organ system independent of apparent external stimuli, such as the beating of the heart, or dependent on external stimuli but not consciously controlled, such as the dilation of the pupil of the eye. **2.** (in philosophy) the theory that the body acts as a machine and that the mind, whose processes depend solely on brain activity, is a noncontrolling adjunct of the body. **3.** (in psychology) mechanical, repetitive, and undirected behavior that is not consciously controlled, as seen in psychomotor epilepsy, hysterical states, and such acts as sleepwalking. Kinds of automatism include **ambulatory automatism, command automatism,** and **immediate posttraumatic automatism.** Also called **automatic behavior.**

**automnesia** /ô′tōmnē′zhə/, the recollection of a previous experience.

**autonomic** /ô′tənom′ik/ [Gk, *autos* + *nomos,* law], **1.** having the ability to function independently without outside influence. **2.** pertaining to the autonomic nervous system.

**autonomic bronchodilators,** a category of drugs with actions that dilate bronchiolar smooth muscle tissue by acting on the autonomic nervous system. Examples include adrenergic drugs, such as epinephrine, and anticholinergic products, such as atropine sulfate.

**autonomic drug,**    any of a large group of drugs that mimic or modify the function of the autonomic nervous system.

**autonomic dysreflexia,**    a syndome affecting persons with a spinal cord lesion above the mid-thoracic level (quadriplegics and some paraplegics) and that is characterized by hypertension, bradycardia, severe headaches, pallor below and flushing above the cord lesions, and convulsions. It is the result of impaired function of the autonomic nervous system caused by simultaneous sympathetic and parasympathetic activity, such as may occur with bowel or bladder distension or a pressure ulcer. A cerebrovascular accident and death may occur during an attack. See also **autonomic hyperreflexia.**

**autonomic epilepsy.**    See **vasomotor epilepsy.**

**autonomic ganglion** [Gk, *autos,* self, *nomos,* law, *ganglion,* knot],    a physical grouping of autonomic neuron cell bodies. It can be near the target organ, as in the parasympathetic division, or more distant, as in the sympathetic division. See also **sympathetic ganglion.**

**autonomic hyperreflexia,**    a neurologic disorder characterized by a discharge of sympathetic nervous system impulses as a result of stimulation of the bladder, large intestine, or other visceral organs. It occurs in persons with certain spinal cord injuries. Symptoms may include bradycardia, profuse sweating, headache, and severe hypertension.

**autonomic imbalance** [Gk, *autos,* self, *nomos,* law; L, *in,* not, *bilanx,* having two scales],    a disruption of a segment of the autonomic nervous system, as in autonomic ataxia.

**autonomic nerve** [Gk, *autos,* self, *nomos,* law, *neuron,* nerve],    a nerve of the autonomic nervous system, which includes both the sympathetic and parasympathetic nervous systems. It possesses the ability to function independently and spontaneously as needed to maintain optimal status of body activities.

**autonomic nervous system,**    the part of the nervous system that regulates involuntary body functions, including the activity of the cardiac muscle, smooth muscles, and glands. It has two divisions: The **sympathetic nervous system** accelerates heart rate, constricts blood vessels, and raises blood pressure; the **parasympathetic nervous system** slows heart rate, increases intestinal peristalsis and gland activity, and relaxes sphincters.

**autonomic reflex,**    any of a large number of normal reflexes governing and regulating the functions of the viscera. Autonomic reflexes control such activities of the body as blood pressure, heart rate, peristalsis, sweating, and urination.

**autonomous** /ôton′əməs/ [Gk, *autos,* self, *nomos,* law],    being functionally independent.

**autonomous bladder.**    See **flaccid bladder.**

**autonomy** /ôton′əmē/ [Gk, *autos* + *nomos,* law],    the quality of having the ability or tendency to function independently. —**autonomous,** *adj.*

**autonomy drive,**    a behavioral trait characterized by the attempt of an individual to master the environment and to impose his or her purposes on it.

**autopentaploid, autopentaploidic.**    See **autopolyploid.**

**autophagia** /-fā′jə/,    **1.** a mental disorder characterized by the biting or eating of one's own flesh, as may occur in Lesch-Nyan syndrome. **2.** the automatic consumption of one's own tissues by fasting or dieting. **3.** the metabolic action of catabolism.

**autoplastic maneuver** /-plas′tik/,    (in psychology) a process that is part of adaptation, involving an adjustment within the self. Compare **alloplastic maneuver.**

**autoplasty** /ô′təplas′tē/ [Gk, *autos* + *plassein,* to mold],    a plastic surgery procedure in which autografts, or parts of the patient's own tissues, are used to replace or repair body areas damaged by disease or injury.

**autoploid** /ô′təploid/,    having homologous chromosome sets, or two or more copies of a single haploid set.

**autopodium** /-pō′dē·əm/,    the distal major subdivision of a hand or foot.

**autopolymer resin.**    See **self-curing resin.**

**autopolyploid** /ô′tōpol′iploid/ [Gk, *autos* + *polyploos,* many times, *eidos* form],    **1.** an individual, organism, strain, or cell that has more than two genetically identical or nearly identical sets of chromosomes that are derived from the same ancestral species. They result from the duplication of the haploid chromosome set and are referred to as autotriploid, autotetraploid, autopentaploid, autohexaploid, and so on, depending on the number of multiples of the haploid chromosomes they contain. **2.** also **autopolyploidic.** pertaining to such an individual, organism, strain, or cell. Compare **allopolyploid.** See also **allodiploid.**

**autopolyploidy** /ô′tōpol′iploi′dē/,    the state or condition of having more than two identical or nearly identical sets of chromosomes. Compare **allopolyploid.**

**autopsy** /ô′topsē/ [Gk, *autos* + *opsis,* view],    a postmortem examination performed to confirm or determine the cause of death. Also called **necropsy** /nek′ropsē/, **thanatopsy** /than′ətop′sē/. —**autopsic, autopsical,** *adj.,* **autopsist,** *n.*

**autopsy pathology,**    the study of disease by the examination of the body after death by a pathologist. The organs and tissues are first described by their appearance at the time of dissection, then by their appearance in the microscopic examination or laboratory analysis of small representative samples of tissue taken for their diagnostic value.

**autoregulation** [Gk, *autos,* self; L, *regula,* rule],    an intrinsic capacity of organs to regulate their own blood flow or metabolic activity. The former process results from the contraction or relaxation of self-excitable smooth muscle, which causes the constriction or dilation vessels. It allows organs to maintain constant blood flow and meet their metabolic needs despite variations in systemic arterial pressure.

**autosensitization** /-sen′sətīzā′shən/ [Gk, *autos,* self; L, *sentire,* to feel],    the sensitization of an individual by humoral antibodies or by a delayed cellular reaction to substances in his or her own body tissues.

**autosepticemia** /-sep′tisē′mē·ə/,    a systemic infection in which pathogens are present in the circulating bloodstream, developing from an infection within the body.

**autoserous treatment** /ô′təsir′əs/ [Gk, *autos* + L, *serum,* whey],    therapy of an infectious disease by inoculating the patient with the patient's own serum.

**autosite** /ô′təsīt/ [Gk, *autos* + *sitos,* food],    the larger, more normally formed member of unequal or asymmetric conjoined twins on whom the other smaller fetus depends for various physiologic functions and for nutrition and growth. Compare **parasitic fetus.** —**autositic.** *adj.*

**autosmia** /ôtoz′mē·ə/ [Gk, *autos,* self, *osme,* smell],    awareness of one's own body odor.

**autosomal** /ô′təsō′məl/ [Gk, *autos* + *soma,* body],    **1.** pertaining to or characteristic of an autosome. **2.** pertaining to any condition transmitted by an autosome.

**autosomal-dominant inheritance,**    a pattern of inheritance in which the transmission of a dominant allele on an autosome causes a trait to be expressed. Males and females are usually affected with equal frequency. If both parents are heterozygous *(Aa),* each of their children has a 50% chance of being heterozygous, a 25% chance of being homozygous for the dominant allele *(AA),* and a 25% chance of being homozygous for the recessive allele *(aa);* children with either of the first two genotypes will express the trait of the dominant allele. If one parent is homozygous for the dominant allele, all of the children will express the trait. Achondroplasia, osteogenesis imperfecta, polydactyly, Marfan's syndrome, and some neuromuscular disorders are transmitted through autosomal-dominant inheritance. Compare **autosomal-recessive inheritance.** See also **dominance.**

**autosomal inheritance,** a pattern of inheritance in which the transmission of traits depends on the presence or absence of certain alleles on the autosomes. The pattern may be dominant or recessive, and males and females are usually affected with equal frequency. The majority of hereditary disorders are the result of a defective gene on an autosome. Kinds of autosomal inheritance are **autosomal-dominant inheritance** and **autosomal-recessive inheritance.** See also **inheritance.**

**autosomal-recessive inheritance,** a pattern of inheritance resulting from the transmission of a recessive allele on an autosome. Males and females are usually affected with equal frequency. If both parents are heterozygous *(Aa),* each of their children has a 25% chance of expressing the trait of the recessive allele. If both parents are homozygous recessive *(aa),* all of the children will express the trait. If one parent is homozygous recessive and the other is homozygous dominant *(AA),* none of the children will express the trait, but all will be carriers *(Aa).* There may be no family history of the trait; it becomes manifest when two carriers have a child who is homozygous recessive. Cystic fibrosis, phenylketonuria, and galactosemia are examples of traits that result from autosomal-recessive inheritance. Compare **autosomal-dominant inheritance.** See also **recessive.**

**autosomatognosis** /-sō′mətognō′sis/, a phantom sensation that an amputated part of the body is still attached.

**autosome** /ô′təsōm/, any chromosome that is not a sex chromosome and that appears as a homologous pair in a somatic cell. Humans have 22 pairs of autosomes, which transmit all genetic traits and conditions other than those that are sex-linked. Also called **euchromosome** /yoo′krəsōm/. Compare **sex chromosome. —autosomal,** *adj.*

**autosplenectomy** /ô′tōsplinek′təmē/ [Gk, *autos* + *splen,* spleen, *ektomē,* excision], a progressive shrinking of the spleen that may occur in sickle cell anemia. The spleen is replaced by fibrous tissue and becomes nonfunctional.

**autosuggestion** [Gk, *autos* + L, *suggerere,* to suggest], an idea, thought, attitude, or belief suggested to oneself, often as a formula or incantation, as a means of controlling one's behavior. Compare **suggestion.**

**autotetraploid, autotetraploidic.** See **autopolyploid.**

**autotopagnosia** /ô′tōtop′əg·nō′zhə/ [Gk, *autos* + *topos,* place, *a* + *gnosis,* without knowledge], the inability to recognize or localize the various body parts because of organic brain damage. It is associated generally with lesions of the dominant hemisphere and may be an effect of some cases of cerebrovascular accident (CVA). It is also characterized by a loss of ability to distinguish left from right, manifested during a neurologic examination when the patient is unable to perform a task such as touching the right ear with the left thumb. Retraining involves touching various parts of the patient's body and asking the patient to identify the area touched and by having the patient assemble human figure puzzles. Also called **body-image agnosia, body-scheme disorder.** See also **agnosia, proprioception.**

**autotoxemia** /-toksē′mē·ə/, a form of poisoning caused by substances generated within the body as a result of the pathologic alteration of the person's own tissues.

**autotoxic,** pertaining to autotoxins.

**autotransfusion[1]** /-transfyōō′zhən/, the collection, anticoagulation, filtration, and reinfusion of blood from an active bleeding site. It may be used in cases of major trauma or in major surgery when blood can be collected from a sterile site. Collection devices can be attached to drains following orthopedic or chest procedures.

**autotransfusion[2],** a nursing intervention from the Nursing Interventions Classification (NIC) defined as collecting and reinfusing blood that has been lost intraoperatively or postoperatively from clean wounds. See also **Nursing Interventions Classification.**

**autotransplantation.** See **autograft, autoplasty.**

**autotriploid, autotriploidic.** See **autopolyploid.**

**autovaccination,** a second vaccination in which a virus from the first vaccine sore is used.

**autozygous** /-zī′gəs/, pertaining to genes in a homozygote that are copies of the same ancestral gene as a result of a mating between related individuals.

**autumn fever.** See **leptospirosis.**

**aux-.** See **auxo-.**

**auxanology** /ôks′ənol′əjē/ [Gk, *auxein,* to grow, *logos,* science], the scientific study of growth and development. **—auxanologic,** *adj.*

**auxcardia** [Gk, *auxein,* increase, *kardia,* heart], an enlarged heart.

**auxesis.** See **hypertrophy.**

**auxiliary** /ôksil′yərē/ [L, *auxilium,* aid], an individual or group serving in assistive, supporting, or complementary tasks in a clinical setting.

**auxiliary enzyme** [L, *auxilium,* assist], an enzyme that links the enzyme being measured with an indicator enzyme. It is a component of the coupled assay system.

**auxiliary storage,** a storage device for adding to the main storage of the computer, using such media as floppy disks, hard disks, compact disks, zip disks, or tapes.

**auxo-, aux-,** prefix meaning 'growth, acceleration, or stimulation': *auxochrome, auxesis.*

**auxotonic** /ôk′sōton′ik/, pertaining to muscle contractions that increase in force as the muscle shortens.

**auxotox** [Gk, *auxein,* increase, *toxikon,* poison], a chemical with a particular atomic grouping that, if added to a relatively benign substance, increases the toxic characteristics of the mixture.

**AV,** abbreviation for *arteriovenous, atrioventricular.*

**available arch length** /əvā′ləbəl/ [ME, *availen,* to be of use], the length or space in a dental arch that is available for all the natural teeth of an individual. See also **arch length, arch length deficiency, arch width.**

**avalvular** /āvalv′yələr/ [Gk, *a,* without; L, *valva,* valve], petaining to an absence of one or more valves.

**Avandia,** trademark for an oral antidiabetic (rosiglitazone).

**avantin.** See **isopropyl alcohol.**

**avascular** /āvas′kyələr/ [Gk, *a,* without; L, *vasculum,* vessel], **1.** pertaining to a tissue area that is not receiving a sufficient supply of blood. The reduced supply may be the result of blockage by a blood clot or of the deliberate stoppage of flow during surgery or during control a hemorrhage. **2.** pertaining to a kind of tissue that does not have blood vessels.

**avascular graft** [Gk, *a,* without; L, *vasculum,* vessel; Gk, *graphion,* stylus], a tissue graft in which there is no infiltration of blood vessels.

**avascularization** [Gk, *a,* without; L, *vasculum,* vessel], a diversion of blood flow away from tissues.

**avascular necrosis.** See **coagulation necrosis.**

**AVB,** abbreviation for **atrioventricular block.**

**average,** (in mathematics) a value established by dividing the sum of a series by the number of its units.

**aversion therapy** /əvur′zhən/ [L, *aversus,* a turning away], a form of behavior therapy in which punishment or unpleasant or painful stimuli, such as electric shock or drugs that induce nausea, are used to suppress undesirable behavior. The procedure is used in treating such conditions as drug abuse, alcoholism, gambling, overeating, smoking, and various sexual deviations. Also called **aversive conditioning.** See also **behavior therapy.**

**aversive stimulus** /əvur′siv/, an undesirable stimulus, such as electric shock, that causes psychic or physical pain. See also **aversion therapy.**

**avian tuberculosis** /ā′vē·ən/, a strain of tuberculosis in birds, caused by *Mycobacterium avium.* The organism is also pathogenic in humans and is especially problematic in the immunocompromised, such as those with human immunodeficiency virus infection.

**aviation medicine** /āv′ē·ā′shən/, a branch of medicine that is concerned with the health effects of travel by aircraft, including such aspects as jetlag, restricted body movement for long periods, and reaction to violent aircraft movement in turbulent weather. Also called **aerospace medicine.** See also **aviation physiology.**

**aviation physiology,** a branch of physiology that is concerned with the effects on humans and animals exposed for long periods to pressurized cabins, radiation hazards at high altitudes, weightlessness, disturbances of biologic rhythms, acceleration, and mental functions under stressful flying conditions.

**avidin,** a glycoprotein in raw egg white that interacts with biotin to make it unavailable to the body. Cooking destroys avidin.

**avidity** /avid′itē/ [L, *avidus,* eager], an inexact measure of the binding strength of antibodies to multiple antigenic determinants on natural antigens.

**A-V interval** [L, *intervallum,* space between ramparts], the time between an atrial polarization and the next ventricular polarization. In His bundle electrograms (HBEs), the A-V interval is the time between the A wave and the V deflection. The A wave is the first deflection on the HBE and represents low right atrial activation. The V deflection is the last deflection on the HBE and represents ventricular activation; it is concurrent with the QRS complex on a surface electrocardiogram.

**avirulent** /āvir′yələnt/ [Gk, *a,* not; L, *virus,* poison], not virulent; not pathogenic.

**avitaminosis** /āvī′təminō′sis/ [Gk, *a,* not; L, *vita,* life, amine, *osis,* condition], a condition resulting from a deficiency of or lack of absorption or use of one or more dietary vitamins. Also called **hypovitaminosis.** Compare **hypervitaminosis.** See also specific vitamins.

**AV nicking,** a vascular abnormality in the retina of the eye, visible on ophthalmologic examination, in which a vein is compressed by an arteriovenous crossing. The vein appears "nicked" as a result of constriction or spasm. It is a sign of hypertension, arteriosclerosis, or other vascular conditions.

**Avogadro's law** /av′ōgad′rōz/ [Amedeo Avogadro, Italian physicist, 1776–1856], a law in physics stating that equal volumes of all gases at a given temperature and pressure contain the identical number of molecules.

**Avogadro's number** [Amedeo Avogadro], the number of atoms in exactly 12 g of the isotope of carbon $^{12}C$, or $6.02 \times 10^{23}$. One mole of any monoatomic element contains this number of atoms and one mole of any polyatomic element or molecule contains this number of molecules.

**avoidance** [ME, *avoiden,* to empty], (in psychiatry) a conscious or unconscious defense mechanism, physical or psychologic, by which an individual tries to avoid or escape

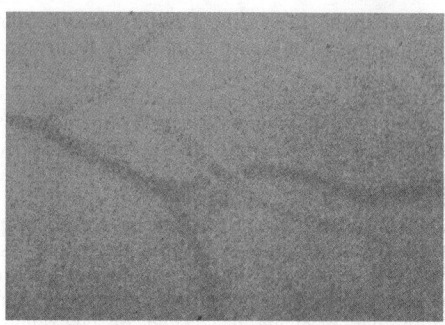

**AV nicking** *(Lemmi and Lemmi, 2000)*

from unpleasant stimuli, conflicts, or feelings, such as anxiety, fear, pain, or danger.

**avoidance-avoidance conflict,** a conflict resulting from the confrontation of two or more alternative goals or desires that are equally aversive and undesirable. Also called **double-avoidance conflict.** See also **conflict.**

**avoidance conditioning,** the establishment of certain patterns of behavior to avoid unpleasant or painful stimuli.

**avoidant personality,** a personality disorder characterized by hypersensitivity to rejection and a reluctance to start a relationship because of a fear of not being accepted uncritically. The person has a strong desire for affection and acceptance and may be distressed by an inability to relate comfortably with others.

**avoirdupois weight** /av′ərdəpoiz′/ [OF, *avoir de pois,* property of weight], the English system of weights in which there are 7000 grains, 256 drams, or 16 ounces to 1 pound. One ounce in this system equals 28.35 g, and 1 pound equals 453.59 g. Compare **apothecaries' weight.** See also **metric system.**

**Avonex,** trademark for an antiviral and immune system regulator (interferon beta-1a) for multiple sclerosis.

**avulse.** See **avulsion.**

**avulsed tooth** /əvulst/ [L, *avulsio,* a pulling away], a tooth that has been forcibly displaced from its normal position. In some cases, if attended to early, it can be surgically reimplanted. Also spelled **evulsed tooth.** See also **avulsion.**

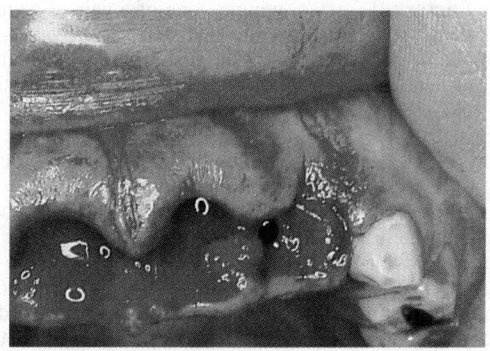

**Avulsed teeth** *(Zitelli and Davis, 1997)*

**avulsion** /əvul′shən/ [L, *avulsio,* a pulling away], the separation, by tearing, of any part of the body from the whole. —**avulse,** *v.*

**avulsion fracture,** a fracture caused by the tearing away of a fragment of bone where a strong ligamentous or tendinous attachment forcibly pulls the fragment away from osseous tissue.

**awake anesthesia** [ME, *awakenen*], an anesthetic procedure in which analgesia and anesthesia are accomplished without loss of consciousness. Dental procedures, surgery on a limb or an extremity, scopic examinations, and certain kinds of head surgery are performed using awake anesthesia. With the patient awake or sedated, muscle relaxation is not required. Various combinations of sedatives, tranquilizers, and low concentrations of anesthetic gas may be used. Also called **conscious sedation.**

**AWHONN,** abbreviation for **Association of Women's Health, Obstetric, and Neonatal Nurses.**

**AWOL** /ā′wôl/, abbreviation for **absent without leave.**

**axetil,** contraction for *L-acetoxyethyl.*

**axi-, axio-, axo-,** prefix meaning 'axis': *axial, axolysis.*

**axial (A)** /ak′sē·əl/ [Gk, *axon,* axle], **1.** pertaining to or situated on the axis of a body structure or part. **2.** (in dentistry) relating to the long axis of a tooth.

**axial current,** the central part of the blood current.

**axial gradient,** **1.** the variation in metabolic rate in different parts of the body. **2.** the development toward the body axis or its parts in relation to the metabolic rate in the various parts.

**axial illumination.** See **illumination.**

**axial neuritis.** See **parenchymatous neuritis.**

**axial skeleton** [L, *axis,* axle; Gk, *skeletos,* dried up], the bones forming the axis of the skeleton, including the skull, vertebrae, ribs, and sternum. See also **appendicular skeleton.**

**axial spillway,** a groove that crosses a cusp ridge or a marginal ridge and extends onto an axial surface of a tooth. Compare **interdental spillway, occlusal spillway.**

**Axid,** trademark for an antiulcerative and antihistaminic agent (nizatidine).

**axifugal** /aksif′yəgəl/ [L, *axis,* axle, *fugere,* to flee], extending away from an axis or axion. Also called **axofugal.** See also **centrifugal.**

**axilla** /aksil′ə/, *pl.* **axillae** [L, wing], a pyramid-shaped space forming the underside of the shoulder between the upper arm and the side of the chest. Also called **armpit.** —**axillary,** *adj.*

**axillary** /ak′siler′ē/ [L, *axilla,* wing], pertaining to the armpit.

**axillary abscess** [L, *axilla,* wing, *abscedere,* to go away], an abscess in the armpit.

**axillary artery** [L, *axilla,* wing], one of a pair of continuations of the subclavian arteries that starts at the outer border of the first rib and ends at the distal border of the teres major, where it becomes the brachial artery. It has three parts and six branches, supplying various chest and arm muscles.

**axillary block anesthesia.** See **brachial plexus block.**

**axillary dissection.** See **axillary node dissection.**

**axillary line,** an imaginary vertical line on the body wall, passing through a point midway between the anterior and posterior folds of the axilla.

**axillary nerve,** one of the last two branches of the posterior cord of the brachial plexus before the posterior cord becomes the radial nerve. It divides into a posterior branch and an anterior branch. The posterior branch innervates the teres minor, part of the deltoideus, and part of the skin overlying the deltoideus; the anterior branch innervates the deltoideus. Some fibers of the nerve also supply the capsule of the shoulder joint.

**axillary node,** one of the lymph glands of the axilla that help fight infections in the chest, armpit, neck, and arm and drain lymph from those areas. The 20 to 30 axillary nodes are divided into the lateral group, the anterior group, the posterior group, the central group, and the medial group. See also **lymphatic system, lymph node.**

**axillary node dissection,** surgical removal of axillary nodes, done as part of radical mastectomy. Also called **axillary dissection.**

**axillary temperature** [L, *axilla,* wing, *temperatura*], the body temperature as recorded by a thermometer placed in the armpit. The reading is generally 0.5° to 1° F less than the oral temperature.

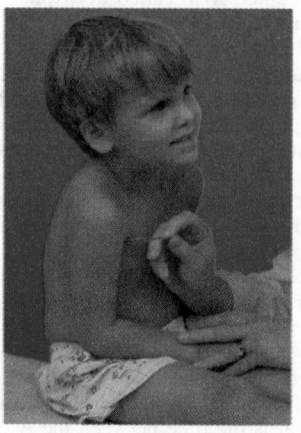

**Axillary temperature measurement** *(Zakus, 1995)*

**axillary vein,** one of a pair of veins of the upper limb that becomes the subclavian vein at the outer border of the first rib. It receives deoxygenated blood from the venous tributaries. Compare **subclavian vein.**

**axillofemoral bypass graft** /ak′silōfem′ərəl/, a synthetic artery that is surgically anastomosed to the axillary and common femoral arteries in cases of peripheral arterial insufficiency. The graft shunts blood between those arteries, increasing blood flow to the lower extremities.

**axio-.** See **axi-.**

**axion** /ak′sē·on/, **1.** the brain and spinal cord. **2.** the cerebrospinal axis.

**axioplasm.** See **axoplasm.**

**axis,** *pl.* **axes** /ak′sēz/ [Gk, *axon,* axle], **1.** (in anatomy) a line that passes through the center of the body, or a part of the body, such as the frontal axis, binauricular axis, and basifacial axis. **2.** the second cervical vertebra, about which the atlas rotates, allowing the head to be turned, extended, and flexed. Also called **epistropheus, odontoid vertebra.**

**axis artery,** one of a pair of extensions of the subclavian arteries, running into and supplying the upper limb, continuing into the forearm as the palmar interosseous artery.

**axis cylinder.** See **axon.**

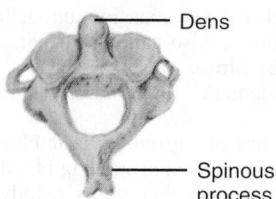

Dens

Spinous process

**Axis** *(Applegate, 2000)*

**axis deviation,** an electrocardiogram trace in which the QRS axis of the heart in the frontal plane lies outside the usual range of −30 to 110 degrees. It represents an abnormal direction of ventricular depolarization.

**axis traction,** 1. the process of pulling a baby's head with obstetric forceps in a direction in line with the path of least resistance, following the curve of Carus through the mother's birth canal. 2. *informal.* any mechanical device attached to obstetric forceps to facilitate pulling in the proper direction.

**axo-.** See **axi-.**

**axoaxonic synapse** /ak′sō·akson′ik/ [Gk, *axon,* axle (to) *axon,* axle], a synapse in which the axon of one neuron comes in contact with the axon of another neuron.

**axodendritic synapse** /-dendrit′ik/ [Gk, *axon* + *dendron,* tree], a synapse in which the axon of one neuron comes in contact with the dendrites of another neuron.

**axodendrosomatic synapse** /-den′drōsōmat′ik/, a synapse in which the axon of one neuron comes in contact with both the dendrites and the cell body of another neuron.

**axofugal.** See **axifugal.**

**axolysis** /aksol′isis/, the degeneration of the axon of a nerve cell.

**axon** /ak′son/ [Gk, axle], an extension, usually long and slender, of a neuron capable of conducting action potentials or self-propagating nervous impulses. Axons can conduct impulses over great distances away from the cell body. Only ends of axons (terminals) can release neurotransmitters and stimulate other neurons/effectors. Also called **axone** /ak′sōn/, **axis cylinder.** Compare **dendrite.** See also **action potential, neurotransmitter.**

**axon flare,** vasodilation, reddening, and increased sensitivity of the skin surrounding an injured area, caused by an axon reflex. It is considered part of a triple response in which injury or stroking of the skin results in local reddening, the release of histamine or a histamine-like substance, a surrounding flare, and wheal formation. A pinprick in the involved area causes more intense pain than a similar stimulus before injury.

**axonography** /ak′sənog′rəfē/, the recording of electrical activity in the axon of a nerve cell. Also called **electroaxonography.**

**axonotmesis** /ak′sənotmē′sis/ [Gk, *axon* + *temnein,* to cut], an interruption of the axon from nerve injury, with subsequent wallerian degeneration of the distal nerve segment. Connective tissue of the nerve, including the Schwann cell basement membranes, may remain intact.

**axon reflex** [Gk, *axon,* axle], a neuron reflex in which an afferent impulse travels along a nerve fiber away from the cell body until it reaches a branching, where it is diverted to an end organ without entering the cell body. It does not involve a complete reflex arc, and therefore it is not a true reflex.

**axon sheath** [Gk, *axon* + AS, *scaeth*], a laminated myelin sheath that is interrupted at intervals by nodes of Ranvier.

**axoplasm** /ak′sōplaz′əm/, cytoplasm of an axon which encloses the neurofibrils.

**axoplasmic flow** /ak′sōplaz′mik/ [Gk, *axon* + *plassein,* to shape], the continuous pulsing, undulating movement of the cytoplasm between the cell body of a neuron, where protein synthesis occurs, and the axon fiber to supply it with the substances vital for the maintenance of activity and for repair. The nerve fiber depends totally on the cell body for metabolites, and any interruption in the axoplasmic flow caused by disease or trauma results in the degeneration of the unsupplied areas of the axon.

**axosomatic synapse** /ak′sōsōmat′ik/ [Gk, *axon* + *soma,* body], a synapse in which the axon of one neuron comes in contact with the cell body of another neuron.

**axotomy** /ak′sōplaz′əm/, surgical transection of an axon.

**Aygestin,** trademark for an oral progestin (norethindrone acetate).

**azatadine maleate** /azat′ədēn/, an antihistamine with antiserotonin, anticholinergic, and sedative effects.

**azathioprine** /az′əthī′ōprēn/, an immunosuppressive.

■ INDICATIONS: It is prescribed to prevent organ rejection after transplantation and to treat lupus erythematosus and other systemic inflammatory diseases, such as rheumatoid arthritis unresponsive to other agents.

■ CONTRAINDICATION: Known hypersensitivity to this drug prohibits its use. It is contraindicated in rheumatoid arthritis in pregnant women.

■ ADVERSE EFFECTS: Among the most serious adverse reactions are bone marrow depression and hepatotoxicity. Nausea and fever are common.

**azelastine,** a leukotriene synthesis inhibitor.

■ INDICATIONS: This drug is used to treat seasonal allergic rhinitis.

■ CONTRAINDICATIONS: Known hypersensitivity, acute asthma attacks, and lower respiratory tract disease prohibit this drug's use.

■ ADVERSE EFFECTS: Side effects include sedation (more common with increased doses), increased drowsiness, weight increase, and myalgia.

**-azepam,** combining form designating a diazepam-type antianxiety agent.

**azidothymidine.** See **zidovudine.**

**azithromycin,** a macrolide antibiotic that suppresses the formation of protein by bacteria, retards bacterial growth, or causes death of the microorganisms.

■ INDICATIONS: It is prescribed in the treatment of mild to moderate infections by certain bacteria in adults, including respiratory tract infections, skin disorders, and sexually transmitted diseases.

■ CONTRAINDICATIONS: The drug should not be given to patients with allergies to erythromycin or any macrolide antibiotics or with kidney or liver diseases. Its safety has not been established for women who are pregnant or breast feeding.

■ ADVERSE EFFECTS: The side effects most often reported include diarrhea, loose stools, nausea, stomach pains, or vomiting.

**Azlin,** trademark for an antibiotic (azlocillin).

**azlocillin sodium** /az′lōsil′in/, a semisynthetic penicillin antibiotic.

■ INDICATIONS: It is prescribed for lower respiratory tract, urinary tract, skin, and bone and joint infections and bacterial septicemia caused by susceptible strains of microorganisms, mainly *Pseudomonas aeruginosa.*

■ CONTRAINDICATION: Hypersensitivity to any of the penicillins prohibits its use.

■ ADVERSE EFFECTS: The most serious adverse reactions are anaphylactic reactions, convulsive seizures, epigastric pain, reduction in blood elements, and elevation in hepatic and renal parameters.

**azo-, az-,** prefix meaning 'containing nitrogen': *azotemia, azine.*

**-azocine,** combining form designating a narcotic agonist or antagonist.

**azo compounds** /ā′zō/ [Fr, *azote,* nitrogen], one of many organic aromatic compounds containing the divalent chromophore, —N═N—. They are produced by the alkaline reduction of nitro compounds among other methods.

**azo dye,** a type of nitrogen-containing compound used in commercial coloring materials. Some forms of the chemical are potential carcinogens.

**azoic** /āzō′ik/ [Gk, *a,* not, *zoe,* life], devoid of life.

**-azoline,** combining form designating an antihistaminic or local vasoconstrictor.

**azoospermia** /āzō′əspur′mē·ə/ [Gk, *a, zoon,* not animal, *sperma* seed], lack of spermatozoa in the semen. It may be caused by testicular dysfunction, cancer chemotherapy, or blockage of the tubules of the epididymis, or it may be induced by vasectomy. Infertility but not impotence is associated with azoospermia. Compare **oligospermia.**

**azoprotein** /ā′zōprō′tēn/, a protein coupled to another substance through a diazo (—N═N—) linkage. Azoproteins are often used in immunochemical procedures.

**Azorean disease.** See **Machado-Joseph disease.**

**-azosin,** combining form designating a prazosin-type antihypertensive agent.

**azotemia** /az′ōtē′mē·ə/ [Fr, *azote,* nitrogen; Gk, *haima,* blood], retention of excessive amounts of nitrogenous compounds in the blood. This toxic condition is caused by failure of the kidneys to remove urea from the blood and is characteristic of uremia. Also spelled **azotaemia.** See also **uremia. —azotemic,** *adj.*

**azoturia** /az′ōtŏŏr′ē·ə/ [Fr, *azote,* nitrogen; Gk, *ouron,* urine], an excess of nitrogenous compounds including urea in the urine.

**AZT,** trademark for a human immunodeficiency virus inhibitor (Zidovudine). Also called Retrovir.

**azul, azula.** See **pinta.**

**Azulfidine,** trademark for a sulfonamide antibacterial (sulfasalazine).

**azure** /āz′hər/, one of a group of basic blue methylthionine or phenothiazine dyes used in staining blood and cell nuclei.

**azurophil,** a substance that stains readily with an azure blue aniline dye.

**azurophilia** /āzh′ŏŏrəfil′yə/, a condition in which the blood contains some cells that have granules that stain readily with azure (blue) dye.

**azygography** /az′īgog′rəfē/, the radiographic imaging of the azygos venous system after injection of a radiopaque contrast medium.

**azygos.** See **azygous.**

**azygospore** /az′igəspôr/ [Gk, *a + zygon,* not yoke, *sporos,* seed], a spore that is produced directly from a gamete that has not undergone conjugation, as in certain algae and fungi.

**azygous** /az′əgəs/ [Gk, *a + zygon,* not yoke], occurring as a single entity or part, such as any unpaired anatomic structure; not part of a pair. Also **azygos. —azygos** /az′əgos′/, *n.*

**azygous lobe,** a congenital anomaly of the lung caused by a fold of pleural tissue carried by the azygous vein during descent into the thorax during embryonic development. It produces an extra lobe in the right upper lung and may appear on x-ray film as a fissure in the shape of an upside-down comma.

**azygous vein,** one of the seven veins of the thorax. Beginning opposite the first or second lumbar vertebra, it rises through the aortic hiatus in the diaphragm and passes to the right of the vertebral column to the fourth thoracic vertebra, then arches ventrally over the root of the right lung, and ends in the superior vena cava. It receives numerous veins, such as the hemiazygous veins, several esophageal veins, and the right bronchial vein. In cases of obstruction to the inferior vena cava it is the principal vein that returns blood to the heart. Compare **internal thoracic vein, left brachiocephalic vein, right brachiocephalic vein.**

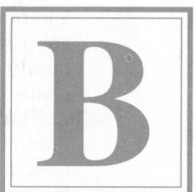

**B,** symbol for the element **boron.**

**B.** See **oxalic acid.**

**B, β.** See **beta.**

**B6 bronchus sign,** an artifact in a lung radiograph in which an air bronchogram appears in the lower lobe as a result of consolidation of atelectasis.

**B19 virus,** a strain of human parvovirus associated with a number of diseases, including hemolytic anemia, erythema infectiosum, fifth disease, and symptoms of arthritis and arthralgia.

**Ba,** symbol for the element **barium.**

**BA,** abbreviation for *Bachelor of Arts.*

**babbling,** a stage in speech development characterized by the production of strings of speech sounds in vocal play, such as "ba-ba-ba."

**Babcock's operation** [William W. Babcock, American surgeon, 1872–1963], the removal of a varicosed saphenous vein by insertion of an acorn-tipped sound, tying the vein to the sound, and drawing it out. Also called **subcutaneous stripping.**

**babesiosis** /bəbē′sē·ō′sis/ [Victor Babés, Romanian bacteriologist, 1854–1926], an infection caused by protozoa of the genus *Babesia.* The parasite is introduced into the host through the bite of ticks of the species *Ixodes dammini* and infects red blood cells. In the United States, incidence of the disease is highest in the Northeast and North Central regions. Symptoms include headache, fever, chills, vomiting, hepatosplenomegaly, hemolytic anemia, fatigue, myalgia, and hemolysis. Treatment is clindamycin or quinone. Also called **babesiasis** /bab′əsī′əsis/.

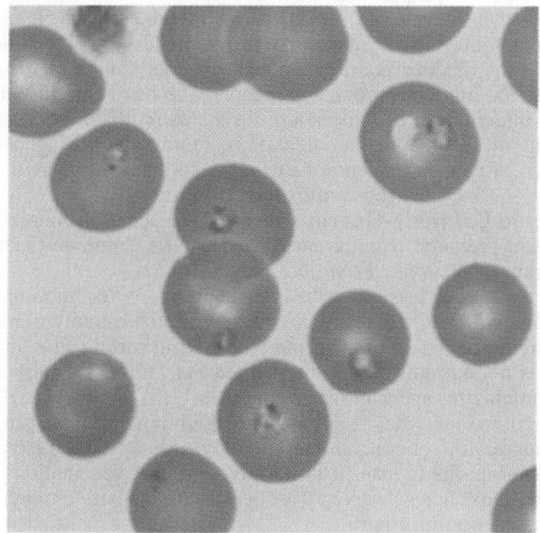

**Babesiosis** *(Carr and Rodak, 1999)*

**Babinski's reflex** /bəbin′skēz/ [Joseph F.F. Babinski, French neurologist, 1857–1932], dorsiflexion of the big toe with extension and fanning of the other toes elicited by firmly stroking the lateral aspect of the sole of the foot. The reflex is normal in newborns and abnormal in children and adults, in whom it may indicate a lesion in the pyramidal tract.

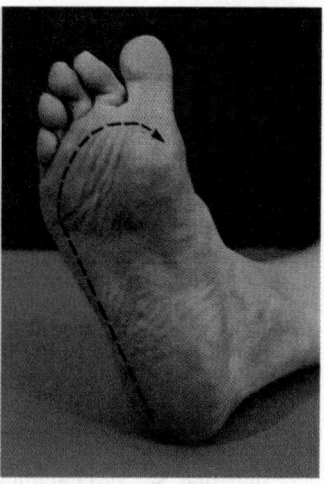

**Babinski's reflex in an adult** *(Seidel et al, 1999)*

**Babinski's sign** [Joseph Babinski], a series of partial responses that are pathognomonic of different degrees of upper motor neuron disease, including (1) absence of an ankle jerk in sciatica; (2) an extensor plantar response, with an extension of the great toe and adduction of the other toes; (3) a more pronounced concentration of platysma on the unaffected side during blowing or whistling; (4) pronation that occurs when an arm affected by paralysis is placed in supination; and (5) when a patient in a supine position with arms crossed over the chest attempts to assume a sitting position, the thigh on the affected side is flexed, and the heel is raised, while the leg on the unaffected side remains flat.

**baby** [ME, *babe*], **1.** an infant or young child, especially one who is not yet able to walk or talk. **2.** to treat gently or with special care.

**baby bottle tooth decay,** a dental condition that occurs in children between 12 months and 3 years of age as a result of being given a bottle at bedtime, resulting in prolonged exposure of the teeth to milk or juice. Caries are formed because pools of milk or juice in the mouth break down to lactic acid and other decay-causing substances. Preventive measures include elimination of the bedtime feeding or substitution of water for milk or juice in the nighttime bottle. Formerly called **nursing bottle caries.**

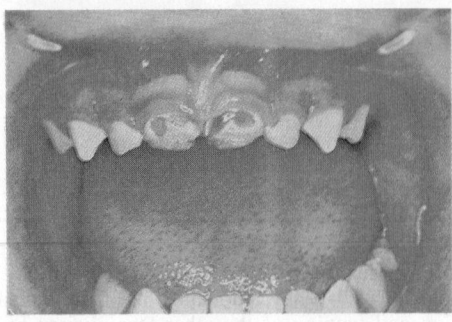

**Baby bottle tooth decay** *(Seidel et al, 1999/courtesy Drs. Abelson and Cameron, Lutherville, MD)*

**Baby Jane Doe regulations,** rules established in 1984 by the U.S. Health and Human Services Department requiring state governments to investigate complaints about parental decisions involving the treatment of handicapped infants. The rules also allowed the federal government to have access to children's medical records and required hospitals to post notices urging physicians and nurses to report any suspected cases of denial of proper medical care to infants. The controversial regulations have been found illegal by a federal court. The popular name for the federal rules was taken from the name "Jane Doe" given to an infant born in New York with an open spinal column and other defects who became the object of a campaign to force lifesaving surgery for the child over parental objections. Also called **Baby Doe rules.**

**baby talk,** **1.** the speech patterns and sounds of young children learning to talk, characterized by mispronunciation, imperfect syntax, repetition, and phonetic modifications, such as lisping or stuttering. See also **lallation. 2.** the intentionally oversimplified manner of speech, imitative of young children learning to talk, used by adults in addressing children or pets. **3.** the speech patterns characteristic of regressive stages of various mental disorders, especially schizophrenia.

**BAC,** abbreviation for **bronchoalveolar carcinoma.**

**bacampicillin hydrochloride,** a semisynthetic penicillin.
- INDICATIONS: It is prescribed in the treatment of respiratory tract, urinary tract, skin, and gonococcal infections.
- CONTRAINDICATIONS: Known sensitivity to this drug or other penicillins prohibits its use.
- ADVERSE EFFECTS: Among the most serious adverse reactions are hypersensitivity reactions, gastritis, enterocolitis, and transient blood disorders.

**Bachelor of Science in Nursing (BSN)** /bach′ələr/, an academic degree awarded on satisfactory completion of a 4-year course of study in a college or university. The recipient is eligible to take the national certifying examination to become a registered nurse. A BSN degree is prerequisite to advancement in nursing education and in most systems and institutions that employ nurses. Compare **Associate Degree in Nursing, diploma program in nursing.**

**bacill-,** combining form meaning 'rod-shaped bacterium': **bacillemia, bacillosis.**

**Bacillaceae** /bas′əlā′si·ē/ [L, *bacillum,* small rod], a family of Schizomycetes of the order Eubacteriales, consisting of gram-positive, rod-shaped cells that can produce cylindric, ellipsoid, or spheric endospores situated terminally, subterminally, or centrally. These cells are chemoheterotrophic

and mostly saprophytic, commonly appearing in soil. Some are parasitic on insects and animals and are pathogenic. The family includes the genus *Bacillus,* which is aerobic, and the genus *Clostridium,* which is facultatively anaerobic.

**bacillary angiomatosis** /bas′əler′ē/, a condition of multiple angiomata caused by an infection of *Bartonella.* The infectious agent is associated with contact with young cats infected with fleas and is also the cause of cat-scratch fever. It is manifested in persons with cellular immunodeficiency such as human immunodeficiency virus (HIV)-infected patients as small hemangioma-like lesions of the skin but may also involve the lymph nodes and viscera. The skin lesions are often mistaken for Kaposi's sarcoma.

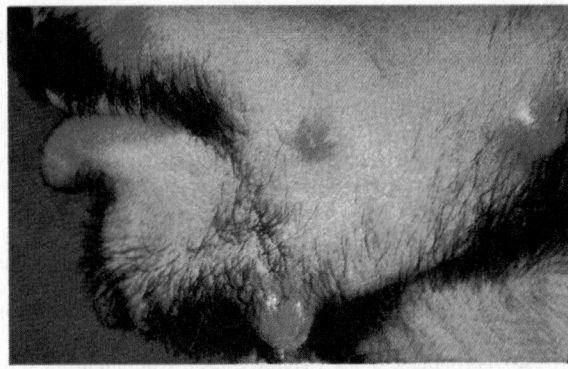

**Bacillary angiomatosis** *(Stone and Gorbach, 2000)*

**bacillary dysentery.** See **shigellosis.**

**bacille Calmette-Guérin (BCG)** /kalmet′gäraN′/ [Léon C.A. Calmette, French bacteriologist, 1863–1933; Camille Guérin, French bacteriologist, 1872–1961], an attenuated strain of tubercle bacilli, used in many countries as a vaccine against tuberculosis, most often administered intradermally, with a multiple-puncture disk. When administered to infants in high-prevalence areas, there is some evidence that it prevents the more serious forms of tuberculosis. It may have some efficacy against leprosy. BCG is also instilled into the bladder as a treatment for bladder cancer to stimulate the immune response in people who have certain kinds of malignancy. It induces a positive tuberculin reaction and may mask early, active infection by removing the diagnostic sign of conversion from the negative to the positive skin reaction. See also **tuberculin test, tuberculosis.**

**bacille Calmette-Guérin vaccine,** an active immunizing agent prepared from an attenuated bacille Calmette-Guérin strain of *Mycobacterium bovis.*
- INDICATION: It is prescribed most commonly for immunization against tuberculosis. It is instilled intravesically to treat carcinoma in situ of the urinary bladder in certain situations. It is not administered in the United States but is a common immunizing agent in many countries.
- CONTRAINDICATIONS: Hypogammaglobulinemia, immunosuppression, or concomitant use of corticosteroids or isoniazid prohibits its use. It is not given after a vaccination for smallpox, nor is it given to patients with a positive tuberculin reaction or a burn.
- ADVERSE EFFECTS: Among the most serious adverse reactions are anaphylaxis and disseminated pulmonary tubercu-

losis. Pain, inflammation, and granuloma may develop at the site of injection.

**bacillemia** /bas′əlē′mē·ə/, a condition in which bacilli are circulating in the blood. See also **bacteremia, sepsis, septicemia.**

**bacilli** /bəsil′ī/, *sing.* **bacillum** [L, *bacillum,* small rod], any rod-shaped bacteria. See **bacillus.**

**bacilliform** /bəsil′ifôrm/, rod-shaped, like a bacillus.

**bacillosis** /bas′əlō′sis/, a condition in which bacilli have invaded tissues, inducing symptoms of an infection.

**bacillum.** See **bacilli.**

**bacilluria** /bas′əlŏŏr′ē·ə/ [L, *bacillum* + Gk, *ouron,* urine], the presence of bacilli in the urine.

**bacillus,** a gram-positive aerobic or facultatively anaerobic, spore-bearing, rod-shaped microorganism of the family Bacillaceae. See also **acid-fast bacillus.**

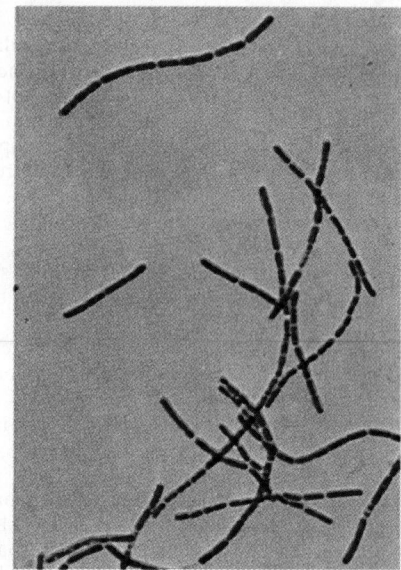

***Bacillus anthracis*** *(Emond, Rowland, and Welsby, 1995)*

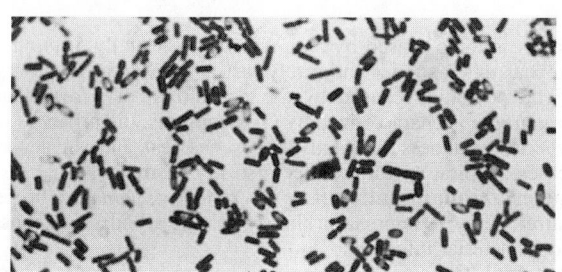

**Bacillus** *(Baron, Peterson, and Finegold, 1994)*

***Bacillus*** /bəsil′əs/, a genus of aerobic, gram-positive spore-producing bacteria in the family Bacillaceae, order Eubacteriales. The genus includes 33 species, 3 of which are pathogenic and the rest saprophytic soil forms. Some species are nonpathogenic, but others cause a wide variety of diseases, ranging from anthrax to tuberculosis. Many microorganisms formerly classified as *Bacillus* are now classified in other genera. See also **Bacillaceae.**

***Bacillus anthracis,*** a species of gram-positive, facultative anaerobe that causes anthrax, a disease primarily of cattle and sheep. The spores of this organism, if inhaled, can cause a pulmonary form of anthrax; spores can live for many years in animal products, such as hides and wool, and in soil. See also **anthrax, woolsorter's disease.**

***Bacillus cereus,*** a species of bacilli found in the soil. It causes food poisoning (an emetic type and a diarrheal type) by the formation of an enterotoxin in contaminated foods. It can also cause infections, such as ocular infections.

**bacitracin** /bas′itrā′sin/ [L, *bacillum* + *Tracy,* surname of patient in whom toxin-producing bacillus species was isolated], an antibacterial.

■ INDICATION: The topical preparation is prescribed for skin infections sensitive to bacitracin. The IM injectable is used to treat infants with pneumonia and empyema caused by susceptible staphylococci.

■ CONTRAINDICATION: Known hypersensitivity to this drug prohibits its use.

■ ADVERSE EFFECTS: Among the more serious adverse reactions are nephrotoxicity and skin rash.

**back** [AS, *baec*], the posterior or dorsal portion of the trunk of the body between the neck and the pelvis. The back is divided by a middle furrow that lies over the tips of the spinous processes of the vertebrae. The skeletal portion of the back includes the thoracic and the lumbar vertebrae and both scapulae. The nerves that innervate the various muscles of the back arise from the segmental spinal nerves.

**backache** /bak′āk/ [AS, *baec* + ME, *aken*], a pain in the lumbar, lumbosacral, or cervical region of the back, varying in sharpness and intensity. Causes may include muscle strain or other muscular disorders or pressure on the root of a nerve, such as the sciatic nerve, caused in turn by a variety of factors, including a herniated vertebral disk. Treatment may include heat, ultrasound, and devices to provide support for the affected area while the individual is in bed or standing or sitting, bed rest, surgical intervention, and medications to relieve pain and relax spasm of the muscle of the affected area.

**back-action condenser,** an instrument for compacting dental amalgams that has a U-shaped shank, which develops the condensing force from a pulling motion rather than from the more common pushing motions.

**backboard,** a long, flat, rigid piece of wood or other material that is placed under an accident victim with possible spinal injury. It is used to transport the patient to a hospital or as a firm surface for CPR.

**backbone,** the vertebral column.

**backcross** [AS, *baec* + *cruc,* cross], **1.** a mating (cross) between a heterozygote and a homozygote. **2.** an organism or strain produced by such a cross. See also **testcross.**

**background radiation** [AS, *baec* + OE, *grund,* ground], naturally occurring radiation emitted by soil, groundwater, building materials, radioactive substances in the body (especially potassium 40, and cosmic rays from outer space. Each year the average person is exposed to 44 millirad (mrad) of external terrestrial radiation, 18 mrad of naturally occurring internal radioaction, and 44 mrad of cosmic radiation. Background radiation levels may vary in different locales.

**backing** /bak′ing/ [AS, *baec*], in dentistry, the piece of metal that supports a porcelain or resin facing on a fixed or removable partial denture.

**back knee.** See **genu recurvatum.**

**back pressure** [AS, *baec* + L, *premere*, to press], pressure that builds in a vessel or a cavity as fluid accumulates. The pressure increases and extends backward if the normal mechanism for egress or passage of the fluid is not restored.

**backscatter radiation.** See **scattered radiation.**

**backup,** **1.** a duplicate computer, data file, equipment, or procedure for use in the event of equipment failure. **2.** The act of creating another copy of a file, group of files, or an entire computer hard drive.

**baclofen,** an antispastic agent.

■ INDICATION: It is prescribed for the alleviation of spasticity.

■ CONTRAINDICATION: Known hypersensitivity to this drug prohibits its use.

■ ADVERSE EFFECTS: Among the more serious adverse reactions are confusion, hypotension, dyspnea, impotence, nausea, and transient drowsiness.

**-bactam,** combining form designating a beta-lactamase inhibitor.

**bacter-.** See **bacterio-.**

**bacteremia** /bak′tirē′mē·ə/ [Gk, *bakterion,* small staff, *haima,* blood], the presence of bacteria in the blood. Undocumented bacteremias occur frequently and usually abate spontaneously. Bacteremia is demonstrated by blood culture. Antibiotic treatment, if given, is specific for the organism found and appropriate to the locus of infection. Also called **bacteriemia.** Also spelled **bacteraemia.** Compare **septicemia.** See also **septic shock. —bacteremic,** *adj.*

**bacteremic shock,** septic shock caused by the release of toxins by bacteria, usually gram-negative bacteria, in the blood.

**bacteria** /baktir′ē·ə/, *sing.* **bacterium** [Gk, *bakterion,* small staff], the small unicellular microorganisms of the class Schizomycetes. The genera vary morphologically, being spheric (cocci), rod-shaped (bacilli), spiral (spirochetes), or comma-shaped (vibrios). The nature, severity, and outcome of any infection caused by a bacterium are characteristic of that species.

**-bacteria,** suffix meaning 'genus of microscopic plants forming the class Schizomycetes': *lysobacteria, streptobacteria.*

**bacterial adherence** /baktir′ēəl/, the process whereby bacteria attach themselves to cells or other surfaces before proliferating.

**bacterial aneurysm,** a localized dilation in the wall of a blood vessel caused by the growth of bacteria. It often follows septicemia or bacteremia and usually occurs in peripheral vessels. See also **mycotic aneurysm.**

**bacterial count.** See **count.**

**bacterial endocarditis,** an acute or subacute bacterial infection of the endocardium or the heart valves or both. The condition is characterized by heart murmur, prolonged fever, bacteremia, splenomegaly, and embolic phenomena. The acute variety progresses rapidly and is usually caused by staphylococci. The subacute variety is usually caused by lodging of *Streptococcus viridans* in heart valves damaged by rheumatic fever. Prompt treatment of both types with antibiotics, such as penicillin, cephalosporin, or gentamicin given intravenously, is essential to prevent destruction of the valves and cardiac failure. See also **endocarditis, subacute bacterial endocarditis.**

**bacterial enzyme,** an enzyme produced by a bacterium.

**bacterial food poisoning,** a toxic condition resulting from the ingestion of food contaminated by certain bacteria. Acute infectious gastroenteritis caused by various species of *Salmonella* is characterized by fever, chills, nausea, vomiting, diarrhea, and general discomfort beginning 8 to 48 hours after ingestion and continuing for several days. Simi-

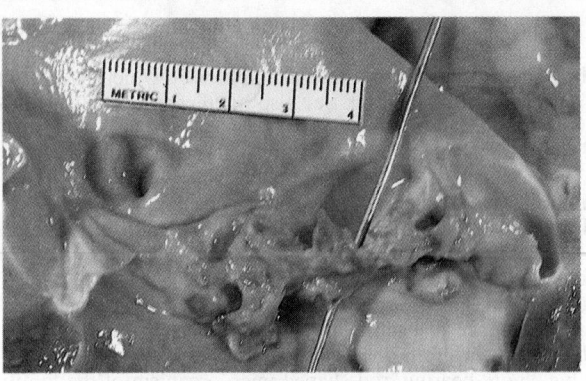

**Acute bacterial endocarditis**
*(Kumar, Cotran, and Robbins, 1997)*

lar symptoms caused by *Staphylococcus,* usually *S. aureus,* appear much sooner and rarely last more than a few hours. Food poisoning caused by the neurotoxin of *Clostridium botulinum* is characterized by GI symptoms, disturbances of vision, weakness or paralysis of muscles, and, in severe cases, respiratory failure. See also **botulism.**

**bacterial inflammation** [L, *bacterium* + *inflammare,* to set afire], any inflammation that is part of a body's response to a bacterial infection.

**bacterial kinase,** **1.** a kinase of bacterial origin. **2.** a bacterial enzyme that activates plasminogen, the precursor of plasmin.

**bacterial laryngitis,** a form of laryngitis caused by a bacterial infection and usually associated with rhinosinusitis or laryngotracheal bronchitis. Signs of a bacterial infection are a cough and purulent rhinorrhea. The infection is treated with any of several antibiotics. See also **laryngitis.**

**bacterial meningitis.** See **meningitis.**

**bacterial overgrowth syndrome.** See **stasis syndrome.**

**bacterial plaque,** a dense, nonmineralized complex composed primarily of colonies of bacteria embedded in a gelatinous matrix. It contains amino acids, carbohydrates, proteins, lipids, and salts from saliva and gingival fluid; soluble food substances; shed leukocytes and epithelial cells; and products of bacterial metabolism. Plaque is the major causitive factor in most dental diseases, including dental caries and inflammatory periodontal diseases. Also called **dental plaque.**

**bacterial pneumonia,** pneumonia caused by bacteria, such as *Klebsiella pneumoniae, Mycoplasma pneumoniae, Staphylococcus aureus, Streptococcus pneumoniae, Streptococcus pyogenes,* and others.

**bacterial prostatitis,** a bacterial infection of the prostate. Acute bacterial infections usually involve gram-negative bacilli, such as *Escherichia coli.* Most cases are treated with broad-spectrum antimicrobial drugs. Abscesses may be associated with anaerobic bacteria. Chronic bacterial prostatitis is usually caused by gram-negative bacilli. It is less common and characterized by low back pain, dysuria, and perineal discomfort. See also **prostatitis.**

**bacterial protein,** a protein produced by a bacterium.

**bacterial resistance,** the ability of certain strains of bacteria to develop a tolerance to specific antibiotics to which they once were susceptible.

**bacterial toxin** [Gk, *bakterion,* small staff, *toxikon,* poison], any poisonous substance produced by a bacterium. Kinds of bacterial toxins include **endotoxins** and **exotoxins.**

**bacterial vaccine,** a saline solution suspension of a strain of attenuated or killed bacteria prepared for injection into a patient to stimulate development of active immunity to that strain.

**bacterial vaginosis** [Gk, *bakterion,* small staff; L, *vagina,* sheath; Gk, *osis,* condition], a chronic inflammation of the vagina caused by a bacterium, *Gardnerella vaginalis.* Also called **vulvovaginitis.**

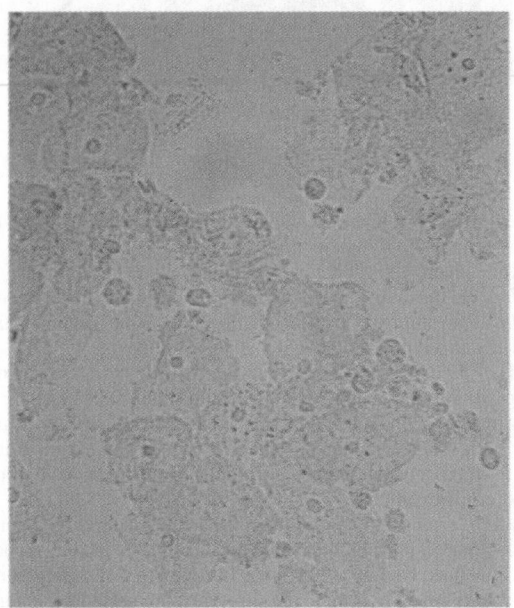

**Bacterial vaginosis** *(Zitelli and Davis, 1997)*

**bacterial virus,** a virus with the ability to destroy bacteria. See also **bacteriophage.**

**bactericidal** /baktir′isī′dəl/, bringing death to bacteria. Also **bacteriocidal.** Compare **bacteriostatic.**

**bactericidal antibiotic** [Gk, *bakterion* + *caedere,* to kill; Gk, *anti,* against, *bios,* life], an antibiotic drug that kills bacteria.

**bactericide** /baktir′əsīd/ [GK, *bakterion* + L, *caedere,* to kill], any drug or other agent that kills bacteria.

**bactericidin** [Gk, *bakterion* + L, *caedere,* to kill], an antibody that kills bacteria in the presence of complement. Also called **bacteriocidin.**

**bacteriemia.** See **bacteremia.**

**bacterio-, bacter-, bacteri-,** combining form meaning 'bacterial microorganism': *bacteriogenic, bacteriod, bactericide.*

**bacteriocidal.** See **bactericidal.**

**bacteriocidal antibiotic.** See **bactericidal antibiotic.**

**bacteriocidin.** See **bactericidin.**

**bacteriocin** /baktir′ē·əsin/, protein produced by certain species of bacteria that are toxic to related strains of those bacteria. Also called **protein antibiotic.**

**bacteriocinogenic** /baktir′ē·əsin′əjen′ik/, pertaining to an organism capable of producing bacteriocins.

**bacteriogenic** /baktir′ē·əjen′ik/, 1. capable of producing bacteria. 2. derived from or originating in bacteria.

**bacterioidal.** See **bacteroid.**

**bacteriologic** /baktir′ē·əloj′ik/ [Gk, *bakterion*], pertaining to **bacteriology.** Also **bacteriological.**

**bacteriologic sputum examination,** a laboratory procedure to determine the presence or absence of bacteria in a specimen of a patient's sputum. Part of the specimen is stained and examined microscopically on a glass slide, and part is mixed with culture medium and allowed to incubate for more specific examination later.

**bacteriologist** /baktir′ē·ol′əjist/, a specialist in the scientific study of bacteria.

**bacteriology** /-ol′əjē/ [Gk, *bakterion* + *logos,* science], the scientific study of bacteria.

**bacteriolysin** /baktir′ē·əlī′sin/ [Gk, *bakterion* + *lyein,* to loosen], an antibody that causes the breakdown of a particular species of bacterial cell. Complement is usually also necessary for this reaction. See also **bacteriolysis.**

**bacteriolysis** /baktir′ē·ol′əsis/, the intracellular or extracellular breakdown of bacteria. See also **bacteriolysin.** —**bacteriolytic,** *adj.*

**bacteriophage** /baktir′ē·əfāj′/ [Gk, *bakterion* + *phagein,* to eat], any virus that causes lysis of host bacteria, including the blue-green algae. Bacteriophages resemble other viruses in that each is composed of either ribonucleic acid (RNA) or deoxyribonucleic acid (DNA). They vary in structure from simple fibrous bodies to complex forms with contractile "tails." Bacteriophages associated with temperate bacteria may be genetically intimate with the host and are named for the bacterial strain for which they are specific, such as coliphage and corynebacteriophage. —**bacteriophagic,** *adj.,* **bacteriophagy** /-of′əjē/, *n.*

**bacteriophage typing,** the process of identifying a species of bacterium according to the type of virus that attacks it.

**bacteriophagic, bacteriphagy.** See **bacteriophage.**

**bacteriospermia** /baktir′ē·əspur′mē·ə/, the presence of bacteria in semen.

**bacteriostasis** /baktir′ē·os′təsis/ [Gk, *bakterion* + Gk, *stasis,* standing still], a state of suspended growth and/or reproduction of bacteria.

**bacteriostatic** /baktir′ē·əstat′ik/ [Gk, *bakterion* + *statikos,* standing], tending to restrain the development or the reproduction of bacteria. Compare **bactericidal.**

**bacterium.** See **bacteria.**

**bacteriuria** /baktir′ēyŏŏr′ē·ə/, the presence of bacteria in the urine. The presence of more than 100,000 pathogenic bacteria per milliliter of urine is usually considered significant and diagnostic of urinary tract infection. See also **urinary tract infection.**

**bacteroid** /bak′təroid/, 1. pertaining to or resembling bacteria. 2. a structure that resembles a bacterium. Also **bacterioid** /baktir′ē·oid/. —**bacteroidal, bacterioidal,** *adj.*

*Bacteroides* /bak′təroi′dēz/ [Gk, *bakterion,* small staff, *eidos,* form], a genus of obligate anaerobic bacilli normally found in the colon, mouth, genital tract, and upper respiratory system. Severe infection may result from the invasion of the bacillus through a break in the mucous membrane into the venous circulation, where thrombosis and bacteremia may occur. Foul-smelling abscesses, gas, and putrefaction are characteristic of infection with this organism. Of the 30 species, *Bacteroides fragilis* is the most common and most virulent.

**Bactrim,** trademark for a fixed-combination drug containing two sulfa antibacterials (sulfamethoxazole and trimethoprim) commonly prescribed to treat urinary tract infection.

**BAER,** abbreviation for **brainstem auditory evoked response.**

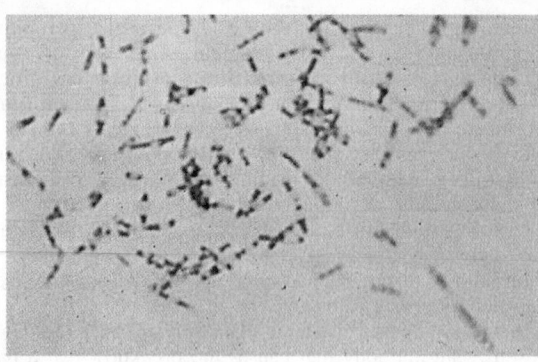

*Bacteroides fragilis* (Baron, Peterson, and Finegold, 1994)

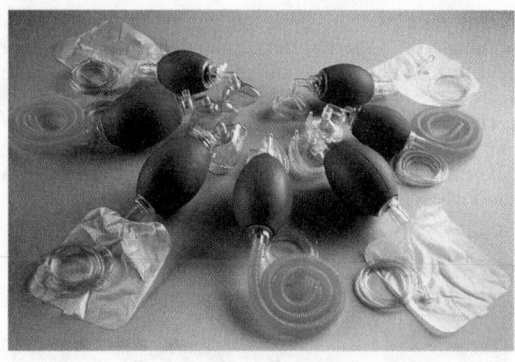

**Bag-valve-mask resuscitators** (Sanders et al, 2000)

**baffling,** the process of removing large water particles from suspension in a jet nebulizer so that the particles entering the patient's airways are of a uniform therapeutic size. The function may be performed in part by a perforated plate against which liquid particles impinge and fracture and are reflected into the vapor chamber of the nebulizer.

**bag** [AS, *baelg*], a flexible or dilatable sac or pouch designed to contain gas, fluid, or semisolid material such as crushed ice. An Ambu bag or breathing bag is used to control the flow of respiratory gases entering the lungs of a patient. Several types of bags are used in medical or surgical procedures to dilate the anus, vagina, or other body openings.

**bagasse** /bəgas'/ [Fr, cane trash], the crushed fibers or the residue of sugarcane, a source of the thermophilic actinomycetes antigen that is a cause of bagassosis hypersensitivity pneumonitis.

**bagassosis** /bag'əsō'sis/, a self-limited lung disease caused by an allergic response to bagasse, the fungi-laden, dusty debris left after the syrup has been extracted from sugarcane. It is characterized by fever, dyspnea, and malaise.

**bagging,** *informal.* the artificial ventilation performed with a ventilator or respirator bag, such as an Ambu bag or the reservoir bag on an anesthesia machine. The bag is squeezed to deliver air to the patient's lungs through a mask or an endotracheal tube. During general anesthesia the anesthetist may also use this technique to assist or control the respiration of an unconscious patient.

**bag lady,** a homeless indigent woman who carries all personal possessions in a portable container.

**bag man,** a homeless indigent man who carries all personal possessions in a portable container.

**bag of waters,** the membranous sac of amniotic fluid surrounding the fetus in the uterus of a pregnant woman. See **amnion.**

**bag-valve-mask resuscitator,** a device consisting of a manually compressible container with a plastic bag of oxygen at one end and at the other a one-way valve and mask that fit over the mouth and nose of the person to be resuscitated. See also **Ambu bag.**

**Bainbridge reflex** [Francis A. Bainbridge, English physiologist, 1874–1921], a cardiac reflex in which stimulation of stretch receptors in the wall of the left atrium causes an increased pulse rate. It may be triggered by the infusion of large amounts of IV fluids or by backflow of blood in congestive heart failure.

**Baker's cyst** [William M. Baker, British surgeon, 1839–1896], a synovial cyst that forms at the back of the knee. It is often associated with rheumatoid arthritis and may appear only when the leg is straightened.

**baker's itch** [AS, *giccan*, to bake], a rash that may develop on the hands and forearms of bakery workers, probably as an allergic reaction to flours or other ingredients in bakery products.

**BAL,** **1.** abbreviation for **British antilewisite.** See **dimercaprol. 2.** abbreviation for **bronchoalveolar lavage.**

**balance**[1] [L, *bilanx,* having two scales], **1.** an instrument for weighing. **2.** a normal state of physiologic equilibrium. **3.** a state of mental or emotional equilibrium. **4.** to bring into equilibrium.

**balance**[2], a nursing outcome from the Nursing Outcomes Classification (NOC) defined as ability to maintain body equilibrium. See also **Nursing Outcomes Classification.**

**balanced anesthesia,** a highly variable technique of general anesthesia in which large doses of narcotic analgesics, muscle relaxation, and minimal inhalation, usually in the form of nitrous oxide only, render the patient unconscious.

**balanced articulation,** simultaneous contact between the upper and lower teeth as they glide over each other when the mandible is moved laterally. See also **balanced occlusion.**

**balanced diet,** a diet containing adequate energy and all of the essential nutrients that cannot be synthesized in adequate quantities by the body, in amounts adequate for growth, energy needs, nitrogen equilibrium, repair, and maintenance of normal health.

**balanced forearm orthosis (BFO).** See **mobile arm support.**

**balanced occlusion,** simultaneous contact between the upper and lower teeth on both sides and in the anterior and posterior occlusal areas of the jaws. An appropriate dental prosthesis develops such an occlusion to prevent the denture base from tipping or rotating in relation to the supporting structures. This term is primarily associated with the mouth but may also be used in relation to testing the occlusion of denture casts with an articulator. See also **balanced articulation.**

**balanced polymorphism,** in a population, the occurrence of a certain proportion of homozygotes and heterozygotes for specific genetic traits, which is maintained from generation to generation by the forces of natural selection. Compare **genetic polymorphism.**

**balanced suspension,** a system of splints, ropes, slings, pulleys, and weights for suspending the lower extremities of the body, used as an aid to realignment and healing from fractures or from surgical intervention. See also **lower extremity suspension, upper extremity suspension.**

**balanced traction,** a system of balanced suspension that supplements traction in the treatment of fractures of the lower extremities or after various operations affecting the lower parts of the body that require traction.

**balanced translocation,** the transfer of segments between nonhomologous chromosomes in such a way that the configuration and total number of chromosomes change but each cell contains the normal amount of diploid or haploid genetic material. Usually the long arm of an acrocentric chromosome is transferred to another chromosome, and the small fragment containing the centromere is lost, leaving only 45 chromosomes. A person with a balanced translocation is phenotypically normal but may produce children with trisomies. Compare **reciprocal translocation, robertsonian translocation.**

**balancing side,** the side of the mouth opposite the working side of dentition or a denture.

**balanic** /bəlan'ik/ [Gk, *balanos,* acorn], pertaining to the glans penis or the glans clitoridis.

**balanic hypospadias.** See **glandular hypospadias.**

**balanitis** /bal'ənī'tis/ [Gk, *balanos + itis*], inflammation of the glans penis.

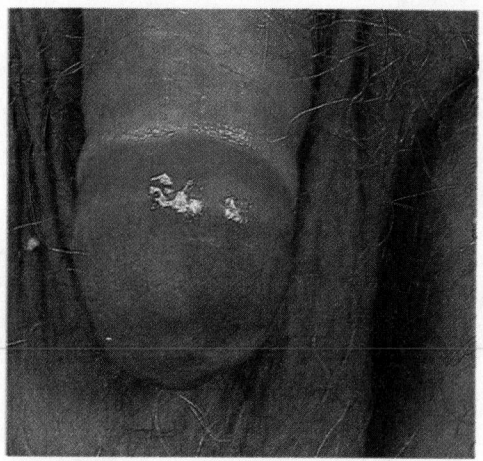

**Balanitis xerotica obliterans** (du Vivier, 1993)

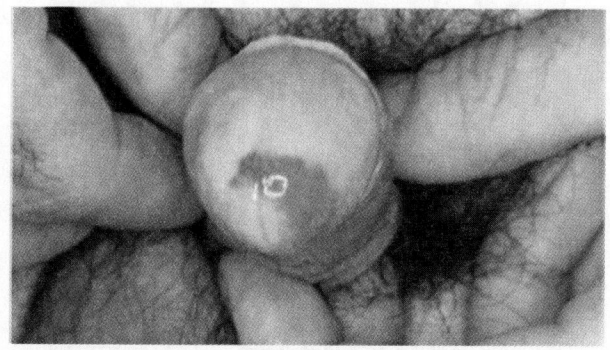

**Balanitis** (Lloyd-Davies et al, 1994)

**balanitis diabetica,** an inflammation of the glans penis or glans clitoridis caused by the sugar content of the urine and commonly seen in diabetics.

**balanitis xerotica obliterans** /zirot'ikə oblit'ərans/ [Gk, *balanos + itis + xeros,* dry, *tokos,* labor; L, *obliterare,* to efface], a chronic skin disease of the penis, characterized by a white indurated area surrounding the meatus. Local antibacterial and antiinflammatory agents are used to treat it.

**balano-, balan-,** combining form meaning 'the head of the penis in males; may also mean the glans clitoris in females': *balanoplasty, balanitis.*

**balanoplasty** /bal'ənōplas'tē/ [Gk, *balanos + plassein,* to mold], an operation involving plastic surgery of the glans penis to correct a congenital defect or to serve an aesthetic purpose.

**balanoposthitis** /bal'ənōposthī'tis/ [Gk, *balanos + posthe,* penis, foreskin, *itis*], a generalized inflammation of the glans penis and prepuce. It is characterized by soreness, irritation, and discharge, which occurs as a complication of bacterial or fungal infection. Smear and culture can determine the causative agent—often a common venereal

disease—so that specific antimicrobial therapy can then be instituted. Circumcision may be considered in severe cases. To relieve discomfort, the inflamed area can be irrigated with a warm saline solution several times a day.

**balanopreputial** /bal'ənōpripyoo'shəl/ [Gk, *balanos +* L, *praeputium,* foreskin], pertaining to the glans penis and the prepuce.

**balanorrhagia** /bal'ənōrā'jē·ə/ [Gk, *balanos + rhegnynai,* to burst forth], balanitis in which pus is discharged copiously from the penis.

**balantidiasis** /bal'əntidī'əsis/, an infection caused by ingestion of cysts of the protozoan *Balantidium coli.* Pigs are the animal reservoir. In some cases the organism is a harmless inhabitant of the large intestine, but infection with *B. coli* usually causes diarrhea. Infrequently the infection progresses, and the protozoan invades the intestinal wall and produces ulcers or abscesses, which may cause dysentery and death. Diagnosis is made by identification of trophozoites in the stool or in sampled colonic tissue. Tetracycline, iodoquinol, or metronidazole is usually prescribed to treat the infection.

***Balantidium coli*** /bal'əntid'ē·əm/ [Gk, *balantidion,* little bag, *kolon,* colon], the largest and the only ciliated protozoan species that is pathogenic to humans, causing balantidiasis. The organism is seen in two life stages: the motile trophozoite and the encysted cercaria. It is a normal inhabitant of the domestic hog and is transmitted to humans by the ingestion of cysts excreted in hog feces.

**baldness** [ME, *balled*], absence of hair, especially from the scalp. See also **alopecia.**

**BAL in Oil,** trademark for a heavy metal antagonist (dimercaprol).

**Balint's syndrome** [Rudolph Balint, Hungarian neurologist, 1874–1929], a group of visual symptoms characterized by agnosia and optic ataxia. The patient experiences nystagmus, or loss of control of eye movements, simultaneously with loss of perceptive ability. The patient may begin to follow a moving object but lose it. The cause is bilateral disease of the parietotemporal areas of the brain.

**Balkan traction frame,** an overhead, rectangular frame attached to the bed and used for attaching splints, suspending or changing the position of immobilized limbs, or providing continuous traction with weights and pulleys.

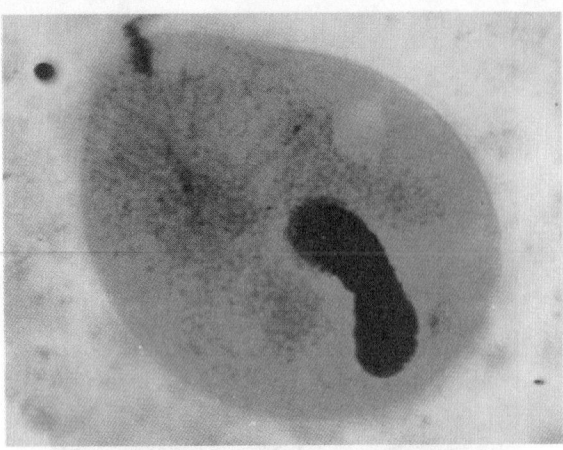

**Trophozoite stage of *Balantidium coli***
*(Baron, Peterson, and Finegold, 1994)*

**ballistics** /bəlis′tiks/ [Gk, *ballein,* to throw], the study of the motion, trajectory, and impact of projectiles, including bullets and rockets.

**ballistocardiograph** [Gk, *ballein,* to throw, *kardia,* heart, *graphein,* to record], an apparatus for recording body movements caused by the thrust of the heart during systolic ejection of the blood into the aorta and the pulmonary arteries. It has been used in measuring cardiac output and the force of contraction of the heart.

**ballistocardiography** /balis′tōkär′dē·og′rəfē/, the recording of body movements in reaction to the beating of the heart and the circulation of the blood.

**ball of the foot,** the part of the foot composed of the distal heads of the metatarsals and their surrounding fatty fibrous tissue pad.

**balloon angioplasty** /bəlo͞on′/, a method of dilating or opening an obstructed blood vessel by threading a small, balloon-tipped catheter into the vessel. The balloon is inflated to compress arteriosclerotic lesions against the walls of the vessel, leaving a larger lumen, through which blood can pass. It is used in treating arteriosclerotic heart disease.

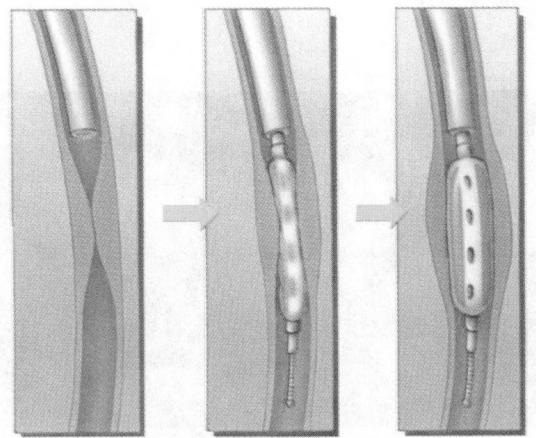

**Balloon angioplasty**
*(Thibodeau and Patton, 1999/Rolin Graphics)*

**Balkan tubulointerstitial nephritis** /to͞o′byəlō· in′tər-stish′-əl/, a chronic kidney disorder marked by renal insufficiency, proteinuria, tubulointerstitial nephritis, and anemia. The onset is gradual, but end-stage disease occurs within 5 years after the first signs. About one third of the patients also suffer from urinary tract cancers. The disease is endemic in the Balkans but is not hereditary.

**ball** [ME, *bal*], spherical object, such as one of the collagen balls embedded in hyaline cartilage.

**Ballance's sign** [Charles A. Ballance, English surgeon, 1856–1936], a dull percussion resonance sound heard on the right flank of a patient lying in the left decubitus position. The sound may shift with the patient's change of position. The condition is attributed to rupture of the spleen, which causes an accumulation of liquid blood on the right side and coagulated blood on the left.

**ball-and-socket joint,** a synovial or multiaxial joint in which the globular (ball-shaped) head of an articulating bone is received into a cuplike cavity, allowing the distal bone to move around an indefinite number of axes with a common center, such as in hip and shoulder joints. Also called **enarthrosis, spheroidea.** Compare **condyloid joint, pivot joint, saddle joint.** See also **joint.**

**ball-bearing feeder.** See **mobile arm support.**

**ball-catcher position,** a position of the hands used in making a radiograph to diagnose rheumatoid arthritis. The hands are held with the palms upward and the fingers cupped, as if to catch a ball.

**Baller-Gerold syndrome** /bä′lər ga′rōlt/ [Friedrich Baller, German physician, 20th century; M. Gerold, German physician, 20th century], an autosomal recessive syndrome characterized by craniosynostosis and absence of the radius.

**ballism,** See **ballismus.**

**ballismus** /bôl′iz′məs/ [Gk, *ballismo,* dancing], an abnormal neuromuscular condition characterized by uncoordinated swinging of the limbs and jerky movements. Ballism is associated with extrapyramidal disorders such as Sydenham's chorea. The condition may occur in a unilateral form as hemiballismus. Also called **ballism.**

**ballistic movement** /bəlis′tik/, a high-velocity musculoskeletal movement, such as a tennis serve or boxing punch, requiring reciprocal coordination of agonistic and antagonistic muscles.

**balloon bezoar** [Fr, *ballon,* a large ball; Ar, *bazahr,* counterpoison], a balloon that is inserted into the stomach and inflated to create a sensation of fullness, used as a therapy for obesity. It is rarely used now because of complications and improved results with gastric bypass.

**balloon compression,** a percutaneous therapy for trigeminal neuralgia. A balloon is inflated to compress the gasserian ganglion and produce trigeminal injury.

**balloon septostomy.** See **Rashkind procedure.**

**balloon tamponade** [Fr, tamponnade], a procedure in which a device consisting of a flexible tube and two balloons is inserted into a passageway and the balloons are expanded to restrict the flow of blood or to force open a stenosis. See also **balloon angioplasty.**

**balloon-tip catheter,** a catheter bearing a nonporous inflatable sac around its far end. After insertion of the catheter the sac can be inflated with air or sterile water, introduced via injection into a special port at the near end of the catheter. The inflated sac secures the catheter in the correct position. See also **Foley catheter, Swan-Ganz catheter.**

**ballottable** /bəlot′əbəl/ [Fr, *balloter,* a shaking about], pertaining to a use of palpation to detect movement of objects suspended in fluid, such as a fetus in amniotic fluid, or the patella bumping against the femur. See **ballottement.**

**ballottable head** [Fr, *ballotage,* shaking up], a fetal head that has not descended and has not become fixed in the maternal bony pelvis.

**ballottement** /bä′lôtmäN′, bəlot′ment/ [Fr, tossing], a technique of palpating an organ or floating structure by bouncing it gently and feeling it rebound. Ballottement of a fetus within a uterus is a probable objective sign of pregnancy. In late pregnancy a fetal head that can be ballotted is said to be **floating** or **unengaged,** as differentiated from a fixed or an engaged head, which cannot be easily dislodged from the pelvis.

**ball thrombus,** a relatively round, coagulated mass of blood, containing platelets, fibrin, and cellular fragments, that may obstruct a blood vessel or an orifice, usually the mitral valve of the heart.

**ball-valve action,** the intermittent opening and closing of an orifice by a buoyant, ball-shaped mass, which acts as a valve. Some kinds of objects that may act in this manner are kidney stones, gallstones, and blood clots.

**balm** /bäm/ [Gk, *balsamon,* balsam], **1.** a healing or a soothing substance, such as any of various medicinal ointments. **2.** an aromatic plant of the genus *Melissa* that relieves pain. Also called **balsam.**

**balneology** /bal′nē·ol′əjē/ [L, *balneum,* bath; Gk, *logos,* science], a field of medicine that deals with the chemical compositions of various mineral waters and their healing characteristics, especially in baths. —**balneologic,** *adj.*

**balneotherapy** /bal′nē-ōther′əpē/ [L, *balneum* + Gk, *therapeia,* treatment], use of baths in the treatment of many diseases and conditions.

**balneum pneumaticum.** See **air bath.**

**balsam** /bôl′səm/ [Gk, *balsamon*], **1.** any of a variety of resinous saps, generally from evergreens, usually containing benzoic or cinnamic acid. Balsam is sometimes used in rectal suppositories and dermatologic agents as a counterirritant. **2.** See **balm.**

**Baltimore Longitudinal Study of Aging (BLSA),** a long-range examination of interrelations between multiple correlates of aging. Although men of varied backgrounds were selected for the original study (1955) in order to explore uncontrolled factors that might lead to new knowledge regarding aging, the BLSA now includes both men and women.

**-bamate,** combining form designating a propanediol or pentanediol derivative.

**Bamberger's sign** [Heinrich Bamberger, Austrian physician, 1822–1888], **1.** a neural disorder characterized by the feeling of a tactile stimulation at a corresponding point on the opposite side of the body (known as allochiria). **2.** pericardial effusion signs at the level of the scapula that disappear when the patient leans forward.

**bamboo spine** /bamboo′/ [Malay, *bambu*], a rigid spine characteristic of advanced ankylosing spondylitis. Also called **poker spine.** See also **ankylosing spondylitis.**

**band** [ME, *bande,* strip], **1.** (in anatomy) a bundle of fibers, as seen in striated muscle, that encircles a structure or binds one part of the body to another. **2.** (in dentistry) a strip of metal that fits around a tooth and serves as an attachment for orthodontic components. **3.** also called **stab form.** *informal,* the immature form of a segmented granulocyte characterized by a sausage-shaped nucleus. It is the only immature leukocyte normally found in the peripheral circulation. Bands represent 3% to 5% of the total white cell volume. An increase in the relative number of bands indicates bacterial infection or acute stress to the bone marrow.

**band adapter,** an instrument for aiding in the fitting of a circumferential orthodontic band to a tooth.

**bandage** /ban′dij/ [ME, *bande,* strip], **1.** a strip or roll of cloth or other material that may be wound around a part of the body in a variety of ways to secure a dressing, maintain pressure over a compress, or immobilize a limb or other part of the body. See also **cravat bandage. 2.** to apply a bandage.

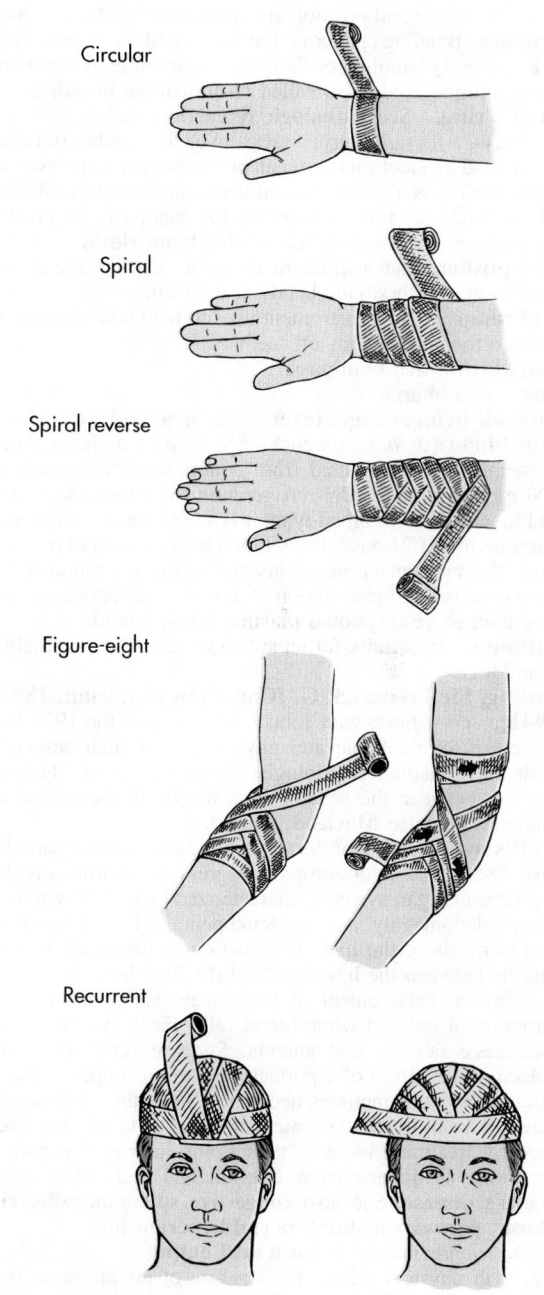

Circular

Spiral

Spiral reverse

Figure-eight

Recurrent

**Types of bandage turns** *(Potter and Perry, 2001)*

**bandage shears,** a sturdy pair of scissors used to cut through bandages. The blades of most bandage shears are angled to the shaft of the instrument, and the lower blade is rounded and blunt to facilitate insertion under the bandage without harming the patient's skin. Also called **bandage scissors.**

**band cell,** a developing granular (immature) leukocyte in circulating blood, characterized by a curved or indented nucleus. Band cells are intermediate leukocytic forms between metamyelocytes and adult leukocytes with segmented nuclei.

**banding** [ME, *bande,* strip], any of several techniques of staining chromosomes with fluorescent stains or chemical dyes that produce a series of transverse light and dark areas whose intensity and position are characteristic of each chromosome. Banding patterns are identified as C-banding, G-banding, Q-banding, or R-banding according to the staining technique used. Also called **chromosome banding.**

**Bandl's ring.** See **pathologic retraction ring.**

**bandpass,** (in radiology) a measure of the number of times per second an electron beam can be modulated, expressed as Hertz (Hz). It is a factor that influences horizontal resolution on a cathode-ray tube. The higher the bandpass, the greater the horizontal resolution. Also called **bandwidth.**

**band pusher,** an instrument used for adapting metal circumferential orthodontic bands to the teeth.

**band remover,** an instrument used to help take circumferential orthodontic bands off teeth.

**bandwidth.** See **bandpass.**

**bang.** See **bhang.**

**Bangkok hemorrhagic fever.** See **dengue fever.**

**bank blood** [It, *banca,* bench; AS, *blod*], anticoagulated preserved blood collected from donors usually in units of 500 ml and stored under refrigeration for future use. Dated and identified as to blood type, it is stored for a usual maximum period of 21 days. Bank blood may be used in transfusion after crossmatching against the recipient's blood or for the extraction and preparation of any of its components. See also **packed cells, pooled plasma, whole blood.**

**Banthine,** trademark for an anticholinergic (methantheline bromide).

**Banting, Sir Frederick G. [Canadian physician, 1891–1941],** co-winner, with John J. Macleod, of the 1923 Nobel prize for medicine and physiology for their research, with the Canadian physiologist Charles H. Best, showing the link between the pancreas and insulin in the control of diabetes. See also **Macleod, John J.**

**Banti's syndrome** /ban'tēz/ [Guido Banti, Italian pathologist, 1852–1925], a chronic, progressive disorder involving several organ systems, characterized by portal hypertension, splenomegaly, anemia, leukopenia, GI tract bleeding, and cirrhosis of the liver. Obstruction of the blood vessels that lie between the intestines and the liver leads to venous congestion, enlargement of the spleen, and abnormal destruction of red and white blood cells. Early symptoms are weakness, fatigue, and anemia. Surgical removal of the spleen and creation of a portacaval shunt to improve portal circulation are sometimes necessary. Since the syndrome is often a complication of alcoholic cirrhosis of the liver, medical treatment includes prescribing improved nutrition, vitamins, abstinence from alcohol, and rest. Also called **Banti's disease.** See also **congestive splenomegalia, cirrhosis, portacaval shunt, portal hypertension.**

**BAO,** abbreviation for **basal acid output.**

**bar,** (in physical science) a measure of air pressure. It is equal to 1000 millibars, or $10^6$ dyne/cm$^2$, or approximately 1 standard atmosphere (1 atm). Also called **barye.**

**bar-.** See **baro-.**

**baralyme** /ber'əlīm/ [Gk, *barys,* heavy; AS, *lim,* lime], a mixture of calcium and barium compounds used to absorb exhaled carbon dioxide in an anesthesia rebreathing system.

**Bárány's test.** See **caloric test.**

**-barb,** combining form designating a barbituric acid derivative.

**Barbados cherry.** See **acerola.**

**barber's itch.** See **sycosis barbae.**

**barbiturate** /bärbich'ŏŏrāt, -'ərit/ [Saint Barbara, drug discovered on day of the saint, 1864], a derivative of barbituric acid that acts as a sedative or hypnotic. These derivatives act by depressing the respiratory rate, blood pressure, temperature, and central nervous system. They have great addiction potential. Some barbiturates are used in anesthesia and in treatment of seizures.

**barbiturate coma** [Ger, Saint Barbara's Day, Gk, *koma,* deep sleep], an effect of barbituric acid or its derivatives, which may be rapid-acting sedatives, hypnotics, and respiratory depressants. Barbituate coma may be intentionally induced for the treatment of some neurologic conditions. Death may result from intentional or accidental overdosage.

**barbiturate poisoning.** See **barbiturism.**

**-barbituric,** combining form used to designate compounds derived from barbituric acid: *dibromobarbituric, isobarbituric.*

**barbiturism** /bärbich'əriz'əm/, **1.** acute or chronic poisoning by any of the derivatives of barbituric acid. Ingestion of such preparations in excess of therapeutic quantities may be fatal or may produce physiologic, pathologic, and psychologic changes, such as depressed respiration, cyanosis, disorientation, and coma. Sometimes referred to as **barbiturate poisoning. 2.** addiction to a barbiturate.

**bar clasp arm,** (in prosthetic dentistry) a clasp arm that originates from a denture base and serves as an extracoronal retainer.

**Bardeleben's bone.** See **os trigonum.**

**Bard-Pic syndrome** /bärd'pik'/ [Louis Bard, French anatomist, 1857–1930; Adrian Pic, French physician, b. 1863], a condition characterized by progressive jaundice, enlarged gallbladder, and cachexia, associated with advanced pancreatic cancer.

**Bard's sign** [Louis Bard], the increased oscillations of the eyeball in organic nystagmus when the patient tries to visually follow a target moved from side to side across the line of sight. Such oscillations usually cease during the same test if the patient has congenital nystagmus.

**bare lymphocyte syndrome,** an immune deficiency condition caused by defective beta-2 microglobulin, one of the major histocompatibility antigens on cell surfaces. It is inherited as an autosomal recessive trait.

**baresthesia** /bär'esthē'zhə/, sensitivity to weight or pressure.

**bar graph** [OF, *barre*], a graph in which frequencies are represented by bars extending from the ordinate or the abscissa, allowing the distribution of the entire sample to be seen at once.

**bariatrics** /ber'ē·at'riks/ [Gk, *baros,* weight, *iatros,* physician], the field of medicine that focuses on the treatment and control of obesity and diseases associated with obesity.

**baritosis** /ber'ətō'sis/, a benign form of pneumoconiosis caused by an accumulation of barium dust in the lungs. Barium does not cause fibrosis and is not a common cause of functional impairment. The condition is most likely to affect persons involved in the mining and processing of barite, a barium-containing compound used in the manufacture of paints.

**barium (Ba)** /ber′ē·əm/ [Gk, *barys,* heavy], a pale yellow, metallic element classified with the alkaline earths. Its atomic number is 56; its atomic mass is 137.36. The acid-soluble salts of barium are poisonous. Barium carbonate, formerly used in medicine, is now used to prepare the cardiac stimulant barium chloride; fine, milky barium sulfate is used as a contrast medium in radiographic imaging of the digestive tract.

**barium enema,** a rectal infusion of barium sulfate, a radiopaque contrast medium, which is retained in the lower intestinal tract during roentgenographic studies for diagnosis of obstruction, tumors, or other abnormalities, such as ulcerative colitis. The procedure is used therapeutically in children to reduce nonstrangulated intussusception. Also called **contrast enema.**

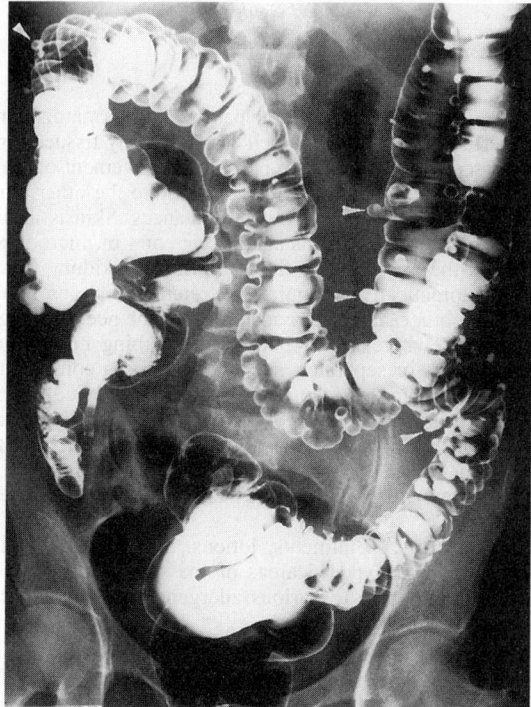

**Barium enema** *(Heuman, Mills, and McGuire, 1997)*

**barium enema with air contrast.** See **double-contrast barium enema.**

**barium meal,** the ingestion of barium sulfate, a radiopaque contrast medium, for the radiographic examination of the esophagus, stomach, and intestinal tract in the diagnosis of such conditions as dysphagia, peptic ulcer, and fistulas. The movement of the barium through the GI tract is followed by fluoroscopy, x-ray studies, or both. Before the test, the patient receives nothing by mouth for at least 8 hours. See also **barium swallow.**

**barium poisoning,** a condition characterized by a severe, rapid decrease in plasma potassium levels and a shift of potassium into cells caused by the ingestion of soluble barium salts. The patient may experience nausea, vomiting, abdominal cramps, bloody diarrhea, dizziness, dysrhythmias, ringing in the ears, cardiac arrest, and respiratory failure.

**barium sulfate,** a radiopaque medium used as a diagnostic aid in roentgenology.

■ INDICATION: It is prescribed for x-ray examination of the GI tract.

■ CONTRAINDICATION: Known hypersensitivity to this drug prohibits its use.

■ ADVERSE EFFECTS: Among the more serious complications is severe constipation.

**barium swallow** [Gk, *barys,* heavy; AS, *swelgan,* to swallow], the oral administration of a radiopaque barium sulfate suspension given to radiographically demonstrate possible defects in the esophagus and abnormal borders of the posterior aspects of the heart. See also **barium meal.**

**Barlow's disease.** See **infantile scurvy.**

**Barlow's syndrome** [John B. Barlow, South African cardiologist, b. 1924], an abnormal cardiac condition characterized by an apical systolic murmur, a systolic click, and an electrocardiogram indicating inferior ischemia. These signs are associated with mitral regurgitation caused by prolapse of the mitral valve. Also called **floppy-valve syndrome.** See also **mitral valve prolapse.**

**Barnard, Kathryn E.,** a nursing theorist who developed the Child Health Assessment Interaction Model. Her model and theory were the outcome of the Nursing Child Assessment Project (1976–1979). Barnard believes that the parent-infant system is influenced by individual characteristics of each member. Those characteristics are modified to meet the needs of the system by adaptive behavior. The interaction between parent (or caregiver) and child is shown in Barnard's model to take place with five cues and activities: (1) the infant's clarity in sending cues, (2) the infant's responsiveness to the parent, (3) the parent's sensitivity to the child's cues, (4) the parent's ability to recognize and alleviate the infant's distress, and (5) the parent's social, emotional, and cognitive growth-fostering activities. A major issue in Barnard's theoretic assertions is that the nurse give support to the mother's sensitivity and response to her infant's cues rather than trying to change her characteristics or mothering style.

**baro-, bar-, bari-** combining form meaning 'pressure, heaviness, weight': *baresthesia, barognosis, bariatrics.*

**barognosis** /ber′əgnō′sis/, *pl.* **barognoses** [Gk, *baros,* weight, *gnosis,* knowledge], the ability to perceive and evaluate weight, especially that held in the hand.

**barograph** /ber′əgraf′/ [Gk, *baros* + *graphein,* to record], an instrument that continually monitors barometric pressure and records pressure changes on paper.

**barometer** /bərom′ətər/ [Gk, *baros* + *metron,* measure], an instrument for measuring atmospheric pressure, commonly consisting of a slender tube filled with mercury, sealed at one end, and inverted into a reservoir of mercury. At sea level the normal height of mercury in the tube is 760 mm. At higher elevations the mercury column height (barometric pressure) is less. Fluctuations in barometric pressure may precede major changes in weather, making a barometer useful in meteorologic forecasting. **—barometric,** *adj.*

**barometric pressure.** See **atmospheric pressure.**

**baroreceptor** /ber′ōrisep′tər/ [Gk, *baros* + L, *recipere,* to receive], one of the pressure-sensitive nerve endings in the walls of the atria of the heart, the aortic arch, and the carotid sinuses. Baroreceptors stimulate central reflex mechanisms that allow physiologic adjustment and adaptation to changes in blood pressure via changes in heart rate, vasodilation, or vasoconstriction. Baroreceptors are essential for homeostasis. Also called **pressoreceptor.**

**barosinusitis.** See **aerosinusitis.**

**Barosperse,**　trademark for a radiopaque medium (barium sulfate).

**barotitis.**　See **aerotitis.**

**barotitis media.**　See **aerotitis media.**

**barotrauma** /ber'ōtrô'mə, -trou'mə/ [Gk, *baros + trauma,* wound],　physical injury sustained as a result of exposure to changing air pressure, or rupture of the tympanic membranes, as may occur among scuba divers or caisson workers or anyone near nuclear or atomic blasts. Barotrauma may be iatrogenic as in the case of excessive ventilator pressures leading to lung injury. Compare **decompression sickness.**

**Barr body.**　See **sex chromatin.**

**barrel chest,**　a large, rounded thorax, as in the inspiratory phase, considered normal in some stocky individuals and certain others who live in high-altitude areas and consequently have increased vital capacity. Barrel chest may also be a sign of pulmonary emphysema. Also called **emphysematous chest.**

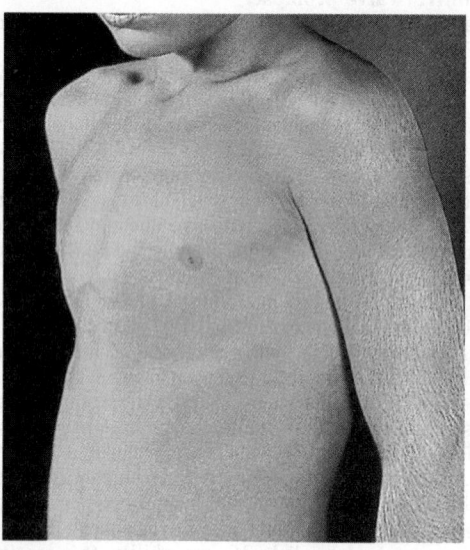

**Barrel chest** *(Zitelli and Davis, 1997/courtesy Dr. Meyer B. Marks)*

**Barr-Epstein virus.**　See **Epstein-Barr virus.**

**Barré's pyramidal sign** /bäräz'/ [Jean A. Barré, French neurologist, 1880–1971],　a diagnostic sign indicating a disease of the pyramidal tracts. The patient lies face down and the legs are flexed at the knee. The patient is unable to maintain this position.

**Barrett's syndrome** [Norman R. Barrett, English surgeon, 1903–1979],　a disorder of the lower esophagus marked by a benign ulcerlike lesion in columnar epithelium, resulting most often from chronic irritation of the esophagus by gastric reflux of acidic digestive juices. Major symptoms include dysphagia, decreased lower esophageal (LES) pressure, and heartburn. Symptoms may be relieved by eating frequent small meals, avoiding foods that produce gas, taking antacid medication, and elevating the head of the bed to prevent passive reflux when lying down. Also called **Barrett's esophagus.**

**barrier** /ber'ē·ər/ [ME, *barrere*],　**1.** a wall or other obstacle that can restrain or block the passage of substances. Barrier methods of contraception, such as the condom or

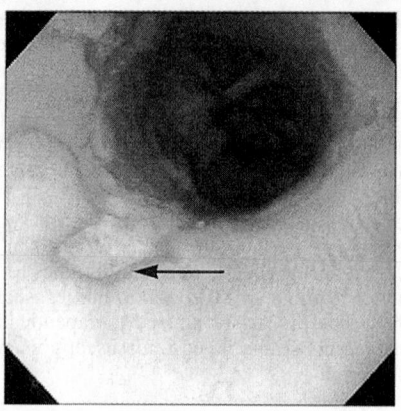

**Barrett's syndrome: endoscopic view**
*(Greig and Garden, 1996)*

cervical diaphragm, prevent the passage of spermatozoa into the uterus. Membranes and cell walls of body tissues function as screenlike barriers to permit the movement of water or certain other molecules from one side to the other while preventing the passage of other substances. Skin is an important barrier that protects against the entry of microorganisms and the exit of body fluids. Barriers in kidney tissues adjust automatically to regulate the retention or excretion of water and other substances according to the needs of organ systems elsewhere in the body. **2.** something nonphysical that obstructs or separates, such as barriers to communication or compliance. **3.** (in radiography) any device that intercepts beams of x-rays. A primary barrier is one that blocks the passage of the useful x-ray beam, such as the walls and floor. A secondary barrier is one that intercepts only leakage and scattered x-ray emissions. An example is the ceiling.

**barrier creams,**　ointments, lotions, and similar preparations applied to exposed areas of the skin to protect skin cells from exposure to various allergens, irritants, and carcinogens, including sunlight.

**barrier-free design** [AS, *freo,* barreres; L, *designare,* to mark out],　the design of homes, workplaces, and public buildings that allows physically challenged individuals to make regular use of such structures.

**Barsony-Koppenstein method,**　a procedure for making radiographic images of the cervical intervertebral foramina.

**Barthel Index (BI)** [D.W. Barthel, twentieth century American psychiatrist],　a disability profile scale developed by D.W. Barthel in 1965 to evaluate a patient's self-care abilities in 10 areas, including bowel and bladder control. The patient is scored from 0 to 15 points in various categories, depending on his or her need for help, such as in feeding, bathing, dressing, and walking.

**bartholinian abscess.**　See **Bartholin's abscess.**

**bartholinitis** /bär'təlinī'tis/ [Caspar T. Bartholin, Danish anatomist, 1655–1738; Gk, *itis*],　an inflammatory condition of one or both Bartholin's glands, caused by bacterial infection. Usually the causative microorganism is a species of *Streptococcus* or *Staphylococcus* or a strain of gonococcus. The condition is characterized by swelling of one or both glands, pain, and development of an abscess in the infected gland. A fistula may develop from the gland to the vagina, anus, or perineum. Treatment includes local application of heat, often by soaking in hot water; antibiotics; or, if necessary, incision of the gland and drainage of the purulent material or excision of the entire gland and its duct.

**Bartholin's abscess** /bär′təlinz/ [Caspar T. Bartholin; L, *abscedere,* to go away], an abscess of the greater vestibular gland of the vagina. Also called **bartholinian abscess.**

**Bartholin's cyst** [Caspar T. Bartholin], a cyst that arises from one of the vestibular glands or from its ducts and fills with clear fluid that replaces the suppurative exudate characteristic of chronic inflammation.

**Bartholin's duct** [Caspar T. Bartholin], the major duct of the sublingual salivary gland.

**Bartholin's gland** [Caspar T. Bartholin], one of two small mucus-secreting glands located on the posterior and lateral aspect of the vestibule of the vagina. Also called **greater vestibular gland.**

**Bartholin's gland carcinoma** [Caspar T. Bartholin], a rare malignancy that occurs deep in the labia majora. The tumor has overlying skin and some normal glandular tissue. The treatment and prognosis are the same as for squamous cell cancer of the vulva.

**Barton, Clara** (1821–1912), an American philanthropist, humanitarian, and founder of the American National Red Cross. During the U.S. Civil War, she was a volunteer nurse, often on the battlefield, and at its end she organized a bureau of records to help in the search for missing men. When the Franco-Prussian War erupted, she assisted in the organization of military hospitals in Europe in association with the International Red Cross. This experience led to her advocacy of establishment of an American Red Cross organization, of which she became the first president.

*Bartonella* /bär′tənel′ə/ [Alberto Barton, Peruvian bacteriologist, 1871–1950], a genus of small gram-negative flagellated pleomorphic coccobacilli. Members of the genus infect red blood cells and the epithelial cells of the lymph nodes, liver, and spleen. They are transmitted at night by the bite of a sandfly of the genus *Phlebotomus. B. bacilliformis,* causes bartonellosis. Because of its distinctive appearance, it is easily identified on microscopic examination of a smear of blood stained with Wright's stain. *B. henselae* is the causative agent of cat-scratch fever and bacillary angiomatosis.

**bartonellosis** /bär′tənəlō′sis/, an acute infection caused by *Bartonella bacilliformis,* transmitted by the bite of a sandfly. It is characterized by fever, severe anemia, bone pain, and, several weeks after the first symptoms are observed, multiple nodular or verrucose skin lesions. The disease is endemic in the valleys of the Andes in Peru, Colombia, and Ecuador. The treatment usually includes chloramphenicol, penicillin, streptomycin, or tetracycline. Untreated, the infection is often fatal. Also called **Carrión's disease, Oroya fever, verruga peruana.**

**Barton forceps.** See **obstetric forceps.**

**Barton's fracture** [John R. Barton, American surgeon, 1794–1871], a break in the distal articular surface of the radius, which may be accompanied by the dorsal dislocation of the carpus on the radius.

**Bartter's syndrome** /bär′tərz/ [Frederick C. Bartter, American physiologist, 1914–1983], a rare hereditary disorder, characterized by hyperplasia of the juxtaglomerular area and secondary hyperaldosteronism. Renin and angiotensin levels may be elevated, but blood pressure usually remains normal. Early signs in childhood are abnormal physical growth and mental retardation, often accompanied by chronic hypokalemia and alkalosis.

**bary-,** combining form meaning 'heavy or difficult': *baryphonia.*

**barye.** See **bar.**

**basal** /bā′səl/ [Gk, *basis,* foundation], pertaining to the fundamental or the basic, as basal anesthesia, which produces the first stage of unconsciousness, and the basal metabolic rate, which indicates the lowest metabolic rate.

**basal acid output (BAO),** the minimum volume of gastric fluid produced by an individual in a given period. Normal adult volume is 2 to 5 mEq/hr. It is used infrequently in the diagnosis of various diseases of the stomach and intestines, such as gastric ulcers and Zollinger-Ellison syndrome.

**basal anesthesia** [Gk, *basis,* foundation, *anaisthesia,* lack of feeling], **1.** a state of unconsciousness just short of complete surgical anesthesia in depth, in which the patient does not respond to words but reacts to pinprick or other noxious stimuli. **2.** narcosis produced by injection or infusion of potent sedatives alone, without added narcotics or anesthetic agents. **3.** also called **narcoanesthesia.** Any form of anesthesia in which the patient is completely unconscious, in contrast to awake anesthesia.

**basal body temperature,** the temperature of the body taken in the morning, orally or rectally, after sleep and before the patient does anything, including getting out of bed, smoking a cigarette, moving around, talking, eating, or drinking.

**basal body temperature method of family planning,** a natural method of family planning that relies on identification of the fertile period of the menstrual cycle by noting the rise in basal body temperature that occurs with ovulation. The progesterone-mediated rise is 0.5° to 1° F; rate and pattern vary greatly from woman to woman, and to some extent from cycle to cycle in any one woman. The woman keeps careful records over several cycles, taking her temperature at the same time every morning, before getting out of bed or doing anything else. She may take her temperature orally or rectally in the same way every day. Talking, getting up, smoking a cigarette, eating, or even moving about in bed may change the temperature. Many other factors may also affect the reading, including infection, stress, a bad night's sleep, medication, or environmental temperature. If any of these factors is present, the woman notes them on her record. The days after that period are considered "safe" infertile days. Abstinence is required to avoid pregnancy from 6 days before the earliest day that ovulation was noted to occur during the preceding 6 months until the third day after the rise in temperature in the current cycle. Another way of calculating the possible beginning of the fertile days is to subtract 19 days from the shortest complete menstrual cycle of the preceding 6 months. The basal body temperature method is more effective when used with the ovulation method than is either method used alone. The combination of these methods is called the symptothermal method of family planning. Compare **calendar method of family planning, ovulation method of family planning.**

**basal bone, 1.** (in prosthodontics) the osseous tissue of the mandible and the maxilla, except for the rami and the processes, which provides support for artificial dentures. **2.** (in orthodontics) the fixed osseous structure that limits the movement of teeth in the creation of a stable occlusion.

**basal cell,** any one of the cells in the deepest layer of stratified epithelium; the base.

**basal cell acanthoma.** See **basal cell papilloma.**

**basal cell carcinoma** [Gk, *basis* + L, *cella,* storeroom; Gk, *karkinos,* crab, *oma,* tumor], a malignant epithelial cell tumor that begins as a papule and enlarges peripherally, developing a central crater that erodes, crusts, and bleeds. Metastasis is rare, but local invasion destroys underlying and adjacent tissue. In 90% of cases the lesion occurs between the hairline and the upper lip. The primary known cause of the cancer is excessive exposure to the sun or to radiation. Treatment is eradication of the lesion, often by electrodesiccation or cryotherapy. Also called **basal cell epithelioma, basaloma, basiloma, carcinoma basocellulare, hair matrix carcinoma.** See also **rodent ulcer.**

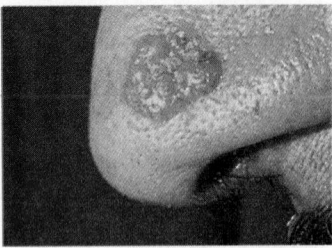

**Basal cell carcinoma** *(Belcher, 1992)*

**basal cell papilloma.** See **seborrheic keratosis.**

**basal energy expenditure (BEE).** See **basal metabolic rate.**

**basal ganglia** [Gk, *basis* + *ganglion,* knot], the islands of gray matter, largely composed of cell bodies, within each cerebral hemisphere. The most important are the caudate nucleus, the putamen, and the pallidum. The basal ganglia are surrounded by the rings of the limbic system and lie between the thalamus of the diencephalon and the white matter of the hemisphere.

**Basaljel,** trademark for an antacid (aluminum carbonate gel).

**basal lamina** [Gk, *basis* + L, *lamina,* plate], a thin, noncellular layer of ground substance lying just under epithelial surfaces. Constituting the uppermost layer of the basement membrane, it can be examined with an electron microscope. Also called **basement lamina.**

**basal layer.** See **stratum basale.**

**basal membrane,** a sheet of tissue that forms the outer layer of the choroid and lies just under the pigmented layer of the retina. It is composed of elastic fibers in an otherwise thin homogenous layer.

**basal metabolic rate (BMR),** the amount of energy used in a unit of time by a fasting, resting subject to maintain vital functions. The rate, determined by the amount of oxygen used, is expressed in Calories consumed per hour per square meter of body surface area or per kilogram of body weight. Also called **basal energy expenditure (BEE).** See also **Calorie (Cal).**

**basal metabolism** [Gk, *basis* + *metabole,* change], the amount of energy needed to maintain essential body functions, such as respiration, circulation, temperature, peristalsis, and muscle tone. Basal metabolism is measured when the subject is awake and at complete rest, has not eaten for 14 to 18 hours, and is in a comfortable, warm environment. It is expressed as a basal metabolic rate, according to Calories per hour per square meter of body surface. See also **Calorie (Cal).**

**basal narcosis** [Gk, *basis,* foundation, *narkosis,* a benumbing], a narcosis induced with sedatives in a surgical patient before general anesthetic is administered. It is less profound than that of general anesthesia. The patient is unresponsive to verbal stimuli but may respond to noxious stimuli. Also called **basis narcosis.**

**basaloid carcinoma** /bā′səloid/ [Gk, *basis* + *eidos,* form, *karkinos* crab, *oma* tumor], a rare transitional malignant neoplasm of the anal canal containing areas that resemble basal cell carcinoma of the skin. Basaloid carcinoma is rapidly invasive. Tumor may spread to the skin of the perineum.

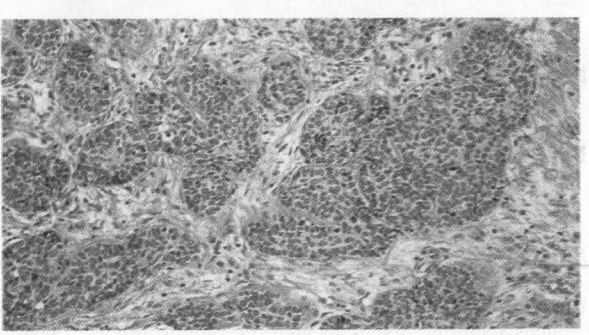

**Basaloid carcinoma** *(Fletcher, 2000)*

**basaloma.** See **basal cell carcinoma.**

**basal seat,** (in dentistry) the oral structures that support a denture. See also **basal seat outline.**

**basal seat area,** the portion of the oral structures that is available to support a denture. Also called **denture-bearing area, stress-bearing area.**

**basal seat outline,** a profile on the oral mucous membrane or on a cast of the entire oral area to be covered by a denture. See also **basal seat.**

**basal temperature.** See **basal body temperature.**

**basal temperature chart** [Gk, *basis,* foundation; L, *temperatura* + *charta,* paper], a daily temperature chart, usually including the temperature on awakening. A basal temperature chart is sometimes used by women to establish a date of ovulation, when the temperature may show a sudden increase.

**basal tidal volume,** the amount of air inhaled and exhaled by a healthy person at complete rest, with all bodily functions at a minimal level of activity, adjusted for age, weight, and sex. See also **tidal volume (TV).**

**base** [Gk, *basis,* foundation], **1.** a chemical compound that increases the concentration of hydroxide ions in aqueous solution. Compare **alkali. 2.** a molecule or radical that takes up or accepts hydrogen ions. **3.** an electron pair donor. **4.** the major ingredient of a compounded material, particularly one that is used as a medication. Petroleum jelly is frequently used as a base for ointments. **5.** (in radiology) the rigid but flexible foundation of a sheet of x-ray film. The base is essentially transparent but is given a bluish tint during manufacture to reduce eyestrain of the radiologist viewing x-ray films.

**base analog** [Gk, *basis* + *analogos,* proportionate], a chemical analog of one of the purine or the pyrimidine bases normally found in RNA or DNA.

**Basedow's goiter** /bä′sədōz/ [Karl A. von Basedow, German physician, 1799–1854], a European name for Graves' disease, which is an enlargement of the thyroid gland, characterized by the hypersecretion of thyroid hormone after iodine therapy. The condition causes increased basal metabolic rate, insomnia, and fine motor tremor.

**base excess,** a measure of metabolic alkalosis or metabolic acidosis (negative value of base excess) expressed as the amount of acid or alkali needed to titrate 1 L of fully oxygenated blood to a pH of 7.40, the temperature being held at a constant 37° C and the $PCO_2$ at 40 mm Hg.

**base-forming food,** a food that increases the pH of the urine. Base-forming foods mainly are fruits, vegetables, and dairy products, which are sources of sodium and potassium. Some foods that are acidic in their natural state may be converted to alkaline metabolites.

**baseline** /bās′līn/ [Gk, *basis* + L, *linea*], **1.** a known value or quantity with which an unknown is compared when mea-

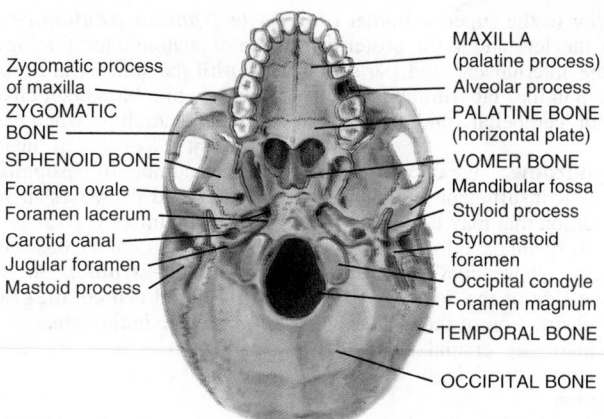

Zygomatic process of maxilla
ZYGOMATIC BONE
SPHENOID BONE
Foramen ovale
Foramen lacerum
Carotid canal
Jugular foramen
Mastoid process

MAXILLA (palatine process)
Alveolar process
PALATINE BONE (horizontal plate)
VOMER BONE
Mandibular fossa
Styloid process
Stylomastoid foramen
Occipital condyle
Foramen magnum
TEMPORAL BONE
OCCIPITAL BONE

**Landmarks on the base of the skull** (Applegate, 2000)

sured or assessed. **2.** (in radiology) any of several basic anatomic planes or locations used for positioning purposes. They include the orbitomeatal, infraorbitomeatal, acanthomeatal, and glabellomeatal lines.

**baseline behavior,** a specified frequency and form of a particular behavior during preexperimental or pretherapeutic conditions.

**baseline condition,** an environmental condition during which a particular behavior reflects a stable rate of response before the introduction of experimental or therapeutic conditions.

**baseline fetal heart rate,** the fetal heart rate pattern between uterine contractions. An electronic fetal monitor is used to detect abnormally rapid or slow rates (less than 110 or more than 160 beats/min) at term.

**basement lamina.** See **basal lamina.**

**basement membrane** [Fr, *soubassement,* under base], the fragile noncellular layer that secures the overlying epithelium to the underlying tissue. It is the deepest layer, may contain reticular fibers, and can be selectively stained with silver stains. Also called **basal lamina, basement lamina.**

**base of the heart,** the portion of the heart opposite the apex. It is superior and medially located. It forms the upper border of the heart, lies just below the second rib, and primarily involves the left atrium, part of the right atrium, and the proximal portions of the great vessels.

**base of the skull,** the floor of the skull, containing the anterior, middle, and posterior cranial fossae and numerous foramina, such as the optic foramen, foramen ovale, foramen lacerum, and foramen magnum.

**base pair,** a pair of nucleotides in the complementary strands of a DNA molecule that interact through hydrogen bonding across the axis of the helix. One of the nucleotides in each pair is a purine (either adenine or guanine), and the other is a pyrimidine (either thymine or cytosine). Because of their spatial configuration, adenine always pairs with thymine, and guanine always pairs with cytosine.

**base pairing,** the formation of base pairs in DNA.

**baseplate** [Gk, *basis* + ME, *plate*], a temporary form that represents the base of a denture, used for making records of maxillomandibular relationships, for arranging artificial teeth, or for ensuring a precise fit of a denture by trial placement in the mouth. Also called **record base, temporary base.**

**baseplate wax,** a dental wax containing about 75 per cent paraffin or ceresin with additions of beeswax and other waxes and resins; used chiefly to establish the initial arch form in making trial plates for the construction of complete dentures.

**base ratio,** the ratio of the molar quantities of purine and pyrimidine bases in DNA and RNA.

**bas-fond** /bäfôN'/ [Fr, bottom], the bottom or fundus of any structure, especially the fundus of the urinary bladder.

**basi-, basio-, bas-, baso-,** prefix meaning 'a foundation or a base': *basicranial, basiotribe, basal, basophil.*

**-basia** /bā'zhə/, suffix meaning 'ability to walk': *brachybasia, dysbasia.*

**BASIC** /bā'sik/, abbreviation for *b*eginner's *a*ll-purpose *s*ymbolic *i*nstruction *c*ode, a computer programming language.

**-basic,** suffix meaning 'relating to or containing alkaline compounds': *ammonobasic, polybasic.*

**basic amino acid,** an amino acid that has a positive electric charge in solution at a pH of 7. The basic amino acids are arginine, histidine, and lysine.

**basic group identity,** (in psychiatry) the shared social characteristics, such as world view, language, values, and ideologic system, that evolve from membership in an ethnic group.

**basic health services,** the minimum degree of health care considered to be necessary to maintain adequate health and protection from disease.

**basic human needs,** the elements required for survival and normal mental and physical health, such as food, water, shelter, protection from environmental threats, and love.

**basic life support (BLS)** [Gk, *basis,* foundation; AS, *lif* + L, *supportare,* to bring up to], emergency treatment of a victim of cardiac or respiratory arrest through cardiopulmonary resuscitation and emergency cardiac care.

**basic salt,** a salt that contains an unreplaced hydroxide ion from the base generating it, such as Ca(OH)Cl.

**basifacial** /bā'sifā'shəl/ [Gk, *basis* + L, *facies,* face], pertaining to the lower portion of the face.

**basilar** /bas'ilər/ [Gk, *basis,* foundation], pertaining to a base or a basal area.

**basilar artery,** the single posterior arterial trunk formed by the junction of the two vertebral arteries at the base of the skull. It extends from the inferior to the superior border of the pons before dividing into the left and right posterior cerebral arteries. It supplies the internal ear and parts of the brain. Its branches are the pontine, labyrinthine, anterior inferior cerebellar, superior cerebellar, and posterior cerebral.

**basilar artery insufficiency syndrome,** the composite of clinical indicators associated with insufficient blood flow through the basilar artery, a condition that may be caused by arterial occlusion. Common signs of this syndrome include dizziness, blindness, numbness, depression, dysarthria, dysphagia, and weakness on one side of the body.

**basilar artery occlusion,** an obstruction of the basilar artery, resulting in dysfunction involving cranial nerves III through XII, cerebellar dysfunction, hemiplegia or quadriplegia, and loss of proprioception.

**basilar membrane,** the cellular structure that forms the floor of the cochlear duct and is supported by bony and fibrous projections from the cochlear wall. It provides a fibrous base for the spiral organ of Corti.

**basilar plexus** [Gk, *basis* + L, braided], the venous network interlaced between the layers of the dura mater over the basilar portion of the occipital bone. It connects the two petrosal sinuses and communicates with the anterior vertebral venous plexus.

**basilar sulcus** [Gk, *basis* + L, furrow], the sulcus that cradles the basilar artery in the midline of the pons.

**basilar vertebra,** the lowest or last of the lumbar vertebrae.

**basilic vein** /bəsil′ik/, one of the four superficial veins of the arm, beginning in the ulnar part of the dorsal venous network and running proximally on the posterior surface of the ulnar side of the forearm. It is often chosen for blood testing. Compare **dorsal digital vein, median antebrachial vein.**

**basiliximab,** an immunosuppressant.

■ INDICATIONS: This drug is used in combination with cyclosporine and corticosteroids to treat acute allograft rejection in renal transplant patients.

■ CONTRAINDICATIONS: Known hypersensitivity to this drug contraindicates its use.

■ ADVERSE EFFECTS: Life-threatening effects of this drug include pulmonary edema and cardiac failure. Other adverse effects include hypotension, headache, constipation, abdominal pain, infection, and moniliasis. Common side effects include pyrexia, chills, tremors, dyspnea, wheezing, chest pain, vomiting, nausea, and diarrhea.

**basiloma.** See **basal cell carcinoma.**

**basiloma terebrans** /ter′əbrənz/ [Gk, *basis* + *oma* + L, *terebare,* to bore], an invasive basal cell epithelioma.

**basin, 1.** a receptacle for collecting or holding fluids. A kidney-shaped basin is commonly used as an emesis receptacle. **2.** term used to describe the shape of the pelvis.

**basio-.** See **basi-.**

**basioccipital** /bā′si·oksip′ətəl/ [Gk, *basis* + L, *occiput,* back of the head], pertaining to the basilar process of the occipital bone.

**basion** /bā′sē·on/ [Gk, *basis,* foundation], the midpoint on the anterior margin of the foramen magnum of the occipital bone.

**basis,** the lower part, designating the base of an organ or other structure, such as the base of the cerebrum.

**basis narcosis.** See **basal narcosis.**

**basis pedunculi cerebri.** See **crus cerebri.**

**basket cell** [L, *bascauda,* dishpan], deep stellate cells (neurons) of the cerebral cortex with a horizontal axon that sends out branches. Each axon branch or collateral breaks up into a basketlike mesh that surrounds a Purkinje cell.

*Basle Nomina Anatomica (BNA),* an international system of anatomic terminology adopted at Basel, Switzerland.

**basophil** /bā′səfil/ [Gk, *basis* + *philein,* to love], a granulocytic white blood cell characterized by cytoplasmic granules that stain blue when exposed to a basic dye. Basophils represent 1% or less of the total white blood cell count. The relative number of basophils increases in myeloproliferative diseases and decreases in severe allergic reactions. An increase in number is seen during the healing phase of inflammation. Also called **basophilic erythrocyte.** Compare **eosinophil, neutrophil.** See also **agranulocyte, differential white blood cell count, granulocyte, leukocyte, polymorphonuclear leukocyte.**

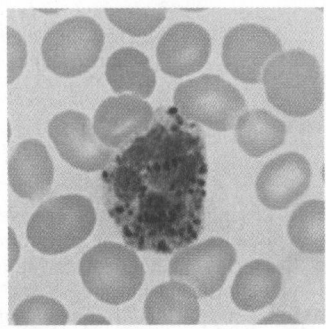

**Basophil** *(Carr and Rodak, 1999)*

**basophilic adenoma** [Gk, *basis* + *philein,* to love, *aden,* gland, *oma*], a tumor of the pituitary gland composed of cells that can be stained with basic dyes. Compare **acidophilic adenoma, chromophobic adenoma.**

**basophilic erythrocyte.** See **basophil.**

**basophilic leukemia** [Gk, *basis* + *philein,* to love, *leukos,* white, *haima,* blood], an acute or chronic malignant neoplasm of blood-forming tissues, characterized by large numbers of immature basophilic granulocytes in peripheral circulation and in tissues. See also **acute myelocytic leukemia.**

**basophilic stippling** [Gk, *basis* + *philein,* to love; D, *stippen,* to prick], the presence of punctate blue nucleic acid remnants in red blood cells, observed under the microscope on a Wright-Giemsa-Gram-stained blood smear. Stippling is characteristic of lead poisoning. See also **basophil, lead poisoning.**

**basosquamous cell carcinoma** /bā′sōskwā′məs/ [Gk, *basis* + L, *squamosus,* scaly], a malignant epidermal tumor composed of basal and squamous cells.

**Bassen-Kornzweig syndrome.** See **abetalipoproteinemia.**

**batch processing** [ME, *baten,* to bake], a processing mode used with computers in which accumulated similar programs and input data are processed simultaneously.

**bath** [AS, *baeth*], (in the hospital) a cleansing procedure performed by or for patients, as needed for hygienic or therapeutic purposes, to help prevent infection, preserve the unbroken condition of the skin, stimulate circulation, promote oxygen intake, maintain muscle tone and joint mobility, and provide comfort.

■ METHOD: The bath may be a bed or tub bath, a shower, or a partial bath, depending on the patient's condition and pref-

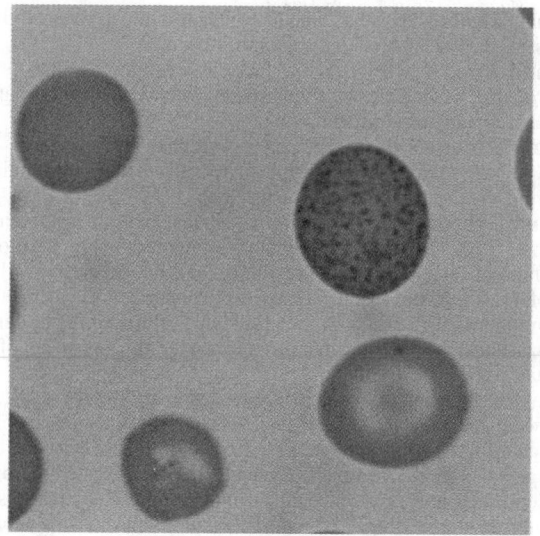

**Basophilic stippling** *(Carr and Rodak, 1999)*

erence and the room temperature. The bath period may be used to instruct the patient on hygienic measures, range of motion exercises, and general measures to promote skin health. Observations are made of the general cleanliness and odor of the patient's body; the color, dryness, turgor, and elasticity and integrity of the skin; and the condition of the hair, hands, joints, feet, fingernails, and toenails. Any discoloration, abrasion, rash, discharge, perineal or rectal irritation, clubbing of the digits, hair loss, or evidence of lice infestation is carefully noted. Mild soap and warm water are used for the bath, and a lanolin-based lotion may be used for an after-bath massage. The patient's hair is combed daily and shampooed as needed; fingernails and toenails are cleaned and trimmed whenever required. The diabetic client may require specialized care of the nails.

■ INTERVENTIONS: The nurse gives the bed bath in a setting that provides privacy for the patient. Firm, gentle strokes are used to wash, dry, and massage the person; vigorous rubbing is avoided. The partial bath is given with the patient seated in or on the side of the bed or in a chair. Self-help is encouraged, and the procedure is completed as quickly as possible to prevent chilling. In preparation for a tub bath, the nurse checks the safety strips in the bottom of the tub and the water temperature and assists the patient into the tub. Precautions are taken to prevent chilling, and on completion of the bath the nurse may help the patient out of the tub. In preparation for a shower, the nurse explains the operation of the dials regulating water temperature and provides a bath mat.

■ OUTCOME CRITERIA: A bath provides an opportunity to assess external signs of disease, effects of therapy, and signs of pressure ulcer development and supports the patient's sense of well-being and self-esteem.

**bath blanket,** a thin, lightweight cloth used to cover a patient during a bath. It absorbs moisture while keeping the patient warm. See also **blanket bath.**

**bathesthesia** /bath'əsthē'zhə/ [Gk, *bathys,* deep, *aisthesia,* feeling], sensitivity to deep pressure. Also called **bathyesthesia.** /bathē·əs-/.

**bathing,** a nursing intervention from the Nursing Interventions Classification (NIC) defined as cleaning of the body

for the purposes of relaxation, cleanliness, and healing. See also **Nursing Interventions Classification.**

**bathmic evolution.** See **orthogenic evolution.**

**bathy-, batho-,** prefix meaning 'depth, deep': *bathycentesis, bathomorphic.*

**bathyanesthesia** /bath'ēan'esthē'zhə/ [Gk, *bathys,* deep, *anaisthesia,* loss of feeling], a loss of deep feeling, such as that associated with organs or structures beneath the body surface, or muscles and joints; a loss of sensitivity to deep structures in the body.

**bathycardia** /bath'ēkär'dē·ə/ [Gk, *bathys,* deep, *kardia,* heart], a condition in which the heart is located at an abnormally low site in the thorax.

**bathyesthesia.** See **bathesthesia.**

**Batten's disease** [Frederick E. Batten, English opthalmologist neurologist, 1865–1918], a progressive childhood encephalopathy characterized by disturbed metabolism of polyunsaturated fatty acids. It occurs in children between 5 and 10 years of age. The child experiences sudden blindness and progressive mental deterioration.

**battered baby syndrome.** See **child abuse.**

**battered woman syndrome (BWS),** repeated episodes of physical assault on a woman by the man with whom she lives and with whom she has a relationship, often resulting in serious physical and psychologic damage to the woman. Not limited to live-in mates. Such violence tends to follow a predictable pattern. The violent episodes usually follow verbal argument and accusation and are accompanied by verbal abuse. Almost any subject—housekeeping, money, childrearing—may begin the episode. Over time, the violent episodes escalate in frequency and severity. Most battered women report that they thought that the assaults would stop; unfortunately, study shows that the longer the women stay in the relationship the more likely they are to be seriously injured. Less and less provocation seems to be enough to trigger an attack once the syndrome has begun. The use of alcohol may increase the severity of the assault. The man is more likely to be abusive as the alcohol wears off. Battering occurs in cycles of violence. In the first phase the man acts increasingly irritable, edgy, and tense. Verbal abuse, insults, and criticism increase, and shoves or slaps begin. The second phase is the time of the acute, violent activity. As the tension mounts, the woman becomes unable to placate the man, and she may argue or defend herself. The man uses this as the justification for his anger and assaults her, often saying that he is "teaching her a lesson." The third stage is characterized by apology and remorse on the part of the man, with promises of change. The calm continues until tension builds again. Battered woman syndrome occurs at all socioeconomic levels, and one half to three quarters of female assault victims are the victims of an attack by a lover or husband. It is estimated that in the United States between 1 and 2 million women a year are beaten by their husbands. Men who grew up in homes in which the father abused the mother are more likely to beat their wives than are men who lived in nonviolent homes. Personal and cultural attitudes also affect the incidence of battering. Aggressive behavior is a normal part of male socialization in most cultures; physical aggression may be condoned as a means of resolving a conflict. A personality profile obtained by psychologic testing reveals the typical battered woman to be reserved, withdrawn, depressed, and anxious, with low self-esteem, a poorly integrated self-image, and a general inability to cope with life's demands. The parents of such women encouraged compliance, were not physically affectionate, and socially restricted their daughters' independence, preventing the widening of social contact that normally occurs in adolescence. Victims of the battered woman syndrome are often afraid to leave the man and the situation; change, loneliness, and the unknown are perceived as more painful than the beatings. Nurses are in an excellent position to offer assistance to battered women in several ways, because encouraging a woman to talk about the battering and the injuries may help her to admit what she may have been too embarrassed to reveal even to her parents. A realistic appraisal of the situation is then possible; the woman wants to hear that the nurse thinks the battering will not recur, but the nurse can tell her only that the usual pattern is for the abuse to continue and to become more severe. The woman may be referred to the social service department or given directions for contacting community agencies such as a battered women's shelter or a hotline to a counseling service. Caring for and counseling a battered woman often require great patience because she is usually ambivalent about her situation and may be confused to the point of believing that she deserves the assaults she has suffered. Written and photographic records are maintained to document the extent of the problem, including the form of abuse reported, the injuries sustained, and a summary of similar incidents and previous admissions.

**battery** [Fr, *batterie*], **1.** a device of two or more electrolytic cells connected to form a single source providing direct current or voltage. **2.** a series or a combination of tests to determine the cause of a particular illness or the degree of proficiency in a particular skill or discipline. **3.** the unlawful use of force on a person. See **assault.**

**Battey bacillus** /bat'ē/ [Battey Hospital, in Rome, Georgia, where bacteria strain first isolated], any of a group of atypical mycobacteria, including *Mycobacterium avium* and *M. intracellulare,* that cause a chronic pulmonary disease resembling tuberculosis. These organisms are resistant to most of the common bacteriostatic and antibiotic medications but may be treated with multiple drug regimens. Surgical resection of involved lung tissue may be necessary and may improve the outcome in serious cases. Rest, good nutrition, and general supportive care are usually recommended. Compare **tuberculosis.**

**battledore placenta** /bat'əldôr'/ [ME, *batyldoure,* a beating instrument; L, *placenta,* flat cake], a condition in which the umbilical cord is attached at the margin of the placenta. It rarely occurs and does not affect placental functioning. Also called **placenta battledore.**

**Battle's sign** [William H. Battle, English surgeon, 1855–1936], a bogginess of the area behind the ear. It may indicate a fracture of a bone of the lower skull.

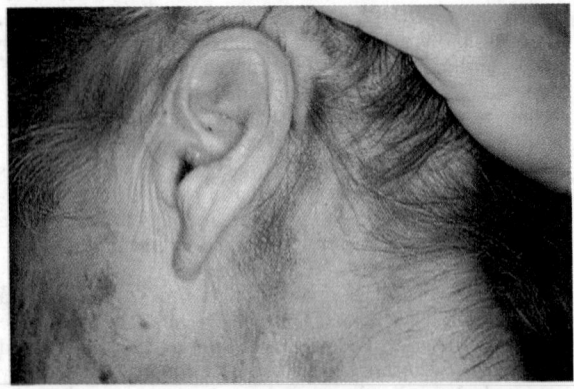

**Battle's sign** *(Bingham, 1992)*

**batyl alcohol** /bat'əl/, an alcohol found in fish liver oil that is used to treat bracken poisoning in cattle.

**baud** /bôd/ [J.M.E. Baudot, French inventor, b. 1845], a measure of data flow or the speed with which a computer device transmits information.

**Baudelocque's diameter.** See **external conjugate.**

**bay,** an anatomic depression or recess, usually containing fluid, as the lacrimal bay of the eye.

**Bayes' theorem** /bāz'/ [Thomas Bayes, British mathematician, 1702–1761], a mathematic statement of the relationships of test sensitivity, specificity, and the predictive value of a positive test result. The predictive value of the test is the number that is useful to the clinician. A positive result demonstrates the conditional probability of the presence of a disease.

**Bayley Scales of Infant Development** [Nancy Bayley, twentieth century American psychologist], a three-part scale for assessing the development of children between the ages of 2 months and 2-1/2 years. Infants are tested for perception, memory, and vocalization on the mental scale; sitting, stair climbing, and manual manipulation on the motor scale; and attention span, social behavior, and persistence on the behavioral scale.

*Baylisascaris* /bā'lis·as'kä·ris/, a genus of nematodes found in the intestines of mammals. *B. columnaris,* infests the central nervous system of dogs. *B. procyonis* is usually found in raccoons and rodents, but fecal contamination from those animals can cause spread to domestic animals and humans, resulting in nervous system infection or larva migrans.

**bayonet angle former.** See **angle former.**

**bayonet condenser** [Fr, *baionette*], an instrument used in dentistry for compacting restorative material. It has an offset nib and a shank with right-angle bends, used primarily for varying the line of force in the compaction of gold. There are many variations in angle, length, and diameter of the nib.

**BBB, 1.** abbreviation for **bundle branch block. 2.** abbreviation for **blood-brain barrier.**

**BCAA,** abbreviation for **branched-chain amino acids.**

**B cell,** a type of lymphocyte that originates in the bone marrow. A precursor of the plasma cell, it is one of the two lymphocytes that play a major role in the body's immune response. Compare **T cell.** See also **plasma cell.**

**B cell growth/differentiation factor,** one of several substances, such as interleukins IL-4, IL-5, and IL-6, that are derived from T cell cultures and are necessary for the differentiation, growth, and maturation of plasma cells and B memory cells.

**B-cell lymphoma,** any in a large group of non-Hodgkin's lymphomas characterized by malignant transformation of the B lymphocytes. See also **non-Hodgkin's lymphoma.**

**B cell–mediated immunity,** the ability to produce an immune response induced by B lymphocytes. Contact with a foreign antigen stimulates B cells to differentiate into plasma cells, which release antibodies. Plasma cells also generate memory cells, which provide a rapid response if the same antigen is encountered again.

**B cell stimulating factor-1.** See **interleukin-4.**

**BCG,** abbreviation for **bacille Calmette-Guérin.**

**BCG vaccine.** See **bacille Calmette-Guérin vaccine.**

**BCNU.** See **carmustine.**

**B complex vitamins,** a large group of water-soluble nutrients that includes thiamine (vitamin $B_1$), cyanocobalamin (vitamin $B_{12}$), niacin (vitamin $B_3$), pyridoxine (vitamin $B_6$), riboflavin (vitamin $B_2$), biotin, folic acid, and pantothenic acid. The B complex vitamins are essential, for example for

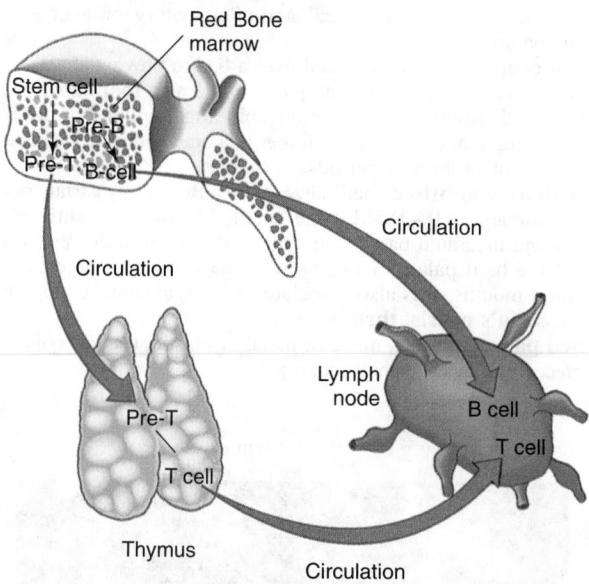

**Development of B and T cells**
*(Thibodeau and Patton, 1999/Network Graphics)*

the conversion of simple carbohydrates like glucose and the carbon skeletons of amino acids into energy, and for the metabolism of fats and proteins. Good sources include brewer's yeast, liver, whole grain cereals, nuts, eggs, meats, fish, and vegetables. Because some B complex vitamins are produced by the intestinal bacteria, taking antibiotics may destroy these bacteria. Symptoms of vitamin B deficiency include nervousness, depression, insomnia, neuritis, anemia, alopecia, acne or other skin disorders, and hypercholesterolemia. See also specific vitamins.

**b.d.** See **b.i.d.**

**B-DNA,** a long, thin form of deoxyribonucleic acid in which the helix is right-handed.

**Be,** symbol for the element **beryllium.**

**beaded** /bē′did/ [ME, *bede*], **1.** having a resemblance to a row of beads. **2.** pertaining to bacterial colonies that develop along the inoculation line in various stab cultures. **3.** pertaining to stained bacteria that develop more deeply stained beadlike granules.

**beak,** **1.** any pointed anatomic structure, as the beak of the sphenoid bone. **2.** a pair of dental pincers used in shaping prostheses. **3.** a radiographic image of a bony protuberance adjacent to a degenerative intervertebral disk.

**beaker cell.** See **goblet cell.**

**beak sign,** the appearance of abnormal structures on radiographic images of the GI tract: of the distal esophagus in achalasia and of the proximal pyloric canal in pyloric stenosis.

**Beals' syndrome** /bēlz/ [Rodney Kenneth Beals, American orthopedic surgeon, b. 1931], a congenital type of bone dysplasia with contractures and arachnodactyly. An autosomal dominant syndrome characterized by long thin extremities with arachnodactyly, multiple joint contractures, kyphoscoliosis, and malformed auricles of the ears; it is a form of hereditary bone dysplasia.

**beam** [ME, *beem*, tree], **1.** a bedframe fitting for pulleys and weights, used in the treatment of patients requiring weight traction. See **Balkan traction frame. 2.** (in ra-

diology) the primary beam of radiation emitted from the x-ray tube.

**BEAM** /bēm, bē′ē′ā′em′/, abbreviation for **brain electrical activity map.**

**beam alignment,** in radiography, the process of positioning the radiographic tube head so it is aligned properly with the x-ray film.

**beam collimation,** the restriction of x-radiation to the area being examined or treated by confining the beam with metal diaphragms or shutters with high radiation-absorption power. In addition to protecting the patient and others from scatter radiation, beam collimation reduces radiographic density.

**beam hardening,** the process of increasing the energy level of an x-ray beam by filtering out the low-energy photons.

**BE amputation,** an amputation of the arm below the elbow.

**beam quality,** the energy of an x-ray beam.

**beam restrictor,** a device that reduces scatter radiation from x-ray equipment. Three basic types of restrictors are variable-aperture collimators, cones or cylinders, and aperture diaphragms.

**beam-splitting mirror,** a device that allows a radiologist to view a fluoroscopic examination of a patient while the same view is being recorded on film. The mirror can be adjusted to reflect from 10% to 90% of the x-ray beam to the fluorescent screen while the rest is directed to the film.

**beam therapy.** See **chromotherapy, external beam radiotherapy.**

**bean** [ME, *bene*], the pod-enclosed flattened seed of numerous leguminous plants. Beans used in pharmacologic preparations are alphabetized by specific name.

**bearing down** /ber′ing/ [OE, *beran*, to bear, *adune,* down], a voluntary effort by a woman in the second stage of labor to aid in the expulsion of a fetus. By applying the Valsalva maneuver, the mother increases intraabdominal pressure.

**bearing down pains** [OE, *beran*, to bear, *adune,* down; L, *poena*, penalty], the pains experienced by a woman during the second stage of labor while performing the Valsalva maneuver to help expel the fetus.

**beat,** the mechanical contraction or electrical activity of the heart muscle, which may be detected and recorded as the pulse or on the electrocardiogram, respectively.

**Beau's lines** /bōz′/ [Joseph H.S. Beau, French physician, 1806–1865], transverse depressions that appear as white lines across the fingernails as a sign of an acute severe illness such as malnutrition, a systemic disease, trauma, or coronary occlusion.

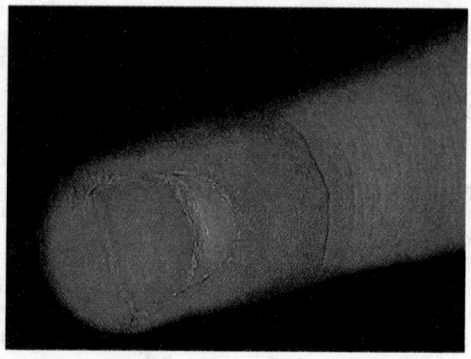

**Beau's lines** *(Habif, 1996)*

**Beck depression inventory (BDI).** See **Beck's Diagnostic Inventory.**

**Becker's muscular dystrophy** [Peter E. Becker, German geneticist, b. 1908], a chronic degenerative disease of the muscles, characterized by progressive weakness. It occurs in childhood between 8 and 20 years of age. It occurs less frequently, progresses more slowly, and has a better prognosis than the more common pseudohypertrophic form of muscular dystrophy. The pathophysiologic characteristics of the disease are not understood; it is transmitted genetically as an autosomal recessive trait. Also called **benign pseudohypertrophic muscular dystrophy.** Compare **Duchenne's muscular dystrophy.**

**Beck's Diagnostic Inventory (BDI)** [Aaron T. Beck, American psychiatrist, b. 1921], a system of classifying a total of 18 criteria of depressive illness. It was developed by A.T. Beck in the 1970s as a diagnostic and therapeutic tool for the treatment of childhood affective disorders. The BDI is similar to the 21-criteria DSM-IV diagnostic system of the 1980s except that the DSM-IV scale includes loss of interest, restlessness, and sulkiness, which are missing from the BDI; the Beck inventory lists somatic complaints and loneliness, which are criteria not included in the DSM-III inventory. Also called **Beck depression inventory (BDI).** See also **DSM.**

**Beck's triad** [Claude Schaeffer Beck, American surgeon, 1894–1971], a combination of three symptoms that characterize cardiac tamponade: high central venous pressure, low arterial pressure, and a small, quiet heart.

**Beckwith's syndrome** [John B. Beckwith, American pathologist, b. 1933], a hereditary disorder of unknown cause associated with neonatal hypoglycemia and hyperinsulinism. Clinical manifestations include gigantism, macroglossia, omphalocele or umbilical hernia, visceromegaly, hyperplasia of the kidney and pancreas, and extreme enlargement of the cells of the adrenal cortex. Treatment consists of adequate glucose, diazoxide, and glucocorticoid therapy. Subtotal pancreatectomy is often necessary in cases of beta cell hyperplasia, nesidioblastosis, or beta cell tumor of the pancreas.

**Beckwith-Wiedemann syndrome.** See **EMG syndrome.**

**beclomethasone dipropionate,** a glucocorticoid.
■ INDICATION: It is prescribed in a metered-dose inhaler in the maintenance treatment of bronchial asthma as prophylactic therapy.
■ CONTRAINDICATIONS: Status asthmaticus, acute asthma, or known hypersensitivity to this drug prohibits its use.
■ ADVERSE EFFECTS: Among the more serious adverse reactions of systemic administration are the symptoms of adrenal insufficiency. Hoarseness, sore throat, and fungal infections of the oropharynx and larynx may occur. Good oral and dental hygiene after each use is requisite.

**becquerel (Bq)** /bekrel′, bek′ərel′/ [Antoine H. Becquerel, French physicist, 1852–1908], the SI unit of radioactivity, equal to one radioactive decay per second. See also **curie.**

**bed** [AS, *bedd*], (in anatomy) a supporting matrix of tissue, such as the nailbeds of modified epidermis over which the fingernails and the toenails move as they grow.

**bed board,** a board that is placed under a mattress to give added support to a patient with back problems.

**bedbug** [AS, *bedd* + ME, *bugge*, hobgoblin], a bloodsucking arthropod of the species *Cimex lectularius* or the species *C. hemipterus* that feeds on humans and other animals. The bedbug can be removed after covering it with petrolatum. The bite, which causes itching, pain, and redness, can be treated with a lotion or cream containing a corticosteroid or other topical antiinflammatory or analgesic preparation.

**bed cradle,** a frame placed over a bed to prevent sheets or blankets from touching the patient. See also **footboard.**

**Bedford finger stall,** a removable finger splint that holds the injured and an adjacent finger in a brace or cast. It can be worn for prolonged periods.

**Bednar's aphthae** /bed′närz/ [Alois Bednar, Austrian pediatrician, 1816–1888], the small, yellowish, slightly elevated ulcerated patches that occur on the posterior portion of the hard palate of infants who place infected objects in their mouths. It is also associated with marasmus. Compare **Epstein's pearls, thrush.**

**bed pan,** a vessel, made of metal or plastic, used to collect feces and urine of bedridden patients.

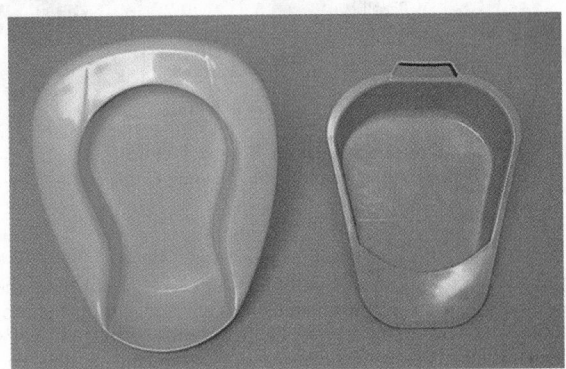

**Bed pans: fracture and regular** *(Potter and Perry, 2001)*

**bed rest,** the restriction of a patient to bed for therapeutic reasons for a prescribed period.

**bed rest care,** a nursing intervention from the Nursing Interventions Classification (NIC) defined as promotion of comfort and safety and prevention of complications for a patient unable to get out of bed. See also **Nursing Interventions Classification.**

**bedridden,** describing a person who is unable or unwilling to leave the bed because of illness or injury.

**bedside laboratory testing,** a nursing intervention from the Nursing Interventions Classification (NIC) defined as performance of laboratory tests at the bedside or point of care. See also **Nursing Interventions Classification.**

**bedside manner,** the behavior of a nurse or doctor as perceived by a patient or peers.

**bedside thermometer.** See **clinical thermometer.**

**bedsore.** See **pressure ulcer.**

**bedwetting.** See **enuresis.**

**BEE,** abbreviation for **basal energy expenditure.**

**bee cell pessary.** See **pessary.**

**beef tapeworm.** See *Taenia saginata.*

**beef tapeworm infection** [OF, *buef,* cow; AS, *taeppe, wyrm*], an infection caused by the tapeworm *Taenia saginata,* transmitted to humans when they eat contaminated beef. The adult worm can live for years in the intestine of humans without causing any symptoms. The infection is rarely found in North America and Western Europe, where beef is carefully inspected before being made available and is often thoroughly cooked before eating, but it is common in other parts of the world. See **tapeworm infection.**

**bee sting** [AS, *beo* + *stingan*], an injury caused by the venom of bees, usually accompanied by pain and swelling. The stinger of the honeybee usually remains implanted and should be removed. Pain may be alleviated by application of an ice pack or a paste of sodium bicarbonate and water. Serious reactions may result from multiple stings, stings on some areas of the head, or the injection of venom directly into the circulatory system. In a hypersensitive person, a single bee sting may result in death through anaphylactic shock and airway obstruction. Hypersensitive individuals are encouraged to carry emergency treatment supplies, including epinephrine, with them when the possibility of bee sting exists. Compare **wasp.**

**behavior** /bihā′vyər/ [ME, *behaven*], **1.** the manner in which a person acts or performs. **2.** any or all of the activities of a person, including physical actions, which are observed directly, and mental activity, which is inferred and interpreted. Kinds of behavior include **abnormal behavior, automatic behavior, invariable behavior,** and **variable behavior.**

**behavioral isolation** /behā′vyərəl/, social isolation that results from a person's socially unacceptable behavior.

**behavioral marital therapy,** a form of marital therapy using principles and techniques from behavior therapy; it attempts to alleviate marital distress by increasing positive, pleasant interactions between the members of a couple.

**behavioral medicine,** a segment of psychosomatic medicine focused on psychological means of influencing physical symptoms, such as biofeedback or relaxation.

**behavioral objective,** a goal in therapy or research that concerns an act or a specific behavior or pattern of behaviors.

**behavioral science,** any of the various interrelated disciplines, such as psychiatry, psychology, sociology, and anthropology, that observe and study human activity, including psychologic and emotional development, interpersonal relationships, values, and mores.

**behavioral systems model,** a conceptual framework describing factors that may affect the stability of a person's behavior. The model examines systems of behavior, not the behavior of an individual at any particular time. In one model, behavior is defined as an integrated response to stimuli. Several subsystems of behavior form the eight human microsystems, which are ingestion, elimination, dependency, sex, achievement, affiliation, aggression, and restoration. Each subsystem comprises several structural components called *imperatives,* which are goal, set, choice, action, and support. The goal of nursing care is to attain, maintain, or restore balance of the subsystems of behavior for the stability of the patient.

**behavior disorder,** any of a group of antisocial behavior patterns occurring primarily in children and adolescents, such as overaggressiveness, overactivity, destructiveness, cruelty, truancy, lying, disobedience, perverse sexual activity, criminality, alcoholism, and drug addiction. Treatment may include psychotherapy, milieu therapy, medication, and family counseling. See also **antisocial personality disorder.**

**behaviorism,** a school of psychology founded by John B. Watson that studies and interprets behavior by observing measurable responses to stimuli without reference to consciousness, mental states, or subjective phenomena, such as ideas and emotions. See also **neobehaviorism.**

**behaviorist,** an advocate of the school of behaviorism.

**behavioristic psychology.** See **behaviorism.**

**behavior management,** a nursing intervention from the Nursing Interventions Classification (NIC) defined as helping a patient to manage negative behavior. See also **Nursing Interventions Classification.**

**behavior management: overactivity/inattention,** a nursing intervention from the Nursing Interventions Classification (NIC) defined as provision of a therapeutic milieu that safely accommodates the patient's attention deficit and/or overactivity while promoting optimal function. See also **Nursing Interventions Classification.**

**behavior management: self-harm,** a nursing intervention from the Nursing Interventions Classification (NIC) defined as assisting the patient to decrease or eliminate self-mutilating or self-abusive behaviors. See also **Nursing Interventions Classification.**

**behavior management: sexual,** a nursing intervention from the Nursing Interventions Classification (NIC) defined as delineation and prevention of socially unacceptable sexual behaviors. See also **Nursing Interventions Classification.**

**behavior modification[1].** See **behavior therapy.**

**behavior modification[2],** a nursing intervention from the Nursing Interventions Classification (NIC) defined as promotion of a behavior change. See also **Nursing Interventions Classification.**

**behavior modification: social skills,** a nursing intervention from the Nursing Interventions Classification (NIC) defined as assisting the patient to develop or improve interpersonal social skills. See also **Nursing Interventions Classification.**

**behavior reflex.** See **conditioned response.**

**behavior therapy,** a kind of psychotherapy that attempts to modify observable maladjusted patterns of behavior by substituting a new response or set of responses to a given stimulus. The treatment techniques involve the methods, concepts, and procedures derived from experimental psychology; they include assertiveness training, aversion therapy, contingency management, flooding, modeling, operant conditioning, and systemic desensitization. Also called **behavior modification.** See also **biofeedback.**

**behaviour.** See **behavior.**

**Behçet's disease** /bā′sets/ [Hulusi Behçet, Turkish dermatologist, 1889–1948], a rare and severe illness of unknown cause, mostly affecting young males and characterized by severe uveitis and retinal vasculitis. Some other signs are optic atrophy and aphthous lesions of the mouth and the genitals, indicating diffuse vasculitis. Also called **Behçet's syndrome.**

**Behla's bodies.** See **Plimmer's bodies.**

**BEI,** abbreviation for **butanol-extractable iodine.**

**bejel** /bej′əl/ [Ar, *bajal*], a nonvenereal form of syphilis prevalent among children in the Middle East and North Africa, caused by the spirochete *Treponema pallidum* subsp. *endemicum.* It is transmitted by person-to-person contact and by the sharing of drinking and eating utensils. The primary lesion is usually on or near the mouth, appearing as a mucous patch, followed by the development of pimplelike sores on the trunk, arms, and legs. Chronic ulceration of the nose and soft palate occurs in the advanced stages of the infection. Destructive changes in the tissues of the heart, central nervous system, and mouth, often associated with the venereal form of syphilis, rarely develop. Intramuscular injection of penicillin is effective in curing the infection, but if extensive tissue destruction has occurred, scar tissue forms and may be permanently disfiguring.

**Békésy audiometry** /bek′əsē/ [George von Békésy, Hungarian-American physicist and Nobel laureate,

1899–1972], a type of hearing test in which the subject controls the intensity of the stimulus by pressing a button while listening to a pure tone whose frequency slowly moves through the entire audible range. The intensity diminishes as long as the button is pressed. When the intensity is too low for the subject to hear the tone, the button is released and the intensity begins to increase. When the subject again hears the tone, the button is again pressed, yielding a zigzag tracing. Continuous and interrupted tones are used, and the tracings of the two are compared. The test may be used to differentiate between hearing losses of cochlear and neural origins.

**Bekhterev-Mendel reflex.** See **Mendel's reflex.**

**bel** [Alexander G. Bell, Canadian inventor, 1847–1922], a unit that expresses intensity of sound. It is the logarithm (to the base 10) of the ratio of the power of any specific sound to the power of a reference sound. The most common reference sound has a power of $10^{-16}$ watts per square centimeter, or the approximate minimum intensity of sound at 1000 cycles per second that is perceptible to the human ear. An increase of 1 bel approximately doubles the intensity or loudness of most sounds. See also **decibel.**

**belching.** See **eructation.**

**belladonna** /bel′ədon′ə, belädôn′ä/ [It, fair lady], the dried leaves, roots, and flowering or fruiting tops of *Atropa belladonna*, a common perennial called deadly nightshade, containing the alkaloids hyoscine and hyoscyamine. Hyoscyamine has anticholinergic and antispasmodic properties.

**belladonna and atropine poisons** [It, *belladonna*, fair lady; Gk, *Atropos*, one of three Fates; L, *potio*, drink], two powerful poisons obtained from solanaceous plants. Atropine, derived from *Atropa belladonna*, blocks the effects of acetylcholine in effector organs supplied by postganglionic cholinergic nerves. Belladonna is obtained from the dried leaves of *Atropa belladonna*, also known as deadly nightshade, or of *Atropa acuminata*, a source of alkaloids that are converted to atropine. Atropine sulfate is commonly used in ophthalmologic applications and as an antispasmodic.

**Bell-Magendie law.** See **Bell's law.**

**bellows murmur** /bel′o͞oz/ [AS, *belg*, bag; L, humming], a blowing sound, such as that of air moving in and out of a bellows.

**bellows ventilator,** a respiratory care device in which oxygen and other gases are mixed in a mechanism that contracts and expands. The system pressure is increased or decreased in the chamber surrounding the bellows. The gases are moved into the patient circuit when the system pressure increases. As the patient exhales, the bellows contracts and fills again with gases from air and oxygen intakes.

**bell-shaped curve,** the curve of the probability density function of the normal distribution. Also called **normal curve.**

**Bell's law** [Charles Bell, Scottish surgeon, 1774–1842], an axiom stating that the anterior spinal nerves contain only motor and the posterior spinal roots are sensory. Also called **Bell-Magendie law, Magendie's law.**

**Bell's palsy** [Charles Bell], a unilateral paralysis of the facial nerve. It results from trauma to the nerve, compression of the nerve by a tumor, or, possibly, an unknown infection. Any or all branches of the nerve may be affected. The person may not be able to close an eye or control salivation on the affected side. The condition is usually unilateral and can be transient or permanent. Also called **Bell's paralysis.**

**Bell's phenomenon** [Charles Bell], a sign of peripheral facial paralysis, manifested by the upward and outward rolling of the eyeball when the affected individual tries to close

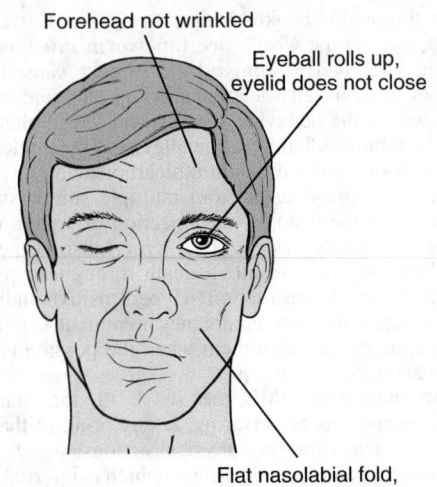

Forehead not wrinkled

Eyeball rolls up, eyelid does not close

Flat nasolabial fold, paralysis of lower face

**Bell's palsy** *(Lewis, Heitkemper, and Dirksen, 2000)*

the eyelid. It occurs on the affected side in peripheral facial paralysis.

**Bell's spasm** [Charles Bell], a convulsive facial tic.

**belly** [AS, *beig*, bag], **1.** the fleshy central bulging portion of a muscle. **2.** Informal term for **abdomen.**

**belly button.** See **umbilicus.**

**belonephobia** /bel′ənəfō′bē·ə/ [Gk, *belone*, needle, *phobos*, fear], a morbid fear of sharp-pointed objects, especially needles and pins.

**belt restraint,** a device used around the waist to secure a patient on a stretcher or in a chair.

**Benadryl,** trademark for a first-generation antihistamine (diphenhydramine hydrochloride).

**Benassi method** /bənas′ē/, a positioning procedure for producing x-ray images of the liver. With the patient in a prone position so that the liver is closer to the x-ray film, two radiographs are made from the angles of 25 degrees caudad and 10 degrees cephalad.

**Bence Jones protein** /bens/ [Henry Bence Jones, English physician, 1814–1873], a protein found almost exclusively in the urine of patients with multiple myeloma. The protein constitutes the light chain component of myeloma globulin; it coagulates at temperatures of 45° to 55° C and redissolves completely or partially on boiling. See also **multiple myeloma, protein.**

**Bence Jones protein test,** a urine test whose positive result most commonly indicates multiple myeloma. The test is used to detect and monitor the treatment and clinical course of multiple myeloma and similar diseases.

**bench research** *informal.* (in medicine) any research done in a controlled laboratory setting using nonhuman subjects.

**-bendazole,** combining form designating a tibendazole-type anthelmintic.

**Bender's Visual Motor Gestalt test** [Lauretta Bender, American psychiatrist, 1897–1987; L, *visus*, vision, *movere*, to move; Ger, *Gestalt*, form; L, *testum*, crucible], a standard psychologic test in which the subject copies a series of patterns.

**bending fracture,** a fracture indirectly caused by the bending of an extremity, such as the foot or the big toe.

**bendrofluazide.** See **bendroflumethiazide.**

**bendroflumethiazide** /ben′drōflo͞o′məthī′əzīd/, a diuretic and antihypertensive.

- INDICATIONS: It is prescribed in the treatment of hypertension and edema.
- CONTRAINDICATIONS: Anuria or known hypersensitivity to this drug, to other thiazide medication, or to sulfonamide derivatives prohibit its use.
- ADVERSE EFFECTS: Among the more serious are hypokalemia, hyperglycemia, hyperuricemia, and hypersensitivity reactions.

**bends.** See **decompression sickness.**

**Benedict's qualitative test** [Stanley R. Benedict, American biochemist, 1884–1936], a test for sugar in the urine based on the reduction by glucose of cupric ions. Formation of an orange or red precipitate indicates more than 2% sugar (called 4+), yellow indicates 1% to 2% sugar (called 3+), olive green indicates 0.5% to 1% sugar (called 2+), and green indicates less than 0.5% sugar (called 1+). It is not in common use. Also called **Benedict's method.**

**Benedict's solution** [Stanley R. Benedict], a term referring to two reagents (a qualitative and a quantitative) used in the examination of urine specimens. Both solutions contain cupric sulfate dissolved in a solution of sodium sulfate and sodium citrate in two different concentrations. When the solution is heated, the color of the resulting mixture depends on the concentration of glucose in the urine. See also **Benedict's qualitative test.**

**beneficiary** /ben′əfish′ərē/, a person or group designated to receive certain profits, benefits, or advantages, as the recipient of a will or insurance policy.

**beneficiary member.** See **enrollee.**

**benefit.** See **covered benefit.**

**Benemid,** trademark for a uricosuric (probenecid).

**benign** /binīn′/ [L, *benignus*, kind], (of a tumor) noncancerous and therefore not an immediate threat, even though treatment eventually may be required for health or cosmetic reasons. See also **benign neoplasm.** Compare **malignant.**

**benign congenital hypotonia,** a condition marked by signs of weakness and floppiness in babies, resulting from nonprogressive weakness of skeletal muscles from birth.

**benign essential tremor.** See **essential tremor.**

**benign familial chronic pemphigus** [L, *benedicere,* to bless, *familia,* household; Gk, *pemphix,* bubble], a hereditary condition of the skin characterized in the early stages by blisters that break, leaving red, eroded areas followed by crusts. Also called **Hailey-Hailey disease.**

**benign familial hematuria,** a rare, usually benign disorder characterized by abnormally thin basement membranes of the glomerular capillaries and persistent hematuria; autosomal dominant inheritance is suspected.

**benign forgetfulness,** a temporary memory block in which some fact from the recent or remote past is forgotten but later recalled.

**benign hypertension,** a misnomer implying a harmless elevation of blood pressure. Because any sustained elevation of blood pressure may adversely affect health, it is incorrect to refer to the condition as "benign." See also **essential hypertension.**

**benign intracranial hypertension.** See **pseudotumor cerebri.**

**benign juvenile melanoma,** a noncancerous pink or fuchsia raised papule with a scaly surface, usually on a cheek. Occurring most commonly in children between 9 and 13 years of age, it may be mistaken for a malignant melanoma. Also called **compound melanocytoma, spindle cell nevus, Spitz nevus.**

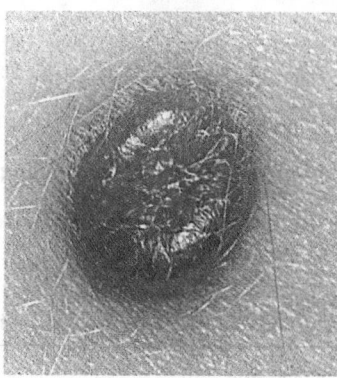

**Benign juvenile melanoma** *(Zitelli and Davis, 1997)*

**benign lymphocytic meningitis.** See **sterile meningitis.**

**benign lymphoreticulosis.** See **cat-scratch fever.**

**benign mesenchymoma** [L, *benignare* + Gk, *meso,* middle, *egchyma,* infusion, *oma,* tumor], a benign neoplasm that has two or more definitely recognizable mesenchymal elements in addition to fibrous tissue.

**benign migratory glossitis.** See **geographic tongue.**

**benign mucosal pemphigoid.** See **cicatricial pemphigoid.**

**benign myalgic encephalomyelitis.** See **postviral fatigue syndrome.**

**benign neoplasm** [L, *benignare* + Gk, *neos,* new, *plasma,* formation], a localized tumor that has a fibrous capsule, limited potential for growth, a regular shape, and cells that are well differentiated. A benign neoplasm does not invade surrounding tissue or metastasize to distant sites. Some kinds of benign neoplasms are **adenoma, fibroma, hemangioma,** and **lipoma.** Also called **benign tumor.** Compare **malignant neoplasm.**

**benign nephrosclerosis,** a renal disorder marked by arteriolosclerotic (arteriosclerosis affecting mainly the arterioles) lesions in the kidney. It is associated with hypertension.

**benign paroxysmal peritonitis.** See **familial Mediterranean fever.**

**benign prostatic hyperplasia (BPH),** nonmalignant, noninflammatory enlargement of the prostate, most common among men over 50 years of age. BPH is usually progressive and may lead to urethral obstruction and to interfer-

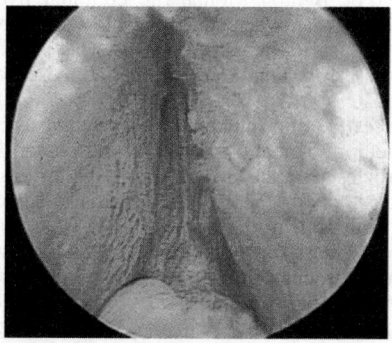

**Benign prostatic hyperplasia** *(Greig and Garden, 1996)*

ence with urine flow, urinary frequency, nocturia, dysuria, and urinary tract infections. Treatment may include medication, localized application of heat, and/or balloon dilation. Surgical resection of the enlarged prostate is sometimes necessary. Compare **prostatitis.** See also **prostatectomy.**

**benign prostatic hypertrophy** See **benign prostatic hyperplasia.**

**benign pseudohypertrophic muscular dystrophy.** See **Becker's muscular dystrophy.**

**benign stupor,** a state of apathy or lethargy, such as occurs in severe depression.

**benign thrombocytosis.** See **thrombocytosis.**

**benign tumor.** See **benign neoplasm.**

**benne oil.** See **sesame oil.**

**Benner, Patricia,** a nursing theorist who confirmed the levels of skill acquisition in nursing practice in *From Novice to Expert: Excellence and Power in Clinical Nursing Practice* (1984). Benner used systematic descriptions of five stages: novice, advanced beginner, competent, proficient, and expert. Thirty-one competencies emerged from an analysis of actual patient care episodes. From this work seven areas of nursing practice having a number of competencies with similar intents, functions, and meanings developed. They are identified as (1) the helping role, (2) the teaching-coaching function, (3) the diagnostic and patient-monitoring function, (4) effective management of rapidly changing situations, (5) administering and monitoring therapeutic interventions and regimens, (6) monitoring and ensuring the quality of health care practices, and (7) organizational work-role competencies. Benner's work describes nursing practice in the context of what nursing actually is and does rather than from context-free theoretic descriptions.

**Bennet's small corpuscle.** See **Drysdale's corpuscle.**

**Bennett angle** [Norman G. Bennett, English dentist, 1870–1947], the angle formed by the sagittal plane and the path of the advancing condyle during lateral mandibular movement, as viewed in the horizontal plane.

**Bennett hand tool test,** a test used in occupational therapy and prevocational testing to measure hand function and coordination and speed in performance.

**Bennett's fracture** [Edward H. Bennett, Irish surgeon, 1837–1907], a fracture that runs obliquely through the base of the first metacarpal bone and into the carpometacarpal joint, detaching the greater part of the articular facet. Bennett's fracture may be associated with dorsal subluxation or with dislocation of the first metacarpal.

**Benoquin,** trademark for a depigmenting agent (monobenzone).

**bent fracture.** See **greenstick fracture.**

**bentonite** [Fort Benton, Montana], colloidal, hydrated aluminum silicate that, when added to water, swells to approximately 12 times its dry size. It is used as a bulk laxative and as a base for skin care preparations. Also called **mineral soap.**

**bentonite test,** a flocculation test for the presence of rheumatoid factor in patient blood samples. After sensitized bentonite particles are added to the serum, the test result is considered positive for rheumatoid arthritis if adsorption has occurred with 50% of the particles.

**Bentyl,** trademark for an anticholinergic antispasmodic (dicyclomine hydrochloride).

**benz,** abbreviation for a *benzoate carboxylate anion.*

**benzalkonium chloride,** a disinfectant and fungicide prepared in an aqueous solution in various strengths.

**benzathine penicillin G.** See **penicillin G benzathine.**

**benzene** /ben′zēn/, a colorless, highly flammable liquid hydrocarbon ($C_6H_6$) derived by fractional distillation of coal tar. The prototypical aromatic compound, it is used in the production of various organic compounds, including pharmaceuticals.

**benzene poisoning,** a toxic condition caused by ingestion of benzene, inhalation of benzene fumes, or exposure to benzene-related products such as toluene or xylene, characterized by nausea, headache, dizziness, and incoordination. In acute cases respiratory failure or ventricular fibrillation may cause death. Chronic exposure may result in aplastic anemia (a form of leukemia). See also **nitrobenzene poisoning.**

**benzethonium chloride** /ben′zəthō′nē·əm/, a topical antiinfective used for disinfecting the skin and for treating some infections of the eye, nose, and throat. It is also used as a preservative in some pharmaceutical preparations.

**benzhexol hydrochloride.** See **trihexyphenidyl hydrochloride.**

**benzo[a]pyrene dihydrodiol epoxide (BPDE-I),** a carcinogenic derivative of benzo[a]pyrene associated with tobacco smoke.

**benzocaine** /ben′zəkān/, an ester-type, local anesthetic agent derived from aminobenzoic acid that is most useful when applied topically. It is used in many over-the-counter compounds for pruritus and pain. Benzocaine has a low incidence of toxicity, but sensitization to it may result from prolonged or frequent use. Topical application of benzocaine may cause methemoglobinemia in infants and small children. A minimum of 5% benzocaine is required in a compound to be effective.

**benzodiazepine derivative** /ben′zōdī·az′əpin/, one of a group of psychotropic agents, including the tranquilizers chlordiazepoxide, diazepam, oxazepam, lorazepam, and chlorazepate, prescribed to alleviate anxiety, and the hypnotics flurazepam and nitrazepam, prescribed in the treatment of insomnia. Tolerance and physical dependence occur with prolonged high dosage. Withdrawal symptoms, including seizures, may follow abrupt discontinuation. Adverse reactions to the benzodiazepines include drowsiness, ataxia, and a paradoxic increase in aggression and hostility; these reactions are not common with the usual recommended dosage.

**benzoic acid** /benzō′ik/, a keratolytic agent, usually used with salicylic acid as an ointment in the treatment of athlete's foot and ringworm of the scalp. It has little antifungal action but makes deep infections accessible to more potent preparation. Mild irritation may occur at the site of application.

**benzonatate** /benzō′nətāt/, a nonopiate antitussive.
- INDICATION: It is prescribed to suppress the cough reflex.
- CONTRAINDICATION: Known hypersensitivity to this drug prohibits its use.
- ADVERSE EFFECTS: Hypersensitivity reactions, such as bronchospasm, laryngospasm, and cardiovascular collapse, may occur and may be serious. Vertigo, sedation, headache, and constipation may sometimes occur.

**benzoyl peroxide** /benzō′il/, an antibacterial, keratolytic drying agent.
- INDICATION: It is prescribed in the treatment of acne.
- CONTRAINDICATIONS: Known hypersensitivity to this drug prohibits its use. It is not used in the eye, on inflamed skin, or on mucous membranes.
- ADVERSE EFFECTS: Among the more serious adverse reactions are excessive drying and allergic contact sensitization.

**benzquinamide** /benzkwin′əmīd/, an antiemetic.
- INDICATIONS: It is prescribed in the treatment of postoperative nausea and vomiting.

- CONTRAINDICATIONS: Known hypersensitivity to this drug prohibits its use. It is not usually administered to children or to pregnant women.
- ADVERSE EFFECTS: Among the most serious adverse reactions are sudden increase in blood pressure and cardiac arrhythmia. Drowsiness, chills, and shivering are commonly noted.

**benzthiazide** /benzthī′əzid/, a diuretic and antihypertensive.

- INDICATIONS: It is prescribed in the treatment of hypertension and edema.
- CONTRAINDICATIONS: Anuria or known hypersensitivity to this drug, to other thiazide medication, or to sulfonamide derivatives prohibits its use.
- ADVERSE EFFECTS: Among the more serious adverse effects are hypokalemia, hyperglycemia, hyperuricemia, and hypersensitivity reactions.

**benztropine mesylate** /benztrō′pēn/, an anticholinergic and antihistaminic agent.

- INDICATIONS: It may be prescribed as adjunctive therapy in the treatment of all forms of parkinsonism.
- CONTRAINDICATIONS: Known sensitivity to this drug prohibits its use, and it is not administered to children less than 3 years of age.
- ADVERSE EFFECTS: Among the most serious adverse reactions are blurred vision, xerostomia, nausea and vomiting, constipation, depression, and skin rash.

**benzyl alcohol** /ben′zil/, a clear, colorless, oily liquid, derived from certain balsams, used as a topical anesthetic and as a bacteriostatic agent in solutions for injection. Also called **phenyl carbinol, phenyl methanol.**

**benzyl benzoate** /benzō′āt/, a clear, oily liquid with a pleasant, pervasive aroma. It is used as an agent to destroy lice and scabies, as a solvent, and as a flavor for gum.

**benzyl carbinol.** See **phenylethyl alcohol.**

**bereavement** /bərēv′mənt/ [ME, bereven, to rob], a form of depression with anxiety symptoms that is a common reaction to the loss of a loved one. It may be accompanied by insomnia, hyperactivity, and other effects. Although bereavement does not necessarily lead to depressive illness, it may be a triggering factor in a person who is otherwise vulnerable to depression. See also **grief, mourning.**

**Berger's disease** [Jean Berger, twentieth century French nephrologist], a kidney disorder characterized by recurrent episodes of macroscopic hematuria, proteinuria, and a granular deposition of immunoglobulin A (IgA) from the glomerular mesangium. The condition may or may not progress to renal failure over a period of many years. A spontaneous remission occurs in some cases. The onset of disease is usually in childhood or early adulthood, and males are affected twice as often as females. Treatment is similar to that of other renal diseases. Also called **mesangial IgA nephropathy** /mesan′jē·əl/.

**Berger's paresthesia** [Oskar Berger, nineteenth century German neurologist; Gk, para, near, aisthesia, sensation], a condition of tingling, prickliness, or weakness and a loss of feeling in the legs without evidence of organic disease. The condition affects young people.

**Berger wave.** See **alpha wave.**

**Bergonié-Tribondeau law** /ber′gônē′tribôdō′/ [Jean A. Bergonié, French radiologist, 1857–1925; Louis F.A. Tribondeau, French physician, 1872–1918], a rule stating that the radiosensitivity of a tissue depends on the number of undifferentiated cells in the tissue, their mitotic activity, and the length of time they are actively proliferating.

**beriberi** /ber′ēber′ē/ [Sinhalese, beri, weakness], a disease of the peripheral nerves caused by a deficiency of or an in-

ability to assimilate thiamine. It frequently results from a diet limited to polished white rice, and it occurs in endemic form in eastern and southern Asia. Rare cases in the United States are associated with stressful conditions, such as hypothyroidism, infections, pregnancy, lactation, and chronic alcoholism. Symptoms are fatigue, diarrhea, appetite and weight loss, disturbed nerve function causing paralysis and wasting of limbs, edema, and heart failure. Kinds of beriberi include alcoholic beriberi, atrophic beriberi, cardiac beriberi, and cerebral beriberi. Administration of thiamine prevents and cures most cases of the disease. Also called **athiaminosis.** See also **thiamine.**

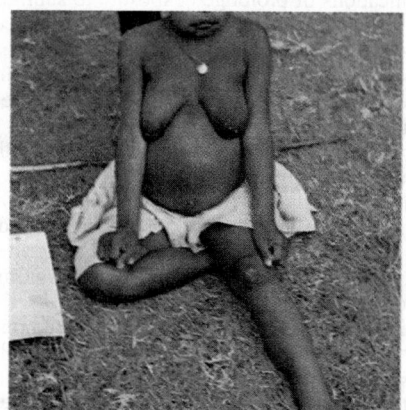

**Cardiac beriberi** (McLaren, 1992)

**berkelium (Bk)** /burk′lē·əm/ [Berkeley, California], an artificial radioactive transuranic element. Its atomic number is 97; the atomic mass of its longest-lived isotope is 247.

**berlock dermatitis** [Fr, breloque, bracelet charm], a temporary skin condition, characterized by hyperpigmentation and skin lesions. It is caused by a unique reaction to psoralen-type photosynthesizers, commonly used in per-

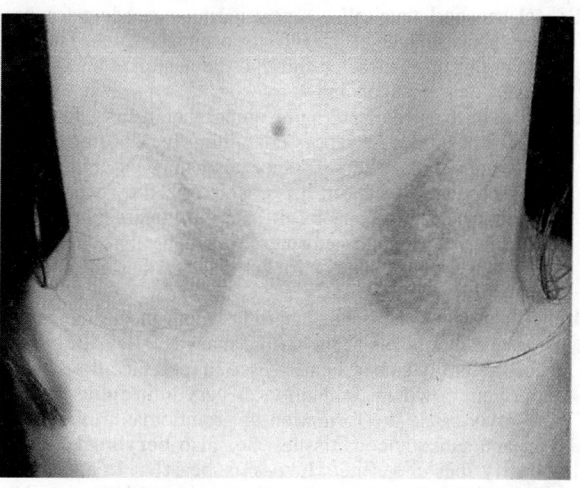

**Berlock dermatitis** (du Vivier, 1993)

fumes, colognes, and pomades, such as oil of bergamot. Also spelled **berloque dermatitis.**

■ OBSERVATIONS: Berlock dermatitis commonly produces an acute erythematous reaction, similar to that associated with sunburn. The area affected becomes hyperpigmented and surrounded by darker pigmentation. Areas of the neck where perfume containing oil of bergamot is applied often become affected by pendantlike lesions. Diagnosis is based on the appearance of such signs and on patient history, which may include recent exposure to psoralens.

■ INTERVENTIONS: Treatment seeks to identify and eliminate the cause of the condition. Topical steroids may be administered to relieve discomfort.

■ NURSING CONSIDERATIONS: Patients benefit from advice about the complications of prolonged exposure to sunlight and ultraviolet light. They also appreciate the reassurance that the lesions will vanish within a few months.

**Bernard-Soulier syndrome** /bernär′soolyā′/ [Jean A. Bernard, French hematologist, b. 1907; Jean-Pierre Soulier, French hematologist, b. 1915], a coagulation disorder characterized by an absence of or a deficiency in the ability of the platelets to aggregate because of the relative lack of an essential glycoprotein in their membranes. On microscopic examination the platelets appear large and dispersed. The use of aspirin may provoke hemorrhage. After trauma or surgery, loss of blood may be greater than normal and a transfusion may be required.

**Bernoulli's principle** /bərnoo′lēz/ [Daniel Bernoulli, Swiss scientist, 1700–1782], (in physics) the principle stating that the sum of the velocity and the kinetic energy of a fluid flowing through a tube is constant. The greater the velocity, the less the lateral pressure on the wall of the tube. Thus, if an artery is narrowed by an atherosclerotic plaque, the flow of blood through the constriction increases in velocity and decreases in lateral pressure. Also called **Bernoulli's law.**

**Bernoulli theorem** /bər·noo′lē/, in an experiment involving probability, the larger the number of trials, the closer the observed probability of an event approaches its theoretical probability.

**berry aneurysm** [ME, berye + Gk, aneurysma, widening], a small, saccular dilation of the wall of a cerebral artery. It occurs most frequently at the junctures of vessels in the circle of Willis. A berry aneurysm may be the result of a congenital developmental defect and may rupture without warning, causing intracranial hemorrhage. Smoking and hypertension increase the likelihood of rupture.

**Bertel method** /bur′təl/, a positioning procedure for producing x-ray images of the inferior orbital fissures. The central x-ray beam is directed through the nasion at an angle of 20 to 25 degrees cephalad.

**berylliosis** /bəril′ē·ō′sis/, poisoning that results from the inhalation of dusts or vapors containing beryllium or beryllium compounds. The substance also may enter the body through or under the skin. It is characterized by granulomas throughout the body and by diffuse pulmonary fibrosis, resulting in a dry cough, shortness of breath, and chest pain. Symptoms may not appear for several years after exposure. See also **inorganic dust.**

**beryllium (Be),** a steel-gray, lightweight metallic element. Its atomic number is 4; its atomic mass is 9.012. Beryllium occurs naturally as beryl and is used in metallic alloys and in fluorescent powders. Inhalation of beryllium fumes or particles may cause the formation of granulomas in the lungs, skin, and subcutaneous tissues. See also **berylliosis.**

**bestiality** /bes′chē·al′itē/ [L, bestia, beast], **1.** a brutal or animal-like character or nature. **2.** conduct or behavior characterized by beastlike appetites or instincts. **3.** also called

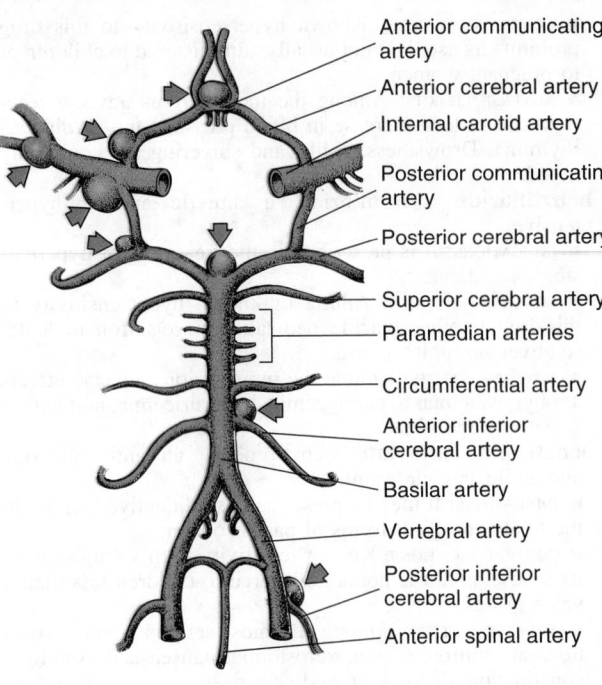

Anterior communicating artery

Anterior cerebral artery

Internal carotid artery

Posterior communicating artery

Posterior cerebral artery

Superior cerebral artery

Paramedian arteries

Circumferential artery

Anterior inferior cerebral artery

Basilar artery

Vertebral artery

Posterior inferior cerebral artery

Anterior spinal artery

**Common sites of berry aneurysms** *(Rudy, 1984)*

**zooerastia** /zoo·əras′tē·ə/. sexual relations between a human being and an animal. **4.** sodomy. See also **zoophilia.**

**besylate,** a contraction for benzenesulfonate.

**beta** /bē′tə, bā′tə/, B, β, the second letter of the Greek alphabet, used in scientific notation to denote position of a carbon atom in a molecule, a type of protein configuration, or identification of a type of activity, as beta blocker, beta particle, or beta rhythm. It is used in statistics to define an error in the interpretation of study results.

**beta-adrenergic blocking agent.** See **antiadrenergic.**

**beta-adrenergic receptor.** See **beta receptor.**

**beta-adrenergic stimulating agent.** See **adrenergic.**

**beta-alaninemia** /-al′əninē′mē·ə/, an inherited metabolic disorder marked by a deficiency of an enzyme, beta-alanine-alpha-ketoglutarate aminotransferase. The clinical signs include seizures, drowsiness, and, if uncorrected, death. The condition is sometimes treated with vitamin $B_6$ (pyridoxine).

**beta-blocker,** a popular term for beta-adrenergic blocking (or beta receptor antagonist) agent. See **antiadrenergic.**

**beta-carotene** [Gk, beta; L, carota, carrot], a vitamin A precursor and ultraviolet screening agent.

■ INDICATION: It is prescribed to ameliorate photosensitivity in patients with erythropoietic protoporphyria.

■ CONTRAINDICATIONS: It is used with caution in patients with impaired renal or hepatic function. Known hypersensitivity to this drug prohibits its use.

■ ADVERSE EFFECTS: No serious adverse reactions have been observed. Diarrhea may occur.

**beta cells,** **1.** insulin-producing cells situated in the islets of Langerhans. Their insulin-producing function tends to accelerate the movement of glucose, amino acids, and fatty acids out of the blood and into the cellular cytoplasm, countering glucagon function of alpha cells. **2.** the basophilic cells of the anterior lobe of the pituitary gland.

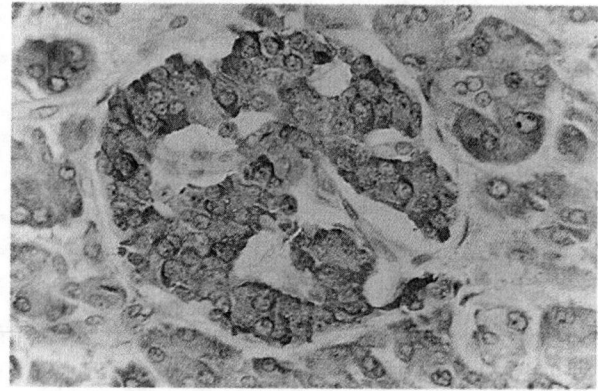

**Beta cells in a normal islet** *(Bloom and Ireland, 1992)*

**beta decay,** a type of radioactivity that results in the emission of beta particles, either electrons or positrons. See **beta particle.**

**Betadine,** trademark for a topical antiinfective (povidone-iodine).

**beta error.** See **type II error.**

**beta-fetoprotein,** a protein found in fetal liver and in some adults with liver disease. It is now known to be identical with normal liver ferritin. See also **alpha-fetoprotein, ferritin, fetoprotein.**

**beta-galactosidase.** See **lactase.**

**Betagan,** trademark for a topical glaucoma drug (levobunolol hydrochloride).

**beta hemolysis,** the development of a clear zone around a bacterial colony growing on blood agar medium, characteristic of certain pathogenic bacteria. Compare **alpha hemolysis.**

**beta-hemolytic streptococci,** the pyogenic streptococci of groups A, B, C, E, F, G, H, K, L, M, and O that cause hemolysis of red blood cells in blood agar in the laboratory. These organisms cause most of the acute streptococcal infections seen in humans, including scarlet fever, many cases of pneumonia and sepsis syndrome, and streptococcal sore throat. Penicillin is usually prescribed to treat these infections when they are suspected, even before the results of the bacteriologic culture are available, because it is known that these organisms as a group are usually sensitive to the effects of penicillin and because the sequelae of untreated streptococcal infection may include glomerulonephritis and rheumatic fever.

**beta-hydroxyisovaleric aciduria,** an inherited metabolic disease caused by a deficiency of an enzyme needed to metabolize the amino acid leucine. The condition results in an accumulation of leucine in the tissues, causing maple sugar odor to the urine, ketoacidosis, retardation, and muscle atrophy. See also **maple syrup urine disease.**

**beta$_2$-interferon.** See **interleukin-6.**

**beta-ketobutyric acid.** See **acetoacetic acid.**

**beta-lactamase** /-lak'təmāz/ [*lactam,* a cyclic amide, *ase,* enzyme], a bacterial enzyme that catalyzes the hydrolysis of the beta-lactam ring of some penicillins and cephalosporins, producing penicilloic acid and rendering the antibiotic ineffective. Also called **cephalosporinase, penicillinase.**

**beta-lactamase resistance.** See **beta-lactamase-resistant antibiotics.**

**beta-lactamase-resistant antibiotics,** antibiotics that are resistant to the enzymatic effects of **beta-lactamase.**

**beta-lactamase-resistant penicillin.** See **beta-lactamase-resistant antibiotics.**

**betamethasone valerate,** a glucocorticoid.

■ INDICATION: It is prescribed for topical corticosteroid-responsive dermatoses.

■ CONTRAINDICATIONS: Systemic fungal infections, dermatologic viral and fungal infections, impaired circulation, or known hypersensitivity to this drug prohibits its use.

■ ADVERSE EFFECTS: Among the more serious adverse reactions associated with prolonged use of the drug are GI, endocrine, neurologic, and fluid and electrolyte disturbances.

**beta-naphthylamine** /-nafthil'əmēn/, an aromatic amine used in aniline dyes and a cause of bladder cancer in humans.

**beta-oxidation,** a catabolic process in which fatty acids are used by the body as a source of energy. The fatty acid molecules are converted through a series of intermediates into acetylcoenzyme A molecules, which then enter the tricarboxylic acid (TCA) cycle along with metabolites of carbohydrates and proteins.

**Betapar,** trademark for a glucocorticoid (meprednisone).

**beta particle,** an electron emitted from the nucleus of an atom during radioactive decay of the atom. Beta particles have a range of 10 m in air and 1 mm in soft tissue. Also called **beta ray.**

**Betapen-VK,** trademark for an antibiotic (penicillin V potassium).

**beta phase,** the period immediately following the alpha, or redistribution, phase of drug administration. During the beta phase the blood level of the drug falls more slowly as it is metabolized and excreted from the body.

**beta rays,** a stream of beta particles, as emitted from atoms of disintegrating radioactive elements. Normally, when the element is a nuclide with a high ratio of neutrons to protons, the beta particle is an electron.

**beta receptor,** any one of the postulated adrenergic (sympathetic fibers of autonomic nervous system) components of receptor tissues that respond to epinephrine and such blocking agents as propranolol. Activation of beta receptors causes various physiologic reactions such as relaxation of the bronchial muscles and an increase in the rate and force of cardiac contraction. Also called **beta-adrenergic receptor.** Compare **alpha receptor.**

**beta rhythm.** See **beta wave.**

**beta-thalassemia,** an anemia that is caused by diminished synthesis of beta chains of hemoglobin. The homozygous form is known as thalassemia major and the heterozygous form is known as thalassemia minor. See **thalassemia.**

**betatron** /bā'tətron/, a cyclic accelerator that produces high-energy electrons for radiotherapy. The magnetic field of the betatron deflects electrons into a circular orbit, and an increasing magnetic orbital flux produces an induced circumferential electric field that accelerates them.

**beta wave,** one of the four types of brain waves, characterized by relatively low voltage and a frequency of more than 13 Hz. Beta waves are the "busy waves" of the brain, recorded by electroencephalograph from the frontal and the central areas of the cerebrum when the patient is awake and alert with eyes open. Also called **beta rhythm.** Compare **alpha wave, delta wave, theta wave.**

**betaxolol hydrochloride** /betak'səlol/, a topical drug for open-angle glaucoma (Betoptic). An oral preparation (Kerlone) is indicated for the management of hypertension.

■ INDICATIONS: It is prescribed for the relief of ocular hypertension and chronic open-angle glaucoma (ophthalmic) and for the management of hypertension (oral).

■ CONTRAINDICATIONS: Betaxolol hydrochloride is contraindicated in patients with sinus bradycardia, greater than first-degree atrioventricular (AV) block, cardiogenic shock, and overt heart failure. The ophthalmic preparation is used with caution by patients who are also receiving oral beta-adrenergic blocking drugs.

■ ADVERSE EFFECTS: Adverse reactions include stinging and tearing of the eyes. Systemic effects are rare. Adverse effects of the oral preparation are bradycardia, fatigue, dyspnea, and lethargy.

**bethanechol chloride** /bethan'əkol/,　a cholinergic.

■ INDICATIONS: It is prescribed in the treatment of fecal and urinary retention and neurogenic atony of the bladder.

■ CONTRAINDICATIONS: Uncertain strength of the bladder, obstruction of the GI or urinary tract, hyperthyroidism, peptic ulcer, bronchial asthma, cardiovascular disease, epilepsy, Parkinson's disease, hypotension, or known hypersensitivity to this drug prohibits its use. It is not given during pregnancy. It is never given intramuscularly or intravenously.

■ ADVERSE EFFECTS: Among the more serious adverse reactions are flushing, headache, GI distress, diarrhea, excessive salivation, sweating, and hypotension.

**Betopic,**　trademark for a topical glaucoma medication (betaxolol hydrochloride).

**Betz cells** [Vladimir A. Betz, Russian anatomist, 1834–1894; L, *cella,* storeroom],　large pyramidal neurons of the motor cortex with axons that form part of the pyramidal tract associated with voluntary movements.

**bevel** /bev'əl/ [OFr, *baif,* open mouth angle],　**1.** any angle, other than a right angle, between two planes or surfaces. **2.** (in dentistry) any angle other than 90 degrees between a tooth cut and a cavity wall in the preparation of a tooth cavity. Compare **cavosurface bevel, contra bevel.**

**bexarotene,**　a second-generation retinoid.

■ INDICATIONS: This drug is prescribed for cutaneous T-cell lymphoma. Investigational uses include treatment of breast cancer.

■ CONTRAINDICATIONS: Pregnancy and known hypersensitivity to retinoids prohibit bexarotene's use.

■ ADVERSE EFFECTS: Life-threatening adverse reactions include acute pancreatitis, leukopenia, and neutropenia. Other serious side effects include asthenia, infection, anemia, and hypothyroidism. Among the drug's common side effects are headache, nausea, abdominal pain, and diarrhea.

**bezoar** /bē'zôr/ [Ar, *bazahr,* protection against poison],　a hard ball of hair or vegetable fiber that may develop within the stomach of humans. More often it is found in the stom-

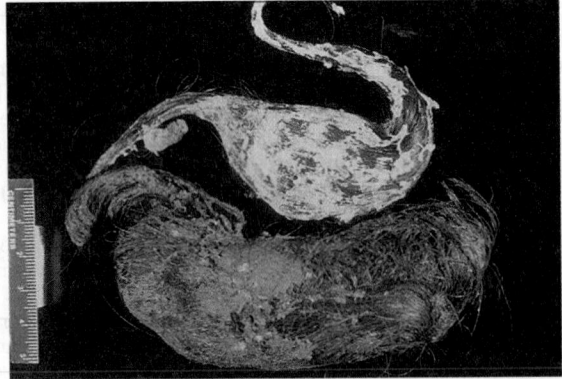

**Bezoar** *(Cotran, Kumar, and Collins, 1999)*

achs of ruminants. In some societies it was formerly considered a useful medicine and possessed of certain magical properties. It is apparently still used as a therapeutic and mystical device by some, especially in the Far East.

**B/F,**　abbreviation for *black female,* often used in the initial identifying statement in a patient record.

**Bg blood group,**　a blood group consisting of the erythrocytic HLA antigens Bg$^a$, Bg$^b$, Bg$^c$, DBG, Ho, Ho-like, Ot, and Sto.

**Bh,**　symbol for the element **Bohrium.**

**bhang** /bang/ [Hindi, *bag*],　an Asian Indian hallucinogenic, composed of dried leaves and the young stems of uncultivated *Cannabis sativa.* It is usually ingested as a boiled mixture with milk, sugar, or water; it produces euphoria. It also may be smoked or chewed. Also spelled **bang.** See also **cannabis.**

**Bi,**　symbol for the element **bismuth.**

**bi-,**　prefix meaning 'twice, two': *biarticular, bicaudal.*

**BIA,**　abbreviation for **bioelectric impedance analysis.**

**-bia,**　suffix meaning 'creature possessing a mode of life': *aerobia.*

**biarticular.**　See **diarticular.**

**bias** /bī'əs/ [MFr, *biais*],　**1.** an oblique or a diagonal line. **2.** a prejudiced or subjective attitude. **3.** (in statistics) the distortion of statistical findings. There can be many kinds of bias; some may be caused by the sampling process, but bias can be caused by other factors. **4.** (in electronics) a voltage applied to an electronic device, such as a vacuum tube or a transistor, to control operating limits. See also **detection bias.**

**biased sample** /bī'əst/ [OFr, *biais,* slant; L, *exemplum,* sample],　(in research) a sample of a group in which all factors or participants are not equally balanced or objectively represented.

**biasing** /bī'əsing/,　a method of treating neuromuscular dysfunction by contracting a muscle against resistance, causing the muscle spindles to readjust to the shorter length and the muscle tissue to be more responsive and sensitive to stretching.

**biauricular** /bī'aw·rik'yōō·lər/ [L, *bis,* twice + *auriculus,* little ear],　pertaining to the two auricles of the ears. Also called **binauricular.**

**Biavax,**　trademark for a rubella and mumps vaccine.

**bibliotherapy**[1],　a type of group therapy in which books, poems, and newspaper articles are read in the group to help stimulate thinking about events in the real world and to foster relations among group members.

**bibliotherapy**[2],　a nursing intervention from the Nursing Interventions Classification (NIC) defined as use of literature to enhance the expression of feelings and the gaining of insight. See also **Nursing Interventions Classification.**

**bicalutamide,**　an anticancer chemotherapy agent.

■ INDICATIONS: It is prescribed in the treatment of metastatic prostate cancer. The drug acts by binding to androgen receptors within target cells, preventing androgens from binding to them.

■ CONTRAINDICATIONS: The drug should not be given to patients who have an allergic reaction to it. Bicalutamide should be used with caution in patients with moderate to severe liver dysfunction.

■ ADVERSE EFFECTS: The side effects most often reported include hot flashes, general body pain, asthenia, constipation, nausea, and diarrhea.

**bicameral** /bī·kam'ər·əl/ [L, *bis,* twice + *camera,* vaulted chamber],　having two chambers.

**bicameral abscess** /bīkam'ərəl/,　an abscess with two pockets.

**bicapsular** /bī·kap′sȳoo·lər/ [L, *bis,* twice + *capsula,* little box], having two capsules, as an articular capsule.

**bicarbonate (HCO₃⁻)** /bīkär′bənāt/ [L, *bis,* twice, *carbo,* coal], an anion of carbonic acid in which only one of the hydrogen atoms has been removed, as in sodium bicarbonate ($NaHCO_3$). It is also called hydrogencarbonate.

**bicarbonate of soda.** See **sodium bicarbonate.**

**bicarbonate precursor,** an injection of sodium lactate used in the treatment of metabolic acidosis. It is metabolized in the body to sodium bicarbonate.

**bicarbonate therapy,** a procedure to increase a patient's stores of bicarbonate when there are signs of severe acidosis. It is usually performed only in certain cases and as a stopgap measure to neutralize acidosis partially when the patient's blood pH has fallen to levels that may be hazardous to the survival of vital tissues.

**bicarbonate transport,** the route by which most of the carbon dioxide is carried in the bloodstream. Once dissolved in the blood plasma, carbon dioxide combines with water to form carbonic acid, which immediately ionizes into hydrogen and bicarbonate ions. The bicarbonate ions serve as part of the alkaline reserve.

**bicellular** /bī·sel′yoo·lər/ [L, *bis,* twice + *cella,* storeroom], made up of two cells, or having two cells.

**biceps brachii** /bī′seps brā′kē·ī/ [L, *bis,* twice, *caput,* head, *bracchii,* arm], the long fusiform muscle of the upper arm on the anterior surface of the humerus, arising in two heads from the scapula. It flexes the arm and the forearm and supinates the hand. Also called **biceps, biceps flexor cubiti.** Compare **brachialis, triceps brachii.**

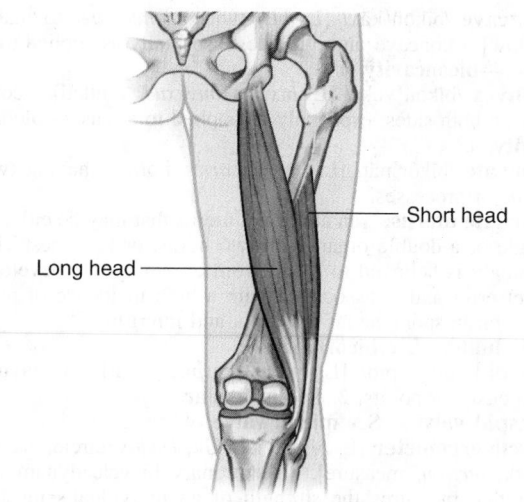

**Biceps femoris**

**biceps flexor cubiti.** See **biceps brachii.**

**biceps reflex,** a contraction of a biceps muscle produced when the tendon is tapped with a percussor in testing deep tendon reflexes. See also **deep tendon reflex.**

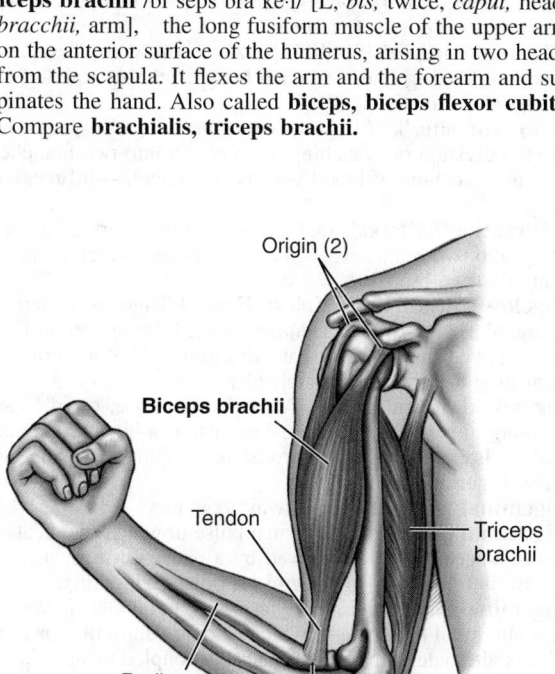

**Biceps brachii** (Herlihy and Maebius, 2000)

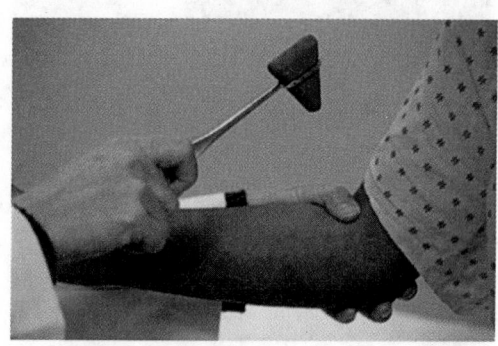

**Biceps reflex testing** (Seidel et al, 1999)

**biceps femoris** [L, *bis,* twice, *caput,* head, *femoris,* thigh], one of the posterior femoral muscles. It has two heads at its origin. The biceps femoris flexes the leg and rotates it laterally and extends the thigh, rotating it laterally. It is one of the **hamstring muscle** group and lies on the posterior, lateral side of the thigh.

**Bichat's membrane** /bishäz/ [Marie F.X. Bichat, French anatomist, 1771–1802], an elastic lining beneath the endothelium of an arterial wall.

**bicipital groove** /bīsip′ətəl/ [L, *bis,* twice, *caput,* head; D, *groeve*], a groove between the greater and lesser tubercles of the humerus for passage of the tendon of the long head of the biceps muscle.

**Bickerdyke** /bik′ərdīk/, **Mary Ann** (1817–1901), an American nurse who, after taking a short course in homeopathy, cared for the sick and wounded on battlefields during the U.S. Civil War. She insisted on cleanliness, good food, and the best of medical care for her patients. At night she searched the battlefield with a lantern for survivors.

**biclor** /bī′klôr/, abbreviation for a *bichloride noncarboxylate anion.*

**biconcave** /bīkon′kāv/ [L, *bis,* twice, *concavare,* to make hollow], concave on both sides, especially as applied to a lens. —**biconcavity,** *n.*

**biconvex** /bīkon′veks/ [L, *bis* + *convexus,* vaulted], convex on both sides, especially as applied to a lens. —**biconvexity,** *n.*

**bicornate** /bīkôr′nāt/ [L, *bis* + *cornu,* horn], having two horns or processes.

**bicornate uterus,** an abnormal uterus that may be either a single or a double organ with two horns, or branches. The anomaly is believed to result from an embryonic development error and is associated with a high incidence of preterm birth, spontaneous abortion, and infertility.

**bicornuate.** See **bicornate.**

**bicuspid** /bīkus′pid/ [L, *bis* + *cuspis,* point], **1.** having two cusps or points. **2.** See **premolar.**

**bicuspid valve.** See **mitral valve.**

**bicycle ergometer** [L, *bis,* twice; Gk, *kyklos,* circle, *ergon,* work, *metron,* measure], a stationary bicycle dynamometer that measures the strength of an individual's muscle contraction.

**b.i.d.,** (in prescriptions) abbreviation for *bis in die* /dē′ā/, a Latin phrase meaning 'twice a day.'

**bidactyly** /bīdak′tilē/ [L, *bis* + Gk, *daktylos,* finger], an abnormal condition in which the second, third, and fourth digits on a hand are missing and only the first and fifth are present. Also called **lobster claw deformity.** —**bidactylous,** *adj.*

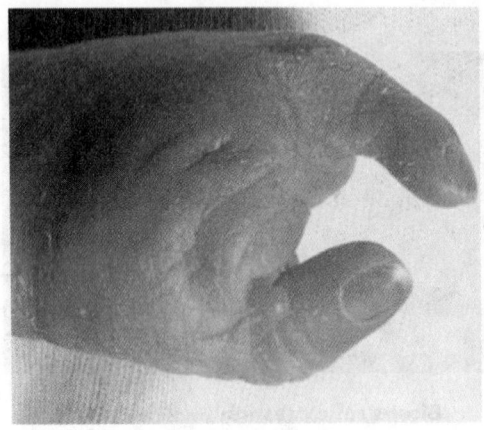

**Bidactyly**
*(Zitelli and Davis, 1997/courtesy Dr. Christine L. Williams, New York Medical College)*

**bidermoma** /bī′dərmō′mə/, *pl.* **bidermomas, bidermomata** [L, *bis* + Gk, *derma,* skin, *oma,* tumor], a teratoid neoplasm composed of cells and tissues originating in two germ layers.

**bidet** /bidā′/ [Fr, pony], a fixture resembling a toilet bowl, with a rim to sit on and usually equipped with plumbing implements for cleaning the genital and rectal areas.

**biduotertian fever** /bī′doo·ətur′shən/ [L, *bis* + *dies,* day, *tertius,* three], a form of malaria characterized by overlapping paroxysms of chills, fever, and other symptoms. It is caused by infection with two strains of *Plasmodium,* each having its own cycle of symptoms, such as in quartan and tertian malaria. Compare **double quartan fever.** See also **malaria.**

**Bier block** /bēr blok/ [August Karl Gustav Bier, German surgeon, 1861−1949], regional anesthesia by IV injection, used for surgical procedures on the arm below the elbow or the leg below the knee; performed in a bloodless field maintained by a pneumatic tourniquet that also prevents the anesthetic from entering the systemic circulation.

**bifid** /bī′fid/ [L, *bis* + *findere* to cleave], cleft, or split into two parts, as in the spinous processes of the cervical vertebrae.

**bifid tongue** [L, *bis* + *findere,* to cleave; AS, *tunge*], a tongue divided by a longitudinal furrow. Also called **cleft tongue.**

**bifocal** /bīfō′kəl/ [L, *bis* + *focus,* hearth], **1.** pertaining to the characteristic of having two foci. **2.** (of a lens) having two areas of different focal lengths.

**bifocal contact lens,** a contact lens that contains corrections for both near and far vision.

**bifocal glasses** [L, *bis,* twice, *focus,* hearth; AS, *glaes*], eyeglasses in which each lens has two foci to permit both near and far vision.

**biforate** /bīfôr′āt/ [L, *bis* + *forare,* to pierce twice], having two perforations or foramina.

**bifrontal suture** /bīfron′təl/ [L, *bis* + *frons,* front, *sutura*], the interlocking lines of fusion between the frontal and parietal bones of the skull.

**bifurcate** /bīfur′kāt/ [L, *bis,* twice, *furca,* fork], pertaining to the division or branching of an object into two branches, as the branching of blood vessels or bronchi. —**bifurcated,** *adj.*

**bifurcation** /bī′fərkā′shən/ [L, *bis* + *furca,* fork], a splitting into two branches, such as the trachea, which branches into the two bronchi.

**Bigelow's lithotrite** /big′əlōz/ [Henry J. Bigelow, American surgeon, 1818–1890; Gk, *lithos,* stone; L, *terere,* to rub], a long-jawed instrument, passed through the urethra, for crushing a calculus in the bladder.

**bigeminal** /bījem′inəl/ [L, *bis,* twice, *geminus,* twin], pertaining to pairs, twins, or dual events, as a bigeminal pulse, which is characterized by two beats in rapid succession. See also **bigeminy.**

**bigeminal pregnancy,** a twin pregnancy.

**bigeminal pulse,** an abnormal pulse in which two beats in close succession are followed by a pause during which no pulse is felt. See also **trigeminal pulse, trigeminy.**

**bigeminal rhythm** [L, *bis* + *geminus,* twin; Gk, *rhythmos*], an abnormal heartbeat in which ectopic ventricular or atrial beats alternate with and are precisely coupled to sinus beats, or in which ventricular ectopic, beats occur in pairs, as in ventricular tachycardia with 3:2 exit block. Also called **bigeminy, coupled rhythm.**

**bigeminy** /bījem′inē/ [L, *bis* + *geminus,* twin], **1.** an association in pairs. **2.** See **bigeminal rhythm.** —**bigeminal,** *adj.*

**bilabe** /bī′lāb/ [L, *bis* + *labium,* lip], a narrow forceps used to remove small calculi from the bladder by way of the urethra.

**bilabial** /bī·lā′bē·əl/, a consonantal speech sound produced using the two lips, such as *b, p,* or *m.* Also called **labial.**

**bilaminar** /bīlam′ənər/ [L, *bis* + *lamina,* plate], pertaining to or having two layers, such as the basal lamina and the reticular lamina that constitute the basement membrane of the epithelium.

**bilaminar blastoderm,** the stage of embryonic development before mesoderm formation in which only the ectoderm and entoderm primary germ layers have formed. Compare **trilaminar blastoderm.**

**bilateral** /bilat′ərəl/ [L, *bis* + *lateralis,* side], **1.** having two sides. **2.** occurring or appearing on two sides. A patient with bilateral hearing loss may have partial or total hearing loss in both ears. **3.** having two layers.

**bilateral carotid artery** [L, *bis,* twice, *latus,* side; Gk, *karos,* heavy sleep], a main artery to the head and neck that divides into left and right branches and again into external and internal branches.

**bilateral lithotomy** [L, *bis,* twice, *latus,* side; Gk, *lithos,* stone, *temnein,* to cut], a surgical procedure for removing urinary tract stones from the bladder by making transverse perineal incisions through the lateral lobes of the prostate.

**bilateral long-leg spica cast,** an orthopedic device of plaster of paris, fiberglass, or other casting material that encases and immobilizes the trunk cranially as far as the nipple line and both legs caudally as far as the toes. A horizontal crossbar to improve immobilization connects the parts of the cast encasing both legs at ankle level. It is used to aid the healing of fractures of the hip, the femur, the acetabulum, and the pelvis and to correct hip deformities. Compare **one-and-a-half spica cast, unilateral long-leg spica cast.**

**bilateral strabismus** [L, *bis* + *latus,* side; Gk, *strabismos*], an eye disorder, characterized by bilateral squint, which is caused by a failure of ocular accommodation.

**bilateral symmetry** [L, *bis* + *latus,* side; Gk, *syn,* together, *metron,* measure], similar structure of the halves of an organism.

**Bilbao tube** /bilbō′ə/, a long, thin, flexible tube that is used to inject barium into the small intestine. The tube is guided with a stiff wire from the mouth to the end of the duodenum under fluoroscopic control.

**bilberry,** an herb found in the central, Northern, and Southeastern regions of Europe.
■ USES: This herb is used for diabetic retinopathy, macular degeneration, glaucoma, cataract, capillary fragility, varicose veins, hemorrhoids, and mild diarrhea.
■ CONTRAINDICATIONS: Bilberry should not be used during pregnancy and lactation or in children until more research is available.

**bile** /bīl/ [L, *bilis*], a bitter, yellow-green secretion of the liver. Stored in the gallbladder, bile receives its color from the presence of bile pigments such as bilirubin. Bile passes from the gallbladder through the common bile duct in response to the cholecystokinin (CCK) produced in the duodenum in the presence of a fatty meal. Bile emulsifies these fats (breaks them into smaller particles and lowers the surface tension), preparing them for further digestion and absorption in the small intestine. Any interference in the flow of bile will result in the presence of unabsorbed fat in the feces and in jaundice. Also called **gall.** See also **biliary obstruction, jaundice. —biliary,** *adj.*

**bile acid,** a steroid acid of the bile, produced during the metabolism of cholesterol. On hydrolysis, bile acid yields glycine and choleic acid.

**bile duct.** See **biliary duct.**

**bile duct abscess,** a cavity containing pus and surrounded by inflamed tissue in the bile duct.

**bile pigments,** a group of substances that contribute to the colors of bile, which may range from a yellowish green to brown. A common bile pigment is bilirubin, which contains a reddish iron pigment derived from the breakdown of old red blood cells.

**bile salts** [L, *bilis,* bile; AS, *sealt*], a mixture of sodium salts of the bile acids and chollic and chenodeoxycholic acids synthesized in the liver as a derivative of cholesterol. Their low surface tension contributes to the emulsification of fats in the intestine and their absorption from the GI tract.

**bile solubility test,** a bacteriologic test used in the differential diagnosis of pneumococcal and streptococcal infection. A broth culture of each organism is placed into two tubes. Ox bile is added to one and salt to the other. Pneumococci dissolve in ox bile, producing a clear solution; because streptococci do not dissolve, the resulting solution is cloudy. The tube with salt is used for comparative purposes.

***Bilharzia.*** See *Schistosoma.*

**bilharziasis.** See **schistosomiasis.**

**bili-,** prefix meaning 'bile': *biliary, bilifuscin.*

**biliary** /bil′ē·er′ē/, pertaining to bile or to the gallbladder and bile ducts, which transport bile. These are often called the **biliary tract** or the **biliary system.** Also **bilious.** See also **bile, biliary calculus.**

**biliary abscess,** an abscess of the gallbladder or liver.

**biliary atresia,** congenital absence or underdevelopment of one or more of the biliary structures, causing jaundice and early liver damage. As the condition worsens, the child's growth may be retarded, and portal hypertension may develop. Surgery can correct the defective ducts in only a small percentage of cases. Liver transplantation is an option. Most infants die in early childhood from biliary cirrhosis. It is essential to distinguish between this condition and neonatal hepatitis, which is treatable. See also **biliary cirrhosis.**

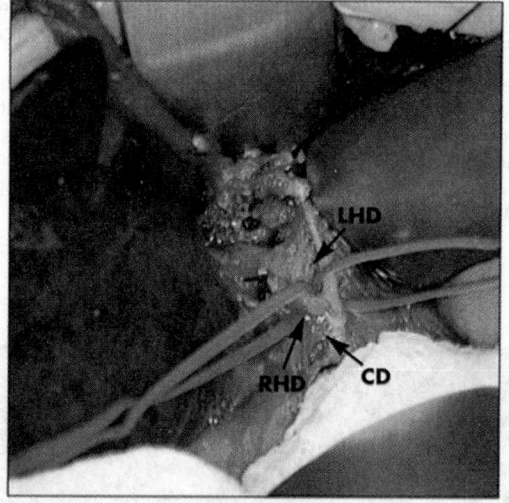

**Biliary atresia: *LHD,* left hepatic duct;**
***RHD,* right hepatic duct**
*(Greig and Garden, 1996)*

**biliary calculus** [L, *bilis,* bile, *calculus,* pebble], a stone formed in the biliary tract, consisting of cholesterol or bile pigments and calcium salts. Biliary calculi may cause jaundice, right upper quadrant pain, obstruction, and inflammation of the gallbladder. If stones cannot pass spontaneously into the duodenum, cholangiography or similar processes

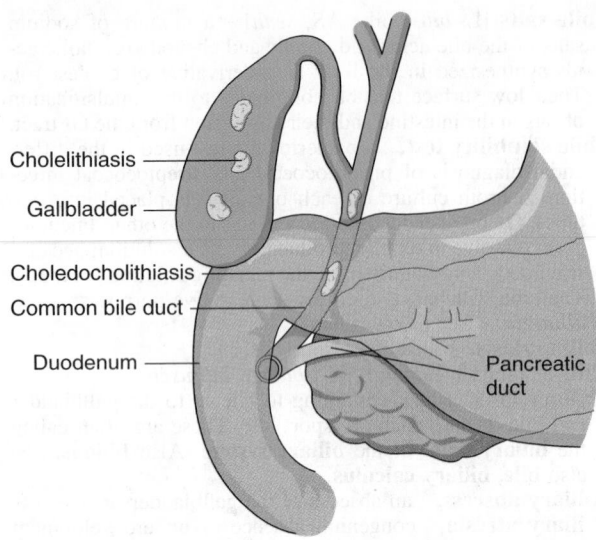

Cholelithiasis

Gallbladder

Choledocholithiasis

Common bile duct

Duodenum

Pancreatic duct

**Common locations of biliary calculi**
*(Beare and Myers, 1998)*

will reveal their location, and they can be removed surgically. Also called **choledocholithiasis, gallstones.** See also **cholangitis, cholecystitis, cholelithiasis.**

**biliary cirrhosis** [L, *bilis* + *kirrhos,* yellow-orange, *osis,* condition], an inflammatory condition in which the flow of bile through the ductules of the liver is obstructed. Primary biliary cirrhosis most commonly affects women in their middle years, and its cause is unknown. It is characterized by itching, jaundice, steatorrhea, and enlargement of the liver and spleen. The disease is slowly progressive. There is no specific medical or surgical treatment. Care must be taken to rule out secondary biliary cirrhosis caused by obstruction of the biliary structures outside the liver, because the latter condition can be treated successfully. Compare **biliary calculus, biliary obstruction.**

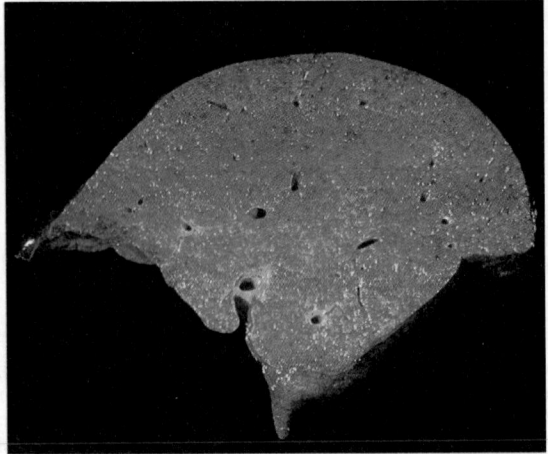

**Biliary cirrhosis** *(Kumar, Cotran, and Robbins, 1997)*

**biliary colic** [L, *bilis* + *kolikos,* colon pain], a type of smooth muscle or visceral pain specifically associated with the passing of stones through the bile ducts. Also called **cholecystalgia.** See also **biliary calculus.**

**biliary duct,** one of the muscular ducts through which bile passes from the liver and gallbladder to the duodenum. See also **common bile duct.**

**biliary dyskinesia,** an abnormal condition caused by a dysfunction of the sphincter of Oddi, disrupting the flow of bile from the gallbladder.

**biliary dyspepsia,** a digestive upset caused by an inadequate flow of bile into the duodenum.

**biliary fistula,** an abnormal passage from the gallbladder, a bile duct, or the liver to an internal organ or the surface of the body. Biliary fistulae into the duodenum may complicate cholelithiasis; a gallstone may become impacted, usually in the ileocecal valve, and cause intestinal obstruction.

**biliary glands.** See **glands of bile duct.**

**biliary obstruction,** blockage of the common or cystic bile duct, usually caused by one or more gallstones. It impedes bile drainage and produces an inflammatory reaction. Less common causes of biliary obstruction include choledochal cysts, pancreatic and duodenal tumors, Crohn's disease, pancreatitis, echinococcosis, ascariasis, and sclerosing cholangitis. Stones, consisting chiefly of cholesterol, bile pigment, and calcium, may form in the gallbladder and in the hepatic duct in persons of either sex at any age but are more common in middle-aged women. Increased amounts of serum cholesterol in the blood, such as occurs in obesity, diabetes, hypothyroidism, biliary stasis, and inflammation of the biliary system, promote gallstone formation. Cholelithiasis may be asymptomatic until a stone lodges in a biliary duct, but the patient usually has a history of indigestion and discomfort after eating fatty foods.

■ OBSERVATIONS: Biliary obstruction is characterized by severe epigastric pain, often radiating to the back and shoulder, nausea, vomiting, and profuse diaphoresis. The dehydrated patient may have chills; fever; jaundice; clay-colored stools; dark, concentrated urine; an electrolyte imbalance; and a tendency to bleed because the absence of bile prevents the synthesis and absorption of fat-soluble vitamin K.

■ INTERVENTIONS: The patient is placed in bed in a semi-Fowler's position and is usually administered intermittent nasogastric suctioning, parenteral fluids with electrolytes and fat-soluble vitamins, and medication for pain. Antibiotics, anticholinergic and antispasmodic drugs, and a cholecystogram or ultrasound scan may be ordered. The blood pressure, temperature, pulse, and respirations are monitored, and the patient is helped to turn, cough, and deep breathe every 2 to 4 hours. Fluid intake and output are measured, and the color and character of urine and stools are noted. When the nasogastric tube is removed, the patient initially receives a low-fat liquid diet and progresses to a soft or normal diet, as tolerated; up to 2500 ml of fluids a day are encouraged or administered intravenously, unless contraindicated. Cholecystectomy is usually the definitive treatment, but in most cases surgery is delayed until the patient's condition is stabilized and any prothrombin deficiency (caused by vitamin K malabsorption) is corrected.

**biliary system.** See **biliary.**

**biliary tract** [L, *bilis,* bile, *tractus*], the pathway for bile flow from the canaliculi in the liver to the opening of the bile duct into the duodenum.

**biliary tract cancer,** a rare adenocarcinoma in a bile duct often causing jaundice, pruritus, and weight loss. The lesion may be papillary or flat and ulcerated. The tumor is often unresectable at diagnosis.

**biligenesis** /bil'ijen'əsis/, the process by which bile is produced.

**bilingulate** /bīling'gyəlit/ [L, *bis*, twice, *lingula*, little tongue], having two tongues or two tonguelike structures.

**bilious** /bil'yəs/ [L, *bilis*, bile], **1.** pertaining to bile. **2.** characterized by an excessive secretion of bile. **3.** characterized by a disorder affecting bile.

**bilirubin** /bil'irōō'bin/ [L, *bilis* + *ruber*, red], the orange-yellow pigment of bile, formed principally by the breakdown of hemoglobin in red blood cells after termination of their normal lifespan. Water-insoluble unconjugated bilirubin normally travels in the bloodstream to the liver, where it is converted to a water-soluble, conjugated form and excreted into the bile. In a healthy person about 250 mg of bilirubin is produced daily. The majority of bilirubin is excreted in the stool. The characteristic yellow pallor of jaundice is caused by the accumulation of bilirubin in the blood and in the tissues of the skin. Testing for bilirubin in the blood provides information for diagnosis and evaluation of liver disease, biliary obstruction, and hemolytic anemia. Normal levels of total bilirubin are 0.1 to 1 mg/dl or 5.1 to 17 μmol/L. See also **jaundice, van den Bergh's test.**

**bilirubinemia** /-ē'mē·ə/ [L, *bilis*, bile, *ruber*, red; Gk, *haima*, blood], the presence of bilirubin in the blood.

**bilirubinuria** /-ōōr'ē·ə/, the presence of bilirubin in urine.

**biliuria** /bil'iyōōr'ē·ə/ [L, *bilis* + Gk, *ouron*, urine], the presence of bile pigments in the urine.

**biliverdin** /bil'ivur'din/ [L, *bilis* + *virdis*, green], a greenish bile pigment formed in the breakdown of hemoglobin and converted to bilirubin. See also **bile, bilirubin.**

**billing limit.** See **limiting charge.**

**Billings method,** a way of estimating ovulation time by changes in the cervical mucus that occur during the menstrual cycle. See also **ovulation method of family planning.**

**Billroth's operation I** [Christian A. Billroth, Austrian surgeon, 1829–1894], the surgical removal of the pylorus in the treatment of gastric cancer or peptic ulcer. The proximal end of the duodenum is anastomosed to the stomach.

**Billroth's operation II** [Christian A. Billroth], the surgical removal of the pylorus and duodenum. The cut end of the stomach is anastomosed to the jejunum through the transverse mesocolon. Also called **gastrojejunostomy.**

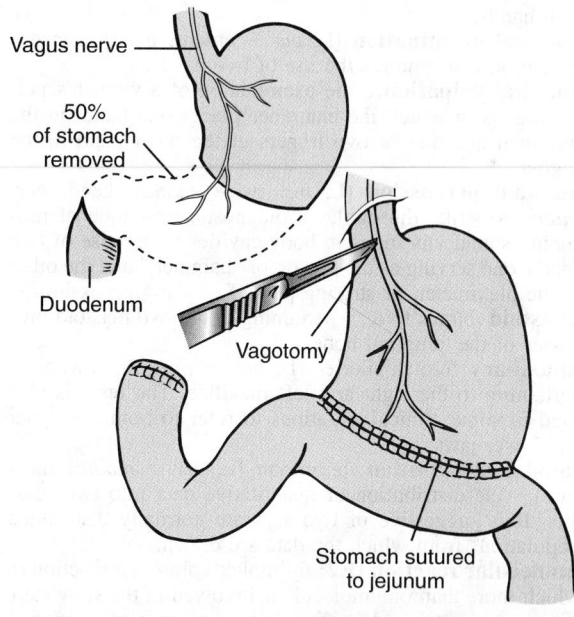

**Billroth's operation II** *(Lewis, Heitkemper, and Dirksen, 2000)*

**Bill's maneuver** [Arthur H. Bill, American obstetrician, 1877–1961], an obstetric procedure in which a forceps is used to rotate the fetal head at midpelvis before extraction of the head during birth.

**bilobate** /bīlō'bāt/ [L, *bis*, twice, *lobus*, lobe], having two lobes.

**bilobate placenta** [L, *bis*, twice, *lobus*, lobe, *placenta*, flat cake], a placenta with two connected lobes. Also called **bilobed placenta, placenta bipartitia.**

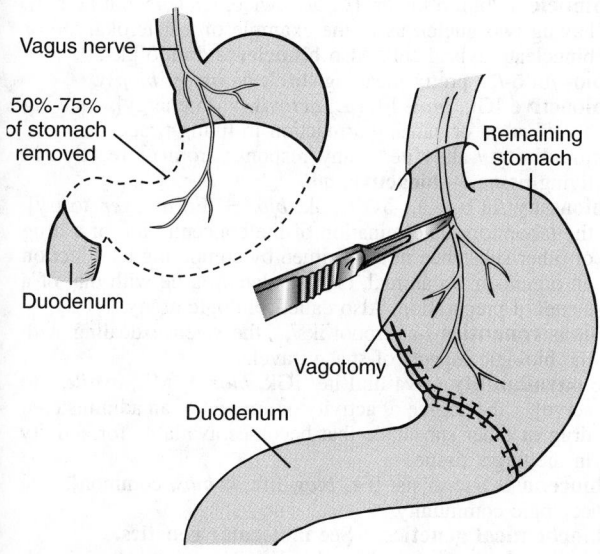

**Billroth's operation I** *(Lewis, Heitkemper, and Dirksen, 2000)*

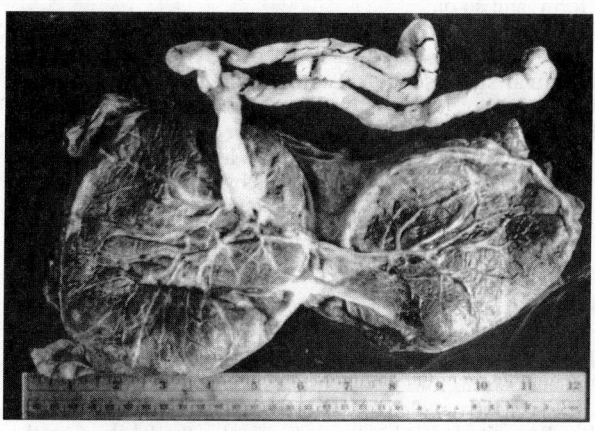

**Bilobate placenta** *(Carlson, 1999)*

**bilobulate** /bīlob′yəlāt/, having two lobules. Also **bilobular.**

**bilocular** /bīlok′yələr/ [L, *bis* + *loculus*, compartment], **1.** divided into two cells. **2.** containing two cells. Also **biloculate.**

**Biltricide,** trademark for an anthelmintic (praziquantel).

**bimanual** /bīman′yŏŏ·əl/ [L, *bis* + *manus*, hand], with both hands.

**bimanual examination** [L, *bis* + *manos*, hand], an examination that requires the use of two hands.

**bimanual palpation,** the examination of a woman's pelvic organs in which the examiner places one hand on the abdomen and one or two fingers of the other hand in the vagina.

**bimanual percussion** [L, *bis*, twice, *manus*, hand, *percutere*, to strike through], a diagnostic technique of producing sound vibrations in body cavities by the use of two hands, one serving as the plexor, or "hammer," and the other as the pleximeter, or striking plate. See also **percussion.**

**bimastoid** /bīmas′toid/, pertaining to the two mastoid processes of the temporal bone.

**bimaxillary** /bīmak′siler′ē/ [L, *bis* + *maxilla*, jawbone], pertaining to the right and left maxillae. The term is also used in some clinical situations to refer to both the upper and lower jaws.

**bimodal distribution** /bīmo′dəl/ [L, *bis* + *modus*, measure], the distribution of quantitative data into two clusters. It is suggestive of two separate normally distributed populations from which the data are drawn.

**bimolecular reaction (E2)** /bī′molek′yələr/, a reaction in which more than one molecule is involved in the slow step. An enzyme-catalyzed reaction usually consists of a series of bimolecular reactions. It may follow second-order, or more complicated chemical kinetics.

**bin-,** prefix meaning 'twice, two': *binocular, binovular.*

**binangle** /bin′ang·gəl/ [L, *bini*, twofold, *angulus*, angle], a double-ended surgical or operative instrument that has a shank with two offsetting angles to keep the cutting edge of the instrument within 3 mm of the shaft axis.

**binary fission** /bī′nərē/ [L, *bini*, twofold, *fissionis*, splitting], the division of a cell or nucleus into two equal parts. It is the common form of asexual reproduction among bacteria, protozoa, and other unicellular organisms. Also called **simple fission.** Compare **multiple fission.**

**binary number,** a number in base 2 represented by 0s and 1s. For example, the number 2 in the decimal form is written as 10 in the binary form, the decimal number 3 is written as 11, the decimal number 4 is written as 100 in the binary form, and so on.

**binaural** /bī·naw′rəl/ [L, *bis*, twice + *auris*, ear], pertaining to both ears.

**binaural stethoscope.** See **diaphragm stethoscope.**

**binauricular.** See **biauricular.**

**bind** [AS, *binden*], **1.** to bandage or wrap in a band. **2.** to join together with a band or with a ligature. **3.** (in chemistry) to combine or unite molecules by using reactive groups within the molecules or by using a binding chemical. Binding is especially associated with chemical bonds that are fairly easily broken, such as in the bonds between toxins and antitoxins.

**binder,** a bandage made of a large piece of material to fit and support a specific body part.

**binding energy, 1.** the amount of energy required to separate a nucleus into its individual nucleons. **2.** the energy released as the nucleus forms from nucleons.

**binding site** [ME, *binden* + L, *situs*], the location on the surface of a cell or a molecule where other cell fragments or molecules attach to initiate a chemical or physiologic action.

**Binet age** /binā′/ [Alfred Binet, French psychologist, 1857–1911], the mental age of an individual, especially a child, as determined by the Binet-Simon tests, which are evaluated on the basis of tested intelligence of the "normal" individual at any given age. The Binet age corresponding to 'profoundly retarded' is 1 to 2 years; to 'severely retarded,' 3 to 7 years; and to 'mildly retarded,' 8 to 12 years.

**binge eating.** See **bulimia.**

**binocular** /bīnok′yələr, bin-/ [L, *bini* + *oculus*, eye], **1.** pertaining to both eyes, especially regarding vision. **2.** a microscope, telescope, or field glass that can accommodate viewing by both eyes.

**binocular fixation,** the process of having both eyes directed at the same object at the same time, which is essential for good depth perception.

**binocular ophthalmoscope,** an ophthalmoscope having two eyepieces used for stereoscopic examination of the eye.

**binocular parallax** /per′ələks/ [L, *bini* + *oculus* + Gk, *parallax*, in turn], the difference in the angles formed by the sight lines to two objects situated at different distances from the eyes. Binocular parallax is a major factor in depth perception. Also called **stereoscopic parallax.**

**binocular perception,** the visual ability to judge depth or distance by virtue of having two eyes.

**binocular vision,** the simultaneous use of both eyes so that the images perceived by each eye are combined to appear as a single image. Compare **diplopia.**

**binomial** /bīno′mē·əl/, containing two names or terms.

**binomial nomenclature** [L, *bis*, twice; Gk, *nomos*, law; L, *nomenclatio*, calling by name], a system of classification of animals, plants, and other life forms (developed by Carl Linné) that assigns a two-part Latinized name to each species, such as *Homo sapiens* for humans.

**binovular** /bīnov′yələr/ [L, *bini* + *ovum*, egg], developing from two distinct ova, as in dizygotic twins. Also **diovular.** Compare **uniovular.**

**binovular twins.** See **dizygotic twins.**

**Binswanger's disease** /bin′swäng·ərz/ [Otto Binswanger, German neurologist, 1852–1929], a degenerative dementia of presenile onset caused by thinning of the subcortical white matter of the brain; some have attributed it to sclerotic changes of blood vessels.

**binuclear** /bīnŏŏ′klē·ər/ [L, *bis*, twice, *nucleus*, nut kernel], having two nuclei, as in the example of a heterokaryon or binucleate hybrid cell. Also **binucleate** /bīnŏŏ′klē·āt/.

**bio-** /bī′ō-/, prefix meaning 'life': *bioassay, biopsy.*

**bioactive** [Gk, *bios*, life; L, *activus*, with energy], having an effect on or causing a reaction in living tissue.

**bioactivity** /-aktiv′itē/, any response from or reaction in living tissue. —**bioactive,** *adj.*

**bioassay** /bī′ō·as′ā, -əsā′/ [Gk, *bios* + Fr, *assayer*, to try], the laboratory determination of the concentration of a drug or other substance in a specimen by comparing its effect on an organism, an animal, or an isolated tissue with that of a standard preparation. Also called **biologic assay.**

**bioastronautics** /-as′trōnôt′iks/, the science dealing with the biologic aspects of space travel.

**bioavailability** /-əvā′libil′itē/ [Gk, *bios* + ME, *availen*, to serve], the degree of activity or amount of an administered drug or other substance that becomes available for activity in the target tissue.

**biocenosis** /-sənō′sis/ [Fk, *bios*, life, *koinos*, common], an ecologic community.

**biochemical genetics.** See **molecular genetics.**

**biochemical marker** /-kem′ikəl/ [Gk, *bios* + *chemeia*, alchemy], any hormone, enzyme, antibody, or other substance that is detected in the urine or other body fluids or tissues that may serve as a sign of a disease or other abnormality. An example is the **Bence Jones protein** that appears in the urine of multiple myeloma patients.

**biochemistry** /-kem'istrē/, the chemistry of organisms and life processes. Also called **biologic chemistry, physiologic chemistry.**

**biochemorphics** /-kemôr'fik/, the study of the relationship between chemical structure and biologic function.

**biochromatic analysis** /-krōmat'ik/ [Gk, *bios + chroma,* color], the spectrophotometric monitoring of a reaction at two wavelengths. It is used to correct for background color.

**bioclimatology** /-klī'mətol'əjē/, the study of the relationship and interactions between climate and organisms.

**biocybernetics** /-sī'bərnet'iks/, the science of communication and control within and among organisms and of the interaction between organisms and mechanical or electronic systems.

**biodegradable** /-digrā'dəbəl/ [Gk, *bios,* life; L, *de,* away, *gradus,* step], the natural ability of a chemical substance to be broken down into less complex compounds or compounds having fewer carbon atoms by bacteria or other microorganisms.

**biodynamics** /-dīnam'iks/, the study of the effects of dynamic processes, such as radiation, on organisms.

**bioelectric impedance analysis (BIA)** /-ilek'trik/, a method of measuring the fat composition of the body, compared to other tissues, by its resistance to electricity. Fat tissue does not conduct electricity; muscle and bone are poor conductors. The method is reported to be 95% accurate, depending on body water content, which may fluctuate with exercise, diet, sweating, and use of alcohol or drugs. See also **total body electric conductivity (TOBEC).**

**bioelectricity** /-ilektris'itē/ [Gk, *bios + elektron,* amber], electrical current that is generated by living tissues, such as nerves and muscles. The electrical potentials of human tissues, recorded by electrocardiograph, electroencephalograph, and similar sensitive devices, are used in diagnosing the condition of various vital organs.

**bioenergetics** /-en'ərjet'iks/ [Gk, *bios + energein,* to be active], a system of exercises based on the concept that natural healing will be enhanced by bringing the patient's body rhythms and the natural environment into harmony.

**bioequivalent** /bī'ō·ikwiv'ələnt/ [Gk, *bios* + L, *aequus,* equal, *valere,* to be strong], **1.** (in pharmacology) pertaining to a drug that has the same effect on the body as another drug, usually one nearly identical in its chemical formulation. **2.** going in and out of the body at the same rate. —**bioequivalence,** *n.*

**bioethics** /bī'ō·eth'iks/ [Gk, *bios,* life + *ethos,* the habits of humans or animals], obligations of a moral nature relating to biological research and its applications.

**biofeedback[1]** /-fēd'bak/ [Gk, *bios* + AS, *faedan,* food, *baec,* back], a process providing a person with visual or auditory information about the autonomic physiologic functions of his or her body, such as blood pressure, muscle tension, and brain wave activity, usually through use of instruments. By trial and error, the person learns consciously to control these processes, which were previously regarded as involuntary. Biofeedback may be used clinically to treat many conditions, such as pain, anxiety, hypertension, insomnia, and migraine headache.

**biofeedback[2],** a nursing intervention from the Nursing Interventions Classification (NIC) defined as assisting the patient to modify a body function using feedback from instrumentation. See also **Nursing Interventions Classification.**

**bioflavonoid** /bī'ōflā'vənoid/ [Gk, *bios* + L, *flavus,* yellow; Gk, *eidos,* form], a generic term for any of a group of colored flavones found in many fruits. Once believed to reduce capillary bleeding, bioflavonoids are now considered nonessential nutrients. Several are being investigated as possible low-calorie sweeteners.

**biogenesis** /bī'ōjen'əsis/ [Gk, *bios + genein,* to produce], **1.** also called **biogeny** /bī·oj'ənē/, the doctrine that living material can originate only from preexisting life and not from inanimate matter. **2.** the origin of life; ontogeny and phylogeny. —**biogenetic,** *adj.*

**biogenetic law.** See **recapitulation concept.**

**biogenic** /bī'ōjen'ik/, **1.** produced by the action of a living organism, such as fermentation. **2.** essential to life and the maintenance of health, such as food, water, and proper rest.

**biogenic amine,** one of a large group of naturally occurring biologically active compounds, most of which act as neurotransmitters. The most dominant, norepinephrine, is involved in such physiologic functions as emotional reactions, memory, sleep, and arousal from sleep. Other biochemicals of the group include three catecholamines: histamine, serotonin, and dopamine. These substances are active in regulating blood pressure, elimination, body temperature, and many other centrally mediated body functions.

**biogenous** /bī·oj'ənəs/, **1.** biogenetic. **2.** biogenic.

**biogeny.** See **biogenesis.**

**biogravics** /-grav'iks/, the study of the effects of gravity, including reduced and increased gravitational forces, on organisms.

**biohazard** /-haz'ərd/ [Gk, *bios,* life; OFr, *hasard*], anything that is a risk to organisms, such as ionizing radiation or harmful bacteria or viruses.

**bioinstrument,** a sensor or other device implanted into or attached to a living organism for the purpose of recording physiologic data, such as brain activity or heart function.

**biokinetics** /-kinet'iks/ [Gk, *bios,* life, *kinetikos,* moving], the study of the movements within developing organisms.

**biologic** /-loj'ik/ [Gk, *bios + logos,* science], **1.** pertaining to organisms and their products. **2.** any preparation made from organisms or their products and used as a diagnostic, preventive, or therapeutic agent. Kinds of biologics include **antigens, antitoxins, sera,** and **vaccines.** Also called **biological.**

**biologic activity,** the inherent capacity of a substance, such as a drug or toxin, to alter one or more chemical or physiologic functions of a cell, tissue, organ, or organism. The biologic activity of a substance is determined not only by the substance's physical and chemical nature but also by its concentration and the duration of cellular exposure to it. Biologic activity may reflect a "domino effect," in which the alteration of one function disrupts the normal activity of one or more other functions.

**biological.** See **biologic.**

**biologic armature,** the connective tissue–rich aggregate of larger ducts, vessels, and autonomic nerves that in many mammalian exocrine glands serves as an internal framework whose function of support, and often anchorage, resembles that of the armature within a clay sculpture.

**biologic assay.** See **bioassay.**

**biologic chemistry.** See **biochemistry.**

**biologic death,** death attributed to natural causes. In CPR terms, *biologic death* refers to permanent cellular damage, resulting from lack of oxygen, that is not reversible.

**biologic dressing,** a dressing for burn injuries that is made from pigskin or synthetic materials with characteristics like those of human skin. The dressing is most effective in treating burns that are of uniform depth and of superficial partial thickness. It should be applied as soon as possible after the injury and should adhere to the wound during healing. Once adherence is established the wound can be left open and the patient can bathe and wear clothing over it.

**biologic half-life,** the time required for the body to eliminate half of an administered dose of any substance by regular physiologic processes. The biologic half-life is approximately the same for stable and radioactive isotopes of a specific element. Also called **metabolic half-life.** See also **effective half-life, half-life.**

**biologic monitoring,** **1.** a process of measuring the levels of various physiologic substances, drugs, or metabolites within a patient during diagnosis or therapy. **2.** the measurement of toxic substances in the environment and the identification of health risks to the population. Biologic monitoring often uses indirect methods of identifying and measuring substances, such as analyses of samples of blood, urine, feces, hair, nails, sweat, saliva, or exhaled air and extrapolation from metabolic effects.

**biologic plausibility,** a method of reasoning used to establish a cause-and-effect relationship between a biologic factor and a particular disease.

**biologic psychiatry,** a school of psychiatric thought that stresses the physical, chemical, and neurologic causes of and treatments for mental and emotional disorders.

**biologic rhythm** [Gk, *bios,* life, *logos,* science, *rhythmos*], the periodic recurrence of a biologic phenomenon, such as the respiratory cycle, the sleep cycle, or the menstrual cycle. Also called **biorhythm.**

**biologic vector.** See **vector.**

**biologist** /bī·ol'əjist/ [Gk, *bios,* life, *logos,* science], a person who studies life.

**biology** /bī·ol'əje/, the scientific study of life. Some branches of biology are **biometry, cell biology, ecology, evolution, genetics, molecular biology,** and **physiology.**

**biolysis** /bī·ol'isis/ [Gk, *bios,* life, *lysis,* loosening], the disintegration or dissolution of organic matter resulting from the activity of organisms, such as bacterial action on living tissue.

**biome** /bī'ōm/ [Gk, *bios* + *oma,* tumor, mass], the collection of biologic communities existing in and characteristic of a broad geographic region, such as desert, tropical forest, or savanna. A biome includes all organisms of a particular region.

**biomechanic.** See **biomechanics.**

**biomechanic adaptation** a process in which a patient with a physical disability adjusts to the use of an orthotic device, such as an ankle-foot brace or a patellar-tendon-bearing prosthesis. Adaptation requires the central nervous system input received during therapeutic exercises with the orthotic appliance.

**biomechanics** [Gk, *bios* + *mechane,* machine], the study of mechanical laws and their application to living organisms, especially the human body and its locomotor system. —**biomechanic, biomechanical,** *adj.*

**biomedical,** pertaining to the biologic aspects of medicine.

**biomedical engineering** /-med'ikəl/ [Gk, *bios* + L, *medicare,* to heal], a system of scientific techniques that is applied to biologic processes to solve practical medical problems or answer questions in biomedical research.

**biometry** /bī·om'ətrē/, the application of statistical methods in analyzing data obtained in biologic or anthropologic research. See also **biology.**

**biomicroscopy** /-mīkros'kəpē/, **1.** microscopic examination of living tissue in the body. **2.** ophthalmic examination of the eye by use of a slit lamp and a magnifying lens. See also **slit lamp, slit-lamp microscope.**

**bionics** /bī·on'iks/, the science of applying electronic principles and devices, such as computers and solid-state miniaturized circuitry, to medical problems. An example of the application of bionics is the development of artificial pacemakers to correct abnormal heart rhythms. —**bionic,** *adj.*

**biopharmaceutics** /-fär'məsoō'tiks/, the study of the chemical and physical properties of drugs, their components, and their activities in living organisms.

**biophore** /bī'əfôr'/ [Gk, *bios* + *phora,* bearer], according to the German biologist A.F.L. Weismann (1834–1914), the basic hereditary unit contained in the germ plasm from which all living cells develop and all inherited characteristics are transmitted. Compare **gemmule.**

**biophysics,** the application of physical laws to life processes of organisms.

**biopotential** /-pəten'shəl/, a voltage produced by a tissue of the body, particularly muscle tissue during a contraction. Electrocardiography depends on measurement of changing potentials in contracting heart muscle; electromyography and electroencephalography function similarly in the diagnosis of neuromuscular and brain disorders, respectively.

**biopsy** /bī'opsē/ [Gk, *bios* + *opsis,* view], **1.** the removal of a small piece of living tissue from an organ or other part of the body for microscopic examination to confirm or establish a diagnosis, estimate prognosis, or follow the course of a disease. **2.** the tissue excised for examination. **3.** *informal,* to excise tissue for examination. Kinds of biopsy include **aspiration biopsy, needle biopsy, punch biopsy,** and **surface biopsy.** —**bioptic** /bī·op'tik/, *adj.*

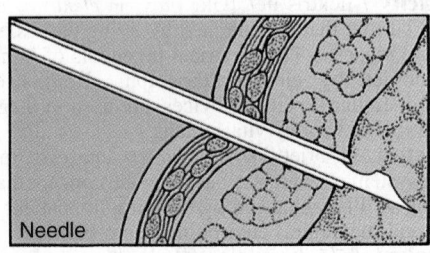

**Aspiration biopsy** *(Belcher, 1992)*

**biopsychic** /bī'ōsī'kik/ [Gk, *bios* + *psyche,* mind], pertaining to mental factors as they relate to living organisms.

**biopsychology.** See **psychobiology.**

**biopsychosocial** /bī'ōsī'kōsō'shəl/ [Gk, *bios* + *psyche,* mind; L, *socius,* companion], pertaining to the complex of biologic, psychologic, and social aspects of life.

**bioptic.** See **biopsy.**

**bioptome tip catheter** /bī·op'tōm/, a catheter with a special end designed for obtaining endomyocardial biopsy samples. It is threaded through a guiding catheter to the right ventricle, where it snips small tissue samples from the septal wall for pathologic examination. The bioptome tip device is used to monitor heart transplantation patients for early signs of tissue rejection.

**biorhythm.** See **biologic rhythm.**

**biosafety,** a system for the safe handling of toxic and dangerous biologic and chemical substances. Guidance in biosafety is offered by the U.S. Centers for Disease Control,

Occupational Safety and Health Administration, and National Institute for Occupational Safety and Health.

**-biosis,** suffix meaning 'a specific way of living': *macrobiosis, otobiosis.*

**biostatistics** /-stətis'tiks/, numeric data on births, deaths, diseases, injuries, and other factors affecting the general health and condition of human populations. Also called **vital statistics.**

**biosynthesis** /-sin'thəsis/ [Gk, *bios* + *synthesis,* putting together], any one of thousands of chemical reactions continually occurring throughout the body in which molecules form more complex biomolecules, especially the carbohydrates, lipids, proteins, nucleotides, and nucleic acids. Biosynthetic reactions constitute the anabolism of the body. —**biosynthetic,** *adj.*

**biosystem,** any organism or complex system of organisms.

**biotaxis** /bī'ōtak'sis/ [Gk, *bios* + *taxis,* arrangement], the ability of cells to develop into certain forms and arrangements. See also **cytoclesis.** —**biotactic,** *adj.*

**biotaxy** /bī'ōtak'sē/, **1.** biotaxis. **2.** the systematic classification of organisms according to their phenotypic characteristics; taxonomy.

**biotechnology** /-teknol'əjē/ [Gk, *bios* + *techne,* art, *logos,* science], **1.** the study of the relationships between humans or other living organisms and machinery, such as the health effects of computer equipment on office workers or the ability of airplane pilots to perform tasks when traveling at supersonic speeds. **2.** the industrial application of the results of biologic research, particularly in fields such as recombinant deoxyribonucleic acids (DNA) or gene splicing, which permits the production of synthetic hormones or enzymes by combining genetic material from different species. See **recombinant DNA.**

**biotelemetry** /-təlem'ətrē/, the transmission of physiologic data, such as electrocardiographic (ECG) and electroencephalographic (EEG) recordings, heart rate, and body temperature by radio or telephone systems. Transmission of such data uses sophisticated electronic devices developed for the study of the effects of space travel on animals and humans; it has progressed to the use of communication satellites for relaying such data from one part of the world to another.

**biotherapy,** a system of cancer therapy that uses alpha- and beta-interferons and mitogen-stimulated lymphocytes.

**-biotic,** suffix meaning 'life': *anabiotic, microbiotic;* also, meaning 'possessing a (specified) mode of life': *endobiotic, photobiotic.*

**biotic factor** /bī·ot'ik/, an environmental influence on living things, as distinguished from climatic or geologic factors.

**biotic potential,** the possible growth rate of a population of organisms under ideal conditions, which include an absence of predators and an unlimited availability of nutrients and space for expansion.

**biotin** /bī'ətin/ [Gk, *bios,* life], a colorless, crystalline, water-soluble B complex vitamin that acts as a coenzyme in fatty acid production and in the oxidation of fatty acids and carbohydrates. It also aids in the use of protein, folic acid, pantothenic acid, and vitamin $B_{12}$. Rich sources are egg yolk, beef liver, kidney, unpolished rice, brewer's yeast, peanuts, cauliflower, and mushrooms. Previously called **vitamin H.** See also **avidin.**

**biotin deficiency syndrome,** an abnormal condition caused by a deficiency of biotin, a B complex vitamin. It is characterized by dermatitis, hyperesthesia, muscle pain, anorexia, slight anemia, and changes in electrocardiographic activity of the heart. The average daily requirement of biotin

for an adult is 100 to 200 μg; the average American diet provides 100 to 300 μg of the vitamin. Because biotin is synthesized by intestinal bacteria, naturally occurring deficiency in adults is unknown, although it can be induced by large quantities of raw egg whites in the diet. Symptoms include scaly dermatitis, grayish pallor, extreme lassitude, anorexia, muscle pains, insomnia, some precordial distress, and slight anemia. Some authorities consider seborrheic dermatitis in infants a form of biotin deficiency.

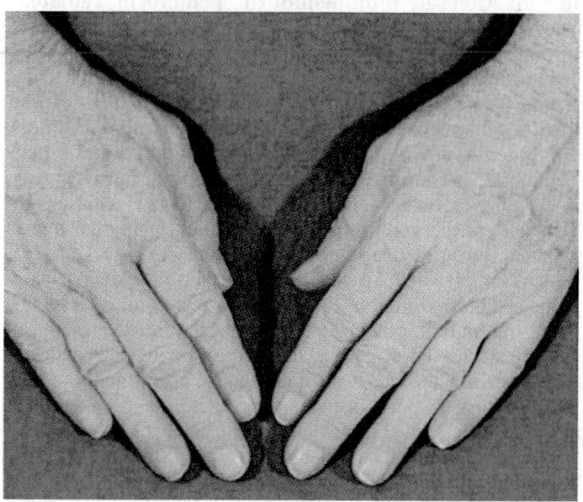

**Scaly dermatitis resulting from biotin deficiency**
(McLaren, 1992/courtesy Dr. C.E. Butterworth, Jr.)

**biotope** /bī'ətōp/ [Gk, *bios* + *topos,* place], a specific biologic habitat or site.

**biotoxin** /bī'ətok'in/, any toxin produced by an organism.

**biotransformation** /-trans'fôrmā'shən/ [Gk, *bios* + L, *trans,* across, *formare,* to form], the chemical changes a substance undergoes in the body, such as by the action of enzymes. See also **metabolic.**

**Biot's respiration** /bē·ōz'/ [Camille Biot, French physician, b. 1878], an abnormal respiratory pattern, characterized by short episodes of rapid, uniformly deep inspirations followed by 10 to 30 seconds of apnea. Biot's respiration is symptomatic of meningitis or increased intracranial pressure.

**biovular twins.** See **dizygotic twins.**

**bipalatinoid** /bī'palat'inoid, -pal'-/, describing a two-compartment capsule with different medications in each side. It is designed so that the two substances become mixed and activated as the gelatin capsule dissolves.

**bipara** /bip'ərə/, a woman who has given birth twice in separate pregnancies.

**biparental inheritance.** See **amphigenous inheritance.**

**biparietal** /bīpərī'ətəl/ [L, *bis,* twice, *paries,* wall], pertaining to the two parietal bones of the head, such as the biparietal diameter.

**biparietal diameter (BPD),** the transverse distance between the protuberances of the two parietal bones of the skull.

**biparietal suture** [L, *bis* + *paries,* wall, *sutura*], the interlocking lines of fusion between two parietal bones of the skull.

**biparous** /bip'ərəs/ [L, *bis,* twice, *parere,* to produce], pertaining to the birth of two infants in separate pregnancies.

**bipartite** /bīpär'tīt/, having two parts.

**biped** /bī'ped/, **1.** having two feet. **2.** any animal with only two feet.

**bipedal** /bīpē'dəl, -ped'əl/ [L, *bis,* twice, *pes,* foot], capable of locomotion on two feet.

**bipenniform** /bīpen'ifôrm'/ [L, *bis* + *penna,* feather, *forma,* form], (of body structure) having the bilateral symmetry of a feather, such as the pattern formed by the fasciculi that converge on both sides of a muscle tendon in the rectus femoris. Compare **multipenniform, penniform, radiate.**

**biperforate** /bī-pər'fə-rāt/ [L, *bis,* twice + *perforatus,* bored through], having two perforations.

**biperiden** /bīper'idən/, a synthetic anticholinergic agent.
■ INDICATIONS: It may be prescribed in the treatment of Parkinson's disease and drug-induced extrapyramidal disorders. Biperiden hydrochloride is administered orally, and biperiden lactate is administered intramuscularly or intravenously.
■ CONTRAINDICATIONS: Narrow-angle glaucoma, asthma, obstruction of the genitourinary or GI tract, or known hypersensitivity to this drug prohibits its use.
■ ADVERSE EFFECTS: Among the more serious adverse reactions are blurred vision, central nervous system effects, urinary retention, postural hypotension, tachycardia, dry mouth, decreased sweating, and hypersensitivity reactions.

**biphasic** /bīfā'zik/ [L, *bis* + Gk, *phasis,* appearance], having two phases, parts, aspects, or stages.

**bipolar** /bīpō'lər/ [L, *bis* + *polus,* pole], **1.** having two poles, such as in certain electrotherapeutic treatments using two poles or in certain types of bacterial staining that affects only the two poles of the microorganism under study. **2.** (of a nerve cell) having an afferent and an efferent process.

**bipolar cell,** a cell, such as a retinal neuron, with two main processes arising from the cell body.

**bipolar disorder,** a major mental disorder characterized by episodes of mania, depression, or mixed mood. One or the other phase may be predominant at any given time, one phase may appear alternately with the other, or elements of both phases may be present simultaneously. Characteristics of the manic phase are excessive emotional displays, such as excitement, elation, euphoria, or in some cases irritability accompanied by hyperactivity, boisterousness, impaired ability to concentrate, decreased need for sleep, and seemingly unbounded energy. In extreme mania, a sense of omnipotence and delusions of grandeur may occur. In the depressive phase, marked apathy and underactivity are accompanied by feelings of profound sadness, loneliness, guilt, and lowered self-esteem. Causes of the disorder are multiple and complex, often involving biologic, psychologic, interpersonal, and social and cultural factors. See also **major depressive disorder.**

**bipolar lead** /lēd/, **1.** an electrocardiographic conductor having two electrodes placed on different body regions, with each electrode contributing to the record. **2.** *informal.* a tracing produced by such a lead on an electrocardiograph.

**bipolar version,** a method for changing the position of a fetus in which one hand is placed on the abdomen of the mother and two fingers of the other hand are inserted into the uterus.

**bipotentiality** /bī'pəten'shē·al'itē/ [L, *bis* + *potentia,* power], the characteristic of acting or reacting according to either of two possible states.

**bird breeder's lung.** See **pigeon breeder's lung.**

**bird face retrognathism.** See **retrognathism.**

**birth** [ME, *burth*], **1.** the event of being born, the entry of a new person out of its mother into the world. Kinds of birth are **breech birth, live birth,** and **stillbirth.** See also **effacement, labor. 2.** the childbearing event, the bringing forth by a mother of a baby. **3.** a medical event, the delivery of a fetus by an obstetric attendant.

**birth canal,** *informal.* the passage that extends from the inlet of the true pelvis to the vaginal orifice through which an infant passes during vaginal birth. See also **clinical pelvimetry.**

**birth center,** a health facility with services limited to maternity care for women judged to be at minimum risk for obstetric complications that would require hospitalization.

**birth certificate,** a legal document recording information about a birth, including, among other details, the date, time, and location of the event; identity of the mother and father; and identity of the attending physician or licensed midwife.

**birth control.** See **contraception.**

**birth defect.** See **congenital anomaly.**

**birthing,** a nursing intervention from the Nursing Interventions Classification (NIC) defined as delivery of a baby. See also **Nursing Interventions Classification.**

**birthing chair,** a special seat used in labor and delivery to promote the comfort of the mother and facilitate the birthing process. The chair may be specially designed, having many technical features, or it may be a simple three-legged stool with a high, slanted back and a circular seat with a large central hole in it. The newer birthing chairs allow women to sit straight up or to recline. The chair has a lower section that may be removed or folded out of the way. Lights, mirrors, and basins may be attached. The upright position appears to shorten the time in labor, particularly the second or expulsive stage of labor, probably because of gravity and increased participation of the mother. The chair is not suitable for use with anesthesia.

**birth injury,** trauma suffered by a baby while being born. Some kinds of birth injury are **Bell's palsy, cerebral palsy,** and **Erb's palsy.**

**birthmark.** See **nevus.**

**birth mother,** the biologic mother or woman who bears a child. The child may have been conceived in a surrogate mother with sperm of the biologic father.

**birth palsy** [ME, *burth* + Gk, *paralyein,* to be palsied], a loss of motor or sensory nerve function in some body part caused by a nerve injury during the birth process. Also called **birth paralysis.**

**birth paralysis.** See **birth palsy.**

**birth parent,** one of an individual's two biologic parents.

**birth rate,** the proportion of the number of live births in a specific area during a given period to the total population of that area, usually expressed as the number of births per 1000 of population. Compare **crude birth rate, refined birth rate, true birth rate.**

**birth trauma, 1.** any physical injury suffered by an infant during the process of delivery. **2.** the supposed psychic shock, according to some psychiatric theories, that an infant suffers during delivery.

**birth weight,** the measured heaviness of a baby when born, usually about 3500 g (7.5 pounds). In the United States, 97% of newborns weigh between 2500 g (5.5 pounds) and 4500 g (10 pounds). Babies weighing less than 2500 g at term are considered **small for gestational age.** Babies weighing more than 4500 g are considered **large for gestational age** and are often infants of mothers with diabetes.

**bis-,** prefix meaning 'twice, two': *bisacromial, bisferious.*

**bisacodyl** /bisak'ōdil/, a cathartic.
■ INDICATIONS: It is prescribed in the treatment of acute or chronic constipation or for emptying of the bowel before or after surgery or before diagnostic radiographic procedures.

■ CONTRAINDICATIONS: Abdominal pain, nausea, vomiting, rectal fissures, ulcerated hemorrhoids, or known hypersensitivity to this drug prohibits its use.

■ ADVERSE EFFECTS: Among the more serious adverse reactions are colic, abdominal pain, and diarrhea.

**bisacromial** /bīsəkrō'mē·əl/, pertaining to both acromions, the triangular, flat, bony plates at the end of the scapula.

**bisalbuminemia** /bis'albyo͞om'inē'mē·ə/, a condition in which two types of albumin exist in an individual. The two types are expressed by heterozygous alleles of the albumin gene and are detected by differences in the mobility of the types on electrophoretic gels.

**bisect** /bīsekt'/ [L, bis + secare, to cut], to divide into two equal lengths or parts.

**bisexual** /bīsek'sho͞o·əl/ [L, bis + sexus, male or female], **1.** hermaphroditic; having gonads of both sexes. **2.** possessing physical or psychologic characteristics of both sexes. **3.** engaging in both heterosexual and homosexual activity. **4.** desiring sexual contact with persons of both sexes.

**bisexual libido,** (in psychoanalysis) the tendency in a person to seek sexual gratification with people of either sex.

**bisferious pulse** /bisfer'ē·əs/ [L, bis + ferire, to beat], an arterial pulse that has two palpable peaks, the second of which is slightly weaker than the first. It may be detected in cases of aortic regurgitation and obstructive cardiomyopathy. Compare **dicrotic pulse.**

**bishydroxycoumarin.** See **dicumarol.**

**bis in die (b.i.d.)** /dē'ā/, a Latin phrase, used in prescriptions, meaning 'twice a day.' It is more commonly used in its abbreviated form.

**bismuth (Bi)** /biz'məth, bis'-/ [Ger, wismut, white mass], a reddish, crystalline, trivalent metallic element. Its atomic number is 83; its atomic mass is 208.98. It is combined with various other elements, such as oxygen, to produce numerous salts used in the manufacture of many pharmaceutic substances.

**bismuth gingivitis,** a dark bluish line along the gingival margin caused by bismuth administered in the treatment of systemic disease. See also **bismuth stomatitis, gingivitis.**

**bismuth stomatitis,** an abnormal oral condition caused by the systemic use of bismuth compounds over prolonged periods. It is characterized by a blue-black line on the inner aspect of the gingival sulcus or dark pigmentation of the buccal mucosa, sore tongue, metallic taste, and burning sensation in the mouth. Compare **arsenic stomatitis, Atabrine stomatitis.**

**bit** /bit/, abbreviation for binary digit, the smallest unit of information in a computer. Bits are the building blocks for all information processing in digital electronics and computers. Eight bits equals one byte. See also **byte.**

**bitart,** abbreviation for a bitartrate carboxylate anion.

**bitartrate** /bītär'trāt/, the monoanion of tartaric acid, $C_4H_5O_6^-$.

**bitartrate carboxylate anion,** an ionotropic agent used in the treatment of cardiovascular patients.

**bite** [AS, bitan], **1.** the act of cutting, tearing, holding, or gripping with the teeth. **2.** the lingual portion of an artificial tooth between its shoulder and its incisal edge. **3.** an occlusal record or relationship between the upper and lower teeth or jaws. Compare **closed bite, open bite.**

**bite block.** See **occlusion rim.**

**bitegauge** /bīt'gāj'/ [AS, bitan + OFr, gauge, measure], a prosthetic dental device that helps attain proper occlusion of the upper and lower teeth.

**biteguard** [AS, bitan + OFr, garder, to defend], a resin appliance that covers the occlusal and incisal surfaces of the teeth. It is used to stabilize the teeth, to provide a platform for the excursive glides of the mandible, and to eliminate the effects of nocturnal grinding of the teeth. Also called **biteplane, night guard.** Compare **mouth guard.**

**biteguard splint,** a device, usually made of resin, for covering the occlusal and incisal surfaces of the teeth and for protecting them from traumatic occlusal forces during immobilization and stabilization processes. See also **Gunning's splint.**

**bitelock** /bīt'lok'/, a dental device for retaining occlusion rims in the same relation outside and inside the mouth.

**bitemporal** /bītem'pərəl/ [L, bis, twice, tempora, temples], pertaining to both temples or both temporal bones.

**bitemporal hemianopia** [L, bis, twice, tempora, temples; Gk, hemi, half, opsis, vision], a loss of the temporal half of the vision in each eye, usually resulting from a lesion in the chiasmal area such as a pituitary tumor.

**biteplane** /bīt'plān/, **1.** See **occlusal plane. 2.** a metal sheet laid across the biting surfaces of the upper or lower teeth to determine the relationship of the teeth to the occlusal plane. **3.** an orthodontic appliance of acrylic resin worn over the maxillary occlusal surfaces and used to treat pain of the temporomandibular joint and adjacent muscles. Although removable, the device is kept in place by labial wires and wrought wire clasps. **4.** See **biteguard.**

**biteplate** /bīt'plāt/, a device used in dentistry as a diagnostic or therapeutic aid prosthodontics or for orthodontics. It is made of wire and plastic and worn in the palate. It may also be used in the correction of temporomandibular joint problems or as a splint in restoring the full mouth.

**bite reflex,** a swift, involuntary biting action that may be triggered by stimulation of the oral cavity. The bite can be difficult to release in some cases, such as when a spoon or tongue depressor is placed in a patient's mouth.

**bite wing film** [AS, bitan + ME, winge], a dental x-ray film on which a tab is placed so the teeth can hold the film in position during exposure. Also called **interproximal film.** See also **bite wing radiograph.**

**bite wing radiograph,** a dental radiograph that reveals the coronal portions of maxillary and mandibular teeth and portions of the interdental septa on the same film. See also **bite wing film.**

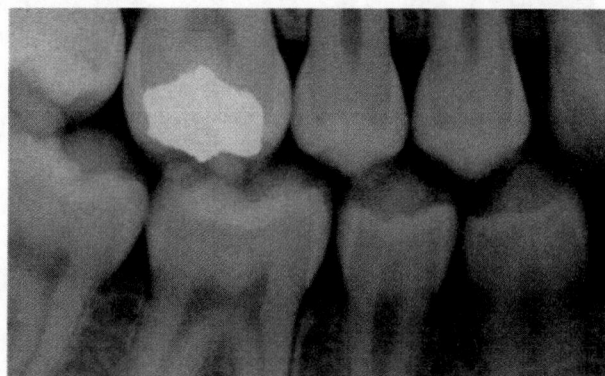

**Bite wing radiograph** (Jordan, 1993)

**bithionol (TBP)** /bithī'ənôl/, a pale gray powder, soluble in acetone, alcohol, or ether, used as a local antiseptic and administered orally in the treatment of infestations of the giant liver fluke *(Fasciola gigantica hepatica)* and of the lung fluke *(Paragonimus westermani),* which cause parasitic hemoptysis in Asiatic countries.

**Bithynia** /bəthin'ē·ə/, a genus of snails, species of which act as intermediate hosts to *Opisthorchis.*

**biting in childhood,** a natural behavior trait and reflex action in infants, acquired at about 5 to 6 months of age in response to the introduction of solid foods in the diet and the beginning of the teething process. The activity represents a significant modality in the psychosocial development of the child, because it is the first aggressive action the infant learns, and through it the infant learns to control the environment. The behavior also confronts the infant with one of the first inner conflicts, because biting can produce both pleasing and displeasing results. Biting during breastfeeding causes withdrawal of the nipple and anxiety in the mother, yet it also serves as a means of soothing teething discomfort. Infants continue to use biting as a mechanism for exploring their surroundings. Toddlers and older children often use biting for expressing aggression toward their parents and other children, especially during play or as a means of gaining attention. Most children normally outgrow the tendency unless they have severe maladaptive or emotional problems. See also **psychosexual development, psychosocial development.**

**bitolterol mesylate** /bitol'tərol mes'ilāt/, an orally inhaled bronchodilator.

■ INDICATIONS: It is used in the treatment of bronchial asthma and reversible bronchospasm.

■ CONTRAINDICATIONS: This product is contraindicated in patients who are known to be hypersensitive to it.

■ ADVERSE EFFECTS: Among adverse reactions reported are tremor, nervousness, headache, dizziness, palpitations, chest discomfort, tachycardia, coughing, and throat irritation.

**Bitot's spots** /bitōz'/ [Pierre Bitot, French surgeon, 1822–1888], white or gray triangular deposits on the bulbar conjunctiva adjacent to the lateral margin of the cornea, a clinical sign of vitamin A deficiency. Also called **Bitot's patches.**

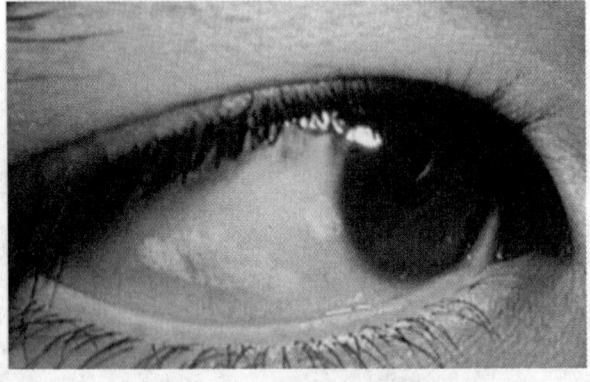

**Bitot's spots** *(McLaren, 1992)*

**bitrochanteric lipodystrophy** /bī'trōkənter'ik/ [L, *bis* + Gk, *trochanter,* runner; *lipos,* fat, *dys,* bad, *trophe,* nourishment], an abnormal and excessive deposition of fat on the buttocks and the outer aspect of the upper thighs, occurring most commonly in women. See also **lipodystrophy.**

**biuret test** /bī'yŏŏret/ [L, *bis* + Gk, *ouron,* urine], a method for detecting proteins in serum. In alkaline solution, copper sulfate ions react with the peptide bonds of proteins to produce a pink to purple color, called the biuret reaction. The amount of serum protein in a sample solution is estimated by comparing its color with that of a standard solution whose protein concentration is known.

**bivalent** /bīvā'lənt/ [L, *bis* + *valere,* to be powerful], **1.** See **divalent.** (in genetics) a pair of synapsed homologous chromosomes that are attached to each other by chiasmata during the early first meiotic prophase of gametogenesis. The structure serves as the basis for the tetrads from which gametes are produced during the two meiotic divisions. **2.** See **valence,** def. 1. —**bivalence,** *n.*

**bivalent antibody,** an antibody that has two or more binding sites that can cross-link one antigen to another.

**bivalent chromosome,** a pair of synapsed homologous chromosomes during the early stages of gametogenesis. See also **bivalent.**

**bivalved cast** [L, *bis* + *valva,* valve], a cast that is cut in half to detect or relieve pressure underneath, especially when a patient has decreased or no sensation in the portion of the body surrounded by the cast. "Windows" are often cut out of the cast over the pressure areas to assess circulation or open wounds under the cast.

**bizarre leiomyoma.** See **epithelioid leiomyoma.**

**Björnstad's syndrome** /byôrn'städz/ [R. Björnstad, Swedish dermatologist, 20th century], an autosomal recessive disorder characterized by congenital sensorineural deafness and kinky hair.

**Bk,** symbol for the element **berkelium.**

**BK,** abbreviation for *below the knee,* referring to amputations, amputees, prostheses, and orthoses.

**black beauties,** *slang,* amphetamines.

**black cohosh,** a perennial herb that grows throughout the United States and in parts of Canada.

■ USES: This herb is used to treat the symptoms of menopause (hot flashes and nervous conditions associated with menopause) and dysmenorrhea (menstrual cramps, pain, inflammation).

■ CONTRAINDICATIONS: Black cohosh should not be used during pregnancy, since uterine stimulation can occur. It also should not be used during lactation or in children.

**black damp.** See **damp.**

**black death.** See **bubonic plague.**

**Blackett-Healy method,** a positioning procedure for producing x-ray images of the subscapularis area. The patient is placed in a supine position with the affected shoulder joint centered on the midline of the film, the arm abducted, and the elbow flexed. The opposite shoulder is raised about 15 degrees and supported with a sandbag.

**black eye,** contusion around the eye with bruising, discoloration, and swelling. It is usually treated for the first 24 hours with ice packs to reduce swelling, then with hot compresses to aid in resorption of blood from the hematoma. Also called **periorbital ecchymosis.**

**Blackfan-Diamond anemia.** See **Diamond-Blackfan syndrome.**

**black fever.** See **kala-azar.**

**black hairy tongue.** See **parasitic glossitis.**

**black haw,** an herb found in the Eastern United States.

■ USES: This herb is used for dysmenorrhea, menstrual cramps and pain, menopausal metrorrhagia, hysteria, asthma, and heart palpitations. It is also used to lower blood pressure.

■ CONTRAINDICATIONS: Black haw should be used with caution in people with kidney stones.

**blackhead.** See **comedo.**

**black light.** See **Wood's light.**

**black lung disease.** See **anthracosis.**

**black measles** [AS, *blac* + OHG, *masala*], hemorrhagic measles characterized by a darkened rash caused by bleeding into the skin and mucous membranes. Also called **hemorrhagic measles.**

**blackout,** *informal.* a temporary loss of vision or consciousness.

**black plague.** See **bubonic plague.**

**Black's Classification of Caries.** See **classification of caries.**

**black spots film fault,** a defect in a radiograph, seen as dark spots throughout the image area. It is caused by dust particles or developer on the x-ray film before development or by outdated film.

**blackwater fever,** a serious complication of chronic falciparum malaria, characterized by jaundice, hemoglobinuria, acute renal failure, and passage of bloody dark red or black urine caused by massive intravascular hemolysis. Death occurs in 20% to 30% of all cases; the mortality rate is particularly high among Europeans. See also **falciparum malaria, malaria,** *Plasmodium.*

**Blackwell, Elizabeth** (1821–1910), a British-born American physician, the first woman to be awarded a medical degree. She established the New York Infirmary, a 40-bed hospital staffed entirely by women, in which she trained nurses in a 4-month course. Her influence helped others establish nursing schools to improve patient care.

**black widow spider** [AS, *blac* + *widewe;* ME, *spithre*], *Latrodectus mactans,* a species of spider found in the United States, whose bite causes pain and sometimes death.

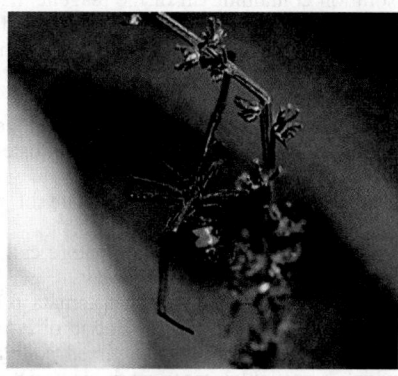

**Black widow spider (*Latrodectus mactans*)**
(Auerbach, 1995/courtesy Paul Auerbach, MD)

**black widow spider antivenin,** a passive immunizing agent.

■ INDICATION: It is prescribed in the treatment of black widow spider bite.

■ CONTRAINDICATIONS: Known hypersensitivity to this drug or to horse serum prohibits its use.

■ ADVERSE EFFECTS: Among the more serious adverse effects are allergic reactions.

**black widow spider bite** [AS, *blac* + *widewe;* ME, *spithre* + AS, *bitan*], the bite of the spider species *Latrodectus*

*mactans,* a poisonous arachnid found in many parts of the world. Black widow venom contains some enzymatic proteins, including a peptide that affects neuromuscular transmission. The bite is perceived as a sharp pinprick pain, followed by a dull pain in the area of the bite; restlessness; anxiety; sweating; weakness; and drooping eyelids. Muscular rigidity starts at the location of the bite and moves in peripherally to the chest. Small children, elderly adults, or persons with heart disorders are most severely affected and may require hospitalization and the administration of an antivenin. Immediate treatment includes keeping the victim quiet and immobilizing the bite area at the level of the heart.

**bladder** [AS, *blaedre*], **1.** a membranous sac serving as a receptacle for secretions, such as the gallbladder. **2.** the urinary bladder.

**bladder cancer,** the most common malignancy of the urinary tract, characterized by multiple growths that tend to recur in a more aggressive form. Bladder cancer occurs 2.3 times more often in men than in women and is more prevalent in urban than in rural areas. The risk of bladder cancer increases with cigarette smoking and exposure to aniline dyes, beta-naphthylamine, mixtures of aromatic hydrocarbons, or benzidine and its salts, used in chemical, paint, plastics, rubber, textile, petroleum, and wood industries and in medical laboratories. Other predisposing factors are chronic urinary tract infections, calculous disease, and schistosomiasis. Symptoms of bladder cancer include hematuria, frequent urination, dysuria, and cystitis. Urinalysis, excretory urography, cystoscopy, or transurethral biopsy are performed for diagnosis. The majority of bladder malignancies are transitional cell carcinomas; a small percentage are squamous cell carcinomas or adenocarcinomas. Superficial or multiple lesions may be treated by fulguration or open loop resection. A segmental resection is usually performed if the tumor is at the dome or in a lateral wall of the bladder. Total cystectomy may be performed for an invasive lesion of the trigone. Radiation therapy and/or chemotherapy may be valuable under certain circumstances, such as unresectable tumor growth. Internal irradiation, the introduction of radioisotopes via a balloon of a catheter, or the implantation of radon seeds may be used in treating small localized tumors on the bladder wall. Medications that are often used as palliatives are BCG, 5-fluorouracil, thio-TEPA, and adriamycin. See also **cystectomy.**

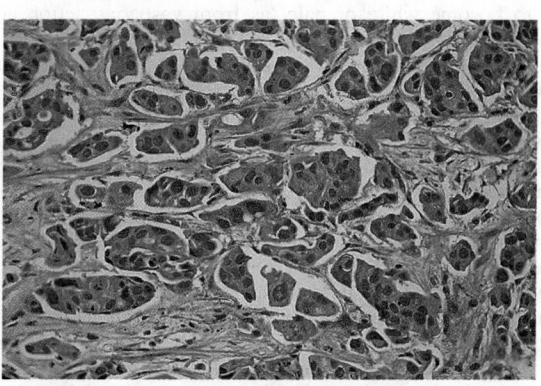

**Transitional cell carcinoma of bladder cancer**
(Fletcher, 2000)

**bladder flap,** *informal.* the vesicouterine fold of peritoneum incised during low cervical cesarean section so the bladder can be separated from the uterus to expose the lower uterine segment for incision. The flap is reapproximated with sutures during closure to cover the uterine incision. See also **cesarean section.**

**bladder hernia,** a protrusion of the bladder through an opening in the abdominal wall.

**bladder irrigation**[1], [AS, *blaedre* + L, *irrigare*, to conduct water], the washing out of the bladder by a continuous or intermittent flow of saline or a medicated solution. The bladder also may be irrigated by an oral intake of fluid.

**bladder irrigation**[2], a nursing intervention from the Nursing Interventions Classification (NIC) defined as instillation of a solution into the bladder to provide cleansing or medication. See also **Nursing Interventions Classification.**

**bladder retraining** [AS, *blaedre* + L, *trahere*, to draw], a system of therapy for urinary incontinence in which a patient practices withholding urine while maintaining a normal intake of fluid. The interval between urination is increased from about 1 hour to 3-4 hours over a period of 10 days. The patient also learns to recognize and react to the urge to urinate.

**bladder sphincter** [AS, *blaedre* + Gk, *sphingein,* to bind], a circular muscle surrounding the opening of the urinary bladder into the urethra.

**bladder stone.** See **vesicle calculus.**

**Blakemore-Sengstaken tube.** See **Sengstaken-Blakemore tube.**

**Blalock-Taussig procedure** /blā′loktô′sig/ [Alfred Blalock, American surgeon, 1899–1964; Helen B. Taussig, American physician, 1898–1986], surgical construction of a shunt as a temporary measure to overcome congenital heart malformations, such as tetralogy of Fallot, in which there is insufficient pulmonary blood flow. Before surgery, a cardiac catheterization is done to identify the defect or defects, and the arterial blood gases are analyzed. Hypothermia anesthesia and a cardiac bypass machine are used. The subclavian artery is joined end to end with the pulmonary artery, directing blood from the systemic circulation to the lungs. Thrombosis of the shunt is the major postoperative complication. Permanent surgical correction is performed in early childhood. See also **heart surgery.**

**blame placing,** the process of placing responsibility for one's behavior on others.

**blanch** /blanch, blänch/ [Fr, *blanchir,* to become white], **1.** to cause to become pale, as a nailbed may be blanched by using digital pressure. **2.** to press blood away and wait for return, such as blanching of fingernails and return of blood. **3.** to become white or pale, as from vasoconstriction accompanying fear or anger.

**blanch test** [Fr, *blanchir,* to become white; L, *testum,* crucible], a test of blood circulation in the fingers or toes. Pressure is applied to a fingernail or toenail until normal color is lost. The pressure is then removed, and, if the circulation is normal, color should return almost immediately, within about 2 seconds. The time may be prolonged by a compromise of circulation, such as arterial occlusion, hypovolemic shock, or hypothermia. Also called **blanching test, capillary refill.**

**bland** [L, *blandus*], mild or having a soothing effect.

**bland aerosols,** aerosols that consist of water, saline solutions, or similar substances that do not have important pharmacologic action. They are primarily used for humidification and liquefaction of secretions.

**bland diet,** a diet that is mechanically, chemically, physiologically, and sometimes thermally nonirritating to the GI

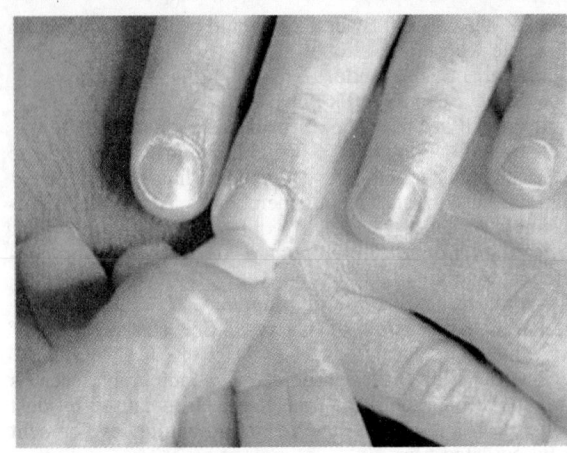

**Blanch test** *(Judd and Ponsell, 1988)*

tract. It is often prescribed in the treatment of peptic ulcer, ulcerative colitis, gallbladder disease, diverticulitis, gastritis, idiopathic spastic constipation, and mucous colitis and after abdominal surgery. Historically, it was first called the "white diet" (or Sippy diet, after Dr. Sippy, who developed it). This allowed the use of only white foods, such as milk, cream, mashed potatoes, and hot cereal (Cream of Wheat). It has progressed to what has been called the "liberal bland diet," which allows all foods except caffeine, alcohol, black pepper, spices, or any other food that could be considered irritating. The clinical value of the traditional bland diet has never been proven.

**blank,** a solution containing all of the reagents needed for analysis of a substance except the substance tested.

**blanket bath** [OFr, *blanchet,* a white garment], the procedure of wrapping the patient in a wet pack and then in blankets.

**blast, 1.** a primitive cell, such as an embryonic germ cell. **2.** a cell capable of building tissue, such as an osteoblast in growing bone.

**-blast,** suffix meaning an 'embryonic state of development': *megaloblast, osteoblast.*

**blast cell** [Gk, *blastos,* germ], any immature cell, such as an erythroblast, lymphoblast, or neuroblast.

**blastema** /blastē′mə/, *pl.* blastemas, blastemata [Gk, bud], **1.** any mass of cells capable of growth and differentiation, specifically the primordial, undifferentiated cellular material from which a particular organ or tissue develops. **2.** in certain animals, a group of cells capable of regenerating a lost or damaged part or creating a complete organism in asexual reproduction. **3.** the budding or sprouting area of a plant. See also **anlage. —blastemal, blastematic, blastemic,** *adj.*

**-blastema** /-blas′təmə/, suffix meaning a 'beginning substance or foundation for new growth': *epiblastema, scytoblastema.*

**blastemata, blastemal, blastematic, blastemic.** See **blastema.**

**blastic transformation,** a late stage in the progress of chronic granulocytic leukemia; the leukemic cells become more undifferentiated and morphologically and genetically more abnormal, with more aggressive growth patterns. Signs of anemia and blood platelet deficiency are present, and half of the blood cells in the bone marrow are immature forms. Blastic transformation indicates that resistance to therapy has developed in the patient who has entered a terminal stage of leukemia.

**blastid** /blas'tid/ [Gk, *blastos,* germ], the site in the fertilized ovum where the pronuclei fuse and the nucleus forms. Also called **blastide.**

**blastin** /blas'tin/ [Gk, *blastanein,* to grow], any substance that provides nourishment for or stimulates the growth or proliferation of cells, such as allantoin.

**blasto-, blast-,** combining form meaning 'an early embryonic or developing stage': *blastocoele, blastema.*

**blastocoele** /blas'tǝsēl'/ [Gk, *blastos,* germ, *koilos,* hollow], the fluid-filled cavity of the blastocyst in mammals and the blastula or discoblastula of lower animals. The cavity increases the surface area of the developing embryo to allow better absorption of nutrients and oxygen. Also spelled **blastocoel, blastocele.** Also called **cleavage cavity, segmentation cavity, subgerminal cavity.**

**blastocyst** /blas'tǝsist/ [Gk, *blastos* + *kystis,* bag], the embryonic form that follows the morula in human development. Implantation in the wall of the uterus usually occurs at this stage, on approximately the eighth day after fertilization. The blastocyst consists of an outer layer (trophoblast) which is attached to the inner cell mass.

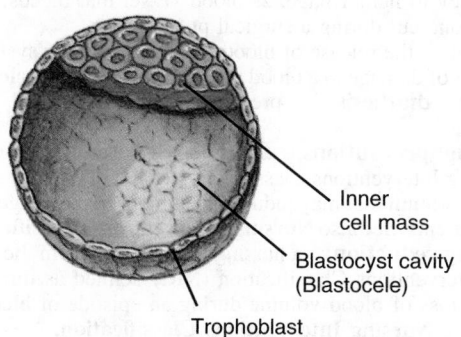

**Blastocyst** *(Applegate, 2000)*

Inner cell mass
Blastocyst cavity (Blastocele)
Trophoblast

**blastocyte** /blas'tǝsīt/ [Gk, *blastos* + *kytos,* cell], an undifferentiated embryonic cell that precedes germ layer formation. —**blastocytic,** *adj.*

**blastocytoma.** See **blastoma.**

**blastoderm** /blas'tǝdurm'/ [Gk, *blastos* + *derma,* skin], the layer of cells forming the wall of the blastocyst in mammals and the blastula in lower animals during the early stages of embryonic development. It is produced by the cleavage of the fertilized ovum and gives rise to the primary germ layers, the ectoderm, mesoderm, and endoderm, from which the embryo and all of its membranes are derived. Kinds of blastoderm are **bilaminar blastoderm, embryonic blastoderm, extraembryonic blastoderm,** and **trilaminar blastoderm.** Also called **germinal membrane.** —**blastodermal, blastodermic,** *adj.*

**blastodisk** /blas'tǝdisk/, the disklike, yolk-free area of cytoplasm surrounding the animal pole in a yolk-rich ovum, such as that of birds and reptiles. The blastodisk is the site where cleavage occurs after fertilization. As cleavage continues, the blastodisk develops into the embryo. Also spelled **blastodisc.**

**blastogenesis** /blas'tōjen'ǝsis/ [Gk, *blastos* + *genein,* to produce], **1.** asexual reproduction by budding. **2.** the transmission of hereditary characteristics by the germ plasm. Compare **pangenesis. 3.** the early development of an embryo during cleavage and formation of the germ layers. **4.** the process of transforming small lymphocytes in tissue culture into large, blastlike cells by exposure to phytohemagglutinin or other substances, often for the purpose of inducing mitosis. —**blastogenetic,** *adj.*

**blastogenic** /-jen'ik/, **1.** originating in the germ plasm. **2.** initiating tissue proliferation. **3.** relating to or characterized by blastogenesis.

**blastogeny** /blastoj'ǝnē/, the early stages in ontogeny; the germ plasm history of an organism or species, which traces the history of inherited characteristics.

**blastokinin** /blas'tǝkī'nin/ [Gk, *blastos* + *kinein,* to move], a globulin, secreted by the uterus in many mammals, that may stimulate and regulate the implantation process of the blastocyst in the uterine wall. Also called **uteroglobulin.**

**blastolysis** /blastol'isis/ [Gk, *blastos* + *lysis,* loosening], destruction of a germ cell or blastoderm. —**blastolytic,** *adj.*

**blastoma** /blastō'mǝ/, *pl.* **blastomas, blastomata** [Gk, *blastos* + *oma,* tumor], a neoplasm of embryonic tissue that develops from the blastema of an organ or tissue. A blastoma derived from a number of scattered cells is pluricentric; one arising from a single cell or group of cells is unicentric. Also called **blastocytoma.** —**blastomatous** /blastom'ǝtǝs/, *adj.*

**blastomatosis** /blast'tōmǝtō'sis/ [Gk, *blastos* + *oma,* tumor, *osis,* condition], the development of many tumors from embryonic tissue.

**blastomatous.** See **blastoma.**

**blastomere** /blas'tǝmēr/ [Gk, *blastos* + *meros,* part], any of the cells formed from the first mitotic division of a fertilized ovum (zygote). The blastomeres further divide and subdivide to form a multicellular morula in the first several days of pregnancy. Also called **segmentation cell.** See also **blastula.** —**blastomeric,** *adj.*

**blastomerotomy** /-merot'ǝmē/ [Gk, *blastos* + *meros,* part, *tome,* cut], the destruction or separation of blastomeres, either caused naturally or induced artificially. Also called **blastotomy** /blastot'ǝmē/. —**blastomerotomic,** *adj.*

*Blastomyces* /blas'tōmī'sēz/ [Gk, *blastos* + *mykes,* fungus], a genus of yeastlike fungus, usually including the species *Blastomyces dermatitidis,* which causes North American blastomycosis, and *Paracoccidioides brasiliensis,* which causes South American blastomycosis.

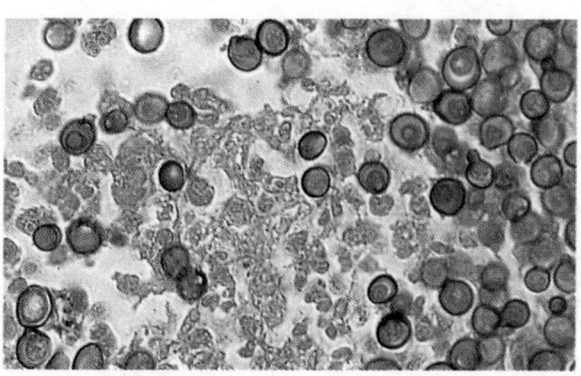

***Blastomyces dermatitidis***
*(Baron, Peterson, and Finegold, 1994)*

**blastomycosis** /blas′tōmīkō′sis/ [Gk, *blastos* + *mykes,* fungus, *osis,* condition], an infectious disease caused by a yeastlike fungus, *Blastomyces dermatitidis.* It usually affects only the skin but may cause acute pneumonitis or disseminated disease and invade the lungs, kidneys, central nervous system, and bones. The disease is most common in river valleys of in North America, particularly the southeastern United States, but outbreaks have occurred in Africa and Latin America. Skin infections are almost always a result of hematogenous seeding from a primary infection and often begin as small papules on the hand, face, neck, or other exposed areas where there has been a cut, bruise, or other injury. The infection may spread gradually and irregularly into surrounding areas. When the lungs are involved, mucous membrane lesions resemble squamous cell carcinoma. The person usually has a cough, dyspnea, chest pain, chills, and a fever with heavy sweating. Diagnosis is made by identification of the disease organism in a culture of specimens from lesions. Treatment usually involves the administration of amphotericin B in pulmonary disease or intraconazole or ketoconazole. Recovery usually begins within the first week of treatment. Also called **Gilchrist's disease.** See also **fungus, mycosis.**

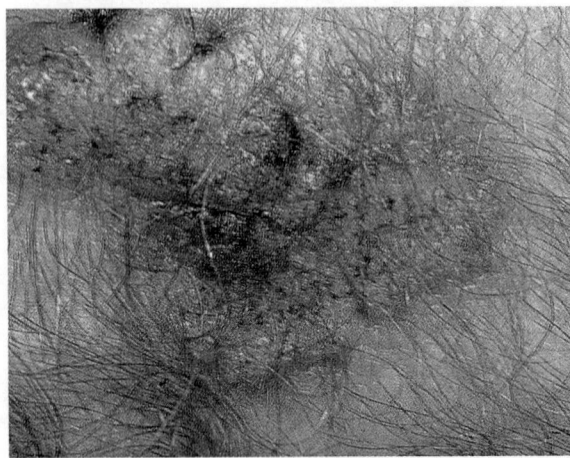

**Blastomycosis: verrucous plaque on the arm**
*(White, 1994)*

**blastopore** /blas′təpôr/ [Gk, *blastos* + *poros,* opening], (in embryology) the opening into the archenteron made by invagination of the blastula.
**blastoporic canal.** See **neurenteric canal.**
**blastosphere.** See **blastula.**
**blastotomy.** See **blastomerotomy.**
**blastula** /blas′tyələ/ [Gk, *blastos,* germ], an early stage of the process through which a zygote develops into an embryo, characterized by a fluid-filled sphere formed by a single layer of cells. The spheric layer of cells is called a blastoderm; the fluid-filled cavity is the blastocoele. The blastula develops from the morula stage and is usually the form in which the embryo becomes implanted in the wall of the uterus. Also called **blastosphere.**
**-blastula,** suffix meaning an 'early embryonic stage in the development of a fertilized egg': *coeloblastula, steroblastula.*
**blastulation,** the transformation of the morula into a blas-

tocyst or blastula by the development of a central cavity, the blastocoele.
**BLB mask,** abbreviation for **Boothby-Lovelace-Bulbulian mask.**
**bleaching** /blēch′ing/ [ME, *blechen*], the act or process of removing stains or color by chemical means.
**bleaching agents,** medications and over-the-counter preparations used to depigment the skin. The products may be used by persons whose skin has become hyperpigmented through exposure to sunlight and particularly for melasma associated with pregnancy or the use of oral contraceptives. Most agents are sold as creams or lotions and contain hydroquinone.
**bleach poisoning,** an adverse reaction to ingestion of hypochlorite salts commonly found in household and commercial bleaches. Symptoms include pain and inflammation of the mouth, throat, and esophagus; vomiting; shock; and circulatory collapse.
**bleb** /bleb/ [ME, blob], an accumulation of fluid under the skin.
**bleed** [AS, *blod,* blood], **1.** to lose blood from the blood vessels of the body. The blood may flow externally through an orifice or a break in the skin or flow internally into a cavity, into an organ, or between tissues. **2.** to cause blood to flow from a vein or an artery.
**bleeder,** *informal.* **1.** a person who has hemophilia or any other vascular or hematologic condition associated with a tendency to hemorrhage. **2.** blood vessel that bleeds, especially one cut during a surgical procedure.
**bleeding,** the release of blood from the vascular system as a result of damage to a blood vessel. See also **blood clotting.**
**bleeding diathesis,** a predisposition to abnormal blood clotting.
**bleeding precautions,** a nursing intervention from the Nursing Interventions Classification (NIC) defined as reduction of stimuli that may induce bleeding or hemorrhage in at-risk patients. See also **Nursing Interventions Classification.**
**bleeding reduction,** a nursing intervention from the Nursing Interventions Classification (NIC) defined as limitation of the loss of blood volume during an episode of bleeding. See also **Nursing Interventions Classification.**
**bleeding reduction: antepartum uterus,** a nursing intervention from the Nursing Interventions Classification (NIC) defined as limitation of the amount of blood loss from the pregnant uterus during third trimester of pregnancy. See also **Nursing Interventions Classification.**
**bleeding reduction: gastrointestinal,** a nursing intervention from the Nursing Interventions Classification (NIC) defined as limitation of the amount of blood loss from the upper and lower gastrointestinal tract and related complications. See also **Nursing Interventions Classification.**
**bleeding reduction: nasal,** a nursing intervention from the Nursing Interventions Classification (NIC) defined as limitation of the amount of blood loss from the nasal cavity. See also **Nursing Interventions Classification.**
**bleeding reduction: postpartum uterus,** a nursing intervention from the Nursing Interventions Classification (NIC) defined as limitation of the amount of blood loss from the postpartum uterus. See also **Nursing Interventions Classification.**
**bleeding reduction: wound,** a nursing intervention from the Nursing Interventions Classification (NIC) defined as limitation of the blood loss from a wound that may be a result of trauma, incisions, or placement of a tube or catheter. See also **Nursing Interventions Classification.**
**bleeding time,** the time required for blood to stop flowing from a tiny wound. A test of bleeding time is the **Ivy method.** See also **hemostasis, simplate bleeding time.**

**bleeding time test,** a blood test used to evaluate the vascular and platelet factors associated with hemostasis. This test is often performed preoperatively to ensure adequate hemostasis.

**blemish** [OFr, *bleme,* to deface], a skin stain, alteration, defect, or flaw.

**blended family** [ME, *blenden,* to mix], a family formed when parents bring together children from previous marriages.

**blending inheritance,** the apparent fusion in offspring of distinct, dissimilar characteristics of the parents. Blended characteristics are usually of a quantitative nature, such as height, and fail to segregate in successive generations. The phenomenon is the result of multiple pairs of genes that have a cumulative effect. See also **polygene.**

**blenno-, blenn-,** combining form meaning 'mucus': *blennemesis, blennothorax.*

**blennorrhea** /blen′ərē′ə/ [Gk, *blennos,* mucus, *rhoia,* flow], excessive discharge of mucus. See also pharyngoconjunctival fever. Also called **blennorrhoea, blennorrhagia** /blen′ôrā′jē·ə/.

**Blenoxane,** trademark for an antineoplastic (bleomycin sulfate).

**bleomycin sulfate** /blē·əmī′sin/, an antineoplastic antibiotic.

■ INDICATIONS: It is prescribed in the treatment of a variety of neoplasms.

■ CONTRAINDICATION: Hypersensitivity to this drug prohibits its use.

■ ADVERSE EFFECTS: Among the most serious adverse reactions are pneumonitis, pulmonary fibrosis, and a syndrome of hyperpyrexia and circulatory collapse. Rashes and skin reactions commonly occur.

**blephar-.** See **blepharo-.**

**blepharal** /blef′ərəl/ [Gk, *blepharon,* eyelid], pertaining to the eyelids.

**blepharedema** /blef′əridē′mə/, a fluid accumulation in the eyelid, causing a swollen appearance.

**-blepharia,** suffix meaning '(condition of the) eyelid': *atretoblepharia, macroblepharia.*

**blepharitis** /blef′ərī′tis/ [Gk, *blepharon* + *itis*], an inflammatory condition of the lash follicles and meibomian glands of the eyelids, characterized by swelling, redness, and crusts of dried mucus on the lids. **Ulcerative blepharitis** is caused by bacterial infection. **Nonulcerative blepharitis** may be caused by psoriasis, seborrhea, or an allergic response.

**blepharo-, blephar-,** combining form meaning 'eyelid or eyelash': *blepharochalasis, blepharelosis.*

**blepharoadenoma** /-ad′inō′mə/, *pl.* **blepharoadenomas, blepharoadenomata,** a glandular epithelial tumor of the eyelid.

**blepharoatheroma** /-ath′ərō′mə/, *pl.* **blepharoatheromas,** blepharoatheromata, a tumor of the eyelid.

**blepharochalasis** /blef′ə·rō·kal′ə·sis/ [Gk, *blepharon,* eyelid + chalasis, relaxation], relaxation of the skin of the eyelid because of atrophy of the intercellular tissue.

**blepharoclonus** /blef′ərok′lōnəs/, a condition characterized by muscle spasms of the eyelid, appearing as increased winking.

**blepharoncus** /blef′əron′kəs/ [Gk, *blepharon* + *onkos,* swelling], a tumor of the eyelid.

**blepharophimosis** /blef′ə·rō·fi·mō′sis/ [Gk, *blepharon,* eyelid + *phimōsis,* a muzzling], abnormal narrowness of the palpebral fissure in the horizontal direction, caused by lateral displacement of the medial canthus.

**blepharoplasty** /blef′əroplas′tē/ [Gk, *blepharon,* eyelid, *plassein,* to mold], the use of plastic surgery to restore or repair the eyelid and eyebrow. Also called **brow lift.**

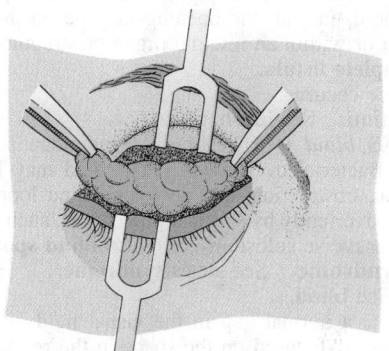

Removal of excess
fat from upper eyelid

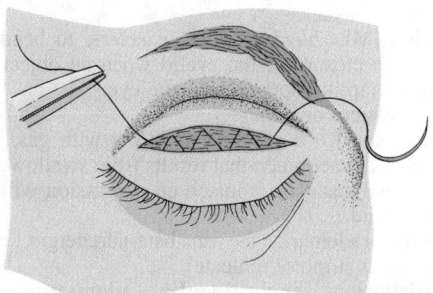

Wound closure

**Blepharoplasty procedure** *(Beare and Myers, 1998)*

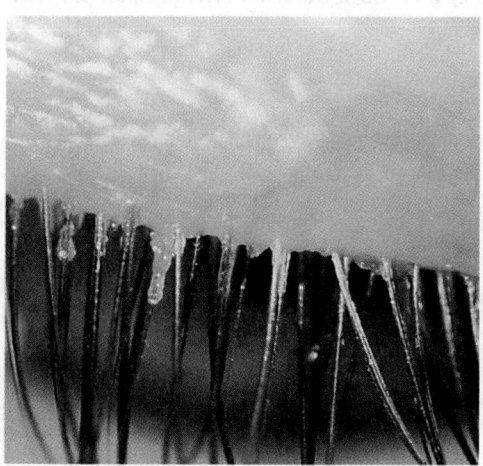

**Blepharitis** *(Zitelli and Davis, 1997)*

**blepharoplegia** /-plē′jē·ə/ [Gk, *blepharon* + *plege,* stroke], paralysis of muscles of the eyelid.

**blepharospasm** /blef′ərōspaz′əm/ [Gk, *blepharon,* eyelid, *spasmos,* spasm], the involuntary contraction of eyelid muscles. The condition may be caused by a local lesion of the eye, a neurologic irritation, or psychologic stress.

**blessed thistle,** an annual herb found in Europe and Asia. ■ USES: This herb is used for loss of appetite, indigestion, and intestinal gas. ■ CONTRAINDICATIONS: Blessed thistle should not be used during pregnancy, in children, or in those with known hypersensitivity to the herb.

**Bleuler, Eugen** /bloi′lər/ [Swiss psychiatrist, 1857–1939], a pioneer investigator in the fields of autism and schizophrenia. Bleuler introduced the term *schizophrenia* to replace *dementia praecox* and identified four primary symptoms of schizophrenia, known as Bleuler's "4 A's": ambivalence, associative disturbance, autistic thinking, and affective incongruity.

**blighted ovum** /blī′tid/, a fertilized ovum that fails to develop. On x-ray or ultrasonic visualization it appears to be a fluid-filled cyst attached to the wall of the uterus. It may be empty, or it may contain amorphous parts. Many first trimester spontaneous abortions represent the expulsion of a blighted ovum. Suction curettage may be necessary if the blighted ovum is retained.

**blind** [AS, *blind*], the absence of sight. The term may indicate a total loss of vision or may be applied in a modified manner to describe certain visual limitations, as in yellow color blindness (tritanopia) or word blindness (dyslexia). Legal blindness is defined as best corrected visual acuity less than 20/200 in the better eye.

**blind fistula** [AS, *blind* + L, pipe], an abnormal passage with only one open end; the opening may be on the body surface or on or within an internal organ or structure. Also called **incomplete fistula.**

**blindgut.** See **cecum.**

**blind intubation.** See **intubation.**

**blind loop** [AS, *blind* + ME, *loupe*], a redundant segment of intestine. Bacterial overgrowth occurs and may lead to malabsorption, obstruction, and necrosis. Blind loops may be created inadvertently by surgical procedures, such as side to side ileotransverse colostomy. See also **blind spot.**

**blind loop syndrome.** See **stasis syndrome.**

**blindness.** See **blind.**

**blind spot,** 1. a normal gap in the visual field occurring when an image is focused on the space in the retina occupied by the optic disc. 2. an abnormal gap in the visual field caused by a lesion on the retina or in the optic pathways or resulting from hemorrhage or choroiditis, often perceived as light spots or flashes.

**blink reflex** [ME, *blenken* + L, *reflectere*, to bend back], the automatic closure of the eyelid when an object is perceived to be rapidly approaching the eye.

**blister,** a vesicle or bulla.

**bloat** [ME, *blout*], a swelling or filling with gas, such as distension of the abdomen that results from swallowed air or from intestinal gas. The stomach on percussion will have a tympanic sound.

**Blocadren,** trademark for a beta-adrenergic receptor blocking agent (timolol maleate).

**Bloch-Sulzberger incontinentia pigmenti, Bloch-Sulzberger syndrome.** See **incontinentia pigmenti.**

**block** [OFr, *bloc*], 1. a stoppage or obstruction. The term is commonly used to indicate an obstruction to the passage of a nerve impulse, as an alpha block of an impulse to an alpha-adrenergic receptor or a beta block of an impulse to a beta-adrenergic receptor. 2. an anesthetic injected in a local area, as a spinal block or mandibular block. 3. a dental device, as a bite block.

**blockade** /blokād′/, an agent that interferes with or prevents a specific action in an organ or tissue, such as a cholinergic blockade that inhibits transmission of acetylcholine-

stimulated nerve impulses along fibers of the autonomic nervous system.

**blockage.** See **obstruction.**

**block anesthesia.** See **conduction anesthesia.**

**blocked communication,** a situation in which communication with a patient is made difficult because of incongruent verbal and nonverbal messages and messages that contain discrepancies and inconsistencies. To clarify blocked communication, therapists may record meetings with patients on videotapes that can be studied for eye contact and other clues to the patient's thinking processes. See also **blocking.**

**blocker.** See **blocking agent.**

**blocking** [ME, *blok*], 1. preventing the transmission of an impulse, such as by an antiadrenergic agent or by the injection of an anesthetic. 2. interrupting an intracellular biosynthetic process, such as by the injection of actinomycin D or the action of an antivitamin. 3. an interruption in the spontaneous flow of speech or thought. 4. repressing an idea or emotion to prevent it from obtruding into the consciousness.

**blocking agent,** a substance administered systemically that blocks or diminishes synaptic efficiency. It is usually specific, as with a beta-adrenergic blocking agent. Also called **blocker.**

**blocking antibody,** an antibody that fails to cross-link and cause agglutination. When such antibodies are present in high concentration, they interfere with the action of other antibodies by occupying all the antigenic sites. See also **antigen-antibody reaction, hapten.**

**blockout** /blok′out/ [OFr, *bloc* + AS, *ūt*], in dentistry, elimination in a cast of undesirable undercut areas by filling them in with a suitable material; this includes all areas that would offer interference to placement of the denture framework and those not crossed by a rigid part of the denture.

**blood** [AS, *blod*], the liquid pumped by the heart through all the arteries, veins, and capillaries. The blood is composed of a clear yellow fluid, called plasma, and the formed elements, and a series of cell types with different functions. The major function of the blood is to transport oxygen and nutrients to the cells and to remove carbon dioxide and other waste products from the cells for detoxification and elimination. Adults normally have a total blood volume of 7% to 8% of body weight, or 70 ml/kg of body weight for men and about 65 ml/kg for women. Blood is pumped through the body at a speed of about 30 cm/second, with a complete circulation time of 20 seconds. Compare **lymph.** See also **blood cell, erythrocyte, leukocyte, plasma, platelet.**

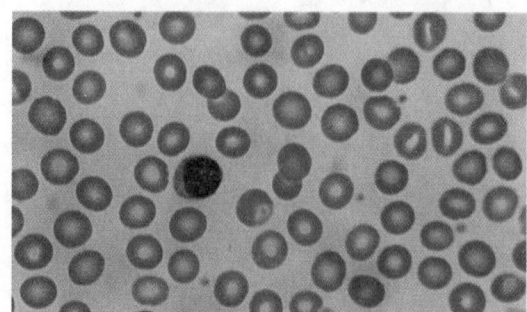

**Blood** *(Carr and Rodak, 1999)*

**blood agar,** a culture medium consisting of blood and nutrient agar, used in bacteriology to cultivate certain microorganisms, including *Staphylococcus epidermidis, Diplococcus pneumoniae,* and *Clostridium perfringens.*

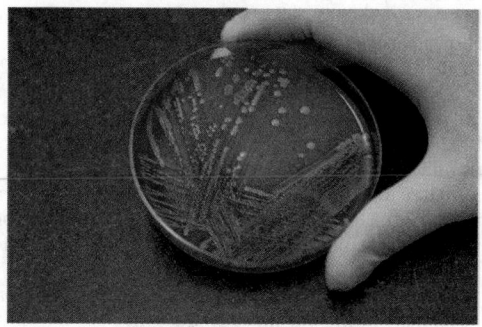

**Blood agar** *(Zakus, 1995)*

**blood albumin** [AS, *blod* + L, *albus*], the plasma protein circulating in blood serum. Also called **serum albumin.**

**blood and urine cortisol,** a blood or urine test that assists in the evaluation of adrenal activity. Adrenal hyperfunction may indicate Cushing's disease, adrenal adenoma or carcinoma, ectopic ACTH-producing tumors, or hyperthyroidism, while hypofunction may indicate congenital adrenal hyperplasia, Addison's disease, hypopituitarism, hypothyroidism, or liver disease.

**blood and urine uric acid,** a blood/urine test that detects levels of uric acid in order to determine the presence of hyperuricemia (elevated uric acid in the blood) and uricosuria (elevated uric acid in the urine). Causes of abnormal uric acid levels may include gout, kidney failure, alcoholism, leukemias, metastatic cancer, multiple myeloma, hyperlipoproteinemia, diabetes mellitus, stress, lead poisoning, and dehydration.

**blood bank,** an organizational unit responsible for collecting, processing, and storing blood for transfusion and other purposes. The blood bank is usually a subdivision of a laboratory in a hospital and is often charged with the responsibility for serologic testing. See also **bank blood, component therapy, transfusion.**

**blood bank technology specialist,** an allied health professional who performs both routine and specialized immunohematologic tests in technical areas of the modern blood bank and who performs transfusion services using methodology that conforms to the *Standards for Blood Banks and Transfusion Services* of the American Association of Blood Banks. The individual may be responsible for testing for blood group antigens, compatibility, and antibody identification; investigating abnormalities such as hemolytic diseases of the newborn, hemolytic anemias, and adverse responses to transfusions; supporting physicians and nurses in transfusion therapy, including that for homologous organ transplantation; collecting and processing blood, including selecting donors, drawing and typing blood, and performing pretransfusion tests to ensure patient safety.

**blood bilirubin test,** a blood test performed in cases of jaundice to help determine whether the jaundice is caused by hepatocellular dysfunction (as in hepatitis) or extrahepatic obstruction of the bile ducts (as with gallstones or tu-

mor blocking the bile ducts). Total serum bilirubin is made up of conjugated (direct) and unconjungated (indirect) bilirubin, with varying ratios of each characterizing different diseases.

**blood blister,** a blister containing blood; it may be caused by a pinch, a bruise, or persistent friction.

**blood-borne pathogens,** pathogenic microorganisms that are transmitted via human blood and cause disease in humans. They include, but are not limited to, hepatitis B virus (HBV) and human immunodeficiency virus (HIV).

**blood-brain barrier (BBB)** [AS, *blod* + *bragen* + ME, *barrere*], an anatomic-physiologic feature of the brain thought to consist of walls of capillaries in the central nervous system and surrounding astrocytic glial membranes. The barrier separates the parenchyma of the central nervous system from blood. The blood-brain barrier prevents or slows the passage of some drugs and other chemical compounds, radioactive ions, and disease-causing organisms such as viruses from the blood into the central nervous system.

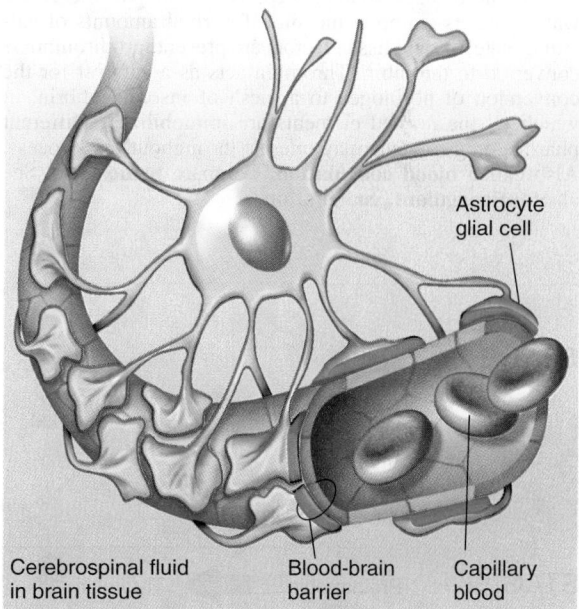

**Blood-brain barrier**

**blood buffers** [AS, *blod* + ME, *buffe,* to cushion], a system of buffers, composed primarily of dissolved carbon dioxide and bicarbonate ions, that functions in maintaining the proper pH of the blood. See also **buffer, arterial pH.**

**blood capillaries** [AS, *blod* + L, *capillaris,* hairlike], the tiny vessels that convey blood between the arterioles and the venules and allow for internal respiration and nourishment of tissues. The capillary wall generally has a thickness of one cell, permitting easy diffusion of gas molecules; occasional tiny openings permit diapedesis of leukocytes, distribution of nutrients to the tissues supplied by the capillary network, and collection of waste products released by the cells.

**blood cell,** any of the formed elements of the blood, including red cells (erythrocytes), white cells (leukocytes), and platelets (thrombocytes). Blood cells constitute about

50% of the total volume of the blood. See also **erythrocyte, leukocyte, platelet.**

**blood cell casts** [AS, *blod* + L, *cella,* storeroom; ONorse, *kasta*],   a mass of blood debris released from a diseased body surface or excreted in the urine.

**blood chloride test,**   a blood test performed as part of multiphasic testing of electrolytes. It is performed along with other electrolyte tests to indicate the patient's acid-base balance and hydrational status.

**blood circulation** [AS, *blod* + L, *circulare,* to go around], the circuit of blood through the body, from the heart through the arteries, arterioles, capillaries, venules, and veins and back to the heart.

**blood clot** [AS, *blod* + *clott,* lump],   a semisolid, gelatinous mass, the final result of the clotting process in blood. Red cells, white cells, and platelets are enmeshed in an insoluble fibrin network of the blood clot. Compare **embolus, thrombus.** See also **blood clotting, fibrinogen.**

**blood clotting,**   the conversion of blood from a free-flowing liquid to a semisolid gel. Although clotting can occur within an intact blood vessel, the process usually starts with tissue damage. Within seconds of injury to the vessel wall, platelets clump at the site. If normal amounts of calcium, platelets, and tissue factors are present, prothrombin is converted to thrombin. Thrombin acts as a catalyst for the conversion of fibrinogen to a mesh of insoluble fibrin, in which all the formed elements are immobilized. Different pharmacologic agents may interact throughout this process. Also called **blood coagulation.** Compare **hemostasis.** See also **anticoagulant, coagulation.**

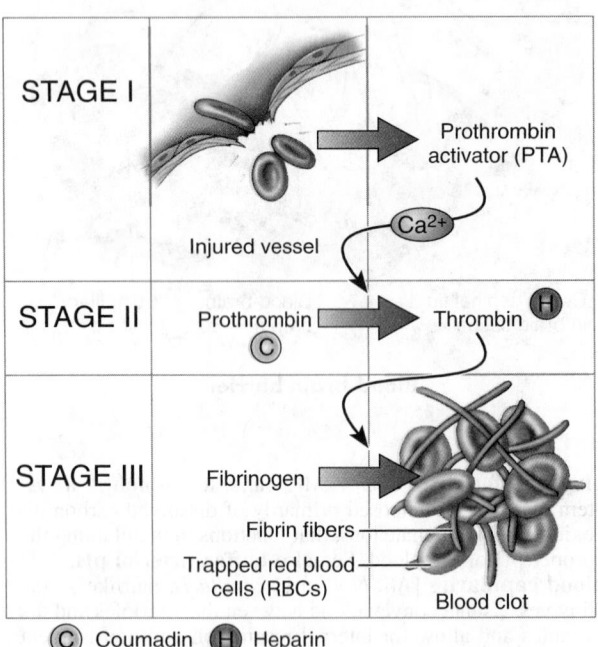

STAGE I

Prothrombin activator (PTA)

Injured vessel

Ca²⁺

STAGE II   Prothrombin   Thrombin

Ⓒ                Ⓗ

STAGE III   Fibrinogen

Fibrin fibers

Trapped red blood cells (RBCs)

Blood clot

Ⓒ Coumadin   Ⓗ Heparin

**Blood clotting** *(Herlihy and Maebius, 2000)*

**blood corpuscle** [AS, *blod* + L, *corpusculum,* little body], an old term for a blood cell, an erythrocyte, a leukocyte, and sometimes a thrombocyte.

**blood count.**   See **complete blood count.**

**blood creatinine test,**   a blood test that measures the amount of creatinine in the blood, in order to diagnose impaired renal function. Elevated creatinine levels suggest a chronic disease process. This test's results are interpreted in conjunction with those for blood urea nitrogen, as part of a renal function study.

**blood crossmatching,**   the direct matching of donor and recipient blood to prevent the transfusion of incompatible blood types. Crossmatching tests for agglutination of (1) donor red blood cells (RBCs) by recipient serum, and (2) recipient RBCs by donor serum.

**blood culture and sensitivity test,**   a blood culture obtained to detect the presence of bacteria in the blood (bacteremia).

**blood culture medium,**   a liquid enrichment medium for the growth of bacteria in the diagnosis of blood infections. It contains a suspension of brain tissue in meat broth with dextrose, peptone, and citrate and has a pH of 7.4.

**blood donor,**   anyone who donates blood or blood components. See also **blood bank, transfusion.**

**blood dyscrasia** [AS, *blod* + Gk, *dys,* bad, *krasis,* mingling],   a pathologic condition in which any of the constituents of the blood are abnormal in structure, function, or quality, as in leukemia or hemophilia.

**blood fluke,**   a parasitic flatworm of the class Trematoda, genus *Schistosoma,* including the species *S. haematobium, S. japonicum,* and *S. mansoni.* See also *Schistosoma,* **schistosomiasis.**

**blood gas,   1.** gas dissolved in the liquid part of the blood. Blood gases include oxygen, carbon dioxide, and nitrogen. **2.** a laboratory test to determine the amount of oxygen, carbon dioxide, and nitrogen in blood.

**blood gas analysis,**   the determination of oxygen and carbon dioxide concentrations and pressures with the pH of the blood by laboratory tests; the following measurements may be made: $PO_2$, partial pressure of oxygen in arterial blood; $PCO_2$, partial pressure of carbon dioxide in arterial blood; $SO_2$, percent saturation of hemoglobin with oxygen in arterial blood; the total $CO_2$ content of (venous) plasma; and the pH.

**blood gas determination,**   an analysis of the pH of the blood and the concentration and pressure of oxygen and carbon dioxide in the blood. It can be performed as an emergency procedure to assess acid-base balance and ventilatory status. Blood gas determination is often important in the evaluation of cardiac failure, hemorrhage, kidney failure, drug overdose, shock, uncontrolled diabetes mellitus, or any other condition of severe stress. The blood for examination is drawn from an artery as ordered in a heparinized syringe, sealed from air, placed in ice, and immediately transported for analysis. Normal adult arterial blood gas values are pH 7.35 to 7.45; $PCO_2$ 35 to 45 mm Hg; $HCO^-_3$ 21 to 28 mEq/L; $PO_2$ 80 to 100 mm Hg; $O_2$ saturation 95% to 100%. See also **acid-base balance, acidosis, alkalosis, oxygenation, PaCO₂, pH, PO₂.**

**blood gas tension,**   the partial pressure of a gas in the blood.

**blood glucose.**   See **blood sugar.**

**blood glucose control,**   a nursing outcome from the Nursing Outcomes Classification (NOC) defined as extent to which plasma glucose levels are maintained in expected range. See also **Nursing Outcomes Classification.**

**blood glucose level** [AS, *blod* + OFr, *livel* + Gk, *glykys,* sweet],   the amount of glucose found in the bloodstream, usually about 70 to 115 mg/dL after an overnight fast. Concentrations higher or lower than these can be a sign of a variety of diseases, such as diabetes mellitus or pancreatic cancer.

**blood glucose test,** a blood test used to detect hyperglycemia or hypoglycemia. This test must be performed frequently in patients with newly diagnosed diabetes mellitus, in order to assist in monitoring and adjusting the insulin dose.

**blood group,** the classification of blood based on the presence or absence of genetically determined antigens on the surface of the red cell. Several different grouping systems have been described. These include ABO, Duffy, high-frequency antigens, I, Kell, Kidd, Lewis, low-frequency antigens, Lutheran, MNS, P, Rh, and Xg. Their relative importance depends on their clinical significance in transfusion therapy, organ transplantation, maternal-fetal compatibility, and genetic studies. See also **ABO blood group.**

**blood island,** one of the clusters of mesodermal cells that proliferate on the outer surface of the embryonic yolk sac and give it a lumpy appearance.

**blood lactate,** lactic acid that appears in the blood as a result of anaerobic metabolism when oxygen delivery to the tissues is insufficient to support normal metabolic demands.

**blood lavage** [AS, *blod* + L, *lavere,* to wash], the removal of toxic elements from the blood by the injection of serum into the veins.

**bloodless, 1.** any organ or body part that lacks blood or appears to lack blood. **2.** a surgical field in which the normal local blood supply has been shunted to other areas.

**bloodless phlebotomy** [AS, *blod* + ME, *les* + Gk, *phleps,* vein, *tomos,* cutting], a technique of trapping blood in a body region by the application of tourniquet pressure that is less than the pressure needed to interrupt arterial blood flow.

**bloodletting,** the therapeutic opening of an artery or vein to withdraw blood from a particular area. It is sometimes performed to treat polycythemia and congestive heart failure. See also **phlebotomy.**

**blood level,** the concentration of a drug or other substance in a measured amount of plasma, serum, or whole blood.

**blood osmolality** [AS, *blod* + Gk, *ōsmos,* impulsion], the osmotic pressure of blood. It measures the amount of solute concentration per unit of total volume of a particular solution. The normal values in serum are 280 to 295 mOsm/L. See also **osmolality.**

**blood osmolality test,** a blood test that measures the concentration of dissolved particles in the blood. It is useful in evaluating patients with fluid and electrolyte imbalance, seizures, coma, and ascites; and in monitoring and evaluating hydration status, acid-base balance, and suspected antidiuretic hormone (ADH) abnormalities.

**blood patch.** See **epidural blood patch.**

**blood pH,** the hydrogen ion concentration of the blood, a measure of blood acidity or alkalinity. The normal pH values for arterial whole blood are 7.35 to 7.454; for venous whole blood, 7.36 to 7.41; for venous serum or plasma, 7.35 to 7.45.

**blood plasma** [AS, *blod* + Gk, *plassein,* to mold], the liquid portion of the blood, free of its formed elements and particles. Plasma represents approximately 50% of the total volume of blood and contains glucose, proteins, amino acids, and other nutritive materials; urea and other excretory products; and hormones, enzymes, vitamins, and minerals. Compare **serum.** See also **blood, plasma protein, pooled plasma.**

**blood platelet.** See **platelet, thrombocyte.**

**blood poisoning.** See **septicemia.**

**blood potassium test (K$^+$),** a blood test that detects the serum concentration of potassium, the major cation within cells. Potassium levels are followed carefully in patients with uremia, Addison's disease, or vomiting and diarrhea; in those on steroid therapy; in those taking potassium-depleting diuretics; and in those taking digitalis-like drugs.

**blood pressure (BP)** [AS, *blod* + L, *premere,* to press], the pressure exerted by the circulating volume of blood on the walls of the arteries and veins and on the chambers of the heart. Blood pressure is regulated by the homeostatic mechanisms of the body by the volume of the blood, the lumen of the arteries and arterioles, and the force of cardiac contraction. In the aorta and large arteries of a healthy young adult, blood pressure is approximately 120 mm Hg during systole and 70 mm Hg during diastole. See also **hypertension, hypotension.**

■ METHOD: The indirect blood pressure is most often measured by auscultation, using an aneroid or mercury sphygmomanometer, a stethoscope, and a blood pressure cuff. With the upper arm at the level of the heart, the cuff is placed around the upper arm and inflated to a pressure greater than the systolic pressure, occluding the brachial artery. The diaphragm of the stethoscope is placed over the artery in the antecubital space, and the pressure in the cuff is slowly released. No sound is heard until the cuff pressure falls below the systolic pressure in the artery; at that point a pulse is heard. As the cuff pressure continues to fall slowly,

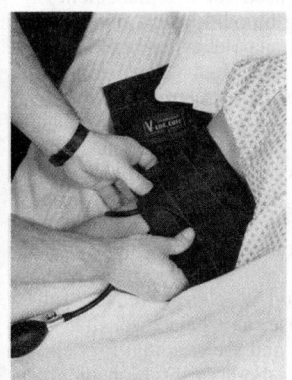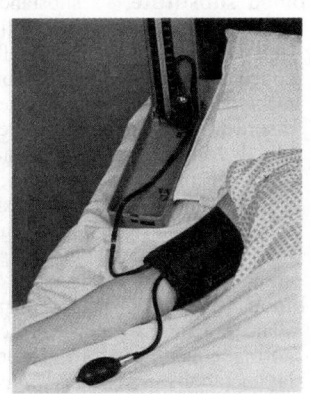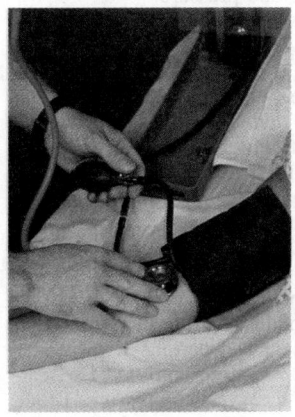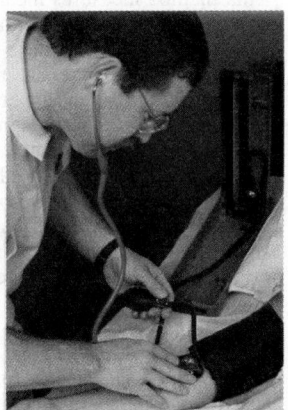

**Measurement of blood pressure** *(Potter and Perry, 1999)*

## Classification of blood pressure for adults ages 18 and older*

| Category | Systolic (mm Hg) | | Diastolic (mm Hg) |
|---|---|---|---|
| Optimal† | <120 | | <80 |
| Normal | <130 | | <85 |
| High normal | 130-139 | | 85-89 |
| Hypertension‡ | | | |
|   Stage 1 (mild) | 140-159 | or | 90-99 |
|   Stage 2 (moderate) | 160-179 | or | 100-109 |
|   Stage 3 (severe) | ≥180 | or | ≥110 |

From Potter PA, Perry AG: *Fundamentals of nursing;* ed 5, St Louis, 2001, Mosby; data from National High Blood Pressure Education Program; National Heart, Lung and Blood Institute; National Institutes of Health: The sixth report of the Joint National Committee on Detection, Evaluation and Treatment of High Blood Pressure, *Arch Intern Med* 157:2413, 2, 1997.

*Not taking antihypertensive drugs and not acutely ill.

†Optimal with respect to cardiovascular risk is below 120/80 mm Hg. Unusually low readings should be evaluated.

‡Based on average of two or more readings.

the pulse continues, first becoming louder, then dull and muffled. These sounds, called **sounds of Korotkoff,** are produced by turbulence of the blood flowing through a vessel that is partially occluded as the arterial pressure falls to the low pressure of diastole. When the cuff pressure is less than the diastolic pressure, no pulse is heard. Thus the cuff pressure at which the first sound is heard is the systolic blood pressure, indicative of the pressure in the large arteries during systole; the cuff pressure at which the sounds stop is the diastolic blood pressure, indicative of the pressure in the arteries during diastole. A variation of this method involves the use of palpation in place of auscultation in the antecubital space to determine the systolic pressure (the pressure at which a pulse is first palpated). Another variation uses a transducer in the cuff to translate changes in ultrasound frequency caused by blood movement within the artery to audible sounds. Blood pressure may be monitored directly by means of a strain gauge or mercury manometer after a cannula has been placed in an artery. The flush method is used when blood pressure is difficult to measure by other methods. The cuff is applied, and complete capillary emptying is performed, usually with an elastic bandage. The cuff is inflated, the elastic bandage is removed, and the earliest discernible flush is observed as the cuff is deflated. This method measures mean blood pressure.

■ INTERVENTIONS: The intervals at which the patient's blood pressure is to be taken are specified. The pressure in both arms is taken the first time the procedure is performed; persistent major differences between the two readings is indicative of a vascular occlusion. Alternatively, the blood pressure may be taken using the thigh and the popliteal space when the leg is at the level of the heart. The width of the cuff should be one third to one half the circumference of the limb used. Thus, a larger cuff is required for a large patient or for any patient if the pressure is taken at the thigh.

■ OUTCOME CRITERIA: Any factor that increases peripheral resistance or cardiac output increases the blood pressure. Therefore, it is important to obtain a blood pressure reading when the patient is at rest. Increased peripheral resistance usually increases the diastolic pressure, and increased cardiac output tends to increase the systolic pressure. Blood pressure increases with age, primarily as a result of the decreased distensibility of the veins. As a person grows older,

an increase in systolic pressure precedes an increase in diastolic pressure.

**blood pressure monitor** [AS, *blod* + L, *premere,* to press, *monere,* to warn], a device that automatically measures blood pressure and records the information continuously. Automatic monitoring of blood pressure is often used in surgery or in an intensive care unit where frequent monitoring is required.

**blood products administration,** a nursing intervention from the Nursing Interventions Classification (NIC) defined as administration of blood or blood products and monitoring of patient's response. See also **Nursing Interventions Classification.**

**blood protein** [AS, *blod* + Gk, *proteios,* of first rank], any of the large variety of proteins normally found in the blood, such as albumin, globulin, hemoglobin, and proteins bound to hormones or other compounds. See also **plasma protein, serum protein.**

**blood protein test (blood albumin),** a blood test that measures levels of albumin, a protein that makes up approximately 60% of the total protein and whose major effect is to maintain colloidal osmotic pressure. Serum protein electrophoresis may assist in diagnosing diseases such as myocardial infarction, chronic infection, granulomatous diseases, cirrhosis, rheumatoid-collagen diseases, nephrotic syndrome, advanced cirrhosis, tuberculosis, endocarditis, and myeloma, among others.

**blood pump,** 1. a device for regulating the flow of blood into a blood vessel during transfusion. 2. a component of a heart-lung machine that pumps the blood through the machine for oxygenation and then through the peripheral circulatory system of the body. Also called **mechanical heartlung.** See also **oxygenation.**

**blood relative,** a related person who shares some of the same genetic material through a common ancestry.

**blood serum.** See **serum.**

**bloodshot,** a redness of the conjunctiva or sclera of the eye caused by dilation of blood vessels in the tissues.

**blood smear,** a blood test used to provide information concerning drugs and diseases that affect the red and white blood cells and to help diagnose certain congenital and acquired diseases. A properly performed and analyzed blood smear is the most informative of all hematologic tests, allowing examination of erythrocytes, platelets, and leukocytes.

**blood sodium test ($Na^+$),** a blood test used to determine the presence of hypo- or hypernatremia by measuring levels of sodium, the major cation in the extracellular space.

**bloodstream,** the blood that flows freely through the circulatory system.

**blood substitute,** a substance used for a replacement or volume expansion for circulating blood. Plasma, human serum albumin, packed red cells, platelets, leukocytes, and concentrates of clotting factors are often administered in place of whole blood transfusions in the treatment of various disorders. Substances that are sometimes used to expand blood volume include dextran, hetastarch, albumin solutions, or plasma protein fraction. Perfluorocarbon emulsions, although potentially toxic, have been tested as blood substitutes; they are able to carry oxygen to tissues, have a long shelf life without refrigeration, and do not induce antigen-antibody reactions.

**blood sugar,** 1. one of a group of closely related substances, such as glucose, fructose, and galactose, that are normal constituents of the blood and are essential for cellular metabolism. 2. *nontechnical.* the concentration of glucose in the blood, represented in milligrams of glucose per deciliter of blood. Home monitoring devices make blood glucose measurement both efficient and accurate. Also called **blood glucose.** See also **hyperglycemia, hypoglycemia.**

**blood test,** any test that yields information about the characteristics or properties of the blood.

**blood transfusion** [AS, *blod* + L *transfundere,* to pour through], the administration of whole blood or a component, such as packed red cells, to replace blood lost through trauma, surgery, or disease.

**blood transfusion reaction control,** a nursing outcome from the Nursing Outcomes Classification (NOC) is defined as extent to which complications of blood transfusions are minimized. See also **Nursing Outcomes Classification.**

**blood typing,** a blood test used to determine the blood type of prospective blood donors and of expectant mothers and newborns. The test detects the presence of ABO antigens as well as the Rh factor.

**blood urea nitrogen (BUN)** [AS, *blod* + Gk, *ouron,* urine, *nitron,* soda, *genein,* to produce], a measure of the amount of urea in the blood. Urea forms in the liver as the end product of protein metabolism, circulates in the blood, and is excreted through the kidney in urine. The BUN, determined by a blood test, is directly related to the metabolic function of the liver and the excretory function of the kidney. Normal findings (in mg/dL) are 10 to 20 for adults, 5 to 18 for children and infants, 3 to 12 for newborns, and 21 to 40 for cord blood. In the elderly, the BUN may be slightly higher than the normal adult range. A critical value of 100 mg/dL indicates serious impairment of renal function. Also called **urea nitrogen, serum urea nitrogen.** See also **azotemia.** Compare **creatinine.**

**blood vessel,** any one of the network of muscular tubes that carry blood. Kinds of blood vessels are **arteries, arterioles, capillaries, veins,** and **venules.**

**blood warming coil,** a device constructed of coiled plastic tubing used for the warming of reserve blood before massive transfusions, such as those often required for patients who experience extensive bleeding. Administration of cold blood in such transfusions may cause the patient to go into a state of shock. The blood warming coil is a prepackaged sterile single-use device. Compare **electric blood warmer.**

**bloody show.** See **vaginal bleeding.**

**bloody sputum** [AS, *blod* + L, *sputum,* spittle], blood-tinged material expelled from the respiratory passages. The amount and color of blood in sputum expelled by coughing or clearing the throat may indicate the cause and location of the bleeding. Swallowed blood regurgitated from the stomach most often loses its vital coloring, however, thus eliminating the opportunity to judge the origin.

**Bloom's syndrome** [David Bloom, American physician, b. 1892], a rare genetic disease occurring mainly in Ashkenazi Jews. It is transmitted as an autosomal recessive trait and is characterized by growth retardation, dilated capillaries of the face and arms, sensitivity to sunlight, and an increased risk of leukemia.

**blot,** **1.** a technique transfering electrophoretically separated components from a gel onto a nitrocellulose membrane, chemically treated paper, or filter for analysis. It is frequently used to analyze genetic material. **2.** the substrate containing the transferred material. See also **Northern blot test, Southern blot test, Western blot test.**

**blotch,** a skin discoloration that may vary in severity from an area of pigmentation to large pustules or blisters.

**blow bottles,** a device used in respiratory care to provide resistance to expiration. The bottles are partially filled with water, and the patient is encouraged to blow the water from one bottle to another, a practice that requires deep inspiration and lung expansion to develop increased lung pressure.

**blow-out fracture,** a break in the floor of the orbit caused by a blow that suddenly increases the intraocular pressure.

**blowpipe** /blō′pīp/ [AS, *blāwan* + *pīpe*], a tube through which a current of air or other gas is forced on a flame to concentrate and intensify the heat.

**BLS,** abbreviation for **basic life support.**

**blue asphyxia.** See **asphyxia livida.**

**blue baby** [OFr, *blou* + ME, *babe*], an infant born with cyanosis caused by a congenital heart lesion, most commonly tetralogy of Fallot. Other causative lesions include transposition of the great vessels, and incomplete expansion of the lungs (congenital atelectasis). Congenital cyanotic heart lesions are diagnosed by cardiac catheterization, angiography, or echocardiography and are corrected surgically, preferably in early childhood. See also **congenital cardiac anomaly, tetralogy of Fallot, transposition of the great vessels.**

**blue cohosh,** a perennial herb found in the midwest and eastern regions of the United States.

■ USES: This herb is used to treat menopausal symptoms and uterine and ovarian pain, to improve the flow of menstrual blood, and as an antiinflammatory and antirheumatic. It is also a popular remedy in African American ethnic medicine.

■ CONTRAINDICATIONS: Blue cohosh should not be used during pregnancy, since the herb is a uterine stimulant. It is also contraindicated during lactation, in children, and in people with cardiac disease.

**Blue Cross,** an independent nonprofit U.S. corporation that functions as a health insurance agency, providing protection for an enrolled patient by covering all or part of the person's hospital expenses. Blue Cross programs vary in different communities because of state laws regulating them.

**blue diaper syndrome** [OFr, *blou;* ME, *diapre,* patterned fabric], a defect of tryptophan absorption in which, because of intestinal bacterial action on the tryptophan, the urine contains abnormal indoles, giving it a blue color. It is similar to Hartnup's disease.

**blue dome cyst,** a spherical dilation of a mammary duct in which bleeding has occurred.

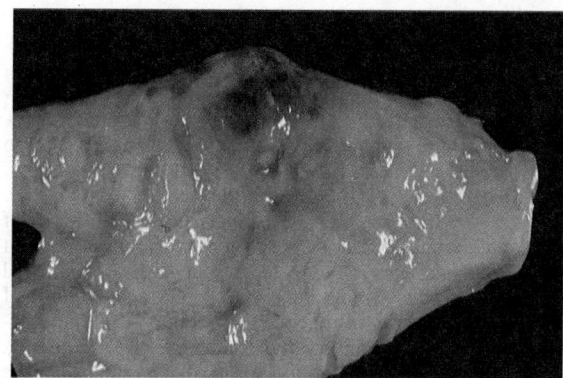

**Blue dome cyst** *(Cotran, Kumar, and Collins, 1999)*

**blue dot sign,** a tender blue or black spot beneath the skin of the testis or epididymis, a sign of testicular torsion of the appendix testis.

**blue fever,** *informal.* Rocky Mountain spotted fever, so named for the dark cyanotic discoloration of the skin after the initial rickettsial infection. See also **rickettsiosis, Rocky Mountain spotted fever, typhus.**

**blue-green algae,** misnomer formerly applied to the group now called the **cyanobacteria.**

**blue-green algae poisoning.** See **cyanobacteria poisoning.**

**blue line,** a bluish discoloration sometimes observed on the gingival side of the mouth in cases of gingivitis. It is a sign of chronic lead or bismuth poisoning.

**blue nevus** [OFr, *blou* + L, *naevus,* mole], a sharply circumscribed, usually benign, steel blue skin nodule with a diameter between 2 and 7 mm. It is found on the face or upper extremities, grows very slowly, and persists throughout life. The dark color is caused by large, densely packed melanocytes deep in the dermis of the nevus. Nodular blue nevi found on the buttocks or in the sacrococcygeal region occasionally become malignant. Any sudden change in the size of such a lesion demands surgical attention and biopsy. Compare **melanoma.**

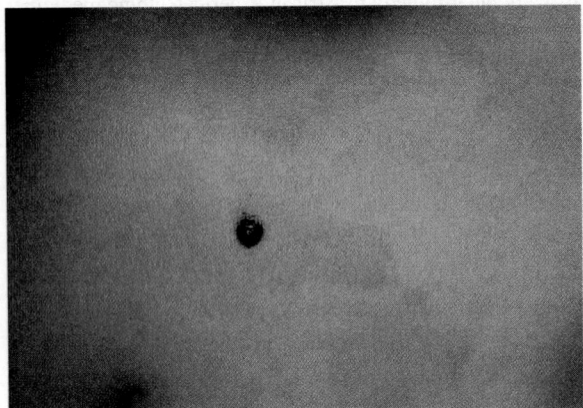

**Blue nevus** *(Weston, Lane, and Morrelli, 1996)*

**blue phlebitis,** a severe form of thrombosis of a deep vein, usually the femoral vein. The condition is acute and fulminating and is usually accompanied by vast edema and cyanosis of the limb distal to the occluding thrombus. Also called **phlegmasia cerulea dolens.**

**blue rubber bleb nevus** [OFR, *blou,* blue; + ME, *rubben,* to scrape; + ME, *bleb,* blob; + L, *naevus,* mole], a type of congenital nevus, transmitted as an autosomal dominant trait, characterized by blue hemangiomas with soft elevated nipple-like centers, found on the skin surface, in the GI tract, and sometimes on mucous membranes; it may be accompanied by pain, regional hyperhidrosis, or GI bleeding.

**blues,** *informal.* a designation for **Blue Cross** (an insurance system that pays the costs of treatment by a hospital or clinic) and **Blue Shield. 2.** *informal.* mild depression.

**Blue Shield,** an independent nonprofit U.S. corporation that offers patient protection for costs of surgery and other medical services. Although Blue Cross and Blue Shield are technically separate organizations, they generally coordinate their functions in providing benefits covering both hospital costs and physician fees.

**blue spot, 1.** also called **macula cerulea** /seroo'le-ə/. one of a number of small grayish blue spots that may appear

near the armpits or around the groins of individuals infested with lice, such as in pediculosis corporis and pediculosis pubis. These spots are usually less than 1 cm in diameter and are caused by a substance in the saliva of lice that converts bilirubin to biliverdin. **2.** one of a number of dark blue round or oval spots that may appear as a congenital condition in the sacral regions of certain children less than 4 or 5 years of age. They usually disappear spontaneously as the affected individual matures. Also called **mongolian spot.**

**blunt dissection** [ME, *blunt* + L, *dissecare,* to cut apart], a dissection performed by separating tissues along natural lines of cleavage without cutting.

**blunt-ended DNA,** a segment of DNA in which the ends of both strands are even with each other.

**blunthook** /blunt'hŏok/ [ME, *blunt* + AS, *hoc*], **1.** a sturdy hook-shaped bar used in obstetrics for traction between the abdomen and the thigh in cases of difficult breech deliveries. **2.** a hook-shaped device with a blunt end used in embryotomy.

**blunting,** a decrease in the intensity of emotional expression from the level one would normally expect as a reaction to a specific situation. It is the opposite of overreaction and may be marked by apathy, minimal response, or indifference.

**blurred film fault** /blurd'/, a defect in a photograph or radiograph that appears as an indistinct or blurred image. It is caused by film movement during exposure, bending of film during exposure, double exposure, or film emulsion flow during processing in excessively warm solutions.

**blush** [ME, *blusshen,* to redden], a brief, diffuse erythema of the face and neck, commonly the result of dilation of superficial small blood vessels in response to heat or sudden emotion.

**BLV-HTLV retroviruses,** a genus similar in morphology and replication to the type C retroviruses; organisms have a long latency and cause B and T cell leukemia and lymphoma and neurological disease. Included in this genus are human T-lymphotropic viruses 1 and 2.

**B lymphocyte.** See **B cell.**

**B/M,** abbreviation for *black male,* often used in the initial identifying statement in a patient record.

**BMA,** abbreviation for **British Medical Association.**

**BMD,** abbreviation for **Bureau of Medical Devices.**

**BMI,** abbreviation for **body mass index.**

**B-mode,** brightness modulation in diagnostic ultrasonography. Bright dots on an oscilloscope screen represent echoes, and the intensity of the brightness indicates the strength of the echo. See also **A-mode, M-mode.**

**BMR,** abbreviation for **basal metabolic rate.**

**BNA,** abbreviation for *Basle Nomina Anatomica.*

**BOA,** abbreviation for **born out of asepsis.**

**board.** See **custodial care.**

**board and care** nonmedical, community-based residential care for individuals who can care for themselves; meals and supervision are provided.

**board certification,** a process by which physicians are certified in a given medical specialty or subspecialty. Certification is awarded by the 23-member boards of the American Board of Medical Specialties on completion of accredited training and examinations and fulfillment of individual requirements of the board.

**board certified,** denoting a physician who has completed the certification requirements established by a medical specialty board and has been certified as a specialist in a particular field of medicine.

**board eligible,** denoting a physician who has completed all of the requirements for admission to a medical specialty board.

**boarder baby,** 1. an infant abandoned to a hospital because the mother is unable to care for him or her. Many infants born with human immunodeficiency virus (HIV) or to a mother with HIV infection or infants delivered to mothers who are drug users are boarder babies. 2. in some hospitals, any infant still in the nursery after the mother's discharge for any reason (even if only very temporarily).

**board of health,** an administrative body acting on a municipal, county, state, provincial, or national level. The functions, powers, and responsibilities of boards of health vary with the locales. Each board is generally concerned with the recognition of the health needs of the people and the coordination of projects and resources to meet and identify these needs. Among the tasks of most boards of health are disease prevention, health education, and implementation of laws pertaining to health.

**bobbing,** the act of moving up and down, usually with a jerking motion.

**Bodansky unit** /bōdăn′skē/ [Aaron Bodansky, American biochemist, 1887–1961], the quantity of alkaline phosphatase that liberates 1 mg of phosphate ion from glycerol 2-phosphate in 1 hour at 37° C and under other standardized conditions.

**body** [AS, *bodig*], 1. the whole structure of an individual with all the organs. 2. a cadaver (corpse). 3. the largest or the main part of any structure, such as the body of the stomach. Also called **corpus, soma.**

**body burden,** the state of activity of a radioactive chemical in the body at a specified time after administration.

**body cast** [AS, *bodig,* body; ONorse, *kasta*], a molded cast that may extend from the chest to the groin to immobilize the spine.

**body cavity,** any of the spaces in the human body that contain organs. One major cavity, the thoracic cavity, is subdivided into a pericardial and two pleural cavities.

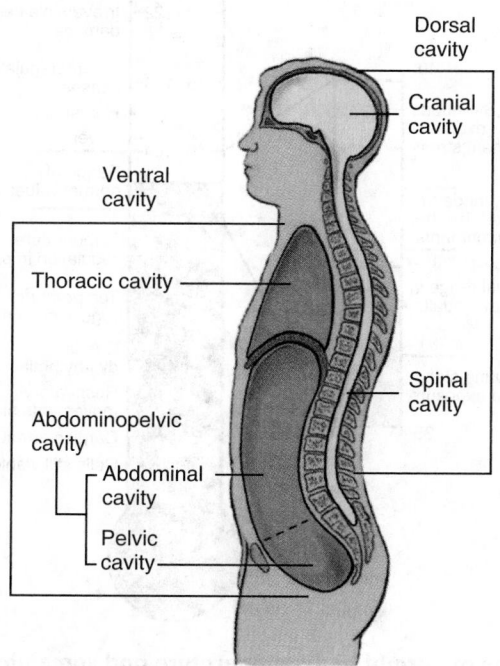

**Major body cavities** *(Applegate, 2000)*

**body composition,** the relative proportions of protein, fat, water, and mineral components in the body. It varies among individuals as a result of differences in body density and degree of obesity. Methods for calculating body composition include underwater weighing and injection of radioactive tracers.

**body fluid** [AS, *bodig* + L, *fluere,* to flow], fluid contained in the three fluid compartments of the body: the plasma of the circulating blood, the interstitial fluid between the cells, and the cell fluid within the cells. See also **blood plasma, interstitial fluid, extracellular fluid (ECF), intracellular fluid.**

**body image**[1] [AS, *bodig* + L, *imago,* likeness], a person's concept of his or her physical appearance. The mental representation, which may be realistic or unrealistic, is constructed from self-observation, the reactions of others, and a complex interaction of attitudes, emotions, memories, fantasies, and experiences, both conscious and unconscious. A marked inability to conceptualize one's personal body characteristics may be caused by organic brain damage, as in autotopagnosia; by a physical disability, such as the loss of a limb; or by psychologic and emotional disturbances, as in anorexia nervosa.

**body image**[2], a nursing outcome from the Nursing Outcomes Classification (NOC) defined as positive perception of own appearance and body functions. See also **Nursing Outcomes Classification.**

**body image agnosia.** See **autotopagnosia.**

**body image, disturbed,** a nursing diagnosis accepted by the Seventh National Conference on the Classification of Nursing Diagnoses. The condition is defined as a disruption in the way one perceives one's body. The cause of a disturbance in body image may be a biophysical, cognitive, perceptual, psychosocial, cultural, or spiritual factor.

■ DEFINING CHARACTERISTICS: Objective characteristics of the deficit include verbal or nonverbal responses to a real or perceived change in structure or function, a missing body part, trauma to a nonfunctioning part, and a change in the ability to estimate spatial relationship of the body to the environment. Subjective characteristics include personalization of the missing part by giving it a name, refusal to look at a part of the body, negative feelings about the body, a change in general social involvement or life-style, and a fear of rejection by others.

■ RELATED FACTORS: Related factors include biophysical, cognitive, perceptual, psychosocial, cultural, and spiritual factors. See also **nursing diagnosis.**

**body image enhancement,** a nursing intervention from the Nursing Interventions Classification (NIC) defined as improving a patient's conscious and unconscious perceptions and attitudes toward his/her body. See also **Nursing Interventions Classification.**

**body jacket,** an orthopedic cast that encases the trunk of the body but does not extend over the cervical area; it may be equipped with shoulder straps. The cast is used to help position and immobilize the trunk for the healing of spinal injuries and scoliosis and after spinal surgery. Compare **Risser cast.** See also **thoracolumbosacral orthosis.**

**body language** [AS, *bodig* + L, *lingua,* tongue], a set of nonverbal signals, including body movements, postures, gestures, spatial positions, facial expressions, and body adornment, that give expression to various physical, mental, and emotional states. See also **kinesics.**

**body louse.** See **lice,** *Pediculus humanus corporis.*

**body mass index (BMI),** a formula for determining obesity. It is calculated by dividing a person's weight in kilo-

## Body mass index calculation

$$BMI = \frac{Weight\ (kg)}{Height\ (m^2)}$$

| Body mass index assessment | |
|---|---|
| 19-25 | Appropriate weight (19-34 years) |
| 21-27 | Appropriate weight (>35 years) |
| 27.5-30 | Mild obesity |
| 30-40 | Moderate obesity |
| >40 | Morbid obesity |

From Thompson JM, Wilson SF: *Health assessment for nursing practice,* St Louis, 1996, Mosby.

grams by the square of the person's height in meters. A BMI of 27 or greater indicates obesity.

**body mechanics,** the field of physiology that studies muscular actions and the function of muscles in maintaining body posture. Knowledge gained from such studies is especially important in the prevention of injury during the performance of tasks that require the body to lift and move.

**body mechanics promotion,** a nursing intervention from the Nursing Interventions Classification (NIC) defined as facilitating the use of posture and movement in daily activities to prevent fatigue and musculoskeletal strain or injury. See also **Nursing Interventions Classification.**

**body movement,** motion of all or part of the body, especially at a joint or joints. Body movements include **abduction, adduction, extension, flexion, rotation,** and **circumduction.**

**body odor,** a fetid smell associated with stale perspiration. Freshly secreted perspiration is odorless, but after exposure to the atmosphere and bacterial activity at the surface of the skin, chemical changes occur to produce the odor. Common body odor usually can be eliminated by bathing with soap and water. Body odors also can be the result of discharges from a variety of skin conditions, including cancer, fungus, hemorrhoids, leukemia, and ulcers. See also **bromhidrosis.**

**body of Retzius** /ret′sē·əs/ [Magnus G. Retzius, Swedish anatomist, 1842–1919], any one of the masses of protoplasm containing pigment granules at the lower end of a hair cell of the organ of Corti in the internal ear.

**body plethysmograph** [AS, *bodig* + Gk, *plethynein,* to increase, *graphein,* to record], a device for studying alveolar pressures, lung volumes, and airway resistance. The patient sits or reclines in an airtight compartment and breathes normally. The pressure changes in the alveoli are reciprocated in the compartment and are recorded automatically.

**body position,** attitude or posture of the body. See **anatomic position, decubitus position, Fowler's position, prone, supine,** and **Trendelenburg position.**

**body positioning: self-initiated,** a nursing outcome from the Nursing Outcomes Classification (NOC) defined as ability to change own body positions. See also **Nursing Outcomes Classification.**

**body righting reflex.** See **righting reflex.**

**body scheme,** a piagetian term for a cognitive structure that develops in infants in the sensorimotor period during the first 2 years of life as they learn to differentiate between themselves and the world around them.

**body-scheme disorder.** See **autotopagnosia.**

**body-section radiography,** a radiographic technique in which the film and x-ray tube are moved in opposite direc-

tions to produce a more distinct image of a selected body plane. The process has the effect of blurring adjacent body structures during exposure. Also called **tomography.**

**body stalk,** the elongated part of the embryo that is connected to the chorion. See also **allantois.**

**body surface area.** See **surface area.**

**body systems model,** (in nursing education) a conceptual framework in which illness is studied in relation to the functional systems of the body, such as the circulatory, nervous, GI, and reproductive. In this model, nursing care is directed to manipulating the patient's environment in such a way that the signs and symptoms of the health problem are alleviated. As the body systems model traditionally focuses on the disease rather than the patient, current educational programs tend to integrate it with other concepts that allow the nurse to approach the patient in a more holistic framework. Also called **medical model.**

**body temperature,** the level of heat produced and sustained by the body processes. Variations and changes in body temperature are major indicators of disease and other abnormalities. Heat is generated within the body through metabolism of nutrients and lost from the body surface through radiation, convection, and evaporation of perspiration. Heat production and loss are regulated and controlled in the hypothalamus and brainstem. Fever is usually a function of an increase in heat generation; however, some abnormal conditions, such as congestive heart failure, produce slight elevations of body temperature through impairment of the heat loss function. Contributing to the failure to dissipate heat are reduced activity of the heart, lower rate of blood flow to the skin, and the insulating effect of edema. Diseases of the hypothalamus or interference with the other regula-

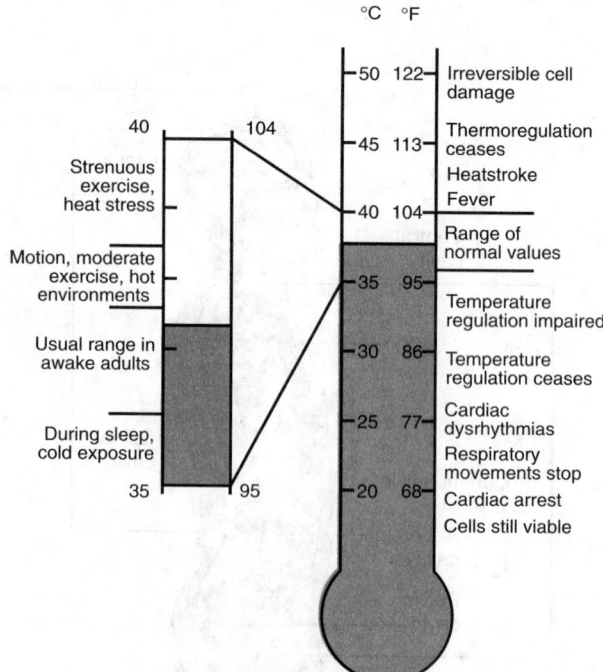

**Range of normal body temperature and some physiologic consequences of abnormal body temperature**
*(Thibodeau and Patton, 1999)*

tory centers may produce abnormally low body temperatures. Normal adult body temperature, as measured orally, is 98.6° F (37° C). Oral temperatures ranging from 96.5° F to 99° F are consistent with good health, depending on the person's physical activity, the environmental temperature, and that person's usual body temperature. Axillary temperature is usually from 0.5° to 1° F lower than the oral temperature. Rectal temperatures may be 0.5° to 1° F higher than oral readings. Body temperature appears to vary 1° to 2° F throughout the day, with lows recorded early in the morning and peaks between 6 PM and 10 PM. This diurnal variation may increase in range during a fever. Whereas adult body temperature, normal and abnormal, tends to vary within a relatively narrow range, children's temperatures respond more dramatically and rapidly to disease, changes in environmental temperature, and levels of physical activity.

**body temperature, imbalanced, risk for,** a nursing diagnosis accepted by the Seventh National Conference on the Classification of Nursing Diagnoses. The condition is a state in which the individual is at risk for failure to maintain body temperature within a normal range.

■ RISK FACTORS: Risk factors are extremes of age; extremes of weight; exposure to cool-to-cold or warm-to-hot environments; dehydration; inactivity or vigorous activity; medications causing vasoconstriction or vasodilation; altered metabolic rate; sedation; clothing inappropriate for environmental temperature; and illness or trauma affecting temperature regulations. See also **nursing diagnosis.**

**body type,** the general physical appearance of an individual human body. Three commonly used terms for body types are ectomorph, describing a thin, fragile physique; endomorph, denoting a round, soft body; and mesomorph, indicating a muscular, athletic body of average size. See also **asthenic habitus, athletic habitus, ectomorph, endomorph, mesomorph, pyknic.**

**body-weight ratio,** a relation expressed by dividing the body weight in grams by the height in centimeters.

**Boeck's disease, Boeck's sarcoid.** See **sarcoidosis.**

**Boerhaave's syndrome** /bôr′hävz/ [Hermann Boerhaave, Dutch physician, 1668–1738], a condition marked by spontaneous rupture of the esophagus, usually preceded by severe vomiting, leading to mediastinitis and pleural effusion. Clinical manifestations are violent retching or vomiting. Emergency care with surgery and drainage is needed to save the life of the patient.

**Bohr effect** [Christian Bohr, Danish physiologist, 1855–1911], the effect of $CO_2$ and $H^+$ on the affinity of hemoglobin for molecular $O_2$. Increasing $PCO_2$ and $H^+$ decrease oxyhemoglobin saturation, whereas decreasing concentrations have the opposite effect. In humans a decrease of pH from 7.4 to 7.3 at 40 mm Hg $PO_2$ decreases oxyhemoglobin saturation by 6%. The Bohr effect is particularly significant in the capillaries of working muscles and the myocardium and in maternal and fetal exchange vessels of the placenta.

**bohrium (Bh).** See **element 107.**

**boil** [AS, *byle*, sore], a skin abscess. See **furuncle.**

**boiling point** [ME, *boilen*, to make bubbles; L, *pungere*, to prick], **1.** the temperature at which a substance passes from the liquid to the gaseous state at a particular atmospheric pressure. **2.** the temperature at which the vapor pressure of a liquid equals the external pressure. See also **evaporation.**

**-bol,** combining form designating an anabolic steroid.

**bole** /bōl/, any of a variety of soft, friable clays of various colors, although usually red from iron oxide. They consist of

hydrous silicate of aluminum, are used as pigments, and were once commonly used as absorbents and astringents.

**Bolivian hemorrhagic fever** /bəliv′ē·ən/, an infectious disease caused by an arenavirus, generally transmitted by contact with or inhalation of aerosolized rodent urine. After an incubation period of from 1 to 2 weeks, the patient experiences chills, fever, headache, muscle ache, anorexia, nausea, and vomiting. As the disease progresses, hypotension, dehydration, bradycardia, pulmonary edema, and internal hemorrhage may occur. The mortality rate may reach 30%; pulmonary edema is the most common cause of death. There is no specific therapy. Peritoneal dialysis is sometimes performed. Also called **Machupo.** See also *Arenavirus,* Argentine hemorrhagic fever, Lassa fever.

**bolus** /bō′ləs/ [Gk, *bolos,* lump], **1.** also called **alimentary bolus.** a round mass, specifically a masticated lump of food ready to be swallowed. **2.** a large round preparation of medicinal material for oral ingestion, usually soft and not prepackaged. **3.** a dose of a medication or a contrast material, radioactive isotope, or other pharmaceutic preparation injected all at once intravenously. **4.** (in radiotherapy) material used to fill in irregular body surfaces to improve dose distribution for hyperthermia or to increase the dose to the skin when high-energy photon beams are used. **5.** a clumping in the stomach of ingested foreign material, often the result of habitual behavior.

**bolus dose,** a relatively large amount of IV medication administered rapidly to decrease the response time. See also **bolus.**

**bombard** /bombärd′/, to shower a drug or tissue sample with radioactive particles from a nuclear isotope source.

**Bombay phenotype** /bombā′/ [Bombay, India, where first reported], a rare genetic trait involving the phenotypic expression of the ABO blood groups. The gene for the H antigen, which in the usual dominant form of HH or Hh is responsible for the precursor necessary for the production of the A and B antigens, is homozygous recessive in individuals with this trait so that the expression of the A, B, and H antigens is suppressed. Cells of such individuals are phenotypically of blood type O, and the serum contains anti-A, anti-B, and anti-H antigens. In such cases the offspring from two phenotypic O blood type parents may be blood type AB. The phenomenon is an example of the intricate interaction of linked genes in which one gene on a chromosome controls the expression or suppression of another gene that is not its allele. See also **ABO blood group.**

**bombesin** /bom′bə·sin/, a neurohormone and pressor substance found in small amounts in brain and intestinal tissue under normal conditions and in increased amounts in certain pulmonary and thyroid tumors; it is a potent mitogen and its effects on gastrin and other hormones are attributed to increased cell numbers.

**bond,** a strong coulombic force between atoms in a substance. See also **coulomb, Coulomb's law.**

**bonding** [ME, *band,* to bind], **1.** (in dentistry) a technique of joining orthodontic brackets or other attachments directly to the enamel surface of a tooth, using orthodontic adhesives. **2.** the reciprocal attachment process that occurs between an infant and the parents, especially the mother. Bonding is significant in the formation of affectionate ties that later influence both the physical and psychologic development of the child. It is usually initiated immediately after birth by placing the nude infant on the mother's abdomen so that both the parents and the child can see and touch one another and begin to interact. The newborn is in an alert, reactive state for about 30 minutes to 1 hour after birth and displays such behaviors as crying, sucking, clinging, grasping, and following with the eyes, which in turn stimulate the expression of parenting instincts. By about the second to third week of the infant's life, a definite, reciprocal pattern of interacting behavior that involves an attention-nonattention cycle occurs during each encounter of parents and child. At the peak of the attention phase, the infant reaches out toward the parent and is very attentive. This peak is followed in a short time by deceleration of excitement in the infant and a turning away from the parent. This nonattentive phase prevents the infant from being overwhelmed by excessive stimuli, and no visual or verbal attempt will regain the infant's attention. Recognizing that the nonattention phase does not represent rejection helps the mother and father develop competence in parenting. Assessment of the attachment process is an important nursing function and requires skillful observation and interviewing. The nurse observes the mother's reactions, especially while feeding, bathing, and comforting her infant, for potential signs of inadequate or delayed mothering. Among the most important actions for bonding are eye contact in the en face position and embracing of the infant close to the body. Many variables determine the development of bonding and parenting, including the parents' fantasies about the child, the conditions surrounding the pregnancy, the arrangements that have been made concerning changes in life-style with the addition of a dependent family member, and the type of parenting the mother and father received as children. Bonding is also seen in adoptive situations and is not limited to the newborn period. Although bonding is considered primarily an emotional response, it is hypothesized that some biochemical and hormonal interaction in the mother may stimulate the response; results of studies testing this hypothesis are inconclusive. Also called **maternal-child attachment.** See also **maternal deprivation syndrome, maternal-infant bonding.**

**bond specificity,** the nature of enzyme action that causes the disruption of only certain bonds between atoms.

**bone** [AS, *ban*], **1.** the dense, hard, and somewhat flexible connective tissue constituting the bones of the human skeleton. It is composed of compact osseous tissue surrounding spongy cancellous tissue permeated by many blood vessels and nerves and enclosed in membranous periosteum. **2.** any single element of the skeleton, such as a rib, the sternum, or the femur. Also called *(Latin)* **os.** See also **connective tissue.**

**bone age** [AS, *ban* + L, *aetas*], the stage of development or decline of the skeleton or its segments, as seen in radiographic examination, when compared with x-ray views of the bone structures of other individuals of the same chronologic age.

**bone cancer** [AS, *ban* + Gk, *karkinos,* crab], a skeletal malignancy occurring as a sarcoma or a myeloma in an area of rapid growth or as metastasis from cancer elsewhere in the body. Primary bone tumors are rare; the incidence peaks during adolescence, decreases, and then rises slowly after 35 years of age. In adults, bone cancer is linked to exposure to ionizing radiation. Paget's disease, hyperparathyroidism, chronic osteomyelitis, old bone infarcts, and fracture callosities increase the risk of many bone tumors. Most osseous malignancies are metastatic lesions found most often in the spine or pelvis and less often in sites away from the trunk. Bone cancers progress rapidly but are often difficult to detect. Alkaline phosphatase levels are elevated in osteoblastic tumors, and serum calcium and urinary calcium levels are increased in highly destructive lesions. X-ray films, radioisotopic scanning, arteriography, and biopsy are diagnostic. Surgical treatment consists of local resection of slow-growing tumors or amputation, including the joint above the tumor, if the lesion is aggressive. Radiotherapy may be

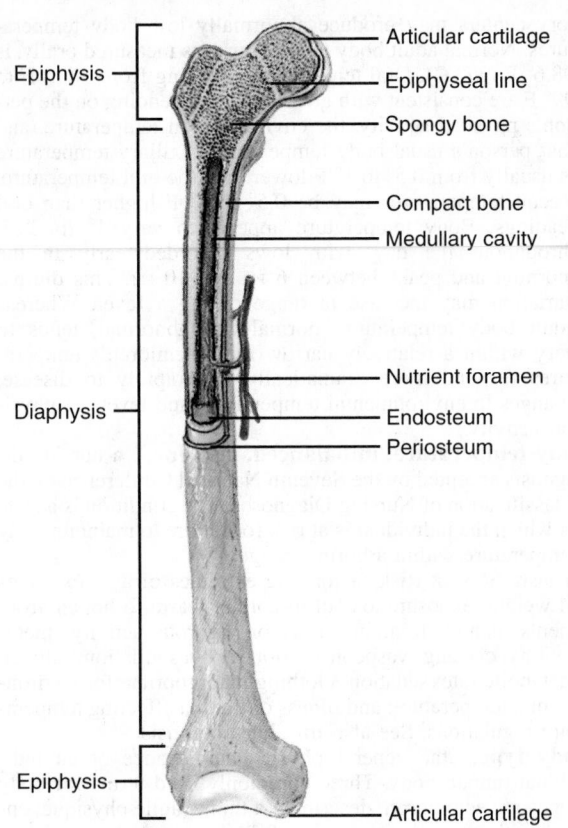

Articular cartilage
Epiphyseal line
Spongy bone
Compact bone
Medullary cavity
Nutrient foramen
Endosteum
Periosteum
Articular cartilage
Epiphysis
Diaphysis
Epiphysis

**Structure of long bones** *(Applegate, 2000)*

given preoperatively or as the primary form of treatment. See also **chondrosarcoma, Ewing's sarcoma, fibrosarcoma, multiple myeloma, osteosarcoma.**

**bone cell** [AS, *ban* + L, *cella,* storeroom], an osteocyte osteoblast, or osteoclast, a cell with myriad spidery processes embedded in the matrix of bone. See also **osteoblast.**

**bone cutting forceps,** a kind of forceps that has long handles, single or double joints, and heavy blades.

**bone cyst** [AS, *ban* + Gk, *kytis,* cyst], **1.** a dilation in the wall of a blood vessel in a bone, usually eccentrically placed. **2.** a sac in bone tissue in the parathyroid disorder osteitis fibrosa.

**bone densitometry,** any of several methods of determining bone mass by measuring radiation absorption by the skeleton. Common techniques include single-photon absorptiometry (SPA) of the forearm and heel, dual-photon absorptiometry (DPA) and dual-energy x-ray absorptiometry (DXA) of the spine and hip, quantitative computed tomography (QCT) of the spine and forearm, and radiographic absorptiometry (RA) of the hand.

**bone graft,** the transplantation of a piece of bone from one part of the body to another to repair a skeletal defect.

**bone healing,** a nursing outcome from the Nursing Outcomes Classification (NOC) defined as the extent to which cells and tissues have regenerated following bone injury. See also **Nursing Outcomes Classification.**

**bone lamella** [AS, *ban,* bone, *lamella,* plate], a thin plate of bone matrix, a basic structural unit of mature bone.

**bone marrow** [AS, *ban* + ME, *marowe*], specialized, semiliquid tissue filling the spaces in cancellous bone of the epiphyses. **Red marrow** is found in many bones of infants

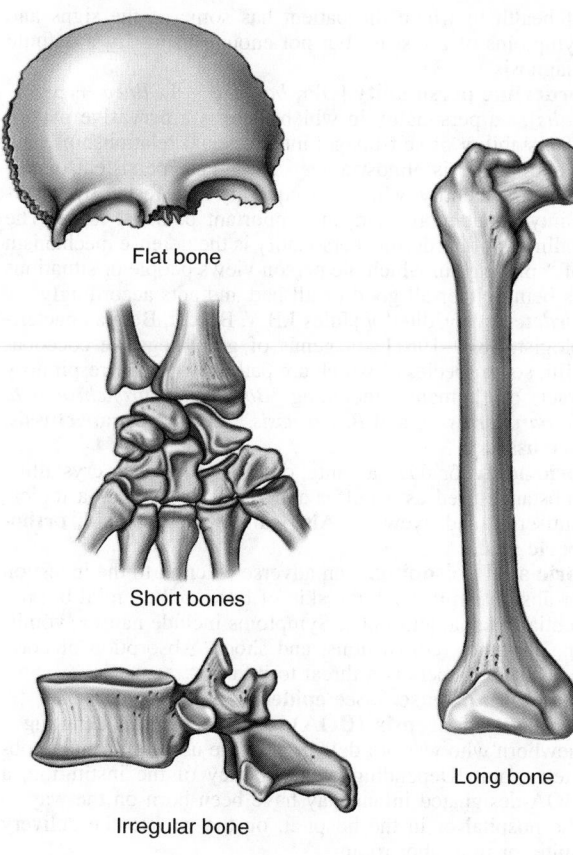

Flat bone

Short bones

Irregular bone

Long bone

**Types of bones** *(Herlihy and Maebius, 2000)*

and children and in the spongy (cancellous) bone of the proximal epiphyses of the humerus and femur and the sternum, ribs, and vertebral bodies of adults. It is known as myeloid tissue and is essential in the manufacture and maturation of red blood cells, most white blood cells, and platelets. Fatty **yellow marrow** is found in the medullary cavity of most adult long bones.

**bone marrow biopsy,** a microscopic tissue examination used to help evaluate patients with hematologic diseases. The biopsy may be done to confirm a diagnosis of megaloblastic anemia, to diagnose leukemia or myeloma, to determine the cause of reduced red blood cells in the peripheral bloodstream, to document deficient iron stores, to document bone marrow infiltrative diseases such as neoplasm or fibrosis, to identify tumors, and to diagnose a variety of other conditions.

**bone marrow failure,** failure of the hematopoietic function of the bone marrow. See also **hematopoietic system.**

**bone marrow infusion,** a method of injecting a fluid substance through an aspiration needle directly into the marrow cavity of a long bone. The substance is absorbed into the general circulation almost immediately.

**bone marrow suppression,** suppression of bone marrow activity, resulting in reduction in the number of platelets, red cells, and white cells, such as in aplastic anemia. Also called **myelosuppression.**

**bone marrow transplant,** the transplantation of bone marrow from a healthy donor to stimulate production of normal blood cells. It is used to treat hematopoietic or lymphoreticular diseases, such as aplastic anemia, leukemia, immune deficiency syndromes, and acute radiation syndrome. The bone marrow is removed from the donor by aspiration and infused intravenously into the recipient. Transplantation is usually preceded by chemotherapy and total body radiation of the recipient.

**bone plate** [AS, *ban,* bone; OFr, *plate*], a metal plate used to reconstruct a bone that has been fractured. The plate is designed to hold bone fragments in apposition.

**bone recession** [AS, *ban* + L, *recedere,* to recede], apical progression of the level of the alveolar crest, resulting in decreased bone support for the teeth. The condition is associated with inflammatory or dystrophic periodontal disease.

**bone scan,** the injection of a radioactive substance to enable visualization of a bone via the image produced by emission of radioactive particles.

**bone tissue** [AS, *ban* + OFr, *tissu*], a hard form of connective tissue composed of osteocytes and a calcified collagenous intercellular substance arranged in thin plates. See **connective tissue.** Also called **bony tissue.**

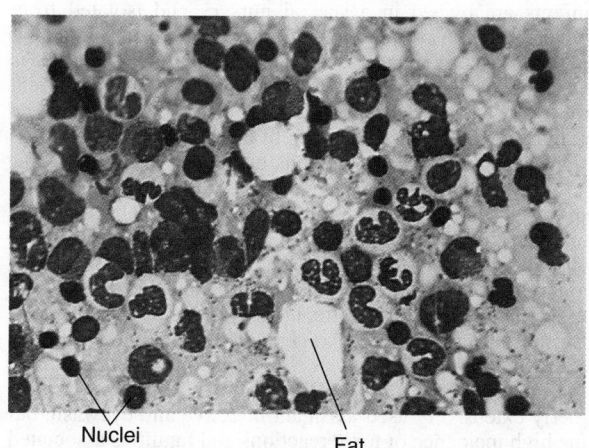

Nuclei

Fat

**Bone marrow** *(© Ed Reschke; used with permission)*

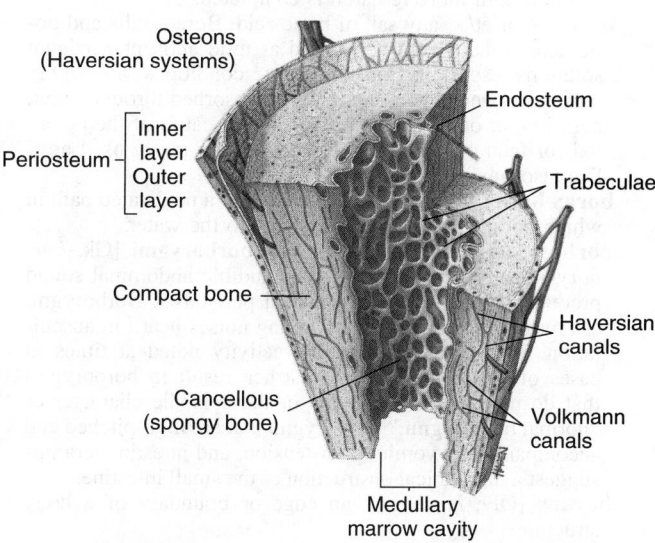

Osteons (Haversian systems)

Endosteum

Periosteum — Inner layer / Outer layer

Trabeculae

Compact bone

Cancellous (spongy bone)

Haversian canals

Volkmann canals

Medullary marrow cavity

**Bone tissue** *(Thibodeau and Patton, 1999/John V. Hagen)*

**Bonine,** trademark for an antiemetic (meclizine hydrochloride).

**Bonnevie-Ullrich syndrome.** See **Turner's syndrome.**

**Bonwill's triangle** [William G.A. Bonwill, American dentist, 1833–1899], an equilateral triangle formed by lines from the contact points of the lower central incisors (or the median line of the residual ridge of the mandible) to the mandibular condyle on each side and from one condyle to the other.

**bony landmark** [AS, *ban* + AS, *land, mearc*], a groove or prominence on a bone that serves as a guide to the location of other body structures. An example is the posterior, superior iliac crest.

**bony palate.** See **hard palate.**

**bony thorax** [AS, *ban* + Gk, *thorax,* chest], the skeletal part of the chest, including the thoracic vertebrae, ribs, and sternum.

**bony tissue.** See **bone tissue.**

**booster injection,** the administration of an additional dose of antigen, such as a vaccine or toxoid, usually in a smaller amount than the original immunization. It is given to maintain the immune response at an appropriate level.

**booster response.** See **secondary antibody response.**

**boot,** 1. a shoelike prosthetic device for holding a leg or arm during treatment. 2. a basketweave bandage that covers the foot and lower leg. 3. an airtight device in which the arm or leg can be inserted and the air pumped out, creating a partial vacuum to divert blood flow from the surrounding area.

**Boothby-Lovelace-Bulbulian (BLB) mask,** an apparatus for the administration of oxygen consisting of a mask fitted with an inspiratory-expiratory valve and a rebreathing bag.

**boracic acid.** See **boric acid.**

**borage,** an annual herb found in North America and Europe.

■ USES: This herb is used as an antiinflammatory for premenstrual syndrome, rheumatoid arthritis, Raynaud's disease, and other inflammatory conditions. It is also used to treat atopic dermatitis, infant cradle cap, cystic fibrosis, high blood pressure, and diabetes.

■ CONTRAINDICATIONS: Borage should not be used during pregnancy and lactation because of the possible presence of pyrrolizidine alkaloids (PAs). It is also contraindicated in children until more research is completed.

**borate** /bôr′āt/, any salt of boric acid. Borate salts and boric acid, although formerly used as mild antiseptic irrigant solutions, especially for ophthalmic conditions, are highly poisonous when taken internally or absorbed through a cut, abrasion, or other wound in the skin. Because of the potential for fatal poisoning, such solutions are rarely used now. See also **boric acid.**

**borax bath** [Ar, *bauraq* + AS, *baeth*], a medicated bath in which borax and glycerin are added to the water.

**borborygmos** /bôr′bərig′məs/, *pl.,* **borborygmi** [Gk, *borborygmos,* bowel rumbling], an audible abdominal sound produced by hyperactive intestinal peristalsis. Borborygmi are rumbling, gurgling, and tinkling noises heard in auscultation. The increased intestinal activity noted at times in cases of gastroenteritis and diarrhea result in borborygmi that do not have the intensity or the episodic character of "normal borborygmi." Borborygmi that are high-pitched and accompanied by vomiting, distension, and intestinal cramps suggest a mechanical obstruction of the small intestine.

**border** [OFr, *bordure*], an edge or boundary of a body structure.

**borderline** [OFr, *bordure* + L, *linea*], pertaining to a state of health in which the patient has some of the signs and symptoms of a disease but not enough to justify a definite diagnosis.

**borderline personality** [OFr, *bordure* + L, *linea* + *personalis*], a personality in which there is a pervasive pattern of instability of self-image, interpersonal relationships, and mood. There is almost always a marked, persistent disturbance of identity, which is frequently manifested by uncertainty about more than one important personal issue. The hallmark of borderline personality is the defense mechanism of "splitting" in which the person views people or situations as being either all good or all bad and acts accordingly.

***Bordetella*** /bôr′ditel′ə/ [Jules J.B.V. Bordet, Belgian bacteriologist, 1870–1961], a genus of gram-negative coccobacilli, some species of which are pathogens of the respiratory tract of humans, including *Bordetella bronchiseptica, B. parapertussis,* and *B. pertussis.* See also **parapertussis, pertussis.**

**boric acid** /bôr′ik/, a white, odorless powder or crystalline substance used as a buffer and formerly used as a topical antiseptic and eyewash. Also called **boracic acid, orthoboric acid.**

**boric acid poisoning,** an adverse reaction to the ingestion or absorption through the skin of boric acid, a mild but potentially lethal antiseptic. Symptoms include nausea, vomiting, diarrhea, convulsions, and shock. Absorption of boric acid from diapers is a threat to infants.

**Bornholm disease.** See **epidemic pleurodynia.**

**born out of asepsis (BOA),** (in a hospital) denoting a newborn who was not delivered in the usual place in an obstetric unit. Depending on the policy of the institution, a BOA-designated infant may have been born on the way to the hospital or in the hospital, on the way to the delivery suite, or in a labor room.

■ OBSERVATIONS: Initial assessment in the admitting unit includes evaluation of respiration, quality of cry, skin color, apical pulse rate, muscle tone, reflexes, temperature, condition of umbilical cord or cord stump, ability to suck, presence of meconium, congenital defect, skin eruption, or signs of sepsis, including jaundice, anorexia, vomiting, diarrhea, irritability or lethargy, high-pitched cry, and hypothermia or hyperthermia.

■ INTERVENTIONS: The usual steps in caring for a newborn are performed. Head and chest circumferences are measured, weight is taken, and the baby is placed in a warmer until the axillary temperature is 36.5° C. Vitamin K and silver nitrate are usually given, and a bath is given when the body temperature is over 36.5° C and stable. In many hospitals BOA infants are placed in a special nursery and isolated from other infants to prevent contagion if they are infected.

■ NURSING CONSIDERATIONS: Daily care for the BOA infant is the same as that given to other newborns, but, in addition, the BOA baby is closely observed for signs of sepsis. The parents are involved in the care of the infant as soon as possible, and the usual instructions are given at discharge for home care of the baby.

**boron (B)** /bôr′on/, a nonmetallic element, whose atomic number is 5; its atomic mass is 10.81. Elemental boron occurs in the form of dark crystals and as a greenish yellow amorphous mass. Certain concentrations of this element are toxic to plant and animal life, but plants need traces of boron for normal growth. It is the characteristic element of boric acid, which is used chiefly as a dusting powder and ointment for minor skin disorders. Boric acid in solution was formerly extensively used as an antiinfective and eyewash, but the high incidence of toxic reactions and fatalities associated with these preparations has greatly reduced their use.

***Borrelia*** /bərel′ē·ə/ [Amédée Borrel, French bacteriologist, 1867–1936], a genus of coarse, unevenly coiled helical spirochetes, several species of which cause tickborne and louseborne relapsing fever. The organism is spread to offspring from generation to generation. This does not occur in lice. Many animals serve as reservoirs and hosts for *Borrelia*. The spirochete may be identified by microscopic examination of a smear of blood stained with Wright's stain; it is also easily inoculated onto culture media for bacterial culture and identification.

***Borrelia burgdorferi*** /burg′dôrfer′ī/, the causative agent in Lyme disease. The organism is transmitted to humans by tick vectors, primarily *Ixodes dammini*. In the United States the disease is found primarily in the Northeast, North-Central, and Northwest.

**boss** [ME, *boce*], a swelling, eminence, or protuberance on an organ, such as a tumor or overgrowth on a bone surface. For example, on the forehead it is often a sign of rickets.

**Boston exanthem** [Boston; Gk, *ex,* out, *anthema,* blossoming], an epidemic disease characterized by scattered, pale red maculopapules on the face, chest, and back, occasionally accompanied by small ulcerations on the tonsils and soft palate. There is little or no adenopathy, and the rash disappears spontaneously in 2 or 3 weeks. It is caused by echovirus 16 and requires no treatment. Compare **herpangina.**

**botox** *(informal).* See **botulinum toxin.**

**bottle feeding**[1], [OFr, *bouteille* + AS, *faeden*], feeding an infant or young child from a bottle with a rubber nipple on the end as a substitute for or supplement to breastfeeding.

■ METHOD: The infant is held on one arm close to the body of the mother or nurse during feeding. The bottle is held at an angle to ensure that the nipple is always filled with liquid so that the infant does not ingest air while feeding. For a newborn, rest periods may be given every several minutes. At least once in the course of the feeding and again at the end the infant is encouraged to burp by being held upright on the mother's or nurse's shoulder or on its stomach on the feeder's lap. Gentle rubbing or patting on the back and pressure on the stomach often help induce burping.

■ INTERVENTIONS: The formula contains protein, fats, carbohydrates, vitamins, and minerals in amounts similar to those in breast milk. The formula may be warmed before feeding by immersing the bottle in warm water for several minutes (although this is not necessary if the formula is kept at room temperature), and the size of the nipple hole is adjusted to the needs of the infant. Smaller infants need larger nipple holes, which require less sucking. Premature or weak infants may be fed by using a long soft nipple through which it is very easy for the infant to feed.

■ OUTCOME CRITERIA: Bottle feeding is used as a substitute for breastfeeding when the mother is unable or unwilling to breastfeed. Bottle feeding can also be substituted for breastfeeding occasionally, once lactation has been established. Bottle feeding is recommended if the mother has active tuberculosis or other active, acute contagious disease; if she has a serious chronic disease, such as cancer or cardiac disease; or if she has recently undergone extensive surgery. Severe mastitis, narcotic addiction, or concurrent use of medication that is secreted in the breast milk usually requires the mother to bottle feed.

**bottle feeding**[2], a nursing intervention from the Nursing Interventions Classification (NIC) defined as preparation and administration of fluids to an infant via a bottle. See also **Nursing Interventions Classification.**

**botulinum toxin** /boch′əlī′nəm/ [L, *botulus,* sausage; Gk, *toxikon,* poison], any of a group of potent bacterial toxins produced by different strains of *Clostridium botulinum.* It may be used therapeutically for blepharospasm or cosmetically to relax facial wrinkles. The strains are sometimes identified by letters of the alphabet, such as A, B, or C. Also called **botox, botulinus toxin.**

**botulism** /boch′əliz′əm/ [L, *botulus,* sausage], an often fatal form of food poisoning caused by an endotoxin produced by the bacillus *Clostridium botulinum.* The toxin is ingested in food contaminated by *C. botulinum,* although it is not necessary for the live bacillus to be present if the toxin has been produced. In rare instances the toxin may be introduced into the human body through a wound contaminated by the organism. Infants may consume spores that produce the toxin, which is associated with eating unpasteurized honey. Botulism differs from most other types of food poisoning in that it develops without gastric distress and occurs from 18 hours up to 1 week after the contaminated food has been ingested. Botulism is characterized by lassitude, fatigue, and visual disturbances, such as double vision, difficulty in focusing the eyes, and loss of ability of the pupil to accommodate to light. Muscles may become weak, and dysphagia often develops. Nausea and vomiting occur in fewer than half the cases. Affected infants are lethargic, feed poorly, are constipated, and have a weak cry and poor muscle tone. Hospitalization is required, and antitoxins are administered. Sedatives are given, mainly to relieve anxiety. Approximately two thirds of the cases of botulism are fatal, usually as a result of delayed diagnosis and respiratory complications. For those who survive, recovery is slow. Most botulism occurs after eating improperly canned or cooked foods. See also *Clostridium.*

**bouba.** See **yaws.**

**Bouchard's node** /bōōshärz′/ [Charles J. Bouchard, French physician, 1837–1915], an abnormal cartilaginous or bony enlargement of a proximal interphalangeal joint of a finger, usually occurring in degenerative diseases of the joints, such as rheumatoid arthritis. Compare **Heberden's node.**

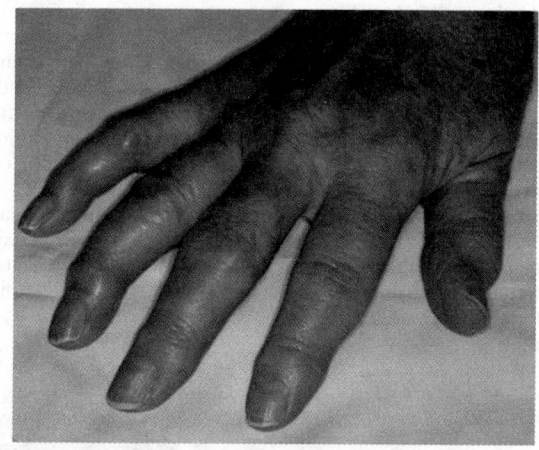

**Bouchard's nodes** *(Lemmi and Lemmi, 2000)*

**Bouchut's tubes** /bōōshōōz′/ [Jean E.W. Bouchut, French physician, 1818–1891], a set of short cylindric devices used for intubation of the larynx.

**bougie** /bōō′zhē, bōōzhē′/ [Fr, candle], a thin cylindric instrument made of rubber, waxed silk, or other flexible material for insertion into canals of the body in order to dilate, examine, or measure them.

**-boulia.** See **-bulia.**

**boulimia.** See **bulimia.**

**boundary** /boun′dərē/, (in psychology) an aspect of family health in which the generations are clearly defined and issues dealt with by the appropriate generation. There are also limits between the family "turf" and the larger society.

**boundary lubrication,** a coating of a thin layer of molecules on each weight-bearing surface of a joint to facilitate a sliding action by the opposing bone surfaces.

**boundary maintenance mechanisms,** (in psychology) behavior and practices that exclude members of some groups from the customs and values of another group.

**bound carbon dioxide,** carbon dioxide that is transported in the bloodstream as part of a sodium bicarbonate molecule, as distinguished from dissolved carbon dioxide or bicarbonate ion.

**bounding pulse** [OFr, *bondir,* to leap; L, *pulsare,* to beat], a pulse that feels full and springlike on palpation as a result of an increased thrust of cardiac contraction or an increased volume of circulating blood within the elastic structures of the vascular system.

**bouquet fever.** See **dengue fever.**

**Bourdon regulator,** a commonly used adjustable device with an attached pressure gauge for controlling the flow of oxygen or other gases from cylinders in medical applications.

**Bourneville's disease.** See **tuberous sclerosis.**

**bouton** /bo͞otôN′, bo͞o′ton/ [Fr, button], **1.** a knoblike swelling, such as the expanded end of an axon at a synapse (terminaux) which comes into contact with cell bodies of other neurons. **2.** a lesion associated with cutaneous leishmaniasis. **3.** a small abscess of the intestinal mucosa in amebic dysentery.

**boutonneuse fever** /bo͞o′təno͞oz′/ [Fr, *bouton,* button; L, *febris*], an infectious disease caused by *Rickettsia conorii,* transmitted to humans through the bite of a tick. The onset of the disease is characterized by a lesion called a *tache noire* /täshnô·är′/, or black spot, at the site of the infection; fever lasting from a few days to 2 weeks; and a papular erythematous rash that spreads over the body to include the skin of the palms and soles. Treatment usually involves administration of antibiotics. There is no prophylactic medication available, and prevention depends primarily on avoiding ticks. See also **rickettsiosis, Rocky Mountain spotted fever.**

**boutonnière deformity** /bo͞o′tônyer′/ [Fr, buttonhole], an abnormality of a finger marked by fixed flexion of the proximal interphalangeal joint and hyperextension of the distal interphalangeal joint. The condition occurs in rheumatoid arthritis.

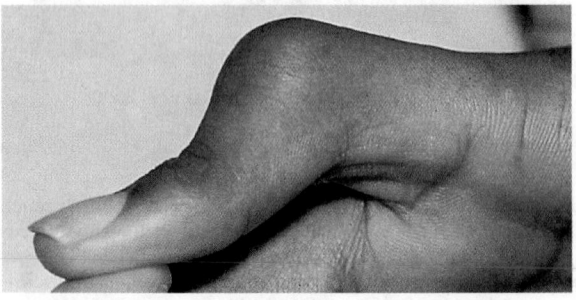

**Boutonnière deformity** *(Zitelli and Davis, 1997)*

**bovine spongiform encephalopathy (BSE),** an infection of cattle characterized by degenerative, clumsy, apprehensive behavior, and death. The BSE brain tissue is perforated and spongy in appearance. The disease was first observed in cattle by veterinarians in 1883. It has been associated with other spongiform encephalopathies such as scrapie and sheep and goats, and Cruetzfeldt-Jakob disease (CJD) in humans. In European "mad cow" disease, it is believed the disease was transmitted to cattle through livestock feed that contained remains of scrapie-infected sheep. The disease was then transmitted to humans who ate BSE-infected beef.

**bovine tuberculosis** /bō′vīn/ [L, *bos,* ox, *tuber,* swelling; Gk, *osis,* condition], a form of tuberculosis caused by *Mycobacterium tuberculosis* that primarily affects cattle. Mastitis and pulmonary symptoms can occur.

**Bowditch's law.** See **all-or-none law.**

**bowel.** See **intestine.**

**bowel bypass syndrome,** a series of adverse effects that may follow bowel bypass surgery, which include chills, fever, joint pain, and skin inflammation on the arms, legs, and thorax.

**bowel continence,** a nursing outcome from the Nursing Outcomes Classification (NOC) defined as control of passage of stool from the bowel. See also **Nursing Outcomes Classification.**

**bowel elimination,** a nursing outcome from the Nursing Outcomes Classification (NOC) defined as ability of the gastrointestinal tract to form and evacuate stool effectively. See also **Nursing Outcomes Classification.**

**bowel incontinence.** See **incontinence, bowel.**

**bowel incontinence care,** a nursing intervention from the Nursing Interventions Classification (NIC) defined as promotion of bowel continence and maintenance of perianal skin integrity. See also **Nursing Interventions Classification.**

**bowel incontinence care: encopresis,** a nursing intervention from the Nursing Interventions Classification (NIC) defined as promotion of bowel continence in children. See also **Nursing Interventions Classification.**

**bowel irrigation,** a nursing intervention from the Nursing Interventions Classification (NIC) defined as instillation of a substance into the lower gastrointestinal tract. See also **Nursing Interventions Classification.**

**bowel management,** a nursing intervention from the Nursing Interventions Classification (NIC) defined as establishment and maintenance of a regular pattern of bowel elimination. See also **Nursing Interventions Classification.**

**bowel training**[1] [OFr, *boel*], a method of establishing regular evacuation by reflex conditioning used in the treatment of fecal incontinence, impaction, chronic diarrhea, and autonomic hyperreflexia. In patients with autonomic hyperreflexia, distension of the rectum and bladder causes paroxysmal hypertension, restlessness, chills, diaphoresis, headache, elevated temperature, and bradycardia.

■ METHOD: The patient's previous bowel habits are assessed, and the necessity of developing a program to induce an evacuation at the same time each day or every other day is explained. Exercises to strengthen abdominal muscles, such as pushing up, bearing down, and contracting the musculature, are demonstrated. The patient is instructed to recognize and respond promptly to signals indicating a full bowel, such as goose pimples, perspiration, and piloerection on arms or legs, and to develop cues to stimulate the urge to defecate, such as drinking coffee, or massaging the abdomen. Fluids to 3000 ml daily are encouraged; exercise is increased as able, and the importance of eating well-balanced meals that include bulk and roughage and of avoiding constipating or gas-producing foods, such as bananas, beans, and cabbage, is discussed. Depending on the patient and the problem, the training program may involve drinking warm fluid, ensuring privacy, and inserting a lubricated glycerin suppository before the set time. The patient is told that no formed stools for 3 days, semiliquid feces, restlessness, and discomfort are signs of impending impaction and that the condition may be treated with a laxative suppository or with a tap water or oil retention enema. The importance of reporting symptoms of autonomic hyperreflexia to the physician is stressed. The possibility that emotional stress or illness may cause accidental incontinence after the program has been established is discussed. Many clients require weeks or months of training to achieve success.

■ INTERVENTIONS: The nurse provides instruction, encourages the patient to establish a program of regular evacuation, and offers positive reinforcement frequently.

■ OUTCOME CRITERIA: Reflex conditioning is often an effective method of developing regular bowel habits for incontinent patients, especially those who are highly motivated and are given good instruction and understanding support. Young persons with spinal cord lesions are able to develop automatic defecation when adequately trained, but some elderly incontinent people may not be able to learn the program.

**bowel training[2],** a nursing intervention from the Nursing Interventions Classification (NIC) defined as assisting the patient to train the bowel to evacuate at specific intervals. See also **Nursing Interventions Classification.**

**bowenoid papulosis.** See **Bowen's disease.**

**Bowen's disease** [John T. Bowen, American dermatologist, 1857–1941], a form of intraepidermal carcinoma (squamous cell). It is characterized by red-brown scaly or crusted lesions that resemble a patch of psoriasis or dermatitis. Treatment includes curettage and electrodesiccation. A corresponding lesion found on the glans penis is called **erythroplasia of Queyrat.** Also called **Bowen's precancerous dermatosis.** See also **intraepidermal carcinoma.**

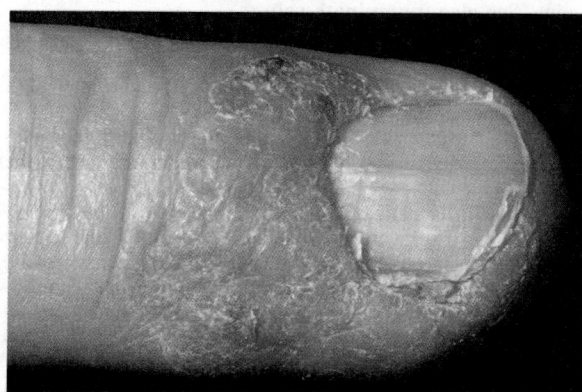

**Bowen's disease**
*(Hordinsky, Sawaya, and Scher, 2000)*

**bowleg.** See **genu varum.**

**Bowman's capsule** /bō'mənz/ [William Bowman, English anatomist, 1816–1892], the cup-shaped end of a renal tubule or nephron enclosing a glomerulus. With the glomerulus, it is the site of filtration in the kidney. Also called **glomerular capsule.**

**Bowman's glands** [William Bowman; L, *glans,* acorn], branched tubuloalveolar glands in olefactory membrane of the mouth. They keep the mouth surfaces moist.

**Bowman's lamina** [William Bowman; L, *lamina,* plate], a tough membrane beneath the corneal epithelium. Also called **anterior elastic lamina, Bowman's layer, Bowman's membrane.**

**bowtie filter** /bō'tī/, a filter shaped like a bow tie that may be used in computed tomography to compensate for the shape of the patient's head or body. It is used with fan-shaped x-ray beams to equalize the amount of radiation reaching the film.

**box bath.** See **cabinet bath.**

**boxer's ear.** See **pachyotia.**

**boxer's fracture** [Dan, *bask,* a blow; L, *fractura,* break], a break in one or more metacarpal bones, usually the fourth or the fifth, caused by punching a hard object. Such a fracture is often distal, angulated, and impacted.

**boxing,** the forming of vertical walls, most commonly made of wax, to produce the desired shape and size of the base of a dental cast.

**boxing wax** [L, *buxis,* box; AS, *weax*], (in dentistry) a wax used for boxing.

**Boyle's law** /boilz/ [Robert Boyle, English scientist, 1627–1691], (in physics) the law stating that the product of the volume and pressure of a gas contained at a constant temperature remains constant.

**BP,** abbreviation for **blood pressure.**

**BPD,** 1. abbreviation for **biparietal diameter. 2.** abbreviation for **bronchopulmonary dysplasia.**

**BPDE-I,** abbreviation for **benzo[a]pyrene dihydrodiol epoxide.**

**BPH,** abbreviation for **benign prostatic hypertrophy.**

**bpm,** abbreviation for *beats per minute.*

**Br,** symbol for the element **bromine.**

**brace** [OFr, *bracier,* to embrace], an orthotic device, sometimes jointed, used to support and hold any part of the body in the correct position to allow function and healing, such as a leg brace that permits walking and standing. Compare **splint.**

**brachi-** /brā'kē-/, prefix meaning 'arm': *brachiation, brachiocyllosis.*

**-brachia** /-brā'kē-ə/, suffix meaning an 'anatomic condition involving an arm': *acephalobrachia, monobrachia.*

**brachial** /brā'kē-əl/ [Gk, *brachion,* arm], pertaining to the arm.

**brachial artery,** the principal artery of the upper arm that is the continuation of the axillary artery. It has three branches and terminates at the bifurcation of its main trunk into the radial artery and the ulnar artery.

**brachialgia** /-al'jē-ə/ [L, *brachium,* arm; Gk, *algos,* pain], a severe pain in the arm, often related to a disorder involving the brachial plexus.

**brachialis** /brā'kē-al'is/ [Gk, *brachion,* arm], a muscle of the upper arm, covering the anterior part of the elbow joint and the distal half of the humerus. It functions to flex the forearm. Compare **biceps brachii, triceps brachii.**

**brachial paralysis** [L, *brachium,* arm; Gk, *paralyein,* to be palsied], paralysis of an arm or a hand as a result of a lesion of the brachial plexus. See also **Erb palsy.**

**brachial plexus** [Gk, *brachion* + L, braided], a network of nerves in the neck, passing under the clavicle and into the axilla, originating in the fifth, sixth, seventh, and eighth cervical and first two thoracic spinal nerves. It innervates the muscles and skin of the chest, shoulders, and arms.

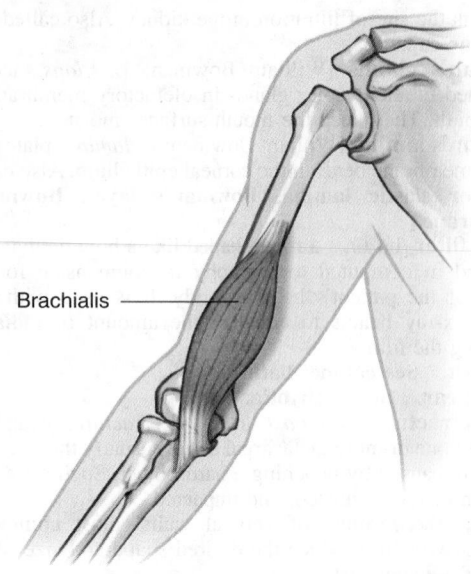

Brachialis

**Brachialis**

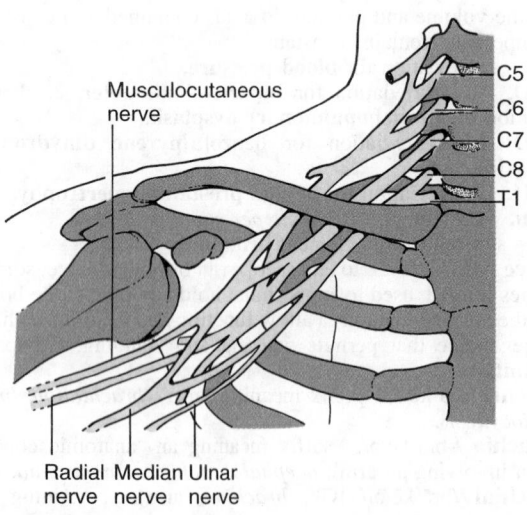

Musculocutaneous
nerve

C5
C6
C7
C8
T1

Radial   Median   Ulnar
nerve    nerve    nerve

**Brachial plexus** *(Crossman and Neary, 1995)*

**brachial plexus anesthesia,** an anesthetic block of the upper extremity, performed by injecting local anesthetic near the plexis formed by the last four cervical and first two thoracic spinal nerves. The plexus extends from the transverse processes of the spine to the apex of the axilla, where the terminal nerves are formed. Because of the anatomy of this area, many approaches are possible. The axillary approach is most common and has the least risk of producing pneumothorax; supraclavicular and interscalene approaches are also used. Various approaches may result in Horner's syndrome, phrenic nerve block, pneumothorax, recurrent laryngeal paralysis, persistent sensory deficits, venous or arterial puncture, subarachnoid injection, paresthesias, or hematoma. Also called **brachial plexus block.** See also **regional anesthesia.**

**brachial plexus block.** See **brachial plexus anesthesia.**
**brachial plexus paralysis.** See **Erb palsy.**
**brachial pulse** [Gk, *brachion* + L, *pulsare,* to beat], the pulse of the brachial artery, palpated in the antecubital space. See also **pulse.**

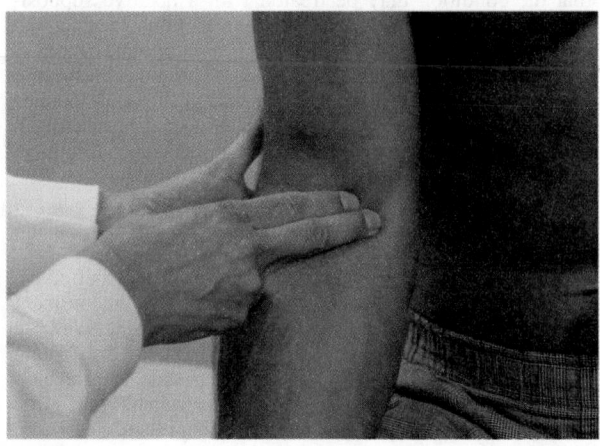

**Assessment of brachial pulse** *(Wilson and Giddens, 2001)*

**brachial region,** an anatomical term used to refer to the arm (shoulder to elbow), divided into anterior and posterior brachial regions.
**brachial vein,** a vein in the arm that accompanies the brachial artery and drains into the axillary vein.
**brachiocephalic,** relating to the arm and head.
**brachiocephalic arteritis.** See **Takayasu's arteritis.**
**brachiocephalic artery,** first branch of the aortic arch. See also **innominate artery.**
**brachiocephalic trunk.** See **innominate artery.**
**brachiocephalic vein,** the vein feeding the superior vena cava, collecting blood from the subclavian and jugular veins. See also **innominate vein.**
**brachiocubital** /-kyōō′bitəl/ [Gk, *brachion* + L, *cubitus,* elbow], pertaining to the arm and forearm.
**brachioplasty,** a surgical procedure to lift and tighten skin of the upper arm.
**brachioradialis** /-rā′dē·al′is/, the most superficial muscle on the radial side of the forearm. It functions to flex the forearm.
**brachioradialis reflex** [Gk, *brachion* + L, *radial, reflectare,* to bend backward], a deep tendon reflex elicited by striking the lateral surface of the forearm proximal to the distal head of the radius, characterized by normal slight elbow flexion and forearm supination. It is accentuated by disease of the pyramidal tract above the level of the fifth cervical vertebra. See also **deep tendon reflex.**
**-brachium** /-brā′kē·əm/, **1.** suffix meaning 'the upper arm from shoulder to elbow.' **2.** suffix meaning 'an arm or armlike growth': *prebrachium, pontibrachium.*
**brachy-** /brak′ē-/, prefix meaning 'short': *brachycheilia, brachyskelous.*
**brachybasia** /-bā′zhə/, abnormally slow walking, with a short, shuffling gait. The condition is associated with cerebral hemorrhage or pyramidal tract disease.
**brachycardia.** See **bradycardia.**
**brachycephaly** /-sef′əlē/ [Gk, *brachys,* short, *kephale,*

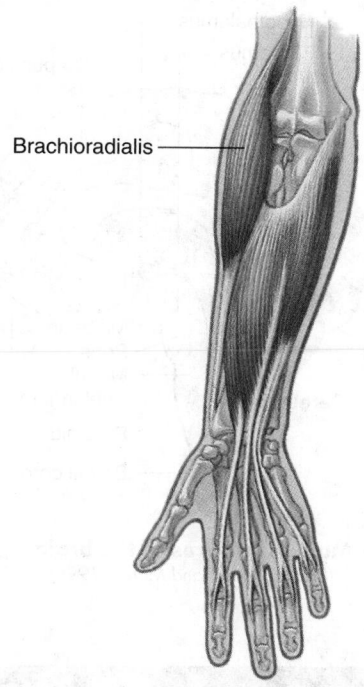

Brachioradialis

**Brachioradialis** *(Thibodeau and Patton, 1999/John V. Hagen)*

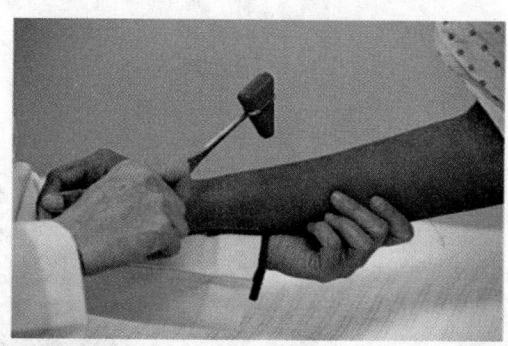

**Brachioradialis reflex testing** *(Seidel et al, 1999)*

head], a congenital malformation of the skull in which premature closure of the coronal suture results in excessive lateral growth of the head, giving it a short, broad appearance. Also called **brachycephalia** /-səfā'lē·ə/, **brachycephalism** /-sef'əlizəm/. See also **craniostenosis.** —**brachycephalic** /-səfal'ik/, **brachycephalous** /-sef'ələs/, *adj.*

**brachydactyly** /-dak'təlē/, a condition in which fingers or toes are abnormally short.

**brachygnathia.** See **micrognathia.**

**brachytherapy** [Gk, *brachys*, short, *therapeia*, treatment], the placement of radioactive sources in contact with or implanted into the tumor tissues to be treated for a specific period. The rationale for this treatment is to provide a high absorbed dose of radiation in the tumor tissues and a very limited absorbed low dose in the surrounding normal tissues. Compare **teletherapy.**

**bracket** /brak'ət/ [Fr, *braguette,* codpiece], a support projecting from the main structure. An **orthodontic bracket** is a small metal attachment soldered or welded to an orthodontic band or cemented directly to the teeth, serving to fasten the arch wire to the band or tooth. Also called **orthodontic attachment.** See **also orthodontic appliance, orthodontic band.**

**Bradford frame** [Edward H. Bradford, American surgeon, 1848–1926], a rectangular orthopedic frame made of pipes to which heavy movable straps of canvas are attached. The straps run from side to side to support a patient in a prone or supine position. They can be removed to permit the patient to urinate or defecate while remaining immobile.

**Bradford solid frame,** a rectangular metal orthopedic device that provides support for the entire body and is especially appropriate for patients who are less than 5 years of age, hyperactive, or mentally retarded. The main purpose of the device is to assist in maintaining proper immobilization, positioning, and alignment by controlling movement. To facilitate nursing care, the Bradford solid frame is not placed directly on a bed but is elevated at both ends by plywood blocks or other suitable devices. It is most often used with Bryant traction but never with balanced suspension traction, cervical traction, cervical tongs, or certain other kinds of traction.

**Bradford split frame,** a rectangular metal orthopedic device covered with two separate pieces of canvas fastened at both ends of the frame. Used especially in pediatrics to aid in the immobilization of children in traction, it is divided in the middle by a large opening designed to accommodate the excretory functions of an incontinent patient in a hip spica cast. The division also allows the upper and lower extremities of the patient to be elevated separately and the cast to be kept clean and dry.

**Bradley method** [Robert Bradley, twentieth century American physician], a method of psychophysical preparation for childbirth, comprising education about the physiologic characteristics of childbirth, exercise and nutrition during pregnancy, and techniques of breathing and relaxation for control and comfort during labor and delivery. The father is extensively involved in the classes and acts as the mother's "coach" during labor. Among the advantages of the method are its simplicity, the father's involvement, and the realistic approach to the efforts and discomfort of labor. Also called **husband-coached childbirth.** Compare **Lamaze method, Read method.**

**brady-** /brad'ē-/, prefix meaning 'slow, dull': *bradycardia, bradydiastalsis, bradyphagia.*

**bradyarrhythmia** /-ərith'mē·ə/ [Gk, *bradys,* slow, *a + rhythmos,* without rhythm], any disturbance of cardiac rhythm in which the heart rate is less than 60 beats/min.

**bradycardia** /-kär'dē·ə/ [Gk, *bradys,* slow, *kardia,* heart], a condition in which the heart rate is less than 60/min. Bradycardia takes the form of sinus bradycardia, sinus arrhythmia, and second- or third-degree atrioventricular block. Sinus bradycardia may be caused by excessive vagal tone, decreased sympathetic tone, or anatomic changes. It is common in athletes and is relatively benign. It may even be beneficial in acute myocardial infarction (especially inferior). Pathologic bradycardia may be symptomatic of a brain tumor, digitalis toxicity, heart block, or vagotonus. Cardiac output is decreased, causing faintness, dizziness, chest pain, and eventually syncope and circulatory collapse. Treatment may include administration of atropine, implantation of a pacemaker, or change in medical treatment. Also called **brachycardia.**

**bradycardia-tachycardia syndrome** [Gk, *bradys* + *kardia*, + *tachys*, fast, *kardia* + *syn*, together, *dromos*, course], a disorder characterized by a heart rate that alternates between being abnormally low (less than 60 beats/min) and abnormally high (greater than 100 beats/min). Also called **bradytachycardia, tachycardia-bradycardia syndrome.** See also **sick sinus syndrome, sinus nodal dysfunction.**

**bradyesthesia** /-esthē′zhə/ [Gk, *bradys*, slow, *aisthesis*, feeling], a slowness in perception.

**bradykinesia** /-kinē′zhə, -kīnē′zhə/ [Gk, *bradys* + *kinesis*, motion], an abnormal condition characterized by slowness of all voluntary movement and speech, such as caused by parkinsonism, other extrapyramidal disorders, and certain tranquilizers.

**bradykinin** /-kī′nin/ [Gk, *bradys* + *kinein*, to move], a peptide containing nine amino acid residues produced from $\alpha_2$-globulin by the enzyme kallikrein. Bradykinin is a potent vasodilator.

**bradylalia.** See **bradyphasia.**

**bradyphagia** /-fā′jə/, a habit of eating very slowly.

**bradyphasia** /-fā′zhə/, an abnormally slow manner of speech, often associated with mental illness. Also called **bradylalia.**

**bradypnea** /-pnē′ə/ [Gk, *bradys* + *pnein*, to breath], an abnormally low rate of breathing. Compare **hypopnea.** See also **respiration rate.**

**bradyspermatism** /-spur′mətiz′əm/, ejaculation that lacks normal force so that semen trickles slowly from the penis.

**bradytachycardia.** See **bradycardia-tachycardia syndrome.**

**bradyuria** /brad′ēyŏŏr′ē·ə/, a condition in which urine is passed very slowly.

**Bragg curve** [William H. Bragg, English physicist, 1862–1942], the path followed by ionizing particles used in a radiation treatment. Because certain particles reach a peak of potential near the end of their path, the Bragg curve can be used to direct the radiation to deep-seated tumors while significantly sparing normal overlying tissues.

**Braille** /brāl, brä′yə/ [Louis Braille, French teacher of the blind, 1809–1852], a system of printing for the blind consisting of raised dots or points that can be read by touch.

**brain** [AS, *bragen*], the portion of the central nervous system contained within the cranium. It consists of the cerebrum, cerebellum, pons, medulla, and midbrain. Specialized cells in its mass of convoluted, soft gray or white tissue coordinate and regulate the functions of the central nervous system, integrating the functions of the body as a whole.

**brain abscess** [AS, *bragen* + L, *abscedere*, to go away], a pocket of infection in a part of the brain. It is usually a result of the spread of an infection from another source, such as the skull, sinuses, or other structures in the head. The infection also may be secondary to a disease in the bones, the nervous system outside the brain, or the heart. Also called **cerebral abscess, intracranial abscess.**

**Brain airway.** See **laryngeal mask airway.**

**brain attack,** term signifying that a stroke is in progress and an emergency situation exists. See also **cerebrovascular accident.**

**brain compression.** See **cerebral compression.**

**brain concussion** [AS, *bragen* + L, *concussus*, a shaking], a bruising to cerebral tissues caused by a violent jarring or shaking or other blunt, nonpenetrating injury to the brain resulting in a sudden change in momentum of the head. Characteristically, after a mild concussion there may be a transient loss of consciousness followed, on awakening, by a headache. Severe concussion may cause prolonged uncon-

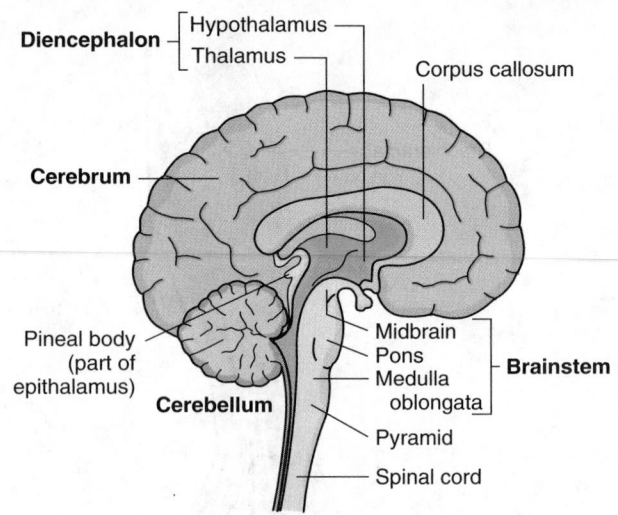

**Major structures of the brain**
*(Phipps, Sands, and Marek, 1999)*

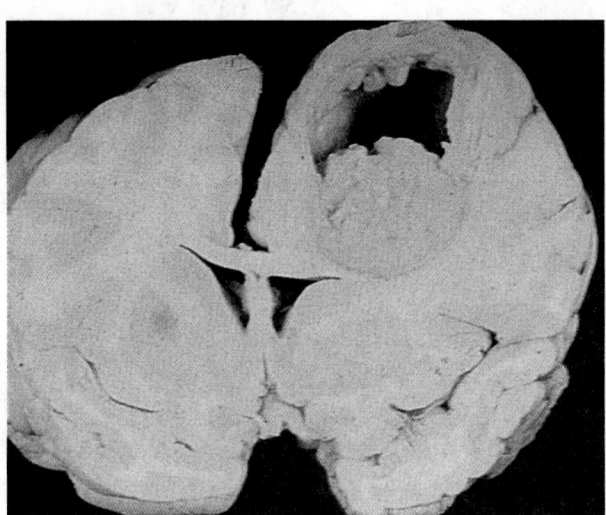

**Brain abscess** *(Farrar, 1993)*

sciousness and disruption of certain vital functions of the brainstem, such as respiration and vasomotor stability. The treatment for a person recovering from a concussion consists principally of observation for signs of intracranial bleeding and increased intracranial pressure. Also called **concussion.**

**brain death** [AS, *bragen* + *death*], an irreversible form of unconsciousness characterized by a complete loss of brain function while the heart continues to beat. The legal definition of this condition varies from state to state. The usual clinical criteria for brain death include the absence of reflex activity, movements, and spontaneous respiration requiring mechanical ventilation or life support to continue any cardiac function. The pupils are dilated and fixed. Because hypothermia, anesthesia, poisoning, or drug intoxication may cause deep physiologic depression that resembles brain death, a diagnosis of brain death may require evaluating and demonstrating that electrical activity of the brain is absent on two electroencephalograms performed 12 to 24 hours apart. Also called **irreversible coma.** Compare **coma, sleep, stupor.**

**brain edema.**    See **cerebral edema.**

**brain electrical activity map (BEAM),**   a topographic map of the brain created by a computer that is able to respond to the electric potentials evoked in the brain by a flash of light. Potentials recorded at 4-msec intervals are converted into a many-colored map of the brain, showing them to be positive or negative. The waves may be observed traveling through the brain. If the wave is disordered, blocked, too small, or too large, a tumor or other lesion may be causing the abnormal pattern.

**brain fever,**   *informal,* any inflammation of the brain or meninges. See also **encephalitis.**

**brain scan** [AS, *bragen* + L, *scandere,* to climb],   a diagnostic procedure using radioisotope imaging to localize and identify intracranial masses, lesions, tumors, or infarcts. Intravenously injected radioisotopes accumulate in abnormal brain tissue and are traced and photographed by a scintillator or scanner. The nature and rate of accumulation of radioisotopes in pathologic tissue are diagnostic of some lesions. Compare **computed tomography.** See also **isotope, radioisotope.**

**Brain's reflex** [Walter R. Brain, English physician, 1895–1966; L, *reflectere,* to bend back],   the reflexive extension of the flexed paralyzed arm of a hemiplegia patient when assuming a quadrupedal posture. Also called **quadrupedal extensor reflex.**

**brainstem** [AS, *bragen* + *stemm*],   the portion of the brain comprising the medulla oblongata, the pons, and the mesencephalon. It performs motor, sensory, and reflex functions and contains the corticospinal and reticulospinal tracts. The 12 pairs of cranial nerves from the brain arise mostly from the brainstem. Compare **medulla oblongata, mesencephalon, pons.**

**brainstem auditory evoked response (BAER),**   the electric activity that may be recorded from the brainstem in the first 10 msec after presentation of an auditory stimulus. In a subject with normal brainstem functioning, seven peaks are observed. A delayed, normally shaped waveform may indicate a hearing loss caused by a middle or inner ear disorder; one or more missing peaks may indicate a neural disorder.

**brain swelling.**    See **cerebral edema.**

**brain syndrome,**   a group of symptoms resulting from impaired function of the brain. It may be acute and reversible, or chronic and irreversible. An organic mental disorder is a specific organic mental syndrome in which the cause is known or presumed. An organic mental syndrome is a temporary or permanent brain dysfunction of any cause.

**brain tumor,**   an invasive neoplasm of the intracranial portion of the central nervous system. Brain tumors cause significant rates of morbidity and mortality but are occasionally treated successfully. In adults 20% to 40% of malignancies in the brain are metastatic lesions from cancers in the breast, lung, GI tract, or kidney or a malignant melanoma. The origin of primary brain tumors is not known, but the risk is increased in individuals exposed to vinyl chloride, in the siblings of cancer patients, and in recipients of renal transplantation being treated with immunosuppressant medication. Symptoms of a brain tumor are often those of increased intracranial pressure, such as headache, nausea, vomiting, papilledema, lethargy, and disorientation. Localizing signs, such as loss of vision on the side of an occipital neoplasm, may occur. Diagnostic measures include visual field and funduscopic examinations, skull x-ray examinations, electroencephalography, cerebral angiography, brain scanning, magnetic resonance imaging, computed tomography, and spinal fluid studies. Gliomas, chiefly astrocytomas, are the most common malignancies. Medulloblastomas occur often in children. Surgery is the initial treatment for most primary tumors of the brain. Radiotherapy is indicated for inoperable lesions, medulloblastomas, and tumors with

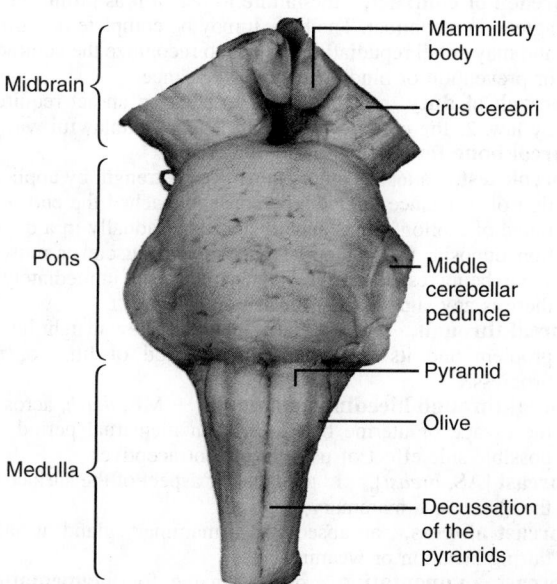

**Brainstem: ventral aspect** *(Crossman and Neary, 1995)*

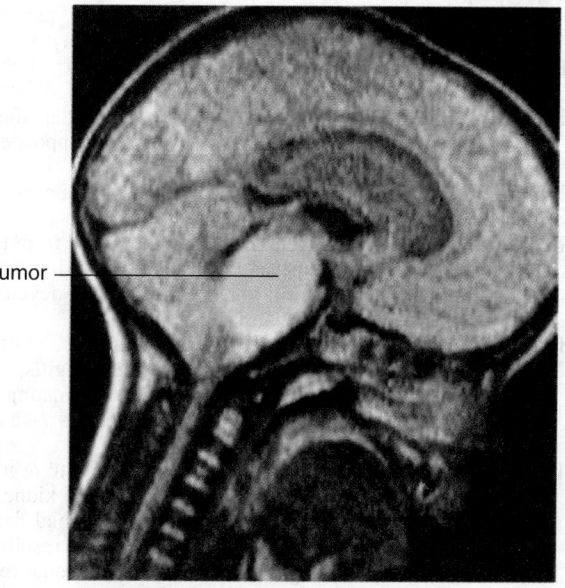

**Brain tumor** *(Ballinger, 1995)*

multiple foci and is used in postoperative treatment of residual tumor tissue. The blood-brain barrier impedes the effect of some antineoplastic agents, but responses are obtained in some cases treated with procarbazine and various nitrosoureas administered alone or with vincristine. Compare **spinal cord tumor.**

**brainwashing,** intensive indoctrination, usually of a political or religious nature, applied to individuals to develop in their minds a specific belief and motivation.

**brain wave** [AS, *bragen* + *wafian*], any of a number of patterns of rhythmic electric impulses produced in different parts of the brain. Most patterns, identified by the Greek letters alpha, beta, delta, gamma, kappa, and theta, are similar for all normal persons and are relatively stable for each individual. Alpha waves are produced when the person is awake but resting, beta waves signal an active phase of cerebral function, delta waves are emitted during deep sleep, and theta waves occur, usually in children but also in adults during emotional stress. Brain waves help in the diagnosis of certain neurologic disorders, such as epilepsy or brain tumors.

**bran,** a coarse outer covering or coat (seed husk) of cereal grain, such as wheat or rye. It is broken or separated from the meal or flour portion of the grain to provide a source of dietary fiber, B vitamins, iron, magnesium, and zinc.

**bran bath** [OFr, *bren* + AS, *baeth*], a bath in which bran has been boiled in the water. It is used for the relief of skin irritation.

**branch,** (in anatomy) an offshoot arising from the main trunk of a nerve or blood vessel.

**branched-chain amino acids,** leucine, isoleucine, and valine; they are incorporated into proteins or catabolized for energy.

**branched chain ketoaciduria.** See **maple syrup urine disease.**

**branched tubular gland** [OFr, *branche*], one of the many multicellular glands with one excretory duct from two or more tube-shaped secretory branches, such as some of the gastric glands.

**brancher glycogen storage disease.** See **Andersen's disease.**

**branchial** /brang′kē·əl/ [Gk, *branchia*, gills], pertaining to body structures of the face, neck, and throat area, particularly the muscles.

**branchial arches** [Gk, *branchia*, gills; L, *arcus*, bow], arched structures in the embryonic pharynx.

**branchial cleft** [Gk, *branchia*, gills; ME, *clift*], a linear depression in the pharynx of the early embryo opposite a branchial or pharyngeal pouch.

**branchial cyst** [Gk, *branchia*, gills, *kystis*, bag], a cyst derived from a branchial remnant in the neck.

**branchial fistula,** a congenital abnormal passage from the pharynx to the external surface of the neck, resulting from the failure of a branchial cleft to close during fetal development. Also called **cervical fistula.**

**branching canal.** See **collateral pulp canal.**

**branchiogenic** /brang′kē·ōjen′ik/ [Gk, *branchia*, gills, *genein*, to produce], pertaining to any tissues originating in the branchial cleft or arch. Also **branchiogenous** /-kē·oj′ənes/.

**branchio-oto-renal syndrome** /brang′kē·ō·ō′tō·rē′nəl/ [Gk, *branchia*, gills + *ous*, ear + L, *ren*, kidney], branchial arch anomalies (preauricular pits, branchial fistulas or pits) associated with congenital deafness resulting from dysgenesis of the organ of Corti, and with renal dysplasia; inherited as an autosomal dominant trait with high penetrance and variable expression.

**brand name.** See **trademark.**

**Brandt-Andrews maneuver** [Thure Brandt, Swedish obstetrician, 1819–1895; Henry R. Andrews, English obstetrician, 1871–1942], a method of expressing the placenta from the uterus in the third stage of labor. One hand grasps the umbilical cord while the other is placed on the mother's abdomen with the fingers over the anterior surface of the uterus. While the hand on the abdomen is pressed backward and slightly upward, the other applies gentle traction on the cord.

**brass founder's ague.** See **metal fume fever.**

**brassy cough** [AS, *brase*, brassy, *cohhetan*, to cough], a high-pitched cough caused by irritation of the recurrent pharyngeal nerve or by pressure on the trachea.

**brassy eye.** See **chalkitis.**

**Braun's canal.** See **neurenteric canal.**

**brawny arm,** a swollen arm caused by lymphedema, usually after a mastectomy.

**Braxton Hicks contractions.** See **preterm contractions.**

**Braxton Hicks version** /brak′stənhiks′/ [John Braxton Hicks, English physician, 1823–1897], one of several types of maneuvers sometimes used to turn the fetus from an undesirable position to one that is more likely to facilitate delivery. See also **version.**

**Brazelton assessment.** See **Neonatal Behavioral Assessment Scale.**

**Brazilian trypanosomiasis.** See **Chagas' disease.**

**BRCA1,** symbol for a breast cancer gene. A healthy BRCA1 gene produces a protein that protects against unwanted cell growth. The protein is packaged by the cell's Golgi apparatus into secretory vesicles, which release their contents on the cell's surface. The protein circulates in the intracellular space, attaching itself to neighboring cell receptors. The receptors signal the cell nuclei to stop growing. When the gene is defective, it produces a faulty protein that is unable to prevent proliferation of abnormal cells as they evolve into potentially deadly breast cancer. BRCA1 may also normally inhibit ovarian cancer.

**BRCA2,** symbol for a breast cancer gene with activity similar to that of BRCA1.

**BRCA3,** symbol for a breast cancer gene.

**breach of contract,** the failure to perform as promised or agreed in a contract. The breach may be complete or partial and may entail repudiation, failure to recognize the contract, or prevention or hindrance of performance.

**breach of duty,** 1. the failure to perform an act required by law. 2. the performance of an act in an unlawful way.

**breakbone fever.** See **dengue fever.**

**break test,** a test of a person's muscle strength by application of resistance after the person has reached the end of a range of motion. Resistance is applied gradually in a direction opposite to the line of pull of the muscle or muscle group being tested. The resistance is released immediately if there is any sign of pain or discomfort.

**breakthrough,** (in psychiatry) a sudden new insight into a problem and its solution after a period of little or no progress.

**breakthrough bleeding** [AS, *brecan* + ME, *thurh*, across], the escape of uterine blood between menstrual periods, a possible side effect of using oral contraceptives.

**breast** [AS, *breast*], 1. the anterior aspect of the surface of the chest. 2. a mammary gland.

**breast abscess,** an abscess of a mammary gland, usually during lactation or weaning.

**breast augmentation,** popular name for **augmentation mammoplasty.**

**breast cancer,** a malignant neoplastic disease of breast tis-

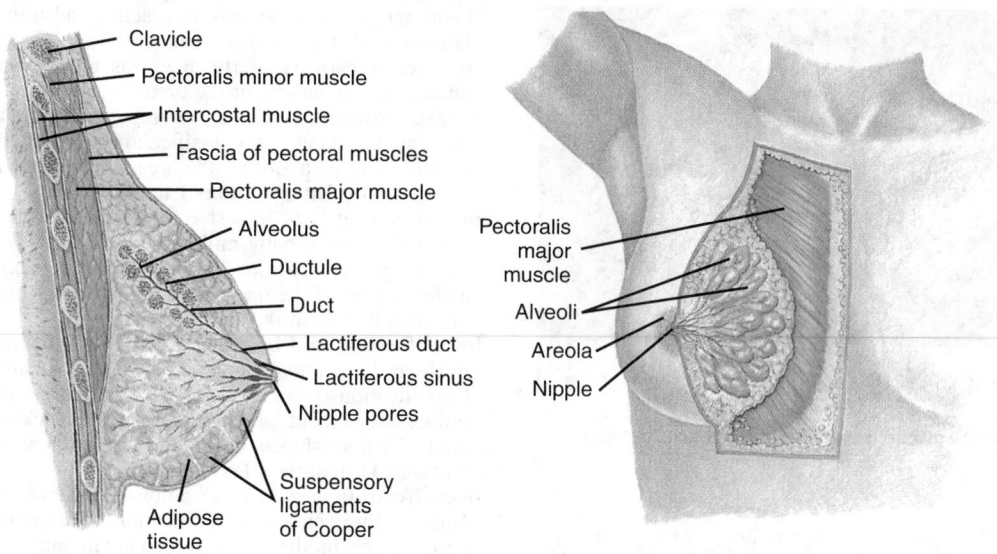

**Female breast** *(Seidel et al, 1999)*

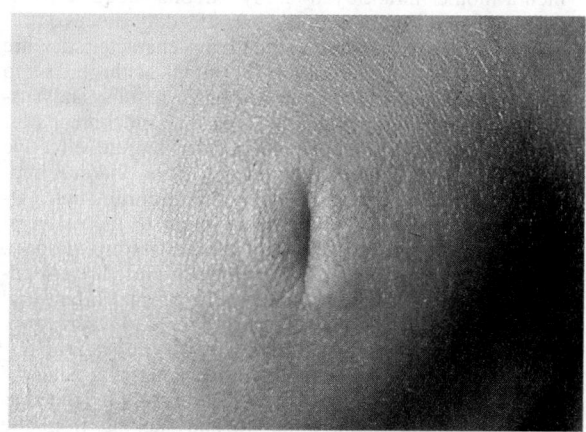

**Breast abscess** *(Zitelli and Davis, 1997)*

sue, a common malignancy in women in the United States. The incidence increases with age from the third to the fifth decade and reaches a second peak at age 65. Risk factors include certain genetic abnormalities, a family history of breast cancer, nulliparity, exposure to ionizing radiation, early menarche, late menopause, obesity, diabetes, hypertension, chronic cystic disease of the breast, and, possibly, postmenopausal estrogen therapy. Women who are above 40 years of age when they bear their first child and individuals who have malignancies in other body sites also have an increased risk of development of breast cancer. Initial symptoms, detected in most cases by self-examination, include a small painless lump, thick or dimpled skin, or nipple retraction. As the lesion progresses, there may be nipple discharge, pain, ulceration, and enlarged axillary glands. The diagnosis may be established by a careful physical examination, mammography, and cytologic examination of tumor cells obtained by biopsy. Infiltrating ductal carcinomas are found in about 75% of cases, and infiltrating lobular, infiltrating medullary, colloid, comedo, or papillary carcinomas in the others. Tumors are more common in the left than in the right breast and in the upper and outer quadrant than in the other quadrants. Metastasis through the lymphatic system to axillary lymph nodes and to bone, lung, brain, and liver is common, but there is evidence that primary carcinomas of the breast may exist in multiple sites and that tumor cells may enter the bloodstream directly without passing through lymph nodes. Surgical treatment may consist of a mastectomy or a lumpectomy, with dissection of axillary nodes. Postoperative radiotherapy, chemotherapy, or both are often prescribed. Chemotherapeutic agents frequently administered in various combinations are cyclophosphamide, methotrexate, 5-fluorouracil, phenylalanine mustard (L-PAM), thio-TEPA, doxorubicin, vincristine, methotrexate, and prednisone. The presence of estrogen receptors in breast tumors is considered an indication for hormonal manipulation such as the administration of antiestrogens. Implantation of a prosthesis after mastectomy is optional and does not appear to decrease survival probability. Reconstructive surgery is also an option. Fewer than 1% of breast cancers occur in men, but those with Klinefelter's syndrome are at much greater risk than other men. See also **lumpectomy, mastectomy, scirrhous carcinoma.**

**breast cancer genetic screening test (BRCA genetic testing),** a blood test used to detect the presence of breast cancer genes, which indicate an increased susceptibility for development of breast cancer. One breast cancer gene also confers an increased susceptibility for ovarian cancer.

**breast examination[1],** a process in which the breasts and their accessory structures are observed and palpated in assessing the presence of changes or abnormalities that could indicate malignant disease. See also **self-breast examination.**

■ METHOD: The breasts are observed with the patient sitting with her arms at her sides; sitting with her arms over her head, back straight, then leaning forward; and, finally, sitting upright as she contracts the pectoral muscles by placing hands on hips. The breasts are observed for symmetry of

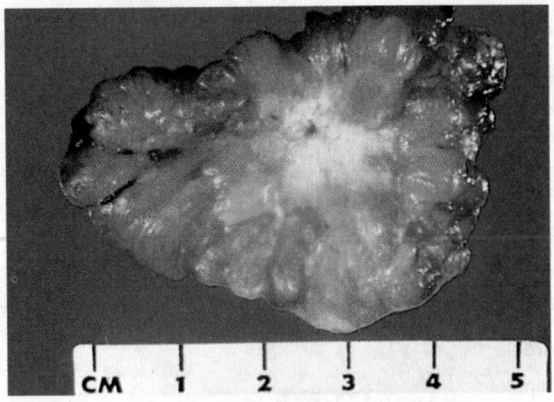

**Breast cancer: invasive ductal carcinoma**
*(Kumar, Cotran, and Robbins, 1997)*

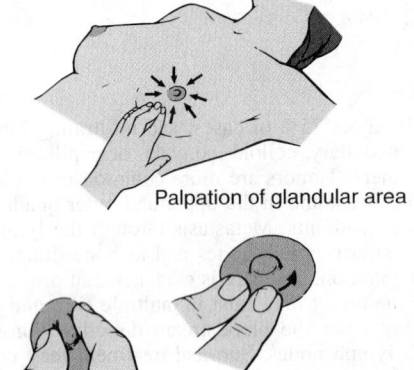

Palpation of glandular area

Palpation of areolar area

Compression of nipple

**Breast examination**

shape and size and for surface characteristics, including moles or nevi, hyperpigmentation, retraction or dimpling, edema, abnormal distribution of hair, focal vascularity, or lesions. With the patient still sitting, the axillary nodes and the supraclavicular and subclavicular areas are palpated. With the patient lying on her back, each breast is shifted medially, and the glandular area in each is palpated with the flat of the fingers of a hand in concentric circles or in a pattern like the spokes of a wheel, from the periphery inward. The areolar areas, the nipples, and the axillary tail of Spence in the upper outer quadrant extending toward the axilla are then palpated. The nipple is squeezed to check for discharge.

■ INTERVENTIONS: The patient should be taught to perform a self-breast examination and encouraged to do it monthly. The American Cancer Society recommends starting at about age 18. Premenopausal women should examine breasts approximately 1 week past the menstrual period, when breasts are less tender and less swollen. Postmenopausal women should choose a specific time each month, such as the first day of the month. Many women find it helpful to check their breasts every time they shower for the first few months after

being taught the procedure to practice and to become very familiar with their own breasts.

■ OUTCOME CRITERIA: Early diagnosis greatly improves the rate of cure in cancer of the breast.

**breast examination**[2], a nursing intervention from the Nursing Interventions Classification (NIC) defined as inspection and palpation of the breasts and related areas. See also **Nursing Interventions Classification.**

**breastfeeding** [AS, **braest** + ME, *feden*], **1.** suckling or nursing, giving a baby milk from the breast. Breastfeeding encourages postpartum uterine involution and slows the natural return of the menses. **2.** taking milk from the breast. See also **breast milk, lactation.**

**breastfeeding and human breastfeeding establishment: maternal,** a nursing outcome from the Nursing Outcomes Classification (NOC) defined as maternal establishment of proper attachment of an infant to and sucking from the breast for nourishment during the first 2 to 3 weeks. See also **Nursing Outcomes Classification.**

**breastfeeding assistance,** a nursing intervention from the Nursing Interventions Classification (NIC) defined as preparing a new mother to breastfeed her infant. See also **Nursing Interventions Classification.**

**breastfeeding, effective,** a nursing diagnosis accepted by the Ninth National Conference on the Classification of Nursing Diagnoses. Effective breastfeeding is a state in which a mother-infant dyad/family exhibits adequate proficiency and satisfaction with the breastfeeding process.

■ DEFINING CHARACTERISTICS: The defining characteristics are the mother's ability to position the infant at the breast to promote a successful latch-on response, regular and sustained suckling/swallowing at the breast, infant content after feeding, appropriate infant weight patterns for age, effective mother-infant communication patterns, signs and/or symptoms of oxytocin release, adequate infant elimination patterns for age, eagerness of the infant to nurse, and maternal verbalization of satisfaction with the breastfeeding process.

■ RELATED FACTORS: Related factors include basic breastfeeding knowledge, normal breast structure, normal infant oral structure, infant gestational age greater than 34 weeks, support sources, and maternal confidence.

**breastfeeding establishment: infant,** a nursing outcome from the Nursing Outcomes Classification (NOC) defined as proper attachment of an infant to and sucking from the mother's breast for nourishment during the first 2 to 3 weeks. See also **Nursing Outcomes Classification.**

**breastfeeding, ineffective,** a nursing diagnosis accepted by the Eighth National Conference on the Classification of Nursing Diagnoses. Ineffective breastfeeding is a state in which a mother, infant, and/or family experiences dissatisfaction or difficulty with the breastfeeding process.

■ DEFINING CHARACTERISTICS: The major defining characteristic is the unsatisfactory breastfeeding process. Other characteristics include an actual or perceived inadequate milk supply, no observable signs of oxytocin release, persistence of sore nipples beyond the infant's first week of life, and maternal reluctance to put the infant to breast as necessary. The infant may be unable to attach to the maternal nipple correctly or may resist latching on, with arching and crying at the breast. Within the first hour after breastfeeding the infant may exhibit fussiness or crying and be unresponsive to other comfort measures. There may also be observable signs of an inadequate infant intake, nonsustained suckling at the breast, suckling at only one breast per feeding, and nursing fewer than seven times in 24 hours.

■ RELATED FACTORS: Related factors in the diagnosis of ineffective breastfeeding are prematurity, infant anomaly, maternal breast anomaly, previous breast surgery, previous history of breastfeeding failure, supplemental feeding of the infant with an artificial nipple, poor infant sucking reflex, nonsupportive partner or family, knowledge deficit, and interruption in breastfeeding. See also **nursing diagnosis.**

**breastfeeding, interrupted,** a nursing diagnosis accepted by the Tenth National Conference on the Classification of Nursing Diagnoses. Interrupted breastfeeding is a break in the continuity of the breastfeeding process as a result of inability or inadvisability of putting the baby to the breast for feeding.

■ DEFINING CHARACTERISTICS: The major defining characteristic is insufficient nourishment by the infant at the breast for some or all feedings. Minor defining characteristics are a maternal desire to maintain lactation and provide her breast milk for her infant's nutritional needs, separation of mother and infant, and lack of knowledge about expression and storage of breast milk.

■ RELATED FACTORS: Related factors include maternal or infant illness, prematurity, maternal employment, contraindications to breastfeeding (e.g., drugs, true breast milk jaundice), or a need to wean the infant abruptly. See also **nursing diagnosis.**

**breastfeeding maintenance,** a nursing outcome from the Nursing Outcomes Classification (NOC) defined as continued nourishment of an infant through breastfeeding. See also **Nursing Outcomes Classification.**

**breastfeeding: weaning,** a nursing outcome from the Nursing Outcomes Classification (NOC) defined as process leading to the eventual discontinuation of breastfeeding. See also **Nursing Outcomes Classification.**

**breast implant,** the surgical placement of prosthetic material in a breast, either to increase the breast's size or for reconstruction after a mastectomy.

**breast milk** [AS, *braest* + *meoluc*], human milk. The nurse should counsel mothers that it is easily digested, clean, and warm and that it confers some immunities (bronchiolitis and gastroenteritis are rare in breastfed babies). Infants fed breast milk are less likely to become obese and to have dental malocclusion. See also **breastfeeding.**

**breast milk jaundice,** jaundice and hyperbilirubinemia in breastfed infants that occur in the first weeks of life as a result of a metabolite in the mother's milk that inhibits the infant's ability to conjugate bilirubin to glucuronide for excretion. See also **hyperbilirubinemia of the newborn.**

■ OBSERVATIONS: Breast milk jaundice usually occurs after the fifth day of life and peaks toward the end of the second or third week. Serum bilirubin levels usually exceed 5 mg/100 ml but rarely reach dangerous levels of 20 mg/100 ml, at which point kernicterus may develop. The infant seems normal and healthy, but the skin, the whites of the eyes, and the serum are jaundiced.

■ INTERVENTIONS: If serum bilirubin exceeds acceptable levels, breastfeeding may be interrupted until they decrease to the normal range, usually a period of 1 to 3 days. During this interval the infant is bottle-fed with a supplemental formula and the mother uses a breast pump or manual device to maintain lactation without engorgement. Phototherapy may be used to accelerate excretion of bilirubin through the skin.

■ NURSING CONSIDERATIONS: The primary concerns of the nurse are to observe for signs of increasing jaundice, to monitor serum bilirubin levels, and usually to reassure the mother that her child is well and that the jaundice resolves slowly but completely in time.

**breast pump,** a mechanical or electronic device for withdrawing milk from the breast.

**breast scintigraphy,** a nuclear scan used to identify breast cancer in patients whose dense breast tissue precludes accurate evaluation by conventional mammography. The test is also used as a second-line imaging modality in patients with an indeterminate mammogram and in women with lumpy breasts.

**breast self-examination.** See **self-breast examination.**

**breast shadows,** artifacts caused by breast tissue that appear on chest radiographs of women. The shadows accentuate the underlying tissue and may cause the appearance of an interstitial disease process. Breast nipples may also appear on the radiograph as "coin lesions," requiring that a second radiograph with special markers attached to the nipples be made so the two films can be compared.

**breast sonogram** an ultrasound test that is used primarily to determine if a mammographic abnormality or a palpable lump is a cyst (fluid-filled) or a solid tumor (benign or malignant). It is also used to examine symptomatic women who should not be exposed to mammographic radiation, such as pregnant women and women under the age of 25.

**breast transillumination** [AS, *braest* + L *trans*, through, *illuminare*, to light up], a method of examining the inner structures of the breast by directing light through the outer wall. See also **diaphanography.**

**breath,** the air inhaled and exhaled during ventilation of the lungs.

**Breathalyzer** /breth′əlī′zər/, trademark for a device that analyzes exhaled air. It is commonly used to test for blood alcohol levels; the test is based on the relationship between alcohol in the breath and alcohol in the blood circulating through the lungs. Also spelled **Breathalyser.**

**breath-holding** /breth-/ [AS, *braeth* + ME, *holden*], a form of voluntary apnea that is usually but not necessarily performed with a closed glottis. Although breath-holding may be prolonged for several minutes, it is invariably terminated either voluntarily or involuntarily.

**breathing.** See **respiration.**

**breathing cycle** /brē′thing/, a ventilatory cycle consisting of an inspiration followed by the expiration of a volume of gas called the tidal volume. The duration or total cycle time of a breathing cycle is the breathing or ventilatory period. Also called **respiratory cycle.**

**breathing frequency (f).** See **respiration rate.**

**breathing nomogram** [AS, *braeth* + Gk, *nomos,* law, *gramma,* a record], a chart that presents scales of data for body weight, breathing frequency, and predicted basal tidal volume arranged so that one can find an unknown value on one scale by drawing a line that connects known values on the other two scales.

**breathing pattern, ineffective,** a nursing diagnosis accepted by the Fourth National Conference on the Classification of Nursing Diagnoses (revised 1998). An ineffective breathing pattern is a state in which inspiration and/or expiration do not provide adequate ventilation for the individual.

■ DEFINING CHARACTERISTICS: Defining characteristics are dyspnea, shortness of breath; respiratory rate (adults [14 years of age or more], 11 or 24; infants, 25 or 60; ages 1 to 4, 20 or 30; ages 5 to 14, 15 or 25); depth of breathing (adults, VT 500 mL at rest; infants, 6 to 8); timing ratio; nasal flaring (infants); use of accessory muscles; altered chest excursion; assumption of three-point position, pursed lip breathing, prolonged expiratory phases, increased anteroposterior diameter; orthopnea; decreased vital capacity; decreased minute ventilation; and decreased inspiratory/expiratory pressure.

■ RELATED FACTORS: Related factors are neuromuscular dysfunction, pain, musculoskeletal impairment, perception/cognitive impairment, anxiety, hyper/hypoventilation, bone deformity, pain, chest wall deformity, obesity, spinal cord injury, body position, neurological immaturity, respiratory muscle fatigue, and decreased energy/fatigue. See also **nursing diagnosis.**

**breathing-related sleep disorder,** any of several disorders characterized by sleep disruption caused by some sleep-related breathing problem, resulting in excessive sleepiness or insomnia; included are central sleep apnea, obstructive sleep apnea, and primary alveolar hypoventilation (Ondine's curse).

**breathing tube.** See **endotracheal tube, nasotracheal tube.**

**breathing work,** the energy required for breathing movements. It is the cumulative product of the instantaneous pressure developed by the respiratory muscles and the volume of air moved during a breathing cycle.

**breathlessness.** See **dyspnea.**

**breath odor,** an odor usually produced by substances or diseases in the lungs or mouth. Certain specific odors are associated with some diseases, such as diabetes, liver failure, uremia, or a lung abscess.

**breath sound** [AS, *braeth* + L, *sonus*], the sound of air passing in and out of the lungs as heard with a stethoscope. Vesicular, bronchovesicular, and bronchial breath sounds are normal. Decreased breath sounds may indicate an obstruction of an airway, collapse of a portion or all of a lung, thickening of the pleurae of the lungs, emphysema, or other chronic obstructive pulmonary disease.

**breath tests,** diagnostic tests for intestinal disorders such as bacterial overgrowth, ileal disease, lactase deficiency, and steatorrhea. Lactose malabsorption is treated by giving the patient 12.5 to 25.0 grams of lactose and measuring the amount of hydrogen excreted in the breath. If lactose absorption is impaired in the small intestine, colonic bacteria ferment the lactose, releasing hydrogen, which is excreted in the breath. Bacterial overgrowth is tested with $^{14}$C-cholylglycine, which is normally absorbed by the ileum and recycled via the enterohepatic circulation. In cases of bacterial overgrowth the labeled glycine is removed by conjugation in the small intestine, absorbed, and metabolized, resulting in an increase of $^{14}CO_2$ in the breath.

**Breckinridge, Mary** (1881–1965), the American nurse who founded the Frontier Nursing Service in Kentucky to improve the obstetric care of women living in remote mountainous areas. The nurses in the service had training in midwifery and reached their patients on horseback and on foot, often encountering personal danger. The service began training midwives and stimulated the establishment of other midwifery schools.

**breech birth** [ME, *brech* + *burth*], parturition in which the infant emerges feet, knees, or buttocks first. Breech birth is often hazardous. The body may deliver easily, but the aftercoming head may become trapped by an incompletely dilated cervix because infants' heads are usually larger than their bodies. See also **assisted breech, breech presentation, complete breech, footling breech, frank breech, version and extraction.**

**breech extraction** [ME, *brech* + L, *ex,* out, *trahere,* to pull], an obstetric operation in which an infant being born feet or buttocks first is grasped before any part of the trunk is born and delivered by traction. Compare **assisted breech.**

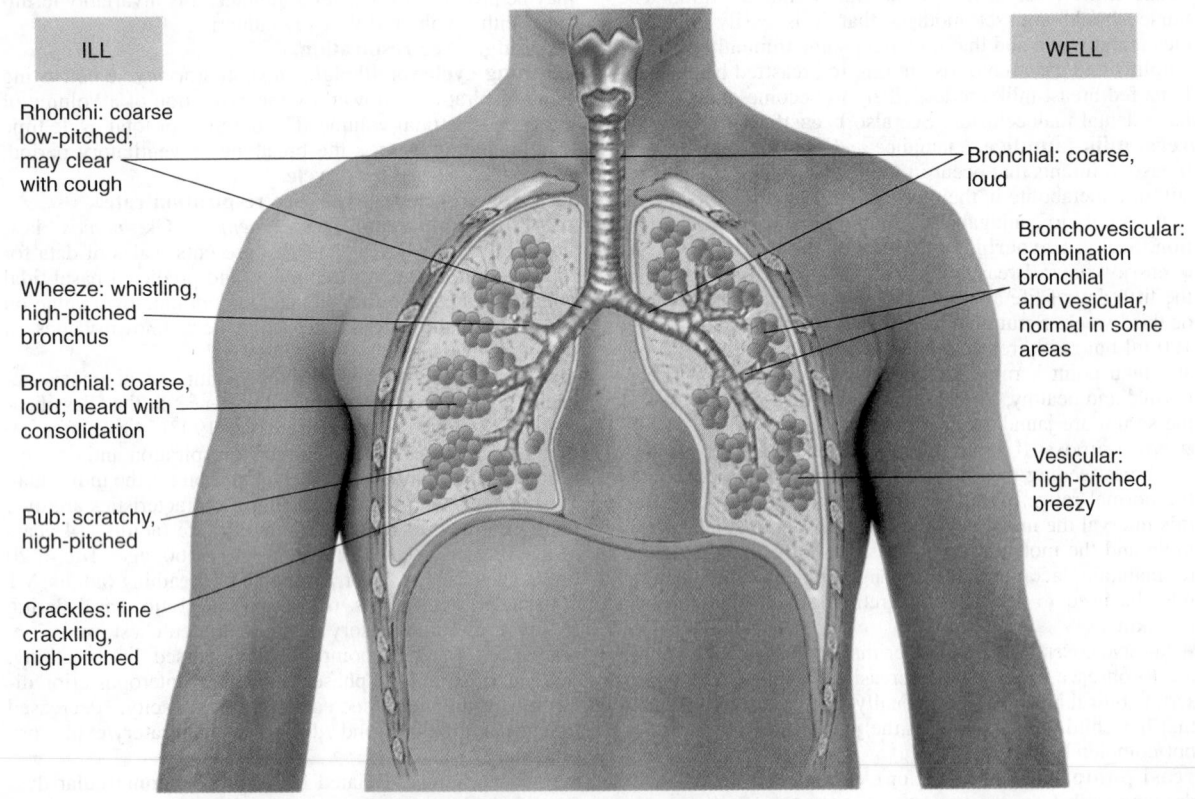

ILL      WELL

Rhonchi: coarse low-pitched; may clear with cough

Wheeze: whistling, high-pitched bronchus

Bronchial: coarse, loud; heard with consolidation

Rub: scratchy, high-pitched

Crackles: fine crackling, high-pitched

Bronchial: coarse, loud

Bronchovesicular: combination bronchial and vesicular, normal in some areas

Vesicular: high-pitched, breezy

**Breath sounds in the ill and well patient** *(Seidel et al, 1999)*

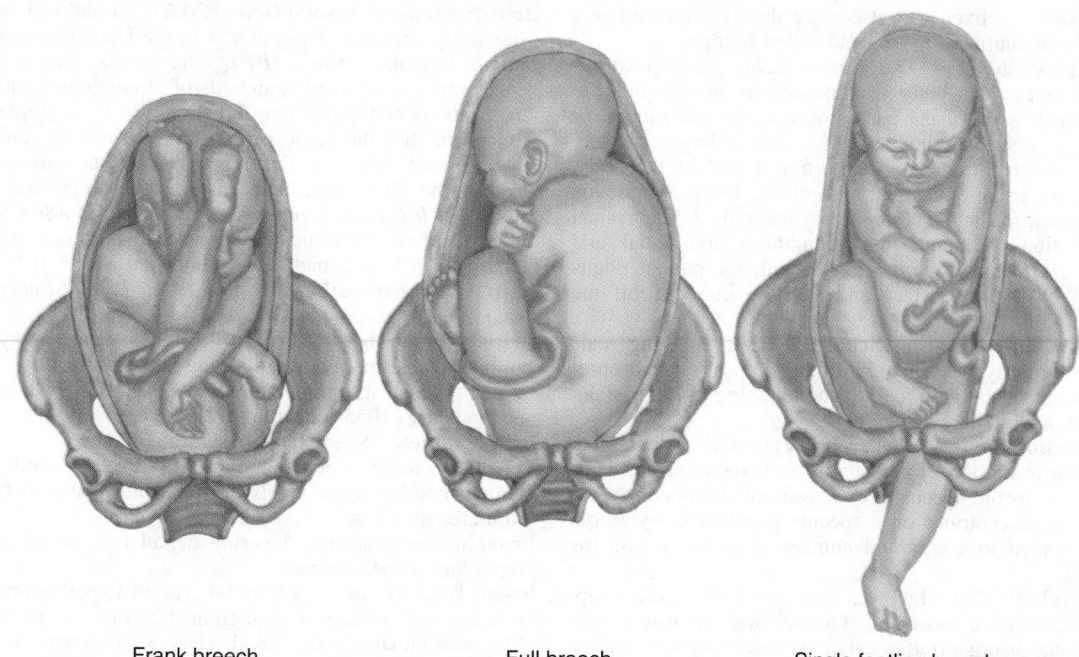

Frank breech       Full breech       Single footling breech

**Breech presentation** (McKinney et al, 2000)

**breech presentation** [ME, *brech* + L, *praesentare,* to show], intrauterine position of the fetus in which the buttocks or feet present. It occurs in approximately 3% of labors. Kinds of breech presentation are **complete breech, footling breech,** and **frank breech.** Compare **vertex presentation.** See also **breech birth.**

**bregma** /breg′mə/ [Gk, the front of the head], the junction of the coronal and sagittal sutures on the top of the skull. —**bregmatic,** *adj.*

**bregmacardiac reflex** /breg′məkär′dē·ək/ [Gk, *bregma,* front of the head], a phenomenon in which pressure on the anterior fontanel of an infant's skull causes the heart to slow.

**bremsstrahlung radiation** /brems′shträ′lŏŏng/ [Ger, braking radiation], a type of x radiation produced by the interaction between electrons and the nuclei of target atoms.

**Brenner tumor** [Fritz Brenner, German pathologist, b. 1877], an uncommon benign ovarian neoplasm consisting of nests or cords of epithelial cells containing glycogen that are enclosed in fibrous connective tissue. The tumor may be solid or cystic and is sometimes difficult to distinguish from certain granulosa-theca cell neoplasms.

**Brethine,** trademark for a beta₂ receptor agonist agent (terbutaline sulfate).

**bretylium tosylate** /britil′ē·əm/, an antiarrhythmic agent.
■ INDICATION: It is prescribed in the treatment of selected life-threatening ventricular arrhythmias when other measures have not been effective.
■ CONTRAINDICATION: Known hypersensitivity to this drug prohibits its use.
■ ADVERSE EFFECTS: Among the more serious adverse reactions are hypotension, nausea and vomiting, anginal pain, and nasal stuffiness.

**Bretylol,** trademark for an adrenergic blocking agent (bretylium tosylate).

**brevi-** /brev′ē-/, prefix meaning 'short': *brevicollis, breviradiate.*

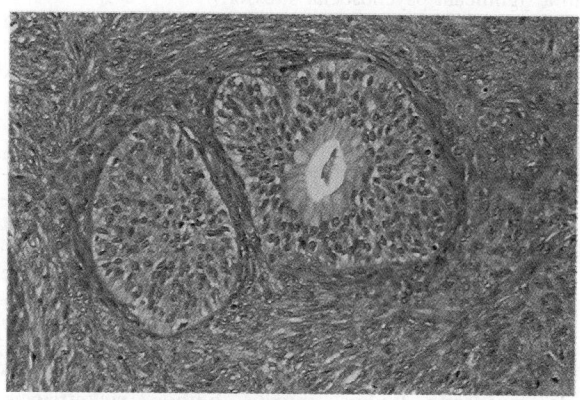

**Brenner tumor** (Fletcher, 2000)

**Brevicon,** trademark for a norethindrone-ethinyl estradiol oral contraceptive.

**Brevital Sodium,** trademark for a barbiturate (methohexital sodium).

**brewer's yeast** /brŏŏ′ərz/ [ME, *brewen,* to boil, *yest,* foam], a preparation containing the dried pulverized cells of a yeast, such as *Saccharomyces cerevisiae,* that is used as a leavening agent and as a dietary supplement. It is one of the best sources of the B complex vitamins and a rich source of many minerals and a high grade of protein.

**Bricanyl,** trademark for a beta₂ receptor agonist agent (terbutaline sulfate).

**brick dust urine,** a reddish discoloration signaling precipitated urates in acidic urine.

**bridge.** See **bridgework.**

**bridge of Varolius.** See **pons.**

**bridgework,** a fixed partial denture that is cemented permanently to abutment teeth. Also called **bridge.**

**bridging** [AS, *brycg*], **1.** a nursing technique of positioning a patient so that bony prominences are free of pressure on the mattress by using pads, bolsters of foam rubber, or pillows to distribute body weight over a larger surface. **2.** a nursing technique for supporting a part of the body, such as the testicles in treating orchitis, using a Bellevue bridge made of a towel or other material. **3.** a physical rehabilitation technique that strengthens abdominal and leg muscles. Reclining with knees bent, the patient plants the feet on a firm surface and lifts the buttocks off the surface.

**Brief Psychiatric Rating Scale (BPRS),** a rating scale for assessing psychopathology on the basis of a small number of items, usually 16 to 24, encompassing psychosis, depression, and anxiety symptoms.

**brief psychotherapy,** (in psychiatry) treatment directed to the active resolution of personality or behavioral problems rather than to the speculative analysis of the unconscious. It usually concentrates on a specific problem or symptom and is limited to a specified number of sessions with the therapist.

**brief psychotic disorder,** an episode of psychotic symptoms (incoherence, loosening of associations, delusions, hallucinations, disorganized or catatonic behavior) with sudden onset, lasting less than one month. If it occurs in response to a stressful life event, it may be called **brief reactive psychosis.**

**brief reactive psychosis,** a short episode, usually less than 2 weeks, of psychotic behavior that occurs in response to a significant psychosocial stressor.

**brightness gain** /brīt'nes/, the increase in illumination level of a radiograph produced by an image intensifier. It is calculated as the minification gain multiplied by the flux gain. The product is the ratio of the number of photons at the output phosphor to the number at the input phosphor.

**Brill-Symmers disease.** See **giant follicular lymphoma.**

**Brill-Zinsser disease** /bril'zin'sər/ [Nathan E. Brill, American physician, 1860–1925; Hans Zinsser, American bacteriologist, 1878–1940], a mild form of epidemic typhus that recurs in a person who appears to have completely recovered from a severe case of the disease years earlier. Some rickettsiae remain in the body after the symptoms of the disease abate, causing the recurrence of symptoms, especially when stress, illness, or malnutrition weakens the person. Treatment with antibiotics may eradicate the organism. See also **epidemic typhus, murine typhus, rickettsiosis, typhus.**

**brim,** **1.** edge or margin. **2.** the edge of the upper border of the true pelvis, or the pelvic inlet. See also **pelvis.**

**brim of true pelvic cavity.** See **iliopectineal line.**

**Brinnell hardness test** [Johann A. Brinnell, Swedish engineer, 1849–1925], a means of determining the surface hardness of a material by measuring the resistance the material offers to the impact of a steel ball. The test result is recorded as the Brinnell hardness number (BHN); harder materials have higher BHNs. The Brinnell hardness test is commonly used to measure abrasion resistance in materials used in dental restorations, such as amalgams, cements, and porcelains. Compare Knoop hardness test.

**Briquet's syndrome.** See **somatization disorder.**

**Brissaud's dwarf** /brisōz'/ [Edouard Brissaud, French physician, 1852–1909], a person affected with infantile myxedema in which short stature is associated with hypothyroidism.

**British antilewisite.** See **dimercaprol.**

**British Medical Association (BMA),** a national professional organization of physicians in the United Kingdom.

*British Pharmacopoeia (BP),* the official British reference work setting forth standards of strength and purity of medications and containing directions for their preparation to ensure that the same prescription written by different doctors and filled by different pharmacists will contain exactly the same ingredients in the same proportions. The first *British Pharmacopoeia* was published in 1864 by the General Medical Council; it superseded the *London Pharmacopoeia,* which had been published since 1618. See also **British Medical Association,** *United States Pharmacopeia* (USP).

**British thermal unit (BTU),** a unit of heat energy. The amount of thermal energy that must be absorbed by 1 lb of water to raise its temperature by 1° at 39.2° F. It is also equivalent to 1055 joules or 252 calories.

**brittle bones.** See **osteogenesis imperfecta.**

**brittle diabetes,** poorly controlled diabetes mellitus in which blood glucose levels are unstable. See also **type 1 diabetes mellitus.**

**broach,** an elongated, tapering dental instrument used in removing pulpal material.

**broad beta disease,** a familial type of hyperlipoproteinemia in which a lipoprotein, high in cholesterol and triglycerides, accumulates in the blood. The condition, which affects males in their twenties and females in their thirties and forties, is characterized by yellowish nodules (xanthomas) on the elbows and knees, peripheral vascular disease, and elevated serum cholesterol levels. Persons with this disease are at risk of development of early coronary disease. Therapy includes dietary measures to reduce weight and levels of serum lipids. Also called **dysbetalipoproteinemia, hyperlipidemia type III.** See also **hyperlipidemia, hyperlipoproteinemia.**

**broad ligament** [ME, *brood* + L, *ligare,* to tie], a folded sheet of peritoneum draped over the uterine tubes, the uterus, and the ovaries. It extends from the sides of the uterus to the sidewalls of the pelvis, dividing the pelvis from side to side and creating the vesicouterine fossa and pouch in front of the uterus and the rectouterine fossa and pouch behind it. Also called **ligamentum latum uteri.** See also **cardinal ligament.**

**broad ligament of liver** [ME, *brod* + L, *ligare,* to bind; AS, *lifer*], a crescent-shaped fold of peritoneum attached to the lower surface of the diaphragm, connecting with the liver and the anterior abdominal wall. Also called **falciform ligament of the liver, ligamentum falciforme hepatis.**

**broad-spectrum antibiotic,** an antibiotic that is effective against a wide range of infectious microorganisms.

**Broca's aphasia** /brō'kəz/ [Pierre P. Broca, French neurologist, 1824–1880], a type of aphasia consisting of nonfluent speech, with a laconic and hesitant, telegraphic quality caused by a large left frontal lesion extending to the central sulcus. The patient's agrammatic speech is characterized by abundant nouns and verbs but few articles and prepositions, the resulting speech is economical but lacking in syntax.

**Broca's area** [Pierre P. Broca], an area involved in speech production situated on the inferior frontal gyrus of the brain. See also **aphasia, Broca's aphasia, motor speech areas, speech centers.**

**Broca's fissure** [Pierre P. Broca], a cleft or groove encircling Broca's area in the left frontal area of the brain.

**Broca's plane** [Pierre P. Broca], a plane that includes the tip of the interalveolar septum between the upper central incisors and the lowest point of the left and right occipital condyles.

**Brodie's abscess** [Benjamin Brodie, English surgeon, 1783–1862], a form of osteomyelitis consisting of an indolent staphylococcal infection of bone, usually in the metaphysis of a long bone of a child, characterized by a necrotic cavity surrounded by dense granulation tissue. See also **osteomyelitis.** Also called **circumscribed abscess of bone.**

**Brodmann's areas** /brod'manz, brŏt'mons/ [Korbinian Brodmann, German anatomist, 1868–1918], the 47 different areas of the cerebral cortex that are associated with specific neurologic functions and distinguished by different cellular components. They control movements of the lips and vocal cords as well as motor speech. Compare **motor area.** See also **cerebral cortex.**

**broken cell preparation.** See **homogenate.**

**brom,** abbreviation for a *bromide noncarboxylate anion.*

**brom-, bromo-,** prefix meaning a compound containing bromine or meaning 'odor, stench': *bromhidrosis, bromoacetophenon.*

**bromelain** /brō'məlān/, any of several enzymes that catalyze cleavage of proteins on the carboxyl side of alanine, glycine, lysine, and tyrosine bonds. Differing forms are derived from the fruit (fruit bromelain) and stem (stem bromelain) of the pineapple plant. The enzyme is administered orally as an anti-inflammatory agent and is also used in immunology to render red cells agglutinable by incomplete antibody.

**Bromfed,** trademark for a fixed-combination decongestant containing brompheniramine maleate and pseudoephedrine maleate.

**bromhidrosis** /brō'midrō'sis/ [Gk, *bromos,* stench, *hidros,* sweat], an abnormal condition in which the apocrine sweat has an unpleasant odor. The odor is usually caused by bacterial decomposition of perspiration on the skin. Treatment includes frequent bathing, changing of socks and underclothes, and use of deodorants, antibacterial soaps, and dusting powders. Also called **body odor.**

**bromide** /brō'mīd/ [Gk, *bromos,* stench], an anion of bromine. Bromide salts, once widely prescribed as sedatives, are now seldom used for that purpose because they may cause serious mental disturbances as side effects.

**bromide poisoning,** an adverse reaction to ingested bromide. Symptoms include nausea, vomiting, an acnelike rash, slurred speech, ataxia, psychotic behavior, and coma.

**bromine (Br)** /brō'mēn/, a toxic red-brown liquid element of the halogen group. Its atomic number is 35; its atomic mass is 79.904. It exists naturally as a diatopic molecule, $Br_2$. Bromine is used in industry, in photography, in the manufacture of organic chemicals and fuels, and in medications. Bromine gives off a red vapor that is extremely irritating to the eyes and the respiratory tract. Liquid bromine causes serious skin burns. Compounds of bromine have been used as sedatives, hypnotics, and analgesics and are still used in some nonprescription, over-the-counter preparations. Prolonged use of these products may cause brominism, a toxic condition characterized by acneiform eruptions, headache, loss of libido, drowsiness, and fatigue. See also **bromide.**

**bromo-.** See **brom-.**

**bromocriptine mesylate** /brō'mōkrip'tēn/, a dopamine receptor agonist.

■ INDICATIONS: It is prescribed for the treatment of amenorrhea and galactorrhea associated with hyperprolactinemia, female infertility, and Parkinson's disease.

■ CONTRAINDICATION: Sensitivity to any ergot alkaloid prohibits its use.

■ ADVERSE EFFECTS: Among the more severe adverse reactions are palpitations, hypotension, bradycardia, hallucinations, syncope, nausea, ataxia, dyspnea, dysphagia, and confusion.

**bromoderma** /brō'mōdur'mə/ [Gk, *bromos,* stench, *derma* skin], an acneiform, bullous, or nodular skin rash, occurring as a hypersensitivity reaction to ingested bromides.

**brompheniramine maleate** /brom'fənir'əmin/, an antihistamine.

■ INDICATIONS: It is prescribed in the treatment of allergic reactions, including rhinitis, skin reactions, and itching.

■ CONTRAINDICATIONS: Asthma or known hypersensitivity to this drug prohibits its use. It is not given to newborns, lactating mothers, or other people for whom anticholinergic medications are contraindicated.

■ ADVERSE EFFECTS: Drowsiness, skin rash, hypersensitivity reactions, dry mouth, and tachycardia commonly occur.

**Brompton's cocktail,** an analgesic solution containing alcohol, morphine or heroin, and, in some cases, a phenothiazine. Formulations vary, and recently cocaine has generally been eliminated from the mixture. The cocktail is administered in the control of pain in the terminally ill patient. Given frequently at the lowest effective dose, it may relieve pain for many months. It was developed at the Brompton Hospital in England. Also called **Brompton's mixture.**

**bronch-, broncho-,** combining form meaning 'bronchus': *bronchiectasis, bronchodilation.*

**bronch(o)-,** prefix meaning relationship to a bronchus. See also **bronchi(o)-.**

**bronchi(o)-,** prefix meaning relationship to a bronchus. See also **bronch(o)-.**

**bronchial** /brong'kē·əl/ [Gk, *bronchos,* windpipe], pertaining to the bronchi or bronchioles.

**bronchial asthma.** See **asthma.**

**bronchial atresia,** atresia of a lobar or segmental bronchus, usually in the left upper lobe; the affected lung segment is often hyperinflated because of leakage of air through the alveolar pores.

**bronchial breath sound** [Gk, *bronchos,* windpipe], a normal sound heard with a stethoscope over the main airways of the lungs, including the trachea. Expiration and inspiration produce noise of equal loudness and duration, sounding like blowing through a hollow tube. The expiratory sound is heard during the greater part of expiration, whereas the inspiratory sound stops abruptly at the height of inspiration, with a pause before the sound of expiration is heard. Also called **tracheal breath sound.**

**bronchial cast,** a cylindrical solid or semisolid plug that blocks a bronchus and is sometimes expectorated.

**bronchial challenge, bronchial challenge test,** a challenge test in which a nonspecific agent such as histamine or methacholine is applied to the bronchi and they are assessed for a bronchoconstriction reaction. Also called **bronchial provocation.** See **inhalational challenge.**

**bronchial cough,** a cough associated with bronchiectasis and heard in early stages as hacking and irritating, becoming looser in later stages.

**bronchial drainage.** See **postural drainage.**

**bronchial fremitus,** a vibration that can be palpated or auscultated on the chest wall over a bronchus. It results from congestion by secretions that rattle as air passes during respiration. See also **fremitus.**

**bronchial hyperreactivity** [Gk, *bronchos* + *hyper,* excess; L, *re,* again, *agere,* to act], an abnormal respiratory condition characterized by reflex bronchospasm in response to histamine or a cholinergic drug, such as methacholine. It is a universal feature of asthma and is used in the differential diagnosis of asthma and heart disease.

**bronchial murmur,** a murmur heard as a blowing sound, caused by air flowing in and out of the bronchial tubes.

**bronchial pneumonia.** See **bronchopneumonia.**

**bronchial provocation.** See **bronchial challenge.**

**bronchial secretion,** a substance produced in the bronchial tree that consists of mucus secreted by the goblet cells and mucous glands of the bronchi, protein salts released from disintegrating cells, plasma fluid, and proteins, including fibrinogen, that have escaped from pulmonary capillaries.

**bronchial spasm.** See **bronchospasm.**

**bronchial toilet,** special care that is given patients with tracheostomies and respiratory disorders, including stimulation of coughing, deep breathing, and suctioning of the respiratory tract with a tracheobronchial aspiration pump.

**bronchial tree,** an anatomic complex of the trachea and bronchi. The bronchi branch from the trachea. The right bronchus is wider and shorter than the left bronchus and branches into three secondary bronchi, one passing to each of the three lobes of the right lung. The left bronchus is smaller in diameter and about twice as long as the right bronchus. It branches into the secondary bronchi for the inferior and the superior lobes of the left lung. The bronchus is sometimes described as a **bronchial tube.**

**bronchial tube.** See **bronchus.**

**bronchial washing** [Gk, *bronchos,* windpipe; ME, *wasshen,* to wash], irrigation of the bronchi and bronchioles performed during bronchoscopy to cleanse the tubes and to collect specimens for laboratory examination.

**bronchiectasis** /brong′kē·ek′təsis/ [Gk, *bronchos + ektasis,* stretching], an abnormal condition of the bronchial tree characterized by irreversible dilation and destruction of the bronchial walls. The condition is sometimes congenital but is more often a result of bronchial infection or of obstruction by a tumor or an aspirated foreign body. Symptoms include a constant cough producing copious purulent sputum, hemoptysis, chronic sinusitis, clubbing of fingers, and persistent moist, coarse crackles. Some of the complications of bronchiectasis are pneumonia, lung abscess, empyema,

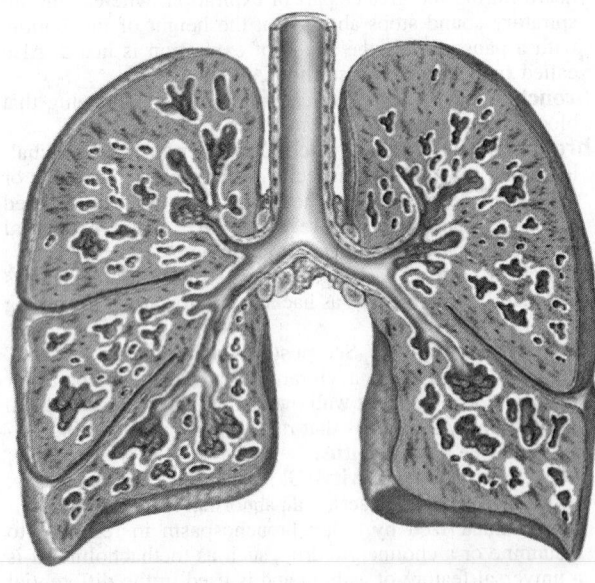

**Bronchiectasis** *(Wilson and Giddens, 2001)*

brain abscess, and amyloidosis. Treatment includes frequent postural drainage, expectorants, antibiotics, and, rarely, surgical resection of the affected part of the lungs.

**bronchioalveolar adenocarcinoma, bronchioalveolar carcinoma.** See **bronchioloalveolar carcinoma.**

**bronchiolar.** See **bronchiole.**

**bronchiolar adenocarcinoma.** See **bronchioloalveolar carcinoma.**

**bronchiolar carcinoma.** See **alveolar cell carcinoma.**

**bronchiolar collapse** /brong′kyələr/ [L, *bronchiolus,* little windpipe, *conlabi,* to fall], a condition in which bronchioles, which are pliable and lack cartilaginous support, become compressed by surrounding structures in the absence of inflowing air needed to keep them inflated. The condition occurs in disorders such as emphysema, cystic disease, and bronchiectasis.

**bronchiole** /brong′kē·ōl/ [L, *bronchiolus,* little windpipe], a small airway of the respiratory system extending from the bronchi into the lobes of the lung. There are two divisions of bronchioles: The terminal bronchioles passively conduct inspired air from the bronchi to the respiratory bronchioles and expired air from the respiratory bronchioles to the bronchi. The respiratory bronchioles function similarly, allowing the exchange of air and waste gases between the alveolar ducts and the terminal bronchioles. —**bronchiolar** /brongkē′ələr/, *adj.*

**bronchiolitis** /brong′kē·ōlī′tis/ [L, *bronchiolus,* little windpipe; Gk, *itis,* inflammation], an acute viral infection of the lower respiratory tract that occurs primarily in infants less than 18 months of age. It is characterized by expiratory wheezing, respiratory distress, inflammation, and obstruction at the level of the bronchioles. The most common causative agents are the respiratory syncytial viruses (RSVs) and the parainfluenza viruses. *Mycoplasma pneumoniae,* rhinoviruses, enteroviruses, and measles virus are less common causative agents. Transmission occurs by infection with airborne particles or by contact with infected secretions. The diagnosis consists of evidence of hyperinflation of the lungs through percussion or chest x-ray.

■ OBSERVATIONS: The condition typically begins as an upper respiratory tract infection with serous nasal discharge and often with low-grade fever. Increasing respiratory distress follows, characterized by tachypnea, tachycardia, intercostal and subcostal retractions, a paroxysmal cough, an expiratory wheeze, and often an elevated temperature. The chest may appear barrel-shaped; x-ray films show hyperinflated lungs and a depressed diaphragm. Respiration becomes more shallow, causing increased alveolar oxygen tension and leading to respiratory acidosis. Complete obstruction and absorption of trapped air may lead to atelectasis and respiratory failure. Blood gas determinations indicate the degree of carbon dioxide retention.

■ INTERVENTIONS: Routine treatment includes administering humidity and oxygen via a mist tent, vaporizer, or Croupette, generally combined with oxygen; ensuring an adequate fluid intake, usually given intravenously because of tachypnea, weakness, and fatigue; suctioning the airways to remove secretions; and promoting rest. Endotracheal intubation is indicated when carbon dioxide retention occurs, when bronchial secretions do not loosen and clear, or when oxygen therapy does not alleviate hypoxia. Such medications as antibiotics, bronchodilators, corticosteroids, cough suppressants, and expectorants are not routinely used. Ribovarin may be used when RSV is the causative agent. Sedatives are contraindicated because of their suppressant effect on the respiratory tract. The infection typically runs its course in 7 to 10 days, with good prognosis. A major complication is bacterial infection, most commonly after prolonged use of a mist tent. The disorder is often confused with asthma. A family history of allergy, the presence of other allergic manifestations, and improvement with epinephrine injection are usually indicative of asthma, not bronchiolitis. Cystic fibrosis, pertussis, the bronchopneumonias, and foreign body obstruction of the trachea are other disorders that may be confused with bronchiolitis.

■ NURSING CONSIDERATIONS: The focus of nursing care is to promote rest and to conserve the child's energy by reducing anxiety and apprehension; to increase the ease of breathing with humidity and oxygen as needed; to aid in changing position for comfort; and to induce drainage of secretions or to suction when necessary. Fever is usually controlled by the cool atmosphere of the mist tent and by administration of antipyretics as needed. Frequent changing of clothing and bed linen is often necessary in a mist environment to reduce chilling. Vital signs and chest and breath sounds are continuously monitored to detect early signs of respiratory distress.

**bronchiolitis obliterans,** a form of bronchiolitis in which the exudate is not expectorated but becomes organized and obliterates the bronchial tubes, causing collapse of the affected part of the lungs.

**bronchioloalveolar carcinoma** /brong′kē·ō′lō·al·vē′ə·lər /, a less common variant of adenocarcinoma of the lung, with columnar to cuboidal epithelial cells lining the alveolar septa and projecting into alveolar spaces in branching papillary formations. Also called **alveolar adenocarcinoma, alveolar carcinoma, alveolar cell carcinoma, bronchioalveolar adenocarcinoma, bronchiolar adenocarcinoma, bronchiolar carcinoma, bronchoalveolar adenocarcinoma, bronchoalveolar carcinoma.**

**bronchiospasm.** See **bronchospasm.**

**bronchitis** /brongkī′tis/ [Gk, *bronchos,* windpipe, *itis,* inflammation], acute or chronic inflammation of the mucous membranes of the tracheobronchial tree. **Acute bronchitis** is characterized by a productive cough, fever, hypertrophy of mucus-secreting structures, and back pain. Caused by the spread of upper respiratory viral infections to the bronchi, it is often observed with or after childhood infections, such as measles, whooping cough, diphtheria, and typhoid fever. Treatment includes bed rest, antipyretics, expectorants, and appropriate antibiotic therapy. See also **chronic bronchitis,**

chronic obstructive pulmonary disease, respiratory syncytial virus.

**bronchoalveolar** /-alvē′ələr/ [Gk, *bronchos,* windpipe; L, *alveolus,* little hollow], pertaining to the terminal air sacs at the ends of the bronchioles.

**bronchoalveolar adenocarcinoma.** See **bronchioloalveolar carcinoma.**

**bronchoalveolar carcinoma (BAC),** a peripheral well-differentiated neoplasm that spreads locally through the air spaces of the alveoli. A variant of adenocarcinoma, BAC constitutes about 5% of all lung cancers.

**bronchoalveolar lavage (BAL),** a diagnostic procedure in which small amounts of physiologic solution are injected through a fiberoptic bronchoscope into a specific area of the lung, while the rest of the lung is sequestered by an inflated balloon. The fluid is then aspirated and inspected for pathogens, malignant cells, and mineral bodies.

**bronchoconstriction** [Gk, *bronchos,* windpipe; L, *constringere,* to draw tight], a narrowing of the lumen of the bronchi, restricting airflow to and from the lungs.

**bronchodilation** /-dil′ətā′shən/ [Gk, *bronchos,* windpipe; L, *dilatare,* to widen], a widening of the lumen of the bronchi, allowing increased airflow to and from the lungs.

**bronchodilator** /-dilā′tər/, a substance, especially a drug, that relaxes contractions of the smooth muscle of the bronchioles to improve ventilation to the lungs. Pharmacologic bronchodilators are prescribed to improve aeration in asthma, bronchiectasis, bronchitis, and emphysema. Commonly used bronchodilators include albuterol, terbutaline, theophylline, and various derivatives and combinations of these drugs. The adverse effects vary, depending on the particular class of the bronchodilating drug. In general, bronchodilators are given with caution to people with impaired cardiac function. Nervousness, irritability, gastritis, or palpitations of the heart may occur.

**bronchofibroscopy.** See **fiberoptic bronchoscopy.**

**bronchogenic** /-jen′ik/ [Gk, *bronchos + genein,* to produce], originating in the bronchi.

**bronchogenic adenocarcinoma,** the more common type of adenocarcinoma of the lung, as distinguished from the type called **bronchioloalveolar carcinoma.**

**bronchogenic carcinoma,** one of the more than 90% of malignant lung tumors that originate in bronchi. Lesions, usually resulting from cigarette smoking, may cause coughing and wheezing, fatigue, chest tightness, and aching joints.

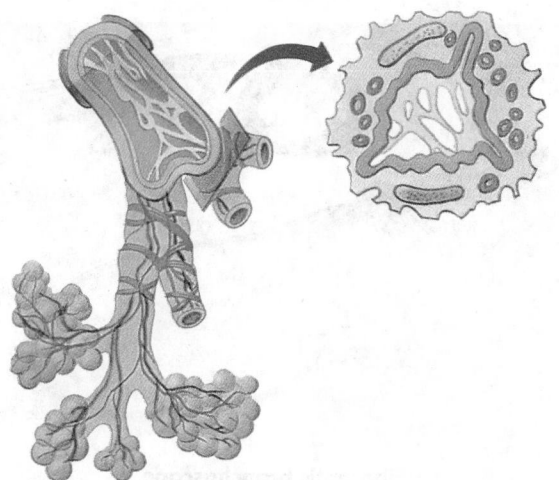

**Chronic bronchitis** *(Thibodeau and Patton, 1999/Rolin Graphics)*

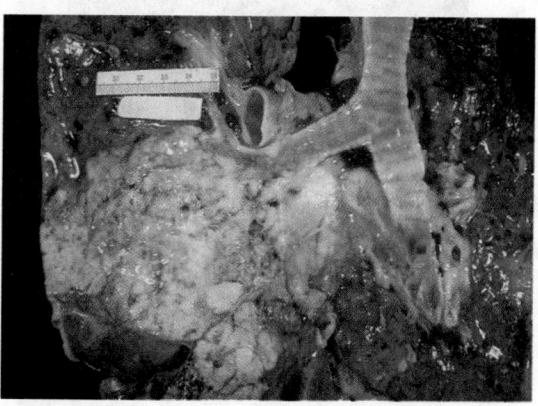

**Bronchogenic carcinoma** *(Kumar, Cotran, and Robbins, 1997)*

In the late stages, bloody sputum, clubbing of the fingers, weight loss, and pleural effusion may be present. Diagnosis is made by bronchoscopy, sputum cytologic examination, lymph node biopsy, radioisotope scanning procedures, or exploratory surgery. Surgery is the most effective treatment, but well over 50% of cases are unresectable when first detected. Palliative treatment includes radiotherapy and chemotherapy.

**bronchogenic cyst,** a cyst that develops in the lungs or mediastinum. It may be asymptomatic or cause cough, stridor, wheezing, or dyspnea. It may also become infected or malignant, requiring surgical removal.

**bronchogram** /brong'kō·gram/ [Gk, *bronchos,* windpipe + *gramma,* something drawn or written], the radiogram obtained by bronchography.

**bronchography** /brongkog'rəfē/, an x-ray examination of the bronchi after they have been coated with a radiopaque substance.

**broncholithiasis** /-lithī'əsis/, inflammation of the bronchi caused by an accumulation of hard concretions or stones on their lining.

**bronchomotor tone,** the state of contraction or relaxation of the smooth muscle in the bronchial walls that regulates the caliber of the airways.

**bronchophony** /brongkof'ənē/ [Gk, *bronchos* + *phone,* voice], an increase in the intensity and clarity of vocal resonance that may result from an increase in lung tissue density, such as in the consolidation of pneumonia.

**bronchopleural fistula** /-ploo͞r'əl/, an abnormal passageway between a bronchus and the pleural cavity.

**bronchopneumonia** [Gk, *bronchos* + *pneumon,* lung], an acute inflammation of the lungs and bronchioles, characterized by chills, fever, high pulse and respiratory rates, bronchial breathing, cough with purulent bloody sputum, severe chest pain, and abdominal distension. The disease is usually a result of the spread of infection from the upper to the lower respiratory tract, caused by the bacterium *Mycoplasma pneumoniae, Staphylococcus pyogenes,* or *Streptococcus pneumoniae.* Atypical forms of bronchopneumonia may occur in viral and rickettsial infections. The most common cause in infancy is the respiratory syncytial virus. Bronchopneumonia causes pleural effusion, empyema, lung abscess, peripheral thrombophlebitis, respiratory failure, congestive heart failure, and jaundice. Treatment includes administration of an antibiotic, oxygen therapy, supportive measures to keep the bronchi clear of secretions, and relief of pleural pain. Also called **bronchial pneumonia, catarrhal pneumonia.** Compare **aspiration pneumonia, eosinophilic pneumonia, interstitial pneumonia.** See also **lobar pneumonia, respiratory syncytial virus.**

**bronchoprovocation inhalation test,** a pulmonary function test performed on patients with a history of asthma who have normal pulmonary function at rest. In a specific test, the patient inhales a particular antigen while the forced expiratory volume (FEV) is measured. In a nonspecific test, the patient inhales a substance such as histamine periodically at increasing concentrations while the FEV is measured.

**bronchopulmonary** /-pul'mōner'ē/ [Gk, *bronchos* + L, *pulmonis,* lung], pertaining to the bronchi and the lungs.

**bronchopulmonary dysplasia (BPD)** /-poo͞l'məner'ē/, a chronic respiratory disorder characterized by scarring of lung tissue, thickened pulmonary arterial walls, and mismatch between lung ventilation and perfusion. It often occurs in infants who have been dependent on long-term artificial ventilation.

**bronchopulmonary hygiene,** the care and cleanliness of the respiratory tract and of ventilatory/respiratory therapy. Hygienic care may include providing assistance with postural drainage and controlled coughing techniques, percussion, vibration, and rib shaking. Respiratory care equipment is a potential source and reservoir of infectious organisms and must be cleaned and sterilized periodically.

**bronchopulmonary lavage** [Gk, *bronchos,* windpipe; L, *pulmonis,* lung; Fr, *lavage,* washing out], the irrigation or washing out of the bronchi and bronchioles to remove pulmonary secretions.

**bronchoscope** /brong'kəskōp'/, a curved, flexible tube for visual examination of the bronchi. It contains fibers that carry light down the tube and project an enlarged image up the tube to the viewer. The bronchoscope is used to examine the bronchi, to secure a specimen for biopsy or culture, or to aspirate secretions or a foreign body from the respira-

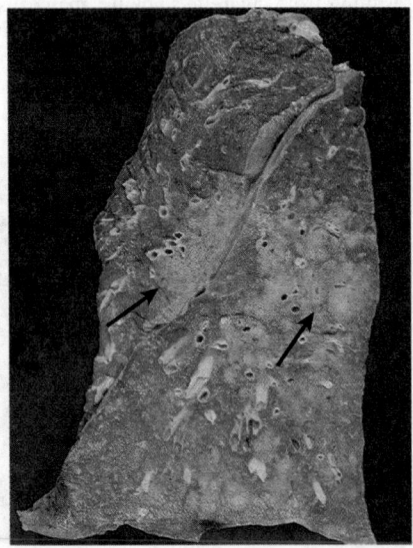

**Bronchopneumonia** *(Cotran, Kumar, and Collins, 1999)*

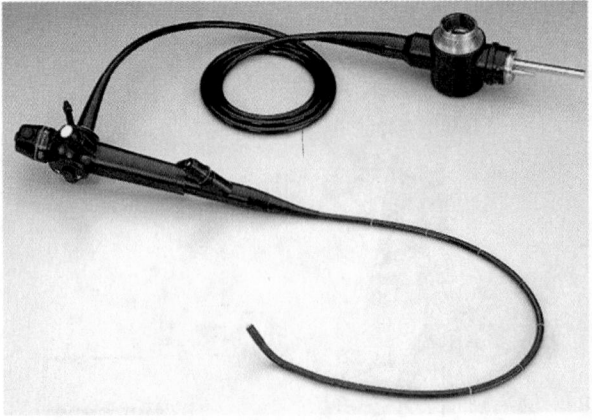

**Fiberoptic bronchoscope**
*(Lewis, Heitkemper, and Dirksen, 2000/courtesy Olympus America, Melville, NY)*

tory tract. See also **fiberoptic bronchoscopy. —broncho-scopic,** *adj.*

**bronchoscopy** /brongkos′kəpē/, the visual examination of the tracheobronchial tree, using the standard rigid, tubular metal bronchoscope or the narrower, flexible fiberoptic bronchoscope. The procedure also may be used for suctioning, for obtaining a biopsy specimen and fluid or sputum for examination, for removing foreign bodies, and for diagnosing such conditions as localized atelectasis, bronchial obstruction, lung abscess, and tracheal extubation. See also **bronchoscope.**

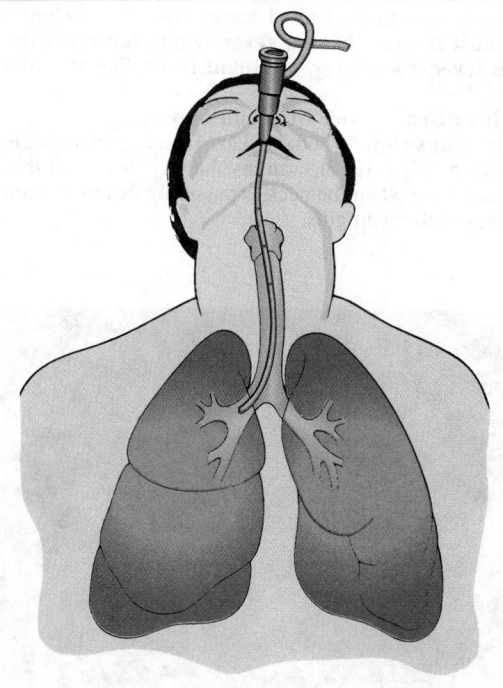

**Bronchoscopy** *(Pagana and Pagana, 1999)*

**bronchospasm** /-spaz′əm/, an excessive and prolonged contraction of the smooth muscle of the bronchi and bronchioles, resulting in an acute narrowing and obstruction of the respiratory airway. The contractions may be localized or general and may be caused by irritation or injury to the respiratory mucosa, infections, or allergies. A cough with generalized wheezing usually indicates the condition. Bronchospasm is a chief characteristic of asthma and bronchitis. Treatment includes the use of active bronchodilators, catecholamines, corticosteroids, or methylxanthines and preventive drugs such as cromolyn sodium. Also called **bronchial spasm, bronchiospasm.** See also **asthma, bronchitis.**

**bronchospirometry** /-spīrom′ətrē/, a technique for the study of the ventilation and gas exchange of each lung separately by the introduction of a catheter into either the left or the right mainstem bronchus. A double-lumen tube permits simultaneous but separate sampling of the gas from both lungs.

**bronchotomogram** /-tom′əgram/, an image of the respiratory system from the trachea to the lower bronchi produced by tomography. The procedure is used to detect tumors or other causes of obstruction of the respiratory tract.

**bronchotracheal.** See **tracheobronchial.**

**bronchovesicular** /-vesik′yələr/, pertaining to the bronchi, bronchioles, and alveoli.

**bronchovesicular sounds** [Gk, *bronchos,* windpipe; L, *vesicula,* small bladder, *sonus,* sound], normal breath sounds that occur between the sounds of the bronchial tubes and those of the alveoli, or a combination of the two sounds.

**bronchus** /brong′kəs/, *pl.* **bronchi** /-kī/ [L; Gk, *bronchos,* windpipe], any one of several large air passages in the lungs through which pass inhaled air and exhaled air. Each bronchus has a wall consisting of three layers. The outermost is made of dense fibrous tissue, reinforced with cartilage. The middle layer is a network of smooth muscle. The innermost layer consists of ciliated mucous membrane. Kinds of bronchi are **lobar bronchus (secondary bronchus), primary bronchus,** and **segmental bronchus (tertiary bronchus).** Also called **bronchial tube.** See also **bronchiole. —bronchial,** *adj.*

**Bronkephrine,** trademark for a sympathomimetic bronchodilator (ethylnorepinephrine hydrochloride).

**Bronkodyl,** trademark for a smooth muscle relaxant (theophylline).

**Bronkosol,** trademark for a bronchodilator (isoetharine hydrochloride).

**Brönsted acid** [Johannes N. Brönsted, Danish physical chemist, 1879–1947], a molecule or an ion that acts as a hydrogen ion donor.

**Brönsted base** [Johannes N. Brönsted], a molecule or an ion that acts as a hydrogen ion acceptor.

**brontophobia.** See **tonitrophobia.**

**bronze diabetes.** See **exogenous hemochromatosis.**

**broth,** **1.** a fluid culture medium, such as a solution of lactose or thioglycollate, used to support the growth of bacteria for laboratory analysis. **2.** a beverage or other clear fluid made with meat extract and water, such as chicken bouillon.

**brow,** the forehead, particularly the eyebrow or ridge above the eye.

**brow lift.** See **blepharoplasty.**

**brown fat** [ME, *broun* + AS, *faett,* filled], a type of fat present in newborns and rarely found in adults. Brown fat is a unique source of heat energy for the infant because it has greater thermogenic activity than ordinary fat. Brown fat deposits occur around the kidneys, neck, and upper chest.

**brownian motion** /brou′nyən/ [Robert Brown, Scottish botanist, 1773–1858], a random movement of microscopic particles suspended in a liquid or gas, such as the continuing erratic behavior of dust particles in still water. The movement is produced by the natural kinetic activity of molecules of the fluid that strike the foreign particles. Also called **brownian movement.**

**brownian movement.** See **brownian motion.**

**brown recluse spider,** a small poisonous arachnid, *Loxosceles reclusa,* also known as the brown or violin spider, found in both North and South America. The bite of the brown or violin spider, *Loxosceles reclusa,* produces a characteristic necrotic lesion. The venom from its bite usually creates a blister surrounded by concentric white and red circles. This so-called bull's-eye appearance is helpful in distinguishing it from other spider bites. There is little or no initial pain, but localized pain develops in about an hour. The patient may experience systemic symptoms; nausea, fever, and chills are common, but the reaction is usually self-limited. Immediate treatment includes keeping the victim quiet and immobilizing the bite area at the level of the heart. A bleb forms, sometimes in a target or bull's-eye pattern.

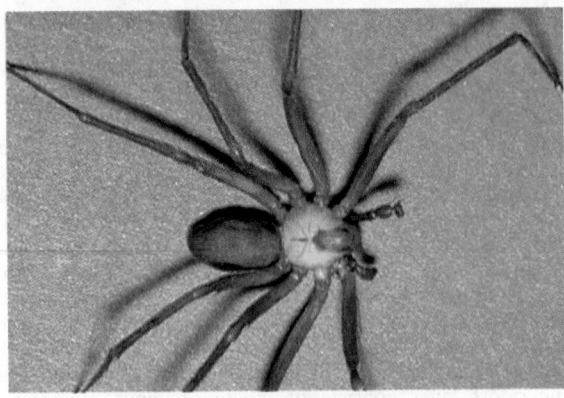

**Brown recluse spider**
*(Auerbach, 1995/courtesy Indiana University Medical Center)*

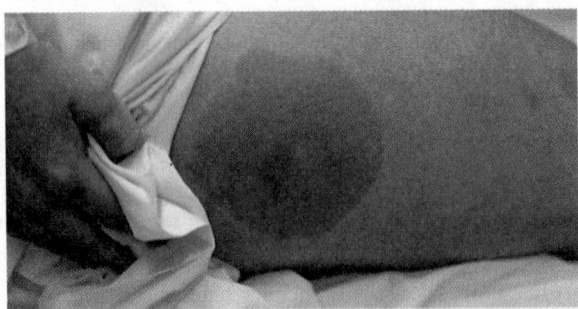

**Brown recluse spider bite after 48 hours**
*(Auerbach, 1995)*

The blood-filled bleb increases in size and eventually ruptures, leaving a black scar. Antivenin is not available in the United States.

**Brown-Séquard's syndrome** /broun'sākärz'/ [Charles E. Brown-Séquard, French physiologist, 1817–1894], a traumatic neurologic disorder resulting from compression of one side of the spinal cord, above the tenth thoracic vertebrae, characterized by spastic paralysis on the body's injured side, loss of postural sense (proprioception), and loss of the senses of pain and heat on the other side of the body.

**Brown-Séquard's treatment.** See **organotherapy**.

**brown spider.** See **brown recluse spider**.

**brow presentation,** an obstetric situation in which the brow, or forehead, of the fetus is the first part of the body to enter the birth canal. Because the diameter of the fetal head at this angle may be greater than that of the mother's pelvic outlet, a cesarean section may be recommended. However, the fetus usually converts to a face presentation.

*Brucella abortus.* See **abortus fever.**

**brucellosis** /broo'səlō'sis/ [David Bruce, English pathologist, 1855–1931], a disease caused by any of several species of the gram-negative coccobacillus *Brucella*. Brucellosis is most prevalent in rural areas among farmers, veterinarians, meat packers, slaughterhouse workers, and livestock producers. Laboratory workers are also at risk. It is primarily a disease of animals (including cattle, pigs, sheep, camels, goats, and dogs); humans usually acquire it by ingestion of contaminated milk or milk products or raw meat or marrow, through a break in the skin, or through inhalation of dust from contaminated soil. It is characterized by fever, chills, sweating, malaise, and weakness. The fever often occurs in waves, rising in the evening and subsiding during the day, at intervals separated by periods of remission. Other signs and symptoms may include anorexia and weight loss, headache, muscle and joint pain, and an enlarged spleen, and orchiepididymitis in young men. In some victims the disease is acute; more often it is chronic, recurring over a period of months or years. Although brucellosis itself is rarely fatal, treatment is important because serious complications such as pneumonia, endocarditis, meningitis, and encephalitis can develop. Tetracycline plus streptomycin is the treatment of choice; bed rest is also important. A vaccine is available outside the United States. Also called **Cyprus fever, dust fever, Gibraltar fever, Malta fever, Mediterranean fever, rock fever, undulant fever.** See also **abortus fever.**

**Bruch's disease.** See **Marseilles fever.**

**Brudzinski's sign** /broodzin'skēz/ [Josef Brudzinski, Polish physician, 1874–1917], an involuntary flexion of the arm, hip, and knee when the neck is passively flexed. It occurs in patients with meningitis.

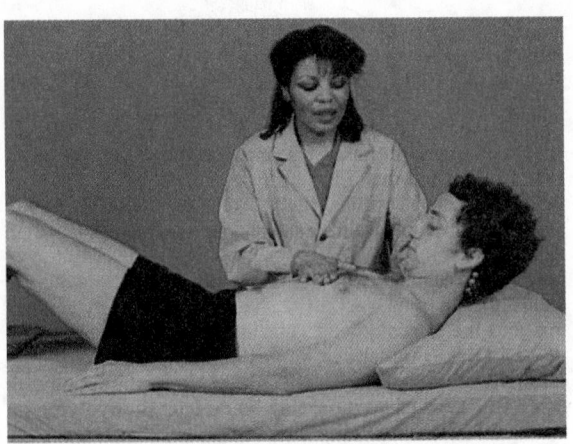

**Elicitation of Brudzinski's sign** *(Barkauskas et al, 1998)*

**Brueghel's syndrome.** See **Meige's syndrome** (def. 1).

*Brugia* /bruj'ə/ [S.L. Brug, Dutch parasitologist in Indonesia, 1879–1946], a genus of nematodes of the superfamily Filarioidea that parasitize humans and other mammals. See also **filariasis.**

**bruise.** See **contusion, ecchymosis.**

**bruit** /broo'ē/ [Fr, noise], an abnormal blowing or swishing sound or murmur heard while auscultating a carotid artery, organ, or gland, such as the liver or thyroid, and resulting from blood flowing through a narrow or partially occluded artery. The specific character of the bruit, its location, and the time of its occurrence in a cycle of other sounds are all of diagnostic importance.

**Brunnstrom hemiplegia classification,** an evaluation procedure that assesses muscle tone and voluntary control of movement patterns in a stroke patient. Results indicate the patient's progress through stages of recovery.

**brush biopsy,** the use of a catheter with bristles that is inserted into the body to collect cells from tissues.

**brush border,** microvilli on the free surfaces of certain epithelial cells, particularly the absorptive surfaces of the intestine and the proximal convoluted tubules of the kidney.

**Brushfield's spots** [Thomas Brushfield, English physician, 1858–1937; ME, *spotte*, stain], pinpoint white or light yellow spots on the iris of a child with Down syndrome. Occasionally, they are seen in normal infants.

**Bruton's agammaglobulinemia** [Ogden C. Bruton, American physician, b. 1908], a sex-linked, inherited condition characterized by the absence of gamma globulin in the blood. Those (usually children) affected by the syndrome are deficient in antibodies and susceptible to repeated infections. Compare **agammaglobulinemia.**

**bruxism** /bruk′sizəm/ [Gk, *brychein*, to gnash the teeth], the compulsive, unconscious grinding or clenching of the teeth, especially during sleep or as a mechanism for releasing tension during periods of extreme stress in the waking hours. Also called **bruxomania.**

**bruxomania.** See **bruxism.**

**bry-,** prefix meaning 'tree moss': *bryocyte, bryocytole.*

**Bryant's traction** [Thomas Bryant, English physician, 1828–1914; L, *trahere*, to pull], an orthopedic mechanism used to immobilize both lower extremities in the treatment of a fractured femur or in the correction of a congenital hip dislocation. The mechanism consists of a traction frame supporting weights, which are connected by ropes that run through pulleys to traction foot plates. The traction pull elevates the lower extremities to a vertical position with the patient supine, the trunk and the lower extremities forming a right angle. The weight applied to the traction mechanism is usually less than 35 pounds. Compare **Buck's traction.**

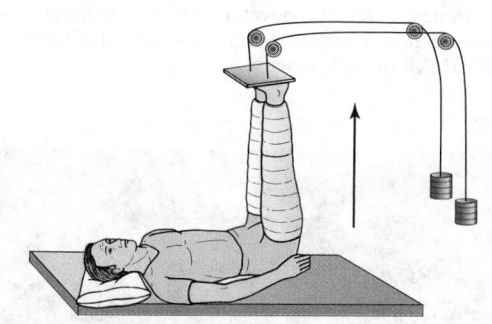

**Bryant's traction** *(Lewis, Heitkemper, and Dirksen, 2000)*

**BSA,** 1. abbreviation for **body surface area.** See **surface area.** 2. abbreviation for *bovine serum albumin.*

**BSE,** 1. abbreviation for **breast self-examination.** See **self-breast examination.** 2. Abbreviation for **bovine spongiform encephalopathy.**

**BSN,** abbreviation for **Bachelor of Science in Nursing.**

**BSP,** abbreviation for **Bromsulphalein.**

**BT,** abbreviation for **bleeding time.**

**BTPD,** abbreviation for *body temperature, ambient pressure, dry.*

**BTPS,** abbreviation for *body temperature, ambient pressure, saturated* (with water vapor). See also **volume BTPS.**

**BTU,** abbreviation for **British thermal unit.**

**buba.** See **yaws.**

**bubble-diffusion humidifier,** a device that provides hu-

midified oxygen or other therapeutic gases by allowing the gas to bubble through a reservoir of water.

**bubble goniometer,** a device used for measuring joint angles, consisting of a spirit level and a pendulum.

**bubble oxygenator,** a heart-lung device that oxygenates the blood while it is diverted outside the patient's body.

**bubo** /byoo′bō/, *pl.* **buboes** [Gk, *boubon*, groin], a greatly enlarged, tender, inflamed lymph node usually in the groin that is associated with diseases such as chancroid, lymphogranuloma venereum, and syphilis. Treatment includes specific antibiotic therapy, application of moist heat, and sometimes incision and drainage.

**bubonic plague** /byoobon′ik/ [Gk, *boubon*, groin; L, *plaga*, stroke], the most common form of plague. It is characterized by painful buboes in the axilla, groin, or neck; fever often rising to 106° F (41.11° C); prostration with a rapid, thready pulse; hypotension; delirium; and bleeding into the skin from the superficial blood vessels. The symptoms are caused by an endotoxin released by a bacillus, *Yersinia pestis,* usually introduced into the body by the bite of a rat flea that has bitten an infected rat. Inoculation with plague vaccine confers partial immunity; infection provides lifetime immunity. Treatment includes antibiotics, supportive nursing care, surgical drainage of buboes, isolation, and stringent precautions against spread of the disease. Conditions favor a plague epidemic when a large infected rodent population lives with a large nonimmune human population in a damp, warm climate. Improved sanitary conditions and eradication of rats and other rodent reservoirs of *Y. pestis* may prevent outbreaks of the disease. Killing the infected rodents, which may include ground squirrels and rabbits, and not the fleas allows a continued threat of human infection. Also called *(informal)* **black death, black plague.** Compare **pneumonic plague, septicemic plague.** See also **bubo, plague,** *Yersinia pestis.*

**bucardia** /bookär′dē-ə/, extreme enlargement of the heart.

**bucca-.** See **bucco-.**

**buccal** /buk′əl/, *pl.* **bucca** [L, *bucca*, cheek], pertaining to the inside of the cheek, the surface of a tooth, or the gum beside the cheek.

**buccal administration of medication,** oral administration of a drug, usually in the form of a tablet, by placing it between the cheek and the teeth or gum until it dissolves.

**buccal bar,** a portion of an orthodontic appliance consisting of a rigid metal wire that extends anteriorly from the buccal side of a molar band. See also **arch bar, labial bar, lingual bar.**

**buccal cavity,** the vestibule of the mouth, specifically the area lying between the teeth and cheeks.

**buccal contour** [L, *bucca* + *cum*, together with, *tornare*, to turn], the shape of the buccal side of a posterior tooth. It is usually characterized by a slight occlusocervical convexity that has its largest prominence at the gingival third of the clinical buccal surface.

**buccal fat pad,** a fat pad in the cheek under the subcutaneous layer of the skin, over the buccinator. It is particularly prominent in infants and is often called a sucking pad.

**buccal flange** [L, *bucca* + OFr, *flanche*, flank], the portion of a denture base that occupies the cheek side of the mouth and extends distally from the buccal notch. Compare **labial flange, lingual flange.** See also **flange.**

**buccal frenum,** a fold of mucous membrane connecting the alveolar ridge to the cheek and separating the labial vestibule from the buccal vestibule.

**buccal glands** [L, *bucca*, cheek, *glans*, acorn], small salivary glands located between the buccinator muscle and the mucous membrane in the vestibule of the mouth.

**buccal mucosa,** the mucous membrane lining the inside of the mouth.

**buccal notch,** a depression in a denture flange that accommodates the buccal frenum. See also **labial notch.**

**buccal smear,** a sample of cells removed from the buccal mucosa for purposes of obtaining a karyotype to determine the genetic sex of an individual.

**buccal splint,** material, usually plaster, that is placed on the buccal surfaces of fixed partial denture units to hold the units in position for assembly.

**buccal vestibule,** that portion of the vestibule of the mouth that lies between the cheeks and the teeth and gingivae or residual alveolar ridges.

**bucci-.** See **bucco-.**

**buccinator** /buk'sinā'tər/ [L, *buccina,* trumpet], the main muscle of the cheek, one of the 12 muscles of the mouth. It is pierced by the duct of the parotid gland opposite the second molar tooth. The buccinator, innervated by buccal branches of the facial nerve, compresses the cheek, acting as an important accessory muscle of mastication by holding food under the teeth.

**bucco-, bucc-, bucca-, bucci-,** combining form meaning 'cheek': *buccodistal, buccal, buccinator.*

**buccoclusion** /buk'ə·klōō'zhən/ [L, *bucca,* cheek + *occludere,* to close up], malocclusion in which the dental arch or a quadrant or group of teeth is buccal to the normal.

**buccogingival** /buk'ōjinjī'vəl/, pertaining to the internal mouth structures, particularly the cheeks and gums.

**buccolinguomasticatory triad** /buk'ōling'wōmas'tək ə-tôr'e/ [L, *bucca,* cheek, *lingua,* tongue, *masticare,* to gnash the teeth], a complex of involuntary lip, tongue, jaw, and head movements seen in tardive dyskinesia.

**buccopharyngeal** /buk'ōfərin'jē·əl/, pertaining to the cheek and the pharynx or to the mouth and the pharynx.

**buccopharyngeal membrane.** See **pharyngeal membrane.**

**buccula** /buk'yələ/ [L, *bucca,* cheek], a fold of fatty tissue, literally a "little cheek" beneath the chin. Also called **double chin.**

**bucket handle fracture** [OFr, *buket,* tub; ME, *handel,* part grasped; L, *fractura,* break], a fracture that produces a tear in a semilunar cartilage along the medial side of the knee joint.

**bucking,** *informal.* **1.** gagging on an endotracheal tube. **2.** involuntarily resisting positive pressure ventilation. Treatment for either is to sedate or extubate as appropriate.

**buck knife,** a periodontal surgical knife with a spear-shaped cutting point, used to make an interdental incision associated with a gingivectomy.

**Buck's fascia** [Gurdon Buck, American surgeon, 1807–1877], the deep fascia encasing the erectile tissue of the penis.

**Buck's skin traction** [Gurdon Buck], an orthopedic procedure that applies traction to the lower extremity with the hips and the knees extended. It is used in the treatment of hip and knee contractures, in postoperative positioning and immobilization, and in disease processes of the hip and the knee. This type of traction may be unilateral, involving one leg, or bilateral, involving both legs.

**Buck's traction** [Gurdon Buck; L, *trahere,* to pull], one of the most common orthopedic mechanisms by which pull is exerted on the lower extremity with a system of ropes, weights, and pulleys. Buck's traction, which may be unilateral or bilateral, is used to immobilize, position, and align the lower extremity in the treatment of contractures and diseases of the hip and knee. The mechanism commonly consists of a metal bar extending from a frame at the foot of the

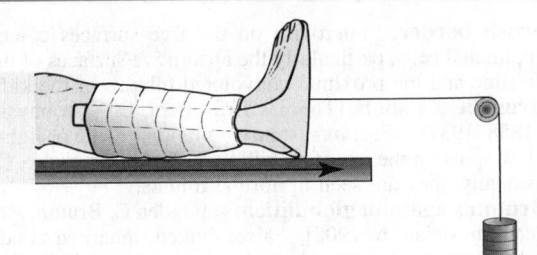

**Buck's traction** *(Lewis, Heitkemper, and Dirksen, 2000)*

patient's bed, supporting traction weights connected by a rope passing through a pulley to a cast or a splint around the affected body structure. Compare **Bryant's traction.**

**Bucky diaphragm** [Gustav P. Bucky, American radiologist, 1880–1963; Gk, *diaphragma,* partition], a moving grid that limits the amount of scattered radiation reaching a radiographic film, thereby increasing the film contrast. Also called **Bucky grid.**

**buclizine hydrochloride** /bōō'kləzēn/, an antiemetic/antivertigo drug derived from piperazine that has anticholinergic and antihistaminic properties. It is used to treat nausea, vomiting, and dizziness of motion sickness.

**bud** [ME, *budde*], any small outgrowth that is the beginning stage of a living structure, as a limb bud from which an arm or leg develops.

**Budd-Chiari syndrome** /bud'kē·är'ē/ [George Budd, English physician, 1808–1882; Hans Chiari, Czech-French pathologist, 1851–1916], a disorder of hepatic circulation, marked by venous obstruction, that leads to liver enlargement, ascites, extensive development of collateral vessels, and severe portal hypertension. Also called **Chiari's syndrome, Rokitansky's disease.**

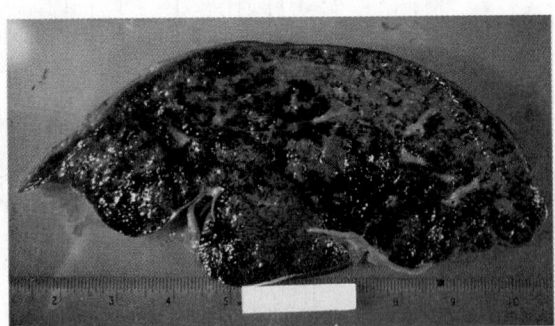

**Budd-Chiari syndrome** *(Kumar, Cotran, and Robbins, 1997)*

**budding** [ME, *budde*], a type of asexual reproduction in which an organism produces a budlike projection containing chromatin that eventually detaches and develops into an independent organism. It is common in simple organisms, such as sponges, yeasts, and molds.

**buddy splint,** a splinting technique commonly used after a finger or toe injury requiring immobilization. The injured and an adjacent digit are typically taped together to limit the range of motion of the affected digit. Also called **buddy tape.**

**buddy tape.** See **buddy splint.**

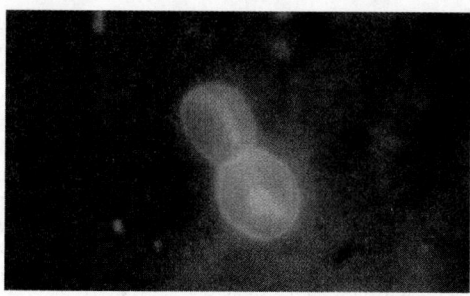

**Budding** (Baron, Peterson, and Finegold, 1994)

**budesonide,** a nasal corticosteroid antiinflammatory agent. It is available in the form of Pulmicort as a turboinhaler (used in the mouth).

■ INDICATIONS: It is prescribed in the management of symptoms of seasonal or perennial allergic rhinitis or perennial nonallergic rhinitis.

■ CONTRAINDICATIONS: The drug should not be given to patients who have an allergic reaction to the drug or to any of its components or to patients with an untreated infection of the mucous membranes.

■ ADVERSE EFFECTS: The side effects most often reported include nasal or throat irritation, stinging, burning, or dryness in the respiratory system, nosebleeds, sneezing, and congestion.

**Buerger's disease.** See **thromboangiitis obliterans.**

**Buerger's postural exercises** [Leo Buerger, American physician, 1879–1943; L, *ponere,* to place, *exercere,* to continue working], exercises designed to maintain circulation in a limb.

**buffalo hump,** an accumulation of fat on the back of the neck associated with the prolonged use of large doses of glucocorticoids or the hypersecretion of cortisol caused by Cushing's syndrome.

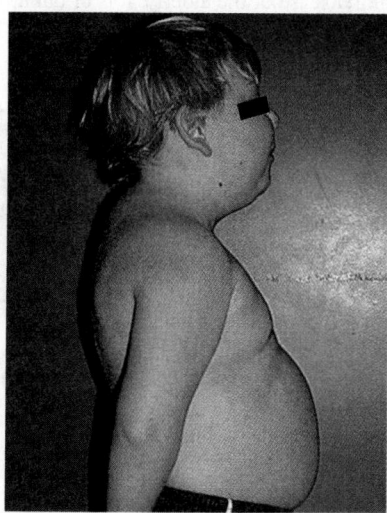

**Buffalo hump** (Zitelli and Davis, 1997)

**buffer** [ME, *buffe,* to cushion], a substance or group of substances that tends to control the hydrogen ion concentration in a solution by reacting with hydrogen ions when an acid is added to the system and releasing hydrogen ions on the addition of a base. Buffers minimize significant changes of pH in a chemical system. Among the functions carried out by buffer systems in the body is maintenance of the acid-base balance of the blood and of the proper pH in kidney tubules. See also **blood buffers, pH.**

**buffer anions,** the negatively charged bicarbonate, protein, and phosphate ions that comprise the buffer systems of the body.

**buffer cations,** the positively charged ions of the body's electrolytes, including sodium, calcium, potassium, and magnesium.

**buffer solution** [ME, *buffet* + L, *solutus,* dissolved], a solution that will minimize changes in pH value despite dilution or addition of a small amount of base or acid.

**buffy coat** [ME, *buffet* + Fr, *cote*], a grayish white layer of white blood cells and platelets, mixed with some red blood cells, that accumulates on the surface of sedimented erythrocytes when blood plasma is allowed to stand.

**buffy coat transfusion.** See **granulocyte transfusion.**

**bug,** an error in a computer program (software bug) or a design flaw in computer hardware (hardware bug), usually causing inability to process data correctly.

**bulb** [L, *bulbus,* swollen root], any rounded structure, such as the eyeball, hair roots, and certain sensory nerve endings.

**bulbar** /bul'bər/ [L, *bulbus*], **1.** pertaining to a bulb. **2.** pertaining to the medulla oblongata of the brain and the cranial nerves.

**bulbar ataxia** [L, *bulbus,* swollen root; Gk, *ataxia,* without order], a loss of motor coordination caused by a lesion in the medulla oblongata or pons.

**bulbar conjunctiva.** See **conjunctiva.**

**bulbar myelitis** [L, *bulbus,* swollen root; Gk, *myelos,* marrow, *itis,* inflammation], an inflammation of the central nervous system involving the medulla oblongata.

**bulbar palsy** [L, *bulbus,* swollen root; Gk, *paralyein,* to be palsied], a form of paralysis resulting from a defect in the motor centers of the medulla oblongata. See also **bulbar poliomyelitis.**

**bulbar paralysis,** a degenerative neurologic condition characterized by progressive paralysis of cranial nerves and involving the lips, tongue, mouth, pharynx, and larynx. The condition occurs most commonly in people above 50 years of age, in multiple sclerosis, and in amyotrophic lateral sclerosis.

**bulbar poliomyelitis** [L, *bulbus,* swollen root; Gk, *polios,* gray, *myelos,* marrow, *itis,* inflammation], a form of poliomyelitis that involves the medulla oblongata and gradually progresses to bulbar paralysis, with respiratory and circulatory failure.

**bulbiform** /bul'bifôrm/, shaped like a bulb.

**bulbocavernosus** /bul'bōkav'ərnō'səs/ [L, *bulbus,* swollen root, *cavernosum,* full of hollows], a muscle that covers the bulb of the penis in the male and the bulbus vestibuli in the female. Also called **accelerator urinae, ejaculator urinae,** *(in females)* sphincter vaginae.

**bulbocavernosus reflex,** the contraction of the bulbospongiosus muscle when the dorsum of the penis is tapped or the glans penis is compressed.

**bulbourethral gland** /-yo͞orē'thrəl/, one of two small glands located on each side of the prostate, draining to the wall of the urethra. Bulbourethral glands secrete a fluid component of the seminal fluid. Also called **Cowper's gland.**

**bulbous** [L, *bulbus,* swollen root],   pertaining to a structure that resembles a bulb or that originates in a bulb.

**bulb syringe,**   a device with a flexible bulb that replaces the plunger for instillation or aspiration. Bulb syringes can be used to irrigate an external orifice, such as the auditory canal. See also **syringe.**

**bulbus oculi.**   See **eye.**

**-bulia, -boulia,**   suffix meaning '(condition of the) will': *abulia, hyperbulia.*

**bulimia** /bo͞olim′ē·ə/ [Gk, *bous,* ox, *limos,* hunger],   a disorder characterized by an insatiable craving for food, often resulting in episodes of continuous eating and often followed by purging, depression, and self-deprivation. Also spelled **boulimia.** Also called **binge eating.** See also **anorexia nervosa.**

**bulimic** /bo͞olim′ik/,   pertaining to bulimia.

**bulk.**   See **dietary fiber.**

**bulk cathartic** [ME, *bulke,* heap; Gk, *kathartikos,* evacuation of bowels],   a cathartic that acts by softening and increasing the mass of fecal material in the bowel. Bulk cathartics contain a hydrophilic agent such as methylcellulose or psyllium seed.

**bulla** /bo͞ol′ə, bul′ə/, *pl.* **bullae** [L, bubble],   a thin-walled blister of the skin or mucous membranes greater than 1 cm in diameter containing clear, serous fluid. Compare **vesicle.** —**bullous,** *adj.*

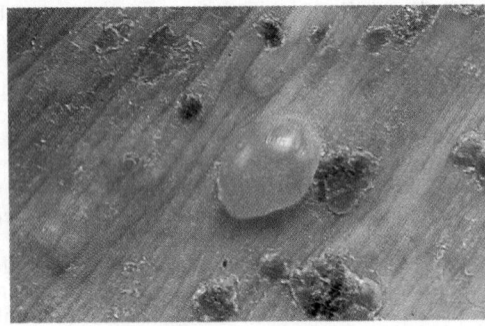

**Bulla** *(du Vivier, 1993)*

**bulldog forceps,**   short spring forceps for clamping an artery or vein for hemostasis. The jaws may be padded to prevent injury to vascular tissue.

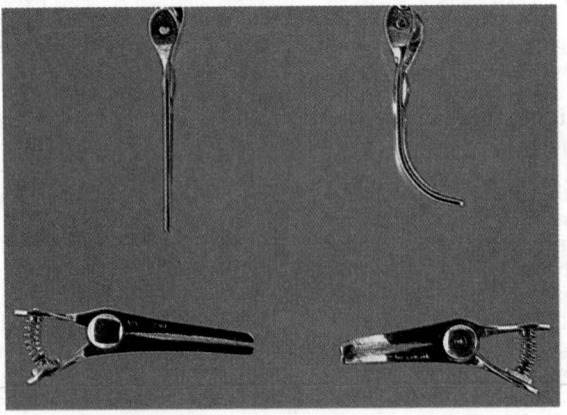

**Bulldog forceps** *(Brooks-Tighe, 1989)*

**bullet forceps,**   a kind of forceps that has thin, curved, serrated blades that are designed for extracting a foreign object, such as a bullet, from the base of a puncture wound.

**bullous.**   See **bulla.**

**bullous disease** /bo͞ol′əs/,   any disease marked by eruptions of blisters, or bullae, filled with fluid, on the skin or mucous membranes. An example is pemphigus.

**bullous emphysema,**   single or multiple large cystic alveolar dilations of lung tissue. Also called **cystic emphysema.**

**bullous impetigo,**   a form of impetigo in which the skin lesions are bullae instead of vesicles. The crusts are thin and greenish yellow.

**bullous myringitis** [L, *bulla* + *myringa,* eardrum],   an inflammatory condition of the ear, characterized by fluid-filled vesicles on the tympanic membrane and the sudden onset of severe pain in the ear. The condition often occurs with bacterial otitis media. Treatment includes administration of antibiotics and analgesics and surgical draining of the vesicles. See also **otitis media.**

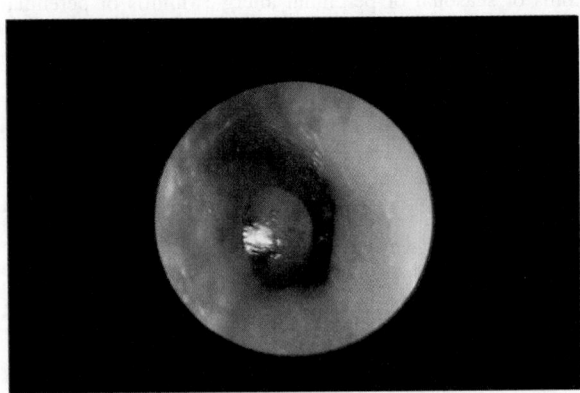

**Bullous myringitis** *(Bingham, 1992)*

**bullous pemphigoid** [L, *bulla,* bubble; Gk, *pemphix,* bubble, *eidos,* form],   a rare, relatively benign subepidermal blistering disease of the elderly. It is of unknown origin.

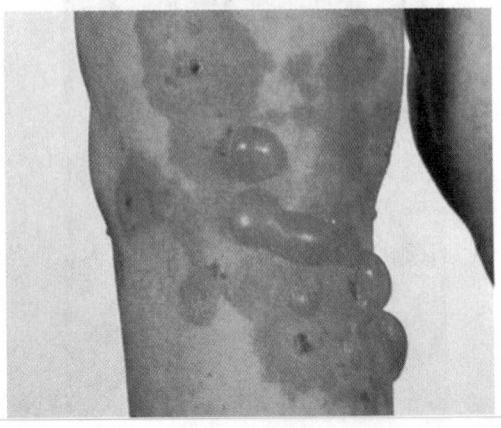

**Bullous pemphigoid, seen on the back of the leg**
*(du Vivier, 1993)*

**bullseye rash.** See **erythema migrans.**

**bumetanide** /bōōmet'ənīd/, a loop diuretic (high ceiling) related to furosemide.

- INDICATIONS: It is prescribed for edema caused by cardiac, hepatic, or renal disease.
- CONTRAINDICATIONS: Anuria, electrolyte depletion, or known sensitivity to this drug prohibits its use.
- ADVERSE EFFECTS: Among the most serious adverse reactions are hypokalemia, hyperuricemia, and azotemia.

**Bumex,** trademark for a diuretic (bumetanide).

**Buminate,** trademark for a blood volume expander (human albumin).

**BUN,** abbreviation for **blood urea nitrogen.**

**-bund,** suffix meaning 'prone to' something specified: *moribund.*

**bundle,** a group of nerve fibers or other threadlike structures running in the same direction. See also **fasciculus.**

**bundle branch** [Dan, *bondel* + Fr, *branche*], a segment of the network of specialized conducting fibers that transmit electrical impulses within the ventricles of the heart. Bundle branches are a continuation of the atrioventricular (AV) bundle, which extends from the upper part of the intraventricular septum. The AV bundle divides into a left and a right branch, each going to its respective ventricle by passing down the septum and beneath the endocardium. Within the ventricles the bundle branches subdivide and terminate in the Purkinje fibers.

**bundle branch block (BBB),** an inability of cardiac impulses to be conducted down the bundle branches, causing a broaded and abnormally shaped QRS complex. BBB is commonly seen in high-risk, acute, anterior wall myocardial infarction. It may be caused by ischemia or necrosis of the bundle branches, trauma (as in surgical manipulation), or mechanical compression of the branches by a tumor. A pacemaker may be inserted if further deterioration of conduction is anticipated. See also **left bundle branch block, right bundle branch block.**

**bundle of His.** See **atrioventricular (AV) bundle.**

**bunion** /bun'yən/ [Gk, *bounion,* turnip], an abnormal, medial enlargement of the joint at the base of the great toe. It is caused by inflammation of the bursa, usually as a result of heredity, degenerative joint disease, or chronic irritation and pressure from poorly fitted shoes. It is characterized by soreness, swelling, thickening of the skin, and lateral displacement of the great toe.

**bunionectomy** /bun'yənek'təmē/, excision of a bunion.

**bunionette** /bun'yənet'/, an abnormal enlargement and inflammation of the joint at the base of the small toe. Also called **tailor's bunion.**

**Bunnell block,** trademark for a small wooden block used in exercise of the fingers after surgery. The exercises with the block allow each joint to be exercised individually with full tendon excursion while the other joints are held extended.

**Bunsen burner** /bōōn'sən, bun'sən/ [Robert E.W. Bunsen, German chemist, 1811–1899], a standard laboratory gas burner designed to produce nearly complete combustion in a smokeless flame.

**Bunyamwera virus infection** /bun'yəmwir'ə/ [Bunyamwera, town in Uganda where the type species was isolated], one of a group of arthropod-borne viruses that infect humans and are carried by mosquitoes from rodent hosts. Related viruses cause California encephalitis, Rift Valley fever, and other diseases characterized by headache, weakness, low-grade fever, myalgia, and a rash. Convalescence is prolonged. Outbreaks have occurred in North America, South America, Africa, and Europe.

**buoyant density,** the thickness or compactness of a substance that allows it to float in a standard fluid.

**buphthalmos.** See **congenital glaucoma.**

**bupivacaine hydrochloride** /byōōpiv'əkān/, a local anesthetic.

- INDICATIONS: It is prescribed for caudal, epidural, peripheral, or sympathetic anesthetic block.
- CONTRAINDICATIONS: Known hypersensitivity to this drug or to any of the amide class of local anesthetics prohibits its use.
- ADVERSE EFFECTS: Among the more serious adverse reactions are central nervous system disturbances, cardiovascular depression, respiratory arrest, cardiac arrest, and hypersensitivity reactions.

**Buprenex,** trademark for a parenteral analgesic (buprenorphine hydrochloride).

**buprenorphine hydrochloride** /bōō'prənôr'fēn/, a parenteral opioid agonist-antagonist analgesic.

- INDICATIONS: It is prescribed for the relief of moderate to severe pain.
- CONTRAINDICATIONS: This Schedule V controlled substance is contraindicated for patients who may be opioid dependent.
- ADVERSE EFFECTS: Among the reported adverse effects are respiratory depression, sedation, nausea, dizziness, vertigo, headache, vomiting, miosis, diaphoresis, and hypotension.

**bupropion** /bōōprō'pē·on/, a heterocyclic mood-elevating drug used to treat some types of depression; trademark: Wellbutrin.

**bur.** see **burr.**

**burden,** a heavy, oppressive load, as a disabling clinical load.

**burdock root,** a perennial herb found in the United States, China, and Europe.

- USES: This herb is used for skin diseases, inflammation, rashes, colds and fever, cancer, gout, and arthritis.
- CONTRAINDICATIONS: Burdock is contraindicated in those who are hypersensitive to this plant. Burdock also should be used cautiously in people with diabetes or cardiac disorders.

**Bureau of Medical Devices (BMD),** an agency of the U.S. Food and Drug Administration organized in 1976 with the responsibility of providing standards for and regulation of the manufacture and uses of medical devices.

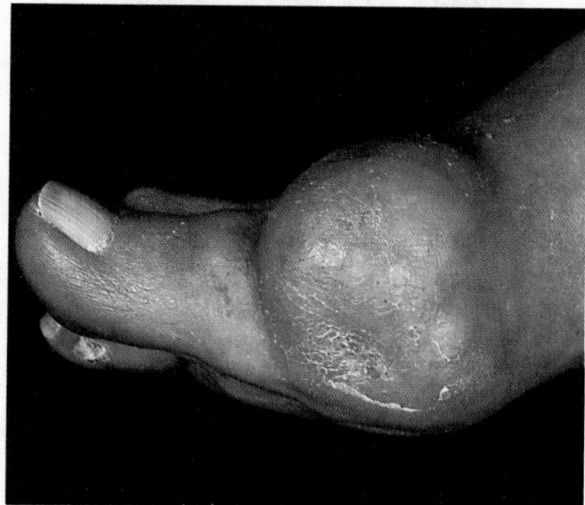

**Bunion** *(du Vivier, 1993)*

**buret** /byŏŏret'/ [Fr, small jug], a laboratory utensil used to deliver a wide range of volumes accurately. Also spelled **burette.**

**buried suture** [L, *sutura*], a suture that is inserted to draw together soft tissues between the viscus and the skin.

*Burkholderia* /bərk'holdēr'ēə/, a genus of gram-negative, rod-shaped bacteria that includes several species formerly classified in the genus *Pseudomonas,* including the agents of glanders and melioidosis.

*Burkholderia mallei,* a nonmotile species that causes glanders. It is pathogenic chiefly for horses, but may also infect humans and other animals.

*Burkholderia pseudomallei,* a species that inhabits water and soil and causes melioidosis.

**Burkitt's lymphoma** /bur'kits/ [Denis P. Burkitt, English surgeon in Africa, b. 1911], a malignant neoplasm composed of undifferentiated lymphoreticular cells that form a large osteolytic lesion in the jaw or, in children, an abdominal mass. The tumor, which is seen chiefly in Central Africa, is characteristically a gray-white mass sometimes containing areas of hemorrhage and necrosis. Central nervous system involvement often occurs, and other organs may be affected. The Epstein-Barr virus (EBV), a herpesvirus, is associated with this lymphoma. Chemotherapy can often cure the disease. Also called **African lymphoma, Burkitt's tumor.**

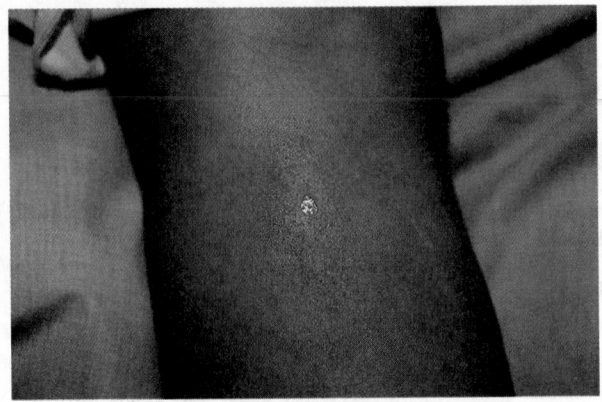

**First-degree burn** *(Sanders et al, 2000)*

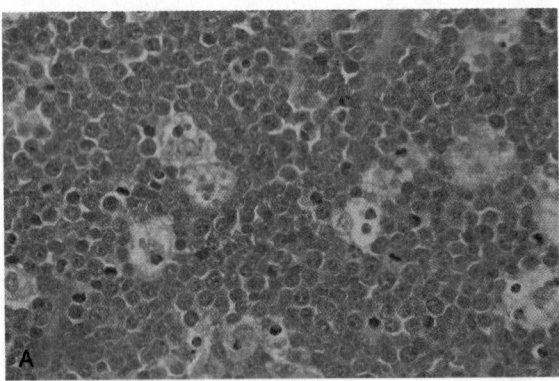

**Burkitt's lymphoma** *(Cotran, Kumar, and Collins, 1999)*

**burn** [AS, *baernan*], any injury to tissues of the body caused by hot objects or flames, electricity, chemicals, radiation, or gases in which the extent of the injury is determined by the nature of the agent, length of time exposed, body part involved, and depth of burn. The treatment of burns includes pain relief, careful asepsis, prevention of infection, regulation of body temperature, maintenance of the balance in the body of fluids and electrolytes, and good nutrition. First priority with burns of the airway is airway control. Severe burns of any origin may cause shock, which is treated before the wound. Burns are sometimes classified as first, second, third, and fourth degree. First-degree burns involve only a superficial layer of epidermal cells. Second-degree burns may be divided into superficial partial-thickness and deep partial-thickness wounds. Damage in second-degree burns extends through the epidermis to the dermis, but is usually not sufficient to prevent skin regeneration. In third-degree burns the entire thickness of the epidermis and dermis is destroyed. Fourth-degree burns are full-thickness injuries that penetrate the subcutaneous tissue, muscle, and periosteum or bone. See also **chemical burn, electrocution, thermal burn.**

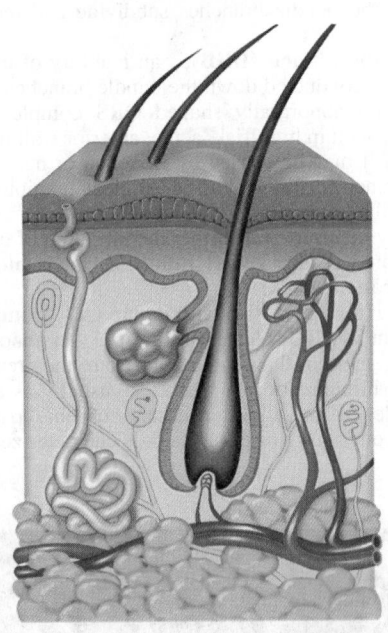

**First-degree burn: damaged epidermis and edema**
*(Thibodeau and Patton, 1996/Jon Henke)*

**burn center,** a health care facility that is designed to care for patients who have been severely burned. A number of burn centers has been established throughout the United States and Canada to provide sophisticated advanced techniques of care for burn victims.

**burner syndrome,** a condition of burning pain, especially in the upper extremities, and sometimes accompanied by shoulder girdle weakness. It may be experienced during contact sports, such as football, as a result of a blow to the head or shoulder. It is attributed to an upper trunk neuropathy of the brachial plexus.

**Burnett's syndrome.** See **milk-alkali syndrome.**

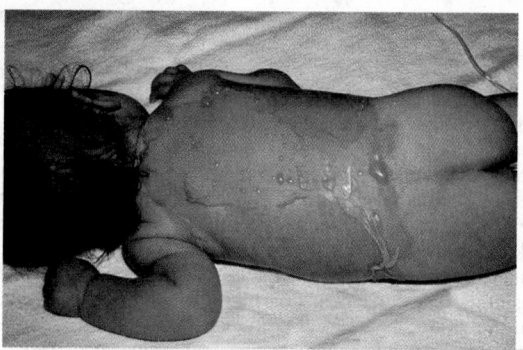

**Superficial partial-thickness second-degree burn**
*(Sanders et al, 2000/courtesy St. John's Mercy Medical Center, St. Louis, MO)*

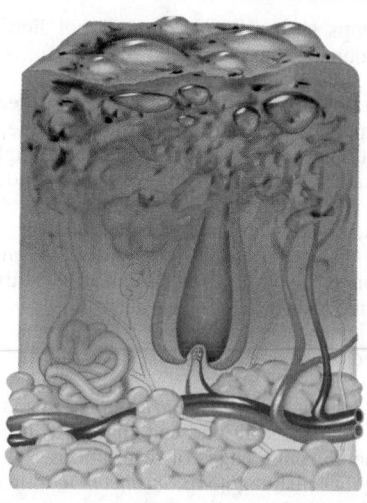

**Deep partial-thickness second-degree burn**

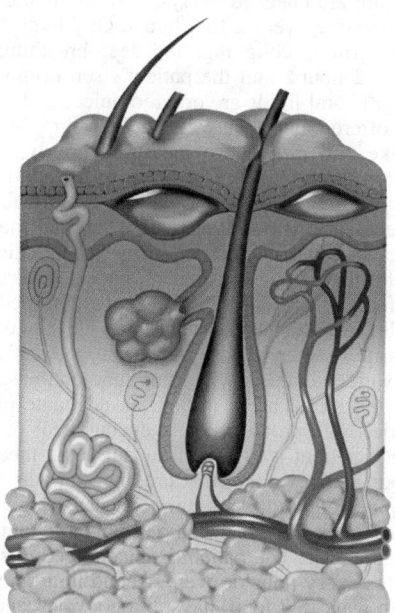

**Superficial partial-thickness second-degree burn**

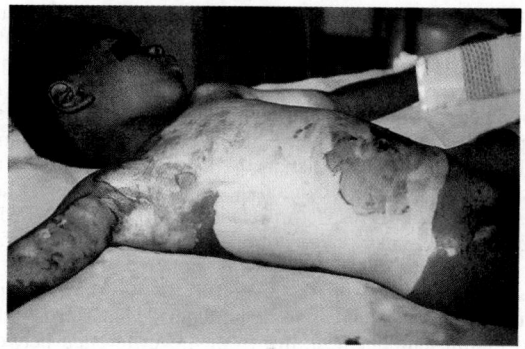

**Third-degree burn**
*(Sanders et al, 2000/courtesy St. John's Mercy Medical Center, St. Louis, MO)*

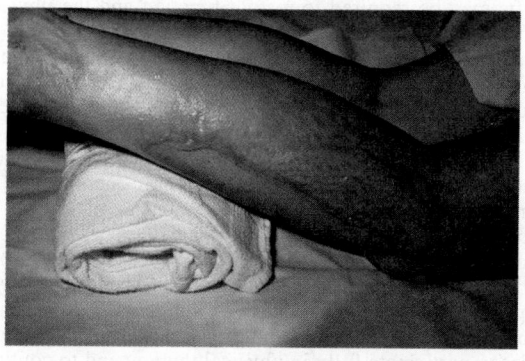

**Deep partial-thickness second-degree burn**
*(Sanders et al, 2000/courtesy St. John's Mercy Medical Center, St. Louis, MO)*

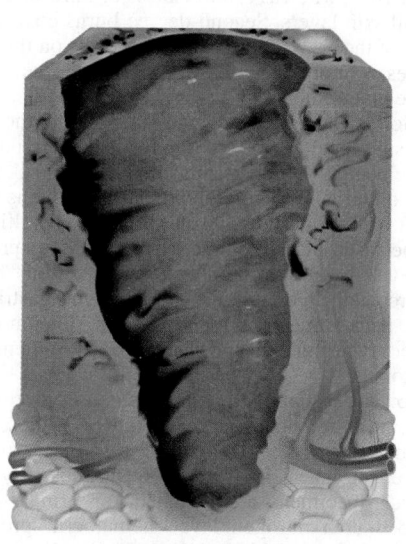

**Third-degree burn**

**burning drops sign,** a sensation of hot liquid dripping into the abdominal cavity caused by a perforated stomach ulcer.

**burning feet syndrome,** a neurologic disorder characterized by symptoms of a burning sensation in the sole of the foot. The burning tends to be more intense at night and may also involve the hands. Possible causes include causalgia from injury to the sciatic nerve, degeneration of the spinal cord, and acute polyneuropathy. The condition is also associated with diabetes mellitus, kidney disease, and a B vitamin deficiency. Also known as **Gopalan's syndrome.**

**burning pain** [AS, *baernan,* to burn; L, *poena,* penalty], the pain experienced as a result of a thermal burn. The term is also used sometimes to describe heartburn or myocardial pain.

**burnisher** /bur′nishər/ [ME, *burnischen,* to make brown], a dental instrument with one end shaped as a beveled nib, used to smooth rough edges of restorations.

**burnishing** /bur′nish·ing/ [ME, *burnischen,* to make brown], **1.** (in dentistry) condensation and polishing under the sliding pressure of a smooth hard instrument, as in finishing the surface of a gold filling. **2.** (in dentistry) smoothing out the margins of a thin, annealed sheet metal to form a band about a tooth root or fit a matrix for porcelain.

**burnout,** a popular term for a mental or physical energy depletion after a period of chronic, unrelieved job-related stress characterized sometimes by physical illness. The person suffering from burnout may lose concern or respect for other people and often has cynical, dehumanized perceptions of people, labeling them in a derogatory manner. Causes of burnout peculiar to the nursing profession often include stressful, even dangerous, work environments; lack of support; lack of respectful relationships within the health care team; low pay scales compared with physicians' salaries; shift changes and long work hours; understaffing of hospitals; pressure from the responsibility of providing continuous high levels of care over long periods; and frustration and disillusionment resulting from the difference between job realities and job expectations.

**burn therapy,** the management of a patient burned by flames, hot liquids, explosives, chemicals, or electric current. Partial thickness burns may be first degree, involving only the epidermis, or second degree, involving the epidermis and dermis, whereas full thickness or third-degree burns involve all skin layers. Second-degree burns covering more than 30% of the body and third-degree burns on the face and extremities, or more than 10% of the body surface, are critical. In the first 48 hours of a severe burn, vascular fluid, sodium chloride, and protein rapidly pass into the affected area, causing local edema, blister formation, hypovolemia, hypoproteinemia, hyponatremia, hyperkalemia, hypotension, and oliguria. The initial hypovolemic stage is followed by a shift of fluid in the opposite direction, resulting in diuresis, increased blood volume, and decreased serum electrolyte level. Potential complications in serious burns include circulatory collapse, renal damage, gastric atony, paralytic ileus, infections, septic shock, pneumonia, and stress ulcer (Curling's ulcer), characterized by hematemesis and peritonitis. ■ METHOD: The extent of the burn, its cause, its time of occurrence, and the patient's age, weight, allergies, and any preexisting illness are recorded. If respiratory distress is present, endotracheal intubation or tracheostomy may be performed. Specimens are obtained for urinalysis, blood type, blood urea nitrogen level, hematocrit, prothrombin time, electrolyte levels, blood gases, and cultures of nasal, throat, wound, and stool organisms. Parenteral fluids and electrolytes, antibiotics, tetanus prophylaxis, and pain medication are administered as ordered; large doses of analgesics and sedatives are avoided when possible to prevent depression of respiration and masking of symptoms. An indwelling urinary catheter is inserted, and a nasogastric tube and catheter for monitoring central venous pressure may be indicated. Local treatment of the burn may use the closed method or the more frequently used open method, in which the injured area is cleaned and exposed to air and the patient is kept warm by a blanket or linen over a bed cradle or by a heater or lamp. In the closed method, a germicidal or bacteriostatic cream, ointment, or solution is applied to the burn, and the wound is covered with a dressing. A porcine heterograft may be used to cover the wound temporarily; this technique prevents fluid loss and reduces the risk of infection, but the graft dries in 1 or 2 days and may pull and cause pain. Newly developed artificial skin holds great promise for treating severe burns. During the acute stage of a burn, the patient's blood pressure, pulse, respiration, and cerebrovascular pressure are checked every 30 to 60 minutes, and the rectal temperature every 2 to 4 hours. Oral hygiene and assistance in turning, coughing, and deep breathing are provided every 2 hours, and the patient's sensorium is evaluated hourly. If oral fluids are ordered, juices and carbonated drinks are offered, but plain water and ice chips are avoided. Fluid intake and output are measured hourly; if a child excretes less than 1 mL/kg of urine or an adult less than 0.5 mL/kg, a diuretic or an increase in IV infusion of fluid may be necessary. Blood transfusions, steroid therapy, and antipyretics may be ordered; aspirin is contraindicated. Excessive chilling and exposure to upper respiratory and wound infections are carefully prevented. Burned extremities are elevated, and contractures are prevented by using firm supports to keep affected areas properly aligned. The patient is weighed daily at the same time on the same scale, and, after the initial acute period, an adequate intake of a high-calorie, high-protein diet is encouraged; to stimulate appetite, the patient is offered frequent small meals of preferred foods and beverages that are high in potassium. Vitamins may be required. Tranquilizers may be given before wound care, but narcotics for pain usually are not needed after the acute phase. The patient is encouraged to stand for a few minutes every hour or every second hour and is generally able to walk in 7 to 10 days, but convalescence may be prolonged. Burn patients often are frightened, withdrawn, and disoriented initially, but after a few days they may become angry, depressed, or rebellious and need emotional support to help them cooperate with their treatment and rehabilitation. Extensive plastic surgery and repeated skin grafts may be required to restore function and the physical appearance of burn patients. ■ INTERVENTIONS: The burn patient requires intensive, prolonged care to prevent complications and disfiguring contractures. The nurse administers parenteral fluids and medication, implements wound care, closely monitors the patient's condition, limits physical discomfort, provides emotional support and diversion, and encourages the family to visit regularly and become involved in the patient's care. ■ OUTCOME CRITERIA: The outcome for the severely burned patient depends greatly on the detailed, near-constant care required during the acute phase of treatment. Scarring may cause residual dysfunction and discouragement. Encouragement to participate fully in physical therapy and to continue treatments may be helpful. Although protection from infection is essential, the nurse does not isolate the patient unless necessary.

**Burow's solution** /byŏŏr'ōz/ [Karl A. Burow, German physician, 1809–1874], a liquid preparation containing aluminum sulfate, acetic acid, precipitated calcium carbonate, and water, used as a topical astringent, antiseptic, and antipyretic for a wide variety of skin disorders. Also called **aluminum acetate solution.**

**burp,** *informal.* **1.** to belch, or eructate; to expel gas from the stomach through the mouth. **2.** a belch, or eructation.

**burr,** a rotary instrument fitted into a handpiece and used to cut teeth or bone. Also spelled **bur.**

**burr cell** [ME, *burre* + L, *cella,* storeroom], a form of mature erythrocyte in which the cells or cell fragments have spicules, or tiny projections, on the surface.

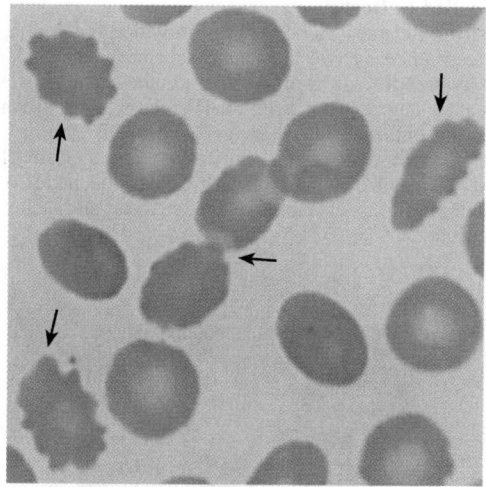

**Burr cell** *(Carr and Rodak, 1999)*

**burr holes,** holes drilled in the skull to drain and irrigate an abscess.

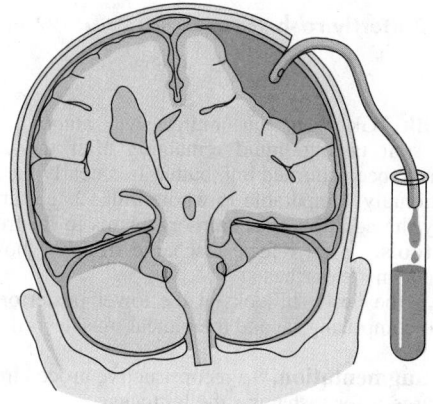

**Burr hole used to drain subdural hematoma**
*(Beare and Myers, 1998)*

**burrowing flea.** See **chigoe.**

**bursa** /bur'sə/, *pl.* **bursae** [Gk, *byrsa,* wineskin], **1.** a fibrous sac between certain tendons and the bones beneath them. Lined with a synovial membrane that secretes synovial fluid, the bursa acts as a small cushion that allows the tendon to move over the bone as it contracts and relaxes. See also **adventitious bursa, bursa of Achilles, olecranon bursa, prepatellar bursa. 2.** a sac or closed cavity. See also **omental bursa, pharyngeal bursa.**

**bursal abscess** /bur'səl/, a collection of pus in the cavity of a bursa.

**bursa of Achilles,** bursa separating the tendon of Achilles and the calcaneus.

**bursectomy** /bərsek'təmē/ [Gk, *byrsa,* wineskin, *ektomē,* cutting out], the excision of a bursa.

**bursitis** /bərsī'tis/, inflammation of the bursa, the connective tissue structure surrounding a joint. Bursitis may be precipitated by arthritis, infection, injury, or excessive or traumatic exercise or effort. The chief symptom is severe pain of the affected joint, particularly on movement. Treatment goals include the control of pain and the maintenance of joint motion. Acute pain is often treated with an intrabursal injection of an adrenocorticosteroid. Other common treatments are analgesics, antiinflammatory agents, cold, and immobilization of the inflamed site. After the inflammation has subsided, heat may be helpful. In chronic cases surgery may be required to remove calcium deposits. Kinds of bursitis include **housemaid's knee, miner's elbow,** and **weaver's bottom.** See also **rheumatism.**

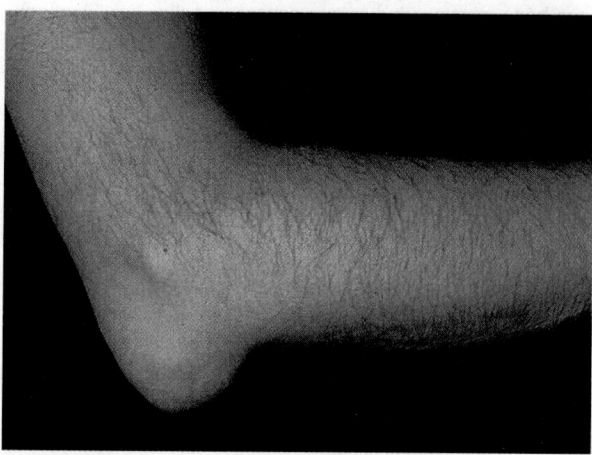

**Bursitis**
*(Reprinted from the Clinical Slide Collection of the Rheumatic Diseases,
© 1991, 1995, 1997. Used with permission of the American College
of Rheumatology)*

**burst,** to break suddenly while under tension or expansion.

**burst fracture** [ME, *bersten* + L, *fractura,* break], any fracture that disperses multiple bone fragments, usually at or near the end of a bone.

**Burton's line** [Henry Burton, English physician, 1799–1849], a dark blue stippled line along the gingival margin, which is a sign of lead poisoning. See also **blue line.**

**Buruli ulcer** /bŏŏ'rə·le/ [Buruli, district in Uganda], a cutaneous infection caused by a species of *Mycobacterium,* manifested by a small, firm, painless, movable subcutaneous nodule that enlarges and ulcerates. It occurs principally in Central Africa, but has also been seen in other tropical areas.

**bus,** a set of parallel wires in a computer to which the central processing unit and all input-output units are connected. Each separate wire carries the electric current representing 1 bit. Buses interconnect the parts of the computer that communicate with each other, such as a video card or modem.

**Buschke's disease.** See **cryptococcosis.**

**BuSpar,** trademark for an oral antianxiety drug (buspirone hydrochloride).

**buspirone hydrochloride** /booˈspirˈōn/, an oral antianxiety drug.

■ INDICATIONS: It is prescribed for anxiety disorders and the short-term relief of anxiety symptoms.

■ CONTRAINDICATIONS: This drug is contraindicated in patients with severe hepatic or renal impairment. Patients taking a benzodiazepine drug should be gradually withdrawn from that medication before starting therapy with buspirone.

■ ADVERSE EFFECTS: Among adverse reactions reported are dizziness, headache, lightheadedness, excitement, and nausea.

**busulfan** /booˈsulˈfan/, an alkylating agent.

■ INDICATION: It is prescribed in the treatment of chronic myelocytic leukemia.

■ CONTRAINDICATIONS: Radiation therapy, depressed neutrophil or platelet counts, concurrent administration of neoplastic medication, or known hypersensitivity to this drug prohibits its use.

■ ADVERSE REACTIONS: Among the more serious adverse reactions are alveolar hyperplasia (busulfan lung), depression of the bone marrow, and severe nausea and diarrhea. Amenorrhea commonly occurs.

**butabarbital sodium** /byooˈtəbärˈbitôl/, a sedative; intermediate-acting barbiturate.

■ INDICATIONS: It is prescribed for the relief of anxiety, nervous tension, and insomnia.

■ CONTRAINDICATIONS: Porphyria, seizure disorders, or known hypersensitivity to this drug prohibits its use.

■ ADVERSE EFFECTS: Among the more serious adverse reactions are jaundice, skin rash, and paradoxical excitement.

**butamben picrate** /byooˈtamˈbən pikˈrāt/, a topical local anesthetic for the temporary relief of pain from minor burns.

**butanamide.** See **acebutolol.**

**butane ($C_4H_{10}$),** a colorless petroleum-based gas. It is the fourth member of the paraffin series of hydrocarbons.

**butanoic acid.** See **butyric acid.**

**butanol.** See **butyl alcohol.**

**Butazolidin,** trademark for an antirheumatic (phenylbutazone).

**Butesin Picrate,** trademark for a local anesthetic (butamben picrate).

**Butisol Sodium,** trademark for a sedative (butabarbital sodium).

**butoconazole nitrate** /byooˈtəkōˈnəzōl/, an intravaginal antifungal cream.

■ INDICATIONS: It is prescribed for the treatment of vulvovaginal fungal infections caused by *Candida* species.

■ CONTRAINDICATIONS: Its use is contraindicated during the first trimester of a pregnancy.

■ ADVERSE EFFECTS: Adverse reactions include vulvar and vaginal burning and itching.

**butorphanol tartrate** /byooˈtôrˈfənôl/, a parenteral agonist/antagonist opioid of the phenanthrene family.

■ INDICATIONS: It is prescribed for surgical premedication, as an analgesic component of balanced anesthesia, and for prompt relief of moderate to severe pain associated with surgical procedures.

■ CONTRAINDICATIONS: Butorphanol tartrate is not given to patients known to be sensitive to phenanthrenes or to persons dependent on opioids because it may provoke withdrawal symptoms.

■ ADVERSE EFFECTS: Toxicity may result from the use of butorphanol with other opioids.

**butt,** **1.** to place two surfaces together to form a joint. **2.** (in dentistry) to place directly against the tissues covering the residual alveolar ridge.

**butter,** a soft, solid substance, such as the oily mass produced by churning cream.

**butterfly bandage** [AS, *buttorfleoge*], a narrow adhesive strip with broader winglike ends used to approximate the edges of a superficial wound and to hold the edges together as they heal. It is used in place of a suture in certain cases. Also called **butterfly.**

**butterfly fracture,** a bone break in which the center fragment contained by two cracks forms a triangle.

**butterfly needle,** a short needle attached to plastic stabilizers at 90 degrees. It is used for IV access of small veins of adults and children. Usual gauge is 25 to 22 length.

**butterfly rash,** an erythematous eruption of both cheeks joined by a narrow band of rash across the nose. It may be seen in lupus erythematosus, rosacea, and seborrheic dermatitis.

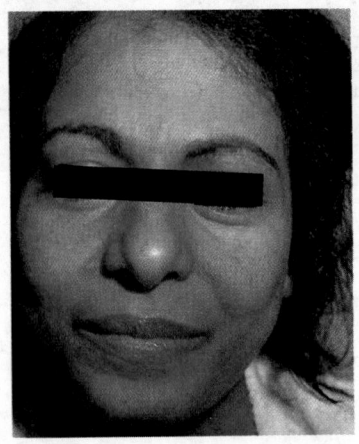

**Butterfly rash** *(Lookingbill and Marks, 1993)*

**buttermilk** [Gk, *boutyron,* butter; AS, *meoluc*], **1.** the slightly sour tasting liquid remaining after the solids in cream have been churned into butter. It is nearly fat free and is nutritionally comparable to whole milk. **2.** cultured milk made by the addition of certain organisms to fat-free milk.

**butter stools,** a fatty fecal discharge from the bowels, as may occur in steatorrhea.

**buttock,** the fleshy hillocks at the lower posterior part of the torso comprising fat and the gluteal muscles. Also called **nates.**

**buttock augmentation,** a reconstructive procedure in cosmetic surgery for reshaping the buttocks.

**button** /butˈən/ [OFr, *boton*]. **1.** a knoblike elevation or structure. **2.** a small appliance shaped like a spool or disk, used in surgery for construction of an intestinal anastomosis.

**buttonhole** [OFr, *boton* + AS, *hol*],   a small slitlike hole in the wall of a structure or a cavity of the body.

**buttonhole fracture,**   a fracture caused by a straight perforation of a bone, such as by a bullet.

**buttonhole stenosis,**   an extreme narrowing of a vessel. The term usually refers to the mitral valve, in which the valve cusps are contracted to form an opening shaped like a buttonhole.

**buttonhook,**   an adaptive device designed to help patients with limited finger range of motion, dexterity, or weakness fastening buttons on clothing.

**button suture,**   a technique in suturing in which the ends of the suture material are passed through buttons on the surface of the skin and tied. It is used to prevent the suture from cutting through the skin.

**buttressing,**   a phenomenon of osteoarthritis in which osteophytes at the hip joint extend across the femoral neck inferior to the femoral head and combine, with a proliferation along the medial aspect of the femoral neck.

**buttress plate,**   a thin, flat metal plate used to provide support in the surgical repair of a fracture.

**butyl** /byōō′til/ [Gk, *boutyron,* butter, *hyle,* matter],   a hydrocarbon radical ($C_4H_9$), the compounds of which are obtained from petroleum. Butyl compounds, some of which are toxic and irritating, are used in a variety of industrial and medical applications, including anesthesia.

**butyl alcohol ($C_4H_9OH$),**   a clear, toxic liquid used as an organic solvent. It exists as four isomers, *n*-butyl, isobutyl, secondary butyl, and tertiary butyl alcohol. Also called **butanol.**

**butyr-,**   combining form meaning 'butter': *butyric, butyrinase.*

**butyric acid ($C_4H_7OOH$)** /byōōtir′ik/,   a fatty acid occurring in rancid butter, feces, urine, perspiration, and, in trace amounts, spleen and blood. Butyric acid is used in the preparation of flavorings, emulsifying agents, and pharmaceutics. Also called **butanoic acid** /byōō′tənō′ik/, **propylformic acid.**

**butyric fermentation,**   the conversion of carbohydrates to butyric acid.

**butyrophenone** /byōō′tərōfē′nōn/,   one of a small group of major tranquilizers. They are used in treating psychosis to decrease the choreic symptoms of Huntington's disease and the tics and coprolalia of Gilles de la Tourette's syndrome and are used as an adjunct in neuroleptanesthesia. Principal butyrophenones are pimozide, haloperidol, and droperidol. Butyrophenones are pharmacologically and clinically similar to phenothiazines.

**Buzzard's maneuver** [Thomas Buzzard, English neurologist, 1831–1919],   a modified patellar reflex in which the patient's toes are firmly pressed on the floor while the quadriceps muscle is tapped.

**BWS,**   abbreviation for **battered woman syndrome.**

**bypass** [AS, *bi,* alongside; Fr, *passer*],   **1.** any one of various surgical procedures to divert or shunt the flow of blood or other natural fluids from normal anatomic courses. A bypass may be temporary or permanent. Bypass surgery is commonly performed in the treatment of cardiac and GI disorders. **2.** a term used by some hospitals to signal that its emergency department lacks the personnel and equipment to handle additional patients, thereby advising that ambulances transporting new patients be diverted to other hospitals.

**by-product material,**   the radioactive waste of nuclear reactors.

**byssinosis** /bis′inō′sis/ [Gk, *byssos,* flax, *osis,* condition],   an occupational respiratory disease characterized by shortness of breath, cough, and wheezing. The condition is an allergic reaction to dust or fungi in cotton, flax, and hemp fibers. The symptoms are typically more pronounced on Mondays when workers return after a weekend break. They are reversible in the early stages, but prolonged exposure results in chronic airway obstruction, bronchitis, and emphysema with fibrosis, leading to respiratory failure, pulmonary hypertension, and cor pulmonale. Treatment is symptomatic for the irreversible changes of emphysema and chronic bronchitis. Compare **pneumoconiosis.** See also **organic dust.**

**byte** /bīt/,   the amount of memory required to encode one character of information (letter, number, or symbol) in a computer system; it is normally 8 bits. See also **bit.**

**Byzantine arch palate** /biz′əntēn/,   a congenital anomaly of the roof of the mouth marked by incomplete fusion of the palatal process and the nasal spine.

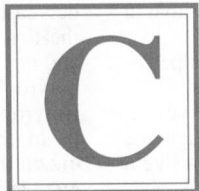

**c,** **1.** symbol for *capillary blood.* **2.** abbreviation for **curie.**

**C,** **1.** (in respiratory physiology) symbol for **compliance.** **2.** symbol for *concentration of gas in the blood.* **3.** symbol for the element **carbon.**

**C1, C2, . . .,** symbols for cervical nerves.

**C3 nephritic factor,** a complement protein that may be deposited in glomerular capillary walls and mesangial tissues, precipitating or contributing to local inflammation and kidney damage.

**Ca,** symbol for the element **calcium.**

**CA 15-3 tumor marker test,** a blood test used to determine the presence of the CA 15-3 tumor-associated serum marker. This serum marker is used for staging breast cancer and monitoring its treatment.

**CA 19-9 tumor marker test,** a blood test used to determine the presence of CA 19-9 antigen. In patients with pancreatic or hepatobiliary cancer, this tumor marker is used in diagnosis, in the evaluation of a patient's response to treatment, and in the surveillance of the disease.

**CA 27.29 tumor marker test,** a blood test used to determine the presence of the CA 27.29 tumor-associated serum marker. This serum marker is used for staging breast cancer and monitoring its treatment.

**CA 125,** abbreviation for *cancer cell surface antigen 125,* a glycoprotein found in the blood serum of patients with ovarian or other glandular cell carcinomas. Increasing levels of the antigen mean continuing tumor growth, which may indicate a poor prognosis.

**CA 125 tumor marker test,** a blood test used to determine the presence of CA 125 serum tumor marker, which has a high degree of sensitivity and specificity for ovarian cancer. It is also used to determine a patient's response to therapy, to predict the outcome of second-look laparotomies, and for posttreatment surveillance.

**CABG,** abbreviation for **coronary artery bypass graft.**

**cabinet bath** [ME, *cabane,* cabin], a bath in which the patient, except his or her head, is enclosed in a cabinet heated by hot air or radiant heat. Also called **box bath.**

**Cabot rings** /kab′ot/ [Richard C. Cabot, American physician, 1868–1939], threadlike figures, often appearing as loops or rings in red blood cells of patients with severe anemia. The inclusions are seen after blood smears are stained with Wright stain. Also called **Cabot bodies.**

**Cabot's splint** [Arthur T. Cabot, American surgeon, b. 1852], a metal splint worn behind the thigh and leg for support.

**cac-.** See **caco-.**

**CaC₂,** the chemical formula for calcium carbide.

**CaC₂O₄,** the chemical formula for calcium oxalate.

**cacao** /kəkā′ō/cacal/, **1.** cocoa. **2.** the substance *Theobroma cacao.* **3.** the seeds of *Theobroma cacao.*

**cacesthesia** /kak′əsthē′zhə/ [Gk, *kakos,* bad, *aisthesis,* feeling], any morbid feeling or disordered sensibility. —**cacesthetic,** *adj.*

**cache** /kash/, (in computer technology) a fast storage buffer in the central processing unit. Also called **cache memory.**

**cachectic** /kəkek′tik/ [Gk, *kakos,* bad, *hexis,* state], pertain-

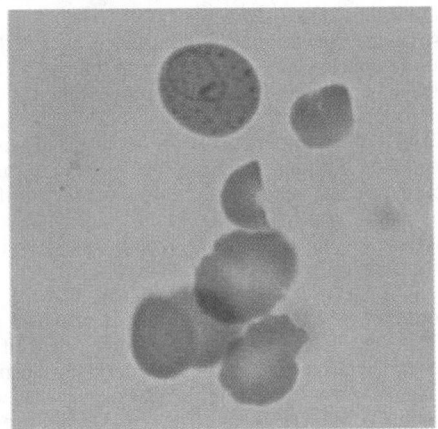

**Cabot rings** *(Carr and Rodak, 1999)*

ing to a state of generally poor health, malnutrition, and weight loss.

**cachet** /käshā′/ [Fr, tablet], any lenticular edible capsule that encloses a dose of medicine.

**cachexia** /kəkek′sē·ə/ [Gk, *kakos,* bad, *hexis,* state], general ill health and malnutrition, marked by weakness and emaciation, usually associated with severe disease, such as tuberculosis or cancer. Also called **cachexy.** —**cachectic,** *adj.*

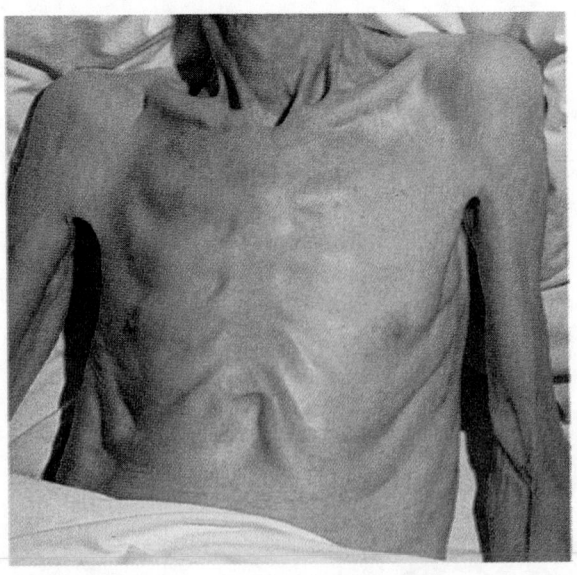

**Cachexia** *(Kamal and Brockelhurst, 1991)*

**cachinnation** /kak′ənā′shən/ [L, *cachinnare,* to laugh aloud], excessive laughter with no apparent cause, often part of the behavioral pattern in schizophrenia. —**cachinnate,** *v.*

**CaCl₂,** the chemical formula for calcium chloride.

**CaCO₃,** the chemical formula for calcium carbonate.

**caco-, cac-,** prefix meaning 'ill, unpleasant, or bad': *cacophony, cachexia.*

**cacodemonomania** /kak′ōdē′mənōmā′nē·ə/ [Gk, *kakos* + *daimon,* spirit, *mania,* madness], an abnormal mental condition in which the patient claims to be possessed by an evil spirit.

**cacophony** /kəkof′ənē/, *pl.* **cacophonies** [Gk, *kakos* + *phone,* voice], a harsh or discordant sound or a mixture of confused, different sounds. —**cacophonic, cacophonous,** *adj.*

**cacoplastic** /kak′əplas′tik/, **1.** pertaining to a low or inferior grade of structure or organization. **2.** pertaining to a state of morbid growth.

**cacosmia** /kakoz′mē·ə/ [Gk, *kakos* + *osme,* odor], the perception of foul odor or stench when none exists. In most instances the condition results from psychologic factors, as in olfactory hallucinations that occur during certain psychoses, although it may be caused by a brain lesion. Also spelled **kakosmia.**

**CAD,** **1.** abbreviation for **coronary artery disease. 2.** abbreviation for *computer-assisted design.*

**cadaver** /kədā′vər/ [L, dead body], a corpse used for dissection and study.

**cadaver graft,** the transfer of tissue from the body of a dead individual to repair a defect in a living person. Also called **postmortem graft.**

**cadaveric** /kad′äver′ik/, pertaining to or resembling a cadaver.

**cadaveric donor transplantation,** allogeneic transplantation of an organ or tissue from a cadaver.

**cadaveric renal transplant (CRT),** a kidney transplant from a dead donor.

**cadence** /kā′dəns/ [L, *cadere,* to fall], a rhythm as in voice, music, or movement.

**cade oil.** See **juniper tar.**

**cadmium (Cd)** /kad′mē·əm/(Cd) [Gk, *kadmeia,* zinc ore], a metallic bluish white element that resembles tin. Its atomic number is 48; its atomic weight (mass) is 112.40. Cadmium has many uses in industry and was formerly included in medications. Such medications have been replaced by less toxic drugs. See also **cadmium poisoning.**

**cadmium poisoning,** poisoning resulting from the inhalation of cadmium in fumes created by welding, smelting, or other industrial processes involving solder. Cadmium bromide, used in engraving, lithography, and photography, can cause severe GI symptoms if swallowed. Cadmium may also cause poisoning by the ingestion of acidic foods prepared and stored in cadmium-lined containers, as lemonade in certain metal cans. The effects may include vomiting, dyspnea, headache, prostration, pulmonary edema, and, possibly, years later, cancer.

**caduceus** /kədōō′sē·əs/ [L; Gk, *karykeion,* herald], the wand of the god Hermes or Mercury, used as the symbol for the U.S. Army Medical Corps. It is represented as a staff with two serpents coiled around it and is often confused with the staff of Æsculapius, a rod with one snake entwined about it.

**caecal.** See **cecal.**

**caec-, caeco-.** See **cec-, ceco-.**

**caecostomy.** See **cecostomy.**

**caenogenesis.** See **cenogenesis.**

**Caesarean hysterectomy.** See **cesarean hysterectomy.**

**Caesarean section.** See **cesarean section.**

**caesium.** See **cesium.**

**café-au-lait spot** /kaf′ā·ōlā′/ [Fr, coffee with milk], a pale tan macule the color of coffee with milk. Simultaneous development of several café-au-lait spots is associated with neurofibromatosis, but occasional café-au-lait spots occur normally. See also **neurofibromatosis.**

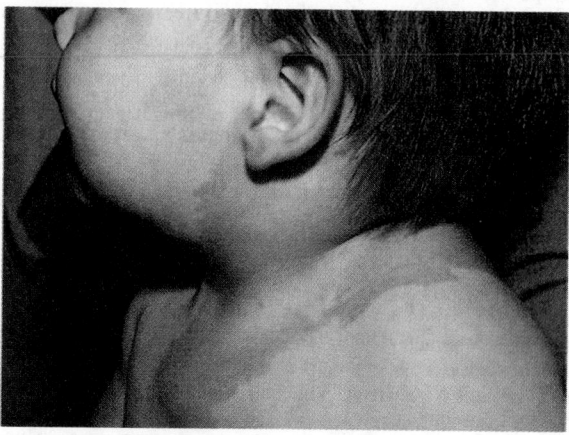

**Café-au-lait spot** *(Weston, Lane, and Morelli, 1996)*

**café coronary** /kəfā′/, a collapse of a person who is eating, caused by asphyxiation that results from obstruction of the glottis by a food bolus. Because the signs are similar to those of a heart attack, such episodes are frequently mistaken for coronary occlusions. See also **Heimlich maneuver.**

**Cafergot,** trademark for a fixed-combination drug containing caffeine and ergotamine, commonly administered in the treatment of migraine headaches.

**caffeine** /kafēn′, kaf′ē·in/ [Ar, *qahwah,* coffee], a central nervous system stimulant.

■ INDICATIONS: It is prescribed to counteract migraine, drowsiness, and mental fatigue.

■ CONTRAINDICATIONS: It is used with caution in patients with heart disease and peptic ulcer. Known hypersensitivity to this drug prohibits its use.

■ ADVERSE EFFECTS: Among the most serious adverse reactions are tachycardia and diuresis. GI distress, restlessness, and insomnia are common.

**caffeine poisoning** [Ar, *qahwah,* coffee; L, *potio,* drink], a toxic condition caused by the chronic ingestion of excessive amounts of caffeine, which is found in coffee, tea, cola beverages, and certain stimulant drugs. Symptoms include restlessness, anxiety, general depression, tachycardia, dysrhythmias (premature atrial contractions), tremors, nausea, diuresis, and insomnia. In cases of caffeine poisoning, death may result from cardiovascular and respiratory collapse. Also called **caffeinism** /kafē′nizəm/, **caffeism** /kaf′ē·izm/. See also **xanthine derivative.**

**Caffey's disease.** See **infantile cortical hyperostosis.**

**Caffey's syndrome** [John Caffey, American pediatrician, 1895–1978], the battered baby syndrome, first described by John Caffey in 1946. See also **child abuse.**

**CAGE** /kāj/, a mnemonic abbreviation formed by the first letters of four questions designed to screen alcoholic patients: *C*utdown, *A*nnoyed by criticism, *G*uilt about drinking, and *E*ye-opener drinks.

**CAH,** **1.** abbreviation for **chronic active hepatitis.** **2.** abbreviation for **congenital adrenal hyperplasia.**

**CAHEA,** abbreviation for **Committee on Allied Health Education and Accreditation.**

**CAI,** abbreviation for **computer-assisted instruction.**

**-caine,** combining form usually indicating a synthetic alkaloid anesthetic: *cocaine, isocaine.*

**caisson disease.** See **decompression sickness.**

**cajeputol.** See **eucalyptol.**

**caked** /kākt/ [ONorse, *kaka*], formed into a compact mass or crust, as the scab of coagulated blood on a healing wound.

**caked breast,** an accumulation of milk in the secreting ducts of the breast after childbirth, causing all or a part of the breast to become hardened and the tissues to become engorged. Also called **lactation mastitis.**

**cal (c),** **1.** abbreviation for **small calorie.** **2.** 4.184 cal = 1 Joule.

**Cal (C),** abbreviation for **kilocalorie, large calorie.** Cal is used to describe the calorie content of food. 1000 cal = 1 Cal.

**calabar swelling** /kal'əbär/ [Calabar, a Nigerian seaport], a localized angioedema and erythema usually on the extremities, characterized by fugitive, swollen lumps of subcutaneous tissue caused by a parasitic filarial worm endemic to Central and West Africa. The swollen areas migrate with the worm through the body at a speed of about 1 cm per minute and may become as large as a small egg. A kind of calabar swelling is *Loa loa.* See also **loiasis.**

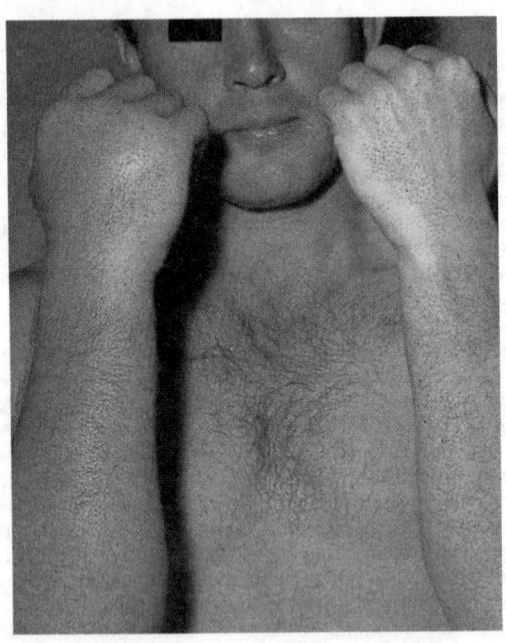

**Calabar swelling on the right arm and hand**
*(du Vivier, 1993/courtesy Dr. Roger Harmon)*

**Caladryl,** trademark for a topical fixed-combination drug containing a skin protective substance (calamine) and an antihistaminic (diphenhydramine hydrochloride).

**calamine** /kal'əmīn/ [Gk, *kadmeia,* zinc ore], a pink odorless powder used as a protectant or as an astringent and sometimes prepared as a lotion. It is composed of zinc oxide with 0.5% ferric oxide.

**Calan,** trademark for a calcium channel blocker (verapamil hydrochloride).

**calc-, calci-,** combining form meaning 'lime or calcium': *calcariuria, calciosis.*

**calcane-, calcaneo-,** combining form meaning 'heel': *calcaneum, calcaneocavus.*

**calcaneal** /kalkā'nē·əl/ [L, *calcaneum,* heel], pertaining to the calcaneus at the back of the tarsus.

**calcaneal epiphysitis,** a painful disorder involving the calcaneus at its epiphysis. The condition tends mainly to affect children who are physically active and whose heel bones are still divided by a layer of cartilage. The stress of jumping and other athletic activities may break the union of the bone segments at the cartilage layer. Treatment may require immobilization of the foot in a cast. Also called **Sever's disease.**

**calcaneal spur,** abnormal, often painful bony outgrowth on the lower surface of the calcaneus, resulting from chronic traumatic pressure on the heel. Also called **heel spur.**

**calcaneal tendon.** See **Achilles tendon.**

**calcaneal tuberosity,** a transverse elevation on the plantar surface of the calcaneus to which are attached the abductor digiti minimi, the long plantar ligament, and various other muscles, including the abductor hallucis and the flexor digitorum brevis.

**calcanean.** See **calcaneus.**

**calcaneodynia** /kalkā'nē·ōdin'ē·ə/ [L, *calcaneum* + Gk, *odyne,* pain], a painful condition of the heel.

**calcaneovalgus, calcaneovarus.** See **clubfoot.**

**calcaneum.** See **calcaneus.**

**calcaneus** /kalkā'nē·əs/ [L, *calcaneum,* heel], the heel bone. The largest of the tarsal bones, it articulates proximally with the talus and distally with the cuboid. —**calcaneal, calcanean,** *adj.*

**calcar** /kal'kär/, *pl.* calcaria, a spur or a structure that resembles a spur.

**calcar avis** /ā'vis/ [L, *calcar,* spur, *avis,* bird], a projection on the medial wall of the posterior horn of the lateral ventricle of the brain. It is associated with the lateral extension of the calcarine fissure. Also called **hippocampus minor.**

**calcareous** /kalker'ē·əs/ [L, *calcar,* spur], pertaining to calcium or lime.

**calcar femorale** /kal'kär fem'ə·rā'lē/ [L], the plate of strong tissue which strengthens the neck of the femur.

**calcaria.** See **calcar.**

**calcarine** /kal'kərīn/, **1.** having the shape of a spur. **2.** pertaining to the calcar.

**calcarine fissure,** a groove between the cuneus and the lingual gyrus on the medial surface of the occipital lobe of the brain. Also called **calcarine sulcus.**

**calcar pedis.** See **heel.**

**calcemia.** See **hypercalcemia, hypocalcemia.**

**calcereous metastasis,** the deposition of calcium salts in visceral organs as a result of hyperparathyroidism, an absorptive disease of the bone, or any cause of hypercalcemia, particularly when associated with hyperphosphatemia. Also called metatastic calcification.

**calcergy** /kal'sərjē/, local calcification of soft tissues at the site of injection of certain types of chemicals.

**calci-.** See **calc-.**

**calcifediol** /kal'sifē'dē·ol/, a major transport form of vitamin D.

■ INDICATION: It is prescribed in the treatment of metabolic bone disease associated with chronic renal failure.

■ CONTRAINDICATIONS: Hypercalcemia, vitamin D toxicity, malabsorption syndrome, decreased renal function, or known hypersensitivity to this drug prohibits its use.

■ ADVERSE EFFECTS: Among the most serious adverse effects are renal toxicity and those reactions associated with hypercalcemia, as soft tissue calcification and GI and central nervous system disturbances.

**calciferol** /kalsif′ərôl/ [L, *calx,* lime, *ferre,* to bear], a fat-soluble, crystalline unsaturated alcohol produced by ultraviolet irradiation of ergosterol in plants. It is used as a dietary supplement in the prophylaxis and treatment of rickets, osteomalacia, and other hypocalcemic disorders. Also called **ergocalciferol, oleovitamin D₂,** vitamin D₂. See also **rickets, viosterol.**

**calcific** /kalsif′ik/ [L, *calx,* lime, *facere,* to make], pertaining to the formation of chalk, lime, or calcium.

**calcific aortic disease** [L, *calx,* lime], an abnormal condition characterized by small deposits of calcium in the aorta.

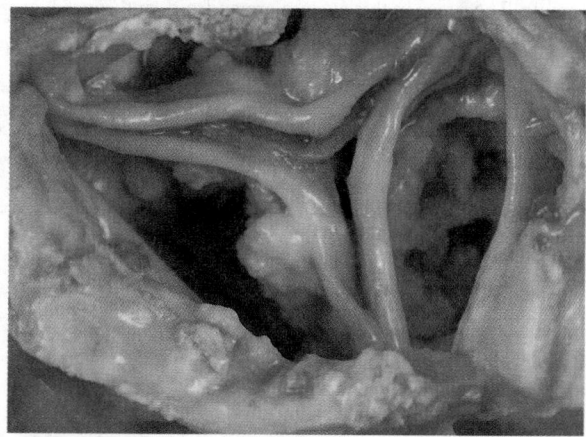

**Calcific aortic stenosis** (Kumar, Cotran, and Robbins, 1997)

**calcification** [L, *calx* + *facere,* to make], the accumulation of calcium salts in tissues. Normally, about 99% of all the calcium entering the human body is deposited in the bones and teeth; the remaining 1% is dissolved in body fluids such as blood. Disorders affecting the delicate balance between calcium and other minerals, parathyroid hormone, and vitamin D can result in calcium deposits in arteries, kidneys, lung alveoli, and other tissues, interfering with normal organ function. See also **calcitonin, calcium, calculus.**

**calcific tendinitis** [L, *calx,* lime, *facere,* to make, *tendo,* tendon; Gk, *itis,* inflammation], a chronic inflammation of a tendon resulting from an accumulation of calcium deposits in the tissue.

**calcified fetus.** See **lithopedion.**

**Calcimar,** trademark for calcitonin.

**calcination** /kal′sinā′shən/ [L, *calcinare,* to burn lime], the heating of inorganic materials to drive off water. It is used in denistry to manufacture plaster and stone from gypsum. Compare **calcification.**

**calcinosis** /kal′sənō′sis/, a condition characterized by abnormal deposits of calcium salts in various tissues. The de-

posits appear as nodules or plaques and may occur in the skin, connective tissue, muscles, or intervertebral disks. Usually the nodules occur secondary to dermatomyositis or to a preexisting inflammatory degenerative or neoplastic dermatosis, primarily scleroderma.

**calcipenia** /kal′sipē′nē·ə/, a deficiency of calcium in the body tissues and fluids.

**calcitonin** /kal′sitō′nin/ [L, *calx* + Gk, *tonos,* tone], a hormone produced in parafollicular cells of the thyroid that participates in regulating the blood level of calcium and stimulates bone mineralization. A synthetic preparation of the hormone is used in the treatment of certain bone disorders. Calcitonin acts to reduce the blood level of calcium and to inhibit bone resorption, whereas parathyroid hormone acts to increase blood calcium level and bone resorption.

**calcitonin test,** a blood test used to evaluate patients who have or are suspected to have medullary carcinoma of the thyroid. It is also used to monitor response to therapy, to predict recurrence of the cancer, and to screen those with a family history of the disease.

**calcitriol** /kalsit′rē·ôl/, the active form of vitamin D, a regulator of calcium metabolism.

■ INDICATION: It is prescribed in the management of hypocalcemia in patients undergoing chronic renal dialysis and in patients with hypoparathyroidism.

■ CONTRAINDICATIONS: Hypercalcemia, evidence of vitamin D toxicity, malabsorption syndrome, decreased renal function, or known sensitivity to this drug prohibits its use.

■ ADVERSE EFFECTS: Among the more serious adverse reactions are renal toxicity and those associated with hypercalcemia, such as soft tissue calcification.

**calcium (Ca)** /kal′sē·əm/ [L, *calx,* lime], an alkaline earth metal element. Its atomic number is 20; its atomic mass is 40.08. Its metallic form is a white flammable solid, somewhat harder than lead. Calcium is commonly produced by the electrolysis or thermal dissociation of calcium chloride. Calcium carbonate is the most common calcium compound. Calcium also occurs as a component of the natural compound gypsum, which forms plaster of paris when heated. It is also a component of calcium cyanamid, a fertilizer and progenitor of other nitrogen compounds. Calcium is the fifth most abundant element in the human body and is mainly present in the bone. The body requires calcium ions for the transmission of nerve impulses, muscle contraction, blood coagulation, cardiac functions, and other processes. It is a component of extracellular fluid and of soft tissue cells. The average daily human intake of calcium varies from 200 to 2500 mg. In the United States dairy products are the major dietary sources of this element. The daily dietary allowances recommended by the Food and Nutrition Board vary from 360 mg for infants to 1200 mg for women 15 to 18 years of age. More than 90% of the calcium in the body is stored in the skeleton, which constantly exchanges its supplies with the calcium of the interstitial fluids. The endocrine system controls the concentration of ionized calcium in the plasma. Only a fraction of this amount is ionized and diffusible; the rest is bound to proteins, especially albumin. It is the ionized, diffusible portion of calcium that participates in the physiologic changes associated with hypocalcemia. About one third of the calcium ingested by humans is absorbed, primarily in the small bowel. Vitamin D, calcitonin, and parathyroid hormone are essential in the metabolism of calcium. The degree of cell permeability varies inversely with calcium ion concentration. Abnormally high levels of ionized calcium in the extracellular fluid can produce muscle weakness, lethargy, and coma. A relatively small decrease from the normal level of this element can produce tetanic seizures. Normal adult blood levels of calcium are 9 to 10.5 mg/dl or 2.25 to 2.75 nmol/L.

**calcium carbide (CaC₂),** a black crystalline compound produced from lime and coke. When mixed with water, it yields acetylene gas ($C_2H_2$), which has been used as an anesthetic.

**calcium carbonate ($CaCO_3$),** precipitated chalk. A white powder sometimes used in antacids.

**calcium channel blocker,** a drug that inhibits the flow of calcium ions across the membranes of smooth muscle cells. By reduction of the calcium flow, smooth muscle tone is relaxed and the risk of muscle spasms is diminished. Calcium channel blockers are used primarily in the treatment of heart diseases marked by coronary artery spasms.

**calcium chloride ($CaCl_2$),** a white granular chemical with an unpleasant taste. It is used in a concentrated solution of the chloride salt of calcium to replenish calcium in the blood and also has uses in cardiac resuscitation.

■ INDICATIONS: It is prescribed for the treatment of hypocalcemic tetany and as an antidote for lead or magnesium poisoning or magnesium sulfate overdose.

■ CONTRAINDICATIONS: Renal insufficiency, ventricular fibrillation, hypercalcemia, or known hypersensitivity to this drug prohibits its use.

■ ADVERSE EFFECTS: Among the more serious adverse reactions is hypercalcemia.

■ CAUTION: Calcium chloride is never injected into tissue.

**calcium gluconate ($C_{12}H_{22}CaO_{14}$),** a white odorless, tasteless powder or granules administered orally or intravenously to replenish the body's calcium stores, as after a transfusion.

**calcium hydroxide (Ca[OH]₂),** a bitter-tasting white powder that may be used in the preparation of treatments for infant diarrhea. Also called **slaked lime.**

**calcium hydroxide solution,** a clear, colorless liquid sometimes used as an alkali and antidote. Also called **lime water.**

**calcium oxalate ($CaC_2O_4$),** a small, colorless crystal that may be present in urine or may be a component of renal calculi.

**calcium oxide (CaO),** a compound formed by the calcination of chalk or marble and sometimes used in the preparation of caustic pastes. Also called **calx, quicklime.**

**calcium phosphate ($Ca_3[PO_4]_2$),** an odorless, tasteless white powder used as a calcium supplement, laxative, and antacid.

**calcium pump,** a theorized, energy-requiring mechanism for transmitting calcium ions across a plasma membrane from a region of low calcium ion concentration to one of higher concentration. Compare **sodium-potassium pump.**

**calcium sulfate ($CaSO_4$),** a white moisture-absorbing powder used for making plaster casts. Also called **plaster of paris.**

**calcium test (Ca),** a blood or urine test used to evaluate parathyroid function and calcium metabolism by directly measuring the total amount of calcium in the blood. It is used to monitor patients with renal failure, renal transplantation, hyperparathyroidism, and various malignancies, as well as to monitor calcium levels during and after large-volume blood transfusions.

**calciuria** /kal′siōōr′ē·ə/ [L, *calx*, lime; Gk, *ouron*, urine], the presence of calcium in the urine.

**calcospherite** /kal′kəsfir′īt/, a spherical mass of calcium salts and organic matter found in an area of calcification.

**calculation for children dosage.** See **Clark's rule.**

**calculogenesis** /kal′kyəlōjen′əsis/, the formation of calculi.

**calculous** /kal′kyələs/, **1.** describing a substance that has the hardness of stone. **2.** pertaining to calculus.

**calculus** /kal′kyələs/, *pl.* **calculi** /kal′kyəlī/ [L, little stone], **1.** an abnormal stone formed in body tissues by an accumulation of mineral salts. Calculi are usually found in biliary and urinary tracts. Kinds of calculi include **biliary calculus** and **renal calculus.** Also called **stone. 2.** a deposit of calcium phosphate, calcium carbonate, and organic matter that accumulates on the teeth or a dental prosthesis. Also called **tartar.** Calculus that forms coronal to the gingival crest, called **supragingival calculus,** is chalky and cream-colored but may be stained by tobacco and food. Calculus that forms in the gingival pocket, or the periodontal pocket, called **serumal calculus, subgingival calculus,** or **veneer,** is usually denser and darker than supragingival calculus; it harbors bacteria, thus contributing to periodontal disease.

**Calderol,** trademark for a transport form of vitamin D (calcifediol).

**Caldwell-Moloy pelvic classification** /kôl′dwelməloi′/ [William E. Caldwell, American obstetrician, 1880–1943; Howard C. Moloy, American gynecologist, 1903–1953], a system for classifying the structure of the bony pelvis of the female. The types in this system are android, anthropoid, gynecoid, and platypelloid. The sacrum, coccyx, sidewalls, sacrosciatic notch, ischial spines, pubic arch, and ischial tuberosities are the anatomic points of reference used to determine pelvic type. The classification system requires that a mixed pelvis be named for the character of its posterior section with the name of the type characterized by the anterior portion after a hyphen, as in a gynecoid-android pelvis. See also **pelvic classification.**

**calefacient** /kal′əfā′shənt/ [L, *calare*, to be warm, *facere*, to make], **1.** making or tending to make anything warm or hot. **2.** an agent that imparts a sense of warmth when applied, such as a hot-water bottle or a hot compress.

**calendar method of family planning.** See **natural family planning method.**

**calf,** *pl.* **calves** [ONorse, *kalfi*], the fleshy mass at the back of the leg below the knee, composed chiefly of the gastrocnemius muscle.

**calfactant,** a natural lung surfactant extract.

■ INDICATIONS: This drug is used in the prevention and treatment (rescue) of respiratory distress syndrome in premature infants.

■ CONTRAINDICATIONS: No contraindications are known at present.

■ ADVERSE EFFECTS: Concurrent illnesses that have occurred during treatment with this drug include pulmonary air leaks, pulmonary interstitial emphysema, apnea, pulmonary hemorrhage, patent ductus arteriosus, intracranial hemorrhage, severe intracranial hemorrhage, necrotizing enterocolitis, posttreatment sepsis, and posttreatment infection. Other serious adverse effects include bradycardia, oxygen desaturation, vasoconstriction, hypotension, and hypertension.

**calf bone.** See **fibula.**

**calf muscle pump,** an action of the calf (soleus) muscles in which the muscles contract and squeeze the popliteal and tibial veins, forcing the blood in those veins to move upward toward the heart. Also called **soleus pump.**

**caliber** /kal′ibər/ [Fr, *calibre*, bore of a gun], the diameter of a tube or a canal, as any of the blood vessels. Also spelled **calibre.**

**calibration** /kal′ibrā′shən/ [Fr, *calibre*, the bore of a gun], the process of measuring or calibrating against an established standard, such as a deciliter or kilogram.

**calibrator,** **1.** an instrument used to measure the size of an opening. **2.** an instrument used to increase the diameter of an opening, as a dilator of a urethral stricture.

**calibre.** See **caliber.**

**calices.** See **calyx.**

**Caliciviridae** /kalis′ivir′idē/, a family of plus-stranded ribonucleic acid viruses that have a nonenveloped virion 35 to 40 nm in diameter. It is associated with episodes of gastroenteritis and hepatitis in humans and animals, including exanthema in swine.

**caliculus** /kalik′yələs/, a cup-shaped structure.

**California encephalitis,** a common acute viral infection that affects the central nervous system. Epidemics occur mainly in the Midwest, on the eastern seaboard, and in Texas and Louisiana. The virus was first isolated in California. The infection generally follows one of two clinical courses. The mild form is characterized by headache, malaise, GI symptoms, and a fever that may reach 104° F. The more severe form may be marked by a sudden onset of fever, vomiting, headaches, lethargy, and signs of neurologic involvement such as loss of reflexes, disorientation, seizure, loss of consciousness, and flaccid paralysis. Recovery usually begins in 1 week. Mortality rate is very low, but a significant number of patients have neurologic sequelae for 1 year or more. Treatment usually involves administration of anticonvulsant and sedative medications. See also **arbovirus, encephalitis.**

**californium (Cf)** [state of California], an artificial element in the actinide group. Its atomic number is 98; the atomic mass of its longest-lived isotope is 251. Californium-252 isotope is a potent source of neutrons.

**caliorraphy** /kal′ə·ôr′əfē/, surgical repair of the calyces of the kidney, usually performed to improve urinary drainage into the ureters.

**calipers** /kal′ipərz/ [Fr, *calibre,* bore of a gun], an instrument with two hinged, adjustable, curved legs, used to measure the thickness or the diameter of a convex or solid body. It is also used to measure space on a graph and in measuring ECG patterns.

**caliper splint,** a leg splint consisting of two metal rods running from the back of a band around the thigh or from a cushioned ring around the lower portion of the pelvis to a metal plate under the shoe below the arch of the foot. Also called **split caliper stirrup.**

**calisthenics** /kal′isthen′iks/, a system of exercise in which emphasis is on movements of muscle groups rather than power and effort. An objective is the acquisition of grace and beauty in exercise.

**calix.** See **calyx.**

**Calliphoridae** /kal′əfôr′ədē/ [Gk, *kallos,* beauty, *pherein,* to bear], a family of medium-sized to large flies that belong to the order Diptera, serve as pathogenic vectors, and may cause intestinal or nasopharyngeal myiasis in humans. These flies include the genera *Auchmeromyia, Calliphora, Cordylobia, Cochliomyia, Chrysomyia, Lucilia, Phaenicia,* and *Phormia.*

**callomania** /kal′ōmā′nē·ə/ [Gk, *kallos,* beauty, *mania,* madness], an abnormal psychologic condition characterized by delusions of personal beauty.

**callosal** /kə·lō′səl/ [L, *callosus,* hard], pertaining to the corpus callosum.

**callosal agenesis,** defect of the callosal structures of the brain.

**callosal fissure** /kəlos′əl/ [L, *callosus,* hard, *fissura,* cleft], a groove following the convex aspect of the corpus callosum.

**callosity.** See **callus.**

**callosomarginal fissure** /kəlō′sōmär′jənəl/, a long, irregular groove on the medial surface of a cerebral hemisphere. It divides the cingulate gyrus from the medial frontal gyrus and from the paracentral lobule. Also called **cingulate sulcus** /sin′gyəlit/.

**callosum.** See **corpus callosum.**

**callous.** See **callus.**

**callous ulcer** /kal′əs/ [L, *callosus,* hard, *ulcus,* ulcer], an ulcer with a hard indurated base and thick inelastic margins. It lacks a blood supply and is frequently associated with edema of the legs.

**callus** /kal′əs/ [L, hard skin], **1.** a common, usually painless thickening of the stratum corneum at locations of external pressure or friction. Compare **corn.** Also called **callosity. 2.** bony deposit formed between and around the broken ends of a fractured bone during healing. Also called **keratoma.** —**callous.** *adj.*

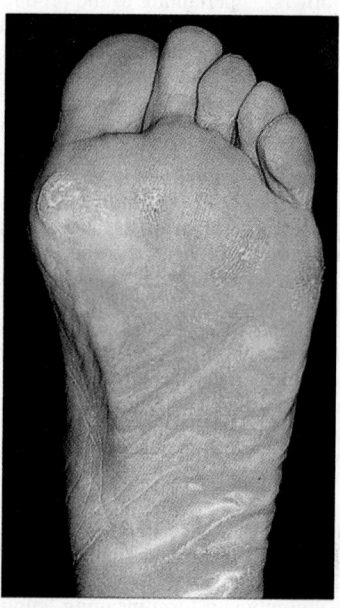

**Callus on the sole of the foot**
*(Lawrence and Cox, 1993)*

**calmative** /kä′mətiv/, having a calming or quieting effect.

**calming technique,** a nursing intervention from the Nursing Interventions Classification (NIC) defined as reducing anxiety in patient experiencing acute distress. See also **Nursing Interventions Classification.**

**calmodulin** /kalmod′yəlin/, a calcium-binding protein that mediates a variety of biochemical and physiologic processes, including the contraction of smooth muscles and the release of norepinephrine. Calmodulin may act independently of, in concert with, or antagonistically to reactions involving cyclic adenosine monophosphate.

**calor** /kal′ôr/ [L, warmth], heat, as that generated by inflammation of tissues or that from the body's normal metabolic processes.

**calor-, calori-,** prefix meaning 'heat': *calorie, calorifacient.*

**caloric** /kalôr′ik/, pertaining to heat or calories.

**caloric test,** a procedure in which the ear canal is alternately irrigated with warm water or air and cold water or air. The warm irrigation produces a rotatory nystagmus toward the irrigated side. Cold irrigation produces a rotatory nystagmus away from the irrigated side. If the vestibular portion of the ear is normal, all irrigations will produce nystagmus that is approximately equal in intensity. If the vestibular portion of the ear is diseased, irrigation may produce less nystagmus than would occur in the normal ear. Also called **Bárány's test.** See also **electronystagmography.**

**calorie (cal)** /kal′ôrē/ [L, *calor,* warmth], the amount of heat required to raise the temperature of 1 g of water 1° C at a pressure of 1 atmosphere. Also called **small calorie.** Compare **Calorie (Cal), kcalorie** —**caloric,** *adj.*

**Calorie (kcal),** **1.** the amount of heat (energy) needed to raise the temperature of 1 kilogram of water 1° C. **2.** a unit, equal to the large calorie, used to denote the heat expenditure of an organism and the fuel or energy value of food. Also called **great calorie, kilocalorie, kilogram calorie, kcalorie, large calorie.** Compare **calorie (cal).**

**calorific** /kal′ərif′ik/, pertaining to the production of heat.

**calorigenic** /kəlôr′ijen′ik/ [L, *calor,* warmth; Gk, *genein,* to produce], pertaining to a substance or process that produces heat or energy or that increases the consumption of oxygen.

**calorimeter** /kal′ərim′ətər/, a device used for measuring quantities of heat generated by friction, chemical reaction, or the human body. —**calorimetric,** *adj.*

**calorimetry** /kal′ərim′ətrē/ [L, *calor,* warmth; Gk, *metron,* measure], the measurement of the amounts of heat radiated and the amounts of heat absorbed. Compare **direct calorimetry, indirect calorimetry.** —**calorimetric,** *adj.*

**calory.** See **calorie.**

**calvaria** /kalver′ē·ə/, the skullcap or superior portion of the skull, which varies greatly in shape from individual to individual. In some persons the calvaria is relatively oval, in others it is more circular. The fontanels, or soft spots, in the skull of an infant are situated on the surface of the calvaria at the junction of the sagittal and coronal sutures and at the junction of the sagittal and lambdoid sutures. See also **bregma.**

**Calvé-Perthes disease.** See **Perthes disease.**

**calvities** /kalvish′i·ēz/ [L, *calvus,* without hair], baldness. —**calvous,** *adj.*

**calyx-, calix-** combining form meaning 'cuplike': *calyces.*

**cambium layer** [L, *cambire,* to exchange], **1.** the loose inner cellular layer of the periosteum that develops during ossification. **2.** a cellular layer of formative tissue that lies between the wood and the bark in plants.

**camera** /kam′ərə/ [L, vaulted chamber], (in anatomy) any compartment, cavity, or chamber, as those of the eye, tooth, or heart.

**camisole restraint.** See **straitjacket.**

**cAMP,** abbreviation for **cyclic adenosine monophosphate.**

**camphor** /kam′fər/ [L, *camphora*], a colorless or white crystalline substance with a penetrating odor and pungent taste, occurring naturally in certain plants, especially *Cinnamomum camphora.* Also called **camphora, gum camphor.**

**camphorated oil** /kam′fərā′tid/ [Malay, *kapur,* chalk; L, *oleum,* oil], a colorless to yellowish liquid with the penetrating, pungent odor of camphor. It is derived from a combination of a dozen organic chemicals, including terpenes, safrole, and acetaldehyde obtained from the camphor laurel plant. It is used mainly as a liniment, counterirritant, and rubefacient.

**camphor bath,** an air bath in which the air is filled with camphor vapor.

**camphor liniment,** a pharmaceutic preparation of 12.5% camphor, with alcohol, lavender oil, and ammonia, used as a rubefacient in the relief of rheumatic symptoms. See also **camphorated oil.**

**camphor poisoning,** a severe toxic condition resulting from the accidental ingestion of camphorated oils. Symptoms may include headache, hallucinations, nausea, vomiting, diarrhea, convulsions, and kidney failure.

**camphor salicylate,** a crystalline substance formed by the fusion of 84 parts of camphor and 65 parts of salicylic acid, previously used in skin ointments and administered internally for diarrhea.

**campimeter** /kampim′ətər/, (in ophthalmology) an instrument for determining the integrity of the central field of vision.

**camptocormia** /kamp′tōkôr′mē·ə/, a condition in which the back is habitually tilted forward although the spinal column remains flexible. It is frequently diagnosed as a psychologic conversion, and there is often a history of trauma.

**camptodactyly** /kamp′tədak′təlē/ [Gk, *kamptos,* bent, *daktylos,* finger], the permanent flexion of one or more fingers. —**camptodactylic,** *adj.*

**camptomelia** /kamp′təmē′lyə/ [Gk, *kamptos,* bent, *melos,* arm], a congenital anomaly characterized by bending of one or more limbs, causing permanent bowing or curving of the affected area. —**camptomelic,** *adj.*

*Campylobacter* [Gk, *campylos,* curved, *bakterion,* small staff], a genus of bacteria found in the family Spirillaceae. The organisms consist of gram-negative, nonspore-forming, spirally curved motile rods that have a single polar flagellum at either or both ends of the cell. They move in a characteristic coillike motion. The organisms require little or no oxygen for growth. The type species is *C. fetus,* which consists of several subspecies that cause human infections, as well as abortion and infertility in cattle. Also called *Vibrio fetus.*

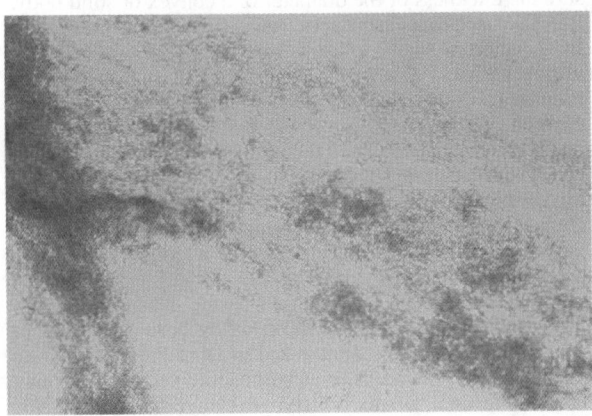

***Campylobacter*** *(Mahon and Manuselis, 2000)*

**campylobacteriosis** /kam′pə·lō·bak·tēr′ē·ō′sis/, infection with organisms of the genus *Campylobacter.*

*Campylobacter pylori.* See *Helicobacter pylori.*

**camsylate,** shortened word form for *camphorsulfonate.*

**Camurati-Engelmann disease** [Mario Camurati, Italian physician, 1896–1948; Guido Engelmann, twentieth-century Czechoslovakian surgeon], an inherited disorder of bone development marked by an onset of symptoms of muscular pain, weakness, and wasting, mainly in the legs, during childhood. The symptoms vary individually from mild to disabling. Radiographic examination usually reveals thickening of the periosteal and medullary surfaces of the diaphyseal edges of the long bones. In some cases compression of nerve tissue may occur. The symptoms usually subside during early adulthood. Also called **diaphyseal dysplasia.**

**Canadian Association of Occupational Therapists.** See **CAOT.**

**Canadian Association of University Schools of Nursing (CAUSN),** a national Canadian organization of baccalaureate and higher degree programs in nursing in Canada. It includes an accreditation system established in 1987.

**Canadian Association of University Teachers (CAUT),** a Canadian national organization representing the interests of all who teach in the universities of the provinces and territories of Canada. The official languages of the CAUT are English and French.

**Canadian crutch,** a wooden or metal device that helps a patient with impaired mobility to stand or walk. It consists of two uprights with a crosspiece to accommodate the hand and a concave crosspiece that fits the upper arm for support.

***Canadian Journal of Public Health (CJPH),*** the official publication of the Canadian Public Health Association.

***Canadian Medical Association Journal (CMAJ),*** the official publication of the Canadian Medical Association.

**Canadian Nurses Association (CNA),** the official national organization for the professional registered nurses of Canada who are members of the nine provincial nurses' associations, the Northwest Territories Registered Nurses Association, and the Yukon Registered Nurses Association. The CNA, a federation of these 11 associations, is supported by membership fees from the association members. The chief objective of the CNA is to promote high standards of nursing practice, education, research, and administration in order to achieve high quality of nursing care in the interest of the people of Canada. It is concerned with the standards of education for nurses, social and economic welfare of nurses, advancement of competence and expertise within the profession, promotion of unity and understanding among the members, and national and international representation of the organized profession of nurses. A board of elected directors and a permanent staff working at CNA House in Ottawa manage the affairs of the organization. Among the services provided are a research and advisory unit that studies trends in nursing and health and prepares briefs, when necessary; a national library containing reference works, the national and international archives of nursing, and up-to-date lists of educational programs in nursing; an information service that collects and disseminates information about nursing and publishes *The Canadian Nurse* and *L'infirmière Canadienne;* a labor relations service; a certification program; a testing service; a governmental liaison service; and an international service that facilitates a working relationship with various organizations such as the World Health Organization and the Pan American Health Organization. All services are provided in the two official languages of Canada, English and French. The CNA is a member of the International Council of Nursing.

**Canadian Nurses Association Testing Service (CNATS),** the organizational affiliate of the Canadian Nurses Association concerned with testing graduates of approved schools of nursing to qualify them as registered nurses.

**Canadian Nurses Foundation (CNF),** a national Canadian foundation organized to support scholarship in nursing. The CNF awards financial support to nurses undertaking baccalaureate and graduate studies in nursing and to nurses conducting research in nursing.

**Canadian Nurses Respiratory Society (CNRS),** an organization of nurses working with or interested in alleviating the problems of respiratory disease. The CNRS is an affiliate of the Canadian Nurses Association, and it is a section of the Canadian Lung Association.

**Canadian Orthopedic Nurses Association (CONA),** a national Canadian organization concerned with the nursing care of orthopedic patients and the continuing education of nurses working in orthopedics. Membership includes orthopedic nurses and other professionals concerned with orthopedics.

**Canadian Public Health Association (CPHA),** a national Canadian organization concerned with issues in public health and epidemiology. Membership is open to professionals and to others interested in these issues.

**canal** /kənal′/ [L, *canalis,* channel], **1.** (in anatomy) a narrow tube or channel. Some kinds of canals are **adductor canal, Alcock's canal,** and **alveolar canal. 2.** (in dentistry) one of the accessory root canals and collateral pulp canals in the teeth.

**canal debridement.** See **epithelial debridement.**

**canalicular** /kan′əlik′yələr/, pertaining to a small canal.

**canaliculus** /kan′əlik′yələs/, *pl.* **canaliculi** [L, little channel], a very small tube or channel, such as the microscopic haversian canaliculi throughout bone tissue.

**canalization** /kan′əlīzā′shən/, the formation of canals or passages through any tissue.

**canal obturation,** in root canal therapy, the filling of the pulp, or root, canal completely and densely with a nonirritating hermetic sealing agent. Also called **root canal filling.** See also **root canal therapy.**

**canal of Corti** [Alfonso Corti, Italian anatomist, 1822–1888], a space between the inner and outer rods and the basilar membrane of the cochlea in the organ of Corti. Also called **Corti's tunnel.**

**canal of Schlemm** /shlem/ [Friedrich Schlemm, German anatomist, 1795–1858], a tiny vein at the angle of the anterior chamber of the eye that connects with the pectinate villi, draining the aqueous humor and funneling it into the bloodstream. Also called **Schlemm's canal.**

**canavanine** /kan′əvan′in/, an amino acid antagonist present in alfalfa sprouts in concentrations of about 15,000 parts per million (ppm), or 1.5% by weight. Canavanine can displace arginine in cellular proteins, thereby rendering them inactive.

**cancellous** /kan′siləs/ [L, *cancellus,* lattice], (of tissue) latticelike, porous, spongy. Cancellous tissue is normally present in the interior of many bones, where the spaces are usually filled with marrow.

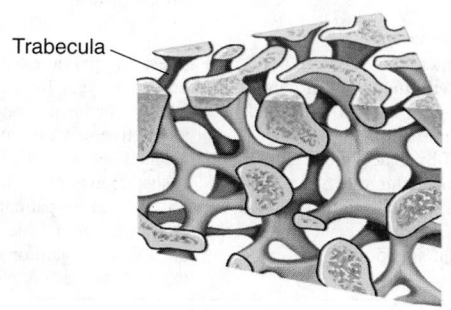

Trabecula

**Cancellous bone**

**cancellous bone,** a reticular latticelike arrangement of bony plates and trabeculae occurring at the ends of the long bones. Also called **spongy bone** spongy tissue of bone.

**cancer** /kan′sər/ [L, crab],    **1.** a neoplasm characterized by the uncontrolled growth of anaplastic cells that tend to invade surrounding tissue and to metastasize to distant body sites. **2.** any of a large group of malignant neoplastic diseases characterized by the presence of malignant cells. Each cancer is distinguished by the nature, site, or clinical course of the lesion. The basis of cancer is believed to reside in alterations in deoxyribonucleic acid (genes), usually at several loci, but many potential causes are recognized. More than 80% of cancer cases are attributed to cigarette smoking, exposure to carcinogenic chemicals, ionizing radiation, and ultraviolet rays. Many viruses induce malignant tumors in animals; an infectious cause is likely in some human cancers and *Helicobacter pylori* bacterium probably causes gastric cancer. An excessive rate of malignant tumors in organ transplantation recipients after immunosuppressive therapy indicates that the immune system plays a major role in controlling the proliferation of anaplastic cells. The incidence of different kinds of cancer varies markedly with gender, age, ethnic group, and geographic location. Cancer is second only to heart disease as a cause of mortality in the United States and is a leading cause of death in children between 3 and 14 years of age. In the United States, common sites for the development of malignant tumors are the skin, lung, prostate, breast, and colon. Surgery remains the major form of treatment, but irradiation is widely used as preoperative, postoperative, or primary therapy; chemotherapy, with single or multiple antineoplastic agents, is often highly effective. Many malignant lesions are curable if detected in the early stage.

### Screening for specific cancer sites

| High-risk profile | Screening | Medium- and low-risk profile | Screening |
|---|---|---|---|
| **Lung cancer** | | | |
| History of 20 pack-years of smoking (1 pack a day for 20 years); exposure to airborne carcinogens, especially asbestos, uranium, hydrocarbons; age range 40 to 80 years; chronic lung disease | Early detection method not available; annual chest x-ray studies (advised by some physicians); observation by patient for change in respiratory status; increased frequency of infections and change in cough, sputum, breathing, voice | History of less than 20 pack-years of smoking, nonsmokers exposed to passive cigarette smoke from smokers, nonsmokers, former smokers after 10 years | Early detection method not available |
| **Colon and rectal cancer** | | | |
| History of familial polyposis, ulcerative colitis, Crohn's disease; personal or family history of colon or rectal cancer; diet high in fat and low in fiber; age range 40 to 75 years | Guaiac test on stools and digital rectal examination annually after age 40; sigmoidoscopic examination every 3 to 5 years with beginning age based on advice of physician; observation by patient for changes in bowel pattern: diarrhea, constipation, pain, flatus, black tarry stools, bleeding | Persons with no known risk factors | Guaiac test on stools and digital rectal examination annually after age 40; sigmoidoscopy, preferably flexible, as a baseline at age 50; after two normal examinations, repeated proctosigmoidoscopic examination every 3 to 5 years |
| **Prostatic cancer** | | | |
| Presence of prostatic hyperplasia, presence of prostatic infection, African-American, increased risk with age | Digital rectal examination and prostate-specific antigen blood test annually age 50 and over; observation by patient for dysuria, blood in urine, difficulty in producing stream of urine | Presence of one risk factor, excluding age | Digital rectal examination and prostate-specific antigen blood test annually age 50 and over |
| **Cervical cancer** | | | |
| Early intercourse (before age 18) with multiple partners or with partners who have had multiple partners, poor personal hygiene, infected with human immunodeficiency virus, genital warts, chlamydia, gonorrhea, cervical dysplasia, smoking | Pap test and pelvic examination every year for women who are or have been sexually active or who have reached age 18; colposcopy if suspicious area is noted; observation by patient for abnormal vaginal bleeding or discharge, pain or bleeding with sexual intercourse | No known risk factors | Pap test and pelvic examination every year after age 18; after 3 or more normal examinations in a row, at least every 3 years. Pap test may be performed less frequently at the discretion of the physician |

From Lewis SL et al: *Medical surgical nursing: assessment & management of clinical problems,* ed 5, St Louis, 2000, Mosby. Based on the American Cancer Society's 1996 recommendations.

## Screening for specific cancer sites—cont'd

| High-risk profile | Screening | Medium- and low-risk profile | Screening |
|---|---|---|---|
| **Endometrial cancer** | | | |
| Infertility, never having children, early menarche, late menopause, ovarian dysfunction, obesity, uterine bleeding, estrogen replacement therapy and tamoxifen over long period of time, diabetes, hypertension, gallbladder disease, exposure to pelvic radiation, over age 50 | Pap test every year; pelvic examination every year; endometrial biopsy for women at menopause and at high risk; observation by patient for abnormal uterine bleeding, pain, change in menstrual pattern | Presence of one risk factor, excluding estrogen therapy, over long period of time | Pap test and pelvic examination, observation by patient for abnormal uterine bleeding, pain, change in menstrual pattern |
| **Skin cancer** | | | |
| Prolonged exposure to sun; three or more blistering sunburns during adolescence; previous radiation exposure; fair, thin skin; positive family history of dysplastic nevus syndrome | Self-examination monthly; physical examination every year; observation by patient for sore that does not heal, change in size, shape, or color of wart or mole | Presence of one risk factor, excluding prolonged exposure to sun | Self-examination, physical examination each year; observation by patient for sore that does not heal, change in size, shape, or color of wart or mole |
| **Breast cancer** | | | |
| Caucasian, early menarche, late menopause, fibrocystic breast disease, infertility, over age 30 for first pregnancy, personal history of breast cancer, mother or sister with history of breast cancer, obesity, age range 35 to 65 | Monthly breast self-examination; breast examination by health professional every 3 years for women age 20 to 40 and every year after age 40; baseline mammogram at age 40; every 1 to 2 years between ages 40 and 49, and every year after age 49; observation by patient for lump or thickening discharge from nipple, pain in breast | Excluding family history of breast cancer, fewer than two risk factors | Monthly breast self-examination; breast examination by health professional every 3 years for women age 20 to 40 and every year after age 40; baseline mammogram at age 40, every 1 to 2 years between ages 40 and 49, and every year after age 49; observation by patient for lump or thickening discharge from nipple, pain in breast |

### Cancer's seven warning signals

- Change in bowel or bladder habits
- A sore that will not heal
- Unusual bleeding or discharge
- Thickening or lump in breast or elsewhere
- Indigestion or difficulty swallowing
- Obvious change in a wart or mole
- Nagging cough or hoarseness

From Cancer facts and figures 1990, Atlanta, 1990, American Cancer Society.

**cancer bodies.** See **Russell's bodies.**

**cancericidal** /kan′sərisī′dəl/ [L, *cancer,* crab, *caedere,* to kill], pertaining to a substance or procedure capable of destroying cancer cells.

**cancerigenic.** See **carcinogenic.**

**cancer in situ.** See **carcinoma in situ.**

**cancer of the small intestine,** a neoplastic disease of the duodenum, jejunum, or ileum. Its characteristics vary, depending on the kind of tumor and the site, but may include abdominal pain, vomiting, weight loss, diarrhea, intermittent bowel obstruction, GI bleeding, or a mass in the right abdomen. Diagnosis typically is made with barium radiographic examination, but results of such studies may be inconclusive until lesions are large. Adenocarcinomas, the most common tumors, occur more frequently in the duodenum or upper jejunum and form polypoid or constricting napkin-ring growths. Lymphomas, found most often in the lower small intestine, may impair bowel motility by invading nerves and in some cases are associated with a malabsorption syndrome. Less common tumors of the small intestine are carcinoids, usually found in the ileum, and sarcomas, including Kaposi's sarcoma, usually seen in the jejunum and ileum. A leiomyosarcoma may sometimes form a large extraluminal mass. Surgery, including a wide resection of mesenteric lymph nodes, is typically indicated for adenocarcinomas and carcinoids. Irradiation occasionally is indicated. Chemotherapy is often useful, particularly for lymphoma.

**cancerous** /kan′sərəs/ [L, crab, *oma,* tumor], pertaining to or resembling a cancer.

**cancer staging,** a system for describing the size and extent of spread of a malignant tumor, used to plan treatment and predict prognosis. Staging may involve a physical examination, diagnostic procedures, surgical exploration, and histologic examination. The system developed by the American Joint Committee for Cancer Staging and End Results Reporting uses the letter $T$ to represent the tumor, $N$ for the regional lymph node involvement, $M$ for distant metastases, and numeric subscripts in each category to indicate the de-

## Risk factors for major cancers

**Lung**
Cigarette smoking
Exposure to some industrial chemicals (e.g., arsenic, asbestos)
Radiation exposure, including radon
Secondhand smoke

**Colon-rectum**
Personal or family history of cancer of polyps of colon or
  rectum
Inflammatory bowel disease
High-fat and/or low-fiber diet

**Breast**
Age over 40
Personal or family history of breast cancer
Early age at menarche
Late age at menopause
Never had children or late age at first birth
Higher education and socioeconomic status
High-fat diet

**Prostate**
Increasing age
Living in northwestern Europe or North America
African-American
Family history of prostate cancer
High-fat diet

**Uterus (cervix)**
Early age at first intercourse
Multiple sex partners
Cigarette smoking
Infection with human papillomavirus
Low socioeconomic status

**Uterus (endometrium)**
Early menarche
Late menopause
History of infertility
Failure to ovulate
Unopposed estrogen therapy (without progesterone)
Obesity, diabetes, gallbladder disease, or hypertension

**Ovary**
Increasing age
Never had children
Personal history of breast cancer
Family history of ovarian cancer

**Mouth**
Cigarette, cigar, pipe smoking
Smokeless tobacco
Excessive drinking of alcohol

**Skin**
Excessive exposure to ultraviolet radiation
Fair complexion
Occupational exposure to coal tar, pitch, creosote, arsenic, or
  radium
Family history of skin cancer

**Bladder**
Cigarette smoking
Urban living
Exposure to dye, rubber, or leather

**Stomach**
Diet heavy in smoked, salted, or pickled foods
Family history of stomach cancer

Harkness GA, Dincher JR: *Medical-surgical nursing,* ed 10, St Louis, 1999, Mosby.

## Summary of American Cancer Society recommendations for the early detection of cancer in asymptomatic people

| Site | Recommendation |
| --- | --- |
| Cancer-related checkup | A cancer-related checkup is recommended every 3 years for people aged 20-40 and every year for people age 40 and older. This examination should include health counseling and depending on a person's age, might include examinations for cancers of the thyroid, oral cavity, skin, lymph nodes, testes, and ovaries, as well as for some nonmalignant diseases. |
| Breast | Women age 40 and older should have an annual mammogram, an annual clinical breast examination by a health care professional and should perform monthly breast self-examination. The CBE should be conducted close to scheduled mammogram. Women ages 20-39 should have a clinical breast examination by a health care professional every 3 years and should perform monthly breast self-examination. |
| Colon and rectum | Beginning at age 50, men and women should follow one of the examination schedules below:<br>• A fecal occult blood test every year and a flexible sigmoidoscopy every 5 years.*<br>• A colonoscopy every 10 years.*<br>• A double-contrast barium enema every 5 to 10 years.* |
| Prostate | The ACS recommends that both the prostate-specific antigen (PSA) blood test and the digital rectal examination be offered annually, beginning at age 50, to men who have a life expectancy of at least 10 years and to younger men who are at high risk. Men in high-risk groups, such as those with a strong familial predisposition (i.e., two or more affected first-degree relatives), or African-Americans may begin at a younger age (i.e., 45 years). |
| Uterus | *Cervix:* All women who are or have been sexually active or who are 18 and older should have an annual Pap test and pelvic examination. After three or more consecutive satisfactory examinations with normal findings, the Pap test may be performed less frequently. Discuss the matter with your physician.<br>*Endometrium:* Women at high risk for cancer of the uterus should have a sample of endometrial tissue examined when menopause begins. |

From Cancer facts and figures 2000, Atlanta, 2000, American Cancer Society.
*A digital rectal examination should be done at the same time as sigmoidoscopy, colonoscopy, or double-contrast barium enema. People who are at moderate or high risk for colorectal cancer should talk with a doctor about a different testing schedule.

gree of dissemination. According to this system $T_1N_0M_0$ designates a small localized tumor; $T_2N_1M_0$ is a larger primary tumor that has extended to regional nodes; and $T_4N_3M_3$ is a very large lesion involving regional nodes and distant sites.

**cancr-, cancri-, cancro-,** combining form meaning 'cancer': *cancriform, cancroid.*

**cancriform** /kang′krifôrm′/ [L, crab, *forma,* form], pertaining to a lesion resembling a cancer.

**cancroid** [L, crab; Gk, *eidos,* form], **1.** pertaining to a lesion resembling a cancer. **2.** a moderately malignant skin cancer.

**cancrum** /kang′krəm/, a gangrenous ulcerative condition, often associated with rhinitis in children.

**candela.** See **candle.**

**candesartan,** an antihypertensive.

■ INDICATIONS: This drug is used to treat hypertension, either alone or in combination with other drugs.

■ CONTRAINDICATIONS: Known hypersensitivity to this drug prohibits its use.

■ ADVERSE EFFECTS: Angioedema is a potentially life-threatening side effect of this drug. Dizziness, diarrhea, cough, and upper respiratory infection are common side effects. Other side effects include fatigue, headache, nausea, arthralgia, and pain.

**Candida** /kan′didə/ [L, *candidus,* white], a genus of yeast-like fungi including the common pathogen *Candida albicans.*

**Candida albicans** /al′bəkanz/, a common budding, yeast-like microscopic fungal organism normally present in the mucous membranes of the mouth, intestinal tract, and vagina of healthy people. Under certain circumstances, it may cause superficial infections of the skin, mouth, or vagina. Infection of the esophagus and severe invasive systemic infections may occur in persons with human immunodeficiency virus (HIV). See also **candidiasis.**

**Candida guilliermondii,** a species that sometimes causes cutaneous candidiasis, onychomycosis, meningitis, and endocarditis.

**Candida krusei,** a species occasionally associated with candidiasis, esophagitis, endocarditis, and vaginitis.

**Candida lusitaniae,** a species that causes opportunistic infections in humans.

**candidal vaginitis, candidal vulvovaginitis.** See **vulvovaginal candidiasis.**

**Candida peritonitis,** peritonitis caused by a species of *Candida,* usually as a complication of peritoneal dialysis; symptoms include abdominal pain with or without mild fever, nausea, and vomiting.

**Candida pneumonia.** See **pulmonary candidiasis.**

**Candida pseudotropicalis,** a species that sometimes causes *Candida* vaginitis.

**Candida stellatoidea,** a species that sometimes causes *Candida* vaginitis or endocarditis; some authorities consider it a variant of *Candida albicans.*

**Candida vaginitis, Candida vulvovaginitis.** See **vulvovaginal candidiasis.**

**candidiasis** /kan′didī′əsis/ [L, *candidus* + Gk, *osis,* condition], any infection caused by a species of *Candida,* usually *Candida albicans.* It is characterized by pruritus, a white exudate, peeling, and easy bleeding. Diaper rash, intertrigo, vaginitis, and thrush are common topical manifestations of candidiasis. Endocarditis and infection of the kidney, spleen, liver, and lungs sometimes occur in debilitated patients. Treatment includes the oral and topical administration of antifungal drugs such as nystatin and clotrimazole and, for more severe infections, amphotericin B or fluconazole. Oral candidiasis without a history of recent antibiotic therapy, cytoxic therapy, corticosteroid therapy, radiation therapy to the head and neck or other immunosuppressive disorder may indicate the possibility of human immunodeficiency virus infection. Also called **candidosis, moniliasis.**

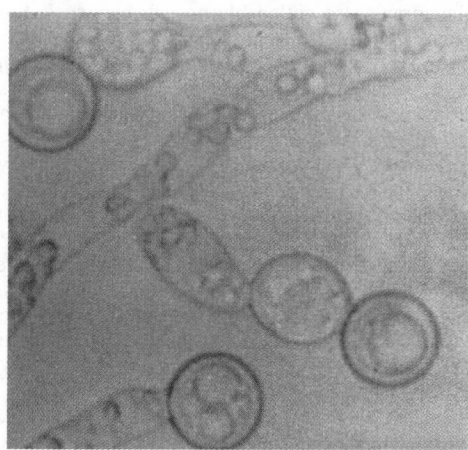

**Candida albicans**
*(Zitelli and Davis, 1997/courtesy Dr. Ellen Wald, Children's Hospital of Pittsburgh)*

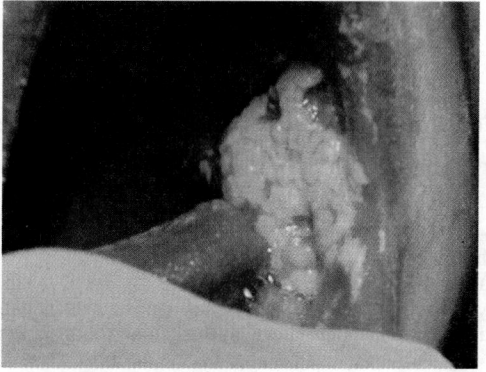

**Oral candidiasis** *(Zitelli and Davis, 1997)*

**Candida endocarditis,** mycotic endocarditis caused by a species of *Candida;* also called **endocardial candidiasis.**

**Candida glabrata.** See *Torulopsis glabrata.*

**Candiru fever** /kan′dirōō′/, an arbovirus infection transmitted to humans by the bite of a sandfly. It is characterized by an acute fever, headache, and muscle aches. Recovery occurs, without treatment, within a few days. The infection occurs mainly in the forests of Brazil. See also **arbovirus, phlebotomus fever.**

**candle** [L, *candela,* light], (in optics) the basic unit of measurement for luminous intensity, equal to 1/60 of the luminous intensity of a square centimeter of a black body heated to 1773.5° C or the solidification temperature of platinum, adopted in 1948 as the international standard of luminous intensity. Also called **candela** /kandē′lə/.

**candle power.**  See **CP.**

**candy-striper,**  *informal,* a hospital volunteer, named for the striped pink and white uniforms traditionally worn by the young people who perform this service.

**cane** [Ar, *qanah,* reed],  a sturdy wooden or metal shaft or walking stick used to give support and mobility during walking to a person with impaired mobility. A cane should be of an appropriate length to allow a person with an injured leg to walk with it held on the side of the sound leg. In walking, the person may rest his or her weight on the cane and the injured leg while moving the unaffected leg forward. To take the next step, the weight is placed on the sound leg while the injured leg and cane are moved forward. The cane should allow 25 degrees of elbow flexion.

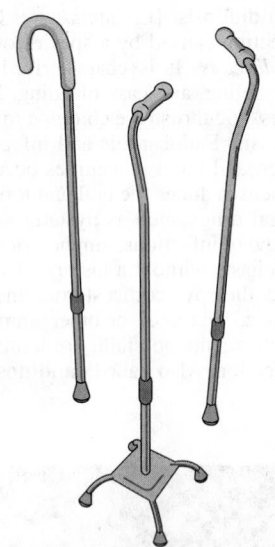

**Single and quad-foot canes** *(Beare and Myers, 1998)*

**cane-cutter's cramp.**  See **heat cramp.**

**canefield fever.**  See **field fever.**

**canine fossa** /kā′nīn/ [L, *canis,* dog; L, ditch],  (in dentistry) either of the wide depressions on the external surface of each maxilla, superolateral to the canine tooth socket. It is the origin of the levator anguli oris muscle. Also called **maxillary fossa.**

**canine tooth,**  any of the four teeth, one on each side of the upper and lower jaws, situated between the lateral incisor and the first premolar. The canine teeth are larger and stronger than the incisors and have characteristics of both anterior and posterior teeth. They project beyond the level of the other teeth in both arches. Their roots sink deeply into the bones, causing marked prominences on the alveolar arch. The upper (maxillary) canine teeth, or eye teeth, are larger and longer than the lower ones and have a distinct basal ridge. The lower (mandibular) canine teeth, or stomach teeth, are situated nearer the midline than the upper ones, and their summits (cuspal edges) correspond to the in-

tervals between the upper canines and incisors. The crowns of the canines are very large and conic and taper to blunted points or cusps. The deciduous canines erupt about 16 to 20 months after birth, whereas the permanent canines errupt during the eleventh or twelfth year of life.

**canities** /kanish′i·ēz/,  loss of pigment, as in the graying of hair or the appearance of white streaks in the nails.

**canker** /kang′kər/ [L, *cancer,* crab],  an ulcer or sore in the mouth or genitals. Also called **aphthous stomatitis, chancre.**

**canker sore,**  an ulcerous lesion of the mouth, characteristic of aphthous stomatitis. See also **aphthous stomatitis.**

**cannabis** /kan′əbis/ [Gk, *kannabis,* hemp],  a psychoactive herb derived from the flowering tops of hemp plants. It has no currently acceptable clinical use in the United States (where is is marketed as marinol) but has been used in the treatment of glaucoma and as an antiemetic in some cancer patients to counter the nausea and vomiting associated with chemotherapy. Cannabis is controlled under Schedule I of the Controlled Substances Act of 1970. All parts of the plant contain psychoactive substances. Cannabinoids, or psychoactive substances synthesized by the hemp plant include cannabinol, cannabidiol, cannabinolic acid, cannabigerol, cannabicyclol, and several isomers of tetrahydrocannabinol (THC). THC is believed to cause the most characteristic psychologic effects, which include alterations of mood, memory, motor coordination, cognitive ability, and self-perception. Low doses of cannabis seldom impair the ability to perform simple motor tasks but commonly hinder more complex actions, as driving and flying, which involve complex sensory perception, concentration, and information processing. Cannabis may also enhance the nondominant senses of touch, taste, and smell. Higher doses in some persons can produce delusions, paranoid feelings, anxiety, and panic. This drug also increases the heart rate and systolic blood pressure. Marijuana is about three times more powerful when smoked than when taken orally. Research indicates that some cannabinoids may be therapeutic as anticonvulsants and helpful in reducing intraocular pressure associated with glaucoma. Also called **bhang, ganja, grass, hashish, marijuana, pot, reefer, tea, weed.**

**cannabism** /kan′əbiz′əm/,  a condition associated with excessive or extended use of cannabis (marijuana) drugs. It is characterized by anxiety, disorientation, hallucinations, memory defects, and paranoia.

**cannon A wave** [L, *cane,* tube; AS, *wafian*],  a powerful atrial wave in the jugular venous pulse, caused by the contraction of the right atrium against a closed tricuspid valve. Rapid, regular cannon A waves (the "frog sign") are diagnostic of paroxysmal supraventricular tachycardia. Irregular cannon A waves are seen in atrioventricular (AV) dissociation and are therefore especially helpful in the diagnosis of ventricular tachycardia, which includes AV dissociation in 50% of cases.

**cannula** /kan′yələ/, *pl.* **cannulas, cannulae** [L, small tube],  a flexible tube that may be inserted into a duct or cavity to deliver medication or drain fluid. It may be guided by a sharp, pointed instrument (trocar). A body fluid may be passed through the cannula to the outside. —**cannular, cannulate,** *adj.* See also **nasal cannula.**

**cannulation** /kan′yələ′shən/,  the insertion of a cannula into a body duct or cavity, as into the trachea, bladder, or a blood vessel. Also called cannulization. —**cannulate, cannulize,** *v.*

**cantering rhythm** [*Canterbury gallop;* Gk, *rhythmos,* beat],  a pattern of three heart sounds in each cardiac cycle, resembling the canter of a horse. See also **gallop rhythm.**

**cantharides.** See **cantharis.**

**cantharis** /kan′thäris/, *pl.* **cantharides** /kanther′idēz/ [Gk, *kantharis,* beetle], the dried insect *Cantharis vesicatoria* which contains cantharidin, formerly used as a topical vesicant. Also called **Spanish fly.**

**canthi, canthic.** See **canthus.**

**cantho-,** combining form meaning 'canthus (the corner of the eye)': *cantholysis, canthotomy.*

**canthoplasty** /kan′thōplas′tē/, a form of plastic surgery used to lengthen the palpebral fissure through the lateral canthus or to restore a defective canthus, which is the juncture of eyelids.

**canthorraphy** /kanthôr′əfē/, surgery to suture the eyelids at either canthus.

**canthus** /kan′thəs/, *pl.* **canthi** [Gk, *kanthus,* corner of the eye], the angle at the medial and the lateral margins of the eyelids. The medial canthus opens into a small space containing the opening to a lacrimal duct. Also called **palpebral commissure.** —**canthic,** *adj.*

**Cantil,** trademark for an anticholinergic antispasmodic (mepenzolate bromide).

**Cantor tube** [Meyer O. Cantor, American physician, b. 1907], a long, single-lumen nasoenteric tube with a small, mercury-filled bag at the distal end, used to relieve obstructions in the small intestine. The tube also contains drainage holes to allow for aspiration of intestinal contents.

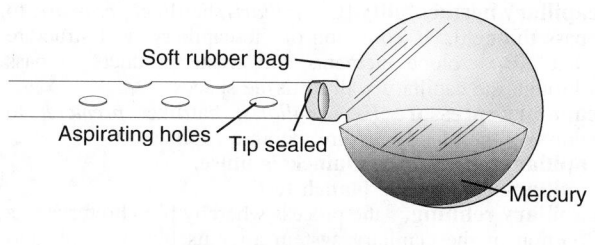

Soft rubber bag
Aspirating holes — Tip sealed
Mercury

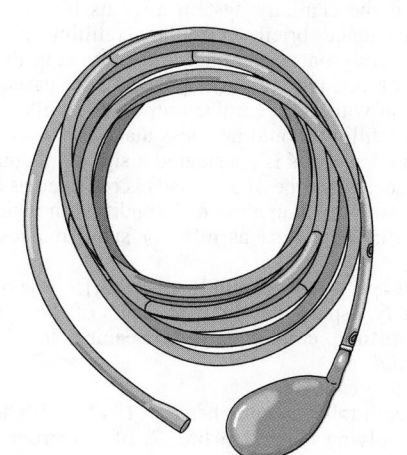

**Cantor tube** *(Lewis, Heitkemper, and Dirksen, 2000)*

**CaO,** chemical formula for calcium oxide.

**Ca(OH)₂,** chemical formula for calcium hydroxide.

**CAOT,** abbreviation for *Canadian Association of Occupational Therapists.*

**cap,** abbreviation for Latin *capiat,* 'let him or her take,' used in prescriptions.

**CAP, 1.** abbreviation for **College of American Pathologists. 2.** (in molecular genetics) abbreviation for **catabolic activator protein.** CAP participates in initiating the transcription of ribonucleic acid in organisms without a true nucleus, as bacteria.

**capacitance** /kəpas′ətəns/, a measure of electrostatic capacity or the amount of stored electrical charge per unit of electrical potential.

**capacitance vessels** [L, *capacitas,* capacity], **1.** the blood vessels that hold the major portion of the intravascular blood volume. **2.** the veins.

**capacitation** /kəpas′itā′shən/, the process in which the spermatozoon, after it reaches the ampulla of the fallopian tube, undergoes a series of changes that lead to its ability to fertilize an ovum.

**capacity** /kə·pas′i·tē/ [L, *capacitas*], **1.** power or ability to hold, retain, or contain, or the ability to absorb. **2.** the volume or potential volume of material (solid, liquid, or gas) that can be held or contained. **3.** see **capacitance,** mental ability to receive, accomplish, endure, or understand.

**capacity factor** /kəpas′itē/ [L, *capacitas + factum,* to make], the ratio of the elution volume of a substance to the void volume in the column.

**Capastat,** trademark for an antibiotic (capreomycin).

**CAPD,** abbreviation for **continuous ambulatory peritoneal dialysis.**

**Capdepont-Hodge syndrome.** See **dentinogenesis imperfecta.**

**capecitabine,** an antineoplastic and antimetabolite.

■ INDICATIONS: This drug is used to treat metastatic breast cancer.

■ CONTRAINDICATIONS: Pregnancy and known hypersensitivity to 5-fluorouracil prohibit this drug's use. Capecitabine also should not be used in infants.

■ ADVERSE EFFECTS: Life-threatening effects of this drug include neutropenia, lymphopenia, thrombocytopenia, and myelosuppression. Other serious adverse effects include anemia, hyperbilirubinemia, and edema. Common side effects include nausea, vomiting, anorexia, diarrhea, and stomatitis.

**capeline bandage** /kap′əlin/ [Fr, hooded cape], a covering applied like a cap. It is used for protecting the head, shoulder, or a stump. Also called **Hippocrates' bandage.**

**Capgras' syndrome** /käp·grä′/ [Jean Marie Joseph Capgras, French psychiatrist, 1873−1950], a form of delusional misidentification in which the patient believes that other persons in the environment are not their real selves but doubles.

*Capillaria* /kap′i·lar′ē·ə/ [L, *capillaris,* hairlike], a genus of nematodes of the family Trichuridae. *C. philippinensis* is a parasite of the human intestine in the Philippines. See **capillariasis.**

**capillariasis** /kap′i·lə·rī′ə·sis/, infection with nematodes of the genus *Capillaria,* species of which attack various different animals; human infection is usually by *C. philippinensis,* which infests the intestines and causes severe diarrhea, malabsorption, and often death.

**capillaries.** See **blood vessel.**

**capillaritis** /kap′ilərī′tis/ [L, *capillaris,* hairlike; Gk, *itis,* inflammation], an abnormal condition characterized by a progressive pigmentary disorder of the skin and of the capillaries without inflammation. It does not involve any systemic problems and runs a benign self-limiting course.

**capillarity.** See **capillary action.**

**capillary** /kap′iler′ē/ [L, *capillaris,* hairlike], one of the microscopic blood vessels (about 0.008 mm in diameter)

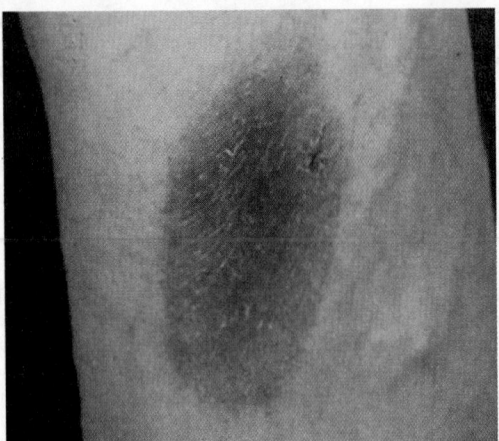

**Capillaritis** *(du Vivier, 1993)*

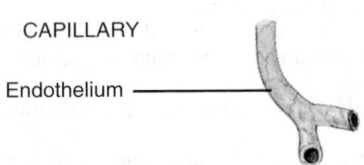

CAPILLARY

Endothelium ————

**Capillary** *(Applegate, 2000)*

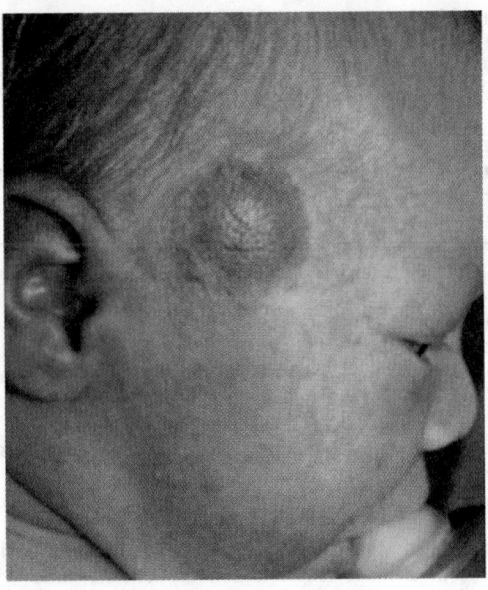

**Capillary hemangioma** *(Weston, Lane, and Morrelli, 1996)*

joining arterioles and venules. The wall consists of a single layer of endothelial cells, which are specialized squamous epithelial cells. Blood and tissue fluids exchange various substances across these walls.

**capillary action,** the process involving molecular adhesion by which the surface of a liquid in a tube is either elevated or depressed, depending on the cohesiveness of the liquid molecules. The more cohesive the molecules, the more depressed will be the surface of the liquid. Less cohesive liquid molecules will adhere to the surfaces of the tube in which they are contained and elevate the surface of the liquid. Also called **capillary attraction, capillarity.**

**capillary angioma.** See **cherry angioma.**

**capillary attraction.** See **capillary action.**

**capillary bed,** a capillary network.

**capillary flames.** See **telangiectatic nevus.**

**capillary fracture,** any thin, hairlike break in a bone.

**capillary fragility,** a condition in which weakened capillaries rupture easily when stressed, observed as bleeding under the skin.

**capillary hemangioma,** a blood-filled birthmark or benign tumor consisting of closely packed small blood vessels. Commonly found during infancy, it first grows, then may spontaneously disappear in early childhood without treatment. Surgical removal is not usually attempted unless frequent trauma and bleeding are present. However, surgery may be performed later for cosmetic reasons. Also called **hemangioma simplex, strawberry hemangioma, strawberry mark, nevus vascularis.** Compare **cavernous hemangioma, nevus flammeus.**

**capillary hemorrhage,** an oozing of blood from the capillaries.

**capillary permeability** [L, *capillaris,* hairlike, *permeare,* to pass through], a condition of the capillary wall structure that allows blood elements and waste products to pass through the capillary wall to tissue spaces.

**capillary pressure** [L, *capillaris,* hairlike, *premere,* to press], the blood pressure within a capillary.

**capillary pulse.** See **Quincke's pulse.**

**capillary refill.** See **blanch test.**

**capillary refilling,** the process whereby blood returns to a portion of the capillary system after its blood supply has been interrupted briefly. Capillary refilling is tested by pressing firmly on a fingernail and estimating the time required for blood to return after pressure is released. In a normal person with good cardiac output and digital perfusion, capillary refilling should take less than 3 seconds. A time of more than 3 seconds is considered a sign of sluggish digital circulation, and a time of 5 seconds is regarded as abnormal.

**capillary tufting,** an abnormal condition in which pulmonary capillaries project as tufts, or small masses, into the alveoli.

**capillus** /kəpil′əs/, *pl.* **capilli** [L, filament], one of the hairs of the body, especially one of the hairs of the scalp.

**capit-, capito-,** combining form meaning 'head': *capitate, capitopedal.*

**capita.** See **caput.**

**capital** /kap′i·təl/ [L, *caput,* head], **1.** of the highest importance; involving danger to life. **2.** of or pertaining to the head of the femur.

**capitate** /kap′itāt/, having the shape of a head.

**capitate bone** [L, *caput,* head; AS, *ban*], one of the largest carpal bones, located at the center of the wrist and having a rounded head that fits the concavity of the scaphoid and the lunate bones. Also called **os capitatum, os magnum.**

**capitation,** a payment method for health care services. The physician, hospital, or other health care provider is paid a contracted rate for each member assigned, referred to as "per-member-per-month" rate, regardless of the number or nature of services provided. The contractual rates are usually adjusted for age, gender, illness, and regional differences.

**capitulum** /kəpich'ələm/, *pl.* **capitula** [L, small head], a small, rounded prominence on a bone where it articulates with another bone.

**capitulum humeri** /hyōō'mərī, hōō'mərē/ [L, small head, *humerus,* shoulder], a rounded eminence at the distal end of the humerus that articulates with the radius.

**Caplan's syndrome** [Anthony Caplan, English physician, 1907–1976], a condition of pneumoconiosis with symptoms of rheumatoid arthritis and radiographic evidence of intrapulmonary nodules. Also called **rheumatoid pneumoconiosis.**

**-capnia,** suffix meaning '(condition of) carbon dioxide content in the blood': *acapnia, hypocapnia.*

**capnograph** /kap'nəgraf'/ [Gk, *kapnos,* smoke, *graphein,* to record], an instrument used in anesthesia, intensive care, and respiratory therapy to produce a capnogram, a tracing that shows the proportion of carbon dioxide in exhaled air.

**capnometry** /kapnom'ətrē/, the measurement of carbon dioxide in a volume of gas. The most common monitoring units are based on the selective absorption of infrared light by carbon dioxide and water vapor. Capnometry may also be performed using mass spectrometry. See also **end-tidal $CO_2$.**

**capotement** /käpōtmäN', kəpōt'mənt/, a splashing sound made by fluid movements in a dilated stomach.

**Capoten,** trademark for an angiotensin-converting enzyme (captopril).

**capping,** a process by which cell-surface molecules aggregate on a plasma membrane.

**capreomycin** /kap'rē·ōmī'sin/, an antibiotic and antitubercular agent.

■ INDICATIONS: It is prescribed in the treatment of pulmonary infections caused by capreomycin-susceptible strains of *Mycobacterium tuberculosis* when the primary agents are ineffective or cannot be used.

■ CONTRAINDICATIONS: Known sensitivity to this drug prohibits its use. It must be used with caution in patients with pre-existing renal or auditory impairment.

■ ADVERSE EFFECTS: Among the most serious adverse reactions are nephrotoxicity, hearing loss, tinnitus, vertigo, leukocytosis, leukopenia, urticaria, and skin rash.

**capric acid ($CH_3(CH_2)_4COOH$)** /kap'rik/ [L, *caper,* goat], a white crystalline carboxylic acid with a rancid odor, occurring as a glyceride in natural oils. Capric acid is used in the production of perfumes, flavors, wetting agents, and food additives. Also called **decanoic acid.**

**caprizant** /kap'rizant/, describing an irregular leaping or bounding pulse.

**caproic acid ($CH_3(CH_2)_4COOH$)** /kaprō'ik/, a carboxylic acid present in milk fat and some plant oils. It is used in the production of artificial flavors. Also called **hexanoic acid.**

**caps-, kaps-, capsul-, capsulo-,** prefix meaning 'capsule or container': *capsitis, capsulation, capsuloplasty.*

**capsaicin** /kap·sa'i·sin/, an alkaloid irritating to the skin and mucous membranes, the pungent active principle in capsicum. See also **capsicum.**

**capsicum,** an herbal product derived from peppers native to tropical areas of the Americas.

■ USES: This herb is used for muscle spasms, the pain of inflammation, neuromas, psoriasis, and dry mouth. It is also used as a food antioxidant and as a food seasoning.

■ CONTRAINDICATIONS: Capsicum peppers are contraindicated in those with known hypersensitivity, women who are preg-

nant or lactating, and in children until more research is available. It should not be used in open wounds or abrasions or near the eyes. Capsicum can cause extreme burns and blisters in its undiluted form.

**capsid** /kap'sid/ [L, *capsa,* box], the layer of protein enveloping the genome of a virion. A capsid is composed of structural units called capsomeres; its symmetry may be cubic or helical.

**capsomere** /kap'səmir/, one of the building blocks of a viral capsid. It consists of groups of identical protein molecules and is visible in an electron microscope.

**capsul-, capsulo-.** See **caps-.**

**capsula.** See **capsule.**

**capsular** /kap'sələr/ [L, *capsula,* little box], pertaining to or resembling a small container.

**capsular cataract** [L, *capsula* + Gk, *katarrhaktes,* waterfall], a visual opacity caused by a thickening of the epithelial cells lining the capsule. The condition is frequently the result of the aging process or a disease that involves surrounding eye tissues.

**capsular pattern,** a series of limitations of joint movement when the joint capsule is a limiting structure. An example is the range in glenohumeral joints, from flexion as the least limited movement to external rotation as the most limited movement. It occurs only in synovial joints that are controlled by muscles and not in joints that depend primarily on ligamentous stability, such as the sacroiliac.

**capsular swelling test.** See **quellung reaction.**

**capsulation** /kap'syōō·lā'shən/ [L, *capsula,* little box], the enclosure of a medicine in a capsule.

**capsule** /kap'syəl, kap'səl/ [L, *capsula,* little box], **1.** a small soluble container, usually made of gelatin, used for enclosing a dose of medication for swallowing. Compare **tablet. 2.** a membranous shell surrounding certain microorganisms, such as the pneumococcus bacterium. **3.** a well-defined anatomic structure that encloses an organ or part, such as the capsule of the adrenal gland. Also called **capsula** (*pl.* **capsuli**).

**capsulectomy** /kap'səlek'təmē/, the surgical excision of a capsule, usually the capsule of a joint or of the lens of the eye.

**capsule of Tenon.** See **fascia bulbi.**

**capsule of the kidney,** the fibrous connective enclosure of the kidney. Fatty tissue covers the fibrous capsule and helps protect the organ from bumps and shocks. It also encloses the adrenal glands. Compare **Bowman's capsule.**

**capsule of the lens.** See **lens capsule.**

**capsuli.** See **capsule.**

**capsulitis** /-ī'tis/ [L, *capsula,* little box; Gk, *itis,* inflammation], an inflammation involving any anatomic capsule.

**capsuloma** /kap'səlō'mə/, *pl.* **capsulomas, capsulomata** [L, *capsula* + Gk, *oma,* tumor], a neoplasm of the capsule or the subcapsular area of the kidney.

**capsuloplasty** /kap'səlōplas'tē/, plastic surgery performed on the capsule of a joint.

**capsulorraphy** /kap'səlôr'əfē/, surgical repair of a tear in the capsule of a joint.

**capsulorrhexis** /kap'səlôrek'sis/, a surgical technique in which a continuous circular tear in the anterior capsule is made in the crystalline lens to allow phacoemulsification of the lens nucleus during cataract surgery.

**capsulotomy** /kap'səlot'əmē/ [L, *capsula* + Gk, *temnein,* to cut], an incision into a capsule, such as in an operation to remove a cataract.

**captain-of-the-ship doctrine,** the historical medicolegal principle that the physician is ultimately responsible for all patient-care activities; he or she thus may be held accountable and may be sued for negligence or malpractice when the act at issue is performed by an employee or other person under the physician's control, even if not ordered by the physician.

**captive reinsurance company,** a reinsurance company organized to serve only one client.

**captopril** /kap′tōpril/, an angiotensin-converting enzyme inhibitor.

■ INDICATION: It is prescribed for the treatment of hypertension and congestive heart failure.

■ CONTRAINDICATION: Known sensitivity to this drug prohibits its use.

■ ADVERSE EFFECTS: Among the most serious adverse reactions are hypotension, proteinuria, renal failure, neutropenia, agranulocytosis, angioneurotic edema, angina, myocardial infarction, Raynaud's disease, cough, hyperkalemia, and congestive heart failure.

**capture** /kap′chər/, **1.** the catching and holding of a nuclear particle, as an electron, or an electrical impulse originating elsewhere. **2.** (in cardiology) the capture of control of the atria or ventricles after a period of independent beating caused by ectopic beats or an atrioventricular block.

**capture beat,** the return of atrial control over ventricular contraction, following a period of atrioventricular dissociation.

**capture-recapture method,** a plan for epidemiologic studies of health problems such as acquired immunodeficiency syndrome, substance abuse, or prostitution. The method provides for comparative analysis of data from various independent sources and adjusting for missing cases.

**caput** /kā′pət, kap′ət/, *pl.* **capita** /cap′itə/ [L, head], **1.** the head. **2.** the enlarged or prominent extremity of an organ or part.

**caput costae** /kos′tē/ [L, head, *costa,* rib], the head of a rib; it articulates with a vertebral body.

**caput epididymidis,** the head of the epididymis.

**caput femoris** /fem′əris/, the head of the femur. It articulates with the acetabulum.

**caput fibulae** /fib′yəlē/, the head of the fibula. It articulates with the lateral condyle of the tibia.

**caput humeri** /hyo͞o′mərī/, the head of the humerus. It articulates with the glenoid cavity of the scapula.

**caput mallei** /mal′ē·ī/, the head of the malleus. It articulates with the incus.

**caput mandibulae** /mandib′yəlē/, the articular process of the ramus of the mandible.

**caput medusae** /mədo͞o′sē/ [L, head of Medusa, a mythical snake-haired Gorgon], a pattern of dilated cutaneous veins radiating from the umbilical area of a newborn. The feature is also observed in adults with cirrhosis of the liver.

**caput ossis metacarpalis,** the metacarpal head. It articulates with the proximal phalanx of the same digit.

**caput phalangis** /falan′jis/, the articular head at the distal end of the proximal and middle phalanges.

**caput radii** /rā′dē·ī/, the head of the radius. It articulates with the capitulum of the humerus.

**caput stapedis** /stape͞′dis/, the head of the stapes.

**caput succedaneum** /suk′sədənē′əm/ [L, *caput,* head, *succeder,* to replace], a localized pitting edema in the scalp of a fetus that may overlie sutures of the skull. It is usually formed during labor as a result of the circular pressure of the cervix on the fetal occiput. On vaginal examination the swelling may be mistaken for unruptured membranes. If the caput enlarges appreciably during labor, it may cause an erroneous impression of fetal descent on successive examinations. At birth the baby's head may appear markedly deformed, but the swelling begins to resolve immediately and

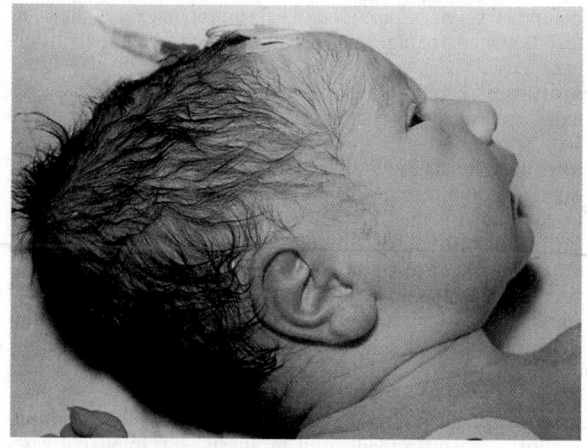

**Caput succedaneum** *(Zitelli and Davis, 1997)*

is usually gone in a few days. Compare **cephalhematoma, molding.**

**Carabelli's cusp** [Georg Carabelli, Austrian dentist, 1787–1842], an accessory cusp found on the mesiolingual cusp of a maxillary first molar. It may be unilateral or bilateral and varies in size. It is commonly seen in persons of Caucasian ancestry but is rarely found in persons of Mongolian or Inuit heritage.

**Carafate,** trademark for an antiulcer drug (sucralfate) that forms a protective layer over the ulcer site.

**carapace** /kar′əpās/ [Sp, *carapacho,* hard shell], a horny shield or shell covering the dorsal surface of an animal, such as a turtle.

**carate.** See **pinta.**

**carb,** abbreviation for a *carbonate noncarboxylate anion.*

**carb-.** See **carbo-.**

**carbam,** abbreviation for a *carbamate carboxylate anion.*

**carbamate** /kär′bəmāt/, any of a group of anticholinesterase enzymes that cause reversible inhibition of cholinesterase. They are used in certain medications and insecticides. Some carbamates are toxic and may cause convulsions and death through ingestion or skin contact. Atropine is a commonly recommended antidote.

**carbamate kinase,** a liver enzyme that catalyzes the transfer of a phosphate group from adenosine triphosphate, associated with ammonia and carbon dioxide, to form adenosine diphosphate and carbamoylphosphate.

**carbamazepine** /kär′bəmaz′əpin/, an anticonvulsant and specific analgesic for trigeminal neuralgia.

■ INDICATIONS: It is prescribed in the treatment of trigeminal neuralgia and certain seizure disorders.

■ CONTRAINDICATIONS: Concomitant use of monoamine oxidase inhibitors, a history of bone marrow depression, or known hypersensitivity to this drug or to any of the tricyclic antidepressants prohibits its use.

■ ADVERSE EFFECTS: Among the more serious adverse reactions are life-threatening blood dyscrasias, drowsiness, dizziness, ataxia, nausea, syndrome of inappropriate diuretic hormone, and dermatologic and hypersensitivity reactions.

**carbamide peroxide** /kär′bəmīd/, a topical antiinfective.

■ INDICATIONS: It is prescribed to treat canker sores and other minor inflammatory conditions of the gums and mouth and to soften impacted earwax.

- CONTRAINDICATION: Perforated eardrum prohibits its use.
- ADVERSE EFFECTS: The most serious adverse reaction is local irritation.

**carbamino compound** /kärbam'inō/, a chemical complex formed by the binding of carbon dioxide molecules to plasma proteins. A small fraction of carbon dioxide binds with protein as it leaves a tissue cell.

**carbaminohemoglobin,** a chemical complex formed by carbon dioxide and hemoglobin after the release of oxygen by the hemoglobin to a tissue cell. The action is similar to that of the formation of a carbamino compound. It accounts for nearly 25% of the carbon dioxide released in the lung. Also spelled **carbaminohaemoglobin.**

**carbenicillin disodium** /kär'bənəsil'in/, a semisynthetic penicillin antibiotic.
- INDICATIONS: It is prescribed in the treatment of certain infections caused by sensitive bacteria.
- CONTRAINDICATIONS: Known hypersensitivity to this drug or to other penicillins prohibits its use.
- ADVERSE EFFECTS: Among the more serious adverse effects are hypersensitivity reactions, neurologic disturbances, and clotting defects. The high sodium content (5.5 to 6.5 mEq/g) may aggravate fluid and electrolyte imbalance in people affected with kidney, heart, or liver disease.

**carbi-.** See **carbo-.**

**carbide,** a binary compound of carbon. The various compounds range in stability from explosive copper or silver carbides to hard abrasive compounds, such as silicon carbide.

**carbidopa** /kär'bidō'pə/, a dopa decarboxylase inhibitor.
- INDICATION: It is prescribed in combination with levodopa in the treatment of idiopathic Parkinson's disease because it inhibits the degradation of levodopa.
- CONTRAINDICATIONS: Glaucoma, hypertension, use of a monoamine oxidase inhibitor within the past 14 days, or known hypersensitivity to this drug prohibits its use.
- ADVERSE EFFECTS: Among the most serious adverse reactions are GI bleeding, cardiac irregularity, hemolytic anemia, tardive dyskinesia, mental depression, blurred vision, and activation of malignant melanoma.

**carbinoxamine maleate** /kär'bənok'səmēn/, an antihistamine.
- INDICATIONS: It is prescribed in the treatment of allergic reactions, including rhinitis, skin reactions, and itching.
- CONTRAINDICATIONS: Asthma or known hypersensitivity to this drug prohibits its use. It should not be administered to infants or lactating mothers.
- ADVERSE EFFECTS: Among the more serious adverse reactions are tachycardia and other side effects of anticholinergic medications. Drowsiness, skin rash, hypersensitivity reactions, and dry mouth commonly occur.

**carbo-, carbon-, carbono-, carb-, carbi-,** combining form meaning 'carbon, carbonic acid, or charcoal': *carbohydrate, carbonate, carbonometry.*

**Carbocaine hydrochloride,** trademark for a local anesthetic (mepivacaine hydrochloride).

**carbocyclic.** See **closed-chain.**

**carbohydrate** /kär'bōhī'drit/ [L, *carbo,* coal; Gk, *hydor,* water], any of a group of organic compounds, the most important of which are the saccharides, starch, cellulose, and glycogen. They are classified according to molecular structure as mono-, di-, tri-, poly-, and heterosaccharides and soon will be classified according to the degree of polymerization. Carbohydrates constitute the main source of energy for all body functions, particularly brain functions, and are necessary for the metabolism of other nutrients. They are synthesized by all green plants and in the body are either ab-

## Summary of carbohydrate classes

| Chemical class name | Class members | Sources |
|---|---|---|
| **Polysaccharides** | | |
| Multiple sugars, complex carbohydrates | Starch | Grains and grain products |
| | | Cereal, bread, crackers, and other baked goods |
| | | Pasta |
| | | Rice, corn, bulgur |
| | | Legumes |
| | | Potatoes and other vegetables |
| | Glycogen | Animal tissues, liver and muscle meats |
| | Dietary fiber | Whole grains |
| | | Fruits |
| | | Vegetables |
| | | Seeds, nuts, skins |
| **Disaccharides** | Sucrose | "Table" sugar: sugarcane, sugar beets |
| Double sugars, simple carbohydrates | | Molasses |
| | Lactose | Milk |
| | Maltose | Starch digestion, intermediate |
| | | Sweetener in food products |
| | | Starch digestion, final |
| **Monosaccharides** | | |
| Single sugars, simple carbohydrates | Glucose (dextrose) | Corn syrup (large use in processed foods) |
| | Fructose | Fruits, honey |
| | Galactose | Lactose (milk) |

From Williams SR: *Basic nutrition and diet therapy,* ed 11, St Louis, 2001, Mosby.

sorbed immediately or stored in the form of glycogen. Current dietary goals of the United States recommend that carbohydrates provide 55% to 60% of total calories. Cereals, vegetables, fruits, rice, potatoes, legumes, and flour products are the major sources of carbohydrates. They can also be manufactured in the body from some amino acids and the glycerol component of fats. Symptoms of deficiency include fatigue, depression, breakdown of essential body protein, and electrolyte imbalance. Muscle protein-sparing amounts of food carbohydrates have been estimated to be 50 to 100 grams per day for most people. Excessive consumption of simple carbohydrates is associated with tooth decay, and is carefully monitored in persons with diabetes.

**carbohydrate intolerance,** inability to properly metabolize one or more carbohydrate(s), as in fructose intolerance and glucose intolerance.

**carbohydrate loading,** a dietary practice of some endurance athletes, such as marathon runners, intended to increase glycogen stores in the muscle tissue. The original, or "classic," carbohydrate loading regimen began with a period of several days on a low-carbohydrate diet designed to deplete stored glycogen, followed by consumption of a diet high in complex carbohydrates for 3 days before the event. A more modern approach advocates that athletes routinely consume the high-carbohydrate diet recommended for the general population (55% to 60% of total calories), and eat extra carbohydrates (70%) for 3 days before an event. The practice is controversial, and is not universally accepted.

**carbohydrate metabolism,** the sum of the anabolic and catabolic processes of the body involved in the synthesis and breakdown of carbohydrates, principally glucosa, fructose, and galactose. Some of the processes are glycogenesis, glyconeogenesis, and glycolysis. Energy-rich phosphate bonds are produced in many metabolic reactions requiring carbohydrates.

**carbohydrate utilization test,** any of several tests for identification of yeasts and certain other organisms according to a profile of carbohydrate assimilation.

**carbolated camphor** /kär′bōlā′tid/ [L, *carbo,* coal, *camphora*], a mixture of 1.5 parts camphor with 1 part each of alcohol and phenol, sometimes used as an antiseptic dressing for wounds.

**carbol-fuchsin solution** /kär′bolfōōk′sin/ [L, *carbo,* coal; Leonard Fuchs, German botanist, 1501–1566], a preparation used in the treatment of superficial fungal infections. It contains boric acid, phenol, resorcinol, fuchsin, acetone, and alcohol in water. Also called **carbolfuchsin, Castellani's paint.**

**carbol-fuchsin stain** [L, *carbo,* coal; Leonard Fuchs], a solution of dilute phenol and basic fuchsin used on microorganisms and cell nuclei for microscopic examination. Also called **Ziehl's stain.**

**carbolic acid ($C_6H_5OH$)** /kärbol′ik/ [L, *carbo,* coal, *acidus,* sour], a poisonous, colorless to pale pink crystalline compound obtained from coal tar distillation and converted to a clear liquid with a strong odor and burning taste by the addition of 10% water. Also called **hydroxybenzene, oxybenzene, phenic acid, phenol, phenylic acid, phenylic alcohol.**

**carbolic acid poisoning.** See **phenol poisoning.**

**carbolism** /kär′bōliz′əm/, poisoning by phenol, also known as carbolic acid. See **phenol poisoning.**

**carbon (C)** /kär′bən/ [L, *carbo,* coal], a nonmetallic, chiefly tetravalent element. Its atomic number is 6; its atomic mass is 12.011. Carbon occurs in pure form in diamonds, graphite, and fullerenes and is a component of all living tissue. The study of organic chemistry focuses on the vast number of carbon compounds. Carbon occurs in impure form in charcoal, coke, and soot, and in the atmosphere as carbon dioxide. Carbon is essential to the chemical mechanisms of the body, participating in many metabolic processes and acting as a component of carbohydrates, amino acids, triglycerides, deoxyribonucleic and ribonucleic acids, and many other compounds. See also **carbon-11, carbon-14.**

**carbon-11,** a radioisotope of carbon with a half-life of 20 minutes. It is produced by a cyclotron and emits positrons. Compare **carbon-14.**

**carbon-14,** a beta-emitter with a half-life of about 5700 years. It occurs naturally, arising from cosmic rays, and is used as a tracer in studying various aspects of metabolism and in dating relics that contain natural carbonaceous materials. Compare **carbon-11.**

**carbon arc lamp,** an electric lamp producing a strong white light of adjustable intensity from an arc of current between carbon electrodes.

**carbonate** /kär′bənāt/, a $CO_3^{2-}$ anion. Carbonates are in equilibrium with bicarbonates in water and frequently occur in compounds as insoluble salts, such as calcium carbonate.

**carbonate dehydratase.** See **carbonic anhydrase.**

**carbon cycle,** the steps by which carbon in the form of carbon dioxide is extracted from and returned to the atmosphere by living organisms, especially human beings. The process starts with the photosynthetic production of carbohydrates by plants, progresses through the consumption of carbohydrates by animals and human beings, and ends with the exhalation of carbon dioxide by those same animals and human beings and with the release of carbon dioxide during the decomposition of dead plants and animals. Various chemical processes intervene between the ingestion of carbohydrates and the release of carbon dioxide. Carbohydrate metabolism starts with the movement of glucose through plasma membranes and subsequently involves glycolysis, the processes of the citric acid cycle, electron transport, and oxidative phosphorylation. See also **citric acid cycle, tricarboxylic acid cycle.**

**carbon damp.** See **damp.**

**carbon dioxide ($CO_2$)** [L, *carbo* + Gk, *dis,* twice, *oxys,* sharp], a colorless, odorless gas produced by the oxidation of carbon; also a "greenhouse" gas. Carbon dioxide, as a product of cell respiration, is carried by the blood to the lungs and is exhaled. The acid-base balance of body fluids and tissues is affected by the level of carbon dioxide and its carbonate compounds. Solid carbon dioxide (dry ice) is used in the treatment of some skin conditions. Normal adult blood levels of carbon dioxide are 23 to 30 mEq/L or 23 to 30 mmol/L (SI units).

**carbon dioxide acidosis.** See **respiratory acidosis.**

**carbon dioxide bath,** a bath taken in water that is saturated with carbon dioxide. See also **Nauheim bath.**

**carbon dioxide content test ($CO_2$ content),** a blood test used to measure $CO_2$ content in the blood. It is used to assist in evaluating the patient's pH status and electrolytes. It is usually performed along with other assessments of electrolytes and is used primarily as a rough guide as to the patient's acid/base balance.

**carbon dioxide inhalation,** a procedure in which high concentrations of carbon dioxide gas are administered to stimulate breathing in a patient, sometimes as a part of resuscitation efforts. The procedure relies on carbon dioxide's excitation of chemoreceptors that trigger an increase in breathing rate.

**carbon dioxide narcosis,** a condition of confusion, tremors, convulsions, and possible coma that may occur if blood levels of carbon dioxide increase to 70 mm Hg or higher. When ventilation is sufficient to maintain a normal oxygen partial pressure in the arteries, the carbon dioxide partial pressure is generally near 40 mm Hg. See also **carbon dioxide poisoning.**

**carbon dioxide poisoning,** a condition of toxic effects caused by inhaling excessive amounts of carbon dioxide. Carbon dioxide is a respiratory stimulant, but it is also an asphyxiant. Concentrations of 10% or greater can cause unconsciousness and death from ventilatory failure. Particularly vulnerable are persons who work in confined spaces with poor air circulation, such as mine shafts, silos, or holds of ships. Faulty home furnaces also have been implicated in many deaths. Home monitors for detection are now available. See also **carbon dioxide narcosis.**

**carbon dioxide pressure.** See **carbon dioxide tension.**

**carbon dioxide response,** the ventilatory reaction to increased concentrations of carbon dioxide in inhaled air. The respiration rate increases linearly up to a concentration of 8% to 10%, rises more gradually up to a concentration of about 20%, and decreases at higher concentrations. At concentrations of around 25%, the person is conscious but unable to perform simple tasks. At concentrations of 30%, carbon dioxide is an anesthetic.

**carbon dioxide retention,** any increased body stores of carbon dioxide resulting from impaired carbon dioxide elimination in conditions such as alveolar hypoventilation, strangulation, apnea, and ventilation-perfusion abnormalities. Respiratory acidosis may result from carbon dioxide retention.

**carbon dioxide stores,** the amount of carbon dioxide contained in the body as a gas and in the form of carbonic acid, carbonate, bicarbonate, and carbaminohemoglobin. During a steady state of ventilation and aerobic respiration, the rat at which carbon dioxide leaves the body equals the rate at which it is produced, and carbon dioxide stores remain constant.

**carbon dioxide tension (PCO$_2$),** the partial pressure of carbon dioxide, a measure of the relative concentration of the gas in air or in a fluid, such as plasma. It is expressed quantitatively in millimeters of mercury (mm Hg). Alveolar PCO$_2$ directly reflects pulmonary gas exchange in relation to blood flow: alveolar PCO$_2$ decreases as the respiration rate increases. Normal values for arterial and alveolar PCO$_2$ are between 35 and 45 mm Hg. Higher levels occur in conditions of slow blood flow and slow respiration. Below-normal values are caused by hyperventilation and lead to respiratory alkalosis. Also called **carbon dioxide pressure.** See also **carbon dioxide, hypercapnia, hyperventilation, hypoventilation.**

**carbon dioxide therapy,** the therapeutic inhalation of a low concentration of carbon dioxide gas. Such therapy may be used to dilate the blood vessels, stimulate the cardiovascular brain centers and central nervous system, overcome hyperventilation, assist in developing a productive cough needed to remove mucous secretions, and control hiccups.

**carbon fiber,** a material consisting of graphite fibers in a plastic matrix. It is used in radiologic devices to reduce patient exposure to x-rays.

**carbonic acid (H$_2$CO$_3$)** /kärbon'ik/ [L, *carbo,* coal, *acidus,* acid], an unstable acid formed by dissolving carbon dioxide in water. It is the basis of carbonated beverages and is related to the carbonate group of compounds.

**carbonic anhydrase** /anhī'drās/, a zinc-containing enzyme in red blood cells that assists in the hydration of carbon dioxide to carbonic acid in the red blood cell so it can be transported from the tissue cell to the lungs. Also called **carbonate dehydratase.**

**carbonic anhydrase inhibitor,** a substance that decreases the rate of carbonic acid and H$^+$ production in the kidney, thereby increasing the excretion of solutes and the rate of urinary output. An example of a carbonic anhydrase inhibitor is acetazolamide. Some carbonic anhydrase inhibitors are used as diuretics, others in the treatment of glaucoma.

**carbon monoxide (CO)** [L, *carbo* + Gk, *monos,* single, *oxys,* sharp], a colorless, odorless, poisonous gas produced by the combustion of carbon or organic fuels in a limited oxygen supply, as in the cylinders of an internal combustion engine. Carbon monoxide combines irreversibly with hemoglobin, preventing the formation of oxyhemoglobin and reducing the oxygen supply to the tissues. Prolonged exposure to high levels of carbon monoxide results in asphyxiation.

**carbon monoxide poisoning,** a toxic condition in which carbon monoxide gas has been inhaled and binds to hemoglobin molecules, thus displacing oxygen from the red blood cells and decreasing the capacity of the blood to carry oxygen to the cells of the body. Characteristically, headache, dyspnea, drowsiness, confusion, cherry-pink skin, unconsciousness, and apnea occur in sequence as the level of carbon monoxide in the blood increases. Cherry-red skin is a late sign most commonly noted in fatalities. The most com-

mon source of carbon monoxide in cases of poisoning is exhaust fumes from an automobile.

**carbon tetrachloride** [L, *carbo* + Gk, *tetra,* four, *chloros,* greenish], a colorless, volatile toxic liquid used as a solvent. Carbon tetrachloride is particularly toxic to the kidneys and liver; permanent damage to these organs may result from exposure.

**carbon tetrachloride poisoning** [L, *carbo,* coal; Gk, *tetra,* four, *chloros,* greenish; L, *potio,* drink], toxic effects of exposure to carbon tetrachloride, a colorless commercial dry cleaning fluid also used in fire extinguishers and industrial solvents. It may attack both liver and kidneys. Symptoms include persistent headache, nausea, vomiting, diarrhea, uremia, lethargy, confusion resulting from central nervous system depression, and degeneration of the liver and kidneys. Ingestion of the liquid or inhalation of the fumes usually results in headaches, nausea, central nervous system depression, abdominal pain, and convulsions. In poisoning by inhalation, ventilatory assistance and oxygen may be necessary.

**carboplatin** /kär'bōplat'in/, one of a series of platinum analog drugs used in cancer therapy. It is commonly administered intravenously for the treatment of ovarian cancer.

**carboxyfluoroquinolone** /kärbok'sēflōō'ərōkwī'nəlōn/, any of a group of oral quinolone antibiotics that are generally effective against Enterobacteriaceae and show varying activity against *Pseudomonas* and other species. The drugs differ in their oral absorption.

**carboxyhemoglobin** /kärbok'sēhē'məglō'bin, -hem'-/ [L, *carbo* + Gk, *oxys,* sharp, *haima,* blood; L, *globus,* ball], a compound produced by the exposure of hemoglobin to carbon monoxide. Carbon monoxide from the environment is inhaled into the lungs, absorbed through the alveoli, and bound to hemoglobin in the blood, blocking the sites for oxygen transport. Oxygen levels decrease; hypoxia and anoxia may result. Also called **carboxyhaemoglobin.** See also **carbon monoxide poisoning, oxyhemoglobin.**

**carboxyl** /kärbok'sil/, a monovalent radical —COOH characteristic of organic acids. The hydrogen of the radical can be replaced by metals to form salts.

**carboxylase** /kär·bok'sə·lās/, an enzyme that catalyzes the addition of a molecule of carbon dioxide to another compound to form a carboxyl group.

**carboxylation** /-lā'shən/, a chemical process in which a carboxyl group (COOH) replaces a hydrogen atom.

**carboxylic acid** /kär'bok·sil'ik as'id/, any of a group of organic acids containing the carboxyl radical —COOH, including amino acids and fatty acids.

**carbuncle** /kär'bungkəl/ [L, *carbunculus,* little coal], a large site of staphylococcal infection containing purulent matter in deep, interconnecting subcutaneous pockets. Pus eventually discharges to the skin surface through openings. Common sites for carbuncles are the back of the neck and the buttocks. Treatment may include the use of antibiotics, hot compresses, and surgical drainage. Compare **furuncle.**

**carbunculosis** /karbung'kyəlō'sis/, an abnormal condition characterized by a cluster of deep painful abscesses that drain through multiple openings onto the skin surface, usually around hair follicles. Carbunculosis is a form of folliculitis, most commonly caused by the coagulase-positive *Staphylococcus aureus.* The lesions caused by this condition may cause fever and malaise.

■ OBSERVATIONS: Carbunculosis commonly follows persistent *S. aureus* infection and furunculosis. Diagnosis is based on obvious skin lesions, a patient history of previous furunculosis, and *S. aureus* in wound culture.

■ INTERVENTIONS: Treatment of carbunculosis requires the administration of systemic antibiotics and surgical drainage.

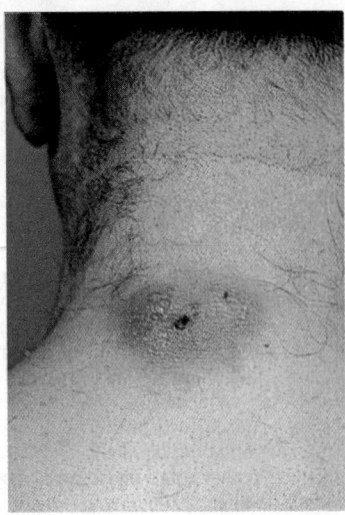

**Carbuncle** *(Lawrence and Cox, 1993)*

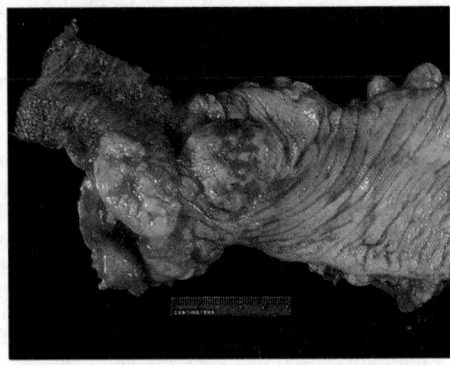

**Carcinoid tumor** *(Kumar, Cotran, and Robbins, 1997)*

Carcinoid tumors spread slowly locally but may metastasize widely. Also called **argentaffinoma, Kulchitsky-cell carcinoma.** See also **argentaffin cell, carcinoid syndrome.**

The prognosis depends on the severity of the infection and the physical condition of the patient.

■ NURSING CONSIDERATIONS: Nursing care for this disorder is mainly supportive and educative to impress the patient with the importance of meticulous personal and family hygiene. Patient teaching includes explaining the importance of reducing sugar and fat intake and cautioning him or her not to squeeze a carbuncle or furuncle because it may rupture into the surrounding area. The patient is also instructed not to share towels and washcloths with other family members because this practice may spread the bacteria. Also stressed are the importance of thoroughly laundering towels and washcloths before reusing them and the need for daily changes of laundered clothes and bedsheets. The patient is additionally encouraged to change dressings frequently and to discard them in paper bags. Because carbunculosis often follows furunculosis, a disorder associated with diabetes, the patient should have a thorough physical examination.

**carcin-, carcino-,** combining form meaning 'cancer': *carcinelcosis, carcinogen.*

**carcinoembryonic antigen (CEA)** /kär′sənō·em′brē·on′ik/ [Gk, *karkinos,* crab, *en,* into, *bryein,* to grow, *anti,* against, *genein,* to produce], an antigen present in very small quantities in adult tissue. A greater than normal amount is suggestive of cancer. Measurement of CEA concentration in blood aids in evaluating recurrent or disseminated disease, and in monitoring treatment effectiveness. Normal serum CEA levels are less than 5 ng/mL or 0 to 2.5 μg/L.

**carcinogen** /kärsin′əjin/ [Gk, *karkinos* + *genein,* to produce], a substance or agent that causes the development or increases the incidence of cancer.

**carcinogenesis** /kär′sinəjen′əsis/, the process of initiating and promoting cancer. Compare **oncogenesis, sarcomagenesis, tumorigenesis.**

**carcinogenic** /kär′sinəjen′ik/, pertaining to the ability to cause the development of a cancer. Also called **cancerigenic, cancerogenic.**

**carcinoid** /kär′sinoid/ [Gk, *karkinos* + *eidos,* form], a small yellow tumor derived from argentaffin cells in the GI mucosa that secrete serotonin and other catecholamines.

**carcinoid syndrome,** the systemic effects of serotonin-secreting carcinoid tumors manifested by flushing, diarrhea, cramps, skin lesions resembling pellagra, labored breathing, palpitations, and valvular heart disease, especially of the tricuspid and pulmonary valve. Treatment includes surgical excision of the tumor, if feasible. Chemotherapy and radiation treatment are occasionally used. Also called **argentaffinoma syndrome.** See also **carcinoid.**

**carcinolysis** /kär′sinol′isis/ [Gk, *karkinos* + *lysis,* loosening], the destruction of cancer cells. See also **cancericidal.** —**carcinolytic,** *adj.*

**carcinoma** /kär′sinō′mə/, *pl.* carcinomas, carcinomata [Gk, *karkinos* + *oma,* tumor], a malignant epithelial neoplasm that tends to invade surrounding tissue and to metastasize to distant regions of the body. Carcinomas develop most frequently in the skin, large intestine, lungs, stomach, prostate, cervix, or breast. The tumor is firm, irregular, and nodular, with a well-defined border. Microscopically, the cells are characterized by anaplasia, abnormal size and shape, disproportionately large nuclei, and clumps of nuclear chromatin. —**carcinomatous,** *adj.*

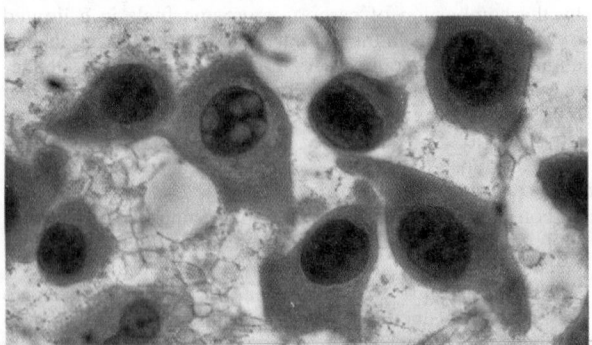

**Carcinoma cells showing loss of cohesion** *(McKee, 1997)*

**-carcinoma,** suffix meaning a 'malignant tumor composed of epithelial cells, with a tendency to metastasize': *ophthalmocarcinoma, phlebocarcinoma.*

**carcinoma basocellulare.** See **basal cell carcinoma.**

**carcinoma cutaneum.** See **basal cell carcinoma, squamous cell carcinoma.**

**carcinoma en cuirasse** /äN'kēräs'/ [Gk, *karkinos + oma +* Fr, breastplate], a rare manifestation of advanced breast cancer characterized by progressive extensive fibrosis and rigidity of the skin of the chest, neck, back, and abdomen.

**carcinoma fibrosum.** See **scirrhous carcinoma.**

**carcinoma gigantocellulare.** See **giant cell carcinoma.**

**carcinoma in situ** /insit'ōō, insī'tōō [Gk, *karkinos + oma + L, in position],* a premalignant neoplasm that has not invaded the basement membrane but shows cytologic characteristics of cancer. Such neoplastic changes in stratified squamous or glandular epithelium frequently occur on the uterine cervix and in the anus, bronchi, buccal mucosa, esophagus, eye, lip, penis, uterine endometrium, and vagina. Also called **cancer in situ, intraepithelial carcinoma, preinvasive carcinoma.** See also **erythroplasia of Queyrat.**

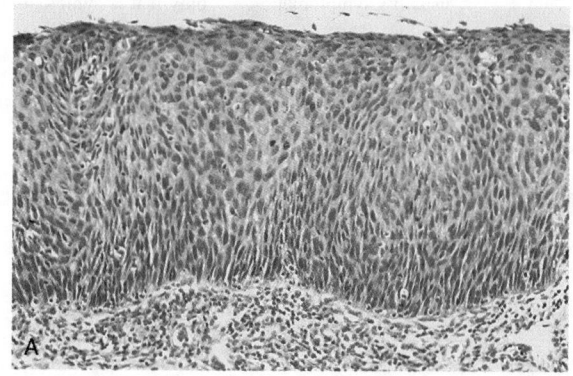

**Carcinoma in situ** *(Cotran, Kumar, and Collins, 1999)*

**carcinoma lenticulare** /len'tikōōlär'ə/ [Gk, *karkinos + oma + L, lens],* a form of carcinoma tuberosum or scirrhous skin cancer characterized by the development of many small, flat nodules that coalesce to form larger areas resembling a fungous infection.

**carcinoma medullare, carcinoma molle.** See **medullary carcinoma.**

**carcinoma mucocellulare.** See **Krukenberg's tumor.**

**carcinoma scroti** /skrō'tī/, an epithelial cell carcinoma of the scrotum.

**carcinoma spongiosum** /spon'jē·ō'səm/, a soft and spongy carcinoma with small and large cavities. See also **medullary carcinoma.**

**carcinomata.** See **carcinoma.**

**carcinoma telangiectaticum** /telan'jē·ektat'ikəm/ [Gk, *karkinos + oma + telos,* end, *angeion,* vessel, *ektasis,* dilation], a neoplasm of the capillaries of the skin causing dilation of the vessels and red spots on the skin that blanch with pressure.

**carcinomatoid** /kär'sinō'mətoid/, resembling a carcinoma.

**carcinomatosis.** See **carcinosis.**

**carcinomatous** /-om'ətəs/, pertaining to carcinoma. Also **carcinous.**

**carcinomatous pericarditis.** See **neoplastic pericarditis.**

**carcinoma tuberosum.** See **tuberous carcinoma.**

**carcinoma villosum.** See **villous carcinoma.**

**carcinophilia** /kär'sinō'fil'yə/ [Gk, *karkinos + philein,* to love], the property in which there is an affinity for carcinomatous tissue. **—carcinophilic,** *adj.*

**carcinosarcoma** /kär'sinōsärkō'mə/, *pl.* **carcinosarcomas, carcinosarcomata** [Gk, *karkinos + sarx,* flesh, *oma,* tumor], a malignant neoplasm composed of carcinomatous and sarcomatous cells. Tumors of this type may occur in the esophagus, thyroid gland, and uterus.

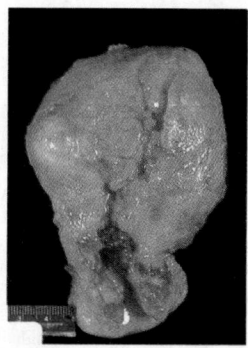

**Carcinosarcoma** *(Fletcher, 2000)*

**carcinosis** /kär'sinō'sis/, *pl.* **carcinoses,** a condition characterized by the development of many carcinomas throughout the body. Kinds of carcinoses are **carcinosis pleurae, miliary carcinosis, pulmonary carcinosis.** Also called **carcinomatosis.**

**carcinosis pleurae** /plōō're/, a secondary malignancy of the pleura in which nodules develop throughout the membranes.

**carcinostatic** /kär'sinōstat'ik/ [Gk, *karkinos + statikos,* causing to stand], pertaining to the tendency to slow or halt the growth of a carcinoma.

**carcinous.** See **carcinomatous.**

**Cardarelli's sign** [Antonio Cardarelli, Italian physician, 1831–1927], a lateral pulsation of the trachea in aneurysm, particularly in dilation of the aortic arch.

**cardia** /kär'dē·ə/ [Gk, *kardia,* heart], **1.** the opening between the esophagus and the cardiac portion of the stomach. **2.** the portion of the stomach surrounding the esophagogastric connection, characterized by the absence of acid cells. **—cardiac,** *adj.*

**cardia-, cardi-, cardio-,** combining form meaning 'heart': *cardiac, cardialgia, cardioclasis.*

**-cardia,** suffix meaning a 'type of heart action or location': *brachycardia, miocardia.*

**cardiac** /kär'dē·ak/ [Gk, *kardia,* heart], **1.** pertaining to the heart. **2.** pertaining to a person with heart disease. **3.** pertaining to the part of the stomach closest to the esophagus.

**-cardiac,** **1.** suffix meaning 'to characterize types and locations of heart ailments': *intracardiac, precardiac.* **2.** suffix meaning 'to identify heart ailment patients': *diplocardiac, hemicardiac.*

**cardiac action potential,** the transmembrane potential in the heart, consisting of five phases: 0, the upstroke or rapid depolarization, which initiates the heartbeat; 1, early rapid repolarization; 2, plateau; 3, final rapid repolarization; and 4, resting membrane potential and diastolic depolarization. Abnormalities of the heart or its conduction system that alter the cardiac action potential lead to the development of cardiac arrhythmias.

**cardiac aneurysm.** See **ventricular aneurysm.**

**cardiac angiography.** See **angiocardiography.**

**cardiac apex.** See **apex cordis.**

**cardiac apnea** [Gk, *kardia + a + pnein,* not to breathe], an abnormal, temporary absence of respiration, such as occurs in Cheyne-Stokes respiration.

**cardiac arrest** [Gk, *kardia* + L, *ad + restare,* to withstand], a sudden cessation of cardiac output and effective circulation. It is usually precipitated by ventricular fibrillation or ventricular asystole. When cardiac arrest occurs, delivery of oxygen and removal of carbon dioxide stop, tissue cell metabolism becomes anaerobic, and metabolic and respiratory acidosis ensue. Immediate initiation of cardiopulmonary resuscitation is required to prevent heart, lung, kidney, and brain damage and death. Also called **cardiopulmonary arrest.** See also **cardiac standstill, cardiopulmonary resuscitation.**

**cardiac arrhythmia** [Gk, *kardia + a + rhythmos,* without rhythm], an abnormal cardiac rate or rhythm. The condition is caused by a failure of the sinus node to maintain its pacemaker function or by a defect in the electrical conduction system. Examples of arrhythmia include **bradycardia, extrasystole, heart block,** and **tachycardia.**

## Common cardiac arrhythmias

| Description | Classic characteristics | Etiology and pathology | Clinical manifestations | Management |
|---|---|---|---|---|
| **Sinus bradycardia** | | | | |
| Heart rate less than 60 beats/min (possibly normal in highly trained athletes and other healthy adults, particularly during sleep) | Pacemaker site: SA node<br>Rhythm: regular<br>Rate <60 beats/min<br>P waves: normal<br>QRS complex: normal<br>Intervals: normal<br>Ectopic beats: possibly present | Inferior wall myocardial infarction<br>Increased intracranial pressure<br>Addison's disease<br>Myxedema<br>Hypothermia<br>Anorexia nervosa<br>Drugs: digitalis, beta blockers (propranolol, nadolol)<br>Vagal stimulation from severe pain, fear, vomiting, bearing down during defecation | This condition is usually asymptomatic but may cause dizziness, angina, disorientation, hypotension, syncope, or heart failure if cardiac output decreases. | This rhythm is treated only if it is symptomatic, and then treatment is directed at increasing heart rate.<br>Causative factor should be removed if possible.<br>Atropine should be administered intravenously.<br>Pacemaker is used in refractory cases. |

Illustrations from Monahan FD, Neighbors M: *Medical-surgical nursing: foundations for clinical practice,* ed 2, Philadelphia, 1998, WB Saunders. *SA,* Sinoatrial; *AV,* atrioventricular.

## Common cardiac arrhythmias—cont'd

| Description | Classic characteristics | Etiology and pathology | Clinical manifestations | Management |
|---|---|---|---|---|
| **Sinus tachycardia** | | | | |
| Heart rate between 100 and 160 beats/min | Pacemaker site: SA node<br>Rhythm: regular<br>Rate: >100 beats/min<br>P waves: normal but in rapid rhythms possibly more peaked or lost in T wave<br>QRS complex: normal<br>Intervals: possible shortening of PR and QT intervals as rate increases | Possible occurrence in normal individuals as a result of fear, anxiety, physical exertion<br>Ingestion of alcohol and caffeine<br>Use of nicotine, atropine, and catecholamines<br>Accompaniment of pathologic processes that raise metabolic rate, such as fever and thyrotoxicosis<br>Short-term compensatory mechanism to maintain circulation of oxygenated blood to tissues during myocardial ischemia and infarction, pulmonary embolism, heart failure, anemia, hypoxemia, and hypovolemia | This condition is often asymptomatic, although it occasionally causes subjective feelings of palpitations.<br>Patients with preexisting heart disease may experience lightheadedness, angina, disorientation, and syncope. | Underlying cause is corrected or eliminated.<br>As indicated, beta-adrenergic blocking agents, calcium channel blockers, digoxin, and adenosine are used to control arrhythmia. |

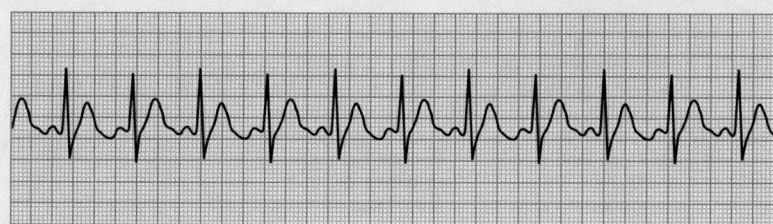

| | | | | |
|---|---|---|---|---|
| **Paroxysmal atrial tachycardia** | | | | |
| Very rapid, regular heart rate of 150-250 beats/min that occurs and stops suddenly | Pacemaker site: atrial tissue<br>Rhythm: regular<br>Rate: 150-25 beats/min<br>P waves: usually hidden in previous T wave<br>QRS complex: normal<br>Intervals: immeasurable PR interval, regular R-R interval | Usual preceding rhythm: frequent premature atrial contractions<br>Possible cause: sympathetic nervous system stimulation or hypermetabolic states<br>Patients at risk: those with ischemic heart disease, rheumatic heart disease, and myocarditis | Patients may experience symptoms of decreased cardiac output.<br>Patients may complain of palpitations, racing heartbeat, dizziness, dyspnea, angina, diaphoresis, and fatigue. | Vagal stimulation by means of Valsalva maneuver or carotid sinus pressure is used.<br>Adenosine, 6-mg intravenous bolus over 1-2 sec, is rapidly administered, followed by 20-mL saline flush.<br>Verapamil, propranolol, or digitalis is administered if adenosine is not effective.<br>Synchronized cardioversion is used if patient not responsive to drug therapy or is hemodynamically unstable. |

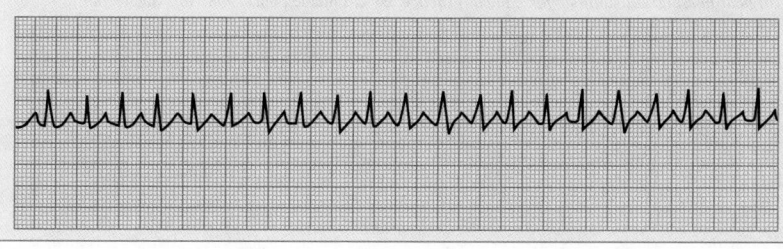

*Continued*

## Common cardiac arrhythmias—cont'd

| Description | Classic characteristics | Etiology and pathology | Clinical manifestations | Management |
|---|---|---|---|---|
| **Atrial flutter** Atrial arrhythmia that occurs when an atrial ectopic pacemaker discharges impulses at 250-400 beats/min (less common than atrial fibrillation) | Pacemaker site: ectopic focus in atrial tissue Rhythm: usually regular but possibly irregular Rate: atrial rate—250-400 beats/min, ventricular rate—depends on AV conduction ratio P waves: presence of flutter waves QRS complex: normal Intervals: immeasurable PR interval, regular or irregular R-R interval | Occurrence in patients with cardiomyopathy, hypoxia, heart failure, pericarditis, myocarditis, hyperthyroidism, pulmonary disease, pulmonary emboli Trigger: reentry conduction Only some impulses from AV node are conducted through to ventricles | This condition may be asymptomatic, or patient may complain of palpitations or fluttering feeling in chest or throat. Patient may become hypotensive and develop cool, clammy skin. | Digitalis, beta-blockers, and calcium channel blockers are administered to slow impulse conduction time. If AV conduction rate is 1:1, immediate synchronized cardioversion is done. Atrial overdrive pacing may be considered if time and patient's condition permit. |

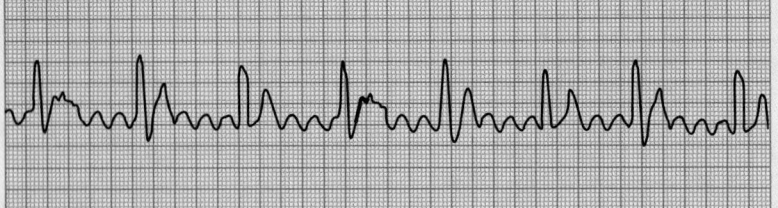

| Description | Classic characteristics | Etiology and pathology | Clinical manifestations | Management |
|---|---|---|---|---|
| **Atrial fibrillation** Arrhythmia in which chaotic ectopic atrial foci cause the atria to quiver rather than contract Atrial rate >400 beats/min | Pacemaker site: many ectopic foci in atrial tissue Rhythm: irregular Rate: atrial rate—>400 beats/min P waves: presence of chaotic F waves QRS complex: normal Intervals: lack of P waves, irregular R-R interval | In healthy people, possible association with stress or excessive alcohol consumption Chronic atrial fibrillation in patients with heart failure, mitral valve disease, rheumatic heart disease, hypertension, and hyperthyroidism Relationship with atrial reentry mechanism Only a few impulses from AV node pass through to the ventricle | Signs and symptoms are related to rate of ventricular response. If ventricular response is rapid, patient experiences manifestations of decreased cardiac output and is at risk for heart failure and myocardial ischemia. Blood pooling in atria places patient at risk for thrombus formation and embolization to the brain and other organs. | Ventricular rate is controlled Anticoagulation therapy is performed. Arrhythmia is converted to sinus rhythm. |

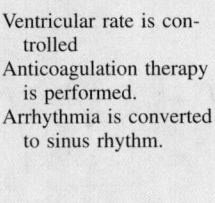

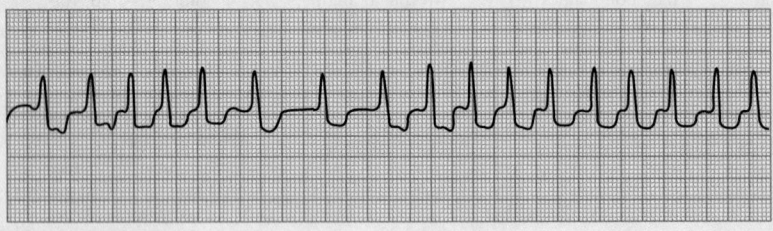

Illustrations from Monahan FD, Neighbors M: *Medical-surgical nursing: foundations for clinical practice*, ed 2, Philadelphia, 1998, WB Saunders. *SA*, Sinoatrial; *AV*, atrioventricular.

## Common cardiac arrhythmias—cont'd

| Description | Classic characteristics | Etiology and pathology | Clinical manifestations | Management |
|---|---|---|---|---|
| **Junctional rhythm** | | | | |
| Rhythm that originates in or around the AV node | Pacemaker site: AV node<br>Rhythm: regular<br>Rate: 40-60 beats/min<br>P waves: possibly present, possibly inverted and found before, in, or after QRS complex<br>QRS complex: usually normal<br>Intervals: shorter-than-normal PR interval, normal R-R interval | Occurrence only when dominant pacemaker of heart fails to function<br>Cause: retrograde stimulation of atria, which do not contract simultaneously with ventricles, reducing cardiac output<br>Possible cause: certain drugs or damage to the AV node secondary to acute myocardial infarction or ischemia | This rhythm is similar to other bradyarrhythmias.<br>Symptoms include manifestations of decreased cardiac output. | Pharmacologic management is used to increase heart rate.<br>Temporary pacemaker may be inserted.<br>Underlying cause is identified and treated. |

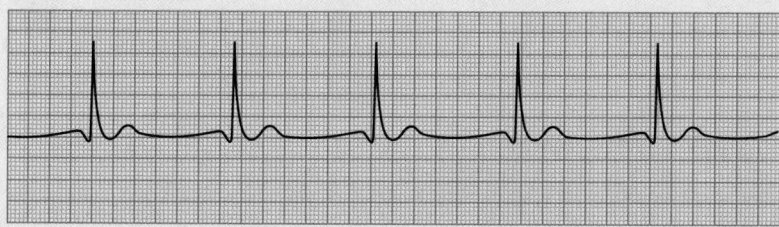

| | | | | |
|---|---|---|---|---|
| **Premature ventricular contractions** | | | | |
| — | Pacemaker site: ventricular tissue (single or multiple foci)<br>Rhythm: irregular<br>Rate: normal 60-100 beats/min<br>P waves: not present because impulses originate in the ventricles<br>QRS complex: usually wide and bizarre, usually no longer than 0.10 sec, possibly with same focus in the ventricles or with variety of configurations if occurring from multiple foci in ventricles<br>Intervals: absent PR intervals | Association with stimulants such as caffeine, alcohol, aminophylline, epinephrine, isoproterenol, and digoxin<br>Associated diseases: acute myocardial infarction, mitral valve prolapse, heart failure, and coronary artery disease<br>Possibly unifocal or multifocal | Most patients are asymptomatic, but some may complain of palpitations and skipped beats. | Treatment is indicated when six or more occur per minute, ventricular couplets or triplets appear, or multifocal premature ventricular contractions occur.<br>Lidocaine is drug of choice; procainamide is second choice if lidocaine is ineffective. |

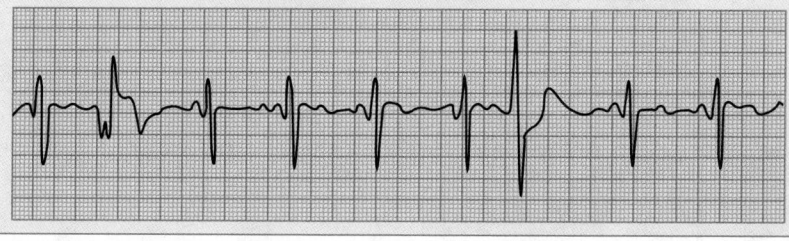

*Continued*

# Common cardiac arrhythmias—cont'd

| Description | Classic characteristics | Etiology and pathology | Clinical manifestations | Management |
|---|---|---|---|---|
| **Ventricular tachycardia** Arrhythmia originating in an ectopic focus in the ventricles | Pacemaker site: ventricular (single or multiple foci) Rhythm: atrial—indeterminable, ventricular—typically regular but possibly slightly irregular Rate: ventricular—100-250 beats/min P waves: usually buried in QRS complex, possible presence of retrograde P waves QRS complex: wide bizarre, and independent of P waves, possibly with same configuration as premature ventricular contractions Intervals: indeterminable | Occurrence when more than three premature ventricular contractions occur in succession with a heart rate of >100 beats/min Usual association: coronary artery disease, acute myocardial infarction, electrolyte imbalances, or cardiomyopathy | Patients may complain of palpitations, dizziness, chest pain, and shortness of breath. Signs and symptoms of decreased cardiac output are present. If this rhythm is rapid or sustained, loss of consciousness may occur. | If rate <100 beats/min and patient is hemodynamically stable, no treatment is necessary. Lidocaine is administered if patient is hemodynamically stable but rate is >100 beats/min. Procainamide is administered if lidocaine is ineffective. Bretylium is third drug of choice. If patient is hemodynamically unstable, immediate synchronized cardioversion is performed. |

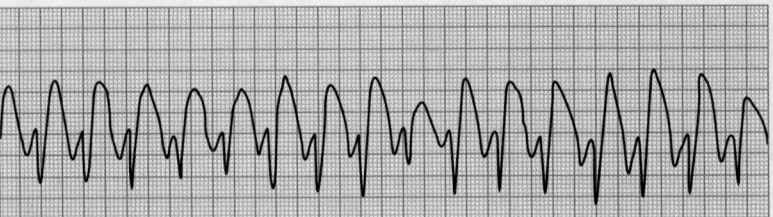

| | | | | |
|---|---|---|---|---|
| **Ventricular fibrillation** Rapid, ineffective, and disorganized depolarization of the ventricles | Pacemaker site: ventricular tissue (multiple foci) Rhythm: irregular, uncoordinated, without specific pattern Rate: rapid, uncoordinated, cannot be determined P waves: none QRS complex: rapid, irregular, not discernible Intervals: not discernible | Characteristics: disorganization of electrical impulses, conduction, and ventricular contraction Occurrence with coronary artery disease, acute myocardial infarction, myocardial ischemia, and cardiomyopathy Possible induction by procedures such as cardiac catheterization or cardiac pacing Possible occurrence with thrombolytic therapy, coronary reperfusion, accidental electrical shock, hyperkalemia, and hypoxia | Loss of consciousness may occur. Pulse, heart sounds, and blood pressure are absent. The patient's pupils are dilated, cyanosis develops rapidly, and seizures are possible. | Immediate CPR and defibrillation are performed after advanced cardiac life-support measures. |

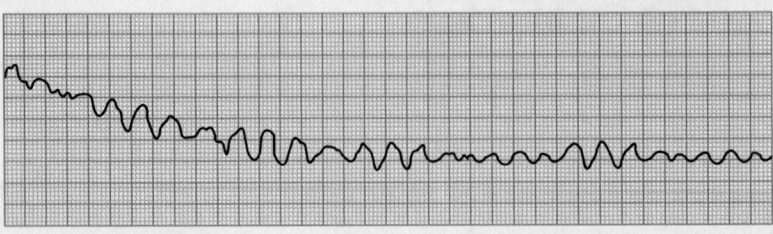

Illustrations from Monahan FD, Neighbors M: *Medical-surgical nursing: foundations for clinical practice,* ed 2, Philadelphia, 1998, WB Saunders. *SA,* Sinoatrial; *AV,* atrioventricular.

## Common cardiac arrhythmias—cont'd

| Description | Classic characteristics | Etiology and pathology | Clinical manifestations | Management |
|---|---|---|---|---|
| **First-degree atrioventricular block** | | | | |
| Block in which every impulse from the SA node is conducted to the ventricles, but a delay occurs at the AV node. | Pacemaker site: SA node<br>Rhythm: regular<br>Rate: 60-100 beats/min<br>P waves: normal<br>QRS complex: normal<br>Intervals: P-R interval >0.20 sec | Association with organic heart diseases such as rheumatic fever, chronic ischemic heart disease, myocardial infarction hyperthroidism, and vagal stimulation<br>Additional association with drugs such as digitalis, beta-blockers, and calcium channel blockers | A soft $S_1$ is heard.<br>Patients may have asymptomatic bradycardia or be otherwise asymptomatic. | Underlying cause is treated.<br>Usually, treatment is not required, but patients should be monitored closely. |

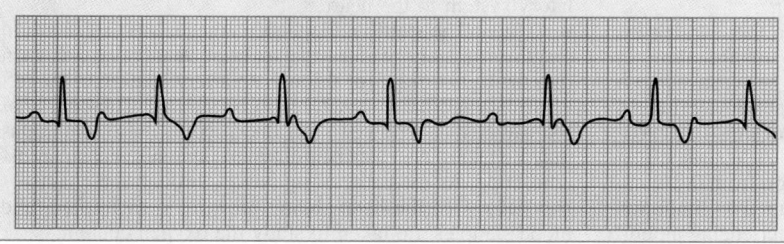

| Description | Classic characteristics | Etiology and pathology | Clinical manifestations | Management |
|---|---|---|---|---|
| **Second-degree atrioventricular block, type I** (also called *Mobitz type I* or *Wenckebach*) | | | | |
| Failure of some of the SA impulses to be conducted to the ventricles | Pacemaker site: SA node<br>Rhythm: atrial—regular, ventricular irregular<br>Rate: atrial—normal, ventricular—normal but possible slower than atrial rate<br>P waves: normal or prolonged<br>QRS complex: normal width with pattern of one nonconducted QRS<br>Intervals: normal | Usual cause: myocardial ischemia in an acute myocardial infarction of inferior wall<br>Possible cause: digitalis toxicity, acute rheumatic fever, electrolyte imbalance, vagal stimulation, or quinidine or procainamide therapy | $S_1$ tends to become progressively softer with intermittent pauses.<br>Otherwise, this rhythm is usually asymptomatic.<br>If ventricular rate is slow, hypotension and syncope can occur. | Usually, no treatment is required if patient is asymptomatic.<br>Underlying cause is treated when necessary.<br>Atropine is administered, temporary pacemaker is inserted, or both treatments are used if patient is symptomatic. |

*Continued*

## Common cardiac arrhythmias—cont'd

| Description | Classic characteristics | Etiology and pathology | Clinical manifestations | Management |
|---|---|---|---|---|
| **Second-degree atrioventricular block, type II** (also called *Mobitz type II*) | | | | |
| Failure of some of the sinus impulses to be conducted to the ventricles | Pacemaker site: SA node<br>Rhythm: atrial regular, ventricular irregular<br>Rate: atrial normal, ventricular normal, but may be slower than atrial rate<br>P waves: occur in multiples<br>QRS complex: widening preceded by two or more P waves<br>Intervals: normal | Association with myocardial infarction of acute anterior or anteroseptal wall, rheumatic and other silent heart diseases, or digitalis toxicity<br>Occurrence lower in the AV node than type I block | This rhythm is more serious than type I second-degree block because a certain number of impulses from the sinus node are not conducted to the ventricles. This almost always occurs in the His-Purkinje system.<br>Patients may be hypotensive, have bradycardia, and exhibit symptoms of decreased cardiac output. | Treatment is necessary even if patient is asymptomatic.<br>If acute myocardial infarction has occurred, pacemaker is inserted.<br>Isoproterenol is last resort in emergency situation. |

Illustrations from Monahan FD, Neighbors M: *Medical-surgical nursing: foundations for clinical practice,* ed 2, Philadelphia, 1998, WB Saunders. *SA,* Sinoatrial; *AV,* atrioventricular.

**cardiac asthma,** an attack of asthma associated with heart disease, such as left ventricular failure, and characterized by predominant pulmonary congestion with some bronchoconstriction.

**cardiac atrophy,** a wasting of heart muscle usually caused by cachexia, aging, or a mediastinal tumor.

**cardiac care,** a nursing intervention from the Nursing Interventions Classification (NIC) defined as limitation of complications resulting from an imbalance between myocardial oxygen supply and demand for a patient with symptoms of impaired cardiac function. See also **Nursing Interventions Classification.**

**cardiac care: acute,** a nursing intervention from the Nursing Interventions Classification (NIC) defined as limitation of complications for a patient recently experiencing an episode of an imbalance between myocardial oxygen supply and demand resulting in impaired cardiac function. See also **Nursing Interventions Classification.**

**cardiac care: rehabilitative,** a nursing intervention from the Nursing Interventions Classification (NIC) defined as promotion of maximum functional activity level for a patient who has suffered an episode of impaired cardiac function that resulted from an imbalance between myocardial oxygen supply and demand. See also **Nursing Interventions Classification.**

**cardiac catheter,** a long, fine catheter designed to be passed into the heart through a blood vessel. Used for diagnosis, it allows the determination of blood pressure and the rate of blood flow in the vessels and chambers of the heart and the identification of abnormal anatomy. Medication may be instilled directly through the catheter into a coronary vessel, often seen by tomography.

**cardiac catheterization,** a diagnostic procedure in which a catheter is introduced through an incision into a large vein, usually of an arm or a leg, and threaded through the circulatory system to the heart.

■ METHOD: The sterile radiopaque catheter 100 to 125 cm in length ultimately reaches the superior vena cava, and then into the right atrium (or through an artery leading to the left ventricle) and other structures to be studied. The course of the catheter is followed with fluoroscopy, and radiographs may be taken. An electrocardiogram is monitored on an oscilloscope. As the catheter tip passes through the chambers and vessels of the heart, blood pressure is monitored, and blood samples are taken to study the oxygen content.

■ NURSING INTERVENTION: An antibiotic is often given the day before the procedure. Cardiac catheterization takes from 1 to 3 hours: the patient has to lie still but may be asked to cough or breathe deeply during the procedure. It is anxiety producing and the patient needs explanation and emotional support. A young child may need a sedative. The pulse on the operative side and the blood pressure on the other side of the body are monitored at least every 15 minutes for 1 hour and every half hour thereafter. During left heart catheterization, peripheral pulses are also monitored. The temperature may be elevated for several hours, and there may be pain at the incision site. The nurse observes the site for bleeding and for signs of infection, thrombophlebitis, and cardiac arrhythmia. Cardiac catheterization is typically performed by a special team in a special laboratory. By offering information and

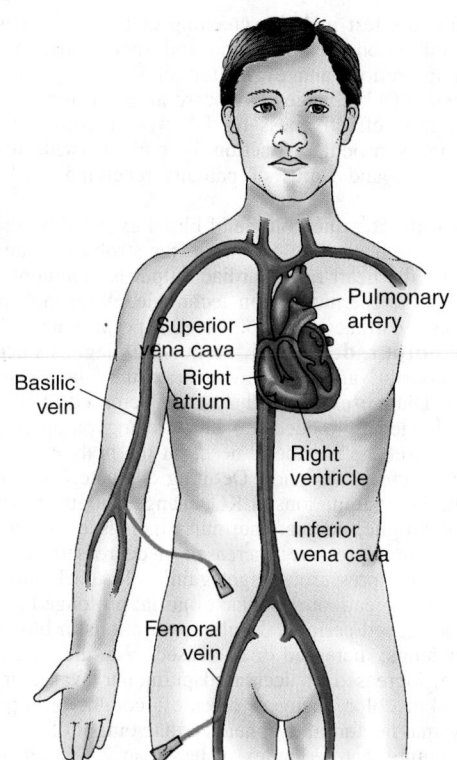

**Right-sided cardiac catheterization**
*(Ignatavicius, Workman, and Mishler, 1999)*

counseling, a member of the team may be of great help to the patient before and after the procedure.

■ OUTCOME CRITERIA: Many conditions may be accurately identified and assessed by using cardiac catheterization, including congenital heart disease, tricuspid stenosis, and valvular incompetence. Among the risks of the procedure are local infection, cardiac arrhythmia, and thrombophlebitis.

**cardiac cirrhosis** [Gk, *kardia,* heart, *kirrhos,* yellow-orange, *osis,* condition], an increase of fibrous tissue in the liver resulting from congestive heart failure, chronic myocarditis, or cardiac fibrosis.

**cardiac compression.** See **cardiac tamponade.**

**cardiac conduction defect,** any impairment of the electrical pathways and specialized muscular fibers that conduct impulses through the heart and result in atrial and ventricular contraction. Conduction defects may develop between the sinus and atrioventricular (AV) nodes, between the SA node and the AV bundle, or within the AV bundle or the left or right bundle branches. Defective transmission of cardiac impulses may be caused by ischemia, necrosis, drugs, electrolyte disturbances, or trauma. See also **heart block.**

**cardiac cycle** [Gk, *kardia* + *kyklos,* circle], the cycle of events in the heart during which an electrical impulse is conducted from the sinus node to the atrioventricular (AV) node, to the AV bundle, to the bundle branches, and to the Purkinje fibers, causing depolarization of the atria followed by depolarization of the ventricles. Depolarization leads to contraction. The contractions of the left and the right atria are nearly simultaneous; they precede the nearly simultaneous contractions of the ventricles. Structural, chemical, or electrical abnormalities may cause a large variety of anomalies in the cardiac cycle.

**cardiac decompensation,** a condition of congestive heart failure in which the heart is unable to ensure adequate cellular perfusion in all parts of the body without assistance. Causes may include myocardial infarction, increased workload, infection, toxins, or defective heart valves.

**cardiac depressant** [L, *deprimere,* to press down], an agent that decreases heart rate and contractility. See also **antiadrenergic, calcium channel blocker.**

**cardiac dyspepsia,** a digestive disorder associated with heart disease.

**cardiac dyspnea** [Gk, *dys,* difficult, *pnoia,* breath], breathing distress caused by heart disease. It is most commonly the result of pulmonary venous congestion.

**cardiac edema** [Gk, *oidema,* swelling], an accumulation of serum fluid from blood plasma in the interstitial tissues as a result of congestive heart failure. In severe cases, the fluid may also accumulate in serous cavities.

**cardiac electrical axis,** the main direction of electrical current flow in the heart. It may be calculated in the frontal plane limb leads or the horizontal plane using precordial leads.

**cardiac exercise stress test,** a noninvasive electrodiagnostic and/or nuclear test used to evaluate chest pain in patients with suspected coronary disease, to determine the safe limits of exercise during a cardiac rehabilitation program, to detect labile or exercise-related hypertension, to detect intermittent claudication, to evaluate the effectiveness of antianginal or antiarrhythmic drugs, and to evaluate the effectiveness of cardiac surgical intervention.

**cardiac failure.** See **heart failure.**

**cardiac hypertrophy,** an abnormal enlargement of the heart muscle. It frequently accompanies long-standing hypertension and congestive heart failure.

**cardiac impulse** [Gk, *kardia* + L, *impellere,* to set in motion], **1.** the mechanical movement of the thorax caused by the beating of the heart. It is readily palpable and easily recorded. See also **point of maximum impulse. 2.** the electrical stimulus generated by the heart for pacing purposes.

**cardiac index,** a measure of the cardiac output of a patient per square meter of body surface area. Its normal range in a healthy adult is 2.8 to 4.2 L/min/m$^2$.

**cardiac insufficiency,** the inability of the heart to pump efficiently. See also **cardiac decompensation.**

**cardiac massage,** repeated, rhythmic compression of the heart applied directly, during surgery, or through the intact chest wall in an effort to maintain circulation after cardiac arrest or ventricular fibrillation. Also called **heart massage.** See also **cardiopulmonary resuscitation.**

**cardiac monitor,** a device for the continuous observation of cardiac function. It may include electrocardiograph and oscilloscope readings, recording devices, and a visual and/or audible record of heart function and rhythm. An alarm system may be set to identify abnormal rhythms or heart rates.

**cardiac monitoring,** a continuous check on the functioning of the heart with an electronic instrument that provides an electrocardiographic reading on an oscilloscope. Each ventricular contraction of the heart is indicated by either a flashing light or an audible sound. The indicator is often integrated with an alarm system that is triggered by a pulse rate above or below predetermined limits. See also **electrocardiograph.**

**cardiac murmur,** an abnormal sound heard during auscultation of the heart, caused by altered blood flow into a chamber or through a valve. A murmur is classified by its time of occurrence during the cardiac cycle, its duration, and its intensity on a scale of I to VI. Also noted are the part of the heart over which the murmur is heard and any parts to which it radiates. In certain age groups, many systolic murmurs are benign and of no significance, while others signal a cardiac disorder. Diastolic murmurs are always pathologic. Also called **heart murmur.**

**cardiac muscle,** a special striated muscle of the myocardium, containing dark intercalated disks at the junctions of abutting fibers. Cardiac muscle is an exception among involuntary muscles, which are characteristically smooth. Its contractile fibers resemble those of skeletal muscle but are only one third as large in diameter, are richer in sarcoplasm, and contain centrally located instead of peripheral nuclei. Compare **smooth muscle, striated muscle.**

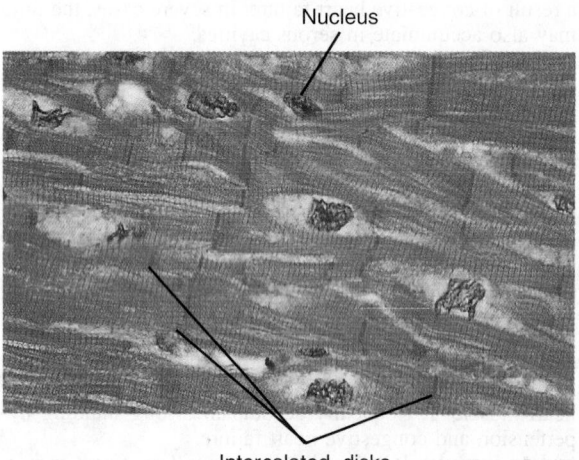

Nucleus

Intercalated disks

**Cardiac muscle** *(© Ed Reschke; used with permission)*

**cardiac nuclear scanning,** a nuclear scan used to detect myocardial ischemia, infarction, wall dysfunction, and decreased ejection fraction. It is commonly used as the imaging method portion of cardiac stress testing. Specific indications for this test include screening of adults for past and recent infarction, quantification and surveillance of myocardial infarction, and evaluation of the following: chest pain and ECG changes, myocardial perfusion pre- and post-surgery, effectiveness of therapy for coronary artery perfusion, ventricular function in patients with myocardial disease, and status of patients receiving cardiotoxic drugs.

**cardiac output,** the volume of blood expelled by the ventricles of the heart with each beat (the stroke volume) multiplied by the heart rate. Cardiac output is commonly measured by the thermodilution technique. A normal, resting adult has a cardiac output of 4 to 8 L per minute.

**cardiac output, decreased,** a nursing diagnosis accepted by the Fourth National Conference on the Classification of Nursing Diagnoses (revised 2000). Decreased cardiac output is defined as inadequate blood being pumped by the heart to meet the metabolic needs of the body.
■ DEFINING CHARACTERISTICS: Defining characteristics include arrhythmias; palpitations; EKG changes; jugular vein distension; fatigue; edema; murmurs; increased or decreased central venous pressure; increased or decreased pulmonary artery wedge pressure; weight gain; cold or clammy skin; shortness of breath or dyspnea; oliguria; prolonged capillary refill; decreased peripheral pulses; variations in blood pressure readings; increased or decreased systemic vascular resistance; increased or decreased pulmonary vascular resistance; skin color changes; crackles; cough; orthopnea or paroxysmal nocturnal dyspnea; cardiac output of less than 4 L per minute; cardiac index of less than 2.5 L per minute; decreased ejection fraction, Stroke Volume Index, or Left Ventricular Stroke Work Index; $S_3$ and $S_4$ heart sounds; anxiety; and restlessness.
■ RELATED FACTORS: Related factors include an altered heart rate or rhythm, altered preload, altered afterload, and altered contractility. See also **nursing diagnosis.**

**cardiac pacemaker.** See **pacemaker.**

**cardiac pain.** See **angina pectoris.**

**cardiac plexus** [Gk, *kardia* + L, pleated], one of several nerve networks situated close to the arch of the aorta. The cardiac plexuses contain sympathetic and parasympathetic nerve fibers that follow the right and left coronary arteries into the heart. Some of these fibers terminate in the sinus node; others terminate in the atrioventricular node and in the atrial myocardium.

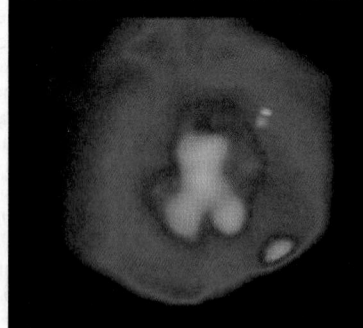
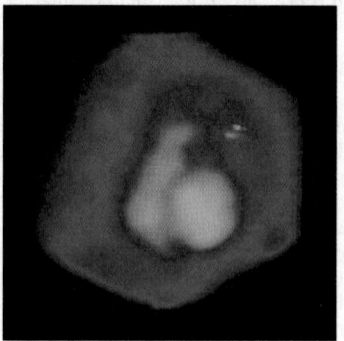

**Determination of ventricular function with cardiac nuclear imaging**
*(Cannobio, 1990)*

**cardiac precautions,** a nursing intervention from the Nursing Interventions Classification (NIC) defined as prevention of an acute episode of impaired cardiac function by minimizing myocardial oxygen consumption or increasing myocardial oxygen supply. See also **Nursing Interventions Classification.**

**cardiac pump effectiveness,** a nursing outcome from the Nursing Outcome Classification (NOC) defined as extent to which blood is ejected from the left ventricle per minute to support systemic perfusion pressure. See also **nursing outcomes classification.**

**cardiac radionuclide imaging** [Gk, *kardia* + L, *radiare,* to shine, *nucleus,* nut kernel, *imago,* image], the noninvasive examination of the heart, using a radiopharmaceutical, such as thallium-201, and a detection device, such as a gamma camera, positron camera, or rectilinear scanner. Clinical applications of cardiac radionuclide imaging are the gated cardiac blood pool scan, myocardial imaging, and detection of myocardial necrosis.

**cardiac reflex** [L, *reflectere,* to bend back], a neural mechanism that automatically increases or reduces the heart rate. Stimulation of stretch receptors in the right side of the heart by increased venous return increases the heart rate, whereas increased arterial blood pressure stimulates nerve endings in the carotid sinus and aortic arch to the heart rate.

**cardiac regurgitation** [Gk, *kardia,* heart; L, *re + gurgitare,* to flow], a backward flow of blood through one or more defective heart valves.

**cardiac rehabilitation** [Gk, *kardia,* heart; L, *re + habilitas,* ability], a supervised program of progressive exercise, psychologic support, education, and training to enable a patient to resume the activities of daily living on an independent basis following a myocardial infarction. The patient may require special training to adapt to a new occupation and life-style.

**cardiac reserve,** the potential capacity of the heart to function well beyond its basal level, in response to alterations in physiologic demands.

**cardiac rhythm** [Gk, *kardia,* heart, *rhythmos*], the recurring beat of the heart.

**cardiac souffle** /soo′fəl/ [Gk, *kardia,* heart; Fr, puff], a heart murmur having a soft, blowing sound.

**cardiac sphincter** [Gk, *kardia* + *sphingein,* to bind], a ring of muscle fibers at the juncture of the esophagus and stomach.

**cardiac standstill,** the complete cessation of ventricular contractions and ejection of blood by the heart. Cardiac standstill requires immediate cardiopulmonary resuscitation and pacing. See also **cardiac arrest.**

**cardiac stenosis** [Gk, *kardia,* heart; Gk, *stenos,* narrow, *osis,* condition], a nonvalvular obstruction of blood flow through any heart chamber. The cause may be a thrombosis or tumor.

**cardiac stimulant,** a pharmacologic agent that increases the action of the heart. Cardiac glycosides increase the force of myocardial contractions and decrease the heart rate and conduction velocity, allowing more time for the ventricles to relax and become filled with blood. These glycosides are used in the treatment of congestive heart failure, atrial flutter and fibrillation, paroxysmal atrial tachycardia, and cardiogenic shock. Toxic signs and symptoms that result from an overdose or the cumulative effect of slowly eliminated digitalis preparations include anorexia, nausea, vomiting, diarrhea, abdominal pain, headache, muscle weakness, confusion, drowsiness, irritability, visual disturbances, bradycardia or tachycardia, ectopic heartbeats, bigeminy, and a pulse deficit. Toxic effects may be attributed to an overdose or decreased growth hormone releasing factor. Epinephrine, a potent vasopressor and cardiac stimulant, is sometimes used to restore heart rhythm in cardiac arrest but is not used in treating heart failure or cardiogenic shock. Isoproterenol hydrochloride, which is related to epinephrine, may be used in treating heart block. Amrinone, dobutamine hydrochloride, and dopamine are used in the short-term treatment of cardiac decompensation resulting from depressed contractility.

**cardiac syncope** /sing′kəpē/ [Gk, *kardia,* heart, *syncope,* fainting], a temporary loss of consciousness caused by inadequate cerebral blood flow, which results from a sudden failure in cardiac output for any reason.

**cardiac tamponade** /tam′pənäd′/, compression of the heart produced by the accumulation of blood or other fluid in the pericardial sac. Also called **cardiac compression, pericardial tamponade.**

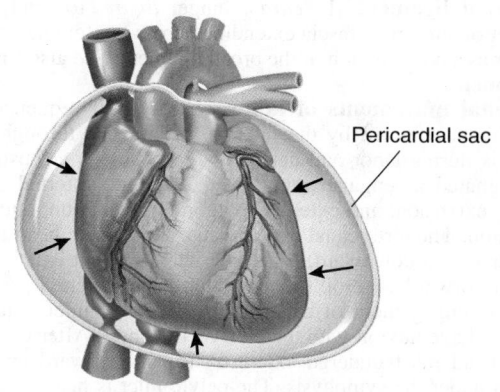

Pericardial sac

**Cardiac tamponade**

■ OBSERVATIONS: Signs of cardiac tamponade may include distended neck veins, hypotension, decreased heart sounds, tachypnea, peripheral pulses that are weak or absent or that fall sharply during inspiration (pulsus paradoxus), reduced left atrial pressure, and pericardial friction rub. The patient, who is usually anxious and restless, may sit upright or lean forward, and the skin may be pale, dusky, or cyanotic. The electrocardiogram generally shows decreased cardiac voltage, and the chest x-ray film may reveal an enlarged heart shadow ("water bottle" heart).

■ INTERVENTIONS: The patient is maintained on bed rest; the head of the bed is elevated 45 degrees, and a defibrillator and emergency drugs are kept at the bedside. Blood pressure, respiration, apical pulse, and atrial and pulmonary wedge pressures are checked every 15 to 30 minutes. Auscultation for pulsus paradoxus is performed, and peripheral pulses are checked every 30 minutes. A 12-lead electrocardiogram is usually ordered, and the patient is placed on a cardiac monitor with the rhythm strip checked every hour. A Doppler echocardiogram is done initially and may be repeated a few days later. Cardiotonic and antiarrhythmic drugs are administered as ordered. Aspiration of the fluid in the pericardial sac (pericardiocentesis) is performed and if surgery is indicated, the patient is prepared for the procedure. In cases where bleeding vessels are the cause of the tamponade, the vessels are ligated.

**cardiac thrombosis** [Gk, *kardia,* heart, *thrombos,* lump, *osis,* condition], a blood clot located at a heart valve or in one of the heart chambers. A left ventricular thrombosis may follow a large myocardial infarction.

**cardiac valve.** See **heart valve.**

**cardiasthenia** /kar′dē·asthē′nē·ə/ [Gk, *kardia,* heart, *a,* without, *sthenos,* strength], a form of neurasthenia in which cardiovascular symptoms are prominent.

**cardiectomy** /kär′dē·ek′təmē/, **1.** removal of the heart. **2.** removal of the cardiac portion of the stomach.

**cardiectopia** /kär′dē·ektō′pē·ə/, abnormal positioning of the heart in the thoracic cavity.

**cardinal** /kär′dənal/ [L, *cardo,* hinge], so fundamental that other things hinge on it, such as a cardinal trait that influences one's total behavior.

**cardinal frontal plane** [L, *cardo,* hinge, *frons,* forehead, *planum,* level ground], the plane that divides the body into front and back portions. Also called **vertical plane.**

**cardinal horizontal plane.** See **transverse plane.**

**cardinal ligament** [L, *cardo,* hinge, *ligare,* to bind], a sheet of subserous fascia extending across the female pelvic floor as a continuation of the broad ligament. See also **broad ligament.**

**cardinal movements of labor,** the typical sequence of positions assumed by the fetus as it descends through the pelvis during labor and delivery. The positions are usually designated as engagement, flexion, descent, internal rotation, extension, and external rotation or restitution, and expulsion. The birth canal is a curved cylinder; the head must enter it in a downward, transverse direction but exit it in a more forward, anteroposterior direction. In a vertex presentation, engagement of the head in the pelvic inlet requires that it have flexion with the chin on the chest. After descent the head must undergo extension to turn forward and be born under the symphysis. The pelvic inlet is heart-shaped, and the fetal head enters it facing obliquely; however, the pelvic outlet is diamond-shaped, and the head usually exits it facing posteriorly and must undergo internal rotation to do so. After delivery of the head, the shoulders remain for a time in the oblique plane, and the head undergoes external rotation or restitution to allow the widest diameter of the shoulders to be delivered from the longer anteroposterior diameter of the pelvic outlet.

**cardinal position of gaze,** (in ophthalmology) one of six positions to which the normal eye may be turned. This test evaluates the functioning of the six extraocular muscles and cranial nerves III, IV, and VI. The positions and the corresponding muscles and nerves are as follows: (1) straight nasal: medial rectus and the third cranial nerve; (2) up nasal: inferior oblique and the third cranial nerve; (3) down nasal: superior oblique and the fourth cranial nerve; (4) straight temporal: lateral rectus and the sixth cranial nerve; (5) up temporal: superior rectus and the third cranial nerve; (6) down temporal: inferior rectus and the third cranial nerve.

**cardinal sagittal plane.** See **median plane.**

**cardinal symptom.** See **symptom.**

**cardioangiography.** See **cardiac angiography.**

*Cardiobacterium,* a gram-negative genus of facultative anaerobic rod-shaped bacteria that is part of the normal flora of the human nasopharynx region. It is associated with endocarditis.

**cardiocatheterization.** See **cardiac catheterization.**

**cardiocele** /kär′dē·ōsēl′/, protrusion of the heart through an opening in the diaphragm or the abdominal wall.

**cardiocirculatory** /kär′dē·ōsur′kyŏŏlətôr′ē/ [Gk, *kardia* heart; L, *circulare,* to go around], pertaining to the heart and the circulation.

**cardioesophageal reflux** /-əsof′əjē′əl/ [Gk, *kardia,* heart, *oisophagos,* gullet; L, *refluere,* to flow back], a backward flow or regurgitation of stomach contents into the esophagus. Repeated episodes of reflux can lead to esophagitis. Among factors contributing to the condition are stomach pressure greater than esophageal pressure, hiatal hernia, and incompetence of the lower esophageal sphincter.

**cardiogenic** /-jen′ik/, originating in the heart muscle.

**cardiogenic shock** [Gk, *kardia* + *genein,* to produce; Fr, *choc*], an abnormal condition often but not always characterized by a low cardiac output associated with acute myocardial infarction and congestive heart failure. Cardiogenic shock is fatal in about 80% of cases, and immediate therapy is necessary. Depending on the signs, therapy may include diuretics, vasoactive drugs, and the application of various devices. Compare **hypovolemic shock.** See also **electric shock, septic shock, shock.**

**cardiogram** See **electrocardiogram.**

**cardiograph.** See **electrocardiograph.**

**cardiography.** See **electrocardiography.**

**cardiohepatomegaly** /-hep′ətōmeg′əlē/, enlargement of the heart and liver.

**cardioinhibitory** /kär′dē·ō′inhib′itôr′ē/, slowing or inhibiting the function of the heart.

**cardiokinetic** /kä′dē·ō·ki·net′ik/ [Gk, *kardia,* heart + *kinesis,* motion], **1.** stimulating the action of the heart. **2.** an agent that stimulates action of the heart.

**cardiologist** /-ol′əjist/, a physician who specializes in the diagnosis and treatment of disorders of the heart.

**cardiology** /-ol′əjē/ [Gk, *kardia* + *logos,* science], the study of the anatomy, normal functions, and disorders of the heart.

**cardiomegaly** /kär′dē·ōmeg′əlē/ [Gk, *kardia* + *megas,* large], enlargement of the heart.

**cardiomyopathy.** See **myocardiopathy.**

**cardiomyopexy** /kär′dē·omī′əpek′sē/ [Gk, *kardia* + *mys,* muscle, *pexis,* fixation], a surgical procedure in which the blood supply from the nearby pectoral muscles of the chest is diverted directly to the coronary arteries of the heart.

**cardiopathy** /kär′dē·op′əthē/ [Gk, *kardia,* heart, *pathos,* disease], a disease of the heart.

**cardiopericarditis** /-per′ikärdī′tis/, inflammation of the heart and the pericardium.

**cardioplasty** /kär′dē·ōplas′tē/, a surgical procedure to correct a defect in the cardiac sphincter of the esophagus that frequently leads to cardiospasm. Cardiospasm is caused by failure of the sphincter to relax so that food can enter the stomach.

**cardioplegia** /-plē′jə/ [Gk, *kardia* + *plege,* stroke], **1.** paralysis of the heart. **2.** the arrest of myocardial contractions

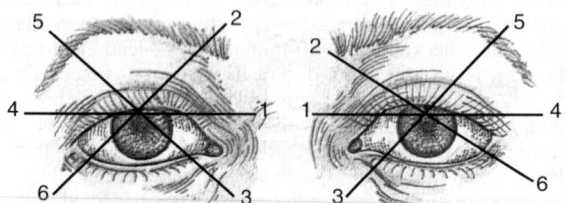

**Cardinal positions of gaze** *(Potter and Perry, 1997)*

by hypothermia, electrical stimuli, or injection of chemicals for the purpose of performing surgery on the heart. See also **cardiac standstill.**

**cardiopulmonary** /-pul′məner′ē/ [Gk, *kardia* + L, *pulmo,* lung],   pertaining to the heart and lungs.

**cardiopulmonary arrest.**   See **cardiac arrest.**

**cardiopulmonary bypass,**   a procedure used in heart surgery in which the blood is diverted from the heart and lungs by means of a pump oxygenator and returned directly to the aorta.

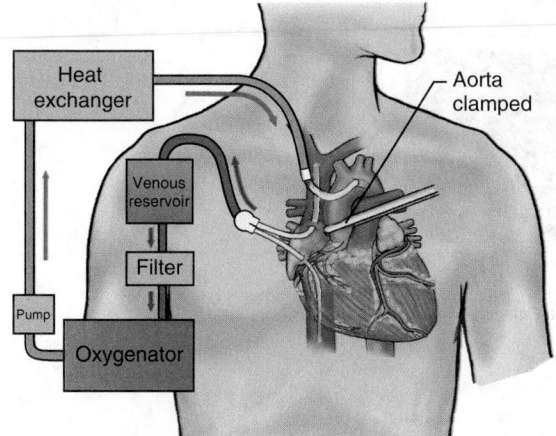

**Components of a cardiopulmonary bypass system**
*(Monahan and Neighbors, 1998)*

**cardiopulmonary murmur** [Gk, *kardia,* heart; L, *pulmo,* lung, *murmur,* humming],   a sound heard over the heart during breathing and during the heartbeat. It is caused by vibrations that result when the heart strikes the lung tissue with every beat. Also called **cardiorespiratory murmur.**

**cardiopulmonary resuscitation (CPR),**   a basic emergency procedure for life support, consisting of artificial respiration and manual external cardiac massage. It is used in cases of cardiac arrest to establish effective circulation and ventilation in order to prevent irreversible cerebral damage resulting from anoxia. External cardiac massage compresses the heart between the lower sternum and the thoracic vertebral column. During compressions, blood is forced into systemic and pulmonary circulation, and venous blood refills the heart when the compression is released. Mouth-to-mouth breathing or a mechanical form of ventilation is used concomitantly with CPR to oxygenate the blood being pumped through the circulatory system.

■ METHOD: Basic cardiopulmonary resuscitation requires no adjunctive equipment, although mechanical devices can be used. It involves three interrelated actions: opening the airway, restoring breathing, and restoring circulation. For an adult, the procedure is performed by one or two rescuers in the following manner:

1. The victim is placed on a hard flat surface, such as a CPR board, a backboard, or, if necessary, the floor. Resuscitation efforts are not delayed while the rescuer is waiting for such a support.
2. The victim is examined closely to determine unresponsiveness and shaken on the shoulder. The rescuer shouts, "Can you hear me? Are you all right?" If there is no response, the victim is assumed to be unconscious.

3. The rescuer (if alone) or someone else activates the emergency medical services system.
4. The rescuer establishes and maintains an open airway. In the supine position the victim's relaxed muscles allow the tongue to drop back in the throat, blocking the airway. This blockage can be relieved easily by tilting the head. One hand is placed on the forehead of the victim, and the other is used to lift the lower jaw or chin, placing the fingers and thumb on top of the jaw, avoiding pressure on the soft tissue below the chin. The head is held in this position, which extends the neck and lifts the tongue from the back of the throat. In a case of suspected cervical spine injury, the neck is not hyperextended. Instead, the lower jaw is lifted by placing the fingers behind the angles of the victim's jaw in front of the ear lobes and displacing it upward. If available, an oropharyngeal airway is inserted; if not, the head is held in position, either tilted back or with jaw lifted, throughout the resuscitation procedure See also **head-tilt, chin-lift airway technique.**
5. The rescuer evaluates the need for artificial respiration by looking, listening, and feeling for signs of air exchange or respiratory effort. If there is no spontaneous exchange and if there is no stoma (artificial airway device) over the larynx, regular artificial respiration is begun immediately. If there is a stoma, mouth-to-stoma respiration is initiated.
6. To begin artificial respiration, the rescuer rotates the hand that has been placed on the victim's forehead and, using the thumb and index finger of this hand, pinches the nostrils closed while continuing to press downward on the forehead. A secretion barrier may be used to prevent contact with the victim's secretions. A tight seal is made with the rescuer's mouth around the mouth of the victim, and two slow, full breaths, lasting 1½ to 2 seconds, are given. The rescuer's mouth is removed, and the victim is allowed to exhale passively. The rescuer watches the chest fall and then breathes in another breath. The cycle is repeated, one breath every 5 seconds, as long as respiratory deficiency exists. If indicated, mouth-to-nose respiration may be used. If the chest does not expand, the head is repositioned and ventilation is again attempted. A second unsuccessful attempt indicates an obstructed airway. See also **Heimlich maneuver.**
7. The rescuer takes the carotid pulse and checks for cardiac arrest. If the pulse is absent or inadequate, the carotid artery is palpated for 5 to 10 seconds immediately after the two initial breaths are given. Absence or questionable pressure of the pulse at that time indicates the need to begin external cardiac compression.
8. To start external massage, the rescuer takes a position facing the side of the victim. To find the correct location for the hands (the landmark position), the chest is uncovered, and the xiphoid process is identified. With the middle finger on the xiphoid process and the index finger beside it, the heel of the other hand is placed on the lower half of the sternum, directly adjacent to the fingers marking the xiphoid. With the fingers extended upward and away from the ribs, the first hand is placed on top of the second and the fingers are interlocked. With arms straight, the rescuer positions the shoulders directly over the hands and rocks up and down from the hip joints, exerting sufficient downward pressure with the forward swing of the body to depress the victim's sternum 1½ to 2 inches. It is extremely important to be positioned properly to prevent depression of the xiphoid process and possibly severe internal injury. After each compression a rest is allowed for a time equal to the time of compression, but the hands are not moved from their position on the chest. The cycle is repeated, using a ratio of 15 compressions to two breaths at the rate of 80 to 100 compressions a minute. The proper rhythm may be achieved by counting "1 and 2 and 3," up to 15. If two rescuers are available, CPR is performed with one rescuer giving compressions and the other giving breaths, at a 5:1 ratio at a rate of 80 to 100 compressions a minute. The proper rhythm can be determined by counting "1-1000, 2-1000," up to "5-1000." Effectiveness of CPR is checked by palpating the carotid artery for the return of a spontaneous heartbeat after the first minute and then

## Basic life support for adults and children

| Objectives | Actions | | |
|---|---|---|---|
| | *Adult* *(over 8 yr)* | *Child* *(1 to 8 yr)* | *Infant* *(under 1 yr)* |
| **A—Airway** | | | |
| 1. Assessment: Determine unresponsiveness. | Tap or gently shake shoulder. | | |
| | Ask, "Are you okay?" | | Observe. |
| 2. Position victim. | Turn on back as unit, supporting head and neck if necessary. | | |
| 3. Open airway. | Open airway with head-tilt/chin-lift. | | |
| **B—Breathing** | | | |
| 4. Assessment: Determine breathlessness. | Maintain open airway. Place ear over mouth, observing chest. Look, listen, feel for breathing (3-5 sec). | | |
| 5. Give two rescue breaths. | Seal mouth-to-mouth with barrier device or bag-valve device. | | Seal mouth-to-mouth/nose with barrier device. |
| | Give two rescue breaths 1½-2 sec each. Observe chest rise. Allow lung deflation between breaths. | | |
| **C—Circulation** | | | |
| 6. Assessment: Determine pulselessness. | Feel for carotid pulse (5-10 sec); maintain head-tilt. | | Feel for brachial pulse maintain head-tilt. |
| 7. If pulseless, begin chest compressions. a. Landmark check. | Run middle finger along bottom edge of rib cage to notch at center (tip of sternum). | | Imagine line drawn between nipples. |

From Sanders MJ: *Mosby's paramedic textbook,* ed 2, St Louis, 2000, Mosby. Illustrations from Stoy WA: *Mosby's first responder textbook,* St Louis, 1997, Mosby.

## Basic life support for adults and children—cont'd

| Objectives | Actions | | |
|---|---|---|---|
| | Adult (over 8 yr) | Child (1 to 8 yr) | Infant (under 1 yr) |
| **C—Circulation—cont'd** | | | |
| b. Hand placement. | Place index finger next to finger on notch. Place two hands next to index finger. Depress 1½-2 inches. | Place heel of one hand next to index finger. Depress 1-1½ inches. | Place 2-3 fingers on sternum, 1 finger's width below line. Depress ½-1 inch. |
| c. Compression rate. | Give 80-100 compressions per min. | Give 100 compressions per min. | |
| **CPR cycles** | | | |
| 8. Compressions to one breath. | Give two breaths every 15 compressions. | Give one breath every five compressions. | |
| 9. Number of cycles. | 4 (52-73 sec) | 10 (60-87 sec) | 20 (approx. 60 sec) |
| 10. Reassessment. | Feel for carotid pulse. If there is no pulse, resume CPR. | | Feel for brachial pulse. |
| **Entrance of second rescuer.** | | | |
| Second rescuer should perform one-rescuer CPR when first rescuer becomes fatigued. Compression rate for two-rescuer CPR is 80-100 per min; compression ratio is five chest compressions to one breath. | | | |
| **Option for pulse return** | | | |
| If not breathing, give rescue breaths. | Give one breath every 5 sec (12 per min). | Give one breath every 3 sec (20 per min). | |

every few minutes thereafter and by watching for "pinking" of the skin, constriction of the pupils, and a return of respiration. If the rescuer doing compressions becomes tired, a switch may be made by changing the counting rhythm to "switch-1000, 2-1000" up to "5-1000." At the end of that cycle, the rescuer giving compressions moves to the victim's head and checks the pulse. The rescuer who has been at the head, after giving a breath, moves to the victim's side and positions hands for administering compressions. If the pulse is absent or its pressure is inadequate, the rescuer at the head says, "No pulse. Continue CPR." The technique for infants up to 1 year of age and for children up to 8 years of age is like that for adults, with the following exceptions. In infants, the neck is not hyperextended because soft cartilage and neck tissues may occlude the airway if the head is tilted too far; placing a hand beneath the shoulders of an infant provides adequate tilt. The rescuer's mouth covers the infant's mouth and nose, and the infant's pulse is checked on the brachial artery. For an infant up to 1 year old, the rescuer imagines a line drawn between the nipples and places an index finger below that line in the center of the chest. The rescuer sets the middle and ring fingers next to the index finger and uses the two fingers to compress the sternum approximately ½ to 1 inch, exerting a downward thrust. For children 1 to 8 years of age, the heel of one hand is used. Because the ventricles of the heart in infants and small children lie higher in the chest cavity than they do in adults, external pressure is applied midsternum and only to a depth of 0.5 to 1 inch for infants, 1 to 1½ inch for young children 1 to 8 years of age, and 1½ to 2 inches for children over 8 years of age. The rate of cardiac compression for infants is at least 100 a minute, with breaths interposed as quickly as possible after each five compressions—approximately one every 3 seconds. The rate of compression for children over 8 years is 100 a minute, with ventilations delivered once every 4 seconds. Less air is necessary for a child than for an adult. For an infant gentle rescue breaths are given. Infants and children are given 20 cycles of compression and rescue breaths before the rescuer quickly phones to activate the emergency medical service system. If a second rescuer is available that person can activate the emergency medical services system while the first rescuer works with the infant or child victim.

■ OUTCOME CRITERIA: To provide adequate basic life support, these rules for correct performance should be followed:
1. CPR should not be interrupted for more than 5 seconds, except for endotracheal intubation or for moving of a victim. In these cases the interruption should not exceed 15 seconds.
2. Compressions should be smooth, regular, and uninterrupted.
3. The victim's condition should be stabilized before transportation to a more convenient site.
4. The pressure on the chest should be completely released after each compression, although the palm of the hand remains in contact with the chest wall.
5. The shoulders of the rescuer should be placed directly above the victim's sternum to provide the most effective thrusts.
6. The sternum should be depressed to the correct degree according to the size and age of the victim.
7. The xiphoid process should not be compressed because of the danger of lacerating the liver or other internal organs.
8. Gastric distension should not be relieved unless it becomes so severe that it interferes with ventilation. CPR is used only in cases of sudden cardiac arrest. Even if it is initiated as soon as possible and all steps are performed correctly, there are some cases, such as those that involve severe emphysema or crushing chest injuries, in which it is not successful. Even properly performed, CPR may cause rib fractures in some victims. Other complications include fracture of the sternum, separation of costochondral cartilage, hepatic hematoma, lung contusions, and fat embolism. The danger of complications is minimized by correct performance. Properly performed, external cardiac massage can produce a systolic blood pressure peaking at more than 100 mm

Hg in the carotid arteries. With no heartbeat the diastolic pressure is 0; thus the mean pressure with CPR is usually about 40 mm Hg, and the flow of arterial blood is approximately 25% to 35% of the normal flow. These figures point out the need for immediate action and for continuous effort to effect a rescue; they also indicate that CPR can be effective and can save lives if properly given in a carefully monitored fashion. CPR is an interim measure used until advanced life support action and definitive measures can be taken. Once initiated, it is continued until one of the following occurs: Spontaneous circulation and respiration are restored; resuscitation efforts are transferred to someone who can continue life-support procedures, either basic or advanced; a physician assumes responsibility for the victim; the victim is handed over to the care of a medical facility; or the rescuer is physically unable to continue.

■ INTERVENTIONS: Cardiopulmonary resuscitation is considered an emergency procedure, and knowledge of the principles, procedures, requirements, and complications of this maneuver is essential. In the hospital, there are additional tasks to perform to implement CPR. Primarily, the nurse evaluates the extent of the emergency and the indications for initiating lifesaving measures. The nurse is also prepared to undertake immediate action should it be necessary to do so before the medical team arrives. If not immediately involved in performing CPR, the nurse prepares for the initiation of definitive therapy by readying equipment, including an electrocardiograph (ECG), a defibrillator, a tracheostomy set, oxygen, and a suction machine. Epinephrine to be directly injected into the heart, sodium bicarbonate to combat acidosis, and calcium chloride to stimulate cardiac contraction are also prepared for injection and properly labeled. While resuscitation proceeds, efforts are made to start an IV infusion, and ECG electrodes are applied to the patient. In the hospital mouth-to-mask ventilation is recommended to protect health care workers from direct contact with oral secretions of the patient. The decision to terminate resuscitation efforts is made by a physician.

**cardiorespiratory.** See **cardiopulmonary.**

**cardiorespiratory murmur.** See **cardiopulmonary murmur.**

**cardiorrhaphy** /kär′dē·ôr′əfē/ [Gk, *kardia* + *rhaphe*, suture], an operation in which the heart muscle is sutured.

**cardioselectivity** /-sel′əktiv′itē/, selectivity of a drug, such as a beta-adrenergic agent, for heart tissue over other tissues of the body.

**cardiospasm** /kär′dē·əspaz′əm/ [Gk, *kardia* + *spasmos*, pull], a form of achalasia characterized by a failure of the cardiac sphincter at the distal end of the esophagus to relax. It causes dysphagia and regurgitation and sometimes requires surgical division of the muscle.

**cardiotachometer** /kär′dē·ō′təkom′ətər/ [Gk, *kardia* + *tachos*, speed, *metron*, measure], an instrument that continually monitors and records the heartbeat.

**cardiotherapy,** treatment of heart disease.

**cardiothoracic ratio** /-thôras′ik/, the ratio of the diameter of the heart at its widest point to the maximum width of the thoracic cavity, assessed by examining a chest x-ray. The normal ratio is 1:2.

**cardiotomy** /kär′dē·ot′əmē/ [Gk, *kardia* + *temnein*, to cut], 1. an operation in which the heart is incised. 2. an operation in which the cardiac end of the stomach or cardiac orifice is incised.

**cardiotonic** /kär′dē·ōton′ik/ [Gk, *kardia* + *tonos*, tone], 1. pertaining to a substance that tends to increase the efficiency of contractions of the heart muscle. 2. a pharmacologic agent that increases the force of myocardial contractions. Cardiac glycosides, derived from certain plant alkaloids, exert a tonic effect by altering the transport of electrolytes across the myocardial membrane, causing an increased influx of sodium and calcium and an increased efflux of potassium. Digitalis, digitoxin, and digoxin, widely used cardiac glycosides obtained from leaves of a species of foxglove, increase the force of myocardial contractions, extend the refractory period of the atrioventricular node, and, to a lesser degree, affect the sinoatrial node and the heart's conduction system.

**cardiotoxic** /-tok′sik/ [Gk, *kardia* + *toxikon,* poison], having a toxic or injurious effect on the heart.

**cardiovascular** /kär′dē·ōvas′kyələr/ [Gk, *kardia* + L, *vasculum,* small vessel], pertaining to the heart and blood vessels.

**cardiovascular assessment,** an evaluation of the condition, function, and abnormalities of the heart and circulatory system.

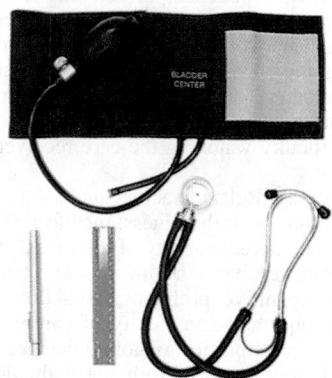

**Equipment for cardiovascular assessment**
*(Canobbio, 1990)*

■ METHOD: The patient is asked to describe the onset, duration, location, and characteristics of any pain present and the occurrence of weakness, fatigue, shortness of breath, fever, coughing, wheezing, and palpitations. Questions are asked about episodes of fainting, indigestion, nausea, edema of extremities, cyanosis, and vision changes, and whether the hands and feet ever feel numb or cold. The person's general appearance, assumed position, rate and rhythm of all arterial pulses, presence of pulsus paradoxus or pulsus alternans, and the distension, pulsation, and pressure of neck veins are observed. Blood pressure, temperature, and rate and character of respirations are checked. The precordium is examined for the point of maximal impulse, symmetry, the cardiac border, pulsations, and evidence of lifts or bulges. Auscultation of the chest is performed to determine the intensity, pitch, duration, timbre, origin, and frequency of heart sounds and murmurs and to identify the location and character of breath sounds, including crackles, rhonchi, and rubs. Color, temperature, turgor, and dryness or sweating of the skin are noted, and the appearance of the extremities, capillary filling time, nails, and lesions are described. The patient's level of consciousness, reflexes, neurologic signs, and responses to pain are recorded, along with data on concurrent hypertension, obesity, diabetes, and any pulmonary and renal conditions. Information is obtained about any previous cardiovascular surgery and illnesses, such as rheumatic fever, myocardial infarction, angina, congenital heart disease, occlusive vascular disease, and lung and kidney disorders. Pertinent background data include the patient's response to stress, coping methods, relationships, occupation, environment, sleep pattern, exercise level, leisure activities, and use of alcohol, tobacco, and other drugs. Other factors considered in the evaluation are the patient's history of medication with digitalis preparations, antihypertensives, diuretics, aspirin, sleeping pills, over-the-counter cold and influenza remedies; use of illegal drugs such as cocaine; and family history of heart disease, hypertension, diabetes, obesity, vascular disorders, stroke, and renal disease. Diagnostic aids are electrocardiogram, chest x-ray film, echocardiogram, radionuclide imaging, coronary arteriogram, cardiac catheterization, and arterial and pulmonary wedge pressure readings. Appropriate laboratory studies include a complete blood count, hemoglobin and hematocrit determinations, electrolyte and clotting profiles, and assays of serum cholesterol, triglycerides, aspartate aminotransferase, alanine aminotransferase, creatine phosphokinase, and lactic acid dehydrogenase.

■ INTERVENTIONS: The nurse usually obtains the patient's history, records the external observations, checks the vital signs, auscultates the chest, and assembles the pertinent background information and reports on diagnostic tests. In specialty areas such as a coronary care unit the nurse may interpret electrocardiographic tracings and adjust medications.

■ OUTCOME CRITERIA: An accurate and complete assessment of cardiovascular function is an essential adjunct to a complete physical examination and is vital to the diagnosis and proper continuing care of a patient with cardiovascular disease.

**cardiovascular disease,** any abnormal condition characterized by dysfunction of the heart and blood vessels. In the United States cardiovascular disease is the leading cause of death. Some common kinds of cardiovascular disease are **atherosclerosis, cardiomyopathy, rheumatic heart disease, syphilitic endocarditis,** and **systemic venous hypertension.**

**cardiovascular reflex,** a reflex in which heart and circulatory functions are altered in response to changes in heart rate, vascular tone, blood volume, or other variables.

**cardiovascular shunt** [Gk, *kardia,* heart; L, *vasculum,* small vessel; ME, *shunten*], any abnormal passage between chambers of the heart or between the systemic and pulmonary circulatory systems.

**cardiovascular system,** the network of anatomic structures, including the heart and blood vessels, that circulate blood throughout the body. The system includes thousands of kilometers of vessels that deliver nutrients and other essential materials to the fluids surrounding the cells and that remove waste products and convey them to excretory organs.

**cardiovascular technologist,** an allied health professional who performs diagnostic examinations at the request or direction of a physician in invasive cardiology, noninvasive cardiology, and/or peripheral vascular study. Through subjective data collection and/or recording, the technologist obtains information from which a correct anatomic and physiologic diagnosis may be established for each patient.

**cardioversion** /-vur′zhən/ [Gk, *kardia* + L, *vertere,* to turn], the restoration of the heart's normal sinus rhythm through an electric shock delivered by a defibrillator. Application of the shock is synchronized to the QRS complex. Cardioversion is used to slow the heart or to restore the heart's normal sinus rhythm when drug therapy is ineffective at doing so. Also called **cardiovert**.

**cardiovert.** See **cardioversion**.

**cardioverter** /-vur'tər/, a defibrillator or other instrument used to convert abnormal heart rhythms into normal rhythms.

**carditis** /kärdī'tis/, inflammation of the heart muscle, usually resulting from infection. In most cases more than one layer of muscle is involved. Chest pain, cardiac arrhythmia, circulatory failure, and damage to the structures of the heart may occur. Kinds of carditis are **endocarditis, myocarditis,** and **pericarditis**.

**Cardizem,** trademark for a calcium channel blocker (diltiazem).

**career ladder, 1.** (in nursing education) a pathway for upward mobility that begins with a course of study in practical nursing or a program that grants an **Associate Degree in Nursing.** On completion of this basic level, the candidate may continue up the ladder, to earn a **Bachelor of Science in Nursing,** and then to the graduate level to earn a master's degree and a doctoral degree in nursing. **2.** a pathway for advancement in the professional nursing role in an institution.

**caregiver,** one who contributes the benefits of medical, social, economic, or environmental resources to a dependent or partially dependent individual, such as a critically ill person.

**caregiver adaptation to patient institutionalization,** a nursing outcome from the Nursing Outcome Classification (NOC) defined as family caregiver adaptation of role when the care recipient is transferred outside the home. See also **nursing outcomes classification.**

**caregiver emotional health,** a nursing outcome from the Nursing Outcome Classification (NOC) defined as feelings, attitudes, and emotions of a family care provider while caring for a family member or significant other over an extended period of time. See also **nursing outcomes classification.**

**caregiver home care readiness,** a nursing outcome from the Nursing Outcome Classification (NOC) defined as preparedness to assume responsibility for the health care of a family member or significant other in the home. See also **nursing outcomes classification.**

**caregiver life-style disruption,** a nursing outcome from the Nursing Outcome Classification (NOC) defined as disturbances in the life-style of a family member due to caregiving. See also **nursing outcomes classification.**

**caregiver-patient relationship,** a nursing outcome from the Nursing Outcome Classification (NOC) defined as positive interactions and connections between the caregiver and care recipient. See also **nursing outcomes classification.**

**caregiver performance: direct care,** a nursing outcome from the Nursing Outcome Classification (NOC) defined as provision by family care provider of appropriate personal and health care for a family member or significant other. See also **nursing outcomes classification.**

**caregiver performance: indirect care,** a nursing outcome from the Nursing Outcome Classification (NOC) defined as arrangement and oversight of appropriate care for a family member or significant other by family care provider. See also **nursing outcomes classification.**

**caregiver physical health,** a nursing outcome from the Nursing Outcome Classification (NOC) defined as physical well-being of a family care provider while caring for a family member or significant other over an extended period of time. See also **nursing outcomes classification.**

**caregiver role strain,** a nursing diagnosis accepted by the Tenth National Conference on the Classification of Nursing Diagnoses (revised 2000). Caregiver role strain is defined as a difficulty in performing the caregiver role.

■ DEFINING CHARACTERISTICS: Defining characteristics include difficulty in performing or completing required tasks; preoccupation with care routine; apprehension about the future regarding the receiver's health and the caregiver's ability to provide care; apprehension about the receiver's care if the caregiver becomes ill or dies; dysfunctional change in caregiving activities; and apprehension about possible institutionalization of care receiver. The caregiver may experience gastrointestinal upset, weight change, rash, hypertension, cardiovascular disease, diabetes, fatigue, headaches, impaired individual coping, feeling depressed, disturbed sleep, anger, stress, somatization, increased nervousness, increased emotional lability, impatience, lack of time to meet personal needs, frustration, withdrawl from social life, change in leisure activities, low work productivity, refusal of career advancement, family conflict, and concerns about family members. The caregiver may also experience grief or uncertainty regarding a changed relationship with the care receiver and difficulty watching the care receiver go through the illness.

■ RELATED FACTORS: Related factors include the severity of illness; the chronicity of the illness; increasing care needs or dependency; the unpredictability of the illness course; instability of the care receiver's health; problem behaviors; psychological or cognitive problems; addiction or codependency; the number and complexity of caregiver activities; 24-hour care responsibilities; ongoing changes in activities; discharge of family members to home with significant care needs; years of caregiving; the unpredictability of the care situation; physical problems; psychological or cognitive problems; marginal coping patterns; urealistic expectations of self; inability to fulfill one's own or other's expectations; isolation from others; competing role commitments; alienation from family, friends, and co-workers; insufficient recreation; history of poor relationship; presence of violence or abuse; unrealistic expectations of caregiver by care receiver; mental status of elder inhibiting conversation; history of marginal family coping; history of family dysfunction; inadequate physical environment for providing care; inadequate equipment for providing care; inadequate transportation; inadequate community resources; insufficient finances; lack of support; caregiver is not developmentally ready for caregiver role; inexperience with caregiving; insufficient time; lack of knowledge about or difficulty accessing community resources; lack of caregiver privacy; emotional strength; physical strength; and assistance and support. See also **nursing diagnosis.**

**caregiver role strain, risk for,** a nursing diagnosis accepted by the Tenth National Conference on the Classification of Nursing Diagnoses. Risk for caregiver role strain is a state of vulnerability to experiencing of difficulty in performing the family caregiver role.

■ RISK FACTORS: Risk factors may be physiologic, developmental, psychosocial, or situational. Physiologic factors include severity of the care receiver's illness, addiction or codependency, premature birth or congenital defect, discharge of a family member with significant home health needs, caregiver health impairment, unpredictable illness course or instability in the care receiver's health, or gender of the caregiver (female). Developmental factors include a developmental inability to fulfill the caregiver role and developmental delay or retardation of the care receiver or caregiver. Psychosocial factors include psychological or cognitive problems in the care receiver, marginal family adaptation or dysfunction before caregiving became necessary, marginal coping patterns of the caregiver, history of a poor relationship with the care receiver, spousal relationship to care receiver, and deviant, bizarre behavior exhibited by the care receiver. Situational factors include the presence of abuse or violence, presence of normal situational stressors, duration of caregiving required, inadequate physical environment for providing care, isolation, lack of respite and recreational, inexperience with caregiving, competing role commitments, and complexity and number of caregiving tasks. See also **nursing diagnosis.**

**caregiver stressor,** a nursing outcome from the Nursing Outcome Classification (NOC) defined as the extent of biopsychosocial pressure on a family care provider caring for a family member or significant other over an extended period of time. See also **nursing outcomes classification.**

**caregiver support,** a nursing intervention from the Nursing Interventions Classification (NIC) defined as provision of the necessary information, advocacy, and support to facilitate primary patient care by someone other than a health care professional. See also **Nursing Interventions Classification.**

**caregiver well-being,** a nursing outcome from the Nursing Outcome Classification (NOC) defined as primary care provider's satisfaction with health and life circumstances. See also **nursing outcomes classification.**

**caregiving endurance potential,** a nursing outcome from the Nursing Outcome Classification (NOC) defined as factors that promote family care provider continuance over an extended period of time. See also **nursing outcomes classification.**

**care of the chronically ill,** medical and nursing services that focus on long-term care of people with chronic diseases or conditions, either at home or in a medical facility. It includes measures specific to the problem, as well as others to encourage self-care, promote health, and prevent loss of function.

**care of the sick,** (in public health nursing) the care of ill patients in their homes, as distinguished from health supervision. Public health nursing agencies are reimbursed for the nursing services rendered by the nurses according to the kind of service rendered, such as a sick visit or a health supervision visit. Compare **health supervision.**

**care plan.** See **nursing care plan.**

**CARF,** abbreviation for *Commission on Accreditation of Rehabilitation Facilities.*

**caries** /ker′ēz/ [L, decay], See **dental caries.**

**carina** /kərē′nə/, *pl.* **carinae** [L, keel], any structure shaped like a ridge, cleft, or keel, such as the carina of the trachea, which projects from the lowest tracheal cartilage.

**caring behaviors,** actions characteristic of concern for the well-being of a patient, such as sensitivity, comforting, attentive listening, and honesty.

**cariocas** /kär′ē-ō′kəs/, a form of lateral movement in a gait cycle in which the side-stepping leg is moved successively behind and then in front of the stance leg.

**cariogenic** /ker′ē-ōjen′ik/, tending to produce dental caries.

**carisoprodol** /ker′isōprō′dol/, a skeletal muscle relaxant.

■ INDICATION: It is prescribed for the relief of muscle spasm.

■ CONTRAINDICATIONS: Porphyria or known hypersensitivity to this drug or to chemically similar drugs, such as meprobamate, prohibits its use.

■ ADVERSE EFFECTS: Among the more serious adverse reactions are ataxia, drowsiness, pronounced weakness, visual disturbances, mental confusion, anaphylactic shock, erythema multiforme, and allergic reactions.

**carmalum.** See **carmine dye.**

**carminative** /kärmin′ətiv/ [L, *carminare,* to cleanse], **1.** pertaining to a substance that relieves flatulence and abdominal distension. **2.** an agent that relieves gaseous distension and painful spasms, especially after meals.

**carmine dye** /kär′min/ [AR, *qirmize* + AS, *deag*], a red coloring substance, produced by the addition of alum to an extract of cochineal, used for staining histologic specimens. Also called **carmalum.**

**carmustine** /kärmus′tin/, a lipid-soluble nitrosourea, 1, 3-bis (2-chloroethyl)-*l*-nitrosourea, used as a single antineoplastic agent or with other approved chemotherapeutic agents in the treatment of brain tumors, multiple myeloma, Hodgkin's disease, and non-Hodgkin's lymphomas. Also called **BCNU.**

**carnal** /kär′nəl/ [L, *caro,* flesh], pertaining to the flesh or body, or worldly things, as distinguished from spiritual.

**carneous** /kär′nē-əs/, having the quality of flesh.

**carnitine** /kär′nitin/, a substance found in skeletal and cardiac muscle and certain other tissues that functions as a carrier of fatty acids across the membranes of the mitochondria. It is used therapeutically in treating angina and certain deficiency diseases, particularly endocardial fibroelastosis, and as an antithyroid agent. It has actions that closely resemble those of amino acids and B vitamins.

**carnitine *O*-palmitoyltransferase** /kär′ni·tēn päl′mi·tō′əl·trans′fər·ās/, an enzyme that catalyzes the transfer between coenzyme A and carnitine of long chain fatty acids; deficiency is a cause of defective fatty acid oxidation. Also written **carnitine palmityltransferase.**

**carnitine palmityltransferase deficiency** /kär′ni·tēn päl′mi·til trans′fər·ās dē·fish′ən·sē/, an autosomal recessive disorder of lipid metabolism, seen more often in men, in which the altered enzyme is abnormally regulated, resulting in muscle aches, fatigability, and myoglobinuria (but without lipid accumulation), occurring after prolonged exercise, particularly in the cold or after fasting.

**Carnitor,** trademark for an amino acid derivative (levocarnitine).

**carnivore** /kär′nivôr/ [L, *caro,* flesh, *vorare,* to devour], an animal belonging to the order Carnivora, classified as a flesh eater, with appropriate teeth and a characteristically simple stomach and a short intestine for such a diet. —**carnivorous** /kärniv′ərəs/, *adj.*

**carnosine** /kär′nō·sēn/ [L, *caro,* flesh], a dipeptide composed of β-alanine and histidine, in humans found in skeletal muscle and in the brain, particularly in the primary olfactory pathways. It may play a role as a neurotransmitter.

**carnosinemia** /kär′nō·si·nē′mē·ə/, **1.** accumulation of carnosine in the blood. **2.** former name for **serum carnosinase deficiency.**

**carob, carob bean** /kar′əb/ [Ar. *al kharrubah*], *Ceratonia siliqua,* a tree native to the Mediterranean basin. The fruit of this tree, whose seed is leguminous. The finely pulverized meal of the dried ripe fruit contains albuminous proteins, carbohydrates, and small amounts of fat and crude fiber, and is used in pharmaceutical formulations as an adsorbent and demulcent in treatment of diarrhea.

**carotene** /kar′ətin/ [L, *carota*, carrot], a red or orange organic compound found in carrots, sweet potatoes, egg yolk, and leafy vegetables, such as beet greens, spinach, and broccoli. Beta-carotene is a provitamin and in the body is converted into vitamin A. See also **vitamin A.**

**carotenemia** /kar′ətinē′mē·ə/, the presence of high levels of carotene in the blood, which result in an abnormal yellow appearance of the plasma and skin. The conjunctivae are not discolored. Also called **pseudojaundice, xanthemia** /zanthē′mē·ə/. See also **jaundice.**

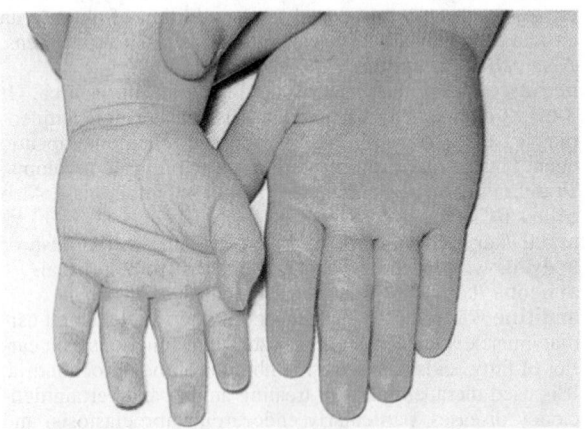

**Carotenemia: yellow-orange pigmentation**
*(Lawrence and Cox, 1993)*

**carotenoid** /kərot′ənoid/, any of a group of red, yellow, or orange highly unsaturated pigments that are found in foods such as carrots, sweet potatoes, and leafy green vegetables. Many of these substances, such as carotene, are used in the formation of vitamin A in the body, whereas others, including lycopene and xanthophyll, show no vitamin A activity. Also spelled **carotinoid.**

**carotenosis.** See **carotenemia.**

**carotid** /kərot′id/ [Gk, *karos*, heavy sleep], pertaining to the arteries that supply the head and neck. See also **carotid body, carotid sinus, common carotid artery.**

**carotid arch** [Gk, *karos*, heavy sleep; L, *arcus*, bow], the third arch of the aorta, the source of the common carotid arteries.

**carotid body** [Gk, *karos* + AS, *bodig*], a small structure containing neural tissue at the bifurcation of the carotid arteries. It monitors the pressure and oxygen content of the blood and therefore assists in regulating respiration.

**carotid-body reflex** [Gk, *karos* + AS, *bodig* + L, *reflectere*, to bend back], a normal chemical reflex initiated by a decrease in oxygen concentration in the blood and, to a lesser degree, by increased carbon dioxide and hydrogen ion concentrations that act on chemoreceptors at the bifurcation of the common carotid arteries. The resulting nerve impulses cause the respiratory center in the medulla to increase respiratory activity. See also **aortic-body reflex.**

**carotid-body tumor,** a benign round, firm growth that develops at the bifurcation of the common carotid artery. The tumor may cause dizziness, nausea, and vomiting, if it im-

pedes the flow of blood and pressure is increased in the vascular system. Surgical excision is the usual treatment in some cases.

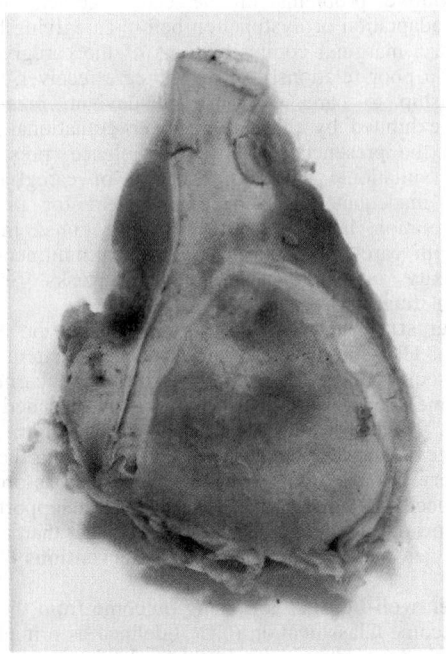

**Carotid-body tumor** *(Skarin, 1996)*

**carotid bruit,** a murmur heard over the carotid artery in the neck, suggesting arterial narrowing and usually secondary to atherosclerosis. Stroke is likely if the narrowing is severe and the condition is untreated.

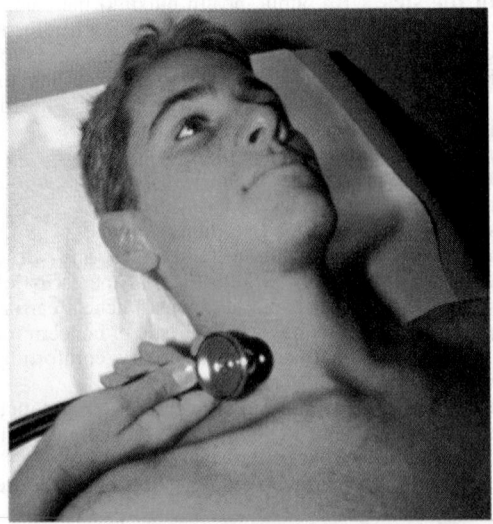

**Auscultation for carotid bruits** *(Lemmi and Lemmi, 2000)*

**carotid duplex scanning,** a noninvasive ultrasound test used on the extracranial carotid artery to detect occlusive disease directly. It is recommended for patients with headaches and with neurologic symptoms such as transient ischemic attacks (TIA), hemiparesis, paresthesia, and acute speech or visual defects.

**carotid endarterectomy,** surgical excision of atheromatous segments of the endothelium and tunica media of the carotid artery, leaving a smooth tissue lining and facilitating blood flow through the vessel. The surgery is done to prevent stroke.

**carotid plexus** [Gk, *karos* + L, pleated], any one of three nerve plexuses associated with the carotid arteries. Compare **common carotid plexus, external carotid plexus, internal carotid plexus.**

**carotid pulse,** the pulse of the carotid artery, palpated by gently pressing a finger in the area between the larynx and the sternocleidomastoid muscle in the neck. See also **pulse.**

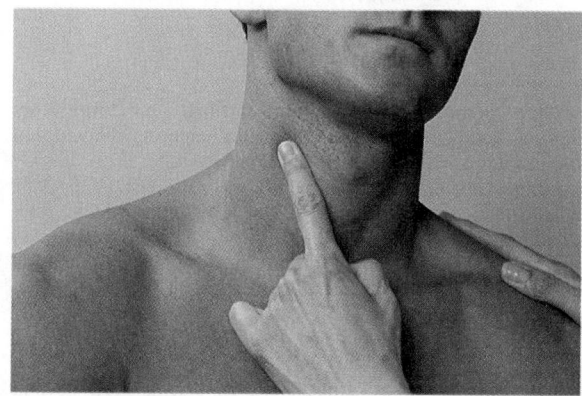

**Assessment of carotid pulse** *(Wilson and Giddens, 2001)*

**carotid sinus** [Gk, *karos* + L, curve], a dilation of the arterial wall at the bifurcation of the common carotid artery. It contains sensory nerve endings from the vagus nerve that respond to changes in blood pressure.

**carotid sinus massage,** firm rubbing at the bifurcation of the carotid artery at the angle of the jaw. It creates an elevation of blood pressure in the carotid sinus that results in reflex slowing of atrioventricular conduction and sinus rate. The technique may be used to reduce the heart rate in tachyarrhythmia.

**carotid sinus reflex,** a neural mechanism in which an increase in blood pressure in the carotid artery at the level of its bifurcation trigger a decrease in heart rate. See also **carotid sinus syndrome.**

**carotid sinus syncope.** See **carotid sinus syndrome.**

**carotid sinus syndrome,** a temporary loss of consciousness that sometimes accompanies convulsive seizures as a result of the intensity of the carotid sinus reflex when pressure builds in one or both carotid sinuses. Also called **carotid sinus syncope.**

**carotidynia** /kərot′idin′ē·ə/ [Gk, *karos* + *odyne*, pain], a pain along the length of the common carotid artery, caused by pressure.

**carp-, carpo-,** combining form meaning 'wrist': *carpal, carpometacarpal.*

**-carp,** suffix meaning 'fruit': *archicarp, pericarp.*

**carpal** /kär′pəl/ [Gk, *karpos*, wrist], pertaining to the carpus, or wrist.

**-carpal,** combining form referring to the wrist: *extracarpal, radiocarpal.*

**carpal ligaments,** four ligaments of the hand: the **dorsal ligament,** a thick band of white fibrous tissue on the dorsum of the wrist, attached to the lower end of the radius and to the styloid process of the ulna; the **radiate ligament of the wrist,** which projects from the head of the capitate bone to the volar aspects of other carpal bones; the broad, flat **transverse ligament,** which is attached to the tubercle of the scaphoid and the crest of the trapezium; and the **volar ligament,** a superficial part of the flexor retinaculum.

**carpal spasm,** a sudden, powerful, involuntary contraction observed as a tetanic flexion of the hands and wrists.

**carpal tunnel** [Gk, *karpos* + Fr, *tonnel*], a conduit for the median nerve and the flexor tendons, formed by the carpal bones and the flexor retinaculum.

**carpal tunnel release,** a surgical procedure for treating carpal tunnel syndrome.

**carpal tunnel syndrome,** a common painful disorder of the wrist and hand, induced by compression on the median nerve between the inelastic carpal ligament and other structures within the carpal tunnel. It is often seen in cumulative trauma to the wrist. Symptoms may result from trauma, synovitis, or tumor or may develop with rheumatoid arthritis, amyloidosis, acromegaly, or diabetes. The median nerve innervates the palm and the radial side of the hand; compression of the nerve causes weakness, pain with opposition of the thumb, and burning, tingling, or aching, sometimes radiating to the forearm and shoulder joint. Weakness and atrophy of muscles may increase from lack of use, as a result of pain that impairs thumb and finger dexterity. Pain may be intermittent or constant and is often most intense at night. Symptomatic treatment usually relieves mild symptoms of recent onset, but if the pain becomes disabling, the injection of corticosteroids often yields dramatic relief. Surgical division of the volar carpal ligament to relieve nerve pressure is usually curative. Treatment includes emotional support, nocturnal splinting of the hand and forearm, elevation of the arm to relieve the swelling of soft tissue, and encouragement of mild wrist and finger movements to prevent atrophy of muscles.

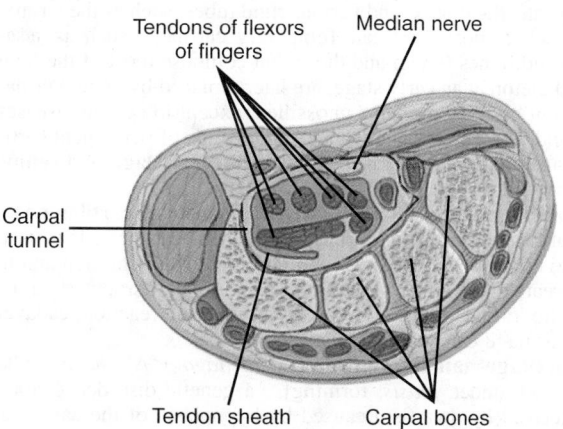

**Carpal tunnel syndrome: compression of the median nerve**
*(Thibodeau and Patton, 1999/Rolin Graphics)*

**Carpenter's syndrome** /kär′pən·tərz/ [George Carpenter, British physician, 1859–1910], an autosomal recessive form of acrocephalopolysyndactyly characterized also by mental retardation and shortened digits. See also **acrocephalopolysyndactyly.**

**carpometacarpal (CMC) joint** /-met′əkär′pəl/ [Gk, *karpos,* wrist, *meta,* next, *karpos*], any of the joints formed by the distal row of carpal bones and the bases of the metacarpals. The joints are essential for prehensile patterns.

**carpopedal** /-ped′əl/ [Gk, *karpos,* wrist; L, *pes,* foot], pertaining to the wrist and foot.

**carpopedal spasm** [Gk, *karpos* + L, *pes,* foot], a spasm of the hand, thumbs, foot, or toes that sometimes accompanies tetany.

**carpus** /kär′pəs/ [Gk, *karpos*], the wrist, made up of eight bones arranged in two rows. The proximal row consists of the scaphoid also called navicular, lunate, triangular, and pisiform. The distal row consists of the greater multiangular, lesser multiangular, capitate, and hamate.

**Carrel-Lindbergh pump.** See **Lindbergh pump.**

**carrier** /ker′ē·ər/ [OFr, *carier*], **1.** a person or animal who harbors and spreads an organism that causes disease in others but does not become ill. **2.** one whose chromosomes carry a recessive gene. **3.** an immunogenic molecule or part of a molecule that is recognized by T cells in an antibody response.

**carrier-free,** **1.** relating to a radioisotope in pure form, free of dilution by stable isotope carriers. **2.** describing a substance in which every molecule is marked by a radioactive tracer or other tag.

**Carrión's disease.** See **bartonellosis.**

**Carroll Quantitative Test of Upper Extremity Function,** a six-part test of a person's ability to grasp and lift objects of different shapes and sizes. It is designed to measure the ability to perform general arm and hand movements required for the activities of daily living.

**carrying angle,** the angle at which the humerus and radius articulate.

**carry-over** [L, *carrus,* wagon; AS *ofer*], contamination of a specimen by the previous one.

**car sickness** [L, *carrus,* wagon; AS, *seoc*], nausea and vomiting caused by the motion of a vehicle. See also **motion sickness.**

**cartilage** /kär′tilij/ [L, *cartilago*], a nonvascular dense supporting connective tissue composed of chondrocytes and various fibers or ground substance. It is found chiefly in the joints, the thorax, and various rigid tubes, such as the larynx, trachea, nose, and ear. Temporary cartilage, such as sesamoid bones (knee) and those that compose most of the fetal skeleton at an early stage, are later replaced by bone. Permanent cartilage remains unossified, except in certain diseases and, sometimes, in advanced age. Kinds of permanent cartilage are **hyaline cartilage, white fibrocartilage,** and **yellow cartilage.** —**cartilaginous,** *adj.*

**cartilage capped exostosis.** See **exostosis cartilaginea.**

**cartilage graft,** the transplantation of cartilage. It is used to correct congenital ear and nose defects in children and to treat severe injuries in adults. Because chondrocytes can be allografted without the risk of an immune reaction, cadaver cartilage can be used for tissue grafts.

**cartilage-hair hypoplasia** [L, *cartilago* + AS, *haer* + Gk, *hypo,* under, *plasis,* forming], a genetic disorder, characterized by dwarfism caused by hypoplasia of the cartilage, multiple skeletal abnormalities, and excessively sparse, short, fine, brittle hair that is usually light colored. It is inherited as an autosomal recessive trait. The condition is found primarily among Amish people in the United States and Canada.

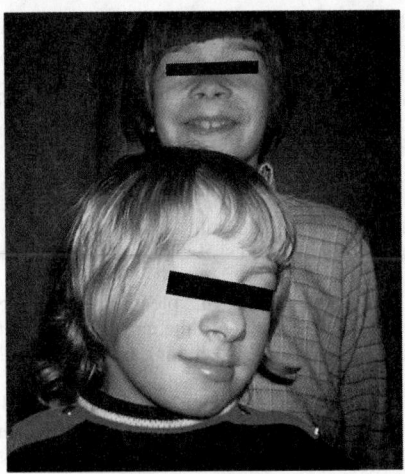

**Cartilage-hair hypoplasia**
*(Hordinsky, Sawaya, and Scher, 2000)*

**cartilage of auditory tube,** the cartilage on the inferomedial surface of the temporal bone that supports the walls of the cartilaginous portion of the auditory tube.

**cartilage tissue.** See **connective tissue.**

**cartilaginous** /kär′tilaj′inəs/ [L, *cartilago,* cartilage], pertaining to cartilage.

**cartilaginous bone,** bone that develops by endochondral ossification in a preexisting cartilage. Also called **endochondral bone.**

**cartilaginous joint** [L, *cartilago* + *junger,* to join], a slightly movable joint in which cartilage unites bony surfaces. Two types of articulation involving cartilaginous joints are synchondrosis and symphysis. Also called **amphiarthrosis, junctura cartilaginea.** Compare **fibrous joint, synovial joint.**

**cartilaginous septum of nose,** the plate of cartilage forming the anterior part of the nasal septum.

**cartilaginous skeleton** [L, *cartilago* + Gk, *skeletos,* dried up], the parts of the skeleton that are formed by cartilage.

**CARTOS** /kär′tos/, abbreviation for *computer-aided reconstruction by tracing of serial sections,* a technique in which serial hand-drawn copies of electron micrographs are programmed on a computer for display on a television screen. The image can be manipulated for study of all dimensions of the structure.

**caruncle** /kär′ungkəl/ [L, *caruncula,* small piece of flesh], a small fleshy projection, as one of the lacrimal caruncles at the inner canthus of the eye or the hymenal caruncles that are the hymenal remnants. Also called **caruncula.**

**carunculae hymenales** [L, *caruncula* + Gk, *hymen,* membrane], remnants of a ruptured hymen that appear as irregular projections of normal skin around the introitus to the vagina. Also called **hymenal tags.**

**carvedilol,** an α-/β-adrenergic blocker.

■ INDICATIONS: This drug is used to treat essential hypertension, either alone or in combination with other antihypertensives.

■ CONTRAINDICATIONS: Known hypersensitivity to this drug, bronchial asthma, class IV decompensated cardiac failure, second- or third-degree heart block, cardiogenic shock, and severe bradycardia prohibit the use of carvedilol.

■ ADVERSE EFFECTS: Life-threatening effects of this drug include atrioventricular block and thrombocytopenia. Other serious adverse effects include somnolence, depression, ataxia, diarrhea, bradycardia, dependent edema, peripheral edema, extrasystoles, hypertension, hypotension, palpitations, peripheral ischemia, urinary tract infection, viral infection, and hypertriglyceridemia.

**carve-out,** a service not covered in a health insurance contract. It is usually reimbursed according to a different arrangement or rate formula than those services specified under the contract umbrella.

**cascade** /kaskād'/ [L, *cadere,* to fall], any process that develops in stages, with each stage dependent on the preceding one, often producing a cumulative effect.

**cascade humidifier,** a bubbling respiratory care device in which gases travel down a tower and pass through a grid into a chamber of heated water. The displaced water rises above the grid, forming a liquid film that is converted to a froth as the gas also rises from the chamber through the grid. The process results in an airflow that can have a relative humidity of up to 100%.

**cascara sagrada,** an herbal product taken from the bark of a tree native to parts of the coast in the Pacific Northwest.
■ USES: This herb is used for chronic constipation, hepatitis, and gallstones.
■ CONTRAINDICATIONS: Cascara should not be used by those who are hypersensitive to this product, by women who are pregnant or lactating, or by children until more research is available. Also, it is contraindicated where GI bleeding, obstruction, abdominal pain, nausea, vomiting, appendicitis, and Crohn's disease are present.

**case** [L, *causus,* a happening], **1.** an episode of illness or injury. **2.** a container.

**caseation** /kā'sē·ā'shən/ [L, *caseus,* cheese], a form of tissue necrosis in which cellular outline is lost and the appearance is that of crumbly or liquified cheese. It is typical of tuberculosis. See also **caseous.** —**caseate,** *v.*

**caseation necrosis** [L, *caseus,* cheese; Gk, *nekros,* dead, *osis,* condition], necrosis that transforms tissue into a dry cheeselike mass. It occurs primarily in tuberculosis.

**case-control study,** an investigation using an epidemiologic approach in which previous cases of the condition are used in lieu of new information gathered from a randomized population. A group of patients with a particular disease or disorder, such as myocardial infarction, is compared with a control group of persons who have not had that medical problem. The two groups, matched for age, sex, and other personal data, are examined to determine which possible factor (e.g., cigarette smoking, coffee drinking) may account for the increased disease incidence in the case group.

**case fatality rate** [L, *causus,* a happening, *fatum,* fate, *(pro) rata*], the number of registered deaths caused by any specific disease, expressed as a percentage of the total number of reported cases of a specific disease.

**case finding,** the act of locating individuals with a disease.

**case history** [L, *causus* + *historia*], a patient's complete medical record before a current illness or injury. The history includes any infectious diseases experienced by the person, all immunizations, hospitalizations or therapies, information relating to deaths or illnesses of parents and other close family members, allergies, and congenital or acquired physical defects.

**casein,** a white powder protein that occurs naturally in milk. It contains phosphorus and sulfur and is regarded as a "complete protein" because it contains all essential amino acids. Casein is precipitated when milk turns sour.

**case management[1], 1.** a problem-solving process through which appropriate services to individuals and families are assured. **2.** a method of structuring acute care for all pa-

tients in three dimensions: work design, clinical management roles, and concurrent monitoring and feedback. **3.** a client-centered goal-oriented process of assessing the need of an individual for particular services and obtaining those services. See also **managed care.**

**case management[2],** a nursing intervention from the Nursing Interventions Classification (NIC) defined as coordinating care and advocating for specified individuals and patient populations across settings to reduce cost, reduce resource use, improve quality of health care, and achieve desired outcomes. See also **Nursing Interventions Classification.**

**case nursing** [L, *casus,* a happening, *nutrix,* nourish], an organizational mode for allocation of nursing staff in which one nurse is assigned to provide total nursing care to one or more patients.

**caseous** /kā'sē·əs/, cottage cheese-like; describing the mixture of fat and protein that appears in some body tissues undergoing necrosis.

**caseous abscess.** See **cheesy abscess.**

**caseous fermentation** [L, *caseus,* cheese, *fermentum,* yeast], the coagulation of soluble casein to form insoluble calcium paracaseinate through the action of rennin.

**caseous necrosis.** See **cheesy necrosis.**

**case rate,** a pricing method in which a flat amount, often a per diem rate, covers a defined group of procedures and services. It is often used in services such as obstetrics and cardiovascular surgery for exceptions to a relative value scale or resource-based relative value scale. Also called **case price.**

**case study,** a study that identifies and samples individuals with a particular disease or condition, noting characteristics of the disease or condition and persons afflicted. Case studies are often used to call attention to new diseases or to diseases entering new populations.

**CaSO$_4$,** the formula for **calcium sulfate.**

**Casodex,** trademark for an anticancer chemotherapy agent (bicalutamide).

**cassette** /kaset'/ [Fr, little box], a device used in radiography for holding a sheet of x-ray film and one or two screens. A cassette also may have a grid to absorb scattered radiation.

**cast** [ONorse, *kasta*], **1.** a stiff, solid dressing formed with plaster of paris or other material around a limb or other body part to immobilize it during healing. Kinds of casts include the **body jacket, long arm cast, long leg cast, short arm cast, short leg cast,** and **spica cast. 2.** a mold of a part or all of a patient's teeth and internal jaw area for fitting prostheses or dentures. **3.** a tiny structure formed by deposits of mineral or other substances on the walls of renal tubules, bronchioles, or other organs. Casts often appear in samples of urine or blood collected for laboratory examination. **4.** the deviation of an eye from the normal parallel lines of vision, such as in strabismus.

**cast brace,** a combination of a brace within a cast at a joint.

**cast care: maintenance,** a nursing intervention from the Nursing Interventions Classification (NIC) defined as care of a cast after the drying period. See also **Nursing Interventions Classification.**

**cast care: wet,** a nursing intervention from the Nursing Interventions Classification (NIC) defined as care of a new cast during the drying period. See also **Nursing Interventions Classification.**

**cast core** [ONorse, *kasta* + L, *cor,* heart], a metal casting, shaped like a stump of a tooth and incorporating a post in the root canal for the retention of an artificial tooth crown. Compare **amalgam core, composite core.** See also **core.**

**Castellani's paint.** See **carbol-fuchsin solution.**

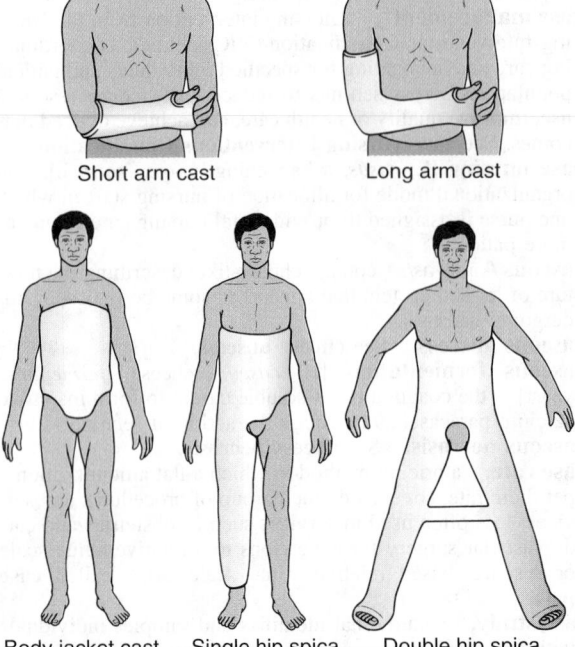

Short arm cast      Long arm cast

Body jacket cast   Single hip spica   Double hip spica

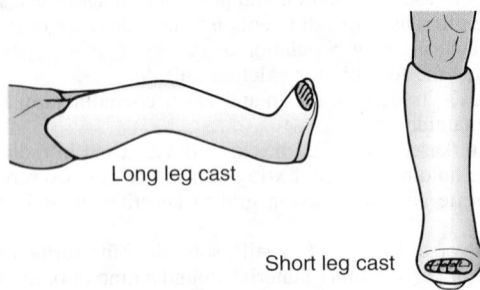

Long leg cast

Short leg cast

**Casts** *(Lewis, Heitkemper and Dirksen, 2000)*

**casting,**   **1.** the act of encasing a body part in a cast. **2.** (in dentistry) the process by which crowns, inlays, and other metallic restorations are produced.

**casting tape,**   an adhesive or resin-impregnated mesh used for shaping lightweight casts.

**Castleman's disease** /kas′əl·mənz/ [Benjamin Castleman, American pathologist, 1906−1982],   a condition resembling lymphoma but without recognizable malignant cells; there are isolated masses of lymphoid tissue and lymph node hyperplasia, usually in the abdominal or mediastinal area. One variety has numerous small germinal centers near blood vessels with vascular proliferation; a second type consists of sheets of plasma cells and fewer but larger germinal centers. The disease may be either benign or premalignant. Also called **giant lymph node hyperplasia.**

**castor oil** /kas′tər/ [L, beaver, *oleum,* olive oil],   an oil derived from *Ricinus communis,* used as a stimulant cathartic.

■ INDICATIONS: It is prescribed for constipation and as a cleansing preparation of the bowel or colon before examination.

■ CONTRAINDICATIONS: Symptoms of appendicitis, intestinal obstruction or perforation, and fecal impaction prohibit its use. It is not to be used during menstruation or pregnancy.

■ ADVERSE EFFECTS: Among the most serious adverse reactions are rectal bleeding and laxative dependence. Nausea, abdominal cramps, and dizziness also may occur.

**castration** /kastrā′shən/ [L, *castrare,* to castrate],   the surgical excision of one or both testicles or ovaries, performed most frequently to reduce the production and secretion of certain hormones that may stimulate the proliferation of malignant cells in women with breast cancer or in men with prostate cancer. The patient must be informed that bilateral excision of the gonads causes sterility. See also **oophorectomy, orchidectomy.**

**castration anxiety,**   **1.** the fantasized fear of injury or loss of the genital organs, often as the reaction to a repressed feeling of punishment for forbidden sexual desires. It may also be caused by some apparently threatening everyday occurrence, such as a humiliating experience, loss of a job, or loss of authority. **2.** a general threat to the masculinity or femininity of a person or an unrealistic fear of bodily injury or loss of power. Also called **anxiety complex.** See also **anxiety disorder.**

**castration complex.**   See **castration anxiety.**

**cast saw,**   a tool used to cut through a cast.

**cast shoe,**   a shoe worn over a foot that is encased in a cast.

**cast stabilization,**   the use of rods, pins, wooden shafts, or other devices to lend stability to a cast.

**casualty** /kazh′əltē/, [L, *casus,* chance],   **1.** a serious or fatal accident. **2.** the victims of a serious or fatal accident. **3.** a person, killed, wounded, or otherwise disabled in war.

**casuistics** /kazh′əwis′tiks/ [L, *casus,* a happening],   the recording and study of the cases of any disease.

**CAT** /kat/,   abbreviation for **computerized axial tomography.** See **computed tomography.**

**cata-, cat-,**   combining form meaning 'down, under, against, lower, with': *catabiosis, catabolic.*

**catabasis** /kətab′əsis/, *pl.* **catabases** [Gk, *kata,* down, *bainein,* to go],   the phase in which a disease declines. —**catabatic** /kat′əbat′ik/, *adj.*

**catabiosis** /kat′əbī·ō′sis/,   the normal aging of cells. —**catabiotic,** *adj.*

**catabolic.**   See **catabolism.**

**catabolic activator protein.**   See **CAP.**

**catabolic illness** /kat′əbol′ik/,   a disorder characterized by weight loss and diminished muscle mass and body fat. Underlying causes include infection, injury, organ system failure, chemotherapy, and uncontrolled diabetes mellitus, particularly type 1.

**catabolism** /kətab′əliz′əm/ [Gk, *kata + ballein,* to throw],   a metabolic process in which complex substances are broken down by living cells into simple compounds. The process liberates energy for use in work, energy storage, or heat production. Carbon dioxide and water are produced, as well as energy. Compare **anabolism.** —**catabolic,** *adj.*

**catachronobiology** /kat′əkrō′nōbī·ol′əjē/,   the study of the harmful effects of time on living systems. See also **chronobiology.**

**catacrotism** /kətak′rətiz′əm/ [Gk, *kata + krotein,* to strike],   an anomaly of the pulse, characterized by one or more small additional waves in the descending limb of the pulse tracing. —**catacrotic,** *adj.*

**catagen.**   See **hair.**

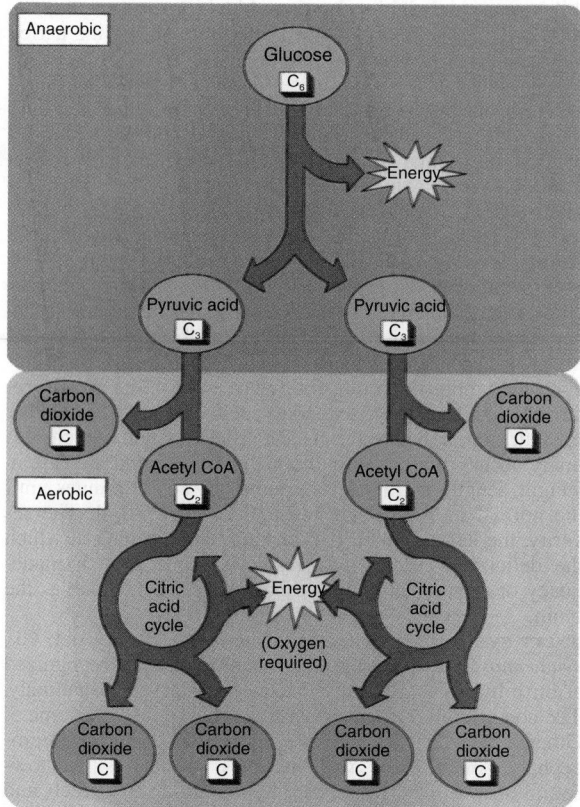

**Catabolism of glucose**
*(Thibodeau and Patton, 1999/Rolin Graphics)*

**catagenesis** /kat′əjen′əsis/ [Gk, *kata,* down, *genein,* to produce], a form of evolution that is retrogressive.

**catalase** /kat′əlās/ [Gk, *katalein,* to dissolve], a heme enzyme, found in almost all biologic cells, that catalyzes the decomposition of hydrogen peroxide to water and oxygen.

**catalepsy** /kat′əlep′sē/ [Gk, *kata* + *lambanein,* to seize], an abnormal state characterized by a trancelike level of consciousness and postural rigidity. It occurs in hypnosis and in certain organic and psychologic disorders such as schizophrenia, epilepsy, and hysteria.

**cataleptic** /kat′əlep′tik/, pertaining to mental illness characterized by maintenance of rigid waxlike postures.

**catalysis** /kətal′əsis/ [Gk, *katalein,* to dissolve], an increase in the rate of a chemical reaction that is caused by a substance that is neither permanently altered nor consumed by the reaction. Compare **negative catalysis.** See also **catalyst. —catalytic.** *adj.*

**catalyst** /kat′əlist/ [Gk, *katalein,* to dissolve], a substance that influences the rate of a chemical reaction without being permanently altered or consumed by the process. Most catalysts, including enzymes in living organisms, accelerate chemical reactions; negative catalysts retard such reactions. See also **enzyme.**

**-catalytic, -catalytical,** suffix meaning 'a chemical reaction caused by an agent unchanged by the reaction': *allelocatalytic, photocatalytic.*

**catalyze,** to produce catalysis, as speeding up a chemical reaction or physical process.

**catamenia.** See **menses.**

**catamnesis** /kat′amnē′sis/ [Gk, *kata* + *men,* month], the medical history of a patient from the onset of an illness. Compare **anamnesis.**

**cataphoria** /kat′əfôr′ē·ə/, a tendency of the visual axes of both eyes to assume a low plane, after the visual fusional stimuli have been eliminated.

**cataphylaxis** /kat′əfəlak′sis/ [Gk, *kata* + *phylax,* guard], **1.** the migration of leukocytes and antibodies to the site of an infection. **2.** the deterioration of the natural defense system of the body. **—cataphylactic,** *adj.*

**cataplexy** /kat′əplek′sē/ [Gk, *kata* + *plexis,* stroke], a condition characterized by sudden muscular weakness and hypotonia, caused by emotions, such as anger, fear, or surprise, often associated with narcolepsy. **—cataplectic,** *adj.*

**Catapres,** trademark for an antihypertensive (clonidine hydrochloride).

**cataract** /kat′ərakt/ [Gk, *katarrhakies,* waterfall], an abnormal progressive condition of the lens of the eye, characterized by loss of transparency. A gray-white opacity can be observed within the lens, behind the pupil. Most cataracts are caused by degenerative changes, often occurring after 50 years of age. The tendency to develop cataracts is inherited. Trauma, such as a puncture wound, may result in cataract formation; less often, exposure to such poisons as dinitrophenol or naphthalene causes them. **Congenital cataracts**

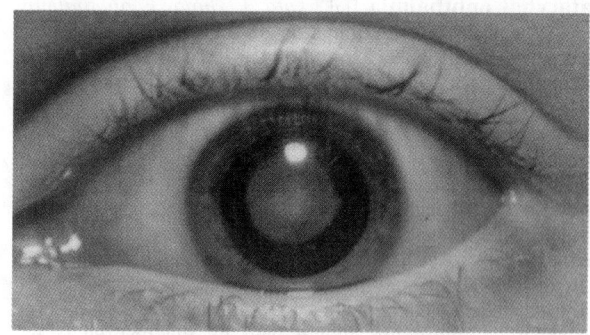

**Appearance of eye with cataract**
*(Black, Hawks, and Keene, 2001/courtesy Ophthalmic Photography, University of Michigan W.K. Kellogg Eye Center, Ann Arbor)*

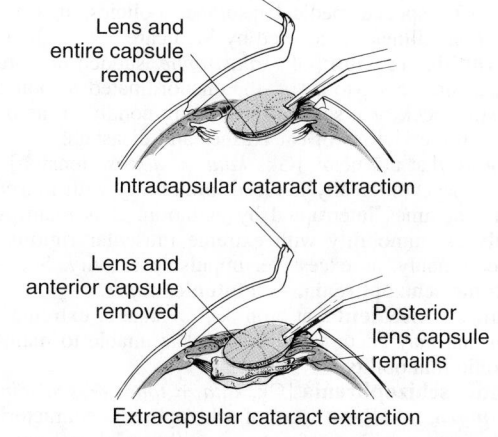

**Cataract removal** *(Black and Matassarin-Jacobs, 1997)*

are usually hereditary but may be caused by viral infection during the first trimester of gestation. If cataracts are untreated, sight is eventually lost. At onset vision is blurred; then bright lights glare diffusely, and distortion and double vision may develop. Uncomplicated cataracts of old age (**senile cataracts**) are usually treated with excision of the lens and either surgical insertion of an intraocular lens (IOL) or prescription of special contact lenses or glasses. The soft cataracts of children and young adults may be either incised and drained or fragmented by ultrasound.

**cataractogenic** /kat′ərak′tōjen′ik/, pertaining to agents that may cause cataracts.

**catarrh** /kətär′/ [Gk, *kata* + *rhoia*, flow], inflammation of the mucous membranes with discharge, especially inflammation of the air passages of the nose and the trachea. See also **rhinitis.** —**catarrhal, catarrhous,** *adj.*

**catarrhal** /kətär′əl/ [Gk, *kata*, down, *rhoia*, flow], pertaining to catarrh, or discharge from an inflamed mucous membrane.

**catarrhal conjunctivitis** [Gk, *kata* + *rhoia* + L, *conjunctivus*, connecting; Gk, *itis*, inflammation], a simple form of inflammation of the conjunctiva, usually associated with an infection, allergy, exposure to pollution, or physical irritation as by an eyelash in the eye. It is accompanied by discharge.

**catarrhal croup** [Gk, *kata* + *rhoia* + Scot, to croak], severe laryngitis accompanied by a croupy cough.

**catarrhal dysentery.** See **sprue.**

**catarrhal ophthalmia** [Gk, *kata* + *rhoia* + *ophthalmos*, eye], a catarrhal inflammation of the conjunctiva with a discharge. See also **catarrhal conjunctivitis.**

**catarrhal pneumonia.** See **bronchopneumonia.**

**catarrhal stomatitis.** See **simple stomatitis.**

**catarrhous.** See **catarrh.**

**catastrophic care** /kat′əstrof′ik/ [Gk, *katastrophe*, sudden downturn; L, *garrire*, to babble], a pattern of medical and nursing care that involves intensive, highly specialized life-support care of an acutely ill or severely traumatized patient.

**catastrophic health insurance,** health insurance that awards benefits to pay for the cost of severe or lengthy disability or illness. Benefits on some policies are not paid until a specified minimum amount paid by the insured is exceeded. Most policies have a limit in total benefits paid, and payment for certain kinds of services may be precluded or limited to a maximum indemnity.

**catastrophic illness,** any illness that requires lengthy hospitalization, extremely expensive therapies, or other care that would deplete a family's financial resources, unless covered by special medical insurance policies. In Canada catastrophic illness is covered by Medicare.

**catastrophic reaction** [Gk, *katastrophe*, sudden downturn; L, *re*, again, *agere*, to act], the uncoordinated response to a drastic shock or a sudden threatening condition, as often occurs in the victims of car crashes and disasters.

**catatonia** /kat′ətō′nē·ə/ [Gk, *kata* + *tonos*, tension], a state of psychologically induced immobility with muscular rigidity at times interrupted by agitation. It is manifested usually as immobility with extreme muscular rigidity or, less commonly, as excessive, impulsive activity. See also **catatonic schizophrenia.** —**catatonic,** *adj.*

**catatonic excitement** /kat′əton′ik/, a state of extreme agitation that may occur when a patient is unable to maintain catatonic immobility.

**catatonic schizophrenia** [Gk, *kata* + *tonos* + *schizein*, to split, *phren*, mind], a form of schizophrenia characterized by alternating periods of extreme withdrawal and extreme excitement. During the withdrawal stage, stupor, waxy flex-

ibility, muscular rigidity, mutism, blocking, negativism, and catalepsy (cerea flexibilitas) may be seen; during the period of excitement, purposeless and impulsive activity may range from mild agitation to violence. See also **catatonia.**

**catatonic stupor,** a form of catatonia characterized by a marked decrease in response to the environment with a reduction in spontaneous movement. These patients sometimes appear unaware of their environment.

**cat-bite fever.** See **cat-scratch fever.**

**CAT-CAM,** abbreviation for **contoured adducted trochanteric controlled alignment method.**

**catchment area** [L, *capere*, to take, *area*, space], the specific geographic area for which a particular institution, especially a mental health center, is responsible.

**catch-up growth** [L, *capere* + As, *uf, gruowan*], an acceleration of the growth rate following a period of growth retardation caused by a secondary deficiency, such as acute malnutrition or severe illness. The phenomenon, which routinely occurs in premature infants, involves rapid increase in weight, length, and head circumference and continues until the normal individual growth pattern is resumed. The severity, the duration, and the developmental timing at which the deficiency occurs may result in some growth inadequacy or permanent deficit, especially in such tissue as the brain.

**cat-cry syndrome** [L, *catta*, cat, *quiritare*, to cry out; Gk, *syndromos*, course], a rare, congenital disorder recognized at birth by a kittenlike cry caused by a laryngeal anomaly. The condition is associated with a defect in chromosome 5. Other characteristics include low birth weight, microcephaly, "moon face," wide-set eyes, strabismus, and low-set misshapen ears. Infants are hypotonic; heart defects and mental and physical retardation are common. Also called **cri-du-chat syndrome, chromosome 5p− syndrome.**

**catecholamine** /kat′əkəlam′in/, any one of a group of sympathomimetic compounds composed of a catechol molecule and the aliphatic portion of an amine. Some catecholamines are produced naturally by the body and function as key neurologic chemicals.

**catechol-o-methyl transferase (COMT)** /kat′əkol′ōmeth′il/, an enzyme that deactivates the catecholamines dopa, dopamine, epinephrine, and norepinephrine.

**categorical variable,** one of the variables that are not continuous but instead put data into categories.

**categoric data** /kat′əgôr′ik/ [Gk, *kategorikos*, affirmation; L, *datus*, giving], (in research) any data that are classified by name rather than by number, such as race, religion, ethnicity, or marital status.

**cat-eye syndrome** [L, *catta* + AS, *eage* + Gk, *syndromos*, course], a rare congenital autosomal anomaly, marked by the presence of an extra, small chromosome 22 and pupils that resemble the vertical pupils of a cat. Anal atresia, heart abnormalities, and severe mental retardation are common.

**catgut** [L, *catta* + AS, *guttas*], an absorbable suture material, prepared from the intestines of sheep, used to close surgical wounds.

**catharsis** /kəthär′sis/, **1.** a cleansing or purging. **2.** the therapeutic release of pent-up feelings and emotions by open discussion of ideas and thoughts. **3.** the process of drawing repressed ideas and feelings into the consciousness by the technique of free association, often in conjunction with hypnosis and use of hypnotic drugs. Also called **psychocatharsis.** See also **abreaction.** —**cathartic,** *n.*

**cathartic** /kəthär′tik/ [Gk, *katharsis*, cleansing], **1.** pertaining to a substance that causes evacuation of the bowel. **2.** an agent that promotes bowel evacuation by stimulating peristalsis, increasing the fluidity or bulk of intestinal contents, softening the feces, or lubricating the intestinal wall. The term *cathartic* implies a fluid evacuation in contrast to *laxative,* which implies the elimination of a soft, formed stool. Cathartics that increase peristalsis, usually by irritating intestinal mucosa, include certain plant substances, such as aloe, colocynth, croton oil, podophyllum senna, phenolphthalein, bisacodyl, and dehydrocholic acid. Saline cathartics, such as sodium sulfate, magnesium sulfate, and magnesium hydroxide, dilute the intestinal contents by retaining water through osmotic forces. Suppositories containing sodium biphosphate, sodium acid pyrophosphate, and sodium bicarbonate induce defecation when the salts react to form carbon dioxide and the expanding gas stimulates peristalsis. Also called **coprogogue** /kop′rəgōg/. See also **laxative.** —**catharsis,** *n.*

**-cathartic,** suffix meaning 'cleaning': *cephalocathartic, emetocathartic.*

**cathectic.** See **cathexis.**

**catheter** /kath′ətər/ [Gk, *katheter,* something lowered], a hollow flexible tube that can be inserted into a vessel or cavity of the body to withdraw or to instill fluids, directly monitor various types of information, and visualize a vessel or cavity. Most catheters are made of soft plastic, rubber, or silicon. Kinds of catheters include **acorn-tipped catheter, angiocatheter, Foley catheter,** and **intrauterine catheter.**

**catheter hub,** a threaded plastic connection at the end of an IV catheter.

**catheterization** /kath′ətur′īzā′shən/, the introduction of a catheter (a hollow flexible tube) into a body cavity or organ to inject or remove a fluid. See also **female catheterization, Foley catheter, male catheterization.** —**catheterize** /kath′ətərīz/, *v.*

**cathexis** /kəthek′sis/ [Gk, *kathexis,* retention], the conscious or unconscious attachment of emotional feeling and importance to a specific idea, person, or object. —**cathectic,** *adj.*

**cathode** /kath′ōd/ [Gk, *kata,* down, *hodos,* way], **1.** the electrode at which reduction occurs. **2.** the negative side of the x-ray tube, which consists of the focusing cup and the filament.

**cathode ray,** a stream of electrons emitted by a negative electrode when it is bombarded by positive ions, in a gaseous discharge device called a cathode ray tube. The ray is focused and deflected by electromagnets that control the position at which it strikes a screen coated with a phosphor, creating a visible pattern.

**cathode ray oscilloscope** [Gk, *kata* + *hodos* + L, *radius* + *ocillare,* to swing; Gk, *skopein,* to view], an instrument that produces a visual representation of electrical variations by means of the fluorescent screen of a cathode ray tube. Oscilloscopes have many applications in medicine and in nursing, such as the displaying of patients' brain waves and heartbeats for monitoring and diagnostic purposes.

**cathode ray tube (CRT),** a vacuum tube that focuses a beam of electrons onto a spot on a screen coated with a phosphor, creating a visible image of information on the face of the tube. The CRT is one type of computer monitor.

**cation** /kat′ī·on/ [Gk, *kata,* down, *ion,* going], a positively charged ion. Compare **anion.**

**cation-exchange resin,** any one of various insoluble organic polymers with high molecular weights that exchange their cations for other ions in solution. Cation-exchange resins are used especially to restrict intestinal sodium absorption in patients with edema. Compare **anion-exchange resin.**

**catling,** a long, sharp double-edged knife used in amputation. Also called **catlin.**

**catoptric** /kətop′trik/ [Gk, *katoptron,* mirror], pertaining to a reflected image or reflected light, such as from a mirror.

**CAT scan.** See **computed tomography.**

**cat's claw,** an herb that belongs to the madder family, found in South America and Southest Asia.

■ USES: This herb is used for cancer, herpes, HIV infection, rheumatoid arthritis, gastritis, gout, wounds, and gastric ulcers.

■ CONTRAINDICATIONS: Cat's claw is contraindicated during pregnancy and lactation and in children younger than 3 years of age until more research is available. It also should not be used in people with muscular sclerosis, tuberculosis, AIDS, or hemophilia; or in those who have had organ transplants.

**cat-scratch disease.** See **cat-scratch fever.**

**cat-scratch fever,** a disease that results from the scratch or bite of a healthy cat. Inflammation and pustules are found on the scratched skin, and lymph nodes in the neck, head, groin, or axilla swell 2 weeks later. Although patients are

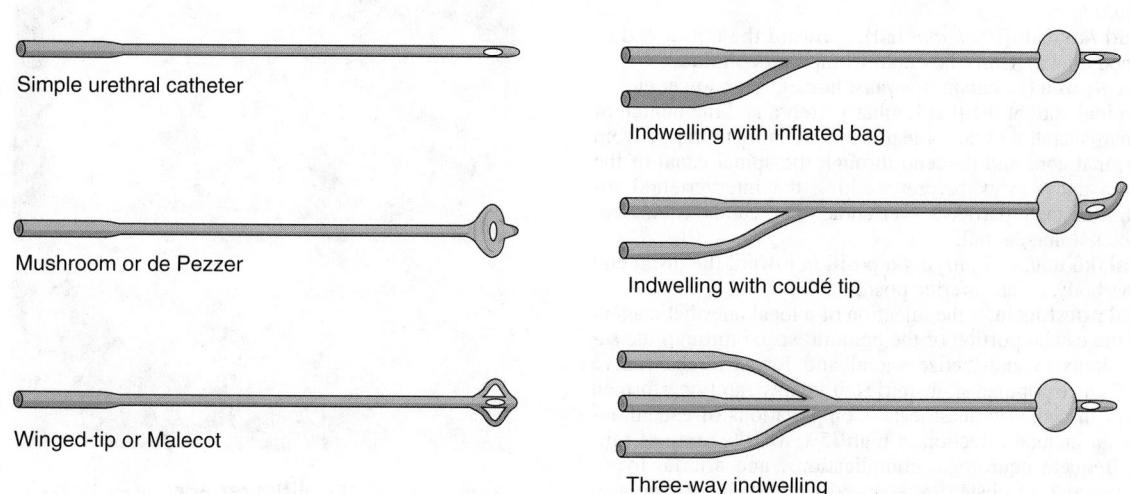

Simple urethral catheter

Mushroom or de Pezzer

Winged-tip or Malecot

Indwelling with inflated bag

Indwelling with coudé tip

Three-way indwelling

**Commonly used catheters** *(Beare and Myers, 1998)*

seldom seriously ill, fever, headache, and malaise may occur and symptoms can persist for months. Tetracycline may aid rapid recovery. The cat scratch skin test is available to help in the diagnosis. There may be spontaneous remission of symptoms in about 2 weeks. Also called **cat scratch disease, benign lymphoreticulosis.**

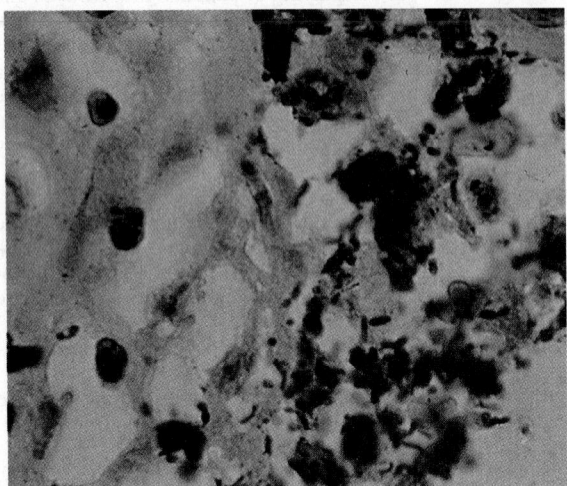

**Cat-scratch fever bacillus in lymph node tissue**
*(Baron, Peterson, and Finegold, 1994/courtesy Dr. Ellen Kahn, North Shore University Hospital, Manhasset, NY)*

**cat's eye amaurosis** [L, *catta* + AS, *aege* + Gk, *amauroin,* to darken], a monocular blindness, with a bright reflection from the pupil caused by a white mass in the vitreous humor resulting from inflammation or a malignant lesion.

**Caucasian,** pertaining to a person whose ancestors were believed to have in ancient times inhabited the geographic region of the Caucasus, in southeastern Europe, or whose ancestors were members of the hypothetical Indo-European cultures identified with the Caucasus.

**caud-,** combining form meaning 'tail': *caudal, caudocephalad.*

**caudad** /kô′dad/ [L, *cauda,* tail], toward the tail or end of the body, away from the head. Compare **cephalad.**

**cauda equina** [L, *cauda* + *equus,* horse], the lower end of the spinal cord at the first lumbar vertebra and the bundle of lumbar, sacral, and coccygeal nerve roots that emerge from the spinal cord and descend through the spinal canal of the sacrum and coccyx before reaching the intervertebral foramina of their particular vertebrae. The cauda equina resembles a horse's tail.

**caudal** /kô′dəl/, signifying a position toward the distal end of the body, or an inferior position.

**caudal anesthesia,** the injection of a local anesthetic agent into the caudal portion of the epidural space through the sacral hiatus to anesthetize sacral and lower lumbar nerve roots. Once popular in obstetrics, it is now rarely performed except in pediatric anesthesia. Complications of caudal anesthesia include infection, a high (5% to 10%) rate of failure, frequent neurologic complications, and arterial hypotension, and, in obstetrics, reduced force of labor. See also **regional anesthesia.**

**caudal ligaments,** bands of fibrous tissue attaching the skin to the coccyx. Remnants of the embryonic notochord, they form a small cup-shaped depression. Also called **caudal retinaculum.**

**caudal regression syndrome,** failure of formation of part or all of the coccygeal, sacral, and occasionally lumbar vertebral units and the corresponding segments of the caudal spinal cord, with resulting neurogenic dysfunction of bowel and bladder. Also called **sacral agenesis.**

**caudate** /kô′dāt/, having a tail.

**caudate lobe of the liver** [L, *cauda,* tail; Gk, *lobos,* lobe; AS, *lifer*], a part of the right lobe of the liver that lies near the vena cava.

**caudate nucleus** [L, *cauda,* tail, *nucleus,* nut kernel], a crescent-shaped mass of gray matter lateral to the thalamus in the floor of the anterior horn and body of the lateral ventricle.

**caudate process** [L, *cauda* + *processus,* projection], a small elevation of tissue that extends obliquely from the lower extremity of the caudate lobe of the liver to the visceral surface of the right lobe. It separates the fossa for the gallbladder from the beginning of the fossa for the inferior vena cava.

**caudocephalad** /kô′dōsef′əlad/ [L, *cauda,* tail; Gk, *kephale,* head; L, *ad,* toward], movement from the tail toward the head.

**caul** /kôl/ [ME, *cawel,* basket], the intact amniotic sac surrounding the fetus at birth. The sac usually ruptures or is ruptured during the course of labor or delivery; when it remains intact, it must be torn or cut to allow the baby to breathe. In the past, pieces of the caul were sold to sailors as a good luck token that would protect the bearer from death by drowning.

**cauliflower ear** [L, *caulis,* cabbage, *fiore,* flower; AS, *eare*], a thickened, deformed pinna and external ear caused by repeated trauma, such as that suffered by boxers. Plastic surgery may be a means of restoring the normal appearance of the ear.

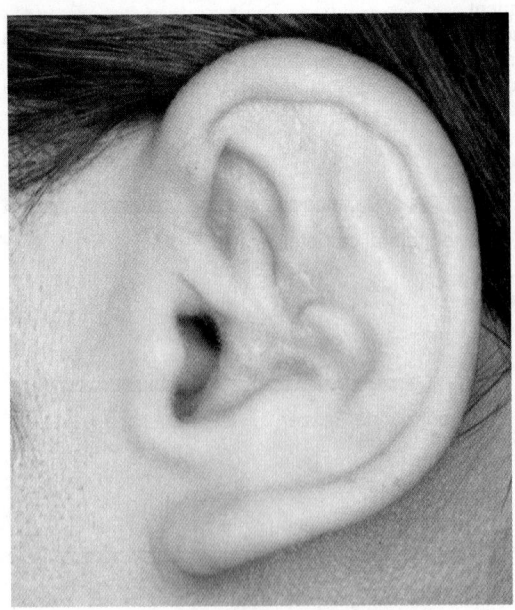

**Cauliflower ear**
*(Bingham, 1992/courtesy Mouth Clinic, Sunnybrook Medical Centre, Toronto)*

**caumesthesia** /kô′məsthē′zhə/ [Gk, *kauma,* heat, *aisthesis,* feeling],    an abnormal condition in which a patient has a low temperature but experiences a sense of intense heat. —**caumesthetic,** *adj.*

**caus-, caut-,** combining form meaning 'burn': *causalgia, cautery.*

**causalgia** /kôzal′jə/ [Gk, *kausis,* burning, *algos,* pain], a severe sensation of burning pain, often in an extremity, sometimes accompanied by local erythema of the skin.

**causal hypothesis** /kô′səl/ [L, *causa,* cause; Gk, *hypotithenia,* foundation], (in research) a hypothesis that predicts a cause-and-effect relationship among the variables to be studied.

**causal hypothesis testing study,** (in nursing research) an experimental design used in testing a hypothesis that predicts a cause-and-effect relationship within the data to be studied.

**causality** /kôsal′itē/, (in research) a relationship between one phenomenon or event (A) and another (B) in which A precedes and causes B. The direction of influence and the nature of the effect are predictable and reproducible and may be empirically observed. Causality is difficult to prove; some social scientists contend that it is impossible to prove a causal relationship.

**causal treatment.** See **treatment.**

**causation** /kôsā′shən/ [L, *causa*], (in law) the existence of a reasonable connection between the misfeasance, malfeasance, or nonfeasance of the defendant and the injury or damage suffered by the plaintiff. In a lawsuit in which negligence is alleged, the harm suffered by the plaintiff must be proved to result directly from the negligence of the defendant; causation must be demonstrated.

**cause** [L, *causa*], any process, substance, or organism that produces an effect or condition.

**CAUSN,** abbreviation for **Canadian Association of University Schools of Nursing.**

**caustic** /kôs′tik/ [Gk, *kaustikos,* burning], **1.** any substance that is destructive to living tissue, such as silver nitrate, nitric acid, or sulfuric acid. **2.** exerting a burning or corrosive effect.

**caustic poisoning,** the accidental ingestion of strong acids or alkalis, resulting in burns and tissue damage to the mouth, esophagus, and stomach. The victim experiences immediate pain, swelling, and edema. The pulse may be weak and rapid. Respirations become shallow, and edema may close the airway. Complications, which include circulatory shock, perforation of the esophagus, and pharyngeal edema leading to asphyxia, can be fatal. See also **acid burn, alkali burn.**

**CAUT,** abbreviation for **Canadian Association of University Teachers.**

**cauterization** /kô′tərīzā′shən/ [Gk, *kauterion,* branding iron], the process of burning a part of the body by cautery.

**cauterize** /kô′tərīz/ [Gk, *kauterion,* branding iron], to burn tissues by thermal heat, including steam, hot metal, or solar radiation; electricity; or another agent such as laser or dry ice, usually with the objective of destroying damaged or diseased tissues, preventing infections, or coagulating blood vessels.

**cautery** /kô′tərē/ [Gk, *kauterion,* branding iron], **1.** a device or agent used in the coagulation of tissue by heat or caustic substances. **2.** a destructive effect produced by a cauterizing agent.

**cautery knife,** a surgical knife that cuts tissue and seals it to prevent bleeding. The knife is connected to an electric source that generates the heat necessary for cauterization.

**cav-, cavo-,** combining form meaning 'hollow': *cavity, cavernome, cavogram.*

**cava.** See **cavum.**

**cavalry bone.** See **rider's bone.**

**Cavell, Edith** /kəvel′/(1865–1915), an English nurse. Trained at London Hospital, in 1907 she was named head of a nurses training school in Brussels, with the task of raising nursing standards to match those of Britain. By 1912, the school offered a 3-year intensive course and was associated with four hospitals in Brussels. After the Germans occupied Belgium in World War I, she nursed or sheltered more than 200 fleeing soldiers and helped them reach Holland; to her, this was an extension of her nursing: helping those in need. For this, she was arrested by the Germans, tried, and shot on October 12, 1915. Her execution, which she met with courage and fortitude, brought her widespread fame.

**caveola** *pl.* **caveolae** [L], a small pit, depression, or invagination, such as any of the minute pits or incuppings of the cell membrane formed during pinocytosis, which close and then pinch off to form small, free, fluid-filled vesicles in the cytoplasm.

**Caverject,** trademark for a prostaglandin-derived drug (alprostadil) for the treatment of male impotence.

**cavernoma.** See **cavernous hemangioma.**

**cavernous** /kav′ərnəs/ [L, *caverna,* hollow place], containing cavities or hollow spaces. See also **cavernous hemangioma.**

**cavernous angioma.** See **cavernous hemangioma.**

**cavernous body of the clitoris, cavernous body of the penis.** See **corpus cavernosum.**

**cavernous hemangioma** [L, *caverna,* hollow place; Gk, *haima,* blood, *oma,* tumor], a benign, congenital tumor consisting of large, blood-filled cystic spaces. The scalp, face, and neck are the most common sites, but these tumors have been found in the liver and other organs. Superficial cavernous hemangiomas are friable and easily infected if the skin is broken. Treatment includes observation, irradiation, sclerosing solutions, and laser surgery and excisional surgery. Also called **angioma cavernosum, cavernoma.** Compare **capillary hemangioma, nevus flammeus.**

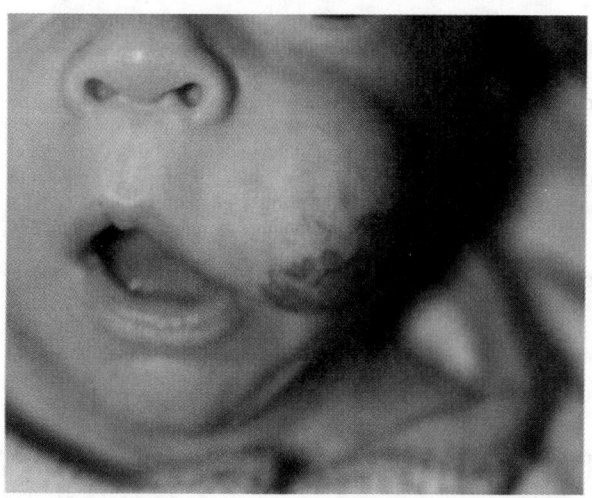

**Cavernous hemangioma**
*(Huether and McCance, 2000/courtesy Department of Dermatology, School of Medicine, University of Utah)*

**cavernous lymphangioma.** See **lymphangioma cavernosum.**

**cavernous sinus** [L, *caverna* + *sinus,* curve], one of a pair of irregularly shaped bilateral venous channels between the sphenoid bone of the skull and the dura mater. It is one of the five anterior inferior venous sinuses that drain the blood from the dura mater into the internal jugular vein.

**cavernous sinus syndrome,** an abnormal condition characterized by edema of the conjunctiva, the upper eyelid, and the root of the nose and by paralysis of the third, fourth, and the sixth cranial nerves. It is caused by a thrombosis of the cavernous sinus.

**cavernous sinus thrombosis,** a syndrome, usually secondary to infections near the eye or nose, characterized by orbital edema, venous congestion of the eye, and palsy of the nerves supplying the extraocular muscles. The infection may spread to involve the cerebrospinal fluid and meninges. Treatment uses antibiotics and sometimes anticoagulants. Prevention includes not squeezing pimples and other skin lesions in the area of the nose and central face.

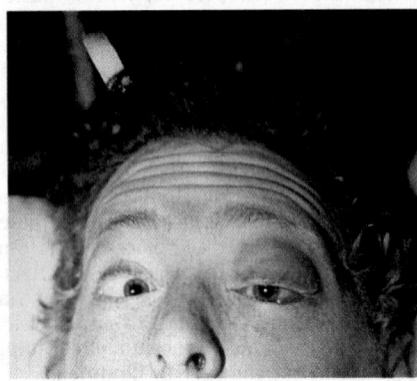

**Cavernous sinus thrombosis** *(Stone and Gorbach, 2000)*

**CAVH,** abbreviation for *continuous arteriovenous hemofiltration.*

**cavitary** /kav'iter'ē/ [L, *cavus,* hollow], **1.** denoting the presence of one or more cavities. **2.** any entozoon having a body cavity or an alimentary canal.

**cavitate** /kav'itāt/ [L, *cavus,* hollow], to rapidly form and collapse vapor pockets or bubbles in a flowing fluid with low pressure areas, often causing damage to surrounding structures.

**cavitation, 1.** the formation of cavities within the body, such as those formed in the lung by tuberculosis. **2.** any cavity within the body, such as the pleural cavities.

**cavity** /kav'itē/ [L, *cavus*], **1.** a hollow space within a larger structure, such as the peritoneal cavity or the oral cavity. See also **body cavity. 2.** *nontechnical.* a space in a tooth formed by dental caries.

**cavity classification,** a method for describing dental caries based on the tooth surfaces on which they occur (labial, buccal, lingual, incisal, occlusal, or root), the type of surface on which they occur (pit and fissure or smooth), their frequency of occurence, and their numeric designation according to the **classification of caries.**

**cavity prep.** See **prepared cavity.**

**cavity preparation,** a procedure for establishing in a tooth the biochemically and mechanically acceptable form necessary to receive and retain a restoration.

**cavogram** /kav'əgram'/ [L, *cavus* + Gk, *gramma,* record], an angiogram of the inferior or superior vena cava.

**cavosurface** /kāv'ō·sur'fəs/ [L, *cavus,* cavity + *superficies,* surface], the surface of a cavity, as of a tooth.

**cavosurface angle** /kāv'ōsur'fəs/, the angle formed by the junction of the wall of a prepared tooth cavity with the external surface of the tooth.

**cavosurface bevel** [L, *cavus* + *superficies,* surface; OFr, *baif,* open mouth], the incline of the cavosurface angle of a prepared tooth cavity wall relative to the enamel wall. Compare **bevel, contra bevel.**

**cavum** /kā'vəm/, *pl.* **cava, 1.** any hollow or cavity. **2.** the inferior or superior vena cava.

**cavus** /kā'vəs/ [L, *cavus,* cavity], an abnormally high or exaggerated arch of the foot. See **pes cavus, talipes cavus.**

**cayenne pepper.** See **capsicum.**

**CBA,** abbreviation for **cost-benefit analysis.**

**CBC,** abbreviation for **complete blood count.**

**CBF,** abbreviation for *cerebral blood flow.*

**cc,** abbreviation for **cubic centimeter.** 1cc = 1 mL.

**CC, 1.** abbreviation for **chief complaint. 2.** abbreviation for *Commission Certified.*

**CCK,** abbreviation for **cholecystokinin.**

**CCP,** abbreviation for **complement control protein.**

**CCPD,** abbreviation for **continuous cycling peritoneal dialysis.**

**CCRN, 1.** abbreviation for *Certified Critical Care Registered Nurse;* **2.** trademark of **American Association of Critical-Care Nurses Certified Corporation.**

**CCU,** abbreviation for **coronary care unit; critical care unit.**

**Cd,** symbol for the element **cadmium.**

**CD,** abbreviation for **compact disc.**

**cdc,** abbreviation for **cell division cycle.**

**CDC,** abbreviation for **Centers for Disease Control and Prevention.**

**CDE, 1.** the major symbols used in one system for the nomenclature of the Rh system, in which D is the same as Rh0, the major determining factor of Rh positivity. **2.** abbreviation for **common duct exploration. 3.** abbreviation for *Certified Diabetes Educator.*

**CD8 cell,** a T lymphocyte that secretes large amounts of gamma-interferon, a lymphokine involved in the body's defense against viruses. CD8 cells prevent the unnecessary formation of antibodies. Also called **cytotoxic T cells.** See also **CD4.**

**CD4,** (cluster of differentiation 4) symbol for a glycoprotein expressed on the surface of helper T lymphocytes and other immune cells. CD4 serves as a receptor for human immunodeficiency virus envelope glycoprotein gp120. Binding of the viral glycoprotein gp120 to CD4 is the first step in viral entry, leading to the fusion of viral and cell membranes.

**CD4/CD8 count,** the ratio of the number of helper T lymphocytes to the number of suppressor and cytotoxic T lymphocytes. The cells are counted with the use of monoclonal antibodies to the surface glycoproteins CD4 on helper T cells and CD8 on suppressor and cytotoxic T cells. In healthy individuals the ratio ranges from 1.6 to 2.2. The ratio is important in monitoring the function of the immune system in patients who have viral infections or who have undergone tissue transplantation, either of which may cause an increase in the number of suppressor T cells.

**CD4 cell count,** a measure of the number of "helper" T cells that carry the CD4 glycoprotein on their cell surface and that help B cells produce certain antibodies. The human immunodeficiency virus (HIV) binds to CD4 and kills T cells bearing this glycoprotein. Thus, the CD4 cell count is an indicator of the progress of an HIV infection and helps measure the effectiveness of anti-HIV drugs. CD4 T cells mainly produce interleukin 2, an autocrine and paracrine T cell growth factor; preactivated or memory CD4 T cells secrete a much larger array of lymphokines on restimulation. See also **CD4, CD8 cell, human immunodeficiency virus, T cell.**

**CDH,** abbreviation for **congenital dislocation of the hip.**

**CDK,** abbreviation for **cyclin-dependent kinase.**

**CDR,** abbreviation for **computed dental radiography.**

**CD/ROM,** abbreviation for **compact disc/read only memory.**

**Ce,** symbol for the element **cerium.**

**CEA,** 1. abbreviation for **carcinoembryonic antigen.** 2. abbreviation for **cost-effectiveness analysis.**

**ceasmic** /sē·az′mik/ [Gk, *keazein*, to split], pertaining to or characterized by a persistent embryonic fissure or abnormal cleavage of parts.

**ceasmic teratism** [Gk, *keazein* + *teras*, monster], a congenital anomaly, caused by developmental arrest, in which body parts that should be fused remain in their fissured embryonic state, such as in cleft palate.

**cec-, ceco-,** combining form meaning 'cecum': *cecitis, cecoplication.*

**cecal** /sē′kəl/ [L, *caecus*, blind, blind gut], 1. pertaining to the cecum. 2. pertaining to the optic disc or the blind spot in the retina. Also spelled **caecal.**

**cecal appendix.** See **vermiform appendix.**

**cecitis** /sē·sī′tis/ [L, *caecus*, blind, blind gut], inflammation of the cecum; also called **typhlitis.**

**Ceclor,** trademark for a cephalosporin antibiotic (cefaclor).

**cecocolostomy** /sē′kōkəlos′təmē/ [L, *caecus*, blind, blind gut; Gk, *kolon*, colon, *stoma*, mouth], 1. a surgical operation that creates an anastomosis between the cecum and the colon. 2. the anastomosis produced by this operation.

**cecofixation.** See **cecopexy.**

**cecoileostomy** /-il′ē·os′təmē/ [L, *caecus* + *ilia*, intestine, *stoma*, mouth], a surgical operation that connects the ileum with the cecum. Also called **ileocecostomy** /il′ē·ōsēkos′təmē/.

**cecopexy** /sē′kōpek′sē/ [L, *caecus* + Gk, *pexis*, fix], a surgical operation that fixes or suspends the cecum to correct its excessive mobility. Also called **cecofixation.**

**cecostomy** /sēkos′təmē/ [L, *caecus* + Gk, *stoma*, mouth], the surgical construction of an opening into the cecum, performed as a temporary measure to relieve intestinal obstruction in a patient who cannot tolerate major surgery. Twenty-four hours before surgery, if time permits, only clear liquids allowed. Cleansing enemas and antibiotics are prescribed to reduce the number of bacteria in the bowel. IV fluids and electrolytes are given, and a nasointestinal tube is inserted. With the patient under local anesthesia, a tube is inserted into the cecum to allow drainage of feces. The procedure may also be done to decompress the large bowel and prevent distension until peristalsis is restored after intestinal surgery. After surgery, the tube is connected to a drainage bag. The nurse irrigates the cecostomy tube with saline solution as necessary, allowing the solution to flow in and out by gravity, if possible. Frequent dressing changes are needed to keep the skin clean and dry. An ileostomy bag may be used. When edema and inflammation have subsided, the obstruction (usually cancer) is resected, the healthy sections of the bowel reconnected, and the cecostomy closed. Also called **caecostomy.** See also **abdominal surgery, intestinal obstruction.**

**cecum** /sē′kəm/ [L, *caecus*, blind, blind gut], a pouchlike structure or cul-de-sac constituting the first part of the large intestine. It is inferior to the junction of the ascending colon and joins the ileum, the last segment of the small intestine, at the ileocecal valve.

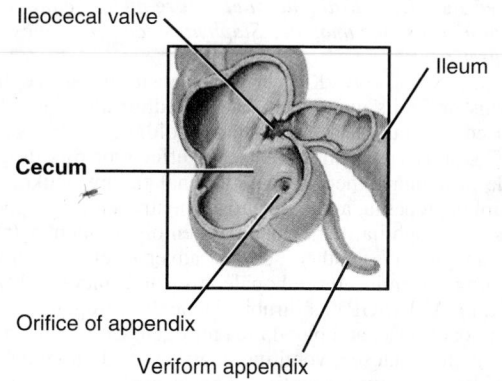

Ileocecal valve

Ileum

Cecum

Orifice of appendix

Veriform appendix

**Cecum** *(Applegate, 2000)*

**Cedax,** trademark for an oral cephalosporin (ceftibuten).

**Cedilanid-D,** trademark for a cardiac glycoside (deslanoside).

**CeeNU,** trademark for an antineoplastic (lomustine).

**cef-,** combining form designating a cephalosporin.

**cefaclor** /sē′fəklôr/, a cephalosporin antibiotic.
  ■ INDICATIONS: It is prescribed in the treatment of selected infections caused by susceptile strains of bacteria.
  ■ CONTRAINDICATIONS: Known hypersensitivity to cephalosporins prohibits its use. It is used with caution in patients who are allergic to penicillin.
  ■ ADVERSE EFFECTS: Among the most serious adverse reactions are hypersensitivity reactions and diarrhea, nausea, and vomiting.

**cefadroxil monohydrate** /sē′fədrok′sil/, a cephalosporin antibiotic.
  ■ INDICATIONS: It is prescribed in the treatment of selected bacterial infections.
  ■ CONTRAINDICATIONS: Known hypersensitivity to cephalosporins prohibits its use. It is administered with caution to patients with a history of allergy to penicillins.
  ■ ADVERSE EFFECTS: Among the most serious adverse reactions are hypersensitivity reactions and severe diarrhea, nausea, and vomiting.

**Cefadyl,** trademark for an antibiotic (cephapirin).

**cefamandole nafate** /sēfəman′dōl naf′āt/, a cephalosporin antibiotic.
  ■ INDICATIONS: It is prescribed in the treatment of infections caused by susceptible bacterial strains.
  ■ CONTRAINDICATIONS: Known hypersensitivity to cephalosporins prohibits its use. It is used with caution in patients who are allergic to penicillin.
  ■ ADVERSE EFFECTS: Among the most serious adverse reactions are hypersensitivity reactions, phlebitis, superinfection, and pain on intramuscular injection.

**cefazolin sodium** /sēfaz′ōlin/, a cephalosporin antibiotic.
- INDICATIONS: It is prescribed in the treatment of infections caused by susceptible bacterial strains.
- CONTRAINDICATIONS: Known hypersensitivity to this drug or to any cephalosporin medication prohibits its use. It is used with caution in patients who are allergic to penicillin.
- ADVERSE EFFECTS: Among the more serious adverse reactions are pain at the site of injection and hypersensitivity reactions.

**cefdinir,** a broad-spectrum antibiotic.
- INDICATIONS: This drug is used to treat *Haemophilus influenzae, H. parainfluenzae, Morganella catarrhalis, Streptococcus pneumoniae, Staphylococcus pyogenes,* and *S. aureus.*
- CONTRAINDICATIONS: Known hypersensitivity to cephalosporins prohibits use of this drug. Cefdinir also should not be used in infants less than 1 month old.
- ADVERSE EFFECTS: Life-threatening effects of this drug include proteinuria, nephrotoxicity, renal failure, leukopenia, thrombocytopenia, agranulocytosis, neutropenia, lymphocytosis, eosinophilia, pancytopenia, hemolytic anemia (rare), and anaphylaxis. Other serious adverse effects include bleeding, anemia, thrombophlebitis, and increased AST (SGOT), ALT (SGPT), bilirubin, lactic dehydrogenase, alkaline phosphatase, and blood urea nitrogen. Common side effects include nausea, vomiting, diarrhea, and anorexia.

**cefepime,** a third-generation cephalosporin.
- INDICATIONS: This drug is used to treat infections caused by gram-negative bacilli, including *Escherichia coli, Proteus,* and *Klebsiella;* gram-positive organisms, including *Streptococcus pneumoniae, S. pyogenes,* and *Staphylococcus aureus*; and infections of the lower respiratory tract, urinary tract, skin, and bone.
- CONTRAINDICATIONS: Known hypersensitivity to cephalosporins prohibits this drug's use. Cefepime also should not be used in infants less than one month old.
- ADVERSE EFFECTS: Life-threatening effects of this drug include nephrotoxicity, renal failure, leukopenia, thrombocytopenia, agranulocytosis, neutropenia, lymphocytosis, eosinophilia, pancytopenia, hemolytic anemia (rare), and anaphylaxis. Other serious effects include GI bleeding; increased AST (SGOT), ALT (SGPT), bilirubin, lactic dehydrogenase, and alkaline phosphatase; proteinuria, candidiasis, increased blood urea nitrogen, and thrombophlebitis. Common side effects include nausea, vomiting, diarrhea, and anorexia.

**Cefizox,** trademark for a cephalosporin antibiotic (ceftizoxime).

**Cefobid,** trademark for a cephalosporin antibiotic (cefoperazone).

**cefonicid sodium** /sēfon′isid/, a parenteral cephalosporin-type antibiotic.
- INDICATIONS: It is prescribed for bacterial infections of the lower respiratory or urinary tract, skin, bones and joints, septicemia, and surgical prophylaxis.
- CONTRAINDICATIONS: A history of allergy to cephalosporins or acute anaphylactic or urticarial reactions to penicillin prohibits its use.
- ADVERSE EFFECTS: Among the more serious adverse reactions are pain and phlebitis at the injection site and occasionally allergic reactions and GI effects.

**cefoperazone sodium** /sē′fōper′əzōn/, a cephalosporin antibiotic.
- INDICATIONS: It is prescribed in the treatment of respiratory tract, intraabdominal, skin, and female genital tract infections and bacterial septicemia.

- CONTRAINDICATIONS: Hypersensitivity to the cephalosporins or known sensitivity to this drug prohibits its use.
- ADVERSE EFFECTS: Among the most serious adverse reactions are pruritus, urticaria, transient eosinophilia, neutropenia, and injection site reactions.

**ceforanide** /sēfôr′ənīd/, a parenteral cephalosporin-type antibiotic.
- INDICATIONS: It is prescribed for infections of the lower respiratory or urinary tract, skin, or bones and joints; septicemia; endocarditis; and surgical prophylaxis.
- CONTRAINDICATIONS: A history of allergy to cephalosporins or acute anaphylactic or urticarial reactions to penicillin prohibit its use.
- ADVERSE EFFECTS: Among the more serious adverse reactions are allergic reactions and GI effects.

**Cefotan,** trademark for a cephalosporin antibiotic (cefotetan disodium).

**cefotaxime sodium** /sēfōtak′zēm/, a cephalosporin antibiotic.
- INDICATIONS: It is prescribed for lower respiratory tract, genitourinary, gynecologic, intraabdominal, skin, bone and joint, and central nervous system infections and bacterial septicemia caused by strains of microorganisms susceptible to ceforanide.
- CONTRAINDICATIONS: Hypersensitivity to the cephalosporins or known hypersensitivity to this drug prohibits its use.
- ADVERSE EFFECTS: The most serious adverse reactions are pruritus, colitis, fungal infections, and injection site reactions.

**cefotetan disodium** /sē′fōtet′ən/, a parenteral cephalosporin antibiotic.
- INDICATIONS: It is prescribed for bacterial infections of the lower resspiratory tract, urinary tract, skin, abdomen, bones or joints, or reproductive organs and for surgical prophylaxis.
- CONTRAINDICATIONS: This drug is contraindicated for patients who are hypersensitive to cefotetan or to other cephalosporin antibiotics.
- ADVERSE EFFECTS: Among adverse reactions reported are skin rash, diarrhea, eosinophilia, positive Coombs' test results, and elevated liver enzyme levels.

**cefoxitin sodium** /sēfok′sitin/, a cephalosporin antibiotic.
- INDICATIONS: It is prescribed in the treatment of certain bacterial infections.
- CONTRAINDICATIONS: Known hypersensitivity to cephalosporins prohibits its use. It is administered with caution to patients who are allergic to penicillin.
- ADVERSE EFFECTS: Among the most serious adverse reactions are hypersensitivity reactions, phlebitis, superinfection, and pain on intramuscular injection.

**ceftazidime** /seftaz′idēm/, a parenteral cephalosporin-type antibiotic.
- INDICATIONS: It is prescribed for treatment of bacterial infections of the lower respiratory tract, urinary tract, skin, abdomen, blood, bones and joints, and central nervous system.
- CONTRAINDICATIONS: This drug is contraindicated in patients who are hypersensitive to this product or to other cephalosporin antibiotics.
- ADVERSE EFFECTS: Among adverse reactions reported are pruritus, fever, skin rash, diarrhea, eosinophilia, thrombocytosis, phlebitis, discomfort at the site of injection, and positive Coombs' test result.

**ceftibuten,** an oral cephalosporin.
- INDICATIONS: It is prescribed in the treatment of chronic bronchitis, acute bacterial otitis media, pharyngitis, and tonsillitis.

■ CONTRAINDICATIONS: The drug should not be given to children with abdominal pain, vomiting, and diarrhea.

■ ADVERSE EFFECTS: The side effects most often reported include nausea, headache, diarrhea, dyspepsia, dizziness, and abdominal pain.

**ceftizoxime sodium** /sef′tizok′zēm/, a cephalosporin antibiotic.

■ INDICATIONS: It is prescribed in the treatment of infections caused by susceptible bacterial strains.

■ CONTRAINDICATIONS: Known sensitivity to this drug prohibits its use. It is used with caution in patients who are allergic to penicillin.

■ ADVERSE EFFECTS: Among the most serious adverse reactions are hypersensitivity reactions, neutropenia, leukopenia, thrombocytopenia, and pain at the injection site.

**ceftriaxone sodium** /sef′trī·ak′sōn/, a parenteral cephalosporin antibiotic.

■ INDICATIONS: It is prescribed for infections of the lower respiratory tract, urinary tract, skin, abdomen, bones, and joints. It is also used to treat gonorrhea, septicemia, and meningitis and in surgical prophylaxis, particularly in coronary bypass operations.

■ CONTRAINDICATIONS: Ceftriaxone sodium is contraindicated in patients who are hypersensitive to this product or to other cephalosporin antibiotics.

■ ADVERSE EFFECTS: Among reported adverse reactions are skin rash, diarrhea, eosinophilia, thrombocytosis, leukopenia, increased liver enzyme and blood urea nitrogen levels, and pain and tenderness at the site of injection.

**cefuroxime sodium** /sef′o͞orok′zēm/, a cephalosporin antibiotic.

■ INDICATIONS: It is prescribed in the treatment of lower respiratory tract, urinary tract, skin, and gonococcal infections; bacterial septicemia; and meningitis and for the prevention of postoperative infections.

■ CONTRAINDICATIONS: Hypersensitivity to the cephalosporins or known sensitivity to this drug prohibits its use.

■ ADVERSE EFFECTS: Among the most serious adverse reactions are pruritus, urticaria, transient eosinophilia, neutropenia, leukopenia, and injection site reactions.

**cel-, coel-,** **1.** combining form meaning 'a cavity of the body': *celarium.* **2.** combining form meaning 'a swelling or tumor, hernia': *celosomia.* **3.** combining form meaning 'belly or abdomen': *coelom.*

**-cele,** suffix meaning 'relating to a hernia or swelling': *rectocele, cystocele.*

**Celestone,** trademark for a glucocorticoid (betamethasone).

**celiac** /sē′lē·ak/ [Gk, *koilia,* belly], pertaining to the abdominal cavity.

**celiac artery** [Gk, *koilia,* belly, *arteria,* airpipe], a thick visceral branch of the abdominal aorta, arising caudal to the diaphragm, usually dividing into the left gastric, common hepatic, and splenic arteries.

**celiac disease** [Gk, *koilia* + L, *dis,* opposite of; Fr, *aise,* ease], an inborn error of metabolism characterized by the inability to hydrolyze peptides contained in gluten. Gluten is found in wheat, oats, and barley. The disease affects adults and young children, who suffer from abdominal distension, vomiting, diarrhea, muscle wasting, and extreme lethargy. A characteristic sign is a pale, foul-smelling stool that floats on water because of its high fat content. There may be a secondary lactose intolerance, and it may become necessary to eliminate all milk products from the diet. Most patients respond well to a high-protein, high-calorie, gluten-free diet. Rice and corn are good substitutes for wheat, and any vita-

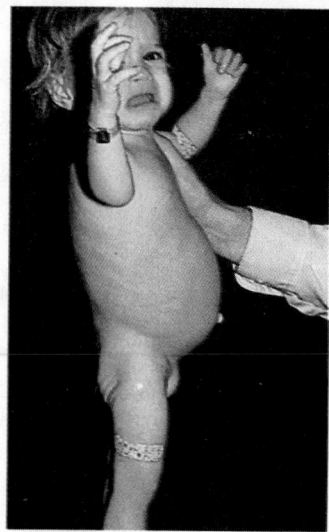

**Celiac disease: abdominal distension**
*(Zitelli and Davis, 1997)*

min or mineral deficiencies can be corrected with oral preparations. Prognosis for full recovery is excellent. Failure to respond generally indicates misdiagnosis. Also called **celiac sprue, gluten-induced enteropathy, nontropical sprue.** Compare **malabsorption syndrome.**

**celiac ganglion,** a group of nerve cells located on each side of the crura of the diaphragm. The cells are connected to the celiac plexus.

**celiac plexus.** See **solar plexus.**

**celiac rickets** [Gk, *koilia* + *rhachis,* spine, *itis,* inflammation], arrested growth and osseous deformities resulting from malabsorption of fat and calcium. See also **celiac disease, rickets.**

**celiac sprue.** See **celiac disease.**

**celio-,** prefix meaning 'belly or abdomen': *celioma, celiorrhaphy.*

**celiocolpotomy** /sē′lē·ōkəlpot′əmē/ [Gk, *koilia* + *kolpos,* vagina, *temnein,* to cut], an incision into the abdomen through the vagina.

**celioscope.** See **endoscope.**

**cell** [L, *cella,* storeroom], the fundamental unit of all living tissue. Eukaryotic cells consist of a nucleus, cytoplasm, and organelles surrounded by a plasma membrane. Within the nucleus are the nucleolus (containing ribonucleic acid) and the chromatin (containing protein and deoxyribonucleic acid), which gives rise to chromosomes, wherein are located the determinants of inherited characteristics. Organelles within the cytoplasm include the endoplasmic reticulum, ribosomes, Golgi apparatus, mitochondria, lysosomes, and the centrosome. Prokaryotic cells are much smaller and simpler than eukaryocytic cells, even lacking a nucleus. The specialized nature of body tissue reflects the specialized structure and function of its constituent cells. See also **cell theory.**

**cella** /sel′ə/, *pl.* **cellae** [L, storeroom], an enclosed space.

**cellae.** See **cella.**

**cell bank,** a storage facility for frozen tissue samples held for research purposes and for surgical reconstruction of damaged body structures.

**cell biology.** See **cytology.**

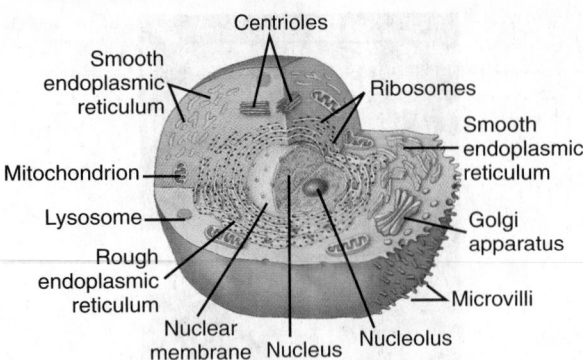

Centrioles

Smooth
endoplasmic
reticulum

Ribosomes

Smooth
endoplasmic
reticulum

Mitochondrion

Lysosome

Golgi
apparatus

Rough
endoplasmic
reticulum

Microvilli

Nuclear
membrane
Nucleus
Nucleolus

**Cell** *(Thibodeau and Patton, 1999/William Ober)*

**cell body** [L, *cella* + AS, *bodig*], the part of a cell that contains the nucleus and surrounding cytoplasm exclusive of any projections or processes, such as the axon and dendrites of a neuron or the tail of a spermatozoon.

**cell culture** [L, *cella*, storeroom, *colere*, to cultivate], living cells that are maintained in vitro in artificial media of serum and nutrients for the study and growth of certain strains or for experiments in controlling diseases, such as cancer.

**cell death,** 1. terminal failure of a cell to maintain essential life functions. See also **necrosis. 2.** the point in the process of dying at which vital functions have ceased at the cellular level.

**cell determination,** the process by which an undifferentiated embryonic cell becomes committed to develop into a specific type of cell. Cell determination appears to involve the selective activation of certain sets of genes and the inactivation of others.

**cell division,** the continuous process by which a cell alternates between a long interphase period and mitosis. Mitosis involves four stages: prophase, metaphase, anaphase, and telophase. Cell division does not occur in discrete steps: each phase is part of a continuous process that may require hours for its completion. During the interphase period new deoxyribonucleic acid, ribonucleic acid, and protein molecules are synthesized before the start of the next prophase. See also **mitosis.** Compare **meiosis.**

**cell division cycle (cdc),** the sequence of events that occur during the growth and division of cells.

**Cellector,** trademark for a device that modifies human blood cells by circulating them through a box containing a number of polystyrene plates. Genetically engineered monoclonal antibodies are permanently attached to the polystyrene plates, which capture specifically targeted cells while the rest of the cells are transfused back into the patient's body. The device is used in bone marrow transplantation.

**cell inclusion** [L, *cella*, storeroom, *in* + *claudere*, to shut], pertaining to any foreign matter that is enclosed within a cell.

**cell line** [L, *cella* + *linea*], a colony of animal cells derived and developed as a subculture from a primary cell culture.

**cell mass** [L, *cella*, storeroom, *massa*], the embryonic cluster of cells that develops into an individual or a part of an organism.

**cell-mediated cytotoxicity,** cytolysis of a target cell by effector lymphocytes, such as cytotoxic T lymphocytes or NK cells; it may be antibody-dependent *(antibody-*

*dependent cell-mediated cytotoxicity)* or independent, as in certain type IV hypersensitivity reactions.

**cell-mediated hypersensitivity,** hypersensitivity initiated by antigen-specific T lymphocytes; unlike forms of hypersensitivity mediated by antibodies, it takes one or more days to develop and can be transferred by lymphocytes but not by serum. The term is often equated with **delayed hypersensitivity,** although the latter is sometimes restricted to hypersensitivity involving cytokine-mediated reactions (as contrasted with direct cytolysis).

**cell-mediated hypersensitivity reaction,** type IV hypersensitivity reaction; see **hypersensitivity reaction.**

**cell-mediated immune response,** a delayed reaction of the immune system, mediated primarily by sensitized T lymphocytes rather than antibodies. Cell-mediated immune responses reactions are responsible for defense against certain bacterial, fungal, and viral pathogens; malignant cells; and other foreign proteins and tissues. Allergic dermatitis is an example of a cell-mediated immune response. Also called **cellular hypersensitivity reaction, delayed hypersensitivity reaction, type IV hypersensitivity.** Compare **anaphylactic hypersensitivity, immune complex hypersensitivity.**

**cell-mediated immunity.** See **cellular immunity.**

**cell membrane.** See **plasma membrane.**

**cell of Corti.** See **auditory hair.**

**cell organelle** [L, *cella*, storeroom; Gk, *organon*, instrument], any of a number of membrane-bound structures within a cell that have specific functions, such as reproduction or metabolism. Examples include mitochondria and Golgi bodies.

**cell receptor,** a protein located either on a cell's surface, in its cytoplasm, or in its nucleus that binds to a specific ligand, initiating signal transduction and a change in cellular activity.

**cells of Paneth** /pä'nət, pan'əth/ [Josef Paneth, Austrian physiologist, 1857–1890], large granular epithelial cells found in intestinal glands. They secrete digestive enzymes and bactericidal lysozyme. Also called **Davidoff's cells.**

**cell theory,** the proposition that cells are the basic units of all living tissues or organisms and that cellular function is the essential process of living things.

**cellular** /sel'yələr/ [L, *cella*, storeroom], pertaining to or consisting of cells.

**cellular hypersensitivity reaction.** See **cell-mediated immune response.**

**cellular immunity** [L, *cellula*, little cell, *immunis*, exempt], the mechanism of acquired immunity characterized by the dominant role of T cell lymphocytes. Cellular immunity is involved in resistance to infectious diseases caused by viruses and some bacteria and in delayed hypersensitivity reactions, some aspects of resistance to cancer, certain autoimmune diseases, graft rejection, and certain allergies. Also called **cell-mediated immunity.** Compare **humoral immunity.**

**cellular infiltration,** the migration and grouping of cells, especially blood cells, within tissues throughout the body.

**cellular pathology.** See **pathology.**

**cellulite** /sel'yəlīt/, a nonmedical term for fat and fibrous tissue deposits that result in dimpling of the skin.

**cellulitis** /sel'yəlī'tis/ [L, *cellula*, little cell; Gk, *itis*, inflammation], a diffuse, acute infection of the skin and subcutaneous tissue characterized most commonly by local heat, redness, pain, and swelling, and occasionally by fever, malaise, chills, and headache. Abscess and tissue destruction usually follow if antibiotics are not taken. The infection is more likely to develop in the presence of damaged skin, poor circulation, or diabetes mellitus. In addition to appropriate antibiotics, treatment includes warm soaks, elevation, and prevention of pressure to the affected areas.

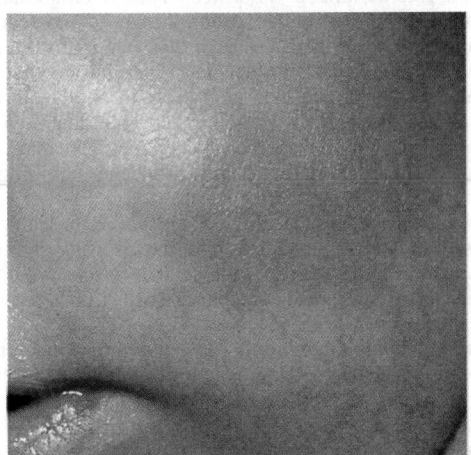

**Cellulitis** *(Zitelli and Davis, 1997)*

**cellulose** /sel'yo͝olōs/ [L, *cellula,* little cell], a colorless, insoluble, indigestible, transparent, solid polysaccharide that is the primary constituent of the cell walls of plants. In the diet it provides the bulk necessary for proper digestive tract functioning. Rich sources are fruits, such as apples and bananas, and legumes, bran, and green vegetables, especially celery. See also **dietary fiber.**

**cell wall,** the structure that covers and protects the plasma membrane in some kinds of cells, such as certain bacteria and all fungi and plant cells. The cell walls of plant cells are composed of cellulose.

**celom, celomic.** See **coelom.**

**Celontin,** trademark for an anticonvulsant (methsuximide).

**celosomia** /sē'ləsō'mē·ə/ [Gk, *kele,* hernia, *soma,* body], a congenital malformation characterized by a fissure or absence of the sternum and ribs and protrusion of the viscera.

**celosomus** /sē'ləsō'məs/, a fetus with celosomia.

**celothelioma.** See **mesothelioma.**

**Celsius (°C)** /sel'sē·əs/ [Anders Celsius, Swedish scientist, 1701–1744], temperature scale in which 0° is the freezing point of water and 100° is the boiling point of water at sea level. To convert to Fahrenheit, multiply the Celsius by 1.8, then add 32. Also called **centigrade.** Compare **Fahrenheit.**

**Celsius thermometer.** See **Celsius.**

**cement** /siment'/ [L, *caementum,* rough stone], **1.** a sticky or mucilaginous substance that hardens into a firm mass and helps neighboring tissue cells stick together. **2.** any of a variety of dental materials used to fill cavities or to hold bridgework or other dental prostheses in place. **3.** a material used in the fixation of a prosthetic joint in adjacent bone, such as methyl methacrylate.

**cemental fiber** /simen'təl/ [L, *caementum,* rough stone, *fibra*], any one of the many fibers of the periodontal membrane that extend from the cementum to the intermediate plexus, where their terminations are mixed with those of the alveolar fibers.

**cementation** /sē'mən·tā'shən/ [L, *caementum,* rough stone], the attachment of anything with cement, such as of restorative material to a natural tooth, or of bands to teeth.

**cement base,** a layer of dental cement material, sometimes medicated, that is pressed into the bottom of a prepared tooth cavity to protect the pulp, reduce the bulk of metallic restoration, or eliminate undercuts in a tapered preparation.

**cementifying fibroma** /-ifī'ing/ [L, *caementum* + *facere,* to make, *fibra,* fiber; Gk, *oma,* tumor], **1.** an intraosseous lesion composed of fibrous connective tissue enclosing foci of calcified material resembling cementum. **2.** a rare odontogenic tumor composed of varying amounts of fibrous connective tissue resembling cementum. **3.** central jaw lesion.

**cementoblast** /simen'təblast/, (in dentistry) one of the large cuboidal cells that are responsible for the formation of cementum on the root dentin of developing teeth.

**cementoblastoma** /simen'tōblastō'mə/, *pl.* **cementoblastomas, cementoblastomata** [L, *caementum* + Gk, *blastos,* germ, *oma,* tumor], an odontogenic fibrous tumor consisting of cells developing into cementoblasts but containing only a small amount of calcified tissue.

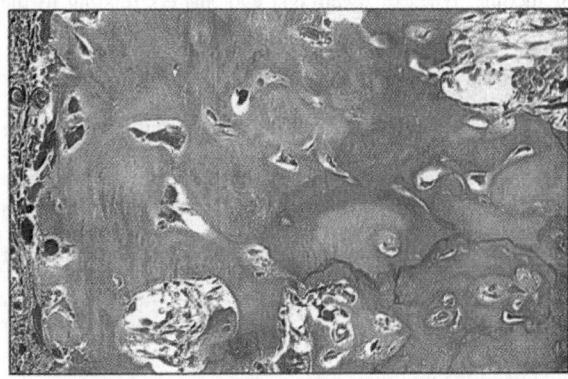

**Benign cementoblastoma** *(Eveson and Scully, 1995)*

**cementocyte** /simen'təsīt/, a cell found in the cementum of teeth.

**cementoma** /sē'mentō'mə/, *pl.* **cementomas, cementomata** [L, *caementum* + Gk, *oma,* tumor], any benign, cementum-producing tumor associated with the apices of teeth. It may be present as a mass of fibrous connective tissue, as fibrous connective tissue with spicules of cementum, or as a calcified mass resembling cementum. Examples are **cementoblastoma** and **cementifying fibroma.**

**cementopathia** /-ōpath'ē·ə/ [L, *caementum* + Gk, *pathos,* disease], an abnormal condition of the teeth caused by cementum that is necrotic and insufficient. The condition is implicated in periodontitis and periodontosis.

**cementum** /simen'təm/, the bonelike connective tissue that covers the roots of the teeth and helps to support them by providing a place of attachment for the periodontal ligament fibers.

**cen,** abbreviation for **centromere.**

**CEN,** abbreviation for **Certified Emergency Nurse.**

**cen-,** combining form meaning 'common': *cenadelphus, cenesthesia, cenesthopathia.*

**cenesthesia** /sē'nesthē'zhə/ [Gk, *kenos,* empty, *aisthesis,* feeling], the general sense of existing, derived as the aggregate of all the various stimuli and reactions throughout the body at any specific moment to produce a feeling of health or of illness. Also called **cenesthesis, coenesthesis.**

**ceno-,** prefix meaning 'new, empty, or having a common feature': *cenogenesis.*

**cenogenesis** /sē'nōjen'əsis/ [Gk, *kenos,* empty, *genein,* to produce], the development of structural characteristics that are absent in earlier forms of a species, as an adaptive response to environmental conditions. Also spelled **coenogenesis, caenogenesis, kenogenesis.** Compare **palingenesis.** —**cenogenetic, coenogenetic, caenogenetic,** *adj.*

**cenophobia.** See **kenophobia.**

**censor** [L, *censere,* to assess], **1.** a person who monitors or evaluates books, newspapers, plays, works of art, speech, or other means of expression in order to suppress certain kinds of information. **2.** (in psychoanalysis) a psychic suppression that allows unconscious thoughts to rise to consciousness only if they are heavily disguised.

**census** [L, *censere,* to assess], an enumeration of the population, usually conducted periodically as a function of an official agency. In addition to counting heads, the census often collects information about members of a household, sources of income, types of dwellings, and matters relating to the health of the community.

**cente-,** combining form meaning 'puncture': *centesis.*

**center** [Gk, *kentron*], **1.** the middle point of the body or geometric entity, equidistant from points on the periphery. **2.** a group of neurons with a common function, such as the accelerating center in the brain that controls the heartbeat.

**center of excellence,** a tertiary or quaternary health care provider that is identified as the most expert and cost efficient and produces the best outcomes. The term often refers to organ transplantation centers. Also called **center of quality.**

**center of gravity,** the midpoint or center of the weight of a body or object. In the standing adult human the center of gravity is in the midpelvic cavity, between the symphysis pubis and the umbilicus.

**center of quality.** See **center of excellence.**

**Centers for Disease Control and Prevention (CDC),** a federal agency of the U.S. government that provides facilities and services for the investigation, identification, prevention, and control of disease. It is concerned with all of the epidemiologic aspects and the laboratory diagnosis of disease. Immunization programs, quarantine regulations and programs, laboratory standards, and community surveillance for disease are among the activities of the CDC, which is located in Atlanta. Many state and local health workers and scientists receive training in specific techniques there. Originally the Communicable Disease Center, it was concerned only with communicable diseases; today its interests include environmental health, smoking, malnutrition, poisoning, and issues in occupational health. The name was changed again in 1992 to indicate its prevention function.

**centesis** /sentē'sis/ [Gk, *kentesis,* pricking], a perforation or a puncture of a cavity, such as paracentesis or thoracocentesis.

**centi-,** combining form meaning 'a hundred or a hundredth': *centibar, centiliter, centipoise.*

**centigrade.** See **Celsius.**

**centigram (cg),** a mass equal to one hundredth of a gram, or 10 milligrams.

**centiliter (cL),** a volume equal to one hundredth of a liter, or 10 milliliters.

**centimeter (cm)** /sen'timē'tər/ [L, *centum,* hundred; Gk, *metron,* measure], the metric unit of measurement equal to one hundredth of a meter, or 0.3937 inch.

**centimeter-gram-second system (cgs, CGS),** the internationally accepted scientific system of expressing length, mass, and time in basic units of centimeters, grams, and seconds. The CGS system is gradually being replaced by the Systeme International d'Unités (SI, or the International System of Units), based on the meter, kilogram, and second.

**centipede bite** /sen'təpēd/ [L, *centum,* hundred, *pes,* foot], a wound produced by the poison claws and the first body segment of a centipede, an elongate arthropod with many pairs of legs. The bite of a few species, including *Scolopendra morsitans* in the southern United States, may cause painful local inflammation, fever, headache, vomiting, and dizziness.

**centipoise** /sen'təpois/ [Jean L.M. Poiseuille, French physiologist, 1797–1869], a measure of the viscosity of a liquid, equal to one hundredth of a poise. The viscosity of glycerin is 1490 centipoise, compared with 1.005 centipoise for water.

**centrad** [L, *centum,* hundred], **1.** pertaining to a central direction, toward the center. **2.** a unit of measure equal to one hundredth part of a radian. **3.** a measure of the refractive strength of a prism.

**central** [Gk, *kentron,* center], pertaining to or situated at a center.

**central amaurosis** [Gk, *kentron* + *amauroein,* to darken], blindness caused by a disease of the central nervous system.

**central anesthesia,** a loss of feeling or sensation as a result of a lesion in the central nervous system.

**central auditory processing disorder (CAPD),** difficulty in processing and interpreting auditory stimuli in the absence of a peripheral hearing loss, usually resulting from a problem in the brainstem or cerebral cortex. Children with CAPD often have difficulty reading and may exhibit other learning disabilities as well.

**central biasing** /bī'əsing/, a theory of pain modulation in which higher centers such as the cerebral cortex influence the perception of and response to pain.

**central canal of spinal cord** [Gk, *kentron* + L, *canalis,* channel], the conduit that runs the entire length of the spinal cord and contains most of the 140 mL of cerebrospinal fluid (CSF) in the body of the average individual. The central canal of the spinal cord lies in the center of the cord between the ventral and the dorsal gray commissures and extends toward the cranium into the medulla oblongata, where it opens into the fourth ventricle of the brain. Lumbar puncture, often performed to obtain samples of CSF for diagnostic purposes, draws fluid from the subarachnoid space around the spinal cord and not from the central canal. See also **lumbar puncture.**

**central catheter** [Gk, *kentron,* central, *katheter,* a thing lowered into], a catheter inserted into either a central artery or a central vein for diagnostic or therapeutic procedures.

**central chemoreceptor,** any of the sensory nerve cells or chemical receptors that are located in the medulla of the brain. Also called **medullary chemoreceptor.**

**central chondrosarcoma** [Gk, *kentron* + *chondros,* cartilage, *sarx,* flesh, *oma,* tumor], a malignant cartilaginous tumor that forms inside a bone. Also called **enchondrosarcoma.**

**central core disease,** an autosomal dominant form of myopathy characterized by dense, amorphous hyaline changes in the central portion of the myofibrils, which lack organelles. Onset is in infancy and causes delayed motor development, especially in the lower limbs. Also called **Shy-Magee syndrome.**

**central deafness.** See **central auditory processing disorder.**

**central electrode,** a key part of a radiation detection instrument. It consists of a positively charged rigid wire in the center of a gas-filled cylinder. The electrode attracts electrons liberated by the ionization effects of radiation and converts them into an electric current.

**central facilitation,** (in chiropractic) a model based on neurophysiologic findings that explains the symptoms of subluxogenic pain and discomfort that arise from nonspinal sites.

**central fissure.** See **central sulcus.**

**central implantation.** See **superficial implantation.**

**central incisor,** one of the two teeth located closest to the sagittal plane in the upper and lower jaws.

**central line,** IV tubing inserted for continuous access to a central vein for administering fluids and medicines and for obtaining diagnostic information. Keeping the central line in place ensures accessibility to the venous system in case the peripheral veins collapse. See also **central venous catheter.**

**central lobe,** one of the lobes constituting each of the cerebral hemispheres, lying hidden in the depths of the lateral sulcus. The central lobe can be seen only if the lips of the sulcus are parted or cut away. Also called **island of Reil.** Compare **frontal lobe, occipital lobe, parietal lobe, temporal lobe.**

**central necrosis** [Gk, *kentron,* central, *nekros,* dead, *osis,* condition], death of the central part of a tissue or organ.

**central nervous system (CNS)** [Gk, *kentron* + L, *nervus,* nerve; Gk, *systema*], one of the two main divisions of the nervous system, consisting of the brain and the spinal cord. The central nervous system processes information to and from the peripheral nervous system and is the main network of coordination and control for the entire body. The brain controls many functions and sensations, such as sleep, sexual activity, muscular movement, hunger, thirst, memory, and emotions. The spinal cord extends various types of nerve fibers from the brain and acts as a switching and relay terminal for the peripheral nervous system. The 12 pairs of cranial nerves emerge directly from the brain. Sensory nerves and motor nerves of the peripheral system leave the spinal cord separately between the vertebrae but unite to form 31 pairs of spinal nerves containing sensory fibers and motor fibers. More than 10 billion neurons constitute but one tenth of the brain cells; the other cells consist of neuroglia that support the neurons. The neurons and the neuroglia form the soft, jellylike substance of the brain, which is supported and protected by the skull. The brain and the spinal cord are composed of gray matter and white matter. The gray matter primarily contains nerve cells and associated processes; the white matter consists predominantly of bundles of myelinated nerve fibers. Compare **peripheral nervous system.** See also **brain, spinal cord.**

**central nervous system depressant,** any drug that decreases the function of the central nervous system, such as alcohol, tranquilizers, barbiturates, and hypnotics. Such drugs can produce tolerance, physical dependence, and compulsive drug use. These substances depress excitable tissue throughout the central nervous system by stabilizing neuronal membranes, decreasing the amount of transmitter released by the nerve impulse, and generally depressing postsynaptic responsiveness and ion movement. Central nervous system depressants elevate the seizure threshold and can produce physical dependence in a relatively short period. The most abused depressants are the short-acting barbiturates, especially pentobarbital, secobarbital, glutethimide, methyprylon, and methaqualone. These substances

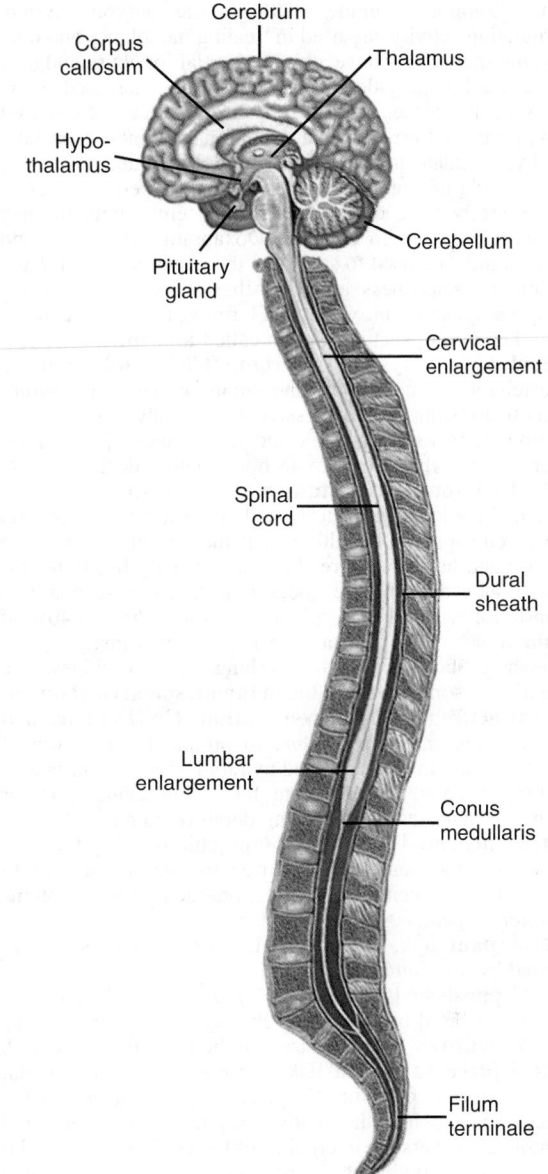

**Central nervous system** *(Chipps, Clanin, and Campbell, 1992)*

have popular street names on the illicit market, such as "reds" (secobarbital) and "yellows" (pentobarbital). Sudden withdrawal of general central nervous system depressants that have been used in high doses for prolonged periods can be fatal to some individuals.

**central nervous system stimulant,** a substance that quickens the activity of the central nervous system by increasing the rate of neuronal discharge or by blocking an inhibitory neurotransmitter. Many natural and synthetic compounds stimulate the central nervous system, but only a few are used therapeutically. Caffeine, a potent central nervous system stimulant, is used to help restore mental alertness and overcome respiratory depression, but it may cause nausea, nervousness, tinnitus, tremor, tachycardia, extra systoles, diuresis, and visual disturbances. Amphetamines, sympathomimetic amines with central nervous system stimulating activity, are used in treating narcolepsy and obesity, but these drugs have a high potential for abuse and may cause dizziness, restlessness, tachycardia, increased blood pressure, headache, mouth dryness, an unpleasant taste, GI symptoms, and urticaria. Various amphetamines, especially methylphenidate and deanol acetamidobenzoate, a precursor of acetylcholine, are prescribed for the hyperkinetic child syndrome because central nervous system stimulants may act as depressants in children. Doxapram, ethamivan, and nikethamide are used to stimulate the respiratory center and restore consciousness after anesthesia and to treat acute sedative-hypnotic intoxication. Flurothyl is used in convulsive therapy in psychiatry. Also called **analeptic.**

**central nervous system syndrome (CNS syndrome),** a constellation of neurologic and emotional signs and symptoms that results from a massive whole-body dosage of radiation. It includes hysteria and disorientation, which increase during the last 24 to 48 hours before death.

**central nervous system tumor,** a neoplasm of the brain or spinal cord that characteristically does not spread beyond the cerebrospinal axis, although it may be highly invasive locally and have widespread effects on body functions. Intracranial neoplasms are about four times more common than those arising in the spinal cord. From 20% to 40% of brain tumors are metastatic lesions from primary cancer elsewhere, such as in the breast, lung, GI tract, kidney, or a site of melanoma. See also **brain tumor, spinal cord tumor.**

**central neurogenic hyperventilation (CNHV)** [Gk, *kentron* + *neuron,* nerve, *genein,* to produce], a pattern of breathing during coma marked by rapid, regular ventilations at a rate of about 25 per minute. Increasing regularity rather than rate indicates an increasing depth of coma.

**central neuronal plasticity,** (in chiropractic) the tendency for the neuronal responses to noxious stimuli to spread to other central pathways, producing the symptoms of referred pain.

**central pain** [Gk, *kentron* + L, *poena,* penalty], pain caused by a lesion in the central nervous system.

**central paralysis** [Gk, *kentron* + *paralyein,* to be palsied], paralysis caused by a lesion in the central nervous system.

**central pathway,** a nerve tract in the brain or spinal cord.

**central placenta previa** [Gk, *kentron* + L, *placenta,* flat cake, *praevius,* preceding], placenta previa in which the placenta is implanted in the lower segment of the uterus and completely covers the internal os of the uterine cervix. In labor, as the cervix dilates, the placenta is gradually separated from the underlying blood vessels in the uterine lining, causing bleeding that usually begins slowly, is painless, and progresses to hemorrhage that is life-threatening to the mother and the baby. Cesarean section is usually performed to save the mother and the baby. The condition may be discovered by ultrasound visualization before any bleeding occurs or by digital palpation in the normal course of prenatal care. Also called **complete previa.** See also **placenta previa.**

**central processing unit (cpu, CPU),** the component of a computer that controls the encoding and execution of instructions, consisting mainly of an arithmetic unit, which performs arithmetic functions, and an internal memory, which controls the sequencing of operations. Also called **processor.**

**central ray (CR),** the portion of an x-ray beam that is directed toward the center of the film or of the object being radiographed.

**central scotoma** [Gk, *kentron* + *skotos,* darkness, *oma,* tumor], an area of blindness or site of depressed vision involving the macula of the retina.

**central sensitization,** (in chiropractic) a state in which neurons activated by noxious mechanical and chemical stimuli are sensitized by such stimuli and become hyperresponsive to all subsequent stimuli delivered to the neurons' receptive fields.

**central sleep apnea,** a form of sleep apnea resulting from decreased respiratory center output. It may involve primary brainstem medullary depression resulting from a tumor of the posterior fossa, poliomyelitis, or idiopathic central hypoventilation.

**central stimulant.** See **central nervous system stimulant.**

**central sulcus** [Gk, *kentron* + L, furrow], a cleft separating the frontal from the parietal lobes of brain. Also called **central fissure, fissure of Rolando.**

**central tendon,** a broad connective tissue sheet that forms the diaphragm. It is composed of interlacing fibers that arise from the lumbar vertebrae, the costal margin, and the xiphoid process of the sternum.

**central venous blood pressure,** the blood pressure in the superior vena cava, measured by inserting a catheter attached to a manometer directly outside the right atrium. It is approximately equal to the right atrial pressure.

**central venous catheter,** a catheter that is threaded through the internal jugular, antecubital, or subclavian vein, usually with the tip resting in the superior vena cava or the right atrium of the heart. It is also used to administer fluids or medications for hemodynamic monitoring and to measure central venous pressure.

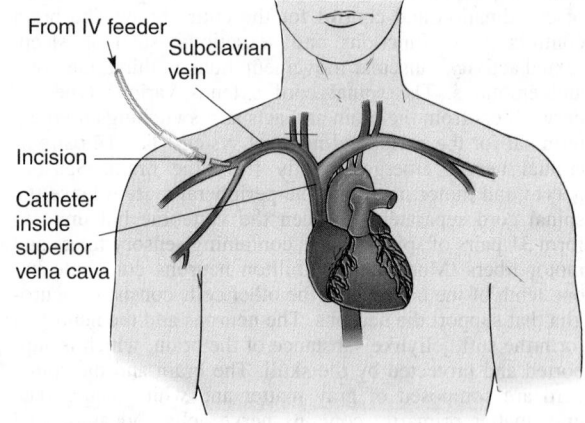

**Central venous catheter placement**
*(Potter and Perry, 2001/Rolin Graphics)*

**central venous oxygen saturation (CVSO₂),** the oxygen saturation in the vena cava. The $CVSO_2$ is measured through a central venous catheter and is useful in measuring cardiac output. A reading of less than 55% usually indicates a falling cardiac output and probable cardiac failure.

**central venous pressure (CVP),** the blood pressure in the large veins of the body, as distinguished from peripheral venous pressure in an extremity. It is measured with a water manometer that may be attached to the head of a patient's bed and to a central venous catheter inserted into the vena cava. The normal CVP values are 2 to 14 cm $H_2O$.

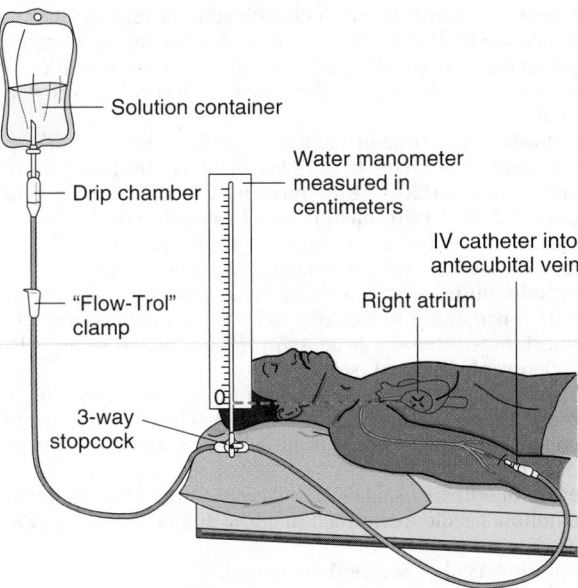

**Measurement of central venous pressure**
*(Phipps, Sands, and Marek, 1999)*

Solution container
Drip chamber
Water manometer measured in centimeters
IV catheter into antecubital vein
"Flow-Trol" clamp
Right atrium
3-way stopcock

**central venous pressure (CVP) monitor,** a device for measuring and recording the venous blood pressure by means of an indwelling venous catheter and a pressure manometer. It is used to evaluate the right ventricular function, the right atrial filling pressure, and the circulating blood volume.

**central venous return,** the blood from the venous system that flows into the right atrium through the vena cava.

**central vertigo** [Gk, *kentron* + L, *vertigo,* dizziness], vertigo that is caused by a central nervous system disorder.

**central vision,** vision that results from images falling on the macula of the retina.

**Centrax,** trademark for a benzodiazepine antianxiety agent (prazepam).

**centre.** See **center.**

**centrencephalic** /sen′trensifal′ik/ [Gk, *kentron* + *enkephalos,* brain], pertaining to the center of the encephalon.

**centri-.** See **centro-.**

**centriacinar emphysema** /sen·trē·ə·sin′ər/, one of the types of emphysema, characterized by enlargement of air spaces in the proximal part of the acinus, primarily at the level of the respiratory bronchioles. Also called **focal emphysema.**

**centric** /sen′trik /, **1.** see **central. 2.** in dentistry, the term is sometimes used as a noun, such as in **power centric.**

**centriciput** /sentris′ipoŏt/, the central part of the head, between the occiput and the sinciput.

**centrifugal** /sentrif′yəgəl/, **1.** denoting a force that is directed outward, away from a central point or axis, such as the force that keeps the moon in its orbit around the earth. **2.** a direction away from the head.

**centrifugal analyzer,** equipment that uses centrifugal force to mix a sample aliquot, or portion, with a reagent and a spinning rotor to pass the reaction mixture through a detector.

**centrifugal current,** an electrical current in the body with the positive pole near the nerve center and the negative pole at the periphery. Also called **descending current.**

**centrifugal force,** an inertial force in a rotating system, directed outward from the axis of rotation and inversely proportional to the distance from the axis of rotation. The force is the product of the mass of an object and its radial acceleration; thus in centrifugation the heavier components of a mixture are separated from the other components by being thrown to the periphery of the orbit.

**centrifuge** /sen′trifyo̅o̅j′/ [Gk, *kentron* + L, *fugere,* to flee], a device for separating components of different densities contained in liquid by spinning them at high speeds. Centrifugal force causes the heavier components to move to one part of the container, leaving the lighter substances in another. **—centrifugal,** *adj.,* **centrifuge,** *v.*

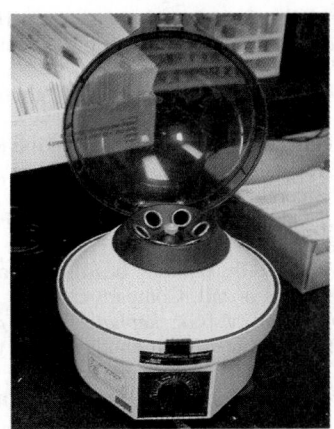

**Centrifuge** *(Zakus, 1995)*

**centrilobular** /sen′trəlob′yələr/ [Gk, *kentron* + L, *lobulus,* small lobe], pertaining to the center of a lobule.

**centrilobular emphysema.** See **centriacinar emphysema.**

**centriole** /sen′trē·ōl′/ [Gk, *kentron*], an intracellular organelle, usually as a component of the centrosome. Often occurring in pairs, centrioles are associated with cell division and can be closely studied only with an electron microscope. They are tiny cylinders positioned at right angles to each other, with walls consisting of nine bundles of fine tubules, three tubules to a bundle. Numerous centrioles occur in some large cells, such as the giant cells in bone marrow. The precise function of centrioles is still a mystery, but they appear to aid in the formation of the spindle that develops during mitosis.

**centripetal** /sentrip′ətəl/ [Gk, *kentron* + L, *petere,* to seek], **1.** denoting an afferent direction, such as that of a sensory nerve impulse traveling toward the brain. **2.** denoting the direction of a force pulling an object toward an axis of rotation or constraining an object to a specific curved path.

**centripetal current,** an electrical current passing through the body from a peripheral positive electrode to a negative pole near the nerve center. Also called **ascending current.**

**centripetal force,** the force, directed toward the axis of rotation, required to keep an object moving in a circular path.

**centro-, centri-,** combining form meaning 'center, central, to the center': *centrocecal, centrocinesia, centrosclerosis.*

**centromere (cen)** /sen′trəmir/ [Gk, *kentron* + *meros,* part], the constricted region of a chromosome that joins the two chromatids to each other and attaches to spindle fibers in mitosis and meiosis. During cell division the centromeres split longitudinally, half going to each of the new daughter chromosomes. The position of the centromere is constant for a specific chromosome and is identified as acrocentric, metacentric, submetacentric, or telocentric. Also called **kinetochore, kinomere, primary constriction. —centromeric,** *adj.*

**centrosome** [Gk, *kentron* + *soma,* body], a self-propagating cytoplasmic organelle present in animal cells and in those of some lower plants. The structure, which consists of the centrosphere and the centrioles, is located near the nucleus of the cell center or attraction sphere and functions as the dynamic center of the cell, especially during mitosis. Also called **cytocentrum, microcentrum, paranuclear body.**

**centrosphere** [Gk, *kentron* + *sphaira,* ball], the condensed area of cytoplasm surrounding the centrioles in the centrosome of a cell.

**centrostaltic** /sen′trōstôl′tik/, pertaining to the center of movement.

**centrum,** *pl.* **centra** [Gk, *kentron*], any kind of center, especially one related to a body structure, as the centrum semiovale of a cerebral hemisphere.

**CEO, C.E.O.,** abbreviation for **chief executive officer.**

**cephal-.** See **cephalo-.**

**cephalad** /sef′əlad/ [Gk, *kephale,* head], toward the head, away from the ends or tail. Compare **caudad.**

**cephalalgia** /sef′əlal′jə/ [Gk, *kephale,* head, *algos,* pain], headache, often combined with another word to indicate a specific type of headache, such as histamine cephalalgia. Also called **cephalea, cephalgia.** See also **histamine headache.**

**cephalea agitata** /sef′əlē′ə/, a violent headache that is frequently an early symptom of an infection.

**cephaledema** /sef′əlidē′mə/, a swelling of the brain caused by fluid accumulation.

**cephalexin** /sef′əlek′sin/, a cephalosporin antibiotic.

■ INDICATIONS: It is prescribed for oral treatment of selected infections caused by susceptible bacterial strains.

■ CONTRAINDICATIONS: Known hypersensitivity to this drug or to any cephalosporin medication prohibits its use. It is used with caution in patients who are allergic to penicillin.

■ ADVERSE EFFECTS: Nausea, diarrhea, and hypersensitivity reactions may occur.

**cephalgia.** See **cephalalgia, headache.**

**cephalhematoma** /sef′əlhē′mətō′mə, -hem′ətō′mə/, swelling caused by subcutaneous bleeding and accumulation of blood. It may begin to form in the scalp of a fetus during labor and enlarge slowly in the first few days after birth. It is usually a result of trauma, often caused by forceps. Large cephalhematomas may become infected, require surgical drainage, and take several months to resolve. Also called **cephalhaematoma.** Compare **caput succedaneum, molding.**

**-cephalia** suffix meaning a specified '(condition of the) head': *hemicephalia, megacephalia, notancephalia.*

**cephalic** /sifal′ik/, pertaining to the head.

**-cephalic,** suffix meaning 'relating to the head': *holocephalic, megalocephalic, postcephalic.*

**cephalic index** [Gk, *kephale,* head, *index,* pointer], a ratio between the breadth and length of the head. It is calculated as 100 times the maximum breadth of the head, measured at the greatest diameter of the cranial vault above the supramastoid crest, divided by the maximum length measured from the most prominent point on the glabella to the opisthocranion.

**cephalic presentation,** a classification of fetal position in which the head of the fetus is at the uterine cervix. Cephalic presentation is usually further qualified by an indication of the part of the head presenting, such as the occiput, brow, or chin.

**cephalic vein,** one of the four superficial veins of the upper limb. It receives deoxygenated blood from the dorsal and palmar surfaces of the forearm. Compare **basilic vein, dorsal digital vein, median antebrachial vein.**

**cephalo-, cephal-,** combining form meaning 'head': *cephalocaudal, cephalocentesis, cephalogenesis.*

**cephalocaudal** /sef′əlōkô′dəl/ [Gk, *kephale* + L, *cauda,* tail], pertaining to the long axis of the body, or the relationship between the head and the base of the spine. Also called **cephalocercal** /sef′əlōsur′kəl/.

**cephalocele** /sef′əlōsēl′/, the protrusion of a part of the brain through an opening in the skull. The opening may be congenital or may result from an injury. Also called **cerebral hernia.**

**cephalocentesis** /-sentē′sis/, the puncture of the skull with a hollow needle, performed to allow drainage of fluid or an abscess.

**cephalocercal.** See **cephalocaudal.**

**cephalogram.** See **cephalometric radiograph.**

**cephalomelus** /sef′əlom′ələs/ [Gk, *kephale* + *melos,* limb], a deformed individual who has a structure resembling an arm or a leg protruding from the head.

**cephalometric radiograph** /sef′ə·lō·met′rik rā′dē·ō·graf/, a radiograph of the head, including the mandible, in full lateral view; used for making cranial measurements. Also called **cephalogram.**

**cephalometric tracing,** a line drawing of structural outlines of craniofacial landmarks and facial bones made directly from a cephalometric radiogram.

**cephalometry** /-ətrē/, scientific measurement of the head, such as that performed in dentistry to determine appropriate orthodontic procedures for correcting malocclusions and other abnormal conditions. —**cephalometric,** *adj.*

**cephalomotor** /sef′ə·lō·mō′tər/ [Gk, *kephale,* head + L, *motare,* to move about], moving the head; pertaining to motions of the head.

**cephalopagus.** See **craniopagus.**

**cephalopelvic** /-pel′vik/, pertaining to a relationship between the fetal head and the maternal pelvis.

**cephalopelvic disproportion (CPD)** [Gk, *kephale* + L, *pelvis,* basin, *dis,* opposite of, *proportio,* similarity], an obstetric condition in which a baby's head is too large or a mother's birth canal too small to permit normal labor or birth. In **relative CPD,** the size of the baby's head is within normal limits but larger than average or the size of the mother's birth canal is within normal limits but smaller than average, or both; relative CPD is often overcome by molding of the head, the forces of labor, or the use of forceps to effect delivery. In **absolute CPD,** the baby's head is markedly or abnormally enlarged or the mother's birth canal is markedly or abnormally contracted, making vaginal delivery impossible. See also **clinical pelvimetry, x-ray pelvimetry.**

**cephalopelvimetry** /-pelvim′ətrē/, radiographic measurement of the fetal head in utero.

**cephalophlebitis,** inflammation of the vena cava.

**cephaloridine** /sef′əlôr′idēn/, a cephalosporin antibiotic.

■ INDICATIONS: It is prescribed in the treatment of bacterial infections.

■ CONTRAINDICATIONS: Concurrent administration of medications that cause nephrotoxicity or known hypersensitivity to this drug or to cephalosporin medication prohibits its use. It is prescribed with caution for patients who are allergic to penicillin.

■ ADVERSE EFFECTS: Among the more serious adverse reactions are nephrotoxicity, pain at the site of injection, and hypersensitivity reactions.

**cephalosporin** /sef'əlōspôr'in/ [Gk, *kephale* + *sporos*, seed], a semisynthetic derivative of an antibiotic originally derived from the microorganism *Cephalosporium falciforme* (*Acremonium kiliense*). Cephalosporins are similar in structure to penicillins except for a beta-lactamdihydrothiazine ring in place of beta-lactamthiazolidin in penicillin. Cephalosporins are used in treating bacterial infections of the respiratory tract, urinary tract, middle ear, and bones, as well as septicemia caused by gram-positive and gram-negative organisms.

**cephalosporinase.** See **beta-lactamase.**

**cephalothin sodium** /sef'əlō'thin/, a cephalosporin antibiotic.

■ INDICATIONS: It is prescribed in the treatment of infections caused by susceptible bacterial strains.

■ CONTRAINDICATIONS: Known hypersensitivity to this drug or to any cephalosporin medication prohibits its use. It is prescribed with caution for patients who are allergic to penicillin.

■ ADVERSE EFFECTS: Among the more serious adverse reactions are pain at the site of injection and hypersensitivity reactions.

**cephalothoracoiliopagus.** See **synadelphus.**

**-cephalus** [Gk, *kephale*, head], suffix meaning *(a)* an abnormal condition of the head, as indicated by the stem to which the ending is attached, such as **hydrocephalus;** *(b)* an individual having an abnormal condition of the head, especially a congenital anomaly of the fetus, such as **dicephalus.**

**-cephaly** [Gk, *kephale*, head], suffix meaning an abnormal condition of the head, as indicated by the stem to which the ending is attached.

**-cephaly, -cephalia,** combining form meaning a '(specified) condition of the head': *macrencephaly, platycephaly, trochocephaly.*

**cephapirin** /sef'əprin/, a cephalosporin antibiotic.

■ INDICATIONS: It is prescribed in the treatment of bacterial infections caused by cephapirin-susceptible strains of a wide variety of microorganisms that cause septicemia, endocarditis, osteomyelitis, and bacterial infections of the respiratory tract, urinary tract, and skin.

■ CONTRAINDICATION: Known sensitivity to cephalosporin antibiotics prohibits its use.

■ ADVERSE EFFECTS: Among the most serious adverse reactions are neutropenia, leukopenia, anemia, bone marrow depression, and allergic reactions.

**cephradine** /sef'rədēn/, a cephalosporin antibiotic.

■ INDICATIONS: It is prescribed in the treatment of certain infections caused by susceptible bacterial strains.

■ CONTRAINDICATIONS: Known hypersensitivity to this drug or to any cephalosporin medication prohibits its use. It is prescribed with caution for patients who are allergic to penicillin.

■ ADVERSE EFFECTS: Nausea, diarrhea, and hypersensitivity reactions may occur.

**-ceptor** [shortened from *receptor;* L, *recipere,* to receive], suffix denoting a receptor, with the root preceding it specifying the type.

**cer-,** combining form meaning 'wax': *ceraceous, cerate, cerumen.*

**cera,** wax. Ordinary yellow beeswax is sometimes identified as cera flava; white beeswax, bleached by exposure to air and sunlight, is known as cera alba.

**ceramics** /səram'iks/, (in dentistry) the process of making dental restorations from fused porcelain and other glasses.

**ceramidase** /sə·ram'i·dās/, an enzyme of the hydrolase class that catalyzes the cleavage of a ceramide to form sphingosine and a fatty acid anion, a step in the degradation of sphingolipids. See also **Farber's disease.**

**ceramidase deficiency.** See **Farber's disease.**

**ceramide** /ser'ə·mīd/, the basic unit of the sphingolipids, consisting of sphingosine or a related base attached via its amino group to a long-chain fatty acyl group.

**cerato-, kerato-,** combining form meaning 'cornea or horny tissue': *ceratocricoid, ceratohyal, ceratopharyngeus.*

**cercaria** /sərker'ē·ə/, *pl.* **cercariae** [Gk, *kerkos,* tail], a minute, wormlike early developmental form of trematode. It develops in a freshwater snail, is released into the water, and swims toward the sun, rising to the surface of the water in the warmest part of the day. Cercariae enter the body of the next host by ingestion, by direct invasion through the skin, or through a cut or other break in the skin. Some cercariae of the genera *Schistosoma, Chlonorchis, Paragonimus, Fasciolopsis,* and *Fasciola* are known to infect humans. They encyst and complete their development in various organs of the body. Each species tends to migrate to one organ, such as *Fasciola hepatica,* which grows to become a liver fluke. See also **fluke, schistosomiasis.**

**cerclage** /serkläzh'/ [Fr, cask hooping], **1.** an orthopedic procedure in which the ends of an oblique bone fracture or the chips of a broken patella are bound together with a wire loop or a metal band to hold them in position until healed. **2.** a procedure in which a taut silicone band is applied around the sclera to restore contact between the retina and the choroid when the retina is detached. **3.** an obstetric procedure in which a nonabsorbable suture is used for holding the cervix closed to prevent spontaneous abortion in a woman who has an incompetent cervix. The band is usually released when the pregnancy is at full term to allow labor to begin. See also **incompetent cervix.**

**cerea flexibilitas** /sirē'ə flek'sibil'itas/ [L, waxlike flexibility], a cataleptic state, frequently observed in catatonic schizophrenia, in which the limbs maintain the positions in which they are placed for an indefinite period. Also called **flexibilitas cerea, waxy flexibility.** See also **catalepsy.**

**cerebella.** See **cerebellum.**

**cerebellar** /ser'əbel'ər/ [L, *cerebellum,* small brain], pertaining to the cerebellum.

**cerebellar angioblastoma** [L, *cerebellum* + Gk, *angeion,* vessel, *blastos,* germ, *oma*], a cystic tumor in the cerebellum composed of a mass of blood vessels. It is frequently associated with von Hippel–Lindau disease.

**cerebellar artery occlusion,** an obstruction of one of the arteries supplying the cerebellum. It can result in ipsilateral ataxia, facial analgesia, contralateral hemiparesis, and loss of temperature and pain sensations.

**cerebellar ataxia** [L, *cerebellum,* small brain; Gk, *ataxia,* without order], a loss of muscle coordination caused by a lesion in the cerebellum.

**cerebellar atrophy** [L, *cerebellum* + Gk, *a* + *trophe,* without nourishment], deterioration and wasting of tissues of the cerebellum. Causes of the condition include nutritional/metabolic factors such as alcohol abuse and degenerative disease. See also **spinocerebellar disorder.**

**cerebellar cortex,** the superficial gray matter of the cerebellum covering the white substance in the medullary core. It consists of two layers, an external molecular layer and an internal granule cell layer. Also called **cortical substance of cerebellum.**

**cerebellar cyst,** a cyst that develops in the white matter of the cerebellum and is often associated with an astrocytoma.

**cerebellar gait** [L, *cerebellum,* small brain; ONorse, *geta,* a way], a staggering gait in which the person walks with a wide base and has difficulty turning. The feet are thrown outward, and the person puts his or her weight first on the heel and then on the toes. The condition is caused by a lesion in the cerebellum or cerebellar pathways. Also called **ataxic gait.**

**cerebellar inferior peduncle** [L, *cerebellum,* small brain, *inferior,* lower, *pes,* foot], a band of nerve fibers that forms the lateral boundary of the bottom part of the fourth ventricle and carries afferent fibers into the cerebellum.

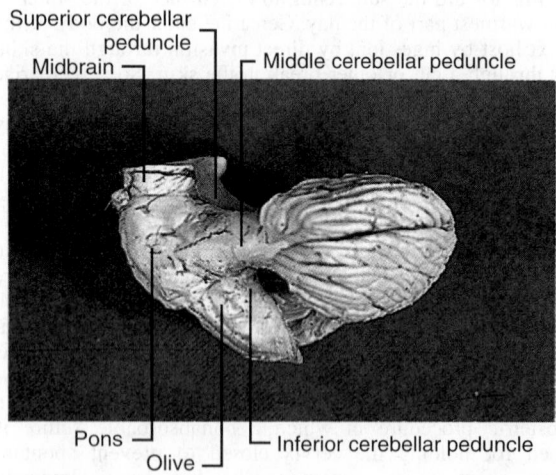

**Cerebellar peduncles** *(Crossman and Neary, 1995)*

Superior cerebellar peduncle
Midbrain
Middle cerebellar peduncle
Pons
Olive
Inferior cerebellar peduncle

**cerebellar middle peduncle** [L, *cerebellum,* small brain, *medius + pes,* foot], a lateral extension of the transverse nerve fibers of the pons. It consists mainly of fibers from the pontine nuclei to the neocerebellum.

**cerebellar notch, 1.** anteriorly, a broad depression that lies dorsal to the midbrain and separates the cerebellar hemispheres rostral to the vermis. **2.** posteriorly, a deep depression adjacent to the falx cerebelli.

**cerebellar rigidity,** a stiffness of the trunk muscles caused by a midline lesion in the cerebellum. In some cases, the limbs may also be rigid and the neck and back arched, as in opisthotonos.

**cerebellar speech** [L, *cerebellum* + AS, *spaec*], abnormal speech seen in diseases of the cerebellum. It is characterized by slow, jerky, and slurred articulation that may be intermittent and explosive or monotonous and unvaried in pitch. See also **ataxic speech.**

**cerebellar superior peduncle** [L, *cerebellum,* small brain, *superior + pes,* foot], a band of nerve fibers that passes from the cerebellum on each side of the superior medullary velum. It includes nerve tracts linking the dentate nucleus to the red nucleus of the midbrain and to the thalamus.

**cerebellar tremor** [L, *cerebellum,* small brain, *tremor,* shaking], an intention tremor or trembling during voluntary movements, caused by lesions in the cerebellum.

**cerebellopontine** /ser′əbel′ōpon′tīn/ [L, *cerebellum* + *pons,* bridge], leading from the cerebellum to the pons varolii.

**cerebellospinal** /ser′əbel′ōspī′nəl/ [L, *cerebellum* + *spina,* backbone], leading from the cerebellum to the spinal cord.

**cerebellum** /ser′əbel′əm/, *pl.* **cerebellums, cerebella** [L, small brain], the part of the brain located in the posterior cranial fossa behind the brainstem. It consists of two lateral cerebellar hemispheres, or lobes, and a middle section called the vermis. Three pairs of peduncles link it with the brainstem. Its functions are concerned primarily with coordinating voluntary muscular activity.

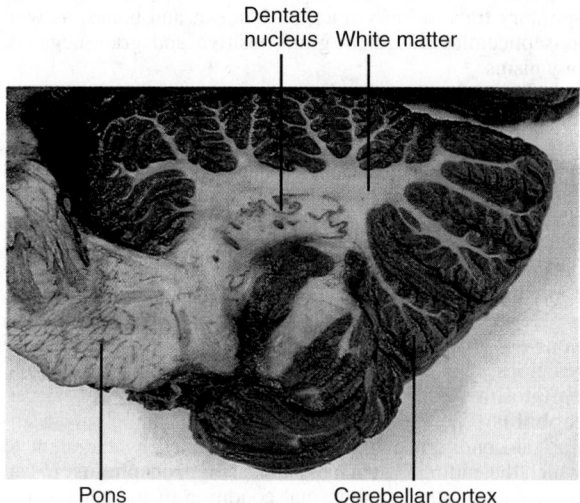

Dentate nucleus   White matter
Pons   Cerebellar cortex

**Cerebellum** *(Crossman and Neary, 1995)*

**cerebr-,** prefix meaning 'cerebrum': *cerebralgia, cerebrocardiac, cerebropathy.*

**cerebra.** See **cerebrum.**

**cerebral** /ser′əbrəl, sərē′brəl/, pertaining to the cerebrum.

**-cerebral,** suffix referring to the brain: *craniocerebral, medicerebral, postcerebral.*

**cerebral abscess.** See **brain abscess.**

**cerebral amyloid angiopathy,** vascular amyloidosis affecting small- and medium-sized arteries of the leptomeninges and cerebral cortex, resulting in microinfarcts or in hemorrhage; it may be asymptomatic or may result in hemorrhagic stroke or dementia. It usually occurs in the elderly and most cases are sporadic. A hereditary form with autosomal dominant inheritance also exists.

**cerebral aneurysm** [L, *cerebrum,* brain; Gk, *aneurysma,* a widening], an abnormal, localized dilation of a cerebral artery. It is most commonly the result of congenital weakness of the tunica media or muscle layer of the arterial wall. Cerebral aneurysms may also be caused by infection, such as occurs in subacute bacterial endocarditis or syphilis, and by neoplasms, arteriosclerosis, and trauma. The most frequent sites are the middle cerebral, internal carotid, basilar, and anterior cerebral arteries, especially at bifurcations of vessels. Cerebral aneurysms may occur in infancy or old age. They may be fusiform dilations of the entire circumference of an artery or saccular outcroppings of the side of a vessel. The outcroppings may be as small as a pinhead or as large as an orange but are usually the size of a pea. Cerebral aneurysms pose a danger of rupture and intracranial hemorrhage.

**cerebral angiography** [L, *cerebrum,* brain; Gk, *angeion,* vessel, *graphein,* to record], a radiographic procedure used to visualize the vascular system of the brain after injection of a radiopaque contrast medium.

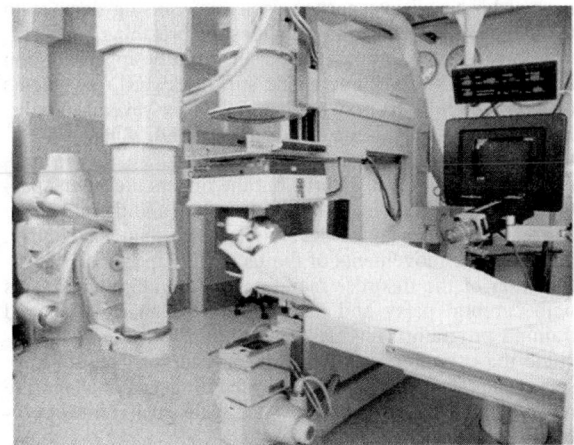

**Positioning of the patient for cerebral angiography**
*(Chipps, Clanin, and Campbell, 1992)*

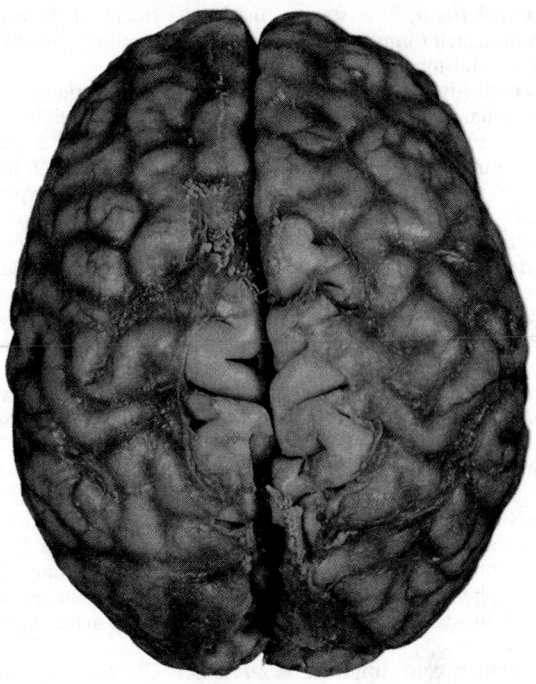

**Cerebral cortex: superior view** *(Crossman and Neary, 1995)*

**cerebral anoxia,** a condition in which oxygen is deficient in brain tissue. This state, which is caused by circulatory failure, can exist for no more than 4 to 6 minutes before the onset of irreversible brain damage.

**cerebral aqueduct** [L, *cerebrum* + *aqueductus,* water canal], the narrow conduit, between the third and the fourth ventricles in the midbrain, that conveys the cerebrospinal fluid. Also called **aqueduct of Sylvius.**

**cerebral arteriovenous malformation.** See **arteriovenous angioma of the brain.**

**cerebral cavity.** See **cranial cavity.**

**cerebral compression** [L, *cerebrum,* brain, *comprimere,* to press together], any abnormal condition, such as hemorrhage, abscess, or tumor, that increases intracranial pressure. If untreated, the compression destroys the brain tissues and causes herniation of the brain. Also called **brain compression.**

**cerebral cortex** [L, *cerebrum* + *cortex,* bark], a layer of neurons and synapses (gray matter) on the surface of the cerebral hemispheres, folded into gyri with about two thirds of its area buried in fissures. It integrates higher mental functions, general movement, visceral functions, perception, and behavioral reactions. It has been classified many different ways. Research has described more than 200 areas on the basis of differences in myelinated fiber patterns and has defined 47 separate function areas with different cell designs. For example, stimulation of the precentral cortex or motor area with electrodes causes contractions of voluntary muscles. Destruction of a motor speech area in the frontal operculum causes motor aphasia or speech defects despite healthy, intact vocal organs. Stimulation of the frontal area affects circulation, respiration, pupillary reaction, and other visceral activity. Also called **pallium.** See also **cerebrum.**

**cerebral deafness.** See **central auditory processing disorder.**

**cerebral depressant** [L, *cerebrum,* brain, *deprimere,* to press down], a drug or other agent that has a sedating effect on the brain, reducing activity and alertness and, in some instances, causing a loss of consciousness.

**cerebral dominance,** the specialization of each of the two cerebral hemispheres in the integration and control of different functions. In 90% of the population, the left cerebral hemisphere specializes in or dominates the ability to speak and write and the capacity to understand spoken and written words. The areas that control these activities are situated in the frontal, parietal, and temporal lobes of the left hemisphere. In the other 10% of the population, either the right hemisphere or both hemispheres dominate the speech and writing abilities. The right cerebral hemisphere dominates the integration of certain sounds other than those associated with speaking, such as sounds of coughing, laughter, crying, and melodies. The right cerebral hemisphere perceives tactual stimuli and visual spatial relationships better than the left cerebral hemisphere. See also **Brodmann's areas.**

**cerebral edema** [L, *cerebrum* + Gk, *oidema,* swelling], an accumulation of fluid in the brain tissues. Causes include infection, tumor, trauma, or exposure to certain toxins. Because the skull cannot expand to accommodate the fluid pressure, brain tissues are compressed. Early symptoms are changes in level of consciousness: sluggishness, then dilation of pupils, and a gradual loss of consciousness. Cerebral edema can be fatal.

**cerebral edema management,** a nursing intervention from the Nursing Interventions Classification (NIC) defined as limitation of secondary cerebral injury resulting from swelling of brain tissue. See also **Nursing Interventions Classification.**

**cerebral embolism** [L, *cerebrum* + *embolos,* plug], a condition in which an embolus blocks blood flow through the vessels of the cerebrum, resulting in tissue ischemia distal to the occlusion. See also **cerebrovascular accident.**

**cerebral fossa,** the stem of the lateral sulcus of the cerebrum, which forms a furrow separating the orbital surface of the frontal lobe from the temporal lobe.

**cerebral gigantism** [L, *cerebrum* + Gk, *gigas,* giant], an abnormal condition characterized by excessive weight and size at birth, accelerated growth during the first 4 or 5 years after birth without any increase in the level of growth hormone, and then reversion to normal growth. Some typical signs of this condition are prognathism, antimongoloid slant, dolichocephalic skull, moderate mental retardation, and impaired coordination. Also called **Sotos' syndrome.**

**cerebral gyrus.** See **gyrus.**

**cerebral hemiplegia** [L, *cerebrum* + Gk, *hemi,* half, *plege,* stroke], paralysis of one side of the body caused by a brain lesion.

**cerebral hemisphere** [L, *cerebrum* + Gk, *hemi,* half, *sphaira,* ball], one of the halves of the cerebrum. The two cerebral hemispheres are divided by a deep longitudinal fissure and are connected medially at the bottom of the fissure by the corpus callosum. Prominent grooves, subdividing each hemisphere into four major lobes, are the central sulcus, the lateral fissure, and the parieto-occipital fissure. Each hemisphere also has a fifth major lobe deep in the brain. The hemispheres consist of an external gray layer and an internal white substance that surrounds islands of gray matter called nuclei.

**cerebral hemorrhage** [L, *cerebrum* + Gk, *haima,* blood, *rhegnynei,* to burst forth], a hemorrhage from a blood vessel in the brain. Three criteria used to classify cerebral hemorrhages are location (subarachnoid, extradural, subdural), kind of vessel involved (arterial, venous, capillary), and origin (traumatic, degenerative). Each kind of cerebral hemorrhage has distinctive clinical characteristics. Most cerebral hemorrhages occur in the region of the basal ganglia and are caused by the rupture of a sclerotic artery as a result of hypertension. Other causes of rupture include congenital aneurysm, cerebrovascular thrombosis, and head trauma. ■ OBSERVATIONS: Bleeding may lead to displacement or destruction of brain tissue. Extensive hemorrhage is usually fatal. Depending on the extent and the location of the damaged tissue, residual effects may include aphasia, diminished mental function, hemiplegia, or disturbance of the function of a special sense. ■ INTERVENTIONS: Lumbar puncture may reveal blood in the spinal fluid. A computed tomography scan may be performed to locate the lesion and to differentiate the hemorrhage from an embolus or thrombus, or cerebral angiography may be used for these purposes. Surgery is sometimes necessary to stop the bleeding and to prevent death from greatly increased intracranial pressure. The person is kept immobile during the acute phase (72 hours), with the body in a position that assures adequate blood flow to and from the head. Physical therapy and speech therapy may be necessary during convalescence.

**cerebral hernia.** See **cephalocele.**

**cerebral infarction.** See **cerebrovascular accident.**

**cerebral lobes,** the well defined areas of the cerebral cortex, demarcated by fissures, sulci, and arbitrary lines; they include the frontal, temporal, parietal, and occipital lobes.

**cerebral localization,** **1.** the determination of various areas in the cerebral cortex associated with specific functions, such as the 47 Brodmann's areas. **2.** the diagnosis of a cerebral condition, such as a brain lesion, by determining the area of the brain affected, through analysis of the signs manifested by the patient.

**cerebral nerve.** See **cranial nerves.**

**cerebral palsy** [L, *cerebrum* + Gk, *para,* beyond, *lysis,*

loosening], a motor function disorder caused by a permanent, nonprogressive brain defect or lesion present at birth or shortly thereafter. The neurologic deficit may result in spastic hemiplegia, monoplegia, diplegia, or quadriplegia; athetosis or ataxia; seizures; paresthesia; varying degrees of mental retardation; and impaired speech, vision, and hearing. The disorder is usually associated with premature or abnormal birth and intrapartum asphyxia, causing damage to the nervous system. Abnormalities in breathing, sucking, swallowing, and responsiveness are usually apparent soon after birth, but the characteristic stiff, awkward movements of the infant's limbs may be overlooked for several months. Beginning to walk is usually delayed, and, when it is attempted, the child manifests a typical scissors gait. The arms may be affected only slightly, but the fingers are often spastic. Deep-tendon reflexes are exaggerated, and there may be slurred speech, delay in development of sphincter control, and athetotic movements of the face and hands. Early identification of the disorder facilitates the handling of infants with cerebral palsy and the initiation of an exercise and training program. Treatment is individualized and may include the use of braces, surgical correction of deformities, speech therapy, and various indicated drugs, such as muscle relaxants and anticonvulsants. Also called **congenital cerebral diplegia, Little's disease.**

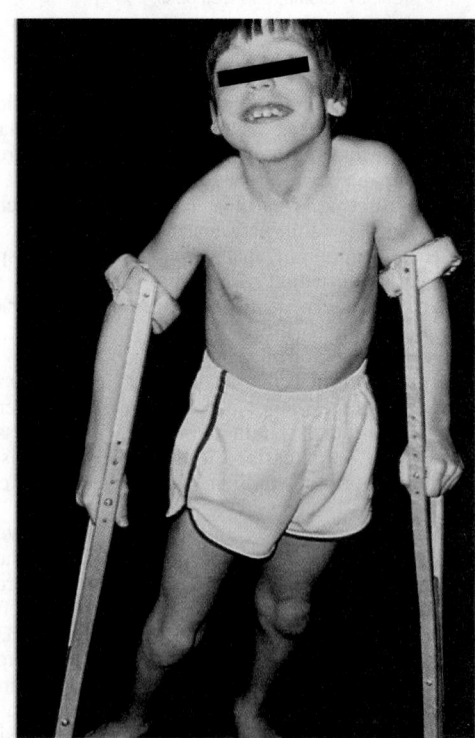

**Cerebral palsy** *(Zitelli and Davis, 1997)*

**cerebral peduncle** [L, *cerebrum,* brain, *pes,* foot], a pair of cylindrical masses of nerve fibers at the upper border of the pons that disappears into the cerebrum left and right hemispheres. It includes corticopontine and pyramidal-tract fibers which constitute the central portion of the midbrain.

**cerebral perfusion pressure (CPP),** a parameter that is related to the amount of blood flow to the brain. It is calculated by subtracting the intracranial pressure from the mean systemic arterial blood pressure.

**cerebral perfusion promotion,** a nursing intervention from the Nursing Interventions Classification (NIC) defined as promotion of adequate perfusion and limitation of complications for a patient experiencing or at risk for inadequate cerebral perfusion. See also **Nursing Interventions Classification.**

**cerebral sulcus,** one of the furrows on the surface of the cerebral cortex between the gyri; see also **gyrus.**

**cerebral thrombosis** [L, *cerebrum* + Gk, *thrombos,* lump, *osis,* condition], an abnormal condition in which a blood clot forms in a cerebral blood vessel.

**cerebral vertigo** [L, *cerebrum,* brain, *vertigo,* dizziness], vertigo that is caused by organic brain disease.

**cerebriform carcinoma.** See **medullary carcinoma.**

**cerebroatrophic hyperammonemia.** See **Rett syndrome.**

**cerebrocerebellar atrophy** /ser′əbrōser′əbel′ər/ [L, *cerebrum,* brain, *cerebellum,* small brain; Gk, *a* + *trophe,* without nourishment], a deterioration of the cerebellum caused by certain abiotrophic diseases.

**cerebrocostomandibular syndrome** /ser′ə·brō·kos′tō·man·dib′yōō·lər/ [L, *cerebrum,* brain + *costa,* rib + *mandibula,* mandible], an autosomal recessive syndrome of severe micrognathia and costovertebral abnormalities, including small bell-shaped thorax, incompletely ossified aberrant rib structure, and abnormal rib attachment to vertebrae. There are also palatal defects, glossoptosis, prenatal and postnatal growth deficiencies, and mental retardation, the last perhaps because of neonatal respiratory distress.

**cerebrohepatorenal syndrome** /ser′ə·brō·hep′ə·tō·rē′nəl /, an autosomal recessive disorder characterized by craniofacial abnormalities, hypotonia, hepatomegaly, polycystic kidneys, jaundice, and death in early infancy, and associated with absence of peroxisomes in the liver and kidneys. Also called **Zellweger syndrome.**

**cerebroid** /ser′əbroid/ [L, *cerebrum* + Gk, *eidos,* form], resembling the substance of the brain.

**cerebroma** /ser′əbrō′mə/, *pl.* **cerebromas, cerebromata,** any unusual mass of brain tissue.

**cerebromedullary tube.** See **neural tube.**

**cerebromeningitis** /-men′injī′tis/, an inflammation of the meninges of the brain, characterized by symptoms of fever, headache, vomiting, slow pulse, and effects of cranial nerve involvement, such as facial paralysis, ptosis, and squint.

**cerebropathia psychia toxemia.** See **Korsakoff's psychosis.**

**cerebroretinal angiomatosis.** See **von Hippel–Lindau disease.**

**cerebroside** /ser′əbrōsīd′/, any of a group of glycolipids found in the brain and other tissue of the nervous system, especially the myelin sheath.

**cerebroside sulfatase** [L, *cerebrum,* brain, *sulfur,* brimstone, *ase,* enzyme], an enzyme of the hydrolase class that catalyzes the reaction of cerebroside 3-sulfate + $H_2O$. A deficiency of the enzyme, which is transmitted through an autosomal recessive gene, causes metachromatic leukodystrophy.

**cerebrospinal** /ser′əbrōspī′nəl, sərē′brō-/, pertaining to or involving the brain and the spinal cord.

**cerebrospinal axis** [L, *cerebrum,* brain, *spina,* spine, *axle*], a line formed by the brain and spinal cord about which the body turns.

**cerebrospinal fever.** See **meningococcal meningitis.**

**cerebrospinal fluid (CSF),** the fluid that flows through and protects the four ventricles of the brain, the subarachnoid spaces, and the spinal canal. It is composed mainly of secretions of the choroid plexi in the lateral ventricles and in the third and the fourth ventricles of the brain and is clear and colorless. Changes in the carbon dioxide content of CSF affect the respiratory center in the medulla, helping to control breathing. A brain tumor may press against the cerebral aqueduct and shut off the flow of the fluid from the third to the fourth ventricle, causing fluid accumulation in the lateral and third ventricles, called internal hydrocephalus. Other blockages of the flow of CSF, such as those caused by blood

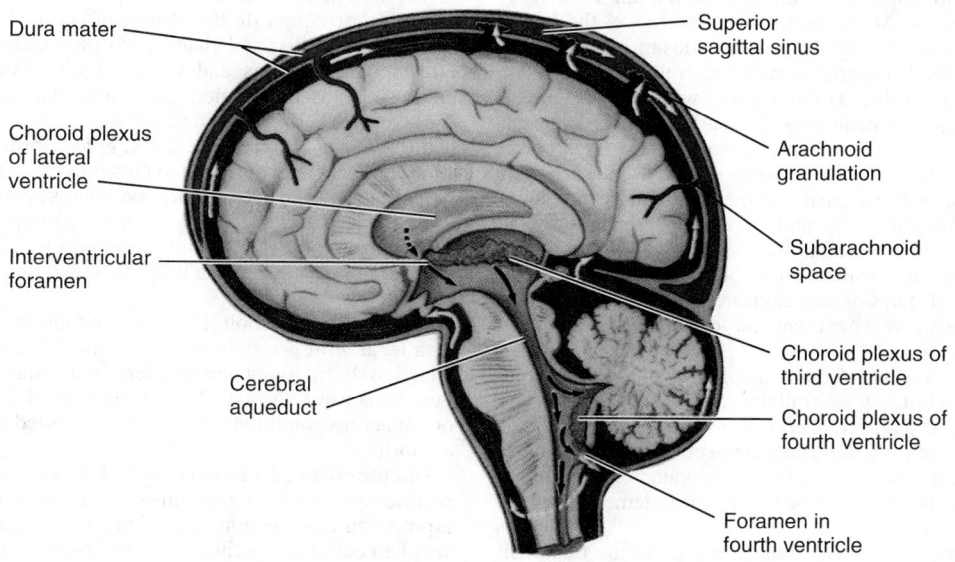

Dura mater

Superior sagittal sinus

Choroid plexus of lateral ventricle

Arachnoid granulation

Interventricular foramen

Subarachnoid space

Cerebral aqueduct

Choroid plexus of third ventricle

Choroid plexus of fourth ventricle

Foramen in fourth ventricle

**Flow of cerebrospinal fluid** *(Applegate, 2000)*

clots, result in serious complications. Certain illnesses and various diagnoses may require microscopic examination and chemical analysis of CSF. Samples of the fluid may be removed by lumbar puncture between the third and the fourth lumbar vertebrae.

**cerebrospinal ganglion,** a cluster of sensory ganglia neurons on roots of cranial and spinal nerve. The neurons lack dendrites and have no synapses on their cell bodies. See also **autonomic ganglion, dorsal root ganglion, ganglion.**

**cerebrospinal nerves,** the 12 pairs of cranial nerves and 31 pairs of spinal nerves that originate in the brain and spinal cord.

**cerebrospinal pressure** [L, *cerebrum* + *spina* + *premere,* to press], the pressure of cerebrospinal fluid in the central nervous system. It usually measures between 100 and 150 mm of $H_2O$ and is measured by a manometer attached to the end of a needle after it has been inserted into the subarachnoid space via lumbar puncture (most commonly).

**cerebrospinal rhinorrhea/otorrhea** [L, *cerebrum,* brain, *spina,* backbone; Gk, *rhis,* nose, *rhoia,* flow], a discharge of cerebrospinal fluid (CSF) from the nose or ear. Basal skull fractures can transverse the paranasal air sinuses of the frontal bone or the middle ear within the temporal bone resulting in a dural tear. CSF can then leak through the dural tear and drain from the nose or ear.

**cerebrotendinous xanthomatosis.** See **van Bogaert's disease.**

**cerebrovascular** /ser′əbrōvas′kyələr, sərē′brō-/ [L, *cerebrum* + *vasculum,* little vessel], pertaining to the vascular system and blood supply of the brain.

**cerebrovascular accident (CVA),** an abnormal condition of the brain characterized by occlusion by an embolus, thrombus, or cerebrovascular hemorrhage or vasospasm, resulting in ischemia of the brain tissues normally perfused by the damaged vessels. The sequelae of a cerebrovascular accident depend on the location and extent of ischemia. Paralysis, weakness, sensory change, speech defect, aphasia, or death may occur. Symptoms remit somewhat after the first few days as brain swelling subsides. Also called **stroke.**

**cerebrum** /ser′əbrəm, sərē′brəm/, *pl.* **cerebrums, cerebra** [L, brain], the largest and uppermost section of the brain, divided by a longitudinal fissure into the left and right cerebral hemispheres. At the bottom of the groove, the hemispheres are connected by the corpus callosum. The internal structures of the hemispheres merge with those of the diencephalon and further communicate with the brainstem through the cerebral peduncles. The surface of the cerebrum is called gyri; each lobe bears the name of the bone under which it lies. The cerebrum performs sensory functions, motor functions, and less easily defined integration functions associated with various mental activities. It generates a variety of electrical waves that may be recorded as an electroencephalogram to localize areas of brain dysfunction, to identify altered states of consciousness, or to establish brain death. See also **cerebral cortex, cerebral hemisphere.** —**cerebral,** *adj.*

**Cerezyme,** trademark for an analog of the human enzyme beta-glucocerebrosiderase (imiglucerase).

**cerium (Ce)** /sir′ē·əm/ [L, *Ceres,* Roman goddess of agriculture], a ductile gray rare earth element. Its atomic number is 58; its atomic mass is 140.13. A compound of cerium, cerium oxalate, is used as a sedative, an antiemetic, and an antitussive.

**cerium nitrate,** a topical antiseptic used in the treatment of burns to control bacterial and fungal infections.

**cerivistatin,** an HMG-CoA reductase inhibitor.

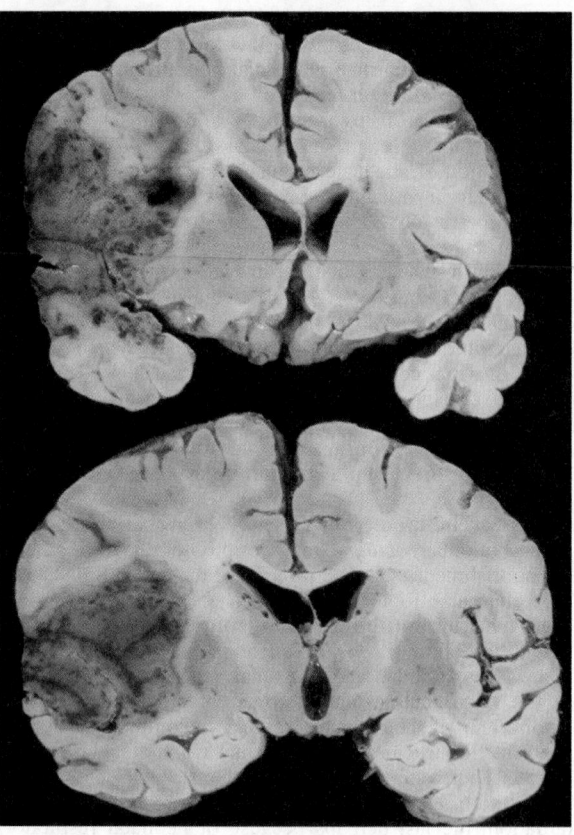

**Effects of a cerebrovascular accident**
*(Cotran, Kumar, and Collins, 1999)*

■ INDICATIONS: This drug is used as an adjunct in primary hypercholesterolemia (types IIa and IIb) and mixed hyperlipidemia.

■ CONTRAINDICATIONS: Known hypersensitivity, pregnancy, lactation, and active liver disease prohibit this drug's use.

■ ADVERSE EFFECTS: Life-threatening effects include liver dysfunction, myositis, and rhabdomyolysis. Common adverse effects include flatus and other GI disturbances, muscle cramps, headache, tremor, rash, pruritus, blurred vision, dysgeusia, and lens opacities.

**ceroid** /sir′oid/ [L, *cera,* wax; Gk, *eidos,* form], a golden, waxy pigment appearing in the cirrhotic livers of some individuals, in the GI tract, in the nervous system, and in the muscles. It is an insoluble, acid-fast, sudanophilic pigment.

**ceroma** /sirō′mə/, *pl.* **ceromas, ceromata** [L, *cera,* wax; Gk, *oma,* tumor], a neoplasm that has undergone waxy degeneration.

**certifiable** /sur′tifī′əbəl/ [L, *certus,* certain, *facere,* to make], **1.** a legal term pertaining to a patient with a mental illness who has been found incompetent and requires care by a guardian or in a hospital. **2.** pertaining to infectious diseases or dangerous conditions that must be reported to local health authorities.

**certificate-of-need or -necessity (CON),** a statement or certificate issued by a governmental agency to the effect that a proposed construction or modification of a health facility will be needed at the time of its completion. The certificate is issued to the individual or group intending to build or modify the facility.

**certification** [L, *certus,* certain, *facere,* to make],   **1.** a process in which an individual, an institution, or an educational program is evaluated and recognized as meeting certain predetermined standards. Certification is usually made by a nongovernmental agency. The purpose of certification is to ensure that the standards met are those necessary for safe and ethical practice of the profession or service. **2.** (in nursing) a process in which the professional organization or association verifies that a person who is licensed has met the standards for specialty practice specified by the profession. The purpose of certification is to assure other professionals and the public that the person has mastered the skills necessary to practice a particular specialty and has acquired the standard body of knowledge common to that specialty. See also **certification in nursing.**

**certification for excellence,**   (in nursing) certification that recognizes professional achievement, advanced education, and superior performance in a specialty or subspecialty field of practice. See also **certification in nursing.**

**certification in nursing,**   one of two processes in which a professional organization formally recognizes the competence of a nurse to practice a subspecialty of nursing. One process, certification for excellence, bases recognition on professional achievement, advanced education, and superior performance. The second process, entry level certification, bases recognition on advanced education in a program approved by the certifying organization. Criteria vary according to the particular requirements of the professional organization but always require current licensure as a registered nurse and usually include an examination and certain educational or practice requirements. Submission and evaluation of documented clinical practice and a statement of a philosophy of practice may also be required by some professional organizations.

**certified dental assistant** /sur′tifīd/,   a person who has successfully completed the education, training, and testing of the Dental Assisting National Examination or of the American Dental Assistants' Association. A dental assistant may also become certified without receiving a formal education by working for 2 years as a full-time chairside dental assistant before taking the certification examination. See also **dental assistant.**

**certified emergency nurse (CEN),**   a nurse who has had training in emergency nursing and successfully completed an examination given by the Board of Certification of Emergency Nursing. To remain certified, a CEN must be reexamined every 4 years (or 8 years if specified educational requirements are met within 4 years).

**certified medical transcriptionist.**   See **medical transcriptionist.**

**certified milk,**   raw milk that is obtained, handled, and marketed in compliance with state health laws. The milk must be produced by disease-free cows that are regularly inspected by a veterinarian and are milked by sterilized equipment in hygienic surroundings. It must contain less than a specified low bacterial count and must be delivered within 36 hours.

**certified nurse administrator (ANCC).**   See **CNA.**

**certified nurse-midwife (CNM),**   (according to the American College of Nurse-Midwives) "an individual educated in the two disciplines of nursing and midwifery, who possesses evidence of certification according to the requirements of the American College of Nurse-Midwives. Nurse-midwifery practice is the independent management of care of essentially normal newborns and women, antepartally, intrapartally, postpartally, and/or gynecologically, occurring within a health care system which provides for medical con-

sultation, collaborative management, or referral and is in accord with the qualifications, standards, and functions for the practice of nurse-midwifery as defined by the American College of Nurse-Midwives." See also **midwife.**

**certified occupational therapy assistant (COTA),**   an allied health paraprofessional who, under the direction of an occupational therapist, directs an individual's participation in selected tasks to restore, reinforce, and enhance performance; facilitates learning of skills and functions essential for adaptation and productivity; diminishes or corrects disorders; and promotes and maintains health.

**certified registered nurse anesthetist.**   See **nurse anesthetist (CRNA).**

**Certified Respiratory Therapy Technician (CRTT),**   a health care professional who performs routine care, management, and treatment of patients with respiratory disorders. Certification requires completion of an approved training course and passing of an examination by the National Board for Respiratory Care.

**certify** /sur′tifī/,   **1.** to guarantee formally that certain requirements based on expert knowledge of significant, pertinent facts have been met. **2.** to attest, by a legal process, that someone is insane. **3.** to attest to the fact of someone's death in writing, usually on a form required by a local authority. **4.** to declare that a person has satisfied certain requirements for membership or acceptance into a professional or other group. See also **board certification. —certification,** *n.,* **certifiable,** *adj.*

**Cerubidine,**   trademark for an antineoplastic (daunorubicin hydrochloride).

**cerulean** /siroo′lē·ən/ [L, *caelum,* sky],   sky-blue in color.

**ceruloplasmin** /siroo′lōplaz′min/ [L, *caelum,* sky; Gk, *plassein,* to shape],   a blue glycoprotein in plasma that transports 96% of the plasma copper. A major decrease is seen in Wilson's disease.

**cerumen** /siroo′mən/ [L, *cera,* wax],   a yellowish or brownish waxy secretion produced by vestigial apocrine sweat glands in the external ear canal. Also called **earwax.**

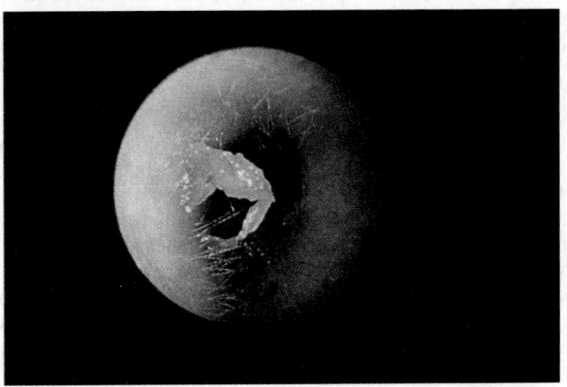

**Cerumen in the external auditory meatus**
*(Bingham, Hawke, and Kwok, 1992/courtesy Dr. Arnold Noyek)*

**ceruminolytic** /siroo′mənōlit′ik/,   pertaining to a drug or other agent that dissolves cerumen (earwax).

**ceruminolytic agent** [L, *cera,* wax; Gk, *lysis,* a loosening; L, *agere,* to do],   a medication that dissolves or loosens cerumen (earwax) to allow for its removal.

**ceruminoma** /seroo′mino′mə/, an adenocarcinoma in the external auditory meatus.

**ceruminosis** /siroo′mino′sis/, excessive buildup of cerumen (earwax) in the external auditory canal. It can cause discomfort, symptoms of hearing loss, and local irritation leading to the development of infection. Removal of excess cerumen is accomplished by the local use of a wax softening agent followed by careful flushing with an ear syringe. A cerumen spoon is sometimes used to scoop out hardened collections of wax.

**ceruminous** /siroo′minəs/, pertaining to earwax.

**ceruminous gland,** one of a number of tiny structures in the external ear canal, believed to be modified sweat glands. They secrete a waxy cerumen instead of watery sweat.

**cervic-,** combining form meaning 'neck': *cervicectomy, cervicitis, cervicobrachial.*

**cervical** /sur′vikəl/ [L, *cervix,* neck], **1.** pertaining to the neck or the region of the neck. **2.** pertaining to the constricted area of a necklike structure, such as the neck of a tooth or the cervix of the uterus.

**cervical abortion** [L, *cervix + ab,* away from, *oriri,* to be born], spontaneous expulsion of a cervical pregnancy.

**cervical adenitis** [L, *cervix + Gk, aden,* gland, *itis,* inflammation], an abnormal condition characterized by enlarged, tender lymph nodes of the neck. It often occurs in association with acute infections of the throat.

**cervical amputation,** the removal of the neck (cervix) of the uterus.

**cervical canal,** the canal within the uterine cervix, which protrudes into the vagina. The uterine end of the canal is closed at the internal os and, in the nullipara, at the distal end by the external os. The canal is a passageway through which the menstrual flow escapes and, vastly dilated and effaced by labor, through which the infant must pass to be delivered vaginally. Various diagnostic and therapeutic procedures require dilation of the muscular cervix surrounding the canal, including endometrial biopsy, suction or surgical curettage, or radium implantation. Pelvic inflammatory disease is the result of the entry of pathogenic bacteria into the uterus through the cervical canal. Sperm must travel upward through the canal to reach the uterus and fallopian tubes.

**cervical cancer,** a neoplasm of the uterine cervix that can be detected in the early, curable stage by the Papanicolaou (Pap) test. Factors that may be associated with the development of cervical cancer are coitus at an early age, relations with many sexual partners, genital herpesvirus infections, multiparity, and poor obstetric and gynecologic care. Early cervical neoplasia is usually asymptomatic, but there may be a watery vaginal discharge or occasional spotting of blood; advanced lesions may cause a dark, foul-smelling vaginal discharge, leakage from bladder or rectal fistulas, anorexia, weight loss, and back and leg pains. Pap smears of cervical cells are highly important in screening, but definitive diagnoses are based on colposcopic examination and cytologic study of specimens obtained by biopsy. Cervical dysplasia may regress, persist, or progress to clinical disease, but carcinoma in situ is considered to be a precursor of invasive carcinoma. About 90% of cervical tumors are squamous cell carcinomas, fewer than 10% are adenocarcinomas, and others are mixtures of these kinds, or, in rare cases, sarcomas. Cervical cancer invades the tissues of adjacent organs and may metastasize through lymphatic channels to distant sites, including the lungs, bone, liver, brain, and paraaortic nodes. Treatment depends on the kind and the extent of the malignancy, the age of the woman, and her general health. Also considered are her wishes in regard to maintaining her reproductive function. Carcinoma in situ may be treated by

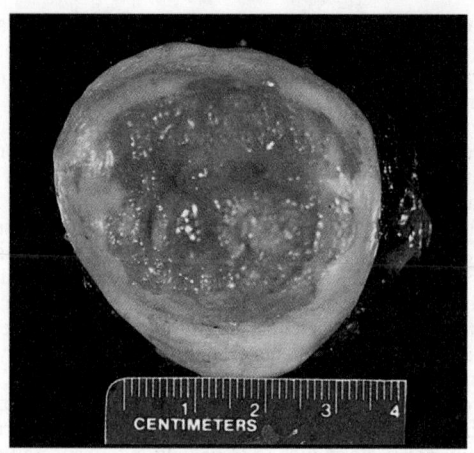

**Invasive carcinoma of the cervix**
*(Cotran, Kumar, and Collins, 1999)*

excisional conization or cryosurgery. Invasive tumors may be treated with radiotherapy or hysterectomy. Chemotherapy has a mainly palliative role.

**cervical cap,** a contraceptive device consisting of a small latex cup fitted over the uterine cervix to prevent spermatozoa from entering the cervical canal.

**cervical cauterization,** the destruction, usually by heat or electrical current, of abnormal superficial tissues of the cervix.

**cervical conization,** the excision of a cone-shaped tissue section from the endocervix, performed to obtain a tissue sample to establish a precise diagnosis. See also **cone biopsy.**

**cervical cyst** [L, *cervix,* neck; Gk, *kystis,* bag], a mucous cyst of the uterine cervix. Also called **nabothian cyst.**

**cervical dilation** /dil′ətā′shən/ [L, *dilatare,* to widen], the diameter of the opening of the cervix in labor as measured on vaginal examination. It is expressed in centimeters or finger breadths; one finger breadth is approximately 2 cm. At full dilation the diameter of the cervical opening is 10 cm.

**cervical disk syndrome,** an abnormal condition characterized by compression or irritation of the cervical nerve roots in or near the intervertebral foramina before the roots divide into the anterior and posterior rami. When it is caused by ruptured intervertebral disks, degenerative cervical disk disease, or cervical injuries, it may produce varying degrees of malalignment, causing nerve root compression. Most cervical disk syndromes are caused by injuries that involve hyperextension. Edema usually occurs in all cases of cervical disk syndrome. Pain, the most common symptom, usually emanates from the cervical area but may radiate down the arm to the fingers and increase with cervical motion. The pain may increase sharply with coughing, sneezing, or any radical movement. Other signs and symptoms may be paresthesia, headache, blurred vision, decreased skeletal function, and weakened hand grip. Physical examination may reveal varying degrees of muscular atrophy, sensory abnormalities, muscular weakness, and decreased reflexes. Radiographic examination may show a loss of normal lordosis associated with the cervical vertebrae and may also reveal some minor malalignment of the vertebrae. Nonsurgical intervention, which is usually a successful treatment, may include immobilization of the cervical vertebrae to decrease irritation and to provide rest for the traumatized area. Other treatment may

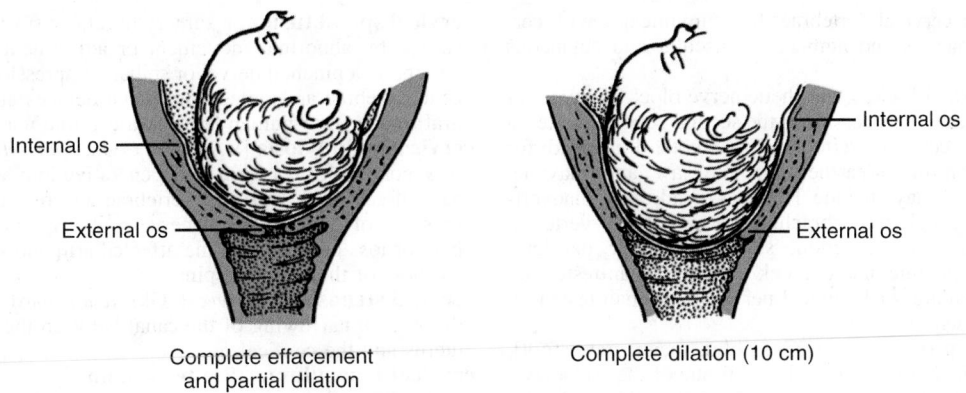

Complete effacement
and partial dilation

Complete dilation (10 cm)

**Cervical dilation** *(Lowdermilk, Perry, and Bobak, 2000)*

include special exercises, heat therapy, and intermittent traction. Mild analgesics are usually successful in controlling the pain associated with cervical disk syndrome, especially when used with immobilization. Surgery is recommended only when signs and symptoms persist despite nonsurgical treatment. The prognosis for this condition is usually good, but recurrence of symptoms is common. Also called **cervical root syndrome.** See also **herniated disk, whiplash injury.**

**cervical dysplasia,** abnormal tissue development of the uterine cervix, with atypical epithelium that may slowly progress to carcinoma.

**cervical erosion** [L, *cervix* + *erodere,* to consume], a condition in which the squamous epithelium of the cervix is abraded as a result of irritation caused by infection or trauma such as childbirth and replaced by columnar epithelium.

**cervical fistula,** an abnormal passage from the cervix to the vagina or bladder. It may be caused by a malignant lesion, radiotherapy, surgical trauma, or injury during childbirth. A cervical fistula communicating with the bladder permits leakage of urine, causing irritation, odor, and embarrassment. See also **branchial fistula.**

**cervical intraepithelial neoplasia (CIN)** /in'trə-ep'ithē'lē·əl/, abnormal changes in the basal layers of the squamous epithelial tissues of the uterus. The disorder is graded according to its pathologic progress, from CIN1 to CIN3; CIN3 represents carcinoma of the cervix. The disorder is associated with human papillomaviruses.

**cervical mucus,** a secretion of the columnar epithelium lining the upper portion of the cervical canal of the uterus. The mucus that is secreted by endocervical glands changes in appearance and consistency through the menstrual cycle. For the first few days after menstruation little mucus is secreted. As ovulation approaches, increasing amounts of sticky cloudy-white or yellowish secretions are seen. Around the time of ovulation, the volume of mucus increases, and it becomes clear, slippery, and elastic, resembling the uncooked white of an egg. After ovulation the mucus becomes cloudy, thick, sticky, and progressively less profuse until menstruation supervenes to begin the cycle again. See also **mucous plug, ovulation method of family planning.**

**cervical mucus method of family planning.** See **ovulation method of family planning.**

**cervical nerves** [L, *cervix,* neck, *nervus,* nerve], the eight pairs of spinal nerves that arise from the cervical segments of the spinal cord, from above the atlas to below the seventh vertebra. The first four supply the head and neck and the other four mainly innervate the upper limbs, scalp, and back. See also **cervical plexus.**

**cervical os.** See **external cervical os, internal cervical os.**

**cervical plexus,** the network of nerves formed by the ventral primary divisions of the first four cervical nerves. Each nerve, except the first, divides into the superior branch and the inferior branch, and both branches unite to form three loops. The plexus is located opposite the cranial aspect of

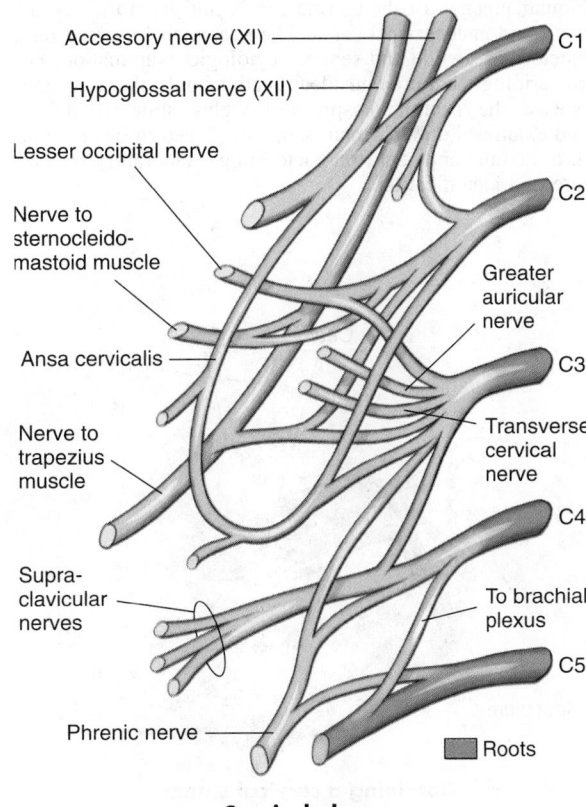

**Cervical plexus**

the first four cervical vertebrae. It communicates with certain cranial nerves and numerous muscular and cutaneous branches.

**cervical plexus block,**   anesthetic nerve block at any point below the mastoid process from the second cervical vertebra to the sixth cervical vertebra. This method is used for operations on the area between the jaw and clavicle. Complications may include Horner's syndrome, inadvertent stellate ganglion or brachial plexus block, vertebral artery bleeding or infection, subarachnoid or peridural penetration, phrenic nerve block or palsy manifested by respiratory failure, or laryngeal nerve block, manifested by sudden hoarseness.

**cervical polyp** [L, *cervix* + Gk, *polys,* mean, *pous,* foot], an outgrowth of columnar epithelial tissue of the endocervical canal. It is usually attached to the canal wall by a slender pedicle. Often there are no symptoms, but multiple or abraded polyps may cause bleeding, especially with contact during coitus. Polyps are most common in women above 40 years of age. The cause is not known. Treatment of a symptomatic polyp is excision. Scant bleeding and prompt healing usually follow.

**cervical regions,**   the various anatomical regions of the neck, including anterior, lateral, and posterior cervical regions and the region over the sternocleidomastoid muscle.

**cervical rib,**   a supernumerary rib that articulates with a cervical vertebra, usually the seventh, but does not reach the sternum.

**cervical root syndrome.**   See **cervical disk syndrome.**

**cervical smear** [L, *cervix* + AS, *smero,* grease],   a small amount of the secretions and superficial cells of the cervix, secured from the external os of the cervix with a sterile applicator or special small wooden or plastic spatula. For a Papanicolaou's (Pap) smear, it is obtained from the squamocolumnar junction of the uterine cervix and from the vaginal vault and endocervical canal. The specimen is spread on a labeled glass slide and sent for cytologic examination. For bacteriologic culture and identification, only the applicator is used; the specimen is spread on a glass slide and stained and examined under a microscope or placed in or on a culture medium and sent to a bacteriologic laboratory for culture and identification.

**cervical spinal fusion,**   surgery to relieve severe neck pain caused by abnormal movement or adjustment of adjacent vertebrae, a pinched nerve, or spinal compression. The adjacent vertebrae are joined with metal devices and/or a bone graft made from human bone or a ceramic material.

**cervical spondylosis** [L, *cervix* + Gk, *spondylos,* vertebra, *osis,* condition],   a form of degenerative joint and disk disease affecting the cervical vertebrae and resulting in compression of the associated nerve roots. Symptoms include pain or loss of feeling in the affected arm and shoulder and stiffness of the cervical spine.

**cervical stenosis** [L, *cervix* + Gk, *stenos,* narrow, *osis,* condition],   a narrowing of the canal between the body of the uterus and the cervical os.

**cervical tenaculum.**   See **tenaculum.**

**cervical traction,**   a system of traction applied to the cervical spine by applying a force to lift the head. Also called **head traction.**

**cervical triangle,**   one of two triangular areas formed in the neck by the oblique course of the sternocleidomastoideus. The anterior triangle is bounded by the midline of the throat anteriorly, the sternocleidomastoideus laterally, and the body of the mandible superiorly. The posterior triangle is bounded by the clavicle inferiorly and by the borders of the sternocleidomastoideus and the trapezius superiorly.

**cervical vertebra,**   one of the first seven segments of the vertebral column. They differ from the thoracic and lumbar vertebrae through the presence of a vertical foramen in each transverse process. The first cervical vertebra (atlas) has no body, supports the head, and contains a smooth, oval facet for articulation with the dens of the second cervical vertebra. The dens extends from the cranial portion of the body of the second cervical vertebra (axis), which has a very large, strong spinous process with a bifid extremity. The seventh cervical vertebra has a very long, prominent spinous process that is nearly horizontal and is often used as a palpable reference for locating the other cervical spines. The bodies of the four remaining cervical vertebrae are small, oval, and broader than the other three in transverse diameter and contain large, triangular foramina within their transverse processes. Their spinous processes are short and bifid. Compare **coccygeal vertebra, lumbar vertebra, sacral vertebra, thoracic vertebra.** See also **vertebra.**

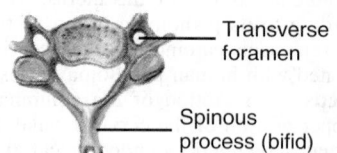

Transverse foramen

Spinous process (bifid)

**Cervical vertebra** *(Applegate, 2000)*

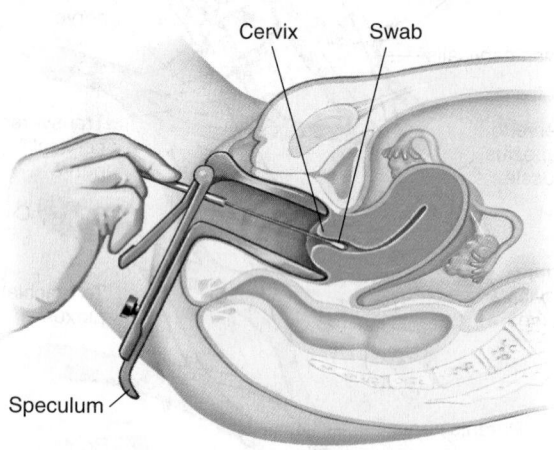

Cervix    Swab

Speculum

**Obtaining a cervical smear**

**cervicitis** /sur′visī′tis/,   acute or chronic inflammation of the uterine cervix. **Acute cervicitis** is infection of the cervix marked by redness, edema, and bleeding on contact. Symptoms do not always occur but may include any or all of the following: copious, foul-smelling discharge from the vagina; pelvic pressure or pain; scant bleeding with intercourse; and itching or burning of the external genitalia. The principal causative organisms are *Trichomonas vaginalis; Candida albicans; Gonococcus, Staphylococcus,* and *Strep-*

*tococcus* species; and *Hemophilus vaginalis.* Diagnosis is by microscopic examination, confirmed in some cases by culture and Papanicolaou (Pap) smear. Specific antimicrobial medication may be effective. Acute cervicitis tends to be a recurrent problem because of reexposure to the germ, undertreatment, or predisposing factors such as human immunodeficiency virus infection, multiple sexual partners, or poor nutrition. **Chronic cervicitis** is a persistent inflammation of the cervix that usually occurs among women in their reproductive years. Symptoms include a thick, irritating, malodorous discharge that may in severe cases be accompanied by significant pelvic pain. The cervix looks congested and enlarged, nabothian cysts are often present, and there are signs of eversion of the cervix and often old lacerations from childbirth. A Pap smear should be performed before treatment. The most effective treatments are hot and cold cautery. See also *Candida albicans,* **cautery, cervical cancer, cervical polyp, condyloma acuminatum, nabothian cyst.**

**cervico** /sur'vikō-/, combining form meaning 'neck': *cervicodynia, cervicolabial, cervicotomy.*

**cervicodynia** /sur'vikōdin'ē·ə/, pain in the neck. Also called **trachelodynia.**

**cervicofacial actinomycosis.** See **actinomycosis.**

**cervicogenic dorsalgia,** back pain caused by a cervical spine disorder.

**cervicogenic headache,** (in chiropractic) a condition in which headaches, particularly those classified as muscle tension headaches involving referred pain, are the result of cervical subluxations.

**cervicogenicity dysfunction** /-jenis'itē/, (in chiropractic) a syndrome of hypomobility, tender points in soft tissues, reduced regional ranges of cervical motion, and static misalignment.

**cervicogenic sympathetic syndrome,** (in chiropractic) any of a large group of bodily disorders involving the cervical spine and the associated sympathetic trunk of nerve fibers. The effects usually include causalgia and reflex sympathetic dystrophy.

**cervicolabial** /sur'vikōlā'bē·əl/ [L, *cervix* + *labium,* lip], pertaining to or situated on the cheek side of the neck of an incisor or a canine tooth.

**cervicoplasty** /sur'vikōplas'tē/, plastic surgery performed on either the uterine cervix or the neck.

**cervicothoracic** /-thôras'ik/, pertaining to the neck and thorax.

**cervicotomy** /sur'vikot'əmē/, a surgical incision into the uterine cervix.

**cervicouterine** /sur'vikōyoo'tərin/, pertaining to or situated at the cervix of the uterus.

**cervicovaginitis** /-vaj'inītis/, an inflammation of the cervix and vagina.

**cervicovesical** /sur'vikōves'ikəl/ [L, *cervix* + *vesica,* bladder], pertaining to the cervix of the uterus and the bladder.

**cervix** /sur'viks/, *pl.* **cervices** /sur'visēz/, **cervixes** [L, neck], the part of the uterus that protrudes into the cavity of the vagina. The cervix is divided into the supravaginal portion and the vaginal portion. The supravaginal portion is separated ventrally from the bladder by the parametrium, which attaches to the sides of the cervix and contains the uterine arteries. The vaginal portion of the cervix projects into the cavity of the vagina and contains the cervical canal and the internal and external os of the canal. The mucous membrane lining the endocervix is broken by numerous oblique ridges, deep glandular follicles, little cysts, and papillae. Also called **neck of uterus.** See also **effacement.**

**ceryl alcohol** /sē'ril/ [L, *cera,* wax; Ar, *alkohl,* essence], a fatty alcohol present in many waxes. Also called **hexacosanol.**

**cesarean hysterectomy** /sizer'ē·ən/ [L, *Caesar lex,* Caesar's law; Gk, *hystera,* womb, *ektomē,* excision], a surgical operation in which the uterus is removed at the time of cesarean section. It is performed most often for complications of cesarean section, usually intractable hemorrhage. Less often it is done to treat preexisting gynecologic disease, such as an intraepithelial cervical neoplasia. It is rarely done electively for sterilization because the danger of hemorrhage is greater when both procedures are performed simultaneously.

**cesarean postmortem section** [Caesar's law; L, *post,* after, *mors,* death, *sectio*], the surgical removal of the fetus immediately after the mother's death.

**cesarean section** [L, *Caesar lex,* Caesar's law, *sectio*], a surgical procedure in which the abdomen and uterus are incised and a baby is delivered transabdominally. It is performed when abnormal maternal or fetal conditions make vaginal delivery hazardous. Approximately 21% of births in the United States are by cesarean section; the operation is performed less frequently in other countries. Maternal indications for the operation include placenta previa or abruptio placentae, and dysfunctional labor. Prior delivery by cesarean section is no longer considered an absolute indication for repeating it in future deliveries. Cesarean birth is less traumatic for babies than difficult midforceps delivery. Fetal indications for the operation include fetal distress, cephalopelvic disproportion, and abnormal presentation, such as breech and transverse lie. The incision in the skin of the abdomen may be horizontal or vertical, regardless of the kind of internal incision into the uterus. Because she must mother while recovering from major surgery, the mother requires special care that provides for both her postoperative medical needs and her need to nurture the baby, who may also be ill or recovering. Also called **cesarean birth.** See also **classic cesarean section, extraperitoneal cesarean section, low cervical cesarean section.**

**cesarean section care,** a nursing intervention from the Nursing Interventions Classification (NIC) defined as preparation and support of patient delivering a baby by cesarean section. See also **Nursing Interventions Classification.**

**cesium (Cs)** /sē'zē·əm/ [L, *caesius,* sky blue], an alkali metal element. Its atomic number is 55; its atomic mass is 132.9. Like other alkali metals cesium emits electrons when exposed to visible light and is used in photoelectric cells and in television cameras. Also called **caesium (Cs).**

**cesium 137,** a radioactive material with a half-life of 30.2 years that is used in radiotherapy as a sealed source of gamma rays intended for application to various malignancies that are treated by brachytherapy. Cesium has replaced radium for such applications. See also **brachytherapy.**

**cesspool fever,** *informal.* typhoid fever.

**cestode.** See **tapeworm.**

**cestode infection, cestodiasis.** See **tapeworm infection.**

**cestoid** /ses'toid/ [Gk, *kestos,* girdle, *eidos,* form], **1.** cestodelike, or resembling a tapeworm. **2.** a tapeworm of the Cestoda subclass.

**CET,** abbreviation for *Certified Enterostomal Therapist.*

**Cetacaine,** trademark for a fixed-combination, anesthetic spray, containing several local anesthetics (benzocaine, butyl aminobenzoate, tetracaine), applied to mucous membranes.

**cetirizine,** an H$_1$-histamine antagonist.

■ INDICATIONS: This drug is used to treat allergy symptoms and rhinitis.

■ CONTRAINDICATIONS: Known hypersensitivity to this drug, lactation, and severe hepatic disease prohibit the use of cetirizine. Cetirizine also should not be used in newborns or premature infants.

■ ADVERSE EFFECTS: Life-threatening effects include hemolytic anemia, thrombocytopenia, leukopenia, agranulocytosis, pancytopenia, and dysrhythmias (rare). Other serious adverse effects include urinary retention, impotence, diarrhea, vomiting, sedation, confusion, blurred vision, tremors, hypotension, palpitations, bradycardia, and tachycardia. Common side effects are thickening of bronchial secretions, nausea, and headache.

**cetyl alcohol ($C_{16}H_{33}OH$)** /sē'til/ [L, *cetus,* whale; Ar, *alkohl,* essence], a fatty alcohol, derived from spermaceti, used as an emulsifier and stiffening agent in creams and ointments. Also called **hexadecanol, palmityl alcohol.**

**cetylpyridinium chloride** /sē'təlpī'ridin'ē·əm/, an antiinfective used as a preservative in pharmaceutical preparations and as a topical cleanser.

■ INDICATIONS: It is prescribed prophylactically to prevent infection of the skin or mucous membranes.

■ CONTRAINDICATIONS: Known hypersensitivity to this drug is the only contraindication.

■ NOTE: It is inactivated by soap, serum, and tissue fluids; therefore the surface of the skin must be clean and well rinsed.

**CEU,** abbreviation for **continuing education unit.**

**Ce-Vi-Sol,** trademark for vitamin C (ascorbic acid) liquid.

**cevitamic acid.** See **ascorbic acid.**

**Cf,** symbol for the element **californium.**

**C-F test,** abbreviation for **complement-fixation test.**

**CGC,** abbreviation for *Certified Gastrointestinal Clinician.*

**CGD,** abbreviation for **chronic granulomatous disease.**

**cGMP,** abbreviation for **cyclic guanosine monophosphate.**

**cgs, CGS,** abbreviation for **centimeter-gram-second system.**

**$C_2H_2$,** chemical formula for acetylene (ethyne).

**$C_2H_4$,** chemical formula for ethylene (ethene).

**$C_6H_6$,** chemical formula for benzene.

**Ch1,** symbol for **Christchurch chromosome.**

**Chaddock reflex** [Charles G. Chaddock, American neurologist, 1861–1936], an abnormal reflex, induced by firmly stroking the ulnar surface of the forearm, characterized by flexion of the wrist and extension of the fingers in fanlike position. It is seen on the affected side in hemiplegia. Compare **Gordon's reflex, Oppenheim reflex.** See also **Babinski's reflex.**

**Chaddock's sign** [Charles G. Chaddock], a variation of Babinski's reflex, elicited by firmly stroking the side of the foot just distal to the lateral malleolus, characterized by extension of the great toe and fanning of the other toes. It is seen in pyramidal tract disease. See also **Babinski's reflex.**

**Chadwick's sign** /chad'wiks/ [James R. Chadwick, American gynecologist, 1844–1905], the bluish coloration of the vulva and vagina that develops after the sixth week of pregnancy as a normal result of local venous congestion. It is an early sign of pregnancy.

**chafe** [L, *calefacere,* to make warm], an irritation of the skin by friction, such as when rough material rubs against an unprotected area of the body.

**chafing,** superficial irritation of the skin by friction.

**Chagas' disease** /chag'əs/ [Carlos Chagas, Brazilian physician, 1879–1934], a protozoal infection caused by *Trypanosoma cruzi,* transmitted to humans by bloodsucking insects. It may occur in acute or chronic form. The acute form, which is common in children and rare in adults, is marked by a lesion at the site of the bite, fever, weakness, enlarged spleen and lymph nodes, edema of the face and legs, and tachycardia. This form resolves within 4 months unless complications, such as encephalitis, develop. The chronic form may be manifested by cardiomyopathy or by dilation of the esophagus or colon. Often, infections are asymptomatic. Treatment with nifurtimox and benznidazole is, at best, only partially effective. Also called **Brazilian trypanosomiasis, Chagas-Cruz disease, Cruz trypanosomiasis, South American trypanosomiasis.** See also **trypanosomiasis.**

**Chagres fever** /chag'ris/ [Chagres River, Panama; L, *febris*], a phlebotomus arbovirus infection transmitted to humans through the bite of a sandfly. The disease is rarely fatal and is characterized by fever, headache, and muscle pains of the chest or abdomen. There may be nausea and vomiting, giddiness, weakness, photophobia, and pain on moving the eyes. The infection subsides within a week. Supportive treatment includes analgesics, bed rest, and adequate fluid intake. The disease is most common in Central America. Also called **Panama fever.**

**chain** [L, *catena*], **1.** a length of several units linked together in a linear pattern, such as a polypeptide chain of amino acids or a chain of atoms forming a chemical molecule. **2.** a group of individual bacteria linked together, such as streptococci formed by a chain of cocci. **3.** the serial relationship of certain structures essential to function, such as the chain of ossicles in the middle ear. Each of the small bones moves successively in response to vibration of the tympanic membrane, thus transmitting the auditory stimulus to the oval window. See also **chain ligature. 4.** a connected series, such as a chain of events.

**chaining,** a system of learning behaviors in which each response is a stimulus for the next response.

**chain ligature** [L, *catena + ligare,* to bind], an interlocking ligature that ties off a pedicle at several places by passing a long thread through the pedicle at different points.

**chain reaction, 1.** (in chemistry) a reaction that produces a compound needed for the reaction to continue, such as in the polymerization of organic monomers into plastics. **2.** (in physics) a reaction that perpetuates itself by the proliferating fission of nuclei and the release of atomic particles that cause more nuclear fissions.

**chain reflex,** a series of reflexes, each stimulated by the preceding one.

**chain-stitch suture,** a continuous surgical stitch in which each loop of the suture is secured by the next loop.

**chalasia** /kəlā'zhə/ [Gk, *chalasis,* relaxation], abnormal relaxation or incompetence of the cardiac sphincter of the stomach, resulting in reflux of the gastric contents into the esophagus with subsequent regurgitation. Conservative treatment in infancy includes feeding several small meals a day to prevent distension of the stomach and holding the baby upright while giving the feeding. The symptoms and treatment are similar to those of a hiatal hernia. See also **gastroesophageal reflux.**

**chalazion** /kəlā'zion/ [Gk, hailstone], a small, localized swelling of the eyelid resulting from obstruction and retained secretions of the meibomian glands. It is a nonmalignant condition that often requires surgery for correction. Compare **hordeolum, sty.**

**chalice cell.** See **goblet cell.**

**chalicosis** /kal'ikō'sis/, a type of fibrosis that results from the inhalation of impure calcium dusts. Pure calcium dusts are soluble and are absorbed. Calcium dusts from marble, limestone, or Portland cement usually do not cause fibrosis.

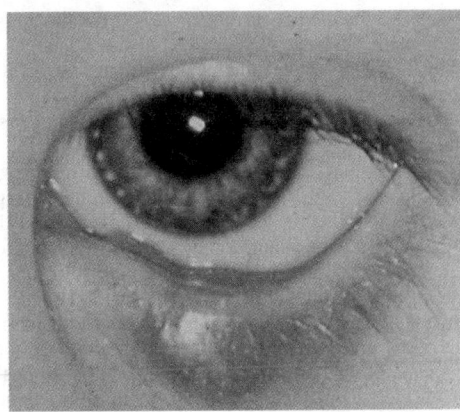

**Chalazion** *(Zitelli and Davis, 1997)*

Respiratory impairment is generally caused by the presence of free silica in the calcium dust.

**chalkitis** /kalkī′tis/ [Gk, *chalkos*, brass, *itis*, inflammation], an abnormal condition characterized by inflammation of the eyes, caused by rubbing the eyes with the hands after touching or handling brass. Also called **brassy eye.**

**challenge,** **1.** a method of testing the sensitivity of an individual to a hormone, allergen, or other substance by administering a sample. A small amount may be injected to determine whether the immune system will react by producing appropriate antibodies. **2.** a term used to describe the rapid or concentrated infusion of a substance such as potassium or magnesium in the face of a life-threatening deficiency or a rapid infusion of IV fluid to differentiate between fluid deficit or renal failure as the cause of severely decreased urine output.

**chalone** /kā′lōn/ [Gk, *chalan*, to relax], any one of numerous polypeptide inhibitors that are elaborated by a tissue and function like hormones on specific target organs.

**chamaeprosopy** /kam′əpros′əpē/ [Gk, *chamai*, low, *prosopon*, face], a facial appearance characterized by a low brow and a broad face. —**chamaeprosopic,** *adj.*

**chamber** [Gk, *kamara*, vaulted enclosure], **1.** a hollow but not necessarily empty space or cavity in an organ, as in the anterior and posterior chambers of the eye or the atrial and ventricular chambers of the heart. **2.** a room or closed space used for research or therapeutic purposes, such as a decompression chamber or hyperbaric oxygen chamber.

**Chamberlain's line** [W.E. Chamberlain, American radiologist, 1891–1947], a line that extends from the posterior of the hard palate to the dorsum of the foramen magnum.

**Chamberlen forceps** [Peter Chamberlen, English obstetrician, 1560–1631], one of the earliest kinds of obstetric forceps, introduced in the seventeenth century.

**chamfer** /cham′fər/, on an extracoronal cavity preparation, a finish on the margin that makes a curve from an axial wall to the cavosurface.

**chamomile** /kam′ə·mēl/, an herb with both annual and perennial forms, native to Germany, Hungary, and other areas of Europe.

■ USES: This herb is used externally as an antiseptic and soothing agent for inflamed skin and minor wounds. Internally, it is used as an antispasmodic, gas-relieving, and antiinflammatory agent for the treatment of digestive problems; as a light sleep aid and sedative for adults and children; and as a possible anticancer agent.

■ CONTRAINDICATIONS: Chamomile should not be used during pregnancy (*Chamaemelum nobile*) and lactation; it may be used in children. Cross-hypersensitivity may result from allergy to sunflowers, ragweed, or members of the aster family (echinacea, feverfew, milk thistle). People with asthma should also avoid its use.

**CHAMPUS,** abbreviation for **Civilian Health and Medical Programs for Uniformed Services.**

**chancr-.** See **cancr-.**

**chancre** /shang′kər/ [Fr, canker], **1.** a skin lesion, usually of primary syphilis, that begins at the infection site as a papule and develops into a red bloodless, painless ulcer with a scooped-out appearance. It heals without treatment and leaves no scar. Two or more chancres may develop at the same time, usually in the genital area but sometimes on the hands, face, or other body surface. The chancre teems with *Treponema pallidum* spirochetes and is highly contagious. Also called **venereal sore. 2.** a papular lesion or ulcerated area of the skin that marks the point of infection of a nonsyphilitic disease, such as tuberculosis. Compare **chancroid.** See also **syphilis.**

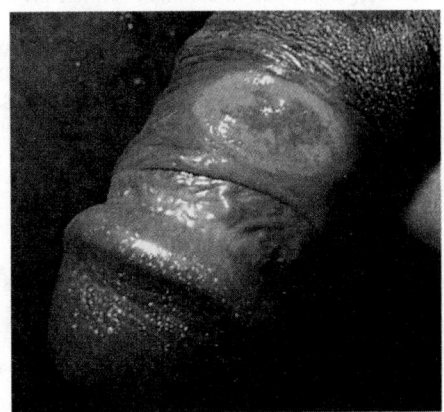

**Chancre of primary syphilis**
*(Morse, Moreland, and Holmes, 1996)*

**chancroid** /shang′kroid/ [Fr, *chancre,* canker; Gk, *eidos,* form], a highly contagious sexually transmitted disease caused by infection with the bacillus *Haemophilus ducreyi.* It characteristically begins as a papule, usually on the skin of the external genitalia; it then grows and ulcerates, other papules form, and, if untreated, the bacillus spreads, causing buboes in the groin. An intradermal skin test is more reliable than smear and culture techniques in diagnosing this condition. Azithromycin or ceftriaxone are prescribed to treat chancroid. Because the lesion resembles syphilis and lymphogranuloma venereum, the diagnosis must be made before treatment to prevent obscuring simultaneous infections. Symptoms may not appear until 10 days after infection. Compare **chancre.**

**chancrous** /shang′krəs/, describing a condition of chancres or lesions resembling chancres.

**change agent,** **1.** a role in which communication skills, education, and other resources are applied to help a client adjust to changes caused by illness or disability. **2.** a role to help members of an organization adapt to organizational change or to create organizational change.

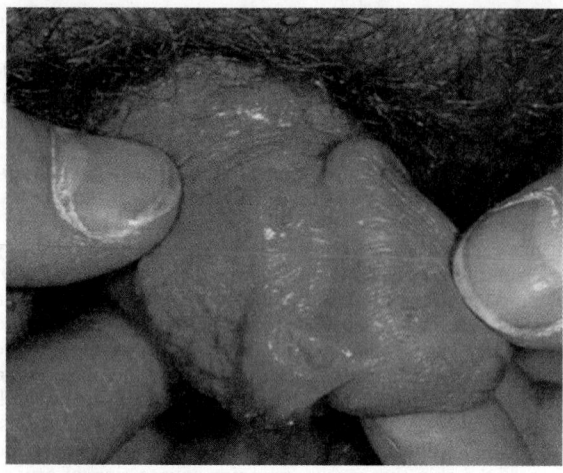

**Chancroid** (Habif, 1996)

**change of life,** *informal.* the female climacteric; menopause.

**channel** [L, *canalis,* pipe], **1.** a passageway or groove that conveys fluid, such as the central channels that connect the arterioles with the venules. **2.** membrane-bound globular proteins that allow diffusion of specific ions and molecules across a cell membrane.

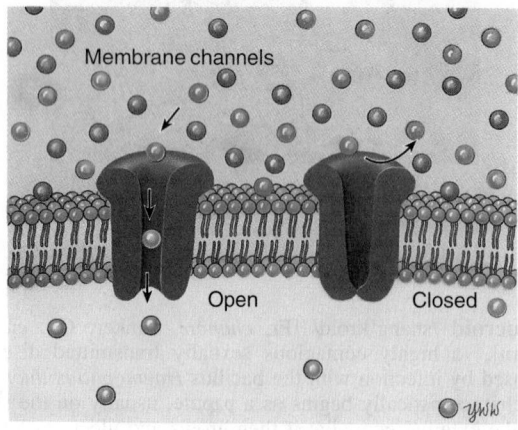

**Membrane channel**
(Thibodeau and Patton, 1999/Yvonne Wylie Walston)

**channeling,** referral of increased numbers of patients in exchange for discounted prices. Does not apply in Canada.

**channel ulcer** [L, *canalis,* pipe, *ulcus,* sore], a rare type of peptic ulcer found in the pyloric canal between the stomach and the duodenum. See also **peptic ulcer.**

**chaos** /kā′əs/, total disorganization with no causal relationships operating.

**chaotic atrial tachycardia** /kā·ot′ik/, an atrial rhythm with a rate exceeding 100/min caused by multifocal atrial activity and characterized by at least three different shapes

of P′ waves on the electrocardiogram. The condition is often associated with chronic obstructive lung disease.

**chaparral,** an herbal product harvested from a shrub found in Mexico and the Southwestern United States.

■ USES: Use of this herb is not recommended because it is potentially toxic to the liver and kidneys.

■ CONTRAINDICATIONS: Do not use chaparral during pregnancy and lactation or in children until more research is completed. Client with liver or renal disease should also avoid the use of this herb. The American Herbal Product Association has recommended that companies not sell chaparral products until the hepatoxicity question has been clarified.

**Chapman lymphatic reflexes,** (in chiropractic) a method of using body wall reflexes to influence the motion of fluids. After a surface locus has been contacted by the tip of the examiner's finger, a firm gentle contact is maintained and a rotary motion is imparted to the finger to express the fluid content of the locus into the surrounding tissues.

**chapped** /chapt/ [ME, *chappen,* cracked], pertaining to skin that is roughened, cracked, or reddened by exposure to cold or excessive moisture evaporation. Stinging or burning sensations often accompany the disorder. Prevention is achieved through protection against exposure to cold and wind. Treatment includes the avoidance of frequent washing, the replacement of soaps and detergents with superfatted soaps, and the application of emollients. Compare **frostbite.** —**chap,** *v.*

**character** [Gk, *charassein,* to engrave], **1.** the integrated composite of traits and behavioral tendencies that enable a person to react in a relatively consistent way to the customs and mores of society. Character, as contrasted with personality, implies volition and morality. Compare **personality. 2.** any letter, number, symbol, or punctuation mark, usually composed of 8 bits or 1 byte, that can be transmitted as output by a computer. See also **bit.**

**character analysis,** a systematic investigation of the personality of an individual with special attention to psychologic defenses and motivations, usually undertaken to improve behavior.

**character disorder,** a chronic, habitual maladaptive and socially unacceptable pattern of behavior and emotional response. The condition is usually accompanied by minimal feelings of anxiety. Also called **personality disorder.**

**characteristic** /kar′ək·tər·is′tik/ [Gk, *charassein,* to engrave], **1.** typical of an individual or other entity. **2.** a trait that distinguishes an individual or entity.

**characteristic curve** /ker′əktəris′tik/, a graphic relationship between the density (blackness) of an x-ray film and the exposure. Also called **sensitometric curve, Hurter and Driffield curve, D log E curve.**

**characteristic radiation,** radiation produced when a projectile electron interacts with and displaces an inner-shell electron of a target atom. It is a key process in x-ray production.

**character printer,** a printer for computers that produces a fully formed character, such as a letter, number, or symbol, with each impression stroke. Compare **dot-matrix printer.**

**charcoal.** See **activated charcoal.**

**Charcot-Bouchard aneurysm** /shärkō′bōōshär′/ [Jean M. Charcot, French neurologist, 1825–1893; Charles J. Bouchard, French physician, 1837–1886], a small, round dilation of a small artery in the cerebral cortex or basal ganglia. Charcot-Bouchard aneurysms often occur in individuals with very high blood pressure.

**Charcot-Leyden crystal** /shärkō′lī′dən/ [Jean M. Charcot; Ernst V. von Leyden, German physician, 1832–1910], any of the proteinaceous crystalline structures shaped like narrow, double pyramids found in the sputum of persons suffering from asthma and found in the feces of dysentery patients. Charcot-Leyden crystals occur in association with the fragmentation of eosinophils. Also called **asthma crystal, leukocytic crystal.**

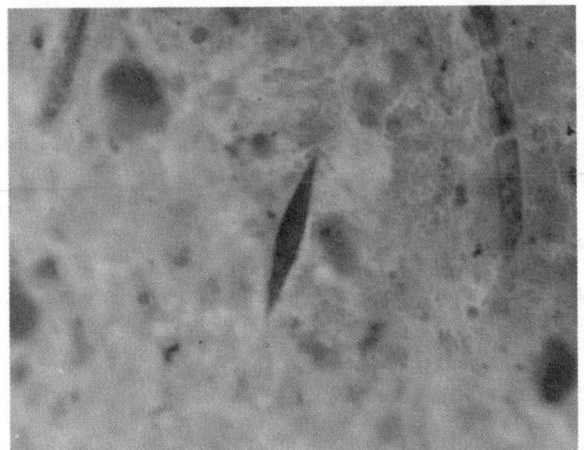

**Charcot-Leyden crystals** *(Baron, Peterson, and Finegold, 1994)*

**Charcot-Marie-Tooth disease** /shärkō'mərē'tooth'/ [Jean M. Charcot; Pierre Marie, French neurologist, 1853–1940; Howard H. Tooth, English neurologist, 1856–1925], a progressive hereditary disorder characterized by degeneration

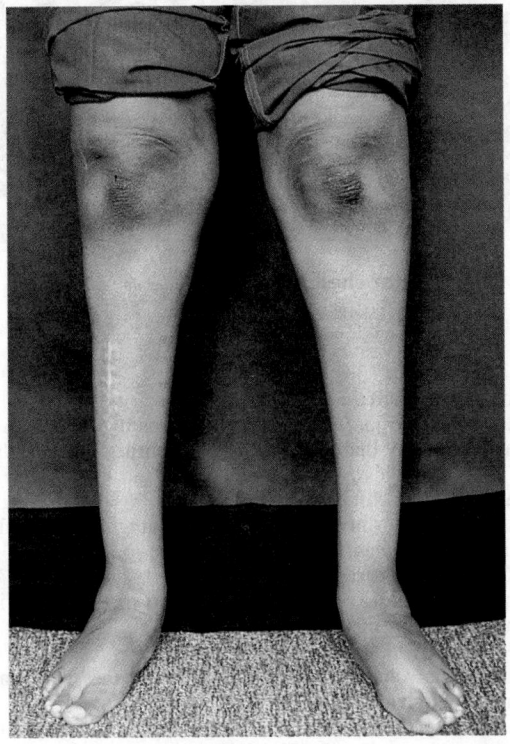

**Charcot-Marie-Tooth disease** *(Zitelli & Davis, 1997)*

of the peroneal muscles of the fibula, resulting in clubfoot, foot drop, and ataxia. Progressive arm weakness can also be present as distal muscles atrophy.

**Charcot's fever** /shärkōz'/ [Jean M. Charcot], a syndrome characterized by recurrent chills and fever, jaundice, and abdominal pain in the right upper quadrant that occurs with inflammation of the bile ducts. It is caused by the intermittent impaction of a stone in the ducts. Also called Charcot's triad.

**Charcot's foot** /shär·kōz'/ [Jean Martin Charcot, French neurologist, 1825–1893], the deformed foot seen in the neuropathic joint disease that accompanies tabes dorsalis.

**Charcot's joint.** See **neuropathic joint disease.**

**Charcot's triad** [Jean M. Charcot; Gk, *trias,* three], a set of three signs of brainstem involvement in multiple sclerosis: intention tremor, nystagmus, and scanning speech.

**CHARGE association,** a syndrome of associated defects, including *c*oloboma of the eye, *h*eart anomaly, choanal *a*tresia, *r*etardation, and *g*enital and *e*ar anomalies. Facial palsy, cleft palate, and dysphagia are often present, and familial transmission has been postulated. Also called **CHARGE syndrome.**

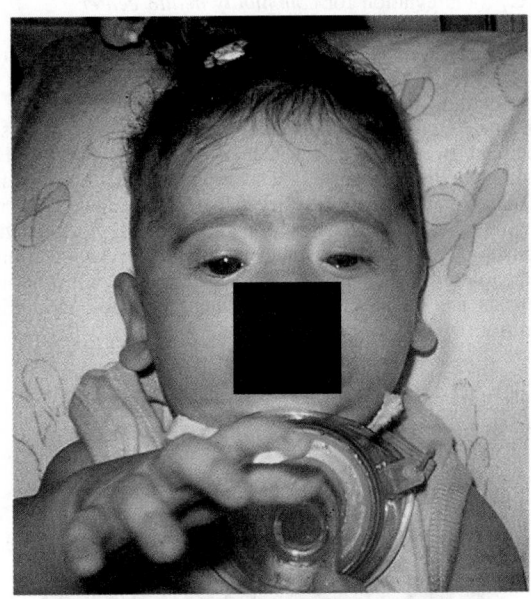

**Infant with CHARGE association**
*(Zitelli and Davis, 1997/courtesy Dr. W. Tunnessen, Children's Hospital of Philadelphia)*

**charge nurse,** the nurse assigned to manage the operations of the patient care area for the shift. Responsibilities may include staffing, admissions and discharge, and coordination of activities in the patient care area in the absence of the head nurse or nurse manager.

**charlatan** /shär'lətən/ [Fr, imposter], a totally unqualified individual posing as an expert, especially an individual pretending to be a physician. Also called **quack. —charlatanical,** *adj.*

**Charles' law.** See **Gay-Lussac's law.**

**charley horse** /chär'lē hôrs'/,   a sudden painful condition of the quadriceps or hamstring muscles characterized by soreness and stiffness. It is the result of a strain, tear, or bruise of the muscle; is aggravated by movement; and is often associated with athletic activity. Treatment includes rest and massage. Compare **cramp.**

**chart** /chärt/ [L, *charta,* paper],   **1.** *informal.* a patient record of data in tabular or graphic form. **2.** to note data in a patient record, usually at prescribed intervals.

**charta** /kär'tə/, *pl.* **chartae** [L, paper],   a piece of paper, especially one treated with medicine, as for external application, or with a chemical for a special purpose, such as litmus paper.

**charting,**   the act of compiling data on clinical records or charts. The charts are updated regularly to keep physicians and other health care workers advised of changes in the patient's condition. The data usually include fluctuations in temperature, pulse, respiration, and other variable factors.

**chauffeur's fracture** /shō'fərz/ [Fr, stoker; L, *fractura,* break],   any fracture of the radial styloid, produced by a twisting or a snapping type of injury.

**Chaussier's areola** /shôsyāz'/ [François Chaussier, French anatomist, 1746–1828; L, little space],   an areola of indurated tissue surrounding a malignant pustule.

**CHB,**   abbreviation for **complete heart block.**

**CHC,**   abbreviation for *community health center.*

**CHD,**   abbreviation for **coronary heart disease.**

**check ligament.**   See **alar ligament.**

**checkup** [Fr, *eschec,* acquire; AS, *uf*],   a thorough study or examination of the health of an individual.

**Chédiak-Higashi syndrome** /ched'ē·ak·higä'shē/ [Moisés Chédiak, twentieth-century Cuban physician; Ototaka Higashi, twentieth-century Japanese physician],   a congenital, autosomal recessive disorder, characterized by partial albinism, photophobia, pale optic fundi, massive leukocytic inclusions, psychomotor abnormalities, recurrent infections, and early death. Antenatal diagnosis can be made by amniocentesis and tissue culture. Treatment includes antibiotics and transfusions.

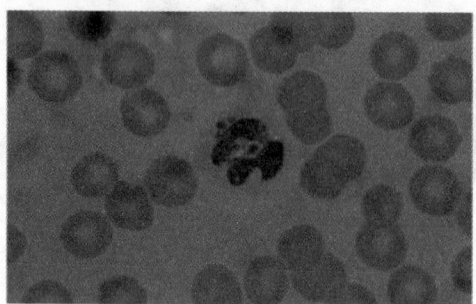

**Chédiak-Higashi syndrome: peripheral blood smear**
*(Zitelli and Davis, 1997/courtesy Dr. William Zinkham, Baltimore)*

**cheek** [AS, *ceace*],   a fleshy prominence, especially the fleshy protuberances on both sides of the face between the eye and the jaw and the ear and the nose and mouth. Also called **bucca.**

**cheekbone.**   See **zygomatic bone.**

**cheesy abscess** [AS, *cese* + L, *abscedere,* to go away],   an abscess that contains a yellowish semisolid, cheeselike ma-

terial. It is found in tuberculous abscesses. Also called **caseous abscess.**

**cheesy necrosis,**   tissue death in which the structures have degenerated into a white, cheesy mass. Also called **caseous necrosis.**

**cheil-.**   See **cheilo-.**

**cheilectomy** /kīlek'təmē/,   surgical removal of irregular surfaces in the lining of a joint.

**-cheilia, -chilia,**   suffix meaning '(condition of the) lips': *atelocheilia, xerocheilia.*

**cheilitis** /kīlī'tis/ [Gk, *cheilos,* lip, *itis,* inflammation],   an abnormal condition of the lips characterized by inflammation and cracking of the skin. There are several forms, including those caused by excessive exposure to sunlight, allergic sensitivity to cosmetics, and vitamin deficiency. Compare **cheilosis.**

**cheilo-, cheil-,**   combining form meaning 'lip': *cheiloangioscopy, cheilocarcinoma, cheiloplasty.*

**cheilocarcinoma** /kī'lōkär'sinō'mə/, *pl.* **cheilocarcinomas, cheilocarcinomata,**   a malignant epithelial tumor of the lip.

**cheiloplasty** /kī'ləplas'tē/ [Gk, *cheilos,* lip, *plassein,* to mold],   surgical correction of a defect of the lip.

**cheilorrhaphy** /kīlôr'əfē/ [Gk, *cheilos,* lip, *raphe,* suture],   a surgical procedure that sutures the lip, such as in the repair of a congenitally cleft lip or a lacerated lip.

**cheilosis** /kīlō'sis/,   a disorder of the lips and mouth characterized by bilateral scales and fissures, resulting from a deficiency of riboflavin in the diet.

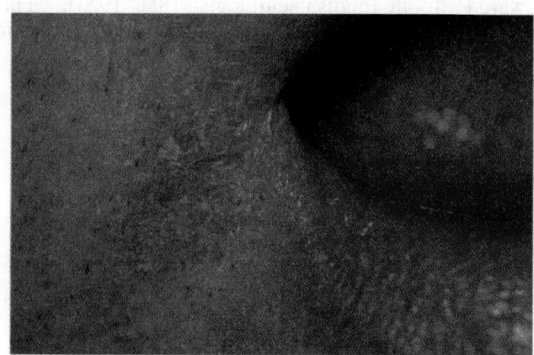

**Angular cheilosis** *(Lemmi and Lemmi, 2000)*

**cheir-.**   See **cheiro-.**

**cheiralgia** /kīral'jə/ [Gk, *cheir + algos,* pain],   a pain in the hand, especially that associated with arthritis. —**cheiralgic,** *adj.*

**-cheiria.**   See **-chiria.**

**cheiro-, cheir-, chir-, chiro-,**   combining form meaning 'hand': *cheiromegaly, cheiroplasty.*

**cheirognostic** /kī'ragnos'tik/ [Gk, *cheir,* hand, *gnostikos,* knowing],   able to distinguish between the left and right hands and sides of the body.

**cheiromegaly** /kī'rōmeg'əlē/ [Gk, *cheir + megas,* large],   an abnormal condition characterized by excessively large hands. —**cheiromegalic,** *adj.*

**cheiroplasty** /kī'rōplas'tē/,   a surgical procedure to restore an injured or congenitally deformed hand to normal use. Also called **chiroplasty. —cheiroplastic,** *adj.*

**chelate** /kē′lāt/ [Gk, *chele,* claw], **1.** to form a bond, thus creating a ringlike complex. An example is the interaction of a metal ion and two or more polar groups of a single molecule. **2.** (in medicine) any coordination compound composed of a central metal ion and an organic molecule with multiple bonds arranged in ring formations, used especially in chemotherapeutic treatments for metal poisoning. **3.** pertaining to chelation.

**chelating agent** /kē′lāting/, a substance that promotes chelation. Chelating agents are used in the treatment of metal poisoning. See also **chelation.**

**chelation** /kēlā′shən/, a chemical reaction in which there is a combination with a metal to form a ring-shaped molecular complex in which the metal is firmly bound and isolated. See also **chelating agent.**

**cheloid, cheloidal.** See **keloid.**

**cheloidosis.** See **keloidosis.**

**chemabrasion** /kem′əbrā′zhən/ [Gk, *chemeia,* alchemy; L, *ab* + *radere,* to scrape off], a method of treating scars, chromatosis, or other skin disorders by applying chemicals that remove the surface layers of skin cells. See also **chemical cauterization, chemosurgery.**

**chemexfoliation.** See **chemical peel.**

**chemical** /kem′əkəl/ [Gk, *chemeia,* alchemy], **1.** a substance composed of chemical elements or a substance produced by or used in chemical processes. **2.** pertaining to chemistry.

**chemical action,** any process in which elements and/or compounds react with each other to produce a chemical change; for example, hydrogen and oxygen combine to produce water.

**chemical affinity** [Gk, *chemeia,* alchemy; L, *affinis,* related], **1.** an attraction that results in the formation of molecules from atoms. **2.** an attraction between chemicals caused by polarity, as used in chromatography.

**chemical agent,** any chemical power, active principle, or substance that can produce an effect in the body by interacting with various body substances, such as aspirin, which produces an analgesic effect.

**chemical antidote** [Gk, *chemeia* + *anti,* against, *dotos,* that which is given], any substance that reacts chemically with a poison to form a compound that is harmless. There are few true antidotes, and treatment of poisoning depends largely on eliminating the toxic agent before it can be absorbed by the body.

**chemical burn,** tissue damage caused by exposure to a strong acid or alkali, such as phenol, creosol, mustard gas, or phosphorus. See also **acid burn, acid poisoning, alkali burn, alkali poisoning.**

**chemical carcinogen** [Gk, *chemeia,* alchemy, *karkinos,* crab, *oma,* tumor, *genein,* to produce], any chemical agent that can induce the development of cancer in living tissue.

**chemical cauterization** [Gk, *chemeia* + *kauterion,* branding iron], the corroding or burning of living tissue by a caustic chemical substance, such as potassium hydroxide. Also called **chemocautery.**

**chemical disaster,** the accidental release of a quantity of toxic chemicals into the environment, resulting in death or injury to workers or members of nearby communities. Examples include the mercury waste poisoning of fish, resulting in 111 human deaths at Minamata, Japan; the release of methyl isocyanate from a chemical plant in Bhopal, India, at a cost of 2000 lives; and a nuclear accident at Chenobyl, Ukraine, requiring the removal of 160,000 people from their homes.

**chemical energy.** See **energy.**

**chemical equivalent,** a drug or chemical containing similar amounts of the same ingredients as another drug or chemical.

**chemical fog,** a curtain effect on x-ray film that causes the loss of image quality. It appears as a dull gray discoloration and is usually caused by chemical contamination of the developer.

**chemical gastritis,** inflammation of the stomach caused by the ingestion of a chemical compound. Treatment is determined by the substance ingested. Compare **corrosive gastritis, erosive gastritis.**

**chemical indicator,** **1.** a commercially prepared device that monitors all or part of the physical conditions of the sterilization cycle. It usually consists of a sensitive ink dye that changes color under certain conditions. **2.** a compound added to a reaction system to show, typically by a change in color, when the process is complete, as in an acid-base titration.

**chemical mediator,** a neurotransmitter chemical, such as acetylcholine.

**chemical name,** the exact designation of the chemical structure of a drug as determined by the rules of accepted systems of chemical nomenclature.

**chemical peel,** a therapy to eliminate wrinkles, blemishes, pigment spots, and sun-damaged areas of the skin. Using a chemical solution of phenol, trichloroacetic acid (TCA), or alpha hydroxy fruit acid, the top skin layers are peeled away, allowing new, smoother skin with tighter cells to occupy the surface. Immediately after the peel, there may be considerable swelling, which subsides after 7 to 10 days as new skin begins to form. Also called **chemexfoliation, chemoexfoliation.**

**chemical peritonitis** [Gk, *chemeia,* alchemy, *peri,* near, *teinein,* to stretch, *itis,* inflammation], an inflammation of the peritoneum resulting from chemicals, including digestive substances, in the peritoneum.

**chemical restraint** [Gk, *chemeia,* alchemy; *restringere,* to confine], the use of psychotropics, hypnotics, or anxiolytics to control a potentially violent patient. Also called **medical restraint.**

**chemical shift,** (in nuclear magnetic resonance spectrometry) the position of a resonance in the substance of interest relative to the position of the resonance of a standard. Nonequivalent atoms of a molecule have different chemical shifts.

**chemical sympathectomy,** the removal of a sympathetic nerve tract or ganglion by injection of a corrosive chemical such as phenol.

**chemical warfare,** the waging of war with poisonous chemicals and gases.

**cheminosis** /kem′ənō′sis/ [Gk, *chemeia* + *osis,* condition], any disease caused by a chemical substance.

**chemist,** **1.** a person with special education and training in the structures, characteristics, and actions of chemicals. **2.** in Great Britain, a pharmacist.

**chemistry** /kem′istrē/ [Gk, *chemeia,* alchemy], the science dealing with the elements, their compounds, and the molecular structure and interactions of matter. Classifications of chemistry include **inorganic chemistry** and **organic chemistry.**

**chemistry, normal values,** the amounts of various substances in the normal human body, determined by testing a large sample of people presumed to be healthy. Normal values are expressed in ranges of numbers, and ranges vary for different age groups and from laboratory to laboratory. For example, a normal concentration of a substance in the blood might be expressed as 5 to 20 mg/dL. Although variations from normal values may be highly significant tools in the diagnoses of certain diseases, in all cases an abnormal result must be cautiously interpreted. See also specific tests.

**chemo-** /kem′ō-, kē′mō-/, combining form meaning 'by chemical reaction' or 'a chemical or chemistry': *chemoantigen, chemobiotic, chemokinesis.*

**chemoattractant** /kē′mō-ə·trak′tənt/ [Gk, *chemeia,* alchemy + L, *attrahere,* to draw to], a chemotactic factor that induces positive chemotaxis.

**chemocautery.** See **chemical cauterization.**

**chemodifferentiation** /-dif′ərən′shē-ā′shən/, a stage in embryonic development that precedes and controls specialization and differentiation of the cells into rudimentary organs.

**chemoexfoliation.** See **chemical peel.**

**chemokine** /kē′mō·kīn/ [Gk, *chemeia,* alchemy + *kinēsis,* movement], any of a group of low-molecular-weight cytokines, such as interleukin-8, identified on the basis of their ability to induce chemotaxis or chemokinesis in leukocytes (or in particular populations of leukocytes) in inflammation, the group now divided into four subgroups on the basis of genetic, structural, and functional criteria. They function as regulators of the immune system and may also play roles in the circulatory and central nervous systems. See also **cytokine.**

**chemokinesis** /kē′mō·ki·nē′sis/ [Gk, *chemeia,* alchemy + *kinesis* movement], increased nondirectional activity of cells caused by the presence of a chemical substance. Compare **chemotaxis.**

**chemonucleolysis** /-nōō′klē·ol′isis-/ [Gk, *chemeia* + L, *nucleus,* nut kernel; Gk, *lysein,* to loosen], a method of dissolving the nucleus pulposus of an intervertebral disk by the injection of a chemolytic agent, such as the enzyme chymopapain. The procedure is used primarily in the treatment of a herniated disk and other intervertebral disk lesions.

**chemoprophylaxis** /-prō′filak′sis/ [Gk, *chemeia* + *prophylax,* advance guard], the use of antimicrobial drugs to prevent the acquisition of pathogens in an endemic area or to prevent their spread from one body area to another.

**chemoreceptor** /-risep′tər/ [Gk, *chemeia* + L, *recipere,* to receive], a sensory nerve cell activated by chemical stimuli. For example, chemoreceptors in the carotid artery are sensitive to the partial pressure of carbon dioxide in the blood; they signal the respiratory center in the brain to increase or decrease the rate of breathing.

**chemoreflex** /-rē′fleks/, any reflex initiated by the stimulation of chemical receptors, such as the carotid and aortic bodies, which respond to changes in carbon dioxide, hydrogen ion, and oxygen concentrations in the blood. See also **chemoreceptor.**

**chemoresistance,** 1. a specific resistance by components of a cell to chemical substances. 2. the resistance of bacteria or a cancer cell to a chemical designed to treat the disorder.

**chemosis** /kimō′sis/ [Gk, *cheme,* cockle, *osis,* condition], an abnormal edematous swelling of the mucous membrane covering the eyeball and lining the eyelids. Usually the result of local trauma or infection, chemosis may also occur in acute conjunctivitis. Obstruction of normal lymph flow, such as might result from growth of a tumor within the eye socket, may less commonly cause chemosis. Systemic disorders, such as angioneurotic edema, anemia, and Bright's disease, may also cause the condition. Also called **conjunctival edema.**

**chemostat** /kē′məstat′/, a device that assures a steady rate of cell division in bacterial populations by maintaining a constant environment.

**chemosurgery** /-sur′jərē/ [Gk, *chemeia* + *cheirourgos,* surgeon], the destruction of malignant, infected, or gangre-

nous tissue by the application of chemicals. The technique is used successfully to remove skin cancers.

**chemotactic** /-tak′tik/ [Gk, *chemeia,* alchemy, *taxis,* arrangement], pertaining to a tendency of cells to migrate toward or away from certain chemical stimuli.

**chemotaxis** /-tak′sis/ [Gk, *chemeia* + *taxis,* arrangement], movement toward or away from a chemical stimulus. Chemotaxis is a cellular function, particularly of neutrophils and monocytes, whose phagocytic activity is influenced by chemical factors released by invading microorganisms. —**chemotactic,** *adj.*

**chemotherapeutic agent** /-ther′əpyōō′tik/, refers to a medication used to treat cancer because it can alter the growth of cancer cells.

**chemotherapeutic index,** a system for judging the safety and effectiveness of a drug as a ratio between a maximum tolerated ($LD_{50}$) dose per kilogram of body weight balanced against a median effective ($ED_{50}$) or minimal curative dose.

**chemotherapy** /-ther′əpē/, the treatment of infections and other diseases with chemical agents. The term has been applied over the centuries to a variety of therapies, including malaria therapy with herbs and use of mercury for syphilis. In modern usage, chemotherapy usually entails the use of chemicals to destroy cancer cells on a selective basis. The cytotoxic agents used in cancer treatments generally function in the same manner as ionizing radiation; they do not kill the cancer cells directly but instead impair their ability to replicate. Most of the commonly used anticancer drugs act by interfering with deoxyribonucleic acid and ribonucleic acid activities associated with cell division. Chemotherapeutic agents are often used in combination with radiation treatments for their synergistic effect. For example, a cytotoxic agent may be used to render a tumor cell more sensitive to the effects of ionizing radiation, thus allowing the cancer to be controlled with smaller doses of radiation.

**chemotherapy management,** a nursing intervention from the Nursing Interventions Classification (NIC) defined as assisting the patient and family to understand the action and minimize side effects of antineoplastic agents. See also **Nursing Interventions Classification.**

**chemotherapy (unsealed radioactive),** the oral or parenteral administration of a radioisotope, such as iodine 131 ($^{131}I$), for the treatment of hyperthyroidism or thyroid cancer or phosphorus 32 ($^{32}P$) for leukemia, polycythemia vera, or peritoneal ascites resulting from widely disseminated carcinoma.

■ METHOD: The patient needs to be isolated during the half-life of the radioisotope (8.1 days for $^{131}I$, 14 days for $^{32}P$, and 2.7 days for $^{198}Au$) to prevent radiation exposure to other persons.

■ INTERVENTION: The nurse wears a radiation badge when entering the patient's room and limits exposure by performing planned procedures efficiently. Routine nursing functions are kept to a minimum. Disposal of urine, feces, and dressings follows a prespecified protocol.

■ OUTCOME CRITERIA: Radioactive iodine usually counteracts hyperthyroidism and is frequently used in conjunction with surgery in the treatment of thyroid cancer. Radioactive phosphorus often controls polycythemia vera, but other agents are generally more effective in leukemia therapy. Radioactive gold is usually administered as a last resort in advanced lung cancer or peritoneal ascites resulting from malignant disease.

**chenodeoxycholic acid** /kē′nōdē·ok′sikō′lik/, a secondary bile acid. It is used in vivo to dissolve cholesterol gallstones, particularly in the elderly and poor-risk patients. See also **ursodeoxycholic acid.**

**cherophobia** /kē′rō′fō′bē·ə/, a morbid aversion to cheerfulness.

**cherry angioma** [L, *cerasus* + *angeion,* vessel, *oma,* tumor], a small, bright red, clearly circumscribed vascular tumor on the skin. It occurs most often on the trunk but may appear anywhere on the body. The lesion is common; more than 85% of people over 45 years of age have several cherry angiomas. Also called **capillary angioma, capillary hemangioma, De Morgan's spots, senile angioma.**

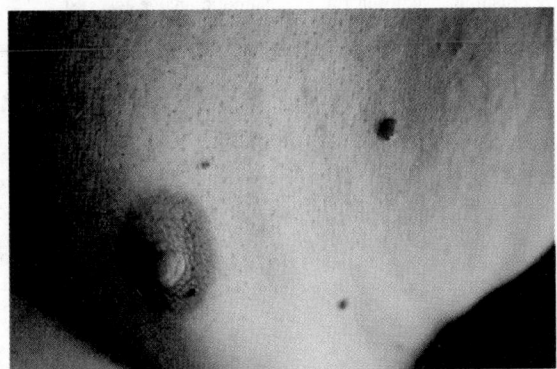

**Cherry angioma** *(Christiansen, 1993)*

**cherry red spot,** an abnormal red circular area of the choroid, visible through the fovea centralis of the eye and surrounded by a contrasting white edema. It is associated with cases of infantile cerebral sphingolipidosis and sometimes appears in the late infantile form of amaurotic familial idiocy. Also called **Tay's spot.**

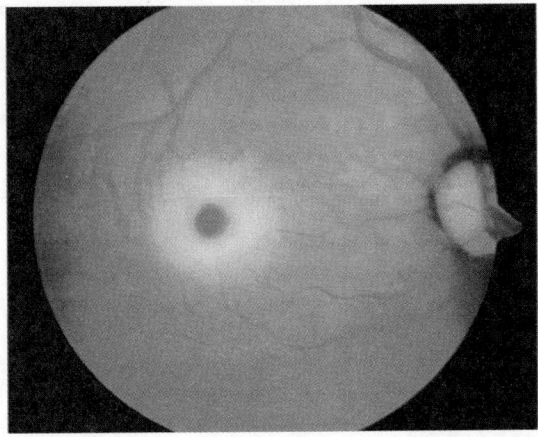

**Cherry red spot** *(Apple and Rabb, 1998)*

**cherubism** /cher′əbiz′əm/ [Heb, *kerubh*], an abnormal hereditary condition characterized by progressive bilateral swelling at the angle of the mandible, especially in children. In some cases of cherubism, the entire jaw swells and the eyes turn up, enhancing the cherubic facial appearance. The condition tends to regress during adult life.

**chest** [AS, *box*], **1.** the thorax, the cavity enclosed by the ribs, sternum, and diaphragm. **2.** the outside front part of the basic thoracic structure. See also **thoracic cage, thoracic cavity, thorax.**

**chest bandage,** any of several types of fabric dressings for chest injuries, including a three-cornered open chest wrapping, a figure-eight roller bandage spica, or a scultetus pattern of narrow strips that can be overlapped and pinned.

**chest binder,** a broad bandage or girdle, with or without shoulder straps, that encircles the chest and aids in supplying heat or other therapies. A chest binder also may be used to support the breasts.

**chest cavity.** See **body cavity.**

**chest drainage,** the withdrawal of air, blood, or fluids from the chest cavity through a tube commonly inserted into the pleural space. The tube may be connected to a suction device that helps reinflate a collapsed lung.

**chest lead** /lēd/, **1.** an electrocardiographic conductor in which the exploring positive electrode is placed on the chest or precordium. The indifferent electrode is placed on the patient's back for a chest back (CB) lead, on the front of the chest for a chest front (CF) lead, on the left arm for a chest left (CL) lead, and on the right arm for a chest right (CR) lead. **2.** *informal.* the tracing produced by such a lead on an electrocardiograph.

**chest pain** [AS, *cest,* box; L, *poena,* punishment], a physical complaint that requires immediate diagnosis and evaluation. Chest pain may be symptomatic of cardiac disease, such as angina pectoris, myocardial infarction, or pericarditis, or of pulmonary disease, such as pleurisy, pneumonia, or pulmonary embolism or infarction. The source of chest pain may also be musculoskeletal, gastrointestinal, or psychogenic; use of illegal drugs such as cocaine may also cause chest pain. Over 90% of severe chest pain is caused by coronary disease, spinal root compression, or psychologic disturbance. Because of its association with life-threatening heart disease, chest pain causes extreme anxiety, which tends to mask other symptoms that would aid in diagnosis and treatment; reassuring the person being examined assists in proper diagnosis. Evaluation of chest pain requires determining the quality of the pain—dull, sharp, or crushing, locating the site of the pain—in the center or side of the chest, and determining how long the pain has persisted, how it has developed, and whether it has occurred in the past. The patient is asked to describe the spread of pain to other parts of the body and to identify such factors as exertion, emotional distress, movement, eating, or deep breathing that aggravate or relieve the pain. Specific cardiovascular conditions associated with chest pain are myocardial infarction, angina pectoris, pericarditis, and a dissecting aneurysm of the thoracic aorta. Musculoskeletal conditions include rib fractures, swelling of the rib cartilage, and muscle strain. GI conditions associated with chest pain include esophagitis, peptic ulcers, hiatal hernia, gastritis, cholecystitis, and pancreatitis.

**chest physiotherapy,** a nursing intervention from the Nursing Interventions Classification (NIC) defined as assisting the patient to move airway secretions from peripheral airways to more central airways for expectoration and/or suctioning. See also **Nursing Interventions Classification.**

**chest physiotherapy**[1]. See **cupping and vibrating, percussion.**

**chest prominences and depressions,** any unnatural surface features of the chest that may be caused by congenital defects, diseases such as emphysema, enlarged organs, tu-

## Differentiating characteristics of chest pain

| Precipitating factors | Character | Relief |
|---|---|---|
| **Cardiovascular** | | |
| *Effort angina* | | |
| Exercise, emotion, extreme temperatures, eating heavy meals | Constricting, squeezing, pressure; usually lasting more than 2 minutes and less than 15 minutes | Rest or nitroglycerin |
| *Rest angina* | | |
| Spontaneous; possible daily cycle | Like effort angina | Nitroglycerin |
| *Acute myocardial infarction* | | |
| Spontaneous | Like angina but more severe, crushing; usually lasting longer than 20 minutes | Narcotic analgesics, rest or glycerin not effective |
| *Pericarditis* | | |
| Deep breath, lying down | Sharp, stabbing; continuous | Antiinflammatories, analgesics; sitting up, leaning forward |
| *Hypertrophic cardiomyopathy* | | |
| Exercise, stress | Anginal pain associated with lightheadedness, dizziness, syncope | Rest, β-blockers |
| *Mitral valve prolapse* | | |
| Spontaneous | Variable in character, possibly migratory | Time |
| *Acute dissecting aortic aneurysm* | | |
| Spontaneous | Sudden, severe, tearing pain in center of chest, radiating to back or abdomen | Large doses of analgesics |
| **Pulmonary** | | |
| *Pulmonary embolism* | | |
| Spontaneous; accentuated by dyspnea and pleuritic respiration | Sharp, stabbing, knifelike; continuous | Time |
| *Pleurisy* | | |
| History of recent respiratory illness; worse with respiratory movement | Sharp, burning, ache or "catch" on one side of the chest | Time |
| **Musculoskeletal** | | |
| Coughing, deep breath, movement | Sharp, stabbing, tenderness, localized; fleeting or lasting for days | Antiinflammatories, analgesics |
| **Gastrointestinal** | | |
| *Gastric or duodenal ulcer* | | |
| Empty stomach | Burning in epigastrium 60 to 90 minutes after eating | Milk or antacids |
| *Esophageal spasm or irritation* | | |
| Spontaneous | Burning deep in throat; accompanying weight loss, dysphagia, regurgitation | Nitroglycerin |
| **Other** | | |
| *Emotional stress* | | |
| Stress stimulus | Tightness, aching; if accompanied by hyperventilation, possible ST-segment and T-wave changes | Stimulus removal |
| *Mediastinitis or mediastinal tumors* | | |
| Spontaneous | Pleuritic, constriction | Time Removal of mass |
| *Tissue rupture or tear* | | |
| Blunt injury | Abrupt, sharp | Time, repair |

From Guzzetta C, Dossey B: *Cardiovascular nursing: holistic practice,* St Louis, 1992, Mosby.

mors, traumas, or occupational hazards. See also **barrel chest, flail chest, funnel chest, pigeon breast.**

**chest regions,** the topographic parts or subdivisions of the chest: presternal, mammary, inframammary, and axillary.

**chest thump** [AS, *cest,* box], a sharp blow delivered to the chest in the precordial area to restore a normal heartbeat after cardiac arrest.

**chest tube,** a catheter inserted through the rib space of the thorax into the pleural space to remove air and/or fluid, thereby restoring negative pressure in the pleural space. It is attached to a water-seal chest drainage device. It is commonly used after chest surgery and lung collapse.

**chest wall percussion.** See **percussion.**

**chewing gum diarrhea.** See **osmotic diarrhea.**

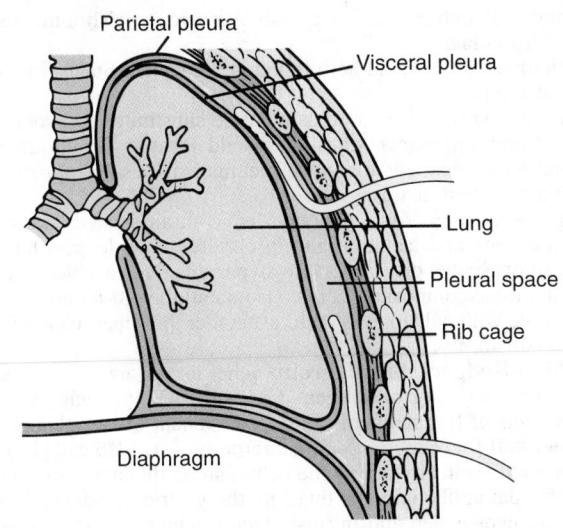

**Placement of chest tubes**
*(Lewis, Heitkemper, and Dirksen, 2000)*

**chewing reflex,** a pathologic sign in brain-damaged adults, characterized by repetitive chewing motions when the mouth is stimulated.

**Cheyne's nystagmus** /shānz/ [John Cheyne, Scottish physician, 1777–1836], an involuntary eyeball movement with a rhythm that resembles that of Cheyne-Stokes respiration.

**Cheyne-Stokes respiration (CSR)** [John Cheyne; William Stokes, Irish physician, 1804–1878; L *respirare* to breathe], an abnormal pattern of respiration, characterized by alternating periods of apnea and deep, rapid breathing. The respiratory cycle begins with slow, shallow breaths that gradually become abnormally rapid and deep. Breathing gradually becomes slower and shallower and is followed by 10 to 20 seconds of apnea before the cycle is repeated. Each episode may last from 45 seconds to 3 minutes. Underlying CSR is a complex alteration in the functioning of the respiratory center in the brain, caused by dysfunction of the diencephalon or by bilateral hemispheric lesions. The respiratory center may have a reduced sensitivity to the concentrations of blood gases, as is seen in cerebral vascular disease, in tumors of the brainstem, and in severe head injury. CSR may be triggered by changes in blood chemical processes, especially in elderly patients with degenerative arterial disease or respiratory diseases, such as bronchopneumonia. In an otherwise healthy person, CSR may occur through hyperventilation, exposure to high altitudes, or an overdose of a narcotic or hypnotic drug. CSR occurs more frequently during sleep. Also called **agonal respiration, periodic breathing.** Compare **Biot's respiration.**

**-chezia, -chesia,** suffix meaning '(condition of) defecation, especially involving the discharge of foreign substances': *dyschezia, hematochezia.*

**CHF,** abbreviation for **congestive heart failure.**

**chi** /kī/, X, χ, **1.** the 22nd letter of the Greek alphabet, sometimes used in scientific notation to designate the 22nd in a series. **2.** in Asian philosophies, energy, whether positive or negative.

**ch'i,** a Chinese concept of a fundamental life energy that flows in orderly ways along meridians, or channels, in the body. See also **acupuncture.**

$\chi^2$ **distribution.** See **chi square distribution.**

**Chiari-Frommel syndrome** /kē·är'ēfrom'əl/ [Johann B. Chiari, German obstetrician, 1817–1854; Richard Frommel, German gynecologist, 1854–1912], a hormonal disorder that occurs after pregnancy in which weaning does not spontaneously end lactation. It is usually the result of a decrease in pituitary gonadotropins and an excess of pituitary prolactin and may be accompanied by amenorrhea. Treatment includes observation, hormonal therapy, and investigation to confirm or rule out pituitary tumor.

**Chiari's malformation** /kē·ä'rēz/ [Hans Chiari, Austrian pathologist, 1851–1916], a congenital anomaly in which the cerebellum and medulla oblongata, which is elongated and flattened, protrude into the spinal canal through the foramen magnum; it is classified into three types according to severity, ranging from prolapse of the cerebellar tonsils into the spinal canal without elongation of the brainstem (type I) to complete herniation of the cerebellum to form an occipital encephalocele (type III). It may be accompanied by hydrocephalus, spina bifida, syringomyelia, and mental defects. The classic form is type II, better known as Arnold-Chiari malformation. Also called **Chiari's deformity.** See also **Arnold-Chiari malformation.**

**Chiari's syndrome.** See **Budd-Chiari syndrome.**

**chiasm** /kī'azəm/ [Gk, *chiasma,* lines that cross], **1.** the crossing of two lines or tracts, as of the optic nerves at the optic chiasm. **2.** (in genetics) the crossing of two chromatids in the prophase of meiosis. —**chiasmal, chiasmic,** *adj.*

**chiasma** /kī·az'mə/, *pl.* **chiasmata** [Gk, lines that cross], a visible connection between homologous chromosomes during the first meiotic division in gametogenesis. Chiasmata appear as X-shaped configurations during the late prophase stage and provide the means by which homologous chromosomes exchange genetic material. See also **crossing over.** —**chiasmatic, chiasmic,** *adj.*

**chiasmal.** See **chiasm.**

**chiasmapexy** /kī·az'məpek'sē/, surgery involving the optic chiasm.

**chiasmatypy.** See **crossing over.**

**chiasmic.** See **chiasm, chiasma.**

**chickenpox** /chik'ənpoks'/ [AS, *cicen* + ME, *pokke*], an acute, highly contagious viral disease caused by a herpesvirus, varicella zoster virus (VZV). It occurs primarily in young children and is characterized by crops of pruritic vesicular eruptions on the skin. The disease is transmitted by direct contact with skin lesions or, more commonly, by droplets spread from the respiratory tract of infected persons, usually in the prodromal period or the early stages of

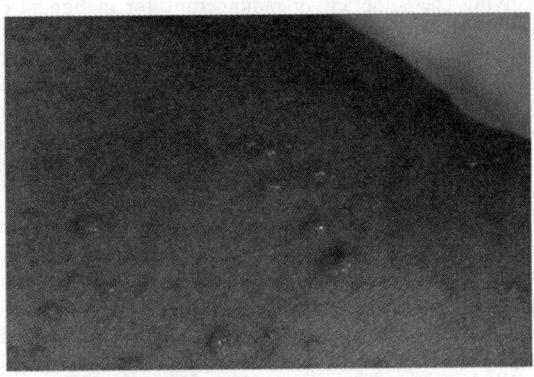

**Chickenpox** *(Lemmi and Lemmi, 2000)*

the rash. The vesicular fluid and the scabs are infectious until entirely dry. Indirect transmission through uninfected persons or objects is rare. The diagnosis is usually made by physical examination and by the characteristic appearance of the disease. The virus may be identified by culture of the vesicle fluid. Also called **varicella.**

■ OBSERVATIONS: The incubation period averages 2 to 3 weeks, followed by slight fever, mild headache, malaise, and anorexia occurring about 24 to 36 hours before the rash begins. The prodromal period is usually mild in children but may be severe in adults. The rash, which is highly pruritic, begins as macules and progresses in 1 or 2 days to papules and, finally, to vesicles surrounding an erythematous base and containing clear fluid. Within 24 to 48 hours the vesicles turn cloudy and become umbilicated, are easily broken, and become encrusted. The lesions, which erupt in crops so that all three stages are present simultaneously, first appear on the back and chest and then spread to the face, neck, and limbs; they occur only rarely on the soles and palms. In severe cases, laryngeal or tracheal vesicles in the pharynx, larynx, and trachea may cause dyspnea and dysphagia. Prolonged fever, lymphadenopathy, and extreme irritability from pruritus are other symptoms. The symptoms last from a few days to 2 weeks.

■ INTERVENTIONS: Routine treatment consists of bed rest; medications to reduce fever; applications of topical antipruritics, such as wet compresses, calamine lotion, or a paste made from baking soda and water; or oral antihistamines, given for the relief of itching. Infected vesicles may be treated with neomycin-bacitracin, and systemic antibiotics may be given if the secondary bacterial infection is extensive. People who are susceptible and at risk for severe disease when exposed to the infection may be passively protected with zoster immune globulin (ZIG), varicella-zoster immune globulin (VZIG), immune serum globulin (ISG), or zoster immune plasma (ZIP). A vaccine for active immunization is available for individuals 12 months of age and older. Babies born to women in whom chickenpox develops within 5 days of delivery are especially likely to have a severe case of the disease. One attack of the disease usually confers permanent immunity, although recurring episodes of herpes zoster occur, especially in elderly or debilitated people, resulting from reactivation of the virus. Herpes zoster virus (HZV), like all herpesviruses, lies dormant in certain sensory nerve roots after primary infection.

■ NURSING CONSIDERATIONS: Chickenpox in childhood is usually benign. Few cases require hospitalization. It may be serious or fatal in immunocompromised people, such as those infected with human immunodeficiency virus (HIV), those receiving chemotherapy or radiotherapy for malignant disease, those who have undergone organ transplantation, those with congenital or acquired defects in cell-mediated immunity, or those receiving high doses of steroids. Common complications are secondary bacterial infections, such as abscesses, cellulitis, pneumonia, and sepsis, and hemorrhagic varicella (tiny hemorrhages that may occur in the vesicles or surrounding skin). Less common complications are encephalitis, Reye's syndrome (associated with the use of aspirin), thrombocytopenia, and hepatitis.

**chiclero ulcer** /chikler′ō/ [Mex, *tzictli,* chicle; L, *ulcus*], a kind of American leishmaniasis caused by *Leishmania mexicana.* It is endemic among the workers in the Yucatan and Central America who harvest chicle from the forest. The disease is characterized by cutaneous ulcers on the head that usually heal spontaneously by 6 months, except for those on the pinna of the ear, which may last for years and cause scar-

ring and deformities. See also **American leishmaniasis, leishmaniasis.**

**chicory,** a perennial herb found in the United States, India, and Egypt.

■ USES: This herb is used as a coffee substitute, as a source of fructo-oligosaccharides, as a mild laxative for children, and as a treatment for gout, rheumatism, loss of appetite, and digestive distress.

■ CONTRAINDICATIONS: Chicory is contraindicated during pregnancy and lactation and in children. People who have cardiovascular disease or are hypersensitive to chicory or asteraceae/compositae herbs, also should avoid its use, and people with gallstones should use under the supervision of a herbalist.

**Chido-Rodgers blood group** /chē′dō roj′ərz/, a blood group consisting of antigens Ch$^a$ and Rg$^a$, antigenic determinants of fragments of the C4 component of complement.

**chief cell** [Fr, *chef;* L, *cella,* storeroom], 1. also called **zymogenic cell.** any one of the columnar epithelial cells or the cuboidal epithelial cells that line the gastric glands and secrete pepsinogen and intrinsic factor, which are needed for the absorption of vitamin B$_{12}$ and the normal development of red blood cells. Anemia may be caused by the absence of intrinsic factor. 2. any one of the epithelioid cells with pale-staining cytoplasm and a large nucleus containing a prominent nucleolus. Cords of such cells form the main substance of the pineal body. 3. also called **principal cell.** Any one of the polyhedral epithelial cells, within the parathyroid glands, which contain pale, clear cytoplasm and a vesicular nucleus.

**chief complaint (CC),** a subjective statement made by a patient describing his or her most significant or serious symptoms or signs of illness or dysfunction. Used most often in a health history.

**Chief Executive Officer (CEO, C.E.O.),** the most senior official of an organization or institution.

**chief resident,** a senior resident physician who acts temporarily as the clinical and administrative director of the house staff in a department of the hospital. The period of duty varies, depending on the size of the department, the length of the residency, and the number of house staff members.

**chief surgeon,** a surgeon appointed or elected head of the surgeons on the staff of a health care facility.

**chigger** /chig′ər/ [Fr, *chique*], the larva of *Trombicula* mites found in tall grass and weeds. It sticks to the skin and causes irritation and severe itching. Also called **harvest mite, red bugs, red mite.** Compare **chigoe.**

**chigoe** /chig′ō/, a flea, *Tunga penetrans,* found in tropical and subtropical America and Africa. The pregnant female flea burrows into the skin of the feet, causing an inflammatory condition that may lead to spontaneous amputation of a toe. Also called **burrowing flea, jigger, sand flea.** Compare **chigger.**

**chikungunya** /chik′un·gun′yə/ [Swahili, that which bends up], a self-limited disease resembling dengue, seen mainly in Africa and Southeast Asia, caused by an alphavirus transmitted chiefly by mosquitoes of the genus *Aedes;* its most prominent symptoms are musculoskeletal and it has occasionally been associated with hemorrhagic fever.

**chikungunya encephalitis** /chik′ən·gun′yə/ [Swahili, that which bends up; Gk, *enkephalos,* brain, *itis,* inflammation], a togavirus infection characterized by a high fever that begins abruptly, muscle aches, a rash, and pain in the joints. It is transmitted by the bite of a mosquito and occurs mainly in Africa, in Asia, and on some of the Pacific islands, including Guam. The fever may last for a week, then rise again after a remission of several days. Pain in the joints may continue after other symptoms have ceased. Supportive nursing care and symptomatic relief are the only treatments.

**chilblain** /chil'blān/ [AS, *cele,* cold, *bleyn,* blister], redness and swelling of the skin caused by excessive exposure to cold. Burning, itching, blistering, and ulceration that are similar to those characteristic of a thermal burn may occur. Treatment includes protection against cold and injury, gentle warming, and avoidance of tobacco. Also called **pernio.** Compare **frostbite.**

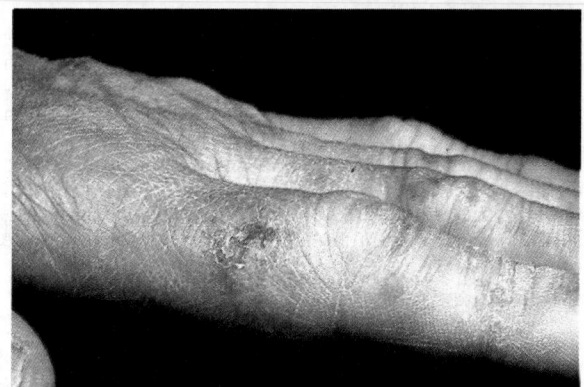

**Chilblain** *(du Vivier, 1993)*

**child** [AS, *cild*],   **1.** a person of either sex between the time of birth and adolescence. **2.** an unborn or recently born human being; fetus, neonate, infant. **3.** an offspring or descendant; a son or daughter or a member of a particular tribe or clan. **4.** one who is like a child or immature.

**child abuse,** the physical, sexual, or emotional maltreatment of a child. Child abuse predominantly affects children less than 3 years of age and is the result of multiple and complex factors involving both the parents and the child, compounded by various stressful environmental circumstances, such as inadequate physical and emotional support within the family and any major life change or crisis, especially those crises arising from marital strife. Parents at high risk for abuse are characterized as having unsatisfied needs, difficulty in forming adequate interpersonal relationships, unrealistic expectations of the child, and a lack of nurturing experience, often involving neglect or abuse in their own childhoods. Predisposing factors among children include the temperament, personality, and activity level of the child; order of birth in the family; sensitivity to parental needs; and requirement for special physical or emotional care resulting from illness, premature birth, or congenital or genetic abnormalities. Identification of abused children or potential child abusers is a major concern for all health care workers. Obvious physical marks on a child's body, as burns, welts, or bruises, and signs of emotional distress, including symptoms of failure to thrive, are common indications of some degree of neglect or abuse. Often, radiograph films to detect healed or new fractures of the extremities or diagnostic tests to identify sexual molestation are necessary. If abuse is suspected, the health care worker is required to make the necessary report. Special counseling services or support groups, such as Parents Anonymous, help families in which a child

**Warning signs of child abuse**

| |
|---|
| Physical evidence of abuse and/or neglect, including previous injuries |
| Conflicting stories about the "accident" or injury from the parents or others |
| Cause of injury blamed on sibling or other party |
| An injury inconsistent with the history, such as a concussion and broken arm from falling off a bed |
| History inconsistent with child's developmental level, such as a 6-month-old turning on the hot water |
| A complaint other than the one associated with signs of abuse (e.g., a chief complaint of a cold when there is evidence of first- and second-degree burns) |
| Inappropriate response of caregiver, such as an exaggerated or absent emotional response; refusal to sign for additional tests or agree to necessary treatment; excessive delay in seeking treatment; absence of the parents for questioning |
| Inappropriate response of child, such as little or no response to pain; fear of being touched; excessive or lack of separation anxiety; indiscriminate friendliness to strangers |
| Child's report of physical or sexual abuse |
| Previous reports of abuse in the family |
| Repeated visits to emergency facilities with injuries |

From Wong DL et al: *Wong's essentials of pediatric nursing,* ed 6, St Louis, 2001, Mosby.

is abused. The nurse can play a significant role in preventing abuse by promoting a positive parent-child relationship, especially in the neonatal period, by teaching parents proper child care and disciplinary techniques; by explaining normal child development and behavior so that parents can formulate realistic guidelines for discipline; and by identifying parents at risk for child abuse. Compare **child neglect.**

**child adaptation to hospitalization,** a nursing outcome from the Nursing Outcome Classification (NOC) defined as child's adaptive response to hospitalization. See also **nursing outcomes classification.**

**childbearing period** [AS, *cild + beran,* to bear; Gk, *peri,* around, *hodos,* way], the reproductive period in a woman's life, from puberty to menopause. It is the time during which she is physiologically able to conceive children.

**childbed fever.** See **puerperal fever.**

**childbirth.** See **birth.**

**childbirth center,** a health facility where prenatal care and delivery services are made available to low-risk pregnant women by a team of nurse-midwives, obstetricians, pediatricians, and ancillary health professionals.

**childbirth preparation,** a nursing intervention from the Nursing Interventions Classification (NIC) defined as providing information and support to facilitate childbirth and to enhance the ability of an individual to develop and perform the role of parent. See also **Nursing Interventions Classification.**

**child development,** the various stages of physical, social, and psychologic growth that occur from birth through young adulthood. See also **adolescence, development, growth, infant, neonatal period, psychosexual development, psychosocial development, toddler.**

**child development: 2 months,** a nursing outcome from the Nursing Outcome Classification (NOC) defined as milestones of physical, cognitive, and psychosocial progression by 2 months of age. See also **nursing outcomes classification.**

**child development: 4 months,** a nursing outcome from the Nursing Outcome Classification (NOC) defined as milestones of physical, cognitive, and psychosocial progression by 4 months of age. See also **nursing outcomes classification.**

**child development: 6 months,** a nursing outcome from the Nursing Outcome Classification (NOC) defined as milestones of physical, cognitive, and psychosocial progression by 6 months of age. See also **nursing outcomes classification.**

**child development: 12 months,** a nursing outcome from the Nursing Outcome Classification (NOC) defined as milestones of physical, cognitive, and psychosocial progression by 12 months of age. See also **nursing outcomes classification.**

**child development: 2 years,** a nursing outcome from the Nursing Outcome Classification (NOC) defined as milestones of physical, cognitive, and psychosocial progression by 2 years of age. See also **nursing outcomes classification.**

**child development: 3 years,** a nursing outcome from the Nursing Outcome Classification (NOC) defined as milestones of physical, cognitive, and psychosocial progression by 3 years of age. See also **nursing outcomes classification.**

**child development: 4 years,** a nursing outcome from the Nursing Outcome Classification (NOC) defined as milestones of physical, cognitive, and psychosocial progression by 4 years of age. See also **nursing outcomes classification.**

**child development: 5 years,** a nursing outcome from the Nursing Outcome Classification (NOC) defined as milestones of physical, cognitive, and psychosocial progression by 5 years of age. See also **nursing outcomes classification.**

**child development: middle childhood (6-11 years),** a nursing outcome from the Nursing Outcome Classification (NOC) defined as milestones of physical, cognitive, and psychosocial progression between 6 and 11 years of age. See also **nursing outcomes classification.**

**child development: adolescence (12-17 years),** a nursing outcome from the Nursing Outcome Classification (NOC) defined as milestones of physical, cognitive, and psychosocial progression between 12 and 17 years of age. See also **nursing outcomes classification.**

**childhood,** 1. the period in human development that extends from birth until the onset of puberty. 2. the state or quality of being a child. See also **development, growth.**

**childhood aphasia,** an inability to process language caused by a brain dysfunction in childhood.

**childhood disintegrative disorder,** pervasive developmental disorder characterized by marked regression in a variety of skills, including language, social skills or adaptive behavior, play, bowel or bladder control, and motor skills, after at least two, but less than ten, years of apparently normal development.

**childhood myxedema** [AS, *cildhad* + Gk, *myxa,* mucus, *oidema,* swelling], a juvenile form of hypothyroidism characterized by atrophy of the thyroid gland after a severe infection of the gland. Also called **juvenile myxedema.**

**childhood-onset pervasive developmental disorders,** disturbances in thought, affect, social relatedness, and behavior that emerge between the ages of 30 months and 12 years of age. An example is autism. See also **pervasive developmental disorder.**

**childhood polycystic disease.** See **polycystic kidney disease.**

**childhood triad,** three types of behavior—fire setting, bedwetting, and cruelty to animals—that may predict emerging sociopathy when they occur consistently or in combination.

**child neglect,** the failure by parents or guardians to provide for the basic human needs of a child by physical or emotional deprivation that interferes with normal growth and development or that places the child in jeopardy. Compare **child abuse.** See also **failure to thrive, maternal deprivation syndrome.**

**child psychology,** the study of the mental, emotional, and behavioral development of infants and children.

**child welfare,** a service agency sponsored by the community or special organizations that provide for the physical, social, or psychologic care of children.

**-chilia.** See **-cheilia.**

**chill** [AS, *cele*], 1. the sensation of cold caused by exposure to a cold environment. 2. an attack of shivering with pallor and a feeling of coldness, often occurring at the beginning of an infection and accompanied by a rapid rise in temperature.

**chilo-,** prefix for medical terms relating to the lips. See also **cheilo-.**

*Chilomastix* /kī′lōmas′tiks/, a genus of flagellate protozoa, as *Chilomastix mesnili,* a nonpathogenic intestinal parasite of humans.

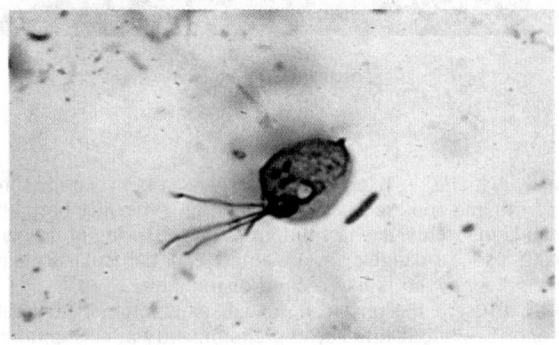

***Chilomastix mesnili* trophozoite**
*(Baron, Peterson, and Finegold, 1994)*

**chimera** /kimir′ə, kīmir′ə/ [Gk, *khimaros,* fire-breathing monster], an organism carrying cell populations derived from two or more different zygotes of the same or different species. Chimeras include recipients of tissue grafts from other individuals. Compare **mosaic.**

**chimerism** /kimir′izəm/, a state in bone marrow transplantation in which bone marrow and host cells exist compatibly without signs of graft-versus-host rejection disease.

**chimney-sweeps' cancer.** See **scrotal cancer.**

**chin,** the raised triangular portion of the mandible below the lower lip. It is formed by the mental protuberance.

**Chinese restaurant syndrome,** a group of transient symptoms consisting of tingling and burning sensations of the skin, facial pressure, headache, and chest pain that occur immediately after eating food containing monosodium glutamate, frequently used in Chinese cooking. It is a pharmacologic reaction and not a allergic reaction

**chin reflex, chin-jerk reflex.** See **mandibular reflex.**

**chinstick.** See **mouthstick.**

**chip** [AS, *kippen,* to slice], 1. a relatively small piece of a bone or tooth. **2.** to break off or cut away a small piece. **3.** a semiconductor in which an integrated circuit is embedded.

**chip fracture,** any small fragmental fracture, usually one involving a bony process near a joint.

**chip graft,** a transplant consisting of small pieces of cartilage or bone that are packed into defective bone structures.

**chir-.** See **cheiro-.**

**chiral,** (in physical science) describing a compound that cannot be superimposed on its mirror image.

**chiralgia** /kəral'jə/, a pain in the hand, particularly one that does not result from a nerve injury or disease.

**chirality.** See **handedness.**

**-chiria, -cheiria, 1.** suffix meaning a '(specified) condition involving hands': *acephalochiria, dichiria.* **2.** suffix meaning a '(specified) condition involving stimulus and its perception': *allochiria, synchiria.*

**chiro-.** See **cheiro-.**

**chiroplasty.** See **cheiroplasty.**

**chiropodist.** See **podiatrist.**

**chiropody.** See **podiatry.**

**chiropractic** /kī'rōprak'tik/ [Gk, *cheir,* hand, *practikos,* efficient], a system of therapy based on the theory that the state of a person's health is determined in general by the condition of his or her nervous system. In most cases treatment provided by chiropractors involves the mechanical manipulation of the spinal column. Some practitioners employ radiology for diagnosis and use physiotherapy and diet in addition to spinal manipulation. Chiropractic does not use drugs or surgery, the primary basis of treatment used by medical physicians. A chiropractor is awarded the degree of Doctor of Chiropractic, or D.C., after completing at least 2 years of premedical studies followed by 4 years of training in an approved chiropractic school. Compare **allopathic physician.**

**chiropractor** /-prak'tər/, a practitioner of **chiropractic.**

**chirospasm.** See **writer's cramp.**

**chisel fracture,** any fracture in which there is oblique detachment of a bone fragment from the head of the radius.

**chi square** ($\chi^2$) /kī/, (in statistics) a statistic test for an association between observed data and expected data represented by frequencies. The test yields a statement of the probability of the obtained distribution having occurred by chance alone.

**chi square distribution** /kī skwar/, a theoretical probability distribution of the sum of the squares of a number *(k)* of normally distributed variables whose mean is 0 and standard deviation is 1; the parameter *k* is the number of degrees of freedom. Also written $\chi^2$ **distribution.**

**Chlamydia** /kləmid'ē-ə/ [Gk, *chlamys,* cloak], **1.** a microorganism of the genus *Chlamydia.* **2.** a genus of microorganisms that live as intracellular parasites, have a number of properties in common with gram-negative bacteria, and are currently classified as specialized bacteria. Three species of *Chlamydia* have been recognized; all are pathogenic to humans. *Chlamydia trachomatis,* an organism that lives in the conjunctiva of the eye and the epithelium of the urethra and cervix, is responsible for inclusion conjunctivitis and the sexually transmitted diseases lymphogranuloma venereum, pelvic inflammatory disease (PID), and trachoma. *Chlamydia* is one of the most common sexually transmitted organisms in North America and a frequent cause of sterility. *Chlamydia psittaci* is an organism that infects birds and causes a type of pneumonia in humans. *Chlamydia pneumoniae* is the causative organism of Taiwan acute respiratory (TWAR) disease, which is responsible for both upper and lower respiratory tract infections and commonly causes community acquired pneumonias. The incubation period ranges from 3 to 21 days. The diagnosis is made by tissue culture or Gram's stain of endocervical or urethral discharge. Treatment consists of one of the following: doxycycline, azithromycin, erythromycin, or ofloxacin. Nursing considerations include encouraging patients to refer for testing any sexual partners of the past 60 days. The nurse should educate the patient about condom use, medications, and avoidance of sexual intercourse until drug therapy is completed and symptoms are gone. See also **psittacosis.** —**chlamydial,** *adj.*

***Chlamydia pneumoniae* pneumonia** /klə·mid'ē·ə nōō·mō'-nē·ē /, a mild form of primary atypical pneumonia caused by infection with *Chlamydia pneumoniae,* characterized by fever, rales, and infiltration of a middle or lower lobe; the recovery period is usually prolonged.

***Chlamydia* test,** a microscopic examination or blood test used to determine the presence of the many *Chlamydia* species that cause human diseases such as respiratory tract infections, sexually transmitted disease, eye disease, genital and urethral infections, and pelvic inflammatory disease.

***Chlamydia trachomatis* pneumonia** /klə·mid'ē·ə trəkom'ə·tis/, a mild type of bacterial pneumonia, usually seen in infants whose mothers are infected with *Chlamydia trachomatis;* characteristics include coughing, tachypnea, and eosinophilia.

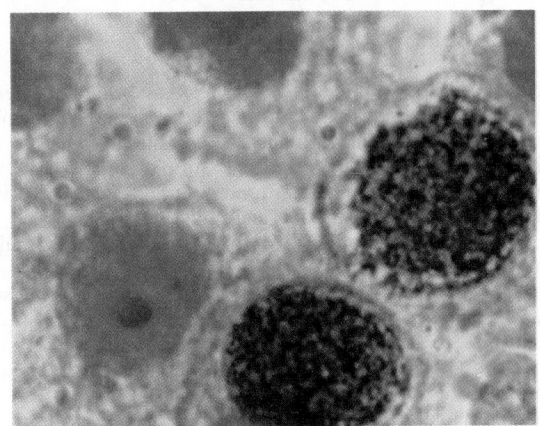

***Chlamydia trachomatis*** *(Tilton, Ballows, and Hohnadel, 1992)*

**chloasma** /klō·az'mə/ [Gk, *chloazein,* to be green], tan or brown pigmentation, particularly of the forehead, cheeks, and nose, commonly associated with pregnancy or the use of oral contraceptives. The hyperpigmentation may be permanent or may disappear, only to recur with subsequent pregnancies or use of oral contraceptives. Also called **mask of pregnancy, melasma.**

**chloasma traumaticum,** a pigmentary discoloration that results from friction on the skin.

**chloasma uterinum,** a skin discoloration that occurs in pregnant women or in diseases of the ovary or uterus.

**chlor-,** combining form meaning 'green': *chloremia, chlorephidrosis, chlorine.*

**chloracne** /klôrak'nē/ [Gk, *chloros,* green, *akme,* point], a skin condition characterized by small, black follicular plugs and papules on exposed surfaces, especially on the arms, face, and neck of workers in contact with chlorinated com-

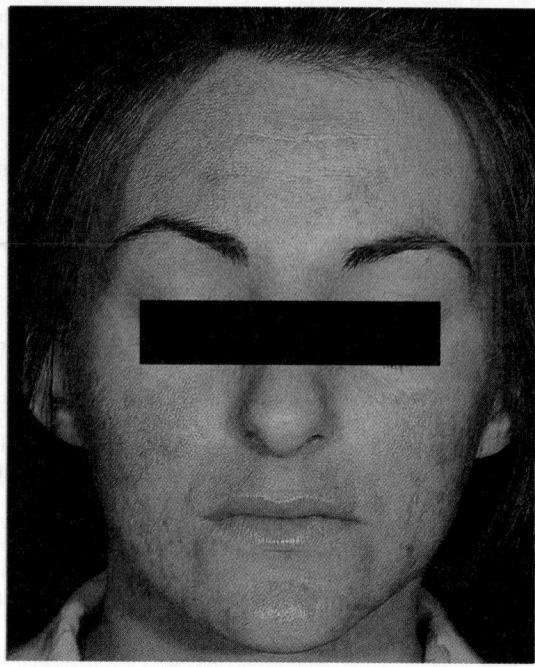

**Chloasma** *(Habif, 1996)*

pounds, such as cutting oils, paints, varnishes, and lacquers. Avoidance of contact with chlorinated compounds or the use of protective garments prevents the condition.

**chloral camphor** /klôr′əl/, a mixture of equal parts of camphor and chloral hydrate, used externally as a sedative.

**chloral hydrate,** a sedative and hypnotic.

■ INDICATIONS: It is prescribed for the relief of insomnia, anxiety, or tension.

■ CONTRAINDICATIONS: Liver or kidney dysfunction or known hypersensitivity to this drug prohibits its use.

■ ADVERSE EFFECTS: Among the more serious adverse reactions are GI disturbances, skin rash, paradoxic excitement, and hypotension.

**chloral hydrate poisoning,** an adverse reaction to ingestion of trichloroethylidine glycol, also known as chloral hydrate, which is sometimes used as a hypnotic because of its depressive effects on the central nervous system. Symptoms include irritation of the digestive tract, vomiting, depressed breathing, shock, confusion, and injury to the liver and kidneys.

**chlorambucil** /klôr′ambo͞o′sil/, an alkylating agent.

■ INDICATIONS: It is prescribed in the treatment of a variety of malignant neoplastic diseases, including chronic lymphocytic leukemia and Hodgkin's disease.

■ CONTRAINDICATIONS: Bone marrow depression or known hypersensitivity to this drug prohibits its use. It is not given during the first trimester of pregnancy or within 28 days of chemotherapy or radiation therapy.

■ ADVERSE EFFECTS: Among the more serious adverse reactions are bone marrow depression, GI disturbance, skin rash, and hepatotoxicity.

**chloramphenicol** /-amfē′nikol/, an antibacterial and antirickettsial.

■ INDICATIONS: It is prescribed in the treatment of a wide variety of serious infections.

■ CONTRAINDICATIONS: Mild or unidentified infections, pregnancy, lactation, or known hypersensitivity to this drug prohibits its use.

■ ADVERSE EFFECTS: Among the more serious adverse reactions are blood dyscrasias, bone marrow depression, and aplastic anemia.

**chlordane poisoning.** See **chlorinated organic insecticide poisoning.**

**chlordiazepoxide** /klôr′dī·az′əpok′sīd/, a minor tranquilizer of the benzodiazepine type.

■ INDICATIONS: It is prescribed in the treatment of anxiety, nervous tension, and alcohol withdrawal symptoms.

■ CONTRAINDICATIONS: Psychosis, acute narrow-angle glaucoma, or known hypersensitivity to this drug prohibits its use.

■ ADVERSE EFFECTS: Among the more serious adverse reactions are withdrawal symptoms that appear on discontinuation of treatment. Drowsiness and fatigue commonly occur.

**chlorhexidine** /-hek′sidēn/, an antimicrobial agent used as a surgical scrub, hand rinse, and topical antiseptic.

**chlorhydria.** See **hyperchlorhydria.**

**-chloric,** suffix meaning 'referring to or containing chlorine': *hydrochloric, hyperchloric, perchloric.*

**chloride** /klôr′īd/ [Gk, *chloros,* green], an anion of chlorine. Metal chlorides are salts of hydrochloric acid; the most common is sodium chloride (table salt).

**chloride shift,** an exchange of chloride ions in red blood cells in peripheral tissues in response to $PCO_2$ of blood. The shift reverses in the lungs.

**chloridometer** /klôr′idom′ətər/, an instrument for measuring the level of chlorides in body fluids.

**chloriduria,** an excessive level of chlorides in the urine.

**chlorinated** /klôr′ənā′tid/ [Gk, *chloros,* greenish], pertaining to material that contains or has been treated with chlorine.

**chlorinated organic insecticide poisoning,** poisoning resulting from the inhalation, ingestion, or absorption of chlorophenothane (DDT) and other insecticides containing chlorophenothane, as heptachlor, dieldrin, and chlordane. It is characterized by vomiting, weakness, malaise, convulsions, tremors, ventricular fibrillation, respiratory failure, and pulmonary edema. Also called **DDT poisoning.**

**chlorination** [Gk, *chloros,* green], the disinfection or treatment of water or other substances with free chlorine.

**chlorine (Cl)** /klôr′ēn/, a yellowish green gaseous element of the halogen group. Its atomic number is 17; its atomic weight (mass) is 35.453. It has a strong, distinctive odor; is irritating to the respiratory tract; and is poisonous if ingested or inhaled. It occurs in nature chiefly as a component of sodium chloride in sea water and in salt deposits. It is used as a bleach and as a disinfectant to purify water for drinking or for use in swimming pools. Chlorine compounds in general use include many solvents, cleaning fluids, and chloroform. Most of the solvents and cleaning fluids containing chlorine are toxic when inhaled or ingested. Chloroform was formerly in general use as an anesthetic.

**chloroform** /klôr′əfôrm′/ [Gk, *chloros* + L, *formica,* ant], a nonflammable volatile liquid that was the first inhalation anesthetic to be discovered. Chloroform has a low margin of safety and significant toxicity. The drug is not used in the United States.

**chloroformism** /-iz′əm/, 1. the habit of inhaling chloroform for its narcotic effect. 2. the anesthetic effect of chloroform.

**chloroleukemia** /klôr′ōlo͞okē′mē·ə/ [GK, *chloros,* green, *leukos,* white, *haima,* blood], a kind of myelogenous leukemia in which specific tumor masses are not seen at autopsy but body fluids and organs are green. See also **myelogenous leukemia.**

**chlorolymphosarcoma** /-lim'fōsärkō'mə/, *pl.* **chlorolymphosarcomas, chlorolymphosarcomata** [Gk, *chloros* + L, *lympha,* water; Gk, *sarx,* flesh, *oma,* tumor], a greenish neoplasm of myeloid tissue occurring in patients with myelogenous leukemia. The mononuclear cells in the peripheral blood are believed to be lymphocytes rather than myeloblasts, such as found with chloroma.

**chloroma** /klôrō'mə/, *pl.* **chloromas, chloromata,** a malignant, greenish neoplasm of myeloid tissue that occurs anywhere in the body of patients who have myelogenous leukemia. The green pigment is primarily myeloperoxidase (verdoperoxidase). The tumor tissue fluoresces bright red under ultraviolet light. Also called **chloromyeloma, granulocytic sarcoma, green cancer.**

**Chloromycetin,** trademark for an antibacterial and antirickettsial (chloramphenicol).

**chloromyeloma.** See **chloroma.**

**chlorophyll** /klôr'əfil/ [Gk, *chloros* + *phyllon,* leaf], one of several pigments that absorb light energy and participate in the production of carbohydrates in photosynthetic organisms. Chlorophylls a and b are found in plants, chlorophyll c occurs in brown algae, and chlorophyll d occurs in red algae. See **photosynthesis.**

**chloroprocaine** /-prō'kān/, a local anesthetic with a chemical structure similar to that of procaine.

**chloroquine** /klôr'əkwīn'/, an antimalarial.

■ INDICATIONS: It is prescribed in the treatment of malaria, extraintestinal amebiasis, rheumatoid arthritis, some forms of lupus erythematosus, and photoallergic reactions.

■ CONTRAINDICATIONS: Retinal or visual field changes, porphyria, or known hypersensitivity to this drug prohibits its use.

■ ADVERSE EFFECTS: Among the more serious adverse reactions are GI disturbances, headache, visual disturbances resulting from retinal damage, and pruritus.

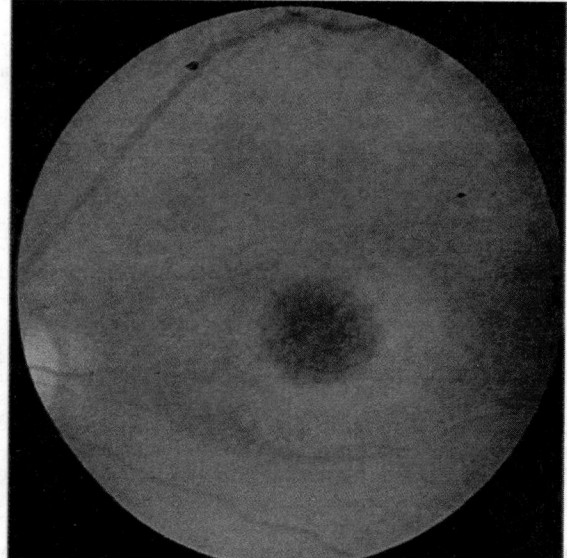

**Retinal damage caused by chloroquine** *(Shipley, 1993)*

**chlorosis** /klôrō'sis/, *obsolete.* an iron deficiency anemia of young women characterized by hypochromic, microcytic erythrocytes and a small reduction in the total number of erythrocytes. See also **anemia.**

**chlorothiazide** /-thī'əzīd/, a thiazide diuretic chemically related to sulfonamides; an antihypertensive.

■ INDICATIONS: It is prescribed in the treatment of hypertension and edema.

■ CONTRAINDICATIONS: Anuria or known hypersensitivity to thiazide medication or to sulfonamide derivatives prohibits its use.

■ ADVERSE EFFECTS: Among the more serious adverse reactions are hypokalemia, hyperglycemia, and hyperuricemia. Hypersensitivity reactions may occur.

**chlorpheniramine maleate** /-fenir'əmēn/, an antihistamine.

■ INDICATIONS: It is prescribed in the treatment of a variety of hypersensitivity reactions, including rhinitis, skin rash, and pruritus.

■ CONTRAINDICATIONS: Asthma or known hypersensitivity to this drug prohibits its use. It is not given to newborns or lactating mothers.

■ ADVERSE EFFECTS: Among the more serious adverse reactions are skin rash, hypersensitivity reactions, and tachycardia. Drowsiness and dry mouth commonly occur.

**chlorpromazine** /-prō'məzēn/, a phenothiazine tranquilizer and antiemetic.

■ INDICATIONS: It is prescribed in the treatment of psychotic disorders, severe nausea and vomiting, and intractable hiccups.

■ CONTRAINDICATIONS: Parkinson's disease, concurrent administration of central nervous system depressants, liver or renal dysfunction, severe hypotension, or known hypersensitivity to this drug or to other phenothiazine medication prohibits its use.

■ ADVERSE EFFECTS: Among the more serious adverse effects are hypotension, liver toxicity, a variety of extrapyramidal reactions, blood dyscrasias, and hypersensitivity reactions.

**chlorpropamide** /-prō'pəmīd/, an oral antidiabetic.

■ INDICATION: It is prescribed in the treatment of non-insulin-dependent diabetes mellitus.

■ CONTRAINDICATIONS: Liver or kidney dysfunction or known hypersensitivity to this drug prohibits its use.

■ ADVERSE EFFECTS: Among the most serious adverse reactions are hematologic derangements and jaundice. Hypoglycemia, GI distress, and rashes are common adverse effects.

**chlortetracycline hydrochloride** /-tet'rəsī'klēn/, a tetracycline antibiotic used as a topical antiinfective.

■ INDICATIONS: It is prescribed in the treatment of bacterial infections.

■ CONTRAINDICATIONS: It is available topically only and has little systemic effect. Known hypersensitivity to this drug or to other tetracycline medication prohibits its use.

■ ADVERSE EFFECTS: Burning, stinging, and yellowing of the skin may occur.

**chlorthalidone** /-thal'idōn/, a diuretic and antihypertensive; a sulfonamide derivative.

■ INDICATIONS: It is prescribed in the treatment of high blood pressure and edema.

■ CONTRAINDICATIONS: Anuria or known hypersensitivity to this drug, to other thiazide medication, or to sulfonamide derivatives prohibits its use.

■ ADVERSE EFFECTS: Among the more serious adverse reactions are hypokalemia, hyperglycemia, hyperuricemia, and hypersensitivity reactions.

**Chlor-Trimeton,** trademark for an older antihistamine (chlorpheniramine maleate).

**chlorzoxazone** /-zok'səzōn/, a skeletal muscle relaxant.

■ INDICATION: It is prescribed for the relief of muscle spasm.

■ CONTRAINDICATION: Impaired liver function and known hypersensitivity to this drug are contraindications.

■ ADVERSE EFFECTS: Among the more serious adverse reactions are jaundice and GI bleeding.

**CHN,** abbreviation for *Certified Hemodialysis Nurse.*

**choana** /kō'ənə/, *pl.* **choanae**, 1. a funnel-shaped channel. 2. See **posterior nares.**

**choanal atresia** /kō'ənəl/ [Gk, *choane,* funnel, *a + tresis,* not hole], a congenital anomaly in which a bony or membranous occlusion blocks the passageway between the nose and pharynx. The condition, which is caused by the failure of the nasopharyngeal septum to rupture during embryonic development, can result in serious ventilation problems in the neonate; therefore providing an oral airway or endotracheal intubation may be necessary. The defect is usually repaired surgically shortly after birth.

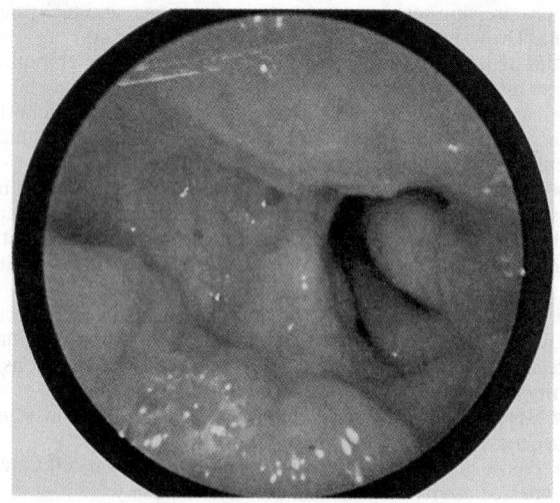

**Unilateral choanal atresia** *(Zitelli and Davis, 1997)*

**chocolate cyst** [Mex, *chocolatl* + Gk, *kystis,* bag], a darkly pigmented cyst sometimes found on the ovaries as a result of endometriosis. It results from an accumulation of extra uterine endometrial tissue.

**choke** [ME, *choken*], to interrupt breathing by compression or obstruction of the larynx or trachea.

**choke damp.** See **damp.**

**choked disc.** See **papilledema.**

**chokes,** a respiratory condition, occurring in decompression sickness, characterized by shortness of breath, substernal pain, and a nonproductive paroxysmal cough caused by bubbles of gas in the blood vessels of the lungs.

**choke-saver,** a curved forceps that can be inserted into the throat of a person who is choking on a food bolus or similar swallowed object. The tweezerlike device can grasp and retrieve the object.

**choking,** the condition in which a respiratory passage is blocked by constriction of the neck, an obstruction in the trachea, or swelling of the larynx. It is characterized by de-

creased movement of air through the airways or sudden coughing and a red face that rapidly becomes cyanotic. The person cannot breathe and clutches his or her throat. Emergency treatment requires removal of the obstruction and resuscitation if necessary. See also **Heimlich maneuver.**

**chol-.** See **chole-.**

**cholagogue** /kō'ləgog/ [Gk, *chole,* bile, *agogein,* to draw forth], a drug that stimulates the flow of bile.

**cholangiectasis** /kōlan'jē·ek'təsis/, dilation of the bile ducts.

**cholangiocarcinoma** /kōlan'jē·ōkär'sinō'mə/, a cancer of the biliary epithelium. Risk factors include ulcerative colitis and infestation of liver flukes. Diagnosis is based on histologic evaluation, and the prognosis is poor.

**cholangiocellular carcinoma.** See **cholangiohepatoma.**

**cholangiogram** /kōlan'jē·əgram'/, an x-ray film of the bile ducts produced after injection of a radiopaque contrast medium. A cholangiogram is routinely performed before or after biliary tract surgery. A postoperative radiogram may be made after injecting an iodinated contrast medium through an indwelling T-tube. The medium also may be introduced directly into the biliary system or intravenously. See also **cholangiography, cholecystography.**

**cholangiography** /kōlan'jē·og'rəfē/, a special roentgenographic test procedure for outlining the major bile ducts by the IV injection or direct instillation of a radiopaque contrast material.

■ METHOD: For IV cholangiography the contrast agent is given slowly by vein, and x-ray films are taken of the region of the gallbladder. Operative and postoperative cholangiography use the injection of contrast material into the common bile duct via a drainage T-tube inserted during surgery to reveal any small, residual gallstones that are present. In percutaneous transhepatic cholangiography the contrast material is injected through a long needle or needle catheter, which is introduced directly through the skin into the substance of the liver. Endoscopic retrograde cholangiography is accomplished by cannulating the ampulla of Vater through a flexible fiberoptic duodenoscope and instilling radiopaque material directly into the common bile duct.

■ INTERVENTIONS: IV cholangiography cannot be used in the presence of severe liver disease or jaundice, because the dye will not be concentrated and excreted into the bile. The patient fasts, and fluids are restricted overnight. An early morning cleansing enema is given, usually followed by a sedative. The patient is warned about a brief burning sensation that occurs as the dye is injected. For percutaneous transhepatic cholangiography, sedative premedication is often ordered and a local anesthetic injected at the site of needle puncture. Appropriate evaluation for bleeding tendencies must be carried out before percutaneous transhepatic cholangiography. Bile peritonitis is occasionally a complication of T-tube or percutaneous cholangiography, and close nursing observation is essential after the test is completed. For endoscopic retrograde cholangiography, nothing is given by mouth after midnight, an explanation is given to the patient, dentures are removed, and, to permit administration of medications, IV infusion is begun. The endoscope is passed with the patient in the left lateral position; then the patient is turned to the prone position, the ampulla is cannulated, the dye is injected, and films are taken. Vital signs are observed and the patient is given a light meal 2 to 4 hours after the procedure.

■ OUTCOME CRITERIA: The resulting cholangiograms from any of these procedures are examined for unobstructed outlining of the biliary system. Calculi may be noted as shadows within the opaque medium. See also **cholecystography.**

**cholangiohepatitis** /kō·lan′jē·ōhep′ə·tī′tis/ [Gk, *chole*, bile +*angeion*, vessel +*hepar*, liver + *-itis*, suffix indicating inflammation], severe inflammation of the bile passages, often associated with liver fluke infestation that causes obstruction of the bile ducts.

**cholangiohepatoma** /kōlan′jē·ōhep′ətō′mə/, *pl.* **cholangiohepatomas, cholangiohepatomata**, a primary carcinoma of the liver that develops in the bile ducts in which an abnormal mixture of liver cord cells and bile ducts exists. Also called **cholangiocarcinoma, cholangiocellular carcinoma.** See also **hepatoma.**

**cholangiolitis** /-lī′tis/, an abnormal condition characterized by inflammation of the fine tubules of the bile duct system, which may cause cholangiolitic cirrhosis. —**cholangiolitic,** *adj.*

**cholangioma** /kōlan′jē·ō′mə/, *pl.* **cholangiomas, cholangiomata**, a neoplasm of the bile ducts.

**cholangioscopy** /kōlan′jē·os′kəpē/, direct examination of the bile ducts with a fiberoptic endoscope.

**cholangiostomy** /kōlan′jē·os′təmē/ [Gk, *chole*, bile, *angeion*, vessel, *stoma*, mouth], a surgical operation performed to form an opening in a bile duct.

**cholangitis** /kō′lanjī′tis/, inflammation of the bile ducts, caused either by bacterial invasion or by obstruction of the ducts by calculi or a tumor. The condition is characterized by severe right upper quadrant pain, jaundice (if an obstruction is present), and intermittent fever. Blood tests reveal an elevated level of serum bilirubin. Diagnosis is made by ultrasound evaluation and cholangiography. Treatment uses antibiotics for infection and surgery for acute obstruction. See also **biliary calculus.**

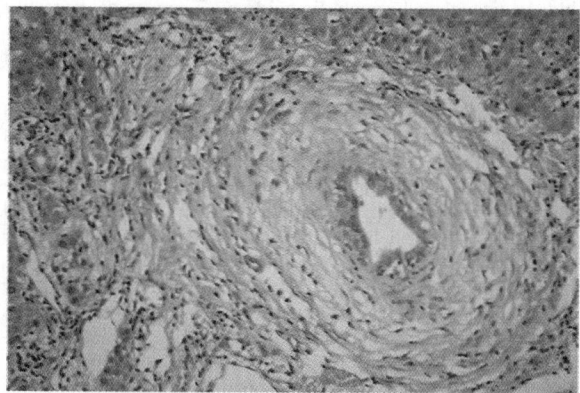

**Primary sclerosing cholangitis**
*(Cotran, Kumar, and Collins, 1999)*

**cholate,** any salt or ester of cholic acid; an anion of cholic acid.

**chole-, chol-, cholo-,** combining form meaning 'bile': *cholecystectomy, cholelithotomy, cholesterase.*

**cholecalciferol.** See **vitamin D₃.**

**cholecystagogue** /kō′ləsis′təgog′/, a drug that stimulates emptying of the gallbladder.

**cholecystalgia.** See **biliary colic.**

**cholecystectomy** /kō′lisistek′təmē/ [Gk, *chole* + *kystis*, bag, *ektomē*, excision], the surgical removal of the gallbladder, performed to treat cholelithiasis and cholecystitis.

Surgery may be delayed while the acute inflammation is treated. Before surgery an electrocardiogram and tests of hepatic function may be ordered. Under general anesthesia, the gallbladder is excised and the cystic duct ligated; the common duct is searched, and any stones found are removed. The most common complication is disruption of the hepatic or other ducts of the biliary system, requiring surgical correction. Wound infection, hemorrhage, bile leakage, and jaundice may also occur. When possible, cholecystectomy is done as a laparoscopic procedure. See also **cholecystitis, cholelithiasis.**

**cholecystic** /kō′lisis′tik/, pertaining to the gallbladder.

**cholecystitis** /kō′lisistī′tis/ [Gk, *chole* + *kystis*, bag, *itis*, inflammation], acute or chronic inflammation of the gallbladder. **Acute cholecystitis** is usually caused by a gallstone that cannot pass through the cystic duct. Pain is felt in the right upper quadrant of the abdomen, accompanied by nausea, vomiting, eructation, and flatulence. The patient may exhibit a positive Murphy's sign. Diagnosis is usually made with ultrasound. Surgery is the preferred mode of treatment. **Chronic cholecystitis,** the more common type, has an insidious onset. Pain, often felt at night, may follow a fatty meal. Complications include biliary calculi, pancreatitis, and carcinoma of the gallbladder. Again surgery is the preferred treatment. See also **biliary calculus, cholecystectomy, cholelithiasis.**

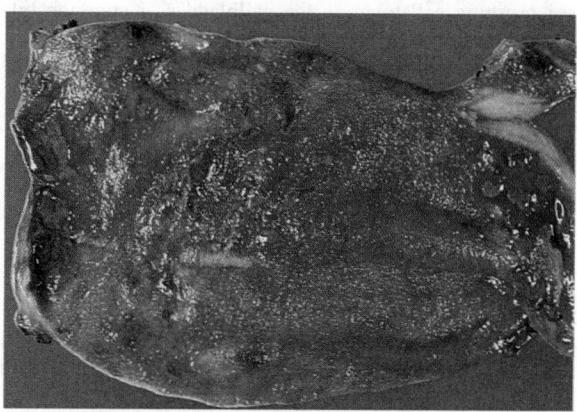

**Acute cholecystitis** *(Damjanov and Linder, 2000)*

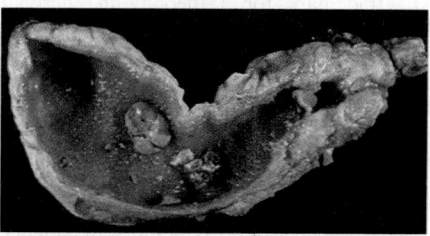

**Chronic cholecystitis** *(Fletcher and McKee, 1987)*

**cholecystoduodenostomy** /kō′lē·sis′tō·dōō′ō·də·nos′tə·mē/ [Gk, *chole* + *kystis* + L, *duodeni,* twelve fingers], surgical anastomosis of the gallbladder and the duodenum.

**cholecystogram** /kō′lisis′təgram′/, an x-ray film of the gallbladder, made after the ingestion or injection of a radiopaque substance, usually a contrast material containing iodine.

**cholecystography** /kō′lisistog′rəfē/, an x-ray examination of the gallbladder. At least 12 hours before the study the patient has a fat-free meal and ingests a contrast material containing iodine, usually in the form of tablets; it may also be given intravenously. The iodine, which is opaque to x-rays, is excreted by the liver into the bile in the gallbladder. After the procedure the patient consumes a fatty meal or cholecystokinin, which stimulates the gallbladder to contract, expelling bile and contrast material into the bile duct. Additional x-ray films are taken about 1 hour later. The test is useful in the diagnosis of cholecystitis, cholelithiasis, and tumors and in the differential diagnosis of a mass in the upper right quadrant of the stomach.

**cholecystoileostomy** /kō′lisis′tō-il′ē-os′təmē/ [Gk, *chole*, bile, *kystis*, bag, *eilein*, to twist, *stoma*, mouth], a surgical procedure performed to connect the gallbladder to the ileum.

**cholecystojejunostomy** /kō′lē-sis′tō-jə-jōō-nos′tə-mē/ [Gk, *chole* + *kystis* + L, *jejunus*, empty], surgical anastomosis of the gallbladder and the jejunum.

**cholecystokinin** /-kī′nin/ [Gk, *chole* + *kystis*, bag, *kinein*, to move], a hormone, produced by the mucosa of the upper intestine, that stimulates contraction of the gallbladder and secretion of pancreatic enzymes.

**cholecystolithiasis** /kō′lisis′tōlithī′əsis/, the presence of gallstones in the gallbladder.

**cholecystolithotripsy** /kō′lisis′tōlith′ətripsē/, a procedure for crushing gallstones in the gallbladder or common bile duct with a lithotrite.

**cholecystosonography** /kō′lisis′tōsōnog′rəfē/, a method of examining the gallbladder using ultrasound.

**choledochal** /-dok′əl/ [Gk, *chole*, bile, *dochus*, containing], pertaining to the common bile duct.

**choledochojejunostomy** /-dok′ōjē′jōōnos′təmē/ [Gk, *chole*, bile, *dochus*, containing; L, *jejunus*, empty; Gk, *stoma*, mouth], a surgical procedure in which the bile duct is connected to the jejunum.

**choledocholith** /kōled′əkōlith′/, a gallstone in the common bile duct.

**choledocholithiasis.** See **biliary calculus.**

**choledocholithotomy** /-lithot′əmē/ [Gk, *chole* + *dochus*, containing, *lithos*, stone, *temnein*, to cut], a surgical operation to make an incision in the common bile duct to remove a stone.

**choledocholithotripsy** /-lith′ətrip′sē/, a procedure for crushing gallstones in the common bile duct with a lithotrite.

**choledocholitis,** an inflammation of the common bile duct.

**Choledyl,** trademark for a theophylline derivative (oxtriphylline).

**choleic** /kōlē′ik/, pertaining to bile.

**cholelithiasis** /-lithī′əsis/ [Gk, *chole* + *lithos*, stone, *osis*, condition], the presence of gallstones in the gallbladder. The condition affects about 20% of the population above 40 years of age and is more prevalent in women and in persons with cirrhosis of the liver. Many patients complain of unlocalized abdominal discomfort, eructation, and intolerance to certain foods; others have no symptoms. In patients with severe attacks of biliary pain associated with cholelithiasis, cholecystectomy is recommended to prevent such complications as cholecystitis, cholangitis, and pancreatitis. Also called **chololithiasis.** See also **biliary calculus, cholecystitis.**

**cholelithic dyspepsia** /kō′lilith′ik/ [Gk, *chole* + *lithos*, stone, *dys*, bad, *peptein*, to digest], an abnormal condition characterized by sudden attacks of indigestion associated with dysfunction of the gallbladder. See **dyspepsia.**

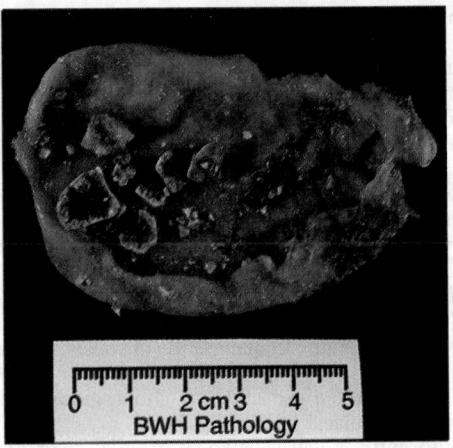

**Cholelithiasis** *(Kumar, Cotran, and Robbins, 1997)*

**cholelithotomy** /-lithot′əmē/, a surgical operation to remove gallstones through an incision in the gallbladder.

**cholera** /kol′ərə/ [Gk, *chole* + *rhein*, to flow], an acute bacterial infection of the small intestine, characterized by severe diarrhea and vomiting, muscular cramps, dehydration, and depletion of electrolytes. The disease is spread by water and food that have been contaminated by feces of persons previously infected. The symptoms are caused by toxic substances produced by the infecting organism, *Vibrio cholerae*. The profuse, watery diarrhea, as much as a liter an hour, depletes the body of fluids and electrolytes. Complications include circulatory collapse, cyanosis, destruction of kidney tissue, and metabolic acidosis. The rate of mortality is as high as 50% if the infection remains untreated. Treatment includes, first and foremost, replacement of fluids and electrolytes (oral rehydration therapy) or IV fluids and, second, the administration of antibiotics. A cholera vaccine is available for people traveling to areas where the infection is endemic but is of limited effacacy. Other preventive measures include drinking only water that has been boiled or decontaminated by iodine or commercially bottled water and eating only cooked foods. See also *Vibrio cholerae, vibrio gastroenteritis*.

**choleragen** /kol′ərəjin/, an exotoxin, produced by the cholera vibrio, that stimulates the secretion of electrolytes and water into the small intestine in Asiatic cholera, draining body fluids and weakening the patient.

**cholera sicca,** a form of cholera in which the patient dies of toxemia before the usual symptoms of vomiting and diarrhea develop. Also called **cholera siderans, dry cholera.**

**cholera vaccine,** an active immunizing agent against cholera.

■ INDICATION: It is prescribed as an immunization against cholera.

■ CONTRAINDICATIONS: Immunosuppression, acute infection, concomitant administration of corticosteroids, or known hypersensitivity to this drug prohibits its use.

■ ADVERSE EFFECTS: The most serious adverse reaction is anaphylaxis.

**choleresis** /kō′lərē′sis/, the secretion of bile by the liver.

**choleretic** /kō′ləret′ik/ [Gk, *chole* + *eresis*, removal], **1.** stimulating the production of bile in the liver either by cholepoiesis or by hydrocholeresis. **2.** a choleretic agent.

**choleric** /kol′ərik, kəler′ik/, having a hot temper or an irritable nature.

**choleriform** /kōler′ifôrm/, resembling cholera. Also **choleroid.**

**cholescintigraphy** /kō′ləsintig′rəfē/, examination of the gallbladder and bile ducts by scanning with radionuclides.

**cholestasis** /-stā′sis/ [Gk, *chole* + *stasis,* standing still], interruption in the flow of bile through any part of the biliary system, from liver to duodenum. It is essential for the physician to discover whether the cause is within the liver (intrahepatic) or outside it (extrahepatic). Intrahepatic causes include hepatitis, drug and alcohol use, metastatic carcinoma, and pregnancy. Extrahepatic causes include presence of an obstructing calculus or tumor in the common bile duct and carcinoma of the pancreas. Symptoms of both types of cholestasis include jaundice, pale and fatty stools, dark urine, and intense itching over the skin. If liver disease is suspected, liver biopsy examination can confirm the suspicion, and attempts can be made to treat the underlying disorder. Extrahepatic cholestasis usually requires surgery. See also **cholestatic hepatitis, hyperbilirubinemia of the newborn. —cholestatic,** *adj.*

**cholestatic hepatitis,** a variant of viral hepatitis. Signs are persistent jaundice, itching, and elevated alkaline phosphatase levels. These signs usually abate when the hepatitis remits. See also **cholestasis, hepatitis.**

**cholestatic jaundice** /-stat′ik/, a yellowing of the skin caused by thickening of bile, obstruction of hepatic ducts, or changes in liver cell function.

**cholesteatoma** /kōles′tē·ətō′mə/ [Gk, *chole* + *stear,* fat, *oma,* tumor], a cystic mass composed of epithelial cells and cholesterol that is found in the middle ear and occurs as a congenital defect or as a serious complication of chronic otitis media. The mass may occlude the middle ear, or enzymes produced by it may destroy the adjacent bones, including the ossicles. Surgery is required to remove a cholesteatoma. See also **otitis media.**

**cholesterase** /kəles′tərās′/ [Gk, *chole* + *aither,* air; Ger, *Saure,* acid; *ase,* enzyme suffix], an enzyme in the blood and other tissues that forms cholesterol and fatty acids by hydrolyzing cholesterol esters.

**cholesteremia.** See **cholesterolemia.**

**cholesterol** /kəles′tərôl/ [Gk, *chole* + *steros,* solid], a waxy lipid soluble compound found only in animal tissues. A member of a group of compounds called sterols, it is an integral component of every cell in the body. It facilitates the absorption and transport of fatty acids. Cholesterol acts as the precursor for the synthesis of various steroid hormones, including cortisol, cortisone, and aldosterone in the adrenal glands; and of the sex hormones progesterone, estrogen, and testosterone. It sometimes precipitates along with

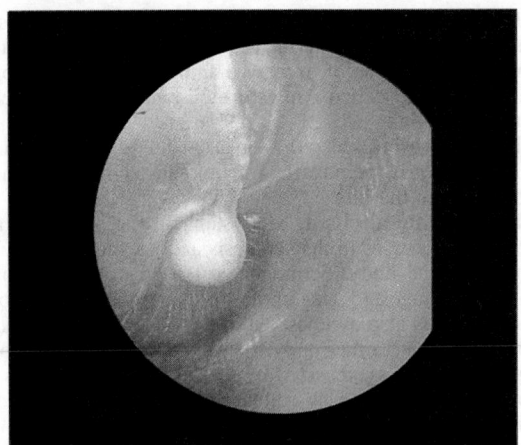

**Cholesteatoma within the eardrum**
*(Zitelli and Davis, 1987/Courtesy Dr. Sylvan Stool)*

other compounds in the gallbladder to form gallstones. Cholesterol is found in foods of animal origin and is continuously synthesized in the body, primarily in the liver. Increased levels of low-density lipoprotein cholesterol may be associated with the pathogenesis of atherosclerosis, whereas higher levels of high-density lipoprotein cholesterol appear to lower the person's risk for heart disease. Normal adult levels of blood cholesterol are 150 to 200 mg/dL or 3.9 to 5.2 mmol/L (SI units). Also called **cholesterin.** See also **high-density lipoprotein (HDL), low-density lipoprotein (LDL), sterol.**

**Chemical structure of cholesterol**
*(Thibodeau and Patton, 1999)*

**Treatment decisions for high blood cholesterol based on LDL cholesterol levels**

| Patient category | Initiation level | LDL goal |
|---|---|---|
| **Dietary therapy** | | |
| Without CAD and with fewer than two risk factors | ≥160 mg/dl (4.1 mmol/L) | ≤160 mg/dL (4.1 mmol/L) |
| Without CAD and with two or more risk factors | ≥130 mg/dl (3.4 mmol/L) | ≤130 mg/dL (3.4 mmol/L) |
| With CAD | >100 mg/dl (2.6 mmol/L) | ≤100 mg/dL (2.6 mmol/L) |
| **Drug treatment** | | |
| Without CAD and with fewer than two risk factors | ≥190 mg/dl (4.9 mmol/L) | ≤130 mg/dL (4.1 mmol/L) |
| Without CAD and with two or more risk factors | ≥160 mg/dl (4.1 mmol/L) | ≤130 mg/dL (3.4 mmol/L) |
| With CAD | ≥130 mg/dl (3.4 mmol/L) | ≤100 mg/dL (2.6 mmol/L) |

From Summary of the Second Report of the National Cholesterol Education Program (NCEP) Expert Panel on Detection, Evaluation, and Treatment of High Cholesterol in Adults (Adult Treatment Panel II), *Circulation* 89:1330, 1996.
*CAD,* Coronary artery disease: *LDL,* low-density lipoprotein.

**cholesterolemia** /-ē′mē·ə/, **1.** the presence of excessive amounts of cholesterol in the blood. **2.** the abnormal condition of the presence of excessive amounts of cholesterol in the blood. Also called **cholesteremia.** See also **hypercholesterolemia.**

**cholesteroleresis** /kəles′tərôler′isis, -erē′sis/ [Gk, *chole, steros + eresis,* removal], the increased elimination of cholesterol in the bile.

**cholesterol metabolism,** the sum of the anabolic and catabolic processes in the synthesis and degradation of cholesterol in the body. Serum cholesterol level is increased when it is ingested and cholestorol is quickly absorbed. Cholesterol is also synthesized in the liver and can be synthesized by most other body tissues. As more cholesterol is ingested, less is synthesized by the body. Cholesterol is removed from the body by conversion in the liver and excretion in the bile.

**cholesterolopoiesis** /kəles′tərō′lōpō·ē′sis/ [Gk, *chole + steros + poiesis,* producing], the elaboration of cholesterol by the liver.

**cholesterolosis** /kəles′tərəlō′sis/, an abnormal condition, found in about 5% of patients with chronic cholecystitis, in which deposits of cholesterol occur within large macrophages in the submucosa of the gallbladder. This produces a spotty appearance, sometimes referred to as a strawberry gallbladder. Cholesterolosis is often associated with gallstones and may be asymptomatic or accompanied by biliary colic. Also called **cholesterosis.** See also **cholecystitis.**

**cholesterol-restricted diet.** See **low-cholesterol diet.**

**cholesterol test,** a blood test used to identify patients who are at risk for arteriosclerotic heart disease. Since cholesterol alone is not a totally accurate predictor of heart disease, this test is usually done as a part of lipid profile testing, which also evaluates levels of lipoproteins and triglycerides.

**cholesteryl ester storage disease** /kōles′təril/, an inherited disorder in which there is an accumulation of neutral lipids, such as cholesterol esters and glycerides, in body tissues. The disease may be asymptomatic or be characterized by hepatosplenomegaly, steatorrhea, and adrenal calcification. The cause is a deficiency of the enzyme cholesterol ester hydrolase. There is no specific treatment. A form of the disorder affecting infants, with symptoms in the first weeks after birth, is Wolman's disease.

**cholestyramine** /-tir′əmēn/, a drug used to treat hypercholesterolemia that acts on the liver's bile acids. It interrupts the bile-acid cycle and increases the function of low-density lipoprotein receptors, thereby increasing cellular cholesterol uptake and lowering blood cholesterol levels.

**cholestyramine resin,** an ion-exchange resin and antihyperlipoproteinemic agent.

■ INDICATIONS: It is prescribed for the treatment of hyperlipoproteinemia and for pruritus resulting from partial biliary obstruction.

■ CONTRAINDICATIONS: Complete biliary obstruction or known hypersensitivity to this drug prohibits its use.

■ ADVERSE EFFECTS: Among the more serious adverse reactions are fecal impaction, GI disturbances, and depletion of vitamins A, D, and K. Constipation is common.

**-cholia, -choly,** suffix meaning '(condition of the) bile': *albuminocholia, syncholia, uricocholia.*

**cholic acid,** a bile acid synthesized in the liver from cholesterol. Cholan-24-oic acid is stored in the liver bound to coenzyme A and converted to glycine and taurine bile salts before secretion into bile.

**choline** /kō′lēn/ [Gk, *chole,* bile], a lipotropic substance that can be synthesized by the body. Under certain circumstances it is considered by some to be essential. Found in most animal tissues, choline is a primary component of acetylcholine, the neurotransmitter, and functions with inositol as a basic constituent of lecithin. It prevents fat deposits in the liver and facilitates the movement of fats into the cells. The richest sources of choline are liver, kidneys, brains, wheat germ, brewer's yeast, and egg yolk. See also **inositol, lecithin.**

**choline esters,** a group of cholinergic drugs that act at sites or organs where acetylcholine is the neurotransmitter. Examples include bethanechol, carbachol, and methacholine.

**cholinergic** /-ur′jik/ [Gk, *chole + ergon,* to work], **1.** pertaining to nerve fibers that liberate acetylcholine at the myoneural junctions. **2.** the tendency to transmit or to be stimulated by or to stimulate the elaboration of acetylcholine. Compare **adrenergic, anticholinergic.**

**cholinergic blocking agent,** any agent that blocks the action of acetylcholine and substances similar to acetylcholine. Such agents, in effect, block the action of cholinergic nerves that transmit impulses by the release of acetylcholine at their synapses.

**cholinergic crisis,** a pronounced muscular weakness and respiratory paralysis caused by excessive acetylcholine, often apparent in patients suffering from myasthenia gravis as a result of overmedication with anticholinesterase drugs.

**cholinergic fibers** [Gr, *chole,* bile, *ergon,* work; L, *fibra*], nerve fibers of the autonomic nervous system that release the neurotransmitter acetylcholine. They include all preganglionic fibers, all postganglionic sympathetic fibers to sweat glands, and efferent fibers innervating skeletal muscle.

**cholinergic nerve,** a nerve that releases the neurotransmitter acetylcholine at its synapse. The cholinergic nerves include all the preganglionic sympathetic and preganglionic parasympathetic nerves, the postganglionic parasympathetic nerves, the somatic motor nerves to skeletal muscles, and some nerves to sweat glands and to certain blood vessels.

**cholinergic receptor** [Gk, *chole,* bile, *ergein,* to work; L, *recipere,* to receive], a specialized sensory nerve ending that responds to the stimulation of acetylcholine.

**cholinergic stimulant.** See **cholinergic.**

**cholinergic urticaria** [Gk, *chole + ergon,* to work; L, *urtica,* nettle], an abnormal and usually temporary vascular reaction of the skin, often associated with sweating in susceptible individuals subjected to stress, strong exertion, or hot weather. The condition is characterized by small, pale, itchy papules surrounded by reddish areas; it is caused by the action of acetylcholine on mast cells.

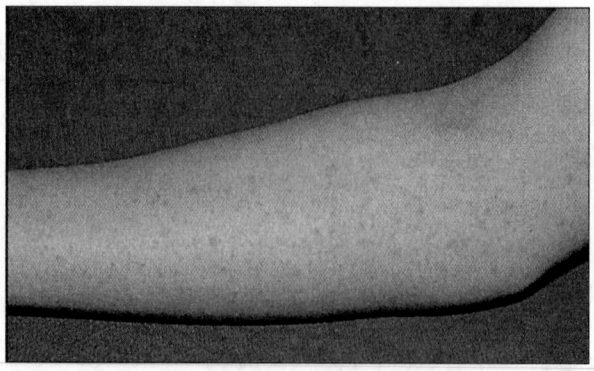

**Cholinergic urticaria** *(Lawrence and Cox, 1993)*

**cholinesterase** /kō'lines'tərās/, an enzyme that acts as a catalyst in the hydrolysis of acetylcholine to choline and acetate.

**cholinesterase test,** a blood test done to identify patients with pseudocholinesterase deficiency before anesthesia or to identify patients who may have been exposed to phosphate poisoning.

**choliopancreatography** /kō'lē·ōpan'krē·ātog'rəfē/ [Gk, chole + pan, all, kreas, flesh, graphein, to record], the radiographic examination of the bile and pancreatic ducts.

**cholo-.** See **chole-.**

**Cholografin,** trade name of a diagnostic contrast medium (iodipamide), used in radiology.

**chololithiasis** /kō'ləlithī'əsis/. See **cholelithiasis.**

**Choloxin,** trademark for an antihyperlipoproteinemic (dextrothyroxine sodium).

**-choly.** See **-cholia.**

**chondr-.** See **chondro-.**

**chondral** /kon'drəl/, pertaining to cartilage.

**chondralgia** /kondral'jə/, pain that appears to originate in cartilage.

**chondrectomy** /kondrek'təmē/, the surgical excision of a cartilage.

**chondri-.** See **chondro-.**

**-chondria,** **1.** suffix meaning a 'condition involving granules in cell composition': *lipochondria, mitochondria, plastochondria.* **2.** combining form from Greek *hypochondrion* ("below the cartilage"). The hypochondriac region was regarded as the seat of emotion.

**chondrial bone** [Gk, *chondros*, cartilage; AS, *ban*, bone], bone that forms under the periosteal membrane. Also called **perichondrial bone.**

**chondriocont** /kon'drē·ōkont'/, a threadlike or rod-shaped mitochondrion.

**chondriome** /kon'drē·ōm/ [Gk, *chondros*, cartilage], the total mitochondrial content of a cell, taken as a unit. Also called **chondrioma.**

**chondriomite** /kon'drē·ōmīt'/ [Gk, *chondros* + *mitos*, thread], a single, granular mitochondrion or a group of such mitochondria that appear in a chain formation.

**chondriosome.** See **mitochondrion.**

**chondritis** /kondrī'tis/, any inflammatory condition affecting the cartilage.

**chondro-, chondr-, chondri-,** combining form meaning 'cartilage': *chondroblast, chondroclast, chondrocostal.*

**chondroadenoma.** See **adenochondroma.**

**chondroangioma** /kon'drō·an'jē·ō'mə/, pl. **chondroangiomas, chondroangiomata** [Gk, *chondros* + *angeion*, vessel, *oma*, tumor], a benign mesenchymal tumor containing vascular and cartilaginous elements.

**chondroblast** /kon'drōblast/ [Gk, *chondros* + *blastos*, germ], any one of the cells that develop from the mesenchyma and form cartilage. Chondroblasts play an important role in endochondrial ossification and especially in longitudinal bone growth. Also called **chondroplast.**

**chondroblastoma** /kon'drōblastō'mə/, pl. **chondroblastomas, chondroblastomata,** a benign tumor, derived from precursors of cartilage cells, that develops most frequently in epiphyses of the femur and humerus, especially in young men. The lesions may contain scattered areas of calcification and necrosis. Also called **Codman's tumor.**

**chondrocalcinosis** /kon'drōkal'sinō'sis/ [Gk, *chondros* + L, *calyx*, lime; Gk, *osis*, condition], an arthritic disease in which calcium deposits are present in the peripheral joints. It resembles gout and often occurs in patients over 50 years of age who have osteoarthritis or diabetes mellitus. It most commonly invades the knee joint. Aspiration of synovial fluid from the affected joints reveals crystals of calcium salts, especially calcium pyrophosphate dihydrate (CPPD). Inflammation and pain may be relieved by intraarticular injections of hydrocortisone and by antiinflammatory medications. Also called **pseudogout.** Compare **gout, gouty arthritis.**

**chondrocarcinoma** /kon'drōkär'sinō'mə/, pl. **chondrocarcinoma, chondrocarcinomata** [Gk, *chondros* + *karkinos*, crab, *oma*, tumor], a malignant epithelial tumor in which cartilaginous metaplasia is present.

**chondroclast** /kon'drōklast'/ [Gk, *chondros* + *klasis*, breaking], a giant multinucleated cell associated with the resorption of cartilage. **—chondroclastic,** *adj.*

**chondrocostal** /kon'drōkos'təl/ [Gk, *chondros* + L, *costa*, rib], pertaining to the ribs and the costal cartilages.

**chondrocyte** /kon'drəsīt/ [Gk, *chondros* + *kytos*, cell], any one of the polymorphic cells that form the cartilage of the body. Each contains a nucleus, a relatively large amount of clear cytoplasm, and the common organelles. **—chondrocytic,** *adj.*

**chondrodysplasia** /kon'drōdisplā'zhə/ [Gk, *chondros* + *dys*, bad, *plassein*, to form], an inherited disease characterized by abnormal growth at the ends of bones, particularly the long bones of the arms and legs. Bones of the hands and feet may be similarly affected.

**chondrodysplasia punctata,** an inherited form of dwarfism characterized by skin lesions, radiographic evidence of epiphyseal stippling, and a pug nose. There are two types of the anomaly: a benign Conradi-Hunermann form marked by mild asymmetric limb shortening and a lethal rhizomelic form with marked proximal limb shortening. The Conradi-Hunermann form of the disorder is transmitted by an autosomal-dominant gene and the rhizomelic form by an autosomal-recessive gene.

**chondrodystrophia calcificans congenita** /-distrō'fē·ə/ [Gk, *chondros* + *dys*, bad, *trophe*, nourishment; L, *calyx*, lime, *congenitus*, born with], an inherited defect characterized by many small opacities in the epiphyses of the long bones. This sign is present on x-ray films of the newborn. Dwarfism, contractures, cataracts, mental retardation, and short stubby fingers develop as the infant grows into childhood. Also called **chondrodystrophia fetalis calcificans, Conradi's disease.**

**chondrodystrophic myotonia.** See **Schwartz-Jampel syndrome.**

**chondrodystrophy** /kon'drōdis'trəfē/ [Gk, *chondros* + *dys*, bad, *trophe*, nourishment], a group of disorders in which there is abnormal conversion of cartilage to bone, particularly in the epiphyses of the long bones. Patients are dwarfed, with normal trunks and shortened extremities. See also **achondroplasia.**

**chondroectodermal dysplasia** /kon'drō·ek'tədur'məl/, an inherited form of dwarfism marked by distal limb shortening, postaxial polydactyly, and cardiovascular abnormalities. It is transmitted by an autosomal recessive gene. Also called **Ellis-van Creveld syndrome.**

**chondroendothelioma** /kon'drō·en'dōthē'lē·ō'mə/, pl. **chondroendotheliomas, chondroendotheliomata** [Gk, *chondros* + *endon*, within, *thele*, nipple, *oma*, tumor], a benign mesenchymal tumor containing cartilaginous and endothelial components.

**chondrofibroma** /kon'drōfībrō'mə/, pl. **chondrofibromas, chondrofibromata,** a fibrous tumor that contains cartilaginous components.

**chondrogenesis** /kon'drōjen'əsis/, the development of cartilage. **—chondrogenetic,** *adj.*

**chondroid** /kon'droid/, resembling cartilage.

**chondrolipoma** /kon'drōlipō'mə/, *pl.* **chondrolipomas, chondrolipomata,** a benign mesenchymal tumor containing fatty and cartilaginous components.

**chondroma** /kondrō'mə/, *pl.* **chondromas, chondromata,** a benign, fairly common tumor of cartilage cells that grows slowly within cartilage (enchondroma) or on the surface (ecchondroma). Kinds of chondromas are **joint chondroma** and **synovial chondroma.** See also **ecchondroma, enchondroma.** —**chondromatous,** *adj.*

**-chondroma,** suffix meaning a 'benign cartilaginous tumor': *hyaloenchondroma, osteochondroma.*

**chondromalacia** /kon'drōmələ'shə/ [Gk, *chondros* + *malakia*, softness], a softening of cartilage. **Chondromalacia fetalis** is a lethal congenital form of the condition in which a stillborn infant has soft and pliable limbs. **Chondromalacia patellae** occurs in young adults after knee injury and is characterized by swelling, pain, and degenerative changes, which are revealed on x-ray examination.

**chondroma sarcomatosum.** See **chondrosarcoma.**

**chondromatosis** /kon'drōmətō'sis/, a condition characterized by the presence of many cartilaginous tumors. A kind of chondromatosis is **synovial chondromatosis.**

**chondromatous.** See **chondroma.**

**chondromere** /kon'drōmir/ [Gk, *chondros* + *meros*, part], a cartilaginous embryonic vertebra and its costal component.

**chondromyoma** /kon'drōmī·ō'mə/, *pl.* **chondromyomas, chondromyomata** [Gk, *chondros* + *mys*, muscle, *oma*, tumor], a benign mesenchymal tumor containing myomatous and cartilaginous tissue.

**chondromyxofibroma** /kon'drōmik'sōfībrō'mə/ [Gk, *chondros* + *myxa*, mucus; L, *fibra*, fiber, *oma*, tumor], a benign tumor that develops from cartilage-forming connective tissue. The lesion, typically a firm, grayish-white mass, tends to occur in the knee and small bones of the foot and may be confused with chondrosarcoma. Also called **chondromyxoid fibroma.**

**chondromyxoid** /kon'drōmik'soid/ [Gk, *chondros* + *myxa*, mucus, *eidos*, form], composed of cartilaginous and myxoid elements.

**chondromyxoid fibroma.** See **chondromyxofibroma.**

**chondrophyte** /kon'drōfīt'/ [Gk, *chondros* + *phyton*, growth], an abnormal mass of cartilage. —**chondrophytic,** *adj.*

**chondroplasia** /-plā'zhə/ [Gk, *chondros*, cartilage, *plassein*, to form], the formation of cartilage.

**chondroplast.** See **chondroblast.**

**chondroplasty** /kon'drōplas'tē/ [Gk, *chondros* + *plassein*, to mold], the surgical repair of cartilage.

**chondrosarcoma** /kon'drōsärkō'mə/, *pl.* **chondrosarcomas, chondrosarcomata** [Gk, *chondros* + *sarx*, flesh, *oma*, tumor], a malignant neoplasm of cartilaginous cells or their precursors that occurs most frequently in long bones, the pelvic girdle, and the scapula. The tumor is a large, smooth, lobulated growth composed of nodules of hyaline cartilage that may show slight to marked calcification. Also called **chondroma sarcomatosum.** —**chondrosarcomatous,** *adj.*

**chondrosarcomatosis** /kon'drōsär'kōmətō'sis/, a condition characterized by multiple malignant cartilaginous tumors.

**chondrosarcomatous.** See **chondrosarcoma.**

**chondrosis** /kondrō'sis/, **1.** the development of the cartilage of the body. **2.** a cartilaginous tumor.

**chondrosternal joint.** See **sternocostal articulation.**

**chondrotomy** /kondrot'əmē/, a surgical procedure for dividing a cartilage.

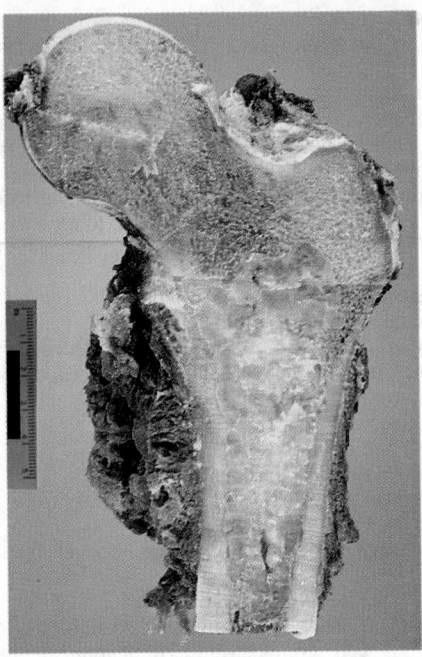

**Chondrosarcoma** *(Kumar, Cotran, and Robbins, 1997)*

**CHOP** /chop/, an abbreviation for an anticancer drug combination that includes cyclophosphamide, doxorubicin, vincristine, and prednisone.

**chopping,** a therapeutic exercise to improve the strength and coordination of upper trunk nerves and muscles by lifting the arms overhead and lowering them in a chopping or slashing movement.

**chord-,** combining form meaning 'string, cord': *chordoblastoma, chordoma, chordotomy.*

**chorda** /kôr'də/, a string filament such as a nerve or tendon.

**chordae tendineae** /kô'dē tendin'i·ē/, *sing.* **chorda tendinea** /kô'dätendin'ē·ä/, the strands of tendon that anchor the cusps of the mitral and tricuspid valves to the papillary muscles of the ventricles of the heart, preventing prolapse of the valves into the atria during ventricular contraction. Also called **chordae tendineae cordis, tendinous cords.**

**chordal canal.** See **notochordal canal.**

**chorda spinalis.** See **spinal cord.**

**chorda umbilicalis.** See **umbilical cord.**

**chordee** /kôr'dē, kôr'dā/ [Gk, *chorde*, cord], a congenital defect of the genitourinary tract resulting in a ventral curvature of the penis, caused by presence of a fibrous band of tissue instead of normal skin along the corpus spongiosum. The condition is often associated with hypospadias and is surgically corrected in early childhood. The goals of surgery are to improve the appearance of the genitalia cosmetically for psychologic reasons, to construct an organ that allows the boy to void in a standing position, and to produce a sexually adequate organ.

**chordencephalon** /kôrd'ensef'əlon/ [Gk, *chorde* + *enkephalos*, brain], the portion of the central nervous system that develops in the early weeks of pregnancy from the neural tube and includes the mesencephalon, the rhombencephalon, and the spinal cord. The chordencephalon is segmented and divided into the alar and basal plates. The alar

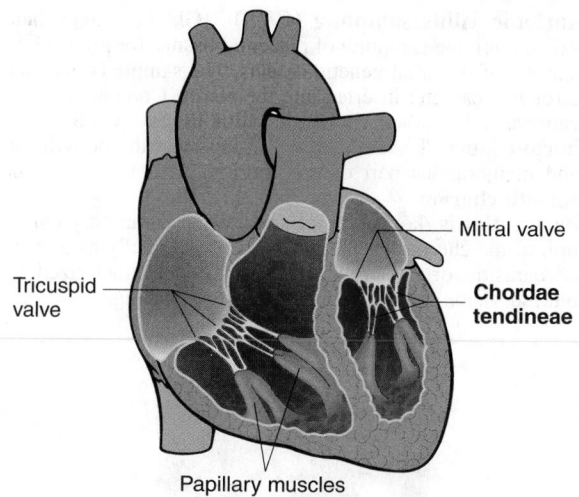

Tricuspid valve

Mitral valve

**Chordae tendineae**

Papillary muscles

**Chordae tendineae** *(Chabner, 2001)*

plate becomes the sensory portion of the gray substance of the spinal cord; the basal plate becomes the motor portion of the gray substance. —**chordencephalic,** *adj.*

**chorditis** /kôrdī′tis/, **1.** inflammation of a spermatic cord. **2.** inflammation of the vocal cords or of the vocal folds.

**chordoid** /kôr′doid/ [Gk, *chorde* + *eidos,* form], resembling the notocord or notochordal tissue.

**chordoma** /kôrdō′mə/, *pl.* **chordomas, chordomata,** a rare tumor that develops from the fetal notochord. It is usually located in the midline, behind the sella; it is slow growing but highly invasive.

**chordotomy** /kôrdot′əmē/ [Gk, *chorde* + *temnein,* to cut], surgery in which the anterolateral tracts of the spinal cord are surgically divided to relieve pain.

**chorea** /kôrē′ə/ [Gk, *choreia,* dance], a condition characterized by involuntary purposeless, rapid motions, as flexing and extending of the fingers, raising and lowering of the shoulders, or grimacing. The movements often appear to be well coordinated. In some forms the person is also irritable, emotionally unstable, physically weak, restless, and fretful. See also **chorea gravidarum, Huntington's chorea, Sydenham's chorea.** —**choreic** /kôrā′ik/, *adj.*

**-chorea,** suffix meaning a '(specified) nervous disorder characterized by involuntary muscle twitching': *hemichorea, monochorea, orthochorea.*

**chorea gravidarum** /kôr′ē·əgrav′idär′əm/, Sydenham's chorea that occurs during the early months of pregnancy with or without a previous history of rheumatic disease. Similar symptoms may develop in a woman who is taking oral contraceptives.

**chorea minor.** See **Sydenham's chorea.**

**choreic.** See **chorea.**

**choreic ataxia** /kôrē′ik/ [Gk, *choreia,* dance, *ataxia,* without order], a form of ataxia in which patients lack muscular coordination and movements are marked by involuntary twitching and abrupt jerking.

**choreiform** /kərē′əfôrm′/, resembling the rapid jerky movements associated with chorea.

**choreiform spasm** [Gk, *chorea,* dance; L, *forma* + Gk, *spasmos*], a condition of involuntary muscle contractions that result in dancing motions. In one type powerful contrac-

tions of the leg muscles cause a leaping, jumping action. It can also involve arm, shoulder, and neck muscles.

**choreoacanthocytosis.** See **neuroacanthocytosis.**

**choreoathetoid cerebral palsy** /kôr′ē·ō·ath′ətoid/, a form of cerebral palsy characterized by choreiform (jerky, ticlike twitching) and athetoid (slow, writhing) movements.

**choreoathetosis** /kôr′ē·ō·ath′ətō′sis/ [Gk, *choreia,* dance, *athetos,* not fixed], irregular involuntary movements that may involve the face, neck, trunk, extremities, or respiratory muscles, giving an appearance of restlessness. The writhing movements may vary from subtle to wild and ballistic and are commonly associated with administration of levodopa in parkinsonism. Levodopa-induced involuntary movement (dyskinesia) occurs most commonly 1 to 3 hours after administration of the drug.

**chorio-,** combining form meaning 'protective fetal membrane': *chorioblastosis, choriocele, chorioma.*

**chorioadenoma** /kərē′ō·ad′inō′mə/, *pl.* **chorioadenomas, chorioadenomata** [Gk, *chorion,* skin, *aden,* gland, *oma,* tumor], an epithelial cell tumor of the outermost fetal membrane that is intermediate in the malignant development of a hydatid mole to invasive choriocarcinoma.

**chorioadenoma destruens** /-des′trōō·əns/ [Gk, *chorion* + *aden* + *oma* + L, *destruere,* to pull down], an invasive hydatidiform mole in which the chorionic villi of the mole penetrate into the myometrium and parametrium of the uterus and metastasize to distant parts of the body, most commonly to the lungs. Also called **metastasizing mole.**

**chorioamnionic** /-am′nē·ot′ik/, pertaining to the chorion and the amnion.

**chorioamnionitis** /-am′nē·ōnī′tis/ [Gk, *chorion* + *amnion,* fetal membrane, *itis,* inflammation], an inflammatory reaction in the amniotic membranes caused by bacteria or viruses in the amniotic fluid. The membranes become infiltrated with polymorphonuclear leukocytes. This term is sometimes used incorrectly to refer to intra-amniotic infection.

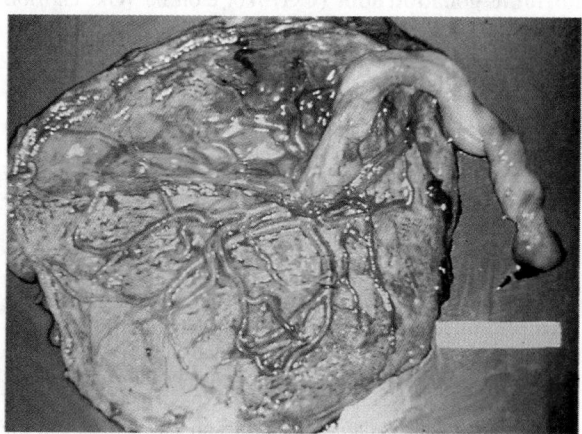

**Chorioamnionitis** *(Zitelli and Davis, 1997)*

**choriocarcinoma** /kôr′ē·ōkär′sinō′mə/, *pl.* **choriocarcinomas, choriocarcinomata,** an epithelial malignancy of fetal origin that develops from the chorionic portion of the products of conception. The primary tumor usually appears in the uterus as a soft dark red, crumbling mass; may invade and destroy the uterine wall; and may metastasize through lymph or blood vessels, forming secondary hemorrhagic and necrotic tumors in the vaginal wall, vulva, lymph nodes, lungs, liver, and brain. The urine often contains much more chorionic gonadotropin than is expected in pregnancy. The hormone level returns to normal when the tumor is completely removed. This form of cancer, which is more common in older women, responds to chemotherapy with cytotoxic drugs such as methotrexate. Rarely a choriocarcinoma may arise in a teratoma of the testis, mediastinum, or pineal gland; chemotherapy is usually not effective in treating these tumors. Also called **chorioblastoma, chorioepithelioma, chorionic carcinoma, chorionic epithelioma.**

**choriocele** /kôr′ē·əsēl′/ [Gk, *chorion* + *kele,* hernia], a hernia or protrusion of the tissue of the choroid layer of the eye.

**chorioepithelioma.** See **choriocarcinoma.**

**choriogenesis** /kôr′ē·ōjen′əsis/, the development of the chorion, which is first evident in the first month of pregnancy. The chorion continues to expand to accommodate the fetus and serves as the outer barrier between the fetus and the uterus. —**choriogenetic,** *adj.*

**choriomeningitis.** See **lymphocytic choriomeningitis.**

**chorion** /kôr′ē·on/ [Gk, *chorion,* skin], (in biology) the outermost extraembryonic membrane composed of trophoblast lined with mesoderm. It develops villi about 2 weeks after fertilization and is vascularized by allantoic vessels 1 week later. It gives rise to the placenta and persists until birth as the outer of the two layers of membrane containing the amniotic fluid and the fetus. Compare **amnion.** See also **amniotic sac.**

**-chorion,** suffix meaning a 'membrane': *allantochorion, omphalochorion, prochorion.*

**chorion frondosum** /kôr′ē·on fron·dō′sum /, the region of the chorion that bears villi; also known as the **shaggy** or **villous chorion.**

**chorionic carcinoma, chorionic epithelioma.** See **choriocarcinoma.**

**chorionic gonadotropin (CG)** /kôr′ē·on′ik/ [Gk, *chorion* + *gone,* seed, *trophe,* nutrition], a chemical component of the urine of pregnant women and pregnant mares. This glycoprotein hormone is secreted by the placental trophoblastic cells. It is composed of two subunits, alpha and beta human chorionic gonadotropin (HCG). The alpha subunit is nearly identical to similar subunits of the follicle-stimulating, luteinizing, and thyroid-stimulating hormones. The specific hormonal effects of chorionic gonadotropin are activated by the beta portion. They include stimulation of the corpus luteum to secrete estrogen and progesterone and to decrease lymphocyte activation. Chorionic gonadotropin is also administered in the treatment of some cases of cryptorchidism and male hypogonadism and in the induction of ovulation in some infertile women. Also called **human chorionic gonadotropin.** See also **gonadotropin.**

**chorionic plate** [Gk, *chorion* + *platys,* flat], the part of the fetal placenta that gives rise to chorionic villi, which attach to the uterus during the early stage of formation of the placenta.

**chorionic sac** [Gk, *chorion,* skin, *sakkos,* sack], the saclike membrane that develops from the blastocyst wall to envelop the embryo.

**chorionic villus** [Gk, *chorion* + L, *villus,* shaggy hair], any of the tiny vascular fibrils on the surface of the chorion that infiltrate the maternal blood sinuses of the endometrium and help form the placenta.

**chorionic villus sampling (CVS)** [Gk, L, shaggy hair, *exemplum*], the sampling of placental tissues for prenatal diagnosis of potential genetic defects. The sample is obtained through a catheter inserted into the uterus. Compare **amniocentesis.** Also called **chorionic villus biopsy (CVB).**

**chorion laeve** /kôr′ē·on lē′vē /, the smooth (nonvillous) and membranous part of the chorion. Also known as the **smooth chorion.**

**chorioretinitis** /kôr′ē·ōret′inī′tis/, an inflammatory condition of the choroid and retina of the eye, usually as a result of parasitic or bacterial infection. It is characterized by blurred vision, photophobia, and distorted images.

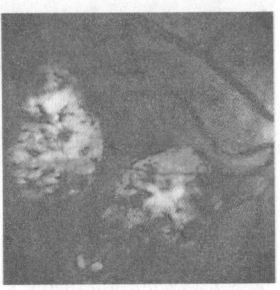

**Chorioretinitis** *(Stein, Slatt, Stein, 1994)*

**chorioretinopathy** /kôr′ē·ōret′ənop′əthē/ [Gk, *chorion* + L, *rete,* net; Gk, *pathos,* disease], a noninflammatory process caused by disease that involves the choroid and the retina. Also called **choroidoretinitis.**

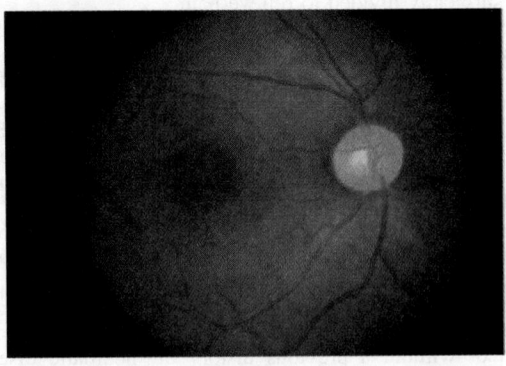

**Chorioretinopathy** *(Lemmi and Lemmi, 2000)*

**choroid** /kôr′oid/ [Gk, *chorion* + *eidos,* form], a thin, highly vascular layer of the eye between the retina and sclera.

**choroidal malignant melanoma** /kôroi′dəl/ [Gk, *chorion* + *eidos* + L, *malignus,* ill-disposed; Gk, *melas,* black, *oma,* tumor], a tumor of the choroid coat of the eye that grows into the vitreous humor, causing detachment and degeneration of the overlying retina. Typically mound-shaped or

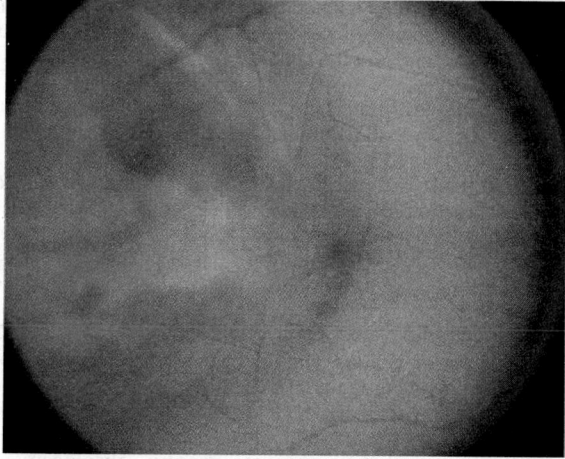

**Choroidal malignant melanoma** *(Michelson, 1996)*

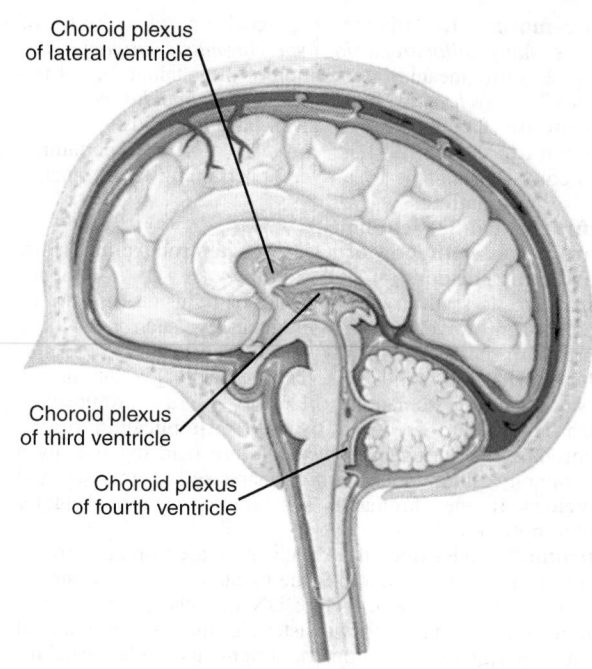

Choroid plexus
of lateral ventricle

Choroid plexus
of third ventricle

Choroid plexus
of fourth ventricle

**Choroid plexus** *(Thibodeau and Patton, 1999/Barbara Cousins)*

mushroom-shaped, the neoplasm may break through the sclera and appear under the conjunctiva.

**choroideremia** /kôr′oid·ər·ē′mē·ə/ [Gk, *chorion,* skin + *eidos,* form + *erēmia,* destitution], hereditary primary degeneration of the choroid, transmitted as an X-linked trait and beginning in the first decade of life. In males, the earliest symptom is usually night blindness, followed by constricted visual field and eventual blindness as the degeneration of the pigment epithelium of the retina progresses to complete atrophy. In females, it is nonprogressive; usually there is normal vision and often an atypical pigmentary retinopathy.

**choroiditis** /kôr′oidī′tis/, an inflammatory condition of the choroid membrane of the eye. See also **chorioretinitis.**

**choroid membrane,** a vascular layer of tissue between the retina and the sclera of the eye.

**choroidocyclitis** /kôroi′dōsiklī′tis/ [Gk, *chorion* + *eidos* + *kyklos,* circle, *itis,* inflammation], an abnormal condition characterized by inflammation of the choroid and the ciliary processes.

**choroidopathy** /kôr′oidop′əthē/, noninflammatory degeneration of the choroid.

**choroidoretinitis.** See **chorioretinopathy.**

**choroid plexectomy** /pleksek′təmē/ [Gk, *chorion* + *eidos* + L, *plexus,* pleated; Gk, *ektomē,* excision], a surgical procedure for the reduction of cerebrospinal fluid production in the ventricles of the brain in hydrocephalus, usually in the newborn. The procedure involves transcortical entry of the lateral ventricles to coagulate or to excise the choroid plexuses and seeks to correct a communicating type of hydrocephalus.

**choroid plexus** [Gk, *chorion* + *eidos* + L, pleated], any one of the tangled masses of tiny blood vessels contained within the lateral, the third, and the fourth ventricles of the brain, responsible for producing cerebrospinal fluid.

**Chotzen's syndrome.** See **Saethre-Chotzen syndrome.**

**Christchurch chromosome (Ch1)** [Christchurch, city in New Zealand], an abnormally small, acrocentric chromosome (either chromosome 21 or chromosome 22), in which the short arm is missing or partially deleted. The aberration is associated with chronic lymphocytic leukemia but has also been found in patients with various other defects. See also **Philadelphia chromosome.**

**Christian Science,** a religious system founded in 1879 by Mary Baker Eddy [1821–1910], based on the metaphysical teachings of Phineas P. Quimby. It holds that healing should be achieved through spiritual means, that sickness and death are illusions, and that one can overcome illness by refusing to think about it.

**Christian-Weber disease** [Henry A. Christian, American physician, 1876–1951; Frederick Parkes Weber, English physician, 1863–1962], a rare form of panniculitis characterized by nodular formations in the subcutaneous tissues and prolonged intermittent relapsing fever.

**Christmas disease.** See **hemophilia B.**

**Christmas factor.** See **factor IX.**

**Christ-Siemens-Touraine syndrome.** See **anhidrotic ectodermal dysplasia.**

**-chroia,** suffix meaning '(condition of) skin coloration': *cacochroia, cyanochroia, xanthochroia.*

**chrom-.** See **chromo-.**

**chromaffin** /krō′məfin/ [Gk, *chroma,* color; L, *affin,* affinity], having an affinity for staining with chromium salts, especially brown staining of the cells of the adrenal, coccygeal, and carotid glands; certain cells of the adrenal medulla; and cells of the paraganglions. Also **chromaphil** /krō′məfil/.

**chromaffin body.** See **paraganglion.**

**chromaffin cell,** any one of the special cells that compose the paraganglia and are connected to the ganglia of the celiac, renal, suprarenal, aortic, and hypogastric plexuses. The chromaffin cells of the adrenal medulla secrete two catecholamines, epinephrine and norepinephrine, which affect smooth muscle, cardiac muscle, and glands (ovary, testes) in the same way as sympathetic stimulation, by increasing and prolonging sympathetic effects.

**chromaffinoma.** See **pheochromocytoma.**

**chromaphil.** See **chromaffin.**

**-chromasia,**   **1.** suffix meaning '(condition of) color (as of cells, skin)': *allochromasia, hyperchromasia, oligochromasia.* **2.** suffix meaning '(condition of the) stainability of tissues': *amblychromasia, anisochromasia, anochromasia.*

**chromate ($CrO_4^{2-}$),**   any salt of chromic acid.

**chromatic** /krōmat'ik/ [Gk, *chroma*, color],   **1.** pertaining to color. **2.** stainable by a dye. **3.** pertaining to chromatin. Also **chromatinic.**

**-chromatic.**   See **-chromic.**

**chromatic asymmetry of iris.**   See **heterochromic iridis.**

**chromatic dispersion** [Gk, *chroma* + L, *dis*, apart, *spargere*, to scatter],   the splitting of light into its various component wavelengths or frequencies, such as with a prism, to separate and study the different colors.

**chromatid** /krō'mətid/ [Gk, *chroma*, color],   one of the two identical, threadlike filaments of a chromosome. Chromatids are produced by the self-replication of the chromosome during interphase and are held together by a common centromere. During anaphase of mitosis and meiosis II, the chromatids separate to become daughter chromosomes.

**chromatid deletion,**   the breakage of a chromatid, sometimes caused by radiation. If the breakage occurs in the $G_1$ phase of the cell cycle, before DNA synthesis, subsequent replication will produce two sister chromatids with material missing and two acentromeric fragments, called isochromatids.

**chromatin** /krō'mətin/ [Gk, *chroma*, color],   the material within a cell nucleus from which the chromosomes are formed. It consists of fine, threadlike strands of DNA attached to proteins called histones and is readily stained with basic dyes. Chromatin occurs in two forms, euchromatin and heterochromatin, which are distinguishable during the phases of the cell cycle by their different degrees of staining, which in turn depends how tightly they are coiled. During cell division, portions of the chromatin condense and coil to form the chromosomes. Also called **chromoplasm, karyotin.** See also **chromatid, euchromatin, heterochromatin, sex chromatin. —chromatinic,** *adj.*

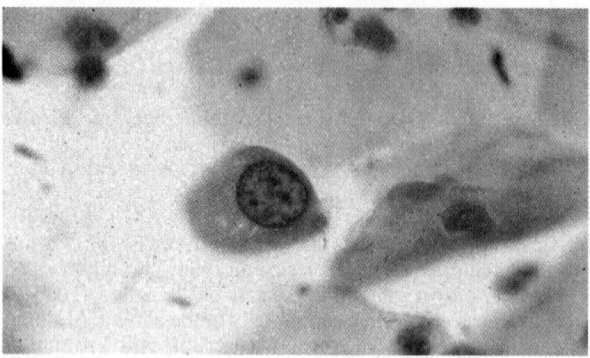

**Rim of chromatin outlining the nuclear membrane**
*(McKee, 1997)*

**chromatinic.**   See **chromatic.**

**chromatin-negative,**   lacking sex chromatin. The term applies to the nuclei of cells in normal males as well as those in individuals with certain chromosomal abnormalities.

**chromatin nucleolus.**   See **karyosome.**

**chromatin-positive,**   containing sex chromatin. The term applies to the nuclei of cells in normal females as well as those in individuals with certain chromosomal abnormalities.

**chromatism** /krō'mətiz'əm/,   **1.** an abnormal condition characterized by hallucinations in which the affected individual sees colored lights. **2.** abnormal pigmentation.

**chromatogram** /krōmat'əgram'/,   **1.** the record produced by the separation of gaseous substances or dissolved chemical substances moving through a column of absorbent material that filters out the various absorbates in different layers. **2.** any graphic record produced by any chromatographic method.

**chromatography** /krō'mətog'rəfē/,   any one of several processes for separating and analyzing various gaseous or dissolved chemical materials according to differences in their absorbency with respect to a specific substance and according to their different pigments. Some kinds of chromatography are **column chromatography, displacement chromatography, gas chromatography, ion-exchange chromatography,** and **paper chromatography. —chromatographic,** *adj.*

**chromatopsia** /krō'mətop'sē·ə/ [Gk, *chroma* + *opsis*, vision],   **1.** an abnormal visual condition that makes colorless objects appear tinged with color. **2.** a form of color blindness characterized by the imperfect perception of various colors. It may be caused by a deficiency in one or more of the retinal cones or by defective nerve circuits that convey color-associated impulses to the cerebral cortex. The most common defect in color sense is the inability to distinguish red from green, a defect evident in about 10% of men and 1% of women. Compare **chromesthesia.**

**chromatosis** /-ō'sis/,   condition of abnormal skin pigmentation in any part of the body. See **chloasma, vitiligo.**

**chromaturia** /-ŏŏr'ē·ə/ [Gk, *chroma*, color, *ouron*, urine],   the production of urine that has an abnormal color.

**-chrome,**   suffix that distinguishes chromium alloys: *hallachrome, nichrome, nicochrome.*

**-chromemia,**   suffix meaning '(condition of the) hemoglobin in the blood': *hyperchromemia, lipochromemia, polychromemia.*

**chromesthesia** /krō'misthē'zhə/ [Gk, *chroma* + *aisthesis*, feeling],   **1.** the color sense that depends on the mixture of wavelengths in the light that enters the eye and the response of the different types of retinal cones associated with color vision. The human eye can distinguish hundreds of different colors that are combinations of the basic light wavelengths for red, green, and blue. Some of the retinal cones can be stimulated by the whole visual spectrum, and variable stimulation of all the cones can produce all the color sensations known to humans. Changes in the pigments within the cones affect color vision, and defects in the cones cause various kinds of color blindness. **2.** an abnormal condition characterized by the confusion of other senses, such as taste and smell, with imagined sensations of color. Compare **chromatopsia.**

**chromhidrosis** /krō'midrō'sis/ [Gk, *chroma* + *hidros*, sweat],   a rare, functional disorder in which apocrine sweat glands secrete colored sweat. The sweat may be yellow, blue, green, or black and often also fluoresces. A known cause is occupational exposure to copper, catechols, or ferrous oxide. Industrial nurses should be aware of this benign condition.

**-chromia,**   suffix meaning a 'state or condition of pigmentation': *metachromia, normochromia, orthochromia.*

**-chromic, -chromatic,**   suffix meaning color: *bichromic, hypochromic.*

**chromic catgut** /krō'mik/ [Gk, *chroma,* color; L, *catta;* AS, *guttas*], surgical catgut that has been treated with chromium trioxide to strengthen it. It is an absorbable suture.

**chromic myopia,** a kind of color blindness characterized by the ability to distinguish colors only of those objects that are close to the eye.

**chromium (Cr)** /krō'mē·əm/ [Gk, *chroma,* color], a hard, brittle metallic element. Its atomic number is 24; its atomic mass is 51.99. It does not occur naturally in pure form but exists in combination with iron and oxygen in chromite, a mineral found chiefly in Africa, Albania, Russia, and Turkey. Chromium strongly resists corrosion and is used extensively to plate other metals, harden steel, and, in combination with other elements, form colored compounds. Stainless steels are more than 10% chromium and strongly resist rusting. Traces of chromium occur in plants and animals, and there is evidence this element may be important in human nutrition, especially in carbohydrate metabolism. Some experts estimate that the safe and adequate daily intake of chromium ranges from 0.1 to 0.2 mg, depending on the age of the individual. Workers in chromite mines are susceptible to pneumoconiosis caused by the inhalation of chromite dust particles that lodge in the lung. Chromium 51 isotope is used in blood studies.

**chromium alum,** a chemical commonly used to fix, or harden, the emulsion of an x-ray film during manual processing.

**chromo-, chrom-, chromat-, chromato-,** combining form meaning 'color': *chromocrinia, chromocyte, chromotrichia.*

**chromobacteriosis** /krō'məbaktir'ē·ō'sis/, an extremely rare, usually fatal systemic infection caused by a gram-negative bacillus *Chromobacterium violaceum.* It is found in fresh water in tropic and subtropic regions and enters the body through a break in the skin. The disease is characterized by sepsis, multiple liver abscesses, and severe prostration. Early diagnosis, surgical drainage of abscesses, and administration of chloramphenicol markedly improve the chance of survival.

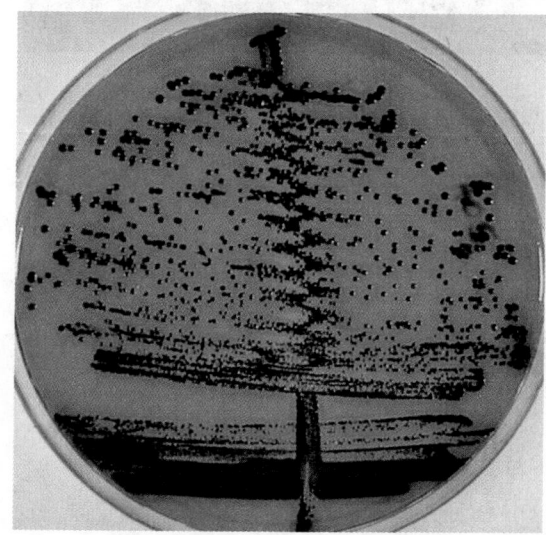

***Chromobacterium violaceum***
*(Baron, Peterson, and Finegold, 1994)*

**chromoblastomycosis** /krō'mōblas'tōmīkō'sis/ [Gk, *chroma + blastos,* germ, *mykes,* fungus, *osis,* condition], a chronic infectious skin disease caused by any of a variety of fungi and characterized by the appearance of pruritic, warty nodules that develop in a cut or other break in the skin. What may first appear as a small dull-red lesion gradually develops into a large ulcerated growth. Over a period of weeks or months additional warty growths may appear elsewhere on the skin along the path of lymphatic drainage. Treatment includes surgical excision and, in some cases, topical application of systemic antibiotics. Also called **chromomycosis, verrucous dermatitis.** See also **mycosis** [and see specific fungal infections].

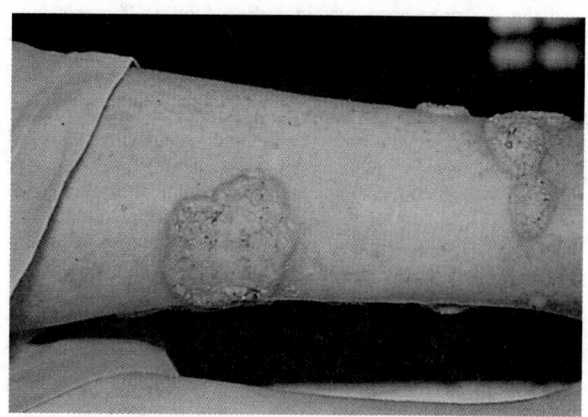

**Chromoblastomycosis** *(Murray et al, 1998)*

**chromocenter.** See **karyosome.**

**chromocystoscopy.** See **cystochromoscopy.**

**chromogen** /krō'mōjən/, a substance that absorbs light, producing color.

**chromolipid, chromolipoid.** See **lipochrome.**

**chromomere** /krō'məmir/ [Gk, *chroma + meros,* part], any of the series of beadlike structures that lie along the chromonema of a chromosome during the early stages of cell division. Chromomeres are most often seen in prophase II of meiosis. The position of each chromomere is relatively constant for each chromosome and probably reflects the chromosome's DNA coiling pattern. Also called **idiomere.**

**chromomycosis.** See **chromoblastomycosis.**

**chromonema** /krō'mənē'mə/, *pl.* **chromonemata** [Gk, *chroma + nema,* thread], the part of a chromosome along which the chromomeres lie during cell division. Also called **chromoneme** /krō'mənēm/. See also **chromosome.** **—chromonemal, chromonematic, chromonemic,** *adj.*

**chromophilic** /krō'məfil'ik/ [Gk, *chroma + philein,* to love], denoting a cell, tissue, or microorganism that is easily stained, particularly certain leukocytes. Compare **chromophobic.**

**chromophobe.** See **chromophobia.**

**chromophobe adenoma.** See **chromophobic adenoma.**

**chromophobia** /krō'məfō'bē·ə/ [Gk, *chroma + phobos,* fear], **1.** the resistance of certain cells and tissues to stains. **2.** a morbid aversion to colors. **—chromophobe,** *n.*

**chromophobic** /krō'məfō'bik/, denoting a cell, tissue, or microorganism that is not easily stained, particularly certain cells of the anterior lobe of the pituitary gland. Compare **chromophilic.**

**chromophobic adenoma,** a tumor of the pituitary gland composed of cells that do not stain with acid or basic dyes. Diabetes insipidus and other conditions resulting from deficiency of one or more pituitary hormones are associated with this tumor. Also called **chromophobe adenoma.**

**chromoplasm.** See **chromatin.**

**chromosensitive,** descriptive of a substance that is affected by and responds to changes in chemical composition.

**chromosomal.** See **chromosome.**

**chromosomal aberration** /-sō'məl/ [Gk, *chroma* + *soma,* body; L, *aberrare,* to wander], any change in the structure or number of any of the chromosomes of a given species. In humans, a number of physical disabilities and disorders are directly associated with aberrations of both the autosomes and the sex chromosomes, including Down, Turner's, and Kleinfelter's syndromes. The incidence of most chromosomal disorders is significantly higher than that of single-gene disorders. See also **trisomy.**

**chromosomal nomenclature,** a standard nomenclature system for identifying chromosomes in an individual as well as any deletions or additions of specific chromosomes or parts of chromosomes. The full complement of human chromosomes is represented as 46, XX for a normal female and 46, XY for a normal male. The pairs of autosomes are numbered from 1 to 22 according to decreasing length and are divided into seven groups: 1 through 3, group A; 4 and 5, group B; 6 through 12, group C; 13 through 15, group D; 16 through 18, group E; 19 and 20, group F; and 21 and 22, group G. Chromosomal aberrations are designated by indicating the total chromosomal number, sex complement, and group or specific chromosome in which the addition or deletion occurs. For example, 47, XY, G+ indicates a male with an extra chromosome in the G group; 47, XX, 21+ indicates a female with an extra chromosome 21, a chromosomal aberration that results in Down syndrome. The short arm of a chromosome is designated by *p,* the long arm by *q,* and a translocation by *t.* See also **Denver classification.**

**chromosomal sex** [Gk, *chroma,* color, *soma,* body; L, *sexus,* male or female], the sex of an individual as determined, in mammals, by the presence or absence of a Y chromosome.

**chromosome** /krō'məsōm/ [Gk, *chroma* + *soma,* body], any of the threadlike structures in the nucleus of a cell that function in the transmission of genetic information. Each consists of a double strand of DNA attached to proteins called histones. The genes, which contain the genetic material that controls the inheritance of traits, are arranged in a linear pattern along the length of each DNA strand. Chromosomes are readily stainable with basic dyes and can be seen easily during cell division, when they are compactly coiled and in their most condensed state. During interphase the chromosomes disperse into chromatin and undergo self-replication, forming identical chromatids that separate during mitosis so that each new cell receives a full set of chromosomes. Each species has a characteristic number of chromosomes in each somatic cell. In humans, there are 46 chromosomes, including 22 homologous pairs of autosomes and 1 pair of sex chromosomes. One member of each pair is derived from each parent. Kinds of chromosomes include **Christchurch chromosomes, daughter chromosomes, gametic chromosomes, giant chromosomes, homologous chromosomes, monosomes, Philadelphia chromosomes, sex chromosomes, somatic chromosomes, W chromosomes,** and **Z chromosomes.** See also **centromere, chromatid, chromatin, Denver classification, gene, karyotype, mitosis.** —**chromosomal,** *adj.*

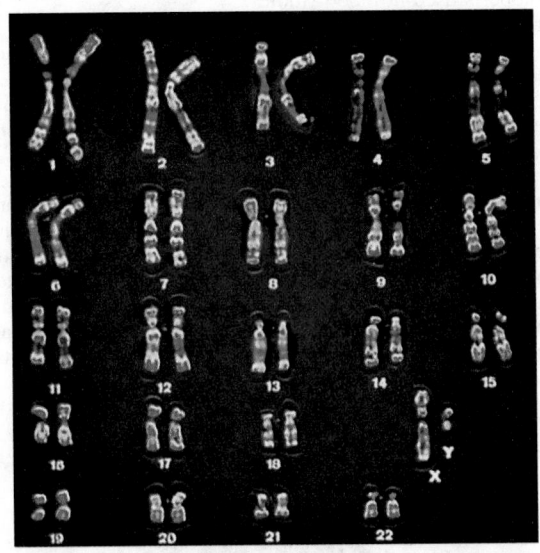

**Human chromosomes**
*(Thibodeau and Patton, 1999/CNRI/Science Photo Library)*

**Analysis of human chromosomes**

| Description of chromosomes | | Group | Autosomes | Sex chromosomes | Number of chromosomes in all body (somatic) cells | |
|---|---|---|---|---|---|---|
| Size | Position of centromere | | | | Male | Female |
| Large | Metacentric or submetacentric | A | 1, 2, 3 | | 6 | 6 |
| Large | Submetacentric | B | 4, 5 | | 4 | 4 |
| Medium | Metacentric and submetacentric | C | 6, 7, 8, 9, 10, 11, 12 | X | 15 | 16 |
| Medium | Acrocentric (subterminal) | D | 13, 14, 15 | | 6 | 6 |
| Small | Metacentric and submetacentric | E | 16, 17, 18 | | 6 | 6 |
| Smallest | Metacentric | F | 19, 20 | | 4 | 4 |
| Small | Acrocentric (subterminal) | G | 21, 22 | Y | 5 | 4 |
| | | | | TOTAL | 46 | 46 |

**chromosome 5p− syndrome.** See **cat-cry syndrome.**

**chromosome banding.** See **banding.**

**chromosome coil,** the spiral formed by the coiling of two or more chromonemata in a chromosome.

**chromosome complement,** the normal number of chromosomes found in the somatic cells of a given species. In humans it is 46, consisting of 22 pairs of homologous autosomes and 1 pair of sex chromosomes.

**chromosome karyotype test,** a blood test used to study an individual's chromosome makeup to determine chromosomal defects associated with disease or the risk of developing disease. It is useful in evaluating congenital anomalies, mental retardation, and delayed puberty, as well as in the prenatal diagnosis of serious congenital diseases such as Klinefelter syndrome and Down syndrome and other suspected genetic disorders.

**chromosome mapping.** See **mapping.**

**chromosome puff,** a band of accumulated chromatin located at a specific site on a giant chromosome. It is indicative of gene activity, specifically DNA and RNA synthesis at that site. Such bands appear at certain chromosomal locations within a given tissue at specific developmental stages in insects and are significant in the study of the mode of genetic transmission.

**chromosome walking,** a molecular genetic technique by which overlapping molecular clones that span large chromosomal intervals are isolated.

**chromotherapy** /krō′məther′əpē/, a system of treating disease with colored lights chosen from specific regions of the spectrum.

**chromotrope** /krō′mətrōp/ [Gk, *chroma* + *trepein,* to turn], **1.** a component of tissue that stains metachromatically with metachromatic dyes. **2.** any one of several dyes differentiated by numeric suffixes. —**chromotropic,** *adj.*

**chron-.** See **chrono-.**

**chronaxy** /krō′naksē/ [Gk, *chronos,* time, *axia,* value], (in electroneuromyography) a measure of the shortest duration of an electrical stimulus needed to excite nerve or muscle tissue.

**-chronia, -chrone,** **1.** suffix meaning '(condition of) processes with respect to time': *isochronia, heterochronia, synchronia.* **2.** suffix meaning '(condition of) chronaxy between muscle and nerve': *isochronia.* **3.** suffix meaning the 'time of formation of a part or tissue': *heterochronia, synchronia.*

**chronic** /kron′ik/ [Gk, *chronos,* time], (of a disease or disorder) persisting for a long period, often for the remainder of a person's lifetime. Compare **acute.**

**chronic abscess** [Gk, *chronos,* time; L, *abscedere,* to go away], a slowly developing abscess that produces pus but shows little or no inflammation, redness, or pain. It is often a tuberculous abscess. Also called **cold abscess.**

**chronic active hepatitis (CAH),** a potentially fatal form of hepatitis complicated by portal inflammation and extending into the parenchyma. There may be progressive destruction of the liver lobule with necrosis and fibrosis leading to scarring and cirrhosis. Possible causes include viral infections, drugs, and autoimmune reactions.

**chronic airway obstruction,** a type of pulmonary disorder, such as ephysema and chronic bronchitis, in which the upper or lower airway is chronically obstructed. The patient, when at rest, breathes at a normal rate and may have prolongation of the expiratory phase with pursed-lip breathing. The patient may be barrel-chested and have large supraclavicular fossae. During inspiration, the intercostal spaces retract, and accessory muscles are used.

**chronic alcoholic delirium.** See also **Korsakoff's psychosis.**

**chronic alcoholism,** a pathologic condition resulting from the habitual use of alcohol in excessive amounts. The syndrome involves complex cultural, psychologic, social, and physiologic factors and usually impairs an individual's health and ability to function normally in society. Symptoms of the disease include anorexia, diarrhea, weight loss, neurologic and psychiatric disturbances (most notably depression), and fatty deterioration of the liver, sometimes leading to cirrhosis. Treatment depends on the severity of the disease and its resulting complications; hospitalization may be necessary. Nutritional therapy, use of tranquilizers in the detoxification process, use of disulfiram as an aid to continued abstinence, and psychotherapy are methods of treatment. Alcoholism often is not detected in patients admitted to the hospital for care after an accident or for esophagitis, gastritis, peripheral neuropathy, anemia, or depression, all of which are secondary effects of alcoholism. If alcoholism is not diagnosed and treated, the patient may not recover. If the patient is to undergo an operation, it is imperative that the anesthesiologist be notified of the condition, which can affect sensitivity to anesthetics. Alcoholism is a family disease, and the health professional can be instrumental in guiding the patient's family to seek treatment. Long-term support for alcoholics and their families is offered by such organizations as Alcoholics Anonymous, Al-Anon, Alateen, and rehabilitation facilities for alcoholism. Compare **acute alcoholism.** See also **alcoholism.**

**chronic anterior poliomyelitis,** an inflammation of the gray matter in the spinal cord, resulting in atrophy of muscles of the upper extremities and neck, with long periods of remission of symptoms. See also **poliomyelitis.**

**chronic appendicitis,** a type of appendicitis characterized by thickening or scarring of the vermiform appendix, caused by previous inflammation.

**chronic bacterial prostatitis,** a prolonged but relatively mild bacterial infection of the prostate. Symptoms may include pain, fever, and dysuria, but they are less intense than in acute prostatitis. Treatment depends on the precise cause of the infection and usually involves administration of antibiotics. See also **prostatitis.**

**chronic bronchitis,** a very common, debilitating pulmonary disease, characterized by greatly increased production of mucus by the glands of the trachea and bronchi and resulting in a cough with expectoration for at least 3 months of the year for more than 2 consecutive years.

■ OBSERVATIONS: The condition has a strong association with smoking. Productive cough, often with wheezing, is a universal feature, followed by progressive dyspnea on exertion, repeated purulent respiratory infections, airway narrowing and obstruction, and often respiratory failure. Cor pulmonale with right ventricular heart failure is a common result. In some patients secondary polycythemia results from chronic hypoxemia. Prolonged expiratory phase, prominent cough, cyanosis, and acute attacks of respiratory distress with rapid, labored respirations may result. Common laboratory findings include elevated hematocrit, with or without respiratory acidosis; abnormal liver function caused by right-sided heart failure and hepatic congestion; pathogenic bacteria in the sputum; abnormal pulmonary function test results; and often chest x-ray signs of increased bronchial markings and emphysema.

■ INTERVENTIONS: Patients with chronic bronchitis should be immunized against influenza and pneumococcal infections. Broad-spectrum antibiotics are usually prescribed during acute exacerbations of symptoms. Bronchodilators, such as albuterol, and sympathomimetic drugs, such as terbutaline and metaproterenol, are prescribed to prevent worsening of the condition. Heart failure is managed with appropriate medication.

■ NURSING CONSIDERATIONS: The nurse encourages the patient to discontinue smoking and to avoid exposure to toxic inhalants, such as hair sprays, aerosol insecticides, and occupational irritants and poisons. The use of low-flow oxygen in the home requires patient/family education and monitoring. Exercise, especially walking, is often indicated. See also **asthma, chronic obstructive pulmonary disease, cor pulmonale, emphysema, respiratory failure.**

**chronic care.** See **care of the chronically ill.**

**chronic carrier,** an individual who acts as host to pathogenic organisms for an extended period without displaying any signs of disease.

**chronic cervicitis.** See **cervicitis.**

**chronic cholecystitis.** See **cholecystitis.**

**chronic chorea.** See **Huntington's chorea.**

**chronic cystic mastitis.** See **fibrocystic disease.**

**chronic delirium** [Gk, *chronos,* time; L, *delirare,* to rave], a form of delirium in which the patient shows signs of psychosis but is afebrile. The condition is sometimes associated with exhaustion, malnutrition, and wasting.

**chronic disease,** a disease that persists over a long period as compared with the course of an acute disease. The symptoms of chronic disease are sometimes less severe than those of the acute phase of the same disease. Chronic disease may be progressive, result in complete or partial disability, or even lead to death. Examples of chronic disease include diabetes mellitus, emphysema, and arthritis.

**chronic endoarteritis** [Gk, *chronos,* time, *endon,* within, *arteria,* airpipe, *itis,* inflammation], persistent inflammation of the tunica intima of an arterial wall. It may be accompanied by fatty degeneration of arterial tissue and calcium deposits. Also called **endarteritis deformans.**

**chronic endocarditis** [Gk, *chronos,* time, *endon,* within, *kardia,* heart, *itis,* inflammation], persistent inflammation of the endocardium and usually follows an attack of acute endocarditis, syphilis, or an atheroma. It frequently involves the cardiac valves, making them incompetent. Also called **valvular endocarditis.**

**chronic fatigue syndrome (CFS),** a condition characterized by disabling fatigue, accompanied by a constellation of symptoms, including muscle pain, multijoint pain without swelling, painful cervical or axillary adenopathy, sore throat, headache, impaired memory or concentration, unrefreshing sleep, and postexertional malaise. The diagnosis is one of exclusion; the cause remains obscure but may be a result of Epstein-Barr virus (EBV), infection, or immune system malfunctioning. Therapy is directed to relief of symptoms. Psychiatric intervention may be helpful if depression or anxiety accompanies the condition. The disorder often persists for years; spontaneous resolution occurs in fewer than 40% of cases. Also called **chronic fatigue and immune dysfunction syndrome (CFIDS).**

**chronic gastritis.** See **gastritis.**

**chronic glaucoma.** See **glaucoma.**

**chronic glomerulonephritis,** a noninfectious disease of the glomeruli of the kidney characterized by proteinuria, hematuria, edema, and decreased production of urine. Of unknown cause, it is asymptomatic for years. The symptoms develop slowly, and the disease progresses to kidney failure. Transplantation and dialysis are the only treatments available. See also **postinfectious glomerulonephritis, subacute glomerulonephritis, uremia.**

**chronic gout** [Gk, *chronos,* time; L, *gutta,* drop], a persistent disorder of purine metabolism, characterized by abnormally high levels of serum uric acid and attacks of arthritis, with deposits of urates in the joints. The disorder may be familial and if untreated can lead to renal failure. See also **gout.**

**chronic granulocytic leukemia.** See **chronic myelocytic leukemia.**

**chronic granulomatous disease (CGD),** any of a group of immunodeficiencies of X-linked or autosomal recessive inheritance, caused by failure of the respiratory or metabolic burst, resulting in deficient microbicidal ability. The clinical picture consists of frequent, severe, prolonged bacterial and fungal infections of the skin, oral and intestinal mucosa, reticuloendothelial system, bones, lungs, and genitourinary tract. The course of the disease varies: symptoms may appear in the neonate, with death during the first decade, or a patient may survive into middle age. There seem to be no physiologic differences between the X-linked and the autosomal recessive types.

**chronic hepatitis** [Gk, *chronos,* time, *hēpar,* liver, *itis,* inflammation], a state in which symptoms of hepatitis continue for several months and may increase in severity. In some cases of hepatitis B, the patient may become a lifelong carrier of the antigen and may show prolonged evidence of the infection. See also **alcoholic hepatitis, anicteric hepatitis, cholestatic hepatitis, hepatitis, hepatitis A, hepatitis B, hepatitis C, hepatitis D, hepatitis E.**

**chronic hyperplastic rhinitis** [Gk, *chronos,* time, *hyper,* excess, *plassein,* to form, *rhis,* nose, *itis,* inflammation], chronic inflammation of the mucous membranes of the nose, with polyp formation.

**chronic hyperplastic sinusitis** [Gk, *chronos,* time, *hyper,* excess, *plassein,* to form; L, *sinus,* hollow; Gk, *itis,* inflammation], chronic sinus inflammation, with polyp formation in the nose and sinuses.

**chronic hypertrophic emphysema.** See **panacinar emphysema.**

**chronic hypertrophic rhinitis** [Gk, *chronos,* time, *hyper,* excess, *trophe,* nourishment, *rhis,* nose, *itis,* inflammation], a condition of chronic inflammation of the nasal mucosa associated with enlargement of the mucous membrane.

**chronic hypoxia,** a usually slow, insidious reduction in tissue oxygenation resulting from gradually destructive or fibrotic lung diseases, congenital or acquired heart disorders, or chronic blood loss. The patient experiences persistent mental and physical fatigue, shows sluggish mental responses, and complains of a loss of ability to perform physical tasks. Unless treated, the condition may lead to disability. There may be some physiologic adjustment to the lack of oxygen as occurs in individuals who move from sea level to mountainous areas, where oxygen pressures are reduced.

**chronic idiopathic thrombocytopenic purpura.** See **idiopathic thrombocytopenic purpura.**

**chronic illness,** any disorder that persists over a long period and affects physical, emotional, intellectual, social, or spiritual functioning.

**chronic inflammatory demyelinating polyradiculoneuropathy,** a rare form of symmetrical motor neuron paralysis similar to Guillain-Barré syndrome but progressing more slowly or in a fluctuating pattern.

**chronic interstitial nephritis.** See **interstitial nephritis.**

**chronic intestinal ischemia.** See **intestinal angina.**

**chronic intractable pain** [Gk, *chronos,* time; L, *intractabilis + poena,* penalty], persistent pain that fails to respond to nonnarcotic analgesics and other treatment measures.

**chronicity** /krōnis'itē/, a state of being chronic.

**chronic leg ulcer** [Gk, *chronos,* time; ONorse, *leggr* + L, *ulcus,* ulcer], a slow-healing ulcer of the leg (usually the lower leg). Typically it is associated with varicose veins, deep venous insufficiency, or a similar circulatory obstacle. Nonvenous causes of leg ulceration include arterial disease; ulcers may also be caused by trauma or have a bacterial, mycotic, hematologic, neoplastic, neurologic, or systemic origin. Treatment includes elevation of the leg two or three times daily, elastic support applied to the limb of the ambulatory patient, and avoidance of maceration of the wound.

**chronic lingual papillitis** [Gk, *chronos* + L, *lingua,* tongue, *papilla,* nipple; Gk, *itis*], an inflammatory disorder of the tongue, sometimes extending to the buccal mucosa and palate. It is characterized by irregularly scattered red patches, thinning of the lingual papillae, severe burning pain, and shedding of epidermal tissue. The disorder affects middle-aged individuals, especially women, and occurs in attacks alternating with remissions that last weeks or months. Also called **Moeller's glossitis.**

**chronic low blood pressure,** a condition in which systolic and diastolic blood pressures are consistently below their normal values (approximately 120 and 70 mm Hg, respectively, in a young adult).

**chronic lymphocytic leukemia (CLL)** [Gk, *chronos* + L, *lympha,* water; Gk, *kytos,* cell, *leukos,* white, *haima,* blood], a neoplasm of blood-forming tissues, characterized by a proliferation of small, long-lived lymphocytes, chiefly B cells, in bone marrow, blood, liver, and lymphoid organs. CLL is rare in persons less than 35 years of age, increases in frequency with age, and is more common in men than in women. The disease has an insidious onset and progresses to cause malaise, ready fatigability, anorexia, weight loss, nocturnal sweating, lymphadenopathy, and hepatosplenomegaly. Most patients can continue normal activities for years; 25 die of unrelated diseases. No treatment is curative, but remissions may be induced by chemotherapy or irradiation. See also **acute lymphocytic leukemia.**

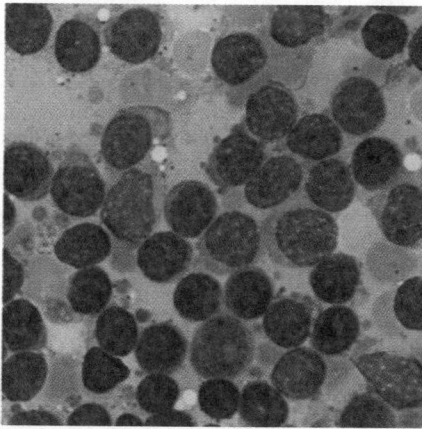

**Chronic lymphocytic leukemia** *(Carr and Rodak, 1999)*

**chronic mastitis.** See **mastitis.**

**chronic mountain sickness** [Gk, *chronos,* time; L, *montana;* AS, *soec*], a form of altitude sickness in which the increased production of red cells results in polycythemia.

Some symptoms, such as headache, weakness, and limb aches, occasionally develop in indigenous mountain dwellers as well as in persons who had become acclimatized to the higher altitudes. See also **altitude sickness.**

**chronic mucocutaneous candidiasis,** a rare form of candidiasis, characterized by candidal infection lesions of the skin, mucous membranes, GI tract, and respiratory tract. This disease usually occurs during the first year of life or with immune system dysfunction but can develop at any time. It affects both males and females and may be associated with an inherited defect of the cell-mediated immune system that allows autoantibodies to develop against target organs. The humoral immune system functions normally in this disease. The onset of infections associated with the disease may precede endocrinopathy.

■ OBSERVATIONS: Chronic mucocutaneous candidiasis may affect the skin, the mucous membranes, the nails, and the vagina, usually causing large, circular lesions. Associated viral infections may lead to endocrinopathy and hepatitis. Infections of the mouth, nose, and palate may cause problems with speech and eating. Tetany and hypocalcemia are the most common symptoms associated with the endocrinopathy and are usually confined to the organ involved. Other complications associated with chronic mucocutaneous candidiasis may include diabetes, Addison's disease, hypothyroidism, and pernicious anemia. In some patients psychiatric problems develop as a result of disfigurements and extensive endocrinal disorders. Diagnosis of this disease usually includes laboratory tests, which commonly show a normal T-cell count and normal immunologic responses to antigens other than *Candida albicans.* The endocrinopathy associated with this disease may include nonimmunologic aberrations, such as hypocalcemia, abnormal hepatic function, hyperglycemia, iron deficiency, and abnormal vitamin $B_{12}$ absorption. Other immunodeficiency diseases associated with chronic *Candida* infection must be excluded by diagnosis. Such immunodeficiency diseases as DiGeorge's syndrome, ataxia-telangiectasia, and severe combined immunodeficiency disease all cause serious immunologic defects. Required after diagnosis of chronic mucocutaneous candidiasis are evaluations of numerous physiologic mechanisms, such as adrenal, gonadal, pancreatic, parathyroid, pituitary, and thyroid functions. Chronic mucocutaneous candidiasis is progressive and usually leads to endocrinopathy.

■ INTERVENTIONS: Chronic mucocutaneous candidiasis resists treatment with topical antifungal agents, miconazole, and nystatin. Endocrinopathies associated with the disease must be treated individually by hormone replacement; some success in this regard has been reported with experimental injections of thymosin and levamisole. Most success in treating severe cases has been achieved with transfer factor from a *Candida*-positive donor, with IV amphotericin B. Some success may also be possible against systemic infection with amphotericin B, but that agent is highly nephrotoxic. Some patients respond fairly well to fetal thymus transplantation. Plastic surgery may aid patients in coping with disfigurements caused by the disease. Treatment may also include oral or intramuscular iron replacement.

■ NURSING CONSIDERATIONS: Patients with chronic mucocutaneous candidiasis must be closely monitored for signs of other associated diseases, as Addison's disease, diabetes, hepatitis, and pernicious anemia. Patients suffering psychologically from disfigurements associated with the disease often respond positively to the counsel, encouragement, and kindness of the nursing staff. Amphotericin B, a nephrotoxin, is involved in the treatment; therefore the patient must be carefully monitored for renal function. Patients benefit from calm explanations of the progressive manifestations of the disease and the importance of regular endocrinologic checkups.

**chronic myelocytic leukemia (CML),** a malignant neoplasm of blood-forming tissues, characterized by a proliferation of granular leukocytes and, often, of megakaryocytes. The disease occurs most frequently in mature adults and begins insidiously. Its progress is marked by malaise, fatigue, heat intolerance, bleeding gums, purpura, skin lesions, weight loss, hyperuricemia, abdominal discomfort, and massive splenomegaly. Differential blood count and bone-marrow biopsies are performed to aid in the diagnosis. The alkaline phosphatase activity of the leukocytes is low, and the Philadelphia chromosome is present in myeloblasts in most patients with CML. Therapy with an oral alkylating agent is usual, but advanced CML is refractory to chemotherapy. Also called **chronic granulocytic leukemia (CGL), chronic myelogenous leukemia (CML), chronic myeloid leukemia, splenomedullary leukemia, splenomyelogenous leukemia.** See also **acute myelocytic leukemia.**

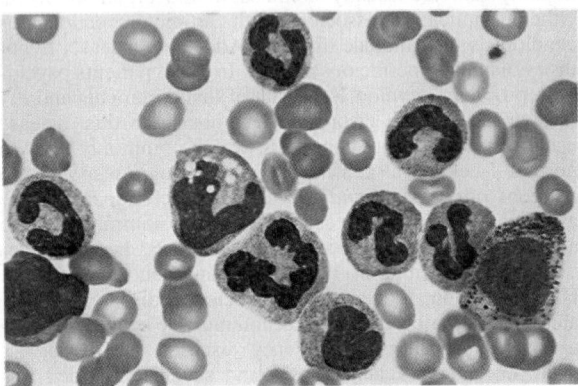

**Chronic myelocytic leukemia**
*(Kumar, Cotran, and Robbins, 1997/courtesy Dr. Robert W. McKenna, Department of Pathology, University of Texas Southwestern Medical School, Dallas)*

phropathy, but the condition can also develop from no known cause. Symptoms include polyuria, renal acidosis, edema, proteinuria, and blood in the urine. Treatment varies with correction of underlying causal factors. See also **kidney disease.**

**chronic obstructive pulmonary disease (COPD),** a progressive and irreversible condition characterized by diminished inspiratory and expiratory capacity of the lungs. The patient complains of dyspnea with physical exertion, difficulty in inhaling or exhaling deeply, and sometimes a chronic cough. The condition is aggravated by cigarette smoking and air pollution. COPDs include asthma, chronic bronchiectasis, chronic bronchitis, and emphysema. Also called **chronic obstructive lung disease.**

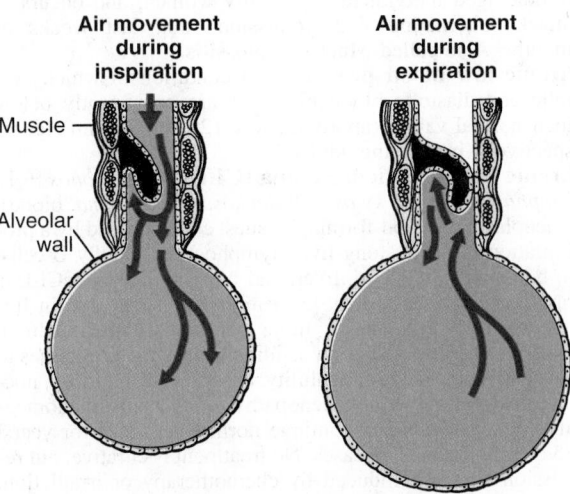

**Mechanisms of air trapping in chronic obstructive pulmonary disease**
*(Huether & McCance, 2000)*

**chronic myocarditis** [Gk, *chronos,* time, *mys,* muscle, *kardia,* heart, *itis,* inflammation], inflammation of the myocardium that persists after an acute bacterial infection. Chronic myocarditis is characterized by degeneration of muscle tissue and fibrosis or infiltration of interstitial tissues.

**chronic nephritis** [Gk, *chronos,* time, *nephros,* kidney, *itis,* inflammation], a form of kidney inflammation usually secondary to another disease, such as chronic pyelonephritis. In chronic interstitial nephritis the kidney becomes small and granular with thickening of arteries and arterioles and proliferation of interstitial tissue. There may be functional abnormalities, such as urea retention, hematuria, and casts.

**chronic nephropathy,** a kidney disorder characterized by generalized or local damage to the tubulointerstitial areas of the kidney. The condition frequently results from more than a single cause, such as diabetes and a bacterial infection. Toxins, in the form of drugs or heavy metals, including cadmium or lead, are common causes, as are gout, cystinosis, and other metabolic disorders. Sickle cell disease is one of several inherited factors that may contribute to chronic ne-

**chronic (open-angle) glaucoma.** See **glaucoma.**

**chronic pain,** pain that continues or recurs over a prolonged period, caused by various diseases or abnormal conditions, such as rheumatoid arthritis. Chronic pain may be less intense than acute pain. The person with chronic pain does not usually display increased pulse and rapid respiration because these autonomic reactions to pain cannot be sustained for long periods. Others with chronic pain may withdraw from their environment and concentrate solely on their affliction, totally ignoring their family, their friends, and external stimuli. Some factors that can complicate the treatment of persons with chronic pain are scarring, continuing psychologic stress, and medication. Compare **acute pain.** See also **pain; pain, chronic; pain intervention; pain pathway.**

**chronic pancreatitis** [Gk, *chronos,* time, *peri,* near, *teinein-all, kreas,* flesh, *itis,* inflammation], chronic inflammation of the pancreas with fibrosis and calcification of the gland. It may follow repeated acute attacks and can lead to diabetes.

**chronic peritonitis** [Gk, *chronos,* time, *peri,* near, *tenein,* to stretch, *itis,* inflammation], a form of peritonitis in which the peritoneum thickens and ascites develop. The condition is usually associated with another disorder, such as pericarditis or polyserositis.

**chronic pharyngitis** [Gk, *chronos,* time, *pharynx,* throat, *itis,* inflammation], persistent throat inflammation that may be associated with the lymphoid granules in the pharyngeal mucosa.

**chronic progressive myelopathy,** gradually progressive spastic paraparesis associated with infection by human T-lymphotropic virus 1, characterized by progressive difficulty in walking and weakness of the lower extremity, sensory disturbances, and urinary incontinence, with no evidence of spinal compression or motor neuron involvement. Also called **HTLV-1−associated myelopathy, tropical spastic paraparesis.**

**chronic prostatitis** [Gk, *chronos,* time, *prostates,* one standing before, *itis,* inflammation], a persistent inflammatory condition of the prostate characterized by dull, aching pain in the lower back or perineal area and dysuria. Other symptoms may include fever and discharge from the penis.

**chronic purulent synovitis.** See **chronic synovitis.**

**chronic pyelonephritis.** See **pyelonephritis.**

**chronic rejection,** immune rejection of transplanted tissue that may continue for several months.

**chronic renal failure.** See **renal failure.**

**chronic rheumatism** [Gk, *chronos,* time, *rheumatismos,* that which flows], a persistent, nonspecific, painful condition of the musculoskeletal tissues, including nonarticular forms of arthritis. See also **rheumatism.**

**chronic synovitis** [Gk, *chronos,* time, *syn,* together; L, *ovum,* egg; Gk, *itis,* inflammation], chronic inflammation of the synovial membrane of a joint. Kinds of chronic synovitis include **chronic purulent synovitis** and **chronic serous synovitis.** See also **synovitis.**

**chronic tetanus** [Gk, *chronos,* time, *tetanos,* convulsive tension], **1.** a form of tetanus with a delayed onset, slow progression of the disease, and milder than usual symptoms. **2.** a reactivated tetanus infection in a healed wound.

**chronic tuberculous mastitis,** a rare infection of the breast resulting from extension of tuberculosis of underlying ribs. The condition is also characterized by multiple sinus tracts and the presence of tuberculosis elsewhere in the body.

**chronic undifferentiated schizophrenia,** a condition marked by the symptoms of more than one of the classic types of schizophrenia—simple, paranoid, or catatonic. See also **acute schizophrenia.**

**chrono-, chron-,** combining form meaning 'time': *chronognosis, chronophobia, chronotropism.*

**chronobiology,** the study of the effects of time on living systems.

**chronograph** /kron′əgraf/ [Gk, *chronos + graphein,* to record], a device that records small intervals of time, such as a stopwatch. **—chronographic,** *adj.*

**chronologic** /kron′əloj′ik/ [Gk, *chronos + logos,* reason], **1.** arranged in time sequence. **2.** pertaining to chronology. Also **chronological.**

**chronologic age,** the age of an individual expressed as time that has elapsed since birth. The age of an infant is expressed in hours, days, or months; the age of children and adults is expressed in years.

**chronopsychophysiology** /kron′ōsī′kofis′ē·ol′əjē/, the science of physiologic cyclic processes in the body.

**chronotherapeutics** /kron′ōther′əpyōō′tiks/, a branch of medicine concerned with effects of circadian rhythms in human health, such as the hour of the day when asthma symptoms or heart attacks are most likely to occur and the best time of day for treating certain complaints. Practitioners of

chronotherapeutics also believe that there is a best time of the month for performing breast cancer surgery and that cholesterol levels are higher and heart attacks are more common during the winter months.

**chronotropism** /krənot′rəpiz′əm/ [Gk, *chronos + trepein,* to turn], the act or process of affecting the regularity of a periodic function, especially interference with the rate of heartbeat. **—chronotropic,** *adj.*

**chrys-,** combining form meaning 'gold': *chrysotherapy, chrysoderma.*

**Chrysanthemum** /kri·san′thə·məm/, a genus of perennial flowering herbs of the family Compositae, native to the Balkans and the Middle East. They are a common cause of contact dermatitis, and their powdered flowers are insecticidal and scabicidal and a source of pyrethrins.

**chrysarobin** /kris′ərō′bin/, a substance obtained from the wood of araboa trees and used as an irritant in the treatment of parasitic skin diseases and psoriasis.

**chrysiasis** /krəsī′əsis/ [Gk, *chrysos,* gold, *osis,* condition], an abnormal condition that may develop after gold therapy. The condition is characterized by the deposition of gold in body tissues. Also called **auriasis.**

**chrysotherapy** /kris′ōther′əpē/ [Gk, *chrysos + therapeia,* treatment], the treatment of any disease with gold salts. **—chrysotherapeutic,** *adj.*

**Chua K'a,** a holistic counseling system of muscle tension release that emphasizes clarification and cleansing of the mind and emotions.

**Churg-Strauss syndrome** /churg′strous′/ [Jacob Churg, twentieth-century American pathologist; Lotte Straus, twentieth-century American pathologist], an allergic disorder marked by granulomatosis, usually of the lungs, and often involving the circulatory system. See also **vasculitis.**

**Chvostek's sign** /khvôsh′teks/ [Franz Chvostek, Austrian surgeon, 1835–1884], an abnormal spasm of the facial muscles elicited by light taps on the facial nerve in patients who are hypocalcemic. It is a sign of tetany.

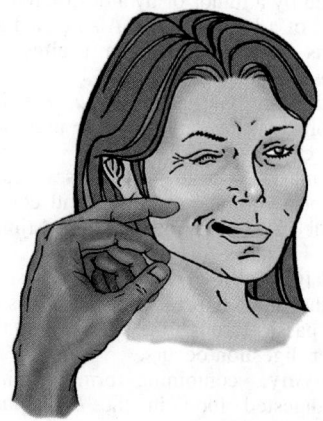

**Chvostek's sign** *(Monahan and Neighbors, 1998)*

**Chvostek-Weiss sign.** See **Chvostek's sign.**

**chyl-.** See **chylo-.**

**chyle** /kīl/ [Gk, *chylos,* juice], the cloudy liquid products of digestion taken up by the small intestine. Consisting mainly of emulsified fats, chyle passes through fingerlike projections in the small intestine, called lacteals, and into the lymphatic system for transport to the venous circulation at the thoracic duct in the neck. Also called **chylus.** —**chylous,** *adj.*

**chylemia** /kīlē′mē·ə/, a condition in which chyle appears in the blood.

**chyli-.** See **chylo-.**

**-chylia,** suffix meaning '(condition of the) digestive juices, or chyle': *dyschylia, euchylia, polychylia.*

**chyliform ascites.** See **chylous ascites.**

**chylo-, chyl-, chyli-,** combining form meaning 'chyle': *chylocyst, chylophonic, chylosis.*

**chylocele** /kī′ləsēl/, a cystic lesion caused by an effusion of chylous fluid into the tunica vaginalis of the testes.

**chyloid** /kī′loid/, resembling the chyle that fills the lacteals of the small intestine during the digestion of fatty foods.

**chylomediastinum** /kī′lōmē′dē·astī′nəm/ [Gk, *chylos,* juice; L, *mediastinus,* midway], the presence of chyle in the mediastinum.

**chylomicron** /kī′lōmī′kron/ [Gk, *chylos* + *mikros,* small], minute lipoproteins measuring less than 0.5 μm in diameter. Chylomicrons consist of about 90 triglycerides with small amounts of cholesterol, phospholipids, fat-soluble vitamins, and protein. They are synthesized in the GI tract and carry dietary fat from the intestinal mucosa via the thoracic lymphatic duct into the plasma and ultimately to the liver and tissues. The remnant chylomicron particles are removed by the liver.

**chylosus ascites.** See **chylous ascites.**

**chylothorax** /kī′lōthôr′aks/ [Gk, *chylos* + *thorax,* chest], a condition marked by the effusion of chyle from the thoracic duct into the pleural space. The cause is usually a traumatic injury to the neck or a tumor that invades the thoracic duct. Treatment is directed at repairing damage to the duct.

**chylous** /kī′ləs/ [Gk, *chylos,* juice], pertaining to or resembling chyle.

**chylous ascites,** an abnormal condition characterized by an accumulation of chyle in the peritoneal cavity. Chylous ascites results from an obstruction in the thoracic duct that may be caused by a tumor or by a destructive lesion, resulting in rupture of a lymph vessel. Also called **ascites adiposus, chylosus ascites, chyliform ascites, fatty ascites, milky ascites.** See also **ascites.**

**chyluria** /kīlŏŏr′ē·ə/ [Gk, *chylos* + *ouron,* urine], a milky appearance of the urine caused by the presence of chyle.

**chylus.** See **chyle.**

**chymase** /kī′mās/, a serine proteinase present in human mast cells, most prominent in skin and connective tissue, where it can cleave angiotensin and stimulate mucous glands.

**chyme** /kīm/ [Gk, *chymos,* juice], the viscous, semifluid contents of the stomach present during digestion of a meal. Chyme then passes through the pylorus into the duodenum, where further digestion occurs.

**-chymia, -chymy,** combining form meaning '(condition of) partly digested food in the duodenum': *achymia, ischochymia, oligochymia.*

**chymopapain** /kī′mōpəpā′ēn/ [Gk, *chymos* + Sp, *papaya*], a proteolytic enzyme isolated from the fruit of *Carica papaya* and related to papain. It is used in the treatment of prolapsed intervertebral or herniated disks.

**chymosin.** See **rennin.**

**chymotrypsin** /kī′mōtrip′sin/ [Gk, *chymos* + *tryein,* to rub, *pepsin,* digestion], **1.** a proteolytic enzyme, produced by the pancreas, that catalyzes the hydrolysis of casein and gelatin. **2.** a yellow crystalline powder prepared from an extract of ox pancreas, which is used in treating digestive disorders in which the enzyme is present in less than normal amounts or is totally lacking.

**chymotrypsinogen** /kī′mōtripsin′əjən/, a substance, produced in the pancreas, that is the zymogen precursor to the enzyme chymotrypsin. It is converted to chymotrypsin by trypsin.

**-chymy.** See **-chymia.**

**Ci,** abbreviation for **curie.**

*CI,* abbreviation for *Colour Index.*

**cibophobia** /sē′bə-/ [L, *cibus,* food; Gk, *phobos,* fear], an abnormal or morbid aversion to food or to eating.

**CIC,** abbreviation for *Certified Infection Control.*

**cicatrices.** See **cicatrix.**

**cicatricial alopecia** /sisətrish′əl/, a form of baldness produced by scar formation in dermatoses such as lupus erythematosus, usually progressing to permanent baldness.

**cicatricial entropion.** See **cicatrix, entropion.**

**cicatricial pemphigoid** [L, *cicatrix,* scar; Gk, *pemphix,* blister or bubble + *eidos,* form], a benign, chronic, usually bilateral, subepidermal blistering disease chiefly involving the mucous membranes, especially those of the mouth and eye; it heals by scarring and may lead to slow shrinkage of the affected tissues, and to blindness if untreated. Also called **benign mucosal pemphigoid.**

**cicatricial scar** [L, *cicatrix,* scar; Gk, *eschara,* scab], a fibrous scar that remains after a wound has healed.

**cicatricial stenosis** [L, *cicatrix,* scar; Gk, *stenos,* narrow, *osis,* condition], the narrowing of a duct or tube caused by the formation of scar tissue.

**cicatrix** /sik′ətriks, sikā′triks/, *pl.* cicatrices /sik′ətrī′sēz/ [L, scar], scar tissue that is avascular, pale, contracted, and firm after the earlier phase of skin healing characterized by redness and softness. —**cicatricial** /sik′ətrish′əl/, *adj.* —**cicatrize,** *v.*

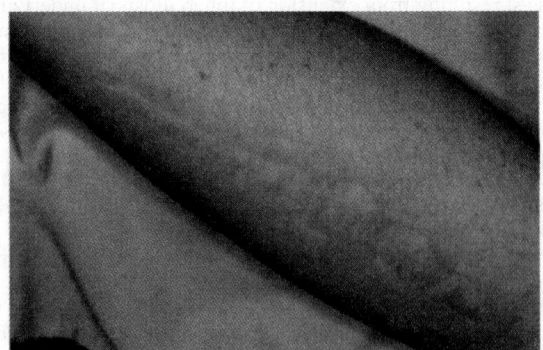

**Cicatrix** *(Lemmi and Lemmi, 2000)*

**cicatrize** /sik′ətrīz/ [L, *cicatrix,* scar], to heal so as to form a scar.

**ciclopirox** /sī′kləpī′roks/, a topical antifungal agent.

■ INDICATIONS: It is prescribed in the treatment of tinea and candidiasis.

■ CONTRAINDICATION: Known sensitivity to this drug prohibits its use.

■ ADVERSE EFFECTS: Among the most serious adverse reactions are local reactions of irritation, pruritus at the application site, burning, and worsening of clinical signs and symptoms.

**ciclosporin.** See **cyclosporine.**

**cicutism** /sik′yo͞otiz′əm/ [L, *Cicuta,* hemlock; Gk, *ismos,* process], poisoning caused by water hemlock, resulting in cyanosis, dilated pupils, convulsions, and coma.

**CID,** abbreviation for **cytomegalic inclusion disease.**

**-cide, -cid,** suffix meaning 'killing': *amebicide, herbicide, protozoacide.*

**-cidin,** combining form designating a natural antibiotic.

**cidofovir,** an antiviral.

■ INDICATIONS: This drug is used to treat cytomegalovirus retinitis in patients with AIDS.

■ CONTRAINDICATIONS: Known hypersensitivity to acyclovir or this drug prohibits its use.

■ ADVERSE EFFECTS: Life-threatening effects include coma, hemorrhage, hematuria, granulocytopenia, thrombocytopenia, irreversible neutropenia, anemia, and eosinophilia. Other serious adverse effects include confusion, psychosis, tremors, somnolence, dysrhythmias, hypertension/hypotension, retinal detachment in cytomegalovirus retinitis, abnormal liver function tests, increased creatinine, increased blood urea nitrogen, and phlebitis.

**cigarette drain** [Sp, *cigarro* + AS, *dranen*], a surgical drain fashioned from a section of gauze or surgical sponge drawn into a tube of gutta-percha.

**cigarette smoking,** the inhalation of the gases and hydrocarbon vapors generated by slowly burning tobacco in cigarettes. The practice stems partly from the effect on the nervous system of the nicotine contained in the smoke. In addition to nicotine, nearly 1000 other chemicals have been identified in cigarette smoke, including carcinogenic polycyclic aromatic alcohols, cocarcinogenic phenols and fatty acids, carbon monoxide, hydrogen sulfide, hydrocyanic acid, nitrogen oxides, and various irritants that suppress protease inhibition and impair alveolar macrophage function. Cigarette smoke is addictive and is considered more dangerous than pipe or cigar smoke because it is less irritating and therefore more likely to be inhaled. See also **lung cancer, nicotine.**

**ciguatera poisoning** /sē′gwəter′ə/ [Sp, *cigua,* sea snail; L, *potio,* drink], a nonbacterial food poisoning that results from eating fish contaminated with the ciguatera toxin. Many of the over 300 varieties of fish from the Caribbean or South Pacific have been implicated; barracuda is a common source. The toxin is believed to block acetylcholinesterase activity. Characteristics of ciguatera poisoning are vomiting, diarrhea, tingling or numbness of extremities and the skin around the mouth, itching, muscle weakness, pain, and respiratory paralysis. Cold liquids feel hot to the surfaces of the mouth and throat. No specific treatment has been developed.

**cili-,** **1.** combining form meaning 'eyelid': *ciliectomy, cilioretinal, cilioscleral.* **2.** combining form meaning 'eyelash': *ciliary, cilium.* **3.** combining form meaning 'minute vibratile': *ciliated, ciliogenesis.*

**cilia** /sil′ē·ə/, *sing.* **cilium** [L, eyelids or eyelashes], **1.** the eyelids or eyelashes. **2.** small, hairlike processes projecting from epithelial cells on the outer surfaces of some cells, aiding metabolism by producing motion, eddies, or current in a fluid. In the lung, cilia wave mucus, pus, and dust upward.

**ciliary** /sil′ē·er′ē/ [L, *cilia*], pertaining to the eyelashes or eyelids.

**ciliary body** [L, *cilia*], the thickened part of the vascular tunic of the eye that joins the iris with the anterior portion of the choroid. It is composed of the ciliary crown, ciliary pro-

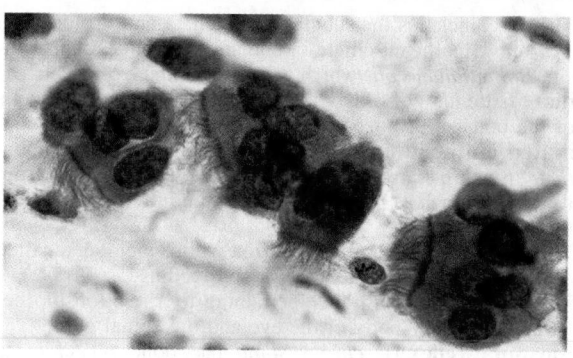

**Cilia** *(McKee, 1997)*

cesses and folds, ciliary orbiculus, ciliary muscle, and a basal lamina.

**ciliary canal,** the spaces of the iridocorneal angle.

**ciliary disk,** the thin part of the ciliary body extending between its crown and the ora serrata retinae.

**ciliary ganglion,** a small parasympathetic ganglion in the orbit of the eye, which controls pupillary and accommodative reflexes.

**ciliary gland,** one of the numerous tiny, modified sweat glands arranged in several rows near the free margins of the eyelids. The apertures of the glands lie near the attachments of the eyelashes. Acute localized bacterial infection of one or more of the ciliary glands causes external sties. Also called **glands of Moll Zeis.** Compare **tarsal gland.**

**ciliary margin,** the peripheral border of the iris, continuous with the ciliary body.

**ciliary movement,** the upward waving motion of the hairlike processes projecting from the epithelium of the respiratory tract and from certain microorganisms.

**ciliary mucus transport,** the movement of mucus-trapped particles from the upper respiratory tract to the lower pharynx, propelled by the motion of microscopic cilia lining the tract.

**ciliary muscle,** a semitransparent circular band of smooth muscle fibers attached to the choroid of the eye, the chief agent in glowing lens adjustment of the eye to assume a more spherical shape. It draws the ciliary process centripetally, relaxing the suspensory ligament of the crystalline lens and allowing the lens to become more convex.

**ciliary process,** any one of about 80 tiny fleshy projections on the posterior surface of the iris, forming a frill around the margin of the crystalline lens of the eye. The processes compose one of the two zones of the ciliary body of the eye and are formed by infolding of the various layers of the choroid. They secrete nutrient fluids to nourish the lens, cornea, and vitreous body. See also **ciliary body.**

**ciliary reflex.** See **accommodation reflex.**

**ciliary ring,** a small grooved band of tissue, about 4 mm wide, that forms the posterior part of the ciliary body of the eye. It extends from the ora serrata of the retina to the ciliary processes and is thicker near the ciliary processes as a result of the thickness of the ciliary muscle.

**ciliary zone,** an outer circular area on the anterior surface of the iris, separated from the inner circular area by the angular line. The ciliary zone contains the stroma of the iris. Also called **zonula ciliaris.**

**Ciliata** /sil′ē·ā′tə/, a class of protozoa of the subphylum Ciliophora, characterized by cilia throughout the life cycle.

The class includes the subclasses Euciliata and Protociliata. The only significant ciliate in humans is the intestinal parasite *Balantidium coli,* which causes dysentery.

**ciliate** /sil′ē·it/, of or having cilia, as certain epithelial cells of the body or protozoa of the class Ciliata.

**ciliated epithelium** /sil′ē·ā′tid/ [L, *cilia* + Gk, *epi,* upon, *thele,* nipple], any epithelial tissue that projects cilia from its surface, such as portions of the epithelium in the respiratory tract.

**Ciliophora,** a phylum of protozoa whose members, called ciliates, use cilia for locomotion and feeding.

**ciliospinal** /sil′ē·ōspī′nəl/, pertaining to a relationship between the ciliary body of the eye and the spinal cord.

**ciliospinal reflex** [L, *cilia* + *spina,* backbone, *reflectere,* to bend back], a normal brainstem reflex initiated by scratching or pinching the skin of the neck or face, causing dilation of the pupil. Also called **pupillary skin reflex.**

**cilium.** See **cilia.**

**-cillin,** suffix designating a penicillin.

**cilostazol,** a platelet aggregation inhibitor.

- INDICATIONS: This drug is used to treat intermittent claudication.

- CONTRAINDICATIONS: Known hypersensitivity to this drug, congestive heart failure, active liver disease, blood dyscrasias, and active bleeding prohibit this drug's use.

- ADVERSE EFFECTS: Life-threatening effects include atrial fibrillation/flutter, cerebral infarct, cerebral ischemia, congestive heart failure, cardiac arrest, myocardial infarction, nodal dysrhythmias, bleeding (epistaxis, hematuria, conjunctival hemorrhage, GI bleeding), agranulocytosis, neutropenia, and thrombocytopenia. Serious adverse effects include palpitations, tachycardia, vomiting, colitis, cholelithiasis, ulcer, and diabetes mellitus. Common side effects include vertigo, diarrhea, rash, back pain, headache, infection, myalgia, peripheral edema, cough, pharyngitis, and rhinitis.

**cimbia** /sim′bē·ə/, a girdlelike band of white fibers that extends across the surface of the cerebral peduncle.

**cimetidine** /simet′idēn/, an H₂-receptor antagonist.

- INDICATIONS: It is prescribed to inhibit the production and secretion of acid in the stomach in the treatment of gastroesophageal reflux disease, pancreatitis, and hypersecretory conditions because of its inhibitory effect on the production and secretion of gastric acid.

- CONTRAINDICATION: Known hypersensitivity to this drug prohibits its use.

- ADVERSE EFFECTS: Among the more serious adverse reactions are diarrhea, dizziness, rash, confusion (usually in elderly patients given large doses), and gynecomastia.

*Cimex lectularius.* See **bedbug.**

**CIN,** abbreviation for **cervical intraepithelial neoplasia.**

**cinchona** /singkō′nə, chinchō′nə/ [countess of Chinchon, Peru], the dried bark of the stem or root of species of *Cinchona,* containing the alkaloids quinine and quinidine.

**cinchonism** /sin′kōniz′əm/, a condition resulting from excessive ingestion of cinchona bark or its alkaloid derivatives. Cinchonism is characterized by hearing loss, headache, ringing in the ears, and signs of cerebral congestion. See also **quinine.**

**cine-, kine-, kinesio-,** prefix meaning 'movement': *cineangiogram, cinefluorography, cineradiography.*

**cineangiocardiogram** /sin′ē·an′jē·ōkär′dē·əgram′/, a radiograph produced by cineangiocardiography.

**cineangiocardiography** /sin′ē·an′jē·ōkär′dē·og′rəfē/ [Gk, *kinesis,* movement, *angeion,* vessel, *kardia,* heart, *graphein,* to record], the production of images of the cardiovascular system by a combination of fluoroscopic, radiographic, and motion-picture techniques. See also **cineradiography.**

**cineangiogram** /sin′ē·an′jē·əgram′/, a motion-picture recording of a blood vessel or of a portion of the cardiovascular system, obtained after injecting a patient with a nontoxic radiopaque medium.

**cineangiograph** /sin′ē·an′jē·əgraf′/, a movie camera used for recording fluorescent images of the cardiovascular system.

**cine film** /sin′ē/, a type of motion picture film used in cineradiography, usually in cardiac catheterization or GI studies.

**cinefluorography.** See **cineradiography.**

**cinematics.** See **kinematics.**

**cineradiography** /sin′irā′dē·og′rəfē/ [Gk, *kinesis,* movement; L, *radiere,* to shine; Gk, *graphein,* to record], the filming with a movie camera of the images that appear on a fluorescent screen, especially images of body structures following injection of a nontoxic radiopaque medium. Cineradiography incorporates the techniques of cinematography, fluoroscopy, and radiography as a diagnostic technique. Also called **cinefluorography, cineroentgenofluorography.** See also **cineangiocardiography.**

**cinesia.** See **kinesia.**

**-cinesis, -cinesia.** See **-kinesis.**

**cingulate** /sing′gyəlit/ [L, *cingulum,* girdle], **1.** having a zone or a girdle, usually with transverse markings. **2.** pertaining to a cingulum.

**cingulate sulcus.** See **callosomarginal fissure.**

**cingulectomy** /sing′gyŏŏlek′təmē/ [L, *cingulum* + Gk, *ektomē,* excision], the surgical excision of a portion of the cingulate gyrus in the frontal lobe of the brain and the immediately surrounding tissue.

**cingulotomy** /sing′gyŏŏlot′əmē/ [L, *cingulum* + *temnein,* to cut], a procedure in brain surgery to alleviate intractable pain by producing lesions in the tissue of the cingulate gyrus of the frontal lobe. The operation interrupts the fibers of the white matter in the gyrus by the stereotactic application of heat or cold.

**cinnamon** /sin′əmən/ [Gk, *kinnamomon*], the aromatic inner bark of several species of *Cinnamomum,* a tree native to the East Indies and China. Saigon cinnamon is commonly used as a carminative, an aromatic stimulant, and a spice. —**cinnamic,** *adj.*

**CIPM,** abbreviation for **Comité International des Poids et Mesures.**

**circa** [L, *circa,* about], approximate, as an approximate date or number.

**circadian dysrhythmia** /sərkā′dē·ən, sur′kədē′ən/ [L, *circa,* about, *dies,* day; Gk, *dys,* bad, *rhythmos*], the biologic and psychologic stress effects of jet lag, or rapid travel through several time zones. In addition to a shift in normal eating and sleeping patterns, disruption of medication schedules and other therapies may occur.

**circadian rhythm** [L, *circa,* about, *dies,* day; Gk, *rhythmos*], a pattern based on a 24-hour cycle, especially the repetition of certain physiologic phenomena, as sleeping and eating.

**circinate** /sur′sināt/ [L, *circinare,* to make round], having a ring-shaped outline or formation; annular.

**circle** [L, *circulus*], (in anatomy) a circular or nearly circular structure of the body, as the circle of Willis and circle of Zinn. —**circular,** *adj.*

**circle of Carus.** See **curve of Carus.**

**circle of least confusion,** (in optics) a disk representing the image of a theoretical point made by a lens.

**circle of Willis** [Thomas Willis, English physician, 1621–1675], a vascular network at the base of the brain. It is formed by the interconnection of the internal carotid, anterior cerebral *(1),* posterior cerebral *(5),* basilar *(6),* ante-

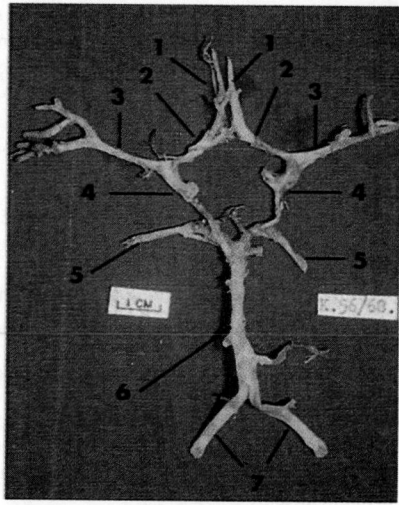

**Circle of Willis** *(Greig and Garden, 1996)*

rior communicating *(2),* and posterior communicating *(4)* arteries.

**CircOlectric (COL) bed,** trademark for an electronically controlled bed that can be vertically rotated 210 degrees and allows a patient to move vertically from the prone to supine position. It is used especially in orthopedics and in the treatment of patients with severe burns and decubitus ulcers. The bed consists of a strong aluminum circular frame supporting an anterior and a posterior straight frame within the exterior aluminum circle. The patient is "sandwiched" and secured between the two straight frames during rotation. Compare **Foster bed, hyperextension bed, Stryker wedge frame.**

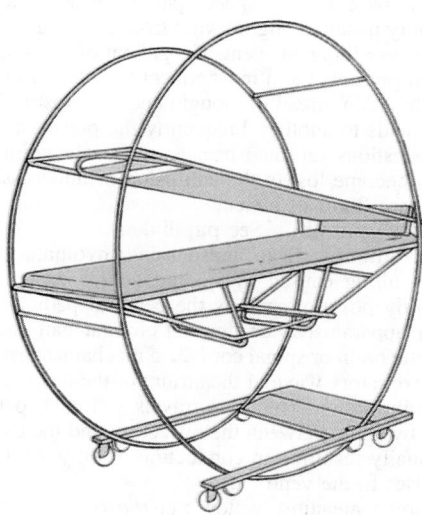

**CircOlectric bed** *(Sorrentino, 1992)*

**circuit** /sur′kit/ [L, *circuitus,* going around], a course or pathway, particularly one through which an electric current passes. Current passes through a closed or continuous circuit and stops if the circuit is open, interrupted, or broken. See also **volt.**

**circuit training,** a method of physical exercise in which activities are arranged in sets and the participant moves quickly from one set to another with a minimum of rest between sets.

**circular.** See **circle.**

**circular bandage** /sur′kyələr/ [L, *circularis,* round], a bandage wrapped around an injured part, usually a limb.

**circular fiber,** any one of the many fibers in the free gingiva that encircle the teeth. Compare **alveolar fiber, apical fiber.**

**circular fold,** one of the numerous annular projections in the small intestine. They vary in size and frequency in the duodenum, the jejunum, and the ileum and are formed by mucous and submucous tissue. Also called **plica circularis, valve of Kerckring.**

**circulation**[1] /sur′kyəlā′shən/ [L, *circulatio,* to go around], movement of an object or substance through a circular course so that it returns to its starting point, such as the circulation of blood through the circuitous network of arteries and veins.

**circulation**[2], a nursing outcome from the Nursing Outcome Classification (NOC) defined as extent to which blood flows unobstructed, unidirectionally, and at an appropriate pressure through large vessels of the systemic and pulmonary circuits. See also **nursing outcomes classification.**

**circulation rate** [L, *circulatio,* to go around, *ratum,* calculation], the rate of blood flow, usually expressed as the amount of blood pumped through the heart per minute. The rate varies with such factors as blood volume and cardiac contractility.

**circulation time,** the time required for blood to flow from one part of the body to another. Timing a particle of blood involves injecting a traceable dye or radioisotope into a vein and timing its reappearance in an artery at the point of injection. Alternatively, a substance that can be tasted, such as saccharin, can be injected and the time it takes to travel to the tongue noted. The resulting time helps determine problems with heart failure and decreased cardiac output.

**circulatory care** /sur′kyələtôr′ē/, a Nursing Interventions Classification defined as promotion of arterial and venous circulation. See also **Nursing Interventions Classification.**

**circulatory care: arterial insufficiency,** a nursing intervention from the Nursing Interventions Classification (NIC) defined as promotion of arterial circulation. See also **Nursing Interventions Classification.**

**circulatory care: mechanical assist device,** a nursing intervention from the Nursing Interventions Classification (NIC) defined as temporary support of the circulation through the use of mechanical devices or pumps. See also **Nursing Interventions Classification.**

**circulatory care: venous insufficiency,** a nursing intervention from the Nursing Interventions Classification (NIC) defined as promotion of venous circulation. See also **Nursing Interventions Classification.**

**circulatory failure** [L, *circulatio* + *fallere,* to deceive], inability of the cardiovascular system to supply the cells of the body with enough oxygenated blood to meet their metabolic demands. The condition may result from abnormal cardiac function, as in myocardial infarction; from an inadequate circulating volume of blood, as occurs in hemorrhage; or from mass systemic vasodilation, as may occur in gram-negative septicemia. See also **shock.**

**circulatory fluid.** See **blood, lymph.**

**circulatory overload** [L, *circulatio,* to go around; AS, *ofer* + ME, *lod*], an elevation in blood pressure caused by an increased blood volume, as by transfusion. The condition can lead to heart failure or pulmonary edema.

**circulatory precautions,** a nursing intervention from the Nursing Interventions Classification (NIC) defined as protection of a localized area with limited perfusion. See also **Nursing Interventions Classification.**

**circulatory system,** the network of channels through which the nutrient fluids (blood) of the body circulate.

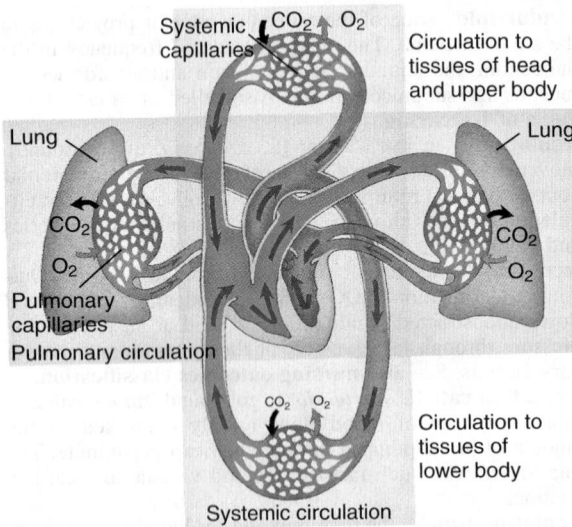

**Circulatory system** *(Thibodeau and Patton, 1999)*

**circulus arteriosus minor** [L, circle; Gk, *arteria,* airpipe; L, less], the small artery encircling the outer circumference of the iris. Also called **circulus arteriosis iridus.**

**circum-** /sur'kəm-/, prefix meaning 'around': *circumanal, circumgemmal, circumvascular.*

**circumanal** /sur'kəmā'nəl/ [L, *circum,* around, *anus*], pertaining to the area surrounding the anus.

**circumcision** /-sizh'ən/ [L, *circum,* around, *cadere,* to cut], a surgical procedure in which the prepuce of the penis or the prepuce of the clitoris is excised. Circumcision is widely performed on newborn boys. The operation is performed on newborns with penile block anesthesia, using one of several kinds of clamp. It is sometimes performed on adult males in the treatment of phimosis and balanitis. Ritual circumcision is required by the religions of approximately one sixth of the world's population.

**circumcorneal** /-kôr'nē·əl/, pertaining to the area of the eye surrounding the cornea.

**circumduction** /sur'kəmduk'shən/ [L, *circum* + *ducere,* to lead], **1.** one of the four basic movements allowed by the various joints of the skeleton. It is a combination of abduction, adduction, extension, and flexion. An example is the motion of a bone whose head articulates with a cavity, such as the femur with the acetabulum. The motion of the bone circumscribes a cone, the apex of which is in the cavity and the base of which is described by the distal end of the bone.

**2.** the circular movement of a limb or of the eye. Compare **angular movement, gliding, rotation.** See also **joint.**

**circumference** /surkum'fərens/ [L, *circum,* around, *ferre,* to bear], **1.** the perimeter or periphery of a circle. **2.** a circular plane surface of a joint.

**circumferential** /sərkum'fəren'shəl/, encircling; pertaining to a circumference or perimeter.

**circumferential fibrocartilage** [L, *circum* + *ferre,* to bring, *fibra,* fiber, *cartilago*], a structure made of fibrocartilage, in which fibrocartilaginous rims surround the margins of various articular cavities, as the glenoid labra of the hip and the shoulder. The rims deepen such cavities and protect their edges. Compare **connecting fibrocartilage, interarticular fibrocartilage, stratiform cartilage.**

**circumferential implantation.** See **superficial implantation.**

**circumflex** /sur'kəmfleks/ [L, *circum,* around, *flexcere,* to bend], winding around; pertaining to blood vessels or nerves that wind around other body structures, as in the circumflex coronary artery.

**circumlocution** /-lōkoo'shən/, the subconscious use of pantomime or nonverbal communication or word substitution by a patient to avoid revealing that a word is difficult to say or has been forgotten.

**circumoral** /sur'kəmôr'əl/ [L, *circum* + *os,* mouth], pertaining to the area of the face around the mouth.

**circumoral pallor** [L, *circum,* around, *os,* mouth, *pallor,* paleness], paleness of the skin area around the mouth, a possible sign of scarlet fever.

**circumscribed** /-skrībd'/ [L, *circum,* around, *scribere,* to draw], within a well-defined area, or in one with definite boundaries or limits.

**circumscribed abscess** [L, *circum,* around, *scribere,* to draw, *abscedere,* to go away], an abscess separated from surrounding tissues by a wall of fibroblasts.

**circumscribed abscess of bone.** See **Brodie's abscess.**

**circumscribed scleroderma.** See **morphea.**

**circum-speech** [L, *circum* + AS, *spaec*], (in psychiatry) behavioral characteristics associated with conversation. The characteristics include body language, maintenance of personal space between individuals, hand sweeps, head nods, and task-oriented activities such as walking or knitting while carrying on a conversation.

**circumstantiality** /-stan'shē·al'itē/ [L, *circum* + *stare,* to stand], (in psychiatry) a speech pattern in which a patient has difficulty in separating relevant from irrelevant information while describing an event. The patient often includes all details and presents them in a sequential order, with the result that the main thread of thought becomes lost as one association leads to another. Frequently the person may need to have questions repeated because the main point of answers has become lost in the confusion of unnecessary detail. Compare **flight of ideas.**

**circumvallate papilla.** See **papilla.**

**circus movement, 1.** an unusual and involuntary rolling or somersaulting caused by injured neural structures that control body posture, such as the cerebral pedicles or the vestibular apparatus. **2.** an unusual circular gait caused by injury to the brain or spinal cord. **3.** a mechanism associated with the excitatory wave of the atrium of the heart and atrial flutter or fibrillation. The wave travels a circular path characterized by a gap between the refractory and the excitatory tissue, usually resulting in conduction of only a fraction of the impulses to the ventricle.

**cirrh-,** prefix meaning 'yellow': *cirrhosis.*

**cirrhosis** /sirō'sis/ [Gk, *kirrhos,* yellow-orange, *osis,* condition], a chronic degenerative disease of the liver in which the lobes are covered with fibrous tissue, the parenchyma degenerates, and the lobules are infiltrated with fat. Gluconeogenesis, detoxification of drugs and alcohol, bilirubin metabolism, vitamin absorption, GI function, hormonal metabolism, and other functions of the liver deteriorate. Blood flow through the liver is obstructed, causing back pressure and leading to portal hypertension and esophageal varices. Unless the cause of the disease is removed, hepatic coma, GI hemorrhage, and kidney failure may occur. Cirrhosis is most commonly the result of chronic alcohol abuse and sometimes nutritional deprivation, hepatitis, cardiac problems, or other causes. The symptoms of cirrhosis are the same regardless of the cause: nausea, fatigue, anorexia, weight loss, ascites, varicosities, and spider angiomas. Diagnosis is made definitively by biopsy, but radiographic and physical examinations and several blood tests of liver function are serially performed to monitor the course of the disease. Treatment depends on the cause. The liver has remarkable ability to regenerate, but recovery may be very slow.

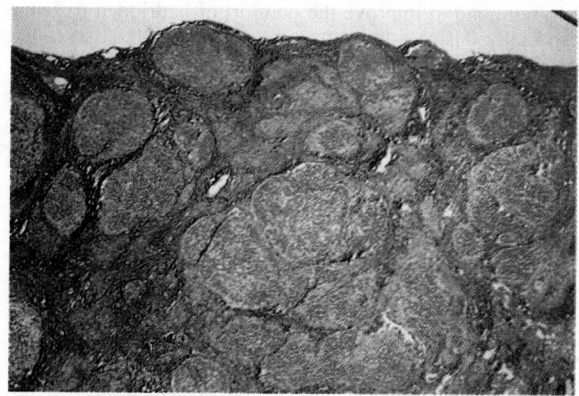

**Alcoholic cirrhosis** *(Kumar, Cotran, and Robbins, 1997)*

**cirsoid aneurysm.** See **racemose aneurysm.**

**cisatracurium,** a nondepolarizing neuromuscular blocker.
- INDICATIONS: This drug is used to facilitate endotracheal intubation and skeletal muscle relaxation during mechanical ventilation, surgery, or general anesthesia.
- CONTRAINDICATIONS: Known hypersensitivity to this drug contraindicates its use.
- ADVERSE EFFECTS: Life-threatening effects of this drug include prolonged apnea, bronchospasm, cyanosis, and respiratory depression. Other serious adverse effects include bradycardia, tachycardia, and increased/decreased blood pressure.

**cis configuration** /sis/, **1.** the presence of the dominant alleles of two or more pairs of genes on one chromosome and the recessive alleles on the homologous chromosome. **2.** the presence of the mutant genes of a pair of pseudoalleles on one chromosome and the wild-type genes on the homologous chromosome. Compare **coupling, trans configuration. 3.** (in chemistry) a form of isomerism in which two substituent groups are on the same side of a double bond. Also called **cis arrangement, cis position.**

**cisplatin** /sisplat′in/, an antineoplastic.
- INDICATIONS: It is prescribed in the treatment of neoplasms, such as metastatic testicular, prostatic, and ovarian tumors.

- CONTRAINDICATIONS: Preexisting renal dysfunction, myelosuppression, hearing impairment, or known hypersensitivity to this drug or other drugs containing platinum prohibits its use.
- ADVERSE EFFECTS: Among the most serious adverse reactions are nephrotoxicity, ototoxicity, myelosuppression, severe nausea, anorexia, vomiting, and allergic reactions.

**cis position.** See **cis configuration.**

**cistern** /sis′tərn/ [L, *cisterna,* vessel], a storage reservoir for fluids.

**cisterna** /sistur′nə/, *pl.* **cisternae** [L, vessel], a cavity that serves as a reservoir for lymph or other body fluids. Kinds of cisternae include **cisterna chyli** and **cisterna subarachnoidea.**

**cisterna chyli** [L, vessel, *chylos,* juice], a dilation at the beginning of the thoracic duct, situated ventral to the body of the second lumbar vertebra, on the right side of and dorsal to the aorta. It receives the two lumbar lymphatic trunks and the intestinal lymphatic trunk.

**cisternal puncture** /sistur′nəl/ [L, vessel, *punctura,* a piercing], the insertion of a needle into the cerebellomedullary cistern to withdraw cerebrospinal fluid for examination. The puncture is made between the atlas and the occipital bone.

**cisterna subarachnoidea** [L, vessel, *sub,* under; Gk, *arachne,* spider, *eidos,* form], any one of many small subarachnoid spaces that serve as reservoirs for cerebrospinal fluid.

**cistron** /sis′tron/ [L, *cis,* this side, *trans,* across], a fragment or portion of DNA that codes for a specific polypeptide. It is the smallest unit functioning as a transmitter of genetic information. In modern molecular genetics the cistron is essentially synonymous with the gene. —**cistronic,** *adj.*

**cisvestitism** /sisves′titiz′əm/ [L, *cis,* this side, *vestis,* garment], the practice of wearing attire appropriate to the sex of the individual involved but not suitable to the age, occupation, or status of the wearer, as when a male bookkeeper impersonates a male police officer by wearing a police uniform.

**cit,** abbreviation for *citrate carboxylate anion.*

**citalopram,** an antidepressant.
- INDICATIONS: This drug is used to treat major depressive disorder.
- CONTRAINDICATIONS: Known hypersensitivity to this drug prohibits its use.
- ADVERSE EFFECTS: Life-threatening effects of this drug include convulsions, hemorrhage, first-degree atrioventricular block, and myocardial infarction. Other serious adverse effects include hallucinations, delusions, psychosis, vomiting, asthma, hyperventilation, respiratory infection, dyspnea, bronchitis, pneumonia, angina pectoris, hypertension, palpitations, tachycardia, bradycardia, thrombophlebitis, arthritis, amenorrhea, cystitis, urine retention, and viral infection. Common side effects are numerous, affecting the GI, integumentary, respiratory, cardiovascular, genitourinary, and central nervous systems. Some are also systemic.

**Citanest Hydrochloride,** trademark for a local anesthetic (prilocaine hydrochloride).

**citicoline** /sit′ikō′lin/, a natural substance that is a component of cell membranes. A pharmaceutic version is used to help stroke victims by inducing injured membranes to repair themselves, limiting cell death. The substance, manufactured by the human body, also helps the brain tissues to repair or replace circuits needed for normal functions. Citicoline treatment can be administered within 24 hours of a stroke.

**citrate** /sit′rāt, sī′trāt/ [L, *kitron,* citron], **1.** an anion of citric acid. **2.** the act of treating with a citrate or citric acid. —**citration,** *n.*

**citric acid** /sit'rik/ [Gk, *kitron,* citron; L, *acidus,* sour], a white, crystalline organic acid soluble in water and alcohol. It is extracted from citrus fruits, especially lemons and limes, or obtained by fermentation of sugars and is used as an acidulating agent, an antioxidant, and a flavoring agent in foods, carbonated beverages, and certain pharmaceutic products, especially laxatives. Compare **ascorbic acid.**

**citric acid cycle** [Gk, *kitron,* citron; L, *acidus,* sour; Gk, *kyklos,* circle], a sequence of enzymatic reactions involving the metabolism of carbon chains of sugars, fatty acids, and amino acids to yield carbon dioxide, water, and high-energy phosphate bonds. The cycle is initiated when pyruvate combines with coenzyme A (CoA) to form a two-carbon unit, acetyl-CoA, which enters the cycle by combining with four-carbon oxaloacetic acid to form six-carbon citric acid. In subsequent steps isocitric acid, produced from citric acid, is oxidized to oxalosuccinic acid, which loses carbon dioxide to form alpha-ketoglutaric acid. Succinic acid, resulting from the oxidative decarboxylation of alpha-ketoglutaric acid, is oxidized to fumaric acid, and its oxidation regenerates oxaloacetic acid, which condenses with acetyl-CoA, closing the cycle. The citric acid cycle provides a major source of adenosine triphosphate energy and also produces intermediate molecules that are starting points for a number of vital metabolic pathways including amino acid synthesis. Also called **Krebs cycle, tricarboxylic acid cycle.** See also **acetylcoenzyme A.**

**citrin** /sit'rin/ [Gk, *kitron,* citron], a crystalline flavonoid concentrate that is used as a source of bioflavonoid.

**citrovorum factor.** See **folinic acid.**

**citrulline** /sitrul'ēn/ [L, *Citrullus,* watermelon], an amino acid produced from ornithine during the urea cycle. It is subsequently transformed to arginine by the transfer of a nitrogen atom from aspartate.

**citrullinemia** /-ē'mē·ə/, a disorder of amino acid metabolism caused by a deficiency of an enzyme, argininosuccinic acid synthetase. The clinical features include vomiting, convulsions, and coma. It is treated with a low-protein diet that provides an essential amino acid mixture, ketoacid analogs of amino acids, and arginine.

**Civilian Health and Medical Programs for Uniformed Services (CHAMPUS),** a health care insurance system for military dependents and members of the military services that covers care not available through the usual U.S. military medical service. CHAMPUS was the first federal third-party reimbursement system to pay for care rendered by nurse-midwives and nurse practitioners.

**CJPH,** abbreviation for *Canadian Journal of Public Health.*

**C/kg,** a unit of radiation exposure in the SI system, coulombs per kilogram of air. 1 roentgen = 2.58 x $10^{-4}$ C/kg.

**CK isoenzyme fraction,** one of several blood-borne enzymes that are released after myocardial necrosis. The isoenzyme of creatine kinase (CK) is identified as MB isomer, or MB-CK, and is a diagnostic clue to heart damage. Also called **creatine phosphokinase (CPK).** See also **lactate dehydrogenase, aspartate aminotransferase.**

**Cl,** symbol for the element **chlorine.**

**Claforan,** trademark for an antibiotic (cefotaxime sodium).

**claim,** a demand for payment from a provider for care that has been rendered.

**claims-made policy** [L, *clamere,* to cry out; ME, *maken* + L, *politicus,* the state], a professional liability-insurance policy that covers the holder for the period in which a claim of malpractice is made. The alleged act of malpractice may have occurred at some previous time, but the policy insures the holder when the claim is made. Compare **occurrence policy.**

**clairvoyance** /klervoi'əns/, the alleged power or ability to perceive or to be aware of objects or events without the use of the physical senses. Also called **clairsentience.** See also **extrasensory perception, parapsychology, telepathy.**

**clamp** [AS, *clam,* to hold together], an instrument with serrated tips and locking handles, used for gripping, holding, joining, supporting, or compressing an organ or vessel. In surgery clamps generally are used for hemostasis.

**clamp forceps.** See **pedicle clamp.**

**clam poisoning.** See **shellfish poisoning.**

**clang association** /klang/ [L, *clangere,* to resound, *associare,* to unite], the mental connection between dissociated ideas made because of similarity in the sounds of the words used to describe the ideas. The phenomenon occurs frequently in schizophrenia. See also **loose association.**

**clap,** a colloquial term for gonorrhea.

**clapping** [AS, *cloeppan,* to beat], (in massage) the procedure of making percussive movements on a patient's body, usually on the chest wall or back, by lowering the cupped palms alternately in a series of rapid, stimulating blows. In this procedure the movement of the hands is from the wrist. Clapping stimulates the circulation and refreshes the skin. It is often done to improve the comfort of bedridden patients, especially during administration of a bed bath. Also called **percussion.**

**Clapton's line** [Edward Clapton, English physician, 1830–1909], a greenish line at the base of the teeth, indicative of copper poisoning.

**clarification** /kler'ifikā'shən/ [L, *clarus,* clear, *facere,* to make], (in psychology) an intervention technique designed to guide the patient in focusing on and recognizing gaps and inconsistencies in his or her statements.

**clarify** /kler'əfī/, (in chemistry) to clear a turbid liquid by allowing any suspended matter to settle, by adding a substance that precipitates any suspended matter, or by heating. —**clarification,** *n.*

**Clark's rule** [Cecil Clark, twentieth century British physician; L, *regula,* model], a method of calculating the approximate pediatric dosage of a drug for a child by using this formula: weight in pounds/150 × adult dose. See also **pediatric dosage.**

**-clasia,** suffix meaning a '(specified) condition involving crushing or breaking up': *aortoclasia, colloidoclasia, osteoclasia.*

**clasmat-, clasmato-,** combining form meaning 'a piece broken off, or fragmentation': *clasmatocyte, clasmatodendrosis, clasmatosis.*

**clasp** [ME, *clippen,* to embrace], **1.** (in dentistry) a sleevelike fitting that is fastened over a tooth to hold a partial denture in place. **2.** (in surgery) any device for holding together tissues, especially bones.

**clasp arm,** an extension, usually from a minor connector, of the clasp of a removable partial denture, that provides retention, reciprocation, or stabilization.

**clasp-knife reflex,** an abnormal sign in which a spastic limb resists passive motion and then suddenly gives way, similarly to the motion of the blade of a jackknife. It is an indication of damage to the pyramidal tract.

**clasp torsion,** the twisting of a retentive clasp arm on a removable partial denture.

**classical conditioning,** a form of learning in which a previously neutral stimulus begins to elicit a given response through associative training. Also called **respondent conditioning.** See also **conditioned reflex.**

**classic cesarean section** [L, *classicus,* first-class, *Caesar lex,* Caesar's law, *sectio,* a cutting], a method for surgically delivering a baby through a vertical midline incision of the upper segment of the uterus. For many practitioners this is the fastest method of cesarean delivery; however, it produces a weaker scar, and, because the upper segment is thicker and more vascular, more bleeding occurs during surgery than from the **low cervical cesarian section.** Compare **extraperitoneal cesarean section.** See also **cesarean section.**

**classic tomography** [L, *classicus* + Gk, *tome,* section, *graphein,* to record], a method that moves the x-ray source and the x-ray plate during an exposure to produce an image in which all but a particular plane is blurred out. This allows an approximate isolation of the image of a detail, which might otherwise be obscured by overlying or underlying structures. This technique is especially valuable in visualizing air-filled structures such as the lungs and paranasal sinuses. See also **computed tomography.**

**classic typhus.** See **epidemic typhus.**

**classification** /klas′ifikā′shən/ [L, *classis,* collection, *facere,* to make], (in research) a process in data analysis in which data are grouped according to previously determined characteristics. —**classify,** *v.*

**classification of caries** [L, *classis,* collection, *facere,* to make, *caries,* decay], a system for dividing dental caries into several classes based on the part of the tooth they affect. Class I caries are pits and fissures in the facial and lingual surfaces of maxillary incisors. Class II caries affect the proximal surfaces of premolars and molars but have not broken through to the occlusal surfaces. Class III caries affect the proximal surfaces of incisors and canines, excluding the incisal angles. Class IV caries affect the proximal surfaces of incisors and canines, including the incisal angles. Class V pertains to caries other than pits and fissures that affect the gingival third of the labial, buccal, and lingual surfaces. Also called **Black's Classification of Caries.** A modification of this classification system adds another group, Class VI, consisting of caries on the incisal edges and cusp tips. See also **cavity classification.**

**classification of malocclusion.** See **Angle's Classification of Malocclusion.**

**classification schemes,** systems of organizing data or information, usually involving categories of items with similar characteristics. Examples of classification schemes include that of the North American Nursing Diagnoses Association (NANDA) and the *Diagnostic and Statistical Manual of Mental Disorders (DSM),* prepared by the American Psychiatric Association.

**classify.** See **classification.**

**class II biologic safety cabinet,** a container that recirculates air through a high-efficiency filter. It is usually located in a hospital pharmacy and is used to prepare chemotherapeutic agents in an environment that protects personnel from exposure.

**-clast,** suffix meaning 'something that breaks': *angioclast, cranioclast, myeloclast.*

**-clastic,** suffix meaning 'causing disintegration': *hemoclastic, histoclastic, lipoclastic.*

**claudication** /klô′dikā′shən/ [L, *claudicatio,* a limping], cramplike pains in the calves caused by poor circulation of the blood to the leg muscles. The condition is commonly associated with atherosclerosis. **Intermittent claudication** is a form of the disorder that is manifested only at certain times, usually after walking, and is relieved by rest. Claudication may require arterial bypass grafting, such as femoral popliteal bypass.

**claustra.** See **claustrum.**

**claustrophobia** /klôs′trə-/ [L, *claustrum,* a closing; Gk, *phobos,* fear], a morbid fear of being in or becoming trapped in enclosed or narrow places. The phenomenon is observed more often in women than in men and can gener-

ally be traced to some traumatic situation involving enclosed spaces, usually occurring in childhood. Treatment consists of psychotherapy to uncover the cause of the phobic reaction, followed by behavior therapy, specifically systematic desensitization or flooding technique.

**claustrum** /klôs′trəm/, *pl.* **claustra** [L, a closing], **1.** a barrier, as a membrane that partially closes an aperture. **2.** a thin sheet of gray matter, composed chiefly of spindle cells, situated lateral to the external capsule of the brain and separating the internal capsule from white matter of the insula. Also called **claustrum of insula.**

**clavicle** /klav′ikəl/ [L, *clavicula,* little key], a long curved, horizontal bone directly above the first rib, forming the ventral portion of the shoulder girdle. It articulates medially with the sternum and laterally with the acromion of the scapula and accommodates the attachment of numerous muscles. It is shorter, thinner, less curved, and smoother in the female than in the male and is thicker, more curved, and more prominently ridged for muscle attachment in persons performing consistent strenuous manual labor. Also called **collarbone** *(informal).*

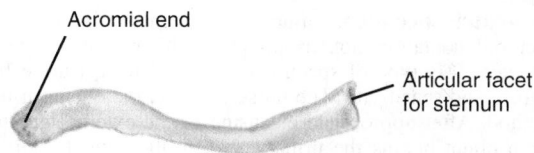

Acromial end

Articular facet for sternum

**Clavicle** *(Applegate, 2000)*

**clavicle strap,** strapping applied to immobilize the clavicle during fracture healing.

**clavicular** /kləvik′yələr/, pertaining to the clavicle (collarbone).

**clavicular notch** [L, *clavicula* + OFr, *enochier*], one of a pair of oval depressions at the superior end of the sternum. A clavicular notch is situated on each side of the sternum and articulates with the clavicle from the same side.

**clavus.** See **corn.**

**clawfoot,** a deformity of the foot characterized by an excessively high arch with hyperextension of the toes at the metatarsophalangeal joints, flexion at the interphalangeal

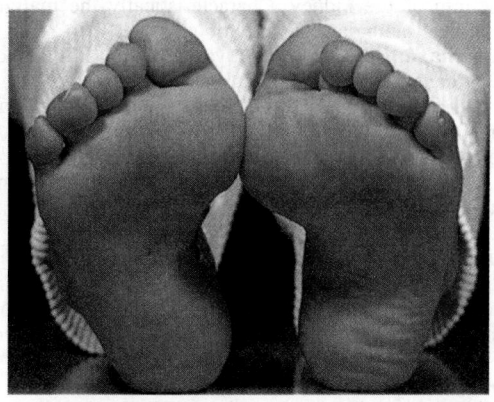

**Clawfoot** *(Perkin, 1998)*

joints, and shortening of the Achilles tendon. The condition may be present at birth or appear later as a result of contractures or an imbalance of the muscles of the foot, as in neuromuscular diseases such as Friedreich's ataxia and peroneal muscular atrophy. Surgical treatment is indicated in severe cases, especially in children. In milder forms the pain from the excessive pressure under the metatarsal heads can be relieved by sponge, rubber, or leather insoles fitted into the shoes. Also called **pes cavus, gampsodactyly, griffe des orteils, talipes cavus.**

**clawhand** [AS, *clawu + hand*], an abnormal condition of the hand characterized by extreme flexion of the middle and distal phalanges and hyperextension of the metacarpophalangeal joints. It is caused by atrophy of the interosseous muscles. Also called **main en griffe.**

**claw-type traction frame,** an orthopedic apparatus that holds various pieces of traction equipment, such as pulleys, ropes, and the weights that suspend or apply traction to various parts of the body. It consists of two metal uprights, one at the head of the bed and the other at the foot. Both uprights are secured to the bed by clawlike attachments and support an overhead metal bar secured to the uprights by metal clamps. Compare **Balkan traction frame, IV-type traction frame.**

**clean-catch specimen,** a urine specimen that is as free of bacterial contamination as possible without the use of a catheter. This type of specimen is needed to test urine for culture and sensitivity. The nurse instructs the client on the method. After appropriate cleansing of the external genitalia, a client begins the urinary stream allowing the initial portion to escape. The initial stream cleans or flushes the urethral orifice and meatus of resident bacteria. During the middle portion of voiding, the client collects the specimen. The procedure is easiest while using toilet facilities.

**cleansing enema,** an enema, usually composed of soapsuds, administered to remove all formed fecal material from the colon. See also **soapsuds enema.**

**clearance** /klir'əns/ [L, *clarus,* clear], the removal of a substance from the blood via the kidneys. Kidney function can be tested by measuring the amount of a specific substance excreted in the urine in a given length of time.

**clear cell** [L, *clarus + cella,* storeroom], **1.** a type of cell found in the parathyroid gland that does not take on a color with the ordinary tissue stains used for microscopic examination. **2.** the principal cell of most renal cell carcinomas and occasionally of ovarian and parathyroid tumors. **3.** a specific type of epidermal cell, probably of neural origin, that has a dark-staining nucleus but clear cytoplasm with hematoxylin and eosin stain.

**clear cell carcinoma, 1.** a malignant tumor of the tubular epithelium of the kidney. Characteristically the malignant cells contain abundant clear cytoplasm. See also **renal cell carcinoma. 2.** an uncommon ovarian neoplasm characterized by cells with clear cytoplasm.

**clear cell carcinoma of the kidney.** See **renal cell carcinoma.**

**clearing agent,** a chemical, such as ammonium thiosulfate, used in the processing of exposed x-ray film to remove unexposed and undeveloped silver halides from the emulsion.

**clearing test,** a range of motion test that moves the joint to its limits, stretching the capsule and other soft tissues in an attempt to reproduce symptoms. If the range of motion is normal and no symptoms are produced, the joint is cleared as a cause of a musculoskeletal disorder.

**clear-liquid diet** [L, *clarus + liquere,* to flow], a diet that supplies fluids and provides minimal fiber primarily to re-

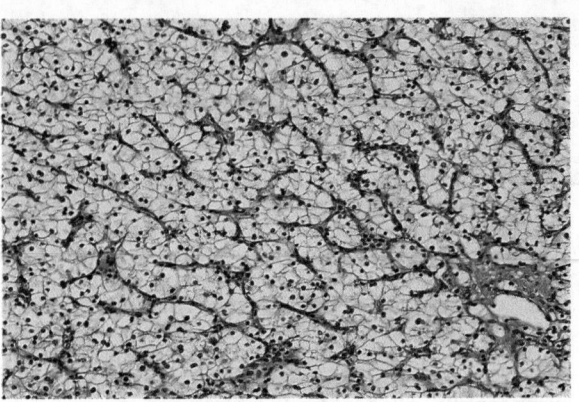

**Clear cell renal cell carcinoma** *(Fletcher, 2000)*

lieve thirst and maintain water balance. Liquid at room temperature, it consists primarily of dissolved sugar and flavored liquids, such as ginger ale, sweetened tea or coffee, fat-free broth, plain gelatin desserts, and strained fruit juices. The diet is nutritionally inadequate and should not be used for more than two days.

**cleavage** /klē'vij/ [AS, *cleofan,* to split], **1.** the series of repeated mitotic cell divisions that occur in an ovum immediately after fertilization. It transforms the single-celled zygote into a multicellular embryo capable of growth and differentiation. During cleavage, the embryo remains uniform in size as its cells, or blastomeres, become smaller with each division. Kinds of cleavage include **determinate cleavage, equal cleavage, indeterminate cleavage, partial cleavage, total cleavage,** and **unequal cleavage. 2.** the act or process of splitting, primarily a complex molecule into two or more simpler molecules.

**cleavage cavity.** See **blastocoele.**

**cleavage cell.** See **blastomere.**

**cleavage fracture,** any fracture that splits cartilage with the avulsion of a small piece of bone from the distal portion of the lateral condyle of the humerus.

**cleavage line,** any one of a number of linear striations in the skin that delineate the general structural pattern, direction, and tension of the subcutaneous fibrous tissue. They correspond closely to the crease lines on the surface of the skin and are present in all areas of the body but are visible only in certain sites, as the palms of the hands and soles of the feet. In general the lines run obliquely, lying in the direction in which the skin stretches the least, perpendicular to the direction of the greatest stretch. Incisions made parallel to these lines heal with much less scarring than those made perpendicular to them. To a certain degree cleavage lines determine the direction and arrangement of lesions in skin diseases. Also called **Langer's line.**

**cleavage nucleus.** See **segmentation nucleus.**

**cleavage plane, 1.** the area in a fertilized ovum where cleavage takes place; the axis along which any cell division occurs. **2.** any plane within the body where organs or structures can be separated with minimal damage to surrounding tissue.

**cleave** /klēv/ [AS, *cleofan*], segment or divide, as in cell division or the splitting of a complex molecule into simpler molecules.

**cleft** [ME, *clift*], **1.** divided. **2.** a fissure, especially one that originates in the embryo, as the branchial cleft or the facial cleft.

**cleft cheek,** a transverse facial cleft, appearing as an abnormally large mouth. It is caused by the failure of the maxillary and mandibular processes to fuse during embryonic facial development.

**cleft foot,** an abnormal condition in which the division between third and fourth toes extends into the metatarsus of the foot.

**cleft hand,** a hand that develops in two parts because of the failure of a digit and metacarpal to form normally during embryonic development.

**cleft jaw,** an abnormal jaw resulting from failure of the left and right mandibles to fuse properly during embryonic development.

**cleft lip,** a congenital anomaly consisting of one or more clefts in the upper lip that result from the failure in the embryo of the maxillary and median nasal processes to close. Treatment is surgical repair in infancy. Also called **harelip.** See also **cleft palate.**

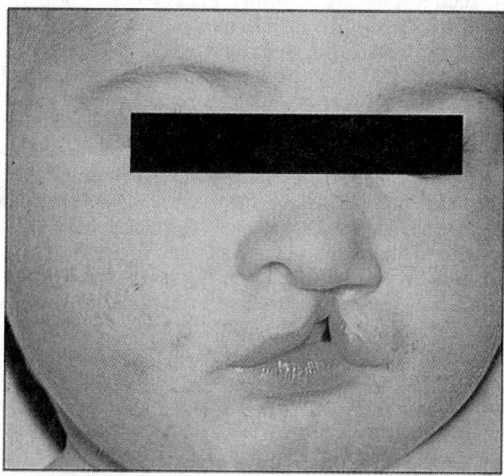

**Unilateral cleft lip** *(Greig and Garden, 1996)*

feeding unit. Parenteral fluids are administered until oral intake is adequate. Milk products, solids, and a nipple or pacifier are not allowed. The diet and manner of feeding may vary, but the infant is fed while held with the head up or is placed in a cardiac chair and burped after the intake of each ounce of food. Fluid intake and output are measured. The elbow restraints are worn at all times except when range-of-motion exercises are performed, one arm at a time, while skin care is administered to that limb.

■ INTERVENTIONS: The nurse provides preoperative and postoperative care and prepares for the infant's discharge by ensuring that the parents understand the proper diet and feeding schedule and technique. The nurse emphasizes the importance of using elbow restraints, maintaining motion and skin integrity of the arms, preventing injury to the surgical area, and reporting symptoms of infection, including separation of the incision, excessive swelling, redness, bleeding, and drainage.

■ OUTCOME CRITERIA: Modern surgical techniques permit remarkable repair of cleft lips. In some cases a second operation is required to eliminate the scar.

**cleft palate,** a congenital defect characterized by a fissure in the midline of the palate, resulting from the failure of the two sides to fuse during embryonic development. The fissure may be complete, extending through both the hard and soft palates into the nasal cavities, or it may show any degree of incomplete or partial cleft. The condition, which occurs approximately once in every 2500 live births and affects females more than males, is often associated with a cleft in the upper lip. Together these abnormalities are the most common of the craniofacial malformations, accounting for half of the total number of defects. Feeding is best accomplished with special devices. Surgical repair of the defect is usually done in the first year of life. Care of the child requires a team approach that includes a plastic surgeon, orthodontist, dentist, nurse, speech and hearing therapists, and social workers. Long-term postoperative problems, including speech impairment and hearing loss, improper tooth development and alignment, chronic respiratory and ear infections, and varying levels of emotional and social maladjustment, may be largely prevented by modern techniques and reconstructive surgery. See also **cleft lip.**

**cleft-lip repair,** the surgical correction of a unilateral or bilateral congenital interruption of the upper lip, usually resulting from the embryologic failure of the median nasal and maxillary processes to unite.

■ METHOD: A cleft lip may sometimes be repaired during the infant's first 48 hours of life, but some surgeons follow a "rule of 10s" and perform the operation when the child is 10 weeks old, weighs 10 or more pounds, and has a hemoglobin level of at least 10 g/dL. Before surgery elbow restraints, used to prevent the infant from touching the incision, are prepared in the proper size and are sent to the operating room with the patient. After surgery the infant is maintained with ventilatory support as necessary until respirations are normal. Essential observations include assessment for respiratory stridor or obstruction, excessive bleeding, separation of the incision, and redness under the elbow restraints used to keep the hands from the mouth. The wire bow applied to the infant's upper lip and taped to the cheeks to prevent tension on the sutures is kept in place; if it becomes loose, it is reapplied with tincture of benzoin. The infant is given clear liquids and juices through a syringe (Asepto) or special

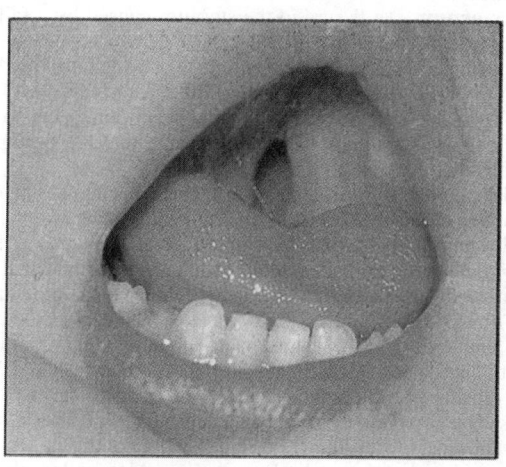

**Cleft palate** *(Greig and Garden, 1996)*

**cleft-palate repair,** the surgical correction of a congenital fissure in the midline of the partition separating the oral and nasal cavities. Palatine clefts range from a simple separation in the uvula to an extensive fissure involving the soft and hard palates and extending forward unilaterally or bilaterally through the alveolar ridge. A cleft lip often accompanies a cleft palate. Repair of a cleft palate is usually undertaken when a child is 6 months old.

■ METHOD: Before surgery properly sized elbow restraints to prevent the child from touching the mouth are prepared and sent to the operating room with the patient. After surgery the youngster is kept in a moist oxygen-rich environment by using a tent device (Croupette) until respirations are normal and is observed for signs of airway obstruction or excessive bleeding. Parenteral fluids are administered until the oral intake is adequate. Clear liquids and juices are given by cup only; straws, nipples, pacifiers, utensils, or toys may not be put into the mouth. Milk products and solids are contraindicated, but the kind of feeding ordered may vary. The child is fed in a high chair when possible, and a bib is used to accommodate drooling. Only circumoral mouth care is administered; the teeth are not brushed. Fluid intake and output are measured. The elbow restraints are worn continuously, except when daily range-of-motion exercises are performed and skin care is administered, to one arm at a time. With improvement the child is permitted to walk as tolerated.

■ INTERVENTIONS: Before discharge the nurse ensures that the parents understand the required diet and the need to feed by cup only, to use elbow restraints, to maintain the motion and skin integrity of the arms, and to prevent injury to the mouth. The nurse reminds the parents to administer the required medication in the proper dosage and on schedule and to report symptoms of incision infection, such as drainage, mouth odor, or bleeding.

■ OUTCOME CRITERIA: Depending on the extent and nature of a cleft palate, it may be repaired in one or in several operations. Some experts believe that early repair of a defect in the bony palate can lead to structural malrelations and advise delaying the operation until the child is between 5 and 7 years of age and has achieved more bone growth. Successful repair often greatly improves the child's oronasopharyngeal physiologic function, speech, and appearance.

**cleft palate speech,** faulty speech due to a cleft palate, often characterized by hypernasality, difficulty with fricatives, and other problems resulting from the velopharyngeal insufficiency.

**cleft sternum,** a fissure in the sternum caused by a failure in embryonic development.

**cleft tongue** [ME, *clift* + AS, *tunge*], a tongue divided by a longitudinal fissure. Also called **bifid tongue.**

**cleft uvula,** an abnormal congenital condition in which the uvula is split into halves as a result of the failure of the posterior palatine folds to unite.

**cleido-, cleid-,** combining form meaning 'clavicle' or collarbone: *cleidocostal, cleidocranial, cleidomastoid.*

**cleidocranial dysostosis** /klī′dōkrā′nē·əl/ [Gk, *kleis*, key, *kranion*, skull, *dys*, bad, *osteon*, bone], a rare abnormal hereditary condition characterized by defective ossification of the cranial bones and by the complete or partial absence of the clavicles. It is transmitted as an autosomal dominant trait. The defective ossification of the cranial bones delays the closing of the cranial sutures and produces large fontanels. The complete or partial absence of the clavicles allows the shoulders to be drawn together. This condition also involves dental and vertebral anomalies. Also called **cleidocranial dysplasia.** See also **dysostosis.**

**cleidocranial dystrophia.** See also **cleidocranial dysostosis.**

**cleidohyoid muscle** /klī′dō·hi′oid/ [Gk, *cleis*, key + *hyoeides*, U-shaped], a slip of muscle sometimes seen augmenting the sternohyoid muscle, extending from the hyoid bone to the clavicle.

**clemastine** /klemas′tēn/, an antihistaminic agent.

■ INDICATIONS: It is prescribed in the treatment of symptoms of allergic rhinitis, pruritus, or lacrimation.

■ CONTRAINDICATIONS: Use by lactating mothers or those undergoing monamine oxidase inhibitor therapy or having known sensitivity to this drug or other antihistamines is contraindicated. It is also contraindicated with narrow-angle glaucoma, asthma, symptomatic prostatic hypertrophy, and bladder-neck destruction.

■ ADVERSE EFFECTS: Among the most serious adverse reactions are hypersensitivity, skin rash, and tachycardia. Transient drowsiness commonly occurs.

**clenching** /klench′ing/ [ME, *clenchen*], the clamping and pressing of the jaws and teeth together in centric occlusion, frequently associated with acute nervous tension or physical effort, such as pushing or lifting a heavy object or performing a difficult task. See also **bruxism.**

**Cleocin,** trademark for an antibacterial (clindamycin).

**cleoid** /klē′oid/ [ME, *cle*, claw + Gk, *eidos*, form], a claw-shaped nib used to carve amalgam restorations.

**cleptomania.** See **kleptomania.**

**click** [Fr, *cliquer*, to clash], an extra heart sound that occurs during systole. See also **ejection click, systolic click.**

**clicking** /klik′ing/ [Fr, *cliquer*, to clash], a series of clicks, such as the snapping, cracking, or crepitant noise evident on excursions of the mandibular condyle.

**click-murmur syndrome.** See **Barlow's syndrome.**

**client** /klī′ənt/ [L, *clinare*, to lean], **1.** a person who is recipient of a professional service. **2.** a recipient of health care regardless of the state of health. **3.** a patient.

**client-centered therapy,** a nondirective method of group or individual psychotherapy, originated by Carl Rogers, in which the therapist's role is to listen to and then reflect or restate without judgment or interpretation the words of the client. The goal of the therapy is personal growth achieved by the client's increased awareness and understanding of his or her attitudes, feelings, and behavior.

**client interview.** See **patient interview.**

**client/server system,** a computer configuration in which the workload is divided between a client computer and a server, as might be used in a health care management plan.

**climacteric.** See **menopause.**

**climate** /klī′mit/ [Gk, *klima*, inclination], **1.** a composite of the prevailing weather conditions that characterize any particular geographic region, including air pressure, temperature, precipitation, sunshine, and humidity. Because these factors affect health, they must be considered in the diagnosis and treatment of certain illnesses, especially those affecting respiration. **2.** the general condition surrounding something, as in a climate of goodwill. —**climatic,** *adj.*

**climax** /klī′maks/ [Gk, *klimax*, ladder], a peak of intensity, such as a sexual orgasm or the high point of a fever.

**climbing fiber** [ME, *climben* + L, *fibra*], a type of nerve fiber that carries impulses to the Purkinje cells of the cerebellar cortex.

**clindamycin hydrochloride** /klin′dəmī′sin/, an antibacterial.

■ INDICATIONS: It is prescribed in the treatment of certain serious bacterial infections (including anaerobic and some gram-positive organisms).

■ CONTRAINDICATION: Hypersensitivity to this drug or to lincomycin prohibits its use.

■ ADVERSE EFFECTS: Among the more serious adverse reactions are pseudomembranous colitis, severe GI disturbances, and hypersensitivity.

**clinic** [Gk, *kline*, bed], **1.** an ambulatory caresite where persons who do not require hospitalization receive medical care. **2.** a group practice of doctors, such as the Mayo Clinic. **3.** a meeting place for doctors and medical students where instruction can be given at the bedside of a patient or in a similar setting. **4.** a seminar or other scientific medical meeting. **5.** a detailed published report of the diagnosis and treatment of a health care problem.

**-clinic,** suffix meaning 'places set aside for medical treatment': *policlinic, polyclinic, psychoclinic.*

**clinical** /klin′ikəl/ [Gk, *kline,* bed], **1.** pertaining to a clinic. **2.** pertaining to direct bedside medical or nursing care. **3.** pertaining to materials or equipment used in the care of a sick person.

**clinical analysis,** the use of laboratory data, including blood tests, urinalysis, and microscopic tissue studies, in determining a diagnosis and treatment regimen.

**clinical assessment,** an evaluation of a patient's physical condition and prognosis based on information gathered from physical and laboratory examinations and the patient's medical history.

**clinical crown,** the portion of the tooth that is occlusal to the deepest part of the gingival crevice. Compare **anatomic crown, artificial crown, partial crown.**

**clinical-crown/clinical-root ratio,** the length of the part of a tooth that is coronal to the junctional epithelium divided by the length of the tooth's root that is apical to the junctional epithelium. The ratio is useful in the diagnosis and prognosis of periodontal disease. Also called **crown/root ratio.**

**clinical cytogenetics,** the branch of genetics that studies the relationship between chromosomal aberrations and pathologic conditions.

**clinical diagnosis,** a diagnosis made on the basis of knowledge obtained by medical history and physical examination alone, without benefit of laboratory tests or x-ray films.

**clinical disease,** a stage in the history of a pathologic condition that begins with anatomic or physiologic changes that are sufficient to produce recognizable signs and symptoms of a disease.

**clinical epidemiology,** the application of the science of epidemiology in a clinical setting. Emphasis is on a medically defined population, as opposed to statistically formulated disease trends derived from examination of larger population categories.

**clinical genetics,** a branch of genetics that studies inherited disorders and investigates the possible factors that may influence the occurrence of pathologic conditions. Also called **medical genetics.**

**clinical horizon,** the imaginary line above which detectable signs and symptoms of a disease first begin to appear. Compare **subclinical.**

**clinical humidity therapy,** respiratory therapy in which water vapor is added to the therapeutic gases to make breathing them more comfortable.

**clinical judgment,** the application of information based on actual observation of a patient combined with subjective and objective data that lead to a conclusion.

**clinical laboratory,** a laboratory in which tests directly related to the care of patients are performed. Such laboratories use material obtained from patients for testing, as compared with research laboratories, where animal and other sources of test material are also used.

**clinical laboratory scientist.** See **clinical laboratory scientist/medical technologist.**

**clinical laboratory scientist/medical technologist,** an allied health professional who, in conjunction with pathologists or other physicians or medical scientists, performs specialized chemical, microscopic, and bacteriologic tests of blood, tissue, and fluids. In addition to possessing the skills of clinical laboratory technicians/medical laboratory technicians, clinical laboratory scientists/medical technologists perform complex analyses, fine-line discrimination, and error correction. They have knowledge of physiologic conditions affecting test results so they can develop data that may be used by a physician in determining the presence, extent, and as far as possible, cause of a disease. They are held accountable for accurate results, establish and monitor quality assurance programs, and modify procedures as necessary. Preparation includes a baccalaureate degree and at least 1 year of professional/clinical education.

**clinical laboratory technician.** See **medical laboratory technician.**

**clinical laboratory technician/medical laboratory technician (MLT)-associate degree,** an allied health professional who, under the supervision of a pathologist or other physician, clinical laboratory scientist/medical technologist, or other medical scientist, performs specialized chemical, microscopic, and bacteriologic tests of blood, tissue, and fluids. The technician can demonstrate discrimination between similar items and correction of errors by the use of preset strategies, is able to recognize factors that directly affect procedures and results, and monitors quality assurance procedures. Preparation is usually 2 academic years, with the graduate receiving an associate's degree.

**clinical laboratory technician/medical laboratory technician (MLT)-certificate,** an allied health professional who, under the supervision of a pathologist or other physician, clinical laboratory scientist/medical technologist, or other medical scientist, performs routine, uncomplicated laboratory tests of blood, tissue, and fluids. Clinical education is usually 12 months, with the graduate receiving a certificate.

**clinical medicine,** a system of health maintenance based on direct observation of and communication with a patient.

**clinical nurse specialist (CNS),** a registered nurse who holds a master's degree in nursing and who has acquired advanced knowledge and clinical skills in a specific area of nursing practice. The CNS, as a practitioner, assumes a leadership role in the distribution of clinical care to a specific patient population while interacting within the total health care system. The unique functions of the CNS are based on clinical expertise and judgment and include caring for patients, delegating responsibility, teaching other staff members, and influencing and effecting change with respect to the needs of the patient and family and the total health care system. Historically, CNS has included research involvement also.

**clinical-pathologic conference,** a teaching exercise in which a case is presented to a clinician, who then demonstrates the process of reasoning that leads to his or her diagnosis. A pathologist then presents an anatomic diagnosis, based on the study of tissue removed at surgery or obtained in autopsy. Often the students will have been asked to suggest a diagnosis based on the same information presented to the clinician. A discussion usually follows and serves to demonstrate the origin of errors present in any of the diagnoses offered. The pathologist's diagnosis is usually the definitive one. The clinical-pathologic conference is the model for the long series called "case report" in the *New England Journal of Medicine* and is a part of the curricula of most medical schools.

**clinical pathology,** the laboratory study of disease by a pathologist using techniques appropriate to the specimen being studied. Among the many branches of clinical pathology are hematology, bacteriology, chemistry, and serology.

**clinical pathway,** a description of practices likely to result in favorable outcomes for a particular diagnosis that uses prospectively defined resources to minimize cost. It may be based on research, literature, or common practice. Also called **critical path.** See also **practice guideline.**

**clinical pelvimetry,** a process used to assess the size of the birth canal by means of the systematic vaginal palpation of specific bony landmarks in the pelvis and an estimation of the distances between them. Internal pelvic diameters are not accessible to direct measurement; they must be inferred. Clinical pelvimetry is usually performed by a midwife or an obstetrician during the first prenatal examination of a pregnant woman. Findings are commonly recorded in terms such as adequate, borderline, or inadequate, rather than in centimeters or inches. Compare **x-ray pelvimetry.** See also **birth canal, cephalopelvic disproportion, contraction, dystocia.**

**clinical psychology,** the branch of psychology concerned with the diagnosis, treatment, and prevention of a wide range of personality and behavioral disorders.

**clinical research center,** an organization, often associated with a medical school or a teaching hospital, that studies, analyzes, correlates, and describes medical cases. Such centers usually have extensive laboratory facilities and specialized staffs of physicians and medical technicians. Clinical research centers often offer free or very inexpensive medical care for patients participating in various research programs and often produce significant new medical information distributed through articles, journals, reports, seminars, and lectures. Funding for such facilities may be generated through minimal fees charged for various medical services and through grants.

**clinical specialist,** a physician or nurse who has advanced training in a particular field of practice, as a nurse-midwife, pediatrician, or radiologist.

**clinical thermometer** [Gk, *kline,* bed, *therme,* heat, *metron,* measure], a thermometer designed for measuring body temperature. Also called **bedside thermometer.**

**clinical thermometry,** a method for determining temperature in heated tissue.

**clinical trial exemption (CTX),** authorization to administer an investigational agent to patients or volunteer subjects under specified conditions of a particular research study in a clinical setting.

**clinical trials,** organized studies to provide large bodies of clinical data for statistically valid evaluation of treatment.

**clinician** /klinish′ən/, a health professional whose practice is based on direct observation and treatment of a patient, as distinguished from other types of health workers, such as laboratory technicians and those employed in research.

**clinic without walls,** a health care system formed by the merger of selected functions, such as administrative, billing and collections, purchasing, personnel, and payroll of various physician groups without the merger of any physical facilities.

**Clinitest,** trademark for reagent tablets used to test for the presence of reducing sugars, such as glucose, in the urine. The tablets contain copper sulfate, and the procedure is a modified version of **Benedict's qualitative test.** It is rarely used in current practice.

**clino-,** combining form meaning 'to bend or make lie down' or a 'sloping shape': *clinodactyl, clinostatic, clinostatism, clinocephaly.*

**clinocephaly** /klī′nōsef′əlē/ [Gk, *klinein,* to bend, *kephale,* head], a congenital anomaly of the head in which the upper surface of the skull is saddle-shaped or concave. Also called **clinocephalism. —clinocephalic, clinocephalous,** *adj.*

**clinodactyly** /klī′nōdak′təlē/ [Gk, *klinein + daktylos,* finger], a congenital anomaly characterized by abnormal lateral or medial bending of one or more fingers or toes. Also called **clinodactylyism. —clinodactylic, clinodactylous,** *adj.*

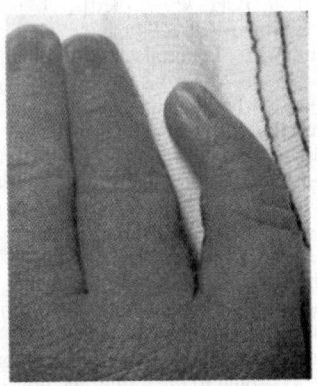

**Clinodactyly**
*(Zitelli and Davis, 1997/courtesy Dr. Christine L. Williams, New York Medical College)*

**clinoid processes** /klī′noid/ [Gk, *kline,* bed, *eidos,* form; L, *processus*], the anterior, middle, and posterior processes of the sphenoid bone at the base of the skull.

**clinometer** /klīnom′ətər/, an instrument used to measure angular convergence of the eyes or the degree of paralysis of extraocular muscles. Also called **clinoscope.**

**Clinoril,** trademark for a nonsteroidal antiinflammatory (sulindac).

**clinoscope.** See **clinometer.**

**clioquinol.** See **iodochlorhydroxyquin.**

**clip** [AS, *clyppan,* to embrace], a surgical device used for grasping the skin to align the edges of a wound and to stop bleeding, especially of the smaller blood vessels. It is also used in radiography for localization.

**Clistin,** trademark for an antihistamine (carbinoxamine maleate).

**clitoridectomy** /klit′əridek′təmē/, the excising of all or part of the clitoris, and sometimes part of the labia, a form of ritual mutilation performed on over 100 million girls and women in more than 40 countries. It is usually performed at 4 to 12 years of age, without anesthesia, with crude cutting tools, and with few or no precautions against infection. The reasons for this ancient practice are very complex, including the male desire to control female sexuality. As of June 1996, the U.S. Board of Immigration Appeals recognized genital mutilation as a form of persecution and a basis for asylum for girls and women. In the United States itself an estimated 40,000 immigrant girls are clitoridectomized every year; federal legislation is pending to prohibit the practice, which several states have outlawed already. Defenders of clitoridectomy sometimes refer to it as "female circumcision," a deliberately misleading euphemism that should be avoided. See also **female genital mutilation.**

**clitoridotomy,** an incision into the clitoris.

**clitoris** /klit′əris/ [Gk, *kleitoris*], the vaginal erectile structure of the female homologous to the corpora cavernosa of the penis. It consists of two corpora cavernosa within a dense layer of fibrous membrane, joined along their inner surfaces by an incomplete fibrous septum. It is situated beneath the anterior labia commissure, partially hidden between the anterior extremities of the labia minora.

**clitoritis** /klit′ôrī′tis/, inflammation of the clitoris.

**clivus** /klī′vəs/ [L, slope], an inclined surface, as on the sphenoid bone.

**CLL,** abbreviation for **chronic lymphocytic leukemia.**

**cloaca** /klō·ā′kə/, *pl.* **cloacae** [L, sewer], **1.** (in embryology) the end of the hindgut before the developmental division into the rectum, the bladder, and the primitive genital structures. **2.** (in pathology) an opening into the sheath of tissue around a necrotic bone.

**cloacal membrane** /klō·ā′kəl/, a thin sheath that separates the internal and external portions of the cloaca in the developing embryo. It is formed from endoderm and ectoderm and closes the fetal anus during early prenatal development; it later ruptures and is absorbed so that the anal canal becomes continuous with the rectum. Also called **anal membrane.**

**cloacal septum.** See **urorectal septum.**

**clobetasol propionate** /klōbet′əsol prō′pyōnāt/, a topical corticosteroid antiinflammatory.

■ INDICATIONS: It is prescribed for the short-term treatment of inflammation and pruritus associated with certain moderate to severe types of dermatitis.

■ CONTRAINDICATIONS: It is contraindicated for prolonged use, for applications to large areas of poor skin integrity, and with the use of occlusive dressing.

■ ADVERSE EFFECTS: Adverse reactions may include hyperglycemia, glycosuria, Cushing's syndrome, and suppression of hypothalamic-pituitary-adrenal functions. Because of the greater ratio of skin surface to body weight in children, they are at risk of absorbing a greater proportion of topical steroid.

**clocortolone pivalate** /klōkôr′təlōn piv′əlāt/, a topical corticosteroid antiinflammatory.

■ INDICATION: It is prescribed for the short-term treatment of inflammation and pruritus associated with certain moderate to severe types of dermatitis.

■ CONTRAINDICATIONS: Viral and fungal diseases of the skin or local impairment of circulation prohibits its use.

■ ADVERSE REACTIONS: Among the more serious adverse reactions are systemic side effects that may as a result from prolonged or excessive application. Local irritation of the skin may occur.

**clofibrate** /klō′fəbrāt/, an antihyperlipidemic.

■ INDICATIONS: It is prescribed in the treatment of high blood levels of cholesterol, triglycerides, or both.

■ CONTRAINDICATIONS: Liver or kidney dysfunction, pregnancy, lactation, biliary cirrhosis, or known hypersensitivity to this drug prohibits its use.

■ ADVERSE EFFECTS: Among the more serious adverse reactions are nausea, diarrhea, weight gain, and a syndrome resembling influenza. This drug interacts with many other drugs.

**Clomid,** trademark for a nonsteroidal fertility drug (clomiphene citrate).

**clomiphene citrate** /klō′məfēn/, a nonsteroidal antiestrogen that acts to stimulate ovulation.

■ INDICATIONS: It is prescribed primarily for the treatment of anovulation and oligoovulation in women.

■ CONTRAINDICATIONS: Abnormal vaginal bleeding, liver dysfunction, or known hypersensitivity to this drug prohibits its use.

■ ADVERSE EFFECTS: Among the more serious adverse reactions are enlargement of the ovaries, blurred vision, gastric upset, rashes, and abdominal pain.

**clomiphene stimulation test,** a test used to evaluate gonadal function in males who show signs of abnormal pubertal development. Clomiphene, a nonsteroidal analog of estrogen, stimulates the hypothalamic-pituitary system to raise follicle stimulating hormone and luteinizing hormone levels of the blood. Failure to respond to clomiphene indicates hypothalamic-pituitary disease, possibly a pituitary tumor. See also **clomiphene citrate, gonadotropin.**

**clonal** /klō′nəl/, pertaining to a clone.

**clonal marker,** a defective or functionally unidentified DNA sequence in a clone of cancer cells. Such sequences are used to monitor the growth of cancer cells after chemical or other treatments.

**clonal selection theory.** See **antibody-specific model.**

**clonazepam** /klōnaz′əpam/, a benzodiazepine anticonvulsant.

■ INDICATIONS: It is prescribed in the prevention of seizures in petit mal epilepsy and other convulsive disorders.

■ CONTRAINDICATIONS: Liver disease, acute narrow-angle glaucoma, or known hypersensitivity to this drug or to other benzodiazepine drugs prohibits its use. It is not given during lactation.

■ ADVERSE EFFECTS: Among the more serious adverse reactions are anemia, coma, palpitations, mental and respiratory depression, muscle weakness, and shortness of breath.

**clone** [Gk, *klon,* a plant cutting], a group of genetically identical cells or organisms derived from a single common cell or organism through mitosis. **—clonal,** *adj.*

**-clonia,** suffix meaning '(condition involving) spasms': *logoclonia, myoclonia, polyclonia.*

**clonic** /klon′ik/ [Gk, *klonos,* tumult], pertaining to increased reflex activity, as in upper motor neuron lesions when repetitive muscular contractions and relaxations in rapid succession are induced by stretching. Also see **clonus.**

**clonic convulsion** [Gk, *klonos,* tumult; L, *convulsio,* cramp], a form of convulsion characterized by rhythmic alternate involuntary contraction and relaxation of muscle groups.

**clonicity** /klōnis′itē/, a state of clonus.

**clonic spasm** [Gk, *klonos,* tumult, *spasmos*], involuntary alternating contractions and relaxations of muscles.

**clonidine hydrochloride** /klō′nədēn/, an antihypertensive.

■ INDICATIONS: It is prescribed for the reduction of high blood pressure.

■ CONTRAINDICATIONS: Known hypersensitivity to this drug prohibits its use.

■ ADVERSE EFFECTS: Among the more serious adverse reactions is a withdrawal syndrome that occurs on discontinuation of the medication, characterized by tachycardia, a rapid increase in blood pressure, and anxiety. Drowsiness, sexual dysfunction, and dry mouth commonly occur.

**cloning** /klō′ning/, a procedure for producing multiple copies of genetically identical organisms or cells or of individual genes. Organisms may be cloned by transplanting blastocysts from one embryo into an empty zona pellucida, or nuclei from the cells of one individual into enucleated oocytes. Cells may be cloned by growing them in culture under conditions that promote cell reproduction. Genes may be cloned by isolating them from the genome of one organism and incorporating them into the genome of an asexually reproducing organism, such as a bacterium or a yeast.

**clonogenic cell** /klō′nōjen′ik/, a cell that can proliferate into a colony of genetically identical cells.

**clonorchiasis** /klō′nôrkī′əsis/, an infestation of liver flukes. See also *Clonorchis sinensis*, **schistosomiasis.**

***Clonorchis sinensis*** /klōnôr′kis sinen′sis/, the Chinese or Oriental liver fluke, a trematode that is acquired by humans who eat raw, imperfectly cooked pickled, salted, or smoked fish that is the intermediate host of the parasite. The fluke exists in a dormant stage as a cercaria, encysted in the skin of a fish and unable to continue its life cycle until ingested by a warm-blooded animal, in which the larvae mature and produce eggs. The eggs are excreted in the feces of the host to enter water, where the new generation evolves first in aquatic snails and then in fish. In human hosts the liver fluke lives in the bile ducts and gallbladder, causing chronic liver disease with enlargement of the liver, diarrhea, edema, and, eventually, death. Cholangitis, cholelithiasis, pancreatitis, and cholangiosarcoma are common complications and may be fatal. Treatment is with praziquantel or albendazole. Also called *Opisthorchis sinensis*.

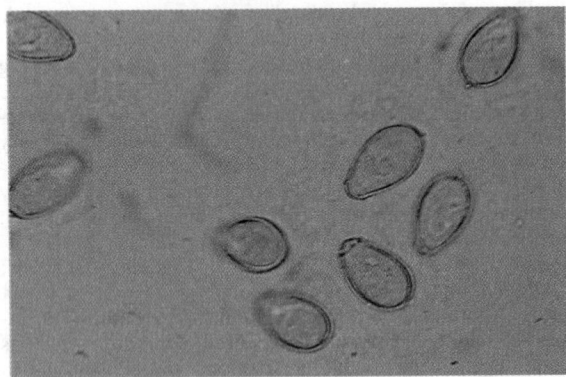

***Clonorchis sinensis* egg** *(Murray et al, 1994)*

**clonus** /klō′nəs/ [Gk, *klonos*, tumult], an abnormal pattern of neuromuscular activity, characterized by rapidly alternating involuntary contraction and relaxation of skeletal muscle. Compare **tonus.** —**clonic,** *adj.*

**C-loop,** a surgically formed loop of bowel with a C-shape.

**clopidogrel,** a platelet aggregation inhibitor.
- INDICATIONS: This drug is used to reduce the risk of stroke in high-risk patients.
- CONTRAINDICATIONS: Known hypersensitivity and active bleeding prohibit this drug's use.
- ADVERSE EFFECTS: Intracranial hemorrhage is a potential life-threatening side effect of this drug. Other adverse effects include rash, pruritus, nausea, vomiting, diarrhea, epistaxis, purpura, edema, hypertension, chest pain, headache, dizziness, musculoskeletal pain, upper respiratory tract infection, bronchitis, urinary tract infection, and hypercholesterolemia.

**Cloquet's hernia.** See **crural hernia.**

**clor,** abbreviation for a *chloride noncarboxylate anion.*

**clorazepate dipotassium** /klôraz′əpāt dī-/, a benzodiazepine tranquilizer.

- INDICATIONS: It is prescribed in the treatment of anxiety, nervous tension, and alcohol withdrawal.
- CONTRAINDICATIONS: Psychosis, acute narrow-angle glaucoma, or known hypersensitivity to this drug prohibits its use.
- ADVERSE EFFECTS: Among the more serious adverse reactions are withdrawal symptoms that occur on discontinuation of treatment. Drowsiness and fatigue commonly occur.

**closed amputation** [L, *claudere*, to shut, *amputare*, to cut away], a kind of amputation in which one or two broad flaps of muscular and cutaneous tissue are retained to form a cover over the end of the bone. It is performed only when no infection is present. Compare **open amputation.**

**closed-angle glaucoma.** See **glaucoma.**

**closed bite** [L, *claudere* + AS, *bitan*], a decrease in the occlusal vertical dimension produced by various factors, such as tooth abrasion and insufficient eruption of supportive posterior teeth. Compare **open bite.**

**closed-cavity tympanomastoidectomy,** tympanomastoidectomy with tympanoplasty and maintenance of an intact posterior wall of the ear canal.

**closed-chain,** (in organic chemistry) pertaining to a compound in which the carbon atoms are bonded to form a closed ring. Also called **carbocyclic.**

**closed-chain exercise,** exercise in which the distal aspect of the extremity is in contact with a support surface such as the floor or a balance board.

**closed-circuit breathing,** rebreathing of a contained gas mixture, either directly or after recirculation of the gas through a water-absorbing or carbon dioxide-absorbing unit. An example is breathing through a spirometer.

**closed-circuit helium dilution,** a technique for measuring residual lung volume and functional residual capacity in which a patient breathes through a spirometer containing a known concentration of helium.

**closed dislocation** [L, *claudere*, to shut, *dis*, apart, *locare*, to place], a joint dislocation not accompanied by a break in the skin.

**closed drainage.** See **drainage.**

**closed fracture** [L, *claudere*, to shut, *fractura*], a bone fracture not accompanied by a break in the skin.

**closed group,** a group in which all members are admitted at the same time and vacancies that occur in the membership are not filled.

**closed loop,** a biologic feedback system in which a substance produced in the body affects the mechanism that causes its own production.

**closed-panel HMO,** (in the United States) a health maintenance organization (HMO) in which physicians have few if any private patients. See also **health maintenance organization.**

**closed physician-hospital organization (PHO),** (in the United States) an organization of selected physicians on a hospital medical staff who have proved to be high-quality, cost-effective practitioners.

**closed reduction of fractures** [L, *claudere*, to shut, *reducere*, to lead back, *fractura*], the manual correction of fractures without incision.

**closed system,** a system that does not interact with its environment.

**closed-system helium dilution method,** a technique for measuring functional residual capacity and residual volume. It is based on the principle that if a known volume and concentration of helium are added to a patient's respiratory system, the helium will be diluted in proportion to the lung volume to which it is added. Helium, an inert gas, is not significantly absorbed from the lungs by the blood.

**closed-wound suction,** any one of several techniques for draining potentially harmful fluids, such as blood, pus, serosanguineous fluid, and tissue secretions, from surgical wounds. Such fluids interfere with wound healing and often promote infection. Postoperative drainage aids the healing process by removing dead spaces where extravascular fluids collect and helps draw healing tissues together. Closed-wound suction is often an important part of postoperative treatment and may be accomplished with a variety of reliable devices that create a gentle negative pressure to drain away undesirable exudates. The technique is used as an aid to many operations, such as mastectomies, augmentations, plastic and reconstructive procedures, and urologic and urogenital procedures. It is generally used whenever the wound drainage is greater than 100 ml in 24 hours. Closed-wound suction devices usually consist of disposable transparent containers attached to suction tubes and portable suction pumps.

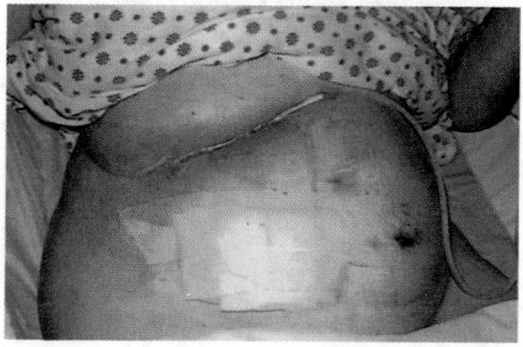

**Closed-wound suction**
*(Bryant, 1992/courtesy Abbott Northwestern Hospital, Minneapolis)*

■ METHOD: After thoroughly irrigating the wound to remove blood clots and debris, the surgeon inserts the perforated tubing into the wound and draws it out through healthy tissue, approximately 5 cm from the incision line. When silicone tubing is used, the tube is passed through a stab wound made adjacent to the surgical wound. With the drainage tubing emerging away from the incision line, the suction system remains completely closed. Air cannot infiltrate the wound and cause contamination. When the suction tube has been inserted, the wound is closed, and a light dressing is applied. Since the tubing drains most fluids, the dressing usually does not require frequent changing. Closed-wound suction usually continues postoperatively for 2 or 3 days or until the wound stops exuding fluid. The surgeon then removes the suction tubing, and all drainage components of the suction device are discarded.
■ INTERVENTIONS: While the suction is functioning the transparent tubing and reservoir are checked regularly as a precaution against clogging and for monitoring of the volume of exudate drawn from the wound. In some individuals closed-wound suction systems can also accommodate antibiotic drips, which are connected to accessory tubing placed within the wound beside the suction tube. Closed-wound suction also allows irrigation of the wound with special flow controls to permit a periodic change in the flow direction of solutions.

**closing capacity (CC),** a measure of lung volume equal to the sum of closing volume and residual volume.

**closing volume (CV),** the volume of gas remaining in the lungs when the small airways begin to close during a controlled maximum exhalation.

**clostridial** /klostrid′ē·əl/ [Gk, *kloster*, spindle], pertaining to anaerobic spore-forming bacteria of the genus *Clostridium.*

**clostridial myonecrosis.** See **myonecrosis.**

***Clostridium*** /-ē·əm/ [Gk, *kloster*, spindle], a genus of spore-forming anaerobic bacteria of the Bacillaceae family: *Clostridium novyi, C. septicum,* and *C. bifermentans* are involved in gas gangrene; *C. botulinum* causes botulism; *C. perfringens* causes food poisoning, cellulitis, and wound infections; *C. tetani* is the cause of tetanus.

***Clostridium botulinum*** [Gk, *kloster*, spindle], a species of anaerobic bacteria that cause botulism in humans and botulism-like diseases in other animals. Botulinus food poisoning results from ingesting food containing preformed toxins produced by the species. It is a proteolytic pathogen commonly present in soil, where its endospores can survive for years. Their resistance to heat makes them an important source of poisoning in improperly cooked or canned foods.

***Clostridium difficile*** /difis′ilē/, a pathogenic species of anaerobic bacteria causing pseudomembranous colitis and diarrhea, particularly after the patient has received antibiotic therapy, and is a frequent cause of nosocomial diarrhea. The species affects guinea pigs and rabbits as well as humans.

***Clostridium perfringens*** [Gk, *kloster*, spindle], a species of anaerobic gram-positive bacteria capable of causing gas gangrene in humans and various digestive and urinary tract diseases in livestock. The oval spores of the bacteria are found in the soil and in the intestinal tracts of humans and animals. Also called *Clostridium welchii.*

***Clostridium perfringens*** *(Cotran, Kumar, and Collins, 1999)*

**closure** /klō′zhər/ [L, *claudere*, to shut], **1.** the surgical closing of a wound by suture or staple. **2.** a visual phenomenon in which the mind sees an entire figure when only a portion is actually visible. See also **flask closure. 3.** the ending of something, as in closure of the grieving process.

**closylate** /klos′ilāt/, a contraction for *p*-chlorobenzenesulfonate.

**clot.** See **blood clot.**

**clothes lice.** See *Pediculus humanus corporis.*

**clot retraction,** the shrinking of a semisolid mass formed by the coagulation of blood, lymph, or other fluid. A normal standing blood clot is completely retracted in about 24 hours, the time depending on such factors as the number of platelets in the clot.

**clot retraction test,** a blood test used to evaluate bleeding disorders such as thrombocytopenia, Glanzmann's thrombasthenia, and others. It measures the time required for blood in a test tube to form a clot and for the clot's edges to retract from the sides of the glass tube.

**clotrimazole** /klōtrim′əzōl/, a broad-spectrum antifungal agent of the imidazole group used in topical applications to treat fungal and yeast infections.
  - INDICATIONS: It is prescribed in the treatment of superficial fungal infections and candidal vulvovaginitis.
  - CONTRAINDICATIONS: Known hypersensitivity to this drug prohibits its use. It is not prescribed for ophthalmic use; contact with eyes is avoided.
  - ADVERSE EFFECTS: The most serious adverse reactions are severe hypersensitivity reactions of the skin.

**clotting.** See **blood clotting.**

**clotting time** [AS, *clott*], the time required for blood to form a clot, tested by collecting 4 ml of blood in a glass tube and examining it for clot formation. The first appearance of a clot is noted and timed. The normal coagulation time in glass tubes is 5 to 15 minutes. This simple test has been used to diagnose hemophilia, but it does not detect mild coagulation disorders. Its chief application is in monitoring anticoagulant therapy. Also called **coagulation time.** Compare **bleeding time.**

**cloud baby** [AS, *clud + babe*], a newborn who appears well and healthy but is a carrier of infectious bacterial or viral organisms. The infant may contaminate the surrounding environment as airborne droplets from the respiratory tract form clouds of the organisms. A cloud baby may be the source of a nursery epidemic, especially one caused by a staphylococcal organism.

**clouding of consciousness,** a mental state in which a patient is confused about or is not fully aware of the immediate surroundings. Also called **sensorium.**

**clove** /klōv/ [L, *clavus*, nail], the dried flower bud of *Eugenia caryophyllata.* It contains the lactone caryophyllin and a volatile oil used as a dental analgesic, a germicide, and a salve. Clove is also used as a spice and a carminative against nausea, vomiting, and flatulence.

**clove-hitch sling,** a bandage that begins with a clove-hitch knot at the center. The loop made is fitted to the hand. The two loose ends are extended over and behind the shoulders and tied beside the neck. Longer ends may be drawn down the back of the shoulders and under each axilla to be tied over the chest. It provides support for an injured upper extremity.

**cloverleaf nail** /klō′vərlēf′/ [AS, *clafre + leaf + nagel*], a surgical nail shaped in cross section like a cloverleaf, used especially in the repair of fractures of the femur.

**cloverleaf skull deformity,** a congenital defect characterized by a trilobed skull resulting from the premature closure of multiple cranial sutures during embryonic development. The condition is associated with hydrocephalus, facial anomalies, and skeletal deformities.

**cloxacillin sodium** /klok′səsil′in/, an antibiotic for bacterial infections.
  - INDICATIONS: It is prescribed in the treatment of serious bacterial infections, primarily those caused by penicillin-resistant strains of staphylococci.
  - CONTRAINDICATION: Known hypersensitivity to this drug or to any penicillin prohibits its use.

  - ADVERSE EFFECT: Among the more serious adverse reactions are GI discomfort, rash, and hypersensitivity.

**clubbed penis** [ME, *clubbe + L, penis*], a penis that is curved or twisted, or both. The abnormality may be accompanied by epispadias or hypospadias.

**clubbing** [ME, *clubbe*], an abnormal enlargement of the distal phalanges. It usually is associated with cyanotic heart disease or advanced chronic pulmonary disease but sometimes occurs with biliary cirrhosis, colitis, chronic dysentery, and thyrotoxicosis. The mechanism whereby diminished oxygen tension in the blood causes clubbing is not understood. Clubbing occurs in all the digits but is most easily seen in the fingers. Advanced clubbing is obvious, but early clubbing may be difficult to diagnose. Clubbing is present if the transverse diameter of the base of the fingernail is greater than the transverse diameter of the most distal joint of the digit. The affected phalanx is full, fleshy, and quite vascular; the skin may be excoriated.

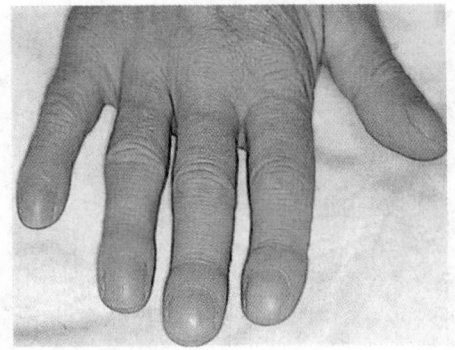

**Clubbing** *(Earis and Pearson, 1995)*

**clubfoot** [ME, *clubbe + AS, fot*], a congenital deformity of the foot, sometimes resulting from intrauterine constriction and characterized by unilateral or bilateral deviation of the metatarsal bones of the forefoot. Ninety-five percent of

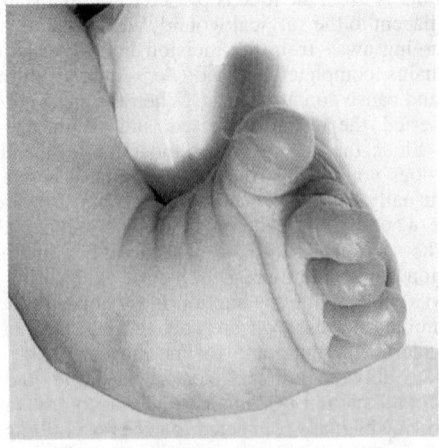

**Clubfoot**
*(Zitelli and Davis, 1997/courtesy Dr. Christine L. Williams, New York Medical College)*

clubfoot deformities are **equinovarus,** characterized by medial deviation and plantar flexion of the forefoot, but a few are **calcaneovalgus,** or **calcaneovarus,** characterized by lateral deviation and dorsiflexion either outward from or inward toward the midline of the body. Treatment depends on the extent and rigidity of the deformity. Splints and casts in infancy may produce complete correction; surgery in several steps may be necessary to achieve normal function. See also **Denis Browne splint, talipes.**

**club hair,** a hair in the resting, or final, stage of the growth cycle. See also **hair.**

**cluster analysis** [AS, *clyster,* growing together; Gk, *analyein,* to loosen], (in statistics) a complex technique of data analysis of numeric scale scores that produces clusters of variables related to one another. The technique is performed with a computer.

**cluster breathing,** a breathing pattern in which a closely grouped series of respirations is followed by apnea. The activity is associated with a lesion in the lower pontine region of the brainstem. See also **Biot's respiration, Cheyne-Stokes respiration.**

**cluster headache,** a migrainelike condition characterized by attacks of intense unilateral pain. The pain occurs most often over the eye and forehead. It is accompanied by flushing and watering of the eyes and nose. The attacks occur in groups with a duration of several hours. See also **histamine headache.**

**cluster-of-differentiation (CD) antigen,** one of a group of cell-surface molecules that are used to classify leukocytes into subsets.

**cluttering** [ME, *clotter*], a speech disorder characterized by a rapid, confused, nervous delivery with uneven rhythmic patterns and omission or transposition of various speech sounds or syllables. The condition is commonly associated with other language disorders, such as difficulty in learning to speak, read, and spell, and with various personality and behavior problems.

**clysis** /klī′sis/ [Gk, *klyster,* washout], the nonoral insertion or injection of a fluid into the body, such as the administration of an enema.

**cm,** abbreviation for **centimeter.**

**Cm,** symbol for the element **curium.**

**cm²,** abbreviation for **square centimeter.**

**cm³,** abbreviation for **cubic centimeter.**

**CMA,** abbreviation for *Canadian Medical Association.*

**CMAJ,** abbreviation for *Canadian Medical Association Journal.*

**CMC,** abbreviation for *carpometacarpal.*

**CMF,** an anticancer drug combination of cyclophosphamide, methotrexate, and fluorouracil.

**CMHC,** abbreviation for **community mental health center.**

**CMI,** abbreviation for **computer-managed instruction.**

**CML,** abbreviation for **chronic myelocytic leukemia.**

**cmm,** abbreviation for **cubic millimeter.**

**c mm,** abbreviation for **cubic millimeter.**

**CMRNG,** abbreviation for *chromosomally mediated resistant Neisseria gonorrhoeae.*

**CMT,** abbreviation for *Certified Medical Transcriptionist.*

**CMV,** abbreviation for **cytomegalovirus.**

**CNA,** 1. abbreviation for **Canadian Nurses Association.** 2. abbreviation for **certified nurse administrator.** 3. Abbreviation for **certified nursing assistant.**

**CNAA,** abbreviation for **certified nurse administrator, advanced.**

**CNATS,** abbreviation for **Canadian Nurses Association Testing Service.**

**-cnemia,** suffix meaning '(condition of the) leg below the knee': *bucnemia, cacocnemia, microcnemia.*

**CNF,** abbreviation for **Canadian Nurses Foundation.**

**CNHV,** abbreviation for **central neurogenic hyperventilation.**

**Cnidaria,** a phylum of invertebrate animals that includes jellyfish, sea anemones, hydroids, and corals. Formerly called **Coelenterata.**

**CNM,** abbreviation for **Certified Nurse-Midwife.**

**CNOR,** abbreviation for *Certified Nurse, Operating Room.*

**CNP,** abbreviation for **community nurse practitioner.**

**CNRN,** abbreviation for *Certified Neuroscience Registered Nurse.*

**CNRS,** abbreviation for **Canadian Nurses Respiratory Society.**

**CNS,** 1. abbreviation for **central nervous system.** 2. abbreviation for **clinical nurse specialist.**

**CNSN,** abbreviation for *Certified Nutrition Support Nurse.*

**CNS sympathomimetic,** a drug, such as cocaine or an amphetamine, whose effects mimic those of sympathetic nervous system stimulation.

**CNS syndrome.** See **central nervous system syndrome.**

**Co,** symbol for the element **cobalt.**

**CO,** 1. formula for **carbon monoxide.** 2. abbreviation for **cardiac output.**

**co-, col-, com-, con-, cor-,** combining form meaning 'together, with': *coadaptation, coagulate, coarctate.*

**CO₂,** formula for **carbon dioxide.**

**CoA,** abbreviation for **coenzyme A.**

**coagglutination** /kō′əglōō′tənā′shən/ [L, *cum* + *agglutinare,* to glue], a clumping of red blood cells by mixtures of protein antigens and their antisera.

**coagulability** /kō·ag′yələbil′itē/ [L, *coagulare,* to curdle], the state of being able to coagulate or form blood clots.

**coagulant** /kō·ag′yələnt/ [L, *coagulare,* to curdle], an agent that causes a coagulum, or blood clot, to form.

**coagulase** /kō·ag′yəlās/ [L, *coagulare,* to curdle], an enzyme produced by bacteria, particularly *Staphylococcus aureus,* that promotes the formation of fibrin from fibrinogen to form thrombi.

**coagulate** /kō·ag′yəlāt/, to undergo or cause to undergo the chemical process whereby a fluid becomes curdled or clotted. —**coagulated,** *adj.*

**coagulated** /kō·ag′yəlā′tid/, curdled; changed to a clotted state.

**coagulation** /kō·ag′yəlā′shən/ [L, *coagulare,* to curdle], 1. the process of transforming a liquid into a solid, especially of the blood. See also **blood clotting.** 2. (in colloid chemistry) the transforming of the liquid dispersion medium into a gelatinous mass. 3. the hardening of tissue by some physical means, as by electrocoagulation or photocoagulation.

**coagulation cascade,** the series of steps beginning with activation of the intrinsic or extrinsic pathways of coagulation, or of one of the related alternative pathways, and proceeding through the common pathway of coagulation to the formation of the fibrin clot; each step involves activation of an enzyme precursor, the activated form catalyzing activation of the following step. See also **common pathway of coagulation, extrinsic pathway of coagulation, intrinsic pathway of coagulation.**

**coagulation current,** an electric current delivered by a needle ball or variously shaped points to bind tissues together. See also **electrocautery, electrocoagulation.**

**coagulation factor,** one of 13 factors in the blood, the interactions of which are responsible for the process of blood clotting. The factors, using standardized numeric nomenclature, are factor I, fibrinogen; factor II, prothrombin; factor III, tissue thromboplastin; factor IV, calcium ions; factors V and VI, proaccelerin or labile factor; factor VII, proconvertin or stable factor; factor VIII, antihemophilic globulin; factor IX, plasma thromboplastin component (PTC); factor X, Stuart-Power factor; factor XI, plasma thromboplastin antecedent (PTA); factor XII, Hageman factor or glass factor or contact factor; factor XIII, fibrin stabilizing factor or fibrinase or Laki-Lorand factor. See also **blood clotting, coagulation, fibrinogen, hemophilia A, hemophilia B, hemophilia C, prothrombin, thromboplastin,** and see **factor IV** through **factor XIII.**

**coagulation factors concentration test,** a set of blood tests used to measure the quantity of a number of specific factors suspected to be responsible for suspected defects in hemostasis, and to help the clinician determine the appropriate treatment. Deficiencies of these factors may result from inherited genetic defects, acquired diseases, or drug therapy.

**coagulation factor VIIa, recombinant,** an antihemophilic.

■ INDICATIONS: This drug is prescribed to prevent the bleeding associated with hemophilia A or B, with inhibitors to Factor VIII or IX.

■ CONTRAINDICATIONS: Factors that prohibit this drug's use include known hypersensitivity to this product or to mouse-, hamster-, or bovine-derived products.

■ ADVERSE EFFECTS: Life-threatening side effects include hemorrhage, hemarthrosis, decreased fibrinogen plasma, diffuse intravascular coagulation, coagulation disorder, and thrombosis. Other adverse effects include fever, headache, hypertension, bradycardia, pain, redness at the injection site, pruritus, purpura, and rash.

**coagulation necrosis,** necrosis in which tissue becomes a dry, opaque, eosinophilic mass containing outlines of anucleated cells; it results from the denaturation of proteins following hypoxic injury, such as that caused by ischemia in infarction. Also called **avascular necrosis** and **ischemic necrosis.**

**coagulation status,** a nursing outcome from the Nursing Outcome Classification (NOC) defined as extent to which blood clots within expected period of time. See also **nursing outcomes classification.**

**coagulation time.** See **clotting time.**

**coagulative** /kō·ag′yəlā′tiv/, **1.** causing blood clot formation. **2.** an agent that assists the formation of blood clots.

**coagulopathy** /kō·ag′yəlop′əthē/, a pathologic condition that affects the ability of the blood to coagulate.

**coalesce** /kō′əles′/ [L, *coalescere,* to grow together], to grow together.

**coal tar,** a topical antieczematic.

■ INDICATIONS: It is prescribed in the treatment of chronic skin conditions, such as eczema and psoriasis.

■ CONTRAINDICATIONS: Known hypersensitivity to this drug prohibits its use.

■ ADVERSE EFFECTS: Among the most serious adverse effects are skin irritation and local hypersensitivity reactions.

**coal worker's pneumoconiosis.** See **anthracosis.**

**Coanda effect,** a phenomenon of fluid movement similar to the Bernoulli effect in which passage of a stream of gas next to a wall results in a pocket of turbulence between the wall and the gas flow. The turbulence forms a low-pressure bubble that makes the gas stream adhere to the wall. The principle is used in fluidic ventilators.

**coaptation splint** /kō′aptā′shən/ [L, *coaptare,* to fit together; ME *splinte*], a small splint fitted to a fractured limb to prevent overriding of the fragments of bone during adjustment of the fracture. A longer splint usually covers the small one to provide more support and fixation of the entire limb.

**coarct** /kō·ärkt′/ [L, *coarctare,* to press together], the act of narrowing or constricting, especially the lumen of a blood vessel.

**coarctate retina** /kō·ärk′tāt/ [L, *coarctare,* to press together, *rete,* net], a funnel-shaped retina caused by a leakage of fluid between the retina and the choroid.

**coarctation** /kō′ärktā′shən/, a compression, shrivelling, or stricture of the walls of a vessel as the aorta.

**coarctation of the aorta,** a congenital cardiac anomaly characterized by a localized narrowing of the aorta. It results in increased pressure proximal to the defect and decreased pressure distal to it. The most common site of coarctation is just beyond the origin of the left subclavian artery from the aorta, resulting in high blood pressure in the upper extremities and head and low blood pressure in the lower extremities. Symptoms are directly related to the pressure changes created by the constriction. Clinical manifestations include dizziness, headaches, fainting, epistaxis, reduced or absent femoral pulses, and muscle cramps in the legs from tissue anoxia during increased exercise. Diagnosis is based on characteristic pressure changes in the upper and lower body and specific radiologic and echocardiographic findings, including notching of the lower ribs, left ventricular hypertrophy, and dilation of the aorta proximal to the stricture. A murmur may or may not be present. Surgical repair is recommended for minor defects because of the high incidence of untreated complications, including aortic rupture, hypertension, infective endocarditis, subarachnoid hemorrhage, and congestive heart failure.

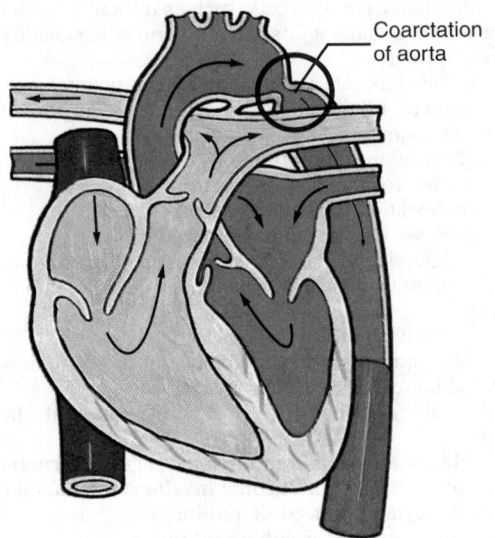

Coarctation
of aorta

**Coarctation of the aorta** *(Wong, 1999)*

**coarse** /kôrs/ [ME, *cors,* common], (in physiology) involving a wide range of movements, such as those associated with tremors and other involuntary motions of the skeletal muscle.

**coarse crackle** [ME, *cors,* common, *krakelen*], an abnormal breathing sound caused by air moving through an excessive amount of fluid in an airway, as in pulmonary edema.

**coarse fremitus,** a rough, loud, tremulous vibration of the chest wall noted on palpation of the chest during a physical examination as the person inhales and exhales. It is most common in pulmonary conditions characterized by consolidation. See also **fremitus.**

**coarse tremor** [ME, *cors,* common; L, *tremor,* shaking], a tremor in which the movements are relatively slow and may involve larger muscle groups.

**coat** [ME, *cote*], **1.** a membrane that covers the outside of an organ or part. **2.** one of the layers of a wall of an organ or part, especially a canal or a vessel.

**coated tablet** [ME, *cote* + Fr, *tablette*], a solid disc of one or more pharmaceutical agents that is coated with sugar or a flavoring to mask the taste or that is enteric-coated, which is when a substance resists dissolution in the stomach but allows release of the medication in the intestine.

**coated tongue** [ME, *cote* + AS, *tunge*], a tongue with a white, yellow, or brown furred surface, representing a possible accumulation of mycelia, bacteria, food debris, or desquamated epithelial cells. There are many possible causes, ranging from a fungal infection to sleeping with the mouth open. Also called **furred tongue.**

**Coats' disease, Coats' retinitis.** See **exudative retinopathy.**

**cobalamin** /kōbôl′əmin/ [Ger, *kobold,* mine goblin], a generic term for a chemical portion of the vitamin $B_{12}$ molecule. See also **cyanocobalamin.**

**cobalt (Co)** /kō′bôlt/ [Ger, *kobold,* mine goblin], a metallic element that occurs in the minerals cobaltite, smaltite, and linnaeite. Its atomic number is 27; its atomic mass is 58.93. Extensive deposits of cobalt minerals are found in Ontario, Canada. Pure cobalt is obtained by reducing the oxide with aluminum or carbon. It is used in special alloys, such as Alnico. Cobalt is a component of vitamin $B_{12}$, is found in most common foods, and is readily absorbed by the GI tract. This element is common in the human diet, but the precise daily intake requirement is not known, and cobalt deficiency in humans has not been seen. Cobaltous chloride has been given to some patients with certain types of anemia because of cobalt's capacity to produce polycythemia. Accidental intoxication by cobaltous chloride, especially by children, may produce cyanosis, coma, and death. Some amounts of cobalt stimulate the production of erythropoietin, by a process not yet understood, but large doses depress erythrocyte production. The only disease for which the use of cobalt is still advocated is normochromic, normocytic anemia associated with renal failure. The radioisotope $^{60}$Co or cobalt-60 emits gamma rays and is often used as an encapsulated radiation source in the treatment of cancer.

**cobalt-60** ($^{60}$**Co),** a radioactive isotope of the element cobalt with a mass of 60 and a half-life of 5.2 years. $^{60}$Co emits high-energy gamma rays and is the most frequently used radioisotope in radiotherapy. It must be stored in a position well shielded by lead or uranium.

**cobalt lung.** See **hard metal disease.**

**cobalt poisoning,** poisoning from long-term excessive exposure to cobalt, seen in those who work with it. It was formerly seen in beer drinkers because cobalt was added to beer as a foam stabilizer. Symptoms include nausea, vomiting, tinnitus, nerve deafness, and cardiomyopathy.

**Coban,** trademark for an elastic pressure wrap applied to reduce edema. It adheres to itself and may be used as a secondary dressing for patients allergic to tape. See also **cohesive bandage.**

**COBOL** /kō′bol/, abbreviation for *common business oriented language,* a high-level compiler computer language for programming.

**COBRA** /kō′brə/, abbreviation for **Consolidated Omnibus Reconciliation Act.**

**cobra venom solution** [L, *colubra,* snake, *venenum,* venom, *solutus,* dissolved], a sterile physiologic salt solution containing minute amounts of cobralysin, the hemolytic substance in cobra venom.

**coca,** a species of South American shrubs, native to Bolivia and Peru and cultivated in Indonesia. The leaves are dried and then chewed for their stimulant effect by some of the people of the region. It is a natural source of cocaine.

**cocaine baby** /kōkān′/, an infant with birth defects caused by exposure to cocaine in utero. Contributing causes may include poor sperm quality of a male cocaine user, poor nutritional habits and/or alcohol or tobacco abuse by the mother during pregnancy, and the direct effect of the drug itself, which can cross the placental barrier.

**cocaine hydrochloride,** a white crystalline powder used as a local anesthetic. It was originally derived from coca leaves but can also be prepared synthetically. Cocaine is a Schedule II drug under the Controlled Substances Act of 1970.

■ INDICATIONS: In solution the drug is sometimes used as a topical anesthetic applied to mucous membranes. Its vasoconstrictive action slows bleeding and limits absorption. Prolonged or frequent use may damage the mucous membranes.

■ CONTRAINDICATIONS: Cocaine is incompatible with all alkaloid precipitants, mercurials, and silver nitrate. Central nervous system overstimulation may result from use with monoamine oxidase inhibitors, amphetamines, or guanethidine. Combination with epinephrine or norepinephrine can lead to cardiac arrhythmias or ventricular fibrillation. Cocaine is not given to patients with severe cardiovascular disease, thyrotoxicosis, hypotension, or hypertension.

■ ADVERSE REACTIONS: Among the most serious adverse reactions are excitement, depression, euphoria, restlessness, tremors, vertigo, nausea, vomiting, hypotension, hypertension, abdominal cramps, exophthalmia, mydriasis, peripheral vascular collapse, tachypnea, tachycardia, chills, fever, coma, and death from respiratory failure.

■ NOTE: Cocaine hydrochloride solution should be freshly made; it deteriorates rapidly on standing and cannot be heat-sterilized.

**cocaine hydrochloride poisoning** [Sp, *coca* + *HCl* + L, *potio,* drink], toxic effects of exposure to the colorless crystalline alkaloid derived from coca leaves. Although used as a local analgesic for a century, cocaine is highly toxic with moderate vasoconstrictor activity and serious psychotropic effects. Symptoms include nervous excitement, restlessness, incoherent speech, fever, hypertension, and cardiac arrhythmias, leading to convulsions, collapse, respiratory arrest, and death. The euphoric effect of cocaine lasts about 30 minutes. A crystalline form of cocaine with the street names **crack** and **rock** is smoked.

**cocarcinogen** /kōkär′sənəjən/ [L, *cum,* together with; Gk, *karkinos,* crab, *genein,* to produce], an agent that alone does not transform a normal cell into a cancerous state but in concert with another agent can effect the transformation.

**coccal.** See **coccus.**

**cocci-, cocco-,** combining form meaning 'seed, berry; or a spherical bacterial cell': *coccobacillus, coccogenous, coccoid.*

**Coccidia,** a subclass of parasitic protozoa found in humans, other vertebrates, and some invertebrates. Among the species of coccidians pathogenic to humans is *Cyclospora cayetanensis.* See also **coccidiosis.**

**coccidian. 1.** pertaining to Coccidia. **2.** a protozoan in the subclass Coccidia.

*Coccidioides* /kok·sid′ē·oi′dēz/, a pathogenic genus of Fungi Imperfecti of the form-class Hyphomycetes, form-family Moniliaceae. In soil it grows as a mycelium with arthrospores; in tissue as a spherule with endospores. *C. immitis* causes coccidioidomycosis and fungal pneumonia.

**coccidioidomycosis** /koksid′ē·oi′dōmīkō′sis/ [Gk, *kokkos,* berry, *eidos,* form, *mykes,* fungus, *osis,* condition], an infectious fungal disease caused by the inhalation of spores of the protozoon *Coccidioides immitis,* which is carried on windborne dust particles. The disease is endemic in hot, dry regions of the southwestern United States and Central and South America and is an opportunistic disease associated with human immunodeficiency virus infection. Primary infection is characterized by symptoms resembling those of the common cold or influenza. Secondary infection, occurring after a period of remission and lasting from weeks to years, is marked by low-grade fever, anorexia and weight loss, cyanosis, dyspnea, hemoptysis, focal skin lesions resembling erythema nodosum, and arthritic pain in the bones and joints. The diagnosis is made by finding that the patient has been living in or visiting an endemic area and by identifying *C. immitis* in sputum, exudate, or tissue. Treatment usually consists of bed rest and the administration of antibiotics, such as amphotericin B or fluconazole. Also called **desert fever, desert rheumatism, San Joaquin fever, valley fever.**

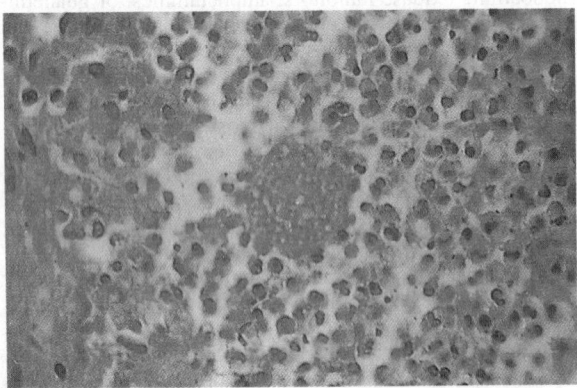

***Coccidioides immitis,* the bacterium that causes coccidioidomycosis**
(Murray et al, 1998)

**coccidiosis** /kok′sidē·ō′sis/ [Gk, *kokkos* + *osis,* condition], a parasitic disease of tropical and subtropical regions caused by the ingestion of oocysts of the protozoon *Isospora belli* or *I. hominis.* Symptoms include fever, malaise, abdominal discomfort, and watery diarrhea. The infection is usually self-limited, lasting 1 to 2 weeks, but occasionally it persists, resulting in malabsorption syndrome and, rarely, death. No specific therapy has been found. Compare **coccidioidomycosis.**

**cocco-.** See **cocci-.**

**coccoid** /kok′oid/ [Gk, *kokkos,* berry, *eidos,* form], having a spherical shape; resembling a micrococcus.

**coccus** /kok′əs/, *pl.* **cocci** /kok′sī, kok′ī/ [Gk, *kokkos,* berry], a bacterium that is round, spheric, or oval, as gonococcus, pneumococcus, staphylococcus, streptococcus. —**coccal,** *adj.*

**-coccus,** suffix meaning a 'berry-shaped organism': *dermococcus, enterococcus, pneumococcus.*

**coccyalgia** /kok′si·al′jə/, a pain in or near the coccyx.

**coccyg-, coccygo-,** combining form meaning 'coccyx': *coccygeal, coccygectomy, coccygodynia.*

**coccygeal.** See **coccyx.**

**coccygeal body** /koksij′ē·əl/ [Gk, *kokkyx,* cuckoo's beak; AS, *bodig*], the coccyx.

**coccygeal vertebra,** one of the four segments of the vertebral column that fuse to form the adult coccyx. They are considered rudimentary vertebrae and have no pedicles, laminae, or spinous processes. Compare **cervical vertebra, lumbar vertebra, sacral vertebra, thoracic vertebra.** See also **coccyx, vertebra.**

**coccyges.** See **coccyx.**

**coccygeus** /koksij′ē·əs/ [Gk, *kokkyx,* cuckoo's beak], one of two muscles in the pelvic diaphragm. Stretching across the pelvic cavity like a hammock, it is a triangular sheet of muscle and tendinous fibers. It acts to draw the coccyx ventrally, helping to support the pelvic floor. Compare **levator ani.**

**coccygodynia** /kok′sigōdin′ē·ə/, a pain in the coccygeal area. Also called **coccyalgia, coccydynia.**

**coccyx** /kok′siks/, *pl.* **coccyges** /koksī′jēz, kok′sijēz/ [Gk, *kokkyx,* cuckoo's beak], the beaklike bone joined to the sacrum by a disk of fibrocartilage at the base of the vertebral column. It is formed by the union of three to five probably vestigial rudimentary vertebrae. The pieces of the coccyx fuse together in males at an earlier period in life than in females. In both the coccyx becomes fused with the sacrum by the sixth decade of life. The coccyx is freely movable on the sacrum during pregnancy. —**coccygeal** /koksij′ē·əl/, *adj.*

**cochineal** /koch′inēl′/ [L, *coccineus,* bright red], a red dye prepared from the dried female insects of the species *Coccus cacti* containing young larvae. During the preparation of the dye the larvae are extracted with an aqueous solution of alum, and the resulting dye has been used in coloring medicines.

**cochlea** /kok′lē·ə/ [L, snail shell], the auditory portion of the inner ear. It is a spiral tunnel about 30 mm long with two full and three quarter-turns, resembling a tiny snail shell and contains the sense organ for hearing. —**cochlear,** *adj.*

**cochlear canal** /kok′lē·ər/ [L *cochlea* + *canalis* channel], a bony spiral tunnel within the cochlea of the internal ear. It contains one opening that communicates with the tympanic cavity, a second that connects with the vestibule, and a third that leads to a tiny canal opening on the inferior surface of the temporal bone.

**cochlear duct.** See **cochlear canal.**

**cochlear hearing loss,** sensorineural hearing loss resulting from a defect in the receptor or transducing mechanisms of the cochlea.

**cochlear implant,** an electronic device that is surgically implanted into the cochlea of a deaf individual. A transmitter placed outside the scalp sends signals to a receiver under the scalp, which in turn transmits an electrical code to the auditory nerve. A microphone is located behind the ear to collect the sound waves that are transmitted through a microprocessor. The microprocessor analyzes the sound waves and relays data back to electrodes in the implanted device. The patient receives electrical pulses that are translated into sound vibrations that can be distinguished as neural sensations. Although the implant does not transmit speech as

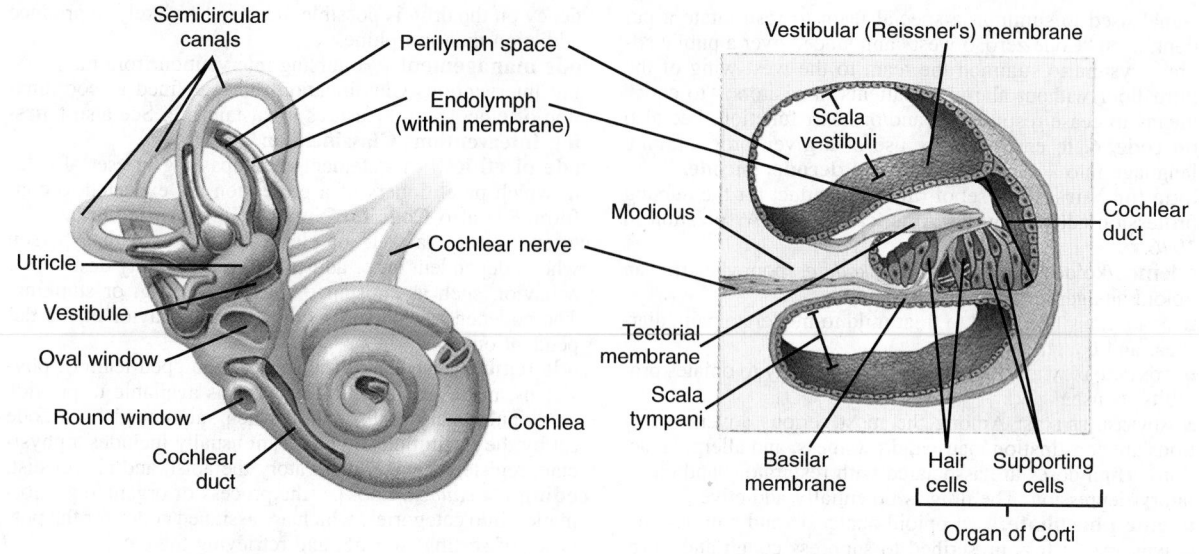

**Position of cochlea within the inner ear**

**Cross section of the cochlea**

**Cochlea** *(Thibodeau and Patton, 1999/Rolin Graphics)*

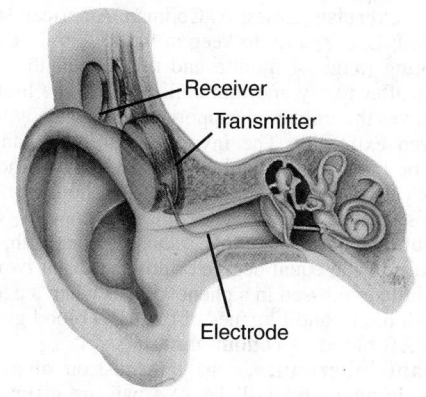

**Cochlear implant** *(Thibodeau and Patton, 1999/Rolin Graphics)*

clearly as it would be perceived by a person with normal hearing, it allows the individual to perceive and distinguish sounds that would not otherwise be audible to him or her and to use those sounds along with other environmental cues to improve communication. Also called **cochlear prosthesis.**

**cochlear nerve** [L, *cochlea,* snail shell, *nervus,* nerve], one of the main divisions of the eighth cranial nerve, with fibers that arise in spiral ganglion cells of the spiral organ and terminate in the dorsal and ventral cochlear nuclei of the brainstem. See also **acoustic nerve.**

**cochlear prosthesis.** See **cochlear implant.**

**cochlear toxicity,** poisonous effects of drugs that may result in hearing disorders, such as sensorineural hearing loss and tinnitus.

**cochlear window.** See **round window.**

**cochleovestibular** /kok′lē-ō′vestib′yələr/, pertaining to the cochlea and vestibule of the ear.

**Cockayne's syndrome** /kok·ānz′/ [Edward Alfred Cockayne, English physician, 1880–1956], an autosomal recessive syndrome of dwarfism with retinal atrophy and deafness, associated with progeria, prognathism, mental retardation, and photosensitivity.

**cockroach,** the common name of members of the Blattidae family of insects that infest homes, workplaces, and other areas inhabited by humans. Cockroaches transmit a number of disease agents, including bacteria, protozoa, and eggs of parasitic worms.

**cockscomb papilloma** /kok′skōm/ [AS, *cocc + camb* + L, *papilla,* nipple; Gk, *oma,* tumor], a benign small red lesion that may project from the uterine cervix during pregnancy; it regresses after delivery.

**cocktail** [AS, *cocc + toegel*], *informal.* an unofficial mixture of drugs, usually in solution, combined to achieve a specific purpose. This term is frequently used when combining medications to treat patients who are HIV positive. See also **Brompton's cocktail.**

**cockup splint,** a splint used to immobilize the wrist and leave the fingers free.

**coconsciousness** /kōkon′shəsnəs/, (in psychiatry) conscious states the patient is not aware of because they are not in the focus of attention but on the fringe of the content of consciousness. Thus something can be recalled and drawn into consciousness only when the conditions of consciousness itself are favorable.

**cocontraction** /kō′kəntrak′shən/, the simultaneous contraction of agonist and antagonist muscles around a joint to hold a position.

**COD,** abbreviation for *cause of death.*

**code** [L, *caudex,* book], **1.** (in law) a published body of statutes, as a civil code. **2.** a collection of standards and rules of behavior, as a dress code. **3.** a symbolic means of representing information for communication or transfer, as a genetic code. **4.** a system of notation that allows information to be transmitted rapidly, such as Morse code, or in secrecy, such as a cryptographic code. **5.** *informal.* a discreet signal used to summon a special team to resuscitate a patient, as in "Code zero, 3 west" announced over a public address system to summon the team to the west wing of the third floor without alarming patients or visitors; "to code" means to cease respirations and/or heart function. See also **no code. 6.** to enter data by use of a given programming language into a computer. Compare **decode, encode.**

**Code for Nurses,** a set of rules of conduct for the nursing profession adopted by the American Nurses Association in 1976.

**codeine** /kō′dēn, kō′dē·in/ [Gk, *kodeia,* poppyhead], an opioid analgesic and antitussive.

■ INDICATIONS: It is used to treat mild to moderate pain, diarrhea, and cough.

■ CONTRAINDICATIONS: Known hypersensitivity to opiates prohibits its use.

■ ADVERSE EFFECTS: Among the most serious adverse reactions are constipation, nausea, drowsiness, and allergic reactions. High doses are associated with respiratory and circulatory depression. The drug is potentially addictive.

**codeine phosphate,** an opioid analgesic and antitussive.

■ INDICATIONS: It is prescribed to suppress cough and to relieve mild to moderate pain.

■ CONTRAINDICATION: Known hypersensitivity to opiates is the only contraindication.

■ ADVERSE EFFECTS: Among the more serious adverse reactions are depression of the central nervous system, paradoxic excitement, and drug dependence.

**codeine sulfate,** a water-soluble salt of monomethylmorphine, an alkaloid derived from opium. It is used as a mild hypnotic, analgesic, and cough reflex suppressant. Dependency on the drug is possible, but it is less likely to produce addiction than morphine.

**code management,** a nursing intervention from the Nursing Interventions Classification (NIC) defined as coordination of emergency measures to sustain life. See also **Nursing Interventions Classification.**

**code of ethics,** a statement encompassing the set of rules to which practitioners of a profession are expected to conform. See also **Code for Nurses, Hippocratic Oath.**

**codependent,** a state of close association with a person who is dependent on or addicted to a potentially destructive behavior, such as substance abuse, gambling, or smoking. The codependent person facilitates the behavior of the dependent one.

**code team,** a specially trained and equipped team of physicians, nurses, and technicians that is available to provide cardiopulmonary resuscitation when summoned by a code set by the institution. A code team usually includes a physician, registered nurse, respiratory therapist, and pharmacist.

**coding** [L, *caudex,* book], the process of organizing information into categories, which are assigned codes for the purposes of sorting, storing, and retrieving the data.

**coding strand.** See **sense strand.**

**cod-liver oil,** a pale-yellow fatty oil extracted from the fresh livers of the cod. It is a rich source of fat-soluble vitamins A and D, useful in the treatment of nutritional deficiency of those vitamins. The oil must be stored in a cool, dark place, or it becomes rancid. See also **osteomalacia, rickets, tetany.**

**Codman's exercise** [Ernest A. Codman, American surgeon, 1869–1940; L, *exercere,* to keep at work], mild exercises for restoring range of motion and function in the arms or shoulders after injury and immobilization of the limbs. The patient flexes the trunk and supports the upper body with the uninvolved extremity. The involved extremity hangs free and can be moved in pendulum fashion through motion of the trunk without active contraction of the shoulder muscles.

**Codman's tumor.** See **chondroblastoma.**

**codominance** /kōdom′ənənt/ [L, *cum,* together with, *dominare,* to rule], the equal degree of dominance of two alleles or traits fully expressed in a phenotype, as when a person inherits both the $I^A$ and $I^B$ genes of the ABO blood group and has type AB blood. —**codominant,** *adj.*

**codominant inheritance,** the transmission of a trait or condition in which both alleles of a pair are given full expression in a heterozygote, as in the alleles for the AB or MNS blood group antigens and the leukocyte antigens.

**codon** /kō′don/, a unit of three adjacent nucleotides along a DNA or messenger RNA molecule that designates a specific amino acid to be incorporated into a polypeptide. The order of the codons along the DNA or messenger RNA determines the sequence of the amino acids in the polypeptide. Also called **trinucleotide.** See also **anticodon, genetic code.**

**coefficient** /kō′efish′ənt/ [L, *cum,* together with, *efficere,* to effect], a mathematic relationship between factors that can be used to measure or evaluate a characteristic under specified conditions. Examples include Henry's law, which measures **solubility coefficient;** Graham's law, which calculates **diffusion coefficient;** and the **oxygen-utilization coefficient,** which measures the amount of oxygen in a patient's venous blood in terms of the proportion of oxygen in his or her arterial blood.

**coel-,** combining form meaning 'colon,' denoting relationship to a cavity or space: *coelarium.*

**-coele,** suffix form of '**coel-**'.

**coelentera.** See **coelenteron.**

---

**Code for Nurses**

1. The nurse provides services with respect for human dignity and the uniqueness of the client unrestricted by considerations of social or economic status, personal attributes, or the nature of health problems.
2. The nurse safeguards the client's right to privacy by judiciously protecting information of a confidential nature.
3. The nurse acts to safeguard the client and the public when health care and safety are affected by the incompetent, unethical, or illegal practice of any person.
4. The nurse assumes responsibility and accountability for individual nursing judgments and actions.
5. The nurse maintains competence in nursing.
6. The nurse exercises informed judgment and uses individual competence and qualification as criteria in seeking consultation, accepting responsibilities, and delegating nursing activities to others.
7. The nurse participates in activities that contribute to the ongoing development of the profession's body of knowledge.
8. The nurse participates in the profession's efforts to implement and improve standards of nursing.
9. The nurse participates in the profession's efforts to establish and maintain conditions of employment conducive to high quality nursing care.
10. The nurse participates in the profession's efforts to protect the public from misinformation and misrepresentation and to maintain the integrity of nursing.
11. The nurse collaborates with members of the health professions and other citizens in promoting community and national efforts to meet the health needs of the public.

From American Nurses' Association: *Code for nurses with interpretive statements,* Kansas City, Mo, 1985, The Association.

**Coelenterata.** See **Cnidaria.**

**coelenteron** /sēlen'tərion/, *pl.* **coelentera** [Gk, *koilos,* hollow, *enteron,* intestine], the digestive cavity of animals in the phylum Cnidaria, such as the hydra and the jellyfish. See also **archenteron.**

**coelom** /sē'ləm/ [Gk, *koilos,* hollow], the body cavity of the developing embryo. It is situated between the layers of lateral mesoderm and in mammals gives rise to the pericardial, pleural, and peritoneal cavities. A kind of coelom is **extraembryonic coelom.** Also called **somatic cavity.** —**coelomic, celomic,** *adj.*

**coelosomy** /sē'ləsō'mē/ [Gk, *koilos* + *soma,* body], a congenital anomaly characterized by protrusion of the viscera from the body cavity.

**coenesthesia, coenesthesis, coenogenesis.** See **cenesthesia.**

**coenogenetic.** See **cenogenesis.**

**coenzyme** /kō·en'zīm/ [L, *cum,* together with, *en,* in, *zyme,* ferment], a nonprotein substance that combines with an apoenzyme to form a complete enzyme or holoenzyme. Coenzymes include some of the vitamins, such as $B_1$ and $B_2$, and have smaller molecules than enzymes. Coenzymes are dialyzable and heat-stable and usually dissociate readily from the protein portions of the enzymes with which they combine. See also **acetylcoenzyme A.**

**coenzyme A (CoA)** [L, *cum* + *en,* into, *zyme,* ferment], an important metabolite in the citric acid cycle. Although not a true enzyme, it plays a significant role in the transfer of acetyl groups and the metabolism of acids and amino acids.

**coenzyme Q (CoQ),** a designation for quinones with polymer side chains that mediate electron transfer between cytochrome beta and cytochrome c. It is chemically similar to tocopherols, including vitamin E.

**coffee** [Ar, *qahwah*], the dried and roasted ripe seeds of *Coffea arabica, C. liberica,* and *C. robusta* trees that may have originated in Africa and now grow in almost all tropical areas. Coffee contains the alkaloid caffeine and is the basis for a stimulating drink that has been used in treating the common headache, chronic asthma, and narcotic poisoning.

**coffee-ground vomitus,** dark brown vomitus the color and consistency of coffee grounds, composed of gastric juices and old blood and indicative of slow upper GI bleeding. Compare **hematemesis.**

**Coffin-Lowry syndrome** /kof'in lou'rē/ [Grange S. Coffin, American pediatrician, b. 1923; R. Brian Lowry, Irish-born Canadian physician, 20th century], a condition with onset in the postnatal period characterized by incapability of speech, severe mental deficiency, and muscle, ligament, and skeletal abnormalities; it is transmitted with X-linked intermediate inheritance.

**Coffin-Siris syndrome** /kof'in sir'is/ [G.S. Coffin; Evelyn Siris, American radiologist, 1914–1987], hypoplasia or absence of the fifth fingers and toenails associated with growth and mental deficiencies, coarse facies, mild microcephaly, hypotonia, lax joints, mild hirsutism, and occasionally cardiac, vertebral, or GI anomalies.

**Cogan's oculomotor apraxia** /kō'gənz/ [David Glendenning Cogan, American ophthalmologist, 1908–1993], an absence or defect of horizontal eye movements, so that when the patient tries to look at an object off to one side, the head must turn to bring the eyes into line with the object and the eyes exhibit nystagmus; the cause is probably a brain lesion. Also called **Cogan's syndrome.**

**Cogentin,** trademark for an antiparkinsonian (benztropine mesylate).

**Cognex,** trademark for cognition enhancer, and analeptic (tacrine). It is a reversible cholinesterase inhibitor. It may have a role in early Alzheimer's disease to improve some cognitive functions. It does not affect the prognosis of the disease.

**cognition** /kognish'ən/ [L, *cognoscere,* to know], the mental process characterized by knowing, thinking, learning, understanding, and judging. Compare **conation.** *cognitive, adj.*

**cognitive** /kog'nitiv/, pertaining to the mental processes of comprehension, judgment, memory, and reasoning, as contrasted with emotional and volitional processes.

**cognitive ability,** a nursing outcome from the Nursing Outcome Classification (NOC) defined as ability to execute complex mental processes. See also **nursing outcomes classification.**

**cognitive development,** the developmental process by which an infant becomes an intelligent person, acquiring knowledge with growth and improving his or her ability to think, learn, reason, and abstract. Jean Piaget demonstrated the orderly sequence of this process from early infancy through childhood. See also **psychosexual development, psychosocial development.**

**cognitive dissonance** [L, *cognoscere,* to know, *dis,* opposite of, *sonare,* to sound], a state of tension resulting from a discrepancy in a person's emotional and intellectual frame of reference for interpreting and coping with his or her environment. It usually occurs when new information contradicts existing assumptions or knowledge.

**cognitive function,** an intellectual process by which one becomes aware of, perceives, or comprehends ideas. It involves all aspects of perception, thinking, reasoning, and remembering. Compare **conation.**

**cognitive learning,** **1.** learning that is concerned with acquisition of problem-solving abilities and with intelligence and conscious thought. **2.** a theory that defines learning as a behavioral change based on the acquisition of information about the environment.

**cognitive orientation,** a nursing outcome from the Nursing Outcome Classification (NOC) defined as ability to identify person, place, and time. See also **nursing outcomes classification.**

**cognitive psychology,** the study of the development of thought, language, and intelligence in infants and children.

**cognitive restoration,** an intervention technique designed to restore cognitive functioning.

**cognitive restructuring**[1], a change in attitudes, values, or beliefs that alters a person's self-expression; it occurs as a result of insight or behavioral achievement.

**cognitive restructuring**[2], a nursing intervention from the Nursing Interventions Classification (NIC) defined as challenging a patient to alter distorted thought patterns and view self and the world more realistically. See also **Nursing Interventions Classification.**

**cognitive stimulation,** a nursing intervention from the Nursing Interventions Classification (NIC) defined as promotion of awareness and comprehension of surroundings by utilization of planned stimuli. See also **Nursing Interventions Classification.**

**cognitive structuring,** the process of reviewing with a patient the changes that have occurred in his or her thinking in order to instill a sense of change, and of his or her role in bringing about that change.

**cognitive therapy,** any of the various methods of treating mental and emotional disorders that help a person change attitudes, perceptions, and patterns of thinking, from rational to realistic thoughts about self and situations. Therapeutic approaches include behavior therapy, existential therapy, Gestalt therapy, and transactional analysis.

**cogwheel respiration,** a breathing pattern characterized by a repeated series of brief interruptions of inhalation and exhalation.

**cogwheel rigidity** [ME, *cugge,* tooth on a gear; AS, *hweol* + L, *rigiditas,* unbending], an abnormal rigor in muscle tissue, characterized by jerky movements when the muscle is passively stretched. The condition is often found in cases of Parkinson's disease.

**cohabitate** /kōhab′itāt/, to live together in a relationship when not married.

**cohere** /kōhir′/ [L, *cohaerere,* to cling together], to stick together, as similar molecules of a common substance.

**coherence** /kōhir′əns/, **1.** the property of sticking together, as the molecules within a common substance. **2.** (in psychology) the logical pattern of expression and thought evident in the speech of a normal, stable individual. —**coherent,** *adj.*

**cohesive bandage** /kōhē′siv/, a dressing material that will adhere to itself but not to other surfaces.

**cohesiveness** /kōhē′sivnəs/ [L, *cohaerere,* to cling together], **1.** (in psychiatry) a force that attracts members to a group and causes them to remain in it. **2.** (in dentistry) a property of annealed pure gold that allows it to be used as a filling material.

**cohesive terminus,** a single-stranded end projecting from a double-stranded DNA segment that can be joined by molecular genetic techniques to an introduced DNA fragment. Also called **sticky end.**

**COHN,** abbreviation for *Certified Occupational Health Nurse.*

**cohort** /kō′hôrt/ [L, *cohortem,* large group], (in statistics) a collection or sampling of individuals who share a common characteristic, such as members of the same age or the same sex.

**cohort study,** (in research) a study concerning a specific subpopulation, such as the children born between December and May in 1975 and those born in the same months in 1955. See also **prospective study.**

**coil.** See **intrauterine device.**

**coiled tubular gland** [L, *colligere,* to gather together, *tubulus,* small tube, *glans,* acorn], one of the many multicellular glands that contain a coiled, tube-shaped secretory portion, such as the sweat glands.

**coil spring contraceptive diaphragm,** a kind of contraceptive diaphragm in which the flexible metal spring that forms the rim is a coiled, circular spring. The rubber dome of the diaphragm is approximately 3.8 cm deep, and the diameter of the rubber-covered rim is from 55 to 100 mm. Seven sizes, in increments of 0.5 cm, allow the clinician to fit the diaphragm to the individual woman. This kind of diaphragm is prescribed for a woman whose vaginal musculature offers good support, whose uterus is not acutely retroflexed or anteflexed, and whose vagina, neither very long nor very short, has a deeper than usual arch behind the symphysis pubis.

**coincidence counting** /kō·in′sidəns/ [L, *coincidere,* to occur together], the detection of two photons that arrive at separate counters simultaneously as the result of annihilation of a positron (created during a radioactive decay) and an electron. Coincidence counting greatly reduces the significance of any background radiation in radiography.

**coinnervation.** See **cocontraction.**

**coital headache** /kō′itəl/, an uncommon type of headache, mainly affecting men, that begins during or immediately after coitus. The complaint may last for several minutes to several hours.

**coitus** /kō′itəs/ [L, *coire,* to come together], the sexual union of two people of opposite sex in which the penis is introduced into the vagina, typically resulting in mutual excitation and usually orgasm. Also called **coition, copulation, sexual intercourse.** —**coital,** *adj.*

**coitus interruptus.** See **withdrawal method.**

**col-, colo-, colon-, colonic-,** combining form meaning 'colon': *colocolic, colodyspepsia, cololysis.*

**Colace,** trademark for a stool softener (docusate sodium sulfosuccinate).

**colation** /kōlā′shən/ [L, *colare,* to strain], the act of filtering or straining, as urine is often strained for medical examination.

**COL bed.** See **CircOlectric (COL) bed.**

**ColBENEMID,** trademark for an antigout medication (probenecid-colchicine combination product).

**colchicine** /kol′chəsēn/ [Gk, *kolchikon*], a gout suppressant.

■ INDICATIONS: It may be prescribed in the treatment of acute gout and prophylaxis of recurrent gouty arthritis.

■ CONTRAINDICATIONS: Ulcer, ulcerative colitis, or known hypersensitivity to this drug prohibits its use. The drug is highly toxic and is not given to elderly, debilitated patients or to those people who have chronic renal, hepatic, cardiovascular, or GI disease.

■ ADVERSE EFFECTS: Among the most serious adverse reactions are severe GI distress including diarrhea with blood, bone marrow depression, peripheral neuritis, liver dysfunction, and alopecia. It is in pregnancy category D.

**cold** [AS, *kald*], **1.** the absence of heat. **2.** a contagious viral infection of the upper respiratory tract, usually caused by a strain of rhinovirus. It is characterized by rhinitis, tearing, low-grade fever, and malaise and is treated symptomatically with rest, mild analgesia, decongestants, and increased fluid intake. Also called **common cold. 3.** a distant method of relating; not friendly.

**COLD** /kōld/, abbreviation for **chronic obstructive lung disease.** See **chronic obstructive pulmonary disease.**

**cold abscess,** a site of infection that does not show common signs of heat, redness, and swelling.

**cold agglutinin,** a nonspecific antibody, found on the surface of red blood cells in certain diseases, that may cause clumping of the cells at temperatures below 36° C and may cause hemolysis. The phenomenon does not occur at body temperature. Mycoplasma pneumonia, infectious mononucleosis, and many lymphoproliferative disorders are associated with cold agglutinins.

**cold agglutinin disease** [AS, *kald* + L, *agglutinare,* to glue, *dis,* without; Fr, *aise,* ease], a disorder characterized by circulating antibodies that can agglutinate red cells at less than normal body temperatures. They occur in the sera of patients with atypical pneumonia and blood diseases, particularly hemolytic anemia. The disease also tends to affect elderly patients.

**cold bath,** a bath in which the water temperature is approximately 50° F (10° C) to 65° F (18° C), used primarily to reduce body temperature.

**cold-blooded,** unable to regulate body heat, as fishes, reptiles, and amphibians, which have internal temperatures that are close to the temperatures of the environments in which they live. Also called **poikilothermic.** Compare **warm-blooded.**

**cold caloric irrigation,** a procedure for testing the integrity of brainstem function. It is carried out by irrigating the external auditory canal of the patient with a cold saline solution while the head is flexed at approximately 30 degrees, after checking the patency of the ear canal. The stimulus results in jerky but regular eye movements (nystagmus) in a normal patient. Absence of the reaction may be a sign of a lesion at the pontine level of the brainstem.

**cold cautery.** See **cryocautery.**

**cold compress** [AS, *kald* + L, *comprimere,* to press together], a pad of damp, thickly folded, soft absorbent cloth, dipped into cold water, wrung out, and applied to a body part for the relief of pain or reduction of inflammation or as a comfort measure.

**cold-curing resin.** See **self-curing resin.**

**cold environment,** a human environment arbitrarily designated as one in which the temperature is below 10° C (50° F). Nearly two thirds of the world population, including most of North America, Europe, and Asia north of the Indian subcontinent, lives in a naturally cold environment for at least a part of each year. The human body generally begins to experience some functional impairment when unprotected in temperatures below 15° C (59° F). The hands and fingers lose sensitivity, and the risk of errors and accidents increases. The body's hemostatic mechanism reacts with vasoconstriction, reducing heat loss to the environment but cooling the skin with a resultant chilling of the extremities. When vasoconstriction no longer eases the thermal strain between the skin and the environment, muscular hypertonus and shivering become mechanisms for maintaining body temperature.

**cold hemoglobinuria.** See **hemoglobinuria.**

**cold injury,** any of several abnormal and often serious physical conditions caused by exposure to cold temperatures. See also **chilblain, frostbite, hypothermia, immersion foot.**

**cold pack** [AS, *kald;* ME, *pakke*], a method of lowering body temperature by wrapping the patient in a blanket or sheet that has been dipped into cold water and wrung out. It is generally no longer done.

**cold-pressor test,** a test for the tendency to develop essential hypertension. One hand of the individual is immersed in ice water for about 60 seconds. An excessive rise in the blood pressure or an unusual delay in the return of normal blood pressure when the hand is removed from the water is believed to indicate that the individual is at risk for hypertension.

**cold-sensitive mutation,** a genetic alteration resulting in a gene that functions only at high temperature.

**cold sore.** See **herpes simplex.**

**cold stress.** See **hypothermia.**

**cold ulcer,** a small gangrenous ulceration on an extremity caused by poor circulation.

**cold urticaria** [AS, *kald* + L, *urtica,* nettle], wheals caused by exposure to cold temperatures.

**cold-wet-sheet pack,** a form of somatic therapy for agitated patients. The patient is swathed in cold, wet sheets, which are then warmed by body heat. The warmth and immobilization are reported to be soothing to very agitated patients.

**colectomy** /kəlek′təmē/ [Gk, *kolon,* colon, *ektomē,* excision], surgical excision of part or all of the colon, performed to treat cancer of the colon, diverticulitis, or severe chronic ulcerative colitis. For several days before surgery a low-residue diet is prescribed. Antibiotics and bowel-cleansing enemas methods are given to reduce the number of bacteria in the bowel. Parenteral fluids and electrolytes are given, and a nasogastric tube is passed. The nurse gives postoperative care as for any abdominal surgery. The nasogastric tube is connected to suction and remains in place until bowel sounds are heard. See **abdominal surgery.**

**coleotomy** /kō′lē·ot′əmē/, a surgical incision into the pericardium or the vagina.

**Colestid,** trademark for an antihyperlipoproteinemic (colestipol hydrochloride).

**colestipol hydrochloride** /kōles′tipol/, an antihyperlipoproteinemic that acts by sequestering bile acids in the intestine, thus reducing plasma levels of cholesterol.

■ INDICATIONS: It is prescribed in the treatment of hypercholesterolemia and xanthoma.

■ CONTRAINDICATIONS: Biliary obstruction or known hypersensitivity to this drug prohibits its use.

■ ADVERSE EFFECTS: Among the more serious adverse reactions are skin rash, fecal impaction, and a deficiency of vitamins A, D, and K.

**colic** /kol′ik/ [Gk, *kolikos,* colon pain], **1.** sharp visceral pain resulting from torsion, obstruction, or smooth muscle spasm of a hollow or tubular organ, such as a ureter or the intestines. Kinds of colic include **biliary colic, infantile colic,** and **renal colic. 2.** pertaining to the colon. —**colicky,** *adj.*

**colicinogen** /kol′isin′əjən/ [(E.) *coli* + L, *caedere,* to kill; Gk, *genein,* to produce], an extrachromosomal segment of DNA in some strains of *Escherichia coli* that induces secretion of a colicin, a protein lethal to other strains of the bacterium. Colicins attach to specific receptors on the cell membrane and impair the synthesis of macromolecules or the production of energy. Also called **colicinogenic factor.**

**colicky.** See **colic.**

**coliform** /kol′ifôrm/ [(E.) *coli* + L, *forma,* form], **1.** pertaining to the colon-aerogenes group, or the *Escherichia coli* species of microorganisms, which comprises most of the intestinal flora in humans and other animals. **2.** having the characteristic of a sieve or cribriform structure, such as some of the porous bones of the skull.

**colistimethate sodium** /kō′listim′əthāt/, an antibiotic. Also called **colistin sulfomethate sodium.**

■ INDICATIONS: It is prescribed in the treatment of GI infections caused by certain gram-negative microorganisms and as a topical medication.

■ CONTRAINDICATIONS: Known hypersensitivity to this drug or to polymyxin B prohibits its use.

■ ADVERSE EFFECTS: Among the more serious adverse reactions are nephrotoxicity and neurotoxicity, including neuromuscular blockade.

**colistin sulfate** /kōlis′tin/, an antibacterial and steroid agent.

■ INDICATIONS: It is prescribed topically in the treatment of infections of the outer ear and systemically for the treatment of serious gram-negative infections and gastroenteritis caused by *Escherichia coli* infections.

■ CONTRAINDICATION: Known hypersensitivity to this drug prohibits its use.

■ ADVERSE EFFECTS: Among the more serious systemic reactions are respiratory arrest, renal toxicity, and neuromuscular blockade.

**colistin sulfomethate sodium.** See **colistimethate sodium.**

**colitis** /kōlī′tis/, an inflammatory condition of the large intestine. Inflammatory bowel disease is characterized by severe diarrhea, bleeding, and ulceration of the mucosa of the intestine. Weight loss and pain are significant. Steroids, fluids, electrolytes, antibiotics, and careful attention to diet are the usual modes of therapy. Most of the diseases of this group are of unknown origin. Kinds of inflammatory bowel disease include **Crohn's disease** and **ulcerative colitis.** —**colitic,** *adj.*

**collaborative power structure** /kəlab′ərativ′/, an arrangement whereby adult members of a functional family make major decisions and are in agreement about power distribution.

**collagen** /kol'əjən/ [Gk, *kolla,* glue, *genein,* to produce], a fibrous insoluble protein consisting of bundles of tiny reticular fibrils that combine to form the white glistening inelastic fibers of the tendons, the ligaments, and the fascia. It is found in connective tissue, including skin, bone, ligaments, and cartilage. It represents 30% of total body protein. —**collagenous,** *adj.*

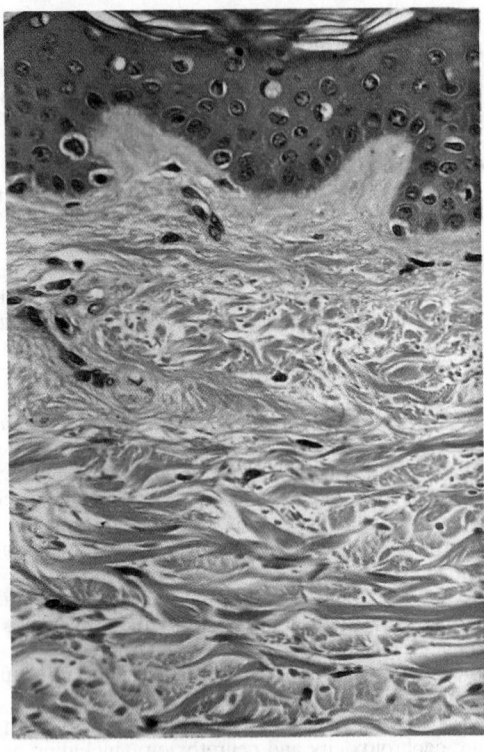

**Collagen** *(du Vivier, 1993)*

**collagenase ointment** /kəlaj'ənās/, a medication used in the treatment of decubitus ulcers, burns, and other epidermal lesions. It is an enzyme preparation derived from the fermentation of *Clostridium histolyticum.*

**collagen disease,** an abnormal condition characterized by extensive disruption of the connective tissue, often involving inflammation and fibrinoid degeneration. Collagen diseases include polyarteritis nodosa, systemic lupus erythematosus, osteoarthritis, and rheumatoid arthritis. See also **collagen vascular disease.**

**collagen injection,** a reconstructive technique in cosmetic surgery to enhance the lips or fatten sunken facial skin.

**collagenoblast** /kəlaj'ənōblast'/ [Gk, *kolla* + *genein* + *blastos,* germ], a cell that differentiates from a fibroblast and functions in the formation of collagen. It can also transform into cartilage and bone tissue by metaplasia.

**collagenous.** See **collagen.**

**collagenous colitis** /kə·laj·ə·nəs ko·lī'tis /, a type of colitis of unknown cause, characterized by deposits of collagenous material beneath the epithelium of the colon, with crampy abdominal pain and marked reduction in fluid and electrolyte absorption, leading to watery diarrhea; there is no mucosal ulceration.

**collagenous fiber** /kəlaj'ənəs/, any one of the tough, white protein fibers that constitute much of the intercellular substance and the connective tissue of the body. Collagenous fibers contain collagen; they are often arranged in bundles that strengthen the tissues in which they are imbedded.

**collagen shield,** a material derived from porcine scleral tissue, used in promotion of corneal healing. The shield enhances the penetration and effective time of subconjunctival antibiotics and corticosteroids. The collagen shield is designed to dissolve within 12 hours.

**collagen vascular disease,** any of a group of acquired disorders that have in common diffuse immunologic and inflammatory changes in small blood vessels and connective tissue. Common features include arthritis, skin lesions, iritis and episcleritis, pericarditis, pleuritis, subcutaneous nodules, myocarditis, vasculitis, and nephritis. Often associated are also Coombs' test–positive hemolytic anemia, thrombocytopenia, leukopenia, B and T cell abnormalities, antinuclear antibodies, cryoglobulins, rheumatoid factors, false-positive serologic test results for syphilis, alterations in serum complement, and immunologic abnormalities. The diseases usually included in this category are mixed connective tissue disease, necrotizing vasculitis, and other vasculopathies; polymyositis; relapsing polychondritis; rheumatic fever; rheumatoid arthritis; scleroderma; and systemic lupus erythematosus. The cause of most of these diseases is unknown. Hereditary factors and deficiencies, autoimmunity, environmental antigens, infections, allergies, and antigen-antibody complexes in various combinations are probably involved. Also called **connective tissue disease.**

**collapse** /kəlaps'/ [L, *collabi,* to fall], **1.** *nontechnical.* a state of extreme depression or a condition of complete exhaustion caused by physical or psychosomatic problems. **2.** an abnormal condition characterized by shock. **3.** the abnormal sagging of an organ or the obliteration of its cavity.

**collapse of the lung** [L, *collabi,* to fall together; AS, *lungen*], a reduction in the volume of a lung. The condition results from increased intrapleural pressure caused by accumulation of air or fluid in the pleural cavity or from a loss of internal pressure and elastic recoil of the lung. See also **atelectasis, hemothorax, pneumothorax.**

**collapsing pulse.** See **Corrigan's pulse.**

**collar** [L, *collum,* neck], any structure that encircles another, usually around its neck, such as the periosteal bone collars that form around the diaphyses of young bones.

**collarbone.** See **clavicle.**

**collateral** /kōlat'ərəl/ [L, *cum,* together with, *lateralis,* side], **1.** secondary or accessory. **2.** (in anatomy) a small branch, such as any one of the arterioles or venules in the body.

**collateral circulation** [L, *cum* + *latus,* side, *circulare,* to go around], an accessory blood pathway developed through enlargement of secondary vessels after obstruction of a main channel.

**collateral fissure,** a fissure separating the subcalcarine and subcollateral gyri of the cerebral hemisphere.

**collateral innervation,** reinnervation of denervated neurons caused by sprouting of uninjured axons in the vicinity.

**collateral ligaments of interphalangeal joints of foot,** fibrous bands, one on either side of each of the interphalangeal joints of the toes.

**collateral ligaments of interphalangeal joints of hand,** massive fibrous bands on each side of the interphalangeal joints of the fingers; they are placed diagonally, the proximal ends being near the dorsal, and the distal ends near the palmar margins of the digits.

**collateral ligaments of metacarpophalangeal joints,**

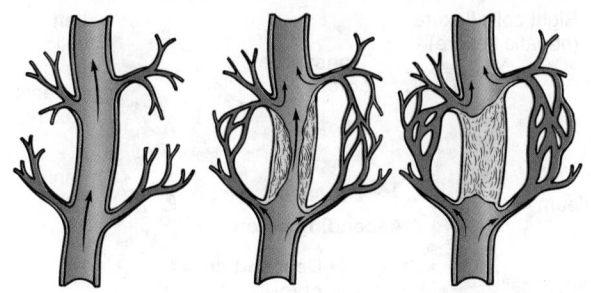

**Collateral circulation forming around a vessel occlusion**
*(Lewis, Heitkemper, and Dirksen, 2000)*

massive, strong fibrous bands on either side of each metacarpophalangeal joint, holding the two bones involved in each joint firmly together.

**collateral ligaments of metatarsophalangeal joints,** strong fibrous bands on either side of each metatarsophalangeal joint, holding the two bones involved in each joint firmly together.

**collateral pulp canal,** a branch of a tooth's pulp canal that emerges from the root at a place other than the apex. Also called **branching canal.** Compare **accessory root canal.**

**collateral ventilation,** the ventilation of alveoli in the lungs through indirect pathways, such as Kohn's pores in alveolar septa or anastomosing bronchioles.

**collateral vessel** [L, *cum* + *latus*, side, *vascellum*, small vase], a branch of an artery or vein used as an accessory to the blood vessel from which it arises.

**collecting tubule** [L, *colligere*, to gather, *tubulus*, small tube], any one of the many relatively straight tubules of the kidney that funnel urine into papillary ducts in the renal pelvis. The small collecting tubules play an important role in maintaining the fluid balance of the body by allowing water to osmose through their membranes into the interstitial fluid in the renal medulla. Antidiuretic hormone in the blood makes the collecting tubules permeable to water. If no antidiuretic hormone is present in the blood, membranes of the collecting tubules are practically impermeable to water. See **Bowman's capsule, kidney.**

**collective bargaining** /kəlek'tiv/, the use of collective action by employees in negotiating working conditions and economic issues with their employer.

**collective hysteria.** See **major hysteria.**

**collective unconscious** [L, *colligere*, to gather; AS, *un*, not; L, *conscious*, aware], (in analytic psychology) that portion of the unconscious common to all humans. Also called **racial unconscious.** See also **analytic psychology.**

**collector,** (in medicine) a device with various modifications, used for gathering secretions from the bronchi and esophagus for bacteriologic and cytologic examination.

**college** [L, *collegium*, society], 1. an institution of higher learning. 2. an organization of individuals with common professional training and interests, as the American College of Nurse-Midwives, the American College of Cardiology, or the American College of Surgeons.

**College of American Pathologists (CAP),** a national professional organization of physicians who specialize in pathology.

**Colles' fascia** /kol'ēz/ [Abraham Colles, Irish surgeon, 1773–1843; L, band], the deep inner layer of the subcutaneous, superficial fascia of the perineum, constituting a dis-

tinctive structure in the urogenital region of the body. It is a strong, smooth sheet of tissue containing elastic fibers that give it a characteristic yellow tint.

**Colles' fracture** [Abraham Colles], a break in the radius at the epiphysis within 1 inch of the joint of the wrist, which causes displacement of the hand to a dorsal and lateral position. Also called **silver-fork fracture.**

**colligative** /kol'igā'tiv/ [L, *colligere*, to gather], (in physical chemistry) pertaining to those properties of matter that depend on the concentration of particles, such as molecules and ions, rather than the chemical properties of any substance. One colligative property is the pressure of a specific volume of gas at a specific temperature. Colligative properties of solutions include boiling point, freezing point, vapor, pressure, and osmotic pressure.

**collimate** [L, *collineare*, to align], to make parallel.

**collimator** /kol'imā'tər/ [L, *collinare*, to bring into alignment], a device for limiting the size and shape of a radiation beam. It is used to reduce scatter radiation, thereby decreasing the patient dose needed and increasing radiographic quality.

**colliquation** /kol'ikwā'shən/ [L, *cum*, together with, *liquifacere*, to make liquid], 1. the degeneration of a body tissue to a liquid state, usually associated with necrotic tissue. 2. abnormal discharge of a body fluid.

**colliquative** /kol'ikwā'tiv/, characterized by a profuse fluid discharge as in suppurating wounds and body structures that are infected.

**collision tumor** /kəlizh'ən/ [L, *cum*, together with, *laedere*, to strike], a tumor formed as two separate growths, developing close to each other, join. See also **carcinoma.**

**collodion** /kəlō'dē·ən/ [Gk, *kolla*, glue, *eidos*, form], a clear or a slightly opaque, highly inflammable liquid composed of pyroxylin, ether, and alcohol. It dries to a strong, transparent film that is used as a surgical dressing.

**collodion baby,** an infant whose skin at birth is covered with a scaly, parchmentlike membrane. See also **harlequin fetus, lamellar exfoliation of the newborn.**

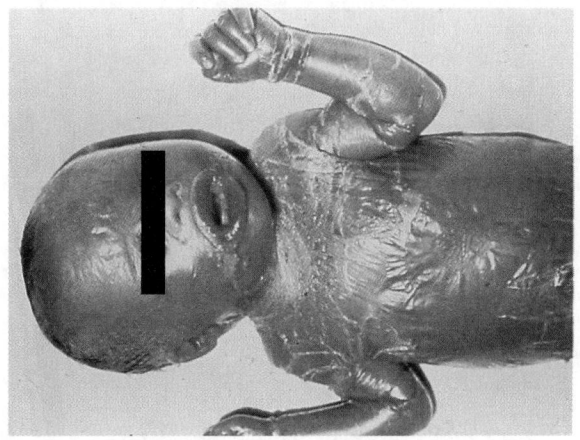

**Collodion baby** *(Zitelli and Davis, 1997)*

**colloid** /kol'oid/ [Gk, *kolla*, glue, *eidos*, form], a state or division of matter in which large molecules or aggregates of molecules (1 to 100 nm in size) do not precipitate and are dispersed in another medium. In a suspension colloid the particles are insoluble and the medium may be solid, liquid, or gas. In an emulsion colloid the particles are usually water, and the medium is any of several complex hydrophilic, organic substances that become evenly dispersed among the particles of water. Compare **solution, suspension.**

**colloidal solution** /koloi′dəl/ [Gk, *kolla,* glue, *eidos,* form; L, *solutus,* dissolved], a solution in which small particles, such as large polymeric molecules, are homogenously dispersed through a liquid medium. See also **colloid.**

**colloidal sulfur,** a form of very finely divided sulfur that is used in the treatment of acne and other skin disorders.

**colloid bath,** a bath taken in water that contains such substances as bran, gelatin, and starch, used to relieve irritation and inflammation. See also **emollient bath.**

**colloid chemistry,** the science dealing with the composition and nature of chemical colloids.

**colloid corpuscle,** a starchlike body. Also called **corpus amylaceum.** See also **amyloid.**

**colloid cyst** [Gk, *kolla,* glue, *eidos,* form, *kystis,* bag], **1.** a thyroid gland follicle distended with thyroid secretion. **2.** a cyst in the third ventricle, leading to hydrocephalus.

**colloid osmotic pressure.** See **oncotic pressure.**

**colloid substance,** a jellylike substance formed in the deterioration of the protoplasm of tissues.

**colloid suspension** [Gk, *kolla,* glue, *eidos,* form; L, *suspendere,* to hang], a system of solids dispersed in a liquid medium, with particles generally smaller than 100 nm.

**collum** /kol′əm/, the anatomic necklike structure between the head and shoulders.

**collyrium** /kolir′ē·əm/, an ophthalmic liquid containing medications to be instilled into the eye.

**coloboma** /kol′əbō′mə/, *pl.* **colobomas, colobomata** [Gk, *koloboma,* defect], a congenital or pathologic defect in the ocular tissue of the body, usually affecting the iris, ciliary body, or choroid by forming a cleft that extends inferiorly. Colobomas are usually the result of the failure of part of the fetal fissure to close. —**colobomatous,** *adj.*

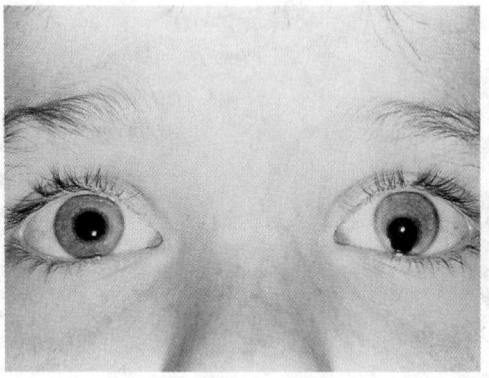

**Coloboma** *(Zitelli and Davis, 1997)*

**coloenteritis.** See **enterocolitis.**

**colon** /kō′lən/ [Gk, *kolon*], the portion of the large intestine extending from the cecum to the rectum. It has four segments: the ascending colon, transverse colon, descending colon, and sigmoid colon. —**colonic** /kəlon′ik/, *adj.*

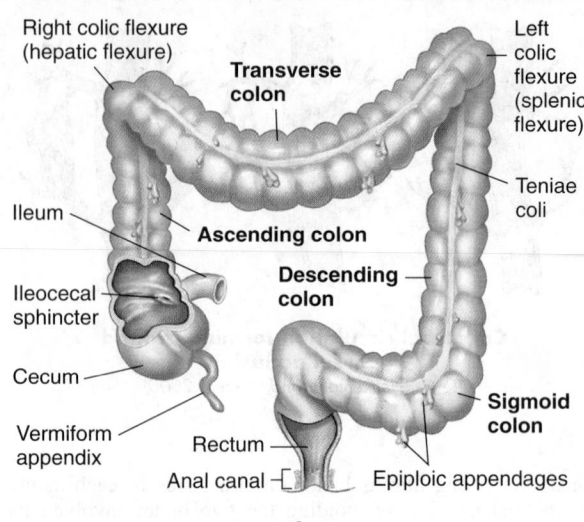

**Colon**

**colon-.** See **colo-.**

**-colon,** suffix meaning the 'part of the large intestine between the cecum and rectum': *cecocolon, megacolon, paracolon.*

**colonic.** See **colon.**

**-colonic** /kōlon′ik/, suffix meaning 'relating to the colon': *pericolonic, rectocolonic, vesicocolonic.*

**colonic fistula** [Gk, *kolon* + L, pipe], an abnormal passage from the colon to the surface of the body or an internal organ or structure. In regional enteritis chronic inflammation may lead to the formation of a fistula between two adjacent loops of bowel. An external opening from the colon to the surface of the abdomen may be created surgically after the removal of a malignant or severely ulcerated segment of the bowel. See also **colostomy.**

**colonic irrigation,** a procedure for washing the inner wall of the colon by filling it with water, then draining it. It is not considered an enema, but rather a technique for removing any material that may be present high in the colon.

**colonization** /kol′ənīzā′shən/, the presence and multiplication of microorganisms without tissue invasion or damage.

**colonoscope** /kō′lənōskōp′/ [Gk, *kolon* + *skopein,* to watch], a long, flexible endoscope, usually fiberoptic, that permits examination of the interior of the entire colon. See also **endoscope.**

**colonoscopy** /kō′lənos′kəpē/, the examination of the mucosal lining of the colon using a colonoscope, an elongated endoscope.

**colon stasis.** See **atonic constipation.**

**colony** /kol′ənē/ [L, *colonia*], **1.** (in bacteriology) a mass of microorganisms in a culture that originates from a single cell. Some kinds of colonies, according to different configurations, are smooth colonies, rough colonies, and dwarf colonies. **2.** (in cell biology) a mass of cells in a culture or in certain experimental tissues, such as a spleen colony.

**colony counter,** a device used for counting colonies of bacteria growing in a culture. It usually consists of an illuminated, transparent plate divided into sections of known area. Petri dishes containing colonies of bacteria are placed over the plate, and the colonies are counted according to the number within the areas viewed.

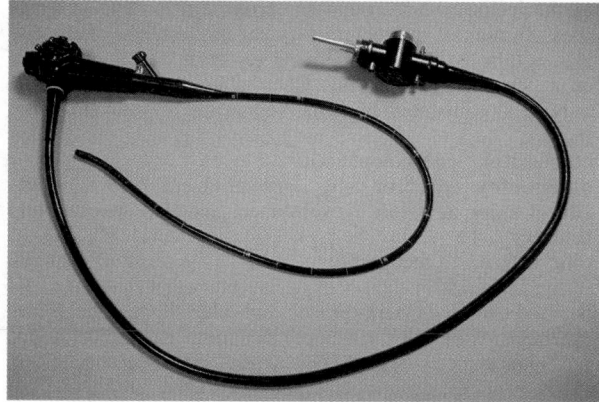

**Fiberoptic flexible colonoscope** *(Zakus, 1995)*

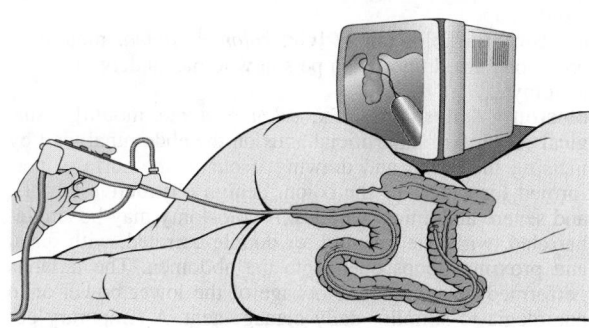

**Colonoscopy** *(Chabner, 2001)*

**colony-stimulating factor (CSF),** a growth factor that allows cells to pass a restriction point in their reproductive cycle. It is no longer needed after cells have entered the DNA synthesis phase.

**coloproctectomy** /kō′ləproktek′təmē/, surgical removal of the colon and rectum.

**coloproctitis** /kō′ləpraktī′tis/, an inflammation of both the colon and rectum. Also called **colorectitis, rectocolitis.**

**coloptosis** /kō′lōptō′sis/ [Gk, *kolon* + *ptosis,* fall], the prolapse or downward displacement of the colon.

**-color,** combining form meaning 'hue or hues': *cuticolor, tricolor, versicolor.*

**Colorado tick fever,** a relatively mild, self-limited arbovirus infection transmitted to humans by the bite of a tick. It is most prevalent in the spring and summer months throughout the Rocky Mountains, particularly in Colorado. Symptoms, occurring in two phases separated by a period of remission, include chills, fever, and headache; pain in the eyes, legs, and back; and sensitivity to light. Treatment is supportive; analgesics can be given for headache and other pains. Also called **American mountain fever, mountain fever, mountain tick fever.** Compare **Rocky Mountain spotted fever.**

**color blindness** [L, color; AS *blint*], an abnormal condition characterized by an inability to distinguish colors of the spectrum clearly. In most cases it is not a blindness but a weakness in perceiving colors distinctly. There are two forms of color blindness: **Daltonism,** the more common form, is characterized by an inability to distinguish reds from greens. It is an inherited, sex-linked disorder. **Total color blindness,** or **achromatic vision,** is characterized by an inability to perceive any color at all. Only white, gray, and black are seen. It may be the result of a defect in or absence of the cones in the retina. Also spelled **colour blindness.**

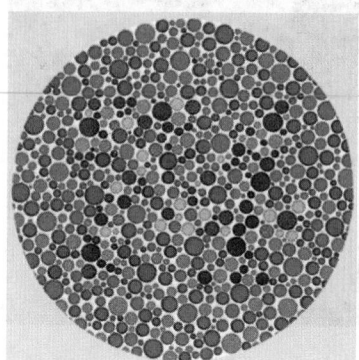

**Color blindness chart**
*(courtesy S. Ishihara; Washington University Dept. of Ophthalmology)*

**color dysnomia** /disnō′mē·ə/ [L, color; Gk, *dys,* difficult, *onoma,* name], an inability to name colors despite an ability to match and distinguish them. It may be caused by expressive dysphasia.

**colorectal** /kō′lō·rek′təl/ [Gk, *kolon,* colon + L, *rectus,* straight], pertaining to or affecting the colon and rectum.

**colorectal cancer** /kō′lərek′təl/ [Gk, *kolon,* colon; L, *rectus,* straight], a malignant neoplastic disease of the large intestine, characterized by a change in bowel habits and the passing of blood (melena) which may be occult initially. Malignant tumors of the large bowel usually occur after 50 years of age, are slightly more frequent in women than in men, and are common in the Western world. They are rare in children; clustering in families is common. The risk of large bowel cancer is increased in patients with chronic ulcerative colitis, villous adenomas, and especially familial adenomatous polyposis of the colon. People who have a high-fat diet, a high consumption of alcohol, and low activity levels; those who smoke tobacco; and those who have inhaled asbestos fibers or who have been irradiated are more likely than others to have colorectal cancer. In the vermiform appendix carcinoid is the most common tumor. Most lesions of the large bowel are moderately differentiated adenocarcinomas. These tumors have a long preinvasive stage, and, when they invade, they tend to grow slowly. Rectal tumors may cause pain, bleeding, and a feeling of incomplete evacuation; they may metastasize slowly through lymphatic channels and veins and occasionally prolapse through the anus. Typical napkin ring tumors in the sigmoid and descending colon grow circumferentially and constrict the intestinal lumen, causing partial obstruction and production of flat or pencil-shaped stools. Manifestations include progressive abdominal distension, pain, vomiting, constipation, cramps, and bright red blood on the stool's surface. Malignant lesions in the ascending colon are usually large growths that may be palpable on physical examination; they generally cause severe anemia, nausea, and alternating constipation

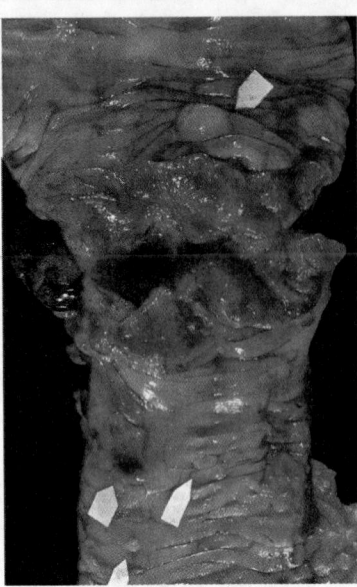

**Colorectal cancer** *(Kumar, Cotran, and Robbins, 1997)*

of the lesion, the surrounding colon, and the attached tissues. Tumors of the rectum may require removal of the entire rectum by abdominoperineal resection and the creation of a permanent colostomy. Chemotherapy and irradiation may be administered as palliative therapy or adjuvant treatment.

**colorectitis.** See **coloproctitis.**

**colorimetry** /kol′ərim′ətrē/, measurement of the intensity of color in a fluid or substance. See also **spectrophotometry.**

**color vision,** a recognition of color as the result of changes in the pigments of the cones in the retina that react to varying intensities of red, green, and blue light. The exact mechanisms of color vision are not completely understood, but some experts believe they depend on three specialized types of cones, each type responding to red, green, or blue light. Some retinal cones respond to the entire visual spectrum. See also **color blindness.**

**colosigmoidoscopy** /kō′ləsig′moidos′kəpē/ [Gk, *kolon* + *sigma,* S-shaped, *eidos,* form, *skopein,* to look], the direct examination of the sigmoid portion of the colon with a sigmoidoscope.

**colostomate** /kəlos′təmāt/ [Gk, *kolon* + *stoma,* mouth; L, *atum,* one acted upon], a person who has undergone a colostomy.

**colostomy** /kəlos′təmē/ [Gk, *kolon* + *stoma,* mouth], surgical creation of an artificial anus on the abdominal wall by incising the colon and drawing it out to the surface, performed for cancer of the colon, benign obstructive tumors, and severe abdominal wounds. A colostomy may be single-barreled, with one opening, or double-barreled, with distal and proximal loops open onto the abdomen. The latter is performed for complete blockage of the lower bowel or in paraplegia to simplify daily management. A temporary colostomy may be done to divert feces after surgery, as in the

and diarrhea. There may be dark red or mahogany-colored blood mixed with the stool. The diagnosis of colorectal cancer is based on digital rectal examination, testing for blood in the stool, proctosigmoidoscopic examination of the sigmoid, and x-ray studies of the GI tract. Suspicious polyps may be removed for histologic study, often through a sigmoidoscope or colonoscope or by laparotomy. Surgical treatment of colorectal cancer may involve a wide resection

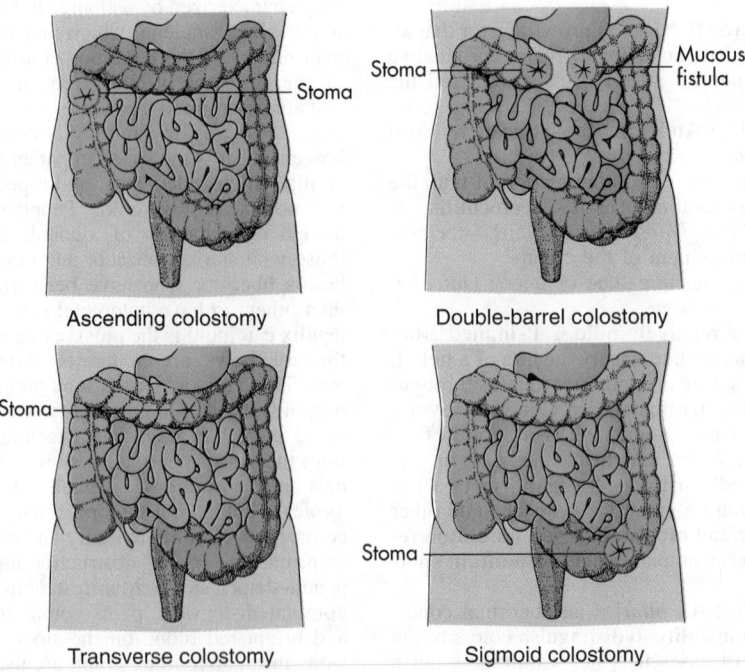

**Types of colostomies** *(Beare and Myers, 1998)*

repair of Hirschsprung's disease, or from an inflamed area; it is repaired when the colon has healed or the inflammation subsides. Preoperative nursing care focuses on teaching the patient what to expect after surgery. A high-calorie, clear liquid diet is given. An antibiotic, usually neomycin, is prescribed to reduce the bacterial count in the bowel, and bowel-cleansing methods are used. Immediate postoperative care is the same as for abdominal surgery. The color of the stoma is checked: a dark blue-black (rather than bright red) indicates a circulation block, and the surgeon is notified. If needed, saline irrigations are begun on the fourth or fifth day. A type of colostomy is **loop colostomy.** Compare **enterostomy.**

**colostomy irrigation,** a procedure used by colostomates to clear the bowel of fecal matter and to help establish an evacuation schedule.

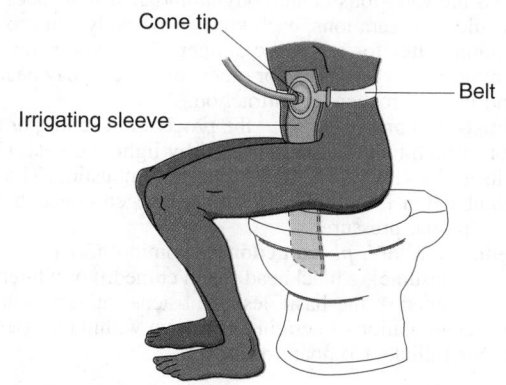

**Colostomy irrigation** *(Phipps, Sands, and Marek, 1999)*

■ METHOD: Daily irrigation may be ordered beginning 7 to 10 days after the surgery, and the patient is involved in assisting in the procedure as soon as possible. In preparation for self-care the technique is explained in a step-by-step manner, and irrigation is carried out with the equipment the patient will use at home. In the hospital the procedure is performed as the patient sits in bed in a semi- or high-Fowler's position or on a commode, if ambulatory; at home the individual will probably find a toilet more convenient. A flexible catheter, lubricated with water-soluble lubricant, is gently inserted into the stoma to a depth of no more than 3 inches; the catheter tip is advanced only as far as it will go easily and is never forced. A cone tip on the tubing controls the depth of insertion and prevents water from coming out of the stoma. An irrigating bag containing 500 to 1000 ml of warm solution is held 12 to 18 inches above the stoma, and the fluid is allowed to flow slowly into the colon. If the patient complains of cramps, the catheter is clamped for a few minutes before the flow is resumed. The fluid is retained for several minutes and then drained through outlet tubing into a basin or commode. From 30 to 45 minutes is allowed for draining; if the return is slow, the patient is asked to lean forward or move from side to side; the abdomen may be massaged. The character and amount of the return flow are noted. The peristomal skin is cleaned, rinsed, and dried well. A dehydrated patient may retain some fluid.

■ INTERVENTIONS: The nurse performs and teaches colostomy irrigation and ensures that the patient knows how to carry out the procedure correctly and where to purchase the necessary equipment. The person is urged to report any symptoms of obstruction or prolapse of the stoma. A home nurse is available in many areas for home visits if help is needed.

■ OUTCOME CRITERIA: Many colostomates establish a regular schedule of evacuation with irrigation; but the procedure may be unsatisfactory for those who have a liquid or semi-soft fecal stream, for patients who before the operation had a tendency to experience diarrhea under stress, or for patients with irregular bowel habits.

**colostrum** /kəlos′trəm/ [L, first milk after birth], the fluid secreted by the breast during pregnancy and the first days after the delivery before lactation begins. It consists of immunologically active substances (maternal antibodies) and white blood cells, water, protein, fat, minerals, vitamins, and carbohydrate in a thin, yellow serous fluid.

**colotomy** /kōlot′əmē/, a surgical incision into the colon, usually performed through the abdominal wall.

**colour blindness.** See **color blindness.**

**Colour Index (C.I.),** a publication of dyers, colorists, and textile chemists that specifies all the standard industrial pigments and stains according to five-digit numbers associated with chemical coloring materials. For example, methylene blue is assigned number 52015.

**colovaginal** /kō′lōvaj′inəl/ [Gk, *kolon*, colon; L, *vagina*, sheath], pertaining to the colon and vagina, or to a communication between the two structures.

**colp-.** See **colpo-.**

**colpalgia** /kolpal′jə/, a pain in the vagina.

**colpectomy** /kolpek′təmē/, the surgical excision of the vagina.

**colpitis** /kolpī′tis/, an inflammation of the vagina.

**colpo-, colp-, kolpo-, kysth-, kystho-,** combining form meaning 'vagina': *colpocele, colpocystitis, colpodynia.*

**colpocystitis** /kol′pōsistī′tis/, an inflammation of the vagina and urinary bladder.

**colpocystocele** /kol′pəsis′təsēl/, the prolapse of the urinary bladder into the vagina, usually through the anterior vaginal wall.

**colpohysterectomy** /-his′tərek′təmē/ [Gk, *kolpos*, vagina, *hystera*, womb, *ektomē*, excision], vaginal hysterectomy. See also **hysterectomy.**

**colporrhaphy** /kolpôr′əfē/ [Gk, *kolpos* + *raphe*, suture], a surgical procedure in which the vagina is sutured to narrow it.

**colposcope** /kol′pəskōp/, a lighted instrument with lenses for direct examination of the surfaces of the vagina and cervix.

**colposcopy** /kolpos′kəpē/ [Gk, *kolpos* + *skopein*, to watch], an examination of the vagina and cervix with an optical magnifying instrument (colposcope). It is commonly performed after a Papanicolaou's (Pap) smear in the treatment of cervical dysplasia and in obtaining biopsy specimens of the cervix.

**colpotomy** /kolpot′əmē/ [Gk, *kolpos* + *temnein*, to cut], any surgical incision into the wall of the vagina.

**columbium,** former name for **niobium.**

**columella,** **1.** a small column. **2.** the fleshy terminal portion of the nasal septum.

**column,** any elongated, cylindrical anatomic structure. It is usually oriented vertically and may provide structural support.

**columna posterior.** See **posterior column.**

**columnar cell** /kəlum′nər/ [L, *columna*, column, *cella*, storeroom], an epithelial cell that appears long and narrow when sectioned along its long axis.

**columnar epithelium** [L, *columna,* column; Gk, *epi,* upon, *thele,* nipple], a type of epithelial cell that resembles a hexagonal prism.

**columnar layer** [L, *columna,* column; AS, *lecgan*], the layer of rods and cones in the retina.

**column chromatography** [L, *columna* + Gk, *chroma,* color, *graphein* to record], the process of separating and analyzing a group of substances according to the differences in their absorption affinities for a given absorbent as evidenced by pigments deposited during filtration through the same absorbent contained in a glass cylinder or tube. The substances are dissolved in a liquid that is passed through the absorbent. The absorbates move down the column at different rates and leave behind a band of pigments that is subsequently washed with a pure solvent to develop discrete pigmented bands that constitute a chromatograph. The cylinder of absorbent is then pushed from the tube, and the individual bands are either separated with a knife or further diluted with the pure solvent and collected in the bottom of the tube for analysis. Effective column chromatography depends on the selection of the appropriate absorbent and solvent and a flow rate that is slow enough to allow complete diffusion of the absorbates from the solvent to the absorbent and the retardation of the absorbates according to their different affinities for the absorbent. Compare **gas chromatography, ion exchange chromatography.**

**Coly-Mycin M,** trademark for a parenteral antibacterial (colistimethate sodium).

**Coly-Mycin S,** trademark for an otic steroid and antibiotic combination containing hydrocortisone, neomycin, and colistin.

**com-.** See **co-.**

**coma** /kō′mə/ [Gk, *koma,* deep sleep], a state of profound unconsciousness, characterized by the absence of spontaneous eye openings, response to painful stimuli, and vocalization. The person cannot be aroused. Coma may be the result of trauma, space-occupying brain tumor, hematoma, cerebral edema, toxic metabolic condition, acute infectious disease with encephalitis, vascular disease, or brain ischemia. See also **Glasgow Coma Scale, unconscious.**

**-coma,** **1.** suffix meaning '(condition of) profound unconsciousness': *narcoma, semicoma.* **2.** combining form meaning '(condition of) torpor': *agrypnocoma.*

**comatose** /kō′mətōs/, pertaining to a state of coma, or abnormally deep sleep, caused by illness or injury.

**combat fatigue** [L, *com,* together, *battuere,* to beat, *fatigare,* to tire], any of a variety of psychoneurotic disorders, usually temporary but sometimes permanent, resulting from exhaustion, the stress of combat, or the cumulative emotions and psychologic strain of warfare or similar situations. It is characterized by anxiety, depression, irritability, memory and sleep disorders, and various related symptoms. Also called **combat neurosis, war neurosis.** See also **posttraumatic stress disorder, shell shock.**

**combination chemotherapy** /kom′binā′shən/, the simultaneous use of two or more anticancer drugs.

**combined anesthesia.** See **balanced anesthesia.**

**combined carbon dioxide** [L, *com,* together, *bini,* twofold], the portion of the total carbon dioxide that is contained in blood carbonate; it can be calculated as the difference between the total and dissolved carbon dioxide.

**combined cycling ventilator,** a mechanical ventilator that has more than one mechanism to recycle gases, such as equipment that may have time cycling or pressure cycling as a backup to a volume cycling control device.

**combined modality treatment,** the use of chemotherapy in combination with surgery or irradiation or both in the treatment of cancer.

**combined oxygen,** the oxygen that is physically bound to hemoglobin as oxyhemoglobin ($HbO_2$). One grammolecular weight of oxygen can combine with 16,700 g of hemoglobin, and each gram of hemoglobin can bind with and carry 1.34 mL of oxygen.

**combined patterns,** a method of evaluating a patient's neuromuscular functions through tests that reveal the degree of coordination between movement patterns of the trunk and the extremities.

**combined system disease,** a disorder of the nervous system caused by a deficiency of vitamin $B_{12}$ that results in pernicious anemia and degeneration of the spinal cord and peripheral nerves, marked by increased difficulty in walking, a feeling of vibration in the legs, and a loss of sense of position. Also known as **subacute combined degeneration of the spinal cord.** See also **pernicious anemia, vitamin $B_{12}$.**

**combining sites,** **1.** concave features on antibody molecules that serve as locations for binding antigens. Because of possible variations in antibody amino acid sequences and molecule configurations, each kind of antibody can provide combining sites for a specific antigen. **2.** locations on protein molecules where drugs or other substances may become bound by electrochemical attraction.

**combustion** /kəmbus′chen/, the process of burning or oxidation, which may be accompanied by light and heat. Oxygen itself does not burn, but it supports combustion. The rate of combustion is influenced by both oxygen concentration and its partial pressure.

**comedo** /kom′idō/, *pl.* **comedones** /komidō′nēz/ [L, *comedere,* to consume], blackhead (open comedo) or whitehead (closed comedo), the basic lesion of acne vulgaris, caused by an accumulation of keratin and sebum within the opening of a hair follicle. Compare **milium.**

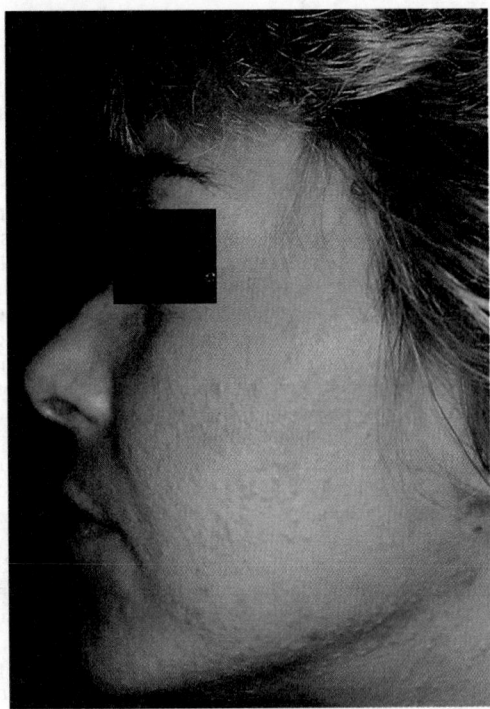

**Comedonal acne**
*(Goldstein and Goldstein, 1997/courtesy Department of Dermatology, Medical College of Georgia)*

**comedocarcinoma** /kom′idōkär′sinō′mə/, *pl.* **comedocarcinomas, comedocarcinomata** [L, *comedere,* to consume; Gk, *karkinos,* crab, *oma,* tumor], a malignant intraductal neoplasm of the breast, in which the central cells degenerate and may be easily expressed from the cut surface of the tumor. Growth confined in the mammary ducts carries a better prognosis than do invasive breast lesions.

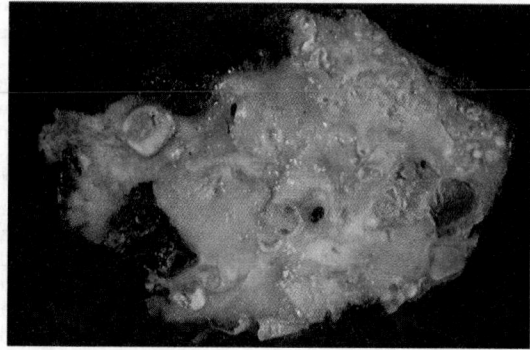

**Comedocarcinoma** *(Cotran, Kumar, and Collins, 1999)*

**comedogenicity** /kom′idōjənis′itē/, the ability of certain drugs or agents, such as anabolic steroids, to produce acne comedones.

**comedone.** See **comedo.**

**comfort level,** a nursing outcome from the Nursing Outcome Classification (NOC) defined as extent of physical and psychological ease. See also **nursing outcomes classification.**

**comfort measure** [L, *com,* together, *fortis,* strong], any action taken to promote the soothing of a patient, such as a back rub, a change in position, or the prewarming of a stethoscope or bedpan.

**comfort zone** [ME, *comforten* + Gk, *zone,* belt], the boundaries of temperature, humidity, wind velocity, and solar radiation within which a person dressed in a specified manner can perform certain tasks without discomfort. Also the psychologic feeling of belonging; being comfortable in a specific area and/or role.

**comfrey,** a perennial herb found in the United States, Australia, and parts of Asia, also cultivated in Japan.
- USES: This herb is used for bruises, sprains, broken bones, acne, and boils.
- CONTRAINDICATIONS: Use of comfrey is not recommended during pregnancy and lactation, in children, and in those with are hypersensitive to this product. Internal use may cause fatal hepatotoxicity. Do not use for more than 6 weeks per year. Do not use topically on broken skin.

**Comité International des Poids et Mesures (CIPM)** /kômitä′ aNternäsyōnäl′ dä pô·ä′ ā mesYr′/, a group of scientists who meet periodically to define the international (SI) units of physical quantities, as the volume of a liter, the length of a meter, or the precise amount of time in a minute. See also **SI units.**

**-comma,** combining form meaning a 'piece of a structure or to cut off a piece': *inocomma, myocomma, osteocomma.*

**command** [L, *commendare,* to protect], an order given to the computer to execute a specific instruction, as a code that evokes a particular program or performs a particular function.

**command automatism,** a condition characterized by an abnormal mechanical responsiveness to commands, usually followed without critical judgment, such as may be seen in hypnosis and certain psychotic states.

**command hallucination,** a condition in which individuals hear and obey voices that command them to perform certain acts. The hallucinations may influence them to engage in behavior that is dangerous to them or to others.

**commensal** /kəmen′səl/ [L, *com,* together, *imensa,* table], (two different species) living together in an arrangement that is not harmful to either and may be beneficial to both. Some bacteria in the digestive tract of humans aid in the processing of food and produce B vitamins needed for normal health while causing no harm (normal flora). Compare **parasite, synergist.**

**commensalism** /kəmen′səliz′əm/, a symbiosis in which one species benefits but the other species is neither helped nor harmed.

**comminuted** /kom′inyōō′tid/ [L, *comminuere,* to break into pieces], crushed or broken into a number of pieces.

**comminuted fracture,** a fracture in which the bone is broken in several places or is shattered, creating numerous fragments. Also called **comminution, fragmented fracture.**

**comminution.** See **comminuted fracture.**

**commissure** /kom′isŏŏr, -syŏŏr/, **1.** a band of nerve fiber or other tissue that crosses from one side of the body to the other, usually connecting two structures or masses of tissue. **2.** a site of union of two anatomic parts, as the corner of the eye, lips, or labia.

**commissurotomy** /kom′ishŏŏrot′əmē/ [L, *commissura,* a connection; Gk, *temnein,* to cut], the surgical division of a fibrous band or ring connecting corresponding parts of a body structure. A commissurotomy is commonly performed to separate the thickened, adherent leaves of a stenosed mitral valve.

**commitment** [L, *committere,* to entrust], **1.** the placement or confinement of an individual in a specialized hospital or other institutional facility. See also **institutionalize. 2.** the legal procedure of admitting a mentally ill person to an institution for psychiatric treatment. The process varies from state to state but usually involves judicial or court action based on medical evidence certifying that the person is mentally ill. See also **certification. 3.** a pledge or contract to fulfill some obligation or agreement, used especially in some forms of psychotherapy or marriage counseling.

**common bile duct** [L, *communis,* common, *bilis,* bile, *ducere,* to lead], the duct formed by the juncture of the cystic and hepatic ducts.

**common carotid artery** [L, *communis* + Gk, *karos,* heavy sleep, *arteria,* airpipe], one of the major arteries supplying blood to the head and neck. Each divides into an external common carotid and an internal common carotid. Branches of the external carotid supply the face, scalp, and most of the neck and throat tissues. The internal common carotids supply the brain and other tissues generally accessible from within the skull, as the eyes.

**common carotid plexus,** a network of nerves on the common carotid artery, supplying sympathetic fibers to the head and the neck, with branches that accompany the cranial blood vessels. The common carotid plexus is formed by the internal and external carotid plexuses and by the cervical ganglia of the sympathetic system.

**common cold.** See **cold.**

**common duct exploration.** See **CDE.**

**common hepatic artery,** the visceral branch of the celiac trunk of the abdominal aorta, passing posterior to the pylorus and dividing into five branches: the gastroduodenal, right gastric, right hepatic, left hepatic, and middle hepatic.

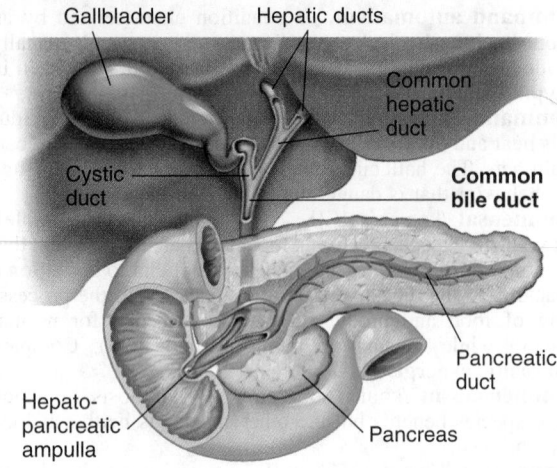

**Common bile duct**

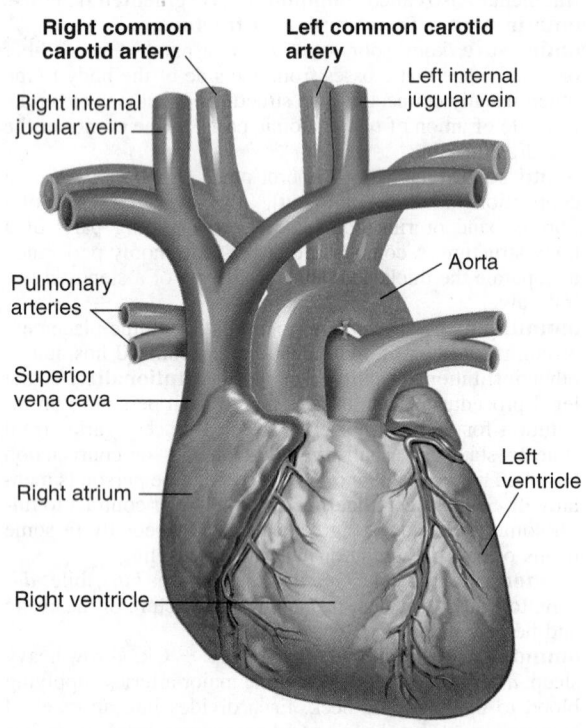

**Common carotid arteries**

**common iliac artery,** a division of the abdominal aorta, starting to the left of the fourth lumbar vertebra, passing caudally about 5 cm, and dividing into external and internal iliac arteries. The right common iliac artery is somewhat longer than the left.

**common iliac node,** a node in one of the seven groups of parietal lymph nodes serving the abdomen and the pelvis. They drain the internal and external iliac nodes and pass their materials to the lateral aortic nodes. Compare **external iliac node, internal iliac node, iliac circumflex node.** See also **lymph, lymphatic system, lymph node.**

**common iliac vein,** one of the two veins that are the sources of the inferior vena cava, formed by the union of the internal and external iliac veins, ventral to the sacroiliac articulation. Each common iliac vein receives the iliolumbar and, in some individuals, the lateral sacral veins. The left common iliac vein also receives the middle sacral vein. Neither of the common iliacs contains valves. Compare **external iliac vein, internal iliac vein.**

**common pathway of coagulation,** the steps in the mechanism of coagulation from the activation of factor X through the conversion of fibrinogen to fibrin. See also **coagulation cascade, intrinsic pathway of coagulation, extrinsic pathway of coagulation.**

**common variable immunodeficiency (CVID),** a heterogeneous group of disorders characterized by hypogammaglobulinemia, decreased antibody production in response to antigenic challenge, and recurrent pyogenic infections, and often associated with hematologic and autoimmune disorders. Most patients have normal numbers of circulating B cells that can identify antigens and proliferate, but they lack plasma cells and may have an intrinsic defect of B cell differentiation. Two less common forms are also recognized, one caused by a disorder of T lymphocyte regulation and one caused by production of autoantibodies against T and B lymphocytes.

**commune** /kom′yo͞on/, a small community of people who share certain social and economic objectives. Members may also share property ownership and control local political leadership.

**communicability period** /kəmyo͞o′nəkəbil′itē/, the usual time span during which contact with an infected person is most likely to result in spread of the infection. For measles the communicability period ranges from 4 days before the appearance of a rash until 5 days after the onset of symptoms.

**communicable** /kəmyo͞o′nəkəbəl/ [L, *communis,* common], contagious; transmissible by direct or indirect means, as a communicable disease.

**communicable disease,** any disease transmitted from one person or animal to another directly, by contact with excreta or other discharges from the body; or indirectly, via substances or inanimate objects, such as contaminated drinking glasses, toys, or water; or via vectors, as flies, mosquitoes, ticks, or other insects. Communicable diseases may be caused by bacteria, chlamydia, fungi, parasites, rickettsiae, and viruses. To control a communicable disease, it is important to identify the organism, prevent its spread to the environment, protect others against contamination, and treat the infected person. Many communicable diseases, by law, must be reported to the local health department. Also called **contagious disease.**

**Communicable Disease Center,** former name of the **Centers for Disease Control and Prevention.**

**communicable disease management,** a nursing intervention from the Nursing Interventions Classification (NIC) defined as working with a community to decrease and manage the incidence and prevalence of contagious diseases in a specific population. See also **Nursing Interventions Classification.**

**communicating hydrocephalus** /kəmyo͞o′nikā′ting/ [L, *communicans* + Gk, *hydor,* water, *kephale,* head], a form of hydrocephalus in which there is an increase in cerebrospinal fluid that involves the entire ventricular system and the subarachnoid space. It is caused by an abnormality in the ability to absorb fluid in the subarachnoid space; no obstruction exists.

**communication** /kəmyo͞o′nikā′shən/ [L, *communis,* common], any process in which a message containing information is transferred, especially from one person to another, via any of a number of media. Communication may be verbal or nonverbal; it may occur directly, such as in a face-to-face conversation or with the observation of a gesture; or it may occur remotely, spanning space and time, such as in writing and reading or in making or playing back of a recording. Communication is basic to all nursing and other health care professions and contributes to the development of all therapeutic relationships. See also **kinesics, therapeutic communication.**

**communication ability,** a nursing outcome from the Nursing Outcome Classification (NOC) defined as ability to receive, interpret, and express spoken, written, and nonverbal messages. See also **nursing outcomes classification.**

**communication channels,** (in communication theory) any gesture, action, sound, written word, or visual image used in transmitting messages.

**communication disorders,** a *DSM-IV* classification defined as mental disorders involving difficulties in speech or language, severe enough to be a problem academically, occupationally, or socially; included are **expressive language disorder, mixed receptive-expressive language disorder, phonological disorder** and **stuttering.**

**communication enhancement: hearing deficit,** a nursing intervention from the Nursing Interventions Classification (NIC) defined as assistance in accepting and learning alternate methods for living with diminished hearing. See also **Nursing Interventions Classification.**

**communication enhancement: speech deficit,** a nursing intervention from the Nursing Interventions Classification (NIC) defined as assistance in accepting and learning alternate methods for living with impaired speech. See also **Nursing Interventions Classification.**

**communication enhancement: visual deficit,** a nursing intervention from the Nursing Interventions Classification (NIC) defined as assistance in accepting and learning alternate methods for living with diminished vision. See also **Nursing Interventions Classification.**

**communication: expressive ability,** a nursing outcome from the Nursing Outcome Classification (NOC) defined as ability to express and interpret verbal and/or non-verbal messages. See also **nursing outcomes classification.**

**communication, impaired verbal,** a nursing diagnosis accepted by the Fourth National Conference on the Classification of Nursing Diagnoses. Impaired verbal communication is defined as the state in which an individual experiences a decreased or absent ability to use or understand language in human interaction.

■ DEFINING CHARACTERISTICS: The defining characteristics include slurring, stuttering, difficulty in forming words or sentences, problem in expressing thoughts verbally, inappropriate verbalization, dyspnea, and disorientation. The critical defining characteristics, one of which must be present for the diagnosis to be made, are an inability to speak the dominant language of the culture, a difficulty in speaking or verbalizing, or the absence of speech.

■ RELATED FACTORS: Related factors include decreased circulation to the brain, a physical barrier (brain tumor, tracheostomy, intubation), psychologic barriers (psychosis, lack of stimuli), cultural differences, and developmentally related or age-related factors. See also **nursing diagnosis.**

**communication: receptive,** a nursing outcome from the Nursing Outcome Classification (NOC) defined as ability to receive and interpret verbal and/or non-verbal messages. See also **nursing outcomes classification.**

**communication theme,** (in psychiatry) a recurrent concept or idea that ties together components of communica-

tion. Kinds of communication themes include **content theme,** in which a single concept links varied topics of discussion; **mood theme,** in which the underlying idea is the emotion communicated by the individual; and **interaction theme,** in which a particular idea best describes the dynamics between communicating participants.

**communication theory,** a hypothesis that describes a model of a system of information transfer consisting of a source of information (the sender), a transmitter, a communication channel, a source of noise (interference), a receiver, and a purpose for the message.

**community** /kəmyoo'nitē/ [L, *communis,* common], a group of species who reside in a designated geographic area and who share common interests or bonds.

**community-acquired infection,** an infection contracted outside of a health care setting. Community-acquired infections are often distinguished from nosocomial, or hospital-acquired, diseases by the types of organisms that affect patients who are recovering from a disease or injury. Community-acquired respiratory infections commonly involve strains of *Haemophilus influenzae* or *Streptococcus pneumoniae* and are usually more antibiotic sensitive.

**community competence,** a nursing outcome from the Nursing Outcome Classification (NOC) defined as the ability of a community to collectively problem solve to achieve goals. See also **nursing outcomes classification.**

**community disaster preparedness,** a nursing intervention from the Nursing Interventions Classification (NIC) defined as preparing for an effective response to a large-scale disaster. See also **Nursing Interventions Classification.**

**community health development,** a nursing intervention from the Nursing Interventions Classification (NIC) defined as facilitating members of a community to identify a community's health concerns, mobilize resources, and implement solutions. See also **Nursing Interventions Classification.**

**community health: immunity,** a nursing outcome from the Nursing Outcome Classification (NOC) defined as resistance of a group to the invasion and spread of an infectious agent. See also **nursing outcomes classification.**

**community health nursing,** a field of nursing that is a blend of primary health care and nursing practice with public health nursing. The community health nurse conducts a continuing and comprehensive practice that is preventive, curative, and rehabilitative. The philosophy of care is based on the belief that care directed to the individual, the family, and the group contributes to the health care of the population as a whole. The community health nurse is not restricted to the care of a particular age or diagnostic group. Participation of all consumers of health care is encouraged in the development of community activities that contribute to the promotion of, education about, and maintenance of good health. These activities require comprehensive health programs that pay special attention to social and ecologic influences and specific populations at risk.

**community health status,** a nursing outcome from the Nursing Outcome Classification (NOC) defined as the general state of well-being of a community or population. See also **nursing outcomes classification.**

**community medicine,** a branch of medicine that is concerned with the health of the members of a community, municipality, or region. The emphasis in community medicine is on the early diagnosis of disease, the recognition of environmental and occupational hazards to good health, and the prevention of disease in the community.

**community mental health,** a treatment philosophy based on the social model of psychiatric care that advocates that a comprehensive range of mental health services be readily accessible to all members of the community.

**community mental health center (CMHC),** a community-based center that provides comprehensive mental health services, including ambulatory and inpatient care. The specific services to be provided are defined in an act of the U.S. Congress, the Community Mental Health Centers Act; these requirements have been updated periodically. The costs of consultation and educational services, instruction, development, and initial operation of the facility are paid for by the federal government. The organization, management, and operation of CMHCs are also specified by the act. Consumer representation in each of these areas is required.

**community nurse practitioner (CNP),** a nurse who has completed a postbaccalaureate program in community nursing.

**community psychiatry,** the branch of psychiatry concerned with the development of an adequate and coordinated program of mental health care for residents of specified catchment areas. See **community mental health center.**

**community rating system,** a program of health maintenance organizations (HMOs) that uses revenues and membership targets to determine health insurance premium rates. The HMO uses its own history in the calculation of rates, rather than any single employer's risk history. See also **health maintenance organization.**

**community reintegration,** the return and acceptance of a disabled person as a participating member of the community.

**community risk control: chronic disease,** a nursing outcome from the Nursing Outcome Classification (NOC) defined as community actions to reduce the risk of chronic diseases and related complications. See also **nursing outcomes classification.**

**community risk control: communicable disease,** a nursing outcome from the Nursing Outcome Classification (NOC) defined as community actions to eliminate or reduce the spread of infectious agents (bacteria, fungi, parasites, and viruses) that threaten public health. See also **nursing outcomes classification.**

**community risk control: lead exposure,** a nursing outcome from the Nursing Outcome Classification (NOC) defined as community actions to reduce lead exposure and poisoning. See also **nursing outcomes classification.**

**Comolli's sign** /kōmō'lēs/ [Antonio Comolli, Italian pathologist, b. 1879], a triangular swelling corresponding to the shape of the scapula after a fracture of that bone.

**comorbidity,** two or more coexisting medical conditions or unrelated disease processes.

**compact bone** /kom'pakt, kompakt'/ [L, *compingere,* to put together], hard, dense bone that is usually found at the periphery of skeletal structures, as distinguished from spongy cancellous bone.

**compact disc (CD),** an optical disc on which computer data are encoded or on which sound is recorded in a digital format. A CD has a capacity of 650 megabytes of data or 75 minutes of recorded music.

**compact disc/read only memory.** See **CD/ROM.**

**companion animal,** a dog, cat, or other pet that provides health benefits to a person. Companion animals may help relieve stress or serve a more active role, as do guide dogs for blind persons and dogs trained to detect telephone or doorbell sounds for deaf persons.

**companionship** /kəmpan'yənship'/ [L, *com,* together, *panis,* food], (in psychiatric nursing) the assignment of a staff

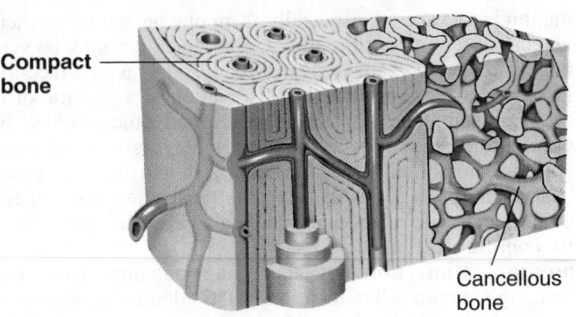

**Compact bone**

member or of another patient to stay with a disturbed patient to provide support and to protect the patient from self-harm or harm to others. In constant companionship the disturbed patient is accompanied in all activities until the companion is convinced the patient has regained control.

**comparative anatomy** /kəmper'ətiv/ [L, *com* + *par,* equal], the study of the morphologic characteristics of all living animals. A comparison of the forms indicates a progression on a scale from the simplest to the most highly specialized animals. The adult stage of animals that are lower in the scale resembles the immature stages of many higher-level animals. See also **applied anatomy, ontogeny, phylogeny.**

**comparative embryology,** the study of the similarities and differences among various organisms during the embryologic period of development.

**comparative method,** the analytic method to which the test method is compared in the comparison-of-methods experiment. This term makes no inference about the quality of the comparative method.

**comparative physiology,** the study of the similarities and differences of the vital processes found in various species of living organisms to determine fundamental physiologic relationships between members of the animal and plant kingdoms.

**comparative psychology, 1.** the study of human behavior as it relates to or differs from animal behavior. **2.** the study of the psychologic and behavioral differences among various peoples.

**compartment model** /kəmpärt'mənt/, a mathematic representation of the body or an area of the body created to study physiologic or pharmacologic kinetic characteristics. A compartment model can simulate all of the biologic processes involved in the kinetic behavior of a drug after it has been introduced into the body, leading to a better understanding of its pharmacodynamic effects. Studies most frequently use one- or two-compartment models. In a one-compartment model the body assumes the characteristics of a homogeneous unit in which an administered drug diffuses instantaneously in the volume of body fluid. In a two-compartment model the body is represented as two distinct compartments, a central and a peripheral compartment, with two separate fluid volumes.

**compartment syndrome** [L, *com* + *partiri,* to share], a pathologic condition caused by the progressive development of arterial compression and consequent reduction of blood supply. The compression may result from an overly restrictive dressing or cast or from nonexpansive muscle fascia.

Clinical manifestations include swelling, restriction of movement, brown urine, myoglobinuria, vascular compromise, and severe pain or lack of sensation. It can result in a permanent contracture deformity of the hand or foot, with or without a fracture. In severe cases, it can lead to necrosis and necessitate the amputation of an extremity. Treatment includes elevation, removal of restrictive dressings or casts, and potentially a surgical decompression. See also **Volkmann's contracture.**

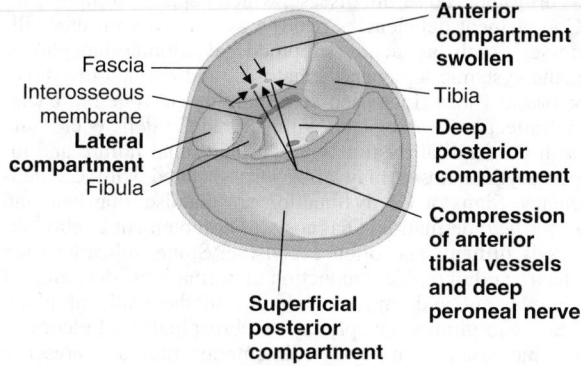

Fascia
Interosseous membrane
**Lateral compartment**
Fibula

Anterior compartment swollen
Tibia
**Deep posterior compartment**
Compression of anterior tibial vessels and deep peroneal nerve

Superficial posterior compartment

**Anterior compartment syndrome**
*(Black, Hawks, and Keene, 2001)*

**compatibility** /kəmpat′əbil′itē/ [L, *compatibilis,* agreeable], **1.** the quality or state of existing together in harmony; congruity. **2.** the orderly, efficient integration of the elements of one system with those of another. **3.** the formation of a stable chemical or biochemical system, specifically in medication, so that two or more drugs can be administered at the same time without producing undesired side effects or without canceling or affecting the therapeutic effects of the others. **4.** (in immunology) the degree to which the body's defense system tolerates the presence of foreign material, such as transfused blood, grafted tissue, or transplanted organs, without an immune reaction. Usually identical twins are completely compatible. **5.** (in blood grouping or crossmatching) the lack of reaction between blood groups so that there is no agglutination when the red blood cells of one sample are mixed with the serum of another sample; no reaction from transfused blood. —**compatible,** *adj.*

**Compazine,** trademark for a phenothiazine (prochlorperazine).

**compendium** /kəmpen′dē·əm/, *pl.* **compendia** [L, *compendere,* to weigh], a collected body of information on the standards of strength, purity, and quality of drugs. The official compendia in the United States are the *United States Pharmacopoeia,* the *Homeopathic Pharmacopoeia of the United States,* and their supplements. See also **formulary.**

**compensated acidosis** /kom′pənsā′tid/ [L, *compensare,* to balance, *acidus,* sour; Gk, *osis,* condition], a condition in which the pH of the blood is maintained within normal limits (adult/child: 7.35 to 7.45) although the blood bicarbonate level is below normal or the $PCO_2$ is above normal.

**compensated alkalosis,** a condition in which the blood bicarbonate is increased or the $PCO_2$ is decreased but buffering keeps the blood pH within the normal range.

**compensated flowmeter** [L, *compensare,* to balance], a gas therapy device with a scale that is calibrated against a constant pressure of 50 psi instead of the atmosphere. It is equipped with a valve distal to the gauge to record the output to the patient accurately.

**compensated gluteal gait,** one of the more common abnormal gaits associated with a weakness of the gluteus medius. It is a variation of the Trendelenburg gait. It involves the dropping of the pelvis on the unaffected side of the body during the walking cycle between the moment of heel strike on the affected side and before the moment of heel strike on the unaffected side. The compensated gluteal gait is also characterized by the dropping of the entire trunk downward and sideways over the affected hip and a short step on the unaffected side. In a compensated gait the trunk is forcibly thrown laterally during the weight-bearing or stance phase in the movement of the affected lower limb. This lateral movement is the result of an attempt to shift a significant portion of body weight above and outside the center of rotation of the affected hip. During this movement the erector spinae and the quadratus lumborum of the involved side function to lift the whole weight of the pelvis and the opposite lower extremity off the ground to allow the uninvolved leg to clear during its swing phase. Also called **gluteal gait.**

**compensated heart failure,** an abnormal cardiac condition in which heart failure is compensated for by such mechanisms as increased sympathetic stimulation of the heart, fluid retention with increased venous return, increased end-diastolic ventricular volume and fiber length, and ventricular hypertrophy. Compensation may be aided by the administration of digitalis glycosides and angiotensin-converting enzyme inhibitors, to improve myocardial function and diuretics to relieve pulmonary and peripheral congestion. See also **heart failure.**

**compensating current** /kom′pənsā′ting/, an electric current that neutralizes the intensity of a muscle current.

**compensating curve,** the curvature of alignment of the occlusal surfaces of the teeth, developed to compensate for the paths of the condyles as the mandible moves from centric to eccentric positions. It is used to maintain posterior tooth contacts on the molar teeth and to provide balancing contacts on dentures associated with a protruding mandible. The compensating curve corresponds to the Spee's curve in natural teeth.

**compensating filter,** a device, such as a wedge of aluminum, clay, or plastic, that is placed over a body area during radiography to compensate for differences in radiopacity. For example, a wedge may be placed over a foot with the thick portion over the toes and the thin edge toward the heel to compensate for the range of thickness of the foot. See also **bowtie filter.**

**compensation** /kom′pənsā′shən/ [L, *compensare,* to balance], **1.** the process of counterbalancing any defect in body structure or function. **2.** the process of maintaining an adequate blood flow through such normal cardiac and circulatory mechanisms as tachycardia, fluid retention with increased venous return, and ventricular hypertrophy. Lack of compensation indicates a diseased heart muscle. See also **compensated heart failure. 3.** a complex defense mechanism that allows one to avoid the unpleasant or painful emotional stimuli that result from a feeling of inferiority or inadequacy. Examples include making an extraordinary effort to overcome a disability, scorning a quality that one lacks ("sour grapes"), and substituting hard work and excellent performance in one field for a lack of ability in another. **4.** changes in structural relationships that accommodate foundation disturbances and maintain balance. See also **overcompensation.**

**compensator** /kom′pənsā′tər/, a device used in radiotherapy to correct for irregularities in body surfaces by providing a differential attenuation of the x-ray beam before it reaches the patient. The result is a more uniform distribution of radiation dose in the tumor. Compensators are generally mounted on the collimator system of a teletherapy unit.

**compensatory hypertrophy** /kəmpen′sətôr′ē/ [L, *compensare,* to balance], an increase in the size or the function of an organ or part to counteract a structural or functional defect. See also **compensated heart failure.**

**compensatory pause,** a pause noted on an electrocardiogram after a premature complex; it precedes the next normal complex.

**competence** /kom′pətəns/[L, *competentia,* capable], **1.** (in embryology) the total capacity of an embryonic cell to react to determinative stimuli in various ways of differentiation. **2.** the ability of bacteria to take up donor deoxyribonucleic acid molecules.

**competent community** /kom′pətənt/, a population that is aware of resources and alternatives, can make reasoned decisions about issues facing the group, and can cope adaptively with problems. It parallels the concept of positive mental health.

**competitive antagonist,** a substance that interferes with usual metabolic activity by competing for binding sites on a substrate (the substance on which an enzyme acts in a chemical reaction) or on an enzyme that ordinarily attacks the substrate. The antagonist is usually an analog of the substrate. See also **antimetabolite.**

**competitive-binding assay** /kompet′itiv/ [L, *competere,* to come together], an analytic procedure based on the reversible binding of a ligand to a binding protein. In proportion to its concentration the ligand competes with a labeled derivative for binding to the limited number of available binding sites.

**competitive displacement,** the tendency of one drug to displace another at a protein-binding site when both drugs are taken at the same time. The bound drug becomes less pharmacologically active than the free drug. An example is phenylbutazone, which has a greater affinity for binding sites than warfarin. As a result, if both drugs are taken at the same time, fewer binding sites are available for warfarin, which remains active in the body, increasing its anticoagulant action.

**competitive identification,** the unconscious modeling of one's personality on that of another as a means of outdoing or bettering the other person. See also **identification.**

**competitive inhibitor,** an inhibitor of an enzyme reaction that competes with the substrate by binding at the active site.

**complaint** [L, *complangere,* to beat the breast], **1.** (in law) a pleading by a plaintiff made under oath to initiate a suit. It is a statement of the formal charge and the cause for action against the defendant. For a minor offense the defendant is tried on the basis of the complaint. A more serious felony prosecution requires an indictment with evidence presented by a state's attorney. **2.** *informal.* any ailment, problem, or symptom identified by the client, patient, member of the person's family, or other knowledgeable person. The chief complaint often causes the person to seek health care.

**complement** /kom′pləmənt/ [L, *complementum,* that which completes], a system of at least 20 complex, enzymatic serum proteins. In an antigen-antibody reaction, complement causes lysis. Complement is also involved in other physiologic reactions, including anaphylaxis and phagocytosis. See also **antibody, antigen, antigen-antibody reaction, immune gamma globulin.**

**complement abnormality,** an unusual condition characterized by deficiencies or by dysfunctions of any of the 11 serum proteins known as complement and designated C1-C11. The most common abnormalities are C2 and C3 deficiencies and C5 familial dysfunction. Patients with complement abnormalities may be more susceptible to infections and to collagen vascular diseases. Primary complement abnormalities may be inherited, while secondary complement abnormalities may stem from immunologic reactions, such as drug-induced serum disease, which depletes complement. Complement deficiencies may be associated with other illnesses, such as acute streptococcal glomerulonephritis, acute systemic lupus erythematosus, and dermatomyositis.

■ OBSERVATIONS: Increased susceptibility to systemic bacterial infection is associated with C2 and C3 deficiencies and with C5 familial dysfunction. Chronic renal failure and lupus erythematosus may also be associated with C2 deficiency. Signs of C5 dysfunction are malaise, diarrhea, and seborrheic dermatitis. Diagnosis of complement abnormalities is difficult and often expensive. Some indications are electrocardiographic conduction abnormalities; detection of complement and immunoglobulins in the walls of blood vessels in glomerulonephritis; cerebrospinal fluid pleocytosis; increased erythrocyte sedimentation rate; and presence in the urine of red blood cells (RBCs), RBC casts, and protein.

■ INTERVENTIONS: Replacement of complement-fixing antibodies and control of infection and associated illnesses are part of standard treatment for complement abnormalities. The patient commonly receives transfusion of fresh plasma to replace antibodies. Bone marrow transplantations and injection of gamma globulin may also be used, but the former carries the risk of a fatal graft-versus-host reaction. Complement abnormalities are usually corrected temporarily by replacement therapy, but no permanent cure is available.

■ NURSING CONSIDERATIONS: Patients should be carefully monitored, especially if they are receiving gamma globulin injections. Gamma globulin is injected into a large muscle mass, which is massaged well after each injection. More than one site is usually selected if the dosage is more than 1.5 mL. If frequent doses are ordered, the injection sites are rotated. With plasma infusions, careful matching of leukocytes for human leukocyte antigen cell types is important to prevent a graft-versus-host reaction and other undesirable responses. Bone marrow transplantation requires close monitoring for transfusion reactions and is usually followed by instructions to the patient for scrupulous hygiene, prompt treatment of even the smallest wounds, and avoidance of crowds or persons with active infections. The nurse should be alert for early signs of ataxia or slight changes in mental activity that may signal neurologic damage caused by infection.

**complemental inheritance** /kom′pləmen′təl/, the expression of a trait as a result of the presence of two independent pairs of nonallelic genes. Both of the genes must be present for the trait to appear in the phenotype.

**complementary feeding** /kom′pləmen′tərē/ [L, *complementum,* that which completes], a supplemental feeding given an infant who is still hungry after breastfeeding.

**complementary gene,** either member of two or more non-allelic gene pairs that interact to produce an effect not expressed in the absence of any of the pairs. Also called **reciprocal gene.**

**complement assay,** a blood test used primarily to measure serum complement in an effort to diagnose angioedema and to monitor the activity of disease in patients with systemic lupus erythematosus nephritis, membranoproliferative nephritis, or poststreptococcal nephritis.

**complement cascade,** a biochemical process involving the C1 to C9 complement proteins in which one protein interacts with another in a specific sequence called a complement pathway. The cascade occurs at the surface of an antigen-bearing cell and causes the cell to accumulate fluid and ultimately rupture.

**complement control protein (CCP),** any of a large family of proteins involved in complement regulation, encoded in a closely linked gene cluster, and having one or more stretches of a common short repeated sequence. See also **complement.**

**complement fixation,** an immunologic reaction in which an antigen combines with an antibody and its complement, causing the complement factor to become inactive or fixed. The complement-fixation reaction can be tested in the laboratory by exposing the patient's serum to antigen, complement, and specially sensitized red blood cells. Complement-fixation tests are used to detect antibodies for infectious diseases, especially syphilis and viral illnesses. See also **complement, immune system, immunity, Wassermann blood test.**

**complement-fixation test (C-F test),** any serologic test in which complement fixation is detected, indicating the presence of a particular antigen. Specific C-F tests are used to aid in the diagnosis of amebiasis, Rocky Mountain spotted fever, trypanosomiasis, and typhus.

**complement protein molecule** [L, *complementum* + *proteios,* first rank], any of the protein molecules that are chief humoral mediators of antigen-antibody reactions in the immune system. Complement proteins stimulate phagocytosis and inflammation. Nine are involved in the "classical pathway" cascade that results in the lysis of antibody-coated bacteria. They are designated *C*1 to *C*9.

**complete abortion** [L, *complere,* to fill up], termination of pregnancy in which the conceptus is expelled or removed in its entirety. Because no products of conception remain in the uterus, surgical evacuation is not necessary. Compare **incomplete abortion.**

**complete bed bath,** a bath in which the entire body of a patient is washed while he or she is in bed. See also **blanket bath.**

**complete blood count (CBC),** a determination of the number of red and white blood cells per cubic millimeter of blood. A complete blood count is one of the most routinely performed tests in a clinical laboratory and one of the most valuable screening and diagnostic techniques. Most laboratories use an electronic counter for reporting numbers of red and white blood cells and platelets. Examining a stained slide of blood yields useful information about red cell morphologic characteristics and types of white blood cells. The normal red blood cell (RBC) count in adult males is 4.7 to 6.1 million/mm$^3$. In adult females the normal RBC is 4.2 to 5.4 million/mm$^3$. Each type of white cell can be represented as a percentage of the total number of white cells observed. This is called a differential count. The normal adult white blood cell count is 5000 to 10,000/cm$^3$. Electronic blood counters also automatically determine hemoglobin or hematocrit and include this value in the complete blood count. See also **differential white blood cell count, erythrocyte, hematocrit, hemoglobin, leukocyte.**

**complete breech,** a fetal presentation in which the buttocks present with the legs folded on the thighs and the thighs on the abdomen. The position of the fetus is the same as in a normal vertex presentation but upside down. Compare **frank breech.** See also **breech birth.**

**complete denture.** See **full denture.**

**complete dislocation** [L, *complere,* to fill up, *dis,* apart, *locare,* to place], a dislocation in which the articular surfaces of the joint are completely separated.

**complete fistula,** an abnormal passage from an internal organ or structure to the surface of the body or to another internal organ or structure.

**complete fracture,** a bone break that completely disrupts the continuity of a bone across its entire width. Also called **100% displaced fracture.**

**complete health history,** a health history that includes a history of the chief complaint, present illness, past and present health history, social history, occupational history, sexual history, and family health history. See also **functional health history, health history.**

**complete heart block (CHB)** [L, *complere,* to fill up; Gk, *kardia,* heart; OFr, *bloc*], total failure of impulses to be conducted from the atria to the ventricles. It causes the atria and ventricles to beat independently. Also called **third-degree AV heart block.**

**complete hernia** [L, *complere,* to fill up, *hernia,* rupture], a hernia characterized by protrusion of the hernial sac and abdominal contents through the abdominal wall.

**complete paralysis** [L, *complere,* to fill up; Gk, *paralyein,* to be palsied], paralysis characterized by a complete loss of motor function.

**complete previa.** See **central placenta previa.**

**complete protein,** a protein that contains all the essential amino acids in appropriate amounts to allow normal growth and tissue maintenance when adequate energy is provided in the diet. Examples are casein (milk protein) and egg whites.

**complete rachischisis,** a rare congenital fissure of the entire vertebral column and spinal cord, resulting from failure of the embryonic neural tube to close. The condition is characterized by flaccid paralysis and impaired sensations. It is often accompanied by other birth defects, such as cleft palate, cleft lip, and hydrocephalus, and is frequently fatal. Also called **rachischisis totalis, holorachischisis.** See also **spina bifida.**

**complete response (CR),** (in oncology) the total disappearance of a tumor.

**complex** /kom'pleks, kəmpleks'/ [L, *complexus,* an embrace], **1.** a group of items, as chemical molecules, that are related in structure or function as are the iron and protein portions of hemoglobin or the cobalt and protein portions of vitamin B$_{12}$. **2.** a combination of signs and symptoms of disease that forms a syndrome. **3.** (in psychology) a group of associated ideas with strong emotional overtones that affect a person's attitudes toward a specific subject.

**complex carbohydrate,** a polysaccharide, such as a carbohydrate that is composed of a large number of glucose molecules, so called to distinguish it from a simple sugar.

**complex cavity,** a cavity that involves more than one surface of a tooth. Compare **gingival cavity.**

**complex fracture,** a closed fracture in which the soft tissue surrounding the bone is severely damaged.

**complex odontoma.** See **composite odontoma.**

**complex protein,** a protein that contains a simple protein and at least one molecule of another substance, as a glycoprotein, lipoprotein, nucleoprotein, or hemoglobin.

**complex relationship building,** a nursing intervention from the Nursing Interventions Classification (NIC) defined as establishing a therapeutic relationship with a patient who has difficulty interacting with others. See also **Nursing Interventions Classification.**

**complex spatial relations,** the perceptual relationship of one figure or part of a figure to another.

**complex sugars,** sugar molecules that can be hydrolyzed or digested to yield two molecules of the same or different simple sugars, such as sucrose, lactose, and maltose. Also called **disaccharide** or **polysaccharide.**

**compliance** /kəmplī′əns/ [L, *complere,* to complete], **1.** fulfillment by a patient of a caregiver's prescribed course of treatment. **2.** (in respiratory physiology) a measure of distensibility of the lung volume produced by a unit pressure change. Abbreviated **C.** Also called **pulmonary compliance.**

**compliance behavior,** a nursing outcome from the Nursing Outcome Classification (NOC) defined as actions taken on the basis of professional advice to promote wellness, recovery, and rehabilitation. See also **nursing outcomes classification.**

**compliance factor,** a measure of the expansion of the flexible tubing in a mechanical ventilating system when pressure is applied.

**complicated dislocation** [L, *complicare,* to fold together, *dis,* apart, *locare,* place], a joint dislocation accompanied by damage to other tissues.

**complicated fracture,** a fracture accompanied by injury to neighboring soft tissues, such as nerves and blood vessels.

**complicated labor** [L, *complicare,* to fold together, *labor,* work], any labor that is made more difficult or complex by a deviation from the normal procedure.

**complication** [L, *complicare,* to fold together], a disease or injury that develops during the treatment of a preexisting disorder. An example is a bacterial infection that is acquired by a person weakened by a viral infection. The complication frequently alters the prognosis.

**component** /kəmpō′nənt/ [L, *componere,* to assemble], a significant part of a larger unit.

**component drip set,** a device used for delivering IV fluids, especially whole blood. It includes plastic tubing and a combination drip-chamber and filter. Compare **component syringe set, microaggregate recipient set, straight line blood set, Y-set.**

**component syringe set,** a device used for delivering IV fluids. It includes plastic tubing, two slide clamps, a Y-connector, and a syringe. The component syringe set may be used in various procedures, as in the transfusion of platelets and cryoprecipitates. In such transfusions the component syringe set is used primarily to prevent clogging the IV line. Compare **component drip set, microaggregate recipient set, straight line blood set, Y-set.**

**component therapy,** a transfusion of specific blood components instead of whole blood. Packed red cells or platelet-rich plasma suspensions may be transfused in larger quantities than would be possible if whole blood were used. More sophisticated processing provides fibrinogen or antihemophilic globulin solutions for administration in therapeutic amounts exceeding what might be given with conventional blood transfusion therapy. Compare **plasmapheresis.** See also **packed cells, pooled plasma.**

**composite core** /kəmpos′it/ [L, *componere,* to assemble], a buildup of composite resin, designed and installed to retain an artificial tooth crown. See also **core.** Compare **amalgam core, cast core.**

**composite graft,** a transplantation that involves more than one type of tissue, such as skin and cartilage. The term may also refer to an artificial vessel graft to replace the aortic arch for a valve in heart surgery.

**composite odontoma,** tumor that develops in tooth-producing tissue and is composed of abnormally arranged calcified enamel and dentin. Also called **complex odontoma.**

**compos mentis** /kom′pōs men′tis/, having a sound mind. Compare **non compos mentis.**

**compound** [L, *componere,* to assemble], **1.** /kom′pound/ (in chemistry) a substance composed of two or more different elements, chemically combined in definite proportions, that cannot be separated by physical means. **2.** /kom′pound/ any substance composed of two or more different ingredients. **3.** /kəmpound′/ to make a substance by combining ingredients, such as a pharmaceutic. **4.** denoting an injury characterized by multiple factors, such as a compound fracture.

**compound aneurysm,** a localized dilation of an arterial wall in which some of the layers of the wall are distended and others are ruptured or dissected.

**compound dislocation.** See **open dislocation.**

**compound fracture,** a fracture in which the broken end or ends of the bone have torn through the skin. Also called **open fracture.**

**compound joint** [L, *componere,* to assemble, *jungere,* to join], a joint that involves more than two bones. The elbow and knee joints are two examples.

**compound melanocytoma.** See **benign juvenile melanoma.**

**compound microscope** [L, *componere,* to assemble; Gk, *mikros,* small, *skopein,* to view], a microscope with two or more simple or complex lens systems.

**compound tubuloalveolar gland** /too͞′byəlō′alvē′ələr/, one of the many multicellular glands with more than one secretory duct that contains both tube-shaped and sac-shaped portions, as the salivary glands.

**comprehensive care.** See **holistic health care.**

**Comprehensive Health Manpower Act of 1971,** legislation passed by the U.S. Congress to provide educational funding for nurse-practitioner (NP) and physician-assistant (PA) programs.

**Comprehensive Health Planning (CHP) and Public Health Services Amendments,** legislation passed by the U.S. Congress in 1966 that emphasized regional planning and introduced the concept that each person has a "right to health care."

**comprehensive medical care,** a health care program that provides for preventive medical care and rehabilitative services in addition to traditional chronic and acute illness services.

**compress** /kom′pres/ [L, *comprimere,* to press together], a soft pad, usually made of cloth, used to apply heat, cold, or medication to the surface of a body area. A compress also may be applied over a wound to help control bleeding. Compare **dressing.**

**compressed air hazards.** See **decompression sickness.**

**compressibility factor** /kəmpres′ibil′itē/, a measure of the amount of tidal volume that may be trapped in a mechanical ventilator system in relation to the water pressure applied. It is expressed in milliliters of gas per centimeter of water pressure.

**compressible volume** /kəmpres′əbəl/, a part of the tidal volume of gas produced by a mechanical ventilator that is prevented from reaching a patient by compression of the gas and expansion of the flexible tubing in the equipment.

**compression** /kəmpresh′ən/ [L, *comprimere,* to press together], the act of pressing, squeezing, or otherwise applying pressure to an organ, tissue, or body area. An intracranial tumor or hemorrhage may cause compression of brain tissue. Kinds of pathologic compression include **compression fracture,** in which bone surfaces are forced against each other, causing a break, and **compression paralysis,** marked by paralysis of a body area caused by pressure on a nerve.

**compression amplification.** See **gray scale display.**

**compression fracture,** a bone break, especially in a short bone, that disrupts osseous tissue and collapses the affected bone. Axial loading is the usual mechanism of injury. The bodies of vertebrae are often sites of compression fractures.

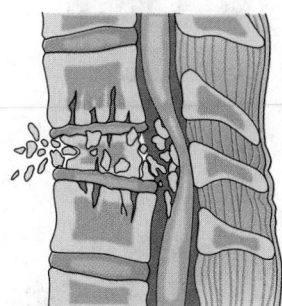

**Compression fracture** (Phipps, Sands, and Marek, 1999)

**compression neuropathy,** any of several disorders involving damage to sensory nerve roots or peripheral nerves, caused by mechanical pressure or localized trauma. It is characterized by paresthesia, weakness, or paralysis. The carpal, peroneal, radial, and ulnar nerves are most commonly involved. Compare **neuritis.** See also **paresthesia.**

**compression paralysis** [L, *comprimere,* to press together; Gk, *paralyein,* to be palsied], a paralysis that is caused by sustained pressure on a peripheral nerve. The condition can be temporary or permanent, depending on the duration and intensity of pressure.

**compressions,** (in physical science) regions of high molecular density, such as a great amount of ultrasound energy, within a longitudinal wave.

**compressive atelectasis** /kəmpres'iv/, a condition in which a region of the lung cannot be ventilated as a result of intrathoracic pressures that compress the alveoli in that region. The condition may result from a pulmonary embolism, which releases chemicals that cause vasoconstriction and bronchospasm, leading to alveolar compression.

**compressor naris** /kompres'ôr när'is/, the transverse part of the nasalis muscle that serves to depress the cartilage of the nose and to draw the ala toward the septum. Compare **dilator naris.**

**compromise** /kom'prəmīs/ [L, *com,* together, *promittere,* to promise], **1.** an action that may involve a change in a person's behavior, as in substituting goals or delaying satisfaction of needs in one area to reduce stress in another. **2.** an illness or condition that can affect another part of the body.

**compromise body image,** a new body image acquired by a patient as part of his or her adjustment to a physical dysfunction. It may harbor important emotional factors for the individual. A compromise body image incorporates and modifies unacceptable features of the condition through psychologic defense mechanisms such as denial, sublimation, repression, and overcompensation.

**compromised host,** a person who is less than normally able to resist infection because of immunosuppressive therapy, immunologic defect, severe anemia, or concurrent disease or condition, including human immunodeficiency

virus infection, metastatic malignancy, cachexia, or severe malnutrition.

**Compton scatter** [Arthur H. Compton, American physicist, 1892–1962], the principal interaction process of photons with tissue in the diagnostic and therapeutic radiology energy range. In this process, the incoming photon transfers energy to an electron in the material and is deflected, with reduced energy, into a path that generally leads to additional interactions.

**compulsion** [L, *compellere,* to urge], an irresistible, repetitive irrational impulse to perform an act that is usually contrary to one's ordinary judgments or standards yet results in overt anxiety if it is not completed; the compulsion also acts to decrease anxiety. The impulse is usually the result of an obsession. Compulsions are characteristic of an obsessive-compulsive disorder. Compare **phobia.** See also **compulsive ritual, obsession, obsessive-compulsive disorder.** —**compulsive,** *adj.*

**compulsion need** [L, *compellere,* to urge; Gk, *neuron,* nerve, *osis,* condition], an irresistible, irrational urge to perform certain acts repeatedly in spite of conscious recognition that doing so is abnormal behavior. The compulsive act may have symbolic significance to the patient.

**compulsive** /kəmpul'siv/ [L, *compellere,* to urge], pertaining to an act repeatedly performed under the stress of pathologic, intense need.

**compulsive idea** [L, *compellere,* to urge], a recurring irrational idea that persists in the mind, usually generating an irresistible urge to perform an inappropriate act. Also called **imperative idea.**

**compulsive personality,** a type of character structure with a pattern of chronic and obsessive adherence to rigid standards of conduct. The person is usually excessively conscientious and inhibited, is extremely inflexible, has an extraordinary capacity for work, and lacks a normal ability to relax and to relate to other people. The compulsive person is likely to follow repetitive patterns of behavior, such as snapping the fingers, crossing the legs, tapping the foot, or refusing to walk on cracks in the sidewalk, and often leads an impoverished emotional life, being dominated by a need for order, cleanliness, punctuality, rules, and systems. See also **compulsive personality disorder.**

**compulsive personality disorder,** a condition in which an irrational preoccupation with order, rules, ritual, and detail interferes with everyday functioning and normal behavior. The disorder is characterized by an excessive devotion to work, a pathologic adherence to a definite set of rules or system of behavior, and a persistent, compulsive following of specific rituals. The person cannot make decisions when faced with unexpected situations and cannot take pleasure in the normal activities of daily life. Psychotherapy is the usual treatment and may include behavior therapy with desensitization and flooding to reduce maladaptive anxiety. See also **compulsive personality.**

**compulsive polydipsia,** a compelling urge to drink excessive amounts of liquid. The condition is psychogenic; it is not caused by any organic dysfunction or physical deprivation. Extreme cases can result in death from water intoxication and electrolyte imbalance. See also **polydipsia.**

**compulsive ritual,** a series of acts a person feels must be carried out even though he or she recognizes that the behavior is useless and inappropriate. Failure to complete the acts causes extreme tension or anxiety.

**computed dental radiography (CDR),** a computer-assisted method for projecting radiographic images of the teeth and jaws on a video monitor. CDR may expose a patient to less radiation than conventional dental radiography.

**computed tomography (CT)** /kəmpyōō'tid/, a radiographic technique that produces an image of a detailed cross section of tissue. The procedure, first used in 1972, is painless and noninvasive and requires no special preparation. It is 100 times more sensitive than conventional radiography. Computed tomography uses a narrowly collimated beam of x-rays that rotates in a full arc around the patient to image the body in cross-sectional slices. An array of detectors, positioned at several angles, records those x-rays that pass through the body. The image is created by a computer that uses multiple attenuation readings taken around the periphery of the body part. The computer calculates tissue absorption and produces a representation of the tissues that demonstrates the densities of the various structures. Tumor masses, infractions, bone displacement, and accumulations of fluid may be detected. For cardiologic examination, ultrafast computed tomography is electrocardiogram-triggered and allows visualization of cardiac function and blood flow. Because modern CT equipment does not involve motion of the x-ray tube, heat loading is not a problem and multilevel images can be acquired in a very short time, sometimes during a single held breath. During a period of two held breaths, as many as 50 continuous tomographic images can be produced in a single-slice mode. Formerly called **computerized axial tomography.**

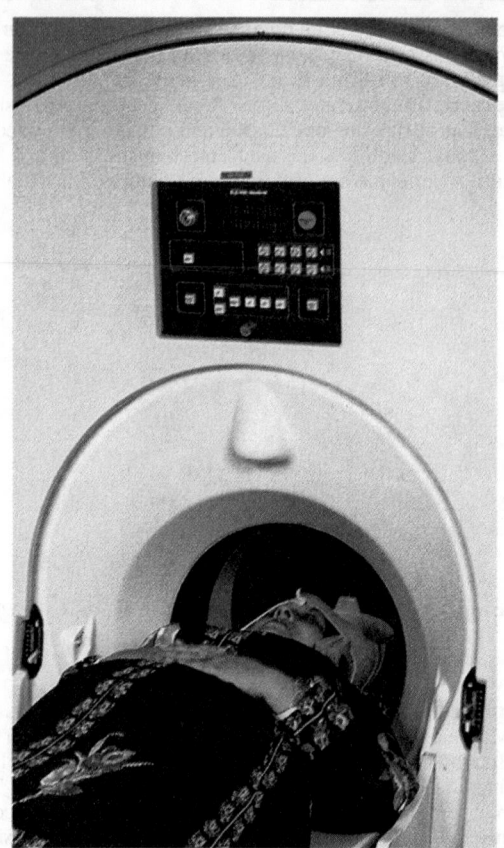

**Positioning of patient for computed tomography**
*(Perkin et al, 1986)*

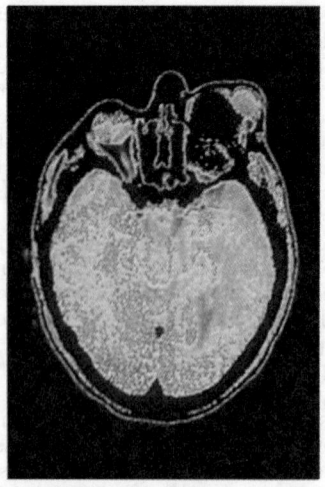

**Computed tomographic scan of the brain**
*(Seeley, Stephens, and Tate, 1995/Howard Sochurek; by permission of The McGraw-Hill Companies)*

**computed tomography portogram,** an x-ray test with contrast dye used to identify tumors of the liver smaller than 2 cm. The contrast medium is injected through a catheter in the splenic artery, rather than through a peripheral vein as in a routine CT scan.

**computer** [L *computare* to calculate], an electronic device that processes and stores large amounts of information very quickly. See also **analog computer, mainframe computer, microcomputer, minicomputer.**

**computer-assisted instruction (CAI),** a teaching process that uses a computer in the presentation of instructional materials, often in a way that requires the student to interact with it. Also called **computer-assisted learning (CAL).**

**computerized axial tomography.** See **computed tomography.**

**computer-managed instruction (CMI),** a system in which a computer is used to manage several aspects of instruction, including learning assessment through administration of pretests and posttests, design and preparation of learning prescriptions, and calculation, analysis, and storage of student scores.

**con-.** See **co-.**

**CONA,** abbreviation for **Canadian Orthopedic Nurses Association.**

**conation** /kōnā'shən/ [L, *conari,* to attempt], the mental process characterized by desire, impulse, volition, and striving. Compare **cognition. —conative,** *adj.*

**-conazole,** suffix designating a miconazole-type systemic antifungal agent.

**concanavalin A** /kon'kənav'əlin/, a protein isolated from the jack bean that reacts with polyglucosans in the blood of mammals and causes blood cells to agglutinate. It has been used in immunology to stimulate T cell production.

**concatenates** /kənkat'ənāts/, long molecules formed by continuous repeating of the same molecular subunit.

**concave** [L, *concavare,* to make hollow], curved like the interior of an arched circle. Compare **convex.**

**concave-convex joint relationship** /kon'kāv, konkāv'/, a relationship in which one of a joint's articulating surfaces is concave and the other is convex.

**concave spherical lens** [L, *concavare,* to make hollow;

Gk, *sphaira,* ball; L, *lentil*], a lens with curved, depressed surfaces that cause light rays to diverge. It is used for the management of myopia (nearsightedness).

**concavity** /kən′kav′itē/, a deep depression or inward curving surface of an organ or body structure.

**concealed accessory pathway** /kənsēld/ [L, *con,* together, *celare,* to hide], a connection between the atria and ventricles that is capable of retrograde conduction only. The electrocardiogram is normal (no delta wave) during sinus rhythm and is not associated with preexcitation, but the patient is prone to paroxysmal supraventricular tachycardia caused by orthodromic circus movement tachycardia. Conduction into the ventricles is normal during atrial fibrillation because the accessory pathway does not conduct in that direction.

**concealed hemorrhage,** the escape of blood from a ruptured vessel into internal organs or cavities.

**concealed junctional extrasystole,** an impulse that arises in and discharges the atrioventricular (AV) node or the AV bundle but fails to reach either the atria or the ventricles. It is identified by its blocking or delaying effect on subsequent AV conduction.

**conceive** /kənsēv′/ [L, *concipere,* to take together], to become pregnant.

**concentrate** /kon′səntrāt/ [L, *con* + *centrum,* center], **1.** to decrease the bulk of a liquid mixture and increase the quantity of dissolved substances per unit of volume by the removal of solvent through evaporation or other means. **2.** a substance, particularly a liquid, that has been strengthened and reduced in volume through such means.

**concentration**[1] /kon′sən·trā′shən/ [L, *concentratio*], **1.** increase in strength by evaporation. **2.** the ratio of the mass or volume of a solute to the mass or volume of the solution or solvent. See also **molality, molarity.**

**concentration**[2], a nursing outcome from the Nursing Outcome Classification (NOC) defined as ability to focus on a specific stimulus. See also **nursing outcomes classification.**

**concentration gradient,** a gradient across a membrane that separates a high concentration of a particular ion from a low concentration of the same ion.

**concentric** /kənsen′trik/ [L, *con* + *centrum,* center], describing two or more circles that have a common center.

**concentric contraction,** a common form of muscle contraction that occurs in rhythmic activities when the muscle fibers shorten as tension develops. See also **isotonic exercise.** Compare **eccentric contraction.**

**concentric fibroma,** a fibrous tumor surrounding the uterine cavity.

**concentric hypertrophy** [L, *con* + *centrum,* center; Gk, *hyper,* excessive, *trophe,* nourishment], a type of tissue overgrowth in which the walls of an organ continue to increase but the exterior size remains the same and the internal size diminishes.

**concept** [L, *concipere,* to take together], a construct or abstract idea or thought that originates and remains within the mind. **—conceptual,** *adj.*

**conception** /kənsep′shən/ [L, *concipere,* to take together], **1.** the beginning of pregnancy, usually taken to be the instant that a spermatozoon enters an ovum and forms a viable zygote. **2.** the act or process of fertilization. **3.** the act or process of creating an idea or notion. **4.** the idea or notion created; a general impression resulting from the interpretation of a symbol or set of symbols.

**conceptional age,** in fetal development the number of weeks since conception. Because the exact time of conception is difficult to determine, conceptional age is assumed to be 2 weeks less than gestational age.

**conception control.** See **contraception.**

**conceptive** /kənsep′tiv/ [L, *concipere,* to take together], **1.** able to become pregnant. **2.** pertaining to or characteristic of the mental process of forming ideas or impressions.

**conceptual.** See **concept.**

**conceptual disorder** /kənsep′choo·əl/ [L, *concipere,* to take together], a disturbance in thought processes, cognitive activities, or ability to formulate concepts.

**conceptual framework,** a group of concepts that are broadly defined and systematically organized to provide a focus, a rationale, and a tool for the integration and interpretation of information. Usually expressed abstractly through word models, a conceptual framework is the conceptual basis for many theories, as communication theory and general systems theory. Conceptual frameworks also provide a foundation and organization for the educational plan in schools of nursing.

**conceptus** /kənsep′təs/ [L, *concipere,* to take together], the product of conception; the fertilized ovum and its enclosing membranes at all stages of intrauterine development, from implantation to birth. See also **embryo, fetus.**

**concha** /kong′kə/, a body structure that is shell-shaped, as the cavity in the external ear that surrounds the external auditory canal meatus or patella or vulva.

**conchitis** /kongkī′tis/, an inflammation of a concha of the ear or nose.

**concoction** /kənkok′shən/ [L, *con* + *coquere,* to cook], a remedy prepared from a mixture of two or more drugs or substances that have been heated.

**concomitant** /konkom′itənt/ [L, *con* + *comitari,* to accompany], designating one or more of two or more things, occurring simultaneously, that may or may not be interrelated or produced as a result of the others; accompanying.

**concomitant strabismus,** a condition of crossed eyes in which the angle of squint is the same in all directions of gaze.

**concomitant symptom,** any symptom that accompanies a primary symptom.

**concordance** /kənkôr′dəns/ [L, *concordare,* to agree], the expression of one or more specific traits in both members of a pair of twins. Compare **discordance. —concordant,** *adj.*

**concrescence** /kən·kres′əns/ [L, *concrescere* to be formed], **1.** a growing together; a union of parts originally separate. **2.** (in embryology) the flowing together and piling up of cells. **3.** (in dentistry) the union of the roots of two adjacent teeth by a deposit of cementum.

**concreteness** /kənkrēt′nes/ [L, *concrescere,* to be formed], the content of a communication that includes specific feelings, behaviors, and experiences or situations.

**concrete operation** /kon′krēt, konkrēt′/, a thought process based on tangible rather than abstract points of reference.

**concrete thinking,** a stage in the development of the cognitive thought processes in the child. During this phase thought becomes increasingly logical and coherent so that the child is able to classify, sort, order, and organize facts while still being incapable of generalizing or dealing in abstractions. Problem solving is accomplished in a concrete, systematic fashion based on what is perceived, keeping to the literal meaning of words, as applying the word *horse* to a particular animal and not to horses in general. In Piaget's classification this stage occurs between 7 and 11 years of age, is preceded by syncretic thinking, and is followed by abstract thinking.

**concretion.** See **calculus.**

**concurrent infection** [L, *concurrere,* to run together, *inficere,* to stain], a condition during which a person has two or more simultaneous infections.

**concurrent nursing audit.** See **nursing audit.**

**concurrent review,** part of a utilization management program in which inpatient or home health care is reviewed as it is provided. Reviewers, usually nurses, monitor appropriateness of the care, the setting, and the progress of discharge plans. The ongoing review is directed at keeping costs as low as possible and maintaining effectiveness of care.

**concurrent sterilization,** a method of preparing an infant-feeding formula in which all ingredients and equipment are sterilized before mixing.

**concurrent validity,** validity of a test or a measurement tool that is established by simultaneously applying a previously validated tool or test to the same phenomenon, or data base, and comparing the results. Concurrent validity is achieved if the results are the same or similar at a statistically significant level. See also **validity.**

**concussion** /konkush′ən/ [L, *concutere,* to shake violently], **1.** damage to the brain caused by a violent jarring or shaking, such as a blow or an explosion. **2.** *informal.* **brain concussion.**

**condensation** /kon′dənsā′shən/ [L, *condensare,* to make thick], **1.** a reduction to a denser form, such as from water vapor to a liquid. **2.** (in psychology) a process often present in dreams in which two or more concepts are fused so that a single symbol represents the multiple components. In some cases of schizophrenia condensation, several thoughts and feelings fuse into a single verbal or nonverbal message and may be expressed in repetitive statements or gestures that can have a variety of meanings.

**condensation nuclei,** neutral particles, such as dust, in the atmosphere that are able to absorb or adsorb water and grow. At relatively high humidities they form fogs or hazes. Condensation nuclei consisting of sulfuric or nitric acid vapors or nitrogen oxides may be a source of respiratory irritants.

**condensed milk,** a thick liquid prepared by the evaporation of half of the water content of cow's milk.

**condenser,** an instrument for compacting restorative material into a prepared tooth cavity. It has a working end, or nib, with a flat or serrated face.

**condition** /kəndish′ən/ [L, *condicere,* to make arrangements], **1.** a state of being, specifically in reference to physical and mental health or well-being. **2.** anything that is essential to or restricts or modifies the appearance or occurrence of something else. **3.** to train a person or an animal, usually through specific exercises and repeated exposure to a particular state or thing. **4.** (in psychology) to subject a person or animal to conditioning or associative learning so that a specific stimulus always elicits a particular response. See also **classical conditioning.**

**conditional discharge** /kəndish′ənəl/, a specified leave of absence or liberty from a psychiatric hospital in which certain behaviors are expected from the patient and the original commitment order remains in effect. It may be referred to as a **pass** or **temporary absence.**

**conditioned avoidance response,** a learned reaction that is performed either consciously or unconsciously to avoid an unpleasant or painful stimulus.

**conditioned escape response,** a learned reaction that is performed either consciously or unconsciously to stop or to escape from an aversive stimulus.

**conditioned orientation response (COR),** the response, in a child under the age of 2 years, to turn his or her head toward the source of a sound. When the child responds appropriately by turning toward the sound, he or she is rewarded by seeing a toy move or light up. See also **visual response audiometry (VRA).**

**conditioned reflex,** a reflex developed gradually by training in association with a specific repeated external stimulus. An example of a conditioned reflex is that in Pavlov's experiment in which a dog salivates at the ringing of a bell if, over a period of time, every feeding is preceded by the bell-ringing stimulus.

**conditioned response,** an automatic reaction to a stimulus that does not normally elicit such response but has been learned through training. Such responses can be physical or psychologic and are produced by repeated association of some physiologic function or behavioral pattern with an unrelated stimulus or event. In Pavlov's classic experiments dogs learned to associate the sound of a ringing bell with feeding time so that they salivated at the sound of the bell, regardless of whether or not food was given to them. Also called **acquired reflex, behavior reflex, conditioned reflex, trained reflex.** Compare **unconditioned response.** See also **classical conditioning, operant conditioning.**

**conditioned stimulus** [L, *conditio* + *stimulus,* goad], any stimulus to which a reflex response has been conditioned by previous training or experience.

**conditioning** /kəndish′əning/ [L, *condicere,* to make arrangements], a form of learning based on the development of a response or set of responses to a stimulus or series of stimuli. Kinds of conditioning are **classical conditioning, instrumental conditioning,** and **operant conditioning.**

**condom** /kon′dəm/, a soft, flexible sheath made of plastic, rubber, or skin that covers the penis. Condoms prevent the exchange of body fluids during sexual activity, thereby preventing infection and conception. Also called **prophylactic,** *(informal)* **rubber.**

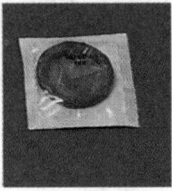

**Condom** *(Edge and Miller, 1994)*

**condom catheter,** a tube attached to a sheath for the penis. It is used to carry urine to a collecting bag.

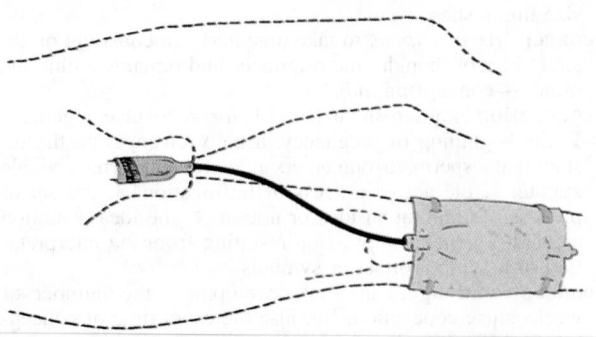

**Condom catheter** *(Elkin, Perry, and Potter, 1996)*

**conduct disorder** /kon′dukt/, (in psychiatry) an enduring set of behaviors that evolves over time. It is characterized by aggression and violations of the rights of others.

**conduction** /kənduk′shən/ [L, *conducere*, to lead], **1.** (in physics) a process in which heat is transferred from one substance to another because of a difference in temperature; a process in which energy is transmitted through a conductor. **2.** (in physiology) the process by which a nerve impulse is transmitted.

**conduction pathway,** the route followed by nerve impulses propagated along synaptically connected neurons.

**conduction system,** specialized tissue that carries electrical impulses, such as bundle branches and Purkinje fibers in the heart.

**conduction system of the heart,** the network of highly specialized muscle tissue that transmits the electrical impulses needed for a heartbeat. It includes the sinus and atrioventricular (AV) nodes, the conducting fibers between the nodes, the AV bundle (bundle of His), the left and right bundle branches, and the Purkinje fibers. See also **cardiac cycle.**

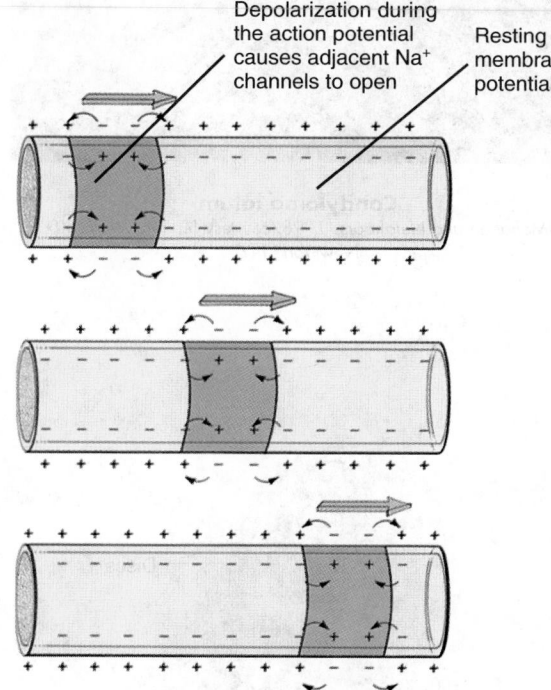

**Conduction of an action potential**
*(Thibodeau and Patton, 1999/Rolin Graphics)*

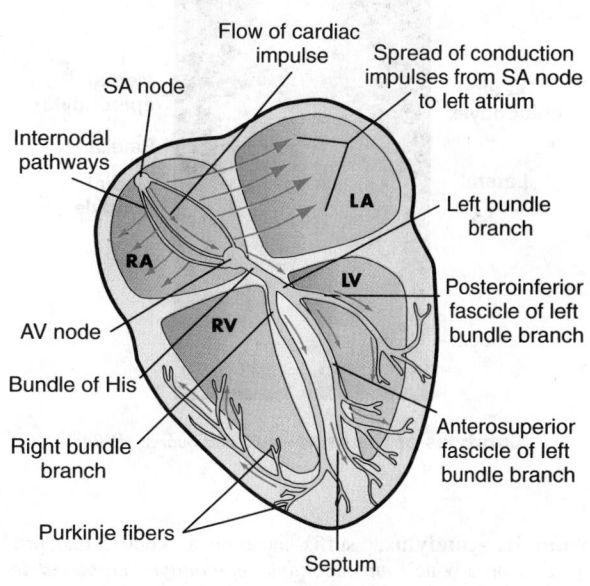

**Conduction system of the heart**
*(Lewis, Heitkemper, and Dirksen, 2000; modified from Kinney et al, 1996)*

**conduction anesthesia,** a loss of sensation, especially pain, in a region of the body, produced by injecting a local anesthetic along the course of a nerve or nerves to inhibit the conduction of impulses to and from the area supplied by that nerve or nerves. Also called **block anesthesia, nerve block anesthesia.** See also **regional anesthesia.**

**conduction aphasia,** a dissociative speech phenomenon in which a patient has no difficulty in comprehending words seen or heard and no dysarthria, yet has problems in self-expression. The patient may substitute words similar in sound or meaning for the correct ones but is unable to repeat from dictation, to spell, and to read aloud. The patient is alert and aware of the deficit. A common cause is an embolus in a branch of the middle cerebral artery. The nurse should try to reduce tension and frustration in the patient, encourage socialization, find alternate means of communication for the patient, use simple language and direct questions requiring simple answers, and help the family to understand the problem and deal with it. See also **aphasia.**

**conduction deafness.** See **conductive hearing loss.**

**conduction velocity,** the speed with which an electrical impulse can be transmitted through excitable tissue, as in the movement of a action potential through His-Purkinje fibers of the heart.

**conductive hearing loss** /kənduk′tiv/ [L, *conducere*, to lead], a form of hearing loss in which sound is inadequately conducted through the external or middle ear to the sensorineural apparatus of the inner ear. Sensitivity to sound is diminished, but clarity (interpretation of the sound) is not changed as long as the sound is sufficiently loud. Compare **sensorineural hearing loss.**

**conductivity,** the ability of an electric or other system to transmit sound, heat, light, or electromagnetic energy.

**conductor,** **1.** any substance through which electrons flow readily. **2.** (in psychiatry) a family therapist who uses his or her own personality to give direction to patients in therapy.

**conduit** /kon′dit, kon′doo·it/, **1.** an artificial channel or passage that connects two organs or different parts of the same organ. **2.** a tube or other device for conveying water or other fluids from one region to another.

**condylar fracture** /kon′dilər/ [Gk, *kondylos*, knuckle], any break in a condyle, a rounded projection on a bone at a hinge joint. Such fractures usually occur at the distal end of the humerus or the femur and frequently detach a bone fragment that includes the condyle.

**condylar guide,** a mechanical device on a dental articulator, designed to guide articular movement similar to that produced by the condyles in the temporomandibular joints. Compare **anterior guide.**

**condyle** /kon′dīl/ [Gk, *kondylos,* knuckle], a rounded projection at the end of a bone that anchors muscle ligaments and articulates with adjacent bones.

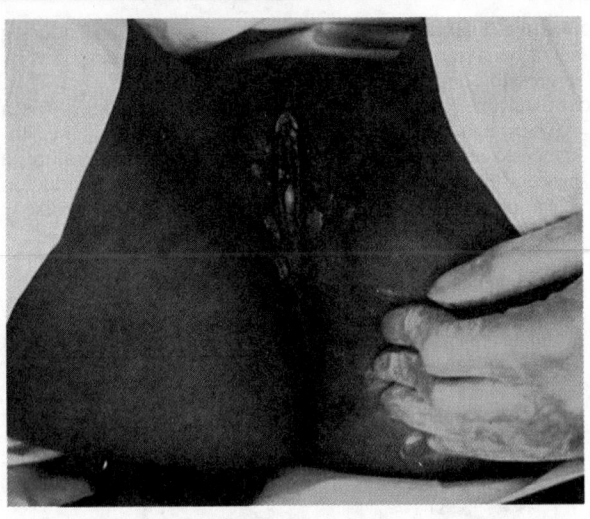

**Condyloma latum**
*(Monahan and Neighbors, 1998/courtesy Leonard Wolf, MD, New York, NY)*

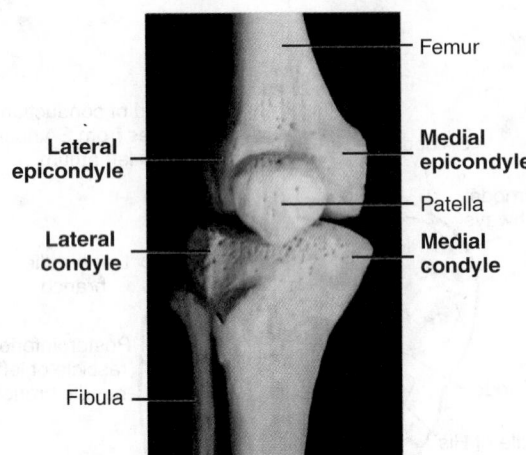

**Condyles of the knee** *(Vidic and Suarez, 1984)*

**-condyle, -condylus,** suffix meaning a 'knucklelike projection on a bone': *entepicondyle, epicondyle, entocondyle.*

**condyloid** /kon′diloid/ [Gk, *kondylos,* knuckle], resembling a knuckle.

**condyloid joint** [L, *kondylos + eidos,* form], a synovial joint in which a condyle is received into an elliptic cavity, as the wrist joint. A condyloid joint permits no axial rotation but allows flexion, extension, adduction, abduction, and circumduction. Also called **articulatio ellipsoidea.** Compare **ball-and-socket joint, pivot joint, saddle joint.** See also **joint.**

**condyloma** /kon′dilō′mə/, *pl.* **condylomas, condylomata** [Gk, *kondyloma,* a knob], a wartlike growth on the anus, vulva, or glans penis, usually sexually transmitted.

**condyloma acuminatum.** See **genital wart.**

**condyloma latum,** *pl.* **condylomata lata,**—a flat, moist papular growth that appears in secondary syphilis in the coronal sulcus of the perineum or on the glans penis.

**condylomatum acuminatum.** See **cervicitis.**

**-condylus.** See **-condyle.**

**cone** /kōn/ [Gk, *konos,* cone], **1.** a photoreceptor cell in the retina of the eye that enables a person to visualize colors. There are three kinds of retinal cones, one each for the colors blue, green, and red; other colors are seen by stimulation of more than one type of cone. **2.** a cone-shaped device attached to radiologic equipment to focus x-rays on a small target of tissue. See also **cone biopsy.** —**conic** /kon′ik/, **conical,** *adj.*

**cone biopsy,** surgical removal of a cone-shaped segment of the cervix, including both epithelial and endocervical tissue. The cone of tissue is excised and examined microscopi-

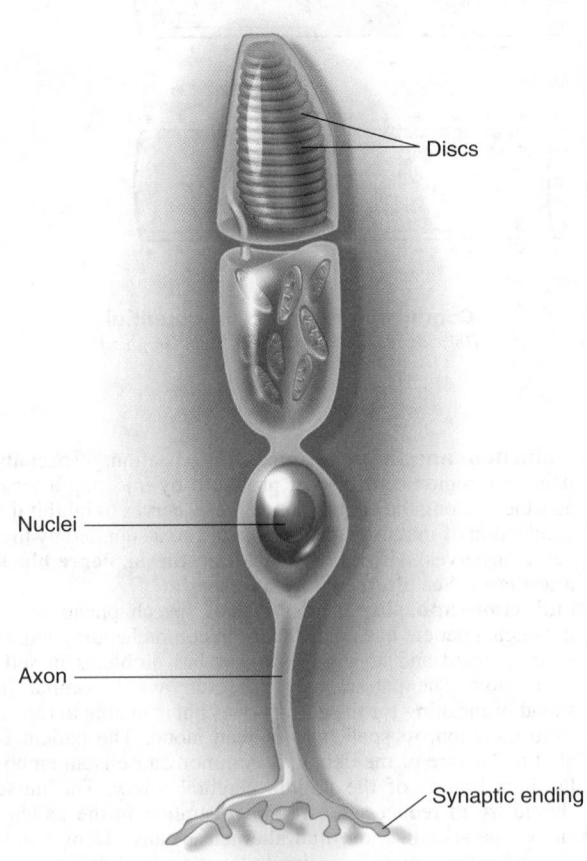

**Cone cell of the retina**

cally to establish a precise diagnosis, usually to confirm or evaluate a positive Papanicolaou's test result. After surgery hemorrhage sometimes occurs. If bleeding occurs 7 to 10 days later, suturing may be required. See also **biopsy, cone.**

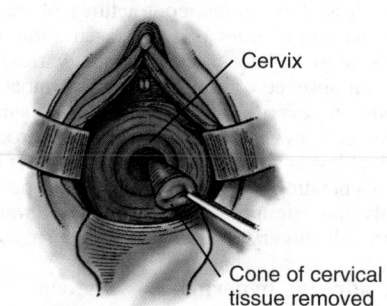

**Cone biopsy** *(Monahan and Neighbors, 1998)*

**cone cutting,** interference with an x-ray beam by a radiographic cone caused by misalignment of the tube, cone, and film. It may result in the loss of one portion of the radiographic image.

**cone of light,** **1.** a triangular reflection observed during an ear examination when the light of an otoscope is focused on the image of the malleus. **2.** the group of light rays entering the pupil of the eye and forming an image on the retina.

**confabulation** /kənfab'yəlā'shən/ [L, *con + fabulari,* to speak], the fabrication of experiences or situations, often recounted in a detailed and plausible way to fill in and cover up gaps in memory. The phenomenon occurs principally as a defense mechanism and is most commonly used by alcoholics, especially those who have Korsakoff's psychosis, and persons with head injuries, amnesic disorders, dementia, or lead poisoning. Also called **fabrication.**

**confession** /kənfesh'ən/, an act of seeking expiation through another from guilt for a real or imagined transgression.

**confidence coefficient** [L, *confidere,* to rely on; L, *coefficiens*], the probability that a confidence interval will contain the true value of the population parameter. For example, if the confidence coefficient is .95, 95 per cent of the confidence intervals so calculated for each of a large number of random samples would contain the parameter.

**confidence interval** [L, *confidere,* to rely on; L, *intervallum,* area within ramparts], a type of statistical interval estimate for an unknown parameter: a range of values believed to contain the parameter, with a predetermined degree of confidence. Its endpoints are the **confidence limits** and it has a stated probability (the **confidence coefficient**) of containing the parameter.

**confidence limits** [L, *confidere,* to rely on; L, *limes,* limit], the endpoints or boundaries of a confidence interval, delineating the minimum and maximum values of the range expected to contain the parameter.

**confidentiality** /kon'fiden'shē·al'itē/, the nondisclosure of information except to another authorized person.

**configuration** /kənfig'yərā'shən/ [L, *configuare,* to form from], the hardware, software, and peripherals assembled to work as a computer unit in a specific situation.

**configurationism.** See **Gestalt psychology.**

**confinement** /kənfīn'mənt/ [L, *confinis,* common boundary], **1.** a state of being held or restrained within a specific place in order to hinder or minimize activity. **2.** the final phase of pregnancy during which labor and childbirth occur. See also **puerperium.**

**confinement deprivation,** an emotional disorder that may result when an individual is separated from familiar surroundings or denied contact with familiar persons or objects. It may occur when one is confined to a single room.

**conflict** /kon'flikt/ [L, *conflictere,* to strike together], **1.** a mental struggle, either conscious or unconscious, resulting from the simultaneous presence of opposing or incompatible thoughts, ideas, goals, or emotional forces, such as impulses, desires, or drives. **2.** a painful state of consciousness caused by the arousal of such opposing forces and the inability to resolve them; a kind of stress found to a certain degree in every person. **3.** (in psychoanalysis) the unconscious emotional struggle between the demands of the id and those of the ego and superego or between the demands of the ego and the restrictions imposed by society. Kinds of conflict include **approach-approach conflict, approach-avoidance conflict, avoidance-avoidance conflict, extrapsychic conflict,** and **intrapsychic conflict.**

**conflict mediation,** a nursing intervention from the Nursing Interventions Classification (NIC) defined as facilitation of constructive dialogue between opposing parties with a goal of resolving disputes in a mutually acceptable manner. See also **Nursing Interventions Classification.**

**confluence of the sinuses** /kon'floo·əns/ [L, *confluere,* to flow together], the wide union of the superior sagittal, the straight, and the occipital sinuses with the two large transverse sinuses of the dura mater. The right transverse sinus usually receives most of the blood from the superior sagittal sinus; the left transverse sinus receives the blood from the straight sinus. The confluence is one of six posterior superior sinuses of the dura matter, draining blood from the section and an inner bulging granular section.

**confluent** /kon'floo·ənt/ [L, *confluere,* to flow together], running together, such as the sinuses of the dura mater, or some skin eruptions.

**confrontation test** /kon'frəntā'shən/ [L, *con + frons,* forehead], a method of assessing a patient's visual field by moving an object into the periphery of each of the visual

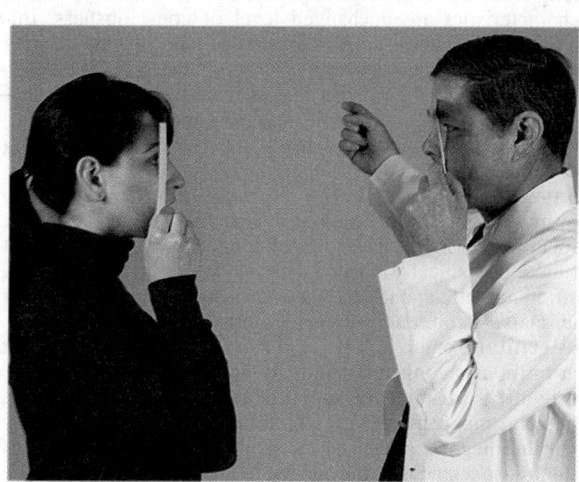

**Confrontation test** *(Seidel et al, 1999)*

quadrants. The test is conducted while one eye is covered and the vision of the other is fixed on a point straight ahead. The patient reports when the moving object, which may be the examiner's finger, is first detected at the edge of the visual field.

**confusion** /kənfyoō'shən/ [L, *confundere,* to mingle], a mental state characterized by disorientation regarding time, place, person, or situation. It causes bewilderment, perplexity, lack of orderly thought, and inability to choose or act decisively and perform the activities of daily living. It is usually symptomatic of an organic mental disorder, but it may accompany severe emotional stress and various psychologic disorders. —**confusional,** *adj.*

**confusion, acute,** a nursing diagnosis accepted by the Eleventh National Conference on the Classification of Nursing Diagnoses. It is defined as the abrupt onset of a cluster of global, transient changes and disturbances in attention, cognition, psychomotor activity, level of consciousness, and/or sleep/wake cycle.
■ DEFINING CHARACTERISTICS: The major defining characteristics are fluctuation in cognition, sleep/wake cycle, level of consciousness, or psychomotor activity; increased agitation or restlessness; misperceptions; and lack of motivation to initiate or follow through with goal-directed or purposeful behavior. A minor defining characteristic is hallucinations.
■ RELATED FACTORS: Related factors include age over 60 years, dementia, alcohol abuse, drug abuse, and delirium. See also **nursing diagnosis.**

**confusional state,** a mild form of delirium. It may occur in any age group or may accompany preexisting brain disease. It may be triggered by a sudden or unexpected change in the person's environment. The confusion may be characterized by failure to perform activities of daily living, memory deficits, disruptive behavior, and inappropriate speech.

**confusion, chronic,** a nursing diagnosis accepted by the Eleventh National Conference on the Classification of Nursing Diagnoses. It is defined as an irreversible long-standing and/or progressive deterioration of intellect and personality characterized by decreased ability to interpret environmental stimuli and decreased capacity to perform intellectual thought processes; it is manifested by disturbances of memory, orientation, and behavior.
■ DEFINING CHARACTERISTICS: The major defining characteristics are clinical evidence of organic impairment, altered interpretation of or response to stimuli, and progressive or long-standing cognitive impairment. The minor defining characteristics are unchanged level of consciousness, impaired socialization, impaired memory (short term and long term), and altered personality.
■ RELATED FACTORS: Related factors include Alzheimer's disease, Korsakoff's psychosis, multi-infarct dementia, cerebrovascular accident, and head injury. See also **nursing diagnosis.**

**congener** /kon'jənər/ [L, *con* + *genus,* origin], one of two or more things that are similar or closely related in structure, function, or origin. Examples of congeners are muscles that function identically, chemical compounds similar in composition and effect, and species of the same genus of plants or animals. —**congenerous** /kənjen'ərəs/, *adj.*

**congenital** /kənjen'itəl/ [L, *congenitus,* born with], present at birth, as a congenital anomaly or defect.

**congenital absence of sacrum and lumbar vertebrae,** an abnormal condition present at birth and characterized by varying degrees of deformity, ranging from the absence of the lower segment of the coccyx to the absence of the entire sacrum and all lumbar vertebrae. Congenital absence of the sacrum and the lumbar vertebrae is relatively rare. Lesser degrees of this anomaly may present so few signs that marked deformities are not present, and the condition may not be diagnosed unless accidentally found on radiographic examination. More severe forms display gross deformities and neurologic deficits. Signs and symptoms of the more severe kinds include short stature, flattened buttocks, muscle paralysis to varying degrees, muscle atrophy in the lower extremities, foot deformities, contractures of the hips and knees, and varying degrees of loss of sensation, especially sensation distal to the knees. The treatment varies greatly for the congenital absence of the sacrum and lumbar vertebrae and depends on severity. Surgical intervention may be reconstructive or may involve disarticulation procedures at various spinal levels and subsequent fusion of the remaining vertebrae. Depending on the severity, many patients with this anomaly gain enough stability to sit and to walk with assistance through surgery. The most severe forms are usually fatal.

**congenital adrenal hyperplasia,** a group of disorders that have in common an enzyme defect resulting in low levels of cortisol and increased secretion of adrenocorticotrophic hormone. The net effects are adrenal gland overgrowth and increased production of cortisol precursors and androgens. During intrauterine life the disorder leads to pseudohermaphroditism in female infants and macrogenitosomia in male infants. Treatment involves hydrocortisone therapy and reconstructive surgery. See also **adrenal virilism, macrogenitosomia, pseudohermaphroditism.**

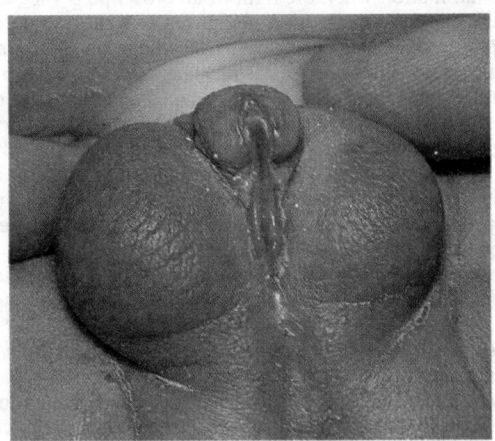

**Congenital adrenal hyperplasia** *(Zitelli and Davis, 1997)*

**congenital amputation,** the absence of a fetal limb or part at birth. The condition previously was attributed to amputation by constricting bands in utero but now is regarded as a developmental defect. See also **amputee.**

**congenital anomaly,** any abnormality present at birth, particularly a structural one, which may be inherited genetically, acquired during gestation, or inflicted during parturition. Also called **birth defect.**

**congenital aspiration pneumonia** [L, *congenitus,* born with, *aspirare,* to breathe upon; Gk, *pneumon,* lung], a neonatal lung inflammation caused by the aspiration of fluid or meconium during labor.

**congenital cardiac anomaly,** any structural or functional abnormality or defect of the heart or great vessels present at birth. Congenital heart anomalies are a major cause of neonatal distress and the most common cause of death in the newborn other than problems related to prematurity. Approximately 90% of all deaths from congenital heart anomalies occur during the first year of life. Congenital heart defects may be inherited or result from environmental factors, such as maternal infection or exposure to radiation or noxious substances during pregnancy. Most defects are probably caused by an interaction between inherited and environmental factors that results in arrested embryonic development. Congenital heart anomalies are classified as broadly cyanotic, in which unoxygenated blood mixes with oxygenated blood in the systemic circulation, and acyanotic, in which such mixing does not occur. The general effects of cardiac malformations on cardiovascular functioning are increased cardiac workload, increased pulmonary vascular resistance, inadequate cardiac output, and, in the case of cyanotic anomalies, decreased oxygen saturation. The general physical symptoms of these pathophysiologic alterations are growth retardation, decreased exercise tolerance, recurrent respiratory infections, dyspnea, tachypnea, tachycardia, cyanosis, tissue hypoxia, and murmurs, all of which vary in severity, depending on the type and degree of the defect. Kinds of congenital cardiac anomalies include **atrial septal defect, coarctation of the aorta, tetralogy of Fallot, transposition of the great vessels, tricuspid atresia,** and **ventricular septal defect.** Also called **congenital heart disease.** See also **aortic stenosis, patent ductus arteriosus, pulmonary stenosis, valvular stenosis.**

**congenital cataracts.** See **cataract.**

**congenital cerebral diplegia.** See **cerebral palsy.**

**congenital cloaca.** See **persistent cloaca.**

**congenital cyanosis** [L, *congenitus,* born with; Gk, *kyanos,* blue, *osis,* condition], cyanosis present at birth caused by a congenital heart disease or atelectasis of the lungs. See also **blue baby.**

**congenital cyst** [L, *congenitus,* born with; Gk, *kystis,* bag], a cyst present at birth, as a dermoid cyst resulting from an embryonic defect in the skin or midline structures.

**congenital cytomegalovirus (CMV) disease.** See **cytomegalic inclusion disease.**

**congenital dermal sinus,** a channel present at birth, extending from the surface of the body and passing between the bodies of two adjacent lumbar vertebrae to the spinal canal.

**congenital dislocation of the hip (CDH),** an orthopedic defect, present at birth, in which the head of the femur does not articulate with the acetabulum as a result of an abnormal shallowness of the acetabulum. Treatment consists of maintaining continuous abduction of the thigh so that the head of the femur presses into the center of the shallow cavity, causing it to deepen. Also called **congenital dysplasia of the hip, congenital subluxation of the hip.** See also **Frejka splint.**

**congenital ectodermal defect.** See **anhidrotic ectodermal dysplasia.**

**congenital erythropoietic porphyria** [L, *congenitus,* born with; Gk, *erythros,* red, *poein,* to make, *porphyros,* purple], a rare autosomal recessive trait caused by a defect in hemoglobin synthesis in erythrocytes and release of porphyrin from normoblasts in the bone marrow. The porphyrin is excreted in the urine. Symptoms may include dermatitis, enlarged spleen, and hemolytic anemia.

**congenital facial diplegia.** See **Möbius' syndrome.**

**congenital generalized fibromatosis,** the presence of small, hard, round fibromas of the subcutaneous and muscle tissues, the viscera, and the osseous systems, usually at

birth. Visceral involvement may cause symptoms such as intestinal obstruction, diarrhea, and respiratory disturbances. Death is usually during the first few months of life.

**congenital glaucoma,** a rare form of glaucoma affecting infants and young children, which results from a congenital closure of the iridocorneal angle by a membrane that obstructs the flow of aqueous humor and increases the intraorbital pressure. The condition is progressive, is usually bilateral, and may damage the optic nerve. It may be corrected surgically. Also called **buphthalmos, hydrophthalmos.**

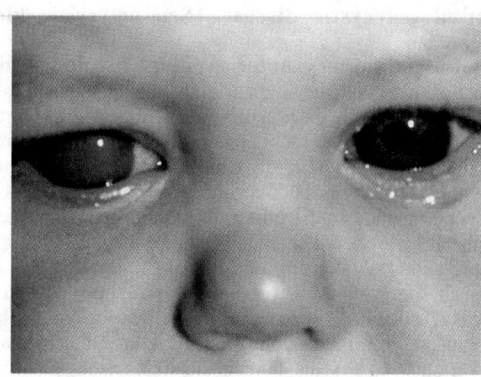

**Congenital glaucoma** (Zitelli and Davis, 1997)

**congenital goiter,** an enlargement of the thyroid gland at birth. It may be caused by a deficiency of enzymes or iodine required for the production of thyroxine.

**congenital heart disease.** See **congenital cardiac anomaly.**

**congenital hernia** [L, *congenitus,* born with, *hernia,* rupture], a hernia caused by a defect present at birth, as an umbilical hernia.

**congenital hypogammaglobulinemia** [L, *congenitus,* born with; Gk, *hypo,* deficiency, *gamma,* third letter of Greek alphabet; L, *globus,* small globe, *haima,* blood], a genetic disease characterized by a deficiency of gamma globulin and antibody in the serum. The cause may be a genetic defect leading to a failure of development of a normal β-lymphocyte system and immune responses.

**congenital hypoplastic anemia.** See **Diamond-Blackfan syndrome.**

**congenital immunity** [L, *congenitus,* born with, *immunis,* free from], the immunity one has at birth that is acquired from the mother's antibodies as they pass through the placenta.

**congenital jaundice** [L, *congenitus,* born with; Fr, *jaune,* yellow], jaundice present at birth or during the first 24 hours of life. It is usually caused by poorly developed bile ducts.

**congenital laryngeal stridor** [L, *congenitus,* born with; Gk, *larynx* + L, *stridens,* a grating noise], a harsh respiratory sound that some infants make the first weeks after birth.

**congenital lobar emphysema** [L, *congenitus,* born with; Gk, *lobos,* lobe; Gk, *en,* in + *physema,* a blowing], a condition characterized by overinflation, commonly affecting one of the upper lobes and causing respiratory distress in early life; also called **congenital lobar overinflation.**

**congenital lymphedema.** See **Milroy's disease.**

**congenital megacolon.** See **Hirschsprung's disease.**

**congenital nonspherocytic hemolytic anemia,** a group of blood disorders made up of a number of similar inherited diseases, each with a deficiency of one of the enzymes of red cell glycolysis. Most are associated with varying degrees of hemolysis, but all are less severe than and are to be differentiated from the more serious disorder associated with spherocytosis. Compare **hemolytic anemia, spherocytic anemia.** See also **elliptocytosis, glucose-6-phosphate dehydrogenase (G-6-PD) deficiency, heme, sickle cell anemia.**

**congenital oculofacial paralysis.** See **Möbius' syndrome.**

**congenital pancytopenia.** See **Fanconi's anemia**.

**congenital polycystic disease.** See **polycystic kidney disease.**

**congenital pulmonary arteriovenous fistula,** a direct connection between the arterial and venous systems of the lung present at birth that results in a right-to-left shunt and permits unoxygenated blood to enter the systemic circulation. The anomaly is probably caused by faulty development of the network of vessels covering the embryonic lungs. It is often accompanied by hereditary hemorrhagic telangiectasis (Rendu-Osler-Weber disease). The fistula may be single or multiple and may occur in any part of the lung; if it is in an accessible site, surgical correction is the method of treatment.

**congenital rubella syndrome,** a collection of birth defects caused by transmission of the rubella virus from an infected mother to a fetus during the first trimester of pregnancy. Anomalies include cataracts, congenital heart disease, and sensorineural hearing loss. The infant may be small for gestational age and exhibit hyperbilirubinemia, thrombocytopenia, and hepatomegaly.

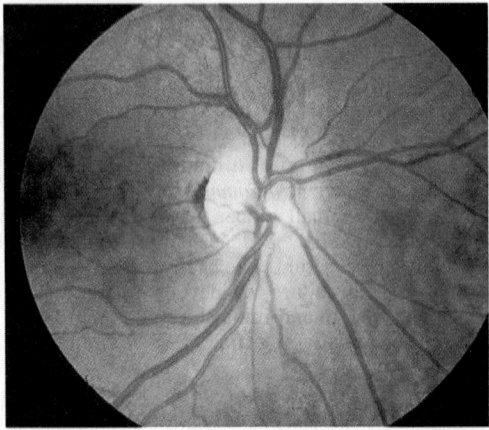

**Hyperpigmentation and hypopigmentation of the retina in congenital rubella syndrome** *(Stone and Gorbach, 2000)*

**congenital scoliosis,** an abnormal condition present at birth, characterized by a lateral curvature of the spine. It results from specific congenital rib and vertebral anomalies. The causative and pathologic characteristics of congenital scoliosis are divided into six categories. Category I is associated with partial unilateral failure of the formation of a vertebra. Category II is associated with complete unilateral failure of the formation of a vertebra. Category III is associ-

ated with bilateral failure of segmentation with the absence of disk space. Category IV is associated with the unilateral failure of segmentation with the unsegmented bar. Category V is associated with the fusion of ribs. Category VI is associated with any condition not covered in the other categories. Category IV scoliosis seems to progress more rapidly and cause the greatest degree of deformity. The degree of obvious deformity caused by congenital scoliosis depends on the cause of the disease. The deformity increases with growth and age, usually progressing slowly during periods of slow growth of the trunk of the body. Treatment of congenital scoliosis may be surgical or nonsurgical. Some kinds of nonsurgical treatment techniques are exercise programs and use of orthotic devices, such as scoliosis splints, a Milwaukee brace, a Risser localizer, or a turnbuckle cast. Surgical intervention in this disease may involve an anterior or a posterior spinal fusion. In a few individuals, additional procedures, such as spinal osteotomy, use of the Harrington rod, or halo traction, may be required. See also **scoliosis.**

**congenital short neck syndrome,** a rare congenital malformation of the cervical spine in which the cervical vertebrae are fused, usually in pairs, into one mass of bone; this fusion causes decreased neck motion and decreased cervical length, sometimes with neurologic involvement. The posterior portion of the laminar arches in the cervical area is not fully developed; the result is spina bifida in the cervical region, usually involving the lower cervical vertebrae and, in some cases, one or more of the upper thoracic vertebrae. Congenital short neck syndrome is often associated with a cervical rib or with hemivertebrae. Neurologic complications, such as nerve-root compression and peripheral nerve symptoms, are secondary to deformities of the vertebral bodies. The extreme shortness of the neck is the most common sign of this deformity, which allows only limited motion, lateral bending, and rotation. When the deformity involves nerve-root compression, symptoms of peripheral nerve involvement, as pain or a burning sensation, may be evident, accompanied by paralysis, hyperesthesia, or paresthesia. Involvement of the spinal cord may present signs of abnormalities of lower extremities with associated signs of an upper motor lesion. Congenital short neck syndrome may require no treatment. Mild associated symptoms may be alleviated with traction, cast application, or cervical collars. Surgery may be required to relieve neurologic manifestations. Also called **Klippel-Feil syndrome.**

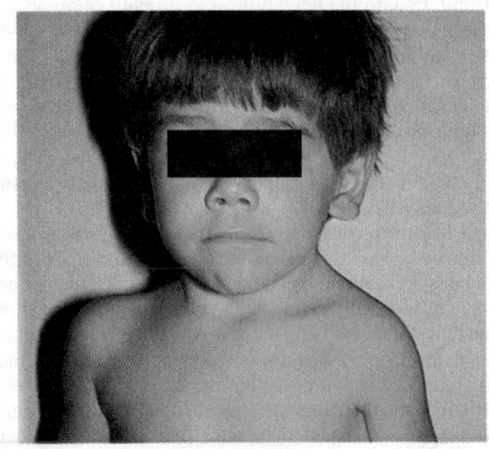

**Congenital short neck syndrome** *(Zitelli and Davis, 1997)*

**congenital subluxation of the hip.** See **congenital dislocation of the hip.**

**congenital syphilis** [L, *congenitus,* born with; Gk, *syn,* together, *philein,* to love], a form of syphilis acquired in utero. It is generally characterized by osteitis, rashes, coryza, and wasting in the first months of life. Later childhood signs of the infection include interstitial keratitis, deafness, and notches in the incisor teeth. Some infected infants may appear disease-free at birth; but typical signs of the disease develop in adolescence. Infants are treated with penicillin; all infected infants require an ophthalmic examination. If untreated, the infection may cause deafness, blindness, crippling, or death.

**congested** /kənjes′tid/, having an excessive accumulation of a substance such as blood. The condition may be the result of increased production of the substance and/or outflow of the substance. It also can result from a decreased ability of the heart to pump.

**congestion** /kənjes′chən/ [L, *congerere,* to accumulate], an abnormal accumulation of fluid in an organ or body area. The fluid is often mucus, but it may be bile or blood.

**congestive** /kənjes′tiv/, pertaining to congestion.

**congestive atelectasis.** See **adult respiratory distress syndrome.**

**congestive cardiomyopathy** [L, *congerere,* to accumulate; Gk, *kardia,* heart, *mys,* muscle, *pathos,* disease], a heart muscle disease characterized by heart failure and enlargement.

**congestive dysmenorrhea** [L, *congerere,* to accumulate; Gk, *dys,* difficult, *men,* month, *rhein,* to flow], a form of secondary dysmenorrhea caused by pelvic congestion, which arises from an increased blood supply in the area caused by pelvic disease.

**congestive heart failure (CHF),** an abnormal condition that reflects impaired cardiac pumping. Its causes include myocardial infarction, ischemic heart disease, and cardiomyopathy. Failure of the ventricles to eject blood efficiently results in volume overload, ventricular dilation, and elevated intracardiac pressure. Increased pressure in the left side of the heart causes pulmonary congestion; increased pressure in the right side causes systemic venous congestion and peripheral edema. See also **heart failure.**

**congestive splenomegalia** [L, *congerere,* to accumulate; Gk, *splen* + *megas,* large], an enlarged spleen associated with gastric hemorrhage, anemia, portal hypertension, and cirrhosis of the liver. Also called **Banti's syndrome, congestive splenomegaly, hepatolienal fibrosis.**

**conglomerate silicosis** /kənglom′ərit/ [L, *con* + *glomerare,* to wind into a ball], a severe form of silicosis marked by conglomerate masses of mineral dust in the lungs, causing acute shortness of breath, coughing, and production of sputum. The conglomerates may encroach on the pulmonary circulation, causing pulmonary hypertension, right ventricular hypertrophy, and complete disability. Cor pulmonale usually develops.

**Congolese red fever.** See **murine typhus.**

**Congress for Nursing Practice,** a unit of the American Nurses Association whose activities concern the scope of nursing practice, legal aspects of nursing practice, public recognition of the significance of nursing practice in health care, and implications of health care trends for nursing practice.

**congruent communication** /kong′groō·ənt/, a communication pattern in which the person sends the same message on both verbal and nonverbal levels.

**-conia,** suffix meaning 'small particles in the (specified) fluid or part of the body': *chondroconia, otoconia, statoconia.*

**conic, conical.** See **cone.**

**conic papilla.** See **papilla.**

**conium.** See **hemlock.**

**conization** /kon′īzā′shən/, the removal of a cone-shaped sample of tissue, as in a cone biopsy.

**conjoined manipulation** /kənjoind′/ [L, *con* + *jungere,* to yoke together], the use of both hands in obstetric and gynecologic procedures, with one positioned in the vagina and the other on the abdomen.

**conjoined tendon.** See **inguinal falx.**

**conjoined twins,** two fetuses developed from the same ovum who are physically united at birth. The defect ranges from a superficial anatomic union of varying extent between equally or nearly equally formed fetuses to one in which only a part of the body is duplicated or in which a small, incompletely developed fetus, or parasite, is attached to a more fully formed one, the autosite. Conjoined twins result when separation of the blastomeres in early embryonic development does not occur until a late cleavage phase and is incomplete, causing the fused condition. Viability depends on the extent of the fusion and the degree of development of the fetuses. See also **Siamese twins.**

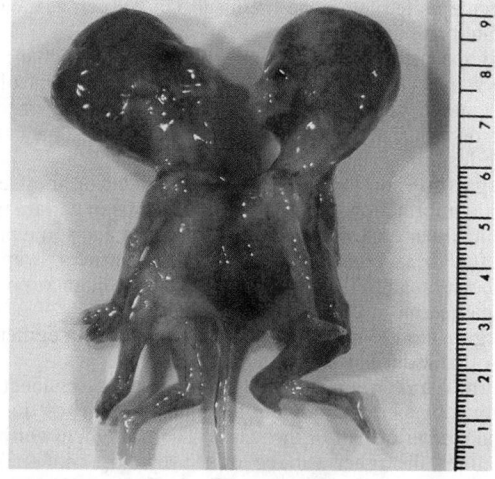

**Conjoined twins at 12 weeks of development**
*(Moore, Persaud, and Shiota, 2000/courtesy Dr. D.K. Kalousek, Department of Pathology, University of British Columbia, Children's Hospital, Vancouver, BC, Canada)*

**conjoint family therapy** /kənjoint′/, a form of psychotherapy in which a therapist sees a single nuclear family and addresses the issues and problems raised by family members.

**conjugata** /kon′jəgā′tə/ [L, *conjugere,* to yoke together], pertaining to the combined diameters of the pelvis, measured from the center of the promontory of sacrum to the back of the symphysis pubis.

**conjugate** /kon′jəgit/ [L, *con* + *jungere,* to yoke together], (in pelvimetry) the measurement of the female pelvis to determine whether the presenting part of a fetus can enter the birth canal. See also **diagonal conjugate, true conjugate.**

**conjugated bilirubin.** See **bilirubin.**

**conjugated estrogen** /kon′jəgā′tid/, a mixture of sodium salts of estrogen sulfates, chiefly those of estrone, equilin, and 17-alpha-dihydroequilin. Conjugated estrogens may be prescribed to relieve postmenopausal vasomotor symptoms, such as hot flushes; to treat atrophic vaginitis, female hypogonadism, primary ovarian failure; and to provide palliation in advanced prostatic carcinoma and metastatic breast cancer in selected patients. The drug is also used to treat and prevent osteoporosis. Continued use of estrogens can increase the risk of endometrial carcinoma, gallbladder disease, and thromboembolic disorders; because of the danger of damage to the fetus all female sex hormones are contraindicated during pregnancy. Among the adverse effects of conjugated estrogens are breakthrough bleeding, breast tenderness, nausea, headache, water retention, and skin eruptions.

**conjugate deviation** [L, *conjugere,* to yoke together, *deviare,* to turn aside], pertaining to movements of the two eyes in which their visual axes function in parallel. The cause is a dysfunction of the ocular muscles, which allows the eyes to diverge to the same side when at rest.

**conjugated hyperbilirubinemia,** hyperbilirubinemia caused by defective excretion of conjugated bilirubin by the liver cells or by anatomic obstruction to bile flow within the liver or in the extrahepatic bile duct system; it includes **Dubin-Johnson syndrome** and **Rotor's syndrome.**

**conjugated protein,** a compound that contains a protein molecule united to a nonprotein substance, such as a carbohydrate or lipid.

**conjugate paralysis** [L, *conjugere,* to yoke together; Gk, *paralyein,* to be palsied], a condition of paralysis of the conjugate movements of the two eyes, up or down, or to the right or left. There is no diplopia. The cause is a cranial nerve lesion.

**conjugation** /kon'jəgā'shən/, an exchange or transfer of genetic information between two individuals in certain types of unicellular organisms, including bacteria and some protozoa. In *Paramecium,* for example, both partners swap micronuclear material. The exchanged material is incorporated and passed on to progeny after replication.

**conjugon** /kon'jo͞ogon/, an extrachromosomal segment of DNA that induces bacterial conjugation.

**conjunctiva** /kon'jungktī'və/ [L, *conjunctivus,* connecting], the mucous membrane lining the inner surfaces of the eyelids and anterior part of the sclera. The **palpebral conjunctiva** lines the inner surface of the eyelids and is thick, opaque, and highly vascular. The **bulbar conjunctiva** is loosely connected, thin, and transparent, covering the sclera of the anterior third of the eye.

**conjunctival burns** /-ī'vəl/, chemical burns of the conjunctiva. Emergency treatment involves irrigating the eye with copious amounts of water until the chemical has been neutralized, as indicated by paper pH indicators. A topical ophthalmic anesthetic may be instilled to relieve pain. Emergency medical care should be sought.

**conjunctival edema.** See **chemosis.**

**conjunctival fornix.** See **inferior conjunctival fornix, superior conjunctival fornix.**

**conjunctival reflex,** a protective mechanism of the eye in which the eyelids close whenever the conjunctiva is touched. Compare **corneal reflex.**

**conjunctival ring,** a narrow ring at the junction of the conjunctiva and the periphery of the cornea. Also called **annulus conjunctivae.**

**conjunctival sac** [L, *conjunctivus,* connecting; Gk, *sakkos*], the potential space enclosed by the conjunctiva and the eyelids.

**conjunctival test,** a procedure used to identify offending allergens by instilling the eye with a dilute solution of the al-

lergenic extract. A positive reaction in the allergic patient causes tearing and redness of the conjunctiva within 5 to 15 minutes. See also **allergy testing.**

**conjunctivitis** /kənjungk'tivī'tis/, inflammation of the conjunctiva, caused by bacterial or viral infection, allergy, or environmental factors. Red eyes, thick discharge, sticky eyelids in the morning, and inflammation without pain are characteristic results of the most common cause, bacteria. The cause may be found by microscopic examination or bacteriologic culture of the discharge. Choice of treatment depends on the causative agent and may include antibacterial agents, antibiotics, or corticosteroids. Also called **pinkeye.** See also **choroiditis, uveitis.**

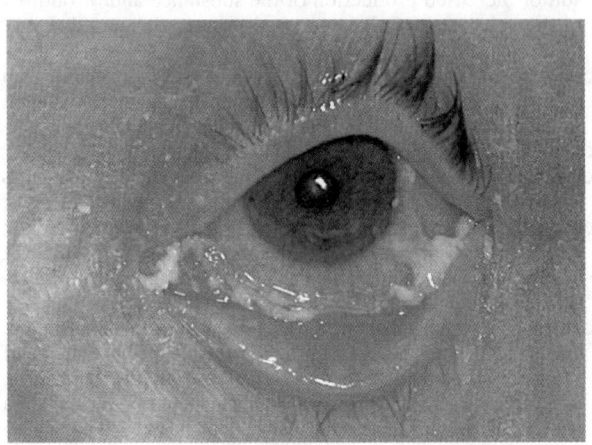

**Acute conjunctivitis** *(Newell, 1996)*

**conjunctivitis of newborn** [L, *conjunctivus,* connecting, *itis,* inflammation; ME, *newe + borne*], a condition characterized by a purulent discharge from the eyes of an infant during the first 3 weeks of life. Frequent causes include gonococcal and chlamydial infections, which may lead to blindness if untreated. Also called **ophthalmia neonatorum.**

**connecting fibrocartilage** [L, *con + nectere,* to bind], a disk of fibrocartilage found between many joints, especially those with limited mobility, such as the spinal vertebrae. Each disk is composed of concentric rings of fibrous tissue separated by cartilaginous laminae. The disk swells outward if it is compressed by the vertebrae above or below. Compare **circumferential fibrocartilage, interarticular fibrocartilage, stratiform fibrocartilage.**

**connective** /kənek'tiv/[L, *cum,* together with, *nectere,* to bind], pertaining to a binding or connection.

**connective tissue,** tissue that supports and binds other body tissue and parts. It derives from the mesoderm of the embryo and is dense, containing large numbers of cells and large amounts of intercellular material. The intercellular material is composed of fibers in a matrix or ground substance that may be liquid, gelatinous, or solid, such as in bone and cartilage. Connective tissue fibers may be collagenous or elastic. The matrix or ground material surrounding fibers and cells is a dynamic substance, susceptible to its own special diseases. Kinds of connective tissue are **bone tissue, cartilage tissue, dense connective tissue, fibrous tissue,** and **loose connective tissue.**

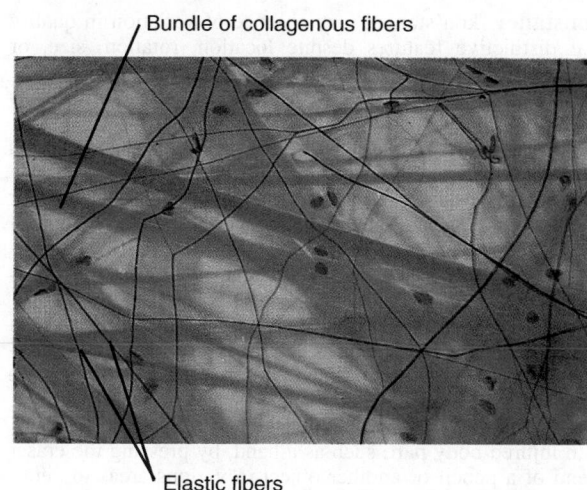

Bundle of collagenous fibers

Elastic fibers

**Loose connective tissue** *(© Ed Reschke; used with permission)*

**connective tissue disease.** See **collagen vascular disease.**

**connector** /kə·nek′tər/ [L, *con* + *nectere,* to bind], **1.** anything serving as a link between two separate objects or units. **2.** (in dentistry) the part of a fixed partial denture that unites the retainer and the pontic; it may be rigid or nonrigid.

**connexon** /kə·nek′son/ [L, *con* + *nectere,* to bind], the functional unit of a gap junction; it is the hexagonal array of membrane-spanning proteins around a central channel that connects with its counterpart in an adjacent cell to form the intercellular pore of the gap junction. See also **gap junction.**

**Conn's syndrome** [Jerome W. Conn, American physician, b. 1907; Gk, *syn,* together, *dromos,* course], primary hyperaldosteronism, characterized by excessive secretion of aldosterone with symptoms of headache, fatigue, nocturia, and increased urination. The patient may also experience hypertension, hypokalemic alkalosis, potassium depletion, and hypervolemia.

**Conor's disease.** See **Marseilles fever.**

**Conradi-Hünermann syndrome** /kon·rä′dē·hu′nər·män/ [Erich Conradi, German physician, 20th century; Carl Hünermann, German physician, 20th century], an autosomal dominant form of chondrodysplasia punctata, characterized by asymmetric shortening of the limbs and scoliosis; intelligence and life expectancy are normal. The syndrome is also associated with maternal use of warfarin sodium during pregnancy.

**Conradi's disease.** See **chondrodystrophia calcificans congenita.**

**consanguinity** /kon′sang·gwin′itē/ [L, *con* + *sanguis,* blood], a hereditary or "blood" relationship between persons that results from having a common parent or ancestor.

**conscience** [L, *conscientia,* to be privy to information], **1.** the moral, self-critical sense of what is right and wrong. **2.** (in psychoanalysis) the part of the superego system that monitors thoughts, feelings, and actions and measures them against internalized values and standards.

**conscious** /kon′shəs/[L, *conscire,* to be aware], **1.** (in neurology) capable of responding to sensory stimuli; awake, alert; aware of one's external environment. **2.** (in psychiatry) that part of the psyche or mental functioning in which thoughts, ideas, emotions, and other mental content are in complete awareness. Compare **preconscious, unconscious.**

**consciousness** /kon′shəsnes/, a clear state of awareness of self and the environment in which attention is focused on immediate matters, as distinguished from mental activity of an unconscious or subconscious nature.

**conscious proprioception,** the conscious awareness of body position and movement of body segments. It is regulated by the lemniscal system through pathways that begin in joint receptors and end in the parietal lobe of the cerebral cortex; it enables the cortex to refine voluntary movements.

**conscious sedation**[1]**,** the administration of central nervous system depressant drugs and/or analgesics to provide analgesia, relieve anxiety, and/or provide amnesia during surgical, diagnostic, or interventional procedures. Consciousness is depressed, and the patient may fall asleep but is not unconscious. A properly trained provider is essential to administration and monitoring of conscious sedation. Oversedation or an adverse patient response to sedation may result in life-threatening complications such as hypotension, loss of airway reflexes, inability to maintain a patent airway, hypoventilation, apnea, or agitation and movement at a critical point in the procedure. Anesthetic monitoring during conscious sedation includes at a minimum monitoring of blood pressure, electrocardiography, and pulse oximetry. See also **awake anesthesia.**

**conscious sedation**[2]**,** a nursing intervention from the Nursing Interventions Classification (NIC) defined as administration of sedatives, monitoring of the patient's response, and provision of necessary physiological support during a diagnostic or therapeutic procedure. See also **Nursing Interventions Classification.**

**consensual light reflex,** a normally present crossed reflex in which light directed at one eye causes the opposite pupil to contract. In monocular blindness the pupil of the blind eye reacts consensually with stimulation of the seeing eye but does not cause constriction of the pupil of either eye. Also called **consensual reaction to light.** See also **light reflex.** Compare **direct light reflex.**

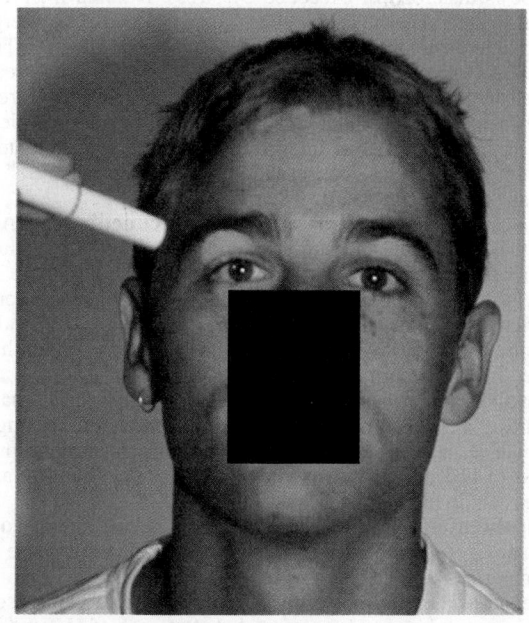

**Assessment of consensual and direct reaction to light**
*(Lemmi and Lemmi, 2000)*

**consensually validated symbols,** symbols that are accepted by enough people that they have an agreed-upon meaning.

**consensual reaction,** contraction of the pupil of one eye when the contralateral retina is stimulated. It is a common reflex.

**consensual reaction to light.** See **consensual light reflex.**

**consensual reflex** /konsen'shoo·əl/ [L, con + sentire, to feel], pertaining to a reflex action in which stimulation of one body part results in a response in another.

**consensual validation,** 1. a mutual agreement by two or more persons about a particular meaning that is to be attributed to verbal or nonverbal behavior. 2. the determination that a measuring tool (e.g., a test) measures what it is supposed to measure.

**consensus sequence** /kənsen'səs/, a sequence of nucleotides in an RNA molecule that serves as a site for the insertion of a splice of a segment of RNA from another source.

**consent** /kənsent'/ [L, consentire, to agree], to give approval, assent, or permission. A person must be of sufficient mental capacity and be of age at which he or she is legally recognized as competent to give consent (age of consent). See also **informed consent.**

**consenting adult,** an adult who willingly agrees to participate in an activity with one or more other adults. The term is usually applied to sexual activity.

**consequences** /kon'səkwen'səs/, stimulus events that follow a behavior that strengthen or weaken it. They may be either reinforcers or punishers.

**conservation of energy** /kon'sərvā'shən/ [L, conservare, to preserve], (in physics) a law stating that in any closed system the total amount of energy is constant.

**conservation of matter,** (in physics) a law stating that matter can be neither created nor destroyed and that the amount of matter in the universe is finite. Also called **conservation of mass.** See also **conservation of energy.**

**conservation principles of nursing,** a conceptual framework for nursing that is directed to maintaining the wholeness or integrity of the patient when the normal ability to cope is disturbed or exceeded by stress. Nursing intervention is determined by the patient's need to conserve energy and to maintain structural, personal, and social integrity. The patient is perceived as a person whose wholeness is threatened by stress. Subjective and objective indicators of stress are assessed by the nurse, the stimuli for the stress are identified, and the level of integrity in each area is evaluated. The nurse acts as a "conservationist."

**conservative treatment.** See **treatment.**

**Consolidated Omnibus Budget Reconciliation Act (COBRA),** legislation that provides for limited continuation of health coverage for individuals and families at the individual's own expense when the individual terminates employment from an organization that provides health insurance. The law applies only to organizations with a specified minimum number of employees.

**consolidation** /kənsol'idā'shən/ [L, consolidare, to make solid], 1. the combining of separate parts into a single whole. 2. a state of solidification. 3. (in medicine) the process of becoming solid, as when the lungs become firm and inelastic in pneumonia.

**consolidation of individuality and emotional constancy,** (in psychiatry) the fourth and final subphase in Mahler's system of the separation-individuation phase of preoedipal development. It begins toward the end of the second year and is seen as open ended. A degree of object constancy is accomplished, and separation of self and object representations is established.

**constancy** /kon'stənsē/, an absence of variation in quality of distinctive features despite location, rotation, size, or color of an object.

**constant positive airway pressure.** See **continuous positive airway pressure.**

**constant positive pressure ventilation.** See **continuous positive pressure ventilation.**

**constant pressure generator,** a machine that provides or generates a constant gas pressure throughout the inspiratory cycle of breathing. The pressure may range from a low value, such as 12 cm $H_2O$, to a high value of as much as 3500 cm $H_2O$, as required.

**constant region,** the part of an immunoglobulin in which the amino acid sequence is relatively constant in all molecules of that class of immunoglobulin. Compare **variable region.**

**constant touch,** a technique to diagnose the sensibility of an injured body part, such as a hand, by pressing the eraser end of a pencil or another object in various areas to determine the person's ability to detect the pressure.

**constipation**[1] /kon'stipā'shən/ [L, constipare, to crowd together], difficulty in passing stools or incomplete or infrequent passage of hard stools. There are many causes, both organic and functional. Among the organic causes are intestinal obstruction, diverticulitis, and tumors. Functional impairment of the colon may occur in elderly or bedridden patients who fail to respond to the urge to defecate. For constipation that is not organically caused the nurse can encourage a liberal diet of fruits, vegetables, and plenty of water. The patient should be encouraged to exercise moderately, if possible, and to develop regular, unhurried bowel habits. See also **atonic constipation. —constipated,** adj.

**constipation/impaction management,** a nursing intervention from the Nursing Interventions Classification (NIC) defined as prevention and alleviation of constipation/impaction. See also **Nursing Interventions Classification.**

**constipation, perceived,** a nursing diagnosis accepted by the Eighth National Conference on the Classification of Nursing Diagnoses. Perceived constipation is a state in which an individual makes a self-diagnosis of constipation and ensures a daily bowel movement through use of laxatives, enemas, and suppositories.

■ DEFINING CHARACTERISTICS: The defining characteristic is an expectation of a daily bowel movement, which may be expected at the same time every day, with the resulting overuse of laxatives, enemas, and suppositories.

■ RELATED FACTORS: Related factors are cultural and family health beliefs, faulty appraisal, and impaired thought processes. See also **nursing diagnosis.**

**constipation, rectal,** a nursing diagnosis accepted by the Eighth National Conference on the Classification of Nursing Diagnoses. Rectal constipation is a state in which an individual's pattern of elimination is characterized by stool retention, normal stool consistency, and delayed elimination that results from biopsychosocial disruptions.

■ DEFINING CHARACTERISTICS: Defining characteristics include stool retention and delayed bowel movements with normal stool consistency. Abdominal discomfort, rectal fullness, and a change in flatus also occur.

■ RELATED FACTORS: Related factors are weak pelvic floor muscles, painful anorectal lesions, self-care deficits, environmental constraints, altered mobility, limited or absent social support, impaired communication, altered awareness; and emotional disturbances. See also **nursing diagnosis.**

**constipation, risk for,** a nursing diagnosis accepted by the Thirteenth National Conference on the Classification of Nursing Diagnoses. The condition is a risk for a decrease in a person's normal frequency of defecation accompanied by difficult or incomplete passage of stool and/or passage or excessively hard, dry stool.

■ RISK FACTORS: Risk factors include habitual denial or ignoring of urge to defecate, recent environmental changes, inadequate toileting, irregular defecation habits, insufficient physical activity, abdominal muscle weakness, emotional stress, mental confusion, depression, insufficient fiber intake, dehydration, inadequate dentition or oral hygiene, poor eating habits, insufficient fluid intake, change in usual foods and eating patterns, decreased motility of GI tract, rectal abcess or ulcer, pregnancy, rectal anal stricture, postsurgical obstruction, rectal anal fissures, megacolon (Hirschsprung's disease), electrolyte imbalance, tumors, prostate enlargement, rectocele, rectal prolapse, neurological impairment, hemorrhoids, obesity, and certain pharmacological agents (phenothiazides, NSAIDs, sedatives, aluminum-containing antacids, laxative overuse, iron salts, anticholinergics, antidepressants, anticonvulsants, antilipemic agents, calcium channel blockers, calcium carbonate, diuretics, sympathomimetics, opiates, and bismuth salts). See also **nursing diagnosis.**

**constitution,** the general bodily health of an individual, expressed by the person's physical and mental abilities to function adequately in adverse circumstances.

**constitutional delay** /kon′stityōō′shənəl/ [L, *constituere,* to establish], a period in a child's development during which growth may be interrupted. In some cases constitutional delay may be associated with an illness or stressful event, and growth resumes later. The lost growth may or may not be regained. A form of constitutional delay is associated with some types of dwarfism.

**constitutional disease** [L, *constituere,* to set up; Gk, *dis,* without; Fr, *aise,* ease], any disease associated with the inborn physical condition of the client, such as a hereditary susceptibility.

**constitutional psychology,** the study of the relationship of individual psychologic makeup to body morphologic characteristics and organic functioning.

**constitutional symptom.** See **symptom.**

**constitutive resistance** /kənstich′ōōtiv/, the bacterial resistance to antibiotics that is contained in the deoxyribonucleic acid molecules of the organism. The trait can be passed on to daughter cells through cell division, but it cannot be transmitted to other species of bacteria.

**constriction** /kənstrik′shən/ [L, *constringere,* to draw tight], an abnormal closing or reduction in the size of an opening or passage of the body, as in vasoconstriction of a blood vessel. See also **stenosis.**

**constriction ring,** a band of contracted uterine muscle that forms a stricture around part of the fetus during labor, usually after premature rupture of the membranes and sometimes impeding labor. The uterine wall is thickened in the zone of the ring and is not prone to rupture. Compare **pathologic retraction ring.**

**constrictive cardiomyopathy** /kənstrik′tiv kär′dē·ōmī·op′əthe/ [L, *constringere,* to draw tight; Gk, *kardia,* heart, *mys,* muscle, *pathos,* disease], a heart disorder characterized by decreased diastolic compliance of the ventricles, imitating constrictive pericarditis. Also called **restrictive cardiomyopathy.**

**constrictive pericarditis,** a fibrous thickening of the pericardium caused by gradual scarring or fibrosis. The pericardium may undergo calcification and gradually becomes rigid, resisting the normal dilation of the heart chambers during the blood-filling phases of the cardiac cycle.

**constrictor** /kənstrik′tər/, a muscle that binds or restricts

an opening, as the ciliary body fibers that control the size of the pupil.

**constructional apraxia** /kənstruk′shənəl/ [L, *construere,* to build], a form of apraxia characterized by the inability to copy drawings or to manipulate objects to form patterns or designs. It is caused by a right hemisphere lesion. The deficit is tested by asking the patient to copy two-dimensional geometric patterns, such as circles, squares, diamonds, and hexagons, and to copy three-dimensional structures constructed of 1-inch building blocks.

**constructive aggression** /kənstruk′tiv/, an act of self-assertiveness in response to a threatening action for purposes of self-protection and preservation. See also **aggression.**

**constructive interference,** (in ultrasonography) an increase in amplitude of sound waves that results when multiple waves of equal frequency are transmitted precisely in phase.

**construct validity** /kon′strəkt/, validity of a test or a measurement tool that is established by demonstrating its ability to identify the variables that it proposes to identify. See also **validity.**

**consultant** /kənsul′tənt/ [L, *consultare,* to deliberate], a person who by training and experience has acquired a special knowledge in a subject area that has been recognized by a peer group.

**consultation**[1] /kon′səltā′shən/ [L, *consultare,* to deliberate], a process in which the help of a specialist is sought to identify ways to handle problems in patient management or in planning and implementation of health care programs.

**consultation**[2], a nursing intervention from the Nursing Interventions Classification (NIC) defined as using expert knowledge to work with those who seek help in problem solving to enable individuals, families, groups, or agencies to achieve identified goals. See also **Nursing Interventions Classification.**

**consultee-centered communication** /kon′sultē′/, expert advice or guidance that is given a consultee (health care worker) to improve the consultee's capacity to function more effectively in working with patients.

**consumption coagulopathy.** See **disseminated intravascular coagulation.**

**contact** [L, *contingere,* to touch], **1.** the touching or drawing together of two surfaces, as those of upper and lower teeth. The term is often used attributively, as in contact dermatitis and contact lens. **2.** the moving together, either directly or indirectly, of two individuals so as to allow the transmission of an infectious organism from one to the other. **3.** a person who has been exposed to an infectious disease.

**contact allergy,** hypersensitivity to a substance that produced a reaction in a previous contact or that is structurally similar to another substance that produced such a reaction. Substances that can cause a contact allergy include poison ivy, metals, detergents, cosmetics, foods, and topical medicines.

**contact dermatitis,** skin rash resulting from exposure to a primary irritant or to a sensitizing antigen. In the first, or nonallergic, type, a primary irritant, such as an alkaline detergent or an acid, causes a lesion similar to a thermal burn. Emergency treatment is to drench liberally and immediately with water. In the second, or allergic, type, sensitizing antigens cause an immunologic change in certain lymphocytes. Subsequent exposure to the antigen causes the lymphocytes to release irritating chemicals, leading to inflammation, edema, and vesiculation. Poison ivy and nickel dermatitis are common examples of this type of delayed hypersensitivity reaction. The diagnosis can be aided by patch testing with suspected antigens. Treatment includes avoidance of the irritant or sensitizer, administration of topical corticosteroid preparations, and use of soothing or drying lotions. In severe cases systemic corticosteroids may be used. Also called **dermatitis venenata.** Compare **atopic dermatitis.** See also **hypersensitivity reaction.**

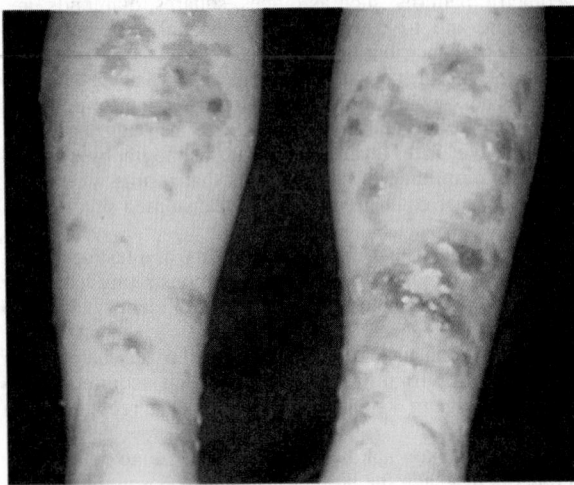

**Contact dermatitis** *(Lewis, Heitkemper, and Dirksen, 2000)*

**contact factor.** See **factor XII.**

**contact hour,** a 50-minute "hour" used to measure time for continuing education programs.

**contact lens,** a small, curved lens, primarily plastic in composition, shaped to fit the person's eye either to correct refractive error or to enhance appearance. The two primary forms of contact lenses are (1) rigid gas-permeable (RGP) lenses, which are small, are durable, and have little to no water absorption; and (2) soft lenses, which are larger, are more fragile, and have a 30% to 70% water content. Contact lenses float on the precorneal tear film and must be inserted, removed, cleaned, and stored to prevent damage or infection to the eyes.

**contact lens care,** a nursing intervention from the Nursing Interventions Classification (NIC) defined as prevention of eye injury and lens damage by proper use of contact lenses. See also **Nursing Interventions Classification.**

**contactor** /kəntak'tər/, a switching device that is part of the timer for the control of voltage across an x-ray tube.

**Contact Precautions,** safeguards designed to reduce the risk of transmission of epidemiologically important microorganisms by direct or indirect contact. Direct-contact transmission involves skin-to-skin contact and physical transfer of microorganisms to a susceptible host from an infected or colonized person (having the presence of microorganisms, but without clinical signs or symptoms of infection). This can occur when health care personnel perform patient-care activities that require physical contact. Direct-contact transmission can also occur between two patients, such as by hand contact, with one patient serving as the source of infectious microorganisms and the other as a susceptible host. Indirect-contact transmission involves contact of a susceptible host with a contaminated intermediate object, usually inanimate, in the patient's environment. Contact Precautions apply to specified patients known or suspected to be infected or colonized with epidemiologically important microorgan-

isms that can be transmitted by direct or indirect contact. See also **Standard Precautions, Transmission-based Precautions.**

**contact shield,** a protective device constructed of lead or other material that is positioned directly over the eyes or gonads of a patient to be exposed to an x-ray beam.

**contagion** /kəntā'jən/ [L, *contingere,* to touch], the transmission of a disease by direct contact with a person who has it or by indirect contact through handling of clothing, bedding, dishes, or other objects the person has used.

**contagious** /kəntā'jəs/ [L, *contingere,* to touch], communicable, such as a disease that may be transmitted by direct or indirect contact. —**contagion,** *n.*

**contagious disease.** See **communicable disease.**

**contagious pustular dermatitis** [L, *contingere,* to touch, *pustula,* pustules; Gk, *derma,* skin, *itis,* inflammation], a skin disease normally affecting sheep and goats but transmitted to humans who handle infected animals. It is caused by a pox virus and results in lesions on the hands, and occasionally on the face. The lesions resolve spontaneously, but slowly. Also called **ecthyma contagiosum, orf.**

**contaminant** /kəntam'inənt/ [L, *contaminare,* to bring in contact], an agent that causes contamination, pollution, or spoilage, such as a mold spore that makes food unsafe to eat.

**contaminated culture** /kəntam'inātid/, a bacterial culture that has acquired unwanted foreign microorganisms.

**contamination** /-ā'shən/[L, *contaminare,* to pollute], a condition of being soiled, stained, touched, or otherwise exposed to harmful agents, making an object potentially unsafe for use as intended or without barrier techniques. An example is entry of infectious or toxic materials into a previously clean or sterile environment.

**content theme.** See **communication theme.**

**content validity,** validity of a test or a measurement as a result of the use of previously tested items or concepts within the tool. See also **validity.**

**context** [L, *contextus,* to weave together], (in communications theory) the setting, meaning, and language of a message. If a message is interpreted without strict regard for these limits, it is taken out of context.

**continence** /kon'tinəns/ [L, *continere,* to contain], **1.** the ability to control bladder or bowel function. **2.** the use of self-restraint, particularly in regard to sexual intercourse.

**continent ileostomy** /kon'tinənt/, an ileostomy that drains into a surgically created pouch or reservoir in the abdomen. Involuntary discharge of intestinal contents is prevented by a nipple valve created from the ileum. This method eliminates the need for the patient to wear an external pouch over the stoma. Also called **Kock's pouch.**

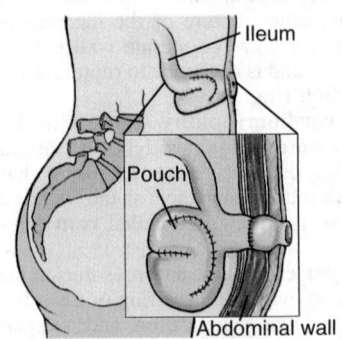

**Continent ileostomy (Kock's pouch)**
*(Monahan and Neighbors, 1998)*

■ METHOD: After surgery the pouch is kept relatively empty by means of a catheter placed in it at surgery. The catheter is removed a week or two afterward, depending on the status of intestinal function and wound healing. Once the indwelling catheter is removed, the pouch is drained by periodically inserting a catheter through the stoma into the pouch through the valve. The time allowed to elapse between catheterizations is gradually lengthened as the capacity of the pouch increases to between 500 and 1000 mL. Six months after surgery drainage may be necessary only three or four times a day. The patient learns to recognize a feeling of fullness that indicates the need for drainage. When the patient is seated on the toilet, the dressing over the stoma is removed, and the tip of a French size 28 to 32 catheter is lubricated and inserted into the stoma. The distal end of the catheter is in a receptacle or in the toilet, at least 30 cm below the stoma. The lubricated tip of the catheter is advanced carefully through the stoma. Resistance is usually felt at a depth of about 5 cm where the valve covers the opening to the pouch. Flow usually begins when the tip of the catheter has passed the valve, at a distance of approximately 7.5 cm from the stoma. Complete drainage may require up to 15 minutes. ■ INTERVENTIONS: After surgery the patient is usually instructed to add foods one at a time. High-fiber foods and those that cause gas formation are particularly likely to be problematic. Thick secretions may be thinned by the injection of a little water into the pouch through the catheter. The stoma may be covered with a stoma cap or dressing. It is important to teach the patient to prevent irritation of the skin around the stoma. Nonallergenic tape may be used to hold the pad in place. After healing, if there is no danger of a blow to the abdomen, a pad is often not necessary. After surgery activity is resumed as the patient is able to tolerate it. There is no reason for activity to be curtailed once healing is complete and the person feels well. ■ OUTCOME CRITERIA: The patient may expect to be able to care for the stoma and to manage the drainage of the pouch. A continent ileostomy has several advantages, including the prevention of unpleasant odors and the convenience of eliminating the need for a colostomy or ileostomy bag.

**contingency contracting** /kəntin′jənsē/ [L, *contingere,* to touch], a formal agreement between a psychotherapist and a patient undergoing behavior therapy regarding the consequences of certain actions by both parties.

**contingency management,** any of a group of techniques used in behavior therapy that attempts to modify a behavioral response by controlling the consequences of that response. Kinds of contingency management include **contingency contracting, shaping,** and **token economy.**

**contingent nurse.** See **float nurse.**

**continua.** See **continuum.**

**continuing care nurse** /kəntin′yoo·ing/ [L, *continuare,* to unite], a nurse who specializes in coordination of the overall needs of the patient with the potential health care resources of the community. Much of the emphasis is on discharge planning and assessment of the availability of participation in the patient's care after discharge by members of the family or other parties. Continuing care nursing responsibilities and discharge planning ideally begin at the time a patient is admitted to a hospital.

**continuing education,** formal educational programs designed to promote knowledge, skills, and professional attitudes. The programs are usually short-term and specific. A certificate may be awarded for completion of a course, and a number of continuing education units or contact hours may be conferred. Continuing education is required for relicensure in many states. It is not to be confused with academic degree-granting programs, such as advanced education or graduate education. See also **contact hour.**

**continuing education unit (CEU),** a point awarded to a professional person by a professional organization for having attended an educational program relevant to the goals of the organization. A value is established for the course and that number of points is given. Many states require professionals in the various fields of medicine and nursing to obtain a specific number of CEUs annually for relicensure. See also **contact hour.**

**continuity theory** /kon′tinyoo′itē/, a concept that an individual's personality does not change as the person ages, with the result that his or her behavior becomes more predictable.

**continuous ambulatory peritoneal dialysis (CAPD)** /kəntin′yoo·əs/ [L, *continuare,* to unite, *ambulare,* to walk about; Gk, *peri,* near, *tenein,* to stretch, *dia,* through, *lysis,* loosening], a maintenance system of peritoneal dialysis in which an indwelling catheter permits fluid to drain into and out of the peritoneal cavity by gravity.

**continuous anesthesia** [L, *continuare,* to unite], a method for maintaining regional nerve block. A local anesthetic solution is infused at intervals or at a slow rate to infiltrate epidural, or, spinal spaces.

**continuous bath.** See **continuous tub bath.**

**continuous bladder irrigation.** See **drainage.**

**continuous cycling peritoneal dialysis (CCPD),** a type of dialysis in which the patient is attached to an automatic cycler for short exchanges while sleeping at night. Mobility is not feasible because of the cumbersome equipment. During waking hours the patient receives long dialysis exchanges but has ambulatory freedom.

**continuous fever,** a fever that persists steadily for a prolonged period. Compare **intermittent fever.**

**continuous flow analyzer,** a device that automatically analyzes a series of samples of biologic materials that are continuously pumped into tubes along with appropriate reagents.

**continuous mandatory ventilation.** See **assist-control mode.**

**continuous murmur** [L, *continuare,* to unite, *murmur,* humming], an uninterrupted heart murmur or cervical venous hum that characteristically begins in systole and persists through diastole. Cervical venous hum is a normal finding in children; other continuous murmurs are always pathologic.

**continuous negative chest wall pressure,** a pressure below ambient pressure that is applied to the chest wall during the entire respiratory cycle, thus increasing transpulmonary pressure.

**continuous passive motion (CPM),** a technique for maintaining or increasing the amount of movement in a joint, using a mechanical device that applies force to produce joint motion without normal muscle function.

**continuous phase** [L, *continuare,* to unite; Gk, *phasis,* appearance], the phase of a colloidal solution corresponding to that of the solvent of a true solution. Also called **external phase, dispersion medium.**

**continuous positive airway pressure (CPAP),** a method of noninvasive ventilation assisted by a flow of air delivered at a constant pressure throughout the respiratory cycle. It is performed for patients who can initiate their own respirations but who are not able to maintain adequate arterial oxygen levels without assistance. CPAP may be given through a ventilator and endotracheal tube, through a nasal cannula, or into a hood over the patient's head. Respiratory distress syndrome in the newborn is often treated with

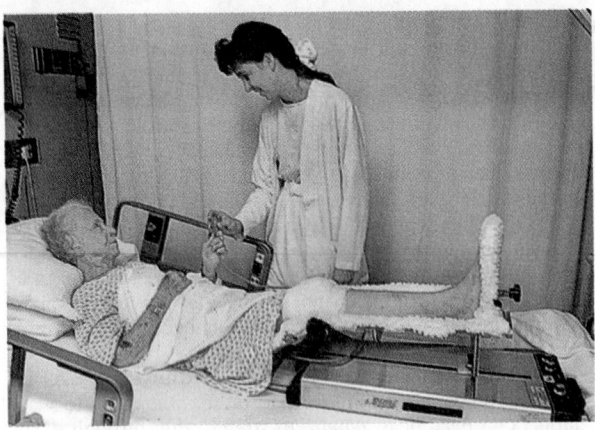

**Continuous passive motion** *(Elkin, Perry, and Potter, 1996)*

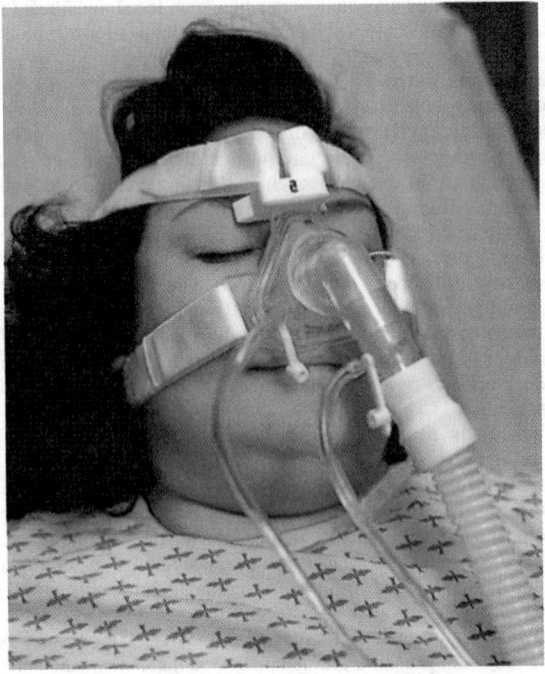

**Continuous positive airway pressure**
*(Elkin, Perry, and Potter, 2000)*

CPAP. Also called **constant positive airway pressure, continuous positive pressure breathing (CPPB).** Compare **positive-end expiratory pressure.**

**continuous positive pressure ventilation (CPPV),** a pressure above ambient pressure maintained in the upper airway throughout the breathing cycle. The term is usually applied to positive-end expiratory pressure and mechanical ventilation. Also called **constant positive pressure ventilation.** See also **continuous positive airway pressure.**

**continuous quality improvement (CQI),** a system that seeks to improve the provision of services with an emphasis on future results. Like total quality management (TQM), CQI uses a set of statistical tools to understand subsystems and uncover problems, but its emphasis is on maintaining quality in the future, not just controlling a process. Once a process that needs improvement is identified, a team of knowledgeable individuals is gathered to research and document each step of that process. Once specific expectations and the means to measure them have established, implementation aims at preventing future failures and involves the setting of goals, education, and the measurement of results. If necessary, the plan may be revised on the basis of the results, so that the improvement is ongoing.

**continuous reinforcement,** a schedule of strengthening or rewarding behavior in which omission of a response is followed by a reinforcing event or behavior.

**continuous tremor,** fine, rhythmic, purposeless movements that persist during rest but sometimes disappear briefly during voluntary movements. The pill-rolling movements and trembling of Parkinson's disease are typical of continuous tremors. Also called **resting tremor.** Compare **intention tremor.** See also **tremor.**

**continuous tub bath,** a therapeutic bath, usually prescribed in the treatment of some dermatologic conditions, in which the patient lies supported in a medicated solution of tepid water.

■ METHOD: The bath is prepared as for a medicated tub bath. The patient is immersed in the water, and a towel saturated with the solution is placed over the torso. The patient may wear a loin cloth, and a harness is fitted comfortably around the chest and under the shoulders and head to hold the head safely out of the water as the patient sleeps or dozes. A pillow or folded towel is placed over the wide supporting straps under the head and neck to add to the patient's comfort. A board is placed on top of the tub from the patient's shoulders to the end of the tub, and a sheet is draped over it. A bell for calling for assistance, a container of drinking water with a flexible straw, and any other materials that may be needed are placed on the board.

■ INTERVENTIONS: The method and the reason for the treatment are explained to the patient. Privacy is maintained; close supervision by a nurse is available throughout the treatment. The procedure is psychologically trying and may be physically unpleasant for the patient. Psychosocial support and attention to maximization of patient comfort improve the patient's tolerance for the procedure.

■ OUTCOME CRITERIA: The patient is observed for any febrile reaction, rapid or weak pulse, faintness, or increased severity of symptoms, as itching, burning, or pain. The solution is changed completely every 4 hours, the linen is changed twice a day, and the harness is changed once a day.

**continuous wave (CW),** 1. an uninterrupted flow of energy, such as a beam of laser light. 2. sound intensity that remains constant while ultrasound is being produced.

**continuum** /kəntin′yo͞o·əm/, *pl.* **continua,** 1. a continuous series or whole. 2. (in mathematics) a system of real numbers.

**contour** /kon′to͞or/ [Fr], 1. the normal outline or configuration of the body or of a part. 2. to shape a solid along certain desired lines.

**contoured adducted trochanteric controlled alignment method (CAT-CAM)** /kon′to͞ord/, a design for an artificial lower limb for persons who have undergone above the knee (AK) amputations.

**contouring** /kon′to͞or·ing/, the process of forming a contour.

**contra-,** prefix meaning 'against': *contraception, contralateral, contraparetic.*

**contra-angle** /kon′trə·ang′gəl/ [L, *contra,* against + *angulus,* angle], an angulation by which the working point of a surgical instrument is brought close to the long axis of its shaft; it may involve two, three, or four bends, or angles, in its shank.

**contra bevel** [L, *contra,* against; OFr, *baif,* open mouth], **1.** the angle between a dental cutting blade and the base of the periodontal pocket when the blade is held so that it separates the sulcular epithelium from the external epithelium of the gingiva. Also called **reverse bevel. 2.** an external bevel of a tooth preparation extending onto a buccal or lingual cusp from an intracoronal restoration.

**contraception** /kon'trəsep'shən/ [L, *contra + concipere,* to take in], a process or technique for preventing pregnancy by means of a medication, device, or method that blocks or alters one or more of the processes of reproduction in such a way that sexual union can occur without impregnation. Kinds of contraception include **cervical cap, condom, contraceptive diaphragm, injectable long-acting progestins, intrauterine device, natural family-planning method, oral contraceptive, spermicide, sterilization** and **subdermal contraceptive implants.** Also called **birth control, conception control, natural family planning method.** See also **basal body temperature method of family planning; injectable contraceptive; planned parenthood.**

**contraceptive** /kon'trəsep'tiv/ [L, *contra + concipere,* to take in], any device or technique that prevents conception. See also **contraception.**

**contraceptive diaphragm,** a contraceptive device consisting of a hemisphere of thin rubber bonded to a flexible ring, inserted into the vagina together with spermicidal jelly or cream up to 2 hours before coitus. Fitted between the pubic symphysis and the posterior fornix of the vagina, the diaphragm cups the cervix in a pool of spermicide so that spermatozoa cannot enter the uterus, thus preventing conception. The rate of failure of the diaphragm method of contraception is approximately 2 unplanned pregnancies in 100 women using the method properly for 1 year. The principal advantage of the diaphragm is that it has no systemic effects. Diaphragms are manufactured in seven standard sizes from 55 to 100 mm in diameter. Kinds of diaphragms are **arcing**

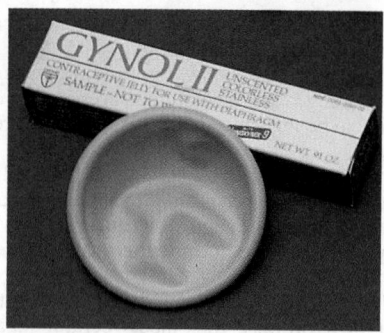

**Contraceptive diaphragm** *(Edge and Miller, 1994)*

**spring, coil spring,** and **flat spring.** Also called **diaphragm.**

**contraceptive diaphragm fitting,** a procedure, performed in an office or clinic, in which a contraceptive diaphragm is selected according to the clinical assessment of anatomic factors specific to the woman being fitted, including size of the vagina, position of the uterus, depth of the arch behind the symphysis pubis, and degree of support afforded by the muscles surrounding the vagina. See also **arcing spring contraceptive diaphragm, coil spring contraceptive diaphragm, flat spring contraceptive diaphragm.**

**contraceptive effectiveness,** the effectiveness of a method of contraception in preventing pregnancy. For clinical purposes it combines the theoretic effectiveness of the device, medication, or method and the use effectiveness. It is sometimes represented as a percentage but more accurately as the number of pregnancies per 100 woman-years. The average pregnancy rate for a couple who are sexually active and do not use contraceptives is equivalent to 85 pregnancies per 100 woman-years. A contraceptive method that results in a pregnancy rate of fewer than 10 pregnancies

## Contraceptive methods: risks, complications, and failure

| Type | Risk/potential complications | Failure rate (%) |
|---|---|---|
| Periodic abstinence | Sexual frustration, STDs | 20 |
| Calendar abstinence | Sexual frustration, unexpected ovulation, STDs | 9 |
| Withdrawal (coitus interruptus) | Anxiety, frustration, inability to relax, pregnancy, STDs | 19 |
| Vasectomy | Bruising, edema, pain, infection, psychologic problems, STDs | 0.15 |
| Tubal ligation | Typical abdominal surgical risks, STDs | 0.40 |
| Norplant implants | Infection, menstrual changes, STDs, tenderness at site, visibility of implants | 0.09 |
| Injectible progestogen | Menstrual changes, weight gain, headaches, STDs | 0.30 |
| Intrauterine devices | Spotting, increased bleeding, uterine cramping, PID, STDs | 0.10-2.0 |
| Oral contraceptive (estrogen/progesterone tablets) | Nausea, headaches, dizziness, spotting, weight gain, breast disease, ovarian cysts, fluid retention, mood changes, cardiovascular problems, STDs | 3 |
| Male condom without spermicide | Allergic reactions, decreased sensitivity, loss of spontaneity, STDs | 12 |
| Female condom | Visibility, loss of spontaneity | 21 |
| Diaphragm with spermicide | Allergy, toxic shock, vaginal irritation, cervical erosion | 18 |
| Cervical cap with spermicide | Allergy, toxic shock, vaginal irritation, cervical erosion | 18 (nulliparous) 36 (parous) |
| Sponge with spermicide | Allergy, toxic shock, vaginal dryness, vaginal irritation | 18 (nulliparous) 36 (parous) |
| Spermicides (alone) | Allergy, unpleasant smell or taste | 21 |
| Douche | Infection, local irritation, STDs | 40 |
| None | Pregnancy, STDs | 85 |

Beare FG, Myers JL: *Adult health nursing,* ed 3, St Louis, 1998, Mosby.
*STD,* Sexually transmitted disease.

per 100 woman-years is considered highly effective. See also **pregnancy rate, woman-year.**

**contraceptive jelly** [L, *contra,* opposed, *concipere,* to take in, *gelare,* to congeal], a gelatinous preparation containing a spermicide to be introduced into the vagina to prevent conception.

**contraceptive method,** any act, device, or medication for avoiding conception or a viable pregnancy. See also **cervical cap, condom, diaphragm, intrauterine device, natural family planning method, oral contraceptive, spermicide, sterilization.**

**contract** [L, *con* + *trahere,* to draw] **1.** /kon′trakt/, an agreement or a promise that meets certain legal requirements, including competence of both or all parties to the contract, proper lawful subject matter, mutuality of agreement, mutuality of obligation, and consideration (the exchange of something of value in payment for the obligation undertaken). **2.** /kəntrakt′/, to make such an agreement or promise. —**contractual,** *adj.*

**contracted kidney,** a kidney that is greatly reduced in size and function as a result of an overgrowth of fibrous tissue and a diminished blood supply. The condition occurs in arteriolar nephrosclerosis and glomerulonephritis.

**contractile** /kəntrak′til/ [L, *con,* with, *trahere,* to draw], capable of becoming reduced in size or length or of being drawn together in response to some stimulus.

**contractile ring dysphagia** [L, *con* + *trahere,* to draw; AS, *hring*], an abnormal condition characterized by difficulty in swallowing caused by an overreactive interior esophageal sphincteric mechanism that induces painful sticking sensations under the lower sternum. Compare **dysphagia lusoria, vallecular dysphagia.**

**contractility** /kon′traktil′itē/, the ability of muscle tissue to contract when its thick (myosin) and thin (actin) filaments slide past each other.

**contraction** /kəntrak′shən/ [L, *con* + *trahere,* to draw], **1.** a reduction in size, especially of muscle fibers. **2.** an abnormal shrinkage. **3.** (in labor) a rhythmic tightening of the musculature of the upper uterine segment that begins as mild tightening and becomes very strong late in labor, occurring as frequently as every 2 minutes and lasting over 1 minute. Contractions decrease the size of the uterus and squeeze the fetus through the birth canal. **4.** abnormal smallness of the birth canal or part of it, a cause of dystocia. **Inlet contraction** exists if the anteroposterior diameter is 10 cm or less or if the transverse diameter is 11.5 cm or less. **Midpelvic contraction** exists if the sum of the measurements in centimeters of the interspinous diameter (normally 10.5 cm) and the posterior sagittal diameter (normally 5 cm) is 13.5 cm or less. **Outlet contraction** exists if the intertuberous diameter is 8 cm or less. See also **clinical pelvimetry, concentric contraction, dystocia, eccentric contraction, x-ray pelvimetry.**

**contractions stress test (CST),** ultrasound monitoring of the fetal heart rate during uterine contractions induced by oxytocin administration or nipple stimulation.

**contract-model HMO,** a model in which the health maintenance organization (HMO) contracts with individual physicians rather than groups of providers for services not produced directly by the HMO.

**contractual.** See **contract.**

**contracture** /kəntrak′chər/ [L, *contractura,* a pulling together], an abnormal, usually permanent condition of a joint, characterized by flexion and fixation. It may be caused by atrophy and shortening of muscle fibers resulting from immobilization or by loss of the normal elasticity of connective tissues or the skin, such as from the formation of exten-

sive scar tissue over a joint. See also **Volkmann's contracture.**

**contraindicate** /kon′trə·in′dikāt/ [L, *contra,* against, *indicare,* to make known], to report the presence of a disease or physical condition that makes it impossible or undesirable to treat a particular client in the usual manner or to prescribe medicines that might otherwise be suitable.

**contraindication** /in′dikā′shən/ [L, *contra,* against, *indicare,* to make known], a factor that prohibits the administration of a drug or the performance of an act or procedure in the care of a specific patient; for example pregnancy is a contraindication for the administration of tetracycline, immunosuppression may be a contraindication for vaccination, and complete placenta previa is a contraindication for vaginal delivery.

**contralateral** /-lat′ərəl/ [L, *contra* + *lateralis,* side], affecting or originating in the opposite side of a point of reference, such as a point on a body.

**contralateral reflexes** [L, *contra,* against, *latus,* side, *reflectere,* to bend back], an overflow phenomenon of the nervous system in which a reflex is elicited on one side of the body by a stimulus to the opposite side.

**contrast** /kon′trast/ [L, *contra,* against, *stare,* to stand], a measure of the difference in optic density, radiation transmission, or other parameters between two adjacent areas in a radiographic image. Contrast plays an important role in the ability of a radiologist to perceive image detail.

**contrast bath,** a bath in which the patient alternately immerses a part of the body, usually the hands or feet, in hot and cold water for a specified period. The procedure is used to increase the blood flow to a particular area.

**contrast enema.** See **barium enema.**

**contrast examination,** the use of radiopaque materials to make internal organs visible on x-ray film. Because of their high atomic numbers, substances such as iodine and barium have an x-ray photoelectrical interaction that is nearly 400 times that of soft tissue. As a result, internal organs or cavities outlined by such substances are more visible.

**contrast medium,** a substance that is injected into the body, introduced via catheter, or swallowed to facilitate radiographic imaging of internal structures that otherwise are difficult to visualize on x-ray films. Contrast media may be either radiopaque or radiolucent.

**contrasuppressor cell** /kon′trəsəpres′ər/, one of a group of T cells that inhibit the function of suppressor T cells.

**contrecoup.** See **coup.**

**contrecoup injury** /kôntrekoo′/ [L, *contra,* against; Fr, *coup,* blow; L, *injuria*], an injury, usually involving the brain, in which the tissue damage is on the side opposite the trauma site, as when a blow to the left side of the head results in brain damage on the right side.

**contributory negligence** /kəntrib′yətôr′ē/, a legal term describing a situation in which both the plaintiff and the defendant share in the negligence that caused injury to the plaintiff.

**control** [Fr, *controler,* to register], **1.** to exercise restraint or maintain influence over a situation, as in self-control, the conscious limitation or suppression of impulses. **2.** a standard against which conclusions may be measured, as in a "control group."

**control cable,** a stainless steel wire, usually contained in a flexible stainless steel housing, used to move or lock a prosthesis into place.

**control gene,** a gene, such as an operator or a regulator, that controls the transcription of a structural gene by either inducing or repressing RNA synthesis.

**control group,** a set of items or people that serves as a standard or reference for comparison with an experimental group. A control group is similar to the experimental group in number and is identical in specified characteristics, such as sex, age, annual income, parity, or other factors.

**controlled area,** a part of a hospital or other health facility that is occupied primarily by personnel who work with radioactive materials. It is designed with barrier shielding to confine the radiation exposure rate in the area to less than 100 milliroentgen per week (mR/wk).

**controlled association,** 1. a direct connection of relevant ideas that results from a specific stimulus. 2. a process of drawing repressed ideas into the consciousness in response to words spoken by a psychoanalyst. Also called **word association.**

**controlled hypotension.** See **deliberate hypotension.**

**controlled oxygen therapy,** the administration of oxygen to a patient on a dose-response basis in which oxygen is regarded as a drug and only the smallest amount of it is used to obtain a desired therapeutic effect.

**controlled substance** [Fr, *controle,* to register; L, *substantia,* essence], any drug defined in the five categories of the federal **Controlled Substances Act of 1970.** The categories, or schedules, cover opium and its derivatives, hallucinogens, depressants, and stimulants.

**controlled substance checking,** a nursing intervention from the Nursing Interventions Classification (NIC) defined as promoting appropriate use and maintaining security of controlled substances. See also **Nursing Interventions Classification.**

**Controlled Substances Act,** a U.S. law enacted in 1970 that regulates the prescribing and dispensing of psychoactive drugs, including stimulants, depressants, and hallucinogens. The act lists five categories of restricted drugs, organized by their medical acceptance, abuse potential, and ability to produce dependence.

**controlled ventilation,** the use of an intermittent positive pressure breathing unit or other respirator that has an automatic cycling device that replaces spontaneous respiration. Some units measure expired volume, nebulize medication or fluids in the air, exert negative pressure at the end of expiration, or have a variety of alarms.

**control of hemorrhage,** the limitation of the flow of blood from a break in the wall of a blood vessel.

■ METHOD: Some of the methods for controlling hemorrhage are direct pressure, use of a tourniquet, and application of pressure on pressure points proximal to the wound. Direct pressure with a thick compress is applied in such a way that the edges of the wound are drawn together. A tourniquet is applied proximal to the site of bleeding only in the most extreme emergency, for the limb may then have to be removed as a result of tissue anoxia stemming from the use of the tourniquet. Firm manual pressure is applied to a pressure point over the main artery supplying the wound. Points used to obtain the pulse may be used as pressure points to stop hemorrhage. See also **tourniquet.**

■ INTERVENTIONS: Blood flow to an area is limited by restricting activity, elevating the part, and applying pressure. Specific treatment depends on the cause of the hemorrhage and the patient's condition. In addition to IV infusion equipment and fluids, the nurse may anticipate the need for vasopressor drugs, ventilatory assistance, central venous pressure monitoring equipment, and materials for obtaining and recording the blood pressure and urinary output. If signs of shock are present, the patient may be placed supine at a 45-degree angle to the pelvis, with the knees straight and the pelvis slightly higher than the chest. The head may be supported with a pillow. The person may be given oxygen, and the central venous pressure may be measured to determine the need for replacement of fluid volume. Sudden, severe hemorrhage with signs of shock usually is treated with IV infusion of fluids and transfusion of blood. The application of additional warmth to the skin is not recommended, because heat increases the metabolism and the need for oxygen.

■ OUTCOME CRITERIA: Signs of continued bleeding, tachycardia, cold sweat, decreasing blood pressure, and patient anxiety alert the nurse to the probability that bleeding has begun again or that replacement fluids administered after the hemorrhage are not adequate. The person is kept calm and quiet; if the fluid balance is promptly restored, recovery is usual. Excessive loss of blood leads to hypoxia of all the tissues of the body, including the brain and vital organs, and causes death.

**Classification of controlled substances**

| Classification | Description | Specific substances |
|---|---|---|
| Schedule I (Schedule H*) | Drugs that have high potential for abuse and no accepted medical use. Containers are marked C-I. | Heroin, LSD, peyote, marijuana |
| Schedule II (Schedule F*) | Drugs that have high potential for abuse but have accepted medical use. Dependence may include strong physical and psychologic dependence. Containers are marked C-II. | Amobarbital, amphetamine, codeine, dextroamphetamine, meperidine, methadone, hydromorphone, morphine, opium, pentobarbital, phenazocine, methylphenidate, secobarbital |
| Schedule III (Schedule F*) | Medically accepted drugs that may cause dependence but are less prone to abuse than drugs in Schedules I and II. Containers are marked C-III. | Codeine-containing medications, butabarbital, paregoric |
| Schedule IV (Schedule F*) | Medically accepted drugs that may cause mild physical or psychologic dependence. Containers are marked C-IV. | Chloral hydrate, chlordiazepoxide, diazepam, meprobamate, phenobarbital |
| Schedule V | Medically accepted drugs with very limited potential for causing mild physical or psychologic dependence. Containers are marked C-V. | Drug mixtures containing small quantities of narcotics, such as over-the-counter cough syrups containing codeine |

Adapted from Clark JF, Queener SF, Karb VB: *Pharmacologic basis of nursing practice,* ed 6, St Louis, 2000, Mosby.
*Canadian classification.

**control process,** a system of establishing standards, objectives, and methods and measuring actual performance, comparing results, reinforcing strengths, and taking necessary corrective action.

**contuse** /kontōōz'/, to injure a body part without breaking the skin.

**contusion** /kənt(y)ōō'zhən/ [L, *contundere,* to bruise], an injury that does not disrupt the integrity of the skin, caused by a blow to the body and characterized by swelling, discoloration, and pain. The immediate application of cold may limit the development of a contusion. Also called **bruise.** Compare **ecchymosis.**

**convalescence** /kon'vəles'əns/ [L, *convalescere,* to grow strong], the period of recovery after an illness, injury, or surgery.

**convalescent carrier,** a person who has recovered from the symptoms of an infectious disease but is still capable of transmitting pathogens to others.

**convalescent home.** See **extended care facility.**

**convection** /kənvek'shən/ [L, *convehere,* to bring together], (in physics) the transfer of heat through a gas or liquid by the circulation of heated particles.

**convergence** /kənvur'jəns/ [L, *convergere,* to bend together], the movement of two objects toward a common point, such as the turning of the eyes inward to see an object close to the face.

**convergent evolution,** the evolution of nonhomologous organs in distantly related species in response to similar environmental conditions. Although of different origin, the organs appear similar in function, shape, or form.

**convergent nystagmus,** an intermittent spasmodic movement of the eyes in which they move rhythmically toward each other and slowly return to the original position. It is usually caused by a tumor of the anterior aqueduct of Silvius, third ventricle, or midbrain.

**convergent squint.** See **esotropia.**

**convergent strabismus.** See **esotropia.**

**conversion** /kənvur'zhən/ [L, *convertere,* to turn around], **1.** changing from one form to another, transmutation. **2.** (in obstetrics) the correction of a fetal position during labor. **3.** (in psychiatry) an unconscious defense mechanism by which emotional conflicts that ordinarily cause anxiety are repressed and transformed into symbolic physical symptoms that have no organic basis. Loss of sensation, paralysis, pain, and other dysfunctions of the nervous system are the most common somatic expressions of conversion.

**conversion disorder,** an abnormality in which repressed emotional conflicts are changed into sensory, motor, or visceral symptoms with no underlying organic cause, such as blindness, anesthesia, hypesthesia, hyperesthesia, paresthesia, involuntary muscular movements (for example, tics or tremors), paralysis, aphonia, mutism, hallucinations, catalepsy, choking sensations, and respiratory difficulties. The person who has a conversion disorder is usually indifferent to the symptoms yet firmly believes the condition exists. Causal factors include a conscious or unconscious desire to escape from or avoid some unpleasant situation or responsibility or to obtain sympathy or some other secondary gain. Treatment usually consists of psychotherapy. Also called **conversion hysteria, conversion reaction, somatoform disorder.**

**conversion dysphonia,** an inability to produce vocal sounds, usually psychogenic in nature. Previously called **hysteric aphonia.**

**conversion factor,** a dollar value multiplied by a procedure's unit value, from the **Current Procedural Terminology (CPT)** codes or a relative value scale, used to calculate the payment amount for contracted services or to set a price for a service. See also **Current Procedural Terminology.**

**conversion hysteria.** See **conversion disorder.**

**conversion reaction,** an ego defense mechanism whereby intrapsychic conflict is expressed symbolically through physical symptoms.

**convex** [L, *convextus,* vaulted], having a surface that curves outward. Compare **concave.**

**convex spherical lens** [L, *convehere,* to bring together; Gk, *sphaira,* ball; L, *lentil*], a lens that has sides that curve outward like a section of the exterior of a sphere; it brings light to a focus. It is used in the treatment of hyperopia (farsightedness).

**convoluted** /kon'vəlōō'tid/, [L, *convolutus,* rolled together], twisted, rolled together, with one part over another in a scroll. Also **convolute.**

**convoluted kidney tubules** [L, *convolutus,* rolled together; ME, *kidenei;* L, *tubulus*], pertaining to the proximal convoluted tubule of the nephron that leads from the glomerulus to the connecting ducts and between the Bowman's capsule and the loop of Henle. The proximal and distal sections are convoluted, whereas the ascending and descending limbs of Henle's loop are relatively straight.

**convoluted seminiferous tubules,** the long threadlike tubes in the areolar tissue of the testes. The testes also contain straight segments of seminiferous tubules.

**convolution** /kon'və·lōō'shən/ [L, *convolutus* rolled together], a tortuous irregularity or elevation caused by a structure being infolded on itself, such as the gyri of the cerebrum. See also **gyrus.**

**convulsion.** See **seizure.**

**convulsive seizure** /kənvul'siv/ [L, *convulsio,* cramp; OFr, *seisir*], a sudden onset of a disease characterized by convulsions, palpitations, and other symptoms. The term is sometimes applied to an attack of an epileptic disorder.

**convulsive syncope.** See **vasovagal.**

**convulsive tic,** a disorder of the facial nerve, causing involuntary spasmodic contractions of the facial muscles supplied by that nerve. Also called **hemifacial spasm.** See also **Gilles de la Tourette's syndrome.**

**Cooley's anaemia, Cooley's anemia.** See **thalassemia.**

**Coolidge tube** [William D. Coolidge, American physician, 1873–1977], a basic type of hot-cathode x-ray tube that, with modern refinements, has been used by radiologists since it was invented in 1913.

**cooling** [AS, *colian,* cool], reducing body temperature by the application of a hypothermia blanket, cold moist dressings, ice packs, or an alcohol bath. Subnormal body temperature may be induced to reduce metabolic function before some kinds of surgery. Very high fevers of any origin may be treated in part by reduction of the fever with cooling techniques. See also **alcohol bath, hypothermia, hypothermia blanket.**

**cooling rate,** the rate at which temperature decreases with time (°C/minute) immediately after the completion of hyperthermia treatment.

**Coombs' positive hemolytic anemia** /kōōmz/ [Robin R.A. Coombs, British immunologist, b. 1921], a form of anemia that results from premature destruction of circulating red blood cells. See also **antiglobulin test.**

**Coombs' test** [Robin R.A. Coombs]. See **antiglobulin test.**

**cooperative play** /kō·op'erətiv'/, any organized recreation among a group of children in which activities are planned for the purpose of achieving some goal. It usually occurs among older children. Compare **associative play, parallel play, solitary play.**

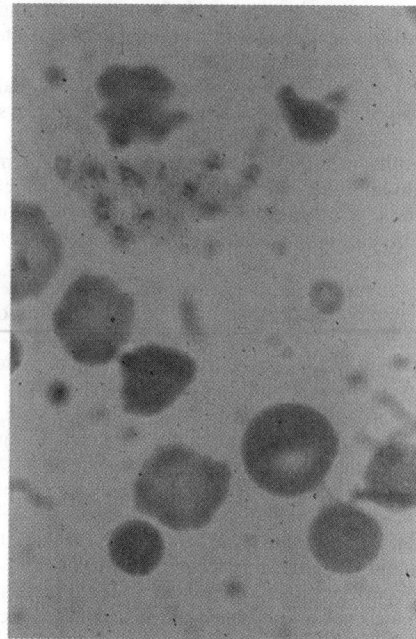

**Coombs' positive hemolytic anemia**
*(Zitelli and Davis, 1997)*

**coordinated reflex** /kō·ôr′dinā′tid/ [L, *coordinare,* to arrange], a sequence of muscular actions that occur in a purposeful, orderly progression, such as the act of swallowing.
**CO-oximeter,** a device that uses spectrophotometry to measure relative blood concentrations of oxyhemoglobin, carboxyhemoglobin, methemoglobin, and reduced hemoglobin.
**copayment** /kō′pāmənt/, (in the United States) an amount paid by a health insurance plan enrollee for each office or emergency department visit or purchase of prescription drugs in addition to the amount paid by the insurance company. See also **deductible.**
**COPD,** abbreviation for **chronic obstructive pulmonary disease.**
**coping**[1] [Gk, *kolaphos,* buffet], a process by which a person deals with stress, solves problems, and makes decisions. The process has two components, cognitive and noncognitive. The cognitive component includes the thought and learning necessary to identify the source of the stress. The noncognitive components are automatic and focus on relieving the discomfort. Many defense mechanisms fall into this category. Although sometimes useful, noncognitive measures may fail to relieve the stress because the response may be inappropriate, may have the wrong effect, and, as it replaces cognitive coping measures, may prevent the person from learning more about the cause and finding a better solution for the problem.
**coping**[2] a nursing outcome from the Nursing Outcome Classification (NOC) defined as actions to manage stressors that tax an individual's resources. See also **nursing outcomes classification.**
**coping, community, ineffective,** a nursing diagnosis accepted by the Eleventh National Conference on the Classification of Nursing Diagnoses. It is defined as a pattern of community activities for adaptation and problem solving

that is unsatisfactory for meeting the demands or needs of the community.
■ DEFINING CHARACTERISTICS: The defining characteristics include a community's inability to meet its own expectations, deficits of community participation, deficits in communication methods, excessive community conflicts, expressed difficulty in meeting demands for change, expressed vulnerability, high illness rates, and stressors perceived as excessive.
■ RELATED FACTORS: The related factors include deficits in social support, inadequate resources for problem solving, and powerlessness. See also **nursing diagnosis.**
**coping, community, readiness for enhanced,** a nursing diagnosis accepted by the Eleventh National Conference on the Classification of Nursing Diagnoses. It is defined as a pattern of community activities for adaptation and problem solving that is satisfactory for meeting the demands or needs of the community but can be improved for management of current and future problems/stressors.
■ DEFINING CHARACTERISTICS: The major defining characteristics include deficits in one or more characteristics that indicate effective coping. The minor defining characteristics include active planning by the community for predicted stressors, active problem solving by the community when faced with issues, agreement that the community is responsible for stress management, positive communication among community members, positive communication between community/aggregates and the larger community, programs available for recreation and relaxation, and resources sufficient for managing stressors.
■ RELATED FACTORS: The related factors include availability of social supports, existence of resources for problem solving, and a community sense of power to manage stressors. See also **nursing diagnosis.**
**coping, defensive,** a nursing diagnosis accepted by the Eighth National Conference on the Classification of Nursing Diagnoses. Defensive coping is a state in which an individual has a falsely positive self-evaluation based on a self-protective pattern that defends against underlying perceived threats to positive self-regard.
■ DEFINING CHARACTERISTICS: Major defining characteristics are denial of obvious problems or weaknesses, projection of blame or responsibility, rationalization of failures, defensiveness and hypersensitivity in response to a slight or criticism, and grandiosity. Minor characteristics are a superior attitude toward others, difficulty in establishing or maintaining relationships, hostile laughter or ridicule of others, difficulty in reality testing perceptions, and lack of follow through or participation in treatment or therapy.
■ RELATED FACTORS: Related factors are to be developed. See also **nursing diagnosis.**
**coping enhancement,** a nursing intervention from the Nursing Interventions Classification (NIC) defined as assisting a patient to adapt to perceived stressors, changes, or threats that interfere with meeting life demands and roles. See also **Nursing Interventions Classification.**
**coping, family, compromised,** a nursing diagnosis accepted by the Fourth National Conference on the Classification of Nursing Diagnoses. The diagnosis refers to a lack or absence of emotional and psychologic support for the client that is usually available from a family member or other supportive person, a deficiency that causes the client further difficulty in coping with the current health problem.
■ DEFINING CHARACTERISTICS: The defining characteristics are divided into subjective and objective categories. Subjectively, the client expresses that support is lacking, or the supportive person expresses that fear, anticipatory grief,

anxiety, or another reaction is interfering with the ability to give support to the client. A frank statement of an inadequate understanding of the health problem from the client or supportive person may be made. Objectively the nurse may observe that the support given is inadequate, that the communication between the parties is limited and unsatisfactory, or that the supportive person offers help that is disproportionate to the need.

■ RELATED FACTORS: Related factors include inadequate or incorrect information or understanding by a primary person; temporary family disorganization and role changes; other situational or developmental crises or situations the significant person may be facing; little support provided by client, in turn, for primary person; and prolonged disease or disability progression that exhausts the supportive capacity of significant people. See also **nursing diagnosis.**

**coping, family, disabled,** a nursing diagnosis accepted by the Fourth National Conference on the Classification of Nursing Diagnoses. The diagnosis refers to the behavior of a significant person (family member or other primary person) who disables his or her own capacities and the capacity to effectively address tasks essential to either the person's adaptation to the health challenge.

■ DEFINING CHARACTERISTICS: The defining characteristics include neglect in the care of the client, intolerance, rejection or abandonment, adoption of the client's symptoms, disregard of the client's needs, and marked distortion of reality in regard to the client's health problem.

■ RELATED FACTORS: Related factors include chronically unexpressed feelings of guilt, anxiety, hostility, and despair in a significant person; highly ambivalent family relationships; arbitrary handling of the family's resistance to treatment, which tends to solidify defensiveness, as it fails to deal adequately with underlying anxiety; and dissonant discrepancy of coping styles for dealing with adaptive tasks by the significant person and client or among significant people. See also **nursing diagnosis.**

**coping, family, readiness for enhanced,** a nursing diagnosis accepted by the Fourth National Conference on the Classification of Nursing Diagnoses. The condition is defined as effective managing of adaptive tasks by the family member involved with the client's health challenge, who now is exhibiting desire and readiness for enhanced health and growth in regard to self and in relation to the client.

■ DEFINING CHARACTERISTICS: The defining characteristics of the family's potential for growth in this area are their expressed wish to discuss the impact of the situation on the client's own life and values, interest in meeting with others in similar situations, and choice of healthful options available to the client.

■ RELATED FACTORS: Related factors are needs sufficiently gratified and adaptive tasks effectively addressed to enable goals of self-actualization to surface. See also **nursing diagnosis.**

**coping, ineffective,** a nursing diagnosis accepted by the Fourth National Conference on the Classification of Nursing Diagnoses. Ineffective individual coping is defined as impairment of a person's adaptive behaviors and problem-solving abilities in meeting life's demands and roles.

■ DEFINING CHARACTERISTICS: The defining characteristics include an inability to meet the expectations of a role, an inability to meet one's basic needs, or an alteration in ability to participate in society. The critical defining characteristics, one of which must be present for the diagnosis to be made, are an inability to ask for help, an inability to solve problems, and verbalization of the inability to cope. Other characteristics that may be present are destructive behavior toward self or others, inappropriate or excessive use of

defense mechanisms, a change in patterns of communication, verbal manipulation, and a greater-than-expected incidence of accidents and illness.

■ RELATED FACTORS: Related factors include situational crises, maturational crises, and vulnerability. See also **nursing diagnosis.**

**coping mechanism,** any effort directed to stress management, including task-oriented and ego defense mechanisms; the factors that enable an individual to regain emotional equilibrium after a stressful experience. It is usually an unconscious process.

**coping resources,** the characteristics of a person, group, or environment that are helpful in assisting individuals in adapting to stress.

**coping style,** the cognitive, affective, or behavioral responses of a person to problematic or traumatic life events.

**copolymer** /kōpol′ə·mər/ [L, co-, together or with + Gk, polys, many + meros, parts], a polymer containing monomers of more than one kind.

**COPP,** an anticancer drug combination of cyclophosphamide, procarbazine, prednisone, and vincristine.

**copper (Cu)** [L, cuprum], a malleable, reddish-brown metallic element. Its atomic number is 29; its atomic mass is 63.55. Copper occurs in a pure state in nature and in many ores. It is a component of several important enzymes in the body and is essential to good health. Copper deficiency is rare because only 2 to 5 mg daily, easily obtained from a variety of foods, is sufficient for a proper balance. Copper accumulates in individuals with Wilson's disease, primary biliary cirrhosis, and, occasionally, chronic extrahepatic biliary tract obstruction. It is an excellent conductor of heat and electricity and a valuable component of numerous alloys, and it may be compounded with arsenic to form insecticides. See also **ceruloplasmin, hepatolenticular degeneration.**

**copperhead** /kop′ərhed′/[L, cuprum + ME, hed], a poisonous pit viper found mainly in the southeastern United States. The reddish brown, darkly banded snake is responsible for nearly 40% of the snakebites in the United States; few bites are fatal. Pain, swelling, fang marks, and a bruise are usually present. Immediate treatment includes keeping the victim quiet and immobilizing the bite area at the level of the heart while seeking medical attention. Antivenin is available but is rarely indicated. See also **coral snake, cottonmouth, rattlesnake.**

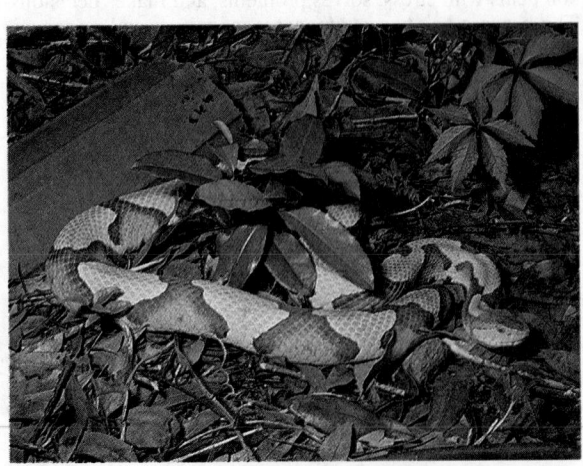

**Copperhead** (Auerbach, 1995/courtesy Sherman Minton, MD)

**Copper T,** trademark for a T-shaped plastic intrauterine device (IUD).

**copro-, copr-, kopr-, kopra-,** combining form meaning 'feces': *coprolalia, coprolith.*

**coprogogue.** See **cathartic.**

**coprolalia** /kop′rōlā′lyə/ [Gk, *kopros*, dung, *lalein*, to babble], the excessive use of obscene language.

**coprolith** /kop′rōlith/, a hard mass of feces in the intestinal tract usually caused by excessive absorption of water from the large intestine.

**coprology.** See **scatology.**

**coproporphyria** /kop′rōpôrfir′ē·ə/ [Gk, *kopros* + *porphyros*, purple], a rare hereditary metabolic disorder in which large quantities of nitrogenous substances, called porphyrins, are excreted in the feces. Attacks, with varying GI and neurologic symptoms, may be precipitated by certain drugs, including barbiturates, sulfonamides, and steroids. Patients are often helped by a high-carbohydrate diet. See also **acute intermittent porphyria, coproporphyrin, porphyria.** Also called **hereditary coproporphyria (HCP).**

**coproporphyrin** /kop′rōpôr′firin/ [Gk, *kopros* + *porphyros*, purple], any of the nitrogenous organic substances normally excreted in the feces that are products of the breakdown of bilirubin from hemoglobin decomposition.

**copula** /kop′ū·lə/ [L], **1.** any connecting part or structure. **2.** a median ventral elevation on the embryonic tongue formed by union of the second pharyngeal arches; it represents the future root of the tongue. Also called **copula linguae.**

**copulation.** See **coitus.**

**CoQ,** abbreviation for **coenzyme Q.**

**cor** /kôr/, **1.** the heart. **2.** relating to the heart.

**cor-.** See **co-.**

**coracoacromial** /kôr′əkō·əkrō′mē·əl/, pertaining to the coracoid process and the acromion of the scapula.

**coracobrachialis** /kôr′əkōbrā′kē·al′is/, a muscle with its origin on the scapula and its insertion on the inner side of the humerus. It functions to adduct the shoulder.

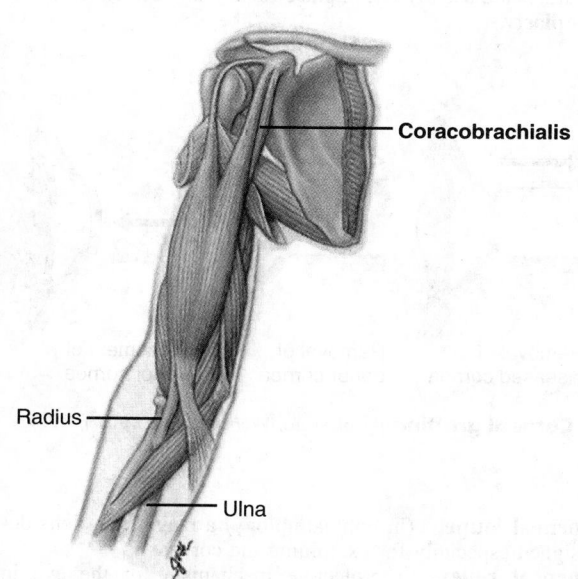

**Coracobrachialis muscle**
*(Thibodeau and Patton, 1999/John V. Hagen)*

**coracoid process** /kôr′əkoid/[Gk, *korax*, crow, *eidos*, form; L, *processus*], the thick, curved extension of the superior border of the scapula, to which the pectoralis minor is attached. Compare **acromion.**

**coral calculus.** See **dendritic calculus.**

**coral snake,** a poisonous snake with transverse red, yellow, and black bands that is native to the southern United States. Bites are rare; pain does not always result, but neuromuscular and respiratory effects may be severe. Immediate treatment includes keeping the victim quiet and immobilizing the bite area at the level of the heart. Ventilatory support should be provided. Antivenin is available.

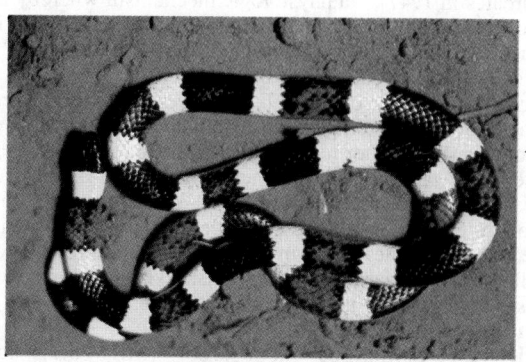

**Coral snake**
*(Sanders et al, 2000/courtesy St Louis Zoo, St Louis, MO)*

**Coramine,** trademark for a respiratory stimulant (nikethamide).

**cord** [Gk, *chorde*, string], any long, rounded, flexible structure. The body contains many different cords, such as the spermatic, vocal, spinal, neural, umbilical, and hepatic cords. Cords serve many different purposes, depending on location, kind of enclosed cells, and body parts or tissue involved.

**cordal,** pertaining to a cord, such as the umbilical cord.

**Cordarone,** trademark for an oral antiarrhythmic (amiodarone hydrochloride).

**cord blood,** blood taken from the umbilical cord vein or artery of the fetus. Like bone marrow, cord blood is rich in blood stem cells. It can be frozen and stored for later transfusion, for example, in cord blood transplant.

**cord blood transplantation,** the removal of blood from the umbilical cord of a fetus or its placenta for the treatment of blood diseases. Cord blood transplantation has been performed successfully in patients with leukemia, aplastic anemia, Fanconi's anemia, immunodeficiency, and genetic and metabolic disorders.

**corditis** /kôrdī′tis/ [Gk, *chorde* + *itis*, inflammation], an inflammation of the spermatic cord, accompanied by pain in the testis, often caused by an infection originating in the urethra or by a tumor, hydrocele, or varicocele. Inflammatory conditions of the testis may lead to swelling and tenderness.

**cord presentation.** See **funic presentation.**

**Cordran,** trademark for a glucocorticoid (flurandrenolide).

**core** [L, *cor*, heart], **1.** a kind of main computer memory. **2.** (in dentistry) a section of a mold, usually of plaster, made over assembled parts of a dental restoration to record and maintain their relationships so that the parts can be reassembled in their original position. Also called **laboratory**

**core. 3.** the center of a structure, as in core temperature of the body.

**core-, coro-,** combining form meaning 'pupil of the eye': *coreclisis, corectasis, corectopia.*

**core gender identity.** See **gender identity.**

**core temperature** [L, *cor,* heart, *temperatura*], the temperature of deep structures of the body, such as the liver, as compared to that of peripheral tissues.

**Corgard,** trademark for a nonselective beta-adrenergic blocking agent (nadolol).

**-coria,** suffix meaning '(condition of the) pupil': *anisocoria, diplocoria, platycoria.*

**Cori cycle** [Carl F. Cori, American physician, 1896–1984; Gerty T. Cori, American biochemist, 1896–1957; co–Nobel laureates in 1947], a physiologic mechanism whereby lactate, produced by glycolysis of glucose in contracting muscle, is converted back to glucose in the liver and returned via the circulation to the muscles.

**Cori's disease** /kôr'ēz/ [Carl F. Cori; Gerty T. Cori], a rare type of glycogen storage disease, in which the lack of an enzyme results in abnormally large deposits of glycogen in the liver, skeletal muscles, and heart. Signs are an enlarged liver, hypoglycemia, acidosis, and, occasionally, stunted growth. Symptoms can be controlled by giving the patient frequent small meals rich in carbohydrate and protein. Also called **Forbes' disease, glycogenosis, glycogen storage disease, type III.** See also **glycogen storage disease.**

**corium.** See **dermis.**

**corkscrew esophagus** /kôrk'skrōō/ [ME *cork,* bark; L, *scrofa,* sow; Gk, *oisophagos,* gullet], a neurogenic disorder in which normal peristaltic contractions of the esophagus are replaced by spastic movements that occur spontaneously or with swallowing or gastric acid reflux. Difficulty in swallowing, weight loss, severe pain over the upper chest, and a characteristic corkscrew image on radiogram are the symptoms usually present. Management may include the use of antispasmodic drugs, avoidance of cold fluids, surgical dilation, or myotomy. Compare **achalasia.** See also **dysphagia.**

**cork worker's lung,** hypersensitivity pneumonitis seen in cork handlers, caused by inhalation of moldy cork dust containing spores of various species of *Penicillium.*

**-cormia, -cormy,** suffix meaning an 'abnormal development of the trunk of the body': *camptocormia, nanocormia, schistocormia.*

**corn** [L, *cornu,* horn], a horny mass of condensed epithelial cells overlying a bony prominence. Corns result from chronic friction and pressure. The conic shape of the corn compresses the underlying dermis, making it thin and ten-

der. Corns can become soft and macerated by perspiration. Treatment includes relief of the mechanical pressure and surgical paring or chemical peeling of the excess keratin. Also called **clavus.** Compare **callus.**

**cornea** /kôr'nē·ə/ [L, *corneus,* horny], the convex, transparent anterior part of the eye, comprising one sixth of the outermost tunic of the eye bulb. It allows light to pass through it to the lens. The cornea is a fibrous structure with five layers: the anterior corneal epithelium, continuous with that of the conjunctiva; the anterior limiting layer (Bowman's membrane); the substantia propria; the posterior limiting layer (Descemet's membrane); and the endothelium of the anterior chamber (keratoderma). It is dense, uniform in thickness, and nonvascular, and it projects like a dome beyond the sclera, which forms the other five sixths of the eye's outermost tunic. The degree of corneal curvature varies among different individuals and in the same person at different ages; the curvature is more pronounced in youth than in advanced age.

**corneal abrasion** /kôr'nē·əl/ [L, *corneus,* horny, *abrasio,* scraping], the rubbing off of the outer layers of the cornea.

**corneal corpuscle,** one of the fixed flattened connective tissue cells between the lamellae of the cornea. Also called **keratocyte.**

**corneal grafting,** transplantation of corneal tissue from one human eye to another, performed to improve vision in corneal scarring or distortion or to remove a perforating ulcer. Preoperative preparation includes constricting the pupil with a miotic drug, such as pilocarpine. With the patient under local anesthesia the affected area is excised, using an operating microscope; an identical section of clear cornea is cut from the donor eye and sutured in place, using an operating microscope. Cataract surgery may be performed at the same time. After surgery the eye is covered with a protective metal shield. The patient is cautioned against coughing, sneezing, vomiting, sudden movement, and lifting. The dressing is changed daily, and antibiotics are instilled. A complication that may occur after several weeks is a clouding over of the graft, a result of the rejection of foreign tissue. Corticosteroid drugs administered immediately postoperatively may prevent the reaction. Healing is slow, and the sutures are usually left in place for 1 year. Also called **keratoplasty.**

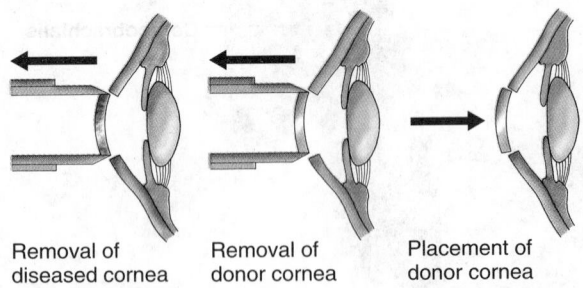

Removal of diseased cornea     Removal of donor cornea     Placement of donor cornea

**Corneal grafting** *(Ignatavicius, Workman, and Mishler, 1999)*

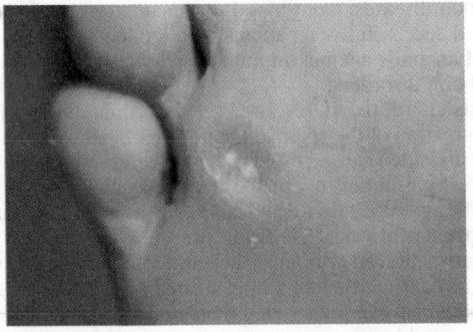

**Corn** *(Weston, Lane, and Morelli, 1996)*

**corneal loupe,** (in ophthalmology) a magnifying lens designed especially for examining the cornea.

**corneal reflex,** a protective mechanism for the eye in which the eyelids close when the cornea is touched. This reflex is mediated by the ophthalmic division of the fifth cranial nerve (sensory) and seventh cranial nerve (motor) and may be used as a test of integrity of those nerves. People who wear contact lenses may have a diminished or absent corneal reflex. Compare **conjunctival reflex.**

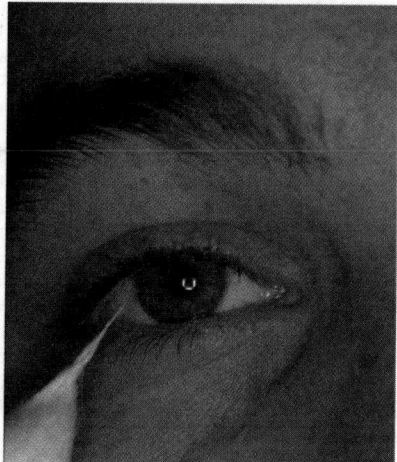

**Assessment of the corneal reflex** *(Lemmi and Lemmi, 2000)*

**corneal transplant.** See **corneal grafting.**

**Cornelia de Lange's syndrome** /kôr·nā′lē·ä dä läng′əz/ [Cornelia de Lange, Dutch pediatrician, 1871−1950], a congenital syndrome of severe mental retardation with many other abnormalities, such as dwarfism, brachycephaly, low-set ears, webbed neck, carp mouth, peculiar shape of the nose, bushy eyebrows meeting at the midline, unruly coarse hair on the forehead and neck, and flat spadelike hands with short tapering fingers.

**corneoblepharon** /kôr′nē·ōblef′əron/, adhesion of the eyelid to the cornea.

**corneous.** See **horny, keratic** (def. 1).

**corneus layer.** See **stratum corneum.**

**cornification** /kôr′nifikā′shən/, the conversion of cells into the horny layer of the skin. Also called **keratinization.**

**corn pad,** a device that helps relieve the pressure and pain of a corn on the toes by transferring the pressure to surrounding unaffected areas. Corn pads are constructed of pliable fabric and fashioned in various ways to accommodate different sites on the feet. See also **corn.**

**cornua** /kôr′nōō·ə/, an anatomic structure that resembles a horn.

**cornual pregnancy** /kôr′nyōō·əl/ [L, *cornu,* horn, *praegnans,* childbearing], an ectopic pregnancy in one of the straight or curved extensions of the body of the uterus. The signs include a uterus that is asymmetric and tender, as well as cramping and spotting. The cornu of the uterus usually ruptures between 12 and 16 weeks of the pregnancy unless the condition is treated surgically to remove the products of conception. In most cases the uterus can be repaired. Also called **interstitial pregnancy.** See also **ectopic pregnancy.**

**cornu posterioris.** See **dorsal horn, posterior horn.**

**coro-.** See **core-.**

**corona** /kərō′nə/ [L, crown], 1. a crown. 2. a crownlike projection or encircling structure, such as a process extending from a bone. —**coronal, coronoid,** *adj.*

**coronal plane.** See **frontal plane.**

**coronal section** [L, *corona,* crown, *sectio*], a section of the body cut in the plane of the coronal suture, or parallel to it.

**coronal suture,** the serrated transverse suture between the frontal bone and the parietal bone on each side of the skull.

**corona radiata,** *pl.* **coronae radiatae** [L, crown; *radiare* to emit rays], 1. a network of fibers that weaves through the internal capsule of the cerebral cortex and intermingles with the fibers of the corpus callosum. 2. an aggregate of cells that surrounds the zona pellucida of the ovum.

**coronary** /kôr′əner′ē/ [L, *corona,* crown], 1. pertaining to encircling structures, such as the coronary arteries. 2. pertaining to the heart. 3. *nontechnical.* a myocardial infarction or occlusion.

**coronary arteriovenous fistula,** an unusual congenital abnormality characterized by a direct communication between a coronary artery, usually the right, and the right atrium or ventricle, the coronary sinus, or the vena cava. There may be a left-to-right shunt of small magnitude causing no symptoms, but a large shunt may result in growth failure, limited exercise tolerance, dyspnea, and anginal pain. Possible complications of a large shunt are bacterial endocarditis, rupture of an aneurysmal fistula, thrombus formation that causes occlusion or distal embolization, and in rare cases pulmonary hypertension and congestive heart failure. A loud continuous murmur heard at the lower or midsternal border of the heart suggests a coronary arteriovenous fistula; the diagnosis may be confirmed by coronary arteriography or aortography. Closure of the fistulous tract is a safe surgical procedure with excellent long-term results.

**coronary artery,** one of a pair of arteries that branch from the aorta, including the left and the right coronary arteries. Because these vessels and their branches supply the heart, any dysfunction or disease that affects them can cause serious, sometimes fatal complications. Coronary arterial anastomoses occur throughout the heart and are especially numerous within the interventricular and interatrial septa, at the apex of the heart, at the crux, over the anterior surface of the right ventricle, and between the sinus-node artery and the other atrial arteries. These anastomoses are more numerous and larger in the epicardium than in the endocardium,

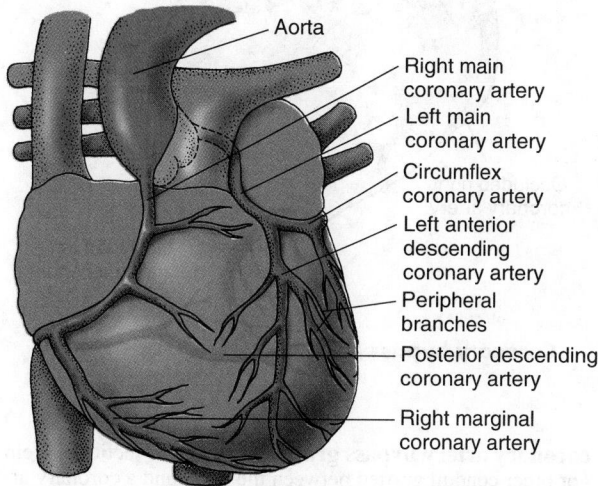

Aorta
Right main coronary artery
Left main coronary artery
Circumflex coronary artery
Left anterior descending coronary artery
Peripheral branches
Posterior descending coronary artery
Right marginal coronary artery

**Coronary artery circulation**
*(Ignatavicius, Workman, and Mishler, 1999)*

and they provide important collateral circulation in the recovery of patients who suffer coronary occlusions. The branches of the coronary arteries are affected by many different disorders, such as embolic, neoplastic, inflammatory, and noninflammatory diseases.

**coronary artery bypass,** open heart surgery in which a prosthesis or a section of a blood vessel is grafted onto one of the coronary arteries, bypassing a narrowing or blockage in a coronary artery. The operation is performed in coronary artery disease to improve the blood supply to the heart muscle and to relieve anginal pain. Coronary arteriography pinpoints the areas of obstruction before surgery. Under general anesthesia and with the use of a cardiopulmonary bypass machine one end of a 15- to 20-cm prosthesis or a segment of saphenous vein from the patient's leg is grafted to the ascending aorta. The other end is sutured to the clogged coronary artery at a point distal to the stoppage. The internal mammary artery may also be used as graft tissue. Usually double or triple grafts are done for multiple areas of blockage. After surgery close observation in an intensive care unit essential to ensure adequate ventilation and cardiac output. The systolic blood pressure is not allowed to drop significantly below the preoperative baseline, nor is it allowed to rise significantly, because hypertension can rupture a graft site. Arrhythmias are treated with medications or by electrical cardioversion. The patient is usually discharged within 5 to 8 days, unless complications occur. In nearly 20% of cases thrombosis occurs within the first year after coronary bypass, making the surgery controversial.

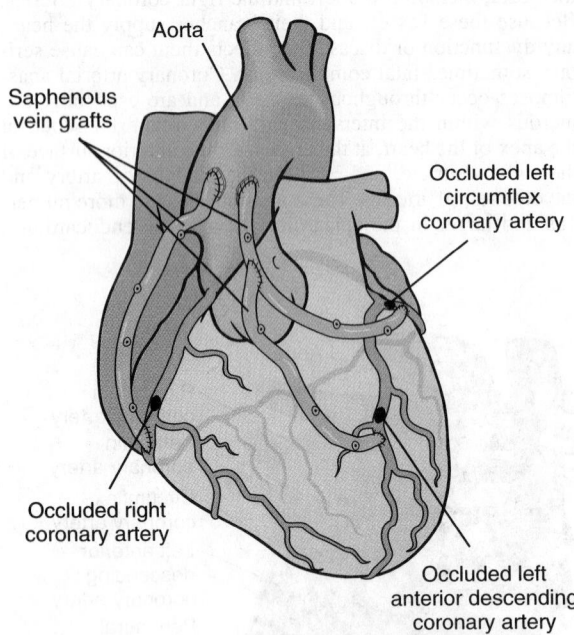

Aorta

Saphenous vein grafts

Occluded left circumflex coronary artery

Occluded right coronary artery

Occluded left anterior descending coronary artery

**Coronary bypass** *(Lewis, Heitkemper, and Dirksen, 2000)*

**coronary artery bypass graft (CABG),** a section of vein or other conduit grafted between the aorta and a coronary artery distal to an obstructive lesion of the coronary artery.

**coronary artery disease (CAD),** an abnormal condition that may affect the heart's arteries and produce various pathologic effects, especially the reduced flow of oxygen and nutrients to the myocardium. The most common kind of coronary artery disease is coronary atherosclerosis, now the leading cause of death in the Western world. Other coronary artery diseases include coronary arteritis and fibromuscular hyperplasia of the coronary arteries. Also called **coronary heart disease.**

■ OBSERVATIONS: Angina pectoris, the classic symptom of coronary artery disease, results from myocardial ischemia. Diagnosis of coronary artery disease is usually based on patient history and tests such as exercise stress tests, electrocardiography, coronary angiography, and myocardial perfusion imaging.

■ INTERVENTIONS: Treatment concentrates on reducing myocardial oxygen demand or on increasing oxygen supply. Therapy commonly includes the administration of nitrates, such as nitroglycerin or isosorbide dinitrate; propranolol, a beta-adrenergic blocker; or calcium channel blockers. Surgical interventions include coronary artery bypass surgery, angioplasty, insertion of cardiac stents, and atherectomy. The prevalence of coronary artery disease highlights the importance of preventive measures, such as reduced of caloric intake by the obese patient; lowered salt, fats, and cholesterol consumption; regular exercise; abstention from the use of tobacco products; and reduction of stress.

■ NURSING CONSIDERATIONS: The nurse monitors of blood pressure and heart rate, records electrocardiograms during anginal episodes, and administers drugs, such as nitroglycerin. The nurse is especially alert to signs of ischemia and arrhythmias and, before the patient is discharged, stresses the importance of following the prescribed regimens of diet, medication, exercise, and cessation of tobacco use.

**coronary artery fistula,** a congenital anomaly characterized by an abnormal communication between a coronary artery and the right side of the heart or the pulmonary artery.

**coronary bypass.** See **coronary artery bypass.**

**coronary care nursing,** the nursing care provided in a hospital in a coronary care unit. Nursing in this setting requires technical knowledge, judgment, and skills, as well as ability to give emotional support to patients and their families during the acute stage of cardiac dysfunction.

**coronary care unit,** a critical care unit used for the treatment and monitoring of patients experiencing acute cardiac episodes.

**coronary collateralization,** the spontaneous development of new blood vessels in or around areas of restricted blood flow to the heart muscle.

**coronary heart disease (CHD).** See **coronary artery disease.**

**coronary occlusion,** an obstruction of an artery that supplies the heart muscle. When complete, it causes myocardial infarction; when incomplete, it may cause angina. The underlying pathophysiologic characteristic is the atherosclerotic plaque, which usually develops slowly by buildup of lipid and macrophage complexes. Rapid plaque accumulation is frequently caused by hemorrhage within a plaque. If the plaque ruptures, platelets aggregate, fibrin is deposited, spasm occurs, and a thrombus develops, resulting in acute myocardial infarction. Treatment includes prompt IV thrombolysis and administration of heparin; primary percutaneous transvenous coronary angioplasty (PTCA) can achieve prompt reperfusion. See also **coronary artery disease.**

**coronary plexus** [L, *corona,* crown, *plexus,* plaited], a network of autonomic nerve fibers located near the base of the heart.

**coronary sinus,** the wide venous channel, about 2.25 cm long, situated in the coronary sulcus and covered by muscular fibers from the left atrium. Through a single semilunar valve it drains five coronary veins: the great cardiac vein, the small cardiac vein, the middle cardiac vein, the posterior vein of the left ventricle, and the oblique vein of the left atrium.

**coronary thrombosis,** development of a thrombus that blocks a coronary artery, often causing myocardial infarction and death. Coronary thromboses commonly develop in segments of arteries with atherosclerotic lesions.

**coronary valve** [L, *corona,* crown, *valva,* folding door], a semicircular fold of endocardium that prevents backflow of blood from the right atrium into the coronary sinus.

**coronary vein,** one of the veins of the heart that drain blood from the capillary beds of the myocardium through the coronary sinus into the right atrium. A few small coronary veins that collect blood from a small area in the right ventricle drain directly into the right atrium.

**Coronaviridae** /kôr′ənəvir′idē/, a family of four antigenic groups of single-stranded ribonucleic acid viruses. Some strains of the organism are associated with upper respiratory infections in humans.

**coronavirus** /kôr′ənəvī′rəs/ [L, *corona* + *virus,* poison], a member of a family of viruses that includes several types capable of causing acute respiratory illnesses.

**coroner** /kôr′ənər/ [L, *corona,* crown], a public official who investigates the causes and circumstances of deaths that occur within a specific legal jurisdiction or territory, especially those that may have resulted from unnatural causes. Also called **medical examiner.**

**coronoid.** See **corona.**

**coronoid fossa** /kô′rənoid/ [L, *corona* + Gk, *eidos,* form; L, *fossa,* ditch], a small depression in the distal dorsal surface of the humerus that receives the coronoid process of the ulna when the forearm is flexed.

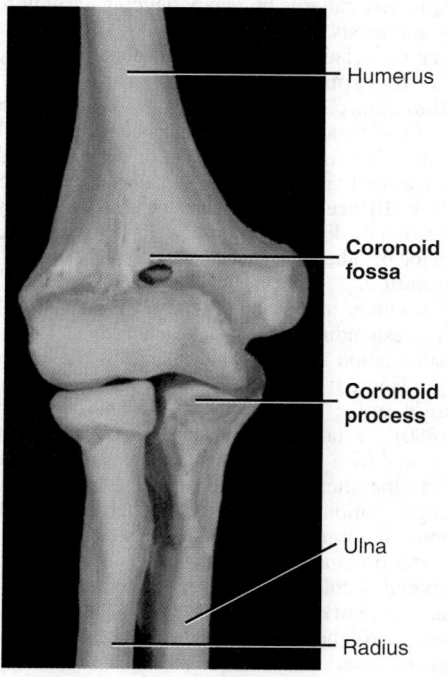

**Coronoid fossa and coronoid process of the elbow**
*(Vidic and Suarez, 1984)*

**coronoid process of mandible,** a prominence on the anterior surface of the ramus of the mandible to which each temporal muscle attaches.

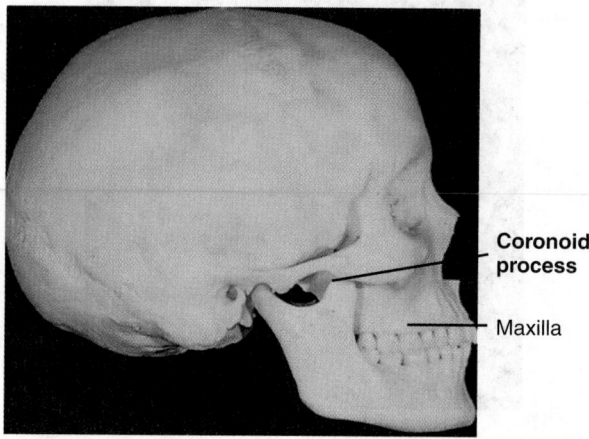

**Coronoid process of the mandible** *(Vidic and Suarez, 1984)*

**coronoid process of ulna,** a wide, flaring projection of the proximal end of the ulna. The proximal surface of the process forms the lower part of the trochlear notch.

**corpor-,** prefix meaning 'body': *corpora, corporeal, corporic.*

**corpora lutea.** See **corpus luteum.**

**corporate practice of medicine,** (in the United States) the role of nonpracticing physicians or nonprofessional corporations in employment relationships with physicians engaged in providing health care. Laws governing corporate practice of medicine vary among different states, but generally they require practitioner control over diagnosis and treatment, practitioner setting of fees, a reasonable relationship between services provided by layperson or corporation and amounts charged to the practitioner, and an unaltered practitioner-patient relationship.

**corpse** /kôrps/ [L, *corpus,* body], the body of a dead human being.

**corpulence** /kôr′pyələns/ [L, *corpus,* body], obesity.

**corpulent** /kôr′pyələnt/, obese.

**cor pulmonale** /kôr pŏŏl′mənal′ē/ [L, heart + *pulmoneus,* lungs], enlargement of the heart's right ventricle caused by primary lung disease. In some patients, the left ventricle also increases in size. Cor pulmonale eventually results in failure of the right ventricle, which cannot accommodate an increase in pressure as easily as the left ventricle. Pulmonary hypertension associated with this condition is caused by some disorder of the pulmonary parenchyma or of the pulmonary vascular system between the origin of the left pulmonary artery and the entry of the pulmonary veins into the left atrium.

**corpus.** See **body.**

**corpus albicans** /kôr′pəs/, a pale white spot on the surface of the ovary that arises from the corpus luteum if conception does not occur. Compare **corpus luteum.**

**corpus amylaceum.** See **colloid corpuscle.**

**corpus callosum** /kôr′pəs kalō′səm/, **1.** a transverse band of nerve fibers joining the cerebral hemispheres. It is located at the bottom of the longitudinal fissure between the two

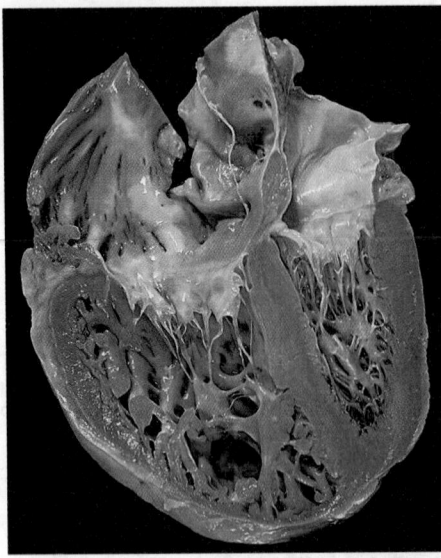

**Cor pulmonale** *(Cotran, Kumar, and Collins, 1999)*

hemispheres and is covered by the cingulate gyrus. **2.** the largest commissure of the brain, connecting the cerebral hemispheres.

**corpus cavernosum** [L, body + *caverna* hollow place], a type of spongy erectile tissue within the penis or clitoris. The tissue becomes engorged with blood during sexual excitement.

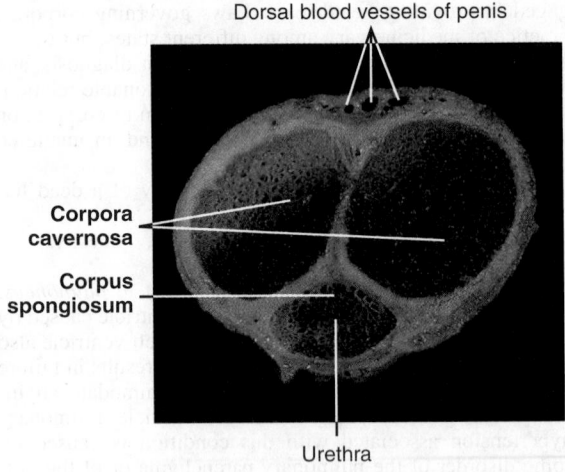

Dorsal blood vessels of penis

Corpora cavernosa

Corpus spongiosum

Urethra

**Corpus cavernosum and corpus spongiosum of the penis**
*(Vidic and Suarez, 1984)*

**corpuscle** /kôr′pəsəl/ [L, *corpusculum*, little body], **1.** any cell of the body. **2.** a red or white blood cell. Also called **corpuscule. —corpuscular,** *adj.*

**corpuscular radiation** /kôrpus′kyələr/ [L, *corpusculum + radiare,* to emit rays], the radiation associated with sub-

atomic particles, such as electrons, protons, neutrons, or alpha particles, which travel in streams at various velocities. All such particles have definite masses and have radiation properties very different from those of electromagnetic radiations, which have no mass and travel as waves at the speed of light. See also **background radiation, leakage radiation, scattered radiation.**

**corpus luteum** /kôr′pəs loo′tē·əm/, *pl.* **corpora lutea** [L, *corpus,* body, *luteus,* yellow], an anatomic structure on the ovary surface, consisting of a spheroid of yellowish tissue 1 to 2 cm in diameter that grows within the ruptured ovarian follicle after ovulation. The pleated wall of the collapsed follicle is made up of several layers of granulosa cells that grow toward the center of the cavity to form the structure. During a woman's reproductive years a corpus luteum forms after every ovulation. It acts as a short-lived endocrine organ that secretes progesterone, which serves to maintain the decidual layer of the uterine endometrium in the richly vascular state necessary for implantation and pregnancy. If conception occurs, the corpus luteum grows and secretes increasing amounts of progesterone. It reaches its maximum function and size (2 to 3 cm) at 10 to 12 weeks of gestation. It persists, slowly diminishing in size and function, until 6 months after the onset of gestation. During the 2 weeks before menstruation the corpus luteum secretes progesterone in decreasing amounts, atrophies, undergoes fibrotic degeneration, and becomes a pale spot on the surface of the ovary. Compare **corpus albicans.**

**corpus spongiosum** /spon′jē·ō′səm/, one of the cylinders of spongy tissue, with the corpora cavernosa, on the dorsum of the penis, erectile tissue.

**corpus vitreum.** See **vitreous humor.**

**corrected pressure** [L, *corrigere,* to make straight], a method of applying Boyle's law of gas pressures to adjust simultaneously for changes in both pressure and humidity.

**corrective emotional experience** /kərek′tiv/, a process by which a patient gives up old behavior patterns and learns or relearns new patterns by reexperiencing early unresolved feelings and needs.

**corrective exercise.** See **therapeutic exercise.**

**corrective therapist.** See **kinesiotherapist.**

**correlation** /kôr′əlā′shən/ [L, *com + relatio,* a carrying back], (in statistics) a relationship between variables that may be negative (inverse), positive, or curvilinear. Correlation is measured and expressed by using numeric scales.

**correlative differentiation** /kərel′ətiv/, (in embryology) specialization or diversification of cells or tissues caused by an inductor or other external factor. Also called **dependent differentiation.**

**correspondence,** (in ophthalmology) the relationship between corresponding points on each retina. The simultaneous stimulation of the points results in the sensation of viewing a single object.

**Corrigan's pulse** [Dominic J. Corrigan, Irish physician, 1802–1880], a bounding pulse in which a great surge is felt, followed by a sudden and complete absence of force or fullness in the artery. This kind of pulse is associated with aortic regurgitation and occurs in excited emotional states; in various abnormal cardiac conditions, including patent ductus arteriosus; and as a result of systemic arteriosclerosis. Also called **collapsing pulse, water-hammer pulse.**

**corrode.** See **corrosive.**

**corrosion** /kərō′zhen/, a result of an oxidation-reduction reaction, or deterioration of a substance by a destructive agent. See also **corrosive.**

**corrosion of surgical instruments** [L, *corrodere,* to gnaw away], the rusting of surgical instruments or the gradual wearing away of their polished surfaces caused by oxidation and the action of contaminants. Though minimized by the use of stainless steel alloys in the fabrication of the instruments, corrosion persists as a problem, even when cleaning procedures seem more than adequate. It usually results from inadequate cleaning and drying of surgical instruments after use, sterilization with solutions that eat into the surface, overexposure to such solutions, or a faulty autoclave. Cleanliness is the single most important factor in preventing corrosion. Any foreign material, either organic or inorganic, on the surface of stainless steel is likely to promote corrosion, and microscopic examinations often reveal foreign material and chlorides from cleaning solutions scattered over the surface of cleaned and sterilized instruments. The more chromium in the stainless steel alloys of which surgical instruments are made, the more resistant the instruments are to corrosion. Carbon, which hardens such alloys, also reduces their resistance to corrosion. Most corrosion of surgical instruments is superficial and may be removed by soaking in a solution of ammonia and alcohol or by repolishing by the manufacturer.

**corrosive** /kərō′siv/ [L, *corrodere,* to gnaw away], **1.** eating away a substance or tissue, especially by chemical action. **2.** an agent or substance that eats away a substance or tissue. —**corrode,** *v.,* **corrosion,** *n.*

**corrosive gastritis,** an acute inflammatory condition of the stomach caused by the ingestion of an acid, alkali, or other corrosive chemical in which the lining of the stomach is eaten away by the corrosive substance. The amount of tissue destruction and recommended treatment depend on the nature of the corrosive agent and the extent of exposure. Compare **chemical gastritis, erosive gastritis.** See also **acid poisoning, alkali poisoning.**

**corrugator supercilii** /kôr′əgā′tər soo′pərsil′ē·ī/ [L, *corrugare,* to wrinkle; *super,* above, *cilium,* eyelash], one of the three muscles of the eyelid. Arising from the medial end of the superciliary arch and inserting into the skin above the or-

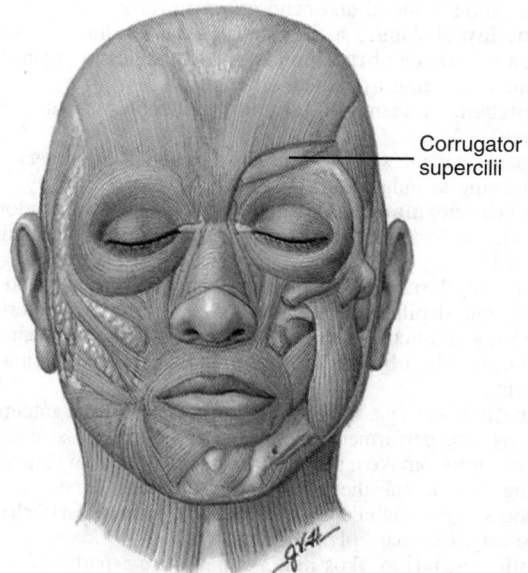

Corrugator supercilii

**Corrugator supercilii**
*(Thibodeau and Patton, 1999/John V. Hagen)*

bital arch, it is innervated by the temporal and zygomatic branches of the facial nerve and functions to draw the eyebrow downward and inward, as if to frown. Also called **corrugator.** Compare **levator palpebrae superioris, orbicularis oculi.**

**-cort,** suffix designating a cortisone derivative.

**cortex,** *pl.* **cortices** /kôr′tisēz/ [L, bark], the outer layer of a body organ or other structure, as distinguished from the internal substance.

**cortic-,** combining form meaning 'cortex or bark': *corticipetal, corticobulbar, corticothalamic.*

**cortical audiometry.** See **audiometry.**

**cortical blindness** /kôr′tikəl/ [L, *cortex* + AS, *blind*], loss of vision that results from a lesion in the visual center of the cerebral cortex of the brain.

**cortical bone,** bone that is 70% to 90% mineralized.

**cortical evoked potential,** an evoked potential recorded from the cerebral cortex.

**cortical fracture** [L, *cortex* + *fractura,* break], a fracture that involves the cortex of a bone.

**corticalization.** See **collapsing pulse.**

**cortical march.** See **jacksonian march.**

**cortical substance of cerebellum.** See **cerebellar cortex.**

**cortices.** See **cortex.**

**corticosteroid** /kôr′tikōstir′oid/ [L, *cortex* + *steros,* solid], any one of the natural or synthetic hormones elaborated by the adrenal cortex (excluding the sex hormones of adrenal origin) that influence or control key processes of the body. These processes include carbohydrate and protein metabolism, maintenance of serum glucose levels, electrolyte and water balance, and functions of the cardiovascular system, the skeletal muscle, the kidneys, and other organs. The corticosteroids synthesized by the adrenal glands include the glucocorticoids and the mineralocorticoids. The principal glucocorticoids are cortisol and corticosterone. The only physiologically important mineralocorticoid in humans is aldosterone. The glucocorticoids tend to cause the cells of the body to shift from carbohydrate catabolism to fat catabolism, to accelerate the breakdown of proteins to amino acids, and to help maintain normal blood pressure. The secretion of these hormones increases during stress, especially that produced by anxiety and severe injury. Chronic overproduction of these substances is associated with various disorders, such as Cushing's syndrome. A high blood level of glucocorticoids markedly increases the number of eosinophils and decreases the size of lymphatic tissues, especially the thymus and the lymph nodes. The decrease in lymphocytes slows antibody formation and affects the body's immune system. Aldosterone is the most powerful of the natural mineralocorticoids in the regulation of electrolyte balance, especially in the balance of sodium and potassium. Cortisol induces sodium retention and potassium excretion, but less effectively than aldosterone. The effects of the corticosteroids on the cardiovascular system, which are not precisely understood, are most evident in hypocortisolism, when the reduction in blood volume, accompanied by increased viscosity, may cause hypotension and cardiovascular collapse. The absence of corticosteroids decreases capillary permeability, decreases vasomotor response of small vessels, and reduces cardiac size and output. The skeletal muscles require adequate amounts of the corticosteroids to function normally; excessive amounts cause them to function abnormally. Cortisol and its synthetic analogs can prevent or reduce inflammation by inhibiting edema, leukocytic migration, and disposition of collagen and by causing other complications associated with inflammatory processes. The antiinflammatory actions of synthetic hormones can be harmful, however, because they mask the disease process and prevent accurate observation of its progress. Toxic effects may result from the too rapid withdrawal of such drugs after prolonged therapy or from the continued use of large doses. Toxic effects associated with prolonged corticosteroid therapy include fluid and electrolyte imbalance, hyperglycemia and glycosuria, increased susceptibility to infections, myopathy, arrested growth, ecchymoses, Cushing's syndrome, acne, and behavioral disturbances. In others receiving large doses of these drugs, myopathy, characterized by weakness of the proximal musculature of the arms and the legs and associated shoulder and pelvic muscles, develops. Corticosteroid therapy may also produce behavioral changes, such as schizophrenia, suicidal tendencies, nervousness, and insomnia. See also **adrenal crisis.**

**corticosteroid-binding globulin.** See **transcortin.**

**corticotroph** /kor'ti·kō·trof'/, a small, irregularly stellate, acidophilic cell of the adenohypophysis, having small, sparsely distributed secretory granules and secreting adrenocorticotropic hormone and β-endorphin. Also called **corticotrope, corticotropic cell.**

**corticotroph adenoma.** See **corticotropinoma.**

**corticotropic cell.** See **corticotroph.**

**corticotropin.** See **adrenocorticotropic hormone.**

**corticotropinoma** /kor'ti·kō·trō'pi·nō'mə/, a pituitary adenoma made up predominantly of corticotrophs; excessive adrenocorticotropic hormone (corticotropin) secretion may cause Cushing's disease or Nelson's syndrome. Also called **corticotropinoma.** See also **Cushing's disease, Nelson's syndrome.**

**corticotropin-releasing hormone (CRH)** /kôr'tikōtrop'in/, a polypeptide hormone secreted by the hypothalamus into the pituitary portal system where it triggers the release of adrenocorticotropic hormone from the pituitary gland.

**cortisol** /kôr'təsôl/, a steroid hormone produced naturally by the adrenal gland.
- INDICATION: It is prescribed topically for inflammation.
- CONTRAINDICATIONS: Fungal infections or known hypersensitivity to this drug prohibits its systemic use. Viral or fungal infections of the skin, impaired circulation, or known hypersensitivity to this drug prohibits its topical use.
- ADVERSE EFFECTS: Among the more serious adverse reactions to the systemic GI of this drug are GI, endocrine, neurologic, fluid, and electrolyte disturbances. Hypersensitivity reactions may result from topical administration.

**cortisone** /kôr'təsōn/, a synthetic glucocorticoid.
- INDICATION: It is topically prescribed for inflammation.
- CONTRAINDICATIONS: Fungal infections or known hypersensitivity to this drug prohibits its systemic use. Viral or fungal infections of the skin, impaired circulation, or known hypersensitivity to this drug prohibits its topical use.
- ADVERSE EFFECTS: Among the more serious adverse reactions to the systemic administration of the drug are GI, endocrine, neurologic, fluid, and electrolyte disturbances. Skin reactions may result from topical administration.

**Corti's organ.** See **organ of Corti.**

**Cortisporin,** trademark for a topical fixed-combination drug that contains a glucocorticoid (hydrocortisone) and three antibacterials (neomycin sulfate, polymyxin B sulfate, and bacitracin zinc).

**Corti's tunnel.** See **canal of Corti.**

**cor triatriatum** /kôr trī·ā'trē·ā'tum/, a congenital anomaly caused by failure of resorption of the embryonic common pulmonary vein, resulting in division of the left atrium by a fibromuscular diaphragm, the posterosuperior chamber receiving the pulmonary venous return and the anteroinferior chamber communicating with the left atrial appendage and mitral orifice. The orifice between the two compartments may be reduced or absent, producing pulmonary venous obstruction.

**Corvert,** trademark for a drug that controls atrial fibrillation and atrial flutter (Ibutilide).

***Corynebacterium*** /kôr'inē'baktir'ē·əm/ [Gk, *koryne,* club, *bakterion,* small staff], a common genus of rod-shaped curved bacilli that includes many species. The most common pathogenic species are *Corynebacterium acnes,* commonly found in acne lesions, and *C. diphtheriae,* the cause of diphtheria. See also *Propionibacterium.*

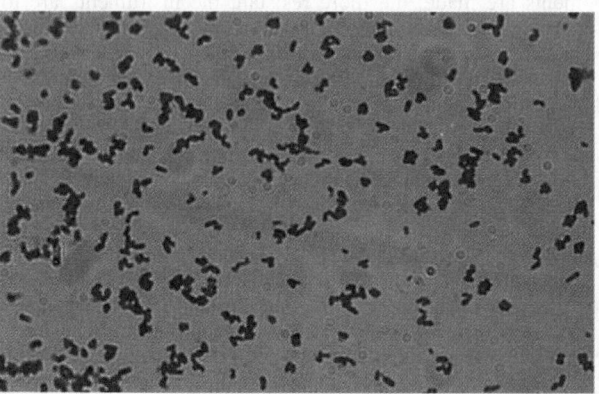

***Corynebacterium diphtheriae* gravis smear from culture**
*(Baron, Peterson, and Finegold, 1994)*

**coryza.** See **rhinitis.**

**coryza spasmodica.** See **hay fever.**

**Corzide,** trademark for a combination antihypertensive medication (nadolol and bendroflumethiazide).

**cosine law** /kō'sīn/, a rule that optimal irradiation occurs when the source of radiation is at right angles to the center of the area being irradiated.

**Cosmegen,** trademark for an antineoplastic (dactinomycin).

**cosmesis** /kosmē'sis/, the use of cosmetics or surgery for preserving or enhancing self-image.

**cosmetic dermatitis,** /kosmet'ik/ [Gk, *kosmesis,* adornment], a form of irritant or allergic contact dermatitis caused by ingredients in cosmetic products. The meaning is commonly broadened to include soaps, shampoos, deodorants, and depilatories in addition to perfumes, coloring agents, and toiletries. This inflammatory skin disease can be manifested in a broad spectrum, ranging from erythema to eczema.

**cosmetic surgery,** reconstruction of cutaneous or underlying tissues, performed to improve and correct a structural defect or to remove a scar, birthmark, or normal evidence of aging. A local anesthetic is usually sufficient. Kinds of cosmetic surgery include **blepharoplasty, rhinoplasty, rhytidoplasty.** Compare **plastic surgery.**

**cosmic radiation** /kos'mik/, high-energy particles with great penetrating power that originate in outer space and reach the earth as normal background radiation. The particles include high-energy atomic nuclei.

**costa** /kos′tə/, *pl.* **costae** /kos′tē/,   a rib.

**costal** /kos′təl/ [L, *costa,* rib],   **1.** pertaining to a rib. **2.** situated near a rib or on a side close to a rib.

**costal arch** [L, *costa* + *arcus,* bow],   an arch formed by the shafts of the ribs.

**costal cartilage,**   the cartilage at the anterior end of each rib.

**costalgia** /kostal′jə·ə/ [L, *costa,* rib; Gk, *algos,* pain],   a pain in the ribs.

**costal notch,**   an indentation beside a costal cartilage on the side of the sternum.

**cost analysis** [L, *costare,* to stand firm; Gk, *ana,* again, *lyein,* to loosen],   an analysis of the disbursements of an activity, agency, department, or program.

**COSTAR** /kō′stär/,   abbreviation for *COmputer STored Ambulatory Record* system, an on-line interactive computerized information system for the public health field.

**cost-based value,**   a relative value scale used to determine the total units of services provided by a medical practice. The total cost of running the practice and the total units of service are then used to calculate the costs for each service provided.

**cost-benefit analysis (CBA),**   a type of economic evaluation of medical care expense. It compares the monetary benefit derived from different health interventions with the cost of providing each of the interventions.

**cost-benefit ratio,**   a mathematic representation of the relationship of the cost of an activity to the benefit of its outcome or product.

**cost cap,**   *informal.* a limit on the amount of money that an agency, department, or institution may spend.

**cost center,**   a department, division, or other subunit of an institution established within its accounting system so that the income and expenses of the subunit can be separated from the income or expenses of other centers and monitored for cost and benefit.

**cost containment,**   a nursing intervention from the Nursing Interventions Classification (NIC) defined as management and facilitation of efficient and effective use of resources. See also **Nursing Interventions Classification.**

**cost control,**   the process of monitoring and regulating the expenditure of funds by an agency or institution. Budgets, reports, and cost-accounting procedures are performed to achieve cost control.

**costectomy** /kostek′təmē/,   surgical removal of a rib.

**cost effectiveness,**   the extent to which an activity is thought to be as valuable as it is expensive. A public-assistance program that issued vouchers for nutritious foods in pregnancy might be considered cost-effective if it lowered the costly incidence of perinatal morbidity.

**cost-effectiveness analysis (CEA),**   a type of economic evaluation used to determine the best use of money available for medical care. It compares different kinds of interventions with similar but not identical effects on the basis of the cost per unit achieved.

**Costen's syndrome.**   See **temporomandibular joint pain dysfunction syndrome.**

**cost-, costi-, costo-,**   prefix meaning 'rib': *costicartilage, costicervical, costifluous.*

**cost model,**   (in the United States) a managed care system in which all components of patient care are defined as costs as opposed to sources of revenue.

**costocervical** /kos′tōsur′vikəl/ [L, *costa,* rib, *cervix,* neck],   pertaining to or involving the ribs and the neck.

**costochondral** /kos′təkon′drəl/ [L, *costa* + Gk, *chondros,* cartilage],   pertaining to a rib and its cartilage.

**costochondritis** /kos′təkondrī′tis/,   an inflammation of the costal cartilage of the anterior chest wall. It is characterized by pain and tenderness.

**costoclavicular** /-klavik′yələr/ [L, *costa* + *clavicula,* little key],   pertaining to or involving the ribs and the clavicle.

**costoclavicular line,**   an imaginary vertical line between the sternal and midclavicular lines. Also called **parasternal line.**

**costophrenic (CP) angle** /-fren′ik/ [L, *costa* + *phrenicus,* diaphragm],   the angle between the diaphragm and the chest wall at the bottom of the lung.

**costosternal** /-stur′nəl/,   pertaining to or involving the ribs and the sternum.

**costotransverse articulation** /-transvurs′/ [L, *costa* + *transversus,* a cross direction],   any of the 20 gliding joints between the ribs and articulating vertebrae, except the eleventh and twelfth ribs. The five ligaments that associate with each costotransverse joint are the articular capsule, the superior costotransverse ligament, the posterior costotransverse ligament, the ligament of the neck of the rib, and the ligament of the tubercle of the rib.

**costovertebral** /-vur′təbrəl/,   of or relating to a rib and the vertebral column.

**costovertebral angle (CVA),**   one of two angles that outline a space over the kidneys. The angle is formed by the lateral and downward curve of the lowest rib and the vertical column of the spine itself. CVA tenderness to percussion is a common finding in pyelonephritis and other infections of the kidney and adjacent structures.

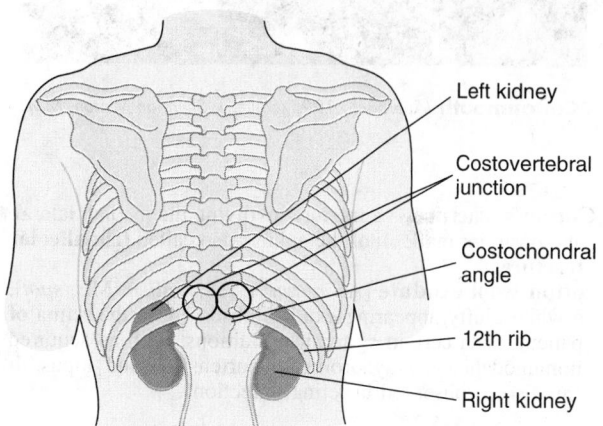

Left kidney

Costovertebral junction

Costochondral angle

12th rib

Right kidney

**Location of the costovertebral angle**
*(Beare and Myers, 1998)*

**cost-sharing program,**   (in the United States) a financial risk-management strategy often used by insurance companies and self-insured employers in which employees share the cost of health services, such as through deductibles and coinsurance.

**cost shifting,**   (in the United States) a mechanism for reducing inpatient costs by providing services in an outpatient setting. The inpatient cost per case is reduced but the overall cost to the organization does not change.

**cost-utility analysis (CUA),**   a type of economic evaluation of different approaches to managed health care costs. It compares the degree to which quality of life is improved per dollar spent. A quality-of-life index is used to compare interventions, including quality adjusted life years.

**cosyntropin** /kō'sintrop'in/, a synthetic form of adrenocorticotropic hormone that is used in the diagnosis and treatment of adrenal hypofunction disorders such as Addison's disease.

**COTA,** abbreviation for **Certified Occupational Therapy Assistant.**

**Cotazym,** trademark for an enzyme (pancrelipase).

**cot death.** See **sudden infant death syndrome.**

**cotton-mill fever.** See **byssinosis.**

**cottonmouth,** a poisonous pit viper commonly found near water and swamps of the southeastern part of the United States. The symptoms of the bite of a cottonmouth are rapid swelling, severe pain, skin discoloration at bite marks, and weakness. Antivenin and ventilatory/circulatory support are the usual treatments. Also called **water moccasin.**

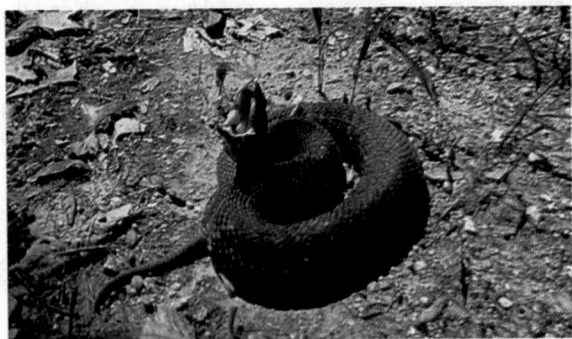

**Cottonmouth** *(Auerbach, 1995/courtesy Sherman Minton, MD)*

**Cotton's fracture,** a fracture involving the medial, lateral, and posterior malleoli of the ankle. Also called **trimalleolar fracture.**

**cotton-wool exudate** [Ar, *qutun* + AS, *wull* + ME, *spot*], a white, fluffy-appearing exudate observed on the retina of patients with certain systemic conditions, such as acquired immunodeficiency syndrome, hypertension, and lupus. It can also be observed in retinal infections.

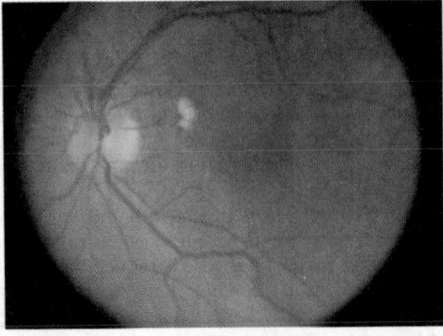

**Cotton-wool exudate** *(Zitelli and Davis, 1997)*

**cotyledon** /kot'ilē'don/ [Gk, *kotyledon*, cup-shaped], one of the visible segments on the maternal surface of the placenta. A typical placenta may have 15 to 28 cotyledons, each consisting of fetal vessels, chorionic villi, and intervillous space.

**cotyloid** /kot'iloid/, cup-shaped, as the acetabulum.

**cotyloid cavity.** See **acetabulum.**

**coudé catheter** /kōōdā'/ [Fr, *coude*, elbow], an elbowed catheter.

**cough** /kôf/ [AS, *cohhetan*], a sudden audible expulsion of air from the lungs. Coughing is preceded by inspiration, the glottis is partially closed, and the accessory muscles of expiration contract to expel the air forcibly from the respiratory passages. Coughing is an essential protective response that serves to clear the lungs, bronchi, and trachea of irritants and secretions or to prevent aspiration of foreign material into the lungs. It is a common symptom of diseases of the chest and larynx. Chronic coughing may be indicative of tuberculosis, lung cancer, bronchiectasis, or bronchitis. Otitis media, subdiaphragmatic irritation, congestive heart failure, and mitral valve disease may be associated with episodes of severe chronic coughing. Coughing is a reflex action that may be induced voluntarily and, to some extent, voluntarily inhibited. The cough-reflex center is located in the medulla of the brain. It responds to stimulation transmitted by the glossopharyngeal or vagus nerve. The reflex is initiated by chemical or mechanical irritation of the pharynx, larynx, or tracheobronchial tree. Because the function of coughing is to clear the respiratory tract of secretions, it is important that the cough expel accumulated debris. If it does not, for example, with weakness or inhibition by pain, instruction in effective coughing and deep-breathing exercises are helpful. Persons with chronic coughs may obtain symptomatic relief through environmental controls that reduce irritants in and humidify air. Medication may help dilate the bronchi, liquefy secretions, and increase expectoration. Antitussive medications are sometimes prescribed even in the absence of mucus or congestion. When congestion is present and the client is unable to cough up the mucus, an expectorant may be prescribed.

**cough enhancement,** a nursing intervention from the Nursing Interventions Classification (NIC) defined as promotion of deep inhalation by the patient with subsequent generation of high intrathoracic pressures and compression of underlying lung parenchyma for the forceful expulsion of air. See also **Nursing Interventions Classification.**

**cough fracture,** a break in a rib, usually the fourth to eighth rib, caused by violent coughing.

**cough syncope** [AS, *cohhetan* + Gk, *syncope*, fainting], a temporary loss of consciousness during coughing. The coughing increases the intrathoracic pressure enough to impede venous return, thereby interfering with normal blood flow to the brain.

**cough variant asthma,** asthma characterized by minimal wheezing and a nonproductive, often severe, cough lasting from a few hours to days.

**coulomb** /kōō'lōm/ [Charles A. de Coulomb, French physicist, 1736–1806], the SI unit of electricity equal to the quantity of charge transferred in 1 second across a conductor in which there is a constant current of 1 ampere, or 1 ampere-second.

**Coulomb's law** [Charles A. de Coulomb], (in physics) a law stating that the force of attraction or repulsion between two electrically charged bodies is directly proportional to the strength of the electrical charges and inversely proportional to the square of the distance between them.

**coulometry** /kōōlom'ətrē/, a type of electroanalytic chemistry in which a reagent generated at the surface of an electrode reacts with a substance to be measured. The substance, usually a metal ion, is measured in terms of the coulombs required for the reaction.

**Coulter counter** /kōl′tər/ [W.H. Coulter, twentieth century American engineer], trademark for an electric device that rapidly identifies and counts red and white blood cells present in a small specimen of human blood.

**Coumadin,** trademark for an anticoagulant (warfarin sodium).

**coumarin** /ko͞o′mərin/, a class of anticoagulant agents.

■ INDICATIONS: It is prescribed for prophylaxis and treatment of thrombosis and embolism.

■ CONTRAINDICATIONS: Known hypersensitivity to the drug prohibits its use. It is not prescribed to patients who are at risk for hemorrhage or who are pregnant.

■ ADVERSE EFFECTS: The most serious adverse reaction is hemorrhage. Many other drugs interact with this drug to increase or decrease its effect.

**counseling**[1] [L, *consulere,* to consult], the act of providing advice and guidance to a patient or his or her family. It is a therapeutic technique that helps the patient recognize and manage stress and that facilitates interpersonal relationships between the patient and the family, significant others, or the health care team. See also **genetic counseling.**

**counseling**[2], a nursing intervention from the Nursing Interventions Classification (NIC) defined as use of an interactive helping process focusing on the needs, problems, or feelings of the patient and significant others to enhance or support coping, problem-solving, and interpersonal relationships. See also **Nursing Interventions Classification.**

**counselor,** a human services professional who deals with human development concerns through support, therapeutic approaches, consultation, evaluation, teaching, and research. Specializations include community counselor, gerontological counselor, marriage and family counselor/therapist, mental health counselor, school counselor, and student affairs practitioner. See also **genetic counselor.**

**count** [L, *computere,* to calculate], a computation of the number of objects or elements present per unit of measurement. Kinds of counts include **Addis count, bacteria count, blood count,** and **platelet count.**

**counterclaim** [L, *contra,* against, *clamere,* to cry out], (in law) a claim made by a defendant establishing a cause for action in his or her favor against a plaintiff. The purpose of a counterclaim is to oppose or detract from a plaintiff's claim or complaint.

**counterconditioning,** a process used in behavioral therapy in which a learned response is replaced by an alternative response that is less disruptive.

**countercurrent,** a change in the direction of flow of a fluid. An example is the countercurrent in the ascending branch of a kidney tubule where osmolality undergoes a reversal after a gradual change in sodium chloride concentrations.

**counterinjunction** /-injungk′shən/, (in transactional analysis) an overt message from the parent ego state of the mother or father that may be difficult to follow if it conflicts with earlier parental instructions. For example, the person may obey an earlier injunction to avoid close relationships, then be instructed later to "grow up and get married."

**counterphobic behavior** /-fō′bik/, an expression of reaction to a phobia by a patient who actively seeks exposure to the type of situation that precipitates phobic symptoms. Examples are thrill-seeking and risk-taking activities.

**counterpulsation** /-pulsā′shən/ [L, *contra* + *pulsare,* to beat], **1.** the action of a circulatory-assist pumping device

that is synchronized with cardiac systole and diastole to decrease the work of the heart. **2.** the process of increasing the intraaortic pressure in diastole by inflation of an intraaortic balloon and deflation of the balloon immediately before the next systole.

**countershock** [L, *contra* + Fr, *choc*], a high-intensity, short-duration electric shock applied to the area of the heart, resulting in total cardiac depolarization. See also **cardioversion, defibrillation.**

**counterstain,** a second stain added to a previously stained tissue sample to make cellular details more distinct.

**countertraction** /-trak′shən/ [L, *contra* + *trahere,* to pull], a force that counteracts the pull of traction, such as the force of body weight resulting from the pull of gravity. Orthopedic countertraction may be obtained by altering the angle of the body-weight force in relation to the pull of traction, such as by elevating the foot of the bed with blocks to attain Trendelenburg's position. The magnitude of countertraction is usually increased gradually by methodically changing the position of a patient and by adding or removing weights from weight hangers.

**countertransference** /-transfur′əns/, the conscious or unconscious emotional response of a psychotherapist or psychoanalyst to a patient, for example, responding as if to a significant person. The response is inappropriate to the content and context of the therapeutic relationship. See also **transference.**

**countertransport** /-trans′pôrt/ [L, *contra* + *trans,* across, *portare,* carry], the simultaneous transport of two different substances across the same membrane, each in the opposite direction.

**counting cell hemocytometer** [OFr, *conter* + L, *cella,* storeroom; Gk, *haima,* blood, *metron,* measure], a device for counting the number of cells in a volume of blood or other fluid. It consists of a microscope slide with a counting chamber. The chamber has a known volume and the slide has a ruled area to help count the cells.

**counts per minute (cpm),** a measure of the rate of ionizing emissions by radioactive substances.

**coup** /ko͞o/ [Fr, blow], any blow or stroke or the effects of such a blow to the body, usually used with a French word identifying a type of stroke: **1. coup de sabre** /ko͞o də säb′-r(ə)/, a wound resembling a sword cut. **2. coup de soleil.** See **sunstroke. 3. coup sur coup** /ko͞o sYr ko͞o′/, administration of a drug in small amounts over a short period rather

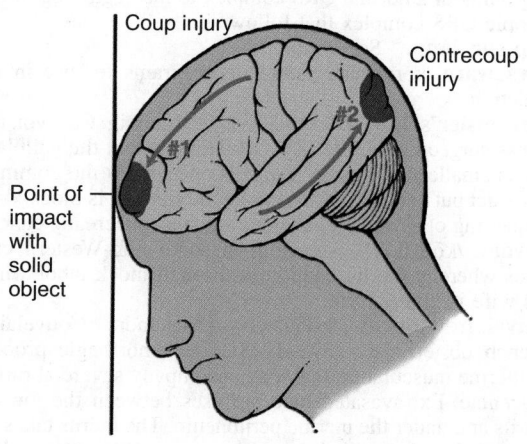

**Contrecoup injury** *(Monahan and Neighbors, 1998)*

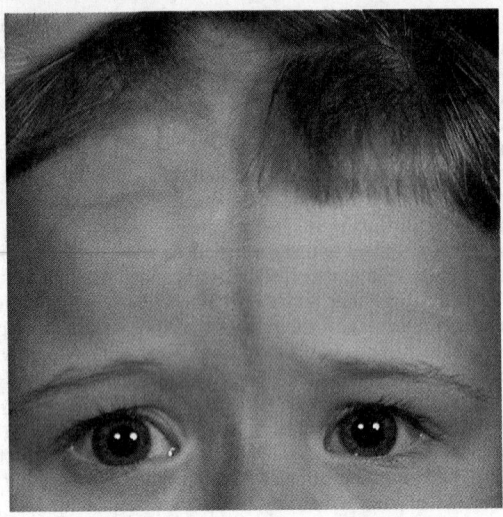

**Coup de sabre** *(du Vivier, 1993)*

**covalent bond,** a chemical bond that forms by the sharing of two electrons between atoms. A double bond is formed when four electrons are shared between two atoms; a triple bond is formed when six electrons are shared between two atoms.

**coverage** /kuv'ərij/, the extent to which services rendered by a health care program cover the potential need for them.

**covered benefit,** a health service included in the premium of a policy paid by or on behalf of the enrolled patient. Also called **benefit, covered service.**

**covered service.** See **covered benefit.**

**Cowden's disease** [Cowden, family name of the first recorded case], an autosomal dominant disorder characterized by hypertrichosis, gingival fibromatosis, facial papules, hemangiomas, and postpubertal fibroadenomatous breast enlargement. Also called **hamartoma syndrome.**

**Cowper's gland** /kou'pərz/ [William Cowper, English surgeon, 1666–1709], either of two round, pea-sized tubular glands embedded in the urethral sphincter of the male beneath the bulb of the male urethra. Normally yellow, they consist of several lobes with ducts that join and form a single excretory duct, emptying mucus into the urethra. Also called **bulbourethral gland.** Compare **Bartholin's gland.**

than in a single larger dose. **4. contre coup** /kôNtrə kōō'/, an injury most often associated with a blow to the skull in which the force of the impact is transmitted through the skull bones to the opposite side of the head, where the bruise, fracture, or other sign of injury appears.

**coupled pacing.** See **pacing.**

**coupled rhythm.** See **bigeminal rhythm.**

**couples therapy,** psychotherapy in which couples, who may be married or unmarried but living together, undergo therapy together.

**coupling** /kup'ling/ [L, *copula,* bonding], **1.** the act of coming together, joining, or pairing. **2.** (in genetics) the situation in linked inheritance in which the nonalleles of two or more mutant genes are located on the same chromosome and are close enough that they are likely to be inherited together. **3.** (in radiation therapy) the efficiency of transfer of power from an applicator to the treatment site. Compare **repulsion.** See also **cis configuration. 4.** (in cardiology) the regular occurrence of a premature beat.

**coupling interval,** the interval between the dominant heartbeat and a linked ectopic beat. It is measured from the beginning of a normal QRS complex to the beginning of the ectopic QRS complex that follows it.

**coup sur coup.** See **coup.**

**courseware** /kôrs'wer/, software programs for use in instruction.

**Courvoisier's law** /kōōrvô·ä·zē·āz'/ [Ludwig Courvoisier, Swiss surgeon, 1843–1918], a statement that the gallbladder is smaller than usual if a gallstone blocks the common bile duct but is dilated if the common bile duct is blocked by something other than a gallstone, such as pancreatic cancer.

**couvade** /kōōväd'/, a custom in some non-Western cultures whereby the husband goes through mock labor while his wife is giving birth.

**Couvelaire uterus** /kōōvəler'/ [Alexandre Couvelaire, French obstetrician, 1873–1948], a hemorrhagic process in uterine musculature that may accompany severe abruptio placentae. Extravasated blood effuses between the muscle fibrils and under the uterine peritoneum. The uterus takes on a purplish color and does not contract well. Also called **uteroplacental apoplexy.** See also **abruptio placentae.**

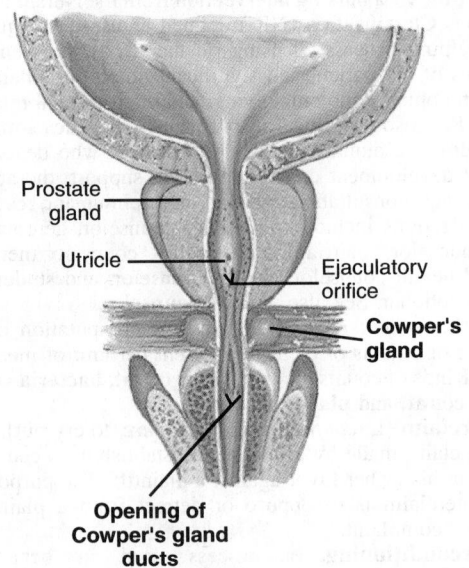

**Cowper's gland** *(Seidel et al, 1999)*

Prostate gland

Utricle

Ejaculatory orifice

**Cowper's gland**

Opening of
Cowper's gland
ducts

**cowpox** /kou'poks/ [AS, *cu* + ME, *pokkes*], a mild infectious disease characterized by a pustular rash, caused by the vaccinia virus transmitted to humans from infected cattle. Cowpox infection usually confers immunity to smallpox, because of the similarity of the variola and vaccinia viruses. See also **smallpox, vaccinia.**

**coxa** /kok'sə/, *pl.* **coxae** [L, hip], the hip joint; the head of the femur and the acetabulum of the innominate bone.

**coxa adducta, coxa flexa.** See **coxa vara.**

**coxal articulation** /kok'səl/ [L, *coxa* + *articularis,* relating to the joints], the ball-and-socket joint of the hip, formed by the articulation of the head of the femur into the cup-shaped cavity of the acetabulum. It involves seven ligaments and permits very extensive movements, such as flexion, ex-

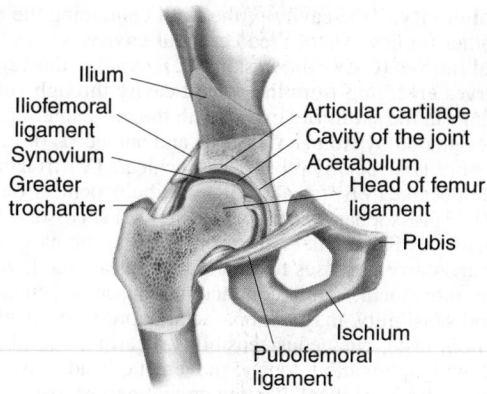

**Coxal articulation** *(Thompson et al, 1997)*

tension, adduction, abduction, circumduction, and rotation. Also called **hip joint.** Compare **shoulder joint.**

**coxa magna,** an abnormal widening of the head and neck of the femur.

**coxa plana.** See **Legg-Calvé-Perthes disease.**

**coxa valga,** a hip deformity in which the angle formed by the axis of the head and neck of the femur and the axis of its shaft is significantly increased.

**coxa vara,** a hip deformity in which the angle formed by the axis of the head and neck of the femur and the axis of its shaft is decreased. Also called **coxa adducta, coxa flexa.**

**coxa vara luxans,** a fissure or crack in the neck of the femur with dislocation of the head, caused by coxa vara.

**coxsackievirus** /koksak′ē-/ [Coxsackie, New York; L, *virus,* poison], any of 30 serologically different enteroviruses associated with a variety of symptoms and primarily affecting children during warm weather. The coxsackieviruses resemble the virus responsible for poliomyelitis, particularly in size; both are picornaviruses. Among the diseases associated with coxsackievirus infections are herpangina, hand-foot-and-mouth disease, epidemic pleurodynia, myocarditis, pericarditis, aseptic meningitis, and several exanthems. There is no known preventive measure except isolation of

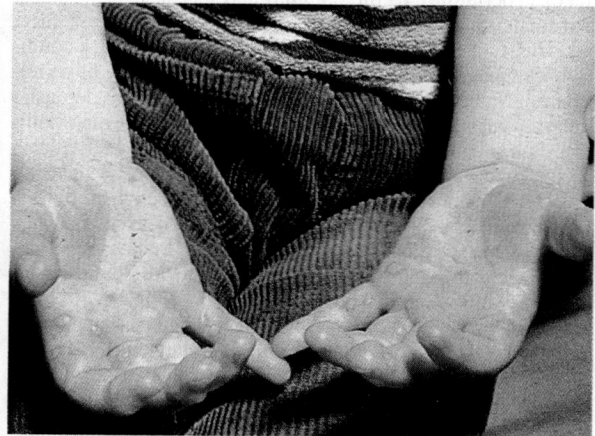

**Coxsackievirus** *(Hart and Broadhead, 1992)*

infected persons, and the treatment is generally directed to relief of symptoms. See also **viral infection.**

**CP,** 1. abbreviation for **candlepower.** 2. abbreviation for **cerebral palsy.** 3. abbreviation for *chemically pure.*

**CPAN,** abbreviation for *Certified Post-Anesthesia Nurse.*

**CPAP,** abbreviation for **continuous positive airway pressure.**

**CPD,** 1. abbreviation for **cephalopelvic disproportion.** 2. abbreviation for **childhood polycystic disease.** See **polycystic kidney disease.** 3. abbreviation for **congenital polycystic disease.** See **polycystic kidney disease.**

**C peptide,** a biologically inactive residue of insulin formation in the beta cells of the pancreas. When proinsulin is converted to insulin, an equal amount of C peptide, a chain of amino acids, is also secreted into the bloodstream. Beta cell secretory function can be determined by measuring the C peptide in a blood sample.

**C-peptide test,** a blood test used to evaluate levels of C-peptide, which correlate with insulin levels in the blood. Direct measurement of C-peptide measures the capacity of the pancreatic beta cells to secrete insulin. It is used to evaluate patients with suspected insulinoma, renal failure, pancreas transplant, factitious hypoglycemia, radical pancreatectomy, and diabetes mellitus.

**CPHA,** abbreviation for the **Canadian Public Health Association.**

**CPK,** abbreviation for *creatine phosphokinase.* See also **creatine kinase (CK).**

**cpm,** abbreviation for **counts per minute.**

**CPNP/A,** abbreviation for *Certified Pediatric Nurse Practitioner/Associate.*

**CPPB,** abbreviation for **continuous positive pressure breathing.**

**CPPD,** abbreviation for *calcium pyrophosphate dihydrate.* See **chondrocalcinosis.**

**CPPV,** abbreviation for **continuous positive pressure ventilation.**

**CPR,** abbreviation for **cardiopulmonary resuscitation.**

**CPRAM,** abbreviation for *controlled partial rebreathing anesthesia method.*

**cps,** abbreviation for **cycles per second.** See **hertz.**

**CPT,** abbreviation for **Current Procedural Terminology.**

**CPT codes,** a coding system, defined in the publication **Current Procedural Terminology (CPT),** for medical procedures that allows for comparability in pricing, billing, and utilization review. See also **Current Procedural Terminology (CPT).**

**cpu, CPU,** abbreviation for **central processing unit.**

**CQI,** abbreviation for **continuous quality improvement.**

**Cr,** symbol for the element **chromium.**

**CR,** abbreviation for *controlled respiration.*

**crab louse** [AS, *crabba + lus*], a species of louse, *Pthirus pubis,* that infests the hairs of the genital area. It is often transmitted between persons by sexual contact. Also called *(informal)* **crab.** Formerly called *Pediculus pubis.* See also **pediculosis.**

**crack** [ME, *craken*], a street drug made by chemically converting cocaine hydrochloride to a form that can be smoked. Smoking crack is a faster, more direct way of getting cocaine molecules into the brain. Because larger amounts of the drug reach the brain more quickly, the effects are more intense than when cocaine, in the white-powder form, is injected, ingested, or inhaled. Also called **crack cocaine, freebase.**

**crack baby,** an infant who was exposed to effects of cocaine in utero by a mother who used the "crack" form of the drug while pregnant. See also **cocaine baby.**

**crack cocaine.** See **cocaine hydrochloride, crack.**

**cracked-pot sound** [ME, *craken* + *pott* + L, *sonus*, sound], a sound sometimes heard on percussion over a cavity with an opening to a bronchus.

**cracked tooth syndrome** [ME, *craken;* AS, *toth*], a group of symptoms caused by presence of a cracked tooth, including pain on pressure or application of cold, with pulpitis if untreated.

**crackle,** a common, abnormal respiratory sound consisting of discontinuous bubbling noises heard on auscultation of the chest during inspiration. Fine crackles have a popping sound produced by air entering distal bronchioles or alveoli that contain serous secretions, as in congestive heart failure, pneumonia, or early tuberculosis. Coarse crackles may originate in the larger bronchi or trachea and have a lower pitch. Crackles are not cleared by coughing. Formerly called **rale.** Compare **rhonchus, wheeze.** See also **coarse crackle.**

**cradle cap** [AS, *cradel* + *caeppe*], a common seborrheic dermatitis of infants, which consists of thick, yellow greasy or waxy scales on the scalp. Treatment includes application of oil or ointment to soften the scales and frequent shampoos. Also called **seborrhea capitis.**

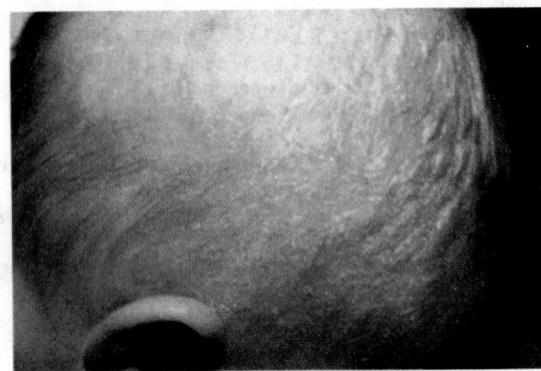

**Cradle cap**
*(Goldstein, 1992/courtesy Dept. of Dermatology, University of North Carolina-Chapel Hill)*

**cramp** [AS, *crammian,* to fill], **1.** a spasmodic and often painful contraction of one or more muscles. **2.** a pain resembling a muscular cramp. Kinds of cramps include **cane-cutter's cramp, fireman's cramp, miner's cramp, stoker's cramp,** and **writer's cramp.** See also **charley horse, dysmenorrhea, heat cramp, wryneck.**

**cranberry,** an herbal product whose berries are harvested from a small shrub found in the United States from Alaska to Tennessee.

■ USES: This herb is used for urinary tract infections (UTIs) and in those with susceptibility to kidney stones.

■ CONTRAINDICATIONS: Those with known hypersensitivity, oliguria, or anuria should not use cranberry.

**-crania,** suffix meaning '(condition of the) skull or head': *diastematocrania, hemicrania, platycrania.*

**cranial.** See **cranium.**

**cranial arteritis.** See **temporal arteritis.**

**cranial bones** /krā′nē·əl/ [Gk, *kranion*, cranium; AS, *ban*], the bones of the skull, particularly the part of the cranium that encloses the brain.

**cranial cavity,** the cavity of the skull containing the brain and other tissues. Also called **cerebral cavity.**

**cranial nerves** [Gk, *kranion*, skull; L, *nervus*], the 12 pairs of nerves emerging from the cranial cavity through various openings in the skull. Beginning with the most anterior, they are designated by Roman numerals and named (I) olfactory, (II) optic, (III) oculomotor, (IV) trochlear, (V) trigeminal, (VI) abducens, (VII) facial, (VIII) vestibulocochlear (acoustic), (IX) glossopharyngeal, (X) vagal, (XI) accessory, (XII) hypoglossal. The cranial nerves originate in the base of the brain and carry impulses for such functions as smell, vision, ocular movement, pupil contraction, muscular sensibility, general sensibility, mastication, facial expression, glandular secretion, taste, cutaneous sensibility, hearing, equilibrium, swallowing, phonation, tongue movement, head movement, and shoulder movement. Certain cranial nerves, particularly V, VII, and VIII, contain two or more distinct functional components considered as independent nerves by some authorities. In this category the masticatory nerve would be separated from the trigeminal (V), the glossopalatine from the facial (VII), and the equilibrium from the vestibulocochlear (VIII), making 15 pairs in all. Some anatomists also classify the terminal nerve as the first cranial. Also called **cerebral nerves.** See also the specific nerves.

**cranial sensory ganglion,** the ganglion found on the root of each cranial nerve, containing the cell bodies of afferent (sensory) neurons.

**cranial sutures,** the interlocking lines of fusion of the bones forming the skull. The lines gradually become less prominent as a person matures. Also called **suturae cranii.**

**craniectomy** /krā′nē·ek′təmē/ [Gk, *kranion*, cranium, *ektomē*, excision], the surgical removal of a portion of the cranium.

**cranio-** /krā′nē·ō-/, prefix meaning 'skull or cranium': *craniobuccal, craniognomy, craniosacral.*

**craniocarpotarsal dystrophy.** See **Freeman-Sheldon syndrome.**

**craniocele.** See **encephalocele.**

**craniocervical** /-sur′vikəl/ [Gk, *kranion* + L, *cervix*, neck], pertaining to the junction of the skull and neck, particularly the area of the foramen magnum. Because of the complex of nerve fibers and blood vessels in the region and the flexibility of the cervical spine, craniocervical tissues are particularly vulnerable to a variety of compression disorders.

**craniodidymus** /krā′nē·ōdid′iməs/ [Gk, *kranion* + *didymos*, twin], a two-headed fetus in which the bodies are fused.

**craniofacial** /-fā′shəl/ [Gk, *kranion*, cranium; L, *facies*, face], pertaining to the cranium and the face.

**craniofacial dysostosis** [Gk, *kranion* + L, *facies*, face; Gk, *dys*, bad, *osteon*, bone], an abnormal hereditary condition characterized by acrocephaly, exophthalmos, hypertelorism, strabismus, parrot-beaked nose, and hypoplastic maxilla with relative mandibular prognathism. This condition is transmitted as an autosomal dominant trait. See also **dysostosis.**

**craniohypophyseal xanthoma** /krā′nē·ōhī′pōfiz′ē·əl/ [Gk, *kranion* + *hypo*, deficient, *phyein*, to grow, *xanthos*, yellow, *oma*, tumor], a condition in which cholesterol deposits are formed around the hypophyses of the bones, as in Hand-Schüller-Christian disease.

**craniology** /krā′nē·ol′əjē/, the study of the shape, size, proportions, and other features of the human skull. It is usually associated with anthropologic research.

**craniometaphyseal dysplasia** /-met′əfiz′ē·əl/, an inherited bone disorder characterized by paranasal overgrowth, thickening of the skull and jaw, and entrapment of cranial nerves. The long bones have widened, club-shaped metaphyses. The patient may experience nasorespiratory infections, associated with bone overgrowth at the sinuses, and malocclusion of the jaws.

**craniopagus** /krā′nē·op′əgəs/ [Gk, *kranion* + *pagos,* fixed], conjoined twins united at the heads. Fusion can occur at the frontal, occipital, or parietal region. Also called **cephalopagus.**

**craniopharyngeal** /krā′nē·ōfərin′jē·əl/ [Gk, *kranion* + *pharynx,* throat], pertaining to the cranium and the pharynx.

**craniopharyngioma** /krā′nē·ōfərin′jē·ō′mə/, *pl.* **craniopharyngiomas, craniopharyngiomata,** a congenital pituitary tumor, appearing most often in children and adolescents, that arises in cells derived from Rathke's pouch or the hypophyseal stalk. The lesion, a solid or cystic body ranging in size from 1 to 8 cm, may expand into the third ventricle or the temporal lobe and frequently becomes calcified. The tumor may interfere with pituitary function, damage the optic chiasm, disrupt hypothalamic control of the autonomic nervous system, and cause hydrocephalus. Increased intracranial pressure, severe headaches, vomiting, stunted growth, defective vision, irritability, somnolence, and infantile genitalia are often associated with the lesion in children. Development of the tumor after puberty usually results in amenorrhea in women and loss of libido and potency in men. Also called **ameloblastoma, craniopharyngeal duct tumor, pituitary adamantinoma, Rathke's pouch tumor.**

**cranioplasty** /krā′nē·ōplast′tē/, plastic surgery performed on the skull.

**craniospinal** /krā′nē·ō·spī′nəl/ [Gk, *kranion,* skull + L, *spina,* backbone or spine], pertaining to the cranium and the vertebral column.

**craniostenosis** /krā′nē·ō′stənō′sis/ [Gk, *kranion* + *stenos,* narrow, *osis,* condition], a congenital deformity of the skull that results from premature closure of the sutures between the cranial bones. The severity of the malformation depends on which sutures close, the point in the developmental process where the closure occurred, and the success or failure of the other sutures to compensate by expansion. Impaired brain growth may or may not be involved. The most common form of the condition is permanent closure of the sagittal suture with anteroposterior elongation of the skull. Surgery is generally indicated when multiple sutures are fused to relieve cerebral pressure and may be performed for cosmetic reasons. See also **brachycephaly, oxycephaly, plagiocephaly, scaphocephaly.** —**craniostenotic,** *adj.*

**craniostosis** /krā′nē·ostō′sis/ [Gk, *kranion* + *osteon,* bone, *osis,* condition], premature ossification of the sutures of the skull, often associated with other skeletal defects. The sutures close before or soon after birth. Without surgical correction the growth of the skull is inhibited, the head is deformed, and the eyes and brain are often damaged. Also called **craniosynostosis.**

**craniosynostosis** [Gk, *kranion,* skull + *syn,* together + *osteon,* bone]. See **craniostosis.**

**craniotabes** /krā′nē·ōtā′bēz/ [Gk, *kranion* + L, *tabes,* wasting], benign congenital thinness of the top and back of the skull of a newborn. The condition is common because the rate of brain growth exceeds the rate of calcification of the skull during the last month of gestation. The bones feel brittle when pressed by an examiner's fingers. Craniotabes disappears with normal nutrition and growth but may persist in infants in whom rickets develops.

**craniotomy** /krā′nē·ot′əmē/ [Gk, *kranion,* cranium, *temnein,* to cut], any surgical opening into the skull, performed to relieve intracranial pressure, to control bleeding, or to remove a tumor. X-ray films of the skull are taken before surgery, and a computed tomographic (CT) scan or an electroencephalogram is done to establish the diagnosis. The operative site is shaved and cleansed. Parenteral corticosteroids are given to reduce cerebral edema. Mannitol and urea are administered to decrease intracranial pressure. Neuroleptic drugs that sedate but do not narcotize the patient may be combined with local anesthesia, or general anesthesia may be given. A semicircular skin incision is made just above the hairline, a series of burr holes are made and connected with a cut, and the flap of bone is removed. The meninges are incised, and the brain is exposed. The flap may be replaced after surgery or left off temporarily to prevent the buildup of pressure from the cerebral edema. After surgery, if the cerebral area is involved, the head of the patient's bed is elevated to 45 degrees to reduce the risk of hemorrhage and edema; if the cerebellum or brainstem is affected, the patient is kept flat. The dressing is checked frequently for yellowish drainage of cerebrospinal fluid. Any moist areas are reinforced with sterile materials to prevent infection. Frequent observation of neurologic signs, including level of consciousness, speech, and strength, is essential. Respirations and vital signs are monitored.

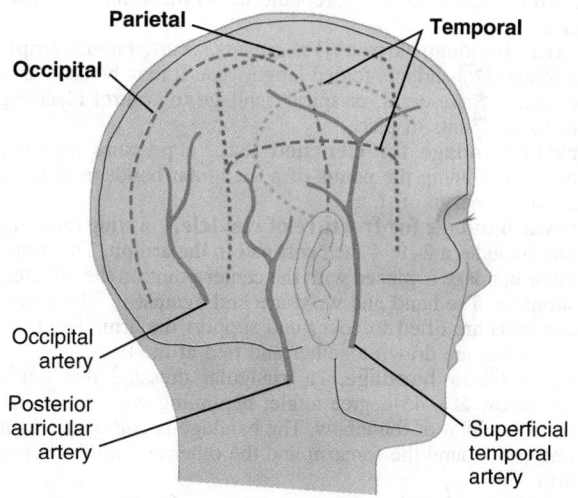

**Basic craniotomy incisions** *(Youmans, 1982)*

**craniotubular** /-toٓob′yələr/, pertaining to a bossing, or overgrowth, of bone that produces an abnormal contour and increased bone density. An example of a craniotubular disorder is craniometaphyseal dysplasia.

**cranium** /krā′nē·əm/ [Gk, *kranion,* skull], the bony skull that holds the brain. It is composed of eight bones: the frontal, occipital, sphenoid, ethmoid, and the paired temporal and parietal bones. —**cranial,** *adj.*

**-cranium,** suffix meaning 'skull': *chondrocranium, desmocranium, endocranium.*

**crankcase-spool catheter** /krangk′kās/, a special elastic catheter stored within a plastic spool to facilitate its insertion, especially for hyperalimentation. When fully inserted, the crankcase-spool catheter is usually lodged in the subclavian vein. The catheter is highly flexible, and each revolution of the spool feeds about 5 inches of the catheter into the vein involved. When the crankcase-spool catheter is fully inserted, a radiographic exposure is made of the insertion area to confirm its correct placement. The crankcase-spool catheter is less irritating than a regular catheter, allows greater limb movement, and minimizes the risk of thrombosis. It may, however, cause complications, such as occlusion, phlebitis, infection, and catheter sensitivity. Occlusion of the vein, a common risk, is usually countered by flushing the vein with dilute streptokinase.

**crash** [ME, *crasschen,* to break violently], a serious malfunction of computer hardware or software.

**crash cart,** a cart carrying emergency equipment and supplies, such as medications, suction devices, sutures, scalpels, surgical needles, sponges, swabs, retractors, hemostats, forceps, airways, $O_2$ supplies, IV supplies, tracheal tubes, and often a cardiac monitor with a defibrillator. Hospital emergency departments and intensive care units usually have several crash carts equipped according to prescribed specifications. Efficient, effective emergency care often depends on the careful provisioning of crash carts and the precise knowledge of their layouts.

**-crasia,** **1.** suffix meaning '(condition of a) mixture, good or bad': *eucrasia, orthocrasia, spermacrasia.* **2.** combining form meaning a '(specified) condition involving loss of control': *copracrasia, uracrasia.*

**crater,** a pitlike depression, as where an ulcer has been surgically removed.

**-cratia,** suffix meaning '(condition of) incontinence': *uracratia.*

**cravat bandage** /krəvat′/[Fr, *cravate,* scarf, *bande,* strip], a triangular bandage, folded lengthwise. It may be used as a circular, figure-eight, or spiral bandage to control bleeding or to tie splints in place.

**cravat bandage for clenched fist,** a pressure dressing made by folding the points of a triangular bandage to form a band about the fist.

**cravat bandage for fracture of clavicle,** a sling dressing that includes a 2- to 4-inch soft pad in the armpit. The triangular bandage is placed with the center point on the affected shoulder. The hand and wrist are laid against it. The opposite ends are lifted to cover and support the arm. The bandage ends are drawn together and tied at the back.

**cravat elbow bandage,** a triangular dressing that holds the elbow at a 45-degree angle, beginning with the center over the point of the elbow. The bandage is completed with one end around the forearm and the other around the upper arm.

**cravat sling bandage,** a support for a fractured arm prepared by laying the wrist on the center of the triangular bandage while the forearm is at a right angle. The two ends of the bandage are carried around the neck and tied.

**crawling reflex.** See **symmetric tonic neck reflex.**

**C-reactive protein (CRP)** /-rē·ak′tiv/, a protein not normally detected in the serum but present in many acute inflammatory conditions and with necrosis. CRP appears in the serum before the erythrocyte sedimentation rate begins to rise, often within 24 to 48 hours of the onset of inflammation. After a myocardial infarction it is present in 24 hours, begins to fall 3 days later, and is absent after 2 weeks. Acute rheumatic fever is monitored with serial estimations of CRP, because the serum level of the protein is the most sensitive indicator of rheumatic activity. Bacterial infections and widespread neoplastic disease are also associated with C-reactive protein in the serum. CRP disappears when an inflammatory process is suppressed by salicylates, steroids, or both. Also called **serum C-reactive protein.**

**C-reactive protein test (CRP),** a blood test used to detect and diagnose bacterial infectious disease, postsurgical wound infection, and inflammatory disorders such as acute rheumatic fever and rheumatoid arthritis. In addition, it is used as an adjunct in detecting acute bacterial meningitis in an acutely febrile child, and as an aid to evaluation of patients with acute myocardial infarction.

**cream** [Gk, *chrisma,* oil], **1.** the portion of milk rich in butterfat. **2.** any fluid mixture of thick consistency. Creams are often used as a method of applying medication to the surface of the body. Compare **ointment.**

**crease** [ME, creste, crest], an indentation or margin formed by a doubling back of tissue, such as the folds on the palm of the hand and sole of the foot.

**creat-,** combining form meaning 'flesh': *creaton, creatorrhea, creatotoxism.*

**creatinase** /krē·at′i·nās/ [Gk, *kreas,* flesh], an enzyme that catalyzes the conversion of creatine to sarcosine and urea.

**creatine** /krē′ətēn, -tin/ [Gk, *kreas,* flesh], an important nitrogenous compound produced by metabolic processes in the body. Combined with phosphorus, it forms high-energy phosphate. In normal metabolic reactions the phosphorus is yielded to combine with a molecule of adenosine diphosphate to produce a molecule of very high–energy adenosine triphosphate. See also **creatinine.**

**creatine kinase (CK),** an enzyme of the transferase class in muscle, brain, and other tissues. It catalyzes the transfer of a phosphate group from adenosine triphosphate to creatine, producing adenosine diphosphate and phosphocreatine. The reaction stores energy in muscle and brain tissue. Also called **creatine phosphokinase (CPK).** See also **Duchenne's muscular dystrophy.**

**creatine phosphate** [Gk, *kreas,* flesh; Du, *potasschen*], an enzyme that increases in blood levels when muscle damage has occurred, as in pseudohypertrophic muscular dystrophy.

**creatine phosphokinase.** See **creatine kinase.**

**creatine phosphokinase test (CPK, CP, or CK),** a blood test used to detect damage to the heart muscle, skeletal muscles, and brain. Serum CPK levels are elevated whenever such damage occurs. CPK is the main cardiac enzyme studied in patients with heart disease.

**creatinine** /krē·at′inēn, -nin/, a substance formed from the metabolism of creatine, commonly found in blood, urine, and muscle tissue. It is measured in blood and urine tests as an indicator of kidney function. Normal adult blood levels of creatinine are 0.5 to 1.1 mg/dL for females and 0.6 to 1.2 mg/dL for males; the numbers decrease in elderly patients because of a smaller muscle mass. See also **creatine.**

**creatinine clearance test,** a diagnostic test for kidney function. It measures the rate at which creatinine is cleared from the blood by the kidney. It is calculated on the basis of a urine volume in milliliters per minute times the amount of milligrams per liter of urinary creatinine excreted in 24 hours. The resulting figure is divided by the amount of serum creatinine in milligrams per deciliter.

**creatinine height index (CHI),** a measurement of a 24-hour urinary excretion of creatinine, which is generally related to the patient's muscle mass and an indicator of malnutrition, particularly in young males.

**creatorrhea,** the presence of undigested muscle fibers in the feces.

**credentialing** /kriden′shəling/, examination and review of the credentials of individuals meeting a set of criteria and therefore being licensed in their field. Strict credentialing is required by both hospital and managed care accreditation bodies. The process is conducted periodically because of the responsibility of the organization for any claims of malpractice by its staff.

**credentials** /kriden′shelz/, a predetermined set of standards, such as licensure or certification, establishing that a person or institution has achieved professional recognition in a specific field of health care.

**Credé's maneuver** /kredā′z/, [Karl S. Credé, German physician, 1819–1892], a technique for aiding the expulsion of the placenta. The uterus is pushed toward the birth canal by pressure exerted by the thumb of one hand on the posterior surface of the abdomen and the other hand on the anterior surface.

**Credé's method** /kredā′z/, [Karl S. Credé], a technique for promoting the expulsion of urine by manual compression of the bladder through external pressure on the lower abdominal wall.

**Credé's prophylaxis** /kredā′z/, [Karl S. Credé], the instillation of a 1% silver nitrate solution into the conjunctiva of newborns to prevent ophthalmia neonatorum.

**creep,** a rheologic effect of metals and other solid materials that may become elongated or deformed as a result of a load being applied for a long period. For example, creep can occur in silver amalgam fillings that have been in place for some time.

**creeping eruption.** See **cutaneous larva migrans.**

**cremaster** /krimas′tər/ [Gk, kremastos, hanging], a thin muscular layer that spreads out over the spermatic cord in a series of loops. It is a continuation of the obliquus internus. The muscle arises from the inguinal ligament and inserts into the crest of the pubis and into the sheath of the rectus abdominis. It is innervated by the genital branch of the genitofemoral nerve and functions to draw the testis up toward the superficial inguinal ring in response to cold or to stimulation of the nerve.

**cremasteric reflex** /krē′məster′ik/, a superficial neural reflex elicited by stroking the skin of the upper inner thigh in a male. This action normally results in a brisk retraction of the testis on the side of the stimulus. The reflex is lost in diseases of the pyramidal tract above the level of the first lumbar vertebra. See also **superficial reflex.**

**crematorium** /krē′mətôrē·əm/, a facility for the disposal of dead bodies by burning.

**crenation** /krinā′shən/ [L, crena, notch], the formation of notches or leaflike scalloped edges on an object. Red blood cells exposed to a hypertonic saline solution acquire a notched, shriveled surface as a result of the osmotic effect of the solution. They are then called crenated red blood cells. **—crenate, crenated,** adj.

**creosol** /krē′əsol/, an oily liquid that is one of the active constituents (phenol) of creosote. It should not be confused with cresol.

**creosote** /krē′əsōt/, a flammable oily liquid with a smoky odor that is used primarily as a wood preservative. It can cause a wide variety of health problems, ranging from cancer and corneal damage to convulsions, dermatitis, and vertigo. Persons who work with treated wood are usually at the greatest risk of exposure. See also **phenol poisoning.**

**crepitant** /krep′itənt/ [L, crepitans, crackling], pertaining to the feel or sound of crackling or rattling, or of rough surfaces being rubbed together.

**crepitant crackle** [L, crepitans, crackling], an abnormal breathing sound produced at the end of inspiration and caused by air entering collapsed alveoli that contain fibrous exudate. It occurs in pneumonia, tuberculosis, and pulmonary edema.

**crepitation.** See **crepitus.**

**crepitus** /krep′itəs/ [L, crackling], **1.** flatulence or the noisy discharge of fetid gas from the intestine through the anus. **2.** a sound or feel that resembles the crackling noise heard when rubbing hair between the fingers or throwing salt on an open fire. Crepitus is associated with gas gangrene, rubbing of bone fragments, air in superficial tissues, or crackles of a consolidated area of the lung in pneumonia. Also called **crepitation,** a clicking sound often heard in movement of joints, for example in temporomandibular joint resulting from joint irregularities.

**cresc-,** combining form meaning 'to grow': crescograph.

**crescendo angina** /krishen′dō/ [L, crescere, to increase], a form of angina pectoris associated with ischemic electrocardiographic changes and marked by increased frequency, provocation, intensity, or character.

**crescendo murmur** [L, crescere, to increase, murmur, humming], a murmur of steadily increasing intensity to a sudden termination.

**crescent** /kres′ənt/ [L, crescere, to increase], **1.** shaped like a new moon. **2.** a structure that has this shape.

**crescent bodies** /kres′ənt/, **1.** (in a blood smear) large, pale, crescent-shaped cells produced from fragile erythrocytes as the blood film preparation is made. **2.** large, round bodies with pink crescentlike margins found in blood of some anemia patients. Also called **achromocytes, selenoid cells.**

**cresol** /krē′sol/, a mixture of three isomers in a liquid with a phenolic odor. It is derived from coal tar and used in synthetic resins and disinfectants. Cresol is a potentially lethal protoplasmic poison that can be absorbed through the skin. Symptoms of chronic poisoning include skin eruptions, digestive disorders, uremia, jaundice, nervous disorders, vertigo, and mental changes. Acute poisoning by oral intake of 8 g or more can cause circulatory collapse and death. See also **phenol poisoning.**

**crest,** a narrow elongated elevation, as the iliac crest.

**CREST syndrome** /krest/, abbreviation for calcinosis, Raynaud's phenomenon, esophageal dysfunction, sclerodactyly, and telangiectasis, which may occur for varying periods in patients with scleroderma.

**cretin.** See **cretinism.**

**cretin dwarf** /krē′tən/, a person in whom short stature is caused by infantile hypothyroidism and severe deficiency of thyroid hormone. Also called **hypothyroid dwarf.** See also **cretinism.**

**cretinism** /krē′təniz′əm/ [Fr, cretin, idiot], a congenital condition characterized by severe hypothyroidism and often associated with other endocrine abnormalities. Myxedema is the acquired form. Typical signs of cretinism include dwarfism, mental deficiency, puffy facial features, dry skin, large tongue, umbilical hernia, and muscular incoordination. The disorder occurs usually in areas where the diet is deficient in iodine and where goiter is common. Early treatment with thyroid hormone generally promotes normal physical growth but may not prevent mental retardation. The use of iodized salt dramatically reduces the incidence of cretinism in a population. The condition is rare in the United States, but in some areas, including parts of Ecuador, the Himalayas, and Zaire, more than 5% of the people are affected. See also **familial cretinism. —cretinoid, cretinous,** adj., **cretin,** n.

**cretinoid,** resembling a cretin or the state of cretinism.

**Creutzfeldt-Jakob disease** /kroits′feltyä′kôp/ [Hans G. Creutzfeldt, German neurologist, 1885–1964; Alfons M. Jakob, German neurologist, 1884–1931], a rare fatal encephalopathy caused by an as yet unidentified slow virus. The disease occurs in middle age. Symptoms are progressive dementia, dysarthria, muscle wasting, and various involuntary movements such as myoclonus and athetosis. Deterioration is obvious week to week. Death ensues, usually within a year. It is the human variant of mad cow disease. Transmission between humans is unusual, but the disease has been observed years after exposure to needles, instruments, and

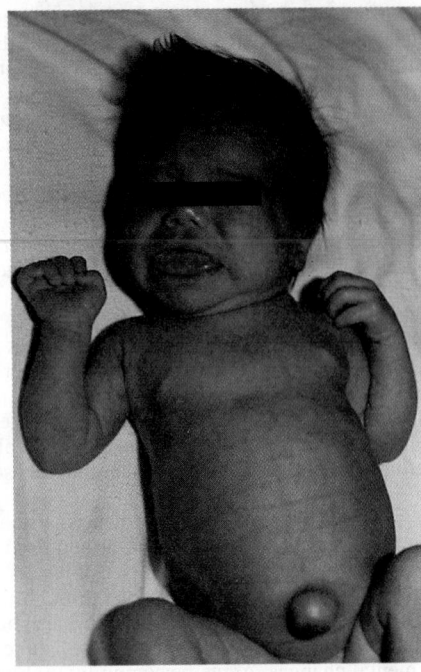

**Cretinism** *(Zitelli and Davis, 1997/courtesy Dr. T.P. Foley, Jr.)*

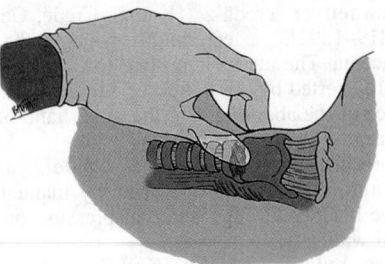

**Cricoid pressure** *(Sanders et al, 2000)*

electrodes previously used in the treatment of a patient with the disease. Isolation is not necessary. Special care in disposal or sterilization of potentially infective items is always necessary. Also called **Jakob-Creutzfeldt disease, spastic pseudoparalysis, spastic pseudosclerosis.**

**crevice** /krev'is/, a cleft or fissure, like that between the gum and the neck of a tooth.

**CRH,** abbreviation for **corticotropin-releasing hormone**.

**crib** /krib/ [L, *cribrum*, sieve], **1.** any racklike structure. **2.** a removable anchorage from an orthodontic appliance. **3.** a habit-breaking orthodontic appliance.

**crib death.** See **sudden infant death syndrome.**

**cribriform** /krib'rifôrm'/ [L, *cribum*, sieve], describing a structure with many perforations or punctures, as in the cribriform plate of the ethmoid bone.

**cribriform carcinoma.** See **adenocystic carcinoma.**

**crico-,** combining form meaning 'ring': *cricoderma, cricoid, cricoidectomy.*

**cricoid** /krī'koid/ [Gk, *krikos*, ring, *eidos*, form], **1.** having a ring shape. **2.** a ring-shaped cartilage connected to the thyroid cartilage by the cricothyroid ligament at the level of the sixth cervical vertebra.

**cricoid cartilage,** a ring-shaped cartilage of the larynx, consisting of a narrow anterior arch and a posterior wide quadrilateral lamina.

**cricoidectomy** /-ek'təmē/ [Gk, *krikos* + *eidos* + *ektomē*, excision], a surgical procedure for removing the cricoid cartilage.

**cricoid pressure,** a technique to reduce the risk of the aspiration of stomach contents during induction of general anesthesia. The cricoid cartilage is pushed against the body of the sixth cervical vertebra, compressing the esophagus to prevent passive regurgitation. The technique cannot, however, stop active vomiting. Cricoid pressure is applied before intubation, immediately after injection of anesthetic drugs; and as a part of "rapid sequence" intubation. Also called **Sellick's maneuver.**

**cricopharyngeal** /krī'kōfərin'jē·əl/ [Gk, *krikos* + *pharynx*, throat], pertaining to the cricoid cartilage and the pharynx.

**cricopharyngeal incoordination,** a defect in the normal swallowing reflex. The cricopharyngeus muscle ordinarily serves as a sphincter to keep the top of the esophagus closed except when the person is swallowing, vomiting, or belching. The trachea remains open for breathing, but air normally does not enter the esophagus during respiration. In swallowing the reverse effect occurs, and the larynx is closed while food slides past it into the esophagus, which is located immediately behind the larynx. When the somewhat complex series of neuromuscular actions is not properly coordinated as a result of disease or injury, the patient may choke, swallow air, regurgitate fluid into the nose, or experience discomfort in swallowing food. See also **dysphagia.**

**cricothyroid membrane** /-thī'roid/, a fibroelastic membrane including the cricothyroid ligament that connects the cricoid and thyroid cartilages. Also called **elastic membrane.**

**cricothyroidotomy** /krī'kō·thī'roi·dot'ə·mē/. See **cricothyrotomy.**

**cricothyrotomy** /krī'kōthīrot'əmē/ [Gk, *krikos* + *thyreos*, shield, *eidos*, form, *temnein*, to cut], an emergency incision into the larynx, performed to open the airway in a person who is choking. A small vertical midline cut is made just below the Adam's apple and above the cricoid cartilage. The incision is opened farther with a transverse cut through the cricothyroid membrane, and the wound is spread open with a knife handle or other dilator. The new opening must be held open with a tube that is open at both ends to allow air to move in and out. The cartridge end of a ballpoint pen will suffice until a tracheostomy can be done. Compare **tracheostomy.**

**cri-du-chat syndrome.** See **cat-cry syndrome.**

**Crigler-Najjar syndrome** /krig'lərnaj'är/ [John F. Crigler, Jr., American pediatrician, b. 1919; Victor A. Najjar, Lebanese-born American microbiologist, b. 1914], a congenital familial autosomal anomaly, in which glucuronyl transferase, an enzyme, is deficient or absent. The condition is characterized by nonhemolytic jaundice, an accumulation of unconjugated bilirubin in the blood, and severe disorders of the central nervous system. See also **hyperbilirubinemia of the newborn.**

**crime** [L, *crimen*], any act that violates a law and may have criminal intent.

**Crimean-Congo hemorrhagic fever** /krīmē'ən/, an arbovirus infection transmitted to humans through the bite of a tick, characterized by fever, dizziness, muscle ache, vomiting, headache, and other neurologic symptoms. After several days in severe cases bleeding from the skin and mucous membranes, particularly from the mouth and nose; bloody sputum or vomit; and blood-tinged feces may be seen. Transfusion may be necessary to replace lost blood; otherwise treatment is symptomatic and supportive. No specific medication or therapy is available for prevention or cure. It occurs mainly in Russia, Asia, and Africa; agricultural workers are most often afflicted. See also **hemorrhagic fever, Omsk hemorrhagic fever.**

**criminal psychology,** the study of the mental processes, motivational patterns, and behavior of criminals.

**crin-,** combining form meaning 'to separate or secrete': *crinin, crinogenic.*

**-crinat,** suffix designating an ethacrynic acid–derived diuretic.

**-crine,** suffix designating an acridine derivative.

**-crine, -crinia,** suffix meaning '(condition of) endocrine secretion': *hypercrinia, neurocrinia.*

**-crisia,** 1. suffix meaning a 'diagnosis or judgment': *acrisia, urocrisia.* 2. combining form meaning a '(specified) condition of endocrine secretion': *hypercrisia, hyperendocrisia, hypocrisia.*

**crisis** /krī'sis/ [Gk, *krisis,* turning point], 1. a transition for better or worse in the course of a disease, usually indicated by a marked change in the intensity of signs and symptoms. A crisis can result in personality growth or personality disorganization. 2. a turning point in events affecting the emotional state of a person, such as death or divorce. 3. a characteristically self-limiting period of from 4 to 6 weeks, that constitutes a transitional phase representing both the danger of increased psychologic vulnerability and an opportunity for personal growth. See also **crisis intervention.**

**crisis intervention**[1], (in psychiatry) a short-term intense therapy that emphasizes identification of the event that triggered the emotional trauma. Focus is on neutralizing the trauma and mobilizing coping skills.

**crisis intervention**[2], a nursing intervention from the Nursing Interventions Classification (NIC) defined as use of short-term counseling to help the patient cope with a crisis and resume a state of functioning comparable to or better than the pre-crisis state. See also **Nursing Interventions Classification.**

**crisis-intervention unit,** a group trained in emergency medical treatment and in various methods for rendering psychiatric therapeutic assistance to a person or group of persons during a period of crisis, especially instances involving suicide attempts or drug abuse. Such networks are found within community hospitals, in health care centers, or as specialized self-contained units, such as suicide-prevention centers, and operate 24 hours a day. The primary objectives of such crisis assistance are to help the person cope with the immediate problem and to offer guidance and support for long-term therapy.

**crisis resolution,** (in psychiatry) the development of effective adaptive and coping devices to resolve a crisis.

**crisis theory,** a conceptual framework for defining and explaining the phenomena that occur when a person faces a problem that appears to be insoluble. The theory is the basis of crisis therapy.

**crisscross inheritance** [*Christ cross;* L, *in + hereditas,* in heredity], the inheritance of characteristics or conditions from the parent of the opposite sex.

**crista.** See **crest.**

**crista ampullaris** /kris'tə am'pə·lar'is/ [L], the most prominent part of a localized thickening of the membrane that lines the ampullae of the semicircular ducts, covered

with neuroepithelium containing endings of the vestibular nerve.

**crista supraventricularis** /kris'tə soō'prəven'trik'yəler'is/ [L, *crista,* ridge; *supra,* above, *ventriculus,* little belly], the muscular ridge on the interior dorsal wall of the right ventricle of the heart. It defines the limit of the arterial cone and extends toward the pulmonary trunk from the ventral cusp of the atrioventricular ring. Compare **moderator band.**

**criterion** /krītir'ē·ən/, *pl.* **criteria** [Gk, *kriterion,* a means for judging], a standard or rule by which something may be judged, such as a health condition, or a diagnosis established. Criteria are sets of rules or principles against which something may be measured, such as health care practices.

**critical care.** See **intensive care.**

**critical care unit (CCU),** a specially equipped hospital area designed for the treatment of patients with sudden, life-threatening conditions. CCUs contain resuscitation and monitoring equipment and are staffed by personnel specially trained and skilled in recognizing and immediately responding to cardiac and other emergencies. See also **intensive care unit.**

**critical organs** /krit'ikəl/ [Gk, *krisis,* turning point, *organon,* instrument], tissues that are the most sensitive to irradiation, such as the gonads, lymphoid organs, and intestine. The skin, cornea, oral cavity, esophagus, vagina, cervix, and optic lens are the next-most sensitive organs to irradiation.

**critical path development,** a nursing intervention from the Nursing Interventions Classification (NIC) defined as constructing and using a timed sequence of patient care activities to enhance desired patient outcomes in a cost-efficient manner. See also **Nursing Interventions Classification.**

**critical pathway.** See **clinical pathway.**

**critical period** [Gk, *kritikos,* critical, *peri,* near, *hodos,* way], a period during a developmental or rehabilitation crisis. Examples are the brief period in which a zygote may be formed, in which a patient may survive a myocardial infarction, or when an embryo is most vulnerable to effects of medications used by the mother.

**critical period of development,** 1. a specific time during which the environment has its greatest impact on an individual's development. 2. time during gestation when critical organ systems are formed.

**critical point,** the temperature and pressure at which, in a sealed system, the densities of the liquid and gas forms of a substance are equal and the two are not visibly separated.

**critical pressure,** the pressure exerted by a vapor in a closed system at the critical temperature.

**critical temperature,** the highest temperature at which a substance can exist as a liquid.

**Crixivan,** trademark for an antiretroviral protease inhibitor (indinavir).

**CRNA,** abbreviation for *certified registered nurse anesthetist.* See also **Nurse Anesthetist.**

**CRNI,** abbreviation for *certified registered nurse, intravenous.*

**crocodile shagreen** /shagrēn'/, a rare degenerative disorder involving either of two membranes of the cornea in which the cornea exhibits opacities separated by clear zones. The disorder may affect Descemet's deep membrane or Bowman's superficial membrane.

**Crohn's disease** /krōnz/ [Burrill B. Crohn, American physician, 1884–1983], a chronic inflammatory bowel disease of unknown origin, usually affecting the ileum, the colon, or another part of the GI tract. Diseased segments may be separated by normal bowel segments, which give it the charac-

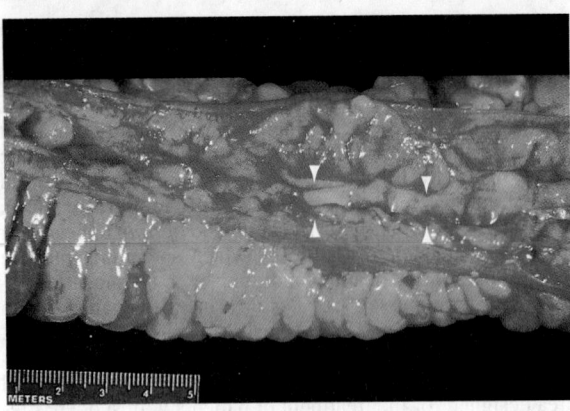

**Crohn's disease** *(Kumar, Cotran, and Robbins, 1997)*

teristic "skip lesions." Also called **regional enteritis.** Compare **ulcerative colitis.** See also **colitis, ileitis.**

**Cromer blood group** /krō'mər /, a blood group consisting of erythrocytic antigens Cr[a], Tc[a], Tc[ab], Dr[a], Es[a], WES[b], UMC, and IFC, which are located on a membrane protein.

**-cromil,** suffix designating a cromoglycic acid–type antiallergic agent.

**cromoglycic acid.** See **cromolyn sodium.**

**cromolyn sodium** /krom'əlin/, an antiasthmatic that acts by inhibiting histamine release from mast cells; a mast cell stabilizer; an antiinflammatory agent.

■ INDICATION: It is prophylactically prescribed to prevent bronchial asthma.

■ CONTRAINDICATION: Known hypersensitivity to this drug prohibits its use.

■ ADVERSE EFFECTS: Bronchospasm, wheezing, nasal congestion, pharyngeal irritation, and other hypersensitivity reactions may occur.

**Cronkhite-Canada syndrome** /krong'kīt/ [Leonard W. Cronkhite, American physician, b. 1919; Wilma J. Canada, twentieth-century American radiologist], an abnormal familial condition characterized by GI polyposis accompanied by ectodermal defects, such as nail atrophy, alopecia, and excessive skin pigmentation. In some individuals it is also accompanied by protein-losing enteropathy, malabsorption, and deficiency of blood calcium, potassium, and magnesium.

**cross** [L, *crux*], (in genetics) **1.** a mating between individuals with different phenotypes. Kinds of crosses include **dihybrid cross, monohybrid cross, polyhybrid cross,** and **trihybrid cross. 2.** any individual, organism, or strain produced from such a mating.

**cross-bite** [L, *crux* + AS, *bitan, toth*], occlusion of the mandibular teeth anterior and/or buccal to the maxillary teeth.

**crossbreeding** [L, *crux* + *bredan*], the production of offspring by the mating of individuals of different varieties, strains, or species; hybridization. See also **inbreeding.** —**crossbred,** *adj.*

**crossed amblyopia** [L, *crux*, cross; Gk, *amblys*, dull, *ops*, eyes], a visual disorder in which the patient is unable to see on one side of the visual field, associated with hemianesthesia of the opposite side of the body. Also called **amblyopia cruciata.**

**crossed extension reflex,** one of the spinally mediated reflexes normally present in the first 2 months of life. It is demonstrated by the adduction and extension of one leg when the foot of the other leg is stimulated.

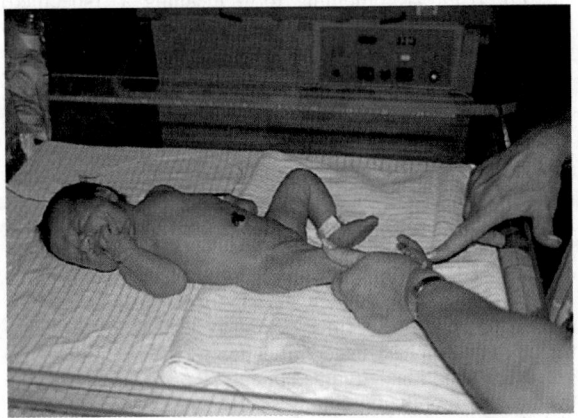

**Crossed extension reflex**
*(Lowdermilk, Perry, and Bobak, 2000)*

**crossed grid,** an assembly of two parallel x-ray grids that are oriented at right angles to each other to eliminate scattered radiation from more than one direction during radiography. Also called **crosshatch grid.** See also **grid.**

**crossed reflex,** any neural reflex in which stimulation of one side of the body results in a response on the other, such as the consensual light reflex.

**cross-eye.** See **esophoria** and **esotropia.**

### Comparison of ulcerative colitis and Crohn's disease

| | Ulcerative colitis | Crohn's disease |
| --- | --- | --- |
| Usual area affected | Left colon, rectum | Distal ileum, right colon |
| Extent of involvement | Diffuse areas, contiguous | Segmental areas, noncontiguous |
| Inflammation | Mostly mucosal | Transmural |
| Mucosal appearance | Ulcerations | Cobblestone effect, granulomas |
| Complications | Toxic megacolon | Fistulas |
| | Pseudopolyps | Perianal disease |
| | Hemorrhoids | Strictures |
| | Hemorrhage | Abscesses |
| | | Perforation |

From Phipps WJ, Sands JK, Marek JF: *Medical surgical nursing concepts and clinical practice,* ed 6, St Louis, 1999, Mosby.

**cross fertilization, 1.** the union of gametes from different species or varieties to form hybrids. **2.** the fertilization of the flower of one plant by the pollen of a different plant. Also called **allogamy.**

**crosshatch grid.** See **crossed grid.**

**cross infection** [L, *crux,* cross, *inficere,* to stain], the transmittal of an infection from one patient in a hospital or health care setting to another patient in the same environment.

**crossing over,** the exchange of sections of chromatids between homologous pairs of chromosomes during the prophase stage of the first meiotic division. Crossing over occurs through the formation of chiasmata and results in the recombination of genes. Also called **chiasmatypy.**

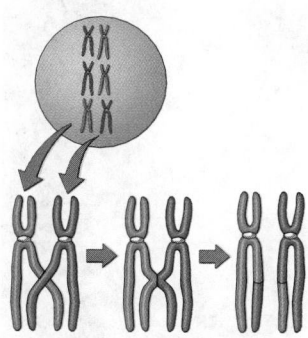

**Crossing over** *(Thibodeau and Patton, 1999/Network Graphics)*

**crossmatching of blood** [L, *crux* + AS, *gemaecca,* matching], a procedure used to determine compatibility of a donor's blood with that of a recipient after the specimens have been matched for major blood type. Serum from the donor's blood is mixed with red cells from the recipient's blood, and cells from the donor are mixed with serum from the recipient. If agglutination occurs, an antigenic substance is present and the bloods are not compatible. If no agglutination occurs, the donor's blood may safely be transfused to the recipient. Compare **blood typing.** See also **ABO blood group, Rh factor, transfusion, transfusion reaction.**

**crossover** /kros'ovər/ [L, *crux* + AS, *ofer*], the result of the recombination of genes on homologous pairs of chromosomes during meiosis. See also **crossing over.**

**cross-reacting antibody** [L, *crux,* cross, *re* + *agere,* to act; Gk, *anti* + AS, *bodig,* body], an antibody that reacts with antigens that are similar to but different than the specific antigens with which it originally reacted.

**cross resistance,** the resistance to a particular antibiotic that also results in resistance to a antibiotic, usually from a similar chemical class, to which the bacteria may not have been exposed. Cross resistance can occur between colistin and polymyxin B or clindamycin and lincomycin.

**cross section, 1.** a transverse section cut through a structure. **2.** (in nuclear physics) of a specific atom or particle at a specific radiation, the area perpendicular to the direction of the radiation that one attributes to the atom or particle.

**cross-sectional** [L, *crux* + *secare,* to cut], (in statistics) pertaining to the comparative data of two groups of persons at one point in time.

**cross-sectional anatomy,** the study of the relationship of the structures of the body by the examination of cross-sections of the tissue or organ. Compare **surface anatomy.**

**cross sensitivity,** a sensitivity to one substance that predisposes an individual to sensitivity to other substances that are related in chemical structure. Cross sensitivity with allergic reactions may develop between antibiotics of similar chemical structures.

**cross-sequential** /-sikwen'shəl/ [L, *crux* + *sequi,* to follow], (in statistics) pertaining to data that compare several cohorts at different points in time.

**cross-species transplant,** a tissue or organ from an animal of one species that has been implanted into an animal of another species. Also called **xenotransplant.**

**Cross syndrome.** See **oculocerebral-hypopigmentation syndrome.**

**cross-tolerance,** a tolerance to other drugs that develops after exposure to a different agent. An example is the cross-tolerance that develops between alcohol and barbiturates.

**crotamiton** /krōtam'iton/, a scabicide.

■ INDICATIONS: It is prescribed in the treatment of scabies and other pruritic skin diseases.

■ CONTRAINDICATIONS: Known hypersensitivity to this drug prohibits its use. It is not applied near the eyes or on the mouth or raw skin.

■ ADVERSE EFFECTS: Among the most serious adverse reactions are irritation and allergic reactions of the skin.

**croup** /kroop/ [Scot, to croak], an acute viral infection of the upper and lower respiratory tract that occurs primarily in infants and young children 3 months to 3 years of age after an upper respiratory tract infection. It is characterized by hoarseness; irritability; fever; a distinctive harsh, brassy cough; persistent stridor during inspiration; and dyspnea and tachypnea, resulting from obstruction of the larynx. Cyanosis or pallor occurs in severe cases. The most common causative agents are the parainfluenza viruses, especially type 1, followed by the respiratory syncytial viruses (RSVs) and in-

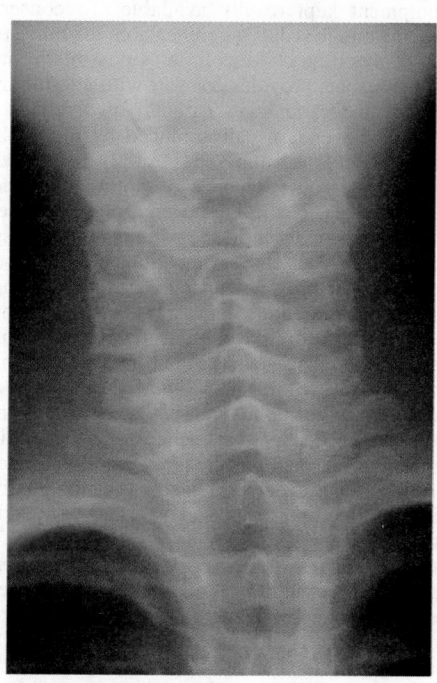

**Subglottic stenosis in croup** *(Stone and Gorbach, 2000)*

fluenza A and B viruses. Also called **angina trachealis, exudative angina, laryngostasis.** Compare **acute epiglottitis.** —**croupous, croupy,** *adj.*

■ OBSERVATIONS: Transmission occurs through infection with airborne particles or with infected secretions. Leukocytosis with an increased proportion of polymorphonuclear cells may be present at first, followed by leukopenia and lymphocytosis. A lateral neck x-ray film shows subepiglottic narrowing and a normal-sized epiglottis, which differentiate the condition from acute epiglottitis. Onset of the acute stage is rapid, usually occurs at night, and may be precipitated by exposure to cold air. The child's condition often improves in the morning, but it may worsen at night.

■ INTERVENTIONS: Routine treatment consists of bed rest, adequate fluid intake, and alleviation of airway obstruction to ensure adequate respiratory exchange. Children with mild infections are usually managed at home with supportive measures, such as use of vaporizers, humidifiers, or steam from hot running water in an enclosed bathroom to reduce the spasm of the laryngeal muscles and to free secretions. Hospitalization is indicated for children with high temperature; progressive stridor and respiratory distress; and hypoxia, cyanosis, or pallor. Endotracheal intubation and tracheostomy may be necessary. Humidity and oxygen are usually prescribed. The vital signs are continuously monitored; changes in pulse and respiration may be early signs of hypoxia and impending airway obstruction. Fluids are often given intravenously to reduce physical exertion and the possibility of vomiting, with its attendant increased risk of aspiration. Corticosteroids and inhaled racemic epinephrine are often used. Other drugs, such as expectorants, bronchodilators, and antihistamines, are rarely used, and sedatives are contraindicated, because they exert a depressant effect on the respiratory tract.

■ NURSING CONSIDERATIONS: The primary focuses of nursing care are to ease breathing by providing humidity and to monitor continuously for signs of respiratory distress and impending airway obstruction, with intubation and tracheostomy equipment kept readily available. To conserve the child's energy and to reduce apprehension, the nurse encourages rest, disturbs the child as little as possible, remains in constant attendance, provides comfort with a familiar toy or other device, and encourages parental involvement whenever possible. Fever is usually reduced by the cool atmosphere of the mist tent; antipyretics are given as needed. To prevent chilling, frequent changes of clothing and bed linen are often necessary in the humid environment. The nurse also explains the condition to the parents and discusses appropriate care after discharge, including continued use of humidity and ensuring of adequate hydration and proper nutrition. In most children the condition is relatively mild and runs its course in 3 to 7 days. The infection may spread to other areas of the respiratory tract and may cause complications, such as bronchiolitis, pneumonia, and otitis media. The most serious complication is laryngeal obstruction, which may cause death. If a tracheostomy is required, as may happen with a small percentage of children, other complications, such as infection, atelectasis, cannula occlusion, tracheal bleeding, granulation, stenosis, and delayed healing of the stoma, may develop.

**Croupette** /krōopet′/, trademark for a device that provides cool humidification with the administration of oxygen or of compressed air. The Croupette consists of a nebulizer with attached tubing that connects with a canopy to enclose the patient and contain the humidifying mist. The patient's environment may be cooled by using a Croupette with its own refrigeration unit. This device is most often used with pediatric patients to relieve hypoxia and liquefy secretions. Also called **cold mist tent.**

**croupous, croupy.** See **croup.**

**Crouzon's disease** /krōozonz′/ [Octave Crouzon, French neurologist, 1874–1938; L, *dis* + Fr, *aise,* ease], a familial disease characterized by a malformed skull and various ocular disorders, including exophthalmos, divergent squint, and optic atrophy.

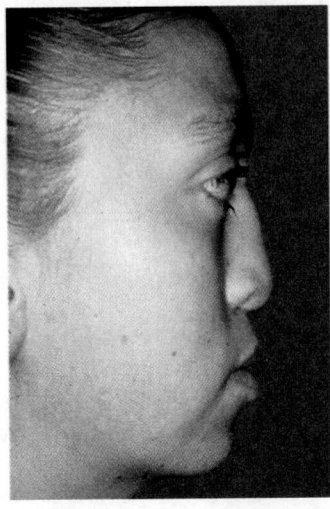

**Crouzon's syndrome: lateral view**
*(Carlson, 1999/courtesy A.R. Burdi, Ann Arbor, Michigan)*

**crowding** /kroud′ing/ [ME, *crowden*], the condition in which the teeth are too close together and have abnormal positions such as overlapping, displacement in various directions, or torsion.

**Crow-Fukase syndrome.** See **POEMS syndrome.**

**crowing inspiration.** See **laryngismus.**

**crown** [L, *corona*], 1. the upper part of an organ or structure, such as the top of the head. 2. the portion of a human tooth that is covered by enamel.

**crown-heel length** [L, *corona* + AS, *hela, lengthu*], the length of an embryo, fetus, or newborn as measured from the crown of the head to the heel. It is compared to the standing height of an older individual.

**crowning** [L, *corona*], (in obstetrics) the phase at the end of labor in which the fetal head is seen at the introitus of the vagina. The labia are stretched in a crown around the head just before birth.

**crown/root ratio.** See **clinical-crown/clinical-root ratio.**

**crown-rump length,** the length of an embryo, fetus, or newborn as measured from the crown of the head to the prominence of the buttocks.

**crown static,** an x-ray film artifact caused by a buildup and discharge of electrons in the film emulsion. It is most likely to appear during periods of low environmental humidity.

**CRP,** abbreviation for **C-reactive protein.**

**CRRN,** abbreviation for *Certified Rehabilitation Registered Nurse.*

**CRT,** 1. abbreviation for **cadaveric renal transplant.** 2. abbreviation for **cathode-ray tube.**

**CRTT,** abbreviation for **Certified Respiratory Therapy Technician.**

**crucial** /krōō′shəl/ [L. *crucialis*], severe and decisive.

**crucial anastomosis** /krōō′shəl/ [L, *crux*, cross; Gk, *anastomoein,* to provide a mouth], an anastomosis in the upper part of the thigh, formed between the first perforating branch of the profunda femoris artery, the inferior gluteal artery, and the lateral and medial circumflex arteries.

**crucial bandage.** See **T bandage.**

**cruciate** /krōō′shē·āt/ [L, *crux,* cross], shaped like a cross.

**cruciate ligament of the atlas** [L, *crux,* cross, *ligare,* to bind], a crosslike ligament attaching the atlas to the base of the occipital bone above and the posterior surface of the body of the axis below.

**crucible** /krōō′səbəl/, a cone-shaped vessel made of a refractory material, used in chemistry to melt or calcine materials at temperatures too high for other laboratory equipment to tolerate.

**cruciform** /krōō′sifôrm/ [L, *crux,* cross], in the shape of a cross.

**cruciform ligament,** any cross-shaped band of white fibrous tissue connecting bones and forming a joint capsule. Examples are the anterior and posterior cruciate ligaments of the knee and the cruciate ligament of the atlas.

**crude birth rate** [L, *crudus,* raw; ME, *burth* + L, *reri,* to reckon], the number of births per 1000 people in a population during 1 year. Compare **birth rate, refined birth rate, true birth rate.**

**cruor** /krōō′ôr/ [L, blood], a blood clot containing erythrocytes.

**crur-,** combining form meaning 'leg or thigh': *crura, crural, crureus.*

**crura.** See **crus.**

**crura anthelicis** /krōōr′ə ant·hē′lisis/ [L, *crus,* leg; Gk, *anti,* against, *helix,* coil], the two ridges on the external ear marking the superior termination of the anthelix and bounding the triangular fossa. Also called **crura of anthelix.**

**crural** /krōō′rəl/, pertaining to the leg, particularly the upper leg or thigh.

**crural hernia** [L, *crus,* leg, *hernia,* rupture], a hernia that protrudes behind the posterior layer of the femoral sheath. Also called **Cloquet's hernia.**

**crural ligament,** a band of fibrous tissue that spans the gap between the anterior superior iliac spine and the pubic tubercle.

**crura of anthelix.** See **crura anthelicis.**

**crureus.** See **vastus intermedius.**

**crus** /krus/, *pl.* **crura** /krōōr′ə/ [L, leg], **1.** the leg, from knee to foot. **2.** a structure resembling a leg, such as the crura anthelicis.

**crus cerebri** /ser′əbrī, -brē/ [L, *crus* + *cerebrum,* brain], either of the two ventral parts of the cerebral peduncle, composed of the descending fiber tracts passing from the cerebral cortex to form the longitudinal fascicles of the pons. Also called **basis pedunculi cerebri.**

**crushing wound** /krush′ing/ [ME, *crushen* + AS, *wund*], a break in the external surface of the body caused by a severe force applied against the tissues. The body structures may be crushed without signs of external bleeding.

**crush syndrome** [ME, *crushen*], a severe, life-threatening condition caused by extensive crushing trauma, characterized by destruction of muscle and bone tissue, hemorrhage, and fluid loss resulting in hypovolemic shock, hematuria, renal failure, and coma. Massive supportive therapy, including fluids, electrolytes, antibiotics, analgesia, oxygen, and intensive care with close monitoring of all vital functions, is usually necessary.

**crust** [L, *crusta,* shell], a solidified, hard outer layer formed by the drying of a body exudate, common in dermatologic conditions such as eczema, impetigo, seborrhea, and favus and during the healing of burns and lesions; a scab.

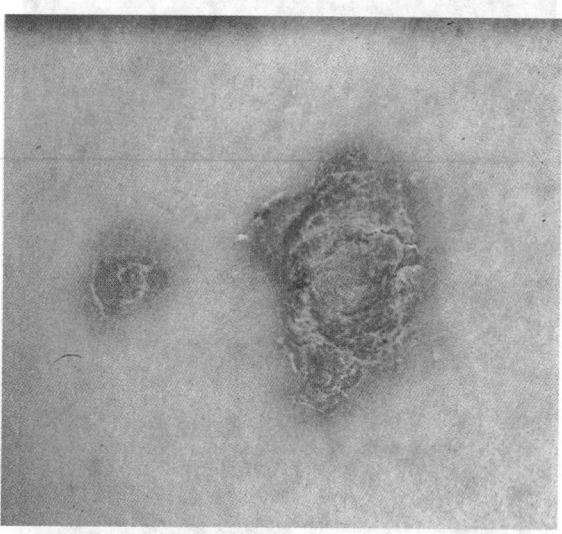

**Crust** *(du Vivier, 1993)*

**crusta.** See **crust.**

**crutch** [AS, *cryce*], a wooden or metal staff that aids a person in walking. The most common kind of crutch is the axillary crutch, which reaches from the ground almost to the axilla. It has a padded, curved surface at the top that fits under the arm and a crossbar that is held in the hand at the level of the palms to support the body. It is important that the crutches be properly fitted and that the person be taught how to use them safely and how to achieve a stable and acceptable gait. See also **Canadian crutch.**

**Crutchfield tongs** [William G. Crutchfield, American neurosurgeon, 1900–1972; ME, *tonges*], an instrument that is attached to the skull to hyperextend the head and neck of patients with fractured cervical vertebrae for the purpose of immobilizing and aligning the vertebrae.

■ METHOD: The tips of the tongs are inserted into small burr holes drilled in each parietal region of the skull; the surrounding skin is sutured and covered with a collodion dressing. A rope tied to the center of the tongs passes over a pulley at the head of the bed and is attached to a weight of 10 to 20 pounds, which hangs freely.

■ INTERVENTIONS: The insertion sites of the tongs are inspected and cleaned every 1 to 2 hours; any formed crusts are removed with hydrogen peroxide twice a day or as required. The patient is turned and assisted in deep breathing every other hour and is given scalp and skin care every 2 to 4 hours. The bed linen is kept dry and smooth, and back rubs are administered to prevent pressure ulcers. Passive range-of-motion exercises of all extremities are performed when prescribed. Sandbags may be used to prevent the patient from sliding to the head of the bed, and the call bell is placed within easy reach. The immobilized patient receives food that is easy to swallow and is fed with care to prevent aspiration; suction apparatus is kept at the bedside as an

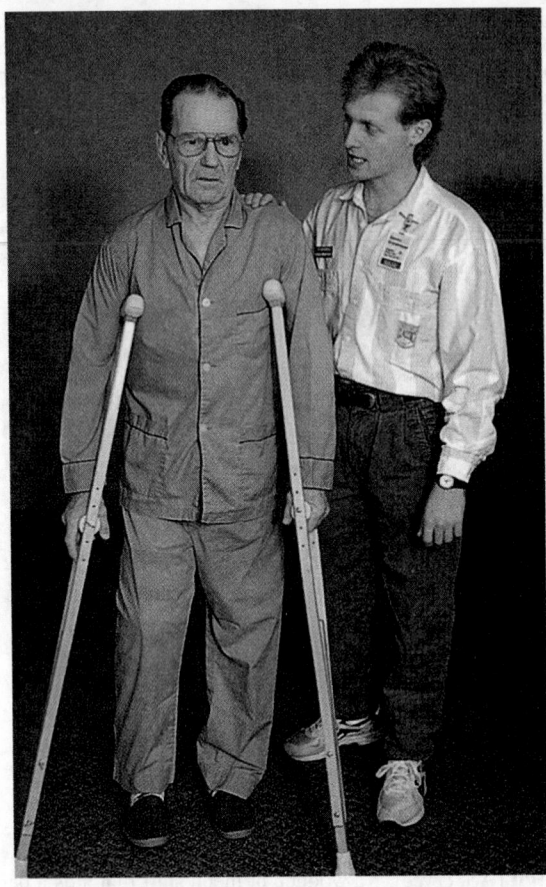

**Axillary crutches** *(Elkin, Perry, and Potter, 2000)*

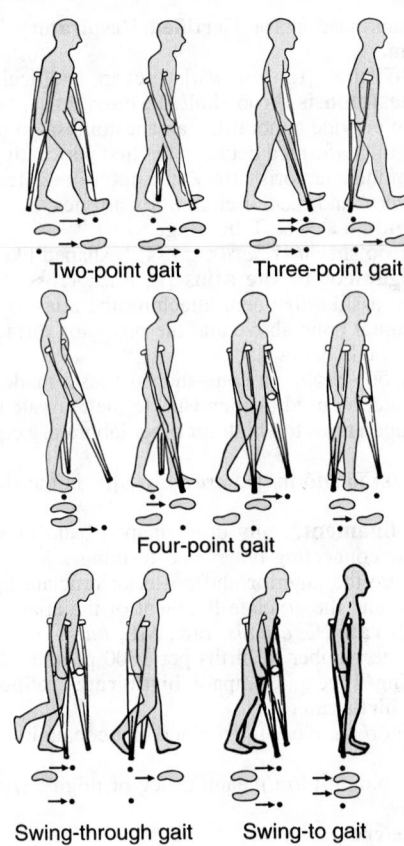

Two-point gait  Three-point gait

Four-point gait

Swing-through gait  Swing-to gait

**Crutch gaits**

emergency measure. The nurse maintains the patient's body alignment and checks that the weights are in the prescribed amount and are hanging freely.

■ OUTCOME CRITERIA: A patient may be immobilized by Crutchfield tongs for weeks before surgery is performed; during an operation on the cervical spine and spinal cord, the tongs may be left in place for proper alignment.

**crutch gait,** a gait achieved by a person using crutches. The gait selected and learned is determined by the physical and functional abilities of the patient and the diagnosis. In a two-point gait, the patient uses each crutch with the opposing leg. In a three-point gait, weight is borne on the noninvolved leg, then on both crutches, and then on the noninvolved leg again; weight-bearing on the involved leg initially is partial or prevented, but the patient usually progresses to full weight-bearing on that leg. A four-point gait gives stability but requires bearing weight on both legs; each leg is used alternately with each crutch. The swing-to and swing-through gaits are often used by paraplegic patients with weight-supporting braces on the legs. Weight is borne on the supported legs; the crutches are placed one stride in front of the person, who then swings to that point or through the crutches to a spot in front of them.

**crutch palsy,** the temporary or permanent loss of sensation or muscle control resulting from pressure on the radial nerve by a crutch. The radial nerve passes under the axillary area superficially. Pressure, often caused by mismatching of the height of the patient and the crutch, can lead to paralysis of the elbow and wrist extensors.

**Cruveilhier-Baumgarten syndrome** /krYvāyā'-boum'gärt ən/ [Jean Cruveilhier, French pathologist, 1791–1874; Paul Baumgarten, German pathologist, 1848–1928], recanalization of the paraumbilical veins with cirrhosis of the liver, portal hypertension, and splenomegaly.

**crux** /kruks, krŏŏks/ [L], **1.** cross. **2.** a difficult problem. **3.** a vital, basic, or decisive point.

**Cruz trypanosomiasis.** See **Chagas' disease.**

**cry** [OFr, *crier*], **1.** a sudden, loud voluntary or automatic vocalization in response to pain, fear, or a startle reflex. **2.** weeping, as a reaction to pain or an emotional response to depression or grief. **3.** See **cri-du-chat syndrome.**

**crying vital capacity (CVC),** a measurement of the tidal volume while an infant is crying. The CVC may be valuable in monitoring infants with lung diseases that cause changes in functional residual capacity.

**cryo-, cry-, crymo-,** prefix meaning 'cold': *cryocautery, cryophilia, cryotolerant.*

**cryoanesthesia** /krī'ō·an'isthē'zhə/ [Gk, *kryos,* cold, *aisthesis,* feeling], freezing of a part the body to deaden neural sensitivity to pain during brief minor surgical procedures.

**cryocautery** /krī'ōkô'tərē/ [Gk, *kryos* + *kauterion,* branding iron], the application of any substance, such as solid carbon dioxide, that destroys tissue by freezing. Also called **cold cautery.**

**cryogen** /krī'əjən/ [Gk, *kryos* + *genein,* to produce], **1.** a chemical that induces freezing, used to destroy diseased tissue without injury to adjacent structures. Cell death is caused by dehydration after cell membranes rupture. **2.** (in magnetic resonance imaging [MRI]) a chemical used to cool the MRI electromagnet so that the magnet remains superconducting and higher magnified strengths can be achieved. Kinds of cryogens include **carbon dioxide, liquid nitrogen, liquid helium,** and **nitrous oxide.** —**cryogenic,** *adj.*

**cryoglobulin** /krī′ōglob′yŏŏlin/ [Gk, *kryos* + L, *globulus,* small sphere], an abnormal plasma protein that precipitates and coalesces at low temperatures and dissolves and disperses at body temperature.

**cryoglobulinemia** /krī′ōglob′yŏŏlinē′mē·ə/ [Gk, *kryos* + L, *globulus,* small sphere; Gk, *haima,* blood], the presence of cryoglobulins in the blood. Presence of cryoglobulins may be associated with Waldenström's macroglobulinemia.

**cryonics** /krī·on′iks/ [Gk, *kryos,* cold], the techniques in which cold is applied for a variety of therapeutic goals, including brief local anesthesia, destruction of superficial skin lesions, and preservation of cells, tissue, organs, or the entire body. —**cryonic,** *adj.*

**cryoprecipitate** /-prisip′itāt/, **1.** any precipitate formed on cooling of a solution. **2.** a preparation rich in factor VIII needed to restore normal coagulation in hemophilia. It is collected from fresh human plasma that has been frozen and thawed.

**cryopreservation** /krī′ōpres′ərvā′shən/, a method of preserving tissues and organs in a viable state at extremely low temperatures.

**cryostat** /krī′ōstat/ [Gk, *kryos* + *statos,* standing], a device used in surgical treatment of pathologic disorders that consists of a special microtome used for freezing and slicing sections of tissue for study by a surgical pathologist. See also **microtome.**

**cryosurgery** /-sur′jərē/ [Gk, *kryos* + *cheirourgos*], use of subfreezing temperature to destroy tissue. Cryosurgery is performed in the destruction of the ganglion of nerve cells in the thalamus in the treatment of Parkinson's disease, in the destruction of the pituitary gland to halt the progress of some kinds of metastatic cancer, and in the treatment of various cancers and lesions of the skin. The process is also used in ophthalmology to cause the edges of a detached retina to heal and to remove cataracts. The coolant is circulated through a metal probe, chilling it to as low as −160° C (−256° F), depending on the chemical used. The moist tis-

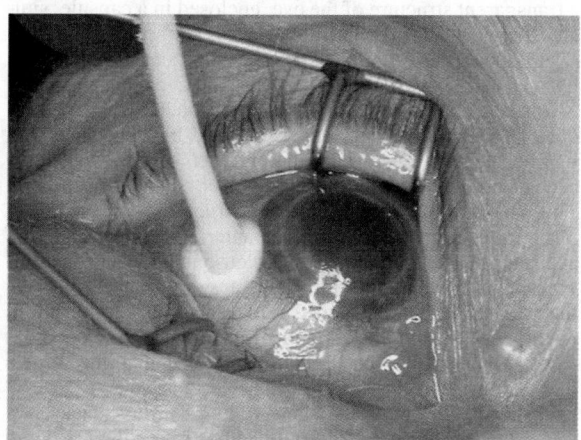

**Cryosurgery** *(Jaffe, 1996)*

sues adhere to the cold metal of the probe and freeze. Cells are dehydrated as their membranes burst; eventually they are discarded or absorbed by the body. No specific postoperative nursing care is required.

**cryotherapy** /krī′ōther′əpē/ [Gk, *kryos* + *therapeia*], a treatment using cold as a destructive medium. Cutaneous tags, warts, condyloma acuminatum, and actinic keratosis are some of the common skin disorders responsive to cryotherapy. Solid carbon dioxide or liquid nitrogen is applied briefly with a sterile cotton-tipped applicator or cryospray instrument. Blistering, followed by necrosis, results. The procedure may be repeated.

**crypt** /kript/ [Gk, *kryptos,* hidden], a blind pit or tube on a free surface. Some kinds of crypts are **anal crypt, dental crypt,** and **synovial crypt.**

**crypt-.** See **crypto-.**

**cryptic** /krip′tik/ [Gk, *kryptos,* hidden], pertaining to something concealed.

**crypto-, crypt-, krypto-,** prefix meaning 'hidden': *cryptocephalus, cryptocrystalline, cryptodidymus.*

**cryptocephalus** /krip′tōsef′ələs/ [Gk, *kryptos* + *kephale,* head], a malformed fetus that has a small, underdeveloped head. —**cryptocephalic, cryptocephalous,** *adj.,* **cryptocephaly,** *n.*

**cryptococcosis** /krip′tōkokō′sis/, an infectious disease caused by a fungus, *Cryptococcus neoformans,* which after inhalation, spreads from the lungs to the brain and central nervous system, skin, skeletal system, and urinary tract. The disease occurs in all parts of the world, but in North America it is most likely to afflict persons with immunodeficiencies such as human immunodeficiency virus (HIV) and middle-aged men in the southeastern United States. It is especially associated with breathing dust from pigeon droppings. It is characterized by the development of nodules or tumors filled with a gelatinous material in visceral and subcutaneous tissues. Initial symptoms may include coughing or other respiratory effects because the lungs are a primary site of infection. After the fungus spreads to the meninges, neurologic symptoms, including headache, blurred vision, and difficulty in speaking, may develop. The diagnosis is made by isolation and identification of the fungus in sputum, pus, or tissue biopsy specimens. Amphotericin B and fluconazole may be administered to control the infection. In patients with HIV, maintenance therapy with fluconazole is indicated. Also called **Buschke's disease, European blastomycosis, torulosis.** See also *Cryptococcus,* and specific fungal infections.

*Cryptococcus* /-kok′əs/, a genus of yeastlike fungi that reproduce by budding rather than by producing spores. Many nonpathogenic species of *Cryptococcus* are commonly found in the soil and on the skin and mucous membranes of people who are well. Certain pathogenic species exist; *C. neoformans* is the most important. See also **fungus, yeast.**

*Cryptococcus neoformans,* a species of yeastlike fungus that causes cryptococcosis, a potentially fatal infection that can affect the lungs, skin, and brain.

**cryptodidymus** /krip′tōdid′əməs/ [Gk, *kryptos* + *didymos,* twin], conjoined twins; one fetus is small, underdeveloped, and concealed within the body of the other, more fully formed autosite.

**crypt of iris,** any one of the small pits in the iris along its free margin encircled by the circulus arteriosus minor. Also called **crypt of Fuchs.**

**crypt of Lieberkühn.** See **Lieberkühn's glands.**

**cryptogenic** /-jen′ik/ [Gk, *kryptos,* hidden, *genein,* to produce], **1.** pertaining to a disease of unknown cause. **2.** a parasitic organism living within another organism.

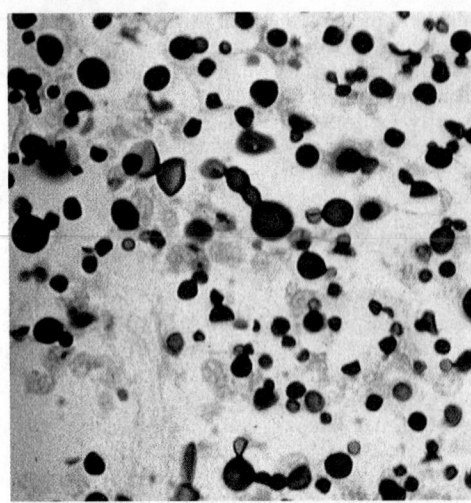

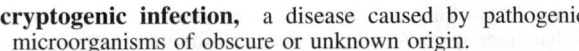

*Cryptococcus neoformans* **in exudate** *(Farrar, 1993)*

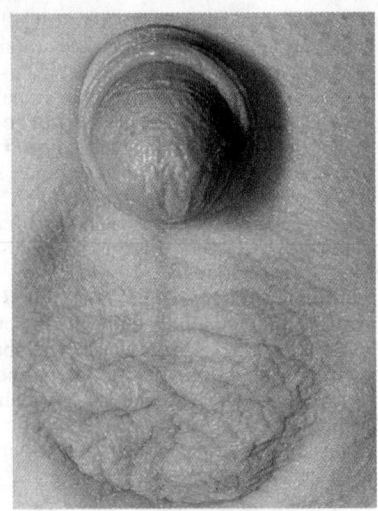

**Cryptorchidism**
*(Zitelli and Davis, 1992/courtesy Dr. Ellen Wald, Children's Hospital of Pittsburgh)*

**cryptogenic infection,** a disease caused by pathogenic microorganisms of obscure or unknown origin.

**cryptogenic septicemia,** a systemic infection in which pathogens are present in the bloodstream but no primary focus of infection can be identified.

**cryptomenorrhea** /krip′tōmenôrē′ə/ [Gk, *kryptos* + L, *mens,* month; Gk, *rhoia,* flow], an abnormal condition in which the products of menstruation are retained within the vagina because of an imperforate hymen, or, less often, within the uterus because of an occlusion of the cervical canal. Cryptomenorrhea is usually accompanied by subjective symptoms of menstruation with scant or absent flow and sometimes by severe pain. If the flow is completely obstructed, uterotubal reflux of menstrual flow into the pelvic cavity may cause peritonitis, pain, adhesions, and endometriosis. —**cryptomenorrheal,** *adj.*

**cryptophthalmos** /krip′təfthal′məs/ [Gk, *kryptos* + *ophthalmos,* eye], a developmental anomaly characterized by complete fusion of the eyelids, usually with defective formation or lack of eyes.

**cryptophthalmos syndrome.** See **Fraser syndrome.**

**cryptorchid.** See **cryptorchidism.**

**cryptorchidism** /kriptôr′kidiz′əm/ [Gk, *kryptos,* hidden, *orchis,* testis], a developmental defect in which one or both testicles fail to descend into the scrotum and are retained in the abdomen or inguinal canal. If spontaneous descent does not occur by the age of 1 year, hormonal injections may be given. If injections are unsuccessful, orchiopexy is usually performed before age 3. Also called **cryptorchis, undescended testis.**

**cryptosporidiosis,** a GI disease caused by a waterborne parasitic protozoon, *Cryptosporidium parvum.* The disease was relatively unknown as a human pathogen before a 1993 epidemic in the Milwaukee, Wisconsin, area, where 400,000 persons were stricken with diarrhea after drinking water contaminated with the parasite. Other sources of infection include raw or undercooked foods contaminated with *Cryptosporidium* oocysts and direct contact with infected humans or animals. Symptoms of watery diarrhea, abdominal cramps, nausea, vomiting, and low-grade fever may appear 2 to 10 days after infection. They may lead to dehydration and weight loss. The symptoms may last 1 or 2 weeks and may be life-threatening to persons with suppressed immune systems. Treatment emphasizes rest, replenishment of body fluids and electrolytes, and medications to control diarrhea. Paromomycin may be partially effective in the treatment of cryptosporidiosis in persons with HIV infection. There is no known safe and effective cure for cryptosporidiosis.

*Cryptosporidium parvum.* See **cryptosporidiosis.**

**cry reflex,** a normal infantile reaction to pain, hunger, or need for attention. The reflex may be absent in an infant born prematurely or in poor health.

**crystal** /kris′təl/ [Gk, *krystallos*], a solid substance, either organic or inorganic, the atoms or molecules of which are arranged in a regular, repeating three-dimensional pattern, which determines the shape of a crystal. —**crystalline,** *adj.*

**crystal gold.** See **mat gold.**

**crystalline,** describing material with a regular geometric shape. Crystalline substances have a very narrow melting point range.

**crystalline lens** /kris′təlin, -līn/ [Gk, *krystallos* + L, lentil], a transparent structure of the eye, enclosed in a capsule, situated between the iris and the vitreous humor, and slightly overlapped at its margin by the ciliary processes. It refracts light to focus images on the retina. The capsule of the lens is a transparent elastic membrane that touches the free border of the iris anteriorly and is secured by the suspensory ligament of the lens. The circumference of the capsule recedes from the iris to form the posterior chamber of the eye. The lens is a transparent biconvex structure with the posterior surface more convex than the anterior. It is composed of a soft cortical material, a firm nucleus, and concentric laminae and is covered anteriorly by transparent epithelium. In the fetus the lens is very soft and has a slightly reddish tint; in the adult it is colorless and firm; in old age it becomes flattened, more dense, slightly opaque, and amber-tinted. See also **eye.**

**crystallization** /kris′təlīzā′shən/ [Gk, *krystallos,* rock crystal], the production of crystals, either by cooling a liquid or gas to a solid state or by cooling a solution until the solute precipitates as a crystalline deposit.

**crystalloid** /kris'təloid/ [Gk, *krystallos* + *eidos,* form], a substance in a solution that can diffuse through a semipermeable membrane. Compare **colloid.**

**crystalluria** /kris'təlŏŏr'ē·ə/, the presence of crystals in the urine. The condition may be a source of urinary tract irritation; adequate intake of alkali can prevent it.

**Crystodigin,** trademark for a cardiac glycoside (digitoxin).

**Cs,** symbol for the element **cesium.**

**CS,** abbreviation for **cesarean section.**

**c-section.** See **cesarean section.**

**CSF,** **1.** abbreviation for **cerebrospinal fluid. 2.** abbreviation for **colony-stimulating factor.**

**CSN,** abbreviation for *certified school nurse.*

**CSR,** abbreviation for **Cheyne-Stokes respiration.**

**c-src,** a cellular oncogene or protooncogene present in some animals. It hybridizes with oncogenes of the highly virulent Rous sarcoma virus.

**CST,** abbreviation for **contraction stress test.**

**CT,** abbreviation for **computed tomography.**

**CT number.** See **Hounsfield unit.**

**Cu,** symbol for the element **copper.**

**CUA,** abbreviation for **cost-utility analysis.**

**Cuban itch.** See **alastrim.**

**cubic centimeter (cm³, cu, cm)** [Gk, *kybos* + L, *centum,* hundred; Gk, *metron,* measure], a theoretical cube or its equivalent, each edge of which is 1 centimeter long. One cubic centimeter is equivalent to 1 milliliter (mL).

**cubic millimeter (cmm, c mm, cu mm, mm³),** a unit of volume equal to one millionth of a liter.

**cubital** /kyōō'bitəl/, pertaining to the elbow or the forearm.

**cubital fossa,** a depression in the front of the elbow, immediately lateral to the tendon of the biceps brachii muscle.

**cubitus** /kyōō'bitəs/, **1.** the elbow. **2.** the forearm.

**cuboidal epithelium** /kyōōboi'dəl/ [Gk, *kybos,* cube, *eidos,* form, *epi,* above, *thele,* nipple], simple epithelial cells that are generally cube-shaped and one layer thick.

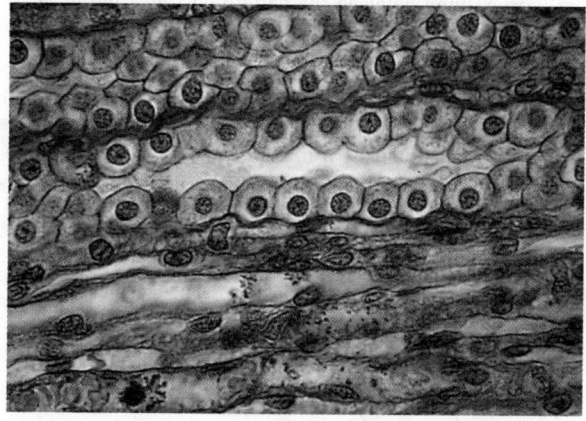

**Simple cuboidal epithelium**
*(© Ed Reschke; used with permission)*

**cuboid bone** /kyōō'boid/ [Gk, *kybos,* cube, *eidos,* form], the outer cuboidal tarsal bone on the lateral side of the foot, proximal to the fourth and fifth metatarsal bones. It articulates with the calcaneus, lateral cuneiform, and fourth and fifth metatarsal bones and occasionally with the navicular. Also called **os cuboideum.**

**cuboidodigital reflex.** See **Mendel's reflex.**

**cu cm,** abbreviation for **cubic centimeter.**

**cue** /kyōō/, a stimulus that determines or may prompt the nature of a person's response.

**cuff [ME],** an inflatable elastic tube that is placed around a limb and inflated with air to restrict arterial circulation during blood pressure examination. See also **cuffed endotracheal tube, Dacron cuff.**

**cuffed endotracheal tube,** an endotracheal tube with a balloon at one end that may be inflated to tighten the fit in the lumen of the airway. The balloon forms a cuff that prevents gastric contents from passing into the lungs and gas from leaking back from the lungs. Both high-pressure and low-pressure cuffs are in use. Overinflation of the cuff can cause contusion, hemorrhage, mucosal sloughing, or stenosis.

**cuffing,** a pathologic condition in which cufflike borders of leukocytes form around small blood vessels, as in certain infections.

**cuirass** /kwiras'/ [Fr, *cuirasse,* breastplate], **1.** a negative-pressure full-body respirator. It consists of a rigid shell that conforms to the surfaces of the body from the neck to the hips. Ventilating pressure is delivered through a flexible hose attached to the top of the device. An electrically driven pump is adjusted to match the timing of the patient's spontaneous breathing. **2.** a tightly fitted chest bandage.

**cuirass ventilator.** See **cuirass** (def. 1).

**cul-de-sac** /kul'dəsak, kYdesok'/, *pl.* **culs-de-sac, cul-de-sacs** [F, bottom of the bag], a blind pouch or cecum, such as the conjunctival cul-de-sac and the dural cul-de-sac.

**cul-de-sac of Douglas** [James Douglas, Scottish anatomist, 1675–1742], a pouch formed by the caudal portion of the parietal peritoneum. Also called **pouch of Douglas, rectouterine excavation, rectouterine pouch.**

**culdocentesis** /kul'dōsentē'sis/, the use of needle puncture or incision through the vagina to remove intraperitoneal fluid, including purulent material.

**culdoplasty** /kul'dōplas'tē/ [Fr, *cul-de-sac,* bottom of the bag; Gk, *plassein,* to mold], plastic surgery to correct a defect in the posterior fornix of the vagina.

**culdoscope** /kul'dəskōp'/, an endoscope with an attached light that can be inserted through the posterior wall of the vagina for examination of the pelvic viscera.

**culdotomy** /kuldot'əmē/, incision or needle puncture of cul-de-sac of Douglas by way of the vagina.

*Culex* /koo'leks/, a genus of humpbacked mosquitoes. It includes species that transmit viral encephalitis and filariasis.

**Cullen's sign** [Thomas S. Cullen, American gynecologist, 1868–1953], the appearance of faint, irregularly formed hemorrhagic patches on the skin around the umbilicus. The discolored skin is usually blue-black and becomes greenish brown or yellow. Cullen's sign may appear 1 to 2 days after the onset of anorexia and the severe, poorly localized abdominal pains that are characteristic of acute pancreatitis. It is also present in massive upper GI hemorrhage and ruptured ectopic pregnancy. Compare **Grey Turner's sign.** See also **pancreatitis.**

**culs-de-sac.** See **cul-de-sac.**

**cult,** a specific complex of beliefs, rites, and ceremonies associated with some particular person or object, which is maintained by a social group. A cult is often considered as having magical significance.

**cultural assimilation** /kul'chərəl/, a process by which members of an ethnic minority group lose cultural character-

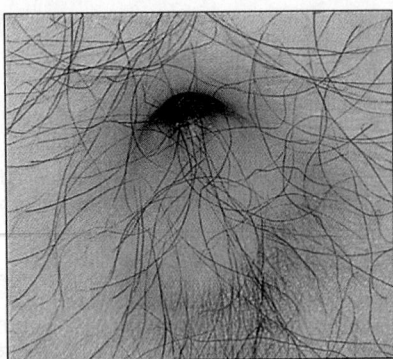

**Cullen's sign** *(Greig and Garden, 1996)*

istics that distinguish them from the dominant cultural group or take on the cultural characteristics of another group.

**cultural event,** a communication of meaning that takes place each time one member of a society interacts with another member.

**cultural healer,** a member of an ethnic or cultural group who uses traditional methods of healing rather than modern scientific methods to provide health care for other members of the group or members of another ethnic minority group.

**culturally relativistic perspective,** an ability to understand the behavior of transcultural patients (those who move from one culture to another) within the context of their own culture. See also **transcultural nursing.**

**cultural relativism,** a concept that health and normality emerge within a social context and that the content and form of mental health will vary greatly from one culture to another. Differences may result from variations in stressors, symbolic interpretation, acceptance of expression and repression, and cohesion and tolerance of deviation of social groups.

**culture** /kul′chər/ [L, *colere,* to cultivate], **1.** (in microbiology) a laboratory test involving the cultivation of microorganisms or cells in a special growth medium. See also **medium. 2.** (in psychology) a set of learned values, beliefs, customs, and behavior that is shared by a group of interacting individuals.

**culture-bound,** pertaining to a health condition that is specific to a particular culture, such as a belief in the effects of certain kinds of prayer or the "evil eye."

**culture brokerage,** a nursing intervention from the Nursing Interventions Classification (NIC) defined as deliberately using culturally competent strategies to bridge or mediate between the patient's culture and the biomedical health care system. See also **Nursing Interventions Classification.**

**culture medium.** See **medium.**

**culture procedure,** (in bacteriology) any of several techniques for growing colonies of microorganisms to identify a pathogen and to determine its sensitivity to various antibiotics. Usually a specimen is secured using sterile technique and a small amount is placed into or on one or more culture media, because different organisms are nourished by different nutrients and grow best at different specific pH levels. The environment in which the media are held during observation is maintained at body temperature, and the ambient oxygen level is adjusted to achieve an aerobic or anaerobic state. All procedures are aseptic, and all equipment is sterile to prevent accidental contamination of the media. As colo-

nies appear in or on the media, small amounts of each (there are often several) are spread onto other media to allow examination of a pure specimen of the microorganisms.

**culture shock,** the psychologic effect of a drastic change in the cultural environment of an individual. The person may exhibit feelings of helplessness, discomfort, and disorientation in attempting to adapt to a different cultural group with dissimilar practices, values, and beliefs.

**cum** /ko͝om/ [L], together with.

**cu mm,** abbreviation for **cubic millimeter.**

**cumulative** /kyo͞o′myəlā′tiv/ [L, *cumulare,* to pile on], increasing by incremental steps with an eventual total that may exceed the expected result.

**cumulative action, 1.** the increased activity of a therapeutic measure or agent when administered repeatedly, as the cumulative action of a regular exercise program. **2.** the increased activity demonstrated by a drug when repeated doses accumulate in the body and exert a greater biologic effect than the initial dose.

**cumulative dose,** the total dose that accumulates as a result of repeated exposure to radiation or a radiopharmaceutic product.

**cumulative gene.** See **polygene.**

**cumulus** /kyo͞o′myo͞o·ləs/ *pl.* **cumuli** [L], a little mound, usually formed by a collection of cells.

**cune-,** combining form meaning 'wedge': *cuneate, cuneiform, cuneus.*

**cuneate** /kyo͞o′nē·āt/ [L, *cuneus,* wedge], (of tissue) wedge-shaped; especially in relation to cells of the nervous system.

**cuneiform** /kyo͞onē′əfôrm′/ [L, *cuneus,* wedge, *forma*], (of bone and cartilage) wedge-shaped.

**cuneiform bone.** See **triangular bone.**

**cuneiform cartilage** [L, *cuneus,* wedge, *forma* + *cartilago*], one of two small pieces of yellow elongated elastic laryngeal cartilage at the edge of the aryepiglottic fold, above and anterior to the corniculate cartilage.

**-cuneo, cuneo-,** combining form meaning 'wedge-shaped structures': *cuneus, cuneiform.*

**cuneus** /kyo͞o′nē·əs/, a wedge-shaped region of the cerebral cortex lying between the parieto-occipital and postcalcarine sulci on the mesial surface of the occipital lobe.

**cunnilingus** /kun′əling′gəs/, the oral stimulation of the female genitalia.

**cup arthroplasty of the hip joint** [L, *cupa,* cask; Gk, *arthron,* joint, *plassein,* to mold], the surgical replacement of the head of the femur by a metal or plastic mold to relieve pain and increase motion in arthritis or to correct a deformity. The damaged or diseased bone is removed, and the acetabulum and the head of the femur are reshaped. A cup is inserted between the two and becomes the articulating surface of the femur. After surgery the patient's leg is placed on an abduction pillow to hold it in a position of abduction extension and internal rotation to keep the disk in place in the acetabulum. Continued abduction may be necessary for 6 weeks. Possible complications include infection, thrombophlebitis, pulmonary embolism, and fat embolism. The patient receives extensive physical therapy. A walker or crutches are necessary to prevent full weight-bearing for 6 months, and an exercise program must be followed for several years. Compare **hip replacement.** See also **arthroplasty, knee replacement, osteoarthritis, plastic surgery.**

**cup/disc ratio,** (in ophthalmology) the mathematic relationship between the horizontal or vertical diameter of the physiologic cup and the diameter of the optic disc.

**cupola.** See **cupula.**

**cupping,** a counterirritant technique of applying a suction device to the skin to draw blood to the surface of the body.

**cupping and vibrating,** a technique for dislodging and removing mucus and fluid from the lungs.

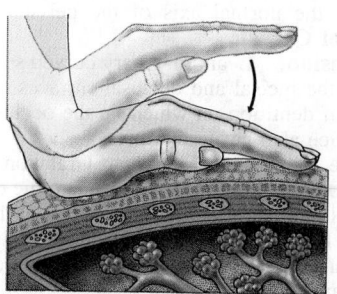

Chest percussion (with cupped hand)

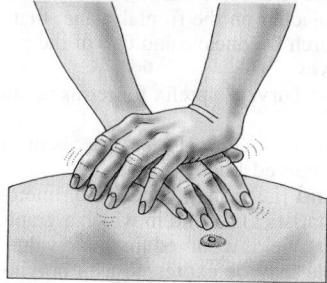

Chest vibration

**Cupping and vibrating**
*(Ignatavicius, Workman, and Mishler, 1999)*

■ METHOD: Cupping consists of the rhythmic percussion of the affected segments of the lungs or bronchi by the practitioner's cupped hands. It is begun gently and is increased in forcefulness as the patient tolerates increased percussion. To perform vibrating, the practitioner places his or her hands over the affected area and alternately tenses and contracts the muscles of the hand, arm, and shoulder. The vibratory movements are transmitted to the patient's chest, increasing the turbulence and velocity of exhaled air in the small bronchi. See also **postural drainage.**

■ INTERVENTIONS: Cupping is never performed over breast tissue, over the spine, or below the ribs because it causes discomfort and can damage soft tissue. After head-down postural drainage with cupping and vibrating, the patient is helped to a position favorable for effective coughing and asked to breathe deeply at least three times and to cough at least twice.

■ OUTCOME CRITERIA: Thick, tenacious mucus is difficult to evacuate from the bronchi, the bronchioles, and the alveoli. As an adjunct to postural drainage, cupping and vibrating may greatly facilitate clearing the passages. The patient can breathe more deeply and with less effort, and the potential for development of pneumonia or atelectasis is reduced.

**cupric** /kyo͞o′prik/ [L, *cuprum,* copper], pertaining to copper in its divalent form, as cupric sulfate. Also termed copper (II), as in copper (II) sulfate.

**Cuprid,** trademark for a copper chelating agent (trientine hydrochloride).

**Cuprimine,** trademark for a chelating agent (D-penicillamine), used in treating poisoning by heavy metals.

**cupula** /kyo͞o′pələ/, any cup- or dome-shaped structure, such as the top of a lymphatic nodule in the small intestine. Also spelled **cupola.**

**cupulolithiasis** /kyo͞o′pyo͞olōlithī′əsis/ [L, *cupula,* little cup; Gk, *lithos,* stone], a severe, long-lasting vertigo brought on by movement of the head to certain positions. Among the many possible causes are otitis media, ear surgery, and injury to the inner ear. In addition to extreme dizziness, signs are nausea, vomiting, and ataxia. There is no treatment except avoidance of the offending head positions. Also called **postural vertigo.**

**curare** /kyo͞orä′rē/ [S. Am. Indian, *ourari*], a substance derived from tropic plants of the genus *Strychnos.* It is a potent neuromuscular blocker that acts by preventing transmission of neural impulses across the myoneural junctions. A large dosage can cause complete paralysis, but action is usually reversible with anticholinergics. Pharmacologic preparations of the substance are used as adjuncts to general anesthesia. The use of curare or other neuromuscular blocking agents requires respiratory and ventilatory assistance by a qualified anesthetist or anesthesiologist. See also **tubocurarine chloride.**

**curariform** /kyo͞orä′rifôrm′/ [*curare* + L, *forma*], **1.** chemically similar to curare. **2.** having the effect of curare.

**curative treatment.** See **treatment.**

**cure** /kyo͞or/ [L, *cura*], **1.** restoration to health of a person afflicted with a disease or other disorder. **2.** the favorable outcome of the treatment of a disease or other disorder. **3.** a course of therapy, a medication, a therapeutic measure, or another remedy used in treatment of a medical problem, as faith healing, fasting, rest cure, or work cure.

**curet** /kyo͞oret′/ [Fr, *curette,* scoop], **1.** a surgical instrument shaped like a spoon or scoop for scraping and removing material or tissue from an organ, cavity, or surface. A curet may be blunt or sharp and is designed in a shape and size appropriate to its use. **2.** to remove tissue or debris with such a device. Kinds of curets include **Hartmann's curet.**

**curettage** /kyo͞or′ətäzh′/ [Fr, *curette,* scoop], scraping of material from the wall of a cavity or other surface, performed to remove tumors or other abnormal tissue or to obtain tissue for microscopic examination. Curettage also refers to clearing unwanted material from fistulas and areas of chronic infection. It may be performed with a blunt or a sharp curet or by suction.

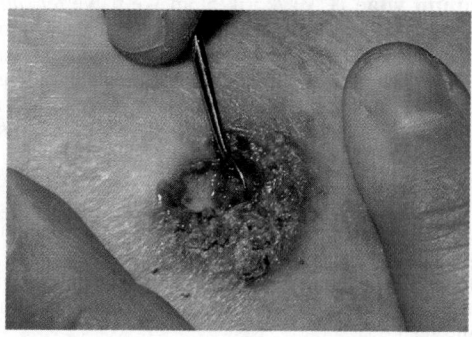

**Curettage** *(Habif, 1996)*

**curie (Ci)** /kyo͞or′ē/ [Marie S. Curie, Polish-born chemist and physicist, 1867–1934; Pierre Curie, French chemist and physicist, 1859–1906; both Nobel laureates], a unit of radioactivity used before adoption of the becquerel (Bq) as the SI unit. It is equal to $3.70 \times 10^{10}$ Bq.

**curing** /kyoor'ing/ [L, *curare,* to take care of or heal], (in dentistry) a method for promoting and accelerating hardening processes by using dampness, heat, cold, chemical agents, electromagnetic radiation, or other agents.

**curium (Cm)** /kyoo're·əm/ [Marie S. Curie; Pierre Curie], a radioactive metallic element. Its atomic number is 96; its atomic mass is 247. Curium is an artificial element produced by bombarding plutonium with helium ions in a cyclotron. Numerous isotopes of curium are produced by bombarding lighter transuranium elements. Curium is so radioactive that it glows in the dark.

**-curium,** suffix designating a neuromuscular blocking agent.

**Curling's ulcer** [Thomas B. Curling, English surgeon, 1811–1888], a duodenal ulcer that develops in people who have suffered severe stress. Curling first diagnosed it in patients who had severe burns. The pathophysiologic characteristics include hypotension from shock, which decreases the blood supply to gastric mucosa, which leads to ischemia. Also called **Curling's stress ulcer.** See also **milk therapy.**

**CURN,** abbreviation for *Certified Urological Registered Nurse.*

**-curonium,** suffix designating a neuromuscular blocking agent.

**currant jelly clot** /kur'ənt/ [ME, *corauns* + L, *gelare,* to congeal; AS, *clott*], a red, jellylike blood clot that is rich in hemoglobin from erythrocytes in the clot.

**current** /kur'ənt/ [L, *currere,* to run], **1.** a flowing or streaming movement. **2.** a flow of electrons along a conductor in a closed circuit; an electric current. **3.** certain physiologic electrical activity and characteristics of blood circulation. Physiologic currents include abnerval current, action current, axial current, centrifugal current, centripetal current, compensating current, demarcation current, and electrotonic current. See also **alternating current, direct current, volt, watt.**

**-current,** suffix meaning 'running, flowing, happening': *concurrent, excurrent, intercurrent.*

**current of injury.** See **demarcation current.**

**Current Procedural Terminology (CPT),** a system developed by the American Medical Association for standardizing the terminology and coding used to describe medical services and procedures. See also **CPT codes.**

**current validity.** See **validity.**

**curriculum vitae (CV)** /kərik'ələm wē'tī, vē'tē/, *pl.* **curricula vitae** [L, *curriculum,* course, *vita,* life], a summary of educational and professional experiences, including activities and honors, to be used in applications for employment, for biographic citations on professional meeting programs, or for related purposes. Also called **résumé, resume.**

**Curschmann's spirals** /koorsh'mon/ [Heinrich Curschmann, German physician, 1846–1910; Gk, *speira,* coil], coiled fibrils of mucus occasionally found in the sputum of persons with bronchial asthma.

**cursor** /kur'sər/, a movable indicator light on a computer monitor that shows the position for entering, modifying, or deleting data.

**curtain effect** /kur'tən/, an artifact produced when chemical processing stains are not properly squeezed from an x-ray film during development of a radiograph.

**curvature** /kur'vəchər/, a bending or curving of a line from the course of a straight line.

**curvature myopia,** a type of nearsightedness caused by

refractive errors associated with an excessive curvature of the cornea.

**curve** [L, *curvare,* to bend], (in statistics) a straight or curved line used as a graphic method of demonstrating the distribution of data collected in a study or survey.

**curve of Carus** [Karl G. Carus, German anatomist, 1789–1869], the normal axis of the pelvic outlet. Also called **circle of Carus.**

**curve of occlusion, 1.** an imaginary curved surface that is described by the incisal and occlusal surfaces of the teeth. **2.** the curve of dentition on which lie the occlusal surfaces of the teeth. See also **reverse curve.**

**curve of Spee** /shpā, spē/ [Ferdinand Graf von Spee, German embryologist, 1855–1937], the anatomic curvature of the occlusal alignment of the teeth. It begins at the tip of the lower canine, follows the buccal cusps of the natural premolars and molars, and continues to the anterior border of the mandibular ramus.

**curve of Wilson** /wil'sən/, the curvature of the cusps of the teeth as projected on the frontal plane; that of the mandibular dental arch is concave and that of the maxillary dental arch is convex.

**curvi-** [L, *curvus,* curve], prefix for terms relating to curvature.

**curvilinear** /cur'vilin'ē·ər/ [L, *curvus,* bent, *linea,* line], pertaining to a curved line.

**curvilinear trend** [L, *curvus,* bent, *linea,* line; AS, *trendan,* to turn], (in statistics) a trend in which a graphic representation of the data yields a curved line. The value of the independent variable may be expressed as a polynomial coefficient; by a more complete mathematic expression, such as a logistic curve; or by a smoothing process, as a moving average.

**cushingoid** /koosh'ingoid/ [Harvey W. Cushing, American surgeon, 1869–1939; Gk, *eidos,* form], having the habitus and facies characteristic of Cushing's disease: fat pads on the upper back and face, ruddy complexion, striae on trunk, thin legs, and excess facial hair.

**Cushing's disease** /koosh'ingz/ [Harvey W. Cushing], a metabolic disorder characterized by abnormally increased secretion of adrenocortical steroids, particularly cortisol, caused by increased amounts of adrenocorticotropic hormone (ACTH) secreted by the pituitary, such as by a pituitary adenoma. Excess adrenocortical hormones result in accumulations of fat on the abdomen chest, upper back, and face and occurrence of edema, hyperglycemia, increased gluconeogenesis, muscle weakness, purplish striae on the skin, decreased immunity to infection, osteoporosis with susceptibility to bone fractures, acne, and facial hair growth in women. Diabetes mellitus may become a chronic condition. Therapy is aimed at removal or destruction of ACTH secreting tissue, most commonly by surgical or radiologic procedures. The adrenal glands may be totally or subtotally removed and pharmacologic preparations of adrenal steroids are administered. Also called **hyperadrenalism.** Compare **Cushing's syndrome.**

**Cushing's syndrome** [Harvey W. Cushing], a metabolic disorder resulting from the chronic and excessive production of cortisol by the adrenal cortex or by the administration of glucocorticoids in large doses for several weeks or longer. When occurring spontaneously, the syndrome represents a failure in the body's ability to regulate the secretion of cortisol or adrenocorticotropic hormone (ACTH). (Normally cortisol is produced only in response to ACTH, and ACTH is not secreted in the presence of high levels of cortisol.) The most common cause of the syndrome is a pitu-

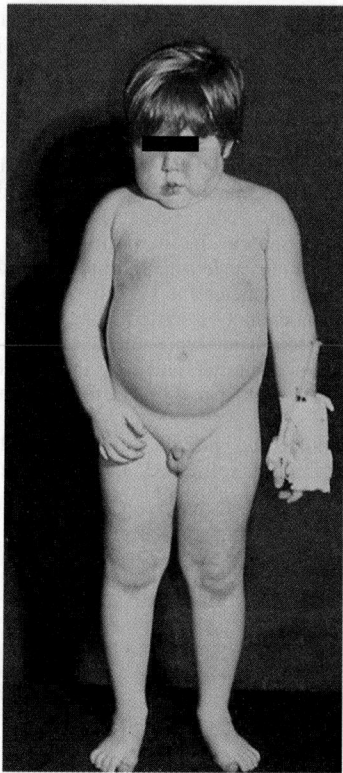

**Cushing's syndrome** *(Zitelli and Davis, 1997)*

itary tumor that increases secretion of ACTH. Also called **hyperadrenocorticism.** See also **Addison's disease, Cushing's disease, Nelson's syndrome.**

■ OBSERVATIONS: Characteristically the patient with Cushing's syndrome has a decreased glucose tolerance; central obesity; round "moon" face; supraclavicular fat pads; an overhanging, striae-covered pad of fat on the chest and abdomen; buffalo hump; scant menstrual periods or decreased testosterone levels; muscular atrophy; edema; hypokalemia; and some degree of emotional change. The skin may be abnormally pigmented and fragile; minor infections may become systemic and long-lasting. Children with the disorder may stop growing. Hypertension, kidney stones, and psychosis may also occur.

■ INTERVENTIONS: The objective of all treatment is decreased cortisol secretion. The source of the excess ACTH is discovered by a series of tests that challenge the function of the adrenal and pituitary glands. If the excess ACTH is caused by an adenoma of the anterior pituitary, irradiation or surgical excision of the tumor corrects the condition. If the condition is the result of medication, decreasing or changing the dosage may alleviate the symptoms.

■ NURSING CONSIDERATIONS: In caring for children the nurse normally observes height and weight, because rapidly developing obesity and failure to grow are suggestive of Cushing's syndrome. Some medications used for some forms of the condition may cause nausea and anorexia, somnolence, and lethargy; the patient is informed of this possibility. Nursing care of the hospitalized patient with Cushing's syndrome is similar to that of patients with Addison's disease,

Cushing's disease, and other endocrinologic disorders. Weight and electrolyte and fluid balance are monitored; an adequate balanced diet is urged; and emotional changes are observed with a goal of maintaining emotional equilibrium.

**cushion** [OFr, *coissin*], any anatomic structure that resembles a pad or pillow.

**cusp** [L, *cuspis,* point], **1.** a sharp projection or a rounded eminence that rises from the chewing surface of a tooth, such as the two pyramidal cusps that arise from the premolars. **2.** any one of the small flaps on the valves of the heart, as the ventral, dorsal, and medial cusps attached to the right atrioventricular valve.

**cuspid** /kus′pid/ [L, *cuspis,* point], a tooth with one cusp, or point; a canine tooth. Also called **unicuspid.**

**cuspless tooth** /kusp′les/, a tooth without cusps, or prominences, on its occlusal surface, possibly as a result of attrition.

**custodial care** /kəstō′dē·əl/ [L, *custodia,* guarding, *garrire,* to chatter], services and care of a nonmedical nature provided on a long-term basis, usually for convalescent and chronically ill individuals. Kinds of custodial care include **board, room,** and **personal assistance.**

**customary and reasonable charge,** (in the United States) a fee usually established by health insurance or government agencies that is considered to be the "usual" cost of a specific medical service. The fee is commonly based on the amount the company or agency will pay for that service and may vary with geographic area.

**cut,** a split in both strands of a DNA molecule. See also **nick.**

**cut-,** prefix meaning 'skin': *cutaneous, cuticle, cuticularization.*

**cutaneous** /kyo͞otā′nē·əs/ [L, *cutis,* skin], pertaining to the skin.

**cutaneous absorption,** the taking up of substances through the skin.

**cutaneous anaphylaxis,** a localized hypersensitivity reaction in the form of a wheal and flare. It occurs in sensitized individuals when, as a test of sensitivity to various allergens, an antigen injected into the skin. See also **antiserum anaphylaxis.**

**cutaneous horn,** a hard, skin-colored projection of the epidermis, usually on the head or face.

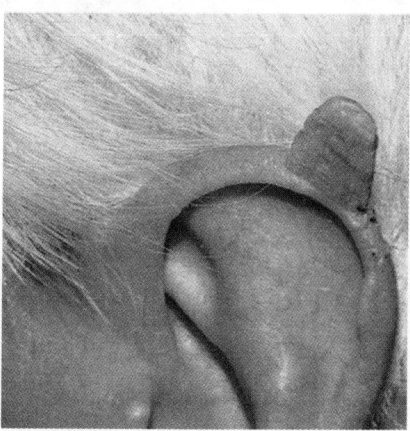

**Cutaneous horn** *(du Vivier, 1993/courtesy St Mary's Hospital)*

**cutaneous larva migrans,** a skin condition caused by a hookworm, *Ancylostoma braziliense,* a parasite of cats and dogs. Its ova are deposited in the ground with the feces of infected animals, develop into larvae, and invade the skin of people, particularly bare feet, although any skin may be involved. The larvae rarely develop into adult hookworms in the human body, but as they migrate through the epidermis, a trail of inflammation follows the burrow, causing severe pruritus. Secondary infections often occur if the skin has been broken by scratching. Topical application of a solution of thiabendazole usually eradicates the larvae. Also called **creeping eruption.**

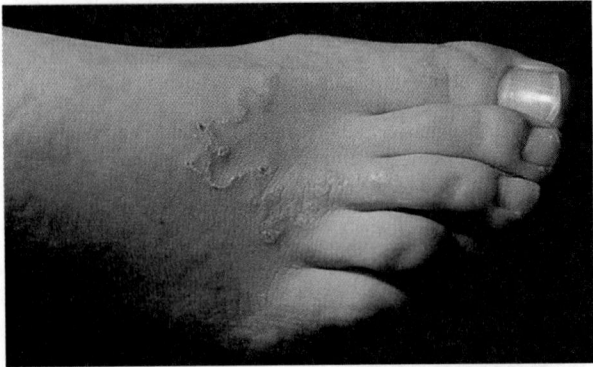

**Cutaneous larva migrans** *(Beeching and Nye, 1994)*

**cutaneous leishmaniasis.** See **oriental sore.**
**cutaneous lupus erythematosus.** See **discoid lupus erythematosus.**
**cutaneous membrane.** See **skin.**
**cutaneous nerve,** any mixed peripheral nerve that supplies a region of the skin.
**cutaneous nevus** [L, *cutis,* skin, *naevus,* birthmark], a congenital discoloration of a skin area, such as a strawberry birthmark.
**cutaneous papilloma,** a small brown or flesh-colored outgrowth of skin, occurring most frequently on the neck of an older person. Also called **cutaneous tag, skin tag.**

**cutaneous sensation** [L, *cutis,* skin, *sentire,* to feel], a sensation experienced in or arising from receptors of the skin.
**cutaneous stimulation,** a nursing intervention from the Nursing Interventions Classification (NIC) defined as stimulation of the skin and underlying tissues for the purpose of decreasing undesirable signs and symptoms such as pain, muscle spasm, or inflammation. See also **Nursing Interventions Classification.**
**cutaneous tag.** See **cutaneous papilloma.**
**cutdown** [ME, *cutten + doun*], an incision into a vein and the insertion of a catheter for IV infusion. It is performed when an infusion cannot be started by venipuncture for total parenteral nutrition. The skin is cleansed before the procedure; the incision is sutured, and a sterile dressing is applied at its conclusion. See also **hyperalimentation, venipuncture.**
**cuticle** /kyo͞o′təkəl/ [L, *cuticula,* little skin], **1.** epidermis. **2.** the sheath of a hair follicle. **3.** the thin edge of cornified epithelium at the base of a nail.

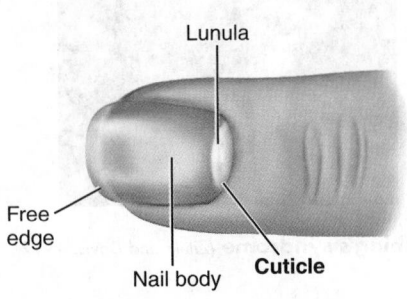

**Cuticle** *(Herlihy and Maebius, 2000)*

**cuticula** /kyo͞otik′yələ/, the cuticle, a narrow region of epidermis that covers the proximal surface of a fingernail or toenail.
**cutis.** See **skin.**
**cutis laxa** /kyo͞o′təs/ [L, skin, *laxus,* loose], abnormally loose, relaxed skin resulting from an absence of elastic fibers in the skin, usually a hereditary condition.

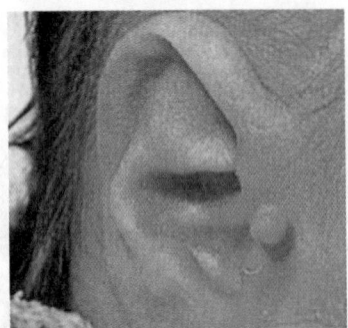

**Cutaneous papilloma**
*(Zitelli and Davis, 1997/courtesy Dr. Christine L. Williams, New York Medical College)*

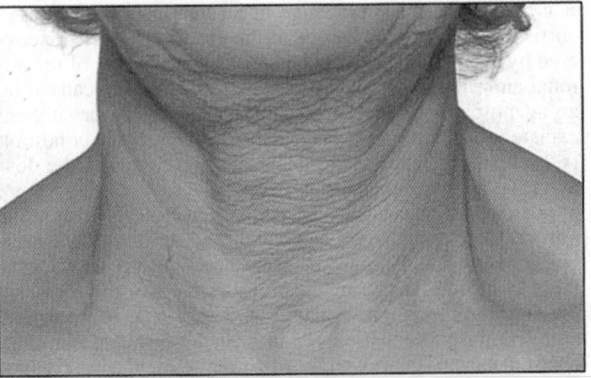

**Cutis laxa** *(Lawrence and Cox, 1993)*

**cutis marmorata,** skin that has a "marbled" appearance caused by conspicuous dilation of small vessels. See **livedo.**

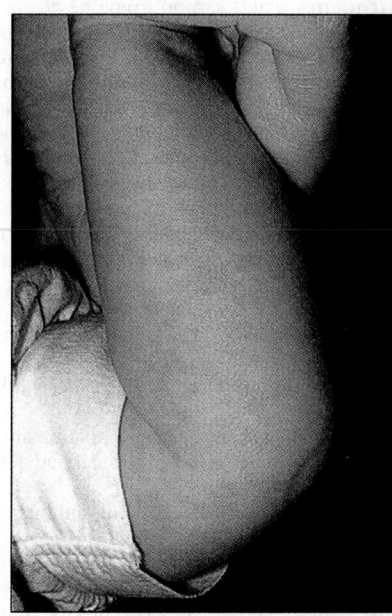

**Cutis marmorata (physiologic)**
*(Lawrence and Cox, 1993)*

**cutting oil dermatitis,** a skin disorder that affects machinists and others who use cutting oils as coolants and lubricants. Exposure to the oil obstructs hair follicles, sweat ducts, and sebaceous glands, leading to development of comedones and folliculitis; sometimes there are secondary infections complicated by minute metal particles in the oil.

**cuvette** /kyo͞ovet′/ [Fr, *cuva,* tub], a small transparent tube or container with specific optical properties. The chemical composition of the container determines the vessel's use, such as Pyrex glass for examining materials in the visible spectrum or silica for those in the ultraviolet range. It is used in laboratory research and analyses, such as photometric evaluations, colorimetric determinations, and turbidity studies.

**CVA,** **1.** abbreviation for **cerebrovascular accident.** **2.** abbreviation for **costovertebral angle.**

**CVB,** abbreviation for **chorionic villus biopsy.**

**CVID,** abbreviation for **common variable immunodeficiency.**

**CVP,** **1.** abbreviation for **central venous pressure. 2.** an anticancer drug combination of cyclophosphamide, vincristine, and prednisone.

**CVP monitor.** See **central venous pressure (CVP) monitor.**

**CW,** abbreviation for **continuous wave.**

**cyan-.** See **cyano-.**

**cyanide poisoning** /sī′ənid, -nīd/ [Gk, *kyanos,* blue], poisoning resulting from the ingestion or inhalation of cyanide from such substances as bitter almond oil, wild cherry syrup, prussic acid, hydrocyanic acid, or potassium or sodium cyanide. Characterized by tachycardia, drowsiness, seizures, headache, apnea, and cardiac arrest, it may cause death within 1 to 15 minutes.

**cyano-, cyan-,** combining form meaning 'blue': *cyanochroia, cyanocrystallin, cyanodermia.*

**cyanobacteria** /sī′ə·nō·bak·tir;′ē·ə/ [Gk, *kyanos,* blue + *bacterion,* small staff], the blue-green bacteria, unicellular or filamentous organisms that fix both carbon dioxide (in the presence of light) and nitrogen. Several species are common causes of water pollution and cause cyanobacteria poisoning. Formerly called **blue-green algae.**

**cyanobacteria poisoning,** poisoning by cyanobacteria, usually as a result of drinking contaminated water. In most cases it is a subacute condition characterized by liver damage with jaundice and sometimes bloody diarrhea and photosensitization. Drinking of heavily contaminated water may cause acute symptoms including muscle tremors, ataxia, dyspnea, cyanosis, and hyperesthesia so that a slight touch may cause convulsions and opisthotonos, which can be fatal. Also called **blue-green algae poisoning.**

**cyanocobalamin** /sī′ənōkōbal′əmin/ [Gk, *kyanos* + Ger, *kobald,* mine goblin], a red crystalline, water-soluble substance that is the common pharmaceutic form of vitamin $B_{12}$. It is involved in the metabolism of protein, fats, and carbohydrates; normal blood formation; and neural function. It is the first substance containing cobalt that is found to be vital to life. It cannot be produced synthetically but can be obtained from cultures of *Streptomyces griseus.* Rich dietary sources are liver, kidney, meats, fish, and dairy products. Deficiency can be caused by the absence of intrinsic factor (produced in the stomach), which is necessary for the absorption of cyanocobalamin from the GI tract. Deficiency can also occur in persons whose diet is strictly vegetarian, thereby excluding meat and dairy sources of the nutrient. Symptoms of deficiency include nervousness, neuritis, numbness and tingling in the hands and feet, poor muscular coordination, and menstrual disturbances. Cyanocobalamin (via injection) is used in the prophylaxis and treatment of pernicious anemia, tropical and nontropical sprue, and other macrocytic and megaloblastic anemias. It is relatively nontoxic, even when administered in amounts greater than those recommended for therapeutic purposes. Also called **antipernicious anemia factor, vitamin $B_{12}$.** See also **intrinsic factor, pernicious anemia.**

**cyanogenic glycosides** /sī′ənōjənet′ik/, chemical compounds contained in foods that release hydrogen cyanide when chewed or digested. The act of chewing or digestion disrupts the structure of the substances, causing cyanide to be released. Cyanogenetic glycosides are present in apples, apricots, cherries, peaches, plums, and quinces, particularly in the seeds of such fruits. The chemicals are also found in almonds, sorghum, lima beans, cassava, corn, yams, chickpeas, cashews, and kirsch. Although human poisoning by cyanogenetic glycosides is rare, cases of cyanide poisoning by certain varieties of lima beans, cassava, and bitter almonds have been reported.

**cyanomethemoglobin** /sī′ənō′met·hē′məglō′bin/ [Gk, *kyanos* + *meta,* together with, *haima,* blood; L, *globus,* ball], a hemoglobin derivative formed during nitrite therapy for cyanide poisoning.

**cyanopsia** /sī′ənop′sē·ə/, a visual condition in which everything appears to have a blue tint.

**cyanosed** /sī′ənōst/, having a bluish discoloration of the skin, fingernails, and mucous membranes caused by a deficiency of oxygen in the blood. Also called **cyanotic.**

**cyanosis** /sī′ənō′sis/ [Gk, *kyanos,* blue, *osis,* condition], bluish discoloration of the skin and mucous membranes caused by an excess of deoxygenated hemoglobin in the blood or a structural defect in the hemoglobin molecule, such as in methemoglobin. —**cyanotic,** *adj.*

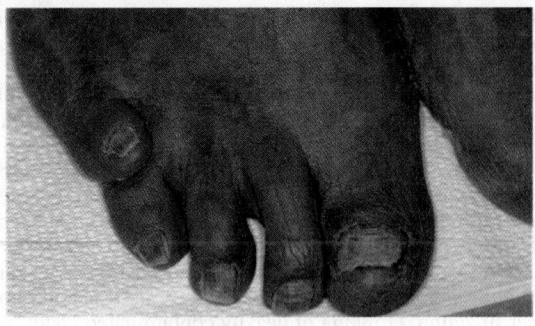

**Cyanosis** *(Lemmi and Lemmi, 2000)*

**cyanotic congenital defect** /sī'ənot'ik/, an inborn heart defect that allows the mixing of unsaturated (venous) blood with saturated (arterial) blood to produce cyanosis.

**cyberknife** /sī'bənīf/, an automated gamma radiation beam used to treat brain tumors. The beam is directed to the tumor from many different angles. The separation of the multiple low-level beams reduces potential for harm to brain tissue as the target is irradiated. The target accumulates a large dose from all the different beams.

**cybernetics** /sī'bərnet'iks/, the science of control and communication in living and nonliving systems, as in comparative study of electronic computers and the living brain.

**cycl-.** See **cyclo-**.

**cyclamate** /sī'kləmāt/, an artificial nonnutritive sweetener formerly used in the form of calcium or sodium salt.

**cyclandelate** /sīklan'dəlāt/, a peripheral vasodilator.

■ INDICATIONS: It is prescribed in the treatment of muscular ischemia and peripheral vascular obstruction or spasm.

■ CONTRAINDICATIONS: Pregnancy or known hypersensitivity to this drug prohibits its use.

■ ADVERSE EFFECTS: Tachycardia, weakness, GI distress, and flushing may occur.

**cyclarthrosis** /sī'klärthrō'sis, sik'-/, a pivot joint, capable of rotation.

**cycle** [Gk, *kyklos,* circle], a series of events that recurs at specified intervals. An example is influenza, which usually occurs in an annual cycle.

**cyclencephaly** /sīk'lənsef'əlē/ [Gk, *kyklos,* circle, *enkephalos,* brain], a developmental anomaly characterized by the fusion of the two cerebral hemispheres. —**cyclencephalic, cyclencephalous,** *adj.,* **cyclencephalus,** *n.*

**cycles per second.** See **hertz**.

**cyclic** /sik'lik, sī'klik/ [Gk, *kyklos,* circle], pertaining to or occurring in a cycle or cycles, such as a chemical compound that contains a ring of atoms in the nucleus. See also **closed-chain**.

**cyclic adenosine monophosphate (cAMP)** /sik'lik, sī'-klik/, a cyclic nucleotide formed from adenosine triphosphate by the action of adenyl cyclase. This cyclic compound, known as the "second messenger," participates in the action of catecholamines, vasopressin, adrenocorticotropic hormone, and many other hormones. Also called **cyclic AMP, adenosine 3′, 5′-cyclic phosphate.**

**cyclic guanosine monophosphate (cGMP),** a substance that mediates the action of certain hormones in a manner similar to that of cyclic adenosine monophosphate (cAMP). In response to the stimulation of cholinergic receptors in a parasympathetic nerve, guanylate cyclase triggers the con-

version of guanosine triphosphate (GTP) to cGMP with the release of various enzymes. Atropine, an anticholinergic drug, can block cholinergic stimulation by means of this process.

**cyclic neutropenia** /sik'lik nōō'trō·pē'nē·ə/, a chronic type of neutropenia that abates and recurs, accompanied by malaise, fever, stomatitis, and various types of infections.

**cyclic phosphate.** See **cyclic adenosine monophosphate**.

**cyclic vomiting,** periodic episodes of vomiting associated with migraine and usually accompanied by headaches and symptoms of ketosis. The episodes may begin in childhood.

**cyclin** /sī'klin/, one of a class of intracellular proteins that appear during the eukaryotic cell cycle. The cyclin concentration increases during the cycle until halfway to the mitosis stage, when it drops to zero. Cyclin may act as a molecular switch that activates mitosis when its concentration reaches a certain point.

**cyclin-dependent kinase (CDK),** a protein kinase that is activated by cyclin.

**-cycline,** suffix designating a tetracycline-derivative antibiotic.

**cyclitis** /siklī'tis/ [Gk, *kyklos + itis*], inflammation of the ciliary body that causes redness of the sclera adjacent to the cornea of the eye.

**cyclizine hydrochloride** /sī'klizēn/, an antihistamine and antiemetic/antivertigo agent.

■ INDICATION: It is prescribed in the treatment or prevention of motion sickness or vertigo.

■ CONTRAINDICATIONS: Known hypersensitivity to this drug prohibits its use. It is not given to newborns or lactating mothers.

■ ADVERSE EFFECTS: Among the more serious adverse reactions are skin rash, hypersensitivity reactions, and tachycardia. Drowsiness and dryness of the mouth occur commonly.

**cyclo-, cycl-,** combining form meaning 'round, recurring,' often with reference to the eye: *cyclodialysis, cycloid, cyclops.*

**cyclobenzaprine hydrochloride** /sī'kləben'zəprēn/, a muscle relaxant.

■ INDICATION: It is prescribed in the short-term treatment of muscle spasm.

■ CONTRAINDICATIONS: Hyperthyroidism, cardiac arrhythmia, cardiac failure, concomitant use of a monoamine oxidase inhibitor, or known hypersensitivity to this drug prohibits its use. It is used with caution in conditions in which anticholinergics are contraindicated.

■ ADVERSE EFFECTS: The most serious adverse effects are hypersensitivity reactions. Drowsiness, dry mouth, and dizziness commonly occur.

**cyclocephaly.** See **cyclopia**.

**Cyclocort,** trademark for a glucocorticoid (amcinonide).

**cyclodestruction** /sī'klədistruk'shən/, (in ophthalmology) a procedure to damage the ciliary body in order to diminish the production of aqueous fluid in the treatment of glaucoma, usually done by cryotherapy.

**cyclodialysis** /-dī·al'isis/, a surgical procedure performed on patients with glaucoma. A pathway is opened between the anterior chamber of the eye and the suprachoroidal space, allowing excess fluid to drain and reducing intraocular pressure.

**cycloduction** /-duk'shən/, (in ophthalmology) the range of rotation of an eye around its visual axis, which allows binocular single vision to be maintained.

**cycloid** /sī'kloid/ [Gk, *kyklos,* circle + *eidos,* form], characterized by alternating moods of elation and depression. The terms cycloid, cyclothymic, and manic-depressive overlap in meaning, although cycloid would generally be used for the least severe, and manic-depressive for the most severe conditions.

**Cyclopar,** trademark for a broad-spectrum antibiotic (tetracycline).

**cyclophosphamide** /-fos′fəmīd/, an alkylating agent.

■ INDICATIONS: It is prescribed in the treatment of neoplasms and as an immunosuppressant in organ transplantation.

■ CONTRAINDICATIONS: This drug is teratogenic in animals. It is not used during pregnancy; adequate methods of contraception should be considered for both males and females who are using it. It is used neither in patients with known hypersensitivity to the drug nor in patients with severely depressed bone marrow function. It is used with caution with impaired renal or hepatic function or with various blood disorders.

■ ADVERSE EFFECTS: Among the more serious adverse reactions are anorexia, vomiting, alopecia, leukopenia, cardiotoxicity, thrombocytopenia, and potentially serious hemorrhagic cystitis.

**cyclopia** /sīklō′pē·ə/ [Gk, *Cyclops,* mythic one-eyed giant], a developmental anomaly characterized by fusion of the orbits into a single cavity containing one eye. The condition is usually combined with various other head and facial defects. Also called **cyclocephaly, synophthalmia. —cyclops,** *n.*

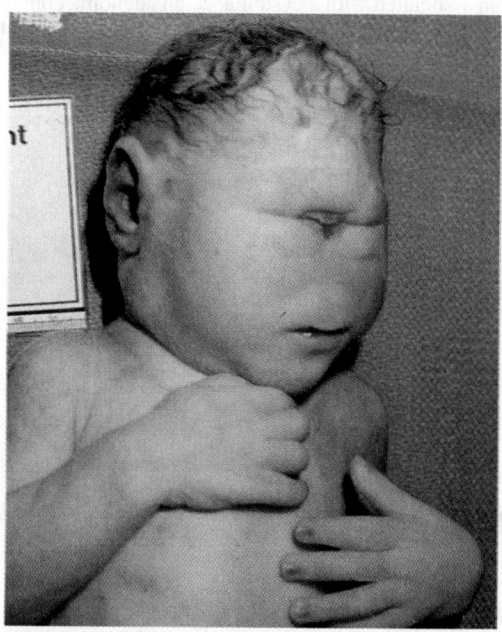

**Cyclopia in a neonate with absence of a proboscis.**
*(Moore, 2000/courtesy Dr. A.E. Chudley, Department of Pediatrics and Child Health, University of Manitoba, Children's Hospital, Winnipeg, Canada)*

**cycloplegia** /sī′kləplē′jə/ [Gk, *kyklos* + *plege,* stroke], paralysis of the ciliary muscles, as induced by certain ophthalmic drugs to allow examination of the eye. See also **cycloplegic.**

**cycloplegic** /sī′kləplē′jik/, **1.** pertaining to a drug or treatment that causes paralysis of the ciliary muscles of the eye. **2.** one of a group of anticholinergic drugs used to paralyze the ciliary muscles of the eye for ophthalmologic examina-

tion or surgery. Any of the cycloplegics may cause adverse effects in persons sensitive to anticholinergics.

**cyclopropane** /sī′klōprō′pān/, an explosive anesthetic gas. It has been replaced by the nonflammable halogenated hydrocarbons and is no longer used in the United States.

**cyclops.** See **cyclopia.**

**cycloserine** /sī′klōser′ēn/, an antibiotic.

■ INDICATIONS: It is prescribed in the treatment of active pulmonary and extrapulmonary tuberculosis.

■ CONTRAINDICATIONS: Epilepsy, depression, severe anxiety, psychosis, severe renal insufficiency, excessive concurrent use of alcohol, or known hypersensitivity to this drug prohibits its use.

■ ADVERSE EFFECTS: Among the most serious reactions are central nervous system toxic effects, including tremor, drowsiness, convulsions, and psychotic changes. Other side effects include arrhythmias and optic neuritis.

**Cyclospora cayetanensis,** a pathogenic protozoon that causes diarrhea, cramps, and fever in humans. The microorganism, a coccidian parasite about 0.01 mm in diameter, was identified in 1979, after the first known cases of the infection were diagnosed. Before 1996 only three outbreaks of *Cyclospora* infection had been reported in the United States. In May and June 1996, several hundred laboratory-confirmed cases were reported in 10 states and in Ontario, Canada. Although *Cyclospora* is transmitted by the fecaloral route, person-to-person transmission is unlikely because oocytes require days to weeks under favorable conditions to become infectious after leaving an infected host.

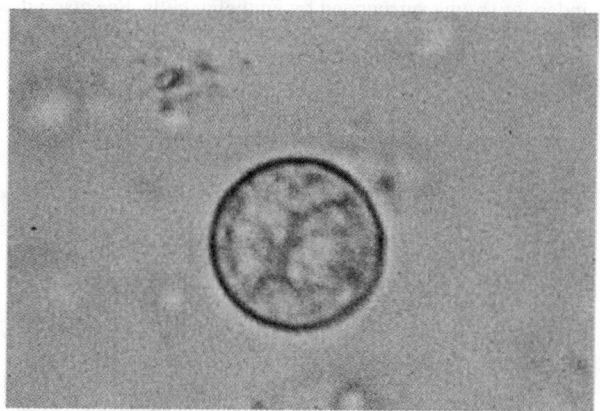

**Cyclospora cayetanensis oocyst**
*(Mahon and Manuselis, 2000)*

**cyclosporin** /-spôr′ēn/, an alternative term for cyclosporin A.

**cyclosporine** /-spôr′in/, any of a group of biologically active metabolites of *Tolypocladium inflatum Gams* and certain other fungi. Nine have been identified and are designated cyclosporin A through I. The major forms are cyclosporin A and C, which are cyclic oligopeptides with immunosuppressive, antifungal, and antipyretic effects. As immunosuppressants, cyclosporins primarily affect T lymphocytes. They are widely used in organ transplantation to suppress rejection. Also spelled **ciclosporin.**

**cyclothymic disorder** /-thīm′ik/ [Gk, *kyklos* + *thymos,* mind], a disorder of mood, wherein the essential feature is a chronic mood disturbance of at least 2 years' duration, involving numerous periods of depression and hypomania, but not of sufficient severity and duration to meet the criteria for a major depressive or manic episode. See also **bipolar disorder, depression, dysthymic disorder.**

**cyclothymic personality,**   a personality characterized by swings in mood from elation to depression.

**cyclotomy** /sīklot'əmē/,   a surgical procedure for the correction of a defect in the ciliary muscle of the eye.

**cyclotron** /sī'klətron/ [Gk, *kyklos + electron,* amber],   a device used to accelerate charged particles or ions. The particles bombard targets where they create radioactive species, which can be used as radiopharmaceuticals or to make neutrons for radiotherapy.

**cyclotropia** /sī'klōtrō'pe·ə/,   (in ophthalmology) a condition in which the ocular position of one eye is rotated around its axis with respect to the other eye.

**cyesis** /sī·ē'sis/ [Gk, *kyesis,* pregnancy],   pregnancy.

**Cylert,**   trademark for a central nervous system stimulant (pemoline).

**cylinder,**   a solid body having a circular transverse section. Exceptions include hollow gas cylinders, crossed cylinders used to measure astigmatism, and terminal cylinders of sensory nerve fibers.

**cylindrical grasp** /silin'drikəl/,   the normal position of the hand and fingers when holding cylindrical objects, such as a glass tumbler, railing, or pot handle. The fingers close and flex around the object, which is stabilized against the palm of the hand. It occurs as a reflex action in infants and later develops into a voluntary gross grasp.

**cylindroma** /sil'indrō'mə/, *pl.* **cylindromas, cylindromata** [Gk, *kylindros,* cylinder],   a tumor that appears to have cylinders of stroma surrounded by epithelial cells. See also **adenocystic carcinoma.**

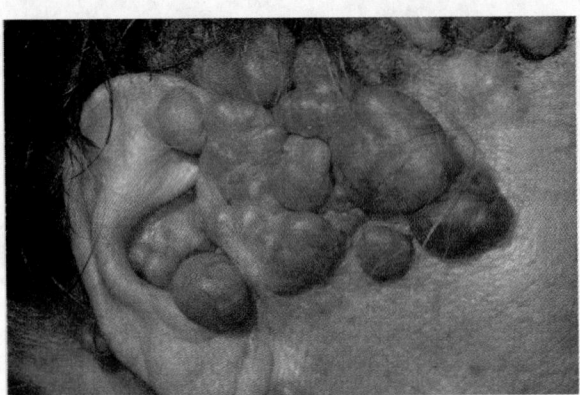

**Cylindroma** *(Hordinsky, Sawaya, and Scher, 2000)*

**cylindromatous spiradenoma.**   See **cylindroma.**

**cyma line** /sī'mə/,   an S-shaped line seen on radiographs at the articulation of the talonavicular and calcaneocuboid bones of the foot. An abnormality in the joint, including pronation or supination of the talar head, appears as a broken cyma line on radiographs.

**cyno-, cyn-,**   combining form meaning 'dog, doglike': *cynobax, cynocephalic, cynophobia.*

**cypionate** /sī'pyōnāt/,   contraction of *cyclopentanepropionate.*

**cyproheptadine hydrochloride** /sī'prōhep'tədēn/,   an antihistamine.

■ INDICATIONS: It is prescribed in the treatment of hypersensitivity reactions, including rhinitis, skin rash, and pruritus.

■ CONTRAINDICATIONS: Asthma or known hypersensitivity to this drug prohibits its use. It is not given to newborns or lactating mothers.

■ ADVERSE EFFECTS: Among the more serious adverse reactions are skin rash, hypersensitivity, and tachycardia. Drowsiness and dry mouth commonly occur.

**Cyprus fever.**   See **brucellosis.**

**Cys,**   abbreviation for the amino acid **cysteine.**

**cyst** /sist/ [Gk, *kystis,* bag],   an uninflamed closed sac in or under the skin lined with epithelium and containing fluid or semisolid material, for example, a **sebaceous cyst.**

**cyst-.**   See **cysto-.**

**-cyst, -cystis,**   suffix meaning a 'pouch or bladder': *enterocyst, microcyst, zoocyst.*

**cystadenocarcinoma** /sis'tədē'nəkär'sinō'mə/,   a type of pancreatic tumor that evolves from a mucus cystadenoma. Clinical features include epigastric pain and a palpable abdominal mass that may also be seen by ultrasonography or computed tomographic scan. It is treated by surgical removal of the tumor or total pancreatectomy.

**cystadenoma** /sis'tədinō'mə/, *pl.* **cystadenomas, cystadenomata** [Gk, *kystis + aden,* gland, *oma,* tumor],   **1.** an adenoma associated with a cystoma. **2.** an adenoma containing multiple cystic structures. The cysts may be serous, containing serum, or pseudomucinous, containing clear serous fluid or thick, viscid fluid.

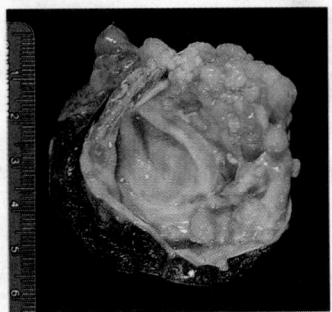

**Serous cystadenoma** *(Kumar, Cotran, and Robbins, 1997)*

**Cystagon,**   trademark for a product (cysteamine bitartrate) used in the treatment of nephropathic cystinosis, a disease in which cysteine accumulates in the cells and can lead to the formation of crystals that can damage various organs, especially the kidneys.

**cystathioninemia** /sis'təthī'əninē'mē·ə/,   an inherited metabolic disorder caused by a deficiency of the enzyme cystathionase that causes an excess of the amino acid methionine. Some patients may be asymptomatic, whereas others show signs of mental retardation. It is treated with large doses of pyridoxine (vitamin $B_6$).

**cysteamine bitartrate,**   a urinary tract product for treatment of kidney disease.

■ INDICATIONS: It is prescribed in the treatment of an inherited amino acid metabolic disease affecting the kidneys.

■ CONTRAINDICATIONS: The drug should not be given to patients with allergy to cysteamine or penicillamine, depression, drowsiness, lethargy, neurologic disorders, or diseases of the liver or digestive tract.

■ ADVERSE EFFECTS: The side effects most often reported include vomiting, diarrhea, constipation, appetite loss, nausea, headaches, convulsions, and seizures.

**cystectomy** /sistek'təmē/ [Gk, *kystis* + *ektomē,* excision], a surgical procedure in which all or a part of the urinary bladder is removed, as may be required in treating bladder cancer.

**cysteine (Cys)** /sis'tēn/, an amino acid found in many proteins in the body, including keratin. It is a metabolic precursor of cystine and an important source of sulfur for various body functions. Compare **cystine.**

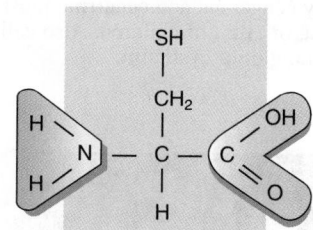

**Chemical structure of cysteine**

**cysti-.** See **cysto-.**

**cystic** /sis'tik/ [Gk, *kystis,* bag], **1.** pertaining to a cyst. **2.** pertaining to a fluid-filled sac, such as the gallbladder or urinary bladder.

**cystic acne.** See **acne conglobata.**

**cystic bile,** concentrated bile stored in the gallbladder.

**cystic carcinoma,** a malignant neoplasm containing closed cavities or saclike spaces. These tumors may occur in the breast and ovary.

**cystic duct,** the duct through which bile from the gallbladder passes into the common bile duct.

**cystic emphysema.** See **bullous emphysema.**

**cysticercosis** /sis'tisərkō'sis/ [Gk, *kystis* + *kerkos,* tail, *osis,* condition], an infection and infestation by the larval stage of the pork tapeworm *Taenia solium* or the beef tapeworm *T. saginata.* The eggs are ingested and hatch in the intestine; the larvae invade the subcutaneous tissue, brain, eye, muscle, heart, liver, lung, and peritoneum. They attach themselves with two rows of hooklets, grow, mature, and become covered with a dense, fibrous capsule. The invasive, early phase of the infection is characterized by fever, malaise, muscle pain, and eosinophilia. Years later seizures and personality change may appear if the brain is affected, and calcification and destruction of local structures are apparent in other infested areas of the body. Prophylaxis depends on eating only thoroughly cooked pork or beef.

**cysticercus** /sis'tisur'kəs/, a larval form of tapeworm. It consists of a single scolex enclosed in a bladderlike cyst.

**cystic fibroma,** a fibrous tumor in which cystic degeneration has occurred.

**cystic fibrosis,** an inherited autosomal-recessive disorder of the exocrine glands, causing those glands to produce abnormally thick secretions of mucus, elevation of sweat electrolytes, increased organic and enzymatic constituents of saliva, and overactivity of the autonomic nervous system. The glands most affected are those in the pancreas and respira-

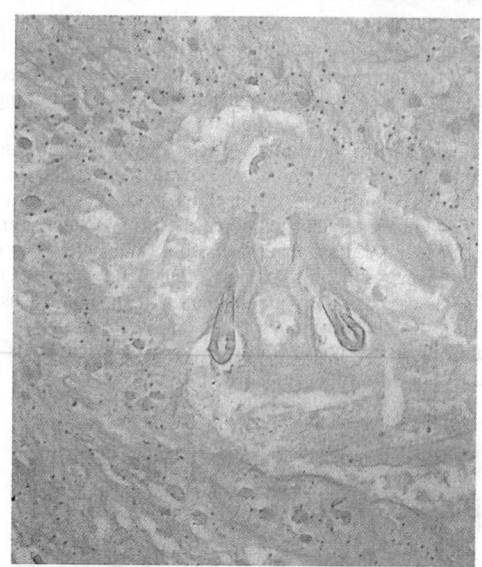

**Cysticercosis** *(Farrar, 1993)*

tory system and the sweat glands. Cystic fibrosis is usually recognized in infancy or early childhood, chiefly among Caucasians. The earliest manifestation is meconium ileus, an obstruction of the small bowel by viscid stool. Other early signs are a chronic cough; frequent, foul-smelling stools; and persistent upper respiratory infections. The most reliable diagnostic tool is the sweat test, which shows elevations of levels of both sodium and chloride. Because there is no known cure, treatment is directed at prevention of respiratory infections, which are the most frequent cause of death. Mucolytic agents and bronchodilators are used to help liquefy the thick, tenacious mucus. Physical therapy measures, such as postural drainage and breathing exercises,

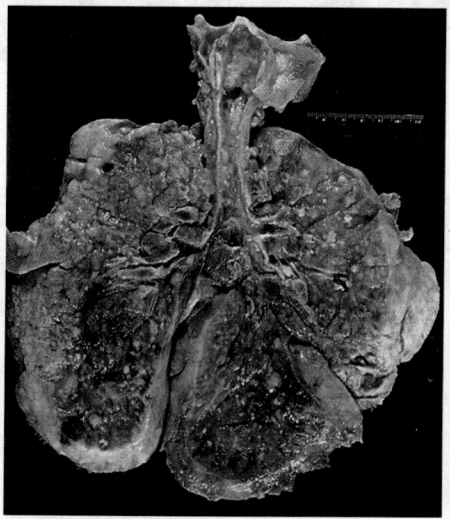

**Cystic fibrosis: lungs of a dying patient**
*(Cotran, Kumar, and Collins, 1999/courtesy Dr. Eduardo Unis, Children's Hospital of Pittsburgh)*

can also dislodge secretions. Broad-spectrum antibiotics may be used prophylactically. The nurse's role is vital in instructing the family in health promotion and in all aspects of the child's care. Particular attention is paid to teaching the child and family the use of pancreatic enzymes, equipment, food selection, prevention of infection, and techniques of expectorating sputum. The nurse can provide emotional support for the family and counsel them on community resources. Life expectancy in cystic fibrosis has improved markedly over the past several decades, and with early diagnosis and treatment most patients can be expected to reach adulthood. Surgery may be indicated for some cases that cannot be treated effectively with medications. Heart-lung and double-lung transplantation have been successful. Also called **fibrocystic disease of the pancreas, mucoviscidosis.**

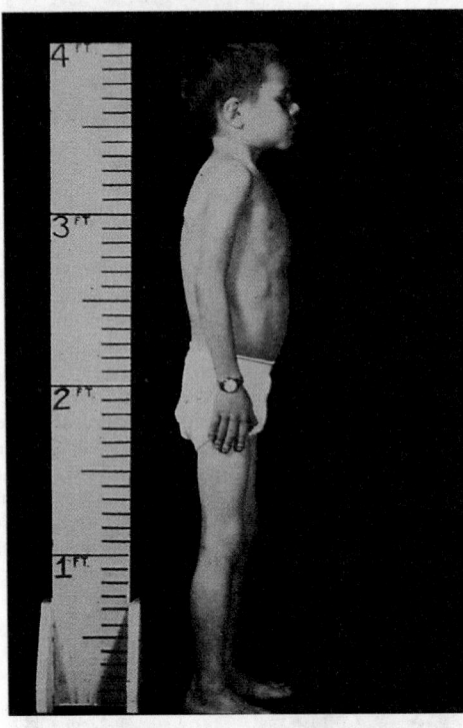

**Cystic fibrosis: poor nutritional status**
*(Zitelli and Davis, 1997)*

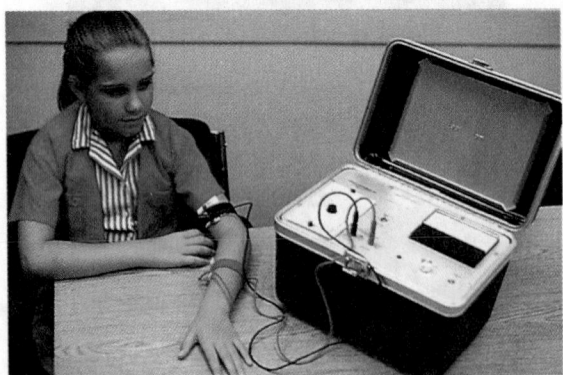

**Sweat test for cystic fibrosis** *(Wilson, 1990)*

**cystic fibrosis transmembrane conductance regulator,** an abnormal protein found in the gene for cystic fibrosis; it causes abnormal chloride channels in cell membranes of the respiratory epithelium, pancreas, salivary glands, sweat glands, intestines, and reproductive tract. Also called **cystic fibrosis transmembrane regulator, cystic fibrosis transmembrane regulator protein.**

**cystic goiter,** an enlargement of the thyroid gland containing cysts resulting from mucoid or colloid degeneration, or liquefaction.

**cystic hygroma.** See **cystic lymphangioma.**

**cystic kidney** [Gk, *kystis,* bag; ME, *kidenei*], pertaining to any of several kidney disorders in which cysts form, including congenital polycystic disease, solitary renal cysts, or cortical cysts associated with nephrosclerosis.

**cystic lymphangioma,** a cystic growth formed by lymph vessels, usually congenital and occurring most frequently in the neck, axilla, or groin of children. Also called **cystic hygroma, lymphangioma cysticum.**

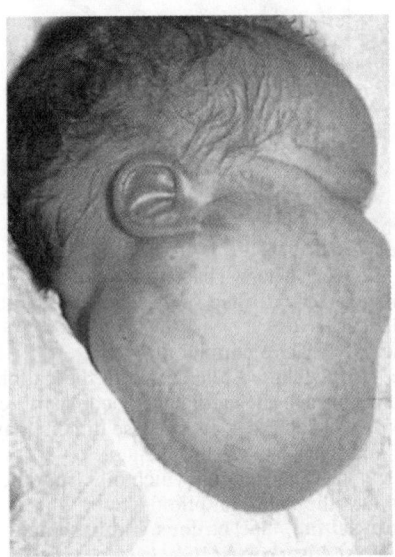

**Cystic lymphangioma** *(Greig and Garden, 1996)*

**cystic mastitis,** a form of mammary dysplasia with inflammation and the formation of nodular cysts in the breast tissue. The cysts contain a turbid fluid. Symptoms may vary with individual breast changes that occur during the menstrual cycle.

**cystic mole.** See **hydatid mole.**

**cystic myxoma,** a tumor of connective tissue that has undergone cystic degeneration.

**cystic neuroma,** a neoplasm of nerve tissue that has degenerated and become cystic. Also called **false neuroma.**

**cystic tumor,** a tumor with cavities or sacs containing a semisolid or a liquid material.

**cystido-.** See **cysto-.**

**cystine** /sis′tin/, a compound consisting of two cysteine residues joined by a disulfide linkage (S–S) linkage. Compare **cysteine (Cys).**

**cystinosis** /sis′tinō′sis/ [*cystine* + Gk, *osis,* condition], a congenital disease characterized by glucosuria; proteinuria;

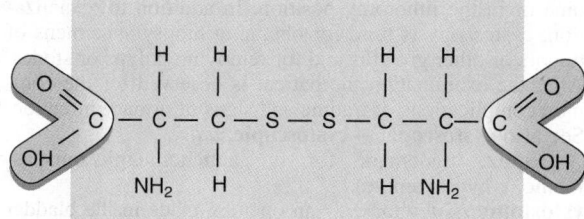

**Chemical structure of cystine**

cystine deposits in the liver, spleen, bone marrow, and cornea; rickets; excessive amounts of phosphates in the urine; and retardation of growth. Also called **cystine storage disease, Fanconi's syndrome.** See also **cystine.**

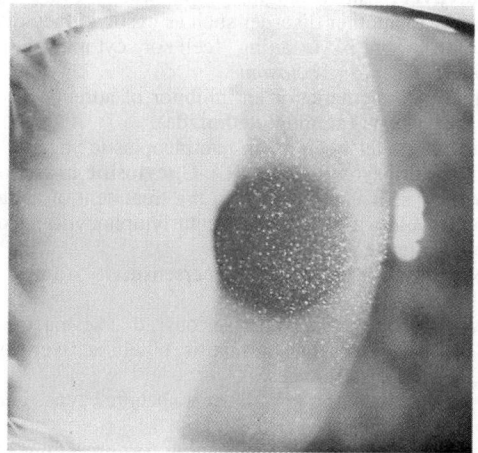

**Cystinosis: deposits of cystine crystals on the cornea**
*(Zitelli and Davis, 1997)*

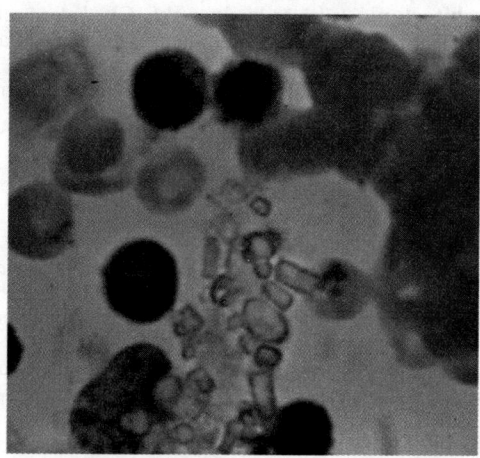

**Cystinosis: deposits of cystine crystals
in the bone marrow**
*(Zitelli and Davis, 1997)*

**cystinuria** /sis'tinŏŏr'ē·ə/ [*cystine* + Gk, *ouron,* urine], **1.** abnormal presence of the amino acid cystine in the urine collected in a 24-hour specimen. **2.** an inherited defect of the renal tubules, characterized by excessive urinary excretion of cystine and several other amino acids. The disorder is caused by an autosomal recessive trait that impairs cystine reabsorption by the kidney tubules. In high concentration cystine tends to precipitate in the urinary tract and form kidney or bladder stones. Treatment attempts to prevent the formation of stones or to dissolve them by increasing the volume of urine flow, decreasing the pH of the urine, and increasing the solubility of cystine. In addition to a large fluid intake, sodium bicarbonate, acetazolamide, and, in refractory cases, D-penicillamine are sometimes prescribed.

**-cystis.** See **-cyst.**

**cystitis** /sistī'tis/ [Gk, *kystis* + *itis,* inflammation], an inflammatory condition of the urinary bladder and ureters, characterized by pain, urgency and frequency of urination, and hematuria. It may be caused by a bacterial infection, calculus, or tumor. Depending on the diagnosis, treatment may include antibiotics, increased fluid intake, bed rest, medications to control bladder wall spasms, and, when necessary, surgery.

**-cystitis,** combining form meaning 'inflammation of the bladder or cyst': *epicystitis, gonecystitis, pericystitis.*

**cysto-, cyst-, cysti-, cystido-,** prefix meaning 'bladder, cyst, or sac': *cystocele, cystodynia, cystomyoma.*

**cystocele** /sis'təsēl'/ [Gk, *kystis* + *kele,* hernia], a herniation or protrusion of the urinary bladder through the wall of the vagina. Compare **rectocele, vesicocele.**

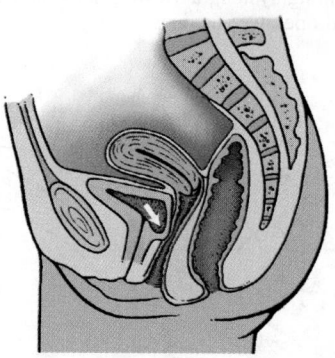

**Cystocele** *(Monahan and Neighbors, 1998)*

**cystochromoscopy** /sis'təkrōmos'kəpē/, examination of the bladder after administration of a colored dye performed as an investigation of renal function and urinary system condition. Also called **chromocystoscopy.**

**cystofibroma** /-fībrō'mə/, a fibrous tumor that contains a cyst.

**cystogram** /sis'təgram'/ [Gk, *kystis* + *gramma,* record], a radiograph produced by cystography.

**cystography** /sistog'rəfē/, the radiographic examination of the urinary bladder after introduction of a radiopaque contrast medium.

**cystoid** /sis'toid/ [Gk, *kystis,* bag + *eidos,* form], pertaining to or resembling a cyst or bladder.

**cystojejunostomy** /-ji'jōōnos'təmē/, drainage of a cyst, such as a pancreatic pseudocyst, into the jejunum.

**cystolith.** See **vesical calculus.**

**cystolithalopexy** /-lith′ələpek′sē/, removal of a kidney stone from the urinary bladder by crushing, followed by extraction of the particles via irrigation.

**cystolithotomy** /-lithot′əmē/, removal of a kidney stone from the urinary bladder following surgical opening of the bladder. Also called **cystolithectomy, vesicle lithotomy.**

**cystoma** /sistō′mə/, *pl.* **cystomas, cystomata** [Gk, *kystis* + *oma,* tumor], any tumor or growth containing cysts, especially one in or near the ovary.

**-cystoma,** combining form meaning a 'cystic tumor': *enterocystoma, hydrocystoma, inocystoma.*

**cystometer** /sistom′ətər/, an instrument that measures bladder capacity in relation to changing urine pressure.

**cystometrography (CMG)** /sis′tōmətrog′rəfē/, a urologic procedure that measures the amount of pressure exerted on the bladder at various bladder volumes. The test helps determine bladder capacity, bladder wall compliance, detrusor stability, and sensations of filling. It is often done in conjunction with electromyography and other urodynamic tests.

**cystometrogram** /sis′tōmet′rəgram′/, the graphic results of the measurements made during cystometrography.

**cystometry** /sistom′ətrē/ [Gk, *kystis* + *metron,* measure], the study of bladder function by use of a cystometer.

**cystoprostatectomy** /-pros′tətek′təmē/, surgical removal of the bladder, prostate gland, and seminal vesicle.

**cystosarcoma phyllodes** /sis′tōsärkō′mə filō′dēs/, a malignant stromal breast tumor that grows rapidly and tends to recur if not adequately excised.

**cystoscope** /sis′təskōp′/ [Gk, *kystis* + *skopein,* to look], an instrument for examining and treating lesions of the urinary tract. It consists of an obdurator for introduction, outer sheath, a lighting system, a viewing lens, and a passage for catheters and operative devices.

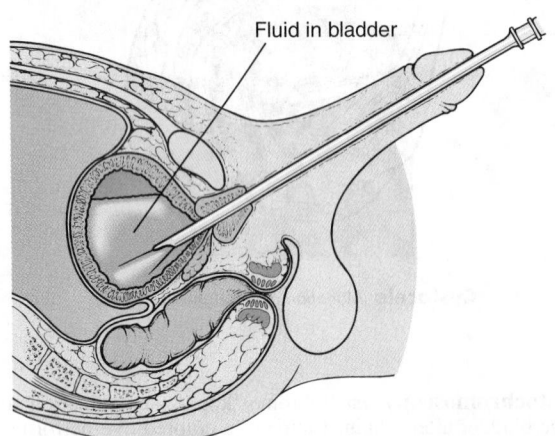
Fluid in bladder

**Cystoscope in the male bladder**
*(Phipps, Sands, and Marek, 1999)*

**cystoscopic.** See **cystoscopy.**
**cystoscopic urography.** See **retrograde cystoscopy.**
**cystoscopy** /sistos′kəpē/, the direct visualization of the urinary tract by means of a cystoscope inserted into the urethra. The procedure is usually performed with the patient in a fasting state and under sedation or local anesthesia. The bladder is distended with air or water while the patient is su-

pine or in the lithotomy position. In addition to visualization, cystoscopy is used for obtaining biopsy specimens of tumors or other growths and for removing polyps or stones. After the examination the patient is observed for the common complications of trauma and signs of urinary infection. See also **cystoscope. —cystoscopic,** *adj.*

**Cystospaz,** trademark for an anticholinergic/antispasmodic (L-hyoscyamine).

**cystostomy** /sistos′təmē/, an opening made in the bladder for drainage, usually through a catheter inserted through the abdominal skin.

**cystotomy** /sistot′əmē/, incision of the urinary bladder, often performed for removal of a calculus.

**cystoureterography** /sis′təyŏŏr′ətərog′rəfē/, the radiographic examination of the bladder and ureters after introduction of a radiopaque contrast medium.

**cystourethrogram** /sis′tə·yŏŏrē′thrəgram′/, a radiograph produced by cystourethrography.

**cystourethrography** /sis′təyŏŏr′ēthrog′rəfē/, the radiographic examination of the urethra and urinary bladder after introduction of a radiopaque contrast medium.

**cysts of liver,** small single, simple watery cysts, usually secondary to another disorder such as cystic kidney disease.

**cyt-, cyto-,** prefix meaning 'cell or cytoplasm': *cytochrome, cytogenesis, cytosome.*

**Cytadren,** trademark for an inhibitor of adrenocorticosteroid biosynthesis (aminoglutethimide).

**cytarabine** /siter′əbēn/, an antineoplastic agent. Also called **arabinosylcytosine, ARA-C, cytosine arabinoside.**
■ INDICATIONS: It is prescribed in the treatment of acute and chronic myelocytic leukemia, acute lymphocytic leukemia, and erythroleukemia.
■ CONTRAINDICATION: Known hypersensitivity to this drug prohibits its use.
■ ADVERSE EFFECTS: The most serious adverse reactions are bone marrow depression, stomatitis, phlebitis, liver toxicity, fever, and GI disturbances.

**-cyte,** suffix meaning a 'cell' of a specified type: *gliacyte, hemocyte, plasmacyte.*

**-cythemia, -cythaemia,** combining form meaning a 'condition involving cells in the blood': *achroiocythemia, rhestocythemia, thrombocythemia.*

**cyto-.** See **cyt-.**

**cytoanalyzer** /sī′tō·an′əlī′zər/, an electronic device that screens samples of smears of suspected malignancies.

**cytoarchitectonic** /sī′tō·är′kitekton′ik/ [Gk, *kytos,* cell; L, *architectura,* architecture], pertaining to the cellular arrangement within a tissue or structure.

**cytoarchitecture** /-är′kitek′chər/, the typical pattern of cellular arrangement within a particular tissue or organ, as in the cerebral cortex. —**cytoarchitectural,** *adj.*

**cytobiotactic, cytobiotaxis.** See **cytoclesis.**

**cytoblast.** See **nucleus.**

**cytocentrum.** See **centrosome.**

**cytocerastic.** See **cytokerastic.**

**cytochemism** /sī′tōkem′izəm/ [Gk, *kytos* + *chemeia,* alchemy], the chemical activity within the living cell, specifically the various reactions to and affinity for chemical substances.

**cytochemistry** /-kem′istrē/, the study of the various chemicals within a living cell and their actions and functions.

**cytochrome** /si′tōkrōm/ [Gk, *kytos,* cell, *chroma,* color], **1.** a class of hemoproteins whose function is electron transport. These proteins have the ability to reverse the valence of heme-iron compounds, alternating between ferrous and ferric states. **2.** proteins involved in mitochondrial exudative electron transport systems associated with adenosine triphosphate production.

**cytochrome-*c* oxidase,** an enzyme complex of the inner mitochondrial membrane that catalyzes the transfer of electrons from cytochrome *c* to oxygen, oxidizing cytochrome and reducing oxygen in the final step of the electron transport chain by which oxygen is used for fuel combustion.

**cytochrome-*c* oxidase deficiency,** a hereditary defect in the cytochrome-*c* oxidase complex that prevents the transfer of electrons from cytochrome *c* to molecular oxygen, ultimately halting the production of ATP. Manifestations are extremely variable and include myopathies, encephalopathies, ocular and cardiac defects, sensorineural deafness, Fanconi syndrome, diabetes mellitus, and short stature. Inheritance may be autosomal recessive, X-linked, or, possibly, maternal (mitochondrial), depending on the part of the cytochrome-*c* oxidase complex that is affected.

**cytochrome P-450** [Gk, *kytos,* cell, *chroma,* color], a protein involved with extramitochondrial electron transport in the liver and during drug detoxification.

**cytocide** [Gk, *kytos* + L, *caedere,* to kill], any substance that is destructive to cells. —**cytocidal,** *adj.*

**cytoclesis** /sī′tōklē′sis/ [Gk, *kytos* + *klesis,* calling for], the influence exerted by one cell on the action of other cells; the vital principle of all living tissue. Also called **cytobiotaxis.** —**cytocletic, cytobiotactic,** *adj.*

**cytoctony** /sītok′tənē/ [Gk, *kytos* + *ktonos,* killing], the destruction of cells in culture by viruses.

**cytode** /sī′tōd/ [Gk, *kytos* + *eidos,* form], the simplest type of cell, consisting of a protoplasmic mass without a nucleus, such as a bacterium.

**cytodendrite** /-den′drīt/. See **dendrite.**

**cytodiagnosis** /-dī′əgnō′sis/, diagnosis of a suspected pathologic tissue by a microscopic examination of the cells in the sample.

**cytodieresis** /sī′tōdī·er′isis/, *pl.* **cytodiereses** [Gk, *kytos* + *diairesis,* separation], cell division, especially the phenomena involving the division of the cytoplasm. See also **cytokinesis, meiosis, mitosis.** —**cytodieretic,** *adj.*

**cytodifferentiation** /-dif′ərən′shē·ā′shən/ [Gk, *kytos* + L, *differentia,* difference], **1.** a process by which embryonic cells acquire biochemical and morphologic properties essential for specialization and diversification. **2.** the total and gradual transformation from an undifferentiated to a fully differentiated state.

**cytofluorograph** /-flôr′əgraf/, a diagnostic instrument used to measure the level of CD4 T lymphocytes in human immunodeficiency virus–positive patients. The lymphocytes are stained with specific monoclonal antibodies.

**cytogene** /sī′təjēn/ [Gk, *kytos* + *genein,* to produce], a self-replicating particle within the cytoplasm of a cell that is derived from genes in the nucleus and is capable of transmitting hereditary information.

**cytogenesis** /sī′tōjen′əsis/ [Gk, *kytos* + *genein,* to produce], the origin, development, and differentiation of cells. —**cytogenetic, cytogenic,** *adj.*

**cytogeneticist** /sī′tōjənet′isist/, a scientist who specializes in cytogenetics.

**cytogenetics** /sī′tōjənet′iks/, the branch of genetics that studies the cellular constituents concerned with heredity, primarily the structure, function, and origin of the chromosomes. One kind of cytogenetics is **clinical cytogenetics.** Also called **cytogenics.** —**cytogenetic,** *adj.*

**cytogenic** /-jen′ik/, pertaining to the formation of cells.

**cytogenic gland,** a glandular organ that secretes living cells, specifically the testes and ovary.

**cytogenic reproduction,** the formation of a new organism from a germ cell, either sexually through the fusion of gametes to form a zygote or asexually by means of spores. Also called **cytogony.**

**cytogenics.** See **cytogenetics.**

**cytogeny** /sītoj′ənē/, **1.** cytogenetics. **2.** the origin and development of cells. —**cytogenic, cytogenous,** *adj.*

**cytogony** /sītog′ənē/. See **cytogenic reproduction.**

**cytohistogenesis** /sī′tōhis′tōjen′əsis/ [Gk, *kytos* + *histos,* tissue, *genein,* to produce], the structural development and formation of cells. —**cytohistogenetic,** *adj.*

**cytohyaloplasm.** See **hyaloplasm.**

**cytoid** /sī′toid/ [Gk, *kytos* + *eidos,* form], like a cell.

**cytoid body,** a small white spot on the retina of each eye seen by using an ophthalmoscope to examine the eyes; often noted in patients affected with systemic lupus erythematosus.

**cytokerastic** /sī′tōkəras′tik/ [Gk, *kytos* + *kerastos,* mixed], pertaining to or characteristic of cellular development from a simple to a more complex arrangement. Also spelled **cytocerastic.**

**cytokine** /sī′təkīn/, one of a large group of low-molecular-weight proteins secreted by various cell types and involved in cell-to-cell communication, coordinating antibody and T cell immune interactions, and amplifying immune reactivity. Cytokines include colony stimulating factors, interferons, interleukins, and lymphokines, which are secreted by lymphocytes.

**cytokine network,** a group of cytokines that modulate and regulate signaling between cells during immune responses. According to the immune network model, T cells and B cells mutually interact, responding to cytokines as well as antigens. This interaction allows the cytokines to direct T cells to antiviral or antitumor functions or to promote allergic reactions.

**cytokinesis** /sī′tōkinē′sis, -kīnē′sis/ [Gk, *kytos* + *kinesis,* movement], the division of the cytoplasm, exclusive of nuclear division, that occurs during the final stages of mitosis and meiosis to form daughter cells. —**cytokinetic,** *adj.*

**cytologic, cytological.** See **cytology.**

**cytologic map** [Gk, *kytos* + *logos,* science; L, *mappa,* table napkin], a graphic representation of the location of genes on a chromosome, based on correlating the genetic recombination results of testcrosses with the structural analysis of chromosomes that have undergone changes, such as deletions or translocations, as detected by banding techniques.

**cytologic sputum examination,** a microscopic examination of a specimen of bronchial secretions, including a search for cells that may be cancerous or otherwise abnormal.

**cytologist** /sītol′əjist/, a biologist who specializes in the study of cells, especially one who uses cytologic techniques in the differential diagnosis of neoplasms.

**cytology** /sītol′əjē/ [Gk, *kytos* + *logos,* science], the study of cells, including their formation, origin, structure, function, biochemical activities, and pathologic characteristics. Kinds of cytology include **aspiration biopsy cytology** and **exfoliative cytology.** Also called **cell biology.** —**cytologic, cytological,** *adj.*

**cytolymph.** See **hyaloplasm.**

**cytolyses.** See **cytolysis.**

**cytolysin** /sītol′isin/ [Gk, *kytos* + *lyein,* to loosen], an antibody that dissolves antigenic cells. Kinds of cytolysin are **bacteriolysin** and **hemolysin.**

**cytolysis** /sītol′isis/, *pl.* **cytolyses** [Gk, *kytos* + *lyein,* to loosen], the destruction or breakdown of cells, primarily by the disintegration of the plasma membrane. A kind of cytolysis is **immune cytolysis.** —**cytolytic,** *adj.*

## Cytokines

| Types | Source | Main functions |
|-------|--------|----------------|
| **Interleukins (IL)** | | |
| IL-1 (α and β) | Predominantly macrophages | ↑ Immune response; inflammatory mediator; activates T cells; activates phagocytes; ↑ |
| Il-2 (T cell growth factor) | Predominantly helper T lymphocytes; NK cells | ↑ T lymphocytes and NK cells; ↑ growth and ↑ T cells |
| IL-3 (multiple colony-stimulating factor) | T lymphocytes, mast cells, NK cells | Hematopoietic growth factor for immature hematopoietic precursor cells, ↑ NK cells |
| IL-4 (B cell growth factor) | T lymphocytes, mast cells | Growth factor for T cells, activated B cells, and mast cells; macrophage-activating factor, ↑ IgE reactions |
| Il-5 | T lymphocytes, macrophages | ↑ Growth and proliferation of activated B cells, ↑ eosinophils, ↑ T cell production |
| IL-6 | Monocytes, T and B lymphocytes, fibroblasts, endothelial cells | B cell stimulatory and differentiation factor; ↑ hematopoiesis, ↑ inflammatory response, fever |
| IL-7 | Bone marrow, thymus | ↑ Lymphoid cells |
| IL-8 (monocyte-derived neutrophil chemotactic factor | Macrophages, monocytes, endothelial cells | Triggers chemotactic activity of neutrophils and lymphocytes |
| IL-9 | Helper T cells | T cell and mast cell growth factor; maturation of erythroid progenitors |
| IL-10 | Helper T cells | ↓ Proliferation of helper T cells; ↑ cytotoxic T cell differentiation; induces MHC antigen expression, ↓ cytokines |
| IL-11 | Fibroblasts | ↑ Monocyte and B cell function, ↓ some inflammatory cytokines |
| IL-12 | Macrophages | ↑ Helper T cells and production of other lymphocytes and cytokines |
| IL-13 | Activated T cells | ↑ Gene expression in nerve and intestinal cells, ↑ osteoclasts, ↑ progenitor cells in bone marrow |
| IL-14 | T cells | B cell growth factor |
| IL-15 | Macrophages | Activity identical to that of IL-2 |
| IL-16 | CD8+ T cells | Chemotactic factor and growth factor for CD4+ T cells, chemotactic for eosinophils |
| IL-17 | Helper T cells | ↑ IL-6 and IL-8 |
| **Interferon (IFN)** | | |
| IFN-α | T and B lymphocytes, macrophages | Provides antiviral protection; ↓ B cell proliferation; ↓ IL-8, ↓ tumor growth, ↑ NK cell |
| IFN-β | Fibroblasts, macrophages, epithelial cells | Provides antiviral protection; ↑ IL-6, ↓ IL-8 |
| IFN-γ | T lymphocytes, NK cells | Activates macrophages; ↑ B cell differentiation and NK cell activity, ↓ tumor growth |
| **Tumor necrosis factor (TNF)** | | |
| TNF-α | Macrophages, lymphocytes, fibroblasts, endothelial cells | ↑ Cytokines, ↑ inflammatory and immune responses |
| TNF-β | T cells | Cytotoxic to tumor cells, ↑ phagocytosis by macrophage and neutrophil, ↑ macrophages, ↑ B cell proliferation |
| **Colony-stimulating factors (CSFs)** | | |
| G-CSF | Monocytes, fibroblasts | Myeloid growth factor |
| GM-CSF | T cells, fibroblasts, monocytes, endothelial cells | Myelocytic growth factor |
| M-CSF | Monocytes, lymphocytes, fibroblasts, endothelial and epithelial cells | Macrophage growth factor |
| **Transforming growth factor (TGF-β)** | | |
| | Lymphocytes, macrophages, platelets, bone | Chemotactic for macrophages, ↑ IL-1 production; stimulates fibroblasts for wound healing; inhibits immune response; potentially inhibits mitotic division in other cells |

From Huether SE, McCance RL: *Understanding pathophysiology,* ed 2, St Louis, 2000, Mosby.
↑, Increased; ↓, decreased; *NK,* natural killer; *MHC,* major histocompatability complex.

**cytomegalic** /sī′tōmegal′ik/, describing a condition characterized by abnormally large cells.

**cytomegalic inclusion disease (CID)** [Gk, *kytos* + *megas,* large; L, *in, claudere,* in enclosure], a viral infection caused by the cytomegalovirus (CMV), a member of the herpesvirus family. It is characterized by malaise, fever, lymphadenopathy, pneumonia, hepatosplenomegaly, and superinfection with various bacteria and fungi as a result of the depression of immune response characteristic of herpesviruses. It is primarily a congenitally acquired disease of newborns, transmitted in utero. Results may range from spontaneous abortion or fatal neonatal illness to birth of a normal infant, depending on such factors as the virulence of the viral strain, fetal age when infected, and primary or recurrent nature of the mother's infection. About 10% of newborns with congenital CMV show clinical signs, such as microcephaly, retarded growth, hepatosplenomegaly, hemolytic anemia, and pathologic fracture of long bones. In 5% to 25% of asymptomatic infections, infants develop significant psychomotor, hearing, ocular, or dental abnormalities. There is no specific treatment. See also **TORCH syndrome.**

**cytomegalovirus (CMV)** /sī′tōmeg′əlōvī′rəs/ [Gk, *kytos* + *megas,* large; L, *virus,* poison], a member of a group of large species-specific herpes-type viruses with a wide variety of disease effects. It causes serious illness in persons with human immunodeficiency virus, in newborns, and in people being treated with immunosuppressive drugs and therapy, especially after organ transplantation. The virus usually causes a retinal or GI infection. See also **cytomegalic inclusion disease, TORCH syndrome.**

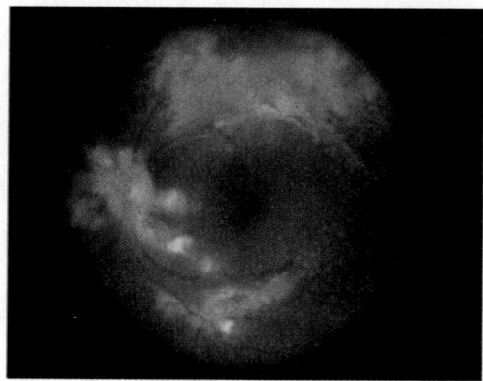

**Cytomegalovirus retinitis**
*(Seidel et al, 1999/courtesy Douglas A. Jabs, MD, The Wilmer Ophthalmological Institute, The Johns Hopkins University and Hospital, Baltimore)*

**cytomegalovirus (CMV) disease.** See **cytomegalic inclusion disease.**

**Cytomel,** trademark for a thyroid hormone (liothyronine sodium).

**cytometer** /sītom′ətər/ [Gk, *kytos* + *metron,* measure], a device for counting and measuring the number of cells within a specified amount of fluid, such as blood, urine, or cerebrospinal fluid.

**cytometry** /sītom′ətrē/, the counting and measuring of cells, specifically blood cells. —**cytometric,** *adj.*

**cytomitome** /sī′təmī′tōm/ [Gk, *kytos* + *mitos,* thread], the fibrillary network within the cytoplasm of a cell, as contrasted with that inside the nucleus. See also **karyomitome.**

**cytomorphology** /-môrfol′əjē/ [Gk, *kytos* + *morphe,* shape, *logos,* science], the study of the various forms of cells and the structures contained within cells. —**cytomorphologic, cytomorphological,** *adj.;* **cytomorphologist,** *n.*

**cytomorphosis** /sī′tōmôr′fəsis/, *pl.* **cytomorphoses** [Gk, *kytos* + *morphosis,* shaping], the various changes that occur within a cell during the entire course of its life cycle.

**cyton.** See **perikaryon.**

**cytopathic** /-path′ik/, pertaining to the effect of disease or another disorder on a cell, such as damage from a virus or nuclear radiation.

**cytopathogenic effect** /-path′əjen′ik/, the morphologic changes in a cultured cell caused by cytopathic damage.

**cytopathology** /-pathol′əjē/, the study of changes at the cellular level caused by disease.

**cytopenia** /-pē′nē·ə/ [Gk, *kytos* + *penes,* poor], a deficiency in numbers of the blood cell elements.

**cytophagy** /sītof′əjē/, cell destruction by phagocytes.

**cytopheresis** /sī′tōfer′əsis/ [Gk, *kytos* + *aphairesis,* withdrawal], **1.** a therapeutic technique to remove red or white blood cells or platelets from patients with certain blood disorders. **2.** a laboratory procedure for separating specific components, such as white blood cells or platelets, from donor blood by centrifugation.

**cytophotometer** /sī′tōfotom′ətər/ [Gk, *kytos* + *phos,* light, *metron,* measure], an instrument for measuring light density through stained portions of cytoplasm, used for locating and identifying chemical substances within cells.

**cytophotometry** /sī′tōfotom′ətrē/, the identification of chemical substances within cells, using a cytophotometer. Also called **microfluorometry.** —**cytophotometric,** *adj.*

**cytophysiology** /-fis′ē·ol′əjē/ [Gk, *kytos* + *physis,* nature, *logos,* science], the study of the biochemical processes involved in the functioning of individual cells. —**cytophysiologic, cytophysiological,** *adj.;* **cytophysiologist,** *n.*

**cytoplasm** /sī′təplaz′əm/ [Gk, *kytos* + *plassein,* to mold], all of the substance of a cell other than the nucleus and the cell wall. See also **cell, nucleus.**

**cytoplasmic bridge.** See **intercellular bridge.**

**cytoplasmic inheritance** /sī′tōplaz′mik/, the acquisition of traits or conditions controlled by self-replicating substances within the cytoplasm, such as mitochondria or chloroplasts, rather than by genes on the chromosomes in the nucleus. The phenomenon occurs in plants and some animals but has not been demonstrated in humans.

**Cytosar-U,** trademark for an antineoplastic (cytarabine).

**cytoscopy** /sītos′kəpē/ [Gk, *kytos* + *skopein,* to watch], the diagnostic study of cells obtained from patient specimens with the aid of microscopes and other laboratory equipment.

**cytosine** /sī′təsin/, a pyrimidine base that is a component of DNA and RNA. In free or uncombined form it occurs in trace amounts in most cells, usually as a product of the enzymatic hydrolysis of nucleic acids and nucleotides. On hydrolysis it is converted to urea and ammonia. See also **thymine, uracil.**

**cytosine arabinoside.** See **cytarabine.**

**cytosis** /sītō′sis/, a condition in which there is a greater than normal number of cells in a tissue or organ.

**cytoskeleton** /-skel′ətən/ [Gk, *kytos* + *skeletos,* dried body], the cytoplasmic elements, including the tonofibrils, keratin, and other microfibrils, that function as a supportive system within a cell, especially an epithelial cell.

**cytosol** /sī′tōsôl/, the liquid medium of the cytoplasm, i.e., cytoplasm minus organelles and nonmembranous insoluble components.

**cytosome** /sī′təsōm/, a multilayered, membrane-bound, lamellar body found in type II pneumocytes. It is a precursor of pulmonary surfactant.

**cytotechnologist,** an allied health professional who works with a pathologist to detect changes in body cells that may be important in early diagnosis of cancer and other diseases. The cytotechnologist prepares cellular samples and examines them under a microscope to evaluate for abnormalities in structure.

**cytotoxic** /tok′sik/ [Gk, *kytos* + *toxikon,* poison], pertaining to a pharmacologic compound or other agent that destroys or damages tissue cells.

**cytotoxic anaphylaxis** [Gk, *kytos* + *toxikon,* poison, *hyper,* above], complement-dependent hypersensitivity to foreign cells or to alterations of cell-surface antigens that is mediated by immunoglobulin G (IgG) or IgM. It causes immediate destruction of cells, as seen in hemolytic disease of the newborn and in severe transfusion reactions. Also called **cytotoxic hypersensitivity, type II hypersensitivity.** Compare **anaphylactic hypersensitivity, immune complex hypersensitivity.** See also **immune gamma globulin.**

**cytotoxic drug,** any pharmacologic compound that inhibits the proliferation of cells within the body. Such compounds as the alkylating agents and the antimetabolites are designed to destroy abnormal cells selectively, while sparing as many normal cells as possible; they are commonly used in chemotherapy. Cytotoxic agents have a potential for producing teratogenesis, mutagenesis, and carcinogenesis.

**cytotoxic hypersensitivity.** See **cytotoxic anaphylaxis.**

**cytotoxic hypersensitivity reaction,** type II hypersensitivity reaction; see **hypersensitivity reaction.**

**cytotoxic killer T cell,** a type of T lymphocyte that has the ability to cause lysis of specific target cells, such as those containing viral antigens. See also **CD4, CD8 cell.**

**cytotoxic T cell.** See **CD8 cell.**

**cytotoxin** /sī′tōtok′sin/ [Gk, *kytos* + *toxikon,* poison], a substance that has a toxic effect on certain cells. An antibody may act as a cytotoxin. —**cytotoxic,** *adj.*

**cytotrophoblast** /sī′tōtrof′əblast′/ [Gk, *kytos* + *trophe,* nutrition, *blastos,* germ], the inner layer of cells of the trophoblast of the early mammalian embryo that gives rise to the outer surface and villi of the chorion. Also called **Langhans′ layer.** Compare **syncytiotrophoblast.** —**cytotrophoblastic,** *adj.*

**cytotropism** /sī′tōtrop′izm/, a characteristic of some cells and agents that enables them to approach other cells or selectively bind them.

**Cytovene,** trademark for an antiviral (ganciclovir).

**Cytoxan,** trademark for an antineoplastic (cyclophosphamide).

**CYVADIC,** an anticancer drug combination of cyclophosphamide, vincristine, doxorubicin, and dacarbazine.

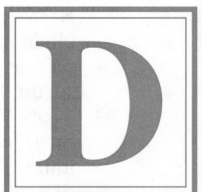

**d,** symbol for one tenth.

**D,** **1.** symbol for *dead space gas.* **2.** symbol for **diffusing capacity.** **3.** abbreviation for *diopter.* **4.** abbreviation for *dexter,* meaning 'right.'

**d4T,** symbol for **dideoxythymidine.**

**da,** symbol for the multiple 10.

**DA,** abbreviation for **developmental age.**

**daboia** /dəboiˈə/ [Hind, *dabna,* to lurk], a local name for Russell's viper, a large, very poisonous snake indigenous to India and Southeast Asia. Its venom is used as a coagulant in cases of hemophilia.

**dacarbazine** /dekärˈbəzēn/, an alkylating agent used as an antineoplastic.

■ INDICATIONS: It is prescribed primarily in the treatment of malignant melanoma and Hodgkin's disease.

■ CONTRAINDICATION: Known hypersensitivity to this drug prohibits its use.

■ ADVERSE EFFECTS: Among the more serious adverse reactions are bone marrow depression, GI symptoms, kidney and liver impairment, alopecia, and fever.

**daclizumab,** an immunosuppressant.

■ INDICATIONS: Daclizumab is used to help prevent acute allograft rejection in renal transplant patients.

■ CONTRAINDICATIONS: Known hypersensitivity to this drug contraindicates its use.

■ ADVERSE EFFECTS: Life-threatening effects of this drug are pulmonary edema, tachycardia, thrombosis, renal tubular necrosis, and hydronephrosis. Other adverse effects include headache, prickly sensation, coughing, atelectasis, congestion, constipation, abdominal pain, pyrosis, hypertension, bleeding, oliguria, dysuria, renal damage, and impaired wound healing. Common side effects include chills, tremors, dyspnea, wheezing, vomiting, nausea, and diarrhea.

**D/A converter.** See **digital-to-analog converter.**

**Dacron cuff,** a sheath of Dacron surrounding an atrial or venous catheter to prevent accidental displacement.

**dacryadenitis.** See **dacryoadenitis.**

**dacryo-, dacry-,** combining form meaning 'tears': *dacryocele, dacryolin, dacryorrhea.*

**dacryoadenitis** /dakˈrē·ō·adˈənīˈtis/, an inflammation of the lacrimal gland. The condition may be seen in mumps infection that involves a lacrimal gland. Also called **dacryadenitis** /-adˈənīˈtis/.

**dacryocyst** /dakˈre·ōsistˈ/ [Gk, *dakryon,* tear, *kytis,* bag], a lacrimal sac at the medial angle of the eye.

**dacryocystectomy** /dakˈrē·ōsistekˈtəmē/ [Gk, *dakryon* + *kytis,* bag, *ektomē,* excision], partial or total excision of the lacrimal sac.

**dacryocystitis** /dakˈrē·ōsistīˈtis/, an infection of the lacrimal sac caused by obstruction of the nasolacrimal duct. It is characterized by tearing and discharge from the eye. In the acute phase the sac becomes inflamed and painful. The disorder is nearly always unilateral and usually occurs in infants. Systemic administration of antibiotics is usual; local topical treatment is seldom effective; rarely a dacryocystorhinostomy may be required. Compare **dacryostenosis.**

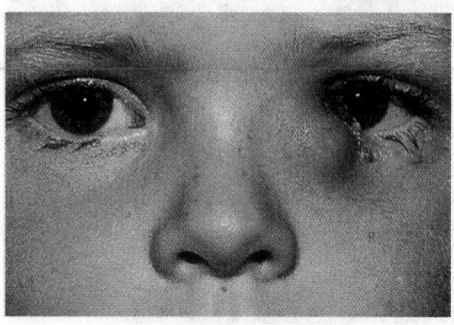

**Dacryocystitis** *(Zitelli and Davis, 1997)*

**dacryocystorhinostomy** /dakˈrē·ōsisˈtôrīnosˈtəmē/ [Gk, *dakryon* + *kytis,* bag, *rhis,* nose, *stoma,* mouth], a surgical procedure for restoring drainage into the nose from the lacrimal sac when the nasolacrimal duct is obstructed.

**dacryon.** See **tears.**

**dacryostenosis** /dakˈrē·ostinōˈsis/ [Gk, *dakryon* + *stenos,* narrow, *osis,* condition], an abnormal stricture of the nasolacrimal duct, occurring either as a congenital condition or as a result of infection or trauma. Dacryocystorhinostomy may be required to correct this condition. Compare **dacryocystitis.**

**dactinomycin** /dakˈtinōmīˈsin/, an antibiotic used as an antineoplastic agent.

■ INDICATIONS: It is prescribed in the treatment of a variety of malignant neoplastic diseases, including Wilms' tumor and rhabdomyosarcoma.

■ CONTRAINDICATIONS: Herpes zoster infection, chicken pox, or known hypersensitivity to this drug prohibits its use.

■ ADVERSE EFFECTS: Among the more serious adverse reactions are bone marrow depression, severe GI disturbances, proctitis, alopecia, and ulcers of the mouth.

**dactyl** /dakˈtil/ [Gk, *daktylos,* finger], a digit (finger or toe). —**dactylic** /daktilˈik/, *adj.*

**dactyl-.** See **dactylo-.**

**-dactyl,** suffix meaning 'digit (finger or toe)': *hermodactyl, pachydactyl, pentadactyl.*

**dactyledema** /dakˈtilidēˈmə/, edema of the fingers or toes.

**-dactylia, -dactyly,** suffix meaning '(condition of the) fingers or toes': *ankylodactylia, heptadactylia, oligodactylia.*

**dactylic.** See **dactyl.**

**dactylion** /daktilˈē·on/, a condition of complete or partial webbing of fingers.

**dactylitis** /dakˈtilīˈtis/, a painful inflammation of the fingers or toes, usually associated with sickle cell anemia or certain infectious diseases, particularly syphilis or tuberculosis.

**dactylo-, dactyl-,** combining form meaning 'finger or toe': *dactylophasia, dactylospasm, dactylosymphysis.*

**dactylus.** See **digit.**

**-dactyly.** See **-dactylia.**

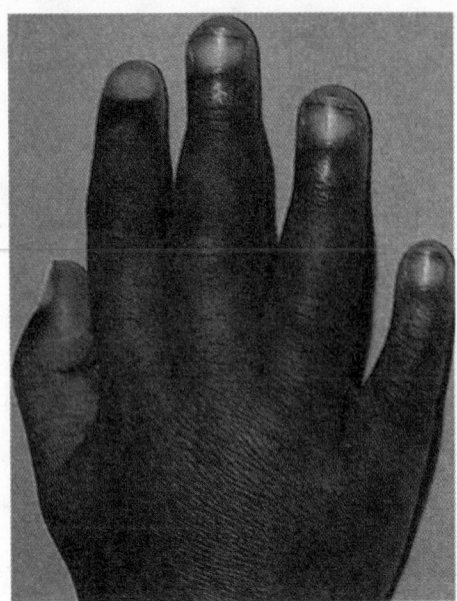

**Dactylitis** *(Zitelli and Davis, 1997)*

**DAI,** abbreviation for **diffuse axonal injury.**

**daily adjusted progressive resistance exercise (DAPRE),** a program of isotonic exercises that allows for individual differences in the rate at which a patient regains strength in an injured or diseased body part.

**daily living skills.** See **activities of daily living.**

**Daily Reference Values (DRVs),** a set of dietary standards for eight nutrients and food compartments: total fat, saturated fat, cholesterol, total carbohydrates, dietary fiber, protein, potassium, and sodium. They are part of the U.S. Food and Drug Administration (FDA) Daily Value (DV) label reference.

**dairy food substitute,** a group of foods that includes imitation cream, coffee whitener, cheese, and ice cream. Although similar in taste and texture to genuine dairy products, nondairy products can differ markedly in composition from products they resemble. Some substitutes may contain milk components despite nondairy claims.

**daisy-wheel printer,** a character printer for computers in which the character dies are on a number of narrow, flexible "fingers" projecting from a central hub, resembling a daisy. Compare **dot-matrix printer, laser printer.**

**Dakin's solution** [Henry D. Dakin, American biochemist, 1880–1952; L, *solutus* dissolved], an antiseptic solution containing boric acid and 0.4% to 0.5% of sodium hypochlorite.

**Dalmane,** trademark for a benzodiazepine sedative-hypnotic (flurazepam hydrochloride).

**dalteparin sodium,** a low–molecular weight heparin.
- INDICATIONS: It is prescribed to prevent deep vein thrombosis in adults undergoing abdominal surgery who are at risk for clotting. It is also used for the treatment of unstable angina and non-Q-wave myocardial infarction to prevent ischemic complications in patients with concurrent aspirin therapy.
- CONTRAINDICATIONS: The drug should not be given to patients with allergy to dalteparin, heparin, or pork products or patients with certain blood disorders.

- ADVERSE EFFECTS: The side effects most often reported include heavy or unusual bleeding, black stools, or bruising or pain at the site of injection.

**dalton** [John Dalton, English chemist and mathematician, 1766–1844], **1.** an unofficial unit of atomic mass, based on 1/16 of the gram mass of hydrogen. **2.** (in biochemistry) unit (kilodaltons) that expresses the molecular weight (mass) of proteins and nucleic acids. See also **atomic weight.**

**daltonism** /dôl′təniz′əm/ [John Dalton], *informal.* a form of red-green color blindness. It is genetically transmitted as a sex-linked autosomal-recessive trait.

**Dalton's law of partial pressures** /dôl′tənz/ [John Dalton], (in physics) a law stating that the total pressure exerted by a mixture of gases is equal to the sum of the pressures that could be exerted by the gases if they were present alone in the container in the same quantity. See also **Avogadro's law, Boyle's law, Gay-Lussac's law.**

**dam,** a barrier to the flow of fluid, as a dam placed around a tooth to protect it from saliva during restoration. See also **rubber dam.**

**damages** /dam′ijəs/ [L, *damnum,* loss], (in law) a sum of money awarded to a plaintiff by a court as compensation for any loss, detriment, or injury to the plaintiff's person, property, or rights caused by the malfeasance or negligence of the defendant. **Actual damages** are awarded to reimburse the plaintiff for the loss or injury sustained. **Nominal damages** are awarded to show that a legal wrong has been committed although no recoverable loss can be determined. **Punitive damages** exceed the actual cost of injury or damage and are awarded when the defendant has acted with malice or reckless disregard of the plaintiff's rights.

**damp** [AS, vapor], a potentially lethal atmosphere in caves and mines. **Black damp** or **choke damp** is caused by absorption of the available oxygen by coal seams. **Fire damp** is composed of methane and other explosive hydrocarbon gases. **White damp** is another name for carbon monoxide.

**damping** [AS, vapor], a gradual decrease in the amplitude of a series of waves or oscillations, such as an arterial pressure waveform.

**danaparoid,** an anticoagulant.
- INDICATIONS: Danaparoid is used to prevent vein thrombosis in hemodialysis, stroke, elective surgery for malignancy or total hip replacement, and hip fracture surgery.
- CONTRAINDICATIONS: Hypersensitivity to this drug, to sulfites, or to pork products prohibits the use of danaparoid. Other factors that contraindicate its use include hemophilia, leukemia with bleeding, thrombocytopenia, purpura, cerebrovascular hemorrhage, cerebral aneurysm, severe hypertension, and other severe cardiac disease.
- ADVERSE EFFECTS: Life-threatening side effects of this drug include hemorrhage and thrombocytopenia. Hypersensitivity reactions and rash are additional adverse effects.

**danazol** /dan′əzol/, a synthetic androgen that acts to suppress the output of gonadotropins from the pituitary.
- INDICATION: It is prescribed in the treatment of endometriosis when alternative hormonal therapy is ineffective, contraindicated, or intolerable.
- CONTRAINDICATIONS: Genital bleeding; cardiac, liver, or kidney dysfunction; or known hypersensitivity to this drug prohibits its use. It is not prescribed during pregnancy or lactation.
- ADVERSE EFFECTS: Among the most serious adverse reactions are muscle spasms, nausea, weight gain, acne, edema, oily skin, voice changes, and other androgenic effects.

**dance reflex** [ME, *dauncen* + L, *reflectere,* to bend back], a normal response in the neonate to simulate walking by a reciprocal flexion and extension of the legs when held in an erect position and inclined forward, with the soles touching a hard surface. The reflex disappears by about 3 to 6 weeks of age and is replaced by controlled, deliberate movement. Also called **step reflex, stepping reflex.**

**dance therapy,** (in psychology) the use of rhythmic body movements or dance to release expression of feelings.

**dander,** dry scales shed from the scalp.

**dandruff** /dan'druf/, an excessive amount of scaly material composed of dead, keratinized epithelium shed from the scalp that may be a mild form of seborrheic dermatitis or psoriasis. Treatment with a keratolytic shampoo is usually recommended to soften and remove the scales.

**dandy fever.** See **dengue fever.**

**Dandy-Walker cyst** [Walter E. Dandy, American neurosurgeon, 1886–1946; Arthur E. Walker, American surgeon, b. 1907], a cystic malformation of the fourth ventricle of the brain, resulting from hydrocephalus. Diagnosis of the defect is made with computed tomographic scan, x-ray films, and less commonly a ventriculogram. See also **hydrocephalus, shunt.**

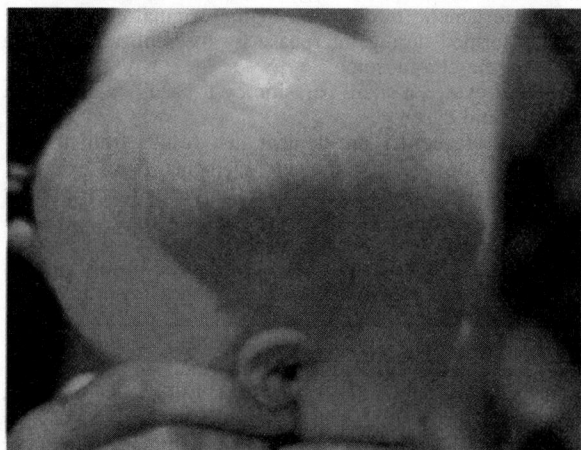

**Dandy-Walker cyst**
*(Zitelli and Davis 1997/courtesy Dr. Michael J. Painter)*

**Dandy-Walker malformation.** See **Dandy-Walker cyst.**

**Danocrine,** trademark for an anterior pituitary suppressant (danazol).

**danthron** /dan'thron/, a stimulant laxative.

■ INDICATIONS: It is prescribed in the treatment of constipation or for bowel evacuation before radiologic or surgical procedures.

■ CONTRAINDICATIONS: Abdominal pain, nausea, vomiting, or other signs and symptoms of appendicitis prohibit its use. It is not recommended for nursing mothers.

■ ADVERSE EFFECTS: Among the most serious adverse reactions are dizziness, palpitations, stomach cramps, and excessive bowel activity.

**Dantrium,** trademark for a skeletal muscle relaxant (dantrolene sodium), used in the treatment of malignant hyperthermia or hyperpyrexia.

**dantrolene sodium** /dan'trəlen/, a skeletal muscle relaxant.

■ INDICATIONS: It is prescribed in the treatment of muscle spasticity resulting from injury to the spinal cord or cere-

brum. It is not indicated in treatment of spasm from rheumatic disorders. It is used intravenously for the management of malignant hyperthermia.

■ CONTRAINDICATIONS: Liver dysfunction or known hypersensitivity to this drug prohibits its use.

■ ADVERSE EFFECTS: The most serious adverse reaction is potentially fatal hepatotoxicity. Common reactions include confusion, drowsiness, diarrhea, dizziness, fatigue, and muscular weakness. Side effects may continue for several days.

**DAP,** abbreviation for **Draw-A-Person Test.**

**DAPRE,** abbreviation for **daily adjusted progressive resistance exercise.**

**dapsone (DDS)** /dap'sōn/, a bacteriostatic and bactericidal sulfone derivative or leptrostatic.

■ INDICATIONS: It is prescribed in the treatment of leprosy and dermatitis herpetiformis.

■ CONTRAINDICATIONS: Pregnancy or known hypersensitivity to this drug prohibits its use.

■ ADVERSE EFFECTS: Among the more serious adverse reactions are hemolysis (particularly in people who have glucose-6-phosphate dehydrogenase deficiency), leprosy reactional state, methemoglobinemia, neuropathy, nausea, anorexia, toxic hepatic aplastic anemia, and skin rash.

**-dapsone,** suffix designating a diaminodiphenylsulfone-derivative antimycobacterial agent.

**Daraprim,** trademark for an antimalarial (pyrimethamine).

**Darbid,** trademark for an anticholinergic (isopropamide iodide).

**Darier's disease.** See **keratosis follicularis.**

**Darier's sign** /däryāz'/ [Jean F. Darier, French dermatologist, 1856–1938], a burning or itching sensation induced by stroking skin lesions in cases of urticaria pigmentosa. The area may become raised and red.

**dark adaptation,** a normal increase in sensitivity of the retinal rod cells of the eye to detect any light that may be available for vision in a dimly lighted environment. The process is accompanied by an adjustment of the pupils to allow more light to enter the eyes.

**darkfield microscopy** [AS, *deorc,* hidden, *feld,* field; Gk, *mikros,* small, *skopein,* to look], examination of a microscopic specimen illuminated by a peripheral light source.

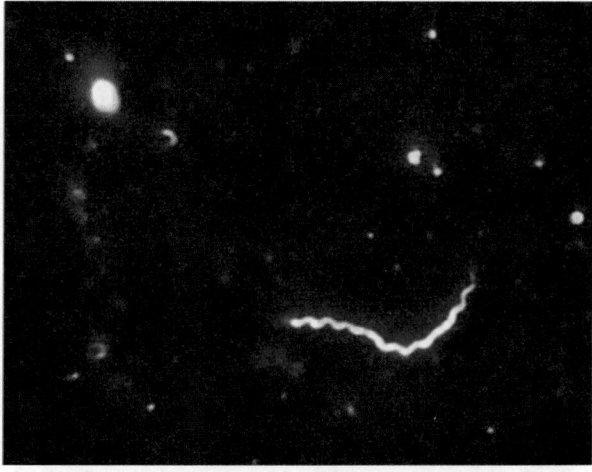

**Darkfield microscopy: positive examination**
*(Morse, Moreland, and Holmes, 1996)*

The illumination causes the specimen to appear to glow against a dark background. In laboratory diagnosis, the technique is used primarily to identify the syphilis spirochete. Also called **darkfield illumination, ultramicroscopy.**

**dark-film fault** [AS, *deorc,* hidden, *filmen,* skin; L, *fallere,* to disappoint], a defect in a photograph or radiograph that appears as an excessively darkened image or image area. It is caused by accidental exposure or overexposure of the film to light or radiation, excessive development, or an unsafe darkroom light.

**darkroom,** a room in a hospital or similar facility for the storage and processing of light-sensitive materials, such as x-ray film.

**Darling's disease.** See **histoplasmosis.**

**dartos.** See **tunica dartos.**

**Darvocet-N,** trademark for a fixed-combination drug containing an analgesic-antipyretic (acetaminophen) and an opioid analgesic (propoxyphene napsylate).

**Darvon,** trademark for an opioid analgesic (propoxyphene hydrochloride).

**Darvon Compound,** trademark for a fixed-combination drug containing an opioid analgesic (propoxyphene hydrochloride) and aspirin, phenacetin, and caffeine (APC).

**Darvon-N,** trademark for an opioid analgesic (propoxyphene napsylate).

**darwinian.** See **darwinian theory.**

**darwinian ear** /därwin′ē·ən/ [Charles R. Darwin, English naturalist, 1809–1882], an external ear with an upper border that projects upward in a flat, sharp edge.

**darwinian reflex.** See **grasp reflex.**

**darwinian theory** [Charles R. Darwin], the theory of Charles Darwin that organic evolution results from the natural selection of those variants of organisms that are best suited to survive in their environment. Also called **darwinism.** Compare **lamarckism.** —**darwinian,** *adj.*

**darwinian tubercle, Darwin's tubercle.** See **auricular tubercle.**

**darwinism.** See **lamarckism.**

**DAS,** abbreviation for **data acquisition system.**

**DASE,** abbreviation for **Denver Articulation Screening Examination.**

**data** /dā′tə, dat′ə, dä′tə/, *sing.* **datum** [L, *datum,* giving], 1. pieces of information, especially those that are part of a collection to be used in an analysis of a problem, such as the diagnosis of a health problem. 2. facts stored and processed by a computer.

**data acquisition system (DAS),** a radiation detection system that measures the amount of radiation passing through a patient. In computed tomography, the system also converts analog signals to digital data that can be analyzed by a computer.

**data analysis,** (in research) the phase of a study that includes classifying, coding, and tabulating information needed to perform quantitative or qualitative analyses according to the research design and appropriate to the data. Data analysis follows collection of information and precedes its interpretation or application.

**data base,** a store or bank of information, especially in a form that can be processed by computer.

**data clustering,** the grouping of related information from a patient's health history, physical examination, and laboratory results as part of the process of making a diagnosis.

**data collection,** (in research) the phase of a study that includes the gathering of information and identification of sampling units as directed by the research design. Data collection precedes data analysis.

**data processing,** the techniques and practices involved in the manipulation of information by a computer.

**data retrieval,** the recovery of information from an organized filing system, such as a computer data base, index card file, or color-coded record folders.

**dataset** /dā′təset/, a collection of similar and related data for processing by computer.

**data source,** the origin of information relevant to a patient's level of wellness and health patterns.

**data validation,** the process of determining whether information gathered during the process of data collection is complete and accurate.

**date/acquaintance rape,** a sexual assault or rape by a person known to the victim, such as a date, employer, friend, or casual acquaintance. See also **rape.**

**datum.** See **data.**

**daughter cell** [ME, *doughter,* female, child; L, *cella,* storeroom], one of the cells produced by the division of a parent cell.

**daughter chromosome** [ME, *doughter,* female, child; Gk, *chroma,* color, *soma,* body], either of the paired chromatids that separate and migrate to the opposite ends of the cell during the anaphase stage of mitosis. Each contains the complete genetic information of the original chromosome and is formed during interphase by the replication of the DNA in the chromosome.

**daughter cyst,** a small parasitic cyst, usually a derivative of a hydatid cyst.

**daughter element,** an element that results from the radioactive decay of another element. For example, technetium-99 is the daughter element created by the decay of molybdenum-99.

**daughter product.** See **decay product.**

**daunorubicin citrate liposomal** /dô′nōr͞oō′bisin/, an anthracycline antibiotic antineoplastic agent.

■ INDICATIONS: It is prescribed in the treatment of cancer, particularly the leukemias and neuroblastoma.

■ CONTRAINDICATIONS: Preexisting drug-induced bone marrow depression or known hypersensitivity to this drug prohibits its use. It is not given to patients who have previously received a complete course of treatment with daunorubicin or doxorubicin.

■ ADVERSE EFFECTS: Among the most serious adverse reactions are bone marrow depression and cardiotoxicity. GI disturbances, stomatitis, and alopecia are common.

**Davidoff's cells.** See **cells of Paneth.**

**Davidson regimen.** See **toilet training.**

**DAWN** /dôn/, abbreviation for **Drug Abuse Warning Network.**

**dawn phenomenon** [ME, *daunen* + Gk, *phainomenon,* anything seen], a tendency for persons with type 1 diabetes mellitus to require an increased insulin dose in the early morning hours as a result of an increase in plasma glucose concentration because of increased cortisol and growth hormone secretion. Compare **Somogyi phenomenon.**

**day blindness.** See **hemeralopia.**

**day care** [OE, *daeg* + *cearu*], a specialized program or facility that provides care for preschool children, usually within a group framework, either as a substitute for or an extension of home care, particularly for single parents or for two parents both employed outside the home. Day-care groups vary in size and function and range from casual neighborhood parent-supervised play groups to formal nursery schools or organized centers run by trained personnel. Most day-care programs incorporate a daily schedule of quiet play, outdoor activities, group games and projects, creative or educational play, and snack and rest periods.

**daydream,** a usually nonpathologic reverie that occurs while a person is awake. The content is usually the imagined fulfillment of wishes that are not disguised.

**day health care services,** the provision of hospitals, nursing homes, or other facilities for health-related services to adult patients who are ambulatory or can be transported and who regularly use such services for a certain number of daytime hours but do not require continuous inpatient care. See also **adult day-care center.**

**day hospital** [OE, *daeg* + L, *hospes,* guest], a psychiatric facility that offers a therapeutic program during daytime hours for patients. See also **partial hospitalization program.**

**day patient.** See **inpatient.**

**day sight.** See **nyctalopia.**

**dB,** abbreviation for **decibel.**

**Db,** symbol for the element **dubnium.**

**DBMS,** abbreviation for *data base management system.*

**DC,** abbreviation for **direct current.**

**d/c,** abbreviation for *discontinue.*

**D&C,** abbreviation for **dilation and curettage.**

**DD,** abbreviation for **developmental disability.**

**DDAVP,** trademark for an antidiuretic (desmopressin acetate).

**ddC,** symbol for 2'3'-dideoxycytidine, an antiretroviral drug used in the treatment of acquired immunodeficiency syndrome. It is related chemically to ddI. Also known as **zalcitabine.**

**DDD pacing,** a specific type of electrical heart pacemaker. The letters indicate Dual pacing for both chambers, Dual chamber activity sensing, and Dual response (triggering and inhibition).

**ddI,** **1.** abbreviation for 2',3'-dideoxyinosine, an antiretroviral medication. Also called **didanosine. 2.** abbreviation for **dideoxyinose.**

**D-dimer test,** a simple and confirmatory test for disseminated intravascular coagulation (DIC) that can also indicate when a clot is lysed by thrombolytic therapy. The fragment D-dimer assesses both thrombin and plasmin activity.

**D.D.S.,** abbreviation for *Doctor of Dental Surgery.*

**DDST,** abbreviation for **Denver Developmental Screening Test.**

**DDT (dichlorodiphenyltrichloroethane),** a nondegradable water-insoluble chlorinated hydrocarbon once used worldwide as a major insecticide, especially in agriculture. In recent years knowledge of its adverse impact on the environment has led to restrictions in its use. In addition, because tolerance in formerly susceptible organisms develops rapidly, DDT has been largely replaced by organophosphate insecticides in the United States, where DDT was banned by the FDA in 1971. It is still used as a pediculicide where epidemic-scale delousing is justified, as in barracks and refugee camps. Its value as a scabicide is marginal, since scabies and crab lice quickly become resistant to it. See also **scabicide.**

**DDT poisoning.** See **chlorinated organic insecticide poisoning.**

**D&E,** abbreviation for **dilation and evacuation.**

**DE,** abbreviation for **dose equivalent.**

**de-,** prefix meaning 'to do the opposite, away, off, to remove entirely, down or from': *decartation, dedentition, decapitation.*

**DEA,** **1.** abbreviation for *Drug Enforcement Administration.* **2.** abbreviation for **Drug Enforcement Agency.**

**deactivation** /dē·ak'tivā'shən/ [L, *de,* from, *activus,* active], the process of becoming or making something inactive or inoperable.

**dead,** pertaining to the absence of all vital functions in a previously living organism.

**dead-end host** [AS, *dead* + *ende* + L, *hospes,* guest], any animal from which a parasite cannot escape to continue its life cycle. Humans are dead-end hosts for trichinosis, because the larvae encyst in muscle and human flesh is unlikely to be a source of food for other animals susceptible to this parasite. Compare **definitive host, intermediate host, reservoir host.**

**dead fetus syndrome,** a condition in which the fetus has died but has remained in the uterus for some time. The condition leads to a blood coagulation disorder, disseminated intravascular coagulation, and the eventual delivery is usually accompanied by massive bleeding. See also **disseminated intravascular coagulation.**

**deadly quartet.** See **syndrome X.**

**dead pulp.** See **nonvital pulp.**

**dead space** [AS, dead; L, *spatium*], **1.** a cavity that remains after the incomplete closure of a surgical or traumatic wound, leaving an area in which blood can collect and delay healing. **2.** the amount of lung in contact with ventilating gases but not in contact with pulmonary blood flow. **Alveolar dead space** is characterized by alveoli that are ventilated by the pulmonary circulation but are not perfused. The condition may exist when pulmonary circulation is obstructed, as by a thromboembolus. **Anatomic dead space** is an area in the trachea, bronchi, and air passages containing air that does not reach the alveoli during respiration. As a general rule, the volume of air in the anatomic dead space in milliliters is approximately equal to the weight in pounds of the individual affected. Certain lung disorders, such as emphysema, increase the amount of anatomic dead space. **Physiologic dead space** is an area in the respiratory system that includes the anatomic dead space together with the space in the alveoli occupied by air that does not contribute to the oxygen-carbon dioxide exchange.

**dead space effect,** any of several potential adverse effects, including hypoxemia and hypercapnia, produced by dead space in the lungs, particularly alveolar dead space.

**deaf** [AS], **1.** unable to hear; hard of hearing. **2.** people who are unable to hear or who have hearing impairment. **—deafness,** *n.*

**deafferentation** /dē·af'ərəntā'shən/ [L, *de,* from, *ad* + *ferre,* to bear], the elimination or interruption of afferent nerve impulses.

**deaf-mute,** a person who is unable to hear or to speak.

**deaf-mutism** [AS, *deaf* + L, *mutus*], a state of being both unable to hear and unable to speak.

**deafness,** a condition characterized by a loss of hearing that makes it impossible for an individual to understand speech through hearing alone. In assessing deafness the ears are examined for drainage, crusts, accumulation of cerumen, or structural abnormality. It is determined whether the hearing loss is conductive or sensory, temporary or permanent, and congenital or acquired in childhood, adolescence, or adulthood. The effect of aging is evaluated. A psychosocial assessment is conducted to ascertain whether the individual is well adjusted to hearing loss or reacts to the disability with fear, anxiety, frustration, depression, anger, or hostility. In all cases the degree of loss and the kind of impairment causing it are determined. See also **conductive hearing loss, sensorineural hearing loss.**

■ OBSERVATIONS: Many conditions and diseases may result in hearing loss. More than 21 million people in the United States have some degree of hearing loss; of them more than 50% are above 65 years of age. The person with a slight hearing loss may be initially unaware of the problem. Recognition, diagnosis, and early treatment may help prevent further impairment and prevent frustration, embarrassment, and danger for the person. An older person with a hearing impairment usually has a sensorineural loss. High-frequency sounds are hard to hear, and discernment of such softer speech sounds as /s/ and /f/ becomes difficult. A severe or sudden hearing loss usually drives the person to seek help. If the loss is sudden, confusion, fear, and even panic are common. The person's speech becomes loud and slurred. There is new danger because the person cannot hear horns, whistles, or sirens and has not developed a way to cope with the impairment safely. The congenitally deaf person needs special speech and language intervention before reaching school age. ■ INTERVENTIONS: The treatment of hearing loss depends on the cause. Merely removing impacted cerumen from the external auditory canal may significantly improve hearing. Hearing aids, amplification of sound, or speech reading may be useful. Speech therapy is useful in teaching a person to speak or helping a person to retain the ability to speak. ■ NURSING CONSIDERATIONS: Caring for a deaf person who is hospitalized for treatment of another problem requires certain adjustments in communication between nurse and patient. If the patient uses a hearing aid, its placement and operation are checked before the speaker begins to talk; the voice is modulated to a level that is comfortable for the patient, and the speaker stands or sits where the lips are visible to the deaf individual. If the patient uses sign language, an interpreter or another means of communication is sought; when a pad and pencil are used, a frequent practice with the newly deaf, the messages are written clearly in short, simple phrases, and adequate time is allowed for the patient to understand and answer. The bed is located so that the patient can see the door.

**deaminase** /dē·am′inās/ [L, *de,* away, *amine,* ammonia; Fr, *diastase,* enzyme], one of the subclasses of enzymes that catalyze the hydrolysis of the $NH_2$ bond in amino compounds. The enzymes are usually named according to the substrate, such as **adenosine deaminase, guanine deaminase,** or **guanosine deaminase.** Also called **aminohydrolase.**

**deamination** /dē′aminā′shən/, the removal, usually by hydrolysis, of the $NH_2$ radical from an amino compound. Also called **deaminization.**

**dean** [L, *decanus,* chief of ten], chief executive and educational officer of a unit of a university, school, or college.

**dean's tax,** a portion of physician practice plan income in an academic medical center that is allocated for the support of the medical school.

**dearterialization** /dē′ärtir′ē·əlīzā′shən/, **1.** conversion of oxygenated arterial blood into venous blood. **2.** interruption of the supply of arterial blood to an organ or body part.

**death** [AS], **1. apparent death,** the cessation of life as indicated by the absence of all vital functions. **2. legal death,** the total absence of activity in the brain and central nervous system, the cardiovascular system, and the respiratory system as observed and declared by a physician. See also **cell death, emotional care of the dying patient, stages of dying, sudden infant death syndrome.**

**death chill.** See **algor mortis.**

**death instinct,** instinctive behavior that tends to be self-destructive.

**death mask** [AS, *death* + Fr, *masque*], a mask made from a plaster of paris cast of the face of a dead person.

**death rate,** the number of deaths occurring within a specified population during a particular period, usually expressed in terms of deaths per 1000 persons per year.

**death rattle,** a sound produced by air moving through mucus that has accumulated in the throat of a dying person who has lost the cough reflex. It is often accompanied by agonal respiration.

**death trance,** a state in which a person appears to be dead.

**"death with dignity"** [AS, *death* + L, *dignus,* worthy], the philosophical concept that a terminally ill client should be allowed to die naturally and comfortably, rather than experience a comatose, vegetative life prolonged by mechanical support systems.

**debilitating** /dibil′itā′ting/, pertaining to a disease or injury that enfeebles, weakens, or otherwise disables a person.

**debility** /dibil′itē/, feebleness, weakness, or loss of strength. See also **asthenia.**

**debride** /dibrēd′/ [Fr, *debridle,* remove], to remove dirt, foreign objects, damaged tissue, and cellular debris from a wound or a burn to prevent infection and to promote healing. In treating a wound, debridement is the first step in cleansing; it also allows thorough examination of the extent of the injury. In treating a burn, debridement of the eschar may be performed in a hydrotherapy bath. —**debridement** /debrēdmäN′/, *n.*

**debris** /dəbrē′/, the dead, diseased, or damaged tissue and any foreign material that is to be removed from a wound or other area being treated.

**Debrox,** trademark for a topical antiinfective (carbamide peroxide).

**debt** /det/ [L, *debere,* to owe], something owed. See also **oxygen debt.**

**debug** /dibug′, dē′bug/ [L, *de* + Welsh, *bwg,* hobgoblin], to find and correct errors in computer software or hardware.

**dec-,** **1.** prefix meaning 'ten': *decagram, decaliter, decipara.* **2.** combining form meaning 'tenth': *decigram, deciliter, decinormal.*

**Decaderm,** trademark for a synthetic analog of cortisol (dexamethasone).

**Decadron,** trademark for a glucocorticoid (dexamethasone).

**Deca-Durabolin,** trademark for an androgen (nandrolone decanoate).

**decalcification** /dēkal′sifikā′shən/ [L, *de* + *calyx,* lime, *facere,* to make], loss of calcium salts from the teeth and bones caused by malnutrition, malabsorption, or other dietary or physiologic factors, such as immobility. It may result, particularly in older people, from a diet that lacks adequate calcium. Malabsorption may be caused by a lack of vitamin D necessary for the absorption of calcium from the intestine; an excess of dietary fats that can combine with calcium to form an indigestible soaplike compound; the presence of oxalic acid, which can combine with calcium to form a relatively insoluble calcium oxalate salt; hormonal changes of menopause; or a relative lack of acid in the digestive tract, which can decrease the solubility of calcium. Other factors include the parathyroid hormone control of the calcium level in the bloodstream, the ratio of calcium to phosphorus in the blood, and the relative activity of osteoblast cells that form calcium deposits in the bones and teeth and osteoclast cells that absorb calcium from bones and teeth. Bone tissue tends to be maintained in quantities no greater than needed to meet current physical stress. Therefore inactive and, particularly, bedridden people lose calcium from their bones; osteoclastic activity exceeds osteoblastic activity, and decalcification occurs. See also **calcium, mineral.**

**decannulation** /dēkan′yəlā′shən/ [L, *de,* from, *cannula,* small reed], the removal of a cannula or tube that may have been inserted during a surgical procedure.

**decanoic acid.** See **capric acid.**

**decant,** the process of separating fluid or solid sediment by pouring off the top liquid layer.

**decapitation** /dēkap′itā′shən/, literally, cutting off the head, as the head of a bone or the head of a fetus when delivery is not possible otherwise. This is no longer used in clinical practice.

**decay** /dikā′/, **1.** a gradual deterioration that accompanies the end of life. **2.** a gradual deterioration, usually caused by bacteria and other decomposers, of the body of an organism after death. **3.** the process of disintegration of a radioactive substance.

**decay product** [L, *de + cadere,* to fall, *producere,* to produce], a stable or radioactive nuclide formed by the disintegration of a radionuclide, either directly or as a result of successive transformation in a radioactive series. Also called **daughter product.**

**decay time,** the period required for a wavelength to go from peak amplitude to 0 volt (V).

**deceleration** /dēsel′ərā′shən/ [L, *de + accelerare,* to hasten], a decrease in the speed or velocity of an object or reaction. Compare **acceleration.**

**deceleration injury,** an injury resulting from a collision between a rapidly moving body part and a stationary object.

**deceleration phase,** (in obstetrics) the latter part of active labor, characterized by a decreased rate of dilation of the cervical os on a Friedman curve.

**decerebrate** /dēser′əbrāt/, **1.** lacking a cerebrum. **2.** lacking neural communication between the cerebrum and lower portions of the central nervous system.

**decerebrate posture** [L, *de + cerebrum,* brain, *ponere* to place], the position of a patient, who is usually comatose, in which the arms are extended and internally rotated and the legs are extended with the feet in forced plantar flexion. It is usually observed in patients afflicted by compression of the brainstem at a low level. Also called **decerebrate rigidity.**

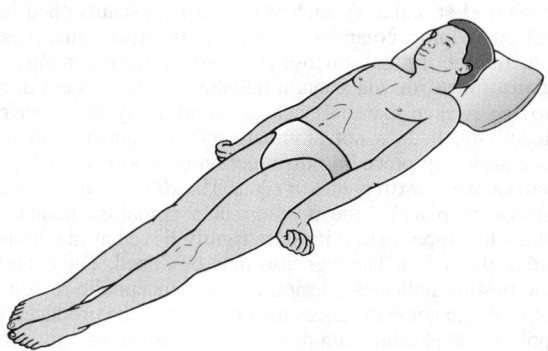

**Decerebrate posture** *(Lewis, Heitkemper, and Dirksen, 2000)*

**decerebrate rigidity.** See **tonic labyrinthine reflex.**

**decerebration** /-brā′shən/ [L, *de,* from, *cerebrum*], the process of removing the brain or of cutting the brainstem above the level of the red nucleus, thus eliminating cerebral function.

**deci-,** combining form indicating one tenth.

**decibel (dB)** /des′əbəl/ [L, *decimus,* one tenth, *bel,* Alexander G. Bell, Canadian inventor, 1847–1922], a unit of measure of the intensity of sound. A decibel is one tenth of 1 bel (B); an increase of 1 B is perceived as a 10-fold increase in loudness, based on a sound-pressure reference level of 0.0002 dyne/cm$^2$, or 20 micropascals.

**decidua** /disij′oo·ə/ [L, *decidere,* to fall off], the epithelial tissue of the endometrium lining the uterus. It envelops the conceptus during gestation and is shed in the puerperium. It is also shed periodically with menstruation. Kinds of decidua are **decidua basalis, decidua capsularis,** and **decidua vera.** See also **amniotic sac.**

**decidua basalis,** the decidua of the endometrium in the uterus that lies beneath the implanted ovum. Also called **decidua serotina.**

**decidua capsularis,** the decidua of the endometrium of the uterus covering the implanted ovum. Also called **decidua reflexa.**

**decidual endometritis** /disij′oo·əl/, an inflammation or infection of any portion of the decidua during pregnancy. See also **endometritis.**

**decidua menstrualis,** the endometrial mucosa shed during menstruation.

**decidua parietalis.** See **decidua vera.**

**decidua reflexa.** See **decidua capsularis.**

**decidua serotina.** See **decidua basalis.**

**decidua vera,** the decidua of the endometrium lining the uterus, except for those areas beneath and above the implanted and developing ovum called, respectively, the decidua basalis and the decidua capsularis. Also called **decidua parietalis.**

**deciduoma** /disij′oo·ō′mə/, a benign or malignant tumor of endometrial tissue. A deciduoma may develop after a pregnancy, regardless of the outcome. It may be detected on a Papanicolaou's (Pap) smear.

**deciduous** /də·sid′yoo·əs/ [L, *decidere,* to fall off], falling off or shed at maturity.

**deciduous dentition,** the set of 20 teeth that appear normally during infancy, consisting of four incisors, two canines, and four molars in each jaw. The teeth start developing at about the sixth week of fetal life as a thickening of the epithelium along the line of the future jaw. During the seventh week the epithelium splits longitudinally into labial and lingual strands. The former becomes the labiodental lamina, and the latter forms the dental lamina, which develops 10 enlargements in each jaw. The enlargements appear at about the ninth week and correspond to the future teeth. In most individuals, the first tooth erupts through the gum about 6

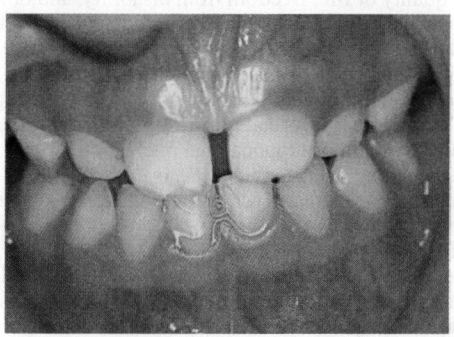

**Deciduous dentition** *(Zitelli and Davis, 1997)*

months after birth. Thereafter one or more teeth erupt about every month until all 20 have appeared. The deciduous teeth are usually shed between the ages of 6 and 13 years, although the timing varies greatly from person to person. Compare **secondary dentition. Also called first dentition, primary dentition, primary teeth.** See also **prediciduous dentition, teething, tooth.**

**deciduous teeth.** See **deciduous dentition.**

**deciduous tooth.** See **deciduous dentition.**

**decigram (dg),** a unit of mass in the metric system equal to 100 milligrams or one tenth of a gram.

**deciliter (dL),** a unit of volume in the metric system equal to 100 milliliters or one tenth of a liter.

**decimeter (dm),** a unit of length in the metric system equal to 10 centimeters or one tenth of a meter.

**decisional conflict,** a nursing diagnosis accepted by the Eighth National Conference on the Classification of Nursing Diagnoses. The condition is a state of uncertainty about the course of action to be taken when choice among competing actions involves risk, loss, or challenge to personal life values. The diagnosis should specify focus of conflict, such as choices regarding health, family relationships, career, finances, or other life events.
■ DEFINING CHARACTERISTICS: Defining characteristics include a verbalized feeling of distress related to uncertainty about choices, reverbalization of undesired consequences of alternative actions being considered, vacillation between alternative choices, delayed decision making, self-focusing, questioning of personal values and beliefs while attempting a decision, and physical signs of distress or tension, such as increased heart rate, increased muscle tension, and restlessness.
■ RELATED FACTORS: Related factors are unclear personal values or beliefs, a perceived threat to one's value system, a lack of experience or interference with decision making, a lack of relevant information, and a support system deficit. See also **nursing diagnosis.**

**decision making[1],** the process of evaluating available information and reaching a judgment or conclusion based on that information.

**decision making[2],** a nursing outcome from the Nursing Outcomes Classification (NOC) defined as ability to choose between two or more alternatives. See also **Nursing Outcomes Classification.**

**decision-making support,** a Nursing Interventions Classification defined as providing information and support for a patient who is making a decision regarding health care. See also **Nursing Interventions Classification.**

**decision tree,** a systematic method of managing a clinical problem by graphically organizing the probabilities of outcomes of alternative treatments. At each decision node or branch a possible alternative is matched with its relative worth, quality of life, freedom from disability, and other factors on which a prognosis may be based.

**declarative memory** /dĕkler'ətiv/, the mental registration, retention, and recall of past experiences, sensations, ideas, knowledge, and thoughts. This memory has a high cognitive basis. The original information must be relayed through either the amygdala or hippocampal nuclear structures before long-term storage is possible.

**Declomycin,** trademark for an antibacterial (demeclocycline hydrochloride).

**decoction** /dikok'shən/ [L, *de* + *coquere,* to cook], a liquid medicine made from an extract of water-soluble substances, usually with the aid of boiling water. Herbal remedies are usually decoctions. See also **concoction.**

**decode** /dikōd'/, to interpret coded information into a form usable by a receiver.

**decoded message,** (in communication theory) a message as translated by a receiver. If it is correctly interpreted within the context of the message as sent by the sender, the decoded message is the same as the encoded message. If it is not understood and interpreted as sent, it is not the same as the encoded message and is potentially misinterpreted.

**decoic acid.** See **capric acid.**

**decoloration,** the natural loss or removal of color, as by bleaching.

**decompensation** /dē'kəmpənsā'shən/ [L, *de* + *compensare,* to balance], **1.** the failure of a system, as cardiac decompensation in heart failure. **2.** (in psychology) the failure of a defense mechanism.

**decomposition** /dē'kəmpəsish'ən/ [L, *de* + *componere,* to put together], the breakdown of a substance into simpler chemical forms.

**decompression** /dē'kəmpresh'ən/ [L, *de* + *comprimere,* to press together], **1.** a technique used to readapt an individual to normal atmospheric pressure after exposure to higher pressures, as in diving. **2.** the removal of pressure caused by gas or fluid in a body cavity, as the stomach or intestinal tract.

**decompression sickness,** a painful, sometimes fatal syndrome caused by the formation of nitrogen bubbles in the tissues of divers, caisson workers, and aviators who move too rapidly from environments of higher to those of lower atmospheric pressures. Nitrogen breathed in air under pressure dissolves in tissue fluids. When ambient pressure is reduced too rapidly, nitrogen goes out of solution faster than it can be circulated to the lungs for expiration. Gaseous nitrogen then accumulates in the joint spaces and peripheral circulation, impairing tissue oxygenation. Disorientation, severe pain, and syncope follow. Treatment entails rapid return of the patient to an environment of higher pressure (hyperbaric therapy) followed by gradual decompression. Death is more often caused by drowning during syncope than by decompression sickness itself. Also called **bends, caisson disease, diver's palsy, diver's paralysis.** Compare **barotrauma.**

**decongestant** [L, *de* + *congerere,* to pile up], **1.** pertaining to a substance or procedure that eliminates or reduces congestion or swelling. **2.** a decongestant drug. Adrenergic drugs (α-1 stimulants), such as ephedrine, pseudoephedrine, and phenylpropanolamine hydrochloride, that cause vasoconstriction of nasal mucosa are used as decongestants.

**decontamination** /dā'kəntam'inā'shən/, the process of removing foreign material such as blood, body fluids, or radioactivity. It does not eliminate microorganisms but is a necessary step preceding disinfection or sterilization.

**decorticate posture** /dēkôr'tikāt/ [L, *de* + *cortex,* bark, *ponere,* to place], the position of a comatose patient in which the upper extremities are rigidly flexed at the elbows and at the wrists. The legs also may be flexed. The decorticate posture indicates a lesion in a mesencephalic region of the brain. In some instances the posture may be produced by applying a painful stimulus to a comatose patient. Also called **decorticate rigidity.**

**decortication** /dēkôr'tikā'shən/ [L, *de* + *cortex,* bark], (in medicine) the removal of portions of the cortex or surface layer of an organ or structure, such as the kidney, the brain, and the lung. —**decorticate,** *v., adj.*

**decrement** /dek'rəmənt/ [L, *de* + *crescere,* to grow], a decrease or stage of decline, as of a uterine contraction.

**decremental conduction** /dek'rəmen'təl/, transmission of an electric impulse in which the amplitude of the impulse decreases with distance.

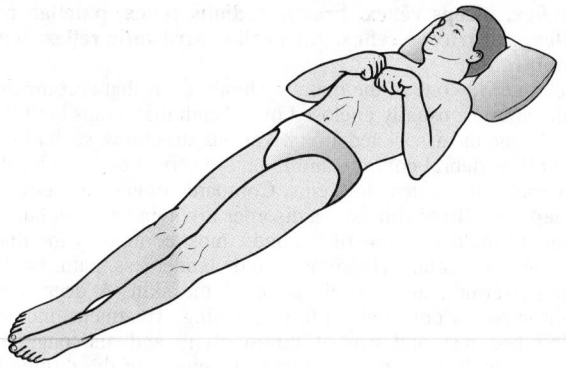

**Decorticate posture** (Lewis, Heitkemper, and Dirksen, 2000)

**decrepitate percussion** /dēkrep′itit/, a crackling noise produced by tapping the thoracic or abdominal wall of a patient with a respiratory disorder.

**decrudescence** /dē′krōōdes′əns/ [L, *de,* from, *crudescere,* to become bad], a decrease in the severity of symptoms.

**decubital** /dikyōō′bitəl/ [L, *decumbere,* to lie down], pertaining to bedsores.

**decubitus** /dikyōō′bitəs/ [L, *decumbere,* to lie down], a recumbent or horizontal position, as lateral decubitus, lying on one side.

**decubitus angina,** a condition characterized by periodic attacks of cardiac pain that occur when a person is lying down.

**decubitus position,** a position used in producing a radiograph of the chest or abdomen of a patient who is lying down, with the central ray horizontal. The patient may be prone (ventral decubitus), supine (dorsal decubitus), or on the left or right side (left or right lateral decubitus). Also called **decubitus projection.**

**decubitus posture,** the position assumed by a bedridden patient to rest on his or her side to relieve the pressure of body weight on the sacrum, heels, or other areas vulnerable to pressure (decubitus) ulcers.

**decubitus projection.** See **decubitus position.**

**decubitus ulcer.** See **pressure ulcer.**

**decubitus ulcer care.** See **pressure ulcer care.**

**decussate** /dəkus′āt/ [L, *decussis,* intersection], to cross in the form of an "X," as certain nerve fibers from the retina cross at the optic chiasm. **—decussation,** *n.*

**decussation** /di′kusā′shən/ [L, *decussare,* to make a cross], a crossing of central nervous system fibers in the brain, as some fibers on the left side cross to the right side, and vice versa.

**decussation of pyramids** [L, *decussare,* to make a cross; Gk, *pyramis*], the crossing of nerve fibers of the corticospinal motor tract at the ventral side on the lower portion of the medulla oblongata.

**dedifferentiation.** See **anaplasia.**

**deductible** /dēduk′tibəl/, an amount paid each year by a health insurance plan enrollee before benefits begin. It is not synonymous with copayment.

**deduction** [L, *deducere,* to lead], a system of reasoning that leads from a known principle to an unknown, or from the general to the specific. Deductive reasoning is used to test diagnostic hypotheses.

**deemed status** /dēmd/ [AS, *deman,* to judge; L, *status,* a standing], a status conferred on a hospital or other organization by a professional standards review organization (PSRO) in formal recognition that the organization's review, continued-stay review, and medical care evaluation programs meet certain effectiveness criteria.

**deep bite.** See **closed bite.**

**deep brachial artery** [As, *dyppan,* to dip; Gk, *brachion,* arm, *arteria,* airpipe], a branch of each of the brachial arteries, arising at the distal border of the teres major, passing deeply into the arm between the long and lateral heads of the triceps brachii, and supplying the humerus and muscles of the upper arm. It has five branches: ascending, radial collateral, middle collateral, muscular, and nutrient. Also called **superior profunda artery.**

**deep breathing and coughing exercises,** movements used to improve pulmonary gas exchange or to maintain respiratory function, especially after prolonged inactivity or general anesthesia. Incisional pain after surgery in the chest or abdomen often inhibits normal respiratory movements. See also **cupping and vibrating, postural drainage.**

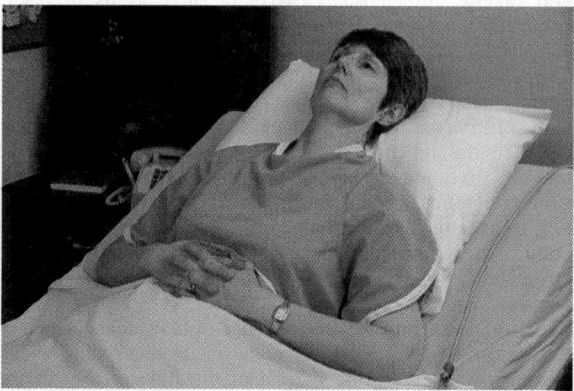

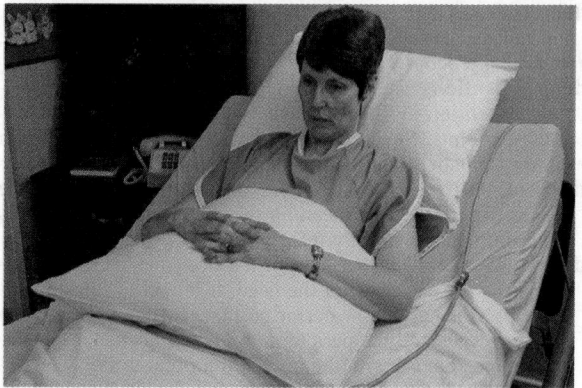

**Deep breathing and coughing exercises**
(Sorrentino 2000)

■ METHOD: The patient is assisted to a comfortable position, supine or sitting up. An analgesic may be given before the exercises if pain is present. Inhalation through the nose and exhalation through the mouth are encouraged. With the incision supported, the patient is asked to cough after a deep inhalation. If pain prevents the patient from producing a deep, effective cough, a series of short barklike coughs may be encouraged.

■ INTERVENTIONS: Simple techniques and encouragement significantly improve the effectiveness of the exercises. Positioning increases comfort, allows the abdominal contents to fall away from the diaphragm, and encourages full expansion of the chest wall on inspiration. If an incision is present, it may be supported with the hands or with a book or pillow held against the abdomen. The patient is often reluctant to breathe deeply or to cough; adequate analgesia, encouragement, and explanation of the benefits of the exercises may overcome that resistance. Various devices are available for use in deep breathing and coughing, such as those used during atelectasis to strengthen the muscles used in expiration and to empty the alveoli of retained gas. Postural drainage is commonly performed concurrently with the exercises.

■ OUTCOME CRITERIA: When shallow breathing replaces deep breathing, mucus tends to dry in the airway, damaging the membranes that line the passages. Coughing and deep breathing improve ventilation and gas exchange by clearing the mucus and allowing moisturized air to enter the bronchi, bronchioles, and alveoli.

**deep fascia,** the most extensive of three kinds of fascia comprising an intricate series of connective sheets and bands that hold the muscles and other structures in place throughout the body, wrapping the muscles in gray, feltlike membranes. The deep fasciae comprise a continuous system, splitting and fusing in an elaborate network attached to the skeleton and divided into the outer investing layer, the internal investing layer, and the intermediate membranes. Compare **subcutaneous fascia, subserous fascia.**

**deep heat,** the application of heat in the treatment of deep body tissues, particularly muscles and tendons. The thermal effects may be produced with shortwave therapy, phonophoresis, or ultrasound.

**deepithelialization.** See **epithelial debridement.**

**deep palmar arch,** the termination of the radial artery, joining the deep palmar branch of the ulnar artery in the palm of the hand.

**deep reflexes** [ME, *dep,* hollow; L, *reflectere,* to bend back], any reflexes caused by stimulation of a deep body structure, such as a tendon reflex.

**deep sensation,** the awareness or perception of pain, pressure, or tension in the deep layers of the skin, muscles, tendons, or joints. Such sensations are conveyed to the brain via the spinal column. Compare **superficial sensation.**

**deep structure,** (in linguistics and neurolinguistics) the deeper experience and meaning to which surface structures in a communication may refer.

**deep temporal artery,** one of the branches of the maxillary artery on each side of the head. It branches into the anterior portion and the posterior portion, both rising between the temporalis and the pericranium to supply the temporalis and to anastomose with the middle temporal artery. The anterior branch communicates with the lacrimal artery by small branches that pierce the zygomatic bone and the great wing of the sphenoid. Compare **middle temporal artery, superficial temporal artery.**

**deep tendon reflex (DTR),** a brisk contraction of a muscle in response to a sudden stretch induced by a sharp tap by a finger or rubber hammer on the tendon of insertion of the muscle. Absence of the reflex may be caused by damage to the muscle, peripheral nerve, nerve roots, or spinal cord at that level. A hyperactive reflex may indicate disease of the pyramidal tract above the level of the reflex arc being tested. Generalized hyperactivity of DTRs may be caused by hyperthyroidism. Kinds of DTRs include **Achilles tendon**

**reflex, biceps reflex, brachioradialis reflex, patellar reflex,** and **triceps reflex.** Also called **myostatic reflex, tendon reflex.**

**deep vein,** one of the many systemic veins that accompany the arteries, usually enclosed in a sheath that wraps both the vein and the associated artery. Various structures, such as the skull, vertebral column, and liver, are served by less closely associated arteries and veins. Compare **superficial vein.**

**deep vein thrombosis,** a disorder involving a thrombus in one of the deep veins of the body, most commonly the iliac or femoral vein. Symptoms include tenderness, pain, swelling, warmth, and discoloration of the skin. A deep vein thrombus is potentially life threatening. Treatment, including bed rest and use of thrombolytic and anticoagulant drugs, is directed to preventing movement of the thrombus toward the lungs.

**deep x-ray therapy,** the treatment of internal neoplasms, such as Wilms' tumor of the kidney, Hodgkin's disease, and other cancers, with ionizing radiation from an external source. The dose delivered is determined according to the radiosensitivity, size, pathologic grade, and differentiation of the tumor; the tolerance of normal surrounding tissue to irradiation; and the patient's condition. Deep x-ray therapy frequently causes nausea, malaise, diarrhea, and skin reactions, such as blanching, erythema, itching, burning, oozing, or desquamation, but with modern techniques the ray is beamed directly to the site, reducing side scatter, and the skin can be spared. Because tumor cells are hypoxic and are more effectively eradicated when they are well oxygenated, the patient may breathe hyperbaric oxygen or atmospheric oxygen with 5% carbon dioxide during therapy.

**deerfly fever.** See **tularemia.**

**defaecation.** See **defecation.**

**defamation** /def′əmā′shən/ [L, *diffamare,* to discredit], any communication, written or spoken, that is untrue and that injures the good name or reputation of another or that in any way brings that person into disrepute.

**default judgment** /difôlt′/ [L, *defallere,* to lack, *judicare,* to decide], (in law) a judgment rendered against a defendant as a result of the defendant's failure to appear in court or to answer the plaintiff's claim within the proper time.

**defecation** /def′ikā′shən/ [L, *defaecare,* to clean], the elimination of feces from the digestive tract through the rectum. Also spelled **defaecation.** See also **constipation, diarrhea, feces.** —**defecate** /def′ikāt/, *v.*

**defecation reflex.** See **rectal reflex.**

**defecography** /def′əkog′rəfē/, the radiographic examination of the rectum and anal canal of patients with defecative dysfunction. A barium sulfate paste is instilled directly into the rectum, and the patient is seated on a radiolucent commode in front of a fluoroscope. Lateral projections of the rectum and anal canal are recorded during defecation.

**defective** /difek′tiv/ [L, *defectus,* a failing], pertaining to something that is imperfect, or, as in an outdated term, to an individual who may be suffering from any disorder.

**defendant** /difen′dənt/, (in law) the party named in a plaintiff's complaint and against whom the plaintiff's allegations are made. The defendant must respond to the allegations.

**defense** /də·fens′/ [L, *defendere,* to ward off], the practice of, or measures taken to ensure, self-protection.

**defense mechanism** [L, *defendere,* to repulse, *mechanicus,* machine], an unconscious intrapsychic reaction that offers protection to the self from stress or a threat. Defense mechanisms are of two types: those that diminish anxiety and are used by an individual to integrate more fully into society, and those that do not reduce anxiety but simply postpone the effects of feeling it. Anxiety-reducing defenses include compensation, identification, introjection, some forms of repression, and sublimation. Defenses that postpone full expression of anxiety include denial, displacement, isolation, projection, reaction formation, rationalization, regression, some forms of repression, suppression, and undoing.

**defense reflex,** an autonomic defensive response by an animal when threatened. The response may consist of dilated pupils, baring of claws, or raising of feathers or hair.

**defensin** /difen′sin/, a peptide with natural antibiotic activity found within human neutrophils. Three types of defensins have been identified, each consisting of a chain of about 30 amino acids. Similar molecules occur in white blood cells of other animal species. They show activity toward viruses and fungi, in addition to bacteria.

**defensive radical therapy** /difen′siv/, (in psychology) a view of the therapeutic process in which as a survival tactic the therapist begins at the patient's present state and encourages the patient to avoid self-defeating behavior. The goal is to create social awareness clients can use in coping with oppressive environments.

**deferens** /def′ərenz/ [L], carrying away. Also **deferent.**

**deferent duct.** See **vas deferens.**

**deferoxamine mesylate** /dē′fərok′səmēn/, a chelating agent with specific affinity for ferric iron and low affinity for calcium.

■ INDICATIONS: It is prescribed in the treatment of acute iron intoxication and chronic iron overload.

■ CONTRAINDICATIONS: Renal disease or anuria prohibits its use.

■ ADVERSE EFFECTS: Among the most serious adverse reactions are hypotension, tachycardia, dysuria, visual difficulties, and anaphylactoid reactions.

**defervescence** /di′fərves′əns/ [L, *defervescere,* to reduce heat], the diminishing or disappearance of a fever. —**defervescent,** *adj.*

**defibrillate** /difī′brilāt, difib′-/ [L, *de* + *fibrilla,* little thread], to stop fibrillation of the ventricles by delivering an electrical shock through the chest wall. See also **defibrillation.**

**defibrillation** /difī′brilā′shən/, the termination of ventricular fibrillation (inefficient, asynchronous contraction) by delivery of an electric shock to the patient's precordium. It is a common emergency measure generally performed by a physician or specially trained nurse or paramedic. The defibrillator paddles are usually applied over special defibrillator pads. In external defibrillation, one paddle is placed to the right of the upper sternum below the clavicle, and the other is applied to the midaxillary line of the left lower rib cage. In internal defibrillation, which may be performed during open-heart surgery, the paddles are placed directly on the heart. The defibrillator, usually a condenser-discharge system, is set to deliver between 200 and 360 J. If shocks fail to restore a perfusion rhythm, cardiopulmonary resuscitation is begun. Repeat shocks also are attempted periodically until ventricular fibrillation ceases. —**defibrillate,** *v.*

**defibrillator** /difī′brilā′tər, difib′-/, a device that delivers an electrical shock at a preset voltage to the myocardium. It is used for restoring the normal cardiac rhythm and rate when the heart has stopped beating or is fibrillating. See also **implantable cardioverter-defibrillator.**

**defibrination,** the removal of fiber from a body fluid, as removal of fibrin from blood to prevent clotting.

**defibrination syndrome.** See **disseminated intravascular coagulation (DIC).**

**deficiency** /difish′ənsē/, a lack or shortage of something.

**deficiency disease** [L, *de* + *facere,* to make, *dis,* opposite

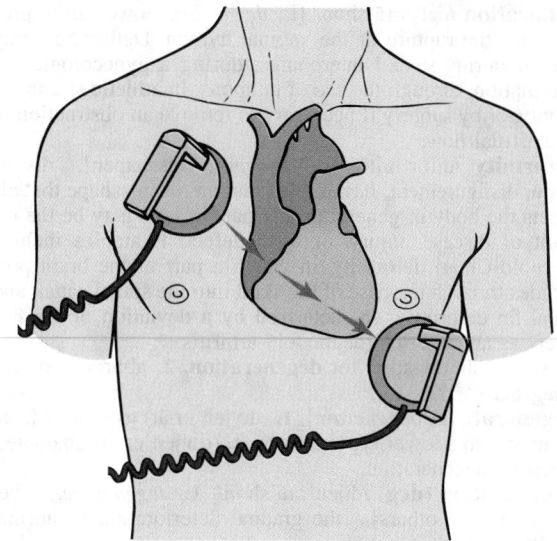

**Paddle placement and current flow in defibrillation**
*(Lewis, Heitkemper, and Dirksen, 2000)*

of; Fr, *aise,* ease], a condition resulting from the lack of one or more essential nutrients in the diet, from metabolic dysfunction, or from impaired digestion or absorption, excessive excretion, or increased biologic requirements. Compare **malnutrition.** See also **avitaminosis.**

**deficiency of sweating** [AS, *swaetan*], a failure of the sweat glands to secrete perspiration in normal amounts. The condition may be the result of a congenital defect, a blockage of the sweat ducts as a sequel to prickly heat, excessive heat, autonomic neuropathy, or conditions such as hemorrhage or diarrhea that cause body fluid loss. Also called **anhidrosis.**

**deficit** /def′isit/, any deficiency or difference from what is normal, such as an oxygen deficit, a cause of hypoxia.

**defined formula diet,** nutritional support provided by simple elemental nutritive components that require no further digestive breakdown and thus are readily absorbed. Examples include free amino acids from hydrolyzed protein and the simple sugar glucose, a carbohydrate. Also called **elemental formula** or **chemically defined formula diet.**

**definitive** /difin′ətiv/ [L, *definitivus,* a limiting], **1.** final; clearly established without doubt or question. **2.** (in embryology) fully formed in the final differentiation of a tissue, structure, or organ. Compare **primitive. 3.** (in parasitology) pertaining to the host in which the parasite undergoes the sexual phase of its reproductive cycle.

**definitive host,** any animal in which the reproductive stages of a parasite develop. The female *Anopheles* mosquito is the definitive host for malaria. Humans are definitive hosts for pinworms, schistosomes, and tapeworms. Also called **primary host.** Compare **dead-end host, intermediate host, reservoir host.** See also **host.**

**definitive prosthesis,** a permanent prosthetic device that replaces an immediate-fit appliance such as a pylon. In some cases a definitive prosthesis is used only when full weight-bearing on an artificial limb is feasible, which may follow amputation by 6 weeks or longer.

**definitive treatment,** any therapy generally accepted as a specific cure of a disease. Compare **expectant treatment, palliative treatment.**

**defloration** /def'lôrā'shən/ [L, *de* + *flos,* flower, *atio,* process],   the rupture of the vaginal hymen. Defloration may occur during sexual intercourse, during a gynecologic examination, through the use of tampons, in athletic sports activity, or by surgery if necessary to remove an obstruction to menstrual flow.

**deformity** /difôr'mitē/ [L, *deformis,* misshapen],   distortion, disfigurement, flaw, malformation, or misshape that affects the body in general or any part of it. It may be the result of disease, injury, or birth defect. Examples include Arnold-Chiari deformity, in which a part of the brain protrudes through the base of the skull into the spinal canal, and seal-fin deformity, characterized by a deviation of the fingers as an effect of rheumatoid arthritis.

**deg,**   **1.** abbreviation for **degeneration. 2.** abbreviation for **degree.**

**degenerate** [L, *degenerare*], **1.** (də·jen'er·āt) to change from a higher to a lower type or form. **2.** (də·jen'er·ət) characterized by degeneration.

**degeneration (deg)** /dijen'ərā'shən/ [L, *degenerare,* to become unlike others],   the gradual deterioration of normal cells and body functions.

**degenerative** /dijen'ərətiv/ [L, *degenerare,* to become unlike others],   pertaining to or involving degeneration or change to a lower or dysfunctional form.

**degenerative chorea.**   See **Huntington's chorea.**

**degenerative disease,**   any disease in which deterioration of structure or function of tissue occurs. Kinds of degenerative diseases include **arteriosclerosis, cancer,** and **osteoarthritis.**

**degenerative joint disease.**   See **osteoarthritis.**

**degenerative lesion** [L, *degenerare,* to become unlike others, *laesio,* hurting],   an injury or disease state that results in loss of function.

**degenerative neuralgia** [L, *degenerare,* to become unlike others; Gk, *neuron,* nerve, *algos,* pain],   a form of neuralgia caused by degenerative changes in nervous tissue, which usually affects older people.

**degenerative neuritis** [L, *degenerare,* to become unlike others; Gk, *neuron,* nerve, *itis,* inflammation],   an inflammation caused by degenerative changes in nervous tissue.

**degloving** /dēglov'ing/ [L, *de* + AS, *glof*],   **1.** an injury to an extremity—finger, hand, arm, leg, or foot—in which the soft tissue down to the bone, including neurovascular bundles and sometimes tendons, is peeled off. **2.** (in dentistry) the exposure of the bony mandibular anterior or posterior regions by oral surgery or trauma. **3.** removal of latex or vinyl hand coverings.

**deglutition** /di'glōōtish'ən/ [L, *deglutire,* to swallow],   swallowing.

**deglutition apnea,**   the normal absence of respiration during swallowing.

**Degos' disease.**   See **malignant atrophic papulosis.**

**degradation** /di'grədā'shən/ [L, *de* + *gradu,* step],   the reduction of a chemical compound to a less complex compound, usually by splitting off one or more groups or subgroups of atoms, as in deamination.

**degranulation** /dēgran'yəlā'shən/,   the release of granules from cells, such as mast cells and basophils.

**degree (deg)** [Fr, *degre*],   one of the divisions or intervals marked on a scale of units of measurement.

**degrees of freedom (df),**   a statistical measure of the number of independent observations or choices among members in a sample. It is used in determining the statistical significance of findings during data analysis.

**degustation** /dē'gəstā'shən/ [L, *degustare,* to taste],   the act of tasting.

**dehiscence** /dihis'əns/ [L, *dehiscere,* to gape],   the separation of a surgical incision or rupture of a wound closure, typically an abdominal incision.

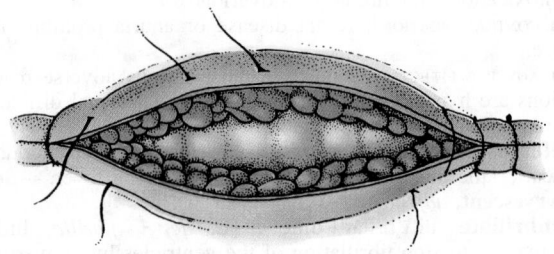

**Wound dehiscence** *(Ignatavicius, Workman, and Mishler, 1999)*

**dehumanization** /dihyōō'mənīzā'shən/ [L, *de,* from, *humanitas,* human nature],   the process of losing altruistic or individual qualities, as may occur in some psychotic states or in enviroments that produce emtional trauma (prisoner-of-war). Maybe influenced by external forces.

**dehumidifier** /dē'yōōmid'ifī'ər/,   an apparatus to remove moisture in the atmosphere.

**dehydrate** /dihī'drāt/ [L, *de* + Gk, *hydor,* water],   **1.** to remove or lose water from a substance. **2.** to lose excessive water from the body.

**dehydrated alcohol,**   a clear, colorless, highly hygroscopic liquid with a burning taste, containing at least 99.5% ethyl alcohol by volume. Also called **absolute alcohol.**

**dehydration** /di'hīdrā'shən/,   **1.** excessive loss of water from body tissues. Dehydration is accompanied by a disturbance in the balance of essential electrolytes, particularly sodium, potassium, and chloride. It may follow prolonged fever, diarrhea, vomiting, acidosis, and any condition in which there is rapid depletion of body fluids. It is of particular concern among infants and young children, because their electrolyte balance is normally precarious. Signs of dehydration include poor skin turgor (not a reliable sign in the elderly), flushed dry skin, coated tongue, dry mucous membranes, oliguria, irritability, and confusion. Normal fluid

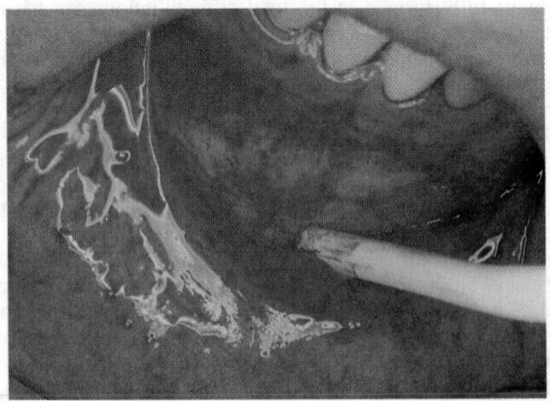

**Degloving injury of the mouth** *(Zitelli and Davis, 1997)*

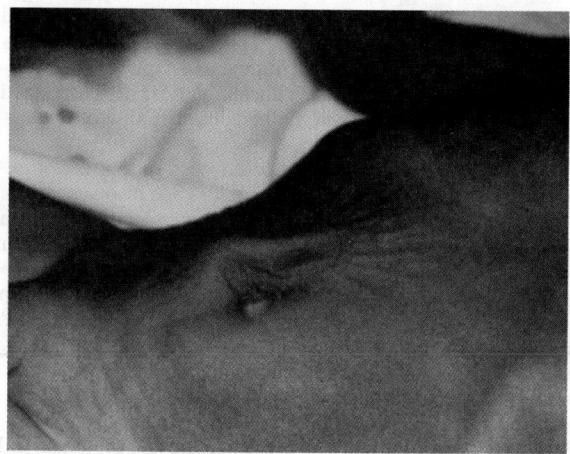

**Dehydration: resulting poor skin turgor**
*(Zitelli and Davis, 1997)*

volume and balanced electrolyte values are the primary goals of therapy. **2.** rendering a substance free from water.

**dehydration fever,** a fever that frequently occurs in newborns, thought to be caused by dehydration. Also called **inanition fever.** Compare **inanition, starvation.**

**dehydration of gingivae,** the drying of gum tissue, often the result of mouth breathing. Dehydration lowers the resistance of the gingivae to infection.

**dehydrogenate,** to remove hydrogen atoms, as in the oxidation processes.

**deinstitutionalization** /dē·in'stityōō'shənal'īzā'shən/ [L, *de* + *instituere,* to put in place], a change in the location and focus of mental health care from an institutional to a community setting.

**Deiters' nucleus** /dī'tərz, dē'terz/ [Otto F.C. Deiters, German anatomist, 1834–1863], one of the vestibular nuclei located in the brainstem.

**DEJ,** abbreviation for **dentinoenamel junction.**

**déjà vu** /dāzhävY', -vē', -vōō'/ [Fr, previously seen], the sensation or illusion that one is encountering a set of circumstances or a place that was previously experienced. The phenomenon, which is normal in everyone but occurs more frequently or continuously in certain emotional and organic disorders, results from some unconscious emotional connection with the present experience. Compare **jamais vu, paramnesia.**

**Déjérine-Klumpke's paralysis.** See **Klumpke's palsy.**

**Déjérine-Roussy syndrome.** See **thalamic syndrome.**

**Déjérine-Sottas disease** /dezh'ərinsot'əz, -sotäz'/ [Joseph J. Dejerine, French neurologist, 1849–1917; Jules Sottas, French neurologist, 1866–1943], a rare congenital spinocerebellar disorder. It is characterized by the development of palpable thickenings along peripheral nerves, degeneration of the peripheral nervous system, pain, paresthesia, ataxia, and diminished sensation and deep tendon reflexes. Diagnosis is made by a histologic examination of a peripheral nerve. There is no specific treatment. Also called **progressive interstitial hypertrophic neuropathy.**

**deka-,** combining form indicating the multiple 10.

**del,** abbreviation for **deletion.**

**Delaney clause,** a 1960 amendment to the 1938 Federal Food, Drug, and Cosmetic Act regulating food additives. It prohibits the use of any food substance found to be carcinogenic in humans or animals. Food products not previously found to be carcinogenic were classified as historically "Generally Regarded As Safe," or *GRAS.*

**Delano, Jane A.** (1862–1919), an American nurse who organized the American Red Cross Nursing Service, an association formed to supply nurses to the military forces. She became director of the Nurses' Training School of the University of Pennsylvania in 1891 and was later appointed director of the Bellevue Hospital Training School for Nurses in New York, where she had been trained. On a trip to survey nursing conditions in Europe, she died after surgery for a mastoid infection at Base Hospital, Savenay, France, in March 1919.

**delavirdine,** a nonnucleoside reverse transcriptase inhibitor (NNRTI).

## Clinical manifestations of dehydration

| | Isotonic (loss of water and salt) | Hypotonic (loss of salt in excess of water) | Hypertonic (loss of water in excess of salt) |
|---|---|---|---|
| **Skin** | | | |
| Color | Gray | Gray | Gray |
| Temperature | Cold | Cold | Cold or hot |
| Turgor | Poor | Very poor | Fair |
| Feel | Dry | Clammy | Thickened, doughy |
| Mucous membranes | Dry | Slightly moist | Parched |
| Tearing and salivation | Absent | Absent | Absent |
| Eyeball | Sunken | Sunken | Sunken |
| Fontanel | Sunken | Sunken | Sunken |
| Body temperature | Subnormal or elevated | Subnormal or elevated | Subnormal or elevated |
| Pulse | Rapid | Very rapid | Moderately rapid |
| Respirations | Rapid | Rapid | Rapid |
| Behavior | Irritable to lethargic | Lethargic to comatose; convulsions | Marked lethary with extreme hyperirritability on stimulation |

From Wong DL: *Whaley and Wong's essentials of pediatric nursing,* ed 5, St Louis, 1997, Mosby.

■ INDICATIONS: Delavirdine is used to treat HIV-1 in combination with zidovudine or didanosine.

■ CONTRAINDICATIONS: Known hypersensitivity to this drug or to atevirdine prohibits the use of delavirdine.

■ ADVERSE EFFECTS: Life-threatening effects are hepatotoxicity, neutropenia, leukopenia, thrombocytopenia, anemia, granulocytopenia, and nephrotoxicity. Other adverse effects include diarrhea, abdominal pain, nausea, fatigue, headache, rash, pain, myalgia, vomiting, and dyspepsia.

**delayed dentition.** See **retarded dentition.**

**delayed development, risk for,** a nursing diagnosis accepted by the Thirteenth National Conference on the Classification of Nursing Diagnoses. It is defined as being at risk for delay of 25% or more in one or more of the areas of social or self-regulatory behavior, or in cognitive, language, gross or fine motor skills.

■ RISK FACTORS: Prenatal risk factors include a maternal age of less than 15 or greater than 35 years of age; substance abuse; infections; genetic or endocrine disorders; unplanned or unwanted pregnancy; lack of, late, or poor prenatal care; inadequate nutrition; illiteracy; and poverty. Individual risk factors include prematurity; seizures; congenital or genetic disorders; positive drug screening test; brain damage; vision impairment; hearing impairment or frequent otitis media; chronic illness; being technology dependent; failure to thrive, inadequate nutrition; foster or adopted child; lead poisoning; chemotherapy; radiation therapy; natural disasters; behavior disorders; and substance abuse. Other risk factors include poverty, violence, abuse, mental illness, mental retardation or severe learning disability. See also **nursing diagnosis.**

**delayed echolalia** [Fr, *delai*, time extension; Gk, *echo*, sound, *lalein*, to babble], a phenomenon, commonly seen in schizophrenia, involving the meaningless automatic repetition of overheard words and phrases. It occurs hours, days, or even weeks after the original stimulus.

**delayed graft** [ME, *delaein*, to leave; Gk, *graphein*, stylus], a type of skin graft that is partially elevated and reinserted later in the same place.

**delayed hypersensitivity,** the type of hypersensitivity which (as opposed to immediate hypersensitivity) takes 24 to 72 hours to develop and is mediated by T lymphocytes rather than by antibodies. Compare **immediate hypersensitivity.**

**delayed hypersensitivity reaction,** a reaction of cellular immunity, named in contrast to immediate hypersensitivity reactions because its onset is 24 to 72 hours after the antigenic challenge; the term is usually used to denote the subset of type IV hypersensitivity reactions (see **hypersensitivity reaction**) involving cytokine release and macrophage activation, as opposed to direct cytolysis, but can be used more broadly, even sometimes being used as a synonym for type IV hypersensitivity reaction. The classic delayed hypersensitivity reaction is the tuberculin reaction observed in skin testing.

**delayed language,** failure of language to develop at the expected age. The cause is often unknown.

**delayed onset muscle soreness,** muscle weakness, restricted range of motion, and tenderness on palpation, occurring 24 to 48 hours after intense or prolonged muscular activity.

**delayed postpartum hemorrhage,** hemorrhage occurring later than 24 hours after giving birth. It is most often caused by retained fragments of the placenta, a laceration of the cervix or vagina that was not discovered or was not completely sutured, or subinvolution of the placental site within the uterus. Characteristics of delayed postpartum hemor-

rhage are heavy bleeding and signs of impending shock and anemia. The cause is diagnosed and treated. A laceration is closed with suture, retained fragments of placenta are removed, infection is treated with antibiotics, or the relaxed uterus is caused to contract by the administration of ergonovine (Ergotrate) or oxytocin.

**delayed sensation,** a feeling or impression that is not experienced immediately after a stimulus. See also **sensation.**

**delayed symptom** [Fr, *delai* + Gk, *symptoma*, that which happens], a symptom such as shock that may not appear until after the precipitating cause.

**delayed treatment seeker,** (in psychology) a person who delays seeking treatment for a problematic life event such as a sexual assault until months or years after the event, usually after a precipitating event such as an anniversary reaction.

**delayed-type hypersensitivity (DTH),** a delayed hypersensitivity. See also **cell-mediated immune response.**

**Delecato-Doman theory,** a therapeutic concept that full neurologic organization of a disabled or mentally retarded child requires that the child pass through developmental patterns covering progressively higher anatomic levels of the nervous system. The first five levels take the child from infantile reflexes through walking; the sixth covers cortical hemispheric dominance.

**delegation,** a nursing intervention from the Nursing Interventions Classification (NIC) defined as transfer of responsibility for the performance of patient care while retaining accountability for the outcome. See also **Nursing Interventions Classification.**

**deleterious** /del′itir′ē·əs/ [Gk, *deleterios*, destroyer], harmful or dangerous.

**deletion (del)** /dilē′shən/ [L, *deletionum*, destruction], the loss of a piece of a chromosome.

**deletion syndrome,** any of a group of congenital autosomal anomalies that result from the loss of part of a chromosome as a result of breakage of a chromatid during meiosis. An example is cat-cry syndrome, which results from the absence of the short arm of chromosome 5.

**Delhi boil.** See **oriental sore.**

**deliberate biologic programming** /dilib′ərit/ [L, *deliberare*, to weigh carefully], the Hayflick theory of aging, based on studies showing that human cells contain biologic clocks that predetermine death after undergoing mitosis a finite number of times.

**deliberate hypotension,** a technique in general anesthesia in which a short-acting hypotensive agent such as sodium nitroprusside; nitroglycerin, or trimethaphan camsylate is given to reduce blood pressure and thus bleeding during surgery. The procedure facilitates surgery by making vessels and tissues more visible and reducing blood loss. Also called **hypotensive anesthesia,** hypotensive technique.

**delinquency** /diling′kwənsē/ [L, *delinquere*, to fail], **1.** negligence or failure to fulfill a duty or obligation. **2.** an offense, fault, misdemeanor, or misdeed; a tendency to commit such acts. See also **juvenile delinquency.**

**delinquent** /diling′kwənt/, **1.** characterized by neglect of duty or violation of law. **2.** one whose behavior is characterized by persistent antisocial, illegal, violent, or criminal acts; a juvenile delinquent.

**délire de toucher** /dālir′ də tŏŏshā′/ [Fr], an abnormal desire or irresistible urge to touch objects.

**delirious.** See **delirium.**

**delirious mania** /dilir′ē·əs/, an extreme form of the manic state in which activity is so frenzied, confused, and incoherent that it is difficult to discern any link between affect and behavior.

**delirium** /dilir′ē·əm/ [L, *delirare*, to rave], **1.** a state of frenzied excitement or wild enthusiasm. **2.** an acute organic mental disorder characterized by confusion, disorientation, restlessness, clouding of the consciousness, incoherence, fear, anxiety, excitement, and often by illusions; hallucinations, usually of visual origin; and at times delusions. The condition is caused by disturbances in cerebral functions that may result from a wide range of metabolic disorders, including nutritional deficiencies and endocrine imbalances; postpartum or postoperative stress; ingestion of toxic substances, as various gases, metals, or drugs, including alcohol; and other causes of physical and mental shock or exhaustion. The symptoms are usually of short duration and reversible with treatment of the underlying cause; in extreme cases, however, in which the toxic condition is exceedingly severe or prolonged, permanent brain damage may occur. Kinds of delirium include **acute delirium, delirium tremens, exhaustion delirium, senile delirium,** and **traumatic delirium.** Compare **dementia. —delirious,** *adj.*

**delirium constantium,** (in psychiatry) a patient's reiteration of a fixed idea.

**delirium management,** a nursing intervention from the Nursing Interventions Classification (NIC) defined as provision of a safe and therapeutic environment for the patient who is experiencing an acute confusional state. See also **Nursing Interventions Classification.**

**delirium of persecution** [L, *delirare,* to rave, *persecutor,* to pursue], a state of clouded consciousness or decreased sensorium in which the person believes others are threatening or conspiring against him or her.

**delirium tremens (DTs),** an acute and sometimes fatal psychotic reaction caused by cessation of excessive intake of alcoholic beverages over a long period. Initial symptoms include loss of appetite, insomnia, and general restlessness, which are followed by agitation; excitement; disorientation; mental confusion; vivid and often frightening hallucinations; acute fear and anxiety; illusions and delusions; coarse tremors of the hands, feet, legs, and tongue; fever; increased heart rate; extreme perspiration; GI distress; and precordial pain. The episode, which usually constitutes a medical emergency, typically lasts from 3 to 6 days and is generally followed by a deep sleep. See also **Korsakoff's psychosis.**

**delivery** /diliv′ərē/ [L, *de* + *liberare,* to free], (in obstetrics) the birth of a child; parturition. See also **Bradley method, Lamaze method, Leboyer method, Read method.**

**delivery room,** a unit of a hospital used for childbirth and infant resuscitation.

**DeLorme technique,** a method of exercise with weights for the purpose of strengthening muscles in which sets of repetitions are repeated with rests between sets. The technique involves isotonic exercise and determination of the maximum level of resistance (RM). See also **progressive resistance exercise.**

**delousing** /dēlou′sing/ [L, *de,* from; AS, *lus*], to rid a person or object of an infestation of lice.

**delta** /del′tə/, Δ, δ, fourth letter of the Greek alphabet.

**delta-1-testolactone.** See **testolactone.**

**delta-9-tetrahydrocannabinol (THC),** a pharmacologically active ingredient of cannabis that has been used in treating some cases of nausea and vomiting associated with cancer chemotherapy. See **cannabis.**

**delta agent hepatitis** [L, *agere,* to do; Gk, *hēpar,* liver, *itis,* inflammation], a disease caused by infection with a ribonucleic acid virus (δ Ag) as a co-infection with hepatitis B virus in cases of chronic hepatitis and progressive liver damage. The delta agent is able to induce infection only when it is a co-infection present along with hepatitis B.

**delta hepatitis.** See **viral hepatitis.**

**delta optical density analysis** [Gk, *delta,* fourth letter of Greek alphabet, *optikos,* of sight; L, *densus,* thick; Gk, a loosening], a technique used to diagnose anemia in a fetus by measuring the proportion of bilirubin decomposition products in the amniotic fluid. The method involves spectrographic examination of a fluid sample. It measures the bilirubin and bilirubin-products concentration according to the wavelengths of light absorbed by the hemolytic products, as the bilirubin products alter the normal color of the amniotic fluid. The data are sometimes expressed in terms of $\delta OD_{450}$, the number representing the wavelength in nanometers at which maximum absorption of light by bilirubin occurs. If the delta optical density analysis indicates the fetus is moderately to severely anemic, immediate delivery is usually recommended when the gestational age permits. Otherwise intrauterine fetal blood transfusions may be recommended.

***Deltavirus*** /del′tə·vī′rəs/ [hepatitis *delta* + *virus*], a genus of satellite viruses that require a helper hepatitis B virus for their replication; an individual consists of spherical virion about 34 nm in diameter with an envelope derived from the helper virus surrounding a spherical core 18 nm in diameter; the genome consists of a single molecule of single-stranded, negative sense, circular RNA (size 1.7 kb). It contains a single species, hepatitis D virus. See also **hepatitis D.**

**delta wave,** **1.** also called **delta rhythm.** The slowest of the four types of brain waves, characterized by a frequency of 4 Hz and a relatively high voltage. Delta waves are "deep-sleep waves" associated with a dreamless state from which an individual is not easily aroused. Compare **alpha wave, beta wave, theta wave. 2.** (in cardiology) a slurring of the QRS portion of an electrocardiogram tracing caused by preexcitation in Wolff-Parkinson-White syndrome.

**deltoid** /del′toid/ [Gk, *delta,* triangular, *eidos,* form], **1.** triangular. **2.** pertaining to the deltoid muscle that covers the shoulder.

**deltoideus.** See **deltoid muscle.**

**deltoid ligament** [Gk, *delta* + L, *ligamentum*], the medial ligament of the ankle joint.

**deltoid muscle,** a large, thick triangular muscle that covers the shoulder joint. It is the prime mover of arm abduction. It is also a synergist of arm flexion, extension, and circumduction. Also called **deltoideus.**

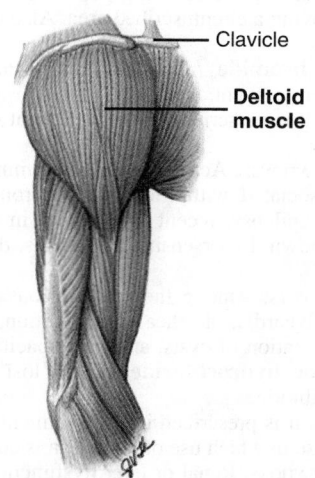

**Deltoid muscle** *(Thibodeau and Patton, 1999/John V. Hagen)*

**delusion** /dilōo′zhən/ [L, *deludere,* to deceive], a persistent aberrant belief or perception held inviolable by a person despite evidence that refutes it. Kinds of delusion include **delusion of being controlled, delusion of grandeur, delusion of persecution, nihilistic delusion, paranoid delusion,** and **somatic delusion.** Compare **illusion.**

**delusion management,** a nursing intervention from the Nursing Interventions Classification (NIC) defined as promoting the comfort, safety, and reality orientation of a patient experiencing false, fixed beliefs that have little or no basis in reality. See also **Nursing Interventions Classification.**

**delusion of being controlled,** the false belief that one's feelings, beliefs, thoughts, and acts are governed by some external force, as experienced in various forms of schizophrenia. See also **delusion.**

**delusion of grandeur** /grän′dyŏor/, the gross exaggeration of one's importance, wealth, power, or talents, as manifested in such disorders as megalomania, general paresis, and paranoid schizophrenia. It may have a somatic or religious theme. See also **delusion.**

**delusion of persecution,** a morbid belief that one is being mistreated, harassed, or conspired against, as seen in paranoia and paranoid schizophrenia. The patient may single out a person or group as the source of persecution. See also **delusion.**

**delusion of poverty,** (in psychology) a false belief of a person that he or she is impoverished or will be deprived of material possessions.

**delusion of reference.** See **idea of reference.**

**demand pacemaker** [L, *demandere,* to give in charge, *passus,* step; ME, *maken*], a device used to stimulate the heart electrically when the heart's own impulses are not sufficient. The device measures the interval between the heart's native beats and delivers a stimulating pulse whenever that interval exceeds a set value.

**demarcation** /dē′märkā′shən/ [L, *de,* from, *marcare,* to mark], the process of setting limits or boundaries.

**demarcation current** [L, *de* + *marcare,* to mark], an electrical current that flows from an uninjured to an injured end of a muscle. Also called **current of injury.**

**Demazin,** trademark for a fixed-combination respiratory drug containing an adrenergic and an antihistaminic (chlorpheniramine maleate).

**deme** /dēm/ [Gk, *demos,* common population], a small, local, closely related, interbreeding population of organisms, usually occupying a circumscribed area. Also called **genetic population.**

**demecarium bromide** /dē′məker′ē·əm/, an ophthalmic anticholinesterase agent.

■ INDICATION: It is prescribed in the treatment of open-angle glaucoma.

■ CONTRAINDICATIONS: Active uveal inflammation and/or glaucoma associated with iridocyclitis, bronchial asthma, peptic ulcer, epilepsy, recent myocardial infarction, pregnancy, or known hypersensitivity to this drug prohibits its use.

■ ADVERSE EFFECTS: Among the most serious adverse reactions are bradycardia, diarrhea, eye irritation, hypotension, headache, formation of cysts, and lens opacities.

**demeclocycline hydrochloride** /dēmek′lōsī′klēn/, a tetracycline antibiotic.

■ INDICATIONS: It is prescribed in the treatment of infections, including those in which use of penicillin is contraindicated.

■ CONTRAINDICATIONS: Renal or liver dysfunction, pregnancy, early childhood, or known hypersensitivity to this drug or to other tetracycline medication prohibits its use.

■ ADVERSE EFFECTS: Among the more serious adverse effects are GI disturbances, phototoxicity, potentially serious superinfections, and hypersensitivity reactions. Discoloration of teeth may occur in children exposed to the drug in utero or before 8 years of age.

**demented** /dimen′tid/ [L, *de,* away from, *mens,* mind], a form of mental disorder in which cognitive functions are affected. Central features are memory loss and inability to learn new material. Common causes are organic brain disorders.

**dementia** /dimen′shə/ [L, *de* + *mens,* mind], a progressive organic mental disorder characterized by chronic personality disintegration, confusion, disorientation, stupor, deterioration of intellectual capacity and function, and impairment of control of memory, judgment, and impulses. Dementia caused by drug intoxication, hyperthyroidism, pernicious anemia, paresis, subdural hematoma, benign brain tumor, hydrocephalus, insulin shock, and tumor of islet cells of the pancreas can be reversed by treating the condition; Alzheimer's disease, Pick's disease, and other organic forms of dementia are generally considered irreversible, progressive, and incurable. However, conditions that cause the decline may be treatable or partially reversible. Kinds of dementia include **dementia paralytica, Pick's disease, secondary dementia, senile dementia, senile dementia–Alzheimer type,** and **toxic dementia.**

**dementia management,** a nursing intervention from the Nursing Interventions Classification (NIC) defined as provision of a modified environment for the patient who is experiencing a chronic confusional state. See also **Nursing Interventions Classification.**

**dementia paralytica.** See **general paresis.**

**dementia praecox.** See **schizophrenia.**

**dementia syndrome of depression,** reversible dementia occurring in association with depression in the elderly, the cognitive deficits resolving with treatment of the depression.

**Demerol,** trademark for an opioid analgesic (meperidine).

**Demerol Hydrochloride,** trademark for an opioid analgesic (meperidine hydrochloride).

**-demic,** suffix meaning 'relating to people or a district': *philodemic, prosodemic, epidemic.*

**demigauntlet bandage** /dem′igônt′lit/ [L, *demidus,* half; Fr, *gant,* glove], a glovelike bandage over the hand that leaves the fingers free. See also **gauntlet bandage.**

**demineralization** /dēmin′əral′īzā′shən/ [L, *de* + *minera,* mine], a decrease in the amount of minerals or inorganic salts in tissues, as occurs in certain diseases.

**demise** /dimīz′/ [OFr, *demettre,* to put away], death, destruction, or end of existence.

**democratic style** /dem′okrat′ik/, people-centered leadership in which the group participates openly in decision making for group goals.

**demography** /dəmog′rəfē/ [Gk, *demos,* people, *graphein,* to record], the study of human populations, particularly the size, distribution, and characteristics of members of population groups. Demography is applied in studies of health problems involving ethnic groups; populations of a specific geographic region; religious groups with special dietary restrictions, such as Mormons (Church of Jesus Christ of Latter-Day Saints) or Seventh-Day Adventists; and members of population groups that may represent a typical cross section of the entire nation, as in the continuing study of residents of Framingham, Massachusetts, by the National Institutes of Health. Compare **epidemiology.**

**demonstrative** /dimon′strətiv/, pertaining to a concept or an action that accompanies and illustrates speech, such as indication of the size of an object with the hands. See also **circum-speech.**

**De Morgan's spots.** See **cherry angioma.**

**de Morsier's syndrome.** See **septo-optic dysplasia.**

**Demser,** trademark for an antihypertensive (metyrosine).

**demulcent** /dimul′sənt/ [L, *demulcere,* to stroke down], **1.** any of several oily substances used for soothing and reducing irritation of surfaces that have been abraded or irritated. **2.** soothing, as a counterirritant or balm.

**Demulen,** trademark for an oral contraceptive containing an estrogen (ethinyl estradiol) and a progestin (ethynodiol diacetate).

**demyelinate** /dēmī′əlināt′/, to remove or destroy the myelin surrounding the axons of nerve cells.

**demyelination** /dimī′əlinā′shən/ [L, *de* + Gk, *myelos,* marrow], the process of destruction or removal of the myelin sheath from a nerve or nerve fiber.

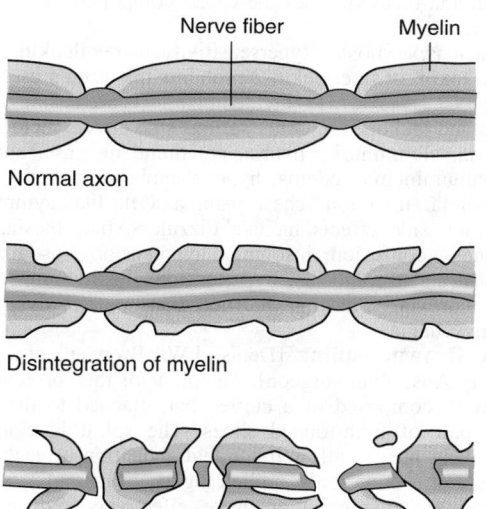

Nerve fiber    Myelin

Normal axon

Disintegration of myelin

Disruption of axon function

**Process of demyelination** *(Phipps, Sands, and Marek, 1999)*

**denasality.** See **hyponasality.**

**denaturation** /dēnā′chərā′shən/ [L, *de* + *natura,* natural], **1.** the alteration of the basic nature or structure of a substance. **2.** the process of making a potential food or beverage substance unfit for human consumption although it may still be used for other purposes, such as a solvent.

**denatured alcohol** /dēnā′chərd/, ethyl alcohol made unfit for ingestion by the addition of acetone or methanol, used as a solvent and in chemical processes.

**denatured protein** [L, *de,* from, *natura, proteios,* first rank], a protein that has undergone change that causes its original properties to be lost. A protein can be denatured by radiation, heat, strong acids, or alcohol.

**dendr-,** combining form meaning 'tree or branches': *dendriceptor, dendroid, dendrophobia.*

**-dendria,** suffix meaning the 'twiglike branching of nerve fibers': *oligodendria, telodendria, zoodendria.*

**dendrite** /den′drīt/ [Gk, *dendron,* tree], a slender branching process that extends from the cell body of a neuron and that is capable of being stimulated by a neurotransmitter. Each neuron usually possesses several dendrites, which receive synapses where chemical transmission occurs from

axons to dendrites (or an axon, in the case of unipolar neurons). The number of dendrites and thus the number of synapses varies with the functions of a neuron. Also called **cytodendrite.** Compare **axon.**

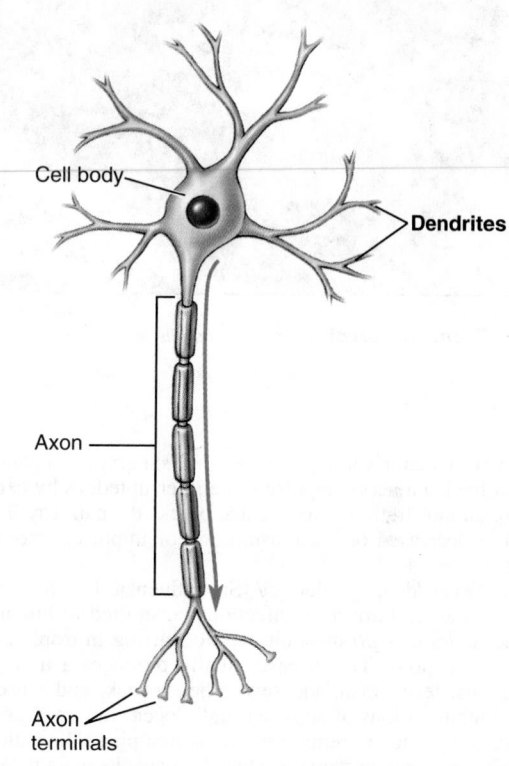

Cell body

Dendrites

Axon

Axon terminals

**Dendrite** *(Herlihy and Maebius, 2000)*

**dendritic** /dendrit′ik/, **1.** treelike, with branches that spread toward or into neighboring tissues, as dendritic keratitis. **2.** pertaining to a dendrite.

**dendritic calculus** [Gk, *dendron,* tree, *calculus,* pebble], a large calculus lodged in the pelvis of the kidney and shaped to fit the branches of the calyx. Also called **coral calculus.**

**dendritic cell,** a cell that captures antigens and migrates to the lymph nodes and spleen, where it presents the processed antigens to T cells.

**dendritic keratitis,** a severe herpesvirus infection of the eye. It is characterized by an ulceration of the surface of the cornea resembling a tree with knobs at the ends of the branches. Photophobia, the sensation of a foreign body in the eye, pain, and conjunctivitis are usual. Treatment entails application of idoxuridine (IDU), chemical debridement with an iodine tincture, or surgical removal of the layer of corneal tissue cells affected. Untreated dendritic keratitis may cause permanent scarring of the cornea with impaired vision or blindness. Also called **herpetic keratitis.**

**dendrodendritic synapse** /den′drōdendrit′ik/ [Gk, *dendron* + *dendron* + *synaptein,* to join], a type of synapse in which a dendrite of one neuron comes in contact with a dendrite of another neuron. Compare **axodendritic synapse.**

**-dendron,** suffix meaning 'the branching portion of a nerve cell receiving an impulse': *neurodendron, telodendron, toxicodendron.*

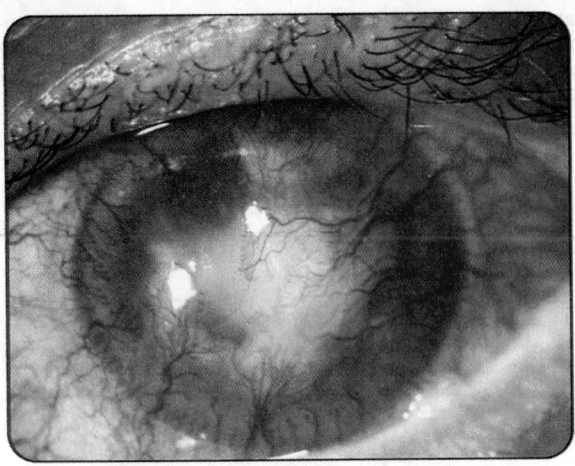

**Dendritic keratitis** *(Kanski and Nischal, 1999)*

**denervated** /dēnur′vātid/ [L, *de* + *nervus,* nerve], a condition of having a nerve impulse route interrupted, as by excision or administration of a drug that blocks the pathway. The result is decreased or no transmission of impulses through this pathway.

**dengue fever** /deng′gē, den′gā/ [Sp, influenza; L, *febris,* fever], an acute *Flavivirus* infection transmitted to humans by the *Aedes aegypti* mosquito and occurring in tropic and subtropic regions. The disease usually produces a triad of symptoms: fever, rash, and severe head, back, and muscle pain. Manifestations of dengue usually occur in two phases, separated by a day of remission. In the first phase the patient experiences fever, extreme weakness, headache, sore throat, muscle pains, and edema of the hands and feet. The second phase is marked by a return of fever and by a bright-red scarlatiniform rash. Dengue is a self-limited illness, although recovery may require several weeks. Treatment is symptomatic; analgesics may be given to relieve headache and other pains. Candidate vaccines are in development. Also called **Aden fever, bouquet fever, breakbone fever, dandy fever, dengue, solar fever.** See also **Aedes, arbovirus.**

**dengue hemorrhagic fever shock syndrome (DHFSS),** a grave form of dengue fever characterized by shock with collapse or prostration; cold, clammy extremities; a weak, thready pulse; respiratory distress; and all of the symptoms of dengue fever. Hemorrhage, bruises, small reddish spots indicating bleeding from skin capillaries, and bloody vomit, urine, and feces may be experienced and may precede circulatory collapse. Treatment includes fluid and electrolyte replacement and blood, fresh frozen plasma, or platelet transfusions as needed. Oxygen and sedatives may be administered. See also **dengue fever.**

**denial** /dinī′əl/ [L, *denegare,* to negate], **1.** refusal or restriction of something requested, claimed, or needed, often causing physical or emotional deficiency. **2.** an unconscious defense mechanism in which emotional conflict and anxiety are avoided by refusal to acknowledge those thoughts, feelings, desires, impulses, or facts that are consciously intolerable.

**denial, ineffective,** a nursing diagnosis accepted by the Eighth National Conference on the Classification of Nursing Diagnoses. Ineffective denial is a conscious or unconscious attempt to disavow the knowledge or meaning of an event to reduce anxiety or fear to the detriment of health.

■ DEFINING CHARACTERISTICS: The defining characteristics include that the individual delays seeking or refuses medical attention and does not perceive the personal relevance of symptoms or danger, the use of home remedies (self-treatment) to relieve symptoms, minimization of symptoms, displacement of the source of symptoms to other organs, and displacement of fear of impact of the condition. The individual does not admit fear of death or invalidism, is unable to acknowledge the impact of disease on his or her life pattern, makes dismissive gestures or comments when speaking of distressing events, and displays inappropriate affect.

■ RELATED FACTORS: The related factors are to be developed. See also **nursing diagnosis.**

**denileukin diftitox,** a miscellaneous antineoplastic.

■ INDICATIONS: This drug is used to treat cutaneous T-cell lymphoma that expresses the CD25 component of the IL-2 receptor.

■ CONTRAINDICATIONS: Hypersensitivity to denileukin, diphtheria toxin, or interleukin-2 prohibits this drug's use.

■ ADVERSE EFFECTS: Life-threatening effects are thrombocytopenia and leukopenia. Other serious side effects include hematuria, albuminuria, pyuria, creatinine increase, anemia, hypoalbuminemia, edema, hypocalcemia, dehydration, hypokalemia, infection, chest pain, and flu-like symptoms. Common side effects include dizziness, paresthesia, nervousness, confusion, insomnia, hypotension, vasodilation, tachycardia, thrombosis, hypertension, dysrhythmias, nausea, anorexia, vomiting, diarrhea, constipation, dyspepsia, and dysphagia.

**Denis Browne splint** [Denis J.W. Browne, twentieth-century Australian surgeon], a splint for the correction of clubfoot, composed of a curved bar attached to the soles of a pair of high-topped shoes. The splint is equipped with wing nuts to allow individual abduction of each foot. The splint is commonly applied nightly in late infancy after casting and manipulation have effectively reduced the deformity.

**denitrogenation** /dēnī′trōjənā′shən/, the elimination of nitrogen from the lungs and body tissues during a period of breathing pure oxygen.

**Denman's spontaneous evolution** [Thomas Denman, English physician, 1733–1815; L, *sponte,* voluntarily, *evolvere,* to roll forth], a natural, unassisted turning of the fetus from the transverse presentation. The head rotates back, and, as the breech descends, the shoulder ascends in the pelvis. The back of the fetus is generally posterior. Also called **Denman's method, Denman's spontaneous version.**

**dens,** *pl.* **dentes** /den′tēz/ [L, tooth], **1.** a tooth or toothlike structure or process. The term is sometimes modified to identify a particular tooth, as dens caninus or dens molaris. **2.** the cone-shaped odontoid process of the axis, or second cervical vertebra. It receives the atlantal ring to act as a pivot for the atlas, or first cervical vertebra. See also **dentition, odontoid process, tooth.**

**dense connective tissue,** connective tissue characterized by dense groups of fibers.

**dense fibrous tissue** [L, *densus,* thick], a fibrous connective tissue consisting of compact, strong, inelastic bundles of mostly parallel collagenous fibers that are glistening white. Dense regular fibrous tissue comprises the tendons, the aponeuroses, and the ligaments; dense irregular fibrous tissue comprises the fascial membranes, the dermis of the skin, the periosteum, and the capsules of organs. Compare **loose fibrous tissue.**

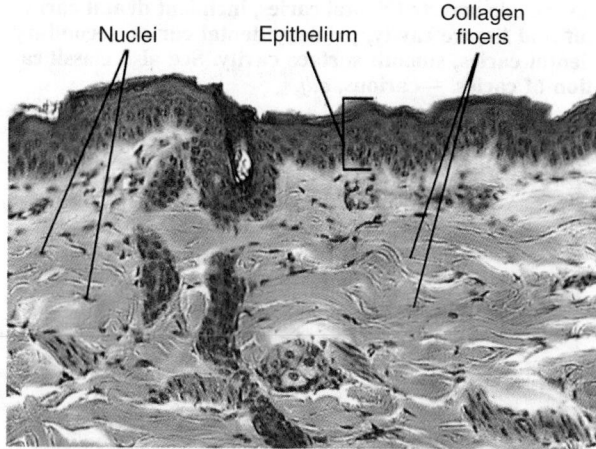

**Dense irregular fibrous tissue**
(© Ed Reschke; used with permission)

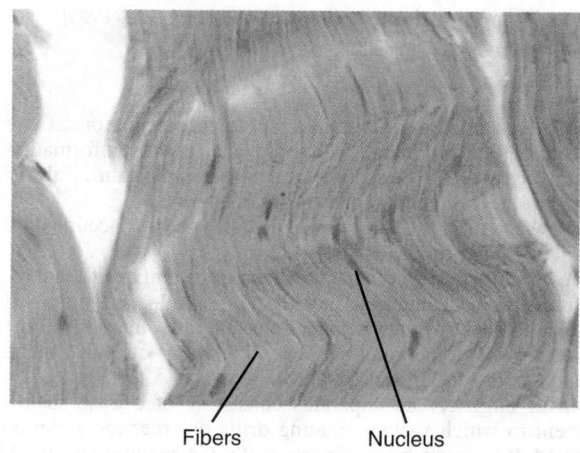

**Dense regular fibrous tissue**
(© Ed Reschke; used with permission)

**dens in dente** /den'tə/, an anomaly of the teeth, found chiefly in the maxillary lateral incisors and characterized by invagination of the enamel. The condition causes a radiographic image suggestive of a tooth within a tooth. Also called **dens invaginatus, gestant odontoma.**

**dens invaginatus.** See **dens in dente.**

**densitometer** /den'sitom'ətər/ [L, *densus* + Gk, *metron,* measure], a device that uses a photoelectric cell to detect differences in the intensity of light transmitted through a substance, such as x-ray film.

**density** /den'sitē/ [L, *densus,* thick], **1.** the amount of mass of a substance in a given volume. The greater the mass in a given volume, the greater the density. See also **mass, volume. 2.** (in radiology) the degree of x-ray film blackening.

**density gradient,** a variation in the density of a solution caused by a change in concentration of a solute in a confined solution.

**dens serotinus.** See **wisdom tooth.**

**dent-, denta-.** See **dento-.**

**dental** [L, *dens,* tooth], pertaining to a tooth or the teeth.

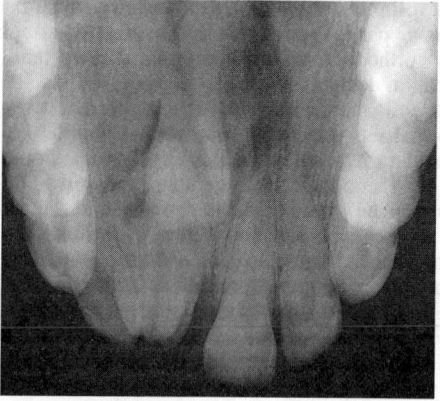

**Dens in dente** *(Regezi, Sciubba, and Pogrel, 2000)*

**dental abscess,** a pus-filled cavity that forms in bone or soft tissues of the jaw as a result of an infection that may follow dental caries or injury to a tooth. Symptoms include pain that may be continuous and exacerbated by hot or cold foods or the pressure of closing the jaws firmly. Untreated, the infection may spread to other structures in the mouth, jaw, and other parts of the body. Treatment may involve the administration of analgesics or antibiotics, root canal therapy, tooth extraction.

**dental alveolus** /alvē'ələs/, a tooth socket in the mandible or maxilla.

**dental amalgam,** an alloy of silver, tin, and mercury with small amounts of zinc and sometimes copper, used for rebuilding tooth surfaces affected by dental caries or trauma.

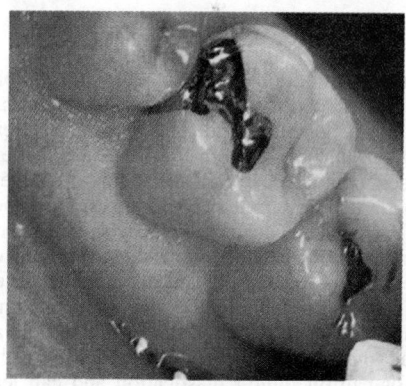

**Dental amalgam** *(Christensen, 1994)*

**dental anesthesia,** any of several methods to reduce or block pain and discomfort during dental procedures. See also **awake anesthesia, inhalational anesthesia, local anesthesia, nitrous oxide, regional anesthesia, topical anesthesia.**

**dental ankylosis,** solid fixation of a tooth resulting from fusion of the cementum and alveolar bone, with obliteration of the periodontal ligament.

**dental anomaly,** an aberration in which one or more teeth deviate from the normal in form, function, or position.

**dental appliance,** any device placed in or on a patient by a dentist as part of a treatment protocol. Dental appliances include orthodontic, prosthetic, retaining, and habit-modification devices.

**dental arch,** the curving shape formed by the arrangement of a normal set of teeth in each jaw.

**dental assistant,** a person who aids a dentist in the performance of generalized tasks, including chairside aid, clerical work, reception, and some radiography and dental laboratory work. See also **certified dental assistant.**

**dental biomechanics,** the study and use of mechanical devices and physical forces to effect desirable changes in oral structures.

**dental calculus,** a salivary deposit of calcium phosphate and calcium carbonate with organic matter on the teeth or a dental prosthesis. See also **calculus, subgingival calculus, supragingival calculus, tartar.**

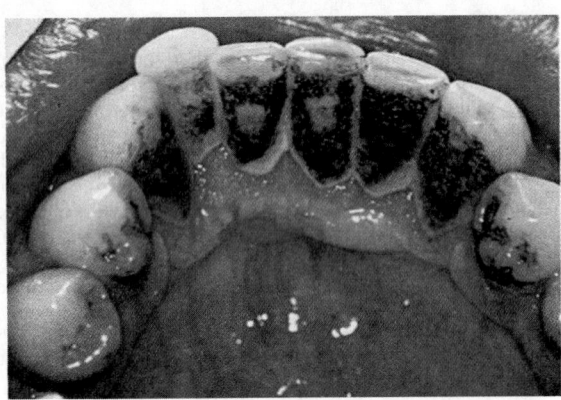

**Dental calculus** *(Grundy and Jones, 1993)*

**dental caries,** a tooth disease caused by the complex interaction of food, especially starches and sugars, with the bacteria that form dental plaque. The term also refers to the tooth cavities that result from the disease. Plaque bacteria produce acids that cause demineralization of enamel and enzymes that attack the protein component of the tooth. This process, if untreated, ultimately leads to the formation of deep cavities and bacterial infection of the pulp chamber, which contains blood vessels and nerves. The development of dental caries in a debilitated patient is a concern because of the danger that infections of the teeth or gingival tissues may spead to the rest of the body. In addition, teeth that are decayed or painful inhibit mastication and can lead to dietary changes, which may in turn cause nutritional and digestive disorders. Dental caries may be prevented by a reduction in the frequency of sugar consumption, use of dental floss between the teeth, regular brushing of the teeth with a fluoridated toothpaste, drinking of fluoridated water, topical application of fluorides to the teeth, and removal of plaque and calculus by a dental hygienist. Treatment of dental caries includes removal of the decayed material and restoration of the surface of the affected tooth with a silver amalgam or other restorative material. If the cavity has reached the pulp chamber, it may be necessary to remove the pulp tissues to alleviate pain, prevent the spread of infection to the rest of the body, and allow the continued use of the tooth. Alternatively, the entire tooth may be extracted. Kinds of dental car-

ies include **arrested dental caries, incipient dental caries, pit and fissure cavity, primary dental caries, secondary dental caries, smooth surface cavity.** See also **classification of caries.** —**carious,** *adj.*

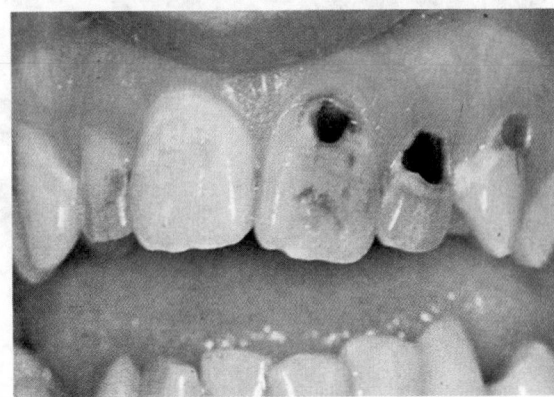

**Recurrent dental caries** *(Grundy and Jones, 1993)*

**dental chart,** a simplified graphic representation of the teeth on which clinical, radiologic, and forensic information may be recorded. See also **FDI numbering system, Palmer notation, universal tooth coding system.**

**dental crypt,** the space in the alveolar process occupied by a developing tooth.

**dental emergency,** an acute disorder of oral health that requires medical attention, including broken, loose, or evulsed teeth caused by traumas; infections and inflammations of the soft tissues of the mouth; and complications of oral surgery, such as dry tooth socket.

**dental engine,** an apparatus consisting of a hand instrument to which various rotating drills or other tools can be fitted. It is driven by an electric motor via a continuous cord-like belt that runs over pulleys.

**dental erosion,** the chemical or mechanochemical destruction of tooth material that causes variously shaped depressions, generally at the cementoenamel junctions of teeth. The surfaces of these depressions, unlike those of dental caries, are hard and smooth.

### Black's system of classification of caries

| | |
|---|---|
| Class I | Located in pits and fissures of the occlusal two thirds of posterior teeth or on the lingual surface of anterior teeth |
| Class II | Located on the proximal surfaces of premolars and molars |
| Class III | Located on the proximal surfaces of central and lateral incisors and cuspids |
| Class IV | Located in the proximal surfaces of incisors and canines and involving the incisal angle |
| Class V | Located in the gingival third on the labial, facial, or lingual surfaces of anterior or posterior teeth |
| Class VI | Located on cusp tips |

Adapted from Woodall IR: *Comprehensive dental hygiene care,* ed 4, St Louis, 1993, Mosby.

**dental ethics** [L, *dens*, tooth; Gk, *ethos*, ethics], a system of moral principles governing the professional conduct of dental and dental hygienic practices.

**dental examination,** an inspection of the teeth and surrounding soft tissues of the oral cavity. The examiner generally uses an explorer, a slender steel instrument with a flexible, sharp point, to probe the minute indentations on tooth surfaces for signs of demineralization and caries development. Fillings are also inspected, and a radiographic record of the teeth is usually made. The examiner may also insert a periodontal probe into the soft-tissue sulcus around each tooth, to measure the depth of each sulcus and to explore for calculus and root defects. Also called **intraoral examination.**

**dental extracting forceps,** a hand instrument used for grasping teeth during their removal from the socket. Most such forceps are designed for the extraction of a particular tooth in the maxilla or mandible.

**dental film,** an x-ray film of the teeth, exposed either intraorally or extraorally. Intraoral films are small, double-emulsion films without screens but with a lead foil backing to reduce patient dose, enclosed in a moisture-resistant envelope. Extraoral films are large, single-emulsion, screen films.

**dental fistula,** an abnormal passage from the apical periodontal area of a tooth to the surface of the oral mucous membrane, permitting the discharge of inflammatory or suppurative material. Also called **alveolar fistula, alveolar sinus.**

**dental floss,** a thread used to clean interproximal tooth surfaces and spaces between the teeth. It may be waxed or unwaxed and flavored or unflavored.

**dentalgia.** See **toothache.**

**dental granuloma,** a pathologic mass of granulation tissue that is attached to the apex of a tooth and is surrounded by a fibrous capsule. On x-ray film it appears as a well-defined radiolucency.

**dental handpiece,** a dental instrument that holds various disks, cups or bits, used to prepare a tooth to receive a restoration or to contour, clean, or polish a tooth or restoration.

**dental history,** a record of a patient's oral health, general health, and medical care, including surgeries and medication use; allergies; childhood diseases; radiographic history; and personal dental care.

**dental hygienist,** an oral health care professional authorized to provide clinical and therapeutic services, including dental prophylaxis, radiography, administration of medications, and dental education at chairside and in the community. In some states, a dental hygienist with additional education may administer local anesthetics and nitrous oxide/oxygen analgesia, place and carve filling materials, conduct additional periodontal procedures, and function as a public health specialist. To practice as a registerd dental hygienist, a person must complete at least 2 years of postsecondary education in an accredited community or dental college or university and be approved by a state or regional board of dental and dental hygiene examiners.

**dental identification** [L, *dens*, tooth, *idem*, the same, *facere*, to make], the process of establishing the unique characteristics of the teeth and dental work of an individual, thereby permitting the identification of the individual by comparison with his or her dental charts and records. See also **forensic dentistry.**

**dental impaction,** the blocking of a tooth by a physical barrier, usually other teeth, so that it cannot erupt. See also **impacted tooth.**

**dental implant,** a plastic or metal anchor that is inserted into a jawbone to provide permanent support for a fixed bridge or denture when the bone itself would provide insufficient support. About 8 weeks after a tooth or teeth are removed, the anchor is screwed into a hole that has been drilled into the jaw. New bone is allowed to grow around and fuse with the anchor for up to 6 months before the bridge or denture is attached.

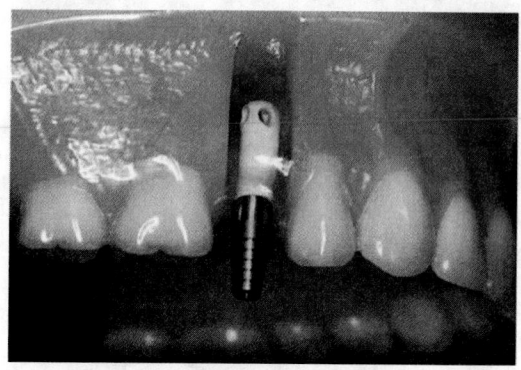

**Dental implant** *(Christensen, 1994)*

**dental jurisprudence** [L, *dens*, tooth, *juris prudentia*, knowledge of the law], the application of the principles of law to the practice of dentistry and of dental hygiene and the relations of dentists and dental hygienists to patients, to society, and to each other.

**dental laboratory technician,** a person who makes dental prostheses and orthodontic appliances as prescribed by a dentist. A dental laboratory technician may have a private laboratory or work in the premises of a dentist. Also called **dental technician.**

**dental operculum** [L, *dens*, tooth, *operculum*, a covering structure], a hood or flap of gingival tissue overlying the crown of an erupting tooth. This tissue is usually chewed away as the tooth erupts.

**dental papilla** [L, *dens*, tooth, *papilla*, nipple], a small mass of mesenchymal tissue in the enamel organ that differentiates into dentin and dental pulp during tooth development. The innermost layer consists of a cell-free zone of reticular fibers that form the basement membrane.

**dental pathology,** the branch of pathology that deals with dental changes that occur in disease.

**dental plaque.** See **bacterial plaque.**

**dental plate** [L, *dens*, tooth; OFr, *plate*, flat structure], a dental prosthesis made to the shape of the maxilla or mandible jaw to support artificial teeth.

**dental porcelain,** a type of porcelain used in dental restorations, either jacket crowns or inlays, artificial teeth, or metal-ceramic crowns. It is essentially a mixture of particles of feldspar and quartz, the feldspar melting first and providing a glass matrix for the quartz.

**dental probe.** See **periodontal probe.**

**dental prophylaxis.** See **oral prophylaxis.**

**dental prosthesis** [L, dens, tooth; Gk, prosthesis, an addition], a fixed or removable appliance used to replace one or more lost or missing natural teeth. See also **denture.**

**dental public health,** the branch of dentistry that is concerned with preventing and controlling dental diseases and promoting dental health through organized community efforts rather than through treatment of individual patients. It

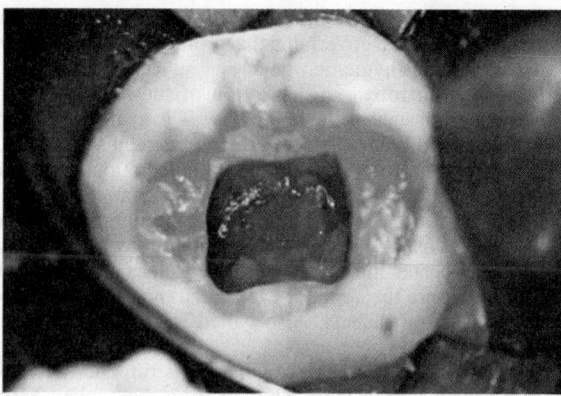

**Dental pulp** *(Grundy and Jones, 1993)*

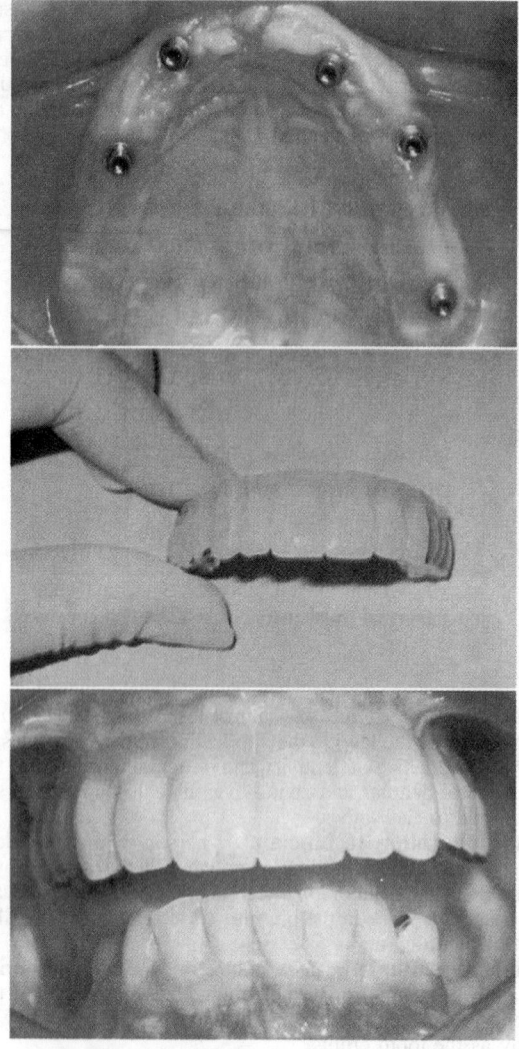

**Dental prosthesis** *(Christensen, 1994)*

is concerned with dental health education, applied dental research, and administration of group dental care programs. Also called **public health dentistry.**

**dental pulp,** a small mass of connective tissue, blood vessels, and nerves located in a chamber within the dentin layer of a tooth. The pulp chamber is found in the crown and the root of a tooth. See also **pulp canal, pulp cavity.**

**dental radiograph** [L, *dens,* tooth; L, *radire,* to shine; Gk, *graphein,* to record], an intraoral and extraoral x-ray film of teeth and the bone surrounding them. See also **bite wing radiograph, periapical radiograph.**

**dental restoration.** See **restoration.**

**dental root cyst.** See **periodontal cyst.**

**dental sealant** /sē′lənt/, a plastic film coating that is applied to and adheres to the caries-free chewing surfaces of teeth to seal pits and fissures where plaque, food, and bacteria usually become trapped. The surface to be treated is isolated to ensure that it is not contaminated with saliva. It is then cleaned with a brush and pumice cleansing agent, dried, and etched with a phosphoric acid solution. After the acid has been washed away and the tooth has been dried, the sealant is applied. Dental sealants are reported to reduce the incidence of caries in children's teeth by 50%. Also called **pit and fissure sealant.**

**dental stone.** See **artificial stone.**

**dental surgeon** [L, *dens,* tooth; Gk, *cheirourgos,* surgeon], a dentist who specializes in surgical procedures involving the teeth and surrounding oral tissues. An **operative dental surgeon** is concerned with the restoration of teeth that have been damaged. An **oral and maxillofacial surgeon** specializes in surgical reconstruction of facial malformations caused by diseases of or trauma to mouth, face, head, or neck. An **exodontist** limits his or her practice to the surgical removal of teeth. An **oral surgeon** specializes in the surgical removal of teeth and surrounding oral tissues.

**dental technician.** See **dental laboratory technician.**

**-dentate,** suffix meaning 'possessing teeth': *edentate, multidentate, tridentate.*

**dentate fracture** /den′tāt/ [L, *dens*], any fracture that causes serrated bone ends that fit together like the teeth of gears.

**dentate nucleus,** a deep cerebellar nucleus. It receives fibers from the lateral zone of the cerebellar cortex and appears to act as a trigger for the motor cortex, governing intentional movements as well as properties of ongoing movements.

**Dentec.** See **xylitol.**

**dentes.** See **dens.**

**denti-, dentia-.** See **dento-.**

**dentibuccal** /den′ti·buk′əl/ [L, *dens,* tooth + *bucca,* cheek], pertaining to the teeth and cheek.

**denticle** /den′tikəl/, a calcified body in the pulp chamber of a tooth. Also called **endolith, pulp stone.** If it is composed of irregular dentin, it is known as a **true denticle.**

**denticulate** /dentik′yəlit/ [L, *denticulus,* little tooth], having very small teeth or toothlike projections.

**dentifrice** /den′tifris/ [L, *dens* + *fricare,* to rub], a pharmaceutic compound used with a toothbrush for cleaning and polishing the teeth. It typically contains a mild abrasive, detergent, flavoring agent, and binder. Other common ingredients are deodorants, humectants, desensitizers, and various medications to prevent dental caries. Also called **toothpaste.**

**dentigerous cyst** /dentij′ərəs/ [L, *dens* + *gerere,* to bear], one of three kinds of follicular cyst, consisting of an

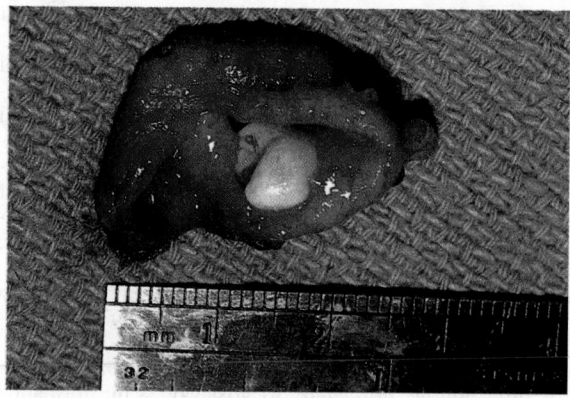

**Dentigerous cyst** *(Regezi, Sciubba, and Pogrel, 2000)*

epithelium-lined sac filled with fluid or viscous material that surrounds the crown of an unerupted tooth or odontoma. Compare **multilocular cyst, primordial cyst.**

**dentin** /den'tin/ [L, *dens*], the chief material of teeth, surrounding the pulp and situated inside the enamel and cementum. Harder and denser than bone, it consists of solid organic substratum infiltrated with lime salts. Also spelled **dentine.**

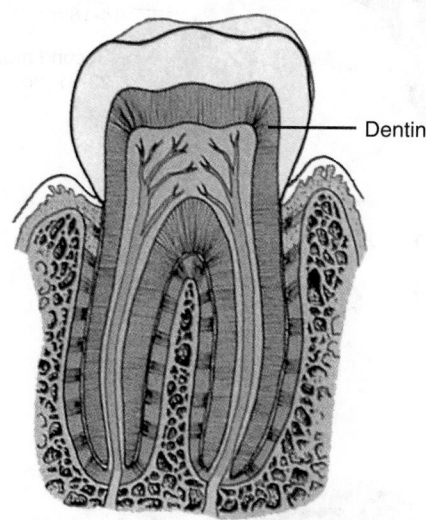

— Dentin

**Position of dentin in a normal mouth**
*(Potter and Perry, 2001)*

**dentin eburnation** /ē'burnā'shən/, a change in carious teeth in which softened and decalcified dentin develops a hard, brown, polished appearance.

**dentin globule,** a small spheric body in peripheral dentin, created by early calcification.

**dentinoenamel** /den'tinō·inam'əl/ [L, *dens* + OFr, *enesmail*, enamel], pertaining to both the dentin and the enamel of the teeth.

**dentinoenamel junction (DEJ),** the interface of the enamel and the dentin of a tooth crown, generally conform-

ing to the shape of the crown. Also called **dentoenamel junction.**

**dentinogenesis** /den'tinōjen'əsis/ [L, *dens* + Gk, *genein*, to produce], the formation of the dentin of the teeth. —**dentinogenic,** *adj.*

**dentinogenesis imperfecta, 1.** a genetic disturbance of the dentin, characterized by early calcification of the pulp chambers, marked attrition, and an opalescent hue of the teeth. **2.** a localized form of mesodermal dysplasia affecting the dentin of the teeth. It may be hereditary and associated with osteogenesis imperfecta. **3.** a genetic condition that produces defective dentin but normal tooth enamel. Also called **hereditary opalescent dentin.**

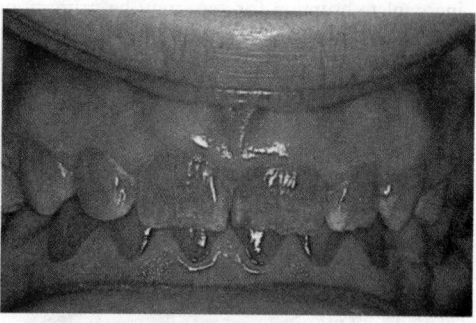

**Dentinogenesis imperfecta** *(Zitelli and Davis, 1997)*

**dentinogenic.** See **dentinogenesis.**

**dentist** [L, *dens*], a person who is qualified by training and licensed by a state or region to diagnose and treat abnormalities of the teeth, gums, and underlying bone, including conditions caused by disease, trauma, and heredity. Required training consists of 2 to 4 years in an undergraduate college, a satisfactory score on a Dental Aptitude Test, and 4 years at an American Dental Association–accredited dental college. After completing dental college, a dentist is awarded a degree of either Doctor of Dental Surgery (D.D.S.) or Doctor of Dental Medicine (D.M.D.); the two degrees are equivalent. A dentist must pass written and practical examinations to obtain a state license. In some states, a dentist can meet licensing requirements by providing a certificate from the National Board of Dental Examiners instead of taking a written test and by taking the practical examination before a Regional Dental Examining Board rather than a state board. Dental internships and residencies are not required for general practice. See also **dentistry.**

**dentistry** /den'tistrē/ [L, *dens*], the art and science of practicing the diagnosis, prevention, and treatment of diseases and disorders of the teeth and surrounding structures of the oral cavity. Responsibilities include the repair and restoration of teeth, the replacement of missing teeth, and the detection of diseases, such as blood dyscrasias and tumors, that would require treatment by a dental specialist or physician. In addition to the general practice of dentistry, there are eight recognized specialties, each requiring additional training after graduation from a dental college: **dental public health, endodontics,** oral and maxillofacial pathology, **oral and maxillofacial surgery, orthodontics and dentofacial orthopedics, pediatric dentistry, periodontics,** and **prosthodontics.**

**dentition** /dentish′ən/ [L, *dentire,* to cut teeth], **1.** the development and eruption of the teeth. See also **teething. 2.** the arrangement, number, and kind of teeth as they appear in the dental arches of the mouth. **3.** the teeth of an individual or species as determined by their form and arrangement. See also **mixed dentition, natural dentition, precocious dentition, predeciduous dentition, deciduous dentition, secondary dentition,** and **retarded dentition.**

**dentition, impaired,** a nursing diagnosis accepted by the Thirteenth National Conference on the Classification of Nursing Diagnoses. The condition is a disruption in tooth development or eruption patterns or a disruption in the structural integrity of individual teeth.

■ DEFINING CHARACTERISTICS: The condition is characterized by excessive plaque, crown or root caries, halitosis, tooth enamel discoloration, toothache, loose teeth, excessive calculus, incomplete eruption for age (may be primary or permanent teeth), malocclusion or tooth misalignment, premature loss of primary teeth, worn down or abraded teeth, tooth

fracture(s), missing teeth or complete absence, erosion of enamel, and assymetrical facial expression.

■ RELATED FACTORS: Related factors include ineffective oral hygiene; sensitivity to heat or cold; barriers to self-care; access or economic barriers to professional care; nutritional deficits; dietary habits; genetic predisposition; selected prescription medications; premature loss of primary teeth; excessive intake of fluorides; chronic vomiting; chronic use of tobacco, coffee, tea, or red wine; lack of knowledge regarding dental health; excessive use of abrasive cleaning agents, and bruxism. See also **nursing diagnosis.**

**dento-, dent-, denta-, denti-, dentia-,** combining form meaning 'tooth or teeth': *dentography, dentoidin, dentonomy.*

**dentoalveolar abscess** /den′tō·alvē′ələr/ [L, *dens + alveolus,* little hollow, *abscedere,* to go away], the formation and accumulation of pus in a tooth socket or the jawbone around the base of a tooth. The pus results from a bacterial infection that is usually secondary to an infection or injury

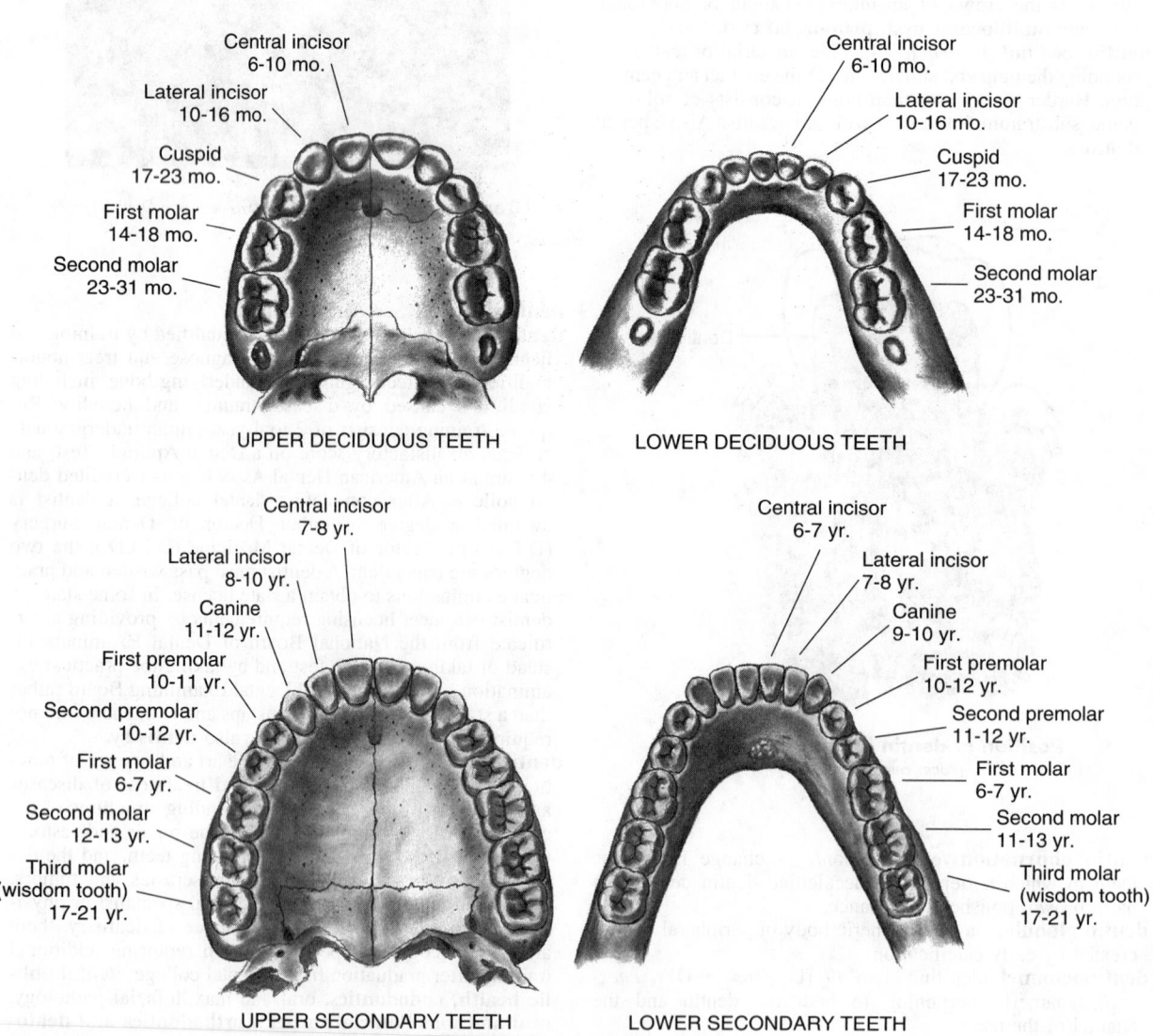

UPPER DECIDUOUS TEETH

Central incisor
6-10 mo.

Lateral incisor
10-16 mo.

Cuspid
17-23 mo.

First molar
14-18 mo.

Second molar
23-31 mo.

LOWER DECIDUOUS TEETH

Central incisor
6-10 mo.

Lateral incisor
10-16 mo.

Cuspid
17-23 mo.

First molar
14-18 mo.

Second molar
23-31 mo.

UPPER SECONDARY TEETH

Central incisor
7-8 yr.

Lateral incisor
8-10 yr.

Canine
11-12 yr.

First premolar
10-11 yr.

Second premolar
10-12 yr.

First molar
6-7 yr.

Second molar
12-13 yr.

Third molar
(wisdom tooth)
17-21 yr.

LOWER SECONDARY TEETH

Central incisor
6-7 yr.

Lateral incisor
7-8 yr.

Canine
9-10 yr.

First premolar
10-12 yr.

Second premolar
11-12 yr.

First molar
6-7 yr.

Second molar
11-13 yr.

Third molar
(wisdom tooth)
17-21 yr.

**Dentition** *(Seidel et al, 1999)*

to the tooth or alveolar tissues. Also called **periapical abscess.**

**dentoalveolar cyst.** See **periodontal cyst.**

**dentoenamel junction.** See **dentinoenamel junction.**

**dentofacial** /-fā'shəl/, pertaining to the mouth or the jaw.

**dentofacial anomaly,** a condition in which a mouth or jaw structure deviates from the normal in form, function, or position.

**dentofacial orthopedics.** See **orthodontics.**

**dentogenesis imperfecta.** See **dentinogenesis imperfecta.**

**dentogingival fiber** /-jinjī'vəl/ [L, *dens* + *gingiva,* gum], any of the many peridental connective tissue fibers that emerge from the supraalveolar part of the cementum of a tooth, spread like a fan, and terminate in the free gingiva.

**dentogingival junction,** the interface between the junctional epithelium and the surface of the teeth.

**dentoperiosteal fiber** /den'tōper'ē·os'tē·əl/ [L, *dens* + Gk, *peri,* around, *osteon* bone], any of the many peridental connective tissue fibers that emerge from the supraalveolar part of the cementum of a tooth and extend apically beyond the alveolar crest into the mucoperiosteum of the attached gingiva.

**dentulous** /den'tyələs/ [L, *dens,* tooth, *-ulosus,* characterized by], possessing one or more natural teeth.

**dentulous dental arch,** a dental arch that contains one or more natural teeth.

**denture** /den'chər/ [L, *dens,* tooth], an artificial tooth or a set of artificial teeth not permanently fixed or implanted. Compare **fixed bridgework, implant denture.**

**denture base,** the part of a denture that covers the soft tissue of the mouth. It is commonly made of resin or a combination of resins and metal.

**denture-bearing area.** See **basal seat area.**

**denture flask,** a sectional metal case in which plaster of paris or artificial stone is molded and in which dentures or other resin restorations are processed.

**denture packing,** the laboratory procedure of filling and compressing a denture-base material into a mold in a denture flask.

**denturist** /den'chərist/, a person other than a dentist who engages in the practice of dentistry, usually only to the extent of providing complete or partial dentures. Most states in the United States have laws restricting such activity. See also **dental laboratory technician.**

**denucleated** /dēnyoo'klē·ā'tid/ [L, *de,* from, *nucleus,* nut kernel], pertaining to a condition in which the nucleus has been removed.

**denudation** /den'oodā'shən/ [L, *denudare,* to make bare], **1.** the process of stripping bare. **2.** a condition of losing an outside layer such as an epithelium.

**Denver Articulation Screening Examination (DASE),** a test for evaluating the clarity of pronunciation in children 2-1/2 to 6 years of age. Each child's performance may be compared with a standardized norm for the age.

**Denver classification,** a system for identifying and classifying human chromosomes according to their size and the position of the centromere as determined during mitotic metaphase. The chromosomes are divided into seven major groups, designated A through G, which are arranged according to decreasing length. See also **chromosomal nomenclature, chromosome, karyotype.**

**Denver Developmental Screening Test (DDST),** a test for evaluating development in children from 1 month to 6 years of age. The developmental level of motor, social, and language skills may be discovered by comparing the child's performance with the average performance of other chil-

dren. The score, or the developmental age, is expressed as a ratio in which the child's age is the denominator, the age at which the norm possesses skills equal to those of the child being tested is the numerator. The **Denver II,** released in 1990, is a major revision and restandardization of the DDST.

**deodorant** /dē·ō'dərənt/ [L, *de* + *odor,* smell], **1.** destroying or masking odors. **2.** a substance that destroys or masks odors. Underarm deodorants are available as sprays, creams, solid gels, and liquids containing an antiperspirant, such as aluminum chloride, aluminum hydroxyl, aluminum sulfate, or aluminum zirconyl hydroxychloride. These aluminum salts form an obstructive hydroxide gel in sweat ducts. Vaginal deodorant sprays contain a fatty ester emollient, a masking fragrance, and an antimicrobial agent, such as benzethonium chloride, chlorhexidine hydrochloride, or triacetin, and are often associated with allergic reactions. Room and breath deodorants contain masking agents, such as mint, pine, eucalyptus, lemon, lavender, rosemary, sassafras, or thyme. Ozone masks odors by decreasing olfactory sensitivity. Chlorophyll has a deodorizing action that is enhanced by crotonic acid. Also called **antibromic.**

**deodorized alcohol** /dē·ō'dərīzd'/, a liquid, free of organic impurities, containing 92.5% absolute alcohol.

**deodorizing douche,** a stream of air or liquid that masks or absorbs foul odors, applied at moderate pressure into a body cavity or onto a body surface. See also **douche.**

**deontologism** /dē'ontol'əgiz'əm/ [Gk, *deon,* obligation, *logos,* science], a doctrine of ethics that states that moral duty or obligation is binding even though a moral action may be different or result in painful consequences; also, that which makes acts right are nonconsequential characteristics such as fidelity, veracity, justice, and honesty. Compare **natural law, utilitarianism.**

**deorsumversion.** See **infraversion** (def. 3).

**deossification** /dē·os'ifikā'shən/, the loss of mineral matter from bones.

**deoxidizer,** an agent that removes oxygen. See also **reducing agent.**

**deoxy-, desoxy-,** prefix meaning 'containing a decreased amount of oxygen': *deoxygenation, desoxymorphine, desoxyribose.*

**deoxygenation** /dē·ok'sijənā'shən/ [L, *de,* from; Gk, *oxys,* sharp, *genein,* to produce], the removal of oxygen from a chemical compound.

**deoxyribonucleic acid (DNA)** /dē·ok'sirī'bōnooklē'ik/, a large, double-stranded, helical molecule that is the carrier of genetic information. In eukaryotic cells, it is found principally in the chromosomes of the nucleus. DNA is composed of four kinds of serially repeating nucleotide bases: adenine, cytosine, guanine, and thymine. Genetic information is coded in the sequence of the nucleotides. Also called **desoxyribonucleic acid.** See also **nucleic acid, ribonucleic acid.**

**deoxyribose** /dē·ok'sē·rī'bōs/, ribose that has been transformed into a deoxy sugar, found in deoxyribonucleic acids (DNA). Compare **ribose.**

**deoxy sugar** /dē·ok'sē shoog'ər/, a sugar in which one or more carbon atoms have been reduced, thus losing their hydroxyl groups.

**Depakene,** trademark for an anticonvulsant (valproic acid).

**Depakote,** trademark for an anticonvulsant drug (divalproex sodium).

**Department of Health and Human Services (DHHS),** a cabinet-level department of the U.S. government with responsibility for the functions of various federal social wel-

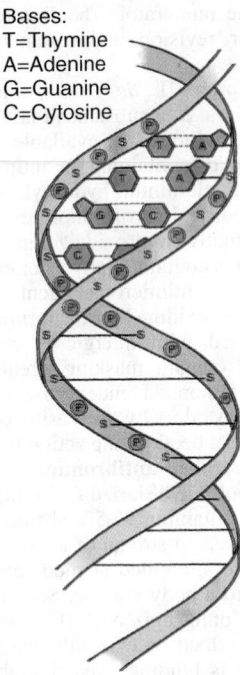

S=Deoxyribose sugar
P=Phosphate group

Bases:
T=Thymine
A=Adenine
G=Guanine
C=Cytosine

**Structure of deoxyribonucleic acid (DNA)**
*(Applegate, 2000)*

fare and health delivery agencies, such as the Food and Drug Administration (FDA). It also directs the U.S. Office of Consumer Affairs, Office of Civil Rights, Administration on Aging, Public Health Service, Indian Health Service, Social Security Administration, and National Institutes of Health.

**Department of Transportation (DOT),** a cabinet-level department of the U.S. government responsible for national transportation policies, including maritime, aviation, railroad, and highway safety and regulation of the transport of hazardous materials, such as medical gases.

**depend.** See **dependent.**

**dependence** /dipen'dəns/ [L, *de* + *pendere*, to hang upon], **1.** the state of being dependent. **2.** the total psychophysical state of one addicted to drugs or alcohol who must receive an increasing amount of the substance to prevent the onset of withdrawal symptoms.

**dependency needs** /dipen'dənsē/, the sum of the physical and emotional requirements of an infant for survival, including parenting, love, affection, shelter, protection, food, and warmth. Reliance on others to satisfy these needs decreases with age and maturity; continuance in later years, in overt or latent form, is indicative of a pathologic emotional disorder. These needs may increase under stress, as during physical illness, in which case they do not reflect a psychopathologic condition. Compare **emotional need.**

**dependent,** pertaining to a condition of being reliant on someone or something else for help, support, favor, and other needs, as a child is dependent on a parent, a narcotics addict is dependent on a drug, or one variable is dependent on another. **—depend,** *v.*

**dependent care,** health care provided for persons, particularly children and handicapped or elderly individuals, who are dependent on others for part or all of the activities of daily living.

**dependent differentiation.** See **correlative differentiation.**

**dependent edema** [L, *de*, from, *pendere*, to hand; Gk, *oidema*, swelling], a fluid accumulation in the tissues that is influenced by gravity. It is usually greater in the lower part of the body than in the part above the level of the heart.

**dependent intervention,** a therapeutic action based on the written or verbal orders of another health professional.

**dependent personality,** behavior characterized by excessive or compulsive needs for attention, acceptance, and approval from other people to maintain security and self-esteem.

**dependent personality disorder,** a mental state characterized by a lack of self-confidence and an inability to function independently.

**dependent variable,** (in research) a factor that is measured to learn the effect of one or more independent variables; for example, in a study of the effect of preoperative nursing intervention on postoperative vomiting, vomiting is the dependent variable measured to determine the effect of the nursing intervention. Compare **independent variable.**

**depersonalization** /dēpur'sənəlīzā'shən/ [L, *de* + *persona*, mask], a feeling of strangeness or unreality concerning oneself or the environment, often resulting from anxiety, stress, or fatigue. See also **alienation, depersonalization disorder.**

**depersonalization disorder,** an emotional disturbance characterized by depersonalization feelings in which a dreamlike atmosphere pervades the consciousness. The body may not feel like one's own, and dramatic and important events may be watched with equanimity. The reaction is commonly seen in various forms of schizophrenia and in severe depression.

**de Pezzer's catheter.** See **Pezzer's catheter.**

**depigmentation.** See **dyspigmentation.**

**depilation** /dep'ilā'shən/ [L, *de* + *pilum,* hair], the removal or extraction of hair from the body, either temporarily by mechanical or chemical means or permanently by electrolysis, which destroys the hair follicle. Also called **epilation. —depilate,** *v.*

**depilatory** /dipil'ətôrē/, **1.** pertaining to a substance or procedure that removes hair. **2.** a depilatory agent.

**depilatory techniques** [L, *depilare,* to deprive of hair; Gk, *technikos,* skillful], methods of removing unwanted body hair, such as plucking, external application of chemicals, electrolysis, or application of melted wax.

**deplete** /də·plēt'/ [L, *deplere,* to empty], to empty or unload; to cause depletion.

**depletion** /də·plē'shən/ [L, *deplere,* to empty], **1.** the act or process of emptying or removing, such as of fluid from a body compartment. **2.** an exhausted state resulting from excessive loss of blood.

**depolarization** /dēpō'lərīzā'shən/, the reduction of a membrane potential to a less negative value. It is caused by the influx of cations, such as sodium and calcium, through ion channels in the membrane. In many neurons and muscle cells, depolarization may lead to an electric impulse called an action potential.

**deposit** /də·poz'it/ [L, *de,* from + *ponere* to place], **1.** sediment or dregs. **2.** extraneous inorganic matter collected in the tissues or in a viscus or cavity. **3.** hard or soft material laid down on a tooth surface, such as dental calculus or plaque.

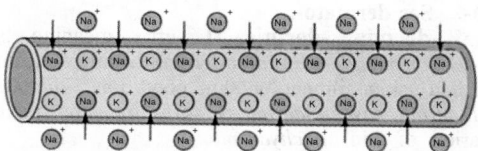

**Depolarization and repolarization**
*(Thibodeau and Patton, 1999/Rolin Graphics)*

**deposition** /dep′əzish′ən/ [L, *deponere,* to lay down], (in law) sworn pretrial testimony given by a witness in response to oral or written questions and cross-examination. The deposition is transcribed and may be used for further pretrial investigation. It may also be presented at the trial if the witness cannot be present. Compare **discovery, interrogatories.**

**depot** /dē′pō, dep′ō/ [Fr, depository], **1.** any area of the body in which drugs or other substances such as fat are stored and from which they can be distributed. **2.** (of a drug) injected or implanted to be slowly absorbed into the circulation.

**depot injection,** an intramuscular injection of a drug in an oil suspension that results in a gradual release of the medication over several days.

**depressant** /dipres′ənt/ [L, *deprimere,* to press down], **1.** (of a drug) tending to decrease the function or activity of a system of the body. **2.** such a drug; for example, a cardiac depressant, central nervous system depressant, or respiratory depressant.

**depressed** [L, *deprimere,* to press down], **1.** pertaining to a body structure that has been forced below the surface of surrounding parts, as in a skull fracture. **2.** pertaining to a condition in which general body activity is diminished, as in depressed urine output during dehydration. **3.** pertaining to an emotional condition, characterized by emotional dejection, loss of initiative, listlessness, loss of appetite, and concentration difficulty. See also **depression.**

**depressed fracture,** a break in the skull in which bone fragments are pushed below the normal surface of the skull.

**depression** /dipresh′ən/ [L, *deprimere,* to press down], **1.** a depressed area, hollow, or fossa; downward or inward displacement. **2.** a decrease of vital functional activity. **3.** a mood disturbance characterized by feelings of sadness, despair, and discouragement resulting from and normally proportionate to some personal loss or tragedy. **4.** an abnormal emotional state characterized by exaggerated feelings of sadness, melancholy, dejection, worthlessness, emptiness, and hopelessness that are inappropriate and out of proportion to reality. The overt manifestations, which are extremely variable, range from a slight lack of motivation and inability to concentrate to severe physiologic alterations of body functions and may represent symptoms of a variety of mental and physical conditions, a syndrome of related symptoms associated with a particular disease, or a specific mental illness. The condition is neurotic when the precipitating cause is an intrapsychic conflict or a traumatic situation or event that is identifiable, even though the person is unable to explain the overreaction to it. The condition is psychotic when there is severe physical and mental functional impairment caused by an unidentifiable intrapsychic conflict; it is often accompanied by hallucinations, delusions, and confusion concerning time, place, and identity. Depression may be expressed in a wide spectrum of affective, physiologic, cognitive, and behavioral manifestations. The varied behav-iors represent the complex actions, reactions, and interactions of the depressed person to stimuli that may be either internal or external. Because the origin of depression can be genetic, pharmacologic, endocrinal, infectious, nutritional, neoplastic, or neurologic, the behavioral effects can appear as aggression or withdrawal, anorexia or overeating, anger or apathy, or any of myriad responses. Kinds of depression include **agitated depression, anaclitic depression, involutional melancholia, reactive depression, major depressive episode,** and **retarded depression.** See also **bipolar disorder. —depressive,** *adj.*

**depression control,** a nursing outcome from the Nursing Outcomes Classification (NOC) defined as personal actions to minimize melancholy and maintain interest in life events. See also **Nursing Outcomes Classification.**

**depression level,** a nursing outcome from the Nursing Outcomes Classification (NOC) defined as severity of melancholic mood and loss of interest in life events. See also **Nursing Outcomes Classification.**

**depression with psychotic features** [L, *deprimere,* to press down; Gk, *psyche,* mind, *osis,* condition], a type of depressive disorder or mood disorder in which there are psychotic features, usually of a paranoid or somatic nature.

**depressive.** See **depression.**

**depressive personality disorder,** a *DSM-IV* psychiatric disorder characterized by a persistent and pervasive pattern of depressive cognitions and behaviors, such as chronic unhappiness, low self-esteem, pessimism, critical and derogatory attitudes toward oneself and others, feelings of guilt or remorse, and an inability to relax or feel enjoyment.

**depressive pseudodementia.** See **dementia syndrome of depression.** This term is discouraged as technically incorrect because the cognitive deficits are now believed to be real, if reversible.

**depressive reaction,** a condition of depressive emotional response to an external situation. The depressive state usually ends when the external situation is resolved.

**depressor** /dipres′ər/ [L, *deprimere,* to press down], any agent that reduces activity when applied to nerves and muscles. See also **depressant.**

**depressor reflex** [L, *deprimere,* to press down, *reflectere,* to bend back], a neural mechanism that produces an involuntary vasodilation and fall in arterial blood pressure in response to mechanical stimulation of the carotid sinus.

**depressor septi** /sep′tī/, one of the three muscles of the nose. Arising from the maxilla and inserting into the septum and the posterior aspect of the ala, it lies between the mucous membrane and the muscular structure of the lip and is a direct antagonist of the other muscles of the nose. It is innervated by buccal branches of the facial nerve and serves to draw down the ala, constricting the nostril. Compare **nasalis, procerus.**

**deprivation** /dep′rivā′shən/ [L, *deprivare,* to deprive], the loss of something considered valuable or necessary by taking it away or denying access to it. In experimental psychology animal or human subjects may be deprived of something desired or expected for study of their reactions.

**deprivation of sleep effects** [L, *deprivare,* to deprive; ME, *slep* + L, *efficere,* to accomplish], the interference with a basic physiologic urge to sleep, which appears to be governed by sleep centers in the hypothalamus and reticular activating system. The loss of sleep for 24 hours usually has no significant effect on physical or mental functioning. However, sleep deprivation results in progressive mental aberrations after 30 to 60 continuous hours. After this point boring tasks become intolerable, speech begins to be slurred, and performance becomes increasingly poor. After a week of sleep deprivation, symptoms of psychosis may appear.

**depth dose** [AS, *diop* + Gk, *dosis*, giving], (in radiotherapy) the relationship between the dose at any depth from a beam of radiation and the dose at the entrance from that beam.

**depth electroencephalography.** See **electroencephalography.**

**depth perception,** the ability to judge depth or the relative distance of objects in space and to orient one's position in relation to them. Binocular vision is essential to this ability.

**depth psychology,** any approach to psychology that emphasizes the study of personality and behavior in relation to unconscious motivation. See also **psychoanalysis.**

**de Quervain's fracture** /də kərvänz'/ [Fritz de Quervain, Swiss surgeon, 1868–1940], a break in the navicular bone of the hand, with dislocation of the lunate bone.

**de Quervain's thyroiditis** [Fritz de Quervain; Gk, *thyreos,* shield, *itis,* inflammation], an inflammatory condition of the thyroid. It is characterized by swelling and tenderness of the gland, fever, dysphagia, fatigue, and severe pain in the neck, ears, and jaw. The disorder often occurs after a viral infection of the upper respiratory tract. It tends to remit spontaneously and to recur several times. The diagnosis may be made by a radiologic scan showing depressed uptake of radioactive iodine in involved areas. Occasionally a fine needle biopsy of the thyroid is performed. Treatment may include antiinflammatory medication, such as aspirin or thyroid hormone, if the condition continues for more than a few days. Corticosteroids are prescribed for prolonged or severe cases. Also called **giant cell thyroiditis, granulomatous thyroiditis, subacute thyroiditis.**

**der,** abbreviation for *derivative chromosome.*

**der-,** prefix meaning 'neck': *deradelphus, deradenitis, deranencephalia.*

**derailment** /dirāl'mənt/, a pattern of speech in which incomprehensible, disconnected, and unrelated ideas replace logical and orderly thought.

**derby hat fracture.** See **dishpan fracture.**

**Dercum's disease** /dur'kəmz/ [Francis X. Dercum, U.S. neurologist, 1856–1931], a potentially fatal disorder characterized by painful localized fatty swellings and nerve lesions. The disease mainly affects menopausal women.

**dereflection** /dē'rəflek'shən/ [L, *de* + *reflectere,* to bend back], a technique of logotherapeutic psychology that is directed to taking a person's mind off a certain goal through a positive redirection to another goal, with emphasis on assets and abilities rather than the problems at hand. Dereflection often results in accomplishment of the original goal.

**dereistic thought, dereism** /dē'rē·is'tik/ [L, *de* + *res,* thing], a type of mental activity in which fantasy is not modified by logic, experience, or reality.

**derivative** /dəriv'ətiv/ [L, *derivare,* to turn away], anything that originates in another substance or object; for example, organs and tissues are derivatives of the primordial germ cells. Chemical derivatives may be produced to confirm identification of a compound.

**derivative chromosome,** a chromosomal aberration caused by translocation.

**derived protein** /dirīvd'/, a small protein obtained by enzymatic or chemical hydrolysis of a larger protein source.

**derived quantity,** any secondary quantity, such as volume, derived from a combination of base quantities, such as mass, length, and time.

**-derm,** suffix meaning 'skin': *angioderm, mucoderm, paraderm.*

**derma-.** See **dermato-.**

**-derma, -dermia, -dermic, 1.** suffix meaning 'skin': *chrysderma, micoderma, sarcoderma.* **2.** suffix meaning a '(specified) skin ailment or skin condition': *rhinoderma, syphiloderma, vaselinoderma.* **3.** suffix meaning 'related to the variety of skin': *pachydermic.*

**dermabrasion** /dur'məbrā'zhən/ [Gk, *derma,* skin; L, *abradere,* to scrape], a treatment for the removal of superficial scars on the skin by the use of revolving wire brushes or sandpaper. An aerosol spray is used to freeze the skin for this procedure. Dermabrasion is performed to reduce facial scars of severe acne.

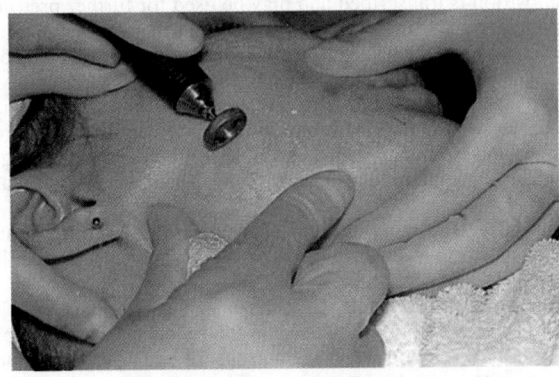

**Dermabrasion** *(Fewkes, 1992)*

***Dermacentor*** /dur'məsen'tər/, a genus of ticks. It includes species that transmit Rocky Mountain spotted fever, tularemia, brucellosis, and other infectious diseases.

**dermal** /dur'məl/ [Gk, *derma,* skin], pertaining to the skin.

**dermal graft** [Gk, *derma,* skin, *graphion,* stylus], the transplantation of any living skin tissue that contains dermis and thus is capable of regenerating and secreting sweat and sebum and generating new hair growth.

**dermal neurofibroma,** a neurofibroma arising within the skin as a small, fleshy nodule that may become pedunculated, overlying a palpable subcutaneous lesion.

**dermal papilla** [Gk, *derma,* skin; L, *papilla,* nipple], any small elevation in the dermis, such as the elongated alpine papilla seen in psoriasis.

**dermat-.** See **dermato-.**

**dermatitis** /dur'mətī'tis/ [Gk, *derma* + *itis,* inflammation], an inflammatory condition of the skin. Various cutaneous eruptions occur and may be unique to a particular allergen, disease, or infection. The condition may be chronic or acute; treatment is specific to the cause. Some kinds of dermatitis are **actinic dermatitis, contact dermatitis, rhus dermatitis,** and **seborrheic dermatitis.**

**dermatitis exfoliativa neonatorum.** See **Ritter's disease.**

**dermatitis herpetiformis,** a chronic, severely pruritic skin disease with symmetrically located groups of red papulovesicular, vesicular, bullous, or urticarial lesions. It is thought to be an immunologic response to dietary gluten. Treatment may include a diet free of gluten and the administration of sulfone, dapsone, sulfapyridine, or antipruritic drugs.

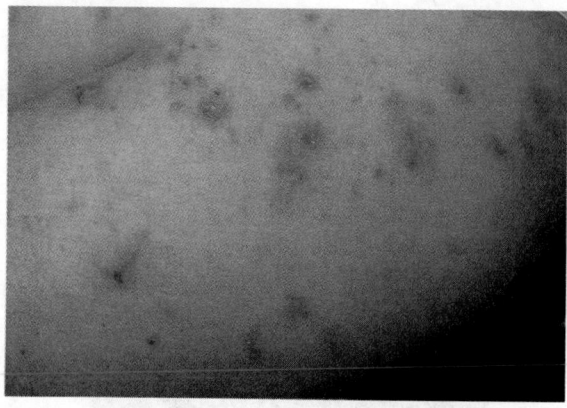

**Dermatitis herpetiformis** *(Cotran, Kumar, and Collins, 1999)*

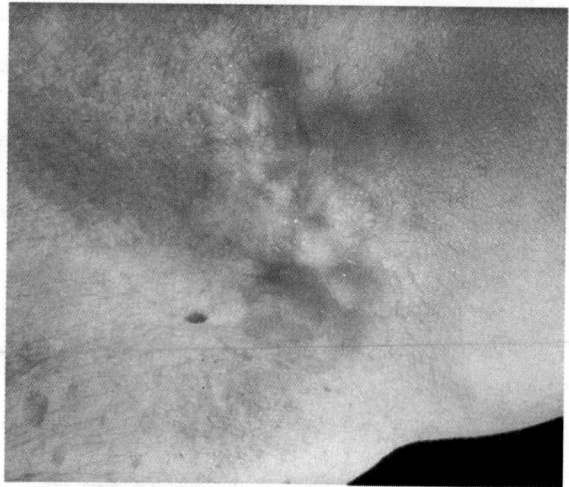

**Dermatofibrosarcomas protuberans**
*(du Vivier, 1993/courtesy Dr. Neil Smith)*

**dermatitis medicamentosa.** See **drug rash.**
**dermatitis papillaris capillitii.** See **keloid acne.**
**dermatitis venenata.** See **contact dermatitis.**
**dermato-, derma-, dermat-, dermo-,** combining form meaning 'skin': *dermatobiasis, dermatocele, dermatocyst.*
**dermatocellulitis** /dur′mətōsel′yəlī′tis/, an inflammation of the skin and subcutaneous connective tissue.
**dermatocyst** /dur′mətōsist′/, a cystic tumor of cutaneous tissues.
**dermatofibroma** /dur′mətōfībrō′mə/, *pl.* **dermatofibromas, dermatofibromata** [Gk, *derma* + L, *fibra,* fiber, *oma,* tumor], a cutaneous nodule that is painless, round, firm, gray or red, elevated, and commonly found on the extremities. No treatment is required. Also called **fibrous histiocytoma.**

**dermatoglyphics** /dur′mətōglif′iks/ [Gk, *derma* + *glyphe,* a carving], the study of the skin ridge patterns on fingers, toes, palms of hands, and soles of feet. The patterns are used as a basis of identification and also have diagnostic value because of associations between certain patterns and chromosomal anomalies.
**dermatographia** /dur′mətōgraf′ē·ə/ [Gk, *derma* + *graphein,* to record], a skin condition characterized by wheals that develop from tracing on the skin with the fingernail or a blunted instrument. This condition makes the patient itch and may be associated with urticaria. Also called **autographism, dermatographism, Ebbecke's reaction.**

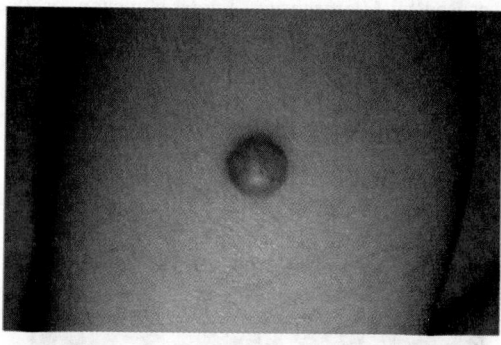

**Dermatofibroma** *(Weston, Lane, and Morelli, 1996)*

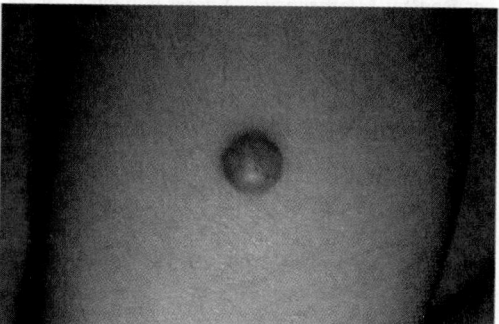

**Dermatographia** *(Weston, Lane, and Morelli, 1996)*

**dermatologic agent** /dur′mətōloj′ik/, a drug used to treat reactions or disorders of the skin.
**dermatologist** /dur′mətol′əjist/, a physician specializing in the skin and its properties of health and disease.
**dermatology** /-ol′əjē/ [Gk, *derma* + *logos,* science], the study of the skin, including its anatomic, physiologic, and pathologic characteristics and the diagnosis and treatment of skin disorders.

**dermatofibrosarcoma** /-fī′brōsärkō′mə/ [Gk, *derma,* skin; L, *fibra,* fiber; Gk, *sarx,* flesh, *oma,* tumor], a specific type of fibrous tumor of the skin.

**dermatoma** /dur′mətō′mə/, **1.** a skin tumor. **2.** a local path of abnormally thick skin.

**dermatome** /dur′mətōm/ [Gk, *derma* + *temnein,* to cut], **1.** (in embryology) the mesodermal layer in the early developing embryo that gives rise to the dermal layers of the skin. **2.** (in surgery) an instrument used to cut thin slices of skin for grafting. **3.** an area on the surface of a body innervated by afferent fibers from one spinal root.

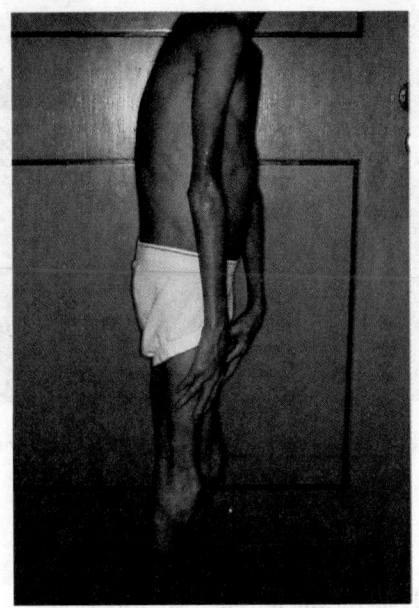

**Dermatomyositis** *(Zitelli and Davis, 1992)*

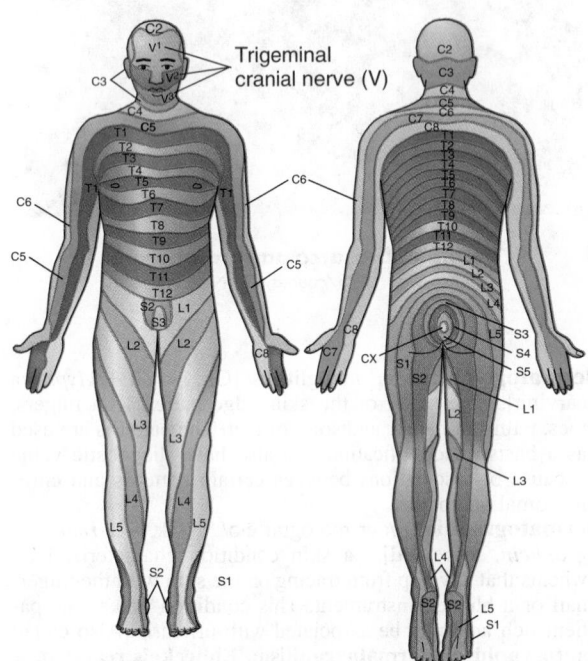

**Dermatome distribution of spinal nerves**
*(Thibodeau and Patton, 1999/Network Graphics)*

**dermatomycosis** /dur′mətō′mīkō′sis/ [Gk, *derma* + *mykes,* fungus, *osis,* condition], a superficial fungal infection of the skin, characteristically found on parts that are moist and protected by clothing, such as the groin or feet. It is caused by a dermatophyte. See also **dermatophytosis. —dermatomycotic,** *adj.*

**dermatomyositis** /dur′mətōmī′ōsī′tis/ [Gk, *derma* + *mys,* muscle, *itis,* inflammation], a disease of the connective tissues, characterized by pruritic or eczematous inflammation of the skin and tenderness and weakness of the muscles. Muscle tissue is destroyed, and loss is often so severe that the person may become unable to walk or to perform simple tasks. Swelling of the eyelids and face and loss of weight are common manifestations. The cause is unknown, but in 15% of cases the condition develops with an internal malignancy. Viral infection and antibacterial medication are also associated with an increased incidence of dermatomyositis.

**dermatopathy** /dur′mətop′əthē/, any disorder of the skin.

*Dermatophagoides* /-fagoi′dēz/ [Gk, *derma* + *phagein,* to eat, *eidos,* form], a genus of household dust mite responsible for allergic reactions in sensitive individuals. Protection against the microscopically small mite includes minimizing dust in the home, especially in the bedroom; encasing pillows and mattresses in allergen-proof coverings; and controlling temperature and humidity. The mites thrive on skin scales, hair, pet foods, carpets, and bedding, in addition to ordinary house dust.

**dermatophyte** /dur′mətōfīt′, dərmat′əfīt/, any of several fungi that cause parasitic skin disease in humans. See also **dermatophytid** and specific fungal infections.

**dermatophytid** /dur′mətof′itid, dur′mətōfī′tid/ [Gk, *derma* + *phyton,* plant], an allergic skin reaction characterized by small vesicles and associated with dermatomycosis. The lesions result from sensitization to the infection elsewhere on the skin and do not contain fungi. See also **dermatomycosis, dermatophyte.**

**dermatophytosis** /dur′mətō′fītō′sis/ [Gk, *derma* + *phyton,* plant, *osis,* condition], a superficial fungus infection of the skin, caused by *Microsporum, Epidermophyton,* or *Trichophyton* species of dermatophyte. On the trunk and upper ex-

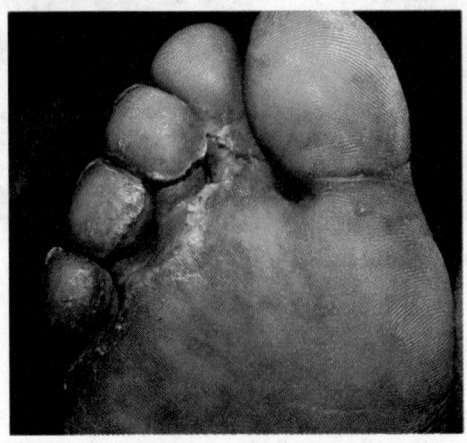

**Dermatophytosis** *(Stone and Gorbach, 2000)*

tremities it is commonly called "ringworm" infection and is characterized by round or oval scaly patches with slightly raised borders and clearing centers. On the feet small vesicles, cracking, itching, scaling, and often secondary bacterial infections occur and are commonly called "athlete's foot." Treatment includes topical antifungal agents, as tolnaftate, clotrimazole, and undecylenic acid, and oral griseofulvin. Fingernails and toenails respond poorly to topical treatment. See also **tinea.**

**dermatoplasty** /dur'mətōplas'tē/, a surgical procedure in which skin tissue is transplanted to a body surface damaged by disease or injury.

**dermatosclerosis** /-sklərō'sis/ [Gk, *derma* + *sklerosis,* hardening], a skin disease characterized by fibrous thickening of the skin. See also **scleroderma.**

**dermatosis** /dur'mətō'sis/ [Gk, *derma* + *osis,* condition], any disorder of the skin, especially those not associated with inflammation. Compare **dermatitis.**

**dermatosis papulosa nigra,** a common condition in individuals with darkly pigmented skin. It consists of multiple tiny, benign skin-colored or hyperpigmented papules on the face, neck, and cheeks. The lesions increase in number with age.

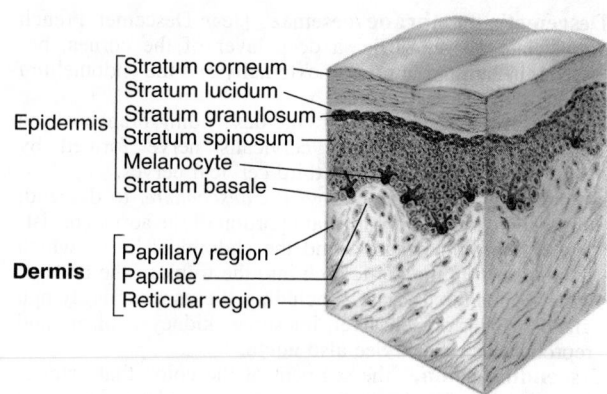

**Dermis** *(Applegate, 2000)*

ity containing fatty material, hair, teeth, bits of bone, and cartilage. Kinds of dermoid cysts are **implantation dermoid cyst, inclusion dermoid cyst, thyroid dermoid cyst,** and **tubal dermoid cyst.** Also called **organoid tumor, teratoid tumor.**

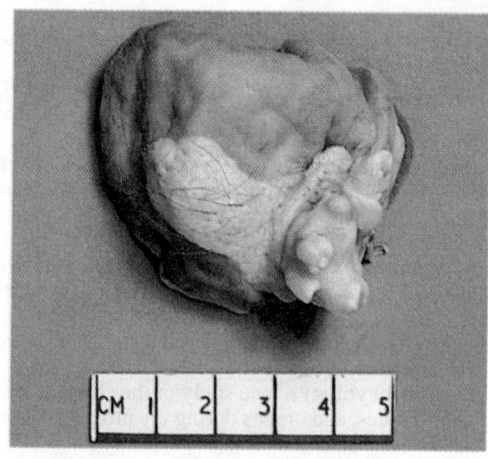

**Dermoid cyst** *(Symonds and MacPherson, 1994)*

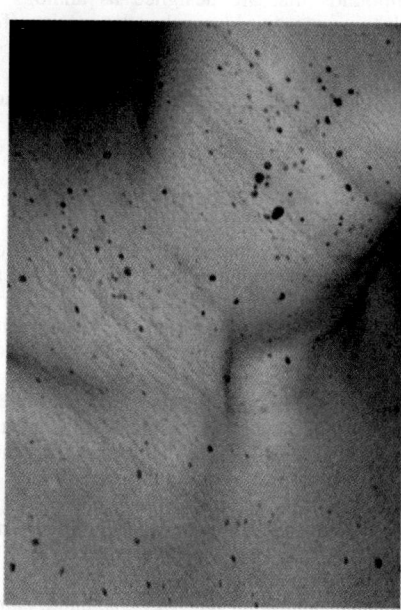

**Dermatosis papulosa nigra** *(Lawrence and Cox, 1993)*

**dermis,** the layer of the skin just below the epidermis, consisting of papillary and reticular layers and containing blood and lymphatic vessels, nerves and nerve endings, glands, and hair follicles. Formerly called **corium.**

**-dermis,** suffix meaning 'tissue or skin': *hypodermis, endepidermis, osteodermis.*

**dermo-.** See **dermato-.**

**dermographism.** See **dermatographia.**

**dermoid** /dur'moid/ [Gk, *derma* + *eidos,* form], **1.** pertaining to the skin. **2.** *informal.* a dermoid cyst.

**dermoid cyst,** a tumor, derived from embryonal tissues, consisting of a fibrous wall lined with epithelium and a cav-

**-dermoma,** suffix meaning a 'tumor of the skin layers': *epidermoma, monodermoma, tridermoma.*

**derotation brace** /dē'rōtā'shən/, a customized orthosis that provides stability at the knee joint. It consists of a single-joint hinged bar on one side and a rotating dial pad on the opposite side. The rotating pad can be placed on either the medial or the lateral side, depending on the location of the primary instability. Each brace is designed individually, based on a negative plaster cast of the knee.

**DES,** abbreviation for **diethylstilbestrol.**

**desalination** /dēsal'inā'shən/ [L, *de,* from, *sal,* salt], the process of removing salt from water or other substances.

**desaturation** /dēsach'ərā'shən/ [L, *de,* from, *saturare,* to fill], the formation of an unsaturated chemical compound from a saturated one.

**Descemet's membrane** /desemāz'/ [Jean Descemet, French physician, 1732–1810], a deep layer of the cornea, between the substantia propria externally and the endothelium internally.

**descendens** /disen'dənz/, **1.** the descending branch of the hypoglossal nerve. **2.** the cervicalis nerve formed by branches of the second and third cervical nerves.

**descending aorta** /disen'ding/ [L, *descendere,* to descend; Gk, *aerein,* to raise], the main portion of the aorta, consisting of the thoracic aorta and the abdominal aorta, which continues from the aortic arch into the trunk of the body. It supplies many structures, including the esophagus, lymph glands, ribs, stomach, liver, intestines, kidneys, spleen, and reproductive organs. See also **aorta.**

**descending colon,** the segment of the colon that extends from the end of the transverse colon at the splenic flexure on the left side of the abdomen down to the beginning of the sigmoid colon in the pelvis. See also **colon.**

**descending current.** See **centrifugal current.**

**descending myelitis** [L, *descendere,* to descend; Gk, *myelos,* marrow, *itis,* inflammation], a form of myelitis in which the pathologic changes spread downward along the spinal cord.

**descending neuritis** [L, *descendere,* to descend; Gk, *neuron,* nerve, *itis,* inflammation], a form of neuritis that spreads downward from the upper part of the nervous system.

**descending neuropathy** [L, *descendere,* to descend; Gk, *neuron,* nerve, *pathos,* disease], a disease of the peripheral nervous system that spreads downward from the upper part of the body.

**descending oblique muscle.** See **external abdominal oblique muscle.**

**descending tract** [L, *descendere,* to descend, *tractus*], a nerve tract in the spinal cord that carries impulses away from the brain axis of the body or body part.

**descending urography.** See **intravenous pyelography.**

**descensus** /disen'səs/, the process of falling or descending; prolapse.

**descent of testis.** See **cryptorchidism.**

**descriptive anatomy** /diskrip'tiv/ [L, *describere,* to write], the study of the morphologic characteristics of the body by systems, such as the vascular system and the nervous system. Each system is composed of similar tissues that are essential to a particular function.

**descriptive embryology,** the study of the changes that occur in cells, tissues, and organs during the progressive stages of prenatal development.

**descriptive epidemiology,** the first stage of epidemiologic investigation. It focuses on describing disease distribution by characteristics relating to time, place, and person.

**descriptive psychiatry,** the study of external, readily observable behavior. Compare **dynamic psychiatry.**

**descriptive statistics,** statistics that measure and describe characteristics of groups without drawing inferences about the population in general.

**DES daughters,** a group of women with increased susceptibility to cancer of the vagina and other reproductive organs because their mothers were given an estrogen medication, diethylstilbestrol (DES), from the 1940s through the 1960s to prevent miscarriage. Several other abnormalities have been reported among the DES daughters, including tissue that covers the cervix or a uterus that is too small to carry a pregnancy. Sons of women who took DES have an increased risk of undescended testes or other genital disorders.

**Desenex,** trademark for a fixed-combination topical drug containing two antifungals (undecylenic acid and zinc undecylenate).

**desensitization.** See **systemic desensitization.**

**desensitize** /dēsen'sitīz/ [L, *de* + *sentire,* to feel], **1.** (in immunology) to render an individual insensitive or less sensitive to any of the various antigens. **2.** (in psychiatry) to relieve an emotionally disturbed person of the stress of phobias and neuroses by encouraging discussion of the anxieties and the stressful experiences that cause the emotional problems involved. **3.** (in dentistry) to remove or reduce the painful response of vital exposed dentin to irritating substances and temperature changes.

**desert fever, desert rheumatism.** See **coccidioidomycosis.**

**Desferal Mesylate,** trademark for an iron chelating agent (deferoxamine mesylate).

**desiccant** /des'ikənt/ [L, *desiccare,* to dry thoroughly], any agent or procedure that promotes drying or causes a substance to dry up. Also called **exsiccant.**

**desiccate** /des'ikāt/, **1.** to dry thoroughly. **2.** to preserve by drying, especially food. Also **exsiccate.**

**designated donor,** a person, usually a friend or relative with the same blood type, who has agreed to donate one or more units of blood in advance of a planned surgery. The designated donor blood must undergo the same tests as anonymous donor blood.

**designer drugs** [L, *de* + *signare,* to mark], synthetic organic compounds that are designed as analogs of illicit drugs, with the same opioid or other dangerous effects. Because designer drugs are generally not listed as controlled substances by the U.S. Drug Enforcement Agency, prosecution of manufacturers, distributors, or users is frequently difficult.

**desipramine hydrochloride** /desip'rəmēn/, a tricyclic antidepressant.

■ INDICATION: It is prescribed in the treatment of mental depression.

■ CONTRAINDICATIONS: Concomitant administration of monoamine oxidase inhibitors, heart block, recent myocardial infarction, or known hypersensitivity to this drug or to tricyclic medication prohibits its use. It is used with caution in patients who have seizure disorders or cardiovascular disease.

■ ADVERSE EFFECTS: Among the more serious adverse reactions are sedation as well as GI, cardiovascular, and neurologic reactions. This drug interacts with many other drugs.

**-desma,** suffix meaning 'something bridging or connecting': *cytodesma, mesodesma, plasmodesma.*

**desmo-,** combining form meaning 'ligament': *desmoma, desmorrhexis, desmotomy.*

**desmocyte.** See **fibroblast.**

**desmoid tumor** /dez'moid/ [Gk, *desmos,* band, *eidos,* form], a fibrous neoplasm that may occur in the head, neck, upper arm, abdomen, or lower extremities. The tumor is usually a firm, rubbery mass.

**desmopressin acetate** /dez'mōpres'in/, a synthetic antidiuretic analog of arginine vasopressin, the naturally occurring human antidiuretic hormone.

■ INDICATION: It is prescribed as an antidiuretic in the treatment of diabetes insipidus.

■ CONTRAINDICATION: Known hypersensitivity to this drug prohibits its use.

■ ADVERSE EFFECTS: Among the most serious adverse reactions are hyponatremia and water intoxication. Mild effects, such as headache, cramps, and nasal congestion, also may occur.

**desmosis** /dezmō'sis/, any disease of the connective tissue.

**desmosome** /dez'məsōm/ [Gk, *desmos,* band, *soma,* body], a small, circular, dense area within the intercellular bridge

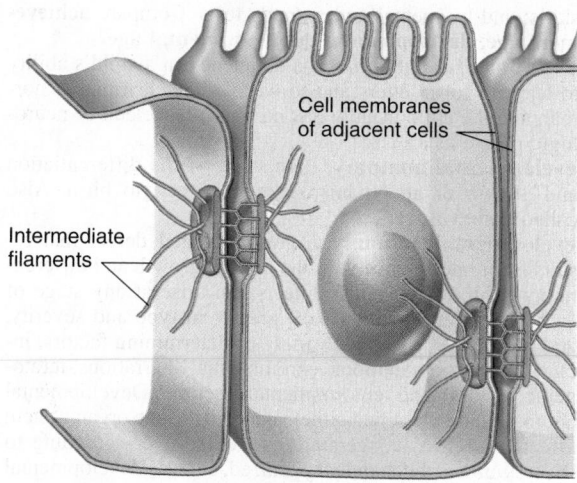

Cell membranes of adjacent cells

Intermediate filaments

**Desmosome**

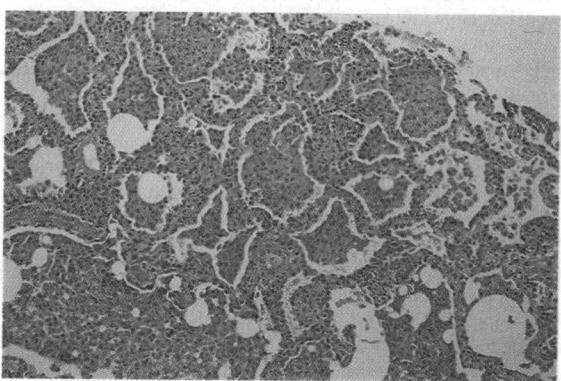

**Desquamative interstitial pneumonia**
*(Cotran, Kumar, and Collins, 1999)*

logic stress, such as trauma to the epithelium. Compare **eruptive gingivitis.**

**desquamative interstitial pneumonia,** a respiratory disease characterized by an accumulation of cellular matter in the alveoli and bronchial tubes. It leads to a fibrotic condition with symptoms of coughing, chest pain, weight loss, and dyspnea. Treatment is with corticosteroids, oxygen, and supportive medical therapy.

that forms the site of adhesion between certain epithelial cells, especially the stratified epithelium of the epidermis. Also called **macula adherens.**

**desonide** /des'ənīd/, a topical corticosteroid.
- INDICATION: It is prescribed for the treatment of skin inflammation.
- CONTRAINDICATIONS: Viral and fungal diseases of the skin, impaired circulation, or known hypersensitivity to this drug or to steroid medication prohibits its use.
- ADVERSE EFFECTS: Among the more serious adverse reactions, usually occurring after prolonged or excessive application, are striae, hypopigmentation or local irritation of the skin, and various systemic effects.

**desoximetasone** /desok'simet'əsōn/, a topical corticosteroid.
- INDICATION: It is prescribed for the treatment of skin inflammation.
- CONTRAINDICATIONS: Viral and fungal diseases of the skin, impaired circulation, or known hypersensitivity to this drug or to other steroid medication prohibits its use. Caution should be used in applying occlusive dressings over topical steroid medications.
- ADVERSE EFFECTS: Among the more serious adverse reactions, usually occurring after prolonged or excessive application, are striae, hypopigmentation, or local irritation of the skin and various systemic effects.

**desoxy-.** See **deoxy-.**

**Desoxyn,** trademark for a central nervous system stimulant (methamphetamine hydrochloride).

**desoxyribonucleic acid.** See **deoxyribonucleic acid.**

**despair,** a feeling of hopelessness and a loss of hope.

**desquamation** /des'kwəmā'shən/ [L, *desquamare*, to take off scales], a normal process in which the cornified layer of the epidermis is sloughed in fine scales. Certain conditions, injuries, and medications accelerate desquamation and may cause peeling and the loss of deeper layers of the skin. Also called **exfoliation. —desquamate,** *v.,* **desquamative,** *adj.*

**desquamative gingivitis** /deskwam'ətiv/, a gingival inflammation characterized by peeling of the epithelium. In its chronic state it is most frequently associated with the hormonal changes of menopause. It may also be caused by bio-

**destructive aggression** /distruk'tiv/ [L, *destruere*, to destroy, *aggressio*, an attack], an act of hostility unnecessary for self-protection or preservation that is directed at an external object or person. See also **aggression, detachment.**

**destructive interference,** a phenomenon that results when propagated waves are out of phase, so that maximum molecular compression for one wave occurs at the same point as maximum rarefaction for the second wave, causing the two waves to cancel each other out.

**destructive lesion** [L, *destruere*, to destroy, *laesio*, a hurting], a disorder that leads to the damage or necrosis of an organ or tissue.

**desudation** /des'ōōdā'shən/, profuse sweating. It is sometimes followed by a skin rash.

**Desyrel,** trademark for an antidepressant (trazodone).

**detached retina.** See **retinal detachment.**

**detachment.** See **destructive aggression.**

**detection bias** /ditek'shən/, a potential artifact in epidemiologic data caused by the use of a particular diagnostic technique or type of equipment. As an example, cancer rates may vary in different regions or periods, not because of an actual difference in the incidence of the disease but because of different diagnostic technologies.

**detergent** /ditur'jənt/ [L, *detergere*, to cleanse], **1.** a cleansing agent. **2.** (in respiratory therapy) a wetting agent that is administered to mediate the removal of respiratory tract secretions from airway walls. Examples include tyloxapol and acetylcysteine. See also **surfactant.**

**deterioration** /ditir'ē·ərā'shən/ [L, *deterior,* worse], a condition that is gradually worsening; retrogression.

**determinant evolution** /ditur'minənt/ [L, *determinare*, to limit], the idea that evolution progresses according to a predetermined course. See also **orthogenesis.**

**determinant of occlusion,** one of the classifiable factors that influence proper closure of the teeth. The common fixed factors are intercondylar distance, anatomic characteristics, mandibular centricity, and the relationship of the jaws. The common changeable factors are tooth shape, tooth position, and vertical dimensions of occlusion, cusp height, and fossa depth.

**determinate cleavage** /ditur′minit/, mitotic division of the fertilized ovum into blastomeres that are each destined to form a specific part of the embryo. Damage to or destruction of any of these cells results in malformation of an organism. Also called **mosaic cleavage.** Compare **indeterminate cleavage.** See also **mosaic development.**

**detoxification** /dētok′sifikā′shən/ [L, *de* + Gk, *toxikon,* poison; L, *facere,* to make], the removal of a poison or its effects from a patient.

**detoxification service,** a hospital service providing treatment to diminish or remove from a patient's body the toxic effects of chemical substances, such as alcohol or drugs, usually as an initial step in the treatment of a chemical-dependent person. The service may also be used to remove poisonous substances to which a person may have been exposed. See also **alcoholism, drug addiction.**

**detoxify** /dētok′sifī/ [L, *de,* from; Gk, *toxikon,* poison], to make a poisonous substance harmless or to overcome the effects of a poison.

**detrition** /də·trish′ən/ [L, *de,* from + *terere* to wear], a wearing away, as of the teeth, by friction. See also **abrasion.**

**detrusor urinae muscle** /ditrōō′zər/ [L, *detruder,* to thrust; Gk, *ouron,* urine; L, *musculus*], a complex of longitudinal fibers that form the external layer of the muscular coat of the bladder.

**deuterium (²H)** /dyōōtir′ē·əm/ [Gk, *deuteros,* second], a stable isotope of the hydrogen atom, used as a kinetic tracer. Also called **heavy hydrogen.** See also **tritium.**

**deutero-, deuto-,** combining form meaning 'second': *deuteroalbumose, deuteroconidium, deuteroelastose.*

**deuteroplasm.** See **deutoplasm.**

**deuto-.** See **deutero-.**

**deutoplasm** /dōō′təplaz′əm/ [Gk, *deuteros* + *plasma,* something formed], the inactive elements of the cytoplasm, primarily the stored nutritive material contained in yolk. Also called **deuteroplasm.**

**DEV,** abbreviation for **duck embryo vaccine.** See also **rabies vaccine.**

**devascularization** /dēvas′kyəler′īzā′shən/ [L, *de,* from, *vasculum,* small vessel], the drawing away of blood from a body part or the stoppage of blood flow to it.

**developer fog,** a defect in a radiographic image characterized by insufficient contrast. Causes include incorrect developer temperature, immersion time, and developer concentration.

**development** [Fr, *developper,* to unfold], **1.** the gradual process of change and differentiation from a simple to a more advanced level of complexity. In humans the physical, mental, and emotional capacities that allow complex adaptation to the environment and function within society are acquired through growth, maturation, and learning. Kinds of development include **arrested development, mosaic development, psychomotor development, psychosexual development, psychosocial development,** and **regulative development. 2.** (in biology) the series of events that occur within an organism from the time of fertilization of the ovum to the adult stage. See also **film development. —developmental,** *adj.*

**developmental age (DA)** /divel′əpmen′təl/, an expression of a child's maturational progress stated in age and determined by standardized measurements, as of body size and dimensions; by social and psychologic functioning; motor

skills; and by mental and aptitude tests. Compare **achievement age, developmental quotient, mental age.**

**developmental agraphia,** a deficiency in a child's ability to learn to form letters and to write. Other learning is normal, and the child usually has no musculoskeletal or neurologic problems.

**developmental anatomy,** the study of the differentiation and growth of an organism from one cell to birth. Also called **embryology.**

**developmental anomaly,** any congenital defect that results from interference with the normal growth and differentiation of the fetus. Such defects can arise at any stage of embryonic development, vary greatly in type and severity, and are caused by a wide variety of determining factors, including genetic mutations, chromosomal aberrations, teratogenic agents, and environmental factors. Developmental anomalies are classified either according to the organ system affected, such as congenital heart defects, or according to the way in which the defect occurred, such as developmental failure or arrest, failure to atrophy or subdivide, fusion, splitting, incorrect migration, and misplacement. Most developmental defects are apparent at birth, especially any structural malformation, but some, especially those involving the organ systems, do not become evident until days, weeks, or even years later.

**developmental apraxia** [L, *developper,* development; Gk, *a,* not, *prassein,* to do], a condition of ineffective motor planning and execution in children caused by immaturity of their central nervous system.

**developmental arrest.** See **arrested development.**

**developmental care,** a nursing intervention from the Nursing Interventions Classification (NIC) defined as structuring the environment and providing care in response to the behavioral cues and states of the preterm infant. See also **Nursing Interventions Classification.**

**developmental crisis,** severe, usually transient, stress that occurs when a person is unable to complete the tasks of a psychosocial stage of development and is therefore unable to move on to the next stage. See also **psychosocial development.**

**developmental disability (DD),** a pathologic condition that starts developing before 18 years of age. Most developmental disabilities persist throughout the individual's life, although many can be effectively treated. See also **congenital anomaly.**

**developmental disorder,** a form of mental retardation that develops in some children after they have progressed normally for the first 3 or 4 years of life. Onset of the mental deterioration usually begins with a vague viral infection or other similar disease symptoms.

**developmental dyspraxia,** a disorder of sensory integration characterized by an impaired ability to plan skilled, nonhabitual coordinated movements.

**developmental enhancement: adolescent,** a nursing intervention from the Nursing Interventions Classification (NIC) defined as facilitating optimal physical, cognitive, social, and emotional growth of individuals during the transition from childhood to adulthood. See also **Nursing Interventions Classification.**

**developmental enhancement: child,** a nursing intervention from the Nursing Interventions Classification (NIC) defined as facilitating or teaching parents/caregivers to facilitate the optimal gross motor, fine motor, language, cognitive, social, and emotional growth of preschool and school-age children. See also **Nursing Interventions Classification.**

**developmental groove,** a fine, recessed line in the enamel of a tooth that marks the union of the lobes of the crown in its development.

**developmental guidance,** comprehensive orthopedic control over the growth of the jaws and the eruption of the teeth. It may require precisely timed therapy with active appliances as well as supervisory examinations, including radiography and other diagnostic records. Guidance may be needed at various developmental stages throughout the entire growth and maturation of the face, beginning at the earliest detection of a developing malformation.

**developmental horizon,** any of 25 stages in the development of the human embryo from the one-cell stage at conception to the morphologically and physiologically complex organism at the end of the seventh week of gestation.

**developmental model,** **1.** a conceptual framework devised to be used as a guide in making a diagnosis, in understanding a developmental process, and in forming a prognosis for continued development. It has five components: The *identifiable state* describes the stage, level, phase, or period of the condition or process; the *shift in state* identifies qualities of change as progressive, sudden, abrupt, or recurrent; and the *form of progression* describes patterns of development as linear, spiral, or oscillating. The *force* that triggers the change or the step in development may be self-actualization or any form of stress. Development is ultimately constrained by the fifth component, *potentiality,* the genetic and environmental possibility of growth. **2.** (in nursing) a conceptual framework describing four stages, or processes, of development in the patient during therapy. In the first stage, called *orientation,* the patient begins a relationship with the nurse or other therapist and begins to clarify the problem with his or her help. In the second stage, called *identification,* the patient develops a sense of closeness and attachment to the therapist. During this period the patient and the therapist work comfortably together. In the third stage, called *exploitation,* the patient makes full use of the nursing services offered, begins to assume some control of the interactions, and becomes more independent. During the last stage, called *resolution,* the therapeutic relationship is terminated; the patient is independent and no longer needs the nurse or therapist. With this model the nurse therapist may plan nursing interventions appropriate to the patient's developmental level. The developmental model is one of the earliest nursing models to be developed. It views the person as a psychobiologic being whose needs are expressed in behavior and who is unique and capable of learning and changing. Health is viewed as a forward movement of personality development and other ongoing processes, reflected by the person's creative, constructive, and productive community living. Thus the focus of nursing is to promote this forward movement by assisting the patient in self-repair and self-renewal.

**developmental physiology,** the study of the physiologic processes as they relate to embryonic development.

**developmental quotient (DQ),** the numeric expression of a child's developmental level as measured by dividing the developmental age by the chronologic age and multiplying by 100. Compare **intelligence quotient.** See also **developmental age.**

**developmental sequence** [Fr, *developper;* L, *sequi,* to follow], the order in which structure and function change during the process of growth and development of an organism. See also **ontogeny, phylogeny.**

**developmental task,** a physical or cognitive skill that a person must accomplish during a particular age period to continue development. An example is walking, which precedes the development of a sense of autonomy in the toddler

period. The nurse may also outline developmental tasks for families.

**developmental theories of aging,** concepts based on the identification of traits and characteristics that may be developed early in life or may change emphasis at different stages of development. Examples are theories of Jung, Erikson, and Havighurst.

**deviance** /dē′vē·əns/ [L, *deviare,* to turn aside], behavior that is contrary to the accepted standards of a community or culture.

**deviant** /dē′vē·ənt/ [L, *deviare,* to turn aside], pertaining to a person or object that departs from what is considered normal or standard.

**deviant behavior,** actions that exceed the usual limits of accepted behavior and involve failure to comply with the social norm of the group.

**deviate** /dē′vē·it/ [L, *deviare,* to turn aside], **1.** a person or an act that varies from that which is considered standard, such as a social or sexual deviate, or that which is within a statistic norm. **2.** to vary from that which is considered standard or within a statistic norm. —**deviant,** *adj.,* **deviation,** *n.*

**deviated septum,** a shifted medial partition of the nasal cavity, a condition affecting many adults. The nasal septum more commonly shifts to the left during normal growth, but this deflection may be aggravated by a blow to the nose or by other trauma. A severe deflection of the septum may significantly obstruct the nasal passages and result in infection, sinusitis, shortness of breath, headache, or recurring nose bleeds. Severe septal deviation may be corrected by various surgical procedures, such as rhinoplasty or septoplasty. Postoperative care in such cases usually includes such measures as the maintenance of nasal packing, the administration of sedatives, and the placement of ice packs around the affected area to reduce swelling.

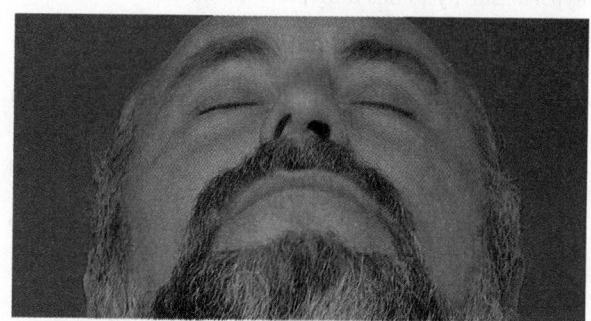

**Deviated septum** *(Monahan and Neighbors, 1998)*

**deviational nystagmus.** See **end-positional nystagmus.**

**deviation, axis** /dē′vē·ā′shən/ [L, *deviare,* to turn aside, *axle*], (in electrocardiography) an abnormal direction of the mean electrical current of the heart.

**deviation from normal,** a quality, characteristic, symptom, or clinical finding that is different from what is commonly regarded as normal, such as an elevated temperature, multiple gestation, or an extra digit.

**deviation of tongue** [L, *deviare,* to turn aside; AS, *tunge*], a tendency of the tongue to turn away from the midline when extended or protruded. The condition is associated with a hypoglossal nerve defect.

**device** /divīs′/ [OFr, *deviser,* to divide], an item other than a drug that has application in the healing arts. The term is sometimes restricted to items used directly by, on, or in the patient, as opposed to surgical instruments or other equipment used for diagnosis and treatment. Devices include orthopedic appliances, crutches, artificial heart valves, pacemakers, prostheses, wheelchairs, cervical collars, hearing aids, and eye glasses.

**Devic's disease** /də·vĕks'/ [Eugène Devic, French physician, 1869–1930], combined, but not usually clinically simultaneous, demyelination of the optic nerve and the spinal cord; it is marked by diminution of vision and sometimes blindness, flaccid paralysis of the extremities, and sensory and genitourinary disturbances.

**devil's grip.** See **epidemic pleurodynia.**

**devitalized** /dēvī'təlīzd/, pertaining to tissues with a reduced oxygen supply and blood flow.

**devital tooth.** See **pulpless tooth.**

**dewar** /dyoo'ər/, a double chamber used to maintain the temperature of superconducting magnet coils near absolute zero. The outer chamber is filled with liquid nitrogen at a temperature of about $-196°$ C ($-321°$ F), and the inner chamber is filled with liquid helium at a temperature of $-270°$ C ($-454°$ F). A dewar is part of magnetic resonance imaging equipment.

**dew point** /dyoo/, the temperature at which air becomes saturated with water vapor and the water vapor condenses to liquid. In aerosol therapy water may condense on containers, tubing, and other surfaces when the dew point is reached.

**DEXA,** abbreviation for **dual-energy x-ray absorptiometry.**

**dexamethasone** /dek'səmeth'əsōn/, a long-acting synthetic adrenocorticoid with intense antiinflammatory activity and mineralocorticoid activity.
- INDICATIONS: It is prescribed topically and systemically in the treatment of inflammatory conditions.
- CONTRAINDICATIONS: Systemic fungal infections or known hypersensitivity to this drug prohibits its use.
- ADVERSE EFFECTS: Among the more serious adverse reactions are GI, endocrine, neurologic, fluid, and electrolyte disturbances.

**dexchlorpheniramine maleate** /deks'klôrfənir'əmēn mal'ē·it/, an antihistamine.
- INDICATIONS: It is prescribed in the treatment of hypersensitivity reactions, including rhinitis, skin rash, and pruritus.
- CONTRAINDICATIONS: Asthma or known hypersensitivity to this drug prohibits its use. It should not be given to newborns or lactating mothers.
- ADVERSE EFFECTS: Drowsiness, skin rash, hypersensitivity reactions, dry mouth, and tachycardia may occur.

**Dexedrine,** trademark for a central nervous system stimulant (dextroamphetamine sulfate) with indications for narcolepsy and attention deficit disorder with hyperactivity.

**dexmedetomidine,** an alpha$_2$ adrenoceptor agonist sedative.
- INDICATIONS: This drug is used to sedate mechanically ventilated and intubated patients in the intensive care unit.
- CONTRAINDICATIONS: Known hypersensitivity to this drug contraindicates its use.
- ADVERSE EFFECTS: Life-threatening effects are atrial fibrillation and infarction. Other serious adverse effects include oliguria, hypertension, pulmonary edema, pleural effusion, hypoxia, leukocytosis, and anemia. Common side effects include nausea, bradycardia, and hypotension.

**dexrazoxane,** a cardioprotective agent.
- INDICATIONS: It is prescribed in the protection of women from heart problems caused by doxorubicin treatment of breast cancer.

- CONTRAINDICATIONS: The drug should not be given to patients with an allergy to dexrazoxane or any of its components or who are receiving chemotherapy that does not contain an anthracycline drug.
- ADVERSE EFFECTS: The side effects most often reported include pain on or at injection site, flushing, bruising, rash, numbness, or general body discomfort.

**dexter** /deks'tər/ [L, *dexter*, right], right side, right.

**dexterity** /dekster'itē/ [L, *dexteritas*], skillfulness in the use of one's hands or body.

**dextrad** /deks'trad/ [L, *dexter*, right], toward the right side.

**dextrad writing** /deks'trad/ [L, *dexter*, right; ME, *writen*], writing that moves from left to right.

**dextrality.** See **right-handedness.**

**dextran fermentation** /dek'strən/ [L, *dexter*, right; *fermentare*, to cause to rise], the conversion of dextrose to dextran by the action of *Leuconostoc mesenteroides* dextran (LMD) bacteria.

**dextran preparation,** any of a group of solutions containing polysaccharides, water, and, in some preparations, electrolytes. These solutions are used as plasma volume extenders in cases of hypovolemia from hemorrhage, dehydration, or another cause and are available for IV administration in several concentrations.

**dextrin,** a glucose polymer formed by the hydrolysis of starch. It is a tasteless, colorless, gummy substance, soluble in water. Dextrin is an intermediate during the conversion of starch into monosaccharides, such as glucose. It is used in a number of pharmaceutic products.

**dextroamphetamine sulfate** /deks'trō·amfet'əmēn/, a central nervous system stimulant.
- INDICATIONS: It is prescribed in the treatment of narcolepsy and hyperkinetic disorders in children and as an anorexiant in treating exogenous obesity.
- CONTRAINDICATIONS: Cardiovascular disease, glaucoma, hypertension, hyperthyroidism, agitation, history of drug abuse, concomitant administration of a monoamine oxidase inhibitor within 14 days, or known hypersensitivity to this drug prohibits its use.
- ADVERSE EFFECTS: Among the more serious adverse reactions are manifestations of central nervous system excitation, increased blood pressure, arrhythmias and other cardiovascular effects, nausea, anorexia, and drug dependence.

**dextrocardia** /-kär'dē·ə/, the location of the heart in the right hemithorax, either as a result of displacement by disease or as a congenital defect.

**dextrocardiogram** /-kär'dē·ōgram'/ [L, *dexter*, right; Gk, *kardia*, heart, *gramma*, record], an electrocardiogram made from a unipolar electrode facing the right ventricle, producing a small R wave and a large S wave.

**dextro-, dextr-,** combining form meaning 'right': *dextrocardia, dextrocerebral, dextrogastria.*

**dextromethorphan hydrobromide** /-methôr'fən/, an antitussive derived from morphine, but lacking opioid effects.
- INDICATION: It is prescribed for the suppression of nonproductive cough.
- CONTRAINDICATIONS: Use of a monoamine oxidase inhibitor within the past 14 days or known hypersensitivity to this drug prohibits its use.
- ADVERSE EFFECTS: The most serious adverse reaction is respiratory depression resulting from large doses.

**dextrose** /dek'strōs/ [L, *dexter*, right], a glucose available in various solutions for IV administration.
- INDICATIONS: It is prescribed for the treatment of calorie deficit, for hypoglycemia, and in solution for fluid deficit.
- CONTRAINDICATIONS: Diabetic coma, intracranial or intraspinal hemorrhage, or delirium tremens prohibits its use.

■ ADVERSE EFFECTS: Among the more serious adverse reactions are hyperglycemia, glycosuria, and phlebitis.

**dextrose and sodium chloride injection,** a fluid, nutrient, and electrolyte replenisher. It is available for parenteral use in a variety of concentrations.

**dextrothyroxine sodium,** an antihyperlipidemic.

■ INDICATION: It is prescribed as an adjunct to other medications in the treatment of primary hypercholesterolemia.

■ CONTRAINDICATIONS: Known organic heart disease, hypertension, advanced liver or kidney disease, pregnancy and lactation, or a history of iodism prohibits its use.

■ ADVERSE EFFECTS: Among the most serious adverse reactions are angina pectoris, supraventricular tachycardia, cardiomegaly, myocardial infarction, insomnia, alopecia, hyperthermia, diuresis, dizziness, paresthesia, gallstones, and psychic changes.

**df,** abbreviation for **degrees of freedom.**

**dg,** abbreviation for **decigram.**

**D gene,** one of a set of genes lying between the V and J genes, which code for the D region of heavy-chain or for the beta or delta chain of the T cell receptor.

**D.H.E.-45,** trademark for a vasodilator that works primarily by stimulating alpha-adrenergic receptors (dihydroergotamine mesylate).

**DHFSS,** abbreviation for **dengue hemorrhagic fever shock syndrome.**

**DHHS,** abbreviation for **Department of Health and Human Services.**

**dhobie itch** /dō′bē/ [Hindi, *dhobie,* laundryman; AS, *giccan*], a form of contact dermatitis associated with the use of laundry marking fluids.

**di-, dia-, 1.** prefix meaning 'two, twice': *diacid, diamide, dimorphic.* **2.** prefix meaning 'apart, through': *diuresia, diactinism.* **3.** prefix meaning 'apart, away from': *diffraction, divergent.*

**di-, dis-, 1.** prefix meaning 'reversal, apart, or to separate': *disacidify, dischronation, disinfect.* **2.** prefix meaning 'two or duplication': *diplegia, dioxide, dissogeny.* **3.** prefix meaning 'opposite': *disease.*

**DiaBeta,** trademark for an oral antidiabetic drug (glyburide).

**diabetes** /dī′əbē′tēz/ [Gk, *diabainein,* to pass through], a clinical condition characterized by the excessive excretion of urine. The excess may be caused by a deficiency of antidiuretic hormone (ADH), as in diabetes insipidus, or it may be the polyuria resulting from the hyperglycemia that occurs in diabetes mellitus. See also **diabetes insipidus, diabetes mellitus.**

**diabetes insipidus** /insip′idəs/, a metabolic disorder caused by injury of the neurohypophyseal system. It is characterized by copious excretion of urine and excessive thirst, caused by deficient production or secretion of the antidiuretic hormone (ADH) or inability of the kidney tubules to respond to ADH. Rarely the symptoms are self-induced by an excessive water intake. The condition may be acquired, familial, idiopathic, neurogenic, nephrogenic, or psychogenic.

■ OBSERVATIONS: The onset may be dramatic and sudden, and urinary output may exceed 10 L in 24 hours. Diagnosis is established by a water deprivation test in which urine volume increases and urine osmolality decreases. A person with diabetes insipidus who is unconscious as result of trauma or surgery continues to produce massive quantities of urine. If fluids are not administered in adequate amounts, the patient becomes severely dehydrated and hypernatremic.

■ INTERVENTIONS: In mild cases no treatment is necessary. Vasopressin in an intramuscular injection or nasal spray is effective. Thiazide diuretics, by inducing a state of salt depletion, sometimes decrease the diuresis of water by as much as 50%.

■ NURSING CONSIDERATIONS: Infants, small children, and the elderly are particularly vulnerable to serious circulatory disturbances when dehydrated; therefore exceedingly careful monitoring is essential when the condition is suspected, especially after head surgery or trauma.

**diabetes mellitus (DM)** /məlī′təs/, a complex disorder of carbohydrate, fat, and protein metabolism that is primarily a result of a deficiency or complete lack of insulin secretion by the beta cells of the pancreas or resistance to insulin. The disease is often familial but may be acquired, as in Cushing's syndrome, as a result of the administration of excessive glucocorticoid. The various forms of diabetes have been organized into categories developed by the Expert Committee on the Diagnosis and Classification of Diabetes Mellitus of the American Diabetes Association. **Type 1 diabetes mellitus** in this classification scheme includes patients with diabetes caused by an autoimmune process, dependent on insulin to prevent ketosis. This group was previously called type I, insulin-dependent diabetes mellitus (IDDM), juvenile-onset diabetes, brittle diabetes, or ketosis-prone diabetes. Patients with **type 2 diabetes mellitus** are those previously designated as having type II, non-insulin-dependent diabetes mellitus (NIDDM), maturity-onset diabetes, adult-onset diabetes, ketosis-resistant diabetes, or stable diabetes. Those with **gestational diabetes mellitus** are women in whom glucose intolerance develops during pregnancy. Other types of diabetes are associated with a pancreatic disease, hormonal changes, adverse effects of drugs, or genetic or other anomalies. A fifth subclass, the impaired glucose tolerance group, includes persons whose blood glucose levels are abnormal although not sufficiently above the normal range to be diagnosed as diabetic. Approximately 95% of the 16 million diabetes patients in the United States are classified as type 2, and more than 70% of those patients are obese. About 650,000 new cases of diabetes mellitus are diagnosed in the United States each year. Contributing factors to the development of diabetes are heredity, obesity, sedentary life-style, high-fat low-fiber diets, hypertension, and aging. Kinds of diabetes mellitus are **gestational diabetes, type 1 diabetes,** and **type 2 diabetes diabetes.** See also **impaired glucose tolerance, potential abnormality of glucose tolerance, previous abnormality of glucose tolerance.**

■ OBSERVATIONS: The onset of type 1 diabetes mellitus is sudden in children. Type 2 diabetes usually begins insidiously. Characteristically the course is progressive and includes polyuria, polydipsia, weight loss, polyphagia, hyperglycemia, and glycosuria. The eyes, kidneys, nervous system, skin, and circulatory system may be affected by the long-term complications of either type of diabetes; infections are common; and atherosclerosis often develops. In type 1 diabetes mellitus, when no endogenous insulin is being secreted, ketoacidosis is a constant danger. The diagnosis is confirmed by fasting plasma glucose and history.

■ INTERVENTIONS: The goal of treatment is to maintain insulin glucose homeostasis. Type 1 diabetes is controlled by insulin, diet and exercise. The Diabetes Control and Complications Trial (DCCT), completed in mid-1993, demonstrated that tight control of blood glucose levels (i.e., frequent monitoring and maintenance at as close as possible to the level of nondiabetics) significantly reduces complications such as eye disease, kidney disease, and nerve damage. Type

## Classification and characteristics of diabetes mellitus

| Name | Previous synonyms | Characteristics |
|---|---|---|
| **Type I: primary beta-cell defect or failure**<br>Immune-mediated diabetes common form | Juvenile diabetes<br>Juvenile-onset diabetes<br>Ketosis-prone diabetes<br>Brittle diabetes<br>Idiopathic diabetes<br>Insulin-dependent diabetes mellitus (IDDM) | Cellular mediated autoimmune destruction of pancreatic B cells<br>Individual prone to ketoacidosis<br>Little or no insulin secretion<br>Insulin dependent<br>75% of individuals develop before 30 yr of age, can occur up to the tenth decade<br>Usually not obese<br>Several syndromes, both primary autoimmune and genetic-environmental |
| Idiopathic | Other types | No defined etiologies; absolute requirement for insulin replacement therapy in affected individuals may come and go |
| **Type II diabetes: insulin resistance with inadequate insulin secretion** | Adult-onset diabetes<br>Maturity-onset diabetes<br>Stable diabetes<br>Ketosis-resistant diabetes<br>Non-insulin-dependent diabetes mellitus (NIDDM) | Usually not insulin-dependent but may be insulin requiring<br>Individual not ketosis prone (but may form ketones under stress)<br>Obesity common in the abdominal region<br>Generally occurs in those older than 40 yr<br>Strong genetic predisposition<br>Frequently associated with hypertension and dyslipidemia |
| **Other forms**<br>Genetic defects of the beta cell | Secondary diabetes<br>Maturity-onset diabetes of the young (MODY) | Genetic abnormalities such as inability to convert proinsulin to insulin, mutation of insulin molecules or mitochondrial deoxyribonucleic acid, glucokinase abnormalities |
| Genetic defects in insulin action | | Mutations in the insulin receptor with hyperinsulinism or hyperglycemia or severe diabetes |
| Pancreatic diseases<br>Drug- or chemical-induced beta-cell dysfunction | Secondary diabetes | Any process that diffusely injures the pancreas<br>Impaired insulin secretion |
| Endocrinopathies<br>Infections | | Inhibition of insulin secretion<br>Beta-cell destruction by viruses: *cytomegalovirus, adenovirus, coxsackievirus B* |
| Uncommon forms of immune-mediated diabetes mellitus | | Few known conditions<br>Anti-insulin receptor antibodies<br>Reported with "stiff man syndrome" and individuals receiving interferon-alpha |
| Other genetic syndromes sometimes associated with diabetes mellitus | | Down, Klinefelter, Turner and Wolfram syndromes |
| **Gestational diabetes mellitus** | Asymptomatic diabetes<br>Subclinical diabetes<br>Latent diabetes | Glucose intolerance first recognized during pregnancy, most likely in the third trimester<br>Following pregnancy, glucose may normalize, remain impaired, or progress to diabetes mellitus<br>Occurs in 1%-14% of all pregnancies; 40%-60% will develop diabetes mellitus within 15 yr after gestation |
| Impaired fasting glucose (IFG)<br>Impaired glucose tolerance (IGT) | | Fasting plasma glucose $\geq$110 and <126 mg/dl<br>Abnormal response to oral glucose tolerance test: 2-hour plasma glucose $\geq$140 and <200 mg/dl<br>10%-25% will convert to type II diabetes within 10 yr<br>Many with IGT are obese |

Data from Gavin J et al: Report of the expert committee on the diagnosis and classification of diabetes mellitus, *Diabetic Care* 20(7):1183, 1997.

2 diabetes is controlled by diet, exercise, one or more oral agents, and insulin in combination with oral agents, and insulin in combination with oral agents. Results of the Kumamoto Study, which studied patients with type 2 diabetes, were comparable to those of the DCCT where a relationship existed between improved glycemic control and reduction in microvascular complications. The United Kingdom Prosepective Diabetes Study is an ongoing study involving more than 5000 people with type 2 diabetes in the United Kingdom. Stress of any kind may require adjustment in the dosage of medication in both type 1 and type 2 diabetes.

**diabetic** /dī′əbet′ik/, **1.** pertaining to diabetes. **2.** affected with diabetes. **3.** a person who has diabetes mellitus.

**diabetic acidosis** [Gk, *diabainein,* to pass through; L, *acidus,* acid; Gk, *osis,* condition], a type of acidosis that may occur in diabetes mellitus as a result of excessive production of ketone bodies during oxidation of fatty acids. See also **diabetic ketoacidosis (DKA).**

## Target nutritional goals for persons with diabetes

**Calories**

Sufficient to achieve and maintain as close to desirable body weight as possible

**Carbohydrate**

Varies in relation to assessment and protein and fat intake; usually 45%-60% calories

Liberalized individualized emphasis on total carbohydrate intake versus eliminating simple sugars only

Carbohydrate consistency at meals

Modest amounts of sucrose and other refined sugars may be acceptable contingent on metabolic control and body weight

**Protein**

Usual dietary intake of protein is double the amount needed

Exact ideal percentage of total calories is unknown; however, usual intake is 12%-20% of total calories

RDA is 0.8 g/kg body weight for adults; it is modified for children, pregnant and lactating women, elderly persons, and those with special medical conditions

Avoidance of excess dietary protein intake is important in renal disease

**Fat**

Usually ≤ 30% of total calories, but may be as high as 40%

Polyunsaturated fats, 6%-8%

Saturated fats, 10%

Monounsaturated fats, remaining percentage

Cholesterol <300 mg/day

May need to be further modified, depending on lipid profile

**Fiber**

Up to 40 g/day

25 g/1000 kcal for low-calorie intakes

**Alternative sweeteners**

Use of various nutritive and nonnutritive sweeteners is acceptable

**Sodium**

≤3000 mg/day

Modified for special medical conditions (e.g., hypertension, edema)

**Alcohol**

≤2 equivalents per day

1 equivalent = 1.5 oz distilled liquor, 4 oz glass of wine, 12 oz glass of beer

**Vitamins/minerals**

No evidence that diabetes mellitus influences need

From Phipps WJ, Sands JK, Marck JF: *Medical-surgical nursing: concepts and clinical practice,* ed 6, St Louis, 1999, Mosby.
*RDA,* Recommended dietary allowances.

**diabetic amaurosis** [Gk, *diabainein,* to pass through, *amaurosis,* to darken], blindness associated with diabetes mellitus, caused by a proliferative hemorrhagic form of retinopathy that is characterized by capillary microaneurysms and hard or waxy exudates. Cataracts are also common in type 2 diabetes; in type 1 diabetes, snowflake cataract may progress until the entire lens is milky white.

**diabetic center,** a cluster of nerve cells on the floor of the fourth ventricle of the brain.

**diabetic coma,** a life-threatening condition occurring in persons with diabetes mellitus. It is caused by undiagnosed diabetes, inadequate treatment, failure to take prescribed insulin, excessive food intake, or, most frequently, infection, surgery, trauma, or other stressors that increase the body's need for insulin. Without insulin to metabolize glucose, fats are used for energy, resulting in ketone waste accumulation and metabolic acidosis. The body's effort to counteract acidosis depletes the alkali reserve; causes a loss of sodium, chloride, potassium, and water; increases respiratory exhalation of carbon dioxide (Kussmaul breathing) and urinary excretion; and leads to dehydration and generalized hypoxia. Warning signs of diabetic coma include a dull headache, fatigue, inordinate thirst, epigastric pain, nausea, vomiting, parched lips, flushed face, and sunken eyes. The temperature usually rises and then falls; the systolic blood pressure drops, and circulatory collapse may occur. Immediate treatment consists of administering short-acting insulin and replacing electrolytes and fluids to correct the acidosis and dehydration. Nonketotic coma may occur in patients with poorly controlled type 2 diabetes mellitus and high levels of blood glucose but no acetone in the urine. The plasma hyperosmolarity causes water to leave cells, and the dehydration of cerebral cells results in coma. See also **diabetic ketoacidosis, insulin shock.**

**diabetic diet,** a diet prescribed in the treatment of type 2 diabetes mellitus. It usually contains limited amounts of simple sugars or readily digestible carbohydrates and increased amounts of proteins, complex carbohydrates, and unsaturated fats. Dietary regulation depends on the severity of the disease and on the type and extent of insulin therapy. The diet should be designed to prevent wide fluctuation in the amount of glucose in the blood, to preserve pancreatic function, and to prevent chronic diabetic complications. See also **diabetes mellitus, Exchange Lists for Meal Planning, insulin.**

**diabetic foot and leg care,** the special attention given to prevent the circulatory disorders and infections that frequently occur in the lower extremities of diabetic patients.

■ METHOD: The patient's legs and feet are examined daily for signs of dry, scaly, red, itching, or cracked skin; blisters; corns; calluses; abrasions; infection; blueness and swelling around varicosities; and thickened, discolored nails. The feet are bathed daily in tepid water with mild or superfatted soap and are dried gently but thoroughly with a soft towel. A lanolin-based lotion is then applied, although not between the toes; excess lotion is removed with a dry towel; vigorous rubbing and use of alcohol preparations are avoided because of drying and irritation of skin which can lead to skin breakdown. The toenails are cut straight across above the level of soft tissue after the feet are soaked for 3 to 5 minutes in tepid water. The feet are also soaked in tepid water for several minutes before hardened areas are treated by applying soft soap and rubbing the area with a washcloth; calluses and corns are removed, and thickened, deformed nails are cut by a podiatrist. Commercial remedies for removing calluses and corns should not be used.

■ INTERVENTIONS: The nurse provides foot and leg care while the diabetic patient is hospitalized. Before discharge the patient is instructed to examine and bathe the feet daily according to the recommended method, to report abnormalities, to keep the feet dry at all times, to wear cotton socks or stockings with cotton feet, and to place clean lamb's wool or cotton between the toes if they perspire. The patient is cautioned to avoid sustaining foot or leg trauma, walking barefoot, scratching insect bites, using a hot-water bottle or heating pad on the lower extremities, getting sunburned, wearing constricting garments, remaining in the same position for long periods, sitting at more than a right-angle bend, and crossing the knees. The diabetic individual is advised to alternate the wearing of two pairs of rubber-soled, well-fitted shoes wide enough to prevent pressure and rubbing; to

air each pair of shoes between use; and to break in new shoes gradually. The patient is urged to walk to tolerance daily, to plan exercise periods after meals, to bend and straighten the knees and rotate the ankles occasionally when sitting, and, when standing, to shift weight from time to time and walk in place. Patients may be referred to a certified diabetic educator (CDE) for initial instruction on care.
■ OUTCOME CRITERIA: Meticulous care of the feet and legs can prevent serious complications, including local infection, skin ulcers, cellulitis, and gangrene.

**diabetic gangrene** [Gk, *diabainein,* to pass through, *gaggraina*], gangrene, usually involving the lower extremities, that develops secondary to sensory peripheal neuropathy and peripheral vascular disease complications related to the diabetic disease process.

**diabetic glycosuria** [Gk, *diabainein,* to pass through, *glykys,* sweet, *ouron,* urine], excessive excretion of glucose into the urine as an effect of diabetes mellitus.

**diabetic ketoacidosis (DKA),** diabetic coma, an acute, life-threatening complication of uncontrolled diabetes mellitus. In this condition urinary loss of water, potassium, ammonium, and sodium results in hypovolemia, electrolyte imbalance, extremely high blood glucose levels, and breakdown of free fatty acids, causing acidosis, often with coma. Compare **insulin shock.**
■ OBSERVATIONS: The person appears flushed; has hot, dry skin; is restless, uncomfortable, agitated, and diaphoretic; and has a fruity odor to the breath. Nausea, confusion, and coma are often noted. Persons with diabetes mellitus whose body produces no natural insulin are most often affected (type 1). Untreated, the condition invariably proceeds to coma and death.
■ INTERVENTIONS: IV insulin and hypotonic saline solution are administered immediately. Nasogastric intubation and bladder catheterization are usual. Blood glucose and ketone levels are determined hourly, and electrolyte and acid-base balance are monitored frequently. Bicarbonate may be given in dosages dependent on the degree of acidosis. Potassium is usually given because of intracellular potassium depletion. Plasma or a plasma expander may be necessary to prevent or correct shock resulting from hypovolemia.
■ NURSING CONSIDERATIONS: The cause of the episode of ketoacidosis is sought. The most common precipitating factors are undiagnosed type 1 diabetes mellitus, infection, GI upset, alcohol consumption, and failure to take insulin. Type 1 diabetes mellitus in childhood characteristically begins suddenly and progresses rapidly; therefore the diagnosis of type 1 diabetes is usually made when the child arrives at the hospital in diabetic ketoacidosis. Inpatient care after an episode of ketoacidosis is the same as for diabetes mellitus.

**diabetic neuropathy,** a noninflammatory disease process associated with diabetes mellitus and characterized by sensory and/or motor disturbances in the peripheral nervous system. Patients commonly experience degeneration of sensory nerves and pathways. Early symptoms, which include pain and loss of reflexes in the legs, may occur in patients with only mild hyperglycemia. Diabetes is associated with a wide range of neuropathies, including mononeuritis multiplex, compression and entrapment mononeuropathies, cranial neuropathies, and autonomic and small fiber neuropathies. Differential diagnosis is difficult because not all sensorimotor neuropathies are caused by diabetes.

**diabetic polyneuritis,** a condition involving many nerves. It usually occurs as a complication in long-term cases of diabetes mellitus.

**diabetic polyneuropathy,** a long-term complication of diabetes mellitus in which a number of nerves are involved

at the same time. Central nervous system, autonomic, and peripheral nerves may be affected. Neuropathic ulcers commonly develop on the feet.

**diabetic retinopathy,** a disorder of retinal blood vessels. It is characterized by capillary microaneurysms, hemorrhage, exudates, and the formation of new vessels and connective tissue. The disorder occurs most frequently in patients with long-standing poorly controlled diabetes mellitus. Repeated hemorrhage may cause permanent opacity of the vitreous humor, and blindness may eventually result. Photocoagulation of damaged retinal blood vessels by a laser beam may be performed to prevent hemorrhage from the vessels.

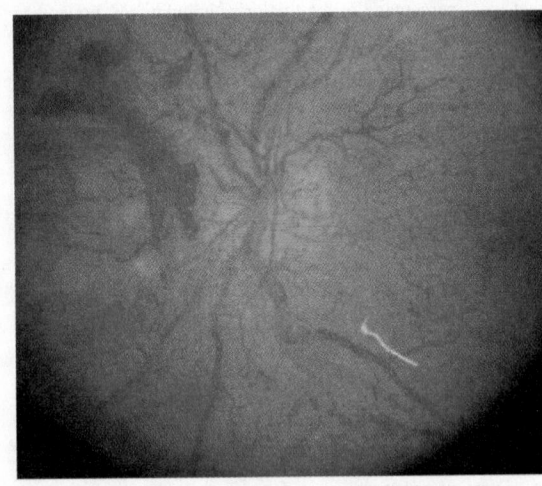

**Diabetic retinopathy** *(Apple and Rabb, 1998)*

**diabetic tabes,** a wasting condition associated with diabetic peripheral neuropathy. It may be accompanied by sharp pain, muscle weakness, atrophy of intrinsic foot muscles, and weakness of the toes' extensors and flexors. It may lead to foot drop because of ankle weakness. When these manifestations coexist with decreased proprioception in the feet, "pseudotabetic" gait may occur.

**diabetic treatment,** management of diabetes mellitus by means of a controlled carbohydrate diet, insulin injections, exercise, low-fat meal plan, blood glucose level monitoring, and or oral agents such as sulfonylureas, alpha-glucosiderase inhibitors, and insulin sensitizers (for patients with type 2 diabetes mellitus).

**diabetic vulvovaginitis** [Gk, *diabainein,* to pass through; L, *vulva,* wrapper, *vagina,* sheath; Gk, *itis,* inflammation], a form of mycotic inflammation of the vulva and vagina that is associated with diabetes.

**diabetic xanthoma,** an eruption of yellow papules or plaques on the skin in uncontrolled diabetes mellitus. The lesion disappears as the metabolic functions are stabilized and the disease is controlled.

**diabetogenic state** /dī′əbet′ōjen′ik/, a health condition manifested by signs and symptoms of diabetes.

**Diabinese,** trademark for an oral antidiabetic (chlorpropamide).

**diacet,** abbreviation for a *carboxylate diacetate anion.*

**diacetic acid.** See **acetoacetic acid.**

**diacetylmorphine.** See **heroin.**

**diacondylar fracture** /dī'əkon'dilər/ [Gk, *dia,* through, *kondylos,* knuckle; L, *fractura,* break], any fracture that runs across the line of a condyle.

**diadochokinesia** /dī·ad'əkōkīnē'zhə/ [Gk, *diadochos,* successor, *kinesis,* motion], the normal ability of the muscles to move a limb alternately in opposite directions by flexion and extension.

**diagnose** /dī'agnōs/, to determine the type and cause of a health condition on the basis of signs and symptoms of the patient; data obtained from laboratory analysis of fluid, tissue specimens, and other tests; and family and occupational background information such as recent injuries or exposure to toxic substances.

**diagnosis** /dī'agnō'sis/, *pl.* **diagnoses** [Gk, *dia* + *gnosis,* knowledge], **1.** identification of a disease or condition by a scientific evaluation of physical signs, symptoms, history, laboratory test results, and procedures. Kinds of diagnoses are **clinical diagnosis, differential diagnosis, laboratory diagnosis, nursing diagnosis,** and **physical diagnosis. 2.** the art of naming a disease or condition. —**diagnostic,** *adj.,* **diagnose,** *v.*

**diagnosis by exclusion** [Gk, *dia,* through, *gnosis,* knowledge; L, *excludere,* to shut out], diagnosis made by eliminating other possible causes of disease symptoms.

**diagnosis-related group (DRG),** a group of patients classified for measuring a medical facility's delivery of care. The classifications, used to determine Medicare payments for inpatient care, are based on primary and secondary diagnosis, primary and secondary procedures, age, and length of hospitalization. See also **prospective payment system.**

**diagnostic** /dī'agnos'tik/, pertaining to a diagnosis.

***Diagnostic and Statistical Manual of Mental Disorders (DSM),*** a manual, published by the American Psychiatric Association, listing the official diagnostic classifications of mental disorders. The *DSM* recommends the use of a multiaxial evaluation system as a holistic diagnostic approach. It consists of five axes, each of which refers to a different class of information, including mental and physical data. Axes I and II include all of the mental disorders, classified broadly as clinical syndromes and personality disorders; axis III contains physical disorders and conditions; and axes IV and V provide a coded outline of supplemental information on, for example, psychosocial stressors and adaptive functioning, which may be useful for planning individual treatment and predicting its outcome. Each of the classifications of the mental disorders contains a code that provides a reference to the WHO *International Classification of Diseases (ICD)* and offers such useful diagnostic criteria as essential and associated features of the disorder, age at onset, course, impairment, complications, predisposing factors, prevalence, sex ratio, familial patterns, and differential diagnoses. *DSM-IV* is the fourth edition of the manual, published in 1994.

**diagnostic anesthesia,** a procedure in which analgesia is induced to a depth adequate to permit comfortable performance of moderately painful diagnostic procedures of short duration. Awake anesthesia is often used for this purpose. See also **awake anesthesia.**

**diagnostician** /dī'agnostish'ən/, a person skilled and trained in making diagnoses.

**diagnostic medical sonographer,** an allied health professional who provides patient services, using diagnostic ultrasound under the supervision of a doctor of medicine or osteopathy responsible for the use and interpretation of ultrasound procedures. The sonographer assists the physician in gathering sonographic data necessary to reach diagnostic decisions.

**diagnostic peritoneal lavage (DPL),** a procedure used to detect intraabdominal bleeding or viscus perforation after abdominal trauma. The open or operative approach allows direct visual examination of the peritoneum when the catheter is inserted. Gastric and bladder decompression must precede performance of DPL.

**diagnostic position of gaze.** See **cardinal position of gaze.**

**diagnostic process,** the act of determining a patient's health status and evaluating the factors influencing that status.

**diagnostic radiology,** medical imaging using external sources of radiation.

**diagnostic radiopharmaceutical,** a radioactive drug administered to a patient as a diagnostic tracer to differentiate normal from abnormal anatomic structures or biochemical or physiologic functions. Most diagnostic radiopharmaceuticals emit gamma rays. A collimated external gamma-ray detector can determine the concentration of the drug in different organs and produce low-resolution images of the organs. Some radiopharmaceuticals, such as those prepared with tritium, carbon-14, or phosphorus-32, do not emit gamma rays. Their diagnostic use involves analyzing the concentration of the isotope in a metabolic end product in the patient's blood, urine, breath, or biopsy samples. For example, when glucose containing $^{14}C$ is administered, the subsequent monitoring of $^{14}CO_2$ in the patient's breath can indicate the absorption of glucose, its metabolism, and its elimination as a metabolic end product.

**diagnostic-related groups (DRG).** See **diagnosis-related group.**

**diagnostic sensitivity,** the conditional probability that a person having a disease will be correctly identified by a clinical test, i.e., the number of true positive results divided by the total number with the disease (which is the sum of the numbers of true positive plus false negative results).

**diagnostic services,** activities related to the diagnosis made by a physician or nurse practitioner, which may also be performed by nurses or other health professionals.

**diagnostic specificity,** the conditional probability that a person not having a disease will be correctly identified by a clinical test, i.e., the number of true negative results divided by the total number of those without the disease (which is the sum of the numbers of true negative plus false positive results).

**diagonal conjugate** /dī·ag'ənəl/, a radiographic measurement of the distance from the inferior border of the symphysis pubis to the sacral promontory. The measurement, which averages around 12.5 to 13.0 cm in adult women, may also be determined by vaginal examination. See also **conjugate, true conjugate.**

**diakinesis** /dī'əkinē'sis, dī'əkī-/ [Gk, *dia* + *kinesis,* motion], the final stage in the first meiotic prophase in gametogenesis, in which the chromosomes achieve their maximum thickness. The chiasmata and nucleolus disappear, the nuclear membrane degenerates, and the spindle fibers form in preparation for the formation of dyads. See also **diplotene, leptotene, pachytene, zygotene.**

**dial,** a circular diagram with black lines radiating outward across a white background from the center, as is used in tests of astigmatism.

**dialect** /dī'əlekt/, a variation of spoken language different from other forms of the same language in pronunciation, syntax, and word meanings. A particular dialect is usually shared by members of an ethnic group, socioeconomic group, or people living together in a geographic area.

**dialogue** /dī'əlog/ [L, *dialogus,* philosophic conversation], a complex form of computer-assisted instruction in which the student is actively engaged in "true conversation" with a computer.

**Dialose,** trademark for a fixed-combination GI drug containing a stool softener (docusate sodium sulfosuccinate) and a laxative (sodium carboxymethylcellulose).

**dialy-,** prefix meaning 'dialysis or dissolution': *dialytic, dialysate.*

**dialysate,** the material that passes through the membrane in dialysis.

**dialysis** /dī·al'isis/ [Gk *dia* + *lysis* a loosening], **1.** the process of separating colloids and crystalline substances in solution by the difference in their rate of diffusion through a semipermeable membrane. **2.** a medical procedure for the removal of certain elements from the blood or lymph by virtue of the difference in their rates of diffusion through an external semipermeable membrane or, in the case of peritoneal dialysis, through the peritoneum. Dialysis may be used to remove poisons and excessive amounts of drugs, to correct serious electrolyte and acid-base imbalances, and to remove urea, uric acid, and creatinine in cases of chronic end-stage renal disease. Dialysis involves diffusion of particles from an area of high to lower concentration, osmosis of fluid across the membrane from an area of lesser to one of greater concentration of particles, and ultrafiltration or movement of fluid across the membrane as a result of an artificially created pressure differential. See also **hemodialysis, peritoneal dialysis.**

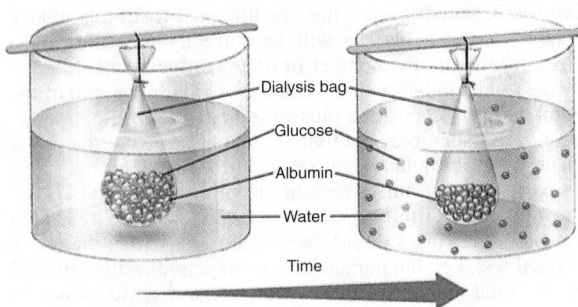

**Dialysis** *(Thibodeau and Patton, 1999/Rolin Graphics)*

**dialysis access integrity,** a nursing outcome from the Nursing Outcomes Classification (NOC) defined as the extent to which a dialysis access site is functional and free of inflammation. See also **Nursing Outcomes Classification.**

**dialysis dementia,** a neurologic disorder that occurs in some patients undergoing dialysis. The precise cause is unknown, but the effect is believed to be related to chemicals in the dialyzing fluid, drugs administered to the dialysis patient, or both.

**dialysis disequilibrium syndrome,** a disorder caused by a rapid change in extracellular fluid composition during dialysis. It may be marked by cerebral or neurologic disturbances, cardiac arrhythmias, and pulmonary edema.

**dialysis fluid.** See **dialysate.**

**dialysis shunt** [Gk, *dia,* through, *lysis,* loosening; ME, *shunten*], an external artificial link between a peripheral artery and a vein, in an arm or leg, for use in hemodialysis.

**dialysis technician** [Gk, *dia,* through, *lysis,* loosening, *technikos,* skillful], an allied health professional who operates and maintains dialysis equipment for patients with kidney diseases.

**dialyzer** /dī'əlī'zər/ [Gk, *dia* + *lysis,* loosening], **1.** a machine used in dialysis. **2.** a semipermeable membrane or porous diaphragm in a dialysis machine. See also **dialysis, hemodialysis, peritoneal dialysis.**

**diameter** /dī·am'ə·tər/ [Gk, *diametros*], the length of a straight line passing through the center of a circle and connecting opposite points on its circumference; hence the distance between two specified opposite points on the periphery of a structure such as the cranium or pelvis.

**Diameter-Index Safety System (DISS),** a system of standardized connections between cylinders of medical gases and flowmeters or pressure regulators. Each gas has connections of a specific size to prevent accidental hookup of the wrong gas. Each type of gas and connector is assigned a DISS number, such as 1040 for nitrous oxide and 1240 for oxygen. See also **Pin-Index Safety System.**

**diameter of fetal skull** [Gk, *diametros* + L, *fetus* + AS, *skulle,* bowl], the average distances between certain landmarks of the fetal skull as measured at term. These measurements include the following: biparietal, the fetal head between the two parietal eminences, 9.25 cm; occipitofrontal, from the external occipital protuberance to the most prominent point of the frontal midline, 11 cm; occipitomental, from the external occipital protuberance to the midpoint of the chin, 13 cm; and suboccipitobregmatic, from the lowest posterior point of the occipital bone to the center of the anterior fontanel, 9.5 cm.

**diamine oxidase.** See **histaminase.**

**diaminovaleric acid.** See **ornithine.**

**Diamond-Blackfan syndrome,** a rare congenital disorder evident in the first 3 months of life, characterized by severe anemia, very low reticulocyte count, but normal numbers of platelets and white cells. It is caused by a deficiency of erythrocyte precursors. Also called **congenital hypoplastic anemia.** See also **anemia.**

**diamond burr** /dī'(ə)mənd/, a rotary device that contains diamond particles and is used as an abrasive in dentistry.

**Diamox,** trademark for a carbonic anhydrase inhibitor (acetazolamide); a diuretic.

**diapedesis** /dī'əpidē'sis/ [Gk, *dia* + *pedesis,* an oozing], the passage of red or white blood corpuscles through the walls of the vessels that contain them without damage to the vessels.

**diaper rash** [ME, *diapre,* patterned fabric], an erythematous, papular, or scaly eruption in the diaper area of infants, caused by irritation from feces, moisture, heat, or ammonia produced by the bacterial decomposition of urine. Secondary infection by *Candida albicans* is common. Principles of treatment include frequent diaper changes, dryness, cleanliness, coolness, and ventilation of the affected area. Specific topical antimicrobial medication may be prescribed for secondary infection. Also called **diaper dermatitis.**

**diaper restraint,** a therapeutic device used for countertraction with lower extremity traction when other methods of countertraction are not effective. One device is used in treating children with orthopedic diseases and abnormalities. It is designed to fit over the pelvic area like diapers, with rings at each of four corners. A webbing strap is threaded through the rings and attached to the top side of the bedspring frame. Diaper restraints are used with Russell traction and with split Russell traction if additional countertraction is required but are not generally used with other kinds of traction. Compare **jacket restraint, sling restraint.**

**diaphanography** /dī·af'ənog'rəfē/ [Gk, *diaphanes,* shining through, *graphein,* to record], a type of transillumination

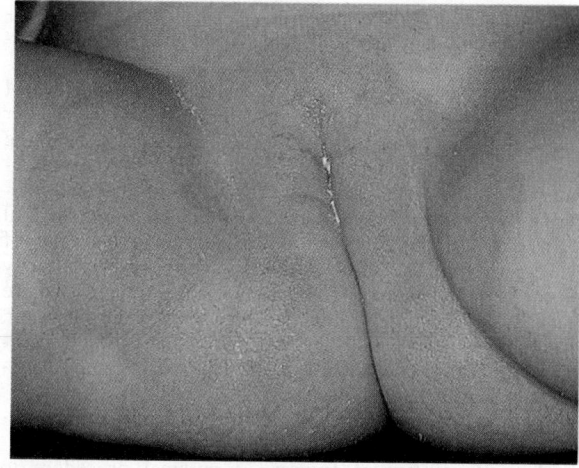

**Diaper rash** (Habif, 1996)

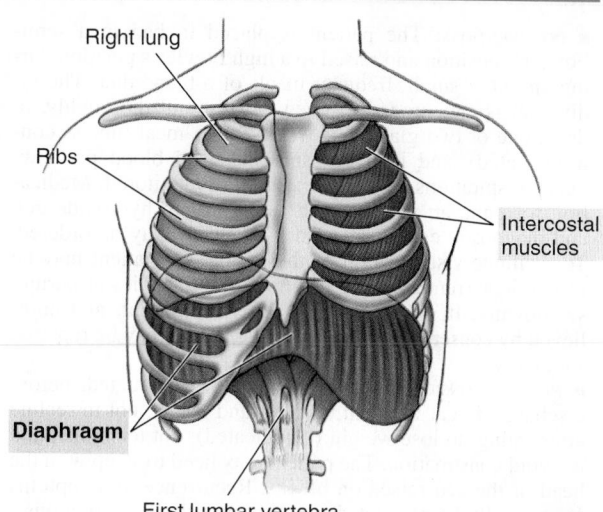

Right lung

Ribs

Intercostal muscles

Diaphragm

First lumbar vertebra

**Diaphragm** (Herlihy and Maebius, 2000)

used to examine the breast, which uses selected wavelengths of light and special imaging equipment. The images are still recordings as in conventional radiography. See also **diaphanoscopy.**

**diaphanoscope,** /dī·af'ənəskōp'/ an instrument that transilluminates body tissues. It is sometimes used in the diagnosis of breast tumors.

**diaphanoscopy** /dī·af'ənos'kəpē/, examination of an internal structure with a diaphanoscope.

**diaphoresis** /dī'əfərē'sis/ [Gk, *dia* + *pherein*, to carry], the secretion of sweat, especially the profuse secretion associated with an elevated body temperature, physical exertion, exposure to heat, and mental or emotional stress. Sweating is centrally controlled by the sympathetic nervous system and is primarily a thermoregulatory mechanism; however, the sweat glands on the palms and soles respond to emotional stimuli and do not always participate in thermal sweating. The rate of sweating is generally not affected by water deficiency, but it may be reduced by severe dehydration; it also diminishes when salt intake exceeds salt loss. Also called **sweating.** See also **sudorific.**

**diaphoretic.** See **sudorific.**

**diaphragm** /dī'əfram/ [Gk, *diaphragma*, partition], **1.** (in anatomy) a dome-shaped musculofibrous partition that separates the thoracic and abdominal cavities. The convex cranial surface of the diaphragm forms the floor of the thoracic cavity; the concave surface forms the roof of the abdominal cavity. This partition is pierced by various openings through which pass the aorta, esophagus, and vena cava. The diaphragm aids respiration by moving up and down. During inspiration it moves down and increases the volume of the thoracic cavity; during expiration it moves up, decreasing the volume. During deep inspiration and expiration the range of diaphragmatic movement in the adult is about 30 mm on the right side and about 28 mm on the left side. The height of this structure also varies with the degree of distension of the stomach and the intestines and with the size of the liver. It is innervated by the phrenic nerve from the cervical plexus. **2.** *informal.* a contraceptive diaphragm. **3.** (in optics) an opening that controls the amount of light passing through an optical network. **4.** a thin, membranous partition, as that used in dialysis. **5.** (in radiography) a metal plate

with a small opening that limits the diameter of the radiographic beam. **—diaphragmatic,** *adj.*

**diaphragmatic breathing** /dī·əfragmat'ik/ [Gk, *diaphragma*, partition], a pattern of exhalation and inhalation in which most of the ventilatory work is done with the diaphragm. Many males normally breathe diaphragmatically, whereas few females do. The technique is taught to patients with chronic obstructive pulmonary disease to facilitate respiration. The patient is trained to strengthen the contractile force of the abdominal wall muscles to elevate the diaphragm and empty the lungs. The patient places a hand on the epigastrium during training to focus attention on that portion of the body. Also called **diaphragmatic respiration.** See also **abdominal breathing.**

**diaphragmatic flutter,** rapid, rhythmic contractions of the diaphragm. The condition may simulate atrial flutter.

**diaphragmatic hernia** [Gk, *diaphragma*, partition; L, rupture], the protrusion of part of the stomach through an opening in the diaphragm, most commonly an abnormally enlarged esophageal hiatus. In some cases the intestines may also herniate into the chest. The enlargement of the normal opening for the esophagus may be caused by trauma, congenital weakness, increased abdominal pressure, or relaxation of ligaments of skeletal muscles, and it permits part of the stomach to slide into the thorax. A sliding hiatal hernia, one of the most common pathologic conditions of the upper GI tract, may occur at any age but is most prevalent in elderly and middle-aged people. A kind of diaphragmatic hernia is **hiatal hernia.**

■ OBSERVATIONS: Symptoms of diaphragmatic hernia vary but usually include heartburn after meals, when the patient is in a supine position, and on exertion, especially when bending forward. Regurgitation of food, dysphagia, abdominal distension after eating, belching, intestinal rumbling, rapid breathing, and a dull epigastric pain radiating to the shoulder may occur. The similarity of some of the symptoms to those of myocardial infarction may make the patient fearful and anxious. Continued reflux of gastric juice into the esophagus may lead to ulceration with bleeding and the formation of fibrous tissue. Gastric contents regurgitated during sleep may be aspirated into the lungs.

■ INTERVENTIONS: The patient is placed in bed in a semi-Fowler's position and raised to a high Fowler's position during and after small, frequent meals of a bland diet. The individual is encouraged to chew slowly and thoroughly, to drink one or two glasses of water with a meal (unless contraindicated), and to avoid smoking. The blood pressure, pulse, respirations, and temperature are monitored. Medication for pain, an antacid such as aluminum hydroxide gel, and diagnostic endoscopy and x-ray films may be ordered. To facilitate visualization of the hernia, the patient may be placed in a Trendelenburg position during studies of barium swallowing. If symptoms are severe, persistent, and unrelieved by conservative measures, the hernia may be repaired surgically.

■ NURSING CONSIDERATIONS: The patient is instructed, before discharge, to eat frequent, small bland meals; not to recline after eating; to lose weight (if indicated); not to smoke; and to avoid constipation. The patient may need to sleep with the head of the bed raised on blocks. Recurrence of symptoms may usually be prevented by observing these instructions.

**diaphragmatic node,** a node in one of three groups of thoracic parietal lymph nodes, situated on the thoracic side of the diaphragm and consisting of the anterior set, the middle set, and the posterior set. The anterior set includes about three nodes dorsal to the base of the xiphoid process. The middle set of about three nodes on each side is close to the diaphragmatic entry of the phrenic nerves. The posterior set of diaphragmatic nodes consists of a few nodes on the crura of the diaphragm, connecting with the lumbar nodes and the posterior mediastinal nodes. Compare **intercostal node, sternal node.** See also **lymphatic system, lymph node.**

**diaphragmatic peritonitis,** an inflammation of the lower surface of the diaphragm.

**diaphragmatic pleurisy,** inflammation of the pleural covering of the diaphragm, which produces severe pain in the epigastric and hypochondrial regions and, occasionally, referred pain via the phrenic nerve to the shoulder.

**diaphragmatic respiration.** See **diaphragmatic breathing.**

**diaphragm pessary.** See **pessary.**

**diaphragm stethoscope,** an instrument for auscultation of bodily sounds. Originally designed by René Laënnec (1781–1826), it consists of a vibrating disk, or diaphragm, which transmits sound waves through tubing to two earpieces. Also called **binaural stethoscope.** See also **stethoscope.**

**diaphyseal aclasis** /dī'əfiz'ē·əl ak'ləsis/ [Gk, *dia + phyein*, to grow, *a, klasis*, not breaking], a relatively rare abnormal condition that affects the skeletal system. Characterized by multiple exostoses or bony protrusions, it is inherited as a dominant trait. Approximately half of the children of an individual with diaphyseal aclasis display varying degrees of its symptoms. The characteristic exostoses are radiographically and microscopically similar to osteochondromas. Evident involvement is diffuse, with the long bones usually affected more severely and more frequently than the short bones. Depending on the specific area involved, various angular or rotational deformities may result. Diaphyseal aclasis is usually bilateral and occurs more frequently in boys than in girls. Although this disease is hereditary, its signs and symptoms are not usually evident until the affected individual is 2 years of age or older. Children of a parent who has the disease are often routinely examined for symptoms. The major signs of the disease are the noticeable protrusions in the areas of the exostoses. Pain is not usually associated with the exostoses and, if present, is usually minimal. Deformities of the extremities may be evident, depending on the

severity and location of the exostoses. Radiographic examination reveals a broadened metaphyseal area, and the specific lesion is identified by abnormal continuity and decreased density. Asymptomatic lesions characteristic of diaphyseal aclasis usually require little or no treatment other than continued observation. The lesions located near the joints that interfere with joint motion or impair neurovascular function may be surgically excised. Angular and rotational deformities caused by the lesions may require surgical correction to facilitate function. Inequalities in the length of lower extremities resulting from unilateral involvement may require epiphysiodesis. A relatively small number of these lesions may become malignant. One form of the disorder, dyschondroplasia, results in dwarfism. Also called **hereditary deforming chondroplasia, multiple cartilaginous exostoses, multiple exostoses.**

**diaphyseal dysplasia.** See **Camurati-Engelmann disease.**

**diaphyseal-epiphyseal fusion,** a surgical procedure to eliminate the epiphyseal line and unite the epiphyseal and diaphyseal bones.

**diaphysis** /dī·af'isis/ [Gk, *dia + phyein*, to grow], the shaft of a long bone, consisting of a tube of compact bone enclosing the medullary cavity.

**diapositive.** See **reversal film.**

**diarrhea**[1] /dī'ərē'ə/ [Gk, *dia + rhein*, to flow], the frequent passage of loose, watery stools. The stool may also contain mucus, pus, blood, or excessive amounts of fat. Diarrhea is usually a symptom of some underlying disorder. Conditions in which diarrhea is an important symptom are dysenteric disorders, malabsorption syndrome, lactose intolerance, irritable bowel syndrome, GI tumors, and inflammatory bowel disease. In addition to stool frequency, patients may complain of abdominal cramps and generalized weakness. Untreated, severe diarrhea may lead to rapid dehydration and electrolyte imbalance; it should be treated symptomatically until proper diagnosis can be made. Antidiarrheal preparations, such as diphenoxylate and paregoric, are helpful. If diarrhea is accompanied by vomiting, IV fluids may be necessary to prevent fluid depletion. Also spelled **diarrhoea.** See also **dehydration. —diarrheal, diarrheic,** *adj.*

**diarrhea**[2], a nursing diagnosis accepted by the Fourth National Conference on the Classification of Nursing Diagnoses. The causes of the condition and related factors were developed at the Fifth National Conference. Diarrhea is the state in which an individual experiences a change in normal bowel habits, characterized by the frequent passage of loose, fluid, unformed stools.

■ DEFINING CHARACTERISTICS: The defining characteristics include abdominal pain, cramping, increased frequency of bowel movements, increased frequency of bowel sounds, loose or liquid stools, urgency of defecation, and a change in the color of the feces.

■ RELATED FACTORS: Related factors include stress and anxiety; dietary intake; side effects of medications; inflammation, irritation, or malabsorption of the bowel; and effects of toxins, contaminants, or radiation. See also **nursing diagnosis.**

**diarrhea management,** a nursing intervention from the Nursing Interventions Classification (NIC) defined as management and alleviation of diarrhea. See also **Nursing Interventions Classification.**

**diarrhoea.** See **diarrhea**[1].

**diarthric.** See **diarticular.**

**diarthrosis.** See **synovial joint.**

**diarticular** /dī'äartik'yələr/ [Gk, *di*, twice; L, *articulare*, to divide into joints], having two joints. Also called **biarticular.**

**Diasone Sodium Enterab,** trademark for a leprostatic antibacterial (sulfoxone sodium).

**diastalsis** /dī′əstal′sis/, a wave of alternating relaxation and contraction of the smooth muscles lining the walls of the small intestine in response to distension of the intestine.

**diastasis** /dī·as′təsis/ [Gk, separation], the forcible separation of two parts that normally are joined, such as parts of a bone at an epiphysis, two bones that lack a synovial joint, or two muscles, as in diastasis recti abdominis.

**diastasis recti abdominis,** the separation of the two rectus muscles along the median line of the abdominal wall. In a newborn the condition is the result of incomplete development. In an adult woman the abnormality is often caused by repeated pregnancies or multiple birth, such as the delivery of triplets.

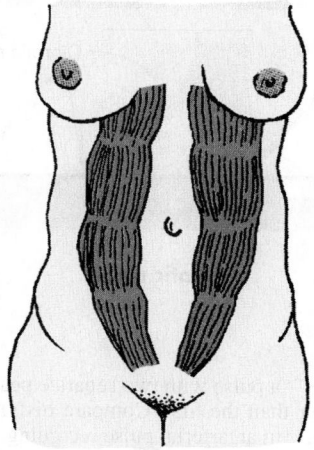

**Diastasis recti abdominis in pregnant woman**
*(Lowdermilk, Perry, and Bobak, 1999)*

**diastatic fermentation** /dī′əstat′ik/ [Gk, *diastasis,* separation; L, *fermentare,* to cause to rise], the conversion of starch to glucose by the enzyme ptyalin.

**diastema** /dī′əstē′mə/ [Gk, interval], an abnormally large space between two teeth in the same dental arch not caused by the loss of a tooth between them. It occurs most commonly between the maxillary central incisors in adults.

**diastole** /dī·as′təlē/ [Gk, *dia* + *stellein,* to set], the period between contractions of the atria or the ventricles during which blood enters the relaxed chambers from the systemic circulation and the lungs. Ventricular diastole begins with the onset of the second heart sound and ends with the first heart sound. Compare **systole.**

**-diastole,** suffix meaning 'the period of dilation of the heart shown as the lower blood pressure measurement': *adiastole, hyperdiastole, prediastole.*

**diastolic** /dī′əstol′ik/, pertaining to diastole, or the blood pressure at the instant of maximum cardiac relaxation.

**diastolic augmentation,** an increase in arterial diastolic blood pressure produced by a counterpulsation device such as an intraaortic balloon pump. A balloon-tipped catheter positioned in the aorta inflates during ventricular diastole, forcing blood back toward the heart, augmenting diastolic pressure, and assisting coronary artery filling. Balloon deflation at the onset of ventricular systole creates suction in the aorta, thereby assisting ventricular ejection and reducing systolic pressure.

**diastolic blood pressure,** the minimum level of blood pressure measured between contractions of the heart. It may vary with age, gender, body weight, emotional state, and other factors.

**diastolic filling pressure,** the blood pressure in a ventricle during diastole.

**diastolic murmur** [Gk, *dia,* between, *stellein,* to set; L, *murmur,* humming], a noise caused by turbulence of blood flow during ventricular relaxation. With few exceptions, diastolic murmurs are caused by organic heart disease.

**diastolic pressure.** See **diastolic blood pressure.**

**diastolic thrill,** a vibration felt over the heart during ventricular diastole. It may be caused by mitral valve stenosis, a patent ductus arteriosus, or severe aortic insufficiency.

**diastrophic** /dī′əstrof′ik/ [Gk, *diastrephein,* to distort], pertaining to a bent or curved condition of bones or distortion of other structures.

**diastrophic dwarf,** a person in whom short stature is caused by osteochondrodysplasia and is associated with various deformities of the bones and joints, including scoliosis, clubfoot, micromelia, hand defects, multiple joint contractures and subluxations, ear deformities, and cleft palate. The condition may be genetically related and transmitted as an autosomal recessive trait.

**diataxia** /dī′ətak′sē·ə/, ataxia affecting both sides of the body.

**diathermal** /dī′əthur′məl/, pertaining to the use of elevated local temperature in the treatment of a disorder. The raised temperature may be produced by high-frequency electric current, ultrasound, or microwave radiation.

**diathermy** /dī′əthur′mē/ [Gk, *dia* + *therme,* heat], the production of heat in body tissues for therapeutic purposes by high-frequency currents that are insufficiently intense to destroy tissues or to impair their vitality. Diathermy is used in treating chronic arthritis, bursitis, fractures, gynecologic diseases, sinusitis, and other conditions.

**diathesis** /dī·əthē′sis/, *pl.* **diatheses** [Gk, arrangement], an inherited physical constitution predisposing to certain diseases or conditions, many of which are believed associated with the Y chromosome because males appear to be more susceptible than females. A diathesis may be bilious, indicating a familial tendency to development of GI distress, or gouty, indicating a predisposition to accumulation of urates in the tissues, particularly in mature males.

**diazepam** /dī·az′əpam/, a benzodiazepine sedative and minor tranquilizer.

■ INDICATIONS: It is prescribed in the treatment of anxiety, nervous tension, and muscle spasm and as an anticonvulsant.

■ CONTRAINDICATIONS: Acute narrow-angle glaucoma, psychosis, or known hypersensitivity to this drug or to any benzodiazepine medication prohibits its use.

■ ADVERSE EFFECTS: Among the more serious adverse reactions are withdrawal symptoms resulting from discontinuation of treatment. Hypotonia, respiratory depression, drowsiness, and fatigue commonly occur.

**diazo-,** prefix indicating a chemical compound containing the group, —N ═ N—; *diazole, diazine.*

**diazoxide** /dī′əzok′sīd/, a vasodilator used as an antihypertensive.

■ INDICATIONS: It is prescribed parenterally for emergency reduction of blood pressure in malignant hypertension and orally in some cases of hypoglycemia.

■ CONTRAINDICATIONS: Compensatory hypertension, cerebral bleeding, or known hypersensitivity to this drug or other thiazides prohibits its use. Caution is advised in heart disease, pregnancy, and impaired kidney function.

■ ADVERSE EFFECTS: Among the more serious adverse reactions are tachycardia, sodium and water retention, hyperglycemia, and severe hypotension.

■ NOTE: This drug is for IV use in hospitalized patients only. Severe hypotension may result from its use.

**Dibenzyline,** trademark for an alpha₁ receptor blocker (phenoxybenzamine hydrochloride).

**dibucaine** /dī′bəkān/, a topical anesthetic ointment.

**dic,** abbreviation for *dicentric.*

**DIC,** abbreviation for **disseminated intravascular coagulation.**

**dicalcium phosphate and calcium gluconate with vitamin D** /dīkal′sē·əm/, a source of calcium and phosphorus.

■ INDICATIONS: It is prescribed for hypocalcemia, especially in pregnancy and lactation.

■ CONTRAINDICATIONS: Hypoparathyroidism or known hypersensitivity to the ingredients of this drug prohibits its use.

■ ADVERSE EFFECTS: There are no known adverse reactions.

**dicarboxylic acid** /dī′kär·sil′ik as′id/, an organic acid containing two carboxyl (COOH) groups.

**dicentric** /desen′trik/ [Gk, *di,* twice, *kentron,* center], (in genetics) pertaining to a structurally abnormal chromosome with two centromeres.

**dicephalus,** a fetus with two heads.

**dicephaly** /dīsef′əlē/ [Gk, *di,* twice, *kephale,* head], a developmental anomaly in which a fetus has two heads. —**dicephalous, dicephalic,** *adj.*

**dichlorodiphenyltrichloroethane.** See **DDT.**

**dichlorphenamide** /dī′klôrfen′əmīd/, a carbonic anhydrase inhibitor.

■ INDICATION: It is prescribed in the treatment of chronic glaucoma.

■ CONTRAINDICATIONS: Liver and adrenocortical insufficiency, kidney failure, hyperchloremic acidosis, depressed sodium or potassium level, pulmonary obstruction, Addison's disease, known or suspected pregnancy, or known hypersensitivity to this drug prohibits its use.

■ ADVERSE EFFECTS: Among the more serious adverse reactions are anorexia, GI disturbances, acidosis, ureteral calculus formation, and aplastic anemia.

**dichorial twins, dichorionic twins.** See **dizygotic twins.**

**dichotomy** /dīkot′əmē/ [Gk, *dicha,* in two, *temnein,* to cut], a division or separation into two equal parts.

**dichroic stain** /dīkrō′ik/, a radiographic film artifact caused by a colored chemical stain. The color may range from yellow to purple and is usually the result of improper processing. See also **curtain effect.**

**dichromatic vision** /dī′kromat′ik/ [Gk, *di,* twice, *chroma,* color; L, *visio*], a form of color vision in which only two of the three primary colors are perceived. Also called **dichromasia, dichromatopsia.**

**Dick-Read method.** See **Read method.**

**Dick test** [George F. Dick, 1881–1967; Gladys R.H. Dick, 1881–1963; American physicians], a skin test for determining sensitivity to an erythrotoxin produced by the group A streptococci that cause scarlet fever. A skin test dose of the toxin is injected intradermally. An area of inflammation 3 to 5 cm in diameter indicates that the person is not immune, has no antitoxin, and therefore is susceptible to the toxin. Larger doses may then be given to induce immunity. Compare **Schultz-Charlton phenomenon.**

**dicloxacillin sodium** /dī′kloksəsil′in/, a penicillinase-resistant penicillin.

■ INDICATIONS: It is prescribed in the treatment of staphylococcal infections, especially those caused by penicillinase-producing strains of staphylococci.

■ CONTRAINDICATIONS: Known hypersensitivity to this drug or to any penicillin medication prohibits its use.

■ ADVERSE EFFECTS: The most serious adverse effect is hypersensitivity reaction. Other side effects include nausea, vomiting, diarrhea, and epigastric distress.

**Dicor,** trademark for a castable ceramic dental material.

**dicrotic** /dī·krot′ik/ [Gk, *dikrotos* double beating], said of a waveform that has two separate peaks.

**dicrotic notch** /dīkrot′ik/, a small, downward deflection observed on the downstroke of an arterial pressure waveform. It represents closure of the aortic or pulmonic valve at the onset of ventricular diastole.

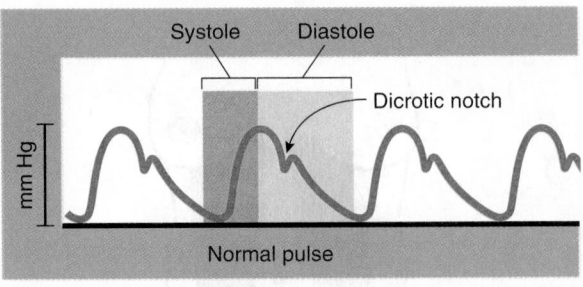

**Dicrotic notch**

**dicrotic pulse,** a pulse with two separate peaks, the second usually weaker than the first. Compare **bisferious pulse.**

**dicrotic wave,** in an arterial pulse recording, the portion of the descending limb following the aortic notch, including a second, smaller peak attributed to the reflected impulse of closure of the aortic valve.

**dicumarol** /dīkyōō′mərol/, an anticoagulant coumarin derivative.

■ INDICATIONS: It is prescribed for the prophylaxis and treatment of thrombosis and embolism.

■ CONTRAINDICATIONS: Risk of hemorrhage, peptic ulcer, ulcerative colitis, or known hypersensitivity to this drug prohibits its use.

■ ADVERSE EFFECTS: Among the more serious adverse reactions are GI disturbances, nausea, bleeding, and diarrhea.

**dicyclomine hydrochloride** /dīsī′kləmīn/, an anticholinergic/antispasmodic.

■ INDICATION: It is prescribed as an adjunct to ulcer therapy. It is prescribed as a treatment for functional/irritable bowel syndrome.

■ CONTRAINDICATIONS: Narrow-angle glaucoma, asthma, obstruction of the genitourinary or GI tract, ulcerative colitis, or known hypersensitivity to this drug prohibits its use.

■ ADVERSE EFFECTS: Among the more serious adverse reactions are blurred vision, central nervous system effects, tachycardia, dry mouth, decreased sweating, and hypersensitivity reactions.

**didactic** /dīdak′tik/ [Gr, *didaskein,* to teach], pertaining to classroom teaching or instruction.

**didanosine.** See **dideoxyinosine.**

**dideoxycytidine (ddC)** /dī′dē·ok′sēsī′tidēn/, an antiretroviral drug that prevents human immunodeficiency virus from multiplying. It is chemically related to **dideoxyinosine (ddI).**

**dideoxyinosine (ddI)** /dī′dē·oks·ē·in′ōsēn/, an antiretroviral drug used in the treatment of human immunodeficiency virus infections. ddI inhibits the enzyme reverse transcriptase, thereby restricting viral replication activity. Inside the body ddI is converted to dideoxyadenosine, which becomes incorporated into the deoxyribonucleic acid chain, interrupting its normal sequence and making viral replication impossible. Also called **didanosine.**

**dideoxythymidine (d4T)** /dīdē′oksēthī′midin/, a drug used in the treatment of acquired immunodeficiency virus. Major clinical toxicity is painful peripheral neuropathy.

**DIDMOAD (*d*iabetes *i*nsipidus, *d*iabetes *m*ellitus, *o*ptic *a*trophy, *d*eafness) syndrome.** See **Wolfram syndrome.**

**Didrex,** trademark for an anorexiant (benzphetamine hydrochloride).

**Didronel,** trademark for a calcium regulator (etidronate disodium).

**didym-,** 1. combining form meaning 'testis': *didymalgia, didymitis, didymodynia.* 2. combining form meaning 'paired or twin': *didymous.*

**-didymis, -didymus,** 1. suffix meaning 'testicles': *epididymis.* 2. suffix meaning 'twins': *atlodidymus, pygodidymus.*

**didymitis** /did′əmī′tis/, an inflammation in a testicle.

**didymus** /did′iməs/, a testis.

**-didymus,** 1. suffix meaning a 'pair of twins joined at a (specified) part of the body': *gastrodidymus, thoracodidymus, vertebrodidymus.* 2. suffix meaning a 'teratic fetus with supernumerary organ(s)': *atlodidymus, opodidymus, pygodidymus.*

**die¹,** to cease living.

**die²,** a model of a prepared tooth made from a hard substance, usually dental stone.

**diecious** /dī·ē′shəs/ [Gk, *di* + *oikos,* house], pertaining to an organism that has either male or female reproductive organs. Also spelled **dioecious.**

**dieldrin** /dī·el′drin/, a highly toxic pesticide that is also poisonous to humans and animals if ingested, inhaled, or absorbed through the skin. It causes dysfunction of the central nervous system and may be a carcinogen.

**diencephalic syndrome** /dis′en·sə·fal′ik/, failure to thrive and emaciation, sometimes with wartlike nevi.

**diencephalon** /dī′ənsef′əlon/ [Gk, *di* + *enkephalon,* brain], the portion of the brain between the cerebrum and the mesencephalon. It consists of the hypothalamus, thalamus, metathalamus, and the epithalamus and includes most of the third ventricle.

**diener** /dē′nər/ [Ger, man-servant], an individual who maintains the hospital laboratory or equipment and facilities. The morgue diener may also assist the pathologist in performing autopsies.

**dienestrol** /dī′ines′trôl/, an estrogen.

■ INDICATIONS: It is prescribed in the treatment of atrophic vaginitis and kraurosis vulvae.

■ CONTRAINDICATIONS: Pregnancy, known or suspected cancer of the breast, thrombophlebitis, unusual vaginal bleeding, or known hypersensitivity to this drug prohibits its use.

■ ADVERSE EFFECTS: Among the more serious adverse reactions are increased risk of cancer, thrombophlebitis, hepatic adenoma, embolism, and gallbladder disease.

**dieresis** /dī·er′əsis/, separation of a structure's parts by surgery or other means.

**diet** /dī′it/ [Gk, *diaita,* way of living], 1. food and drink considered with regard to their nutritional qualities, composition, and effects on health. 2. nutrients prescribed, regulated, or restricted as to kind and amount for therapeutic or other purposes. 3. the customary allowance of food and drink regularly provided or consumed. Compare **nutrition.** See also specific diets. —**dietetic,** *adj.*

**dietary** /dī′əter′ē/, pertaining to diet.

**dietary allowances.** See **recommended dietary allowances (RDA).**

**dietary amenorrhea** [Gk, *diaita,* way of living, *a,* absence, *men,* month, *rhoia,* to flow], an interruption of menstruation caused by malnutrition, starvation, or excessive voluntary dieting.

**dietary fiber,** a generic term for nondigestible carbohydrate substances found in plant cell walls and surrounding cellular material, each with a different effect on the various GI functions, such as colon transit time, water absorption, and lipid metabolism. Dietary fiber may be water soluble or insoluble. The soluble fibers include pectins, gums, mucilages, and algal products. They impact nutrient absorption and regulation. The insoluble fibers include cellulose, hemicellulose, and lignin and promote stool bulk and caloric motility. The main dietary fiber components are cellulose, lignin, hemicellulose, pectin, and plant gums. Foods high in dietary fiber are fruits; green leafy vegetables, such as lettuce, spinach, celery, and cabbage; root vegetables, such as carrots, turnips, and potatoes; legumes; and whole-grain cereals and breads. The risk of development of constipation, hemorrhoids, diverticular disease, and colon cancer may be decreased by regular consumption of sufficient amounts of fiber. Most experts recommend intake of 20 to 30 g per day. Also called **bulk, roughage.**

**dietetic.** See **diet.**

**dietetic food,** 1. a specially prepared low-calorie food, often containing natural or artificial sweeteners. 2. a food prepared for any specific dietary need or restriction, such as salt-free or vegetarian food. See also **dietetics.**

**dietetic food diarrhea.** See **osmotic diarrhea.**

**dietetics** /dī′itet′iks/, the science of applying nutritional principles to the planning and preparation of foods and regulation of the diet in relation to both health and disease.

**dietetic technician,** a person trained in food and nutrition who may work independently or in a team with a registered

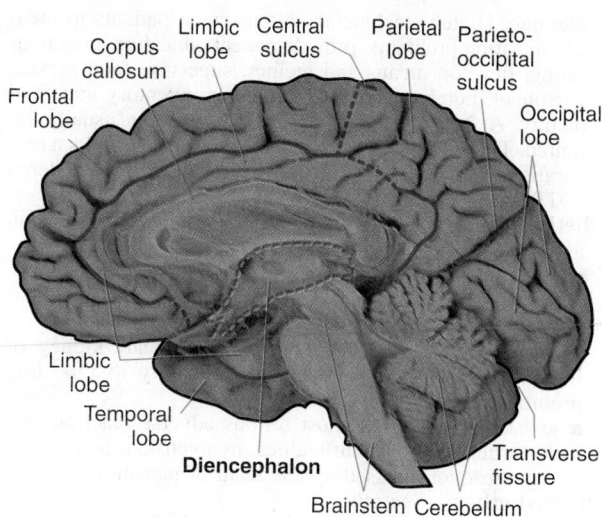

Limbic lobe · Central sulcus · Parietal lobe · Parieto-occipital sulcus
Corpus callosum
Frontal lobe
Occipital lobe
Limbic lobe
Temporal lobe
**Diencephalon**
Transverse fissure
Brainstem Cerebellum

**Diencephalon** *(Nolte and Angevine, 2000)*

dietitian. Dietetic technicians often screen patients to identify nutrition problems, provide patient education and counseling, develop menus and recipes, supervise food service personnel, purchase food, and monitor inventory and food quality. A 2-year associate degree program is usually required. Those who complete the AD program and pass a registration exam become a Dietetic Technician, Registered (DTR).

**diethylcarbamazine citrate** /dī·eth′əlkärbam′əzēn/, an anthelmintic.
■ INDICATIONS: It is prescribed in the treatment of ascariasis, Bancroft's filariasis, onchocerciasis, loiasis, and tropical eosinophilia.
■ CONTRAINDICATIONS: Hypertension; severe heart, kidney, or liver impairment; or known hypersensitivity to this drug prohibits its use.
■ ADVERSE EFFECTS: The most serious adverse reactions are tachycardia, breathing difficulties, hypotension, and severe allergic reactions caused by the death of parasites.

**diethyl ether.** See **ether.**

**diethylpropion hydrochloride** /dī·eth′ilprō′pē·on/, an appetite suppressant; a central nervous system stimulant.
■ INDICATION: It is prescribed in the treatment of exogenous obesity.
■ CONTRAINDICATIONS: Arteriosclerosis, hyperthyroidism, glaucoma, history of drug dependence or drug abuse, hypertension, concomitant administration of a monoamine oxidase inhibitor within 14 days, or known hypersensitivity to this drug prohibits its use.
■ ADVERSE EFFECTS: Among the more serious adverse reactions are restlessness and insomnia, increased blood pressure, arrhythmias, cardiovascular effects, nausea, dry mouth, and drug dependence.

**diethylstilbestrol (DES)** /-stilbes′trol/, synthetic hormone with estrogenic properties. Also called **stilbestrol.**

**diethylstilbestrol diphosphate,** an antineoplastic agent.
■ INDICATION: It is prescribed for inoperable, progressing prostatic cancer.
■ CONTRAINDICATIONS: Present or previous condition of markedly impaired liver, thrombophlebitis, thromboembolic disorders, or cerebral apoplexy prohibits its use.
■ ADVERSE EFFECTS: The most serious adverse reactions are thrombophlebitis, pulmonary embolism, cerebral thrombosis, cholestatic jaundice, mental depression, erythema nodosum and erythema multiforme, changes in libido, and dizziness.

**dieting syndrome,** the extreme practice of following fad diets, often leading to harmful physical and psychologic effects.

**dietitian.** See **registered dietitian, nutritionist.**

**Dietl's crisis** /dē′təlz/ [Joseph Dietl, Polish physician, 1804–1878; Gk, krisis, turning point], a sudden excruciating pain in the kidney, caused by distension of the renal pelvis, rapid ingestion of very large amounts of liquid, or kinking of a ureter that produces temporary occlusion of the flow of urine from the kidney. The pain may be accompanied by nausea, vomiting, hematuria, and general collapse. See also **hydronephrosis.**

**diet staging,** a nursing intervention from the Nursing Interventions Classification (NIC) defined as instituting required diet restrictions with subsequent progression of diet as tolerated. See also **Nursing Interventions Classification.**

**diet therapy, 1.** the branch of dietetics concerned with the use of foods for therapeutic purposes. **2.** a nutritional therapy based on a person's normal nutritional requirements, but modified for a disease or disorder to provide appropriate

changes in amount and form of nutrients, energy value, and texture of solids and liquids.

**differential** /dif′əren′shəl/, pertaining to or creating a difference.

**differential absorption** [L, differentia, difference], the difference in absorption of x-rays by different body tissues. In a radiograph of a body part, such as an arm, the image of the bone is produced because more x-rays are absorbed by bone than by the surrounding soft tissue. Lowering the kilovolt peak of an x-ray beam increases differential absorption, but it also increases the patient dose. Also called **selective absorption.**

**differential blood count.** See **differential white blood cell count.**

**differential diagnosis,** the distinguishing between two or more diseases with similar symptoms by systematically comparing their signs and symptoms. See also **diagnosis.**

**differential growth,** a difference in the size or rate of growth of dissimilar organisms, tissues, or structures.

**differential leukocyte count.** See **differential white blood cell count.**

**differential threshold,** the lowest limit at which two stimuli can be differentiated or distinguished.

**differential white blood cell count,** an examination and enumeration of the distribution of leukocytes in a stained blood smear. The different kinds of white cells are counted and reported as percentages of the total examined. Differential white blood cell count provides more specific information related to infections and diseases. Compare **complete blood count.** See also **leukocyte.**

**differentiating agent,** a substance, such as a retinoid, that induces a cell to stop dividing and to differentiate. Such agents may be capable of halting the proliferation of cancer cells.

**differentiation** /dif′əren′shē·ā′shən/ [L, differentia, difference], **1.** (in embryology) a process in development in which unspecialized cells or tissues are systemically modified and altered to achieve specific and characteristic physical forms, physiologic functions, and chemical properties. Kinds of differentiation are **correlative differentiation, functional differentiation, invisible differentiation,** and **self-differentiation. 2.** progressive diversification leading to complexity. **3.** acquisition of functions and forms different from those of the original. **4.** distinguishing of one thing or disease from another, as in differential diagnosis. **5.** (in psychology) mental autonomy or separation of intellect and emotions so that one is not dominated by reactive anxiety of a family or group emotional system. **6.** the first subphase of the separation-individuation phase in Mahler's system of preoedipal development. It generally occurs between 5 and 9 months of age, coinciding with the maturation of partial locomotor functioning and the beginning of the child's viewing the mother as a separate being. —**differentiate,** v.

**differentiation therapy,** a cancer therapy technique in which the malignant cell is regarded as having escaped the normal controls of cell growth and differentiation. The cancer cell is regarded as pathologically arrested at an early stage of differentiation, retaining the ability to proliferate. It is treated with agents that remove this block and allow the cells to differentiate along more normal lines until they eventually lose their ability to divide and replicate.

**diffraction** /difrak′shən/ [L, dis, opposite of, frangere, to break], the bending and scattering of wavelengths of light or other radiation as the radiation passes around obstacles or through narrow slits. X-ray diffraction is used in the study of the internal structure of cells. See also **refraction.**

**diffuse** /dify$\overline{oo}$z′/ [L, *diffundere,* to spread out], becoming widely spread, such as through a membrane or fluid.

**diffuse abscess,** an abscess that spreads into neighboring tissues beyond fibrous walls.

**diffuse axonal injury (DAI),** a type of brain injury caused by shearing forces that occur between different parts of the brain as a result of rotational acceleration. The corpus callosum and the brainstem are often affected. DAI most commonly occurs in motor vehicle crashes when the vehicle suddenly stops.

**diffused light,** light in which the precise source cannot be seen while the apparent area of the source is increased.

**diffuse emphysema.** See **panacinar emphysema.**

**diffuse erythema,** skin redness or inflammation that is spread over a large body surface.

**diffuse esophageal spasm,** abnormal contractions of the esophagus leading to difficult or painful swallowing and chest pain.

**diffuse fibrosing alveolitis.** See **interstitial pneumonia.**

**diffuse goiter,** an enlargement of all parts of the thyroid gland. Symptoms are those of hyperthyroidism.

**diffuse hypersensitivity pneumonia,** an immunologically mediated inflammatory reaction in the lungs induced by exposure to an allergen or a drug. Allergens that trigger the reaction may be derived from fungi; bird excreta; piscine, porcine, or bovine proteins; wood dust; and fur. Drugs that induce hypersensity pneumonia include chlorpropamide, hydrochlorothiazide, mecamylamine, mephenesin, methotrexate, nitrofurantoin, paraaminosalicylic acid, and penicillin. The disorder is characterized by cough, fever, dyspnea, malaise, pulmonary edema, and infiltration of the alveoli with eosinophils and large mononuclear cells. Also called **allergic alveolitis, allergic interstitial pneumonitis, extrinsic allergic pneumonia.** See also **bagassosis, pulmonary infiltrate with eosinophilia.**

**diffuse idiopathic skeletal hyperostosis,** a form of degenerative joint disease in which the ligaments along the spinal column become calcified and lose their flexibility.

**diffuse lipoma, diffuse lipomatosis.** See **multiple lipomatosis.**

**diffuse myelitis.** See **disseminated myelitis.**

**diffuse myocardial fibrosis,** a type of heart disease characterized by a generalized distribution of fibrous tissue that replaces normal heart muscle cells.

**diffuse peritonitis** [L, *diffundere,* to spread out; Gk, *peri,* near, *teinein,* to stretch, *itis,* inflammation], widespread peritonitis, affecting most of the peritoneum, usually caused by a ruptured stomach or appendix. See also **generalized peritonitis, peritonitis.**

**diffuse sclerosis** [L, *diffundere,* to spread out; Gk, *sklerosis,* hardening], a form of sclerosis that extends through much of the central nervous system.

**diffusing capacity** /dify$\overline{oo}$′sing/, the rate of gas transfer through a unit area of a permeable membrane per unit of gas pressure difference across it. It is affected by specific chemical reactions that may occur in the blood. Also called **diffusion factor, transfer factor of lungs.**

**diffusing capacity of lungs ($D_L$),** the volume of a gas that diffuses from the lung across the alveolar-capillary membrane into the bloodstream per minute per mm Hg difference in pressure across the membrane. The normal $D_L$ for oxygen averages 20 mL/min/mm Hg. Also called **transfer factor of lungs.**

**diffusion** /dify$\overline{oo}$′zhən/ [L, *diffundere,* to spread out], the process in which particles in a fluid moves from an area of higher concentration to an area of lower concentration, re-

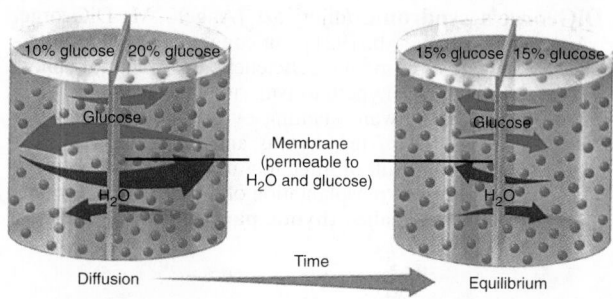

**Diffusion** *(Thibodeau and Patton, 1999/Rolin Graphics)*

sulting in an even distribution of the particles in the fluid. Little or no energy is required.

**diffusion coefficient.** See **coefficient.**

**diffusion constant,** a mathematical constant relating to the ability of a substance to spread widely.

**diffusion defect,** any impairment in the diffusion of oxygen across the alveolar-capillary membrane caused by pathologic changes in any of the structures of the membrane. Specific causes may include fibrosis, granuloma, interstitial edema, and proliferation of connective tissue.

**diffusion deposition,** the adsorption of an aerosol particle on the surface of an alveolar membrane or other airway structure.

**diffusion factor.** See **diffusing capacity.**

**diffusion of gases,** a natural process, essential in respiration, in which molecules of a gas pass from an area of high concentration to one of lower concentration.

**diflorasone diacetate** /dīflôr′əsōn dī·as′ətāt/, a topical corticosteroid.

■ INDICATION: It is prescribed for the treatment of skin inflammation.

■ CONTRAINDICATIONS: Viral and fungal diseases of the skin, impaired circulation, or known hypersensitivity to this drug or to other steroidal medication prohibits its use.

■ ADVERSE EFFECTS: Among the more serious adverse reactions, usually occurring after prolonged or excessive application, are striae, hypopigmentation, local irritation of the skin, and various systemic effects.

**Diflucan,** trademark for a broad-spectrum bis-triazole antifungal agent (fluconazole).

**diflunisal** /dīfl$\overline{oo}$′nisal/, a nonsteroidal antiinflammatory agent.

■ INDICATIONS: It is prescribed for the treatment of mild to moderate pain and inflammation in osteoarthritis and other musculoskeletal disorders.

■ CONTRAINDICATIONS: Hypersensitivity to aspirin and other nonsteroidal antiinflammatory drugs or known sensitivity to this drug prohibits its use.

■ ADVERSE EFFECTS: The most serious adverse reactions are GI pain, diarrhea, peptic ulcer, anorexia, anaphylactoid reactions with bronchospasm, and edema.

**digastricus** /dīgas′trikəs/ [Gk, *di,* twice, *gaster,* stomach], one of four suprahyoid muscles having two parts, an anterior belly and a posterior belly. The anterior belly acts to open the jaw and to draw the hyoid bone forward. The posterior belly acts to draw back and to raise the hyoid bone. Also called **digastric muscle.** Compare **geniohyoideus, mylohyoideus, stylohyoideus.**

**DiGeorge's syndrome** /dijôrj′əz/ [Angelo M. DiGeorge, American physician, b. 1921], a congenital disorder characterized by severe immunodeficiency and structural abnormalities, including hypertelorism; notched, low-set ears; small mouth; downward slanting eyes; cardiovascular defects; and absence of the thymus and parathyroid glands. Death, often as a result of infection, usually occurs before 2 years of age. Rarely transplantation of a human fetal thymus is performed. Also called **thymic parathyroid aplasia.**

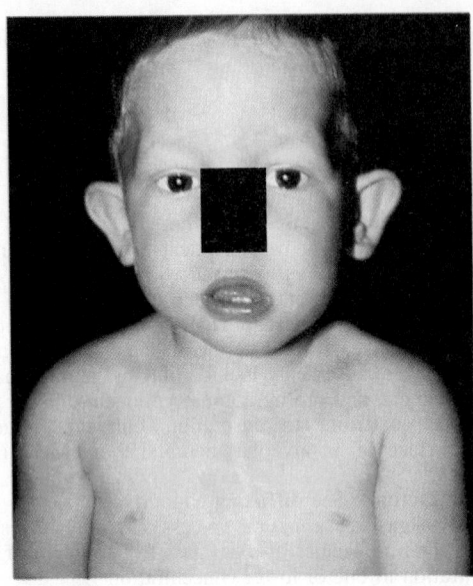

**DiGeorge's syndrome** *(Zitelli and Davis, 1997)*

**digest** [L, *digerere,* to break down], **1.** /dijest′/ to soften by heat and moisture. **2.** /dijest′/, to break into smaller parts and simpler compounds by mastication, hydrolysis, and action of intestinal secretions and enzymes, especially in the way the body digests food for the absorption of nutrients required in metabolism. The small intestine digests food by enzymatic actions that produce absorbable amino acids, emulsified fat particles, and monosaccharides. **3.** /dī′jəst/, any material that results from digestion or hydrolysis.

**digestant** /dijes′tənt/, a substance, such as pepsin, that is added to the diet as an aid to the digestion of food.

**digestible** /dijes′tibəl/, capable of being digested.

**digestion** /dijes′chən/ [L, *digerere,* to break down], the conversion of food into absorbable substances in the GI tract. Digestion is accomplished through the mechanical and chemical breakdown of food into smaller and smaller molecules, with the help of glands located both inside and outside the gut. —**digestive,** *adj.*

**digestive enzyme** /dijes′tiv/ [L, *digerere,* to break down; Gk, *en* + *zyme,* ferment], any digestive system enzyme that hydrolyzes fats, proteins, and carbohydrates for absorption.

**digestive fever,** a slight rise in body temperature that normally accompanies the digestive process.

**digestive gland,** any one of the many structures that secrete agents involved in the breaking down of food into the constituent absorbable substances needed for metabolism. Some kinds of digestive glands are the salivary glands, gastric glands, intestinal glands, liver, and pancreas. Among important secretions produced by different digestive glands are hydrochloric acid, bile, mucus, and various enzymes.

**digestive juice,** a thin, colorless secretion of the glands of the human stomach, composed mainly of hydrochloric acid, chymosin, pepsinogen, intrinsic factor, and mucus. Also called **digestive secretion.**

**digestive system,** the organs, structures, and accessory glands of the digestive tube of the body through which food passes from the mouth to the esophagus, stomach, and intestines. The accessory glands secrete the digestive enzymes, which break down food substances in preparation for absorption into the bloodstream. See also the Color Atlas of Human Anatomy.

**digestive tract,** a musculomembranous tube, about 9 m long, extending from the mouth to the anus and lined with mucous membrane. Its various portions are the mouth, pharynx, esophagus, stomach, small intestine, and large intestine. The tube, which is part of the digestive system, includes numerous accessory organs. Also called **alimentary canal, alimentary tract, digestive tube, gastrointestinal tract, intestinal tract, intestinal tube.** See also **digestive system.**

**Digibind,** trademark for the antibody used in the treatment of digoxin toxicity (digoxin immune Fab, ovine).

**digit** /dij′it/ [L, *digitus*], a finger or toe. Also called **dactylus.**

**digit-,** combining form meaning 'finger or toe': *digitate, digitigrade, digitoplantar.*

**digital**[1] /dij′itəl/ [L, *digitus,* finger], **1.** pertaining to a digit, that is, a finger or toe. **2.** resembling a finger or toe. See also **digitate.**

**digital**[2], **1.** the characterization or measurement of a signal in terms of a series of numbers rather than some continuously varying value. **2.** use of the binary system in computer technology, or computerized communications, such as digital telephone, pagers, and cellular telephones.

**digital angiography,** a technique of producing computer-enhanced radiographic images of the heart and great vessels. Before injection of contrast material through a large vein, a mask image is digitized and stored in the computer. Successive digitized images made after injection are electronically subtracted from the mask image, and the result is amplified and displayed on a video monitor. The displayed images can be recorded on videotape and stored on disk.

**digital compression** [L, *digitus,* finger, *comprimere,* to press together], the act of pressing with the fingers, as when arresting the blood flow from a wound.

**digital computer,** a computer that processes information in numeric form. Compare **analog computer, hybrid computer.**

**digital fluoroscopy,** the projection of a radiographic image on an image-intensifying fluorescent screen coupled to a digital video image processor. The screen has an input surface coated with a phosphor that is twice as sensitive to x-rays as conventional x-ray film. The visible light from the energized phosphor is electronically amplified and directed into a video camera. The video image is divided into pixels, which are in turn converted or digitized for storage or reproduction through an image processor.

**digitalis** /dij′ital′is/ [L, *digitus,* finger or toe], a general term for cardiac glycoside.

■ INDICATIONS: It is prescribed in the treatment of congestive heart failure and certain cardiac arrhythmias.

■ CONTRAINDICATIONS: Ventricular fibrillation, ventricular tachycardia, or known hypersensitivity to this drug prohibits its use.

■ ADVERSE EFFECTS: The most serious reactions are cardiac arrhythmias that are more common with concomitant diuretics; disorientation; and visual distubances.

**digitalis glycoside.** See **glycoside.**

**digitalis poisoning** [L, *digitalis,* of the fingers, *potio,* drink], the toxic effects of digitalis medications prescribed for heart disorders such as heart failure and atrial fibrillation. Toxicity may result from the cumulative effect of the drug or from hypokalemia. Symptoms include vomiting, headache, heartbeat abnormalities, disorientation, and visual color distortions.

**digitalis therapy,** the administration of a digitalis preparation to a person with a heart disorder to increase the force of myocardial contractions; produce a slower, more regular apical rate; and slow the transmission of impulses through the conduction system. It may be used in treating many cardiac disorders, including atrial fibrillation, atrial septal defect, coarctation of the aorta, congenital heart block, congestive heart failure, endocardial fibroelastosis, great vessel transposition, malformation of the tricuspid valve, myocarditis, paroxysmal atrial tachycardia, and patent ductus arteriosus.

■ METHOD: Complete orders include the name of the digitalis preparation, the dosage in milligrams, the route and intervals of administration, and the pulse rate under which the drug is to be withheld. It is administered before feeding and is never mixed with the formula or food. Before each administration the person's resting apical pulse is checked for rate and rhythm for a full minute. If the rate is slower than desired; if it is irregular or shows a rapid rise or fall; if there are any signs of toxicity such as anorexia, nausea, or vomiting; or if there are visual disturbances, the drug is withheld and the problem is reported.

■ INTERVENTIONS: The nurse participates in calculating the dosage volume ordered, administers the drug, and observes for and reports any undesirable effects. Once the dosage is stabilized and before discharge, the nurse or pharmacist ensures that the patient understands the proper method, time, and purpose of administering the drug, as well as the need and the time to give the complete dose, when to withhold medication, and how to recognize and report signs of toxicity to the drug.

■ OUTCOME CRITERIA: In addition to promoting more forceful myocardial contractions and a slower, more regular apical beat, digitalis therapy can reduce venous pressure, improve pulmonary and systemic circulation, increase urinary output, reduce edema, and stop paroxysmal atrial tachycardia and atrial fibrillation.

**digitalization** /dij'ətal'īzā'shən/, the administration of digitalis in doses sufficient to achieve maximum pharmacologic effects without producing toxic symptoms.

**digitalized** /dij'ətəlīzd'/, having a therapeutic total body level of digitalis, a cardiac glycoside.

**digitalizing dose,** the amount of digitalis needed to achieve a desired therapeutic effect.

**digital radiography (DR)** /dij'itəl/, any method of radiographic image formation that uses a computer to store and manipulate data. See also **digital angiography, digital fluoroscopy, digital tomosynthesis.**

**digital reflex, 1.** a finger-jerk reaction produced by tapping the palmar aspect of the terminal phalanges of the fingers when they are slightly flexed. **2.** sudden flexion of the terminal phalanx of the thumb produced by tapping the terminal phalanx of the middle finger.

**digital subtraction angiography (DSA),** a method in which radiographic images of blood vessels filled with contrast material are digitized and then subtracted from images

obtained before administration of the material. The method increases the contrast between the vessels and the background.

**digital thermometer.** See **thermometer.**

**digital-to-analog converter,** a device for translating digital information into a continuous form, as from an ohmmeter or thermometer. They are widely used in CD players, digital audio and videotape players, and in digital signal processing audio and video equipment. Also called **D/A converter.**

**digital tomosynthesis,** a system of tomography using a computer and a digital fluoroscopy unit, which can synthesize any tomographic plane from a single tomographic pass. As only one tomographic pass is required, patient radiation exposure is reduced. Patient time in examination is also reduced as the recorded images can be synthesized and manipulated at a later time. See also **digital fluoroscopy.**

**digitate** /dij'itāt/ [L, *digitatus,* having fingers], having fingers or fingerlike projections. See also **digital.**

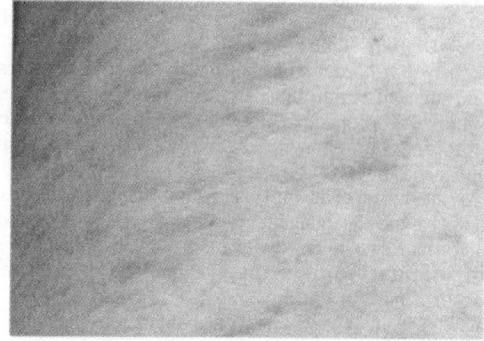

**Digitate dermatosis** *(du Vivier, 1993)*

**digitate wart,** a fingerlike horny projection that arises from a pea-shaped base. It is a benign viral infection of the skin and the adjacent mucous membrane. It may disappear spontaneously as an immune response develops in the host, or it may require treatment, such as by electrodesiccation and curettage. Also called **filiform warts.**

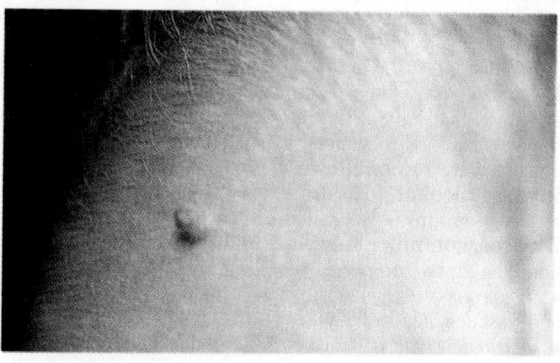

**Digitate wart** *(Weston, Lane, and Morrelli, 1996)*

**digitoxin** /dij'itok'sin/, a cardiac glycoside obtained from leaves of *Digitalis purpurea.* Digitoxin differs in many ways from digoxin, including having a far greater half-life and a different route of elimination.

■ INDICATIONS: It is prescribed in the treatment of congestive heart failure and certain cardiac arrhythmias.

■ CONTRAINDICATIONS: Ventricular fibrillation, ventricular tachycardia, or known hypersensitivity to this drug prohibits its use.

■ ADVERSE EFFECTS: The most serious adverse reactions are cardiac arrhythmias and heart block, disorientation, and visual disturbances.

**digit span test,** an examination of the ability of a child to recall a sequence of numbers just spoken.

**diglyceride** /dīglis'ərīd/, a chemical compound, an ester of glycerol in which the hydrogen in two of the hydroxyl groups is replaced by an acyl radical.

**dignathus** /dīnath'əs, dignā'thəs/, **1.** a fetus with a double lower jaw. **2.** a person with a cleft of the mandible.

**dignified dying,** a nursing outcome from the Nursing Outcomes Classification (NOC) defined as maintaining personal control and comfort with the approaching end of life. See also **Nursing Outcomes Classification.**

**digoxin** /digok'sin/, a cardiac glycoside obtained from leaves of *Digitalis lanata.*

■ INDICATIONS: It is prescribed in the treatment of congestive heart failure and certain cardiac arrhythmias.

■ CONTRAINDICATIONS: Ventricular fibrillation, ventricular tachycardia, or known hypersensitivity to this drug prohibits its use.

■ ADVERSE EFFECTS: The most serious adverse reactions are cardiac arrhythmia and heart block, disorientation, and visual disturbances.

**digoxin immune Fab, ovine,** a parenteral antidote for digoxin or digitoxin toxicity.

■ INDICATIONS: It is prescribed for the treatment of life-threatening digoxin or digitoxin toxicity.

■ CONTRAINDICATIONS: Use of this product should be restricted to patients who are in shock or cardiac arrest or show signs of severe ventricular arrhythmias, progressive bradycardia, or potassium concentrations exceeding 5 mEq/L.

■ ADVERSE EFFECTS: Among reported adverse reactions are low cardiac output, congestive heart failure exacerbated by withdrawal of the inotropic effect of digoxin, rapid ventricular response caused by withdrawal of the digitalis effect, and possible hypokalemia.

**di Guglielmo's disease, di Guglielmo's syndrome.** See **erythroleukemia.**

**dihybrid** /dī'hī'brid/ [Gk, *di,* twice; L, *hybrida,* mongrel offspring], pertaining to an individual, an organism, or a strain that is heterozygous for two specific traits, that is the offspring of parents differing in two specific gene pairs, or that is heterozygous for two particular traits or gene loci being followed.

**dihybrid cross,** the mating of two individuals, organisms, or strains that have different gene pairs that determine two specific traits or in which two particular characteristics or gene loci are being followed.

**dihydric alcohol** /dīhī'drik/, an alcohol containing two hydroxyl groups. Also called **diol.**

**dihydroergotamine mesylate** /dīhī'drō·ərgot'əmēn me'si lāt/, an alpha-adrenergic blocking agent.

■ INDICATIONS: It is prescribed for the treatment of migraine and vascular headache.

■ CONTRAINDICATIONS: Cardiovascular disease, hypertension, liver or kidney dysfunction, sepsis, pregnancy, or known hypersensitivity to this drug prohibits its use.

■ ADVERSE EFFECTS: Among the more serious adverse reactions are gangrene and the toxicity of the ergot alkaloids.

**dihydrotachysterol** /dīhī'drōtəkis'tərol/, a rapid-acting form of vitamin D.

■ INDICATIONS: It is prescribed in the treatment of hypocalcemia resulting from hypoparathyroidism and pseudohypoparathyroidism.

■ CONTRAINDICATIONS: Hypercalcemia, hypocalcemia with kidney insufficiency, hyperphosphatemia, or known hypersensitivity to this drug or to vitamin D prohibits its use. Caution is advised for lactating mothers.

■ ADVERSE EFFECTS: The most serious adverse reaction is hypercalcemia. With overdosage calcification of soft tissues, including those of the heart, or cardiovascular or kidney failure may occur.

**diiodohydroxyquin.** See **iodoquinol.**

**dil-, -dil,** combining form for the name of a vasodilator.

**dilaceration** /dī·las'ər·ā'shən/ [L. *di-,* apart or through + *lacerare,* to tear], **1.** a tearing apart, as of a cataract. **2.** (in dentistry) a condition resulting from injury to a tooth during its developmental period, with a crease or band at the junction of the crown and root, or with tortuous roots having abnormal curvatures.

**Dilantin,** trademark for an anticonvulsant (phenytoin) used to control tonic-clonic and psychomotor seizures.

**dilatancy** /dī·lā'tən·sē/ [L, *dilatare,* to widen], an unusual behavior observed in cytoplasm (and in some physical systems) during which its viscosity and applied force both increase.

**dilatant,** exhibiting dilatancy.

**dilatation.** See **dilation.**

**dilate** /dī'lāt/, to cause a physiologic increase in the diameter of a body opening, blood vessel, or tube, such as the widening of the pupil of the eye in response to decreased light or the widening of the uterine cervix during labor.

**dilation** [L, *dilatare,* to widen], **1.** the condition of being dilated or stretched. **2.** the process of causing a physiologic increase in the diameter of a body opening, blood vessel, or tube. Examples include the widening of the pupil of the eye by the use of cycloplegic eyedrops for examination of the retina and opening of the uterine cervix to facilitate curettage by the use of a dilator. Also called *dilatation.*

**dilation and curettage (D&C),** widening of the uterine cervix and scraping of the endometrium of the uterus. It is done to diagnose disease of the uterus, to correct heavy or prolonged vaginal bleeding, or to empty the uterus of the products of conception. It is also performed to remove tumors, to rule out carcinoma of the uterus, to remove retained placental fragments after delivery or after an incomplete abortion, and to find the cause of infertility. The cervix is dilated with a series of dilators of increasing size to allow the insertion of a curet into the uterus. Vaginal packing may sometimes be inserted for up to 24 hours to slow bleeding but is not usually recommended. A perineal pad is applied. Postoperative care requires emotional support appropriate to the clinical situation and close observation for hemorrhage, infection, or dysuria. See also **abortion, fractional dilation and curettage.**

**dilation and evacuation (D&E)** /dīlā'shən/ [L, *dilatare,* to widen, *evacuare,* to empty], the removal of the products of conception, using suction curettage and forceps, during the second trimester of pregnancy; a type of abortion.

**dilation of the heart** [L, *dilatare,* to widen; AS, *heorte*], an enlargement of the heart caused by stretching of a weakened myocardium. The condition is associated with acute pulmonary embolism and heart failure.

**dilator** /dī'lātər/ [L, *dilatare*, to widen], a device for expanding a body opening or cavity. Examples include a tent dilator, consisting of a sponge or bundle of seaweed that expands the cervical os, and a Barnes' bag (dilator), a rubber bag that can be inserted into a body cavity and filled with water to produce pressure on the cavity walls.

**dilator naris,** the alar portion of the nasalis muscle that dilates the nostril. Compare **compressor naris.**

**dilator pupillae,** a muscle that contracts the iris of the eye and dilates the pupil. It is composed of radial fibers, like spokes of a wheel, that converge from the circumference of the iris toward the center and blend with fibers of the sphincter pupillae near the margin of the pupil. The dilator pupillae is innervated primarily by nerve fibers from the sympathetic system through the oculomotor nerve. Compare **sphincter pupillae.**

**Dilaudid Hydrochloride,** trademark for an opioid analgesic (hydromorphone hydrochloride).

**Dilor,** trademark for a bronchodilator (dyphylline).

**diltiazem** /diltī'əzam/, a calcium channel blocker or calcium antagonist.

■ INDICATIONS: It is prescribed for the treatment of vasospastic and effort-associated angina, in addition to hypertension.

■ CONTRAINDICATIONS: Sick sinus syndrome, second- or third-degree atrioventricular block, or hypotension prohibits its use.

■ ADVERSE EFFECTS: Among the more serious adverse reactions are edema, arrhythmia, bradycardia, hypotension, syncope, rash, headache, and dizziness.

**diluent** /dil'ōō·ənt, dil'yōō·ənt/ [L, *diluere*, to wash], a substance, generally a fluid, that makes a solution or mixture less concentrated, less viscous, or more liquid.

**dilute** /dilōōt', dī'lōōt/ [L, *diluere*, to wash], **1.** pertaining to a solution that contains a relatively small amount of solute in proportion to solvent. **2.** to make a more concentrated solution less concentrated.

**diluting agent** /dilōō'ting/, a substance used to reduce the viscosity of respiratory tract secretions so they can be removed easily. Examples include water and hypotonic saline solution, which can be aerosolized or nebulized.

**dimenhydrinate** /dim'ənhī'drināt/, an antiemetic.

■ INDICATIONS: It is prescribed in the treatment of nausea and motion sickness.

■ CONTRAINDICATIONS: Asthma or known hypersensitivity to this drug prohibits its use. It is not given to newborns or lactating mothers.

■ ADVERSE EFFECTS: Among the more serious adverse reactions are skin rash, hypersensitivity reactions, and tachycardia. Drowsiness and dry mouth are common.

**dimension,** a measure of the width, length, or height of a space, usually described in units of a linear scale.

**dimensional stability** /dimen'shənəl/, the resistance of radiographic film to image distortion from warping or changing size or shape during processing.

**dimer** /dī'mər/ [Gk, *di*, twice, *meros*, parts], a compound formed by the union of two radicals or two molecules of a simpler compound, as a polymer formed from two or more molecules of a monomer.

**dimercaprol** /dī'mərkap'rol/, a heavy-metal antagonist. Previously called **British antilewisite (BAL).**

■ INDICATIONS: It is prescribed in the treatment of Wilson's disease and in the treatment of acute arsenic, mercury, or gold poisoning, as from an overdosage with mercurial diuretics, arsenics, or gold salts.

■ CONTRAINDICATIONS: Hepatic or renal insufficiency; poisoning with cadmium, iron, or selenium; or known hypersensitivity to the drug prohibits its use.

■ ADVERSE EFFECTS: Among the most serious adverse reactions are nephrotoxicity, acidosis, convulsions, and abnormal cardiovascular functions. Mild reactions include pain at the injection site, nausea, excessive salivation, and paresthesia.

**Dimetane,** trademark for an antihistamine (brompheniramine maleate).

**Dimetapp,** trademark for a fixed-combination drug containing a decongestant (phenylpropanolamine hydrochloride) and an antihistamine (brompheniramine maleate).

**dimethisterone** /dī'məthis'tərōn/, an orally active progestational agent with no androgenic, estrogenic, or anabolic activity.

**dimethoxymethylamphetamine (DOM)** /dī'məthok'sēmeth'iləmfet'əmēn/, a psychoactive or hallucinogenic agent.

**dimethylamine [$(CH_3)_2NH$],** a secondary amine found in guano and decomposing fish.

**dimethylaniline.** See **auramine.**

**dimethyl carbinol.** See **isopropyl alcohol.**

**dimethyl sulfoxide (DMSO)** /dīmeth'il/, an antiinflammatory agent and organic solvent.

■ INDICATIONS: It is prescribed in the treatment of interstitial cystitis.

■ CONTRAINDICATION: Known hypersensitivity to this drug prohibits its use.

■ ADVERSE EFFECTS: Among the most serious adverse reactions are GI disturbances, photophobia, disturbance of color vision, and headache. A garliclike body odor and taste in the mouth may occur. When applied topically, it can cause local irritations and carry toxins into the systemic circulation.

**dimethyl tubocurarine iodide.** See **metocurine iodide.**

**Dimitri's disease.** See **Sturge-Weber syndrome.**

**dimorphous** /dīmôr'fəs/ [Gk, *di*, twice, *morphe*, form], pertaining to an organism or substance that exists in two distinct forms.

**dimoxyline phosphate.** See **dioxyline phosphate.**

**dimple, 1.** a slight natural indentation or depression on a body surface, such as on the cheek. **2.** a depression on a body surface resulting from contracting scar tissue or trauma.

**dimpled sign,** a physical diagnostic test to differentiate between a benign dermatofibroma lesion and a nodular melanoma. On pressure of the examiner's thumb and index finger benign tumors dimple, but malignant growths do not.

**dimpling** [ME, *dympull*], small, abnormal indentations or depressions on the surface of a body or organ.

**dinitrochlorobenzene (DNCB)** /dīnī'trōklôr'ōben'zēn/, a substance applied topically as a test for delayed hypersensitivity reactions. The compound has also been used as an immunotherapeutic agent to treat skin tumors.

**2, 4-dinitrophenol (DNP), 1.** a dye used in biochemical research into oxidative processes. **2.** a hapten commonly used to induce immune response.

**dinucleotide,** a compound containing two nucleotides.

**dioctyl calcium sulfosuccinate, dioctyl potassium sulfosuccinate, dioctyl sodium sulfosuccinate.** See **docusate.**

**diode** /dī'od/, **1.** an electron tube or x-ray tube having a cathode and an anode. **2.** an electrical device that has a higher conductance for current flowing in one direction than for current flowing in the opposite direction.

**diode laser,** a solid-state semiconductor used as a lasering medium.

**dioecious.** See **diecious.**

**diol.** See **dihydric alcohol.**

**diolamine** /dī·ol'əmēn/, abbreviated form for *diethanolamine.*

**Dionysian** /dē·onis′ē·ən/ [Gk, *Dionysos,* Greek god of wine], the personal attitude of one who is uninhibited, mystic, sensual, emotional, and irrational and who may seek to escape from the boundaries imposed by the limits of the senses.

**diopter** /dī·op′tər/ [Gk, *dioptra,* optical measuring instrument], a metric measure of the refractive power of a lens. It is equal to the reciprocal of the focal length of the lens in meters. For example, a lens with a focal length of 0.5 m has a diopter measure of 2.0 (1/0.5) and when prescribed as a corrective lens for the eye should make printed matter most clearly focused when it is held 0.5 m from the eyes.

**dioptric power** /dī·op′trik/, the refractive power of an optic lens as measured in diopters.

**Diothane,** trademark for a local anesthetic (diperodon monohydrate).

**diovular.** See **binovular.**

**diovulatory** /dī·ov′yələtôr′ē/ [Gk, *di,* twice; L, *ovum,* egg], routinely releasing two ova during each ovarian cycle. Compare **monovulatory.**

**dioxide** /dī·ok′sīd/ [Gk, *di,* twice, *oxys,* sharp, *genein,* to produce], an oxide that contains two oxygen atoms.

**dioxin** /dī·ok′sin/, a contaminant of the herbicide 2,4,5-trichlorophenoxyacetic acid (2,4,5-T), widely used throughout the world in forestry, on grassland, against woody shrubs and trees on industrial sites, and for rice and sugarcane weed control. Because of its toxicity it is no longer manufactured in the United States. Exposure to dioxin is associated with chloracne and porphyria cutanea tarda. Dioxin was a contaminant of the jungle defoliant Agent Orange sprayed by the U.S. military aircraft over areas of Southeast Asia from 1965 to 1970. Also called **TCDD (2,3,7,8-tetrachlorodibenzoparadioxin).**

**dioxyline phosphate,** a synthetic analog of papaverine, used as a vasodilator, mainly in the treatment of vascular spasm associated with acute myocardial infarction. Also called **dimoxyline phosphate.**

**DIP,** abbreviation for **desquamative interstitial pneumonia.**

**dipeptidases** /dīpep′tidāz/, the final enzymes in the protein splitting system of digestion. They complete the task of breaking two-amino-acid dipeptides into single amino acids.

**dipeptide,** an organic compound formed by the union of two amino acids, with the link provided by the carboxyl group of one molecule and the amine group of the other.

**diphasic** /dīfā′zik/ [Gk, *di,* twice, *phasis,* appearance], pertaining to something that occurs in two stages or phases.

**diphenhydramine** /dī′fenhī′drəmēn/, an antihistamine that works both centrally and peripherally. A drug with potent anticholinergic effects, it is one of the most commonly used over-the-counter antihistamines. It is sedating.

**diphenhydramine hydrochloride,** an antihistamine.

■ INDICATIONS: It is prescribed in the treatment of hypersensitivity reactions, including rhinitis, skin rash, and pruritus, and in the treatment of motion sickness.

■ CONTRAINDICATIONS: Asthma or known hypersensitivity to this drug prohibits its use. It is not given to newborns or lactating mothers.

■ ADVERSE EFFECTS: Among the more serious adverse reactions are skin rash, hypersensitivity reactions, and tachycardia. Drowsiness and dry mouth commonly occur.

**diphenidol** /dīfē′nidol/, an antiemetic, antivertigo agent.

■ INDICATIONS: It is prescribed in the treatment of vertigo and vomiting.

■ CONTRAINDICATIONS: Anuria, nausea and vomiting as a result of pregnancy, or known sensitivity to this drug prohibits its use.

■ ADVERSE EFFECTS: Among the most serious adverse reactions are transient hypotension, hallucinations, disorientation, drowsiness, sleep disturbances, and mental confusion.

**diphenoxylate hydrochloride** /dī′fənok′silāt/, an antidiarrheal that contains atropine sulfate.

■ INDICATIONS: It is prescribed in the treatment of noninfectious diarrhea and intestinal cramping.

■ CONTRAINDICATIONS: Liver disease, antibiotic-associated diarrhea, or known hypersensitivity to this drug prohibits its use. It is not given to children less than 2 years of age.

■ ADVERSE EFFECTS: Among the more serious adverse reactions are abdominal discomfort, intestinal obstruction, skin rash, tachycardia, urinary retention, and nausea. Addiction is possible.

**diphenylhydantoin.** See **phenytoin.**

**2,3-diphosphoglycerate test,** a blood test used in the evaluation of nonspherocytic anemia.

**2,3-diphosphoglyceric acid (DPG)** /dīfos′fōgliser′ik/, a substance in the erythrocyte that affects the affinity of hemoglobin for oxygen. It is a chief end product of glucose metabolism and a link in the biochemical feedback control system that regulates the release of oxygen to the tissues.

**diphtheria** /difthir′ē·ə, dipthir′ē·ə/ [Gk, *diphthera,* leather membrane], an acute contagious disease caused by the bacterium *Corynebacterium diphtheriae.* It is characterized by the production of a systemic toxin and an adherent false membrane lining of the mucous membrane of the throat. The toxin is particularly damaging to the tissues of the heart and central nervous system, and the dense pseudomembrane in the throat may interfere with eating, drinking, and breathing. The membrane may be present in other body tissues. Lymph glands in the neck swell, and the neck becomes edematous. Untreated, the disease is often fatal from respiratory obstruction or heart and kidney failure. Patients are usually hospitalized in isolation rooms. Treatment of the isolated patient may include administration of diphtheria antitoxin, antibiotics, bed rest, fluids, and an adequate diet. Tracheostomy is sometimes necessary. Recovery is slow, but it is usually uneventful. Immunization against diphtheria is available to all children in the United States and is usually given in conjunction with pertussis and tetanus immunization early in infancy. See also **Schick test.**

**diphtheria and tetanus toxoids (DT),** an active immunizing agent.

■ INDICATIONS: It is prescribed for immunization against diphtheria and tetanus.

■ CONTRAINDICATIONS: Immunosuppression, acute infection, or concomitant use of corticosteroids prohibits its use.

■ ADVERSE EFFECTS: The most serious adverse reaction is anaphylaxis.

**diphtheria and tetanus toxoids and pertussis vaccine (DTP),** an active immunizing agent.

■ INDICATIONS: It is prescribed for the routine immunization of children less than 6 years of age against diphtheria, tetanus, and pertussis.

■ CONTRAINDICATIONS: Immunosuppressive therapy, active infection, or neurologic disorders prohibit its use.

■ ADVERSE EFFECT: The most serious adverse reaction is anaphylaxis.

**diphtheria antitoxin** [Gk, *diphtheria,* leather membrane, *anti,* against, *toxikon,* poison], an antitoxin prepared by immunizing horses with diphtheria toxoid and extracting serum from the animal. The serum is standardized for strength and quality.

**diphtherial cough** /difthir′ē·əl/, a brassy, noisy, crouplike cough accompanied by stridor, observed mainly in children with laryngeal diphtheria.

**diphtheria toxin** [Gk, *diphtheria* + *toxikon,* poison], the filtrate of a broth culture used to prepare an intradermal injectable form of toxin for Schick tests. A positive test result is characterized by an inflammatory reaction at the point of injection, whereas circulating antibodies in the blood cause a negative test result, indicating immunity.

**diphtheritic croup** /dif'thirit'ik/ [Gk, *diphtheria* + Scot, *croak,* to speak hoarsely], a diphtheritic inflammation of the larynx. Also called **laryngeal diphtheria.** See **diphtheritic laryngitis.**

**diphtheritic laryngitis** [Gk, *diphtheria, larynx, itis,* inflammation], inflammation of the larynx caused by the bacterium *Corynebacterium diphtheriae.* A serious complication is the formation of a false membrane. Also called **diphtheritic croup, laryngeal diphtheria.**

**diphtheritic membrane,** a membrane of coagulated fiber with bacteria and leukocytes. It is usually white or grayish yellow with well-defined margins.

**diphtheritic pharyngitis** [Gk, *diphtheria* + *pharynx,* throat, *itis,* inflammation], an inflammation of the pharynx caused by the bacterium *Corynebacterium diphtheriae* and associated with the formation of a false membrane.

**diphtheritic sore throat,** an inflammation of the pharynx or larynx caused by an infection of *Corynebacterium diphtheriae.*

**diphtheritic stomatitis,** an inflammation of the mucous membrane of the mouth, caused by *Corynebacterium diphtheriae.*

**diphtheroid** /dif'thəroid'/ [Gk, *diphthera,* leather membrane, *eidos,* form], **1.** pertaining to diphtheria. **2.** resembling the bacillus *Corynebacterium diphtheriae.*

**diphyllobothriasis.** See **fish tapeworm infection.**

*Diphyllobothrium* /dəfil'ōboth'rē·əm/ [Gk, *di,* twice, *phyllon,* leaf, *bothrion,* pit], a genus of large parasitic intestinal flatworms having a scolex with two slitlike grooves. The species that most often infects humans is *Diphyllobothrium latum,* a giant freshwater fish tapeworm of North America and Europe. See also **fish tapeworm infection.**

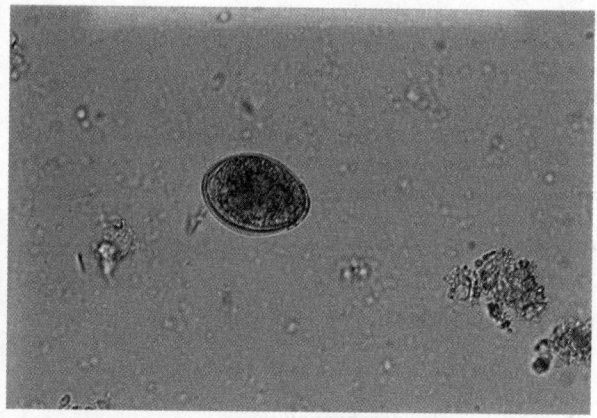

***Diphyllobothrium latum* egg** *(Mahon and Manuselis, 2000)*

*Diphyllobothrium latum.* See **tapeworm.**

**-dipine,** suffix for the name of a phenylpyridine vasodilator.

**dipivefrin** /dī'pivef'rin/, an ophthalmic sympathomimetic agent.

■ INDICATION: It is prescribed in the treatment of open-angle glaucoma.

■ CONTRAINDICATIONS: Narrow-angle glaucoma or known hypersensitivity to this drug prohibits its use.

■ ADVERSE EFFECTS: Among the most serious adverse effects are reactive hyperemia, conjunctivitis, allergic reactions, macular edema, tachycardia, arrhythmia, and hypertension.

**diplegia** /dīplē'jē·ə/ [Gk, *di,* twice, *plege,* stroke], paralysis of both sides of any body part or of like parts on the opposite sides of the body. A kind of diplegia is **facial diplegia.** Compare **hemiplegia.** —**diplegic,** *adj.*

**diplo-,** combining form meaning 'double': *diplobacilli, diplococcus, diplokaryon.*

**diplococcus** /dip'lōkok'əs/, *pl,* diplococci /-kok'sī/ [Gk, *diploos,* double, *kokkos,* berry], **1.** a member of the Coccaceae family that occurs in pairs because of incomplete cell division. Diplococci are often found as parasites or saprophytes. **2.** describing bacteria of the Coccaceae family, which occur as pairs of cocci.

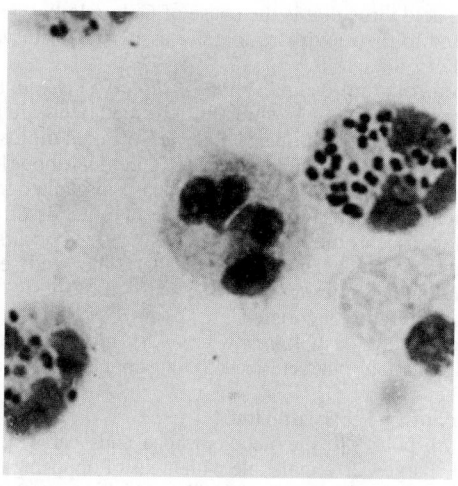

**Diplococci** *(Baron, Peterson, and Finegold, 1994)*

**diploë** /dip'lō·ē/, the loose tissue filled with red bone marrow between the two layers of the cranial bones.

**diploid** /dip'loid/ [Gk, *diploos* + *eidos,* form], having two complete sets of homologous chromosomes, such as are normally found in somatic cells and primordial germ cells before maturation. In humans the normal diploid number is 46. Also called **diploidic.** Compare **haploid, tetraploid, triploid.**

**diploid nucleus,** nucleus having two sets of chromosomes, as normally found in the somatic cells of higher organisms.

**diploidy** /dip'loidē/, the state or condition of having two complete sets of homologous chromosomes.

**diplokaryon** /dip'lōker'ē·on/ [Gk, *diploos* + *karyon,* nut], a nucleus that contains twice the diploid number of chromosomes.

**diploma program in nursing,** a basic educational program that is designed to prepare nursing students for entry into practice, usually in 2 or 3 years. The recipient of a diploma is eligible to take the national certifying registration examination to become a registered nurse. In the United States, most diploma programs are conducted in hospitals, although some are located in community colleges. In Canada diploma programs are conducted in community colleges or CEGEPS (in Quebec), as well as in a few hospital schools of nursing in the western provinces. These schools are negotiating collaboration with university schools of nursing. Many diploma programs are closing.

**diplomate** /dip'ləmāt/, an individual who has earned a diploma or certificate, especially a physician who has been certified by a specialty board. See also **board certified.**

**diplonema** /dip'lənē'mə/ [Gk, *diploos,* + *nema,* thread], the looplike formation of the chromosomes in the diplotene stage of the first meiotic prophase in gametogenesis.

**diplopagus** /diplop'əgəs/ [Gk, *diploos* + *pagos,* something fixed], conjoined twins that are more or less equally developed, although one or several internal organs may be shared.

**diplopia** /diplō'pē·ə/ [Gk, *diploos* + *opsis,* vision], double vision caused by defective function of the extraocular muscles or a disorder of the nerves that innervate the muscles. Also called **ambiopia.** Compare **binocular vision.**

**-diplopia,** suffix meaning '(condition of) double vision': *amphodiplopia, amphoterodiplopia, monodiplopia.*

**diplornavirus** /dī'plôrnəvī'rəs/, a double-stranded ribonucleic acid virus that is the cause of Colorado tick fever. It is related to the reoviruses that are associated with various respiratory infections.

**diplosomatia** /dip'lōsōmā'shə/ [Gk, *diploos* + *soma,* body], a congenital anomaly in which fully formed twins are joined at one or more areas of their bodies. Also called **diplosomia.**

**diplotene** /dip'lətēn/ [Gk, *diploos* + *tainia,* ribbon], the fourth stage in the first meiotic prophase in gametogenesis, in which chiasmata form between the chromatids of paired homologous chromosomes and crossing over occurs. The chromosomes then begin to repel each other and separate longitudinally, forming loops. See also **diakinesis, leptotene, pachytene, zygotene.**

**dipodia** /dīpō'dē·ə/ [Gk, *di,* twice, *pous,* foot], a developmental anomaly characterized by the duplication of one or both feet.

**dipolar ion.** See **zwitterion.**

**dipole** /dī'pōl/, **1.** a molecule whose ends carry opposite partial charges. **2.** a molecule with areas of opposing electrical charges, as hydrogen chloride, which has a predominance of electrons about the chloride portion and a positive charge on the hydrogen side.

**diprop,** abbreviation for a *carboxylate dipropionate anion.*

**diprosopus** /dīpros'əpəs, dī'prəsō'pəs/ [Gk, *di,* twice, *prosopon,* face], a malformed fetus that has a double face showing varying degrees of development.

**dipsesis** /dipsē'sis/, extreme thirst.

**-dipsia, -dipsy,** combining form meaning '(condition of) thirst': *hydroadipsia, oligodipsia, polydipsia.*

**dipsomania** /dip'sōmā'nē·ə/ [Gk, *dipsa,* thirst, *mania,* madness], an uncontrollable, often periodic craving for and indulgence in alcoholic beverages; alcoholism.

**dipstick,** a chemically treated strip of paper used in the analysis of urine or other fluids.

**-dipsy.** See **-dipsia.**

**dipus** /dī'pəs/, conjoined twins that have only two feet.

**dipygus** /dīpī'gəs, dip'əgəs/ [Gk, *di,* twice, *pyge,* rump], a malformed fetus that has a double pelvis, one of which is usually not fully developed.

**dipyridamole** /dī'pirid'əmōl/, an antiplatelet agent.

■ INDICATION: When used in combination with coumarin anticoagulants, it is used to prevent postoperative thromboembolic complications of cardiac valve replacement.

■ CONTRAINDICATIONS: The drug should be used with caution in hypotension.

■ ADVERSE EFFECTS: The adverse reactions are mild and transient, such as headache, dizziness, rash, nausea, and flushing.

**direct-access memory,** access to computerized data independent of previously obtained data. The data transfer occurs directly between the computer memory and peripheral devices. See also **random-access memory.**

**direct agglutination test,** a test for the presence of antibodies to a specific antigen in which a dilute antiserum is mixed with the antigen in question.

**direct antagonist** [L, *diregere,* to direct; Gk, *antagonisma,* struggle], one of a pair or a group of muscles that pull in opposite directions, whose combined action prevents the part from moving.

**direct blood donation,** the donation of a unit of blood for transfusion into a specific individual.

**direct calorimetry,** the measurement of the amount of heat directly generated by reaction. Compare **indirect calorimetry.**

**direct causal association,** a cause-and-effect relationship between a causative factor and a disease with no other factors intervening in the process.

**direct contact,** mutual touching of two individuals or organisms. Many communicable diseases may be spread by direct contact between an infected and a healthy person.

**direct Coombs' test,** a blood test performed to identify hemolysis or to investigate hemolytic transfusion reactions. This test demonstrates whether the patient's red blood cells have been attacked by antibodies in the patient's own bloodstream.

**direct costs,** in managed care the costs of labor, supplies, and equipment to provide direct patient care services.

**direct current (DC),** an electric current that flows in one direction only and is substantially constant in value. Compare **alternating current.**

**direct-exposure film,** a type of radiograph film that is directly exposed by x-rays. It is used most often in dental radiography.

**direct fracture,** any fracture occurring at a specific point of injury that is a direct result of that injury.

**direct generation.** See **asexual reproduction.**

**direct gold,** any form of pure gold that may be compacted or condensed directly into a prepared tooth cavity to form a restoration. See also **gold foil.**

**direct illumination.** See **illumination.**

**direct intervention,** hands-on therapy to increase the potential for new motor learning when there are deficits in movement and postural control.

**directional atherectomy,** atherectomy done with a directional atherectomy catheter.

**directional atherectomy catheter,** a type of atherectomy catheter whose direction can be shifted to shave off additional plaque.

**directive therapy** [L, *diregere,* to direct, *therapeia,* treatment], a psychotherapeutic approach in which the psychotherapist directs the course of therapy by intervening to ask questions and offer interpretations. Compare **nondirective therapy.** See also **psychoanalysis.**

**direct laryngoscopy** [L, *diregere,* to direct; Gk, *larynx* + *skopein,* to watch], an examination of the larynx by means of a lighted instrument inserted through the mouth.

**direct lead** /lēd/, **1.** an electrocardiographic conductor in which the exploring electrode is placed directly onto the surface of the exposed heart. **2.** *informal.* a tracing produced by such a lead on an electrocardiograph.

**direct light reflex,** the constriction of a pupil receiving increased illumination, as by a light source during an ophthalmologic examination. Also called **direct reaction to light.** Compare **consensual reaction to light.**

**direct measurement of blood pressure** [L, *diregere*, to direct, *mensura*, to measure; ME, *blod* + L, *premere*, to press], measurement of blood pressure by means of a catheter inserted into an artery. The catheter is connected to a pressure transducer.

**direct nursing care functions,** liaison nursing activities that are focused on a particular patient, a patient's family, or a group for whom the nurse is directly responsible and accountable.

**directory** /direk'tərē/, a listing of the files in a computer storage device, such as an area of a hard drive or other storage device. A device may contain many directories to facilitate organization of files.

**direct patient care,** (in nursing) care of a patient provided personally by a staff member. Direct patient care may involve any aspects of the health care of a patient, including treatments, counseling, self-care, patient education, and administration of medication.

**direct percussion.** See **percussion.**

**direct provider reimbursement,** a method of direct payment for health care services, as fee-for-service.

**direct-question interview,** an inquiry that usually requires simple one- or two-word responses.

**direct reaction to light.** See **direct light reflex.**

**direct reflex,** a response that occurs on the same side of the body as the stimulus.

**direct relationship.** See **positive relationship.**

**direct retainer,** a clasp, attachment, or assembly fastened to an abutment tooth for the purpose of maintaining a removable restoration in its planned position in relation to oral structures. See also **precision rest.**

**direct self-destructive behavior (DSDB),** any form of suicidal activity such as suicide threats, attempts, or gestures and the act of suicide itself. The person is aware that death is the desired outcome of his or her act.

**direct transfusion** [L, *dirigere*, to direct, *transfundere*, to pour through], the transfer of whole blood directly from a vein of the donor to a vein of the recipient.

**dirithromycin,** an antiinfective.

■ INDICATIONS: This drug is used to treat infections of the respiratory tract caused by *Moraxella catarrhalis, Streptococcus* sp. (*S. pneumoniae, S. agalactiae, S. viridans*), *Legionella pneumophilia, Mycoplasma pneumoniae, Streptococcus pyogenes, Staphylococcus aureus, Bordetella pertussis,* and *Propionibacterium acnes.*

■ CONTRAINDICATIONS: Factors that prohibit the use of this drug are bacteremia and known hypersensitivity to erythromycin or to dirithromycin or any other macrolide.

■ ADVERSE EFFECTS: Pseudomembranous colitis is a life-threatening effect of this drug. Other adverse effects are GI disorders, flatulence, abnormal stools, anorexia, constipation, increased platelet count, increased eosinophils, cough, dyspnea, pruritus, and urticaria. Common side effects are abdominal pain, nausea, diarrhea, vomiting, dyspepsia, headache, dizziness, and insomnia.

**dirofilariasis** /dī'rōfil'ərī'əsis/, a human infestation of the dog heartworm, *Dirofilaria immitis,* which may be transmitted through the bite of any of several species of mosquitoes. The filaria migrate through the bloodstream to the lung, producing pulmonary nodules and causing chest pain, coughing, and hemoptysis. The disease is rare among humans.

**dis-.** See **di-, dis-.**

**disability** /dis'əbil'itē/ [L, *dis,* opposite of, *habilis,* fit], the loss, absence, or impairment of physical or mental fitness. Compare **handicapped.**

**disablement model** /disā'bəlmənt/, an evaluation and treatment model based on specific impairment, functional loss, and attainable quality of life, rather than on a medical diagnosis.

**disaccharidase deficiency.** See **lactase deficiency.**

**disaccharide** /dīsak'ərīd/ [Gk, *di,* twice, *sakcharon,* sugar], a general term for simple carbohydrates formed by the union of two monosaccharide molecules.

**disadvantaged** /dis'ədvan'tijd/ [L, *dis* + *abante,* superior position], 1. any group of people who lack money, education, literacy, or another status advantage. 2. a euphemism for "poor."

**disarticulation** /dis'ärtik'yəlā'shən/ [L, *dis, articulare,* to divide into joints], separation of a joint without cutting through a bone.

**disaster** [L, *dis,* apart, *astrum.* a star], any mishap or misfortune that is ruinous, distressing, or calamitous.

**disaster-preparedness plan** [L, *dis* + *astrum,* favorable stars, *praeparare,* to prepare], a formal plan of action, usually prepared in written form, for coordinating the response of a hospital staff in the event of a disaster within the hospital or the surrounding community.

**disc.** See **disk.**

**discectomy.** See **diskectomy.**

**discharge** /dis'chärj/ [OFr, *deschargier,* to expel], 1. to release a substance or object. Also **evacuate, excrete, secrete.** 2. to release a patient from a hospital. 3. to release an electric charge, which may be manifested by a spark or surge of electricity, from a storage battery, condenser, or other source. 4. to release a burst of energy from or through a neuron. 5. a release of emotions, often accompanied by a wide range of voluntary and involuntary reflexes, weeping, rage, or other emotional displays, called **affective discharge** in psychology. 6. a substance or object discharged. 7. the flow of a secretion or an excretion.

**discharge abstract,** items of information compiled from medical records of patients discharged from a hospital, organized and recorded in a uniform format to provide data for statistical studies, reports, or research.

**discharge coordinator,** an individual who arranges with community agencies and institutions for the continuing care of patients after their discharge from a hospital or another health care facility.

**discharge planning[1],** the activities that facilitate a client's movement from one health care setting to another, or to home. It is a multidisciplinary process involving physicians, nurses, social workers, and possibly other health professionals; its goal is to enhance continuity of care.

**discharge planning[2],** a nursing intervention from the Nursing Interventions Classification (NIC) defined as preparation for moving a patient from one level of care to another within or outside the current health care agency. See also **Nursing Interventions Classification.**

**discharge summary,** a clinical report prepared by a physician or other health professional at the conclusion of a hospital stay or series of treatments. It outlines the patient's chief complaint, the diagnostic findings, the therapy administered and the patient's response to it, and recommendations on discharge.

**discharging lesion** [OFr, *deschargier* + L, *laesio,* hurting], an injury or infection of the central nervous system that causes sudden abnormal episodes of discharging nerve impulses.

**dischronation** /dis'krōnā'shən/, a disorder of time awareness. Also called **time agnosia.**

**disciform keratitis** /dis'ifôrm/ [Gk, *diskos,* flat plate; L, *forma,* form; Gk, *keras,* horn, *itis,* inflammation], an inflammatory condition of the eye that often follows an attack of dendritic keratitis; it is believed to be an immunologic response to an ocular herpes simplex infection. The condition is characterized by disclike opacities in the cornea, usually with inflammation of the iris. See also **herpes simplex.**

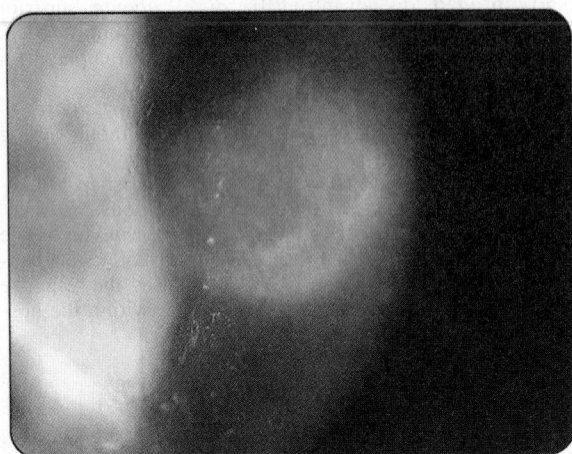

**Disciform keratitis** *(Kanski and Nischal, 1999)*

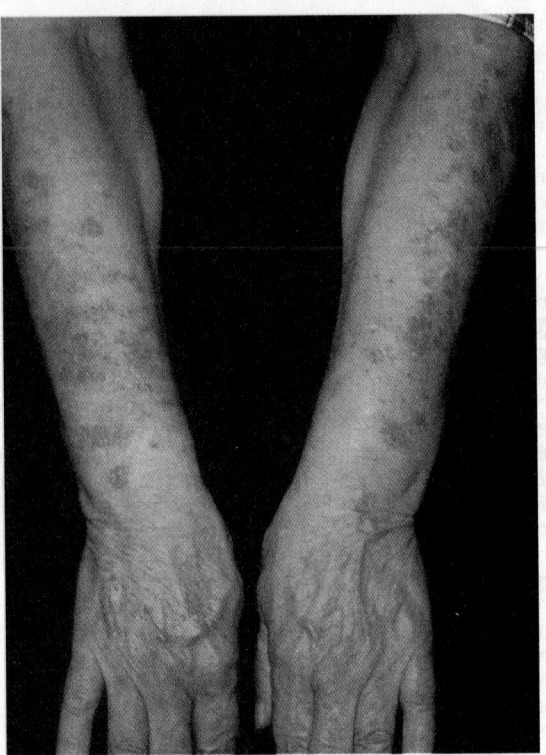

**Discoid lupus erythematosus**
*(Huether and McCance, 2000/courtesy Department of Dermatology, School of Medicine, University of Utah)*

**disclosing solution** [L, *dis* + *claudere,* to close, *solutus,* dissolved], a topically applied dye solution used to stain and reveal plaque and other deposits on teeth.

**disco-,** combining form meaning 'disk, disk-shaped': *discophorous, discopathy, discoplacenta.*

**discoblastula** /dis′kōblas′tyələ/ [Gk, *diskos,* flat plate, *blastos,* germ], a blastula formed from the partial cleavage that occurs in a fertilized ovum containing a large amount of yolk. It develops from the blastodisc and consists of a cellular cap, or blastoderm, separated from the uncleaved yolk mass by a small cavity, the blastocele.

**discocyte** /dis′kəsīt/ [Gk, *diskos* + *kytos,* cell], a mature normal erythrocyte, exhibiting one of many steady-state configurations, such as a biconcave disk without a nucleus.

**discoid** /dis′koid/ [Gk, *diskos,* flat plate, *eidos,* form], having a flat, round shape.

**discoid lupus erythematosus (DLE)** [Gk, *diskos* + *eidos,* form; L, *lupus,* wolf; Gk, *erythema,* redness, *osis,* condition], a chronic, recurrent disease, primarily of the skin, characterized by lesions that are covered with scales and extend into follicles. The lesions are typically distributed on the face but may also be present on other parts of the body. On healing the lesions often leave atrophic, hyperpigmented, or hypopigmented scars; if hairy areas are involved, alopecia may result. The cause of the disease is not established, but there is evidence that it may be an autoimmune disorder, and some cases seem to be induced by certain drugs. It is at least five times more common in women than in men and occurs most frequently in the third and fourth decades of life. Treatment includes use of a sunblock when exposure to sunlight cannot be avoided, application of steroids to the lesions, and use of systemic antimalarial drugs such as hydroxychloroquine; systemic corticosteroid agents may be used in severe cases. Also called **cutaneous lupus erythematosus.** See also **systemic lupus erythematosus.**

**discoid meniscus,** an abnormal condition characterized by a discoid rather than a semilunar shape of the cartilaginous meniscus of the knee. The lateral meniscus is usually affected, although the medial meniscus may also become involved. The condition is a developmental anomaly that is asymptomatic in infants and young children; it appears most often between 6 and 8 years of age. Common complaints are that the knee joint clicks or gives way. These characteristics are often but not always associated with an injury to the knee. Examination demonstrates the clicking, usually during the last 15 to 20 degrees, when the knee is moved from flexion to extension. Surgical excision of the meniscus is seldom warranted in treating this benign condition.

**discoid placenta** [Gk, *diskos,* quoit, *eidos,* form; L, *placenta,* flat cake], a round placenta.

**disconfirmation** /diskon′fərmā′shən/, a dysfunctional communication that negates, discounts, or ignores information received from another person.

**discordance** /diskôr′dəns/ [L, *discordare,* to disagree], the expression of one or more specific traits in only one member of a pair of twins. Compare **concordance. —discordant,** *adj.*

**discordant twins,** twins showing a marked difference in size (greater than 10% in weight) at birth. The condition is usually caused by overperfusion of one twin and underperfusion of the other. It is fairly common in identical twins but may also occur in dizygotic twins.

**discovery** /diskov′ərē/ [L, *dis* + *coopiere,* to cover], (in law) a pretrial procedure that allows one party to examine vital witnesses and documents held exclusively by the ad-

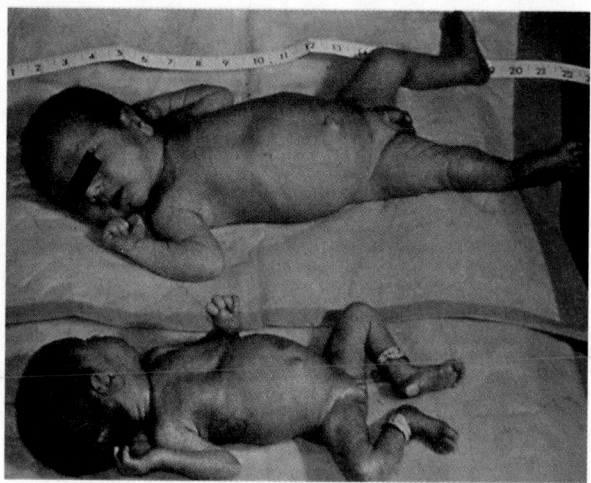

**Discordant twins** *(Zitelli and Davis, 1997)*

verse party. Discovery is limited to materials, facts, and other resources that could not otherwise be reasonably expected to be discovered and that are necessary to the preparation of the case for trial. Also called **pretrial discovery.** Compare **deposition, interrogatories.**

**discrete** /diskrēt′/ [L, *discretus,* separated], **1.** individually distinct. **2.** composed of distinct parts.

**discrete x-rays.** See **x-ray.**

**discrimination** /diskrim′inā′shən/ [L, *discrimen,* division], the act of distinguishing or differentiating. The ability to distinguish between touch or pressure at two nearby points on the body is known as two-point discrimination.

**discriminator** /diskrim′inā′tər/, an electronic device capable of accepting or rejecting a pulse of energy on the basis of the pulse's amplitude. It is used to separate low-energy from high-energy radionuclides.

**discus.** See **disk.**

**discus articularis** /dis′kəs/, a small oval plate between the condyle of the mandible and the mandibular fossa. Displacement of or injury to the plate may be a cause of temporomandibular joint (TMJ) pain.

**discus interpubicus.** See **interpubic disk.**

**discus nervi optici.** See **optic disc.**

**disease** [L, *dis* + Fr, *aise,* ease], **1.** a condition of abnormal vital function involving any structure, part, or system of an organism. **2.** a specific illness or disorder characterized by a recognizable set of signs and symptoms, attributable to heredity, infection, diet, or environment. Compare **condition, diathesis.**

**disease prevention,** activities designed to protect patients or other members of the public from actual or potential health threats and their harmful consequences.

**disengagement** /dis′engāj′mənt/ [Fr, *disengager,* to release from engagement], **1.** an obstetric manipulation in which the presenting part of the baby is dislodged from the maternal pelvis as part of an operative delivery. See also **Kielland's rotation, version and extraction. 2.** the release or detachment of oneself from other persons or responsibilities. **3.** (in transactional family therapy) a role assumed by a nurse or other therapist in observing and restructuring intervention without becoming actively and directly involved in the problem.

**disengagement theory,** the psychosocial concept that normally aging individuals and society mutually withdraw from normal interaction. The theory also assumes that older adults are a homogenous group whose members prefer the company of others of their own age. See also **activity theory.**

**disequilibrium** /disē′kwilib′rē·əm/ [L, *dis,* apart, *aequilibrium*], the loss of balance or adjustment, particularly mental or psychologic balance.

**dishpan fracture** [AS, *disc,* plate; L, *patina,* dish; *fractura,* break], a fracture that depresses the skull. Also called **derby hat fracture.**

**disinfect** /dis′infekt′/ [L, *dis,* apart, *inficere,* to infect], to eliminate many or all pathogenic microorganisms with the exception of bacterial spores.

**disinfectant** /dis′infek′tənt/, a liquid chemical that can be applied to objects to eliminate many or all pathogenic microorganisms with the exception of bacterial spores.

**disinfection** /dis′infek′shən/, the process of killing pathogenic organisms or rendering them inert.

**disinfestation** /dis′infestā′shən/ [L, *dis,* apart, *infestare,* to infest], elimination of a threat of infestation by vermin, rodents, lice, or other noxious organisms.

**disinhibition** /dis′inhibish′ən/ [L, *dis,* apart, *inhibere,* to restrain], the removal of inhibition. See **inhibition.**

**disintegrative psychosis** /disin′təgrā′tiv/, a mental disorder of childhood that usually has an onset after 3 years of age and after normal development of speech, social behavior, and other traits. After a vague illness the child becomes irritable and undergoes mental deterioration, eventually reaching a stage of severe mental retardation. The cause may be a viral infection. There is no specific treatment.

**disjunction** /disjungk′shən/ [L, *disjungere,* to disjoint], the separation of paired homologous chromosomes during anaphase of the first meiotic division, or the separation of the chromatids of a chromosome during anaphase of mitosis and the second meiotic division. Compare **nondisjunction.**

**disk** [Gk, *diskos,* flat plate], **1.** a flat, circular platelike structure, as an articular disk or an optic disc. Also spelled (chiefly in ophthalmology) **disc. 2.** *informal.* an intervertebral disk. Also called *(Latin)* **discus.**

**disk drive,** a computer device containing a disk that spins at high speeds that allows magnetic impulses to be written onto and read from the electromagnetic surface. Most computers contain a hard disk drive, a compact disk–read only memory (CD-ROM) drive, and one or more diskette drives.

**diskectomy** /dis·kek′tə·me/ [Gk, *diskos,* flat plate + *ektome,* incision], excision of an intervertebral disk. Also called **discectomy.**

**diskette,** a semiflexible plastic, oxide-coated disk contained in a special flat plastic box or jacket that is used in a computer disk drive. Diskettes for most personal computers are 3-1/2 inches in diameter.

**diskography** /diskog′rəfē/, the radiographic examination of individual intervertebral disks after introduction of a radiopaque contrast medium into the center of the disk. It is used in the investigation of ruptured disks but has largely been replaced by MRI and CT myelography.

**dislocation** /dis′lōkā′shən/ [L, *dis* + *locare,* to place], the displacement of any part of the body from its normal position, particularly a bone from its normal articulation with a joint. See also **subluxation. —dislocate,** *v.*

**dislocation fracture,** a fracture of the bony components of a joint associated with a displacement of a bone from its normal articulation with the joint.

**dislocation of clavicle** [L, *dis,* apart, *locare,* to place, *clavicula,* little key], displacement of the collarbone. It may occur either at the sternal end or at the acromial or scapular extremity.

**dislocation of finger** [L, *dis*, apart, *locare*, to place; AS, *finger*], displacement of a finger at a joint, as a result of trauma. In the absence of an accompanying fracture the dislocated finger can usually be reduced by steadying the hand at the wrist and maneuvering the dislocated bone back into place. After reduction, a splint is applied from the fingertip to the palm of the hand, and an x-ray film is obtained.

**dislocation of hip** [L, *dis*, apart, *locare*, to place; AS, *hype*], displacement of the femoral head out of the hip joint, usually accompanied by pain, edema, rigidity, shortening of the leg, and loss of function. It may be congenital or acquired. Types of hip dislocation include **obturator dislocation,** in which the femoral head lies in the obturator foramen; **perineal dislocation,** in which the femoral head is displaced into the perineum; **sciatic dislocation,** in which the femoral head lies in the sciatic notch; or **subpubic dislocation,** in which the femoral head is displaced anteriorly.

**dislocation of jaw** [L, *dis,* apart, *locare,* to place; ME, *jowe*], unilateral or bilateral displacement of the mandible, typically as a result of a blow, a fall, or yawning. The mandible is fixed in an open position with only the back teeth in contact. If the mandible appears deviated to one side, the dislocation involves only one side. The dislocation is reduced manually, with or without injection of a local anesthetic.

**dislocation of knee** [L, *dis,* apart, *locare,* to place; AS, *cneow*], displacement of one of the bones of the knee joint. First aid treatment for the dislocation is the same as for a fracture: the joint is immobilized with splints, and the patient is moved quickly to a health care facility.

**dislocation of shoulder** [L, *dis* + *locare* + AS, *sculder*], any of several kinds of displacement of the bones of the shoulder joint, including acromial joint disruption and separation and dislocation of the glenohumeral joint with the humeral head displaced anteriorly and inferiorly.

**dislocation of toe,** displacement of a metatarsal bone at a joint.

**dismiss** [L, *dis* + *mittere*, to send], (in law) to discharge or dispose of an action, suit, or motion trial. **—dismissal,** *n.*

**disobliterative endarterectomy.** See **endarterectomy.**

**disodium edetate.** See **edetate disodium.**

**Disophrol,** trademark for a fixed-combination respiratory drug containing an antihistamine (dexbrompheniramine maleate) and an adrenergic bronchodilator (pseudoephedrine sulfate).

**disopyramide phosphate** /dī′sōpir′əmīd/, a cardiac antiarrhythmic.

■ INDICATIONS: It is prescribed in the treatment of documented ventricular arrhythmias considered to be life-threatening.

■ CONTRAINDICATIONS: Cardiogenic shock, heart failure, pre-existing second- or third-degree heart block in the absence of a pacemaker, sick sinus syndrome, or known hypersensitivity to this drug prohibits its use.

■ ADVERSE EFFECTS: Among the more serious adverse reactions are severe hypotension, precipitation of heart failure, and aggravation of heart block. Urinary retention, dry mouth, and constipation commonly occur.

**disorder** [L, *dis*, apart, *ordo*, rank], a disruption of or interference with normal functions or established systems, as a mental disorder or nutritional disorder.

**disordered metabolism,** changes in metabolism that result from disease and medications administered to control diseases. Acquired immunodeficiency syndrome patients, for example, may experience severe malnutrition, wasting, weight loss, hypermetabolism, and altered energy metabolism. Human immunodeficiency virus causes blunting of intestinal villi and secretion of abnormal intestinal enzymes, resulting in severe diarrhea and malabsorption.

**disorder of movement** [L, *dis*, apart, *ordo*, rank, *movere*, to move], any perverse or abnormal function of muscular action that may result from infection, injury, or congenital disability, such as ataxia, involuntary grimacing, and chorea.

**disorder of sleep** [L, *dis* + *ordo* + AS, *slaep*], any condition that interferes with normal sleep patterns, such as sleep apnea, phase shift, use of alcohol and certain drugs, excessive sleepiness, sleep walking, nightmares, sleep paralysis, and narcolepsy. Treatment may include medications, relaxation, avoidance of stimulants, and referral to sleep disorder clinics.

**disorder of written expression,** a learning disorder in which the affected skill is written communication, characterized by errors in spelling, grammar, or punctuation, by poor paragraph organization, or by poor story composition or thematic development.

**disorganized schizophrenia** /disôr′gənīzd/ [L, *dis* + Gk, *organon*, organ], a subtype of schizophrenia characterized by an earlier age of onset, usually at puberty, and a more severe disintegration of the personality than occurs in other forms of the disease. The essential features include incoherence, loose associations, gross disorganization of behavior, and flat or inappropriate affect. See also **schizophrenia.**

**disorient** /disôr′ē·ənt/, to cause to lose awareness or perception of space, time, or personal identity and relationships.

**disorientation** /-ā′shən/ [L, *dis* + *orienter*, to proceed from], a state of mental confusion characterized by inadequate or incorrect perceptions of place, time, or identity. Disorientation may occur in organic mental disorders, in drug and alcohol intoxication, and, less commonly, after severe stress.

**disparate twins** /dis′pərāt, disper′it/, twins who are distinctly different from each other in weight and other features.

**dispense** /dispens′/ [L, *dis*, apart, *pensare*, to weigh], to prepare and issue drugs or drug mixtures from a pharmaceutical outlet or department.

**disperse** /dis·pers′/ [L, *dis* + *spargere* to scatter], to scatter the component parts, as of a tumor or of the fine particles in a colloid system; also the particles so scattered.

**dispersing agent** /dispur′sing/ [L, *dis* + *spargere*, to scatter, *agere*, to do], a chemical additive used in pharmaceutics to cause the even distribution of the ingredients throughout the product, such as in dermatologic emulsions containing both oil and water. Dispersing agents commonly used in skin creams, lotions, and ointments include glyceryl monostearate, sodium lauryl sulfate, and polyethylene glycol derivatives. A dispersing agent may cause an allergic reaction or adverse effect in a hypersensitive person.

**dispersion** /dispur′shən/, the scattering or dissipation of finely divided material, as when particles of a substance are scattered throughout the volume of a fluid. Examples include colloids and gels, such as egg white, soap, and gelatin, which consist of large molecules or clumps of molecules that are able to attract and hold large numbers of water molecules.

**dispersion forces.** See **van der Waals forces.**

**dispersion medium.** See **continuous phase.** See also **medium.**

**displaced fracture** /displāst/ [Fr, *deplacement*, to remove], a traumatic bone break in which two ends of a fractured bone are separated and out of their normal positions. The ends may pierce surrounding skin, as in a compound fracture, or may be contained within the skin, as in a closed fracture.

**100% displaced fracture.** See **complete fracture.**

**displaced testis** [Fr, *deplacement* + L, *testis,* testicle], a testis that is located in the pelvis, inguinal canal, or elsewhere after it normally would have descended into the scrotum.

**displacement** /displās'mənt/ [Fr, *deplacement,* to remove], **1.** the state of being displaced or the act of displacing. **2.** (in chemistry) a reaction in which an atom, molecule, or radical is removed from combination and replaced by another. **3.** (in physics) the displacing in space of one mass by another, as when the weight or volume of a fluid is displaced by a floating or submerged body. **4.** (in psychiatry) an unconscious defense mechanism for avoiding emotional conflict and anxiety by transferring emotions, ideas, or wishes from one object to a substitute that is less anxiety-producing. Compare **sublimation.** See also **percolation.**

**displacement chromatography.** See **chromatography.**

**DISS,** abbreviation for **Diameter-Index Safety System.**

**dissect** /disekt'/ [L, *dissecare,* to cut apart], to cut apart tissues for visual or microscopic study using a scalpel, a probe, or scissors. Compare **bisect. —dissection,** *n.*

**dissecting aneurysm** [L, *dissecare,* to cut apart; Gk, *aneurysma,* a widening], a localized dilation of an artery, most commonly the aorta, characterized by a longitudinal separation of the outer and middle layers of the vascular wall. Aortic dissecting aneurysms occur most frequently in men between 40 and 60 years of age and are preceded by hypertension in more than 90% of cases. Blood entering a tear in the intimal lining of the vessel causes a separation of weakened elastic and fibromuscular elements in the medial layer and leads to the formation of cystic spaces filled with matrix. Dissecting aneurysms in the thoracic aorta may extend into blood vessels of the neck. Rupture of a dissecting aneurysm may be fatal in less than 1 hour. Treatment consists of resection and replacement of the excised section of aorta with a synthetic prosthesis. See also **aortic aneurysm.**

**dissection.** See **dissect.**

**disseminated** /disem'inā'tid/, dispersed or spread throughout, as in an organ or the whole body.

**disseminated intravascular coagulation (DIC)** [L, *dis* + *seminare,* to sow, *intra,* within, *vasculum,* little vessel, *coagulare,* to curdle], a grave coagulopathy resulting from the overstimulation of clotting and anticlotting processes in response to disease or injury, such as septicemia, acute hypotension, poisonous snakebites, neoplasms, obstetric emergencies, severe trauma, extensive surgery, and hemorrhage. The primary disorder initiates generalized intravascular clotting, which in turn overstimulates fibrinolytic mechanisms; as a result the initial hypercoagulability is succeeded by a deficiency in clotting factors with hypocoagulability and hemorrhaging. Diagnosis is based on the presence of degradation products. Also called **consumption coagulopathy, defibrination syndrome.**

■ OBSERVATIONS: Purpura on the lower extremities and abdomen, reflecting fibrin deposits in capillaries, is a common first sign of DIC. Hemorrhagic bullae, acral cyanosis, and focal gangrene in the skin and mucous membranes may follow. Hemorrhages from incisions, catheter or injection sites, GI bleeding, hematuria, pulmonary edema, pulmonary embolism, progressive hypotension, tachycardia, absence of peripheral pulses, restlessness, convulsions, or coma may occur. Laboratory studies generally show a marked deficiency of blood platelets, low levels of fibrinogen and other clotting factors, prolonged prothrombin and partial throm-

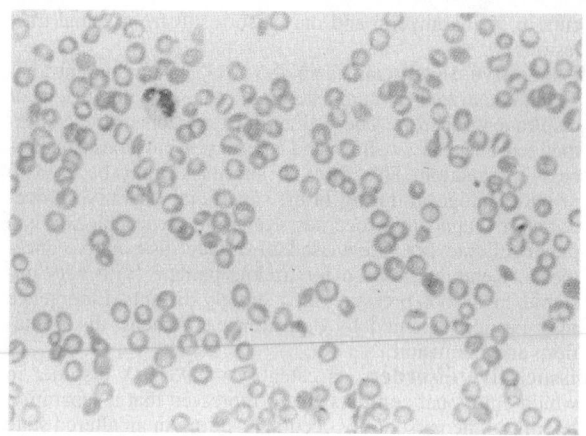

**Disseminated intravascular coagulation**
*(Zitelli and Davis, 1997)*

boplastin times, and abnormal erythrocyte morphologic characteristics.

■ INTERVENTIONS: Treatment of the primary disorder is essential in the management of DIC or patients actively bleeding into a closed space, for example the head or the chest. Use of heparin is controversial; it may be infused intravenously to prevent clot formation but may increase bleeding. Heparin is not always used for surgical patients with DIC or patients actively bleeding into a closed space, for example the head or the chest. Transfusions of whole blood, plasma, platelets, cryoprecipitate, and other blood products are administered to replace depleted factors. Patients are maintained in a quiet, nonstressful environment and are protected from trauma and bleeding. The side rails of the bed are padded. Foam or cotton swabs are used for mouth care.

■ NURSING CONSIDERATIONS: The care of a patient with life-threatening DIC requires monitoring of vital signs, observation for evidence of bleeding, extremely gentle handling, maintenance of a safe environment, and emotional support.

**disseminated lupus erythematosus.** See **systemic lupus erythematosus.**

**disseminated multiple sclerosis.** See **multiple sclerosis.**

**disseminated myelitis,** an inflammation of the spinal cord. Also called **diffuse myelitis.**

**disseminated neuritis,** inflammation of peripheral nerves, with pain, tenderness, and loss of function. Lesions may affect the parenchyma of peripheral sensory and motor tracts. The condition may be caused by alcohol, infectious agents, or exposure to heavy metals.

**dissent** /disent'/ [L, *dis* + *sentire,* to feel], **1.** to differ in belief or opinion; disagree. **2.** (in law) a statement written by a judge who disagrees with the decision of the majority of the court. The dissent states explicit reasons for the contrary opinion. **—dissenting,** *adj.*

**dissimilar twins.** See **dizygotic twins.**

**dissociation** /disō'shē·ā'shən/ [L, *dis* + *sociare,* to unite], **1.** the act of separating into parts or sections. **2.** an unconscious defense mechanism by which an idea, thought, emotion, or other mental process is separated from the consciousness and thereby loses emotional significance. See **dissociative disorder. —dissociative** /disō'shē·ətiv/, *adj.*

**dissociation syndrome,** a loss of the ability to sense painful and thermal stimuli, while retaining the sense of touch, tactile discrimination, and position sense. The disorder occurs in syringomyelia and may also result from spinal tract lesions.

**dissociative anesthesia** /disō'shē·ətiv/, a unique anesthesia characterized by analgesia and amnesia without loss of respiratory function. The patient does not appear to be anesthetized and can swallow and open eyes but does not process information. This form of anesthesia may be used to provide analgesia during brief, superficial operative procedures or diagnostic processes. Ketamine hydrochloride is a phencyclidine derivative used to induce dissociative anesthesia. Ketamine is used for trauma patients with very unstable, low blood pressure or for elderly patients. Emergence may be accompanied by delirium, excitement, disorientation, and confusion.

**dissociative disorder,** a category of *DSM-IV* disorder in which emotional conflicts are so repressed that a separation or split in the personality occurs, resulting in an altered state of consciousness or a confusion in identity. Symptoms may include amnesia, somnambulism, fugue, dream state, and dissociative identity disorder. It is caused by an inability to cope with severe stress or conflict and usually occurs suddenly, after a situation catastrophic to the person. Treatment may include hypnosis, especially when amnesia is the primary symptom; psychotherapy; and use of antianxiety medication. Also called **dissociative reaction.** Compare **conversion disorder.** See also **dissociation.**

**dissociative identity disorder,** a psychiatric disorder characterized by the existence of two or more distinct, clearly differentiated personality structures within the same individual, any of which may dominate at a particular time. Each personality is a complex unit with separate well-developed emotional and thought processes, behavior patterns, and social relationships. The various subpersonalities are usually dramatically different and may or may not be aware of the existence of the others. Formerly called **multiple personality disorder.**

**dissociative reaction.** See **dissociative disorder.**

**dissolution** /dis'əloo'shən/ [L, *dis + solvere,* to loosen], **1.** the separation of a complex chemical compound into simpler molecules. **2.** the dissolving of chemical substances into a homogenous solution. **3.** the loss of mental powers.

**dissolve,** to disperse the molecules or ions of one substance throughout the bulk of another substance.

**dissolved gas** /disolvd'/ [L, *dis + solvere,* to loosen], gas in a simple physical solution, as distinguished from gas that has reacted chemically with a solvent or other solutes and is chemically combined.

**dissonance,** the interference between sound waves of a different pitches.

**distal** /dis'təl/ [L, *distare,* to be distant], **1.** away from or the farthest from a point of origin or attachment. **2.** away from or the farthest from the midline or a central point, as a distal phalanx. Compare **proximal.**

**distal acinar emphysema,** one of the principal types of emphysema, limited to the distal ends of the alveoli along the interlobular septa and beneath the pleura, forming bullae (see also **bullous emphysema**). Also called **interlobular emphysema** and **paraseptal emphysema.**

**distal convoluted tubule.** See **distal tubule.**

**distal latency,** (in electroneuromyography) the interval between the stimulation of a compound muscle and the observed response. Normal nerve conduction velocity is above 40 m/sec in the lower extremities and above 50 m/sec in the upper extremities, but age, muscle disease, temperature, and other factors can influence the velocity.

**distal muscular dystrophy,** a rare form of muscular dystrophy that usually affects adults. It is characterized by moderate weakness and by wasting that begins in the arms and legs and then extends gradually to the proximal and facial muscles. Also called **Gowers' muscular dystrophy.**

**distal phalanx,** any one of the small distal bones in the third row of phalanges of the hand or the foot (second phalanx in the thumb and great toe). Each one at the end of the finger has a convex dorsal surface and a flat palmar surface, with a rough elevation at the end of the palmar surface that supports a fingernail and its sensitive pulp. The distal phalanx of each of the toes is smaller and more flattened than that of a finger; it also has a rough elevation to support the toenail and its pulp. Also called **ungual phalanx.**

**distal radioulnar articulation,** the pivotlike articulation of the head of the ulna and the ulnar notch on the lower end of the radius, involving two ligaments. The joint allows rotation of the distal end of the radius around an axis that passes through the center of the head of the ulna. Also called **inferior radioulnar joint.** Compare **proximal radioulnar articulation.**

**distal renal tubular acidosis (distal RTA),** an abnormal condition characterized by excessive acid accumulation and bicarbonate excretion. It is caused by the inability of the kidney's distal tubules to secrete hydrogen ions, thus decreasing the excretion of titratable acids and ammonium and increasing the urinary loss of potassium and bicarbonate. The condition may cause hypercalciuria and the formation of kidney stones. Treatment is the same as for renal tubular acidosis. **Primary distal RTA** occurs mostly in females, adolescents, older children, and young adults. It may occur sporadically or result from hereditary defects. **Secondary distal RTA** is associated with numerous disorders, such as cirrhosis of the liver, malnutrition, starvation, and various genetic abnormalities. Compare **proximal renal tubular acidosis.**

**distal sparing,** a condition in which the spinal cord remains intact below a lesion. The reflex arc remains but is not modified by supraspinal influences. As a result, spastic movements may occur distal to the level of the lesion.

**distal tubule,** the portion of the nephron lying between the descending Henle's loop and the collecting duct in the kidney. Also called **distal convoluted tubule.**

**distance regulation** [L, *distantia + regula,* rule], behavior that is related to the control of personal space. Most humans establish a quantum of space between themselves and others that offers security from either psychologic or physical threat while not creating a feeling of isolation. The amount of social distance thus maintained varies with different individuals and in different cultures. A wild animal generally maintains a flight distance, the minimum it will allow between itself and a potential enemy before fleeing. Animals of the same species also maintain a personal distance from each other.

**distance vision,** the ability to see objects clearly from a distance, usually from 20 feet or 6 m or more.

**distemper** /distem'pər/ [L, *dis,* apart, *temperare,* to regulate], **1.** any mental or physical disorder or indisposition. **2.** a potentially fatal viral disease of animals, characterized by rhinitis, fever, and a loss of appetite.

**distend** /distend'/ [L, *distendere,* to stretch], to enlarge or dilate something.

**distensibility** /disten'sibil'itē/ [L, *distendere,* to stretch], the ability of something to become stretched, dilated, or enlarged.

**distension** /disten'shən/, the state of being distended or swollen.

**distillate** /distil'it/ [L, *distillare,* to drop down], the liquid vaporized, condensed, and collected in a distillation.

**distillation** /dis'tilā'shən/ [L, *distillare*, to drop down], the process of vaporization followed by condensation in another part of the system.

**distilled water** /distild'/ [L, *distillare*, to drop down; AS, *waeter*], water that has been purified by being heated to a vapor form and then condensed into another container as liquid water free of nonvolatile solutes.

**distoclusion** /dis'tə·klōō'zhən/ [L, *distare*, to be distant + *occludere*, to close up], malocclusion in which the mandibular arch is in a posterior position in relation to the maxillary arch. Generally considered as identical with Class II in Angle's classification of malocclusion. Also called **distoocclusion, posterior occlusion.** See also **Angle's Classification of Malocclusion.**

**distogingival** /dis'tōjinjī'vəl/, pertaining to the surfaces of a tooth nearest the gum and the back of the mouth.

**distolabial** /dis'tōlā'bē·əl/, pertaining to the surfaces of a tooth nearest the lips and back of the mouth.

**disto-occlusion.** See **distoclusion.**

**distorted thought control,** a nursing outcome from the Nursing Outcomes Classification (NOC) defined as self-restraint of disruption in perception, thought processes, and thought content. See also **Nursing Outcomes Classification.**

**distortion** /distôr'shən/ [L, *dis* + *torquere*, to twist], **1.** (in psychology) the process of shifting experience in one's perceptions. Distortions represent personal constructs of truth, validity, and right and wrong. The distortions of patients tend to influence their views of the world and themselves, as by altering a negative perception to one more favorable. **2.** (in radiology) radiographic image artifacts that may be caused by variations in the size and shape or position of the object. Thick or curved objects cause greater distortion than thin, flat objects because of unequal magnification.

**distoversion** /dis'tō·vər'zhən/ [L, *distare*, to be distant + *vertere*, to turn], the position of a tooth which is farther than normal from the median line of the face along the dental arch.

**distractibility** /distrak'tibil'itē/ [L, *dis* + *trahere*, to draw apart], a mental state in which attention does not remain fixed on any one subject but wavers or wanders.

**distraction**[1] /distrak'shən/ [L, *dis* + *trahere*, to draw apart], **1.** a procedure that prevents or lessens the perception of pain by focusing attention on sensations unrelated to pain. **2.** a method of straightening a spinal column by the forces of axial tension pulling on the joint surfaces, such as applied by a Milwaukee brace.

**distraction**[2], a nursing intervention from the Nursing Interventions Classification (NIC) defined as purposeful focusing of attention away from undesirable sensations. See also **Nursing Interventions Classification.**

**distraught** /distrôt'/ [OFr, *destrait*, inattentive], pertaining to a mental state of confusion, distraction, or absentmindedness.

**distress** /distres'/ [ME, *distressen*, to cause sorrow], an emotional or physical state of pain, sorrow, misery, suffering, or discomfort.

**distress of the human spirit.** See **spiritual distress.**

**distributed processing** /distrib'yətid/ [L, *distribuere*, to distribute], a combination of local and remote computer terminals in a network connected to a central computer to divide the workload.

**distributing artery,** an artery with a tunica media composed of circularly arranged smooth muscle. It receives blood from conducting arteries and distributes the blood to organs and tissues. Also called **muscular artery.**

**distribution,** the location of medications in various organs and tissues after administration. The concentration of highly water-soluble drugs may be greater in persons who are elderly, dehydrated, or febrile because they have less total body water for dilution of the substance. As the lean muscle mass decreases and body fat increases, drugs that are distributed primarily in body fat have a more prolonged effect.

**distributive analysis and synthesis** /distrib'yətiv/, the system of psychotherapy used by the psychobiologic school of psychiatry. It involves an extensive and systematic investigation and analysis of a person's total past experiences to discover the emotional factors underlying personality problems and ways they can be synthesized into constructive behavioral patterns.

**distributive care,** a pattern of health care that is concerned with environment, heredity, living conditions, lifestyle, and early detection of pathologic effects. The system is usually directed to continuous care of persons not confined to hospitals or other health care facilities.

**district** [L, *distringere*, to compel], **1.** (in hospital nursing) a group of patients in an area of the unit, usually a subdivision of a ward, for whom a nurse manager or primary nurse is responsible. Patients are customarily assigned to a district on the basis of certain shared needs for nursing care. **2.** the area of a city or town assigned to a public health nurse.

**district nurse.** See **public health nursing.**

**disulfiram** /dīsul'firam/, an alcohol-use deterrent.

■ INDICATIONS: It is prescribed as a deterrent to drinking alcohol in the treatment of chronic alcoholism. It causes severe intestinal cramping, diaphoresis, and nausea and vomiting if alcohol is ingested. It requires that the patient explicitly know that, when combined with alcohol intake, death may occur.

■ CONTRAINDICATIONS: Alcoholic intoxication; recent or concomitant administration of metronidazole, paraldehyde, or alcohol; severe myocardial disease; coronary occlusion; psychosis; or known hypersensitivity to this drug prohibits its use.

■ ADVERSE EFFECTS: The most serious adverse reactions, which include optic neuritis, psychotic reaction, and polyneuritis, result from alcohol ingestion. Drowsiness, headache, and skin rash may occur. This drug interacts with several other drugs, such as metronidazole and warfarin.

**disuse phenomena** /disyōōs'/ [L, *dis* + *usus*, to make use of; Gk, *phainein*, to show], the physical and psychologic changes, usually degenerative, that result from the lack of use of a body part or system. Disuse phenomena are associated with confinement and immobility, especially in orthopedics. Individuals treated for fractures and other orthopedic disorders must often be immobilized in traction for long periods. They are often deprived of sufficient interaction with the world around them and lose motivation, expectation, and even acquired abilities because of lack of practice. This disorientation is compounded by pain and therapeutic narcotic drugs commonly associated with the treatment of many illnesses and abnormal conditions. The physical changes often induced by continued bed rest constitute problems that affect many key areas and systems of the body, such as the skin, the musculoskeletal system, the GI tract, the cardiovascular system, and the respiratory system. Prolonged bed rest commonly subjects the patient's skin to abnormal pressure, moisture, and friction. Pressure exerted on the skin by the bed is slightly higher than capillary hydrostatic pressure and may cause collapse of the superficial capillaries and lead to ischemia and eventual tissue necrosis. A burning pain or absence of feeling may be the first sign of ischemia, followed by a rapid breakdown of the skin. Some indications of skin ischemia are redness, pain, edema, and skin breakdown. Unused muscles lose size and strength, often wasting until they are unable to perform their functions of support and contraction. Contractures are usually caused by flexion, because patients flex knees and hips whenever possible to relax muscles, especially when cold or in pain. The immobilized patient may experience bone demineralization caused by a restricted diet and decreased motility. Calcium and phosphorus are dependent on vitamin D for absorption from the gut and movement into the bones, and some nutrition experts describe calcium loss as a natural disuse phenomenon of bed rest. Muscle action is required to maintain blood flow to the bones, and the immobilized patient may not be capable of sufficient muscular activity to assure such blood flow, with its attendant delivery of critical nutrients and oxygen. The pooling of respiratory secretions is another disuse phenomenon caused by immobility and the horizontal position of the bed-rest patient. Some common therapeutic measures to deal with disuse phenomena are improvement of diet and nutrition, proper positioning and regular movement of the patient, meticulous hygiene, scrupulous skin care, and positive social interaction with the patient. See also **hypostatic pneumonia.**

**disuse syndrome.** In nursing, **disuse syndrome** is a term that encompasses similar concepts and includes nursing diagnoses related to inactivity. Risks for disuse syndrome include impaired skin integrity, constipation, altered respiratory function, altered peripheral tissue perfusion, activity intolerance, impaired physical mobility, injury, altered sensory perception, powerlessness, and body image disturbance.

**disuse syndrome, risk for,** a nursing diagnosis accepted by the Eighth National Conference on the Classification of Nursing Diagnoses. Risk for disuse syndrome is a state characterized by potential for deterioration of body systems as the result of prescribed or unavoidable inactivity.
■ RISK FACTORS: Risk factors include paralysis, mechanical immobilization, prescribed immobilization, severe pain, and altered level of consciousness. See also **nursing diagnosis.**

**Ditropan,** trademark for an antispasmodic (oxybutynin chloride).

**Diucardin,** trademark for an antihypertensive and diuretic (hydroflumethiazide).

**Diupres,** trademark for a fixed-combination drug containing a diuretic (chlorothiazide) and an antihypertensive (reserpine).

**diurese** /dī′yŏorēs/, the act of effecting diuresis.

**diuresis** /dī′yŏorē′sis/ [Gk, *dia,* through, *ouron,* urine], increased formation and secretion of urine. Diuresis occurs in conditions such as diabetes mellitus, diabetes insipidus, and acute renal failure. It is normal in the first 48 hours after giving birth. Coffee, tea, certain foods, diuretic drugs, anxiety, fear, and some steroids cause diuresis. Water is considered the least expensive diuretic.

**diuretic** /dī′yŏoret′ik/, **1.** (of a drug or other substance) tending to promote the formation and excretion of urine. **2.** a drug that promotes the formation and excretion of urine. The more than 50 diuretic drugs available in the United States and Canada are classified by chemical structure and pharmacologic activity into groups: aldosterone antagonists, carbonic anhydrase inhibitors, loop diuretics, mercurials, osmotics, potassium-sparing diuretics, and thiazides. A diuretic medication may contain drugs from one or more of these groups. Diuretics are prescribed to reduce the volume of extracellular fluid in the treatment of many disorders, including hypertension, congestive heart failure, and edema. The specific drug to be prescribed is selected according to the action desired and the patient's physical status. Hypersensitivity to sulfonamides prohibits use of this class of drug, and diabetes mellitus may be aggravated by thiazide

medications; thus the presence of a particular condition may prohibit the use of a particular agent. Several adverse reactions, including hypovolemia and electrolyte imbalance, are common to all diuretics. Mercurial diuretics are rarely used because of their nephrotoxicity, and carbonic anhydrase inhibitors have only weak diuretic activity.

**diuretic ceiling effect,** the effect of possible increased drug toxicity without additional clinical benefit with the administration of more than a certain amount of diuretic drugs in a 24-hour period. Different diuretic drugs have different ceilings.

**Diuril,** trademark for a thiazide diuretic (chlorothiazide).

**diurnal** /dīyŏor′nəl/ [L, *diurnalis,* of a day], happening daily, as sleeping and eating.

**diurnal enuresis** [L, *diurnalis,* of a day; Gk, *enourein,* to urinate], involuntary voiding of urine during daylight hours.

**diurnal mood variation,** a change in mood that is related to the time of day. Examples are commonly found in differences between "night people" and "morning people."

**diurnal rhythm** [L, *diurnalis,* of a day; Gk, *rhythmos*], patterns of activity or behavior that follow day-night cycles, such as breakfast-lunch-dinner schedules.

**diurnal variation,** the range of the output or excretion rate of a substance in a specimen being collected for laboratory analysis over a 24-hour period.

**divalent,** referring to a chamical valency of two. Also called **bivalent.**

**divalproex sodium,** an anticonvulsant drug used to treat epilepsy and seizures, controlling simple and complex absence seizures alone or in combination with other anticonvulsant drugs. It is also approved for the treatment of migraines.
■ INDICATIONS: It is prescribed to prevent or reduce the number of seizures by decreasing the activity of nerve impulses in the brain and central nervous system. Divalproex sodium is converted to valproic acid in the body.
■ CONTRAINDICATIONS: The drug should not be given to patients with an allergy to valproic acid, sodium valproate, or divalproex or to those with liver disease.
■ ADVERSE EFFECTS: The side effects most often reported include changes in appetite, nausea, vomiting, stomach cramps, diarrhea, constipation, weakness, tiredness, clumsiness, drowsiness, or behavioral changes.

**divergence** /divur′jəns/ [L, *di* + *vergere,* to incline], a separation or movement of objects away from each other, as in the simultaneous turning of the eyes outward as a result of an extraocular muscle defect.

**divergent dislocation** /divur′jənt/, the temporary displacement of two bones, such as the radius and ulna.

**divergent squint.** See **exotropia.**

**divergent strabismus.** See **exotropia.**

**diversional activity, deficient,** a nursing diagnosis accepted by the Fourth National Conference on the Classification of Nursing Diagnoses. Diversional deficit is a state in which an individual experiences decreased stimulation from or interest or engagement in recreational or leisure activities.
■ DEFINING CHARACTERISTICS: The defining characteristics are boredom, a desire for something to do, and an inability to participate in usual hobbies.
■ RELATED FACTORS: Related factors include an environmental lack of diversional activity, long-term hospitalization, and frequent, lengthy treatments. See also **nursing diagnosis.**

**diver's palsy, diver's paralysis.** See **decompression sickness.**

**diverticula, diverticular.** See **diverticulum.**

**diverticular disease.** See **diverticulitis, diverticulosis.**

**diverticular hernia** /dīvurtik′yo͞olər/, the protrusion of a congenital intestinal diverticulum through an opening in the abdominal cavity.

**diverticulectomy** /dī′vurtik′yo͞olek′təmē/, surgical removal of a diverticulum.

**diverticulitis** /dī′vurtik′yo͞olī′tis/ [L, *diverticulare,* to turn aside; Gk, *itis,* inflammation], inflammation of one or more diverticula. The penetration of fecal matter through the thin-walled diverticula causes inflammation and abscess formation in the tissues surrounding the colon. With repeated inflammation the lumen of the colon narrows and may become obstructed. During periods of inflammation the patient experiences crampy pain, particularly over the sigmoid colon; fever; and leukocytosis. Barium enemas and proctoscopy are used to rule out carcinoma of the colon, which exhibits some of the same symptoms. Conservative treatment includes bed rest, IV fluids, antibiotics, and abstaining from eating and drinking. In acute cases bowel resection of the affected part greatly reduces mortality and morbidity rates. Compare **diverticulosis.**

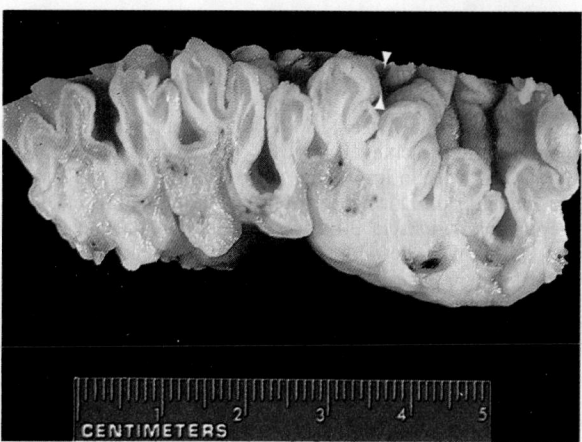

**Diverticulosis** *(Kumar, Cotran, and Robbins, 1997)*

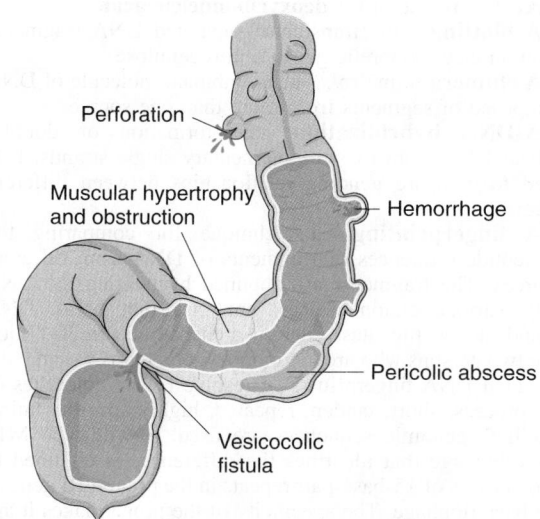

**Complications of diverticulitis** *(Beare and Myers, 1998)*

**diverticulosis** /dī′vurtik′yo͞olō′sis/ [L, *diverticulare,* to turn aside; Gk, *osis,* condition], the presence of pouchlike herniations through the muscular layer of the colon, particularly the sigmoid colon. Diverticulosis affects increasing numbers of people over 50 years of age and may be the result of the modern highly refined low-residue diet. Most patients with this condition have few symptoms except occasional bleeding from the rectum. Other reasons for bleeding, such as hemorrhoids, carcinoma, and inflammatory bowel disease, must be ruled out. Barium enemas and proctoscopic examination are used in establishing diagnosis. An increase in dietary fiber intake can aid in propelling the feces through the colon. Avoidance of foods with seeds and nuts decreases the risk of fecal material lodging in the diverticula. Hemorrhage from bleeding diverticula can become quite severe, and the patient may require surgery. Diverticulosis may lead to diverticulitis. See also **diverticulitis.**

**diverticulum** /dī′vurtik′yo͞oləm/, *pl.* **diverticula** [L, *diverticulare,* to turn aside], a pouchlike herniation through the muscular wall of a tubular organ. A diverticulum may be present in the stomach, the small intestine, or, most commonly, the colon. It is typically detected by radiography after the ingestion of a radiopaque substance. See also **diverticulitis, diverticulosis, Meckel's diverticulum. —diverticular,** *adj.*

**divided dose,** a measured fraction of a full dose of a medication, given at short intervals so that the full dose is eventually taken within a specified period.

**diving,** the act of work or recreation in an underwater environment. The main health effects are related to the increased pressure to which the person is subjected as the ambient pressure generally increases by 1 atm (14.7 pounds per square inch) for each 33 feet of descent below the water surface. Conditions that warrant caution about diving include obesity, diabetes, alcoholism, epilepsy, drug abuse, and respiratory disorders, including allergic rhinitis. See also **decompression sickness, diving reflex.**

**diving goiter** [AS, *dyypan,* to dip; L, *guttur,* throat], a large movable thyroid gland located at times above the sternal notch and at other times below the notch. Also called **plunging goiter, wandering goiter.**

**diving reflex,** a neural mechanism that produces an automatic change in the cardiovascular system when the face and nose are immersed in cold water. The heart rate decreases and the blood pressure remains stable or increases slightly, while blood flow to all parts of the body except the brain is reduced, thereby helping the body to conserve oxygen. The reflex occurs in humans and other mammals. It is sometimes used in the treatment of paroxysmal tachycardias. The reflex extends the duration of the viability of brain cells during apnea beyond the usual period of 5 to 10 min. For this reason, cardiopulmonary resuscitation should always be attempted in drowning victims regardless of their time under water.

**division** [L, *dividere,* to divide], **1.** an administrative subunit in a hospital, such as a division of medical nursing or a division of surgical nursing. **2.** (in public health nursing) an area that encompasses several geographic districts. **3.** the separation of something into two or more parts or sections, such as **cell division.**

**divorce therapy,** a type of counseling that attempts to help divorced couples disengage from their former relationship and malicious behavior toward each other or their children.

**Dix, Dorothea Lynde (1802–1887),** an American humanitarian who achieved fame as a social reformer, primarily for her work in improving prison conditions and care of the mentally ill. During her lifetime she helped to establish mental institutions in 30 states and in Canada. During the U.S. Civil War she was appointed superintendent of army nurses for government hospitals.

**Dix-Hallpike test,** /hôl'pīk/, a method for evaluating the function of the vestibule of the ear in patients with vertigo or hearing loss. The patient's position is quickly changed from sitting to lying down with the neck hyperextended, and then returned to sitting. Nystagmus can then be evaluated, and specific disorders of the vestibule may be diagnosed. See also **caloric test, electronystagmography, nystagmus.**

**dizygotic** /dī'zīgot'ik/ [Gk, *di,* twice, *zygotos,* yolked together], pertaining to twins from two fertilized ova. Compare **monozygotic.** See also **twinning.**

**dizygotic twins,** two offspring born of the same pregnancy and developed from two ova that were released from the ovary simultaneously and fertilized at the same time. They may be of the same or opposite sex, differ both physically and genetically, and have two separate and distinct placentas and membranes, both amnion and chorion. The frequency of dizygotic twinning varies according to ethnic origin: the highest incidence occurs in African-Americans, the lowest in Asian-Americans, with Caucasians intermediate; maternal age: the highest rate occurs when the mother is 35 to 39 years of age; and heredity: showing an increase in the female genetic line rather than the male, although fathers may

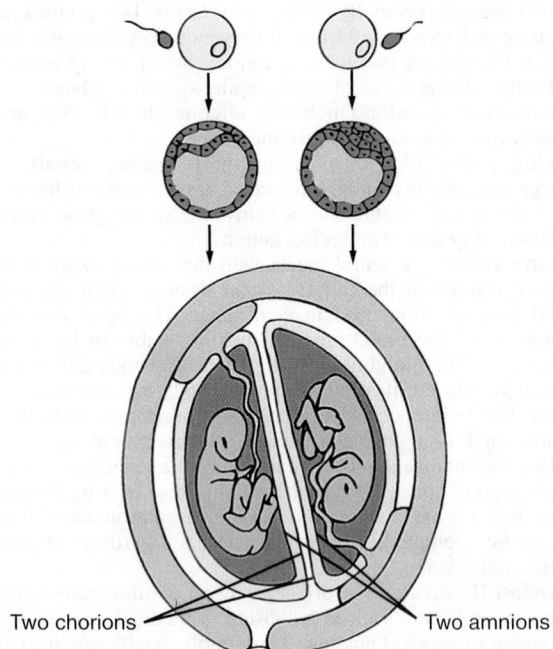

**Development of dizygotic twins**
*(Lowdermilk, Perry, and Bobak, 2000)*

Two chorions        Two amnions

transmit the disposition to double ovulation to their daughters. In general the overall ratio is two thirds dizygotic twinning to one third monozygotic. Also called **binovular twins, dissimilar twins, false twins, fraternal twins, heterologous twins.** Compare **monozygotic twins.**

**dizziness** [AS, *dysig,* stupid], a sensation of faintness and whirling or an inability to maintain normal balance in a standing or seated position, sometimes associated with giddiness, mental confusion, nausea, and weakness. Sometimes the room seems to spin, sometimes the individual. A person who experiences dizziness should be carefully lowered to a safe position on a bed, chair, or floor because of the danger of injury from falling. Compare **syncope.**

**DKA,** abbreviation for **diabetic ketoacidosis.**

**dL,** abbreviation for **deciliter.**

**DLE,** abbreviation for **discoid lupus erythematosus.**

**D log E curve.** See **characteristic curve.**

**DM,** abbreviation for **diabetes mellitus.**

**D.M.D.,** abbreviation for *Doctor of Dental Medicine.* It is equivalent to a **D.D.S.** degree. Programs that offer the degree tend to emphasize the relationship of the mouth to the entire body.

**DMSO,** abbreviation for **dimethyl sulfoxide.**

**DNA,** abbreviation for **deoxyribonucleic acid.**

**DNA blotting,** the transfer of separated DNA fragments from an electrophoretic gel to a nitrocellulose.

**DNA chimera** /kīmē'rə/, a recombinant molecule of DNA composed of segments from more than one source.

**DNA-DNA hybridization,** the formation of double-helical DNA from two complementary single strands. It is used to compare genome relationships between different species.

**DNA fingerprinting,** a technique for comparing the nucleotide sequences of fragments of DNA from different sources. The fragments are obtained by treating the DNA with various endonucleases, enzymes that break DNA strands at specific sites. There is a chance of 1 in 30 billion that two persons who are not monozygotic twins would have identical DNA fingerprints. To resolve the complexities of the process, short, tandem-repeated, highly specific "minisatellite" genomic sequences are used. A wild-type M13 bacteriophage that identifies the differences is confined to two clusters of 15-base-pair repeats in the protein III gene of the bacteriophage. The specificity of the probe makes it applicable to questions of forensic science.

**DNA gyrase,** an enzyme that catalyzes the breakage and rejoining of DNA.

**DNA helicase,** an enzyme that catalyzes the energy-dependent unwinding of the DNA double helix during DNA replication.

**DNA library,** a collection of DNA fragments of one organism, each carrried by a plasmid or virus and cloned in an appropriate host. A DNA probe is used to locate a specific DNA sequence in the library. A collection representing the entire genome is called a genomic library. An assortment of DNA copies of messenger RNA produced by a cell is known as a complimentary DNA (cDNA) library. Also called **gene library.** See also **DNA probe.**

**DNA ligase,** an enzyme that can repair breaks in a strand of deoxyribonucleic acid (DNA) by synthesizing a bond between adjoining nucleotides. Under some circumstances the enzyme can join together loose ends of DNA strands, and in some cases it can repair breaks in ribonucleic acid (RNA). It serves as a catalyst.

**DNA polymerase,** (in molecular genetics) an enzyme that catalyzes the assembly of deoxyribonucleoside triphosphates into deoxyribonucleic acid, with single-stranded

DNA serving as the template. The enzyme is often found in tumor cells. Also called **DNA nucleotidyltransferase.**

**DNA probe,** a labeled segment of DNA or RNA used to find a specific sequence of nucleotides in a DNA molecule. Probes may be synthesized in the laboratory, with a sequence complementary to the target DNA sequence.

**DNAR,** abbreviation for *do not attempt resuscitation.*

**DNCB,** abbreviation for 2,4-*dinitrochlorobenzene.*

**DNP,** abbreviation for 2,4-**dinitrophenol.**

**DNR,** abbreviation for *do not resuscitate.* See **DNAR, no code.**

**D.O.,** abbreviation for *Doctor of Osteopathy.* See **physician.**

**DOA,** abbreviation for *dead on arrival.*

**Dobie's globule** /dō′bēz/ [William M. Dobie, English physician, 1828–1915], a very small stainable body in the transparent disk of a striated muscle fiber.

**dobutamine hydrochloride** /dōbyoō′təmēn/, a beta-adrenergic stimulating agent.
- INDICATIONS: It is prescribed to increase cardiac output in severe chronic congestive heart failure and to provide adjunct in cardiac surgery.
- CONTRAINDICATIONS: Idiopathic hypertrophic subaortic stenosis or known hypersensitivity to this drug prohibits its use. It is not recommended for use in pregnancy.
- ADVERSE EFFECTS: Among the most serious adverse reactions are cardiovascular effects, including tachycardia, hypertension, arrhythmias, and precipitation of angina. Nausea, vomiting, and headache may also occur.

**Dobutrex,** trademark for a synthetic catecholamine (dobutamine hydrochloride), which stimulates beta-adrenergic receptors. It has many drug interactions.

**Dock, Lavinia Lloyd (1858–1956),** an American public health nurse. A graduate of the Bellevue Hospital Training School for Nurses in New York in 1886, she started a visiting nurse service in Norwalk, Connecticut. She then joined the New York City Mission before becoming an assistant to Isabel Hampton Robb at Johns Hopkins Hospital in Baltimore. She returned to public health nursing when she joined the Henry Street Settlement in New York to work with Lillian Wald. She advocated an international public health movement and the improvement of education for nurses. With M. Adelaide Nutting, she wrote *History of Nursing,* a classic in nursing literature.

**doctoral program in nursing,** an educational program that offers preparation for a doctoral degree in the field of nursing designed to prepare nurses for advanced practice, academia, and research. On satisfactory completion of the course of study, the Ph.D. with a major in nursing, D.N.Sc. (Doctor of Nursing Science), or D.S.N. (Doctor of Science in Nursing) degree is awarded.

**Doctor of Medicine, Doctor of Osteopathy.** See **physician.**

**documentation**[1] /dok′yəmentā′shən/ [L, *documentum,* proof], written material associated with a computer or a program. Kinds of documentation include **user documentation,** an instruction manual that provides enough information to allow an individual to use the system; **system documentation,** a complete description of the hardware and software that make up a system; and **program documentation,** a general and specific description of what a program does and how it does it.

**documentation**[1], a nursing intervention from the Nursing Interventions Classification (NIC) defined as recording of pertinent patient data in a clinical record. See also **Nursing Interventions Classification.**

**docusate** /dok′yoōsāt/, a stool softener. Also called **dioctyl**

calcium sulfosuccinate, dioctyl potassium sulfosuccinate, dioctyl sodium sulfosuccinate.
- INDICATION: It is prescribed in the treatment of constipation.
- CONTRAINDICATIONS: Signs or symptoms of appendicitis, concomitant administration of mineral oil, or known hypersensitivity to the drug prohibits its use.
- ADVERSE EFFECTS: No serious adverse reactions are known.

**Döderlein's bacillus** /dā′dərlīnz, dō′dərlēnz/ [Albert S. Döderlein, German physician, 1860–1941], a gram-positive bacterium present in normal vaginal secretions.

**dofetilide,** a class III antidysrhythmic.
- INDICATIONS: This drug is used to treat atrial fibrillation and flutter.
- CONTRAINDICATIONS: Known hypersensitivity to this drug, digitalis toxicity, aortic stenosis, pulmonary hypertension, QT syndromes, and severe renal disease prohibit the use of dofetilide. This drug is also contraindicated in children.
- ADVERSE EFFECTS: Serious adverse effects of this drug include severe diarrhea, anorexia, angina, premature ventricular contractions, substernal pressure, transient hypertension, and precipitation of angina. Common side effects include syncope, dizziness, nausea, vomiting, hypotension, postural hypotension, and bradycardia.

**Döhle-Heller disease.** See **syphilitic aortitis.**

**Döhle's inclusion bodies** /dā′les, dōls/ [Karl G.P. Döhle, German pathologist, 1855–1928], blue inclusions in the cytoplasm of some leukocytes in May-Hegglin anomaly and in blood smears from patients with acute viral infections.

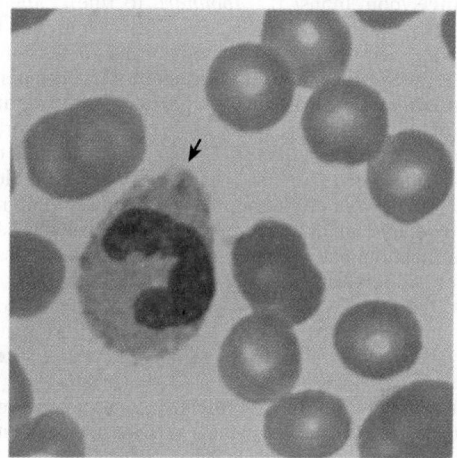

**Döhle's body** *(Carr and Rodak, 1999)*

**dolasetron,** an antiemetic.
- INDICATIONS: Dolasetron is used to prevent the nausea and vomiting associated with cancer chemotherapy and radiotherapy, and to prevent postoperative nausea and vomiting.
- CONTRAINDICATIONS: Known hypersensitivity prohibits the use of this drug.
- ADVERSE EFFECTS: Bronchospasm and dysrhythmias are life-threatening effects of this drug. Other adverse reactions include constipation, increased AST and ALT, abdominal pain, anorexia, dizziness, fatigue, drowsiness, rash, urinary retention, oliguria, electrocardiogram changes, hypotension,

tachycardia, and hypertension. Common side effects include diarrhea and headache.

**Dolene,** trademark for an analgesic (propoxyphene hydrochloride).

**dolicho-,** combining form meaning 'long': *dolichocephaly, dolichocolon, dolichomorphic.*

**dolichocephaly.** See **scaphocephaly.**

**doll's-eye reflex,** a normal response in newborns to keep the eyes stationary as the head is moved to the right or left. The reflex disappears as ocular fixation develops. It is also evaluated in comatose children for assessment of cranial nerve (III, IV, VI) function.

**doll's head maneuver,** a test for central nervous system brainstem damage in a comatose patient. The head is quickly rotated from side to side. Normally the eyes deviate to the opposite direction. Failure of the eyes to make the movement is an indication of severe brainstem damage.

**Dolobid,** trademark for a nonsteroidal antiinflammatory agent (diflunisal).

**Dolophine Hydrochloride,** trademark for an opioid agonist analgesic (methadone hydrochloride).

**dolor** /dō'lôr/ [L, pain], any condition of physical pain, mental anguish, or suffering from heat. It is one of the four signs of inflammation. The others are calor (heat), rubor (redness), and tumor (swelling).

**DOM,** abbreviation for **dimethoxymethylamphetamine.**

**domain,** a region of a protein or polypeptide whose three-dimensional configuration enables it to interact specifically with particular receptors, enzymes, or other proteins.

**dome fracture** [L, *domus,* house, *fractura,* break], a break in the acetabulum, specifically one involving a weight-bearing surface.

**dominance** /dom'inəns/ [L, *dominari,* to rule], the property of an allele in which the allele is fully expressed in the phenotype, even when only one copy of the allele is present. See also **autosomal-dominant inheritance, independent assortment, recessive allele, segregation. —dominant,** *adj.*

**dominant** /dom'i·nənt/ [L, *dominari,* to rule], **1.** exerting a ruling or controlling influence. **2.** in genetics, capable of expression when carried by only one of a pair of homologous chromosomes. **3.** in coronary artery anatomy, supplying the posterior diaphragmatic part of the interventricular septum and the diaphragmatic surface of the left ventricle; said of the right and left coronary arteries.

**dominant allele** [L, *dominari,* to rule; Gk, *genein* to produce], one of two or more alternative forms of a gene that is fully expressed in a heterozygote. Compare **recessive allele.**

**dominant eye** /dom'inənt/, the eye that is customarily used for monocular tasks. It may or may not be related to hand preference.

**dominant group,** a social group that controls the value system and rewards in a particular society.

**dominant idiotype,** a segment of an immunoglobulin molecule that is present on a large proportion of the immunoglobulins generated in response to a particular antigen. See also **idiotype.**

**dominant trait,** an inherited characteristic that is determined by a dominant allele. Polydactyly is an example of a dominant trait; individuals with either one or two copies of the polydactyly allele have extra fingers or toes.

**Donath-Landsteiner syndrome** /dō'notland'stīnər/ [Julius Donath, Austrian physician, 1870–1960; Karl Landsteiner, Austrian-American pathologist, 1868–1943], a rare blood disorder marked by hemolysis minutes or hours after exposure to cold. Systemic symptoms include the passage of dark urine, severe pain in the back and legs, headache, vom-

iting, diarrhea, and moderate reticulocytosis. Temporary hepatosplenomegaly and mild hyperbilirubinemia may follow the onset of an attack. The condition may occur with congenital or acquired syphilis, in which case antisyphilitic treatment is used. Also called **paroxysmal cold hemoglobinuria.**

**Done nomogram,** a graph on which a number of variables are plotted so that the value of a dependent variable can be read on the appropriate line when the values of the other variables are given.

**donepezil,** a reversible cholinesterase.

■ INDICATIONS: This drug is used to treat mild to moderate dementia in Alzheimer's disease.

■ CONTRAINDICATIONS: Known hypersensitivity to this drug or to piperidine derivatives prohibits its use.

■ ADVERSE EFFECTS: Life-threatening effects of donepezil include seizures and atrial fibrillation. Other adverse effects are dizziness, somnolence, fatigue, abnormal dreams, syncope, hypotension or hypertension, anorexia, urinary frequency, urinary tract infection, incontinence, rash, flushing, rhinitis, upper respiratory infection, cough, pharyngitis, cramps, and arthritis. Common side effects include insomnia, headache, nausea, vomiting, and diarrhea.

**dong quai,** a perennial herb found in Japan, China, and Korea.

■ USES: This herb is used to restore vitality in tired women; for a variety of gynecologic, menstrual, and menopausal symptoms; and to treat cirrhosis of the liver.

■ CONTRAINDICATIONS: Dong quai should not be used during pregnancy, in children, or in those with known hypersensitivity. In Chinese medicine, dong quai has been used during pregnancy, but it must be monitored by an herbalist. It is contraindicated in people with bleeding disorders, excessive menstrual flow, or acute illness.

**Don Juan,** a legendary Spanish libertine cited in many works of literature as a seductive and sexually promiscuous man. See also **satyriasis.**

**Donnatal,** trademark for a GI fixed-combination drug containing a sedative (phenobarbital) and three anticholinergics (hyoscyamine sulfate, atropine sulfate, and hyoscine hydrobromide), used to decrease the motility of the GI tract.

**Donohue's syndrome.** See **leprechaunism.**

**donor** /dō'nər/ [L, *donare,* to give], **1.** a human or other organism that gives living tissue to be used in another body, for example, blood for transfusion or a kidney for transplantation. **2.** a substance or compound that gives part of itself to another substance. Compare **acceptor.** See also **universal donor.**

**donor card** [L, *donare,* to give, *charta*], a document in which a person offers to make an anatomic gift of body parts, at the time of death, for transplantation to recipients needing replacement of vital organs or tissues. The card is often incorporated into a state driver's license so the authorization will be immediately available if the donor dies in a traffic accident.

**do not attempt resuscitation (DNAR),** an advisory that resuscitation of a patient should not even be attempted. The order is more strictly defined than the **DNR** (do not resuscitate), which may be interpreted as authorizing an attempt at resuscitation.

**Donovan bodies** /don'əvan/ [Charles Donovan, Irish physician, 1863–1951], encapsulated gram-negative rods of the species *Calymmatobacterium granulomatis,* present in the cytoplasm of mononuclear phagocytes obtained from the lesions of granuloma inguinale. They may be seen under the microscope in a Wright-stained smear of infected tissue. See also **granuloma inguinale.**

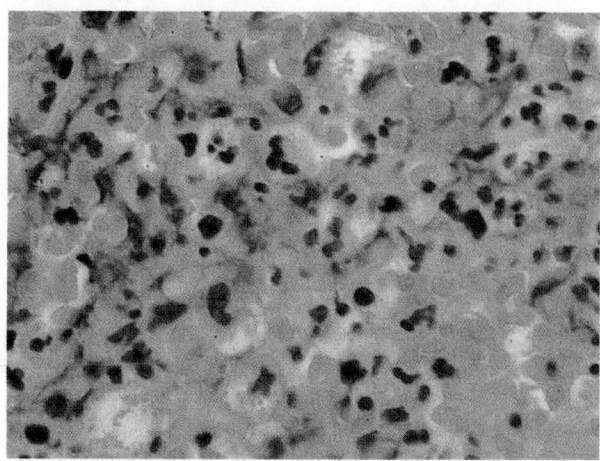

**Donovan bodies** *(Morse, Moreland, and Holmes, 1996)*

**donut pad** /dō′nut/, a pad designed to protect an injured joint. Cut to fit over the site of the injury, it causes the force on the body part to be transferred to surrounding areas. It is most effective for protecting small areas, such as heels or elbows.

**DOOR syndrome,** a rare syndrome of congenital *deaf*ness, *o*nycho-*o*steodystrophy, and mental *r*etardation, existing in autosomal dominant and recessive forms.

**dopa** /dō′pə/, an amino acid, produced by oxidation of tyrosine, that occurs naturally in plants and animals. It is a precursor of dopamine, epinephrine, norepinephrine, and melanin. See also **dopamine hydrochloride, levodopa.**

**dopamine** /dō′pəmin/, a naturally occurring sympathetic nervous system neurotransmitter that is the precursor of norepinephrine. It is produced in the substantia nigra and transmitted to the putamen and caudate nucleus. It has an inhibitory effect on movement. A depletion of dopamine produces the symptoms of rigidity, tremors, and bradykinesia that are characteristic of Parkinson's disease. It is available as an intravenously injectable drug. Dopamine has potent dopaminergic, beta-adrenergic, and alpha-adrenergic receptor activity. See also **dopamine hydrochloride.**

**dopamine hydrochloride,** a sympathomimetic catecholamine.

■ INDICATIONS: It is prescribed in the treatment of shock, hypotension, and low cardiac output.

■ CONTRAINDICATIONS: Pheochromocytoma, tachyarrhythmias, ventricular fibrillation, or known hypersensitivity to this drug prohibits its use.

■ ADVERSE EFFECTS: Among the more serious adverse reactions are arrhythmias, hypotension, hypertension, and tachycardia.

**dopaminergic** /dō′pəminur′jik/, having the effect of dopamine.

**dopaminergic receptor,** a protein on the surfaces of certain cells that binds specifically to the neurotransmitter dopamine. Such receptors on vascular epithelial cells, when stimulated by dopamine, cause the renal mesenteric, coronary, and cerebral arteries to dilate and the flow of blood to increase.

**dope** [AS, *dyppan,* to dip], *slang,* morphine, heroin, or another opioid; marijuana; or another substance illicitly

bought or sold and often self-administered for sedative, hypnotic, euphoric, or other mood-altering purposes.

**Doppler color flow** /dop′lər/ [Christian J. Doppler, Austrian physicist and mathematician, 1803–1853], an ultrasonic technique for detecting anatomic details by color coding of velocity shifts. In cardiography blood flowing in one direction appears red, and blood flowing in the opposite direction appears blue. The technique can also indicate the velocity of red blood corpuscles moving through the circulatory system, which makes it possible to quantify the flow, measure the pressures within the heart chambers, and calculate the stroke volume. In laparoscopy, Doppler color flow allows for rapid identification and differentiation of ducts and valves in the viscera, particularly in detection and diagnosis of pancreatic and liver tumors and colorectal liver metastases. See also **Doppler ultrasonography.**

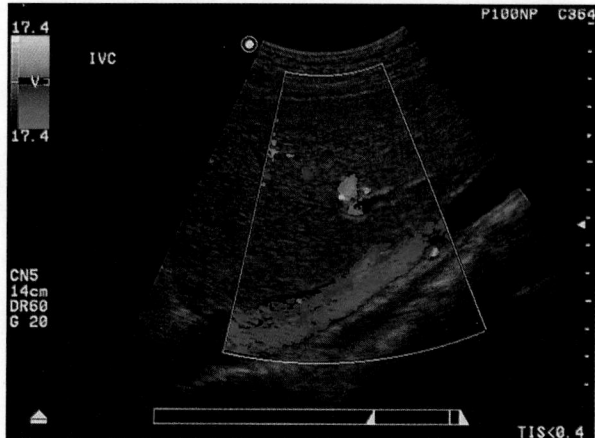

**Image of inferior vena cava produced by Doppler scanning**
*(Gill, 2001)*

**Doppler echocardiography** [Christian J. Doppler], a technique in which Doppler ultrasonography is used to evaluate the direction and pattern of blood flow within the heart.

**Doppler effect** [Christian J. Doppler; L, *effectus*], the apparent change in frequency of sound or light waves emitted by a source as it moves away from or toward an observer. The frequency increases as the source moves toward the observer and decreases as it moves away, as the rising pitch of the whistle of an approaching train and the falling pitch of a departing train. The Doppler effect is also observed in electromagnetic radiation, such as light and radio waves. Also called **Doppler shift.** See also **electromagnetic radiation, ultrasonography, wavelength.**

**Doppler-guided injection** [Christian J. Doppler], the use of a hand-held ultrasound detector in sclerotherapy to guide a needle or syringe for injecting sclerosing fluid.

**Doppler probe** [Christian J. Doppler], a hand-held diagnostic device that emits ultrasonic waves into the body. Reflection of the waves by a moving structure causes a change in their frequency. The Doppler probe has been used as a diagnostic tool since 1960 to study changes in blood flow in arteries and veins.

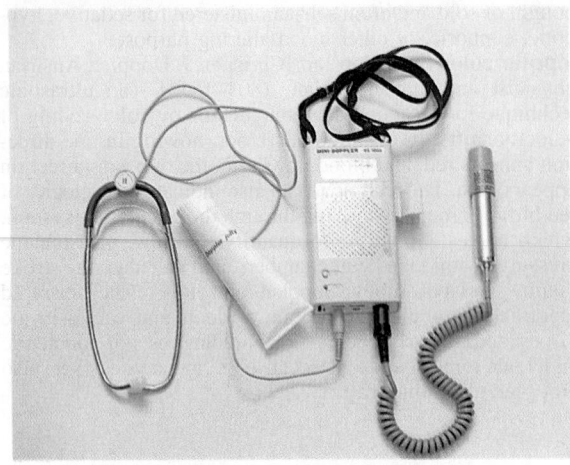

**Doppler flow detector** *(Seidel et al, 1999)*

**Doppler scanning.** See **Doppler ultrasonography.**
**Doppler shift.** See **Doppler effect.**
**Doppler ultrasonography** [Christian J. Doppler], a technique used in ultrasound imaging to monitor moving substances or structures, such as flowing blood or a beating heart. The frequency of ultrasonic waves reflected by a moving surface is slightly different from that of the incident waves. The detected frequency shift yields information about the moving surface. The technique can be used to locate vessel obstructions, observe fetal heart sounds, localize the placenta, and image heart functions. Also called **Doppler scanning.**
**Dorantamin,** trademark for an antihistamine (pyrilamine maleate).
**dornase alfa** /dôr′nās/, a natural proteolytic substance that depolymerizes deoxyribonucleic acid (DNA) molecules. Because as much as 70% of the solid matter of purulent material consists of DNA, dornase is used in respiratory therapy to help break off sputum accumulation in the airways. A principal source of dornase is beef pancreas.
**dorsal** /dôr′səl/ [L, *dorsum,* the back], pertaining to the back or posterior. Compare **ventral.** See also **dorsiflect.** —**dorsum,** *n.*
**-dorsal,** suffix meaning 'the back of something' or 'the back': *predorsal, thoracodorsal, ventrodorsal.*
**dorsal carpal ligament.** See **retinaculum extensorum manus.**
**dorsal column.** See **dorsal horn.**
**dorsal decubitus position.** See **supine.**
**dorsal digital vein,** one of the communicating veins along the sides of the fingers. The veins from the adjacent sides of the fingers unite to form three dorsal metacarpal veins, which end in a dorsal venous network on the back of the hand. Compare **basilic vein, cephalic vein, median antebrachial vein.**
**dorsal flexure** [L, *dorsalis,* back, *flectere,* to bend], the dorsal convexity of the thoracic region of the spine.
**dorsalgia.** See **dorsodynia.**
**dorsal horn** [L, *dorsalis,* back; AS, horn], See **posterior horn.**
**dorsal impaction syndrome,** dorsal wrist pain after weight-bearing activities involving hyperextension, as may occur in weight lifting and gymnastics. Treatment includes

rest, ice, antiinflammatory drugs, and technique modification.
**dorsal inertia posture,** a tendency of a debilitated or weak person to slip downward in bed when the head of the bed is raised. Because of loss of muscular strength or mental apathy the person seems unable to adjust to a new position in bed.
**dorsal interventricular artery,** the arterial branch of the right coronary artery, branching to supply both ventricles. It runs down the dorsal sulcus two thirds of the way to the apex of the heart. Also called **right interventricular artery.**
**dorsalis pedis artery,** the continuation of the anterior tibial artery, starting at the ankle joint, dividing into five branches, and supplying various muscles of the foot and toes. Its branches are the lateral tarsal, medial tarsal, arcuate, first dorsal metatarsal, and deep plantar.
**dorsalis pedis pulse,** the pulse of the dorsalis pedis artery, palpable between the first and second metatarsal bones on the top of the foot. It can be felt in approximately 90% of people.

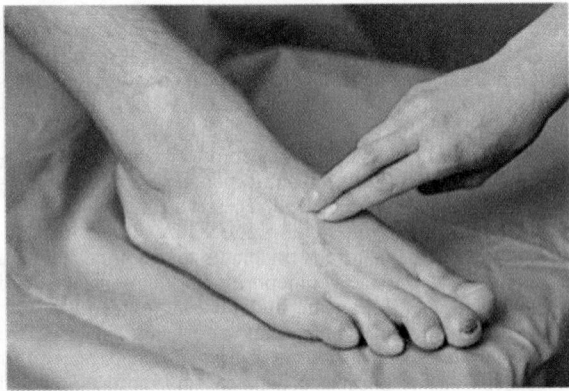

**Palpation of the dorsalis pedis pulse** *(Seidel et al, 1999)*

**dorsal lip,** the marginal fold of the blastopore during gastrulation in the early stages of embryonic development of many animals. It marks the dorsal limit of the developing embryo, constitutes the primary organizer, gives rise to neural tissue, and corresponds to the primitive node in humans and higher animals.
**dorsal recumbent** [L, *dorsalis,* back; *recumbere,* to lie down], lying on the back, as in a supine position.
**dorsal recumbent position** [L, *dorsalis,* back, *positio*], the supine position with the person lying on the back, head, and shoulders.

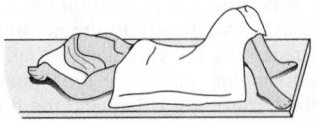

**Dorsal recumbent position** *(Potter and Perry, 2001)*

**dorsal reflex.** See **erector spinae reflex.**

**dorsal rigid posture,** a position in which a patient lying in bed holds one or both legs drawn up to the chest. It often involves only the right leg and is intended to relieve the pain of appendicitis, peritonitis, kidney stones, or pelvic inflammation.

**dorsal root** [L, *dorsalis,* back; AS, *rot*], the sensory component or posterior root of a spinal nerve, attached centrally to the spinal cord.

**dorsal root ganglion** [L, *dorsalis* + AS, *rot* + Gk, *ganglion,* knot], a swelling consisting of sensory neuron cell bodies whose axons constitute the dorsal root of a spinal nerve.

**dorsal scapular nerve,** one of a pair of supraclavicular branches from the roots of the brachial plexus. It supplies the rhomboideus major and the rhomboideus minor and sends a branch to the levator.

**dorsi-.** See **dorso-.**

**dorsiflect** /dôr'siflekt/ [L, *dorsum* + *flectere,* to bend], to bend or flex backward, as in the upward bending of the fingers, wrist, foot, or toes.

**dorsiflexion** /dôr'siflek'shən/, upward or backward flexion of a part of the body. See also **dorsiflexor.**

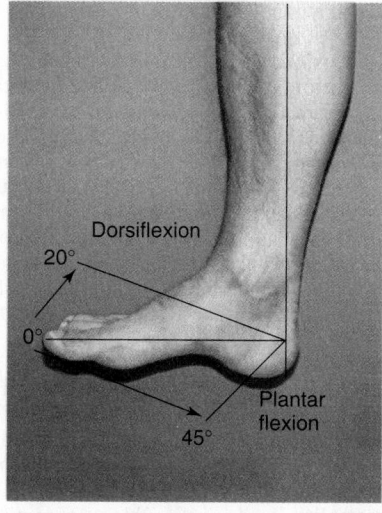

**Dorsiflexion and plantar flexion of the foot**
*(Seidel et al, 1999/Patrick Watson)*

**dorsiflexor** /dôr'siflek'sər/, a muscle causing backward flexion of a part of the body, as the hand or foot.

**dorsiflexor gait,** an abnormal gait caused by the weakness of the dorsiflexors of the ankle. It is characterized by footdrop during the entire gait cycle and excessive knee and hip flexion to allow clearance of the involved extremity during the swing phase. The sole of the affected foot also slaps forcibly against the ground at the moment of heel strike because of the inability of the dorsiflexor to decelerate the body weight as the heel strikes the ground. Compare **Trendelenburg gait.**

**dorsocuboidal reflex.** See **Mendel's reflex.**

**dorso-, dorsi-,** combining form meaning 'dorsum or back': *dorsocephalad, dorsomesial, dorsoscapular.*

**dorsodynia** /dôr'sōdin'ē·ə/, back pain, particularly in the muscles of the upper back area. Also called **dorsalgia.**

**dorsolateral** /dôr'sōlat'ərəl/, pertaining to the back of the body and the two sides.

**dorsolumbar** /dôr'sōlum'bər/, pertaining to the back of the body and the lumbar region.

**dorsosacral** /dôr'sōsā'krəl/, pertaining to the back of the body and the sacrum.

**dorsosacral position.** See **lithotomy position.**

**dorsoventral** /dôr'sōven'trəl/ [L, *dorsum,* back, *venter,* belly], pertaining to the axis that passes through the back of the body and the abdomen.

**dorsum** /dôr'səm/ [L, *dorsum,* back], the back of the body; the posterior or upper surface of a body part.

**dorsum sellae** /sel'ē/, the posterior boundary of the sella turcica of the sphenoid bone. It bears the posterior clinoid process and is an anatomic marker for the location of the pituitary gland at the base of the skull.

**dorzolamide hydrochloride,** a carbonic anhydrase inhibitor.

■ INDICATIONS: It is prescribed in the treatment of glaucoma. It reduces intraocular pressure by decreasing the rate of fluid production.

■ CONTRAINDICATIONS: The drug should not be given to patients wearing soft contact lenses or those with allergy to dorzolamide or its components or related substances.

■ ADVERSE EFFECTS: The side effects most often reported include ocular burning, stinging or discomfort following use, tearing, blurred vision, or light sensitivity.

**DOS** /dos/, abbreviation for *disk operating system.* a generic term describing any operating system that is loaded from disk devices when the system is started or rebooted.

**dosage** /dō'sij/ [Gk, *didonai,* to give], the regimen governing the size, amount, frequency, and number of doses of a therapeutic agent to be administered to a patient.

**dosage compensation,** a mechanism by which the expression of X-linked traits is equalized in males, which have one X chromosome, and females, which have two. In mammals it is accomplished by the inactivation of one of the X chromosomes in the somatic cells of females. See also **Lyon hypothesis.**

**dose** /dōs/ [GK, *didonai,* to give], the amount of a drug or other substance to be administered at one time. See also **absorbed dose.**

**dose calculations,** formulas for adjusting drug dosages for children, elderly adults, or other patients who may lack mechanisms for metabolizing and excreting average adult levels of medications. Infants, for example, have skin that is thin and permeable, a stomach that lacks gastric acid, body temperature that is poorly regulated, and immature liver and kidney. See also **pediatric dosage.**

**dose equivalent (DE),** a quantity used in radiation-safety work that expresses the amount of radiation dose and the physical damage that it may produce. It is the product of the dose (in rad or gray) and a quality factor specific to the type and energy of the radiation delivering that dose. The unit of dose equivalent is the sievert (Sv) or the rem.

**dose fractionation.** See **fractionation,** def. 5.

**dose-limited side effects,** drug effects that prevent a drug from being administered in higher doses.

**dose-limiting recommendations,** the absorbed dose equivalent limit of radiation exposure, which may vary for different body or organ exposures. For example, the absorbed dose equivalent limit for the skin or forearms of a radiation worker is much higher than the whole-body exposure.

**dose rate,** the amount of delivered radiation absorbed per unit time.

**dose ratemeter** /rāt'mētər/, an instrument for measuring the dose rate of radiation.

**dose response,** a range of drug effects between the minimum dose needed to reach the threshold level at which an effect is first observed and a toxic dose level at which adverse effects result.

**dose-response relationship,** a mathematic relationship between the dose of a drug or radiation and the body's reaction to it. In a linear dose-response relationship, the response is proportional to the dose. Thus, if the dose is doubled, the response is also doubled. In a linear nonthreshold relationship, any dose, regardless of size, can theoretically cause a response.

**dose threshold,** the minimum amount of a drug or absorbed radiation that produces a detectable effect.

**dose to skin,** the amount of absorbed radiation at the center of the irradiation field on the skin. It is the sum of the dose in the air and the scatter from body parts.

**dosimeter** /dōsim'ətər/ [L, *dosis* + Gk, *metron*, measure], an instrument used to detect and measure accumulated radiation exposure. It consists of pencil-sized ionization chamber with a self-reading electrometer.

**dosimetry** /dōsim'ətrē/ [Gk, *dosis*, giving, *metron*, measure], **1.** the determination of the amount, rate, and distribution of radiation or radioactivity from a source of ionizing radiation. **2.** the accurate determination of medicinal doses based on body size, sex, age, and other factors.

**DOT,** abbreviation for **Department of Transportation.**

**dot-matrix printer,** a printer that imprints a character by creating it from a pattern of dots, each of which is produced by activating selected wires in a set so that their ends strike the paper through an inked ribbon. Compare **character printer, daisy-wheel printer, laser printer.**

**double** [L, *duplus*], twice as much in strength, size, or amount.

**double-approach conflict.** See **approach-approach conflict.**

**double-avoidant conflict.** See **avoidance-avoidance conflict.**

**double-barrel colostomy.** See **loop colostomy.**

**double bind** /bīnd/ [L, *duplus*, double; AS, *bindan*, to bind], a "no win" situation resulting from two conflicting messages from a person who is crucial to one's survival, such as a verbal message that differs from a nonverbal message. An example is the insistence of a mother that she is not angry about a child's behavior although she is perceived as being obviously angry and hostile.

**double-blind study,** an experiment designed to test the effect of a treatment or substance by using groups of experimental and control subjects in which neither the subjects nor the investigators know which treatment or substance is being administered to which group. In a double-blind test of a new drug, the substance may be identified to the investigators by only a code. The purpose of a double-blind study is to eliminate the risk of prejudgment by the participants, which could distort the results. A double-blind study may be augmented by a **cross-over experiment,** in which experimental subjects unknowingly become control subjects, and vice versa, at some point in the study. See also **placebo.**

**double-blind test** [L, *duplus*, double; AS, *blind, testum*, crucible], an experimental design for drug testing in which neither the clients receiving the drugs nor the persons conducting the test know which subjects are receiving a new drug and which are getting a placebo, or sugar pill.

**double-channel catheter** [L, *duplus*, double; ME, *chanel* + Gk, *katheter*, a thing lowered into], a catheter with two lumens (channels) used to irrigate an internal cavity, with fluid entering one lumen and draining through the other. Also called **two-way catheter.**

**double chin.** See **buccula.**

**double-contrast arthrography,** a method of making a radiographic image of a joint by injecting two contrast agents, usually a gaseous medium and a water-soluble iodinated agent, into the capsular space. The technique is most commonly used in radiography of the knee.

**double-contrast barium enema** [L, *duplus*, double, *contra*, against, *stare*, to stand; Gk, *barys*, heavy, *enienai*, to inject], an enema of radiopaque barium followed by evacuation and injection of air. The purpose is to detail radiographically the mucosal lining of the large intestine. Also called **double-contrast enema.**

**double-contrast enema.** See **double-contrast barium enema.**

**double-emulsion film,** x-ray film that is coated with emulsion on both sides.

**double-flap amputation** [L, *duplus*, double; ME, *flappe*, flap; L, *amputare*], an amputation in which two flaps are made from the soft tissues to cover an area that has lost its integument in surgery or accident.

**double fracture,** a fracture consisting of breaks or cracks in two places in a bone, producing more than two bone segments.

**double gel diffusion.** See **immunodiffusion.**

**double innervation,** innervation of effector organs by fibers of the sympathetic and parasympathetic divisions of the autonomic nervous system. The pelvic viscera, bronchioles, heart, eyes, and digestive system are all doubly innervated. The fibers of the two divisions operate at cross-purposes to achieve a state of balance and maintain constancy in the body's internal environment. The mode of action of each division varies. In some structures one division is stimulating and the other inhibiting; in others, separate fibers from each division act to stimulate and inhibit complementary function.

**double-needle entry,** a technique for injecting a contrast medium or other agent with two needles, one with a larger bore. In diskography a 20-gauge needle is used to perform a spinal puncture and reach the annulus fibrosus of the disk, after which a longer, 26-gauge needle is passed through the guide needle to the injection target area.

**double personality** [L, *duplus*, double, *personalis*, of a person], a state of dissociation in which the individual presents personas to associates at different times as two different persons, each with a different name and different personality traits. The two personalities are generally independent, contrasting, and unaware of the existence of the other. Also called **dual personality.** See also **dissociative identity disorder.**

**double pneumonia,** acute lobar pneumonia affecting both lungs.

**double quartan fever,** a form of malaria in which paroxysms of fever occur in a repeating pattern of 2 consecutive days followed by 1 day of remission. The pattern is usually the result of concurrent infections by two species of the genus *Plasmodium*, one causing paroxysms every 72 hours and the other every 48 hours. Compare **biduotertian fever.**

**double setup,** a nursing procedure in which an obstetric operating room is prepared for both vaginal delivery and cesarean section. The circulating and scrub nurses lay out the equipment required for both procedures, which may include a vacuum extractor, forceps, and cesarean section packs.

The scrub nurse remains scrubbed until the infant is delivered but does not participate unless a cesarean section is performed.

**double vision.** See **diplopia.**

**double-void,** a urinalysis procedure in which the first specimen is discarded and a second, obtained 30 to 45 minutes later, is tested. This method gives a more accurate measure of the amount of glucose in the urine at that particular time.

**douche** /dōōsh/ [Fr, shower-bath], **1.** a procedure in which a liter or more of a solution of a medication or cleansing agent in warm water is introduced into the vagina under low pressure. The woman often performs the procedure herself. Sitting on a toilet seat or semisitting in a bathtub, she introduces the douche tip into the vagina and releases a clamp on the tubing connected to the douche bag, which is suspended 2 feet above the introitus. She allows the solution to flow in, while holding the lips of the vagina closed to retain the fluid. As the accumulation of fluid distends the vagina, she clamps the tubing and, after a few minutes, allows the fluid to flow out. The process is repeated until the entire quantity of solution in the douche bag has been used. Douches also are administered via prepackaged preparations in flexible plastic bottles. Douching may be recommended in the treatment of various pelvic and vaginal infections. **2.** to perform a douche.

**doughnut pessary.** See **pessary.**

**Douglas's cul-de-sac** [James Douglas, Scottish anatomist, 1675–1742; Fr, bottom of the bag], a rectouterine pouch or recess formed by a fold of peritoneum that extends between the rectum and the uterus. Also called **excavatio rectouterina.**

**doula.** See **labor coach.**

**dowager's hump** /dow′ijərz/, an abnormal backward curvature of the cervical spine that afflicts some older women as a result of compression fractures of osteoperosis.

**dowel** /dow′əl/ [ME, *doule,* part of a wheel], a small rod or pin, usually metal, fitted into a prepared hole within the root canal and cemented in place, serving to retain a dental restoration, such as a crown. Also called **post.**

**down** [AS, *adune,* off hill], (of a computer) not operating as a result of malfunction or maintenance or for other reasons.

**Downey cells** [Hal Downey, American hematologist, 1877–1959], lymphocytes identified in one system of classification of the blood cells of patients with infectious mononucleosis and hepatitis. The cells are designated as Downey I, II, or III lymphocytes.

**download,** to transfer data or programs from a central computer to a peripheral unit.

**Down syndrome** [John L. Down, English physician, 1828–1896], a congenital condition characterized by varying degrees of mental retardation and multiple defects. It is the most common chromosomal abnormality of a generalized syndrome and is caused by the presence of an extra chromosome 21 in the G group or, in a small percentage of cases, by the translocation of chromosome 14 or 15 in the D group and chromosome 21 or 22. Down syndrome occurs in approximately 1 in 600 to 650 live births and is associated with advanced maternal age, particularly over 35 years of age. The incidence is as high as 1 in 80 for offspring of women above 40 years of age. In cases caused by translocation, which is a genetic aberration that is hereditary rather than a chromosomal aberration caused by nondisjunction during cell division, the incidence is not associated with maternal age, and the risk is low, about 1 in 5 if the mother is the carrier and 1 in 20 if the father is the carrier. The condi-

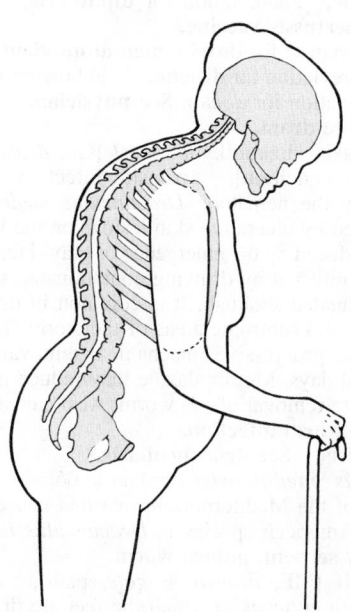

**Dowager's hump** *(Seidel et al, 1999)*

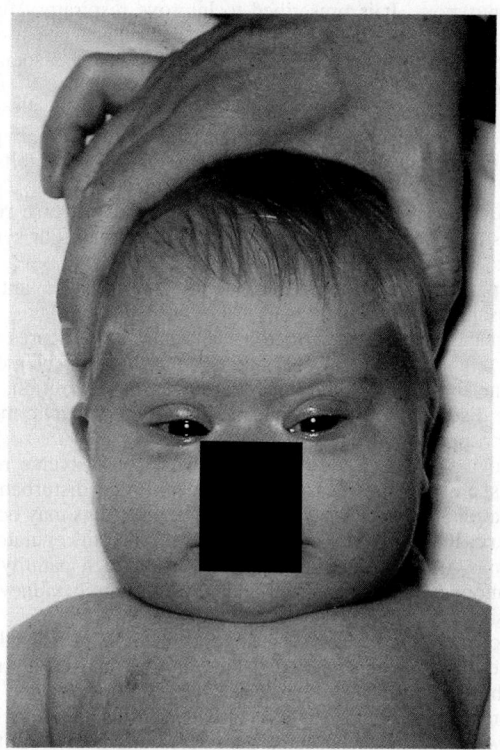

**Typical face seen in Down syndrome**
*(Zitelli and Davis, 1997)*

tion can be diagnosed prenatally by amniocentesis. A mosaic variant, in which there is a mixture of trisomy 21 and normal cells, causes fewer physical defects and less severe retardation, depending on the degree of mosaicism. Infants with the syndrome are small and hypotonic, with characteristic microcephaly, brachycephaly, a flattened occiput, and typical facies with a mongoloid slant to the eyes, depressed nasal bridge, low-set ears, and a large, protruding tongue that is furrowed and lacks a central fissure. The hands are short and broad with a transverse palmar or simian crease; the fingers are stubby and show clinodactyly, primarily of the fifth finger. The feet are broad and stubby with a wide space between the first and second toes and a prominent plantar crease. Other anomalies associated with the disorder are bowel defects, congenital heart disease (primarily septal defects), chronic respiratory infections, visual problems, abnormalities in tooth development, and susceptibility to acute leukemia. The most significant feature of the syndrome is mental retardation, which varies considerably. The average IQ is in the range of 50 to 60, so that the child is generally trainable and in most instances can be reared at home. The mortality rate is high within the first few years, especially in children with cardiac anomalies. Those who survive tend to be shorter than average and stocky in build; they show delayed or incomplete sexual development and can live to middle or old age, although adults with Down syndrome are prone to respiratory infections, pneumonia, and lung disease. Formerly called **mongolism.** Also called **trisomy 21.** See also **nondisjunction.**

**down-time,** a period during which a computer system is inoperable, for maintenance, as a result of malfunction, or for other reasons.

**doxapram hydrochloride** /dok′səpram/, a respiratory stimulant.
- INDICATIONS: It is prescribed to improve respiratory function after anesthesia, in drug-induced central nervous system depression, and for chronic pulmonary disease associated with acute hypercapnia.
- CONTRAINDICATIONS: Seizure disorder, pulmonary disease, coronary artery disease, uncompensated heart failure, hypertension, or known hypersensitivity to this drug prohibits its use.
- ADVERSE EFFECTS: Among the more serious adverse reactions are convulsions, bronchospasm, cardiovascular symptoms, and phlebitis.

**doxepin hydrochloride** /dok′səpin/, a tricyclic antidepressant.
- INDICATION: It is prescribed in the treatment of depression.
- CONTRAINDICATIONS: Concomitant administration of monoamine oxidase inhibitors, recent myocardial infarction, seizure disorders, or known hypersensitivity to tricyclic medication prohibits its use.
- ADVERSE EFFECTS: Among the more serious adverse reactions are GI, cardiovascular, and neurologic disturbances. Sedation, dry mouth, and many drug interactions may occur.

**doxercalciferol,** a parathyroid agent (calcium regulator).
- INDICATIONS: This drug is used to lower high parathyroid hormone levels in patients undergoing chronic kidney dialysis.
- CONTRAINDICATIONS: Known hypersensitivity to this drug, hyperphosphatemia, hypercalcemia, and vitamin D toxicity prohibit the use of doxercalciferol.
- ADVERSE EFFECTS: Adverse effects of this drug include drowsiness, headache, lethargy, nausea, diarrhea, vomiting, anorexia, dry mouth, constipation, cramps, metallic taste, myalgia, arthralgia, decreased bone development, polyuria,

hypercalciuria, hyperphosphatemia, hematuria, and shortness of breath.

**doxorubicin hydrochloride** /dok′səroo′bisin/, an anthracycline antibiotic.
- INDICATIONS: It is prescribed in the treatment of malignant neoplastic diseases.
- CONTRAINDICATIONS: Myelosuppression, heart disease, concurrent administration of daunorubicin, or known hypersensitivity to this drug prohibits its use.
- ADVERSE EFFECTS: Among the more serious adverse reactions are myelosuppression and cardiomyopathy. Stomatitis, GI disturbances, and alopecia commonly occur.

**doxycycline** /dok′sisī′klēn/, a tetracycline antibiotic.
- INDICATIONS: It is prescribed in the treatment of infections caused by susceptible bacterial strains.
- CONTRAINDICATIONS: Renal or liver dysfunction or known hypersensitivity to this drug or to other tetracycline medication prohibits its use. It is not given during pregnancy or to children less than 8 years of age.
- ADVERSE EFFECTS: Among the more serious adverse reactions are GI disturbances, phototoxicity, potentially serious superinfections, and hypersensitivity reactions. Discoloration of teeth may occur in children exposed to the drug in utero or under 8 years of age.

**doxylamine succinate** /dok′silam′ēn/, an antihistamine.
- INDICATIONS: It is prescribed for the treatment of acute allergic symptoms produced by the release of histamine.
- CONTRAINDICATIONS: Known hypersensitivity to this drug prohibits its use. It is not recommended for use during pregnancy or lactation and is not given to children less than 6 years of age.
- ADVERSE EFFECTS: Among the more serious reactions are sedation, ataxia, tachycardia, hemolytic anemia, and thrombocytopenia.

**dP/dt,** the rate of change of pressure with respect to time.

**DPG,** abbreviation for **2,3-diphosphoglyceric acid.**

**D.P.H.,** abbreviation for *Diploma in Public Health.*

**DPL,** abbreviation for **diagnostic peritoneal lavage.**

**D.P.M.,** abbreviation for *Doctor of Podiatric Medicine.* See also **podiatrist.**

**DPT vaccine,** abbreviation for **diphtheria, tetanus toxoids, and pertussis vaccine.**

**DQ,** abbreviation for **developmental quotient.**

**dr.,** 1. abbreviation for **drachm.** 2. abbreviation for **dram.**

**Dr.,** abbreviation for *doctor.* See **physician.**

**drachm.** See **dram.**

**dracunculiasis** /drakun′kyoōlī′əsis/ [Gk, *drakontion,* little dragon, *osis,* condition], a parasitic infection caused by infestation by the nematode *Dracunculus medinensis.* It is characterized by ulcerative skin lesions on the legs and feet that are produced by the emergence of gravid female worms. People are infected by drinking contaminated water or eating contaminated shellfish. It is common in densely populated tropic and subtropic areas of the world. Treatment involves slow, progressive, mechanical removal of a worm over several days. Metronidazole may reduce inflammation and facilitate removal of the worm. Also called **dracontiasis, guinea worm infection.**

**dracunculosis.** See **dracunculiasis.**

***Dracunculus medinensis*** /drakun′kyoōləs/, a parasitic nematode of the Mediterranean area that causes dracunculiasis. An American species is *Dracunculus insignis.* Also called **fiery serpent, guinea worm.**

**drag-to gait** [ME, *dragen* + *gate,* path], a method of walking with crutches in which the feet are dragged rather than lifted with each step. See also **crutch gait.**

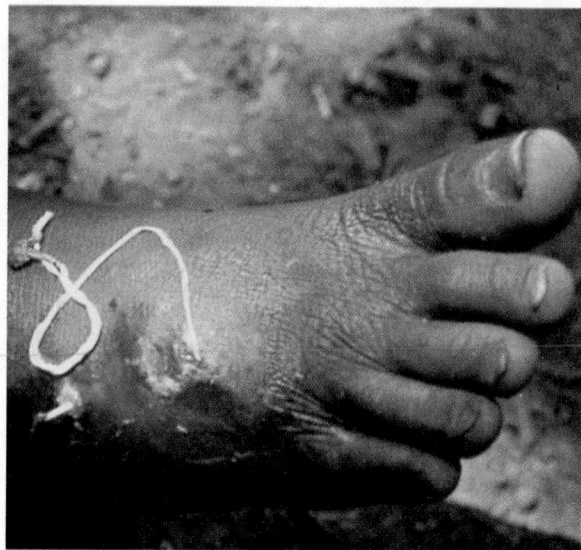

**Dracunculiasis** *(du Vivier, 1993/courtesy Dr. R. Muller)*

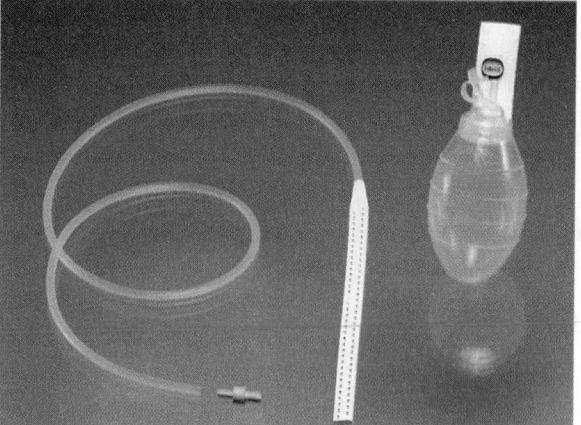

**Jackson-Pratt silicon suction drain**
*(Ignatavicius, Workman, Mishler, 1999/courtesy*
*C.R. Bard Inc., Covington, Ga)*

**drain,** a tube or other device used to remove air or a fluid from a body cavity or wound. The drain may be a closed system, designed to provide complete protection against contamination, or an open system in which there is a continual exchange of material.

**drainage** /drā′nij/ [AS, *drachen*, teardrop], the removal of fluids from a body cavity, wound, or other source of discharge by one or more methods. **Closed drainage** is a system of tubing and other apparatus attached to the body to remove fluid in an airtight circuit that prevents environmental contaminants from entering the wound or cavity. **Continuous bladder irrigation** is drainage in which a body area is washed out by alternately flooding and then emptying it with the aid of gravity, a technique that may be used in treating a urinary bladder disorder. See also **postural drainage**. **Open drainage** is drainage in which discharge passes through an open-ended tube into a receptacle. **Suction drainage** uses a pump or other mechanical device to assist in extracting a fluid.

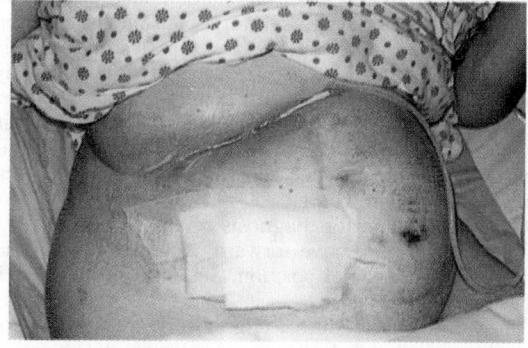

**Closed wound drainage system**
*(Bryant, 1992/courtesy Abbot Northwestern Hospital, Minneapolis)*

**drainage tube,** a heavy-gauge catheter used for the evacuation of air or a fluid from a cavity or wound in the body. The tube may be attached to a suction device or may allow flow by gravity into a receptacle.

**draining sinus** [AS, *drachen*, teardrop; L, *sinus*, hollow], an abnormal channel or fistula permitting the escape of exudate to the outside of the body.

**Draize test** /drāz/, a controversial method of testing the toxicity of pharmaceutic and other products to be used by humans by placing a small amount of the substance in the eyes of rabbits. The eye-irritancy potential of a substance is considered a measure of the possible effect of the product on similar human tissues. The Draize in vivo test is recognized by the U.S. Food and Drug Administration as a reliable method of predicting the risk of new products to human eyesight, although alternative testing methods are being sought.

**-dralazine,** suffix for the name of an antihypertensive.

**dram (dr.)** /dram/ [Gk, *drachme*, weight of the same value], a unit of mass equivalent to an apothecary's measure of 60 grains or ⅛ ounce and to 1/16 ounce or 27.34 grains avoirdupois. Also spelled **drachm (dr.)**.

**Dramamine,** trademark for an antiemetic (dimenhydrinate).

**dramatic play** /dramat′ik/ [Gk, *drama*, deed; AS, *plegan*, game], an imitative activity in which a child fantasizes and acts out various domestic and social roles and situations, as rocking a doll, pretending to be a doctor or nurse, or teaching school. It is the predominant form of play among preschool children.

**drape** [ME, *drap*, cloth], a sheet of fabric or paper, usually the size of a small bed sheet, for covering all or a part of a person's body during a physical examination or treatment. **—drape,** *v.*

**Drash syndrome** /drash/ [Allan Lee Drash, American pediatrician, b. 1931], a syndrome of male pseudohermaphroditism, nephropathy leading to renal failure, and, in most cases, Wilms' tumor, caused by a genetic abnormality in chromosome 11.

**Draw-a-Person Test (DAP)** [AS, *dragan* + L, *personalis* + *testum*, crucible], a test developed by Karen Machover [American psychologist, b. 1902] based on the interpretation of drawings of human figures of both sexes. Interpretation depends on the subject's verbalizations, self-image, anxiety, and sexual conflicts and other factors. Also called **Machover Draw-a-Person Test.**

**drawer sign** [AS, *dragan,* to drag], a diagnostic sign of a ruptured or torn knee ligament. Testing involves having the patient flex the knee at a right angle while the lower leg is grasped just below the knee and moved first toward, then away from the examiner. The test result is positive for the knee injury if the head of the tibia can be moved more than a half inch from the joint.

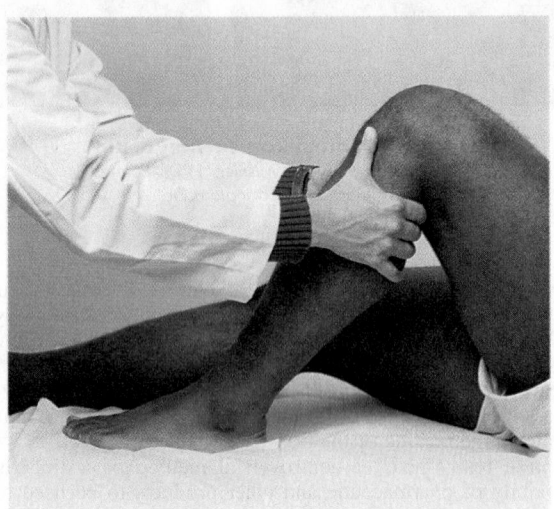

**Drawer sign** *(Seidel et al, 1999)*

**drawing,** *informal.* a vague sensation of muscle tension.

**drawsheet,** a sheet that is smaller than a bottom or top sheet of a bed and is usually placed over the middle of the bottom sheet to keep the mattress and bottom linens dry. The draw-sheet can also be used to turn or move a patient in bed. Also called **pull sheet, turning sheet.**

**dream** [ME, *dreem,* joyful noise], **1.** a sequence of ideas, thoughts, emotions, or images that pass through the mind during the rapid-eye-movement stage of sleep. **2.** the sleeping state in which this process occurs. **3.** a visionary creation of the imagination experienced during wakefulness. **4.** (in psychoanalysis) the expression of thoughts, emotions, memories, or impulses repressed from the consciousness. **5.** (in analytic psychology) the wishes, emotions, and impulses that reflect the personal unconscious and the archetypes that originate in the collective unconscious. See also **dream analysis, dream state.**

**dream analysis,** a process of gaining access to the unconscious mind by means of examining the content of dreams, usually through the method of free association.

**dream association,** a relationship of thoughts or emotions discovered or experienced when a dream is remembered or analyzed. See also **dream analysis.**

**dream state,** a condition of altered consciousness in which a person does not recognize the environment and reacts in a manner opposed to his or her usual behavior, as by flight or an act of violence. The state is seen in epilepsy and certain disorders. See also **automatism, fugue.**

**drepanocytic anemia** /drep′ənōsit′ik/ [Gk, *drepane,* sickle, *kytos,* cell], sickle cell anemia.

**dress code** [OFr, *dresser,* to arrange; L, *codex,* book], the standards set by an institution for the appropriate attire of its members.

**dressing**[1] [OFr, *dresser,* to arrange], a clean or sterile covering applied directly to wounded or diseased tissue for absorption of secretions, protection from trauma, administration of medications, maintaining wound cleanliness, or stopping bleeding. Kinds of dressings include **absorbent dressing, antiseptic dressing, occlusive dressing, pressure dressing,** and **wet dressing.**

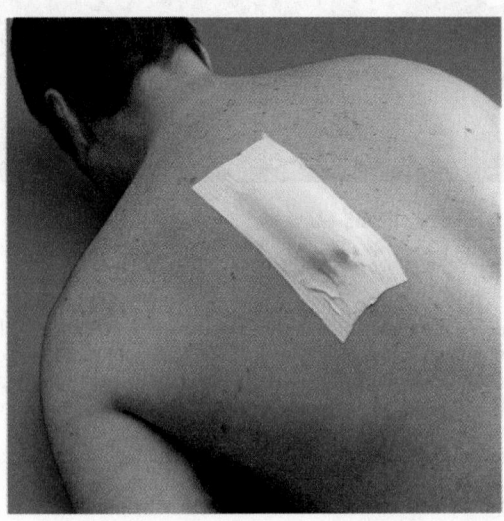

**Simple dressing** *(Sanders et al, 2000)*

**dressing**[2], a nursing intervention from the Nursing Interventions Classification (NIC) defined as choosing, putting on, and removing clothes for a person who cannot do this for self. See also **Nursing Interventions Classification.**

**dressing forceps,** a kind of forceps that has narrow blades and blunt or notched teeth, designed for dressing wounds, removing drainage tubes, or extracting fragments of necrotic tissue.

**Dressler's syndrome** /dres′lərz/ [William Dressler, American physician, 1890–1969], an autoimmune disorder that may occur several days to several months after acute coronary infarction, characterized by fever, pericarditis, pleurisy, pleural effusions, and joint pain. It results from the body's immunologic response to a damaged myocardium and pericardium. Treatment usually includes intensive aspirin therapy and, in severe cases, use of corticosteroids. A similar syndrome may occur after cardiac surgery. See **postmyocardial infarction syndrome.**

**DRG,** abbreviation for **diagnosis related group.**

**drift** [AS, *drifan,* to move forward], a gradual movement away from the original position. See also **antigenic drift, genetic drift.**

**drifting tooth,** a tooth that migrates from its normal position. Causes include a loss of proximal support or functional antagonists, occlusal traumatic tooth relationships, inflammatory and retrograde changes in the attachment apparatus, and oral habits, such as thumb-sucking and bruxism.

**drill** /dril/ [Dutch *drillen*, to bore], **1.** a rotating cutting instrument for making holes in hard substances, such as bones or teeth. **2.** see **burr.**

**Drinker respirator** [Philip Drinker, American engineer, 1894–1972], an airtight respirator consisting of a metal tank that encloses the entire body, except the head. Used for long-term therapy, it alternates positive and negative air pressure within the tank, providing artificial respiration by contracting and expanding the walls of the chest. Also called **artificial lung, iron lung.**

**drip** [AS, *dryppan*, to fall in drops], **1.** the process in which a liquid or moisture forms and falls in drops. Kinds of drip include **nasal drip** and **postnasal drip. 2.** the slow but continuous infusion of a liquid into the body, as into the stomach or a vein. **3.** to infuse a liquid continuously into the body.

**drip gavage,** a method of feeding a liquid formula diet through a tube inserted through the nostrils to the stomach. The formula may be heated to about 100° F (37.8° C) or administered at room temperature and is contained in a bag suspended from a stand. It may also be administered with a feeding pump. See also **enteral tube feeding, tube feeding.**

**drip system,** (in IV therapy) an apparatus for delivering specific volumes of IV solutions within predetermined periods and at a specific flow rate. See also **macrodrip, microdrip.**

**drive** [AS, *drifan*, to move forward], **1.** a basic, compelling urge. **Primary drive** refers to one that is innate and in close contact with physiologic processes. A **secondary drive** is one that evolves during the process of growth and that incites and directs behavior. **2.** an electromechanical device that holds a secondary-storage medium and allows for the transfer of data to and from the computer, such as a disk drive or tape drive.

**Drixoral,** trademark for a fixed-combination drug containing an antihistamine (dexbrompheniramine maleate) and a vasoconstrictor (pseudoephedrine sulfate), used for the relief of congestion of the upper respiratory tract.

**-drome,** suffix meaning 'that which runs or moves together' in a specified way: *dermadrome, heterodrome, syndrome.*

**dromo-,** combining form meaning 'running or conduction': *dromomania, dromophobic, dromotropic.*

**dromostanolone propionate** /drō'mostan'əlōn/, a synthetic androgen.
■ INDICATION: It is prescribed for the treatment of female breast cancer.
■ CONTRAINDICATIONS: It is not used for male breast cancer or in premenopausal women.
■ ADVERSE EFFECTS: Among the more serious adverse reactions are masculinization, edema, and hypercalcemia.

**dromotropic,** an agent that influences the conduction of electrical impulses. A positive dromotropic agent enhances the conduction of electrical impulses to the heart.

**dronabinol** /drōnab'inol/, an oral antiemetic that is a synthetic derivative of THC, the principal psychotropic constituent of marijuana.
■ INDICATIONS: It is prescribed for the treatment of refractory nausea and vomiting caused by cancer chemotherapy.
■ CONTRAINDICATIONS: Dronabinol should not be given to persons with known hypersensitivity to the drug or to tetrahydrocanabinol, its active ingredient.
■ ADVERSE EFFECTS: Among adverse effects reported are drowsiness, dizziness, impaired coordination, and hallucinations. Dronabinol is a Schedule III controlled substance with a high potential for abuse. It can produce both physical and psychologic dependence. It is not recommended for patients

who are using a central nervous system depressant or other psychoactive drugs.

**drooping eyelid.** See **ptosis.**

**drop** [AS, *dropa*], a small spherical mass of liquid. A drop may vary in size with differences in temperature, viscosity, and other factors. For therapeutic purpose, a drop is regarded as having a volume of 0.06 to 0.1 ml, or 1 to 1.5 minims; 1.5 drops = 1 ml. Drop is abbreviated *gtt.*

**drop arm test,** a diagnostic test for a tear in the supraspinatus tendon. The result is positive if the patient is unable to lower the affected arm from a position of 90 degrees of abduction slowly and smoothly.

**drop attack,** a form of transient ischemic attack in which a brief interruption of cerebral blood flow causes a person to fall to the floor without losing consciousness. The fall may be caused by a disrupted sense of balance or decreased leg muscle tone. Weakness of the leg muscles or a hip or knee joint dysfunction may be a contributing factor.

**droperidol** /drəper'ədol/, an antipsychotic, sedative drug of the butyrophenone group, used most commonly with an opioid analgesic (fentanyl) in neuroleptanesthesia.

**drop foot.** See **footdrop.**

**droplet infection** [AS, *dropa* + L, *inficere*, to infect], an infection acquired by the inhalation of pathogenic microorganisms suspended in particles of liquid exhaled, sneezed, or coughed by another infected person or animal. Some diseases spread by droplets are chickenpox, common cold, influenza, measles, and mumps.

**Droplet Precautions,** safeguards designed to reduce the risk of droplet transmission of infectious agents. Droplet transmission involves contact of the conjunctivae or the mucous membranes of the nose or mouth of a susceptible person with large-particle droplets (larger than 5 μm in size) containing microorganisms generated from a person who has a clinical disease or is a carrier of the disease. Droplets are generated from the source person primarily during coughing, sneezing, talking, and performance of certain procedures such as suctioning and bronchoscopy. Large-particle droplet transmission requires close contact between source and recipient persons because droplets do not remain suspended in the air and generally travel only short distances (usually 3 feet or less). Special air handling and ventilation are not required to prevent droplet transmission. Droplet Precautions apply to any patient known or suspected to be infected with epidemiologically important pathogens that can be transmitted by infectious droplets. See also **Standard Precautions, Transmission-based Precautions.**

**dropped-beat pulse.** See **intermittent pulse.**

**dropped wrist.** See **radial paralysis.**

**dropper,** a glass or plastic tube narrowed at one end with a rubber bulb at the other end to dispense a liquid medication one drop at a time.

**dropsy.** See **hydrops.**

***Drosophila*** /drōsof'ilə/ [Gk, *drosos*, dew, *philein*, to love], a genus of fly, which includes *Drosophila melanogaster,* the Mediterranean fruit fly. It is useful in genetic experiments because of the large chromosomes found in its salivary glands and its sensitivity to environmental effects, as exposure to radiation.

**drowning** [ME, *drounen*], asphyxiation caused by submersion in a liquid. See also **near drowning.**

**drowsiness,** a decreased level of consciousness characterized by sleepiness and difficulty in remaining alert. It may be caused by a lack of sleep, medications, substance abuse, or a cerebral disorder.

**drox,** abbreviation for a *noncarboxylate hydroxide anion.*

**Dr. P.H.,** abbreviation for *Doctor of Public Health.*

**DRSP,** abbreviation for **drug-resistant** *Streptococcus pneumoniae.*

**drug** [Fr, *drogue*], **1.** also called **medicine.** any substance taken by mouth; injected into a muscle, the skin, a blood vessel, or a cavity of the body; or applied topically to treat or prevent a disease or condition. **2.** *informal.* an opioid substance.

**drug absorption,** the process whereby a drug moves from the muscle, digestive tract, or other site of entry into the body toward the circulatory system.

**drug abuse,** the overuse of a drug for a nontherapeutic effect. Some of the most commonly abused drugs are alcohol, amphetamines, barbiturates, cocaine, methaqualone, opium alkaloids, and minor tranquilizers (benzodiazepine). Drug abuse may lead to organ damage, addiction, and disturbed patterns of behavior. Some illicit drugs, such as heroin, lysergic acid diethylamide (LSD), and phencyclidine hydrochloride (PCP), have no recognized therapeutic effect in humans. Use of these drugs often incurs criminal penalty in addition to the potential for physical, social, and psychologic harm. See also **drug addiction.**

**Drug Abuse Warning Network (DAWN),** a system of collecting information about admissions to emergency treatment facilities for drug abuse.

**drug action,** the means by which a drug exerts a desired effect. Drugs are usually classified by their actions; for example, a vasodilator, prescribed to decrease the blood pressure, acts by dilating the blood vessels.

**drug addiction,** a condition characterized by an overwhelming desire to continue taking a drug to which one has become habituated through repeated consumption because it produces a particular effect, usually an alteration of mental status. Addiction is usually accompanied by a compulsion to obtain the drug, a tendency to increase the dose, a psychologic or physical dependence, and detrimental consequences for the individual and society. Common addictive drugs are barbiturates, alcohol, and morphine and other opioids, especially heroin, which has slightly greater euphorigenic properties than other opium derivatives. See also **alcoholism, drug abuse.**

**drug agonist,** one of two similar drugs that may affect the same target organ or tissue, producing the same or a similar response. If the drugs compete for the same receptor sites, the two products may act as competitive antagonists, requiring larger than usual doses to achieve a desired effect.

**drug allergy,** hypersensitivity to a pharmacologic agent. Manifestions range from a mild rash to anaphylactic shock, depending on the dose, and the allergen sensitivity of the individual. The primary drug that produces allergy is penicillin. Others include aspirin, phenylbutazone, novobiocin, other antibiotics and radiopaque contrast media containing iodine. See also **anaphylactic shock.**

**drug clearance,** the elimination of a drug from the body. Common methods of excretion are by the kidneys, liver, and lungs. The rate of clearance helps determine the size and frequency of a dosage of a particular medication.

**drug compliance,** the reliability of the patient in using a prescribed medication exactly as ordered by the physician. Noncompliance occurs when a patient forgets or neglects to take the prescribed dosages at the recommended times or decides to discontinue the drug without consulting the physician.

**drug concentration,** the amount of drug in the blood or plasma. Toxic drug levels may be observed when the body's normal mechanisms for metabolizing and excreting drugs are impaired, as commonly occurs in patients with liver or kidney disorders and in infants with immature organs. Dos-

age adjustments should be made in such individuals to accommodate their impaired metabolism and excretion.

**drug dependence,** a psychologic craving for, habituation to, abuse of, or physiologic reliance on a chemical substance. See also **drug abuse, drug addiction.**

**drug dispensing,** the preparation, packaging, labeling, record keeping, and transfer of a prescription drug to a patient or an intermediary, who is responsible for administration of the drug.

**drug disposition,** the absorption, distribution, metabolism, and excretion of drugs.

**drug distribution,** the pattern of distribution of drug molecules by various tissues after the chemical enters the circulatory system. Because of differences in pH, cell membrane functions, and other individual tissue factors, most drugs are not distributed equally in all parts of the body. For example, the acidity of aspirin influences a distribution pattern that is different from that of an alkaline product such as amphetamine.

**drug-drug interaction,** a modification of the effect of a drug when administered with another drug. The effect may be an increase or a decrease in the action of either substance, or it may be an adverse effect that is not normally associated with either drug. The particular interaction may be the result of a chemical-physical incompatibility of the two drugs or a change in the rate of absorption or the quantity absorbed in the body, the binding ability of either drug, or an alteration in the ability of receptor sites and cell membranes to bind either drug. Most adverse drug-drug interactions are either pharmacodynamic or pharmacokinetic in nature.

**Drug Enforcement Agency (DEA),** an agency of the Drug Enforcement Administration of the federal government, empowered to enforce regulations that control the import or export of narcotic drugs and certain other substances or the traffic of these substances across state lines.

**drug eruption.** See **drug rash.**

**drug fever,** a fever caused by the pharmacologic action of a medication, its thermoregulatory action, a local complication of parenteral administration, or, most commonly, an immunologic reaction mediated by drug-induced antibodies. The onset of fever occurs usually between 7 and 10 days after the medication is begun; a return to normal is ordinarily seen within 2 or 3 days of discontinuance of the drug. The correct diagnosis of drug fever and the discontinuance of the medication are important to prevent further adverse reactions and possibly dangerous and expensive diagnostic and therapeutic interventions. See also **Jarisch-Herxheimer reaction.**

**drug-food interaction,** the effect produced when some drugs and certain foods or beverages are taken at the same time.

**drug holiday,** a period of drug withdrawal to reverse ineffectiveness of a drug resulting from receptor desensitization or adverse effects that may result from chronic treatment. For example, after a 7- to 10-day drug holiday, levodopa responsiveness appears to be enhanced, and lower doses are required to produce a therapeutic effect.

**drug-induced parkinsonism,** a reversible syndrome with the clinical features of Parkinson's disease but caused by the acetylcholine-dopamine imbalance of antipsychotic drugs. See also **parkinsonism.**

**drug-induced teratogenesis,** congenital anomalies that reflect toxic effects of drugs on the developing fetus. See also **fetal alcohol syndrome, thalidomide.**

**drug metabolism,** the transformation of a drug by the body tissues into a metabolite as the body readies the agent for elimination.

**drug monograph,** a statement that specifies the kinds and amounts of ingredients a drug or class of drugs may contain, the directions for the drug's use, the conditions in which it may be used, and the contraindications to its use.

**drug overdose (O.D.)** [Fr, *drogue,* drug; AS, *ofer;* Gk, *dosis,* giving], an accidental or purposeful dose of a drug large enough to cause severe adverse reactions. See also **dose-response relationship.**

**drug potency,** a measure of the effect of one drug as compared with a similar medication of the same dosage. The drug that produces the maximum effect with the smallest dose has the greater potency.

**drug profile,** an outline or summary of the characteristics of a drug or drug family, listing dosage types, pregnancy category, prescription or over-the-counter forms, generics if available, contraindications, and classification if covered by controlled-substance laws.

**drug psychosis** [Fr, *drogue,* drug; Gk, *psyche,* mind, *osis,* condition], a psychotic state induced by excessive dosage of certain therapeutic drugs as well as drugs of abuse. Therapeutic drugs often associated with drug-induced psychosis include belladonna, chloral hydrate, steroids, and isoniazid.

**drug rash,** a skin eruption, usually an allergic reaction, that is caused by a particular drug. Nearly any drug can produce a skin reaction as a result of gradual accumulation of the drug or development of antibodies that reject a component of the medication. A drug rash that is a sensitivity reaction does not occur the first time the drug is taken; the effect is observed with subsequent uses. Also called **dermatitis medicamentosa.** See also **fixed drug eruption.**

**drug reaction.** See **adverse drug reaction.**

**drug receptor,** any part of a cell, usually a large protein molecule, with which a drug molecule interacts to trigger a response or effect on the cell surface or in the cytoplasm.

**drug rehabilitation center,** an agency that provides treatment for a person with a chemical or drug dependency.

**drug resistance,** the ability of disease organisms to resist effects of drugs that previously were toxic to them. Bacterial resistance to an antibiotic can result from mutation of a strain that has been exposed to an antibiotic or similar agent. Such acquired resistance may result from a chromosomal disruption or acquisition of a stray bit of deoxyribonucleic acid (DNA) on a resistant plasmid. It can also be caused by extrachromosomal pieces of DNA that carry codes for antibiotic-resistant genes from a transposon, a DNA segment capable of insertion into a bacterial chromosome-resistant plasmid, or both. Decreased permeability to an antimicrobial is a common form of intrinsic resistance. Alteration or inactivation of the antibiotic is perhaps the most common mechanism of drug resistance. Acquired resistance to beta-lactam antibiotics is determined by the production of enzymes that inactivate the antibiotic. Drug resistance may also result from a change in the target site on which it acts.

**drug-resistant *Streptococcus pneumoniae* (DRSP),** a widespread strain of respiratory pathogen that is drug resistant. Until the 1960s *S. pneumoniae* was almost uniformly susceptible to penicillin alone. In 1967 resistance to penicillin and other microbial drugs was first reported in Australia; it has since spread worldwide.

**drug-seeking behavior (DSB),** a pattern of seeking narcotic pain medication or tranquilizers with forged prescriptions, false identification, repeated requests for replacement of "lost" drugs or prescriptions, complaints of severe pain without an organic basis, and abusive or threatening behavior manifested when denied drugs.

**drug sequestration,** the process by which certain drugs are stored in the body tissues. Examples include tetracycline, which may be stored in bone tissue, and chloroquine, which is stored in the liver. Certain vitamins and other substances are stored in fat deposits.

**drug tolerance,** a condition of cellular adaptation to a pharmacologically active substance so that increasingly larger doses are required to produce the same physiologic or psychologic effect obtained earlier with smaller doses.

**drug trial,** the process of determining an adequate and effective therapeutic dose or duration of treatment of a specific drug for a particular disease state. The trial culminates with (1) an acceptable clinical result, (2) intolerable adverse effects, (3) a poor response after an appropriate blood level is reached, or (4) administration of the drug for a specific time.

**drum cartridge catheter technique,** a method used in central vein cannulation. The vein is cannulated with an introducer cannula. The needle is removed and is replaced by the drum cartridge catheter, which is left in place.

**drum electrode,** an induction electrode that produces a strong magnetic field, used primarily with pulsed short-wave diathermy.

**drusen** /drōo′zən/ [Ger, *Drüse,* stony granule], small yellowish hyaline deposits that develop beneath the retinal pigment epithelium, sometimes appearing as nodules within the optic nerve head. They tend to occur most frequently in persons older than 60 years of age.

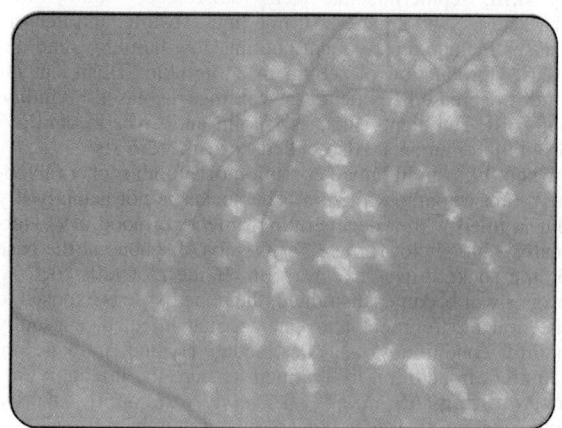

**Retinal drusen** *(Kanski and Nischal, 1999)*

**DRV,** abbreviation for **Daily Reference Values.**

**dry abscess,** a collection of pus that disperses without reaching a point of bursting.

**dry catarrh** [AS, *dryge* + Gk, *kata,* down, *rhoia,* flow], a dry cough, accompanied by almost no expectoration, that occurs in severe coughing spells. It is associated with asthma and emphysema in older people.

**dry cholera.** See **cholera sicca.**

**dry cough,** a cough that does not produce sputum.

**dry crackle,** an abnormal chest sound produced by air passing through a constricted bronchial tube.

**dry dressing,** a plain dressing containing no medication, applied directly to an incision or a wound to prevent contamination or trauma or to absorb secretions.

**dry eye syndrome,** a dryness of the cornea and conjunctiva caused by a deficiency in tear production or altered tear film composition. The condition mainly affects women during and after menopause. It results in a sensation of a foreign body in the eye, burning eyes, keratitis, and erosion of the epithelial layers of the cornea and conjunctiva. See also **Sjögren's syndrome.**

**dry gangrene.** See **gangrene.**

**dry gas (D),** a gas that contains no water vapor.

**dry heat,** a thermal effect produced by adding dry air or reducing the humidity of the environment.

**dry heat sterilization** [AS, *dryge* + *haetu* + L, *sterilis*], a method of sterilization that uses heated dry air at a temperature of 320° to 356° F (160° to 180° C) for 90 minutes to 3 hours.

**dry ice,** solid carbon dioxide, with a temperature of about −140° F. It is used in cryotherapy of various skin disorders, such as the removal of warts.

**dry labor,** *informal.* labor in which amniotic fluid has already escaped. As amniotic fluid is continually produced, no labor is really dry.

**dry mouth.** See **xerostomia.**

**dry pleurisy** [AS, *dryge,* dry; Gk, *pleuritis*], inflammation of the pleura without effusion of serum. The cause may be a localized injury. Dry pleurisy may also be an early sign of tuberculosis.

**Drysdale's corpuscle** /drīz'dālz/ [Thomas M. Drysdale, American gynecologist, 1831–1904], one of a number of transparent cells in the fluid of some ovarian cysts. Also called **Bennet's (small) corpuscle.**

**dry skin,** epidermis that lacks moisture or sebum, often characterized by a pattern of fine lines, scaling, and itching. Causes include too frequent bathing, low humidity, and decreased production of sebum in aging skin. Treatment includes decreased frequency of bathing, increased humidity, bath oils, emollients such as lanolin and glycerin, and hydrophilic ointments. Also called **xerosis** /zēr̄o'sis/.

**dry socket,** an inflamed condition of a tooth socket (alveolus) after a tooth extraction. The socket is not actually dry but is filled with a degenerating, infective blood clot. Normally a blood clot forms over the alveolar bone at the base of the socket after an extraction. If the clot fails to form properly or becomes dislodged, the bone tissue is exposed to the oral environment and can become infected, a usually painful condition. Analgesics, sedatives, and drainage are required, in addition to treatment to cure the infection.

**dry vomiting** [AS, *dryge* + L, *vomere,* to vomit], nausea with retching that does not produce vomitus.

**DSA,** abbreviation for **digital subtraction angiography.**

**DSB,** abbreviation for **drug-seeking behavior.**

**DSDB,** abbreviation for **direct self-destructive behavior.**

**DSM,** abbreviation for *Diagnostic and Statistical Manual of Mental Disorders.*

**DSN,** abbreviation for *Doctor of Science in Nursing.*

**DSR,** abbreviation for **dynamic spatial reconstructor.**

**DT,** abbreviation for **diphtheria and tetanus toxoids.**

**dTc,** abbreviation for *d-tubocurarine.*

**DTH,** abbreviation for **delayed-type hypersensitivity.**

**DTIC-Dome,** trademark for an antineoplastic (dacarbazine).

**DTP vaccine,** a combination of diphtheria and tetanus toxoids and killed pertussis vaccine that is administered intramuscularly for active immunization against those diseases.

**DTR,** abbreviation for **deep tendon reflex.**

**DTs,** abbreviation for **delirium tremens.**

**dual-energy imaging** /dyōo'əl/, a radiographic imaging technique in which two radiographs are taken of the same target area using two different kilovoltages. Because the radiographic image of soft tissue and bone varies with the kilovoltage, one radiograph isolates bone contrast and the other isolates soft tissue contrast. The combined x-ray films can facilitate a more precise identification of an abnormality, such as a lung nodule calcification.

**dual-energy x-ray absorptiometry (DEXA),** an imaging technique for quantifying bone density. It is used in the diagnosis and management of osteoporosis.

**dual-focus tube,** an x-ray tube used for diagnostic imaging. It has one large and one small focal spot. The large focal spot is used when techniques that produce high heat are required; the small focal spot is used to produce fine, detailed images.

**duality of central nervous system control** /dyōo·al'itē/, a theory that the normal central nervous system is regulated by a check-and-balance feedback program. The theory is based on studies of posture-movement, mobility-stability, flexion-extension synergies, and similar action-reaction examples related to laws of basic physics. Duality theorists suggest that central nervous system disorders result from imbalances in the feedback system.

**dual personality.** See **double personality.**

**Duane's syndrome** /dwānz/ [Alexander Duane, American ophthalmologist, 1858−1926], an autosomal dominant syndrome in which the affected eye shows limitation or absence of abduction, restriction of adduction, retraction of the globe on adduction, narrowing of the palpebral fissure on adduction and widening on abduction, and deficient convergence.

**DUB,** **1.** abbreviation for **dysfunctional uterine bleeding.** **2.** a genetically determined human blood factor that is associated with immunity to certain diseases.

**Dubin-Johnson syndrome** /dōo'binjon'sən/ [Isadore N. Dubin, American pathologist, 1913–1980; Frank B. Johnson, American pathologist, b. 1919], a rare chronic hereditary hyperbilirubinemia, characterized by nonhemolytic jaundice, abnormal liver pigmentation, and abnormal function of the gallbladder. It is caused by inability of the liver to excrete several organic anions. See also **hyperbilirubinemia of the newborn, rotor syndrome.**

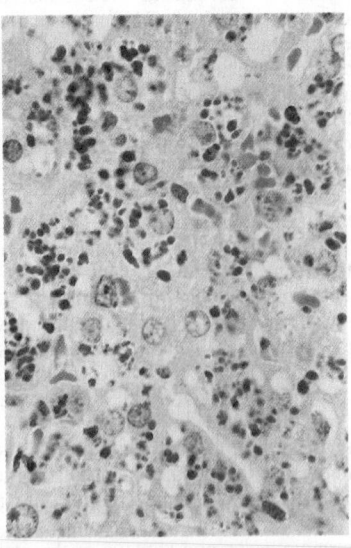

**Dubin-Johnson syndrome** *(Cotran, Kumar, and Collins, 1999)*

**dubnium (Db)** [Joint Institute for Nuclear Research at Dubna, Russia], a transuranic element. Its atomic number is 104; its atomic weight (mass) is 260. It is produced by an induced nuclear reaction. Also called **element 105;** formerly known as hahnium.

**DuBois formula** /d$\overline{oo}$boiz'/, a logarithmic method of calculating the number of square meters of body surface area (BSA) of an individual from the height in centimeters, the weight in kilograms, and a constant, 0.007184.

**Dubowitz assessment** [Victor Dubowitz, South African-English pediatrician, b. 1931], a system of estimating the gestational age of a newborn according to such factors as posture, ankle dorsiflexion, and arm and leg recoil.

**Duchenne-Aran disease** /d$\overline{oo}$shen'äräN'/ [Guillaume B.A. Duchenne; François A. Aran, French physician, 1817–1861], muscular atrophy caused by degeneration of the anterior horn cells of the spinal cord and primarily affecting the upper extremities. Chronic muscle wasting and weakness first appear in the hands and advance progressively to the arms and shoulders, eventually affecting the legs and other body areas. Several conditions may lead to this disease, such as the injection of toxins.

**Duchenne-Erb paralysis.** See **Erb palsy.**

**Duchenne's disease** /d$\overline{oo}$shenz'/ [Guillaume B.A. Duchenne, French neurologist, 1806–1875], a series of three different neurologic conditions: **spinal muscular atrophy, bulbar paralysis,** and **tabes dorsalis.** See also **muscular dystrophy.**

**Duchenne's muscular dystrophy** [Guillaume B.A. Duchenne], an abnormal congenital condition characterized by progressive symmetric wasting of the leg and pelvic muscles. This disease predominantly affects males and accounts for 50% of all muscular dystrophy diseases. It is an X-linked recessive disease that appears insidiously between 3 and 5 years of age and spreads from the leg and pelvic muscles to the involuntary muscles. Associated muscle weakness produces a waddling gait and pronounced lordosis. Muscles rapidly deteriorate, and calf muscles become firm and enlarged as a result of fatty deposits. Affected children experience contractures, have difficulty climbing stairs, often stumble and fall, and display wing scapulae when they raise their arms. Such persons are usually confined to wheelchairs by 12 years of age, and progressive weakening of cardiac muscle causes tachycardia and pulmonary problems. The patients affected may also have cardiac murmurs, faint heart sounds, and chest pain and may suffer arrhythmias or infections that produce overt heart failure. Such complications, especially in the later stages of this disease, can cause sudden death. Duchenne's muscular dystrophy usually causes death within 10 to 15 years of symptom onset. There is no successful treatment of the disease. Orthopedic appliances, exercise, physical therapy, and surgery to correct contractures can help preserve mobility. Nursing care involves psychologic support of the patient and family and encouragement of the patient to prevent long periods of bed rest and inactivity and ensure maximum physical activity. Splints, braces, grab bars, and overhead slings help the patient exercise. A wheelchair helps preserve mobility. Other devices that can increase comfort and help prevent footdrop include footboards, high-topped sneakers, and foot cradles. Also called **pseudohypertrophic muscular dystrophy.**

**Duchenne's paralysis** [Guillaume B.A. Duchenne; Gk, *paralyein,* to be palsied], a form of motor neuron disease characterized by wasting and weakness in the laryngeal, pharyngeal, tongue, and facial muscles, leading to dysarthria and dysphagia. There may also be pyramidal tract involve-

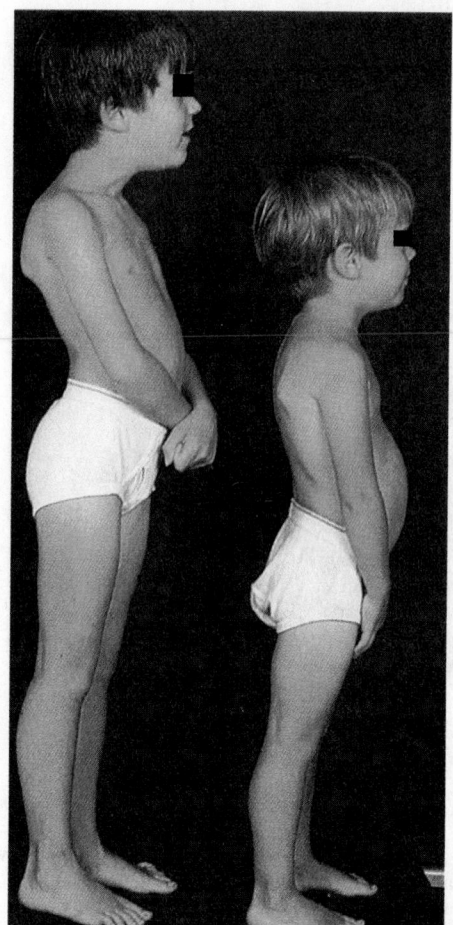

**Duchenne's muscular dystrophy: postural adjustments**
*(Zitelli and Davis, 1997)*

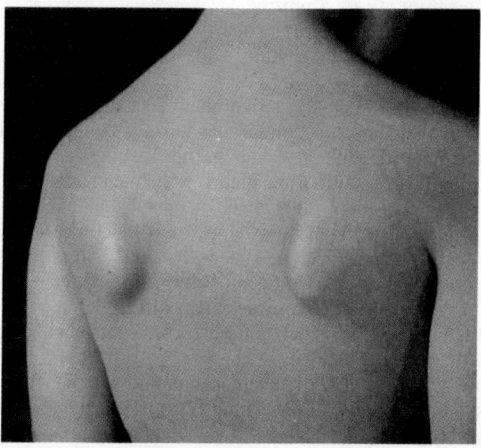

**Duchenne's muscular dystrophy: winged scapulae**
*(Zitelli and Davis, 1997)*

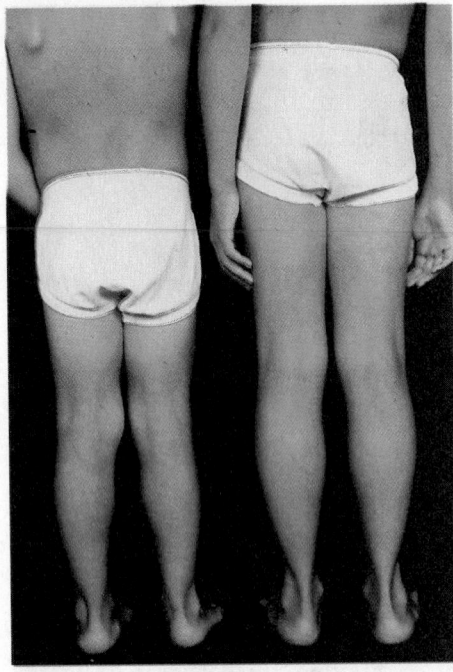

**Duchenne's muscular dystrophy: enlargement of calves**
*(Zitelli and Davis, 1997)*

ment. Also called *Duchenne's syndrome,* **progressive bulbar paralysis.**

**duck embryo vaccine.** See **rabies vaccine.**

**duck walk.** See **metatarsus valgus.**

**duct** [L, *ducere,* to lead], a narrow tubular structure, especially one through which material is secreted or excreted.

**duct carcinoma,** a neoplasm of the epithelium of ducts, especially in the breast or pancreas.

**duct ectasia,** an abnormal dilation of a duct by lipids and cellular debris. In a mammary duct the condition, which tends mainly to affect postmenopausal women, may be accompanied by inflammation and infiltration by plasma cells.

**ductile,** having the property of allowing metals to be drawn into the thinness of a wire.

**ductility** /duktil'itē/, the property of a material of having a large elastic range and tending to deform before failing from stress.

**duction** /duk'shən/, the movement of an individual eyeball from the primary to secondary or tertiary position of gaze.

**ductless gland** /dukt'les/, a gland lacking an excretory duct, such as an endocrine gland, which secretes hormones directly into blood or lymph.

**duct of Rivinus** /rivē'nəs/ Augustus Q. Rivinus, German anatomist, 1652–1723; [L, *ducere,* to lead], one of the minor sublingual ducts. Compare **Bartholin's duct.**

**duct of Wirsung.** See **pancreatic duct.**

**ductus** /duk'təs/, *pl.* **ductus** /duk'tōōs/, the Latin term for *duct.*

**ductus arteriosus,** a vascular channel in the fetus that joins the pulmonary artery directly to the descending aorta. It normally closes after birth.

**ductus deferens.** See **vas deferens.**

**ductus epididymidis,** a tube into which the efferent ductules of the testes empty.

**ductus venosus,** the vascular channel in the fetus passing through the liver and joining the umbilical vein with the inferior vena cava. Before birth it carries highly oxygenated blood from the placenta to the fetal circulation. It closes shortly after birth as pulmonary circulation is established and as the vessels in the umbilical cord collapse and become occluded. See also **ductus arteriosus, foramen ovale.**

**due diligence,** efforts made by responsible persons to prevent causing harm to others or their property or organization.

**Duhring's disease.** See **dermatitis herpetiformis.**

**Duke diet.** See **rice diet.**

**Duke longitudinal study,** long-range in-depth research into the normal aging process of middle-aged and older men and women conducted at Duke University Medical Center, Durham, NC. The Duke studies led to development of the "longevity quotient" (LQ) used to evaluate an individual's rate of aging. It is calculated by the number of years a person survives beyond a given time divided by the expected number of years derived from actuarial tables.

**Dukes' classification,** a staging system for colorectal tumors, from A to D, according to the degree of tissue invasion and metastasis. A Dukes' A tumor is one that is confined to the mucosa and submucosa. A B tumor is one that has invaded the musculature but has not involved the lymphatic system. C tumors have invaded the musculature with metastatic involvement of the regional lymph nodes. D tumors are those that have metastasized to distant organ tissues.

**Dulcolax,** trademark for a stimulant laxative (bisacodyl).

**dull,** 1. blunt. 2. sluggish. 3. not sharp, vivid, or intense.

**dull pain** [ME, *dul,* not sharp; L, *poena,* penalty], a mildly throbbing acute or chronic pain, which may not deter the patient from expected or desired activity.

**dumb terminal** [AS, *tumb,* mute; L, *terminalis,* end], a computer terminal, that serves as an input or output device only and is incapable of performing any data-processing functions by itself. Compare **intelligent terminal.**

**dumdum fever.** See **kala-azar.**

**dump** [ME, *dumpen,* to throw down], 1. to print out the contents of a computer memory or other computer-storage medium. 2. the printout resulting from such an operation.

**dumping syndrome** [ME, *dumpen,* to throw down], the combination of profuse sweating, nausea, dizziness, and weakness experienced by patients who have had a subtotal gastrectomy. Symptoms are felt soon after eating, when the contents of the stomach empty too rapidly into the duodenum. The entrance of this hypertonic material into the small intestine causes fluid to shift into the intestine via osmosis. This increased volume causes peristalsis and diarrhea. The loss of fluid from capillaries causes hypotension with resulting weakness and dizziness. A high-protein, high-calorie diet, with small, dry meals taken frequently, should prevent discomfort and ensure adequate nutrition. See also **gastrectomy.**

**Duncan's mechanism** [James M. Duncan, English obstetrician, 1826–1890; Gk, *mechane,* machine], a technique for delivery of the placenta with the maternal surface rather than the fetal surface presenting.

**Dunlop skeletal traction,** an orthopedic mechanism that helps immobilize the upper limb in the treatment of contracture or supracondylar fracture of the elbow. The mechanism uses a system of traction weights, pulleys, and ropes and may be accompanied by skin traction. Dunlop skeletal traction is usually applied unilaterally but may also be applied bilaterally. Compare **Dunlop skin traction.**

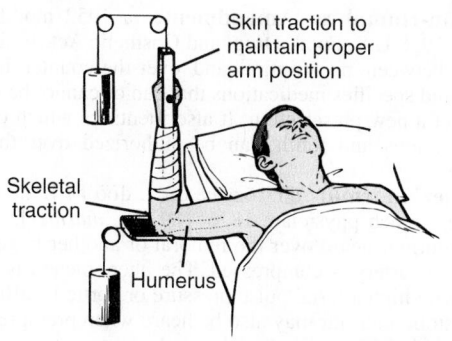

**Dunlop skeletal traction**

**Dunlop skin traction,** an orthopedic mechanism consisting of adhesive or nonadhesive skin traction that helps immobilize the upper limb in the treatment of contracture or supracondylar fracture of the elbow. The mechanism uses a system of traction weights, pulleys, and ropes, usually applied unilaterally but sometimes bilaterally. Compare **Dunlop skeletal traction.**

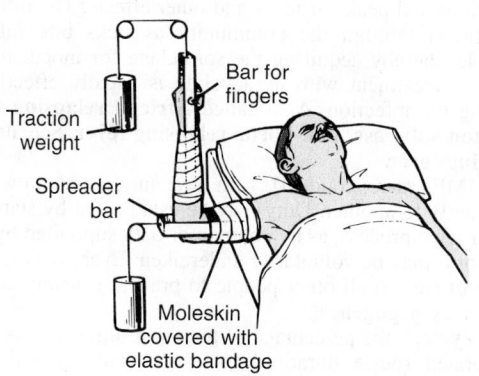

**Dunlop skin traction**

**duodena.** See **duodenum.**
**duodenal** /dōō'ədē'nəl/ [L, *duodeni,* 12 fingers], pertaining to the duodenum.
**duodenal atresia,** congenital absence or occlusion of a portion of the duodenum, characterized by vomiting a few hours after birth, cessation of bowel movements after one to three days, and usually distension of the epigastrium. It is often associated with Down syndrome.
**duodenal bulb,** the first part of the superior portion of the duodenum, which has a bulblike appearance on radiographic views of the small intestine.
**duodenal digestion** [L, *duodeni,* 12 fingers, *digere,* to separate], digestion that occurs in the first intestinal segment beyond the pylorus, where secretions of the liver and pancreas are received and mixed with the partially digested food from the stomach. Chyle is formed, fats are emulsified, starch is hydrolyzed, and proteolytic enzymes begin to break down proteins.
**duodenal mesentery.** See **mesoduodenum.**

**duodenal ulcer,** an ulcer in the duodenum, the most common type of peptic ulcer. See also **peptic ulcer.**
**duodenectomy** /dōō'ədēnek'təmē/ [L, *duodeni,* 12 fingers, Gk, *ektomē,* excision], the total or partial excision of the duodenum.
**duodenitis** /dōō'ədēnī'tis/ [L, *duodeni,* 12 fingers; Gk, *itis,* inflammation], a condition of inflammation of the duodenum.
**duodeno-,** combining form meaning 'duodenum': *duodenocolic, duodenohepatic, duodenostomy.*
**duodenogastric reflux** /dōō'ə·dē'nō·gas'trik/ [L, *duodeni,* 12 fingers + Gk, *gaster,* stomach; L, *refluere,* to flow back], reflux of the contents of the duodenum into the stomach; it may occur normally, especially during fasting.
**duodenogastroesophageal reflux.** See **gastroesophageal reflux.**
**duodenography** /dōō'ədənog'rəfē/ [L, *duodeni,* 12 fingers; Gk, *graphein,* to record], the radiographic examination of the duodenum and pancreas. It usually requires drug-induced paralysis of the duodenum to prevent peristaltic activity, use of a double-contrast medium, and maximum distension with the contrast medium so that the duodenum presses against and outlines the head of the pancreas. Also called **hypotonic duodenography.**
**duodenojejunal flexure.** See **angle of Treitz.**
**duodenoscope** /dōō'ədē'nəskōp'/, an endoscopic instrument, usually fiberoptic, inserted via the mouth for the visual examination of the duodenum.
**duodenoscopy** /dōō'ədēnos'kəpē/, the visual examination of the duodenum by means of an endoscope.
**duodenostomy** /dōō'ədēnos'təmē/ [L, *duodeni,* 12 fingers; Gk, *stoma,* mouth], the surgical creation of a direct opening to the duodenum through the abdominal wall.
**duodenum** /dōō'ədē'nəm, dōō·od'inəm/, *pl.* **duodena, duodenums** [L, *duodeni,* 12 fingers], the shortest, widest, and most fixed portion of the small intestine, taking an almost circular course from the pyloric valve of the stomach so that its termination is close to its starting point. It is about 25 cm long and is divided into superior, descending, horizontal, and ascending portions. The superior portion extends from the pylorus to the neck of the gallbladder. The descending portion extends from the neck of the gallbladder at the level of the first lumbar vertebra to the cranial border of the fourth lumbar vertebra. The horizontal portion passes from right to left, from the level of the fourth lumbar vertebra to the diaphragm. The ascending portion rises on the left side of the aorta to the level of the second lumbar vertebra, turning ventrally to become the jejunum at the duodenojejunal flexure. Compare **jejunum, ileum.**
**dup,** (in cytogenetics) abbreviation for *duplication.*
**duplex inheritance.** See **amphigenous inheritance.**
**duplex scanner** /dōō'pleks/, an ultrasound machine that generally combines a 7.5- or 10-MHz imaging probe with a 3-MHz pulsed Doppler to allow visualization of a portion of the venous system. The scanner can determine the direction of blood flow within the veins.
**duplex transmission** [L, *duplex,* twofold], the passage of a neural impulse in both directions along a nerve fiber.
**duplex ultrasonography,** a combination of real-time and Doppler ultrasonography. See also **duplex scanner.**
**duplicating film** /dōō'plikā'ting/, a single-emulsion film used to copy an existing radiographic image by exposing it to ultraviolet light.
**duplicatus anterior.** See **anadidymus.**
**dupp** /dup/, a syllable used to represent the second heart sound in auscultation; it is shorter and higher pitched than the first heart sound. See **heart sound.**

**Dupuytren's contracture** /dYpY·itraNs', dēpē·itranz'/ [Guillaume Dupuytren, French surgeon, 1777–1835; L *contractura* drawing together], a progressive painless thickening and tightening of subcutaneous tissue of the palm, causing the fourth and fifth fingers to bend into the palm and resist extension. Tendons and nerves are not involved. Although the condition begins in one hand, both become symmetrically affected. Of unknown cause, it is most frequent in middle-aged males. Early surgical removal of the excess fibrous tissue under general anesthesia restores full use of the hand. An incision is made in the palm, and the thickened tissue is excised carefully to prevent injury to adjacent ligaments.

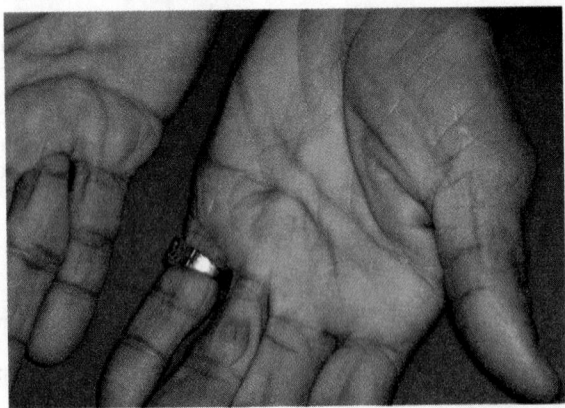

**Dupuytren's contracture** *(Lemmi and Lemmi, 2000)*

**Dupuytren's fracture.** See **Galeazzi's fracture.**
**dura.** See **dura mater.**
**durable power of attorney for health care** /dyŏŏr'əbəl/, a document that designates an agent or proxy to make health care decisions if the patient is no longer able to make them. The document directs the surrogate person to function as "attorney-in-fact" and make decisions regarding all treatment, including the final decision about cessation of treatment.
**Durabolin,** trademark for an anabolic steroid (nandrolone phenpropionate).
**dural sac** /dyŏŏr'əl/, the blind pouch formed by the lower end of the dura mater, at the level of the second sacral segment.
**dural sheath,** an extension of the dura mater covering the optic nerve and spinal nerve roots.
**dura mater** /dŏŏ'rə mā'tər, dyŏŏ'rə/ [L, *durus,* hard, *mater,* mother], the outermost and most fibrous of the three membranes surrounding the brain and spinal cord. The **dura mater encephali** covers the brain, and the **dura mater spinalis** covers the cord. See also **meninges.**
**Duranest,** trademark for a local anesthetic (etidocaine hydrochloride).
**duration,** the length of time a current is flowing. Also called **pulse width.**
**duration tetany.** See **tetany.**
**duress** /dyŏŏres'/ [L, *durus,* hard], (in law) an action compelling another person to do what he or she would not do voluntarily. A consent form signed under duress is not valid.

**Durham-Humphrey Amendment,** a 1952 modification of the 1938 U.S. Food, Drug, and Cosmetic Act. It differentiates between prescription and over-the-counter medications and specifies medications that can or cannot be refilled without a new prescription. It also identifies which original prescriptions and refills can be authorized over the telephone.
**Duroziez' murmur** /dY'rōzyās, dir'-, dōō'r-/ [Paul L. Duroziez, French physician, 1826–1897; L, *murmur*], a systolic murmur heard over the femoral or another large artery when the artery is compressed. The phenomenon is associated with high arterial pulse pressure or aortic insufficiency. A diastolic murmur may also be heard when pressure on the artery is increased distal to the stethoscope.
**dust** [AS], any fine, particulate, dry matter. Kinds of dust include **inorganic dust** and **organic dust.**
**dustborne infection,** a disease in which the pathogenic organism is airborne in dust particles, as in coccidioidomycosis.
**dust fever.** See **brucellosis.**
**Dutton's relapsing fever** [Joseph E. Dutton, English pathologist, 1877–1905], an infection caused by a spirochete, *Borrelia duttonii,* which is transmitted by a soft tick, *Ornithodoros moubata,* found in human dwellings in tropical Africa. The spirochete enters the lesion through a tick bite, characteristically producing a high fever, chills, rapid heartbeat, headache, joint and muscle pain, vomiting, and neurologic disorders. The symptoms recur in a pattern of remissions and peaks of fever and other effects. The infection is spread through the community as ticks bite infected people, thereby acquiring the spirochete for inoculation in others. Treatment with tetracycline is usually effective in curing the infection. Also called **African relapsing fever, Dutton's disease, tick-borne relapsing fever.** See also **relapsing fever.**
**duty** [ME, *duete,* conduct], (in law) an obligation owed by one party to another. Duty may be established by statute or other legal process, as by contract or oath supported by statute, or it may be voluntarily undertaken. Every person has a duty of care to all other people to prevent causing harm or injury by negligence.
**duty cycle,** the percentage of time that ultrasound is being generated (pulse duration) over one pulse period. Also called **duty factor, mark:space ratio.**
**Duverney's fracture** /dōō'vərnāz'/ [Joseph G. Duverney, French anatomist, 1648–1730], a break in the ilium just below the anterior superior spine.
**Duvoid,** trademark for a cholinergic receptor agonist (bethanechol chloride) available only in Canada.
**dV/dt,** the rate of change of voltage with respect to time.
**D.V.M.,** abbreviation for *Doctor of Veterinary Medicine.*
**dwarf** /dwôrf/ [AS, *dweorge*], **1.** also called **nanus.** an abnormally short, undersized person, especially one whose body parts are not proportional. Kinds of dwarfs include **achondroplastic dwarf, asexual dwarf, ateliotic dwarf, Brissaud's dwarf, cretin dwarf, diastrophic dwarf, nanocephalic dwarf, phocomelic dwarf, pituitary dwarf, primordial dwarf, rachitic dwarf, renal dwarf, Russell dwarf, sexual dwarf, Silver dwarf,** and **thanatophoric dwarf. 2.** to prevent or retard, for example, normal growth.
**dwarfism** /dwôrf'izəm/, the abnormal underdevelopment of the body, characterized predominantly by extreme shortness of stature, although the condition is associated with numerous other defects and may involve varying degrees of mental retardation. Dwarfism has multiple causes, including genetic defects, endocrine dysfunction involving either the pituitary or thyroid gland, chronic diseases such as rickets,

renal failure, intestinal malabsorption defects, and psychosocial stress, as in the maternal deprivation syndrome. See also **dwarf.**

**dwarf tapeworm infection,** a type of intestinal parasitic disease caused by an infestation of *Hymenolepis nana.* It occurs mainly in the southern United States and usually affects children who ingest eggs by placing contaminated materials into the mouth. The disease may be asymptomatic or may result in abdominal complaints and diarrhea. An infection may be treated with niclosamide or paromomycin. See also *Hymenolepis.*

**Dwayne-Hunt law** /dwān′hunt′/, the principle that x-ray energy is inversely proportional to the photon wavelength. Thus, as the photon wavelength increases, photon energy decreases, and vice versa.

**dwindles,** *informal.* a condition of physical deterioration involving several body systems, usually in an elderly person.

**Dwyer instrumentation** /dwī′ər/, one method for correcting the spinal curvature associated with scoliosis. The Dwyer cable method uses a mechanical device that assists in correcting the curvature. The device is inserted to assist in maintaining the corrected curvature while the fusion heals; it is not usually removed unless there is postoperative indication of displacement or a pattern of associated symptoms. Dwyer cable instrumentation involves surgical intervention through the pulmonary cavity and the rib cage and is accompanied by a relatively greater surgical risk than a posterior approach. It is often inadequate to correct the spinal curvature involved and must frequently be followed several weeks later by a posterior spinal fusion.

**D-xylose absorption test,** a blood or urine test whose results reflect intestinal absorption, since the monosaccharide D-xylose is not metabolized by the body. In patients with malabsorption, intestinal D-xylose absorption is diminished, and as a result, blood levels and urine excretion are reduced. The test is used to separate patients with diarrhea caused by maldigestion (pancreatic/biliary dysfunction) from those with diarrhea cause by malabsorption (sprue, Whipple's disease, Crohn's disease).

**Dy,** symbol for the element **dysprosium.**

**dyad** /dī′ad/ [Gk, *dyas,* two], one of the paired homologous chromosomes, consisting of two chromatids, which result from the division of a tetrad in the first meiotic division of gametogenesis. —**dyadic,** *adj.*

**dyadic interpersonal communication** /dī·ad′ik/, a process in which two people interact face to face as senders and receivers, as in a conversation.

**Dyazide,** trademark for a fixed-combination drug containing two diuretic agents (triamterene and hydrochlorothiazide).

**Dyclone,** trademark for a local anesthetic (dyclonine hydrochloride).

**dyclonine hydrochloride** /dī′klōnīn/, a local anesthetic, with bactericidal and fungicidal properties, for oral pain, pruritis, insect bites, and minor skin burns and injuries.

**dye** /dī/ [AS, *deag*], **1.** to apply coloring to a substance. **2.** a chemical compound capable of imparting color to a substance to which it is applied. Various dyes are used in medicine as stains for tissues, test reagents, therapeutic agents, and coloring agents in pharmaceutic preparations.

**dye laser,** a system of highly selective laser destruction of skin blemishes using various dyes at wavelengths at the longer oxygenated hemoglobin absorption peaks to overcome interference from overlying melanin.

**dying care,** a nursing intervention from the Nursing Interventions Classification (NIC) defined as promotion of physi-

cal comfort and psychological peace in the final phase of life. See also **Nursing Interventions Classification.**

**Dymelor,** trademark for an antidiabetic (acetohexamide).

**-dynamia, -dynamy,** suffix meaning '(condition of) strength': *ataxiadynamia, hyperdynamia, plastodynamia.*

**dynamic** /dīnam′ik/ [Gk, *dynamis,* force], **1.** tending to change or to encourage change, such as a dynamic nurse-patient relationship. **2.** (in respiratory therapy) a condition of changing volume. Compare **static.**

**dynamic cardiac work,** the energy transfer that occurs during the ventricular ejection of blood.

**dynamic compliance,** the distensibility of the lungs, as measured by plethysmography during the breathing cycle. See also **lung compliance.**

**dynamic equilibrium,** the ability of a person to adjust to displacements of the body's center of gravity by changing its base of support.

**dynamic ileus,** an intestinal obstruction with associated recurrent and continuous muscle spasms. Also called **spastic ileus.**

**dynamic imaging,** the ultrasonographic imaging of an object in motion at a frame rate that does not cause significant blurring of images and at a repetition rate sufficient to represent the movement pattern adequately. Also called **real-time imaging.**

**dynamic nurse-patient relationship,** a conceptual framework in which the interpersonal aspects of the nurse-patient relationship are analyzed. Many factors affect the relationship. Elements in the process include the behavior of the patient, the reaction of the nurse, and the actions of the nurse that are intended to aid the patient. Also examined are the means for validating nurses' perceptions and interpretations and for evaluating the effects of the nursing actions taken.

**dynamic psychiatry,** the study of motivational, emotional, and biologic factors as determinants of human behavior.

**dynamic range,** **1.** in radiology, the range of voltage or input signals that result in a digital output. **2.** the range of sound intensity from the faintest sound a person can hear to the level that causes pain.

**dynamic response,** the accuracy with which a physiologic monitoring system such as an electrocardiograph simulates the actual event being recorded.

**dynamic spatial reconstructor (DSR),** a radiographic device that allows moving, three-dimensional images of organs to be examined from any direction. It is used in research.

**dynamic splint** [Gk, *dynamis,* force; D, *splinte*], any splint that incorporates springs, elastic bands, or other materials that produce a constant active force to counteract deforming forces of a splint.

**dynamo-,** combining form meaning 'power or strength': *dynamogenesis, dynamometer, dynamophore.*

**dynamometer** /dī′nəmom′ətər/ [Gk, *dynamis,* force, *metron,* measure], a device for measuring the degree of force used in the contraction of a group of muscles, such as a squeeze dynamometer, which measures the gross grip strength of the hand muscles. Also called **ergometer.**

**-dynamy.** See **-dynamia.**

**Dynapen,** trademark for an antibiotic (dicloxacillin sodium).

**dyne** /dīn/, a unit of force, specifically the force required to accelerate a free mass of 1 g at 1 cm/sec. One dyne equals $10^{-5}$ newton.

**-dynia,** suffix meaning 'pain': *cephalodynia, gastrodynia.*

**dynode** /dī′nōd/, one of a series of platelike elements that amplify electron pulses in a photomultiplier tube. Each electron that strikes a dynode, causes several secondary electrons to be emitted. The dynode gain is the ratio of the number of secondary electrons to the number of incident electrons.

**dynorphin** /dīnôr′fən/, an endogenous opioid derived from the prohormone prodynorphin. It is a neuroactive peptide with potent analgesic effects.

**dyphylline** /dīfil′in/, a bronchodilator.

■ INDICATIONS: It is prescribed in the treatment of bronchospasm in acute bronchial asthma, bronchitis, and emphysema.

■ CONTRAINDICATIONS: It is used with caution in patients with peptic ulcer or cardiovascular disease. Known hypersensitivity to this or to other xanthines prohibits its use.

■ ADVERSE EFFECTS: Among the more serious adverse reactions are GI distress, dizziness, tachycardia, headache, and palpitations.

**Dyrenium,** trademark for a potassium-sparing diuretic (triamterene).

**dys-,** prefix meaning 'bad, painful, disordered': *dysadrenia, dysbolism, dysmnesia.*

**dysacusis** /dis′əkoo′sis/ [Gk, *dys,* difficult, *akouein,* to hear], a condition in which loud sounds can cause pain or discomfort. It is usually the result of damage to the cochlea. Also called **dysacousia, dysacousma.**

**dysadrenia** /dis′adrē′nē·ə/ [Gk, *dys,* bad; L, *ad,* to, *ren,* kidney], abnormal adrenal function characterized by decreased hormone production, as in hypoadrenalism or hypoadrenocorticism, or by increased secretion of the products of the gland, as in hyperadrenalism or hyperadrenocorticism. Also called **dysadrenalism.**

**dysaesthesia.** See **dysesthesia.**

**dysaphia.** See **paraphia.**

**dysarthria** /disär′thrē·ə/ [Gk, *dys* + *arthroun,* to articulate], difficult, poorly articulated speech, resulting from interference in the control and execution over the muscles of speech, usually caused by damage to a central or peripheral motor nerve.

**dysarthrosis** /dis′ärthrō′sis/ [Gk, *dys,* difficult, *arthron,* joint], any disorder of a joint, including disease, dislocation, or deformity, that makes movement of the joint difficult.

**dysautonomia** /disô′tənō′mē·ə/ [Gk, *dys* + *autonomia,* self-government], an autosomal recessive disease of childhood characterized by defective lacrimation, skin blotching, emotional instability, motor incoordination, total absence of pain sensation, and hyporeflexia; seen almost exclusively in Ashkenazi Jews. Also called **familial autonomic dysfunction, familial dysautonomia, Riley-Day syndrome.**

**dysbarism** /dis′bäriz′əm/, a reaction to a sudden change in environmental pressure, such as rapid exposure to the lower atmospheric pressures of high altitudes. It is marked by symptoms similar to those of decompression sickness.

**dysbasia** /disbā′zhə/, difficulty in walking caused by a nerve lesion or lameness associated with atherosclerosis.

**dysbetalipoproteinemia** /disbet′əlip′əprō′tinē′mē·ə/, an accumulation of abnormal beta-lipoprotein in the blood. See **broad beta disease.**

**dyscholia** /diskō′lē·ə/ [Gk, *dys* + *chole,* bile], any abnormal condition of the bile, related to either the quantity secreted or the condition of the constituents.

**dyschondroplasia.** See **enchondromatosis.**

**dyschroic film fault** /diskrō′ik/, a defect in a photograph or radiograph that appears as a pinkish coloration when the film is viewed by transmitted light and as a green coloration when the film is viewed by reflected light. It is usually caused by incomplete fixation of the film or by an overused fixing solution with a depleted acid concentration.

**dyscrasia** /diskrā′zhə/ [Gk, *dys* + *krasis,* mingling], pertaining to an abnormal condition of the blood or bone marrow, such as leukemia, aplastic anemia, or prenatal Rh incompatibility.

**dyscrastic fracture** /diskras′tik/, any fracture caused by the weakening of a specific bone as a result of a debilitating disease.

**dysdiadochokinesia** /dis′dī·ədō′kōkinē′zhə/ [Gk, *dys* + *diadochos,* working in turn, *kinesis,* movement], an inability to perform rapidly alternating movements, such as rhythmically tapping the fingers on the knee. The cause is a cerebellar lesion and is related to dysmetria, which also involves inappropriate timing of muscle activity. Also called **dysdiadochokinesis.**

**dysenteric** /dis′enter′ik/ [Gk, *dys* + *enteron,* intestine], pertaining to or resembling dysentery.

**dysentery** /dis′inter′ē/ [Gk, *dys* + *enteron,* intestine], an inflammation of the intestine, especially of the colon, that may be caused by chemical irritants, bacteria, protozoa, or parasites. It is characterized by frequent and bloody stools, abdominal pain, and tenesmus. Dysentery is common in underdeveloped areas of the world and in times of disaster and social disorganization when sanitary living conditions, clean food, and safe water are not available. See also **amebic dysentery, shigellosis.**

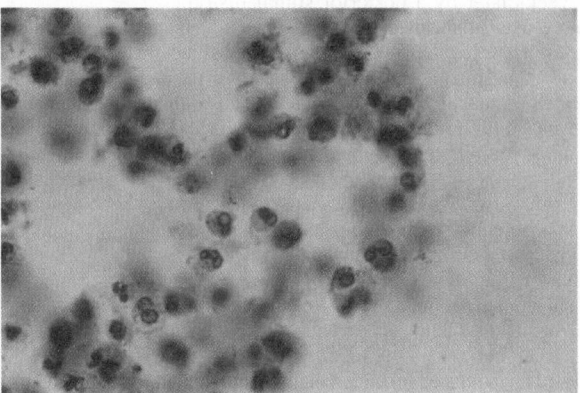

**Fecal smear from a patient with bacillary dysentery**
*(Auerbach, 1995)*

**dysentery toxin,** an exotoxin produced by *Shigella dysenteriae.*

**dysentry.** See **dysentery.**

**dysergia** /disur′jē·ə/ [Gk, *dys* + *ergon,* work], a condition characterized by lack of muscle coordination caused by a defect of efferent nerve impulses.

**dysesthesia** /dis′esthē′zhə/, a common effect of spinal cord injury characterized by sensations of numbness, tingling, burning, or pain felt below the level of the lesion. Also spelled **dysaesthesia.**

**dysfluency** /dis·floo′ən·sē/ [Gk, *dys-,* difficult + L, *fluere,* to flow], difficulty of proceeding, said of speech disorders such as stuttering. —**dysfluent,** *adj.*

**dysfunctional** /disfungk'shənəl/ [Gk, *dys* + L, *functio*, performance], (of a body organ or system) unable to function normally. —**dysfunction,** *n.*

**dysfunctional communication,** a communication that results from inaccurate perceptions, faulty internal filters (personal interpretations of information), and social isolation. Communication behaviors of emotionally ill persons may have characteristics that prevent their establishing and maintaining relationships with others.

**dysfunctional stereotype,** a stereotype in which abnormal or impaired aspects of a culture are emphasized.

**dysfunctional uterine bleeding (DUB),** abnormal uterine bleeding that is not caused by a tumor, inflammation, or pregnancy. It may be characterized by painless, irregular heavy bleeding or intermenstrual spotting or periods of amenorrhea. The condition is associated with anovulation and unopposed estrogen stimulation. The plan of treatment depends on the patient's age and may include dilation and curettage and use of hormones and other medications.

**dysgammaglobulinemia** /disgam'əglob'yəline'me·ə/, an inherited immunodeficiency disease. Affected individuals do not produce adequate numbers of immunoglobulins, including antibodies, and therefore are susceptible to infection, cancer, and other diseases. Also spelled **dysgammaglobulinaemia.**

**dysgenesis** /disjen'əsis/ [Gk, *dys* + *genein*, to produce], **1.** also called **dysgenesia.** defective or abnormal formation of an organ or part, primarily during embryonic development. **2.** impairment or loss of ability to procreate. A kind of dysgenesis is **gonadal dysgenesis.** Compare **agenesis.** —**dysgenic,** *adj.*

**dysgenics** /disjen'iks/, the study of factors or situations that are genetically detrimental to the future of a race or species. Compare **eugenics.**

**dysgenitalism** /disjen'itəliz'əm/ [Gk, *dys* + L, *genitalis*, belonging to birth], any condition involving the abnormal development of the genital organs.

**dysgerminoma** /dis'jərmino'mə/, *pl.* **dysgerminomas, dysgerminomata** [Gk, *dys* + L, *germen*, germ; Gk, *oma*, tumor], a rare malignant tumor of the ovary, which occurs in young women and is believed to arise from the undifferentiated germ cells of the embryonic gonad. The tumor is histologically identical to seminoma. Dysgerminomas are extremely sensitive to irradiation and chemotherapy, and most patients retain their fertility. Also called **embryoma of the ovary, ovarian seminoma.**

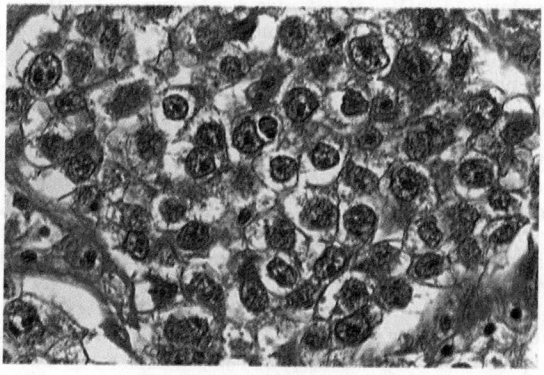

**Dysgerminoma** *(Fletcher, 2000)*

**dysgeusia** /disgoo'zhə/ [Gk, *dys* + *geusis*, taste], an abnormal or impaired sense of taste.

**dysglandular** /disglan'dyələr/, caused by or related to excessive or inadequate secretion by a gland.

**dysgnathia.** See **dysgnathic anomaly.**

**dysgnathic anomaly** /disnath'ik/ [Gk, *dys* + *gnathos*, jaw], an abnormality that affects one or both jaws.

**dysgraphia** /disgraf'e·ə/ [Gk, *dys* + *graphein*, to write], an impairment of the ability to write. Compare **agraphia.**

**dyshidrosis** /dis·hī·drō'sis/ [Gk, *dys*, difficult + *hidros*, sweat], any disorder of the eccrine sweat glands. Spelled also **dyshydrosis.**

**dyskeratosis** /dis'kerətō'sis/ [Gk, *dys* + *keras*, horn, *osis*, condition], an abnormal or premature keratinization of epithelial cells.

**dyskeratosis congenita,** an X-linked syndrome with onset in childhood, characterized by nail dystrophy, reticular cutaneous hyperpigmentation, mucosal leukokeratosis, and pancytopenia resembling that of Fanconi's syndrome.

**dyskinesia** /dis'kine'zhə/ [Gk, *dys* + *kinesis*, movement], an impairment of the ability to execute voluntary movements. Tardive dyskinesia is caused by an adverse effect of prolonged use of phenothiazine medications in elderly patients or those with brain injuries. See also **tardive dyskinesia.** —**dyskinetic** /-et'ik/, *adj.*

**dyskinesia intermittens,** a condition of intermittent limping caused by circulatory impairment.

**dyskinetic syndrome** /dis'kinet'ik/, a form of cerebral palsy involving a basal ganglion disorder. Clinical features include athetoid movements of the extremities and sometimes the trunk. There may also be choreiform movements that tend to increase with emotional tension and diminish during sleep.

**dyslexia** /dislek'se·ə/ [Gk, *dys* + *lexis*, word], an impairment of the ability to read, as a result of a variety of pathologic conditions, some of which are associated with the central nervous system. Dyslexic persons often reverse letters and words, cannot adequately distinguish the letter sequences in written words, and have difficulty determining left from right. Compare **alexia.** —**dyslexic,** *adj.*

**dyslipidemia** /dis·lip'id·ē'mē·ə/ [Gk, *dys*, difficult + *lipid* + Gk, *haima*, blood], abnormality in, or abnormal amounts of, lipids and lipoproteins in the blood. See also **hyperlipidemia** and **hypolipoproteinemia.**

**dysmaturity** /dis'machoŏr'ite/ [Gk, *dys* + L, *maturare*, to make ripe], **1.** the failure of an organism to develop, ripen, or otherwise achieve maturity in structure or function. **2.** the condition of a fetus or newborn that is abnormally small or large for its age of gestation. Kinds of dysmaturity are **small for gestational age** and **large for gestational age.** Compare **postmature, premature.** —**dysmature,** *adj.*

**dysmegalopsia** /dis'megəlop'se·ə/ [Gk, *dys* + *megas*, large, *opsis*, appearance], an inability to judge the size or measure of an object accurately. Also called **dysmetropsia.**

**dysmelia** /dismē'lyə/ [Gk, *dys* + *melos*, limb], an abnormal congenital condition characterized by missing or shortened extremities of the body and associated with abnormalities of the spine in some individuals. It is caused by abnormal metabolism during the embryonic development of the limbs. See also **phocomelia.**

**dysmenorrhea** /dis'menəre'ə/ [Gk, *dys* + *men*, month, *rhein*, to flow], pain associated with menstruation. Primary dysmenorrhea is menstrual pain that results from factors intrinsic to the uterus and the process of menstruation. It is extremely common, occurring at least occasionally in almost all women. If the painful episode is mild and brief, it is considered functional and normal and requires no treatment. In approximately 10% of women dysmenorrhea is sufficiently severe to cause episodes of partial or total disability. The cause in most cases is poorly understood; various anatomic, neurohormonal, and psychosomatic abnormalities have been suggested. Pain occurs typically in the lower abdomen or back and is crampy, occurring in successive waves —apparently in conjunction with intense uterine contractions and slight cervical dilation. Pain usually begins just before, or at the onset of, menstrual flow and lasts from a few hours to 1 day or more; it may persist through the entire period in a few women. Pain is frequently associated with nausea, vomiting, and frequent bowel movements with intestinal cramping. Dizziness, fainting, pallor, and obvious distress may also be observed. Treatment with an antiprostaglandin provides relief for many women if begun 1 to 3 days before menstruation and continued through the first day of the menses. Oral contraceptive steroids are also effective for many women and are taken through the full monthly cycle. Potent analgesics or narcotics may be required by a few women. Secondary dysmenorrhea is menstrual pain that occurs secondary to specific pelvic abnormalities, such as endometriosis, adenomyosis, chronic pelvic infection, chronic pelvic congestion, or degenerating fibroid tumors. Typically the pain begins earlier in the cycle and lasts longer than the pain of primary dysmenorrhea. Painful bowel or bladder function may accompany the condition, depending on the location of the specific lesions. Diagnosis of the chief cause is made by pelvic examination, ultrasonography, laparoscopy, or laparotomy. Treatment is directed at the specific organic disease involved. Also spelled **dysmenorrhoea.** Also called **menorrhalgia.**

**dysmetria** /dismē′trē·ə/ [Gk, *dys* + *metron,* measure],   an abnormal condition that prevents the affected individual from properly measuring distances associated with muscular acts and from controlling muscular action. It is associated with cerebellar lesions and typically characterized by overestimating or underestimating the range of motion needed to place the limbs correctly during voluntary movement. A normal person with eyes closed can move the arms from a position of 90 degrees of flexion to a position over the head and then return them to the 90-degree position; a person with dysmetria is unable to perform this test accurately. See also **hypermetria, hypometria.**

**dysmetropsia.**   See **dysmegalopsia.**

**dysmnesic syndrome** /disnē′sik/,   a memory disorder characterized by an inability to learn simple new skills although the person can still perform highly complex skills learned before the onset of the condition. The cause is a disease or injury that affects only certain brain tissues associated with memory. The victim often confabulates about events of the recent past for which there is no clear memory. Also called **dysmnesia.**

**dysmorphogenesis** /dis′môrfōjen′əsis/,   the development of ill-shaped or otherwise malformed body structures.

**dysmorphophobia** /-fō′bē·ə/ [Gk, *dys* + *morphe,* form, *phobos,* fear],   **1.** a fundamental delusion of body image. **2.** the morbid fear of deformity.

**dysorexia** /dis′ôrek′sē·ə/,   an eating disorder associated with emotional or psychologic impairment.

**dysostosis** /dis′ostō′sis/ [Gk, *dys* + *osteon,* bone, *osis*],   an abnormal condition characterized by defective ossification, especially defects in the normal ossification of fetal cartilages. Kinds of dysostoses include **cleidocranial dysostosis, craniofacial dysostosis, mandibulofacial dysostosis, metaphyseal dysostosis,** and **Nager's acrofacial dysostosis.**

**dysostosis mandibularis.**   See **Nager's acrofacial dysostosis.**

**dyspareunia** /dis′pəroo̅′nē·ə/ [Gk, *dys* + *pareunos,* mating],   an abnormal pain during sexual intercourse. It may result from abnormal conditions of the genitalia, dysfunctional psychophysiologic reaction to sexual union, forcible coition, or incomplete sexual arousal. Dyspareunia is also associated with hormonal changes of the menopause and lactation that result in drying of the vaginal tissues as well as with endometriosis. Painful adhesions around the vagina and ligaments may result, decreasing their flexibility during intercourse. Dryness is commonly relieved by the local application of water-soluble lubricants. See also **vaginismus.**

**dyspepsia** /dispep′sē·ə/ [Gk, *dys* + *peptein,* to digest],   a vague feeling of epigastric discomfort after eating. There is an uncomfortable feeling of fullness, heartburn, bloating, and nausea. Dyspepsia is not a distinct condition, but it may be a sign of an underlying intestinal disorder such as peptic ulcer, gallbladder disease, or chronic appendicitis. Symptoms usually increase in times of stress. —**dyspeptic,** *adj.*

**dysphagia** /disfā′jē·ə/ [Gk, *dys* + *phagein,* to swallow],   difficulty in swallowing, commonly associated with obstructive or motor disorders of the esophagus. Patients with obstructive disorders such as esophageal tumor or lower esophageal ring are unable to swallow solids but can tolerate liquids. Persons with motor disorders, such as achalasia, are unable to swallow solids or liquids. Diagnosis of the underlying condition is made through barium studies, the observed clinical signs, and evaluation of the patient's symptoms. See also **achalasia, aphagia, corkscrew esophagus.**

**dysphagia lusoria,**   an abnormal condition, characterized by difficulty in swallowing, caused by the compression of the esophagus from an anomalous right subclavian artery that arises from the descending aorta and courses behind or in front of the esophagus. Compare **contractile ring dysphagia, vallecular dysphagia.**

**dysphasia.**   See **aphasia.**

**dysphonia** /disfō′nē·ə/ [Gk, *dys* + *phone,* voice],   any abnormality in the speaking voice, such as hoarseness. Dysphonia puberum identifies the voice changes that occur in adolescent boys.

**dysphoria** /disfôr′ē·ə/,   a disorder of affect characterized by depression and anguish.

**dysphrasia.**   See **dysphasia.**

**dysphylaxia** /dis′filek′sē·ə/,   a sudden awakening from deep sleep or a condition marked by too early awakening.

**dyspigmentation** /dispig′məntā′shən/,   any abnormality in the production or distribution of skin pigment. See also **depigmentation.**

**dysplasia** /displā′zhə/ [Gk, *dys* + *plassein,* to form],   any abnormal development of tissues or organs. An alteration in cell growth results in cells that differ in size, shape, and appearance often as a result of chronic irritation. Common sites for dysplasia are the respiratory tract in smokers and the cervix.

**-dysplasia,**   combining form meaning '(condition of) abnormal development': *chondrodysplasia, epidermodysplasia, osteomyelodysplasia.*

**dysplasia epiphysealis hemimelica,**   a rare condition characterized by swellings in the extremities, usually on the inner and outer aspects of the ankles and knees, consisting of bone covered with epiphyseal cartilage, leading to limitation of motion of the joints. Also called **Trevor's disease.**

**dysplastic nevus,**   an acquired atypical nevus with an irregular border, indistinct margin, and mixed coloration, often occurring in large numbers and often a precursor of malignant melanoma.

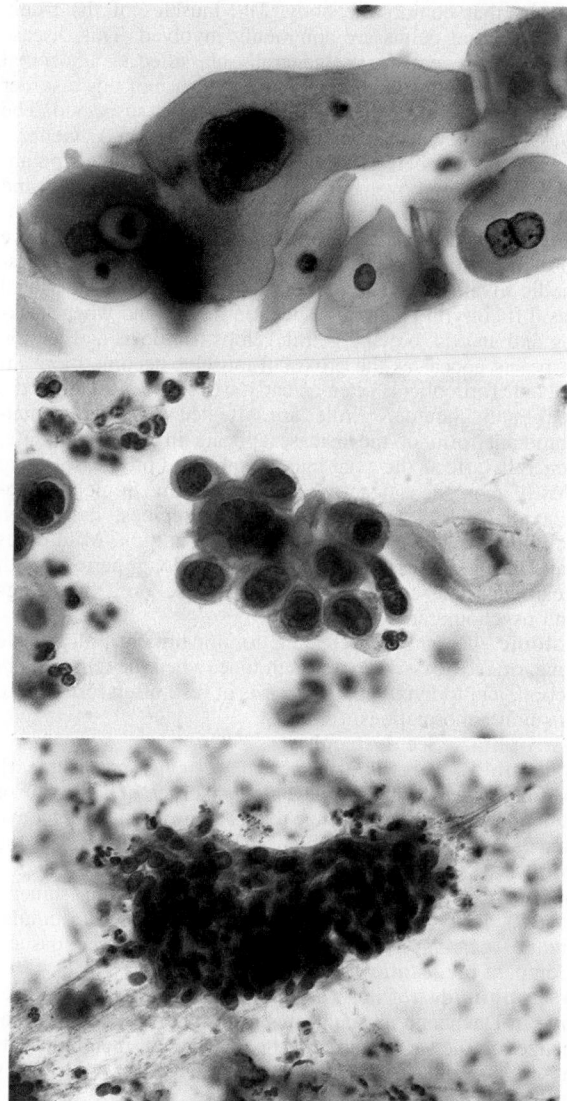

*Top,* Mild dysplasia. *Center,* Severe dysplasia. *Bottom,* Carcinoma in situ.
*(Damjanov and Linder, 1996)*

**dysplastic nevus syndrome,**   the occurrence of dysplastic nevi in persons with or at risk for familial or nonfamilial malignant melanoma.

**dyspnea** /dispnē′ə/ [Gk, *dys + pnoia,* breathing],   a distressful sensation of uncomfortable breathing that may be caused by certain heart conditions, strenuous exercise, or anxiety. Also spelled **dyspnoea.** Also called **breathlessness.** Compare **hyperpnea.** —**dyspneal, dyspneic,** *adj.*

**dyspraxia** /disprak′sē·ə/ [Gk, *dys + prassein,* to do],   a partial loss of the ability to perform skilled, coordinated movements in the absence of any associated defect in motor or sensory functions. See also **apraxia.**

**dysprosium (Dy)** /disprō′sē·əm/ [Gk, *dys + prositos,* to approach],   a rare-earth metallic element. Its atomic number is 66; its atomic mass is 162.50. Radioactive isotopes of dysprosium are used in radioisotope scanning, particularly in studies of the bones and joints.

**dysproteinemia** /disprō′tēnē′mē·ə/ [Gk, *dys + protos,* first, *haima,* blood],   an abnormality of the protein content of the blood, usually involving the immunoglobulins.

**dysraphia** /disrā′fē·ə/ [Gk, *dys + raphe,* seam],   failure of a raphe to fuse completely, as in incomplete closure of the neural tube. Also called **status dysraphicus.**

**dysraphic syndrome** /disraf′ik/,   a developmental disorder, usually involving the spinal cord, such as encephalocele or myelomenigocele. See also **Arnold-Chiari malformation.**

**dysreflexia, autonomic** /dis′riflek′sē·ə/ [Gk, *dys + L, reflectere,* to bend back],   a nursing diagnosis accepted by the Eighth National Conference on the Classification of Nursing Diagnoses. The condition is a state in which an individual with a spinal cord injury at T7 or above experiences or is at risk to experience a life-threatening uninhibited sympathetic response of the nervous system to a noxious stimulus.

■ DEFINING CHARACTERISTICS: The defining characteristics of the diagnosis of an individual with spinal cord injury (T7 or above) are paroxysmal hypertension (sudden periodic elevated blood pressure in which systolic pressure is above 140 mm Hg and diastolic above 90 mm Hg), bradycardia or tachycardia (pulse rate of less than 60 or more than 100 beats/min), diaphoresis above the injury, red splotches on the skin above the injury, and pallor below the injury. A headache that is a diffuse pain in different parts of the head and not confined to any nerve distribution area occurs. Other characteristics include chilling (shivering accompanied by the sensation of coldness or pallor of the skin), conjunctival congestion (excessive amount of blood and tissue fluid in the conjunctiva), blurred vision, chest pain, metallic taste in the mouth, nasal congestion, and pilomotor reflex (gooseflesh formation when skin is cooled). There can also be paresthesia (abnormal sensation such as numbness, prickling or tingling, and increased sensitivity). Horner's syndrome caused by paralysis of the cervical sympathetic nerve trunk can also be a characteristic with contraction of the pupil, partial ptosis of the eyelid, enophthalmos, and sometimes sweating over the affected side of the face.

■ RELATED FACTORS: Related factors include bladder and bowel distension, skin irritation, and lack of patient and caregiver knowledge. See also **nursing diagnosis.** —**dysreflexic,** *adj.*

**dysreflexia, autonomic, risk for,**   a nursing diagnosis accepted by the Thirteenth National Conference on the Classification of Nursing Diagnoses (revised 2000). The condition is defined as being a life-threatening uninhibited response of the sympathetic nervous system, post spinal shock, in an individual with a spinal cord injury or lesion at T6 or above.

■ DEFINING CHARACTERISTICS: The condition is defined by having an injury at T6 or above and experiencing at least one of the following stimuli: painful or irritating stimuli below the level of the injury; bladder distension; detrusor sphincter dyssynergia; bladder spasm; instrumentation or surgery; epididymitis; urethritis; urinary tract infection; calculi; cystitis; catheterization; bowel distension; fecal impaction; digital stimulation; suppositories; hemorrhoids; difficult passage of feces; constipation; enemas; GI system pathology; gastric ulcers; esophageal reflux; gallstones; menstruation; sexual intercourse; pregnancy; labor and delivery; ovarian cyst; ejaculation; cutaneous stimulation; pressure over bony prominences; or genitalia; heterotrophic bone; spasms; fractures; range-of-motion exercises; wounds; sunburns; temperature fluctuations; extreme environmental temperatures; positioning; constrictive clothing; drug reactions; surgical procedures; pulmonary emboli; and deep vein thrombosis. See also **nursing diagnosis.**

**dysreflexia management,** a nursing intervention from the Nursing Interventions Classification (NIC) defined as prevention and elimination of stimuli that cause hyperactive reflexes and inappropriate autonomic responses in a patient with a cervical or high thoracic cord lesion. See also **Nursing Interventions Classification.**

**dysregulation hypothesis** /disreg'yəlā'shən/, the view that depression and affective disorders do not simply reflect decreased or increased catecholamine activity but that they are failures of the regulation of these systems.

**dysrhythmia** /disrith'mē·ə/, any disturbance or abnormality in a normal rhythmic pattern, specifically, irregularity in the brain waves or cadence of speech. Compare **arrhythmia.**

**dysrhythmia management,** a nursing intervention from the Nursing Interventions Classification (NIC) defined as preventing, recognizing, and facilitating treatment of abnormal cardiac rhythms. See also **Nursing Interventions Classification.**

**dyssebacea** /disibā'shē·ə/ [Gk, *dys* + L, *sebum,* suet], a skin condition characterized by red, scaly, greasy patches on the nose, eyelids, scrotum, and labia. It results from a deficiency of vitamin $B_2$ and is most commonly associated with chronic alcoholism, liver disease, chronic diarrhea, and protein malnutrition. Also called *(informal)* **shark skin.**

**dyssynergia** /dis'inur'jē·ə/ [Gk, *dys* + *syn,* together, *ergein,* work], any disturbance in muscular coordination, as in cases of ataxia.

**dystaxia** /distak'sē·ə/ [Gk, *dys* + *taxis,* order], partial ataxia, such as dystaxia agitans, in which a spinal cord irritation causes a tremor but no paralysis.

**dysthymia** /disthim'ē·ə/ [Gk, *dys* + *thymos,* mind], a form of chronic unipolar depression that tends to occur in elderly persons with debilitating physical disorders, multiple interpersonal losses, and chronic marital difficulties. Several depressive episodes may merge into a low-grade chronic depressive state.

**dysthymic disorder** /disthim'ik/ [Gk, *dys* + *thymos,* mind], a disorder of mood in which the essential feature is a chronic disturbance of mood of at least 2 years' duration. It involves either depressed mood or loss of interest or pleasure in all or almost all usual activities and pastimes, and associated symptoms, but not of sufficient severity and duration to meet the criteria for a major depressive episode.

**dysthyroid orbitopathy** /dis·thī'roid or'bi·top'ə·thē/ [Gk, *dys-,* difficult + *thyreos,* shield + *eidos,* form; L, *orbita,* wheel track + Gk, *pathos,* disease], the ocular changes associated with thyroid dysfunction, usually in Graves' disease. Also called **dysthyroid ophthalmopathy.**

**dystocia** /distō'shə/ [Gk, *dys* + *tokos,* birth], pathologic or difficult labor, which may be caused by an obstruction or constriction of the birth passage or abnormal size, shape, position, or condition of the fetus. See also **clinical pelvimetry, fetal presentation, x-ray pelvimetry.**

**dystonia** /distō'nē·ə/ [Gk, *dys* + *tonos,* tone], any impairment of muscle tone. The condition commonly involves the head, neck, and tongue and often occurs as an adverse effect of a medication.

**dystonia musculorum deformans,** a rare abnormal condition characterized by intense, irregular torsion muscle spasms that contort the body. The muscles of the trunk, shoulder, and pelvis are commonly involved. This disease appears in several forms, generally classified as autosomal recessive or autosomal dominant. The cause of this disorder is not known; a biochemical dysfunction is suspected. The autosomal-recessive form appears most often in Ashkenazic Jews and starts between 5 and 15 years of age, causing abnormalities of movement and speech. Muscle power and tone appear normal, but convulsive spasms make the involved muscles relatively useless. The autosomal-recessive form of the disease commonly begins with intermittent spasmodic inversion of the foot, so that the affected individual has difficulty in placing the heel on the ground when walking and an odd, bowing gait develops. Lordosis and torsion of pelvis appear as the proximal muscles become more involved. Torticollis is often an early sign if the muscles of the neck and shoulder girdle are affected. The autosomal-dominant form of the disease appears in early adult life, generally affects the axial musculature, and progresses more slowly than the autosomal recessive form. Some muscle-relaxing drugs, such as the benzodiazepines, have been helpful in treating both forms of the condition. Mild cases have been successfully controlled for long periods with treatments that combine the use of muscle-relaxing drugs and psychotherapy.

**dystonic** /diston'ik/, referring to impairments of muscle tone, often excessive increase in tone, when the muscle is in action, and to hypotonia when it is at rest, often resulting in postural abnormalities.

**dystrophia.** See **dystrophy.**

**dystrophic** /distrof'ik/ [Gk, *dys* + *trophe,* nourishment], pertaining to a usually congenital disorder of structure or function of an organ or tissue that is aggravated by defective nutrition, such as accumulation of calcium salts in the cornea.

**dystrophic calcification** [Gk, *dys* + *trophe,* nourishment; L, *calx,* lime, *facere,* to make], the pathologic accumulation of calcium salts in necrotic or degenerated tissues. Compare **metastatic calcification.**

**dystrophin** /distrof'in/, a protein that is missing or defective in Duchenne muscular dystrophy (DMD), which is localized to the sarcolemma of the muscle cell membrane. Its absence results in abnormal cell permeability, which may lead to cell destruction.

**dystrophy** /dis'trəfē/ [Gk, *dys* + *trophe,* nourishment], any abnormal condition caused by defective nutrition. It often entails a developmental change in muscles that does not involve the nervous system, such as fatty degeneration associated with increased size but decreased strength. Also called **dystrophia.**

**dysuria** /disyoor'ē·ə/ [Gk, *dys* + *ouron,* urine], painful, burning urination, usually caused by a bacterial infection or obstruction of the urinary tract. Laboratory examination of the urine may reveal the presence of blood, bacteria, or white blood cells. Dysuria is a symptom of cystitis, urethritis, prostatitis, urinary tract tumors, and some gynecologic disorders and of the use of certain medications, such as opiates. Compare **hematuria, pyuria.**

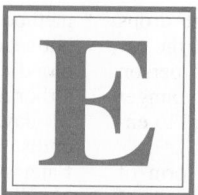

**E,** symbol for **expired gas.**

**E, ε.** See epsilon.

**e-,** prefix meaning 'out from': *ebonation, egesta, emollient.*

**E1,** symbol for **monomolecular elimination reaction.**

**E2,** symbol for **bimolecular elimination reaction.**

**E2-Mycin,** trademark for an antibiotic (erythromycin).

**ea,** abbreviation for *each.*

**Eales' disease** /ēlz/ [Henry Eales, British physician, 1852–1913], a condition marked by recurrent hemorrhages into the retina and vitreous, affecting mainly males in the second and third decades of life.

**E and GW,** abbreviation for **Economic and General Welfare.**

**ear** [AS, *eare*], one of two organs of hearing and balance, consisting of the external, middle, and internal ear. The external ear includes the skin-covered cartilaginous auricle visible on either side of the head and the part of the external auditory canal outside the skull. Together they form a funnel that directs sound waves toward the eardrum, or tympanic membrane, which marks the boundary between the external ear and the air-filled middle ear. The middle ear contains three very small bones, the malleus, incus, and stapes, which transmit vibrations caused by sound waves reaching the tympanic membrane to the oval window of the inner ear. The leverage of the ossicles, or middle-ear bones, increases the intensity of sound vibrations by more than 25 dB. Because the inner ear is filled with fluid, the increased intensity helps compensate for the loss of signal normally caused by sound-wave reflection of the fluid. The inner ear contains two separate organs: the vestibular apparatus, which provides the sense of balance, and the organ of Corti, which receives vibrations from the middle ear and translates them into nerve impulses, which are again interpreted by brain cells as specific sounds.

**earache** /ir'āk/ [AS, *eare* + *acan,* to hurt], a pain in the ear, sensed as sharp, dull, burning, intermittent, or constant. The cause is not necessarily a disease of the ear, because infections and other disorders of the nose, oral cavity, larynx, and temporomandibular joint can produce referred pain in the ear. Also called **otalgia, otodynia.**

**ear care,** a nursing intervention from the Nursing Interventions Classification (NIC) defined as prevention or minimization of threats to ear or hearing. See also **Nursing Interventions Classification.**

**eardrop instillation,** the instillation of a medicated solution into the external auditory canal of the ear. The patient is asked to turn the head to the side so that the ear being

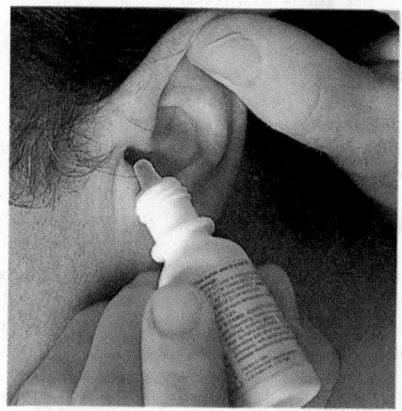

Instilling drops into the ear canal

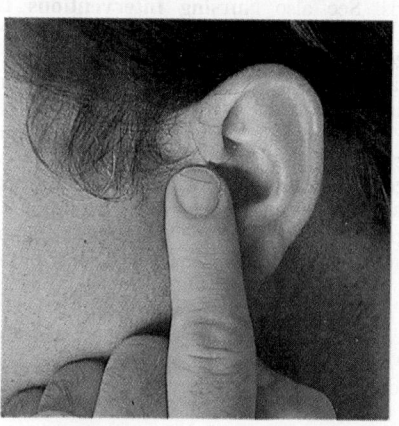

Pushing the tragus against the ear canal

**Eardrop instillation** *(Potter and Perry, 2001)*

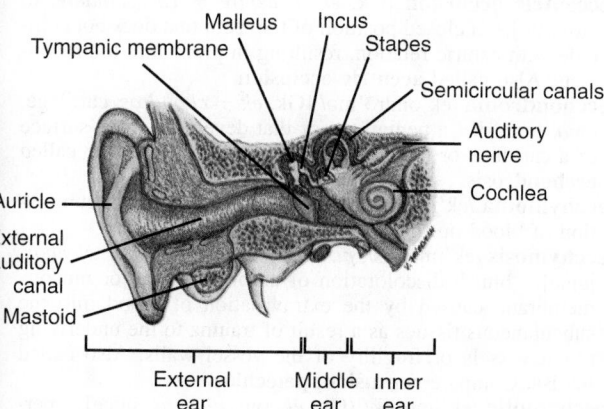

**Structures of the ear** *(Potter and Perry, 2001)*

treated faces upward. The orifice is exposed, and the drops of medicine are directed toward the internal wall of the canal. The pinna is pulled upward and outward in a person more than 3 years of age and down and back in a younger child. The tragus is then pushed against the ear canal to ensure that the drops stay in the canal.

**eardrops** [AS, *eare* + *dropa*], a topical, liquid form of medication for the local treatment of various conditions of the ear, such as inflammation or infection of the lining of the external auditory canal or impacted cerumen (earwax).

**eardrum.** See **tympanic membrane.**

**Early and Periodic Screening Diagnosis and Treatment (EPSDT),** a section of the Medicaid program that requires all states to maintain a program to determine the physical and mental defects of persons who are covered by the program and to provide short- and long-range treatment. See also **Medicaid.**

**ear oximeter** [AS, *eare* + Gk, *oxys,* sharp, *genein,* to produce, *metron,* measure], a device placed over the ear lobe that transmits a beam of light through the ear lobe tissue to a receiver. It is a noninvasive method of measuring the level of saturated hemoglobin in the blood. As the amount of saturated hemoglobin alters the wavelengths of light transmitted through the ear lobe, analysis of the light received is translated into percentage of oxygen saturation ($SO_2$) of the blood. See also **pulse oximeter.**

**ear speculum** [AS, *eare* + L, *speculum,* mirror], a short, funnel-shaped tube attached to an otoscope for examining the ear canal.

**ear thermometry,** the measurement of the temperature of the tympanic membrane by detection of infrared radiation from the eardrum. See also **tympanic membrane thermometer.**

**earwax.** See **cerumen.**

**East African sleeping sickness.** See **Rhodesian trypanosomiasis.**

**eastern equine encephalitis.** See **equine encephalitis.**

**eating disorders,** a group of behaviors often fueled by unresolved emotional conflicts symptomized by altered food consumption. Disorders include anorexia nervosa, bulimia nervosa, and binge eating. Compare **pica.**

**eating disorders management,** a nursing intervention from the Nursing Interventions Classification (NIC) defined as prevention and treatment of severe diet restriction and overexercising or binging and purging of food and fluids. See also **Nursing Interventions Classification.**

**Eaton agent,** an alternative name for *Mycoplasma pneumoniae,* a common cause of atypical pneumonia in humans. It is distinguished from other *Mycoplasma* organisms by its lack of a "fried egg" appearance when cultured on agar. See also *Mycoplasma.*

**Eaton agent pneumonia.** See **mycoplasma pneumonia.**

**Eaton-Lambert syndrome,** [Lee M. Eaton, American neurologist; Edward H. Lambert, twentieth-century American physiologist], a form of myasthenia that tends to be associated with lung cancer.

**Ebbecke's reaction.** See **dermatographia.**

**Ebner's glands** [Victor von Ebner, Austrian histologist, 1842–1925], serous glands of the tongue, opening at the bottom of the trough surrounding the circumvallate papillae.

**Ebola hemorrhagic fever.** See **Ebola virus disease.**

**Ebola virus disease** /ēbō′lə/ [Ebola River District, Congo], an infection caused by a species of ribonucleic acid viruses of the *Filovirus* genus. The usually lethal disease is characterized by hemorrhage and fever. The natural reservoir and method of transmission of primary infections are unknown, but secondary infection is by direct contact with infectious blood or other body secretions, in research settings, or by airborne particles. The incubation period ranges from 2 to 21 days. Initial symptoms include high fever, headache, chills, myalgia, sore throat, red itchy eyes, and malaise. Later symptoms include severe abdominal pain, chest pain, bleeding, shock, vomiting, and diarrhea. Maculopapular rash may occur in some patients. Treatment is supportive; in nearly 90% of cases, death occurs within 1 week. The Ebola virus is related to the Marburg virus. See also **Marburg virus disease.**

**EBP,** abbreviation for **epidural blood patch.**

**Ebstein's anomaly** [Wilhelm Ebstein, German physician, 1836–1912; Gk, *anomalia,* irregularity], a congenital heart defect in which the tricuspid valve is displaced downward into the right ventricle. The abnormality is often associated with right-to-left atrial shunting and Wolff-Parkinson-White syndrome.

**eburnation of dentin.** See **arrested dental caries.**

**EBV,** abbreviation for **Epstein-Barr virus.**

**ec-,** prefix meaning 'out of': *ecbolic, eccephalosis, ecchondroma.*

**ECC,** **1.** abbreviation for **emergency cardiac care. 2.** abbreviation for *external cardiac compression.*

**eccentric** /eksen′trik/ [Gk, *ek,* out, *centre,* center], **1.** pertaining to an object or activity that departs from the usual course or practice. **2.** pertaining to behavior that may appear to be odd or unconventional but does not necessarily reflect a disorder.

**eccentric contraction,** a type of muscle contraction that occurs as the muscle fibers lengthen, such as when a weight is lowered through a range of motion. The contractile force generated by the muscle is weaker than an opposing force, which causes the muscle to stretch. Compare **concentric contraction.**

**eccentric exercise,** a voluntary muscle activity in which there is an overall lengthening of the muscle in response to external resistance.

**eccentric implantation** [Gk, *ek,* out, *centre,* center], (in embryology) the embedding of the blastocyst within a fold or recess of the uterine wall, which then closes off from the main cavity.

**eccentricity** /ek′sentris′itē/, behavior that is regarded as odd or peculiar for a particular culture or community although not unusual enough to be considered pathologic.

**eccentric jaw relation,** any jaw relation other than centric relation.

**eccentric occlusion** [Gk, *ek* + *centre* + L, *occludere,* to close up], a closed position of the teeth that does not coincide with centric relation, resulting in premature tooth contacts. Also called **acentric occlusion.**

**ecchondroma** /ek′əndrō′mə/ [Gk, *ek* + *chondros,* cartilage, *oma,* tumor], a benign tumor that develops on the surface of a cartilage or under the periosteum of bone. Also called **ecchondrosis.**

**ecchymoma** /ek′imō′mə/, a swelling caused by accumulation of blood on the site of a bruise.

**ecchymosis** /ek′imō′sis/, *pl.* **ecchymoses** [Gk, *ek* + *chymos,* juice], bluish discoloration of an area of skin or mucous membrane caused by the extravasation of blood into the subcutaneous tissues as a result of trauma to the underlying blood vessels or fragility of the vessel walls. Also called **bruise.** Compare **contusion, petechiae.**

**ecchymotic** /ek′imot′ik/ [Gk, *ek,* out, *chymos,* juice], pertaining to a discolored area on the skin or membrane caused by blood seeping into the tissue as a result of a contusion.

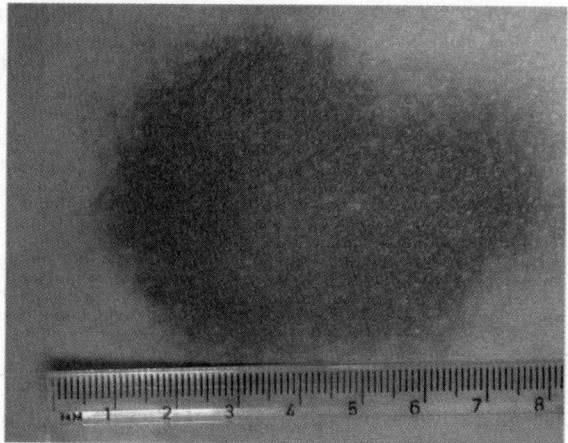

**Ecchymosis** (Lemmi and Lemmi, 2000)

nus *Echinococcus*. Dogs are the principal hosts of the adult worm; sheep, goats, horses, camels, cattle, rodents, and deer are the natural intermediate hosts for the larvae. Humans, especially children, can become infested with larvae by ingesting eggs shed in the stool of infected dogs and cats or by petting or handling household dogs or cats. The disease is most common in countries where livestock is raised with the help of dogs. Fluid-filled cysts form in affected organs such as the liver, lungs, brain, bones, or heart. Clinical manifestations and prognosis vary, depending on the tissue invaded and the extent of infestation. Diagnosis is made by skin tests for sensitivity, serologic tests, radiologic evidence of cyst formation, and identification of larval cysts in infected tissue. Treatment is an extended course of benzimidazole; puncture, aspiration, injection, and reaspiration (PAIR) of cysts; or careful removal of cysts, avoiding rupture of a cyst, which could cause severe allergic reactions or disseminate infection. The disease can be prevented by avoiding contact with infected dogs, deworming pet animals, and preventing dogs from eating carcasses of infected intermediate hosts. Also called **hydatid disease, hydatidosis.** See also **cysticercosis, tapeworm infection.**

**ecchymotic mask** [Gk, *ek* + *chymos* + Fr, *masque*], a cyanotic or bluish discoloration of the face of a victim of traumatic asphyxia, as in strangulation or choking. The color is the result of petechial hemorrhages.

**ecchymotic rash** [Gk, *ek* + *chymos,* juice; OFr, *rasche, scurf*], a skin eruption characterized by black-blue spots caused by extravasation of blood into the tissues, usually as a result of a contusion.

**eccrine** /ek′rin/ [Gk, *ekkrinein,* to secrete], pertaining to a sweat gland that secretes outwardly through a duct to the surface of the skin. See also **exocrine.**

**eccrine gland,** one of two kinds of sweat glands in the dermis. Such glands are unbranched, coiled, and tubular, and they are distributed throughout the dermal covering of the body. They promote cooling by evaporation of their secretion, which is clear, has a faint odor, and contains water, sodium chloride, and traces of albumin, urea, and other compounds. Compare **apocrine gland.**

**eccyesis.** See **ectopic pregnancy.**

**ECF, 1.** abbreviation for **extended care facility. 2.** abbreviation for **extracellular fluid.**

**ECG, 1.** abbreviation for **electrocardiogram. 2.** abbreviation for **electrocardiograph. 3.** abbreviation for **electrocardiography.**

**-echia,** suffix meaning a 'condition of holding': *asynechia, blepharosynechia, synechia.*

**echinacea,** a perennial herb found only in Missouri, Nebraska, and Kansas in the United States.

■ USES: This herb is used for those with low immune status, for hard-to-heal superficial wounds, and as a sun protectant.

■ CONTRAINDICATIONS: Echinacea is not recommended during pregnancy and lactation or in children. It is also contraindicated in people who have autoimmune diseases such as lupus erythematosus, multiple sclerosis, HIV/AIDS, or collage disease, and in people with tuberculosis or hypersensitivity to *Bellis* species, or the Compositae family of herbs. Immunosuppression may occur after extended therapy with this herb. It should not be used for more than 8 weeks.

**echino-,** combining form meaning 'spine or spiny': *echinochroma, echinosis, echinostomiasis.*

**echinococcosis** /ekī′nōkokō′sis/ [Gk, *echinos,* prickly husk, *kokkos,* berry, *osis,* condition], an infestation, usually of the liver, caused by the larval stage of a tapeworm of the ge-

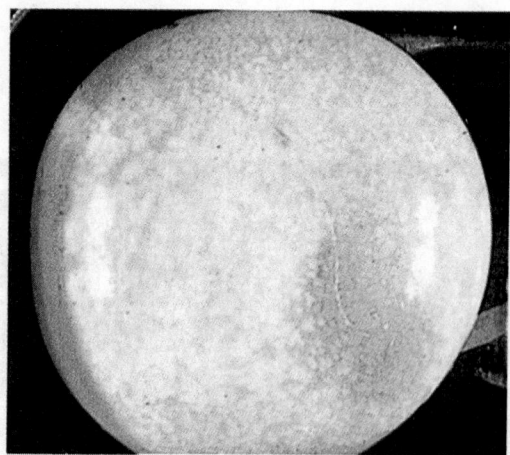

**Echinococcosis** (Farrar, 1993/courtesy Dr. H. Whitwell)

***Echinococcus*** /ekī′nōkok′əs/ [Gk, *echinos,* prickly husk, *kokkos,* berry], a genus of small tapeworms that primarily infect canines. See also **echinococcosis, hydatid cyst.**

**echinocyte.** See **burr cell.**

**echo** /ek′ō/, **1.** the reflection of an ultrasound wave back to the transducer from a structure in the plane of the sound beam. **2.** (informal) echoradiography.

**echo beat.** See **reciprocal beat.**

**echocardiogram** /ek′ōkär′dē·əgram′/ [Gk, *echo,* sound, *kardia,* heart, *gramma,* record], a graphic outline of the movements of heart structures produced by ultrasonography.

**echocardiography** /ek′ōkär′dē·og′rəfē/ [Gk, *echo* + *kardia,* heart, *graphein,* to record], a diagnostic, noninvasive procedure for studying the structure and motion of the heart. Ultrasonic waves directed through the heart are reflected backward, or echoed, when they pass from one type of tissue to another, such as from cardiac muscle to blood. The sound waves are transmitted from and received by a transducer and are recorded on a strip chart. Major diagnostic uses include the detection of atrial tumors and pericardial effusion, measurement of the ventricular septa and ventricular chambers, evaluation or monitoring of prosthetic valve function, and determination of mitral valve motion abnormalities and congenital lesions. Also called **ultrasonic cardiography.** See also **phonocardiograph, ultrasonography.**

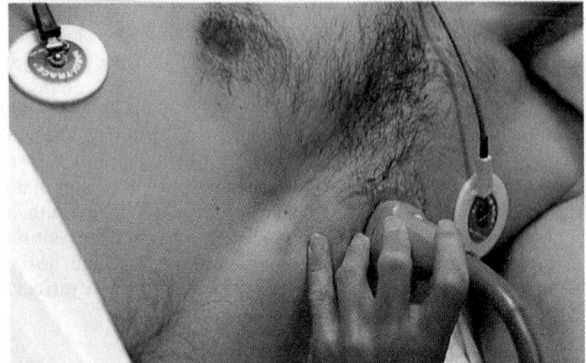

**Echocardiography: placement of chest leads and transducer**
*(Canobbio, 1990)*

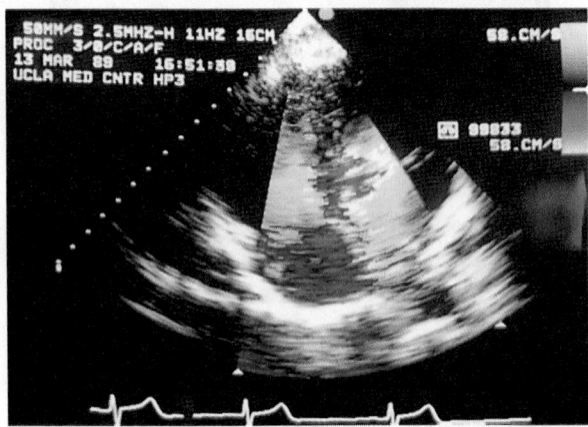

**Color flow Doppler echocardiography** *(Canobbio, 1990)*

**echoencephalogram (EEG)** /ek′ō·ensef′ələgram′/ [Gk, *echo* + *enkephalos,* brain, *gramma,* record], a recording produced by an echoencephalograph.

**echoencephalography** /ek′ō·ensef′əlog′rəfē/, the use of ultrasound to study the intracranial structures of the brain. The technique is useful for showing ventricular dilation and a major shift of midline structures caused by an expanding lesion. See also **ultrasonography.** —**echoencephalographic,** *adj.*

**echogram** /ek′ōgram/ [Gk, *echo,* sound, *gramma,* record], a recording of ultrasound echo patterns of a body structure, such as a gravid uterus.

**echographia.** See **pseudoagraphia.**

**echography.** See **ultrasonography.**

**echo home,** an independent housing facility for an older person in or near the family home.

**echolalia** /ek′ōlā′lyə/ [Gk, *echo* + *lalein,* to babble], **1.** (in psychiatry) the automatic and meaningless repetition of another's words or phrases, especially as seen in schizophrenia. A kind of echolalia is **delayed echolalia. 2.** (in pediatrics) a baby's imitation or repetition of sounds or words produced by others. It occurs normally in early childhood development. Also called **echophrasia, echo speech.** —**echolalic,** *adj.*

**echopraxia** /ek′ōprak′sē·ə/ [Gk, *echo* + *prassein,* to practice], imitation or repetition of the body movements of another person, sometimes practiced by schizophrenic patients.

**echoradiography** /ek′ōrā′dē·og′rəfē/ [Gk, *echo* + L, *radius,* ray; Gk, *graphein,* to record], a diagnostic procedure using ultrasonography and various devices for the visualization of internal structures of the body.

**echo sign, 1.** a repeated sound heard on percussion of a hydatid cyst. **2.** an involuntary repetition of words heard **(echolalia).**

**echo speech.** See **echolalia.**

**echothiophate iodide** /-thī′ōfāt/, an anticholinesterase used for ophthalmic purposes.

■ INDICATIONS: It is prescribed for the treatment of chronic open-angle glaucoma and accommodative esotropia.

■ CONTRAINDICATIONS: Uveal inflammation, most types of angle-closure glaucoma, or known hypersensitivity to this drug prohibits its use.

■ ADVERSE EFFECTS: Among the more serious adverse reactions are retinal detachment, nonreversible cataract, lens opacity, activation of iritis or uveitis, and iris cysts.

**ECHO virus** /ek′ōvī′rəs/ [*enteric cytopathogenic human orphan* + L, *virus,* poison], a picornavirus associated with many clinical syndromes but not identified as the causative organism of any specific disease. There are many ECHO viruses. More than 30 serotypes have been identified; many are harmless. Bacterial or viral disease may be complicated by ECHO virus infection, as aseptic meningitis accompanying some severe bacterial and viral infections.

**Eck's fistula** [Nikoli V. Eck, Russian physiologist, 1849–1917], an artificial passage between the end of the hepatic portal vein and the side of the inferior vena cava. It is used to treat esophageal varices in portal hypertension.

**eclampsia** /iklamp′sē·ə/ [Gk, *ek,* out, *lampein,* to flash], the gravest form of pregnancy-induced hypertension. It is characterized by grand mal seizure, coma, hypertension, proteinuria, and edema. The symptoms of impending seizure often include body temperature of up to 104° F, anxiety, epigastric pain, severe headache, and blurred vision. The nurse is alert to persistently and extremely high blood pressure and to increasingly hyperactive deep-tendon reflexes, or clonus. Convulsions may be prevented by bed rest in a quiet, dimly lit room and parenteral administration of magnesium sulfate and antihypertensive medications. The nurse attentively monitors the mother's general condition, including respiration, deep tendon reflexes, blood pressure, magnesium sulfate levels, and urine and protein excretion, and the baby's heart rate. Treatment of a convulsion must include maintenance of the mother's airway, protection of the mother against self-injury, and administration of medication to check the convulsion and decrease the blood pressure. Once this is accomplished, delivery is indicated. Convulsions rarely occur in the puerperium. Complications of eclampsia include cerebral hemorrhage, pulmonary edema, renal failure, liver necrosis, abruptio placentae, hypofibrinogenemia, hemolysis, and retinal hemorrhages, sometimes with temporary blindness. The maternal mortality rate in eclampsia is 10%; the fetal mortality rate is 25%. Eclampsia occurs in 0.2% of pregnancies. The cause is not known.

**eclectic** /iklek'tik/ [Gk, *eklektikos*, selecting], pertaining to a therapy that selects, combines, and incorporates diverse techniques from several systems or theories into an integrated approach.

**eclipse scotoma** /iklips'/ [Gk, *ekleipsis*, abandoning, *skotos*, darkness, *oma*, tumor], a small central area of depressed or lost vision caused by looking directly at the sun without adequate protection.

**ECM**, abbreviation for **erythema chronicum migrans.**

**ECMO**, abbreviation for **extracorporeal membrane oxygenator.**

**-ecoia**, suffix meaning '(condition of the) sense of hearing': *bradyecoia, dysecoia, oxyecoia.*

**E. coli**, abbreviation for *Escherichia coli.*

**ecologic chemistry** /ikəloj'ik/, the study of chemical compounds synthesized by plants that influence ecologic characteristics through chemical communication or toxic effects.

**ecologic fallacy**, a false assumption that the presence of a pathogenic factor and a disease in a population can be accepted as proof that a particular individual is the cause of the disease.

**ecology** /ikol'əjē/ [Gk, *oekos*, house, *logos*, science], the study of the interaction between organisms and their environment.

**econazole** /ikon'əzōl/, a topical antifungal agent.
- INDICATIONS: It is prescribed in the treatment of tinea pedis, tinea cruris, tinea corporis, tinea versicolor, and candidiasis.
- CONTRAINDICATION: Known sensitivity to this drug prohibits its use.
- ADVERSE EFFECTS: Among the most serious adverse reactions are local irritation and hypersensitivity of the skin.

**Economic and General Welfare (E and GW),** a structural unit of the American Nurses Association and state nurses' associations whose major goal is to upgrade the salaries, benefits, and working conditions of nurses.

**ecosystem** /ek'ōsis'təm/, the total of all living things within a particular area and the nonliving things with which they interact.

**EC space,** abbreviation for *extracellular space.* See **extracellular.**

**ecstasy** /ek'stəsē/ [Gk, *ekstasis*, derangement], an emotional state characterized by exultation, rapturous delight, or frenzy. Compare **euphoria, mania. —ecstatic,** *adj.*

**ECT,** abbreviation for **electroconvulsive therapy.**

**-ectas** combining form meaning 'dilatation, dilation, extension, or distension of an organ': *esophagectasia, lymphectasia, pharyngectasia.*

**ectatic emphysema.** See **panacinar emphysema.**

**ecthyma** /ek'thimə/ [Gk, *ek*, out, *thyein*, to rush], an ulcerative pyoderma characterized by large pustules, crusts, and ulcerations surrounded by erythema. It is caused by a streptococcal infection after a minor trauma. The skin of the legs is most frequently affected. Treatment includes vigorous cleansing, application of compresses of cool Burow's solution to soften and remove crusts, and systemic administration of antibiotics. Compare **folliculitis, impetigo.**

**ecthyma contagiosum.** See **contagious pustular dermatitis.**

**ecto-,** prefix meaning 'outside': *ectoblast, ectocolon, ectodermal.*

**ectocytic** /ek'təsit'ik/ [Gk, *ektos*, outside, *kytos*, cell], outside a cell and not part of its organization.

**ectoderm** /ek'tədurm/ [Gk, *ektos*, outside, *derma*, skin], the outermost of the three primary cell layers of an embryo.

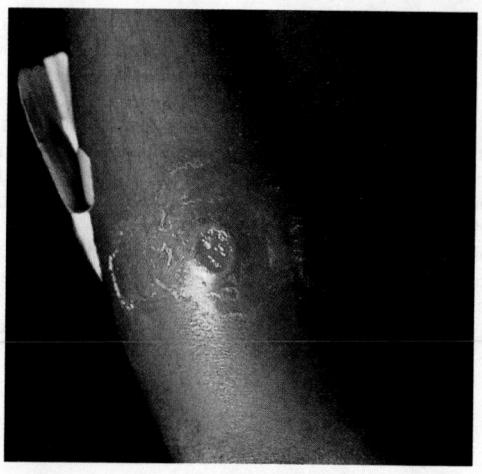

**Ecthyma**
*(Zitelli and Davis, 1997/courtesy Dr. Ellen Wald, Children's Hospital of Pittsburgh)*

The ectoderm gives rise to the nervous system; the organs of special sense, such as the eyes and ears; the epidermis and epidermal tissue, such as fingernails, hair, and skin glands; and the mucous membranes of the mouth and anus. See also **embryo, endoderm, mesoderm. —ectodermal, ectodermic,** *adj.*

**ectodermal cloaca** /ek'tədur'məl/, a part of the cloaca in the developing embryo that lies external to the cloacal membrane and eventually gives rise to the anus and anal canal. Compare **endodermal cloaca.**

**ectodermal dysplasias,** a group of hereditary disorders involving tissues and structures derived from the embryonic ectoderm; ectodermal dysplasia is a component of various syndromes, including **anhidrotic ectodermal dysplasia** and **EEC syndrome.**

**ectodermic.** See **ectoderm.**

**ectodermoidal** /ek'tədərmoi'dəl/ [Gk, *ektos*, outside, *derma*, skin, *eidos*, form], resembling or having the characteristics of ectoderm.

**ectomorph** /ek'təmôrf'/ [Gk, *ektos + morphe*, form], a person whose physique is characterized by slenderness, fragility, and a predominance of structures derived from the ectoderm. Compare **endomorph, mesomorph.** See also **asthenic habitus.**

**-ectomy,** suffix meaning the 'surgical removal' of something specified: *lobectomy, thrombectomy, thyroidectomy.*

**ectoparasite** /ek'tōper'əsīt/ [Gk, *ektos + parasitos*, guest], (in medical parasitology) an organism that lives on the outside of the body of the host, such as a louse.

**-ectopia,** combining form meaning a 'condition in which a (specified) organ or part is out of its normal place': *corectopia, osteectopia, tarsectopia.*

**ectopic** /ektop'ik/ [Gk, *ek + topos*, place], **1.** (of an object or organ) situated in an unusual place, away from its normal location, for example, an ectopic pregnancy, which occurs outside the uterus. **2.** (of an event) occurring at the wrong time, as a premature heartbeat or premature ventricular contraction.

**ectopic beat** [Gk, *ek*, out, *topos*, place; AS, *beatan*], an impulse that originates in the heart at a site other than the sinus node. Also called **extrasystole.**

**ectopic focus,**   an area in the heart that initiates abnormal beats. Ectopic foci may occur in both healthy and diseased hearts and are usually associated with irritation of a small area of myocardial tissue. They are produced in association with myocardial ischemia, drug (catecholamine) effects, emotional stress, and stimulation by foreign objects, including pacemaker catheters. Also called **ectopic pacemaker.**

**ectopic myelopoiesis.**   See **extramedullary myelopoiesis.**

**ectopic pacemaker.**   See **ectopic focus.**

**ectopic pregnancy,**   an abnormal pregnancy in which the conceptus implants outside the uterine cavity. Kinds of ectopic pregnancy are **abdominal pregnancy, ovarian pregnancy,** and **tubal pregnancy.** Also called **eccyesis** /ek'sī·ē'sis/.

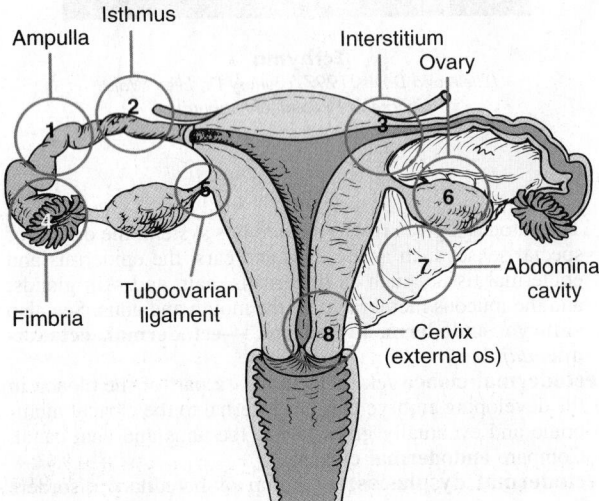

**Ectopic pregnancy implantation sites: numbers indicate order of frequency of occurrence (1, Most common; 8, least common)**
*(Lewis, Heitkemper, and Dirksen, 2000)*

**ectopic rhythm**   [Gk, *ek* + *topos*, place, *rhythmos*, beat], an abnormal heart rhythm caused by the formation of impulses in a focus outside the sinus node. Such a rhythm may be protective in cases of failure of the sinus node or excessive slowing of its rhythm, or it may indicate an active abnormal focus.

**ectopic tachycardia**   [Gk, *ek* + *topos*, place, *tachys*, swift, *kardia*, heart], an abnormally rapid heartbeat caused by excitation arising from a focus outside the sinus node.

**ectopic teratism,**   a congenital anomaly in which one or more parts are misplaced, such as dextrocardia, palatine teeth, and transposition of the great vessels.

**ectopic testis,**   a testis that has descended from the abdominal cavity and settled in the suprapubic area, the thigh, or the perineum instead of the scrotum. Therapy requires surgery.

**ectoplasm,**   the compact, peripheral portion of the cytoplasm of a cell.

**ectopy** /ek'təpē/   [Gk, *ek*, out, *topos*, place], a condition in which an organ or substance is not in its natural or proper place, such as an ectopic pregnancy that develops outside the uterus or an ectopic heartbeat.

**ectotoxin.**   See **exotoxin.**

**ectro-,**   prefix meaning 'loss or absence of, miscarriage, abortion'; used primarily to indicate a loss of limbs or body parts: *ectrodactyly, ectromelia.*

**ectrodactyly** /ek'trōdak'təlē/   [Gk, *ektrosis*, miscarriage, *daktylos*, finger], a congenital anomaly characterized by the absence of part or all of one or more of the fingers or toes. Also called **ectrodactylia, ectrodactylism.**

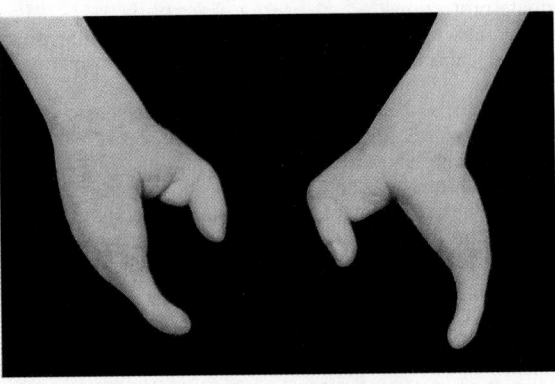

**Ectrodactyly involving the hands**
*(Moore, Persaud, and Shiato/courtesy Dr. A.E. Chudley, Department of Pediatrics and Child Health, University of Manitoba, Children's Hospital, Winnipeg, Canada)*

**ectrodactyly−ectodermal   dysplasia−clefting   syndrome.**   See **EEC syndrome.**

**ectrogenic.**   See **ectrogeny.**

**ectrogenic teratism** /-jen'ik/   [Gk, *ektrosis* + *genein*, to produce, *teras*, monster], a congenital anomaly caused by developmental failure in which one or more parts or organs are missing.

**ectrogeny** /ektroj'ənē/   [Gk, *ektrosis* + *genein*, to produce], the congenital absence or defect of any organ or part of the body. —**ectrogenic,** *adj.*

**ectromelia** /ek'trōmē'lyə/   [Gk, *ektrosis* + *melos*, limb], the congenital absence or incomplete development of the long bones of one or more of the limbs. Kinds of ectromelia are **amelia, hemimelia,** and **phocomelia.** —**ectromelic,** *adj.,* **ectromelus,** *n.*

**ectropic** /ektrop'ik/,   inside-out.

**ectropion** /ektrō'pē·on/   [Gk, *ek* + *trepein*, to turn], eversion, most commonly of the eyelid, exposing the conjunctival membrane lining the eyelid and part of the eyeball. The

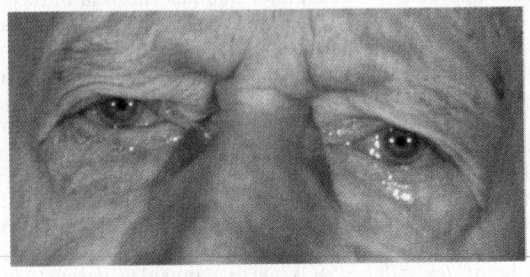

**Ectropion** *(Lemmi and Lemmi, 2000)*

condition may involve only the lower eyelid or both eyelids. The cause may be paralysis of the facial nerve or, in an older person, atrophy of the eyelid tissues. Compare **entropion.**

**ectrosyndactyly** /ek′trōsindak′tǝlē/ [Gk, *ektrosis* + *syn,* together, *daktylos,* finger], a congenital anomaly characterized by the absence of some but not all of the digits, with those that are formed webbed so as to appear fused. Also called **ectrosyndactylia.**

**eczema** /ek′simǝ/ [Gk, *ekzein,* to boil over], superficial dermatitis of unknown cause. In the early stage it may be pruritic, erythematous, papulovesicular, edematous, and weeping. Later it becomes crusted, scaly, thickened, or lichenified. Exacerbating factors include sudden temperature changes, humidity, psychologic stress, illness, allergies, fibers, detergents, and perfumes. Eczema is not a distinct disease entity. See also **atopic dermatitis, nummular dermatitis. —eczematous,** *adj.*

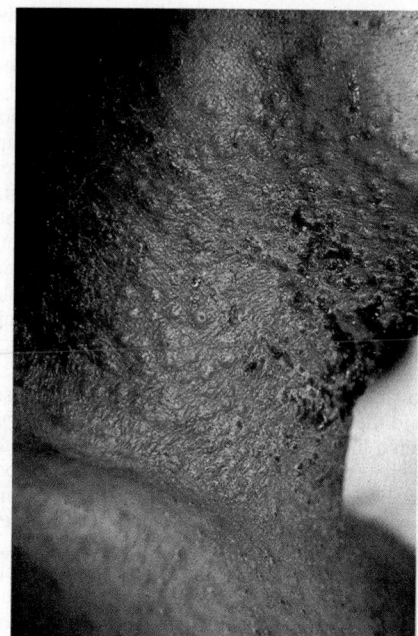
**Eczema herpeticum** *(Stone and Gorbach, 2000)*

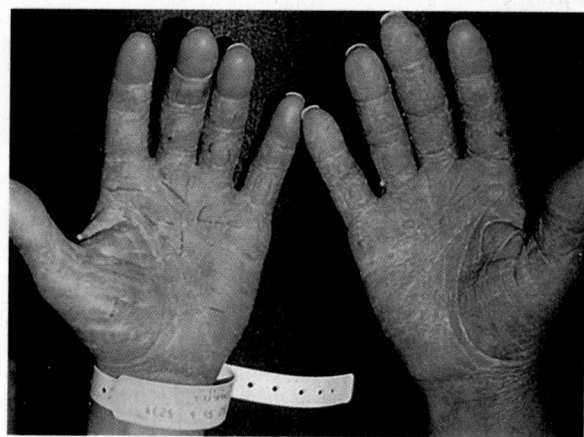
**Eczema** *(Hill, 1994)*

**eczema herpeticum,** a generalized vesiculopustular rash caused by herpes simplex virus or vaccinia virus infection of a preexisting rash such as atopic dermatitis. Also called **Kaposi's varicelliform eruption.**

**eczema marginatum.** See **tinea cruris.**

**eczematous.** See **eczema.**

**eczematous conjunctivitis** /eksem′ǝtǝs/, conjunctival and corneal inflammation associated with multiple tiny ulcerated vesicles. The cause is believed to be a delayed hypersensitivity to bacterial protein. If untreated, the condition may lead to ingrowth of small blood vessels in the cornea, eventually obscuring vision. Treatment usually includes topical instillation of corticosteroids.

**ED,** **1.** abbreviation for **effective dose. 2.** abbreviation for **emergency department.**

**ED₅₀,** symbol for **median effective dose.**

**edaphon** /ed′ǝfon/, the composite of organisms that live in the soil. **—edaphic,** *adj.*

**EDB,** **1.** abbreviation for **ethylene dibromide. 2.** abbreviation for *expected date of birth.* See **expected date of delivery.**

**EDC,** abbreviation for *expected date of confinement.*

**EDD,** abbreviation for **expected date of delivery.**

**eddy currents,** small circular electric fields induced when a magnetic field is created. They result in intramolecular os-

cillation or vibration of tissue contents, causing generation of heat.

**Edecrin,** trademark for a diuretic (ethacrynic acid).

**Edecrin Sodium,** trademark for a loop diuretic (ethacrynate sodium).

**edema** /idē′mǝ/ [Gk, *oidema,* swelling], the abnormal accumulation of fluid in interstitial spaces of tissues, such as in the pericardial sac, intrapleural space, peritoneal cavity, or joint capsules. Edema may be caused by increased capillary fluid pressure; venous obstruction such as occurs in varicosities; thrombophlebitis; pressure from casts, tight ban-

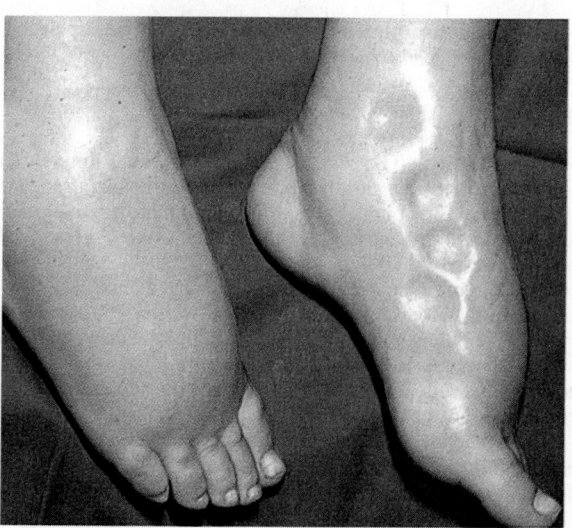
**Pitting edema** *(Bloom and Ireland, 1992)*

dages, or garters; congestive heart failure; overloading with parenteral fluids; renal failure; hepatic cirrhosis; hyperaldosteronism such as in Cushing's syndrome; corticosteroid therapy; and inflammatory reactions. Edema may also result from loss of serum protein in burns, draining wounds, fistulas, hemorrhage, nephrotic syndrome, or chronic diarrhea; in malnutrition, especially kwashiorkor; in allergic reactions; and in blockage of lymphatic vessels caused by malignant diseases, filariasis, or other disorders. Treatment of edema focuses on correcting the underlying cause. Potassium-sparing diuretics may be administered to promote excretion of sodium and water. Edematous parts of the body should be protected from prolonged pressure, injury, and temperature extremes. In the evaluation of tissue turgor, edema may be evaluated by position change, specific location, and response to pressure, as in pitting edema when pressing the fingers into the edematous area causes a temporary indentation. When a limb is edematous as a result of venous stasis, elevating the extremity and applying an elastic stocking or sleeve facilitate venous return. Also spelled **oedema.** See also **anasarca, lymphedema. —edematous, edematose,** *adj.*

**-edema, -edem,** combining form meaning 'swelling resulting from an excessive accumulation of serous fluid in the tissues of the body in (specified) locations': *cephaledema, dactyledema, papilledema.*

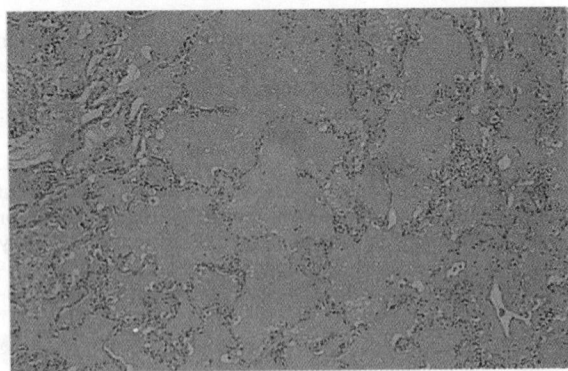

**Edema: accumulation of fluid in interstitial spaces**
*(Christiansen and Grzybowski, 1993)*

**edema of glottis** [Gk, *oidema,* swelling, *glossa,* tongue], a swelling caused by fluid accumulation in the soft tissues of the larynx. The condition, usually inflammatory, may result from infection, injury, or inhalation of toxic gases. Also called **laryngeal edema.**

**edematogenic** /ēdem′ətōjen′ik/, causing edema.

**edematous** /ēdem′ətəs/ [Gk, *oidema,* swelling], pertaining to or resembling edema, or excessive fluid accumulation in the tissues, causing swelling.

**edentulous** /ēden′chələs/, lacking natural teeth.

**edetate calcium disodium (EDTA)** /ed′ətāt/, calcium disodium edetate and edetate disodium, used as a chelating agent in treating lead poisoning.

**edetate disodium,** a parenteral chelating agent.

■ INDICATIONS: It is prescribed for hypercalcemic crisis, for ventricular arrhythmia and heart block resulting from digitalis toxicity, and for lead poisoning.

■ CONTRAINDICATIONS: Hypocalcemia, kidney disease, or known hypersensitivity to this drug prohibits its use.

■ ADVERSE EFFECTS: Among the more serious adverse reactions are hypocalcemia, thrombophlebitis, kidney damage, and hemorrhage associated with hypocoagulability.

**edetic acid (EDTA)** /idet′ik/, a chelating agent.

**EDG,** abbreviation for **electrodynograph.**

**edge** /ej/ [ME, *egge*], a thin side or border.

**edge response function (ERF),** the ability of a computed tomography system to produce a sharp image of a high-contrast edge, such as the edge of the heart.

**edgewise appliance,** a fixed orthodontic appliance whose attachment brackets have a rectangular slot that engages a round or rectangular arch wire. The most widely prescribed orthodontic appliance, it is used to correct or improve malocclusion.

**EDI,** abbreviation for **Electronic Data Interchange.**

**edible,** pertaining to a substance that can be eaten.

**EDRF,** abbreviation for **endothelial-derived relaxing factor.**

**edrophonium chloride** /ed′rōfō′nē·əm/, a cholinesterase inhibitor that acts as an antidote to curare and is an aid in the diagnosis of myasthenia gravis.

■ INDICATIONS: It is prescribed in the treatment of curare toxicity, the diagnosis of suspected myasthenia gravis, and the termination of paroxysmal supraventricular tachycardia.

■ CONTRAINDICATIONS: Obstruction of the GI or urinary tract, hypotension, bradycardia, or known hypersensitivity to this drug prohibits its use.

■ ADVERSE EFFECTS: Among the most serious adverse reactions are respiratory paralysis, hypotension, bradycardia, and bronchospasm.

**edrophonium test,** a test for myasthenia gravis in which an IV solution of edrophonium chloride is injected into a patient. A total of 10 mg of the cholinergic drug is prepared and a 2 mg dose is injected. If there is no reaction in 30 seconds, the remaining 8 mg is administered. A brief improvement in muscle activity is regarded as a positive result. Edrophonium chloride is also used to distinguish between myasthenia gravis and a cholinergic crisis. Because edrophonium chloride can precipitate respiratory depression, the test should not be performed unless an anticholinergic antidote, such as atropine, and respiratory resuscitation equipment are available. For further explanation of electroencephalographic recording of brain waves, see **alpha wave, beta wave, delta wave, theta wave.**

**Edsall's disease** [David L. Edsall, American physician, 1869–1945], a cramping condition that is the result of excessive exposure to heat. Also called **heat cramp.**

**EDTA, 1.** abbreviation for **edetate calcium disodium. 2.** abbreviation for **edetic acid.**

**educational psychology** /ej′əkā′shənəl/ [L, *educatus,* to rear; Gk, *psyche,* mind, *logos,* science], the application of psychologic principles, techniques, and tests to educational problems, such as the determination of more effective instructional methods, the assessment of student advancement, and the selection of students for specialized programs.

**Edwards' syndrome.** See **trisomy 18.**

**EEC syndrome,** an autosomal dominant syndrome involving both ectodermal and mesodermal tissues, with ectodermal dysplasia associated with hypopigmentation of skin and hair, scanty hair and eyebrows, absence of lashes, nail dystrophy, small or missing teeth, missing digits, and cleft lip and palate. Also called **ectrodactyly—ectodermal dysplasia—clefting syndrome.**

**EEE,** abbreviation for **eastern equine encephalitis.** See **equine encephalitis.**

**EEG,** **1.** abbreviation for **electroencephalogram. 2.** abbreviation for **electroencephalograph. 3.** abbreviation for **electroencephalography.**

**EENT,** abbreviation for *eyes, ears, nose, and throat.*

**EEOC,** abbreviation for **Equal Employment Opportunity Commission.**

**ef-.** See **ex-.**

**EFA,** abbreviation for **essential fatty acid.**

**efavirenz,** an antiviral.

■ INDICATIONS: Efavirenz is used to treat HIV-1 in combination with other antiretroviral agents.

■ CONTRAINDICATIONS: Known hypersensitivity to this drug prohibits its use.

■ ADVERSE EFFECTS: Adverse reactions to this drug include abdominal pain, headache, dizziness, fatigue, impaired concentration, insomnia, abnormal dreams, and depression. Common side effects include diarrhea, nausea, and rash.

**effacement** /ifās′mənt/ [Fr, *effacer,* to erase], the shortening of the vaginal portion of the cervix and thinning of its walls as it is stretched and dilated by the fetus during labor. When the cervix is fully effaced, the constrictive neck of the uterus is obliterated; the cervix is then continuous with the lower uterine segment. The extent of effacement, determined by vaginal examination, is expressed as a percentage of full effacement. See also **birth, cervix, dilation, station.**

**effect,** *n.* the result of an agent or cause.

**effective compliance** /ifek′tiv/ [L, *effectus,* performance], the ratio of tidal volume to peak airway pressure.

**effective dose (ED),** the dosage of a drug that may be expected to cause a specific effect of desired intensity in the people to whom it is given.

**effective half-life (ehl),** the time required for a radioactive element in an animal body to be diminished by 50% as a result of radioactive decay and biologic elimination. The effective half-life is equal to the product of the biologic half-life *(bhl)* and the radioactive half-life *(rhl)* divided by the sum of the *bhl* and the *rhl: ehl = (bhl × rhl)/(bhl + rhl).* See also **biologic half-life.**

**effective osmotic pressure,** the part of total osmotic pressure of a solution that determines the tendency of the solvent to pass through a boundary, such as a semipermeable membrane.

**effective radiating area,** the total area of the surface of the transducer that actually produces the sound wave.

**effective refractory period.** See **refractory period.**

**effector** /ifek′tər/ [L, *efficere,* to accomplish], **1.** an organ that produces an effect, such as glandular secretion, as a result of nerve stimulation. **2.** a molecule, such as an enzyme, that can start or stop a chemical reaction.

**effector cell, 1.** a terminally differentiated leukocyte that performs more than one specific function. **2.** a muscle cell or gland cell.

**effeminate** /ifem′init/ [L, *effeminare,* to make womanish], womanly or female in physical and mental characteristics, regardless of biologic sex.

**efferent** /ef′ərənt/ [L, *effere,* to carry out], directed away from a center, such as certain arteries, veins, nerves, kidney, and lymphatics. Compare **afferent.**

**efferent duct,** any duct through which a gland releases its secretions.

**efferent nerve,** a nerve that transmits impulses away or outward from a nerve center such as the brain or spinal cord, usually causing a muscle contraction or release of a glandular secretion.

**efferent pathway** [L, *effere,* to carry out; ME, *paeth + weg*], **1.** the route of nerve fibers carrying impulses away from a nerve center. **2.** the system of blood vessels that convey blood away from a body part. Compare **afferent.**

**effervesce** [Gk, *effervescere,* to foam up], to produce small bubbles or foam on the release of gas from a fluid.

**effervescence** /ef′ərves′əns/ [L, *effervescere,* to foam up], the production of small bubbles or foam associated with the escape of gas from a fluid.

**effervescent** /ef′ərves′ənt/, producing and releasing gas bubbles.

**efficacy** /ef′əkəsē/ [L, *effectus,* performance], (of a drug or treatment) the ability of a drug or treatment to produce a specific result, regardless of dosage. Opioids have a nearly identical efficacy but require various dosages to obtain the effect.

**efficiency** /ifish′ənsē/, **1.** the production of desired results with the minimum waste of time and effort. **2.** the amount of achievement compared with the effort expended. **3.** (in radioassay) the counts perceived by a beta or gamma counter relative to the known disintegration rate of a comparable standard radioactive source.

**effleurage** /ef′ləräzh′/ [Fr, skimming the surface], a technique in massage in which long, light, or firm strokes are used, usually over the spine and back. Fingertip effleurage is a light technique performed with the tips of the fingers in a circular pattern over one part of the body or in long strokes over the back or an extremity. Fingertip effleurage of the abdomen is a technique commonly used in the Lamaze method of natural childbirth. Compare **pétrissage, rolling effleurage.**

**effluent** /ef′loō·ənt/, a liquid, solid, or gaseous emission, such as the discharge or outflow from a machine or an industrial process.

**effluvium** /ifloō′vē·əm/ [L, *effluvium,* a flowing out], an outflow of gas or vapor, usually malodorous or toxic.

**effort syndrome** [Fr, exertion; Gk, *syn,* together, *dromos,* course], an abnormal condition characterized by chest pain, dizziness, fatigue, palpitations, cold, moist hands, and sighing respiration. The condition is often associated with

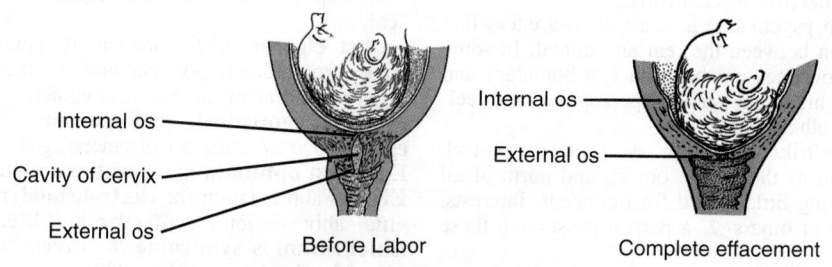

Internal os — Cavity of cervix — External os — Before Labor

Internal os — External os — Complete effacement

**Cervical effacement** *(Lowdermilk, Perry, and Bobak, 2000)*

soldiers in combat but occurs also in other individuals. The pain often mimics angina pectoris but is more closely connected to anxiety states and occurs after rather than during exercise. Because angina may also be associated with anxiety, positive diagnosis of effort syndrome may require an exercise electrocardiogram. Other chest pains that mimic effort syndrome and angina may be caused by musculoskeletal problems, such as inflammation of the costochondral junctions, fractured ribs, or cervical spondylosis. Also called **neurocirculatory asthenia.**

**effort thrombosis,** an abnormal condition in which a clot develops within the subclavian or axillary vein following strenuous exercise. The condition is accompanied by pain, edema, and skin discoloration in the shoulder and upper arm. Also called **Paget-Schroetter syndrome, Paget-von Schroetter syndrome.**

**effraction** /ifrak′shən/, a breaking open or weakening.

**effusion** /ifyōō′zhən/ [L, *effundere,* to pour out], **1.** the escape of fluid, for example, from blood vessels as a result of rupture or seepage, usually into a body cavity. The condition is usually associated with a circulatory or renal disorder and is often an early sign of congestive heart disease. The term may be associated with an affected body area, as pleural or pericardial effusion. See also **edema, transudate. 2.** the outward spread of a bacterial growth.

**eflornithine hydrochloride** /eflôr′nithēn/, an antiprotozoal used to treat the meningoencephalitic stage of *Trypanosoma brucei* (sleeping sickness) infection.

**EFM,** abbreviation for **electronic fetal monitor.**

**Efudex,** trademark for an antineoplastic (fluorouracil).

**EGD,** abbreviation for **esophagogastroduodenoscopy.**

**egest** /ijest′/ [L, *egerere,* to expel], to discharge or evacuate a substance from the body, especially to evacuate unabsorbed residue of foods from the intestines. **—egesta,** *n. pl.,* **egestive,** *adj.*

**EGF,** abbreviation for **epidermal growth factor.**

**egg** /eg/ [ONorse], a female reproductive cell at any stage before fertilization; after fertilization and fusion of the pronuclei, it is called a zygote. Also called **ovum.**

**eglandulous** /ēglan′dyələs/, describing an absence of glands.

**ego** /ē′gō, eg′ō/ [Gk, I or self], **1.** the conscious sense of the self; those elements of a person, such as thinking, feeling, and willing that distinguish him or her as an individual. **2.** (in psychoanalysis) the part of the psyche that experiences and maintains conscious contact with reality and tempers the primitive drives of the id and the demands of the superego with the social and physical needs of society. It represents the rational element of the personality, is the seat of such mental processes as perception and memory, and develops defense mechanisms against anxiety. See also **id, superego.**

**ego-alien.** See **ego-dystonic.**

**ego analysis,** (in psychoanalysis) the intensive study of the ego, especially the defense mechanisms.

**ego boundary,** (in psychiatry) a sense or awareness that there is a distinction between the real and unreal. In some psychoses the person does not have an ego boundary and cannot differentiate his or her personal perceptions and feelings from those of other people.

**egocentric** /ē′gōsen′trik/ [Gk, *ego* + *kentron,* center], **1.** regarding the self as the center, object, and norm of all experience and having little regard for the needs, interests, ideas, and attitudes of others. **2.** a person possessing these characteristics.

**ego-defense mechanism.** See **defense mechanism.**

**ego-dystonic** /ē′gōdiston′ik/, describing elements of a person's behavior, thoughts, impulses, drives, and attitudes that are unacceptable to him or her and cause anxiety. Also called **ego-alien, self-alien.** Compare **ego-syntonic.**

**ego-dystonic homosexuality,** a psychosexual disorder characterized by discomfort with one's sexuality and a persistent desire to change sexual orientation to heterosexuality. See also **homosexual.**

**ego ideal,** the image of the self to which a person aspires both consciously and unconsciously and against which he measures himself or herself and judges personal performance. It is usually based on a positive identification with the significant and influential figures of the early childhood years. See also **identification.**

**ego-integrity,** an acceptance of self, both successes and failure. It implies a healthy psychologic state. Despair often precedes ego-integrity.

**egoism** /ē′gō·iz′əm, eg′-/, **1.** selfishness, an overvaluation of the importance of the self, expressed as a willingness to gain an advantage at the expense of others. See also **egotism. 2.** the belief that individual self-interest is, or ought to be, the basic motive for all conscious behavior.

**egoist** /ē′gō·ist, eg′-/, **1.** a selfish person, one who seeks to satisfy his or her own interests at the expense of others. See also **egotist. 2.** a person who believes in or acts in accordance with the concept that all conscious action is justifiably motivated by self-interest. **—egoistic, egoistical,** *adj.*

**ego libido,** (in psychoanalysis) concentration of the libido on the self; self-love, narcissism.

**egomania** /ē′gōmā′nē·ə/ [Gk, *ego,* I, *mania,* madness], a pathologic preoccupation with the self and an exaggerated sense of one's own importance.

**egophony** /ēgof′ənē/, a change in the voice sound of a patient with pleural effusion as heard on auscultation. When the patient is asked to make /ē-ē-ē/ sounds, they are heard over the peripheral chest wall as /ä-ä-ä/, particularly over an area of consolidated or compressed lung above the effusion. Also called **tragophony.**

**ego strength,** (in psychotherapy) the ability to maintain the ego by a cluster of traits that together contribute to good mental health. The traits usually considered important include tolerance of the pain of loss, disappointment, shame, or guilt; forgiveness of those who have caused an injury, with feelings of compassion rather than anger and retaliation; acceptance of substitutes and ability to defer gratification; persistence and perseverance in the pursuit of goals; openness, flexibility, and creativity in learning to adapt; and vitality and power in the activities of life. The psychiatric prognosis for a client correlates positively with ego strength.

**ego-syntonic** /ē′gōsinton′ik/, describing those elements of a person's behavior, thoughts, impulses, drives, and attitudes that are acceptable to him or her and are consistent with the total personality. Compare **ego-dystonic.**

**egotism** /ē′gətiz′əm, eg′-/, vanity, conceit, or overvaluation of the importance of the self and undervaluation or contempt of others. See also **egoism. —egotistic, egotistical,** *adj.*

**egotist** /ē′gətist, eg′-/, one who is vain or conceited or who places too much importance on the self and is boastful, egocentric, and arrogant. See also **egoist.**

**egotistic, egotistical.** See **egotism.**

**egress** /ē′gres/, the act of emerging or moving forward.

**Egyptian ophthalmia.** See **trachoma.**

**EHD,** abbreviation for **electrohemodynamics.**

**ehl,** abbreviation for **effective half-life.**

**Ehlers-Danlos syndrome** /ā′lərzdan′ləs/ [Edward Ehlers, Danish physician, 1863–1937; Henri A. Danlos, French physician, 1844–1912], a hereditary disorder of connective tissue, marked by hyperplasticity of skin, tissue fragility, and hypermotility of joints. Minor trauma may cause a gaping wound with little bleeding. Sprains, joint dislocations, and synovial effusions are common. However, life expectancy is usually normal. Treatment includes symptomatic therapy, emotional support for the patient and family, and emphasis on avoiding trauma in childhood.

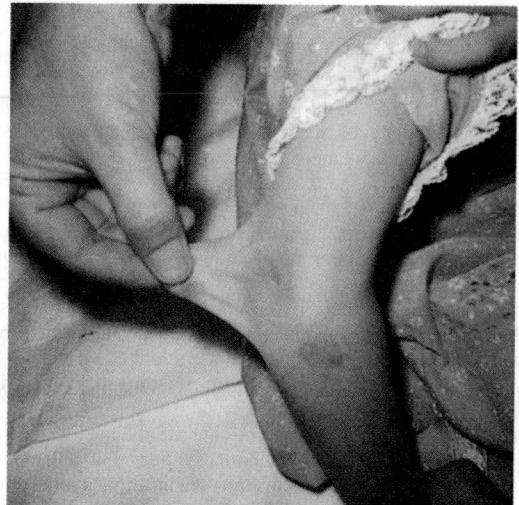

**Ehlers-Danlos syndrome: hyperplasticity of skin**
*(Weston, Lane, and Morelli, 1996)*

*Ehrlichia*, a genus of small spherical to ellipsoidal, nonmotile gram-negative bacteria. They occur singly or in compact inclusions in circulating mammalian leukocytes. Some species are the causative agents of ehrlichiosis and are transmitted by ticks. Two human tickborne diseases have been associated with *Ehrlichia* species: human monocytic ehrlichiosis caused by *E. chaffeensis,* and human granulocytic ehrlichiosis caused by *E. equi.*

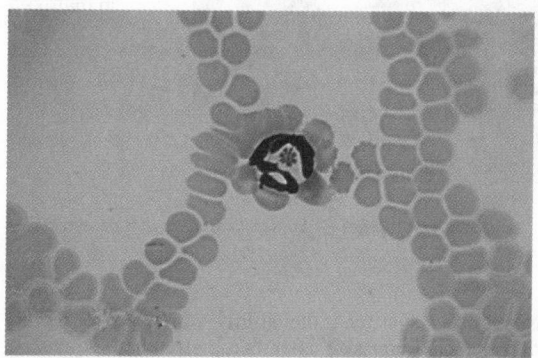

**Inclusion body of *Ehrlichia* within a neutrophil**
*(Cotran, Kumar, and Collins, 1999/courtesy Dr. Sam Telford, Harvard School of Public Health)*

**ehrlichiosis,** a sometimes fatal tickborne infection with symptoms similar to but more severe than those of Lyme disease. The disease usually begins about 10 days after the bite of an infected tick, although some cases have begun abruptly, within hours, with influenza-like symptoms, including painful muscle aches, headaches, fever, chills, loss of appetite, and depressed blood cell counts. Although similar to Lyme disease, the infection does not respond to antibiotics used to treat Lyme disease. However, ehrlichiosis does respond to early treatment with tetracycline antibiotics. The tick that carries the ehrlichiosis infection is the same species as the vector of Lyme disease, *Borrelia burgdorferi,* but the patient usually recovers within 8 weeks without the chronic arthritis symptoms associated with Lyme disease. Diagnosis is difficult because of the similarities with Lyme disease, and cases of simultaneous infections of both types of bacteria have been reported. Also, one of the organisms associated with ehrlichiosis, *Ehrlichia equi,* is nearly identical to a bacterium that causes fevers in horses. Also called **human granulocytic ehrlichiosis (HGE), human monocytic ehrlichiosis (HME).** See also *Ehrlichia.*

**eicosanoic acid** /ī′kōsənō′ik/ [Gk, *eikosa,* twenty], a saturated fatty acid containing 20 carbon atoms in a straight chain, found in peanut oil, butter, and other fats. Also called **arachidic acid.**

**eicosapentaenoic acid** /ī·kō′sə·pen′tə·ē·nō′ik /, a 20-carbon fatty acid found almost exclusively in fish and marine animal oils.

**EID,** abbreviation for **electronic infusion device.**

**eidetic** /īdet′ik/ [Gk, *eidos,* a form or shape seen], **1.** pertaining to or characterized by the ability to visualize and reproduce accurately the image of objects or events previously seen or imagined. **2.** a person possessing such ability.

**eidetic image,** an unusually vivid, elaborate, and apparently exact mental image resulting from a visual experience and occurring as a fantasy, dream, or memory. See also **image.**

**eighth cranial nerve.** See **vestibulocochlear nerve.**

**einsteinium (Es)** /īnstī′nē·əm/ [Albert Einstein, German-born physicist and Nobel laureate, 1879–1955], a synthetic transuranic metallic element. Its atomic number is 99; its atomic mass is 254. Einsteinium was first found in the debris from a hydrogen bomb explosion. It decays rapidly into berkelium.

**Einthoven's formula** /īnt′hōvənz/ [Willem Einthoven, Dutch physiologist, scientist, and Nobel laureate, 1860–1927; L, *forma,* pattern], a mathematical expression relating the voltages measured by electrocardiographic leads. The formula states that the sum of the voltages from lead I plus those from lead III minus those from lead II equals zero (I + III − II = 0). This formula is based on the principle that the sum of the voltages in any closed path equals zero. Because the positive and negative electrodes of lead II are reversed, the voltage from lead II is subtracted instead of added to the voltages from leads I and III. See also **Einthoven's triangle.**

**Einthoven's triangle** [Willem Einthoven], an equilateral triangle whose vertices lie at the left and right shoulders and the pubic region and whose center corresponds to the vector sum of all electric activity occurring in the heart at any given moment. Einthoven's triangle is approximated by the triangle formed by the axes of the bipolar electrocardiographic (ECG) limb leads I, II, and III. The center of the triangle offers a reference point for the unipolar ECG leads.

**Eisenmenger's complex** /ī′sənmeng′ərz/ [Victor Eisenmenger, German physician, 1864–1932; L, *complexus,* encirclement], a congenital heart disease characterized by a defect of the ventricular septum, a malpositioned aortic root that overrides the interventricular septum, and a dilated pulmonary artery.

**Eisenmenger's syndrome** /i'sən·meng'ərz/ [Victor Eisenmenger, German physician, 1864–1932], ventricular septal defect with pulmonary hypertension and cyanosis resulting from right-to-left (reversed) shunt of blood. Sometimes defined as pulmonary hypertension and cyanosis with the shunt being at the atrial, ventricular, or great vessel area.

**ejaculate** /ijak'yəlit/, *n.* the semen discharged in a single emission. See also **ejaculation.** —**ejaculate** /ijak'yəlāt/, *v.*

**ejaculation** /-ā'shən/ [L, *ejaculari,* to hurl out], the sudden emission of semen from the male urethra, usually during copulation, masturbation, or nocturnal emission. It is a reflex action in two phases. In the first phase, sperm, seminal fluid, and prostatic and bulbourethral gland secretions are moved into the urethra. In the second phase, strong spasmodic peristaltic contractions force ejaculation. The sensation of ejaculation is commonly also called orgasm. The fluid volume of the ejaculate is usually between 2 and 5 mL; each milliliter usually contains 50 million to 150 million spermatozoa. —**ejaculatory** /ijak'yələtôr'ē/, *adj.*

**ejaculator urinae.** See **bulbocavernosus.**

**ejaculatory duct** /ijak'yələtôr'ē/, the passage formed by the junction of the duct of the seminal vesicles and ductus deferens through which semen enters the urethra.

**ejection** /ijek'shən/ [L, *ejicere,* to cast out], forceful expulsion, as of blood from a ventricle of the heart.

**ejection click,** a sharp, clicking sound arising from near the heart. It may be caused by sudden swelling of a pulmonary artery, abrupt dilation of the aorta, or forceful opening of the aortic cusps. Ejection clicks are often heard during examination of individuals with septal defects or patent ductus arteriosus. Although they are associated with high pulmonary resistance and hypertension, they are common and of no clinical significance in pregnant women and in many other healthy people. See also **ejection sound.** Compare **systolic click.**

**ejection fraction (EF),** the fraction of the total ventricular filling volume that is ejected during each ventricular contraction. The normal EF of the left ventricle is 65%.

**ejection murmur.** See **systolic murmur.**

**ejection period,** the second phase of ventricular systole, when the semilunar valves are open and blood is being discharged into the aortic and pulmonary arteries. Also called **sphygmic interval.**

**ejection sound,** a sharp, clicking sound heard early in systole, coinciding with the onset of either right or left ventricular ejection. Aortic ejection sounds are commonly heard in aortic valvular stenosis, aortic insufficiency, coarctation of the aorta, and hypertension with aortic dilation. Pulmonary ejection sounds are heard in mild to moderate pulmonary stenosis, pulmonary hypertension, and dilation of the pulmonary artery. See also **ejection click.**

**Ekbom's syndrome.** See **restless legs syndrome.**

**EKC,** abbreviation for **epidemic keratoconjunctivitis.**

**EKG,** abbreviation for **electrocardiogram.**

**elaborate** /ilab'ərāt/ [L, *elaborare,* to work out], (in endocrinology) a process by which a gland synthesizes a complex substance from simpler substances and secretes it, usually under the stimulation of a tropic hormone from the pituitary gland. This process, regulated by a negative feedback system, which includes the hypothalamus, pituitary, and target gland, serves to maintain homeostasis in body function. —**elaboration,** *n.*

**elaio-.** See **eleo-.**

**Elase,** trademark for a topical fixed-combination drug containing enzymes (fibrinolysin and desoxyribonuclease).

**Elase with Chloromycetin,** trademark for a topical fixed-combination drug containing two lytic enzymes (fibrinolysin and desoxyribonuclease) and an antibacterial (chloramphenicol).

**elastance** /ilas'təns/ [Gk, *elaunein,* to drive], **1.** the quality of recoiling or returning to an original form after the removal of pressure. **2.** the degree to which an air- or fluid-filled organ, such as a lung, bladder, or blood vessel, can return to its original dimensions when a distending or compressing force is removed. **3.** the measurement of the unit volume of change in such an organ per unit of decreased pressure change. **4.** the reciprocal of compliance.

**elastase,** an enzyme that cleaves bonds adjacent to neutral amino acids in elastin.

**elastic bandage** /ilas'tik/ [Gk, *elaunein,* to drive; Fr, *bande,* strip], a bandage of stretchable fabric that provides support and allows movement. Among its uses is application to swollen extremities, such as knees or wrists; varicose veins; and broken ribs.

**elastic-band fixation,** a method of treatment of fractures of the jaw using rubber bands to connect metal splints or wires that are attached to the maxilla and mandible. The rubber bands produce traction and draw the teeth into occlusion and proper alignment while the fracture is healing. Rubber bands are safer than rigid wires in the event of vomiting. See also **maxillomandibular fixation, nasomandibular fixation.**

**elastic bougie,** a flexible bougie that can be passed through angular or winding channels. See also **bougie.**

**elastic cartilage,** the most pliant of the three kinds of cartilage, consisting of elastic fibers in a flexible fibrous matrix. It is yellow and is located in various parts of the body, such as the external ear, the auditory tube, and the epiglottis. Also called **yellow cartilage.** Compare **hyaline cartilage, white fibrocartilage.**

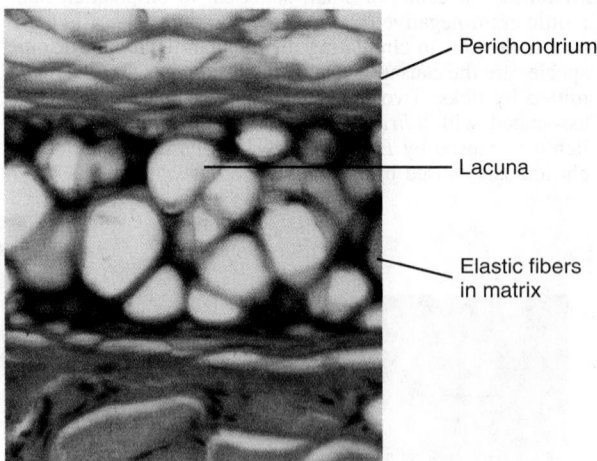

**Elastic cartilage** *(© Ed Reschke; used with permission)*

Perichondrium

Lacuna

Elastic fibers in matrix

**elasticity** /i'lastis'itē/, the ability of tissue to regain its original shape and size after being stretched, squeezed, or otherwise deformed. Muscle tissue is generally regarded as elastic because it is able to change size and shape and return to its original condition.

**elastic membrane.** See **cricothyroid membrane.**

**elastic recoil** /rē'koil/, the difference between intrapleural pressure and alveolar pressure at a given lung volume under static conditions.

**elastic stocking,** a type of hosiery that applies gradient pressure to the legs to prevent excessive blood accumulation in the lower extremities caused by faulty vein valves. The stockings are commonly prescribed for patients with varicose veins. Compare **antiembolism hose.**

**elastic tissue** [Gk, *elaunein,* to drive; OFr, *tissu*], a type of connective tissue containing elastic fibers. It is found in ligaments of the spinal column, in the cartilage of the external ear, and in the walls of some large blood vessels.

**elastic traction** [Gk, *elaunein* + L, *trahere,* to draw], any therapeutic apparatus that uses an elastic device to pull on a limb.

**elastin** /ilas′tin/ [Gk, *elaunein,* to drive], a protein that forms the principal substance of yellow elastic tissue fibers.

**elastofibroma** /ilas′tōfībrō′mə/, a benign nonencapsulated mass of collagenous, fibrous, and elastic tissue that develops in subscapular fatty tissue in older persons.

**elastomer** /i·las′tō·mər/ [Gk, *elaunein,* to drive + *meros,* part], a synthetic rubber; any of various soft, elastic, rubberlike polymers; used in dentistry as an impression material and for maxillofacial extraoral prostheses. **—elastomeric,** *adj.*

**elation** /ilā′shən/ [L, *elatus,* a lifting up], an emotional reaction characterized by euphoria, excitement, extreme joyfulness, optimism, and self-satisfaction. It is considered to be of pathologic origin when such a response does not realistically reflect a person's actual circumstances. Thus an elated mood may be characteristic of a manic state.

**Elavil,** trademark for a tricyclic antidepressant (amitriptyline hydrochloride).

**elbow** [AS, *elboga*], the bend of the arm at the joint that connects the upper arm and the forearm. It is a common site of inflammation and injuries, such as those incurred during participation in various sports. See also **elbow joint.**

Lateral epicondyle
Capitulum
Head of radius
Radial neck
Humerus
Coronoid fossa
Medial epicondyle
Trochlea
Semilunar notch
Coronoid process
Radial notch
Radial tuberosity
Ulna
Radius

**Elbow joint** *(Vidic and Saurez, 1984)*

**elbow bone.** See **ulna.**

**elbow jerk.** See **triceps reflex.**

**elbow joint,** the hinged articulation of the humerus, the ulna, and the radius. It is covered by a protective capsule associated with three ligaments and an extensive synovial membrane. The elbow joint allows flexion and extension of the forearm and accommodates the radioulnar articulation. Also called **articulatio cubiti.**

**elbow reflex.** See **triceps reflex.**

**elder,** an herb found in the United States and Europe as a tall shrub.

■ USES: This herb may be useful for those with susceptibility to colds, flu, and yeast infections; it is also used for nasal and chest congestion, earache associated with chronic congestion, and hay fever.

■ CONTRAINDICATIONS: Elderberry is not recommended during pregnancy and lactation, in children, or in those with known hypersensitivity to this plant or similar plants.

**elder abuse,** a reportable offense of physical, psychologic, or material abuse, as well as violation of the rights of safety, security, and adequate health care of older adults. Contributing factors may include economic considerations, interpersonal conflicts, health, and dependency. Often the abused person denies that abusive acts occur and feels helpless and resigned to abuse. Health care workers are expected to report suspected abuse. Also called **abuse of the elderly.**

**elderly primigravida,** a woman who becomes pregnant for the first time after the age of 34. Although an elderly primigravida was in the past at greater risk of adverse complications of a pregnancy, newer techniques and drugs have eliminated most of the risk and made it possible even for women of menopausal age to bear children.

**Eldopaque,** trademark for a dermatologic bleaching agent (hydroquinone).

**elective** /ilek′tiv/ [L, *eligere,* to choose], pertaining to a procedure that is performed by choice and is not essential, such as elective surgery.

**elective abortion,** induced termination of a pregnancy **(TOP),** usually before the fetus has developed enough to live if born, deemed necessary by the woman carrying it and performed at her request. Commonly (but incorrectly) called **therapeutic abortion.** See also **induced abortion, therapeutic abortion.**

**elective induction of labor.** See **induction of labor.**

**Electra complex** /ilek′trə/, (in psychiatry) the libidinous desire of a daughter for her father.

**electret** /ilek′trət/, an insulator carrying a permanent charge similar to a permanent magnet.

**electrically stimulated osteogenesis** /ilek′triklē/ [Gk, *elektron,* amber; L, *stimulare,* to incite; Gk, *osteon,* bone, *genein,* to produce], a bone regeneration process induced by surgically implanted electrodes conveying electric current, especially at nonunion fracture sites. The process is effective because of the different electric potentials within bone tissue. Viable nonstressed bone is electronegative in the metaphyseal regions and over a fracture callus and electropositive in the diaphyses and other less active regions. Electric stimulation of fractures can accelerate osteogenesis, forming bone more quickly in the area of a surgically inserted negative electrode. The precise mechanisms by which electricity induces osteogenesis are not understood, but research shows that when cathodes are implanted at a fracture site and an electric potential of less than 1 volt is applied, oxygen is consumed at the cathode, and hydroxyl ions are produced, decreasing the oxygen tension of the local tissue and increasing the alkalinity. Low tissue oxygen tension encourages bone formation, which follows a predominantly anaerobic metabolic pathway. Studies of bone-forming junctions demonstrate that an alkaline pH exists in the zone of hypertrophic cells of the bone growth plate when calcification starts. Electrically stimulated osteogenesis can be achieved with a device that stimulates the fracture site electrically by means of several surgically implanted cathodes. Cathode pins are connected to an external power supply that delivers 20 μA to each pin. The cathodes are inserted and positioned in the fracture space with the aid of image intensification or other radiographic techniques. Other methods for applying electrical current to fractured bone involve open surgical procedures and implantation of electrodes. The percutaneous technique involving the insertion of cathode pins is performed with a local anesthetic and usually involves less postoperative pain than open surgery methods. The number and the position of the cathodes in the percutaneous technique vary, depending on the bone involved. Generally two cathodes are used for nonunion fractures of small bones, such as the medial malleolus or the carpal navicular. Three or more cathodes are used in the clavicle and the bones of the forearm. Four cathodes are used in the treatment of large bones, such as the tibia, the femur, and the humerus. Cathodes are generally inserted from opposite directions into the nonunion site. If four cathodes are used, two are placed above, and two below the fracture site; the exposed tips of the cathodes rest directly in the nonunion space. Patients who receive such treatment are routinely released from the hospital the day after the procedure, and the stimulation of their fractures by a portable power supply strapped to the skin over the fracture site continues during the healing period. The osteogenesis is radiographically monitored, and after about 12 weeks the cathode pins are removed and the affected portion of the limb involved is placed in a weight-bearing cast. Use of the cathode-pin method of electrically stimulated osteogenesis is contraindicated in the treatment of pathologic fractures associated with benign or malignant tumors and in the treatment of congenital conditions, such as congenital pseudarthrosis and osteogenesis imperfecta. The cathode-pin method is also contraindicated in the presence of active systemic infections, clinically active osteomyelitis, proven patient sensitivity to the nickel or chromium from which the pins are made, or synovial pseudarthrosis, unless the fluid-filled cavity at the nonunion site is excised before the cathode pins are inserted. The success rate of treatment with the percutaneous method of electrically stimulated osteogenesis is significantly reduced in nonunions in which the gap is wider than one half the diameter of the bone involved.

**electric blood warmer,** a device for heating blood before infusions, especially massive transfusions in which cold blood may cause a state of shock. The electric blood warmer includes a receptacle containing an electric heater and space for the insertion of a disposable blood-warming bag composed of parallel plastic tubes. The warmer is also equipped with a temperature indicator, which shows when the heating bag reaches the proper temperature of 99° F (37.6° C). An IV Y-set is commonly used in transfusions involving the electric blood warmer.

**electric burn,** the tissue damage resulting from heat of up to 5000° C generated by an electric current. The points of entrance and exit on the skin are burned, along with the muscle and subcutaneous tissues through which the current passes. Fatal cardiac arrhythmia may result.

**electric cautery.** See **electrocautery.**

**electric circuit,** the path of the electron flow from a generating source through various components and back to the generating source.

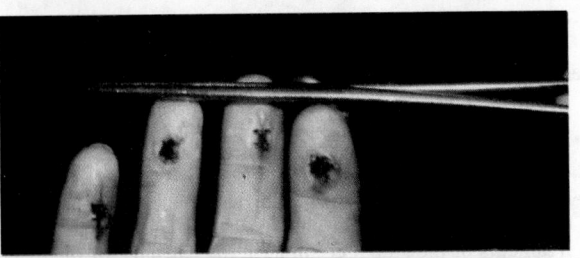

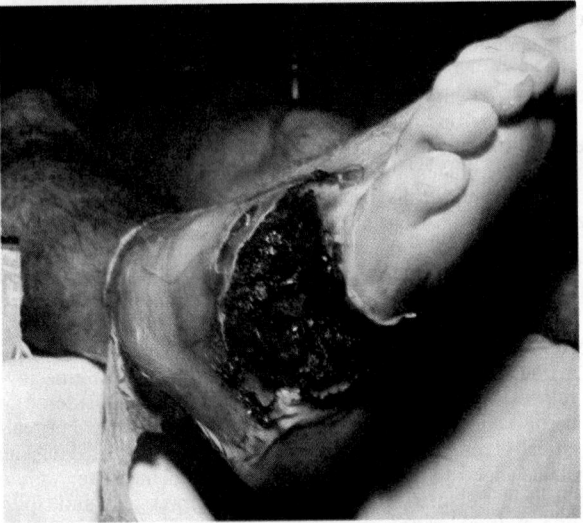

**Entry site *(top)* and exit site *(bottom)* of an electric burn**
*(Sanders, 2000)*

**electric current,** the net movement of electrons along a conducting medium.

**electric field,** the lines of force exerted on charged ions in the tissues by the electrodes that cause charged particles to move from one pole to another.

**electric impedance,** an opposition to electron flow in a conducting material.

**electricity** /i′lektris′itē/ [Gk, *elektron,* amber], a form of energy expressed by the activity of electrons and other subatomic particles in motion, as in dynamic electricity, or at rest, as in static electricity. Electricity can be produced by heat; generated by a voltaic cell; or produced by induction, rubbing of nonconductors with dry materials, or chemical activity. Electricity may be negative, when there is a surplus of electrons, or positive, when there is a surplus of protons or a deficiency of electrons.

**electric muscle stimulator (EMS),** a therapeutic electric current used to stimulate muscle directly, such as when the muscle is denervated and peripheral nerves are not functioning. See also **electrostimulation.**

**electric potential,** the potential difference between charged particles. See also **potential.**

**electric potential gradient.** See **membrane potential.**

**electric shock,** a traumatic physical state caused by the passage of electric current through the body. It usually involves accidental contact with exposed parts of electric circuits in home appliances and domestic power supplies but may also result from lightning or contact with high-voltage wires. The resultant damage depends on the intensity of the electric current, the type of current, and the duration and the frequency of current flow. Alternating current (AC), direct current (DC), and mixed current cause different kinds and degrees of damage. High-frequency current produces more heat than low-frequency current and can cause burns, coagulation, and necrosis of affected body parts. Low-frequency current can burn tissues if the area of contact is small and concentrated. Severe electric shock commonly causes unconsciousness, respiratory paralysis, muscle contractions, bone fractures, and cardiac disorders. Even passage of small electric currents through the heart can cause fibrillation. About 1000 persons in the United States die from electric shock each year. Treatment may involve such measures as cardiopulmonary resuscitation, defibrillation, and IV administration of electrolytes to help stabilize vital functions. See also **cardiogenic shock, hypovolemic shock.**

**electric shock therapy.** See **electroconvulsive therapy.**

**electric spinal orthosis,** an electric device that helps control curvature of the spine by stimulating back muscles. The portable battery-powered machine does not correct scoliosis but prevents it from worsening.

**electro-,** prefix meaning 'electricity': *electrobiology, electrocatalysis, electrolepsy.*

**electroanalgesia** /ilek′trō·an′əljē′sē·ə/, the use of an electric current to relieve pain. See also **transcutaneous electrical nerve stimulation.**

**electroanalytic chemistry** /-an′əlit′ik/ [Gk, *elektron* + *analysis,* a loosening, *chemeia,* alchemy], the branch of chemistry concerned with the analysis of compounds by use of electrical properties to produce characteristic observable change in the substance being studied. See also **chemistry.**

**electroanesthesia** /-an′esthē′zhə/, the use of an electric current to produce local or general anesthesia.

**electroaxonography.** See **axonography.**

**electrocardiogram (ECG, EKG)** /-kär′dē·əgram′/ [Gk, *elektron* + *kardia,* heart, *gramma,* record], a graphic record produced by an electrocardiograph, a device for recording electrical conduction through the heart.

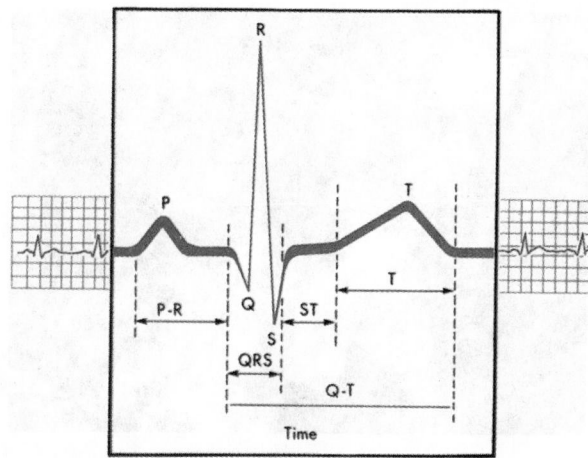

**Usual waveform of an electrocardiogram**
(Berne and Levy, 1997)

**electrocardiograph (ECG, EKG)** /-kär′dē·əgraf′/, a device used for recording the electrical activity of the myocardium to detect transmission of the cardiac impulse through

the conductive tissues of the muscle. Electrocardiography allows diagnosis of specific cardiac abnormalities. Leads are affixed to certain anatomic points on the patient's chest, usually with an adhesive gel that promotes transmission of the electric impulse to the recording device. **—electrocardiographic,** *adj.*

**electrocardiographic technician** /-kär′dē·ōgraf′ik/, an allied health worker with special training and experience in operating and maintaining electrocardiographic equipment and providing recorded data for diagnostic review by a physician.

**electrocardiograph lead** /lēd/, **1.** an electrode placed on part of the body and connected to an electrocardiograph. **2.** a record, made by the electrocardiograph, that varies with the site of the electrode. Electrocardiography is generally performed with the use of six limb leads and six leads placed on the precordium. The peripheral or extremity leads are designated I, II, III, AVR, AVL, and AVF. The chest leads are designated $V_1$, $V_2$, $V_3$, $V_4$, $V_5$, and $V_6$ to indicate the points on the precordium on which the electrodes are placed.

**electrocardiography (ECG, EKG)** /-kär′dē·og′rəfē/ [Gk, *elektron* + *kardia,* heart, *graphein,* to record], the study of records of electric activity generated by the heart muscle. Also called **cardiography.**

**electrocardiophonograph.** See **phonocardiograph.**

**electrocatalysis,** the chemical decomposition of tissues caused by the application of electric current to the body.

**electrocautery** /ilek′trōkô′tərē/ [Gk, *elektron* + *kauterion,* branding iron], the application of a needle or snare heated by electric current for the destruction of tissue, such as for removing warts or polyps and cauterizing small blood vessels to limit blood loss during surgery. Also called **electric cautery, galvanic cautery, galvanocautery.** See also **diathermy.**

**electrochemistry,** the study of the electric effects that accompany chemical action and the chemical activity produced by electric influence.

**electrocoagulation** /-kō·ag′yəlā′shən/ [Gk, *elektron* + L, *coagulare,* to curdle], a therapeutic destructive form of electrosurgery in which tissue is hardened by the passage of high-frequency current from an electric cautery device. Also called **surgical diathermy.** Compare **electrodesiccation.**

**electroconvulsive therapy (ECT)** /-kənvul′siv/, the induction of a brief convulsion by passing an electric current through the brain for the treatment of affective disorders, especially in patients resistant to psychoactive-drug therapy. ECT is primarily used when rapid definitive response is required for either medical or psychiatric reasons, such as for a patient who is extremely suicidal and when the risks of other treatments outweigh the risk of ECT. A secondary use of ECT is treatment failure of other choices. Also called **electric shock therapy (EST), electroshock therapy (EST), electrotherapy.**

**electrocution** /-kyōō′shən/, death caused by the passage of electric current through the body. See also **electric shock.**

**electrode** /ilek′trōd/ [Gk, *elektron* + *hodos,* way], **1.** a contact for the induction or detection of electrical activity. **2.** a medium for conducting an electrical current from the body to physiologic monitoring equipment.

**electrodermal** /-dur′məl/, pertaining to electrical properties of the skin, particularly altered resistance.

**electrodermal audiometry** [Gk, *elektron* + *derma,* skin; L, *audire,* to hear; Gk, *metron,* measure], a method for determining hearing thresholds in which a harmless electric shock is used to condition the subject to a pure tone; thereafter the tone, coupled with the anticipation of a shock, elicits a brief electrodermal response. The lowest intensity of the sound that produces the skin response is considered the subject's hearing threshold. It is a very old procedure and rarely used today.

**electrodesiccation** /-des′ikā′shən/ [Gk, *elektron* + *desiccare,* to dry up], a technique in electrosurgery in which tissue is destroyed by burning with an electric spark. It is used primarily for eliminating small superficial growths but may be used with curettage for eradicating abnormal tissue deeper in the skin. In the latter case, layers of skin may be burned, then successively scraped away. The procedure is performed under local anesthesia.

**electrodiagnosis** /-dī′agnō′sis/ [Gk, *elektron* + *dia,* twice, *gnosis,* knowledge], the diagnosis of disease or injury by electric stimulation of various nerves and muscles.

**electrodynamics** /-dīnam′iks/, the study of electrostatic charges in motion, such as the flow of electrons in an electric current. Compare **electrohemodynamics.**

**electrodynograph (EDG)** /-din′əgraf′/ [Gk, *elektron* + *dynamis,* force, *graphein,* to record], an electronic device used to measure pressures exerted in biologic activity, such as those exerted by the human foot in walking, running, jogging, or climbing stairs.

**electroencephalogram (EEG)** /ilek′trō·ensef′ələgram′/ [Gk, *elektron* + *enkephalos,* brain, *gramma,* record], a graphic chart on which is traced the electric potential produced by the brain cells, as detected by electrodes placed on the scalp. The resulting brain waves are called alpha, beta, delta, and theta rhythms, according to the frequencies they produce, which range from 2 to 12 cycles per second with an amplitude of up to 100 μV. Variations in brain wave activity are correlated with neurologic conditions, psychologic states, and level of consciousness. See also **encephalography.**

**electroencephalograph (EEG)** /ilek′trō·ensef′ələgraf′/, an instrument for receiving and recording the electric potential produced by the brain cells. It consists of a vacuum tube amplifier that magnifies the electrical currents received through electrodes placed on the scalp and electromagnetically records the patterns on a graphic chart. See also **electroencephalography.**

**electroencephalographic technologist** /ilek′trō·ensef′əl əgraf′ik/, a person trained in the management of an electroencephalographic laboratory. The technologist may supervise electroencephalographic technicians, who are generally responsible for the operation and maintenance of the equipment.

**electroencephalography (EEG)** /ilek′trō·ensef′əlog′rəfē/, the process of recording brain wave activity. Electrodes are attached to various areas of the patient's head with collodion. During the procedure the patient remains quiet, with eyes closed, and refrains from talking or moving; in certain cases prescribed activities, especially hyperventilation, may be requested. The test is used to diagnose seizure disorders, brainstem disorders, focal lesions, and impaired consciousness. During neurosurgery the electrodes can be applied directly to the surface of the brain (intracranial electroencephalography) or placed within the brain tissue (depth electroencephalography) to detect lesions or tumors. See also **electroencephalogram. —electroencephalographic,** *adj.*

**electrogram** /ilek′trōgram′/ [Gk, *elektron* + *gramma,* record], a unipolar or bipolar record of the electric activity of the heart as recorded by electrodes within the cardiac chambers or on the epicardium. Examples are the atrial electrogram, ventricular electrogram, and His bundle electrogram.

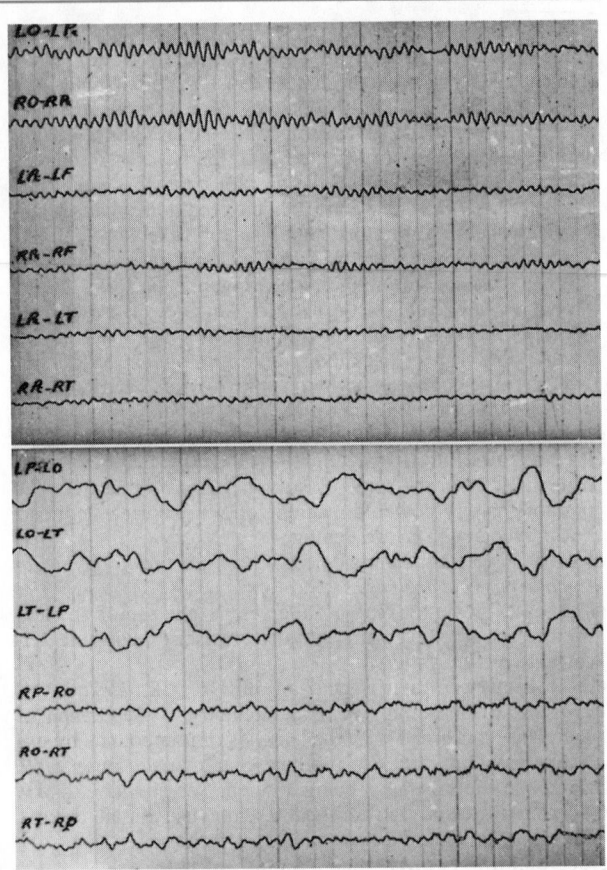

**Electroencephalogram:** *top:* **normal;** *bottom,* **intracranial tumor**
*(Thompson et al, 1996)*

**Electroencephalography** *(Chipps, Clanin, and Campbell, 1992)*

**electrohemodynamics (EHD)** /ilek′trōhē′mōdīnam′iks/ [Gk, *elektron* + *haima,* blood, *dynamis,* force], a technique for noninvasively measuring the mechanical properties and hemodynamic characteristics of the vascular system, including arterial blood pressure, electric impedance, blood flow, and resistance to blood flow.

**electroimmunodiffusion.** See **immunodiffusion.**

**electrolarynx** /i·lek′trō·ler′ingks/ [Gr, *elektron,* amber + *larynx*], an electromechanical device that enables a laryngectomized person to speak. When it is placed against the region of the laryngectomy a buzzing sound is produced, which is converted into simulated speech by movements of the organs of articulation (lips, tongue, glottis).

**electrolysis** /il′ektrol′isis/ [Gk, *elektron* + *lysis,* loosening], a process in which electric energy causes a chemical change in a conducting medium, usually a solution or a molten substance, or the decomposition of a substance such as hair follicles. **—electrolytic,** *adj.*

**electrolyte** /ilek′trōlīt/ [Gk, *elektron* + *lytos,* soluble], an element or compound that, when melted or dissolved in water or another solvent, dissociates into ions and is able to conduct an electric current. Electrolytes differ in their concentrations in blood plasma, interstitial fluid, and cell fluid and affect the movement of substances between those compartments. Proper quantities of principal electrolytes and balance among them are critical to normal metabolism and function. For example, calcium ($Ca^{++}$) is necessary for relaxation of skeletal muscle and contraction of cardiac muscle; potassium ($K^+$) is required for contraction of skeletal muscle and relaxation of cardiac muscle. Sodium ($Na^+$) is essential in maintaining fluid balance. Certain diseases, conditions, and medications may lead to a deficiency of one or more electrolytes and to an imbalance among them; for example, certain diuretics and a low-sodium diet prescribed in hypertension may cause hypokalemic shock as a result of a loss of potassium. Diarrhea may cause a loss of many electrolytes, leading to hypovolemia and shock, especially in infants. Careful and regular monitoring of electrolytes and IV replacement of fluid and electrolytes are aspects of acute care in many illnesses. **—electrolytic,** *adj.*

**electrolyte & acid/base balance,** a nursing outcome from the Nursing Outcomes Classification (NOC) defined as balance of electrolytes and non-electrolytes in the intracellular and extracellular compartments of the body. See also **Nursing Outcomes Classification.**

**electrolyte balance,** the equilibrium between electrolytes in the body.

### Normal electrolyte content of body fluids*

| Electrolytes (anions and cations) | Extracellular | | Intracellular (mEq/L) |
|---|---|---|---|
| | Intravascular (mEq/L) | Interstitial (mEq/L) | |
| Sodium ($Na^+$) | 142 | 146 | 15 |
| Potassium ($K^+$) | 5 | 5 | 150 |
| Calcium ($Ca^{++}$) | 5 | 3 | 2 |
| Magnesium ($Mg^{++}$) | 2 | 1 | 27 |
| Chloride ($Cl^-$) | 102 | 114 | 1 |
| Bicarbonate ($HCO_3^-$) | 27 | 30 | 10 |
| Protein ($Prot^-$) | 16 | 1 | 63 |
| Phosphate ($HPO_4^=$) | 2 | 2 | 100 |
| Sulfate ($SO_4^=$) | 1 | 1 | 20 |
| Organic acids | 5 | 8 | 0 |

From Phipps WJ, Sands JK, Marek JF: *Medical-surgical nursing: concepts and clinical practice,* ed 6, St Louis, 1999, Mosby.

*Note that the electrolyte level of the intravascular and interstitial fluids (extracellular) is approximately the same and that sodium and chloride contents are markedly higher in these fluids, whereas potassium, phosphate, and protein contents are markedly higher in intracellular fluid.

**electrolyte management,** a nursing intervention from the Nursing Interventions Classification (NIC) defined as promotion of electrolyte balance and prevention of complications resulting from abnormal or undesired serum electrolyte levels. See also **Nursing Interventions Classification.**

**electrolyte management: hypercalcemia,** a nursing intervention from the Nursing Interventions Classification (NIC) defined as promotion of calcium balance and prevention of complications resulting from serum calcium levels higher than desired. See also **Nursing Interventions Classification.**

**electrolyte management: hyperkalemia,** a nursing intervention from the Nursing Interventions Classification (NIC) defined as promotion of potassium balance and prevention of complications resulting from serum potassium levels higher than desired. See also **Nursing Interventions Classification.**

**electrolyte management: hypermagnesemia,** a nursing intervention from the Nursing Interventions Classification (NIC) defined as promotion of magnesium balance and prevention of complications resulting from serum magnesium levels higher than desired. See also **Nursing Interventions Classification.**

**electrolyte management: hypernatremia,** a nursing intervention from the Nursing Interventions Classification (NIC) defined as promotion of sodium balance and prevention of complications resulting from serum sodium levels higher than desired. See also **Nursing Interventions Classification.**

**electrolyte management: hyperphosphatemia,** a nursing intervention from the Nursing Interventions Classification (NIC) defined as promotion of phosphate balance and prevention of complications resulting from serum phosphate levels higher than desired. See also **Nursing Interventions Classification.**

**electrolyte management: hypocalcemia,** a nursing intervention from the Nursing Interventions Classification (NIC) defined as promotion of calcium balance and prevention of complications resulting from serum calcium levels lower than desired. See also **Nursing Interventions Classification.**

**electrolyte management: hypokalemia,** a nursing intervention from the Nursing Interventions Classification (NIC) defined as promotion of potassium balance and prevention of complications resulting from serum potassium levels lower than desired. See also **Nursing Interventions Classification.**

**electrolyte management: hypomagnesemia,** a nursing intervention from the Nursing Interventions Classification (NIC) defined as promotion of magnesium balance and prevention of complications resulting from serum magnesium levels lower than desired. See also **Nursing Interventions Classification.**

**electrolyte management: hyponatremia,** a nursing intervention from the Nursing Interventions Classification (NIC) defined as promotion of sodium balance and prevention of complications resulting from serum sodium levels lower than desired. See also **Nursing Interventions Classification.**

**electrolyte management: hypophosphatemia,** a nursing intervention from the Nursing Interventions Classification (NIC) defined as promotion of phosphate balance and prevention of complications resulting from serum phosphate levels lower than desired. See also **Nursing Interventions Classification.**

**electrolyte monitoring,** a nursing intervention from the Nursing Interventions Classification (NIC) defined as collection and analysis of patient data to regulate electrolyte balance. See also **Nursing Interventions Classification.**

**electrolyte solution,** any solution containing electrolytes prepared for oral, parenteral, or rectal administration for the replacement or supplementation of ions necessary for homeostasis. The loss of potassium ion ($K^+$) by vomiting, by diarrhea, or by the action of certain medications, including diuretics and corticosteroids, may be corrected by administering a solution high in potassium. Other electrolyte solutions containing combinations of calcium, sodium, phosphate, chloride, or magnesium may be given to treat acid-base disturbance, as seen in chronic renal dysfunction or diabetic ketoacidosis. The solutions are available in a wide range of balanced formulas for replacement or maintenance, and most include various trace minerals.

**electrolytic.** See **electrolysis.**

**electromagnetic** /-magnet′ik/ [Gk, *elektron, Magnesia*, ancient source of lodestone], **1.** pertaining to magnetism that is induced by an electric current. **2.** pertaining to radiation such as light, microwaves, x-rays, γ-rays, or radio waves.

**electromagnetic induction** [Gk, *elektron + magnes*, lodestone; L, *inducere*, to bring in], the production of electric current in a circuit when it is passed through a changing magnetic field.

**electromagnetic radiation,** radiation that is produced with a combination of magnetic and electric forces. It exists as a continuous spectrum of radiation, from that with the highest energy level and shortest wavelength (gamma rays) to that with the lowest energy and longest wavelength (long radio waves). The visible part of the electromagnetic spectrum has a wavelength between 400 and 700 nm. Ultraviolet and infrared radiation have wavelengths just below the short end and above the long end of the visible spectrum, respectively. X-rays have wavelengths from about 0.005 to 10 nm. All forms of electromagnetic radiation travel at the speed of light.

**electromagnetic spectrum,** the range of frequencies and wavelengths associated with radiant energy.

**electromallet condenser** /-mal′ət/ [Gk, *elektron* + OFr, *mail*, maul; L, *condensare*, to make dense], an electromechanical device formerly used for compacting direct-filling gold, such as gold foil restorations in prepared tooth cavities.

**electromotive force (EMF)** /-mō′tiv/, the electric potential, or ability of electric energy to perform work. EMF is usually measured in joules per coulomb, or volts (V). The higher the voltage, the greater the potential of electric energy. Any device, such as a storage battery, that converts some form of energy into electricity is a source of EMF.

**electromyogram (EMG)** /ilek′trōmī′əgram′/, a record of the intrinsic electric activity in a skeletal muscle. Such data aid the diagnosis of neuromuscular problems and are obtained by applying surface electrodes or by inserting a needle electrode into the muscle and observing electric activity with an oscilloscope and a loudspeaker. Some electromyograms show abnormalities, such as spontaneous electric potentials within the muscle under study, and help pinpoint lesions of motor nerves. Electromyograms also measure electric potentials induced by voluntary muscular contraction. See also **electroneuromyography.**

**electromyographic biofeedback** /-mī′əgraf′ik/, a therapeutic procedure that uses electronic or electromechanical instruments to measure, process, and feed back reinforcing information with auditory and visual signals accurately. It is used to provide information about muscle activity during ambulation, for example, in clients with brain injury, stroke, or cerebral palsy.

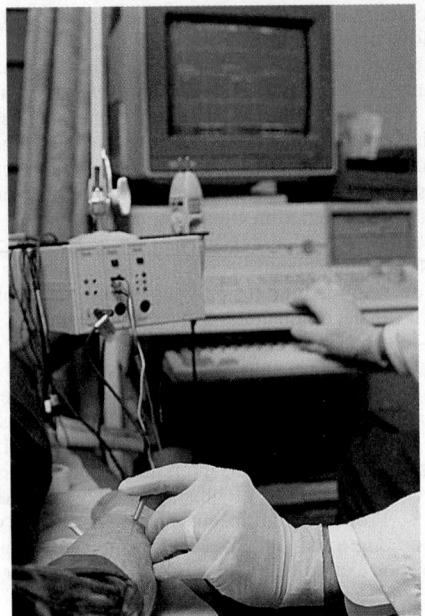

**Electromyogram** *(Mourad, 1991)*

**electromyographic technician** /-mī′əgraf′ik/, a health care provider with special training and experience to assist the physician in recording and analyzing muscle action potentials with the use of various electronic devices.

**electromyography (EMG)** /-mī·og′rəfē/, the electrical recording of muscle action potentials.

**electromyography of pelvic floor sphincter,** an electrodiagnostic test performed to evaluate the neuromuscular function of the urinary or anal sphincter. It is done most often in patients with urinary or fecal incontinence.

**electron** /ilek′tron/ [Gk, *elektron*, amber], **1.** a negatively charged elementary particle that has a specific charge, mass, and spin. The number of electrons associated with the nucleus of an atom is equal to the atomic number of the substance. **2.** a negative beta particle emitted from a radioactive substance. See also **atom, element, ion, neutron, proton.**

**electronarcosis** /ilek′trōnärkō′sis/ [Gk, *elektron + narkosis*, numbness], anesthesia produced by passing an electric current through the brain. The experimental procedure has been used in the former USSR. Compare **electrosleep therapy.**

**electron beam computed tomography (EBCT),** ultrafast computed tomography done with a scanner in which the patient is surrounded by a large circular anode that emits x-rays as the electron beam is guided around it.

**electron capture,** a radioactive decay process in which an atomic nucleus with an excess of protons draws an electron into itself, creating a neutron out of a proton and thus decreasing the atomic number by 1. Often the resulting nucleus is unstable and achieves stability by giving off a gamma ray.

**electroneurodiagnostic technologist,** an allied health professional who, in collaboration with an electroencephalographer, obtains interpretable recordings of a patient's nervous system function. The electrodiagnostic technologist takes a patient history; applies adequate recording electrodes and uses optimal EEG, EP, and PSG techniques; and documents the clinical condition of patients.

**electroneurography,** an electrodiagnostic test that assists in detecting and locating peripheral nerve injury or disease. This study is usually done in conjunction with electromyography and may also be called electromyoneurography.

**electroneuromyography** /ilek′trōnŏŏr′ōmī·og′rəfē/ [Gk, *elektron* + *neuron*, nerve, *mys*, muscle, *graphein*, to record], a procedure for testing and recording neuromuscular activity by electric stimulation of nerves. Needle electrodes are inserted into any skeletal muscle being studied, electric current is applied to the electrodes, and neuromuscular functions are observed and recorded by means of instruments, such as a cathode-ray oscilloscope and an appropriate recording device. The procedure is helpful in the study of neuromuscular conduction, the extent of nerve lesions, and reflex responses. See also **electromyogram.**

**electronic bulletin board** /ilektron′ik/, a computerized communication system that allows users to compose and store information to be retrieved by other users of the system.

**Electronic Data Interchange (EDI),** a method by which two or more autonomous computer systems exchange computer-readable transaction data. It is possible even when the computers use different operating systems. It is the key factor in achieving automated medical records that can be shared electronically among providers.

**electronic fetal monitor (EFM)** [Gk, *elektron* + L, *fetus* + *monere,* to warn], a device that allows observation of the fetal heart rate and the maternal uterine contractions. It may be applied externally or internally. With an external monitor the fetal heart is detected by an ultrasound transducer positioned on the abdomen. Internal monitoring of the fetal heart rate is accomplished via an electrode clipped to the fetal scalp.

**electronic fetal monitoring: antepartum,** a nursing intervention from the Nursing Interventions Classification (NIC) defined as electronic evaluation of fetal heart rate response to movement, external stimuli, or uterine contractions during antepartal testing. See also **Nursing Interventions Classification.**

**electronic fetal monitoring: intrapartum,** a nursing intervention from the Nursing Interventions Classification (NIC) defined as electronic evaluation of fetal heart rate response to uterine contractions during intrapartal care. See also **Nursing Interventions Classification.**

**electronic infusion device (EID),** an automated system of introducing a fluid other than blood into a vein. The device may have programmable settings that control the amount of fluid to be infused, rate, low-volume notification level, and a keep-vein-open rate. Some EIDs have titration modes that allow a change in the delivery rate without interrupting fluid flow. They also allow delivery in milliliters per hour. Often called an IV pump.

**electronic mail (email, E-mail),** messages sent by one user of a computerized communications system and retrieved almost instantaneously by other users. The messages may be transmitted via modem through telephone lines or, in some instances, by shortwave radio. See also **electronic bulletin board.**

**electronic stethoscope,** a stethoscope designed and equipped to detect and amplify body sounds.

**electronic thermometer,** a battery-powered thermometer that registers temperature by electronic means.

**electron microscope,** an electronic instrument that scans cell and tissue sections with a beam of electrons, instead of visible light. The specimen is stained with electron-opaque

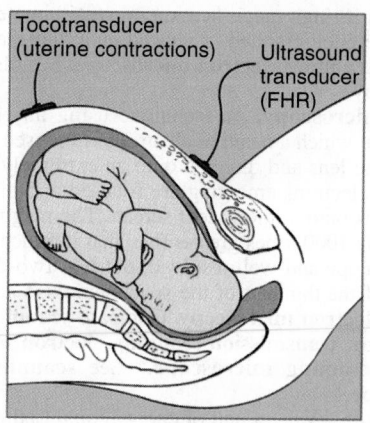

External fetal monitoring

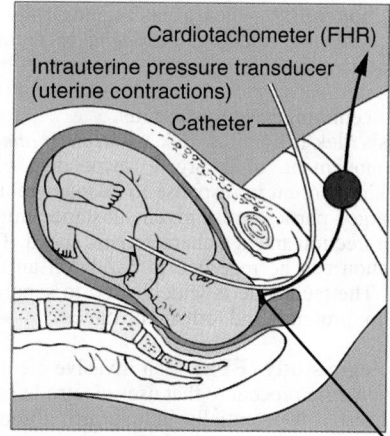

Internal fetal monitoring   Electrode

**Electronic fetal monitor** *(Lowdermilk, Perry, and Bobak, 2000)*

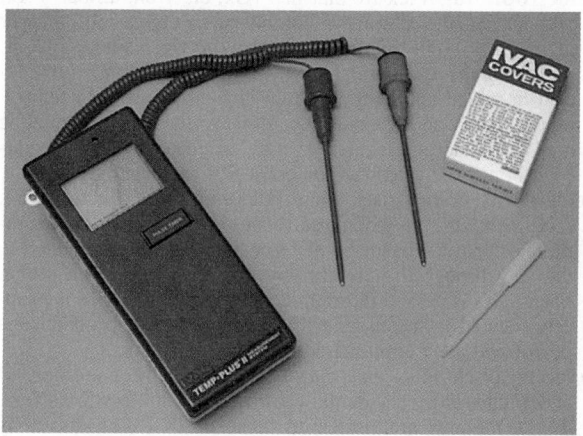

**Electronic thermometer** *(Potter and Perry, 2001)*

dyes. With its high magnification power, it creates an image that can be photographed or viewed on a fluorescent screen. Compare **scanning electron microscope.** See also **electron microscopy.**

**electron microscopy,** a technique using an electron microscope in which a beam of electrons is focused by an electromagnetic lens and directed onto an extremely thin specimen. The electrons emerging are focused and directed by a second lens onto a fluorescent screen. The magnified image produced is 1000 times greater than that produced by an optic microscope and well resolved, but it is two-dimensional because of the thinness of the specimen. Also called **transmission electron microscopy.** Compare **scanning electron microscopy, transmission scanning electron microscopy.**

**electron scanning microscope.** See **scanning electron microscope.**

**electron volt (eV),** a unit of energy equal to the energy acquired by an electron falling through a potential difference of 1 volt. One electron volt equals $1.6 \times 10^{-12}$ erg or $1.6 \times 10^{-19}$ J.

**electronystagmography** /ilek′trōnis′tagmog′rəfē/ [Gk, *elektron* + *nystagmos,* nodding, *graphein,* to record], a method of assessing and recording eye movements by measuring the electric activity of the extraocular muscles. See also **electroencephalogram, nystagmus.**

**electrophoresis** /ilek′trōfərē′sis/ [Gk, *elektron* + *pherein,* to bear], the movement of charged suspended particles through a liquid medium in response to changes in an electric field. Charged particles of a given substance migrate in a predictable direction and at a characteristic speed. The pattern of migration can be recorded in bands on an electrophoretogram. The technique is widely used to separate and identify serum proteins and other substances. —**electrophoretic,** *adj.*

**electrophysiologic study (EPS),** an invasive electrodiagnostic or manometric procedure that uses electrode catheters to pace the heart and potentially induce arrhythmias. The test identifies defects in the heart conduction system and arrhythmias that are otherwise inapparent; it also is used to assess the effectiveness of antiarrhythmic drugs.

**electrophysiology** /-fis′ē·ol′əjē/ [Gk, *elektron* + *physis,* nature, *logos,* science], a branch of biology concerned with the relationship between electric phenomena and biologic function.

**electropiezo activity.** See **piezoelectric activity.**

**electroplating** /i·lek′trō·plāt′ing/ [Gk, *electron,* amber + Fr, *plat,* flat dish], plating or coating of an object with a layer of metal through the use of electrolytic processes.

**electroporation** /-pōrā′shən/, a type of osmotic transfection in which an electric current is used to produce temporary holes in cell membranes allowing the entry of nucleic acids or macromolecules (a way of introducing new deoxyribonucleic acid into the cell). See also **transfection.**

**electroresection** /-risek′shən/ [Gk, *elektron* + L, *re,* again, *secare* to cut], a technique for the removal of bladder tumors or prostate tissue by electrocautery. A wire is guided to the site through the urethra with the aid of an optic probe. Electricity is passed through the wire when the wire is properly located in the tissue to be destroyed. The procedure is performed after administration of an anesthetic.

**electroshock** [Gk, *elektron* + Fr, *choc*], a condition of shock caused by accidental contact with an electric current. The symptoms are similar to those of shock produced by thermal burns, trauma, or coronary thrombosis.

**electroshock therapy.** See **electroconvulsive therapy.**

**electrosleep therapy** [Gk, *elektron* + AS, *slaep* + Gk, *therapeia,* treatment], a technique designed to induce sleep, especially in psychiatric patients, by administering a low-amplitude pulsating current to the brain. The cathode is placed supraorbitally, and the anode is placed over the mastoid process. The current, which is discharged for 15 to 20 minutes, produces a tingling sensation but does not always induce sleep. The procedure is repeated from 5 to 30 times. Electrosleep therapy is said to be beneficial for patients with anxiety, depression, gastric distress, insomnia, personality disorders, and schizophrenia. Compare **electronarcosis.**

**electrostatic imaging** /-stat′ik/ [Gk, *elektron* + *stasis,* standing still; L, *imago,* image], a radiographic technique in which the ionic charge liberated during the irradiation process is converted into a visible image. The image may be produced by an electronic read-out device or by liquid or powdered toner.

**electrostimulation** /-stim′yəlā′shən/, the application of electric current to stimulate bone or muscle tissue for therapeutic purposes, such as facilitation of muscle activation and muscle strengthening. See also **electric muscle stimulator.**

**electrosurgery** /-sur′jərē/ [Gk, *elektron* + *cheiourgos,* surgeon], surgery performed with various electric instruments that operate on high-frequency electric current. Kinds of electrosurgery include **electrocoagulation, electrodesiccation.**

**electrotherapeutic current,** any of three types of electric current, which, when introduced into biologic tissue, is capable of producing specific physiologic changes. The three types are direct monophasic, alternating biphasic, and pulsed polyphasic electric current.

**electrotherapist** /-ther′əpist/, a health care provider who has specific training and experience in the therapeutic uses of electricity.

**electrotherapy.** See **electroconvulsive therapy.**

**electrotonic current** [Gk, *elektron* + *tonos,* tension], a current induced in a nerve sheath without the generation of new current by an action potential.

**electrotonic synapse,** a gap junction in electrically excitable tissue, transmitting electrical impulses; see also **gap junction.**

**electrovalence,** the valence of an ion, equal to the absolute value of its charge. See also **valence, valence electron.**

**eleidin** /əlē′ədin/ [Gk, *elaia,* olive tree], a transparent, proteinaceous substance, resembling keratin, found in the outer stratum lucidum of the epidermis.

**element** [L, *elementum,* first principle], one of more than 100 primary, simple substances that cannot be broken down by chemical means into any other substance. Each atom of any element contains a specific number of protons in the nucleus and an equal number of electrons outside the nucleus. The nucleus contains a variable number of neutrons. An element with a disproportionate number of neutrons may be unstable, in which case the nucleus undergoes radioactive decay into a more stable elemental form. See also **atom, compound, molecule, radioactivity.**

**element 104.** See **rutherfordium.**

**element 105.** See **dubnium.**

**element 106.** See **seaborgium.**

**element 107,** an element reportedly synthesized in 1976 by Russian scientists who bombarded isotopes of bismuth with heavy nuclei of chromium-54. The finding was not confirmed by scientists of other nations. Its proposed name is **bohrium (Bh).**

**elemental formula.** See **defined formula diet.**

**elementary particle,** (in physics) a subatomic particle, such as an electron, neutron, or proton.

**eleo-,** combining form meaning 'oil': *eleoma, eleomyenchysis, eleopten.*

**eleoma** /ē′lē·ō′mə/, a lipogranuloma, or swelling, usually caused by subcutaneous injection of oil.

**elephantiasis** /el′əfəntī′əsis/ [Gk, *elephas,* elephant, *osis,* condition], the end-stage lesion of filariasis, characterized by extensive swelling, usually of the external genitalia and the legs resulting from obstruction of the lyphatics by filariae. The overlying skin becomes dark, thick, and coarse. Elephantiasis results from filariasis of many years' duration. See also **filariasis.**

**elephantine psoriasis** /el′əfan′tīn/, a rare form of psoriasis that is characterized by thick, scaly plaques on the hips, thighs, and back.

**elephantoid fever.** See **elephantiasis, filariasis.**

**elevation** /el′ə·va·shən/ [L, *elevare,* to lift], a raised area, or point of greater height.

**elevator** /el′ə·vā′tər/ [L, *elevare,* to lift], an instrument for lifting tissues, removing bony fragments, or removing roots of teeth.

**eleventh cranial nerve.** See **accessory nerve.**

**elfin facies syndrome.** See **Williams' syndrome.**

**eligibility** /el′əjəbil′itē/, entitlement of an individual to receive services based on that individual's enrollment in a health care plan.

**Eligibility Guarantee Payment,** a contract provision for guaranteeing payment from the health maintenance organization to the provider for services already delivered to enrollees whose coverage is terminated retroactively. Not applicable in Canada.

**elimination** /i·lim′i·nā′shən/ [L, *ex,* out + *limen,* threshold], **1.** the act of expulsion or of extrusion, especially of expulsion from the body. See also **clearance, defecation, excretion, urination. 2.** omission or exclusion, as in an **elimination diet.**

**elimination diet** /ilim′inā′shən/ [L, *eliminare,* to expel; Gk, *diata,* way of living], a procedure for identifying a food or foods to which a person is allergic by successively omitting from the diet certain foods in order to detect those responsible for the symptoms.

**ELISA** /əlī′zə/, abbreviation for **enzyme-linked immunosorbent assay.**

**elixir** /ilik′sər/ [Ar, *il-iksir,* seen as the philosopher's stone], a clear liquid containing water, alcohol, sweeteners, or flavors, used primarily as a vehicle for the oral administration of a drug.

**Elixophyllin,** trademark for a bronchodilator (theophylline), used as a bronchodilator.

**Elliot forceps.** See **obstetric forceps.**

**Elliot's position** [John W. Elliott, American surgeon, 1852–1925], a supine posture assumed by the patient on the operating table, with a support placed under the lower costal margin to elevate the chest. The position is used in gallbladder surgery.

**ellipsis** /ilip′sis/, (in psychiatry) the omission by a patient of meaningful thoughts and ideas while undergoing therapy.

**ellipsoidal,** describing an object that has the shape of a spindle or an ellipse.

**elliptocyte** /ilip′təsīt/ [Gk, *elleipsis,* ellipse, *kytos,* cell], an oval red blood cell. See also **elliptocytosis.**

**elliptocytic anemia,** hereditary elliptocytosis; see **elliptocytosis.**

**elliptocytosis** /ilip′tōsītō′sis/ [Gk, *elleipsis* + *kytos* + *osis,* condition], an abnormal condition of the blood characterized by increased numbers of elliptocytes or oval erythrocytes. Less than 15% of the red cells appear in this form in normal blood; modest increases occur in a variety of anemias, including a rare congenital disorder, hereditary elliptocytosis. Also called **ovalocytosis.** Compare **spherocytosis.**

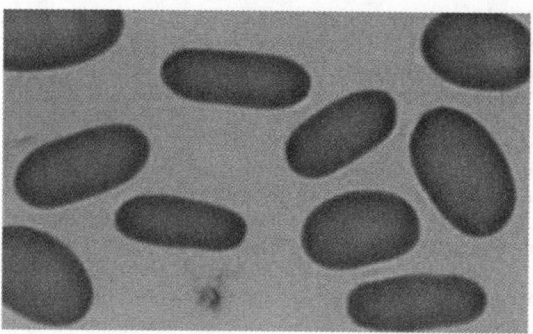

**Elliptocytosis** *(Carr and Rodak, 1999)*

See **acanthocytosis, congenital nonspherocytic hemolytic anemia, sickle cell anemia, spherocytic anemia.**

**Ellis-van Creveld syndrome.** See **chondroectodermal dysplasia.**

**elongation** /i′longā′shən/ [L, *elongatio,* a prolonging], a state of being lengthened or extended.

**elope** /ilōp′/ [ME, *gantlopp,* to run away], *informal.* to leave a locked or secured psychiatric institution without notice or permission.

**elopement precautions,** a nursing intervention from the Nursing Interventions Classification (NIC) defined as minimizing the risk of a patient leaving a treatment setting without authorization when departure presents a threat to the safety of patient or others. See also **Nursing Interventions Classification.**

**Elspar,** trademark for an antineoplastic (asparaginase).

**eluate** /el′yoo·āt/ [L, *eluere,* to wash out], a solution or substance that results from an elution process. In column chromatography the eluate is collected as it drips from the column.

**eluent** /el′yoo·ənt/, a solvent or solution used in an elution process, such as column chromatography.

**elution** /eloo′shən/, the removal of an absorbed substance from a porous bed or chromatographic column by means of a stream of liquid or gas or the application of heat. The technique may consist of washing a material that dissolves out just one component of a mixture. The term is also applied to the removal of antibodies or radioactive tracers from erythrocytes. In heat elution of antibodies red cells in a saline solution are heated to 56° C and then centrifuged. Liquid elution of antibodies usually uses ether as the solvent.

**em,** abbreviation for **extrinsic muscles.**

**EM,** abbreviation for **erythema multiforme.**

**em-,** prefix meaning 'in, on': *embolism, empasma.*

**emaciated** /imā′shē·ā′tid/, characterized by an extreme loss of subcutaneous fat that results in an abnormally lean body, such as with starvation.

**emaciation** /imā′shi·ā′shən/ [L, *emaciare,* to make lean], excessive leanness caused by disease or lack of nutrition.

**E-mail.** See **electronic mail.**

**emancipated minor** /iman′sipā′tid/ [L, *emancipare,* to set free], a person who is not legally an adult but who, because he or she is married, in the military, or otherwise no longer dependent on the parents, may not require parental permission for medical or surgical care. State and national laws vary in specific interpretations of the rule.

**emasculation** /imas′kyəlā′shən/, a loss of the testes or penis or both. See also **castration.**

**embalming** /embä′ming/, the practice of applying antiseptics and preservatives to a corpse to retard the natural decomposition of tissues.

**Embden-Meyerhof defects** /emb′denmī′ərhof/ [Gustav G. Embden, German biochemist, 1874–1933; Otto F. Meyerhof, German biochemist, 1884–1951], a group of hereditary hemolytic anemias caused by enzyme deficiencies. The most common form of the disorder is a pyruvate kinase deficiency. The condition is characterized by an absence of spherocytes and the presence of small numbers of crenated erythrocytes. The trait is transmitted as an autosomal recessive gene, and the hemolytic anemia occurs only in homozygotes.

**Embden-Meyerhof pathway.** See **glycolysis.**

**embedded tooth,** an unerupted tooth, usually completely covered with bone. Also called **imbedded tooth.** Compare **impacted tooth.**

**embol-** **1.** prefix meaning 'to insert': *embolia, embole.* **2.** prefix meaning 'embolus or plug': *embolectomy.*

**embolectomy** /em′bəlek′təmē/ [Gk, *embolos,* plug, *ektomē,* excision], a surgical incision into an artery for the removal of an embolus or clot, performed as emergency treatment for arterial embolism. The operation is done as soon as possible after a decrease in perfusion is detected. When the thrombi have broken away from a thrombophlebitis, they tend to lodge at the juncture of major arteries. More than half lodge in the aorta, in arteries of the lower extremities, in the common carotid arteries, or in the pulmonary arteries. Before surgery, heparin may be administered, and an arteriogram may be used to identify the affected artery. A longitudinal incision is made in the artery, and the embolus is removed. After surgery the blood pressure is maintained close to the level of the preoperative baseline, as a decrease might predispose to new clot formation. A frequent complication of the procedure is hemorrhage from small arteries that may have been clogged with the embolus but overlooked during tying of larger bleeding vessels.

**embolic** /embol′ik/ [Gk, *embolos,* plug], pertaining to or resembling an embolus or embolism.

**embolic gangrene** [Gk, *embolos* + *gaggraina*], the death and decay of body tissues caused by an embolus blocking the blood supply to that part.

**embolic necrosis,** death of a portion of tissue that results from an infarction caused by an embolus.

**embolic thrombosis** [Gk, *embolos,* plug, *thrombos,* lump, *osis,* condition], a clot that develops at the site of an impacted embolus (foreign body) in a blood vessel.

**embolism** /em′bəliz′əm/, an abnormal condition in which an embolus travels through the bloodstream and becomes lodged in a blood vessel. Symptoms vary with the character of the embolus, the degree of occlusion that results, and the size, nature, and location of the occluded vessel. Kinds of embolism include **air embolism, fat embolism,** and **gas embolism. —embolic,** *adj.*

**embolization agent,** a substance used to occlude or drastically reduce blood flow within a vessel. Examples include vasoconstrictors, microfibrillar collagen, absorbable gelatin sponge (Gelfoam), polyvinyl alcohol, and silicone beads.

**embolized atheroma,** a fat particle lodged in a blood vessel.

**emboloid.** See **embolus.**

**embolotherapy** /em′bəlōther′əpē/, a technique of blocking a blood vessel with a balloon catheter. It is used for treating bleeding ulcers and blood vessel defects and for stopping blood flow to a tumor during surgery.

**embolus** /em′bələs/, *pl.* **emboli** [Gk, *embolos,* plug], a foreign object, quantity of air or gas, bit of tissue or tumor, or

piece of a thrombus that circulates in the bloodstream until it becomes lodged in a vessel. **—embolic, emboloid,** *adj.*

**embolus care: peripheral,** a nursing intervention from the Nursing Interventions Classification (NIC) defined as limitation of complications for a patient experiencing, or at risk for, occlusion of peripheral circulation. See also **Nursing Interventions Classification.**

**embolus care: pulmonary,** a nursing intervention from the Nursing Interventions Classification (NIC) defined as limitation of complications for a patient experiencing, or at risk for, occlusion of pulmonary circulation. See also **Nursing Interventions Classification.**

**embolus precautions,** a nursing intervention from the Nursing Interventions Classification (NIC) defined as reduction of the risk of an embolus in a patient with thrombi or at risk for developing thrombus formation. See also **Nursing Interventions Classification.**

**embolysis** /embol′isis/, the dissolution of an embolus, especially one caused by a blood clot. See also **thrombolysis.**

**embrasure** /embrā′zhər/, a normally occurring space between adjacent teeth resulting from variations in the positions and contours of teeth. Embrasures provide a spillway for the escape of food during mastication. See also **spillway.**

**embryatrics.** See **fetology.**

**embryectomy** /em′brē·ek′təmē/ [Gk, *en,* in, *bryein,* to grow, *ektomē,* excision], the surgical removal of an embryo, most commonly in an ectopic pregnancy.

**embryo** /em′brē·ō/ [Gk, *en,* in, *bryein,* to grow], **1.** any organism in the earliest stages of development. **2.** in humans the stage of prenatal development from the time of implantation of the fertilized ovum about 2 weeks after conception until the end of the seventh or eighth week. The period is characterized by rapid growth, differentiation of the major organ systems, and development of the main external features. Compare **fetus, zygote. —embryonal, embryonoid, embryonic,** *adj.*

**embryo-,** combining form meaning 'fetus': *embryoctony, embryology.*

**embryocidal** /em′brē·əsī′dəl/, pertaining to the killing of an embryo.

**embryoctony** /em′brē·ok′tənē/ [Gk, *en* + *bryein* + *kteinein,* to kill], the intentional destruction of a living embryo or fetus in utero. Also called **feticide.** See also **abortion.**

**embryogenesis** /em′brē·ō·jen′əsis/ [Gk, *en* + *bryein* + *genein,* to produce], the process in sexual reproduction by which an embryo forms from the fertilization of an ovum. Also called **embryogeny** /em′brē·oj′ənē/. See also **heterogenesis, homogenesis. —embryogenetic, embryogenic.** *adj.*

**embryologic, embryological.** See **embryology.**

**embryologic development** /-loj′ik/, the various intrauterine stages and processes involved in the growth and differentiation of the conceptus from the time of fertilization of the ovum until the eighth week of gestation. The stages are related to the biologic status of the unborn child and involve the differentiation of the various cells, tissues, and organ systems and the development of the main external features of the embryo. It occurs from approximately the end of the second week to the eighth week of intrauterine life. The fetal stage follows these stages, beginning at about the ninth week of gestation. The entire process of growth and development of the embryo and fetus is loosely called prenatal development. See also **prenatal development.**

**embryologist** /em′brē·ol′əjist/, one who specializes in embryology.

**embryology** /em′brē·ol′əjē/ [Gk, *en, bryein* + *logos,* science], the study of the origin, growth, development, and function of an organism from fertilization to birth. Kinds of embryology include **comparative embryology, descriptive embryology,** and **experimental embryology.** —**embryologic, embryological,** *adj.*

**embryoma** /em′brē-ō′mə/, *pl.* **embryomas, embryomata** [Gk, *en + bryein + oma,* tumor], a tumor that arises from embryonic cells or tissues.

**embryoma of the ovary.** See **dysgerminoma.**

**embryomorph** /embrē′əmôrf′/ [Gk, *en + bryein + morphe,* form], any structure that resembles an embryo, especially a mass of tissue that may represent an aborted conceptus. —**embryomorphous,** *adj.*

**embryonal.** See **embryo.**

**embryonal adenomyosarcoma, embryonal adenosarcoma.** See **Wilms' tumor.**

**embryonal carcinoma** /em′brē·ənəl/, a malignant neoplasm derived from germinal cells that usually develops in gonads, especially the testes. The tumor, a firm nodular mass with hemorrhagic areas, is characterized histologically by large, undifferentiated cells with indistinct borders, eosinophilic cytoplasm, and prominent nucleoli in pleomorphic nuclei. Bodies resembling a 1- or 2-week-old embryo are occasionally seen in these tumors. The neoplasm is relatively resistant to radiation therapy. The tumor metastasizes by way of lymph channels. Surgery and chemotherapy are usually used in the treatment. See also **choriocarcinoma.**

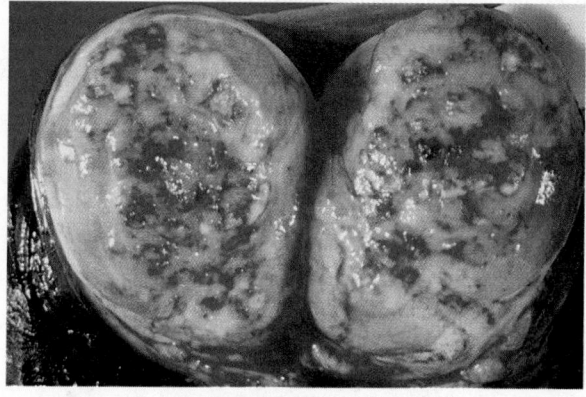

**Embryonal carcinoma**
*(Kumar, Cotran, and Robbins, 1997/courtesy Dr. Kyle Molberg, Department of Pathology, University of Texas Southwestern Medical Center, Dallas)*

**embryonal leukemia.** See **stem cell leukemia.**

**embryonate** /em′brē·ənāt′/ [Gk, *en + bryein + L, atus,* shaped like], **1.** impregnated; containing an embryo. **2.** pertaining to or resembling an embryo.

**embryonic** /em′brē·on′ik/ [Gk, *en + bryein,* to grow], pertaining to or resembling an embryo.

**embryonic abortion, 1.** termination of pregnancy before the twentieth week of gestation. **2.** products of conception expelled before the twentieth week. Compare **fetal abortion.**

**embryonic anideus** [Gk, *en + bryein + an,* not, *eidos,* form], a blastoderm in which the axial elongation of the primitive streak and primitive groove fail to develop.

**embryonic blastoderm,** the area of the blastoderm that gives rise to the primitive streak from which the embryonic body develops. Compare **extraembryonic blastoderm.**

**embryonic competence,** the ability of an embryonic cell to react normally to the stimulation of an inductor, allowing continued normal growth or differentiation of the embryo.

**embryonic disk,** the thickened plate from which the embryo develops in the second week of pregnancy. Scattered cells from the border of the disk migrate to the space between the trophoblast and yolk sac and become the embryonic mesoderm. The disk develops from the ectoderm and endoderm. Also called **gastrodisk, germ disk.**

**embryonic layer,** one of the three layers of cells in the embryo: the endoderm, the mesoderm, and the ectoderm. From these layers of cells arise all of the structures and organs and parts of the body. The endoderm is the first to develop, followed by the ectoderm. During the third week of gestation the mesoderm arises between the ectoderm and the endoderm.

**embryonic rest,** a portion of embryonic tissue that remains in the adult organism. Also called **epithelial rest, fetal rest.**

**embryonic stage,** (in embryology) the interval of time from the end of the germinal stage, at 10 days of gestation, to the eighth week.

**embryonic tissue** [Gk, *en + bryein,* to grow; OFr, *tissu*], **1.** a loose, gelatinous mass of connective tissue cells. The gelatinous matrix is caused by the presence of mucopolysaccharides. Also called **mucous tissue, mucoid tissue. 2.** pertaining to tissue of an embryo.

**embryoniform** /em′brē·on′ifôrm′/ [Gk, *en + bryein + L, forma,* form], resembling an embryo.

**embryonoid.** See **embryo.**

**embryopathy** /em′brē·op′əthē/ [Gk, *en + bryein + pathos,* disease], any anomaly occurring in the embryo or fetus as a result of interference with normal intrauterine development. A kind of embryopathy is **rubella embryopathy.**

**embryoplastic** /em′brē·ōplas′tik/ [Gk, *en + bryein + plassein,* to mold], pertaining to the formation of an embryo, usually with reference to cells.

**embryoscopy** /em′brē·os′kəpē/, the direct examination of an embryo by insertion of a lighted instrument through the mother's abdominal wall and uterus. The technique may be used to obtain tissue specimens for analysis or to perform needed surgery.

**embryotome** /em′brē·ətōm′/ [Gk, *en + bryein + temnein,* to cut], a cutting instrument for the removal of a fetus when normal birth is not possible. See also **embryotomy.**

**embryotomy** /em′brē·ot′əmē/ [Gk, *en + bryein + temnein,* to cut], **1.** the dismemberment or mutilation of a fetus for removal from the uterus when normal delivery is not possible. **2.** the dissection of an embryo for examination and analysis.

**embryo transfer,** a process of implanting a fertilized ovum in a uterus.

**embryotroph** /em′brē·ətrof′/ [Gk, *en + bryein + trophe,* nourishment], the liquefied uterine nutritive material, composed of glandular secretions and degenerative tissue, that nourishes the mammalian embryo until placental circulation is established. Also called **embryotrophe** /-trōf′/, **histotroph, histotrophic nutrition.** Compare **hemotroph.**

**embryotrophy** /em′brē·ot′trəfē/, the nourishment of the embryo. See also **embryotroph, hemotroph.** —**embryotrophic,** *adj.*

**embryulcia** /em′brē·ul′sē·ə/ [Gk, *en + bryein + elkein,* to draw], the surgical extraction of the embryo or fetus from the uterus.

**Emcyt,** trademark for an antineoplastic agent (estramustine phosphate sodium).

**eme-,** combining form meaning 'to vomit': *emetocathartic, emetine.*

**emergence** /imur′jəns/ [L, *emergere,* to come forth], the point in the process of recovery from general anesthesia at which a return of spontaneous respiration, airway reflexes, and consciousness occurs. See also **postanesthesia care.**

**emergency** /imur′jənsē/ [L, *emergere,* to come forth], a perilous situation that arises suddenly and threatens the life or welfare of a person or a group of people, as a natural disaster, medical crisis, or trauma situation.

**emergency cardiac care (ECC)** [L, *emergeere,* to come forth; Gk, *kardia* + ME, *caru,* sorrow], the concentration of personnel and facilities organized to sustain the cardiovascular and pulmonary systems when a myocardial infarction or cardiac arrest occurs. The interventions assure prompt availability of basic life support (BLS), monitoring and treatment facilities, prevention of complications, and psychologic reassurance. If cardiac arrest occurs outside a hospital, efforts are devoted to stabilizing the patient's cardiovascular and pulmonary systems before removing the individual to a hospital.

**emergency care,** a nursing intervention from the Nursing Interventions Classification (NIC) defined as providing lifesaving measures in life-threatening situations. See also **Nursing Interventions Classification.**

**emergency cart checking,** a nursing intervention from the Nursing Interventions Classification (NIC) defined as systematic review of the contents of an emergency cart at established time intervals. See also **Nursing Interventions Classification.**

**emergency childbirth,** a birth that occurs accidentally or precipitously in or out of the hospital, without standard obstetric preparations and procedures. Signs and symptoms of impending delivery include increased bloody show, frequent strong contractions, the mother's desire to bear down forcibly or her report that she feels as though she is going to defecate, visible bulging of the bag of waters, and crowning of the baby's head at the vaginal introitus.

■ METHOD: If time permits, equipment is readied, but the delivery is not delayed for such preparations. Useful equipment includes sterile gloves, towels, bulb syringe, receiving blankets, scissors, two Kelly clamps, cord clamp or tie, and a basin for the placenta. The mother's vital signs are taken, and the fetal heart sounds are listened to if time permits and if equipment is available. The mother is reassured that emergency deliveries are usually simple and that all procedures and events will be explained. Despite her compelling urge to push and to deliver quickly, the mother is encouraged to ease the baby out slowly by not pushing and by blowing air forcibly out through pursed lips as she feels the strength of the urge building. As the head emerges, it is supported but allowed to rotate naturally. A check is made immediately to determine whether or not the umbilical cord is wound around the neck. If it is, a gentle attempt is made to slip it over the baby's head; if it is too tight, it is immediately clamped with two Kelly clamps placed 2 or 3 inches apart, cut between the clamps, and unwound from the neck. If the baby does not deliver immediately, mucus and fluid in the nose and mouth are sucked out with a bulb syringe. The shoulders are delivered one at a time by guiding the head downward to deliver the anterior (upper) shoulder under the symphysis pubis, and then upward to deliver the posterior (lower) shoulder over the perineum. The rest of the baby is quickly born. If the membranes of the amniotic sac are intact, the sac is snipped or torn behind the baby's neck and

peeled away from the face so that the baby can breathe. If necessary, the nares, nasopharynx, and mouth may be suctioned with the bulb syringe, taking care not to slow the heart rate by stimulating the vagus nerve with the tip of the syringe on the back of the throat. The baby is kept warm and held with the head lower than the chest; it may be laid skinto-skin on the mother's abdomen. The baby may thus be positioned, observed, and warmed in one place as the nurse or other helper covers the mother and baby with a dry blanket or towel and continues to provide emergency care as necessary through the third stage of labor. There is no urgent need to cut the cord or to deliver the placenta. When it is desired, the cord may be cut by clamping it in two places several inches from the baby and cutting it between the clamps with sterile scissors. The cord clamp may be put on later. If possible, an Apgar score is taken first at 5 minutes of age, then at 10. The placenta is ready to be delivered when the cord is seen to advance a few inches, the uterus becomes firmer and rises in the abdomen, and a small gush of bright red blood emerges from the vagina. The mother may help expel it by bearing down. The placenta is lifted out of the vagina slowly, with care, so that all of the membranes are drawn out with it. The placenta and membranes are kept for further evaluation. The uterus is massaged to ensure that it is well contracted, and the baby is put to breast if the mother wishes. The uterus is palpated frequently, and it is massaged when necessary. The baby is kept with the mother and observed for warmth, color, activity, and respiration. After delivery of the placenta, the perianal area is rinsed with warm sterile water and dried with a clean towel or cloth, and an ice pack and a sanitary pad or small towel are applied in such a way that the mother can hold them in place by drawing her legs together.

■ OUTCOME CRITERIA: Almost all births are normal and do not constitute true medical emergencies. If a mother is healthy and is not bleeding, if her vital signs are normal, and if the fetal heart sounds are normal, there is no immediate cause for alarm, even if the birth is imminent. Emergency care is directed to ensuring that the newborn breathes well and is kept warm, that the mother is protected from hemorrhage, and that the mother's privacy is maintained. The nurse is likely to be the person who must initially evaluate the situation and decide whether to attempt to transfer or transport the mother or to prepare for emergency delivery. If a mother says the baby is coming, the attendant is advised to believe her and to act accordingly. Throughout the delivery and the third stage of labor, the nurse works to help the mother to feel calm, confident, and well cared for.

**emergency department (ED),** (in a health care facility) a section of an institution that is staffed and equipped to provide rapid and varied emergency care, especially for those who are stricken with sudden and acute illness or who are the victims of severe trauma. The emergency department may use a triage system of screening and classifying clients to determine priority needs for the most efficient use of available personnel and equipment. Also called **emergency room.**

**emergency doctrine,** (in law) a doctrine that assumes a person's consent to medical treatment when the he or she is in imminent danger and unable to give informed consent to treatment. Emergency doctrine assumes that the person would consent if able to do so. Commonly known as **implied consent.**

**emergency handling of radiation accidents.** See **radiation exposure.**

**emergency medical identification.** See **Medic Alert.**

**emergency medical service (EMS),** a network of services coordinated to provide aid and medical assistance from primary response to definitive care, involving personnel trained in the rescue, stabilization, transportation, and advanced treatment of traumatic or medical emergencies. Linked by a communication system that operates on both a local and a regional level, EMS is a tiered system of care, which is usually initiated by citizen action in the form of a telephone call to an emergency number. Subsequent stages include the emergency medical dispatch (EMD), first medical responder, ambulance personnel, medium and heavy rescue equipment, and paramedic units, if necessary. In the hospital, service is provided by emergency department nurses, emergency department physicians, specialists, and critical care nurses and physicians. See also **emergency medical technician, emergency medical technician–advanced life support, emergency medical technician–intermediate, emergency medical technician–intravenous, emergency medical technician–paramedic.**

**emergency medical technician (EMT),**   a person trained in and responsible for the administration of specialized emergency care and the transportation of victims of acute illness or injury to a medical facility, based on national standards developed by the U.S. Department of Transportation. In addition to basic life-support skills, the EMT is trained in extrication, operation of emergency vehicles, basic anatomy, basic assessment of injury or illness, triage, care for specific injuries and illnesses, environmental emergencies, childbirth, and transport of the patient. Certification varies from 2 to 4 years, depending on the state. EMTs receive ongoing training in new procedures and must qualify for national recertification every 2 years. See also **emergency medical service.**

**emergency medical technician–advanced life support (EMT-ALS),**   a third-level EMT. The EMT-ALS is locally certified in all the skills of the basic-level EMT and EMT-IV. The EMT-ALS may also administer certain medications following the protocols or orders of the hospital physician, with whom radio contact is maintained. An EMT-ALS is also trained in the use of advanced life support systems, including electrical defibrillation equipment. See also **emergency medical service.**

**emergency medical technician–intermediate (EMT-I),** a second-level emergency medical technician nationally certified as both an EMT-ALS and an EMT-IV. See also **emergency medical service.**

**emergency medical technician–intravenous (EMT-IV),** a second-level emergency medical technician. The EMT-IV is trained and locally certified in IV therapy, endotracheal intubation, and use of other antishock techniques. See also **emergency medical service.**

**emergency medical technician–paramedic (EMT-P),** an advanced-level emergency medical technician who works in prehospital care settings under the direction of a physician, often through radio contact. The EMT-P is nationally certified in all the skills of EMTs of other levels and has additional training in pharmacology and administration of emergency drugs. See also **emergency medical service.**

**emergency medicine,**   a branch of medicine concerned with the diagnosis and treatment of conditions resulting from trauma or sudden illness. The patient's condition is stabilized, and care is transferred to the primary physician or to a specialist. Emergency medicine requires broad interdisciplinary training in the physiologic and pathologic characteristics of all body systems.

**Emergency Nurses' Association (ENA),**   a national professional organization of emergency department nurses that defines and promotes emergency nursing practice. The association, which was founded in 1970 and has more than 11,000 members, has written and implemented the Standards of Emergency Nursing Practice. The association offers a certification examination and awards the designation Certified Emergency Nurse (CEN) to nurses who successfully complete it. ENA publishes the *Journal of Emergency Nursing (JEN)* and *Continuing Education Core Curriculum of Emergency Nursing Practice.* The association, which has headquarters in Chicago, works closely with its members and with related associations to define practice and to prepare professionals to deliver emergency care.

**emergency nursing,**   nursing care provided to prevent imminent severe damage or death or to avert serious injury. Activities that exemplify emergency nursing are basic life support, cardiopulmonary resuscitation, and control of hemorrhage.

**emergency preparation of safe drinking water.**   See **water purification, emergency.**

**emergency readiness,**   a state of having made advance plans for coping with an unexpected natural disaster, civil disturbance, or military attack that may threaten death and injury to a local population. The planning includes educating the population about location of shut-off valves for utilities and about first aid, including cardiopulmonary resuscitation; ensuring that adequate sources of food, water, basic medical supplies, and bedding materials will be available; arranging for the disposal of human wastes when toilets are not functional; and establishing procedures for emergency care of the elderly, infants, small children, and women who may be pregnant. Plans for communication systems also may be part of emergency readiness.

**emergency room.**   See **emergency department.**

**emergent** /imur'jənt/ [L, *emergens,* emerging],   arising, often unexpectedly, or improving or modifying an existing thing.

**emergent evolution,**   the theory that evolution occurs in a series of major changes at certain critical stages and results from the total rearrangement of existing elements so that completely new and unpredictable characteristics appear within the species. See also **saltatory evolution.**

**Emery-Dreifuss syndrome** /em'ərēdrī'fəs/ [Alan E.H. Emery, British geneticist, b. 1928; Fritz E. Dreifuss, twentieth-century British physician, b. 1926],   an X-linked recessive form of muscular dystrophy that begins in early childhood and is characterized by joint contractures and cardiac conduction disorders. Patients who reach adulthood are often unable to work and require cardiac pacemakers to control arryhthmias.

**emesis.**   See **vomit,** def. 2.

**-emesis,**   combining form meaning 'to vomit': *hyperemesis.*

**emesis basin** /em'əsis, əmē'sis/ [Gk, *emesis,* vomiting; Fr, *bassin,* hollow vessel],   a kidney-shaped bowl or pan that fits against the neck to collect vomitus.

**emesis gravidarum,**   vomiting associated with pregnancy.

**Emete-con,**   trademark for an antiemetic (benzquinamide hydrochloride).

**emetic** /imet'ik/,   **1.** pertaining to a substance that causes vomiting. **2.** an emetic agent. Apomorphine hydrochloride, acting through the central nervous system, induces vomiting 10 to 15 minutes after parenteral administration. Syrup of ipecac is used in the emergency treatment of drug overdosage and in certain cases of poisoning.

**-emetic, -emetical,**   combining form meaning 'to cause vomiting': *antiemetic, hematemetic, hyperemetic.*

**Emetrol,**   trademark for a fixed-combination drug containing fructose, glucose, and orthophosphoric acid, used to treat nausea and vomiting.

**EMG,**   **1.** abbreviation for **electromyogram. 2.** abbreviation for **electromyography, 3.** abbreviation for **exophthalmos, macroglossia,** and **gigantism.**

**EMG syndrome,**   a hereditary disorder transmitted as an autosomal recessive trait. Clinical manifestations include umbilical hernia (examphalos), macroglossia, and gigantism, often accompanied by visceromegaly, dysplasia of the renal medulla, and enlargement of the cells of the adrenal cortex. Also called **Beckwith-Wiedemann syndrome, exophthalmos-macroglossia-gigantism syndrome.**

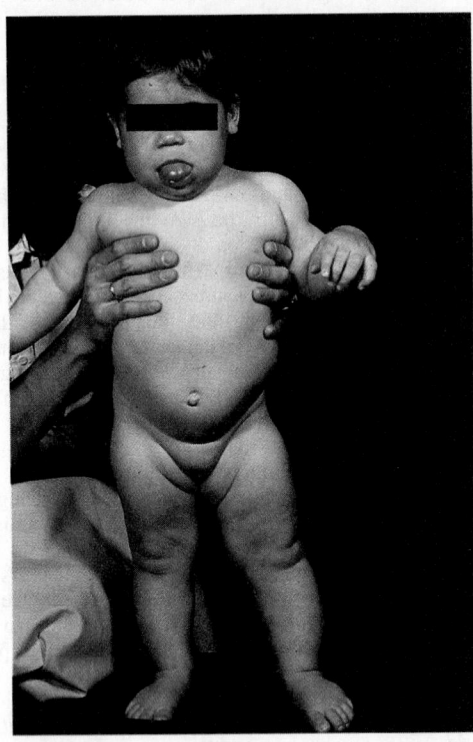

**EMG syndrome** *(Zitelli and Davis, 1997/courtesy Dr. D. Becker)*

**-emia, -aemia, -hemia, -haemia,**   suffix meaning 'blood condition': *anemia, polycythemia, hyperemia.*

**emissary veins** /em′əser′ē/ [L, *emittere,* to send forth],   the small vessels in the skull that connect the sinuses of the dura mater with the veins on the exterior of the skull through a series of anastomoses.

**emission** /imish′ən/ [L, *emittere,* to send out],   a discharge or release of something, as a fluid from the body, electronic signals from a radio transmitter, or an alpha or beta particle from an atomic nucleus during radioactive decay.

**emission computed tomography (ECT)** [L, *emittere,* to send forth; *computare,* to count; Gk, *tome,* section, *graphein,* to record],   a form of tomography in which the emitted decay products, as positrons or gamma rays, of an ingested radioactive pharmaceutical are recorded in detectors outside the body. Computer reconstruction of the data yields a cross-sectional image of the body.

**emit** [L, *emittere,* to send out],   to give or send out something, such as energy, sound, heat, or radiation.

**Emivan,**   trademark for an analeptic agent (ethamivan).

**emmetr-,**   combining form meaning 'the correct measure': *emmetropia, emmetrope.*

**emmetropia** /em′ətrō′pē·ə/ [Gk, *emmetros,* proportioned, *opsis,* vision],   a state of normal vision characterized by the proper relationship between the refractive system of the eyeball and its axial length. This correlation ensures that light rays entering the eye parallel to the optic axis are focused exactly on the retina. Compare **amblyopia, hyperopia, myopia. —emmetropic,** *adj.*

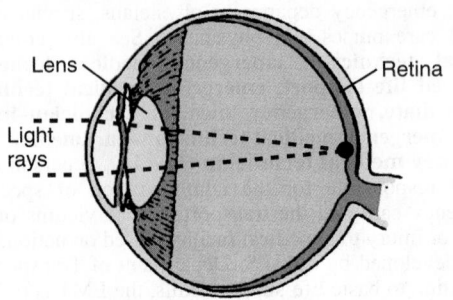

**Emmetropia** *(Monahan and Neighbors, 1998)*

**Emmet's operation,**   a surgical procedure for repair of a lacerated perineum or ruptured uterine cervix.

**emollient** /imol′yənt/ [L, *emolliere,* to soften],   a substance that softens tissue, particularly the skin and mucous membranes.

**emollient bath,**   a bath taken in water containing an emollient, such as bran, to relieve irritation and inflammation. See also **colloid bath.**

**emotion** /imō′shən/ [L, *emovere,* to disturb],   the outward expression or display of mood or feeling states. Also, the affective aspect of consciousness as compared with volition and cognition. Physiologic alterations often occur with a marked change of emotion regardless of whether the feelings are conscious or unconscious, expressed or unexpressed. See also **emotional need, emotional response.**

**emotional abuse** /imō′shənəl/,   the debasement of a person's feelings that causes the individual to perceive himself or herself as inept, not cared for, and worthless.

**emotional age** [L, *emovere,* to disturb; L, *aetas,* age],   the age of an individual as determined by the stage of emotional development reached.

**emotional amalgam,**   an unconscious effort to deny or counteract anxiety.

**emotional amenorrhea,**   a suppression of menstrual discharge from the uterus caused by psychologic factors.

**emotional care of the dying patient,**   the compassionate, consistent support offered to help the terminally ill patient and the family cope with impending death. See also **hospice, stages of dying.**

■ METHOD: The professional person providing emotional support for the terminally ill encourages the expression of personal feelings, anxieties, and experiences regarding death and empathizes with the patient and the family. To prevent conflicting statements, it is essential to know what the physician, other professionals, and family members tell the patient about the outcome. Effective support in terminal illness involves a nonjudgmental approach to the patient's relatives and significant others, an understanding of their problems,

and efforts to assist them in the grieving process. The patient needs relief from pain, tender care, and continued attention through all the stages of dying: characteristically, a period of denial, followed by anger, bargaining, depression, and, finally, acceptance. A patient may not progress through all of these stages, and they may progress through them in a different order. When the patient denies the prognosis and refuses to follow directions, the nursing staff does not interfere with or support the denial mechanism but spends time with the sick person and encourages self-care. During the stage of anger, often manifested by refusal of care and food and by abusive language and negative criticism of the staff, the patient is not allowed to indulge in physically harmful behavior but is encouraged to verbalize his or her anger. In the period in which the patient tries to make bargains, such as "If I could live until. . .," it should be recognized that time is needed to accept death and that the person may appreciate discussing the importance of various events and people in earlier life. When depression, marked by apathy, insomnia, inability to concentrate, poor appetite, and weariness, sets in, efforts to cheer the patient or interrupt crying are inappropriate; the patient may want only the most beloved person to be present. In the final stage of acceptance the patient usually experiences less pain and discomfort, seems peaceful and lacking in emotional affect, and appreciates care from people who are close and familiar.
■ INTERVENTIONS: The nurse has the major role in providing emotional care for the hospitalized terminally ill patient and may help the family arrange for hospice care or home care when it is possible and desirable. The nurse may teach methods of care required at home, may assist the family in realizing the patient's need to live as normally and as long as possible, and may refer the family to the social service department and to community resources for assistance.
■ OUTCOME CRITERIA: Sensitive emotional support appropriate to the stages of dying may help the person to move more rapidly to acceptance. The family usually goes through similar stages; therefore support and counseling by an experienced person may greatly enhance the quality of life of the patient and family.

**emotional deprivation** [L, *emovere,* to disturb, *deprivare,* to deprive], a lack of adequate warmth, affection, and interest, especially of a parent or significant nurturer. It is a relatively common problem among institutionalized persons or children from broken homes.

**emotional diarrhea,** the frequent passage of liquid stools caused by extreme emotional stress.

**emotional glycosuria,** a temporary increase in the level of sugar excretion in the urine resulting from extreme emotional disturbances.

**emotional illness.** See **mental disorder.**

**emotional lability,** a condition of excessive emotional reactions and frequent mood changes.

**emotional need,** a psychologic or mental requirement of intrapsychic origin. It usually centers on such basic feelings as love, fear, anger, sorrow, anxiety, frustration, and depression and involves the understanding, empathy, and support of one person for another. Such needs normally occur in everyone but usually increase during periods of excessive stress or physical and mental illness and during various stages of life, as infancy, early childhood, and old age. If these needs are not routinely met by appropriate, socially accepted means, they can precipitate psychopathologic conditions. Appropriate measures common in nursing for anticipating and satisfying the emotional needs of patients in stress include physical closeness, especially remaining with the person during periods when the feeling is acute; empa-

thetic listening as the patient discusses the feeling; encouragement to verbalize feelings; and planning activities that provide a constructive outlet for the feeling or the situation causing it. Compare **dependency needs.** See also **emotion.**

**emotional response,** a reaction to a particular intrapsychic feeling or feelings, accompanied by physiologic changes that may or may not be outwardly manifested but that motivate or precipitate some action or behavioral response. See also **emotion.**

**emotional support**[1], the sensitive, understanding approach that helps patients accept and deal with their illnesses; communicate their anxieties and fears; derive comfort from a gentle, sympathetic, caring person; and increase their ability to care for themselves.
■ METHOD: Essential in providing emotional support are recognizing and respecting the individuality, personal preferences, and human needs of each patient. Understanding the sick and appreciating the psychologic effects on the patient of the transition from health to illness are also important. The patient is encouraged to verbalize feelings and concerns, and the attentive listener avoids interjecting clichés, such as "Don't worry," "Take it easy," or "Everything will be all right." The nurse and other health team members realize that the patient may express some fears but may act out others through anger, hostility, silence, or assumed joviality. Efforts to change the patient, negative criticism, a judgmental attitude, and facial expressions that may indicate rejection are carefully avoided. Opportunities to listen to the troubled patient and provide compassionate and realistic counseling and care are sought.
■ INTERVENTIONS: The nurse establishes means of communication, provides an atmosphere that invites the patient to discuss worrisome feelings, and presents a caring attitude. This is especially important when the illness damages the person's body image or self-concept.
■ OUTCOME CRITERIA: Emotional support frequently improves the patient's psychologic and physical state, often enabling him or her to accept the illness and to adjust with less anxiety to the changes required.

**emotional support**[2], a nursing intervention from the Nursing Interventions Classification (NIC) defined as provision of reassurance, acceptance, and encouragement during times of stress. See also **Nursing Interventions Classification.**

**empathic** /empath′ik/ [Gk, *en,* into, *pathos,* feeling], pertaining to or involving the entering of one person into the emotional state of another while remaining objective and distinctly separate.

**empathy** /em′pəthē/ [Gk, *en,* in, *pathos,* feeling], the ability to recognize and to some extent share the emotions and states of mind of another and to understand the meaning and significance of that person's behavior. It is an essential quality for effective psychotherapy. Compare **sympathy.** —**empathic,** *adj.,* **empathize,** *v.*

**emphysema** /em′fəsē′mə/ [Gk, *en + physema,* a blowing], an abnormal condition of the pulmonary system, characterized by overinflation and destructive changes in alveolar walls. It results in a loss of lung elasticity and decreased gas exchange. When emphysema occurs early in life, it is usually related to a rare genetic deficiency of serum alpha-1-antitrypsin, which inactivates the enzymes leukocyte collagenase and elastase. Acute emphysema may be caused by the rupture of alveoli during severe respiratory efforts, as may occur in acute bronchopneumonia, suffocation, whooping cough, and occasionally, labor. Patients with chronic emphysema may also have a component of chronic bronchitis. Emphysema also occurs after asthma or tuberculosis, conditions in which the lungs are overstretched until the elastic fibers of the alveolar walls are destroyed. In old age the alveolar membranes atrophy and may collapse, producing large, air-filled spaces and a decreased total surface area of the pulmonary membranes. There are 3 primary types: centriacinar emphysema, distal acinar emphysema, and panacinar emphysema. **emphysematous,** *adj.*

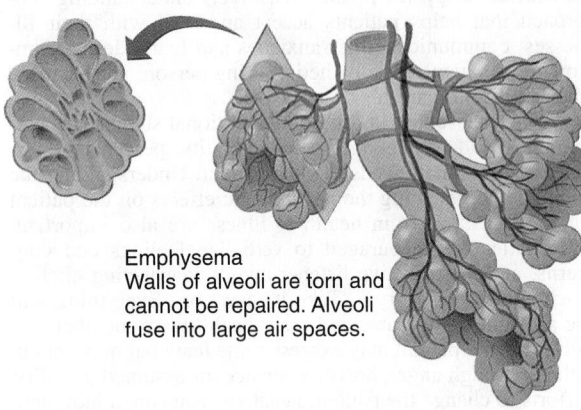

Emphysema
Walls of alveoli are torn and cannot be repaired. Alveoli fuse into large air spaces.

**Emphysema** *(Thibodeau and Patton, 1999/Rolin Graphics)*

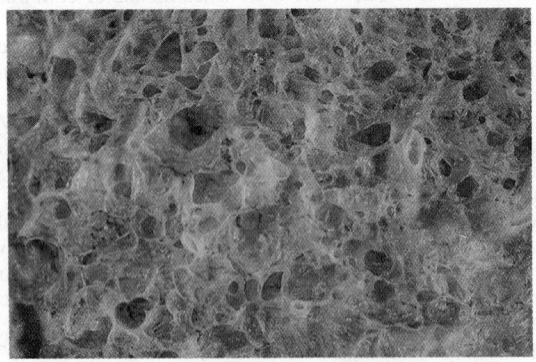

**Panacinar emphysema: ruptured alveoli**
*(Cotran, Kumar, and Collins, 1999)*

■ OBSERVATIONS: The patient may have dyspnea on exertion or at rest, cough, orthopnea, unequal chest expansion, tachypnea, tachycardia, and an elevated temperature if there is an infection. Anxiety, increased $PaCO_2$, restlessness, confusion, weakness, anorexia, hypoxemia, and respiratory failure are common in advanced cases.

■ INTERVENTIONS: The airway is kept open, and oxygen is administered to maintain an arterial oxygen saturation of 92%. Bronchodilators, antibiotics, expectorants, methylxanthines, and corticosteroids may be prescribed. Sedation is to be avoided because sedatives depress respiratory function.

■ NURSING CONSIDERATIONS: The patient is taught breathing exercises and encouraged to drink between 2 and 3 L of fluids daily, if not contraindicated by cardiac function. Activity is encouraged to the limit of the patient's tolerance. Fatigue, constipation, and upper respiratory tract infection and irrita-

tion are to be avoided. Mechanical ventilation and oxygen therapy may be prescribed for use at home. The patient is taught the adverse role that smoking plays in the disease and is encouraged to stop smoking.

**emphysematous** /em′fisem′ətəs/ [Gk, *en,* in, *physema,* a blowing], pertaining to or affected with emphysema.

**emphysematous abscess,** an abscess in which air or gas is present.

**emphysematous chest.** See **barrel chest.**

**empiric** /empir′ik/ [Gk, *empeirikos,* experimental], pertaining to a method of treating disease based on observations and experience without an understanding of the cause or mechanism of the disorder or the way the therapeutic agent or procedure effects improvement or cure. The empiric treatment of a new disease may be based on observations and experience gained in the management of analogous disorders. —**empirical,** *adj.*

**empirical formula,** a chemical formula that shows the smallest whole number ratio of atoms of different elements in a molecule. It does not indicate structural linkage. An example is $CH_2O$, a carbohydrate.

**empiricism** /empir′isiz′əm/, a form of therapy based on the therapist's personal experience and that of other practitioners. —**empiricist,** *n.*

**empiric treatment.** See **treatment.**

**Employment Retirement Income Security Act (ERISA),** a federal law, enacted in 1974, regulating employee welfare benefit plans, including group health plans.

**emprosthotonos** /em′prosthot′ənəs/ [Gk, *emprosthen,* forward, *tenein,* to cut], a position of the body characterized by forward, rigid flexure at the waist. The position is the result of a prolonged involuntary muscle spasm that is most commonly associated with tetanus infection or strychnine poisoning.

**empty end-feel.** See **end-feel.**

**empty follicle syndrome,** a condition in which oocytes are absent from stimulated follicles.

**empty sella syndrome** [AS, *oemettig,* unoccupied; L, *sella,* saddle], an abnormal enlargement of the sella turcica; the pituitary gland may be smaller than normal, or it may be absent. Signs and symptoms of hormonal imbalance (for example, hypopituitarism) may be present, but some patients may be asymptomatic. The diagnosis may be made by computed axial tomography scan, skull radiographic study, or pneumoencephalography.

**empyema** /em′pī·ē′mə, em′pē·ē′mə/ [Gk, *en* + *ipyon,* pus], an accumulation of pus in a body cavity, especially the pleural space, as a result of bacterial infection, such as pleurisy or tuberculosis. It is usually removed by surgical incision, aspiration, and drainage. Antibiotics are administered to correct the cause of the underlying infection.

**-empyema,** combining form meaning an 'accumulation of pus': *arthroempyema, pneumoempyema, typhloempyema.*

**EMS,** 1. abbreviation for **electric muscle stimulator.** 2. abbreviation for **emergency medical service.** 3. abbreviation for **eosinophilia-myalgia syndrome.**

**EMS standing orders,** routine medical procedures approved in advance for emergency medical service (EMS) crews to perform before consulting a physician.

**EMT,** abbreviation for **emergency medical technician.**

**EMT-A,** abbreviation for *emergency medical technician–ambulance,* a member of an emergency medical services crew.

**EMT-ALS,** abbreviation for **emergency medical technician–advanced life support.**

**EMT-B,** abbreviation for *emergency medical technician–basic,* an entry-level emergency medical technician who is

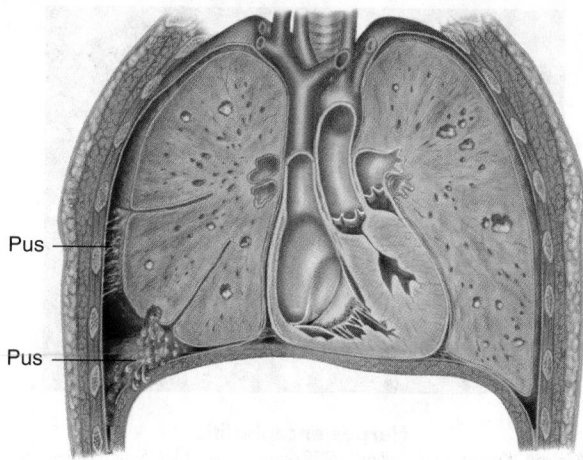

Pus

Pus

**Empyema** *(Seidel et al, 1999)*

trained in basic emergency care skills, such as defibrillation, airway maintenance, CPR, spinal immobilization, bleeding control, and fracture management. Often used interchangeably with **emergency medical technician.**

**EMT-D,** abbreviation for *emergency medical technician–defibrillator,* a member of an emergency medical services crew with special training in the use of cardiac defibrillating equipment.

**EMT-I,** abbreviation for **emergency medical technician–intermediate.**

**EMT-IV,** abbreviation for **emergency medical technician–intravenous.**

**EMT-P,** abbreviation for **emergency medical technician–paramedic.**

**emulsification** /imul′sifikā′shən/, the breakdown of large fat globules into smaller, uniformly distributed particles. It is accomplished mainly by bile acids in the small intestine. Emulsification is the first preparation of fat for chemical digestion by specific enzymes. See also **emulsify.**

**emulsifier** /imul′sifī′ər/ [L, *emulgere,* to milk out, *facere,* to make], a substance such as egg yolk or gum arabic that can cause oil to be suspended in water.

**emulsify** [L, *emulgere,* to milk out, *facere,* to make], to disperse a liquid into another liquid, making a colloidal suspension. Soaps and detergents emulsify by surrounding small globules of fat, preventing them from settling out. Bile acts as an emulsifying agent in the digestive tract by dispersing ingested fats into small globules. —**emulsification,** *n.*

**emulsion** /imul′shən/ [L, *emulgere,* to milk out], **1.** a system consisting of two immiscible liquids, one of which is dispersed in the other in the form of small droplets. **2.** (in photography) a composition sensitive to actinic rays of light, consisting of one or more silver halides suspended in gelatin applied in a thin layer to film.

**en-,** prefix meaning 'in, on': *enanthema, encelialgia, enostosis.*

**ENA,** abbreviation for **Emergency Nurses' Association.**

**enabler** /enā′blər/, a significant other of a substance abuser who provides covert support of substance-abusing behavior.

**enalapril maleate** /enal′əpril/, an angiotensin-converting enzyme (ACE) inhibitor used as an oral antihypertensive drug.

■ INDICATIONS: It is prescribed in the treatment of hypertension or heart failure.

■ CONTRAINDICATIONS: Enalapril maleate should be used with caution in patients suffering severe salt or fluid depletion or when used with a potassium-sparing diuretic.

■ ADVERSE EFFECTS: Among the more serious adverse reactions are hyperkalemia, cough, hypotension, dizziness, and headache.

**enamel** /inam′əl/ [OFr, *esmail*], the hard, white substance that forms the outermost covering of the clinical and anatomic crown of a tooth. It is produced by epithelial cells called ameloblasts.

**enamel hypocalcification,** a defect in which the enamel of the teeth is soft and undercalcified but normal in quantity. It is caused by defective maturation of ameloblasts. The teeth are chalky in consistency, their surfaces wear down rapidly, and a yellowish-brown stain appears on the teeth as the underlying dentin is exposed. The condition affects both primary and secondary teeth. Compare **enamel hypoplasia.** See also **amelogenesis imperfecta.**

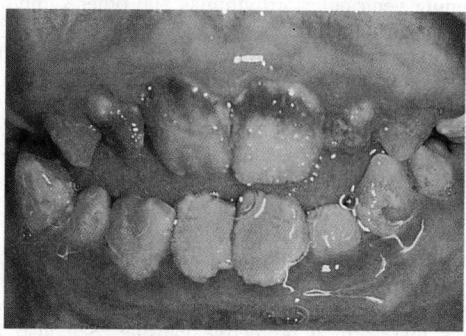

**Enamel hypocalcification** *(Zitelli and Davis, 1997)*

**enamel hypoplasia,** a defect in which the enamel of the teeth is hard but thin and deficient in amount as a result of defective enamel matrix formation with a shortage of the cementing substance. It is characterized by lack of contact between teeth, rapid breakdown of occlusal surfaces, and a yellowish-brown stain that appears where the dentin is exposed. The condition, affects both deciduous and secondary dentition. It is transmitted genetically or caused by environmental factors such as vitamin A, C, or D deficiency; fluorosis; rash-producing childhood diseases; congenital syphilis; injury or trauma to the mouth; or administration of tetracyclines during the second half of pregnancy or during early tooth development. Compare **enamel hypocalcification.** See also **amelogenesis imperfecta.**

**enamel niche,** either of two depressions on a tooth, located between the lateral dental lamina and the developing dental germ.

**enamel organ,** a complex epithelial structure on the dental papilla. It produces enamel for the developing tooth.

**enanthema** /en′anthē′mə/ [Gk, *en* + *anthema,* blossoming], a sudden eruptive lesion of the surface of a mucous membrane. Also called **enanthem** /ənan′thəm/.

**enantiomer,** (in physical science) the nonsuperimposable mirror image of a chiral compound.

**enarthrosis.** See **ball-and-socket joint.**

**en bloc** /enblok′, äNblôk′/ [Fr, in a block], all together, or as a whole.

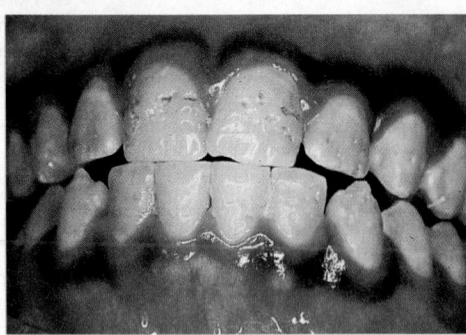

**Enamel hypoplasia** *(Zitelli and Davis, 1997)*

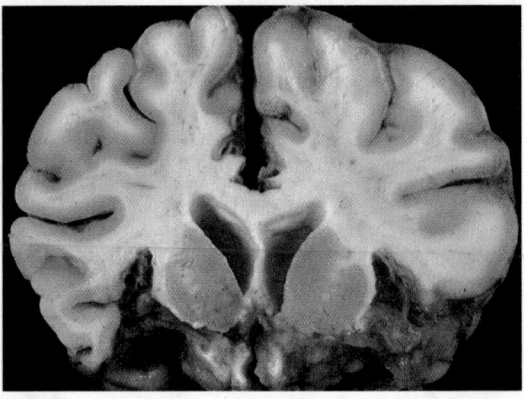

**Herpes encephalitis**
*(Cotran, Kumar, and Collins, 1999/courtesy Dr. T.W. Smith, University of Massachusetts Medical School, Worcester, Massachusetts)*

**encainide** /en′kānīd/, a sodium channel antagonist used as an antiarrhythmic agent.

■ INDICATIONS: It is prescribed in the treatment of life-threatening ventricular arrhythmias and other symptomatic ventricular arrhythmias.

■ CONTRAINDICATIONS: The product should not be given to patients with a known hypersensitivity to encainide or to similar sodium channel antagonists.

■ ADVERSE EFFECTS: Among the most common side effects are dizziness and blurred vision. Fatal ventricular tachycardia can occur. Encainide potentiates other antiarrhythmics, and the dose of each may need to be adjusted to reduce adverse effects.

**encapsulated** /enkaps′yəlā′tid/ [Gk, *en* + L, *capsula,* little box], (of arteries, muscles, nerves, and other body parts) enclosed in fibrous or membranous sheaths. It refers to organisms that form a protective capsule. See also **fascia bulbi, synovial sheath.**

**-ence.** See **-ency.**

**encephal-,** combining form meaning 'the brain': *encephalopathy, encephalitis.*

**encephalalgia** /ənsef′əlal′jə/, headache. See also **cephalalgia.**

**-encephalia, -encephaly,** suffix meaning '(condition of the) brain': *amyelencephalia, rhinencephalia, synencephalia.*

**encephalitis** /ensef′əlī′tis/, *pl.* **encephalitides** /-tidēz/ [Gk, *enkephalos,* brain, *itis,* inflammation], an inflammatory condition of the brain. The cause is usually an arbovirus infection transmitted by the bite of an infected mosquito, but it may be the result of lead or other poisoning or of hemorrhage. **Postinfectious encephalitis** occurs as a complication of another infection, such as chickenpox, influenza, or measles, or after smallpox vaccination. The condition is characterized by headache, neck pain, fever, nausea, and vomiting. Neurologic disturbances, including seizures, personality change, irritability, lethargy, paralysis, weakness, and coma, may occur. The outcome depends on the cause, the age and condition of the person, and the extent of inflammation. Severe inflammation with destruction of nerve tissue may result in a seizure disorder, loss of a special sense or other permanent neurologic problem, or death. Usually the inflammation involves the spinal cord and brain; hence in most cases a more accurate term is *encephalomyelitis.* Compare **meningitis.** See also **encephalomyelitis, equine encephalitis.**

**encephalitis lethargica.** See **epidemic encephalitis.**

**encephalitis neonatorum.** See **neonatorum encephalitis.**

**encephalitis periaxialis diffusa.** See **Schilder's disease.**

**encephalocele** /ensef′ələsēl′/ [Gk, *enkephalos* + *koilia,* cavity], protrusion of the brain through a congenital defect in the skull; hernia of the brain. See also **neural tube defect.**

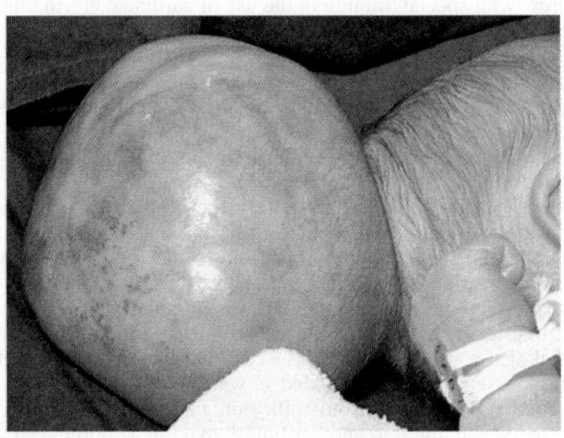

**Encephalocele**
*(Zitelli and Davis, 1997/courtesy Dr. Christine L. Williams, New York Medical College)*

**encephalodysplasia,** any congenital anomaly of the brain.

**encephalogram** /ensef′ələgram′/ [Gk, *enkephalos* + *gramma,* record], a radiograph of the brain made during encephalography.

**encephalography** /ensef′əlog′rəfē/, radiographic delineation of the structures of the brain containing fluid after the cerebrospinal fluid is withdrawn and replaced by a gas, such as air, helium, or oxygen. The procedure is used mainly for indicating the site of cerebrospinal fluid obstruction in hydrocephalus or structural abnormalities of the posterior fossa. Because of the risks involved, it is used only when results of computed tomography are not definitive. Kinds of encephalography are **pneumoencephalography** and **ventriculography.** Also called **air encephalography.** Compare echoencephalography, electroencephalography. **—encephalographic,** *adj.*

**encephaloid carcinoma.** See **medullary carcinoma.**

**encephalomeningitis** /-men′inji′tis/ [Gk, *enkephalos*, brain, *meninx*, membrane, *itis*, inflammation], an inflammation of the brain and meninges.

**encephalomeningocele.** See **meningoencephalocele.**

**encephalomyelitis** /ensef′əlōmī′əli′tis/ [Gk, *enkephalos* + *myelos*, marrow, *itis*], an inflammatory condition of the brain and spinal cord characterized by fever, headache, stiff neck, back pain, and vomiting. Depending on the cause, the age and condition of the person, and the extent of the inflammation and irritation to the central nervous system, seizures, paralysis, personality changes, a decreased level of consciousness, coma, or death may occur. Sequelae, such as seizure disorders or decreased mental ability, may occur after severe inflammation that causes extensive damage to the cells and tissues of the nervous system. See also **encephalitis, equine encephalitis.**

**encephalomyocarditis** /ensef′əlōmī′ōkärdi′tis/ [Gk, *enkephalos* + *mys*, muscle, *kardia*, heart, *itis*, inflammation], an infectious disease of the central nervous system and heart tissue caused by a group of small ribonucleic acid picornaviruses. Rodents are a major reservoir of the infection. Human illness ranges from asymptomatic infection to severe encephalomyelitis. Symptoms are generally similar to those of poliomyelitis. Myocarditis is not a feature of infection in humans, and most victims recover promptly without sequelae. Treatment is supportive. See also **picornavirus.**

**encephalon** [Gk, *enkephalos*, brain], **1.** the cerebrum and its related structures of cerebellum, pons, and medulla oblongata. **2.** the contents of the cranium.

**encephalopathy** /ensef′əlop′əthē/ [Gk, *enkephalos* + *pathos*, disease], any abnormal condition of the structure or function of brain tissues, especially chronic, destructive, or degenerative conditions, as Wernicke's encephalopathy or Schilder's disease.

**encephalotrigeminal angiomatosis.** See **Sturge-Weber syndrome.**

**-encephaly.** See **-encephalia.**

**enchondroma** /en′kəndrō′mə/, *pl.* **enchondromas, enchondromata** [Gk, *en* + *chondros*, cartilage, *oma*, tumor], a benign, slowly growing tumor of cartilage cells that arises in the extremity of the shaft of tubular bones in the hands or feet. The growth of the neoplasm may distend the bone. Also called **enchondrosis, true chondroma.**

**enchondromatosis** /en′kəndrō′mətō′sis/ [Gk, *en* + *chondros*, cartilage, *oma*, tumor, *osis*, condition], a congenital disorder characterized by the proliferation of cartilage within the extremity of the shafts of bones, causing thinning of the cortex and distortion in length. Also called **dyschondroplasia, Ollier's disease.** Compare **Maffucci's syndrome.**

**enchondromatous myxoma** /en′kondrō′mətəs/, a tumor of the connective tissue, characterized by the presence of cartilage between the cells of connective tissue. See also **myxoma.**

**enchondrosarcoma.** See **central chondrosarcoma.**

**enchondrosis.** See **enchondroma.**

**enchylema.** See **hyaloplasm.**

**-enchyma,** combining form meaning the 'liquid that nourishes tissue, or tissue itself': *karyenchyma, mesenchyma, sclerenchyma.*

**enclave** /en′klāv, enklāv′/, a detached mass of tissue enclosed in an organ or in a different kind of tissue.

**encode** /enkōd′/ [Gk, *en* + L, *caudex*, book], **1.** to translate a message, signal, or stimulus into a code. **2.** to rewrite information into a form that can be interpreted by a computer manually or automatically, as by a computer program.

**encoded message,** (in communication theory) a message as transmitted by a sender to a receiver.

**encopresis** /en′kōprē′sis/, fecal holding with constipation and fecal soiling. **—encopretic,** *adj.*

**encounter** [Gk, *en* + L, *contra*, against], (in psychotherapy) the interaction between a patient and a psychotherapist, such as occurs in existential therapy, or among several members of a small group such as encounter or sensitivity training groups. In an encounter emotional change and personal growth are effected by participants' expression of strong feelings.

**encounter data,** information showing use of provider services by health plan enrollees that is used to develop cost profiles of a particular group of enrollees and then to guide decisions about or provide justification for the maintenance or adjustment of premiums.

**encounter group,** (in psychology) a small group of people who meet to increase self-awareness, promote personal growth, and improve interpersonal communication. Members focus on becoming aware of their feelings and on developing the ability to express those feelings openly, honestly, and clearly. See also **group therapy, psychotherapy, sensitivity training group.**

**enculturation** /enkul′chərā′shən/ [Gk, *en* + L, *cultura*, cultivation], the process of learning the concepts, values, and behavioral standards of a particular culture.

**-ency, -ance, -ancy, -ence, 1.** suffix meaning a 'quality or state': *deficiency, dependency.* **2.** suffix meaning a 'person or thing in a state': *latency.* **3.** suffix meaning an 'instance of a quality or state': *emergency.*

**encyst** /ensist′/, to form a cyst or capsule. See also **cyst.** **—encysted,** *adj.*

**end** /ē′en′dē′, end/, (in cytogenetics) abbreviation for *endoreduplication.*

**end-.** See **endo-.**

*Endameba.* See *Entamoeba.*

**endamebiasis.** See **amebiasis.**

*Endamoeba.* See *Entamoeba.*

**endamoebiasis.** See **amebiasis.**

**endarterectomy** /en′därtərek′təmē/ [Gk, *endon*, within, *arteria*, airpipe, *ektomē*, excision], the surgical removal of the intimal lining of an artery. The procedure is done to clear

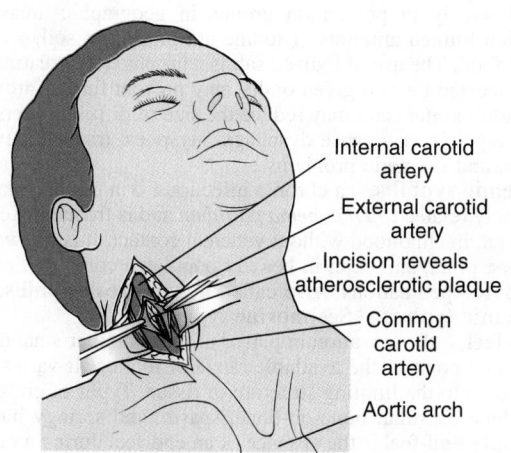

Internal carotid artery

External carotid artery

Incision reveals atherosclerotic plaque

Common carotid artery

Aortic arch

**Endarterectomy of the carotid artery**
*(Lewis, Heitkemper, and Dirksen, 2000)*

a major artery that may be blocked by plaque accumulation. Kinds of endarterectomy include **disobliterative endarterectomy** and **gas endarterectomy.**

**endarteritis** /en'därtərī'tis/ [Gk, *endon* + *arteria* + *itis*, inflammation], inflammation of the inner layer of one or more arteries, which may become partially or completely occluded.

**endarteritis deformans.** See **chronic endoarteritis.**

**endarteritis obliterans,** an inflammatory condition of the lining of the arterial walls in which the intima proliferates, narrowing the lumen of the vessels and occluding the smaller vessels. Also called **arteritis obliterans.**

**end artery,** a blood vessel that does not join with any other vessel. Also called **terminal artery.**

**end bud** [AS, *ende* + Gk, *bolbos,* onion], a mass of undifferentiated cells produced from the remnants of the primitive node and the primitive streak at the caudal end of the developing embryo after formation of the somites is completed. In lower animals it gives rise to the tail or any other caudal appendage and part of the trunk; in humans it forms the caudal portion of the trunk. Also called **tail bud.**

**end bulbs of Krause.** See **Krause's corpuscles.**

**end-diastolic pressure** /-dī·əstol'ik/ [AS, *ende* + Gk, *dia* + *stellein,* to set; L, *premere,* to press], the pressure of the blood in the ventricles at the end of diastole.

**endemic** /endem'ik/ [Gk, *endemos,* native], (of a disease or microorganism) the expected or "normal" incidence indigenous to a geographic area or population. See also **epidemic, pandemic.**

**endemic disease,** a physical or mental disorder caused by health conditions constantly present within a community. It usually describes an infection that is transmitted directly or indirectly between humans and is occurring at the usual expected rate.

**endemic goiter,** an enlargement of the thyroid gland caused by the intake of inadequate amounts of dietary iodine. Iodine deprivation leads to diminished production and secretion of thyroid hormone by the gland. The pituitary gland, operating on a negative feedback system, senses the deficiency and secretes increased amounts of thyroid-stimulating hormone (TSH), causing hyperplasia and hypertrophy of the thyroid gland. The goiter may grow during the winter months and shrink during the summer months when the person eats more iodine-containing fresh vegetables. Initially the goiter is diffuse; later it becomes multinodular. Endemic goiter occurs occasionally in adolescents at puberty and widely in population groups in geographic areas in which limited amounts of iodine are present in soil, water, and food. The use of iodized salt is a prophylactic treatment. Desiccated thyroid given orally may prevent further growth of adult goiters and may reduce the size of diffuse goiters. A large goiter may cause dysphagia, dyspnea, tracheal deviation, and cosmetic problems.

**endemic syphilis,** a chronic infectious skin disease that is closely related to *Treponema pallidum* and is frequently contracted in childhood without venereal contact. It is known as yaws, pinta, and bejel in heavily populated communities of undeveloped nations. Also called **nonvenereal syphilis.**

**endemic typhus.** See **murine typhus.**

**end-feel,** the sensation imparted to the examiner's hands at the end point of the available range of motion. It varies according to the limiting structure or tissue. Types of end-feel include capsular, bone-on-bone, spasm, and springy block. **Empty end-feel** is the absence of an end-feel during a range of motion examination when the patient stops further movement of a joint before the examiner senses any organic resistance to the movement.

**endo-, end-, ent-, ento-,** prefix meaning 'inward, within': *endobiotic, endocranial, endognathion.*

**endobronchitis** /en'dōbrongkī'tis/, inflammation of the smaller bronchi, often caused by a bronchial mucosal infection.

**endocardia.** See **endocardium.**

**endocardial,** pertaining to the **endocardium.**

**endocardial candidiasis.** See *Candida* endocarditis.

**endocardial cushion defect** /en'dōkär'dē·əl/, any cardiac defect resulting from the failure of the endocardial cushions in the embryonic heart to fuse and form the atrial septum. See also **atrial septal defect, congenital cardiac anomaly.**

**endocardial cushions,** a pair of thickened tissue sections in the embryonic atrial canal. During embryonic development they meet and fuse to form a septum dividing the canal into two channels which eventually become the atrioventricular orifices.

**endocardial fibroelastosis** /fī'brō·ē'lastō'sis/ [Gk, *endon* + *kardia,* heart; L, *fibra,* fiber; Gk, *elaunein,* to drive, *osis,* condition], an abnormal condition characterized by the development of a thick, fibroelastic endocardium that can cause failure of the heart to pump blood.

**endocardial murmur,** a continuous, soft sound made by an abnormality within the heart.

**endocardial pacing.** See **pacing.**

**endocarditis** /en'dōkärdī'tis/ [Gk, *endon* + *kardia,* heart; *itis,* inflammation], inflammation of the endocardium and heart valves. The condition is characterized by lesions caused by a variety of diseases. Kinds of endocarditis are bacterial endocarditis, nonbacterial thrombotic endocarditis, and Libman-Sacks endocarditis. All types of endocarditis are rapidly lethal if untreated, but most patients with endocarditis are successfully treated by various antibacterial and surgical measures. See also **bacterial endocarditis, subacute bacterial endocarditis.**

**endocardium** /en'dōkär'dē·əm/, *pl.* **endocardia,** the lining of the heart chambers, containing small blood vessels and a few bundles of smooth muscle. It is continuous with the endothelium of the great blood vessels. Compare **epicardium, myocardium.**

**endocervical** /-sur'fikəl/ [Gk, *endon* + L, *cervix,* neck], pertaining to the interior of the cervix. Also called **intracervical.**

**endocervicitis** /en'dōsur'visī'tis/, an abnormal condition characterized by inflammation of the epithelium and glands of the canal of the uterine cervix. See also **cervicitis.**

**endocervix** /en'dōsur'viks/, **1.** the membrane lining the canal of the uterine cervix. **2.** the opening of the cervix into the uterine cavity.

**endochondral** /-kon'drəl/ [Gk, *endon,* within, *chondros,* cartilage], pertaining to something within the cartilage.

**endochondral bone.** See **cartilaginous bone.**

**endocrinasthenia** /-krin'asthē'nē·ə/, a neural deficit caused by an alteration of the endocrine system.

**endocrine** /en'dəkrēn, -krīn/ [Gk, *endon* + *krinein,* to secrete], pertaining to a process in which a group of cells secrete into the blood or lymph circulation a substance (for example, hormone) that has a specific effect on tissues in another part of the body.

**endocrine diabetes mellitus** [Gk, *endon,* within, *krinein,* to secrete, *diabainein,* to pass through, *mellitus,* honeyed], a form of diabetes associated with diseases of other glands, such as the adrenals, pituitary, or thyroid.

**endocrine fracture** /-krēn/, any fracture that results from weakness of a specific bone caused by an endocrine disorder such as hyperparathyroidism.

**endocrine gland,** a ductless gland that produces and secretes hormones into the blood or lymph nodes. The hormones exert powerful effects on specific target tissues throughout the body. The endocrine glands include the pituitary, pineal, hypothalamus, thymus, thyroid, parathyroid, adrenal cortex, medulla islands of Langerhans, and gonads. Cells in other structures, such as the GI mucosa, the kidneys, and the placenta, also have endocrine functions.

**endocrine system** [Gk, *endon* + *krinein*, to secrete; *systema*], the network of ductless glands and other structures that elaborate and secrete hormones directly into the bloodstream, affecting various processes throughout the body, such as metabolism, growth, and secretions from other organs. Glands of the endocrine system include the thyroid, the parathyroid, the anterior pituitary, the posterior pituitary, the pancreas, the suprarenal glands, and the gonads. The pineal gland is also considered an endocrine gland because it is ductless, although its precise endocrine function is not established beyond its involvement in daily, monthly, and annual rhythms. Various other organs have some endocrinologic function. Compare **exocrine.** See also the Color Atlas of Human Anatomy.

**endocrine therapy.** See **hormone therapy.**

**endocrino-** [Gk, *endon,* within, *krinein,* to secrete], combining form meaning 'endocrine system, endocrine structures or function': *endocrinology, endocrinopathy.*

**endocrinologist** /en'dōkrinol'əjist/, a physician who specializes in the endocrine system and its disorders.

**endocrinology** /-krinol'əjē/ [Gk, *endon* + *krinein,* to secrete, *logos,* science], the study of the anatomic, physiologic, and pathologic characteristics of the endocrine system and of the treatment of endocrine problems.

**endocrinopathy** /-krinop'əthē/ [Gk, *endon,* within, *krinein,* to secrete, *pathos,* disease], a disease involving an endocrine gland or a dysfunction that decreases the quality or quantity of its secretion.

**endocytosis** /en'dō·sī·tō'sis/ [Gk, *endon,* within, + *kytos,* cell], uptake by a cell of material from the environment by invagination of its plasma membrane, which may be either phagocytosis or pinocytosis. Compare **exocytosis.**

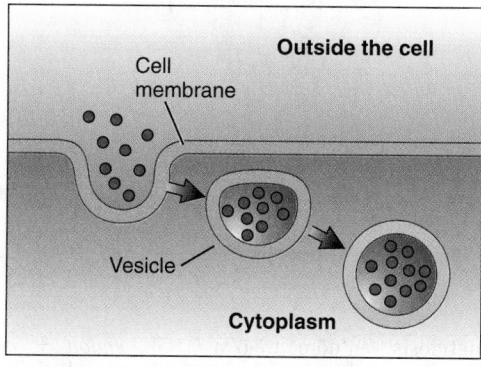

**Endocytosis** *(Herlihy and Maebius, 2000)*

**endoderm** /en'dədurm/ [Gk, *endon* + *derma,* skin], (in embryology) the innermost of the cell layers that develop from the embryonic disk of the inner cell mass of the blastocyst. From the endoderm arises the epithelium of the trachea, bronchi, lungs, GI tract, liver, pancreas, urinary bladder and canal, pharynx, thyroid, tympanic cavity, tonsils, and parathyroid glands. The endoderm thus comprises the lining of the cavities and passages of the body and the covering of most of the internal organs. Compare **ectoderm, hypoblast, mesoderm.**

**endodermal** /-dur'məl/ [Gk, *endon,* within, *derma,* skin], pertaining to the inner of the three layers of the embryo, the epithelial lining of the respiratory system, the digestive tract, and other tissues. Also spelled **entodermal.** See also **endoderm.**

**endodermal cloaca,** a part of the cloaca in the developing embryo that lies internal to the cloacal membrane and gives rise to the bladder and urogenital ducts. Compare **ectodermal cloaca.** See also **urogenital sinus.**

**endodontia.** See **endodontics.**

**endodontics** [Gk, *endon,* within, *odous,* tooth], the branch of dentistry that specializes in the diagnosis and treatment of diseases of the dental pulp, tooth root, and surrounding tissues and in the associated practice of root canal therapy. Also called **endodontia, endodontology, pulpodontia.**

**endodontist** /-don'tist/ [Gk, *endon,* within, *odous,* tooth], a dentist who specializes in endodontics.

**endodontology.** See **endodontics.**

**endogenous** /endoj'ənəs/ [Gk, *endon* + *genein,* to produce], **1.** growing within the body. **2.** originating from within the body or produced from internal causes, such as a disease caused by the structural or functional failure of an organ or system. Compare **exogenous. —endogenic,** *adj.*

**endogenous carbon dioxide,** carbon dioxide produced within the body by metabolic processes.

**endogenous hypertriglyceridemia.** See **hyperlipidemia type IV.**

**endogenous infection,** an infection caused by the reactivation of previously dormant organisms, as in coccidioidomycosis, histoplasmosis, and tuberculosis. Compare **germinal infection, mixed infection, retrograde infection, secondary infection.**

**endogenous iritis.** See **primary iritis.**

**endogenous obesity,** obesity resulting from dysfunction of the endocrine or metabolic system. Compare **exogenous obesity.** See also **obesity.**

**endogenous opioid,** an opiate-like substance, such as an endorphin, produced by the body.

**endogenous uric acid** [Gk, *endon,* within + *genein,* to produce + *ouron,* urine; L, *acidus*], uric acid produced by the metabolism of purines in the body's own nucleoproteins, as distinguished from metabolism of purine products in foods.

**endointoxication** /en'dō·intok'sikā'shən/, poisoning caused by a toxin produced within the body, such as from dead and infected tissue in gangrene.

**endolith.** See **denticle.**

**endolymph** /en'dəlimf/ [Gk, *endon* + *lympha,* water], the pale fluid in the membranous labyrinth (cochlear duct) of the internal ear. Compare **perilymph.**

**endolymphatic duct** /-limfat'ik/, a labyrinthine passage joining an endolymphatic sac with the utricle and saccule.

**endolymphatic sac,** the blind end of an endolymphatic duct.

**endomastoiditis** /-mas'toidī'tis/, an inflammation within the mastoid cavity and cells.

**endometrial** /en'dōmē'trē·əl/ [Gk, *endon* + *metra,* womb], **1.** pertaining to endometrium. **2.** pertaining to the uterine cavity.

**endometrial biopsy,** a microscopic examination of a sample of endometrial tissue to assess corpus luteum function. It is performed in infertile women with regular ovulatory cycles and no identifiable reason for infertility; in women with repeated first trimester abortions; in cases of abnormal vaginal bleeding; and during ovulation induction therapy.

**endometrial cancer,** an adenocarcinoma of the endometrium of the uterus. It is the most prevalent gynecologic malignancy, most often occurring in the fifth or sixth decade of life. Although the cause of endometrial cancer is not clear, some of the risk factors associated with an increased incidence of the disease are a medical history of infertility; anovulation, late menopause (52 years); administration of exogenous estrogen; uterine polyps; and a combination of diabetes, hypertension, and obesity. Abnormal vaginal bleeding, especially in a postmenopausal woman, is the cardinal symptom. Lower abdominal and low back pain may also be present; a large, boggy uterus is often a sign of advanced disease. Fewer than half the patients with endometrial cancer have a positive finding of a Papanicolaou's (Pap) test of the cervix and vagina, because the tumor cells rarely exfoliate in early stages of the lesion. A Pap test of cells removed from the endometrium obtained from jet washings of the uterine cavity provides more accurate data. Vacuum curettage is also used to extract endometrial cells for study, but the diagnostic technique most frequently recommended is dilation and curettage, in which each section of the uterus is examined and curetted for biopsy specimens. Adenocarcinomas constitute roughly 90% of all endometrial tumors; the remaining 10% comprises mixed carcinomas, sarcomas, and benign adenoacanthomas. Endometrial lesions may spread to the cervix but rarely invade the vagina. They metastasize to the broad ligaments, fallopian tubes, and ovaries so frequently that bilateral salpingo-oophorectomy with abdominal hysterectomy is the usual treatment. Radiotherapy is usually administered before and after surgery. High doses of a progestogen may be prescribed for palliation in advanced or inoperable cases. Chemotherapy may also be used.

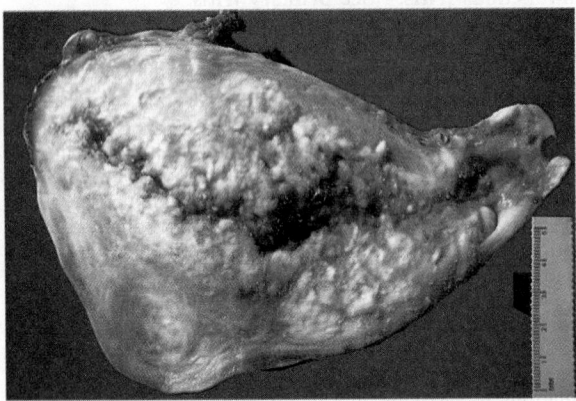

**Endometrial cancer**
*(Kumar, Cotran, and Robbins, 1997/courtesy Dr. Kyle Molberg, Department of Pathology, University of Texas Southwestern Medical Center, Dallas)*

**endometrial cyst** [Gk, *endon,* within, *metra,* womb, *kystis,* bag], **1.** an endometrial tumor. **2.** an ovarian cyst that develops as a distension of an endometrial gland.
**endometrial hyperplasia,** an abnormal condition characterized by overgrowth of the endometrium resulting from sustained stimulation by estrogen (of endogenous or exogenous origin) that is not opposed by progesterone. Estrogen

acts as a growth hormone for the endometrium. Through a complex intercellular mechanism, endometrial cells bind estrogen preferentially and undergo changes characteristic of the proliferative phase of the menstrual cycle. If estrogen stimulation continues for 3 to 6 months without periodic cessation or counteractive progesterone stimulation, as occurs in anovulation or perimenopausal women and in those receiving replacement estrogen without added progestogen, the endometrium becomes abnormally thickened and glandularized. Unremitting estrogen stimulation eventually causes cystic or adenomatous endometrial hyperplasia. The latter is a premalignant lesion that undergoes malignant degeneration in approximately 25% of cases. The causative relationship between estrogen and endometrial hyperplasia is well established; there is some indication but no proof that estrogen also provokes the change from hyperplasia to neoplasia and malignancy. Endometrial hyperplasia often results in abnormal uterine bleeding; such bleeding, particularly in older women, constitutes an indication for biopsy or curettage of the endometrium to establish histopathologic diagnosis and to rule out malignancy. A functioning estrogen-secreting tumor is suspected if the woman is not taking estrogen medication. Progestogen therapy is effective in reversing the abnormal histopathologic changes of endometrial hyperplasia; if hyperplasia is adenomatous, hysterectomy is commonly performed.
**endometrial polyp,** a pedunculated overgrowth of endometrium, usually benign. Polyps are a common cause of vaginal bleeding in perimenopausal women and are often associated with other uterine abnormalities, such as endometrial hyperplasia or fibroids. They may occur singly or in clusters and are usually 1 cm or less in diameter, but they may become much larger and prolapse through the cervix. Treatment for the condition includes surgical dilation and curettage.

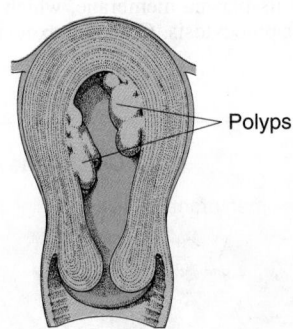

**Endometrial polyps** *(Beare and Myers, 1998)*

**endometriosis** /en′dōmē′trē·ō′sis/ [Gk, *endon* + *metra,* womb, *osis,* condition], an abnormal gynecologic condition characterized by ectopic growth and function of endometrial tissue. Precise incidence of the disease is unknown, but evidence of it is found in approximately 15% of women who undergo pelvic laparotomy for other indications. The average age of women found to have endometriosis is 37 years. Pregnancy may have an influence in preventing or ameliorating the disease. The causes of endometriosis are unknown; evidence suggests that the ectopic endometrium of endometriosis develops from vestigial tissue of the wolffian or müllerian duct; other evidence strongly suggests that fragments of endometrium from the lining of the uterus are refluxed during menstruation backward through the fallopian tubes into the peritoneal cavity, where they attach, grow, and function. The tissue is microscopically similar to or identical with endometrium, having glands or glandlike structures, stroma, and areas of hemorrhage. Fragments may be found in the wall of the uterus or on its surface; in or on the tubes, ovaries, rectosigmoid, or pelvic peritoneum; or occasionally in remote extrapelvic areas. Foci of endometriosis have been found in surgical scars, the umbilicus, the bowel, the lung, the eye, and the brain. When endometriosis occurs in a critical location it may cause grave dysfunction of the organ involved or, rarely, death; intestinal obstruction is a common complication. The lesions of pelvic endometriosis are typically small cystic structures a few millimeters in diameter that appear individually or in clusters as black nodules on the visceral and parietal peritoneum.

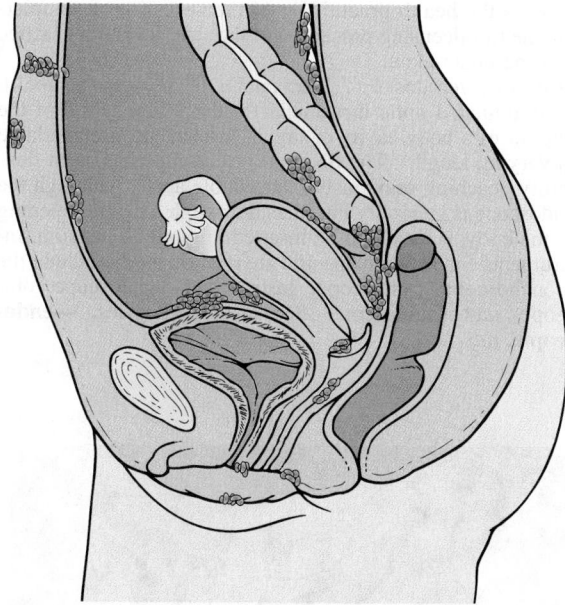

**Common sites of endometriosis**
*(Lewis, Heitkemper, and Dirksen, 2000)*

**endometriosis interna.** See **primary endometriosis.**
**endometritis** /en′dōmitrī′tis/ [Gk, *endon*, within, + *metra*, womb, *itis*, inflammation], an inflammatory condition of the endometrium. It is usually caused by bacterial infection, commonly by gonococci or hemolytic streptococci. The condition is characterized by fever, abdominal pain, malodorous discharge, and enlargement of the uterus. It occurs most frequently after childbirth or abortion and is associated with the use of an intrauterine contraceptive device. Diagnosis may be made by physical examination, history, laboratory analysis revealing an elevated white blood cell count, ultrasound, and bacteriologic identification of the pathogen. Treatment includes antibiotics, rest, analgesia, adequate fluid intake, and, if necessary, surgical drainage of a suppurating abscess, hysterectomy, or salpingo-oophorectomy. Endometritis may be mild and self-limited, chronic or acute, and unilateral or bilateral. It may cause sterility if scar for-

mation occludes the passage of the fallopian tubes. Septic abortion and puerperal fever are forms of endometritis that caused many deaths before asepsis and antibiotics became commonly available. A kind of endometritis is **decidua endometritis.** See also **pelvic inflammatory disease.**
**endometrium** /en′dōmē′trē·əm/ [Gk, *endon* + *metra*, womb], the mucous membrane lining of the uterus, consisting of the stratum compactum, the stratum spongiosum, and the stratum basale. The endometrium changes in thickness and structure with the menstrual cycle. The stratum compactum and the stratum spongiosum constitute the pars functionalis and are shed with each menstrual flow. The pars functionalis is known as the decidua during pregnancy, when it underlies the placenta. Compare **myometrium, parametrium.**
**endomorph** /en′dəmôrf′/ [Gk, *endon* + *morphe*, form], a person whose body build is characterized by a soft, round physique with a large trunk and thighs, tapering extremities, an accumulation of fat throughout the body, and a predominance of structures derived from the endoderm. Compare **ectomorph, mesomorph.** See also **pyknic.**
**endomyocardial fibrosis** [Gk, *endon*, within + *mys*, muscle + *kardia*, heart; L, *fibra*, fiber + *osis*, condition], idiopathic myocardiopathy occurring endemically in various parts of Africa and rarely in other areas, characterized by cardiomegaly, marked thickening of the endocardium with dense, white fibrous tissue that frequently extends to involve the inner third or half of the myocardium, and congestive heart failure.
**endomyocarditis** /-mī′ōkärdī′tis/ [Gk, *endon*, within, *mys*, muscle, *kardia*, heart, *itis*, inflammation], an inflammation of the lining of the heart.
**endoneurial nerve sheath.** See **nerve sheath.**
**endoparasite** /en′dōper′əsīt/ [Gk, *endon* + *parasitos*, guest], (in medical parasitology) an organism that lives within the body of the host, such as a tapeworm.
**endopathy** /endop′əthē/, any disease originating within the person.
**endopeptidase** /en′dō·pep′ti·dās/ [Gk, *endon*, within + Gk, *peptein*, to digest + *ase*, enzyme suffix], any peptidase that catalyzes the cleavage of internal peptide bonds in a polypeptide or protein; they are divided into subclasses on the basis of catalytic mechanism and comprise the serine endopeptidases, cysteine endopeptidases, aspartic endopeptidases, metalloendopeptidases, and other endopeptidases.
**endophthalmitis** /endof′thalmī′tis/ [Gk, *endon* + *ophthalmos*, eye, *itis*], an inflammatory condition of the internal eye in which the primary signs are decreased vision, vitritis, and development of a hypopyon. Patients may or may not complain of pain. Other symptoms include erythema and edema. It may result from bacterial or fungal infection, trauma, allergy, drug or chemical toxicity, or vascular disease. Depending on the cause, therapy requires surgical intervention or administration of an antibiotic, atropine, or a corticosteroid. Also called **endophthalmia.**
**endophthalmitis phacoanaphylactica** /fak′ō·an′əfilak′-təkə/, an abnormal condition characterized by an acute autoimmune reaction of the eye. It is caused by hypersensitivity of the eye to the protein of the crystalline lens and commonly follows trauma to the crystalline lens or cataract surgery. Associated symptoms include swelling and inflammation of the eye, severe pain, and blurred vision. The substance of the lens is invaded by polymorphonuclear cells and mononuclear phagocytes. Sensitization of one eye often follows the extracapsular removal of the lens of the eye on the opposite side. Accurate diagnosis must differentiate between this condition and infectious endophthalmitis.

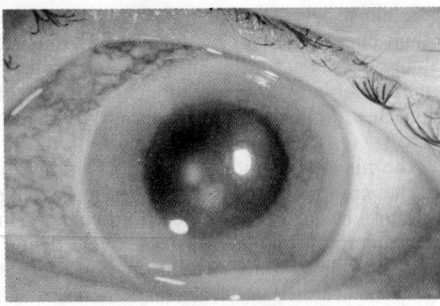

**Bacterial endophthalmitis**
*(Stone and Gorbach, 2000/courtesy Dr. Jay Duker, New England Medical Center, Boston)*

Therapy is supportive and commonly includes the administration of corticosteroids and atropine. Refractory cases may require surgical removal of the lens. Compare **uveitis.**

**endophytic** /en'dōfit'ik/ [Gk, *endon* + *phyton*, plant], pertaining to the tendency to grow inward, such as a tumor that grows into the wall of a hollow organ.

**endoplasm** /en'doplaz'əm/ [Gk, *endon*, within, *plasma*, plasm], the inner portion of cytoplasm.

**endoplasmic reticulum** /-plaz'mik/ [Gk, *endon* + *plassein*, to mold], an extensive network of membrane-enclosed tubules in the cytoplasm of cells. The structure functions in the synthesis of proteins and lipids and in the transport of these metabolites within the cell.

**end-organ** [AS, *ende* + Gk, *organon*, instrument], a nerve ending in which the terminal nerve filaments are encapsulated.

**endorphin** /endôr'fin/ [Gk, *endon* + *morphe*, shape], any of the neuropeptides composed of many amino acids, elaborated by the pituitary gland and other brain areas, and acting on the central and the peripheral nervous systems to reduce pain. There are several types, designated alpha, beta, and gamma. Beta-endorphin has been isolated in the brain and in the GI tract and seems to be the most potent of the endorphins. Beta-endorphin is composed of 31 amino acids that are identical to part of the sequence of 91 amino acids of the hormone beta-lipotropin, also produced by the pituitary gland. Behavioral tests indicate that beta-endorphin is a powerful analgesic in humans and animals. Brain-stimulated analgesia in humans releases beta-endorphin into the cerebrospinal fluid. Compare **enkephalin.**

**endorsement** /endôrs'mənt/ [Gk, *en* + L, *dorsum*, the back], a statement of recognition of the license of a health practitioner in one state by another state. An endorsement relieves the health practitioner of the necessity of completing the full licensing procedure of the state in which practice is to be undertaken.

**endoscope** /en'dəskōp'/ [Gk, *endon* + *skopein*, to look], an illuminated optic instrument for the visualization of the interior of a body cavity or organ. Instruments are available in varying lengths. The fiberoptic endoscope has great flexibility, reaching previously inaccessible areas. Although the endoscope is generally introduced through a natural opening in the body, it may also be inserted through an incision. Instruments for viewing specific areas of the body include the bronchoscope, cystoscope, gastroscope, laparoscope, otoscope, and vaginoscope. See also **fiberoptics.** —**endoscopic,** *adj.*

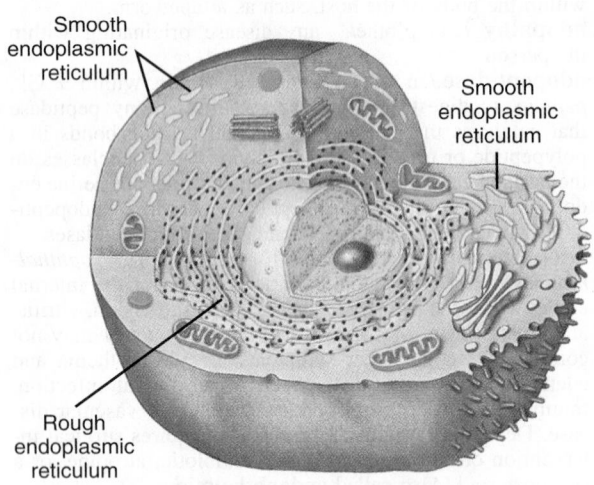

Smooth endoplasmic reticulum

Smooth endoplasmic reticulum

Rough endoplasmic reticulum

**Endoplasmic reticulum**
*(Thibodeau and Patton, 1999/William Ober)*

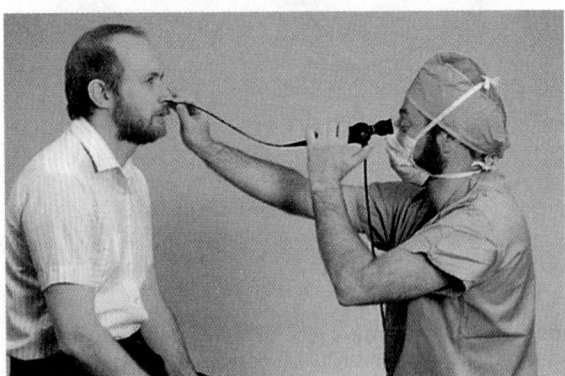

**Endoscope** *(Bingham, Hawke, and Kwok, 1992)*

**endoprosthesis** /-prosthē'sis, -pros'thəsis/ [Gk, *endon* + *prosthesis*, addition], a prosthetic device installed within the body, such as an internal cardiac pacemaker.

**endoreduplication** /en'dō·ridoo'plikā'shən/ [Gr, *endon* + L, *re-*, again, *duplicare*, to duplicate], replication of the chromosomes without subsequent cell division.

**endoscopic laser cholecystectomy.** See **cholecystectomy.**

**endoscopic retrograde cholangiopancreatography (ERCP),** an endoscopic test that provides radiographic visualization of the bile and pancreatic ducts. A flexible fiberoptic duodenoscope is placed into the common bile duct. A radiopaque substance is instilled directly into the duct, and serial x-ray films are taken. It is useful in identifying partial or total obstruction of these ducts, as well as stones, benign strictures, cysts, ampullary stenosis, anatomic variations, and malignant tumors. See also **cholangiography.**

**endoscopy** /endos′kəpē/, the visualization of the interior of organs and cavities of the body with an endoscope. The GI structures that can be examined through this procedure include the esophagus, stomach, duodenum, colon, and pancreas and biliary tract with the aid of x-ray film and fluoroscopy. Endoscopy can also be used to obtain samples for cytologic and histologic examination and to follow the course of a disease, as the assessment of the healing of gastric and duodenal ulcers. See also **bronchoscopy, cystoscopy, gastroscopy, laparoscopy.**

**endoskeletal prosthesis** /-skel′ətəl/ [Gk, *endon* + *skeletos,* dried up, *prosthesis,* addition], a lower-limb support consisting of an internal pylon usually covered with a lightweight material, such as plastic foam. See also **pylon.**

**endoskeleton,** the internal network of bones to which muscles are attached. Compare **exoskeleton.**

**endosteal hyperostosis** /endos′tē·əl/, an inherited bone disorder characterized by an overgrowth of the mandible and brow areas. The excessive bone growth can lead to entrapment of cranial nerves, causing facial palsy and loss of hearing. Also called **Van Buchem's syndrome.**

**endosteal implant** [Gk, *endon,* within + *osteon,* bone], a dental implant made of metal, ceramic, or polymeric material, consisting of a blade, screw, pin, or vent, inserted into the jaw bone through the alveolar or basal bone, with a post protruding through the mucoperiosteum into the oral cavity to serve as an abutment for dentures or orthodontic appliances, or to serve in fracture fixation.

**endostomy therapist.** See **enterostomal therapist.**

**endothelial** /en′dōthē′lē·əl/ [Gk, *endon,* within, *thele,* nipple], pertaining to endothelium.

**endothelial cell** [Gk, *endon,* within, *thele,* nipple; L, *cella,* storeroom], a lining cell of a body cavity or of the cardiovascular system. It is usually seen as a flat nucleated cell.

**endothelium** /en′dōthē′lē·əm/ [Gk, *endon* + *thele,* nipple], the layer of simple squamous epithelial cells that lines the heart, the blood and lymph vessels, and the serous cavities of the body. It is highly vascular, heals quickly, and is derived from the mesoderm.

**endothoracic fascia** /-thôras′ik/, a sheet of connective tissue within the thorax. It separates the parietal pleura from the chest wall and the diaphragm. A thickened portion also attaches to the medial border of the first rib.

**endotoxin** /en′dōtok′sin/ [Gk, *endon* + *toxikon,* poison], a toxin contained in the cell walls of some microorganisms, especially gram-negative bacteria, that is released when the bacterium dies and is broken down in the body. Fever, chills, shock, leukopenia, and a variety of other symptoms result, depending on the particular organism and the condition of the infected person. Compare **exotoxin.**

**endotoxin shock** [Gk, *endon,* within, *toxikon,* poison; Fr, *choc*], a septic shock in response to the release of endotoxins produced by gram-negative bacteria. The toxin is released on the death of the bacterial cell.

**endotracheal** /en′dōtrā′kē·əl/ [Gk, *endon* + *tracheia* + *arteria,* airpipe], within or through the trachea.

**endotracheal anesthesia,** anesthesia that is achieved by the inhalation of an anesthetic gas or mixture of gases through an endotracheal tube into the lungs, where it is absorbed into the bloodstream.

**endotracheal extubation,** a nursing intervention from the Nursing Interventions Classification (NIC) defined as purposeful removal of the endotracheal tube from the nasopharyngeal or oropharyngeal airway. See also **Nursing Interventions Classification.**

**endotracheal intubation,** the management of the patient with an airway catheter inserted through the mouth or nose into the trachea. An endotracheal tube may be used to maintain a patent airway, to prevent aspiration of material from the digestive tract in the unconscious or paralyzed patient, to permit suctioning of tracheobronchial secretions, or to administer positive-pressure ventilation that cannot be given effectively by a mask. Endotracheal tubes may be made of rubber or plastic and usually have an inflatable cuff to maintain a closed system with the ventilator.

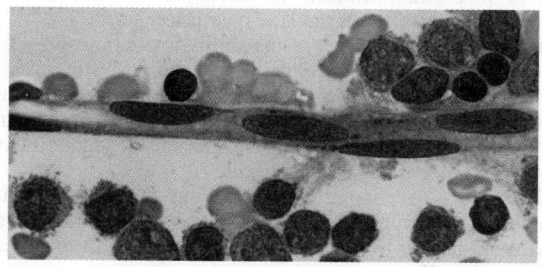

**Endothelial cells** *(Carr and Rodak, 1999)*

**endothelial-derived relaxing factor (EDRF),** an agent that relaxes smooth muscles and stimulates blood flow in veins.

**endothelial myeloma.** See **Ewing's sarcoma.**

**endothelin (ET)** /-thē′lin/, any of a group of vasoconstrictive peptides produced by endothelial cells. Three known endothelins, designated ET-1, ET-2, and ET-3, are chemically related to asp venom. ET-1 is the most potent vasoconstrictor yet discovered, being 10 times stronger than the second-most potent vasoconstrictor known, angiotensin II.

**-endothelioma,** combining form meaning 'a tumor of endothelial tissue': *hemendothelioma, lymphendothelioma.*

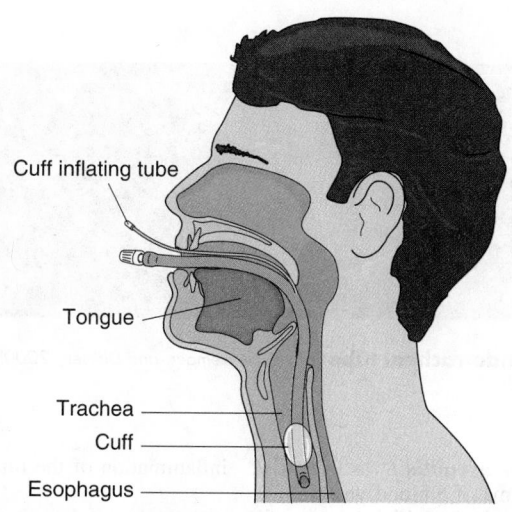

**Endotracheal intubation** *(Phipps, Sands, and Marek, 1999)*

■ METHOD: With the aid of paralytic agents to ease the passage, the endotracheal tube is inserted via the mouth or nose through the larynx into the trachea; if the oral route is used, a bite block may be required to prevent the patient from biting and obstructing the tube. Breath sounds are auscultated immediately after insertion and every 1 or 2 hours thereafter to make certain the tube is properly positioned and is not obstructing one of the mainstem bronchi. Once the tube is correctly positioned, it is taped securely in place and checked for patency and slippage every 15 to 60 minutes or per institutional protocol. The trachea is suctioned every hour and as needed, as indicated by patient assessment (dyspnea, gurgling, respirations, activation of ventilator pressure alarms). If so ordered, the trachea is irrigated with normal saline solution. The patient is usually on intermittent positive-pressure breathing (IPPB) or a volume respirator with the cuff of the endotracheal tube inflated; if the patient can breathe independently, the trachea and mouth are suctioned, the cuff is deflated, and the respiratory rate and quality are checked hourly. The patient is turned every 1 to 2 hours, and the blood pressure and pulse checked every 2 to 4 hours or according to institutional protocol. Parenteral fluids are administered as ordered; nothing is given orally; fluid intake and output are measured and recorded. The patient's level of consciousness is determined hourly, and, if he or she is sufficiently conscious, a method of communication is established.
■ NURSING ORDERS: The nurse monitors the position and patency of the endotracheal tube, performs the necessary suctioning, inflates and deflates the cuff at appropriate times, and administers IPPB or support with the volume respirator. The nurse checks the vital signs at specified intervals and provides emotional support and physical care for the patient, who is usually acutely ill, unable to communicate, and suffering from the discomfort of an endotracheal tube.
■ OUTCOME CRITERIA: Meticulous assessment of the patient with an endotracheal tube can promote the survival of a critically ill person.

**endotracheal tube,** a large-bore catheter inserted through the mouth or nose and into the trachea to a point above the bifurcation of the trachea. It is used for delivering oxygen under pressure when ventilation must be totally controlled and in general anesthetic procedures. See also **endotracheal intubation.**

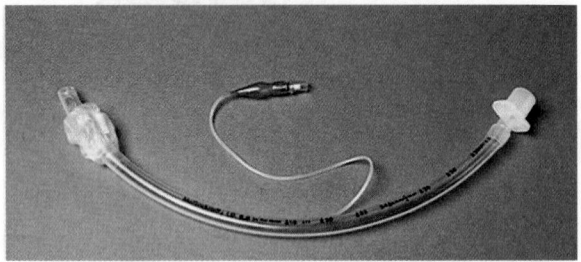

**Endotracheal tube** *(Lewis, Heitkemper, and Dirksen, 2000)*

**endovasculitis** /-vas'kyəlī'tis/, inflammation of the tunica intima of a blood vessel.

**endoxin** /endok'sin/, an endogenous analog of digoxin that occurs naturally in humans. It is a hormone that may regulate the excretion of salt.

**endplate** [AS, *ende* + ME, *plat*], the motor endplate in the nervous system, located at the terminal membrane of an axon and the postjunctional membrane of the adjoining muscle tissue. Also called **myoneural junction.**

**end point,** 1. (in chemistry) the point at which a physical change associated with the condition of equivalence is observed during a titration. 2. the point or time at which an activity is finished. 3. the point at which a chemical indicator changes color, for example, in an acid-base titration.

**end-positional nystagmus,** a horizontal rhythmic oscillation of the eyes on extreme lateral gaze. It occurs in normal eyes when the fixation point is outside the binocular field. Also called **deviational nystagmus, pseudonystagmus.**

**end product** /end prod'əkt /, the chemical compound resulting from completion of a sequence of metabolic reactions.

**end-stage disease** [AS, *ende* + OFr, *estage* + L, *dis* + Fr, *aise,* ease], a disease condition that is essentially terminal because of irreversible damage to vital tissues or organs. Kidney or renal end-stage disease is defined as a point at which the kidney is so badly damaged or scarred that dialysis or transplantation is required for patient survival.

**end-tidal capnography** /end'tīdəl/, the process of continuously recording the level of carbon dioxide in expired air. The percentage of carbon dioxide at the end of expiration can be estimated and gives a close approximation of the alveolar carbon dioxide concentration. The process, which requires the use of infrared spectroscopy, is used to monitor critically ill patients and in pulmonary function testing. The data are typically recorded automatically on a strip of graph paper.

**end-tidal $CO_2$.** See **capnometry.**

**end-tidal $CO_2$ determination,** the concentration of carbon dioxide in a patient's end-tidal breath, assumed to reflect arterial carbon dioxide tension. A significant difference may indicate a change in ventilation/perfusion matching.

**end-to-end anastomosis.** See **anastomosis.**

**end-to-side anastomosis,** an anastomosis connecting the end of one vessel with the side of a larger one.

**endurance**[1] /endyŏŏr'əns/, the ability to continue an activity despite increasing physical or psychologic stress, as in the effort to perform additional numbers of muscle contractions before the onset of fatigue. Although endurance and strength are different qualities, weaker muscles tend to have less endurance than strong muscles.

**endurance**[2], a nursing outcome from the Nursing Outcomes Classification (NOC) defined as extent that energy enables a person to sustain activity. See also **Nursing Outcomes Classification.**

**Enduron,** trademark for a thiazide diuretic and antihypertensive (methyclothiazide).

**Enduronyl,** trademark for a fixed-combination cardiovascular drug containing a diuretic (methyclothiazide) and an antihypertensive (deserpidine).

**-ene,** suffix used for naming hydrocarbons: *ethidene, xanthene.*

**enema** /en'əmə/ [Gk, *enienai,* to send in], the introduction of a solution into the rectum for cleansing or therapeutic purposes. Enemas may be commercially packed disposable units or reusable equipment prepared just before use.
■ METHOD: The equipment is assembled. If disposable equipment is to be used, an 18- to 20- French catheter, a 2- to 3-foot length of tubing, an enema bag, the solution, and a clamp are collected and taken to the bedside. If a disposable

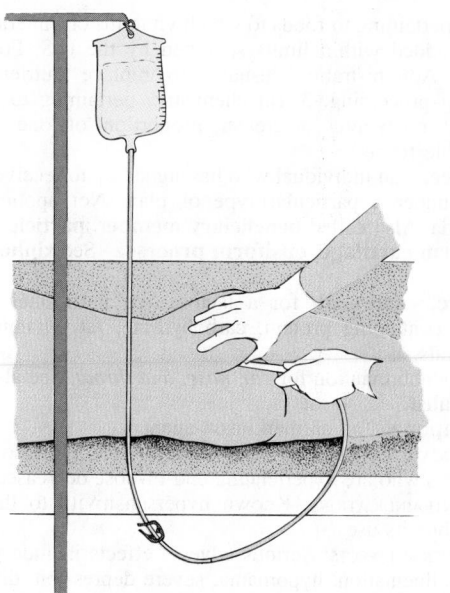

**Enema administration** (Potter and Perry, 2001)

set is to be used, no other equipment is necessary. The patient is positioned in the left lateral or dorsal position. After air is expelled from the tubing, the tip of the catheter is lubricated. (Disposable units usually have prelubricated tips.) The patient is asked to bear down, as if to defecate, and the tip of the catheter is gently inserted 3 to 4 inches into the rectum, depending on the size of the patient and the purpose of the enema. The solution is allowed to flow from a height of 18 to 20 inches above the level of the hips. The tip of the catheter or squeeze bottle is withdrawn when most of the solution has been administered. Some solution is left in the tubing to prevent air from entering the rectum. Light pressure is applied over the anus with toilet tissue or a gauze pad. The fluid is held in by the patient for the prescribed length of time. It is then expelled as the patient sits on the toilet.
■ INTERVENTIONS: The reasons for performing the procedure and the steps to be taken are explained to the patient. The solution is warmed to 99° to 105° F (37.8° to 40.6° C) to reduce the stimulation of intestinal peristalsis by a sudden temperature change in the colon. The patient is warned that some discomfort may occur because the colon tends to contract when distended by the fluid. The enema is given slowly to prevent sudden distension that would cause peristalsis or spasm and greater discomfort. A call bell is kept within reach of the patient during expulsion of the enema because the discomfort of the procedure and the effort required to expel the enema may cause faintness. The color, consistency, and amount of material evacuated are evaluated. If nondisposable equipment is used, it is rinsed in cold water before being washed with warm soapy water and sterilized.
■ OUTCOME CRITERIA: A thorough explanation to the patient of all aspects of the procedure, careful observation of the patient during the procedure, slow and gentle administration of the enema, and evaluation of the results of the procedure are important to achieve the desired effect.

**energy** /en′ərjē/ [Gk, *energia*], the capacity to do work or to perform vigorous activity. Energy may occur in the form of heat, light, movement, sound, or radiation. Human energy is usually expressed as muscle contractions and heat production, made possible by the metabolism of food that originally acquired the energy from sunlight. Chemical energy is that released as a result of a chemical reaction, as in the metabolism of food. Compare **anergy. —energetic,** *adj.*

**energy conservation**[1], a principle that energy cannot be created or destroyed although it can be changed from one form into another, as when heat energy is converted to light energy.

**energy conservation**[2], a nursing outcome from the Nursing Outcomes Classification (NOC) defined as extent of active management of energy to initiate and sustain activity. See also **Nursing Outcomes Classification.**

**energy cost of activities,** the metabolic cost in calories or kilojoules of various forms of physical activity. For example, the average metabolic (MET) equivalent of walking at a rate of 3 km/hr is 2 METs per minute, and the energy cost of walking at a speed of 6 km/hr is 5 METs per minute. See also **MET.**

**energy field, disturbed,** a nursing diagnosis accepted by the Eleventh National Conference on the Classification of Nursing Diagnoses. It is defined as a disruption of the flow of energy surrounding a person's being, which causes a disharmony of the body, mind, or spirit.
■ DEFINING CHARACTERISTICS: The defining characteristics include temperature change (warmth or coolness), visual changes (image or color), disruption of the field (vacant/hold/spike/bulge), movement (wave/spike/tingling/dense/flowing), and sounds (tone or words). See also **nursing diagnosis.**

**energy management,** a nursing intervention from the Nursing Interventions Classification (NIC) defined as regulating energy use to treat or prevent fatigue and optimize function. See also **Nursing Interventions Classification.**

**energy output,** the amount of energy expended by work or activity by the body per specified period.

**energy-protein malnutrition,** See **protein-energy malnutrition.**

**energy subtraction,** a radiographic technique in which two different x-ray beams are used alternately to provide a subtraction image resulting from differences in photoelectrical interaction.

**enervation** /en′ərvā′shən/ [L, *enervare,* to weaken], **1.** reduction or lack of nervous energy; weakness; lassitude; languor. **2.** removal of a complete nerve or a section of nerve.

**en face** /äNfäs′, enfäs′/, "face-to-face"; a position in which the mother's face and the infant's face are approximately 8 inches apart and on the same plane, as when the mother holds the infant up in front of her face or when she nurses the child. Studies of maternal and infant bonding have shown that mothers seek eye-to-eye contact and that they will instinctively move the baby to an en face position. In addition, infants have been shown to prefer a human face to other visual stimuli and to be best able to focus at a distance of 8 to 10 inches.

**enflurane** /en′flŏŏrān/, a nonflammable anesthetic gas of the ether family.
■ INDICATIONS: It is used for maintenance of general anesthesia. A halogenated volatile liquid, enflurane is administered through calibrated vaporizers, permitting close control of dosage.

■ CONTRAINDICATIONS: Because excitement may occur on induction, a hypnotic dose of short-acting barbiturate is used for premedication.

■ ADVERSE EFFECTS: Adverse reactions may include seizures, hypotension, cardiac arrhythmia, shivering, nausea, and vomiting on emergence.

**engagement** /engāj′mənt/ [Fr, a bonding], **1.** fixation of the presenting part of the fetus in the maternal true pelvis. The largest diameter of the presenting part is at or below the level of the ischial spines. **2.** fixation of the fetal head in the maternal midpelvis with the biparietal diameter of the head level with the ischial spines.

**English position.** See **lateral recumbent position.**

**engorged** /in·gÔrjd′/ [Fr, *engorger,* to fill up], distended or swollen with fluids.

**engorgement** /engôrj′mənt/ [Fr, *engorger,* to fill up], distension or vascular congestion of body tissues, such as the swelling of breast tissue caused by an increased flow of blood and lymph before true lactation.

**engram** /en′gram/, **1.** a hypothetical neurophysiologic storage unit in the cerebrum that is the source of a particular memory. **2.** an interneuronal circuit involving specific neurons and muscle fibers that can be coordinated to perform specific motor activity patterns. Thousands of repetitions may be needed to establish an engram. **3.** the permanent trace left by a stimulus in nerve tissue.

**engrossment.** See **bonding.**

**enhancement** /enhans′mənt/ [ME, *enhauncen,* to raise], to improve, heighten, or augment.

**Enkaid,** trademark of a sodium channel antagonist antiarrhythmic drug (encainide).

**enkephalin** /enkef′əlin/ [Gk, *enkepalos,* brain, *in,* within], one of two pain-relieving pentapeptides produced in the body. Enkephalins are located in the pituitary gland, brain, and GI tract. Axon terminals that release enkephalins are concentrated in the posterior horn of the gray matter of the spinal cord, in the central part of the thalamus, and in the amygdala of the limbic system of the cerebrum. Enkephalins inhibit neurotransmitters in the pathway for pain perception, thereby reducing the emotional as well as the physical impact of pain. Methionine-enkephalin and isoleucine-enkephalin are each composed of five amino acids, four of which are identical in both compounds. These two neuropeptides can depress neurons throughout the central nervous system. Although it is not known exactly how these two neuropeptides function, the enkephalins are natural pain killers and may be involved, with other neuropeptides, in the development of psychopathologic behavior in some cases. Compare **endorphin.**

**enkephalinergic neuron** /enkef′əlinur′jik/, a nerve cell that releases the peptide neurotransmitter enkephalin. Such neurons are widespread in the central nervous system.

**enol** /ē′nol/, an organic compound with an alcohol or hydroxyl group directly attached (bonded) to a double bond. By transfer of the hydrogen atom from oxygen to carbon the enol form becomes the keto form. Such compounds usually exist as enol-keto tautomers.

**enophthalmos** /en′əfthal′məs/ [Gk, *en,* in, *ophthalmos,* eye], backward displacement of the eye in the bony socket, caused by traumatic injury or developmental defect. Ptosis may cause an incorrect diagnosis of enophthalmos. —**enophthalmic,** *adj.*

**Enovid,** trademark for an oral contraceptive containing an estrogen (mestranol) and a progestin (norethynodrel).

**enriched,** **1.** (in chemistry) pertaining to a substance containing a proportion of isotope greater than that found in the naturally occurring form of the same element. **2.** (in nutri-

tion) pertaining to foods to which vitamins or minerals have been added within limits specified by the U.S. Food and Drug Administration, usually to replace nutrients lost during processing. **3.** (in chemistry) pertaining to a compound containing a greater proportion of one of two possible forms.

**enrollee,** an individual who has signed up to receive health care under a particular type of plan. Not applicable in Canada. Also called **beneficiary member, participant.**

**ensiform cartilage, ensiform process.** See **xiphoid process.**

**Ensure,** trademark for a lactose-free nutritional supplement containing protein, carbohydrate, fat, vitamins, and minerals.

**ENT,** abbreviation for *ear, nose, and throat.* See also **ENT specialist.**

**entacapone,** an antiparkinson agent.

■ INDICATIONS: Entacapone is used to treat parkinsonism in patients who are experiencing end-of-dose decreased effect.

■ CONTRAINDICATIONS: Known hypersensitivity to this drug prohibits its use.

■ ADVERSE EFFECTS: Serious adverse effects include psychosis, hallucination, hypomania, severe depression, dizziness, gastritis, GI disorders, alopecia, dark urine, back pain, dyspnea, purpura, fatigue, asthenia, and bacterial infection. Common side effects include involuntary choreiform movements, hand tremors, fatigue, headache, anxiety, twitching, numbness, dyskinesia, hypokinesia, hyperkinesia, weakness, confusion, agitation, nightmares, nausea, vomiting, anorexia, abdominal distress, dry mouth, flatulence, bitter taste, diarrhea, constipation, dyspepsia, and orthostatic hypotension.

**ental** /en′tal/ [Gk, *entos,* within], central or inner; interior or inside.

**Entameba.** See *Entamoeba.*

**entamebiasis.** See **amebiasis.**

**Entamoeba** /en′təmē′bə/ [Gk, *entos,* within, *amoibe,* change], a genus of intestinal amebic parasites of which several species are pathogenic to humans. Also spelled *Entameba.* See also *Entamoeba histolytica.*

*Entamoeba coli,* a common nonpathogenic amebic parasite found in the intestines of humans and other mammals. It is similar to and sometimes confused with *E. histolytica,* the causal agent of amebic dysentery. However, *E. coli* organisms tend to be slightly larger, have more pseudopods, and are sluggish in movement.

*Entamoeba gingivalis,* a temperature-resistant species of ameba found in the mouth of humans and other mammals. As a causal agent of gingivitis, it is associated with poor dental hygiene.

*Entamoeba histolytica* /his′təlit′ikə/, a pathogenic species of ameba that causes amebic dysentery and hepatic amebiasis in humans. See also **amebiasis, amebic dysentery, hepatic amebiasis.**

**entamoebiasis.** See **amebiasis.**

**enter-.** See **entero-.**

**enteral** /en′tərəl, enter′əl/ [Gk, *enteron,* bowel], within the small intestine, or via the small intestine.

**enteral feeding,** a mode of feeding that uses the GI tract, such as oral or tube feeding.

**enteral nutrition,** the provision of nutrients through the GI tract when the client cannot ingest, chew, or swallow food but can digest and absorb nutrients.

**enteral tube feeding**[1] [Gk, *enteron,* bowel; L, *tubus* + AS, *faedan*], the introduction of nutrients directly into the GI tract by feeding tube. Routes include both nonsurgical and surgically placed: nasogastric, nasoduodenal, nasojejunal,

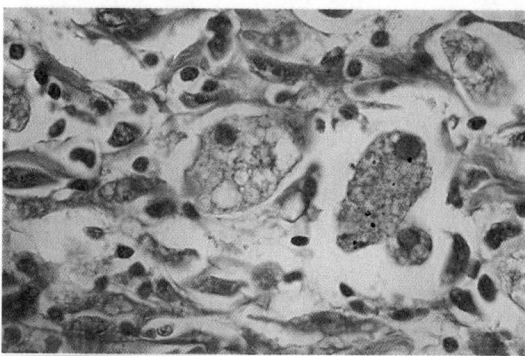

**Entamoeba histolytica trophozoites**
*(Kumar, Cotran, and Robbins, 1997)*

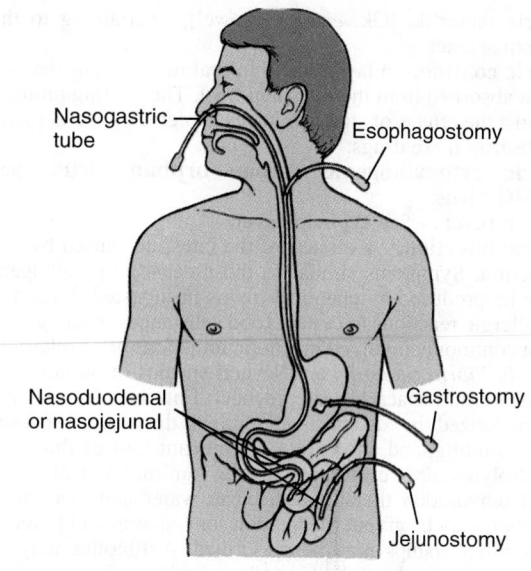

Nasogastric tube

Esophagostomy

Nasoduodenal or nasojejunal

Gastrostomy

Jejunostomy

**Common placement locations
for enteral feeding tubes**
*(Lewis, Collier, and Heitkemper, 1996)*

esophagostomy, gastrostomy, and jejunostomy. See also **drip gavage. tube feeding.**

**enteral tube feeding**[2], a nursing intervention from the Nursing Interventions Classification (NIC) defined as delivering nutrients and water through a gastrointestinal tube. See also **Nursing Interventions Classification.**

**enterectomy** /en'tərek'təmē/ [Gk, *enteron*, intestine, *ektomē*, excision], the surgical removal of a portion of intestine.

## Common problems of patients receiving enteral tube feedings

| Problems and possible causes | Corrective measures |
|---|---|
| **Vomiting** | |
| Improper placement of tube | Replace tube in proper position. Check tube position before beginning feeding and every 4 hr if continuous feedings. |
| Initiation of feeding too soon after placement | Give patient time to get adjusted to tube before feeding. |
| Feeding too fast | Hold feeding 2-8 hr, then resume at slower rate. Give feeding by slow drip or via pump slowly. Avoid use of force. |
| Patient in wrong position | Keep head of bed elevated to 30- to 45-degree angle. Have patient lie on right side for ½ hr after feeding. Have patient sit up on side of bed or in chair. Encourage ambulation unless contraindicated. |
| Contamination of formula | Refrigerate unused formula and record date opened. Discard outdated formula every 24 hr. Discard formula left standing for a long time. |
| Air in stomach | Clear tubing of air before feeding. Keep tube feeding container filled so air does not enter through feeding set. |
| **Diarrhea** | |
| Feeding too fast, high concentration of formula | Decrease rate of feeding. Change to continuous drip feedings. Check for drugs that may cause diarrhea (e.g., antibiotics) |
| Lactose intolerance | Consult physician for change in formula to lactose-free solution. |
| Contamination of formula or tubing | Discard old tubing or other equipment. Change tubing every 24 hr. |
| **Constipation** | |
| No fiber in diet | Consult physician for change in formula to one with more fiber content. Obtain laxative order. |
| Inadequate fluid intake | Increase fluid intake if not contraindicated. Give free water as well as formula. |
| Drugs | Check for drugs that may be constipating. |
| **Dehydration** | |
| Excessive diarrhea, vomiting | Decrease rate or change formula. Check drugs patient is receiving, especially antibiotics. Take care to prevent bacterial contamination of formula and equipment. |
| Poor fluid intake | Increase intake and check amount and number of feedings. Increase amount of intake if appropriate. |
| High protein formula | Change formula. |

From Lewis SM, Collier LC, Heitkemper MM: *Medical-surgical nursing: assessment and management of clinical problems,* ed 4, St Louis, 1996, Mosby.

**enteric** /enter′ik/ [Gk, *enteron,* bowel], pertaining to the intestinal tract.

**enteric coating,** a layer added to oral medications that are to be absorbed from the intestinal tract. The coating protects against the effects of stomach juices, which can interact with or destroy these drugs.

**enteric cytopathogenic human orphan virus.** See **ECHO virus.**

**enteric fever.** See **typhoid fever.**

**enteric infection,** a disease of the intestine caused by any infection. Symptoms similar to those caused by pathogens may be produced by chemical toxins in ingested foods and by allergic reactions to certain food substances. Among bacteria commonly involved in enteric infections are *Escherichia coli, Vibrio cholerae,* and several species of *Salmonella, Shigella,* and anaerobic streptococci. Enteric infections are characterized by diarrhea, abdominal discomfort, nausea and vomiting, and anorexia. A significant loss of fluid and electrolytes may result from severe vomiting and diarrhea. Oral rehydration therapy with clean water and electrolyte solution may be given. Medication for sedation and relief of abdominal cramps may be prescribed. Antibiotics may be recommended, depending on the specific microorganism causing the infection.

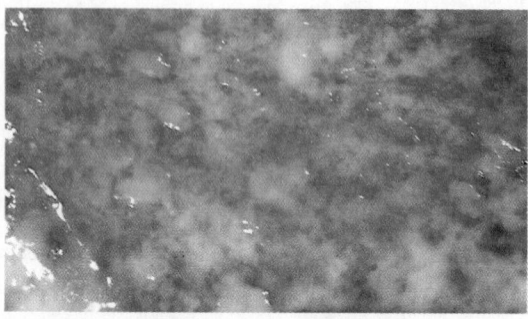

**Colonic mucosa in enteric infection**
*(Cotran, Kumar, and Collins, 1999)*

**entericoid fever** /enter′ikoid/ [Gk, *enteron + eidos,* form], a typhoidlike febrile disease characterized by intestinal inflammation and dysfunction. See also **enteric infection, typhoid fever.**

**enteric orphan virus** [Gk, *enteron,* bowel, *orphanos,* bereft; L, *virus,* poison], a GI disease virus that has been identified and isolated but was not originally associated with the disease. See also **ECHO virus.**

**enteritis** /en′tərī′tis/, inflammation of the mucosal lining of the small intestine, resulting from a variety of causes—bacterial, viral, functional, and inflammatory. Involvement of both small and large intestines is called **enterocolitis.** Compare **gastroenteritis.**

**entero-, enter-,** combining form meaning 'intestines': *enteric, enterobiliary, enteroptosis.*

**Enterobacter cloacae** /en′tirōbak′tər klō·ā′kē, klō·ā′sē/ [Gk, *enteron + bakterion,* small staff; L, *cloaca,* sewer], a common species of bacteria found in human and animal feces, dairy products, sewage, soil, and water. It is rarely the cause of disease. Also called *Aerobacter aerogenes, Enterobacter aerogenes.*

**Fungal enteritis** *(Damjanov, 2000)*

**Enterobacteriaceae** /en′tirōbaktir′ē·ā′si·ē/ [Gk, *enteron + bakterion,* small staff], a family of aerobic and anaerobic bacteria that includes both normal and pathogenic enteric microorganisms. Among the significant genera of the family are *Escherichia, Klebsiella, Proteus,* and *Salmonella.*

**enterobacterial** /-baktir′ē·əl/ [Gk, *enteron + bakterion,* small staff], pertaining to a species of bacteria found in the digestive tract.

**enterobiasis** /en′tirōbī′əsis/ [Gk, *enteron + bios,* life, *osis,* condition], a parasitic infestation with *Enterobius vermicularis,* the common pinworm. The worms infect the large intestine, and the females deposit eggs in the perianal area, causing pruritus and disturbed sleep. Reinfection commonly results from transfer of eggs to the mouth by contaminated fingers. Airborne transmission is possible because eggs remain viable for 2 weeks in contaminated clothing, bedding, or objects. Diagnosing enterobiasis requires the sticky side of an adhesive cellophane tape swab to be pressed against the perianal skin and examined for eggs under a microscope. Therapy for the whole family may be necessary. Effective anthelmintics include pyrantel pamoate, mebendazole, albendazole, and thiabendazole. Personal hygiene, including handwashing, is the best preventive measure. There appears to be little benefit derived from disinfection procedures for the home. Also called **oxyuriasis.**

**Enterobius vermicularis** /en′tərō′bē·əs/ [Gk, *enteron + bios,* life; L, *vermiculus,* small worm], a common parasitic nematode that resembles a white thread between 0.5 and 1 cm long. Also called **pinworm, seatworm, threadworm.**

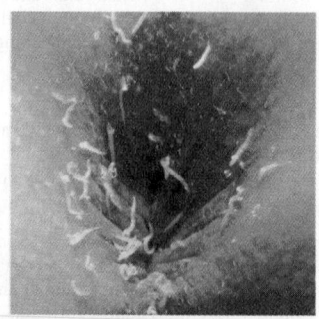

**Enterobiasis** *(Weber, 1993)*

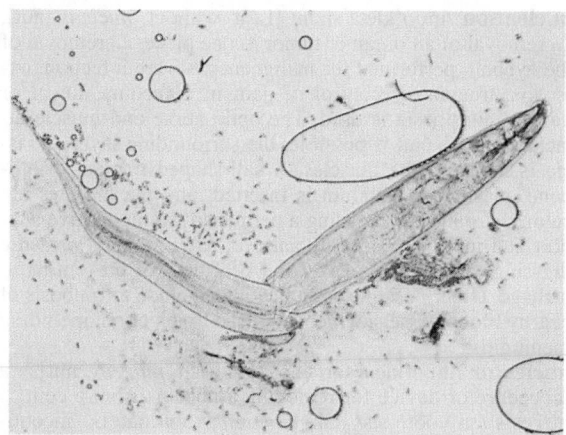

***Enterobius vermicularis*: mature worm surrounded by eggs**
*(Zitelli and Davis, 1997)*

**enterocele** /en′tirōsēl′/,   1. a hernia of the intestine. 2. posterior vaginal hernia. Compare **enterocoele**.

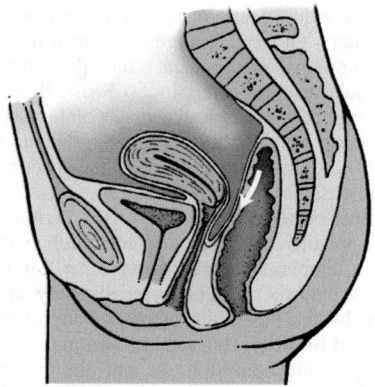

**Enterocele** *(Monahan and Neighbors, 1998)*

**enterochromaffin cell.**   See **argentaffin cell**.

**enteroclysis** /en′tərok′lisis/,   a radiographic procedure in which a contrast medium is injected into the duodenum to permit examination of the small intestine. To improve visualization of the bowel wall, air is sometimes injected into the small intestine after the contrast medium has reached the cecum.

**enterococcus** /-kokəs/, *pl.* **enterococci** /-kok′sī, -kôk′ē/ [Gk, *enteron* + *kokkos,* berry],   any *Streptococcus* that inhabits the intestinal tract.

**enterocoele,**   the abdominal cavity. Compare **enterocele**.

**enterocolitis** /-kōlī′tis/ [Gk, *enteron* + *kolon,* bowel, *itis*],   an inflammation involving both the large and small intestines. Also called **coloenteritis**.

**enterodynia** /-din′ē·ə/,   intestinal pain.

**enteroenterostomy** /en′tərō·en′təros′təmē/,   the surgical creation of an artificial connection between two segments of the intestine.

**enterogastritis.**   See **gastroenteritis**.

**enteroglucagon** /-gloo′kəgon/,   any of a group of glucagon-like hyperglycemic peptides, released by cells in the mucosa in the upper intestine in response to the ingestion of carbohydrates and fat and stimulating intestinal epithelial cell preparation and renewal. Enteroglucagon is similar to pancreatic glucagon but immunologically different. Glicentin is the principal enteroglucagon.

**enterohemorrhagic *Escherichia coli*** /-hem′ôraj′ik/,   a strain of *E. coli* that causes hemorrhage in the intestines. The organism produces a toxin that damages bowel tissue, causing intestinal ischemia and colonic necrosis. Spread by contaminated beef, the infection can be serious although there may be no fever. Treatment consists of antibiotics and maintenance of fluid and electrolyte balance.

**enterohepatic circulation** /en′tərōhəpat′ik/,   a route by which part of the bile produced by the liver enters the intestine, is resorbed by the liver, and then is recycled into the intestine. The remainder of the bile is excreted in feces.

**enterokinase** /en′tirōkī′nās/ [Gk, *enteron* + *kinesis,* movement, *ase,* enzyme],   an intestinal juice enzyme that activates the proteolytic enzymes in pancreatic juice as they enter the duodenum.

**enterolith** /en′tərōlith′/ [Gk, *enteron* + *lithos,* stone],   a stone consisting of ingested material found within the intestine. See also **calculus**.

**enterolithiasis** /en′tərōlithī′əsis/,   the presence of enteroliths in the intestine.

**enteron.**   See **digestive tract, small intestine**.

**enteropathic *Escherichia coli*** /-path′əjen′ik/,   a strain of *E. coli* that is the cause of epidemic infantile diarrhea. See also **epidemic diarrhea in newborn**.

**enteropathy** /en′tərop′əthē/,   a disease or other disorder of the intestines.

**enterostomal therapist** /-stō′məl/,   a registered nurse who is qualified by education in an accredited program in enterostomal therapy to provide care for persons with stomas, draining wounds, fistulae, incontinence, and actual or potential alterations in tissue integrity. Also called **endostomy therapist**. See **WOCN**.

**enterostomy** /en′təros′təmē/ [Gk, *enteron* + *stoma,* mouth],   a surgical procedure that produces an artificial anus or fistula in the intestine by incision through the abdominal wall. Compare **colostomy**.

**enterotoxigenic** /-tok′sijen′ik/,   producing an enterotoxin.

**enterotoxigenic *Escherichia coli*,**   a strain of *E. coli* that is a frequent cause of diarrhea in travelers. See also **traveler's diarrhea**.

**enterotoxin** /-tok′sin/,   a toxic substance that causes an adverse reaction by cells of the intestinal mucosa. Most enterotoxins are produced by certain species of bacteria, such as *Staphylococcus*.

**enterovirus** /-vī′rəs/ [Gk, *enteron* + L, *virus,* poison],   a virus that multiplies primarily in the intestinal tract. Kinds of enteroviruses are **coxsackievirus, ECHO virus,** and **poliovirus. —enteroviral,** *adj.*

**enthesitis** /en′thəsī′tis/,   an inflammation of the insertion of a muscle with a strong tendency toward fibrosis and calcification. It is usually only painful when the involved muscle is activated.

**enthesopathy** /en′thəsop′əthē/,   an arthritic condition affecting tendons and ligaments rather than joint membranes.

**ento-.**   See **endo-**.

**entoderm, entodermal.**   See **endodermal**.

**entopic** /entop′ik/,   occurring in the proper place. Compare **ectopic**.

**entoptic phenomena,** sensations perceived for mechanical reasons within the eye, such as floaters or flashes caused by retinal changes.

**Entozyme,** trademark for a GI fixed-combination drug containing bile salts and the digestive enzymes pancreatin and pepsin.

**entrainment** /entrān'mənt/ [Fr, *entrainer*, to drag along], a phenomenon observed in the microanalysis of sound films in which the speaker moves several parts of the body and the listener responds by moving in ways that are coordinated with the rhythm of the sounds. Infants have been observed to move in time to the rhythms of adult speech but not to random noises or disconnected words or vowels. Entrainment is thought to be an essential factor in the process of maternal-infant bonding.

**entrance block** [Fr, *entrer*, to enter; AS, *blok*], a theoretic zone that surrounds a pacemaker focus and protects it from discharge by an extraneous impulse that might trigger ectopic ventricular contractions.

**entrance exposure,** the skin dose of radiation. It may be expressed in milliroentgens.

**entrapment neuropathy** /entrap'mənt/ [OFr, *entraper*, to catch in a trap; Gk, *neuron*, nerve, *pathos*, disease], injury or inflammation of single nerves caused by pressure from surrounding tissues, such as ligaments and fascia.

**entropion** /entrō'pē·on/ [Gk, *en* + *tropos*, a turning], turning inward or turning toward, usually a condition in which the eyelid turns inward toward the eye. In either the upper or lower eyelid **cicatricial entropion** can result from scar tissue formation. **Spastic entropion** results from an inflammation or other factor that affects tissue tone. An inflammation of the eyelid may be the result of an infectious disease or irritation from an inverted eyelash. Compare **ectropion.** See also **blepharitis.**

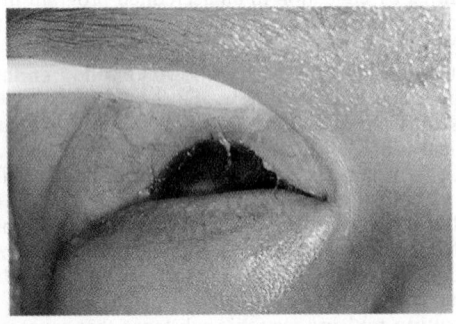

**Entropion** *(Zitelli and Davis, 1997)*

**entropy** /en'trəpē/ [Gk, *en* + *tropos*, a turning], the tendency of a system to change from a state of order to a state of disorder, expressed in physics as a measure of the part of the energy in a thermodynamic system that is not available to perform work. According to the principles of evolution, living organisms tend to go from a state of disorder to a state of order in their development and thus appear to reverse entropy. However, maintaining a living system requires the expenditure of energy, leaving less energy available for work, with the result that the entropy of the system and its surroundings increases.

**ENT specialist,** a physician who specializes in the treatment of the ear, nose, and throat. See also **otolaryngologist.**

**enucleation** /inoo'klē·ā'shən/ [L, *e*, without, *nucleus*, nut], **1.** removal of an organ or tumor in one piece. **2.** removal of the eyeball, performed for malignancy, severe infection, extensive trauma, or control of pain in glaucoma. Local or general anesthesia is used. The optic nerve and muscle attachments are cut; if possible, the surrounding layer of fascia is left with the muscles. A ball-shaped implant of silicone, plastic, or tantalum is inserted, and the muscles are sutured around it, providing a permanent stump to give support and motion to an artificial eye. After surgery, pressure dressings are kept in place for 1 or 2 days to prevent hemorrhage. Other possible complications include thrombosis of nearby blood vessels, which may lead to infection, including meningitis.

**enucleator** /inoo'klē·ā'tər/ [L, *e*, without, *nucleus*, nut], a procedure or device for removing a nucleus from a cell.

**enuresis** /en'yŏōrē'sis/ [Gk, *enourein*, to urinate], incontinence of urine, especially nocturnal bed-wetting.

**envenomation** /enven'əmā'shən/, the injection of snake, arachnid, or insect venom into the body.

**environment** [Gk, *en*, in; L, *viron*, circle], all of the many factors, as physical and psychologic, that influence or affect the life and survival of a person. See also **biome, climate.**

**environmental carcinogen** /envī'rənmen'təl/, any of the natural or synthetic substances that can cause cancer. Such agents may be divided into chemical agents, physical agents, hormones, and viruses. Some environmental carcinogens are arsenic, asbestos, uranium, vinyl chloride, ionizing radiation, ultraviolet rays, x-rays, and coal tar derivatives. Carcinogenic effects of chemicals may be delayed as long as 30 years. Other carcinogens produce more immediate effects. Some studies indicate that the carcinogens in cigarette smoke are involved in 80% of all lung cancer. Most carcinogens are unreactive or secondary carcinogens but are converted to primary carcinogens in the body. Numerous factors, such as heredity, affect the susceptibilities of different individuals to cancer-causing agents.

**environmental control units (ECUs),** various apparatus for disabled persons that control devices such as lamps, television, radio, telephone, and alarm systems. Similar to television remote control devices, typically they are switches manipulated by the lips, chin, or other body movements.

**environmental health,** the total of various aspects of substances, forces, and conditions in and about a community that affect the health and well-being of the population.

**environmental health technician,** a health care professional who performs technical assistance under professional supervision in monitoring environmental health hazards such as radioactive contamination, air and water pollution, and disposal of chemical wastes of industry.

**environmental interpretation syndrome, impaired,** a nursing diagnosis accepted by the Eleventh National Conference on the Classification of Nursing Diagnoses. It is defined as a consistent lack of orientation to person, place, time, or circumstances over more than 3 to 6 months, necessitating a protective environment.

■ DEFINING CHARACTERISTICS: The major defining characteristics include consistent disorientation in known or unknown environments and chronic confusional states. The minor defining characteristics include loss of occupation or social functioning resulting from memory decline; inability to follow simple directions or instructions; inability to reason; inability to concentrate; and slowness in responding to questions.

■ RELATED FACTORS: The related factors include dementia (Alzheimer's disease, multi-infarct dementia, Pick's disease, acquired immunodeficiency syndrome dementia); Parkinson's disease; Huntington's disease; depression; and alcoholism. See also **nursing diagnosis.**

**environmental management,** a nursing intervention from the Nursing Interventions Classification (NIC) defined as manipulation of the patient's surroundings for therapeutic benefit. See also **Nursing Interventions Classification.**

**environmental management: attachment process,** a nursing intervention from the Nursing Interventions Classification (NIC) defined as manipulation of the patient's surroundings to facilitate the development of the parent-infant relationship. See also **Nursing Interventions Classification.**

**environmental management: comfort,** a nursing intervention from the Nursing Interventions Classification (NIC) defined as manipulation of the patient's surroundings for promotion of optimal comfort. See also **Nursing Interventions Classification.**

**environmental management: community,** a nursing intervention from the Nursing Interventions Classification (NIC) defined as monitoring and influencing of the physical, social, cultural, economic, and political conditions that affect the health of groups and communities. See also **Nursing Interventions Classification.**

**environmental management: home preparation,** a nursing intervention from the Nursing Interventions Classification (NIC) defined as preparing the home for safe and effective delivery of care. See also **Nursing Interventions Classification.**

**environmental management: safety,** a nursing intervention from the Nursing Interventions Classification (NIC) defined as monitoring and manipulation of the physical environment to promote safety. See also **Nursing Interventions Classification.**

**environmental management: violence prevention,** a nursing intervention from the Nursing Interventions Classification (NIC) defined as monitoring and manipulation of the physical environment to decrease the potential for violent behavior directed toward self, others, or environment. See also **Nursing Interventions Classification.**

**environmental management: worker safety,** a nursing intervention from the Nursing Interventions Classification (NIC) defined as monitoring and manipulation of the worksite environment to promote safety and health of workers. See also **Nursing Interventions Classification.**

**environmental risk protection,** a nursing intervention from the Nursing Interventions Classification (NIC) defined as preventing and detecting disease and injury in populations at risk from environmental hazards. See also **Nursing Interventions Classification.**

**environmental services,** a functional unit of a health care facility. It has the responsibility for laundry, liquid and solid waste control, safe disposal of materials contaminated by radiation or pathogenic organisms, and general maintenance of safety and housekeeping.

**Enzactin,** trademark for a topical antifungal (triacetin).

**enzygotic twins.** See **monozygotic twins.**

**enzymatic debridement** /en'zīmat'ik/, the use of nonirritating, nontoxic vegetable enzymes to remove dead tissue from a wound without destroying normal tissue.

**enzymatic detergent asthma,** an allergic reaction experienced by persons who have become sensitized to alcalase, an enzyme contained in some laundry detergents. Alcalase is produced by the bacterium *Bacillus subtilis,* and persons sensitive to the enzyme are also usually allergic to the bacterium. Asthmatic symptoms may progress in severe cases to an allergic alveolitis. The most serious cases were originally among workers in plants that manufacture laundry detergents.

**enzyme** /en'zīm/ [Gk, *en,* in, *zyme,* ferment], a complex produced by living cells that catalyzes chemical reactions in organic matter. Most enzymes are produced in tiny quantities and catalyze reactions that take place within the cells. Digestive enzymes, however, are produced in relatively large quantities and act outside the cells in the lumen of the digestive tube. The substance that is acted on by an enzyme is called a **substrate.**

**Enzyme Commission (EC),** a body, formed in 1956 by the International Union of Biochemistry, that has standardized the nomenclature for enzymes.

**enzyme deficiency anemia,** a deficiency of enzymes in the pathways that metabolize glucose and adenosine triphosphate (Embden-Meyerhof and pentose phosphate shunt pathways), which frequently leads to premature red blood cell destruction.

**enzyme induction** [Gk, *en* + *zyme,* ferment; L, *inducere,* to lead in], the increase in the rate of a specific enzyme synthesis from basal to maximum level caused by the presence of a substrate or substrate analog that acts as an inducer. The inducer may be a substance that inactivates a repressor chemical in the cell.

**enzyme-linked immunosorbent assay (ELISA),** a laboratory technique for detecting specific antigens or antibodies, using enzyme-labeled immunoreactants and a solid-phase binding support, such as a test tube. A number of different enzymes can be used, including carbonic anhydrase, glucose oxidase, and alkaline phosphatase. Labeling is done by covalently binding the enzyme to the test substance through an enzyme-protein coupling agent such as glutaraldehyde. Products of the reaction may be detected by fluorometry or photometry. ELISA is nearly as sensitive as radioimmunoassay and more sensitive than complement fixation, agglutination, and other techniques. It is commonly used in the diagnosis of human immunodeficiency virus infections.

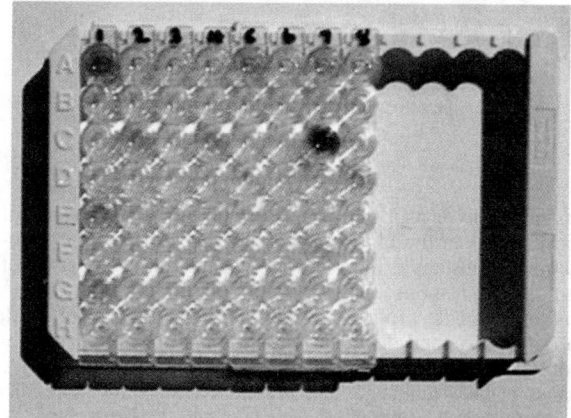

**Enzyme-linked immunosorbent assay**
*(Hart and Broadhead, 1992)*

**enzymology** /en'zīmol'əjē/, the study of enzymes and their actions.

**enzymolysis** /en'zīmol'isis/ [Gk, *en,* in, *zyme,* ferment, *lysis,* loosening], destruction or change of a substance caused by means of enzymatic action.

**enzymopenia** /en'zīmōpē'nē·ə/, the deficiency of an enzyme.

**enzymuria** /en'zīmŏŏr'ē·ə/, the presence of enzymes in urine.

**EOA,** abbreviation for **esophageal obturator airway.**

**EOM,** abbreviation for **extraocular muscle.**

**eosin** /ē'əsin/, a group of red acidic xanthine dyes often used in combination with a blue-purple basic dye such as hematoxylin to stain tissue slides in the laboratory.

**eosin-,** combining form meaning 'a rose, red, or dawn color': *eosinophil, eosinopenia, eosinophilic.*

**eosinoblast.** See **myeloblast.**

**eosinopenia** /ē'əsinəpē'nē·ə/, an abnormally low number of eosinophil leukocytes in the blood.

**eosinophil** /ē'əsin'əfil/ [Gk, *eos,* dawn, *philein,* to love], a granulocytic bilobed leukocyte somewhat larger than a neutrophil. It is characterized by large numbers of coarse refractile cytoplasmic granules that stain with the acid dye eosin. Eosinophils constitute 1% to 3% of the white blood cells of the body. They increase in number with allergy and some parasitic conditions and decrease with steroid administration. Compare **basophil, neutrophil. —eosinophilic,** *adj.*

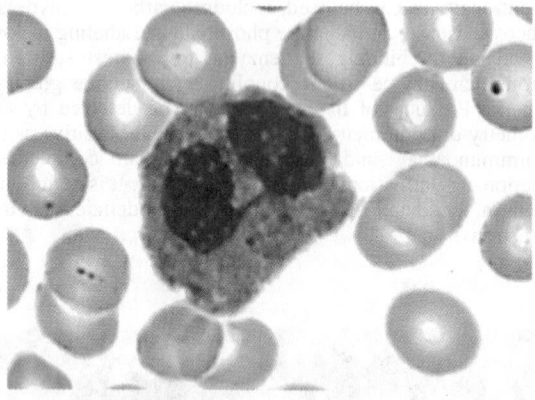

**Eosinophil** *(Carr and Rodak, 1999)*

**eosinophilia** /ē'əsin'ōfil'yə/, an increase in the number of eosinophils in the blood, accompanying inflammatory conditions. Substantial increases are considered a reflection of an allergic response.

**eosinophilia-myalgia syndrome, tryptophan-induced,** a potentially fatal disorder resulting from ingestion of tryptophan. It is characterized by a symptom complex of severe muscle pain, tenosynovitis, muscle edema, and skin rash lasting several weeks.

**eosinophilic** /ē'əsin'əfil'ik/, **1.** the tendency of a cell, tissue, or organism to be readily stained by the dye eosin. **2.** pertaining to an eosinophilic leukocyte.

**eosinophilic adenoma.** See **acidophilic adenoma.**

**eosinophilic cellulitis.** See **Wells' syndrome.**

**eosinophilic enteropathy,** a rare form of food allergy that is characterized by nausea, crampy abdominal pain, diarrhea, urticaria, an elevated eosinophil count in the blood, and eosinophilic infiltrates in the intestine. Diagnosis is made by an elimination diet; symptoms usually disappear when the offending food is removed from the diet.

**eosinophilic fasciitis,** inflammation of fasciae of the limbs, associated with eosinophilia, edema, and swelling; the cause is unknown, but the condition often occurs after strenuous exercise. Also called **Shulman's syndrome.**

**eosinophilic gastroenteritis,** a disorder marked by infiltration of the mucosa of the small intestine by eosinophils, with edema but without vasculitis, and by eosinophilia of the peripheral blood. Symptoms, including abdominal pain, diarrhea, nausea, fever, and malabsorption, depend on the site and extent of the disorder. The stomach is also frequently involved. The disorder is commonly associated with intolerance to specific foods.

**eosinophilic granuloma,** a simple or multiple growth in the bone or lung characterized by numerous eosinophils and histiocytes. Eosinophilic granulomas occur most frequently in children and adolescents.

**eosinophilic leukemia,** a malignant neoplasm of the blood-forming tissues in which eosinophils are the predominant cells. The disease resembles chronic myelocytic leukemia but may have an acute course, even when no blast forms are present in the peripheral blood.

**eosinophilic leukocyte.** See **eosinophil.**

**eosinophilic meningitis,** meningitis with an increase in lymphocytes and a high percentage of eosinophils in the cerebrospinal fluid; it usually results from infection with *Angiostrongylus cantonensis.*

**eosinophilic myeloencephalitis,** a complex of neurologic symptoms produced by invasion of the central nervous system by *Gnathostoma spinigerum,* including severe nerve root pain, followed by paralysis of extremities and sudden sensorial impairment, accompanied by increased number of eosinophils in the cerebrospinal fluid, which is often bloody or yellowish.

**eosinophilic pneumonia,** inflammation of the lungs, characterized by infiltration of the alveoli with eosinophils and large mononuclear cells, pulmonary edema, fever, night sweats, cough, dyspnea, and weight loss. The disease may be caused by a hypersensitivity reaction to fungi spores; plant fibers; wood dust; bird droppings' porcine, bovine, or piscine proteins; *Bacillus subtilis* enzyme in detergents; or certain drugs. Treatment consists of removal of the offending allergen and symptomatic and supportive therapy. Compare **bronchopneumonia.** See also **asthmatic eosinophilia.**

**-eous,** suffix meaning 'like' or 'composed of' or 'relating to' something specified: *cutaneous, osseous.*

**EP,** abbreviation for **evoked potential.**

**ep-.** See **epi-.**

**EPA,** abbreviation for *Environmental Protection Agency.*

**ependyma** /ipen'dimə/ [Gk, an upper garment], a layer of ciliated epithelial membrane that lines the central canal of the spinal cord and the ventricles of the brain. —**ependymal** /ipen'diməl/, *adj.*

**ependymal glioma,** a large vascular fairly solid tumor in the fourth ventricle, composed of malignant glial cells.

**ependymitis** /ipen'dimī'tis/, an inflammation of the ependymal tissue.

**ependymoblastoma** /ipen'dimōblastō'mə/, a malignant neoplasm composed of primitive cells of the ependyma. Also called **malignant ependymoma.**

**ependymoma** /ipen'dimō'mə/ [Gk, *ependyma,* an upper garment, *oma,* tumor], a neoplasm composed of differentiated cells of the ependyma. The tumor, which is usually a benign pale, firm, encapsulated, somewhat nodular mass, commonly arises from the roof of the fourth ventricle and may extend to the spinal cord. Primary lesions may also develop in the spinal cord. Also called **ependymocytoma.**

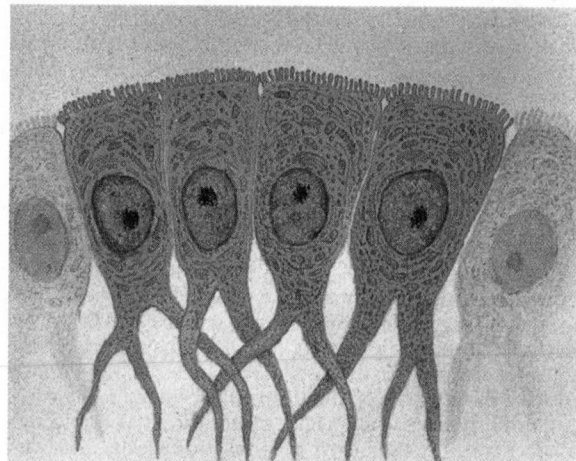

**Ependyma cells** *(Chipps, Clanin, and Campbell, 1992)*

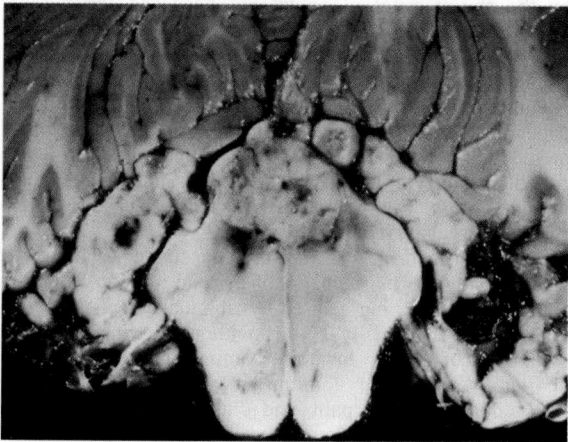

**Ependymoma** *(Cotran, Kumar, and Collins, 1999)*

**ephapse** /ef'aps/ [Gk, *ephasis,* a touching], a point of lateral contact between nerve fibers across which impulses may be transmitted directly through the cell membranes rather than across a synapse. Compare **synapse.** —**ephaptic,** *adj.*

**ephaptic transmission** /ifap'tik/, the passage of a neural impulse from one nerve fiber, axon, or dendrite to another through the membranes. The mechanism may be a factor in epileptic seizures. Compare **synaptic transmission.**

**ephebiatrics** /ēfeb'ē·at'riks/ [Gk, *ephebos,* puberty, *iatros,* physician], a branch of medicine that specializes in the health of adolescents.

**ephedra,** an evergreen herb found throughout the world. Also called *ma huang.*
- USES: This herb is used for seasonal and chronic asthma, nasal congestion, and cough.
- CONTRAINDICATIONS: Ephedra is contraindicated in those with known hypersensitivity to sympathomimetics, women who are pregnant or lactating, children less than 12 years of age, and people with narrow-angle glaucoma, seizure disorders, hyperthyroidism, diabetes mellitus, prostatic hypertro-

phy, arrhythmias, heart block, hypertension, psychosis, tachycardia, and angina pectoris.

**ephedrine** /ef'ədrēn/, an adrenergic bronchodilator.
- INDICATIONS: It is prescribed in the treatment of asthma and bronchitis and is used topically as a nasal decongestant.
- CONTRAINDICATIONS: Concomitant administration of monoamine oxidase inhibitors, hypertension, cardiac artery disease, cardiac arrhythmia, or known hypersensitivity to this drug prohibits its use.
- ADVERSE EFFECTS: Among the more serious adverse reactions are nervousness, insomnia, anorexia, and increased blood pressure.

**ephemeral** /ifem'ərəl/ [Gk, *epi,* above, *hemera,* day], pertaining to a short-lived condition, such as a fever.

**ephemeral fever,** any febrile condition lasting only 24 to 48 hours that is uncomplicated and of unknown origin.

**epi-, ep-,** prefix meaning 'on, upon': *epicanthus, epicostal, epidural.*

**epiblast** /ep'iblast'/ [Gk, *epi,* upon, *blastos,* germ], the primordial outer layer of the blastocyst or blastula, before differentiation of the germ layers, that gives rise to the ectoderm and contains cells capable of forming the endoderm and mesoderm. See also **ectoderm.** —**epiblastic,** *adj.*

**epicanthus** /ep'ikan'thəs/ [Gk, *epi* + *kanthos,* lip of a vessel], a vertical fold of skin over the angle of the inner canthus of the eye. It may be slight or marked, covering the canthus and the caruncle. It is a hereditary trait in Asian people and is of no clinical significance. Some infants with Down syndrome have marked epicanthal folds. Also called **epicanthal fold, epicanthic fold.** —**epicanthal, epicanthic,** *adj.*

**epicardia** /-kär'dē·ə/ [Gk, *epi,* above, *kardia,* heart], the part of the esophagus that lies between the cardiac orifice of the stomach and the esophageal opening of the diaphragm.

**epicardial.** See **epicardium.**

**epicardial pacing.** See **pacing.**

**epicardium** /ep'ikär'dē·əm/ [Gk, *epi* + *kardia,* heart], the outermost of the three layers of tissue that form the heart wall. It is composed of a single sheet of squamous epithelial cells overlying delicate connective tissue. The epicardium is the visceral portion of the serous pericardium and folds back on itself to form the parietal portion of the serous pericardium. Compare **myocardium.** See also **pericardium.**—**epicardial,** *adj.*

**epicondylar.** See **epicondyle.**

**epicondylar fracture** /-kon'dilər/, any fracture that involves the medial or lateral epicondyle of a specific bone, such as the humerus.

**epicondyle** /ep'ikon'dəl/ [Gk, *epi* + *kondylos,* knuckle], a projection on the surface of a bone above its condyle. —**epicondylar,** *adj.*

**epicondylitis** /ep'ikon'dilī'tis/, a painful and sometimes disabling inflammation of the muscle and surrounding tissues of the elbow, caused by repeated strain on the forearm near the medial or lateral epicondyle of the humerus. The strain may result from violent extension or supination of the wrist against a resisting force, such as may occur in playing tennis or golf, twisting a screwdriver, or carrying a heavy load with the arm extended. Treatment usually includes rest, injection of procaine with or without hydrocortisone, stretching and strengthening of the muscle, and, in some cases, surgery to release part of the muscle from the epicondyle. See also **golfer's elbow, lateral humeral epicondylitis.**

**epicranial.** See **epicranium.**

**epicranial aponeurosis** /-krā'nē·əl/ [Gk, *epi* + *kranion,* skull, *apo,* away, *neuron,* tendon], a fibrous membrane that covers the cranium between the occipital and frontal muscles of the scalp. Also called **galea aponeurotica.**

**epicranium** /-krā'nē·əm/ [Gk, *epi + kranion,* skull], the complete scalp, including the integument, the muscular sheets, and the aponeuroses. Compare **epicranius. —epicranial,** *adj.*

**epicranius** [Gk, *epi + kranion,* skull], the broad muscular and tendinous layer of tissue covering the top and sides of the skull from the occipital bone to the eyebrows. It consists of broad, thin muscular bellies, connected by an extensive aponeurosis. Innervation of the epicranius by branches of the facial nerves can draw back the scalp, raise the eyebrows, and move the ears. Compare **epicranium.** See also **epicranial aponeurosis, occipitofrontalis, temporoparietalis.**

**epicritic** /-krit'ik/, pertaining to the somatic sensations of fine discriminative touch, vibration, two-point discrimination, stereognosis, and conscious and unconscious proprioception.

**epidemic** /-dem'ik/ [Gk, *epi + demos,* people], **1.** affecting a significantly large number of people at the same time. **2.** a disease that spreads rapidly through a demographic segment of the human population, such as everyone in a given geographic area, a military base, or similar population unit, or everyone of a certain age or sex, such as the children or women of a region. **3.** a disease or event whose incidence is beyond what is expected. Compare **endemic, epizootic, pandemic.**

**epidemic cerebrospinal meningitis.** See **meningococcal meningitis.**

**epidemic diarrhea in newborns** [Gk, *epi,* above, *demos,* the people, *dia,* through, *rhein,* flow; ME, *newe + beren*], any severe gastroenteritis epidemic among a community of newborns, as may occur in a hospital nursery.

**epidemic encephalitis,** any diffuse inflammation of the brain occurring in epidemic form. Two kinds of epidemic encephalitis are **Japanese encephalitis** and **St. Louis encephalitis.** See also **encephalitis.**

**epidemic hemoglobinuria.** See **hemoglobinuria.**

**epidemic hemorrhagic conjunctivitis** [Gk, *epi,* above, *demos,* the people, *haima,* blood, *rhegnynei,* to gush; L, *conjunctivus,* connecting; Gk, *itis,* inflammation], a highly contagious infection, commonly involving an enterovirus, that begins with eye pain accompanied by swollen eyelids and hyperemia of the conjunctiva. It is a self-limiting disorder that has no specific remedy.

**epidemic hemorrhagic fever,** a severe viral infection marked by fever and bleeding. The disorder develops rapidly and is characterized initially by fever and muscle ache, possibly followed by hemorrhage, peripheral vascular collapse, hypovolemic shock, and acute kidney failure. The arbovirus or other pathogen is believed to be transmitted by mosquitoes, ticks, or mites. The pathophysiologic characteristics of the hemorrhagic effect are uncertain, although it is assumed the disease organism causes damage to the lining of the capillaries. Among the various forms of epidemic hemorrhagic fevers are **Argentine hemorrhagic fever, Bolivian hemorrhagic fever, dengue hemorrhagic fever, Lassa fever,** and **yellow fever.** See also specific viral infections.

**epidemic hysteria.** See **major hysteria.**

**epidemic keratoconjunctivitis (EKC)** [Gk, *epi,* above, *demos,* the people, *keras,* horn; L, *conjunctivus;* Gk, *itis,* inflammation], an acute complex of keratitis and conjunctivitis transmitted by an adenovirus. A highly contagious form of keratoconjunctivitis, it often includes lymph node involvement.

**epidemic myalgia,** a disease caused by coxsackie B virus. It is characterized by sudden acute chest or epigastric pain and fever lasting a few days, followed by complete spontaneous recovery. Also called **devil's grip, epidemic myositis, epidemic pleurodynia.**

**epidemic myositis.** See **epidemic myalgia, epidemic pleurodynia.**

**epidemic parotitis.** See **mumps.**

**epidemic pleurodynia,** an infection caused by a coxsackievirus, mainly affecting children. It is characterized by severe intermittent pain in the abdomen or lower chest, fever, headache, sore throat, malaise, and extreme myalgia. The symptoms may continue for weeks or subside after a few days and recur for a period of weeks. Treatment is symptomatic; complete recovery is usual. Also called **Bornholm disease, devil's grip, epidemic myalgia, epidemic myositis.**

**epidemic typhus,** an acute severe rickettsial infection characterized by prolonged high fever, headache, and dark maculopapular rash that covers most of the body. The causative organism, *Rickettsia prowazekii,* is transmitted indirectly as a result of the bite of the human body louse; the pathogen is contained in feces of the louse and enters the body tissues as the bite is scratched. Disease is manifested by the abrupt onset of an intense headache and a fever reaching 40° C (104° F) beginning after an incubation period of 1 week. The rash follows on the fifth day of onset. Complications may include vascular collapse, renal failure, pneumonia, or gangrene. Mortality rate is as high as 40% depending on preexisting clinical conditions. Treatment may include antipyretics and supportive symptomatic care. Also called **classic typhus, European typhus, jail fever, louse-borne typhus.** Compare **murine typhus.** See also **Brill-Zinsser disease, rickettsia, typhus.**

**epidemic vomiting,** an episode of sudden ejection of stomach contents by members of a group of people in close contact. The vomiting, caused by ribonucleic acid Norwalk virus infection, usually begins without previous signs or symptoms of illness and may continue for several hours, ending abruptly. The vomiting may be accompanied by headache, abdominal pain, and diarrhea. The patients are frequently children who are attending the same school.

**epidemiologic.** See **epidemiology.**

**epidemiologist** /-dē'mē·ol'əjist/, a physician or medical scientist who studies the incidence, prevalence, spread, prevention, and control of disease in a community or a specific group of individuals. In a hospital a physician may be assigned as a staff epidemiologist with responsibility for directing infection control programs within the facility.

**epidemiologist nurse,** a registered nurse with special education and experience in the control of infections in the health care facility and community.

**epidemiology** /-dē'mē·ol'əjē/ [Gk, *epi + demos,* people, *logos,* science], the study of the determinants of disease events in populations. —**epidemiologic,** *adj.*

**epiderm-, epidermo-,** combining form meaning 'epidermis': *epidermoid, epidermolysis, epidermolytic.*

**epidermal growth factor (EGF)** /ep'i·dur'məl /, a mitogenic polypeptide produced by many cell types and made in large amounts by some tumors. It promotes growth and differentiation, is essential in embryogenesis, and is also important in wound healing. It has been found to be part of a family of compounds that includes also **transforming growth factor.**

**epidermal nevus** /-dur'məl/ [Gk, *epi + derma,* skin; L, *naevus,* birthmark], a discrete discolored congenital lesion caused by an overgrowth of epidermis. It may be seen in newborns. Also called **epithelial nevus, hard nevus.**

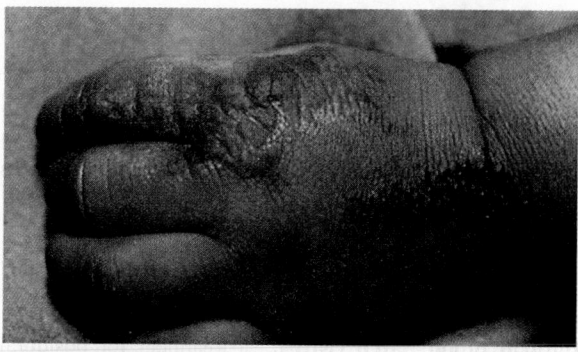

**Epidermal nevus** *(Weston, Lane, and Morrelli, 1996)*

**epidermis** /ep'idur'mis/ [Gk, *epi* + *derma*, skin], the superficial avascular layers of the skin, made up of an outer dead, cornified part and a deeper living, cellular part. Each layer is named for its unique function, texture, or position. The deepest layer is the stratum basale. It anchors the more superficial layers to the underlying tissues, and it provides new cells to replace those lost by abrasion from the outermost layer. The cells of each layer migrate upward as they mature. Above the stratum basale lies the stratum spinosum. As the cells migrate to the next layer, the stratum granulosum, they become flat, lying parallel with the surface of the skin. Over this layer lies a clear, thin band of homogenous tissue called the stratum lucidum. The outermost layer, the stratum corneum, is composed of scaly, squamous plaques of dead cells that contain keratin, a waterproofing protein that hardens over several days. This horny layer is thick over areas of the body subject to abrasion, such as the palms of the hands, and thin over other more protected areas. Altogether these layers are between 0.5 and 1.1 mm in thickness. Also called **cuticle.** See also **skin.** —epidermal, epidermoid, *adj.*

Stratum corneum
Stratum lucidum
Stratum granulosum
Stratum spinosum
Melanocyte
Stratum basale

epidermis

Papillary region
Papillae

ermis

Reticular region

**Epidermis** *(Applegate, 2000)*

**epidermitis** /ep'idurmī'tis/, an inflammation of the epidermis, the outer layer of the skin.

**epidermoid carcinoma** /-dur'moid/ [Gk, *epi* + *derma* +

*eidos,* form], a malignant neoplasm in which the tumor cells tend to differentiate in the manner of epidermal cells, then form horny cells called prickle cells.

**epidermoid cyst,** a common benign cavity lined by keratinizing epithelium and filled with a cheesy material composed of sebum and epithelial debris. The cyst is in the skin, connected to the surface by a pore. Treatment is surgical excision. Also called **sebaceous cyst.** Compare **pilar cyst.**

**epidermolysis bullosa** /ep'idərmol'isis/ [Gk, *epi* + *derma* + *lysis,* loosening], a group of rare hereditary skin diseases in which vesicles and bullae develop, usually at sites of trauma. Severe forms may also involve mucous membranes and may leave scars and contractures on healing. Basal cell and squamous cell carcinomas sometimes develop in the scar tissue.

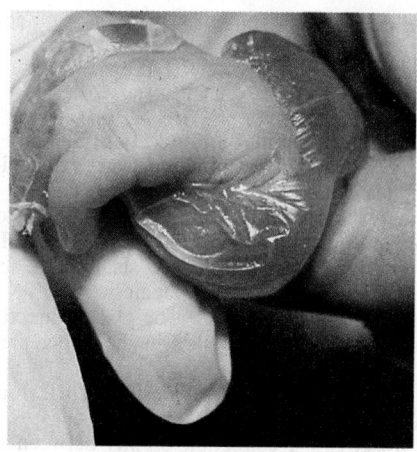

**Junctional epidermolysis bullosa** *(Zitelli and Davis, 1997)*

**epidermolytic hyperkeratosis** [Gk, *epi* + *derma,* skin + *lysis,* loosening; Gk, *hyper,* excess + *keras,* horn + *osis,* condition], an autosomal dominant form of ichthyosis, present at birth, characterized by generalized erythroderma and severe hyperkeratosis with small wartlike scales over the entire body, especially in body folds, and sometimes on the palms and soles; there are also recurrent bullae on the lower limbs. See also **ichthyosis.**

**epidermophytosis** /ep'idur'mōfītō'sis/, a superficial fungus infection of the skin.

**epididym-,** combining form meaning 'epididymis': *epididymectomy, epididymitis.*

**epididymis** /ep'idid'imis/, *pl.* **epididymides** [Gk, *epi* + *didymos,* pair], one of a pair of long tightly coiled ducts that carry sperm from the seminiferous tubules of the testes to the vas deferens.

**epididymitis** /ep'idid'imī'tis/ [Gk, *epi* + *didymos* + *itis,* inflammation], acute or chronic inflammation of the epididymis. It may result from venereal disease, urinary tract infection, prostatitis, prostatectomy, or prolonged use of indwelling catheters. Symptoms include fever and chills, pain in the groin, and tender, swollen epididymides. Treatment includes bed rest, scrotal support, and antibiotics, as appropriate.

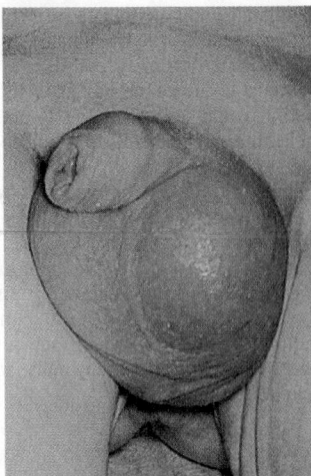

**Epididymitis** (Lloyd-Davies, Gow, and Davies, 1994)

**epididymoorchitis** /ep′idid′imō′ôrkī′tis/ [Gk, *epi +, didymos + orchis*, testis, *itis*], inflammation of the epididymis and of the testis. See also **epididymitis, orchit is.**

**epididymovesiculography** /ep′idid′imōves′ikyəlog′rəfē/, the radiographic examination of the seminal ducts. It is usually performed in cases of sterility, cysts, tumors, abscesses, or inflammation. The contrast medium may be injected through a catheter in the urethra or placed directly in the ducts through a surgical incision in the upper part of the scrotum.

**epidural** /ep′idoŏr′əl/ [Gk, *epi + dura*, hard], outside or above the dura mater.

**epidural abscess,** a collection of pus between the dura mater of the brain and skull, or between the dura mater of the spinal cord and the vertebral canal.

**epidural anesthesia/analgesia,** a type of anesthesia block in which a local anesthetic is injected into the epidural space surrounding the dural membrane, which contains cerebrospinal fluid and spinal nerves. Epidurals are most commonly performed in the lumbar area by an injection of medication through a catheter placed in the space. Analgesia is maintained by either intermitted dosing or a titrated infusion. Close monitoring of vital signs, respirations, pain and extremity is important. Epidurals have a wide application in anesthesia and pain management because of their safety and versatility. Epidural anesthesia or analgesia can be tailored to affect an area of the body from the lower extremities up to the upper abdomen. Epidurals are often used in labor and birth and postoperative pain management. The most common adverse effects include unintentional dural membrane puncture, postdural puncture headache, unintentional and hypotension from sympathetic nerve block and vascular dilation. See also *regional anesthesia.*

**epidural blood patch (EBP),** a treatment for postdural puncture headache in which 15 to 20 mL of a patient's blood is injected into the epidural space at or near the location of a dural puncture. The volume injected displaces cerebrospinal fluid (CSF) from the lumbar CSF space into the area surrounding the brain, often yielding immediate relief. When the blood clots, it seals the dural puncture, prohibiting further leakage of CSF from the subarachnoid space.

**epidural hematoma,** accumulation of blood in the epidural space, caused by damage to and leakage of blood from the middle meningeal artery, producing compression of the dura mater and thus of the brain. Unless evacuated, it may result in herniation through the tentorium, and death.

**epidural hemorrhage,** a hemorrhage that produces a collection of blood outside the dura mater of the brain or spinal cord. It usually results from tearing of the middle meningeal artery and may be rapidly life-threatening. Also called **extradural hemorrhage.**

**epidural space,** the space immediately above and surrounding the dura mater of the brain or spinal cord, beneath the endosteum of the cranium and the spinal column.

**epifascial** /ep′i·fash′ē·əl/ [Gk, *epi + L, fascia*, band], on a fascia.

**epifolliculitis** /ep′ifolik′yəlī′tis/, an inflammation of the hair follicles of the head. See also **folliculitis.**

**epigastric** /-gas′trik/ [Gk, *epi*, above, *gaster*, stomach], pertaining to the epigastrium, the area above the stomach.

**epigastric hernia,** the protrusion of an internal organ through the linea alba.

**epigastric node** [Gk, *epi + gaster*, stomach; L, *nodus*, knot], a node in one of the seven groups of parietal lymph nodes serving the abdomen and the pelvis, comprising about four nodes along the caudal portion of the inferior epigastric vessels. See also **lymph, lymphatic system, lymph node.**

**epigastric pain** [Gk, *epi*, above, *gaster*, stomach; L, *poena*, penalty], pain in the upper middle part of the abdomen.

**epigastric reflex** [Gk, *epi*, above, *gaster*, stomach; L, *reflectere*, to bend back], a contraction of the rectus abdominis muscle that occurs when the skin surface in the upper and middle abdominal region is stimulated. The reflex also may be induced by stimulation of the axillary region of the fifth and sixth dorsal nerves.

**epigastric region,** the part of the abdomen in the upper zone between the right and left hypochondriac regions. Also called **antecardium, epigastrium.** See also **abdominal regions.**

**epigastric sensation,** a weak, sinking feeling of undefined nature that is usually localized in the pit of the stomach but may occur throughout the abdominal region. See also **sensation,** def. 1.

**epigastrium.** See **epigastric region.**

**epigenesis** /ep′ijen′əsis/ [Gk, *epi + genein*, to produce], (in embryology) a theory of development in which the or-

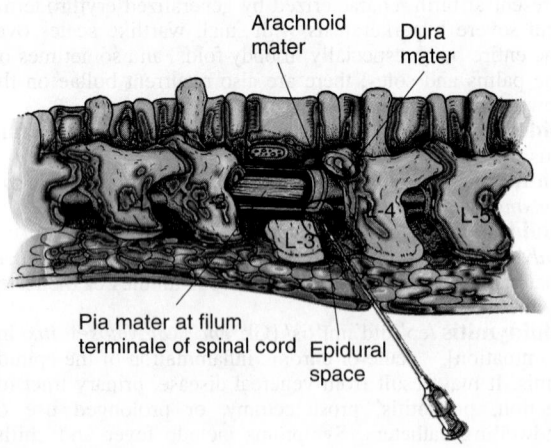

Arachnoid mater  Dura mater

L-3  L-4  L-5

Pia mater at filum terminale of spinal cord  Epidural space

**Epidural anesthesia** (Ignatavicius, Workman, and Mishler, 1999)

ganism grows from a simple to more complex form through the progressive differentiation of an undifferentiated cellular unit. Compare **preformation.** —**epigenesist,** *n.,* **epigenetic,** *adj.*

**epigenetic.** See **epigenesis, extrachromosomal.**

**epiglott-,** combining form meaning 'epiglottis': *epiglottitis.*

**epiglottiditis.** See **epiglottitis.**

**epiglottis** /ep'iglot'is/ [Gk, *epi* + *glossa,* tongue], the thin, leaf-shaped cartilaginous structure that overhangs the larynx like a lid and prevents food from entering the larynx and the trachea while swallowing.

**epiglottitis** /ep'iglotī'tis/ [Gk, *epi* + *glossa,* tongue, *itis,* inflammation], an inflammation of the epiglottis. Acute epiglottitis is a severe form of the condition, which primarily affects children. It is characterized by fever, sore throat, stridor, croupy cough and an erythematous, swollen epiglottis. The patient may become cyanotic and require an emergency tracheostomy to maintain respiration. The causative organism is usually *Haemophilus influenzae,* type B. Antibiotics, rest, oxygen, and supportive care are usually included in treatment. Also called **epiglottiditis.** See also **acute epiglottitis.**

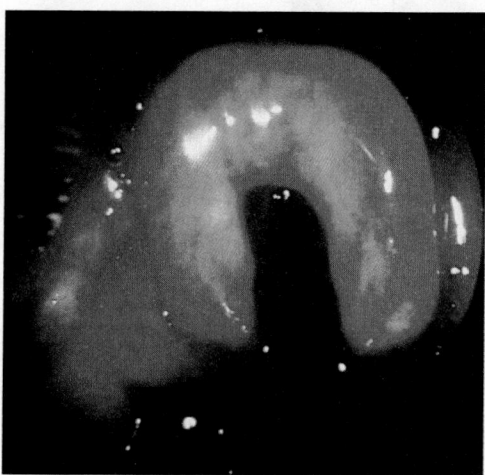

**Acute epiglottitis** *(Zitelli and Davis, 1997)*

**epilating forceps** /ep'ilā'ting/ [L, *e* + *pilus,* without hair], a kind of small spring forceps, used for removing unwanted hair.

**epilation.** See **depilation.**

**epilepsy** /ep'ilep'sē/ [Gk, *epilepsia,* seizure], a group of neurologic disorders characterized by recurrent episodes of convulsive seizures, sensory disturbances, abnormal behavior, loss of consciousness, or all of these. Common to all types of epilepsy is an uncontrolled electrical discharge from the nerve cells of the cerebral cortex. Although most epilepsy is of unknown cause, it is sometimes associated with cerebral trauma, intracranial infection, brain tumor, vascular disturbances, intoxication, or chemical imbalance. See also **absence seizure, focal seizure, tonic-clonic seizure, psychomotor seizure.**

■ OBSERVATIONS: The frequency of attacks may range from many times a day to intervals of several years. In predis-

### Classification of seizures

**Generalized seizures**

Tonic-clonic seizures
Absence seizures
  Simple
  Complex or atypical (with myoclonic jerks, change in postural tone, automatisms)
  Myoclonic seizures
  Infantile spasms
  Tonic seizures
  Atonic seizures

**Partial seizures**

Simple partial (consciousness preserved)
  Motor symptoms
  Somatosensory symptoms
  Special sensory (visual, auditory) symptoms
  Autonomic features
  Psychic symptoms
Complex partial (consciousness impaired)
  Cognitive
  Affective

**Secondarily generalized seizures**

Simple partial evolving to generalized seizure
Complex partial evolving to generalized seizure
Simple partial evolving to complex partial, then to generalized seizures

From Weisberg LA, Garcia C, Strub R: *Essentials of clinical neurology,* ed 3, St Louis, 1996, Mosby.

posed individuals, seizures may occur during sleep or after physical stimulation, such as by a flickering light or sudden loud sound. Emotional disturbances also may be significant triggers. Some seizures are preceded by an aura, but others have no warning symptoms. Most epileptic attacks are brief. They may be localized or general, with or without clonic movements, and are often followed by drowsiness or confusion. Diagnosis is made by observation of the pattern of seizures and abnormalities on an electroencephalogram. Diagnosis is also aided by a system of classification of the criteria that characterize the different types of epileptic seizures. One major category in the classification scheme encompasses the partial seizures, which often begin focally, then spread to other brain areas. A second major category includes the generalized seizures, which usually begin deep in the brain and impair consciousness.

■ INTERVENTIONS: The kind of epilepsy determines the selection of preventive medication. Correctable lesions and metabolic causes are eliminated when possible. During a seizure the patient should be protected from injury without being severely restrained.

■ NURSING CONSIDERATIONS: In addition to protecting the patient from injury, a nurse observing an epileptic seizure should carefully note and accurately describe the sequence of seizure activity. The patient and family must be fully informed and counseled about the disorder; the importance of regularly taking prescribed medication, never discontinuing treatment without professional advice, and using a medical identification tag; the toxic effects of medication, and the maintenance of the most normal life-style possible. Nurses also have a responsibility to help improve the public's attitude toward epilepsy and to correct misunderstanding that limits educational and occupational opportunities for individuals affected by this condition. See also **anticonvulsant, aura, central nervous system stimulant, clonus, ictus, tonic. —epileptic,** *adj., n.*

**epileptic cry** /ep′ilep′tik/, a loud vocalization by a person with epilepsy, often immediately before onset of a seizure.

**epileptic dementia** [Gk, *epilepsia,* seizure; L, *de* + *mens,* mind], a loss of cognitive and intellectual functions that develops in some cases of incompletely controlled epilepsy. Symptoms include slowness and circumstantiality of speech and narrowed attention span.

**epileptic march.** See **jacksonian march.**

**epileptic stupor,** the state of unawareness and unresponsiveness that follows an epileptic seizure.

**epileptic vertigo** [Gk, *epilepsia,* seizure; L, *vertigo,* dizziness], an aura of dizziness that may precede, accompany, or follow an epileptic seizure.

**epileptogenic** /ep′ilep′tōjen′ik/, causing epileptic seizures.

**epiloia.** See **tuberous sclerosis.**

**epimysium** /ep′imiz′ē·əm/ [Gk, *epi* + *mys,* muscle], the outermost fibrous sheath that enfolds a muscle and extends between bundles of muscle fibers, as the perimysium. It is sturdy in some areas but more delicate in others, such as those areas where the muscle moves freely under a strong sheet of fascia. The epimysium may also fuse with fascia that attaches a muscle to a bone.

**epinephrine** /ep′ənef′rin/ [Gk, *epi* + *nephros,* kidney], an endogenous adrenal hormone and synthetic adrenergic agent. It acts as an agonist at alpha-1, beta-1, and beta-2 receptors.

■ INDICATIONS: It is prescribed to treat anaphylaxis, acute bronchial spasm, and nasal congestion and to increase the effectiveness of a local anesthetic.

■ CONTRAINDICATION: Known hypersensitivity to this drug prohibits its use.

■ ADVERSE EFFECTS: Among the most serious adverse reactions are arrhythmias, increases in blood pressure, rebound congestion (when it is used as a decongestant), tachycardia, and nervousness.

**epinephryl borate** /-nef′ril/, a sympathomimetic.

■ INDICATIONS: It is prescribed in the treatment of primary open-angle glaucoma.

■ CONTRAINDICATIONS: Narrow-angle glaucoma, aphakia, or known hypersensitivity to this drug prohibits its use. It should not be given before peripheral iridectomy and should not be administered to eyes that are capable of angle closure.

■ ADVERSE EFFECTS: Among the more serious adverse reactions are tachycardia, hypertension, headache, blurred vision, and allergic reaction.

**epiotic** /ep′ē·ot′ik/, pertaining to the portion of the temporal bone that is the ossification center for the mastoid; above the ear.

**epipastic** /ep′ipas′tik/ [Gk, *epipassein,* to sprinkle about], dusting powder.

**epiphora.** See **tearing.**

**epiphyseal** /ep′fiz′ē·əl, ipif′əsē′əl/ [Gk, *epi,* above, *phyein,* to grow], pertaining to or resembling the epiphysis. Also spelled **epiphysial.**

**epiphyseal fracture** [Gk, *epi* + *phyein,* to grow, *fractura,* break], a fracture involving the epiphyseal plate of a long bone, which causes separation or fragmentation of the plate. Also called **Salter fracture.**

**epiphyseal plate** [Gk, *epi,* above, *phyein,* to grow, *platys,* flat], a thin layer of cartilage between the epiphysis, a secondary bone-forming center, and the bone shaft. The new bone forms along the plate.

**epiphysial.** See **epiphyseal.**

**epiphysis** /epif′isis/, *pl.* **epiphyses** [Gk, *epi* + *phyein,* to grow], the enlarged proximal and distal ends of a long bone. See also **epiphyseal plate. —epiphysial** /ipif′əsē′əl/, *adj.*

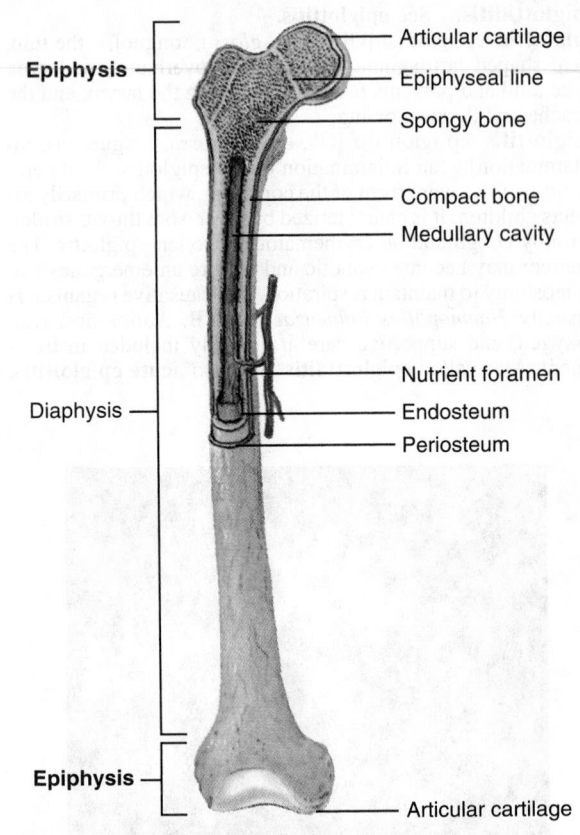

**Epiphysis** *(Applegate, 2000)*

**epiphysis cerebri.** See **pineal body.**

**epiphysitis** /ipif′isī′tis/, an inflammation of the epiphysis, usually of a long bone, such as the femur or humerus. The disorder mainly affects children.

**epipial** /ep′i·pi′əl/ [Gk, *epi* + L, *pia,* soft or tender], situated on the pia mater.

**epiploic** /ep′iplō′ik/, pertaining to the omentum.

**epiploic foramen** [Gk, *epiploon,* caul; L, *foramen,* a hole], an opening between the greater and lesser omentum. It is lined with peritoneum and is approximately 3 cm in diameter.

**epipygus.** See **pygomelus.**

**epirubicin,** an antibiotic antineoplastic.

■ INDICATIONS: This drug is used as an adjuvant therapy to treat breast cancer with axillary node involvement following resection.

■ CONTRAINDICATIONS: Factors that prohibit the use of this drug include severe hepatic disease, baseline neutrophil count less than 1500 cells/mm$^3$, severe myocardial insufficiency, recent myocardial infarction, pregnancy, lactation, systemic infections, and known hypersensitivity to this drug, anthracyclines, or anthracenediones.

■ ADVERSE EFFECTS: Life-threatening effects of this drug are thrombocytopenia, leukopenia, anemia, neutropenia, secondary acute myelocytic leukemia, sinus tachycardia, premature ventricular contractions, bradycardia, and extrasystoles. Other serious adverse effects include increased blood pressure and chest pain. Common side effects include nausea, vomiting, anorexia, mucositis, diarrhea, amenorrhea, hot flashes, hyperuricemia, rash, necrosis at the injection site, reversible alopecia, infection, febrile neutropenia, lethargy, fever, and conjunctivitis.

**episcleritis** /ep'isklərī'tis/, inflammation of the outermost layers of the sclera and the tissues overlying its posterior parts.

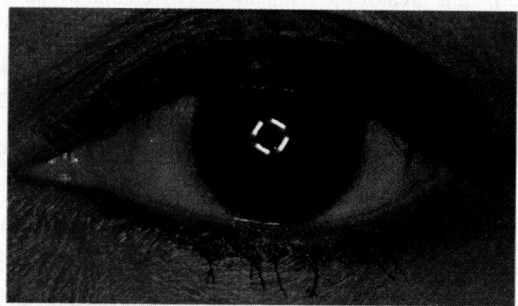

**Episcleritis** *(Lemmi and Lemmi, 2000)*

**episcope,** a skin surface microscope that uses the technology of epiluminescence microscopy (ELM) (the application of oil to produce translucence of the epidermis on a skin lesion). The episcope is placed gently over the lesion to observe its general appearance, surface, pigment pattern, border, and depigmentation.

**episi-,** combining form meaning 'vulva': *episioplast, episiotomy.*

**episiotomy** /epē'zē·ot'əmē/ [Gk, *episeion,* pubic region, *temnein,* to cut], a surgical procedure in which an incision is made in a woman's perineum to enlarge her vaginal opening for delivery. It is performed most often electively to prevent tearing of the perineum, to hasten or facilitate birth of the baby, or to prevent stretching of perineal muscles and connective tissue thought to predispose to subsequent abnormalities of pelvic outlet relaxation, as cystocele, rectocele, and uterine prolapse; its prophylactic efficacy is debated. It is usually required for a forceps delivery. The incision into the vaginal and perineal tissue is closed with absorbable sutures that need not be removed. Deep incisions require closure in two or more layers. Immediate complications include hemorrhage and extension of the incision along the vaginal sulcus or into the anal sphincter or rectum. Delayed complications include hematoma and abscess. Application of cold packs to the perineum for several hours immediately after delivery minimizes swelling. Later alternating applications of heat and cold and warm sitz baths reduce discomfort, but sitz baths longer than 10 minutes soften tissue and prolong healing time. A mediolateral episiotomy is an episiotomy cut at an angle of approximately 45 degrees with the midline. Although it affords wide exposure for delivery, it is painful after delivery and is prone to hematoma and infection. A median or midline episiotomy is an incision in the perineum in the midline; although less painful after delivery, it affords

less exposure for delivery and may extend into or through the anal sphincter and into the rectum.

**episode** /ep'isōd/ [Gk, *episodion,* coming in besides], an incident or event that stands out from the continuity of everyday life, such as an episode of illness or a traumatic event in the course of a child's development. —**episodic,** *adj.*

**episode of hospital care,** the services provided by a hospital in the continuous course of care of a patient with a health condition. It may cover a sequence from emergency through inpatient to outpatient services.

**episodic.** See **episode.**

**episodic care** /-sod'ik/, a pattern of medical and nursing care in which services are provided to a person for a particular problem, without an ongoing relationship being established between the person and health care professionals. Emergency departments provide episodic care.

**episome** /ep'isōm/ [Gk, *epi* + *soma,* body], an extrachromosomal replicating unit that exists autonomously or functions with a chromosome. See also **colicinogen, conjugon, F factor, plasmid, R factor.**

**epispadias** /ep'ispā'dē·əs/ [Gk, *epi* + *spadon,* a rent], a congenital defect in which the urethra opens on the dorsum of the penis proximal to the glans. Other pelvic abnormalities may be present. Treatment focuses on correcting or managing urinary incontinence, which occurs because the urinary sphincters are defective, and on permitting sexual function. The corresponding defect in women, in which the urethra opens by the separation of the labia minora and a fissure of the clitoris, is quite rare.

**epistasis** /epis'təsis/ [Gk, a standing], an interaction between genes at different loci in which one gene masks or suppresses the expression of the other. Epistasis, which is nonallelic and therefore different from dominance, may be caused by the presence of homozygous recessive alleles at one gene pair, as occurs in the Bombay phenotype, or by the presence of a dominant allele at one locus that counteracts the expression of a dominant allele at the other locus. Compare **dominance.** —**epistatic,** *adj.*

**epistaxis** /ep'istak'sis/ [Gk, a dropping], bleeding from the nose caused by local irritation of mucous membranes, violent sneezing, fragility of the mucous membrane or of the arterial walls, chronic infection, trauma, hypertension, leukemia, vitamin K deficiency, or, most often, picking the nose. Also called **nose-bleed.**

■ OBSERVATIONS: Epistaxis may result from the rupture of tiny vessels in the anterior nasal septum; this occurs most frequently in early childhood and adolescence. In adults it occurs more commonly in men than in women; may be severe in elderly persons; may be accompanied by respiratory distress, apprehension, restlessness, vertigo, and nausea; and may lead to syncope.

■ INTERVENTIONS: The patient suffering epistaxis is instructed to breathe through the mouth, to sit quietly with the head tilted slightly forward to prevent blood from entering the pharynx, and to avoid swallowing blood. The bleeding may be controlled by pinching the soft part of the nose firmly with the fingers; by inserting a cotton ball soaked in a topical vasoconstrictor and applying pressure to the skin on both sides of the nose, occluding the blood supply to the nostrils; or by placing an ice compress over the nose. If bleeding continues, the clots may be removed by suction. The nasal mucosa may be anesthetized with topical lidocaine, cauterized with a silver nitrate stick or an electrical cautery, and then sprayed with epinephrine. Cocaine derivative may be used as a potent temporary vasoconstrictor. Severe bleeding, especially from the posterior nasal septum, may be treated by inserting packing, which generally is left in place for 1 to

3 days. Persistent or recurrent profuse epistaxis may be treated by ligating an artery supplying the nose, such as the external carotid, ethmoid, or internal maxillary artery.

■ NURSING CONSIDERATIONS: The nurse administers first aid and ordered medication; assists in cauterization and nasal packing; checks the patient's blood pressure, pulse, and respiration every half hour until bleeding subsides; and then continues to check them every 4 hours. The nurse limits the patient's activity, avoids serving milk and hot liquids, encourages expectoration rather than swallowing of blood, and reports symptoms of respiratory distress, vertigo, and bleeding. Before the patient is discharged, the nurse provides instruction on the prevention of epistaxis by using a vaporizer and applying a water-soluble gel with a cotton swab gently to the mucous membrane lining the nostrils.

**episternal** /ep′istur′nəl/, situated on or over the sternum.

**epistropheus.** See **axis.**

**epithalamus** /ep′ithal′əməs/ [Gk, *epi* + *thalamos*, chamber], the uppermost portion of the diencephalon. It includes the trigonum habenulae, the pineal body, and the posterior commissure, and the medullares thalmi. Compare **hypothalamus, metathalamus, subthalamus, thalamus.** —**epithalamic,** *adj.*

**epithelial** /-thē′lē·əl/ [Gk, *epi*, above, *thele*, nipple], pertaining to or involving the outer layer of the skin.

**epithelial cancer** [Gk, *epi*, above, *thele*, nipple; L, *cancer,* crab], a carcinoma that develops from epithelium or related tissues in the skin, hollow viscera, and other organs. Also called **epithelioma.**

**epithelial cells,** cells arranged in one or more layers that form part of a covering or lining of a body surface. The cells usually adhere to each other along their edges and surfaces. One surface is free; the other rests on a noncellular basement membrane. See also **epithelial tissue.**

**epithelial cuff.** See **junctional epithelium.**

**epithelial debridement** [Gk, *epi*, above, *thele*, nipple; Fr, *debridement,* incision], the removal of the entire inner lining and the attachment from the gingival or periodontal pocket in gingival curettage. Also called **canal debridement, deepithelialization.**

**epithelialization** /-thē′lē·al′izā′shən/ [Gk, *epi*, above, *thele*, nipple; L, *ization,* process], the regrowth of skin over a wound.

**epithelial nevus.** See **epidermal nevus.**

**epithelial peg** [Gk, *epi* + *thele*, nipple], any of the papillary projections of the epithelium that penetrate the underlying stroma of connecting tissue and normally develop in mucous membranes and dermal tissues. Also called **rete peg.**

**epithelial rest.** See **embryonic rest.**

**epithelial tissue** [Gk, *epi*, above, *thele*, nipple; OFr, *tissu*], a closely packed single or stratified layer of cells covering the body and lining its cavities, with the exception of the blood and lymph vessels.

**epithelioblastoma** /ep′ithē′lē·ō′blastō′mə/, a tumor composed of epithelial cells.

**epitheliofibril.** See **tonofibril.**

**epithelioid leiomyoma** /ep′ithē′lē′oid/ [Gk, *epi* + *thele* + *eidos,* form], an uncommon neoplasm of smooth muscle in which the cells are polygonal in shape. It usually develops in the stomach. Also called **bizarre leiomyoma, leiomyoblastoma.**

**epithelioma** /-thē′lē·ō′mə/ [Gk, *epi* + *thele* + *oma,* tumor], a neoplasm derived from the epithelium.

**-epithelioma,** combining form meaning a 'tumor of epithelial tissue': *inoepithelioma, periepithelioma, trichoepithelioma.*

**epithelioma adamantinum.** See **ameloblastoma.**

**epithelioma adenoides cysticum.** See **trichoepithelioma.**

**epithelium** /-thē′lē·əm/ [Gk, *epi* + *thele*, nipple], the covering of the internal and external organs of the body and the lining of vessels, body cavities, glands, and organs. It consists of cells bound together by connective material and varies in the number of layers and the kinds of cells. The stratified squamous epithelium of the epidermis comprises five different cellular layers. —**epithelial,** *adj.*

**epitope** /ep′itōp/ [Gk *epi* + *topos,* place], an antigenic determinant that causes a specific reaction by an immunoglobulin. It consists of a group of amino acids on the surface of the antigen. See also **antibody.**

**epitympanic recess** /-timpan′ik/ [Gk, *epi* + *tympanon,* drum], the area of the tympanic cavity cranial to the tympanic membrane, which contains the upper half of the malleus and greater part of the incus. Also called **attic.**

**epizootic** /ep′izō·ot′ik/, a disease or condition that occurs at about the same time in many individuals of the same species in a geographic area.

**EPO, 1.** abbreviation for **erythropoietin. 2.** abbreviation for **Exclusive Provider Organization.**

**eponychium.** See **cuticle,** definition 3.

**eponym** /ep′ənim/ [Gk, *epi*, above, *onyma,* name], a name for a disease, organ, procedure, or body function that is derived from the name of a person, usually a physician or scientist who first identified the condition or devised the object bearing the name. Examples include fallopian tube, Parkinson's disease, and Billing's method.

**epoophoron** /ep′ō·of′əron/ [Gk, *epi* + *oophoron,* ovary], a rudimentary structure that is situated in the mesosalpinx between the ovary and the uterine tube. The epoophoron is a persistent portion of the embryonic mesonephric duct. Also called **parovarium.**

**epoxy,** an organic chemical formula derived from the union of an oxygen atom and two carbon atoms. Epoxy resins are used as bonding agents. Also called **epoxide.**

**EPP,** abbreviation for *erythropoietic porphyria.*

**EPSDT,** abbreviation for **Early and Periodic Screening Diagnosis and Treatment.**

**epsilon** /ep′silon/, E, ∈, the fifth letter of the Greek alphabet.

**Epsom salt.** See **magnesium sulfate.**

**EPSP,** abbreviation for *excitatory postsynaptic potential.*

**Epstein-Barr virus (EBV)** /ep′stīnbär′/ [Michael A. Epstein, b. 1921, English pathologist; Yvonne M. Barr, twentieth-century English virologist; L, *virus,* poison], the herpesvirus that causes infectious mononucleosis and is associated with nasopharyngeal sarcoma, Hodgkin's disease, B cell lymphoma, leukoplakia, central nervous system lymphoma in AIDS, and Burkitt's lymphoma, especially in immunodeficient patients such as posttransplantation patients on immunosuppressive therapy. It is also thought to cause oral hairy leukoplakia. The virus resides in the salivary glands, is transmitted with saliva, and continues to be shed. EBV is ubiquitous; by 40 years of age 99% of the U.S. population has serologic evidence of EBV infection.

**Epstein's pearls** [Alois Epstein, Czechoslovakian physician, 1849–1918; L, *perla,* a mussel], small white pearl-like epithelial cysts that occur on both sides of the midline of the hard palate of the newborn. They are normal and usually disappear within a few weeks. Compare **Bednar's aphthae, thrush.**

**e.p.t.,** trademark for a human pregnancy test kit that uses monoclonal antibody technology to detect the presence of human chorionic gonadotropin in urine.

**Cell Shapes:**

**Types of cell layers:**

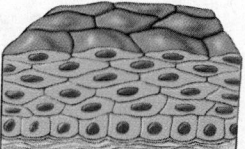

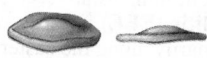

Squamous     Simple     Stratified

Ovary surface:
Simple cuboidal

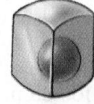 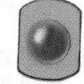

Cuboidal

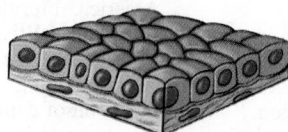

Digestive tract:
Simple columnar

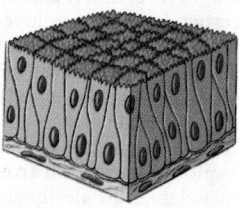

Respiratory airways:
Pseudostratified columnar

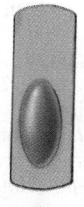

Columnar

**Classification of epithelium** *(Herlihy and Maebius, 2000)*

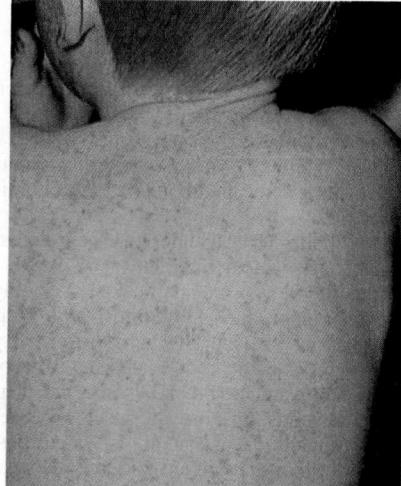

**Maculopapular rash commonly
seen in Epstein-Barr virus**
*(Zitelli and Davis, 1997/courtesy Dr. M. Sherlock)*

**eptifibatide,** an antiplatelet agent.

■ INDICATIONS: Eptifibatide is used to treat acute coronary syndrome, including patients with percutaneous coronary intervention (PCI).

■ CONTRAINDICATIONS: The following factors prohibit the use of eptifibatide: known hypersensitivity to this drug, active internal bleeding, history of bleeding, stroke within 1 month, major surgery with severe trauma, severe hypotension, history of intracranial bleeding, intracranial neoplasm, arteriovenous malformation/aneurysm, aortic dissection, and dependence on renal dialysis.

■ ADVERSE EFFECTS: Life-threatening effects of this drug are stroke and bleeding. Hypotension is another serious adverse reaction.

**epulis** /epyo͞o′lis/, *pl.* **epulides** [Gk, *epi* + *oulon,* gum], any tumor or growth on the gingiva.

**epulosis** /ep′yəlō′sis/, a healing process by scar formation, resulting in the production of a cicatrix.

**Equagesic,** trademark for a fixed-combination central nervous system drug that contains an analgesic (aspirin) and a sedative (meprobamate).

**equal cleavage** /ē′kwəl/ [L, *aequare,* to make alike; AS, *cleofan*], mitotic division of the fertilized ovum into blastomeres of identical size, as occurs in humans and most other mammals. Compare **unequal cleavage.**

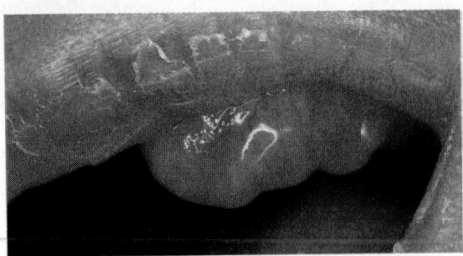

**Epulis** *(Zitelli and Davis, 1997)*

**equal distribution,** a capitation method in which income is distributed equally among providers. It is used when the patient population is geographically and clinically homogeneous. Not applicable in Canada. See also **capitation.**

**Equal Employment Opportunity Commission (EEOC),** a body appointed by the president of the United States to administer the Civil Rights Act of 1964, particularly to investigate complaints of discrimination in employment in businesses engaged in interstate commerce. Discrimination based on race, color, creed, or national origin is forbidden, but certain kinds of employers and certain conditions of employment allow exceptions to the act.

**Equanil,** trademark for a sedative (meprobamate).

**equation** [L, *aequare,* to make equal], an expression in symbols of equality or equivalence.

**equator** /ē·kwā'tər/ [L, *aequator,* equalizer], an imaginary line encircling a globe, equidistant from the poles. Used in anatomical nomenclature to designate such a line on a spherical organ, dividing the surface into two approximately equal parts. Also spelled **aequator.**

**equatorial plate** /ēk'wətôr'ē·əl/ [L, *aequare,* to make alike; Fr, *flat + vessel*], the plane at the center of the spindle in which the chromosomes are arranged during metaphase of mitosis and meiosis.

**equi-,** prefix meaning 'equal' or 'equality': *equilibrate, equilibrium.*

**equianalgesic dose** /ē'kwē·an'əljē'sik/, a dose of one analgesic that is equivalent in pain-relieving effects to another analgesic. This equivalence permits substitution of medications to prevent possible adverse effects of one of the drugs. The term is also applied to equivalent alternative dose sizes and routes of administration.

**equilibration** /ē'kwilibrā'shən/ [L, *aequus,* equal, *libra,* balance], the balancing and integrating of new experiences with those of the past in the psychologic development of an individual.

**equilibrium** /ē'kwilib're·əm/ [L, *aequilibrium*], **1.** a state of balance or rest resulting from the equal action of opposing forces such as calcium and phosphorus in the body. **2.** (in psychiatry) a state of mental or emotional balance. **3.** (in radiotherapy) a point at which the rate of production of a daughter element is equal to the rate of decay of the parent element and the activities of parent and daughter are identical.

**equilibrium reaction,** any of several reflexes that enable the body to recover balance. Equilibrium reactions begin to develop around 6 months of age. See also **local adaptation syndrome, general adaptation syndrome.**

**equin-, equino-,** combining form meaning 'characteristic of a horse': *equinovarus.*

**equine encephalitis** /ē'kwīn, ek'win/ [L, *equus,* horse; Gk, *enkephalon,* brain, *itis,* inflammation], an arbovirus infec-

tion, characterized by inflammation of the nerve tissues of the brain and spinal cord. Other characteristics include high fever, headache, nausea, vomiting, myalgia, and neurologic symptoms, such as visual disturbances, tremor, lethargy, and disorientation. The virus is transmitted by the bite of an infected mosquito. Horses are the primary host of the viruses that cause the infection; humans are secondary hosts. **Eastern equine encephalitis (EEE)** is a severe form of the infection. It occurs primarily along the eastern seaboard of the United States and lasts longer and causes more deaths and residual morbidity than **western equine encephalitis (WEE),** which occurs throughout the United States and produces a mild, brief illness, as does **Venezuelan equine encephalitis (VEE),** which is common in Central and South America, Florida, and Texas. See also **encephalitis, encephalomyelitis.**

**equine gait** [L, *equus,* horse; ONorse, *gate,* a way], a manner of walking characterized by footdrop. The condition is the result of damage to the peroneal nerve, which causes the foot to hang in a toes-downward position.

**equinovarus.** See **clubfoot.**

**equinus** /ēkwī'nəs/ [L, horse], a condition characterized by tiptoe walking on one or both feet. It is usually associated with clubfoot.

**equipotential, 1.** (in physics) indicating bodies that have the same electrical potential. **2.** lines of force that have the same electrical potential.

**equity model** /ek'witē/, an organizational model for medical providers that offers the provider equity in the company instead of cash payments. Not applicable in Canada.

**equivalence** /ikwiv'ələns/, a state of being equal in value.

**equivalent weight** [L, *a + aequus + valere,* equal value; AS, *gewiht*], **1.** the weight of an element in any given unit (such as grams) that will displace a unit weight of hydrogen from a compound or combine with or replace a unit weight of hydrogen. **2.** the weight of an acid or base that will produce or react with 1.008 grams of hydrogen ion. **3.** the weight of an oxidizing or reducing agent that will produce or accept one electron in a chemical reaction.

**equivocal symptom** [L, *aequus,* equal, *vocare,* to call; Gk, *symptoma,* that which happens], a symptom that may be attributed to more than one cause or that may occur in several diseases.

**Er,** symbol for the element **erbium.**

**ER, E.R.,** abbreviation for *emergency room.*

**eradication** /irad'ikā'shən/, the process of completely removing or destroying something.

**Erb-Duchenne paralysis.** See **Erb palsy.**

**erbium (Er)** /ur'bē·əm/ [Ytterby, Sweden], a metallic rare earth element. Its atomic number is 68; its atomic weight (mass) is 167.26.

**Erb palsy** [Wilhelm H. Erb, German neurologist, 1840–1921], a kind of paralysis caused by traumatic injury to the upper brachial plexus. It occurs most commonly as a result of forcible traction during childbirth, with injury to one or more cervical nerve roots. The signs of Erb palsy include loss of sensation in the arm and paralysis and atrophy of the deltoid, the biceps, and the brachialis muscles. The arm on the affected side hangs loosely with the elbow extended and the forearm pronated. Treatment initially requires that the arm and shoulder be immobilized to allow the swelling and inflammation of the associated neuritis to resolve. Physical therapy and splinting may be necessary to improve muscle function and to prevent flexion contracture of the elbow. Also called **Erb-Duchenne paralysis.**

**Erb's muscular dystrophy** [Wilhelm H. Erb], a form of muscular dystrophy that first affects the shoulder girdle and later often involves the pelvic girdle. It is a progressively crippling disease with onset in childhood or adolescence and is usually inherited as an autosomal recessive trait. It affects both sexes. In males differential diagnosis of Erb's muscular dystrophy and Duchenne's muscular dystrophy may be difficult. Also called **scapulohumeral muscular dystrophy.**

**Erb's point** [Wilhelm H. Erb], a landmark of the brachial plexus on the upper trunk, located about 1 inch (2.5 cm) above the clavicle at about the level of the sixth cervical vertebra. The point is the location of an angle between the posterolateral border of the sternocleidomastoid muscle and the clavicle. Electrical stimulation at Erb's point causes contractions of the biceps, deltoid, and other arm muscles.

**erectile** /irek'til, -tīl/ [L, *erigere*, to erect], capable of being erected or raised to an erect position. The term is usually used to describe spongy tissue of the penis or clitoris that becomes turgid and erectile when filled with blood. It also may be used when referring to the epidermal tissue involved in the appearance of "goose bumps" (piloerection) in response to fear, anger, cold, or other stimuli.

**erectile dysfunction.** See **impotence** (def. 2).

**erectile myxoma,** an angioma that contains areas of myxomatous tissue.

**erection** /irek'shən/ [L, *erigere,* to erect], the condition of hardness, swelling, and elevation observed in the penis and to a lesser degree in the clitoris, usually caused by sexual arousal but also occurring during sleep or after physical stimulation. It results when additional blood enters the organ and blood pressure within the organ increases, and it is influenced by psychic and nerve stimulation. Erection enables the penis to enter the vagina and to emit semen. See also **ejaculation, nocturnal emission, priapism.**

**erector spinae.** See **sacrospinalis.**

**erector spinae reflex** [L, *erigere,* to erect, *spina,* spine, *reflectere,* to bend back], a reflex characterized by contraction of the sacrospinalis and other back muscles when the overlying skin is stimulated. Also called **dorsal reflex, lumbar reflex.**

**erg** /urg, erg/, a unit of energy in the centimeter-gram-second (CGS) system equal to the work done by a force of 1 dyne through a distance of 1 cm. 1 erg $= 10^{-7}$J. See also **joule.**

**-erg-,** combining form denoting an ergot alkaloid derivative.

**ergastoplasm** /ərgas'təplaz'əm/ [Gk, *ergaster,* worker, *plassein,* to mold], a network of cytoplasmic structures that show basophilic staining properties; granular endoplasmic reticulum. See **endoplasmic reticulum.**

**-ergic, -ergetic,** combining form meaning an 'effect of activity': *allergic, pathergic, telergic.*

**ergo-,** combining form meaning 'work': *ergodermatosis, ergomaniac, ergotropy.*

**ergocalciferol.** See **calciferol.**

**ergogenic** /ur'gōjen'ik/, a tendency to increase work output.

**ergogenic aid,** a substance, such as a steroid, used by athletes with the expectation that it will provide a competitive edge.

**ergoloid mesylate** /ur'gōloid/, an adrenergic with psychotropic actions.

■ INDICATIONS: It is prescribed in the treatment of symptomatic age-related decline in mental capacity with an unknown cause, as in senile dementia.

■ CONTRAINDICATIONS: Psychosis or known sensitivity to this drug prohibits its use.

■ ADVERSE EFFECTS: Among the most serious adverse reactions are sublingual irritation, transient nausea, and gastric disturbance.

**Ergomar,** trademark for an ergot alkaloid (ergotamine tartrate).

**ergometer.** See **dynamometer.**

**ergometrine maleate.** See **ergonovine maleate.**

**ergometry** /ərgom'ətre/, the study of physical work activity, including that performed by specific muscles or muscle groups. The studies may involve testing with equipment such as stationary bicycles, treadmills, or rowing machines.

**ergonomics** /ur'gōnom'iks/ [Gk, *ergon,* work, *nomos,* law], a scientific discipline devoted to the study and analysis of human work, especially as it is affected by individual anatomic, psychologic, and other human characteristics. **—ergonomic,** *adj.*

**ergonovine maleate** /ur'gōnō'vēn/, an oxytocic ergot alkaloid. Also called **ergometrine maleate.**

■ INDICATIONS: It is prescribed to contract the uterus in the treatment or prevention of postpartum or postabortion hemorrhage caused by uterine atony.

■ CONTRAINDICATIONS: Pregnancy, peripheral vascular disease, elevated blood pressure, or known hypersensitivity to this drug prohibits its use.

■ ADVERSE EFFECTS: Among the more serious adverse effects are hypertension, nausea, headache, blurred vision, and hypersensitivity reactions. Fetal death may result from use of the drug in pregnancy.

**ergosome.** See **polysome.**

**ergosterol** /ərgos'tərôl/, an unsaturated hydrocarbon of the vitamin D group isolated from yeast, mushrooms, ergot, and other fungi. When treated with ultraviolet irradiation it is converted into vitamin D$_2$. See also **calciferol, viosterol, vitamin D.**

**ergot** /ur'gət/ [L, *ergota,* a grain fungus], (in pharmacology) the food storage body of a fungus, *Claviceps purpurea,* that commonly infects rye and other cereal grasses. It contains ergot alkaloids.

**ergot alkaloid,** one of a large group of alkaloids derived from a common fungus, *Claviceps purpurea.* The alkaloids comprise three groups: the amino acid alkaloids typified by ergotamine, the dihydrogenated amino acid alkaloids such as dihydroergotamine, and the amine alkaloids such as ergonovine.

■ INDICATIONS: Ergotamine and dihydroergotamine are less effective oxytocics than ergonovine; therefore ergonovine, given orally or intravenously, is currently used in obstetrics to treat or prevent postpartum uterine atony and to complete an incomplete or missed abortion. Ergotamine is prescribed to relieve migraine headache. It acts by reducing the amplitude of arterial pulsations in the external carotid branches of the cranial arteries. See also **missed abortion.**

■ CONTRAINDICATIONS: Contraindications to the use of any of the ergot alkaloids include peripheral vascular disease, coronary artery disease, hypertension, renal or hepatic dysfunction, and sepsis. Pregnancy prohibits their use because they may cause contractions of the uterus, decreased blood flow to the fetus, and fetal death.

■ ADVERSE EFFECTS: Ergot poisoning may result from prolonged or excessive use of the drug or accidental ingestion of contaminated grain. Signs of toxicity are thirst, diarrhea, dizziness, chest pain, abnormal and variable rate of cardiac contraction, nausea and vomiting, digital paresthesia, severe cramping, and seizures. Tissue anoxia and gangrene of the extremities may occur as a result of prolonged vasoconstriction, if poisoning is severe.

**ergotamine tartrate** /ərgot'əmēn/, a vasoconstrictor.

■ INDICATIONS: It is prescribed to abort or prevent vascular headaches such as migraines.

■ CONTRAINDICATIONS: Pregnancy, peripheral vascular disease, infectious disease, or known hypersensitivity to this drug prohibits its use.

■ ADVERSE EFFECTS: Among the more serious adverse reactions are vomiting, diarrhea, thirst, tingling of fingers and toes, and increased blood pressure. Fetal death may occur if the drug is used during pregnancy.

**ergotherapy** /ur'gōther'əpē/ [Gk, *ergon,* work, *therapeia,* treatment], the use of physical activity and exercise in the treatment of disease. By extension the therapy includes any procedure that increases the blood supply to a diseased or injured part, such as massage or various types of hot baths. —**ergotherapeutic,** *adj.*

**ergotism** /ur'gətiz'əm/ [L, *argota,* a grain fungus], **1.** an acute or chronic disease caused by excessive dosages of medications containing ergot. Symptoms may include cerebrospinal manifestations such as spasms, cramps, and dry gangrene. **2.** a chronic disease caused by ingestion of cereal products made with rye flour contaminated by ergot fungus.

**ergot poisoning** [L, *argota,* a grain fungus; L, *potio,* drink], the toxic effects of ingesting food or medications containing ergot alkaloids, particularly ergotamine. See **ergotism.**

**ergotropic** /ur'gōtrop'ik/, **1.** pertaining to an activity or work state involving somatic muscle, sympathetic nervous system, and cortical alpha rhythm activity. **2.** pertaining to the administration of medications or other therapies to energize the power of the body's blood and other tissues to resist infections.

**-ergy, 1.** suffix meaning an 'action': *leukergy, synergy.* **2.** combining form meaning an 'effect or result': *allergy, anabolergy, pathergy.*

**Erickson, Helen C.** See **Modeling and Role Modeling.**

**-eridine,** combining form denoting an analgesic of the meperidine group.

**Erikson, Erik,** a psychologist who described the development of identity of the self and the ego through successive stages that naturally unfold throughout the lifespan. The eight stages are trust vs. mistrust (infancy); autonomy vs. shame and doubt (toddler-hood); initiative vs. guilt (preschool); industry vs. inferiority (middle childhood); identity vs. role confusion (adolescence); intimacy vs. isolation (young adulthood); generativity vs. stagnation (middle adulthood); and ego integrity vs. despair (older adulthood).

**ERISA,** abbreviation for **Employment Retirement Income Security Act.**

**erogenous** /iroj'ənəs/ [Gk, *eros,* love, *genein,* to produce], pertaining to the production of erotic sensations or sexual excitement. Also called **erotogenic** /irot'ōjen'ik/.

**erogenous zones,** areas of the body in which sexual tension tends to become concentrated and can be relieved by manipulation of the region. The areas include the mouth, anus, and genitals.

**Eros** /ir'os, er'os/ [Gk, mythic love-inciting son of Aphrodite], a freudian term for the drive or instinct for survival, including self-preservation and continuation of the species through reproduction.

**erosion** /irō'zhən/ [L, *erodere,* to consume], the wearing away or gradual destruction of a surface. For example, a mucosal or epidermal surface may erode as a result of inflammation, injury, or other causes, usually marked by the appearance of an ulcer. See also **necrosis.**

**erosive gastritis** /irō'siv/, an inflammatory condition characterized by multiple erosions of the mucous membrane lining the stomach. Nausea, anorexia, pain, and gastric hemorrhage may occur. See also **chemical gastritis, corrosive gastritis.**

**erosive osteoarthritis.** See **Kellgren's syndrome.**

**-erotic,** combining form meaning 'sexual love or desire': *anterotic, homoerotic, hysteroerotic.*

**eroticism** /irot'isiz'əm/ [Gk, *erotikos,* sexual love], **1.** sexual impulse or desire. **2.** the arousal or attempt to arouse the sexual instinct through suggestive or symbolic means. **3.** the expression of sexual instinct or desire. **4.** an abnormally persistent sexual drive. Also called **erotism.** See also **anal eroticism, oral eroticism.**

**eroto-** /irot'ə-/, combining form meaning 'sexual love or desire': *erotogenic, erotopath, erotophobia.*

**erotogenic.** See **erogenous.**

**erratic** /irat'ik/ [L, *erraticus,* wandering], deviating from the normal but with no apparent fixed course or purpose.

**error** [L, *errare,* to wander], (in research) a defect in the design of a study, in the development of measurements or instruments, or in the interpretation of findings.

**error message,** a brief statement delivered by a computer via a peripheral device, such as a monitor or printer, that a procedure has been done incorrectly.

**error of the first kind.** See **type I error.**

**error of the second kind.** See **type II error.**

**ERT,** abbreviation for **external radiation therapy.**

**erucic acid** /erōō'sik/, a fatty acid that has been associated with heart disease. It is present in rapeseed oil that is used in some countries as a vegetable oil for salad dressings, margarines, and mayonnaise. Canola oil is a rapeseed oil from which virtually all erucic acid has been removed through breeding.

**eructation** /ē'ruktā'shən/ [L, *eructare,* to belch], the act of drawing up air from the stomach with a characteristic sound through the mouth. Also called **belching.**

**eruption** /irup'shən/ [L, *eruptio,* bursting forth], the appearance of the rapidly forming skin lesion, especially of a viral exanthem, or of a rash that commonly accompanies a drug reaction.

**eruptive fever** /irup'tiv/ [L, *eruptio,* bursting forth; *febris*], any disease characterized by fever and a rash.

**eruptive gingivitis,** inflammation of the gums that may occur when the secondary teeth break through. Compare **desquamative gingivitis.**

**eruptive xanthoma,** a skin disorder associated with elevated triglyceride levels in the blood. Numerous erythematous or pale raised papules suddenly appear on the trunk, legs, arms, and buttocks.

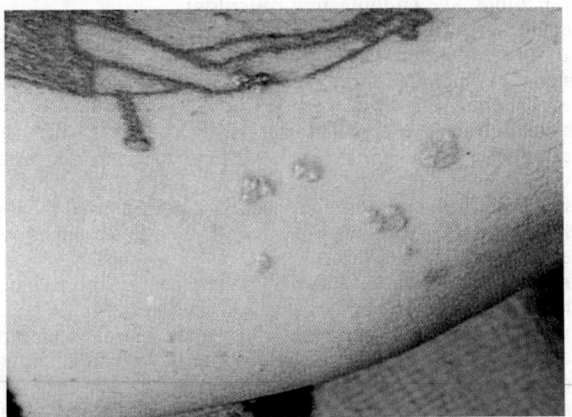

**Eruptive xanthoma** *(Bloom and Ireland, 1992)*

**ERV,** abbreviation for **expiratory reserve volume.**

**erysipelas** /er'isip'ələs/ [Gk, *erythros,* red, *pella,* skin], an infectious skin disease characterized by redness, swelling, vesicles, bullae, fever, pain, and lymphadenopathy. It is caused by a species of group A beta-hemolytic streptococci. Treatment includes antibiotics, analgesics, and packs or dressings applied locally to the lesions.

rash may reappear whenever the skin is irritated. It is caused by parvovirus $B_{19}$. No treatment is necessary, and prognosis is excellent. Isolation of patients is not required. Also called **fifth disease.**

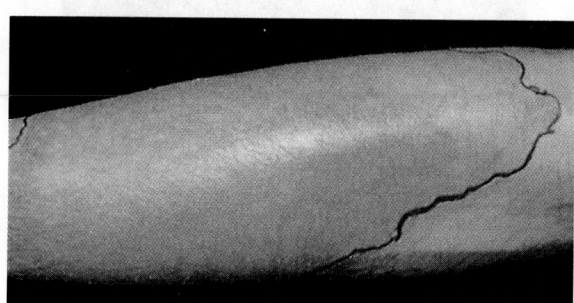

**Erysipelas**
*(Goldstein, 1997/courtesy Department of Dermatology, University of North Carolina at Chapel Hill)*

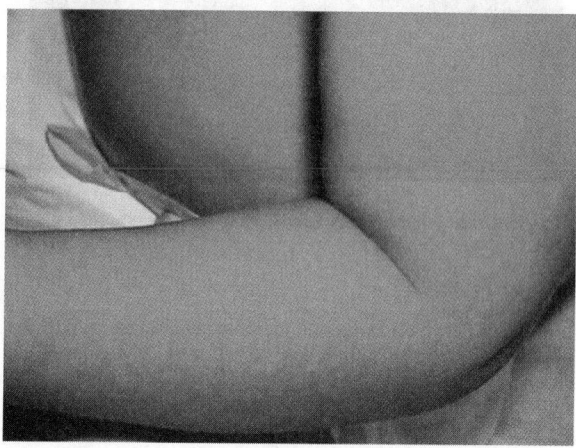

**Erythema infectiosum**
*(Zitelli and Davis, 1997/courtesy Dr. M. Sherlock)*

**erysipeloid** /er'isip'əloid/ [Gk, *erhthros + pella + eidos,* form], an infection of the hands characterized by blue-red patches and occasionally by erythema. It is acquired by handling meat or fish infected with *Erysipelothrix rhusiopathiae.* The disease is self-limited, lasting about 3 weeks, but responds to penicillin. Also called **fish-handler's disease.** Compare **erysipelas.**

**erythema marginatum,** a skin disorder seen in acute rheumatic fever characterized by temporary disk-shaped nonpruritic reddened macules that fade in the center, leaving raised margins.

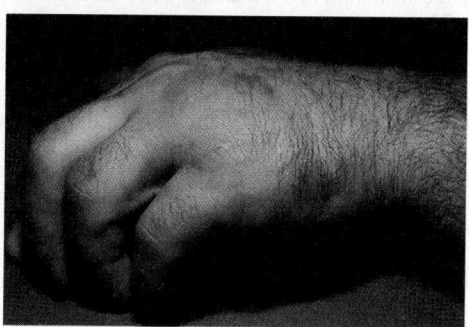

**Erysipeloid** *(Auerbach, 1995)*

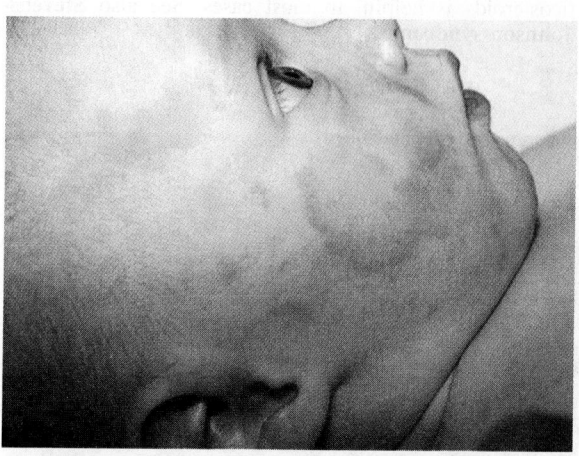

**Erythema marginatum** *(Weston, Lane, and Morelli, 1996)*

**erythema** /er'ithē'mə/ [Gk, *erythros,* red], redness or inflammation of the skin or mucous membranes that is the result of dilation and congestion of superficial capillaries. Examples of erythema are nervous blushes and mild sunburn. See also **erythroderma, rubor. —erythematous,** *adj.*

**erythema infectiosum,** an acute benign infectious disease, mainly of childhood. It is characterized by fever and an erythematous rash that begins on the cheeks and later appears on the arms, thighs, buttocks, and trunk. As the rash progresses, earlier lesions fade. Sunlight aggravates the eruption, which usually lasts about 10 days. For a period the

**erythema migrans (EM),** a skin lesion that begins as a small papule and spreads peripherally; it is characterized by a raised, red margin and clearing in the center. It may mark the site of a tick bite and is a diagnostic sign of **Lyme disease.** Also called **bullseye rash.**

**erythema multiforme (EM)** /mul'tifôr'mē, mŏŏl'tēfôr'mā/, any of three major clinical syndromes characterized by lymphocytic infiltrates in the skin that cause keratinocyte necrosis. The patient may experience polymorphous

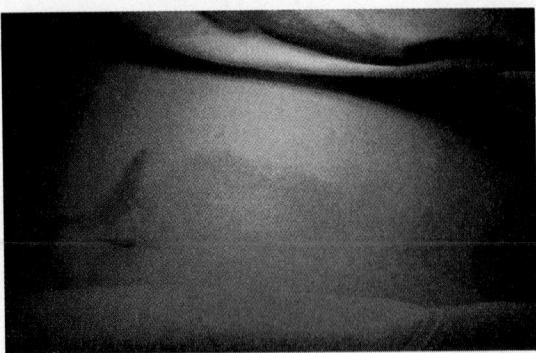

**Erythema migrans in Lyme disease** *(Auerbach, 1995)*

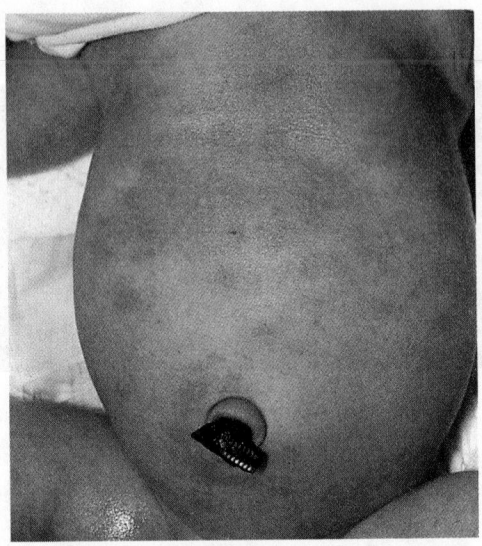

**Erythema neonatorum** *(Zitelli and Davis, 1997)*

24 to 48 hours after birth and disappears spontaneously after several days. A smear of the papules that reveals the presence of eosinophils rather than neutrophils differentiates the condition from neonatal pustular melanosis.

eruption of skin and mucous membranes. Macules, papules, nodules, vesicles or bullae, and target (bull's-eye-shaped) lesions are seen. The three major classifications of erythema multiforme are EM minor, EM major, and pure plaque toxic epidermal necrosis. EM minor is an acute form of the disease, characterized by three-ring target lesions on the extremities. Symptoms often follow an infection of herpes simplex. The patient may have raised lesions but no fever and no blistering. EM major, also called Stevens-Johnson syndrome, is characterized by the presence of target lesions, blistering, and detachment of the skin and mucous membranes. EM major also tends to follow herpes simplex virus infections. Plaque toxic epidermal necrolysis may not be associated with target lesions. However, the condition is associated with detachment of large sheets of skin. It is generally drug induced. Definitive and preventive treatment depends on finding the specific cause; use of topical or systemic corticosteroids is helpful in most cases. See also **Stevens-Johnson syndrome.**

**erythema nodosum,** a hypersensitivity reaction characterized by reddened, tender subcutaneous nodules on the extensor aspects of the extremities, such as the shins. The nodules last for several days or weeks; never ulcerate; and are often associated with mild fever, malaise, and pain in muscles and joints. This condition may accompany streptococcal infections, tuberculosis, sarcoidosis, drug sensitivity, ulcerative colitis, and pregnancy. The prognosis is good with appropriate treatment of the underlying disease. A course of corticosteroids is usually effective in diminishing the symptoms.

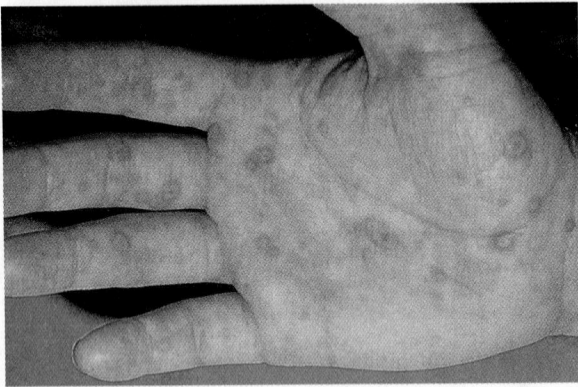

**Mild erythema multiforme**
*(Goldstein, 1997/courtesy Department of Dermatology, University of North Carolina at Chapel Hill)*

**erythema neonatorum,** a common skin condition of neonates characterized by a pink papular rash frequently superimposed with vesicles or pustules. The rash appears within

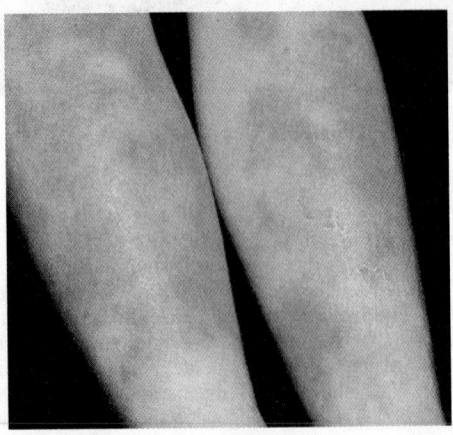

**Erythema nodosum** *(Zitelli and Davis, 1997)*

**erythema perstans,** a persistent local redness of the skin, characteristically annular.

**erythematous.** See **erythema.**

**erythematous pemphigus** [Gk, *erythros,* red, *pemphix,* bubble], a skin disorder characterized by bullous eruptions on the trunk and a facial eruption that resembles that of lupus erythematosus. The condition may be accompanied by seborrheic dermatitis. Also called **pemphigus erythematosus.**

**erythemo-,** combining form meaning 'red': *erythematous, erythemogenic.*

**erythralgia** /er′ithral′jə/ [Gk, *erythros,* red, *algos,* pain], a skin disorder characterized by a painful burning sensation, raised skin temperature, and redness, generally of the lower limbs.

**erythrasma** /er′ithraz′mə/ [Gk, *erythros,* red], a bacterial skin infection common in the axillary or inguinal region, characterized by irregular reddish-brown areas. An asymptomatic disease, it is more common in diabetics and responds quickly to oral erythromycin. Compare **intertrigo, tinea cruris.**

**erythremia** /er′ithrē′mē·ə/ [Gk, *erythros* + *haima,* blood], an abnormal increase in the number of red blood cells.

**erythro-,** combining form meaning 'red': *erythroblast, erythroclast, erythrocyte.*

**erythroblast** /erith′rəblast′/, an immature form of a red blood cell. It is normally found only in bone marrow and contains hemoglobin.

**erythroblastoma** /-blastō′mə/ [Gk, *erythros,* red, *blastos,* germ, *oma,* tumor], a myeloma tumor (osteolytic neoplasm) in which the cells resemble erythroblasts.

**erythroblastosis fetalis** /-blastō′sis/ [Gk, *erythros* + *blastos,* germ, *osis,* condition; L, *fetus,* bringing forth], a type of hemolytic anemia in newborns that results from maternal-fetal blood group incompatibility, specifically involving the Rh factor and the ABO blood groups. The condition is caused by an antigen-antibody reaction in the bloodstream of the infant caused by placental transmission of maternally formed antibodies against the incompatible antigens of the fetal blood. In Rh factor incompatibility the hemolytic reaction occurs only when the mother is Rh negative and the infant is Rh positive. The isoimmunization process rarely occurs in the first pregnancy, but there is increased risk with each succeeding pregnancy. However, maternal sensitization to the Rh factor can be prevented by injection of a high-titer anti-Rh gamma globulin preparation after delivery or abortion of an Rh positive fetus. No sensitization may occur in situations in which a strong placental barrier prevents transfer of fetal blood into the maternal circulation. In about 10% to 15% of sensitized mothers, no hemolytic reaction occurs in the newborn. Clinical manifestations of the condition include severe anemia, jaundice, and enlargement of the liver and spleen, which, without intervention, can lead to hypoxia, cardiac failure, generalized edema, respiratory distress, and death. Prenatal diagnosis of the disease is confirmed through amniocentesis and analysis of bilirubin levels in amniotic fluid. Higher than normal levels result from the breakdown of hemoglobin from the lysed erythrocytes. Treatment consists of intrauterine transfusion when placental bilirubin levels progressively increase or immediate exchange transfusions after birth. Hemolytic reactions involving the ABO blood groups have similar manifestations but are generally less severe. See also **hydrops fetalis, hyperbilirubinemia of the newborn, Rh factor.**

**erythrochromia** /-krō′mē·ə/, **1.** a red coloration or stain. **2.** red pigmentation in spinal fluid caused by the presence of blood.

**Erythrocin,** trademark for an antibiotic (erythromycin).

**erythrocyanosis** /-sī′ənō′sis/, a condition characterized by bluish-red discoloration of skin, accompanied by swelling, burning, and itching.

**erythrocyte** /erith′rəsīt′/ [Gk, *erythros* + *kytos,* cell], mature red blood cell; a biconcave disk about 7 μm in diameter that contains hemoglobin confined within a lipoid membrane. It is the major cellular element of the circulating blood and transports oxygen as its principal function. The number of cells per cubic millimeter of blood is usually maintained between 4.5 and 5.5 million in men and between 4.2 and 4.8 million in women. It varies with age, activity, and environmental conditions. For example, an increase to a level of 8 million/mm$^3$ can normally occur at over 10,000 feet above sea level. An erythrocyte normally lives for 110 to 120 days, when it is removed from the bloodstream and broken down by the reticuloendothelial system. New erythrocytes are produced at a rate of slightly more than 1% a day; thus a constant level is usually maintained. Acute blood loss, hemolytic anemia, or chronic oxygen deprivation may cause erythrocyte production to increase greatly. Erythrocytes originate in the marrow of the long bones. Maturation proceeds from a stem cell (promegaloblast) through the pronormoblast stage to the normoblast, the last stage before the mature adult cell develops. Kinds of erythrocytes include the **burr cell, discocyte, macrocyte, meniscocyte,** and **spherocyte.** Also called **red blood cell (RBC), red cell, red corpuscle.** Compare **normoblast, reticulocyte.** See also **erythropoiesis, hemoglobin, red cell indexes.**

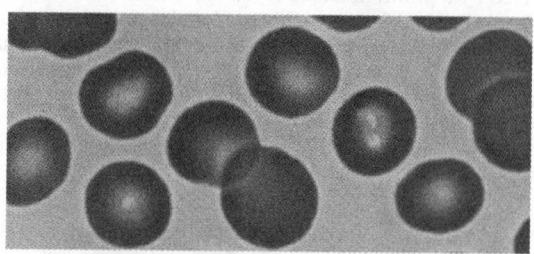

**Erythrocytes** *(Carr and Rodak, 1999)*

**erythrocyte fragility.** See **osmotic fragility.**

**erythrocyte reinfusion,** the process of injecting into an individual's bloodstream red blood cells previously taken from that individual and preserved temporarily by freezing. The process is managed in the same manner as when an individual donates his or her own blood for later retransfusion (autologous transfusion).

**erythrocyte sedimentation rate (ESR),** the rate at which red blood cells settle out in a tube of unclotted blood, expressed in millimeters per hour. Blood is collected in an anticoagulant and allowed to form a sediment in a calibrated glass column. At the end of 1 hour the laboratory technician measures the distance the erythrocytes have fallen in the tube. Elevated sedimentation rates are not specific for any disorder but indicate the presence of inflammation. Inflammation causes an alteration of the blood proteins, which makes the red blood cells aggregate, becoming heavier than normal. The speed with which they fall to the bottom of the tube corresponds to the degree of inflammation. Serial evaluations of erythrocyte sedimentation rate are useful in monitoring the course of inflammatory activity in rheumatic diseases and, when performed with a white blood cell count, can indicate infection. Certain noninflammatory conditions, such as pregnancy, are also characterized by high sedimentation rates. The Westergren ESR is determined with a 200-mm Westergren tube. Values are higher for women in both methods and vary according to the method used. Normal findings by the Westergren method are up to 20 mm/hr for females and up to 15 mm/hr for males. Also called *(informal)* **sed. rate.** See also **inflammation.**

**erythrocythemia** /erith′rōsīthē′mē·ə/ [Gk, *erythros* + *kytos* + *haima*, blood], an increase in the number of erythrocytes circulating in the blood.

**erythrocytopenia** /-sī′təpē′nē·ə/ [Gk, *erythros*, red, *kytos*, cell, *penes*, poor], a condition characterized by a deficiency or decrease in number of erythrocytes.

**erythrocytopoiesis.** See **erythrogenesis, erythropoiesis.**

**erythrocytosis** /erith′rōsītō′sis/ [Gk, *erythros* + *kytos* + *osis*, condition], an abnormal increase in the number of circulating red cells. See also **polycythemia.**

**erythroderma** /erith′rōdur′mə/ [Gk, *erythros* + *derma*, skin], an abnormal redness of the skin. Compare **erythema, rubor.**

**erythroderma desquamativum.** See **Leiner's disease.**

**erythroderma polyneuropathy.** See **acrodynia.**

**erythrogenesis,** the creation of red blood cells. See also **erythropoiesis.**

**erythroid** /erith′roid/, 1. reddish in color. 2. pertaining to erythrocytes.

**erythroleukemia** /-lōōkē′mē·ə/ [Gk, *erythros* + *leukos*, white, *haima*, blood], a malignant blood disorder characterized by a proliferation of erythropoietic elements in bone marrow, erythroblasts with bizarre lobulated nuclei, and abnormal myeloblasts in peripheral blood. The disease may have an acute or chronic course. Also called **diGuglielmo's disease** /di′gōōlyel′mōs/, **diGuglielmo's syndrome, erythromyeloblastic leukemia.**

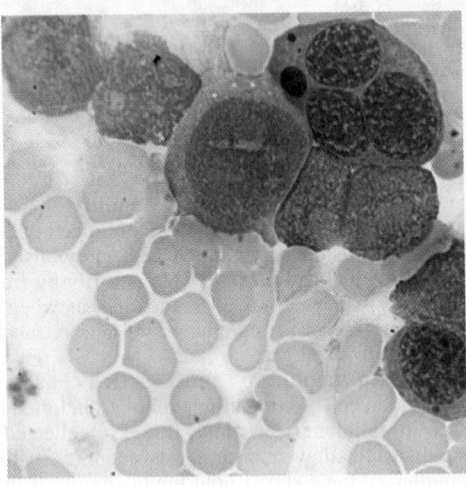

**Erythroleukemia** *(Carr and Rodak, 1999)*

**erythroleukosis,** an abnormal increase in numbers of granulocytes and red blood cells.

**erythromelalgia** /erith′rōmilal′jə/ [Gk, *erythros* + *melos*, limb, *algos*, pain], a rare disorder characterized by a paroxysmal dilation of the peripheral blood vessels. It occurs

bilaterally, usually in the extremities, and is associated with burning, redness of the skin, and pain. —**erythromelalgic,** *adj.*

**erythromycin** /erith′rōmī′sin/, an antibiotic (of the macrolide type).

■ INDICATIONS: It is prescribed in the treatment of many bacterial and mycoplasmic infections, particularly those that cannot be treated by penicillins.

■ CONTRAINDICATIONS: Liver disease or known hypersensitivity to this drug prohibits its use.

■ ADVERSE EFFECTS: Among the more serious adverse effects are cholestatic hepatitis, hypersensitivity reactions, GI discomfort, and serious interactions with other drugs.

**erythromyeloblastic leukemia.** See **erythroleukemia.**

**erythron** /erith′ron/, the total mass of circulating red blood cells and the red-blood-cell-forming tissues from which they are derived.

**erythropathy** /er′ithrop′əthē/, any disease involving the red blood cells (erythrocytes).

**erythrophage** /erith′rəfāj/, a phagocyte that ingests red blood cells or blood pigment.

**erythrophobia** /-fō′bē·ə/ [Gk, *erythros* + *phobos*, fear], 1. an anxiety disorder characterized by an irrational fear of blushing or of displaying embarrassment. 2. a symptom manifested by blushing at the slightest provocation. 3. a morbid fear of or aversion to the color red. —**erythrophobic,** *adj.*

**erythrophthisis** /erith′rōtī′sis/, grave damage to the restorative power of red corpuscles. See also **anemia.**

**erythroplasia of Queyrat** /erith′rōplā′zhə/ [Gk, *erythros* + *plasis*, forming; Louis A. Queyrat, French dematologist, 1856–1933], a premalignant lesion on the glans or corona of the penis. It is a shiny, velvety, well-circumscribed reddish patch on the skin. It is usually excised surgically. See also **Bowen's disease.**

**erythropoiesis** /erith′rōpō·ē′sis/ [Gk, *erythros* + *poiein*, to make], the process of erythrocyte production in the bone marrow involving the maturation of a nucleated precursor into a hemoglobin-filled, nucleus-free erythrocyte that is regulated by erythropoietin, a hormone produced by the kidney. Also called **erythrocytopoiesis, erythrogenesis.** See also **erythrocyte, erythropoietin, hemoglobin, leukopoiesis.** —**erythropoietic,** *adj.*

**erythropoietic porphyria.** See **porphyria.**

**erythropoietin (EPO)** /erith′rōpō·ē′tin/ [Gk, *erythros* + *poiein*, to make], a glycoprotein hormone synthesized mainly in the kidneys and released into the bloodstream in response to anoxia. The hormone acts to stimulate and to regulate the production of erythrocytes and thus increases the oxygen-carrying capacity of the blood. See also **erythropoiesis.**

**Es,** symbol for the element **einsteinium.**

**ESADDI,** abbreviation for **Estimated Safe and Adequate Daily Dietary Intake.**

**escape beat** [ME, *escapen*, to flee; *beten*, to beat], an automatic beat of the heart that occurs after an interval equal to or longer than the duration of its normal cycle. Escape beats function as safety mechanisms, and anything that produces a long pause in the prevailing heart cycle may allow an escape to occur. Pauses in which escape beats occur may be caused by sinoatrial block, atrioventricular (AV) block, or sinus bradycardia. Escape beats may arise from the atria, the AV junction, or the ventricles.

**escape rhythm** [OFr, *escaper* + Gk, *rhythmos*, beat], a sustained heartbeat that occurs when the sinus or atrioventricular (AV) node is depressed or blocked. Under such conditions, the heart rate is controlled by the AV junction or the His-Purkinje system.

escarronodulaire. See **Marseilles fever.**

**-escent,** suffix meaning 'beginning to be': *alkalescent, convalescent, turgescent.*

**eschar** /es'kär/ [Gk, *eschara,* scab], a scab or dry crust that results from trauma, such as a thermal or chemical burn, infection, or excoriating skin disease. **—escharotic,** *adj.*

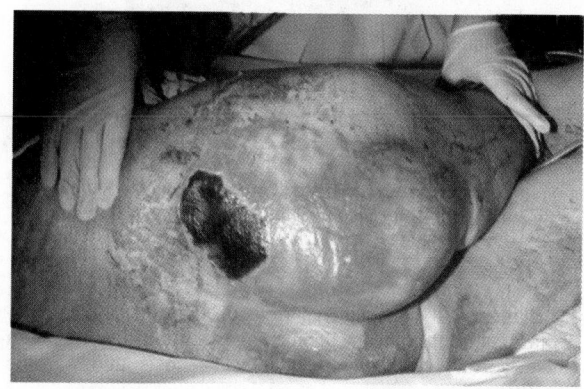

**Stage III pressure ulcer with eschar**
*(Monahan and Neighbors, 1998)*

**escharotic.** See **eschar.**

**escharotomy** /es'kärot'əmē/, a surgical incision into necrotic tissue resulting from a severe burn. The procedure is sometimes necessary to prevent edema from generating sufficient interstitial pressure to impair capillary filling, causing ischemia.

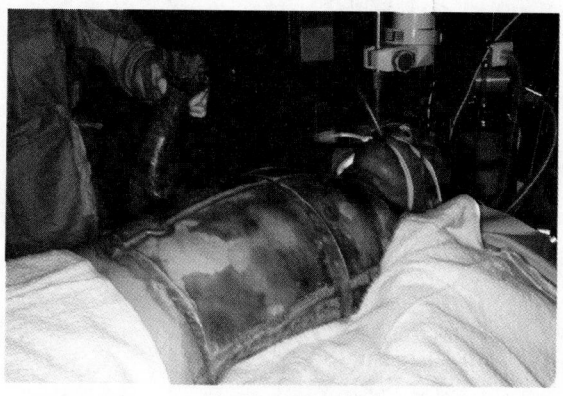

**Linear escharotomy**
*(Phipps, Sands, and Marek/courtesy Burn Center, MetroHealth Medical Center, Cleveland)*

**escharronodulaire.** See **Marseilles fever.**

*Escherichia coli* (E. coli) /eshirī'kē-ə kō'lī/ [Theodor Escherich, German physician, 1857–1911; Gk, *kolon,* colon], a species of coliform bacteria of the family Enterobacteriaceae, normally present in the intestines and common in wa-

ter, milk, and soil. *E. coli* is the most frequent cause of urinary tract infection and is a serious gram-negative pathogen in wounds. *E. coli* septicemia may rapidly result in shock and death through the action of an endotoxin released from the bacteria.

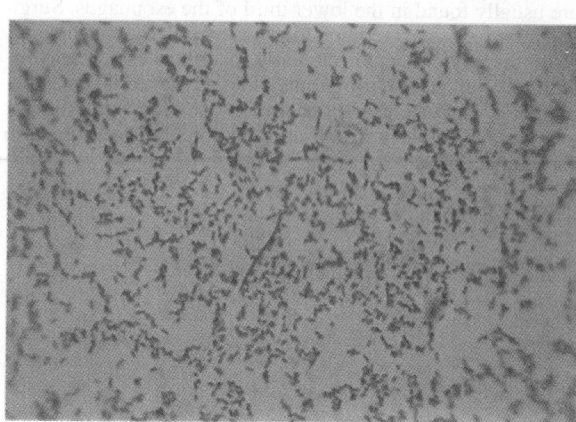

***Escherichia coli***
*(Mahon and Menuselis, 2000/courtesy Andrew G. Smith, Baltimore)*

**Escobar syndrome.** See **multiple pterygium syndrome.**

**escutcheon** /eskuch'ən/ [L, *scutum,* shield], the shieldlike pattern of distribution of coarse, adult pubic hair.

**Esidrix,** trademark for a thiazide diuretic (hydrochlorothiazide).

**-esis,** suffix meaning an 'action, process, or result of': *enuresis, oxydesis, synthesis.*

**Eskalith,** trademark for a medication used to treat bipolar affective disorders (lithium carbonate).

**Esmarch's bandage** /es'märks/ [Johann F. A. von Esmarch, German surgeon, 1823–1908], a broad, flat elastic bandage wrapped around an elevated limb to force blood out of the limb. It is used before certain surgical procedures to create a blood-free field.

**eso-,** combining form meaning 'within': *esogastritis, esotropia, esophagus.*

**esophageal.** See **esophagus.**

**esophageal atresia** /əsof'əjē'əl, es'ofā'jē-əl/ [Gk, *oisophagos,* gullet], an abnormal esophagus that ends in a blind pouch or narrows to a thin cord and thus does not provide a continuous passage to the stomach. It usually occurs as a congenital anomaly. Thoracotomy can effect repair.

**esophageal cancer,** a rare malignant neoplastic disease of the esophagus that peaks at about 60 years of age, occurs three times more frequently in men than in women, and is found more often in Asia and Africa than in North America. Risk factors associated with the disease are heavy consumption of alcohol, tobacco smoking, betel-nut chewing, Plummer-Vinson syndrome, Barrett's esophagus, and achalasia. Aflatoxin in moldy grain and peanuts or a dietary deficiency, especially of molybdenum, may be involved. Esophageal cancer does not often cause any symptoms in the early stages but in later stages produces painful dysphagia, chest pain, anorexia, weight loss, regurgitation, cervical adenopathy, and, in some cases, persistent cough. Left vocal cord paralysis and hemoptysis indicate an advanced state of the disease. Esophageal cancer metastasizes rapidly and thus has a poor prognosis. The tumor may spread locally to invade the trachea, bronchi, pericardium, great blood vessels, and thoracic vertebrae or may metastasize to lymph nodes, the lungs, and the liver. Diagnostic measures include barium swallow, fiberoptic esophagoscopy, and biopsy and cytologic examination of the primary lesion and regional nodes. Most esophageal tumors are poorly differentiated squamous cell carcinomas; adenocarcinomas occur less frequently and are usually found in the lower third of the esophagus. Surgical treatment may require total or partial esophagectomy. Radiotherapy may eradicate early local tumors and may effectively palliate the symptoms of an advanced lesion. Chemotherapy may be used in palliation of advanced disease or as an adjuvant to surgery or radiation therapy. See also **esophagectomy.**

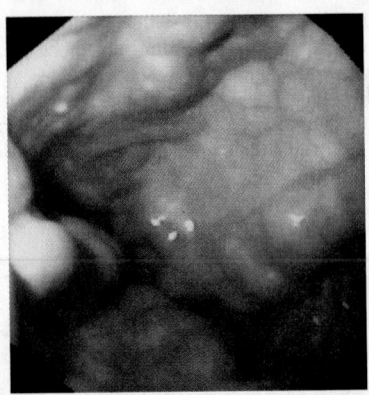

**Esophageal varices: endoscopic view**
*(Gitlin and Strauss, 1995)*

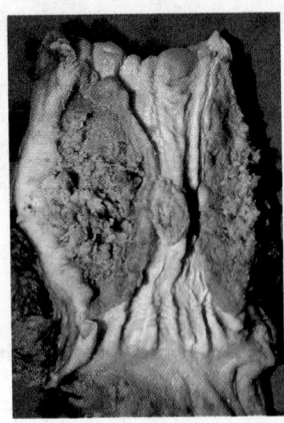

**Esophageal cancer** *(Fletcher, 2000)*

len as the result of portal hypertension. These vessels are especially susceptible to hemorrhage. Conditions that can cause portal hypertension include cirrhosis and chronic hepatitis.

**esophageal web,** a thin membrane that may develop across the lumen of the esophagus, usually near the level of the cricoid cartilage. The abnormal condition is generally associated with iron deficiency anemia and usually disappears when the underlying problem is resolved. See also **Plummer-Vinson syndrome.**

**esophagectomy** /esof′əjek′təmē/ [Gk, *oisophagos* + *ektomē,* excision], a surgical procedure in which all or part of the esophagus is removed, as may be required to treat severe recurrent bleeding esophageal varices or esophageal cancer. Also spelled **oesophagectomy.**

**esophageal dysfunction,** any disturbance, impairment, or abnormality that interferes with the normal functioning of the esophagus, such as dysphagia, esophagitis, or sphincter incompetence. The condition is one of the primary symptoms of scleroderma.

**esophageal lead** /lēd/, **1.** an electrocardiographic conductor in which the exploring electrode is placed within the lumen of the esophagus. It is used to detect sizable atrial deflections as an aid in identifying cardiac arrhythmias. **2.** *informal.* a tracing produced by such a lead on an electrocardiograph.

**esophageal obturator airway,** an emergency device that consists of a large tube that is inserted into the mouth through an airtight face mask. Holes in the tube open into the oropharynx when properly placed. The esophagus is blocked by inflating a balloon at the end of the tube. Because of the design, air passes only into the trachea.

**esophageal peristalsis** strong, uncoordinated nonpropulsive contractions of the esophagus evoked by swallowing, especially in the elderly. On barium radiography, the lumen of the esophagus appears as a series of concentric narrowings or as a spiral coil.

**esophageal spasm.** See **esophageal peristalsis.**

**esophageal speech** /isofəjēl/ [Gk, *oisophagos,* gullet; AS, *spaec*], alaryngeal sounds made by forcing air into and out of the esophagus, causing it to vibrate. See **alaryngeal speech.**

**esophageal varices,** a complex of longitudinal tortuous veins at the lower end of the esophagus, enlarged and swol-

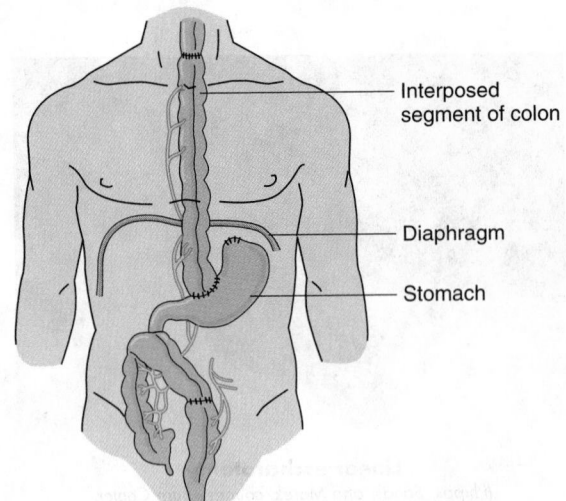

**Esophagectomy with colon interposition**
*(Phipps, Sands, and Marek, 1999)*

**esophagitis** /esof′əjī′tis/ [Gk, *oisophagos* + *itis*], inflammation of the mucosal lining of the esophagus, caused by infection, irritation from a nasogastric tube, or, most commonly, backflow of gastric juice from the stomach. Also spelled **oesophagitis.** See also **gastroesophageal reflux.**

**esophagocele** /esof'əgōsēl'/, a hernia of the mucous membrane through a weakened area in the wall of the esophagus.

**esophagogastroduodenoscopy (EGD),** /ə·sof'ə·gō·gas'-trō·dōō'od·ə·nos'kə·pe/, an endoscopic test that permits direct visualization of the upper GI tract. Insertion of a long, flexible, fiberoptic-lighted scope allows examination of tumors, varices, mucosal inflammations, hiatal hernias, polyps, ulcers, and obstructions. This test evaluates patients with dysphagia, weight loss, early satiety, upper abdominal pain, ulcer symptoms, or dyspepsia, and is also used therapeutically for electrocoagulation, laser coagulation, or injection of sclerosing agents.

**esophagogastronomy** /esof'əgō'gastron'əmē/ [Gk, oisophagos, gullet, gaster, stomach, stoma, mouth], the surgical creation of a passage between the esophagus and the stomach.

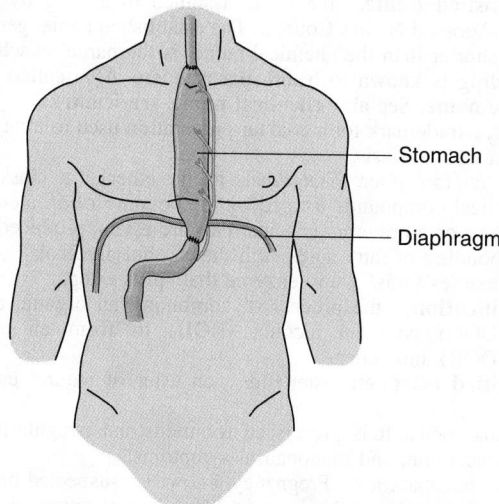

**Esophagogastrostomy for esophageal cancer**
(Phipps, Sands, and Marek, 1999)

**esophagogastroscopy** /-gastros'kəpē/ [Gk, oisophagos, gullet, gaster, stomach, skopein, to watch], the examination of the esophagus and stomach using an endoscope.

**esophagogastrostomy** /-gastros'təmē/, an artifical anastomosis of the esophagus to the stomach.

**esophagojejunostomy** /-jij'ōōnos'təmē/ [Gk, oisophagos, gullet; L, jejunum, empty, stoma, mouth], the surgical creation of a direct passage from the esophagus to the jejunum, bypassing the stomach. The procedure is used after total gastrectomy.

**esophagomyotomy** /-mī'ot'·mē/, a longitudinal incision in the lower part of the esophageal muscle made to treat esophageal achalasia, an obstruction to the passage of food.

**esophagoscopy** /esof'əgos'kəpē/ [Gk, oisophagos + skopein, to look], examination of the esophagus with an endoscope. Also spelled **oesophagoscopy.**

**esophagospasm** /esof'əgōspaz'əm/ [Gk, oisophagos, gullet, spasmos], spasmodic contractions of the walls of the esophagus. The symptoms are substernal chest pain similar to angina pectoris and dysphagia for both liquids and solid food.

**esophagostomy** /esof'əgos'təmē/, a surgical opening into the esophagus for enteral tube feeding.

**esophagus** /esof'əgəs/ [Gk, oisophagos], the musculo membranous canal, about 24 cm long, extending from the pharynx to the stomach. It begins in the neck at the inferior border of the cricoid cartilage, opposite the sixth cervical vertebra, and descends to the cardiac sphincter of the stomach in a vertical path with two slight curves. The esophagus is composed of a fibrous coat, a muscular coat, and a submucous coat and is lined with mucous membrane. Also spelled **oesophagus.** Also called **gullet. —esophageal,** adj.

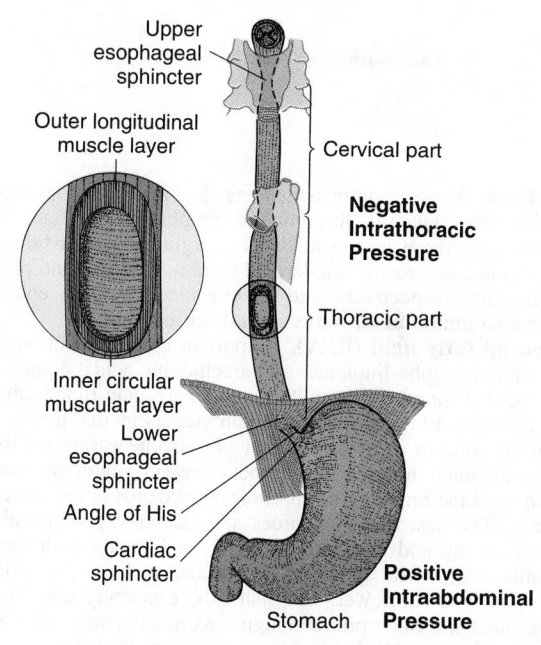

**Esophagus** (Beare and Myers, 1998)

**esophoria** /es'əfôr'ē·ə/ [Gk, eso, inward, pherein, to bear], the latent medial deviation of the visual axis of one eye in the absence of visual stimuli for fusion. Also called **cross-eye.** Compare **esotropia, exophoria. —esophoric,** adj.

**esotropia** /es'ətrō'pē·ə/ [Gk, eso + tropos, turning], a medical deviation of one eye relative to the other fixating eye. Also called **convergent strabismus, convergent squint, internal strabismus.** Compare **esophoria, exotropia.** See also **strabismus. —esotropic,** adj.

**ESP,** abbreviation for **extrasensory perception.**

**espundia** /espun'dē·ə/ [Sp, cancerous ulcer], a cutaneous form of American leishmaniasis most common in Brazil, caused by Leishmania brasiliensis. The primary lesion often disappears spontaneously, followed by mucocutaneous lesions that destroy the mucosal surface of the nose, pharynx, and larynx. If the condition is untreated, potentially fatal secondary bacterial infections may occur.

**ESR,** abbreviation for **erythrocyte sedimentation rate.**

**essential** /esen'shəl/, a necessary part of a thing without which it could not exist.

**essential amino acid** [L, essentia, quality], an organic compound not synthesized in the body that is essential for protein synthesis in adults and optimal growth in infants and

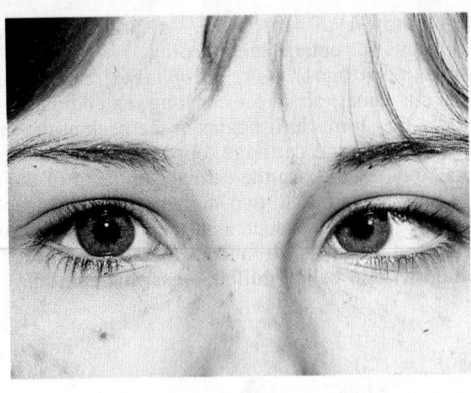

**Esotropia** *(Zitelli and Davis, 1997)*

children. Adults require isoleucine, leucine, lysine, methionine, phenylalanine, threonine, tryptophan, and valine. Infants need these amino acids plus arginine and histidine. Cysteine and tyrosine are derived from methionine and phenylalanine, respectively, and are considered semi-essential. See also **amino acid, nonessential amino acid.**

**essential fatty acid (EFA),** a polyunsaturated acid, such as linoleic, alpha-linolenic, and arachidonic acids, essential in the diet for proper growth, maintenance, and functioning of the body. EFAs are prostaglandin precursors that play important roles in metabolism They are also necessary for the normal functioning of the reproductive and endocrine systems and the breaking up of cholesterol deposits on arterial walls. The best dietary sources are natural vegetable oils, such as soy and corn oils; margarines blended with vegetable oils; wheat germ; edible seeds, such as pumpkin, sesame, and sunflower; and fish oils, especially cod liver and other fish body oil. Although rare, a deficiency of EFAs causes changes in cell structure and enzyme function, resulting in decreased growth and other disorders. Symptoms include brittle and lusterless hair, nail problems, dandruff, allergic conditions, and dermatoses, especially eczema in infants. Also excessive amounts may reduce the level of vitamin E in tissues and cause other metabolic disturbances.

**essential fever,** any fever of unknown origin.

**essential hypertension,** an elevated systemic arterial pressure for which no cause can be found. It is often the only significant clinical finding. Individuals with elevated blood pressure are at risk for cardiovascular disease. In examining patients with essential hypertension, clinicians consider the complex mechanisms that control blood pressure, such as the arterial baroreflex, body fluid regulators, the renin-angiotensin system, and vascular autoregulation. Also called **primary hypertension.** See also **benign hypertension, malignant hypertension.**

**essential mixed cryoglobulinemia,** a rare condition characterized by deposition of type II cryoglobulins without a detectable cause, inducing cutaneous vasculitis, synovitis, and glomerulonephritis. See also **cryoglobulin.**

**essential nutrient,** the carbohydrates, proteins, fats, minerals, vitamins, and water necessary for growth, normal function, and body maintenance. These substances must be supplied by food, because most are not synthesized by the body in the quantities required for normal health.

**essential oil,** a class of generally aromatic volatile oil extracted from plants for use in flavoring foods, perfumes, and medicines. Some have been used therapeutically for thousands of years.

**essential pruritis** [L, *essentia,* quality, *prurire,* to itch], localized or general pruritis that begins without preexisting skin disorder.

**essential thrombocythemia.** See **thrombocytosis.**

**essential tremor,** an involuntary fine shaking of the hand, the head, and the face, especially during routine body movements. It is a familial disorder inherited as an autosomal dominant trait and appears during adolescence or in middle age, slowly progressing as a more pronounced disorder. The precise cause of this condition is not known. Essential tremor is aggravated by activity and emotion and can be reduced in some patients by the administration of mild sedatives, such as propranolol and diazepam. Also called **benign essential tremor, familial tremor.** Compare **parkinsonism.**

**essential vertigo** [L, *essentia,* quality, *vertigo,* dizziness], a form of vertigo for which no organic cause has been found.

**EST.** See **electroconvulsive therapy.**

**established name,** the name assigned to a drug by the U.S. Adopted Names Council. The established name, generally shorter than the chemical name, is the name by which the drug is known to health practitioners. Also called **generic name.** See also **chemical name, trademark.**

**Estar,** trademark for a coal tar preparation used to treat eczema and psoriasis.

**ester** /es'tər/ [Ger, *Essigäther,* acetic ether], a class of chemical compounds formed by the bonding of an alcohol and one or more organic acids. Fats are esters, produced by the bonding of fatty acids with the alcohol glycerol.

**esterase** /es'tərās/, any enzyme that splits esters.

**esterification,** the process of combining an organic acid (RCOOH) with an alcohol (ROH) to form an ester (RCOOR) and water.

**esterified estrogen** /ester'ifīd/, an ester of natural estrogen.

■ INDICATIONS: It is prescribed for menstrual irregularities, contraception, and menopausal symptoms.

■ CONTRAINDICATIONS: Pregnancy, known or suspected breast cancer, thrombophlebitis, vaginal bleeding of unknown origin, or known hypersensitivity to this drug prohibits its use.

■ ADVERSE EFFECTS: Among the more serious adverse reactions are gallbladder disease, thromboembolic disease, and a possible increase in risk of cancer.

**esterify,** to convert into an ester.

**ester local anesthetic,** a class of local anesthetics with an ester group that differentiates it from the amide group of local anesthetics. Ester local anesthetics include **chloroprocaine, benzocaine, cocaine,** and **procaine hydrochloride.**

**esthesia** /esthē'zhə/, **1.** capacity for perception. **2.** sensitivity or feeling. **3.** any disorder of the nervous system that affects perception or sensitivity.

**esthesio-,** combining form meaning 'feeling or perceptive faculties': *esthesiogenic, esthesioneure, esthesioscopy.*

**esthesiophysiology** /esthē'zē·ōfiz'ē·ol'əjē/, the study of sense organ function.

**-esthetic, -esthetical, -esthes, -aesthetic, -aesthetical,** combining form meaning 'a person's consciousness of a sensation or something': *anesthesia, cenesthetic, photoesthetic, somatesthetic.*

**esthetics** /esthet'iks/ [Gk, *aisthetikos,* sensitivity], the branch of philosophy dealing with the forms and psychologic effects of beauty. In medicine, esthetics may be applied to dental reconstruction and plastic surgery.

**Estimated Safe and Adequate Daily Dietary Intake (ESADDI),** nutrient intake recommendations, made by the National Academy of Sciences' Food and Nutrition Board, that give what is considered a safe range of intake for some nutrients because not enough information is available to set recommended dietary allowance values for them.

**Estinyl,** trademark for an estrogen (ethinyl estradiol).

**estr-,** combining form for the name of an estrogen, a female hormone.

**Estrace,** trademark for an estrogen (estradiol).

**estradiol** /es'trədī'ôl/, the most potent naturally occurring human estrogen.

**Estradurin,** trademark for an antineoplastic estrogen (polyestradiol phosphate).

**estramustine phosphate sodium** /es'trəmus'tēn/, an antineoplastic agent.

■ INDICATIONS: It is prescribed for palliative treatment of metastatic or progressive carcinoma of the prostate.

■ CONTRAINDICATIONS: Thromboembolytic disorders or known hypersensitivity to this drug prohibits its use.

■ ADVERSE EFFECTS: The most serious adverse reactions are cerebrovascular accident, myocardial infarction, thrombophlebitis, pulmonary emboli, and congestive heart failure.

**estrangement** /estrānj'mənt/ [L, *extraneus,* not belonging], **1.** a psychologic effect of the separation of a mother from her newborn required when the infant is ill or premature or has a congenital defect, thereby diverting the mother from establishing a normal relationship with her child. **2.** the feeling that external objects have a strange, unfamiliar, or unreal quality, caused by a failure of cathexis of the external ego boundary, one of whose functions is to identify external objects as real and familiar.

**Estratab,** trademark for esterified estrogens.

**Estraval,** trademark for an estrogen (estradiol valerate).

**estrin,** the former name of estrogen.

**estriol** /es'trē·ôl/, a relatively weak naturally occurring human estrogen found in high concentrations in urine. Also spelled **oestriol.** See also **estrogen.**

**estrogen** /es'trojən/ [Gk, *oistros,* gadfly, *genein,* to produce], one of a group of hormonal steroid compounds that promote the development of female secondary sex characteristics. Human estrogen level is elaborated in the ovaries, adrenal cortices, testes, and fetoplacental unit. During the menstrual cycle estrogen renders the female genital tract suitable for fertilization, implantation, and nutrition of the early embryo. Pharmaceutic preparations of estrogen are used in oral contraceptives to prevent pregnancy; palliate certain types of postmenopausal breast cancer and prostatic cancer; inhibit lactation; and treat threatened abortion, osteoporosis, and ovarian disease. Estrogen replacement therapy may be prescribed to relieve the vasomotor symptoms of menopause; its long-term continued use increases the risk of endometrial carcinoma. Kinds of estrogen are **conjugated estrogen, esterified estrogen, estradiol, estriol,** and **estrone.** Also spelled **oestrogen. —estrogenic,** *adj.*

**estrogen fractions test,** a 24-hour urine or blood test that measures levels of the three major estrogens. Test results aid in the evaluation of menopausal status, sexual maturity, gynecomastia or feminization syndromes, certain ovarian tumors, and placental function and fetal normality in high-risk pregnancies.

**estrone** /es'trōn/, a relatively potent estrogen. Also spelled **oestrone.**

**estropipate** /es'trəpip'āt/, an estrogen.

■ INDICATIONS: It is prescribed in the treatment of vasomotor symptoms of menopause, atrophic vaginitis, kraurosis vulvae, female hypogonadism, female castration, and primary ovarian failure.

■ CONTRAINDICATIONS: Known or suspected cancer of the breast or estrogen-dependent neoplasia, pregnancy, thrombophlebitis or thromboembolic disorders, undiagnosed abnormal genital bleeding, or complications of previous administration of estrogen prohibit its use.

■ ADVERSE EFFECTS: Among the most serious adverse reactions are a possible increased risk of cancer, gallbladder disease, and thromboembolic disorders.

**estrus** /es'trəs/, the cyclic period of sexual receptivity in mammals other than primates, marked by intense sexual urge and coinciding with the time that fertilization can take place.

**estrus cycle** [Gk, *oistros,* gadfly, *kyklos,* circle], the periodic changes in the female body that occur under the influence of sex hormones.

**ESWL,** abbreviation for **extracorporeal shock-wave lithotripsy.**

**eta** /ē'tə, ā'tə/, H, η, the seventh letter of the Greek alphabet.

**etanercept,** a biologic agent.

■ INDICATIONS: Etanercept is used to treat acute, chronic rheumatoid arthritis that has not responded to other treatments.

■ CONTRAINDICATIONS: Known hypersensitivity and sepsis prohibit the use of this drug.

■ ADVERSE EFFECTS: Adverse reactions to this drug include abdominal pain, dyspepsia, headache, asthenia, dizziness, injection site reaction, cough, upper respiratory infection, non-upper respiratory infection, and sinusitis. Common side effects include rash, pharyngitis, and rhinitis.

**-etanide.** See **-eridine.**

**état criblé** /ātä'krēblā'/ [Fr, sievelike state], a condition or state of multiple sievelike perforations in swollen lymphatic nodules in the intestine. It is a frequently fatal complication of untreated typhoid fever.

**ethacrynate sodium.** See **ethacrynic acid.**

**ethacrynic acid** /eth'əkrin'ik/, a loop diuretic.

■ INDICATIONS: It is prescribed as a treatment for severe edema, such as nephrotic syndrome, hepatic cirrhoses, and ascites of malignancy.

■ CONTRAINDICATIONS: Pregnancy, anuria, or known hypersensitivity to this drug prohibits its use. It is not given to infants.

■ ADVERSE EFFECTS: Among the more serious adverse reactions are tetany, muscle weakness, cramps, and excessive diuresis. Hearing loss may occur.

**ethambutol hydrochloride** /eth'əmbyo͞o'təl/, a tuberculostatic antibiotic.

■ INDICATION: It is prescribed in the treatment of pulmonary tuberculosis.

■ CONTRAINDICATIONS: Optic neuritis or known hypersensitivity to this drug prohibits its use. It is not recommended for small children.

■ ADVERSE EFFECTS: Among the most serious adverse reactions are diminished visual acuity and allergic reactions, such as rashes.

**ethanedioic acid.** See **oxalic acid**

**ethanoic acid.** See **acetic acid.**

**ethanol** /eth'ənol/, ethyl alcohol. See also **alcohol.**

**ethanolamine.** See **monoethanolamine.**

**ethanol test,** a blood, urine, gastric, or breath test usually performed to evaluate alcohol-impaired drivers or those with alcohol overdose.

**ethaverine hydrochloride** /eth'əver'ēn/, a smooth muscle relaxant.

■ INDICATIONS: It is prescribed to relieve spasm of the GI or genitourinary tract, arterial vasospasm, cerebral insufficiency, and peripheral and cerebrovascular insufficiency.

- CONTRAINDICATIONS: Liver disease, atrioventricular dissociation, or known hypersensitivity to this drug prohibits its use. It is prescribed with caution to patients who have glaucoma.
- ADVERSE EFFECTS: Among the more serious adverse reactions are hypotension, abdominal distress, cardiac arrhythmia, and headache.

**ethchlorvynol** /ethklôr′vənôl/,  a sedative and hypnotic.
- INDICATIONS: It is prescribed in the treatment of insomnia.
- CONTRAINDICATIONS: Porphyria or known hypersensitivity to this drug prohibits its use.
- ADVERSE EFFECTS: Among the most serious adverse reactions are allergic effects, nausea, dizziness, aftertaste, and drug hangover.

**ethene.**  See **ethylene.**

**ether** /ē′thər/ [Gk, *aither,* air],  **1.** any of a class of organic compounds in which two hydrocarbon groups are linked by an oxygen atom. **2.** a nonhalogenated volatile liquid no longer used in clinical practice as a general anesthetic. Also called **diethyl ether.**

**ethereal** /ithir′ē·əl/ [Gk, *aither,* air],  pertaining to or resembling ether.

**ethics** /eth′iks/ [Gk, *ethikos,* moral duty],  the science or study of moral values or principles, including ideals of autonomy, beneficence, and justice.

**Ethics in Patient Referrals Act,**  a federal law, the Stark Law, enacted in 1989, that prohibits referrals by a physician to a clinical laboratory in which the physician has a financial interest. A 1994 amendment includes other services and equipment such as physical and occupational therapy; radiology and other diagnostic services; radiation therapy; parenteral and enteral nutrients, equipment, and supplies; and home health services.

**ethinamate** /ethin′əmāt/,  a sedative.
- INDICATION: It is prescribed in the treatment of insomnia.
- CONTRAINDICATIONS: Known hypersensitivity to this drug prohibits its use. It is not recommended for pregnant women, for people less than 15 years of age, or for persons with a history of drug abuse.
- ADVERSE EFFECTS: Among the more serious adverse reactions are thrombocytopenic purpura, physical and psychologic dependence, and skin rash.

**ethinyl estradiol** /eth′inil/,  an estrogen.
- INDICATIONS: It is prescribed in the treatment of postmenopausal breast cancer, menstrual cycle irregularities, prostatic cancer, and hypogonadism and for contraception and relief of menopausal vasomotor symptoms.
- CONTRAINDICATIONS: Thrombophlebitis, abnormal genital bleeding, known or suspected pregnancy, or known hypersensitivity to this drug prohibits its use.
- ADVERSE EFFECTS: Among the more serious adverse reactions are thrombophlebitis, embolism, and hypercalcemia. See also **estrogen.**

**ethionamide** /eth′ē·ənam′īd/,  a tuberculostatic antibacterial.
- INDICATION: It is prescribed for the treatment of tuberculosis when frontline therapy has failed.
- CONTRAINDICATIONS: Existing liver damage or known hypersensitivity to this drug prohibits its use.
- ADVERSE EFFECTS: Among the more serious adverse reactions are skin rash, jaundice, mental depression, and GI side effects.

**ethmocarditis** /eth′mōkärdī′tis/,  a chronic inflammation of the cardiac connective tissue.

**ethmoid** /eth′moid/ [Gk, *ethmos,* sieve, *eidos,* form],  **1.** pertaining to the ethmoid bone. **2.** having a large number of sievelike openings.

**ethmoidal air cell** /ethmoi′dəl/ [Gk, *ethmos,* sieve, *eidos,* form],  one of the numerous small thin-walled cavities in the ethmoid bone of the skull. The cavities are lined with mucous membrane continuous with that of the nasal cavity and lie between the upper part of the nasal cavities and the orbits. Compare **frontal sinus, maxillary sinus, sphenoidal sinus.**

**ethmoidal process,**  an outgrowth on the superior border of the inferior concha that articulates with the uncinate process of the ethmoid.

**ethmoid bone,**  the very light, sievelike, and spongy bone at the base of the cranium, also forming the roof and most of the walls of the superior part of the nasal cavity. It consists of four parts: a horizontal plate, a perpendicular plate, and two lateral labyrinths.

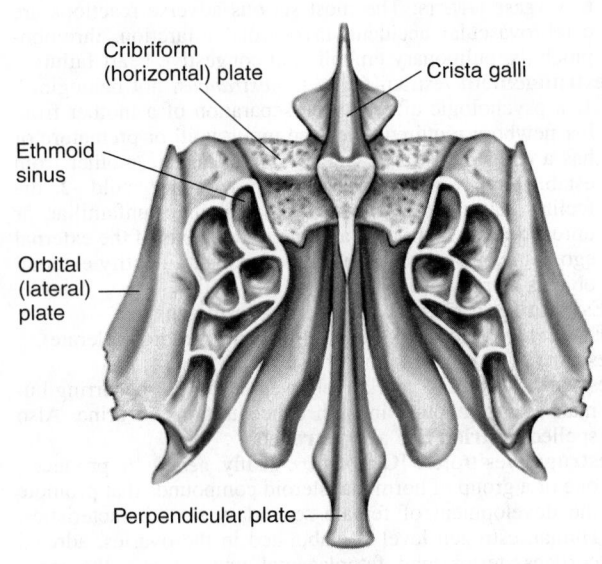

**Ethmoid bone**

**ethmoidofrontal suture** /ethmoi′dōfron′təl/,  a line in the skull between the cribriform plate of the ethmoid and the orbital plate and posterior margin of the nasal process. Also called **frontoethmoidal suture.**

**ethmoidolacrimal suture** /-lak′riməl/,  a line in the skull between the orbital plate of the ethmoid and the posterior margin of the lacrimal bone.

**ethmosphenoid suture** /eth′mōsfē′noid/,  a line in the skull between the crest of the sphenoid bone and the perpendicular and cribriform plates of the ethmoid. Also called **sphenoethmoidal suture.**

**ethnic group** /eth′nik/,  a population of individuals organized on the basis of an assumed common cultural origin.

**ethnocentrism** /eth′nōsen′trizm/ [Gk, *ethnos,* nation, *kentron,* center],  **1.** a belief in the inherent superiority of the "race" or group to which one belongs. **2.** a proclivity to consider other ethnic groups in terms of one's own racial origins.

**ethnography** /ethnog′rəfē/ [Gk, *ethnos,* nation, *graphein,* to record],  a branch of anthropology that is concerned with the history of nations and ethnic populations.

**ethology** /ethol′əjē/ [Gk, *ethos,* character, *logos,* science], **1.** (in zoology) the scientific study of the behavioral patterns of animals, specifically in their native habitat. **2.** (in psychology) the empiric study of human behavior, primarily social customs, manners, and mores. —**ethologic, ethological,** *adj.,* **ethologist,** *n.*

**ethosuximide** /eth′ōsuk′simīd/, an anticonvulsant.
■ INDICATION: It is prescribed in the treatment of petit mal epilepsy.
■ CONTRAINDICATIONS: Known hypersensitivity to this drug or to any succinimide medication prohibits its use.
■ ADVERSE EFFECTS: Among the more serious adverse reactions are blood dyscrasias, GI disturbance, and hematopoietic complications.

**ethotoin** /eth′ōtō′in/, an anticonvulsant.
■ INDICATIONS: It is prescribed in the treatment of generalized tonic-clonic and complex-partial seizures.
■ CONTRAINDICATIONS: Liver disease, hematologic disorders, or known hypersensitivity to this drug or to any hydantoin prohibits its use. It is not recommended for use during pregnancy or lactation.
■ ADVERSE EFFECTS: Among the more serious adverse reactions are blood disorders, nausea, fatigue, skin rash, alopecia, erythema multiforme, exfoliative dermatitis, and chest pain.

**Ethrane,** trademark for an inhalational general anesthetic (enflurane).

**Ethril,** trademark for an antibacterial (erythromycin stearate).

**ethyl alcohol.** See **alcohol.**

**ethyl aminobenzoate.** See **benzocaine.**

**ethyl chloride** /eth′il/, a topical anesthetic used in short operations.
■ INDICATIONS: It is prescribed in the treatment of skin irritations and in minor skin surgery.
■ CONTRAINDICATIONS: Known hypersensitivity to this drug prohibits its use. It is not used on broken skin or on mucous membrane.
■ ADVERSE EFFECTS: Among the more serious adverse reactions are pain, muscle spasm, and, as a result of excessive use, frostbite.
■ NOTE: It is highly flammable.

**ethylene** /eth′əlēn/ [Gk, *aither,* air, *hyle,* stuff], a colorless flammable gas that is lighter than air and has a slightly sweet odor and taste. It was previously used as a general anesthetic and is slightly more potent than nitrous oxide. Also called **ethene, olefiant gas.**

**ethylenediamine** /eth′əlēndi·am′ēn/, a clear thick liquid having the odor of ammonia. It is used as a solvent, an emulsifier, and a stabilizer with aminophylline injections.

**ethylene dibromide (EDB),** a volatile liquid used as an insecticide and gasoline additive. Because it has been found to be a cause of cancer in animals, the Environmental Protection Agency has restricted the use of EDB to control insect pests in grains and fruits intended for human use.

**ethylene dichloride poisoning,** the toxic effects of exposure to ethylene dichloride, a hydrocarbon solvent, diluent, and fumigant, which is one of the most abundant of all chlorinated organic chemicals. It is an eye, ear, nose, throat, and skin irritant and has produced cancers in laboratory animals. Inhalation or ingestion can lead to serious illness or death. The compound is metabolized into 2-chloroethanol and monochloroacetic acid, both more toxic than the original chemical.

**ethylene glycol poisoning,** the toxic reaction to ingestion of ethylene glycol or diethylene glycol, chemicals used in automobile antifreeze preparations. Symptoms in mild cases may resemble those of alcohol intoxication but without the breath odor produced by alcoholic beverages. Vomiting, carpopedal spasm, lumbar pain, renal failure, respiratory distress, convulsions, and coma may also occur.

**ethylene oxide ($CH_2CH_2O$),** a highly flammable gas used to sterilize surgical instruments and other supplies.

**ethylestrenol,** an anabolic steroid.

**ethyl oxide,** an alternative name for diethyl ether.

**ethynodiol diacetate and ethinyl estradiol,** an oral contraceptive.
■ INDICATION: It is prescribed for prevention of pregnancy.
■ CONTRAINDICATIONS: Thrombophlebitis, cardiovascular disease, breast or reproductive organ cancer, or known hypersensitivity to either ingredient prohibits its use.
■ ADVERSE EFFECTS: Among the more serious adverse reactions are thrombophlebitis, uterine fibroma, gallbladder disease, embolism, and hepatic lesions.

**ethynodiol diacetate and mestranol,** an oral contraceptive.
■ INDICATION: It is prescribed for contraception.
■ CONTRAINDICATIONS: Thrombophlebitis, cardiovascular disease, breast or reproductive organ cancer, or known hypersensitivity to either ingredient prohibits its use.
■ ADVERSE EFFECTS: Among the more serious adverse reactions are thrombophlebitis, uterine fibroma, gallbladder disease, embolism, and hepatic lesions.

**-etic,** suffix used as the equivalent of *-ic* in forming adjectives: *enuretic, genetic, kinetic.*

**etidocaine.** See **amide local anesthetic.**

**etidronate disodium** /etid′rənāt/, a regulator of calcium metabolism. Also called **sodium etidronate.**
■ INDICATIONS: It is prescribed in the treatment of Paget's disease and heterotopic ossification caused by injury to the spinal cord, and after total hip replacement.
■ CONTRAINDICATIONS: There are no known contraindications.
■ ADVERSE EFFECTS: Among the more serious adverse reactions are bone pain both at pagetic sites and at previously asymptomatic sites, GI disturbances, and elevated serum phosphate concentrations.

**etio-,** prefix meaning 'causation': *etiology.*

**etiology** /ē′tē·ol′əjē/ [Gk, *aitia,* cause, *logos,* science], **1.** the study of all factors that may be involved in the development of a disease, including the susceptibility of the patient, the nature of the disease agent, and the way in which the patient's body is invaded by the agent. **2.** the cause of a disease. Compare **pathogenesis.** —**etiologic,** *adj.*

**etomidate** /etom′idāt/, a short-acting and hypnotic nonbarbiturate IV agent for induction of general anesthesia. It has minimal adverse cardiovascular and respiratory effects, thus providing a greater margin of safety in patients at risk because of heart disease. Adverse effects include transient interference with adrenal releasing cortisol and perhaps postoperative stimulates more than barbiturates.

**etoposide,** an antineoplastic or chemotherapeutic agent and mitotic inhibitor.
■ INDICATIONS: It is prescribed in the treatment of cancer of the testicles and small cell lung cancer to prevent tumor cells from dividing and spreading.
■ CONTRAINDICATIONS: The drug should not be used if there is an allergy to etoposide or podophyllum. The safety of the drug in breastfeeding women and in children has not been established. There is a potential adverse effect to the fetus if used by a pregnant patient.
■ ADVERSE EFFECTS: The side effects most often reported include chills, rapid heartbeat, painful or difficult breathing, decreased blood pressure, hair loss, rash, itching, skin discoloration, and digestive disorders.

**Etrafon,** trademark for a central nervous system fixed-combination drug containing a tranquilizer (perphenazine) and an antidepressant (amitriptyline hydrochloride).

**etretinate** /etret'ināt/, a synthetic derivative of vitamin A used as an oral drug to treat psoriasis.

■ INDICATIONS: Etretinate is prescribed for severe recalcitrant psoriasis, including generalized pustular and erythrodermic psoriasis.

■ CONTRAINDICATIONS: It is contraindicated for women who are of childbearing age unless a pregnancy test within 2 weeks of the start of therapy has negative results. Because of the risk of hyperostosis, the drug should not be given to children unless all alternative therapies have been exhausted. Intolerance to vitamin A derivative is another contraindication

■ ADVERSE EFFECTS: Adverse reactions may include benign intracranial hypertension, hepatitis, visual abnormalities including corneal damage, skeletal hyperostosis, peeling skin, alopecia, muscle cramps, and headache.

**etymology** [Gk, *etymos,* base; L, *logos,* words], the study of the origin and development of words. An **etymon** (*pl.* **etyma**) is an earlier form of a word.

**Eu,** symbol for the element **europium.**

**eu-,** prefix meaning 'well, easily, good, true': *euangiotic, eucrasia, euthyroid.*

**Eubacterium** /yōo'baktir'ē·əm/, a genus of gram-positive anaerobic rod-shaped bacteria normally found in soil and water. The organisms are also found in the skin and cavities of humans and other mammals, where they may cause soft-tissue infections. One species has been found in dental tartar; another synthesizes vitamin $B_{12}$.

**eubiotics** /yōo'bī·ot'iks/ [Gk, *eu,* well, *bios,* life], the science of healthy living.

**eucalyptol** /yōo'kəlip'tol/, a substance with an aromatic odor obtained from the volatile oil of *Eucalyptus* and used in nasal emollients. Also called **cajeputol.**

**eucaryocyte.** See **eukaryocyte.**

**eucaryon.** See **eukaryon.**

**eucaryosis.** See **eukaryosis.**

**eucaryote, eucaryotic.** See **eukaryote.**

**eucatropine hydrochloride** /yōokat'rəpin/, an ophthalmic anticholinergic.

■ INDICATION: It is prescribed for dilating the pupil in an ophthalmoscopic examination of the eye.

■ CONTRAINDICATIONS: Known hypersensitivity to this drug or to other anticholinergics prohibits its use.

■ ADVERSE EFFECTS: Among the most serious adverse reactions are tachycardia and severe constipation. Dry mouth, heat intolerance, and other effects associated with systemic absorption of an anticholinergic agent may also occur.

**eucholia** /yōokō'lyə/ [Gk, *eu,* well, *chole,* bile], the normal state of the bile as to the quantity secreted and the condition of the constituents.

**euchromatin** /yōokrō'mətin/ [Gk, *eu* + *chroma,* color], the part of a chromosome that is active in gene expression. It stains most deeply during mitosis, when it is in a coiled, condensed state; during each repetition of the cell cycle, it alternates between condensation and dispersion. Compare **heterochromatin.** See also **chromatin.** —**euchromatic,** *adj.*

**euchromosome.** See **autosome.**

**eugamy** /yōo'gəmē/ [Gk, *eu* + *gamos,* marriage], the union of gametes that contain the same haploid number of chromosomes. —**eugamic,** *adj.*

**eugenics** /yōojen'iks/ [Gk, *eu* + *genein,* to produce], the study of methods for controlling the characteristics of populations through selective breeding.

**euglobulin** /yōoglob'yəlin/ [Gk, *eu* + L, *globulus,* small sphere], that fraction of serum globulin that is insoluble in distilled water but soluble in saline solutions. This is one of a number of different properties used to classify proteins. Compare **albumin, cryoglobulin.** See also **plasma protein, electrophoresis.**

**euglobulin lysis time test,** a blood test used to identify primary and secondary systemic fibrinolysis, and to monitor streptokinase or urokinase therapy in patients with acute myocardial infarction.

**eugnathia** /yōo·na'thē·ə/ [Gk, *eu,* well + *gnathos,* jaw], an abnormality of the oral cavity that is limited to the teeth and their immediate alveolar supports and does not include the jaws. Compare **dysgnathic anomaly.**

**eugnathic anomaly** /yōonath'ik/ [Gk, *eu* + *gnathos,* jaw; *anomalia,* irregularity], an abnormality of the teeth and their alveolar supports. Compare **dysgnathic anomaly.**

**eukaryocyte** /yōoker'ē·ōsīt'/ [Gk, *eu* + *karyon,* nut, *kytos,* cell], a cell that has a true nucleus, found in all organisms except bacteria. Also spelled **eucaryocyte.**

**eukaryon** /yōoker'ē·on/ [Gk, *eu,* good, *karyon,* nut], a cell nucleus that is highly complex and organized and is surrounded by a double membrane. Also spelled **eucaryon.** Compare **prokaryon.**

**eukaryosis** /yōoker'i·ō'sis/ [Gk, *eu* + *karyon,* nut, *osis,* condition], the state of having a eukaryon. Compare **prokaryosis.**

**eukaryote** /yōoker'ē·ot/ [Gk, *eu* + *karyon,* nut], an organism whose cells contain a true nucleus. All organisms except bacteria are eukaryotes. Also spelled **eucaryote.** —**eukaryotic, eukaryotic,** *adj.*

**Eulexin,** trademark for a hormonal antineoplastic agent (flutamide).

**eunuch** /yōo'nək/ [Gk, *eune,* couch, *echein,* to guard], a male whose testicles have been destroyed or removed. If this occurs before puberty, secondary sex characteristics fail to develop, and symptoms such as a feminine voice and absence of facial hair can result from the reduced level of male hormones in the blood. See also **secondary sex characteristic.**

**eunuchism** /yōo'nəkiz'əm/, the condition of being a eunuch with the lack of male hormones caused by castration.

**eunuchoidism** /yōo'nəkoidiz'əm/, a condition resulting from a deficiency in the production or effectiveness of male hormones. The deficiency leads to sterility, abnormal tallness, small testes, and impaired development of secondary sexual characteristics, libido, and sexual potency.

**euphoretic** /yōo'fəret'ik/ [Gk, *eu* + *pherein,* to bear], **1.** (of a substance or event) tending to produce a condition of well-being or elation. **2.** a substance tending to produce a feeling of well-being or elation, as lysergic acid diethylamide (LSD), mescaline, marijuana, and other hallucinogenic drugs.

**euphoria** /yōofôr'ē·ə/ [Gk, *eu* + *pherein,* to bear], **1.** a feeling or state of well-being or elation. **2.** an exaggerated or abnormal sense of physical and emotional well-being not based on reality or truth, disproportionate to its cause, and inappropriate to the situation, as commonly seen in the manic stage of bipolar disorder, in some forms of schizophrenia, in organic mental disorders, and in toxic and drug-induced states. Compare **ecstasy.**

**euploid** /yōo'ploid/ [Gk, *eu* + *ploos,* multiple], **1.** an individual, organism, strain, or cell whose chromosome number is an integral multiple of the normal haploid number characteristic of the species. Euploids may be as diploid, triploid, tetraploid, or polyploid. **2.** pertaining to such an individual, organism, strain, or cell. **—euploidy,** *n.* Compare **aneuploid.**

**euploidy** /yo͞o′ploidē/, the state or condition of having a variation in chromosome number that is an exact multiple of the characteristic haploid number. Compare **aneuploidy.**

**eupnea** /yo͞op·nē′ə/ [Gk, *eu,* well, *pnein,* to breathe], normal, quiet breathing at a rate of 12 to 20 breaths per minute in adults.

**Eurax,** trademark for a scabicide (crotamiton).

**European blastomycosis.** See **cryptococcosis.**

**European typhus.** See **epidemic typhus.**

**europium (Eu)** /yo͞oro͞o′pē·əm/ [Europe], a metallic rare earth element. Its atomic number is 63; its atomic weight (mass) is 151.96.

**eury-,** combining form meaning 'wide, broad': *eurycephalic, eurygnathic, euryopia.*

**eustachian salpingitis,** an inflammation of the eustachian tube.

**eustachian tube** /yo͞ostā′shən/ [Bartolomeo Eustachio, Italian anatomist, 1524–1574; L, *tubus*], a tube lined with mucous membrane that joins the nasopharynx and the middle ear cavity. It is normally closed but opens during yawning, chewing, and swallowing to allow equalization of the air pressure in the middle ear with atmospheric pressure.

**eustress** /yo͞o′stres/, **1.** a positive form of stress. **2.** a balance between selfishness and altruism through which an individual develops the drive and energy to care for others.

**euthanasia** /yo͞o′thənā′zhə/ [Gk, *eu,* good; *thanatos,* death], **1.** the deliberate causing of the death of a person who is suffering from an incurable disease or condition. It may be active such as by administration of a lethal drug or passive by withholding of treatment. Legal authorities, church leaders, philosophers, and commentators on ethics and morality usually distinguish passive euthanasia from active euthanasia. Also called **mercy killing. 2.** a easy, quiet, painless death.

**euthenics** /yo͞othen′iks/ [Gk, *eu* + *tithenai,* to place], the science that deals with improvement of the human species through the control of environmental factors, as pollution, malnutrition, disease, and drug abuse. Compare **eugenics.**

**Euthroid,** trademark for a thyroid hormone preparation (liotrix, a combination of levothyroxine sodium and liothyronine sodium).

**euthymia,** a pleasant relaxed state of tranquility.

**euthymic,** pertaining to a normal mood in which the range of emotions is neither depressed nor highly elevated.

**euthymism** /yo͞othī′mizəm/ [Gk, *eu* + *thymos,* thyme flowers], the characteristic of normal mood responses.

**euthyroid** /yo͞othī′roid/ [Gk, *eu,* well, *thyreos,* oblong shield], pertaining to a normal thyroid gland and normal thyroid gland function.

**evacuant** /ivak′yo͞o·ənt/ [L, *evacuare,* to empty], any medicine or other agent that causes an organ to discharge its contents, as an emetic or laxative.

**evacuate** /ivak′yo͞o·āt/ [L, *evacuare,* to empty], **1.** to discharge or to remove a substance from a cavity, space, organ, or tract of the body. **2.** a substance discharged or removed from the body, such as evacuation of stool. **—evacuation,** *n.*

**evacuator** /ivak′yo͞o·ā′tər/, an instrument for emptying a cavity, such as removing a calculus from the urinary bladder.

**evagination** /ēvaj′inā′shən/, the turning inside-out or protrusion of a body part or organ.

**evaluating** /ival′yo͞o·ā′ting/ [L, *ex,* away, *valare,* to be strong], (in five-step nursing process) a category of nursing behavior in which the extent to which the established goals of care have been met is determined and recorded. To make this judgment, the nurse estimates the degree of success in meeting the goals, evaluates the implementation of nursing measures, investigates the patient's compliance with therapy, and records the patient's response to therapy. The nurse evaluates effects of the measures used, the need for change in goals of care, the accuracy of the implementation of nursing measures, and the need for change in the patient's environment or in the equipment or procedures used. The impact of the care or treatment on the patient, the patient's family, and the staff is evaluated; the accuracy of tests and measurements is checked; and the patient's and family's understanding of the information given them is evaluated. The patient's expressed and observed response to care is recorded. Although evaluation is considered the final step of the five-step nursing process, in practice it is integral to effective nursing practice at all steps of the process. See also **analyzing, assessing, implementing, nursing process, planning.**

**Evans blue** [Herbert Evans, American anatomist, 1882–1971], a nontoxic blue-green dye. It has been used to determine blood and plasma volumes.

**evaporate.** See **evaporation.**

**evaporated milk** /ivap′ərā′tid/, homogenized whole milk from which 50% to 60% of the water content has been evaporated. It is fortified with vitamin D, canned, and sterilized. When it is diluted with an equal amount of water, its nutritional value is comparable to that of fresh whole milk.

**evaporation** /ivap′ərā′shən/ [L, *ex* + *vapor,* steam], the change of a substance from a liquid state to a gaseous state. The process of evaporation is hastened by an increase in temperature and a decrease in atmospheric pressure. See also **boiling point. —evaporate,** *v.*

**eventration** /ē′vəntrā′shən/, the protrusion of the intestines from the abdomen.

**event-related potential (ERP)** [L, *evenire,* to happen, *relatus,* carry back, *potentia,* power], a type of brain wave that is associated with a response to a specific stimulus, such as a particular wave pattern observed when a patient hears a clicking sound. See also **evoked potential.**

**evergreen contract,** a health care contract that is automatically renewed for the term of the contract unless it is renegotiated. Not applicable in Canada.

**eversion** /ivur′zhən/, a turning outward or inside-out, such as a turning of the foot outward at the ankle.

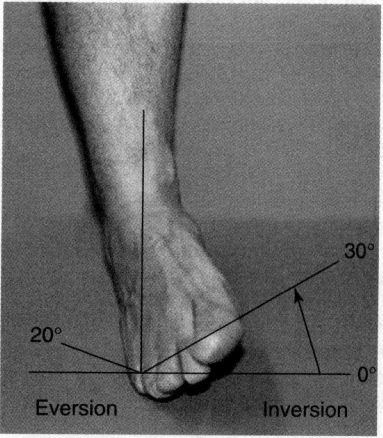

**Eversion and inversion of the foot**
*(Seidel et al, 1995/Patrick Watson)*

**everywhere lines.** See **Kerley lines.**

**evisceration** /ivis′ərā′shən/ [L, *ex* + *viscera,* entrails],
**1.** the removal of the viscera from the abdominal cavity;
disembowelment. **2.** the removal of the contents from an organ or an organ from its cavity. **3.** the protrusion of an internal organ through a wound or surgical incision, especially in
the abdominal wall. —**eviscerate,** *v.*

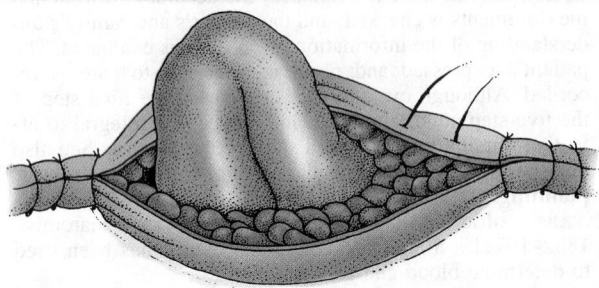

**Evisceration** *(Ignatavicius, Workman, and Mishler, 1999)*

**evocation** /ev′ōkā′shən/ [L, *evocare,* to call forth], a specific morphogenetic change within a developing embryo
that results from the action of a single hormone or other
chemical. See also **induction.**

**evocator** /ev′ōkā′tər/ [L, *evocare,* to call forth], a specific
chemical substance or hormone that is emitted from the organizer part of the embryonic tissue and acts as a morphogenetic stimulus in the developing embryo.

**evoked potential (EP)** /ivōkt′/ [L, *evocare,* to call forth, *potentia,* power], an electrical response in the brainstem or
cerebral cortex that is elicited by a specific stimulus. The
stimulus may affect the visual, auditory, or somatosensory
pathway, producing a characteristic brain wave pattern. The
activity and function of the system may be monitored during
surgery while the patient is unconscious. The surgeon is thus
able to prevent damage to the nerves during operative procedures. Evoked potentials are also used to diagnose multiple
sclerosis and various disorders of hearing and of sight.
Kinds of evoked potentials include **brainstem auditory
evoked potential, somatosensory evoked potential,** and
**visual evoked potential.** See also **brain electrical activity
map.**

**evoked potential studies (EP),** an electrodiagnostic test
indicated for patients with suspected sensory deficit who are
unable to or unreliable in indicating stimulus recognition.
Evoked potential studies are used to evaluate areas of the
cortex that receive incoming stimulus from the eyes, ears, and
lower/upper extremity sensory nerves; to monitor natural
progression or treatment of deteriorating neurologic diseases;
and to identify histrionic or malingering patients with sensory
deficit complaints. These studies include visual-evoked responses (VERs), auditory brainstem-evoked potentials
(ABEPs), and somatosensory-evoked responses (SERs).

**evoked response audiometry,** a method of testing hearing ability at the level of the brainstem and auditory cortex.
Evoked response audiometry is useful in diagnosing possible defects in the vestibulocochlear nerve and brainstem
auditory pathways.

**evolution** /ev′əlōō′shən/ [L, *evolvere,* to roll forth], **1.** a
gradual, orderly, and continuous process of change and development from one condition or state to another. It encompasses all aspects of life, including physical, psychologic,
sociologic, cultural, and intellectual development, and involves a progressive advancement from a simple to a more
complex form or state through the processes of modification, differentiation, and growth. **2.** a change in the genetic
composition of a population of organisms over time. **3.** the
appearance over long periods of time of new taxonomic
groups of organims from preexisting groups. Kinds of evolution are **convergent evolution, determinant evolution,
emergent evolution, organic evolution, orthogenic evolution,** and **saltatory evolution.** —**evolutionist,** *n.*

**evolution of infarction,** the normal healing process after a
myocardial infarction, as demonstrated on successive electrocardiograms.

**evulsed tooth.** See **avulsed tooth.**

**Ewing's sarcoma** /yōō′ingz/ [James Ewing, American pathologist, 1866–1943], a malignant tumor that develops
from bone marrow, usually in long bones or the pelvis. It occurs most frequently in adolescent boys and is characterized
by pain, swelling, fever, and leukocytosis. The tumor, a soft,
crumbly grayish mass that may invade surrounding soft tissues, may be difficult to distinguish histologically from a
neuroblastoma or a lymphoma. Surgery, chemotherapy, and
radiotherapy are often used in treatment. Also called **endothelial myeloma,** *Ewing's tumor.* See also **neuroblastoma,
reticulum cell sarcoma.**

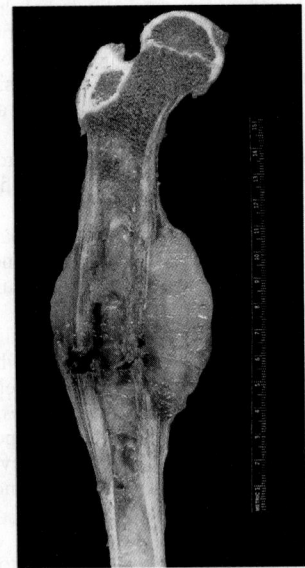

**Ewing's sarcoma** *(Fletcher, 2000)*

**ex-,** prefix meaning 'away from, outside, without': *excoriation, exfoliatio, exocrinous.*

**exa-,** prefix of a Standard International unit that indicates
$10^{18}$.

**exacerbation** /igzas′ərbā′shən/ [L, *exacerbare,* to provoke],
an increase in the seriousness of a disease or disorder as
marked by greater intensity in the signs or symptoms of the
patient being treated.

**examination,** a critical inspection and investigation, usually following a particular method, performed for diagnostic or investigational purposes.

**examination assistance,** a nursing intervention from the Nursing Interventions Classification (NIC) is defined as providing assistance to the patient and another health care provider during a procedure or exam. See also **Nursing Interventions Classification.**

**exanthem** /ig′zan′thəm/ [Gk, eruption], a rapidly erupting rash that may have specific diagnostic features of an infectious disease. Chickenpox, measles, roseola infantum, and rubella are usually characterized by a particular type of exanthem. Also called **exanthema.** Compare **enanthem.** —**exanthematous,** *adj.*

**exanthema subitum.** See **roseola infantum.**

**exanthematous** /ig′zənthem′ətəs/ [Gk, *ex,* out, *anthema,* blossoming], pertaining to the skin rash that accompanies an infectious disease.

**exanthem subitum.** See **roseola infantum.**

**excavatio rectouterina.** See **Douglas's cul-de-sac.**

**excavator** /eks′kə·vāt′ər/ [L, *ex,* out + *cavus,* hollow], **1.** an instrument for hollowing out something by removing the center or inner part, or for making a hole or cavity. **2.** a scoop or gouge for surgical use.

**excessive sweat** /ikses′iv/ [L, *excedere,* to go out; AS, *swaeaten*], perspiration greater than normal for the ambient environment. It is usually a sign of septic fever, pulmonary tuberculosis, hyperthyroidism, chronic renal disease, or malaria. Abnormal sweating of the hands and feet is often a sign of nervous irritability or other emotional stress.

**excess mortality** /ikses′/ [L, *excedere,* to go out, *mortalis,* mortal], a premature death, or one that occurs before the average life expectancy for a person of a particular demographic category.

**Exchange Lists for Meal Planning,** a grouping of foods in which the carbohydrates, fats, proteins, and calories are similar for the serving sizes listed. The lists, published by the American Dietetic Association and the American Diabetes Association, are used in meal planning for various diseases as well as for weight reduction. Foods are divided into three different groups or lists: carbohydrates, meat and meat substitutes, and fats. The carbohydrate group is subdivided into lists of starch, fruit, milk, other carbohydrates, and vegetables. A dietitian can create an appropriate dietary program prescribing the number of calories and units of each exchange category to be consumed daily, as well as a plan for when they should be eaten. The patient selects preferred foods from the lists. Other countries such as Canada use similar lists, for example Food Choices.

**exchange transfusion in the newborn** /iks·chāng′/ [L, *ex* + *cambire,* to change], the introduction of whole blood in exchange for 75% to 85% of an infant's circulating blood that is repeatedly withdrawn in small amounts and replaced with equal amounts of donor blood. The procedure is performed to improve the oxygen-carrying capacity of the blood in the treatment of erythroblastosis neonatorum by removing Rh and ABO antibodies, sensitized erythrocytes that produce hemolysis, and accumulated bilirubin.

■ METHOD: A radiant heat warmer, pacifier, and cardiac and respiratory monitors are prepared, and resuscitative equipment and drugs, including oxygen, a mask, a bag, suction apparatus, glucose, calcium, and sodium bicarbonate, are made readily available. The results of laboratory studies of the infant's bilirubin, hemoglobin, and calcium levels; hematocrit; blood culture; and random blood glucose test and the donor blood culture are checked. The donor blood is checked to make certain that it is not more than 48 hours old; if fresh whole blood is not used, stored blood is mixed in amounts as ordered with frozen plasma or human plasma protein fraction (Plasmanate). Before exchange transfusion nothing is administered by mouth for 3 to 4 hours, or the contents of the infant's stomach are aspirated. The baby's extremities are restrained; the blood is warmed as ordered, and the physician is assisted with the insertion of an umbilical venous line, if one is not in place. The physician may administer albumin with the donor blood. The procedure may be carried out under phototherapy lights; unless contraindicated, the infant's parents may be present. During the procedure the young patient is observed for bradycardia with less than 100 beats a minute, cyanosis, hypothermia, vomiting, aspiration, apnea, an air embolus, abdominal distension, or cardiac arrest. The respiratory and cardiac rates are checked every 5 minutes, the axillary temperature every 15 to 30 minutes. The integrity of all blood tubing connections is inspected periodically. The amount of blood withdrawn and infused is recorded, and the physician is notified when each 100 mL of blood has been exchanged. A repetition of laboratory studies is requested as ordered for the last amount of blood removed from the infant. After the procedure the infant is observed for signs of tachycardia or bradycardia, tachypnea or bradypnea, hypothermia, lethargy, jitteriness, increasing jaundice, cyanosis, edema, dark urine, bleeding from the cord, convulsions, or complications, such as hemorrhage, hypocalcemia, heart failure, hypoglycemia, sepsis, acidosis, hyperkalemia, thrombus formation, or shock. The infant is maintained in a neutral thermal environment and is handled gently and minimally for the next 2 to 4 hours. The cardiac and respiratory rates are monitored every 15 minutes for 4 hours, then every 30 to 60 minutes for 24 to 48 hours or as ordered. The axillary temperature is checked every 1 to 3 hours for 48 hours, and the cord is observed for bleeding every 5 to 15 minutes for 1 to 2 hours after the procedure. Feeding by gavage or a bottle with a soft nipple with a large enough hole to ensure adequate intake is initiated 4 to 6 hours after the transfusion, as ordered; the infant is fed slowly and repositioned after each feeding. Fluid intake and output are measured, and ongoing care is provided as for all high-risk infants.

■ INTERVENTIONS: The nurse prepares the equipment and infant for the exchange transfusion, assists the physician in the insertion of the umbilical venous line, and monitors the baby during and after the procedure.

■ OUTCOME CRITERIA: An exchange transfusion is usually administered only to a high-risk infant, but the procedure often effectively counteracts the hemolytic anemia and hyperbilirubinemia associated with erythroblastosis neonatorum.

**excimer laser** /ek′simər/, one of a class of lasers with output in the ultraviolet range of the electromagnetic spectrum. The name is derived from the symbol formed by the combination of xenon atoms (Xe) and halogen atoms (X) to yield xenon-halide compounds as XEX.

**excise** /iksīz′/ [L, *ex* + *caedere,* to cut], to remove completely, as in the surgical excision of the palatine tonsils. Compare **resect.**

**excision** /iksish′ən/ [L, *ex* + *caedere,* to cut], **1.** the process of excising or amputating. **2.** (in molecular genetics) the process by which a genetic element is removed from a strand of deoxyribonucleic acid.

**excitability** /iksī′təbil′itē/ [L, *excitare,* to arouse], the property of a cell that enables it to react to irritation or stimulation, such as the ability of a nerve or muscle cell to react to an electric stimulus.

**excitant** /eksī′tənt/, a drug or other agent that arouses the central nervous system or other body system in a particular manner. Excitants may be drugs or other substances, such as caffeine, or visual or auditory stimuli.

**excitation** /ek′sitā′shən/ [L, *excitare,* to rouse], a state of mental or physical excitement; nerve or muscle action on impulse.

**excitatory amino acids** /eksī′tətôr′ē/, one of a group of amino acids that affect the central nervous system by acting as neurotransmitters and in some cases as neurotoxins. Examples include glutamate and aspartate, which cause depolarization but may also trigger the death of neurons. Some excitatory amino acids are produced by plants and fungi and may be responsible for hypoxic or hypoglycemic brain damage.

**excitatory impulse,** a sudden force that stimulates activity.

**excited state** /eksī′tid/ [L, *excitare,* to rouse, *status*], (in chemistry and physics) an energy level of a system that is higher than the ground state. The system decays to the ground state and emits the energy difference, usually in the form of photons.

**excitement** /eksīt′mənt/, (in psychiatry) a pathologic state marked by emotional intensity, impulsive behavior, anticipation, and arousal. Excitement in schizophrenic patients tends to result from blocked communications and hostile feelings between the patients and the hospital staff.

**exciting eye,** (in sympathetic ophthalmia) the eye that sustains a penetrating injury and causes an inflammatory reaction in the fellow eye. Also called **inciting eye.**

**exclusion from base price,** a health care contract provision in which high-cost variable items beyond the control of the provider, such as organ procurement costs, are excluded from the base price. Not applicable in Canada.

**Exclusive Provider Organization (EPO),** a type of managed health care organization in which no coverage is typically provided for services received outside the EPO. However, some EPOs incorporate the primary care physician gatekeeper concept along with prospective approval of referrals to specialists of providers outside the EPO.

**excoriation** /ekskôr′ē·ā′shən/ [L, *excoriare,* to flay], an injury to a surface of the body caused by trauma, such as scratching, abrasion, or a chemical or thermal burn.

**excrement** /eks′krəmənt/, any waste matter, particularly feces, discharged from the body.

**excreta** /ekskrē′tə/ [L, *excernere,* to separate], any waste matter discharged from the body.

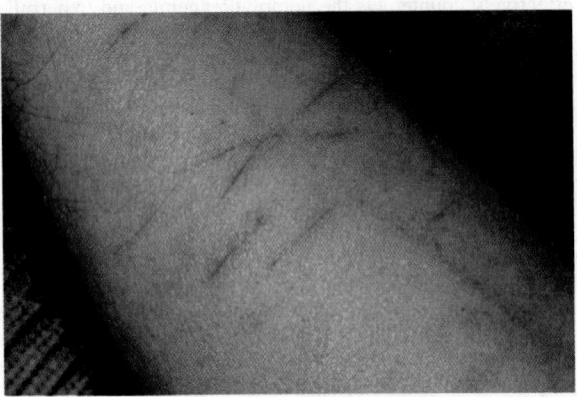

**Excoriations from tree branch scratches**
*(Lemmi and Lemmi, 2000)*

**excrete** /ekskrēt′/ [L, *excernere,* to separate], to evacuate a waste substance from the body, often via a normal secretion; for example, a drug may be excreted in breast milk.

**excretion** /ekskrē′shən/, the process of eliminating, shedding, or getting rid of substances by body organs or tissues, as part of a natural metabolic activity. Excretion usually begins at the cellular level, where water, carbon dioxide, and other waste products of cellular life are emptied into the capillaries. The epidermis excretes dead skin cells by shedding them daily.

**excretory** /eks′krətôr′ē/ [L, *excernere,* to separate], relating to the process of excretion, often used in combination with a term to identify an object or procedure associated with excretion, such as **excretory urography.**

**excretory duct,** a duct that is conductive but not secretory.

**excretory organ,** an organ that is concerned primarily with the production and discharge of body wastes.

**excretory urography** [L, *excernere,* to separate; Gk, *ouron,* urine, *graphein,* to record], the radiographic examination of the urinary tract. It is accomplished with the use of contrast medium that is injected into the blood, filtered by the kidneys, and passed through the tract. Also called **intravenous pyelography (IVP).**

**excursion** /ikskur′zhən/ [L, *ex,* out, *currere,* to run], a departure or deviation from a direct or normal course.

**execute** /ek′səkyoot/, (of a computer) to follow a set of instructions to complete a program or specified function.

**executive physical** /iksek′yətiv/, a physical examination that includes extensive laboratory, radiographic, and other tests that may be provided periodically to management level personnel at employer expense. Such examinations may be detailed, expensive, and overly complete.

**exemestane,** an antineoplastic.

■ INDICATIONS: Exemestane is used to treat advanced breast cancer in postmenopausal patients whose cancer is unresponsive to other therapies.

■ CONTRAINDICATIONS: Use of this drug is prohibited in premenopausal women, pregnant women, and clients with known hypersensitivity to this drug.

■ ADVERSE EFFECTS: Adverse effects of this drug include fatigue, diarrhea, constipation, abdominal pain, increased appetite, hypertension, depression, insomnia, anxiety, cough, and dyspnea. Common side effects include nausea, vomiting, hot flashes, and headache.

**exencephaly** /ek′sən·sef′ə·lē/ [L, *ex,* out + Gk, *enkephalos,* brain], a developmental anomaly characterized by lack of all or part of the skull, so that the brain is exposed.

**exercise** /ek′sərsiz/ [L, *exercere,* to exercise], **1.** the performance of any physical activity for the purpose of conditioning the body, improving health, or maintaining fitness or as a means of therapy for correcting a deformity or restoring the organs and body functions to a state of health. **2.** any action, skill, or maneuver that causes muscle exertion and is performed repeatedly to develop or strengthen the body or any of its parts. **3.** to use a muscle or part of the body in a repetitive way to maintain or develop its strength. Exercise has a beneficial effect on each of the body systems, although in excess it can lead to the breakdown of tissue and cause injury. Kinds of exercise are **active assisted exercise, active exercise, active resistance exercise, aerobic exercise, anaerobic exercise, corrective exercise, isometric exercise, isotonic exercise, muscle-setting exercise, passive exercise, progressive resistance exercise, range of motion exercise,** and **underwater exercise.**

**exercise amenorrhea,** a suppression of ovulation and thus menstruation that affects some women who participate in high-intensity athletics. See also **stress amenorrhea.**

**exercise electrocardiogram (exercise ECG),** an electrocardiogram that is recorded as a person walks on a treadmill or pedals a stationary bicycle for a given length of time at a specific rate of speed. It is important in the diagnosis of coronary artery disease. Abnormal changes in cardiac function that are absent during rest may occur with exercise. See **stress test.**

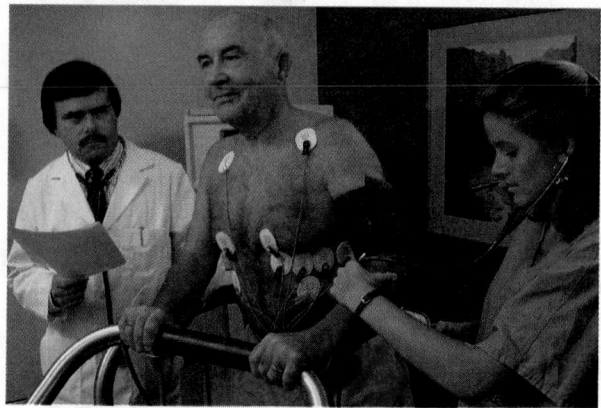

**Exercise electrocardiogram** *(Zakus, 1995)*

**exercise-induced anaphylaxis,** a severe allergic reaction brought on by strenuous exercise. See also **anaphylaxis.**

**exercise-induced asthma** /-indyo͞ost′/, a form of asthma that produces symptoms after strenuous exercise. The condition usually occurs in persons who already have asthma, hay fever, or related hypersensitivity reactions. The effect may be acute but is reversible.

**exercise prescription** [L, *exercere + prae + scribere,* to write], an individualized schedule for physical fitness exercises.

**exercise promotion,** a nursing intervention from the Nursing Interventions Classification (NIC) defined as facilitation of regular physical exercise to maintain or advance to a higher level of fitness and health. See also **Nursing Interventions Classification.**

**exercise promotion: strength training,** a nursing intervention from the Nursing Interventions Classification (NIC) defined as facilitation of regular resistive muscle training to maintain or increase muscle strength. See also **Nursing Interventions Classification.**

**exercise promotion: stretching,** a nursing intervention from the Nursing Interventions Classification (NIC) defined as facilitation of systematic slow-stretch-n-hold muscle exercises to induce relaxation, to prepare muscles/joints for more vigorous exercise, or to increase or maintain body flexibility. See also **Nursing Interventions Classification.**

**exercise therapy: ambulation,** a nursing intervention from the Nursing Interventions Classification (NIC) defined as promotion and assistance with walking to maintain or restore autonomic and voluntary body functions during treatment and recovery from illness or injury. See also **Nursing Interventions Classification.**

**exercise therapy: balance,** a nursing intervention from the Nursing Interventions Classification (NIC) defined as use of specific activities, postures, and movements to maintain, enhance, or restore balance. See also **Nursing Interventions Classification.**

**exercise therapy: joint mobility,** a nursing intervention from the Nursing Interventions Classification (NIC) defined as use of active or passive body movement to maintain or restore joint flexibility. See also **Nursing Interventions Classification.**

**exercise therapy: muscle control,** a nursing intervention from the Nursing Interventions Classification (NIC) defined as use of specific activity or exercise protocols to enhance or restore controlled body movement. See also **Nursing Interventions Classification.**

**exercise tolerance,** the level of physical exertion an individual may be able to achieve before reaching a state of exhaustion. Exercise tolerance tests are commonly performed on a treadmill under the supervision of a health professional who can stop the test if signs of distress are observed.

**exeresis** /ekser′əsis/ [Gk, *ex + eresis,* removal], the surgical removal of a part, organ, or body structure.

**exertional headache** /igzur′shənəl/ [L, *exserere,* to stretch out; AS, *heafod + acan,* headache], an acute headache that occurs during strenuous exercise. It usually recedes when the level of effort is reduced, when an analgesic medication is taken, or both.

**exfoliation** /eksfō′lē·ā′shən/ [L, *ex + folium,* leaf], peeling and sloughing off of tissue cells. This is a normal process that may be exaggerated in certain skin diseases or after a severe sunburn. See also **desquamation, exfoliative dermatitis. —exfoliative,** *adj.*

**exfoliative cytology** /eksfō′lē·ətiv/, the microscopic examination of desquamated cells for diagnostic purposes. The cells are obtained from lesions, sputum, secretions, urine, and other material by aspiration, scraping, a smear, or washings of the tissue. Compare **aspiration biopsy cytology.**

**exfoliative dermatitis,** any inflammatory skin disorder characterized by excessive peeling or shedding of skin. The cause is unknown in about half of cases. Known causes include drug reactions, scarlet fever, leukemia, lymphoma, and generalized dermatitis. Treatment is individualized, but care is essential to prevent secondary infection, avoid further irritation, maintain fluid balance, and stabilize body temperature.

**exhalation.** See **expiration.**

**exhale.** See **expire.**

**exhaustion** /igzôs′chən/ [L, *exhaurire,* to drain away], a state of extreme loss of physical or mental abilities caused by fatigue or illness.

**exhaustion delirium,** a delirium that may result from prolonged physical or emotional stress, fatigue, or shock associated with severe metabolic or nutritional problems. See also **delirium.**

**exhaustion psychosis** [L, *exhaurire,* to drain out; Gk, *psyche,* mind, *osis,* condition], an abnormal mental condition attributed to physical exhaustion. The main symptom, a delirious state, may develop in some explorers, mountain climbers, persons lost in the wilderness, and terminally ill patients. See also **exhaustion delirium.**

**exhibitionism** /ek′sibish′əniz′əm/ [L, *exhibere,* to exhibit], **1.** the flaunting of oneself or one's abilities to attract attention. **2.** (in psychiatry) a psychosexual disorder that occurs primarily in men in which the repetitive act of exposing the genitals in socially unacceptable situations is the preferred means of achieving sexual excitement and gratification. See also **paraphilia, scopophilia. —exhibitionist,** *n.*

**eximer laser** /ek′simir/, a small laser designed to break up organic molecules, such as cholesterol deposits, without producing intense heat.

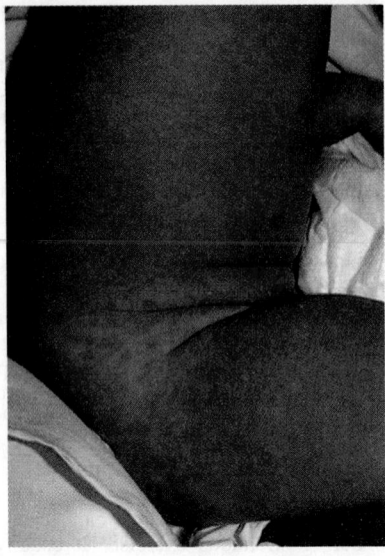

**Exfoliative dermatitis** *(Weston, Lane, and Morelli, 1996)*

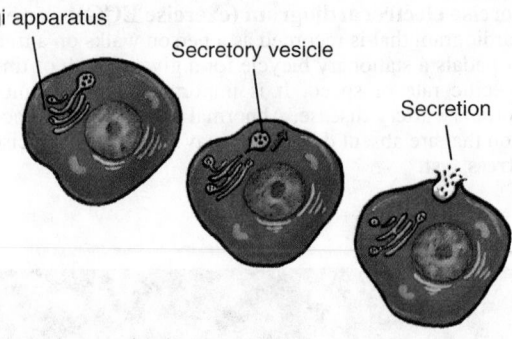

**Exocytosis** *(Applegate, 2000)*

**existential humanistic psychotherapy.** See **humanistic existential therapy.**

**existential psychiatry** /eg'zisten'shəl/ [L, *existere*, to spring forth; Gk, *psyche*, mind, *iatreia*, medical care], a school of psychiatry based on the philosophy of existentialism that emphasizes an analytic, holistic approach in which mental disorders are viewed as deviations within the total structure of an individual's existence rather than as results of any biologically or culturally related factors.

**existential therapy,** a kind of psychotherapy that emphasizes the development of a sense of self-direction through choice, awareness, and acceptance of individual responsibility.

**exit block** [L, *exire*, to depart; Fr, *bloc*], the failure of an expected impulse to emerge from its focus of origin and cause depolarization of cardiac muscle.

**exit dose,** the amount of radiation at the surface of the body opposite that to which the radiation is directed.

**Exna,** trademark for a diuretic and antihypertensive (benzthiazide).

**exo-,** prefix meaning 'outside, outward': *exocataphoria, exohysteropexy, exotoxin.*

**exocoelom.** See **extraembryonic coelom.**

**exocrine** /ek'səkrin/ [Gk, *exo*, outside, *krinein*, to secrete], pertaining to the process of secreting outwardly through a duct to the surface of an organ or tissue or into a vessel, such as a gland that secretes through a duct. Compare **endocrine system.** See also **eccrine.**

**exocrine gland,** any external secretory gland that opens onto the skin surface through ducts in the epithelium, as the sweat glands and the sebaceous glands. Exocrine glands include simple glands having only one duct and compound glands having more than one duct. See also **apocrine gland, endocrine system.**

**exocytosis** /ek'sō-sī·tō'sis/ [Gk, *exos*, outside + *kytos*, a hollow vessel], **1.** discharge from a cell of particles that are too large to diffuse through the wall. Compare **endocytosis. 2.** aggregation of migrating leukocytes in the epidermis as part of the inflammatory response.

**exodondist** See **dental surgeon.**

**exoenzyme** /ek'sō·en'zīm/, an enzyme that does not function within the cells from which it is secreted.

**exogenous** /igzoj'ənəs/ [Gk, *exo* + *genein*, to produce], **1.** outside the body. **2.** originating outside the body or an organ of the body or produced from external causes, such as a disease caused by a bacterial or viral agent foreign to the body. Compare **endogenous. —exogenic,** *adj.*

**exogenous hemochromatosis** [Gk, *exo*, outside, *genein*, to produce, *haima*, blood, *chroma*, color, *osis*, condition], a condition of bronzed pigmentation of the skin caused by accumulation of an iron pigment from excessive intake of iron-rich foods or blood transfusions. Also called **bronze diabetes.**

**exogenous hypertriglyceridemia.** See **hyperlipidemia type I.**

**exogenous infection** [Gk, *exo*, outside, *genein*, to produce; L, *inficere*, to infect], an infection that develops from bacteria normally outside the body that have gained access to the body.

**exogenous obesity,** obesity caused by a caloric intake greater than needed to meet the metabolic needs of the body. Compare **endogenous obesity.** See also **obesity.**

**exogenous uric acid** [Gk, *exo*, outside, *genein*, to produce, *ouron*, urine; L, *acidus*], the accumulation of uric acid in the body produced by the metabolism of purine-rich foods.

**exon** /ek'son/ [Gk, *exo* + *genein*, to produce], the part of a DNA molecule that contains the code for the final messenger RNA.

**exonuclease** /ek'sōnoo'klē·ās/ [Gk, *exo* + L, *nucleus*, nut; *ase*, enzyme], an enzyme that digests DNA or RNA from the ends of the strands.

**Exophiala** /ek'so·fī'ə·lə /, a widespread genus of saprobic Fungi Imperfecti. *E. jeanselmei* is commonly found in soil and sewage and causes mycetoma and opportunistic infections in humans. *E. werneckii* is the cause of tinea nigra; because it is so variable, some authorities have proposed dividing it into more than one species.

**exophoria** /ek'səfôr'ē·ə/ [Gk, *exo* + *pherein*, to bear], the latent lateral deviation of the visual axis of one eye outward. It occurs in the absence of visual stimuli for fusion. Also called **divergent strabismus.** Compare **exotropia. —exophoric,** *adj.*

**exophthalmia** /ek'softhal'mē·ə/ [Gk, *exo* + *ophthalmos*, eye], an abnormal condition characterized by a marked protrusion of the eyeballs (**exophthalmos, exophthalmus**), usually resulting from the increased volume of the orbital contents caused by a tumor; swelling associated with cerebral, intraocular, or intraorbital edema or hemorrhage; paralysis of or trauma to the extraocular muscles; or cavernous sinus thrombosis. It may also be caused by endocrine disorders such as hyperthyroidism and Graves' disease, varicose veins within the orbit, or injury to orbital bones. Visual acuity may be impaired in exophthalmia; keratitis, ulceration, infection, and blindness may also occur. Treatment depends on the underlying cause. Acute advanced exophthalmia is often irreversible. Also called **protrusio bulbi.** See also **proptosis. —exophthalmic,** *adj.*

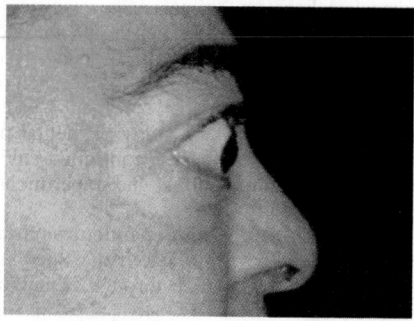

**Exophthalmia** *(Stein, Slatt, and Stein, 1994)*

**exophthalmic goiter** /ek'softhal'mik/, exophthalmos that occurs in association with goiter, as in Graves' disease.

**exophthalmometer** /ek'səfthalmom'ətər/ [Gk, *exo* + *ophthalmos,* eye, *metron,* measure], an instrument used for measuring the degree of forward displacement of the eye in exophthalmos. The device allows measurement of the distance from the center of the cornea to the lateral orbital rim.

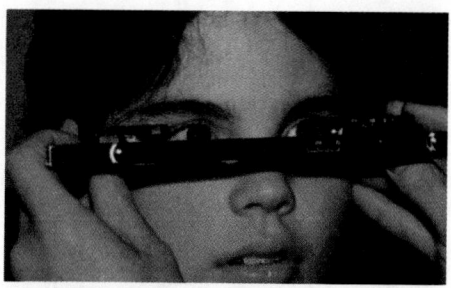

**Exophthalmometer** *(Zitelli and Davis, 1992)*

**exophthalmos.** See **exophthalmia.**

**exophthalmos-macroglossia-gigantism syndrome.** See **EMG syndrome.**

**exophytic** /ek'səfit'ik/ [Gk, *exo* + *phyton,* plant], pertaining to the tendency to grow outward, such as a tumor that grows into the lumen of a hollow organ rather than into the wall.

**exophytic carcinoma,** a malignant epithelial neoplasm that resembles a papilloma or wart.

**exoskeletal prosthesis** /ek'səskel'ətəl/ [Gk, *exo* + *skeletos,* dried up, *prosthesis,* addition], a prosthetic device in which support is provided by an outside structure (not an implant), such as an artificial limb. See also **prosthesis.**

**exoskeleton** /ek'səskel'ətən/ [Gk, *exo,* outside, *skeletos,* dried up], the hard outer covering of many invertebrates, such as crustaceans, which lack the bony internal skeleton of vertebrates. Compare **endoskeleton.**

**exostosis** /ek'sostō'sis/ [Gk, *exo* + *osteon,* bone], an abnormal benign growth on the surface of a bone. Also called **hyperostosis. —exostosed, exostotic,** *adj.*

**exostosis cartilaginea** [Gk, *ex,* out, *osteon,* bone; L, *cartilago,* cartilage], an outgrowth of cartilage at the ends of long bones. Also called **cartilage capped exostosis.**

**exostotic.** See **exostosis.**

**exoteric** /ek'səter'ik/ [Gk, *exoterikos,* external], lying outside an organism.

**exothermic,** indicating a chemical process accompanied by the release of heat, such as the loss of body surface heat.

**exotoxin** /ek'sətok'sin/ [Gk, *exo* + *toxikon,* poison], a toxin that is secreted or excreted by a living microorganism. Compare **endotoxin.**

**exotropia** /ekstrō'fēə/, a visual disorder in which a deviating eye looks outward. The eye often is blind or has defective vision. Also called **divergent squint, divergent strabismus.**

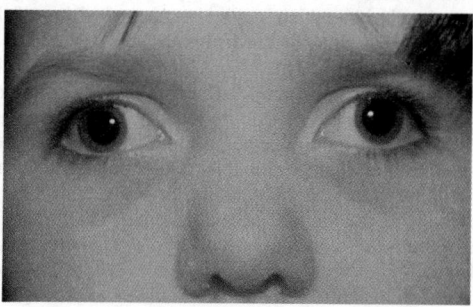

**Exotropia** *(Zitelli and Davis, 1997)*

**expanded role** [L, *expandere,* to spread out; OFr, *rolle,* an assumed character], the functions of a nurse that are not specified in the traditional limits of nursing practice legislation. Common roles are primary nurse and nurse practitioner, necessitating legal coverage through the establishment of standardized procedures or amendments or changes in nursing practice acts.

**expansion** /ek·span'shən/ [L, *expandere,* to spread out], **1.** the process or state of being increased in extent, surface, or bulk. **2.** a region or area of increased bulk or surface.

**expectant treatment** /ekspek'tənt/ [L, *exspectare,* to wait for; Fr, *traitment*], application of therapeutic measures to relieve symptoms as they arise in the course of a disease, rather than treatment of the cause of illness. Some kinds of expectant treatment are amputations for gangrene in a patient with diabetes, coronary bypass procedures in a patient with generalized atherosclerosis, and transplantation of tendons in a patient with severe rheumatoid arthritis. Compare **definitive treatment, palliative treatment, treatment.**

**expectation** /eks'pektā'shən/ [L, *exspectare,* to wait for], **1.** (in nursing) anticipation by the staff of a patient's behavior that is based on a knowledge and understanding of the person's abilities and problems. **2.** anticipation of the performance of the nursing staff in defined roles, as role expectation.

**expectation of life.** See **life expectancy.**

**expected date of delivery (EDD),** the predicted date of a pregnant woman's delivery. Pregnancy lasts approximately 266 days, or 38 weeks from the day of fertilization, but is considered clinically to last 280 days, or 40 weeks, or 10 lunar months, or 9⅓ calendar months from the first day of the last menstrual period (LMP). The EDD is usually calculated on the basis of 9⅓ calendar months, but if a woman is certain that coitus occurred only once during the month and if she knows the date on which it occurred, the EDD may be calculated as 38 weeks from that date. In the absence of a special calendar or device for calculating the EDD, it is arrived at by counting back 3 months from the first day of the LMP and then adding 7 days and 1 year; thus, if the first day of a woman's LMP was July 18, 1997, one counts back 3 months to April 18, 1997, then adds 7 days and 1 year to arrive at an EDD of April 25, 1998 (Nägele's rule). Because calendar months differ in length, this calculation may give a date that is a few days more or less than 280 days from the first day of the LMP, but it provides a very close approximation, and a trivial error will not be of clinical significance because of the variability of the actual durations of normal pregnancies. The expectant mother is advised that the EDD is only an estimate and that the chances are that she will give birth within 2 weeks before or, more commonly, after the calculated date. Also called **expected date of birth (EDB), expected date of confinement (EDC).**

**expectorant** /ikspek′tərənt/ [Gk, *ex,* out, *pectus,* breast], **1.** pertaining to a substance that promotes the ejection of mucus or other exudates from the lung, bronchi, and trachea. **2.** an agent that promotes expectoration by reducing the viscosity of pulmonary secretions or by decreasing the tenacity with which exudates adhere to the lower respiratory tract. Expectorant drugs include acetylcysteine, guaifenesin, and terpin hydrate. Also called **mucolytic. —expectorate,** *v.*

**expectoration** /ikspek′tərā′shən/, the ejection of mucus, sputum, or fluids from the trachea and lungs by coughing or spitting.

**experience rating** /ikspir′ē·əns/ [L, *experientia,* testing, *rata,* proportion], a system used by insurance companies in the United States to set the premium to be paid by the insured based on the risk to the company of providing the insurance. Experience rating may lead to very high malpractice premiums in some medical specialties, for the insurance company calculates the premium based on settlements made in related malpractice cases during a specified period. Experience rating is also used to set annual membership health maintenance fees in organizations in which the cost of providing the services in a previous accounting period is used to determine the premiums for the next fiscal year.

**experiment,** an investigation in which one or more variables may be altered under controlled circumstances to study the effects of altering variables.

**experimental design** /eksper′imen′təl/ [L, *experimentum + designare,* to mark out], (in research) a study design used to test cause-and-effect relationships between variables. The classic experimental design specifies an experimental group and a control group. The independent variable is administered to the experimental group and not to the control group, and both groups are measured on the same dependent variable. Subsequent experimental designs have used more groups and more measurements over longer periods.

**experimental embryology,** the study and analysis through experimental techniques of the factors, mechanisms, and relationships that determine and influence prenatal development.

**experimental epidemiology,** a type of epidemiologic investigation that uses an experimental model for studies to confirm a causal relationship suggested by observational studies.

**experimental group,** a set of items or people under study to determine the effect of an event, a substance, or a technique

**experimental medicine,** a branch of the practice of medicine in which new drugs or treatments are evaluated for safety and efficacy in a clinical laboratory setting by using animals or, in certain cases, human subjects.

**experimental pathology,** the study of diseases deliberately induced in laboratory animals.

**experimental physiology,** a branch of the study of physiology in which the functions of various body systems are evaluated in a clinical laboratory setting by using animals or, in some cases, human subjects.

**experimental psychology,** the study of mental processes and phenomena by observation in a controlled environment using various tests, manipulations, and experiments. Compare **analytic psychology.**

**experimental variable.** See **independent variable.**

**expertise** /eks′pərtēz′/ [L, *experiri,* to try], special skills or knowledge acquired by a person through education, training, or experience.

**expert witness** /ikspurt′, ek′spərt/ [L, *experiri,* to try; AS, *witnes,* knowledge], a person who has special knowledge of a subject about which a court requests testimony. Special knowledge may be acquired by experience, education, observation, or study but is not possessed by the average person. An expert witness gives expert testimony or expert evidence. This evidence often serves to educate the court and the jury in the subject under consideration.

**expiration** /ik′spirā′shən/ [L, *expirare,* to breathe out], **1.** breathing out, normally a passive process, depending on the elastic qualities of lung tissue and the thorax. Also called **exhalation.** Compare **inspiration. 2.** termination or death.

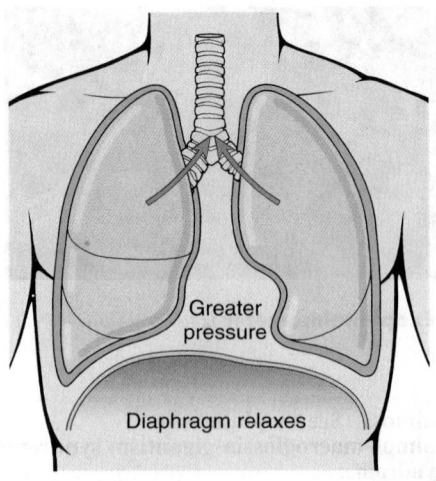

**Expiration** *(Chabner, 2001)*

**expiratory** /ikspī′rətôr′ē/ [L, *expirare,* to breathe out], pertaining to the exhalation of air from the lungs.

**expiratory center** [L, *expirare,* to breath out; Gk, *kentron,* center], one of several regions of the medulla responsible for control of respiration. It is a subregion specifically involved in carrying out the activity of expiration.

**expiratory phase,** the portion of the respiratory cycle that involves exhalation, or moving air out of the lungs. In a ventilated patient the expiratory phase may be passive, depending on the recoil of elastic tissues in the lung to move air out, or active, applying positive pressure to the abdominal area or negative pressure to the upper airway.

**expiratory reserve volume (ERV),** the maximum volume of gas that can be exhaled after a resting volume exhalation. See also **vital capacity.**

**expiratory retard,** (in respiratory care) a mode of mechanical ventilation that mimics the prolonged expiratory phase and pursed-lip breathing of emphysema. The method adds some resistance to expiration. Low levels of positive end-expiratory pressure may produce a similar effect. Also called *expiratory resistance.*

**expire** /ikspī′ər/ [L, *expirare,* to breathe out], **1.** Also called **exhale.** To breathe out. **2.** to die.

**expired gas (E),** any gas exhaled from the lungs.

**exploratory** /iksplôr′ətôr′ē/ [L, *explorare,* to search out], pertaining to investigation, as in exploratory surgery.

**exploratory operation** [L, *explorare,* to search out, *operari,* to work], surgical intervention to find the cause of a disorder by opening a body cavity or organ and examining the interior.

**explosion,** **1.** a sudden and violent decomposition of a chemical compound. **2.** a sudden radical breakout.

**explosive personality** /iksplō′siv/ [L, *ex,* out, *plaudere,* to clap], behavior characterized by episodes of uncontrolled rage and physical abusiveness in reaction to relatively minor stressors.

**explosive speech,** abnormal speech characterized by slow, jerky articulation interspersed with sudden loud enunciation of words, often seen in brain disorders. The term is less often used by speech-language pathologists.

**exponent** /ikspō′nənt/, a superscript on a number that indicates how many times a number is to be multiplied by itself (for example, $3^4 = 3 \times 3 \times 3 \times 3 = 81$). In medical or scientific reports, powers of 10 are commonly used to indicate very large or very small numbers, such as in the examples $10^6$ representing 1,000,000 or $10^{-6}$ representing 1/1,000,000. Exponents also are indicated by prefixes, such as mega- for $10^6$ and micro- for $10^{-6}$.

**exposed pulp** [L, *exponere,* to lay out, *pulpa,* flesh], dental pulp that becomes exposed to the oral environment and potential bacterial infection. Causes include fracture of the crown through trauma and loss of a tooth crown or penetration of the dentin during restorative preparation.

**exposure** /ikspō′zhər/ [L, *exponere,* to lay out], a measure of the ionization of air produced by a beam of radiation. It is expressed as coulombs per kilogram of air.

**exposure angle,** the angle of the arc described by the movement of a radiographic tube and film during a tomographic exposure. It is usually less than the tomographic angle. The exposure angle influences the thickness of the tomographic section: smaller angles produce thicker sections.

**exposure switch,** (in radiology) a control device designed to interrupt the power automatically when pressure by the operator's hand or foot is released. The purpose is to prevent accidental continuing exposure of the patient to radiation. A common exposure switch is a foot pedal.

**exposure unit,** any of the conventional or SI units used to measure radiation exposure: roentgen (R), rad, rem, curie (Ci), gray (Gy), sievert (Sv), and becquerel (Bq).

**expression** /ikspresh′ən/ [L, *exprimere,* to express], **1.** the indication of a physical or emotional state through facial appearance or vocal intonation. **2.** the act of pressing or squeezing to expel something, such as milk from the breast when lactating or the fetus from the uterus by exertion of pressure on the abdominal wall. **3.** (in genetics) the detectable effect or appearance in the phenotype of a particular trait or condition. See also **expressivity. —express,** *v.*

**expressive aphasia.** See **motor aphasia.**

**expressive language disorder,** a communication disorder in children and adults, characterized by problems with expression of language, either oral or signed. It includes difficulties such as limited speech or vocabulary, vocabulary errors, difficulty or hesitation in word selection, oversimplification of grammatical or sentence structure, omission of parts of sentences, unusual word order, and slowed acquisition of language skills. Two types are recognized, *acquired* and *developmental.*

**expressivity** /eks′presiv′itē/ [L, *exprimere,* to make clear], the variability with which basic patterns of inheritance are modified, both in degree and in variety, by the effect of a given gene in people of the same genotype. For example, polydactyly may be expressed as extra toes in one generation and extra fingers in another.

**expulsive stage of labor** /ikspul′siv/ [L, *expellere,* to drive out, *stare,* stand, *labor,* work], the second stage of labor, during which the mother's uterine contractions are accompanied by a bearing-down reflex. It begins after full dilation of the cervix and continues to the complete birth of the infant.

**exsanguinate** /eksang′gwināt/ [L, *ex, sanguis,* blood], to drain away or deprive an organ of blood.

**exsanguination** /eksang′gwinā′shən/, a loss of blood.

**exsiccant.** See **desiccant.**

**exsiccate.** See **desiccate.**

**exstrophy** /ek′strōfē/ [Gk, *ekstrephein,* to turn inside out], a congenital malformation in which a hollow organ has its wall turned inside-out, establishing a communication with the exterior. An example is exstrophy of the bladder with eversion of the posterior bladder wall, which causes urine to drain to the exterior.

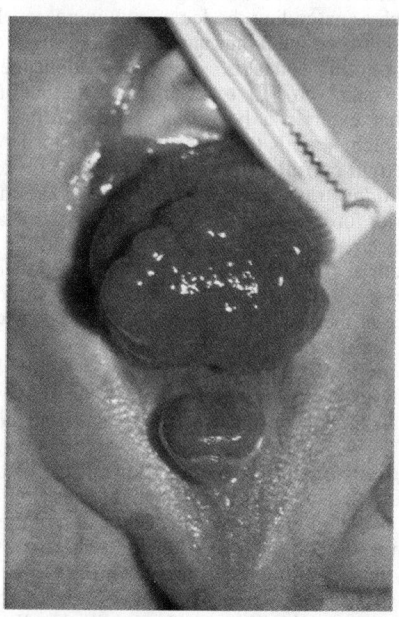

**Exstrophy of the bladder**
*(Cotran, Kumar, and Collins, 1999/courtesy Dr. Hardy Hendren, Surgeon-in-Chief, Children's Hospital, Boston)*

**exstrophy of the bladder,** a developmental anomaly marked by absence of part of the lower abdominal wall and the anterior wall of the urinary bladder, with eversion of the posterior wall of the bladder through the defect, as well as an open pubic arch and widely separated ischia connected by a fibrous band.

**extended arm.** See **reacher.**

**extended care facility** [L, *extendere,* to stretch], an institution devoted to providing medical, nursing, or custodial care for an individual over a prolonged period, such as during the course of a chronic disease or the rehabilitation phase after an acute illness. Kinds of extended care facilities are **intermediate care facility** and **skilled nursing facility.** Also called **convalescent home, nursing home.**

**extended family,** a family group consisting of the biologic or adoptive parents, their children, the grandparents, and other family members. The extended family is the basic family group in many societies. Among its characteristics are exchange of information from experienced older members to less experienced younger ones, care of the older family members in the home by the younger ones, and care of younger members' children by older members. Compare **nuclear family.**

**extended insulin-zinc suspension,** a long-acting insulin that is slowly absorbed and slow to act.

**extended wear contact lens,** a refractive index device that fits over the cornea, designed to permit air permeation. Oxygen may pass between the lens and the cornea, thereby reducing the risk of corneal irritation.

**extender,** something that causes an increase in time or size, such as a substance added to a medication to stretch the time required for the drug to be absorbed. A kind of extender is **plasma volume extender.**

**Extendryl,** trademark for a fixed-combination nasal decongestant drug containing an adrenergic (phenylephrine hydrochloride), an antihistaminic (chlorpheniramine maleate), and an anticholinergic (methscopolamine nitrate).

**extension** /iksten′shən/ [L, *extendere,* to stretch], a "straightening" movement allowed by certain joints of the skeleton that increases the angle between two adjoining bones, such as extending the leg, which increases the posterior angle between the femur and the tibia. Compare **flexion.**

**extension partial denture.** See **partial denture.**

**extensor** /iksten′sər/ [L, *extendere,* to stretch out], any muscle that extends a body part, such as the **extensor indicis,** which extends the index finger.

**extensor carpi radialis brevis** [L, *extendere* + Gk, *karpos,* wrist; L, *radius,* ray, *brevis,* short], one of the muscles of the posterior forearm. It inserts into the dorsal surface of the third metacarpal bone and functions to extend the hand.

**extensor carpi radialis longus,** one of the seven superficial muscles of the posterior forearm. It inserts into the dorsal surface of the second metacarpal bone and serves to extend and flex the hand radially.

**extensor carpi ulnaris,** one of the muscles of the lateral forearm. It inserts by a tendon into the ulnar side of the fifth metacarpal bone and functions to extend and adduct the hand.

**extensor digiti minimi,** an extensor muscle of the posterior forearm. It is a slender muscle that arises from the common extensor tendon and joins the expansion of the extensor digitorum tendon on the back of the first phalanx of the little finger. It functions to extend the little finger.

**extensor digitorum,** the principal muscle of the medial digits of the posterior forearm. It divides distally into four tendons that pass through the extensor retinaculum and diverge on the back of the hand, inserting into the second and

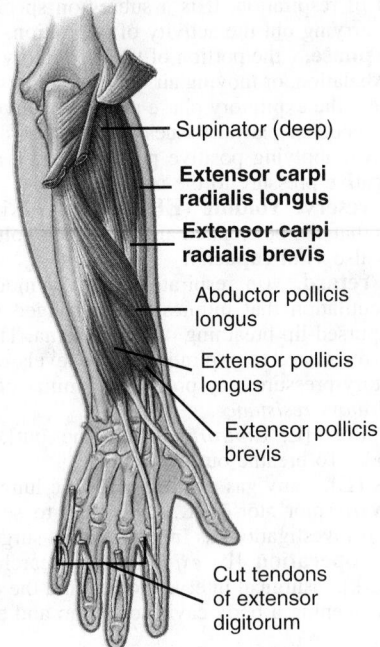

- Supinator (deep)
- **Extensor carpi radialis longus**
- **Extensor carpi radialis brevis**
- Abductor pollicis longus
- Extensor pollicis longus
- Extensor pollicis brevis
- Cut tendons of extensor digitorum

**Extensor carpi radialis**
*(Thibodeau and Patton, 1999/John V. Hagen)*

third phalanges of the fingers. It functions to extend the phalanges and, by continued action, the wrist. Also called *extensor digitorum communis.*

**extensor digitorum longus,** a penniform muscle located at the lateral part of the anterior leg. It is one of three anterior crural muscles. It extends the proximal phalanges of the four small toes and dorsally flexes and pronates the foot.

**extensor indicis.** See **extensor.**

**extensor retinaculum of ankle,** either of two thick layers of fascia holding tendons in the ankle.

**extensor retinaculum of hand,** the thick band of antebrachial fascia that wraps tendons of the extensor muscles of the forearm at the distal ends of the radius and the ulna. Also called **dorsal carpal ligament, retinaculum extensorum manus.**

**extensor retinaculum of wrist,** a broad thickening of deep fascia over the back of the wrist, over the extensor tendons.

**extensor thrust,** a spinal-level reflex present in a human in the first 2 months of life. It is an exaggeration of the positive support reflex and consists of an uncontrolled extension of a flexed leg when the sole of the foot is stimulated.

**extern** /eks′turn/ [L, *externus,* outward], a medical or dental student who lives outside the institution but provides medical or dental care to patients as an extracurricular activity under the professional supervision of hospital staff members. Compare **intern.**

**external** /ikstur′nəl/ [L, *externus,* outward], **1.** being on the outside or exterior of the body or an organ. **2.** acting from the outside, such as an external influence or exogenous factor. **3.** pertaining to the outward or visible appearance. Compare **internal.**

**external abdominal oblique muscle,** one of a pair of muscles that are the largest and the most superficial of the five anterolateral muscles of the abdomen. It is a broad, thin four-sided muscle, which acts to compress the contents of the abdomen and assists in micturition, defecation, emesis, parturition, and forced expiration. Both sides acting together serve to flex the vertebral column, drawing the pubis toward the xiphoid process. One side alone functions to bend the vertebral column laterally and to rotate it, drawing the shoulder of the same side forward. Also called **obliquus externus abdominis.** Compare **internal abdominal oblique muscle.**

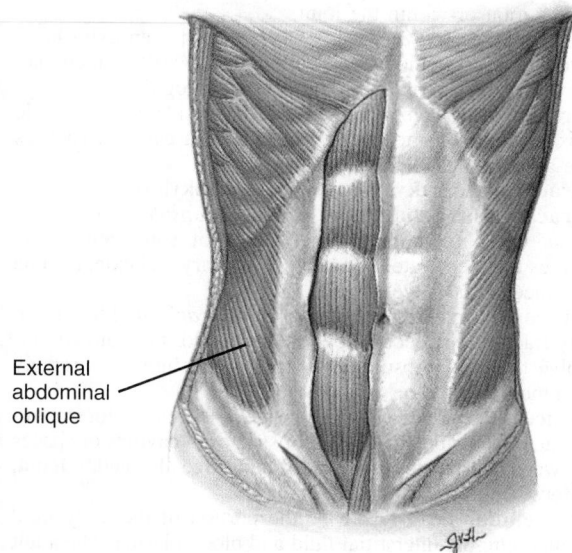

External abdominal oblique

**External abdominal oblique muscle**
*(Thibodeau and Patton, 1999/John V. Hagen)*

**external abdominal region.** See **lateral region.**

**external absorption,** the taking up of substances through the mucous membranes or the skin.

**external acoustic meatus,** the canal of the external ear, composed of bone and cartilage, extending from the auricle to the tympanic membrane. Also called **external auditory canal.**

**external aperture of aqueduct of vestibule,** an external opening for the small canal extending from the vestibule of the inner ear, located on the internal surface of the petrous part of the temporal bone lateral to the opening for the internal acoustic passage.

**external aperture of canaliculus of cochlea,** an external opening of the cochlear channel on the margin of the jugular opening in the temporal bone.

**external aperture of tympanic canaliculus,** the lower opening of the tympanic channel on the inferior surface of the petrous part of the temporal bone.

**external auditory canal, external auditory meatus.** See **external acoustic meatus.**

**external beam radiotherapy,** treatment by radiation emitted from a source located at a distance from the body; also called **beam therapy,** *external beam therapy.*

**external carotid artery,** one of a pair of arteries with eight major temporal or maxillary branches, rising from the common carotid arteries. It supplies various parts and tissues of the head and neck.

**external carotid plexus,** a network of nerves around the external carotid artery, formed by the external carotid nerves from the superior cervical ganglion. It supplies sympathetic fibers associated with branches of the external carotid artery. Compare **common carotid plexus, internal carotid plexus.**

**external cervical os,** an external opening of the uterus that leads into the cavity of the cervix. Compare **internal cervical os.**

**external conjugate,** the distance measured with obstetric calipers from the depression below the lowest lumbar vertebra posteriorly to the upper border of the symphysis anteriorly (usually about 21 cm). Also called **Baudelocque's diameter.**

**external counterpulsation,** a noninvasive technique for providing counterpulsation (assisted heart pumping). In one technique the limbs are placed in inflatable trousers. Inflation and deflation are synchronized with the cardiac cycle, generating augmented blood flow during diastole and assisted ejection during systole.

**external cuneiform bone.** See **lateral cuneiform bone.**

**external ear,** the outer structure of the ear, consisting of the auricle and the external acoustic meatus. Sound waves are funneled through the external ear to the middle ear. Compare **internal ear, middle ear.**

**external fertilization,** the union of male and female gametes outside the bodies from which they originated, such as occurs in frogs and most fish.

**external fistula,** an abnormal passage between an internal organ or structure and the cutaneous surface of the body. It can be surgically created or caused by delayed wound healing or necrotizing tumors.

**external fixation,** a method of holding together the fragments of a fractured bone by using transfixing metal pins through the fragments and a compression device attached to the pins outside the skin surface. Nursing care includes regular cleansing of the skin around the pins and, in certain cases, application of antibiotic solutions or ointments. The pins are removed at a later procedure when the fracture is healed. Compare **internal fixation.**

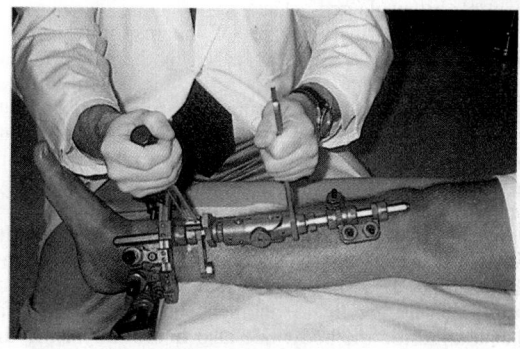

**External fixation**
*(Monahan and Neighbors, 1998/courtesy Zimmer, Inc., Warsaw, Indiana)*

**external iliac artery,** the larger, more superficial division of the common iliac artery, which descends into the thigh and becomes the femoral artery. The external iliac supplies the lower limb. Compare **internal iliac artery.**

**external iliac node,**  a node in one of the seven groups of parietal nodes serving the lymphatic system in the abdomen and the pelvis. Compare **common iliac node, iliac circumflex node, internal iliac node.** See also **lymph, lymphatic system, lymph node.**

**external iliac vein,**  one of a pair of veins in the lower body that join the internal iliac vein to form the two common iliac veins. Compare **internal iliac vein.**

**external jugular vein,**  the more superficial and lateral of a pair of large vessels on each side of the neck that receive most of the blood from the exterior of the cranium and the deep tissues of the face. Compare **internal jugular vein.**

**external locus of control.**  See **locus of control.**

**external malleolus** /male′ōlas/ [L, *externus,* outward, *malleolus,* little hammer],  a rounded bony prominence on either side of the ankle joint. Also called **malleolus fibulae.**

**external pacemaker** [L, *externus,* outward, *passus,* step; ME, *maken,* to make],  **1.** a device used to stimulate the heartbeat electrically by means of impulses conducted through the chest wall, as used in emergency care of significant bradyarrhythmias. **2.** a similar device in which the impulse generator is outside the chest but is connected with the heart by wires that pass under the skin. The wires are placed during open-heart surgery and are removed after surgery, when the risk of bradycardia has diminished.

**external perimysium.**  See **epimysium.**

**external phase.**  See **continuous phase.**

**external pin fixation.**  A method of holding together the fragments of a fractured bone by means of pins that are attached to the bone and that protrude from the skin. See also **skeletal fixation.**

**external pterygoid muscle,**  one of the four short, thick, somewhat conical muscles of mastication. It functions to open the jaws, protrude the mandible, and move the mandible from side to side. Also called **pterygoideus lateralis.**

**external radiation therapy (ERT),**  the therapeutic application of ionizing radiation from an external beam of a kilovoltage radiographic machine, a megavoltage cobalt 60 machine, or a supervoltage linear accelerator, cyclotron, or betatron. ERT is used most frequently in the treatment of cancer but also in the therapy of keloids and some dermatologic conditions and in counteracting the body's physiologic rejection of transplanted organs.

**external respiration,**  the part of the respiratory process that involves the exchange of gases in the alveoli of the lungs.

**external rotation,**  turning outwardly or away from the midline of the body, such as when a leg is externally rotated with the toes turned outward or away from the body's midline.

**external secretion.**  See **exocrine gland.**

**external shunt,**  a device for the passage of body fluid from one compartment to another. It consists of a tube or catheter (or a series of such containers) that passes from one compartment or cavity to another over the body surface rather than inside the body. See also **hemodialysis, hydrocephalus.**

**external version,**  an obstetric procedure in which a fetus is turned, usually from a breech to a vertex presentation, by external manipulation through the abdominal wall. Compare **version and extraction.**

**exteroceptive** /ek′stərōsep′tiv/ [L, *externus,* outside, *recipere,* to receive],  pertaining to stimuli that originate from outside the body or to the sensory receptors that they activate. Compare **interoceptive, proprioception.**

**exteroceptor** /ek′stərōsep′tər/ [L, *externus,* outside, *recipere,* to receive],  any sensory nerve ending, as those located in the skin, mucous membranes, or sense organs, that responds to stimuli originating outside the body, such as touch, pressure, or sound. Compare **interoceptor, proprioceptor.** See also **chemoreceptor.**

**extinction** /iksting′shən/,  a state of being lost or destroyed.

**extirpation** /ek′stərpā′shən/ [L, *extirpare,* to root out],  the total removal of a diseased organ or body part.

**extra-, extro-,**  combining form meaning 'outside, beyond, in addition to': *extrabronchial, extradural, extramarginal, extroversion.*

**extraarticular** /ek′strə·ärtik′yələr/ [L, *extra,* outside, *articulare,* to divide into joints],  pertaining to the area outside a joint or within the joint.

**extra beat** [L, *extra,* outside; AS, *beatan*],  an extra heart contraction. It is indicated by a premature atrial, junctional, or ventricular complex on an electrocardiogram.

**extracapsular** /-kaps′yələr/ [L, *extra,* outside, *capsula,* little box],  pertaining to something outside a capsule, such as the articulare capsule of the knee joint.

**extracapsular ankylosis.**  See **false ankylosis.**

**extracapsular dendrite** [L, *extra* + *capsula* + Gk, *dendron,* tree],  pertaining to dendrites of some autonomic nerves that penetrate the capsule boundary and extend some distance from the cell body.

**extracapsular fracture** [L, *extra* + *capsula,* little box],  any fracture that occurs near a joint but does not directly involve the joint capsule. This type of fracture is extremely common in the hip.

**extracellular** /-sel′yələr/ [L, *extra* + *cella,* storeroom],  occurring outside a cell or cell tissue or in cavities or spaces between cell layers or groups of cells. See also **cell, edema, interstitial.**

**extracellular fluid (ECF),**  the portion of the body fluid comprising the interstitial fluid and blood plasma. The adult body contains about 11.2 L of interstitial fluid, constituting about 16% of body weight, and about 2.8 L of plasma, constituting about 4% of body weight. Plasma and interstitial fluid are very similar chemically and, in conjunction with intracellular fluid, help control the movement of water and electrolytes throughout the body. Some of the important ionized components of extracellular fluid are protein, magnesium, potassium, chlorine, calcium, and certain sulfates.

**extracellular matrix,**  a substance containing collagen, elastin, proteoglycans, glycosaminoglycans, and fluid, produced by cells and in which the cells are embedded. The matrix secreted by chondroblasts, for example, is responsible for the properties of cartilage.

**extracellular space.**  See **extracellular.**

**extrachromosomal** /-krō′məsō′məl/,  occurring without direct involvement of the chromosomes. Also **epigenetic.**

**extracoronal** /eks′trə·kor′ə·nəl/ [L, *extra* + *corona,* crown],  outside the crown of a tooth.

**extracoronal retainer** /-kôr′ənəl/ [L, *extra* + *corona,* crown, *retinere,* to hold],  **1.** a dental anchor that incorporates a cast restoration lying largely external to the coronal portion of a tooth and complements the contour of the tooth crown. Resistance to displacement is developed between the inner surfaces of the casting and the external walls of the prepared tooth. The restoration incorporating an extracoronal retainer may be a complete or partial crown. **2.** a direct clasp-type retainer that engages an abutment tooth on its external surface, used to retain and stabilize a removable partial denture. **3.** a manufactured direct retainer, the protruding portion of which is attached to the external surface of a cast crown on an abutment tooth.

**extracorporeal** /ek′strakôr′pôr′ē·əl/ [L, *extra* + *corpus,* body],  something that is outside the body, such as extracorporeal circulation in which venous blood is diverted outside the body to a heart-lung machine and returned to the body through a femoral or other artery.

**extracorporeal membrane oxygenator (ECMO),** a device that oxygenates a patient's blood outside the body and returns the blood to the patient's circulatory system. The technique may be used to support an impaired respiratory system.

**extracorporeal oxygenation,** the use of an artificial membrane outside the body to provide for oxygenation of the blood in a patient with severe lung disease.

**extracorporeal photochemotherapy,** a procedure for treating pemphigus vulgaris by treating the patient's blood outside the body. Certain drugs are first administered to the patient. Some of the patient's blood is then removed temporarily for exposure to ultraviolet light outside the body. The blood, after treatment, is returned to the patient. See also **photochemotherapy.**

**extracorporeal shock-wave lithotripsy (ESWL)** [L, *extra,* outside, *corpus,* body; Fr, *choc* + AS, *wafian* + Gk, *lithos,* stone, *tribein,* to wear away], use of vibrations of powerful sound waves to break up calculi in the urinary tract or gallbladder.

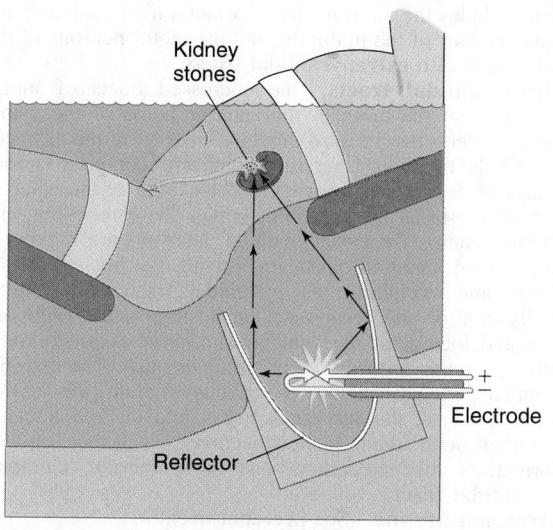

**Extracorporeal shock-wave lithotripsy**
*(Beare and Myers, 1998)*

**extracorporeal technician.** See **perfusion technologist.**

**extracranial** /-krā′nē·əl/ [L, *extra,* outside; Gk, *kranion,* skull], pertaining to something outside or unconnected with the skull.

**extract** [L, *ex,* out, *trahere,* to draw], **1.** /ek′strakt/ a substance, usually a biologically active ingredient of a plant or animal tissue, prepared by the use of solvents or evaporation to separate the substance from the original material. Beef extract, belladonna, and cascara are examples of extracts. **2.** /ikstrakt′/ to remove a tooth from the oral cavity by means of elevators or forceps or both.—**extraction,** *n.*

**extractor** /ikstrak′tər/, a medical instrument, such as a forceps, used to remove a foreign body, tissue sample, or medical device placed in a body cavity.

**extradural** /ek′trədŏŏr′əl/ [L, *extra* + *dura,* hard], outside the dura mater.

**extradural anesthesia,** anesthetic nerve block achieved by the injection of a local anesthetic solution into the space in the spinal canal outside the dura mater of the spinal cord, as in **epidural, caudal,** or **paravertebral anesthesia.**

**extradural hemorrhage.** See **epidural hemorrhage.**

**extraembryonic blastoderm** /-em′brē·on′ik/ [L, *extra* + Gk, *en,* in, *bryein,* to grow], the area of the blastoderm outside the embryo that gives rise to the membranes that surround the embryo during gestation. Compare **embryonic blastoderm.** See also **allantois, amnion, chorion, yolk sac.**

**extraembryonic coelom,** a cavity external to the developing embryo that forms between the mesoderm of the chorion and that covers the amniotic cavity and yolk sac. Also called **exocoelom.**

**extraembryonic mesoderm** [L, *extra,* outside; Gk, *en* + *bryein,* to grow, *mesos,* middle, *derma,* skin], any mesoderm in the uterus that is not involved with the embryo itself. Included are mesoderms in the amnion, chorion, and yolk sac.

**extramammary Paget's disease** /-mam′ərē/ [L, *extra,* outside, *mamma,* breast; James Paget, English surgeon, 1814–1899; L, *dis* + Fr, *aise,* ease], a gradually spreading red, scaly and crusted lesion resembling that of Paget's disease, but not occurring on the breast. A common area is the vulva. The lesions give rise to carcinoma in approximately 50% of the cases.

**extramarital** /-mer′itəl/, happening outside a marriage, such as an extramarital affair.

**extramedullary** /-med′yələr′ē/ [L, *extra* + *medulla,* marrow], pertaining to something outside or unrelated to any medulla.

**extramedullary myeloma** [L, *extra* + *medulla,* marrow], a plasma cell tumor that occurs outside the bone marrow, usually affecting the visceral organs or the nasopharyngeal and oral mucosa. Also called **extramedullary plasmacytoma, peripheral plasma cell myeloma, plasma cell tumor.**

**extramedullary myelopoiesis,** the formation and development of myeloid tissue outside the bone marrow. Also called **ectopic myelopoiesis.**

**extramedullary plasmacytoma.** See **extramedullary myeloma.**

**extraneous** /exstrā′nē·əs/ [L, *strange*], exogenous; originating or entering from outside the organism.

**extraocular** /-ok′yŏŏlər/ [L, *extra* + *oculus,* eye], outside the eye.

**extraocular muscle palsy,** an abnormal condition characterized by paralysis of the extrinsic muscles of the eye, such as the superior, inferior, medial, and lateral rectus muscles, and the superior and the inferior oblique muscles. See also **strabismus.**

**extraocular muscles (EOMs)** the six sets of muscles that control movements of the eyeball. They are the superior rectus and inferior rectus, which move the eye up and down; the medial rectus and the lateral rectus, which move the eye to either side; and the superior oblique and inferior oblique, which move the eye downward and inward, and upward and inward, respectively.

**extraoral anchorage** /-ôr′əl/ [L, *extra* + *oralis,* mouth, *ancora,* hook], an orthodontic holding device outside the mouth, typically linking dental attachments to a wire bow or to hooks extending between the lips and attached by elastic to a cap, neck strap, or other device outside the mouth. Also called **extraoral orthodontic appliance.**

**extraoral orthodontic appliance.** See **extraoral anchorage.**

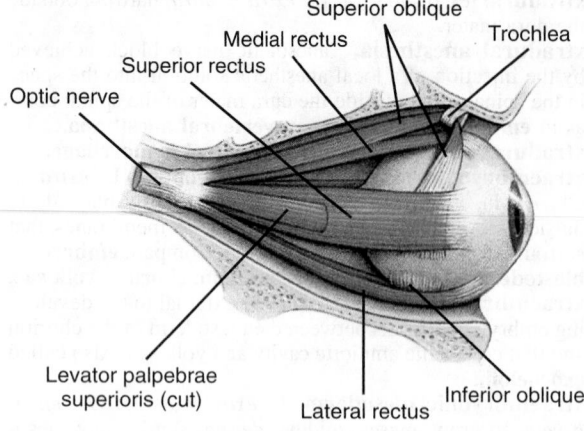

Superior oblique
Medial rectus
Superior rectus
Trochlea
Optic nerve

Levator palpebrae
superioris (cut)
Lateral rectus
Inferior oblique

Superior view

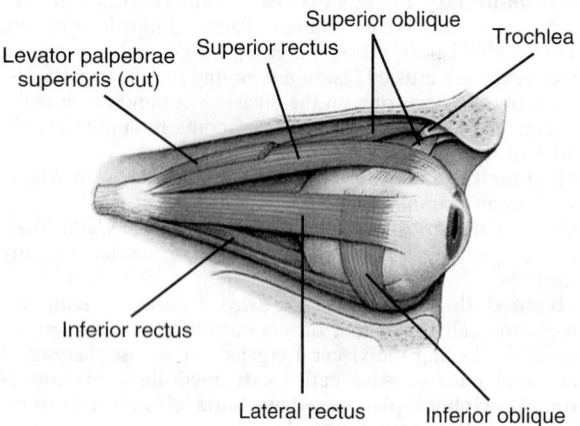

Superior oblique
Levator palpebrae
superioris (cut)
Superior rectus
Trochlea

Inferior rectus

Lateral rectus
Inferior oblique

Inferior view

**Extrinsic muscles of the eye**
*(Thibodeau and Patton, 19995/John V. Hagen)*

**extraperitoneal** /-per′itənē′əl/ [L, *extra* + Gk, *peri*, near, around, *teinein*, to stretch], occurring or located outside the peritoneal cavity.

**extraperitoneal cesarean section,** a method for surgically delivering a baby through an incision in the lower uterine segment without entering the peritoneal cavity. The uterus is approached through the paravesical space. This procedure is performed most often to prevent spread of infection from the uterus into the peritoneal cavity. It takes longer to perform than the low cervical or classic cesarean operation. Compare **classic cesarean section, low cervical cesarean section.** See also **cesarean section.**

**extrapleural** /-ploor′əl/, outside the pleural cavity.

**extrapleural pneumothorax,** a condition in which a pocket of air or gas forms between the endothoracic fascia-pleura layer and the adjacent chest wall. See also **pneumothorax.**

**extrapsychic conflict** /-sī′kik/ [L, *extra* + Gk, *psyche*, mind; L, *confligere*, to strike together], an emotional conflict that usually occurs when one's inner needs and desires do not coincide with the restrictions of the environment or society. Compare **intrapsychic conflict.** See also **conflict.**

**extrapulmonary** /-pul′məner′ē/, outside of or unrelated to the lungs.

**extrapulmonary small cell carcinoma,** a primary small cell cancer with a histologic diagnosis of small cell carcinoma but located in body areas outside the lungs. It occurs most frequently around the head and neck; in the pancreas, colon, and rectum; and in the genitourinary tract.

**extrapyramidal** /ek′strəpiram′ədəl/ [L, *extra* + Gk, *pyramis,* pyramid], **1.** pertaining to the tissues and structures outside the cerebrospinal pyramidal tracts of the brain that are associated with movement of the body, excluding motor neurons, the motor cortex, and the corticospinal and corticobulbar tracts. **2.** pertaining to the function of these tissues and structures.

**extrapyramidal disease,** any of a large group of conditions affecting the extrapyramidal tracts and characterized by involuntary movement, changes in muscle tone, and abnormal posture. Examples include tardive dyskinesia, chorea, athetosis, and Parkinson's disease.

**extrapyramidal side effects,** side effects that mimic extrapyramidal disease and are caused by drugs that block dopamine receptor sites in the extrapyramidal system tract.

**extrapyramidal system,** the part of the nervous system that includes the basal nuclei, substantia nigra, subthalamic nucleus, part of the midbrain, and the motor neurons of the spine. See also **extrapyramidal tracts.**

**extrapyramidal tracts,** the uncrossed tracts of motor nerves from the brain to the anterior horns of the spinal cord, except the crossed fibers of the pyramidal tracts. Within the brain, extrapyramidal pathways comprise various relays of motoneurons between motor areas of the cerebral cortex, the basal nuclei, the thalamus, the cerebellum, and the brainstem. The extrapyramidal pathways are functional rather than anatomic units, comprising the nuclei and the fibers and excluding the pyramidal tracts. They especially control and coordinate the postural, static, supporting, and locomotor mechanisms and cause contractions of muscle groups sequentially or simultaneously. The extrapyramidal pathways include the corpus striatum, the subthalamic nucleus, the substantia nigra, and the red nucleus, together with their interconnections with the reticular formation, the cerebellum, and the cerebrum. Compare **pyramidal tract.**

**extrarenal uremia** See **prerenal uremia.**

**extrasensory** /-sen′sərē/ [L, *extra* + *sentire,* to feel], pertaining to alleged awareness of events that cannot be observed by any of the five basic senses. It includes telepathy, clairvoyance, and psychokinesis.

**extrasensory perception (ESP)** [L, *extra* + *sentire,* to feel, *percipere,* to perceive], alleged awareness or knowledge acquired without using the physical senses. See also **clairvoyance, parapsychology, telepathy.**

**extrasystole.** See **ectopic beat.**

**extrauterine** /-yoō′tərin/ [L, *extra* + *uterus,* womb], occurring or located outside the uterus, as an ectopic pregnancy.

**extravasation** /ikstrav′əsā′shən/ [L, *extra* + *vas,* vessel], **1.** a passage or escape into the tissues, usually of blood, serum, or lymph. Compare **bleeding. 2.** passage or escape into tissue of antineoplastic chemotherapeutic drugs. Signs and symptoms may be sudden onset of localized pain at an injection site, sudden redness or extreme pallor at an injection site, or loss of blood return in an IV needle. Tissue slough and necrosis may occur if the condition is severe.

Treatment depends on the causative agent. Nursing responsibilities include maintaining the patient IV line, elevating the affected area, applying ice packs, and notifying the physician of the need for antidote injections, if applicable. See also **exudate, transudate. —extravasate,** *v.*

**extravascular fluid** /-vas′kyələr/ [L, *extra,* outside, *vasculum,* small vessel, *fluere,* to flow], fluid in the body that is outside the blood vessels. Examples include lymph and cerebrospinal fluid.

**extraventricular hydrocephalus.** See **hydrocephalus.**

**extraversion.** See **extroversion.**

**extravert.** See **extrovert.**

**extraverted personality.** See **extroverted personality.**

**extremity** /ikstrem′itē/ [L, *extremitas*], an arm or a leg. The arm may be identified as an upper extremity and the leg as a lower extremity.

**extrinsic** /ikstrin′sik/ [L, *extrinsecus,* on the outside], pertaining to anything external or originating outside a structure or organism, including parts of an organ that are not wholly contained within it, as an extrinsic muscle.

**extrinsic allergic alveolitis.** See **hypersensitivity pneumonitis.**

**extrinsic allergic pneumonia.** See **diffuse hypersensitivity pneumonia.**

**extrinsic asthma.** See **allergic asthma.**

**extrinsic factor.** See **cyanocobalamin.**

**extrinsic muscle (em)** [L, *extrinsecus,* on the outside], **1.** muscle that is outside the organ it controls, as the extraocular muscles that control eye movements. **2.** muscle that links a limb to the trunk of the body.

**extrinsic pathway of coagulation,** the mechanism that produces fibrin following tissue injury, beginning with formation of an activated complex between tissue factor and activated factor VII and leading to activation of factor X, which induces the reactions of the common pathway of coagulation. Compare **intrinsic pathway of coagulation.** See also **coagulation cascade, common pathway of coagulation.**

**extro-.** See **extra-.**

**extroversion** /-vur′zhən/ [L, *extra* + *vertere,* to turn], **1.** the tendency to direct one's interests and energies toward external values or things outside the self. **2.** the state of being totally or primarily concerned with what is outside the self. Also spelled **extraversion.** Compare **introversion.**

**extrovert** /ik′strəvurt′/, **1.** a person whose interests are directed away from the self and concerned primarily with external reality and the physical environment rather than with inner feelings and thoughts. This person is usually highly sociable, outgoing, impulsive, and emotionally expressive. **2.** a person characterized by extroversion. Also spelled **extravert.** Compare **introvert.**

**extroverted personality** /-vur′tid/ [L, *extra,* outside, *vertere,* to turn, *personalis,* of a person], a persona that is directed to a greater degree toward the outer world of people and events rather than the subjective inner world experience. Also called **extraverted personality.**

**extrude** /ekstrōod′/ [L, *extrudere,* to push out], to thrust out from a surface or from alignment.

**extrusion** /ek·strōo′zhən/ [L, *extrudere,* to push out], **1.** thrusting or pushing out; expulsion by force. **2.** the overeruption or movement of a tooth beyond its normal occlusal plane in the absence of opposing occlusal force. **3.** an orthodontic technique for the elongation or elevation of a tooth. Compare **intrusion.**

**extrusion reflex** /ekstrōo′zhən/ [L, *extrudere,* to push out, *reflectere,* to bend back], a normal response in infants to force the tongue outward when touched or depressed. The reflex begins to disappear by about 3 or 4 months of age. Constant protrusion of a large tongue may be a sign of Down syndrome.

**extubation** /iks′t(y)ōobā′shən/ [L, *ex,* out, *tuba,* tube], the process of withdrawing a tube from an orifice or cavity of the body. —**extubate,** *v.*

**exuberant callus.** See **heterotopic ossification.**

**exudate** /eks′yōodāt/ [L, *exsudare,* to sweat out], fluid, cells, or other substances that have been slowly exuded, or discharged, from cells or blood vessels through small pores or breaks in cell membranes. Perspiration, pus, and serum are sometimes identified as exudates.

**exudation** /eks′yədā′shən/ [L, *exudare*], the oozing of fluid, pus, or serum. The exudate may or may not contain fibrous or coagulated material.

**exudative** /igzōo′dətiv/, relating to the oozing of fluid and other materials from cells and tissues, usually as a result of inflammation or injury.

**exudative angina.** See **croup.**

**exudative enteropathy,** diarrhea that occurs in diseases characterized by inflammation or destruction of intestinal mucosa. Crohn's disease, ulcerative colitis, tuberculosis, and some lymphomas cause an increased amount of plasma, blood, mucus, and protein to accumulate in the intestine, adding to fecal bulk and frequency. See also **diarrhea.**

**exudative inflammation** [L, *exudare,* to sweat out, *inflammare,* to set afire], an inflammation of a serous or raw cavity in which fluid is released from the inflamed surface.

**exudative retinopathy,** a condition marked by masses of white or yellowish exudate in the posterior part of the fundus oculi, with deposit of cholesterin and blood debris from retinal hemorrhage, and leading to destruction of the macula and blindness. Also called **Coats' disease, Coats' retinitis, exudative retinitis.**

**eye** [AS, *eage*], one of a pair of organs of sight, contained in a bony orbit at the front of the skull, embedded in orbital fat, and innervated by four cranial nerves: optic, oculomotor, trochlear, and abducens. Associated with the eye are certain accessory structures, such as the muscles, the fasciae, the eyebrow, the eyelids, the conjunctiva, and the lacrimal gland. The bulb of the eye is composed of segments of two spheres with nearly parallel axes that constitute the outside tunic and one of three fibrous layers enclosing two internal cavities separated by the crystalline lens. The smaller cavity anterior to the lens is divided by the iris into two chambers, both filled with aqueous humor. The posterior cavity is larger than the anterior cavity and contains the jellylike vit-

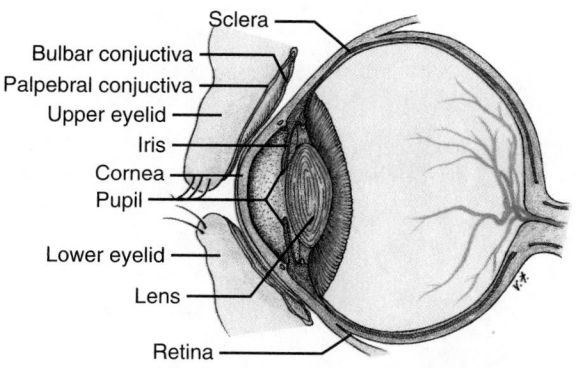

Sclera
Bulbar conjuctiva
Palpebral conjuctiva
Upper eyelid
Iris
Cornea
Pupil
Lower eyelid
Lens
Retina

**Cross section of the eye** *(Potter and Perry, 2001)*

reous body that is divided by the hyaloid canal. The outside tunic of the bulb consists of the transparent cornea anteriorly, constituting one fifth of the tunic, and the opaque sclera posteriorly, constituting five sixths of the tunic. The intermediate vascular, pigmented tunic consists of the choroid, the ciliary body, and the iris. The internal tunic of nervous tissue is the retina. Light waves passing through the lens strike a layer of rods and cones in the retina, creating impulses that are transmitted by the optic nerve to the brain. The transverse and the anteroposterior diameters of the eye bulb are slightly greater than the vertical diameter; the bulb in women is usually smaller than the bulb in men. Eye movement is controlled by six muscles: the superior and inferior oblique muscles and the superior, inferior, medial, and lateral rectus muscles. Also called **bulbus oculi, eyeball.**

**eye bank** [AS, *eage* + It, *banca,* bench], a facility for collecting and storing corneas and other ocular tissues for transplantation to recipients.

**eyebrow** [AS, *eage* + *bru*], **1.** the supraorbital arch of the frontal bone that separates the orbit of the eye from the forehead. **2.** the arch of hairs growing along the ridge formed by the supraorbital arch of the frontal bone.

**eye care,** a nursing intervention from the Nursing Interventions Classification (NIC) defined as prevention or minimization of threats to eye or visual integrity. See also **Nursing Interventions Classification.**

**eye-closure reflex.** See **wink reflex**.

**eyecup,** a small vessel or cup that is shaped to fit over the eyeball and used to bathe the exposed surface of the eye.

**eye deviation** [AS, *eage* + L, *deviare,* to turn aside], **1.** a movement of one or both eyes, singly or jointly, from the median line or from the original direction of fixation. **Manifest deviation** is the number of degrees by which the visual axis of one eye deviates from that of the other in cases of squint, when both eyes are open. **2.** (in strabismus) the departure of the foveal line of sight of one eye from the point of fixation.

**eye dominance,** an unconscious preference to use one eye rather than the other for certain purposes, such as sighting a rifle or looking through a telescope.

**eyedrops,** a liquid medicine that is administered by allowing it to fall in drops onto the conjunctival surface.

**eye glasses,** transparent lenses held in metal or plastic frames in front of the eyes to correct refractive errors or to protect the eyes from harmful electromagnetic waves or flying objects.

**eyeground,** the fundus of the eye as revealed by ophthalmoscopic examination.

**eyelash** [AS, *eage* + ME, *lasche*], one of many stiff hairs

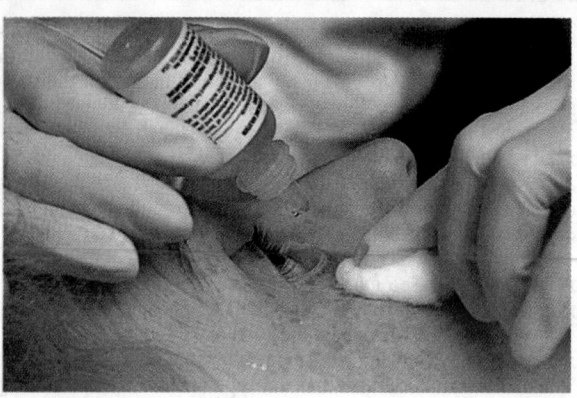

**Eyedrop administration** *(Potter and Perry, 2001)*

growing in double or triple rows along the border of the eyelids in front of a row of ciliary glands that are in front of a row of meibomian glands.

**eyelid** [AS, *eage* + *hlid*], one of two movable folds of protective thin skin over the eye, with eyelashes and ciliary and meibomian glands along its margin. It consists of loose connective tissue containing a thin plate of fibrous tissue lined with mucous membrane (conjunctiva). The orbicularis oculi muscle and the oculomotor nerve control the opening and closing of the eyelid. The upper and lower eyelids are separated by the palpebral fissure. Also called **palpebra** /pal'-pəbrə/.

**eye memory.** See **visual memory.**

**eye patching,** **1.** placement of a soft patch over a closed eye to restrict lid movement during corneal reepithelialization or a similar healing procedure in progress. **2.** occlusion of the better eye by patch placement in young patients with strabismic amblyopia to force greater use of the amblyopic eye. **3.** patching used in cases of diplopia (double vision).

**eye shielding,** protection of an injured eye by securing a metal or plastic eye shield or a disposable cup to prevent further injury.

**eye shower,** an apparatus for irrigating the eyes after exposure to dust or other debris or chemical contamination. The shower directs one or two streams of water so that they flush over the eyes and lids. The patient should blink the eyes and move the head in different directions with the eyes open, continuing the irrigation as needed.

**eye worm.** See *Loa loa.*

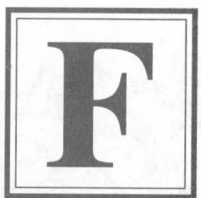

**f,** 1. symbol for *breaths per unit time.* 2. symbol for *respiratory frequency.*

**F,** 1. abbreviation for **Fahrenheit.** 2. abbreviation for **farad.** 3. symbol for **fluorine.** 4. abbreviation for **frequency.**

**F₁,** the symbol for **first filial generation.**

**F₂,** the symbol for **second filial generation.**

**F²ARV,** abbreviation for Fear/Frustration (F²), Anger, Rage, and Violence, a highly volatile emotional reaction that escalates from fear or frustration and proceeds sequentially through anger and rage to violence.

**Fₐb,** the fragment of an antibody molecule that contains the antigen-binding site, consisting of a light chain and part of a heavy chain. Such fragments are produced when antibodies are digested by enzymes, such as the protease papain. $F_{ab}$ fragments are used as an antidote for treating toxicity caused by digoxin, digitoxin, and oleander tea. See also **Fₑ, Digibind.**

**Fₑ,** a part of a molecule of an antibody that has been split by a proteolytic enzyme. It represents the relatively constant region, as distinguished from the $F_{ab}$ portion, that contains the binding sites. The $F_c$ portion is sometimes identified as the crystallizable fragment.

**FA,** 1. abbreviation for **fatty acid.** 2. abbreviation for **femoral artery.** 3. abbreviation for **folic acid.**

**F.A.A.N.,** abbreviation for **Fellow of the American Academy of Nursing.**

**fabere** abbreviation for *f*lexion, *ab*duction, *e*xternal *rota*tion, then *e*xtension. See **Patrick test.**

**fabere sign.** See **Patrick test.**

**fabrication** /fab′rikā′shən/, a psychologic reaction in which false statements are contrived to mask memory defects. It is a clinical feature of Korsakoff's syndrome and other disorders. See also **confabulation.**

**Fabry's disease, Fabry's syndrome.** See **angiokeratoma corporis diffusum.**

**FAC,** an anticancer drug combination of fluorouracil, doxorubicin, and cyclophosphamide.

**F.A.C.C.P.,** abbreviation for *Fellow of the American College of Chest Physicians.*

**F.A.C.D.,** abbreviation for *Fellow of the American College of Dentists.*

**face** [L, *facies*], 1. the front of the head from the chin to the brow, including the skin and muscles and structures of the forehead, eyes, nose, mouth, cheeks, and jaw. 2. the visage or countenance. 3. to direct the face toward something. See also **en face. —facial,** *adj.*

**face-bow** [L, *facies* + AS, *boga*], a device resembling a caliper for measuring the relationship of the maxilla to the temporomandibular joints. The measurement is used in the fabrication of denture casts and major restorative procedures involving natural teeth.

**face lift,** a plastic surgery procedure in which wrinkles and other signs of aging skin are eliminated. Also called **rhytidoplasty, rhytidectomy.**

**face presentation** [L, *facies,* face, *praesentare,* to show],

an obstetric presentation in which the chin of the fetus is the first feature to appear in labor.

**facet** /fas′it/ [Fr, *facette,* little face], 1. (in dentistry) a flattened, highly polished wear pattern on a tooth. 2. a small, smooth-surfaced process for articulation.

**facetectomy** /fas′itek′təmē/, surgical removal of a facet, particularly the articular facet of a vertebra.

**facet joint,** synovial joint between articular processes (zygapophytes) of the vertebrae. Also called **zygapophyseal joint.**

**facial.** See **face.**

**facial angle** /fāshəl/ [L, *facies* + *angulus,* a corner], the degree of protrusion of the lower face, assessed by measuring the inclination of the facial plane relative to the horizontal reference plane.

**facial artery,** one of a pair of tortuous arteries that arise from the external carotid arteries, divide into four cervical and five facial branches, and supply various organs and tissues in the head. The cervical branches of the facial artery are the ascending palatine, tonsillar, glandular, and submental. The facial branches are the inferior labial, superior labial, lateral nasal, angular, and muscular.

**facial bones,** the 14 bones that form the face of the skull. They include two each of the nasal, palatine, inferior nasal concha, maxilla, lacrimal, and zygomatic bones, plus the mandible and vomer.

**facial diplegia,** a rare neuromuscular condition characterized by bilateral paralysis of various muscles of the face. See also **Möbius' syndrome.**

**facial hemiplegia,** paralysis of the muscles of one side of the face.

**facial hemispasm.** See **Bell's spasm.**

**facial muscle,** one of numerous muscles of the face that seldom remains distinct over its entire length because of a tendency to merge with a neighboring muscle at its termination or its attachment. The five groups of facial muscles are the muscles of the scalp, the extrinsic muscles of the ear, the muscles of the nose, the muscles of the eyelid, and the muscles of the mouth. The platysma is one of the facial group but is classified among the muscles of the neck. Also called **muscle of expression.**

**facial nerve,** either of a pair of mixed sensory and motor cranial nerves that arise from the brainstem at the base of the pons and divide immediately in front of the ear into six branches, innervating the scalp, forehead, eyelids, muscles of facial expression, cheeks, and jaw. Also called **seventh cranial nerve.**

**facial nerve paralysis,** a loss of voluntary control of the muscles of the face, usually on one side. The condition may be caused by a lesion involving the facial muscles or a nerve peripheral to the nucleus or by damage elsewhere in the brainstem or cerebrum. Weakness may be limited to the lower portion of the face, depending on the site of the lesion and the tracts involved.

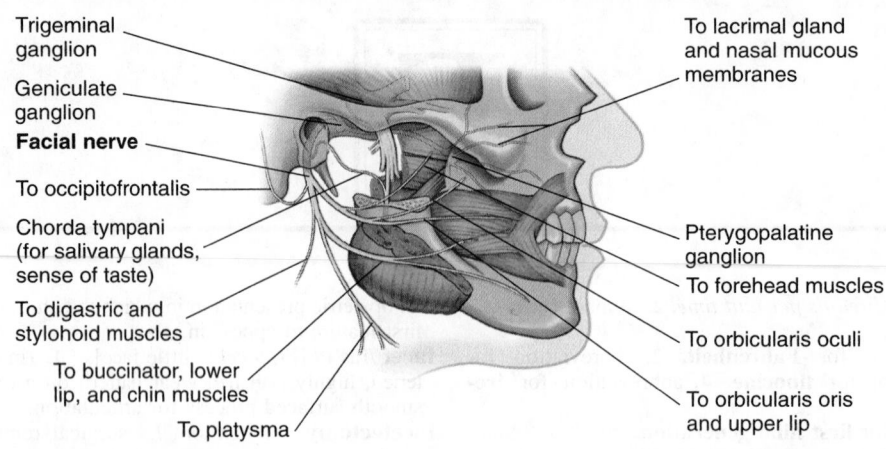

Trigeminal ganglion

Geniculate ganglion

**Facial nerve**

To occipitofrontalis

Chorda tympani (for salivary glands, sense of taste)

To digastric and stylohoid muscles

To buccinator, lower lip, and chin muscles

To platysma

To lacrimal gland and nasal mucous membranes

Pterygopalatine ganglion

To forehead muscles

To orbicularis oculi

To orbicularis oris and upper lip

**Facial nerve**

**facial neuralgia,** the occurrence of pain in the middle ear and auditory canal caused by inflammation of the otic ganglion.

**facial palsy** [L, *facies,* face; Gk, *paralyein,* to be palsied], a loss of motor nerve function in the muscles of the face. See also **Bell's palsy.**

**facial paralysis,** an abnormal condition characterized by the partial or total loss of the functions of the facial muscles or the loss of sensation in the face. It may be caused by disease or by trauma. The degree of paralysis depends on the nerves affected. Brain injury above the facial nerve nucleus usually does not block the innervation of the brow and the forehead muscles. Injury to the nucleus of the facial nerve or injury to its peripheral neurons paralyzes all the ipsilateral facial muscles. See also **Bell's palsy.**

**facial perception,** the ability to judge the distance and direction of objects through the sensation felt in the skin of the face. The phenomenon is commonly experienced by those who are blind and rarely experienced in the dark by those with sight. Also called **facial vision.**

**facial tic** [L, *facies,* face; Fr, *tic,* twitching], any repetitive, spasmodic, and involuntary contraction of groups of facial muscles. See also **tic douloureux.**

**facial vein,** one of a pair of superficial veins that drain deoxygenated blood from the superficial structures of the face. The facial vein anastomoses with the cavernous sinus through various veins, such as the angular, the supraorbital, and the superior ophthalmic. Because the vein has no valves that prevent the backflow of blood, infections of the skin near the nose and mouth may progress into deeper tissues and lead to meningitis. Blood-borne organisms can reach the cavernous sinus through the anastomoses.

**facial vision.** See **facial perception.**

**facies** /fā'shē-ēs/, *pl.* **facies** /fā'shē-ēs/ [L, face], **1.** the face. **2.** the surface of any body structure, part, or organ. **3.** facial expression or appearance.

**facilitation** /fəsil'itā'shən/ [L, *facilitas,* easiness], **1.** the enhancement or reinforcement of any action or function so that it can be performed more easily. Compare **inhibition.** See also **summation. 2.** (in neurology) the phenomenon whereby two or more afferent impulses that individually are not strong enough to elicit a response in a neuron can collectively produce a reflex discharge greater than the sum of the separate responses.

**facilitory casting** /fəsil'itôr'ē/, a method of making pros-

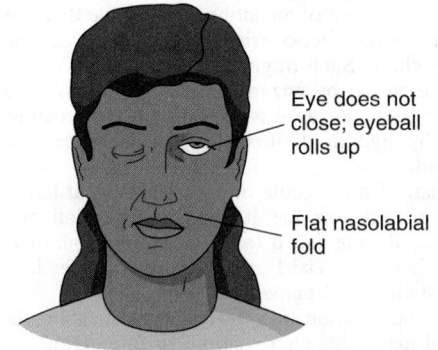

Eye does not close; eyeball rolls up

Flat nasolabial fold

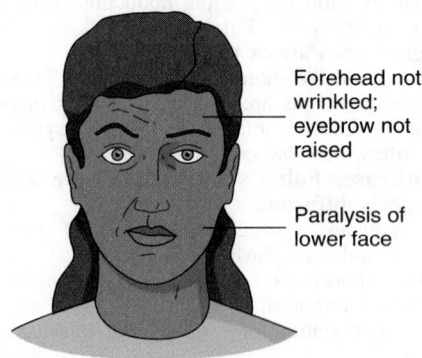

Forehead not wrinkled; eyebrow not raised

Paralysis of lower face

**Clinical manifestations of facial nerve paralysis**
(Beare and Myers, 1998)

thetic casts with materials that increase muscle tone in a specific group while increasing or decreasing range of motion.

**facio-,** combining form meaning 'face': *faciocervical, faciolingual, facioplegia.*

**faciodigitogenital syndrome, faciogenital dysplasia.** See **Aarskog syndrome.**

**faciolingual** /fā'shōling'gwəl/, pertaining to the face and tongue.

**F.A.C.O.G.,** abbreviation for *Fellow of the American College of Obstetricians and Gynecologists.*

**F.A.C.P.,** abbreviation for *Fellow of the American College of Physicians.*

**F.A.C.S.,** abbreviation for *Fellow of the American College of Surgeons.*

**facsimile (fax),** a method of transmitting images or printed matter by electronic means. Images are scanned, converted into electronic signals, and sent over telephone lines to a fax receiver, which reconverts the electronic data into a duplicate of the original image.

**F.A.C.S.M.,** abbreviation for *Fellow of the American College of Sports Medicine.*

**-faction,** suffix meaning a 'process of making': *bilifaction, chylifaction, liquefaction.*

**factitial** /fakti'shəl/ [L, *facticius,* artificial], artificial or self-induced, such as a factitial dermatitis.

**factitial dermatitis,** a skin rash caused by the patient, usually for secondary gain or as a manifestation of a psychiatric illness.

**factitious disorder** /faktish'əs/, a *DSM-IV* diagnosis marked by disease symptoms caused by deliberate efforts of a person to gain attention. Such actions may be repeated, even when the individual is aware of the hazards involved. See also **Munchausen's syndrome.**

**-factive, -fying,** suffix meaning 'making': *liquefactive, stupefactive, vasofactive.*

**factor,** 1. one of a number of elements contributing to a whole. 2. a number by which another number is exactly divisible. 3. one of a number of elements that affect a specific result.

**factor I.** See **fibrinogen.**

**factor II,** a plasma protein precursor of thrombin. It is synthesized in the liver in the presence of vitamin K and is converted to thrombin by activated Factor X. Also called **prothrombin.**

**factor III.** See **thromboplastin.**

**factor IV,** a designation for calcium that is involved in the process of the blood coagulation.

**factor V,** an unstable procoagulant needed to convert prothrombin rapidly to thrombin. Research indicates that during coagulation factor V changes from an inactive agent to an active prothrombin accelerator. Also called **proaccelerin.**

**factor VI,** a hypothetic chemical agent that some suggest is derived from proaccelerin, or factor V, in the process of blood coagulation.

**factor VII,** a blood procoagulant present in the blood plasma and synthesized in the liver in the presence of vitamin K. Also called **proconvertin.**

**factor VIII,** a coagulation factor present in normal plasma but deficient in the blood of persons with hemophilia A. It is a macromolecular complex composed of two separate entities, one of which, when deficient, results in hemophilia A, and the other, when deficient, results in Von Willebrand's disease. See also **antihemophilic factor.**

**factor IX,** a coagulation factor present in normal plasma but deficient in the blood of persons with hemophilia B. Also called **Christmas factor.**

**factor X,** a coagulation factor that occurs in normal plasma but is deficient in some inherited defects in coagulation. Factor X and prothrombin are closely related; both are synthesized in the liver in the presence of vitamin K. Also called **Stuart-Prower factor,** *(formerly)* **thrombokinase.**

**factor XI,** a coagulation factor present in normal plasma. Deficiency results in hemophilia C.

**factor XII,** a coagulation factor present in normal plasma that triggers the formation of bradykinin and associated enzymatic reactions. Factor XII is required for rapid coagulation in vitro but is apparently not needed for hemostasis in vivo. It can be activated in the laboratory by contact with negatively charged surfaces, which can develop on glass and kaolin or on biologic material, such as collagen. Also called **activation factor, contact factor, glass factor, Hageman factor.**

**factor XIII,** a coagulation factor present in normal plasma that acts with calcium to produce an insoluble fibrin clot. Also called **fibrinase, fibrin stabilizing factor, Laki-Lorand factor.**

**factor IX complex,** a hemostatic containing factors II, VII, IX, and X.
- INDICATION: It is prescribed in treatment of hemophilia B.
- CONTRAINDICATION: Liver disease with associated intravascular coagulation and fibrinolysis is contraindicated.
- ADVERSE EFFECTS: Among the more serious adverse reactions are hepatitis, intravascular coagulation, circulatory collapse, and hypersensitivity reaction.

**factor-searching study,** (in nursing research) a study design that produces a qualitative narrative description that includes categories or classifications of phenomena. It may be used to describe various aspects of nursing practice, characteristics of a population, or both. Factor searching is often a preliminary step in a study at a higher level of inquiry.

**facultative** /fak'əltā'tiv/ [L, *facultas,* capability], not obligatory; having the ability to adapt to more than one condition, such as a facultative anaerobe.

**facultative aerobe,** an organism able to grow under anaerobic conditions but develops most rapidly in an aerobic environment. Compare **obligate aerobe.** See **aerobe.**

**facultative anaerobe,** an organism that is able to grow under aerobic conditions but that develops most rapidly in an anaerobic environment. Compare **obligate anaerobe.** See also **anaerobe, anaerobic infection.**

**facultative parasite.** See **parasite.**

**faculty** /fak'əltē/ [L, *facultas,* capability], 1. any normal physiologic function or natural ability of a living organism, such as the digestive faculty or the ability to perceive and distinguish sensory stimuli. 2. an ability to do something specific, such as learn languages or remember names. 3. any mental ability or power, such as memory or thought. 4. a department in an institution of learning or the people who teach in a department of such an institution.

**FAD.** See **nonstress test.**

**fading time,** the time required for a constant stimulus applied to a fixed area of the peripheral visual field to stop.

**faecal.** See **fecal.**

**faeces, faex** See **feces.**

**Faget's sign** /fazhäz'/ [Jean C. Faget, French physician, 1818–1884], a falling pulse rate associated with a constant temperature, or a constant pulse associated with a rising temperature. It is an unusual sign found in yellow fever. Also called *Faget's law.*

**fagicladosporic acid** /faj'iklad'ōspôr'ik/, a toxin produced by *Cladosporium epiphyllum,* a member of a genus of fungi that cause "black spot" in stored meat, tinea nigra, and black degeneration of the brain.

**Fahrenheit (F)** /fer'ənhīt/ [Daniel G. Fahrenheit, German physicist, 1686–1736], a scale for the measurement of temperature in which the boiling point of water is 212° and the freezing point of water is 32° at sea level. To convert to Celsius, subtract 32, then divide by 1.8. Compare **Celsius.**

**failed forceps,** an attempted midforceps operation that is abandoned because there is a greater degree of resistance to rotation or traction than anticipated, as a result of cephalopelvic disproportion. Cesarean section is performed to deliver the infant. Compare **trial forceps.** See also **cephalo-pelvic disproportion.**

**failure to thrive (FTT)** /fāl′yər/ [L, *fallere,* to deceive; ME, *thriven,* to grasp], the abnormal retardation of growth and development of an infant resulting from conditions that interfere with normal metabolism, appetite, and activity. Causative factors include chromosomal abnormalities, as in Turner's syndrome and the various trisomies; major organ system defects that lead to deficiency or malfunction; systemic disease or acute illness; physical deprivation, primarily malnutrition; and various psychosocial factors, as in severe cases of maternal deprivation syndrome. Metabolic disturbances of short duration, as occur during acute illness, usually have no long-term effects on development and are usually followed by a period of rapid growth. Prolonged nutritional deficiency may cause permanent and irreversible retardation of physical, mental, or social development.

**faint** [OFr, *faindre,* to feign] *(nontechnical)* **1.** to lose consciousness, as in a syncopal attack. **2.** a syncopal attack. See also **syncope.**

**fainting.** See **syncope.**

**faith healing** [L, *fidere,* to trust; AS, *hoelen,* to make whole], alleged healing through the power to cause a cure or recovery from an illness or injury without the aid of conventional medical treatment. The healer is believed to have been given that power by a supernatural force.

**falciform body.** See **sporozoite.**

**falciform ligament** /fal′sifôrm/, a triangular or sickle-shaped ligament of the body, such as the ligamentum falciform hepatis. See also **broad ligament of liver.**

**falciform ligament of liver.** See **broad ligament of liver.**

**falciparum malaria** /falsip′ərəm/ [L, *falx,* sickle, *forma,* form; It, *mal,* bad *aria,* air], the most severe form of malaria, caused by the protozoon *Plasmodium falciparum.* The condition is characterized by extremely grave systemic symptoms, mental confusion, enlarged spleen, edema, GI symptoms, and anemia. The parasite replicates so rapidly in erythrocytes that cerebral vessels may be obstructed. Falciparum malaria episodes do not last as long as other forms of malaria; if treatment is begun promptly, the disease may be mild and the recovery uneventful. Relapses are uncommon, but death may result from dehydration and anemia. The usual treatment is chloroquine, but patients known to have contracted malaria in an area that harbors drug-resistant *P. falciparum* are often treated with a combination of quinine, pyrimethamine, and mefloquine. Compare **quartan malaria, tertian malaria.** See also **algid malaria, blackwater fever, malaria.**

**fallectomy** /fəlek′təmē/, the surgical removal of one or both of the fallopian tubes. See **salpingectomy.**

**fallen arch,** a broken down foot arch, which often results in a flat deformity or splay foot. The condition may involve the longitudinal arch, the transverse arch, or both. When the longitudinal arch is involved, the condition is called **flatfoot** or **pes planus.**

**fallopian canal** [Gabriello Fallopio, Italian anatomist, 1523–1562; L, *canalis*], a passageway for the facial nerve through the petrous bone.

**fallopian tube** /fəlō′pē·ən/ [Gabriello Fallopio], one of a pair of ducts opening at one end into the uterus and at the other end into the peritoneal cavity, over the ovary. Each tube serves as the passage through which an ovum is carried to the uterus and through which spermatozoa move out toward the ovary. The tube lies in the upper border of the broad ligament (the mesosalpinx). Each tube has four parts: the fimbriae, the infundibulum, the ampulla, and the isthmus. The fimbriae drape in fingerlike projections from the

infundibulum over the ovary. Immediately proximal to the infundibulum is the ampulla, the widest portion of the tube. The ampulla is connected to the fundus of the uterus by the isthmus. Also called **oviduct, uterine tube.** See **tubal ligation.**

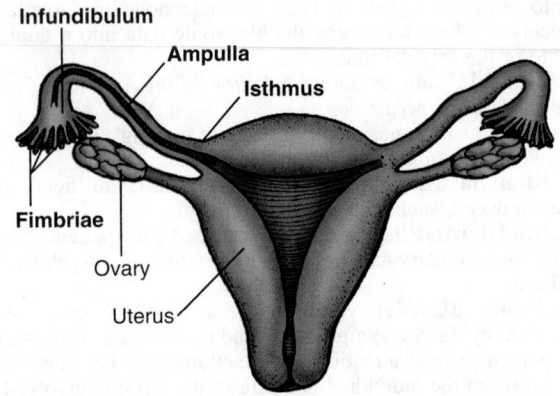

**Parts of the fallopian tube** (Monahan and Neighbors, 1998)

**Fallot's syndrome.** See **tetralogy of Fallot.**

**fallout** [AS, *feallan,* to fall, *ut*], the deposition of radioactive debris after a nuclear explosion. The waste products of an atmospheric explosion of an atomic bomb may travel thousands of miles in the atmosphere and be deposited over a large geographic area.

**fall prevention,** a nursing intervention from the Nursing Interventions Classification (NIC) defined as instituting special precautions with patient at risk for injury from falling. See also **Nursing Interventions Classification.**

**falls, risk for,** a nursing diagnosis accepted by the Fourteenth National Conference on the classification of nursing diagnoses. The state is a defined as an increased susceptibility to falling that may cause physical harm.

■ RISK FACTORS: In adults, risk factors include a history of falls, wheelchair use, being an elderly female, being over 65 years of age, living alone, use of assistive devices, presence of acute illness, postoperative conditions, visual difficulties, arthritis, hearing difficulties, orthostatic hypotension, sleeplessness, faintness when turning or extending neck, anemias, vascular disease, neoplasms, urgency or incontinence, diarrhea, decreased lower extremity strength, postprandial blood sugar changes, foot problems, impaired physical mobility, impaired balance, difficulty with gait, proprioceptive deficits, neuropathy, diminished mental status, antihypertensive agents, ACE inhibitors, diuretics, tricyclic antidepressants, alcohol use, antianxiety agents, narcotics, hypnotics or tranquilizers, restraints, weather conditions, throw rugs, cluttered environment, unfamiliar or dimly lit rooms, and lack of antislip material in the bath or shower. In children, risk factors include age younger than 2 years; male gender when under 1 year of age; lack of automobile restraints; lack of gate for stairs; lack of window guards, bed located near a window; lack of supervision while infant is on a bed, changing table or sofa; and lack of parental supervision. See also **nursing diagnosis.**

**false ankylosis** [L, *fallere,* to deceive; Gk, *agkylosis,* joint stiffness], a type of joint immobility that results from abnormal inflexibility of body parts outside the joint. Also called **extracapsular ankylosis.**

**false anorexia.**   See **pseudoanorexia.**

**false diverticulum** [L, *fallere,* to deceive, *diverticulare,* to turn aside], a protrusion of mucous membrane through a muscular coat defect of a hollow organ.

**false imprisonment** [L, *falsus,* deceptive; ME, *imprisonen*], (in law) the intentional unjustified, nonconsensual detention or confinement of a person for any length of time.

**false joint** [L, *fallere,* to deceive, *jungere,* to join], a joint that develops at the site of a former fracture. Also called **pseudarthrosis.**

**false labor.**   See **preterm contractions.**

**false negative,** an incorrect result of a diagnostic test or procedure that falsely indicates the absence of a finding, condition, or disease. The rate of occurrence of false-negative results varies with the diagnostic accuracy and specificity of the test or procedure. As the accuracy and specificity of a test increase, the rate of false negatives decreases. Certain tests are known to yield false negative results at a certain rate; in all tests a small number will occur by chance alone. False negative results are more common than false positive results, because the person conducting the test is more likely to fail to observe a finding than to imagine seeing something that does not exist. Compare **false positive.**

**false-negative rate** [L, *fallere,* to deceive, *negare,* to deny, *ratum,* calculate], the rate of occurrence of negative test results in subjects known to have the disease or behavior for which an individual is being tested.

**false neuroma,** **1.** a neoplasm that does not contain nerve elements. **2.** a cystic neuroma.

**false nucleolus.**   See **karyosome.**

**false pelvis,** the part of the pelvis superior to a plane passing through the linea terminalis.

**false personification,** (in psychiatry) the labeling and prejudgment of others without validating evidence.

**false positive,** a test result that wrongly indicates the presence of a disease or other condition the test is designed to reveal. Compare **false negative.**

**false-positive rate** [L, *fallere,* to deceive, *positivus* + *ratum,* calculate], the rate of occurrence of positive test results in subjects known to be free of a disease or disorder for which an individual is being tested.

**false pregnancy.**   See **pseudocyesis.**

**false rib.**   See **rib.**

**false suture,** an immovable fibrous joint in which rough articulating surfaces form the connection between certain bones of the skull. Two kinds of false sutures are **sutura plana** and **sutura squamosa.** Compare **true suture.**

**false transactions,** (in transactional analysis), transactions in which communication is stopped or distorted when one individual relates from a different ego state than expected.

**false twins.**   See **dizygotic twins.**

**false vertebra,** one of the vertebral segments that form the sacrum and the coccyx. Also called **fixed vertebra.**

**false vocal cord,** either of two thick folds of mucous membrane in the larynx separating the ventricle from the vestibule. Each fold encloses a narrow band of fibrous tissue (the ventricular ligament). Compare **vocal cord.**

**falx** /falks, fôlks/, *pl.* **falces** /fal′sēz, fôl′sēz/ [L, sickle], **1.** a sickle-shaped structure. **2.** sickle-shaped.

**falx cerebelli** /ser′əbel′ī/, a small sickle-shaped process of the dura mater attached to the occipital bone above and projecting into the posterior cerebellar notch between the two cerebellar hemispheres.

**falx cerebri** /ser′əbrī/, a sickle-shaped fold of dura mater membrane extending into and following along the longitudinal fissure and separating the two hemispheres of the cerebrum.

**falx inguinalis,** transverse and internal oblique muscles.

**falx ligamentosa,** the broad ligament of the liver.

**FAM,** an anticancer drug combination of fluorouracil, doxorubicin, and mitomycin.

**famciclovir,** an antiviral drug.

■ INDICATIONS: It is prescribed in the treatment of acute herpes zoster.

■ CONTRAINDICATIONS: The drug should not be given to patients with kidney disease or an allergy to famciclovir. The safety of the drug in children or in women who are pregnant or breastfeeding has not been established.

■ ADVERSE EFFECTS: The side effects most often reported include fatigue, fever, pain, chills, headache, dizziness, nausea, diarrhea, vomiting, or constipation.

**familial** /fəmil′yəl/ [L, *familia,* household], pertaining to a characteristic, condition, or disease that is present in some families and not others or that occurs in more family members than would be expected by chance. It is usually but not always hereditary. Compare **acquired, congenital, hereditary.**

**familial adenomatous polyposis.**   See **adenomatous polyposis coli.**

**familial autonomic dysfunction.**   See **dysautonomia.**

**familial centrolobar sclerosis.**   See **Pelizaeus-Merzbacher disease.**

**familial cretinism,** a rare genetic disorder caused by an inborn error of metabolism resulting from an enzyme deficiency that interferes with thyroid hormone biosynthesis. Clinical manifestations include lethargy, stunted growth, and mental retardation. The condition is transmitted as an autosomal recessive trait and is treated by early administration of thyroid hormone, if possible in utero, to reduce the abnormalities of mental development. See also **cretinism.**

**familial dysautonomia**   See **dysautonomia.**

**familial histiocytic reticulosis** [L, *familia,* household; Gk, *histion,* web, *kytos,* cell; L, *reticulum,* little net; Gk, *osis,* condition], a hereditary disease, transmitted as an autosomal recessive trait, characterized by anemia, granulocytopenia, and thrombocytopenia. Phagocytosis of blood cells and infiltration of bone marrow by histocytes commonly cause death in childhood. Also called *familial hemophagocytic reticulosis.*

**familial hypercholesterolemia,** an inherited disorder transmitted as a dominant trait and characterized by a high level of serum cholesterol, tendinous xanthomas, and early evidence of atherosclerosis, especially of the coronary arteries. Affected individuals at 50 years of age have 3 to 10 times greater risk of ischemic heart disease than the general population. Cholesterol levels are elevated at birth, increase with age, and average 250 to 500 mg/dL in heterozygous adults and 500 to 1000 mg/dL in adults who are homozygous for the gene. Xanthomas begin to appear at 20 years of age and occur most frequently on the Achilles tendon, extensor tendons of the hands, elbows, and tibial tuberosities. In type IIA familial hypercholesterolemia, only low-density lipoprotein (LDL) level is elevated, whereas in type IIB LDL and very low-density lipoprotein (VLDL) levels are increased. The disorder occurs in Caucasians, African-Americans, and Asian-Americans; the prevalence of the gene in the United States is 1:1000. Treatment includes a low-cholesterol and low-saturated-fat diet. Cholestyramine may be given to patients with type IIA familial hypercholesterolemia but not to those with type IIB. Also called **hypercholesterolemic xanthomatosis, hyperlipidemia type IIA.**

**familial hyperglyceridemia.** See **hyperlipidemia type I.**

**familial iminoglycinuria.** See **iminoglycinuria.**

**familial juvenile nephronophthisis.** See **medullary cystic disease.**

**familial lipoprotein lipase deficiency.** See **hyperchylomicronemia.**

**familial Mediterranean fever,** an autosomal recessive disease usually occurring in Armenians and Sephardic Jews, characterized by short recurrent attacks of fever with pain in the abdomen, chest, or joints and erythema resembling that seen in erysipelas; it is sometimes complicated by secondary amyloidosis. Also called **benign paroxysmal peritonitis, familial recurrent polyserositis, periodic peritonitis, periodic polyserositis, recurrent polyserositis.**

**familial multiple endocrine.** See **multiple endocrine adenomatosis (MEA).**

**familial osteochondrodystrophy.** See **Morquio's disease.**

**familial periodic paralysis** [L, *familia,* household; Gk, *peri,* near, *hodos,* way, *paralysein,* to be palsied], a rare inherited disorder in which clients suffer attacks of general flaccid paralysis after attacks of hypokalemia (potassium depletion). The episodes may follow administration of glucose and are relieved by administration of potassium chloride.

**familial polyposis,** an abnormal condition characterized by multiple polyps in the colon and rectum. The disease has high malignancy potential and is inherited as a heterozygous, autosomal-dominant trait. Total proctocolectomy eliminates the risk of cancer, which, if untreated, occurs before 40 years of age. Genetic counseling is advised. A kind of familial polyposis is **Gardner's syndrome.** See also **polyposis.**

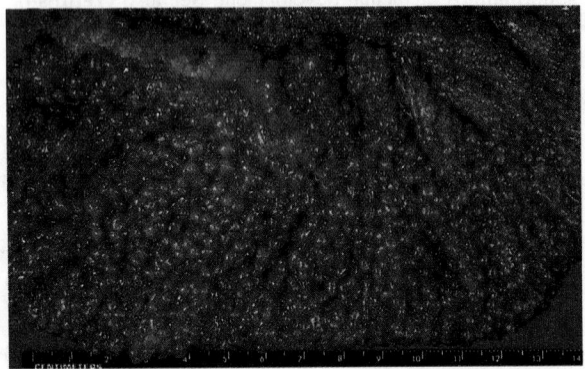

**Familial polyposis** *(Kumar, Cotran, and Robbins, 1997)*

**familial recurrent polyserositis.** See **familial Mediterranean fever.**

**familial spinal muscular atrophy.** See **Werdnig-Hoffmann disease.**

**familial tremor.** See **essential tremor.**

**family** [L, *familia,* household], a group of people related by heredity, such as parents, children, and siblings. The term sometimes is broadened to include persons related by marriage or those living in the same household, who are emotionally attached, interact regularly, and share concerns for the growth and development of the group and its individual members.

**family Apgar,** a family therapy rating system in which the name Apgar contains the first letters of five words–*adaptability, partnership, growth, affection,* and *resolve*—that represent the questionnaire categories. Each family member indicates a degree of satisfaction in each of the five categories on a scale of 0 to 2. The system is used most frequently in studies of families with a geriatric member. See also **Apgar score.**

**family care leave,** absence from a job that is permitted for an employee to care for a family member who is ill, disabled, or pregnant. The U.S. Family and Medical Leave Act of 1993 provides 12 weeks of unpaid leave per year from a job for the birth or adoption of a child; for the care of a seriously ill child, spouse, or parent; or for a serious illness affecting the employee. The law applies only to companies with 50 or more employees. Employers must guarantee that a worker can return to the same or a comparable job.

**family-centered care,** primary health care that includes an assessment of the health of an entire family, identification of actual or potential factors that might influence the health of its members, and implementation of interventions needed to maintain or improve the health of the unit and its members.

**family-centered maternity care,** a system for the delivery of safe, high-quality health care adapted to the physical and psychosocial needs of the patient, the patient's entire family, and the newly born offspring.

**family-centered nursing care,** nursing care directed to improving the potential health of a family or any of its members by assessing individual and family health needs and strengths, by identifying problems influencing the health care of the family as a whole and those influencing the individual members, by using family resources, by teaching and counseling, and by evaluating progress toward stated goals.

**family coping,** a nursing outcome from the Nursing Outcomes Classification (NOC) defined as family actions to manage stressors that tax family resources. See also **Nursing Outcomes Classification.**

**family counseling,** a program of providing information and professional guidance to members of a family concerning specific health matters, such as the care of a severely retarded child or the risk of transmitting a known genetic defect.

**family disorganization,** a breakdown of a family system. It may be associated with parental overburdening or loss of significant others who served as role models for children or support systems for family members. Family disorganization can contribute to the loss of social controls that families usually impose on their members.

**family dynamics,** the forces at work within the family that produce particular behaviors or symptoms.

**family environment: internal,** a nursing outcome from the Nursing Outcomes Classification (NOC) defined as social climate as characterized by family member relationships and goals. See also **Nursing Outcomes Classification.**

**family functioning,** a nursing outcome from the Nursing Outcomes Classification (NOC) defined as ability of the family to meet the needs of its members through developmental transitions. See also **Nursing Outcomes Classification.**

**family functions,** processes by which the family operates as a whole, including communication and manipulation of the environment for problem solving.

**family health.** See **family history.**

**family health status,** a nursing outcome from the Nursing Outcomes Classification (NOC) defined as overall health status and social competence of family unit. See also **Nursing Outcomes Classification.**

**family history,** an essential part of a patient's medical history in which he or she is asked about the health of members of the immediate family in a series of specific questions to discover any disorders to which the patient may be particularly vulnerable, such as "Has anyone in your family had tuberculosis? diabetes mellitus? breast cancer?" Hereditary and familial diseases are especially noted. The age and health of each person, age at death, and causes of death are charted. Often a genogram is developed for pictoral documentation. The family health history is obtained from the patient or family in the initial interview and becomes a part of the permanent record. Other questions, such as those concerning the age, sex, relationships of others in the household, and marital history of the patient, may also be asked if the information has not already been secured.

**family integrity,** a nursing outcome from the Nursing Outcomes Classification (NOC) defined as extent that family members' behaviors collectively demonstrate cohesion, strength, and emotional bonding. See also **Nursing Outcomes Classification.**

**family integrity promotion,** a nursing intervention from the Nursing Interventions Classification (NIC) defined as promotion of family cohesion and unity. See also **Nursing Interventions Classification.**

**family integrity promotion: childbearing family,** a nursing intervention from the Nursing Interventions Classification (NIC) defined as facilitation of the growth of individuals or families who are adding an infant to the family unit. See also **Nursing Interventions Classification.**

**family involvement promotion,** a nursing intervention from the Nursing Interventions Classification (NIC) defined as facilitating family participation in the emotional and physical care of the patient. See also **Nursing Interventions Classification.**

**family medicine,** the branch of medicine that is concerned with the diagnosis and treatment of health problems in people of either sex and any age. Practitioners of family medicine are often called family practice physicians, family physicians, or, formerly, general practitioners. They often act as the primary health care providers, referring complex disorders to a specialist.

**family mobilization,** a nursing intervention from the Nursing Interventions Classification (NIC) defined as utilization of family strengths to influence patient's health in a positive direction. See also **Nursing Interventions Classification.**

**family myths,** myths that are constructed to deny the reality of family situations.

**family normalization,** a nursing outcome from the Nursing Outcomes Classification (NOC) defined as ability of the family to develop and maintain routines and management strategies that contribute to optimal functioning when a member has a chronic illness or disability. See also **Nursing Outcomes Classification.**

**family nurse practitioner (FNP),** a nurse practitioner possessing skills necessary for the detection and management of acute self-limiting conditions and management of chronic stable conditions. An FNP provides primary ambulatory care for families in collaboration with primary care physicians. The FNP gives direct health care and guides or counsels families as required. Consultation, copractice, and referral to associated physicians are aspects of the FNP's practice.

**family of origin,** the family into which a person is born.

**family of procreation,** the family a person forms through marriage and/or childbearing.

**family participation in professional care,** a nursing outcome from the Nursing Outcomes Classification (NOC) defined as family involvement in decision making, delivery, and evaluation of care provided by health care personnel. See also **Nursing Outcomes Classification.**

**family physician,** **1.** a medical practitioner of the specialty of family medicine. **2.** *(formerly)* practitioner. **3.** a family practice physician. See also **family medicine.**

**family planning.** See **contraception.**

**family planning: contraception,** a nursing intervention from the Nursing Interventions Classification (NIC) defined as facilitation of pregnancy prevention by providing information about the physiology of reproduction and methods to control conception. See also **Nursing Interventions Classification.**

**family planning: infertility,** a nursing intervention from the Nursing Interventions Classification (NIC) defined as management, education, and support of the patient and significant other undergoing evaluation and treatment for infertility. See also **Nursing Interventions Classification.**

**family planning: unplanned pregnancy,** a nursing intervention from the Nursing Interventions Classification (NIC) defined as facilitation of decision making regarding pregnancy outcome. See also **Nursing Interventions Classification.**

**family practice** [L, *familia,* household; Gk, *praktikos,* ready for action], a medical specialty that encompasses several branches of medicine, including internal medicine, preventive medicine, pediatrics, surgery, psychiatry, and obstetrics and gynecology; includes client management, counseling, and problem solving; and coordinates total health care delivery to all members of a family, regardless of sex or age.

**family practice physician,** a practitioner of family medicine, usually one who has completed a residency program in the specialty. See also **family medicine.**

**family processes, dysfunctional: alcoholism,** a nursing diagnosis accepted by the Eleventh National Conference on the Classification of Nursing Diagnoses. It is defined as the state in which the psychosocial, spiritual, and physiologic functions of the family unit are chronically disorganized, leading to conflict, denial of problems, resistance to change, ineffective problem solving, and a series of self-perpetuating crises.

■ DEFINING CHARACTERISTICS: Major defining characteristics include a wide range of feelings, roles and relationships, and behaviors. Feelings include decreased self-esteem or sense of worthlessness, anger or suppressed rage, frustration, powerlessness, anxiety, tension, distress, insecurity, repressed emotions, responsibility for the alcoholic's behavior, lingering resentment, and shame or embarrassment. Roles and relationships include deterioration in family relationships or disturbed family dynamics, ineffective spouse communication or marital problems, altered role function or disruption of family roles, inconsistent parenting or low perception of parental support, family denial, intimacy dysfunction, chronic family problems, and closed communication systems. Behaviors include inappropriate expression of anger, difficulty with intimate relationships, loss of control of drinking, impaired communication, ineffective problem-solving skills, enabling of alcoholic to maintain drinking, inability to meet emotional needs of its members, manipulation, dependency, criticizing, and inadequate understanding or knowledge of alcoholism. Some minor defining characteristics are feelings of being different from other people, depression, hostility, fear, emotional control by others, confusion, dissatisfaction, and lack of identity. Some minor defining characteristics in roles and relationships are triangulating family relationships, reduced ability of family members to relate to each other for mutual growth and maturation, lack of skills necessary for relationships, lack of cohesiveness, and neglected obligations. Some minor defining characteristics of behaviors are inability to meet spiritual needs of its members, inability to express or accept a wide range of feelings, orientation toward tension relief rather than achievement of goals, and family special occasions that are alcoholic-centered.

■ RELATED FACTORS: Related factors include abuse of alcohol; family history of alcoholism, resistance to treatment; inadequate coping skills; genetic predisposition; addictive personality; lack of problem-solving skills; and biochemical influences. See also **nursing diagnosis.**

**family processes, interrupted,** a nursing diagnosis accepted by the Fifth National Conference on the Classification of Nursing Diagnoses. Altered family processes is the state in which a family that normally functions effectively experiences a dysfunction.

■ DEFINING CHARACTERISTICS: The defining characteristics include the inability of the family system to meet the physical, emotional, spiritual, or security needs of its members; the inability of family members to communicate adequately, to express or accept a wide range of feelings, or to relate to each other for mutual growth and maturation; the parents' disrespect for each other's views on child-rearing practices; family rigidity in function and roles and its noninvolvement in community activities; inability of the family to accept or receive appropriate help, to adapt to change, or to deal with traumatic experience constructively; disrespect for individuality and autonomy; failure to accomplish current or past developmental tasks; ineffective decision-making processes; inappropriate or poorly communicated family rules, rituals, or symbols; and unexamined family myths.

■ RELATED FACTORS: Related factors include a situation transition and/or crisis and developmental transition and/or crisis. See also **nursing diagnosis.**

**family process maintenance,** a nursing intervention from the Nursing Interventions Classification (NIC) defined as minimization of family process disruption effects. See also **Nursing Interventions Classification.**

**family structure,** the composition and membership of the family and the organization and patterning of relationships among individual family members. In planning health care for a family member or the entire family, an awareness of that family's structure may be important.

**family support,** a nursing intervention from the Nursing Interventions Classification (NIC) defined as promotion of family values, interests, and goals. See also **Nursing Interventions Classification.**

**family therapy**[1] (in psychiatry) a therapy modality that focuses treatment on the process between family members that supports and perpetuates symptoms; a way of conceptualizing human relationship problems that focuses on the context in which an emotional problem is generated.

**family therapy**[2], a nursing intervention from the Nursing Interventions Classification (NIC) defined as assisting family members to move their family toward a more productive way of living. See also **Nursing Interventions Classification.**

**famine fever.** See **relapsing fever.**

**famotidine** /famot'idēn/, an oral and parenteral antiulcer drug; an $H_2$-receptor agonist.

■ INDICATIONS: It is prescribed in treatment of duodenal ulcer and pathologic hypersecretory conditions such as Zollinger-Ellison syndrome.

■ CONTRAINDICATIONS: Famotidine should be used with caution in patients with impaired kidney function.

■ ADVERSE EFFECTS: Among adverse reactions reported are headache, dizziness, constipation, diarrhea, and temporary irritation of the injection site.

**Famvir,** trademark for an antiviral drug (famciclovir).

**fan beam,** a geometric pattern produced by collimating a spatially extended x-ray beam with a long, narrow slit. Also called *fan x-ray beam.*

**FANCAP,** *U.S.* a mnemonic device for helping student nurses learn to assess, provide, and evaluate direct patient care. It stands for fluids, aeration, nutrition, communication, activity, and pain. Occasionally a variant, FANCAS, in which S represents stimulation, is substituted.

**Fanconi's anemia** /fankō'nēs/ [Guido Fanconi, Swiss pediatrician, 1892–1979], a rare, usually congenital disorder transmitted as an autosomal-recessive trait, characterized by aplastic anemia in childhood or early adult life, bone abnormalities, chromatin breaks, and developmental anomalies. Children begin to show symptoms between 4 and 12 years of age. Also called **congenital pancytopenia, pancytopenia-dysmelia.** Also spelled *Fanconi's anaemia.*

**Fanconi's syndrome** [Guido Fanconi], a group of disorders that includes pancytopenia, renal tubular dysfunction, glycosuria, phosphaturia, and bicarbonate wasting. The condition is often marked by osteomalacia, acidosis, rickets, and hypokalemia. Two main types of the syndrome have been differentiated. Idiopathic Fanconi's syndrome is inherited and usually accompanies other genetic disorders such as Wilson's disease, galactosemia, or glycogen storage disease. Acquired Fanconi's syndrome is usually the result of toxicity from various sources, including ingestion of outdated tetracycline, heavy metal poisoning, or vitamin D deficiency. Because of numerous variations of the syndrome, different alleles are believed responsible for the different recessively inherited factors expressed as signs and symptoms of the group of disorders.

**fango** /fän'gō/ [It, mud], mud taken from thermal springs at Battaglia, Italy, and used to treat gout and other rheumatic diseases.

**fan lateral projection,** a technique for making a radiographic image of the hand without superimposition of the phalanges. The patient places the fingers around a sponge wedge shaped so that each finger appears separately, in a fanlike pattern, on the x-ray film.

**Fansidar,** trademark for a fixed-combination antimalarial agent (pyrimethamine and sulfadoxine).

**fantasy** /fan'təsē/ [Gk, *phantasia,* imagination], **1.** the unrestrained free play of the imagination; fancy. **2.** a mental image, usually distorted or grotesque, that is often the result of the action of drugs or a disease of the central nervous system. **3.** the mental process of transforming undesirable experiences into imagined events or into a sequence of ideas in order to fulfill an unconscious wish, need, or desire or to give expression to unconscious conflicts, such as a daydream.

**F.A.O.T.A.,** abbreviation for *Fellow of the American Occupational Therapy Association.*

**F.A.P.T.A.,** abbreviation for *Fellow of the American Physical Therapy Association.*

**farad (F)** /fer'əd/ [Michael Faraday, English scientist, 1791–1871], a unit of capacitance that increases the potential difference between the plates of a capacitor by 1 volt with a charge of 1 coulomb.

**Faraday cage** /fer'ədā/, a wire-mesh cage that surrounds a magnetic resonance (MR) scanner and shields it from stray radiofrequency waves. Such waves would otherwise distort the results of MR imaging.

**Farber's disease, Farber's lipogranulomatosis** /fär'bərz/ [Sidney Farber, American pediatrician, 1903–1973], a lysosomal storage disease of ceramide metabolism resulting from defective ceramidase, marked by hoarseness, aphonia, a brownish desquamating dermatitis that begins at about three months of age, foam cell infiltration of bones and joints that causes deformations, granulomatous reaction in lymph nodes, heart, lungs, and kidneys, and psychomotor retardation. Also called **ceramidase deficiency.**

**Farber test,** a microscopic examination of newborn meconium for lanugo and squamous cells. The fetus normally swallows amniotic fluid containing these large proteins, which then pass through the digestive system to be excreted, usually after birth, in the first stools. The absence of hair or skin cells is suggestive of intestinal obstruction or atresia and requires further evaluation.

**Far Eastern hemorrhagic fever,** a form of epidemic hemorrhagic fever, indigenous to Asia, that is transmitted by a virus carried by Asian rodents and causes hemorrhagic fever with renal syndrome. The infection is characterized by four phases: febrile phase, hypotensive phase, oliguric phase, and polyuric phase. Hypotensive shock may occur as the fever subsides. Thirst continues into the second week, oliguria develops, and the blood pressure returns to normal. Blood urea nitrogen levels increase hyperphosphatemia and hypercalcemia, and other complications occur. Diuresis follows the oliguric phase, generating an output of as much as 8 L a day of urine and causing electrolyte imbalance. The mortality rate may be as high as 33%. There is no specific treatment.

**far field.** See **Fraunhofer zone.**

**farmer's lung** [L, *firmare,* to make firm], a respiratory disorder caused by the inhalation of actinomycetes or other microbes in dusts from moldy hay. It is a form of hypersensitivity pneumonitis, which affects individuals in whom antibodies to the mold spores have developed. It is characterized by coughing, dyspnea, cyanosis, tachycardia, nausea, chills, and fever. Treatment may include cromolyn sodium and a corticosteroid.

**far point** [ME, *farr* + L, *punctus,* pricked], **1.** the farthest distance from the eye at which an object can be seen clearly when the eye is at rest and accommodation is fully relaxed. **2.** the point at which the visual axes of the two eyes meet when at rest.

**farsightedness.** See **hyperopia.**

**FAS,** abbreviation for **fetal alcohol syndrome.**

**fasci-,** combining form meaning 'band or bundle of fibrous tissue': *fasciagram, fascicular, fasciitis.*

**fascia** /fash′ē-ə/, *pl.* **fasciae** [L, band], the fibrous connective membrane of the body that may be separated from other specifically organized structures, such as the tendons, the aponeuroses, and the ligaments, and that covers, supports, and separates muscles. It varies in thickness and density and in the amounts of fat, collagenous fiber, elastic fiber, and tissue fluid it contains. Kinds of fasciae are **deep fascia, subcutaneous fascia,** and **subserous fascia.** —**fascial,** *adj.*

**fascia bulbi,** a thin membranous socket that envelops the eyeball from the optic nerve to the ciliary region and allows it to move freely. The fascia bulbi has a smooth inner surface, pierced by vessels and nerves, and fuses with the sheath of the optic nerve and with the sclera. The lower part of the membrane thickens into the suspensory ligament, which attaches to the zygomatic arch and the lacrimal bones. Also called **Tenon's capsule.**

**fasciae, fascial.** See **fascia.**

**fascial cleft** /fash′ē-əl/ [L, *fascia* + ME, *clift*], a place of cleavage between two contiguous fascial surfaces, such as the deep fasciae and the subcutaneous fasciae. A fascial cleft is rich in fluid but poor in traversing fibers; thus two fascial

surfaces may move or be separated easily. Compare **fascial compartment, fascial membrane lamination.**

**fascial compartment,** a part of the body that is walled off by fascial membranes, usually containing a muscle or group of muscles or an organ, just as the heart is contained by the mediastinum. Compare **fascial cleft, fascial membrane lamination.**

**fascial membrane lamination,** a pad of connective tissue that contains fat and an occasional blood vessel or lymph node. It is found where a fascial membrane splits into two sheets, such as at the division of the outer cervical fascia above the sternum. Compare **fascial cleft, fascial compartment.**

**fascia thoracolumbalis,** the extensive subdivision of the vertebral fascia that sheaths the sacrospinalis muscle. It spreads caudally to become the glistening white lumbar aponeurosis and the origin of the latissimus dorsi. Medially it attaches to the sacrum, laterally to the ribs and the intercostal fascia, and cranially to the ligamentum nuchae. Also called **lumbodorsal fascia.**

**fascicle.** See **fasciculus.**

**fascicular** /fəsik′yələr/ [L, *fasciculus,* little bundle], pertaining to something arranged as a bundle of rods, such as groups of nerve or muscle fibers.

**fascicular neuroma,** a neoplasm composed of myelinated nerve fibers. Also called **medullated neuroma.**

**fascicular twitching.** See **twitching.**

**fasciculation** /fasik′yŏŏlā′shən/ [L, *fasciculus,* little bundle, *atio,* process], a localized uncoordinated, uncontrollable twitching of a single muscle group innervated by a single motor nerve fiber or filament that may be palpated and seen under the skin. In anesthesia it refers to muscle twitches that occur with administration of the depolariatng muscle relevant succinyl choline. It also may be symptomatic of a number of disorders, including dietary deficiency, cerebral palsy, fever, neuralgia, polio, rheumatic heart disease, sodium deficiency, tic, or uremia. Fasciculation of the heart muscle is known as fibrillation. —**fascicular,** *adj.,* **fasciculate,** *v.*

**fasciculus** /fəsik′yələs/, *pl.* **fasciculi** [L, little bundle], a small bundle of muscle, tendon, or nerve fibers wrapped by a layer of connective tissue called the perimysium (muscle) or perineurium (nerve fiber). The arrangement of fasciculi in a muscle is correlated with the power of the muscle and its range of motion. The patterns of muscular fasciculi are penniform, bipenniform, multipenniform, and radiated. Also called **fascicle.** —**fascicular,** *adj.*

**fasciitis** /fas′ē-ī′tis/, **1.** an inflammation of the connective tissue that may be caused by streptococcal or other types of infection, an injury, or an autoimmune reaction. **2.** an abnormal benign growth (*Pseudosarcomatous fasciitis*) resembling a tumor that develops in the subcutaneous oral tissues, usually in the cheek. Commonly growing rapidly and then regressing, it consists of young fibroblasts and many capillaries and may be mistaken for fibrosarcoma. Also spelled **fascitis** /fasī′tis/.

**fasciodesis** /fā′sē-ōdē′sis/, a surgical procedure in which a fascia is attached to another fascia or to a tendon.

**fascioliasis** /fas′ē-ōlī′əsis/ [L, *fasciola,* little band; Gk, *osis,* condition], infection by the river fluke *Fasciola hepatica.* It is characterized by epigastric pain, fever, hepatomegaly, jaundice, eosinophilia, urticaria, and diarrhea; fibrosis of the liver is a consequence of prolonged infection. It is acquired by ingestion of encysted forms of the fluke found on aquatic plants, such as raw watercress grown in water contaminated by sheep or cattle dung. The disease is prevalent in many parts of the world, including the southern and western

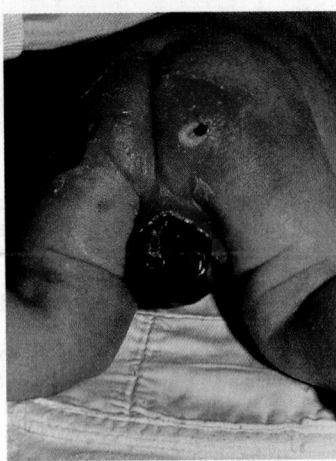

**Necrotizing fasciitis**
(Zitelli and Davis, 1997/courtesy Dr. Michael Sherlock)

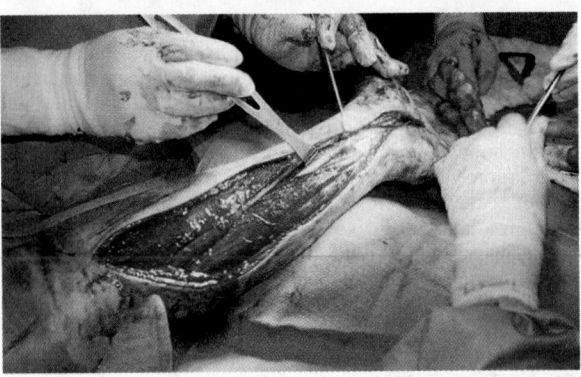

**Fasciotomy** (Auerbach, 1995/courtesy Robert Norris, MD)

United States. Bithionol or triclabendazole, given orally, is the usual treatment.

**fasciolopsiasis** /fas′ē-ōlopsī′əsis/ [L, *fasciola,* little band; Gk, *opsis,* appearance, *osis,* condition], an intestinal infection of humans and pigs, prevalent in Asia. It is characterized by abdominal pain, diarrhea, constipation, eosinophilia, ascites, and sometimes edema. It is caused by the fluke *Fasciolopsis buski.* The disease is usually acquired by eating contaminated water plants such as raw water chestnuts. Most infections are light and asymptomatic. Symptomatic infection is easily treated with anthelmintics, such as praziquantel.

**Fasciolopsis buski** /fas′ē-əlop′sis bus′kē/, a species of fluke that is an important intestinal parasite endemic in Asia and the tropics. In the United States and other countries, it is occasionally found in imported food products. See also **fasciolopsiasis.**

**fascioscapulohumeral muscular dystrophy** /fas′ē-ō-skap′yəlōhyoō′mərəl/ [L, *fasciculus,* little bundle, *scapula,* shoulderblade, *humerus,* shoulder], an abnormal congenital condition that is one of the main types of muscular dystrophy. It is characterized by progressive symmetric wasting of the skeletal muscles, especially the muscles of the face, the shoulders, and the upper arms, without any associated neural or sensory disorders. This disease is not usually fatal but spreads to all the voluntary muscles and commonly produces a pendulous lower lip and the absence of the nasolabial fold. It is an autosomal dominant disease that may be transmitted to males and females. Also called **Landouzy-Dejerine muscular dystrophy.** Compare **Duchenne's muscular dystrophy.**

**fasciotomy** /fas′ē-ot′əmē/, a surgical incision into an area of fascia.

**fascitis.** See **fasciitis.**

**F.A.S.R.T.,** abbreviation for *Fellow of the American Society of Radiologic Technologists.*

**fast,** 1. resistant to change, especially to the action of a specific drug or chemical, as a staining agent. 2. abstinence from all or certain foods. See also **fasting.**

**fast-acting insulin,** See **short-acting insulin.**

**fast brushing,** the use of a battery-powered brush to stimulate C fibers (group IV afferent neurons), which send many collaterals to the reticular activating system.

**fastigial nucleus** /fastij′ē-əl/, one of a group of deep cerebellar nuclei that receive input from the medial zone of the cerebellum. It is involved in the control of posture and equilibrium.

**fastigium** /fastij′ē-əm/ [L, ridge], 1. the highest point in the course of a fever, or the most symptomatic point in the course of an illness. 2. the angle at the top of the roof of the fourth ventricle in the brain. 3. the highest point.

**Fastin,** trademark for an anorexiant (phentermine hydrochloride).

**fasting** [AS, *foestan,* to observe], the act of abstaining from food for a specific period, usually for therapeutic or religious purposes.

**fasting plasma glucose (FPG),** a measurement of the concentration of glucose in the plasma after the patient has not eaten for at least 8 hours.

**fast neutron therapy,** a radiotherapeutic technique used in the treatment of certain soft tissue sarcomas.

**fast pain,** a localized sensation of discomfort felt immediately after a noxious stimulus is delivered. It usually disappears when the stimulus ceases.

**fast smear,** a cytologic sample of tissue scrapings from the vaginal-cervical area, smeared on a microscope slide and fixed immediately for routine screening of female reproductive function.

**fast-twitch (FT) fiber,** a muscle fiber that can develop high tension rapidly. It is usually innervated by a single alpha neuron and has low fatigue resistance, low capillary density, low levels of aerobic enzymes, and low oxygen availability. FT fibers are used in such activities as sprinting, jumping, and weight lifting. Also called *fast-twitch muscle fiber.* See also **slow-twitch (ST) fiber.**

**fat** [AS, *faett*], 1. a substance composed of lipids or fatty acids and occurring in various forms or consistencies ranging from oil to tallow. 2. a type of body tissue composed of cells containing stored fat (depot fat). Stored fat is usually identified as white fat, which is found in large cellular vesicles, or brown fat, which consists of lipid droplets. Stored fat contains more than twice as many calories per gram as sugars and serves as a source of body energy. In addition, stored fat helps cushion and insulate vital organs. See also **adipose, obesity.**

**fatal** /fā′təl/ [L, *fatum,* what has been spoken], causing death.

**fatality** /fātal′itē/ [L, *fatalis,* preordained], 1. an individual case of death. 2. a condition, disease, or disaster resulting in death.

**fatality rate,** the death rate observed in a specified group of people involved in a simultaneous event such as a disaster.

**fat cell lipoma.** See **hibernoma.**

**fat embolism,** a circulatory condition characterized by the blocking of an artery by a plug of fat. The plug enters the circulatory system after the fracture of a long bone or, less commonly, after traumatic injury to adipose tissue or to a fatty liver. Fat embolism usually occurs suddenly 12 to 36 hours after an injury and is characterized by symptoms related to the site occluded, such as severe chest pain, pallor, dyspnea, tachycardia, delirium, prostration, and in some cases coma. Anemia and thrombocytopenia are common. Systemic fat embolism may occur after extensive trauma, since lipid metabolism is altered by the injury and free fatty acids are released, resulting in vasculitis with obstruction of many small pulmonary and cerebral arteries. Classic signs of systemic fat embolism are petechial hemorrhages on the neck, shoulders, axillae, and conjunctivae that appear 2 or 3 days after the injury. There is no specific therapy for systemic fat embolism; the patient is placed in a high Fowler's position and given oxygen, corticosteroids, blood transfusion, respiratory assistance, or other supportive care as needed.

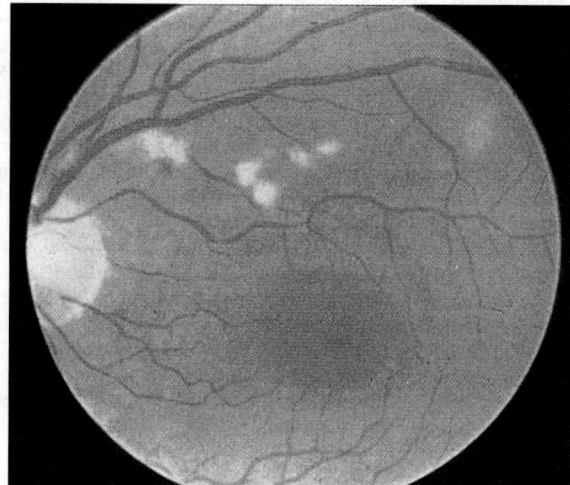

**Fat embolism** *(Michelson and Friedlaender, 1996)*

**FA test.** See **fluorescent antibody test.**

**father complex** [L, *pater* + *complecti,* to embrace], *(nontechnical)* a repressed desire for an incestuous relationship with one's father.

**father fixation,** an arrest in psychosexual development characterized by an abnormally persistent, close, and often paralyzing emotional attachment to one's father. Compare **mother fixation.** See also **freudian fixation.**

**fatigability** /fat′igəbil′itē/, a tendency to become tired or exhausted quickly or easily. It may occur in certain types of cells that undergo periods of excessive activity.

**fatigue¹** /fətēg′/ [L, *fatigare,* to tire], **1.** a state of exhaustion or a loss of strength or endurance, such as may follow strenuous physical activity. **2.** loss of ability of tissues to respond to stimuli that normally evoke muscular contraction or other activity. Muscle cells generally require a refractory or recovery period after activity, when cells restore their en-ergy supplies and excrete metabolic waste products. **3.** an emotional state associated with extreme or extended exposure to psychic pressure, as in battle or combat fatigue.

**fatigue²,** a nursing diagnosis accepted by the Eighth National Conference on the Classification of Nursing Diagnoses. It is defined as an overwhelming sense of exhaustion and decreased capacity for physical and mental work regardless of adequate sleep.

■ DEFINING CHARACTERISTICS: The major defining characteristics are verbalization of fatigue or lack of energy and inability to maintain usual routines. Minor characteristics include a perceived need for additional energy to accomplish routine tasks, an increase in physical complaints, impaired ability to concentrate, decreased performance, and decreased libido. The individual with fatigue can also be emotionally labile or irritable, lethargic or listless; have disinterest in surroundings or introspection; and be accident-prone.

■ RELATED FACTORS: Related factors include overwhelming psychologic or emotional demands, increased energy requirements to perform activity of daily living, excessive social or role demands, states of discomfort, decreased metabolic energy production, and altered body chemical characteristics such as from medications or drug withdrawal. See also **nursing diagnosis.**

**fatigue fever,** a benign episode of fever and muscle pain after overexertion. The symptoms are caused by an accumulation of the metabolic waste products of muscle contractions and may persist for several days.

**fatigue fracture,** any fracture that results from excessive physical activity and not from any specific injury, as commonly occurs in the metatarsal bones of runners. See also **stress fracture.**

**fatigue state** [L, *fatigare,* to tire, *status,* condition], the state of lowest energy of a system. See also **ground state.**

**fat-induced hyperlipidemia.** See **hyperlipidemia type I.**

**fat injection,** transplantation of a patient's own fat to other areas on the body, as to the face to minimize wrinkles or to the lips or penis to augment size. The procedure is discouraged in breast augmentation, because it can hamper the detection of early breast cancer, causing false-positive test results.

**fat metabolism,** the biochemical process by which fats are broken down, incorporated, and used by the cells of the body. Fats provide more food energy (9 kcal/g) than carbohydrates (4.1 kcal/g). Fat catabolism begins with the hydrolysis of fats (triglycerides) into glycerol and fatty acids. Glycerol is converted into a compound that can enter the citric acid cycle. Catabolism of fatty acids continues by beta-oxidation to produce acetyl-coenzyme A, which also enters the citric acid cycle. The body synthesizes fats from fatty acids and glycerol or from compounds derived from excess glucose or from amino acids. The body can synthesize only saturated fatty acids; essential unsaturated fatty acids can be supplied only by diet. Fat metabolism is controlled by hormones such as insulin, growth hormone, adrenocorticotropic hormone, and glucocorticoids. The rate of fat catabolism is inversely related to the rate of carbohydrate catabolism, and in some conditions, such as diabetes mellitus, the secretion of these hormones increases to counter a decrease in carbohydrate catabolism.

**fat necrosis** [AS, *faett* + Gk, *nekros,* dead, *osis,* condition], a condition caused by trauma or infection in which neutral tissue fats are broken down into fatty acids and glycerol. Fat necrosis occurs most commonly in the breasts and subcutaneous areas. It also may develop in the abdominal cavity after an episode of pancreatitis causes a release of enzymes from the pancreas.

**fat overload syndrome,** a condition of hepatosplenomegaly, anemia, GI disturbances, and very high triglyceride levels resulting from IV administration of fat emulsion.

**fat pad,** a mass of closely packed fat cells surrounded by fibrous tissue septa. Fat pads may be generously supplied with capillaries and nerve endings. Intraarticular fat pads are also covered by a layer of synovial cells. An example is the buccal pad of fat seen in nursing babies.

**fat solvent.** See **nonpolar solvent.**

**fatty acid** [AS, *faett* + L, *acidus,* sour], any of several organic acids produced by the hydrolysis of neutral fats and consisting of a long hydrocarbon chain ending in a carboxyl group. In cells, fatty acids usually occur in combination with another molecule rather than in a free state. Essential fatty acids, including **linoleic acid** and **linolenic acid,** are unsaturated molecules that cannot be produced by the body and must therefore be included in the diet. See also **saturated fatty acid, unsaturated fatty acid.**

**fatty alcohol,** a hydroxy derivative of a hydrocarbon from the paraffin series.

**fatty ascites.** See **chylous ascites.**

**fatty cirrhosis** [AS, *faett* + Gk, *kirrhos,* yellow-orange, *osis,* condition], a form of cirrhosis that develops over a long period of poor nutrition resulting in fatty infiltration of the liver. See also **cirrhosis.**

**fatty degeneration** [AS, *faett* + L, *degenerare,* to deviate], the abnormal deposition of fat within cells or the invasion of organs by fatty tissue. Also called **adipose degeneration.**

**fatty diarrhea,** the excretion of fatty, foul-smelling stools that float on water. The condition is associated with chronic pancreatic disease and other malabsorption disorders. Also called **pimelorrhea.**

**fatty infiltration,** a normal phase of breast development, characterized by accumulation of increased amounts of fat around the parenchymal breast tissue. It is normally followed later in life by involution.

**fatty infiltration of heart** [AS, *faett* + L, *in* + *filtrare* + AS, *heorte*], an accumulation of large amounts of fat within the cells of the heart. The heart muscle may be marked by irregular, pale streaks representing areas of fatty infiltration. The condition is sometimes associated with severe and prolonged anemia.

**fatty liver,** an accumulation of triglycerides in the liver. The causes include obesity, diabetes, excessive consumption of alcohol, IV administration of drugs such as tetracycline and corticosteroids, and exposure to toxic substances, such as carbon tetrachloride and yellow phosphorus. Fatty liver is also seen in kwashiorkor and is a rare complication of un-

known origin in late pregnancy. The symptoms are anorexia, hepatomegaly, and abdominal discomfort; fat cells can be seen under the microscope after liver biopsy. The condition is usually reversible after the underlying condition is corrected or the offending drug is withdrawn. See also **cirrhosis.**

**fatty stool** [AS, *faett* + *stol,* seat], feces containing an abnormally large amount of fat, as indicated by their floating on water. See also **celiac disease, steatorrhea.**

**fatty tissue** [AS, *faett* + OFr, *tissu*], loose connective tissue with many cells that contain fat vacuoles. Also called **adipose tissue.**

**fauces** /fô′sēz/ [L, *faux,* throat], the aperature of the mouth into the pharynx. The anterior pillars of the fauces form the glossopalatine arch; the posterior pillars form the pharyngopalatine arch.

**faucial isthmus** /fô′shəl/, an aperture between the pharynx and the mouth.

**faulty restoration** /fôl′tē/ [L, *fallere,* to deceive, *restaurare,* to renew], any dental filling or fabrication that contains flaws, such as overhanging or incomplete fillings and incorrect anatomic characteristics of occlusal and marginal ridge areas. Such flaws may mar individual tooth fillings and fixed bridges or clasps of removable prosthetics and may cause inflammatory and dystrophic diseases of the teeth and periodontium. See also **restoration.**

**favism** /fā′vizəm/ [It, *fava,* bean], an acute hemolytic anemia caused by ingestion of the beans or inhalation of the pollen from the *Vicia faba* (fava) plant. Sensitive individuals have a genetic deficiency of glucose-6-phosphate dehydrogenase, usually the result of a hereditary biochemical abnormality of the erythrocytes. Symptoms include dizziness, headache, vomiting, fever, jaundice, eosinophilia, and often diarrhea. The condition occurs primarily in persons of southern Italian extraction and is treated by blood transfusion and avoidance of fava beans and pollen. See also **glucose-6-phosphate dehydrogenase (G-6-PD) deficiency.**

**favus** /fā′vəs/ [L, honeycomb], a fungal infection of the scalp, skin, or nails, more common in children than adults. It is caused by *Trichophyton* fungi. Favus is characterized by thick yellow crusts with suppuration, a honeycomb appearance, a distinct "mousy" odor, permanent scars, and alopecia. It is rarely seen in North America, common in the Middle East and Africa.

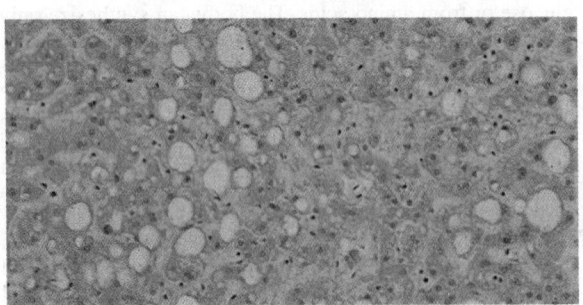

**Fatty liver in kwashiorkor**
*(McLaren, 1992/courtesy Professor J.D.L. Hansen)*

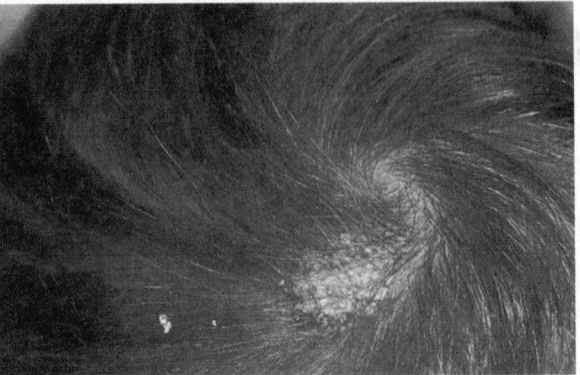

**Favus** *(Hordinsky, Sawaya, and Scher, 2000)*

**fax,** abbreviation for **facsimile.**

**F.C.A.P.,** abbreviation for *Fellow of the College of American Pathologists.*

**FCC,** abbreviation for **Federal Communications Commission.**

**FDA,** abbreviation for **Food and Drug Administration.**

**FDI numbering system** [Fr, Féderation Dentaire Internationale], an internationally used two-digit system for identifying and referring to teeth established through the FDI, headquartered in Paris, France. See also **Palmer notation, universal tooth coding system.**

**Fe,** symbol for the element **iron.**

**fear,** a nursing diagnosis accepted by the Fourth National Conference on the Classification of Nursing Diagnoses (revised 2000). Fear is defined as a response to perceived threat that is consciously recognized as a danger.

■ DEFINING CHARACTERISTICS: Defining characteristics include a report of apprehension, increased tension, decreased self-assurance, excitement, being scared, jitteriness, dread, alarm, terror, or panic. Further defining characteristics include an ability to identify the object of fear; a stimulus believed to be a threat; diminished productivity, learning ability, and problem-solving ability; increased alertness; avoidance or attack behaviors; impulsiveness; narrowed focus on the object of fear; increased pulse; anorexia; nausea; vomiting; diarrhea; muscle tightness; fatigue; increased respiratory rate and shortness of breath; pallor; increased perspiration; increased systolic blood pressure; pupil dilation; and dry mouth.

■ RELATED FACTORS: Related factors include a natural or innate origin; a learned response; separation from support system in a potentially stressful situation; unfamiliarity with environmental experiences; language barrier; sensory impairment; innate releasers; and phobic stimulus. See also **nursing diagnosis.**

**fear control,** a nursing outcome from the Nursing Outcomes Classification (NOC) defined as personal actions to eliminate or reduce disabling feelings of alarm aroused by an identifiable source. See also **Nursing Outcomes Classification.**

**fear-tension-pain syndrome,** a concept formulated by Grantly Dick-Read, M.D., to explain the pain commonly expected and reported in childbirth. The concept proposes that attitudes induce anxiety before labor and cause fear in labor. This fear causes muscular and psychologic tension that interferes with the natural processes of dilation and delivery, resulting in pain. He advocated education, exercise, and warm emotional and physical support in labor to counteract the syndrome and coined the term *natural childbirth* for a labor or delivery in which the well-trained woman joyfully, comfortably, and with a calm, cooperative attitude participates in a natural experience. Elements of his method of psychophysical preparation for childbirth are incorporated into most other methods of natural childbirth. See also **Bradley method, Lamaze method, Read method.**

**febri-,** combining form meaning 'fever': *febricant, febrifugal, febriphobia.*

**febrifacient** /feb′rifā′shənt/, an agent that induces a fever.

**febrifuge.** See **antipyretic.**

**febrile** /fē′bril, feb′ril/ [L, *febris,* fever], pertaining to or characterized by an elevated body temperature, such as a febrile reaction to an infectious agent. A body temperature above 100° F (37.8° C), or 99.6° F (37.6° C) rectally, is commonly regarded as febrile. —**febrility,** *n.*

**-febrile,** combining form meaning 'fever': *afebrile, nonfebrile, subfebrile.*

**febrile/cold agglutinins test,** blood tests used to diagnose infectious diseases and some neoplastic diseases. The febrile agglutinins serologic studies are used to diagnose salmonellosis, rickettsial diseases, brucellosis, tularemia, and some leukemias and lymphomas, while cold agglutinins are found in patients infected by *Mycoplasma pneumoniae,* influenza, mononucleosis, rheumatoid arthritis, and lymphomas.

**febrile delirium** [L, *febris,* fever, *delirare,* to rave], a symptom of disordered central nervous system function, with excitement, restlessness, and disorientation, accompanying some acute fevers.

**febrile seizure,** a seizure associated with a febrile illness. Treatment depends on the age of the patient and the number of seizures. Generalized recurrent febrile seizures in children may be treated as grand mal epilepsy.

**febrile state** [L, *febris,* fever, *status,* condition], a significant increase in body temperature accompanied by increased pulse and respiration rates, anorexia, constipation, insomnia, headache, pains, and irritability.

**febrile urine,** a deep orange–colored strong smelling urine of a patient with a fever, usually caused by concentration of the urine as a result of dehydration.

**febrility.** See **febrile.**

**fecal** /fē′kəl/ [L, *faex,* waste matter], pertaining to the nature of feces or excrement. Also spelled **faecal.**

**fecal fat test,** a stool test performed to confirm the diagnosis of steatorrhea.

**fecal fistula** [L, *faex,* waste matter, *fistula,* pipe], an abnormal passage from the colon to the external surface of the body, discharging feces. Fistulas of this kind are usually created surgically in operations involving the removal of malignant or severely ulcerated bowel segments. See also **colostomy.**

**fecal impaction,** an accumulation of hardened or inspissated feces in the rectum or sigmoid colon that the individual is unable to move. Diarrhea may be a sign of fecal impaction, since only liquid material is able to pass the ob-

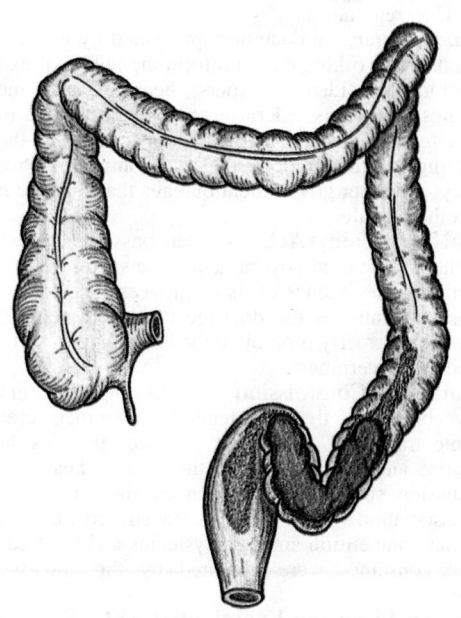

**Fecal impaction** *(Potter and Perry, 1999)*

struction. Occasionally fecal impaction may cause urinary incontinence through pressure on the bladder. Treatment includes oil and cleansing enemas and manual breaking up and removal of the stool by a gloved finger. Persons who are dehydrated, nutritionally depleted, on long periods of bed rest; receiving constipating medications such as iron or opiates; or undergoing barium radiographic studies are at risk of developing fecal impaction. Prevention includes adequate ingestion of bulk food, fluids, exercise, regular bowel habits, privacy for defecation, and occasional stool softeners or laxatives. See also **constipation, obstipation.**

**fecalith** /fē′kəlith/ [L, *faex* + Gk, *lithos,* stone], a hard, impacted mass of feces in the colon. To allow evacuation, an oil retention enema is usually administered; if it is ineffective, manual removal can be performed. See also **atonic constipation, constipation.**

**fecal softener,** a drug that lowers the surface tension of the fecal mass, allowing the intestinal fluids to penetrate and soften the stool. Also called **stool softener.**

**feces** /fē′sēz/, *sing.* **faex** /feks/ [L, *faex,* waste matter], waste or excrement from the digestive tract that is formed in the intestine and expelled through the rectum. Feces consist of water, food residue, bacteria, and secretions of the intestines and liver. Gross examination of feces for color, odor, quantity, and consistency and microscopic examination for the presence of blood, fat, mucus, or parasites are common diagnostic procedures. Also spelled **faeces.** Also called **stool.** See also **defecation.** —**fecal,** *adj.*

**fecund.** See **fecundity.**

**fecundation** /fē′kəndā′shən, fek′-/ [L, *fecundare,* to make fruitful], impregnation or fertilization; the act of fertilizing. See also **artificial insemination.** —**fecundate,** *v.*

**fecundity** /fikun′ditē/, the ability to produce offspring, especially in large numbers and rapidly; fertility. —**fecund** /fek′ənd, fē′kənd/, *adj.*

**Federal Communications Commission (FCC),** a U.S. federal agency that assigns frequencies for all radio transmitters in the United States, including diathermies.

**federally qualified HMO,** a health maintenance organization that is qualified to receive federal funding as defined under U.S. regulations.

*Federal Register*, a document published by the U.S. government each working day to inform the public of executive regulations, presidential orders, hearings and meetings schedules of various federal agencies, and related matters. The *Federal Register* contains announcements of the Food and Drug Administration, the Environmental Protection Agency, and other government bureaus that regulate matters of health and safety.

**Federal Tort Claims Act,** a statute passed in 1946 that allows the U.S. federal government to be sued for the wrongful action or negligence of its employees. The act, for most purposes, eliminates the doctrine of governmental immunity, which formerly prohibited the bringing of a suit against the federal government.

**Federal Trade Commission (FTC),** an agency in the executive branch of the U.S. federal government created to promote trade and to prevent practices that restrain free enterprise and competition. In the area of health care the commission successfully challenged the American Medical Association's ban on physician advertising. The FTC held that competition among physicians and the free choice of the consumer were impaired by the antiadvertising policy.

**Federation Licensing Examination (FLEX),** the standardized licensing examination for state licensure of physicians. Developed by the U.S. Federation of State Medical Boards, the examination is based on National Board of Medical Examiners test materials.

**Fede's disease.** See **Riga-Fede disease.**

**feedback** [AS, *faedan* + *baec*], (in communication theory) **1.** information produced by a receiver and perceived by a sender that informs the sender of the receiver's reaction to the message. Feedback is a cyclic part of the process of communication that regulates and modifies the content of messages. **2.** the return of some of the output so as to exert some control in the process.

**feedback loop,** the circular path seen in a system that has feedback, such that the output of the system participates in the control of the system.

**feedforward control,** an anticipatory correction in motor behavior. During movement, various brain centers depend on feedback from receptors to control motor behavior. If the actual and intended motor behaviors do not match, an error signal is generated and alterations are made. In some instances the control system anticipates an error and makes the corrective change in advance of the start of movement.

**feeding**[1] [AS, *faedan*], the act or process of taking or giving food or nourishment. Kinds of feeding include **breastfeeding** and **tube feeding.** See also **alimentation, parenteral nutrition.**

**feeding**[2], a nursing intervention from the Nursing Interventions Classification (NIC) defined as providing nutritional intake for patient who is unable to feed self. See also **Nursing Interventions Classification.**

**feeding tube,** a tube for introducing fluids of high caloric value into the stomach. See also **tube feeding.**

**fee-for-service** [AS, *feoh,* property; L, *servitum,* slavery], **1.** a charge made for a professional activity, such as a physical examination, the fitting of a contraceptive diaphragm, or the monitoring of a person's blood pressure. **2.** a system for the payment of professional services in which the practitioner is paid for the particular service rendered, rather than receiving a salary for providing professional services as needed during scheduled hours of work or time on call.

**fee-for-service equivalent,** (in U.S. managed care) a specialty capitation method in which a fee schedule is developed for service and providers are paid a percentage of the fee schedule. Periodically the overall value of services provided is compared with payments received and the balance is distributed proportionally to participating providers.

**feeling,** **1.** a quality of mood. **2.** a subjective experience caused by stimulation of a sensory nerve.

**Feer's disease.** See **acrodynia.**

**fee schedule,** (in U.S. managed care) the specific dollar amount to be charged for each service offered.

**fee screen system,** a method of establishing payment for physician services that is based on the usual, customary, or reasonable charge according to a regional evaluation. It allows physicians to establish their own reimbursement level for units of service.

**feet.** See **foot.**

**FEF,** abbreviation for **forced expiratory flow.**

**Fehling's solution** /fā′lingz/ [Hermann C. von Fehling, German chemist, 1812–1885], a solution containing cupric sulfate with sodium hydroxide and potassium sodium tartrate, used for testing for the presence of glucose and other reducing substances in the urine. Also called *Fehling's reagent.*

**Feingold diet** /fīn′gōld/, [Benjamin Feingold, American pediatrician, 1900–1982], a diet developed to treat hyperactive children. The diet excludes foods manufactured with synthetic colorings, flavorings, and preservatives and limits the intake of fruits and vegetables that contain salicylates such as oranges, apricots, peaches, cucumbers, and tomatoes. Studies have shown the Feingold diet to be ineffective.

**Feldene,** trademark for an antiinflammatory agent (piroxicam).

**Feldenkrais therapy** /fel′dənkrīs/, (in psychiatry) an alternative therapy based on establishment of a good self-image through awareness and correction of body movements.

**feldspar** /feld′spär/ [Ger, *feld,* field, *spath,* spar], a crystalline mineral of aluminum silicate with potassium, sodium, barium, and calcium. It melts over a range of 593.5° C to 1093° C (1100° F to 2000° F) and is an important component of dental porcelain.

**F element.** See **F factor.**

**fellatio** /fəlā′shō/, oral stimulation of the male genitalia.

**fellow** [AS, *feolaga,* friendly association], **1.** a member of a learned society. **2.** a graduate student who holds a position in a university or college. **3.** a peer, associate, or person of the same class or rank.

**Fellow of the American Academy of Nursing (F.A.A.N.),** a member of the American Academy of Nursing. The Academy was established in 1966 by the House of Delegates of the American Nurses Association (ANA) to recognize significant contributions of individuals to the nursing profession. See also **American Academy of Nursing.**

**fellowship** /fel′ōship/ [As, *feolaga,* friendly association], a grant given to a person to pay for study or training or to allow payment for work on a special project. It provides a stipend and in some cases the miscellaneous expenses involved in the study, training, or project.

**felon** /fel′ən/ [L, *fel,* venom], a suppurative abscess on the distal phalanx of a finger.

**felonious assault.** See **felony.**

**felony** /fel′ənē/, (in criminal law) a crime declared by statute to be more serious than a misdemeanor and deserving of a more severe penalty. Conviction usually requires imprisonment in a penitentiary for longer than 1 year. Crimes of murder, rape, burglary, and arson are tried as felonies in most cases. In many states there is current, pending, or new legislation that essentially bars applicants from taking the nursing licensure exam NCLEX-RN or PN if certain felonies exist in their history. Criminal background checks, state and federal, are being required of all graduate nurses.

**Felty's syndrome** /fel′tēz/ [Augustus R. Felty, American physician, 1895–1963], a group of pathologic changes that occurs with adult rheumatoid arthritis, characterized by splenomegaly, leukopenia, frequent infections, and sometimes thrombocytopenia and anemia. The cause of the syndrome is unknown. Surgical resection of the spleen offers temporary improvement in about one half of the cases. See also **hypersplenism.**

**female** [L, *femella,* young woman], **1.** pertaining to the sex that has the ability to become pregnant and bear children; feminine. **2.** a female person.

**female catheterization,** a procedure for removing urine by means of a urinary catheter introduced through the urinary meatus and urethra into the bladder. The procedure is performed for relief of distension if voluntary micturition is not possible (such as after trauma or surgery), as a preparation for and during anesthesia, or if a specimen of urine from the bladder is required or medication is to be instilled into the bladder. A straight catheter or a retention catheter with a balloon may be used. A French size 12 to 16 is usually selected for straight drainage. See also **catheterization, male catheterization.**

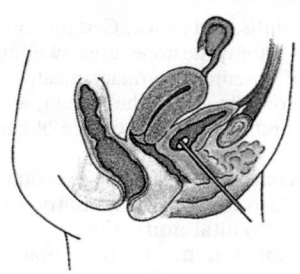

**Female catheterization** *(Potter and Perry, 2001)*

■ METHOD: The necessary sterile equipment is usually available in a sterile catheterization kit and includes cotton swabs, a bowl for collecting urine, a disposable catheter, a sponge stick for holding the swabs, a disinfectant for washing the urinary meatus and the perineal area adjacent to it, gloves, a lubricant for the catheter tip, and a drape. Often a preassembled kit of disposable sterile equipment is available, leaving only the separately packaged catheter to be selected. The patient is positioned on her back, with knees flexed and legs abducted, and is then draped. A bright light is directed at the perineum. The nurse then scrubs the hands, dries them well, and opens the catheterization kit or tray carefully, not touching the inside of the wrapper or the contents. Sterile gloves are put on, and the tray is lifted and placed between the patient's legs. The small sterile drape in the kit is placed over the patient so that the window in it allows access to the urinary meatus. With the thumb and the forefinger of the nurse's nondominant hand the labia are separated and the tissues are retracted, exposing the meatus. The area is cleansed from the front to the back, using one pledget or swab for each stroke. Each pledget is discarded before beginning another stroke; three or more strokes are made, and the location of the meatus is verified while the area is cleaned. The catheter is picked up approximately 1.5 inches from its tip with the sterile hand, the tip is lubricated, and the end is placed in the basin. The catheter is inserted approximately 3 inches until the urine begins to flow. When the urine stops flowing, the catheter is slowly withdrawn or left indwelling as ordered. A sterile sponge is gently pressed to the meatus to remove any lubricant and to dry the area. The urine is measured, and the odor, color, and any abnormal precipitate are noted. A specimen for bacteriologic culture and antibiotic sensitivity is often secured, labeled, and sent to the laboratory.

■ INTERVENTIONS: Catheterization is ordered by a physician for an individual patient, or the conditions under which a catheterization is to be performed are stated in written standing orders. Careful explanation of the procedure ensures the patient's cooperation. Having the woman take a deep breath through the mouth may cause the meatus to open slightly, revealing its presence, and asking her to bear down slightly may minimize the momentary discomfort that commonly accompanies the insertion of the catheter into the bladder. Voluntary micturition is almost always preferable, and the nurse encourages the woman to try to void spontaneously. Signs of infection are carefully observed. If a woman is to be catheterized more than twice, an indwelling catheter is usually preferred to a third catheterization.

■ OUTCOME CRITERIA: Catheterization predisposes the urinary tract to infection, and traumatic catheterization further increases the risk. Care, gentleness, and asepsis are essential. If the bladder is distended with urine, it may cause damage to the bladder, chills, and shock. Certain conditions, including radical vulvectomy, postoperative swelling, or structural anomalies, may obscure the urinary meatus. The indication for catheterization, the age of the patient, and the condition and size of the urethra affect the choice of catheter style and size.

**female circumcision,** the surgical excision of the prepuce of the clitoris. Also called **clitoridotomy.** Compare **clitoridectomy, female genital mutilation.**

**female genital mutilation,** the ritual practice in some cultures of excising the entire clitoris without anesthetic, sometimes as part of a maturity initiation rite. The procedure may be performed in support of a mistaken belief that the absence of a clitoris will prevent a woman from experiencing orgasm or control masturbation and nymphomania. Also called **clitoridectomy.**

**female pseudohermaphroditism,** a form of the congenital gonadal disorder in which ovaries are present, irrespective of the condition of the external genitals. See also **pseudohermaphroditism.**

**female reproductive system assessment,** an evaluation of a patient's genital tract and breasts with an investigation of past and present disorders that may be factors in the individual's current gynecologic condition. See also **pelvic examination.**

■ METHOD: In a relaxed professional interview the procedures to be conducted are explained and the patient is reassured that her privacy will be scrupulously maintained. The patient is interviewed to determine whether she has lower abdominal pain, cramps, vaginal bleeding, itching, swelling, redness, or a vaginal discharge that is mucoid, watery, frothy, or thick in consistency and white, yellow, greenish, bloody, or brown, or that has an odor. She is asked whether she experiences pain on intercourse and pain or burning on urination. Observations are recorded of her general appearance; vital signs; weight; breast symmetry, texture, and lumps or bumps; nipple color; and the presence of a serous, bloody, or purulent nipple discharge. The abdomen is examined for contour, symmetry, stretch marks, scars, lesions, and visible pulsations and peristaltic waves and is auscultated for bowel sounds in each quadrant. Carefully noted are edema or redness of the external genitalia, cervix, and perineum; lumps or lesions on the labia majora, the size of the urethral orifice; the presence or absence of the hymenal ring, hymenal tags, and perineal scars or excoriation; and a bloody, purulent, or odoriferous discharge. The normal mucoid secretion is distinguished from the thick, white, cheesy discharge typical of candidiasis; the frothy, yellow-green, watery liquid characteristic of trichomoniasis; and the thick, yellow-green or brown, and bloody drainage typical of upper genital tract infection. The patient's age at onset of menses; the duration, spacing, and regularity of cycles; the amount and character of the flow; the date of the last menstrual period; and associated symptoms such as pain and menorrhagia are investigated. The complications and outcome of each of the patient's pregnancies, the kind of delivery, the incidence and outcome of any abortion, and the date of menopause and associated symptoms, such as hot flashes and dry vaginal mucosa, are explored. It is determined whether the patient suffers from a sexually transmitted disease, constipation, hemorrhoids, hypothyroidism or hyperthyroidism, polycystic ovary syndrome, hypertension, or blood dyscrasias or has a history of gynecologic or other major abdominal surgery or a serious illness, especially one related to the endocrine system. The patient's smoking habits, sexual activity, use of oral contraceptives or an intrauterine device; her experience with estrogen therapy; and family history of gynecologic diseases and deaths are reported in the assessment. Diagnostic procedures indicated by the history may include a manual examination, Papanicolaou's (Pap) test, basal body temperature determination, culture of vaginal discharge, punch biopsy, endometrial biopsy, dilation and curettage, cold-knife conization, laparoscopy, ultrasound study, and tubal insufflation. Laboratory studies that may be performed include determinations of levels of human chorionic gonadotropin, serum luteinizing and follicle-stimulating hormones, 17-ketosteroids, and corticosteroids; tests for sexually transmitted diseases; and thyroid function tests such as the basal metabolic rate and protein-bound iodine level.

■ INTERVENTIONS: The nurse conducts the interview, records observations of the patient, and collects the pertinent background information and the results of diagnostic procedures and laboratory studies. Throughout the assessment the nurse recognizes that the patient may be reluctant to discuss her symptoms and activities and may be sensitive about the necessary procedures.

■ OUTCOME CRITERIA: A careful assessment of the patient's reproductive system is essential in establishing the diagnosis.

**female sexual dysfunction,** impaired or inadequate ability of a woman to engage in or enjoy satisfactory sexual intercourse and orgasm. Symptoms, usually psychologic in origin, include dyspareunia, vaginismus, persistent inability to reach orgasm, and inhibition in sexual arousal, so that congestion and vaginal lubrication are minimal or absent. Causes include anxiety, fear, negative emotions associated with sexual arousal and intercourse, and interpersonal problems. Treatment is focused on eliminating physical problems and sexual anxieties and on enhancing erotic sensitivities. Compare **male sexual dysfunction.** See also **sexual dysfunction.**

**female sterility** [L, *femella,* young woman, *sterilis,* barren], a condition of being an infertile woman. The inability to reproduce may result from congenital defects in the reproductive system, such as failure of the uterus to develop normally, or disease, injury, or corrective surgery that affects functioning of the ovaries, fallopian tubes, uterus, cervix, or vagina.

**feminist therapy,** an alternative therapy that is both a philosophical approach to the conduct of therapy and a specific type of therapy. The focus of both types is a consciousness raising that focuses on the presence of sexism and sex role stereotyping in society.

**feminization** /fem'inīzā'shən/ [L, *femina,* woman], **1.** the normal development or induction of female secondary sex characteristics. **2.** the induction of female sex characteristics in a genotypic male. Testicular feminization may be caused by the inability of target tissues to respond to endogenous or administered androgen; some cases seem related to an absent or inadequate conversion of testosterone to dihydrotestosterone, which is the active form of the androgen. Testicular feminization in males with an X and a Y chromosome and a female phenotype may be caused by fetal hypogonadism and is often familial. Individuals with this defect usually have undescended or labial testes, a short blind vaginal pouch; no uterus, well-developed breasts, sparse or absent axillary and pubic hair, normal plasma levels of testosterone and follicle-stimulating hormone, and increased concentrations of estradiol and luteinizing hormone. Treatment consists of orchiectomy because of the risk of cancer in gonads of these patients. Feminization may also be caused by adrenocortical estrogen-secreting tumor, failure of the liver to inactivate endogenous estrogens such as in advanced alcoholism, or the administration of estrogen therapy for androgen-dependent neoplasms. Some testicular tumors may produce feminizing symptoms, and gynecomastia may be caused by Klinefelter's syndrome and by certain drugs, such as reserpine, digitalis, meprobamate, and cimetidine. Compare **virilization.** See also **pseudohermaphroditism.**

**feminizing adrenal tumor** /fem′inī′zing/, a rare neoplasm of the adrenal cortex, characterized in males by gynecomastia, hypertension, diffuse pigmentation, a high level of estrogen in urine, and loss of potency. Testicular atrophy frequently occurs, but the prostate and penis are usually normal in size. The tumor may be large enough to be palpated or to be diagnosed by IV urography or arteriography. In most cases it is a carcinoma. Treatment includes surgical resection and chemotherapy with mitotane. In women these tumors, which are extremely rare, are associated with precocious puberty.

**femora.** See **femur.**

**femoral** /fem′ərəl/ [L, *femur,* thigh], pertaining to the femur or the thigh.

**femoral angle.** See **neck shaft angle.**

**femoral artery,** an extension of the external iliac artery into the lower limb, starting immediately distal to the inguinal ligament and ending at the junction of the middle and lower thirds of the thigh. It divides into seven branches and supplies various parts of the lower limb and trunk, such as the groin and its organs.

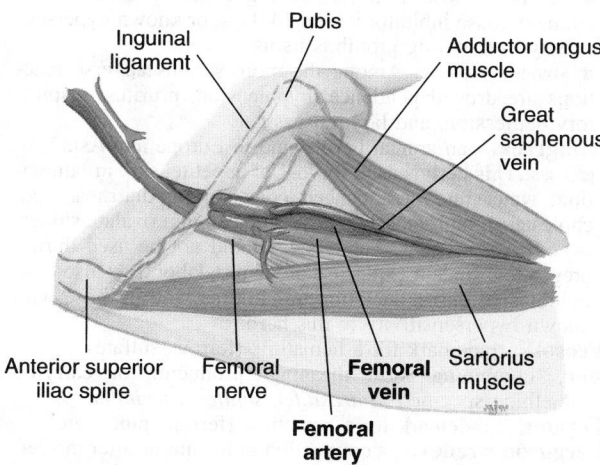

Femoral artery and femoral vein *(Sanders et al, 2000)*

**femoral condyle,** one of a pair of large flared prominences on the distal end of the femur. Identified as lateral and medial femoral condyles, they are covered with a thick layer of hyaline cartilage and articulate with the patella and the tibia at the knee joint.

**femoral epiphysis,** a secondary bone-forming center of the femur, separated from the main part of the bone by cartilage during the period of bone immaturity. In overweight adolescents, there may be bone slippage along the femoral capital epiphysis, marked by pain and loss of range of motion.

**femoral hernia,** a hernia in which a loop of intestine descends through the femoral canal into the groin. Surgical repair, herniorrhaphy, is the usual treatment. See **hernia.**

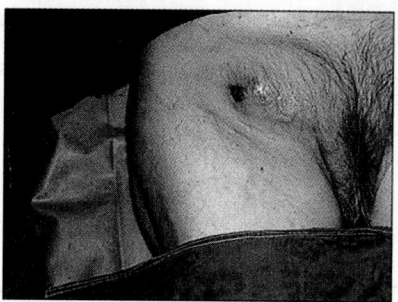

**Femoral hernia** *(Greig and Garden, 1996)*

**femoral nerve,** the largest of the seven nerves stemming from the lumbar plexus and the main nerve of the anterior part of the thigh. Also called **anterior crural nerve.**

**femoral pulse,** the pulse of the femoral artery, palpated in the groin.

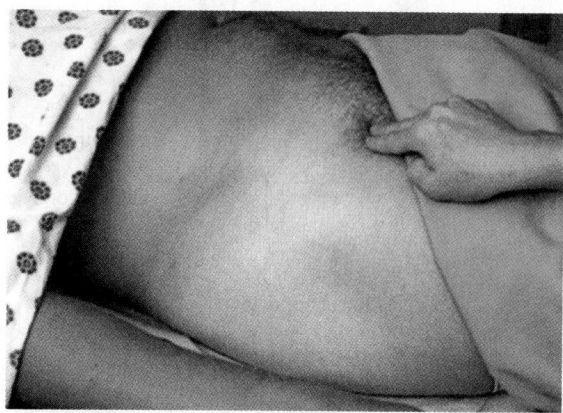

**Palpation of femoral pulse** *(Potter and Perry, 2001)*

**femoral reflex** [L, *femur,* thigh, *reflectere,* to bend back], an extension of the knee and a plantar flexion of the toes of the foot that occurs when the skin on the upper anterior third of the thigh is stimulated.

**femoral torsion,** an extreme lateral or medial twisting rotation of the femur on its longitudinal axis, which may be caused by the action of the gluteal or other muscles. Compare **tibial torsion.**

**femoral vein,** a large vein in the thigh originating in the popliteal vein and accompanying the femoral artery in the proximal two thirds of the thigh. Its distal portion lies lateral to the artery; its proximal portion, deeper to the artery. Near its termination, it is joined by the great saphenous vein. At the inguinal ligament it becomes the external iliac vein.

**femoro-** [L, *femora,* plural of *femur*], a prefix meaning relationship to the femur.

**Femstat,** trademark for an antifungal drug (butoconazole nitrate).

**femur** /fē′mər/, *pl.* **femora, femurs** /fem′ərə/ [L, thigh], the thigh bone, which extends from the pelvis to the knee. It is largely cylindric and is the longest and strongest bone in the body. It has a large round head that fits the acetabulum of the hip, and it displays a large neck and several prominences and ridges for muscle attachments. In an erect posture it inclines medially, drawing the knee joint near the line of gravity of the body.

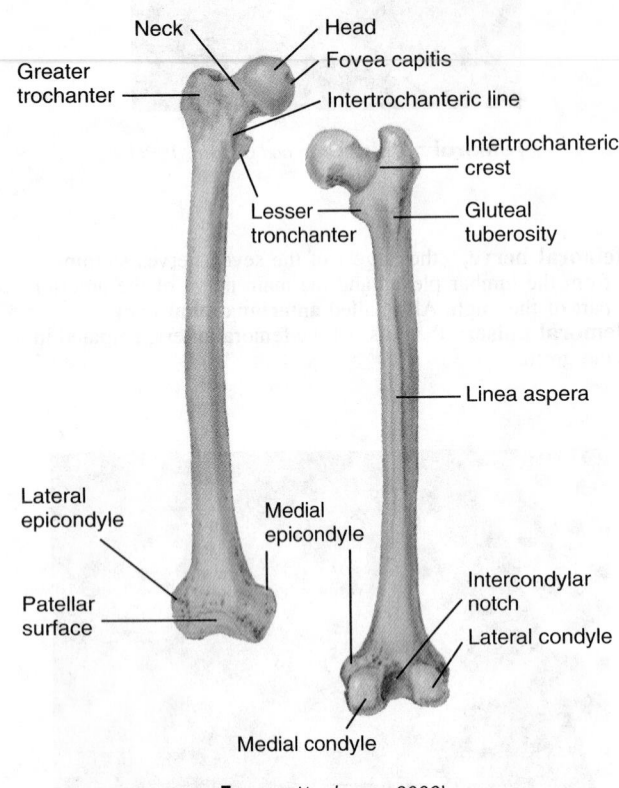

**Femur** *(Applegate, 2000)*

Labels: Neck · Head · Fovea capitis · Greater trochanter · Intertrochanteric line · Intertrochanteric crest · Lesser trochanter · Gluteal tuberosity · Linea aspera · Lateral epicondyle · Medial epicondyle · Patellar surface · Intercondylar notch · Lateral condyle · Medial condyle

**fenestra** /fines′trə/, *pl.* **fenestrae** [L, window], **1.** an aperture, as in a bandage or cast, that is cut out to relieve pressure or to administer regular skin care. **2.** a microscopic opening in certain capillaries specialized in filtration, as in the glomerular capillaries of the kidney often covered by membrane.

**fenestra cochlea.** See **round window.**

**fenestrae.** See **fenestra.**

**fenestra rotunda.** See **round window.**

**fenestrate.** See **fenestration.**

**fenestrated** /fen′əstrā′tid/ [L, *fenestra*, window], having numerous small holes or openings.

**fenestrated drape,** a drape with a round or slitlike opening in the center.

**fenestration** /fen′əstrā′shən/ [L, *fenestra*, window], **1.** a surgical procedure in which an opening is created to gain access to the cavity within an organ or a bone. **2.** an opening created surgically in a bone or organ of the body. **3.** (in dentistry) a procedure to expose a root tip of a tooth to permit drainage of exudate. Also called **window. –fenestrate,** *v.*

**fenoldopam,** an antihypertensive.

■ INDICATIONS: Fenoldopam is used to treat hypertensive crisis when an urgent decrease of pressure is required, including malignant hypertension.

■ CONTRAINDICATIONS: Known hypersensitivity to this drug and sulfite sensitivity prohibit fenoldopam's use.

■ ADVERSE EFFECTS: Life-threatening effects of this drug are hypotension, myocardial infarction, ischemic heart disease, and leukocytosis. Other adverse effects include anxiety, dizziness, ST-T wave changes, angina pectoris, palpitations, nausea, vomiting, constipation, diarrhea, bleeding, and increased levels of blood urea nitrogen, glucose, lactic dehydrogenase, creatinine, and hypokalemia. Headache is a common side effect.

**fenoprofen calcium** /fē′nəprō′fen/, a nonsteroidal antiinflammatory agent and analgesic.

■ INDICATIONS: It is prescribed in the treatment of arthritis and other painful inflammatory conditions.

■ CONTRAINDICATIONS: Renal dysfunction, upper GI disease, or known hypersensitivity to this drug, to aspirin, or to nonsteroidal antiinflammatory medication prohibits its use.

■ ADVERSE EFFECTS: Among the more serious adverse reactions are GI disturbances, gastric or duodenal ulceration, dizziness, skin rash, and tinnitus.

**fenoterol** /fen′ōter′ol/, an investigational beta-adrenergic drug used in respiratory therapy.

**fentanyl** /fen′tənil/, a potent opioid analgesic, used most commonly with the sedative and antipsychotic drug droperidol as an adjunct in anesthesia.

**fentanyl citrate,** a general anesthetic.

■ INDICATIONS: It is prescribed as an adjunct to general anesthesia, as a preoperative and postoperative analgesic, and as a component in neuroleptanesthesia and analgesia.

■ CONTRAINDICATIONS: Myasthenia gravis, use of a monoamine oxidase inhibitor within 14 days, or known hypersensitivity to this drug prohibits its use.

■ ADVERSE EFFECTS: Among the more serious adverse reactions are drug dependence, hypotension, pruritus, respiratory depression, and laryngospasm.

**fenugreek,** an annual herb found in Europe and Asia.

■ USES: This herb is used for loss of appetite, skin inflammation, water retention, cancer, constipation, diarrhea, high cholesterol, high blood glucose, and calcium oxalate stones.

■ CONTRAINDICATIONS: Fenugreek should not be used during pregnancy, since it can cause premature labor. It is also contraindicated during lactation, in children, and in those with known hypersensitivity to this herb.

**Feosol,** trademark for a hematinic (ferrous sulfate).

**-fer,** combining form meaning 'producing or carrying something specified': *parasitifer, sonifer, vaccinifer.*

**Fergon,** trademark for a hematinic (ferrous gluconate).

**Ferguson's reflex,** a contraction of the uterus after the cervix is stimulated. The reflex is an important function of labor.

**fermentation** /fur′məntā′shən/ [L, *fermentare,* to cause to rise], a chemical change that is brought about in a substance by the action of an enzyme or microorganism, especially the anaerobic conversion of foodstuffs to certain products. Kinds of fermentation are **acetic fermentation, alcoholic fermentation, ammoniacal fermentation, amylic fermentation, butyric fermentation, caseous fermentation, dextran fermentation, diastatic fermentation, lactic acid fermentation, propionic fermentation, storing fermentation,** and **viscous fermentation.**

**fermentative dyspepsia** /fərmen′tətiv/, an abnormal condition characterized by impaired digestion associated with the fermentation of digested food. See also **dyspepsia.**

**fermium (Fm)** /fur′mē·əm/ [Enrico Fermi, Italian physicist, 1901–1954], a synthetic transuranic metallic element. Its atomic number is 100; its atomic mass is 257. Fermium was first detected in the debris from a hydrogen bomb explosion and later produced in a reactor.

**ferning test** /fur′ning/ [AS, *faern,* fern; L, *testum,* crucible], a technique used to determine the presence of estrogen in the uterine cervical mucus. It is often used to test for ovulation; high levels of estrogen cause the cervical mucus to dry in a fernlike pattern on a slide. Also called **arborization test.**

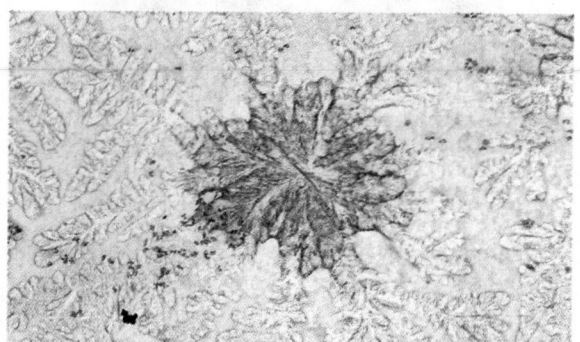

**Ferning** *(McKee, 1997)*

**-ferous,** suffix meaning 'producing or carrying' something specified: *lactiferous, sebiferous, tubiferous.*

**ferr-, ferri-.** See **ferro-.**

**ferredoxin,** a nonheme protein containing equal amounts of iron and sulfur. Ferredoxins are involved in electron transport in photosynthesis and nitrogen fixation.

**ferric** /fer′ik/, pertaining to a cation of iron in which the metal is trivalent, as in ferric chloride and ferric hydroxide. Also called **iron (III).**

**ferritin** /fer′itin/ [L, *ferrum,* iron], an iron compound formed in the intestine and stored in the liver, spleen, and bone marrow for eventual incorporation into hemoglobin. Serum ferritin levels are used as an indicator of the body's iron stores. Normal adult findings are 12 to 300 ng/mL for males and 10 to 150 ng/mL for females.

**ferritin test,** a blood test used to determine available iron stores in the body. It is used to diagnose iron deficiency anemia, and when combined with the serum iron level and total iron-binding capacity tests, can differentiate and classify various kinds of anemias.

**ferro-, ferr-, ferri-,** combining form meaning 'iron': *ferrocyanide, ferropectic, ferrosilicon.*

**ferrokinetics** /fer′ōkinet′iks/, the study of iron metabolism.

**ferromagnetic** /fer′ōmagnet′ik/, pertaining to substances, such as iron, nickel, and cobalt, that are strongly affected by magnetism and may become magnetized by exposure to a magnetic field.

**ferrotherapy** /fer′ōther′əpē/, the use of iron and iron compounds in the treatment of illness.

**ferrous** /fer′əs/, pertaining to a compound of iron in which the metal is divalent, such as ferrous ammonium sulfate. Also called **Fe (II).**

**ferrous sulfate,** a hematinic agent.
- INDICATION: It is prescribed in the treatment of iron deficiency anemia.

- CONTRAINDICATIONS: Hemochromatosis, hemosiderosis, hemolytic anemias, and hypersensitivity to any of the ingredients prohibit its use.
- ADVERSE EFFECTS: Among the most serious adverse reactions are GI irritation, diarrhea, and constipation.

**fertile** /fur′təl/ [L, *fertilis,* fruitful], **1.** capable of reproducing or bearing offspring. **2.** (of a gamete) capable of inducing fertilization or being fertilized. **3.** prolific; fruitful; not sterile. —**fertility,** *n.,* **fertilize,** *v.*

**fertile eunuch syndrome,** a hypogonadotropic hormonal disorder of males in which the levels of testosterone and follicle stimulating hormone are inadequate to induce spermatogenesis and the development of secondary sexual characteristics. If supplemental hormones are not prescribed, the affected person acquires the appearance of a eunuch.

**fertile period,** the time in the menstrual cycle during which fertilization may occur. Spermatozoa can survive for 5 days; the ovum lives for 24 hours. Thus the fertile period begins up to 6 days before ovulation and lasts for 1 day afterward. It may be identified by observation of the changes in the quantity and character of the cervical mucus or changes in the basal body temperature, or it may be determined from a calendar record of six or more menstrual cycles, applying the knowledge that ovulation usually occurs 14 days before menstruation.

**fertility** /fərtil′itē/, the ability to reproduce.

**fertility factor.** See **F factor.**

**fertility preservation,** a nursing intervention from the Nursing Interventions Classification (NIC) defined as providing information, counseling, and treatment that facilitate reproductive health and the ability to conceive. See also **Nursing Interventions Classification.**

**fertility rate,** the number of live births divided by the number of females aged 15 through 44 years of age. It is usually expressed as the number per 1000 women.

**fertilization** /fur′tilīzā′shən/ [L, *fertilis,* fruitful], the union of male and female gametes to form a zygote from which the embryo develops. The process usually takes place in the outer one third of the fallopian tube of the female when a spermatozoon, carried in the seminal fluid discharged during coitus, comes in contact with and penetrates the ovum. Rapid chemical changes in the membrane of the ovum prevent the entrance of additional spermatozoa. Penetration by the spermatozoon stimulates the completion of the second meiotic division and formation of the pronucleus in the ovum. Fusion and synapsis of the male and female pronuclei restore the diploid number of chromosomes to the germ cell, thereby determining the sex of the zygote and of

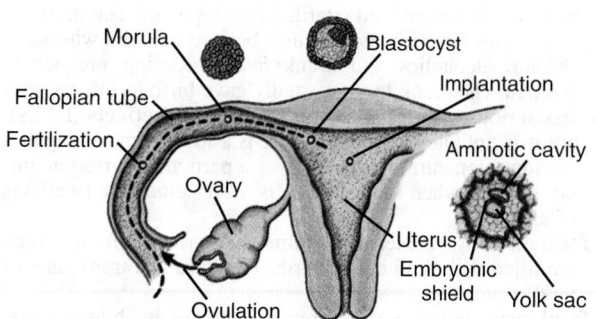

**Fertilization cycle** *(Potter and Perry, 1995)*

the characteristics inherited from each parent and stimulating the initiation of development through cleavage. Kinds of fertilization include **cross-fertilization, external fertilization,** and **internal fertilization.** See also **in vitro fertilization, oogenesis, spermatogenesis.**

**fertilization age.** See **fetal age.**

**fertilization membrane,** a viscous membrane surrounding a fertilized ovum that prevents penetration of additional spermatozoa. It is formed by granules that are released by the fertilized ovum and adhere to the vitelline membrane.

**fertilize.** See **fertile.**

**fertilizin** /fərtil′izin/, a glycoprotein found on the plasma membrane of the ovum in various species. See also **acrosomal reaction.**

**Festal,** trademark for a fixed-combination GI drug that contains a group of digestive enzymes and bile constituents.

**fester, 1.** to become superficially inflamed and pus-producing. **2.** to become increasingly virulent.

**festinant** /fes′tinənt/, pertaining to a gait pattern that accelerates involuntarily as a result of a nervous system disorder. The increased rate of walking represents an automatic attempt by the body to overtake a displaced center of gravity. See also **festinating gait.**

**festinating gait** /fes′tinā′ting/ [L, *festinare,* to hasten], a manner of walking in which a person's speed increases in an unconscious effort to "catch up" with a displaced center of gravity. It is a common characteristic of Parkinson's disease.

**festoon** [Fr, *feston,* scallop], a carving in the base material of a denture that simulates the contours of the natural gingival tissues. See also **gingival festoon, McCall's festoon.**

**FET,** abbreviation for **forced expiratory time.**

**fetal** /fē′təl/ [L, *fetus,* fruitful], pertaining to the final stage of development of an embryonic mammal. In humans the fetal period extends from the end of the eighth week of intrauterine life until birth.

**fetal abortion** [L, *fetus*], termination of pregnancy after the twentieth week of gestation but before the fetus has developed enough to live outside the uterus. Compare **embryonic abortion.**

**fetal activity determination.** See **nonstress test.**

**fetal advocate,** a person who regards the health and well-being of the fetus as a matter of top priority.

**fetal age,** the age of the conceptus computed from the time elapsed since fertilization. Also called **fertilization age.** Compare **gestational age.**

**fetal alcohol syndrome (FAS)** [L, *fetus* + Ar, *alkohl,* essence; Gk, *syn,* together, *dromos,* course], a set of congenital psychologic, behavioral, and physical abnormalities that tend to appear in infants whose mothers consumed alcohol during pregnancy. It is characterized by typical craniofacial and limb defects, cardiovascular defects, intrauterine growth retardation, and retarded development. The most serious cases have involved infants born to mothers who were chronic alcoholics and drank heavily during pregnancy. Women who drank less reportedly gave birth to infants with less serious malformations, or **fetal alcohol effects (FAEs),** but it is not known whether there is a lower limit to alcohol consumption during pregnancy or a particular period in embryonic life when the offspring is most vulnerable to effects of alcohol.

**fetal alveoli,** the terminal pulmonary sacs of a fetus, which are filled with fluid before birth. The fluid is a transudate of fetal plasma.

**fetal asphyxia,** a condition of hypoxemia, hypercapnia, and respiratory and metabolic acidosis that may occur in the uterus. Among possible causes are uteroplacental insufficiency, abruptio placentae, placenta previa, uterine tetany,

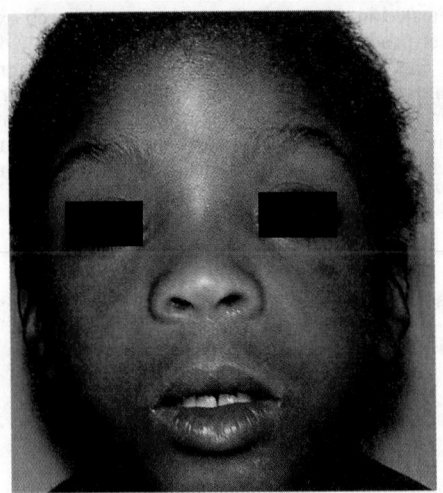

**Fetal alcohol syndrome** *(Zitelli and Davis, 1997)*

maternal hypotension, and compression of the umbilical cord.

**fetal attitude,** the relationship of the fetal parts to each other. An example is the "military" attitude, in which the fetal head is not flexed and the chin is not on the chest as usual but is held straight up. Compare **fetal position, fetal presentation.**

**fetal biophysical profile,** an ultrasound method of evaluating fetal status during the antepartal period based on five variables originating within the fetus: fetal heart rate, breathing movement, gross movements, muscle tone, and amniotic fluid volume. It is indicated in cases of postdate pregnancy, maternal hypertension, diabetes mellitus, vaginal bleeding, maternal Rh sensitization, maternal history of stillbirth, and premature membrane rupture.

**fetal bradycardia,** an abnormally slow fetal heart rate, usually below 100 beats/min.

**fetal circulation,** the pathway of blood circulation in the fetus. Oxygenated blood from the placenta travels through the umbilical vein to the heart. The blood enters the right atrium at a pressure sufficient to direct most of the flow across the atrium and through the foramen ovale into the left atrium; thus oxygenated blood is available for circulation through the left ventricle to the head and upper extremities. The blood returning from the head and arms enters the right atrium via the superior vena cava. It flows through the atrium at a relatively low pressure; passing the tricuspid valve, it falls into the right ventricle, from which most of it is pumped through the pulmonary artery and the ductus arteriosus into the descending aorta for circulation to the lower parts of the body. A small amount of blood in the pulmonary artery is not shunted through the ductus and is carried to the lungs. The blood is returned to the placenta through the umbilical arteries.

**fetal death,** the intrauterine death of a fetus, or the death of a fetus weighing at least 500 g or after 20 or more weeks of gestation.

**fetal distress,** a compromised condition of the fetus, usually discovered during labor, characterized by a markedly abnormal rate or rhythm of myocardial contraction. Some patterns, such as late decelerations of the fetal heart rate seen on records of electronic fetal monitoring, are indicative

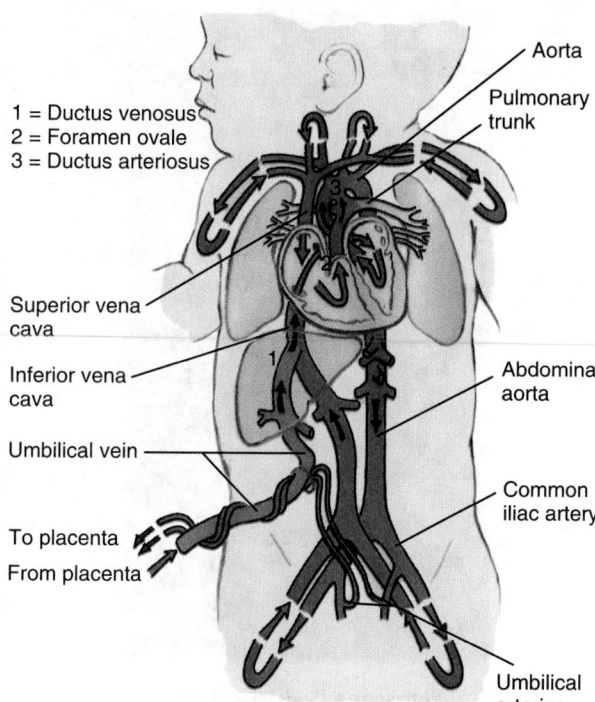

1 = Ductus venosus
2 = Foramen ovale
3 = Ductus arteriosus

Aorta

Pulmonary trunk

Superior vena cava

Inferior vena cava

Umbilical vein

Abdominal aorta

Common iliac artery

To placenta

From placenta

Umbilical arteries

**Fetal circulation** *(Applegate, 2000)*

of fetal distress. If possible, the cause of the situation is identified and corrected and the acid-base balance of the fetal blood is tested. Labor is allowed to continue if the pH is within normal range and if the abnormal pattern does not recur or persist. Cesarean section may be necessary if the fetus is markedly alkalotic or acidotic or if the cause of the problem cannot be corrected. If possible, the condition of the baby is stabilized before delivery by giving the mother oxygen, increased fluids, or a narcotic antagonist, a vasopressor, or an agent to relax the uterus. A pediatrician or neonatologist is required to attend the birth of a distressed baby to manage resuscitation and care immediately after delivery.

**fetal dose,** the estimated amount of radiation received by a fetus during a radiographic examination of a pregnant woman. It is expressed in millirad per 1000 milliroentgens of skin exposure and varies from less than 1 when an extremity is being examined to nearly 300 when the beam is directed toward the pelvis.

**fetal face syndrome.** See **Robinow's syndrome.**

**fetal heart rate (FHR),** the number of heartbeats in the fetus that occur in a given unit of time. The FHR varies in cycles of fetal rest and activity and is affected by many factors, including maternal fever, uterine contractions, maternal-fetal hypotension, and many drugs. The normal FHR is between 110 beats/min and 160 beats/min. In labor the FHR is monitored with a fetoscope, an electronic fetal monitor for detecting abnormal alterations in the rate, especially recurrent decelerations that continue past the end of uterine contractions.

**fetal heart sound** [L, *fetus,* fruitful; AS, *heorte* + L, *sonus,* sound], a sound produced by the heart of a fetus, as detected by auscultation or by electronic fetal monitoring. The heart begins beating at about 14 days of intrauterine life.

**fetal hemoglobin,** hemoglobin F, the major hemoglobin present in the blood of a fetus and neonate. Hemoglobin F

is present in only trace amounts in the blood of normal adults.

**fetal hydantoin syndrome (FHS),** a complex of birth defects associated with prenatal maternal ingestion of hydantoin derivatives. Symptoms of FHS include microcephaly, hypoplasia or absence of nails on the fingers or toes, abnormal facies, mental and physical retardation, and cardiac defects. The syndrome occurs to some degree in 10% to 40% of infants born of mothers who use this anticonvulsant. Hydantoin is sometimes associated with hemorrhage and, more rarely, with neural crest tumors in the newborn.

**fetal hydrops.** See **hydrops fetalis.**

**fetal lie,** the relationship of the long axis of the fetus to the long axis of the mother. See also **fetal presentation.**

**fetal lipoma.** See **hibernoma.**

**fetal membranes,** the structures that protect, support, and nourish the embryo and fetus, including the yolk sac, allantois, amnion, chorion, placenta, and umbilical cord.

**fetal monitor.** See **electronic fetal monitor.**

**fetal mortality,** the number of fetal deaths per 1000 births, or per live births.

**fetal movements** [L, *fetus* + *movere,* to move], muscular motions produced by the fetus in utero beginning around the fifth month of life. The early fetal movements can be felt by the mother.

**fetal placenta** [L, *fetus* + *placenta,* flat cake], the portion of the placenta that is formed from the shaggy chorion frondosum, the villi of which invade the decidua basalis. Also called **pars fetalis.**

**fetal position,** the relationship of the part of the fetus that presents in the pelvis to four quadrants of the maternal pelvis, identified by initial L (left), R (right), A (anterior), and P (posterior). The presenting part is also identified by initial O (occiput), M (mentum), and S (sacrum). If a fetus presents with the occiput directed to the posterior aspect of the mother's right side, the fetal position is right occiput posterior (ROP). Compare **fetal attitude, fetal presentation.**

**fetal presentation,** the part of the fetus that lies closest to or has entered the true pelvis. Cephalic presentations are vertex, brow, face, and chin. Breech presentations include frank breech, complete breech, incomplete breech, and single or double footling breech. Shoulder presentations are rare and require cesarean section or turning before vaginal birth. Compound presentation involves the entry of more than one part in the true pelvis, most commonly a hand next to the head. See also **fetal attitude, fetal lie, fetal position.**

**fetal respiration,** the exchange of gases between the blood of the mother and that of the fetus through the placenta.

**fetal rest.** See **embryonic rest.**

**fetal rickets.** See **achondroplasia.**

**fetal rotation** [L, *fetus* + *rotare,* to rotate], the turning of the head of the fetus as it begins the descent through the birth canal. The fetal head may be rotated by hand or with forceps if needed to guide the body in a proper position for delivery.

**fetal stage,** (in embryology) the interval from the end of the embryonic stage, at the end of the seventh or eighth week of gestation, to birth, 38 to 42 weeks after the first day of the last menstrual period.

**fetal status: antepartum,** a nursing outcome from the Nursing Outcomes Classification (NOC) defined as conditions indicative of fetal physical well-being from conception to the onset of labor. See also **Nursing Outcomes Classification.**

**fetal status: intrapartum,** a nursing outcome from the Nursing Outcomes Classification (NOC) defined as conditions and behaviors indicative of fetal well-being from onset of labor to delivery. See also **Nursing Outcomes Classification.**

**fetal tachycardia,** a fetal heart rate that continues at 160 beats/min or more for more than 10 minutes.

**fetal viability.** See **viable infant.**

**feti-, feto-, foeti-, foeto-,** combining form meaning 'fetus or fetal': *feticide, fetochorionic, fetoscope.*

**feticide.** See **embryoctony.**

**fetid** /fet′id, fē′tid/ [L, *fetere,* to stink], pertaining to something that has a foul or putrid odor.

**fetish** [Fr, *fetiche,* artificial], **1.** any object or idea given unreasonable or excessive attention or reverence. **2.** (in psychology) any inanimate object or any body part not of a sexual nature that arouses erotic feelings or fixation. The erotic symbolism is unique to the fetishist and results from unconscious associations. See also **paraphilia.** —**fetishism,** *n.*

**fetishist** /fet′ishist/, a person who believes in or receives erotic gratification from fetishes.

**feto-** [L. *fetus,* q.v.], a prefix meaning relationship to the fetus.

**fetochorionic** /fē′tōkôr′ē·on′ik/ [L, *fetus,* fruitful; Gk, *chorion,* skin], pertaining to the fetus and the chorion.

**fetofetal transfusion.** See **parabiotic syndrome.**

**fetoglobulins** /fē′tōglob′yəlinz/, proteins found in large amounts in fetal blood and normally in very small amounts in adult blood. The group includes alpha-fetoprotein (AFP). In certain diseases fetoglobulins may be present in adult blood in larger amounts.

**fetography** /fētog′rəfē/ [L, *fetus* + Gk, *graphein,* to record], roentgenography of the fetus in utero. See also **fetometry.**

**fetology** /fētol′əjē/ [L, *fetus* + Gk, *logos,* science], the branch of medicine that is concerned with the fetus in utero, including the diagnosis of abnormalities, congenital anomalies, the prevention of teratogenic influences, and the treatment of certain disorders. Also called **embryatrics.**

**fetometry** /fētom′ətrē/ [L, *fetus* + Gk, *metron,* measure], the measurement of the size of the fetus, especially the diameter of the head and circumference of the trunk. A kind of fetometry is **roentgen fetometry.**

**fetoplacental** /-pləsen′təl/ [L, *fetus* + *placenta,* flat cake], pertaining to the fetus and the placenta.

**fetoprotein** /-prō′tēn/ [L, *fetus* + Gk, *proteios,* first rank], an antigen that occurs naturally in fetuses and occasionally in adults as the result of certain diseases. An increased amount of **alpha-fetoprotein** in the fetus is diagnostic for neural tube defects. The presence of **beta-fetoprotein** in the blood of adults is associated with leukemia, hepatoma, sarcoma, and other neoplasms.

**fetor ex ore.** See **halitosis.**

**fetor hepaticus** [L, stench, *hēpar,* liver], foul-smelling breath associated with severe liver disease. Also called **liver breath.**

**fetor oris.** See **halitosis.**

**fetoscope** /fē′təskōp′/ [L, *fetus* + Gk, *skopein,* to look], a stethoscope for monitoring the fetal heartbeat through the mother's abdomen.

**fetoscopy** /fētos′kəpē/, a procedure in which a fetus may be directly observed in utero, using a fetoscope introduced through a small incision in the abdomen under local anesthesia. Photographs may be taken, and amniotic fluid, fetal cells, or blood may be sampled for prenatal diagnosis of many congenital anomalies or genetic defects.

**fetotoxic** /-tok′sik/ [L, *fetus* + Gk, *toxikon,* poison], pertaining to anything that is poisonous to a fetus.

**fetus** /fē′təs/ [L, fruitful], the unborn offspring of any vi-

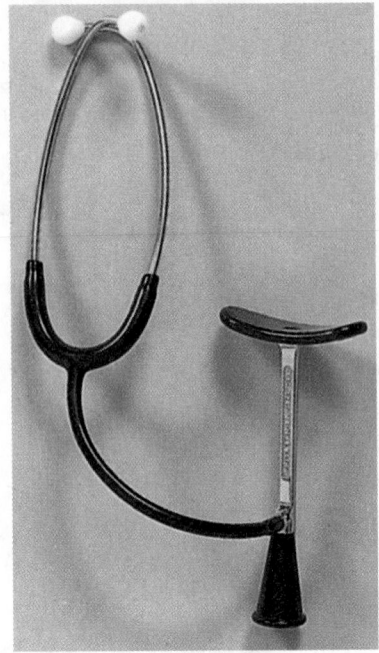

**Fetoscope** *(Seidel et al, 1999)*

viparous animal after it has attained the particular form of the species; more specifically the human being in utero after the embryonic period and the beginning of the development of the major structural features, usually from the eighth week after fertilization until birth. Kinds of fetal anomalies include **anideus, lithopedion, mummified fetus, parasitic fetus,** and **sirenomelia.** Also spelled **foetus.** Compare **embryo.** See also **prenatal development.** —**fetal, foetal,** *adj.*

**fetus acardiacus, fetus acardius.** See **acardia.**

**fetus amorphus,** a shapeless conceptus that has no formed or recognizable parts.

**fetus anideus.** See **anideus.**

**fetus in fetu** /infē′tōō/, a fetal anomaly in which a small, imperfectly formed twin, incapable of independent existence, is contained within the body of the normal twin, the autosite.

**fetus papyraceus,** a twin fetus that has died in utero early in development and has been pressed flat against the uterine wall by the living fetus. Also called **paper-doll fetus, papyraceous fetus.**

**fetus sanguinolentis** /sang′gwinəlen′tis/, a darkly colored, partly macerated fetus that has died in utero.

**FEV,** abbreviation for **forced expiratory volume.**

**FEVC,** abbreviation for **forced expiratory vital capacity.**

**fever** [L, *febris*], an elevation of body temperature above the normal circadian range as a result of an increase in the body's core temperature. Fever is a temperature above 37.2° C (98.9° F) in the morning or above 37.7° C (99.9° F) in the evening. Fever results from an imbalance between the elimination and the production of heat. Exercise, anxiety, and dehydration may increase the temperature of healthy people. Infection, neurologic disease, malignancy, pernicious anemia, thromboembolic disease, paroxysmal tachycardia, congestive heart failure, crushing injury, severe trauma, and many drugs may cause fever. No single theory explains the mechanism whereby the temperature is increased. Fever has no recognized function in conditions other than infection. It increases metabolic activity by 7% per degree Celsius, requiring a greater intake of food. Convulsions may occur in children whose fevers tend to rise abruptly, and delirium is seen with high fevers in adults and in children. Very high temperatures, as in heatstroke, may be fatal. The course of a fever varies with the cause and condition of the patient and the treatment given. The onset may be abrupt or gradual, and the period of maximum elevation, called the stadium or fastigium, may last for a few days or up to 3 weeks. The fever may resolve suddenly, by crisis, or gradually, by lysis. Certain diseases and conditions are associated with fevers that begin, rise, and fall in such characteristic curves that diagnosis may be made by studying a graphic record of the course of the fever. Kinds of hyperthermia include **habitual fever, intermittent fever,** and **relapsing fever.** See also **fever treatment, hyperpyrexia, quartan malaria, remittent fever, septic fever, tertian malaria.**

**fever blister,** a cold sore caused by herpesvirus I or II. It generally appears around the mouth or nasal mucous membranes following a febrile episode or cold. See **herpes simplex.**

**feverfew,** a perennial herb found throughout the world.
■ USES: This herb is used for migraines, cluster headaches, fever, psoriasis, and inflammation.
■ CONTRAINDICATIONS: Feverfew should not be used during pregnancy and lactation, in children, or in those with known hypersensitivity to this herb.

**fever of unknown origin (FUO),** a fever of any duration that proves to be a cause for study and for which there is at least at first no discovery of the cause despite intensive search.

**fever therapy.** See **artificial fever.**

**fever treatment[1],** the care and management of a person who has an elevated temperature.
■ METHOD: The patient is observed for symptoms of fever, such as tachycardia; a full, bounding pulse or a weak, thready pulse; rapid breathing; hot, dry, hyperemic skin; chills; headache; diaphoresis; restlessness; delirium; dehydration; tremors; convulsions; and coma. Diagnostic studies such as blood, urine, and sputum cultures and visualization procedures may be ordered to determine fever causation. Treatment may include the administration of antibiotic, antipyretic, and sedative drugs. If the temperature is extremely high, a cooling tub bath, cold wet sheet, ice packs, or hypothermia blanket may be ordered. The patient's temperature is checked every 2 to 4 hours or as condition and protocol indicate. Antipyretic and sedative therapy is continued as ordered, and, if necessary, cooling measures are reinstituted; the room temperature is reduced, and air currents are increased by a fan. Increased amounts of fluids are given orally or parenterally, physical activity is reduced, and the skin is exposed to air, with care taken to prevent chilling.
■ INTERVENTIONS: The nurse observes and records the symptoms accompanying fever, administers the ordered medication and cooling measures, reassures the patient, and explains the importance of therapy and adequate fluid intake.
■ OUTCOME CRITERIA: Antipyretic drugs and cooling measures usually reduce the temperature, but the patient may require additional fluids and treatment for the underlying cause of the fever.

**fever treatment[2],** a nursing intervention from the Nursing Interventions Classification (NIC) defined as management of a patient with hyperpyrexia caused by nonenvironmental factors. See also **Nursing Interventions Classification.**

**Fèvre-Languepin syndrome.** See **popliteal pterygium syndrome** (def. 2).

**fexofenadine,** an antihistamine.
■ INDICATIONS: This drug is used to treat rhinitis and allergy symptoms.
■ CONTRAINDICATIONS: Known hypersensitivity to this drug and severe hepatic disease prohibit the use of fexofenadine. Its use is also contraindicated in lactating women and in newborn or premature infants.
■ ADVERSE EFFECTS: Life-threatening effects are hemolytic anemia, thrombocytopenia, leukopenia, agranulocytosis, pancytopenia, and dysrhythmias (rare). Other adverse effects are urinary frequency, dysuria, urinary retention, impotence, thickening of bronchial secretions, dry nose and throat, nausea, diarrhea, abdominal pain, vomiting, constipation, headache, stimulation, drowsiness, sedation, fatigue, confusion, blurred vision, tinnitus, restlessness, tremors, paradoxical excitation in children or the elderly, rash, eczema, photosensitivity, urticaria, hypotension, palpitations, bradycardia, and tachycardia.

**FFA,** abbreviation for **free fatty acid.**

**F factor,** an extrachromosomal segment of DNA that is present in conjugating male bacteria but absent in females. Also called **F element, fertility factor, sex factor.**

**$^{18}$F-FDG,** symbol for $[^{18}F]$-2-fluoro-2-deoxy-D-glucose, a sugar analog used in positron emission tomography to determine the local cerebral metabolic rate of glucose as a measure of neural activity in the brain.

**FG syndrome** [FG, initials of family names of patients in whom it was first observed], an X-linked recessive syndrome of mental retardation, megalencephaly, imperforate anus and other GI defects, delayed motor development, congenital hypotonia, characteristic facies and personality, short stature, skeletal anomalies, and congenital cardiac defects.

**FGT cytologic smear,** abbreviation for *female genital tract cytologic smear,* any sample of tissues from the female reproductive tract smeared on a microscope slide for examination.

**FHR,** abbreviation for **fetal heart rate.**

**FHS,** abbreviation for **fetal hydantoin syndrome.**

**fiber** /fī′bər/, **1.** a long, filmlike, threadlike, acellular structure found in plant and animal tissues. Plant fibers usually consist of structural carbohydrates such as cellulose in cell walls. Composed of repeating glucose units in long, single strands, cellulose cannot be digested by enzymes in the human intestine. Other plant fiber components include hemicellulose and pectin. Animal fibers are composed mainly of the protein collagen, which forms elastic threads of loose connective tissue in skin and other organs. **2.** a skeletal muscle cell. **3.** the axon of a nerve cell. See also **dietary fiber.**

**fiberglass dermatitis,** a pruritic papular skin disease produced by mechanical irritation from glass fibers. Body folds and areas covered by tight-fitting clothing are among common sites of the pruritic dermatitis. Hardening of the sites usually occurs after several weeks.

**fiber modified diet.** See **dietary fiber.**

**fiberoptic bronchoscopy** /-op′tik/ [L, *fibra* + Gk, *optikos,* sight], the visual examination of the tracheobronchial tree through a fiberoptic bronchoscope. Also called **bronchofibroscopy.** See also **bronchoscopy, fiberoptics.**

**fiberoptic duodenoscope,** an instrument for visualizing the interior of the duodenum, consisting of an eyepiece, a flexible tube incorporating bundles of coated glass or plastic fibers with special optic properties, and a terminal light. When the duodenoscope is introduced into the patient's mouth and threaded through the upper digestive tract to the duodenum, the light illuminates the internal structures and

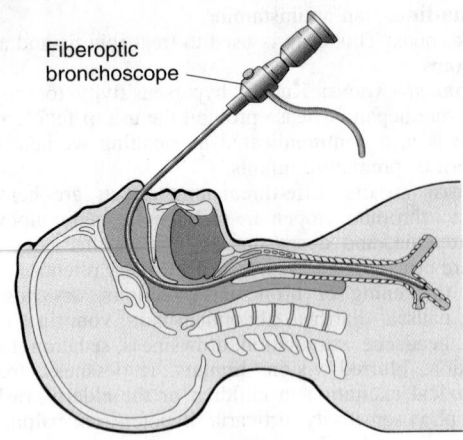

Fiberoptic
bronchoscope

**Fiberoptic bronchoscopy** *(Chabner, 2001)*

any lesions present, and the fiberoptic bundles transmit the image to the observer's eyepiece.

**fiberoptics** /-op'tiks/, the technical process by which an internal organ or cavity can be viewed, using glass or plastic fibers to transmit light through a specially designed tube and reflect a magnified image. Also spelled **fibreoptics. —fiberoptic,** *adj.*

**fiberscope** /fī'bərskōp/ [L, *fibra* + Gk, *skopein,* to look], a flexible fiberoptic instrument having an inner shaft coated with light-conveying glass or plastic fibers for visualization of internal structures. Fiberscopes are specially designed for the examination of particular organs and cavities of the body and are used in bronchoscopy, endoscopy, and gastroscopy.

**-fibrate,** combining form for clofibrate-type compounds.

**fibreoptics.** See **fiberoptics.**

**fibril** /fī'bril/ [L, *fibrilla,* small fiber], a small filamentous fiber that often is a component of a cell, as in a mitotic spindle or a myofibril.

**fibrillation** /fī'brilā'shən/ [L, *fibrilla,* small fiber, *atio,* process], involuntary recurrent contraction of a single muscle fiber or of an isolated bundle of nerve fibers. Fibrillation of a chamber of the heart results in inefficient random contraction of that chamber and disruption of the normal sinus rhythm of the heart. Fibrillation is usually described by the part that is contracting abnormally, such as atrial fibrillation or ventricular fibrillation.

**fibrillin** /fibri'lin/ [L, *fibrilla,* small fiber], a major component of elastin-associated microfibrils. It is linked to **Marfan's syndrome** by findings of immunohistochemical studies and is associated with **arachnodactyly,** a disease similar to Marfan syndrome.

**fibrin** /fī'brin/ [L, *fibra,* fiber], a stringy insoluble protein produced by the action of thrombin on fibrinogen in the clotting process. Fibrin is responsible for the semisolid character of a blood clot. Compare **fibrinogen.** See also **blood clotting, coagulation, fibrinolysis, thrombin.**

**fibrinase.** See **factor XIII.**

**fibrinocellular** /fī'brinōsel'yələr/, composed of fibrin and cells, as occurs in some exudates that result from inflammation.

**fibrinogen** /fībrin'əjən/ [L, *fibra,* fiber; Gk, *genein,* to produce], a plasma protein that is converted into fibrin by thrombin in the presence of calcium ions. Also called **factor I.** Compare **fibrin.** See also **afibrinogenemia, blood clotting, fibrinolysis, thrombin.**

**fibrinogenic.** See **fibrinogenous.**

**fibrinogenopenia** /fī'brinōjen'ōpē'nē·ə/ [L, *fibra* + Gk, *genein,* to produce, *penia,* poverty], a deficiency of fibrinogen in the blood.

**fibrinogenous** /fī'brinoj'ənəs/ [L, *fibra,* fiber; Gk, *genein,* to produce], pertaining to the characteristics or properties of fibrinogen or the production of fibrin. Also spelled **fibrogenous.** Also **fibrinogenic.**

**fibrinogen test,** a blood test that evaluates the blood clotting mechanism. Elevated levels of fibrinogen may indicate tissue inflammation or necrosis and may predict increased risk of coronary artery or cerebrovascular disease. Low levels are seen with liver disease, malnutrition, and consumptive coagulopathy.

**fibrinokinase** /fī'brinōkī'nās/ [L, *fibra* + Gk, *kinesis,* motion], a non-water-soluble enzyme in animal tissue that activates plasminogen. Also called **tissue plasminogen activator (TPA), tissue kinase.**

**fibrinolysin** /fī'brinol'isin/ [L, *fibra* + Gk, *lysein,* to loosen], a proteolytic enzyme that dissolves fibrin. It is formed from plasminogen in the blood plasma. Also called **plasmin.** See also **fibrinolysis.**

**fibrinolysis** /fī'brinol'isis/, the continual process of fibrin decomposition by fibrinolysin that is the normal mechanism for the removal of small fibrin clots. It is stimulated by anoxia, inflammatory reactions, and other kinds of stress. **—fibrinolytic,** *adj.*

**fibrinopeptide** /fī'brinōpep'tīd/ [L, *fibra* + Gk, *peptein,* to digest], a product of the action of thrombin on fibrinogen. The enzymatic cleavage responsible for the release of this protein fragment produces fibrin as well as the fibrinopeptides A and B. The latter consist of short peptides derived from the N-terminal ends of the alpha and beta chains of the fibrinogen molecule. See also **fibrinogen, thrombin.**

**fibrinous pericarditis** [L, *fibra,* fiber; Gk, *peri,* near, *kardia,* heart, *itis,* inflammation], a condition in which a lymphoid exudate accumulates on the pericardium and coagulates. The coagulated exudate may acquire a thick, buttery appearance.

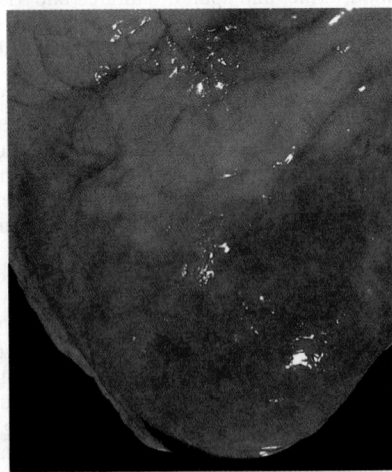

**Fibrinous pericarditis** *(Cotran, Kumar, and Collins, 1999)*

**fibrin-stabilizing factor.** See **factor XIII.**

**fibro-** /fī'brō-/, combining form meaning 'fiber': *fibroadipose, fibroblast, fibroelastosis.*

**fibroadenoma** /fī'brō·ad'inō'mə/, *pl.* **fibroadenomas, fi-**

broadenomata [L, *fibra* + Gk, *aden,* gland, *oma*], a benign tumor composed of dense epithelial and fibroblastic tissue. A fibroadenoma of the breast is nontender, encapsulated, round, movable, and firm. It occurs most frequently in women less than 25 years of age. Surgical excision is usually performed to ensure that it is not cancerous.

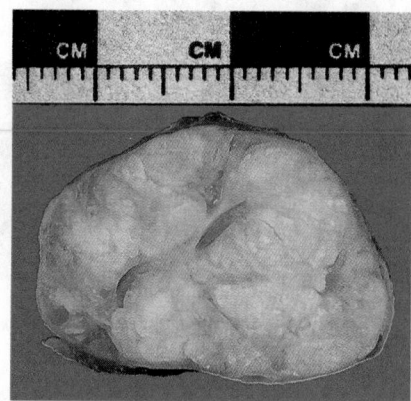

**Fibroadenoma** *(Fletcher, 2000)*

**fibroangioma.** See **angiofibroma.**
**fibroareolar tissue.** See **areolar tissue.**
**fibroblast** /fī'brəblast/ [L, *fibra* + Gk, *blastos,* germ], a flat, elongated undifferentiated cell in the connective tissue that gives rise to various precursor cells such as the chondroblast, collagenoblast, and osteoblast, which form the fibrous, binding, and supporting tissue of the body. Also called **desmocyte, fibrocyte. —fibroblastic,** *adj.*
**fibroblastoma** /-blastōma/, *pl.* **fibroblastomas, fibroblastomata** [L, *fibra* + Gk, *blastos,* germ, *oma*], a tumor derived from a fibroblast, now differentiated as a fibroma or a fibrosarcoma.
**fibrocarcinoma.** See **scirrhous carcinoma.**
**fibrocartilage** /-kär'tilij/ [L, *fibra* + *cartilago*], cartilage that consists of a dense matrix of white collagenous fibers. Of the three kinds of cartilage in the body, fibrocartilage has

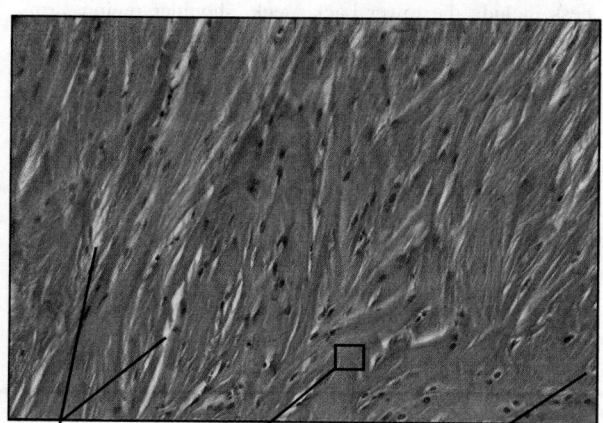

Matrix  Collagenous fibers  Cartilage cell in lacuna
**Fibrocartilage**
*(Thibodeau, 1999/Rob Callantine and James M. Kron)*

the greatest tensile strength. Fibrocartilaginous disks between the vertebrae help cushion the jolts to which the vertebral column is continually subjected. See also **hyaline cartilage. —fibrocartilaginous,** *adj.*
**fibrocartilaginous joint.** See **symphysis.**
**fibrochondritis** /-kondrī'tis/, an inflammation of fibrocartilage.
**fibrochondroma** /-kondrō'mə/, a tumor composed of mixed fibrous and cartilaginous tissues.
**fibrocyst** /fī'brəsist/, **1.** any cystic lesion within a fibrous connective tissue. **2.** a cystic fibroma.
**fibrocystic** /-sis'tik/, pertaining to a fibrocyst or cystic fibroma.
**fibrocystic disease of the breast** /-sis'tik/ [L, *fibra* + Gk, *kystis,* bag], the presence of single or multiple cysts that are palpable in the breasts. The cysts are benign and fairly common, yet must be considered potentially malignant and observed carefully for growth or change. The client may report unilateral or bilateral breast pain and tenderness that frequently begin 7 to 10 days before menses and resolve as the menses progresses. The cysts can be aspirated and a biopsy performed. In most cases no treatment is required. Decreasing caffeine in the diet and taking supplemental vitamin E have been effective in helping to alleviate breast tenderness. The nurse must vigorously counsel women who have fibrocystic disease to examine their own breasts frequently. A woman is shown any cysts present and is taught palpation, and the importance of any change is emphasized. Reassurance should also be given that the condition is very common and generally not associated with cancer. Only about 5% of fibrocystic conditions could be considered a risk factor for later development of cancer. Also called **chronic cystic mastitis.** See also **cystic fibrosis.**

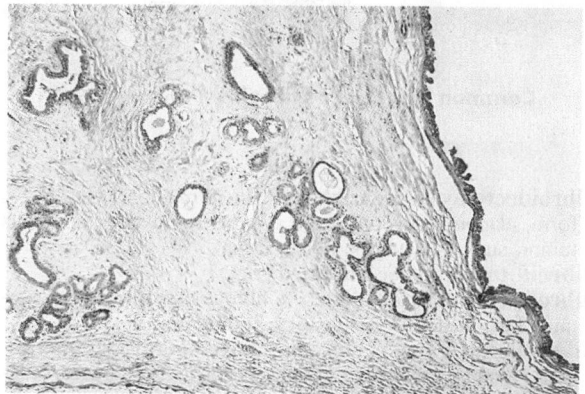

**Fibrocystic disease of the breast**
*(Kumar, Cotran, and Robbins, 1997/courtesy Dr. Kyle Molberg, Department of Pathology, University of Texas Southwestern Medical Center, Dallas)*

**fibrocystic disease of the pancreas.** See **cystic fibrosis.**
**fibrocyte.** See **fibroblast.**
**fibrodysplasia ossificans progressiva.** See **myositis ossificans progressiva.**
**fibroelastic tissue.** See **fibrous tissue.**
**fibroepithelial papilloma** /-ep'ithē'lē-əl/ [L, *fibra* + Gk, *epi,* above, *thele,* nipple; L, *papilla,* nipple; Gk, *oma,* tumor], a benign epithelial tumor containing extensive fibrous tissue. Also called **fibropapilloma.**

**fibroepithelial polyp.** See **acrochordon.**

**fibroepithelioma** /fī′brō·ep′ithē′lē·ō′mə/, *pl.* **fibroepitheliomas, fibroepitheliomata** [L, *fibra* + Gk, *epi,* above, *thele,* nipple, *oma,* tumor], a neoplasm consisting of fibrous and epithelial components.

**fibrofolliculoma** /-folik′yəlō′mə/, a benign tumor derived from the dermal part of a hair follicle. It may appear as a dome-shaped yellowish papule on the skin, accompanied by strands of follicular epithelium.

**fibrogenous.** See **fibrinogenous.**

**fibrogliosis** /-glī·ō′sis/, the formation of scar tissue in the brain in reaction to a penetrating injury. The scar is produced by fibroblasts and astrocytes, a type of glial cell.

**fibroid** /fī′broid/ [L, *fibra* + Gk, *eidos,* form], **1.** having fibers. **2.** *(informal)* a fibroma or myoma, particularly of the uterus.

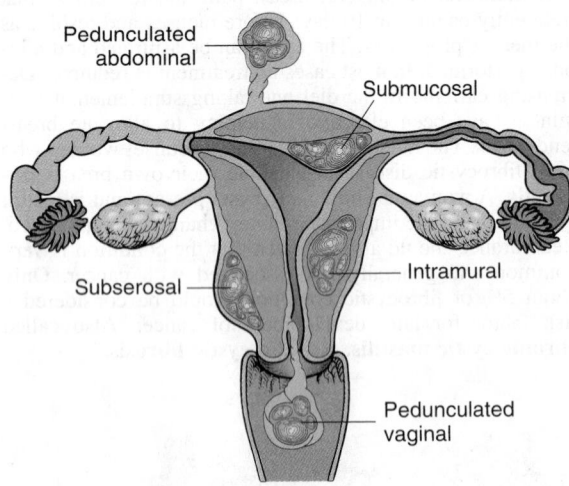

**Common locations of fibroids** *(Damjanov, 1996)*

**fibroidectomy** /fī′broidek′təmē/ [L, *fibra,* fiber; Gk, *eidos,* form, *ektomē,* excision], the surgical removal of a fibrous tumor, such as a uterine fibromyoma.

**fibroid tumor.** See **fibroma.**

**fibrolipoma** /fī′brōlipō′mə/, a fibrous tumor that also contains fatty material. Also called **lipofibroma.**

**fibroma** /fībrō′mə/, *pl.* **fibromas, fibromata** [L, *fibra* + Gk, *oma,* tumor], a benign neoplasm consisting largely of fibrous or fully developed connective tissue. See also specific fibromas.

**fibroma cavernosum,** a tumor that contains large vascular spaces, an excessive amount of fibrous tissue, and blood or lymph vessels.

**fibroma cutis,** a fibrous tumor of the skin.

**fibroma durum.** See **hard fibroma.**

**fibroma molle.** See **soft fibroma.**

**fibroma mucinosum,** a fibrous tumor in which degenerating mucoid material is present.

**fibroma myxomatodes.** See **myxofibroma.**

**fibroma of breast** [L, *fibra,* fiber; Gk, *oma,* tumor; AS, *braest*], a connective tissue tumor of the breast. It is usually benign and painless.

**fibroma pendulum,** a pendulous fibrous tumor of the skin.

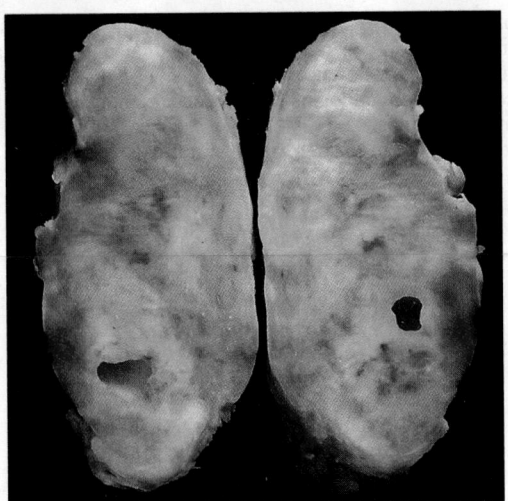

**Cardiac fibroma** *(Fletcher, 2000)*

**fibroma sarcomatosum.** See **fibrosarcoma.**

**fibromata.** See **fibroma.**

**fibroma thecocellulare xanthomatodes.** See **theca cell tumor.**

**fibromatosis** /-mətō′sis/ [L, *fibra* + Gk, *oma,* tumor, *osis,* condition], a gingival enlargement believed to be hereditary, manifested in the secondary dentition. It is characterized by a firm hyperplastic tissue that covers the surfaces of the teeth. Differentiation between this condition and phenytoin hyperplasia is based on a history of phenytoin ingestion.

**fibromuscular dysplasia (FMD)** /-mus′kyələr/, an arterial disorder sometimes associated with strokes or transient ischemic attacks (TIAs). The condition, which may appear as either fibromuscular hyperplasia or perimuscular fibrosis, is characterized by intraluminal folds of fibrous endothelial tissue. They appear as vertical bars on angiography and become the originating site of platelet adherence aggregation and thrombus formation. The condition commonly involves the renal arteries and is associated with hypertension.

**fibromyalgia,** a form of nonarticular rheumatism characterized by musculoskeletal pain, spasms, stiffness, fatigue, and severe sleep disturbance. Common sites of pain or stiffness include the lower back, neck, shoulder region, arms, hands, knees, hips, thighs, legs, and feet. These sites are known as trigger points. Physical therapy, nonsteroidal antiinflammatory drugs, and muscle relaxants provide temporary relief. Also called **fibrositis.**

**fibromyoma uteri.** See **leiomyoma uteri.**

**fibromyomectomy** /fī′brōmī′ōmek′təmē/, a surgical procedure for removing a uterine fibroma or other type of fibromyoma.

**fibromyositis** /fī′brōmī′əsī′tis/ [L, *fibra* + Gk, *mys,* muscle, *itis,* inflammation], any one of a large number of disorders characterized by stiffness and joint or muscle pain, accompanied by localized inflammation of muscle and fibrous connective tissues. The condition may develop after climatic change, infection, or physical or emotional trauma. It may recur and become chronic. Treatment includes rest, heat, massage, salicylates, and, in severe cases, intraarticular injections of a corticosteroid and procaine. Kinds of fibromyositis include **lumbago, pleurodynia,** and **torticollis.** See also **rheumatism.**

**fibropapilloma.** See **fibroepithelial papilloma.**

**fibroplasia** /-plā′zhə/,  the formation of a scar during the fibroblastic repair phase of healing.

**fibrosarcoma** /-särkō′mə/, *pl.* **fibrosarcomas, fibrosarcomata** [L, *fibra* + Gk, *sarx,* flesh, *oma,* tumor],  a sarcoma that contains fibrous connective tissue.

**fibrosing alveolitis** /fī′brōsing/ [L, *fibra* + *alviolus,* small hollow; Gk, *itis,* inflammation],  a severe form of alveolitis characterized by dyspnea and hypoxia. It occurs in advanced rheumatoid arthritis and other autoimmune diseases. X-ray films show thickening of the alveolar septa and diffuse pulmonary infiltrates. See also **alveolitis.**

**fibrosis** /fībrō′sis/ [L, *fibra* + Gk, *osis,* condition],  **1.** a proliferation of fibrous connective tissue. The process occurs normally in the formation of scar tissue to replace tissue lost through injury or infection. **2.** an abnormal condition in which fibrous connective tissue spreads over or replaces normal smooth muscle or other normal organ tissue. Fibrosis is most common in the heart, lung, peritoneum, and kidney. See also **cystic fibrosis, fibrositis.**

**fibrosis of the lungs** [L, *fibra* + Gk, *osis,* condition; AS, *lungen*],  the formation of scar tissue in the connective tissue of the lungs as a sequel to any inflammation or irritation caused by tuberculosis, bronchopneumonia, or a pneumoconiosis. Localized fibrosis may be complicated by infarction, abscess, or bronchiectasis. Also called **pulmonary fibrosis.**

**fibrositis.** See **fibromyalgia.**

**fibrothorax** /-thôr′aks/,  fibrosis of the pleural membranes.

**fibrous** /fī′brəs/ [L, *fibra,* fiber],  consisting mainly of fibers or fiber-containing materials, such as fibrous connective tissue. See also **fibrosis.**

**-fibrous,**  combining form meaning 'composed of fibrous tissue': *cellulofibrous, fibrofibrous, interfibrous.*

**fibrous astrocyte,**  a glial cell with long, fibrous processes found in the white matter of the brain and spinal cord. Its cytoplasm contains bundles of glial filaments.

**fibrous connective tissue.** See **connective tissue.**

**fibrous dysplasia,**  an abnormal condition characterized by the fibrous displacement of the osseous tissue within the bones affected. The specific cause of fibrous dysplasia is unknown, but indications are that the disease is of developmental or congenital origin. The distinct kinds of fibrous dysplasia are monostotic fibrous dysplasia, polyostotic fibrous dysplasia, and polyostotic fibrous dysplasia with associated endocrine disorders. Any bone may be affected with monostotic fibrous dysplasia. The polyostotic type usually displays a segmental distribution of the involved bones, all of which show varying degrees of the characteristic fibrous replacement of the osseous tissue. The onset of fibrous dysplasia is usually during childhood, and the disorder progresses beyond puberty and through adulthood. The onset of symptoms is usually during childhood, although diagnosis may be delayed until adolescence or even early adulthood if symptoms are minimal. The initial signs may be a limp, a pain, or a fracture on the affected side. Girls affected may have an early onset of menses and breast development and early epiphyseal closure. Albright's syndrome is usually diagnosed on the basis of a triad of symptoms, including the polyostotic type of fibrous dysplasia, café-au-lait patches on the skin, and precocious puberty. Pathologic fractures are frequently associated with this process, and angulation deformities may follow. The involved extremity may be shortened, and the classic "shepherd's crook" deformity is common. Radiographic examination usually reveals a well-circumscribed lesion occupying all or a portion of the shaft of the long bone involved. Pathologic fractures in patients with fibrous dysplasia usually heal with conservative treatment, but residual deformities often remain. When symptoms are mild and limited, this disease usually progresses slowly. Radiation therapy is not used because it may provoke malignant degeneration. Biopsies are commonly performed if pain increases or if alterations are seen on radiographic examination.

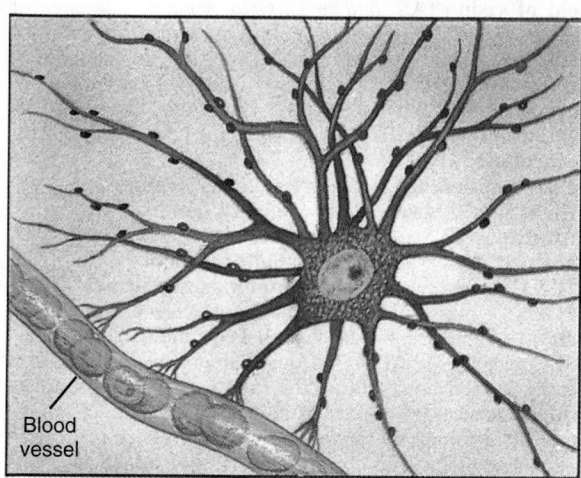

**Fibrous astrocyte** *(Chipps, Clanin, and Campbell, 1992)*

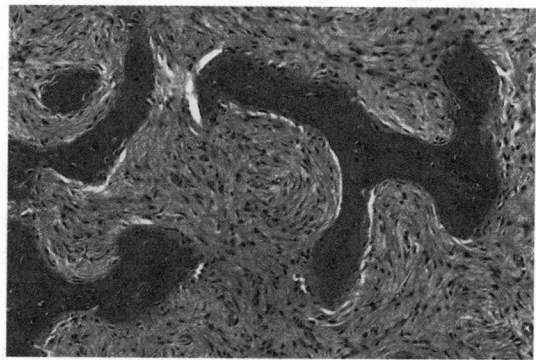

**Fibrous dysplasia** *(Fletcher, 2000)*

**fibrous capsule,**  **1.** the external layer of an articular capsule. It surrounds the articulation of two adjoining bones. **2.** the external, tough membranous envelope surrounding some visceral organs, such as the liver. Compare **synovial membrane.**

**fibrous goiter,**  an enlargement of the thyroid gland, characterized by hyperplasia of the capsule and connective tissue.

**fibrous histiocytoma.** See **dermatofibroma.**

**fibrous joint,**  any one of many immovable joints, such as those of the skull segments, in which a fibrous tissue or sometimes a form of cartilage connects the bones. The three kinds of articulation associated with fibrous joints are syndesmosis, sutura, and gomphosis. Also called **junctura fibrosa, synarthrosis.** Compare **cartilaginous joint, synovial joint.**

**fibrous thyroiditis,** a rare disorder characterized by slowly progressive fibrosis of an enlarged thyroid with replacement of normal thyroid tissue by dense fibrous tissue. The gland eventually becomes fixed to the adjacent muscles, nerves, blood vessels, and trachea by means of this fibrous tissue. The disease occurs more frequently in women than in men and usually arises after 40 years of age. Obstrive symptoms are uncommon but can include a choking sensation, dyspnea, and dysphagia. Hypothyroidism may occur, but in most patients the gland functions normally. Treatment includes surgical excision and thyroid hormone administered postoperatively, as required. Also called **ligneous thyroiditis, Riedel's struma, Riedel's thyroiditis.**

**fibrous tissue,** the connective tissue of the body, consisting of closely woven elastic fibers and fluid-filled areolae. Also called **fibroelastic tissue.** Compare **areolar tissue.** See **connective tissue.**

**fibrovascular proliferation** /-vas′kyələr/, the growth of new blood vessels and fibrous tissues on the surface of the retina and optic nerve in diabetic retinopathy. The growths can vary from barely visible vessels to dense sheets of avascular fibrous tissue.

**fibula** /fib′yələ/ [L, buckle], one of the two bones of the lower leg, lateral to and smaller in diameter than the tibia. In proportion to its length, it is the most slender of the long bones and presents three borders and three surfaces for attaching various muscles, including the peronei longus and brevis and the soleus longus. Also called **calf bone.**

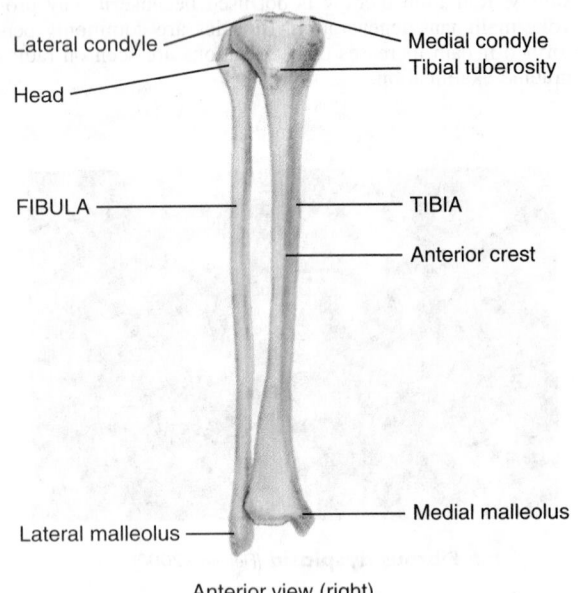

Lateral condyle — Head —

Medial condyle — Tibial tuberosity

FIBULA — TIBIA

Anterior crest

Lateral malleolus —

Medial malleolus

Anterior view (right)

**Fibula and tibia** *(Applegate, 2000)*

**fibular** /fib′yələr/ [L, *fibula,* clasp], pertaining to the fibula.

**fibular notch,** a depression on the lateral surface of the lower end of the tibia, which articulates with the lower end of the fibula.

**Fick's law** [Adolf E. Fick, German physiologist, 1829–1901], **1.** (in chemistry and physics) an observed law stating that the rate at which one substance diffuses through another is directly proportional to the concentration gradient of the diffusing substance. **2.** (in medicine) an observed law stating that the rate of diffusion across a membrane is directly proportional to the concentration gradient of the substance on the two sides of the membrane and inversely related to the thickness of the membrane.

**Fick's principle,** a method for making indirect measurements, based on the law of conservation of mass. It is used specifically to determine cardiac output, in which the amount of oxygen uptake of each unit of blood as it passes through the lungs is equal to the oxygen concentration difference between arterial and mixed venous blood. Cardiac output is calculated by measuring the uptake of oxygen for a given period, noted as milliliters per minute, then dividing that ratio by the difference in oxygen saturation of arterial and mixed venous blood samples in milliliters per 100 ml of blood and multiplying the total by 100.

**F.I.C.S.,** abbreviation for *Fellow of the International College of Surgeons.*

**fictive kin** /fik′tiv/, people who are regarded as being part of a family even though they are not related by either blood or marriage bonds. Fictive kinship may bind people together in ties of affection, concern, obligation, and responsibility.

**FID,** abbreviation for **free-induction decay.**

**field** [AS, *feld*], **1.** a defined space, area, or distance. The field of vision represents the total area that can be seen with one fixed eye. The binocular field is the area that can be seen with both eyes. **2.** an area within a computer record where a specified type of data is stored.

**field fever,** a form of leptospirosis caused by *Leptospira grippotyphosa,* which primarily affects agricultural workers. It is characterized by fever, abdominal pain, diarrhea, vomiting, stupor, and conjunctivitis. Also called **canefield fever, harvest fever.** See also **leptospirosis.**

**field of vision** [AS, *feld* + L, *visio,* seeing], the area of space in which objects are visible at the same time when the eye is fixed and the face is turned so as to exclude the limiting effects of the orbital margins and nose.

**fiery serpent** /fī′ərē/ [AS, *fyre* + L, *serpere,* to creep], an informal term for *Dracunculus medinensis.* See also **dracunculiasis.**

**fièvre boutonneuse.** See **African tick typhus.**

**fifth cranial nerve.** See **trigeminal nerve.**

**fifth disease.** See **erythema infectiosum.**

**fight-or-flight.** See **flight-or-fight reaction.**

**FIGLU,** abbreviation for **formiminoglutamic acid.**

**FIGO,** a classification system for cancers of the uterine cervix established by the French Fédération Internationale de Gynécologie et d'Obstétrique. Tumors are classified as 0 or by Roman numerals from I to IV, representing a range from precancerous or in situ to highly malignant. Classification subdivisions are represented by letters, such as IA, IIB, and so on.

**figure-eight bandage,** a bandage with successive laps crossing over and around each other to resemble the numeric figure eight. See also **bandage.**

**figure-eight suture** [L, *sutura*], a suture that begins at the deepest layer on each side of a wound, then crosses over to pass through the superficial layers on the opposite side before being tied.

**figure-four test.** See **Patrick test.**

**figure-ground relationship** /fig′(y)ər/ [L, *figura,* form; AS, *grund* + L, *relatus,* carry back], a perceptual field that is divided into a figure, which is the object of focus, and a diffuse background. See also **ground.**

**fila-,**   combining form meaning 'thread or threadlike': *filaceous, filamentous, filaria.*

**filament** /fil′əmənt/ [L, *filare,* to spin],   a fine threadlike fiber. Filaments are found in most tissues and cells of the body and serve various morphologic or physiologic functions.

**filamentous** /fil′əmen′təs/ [L, *filare,* to spin],   pertaining to something that is threadlike or capable of being drawn out into a threadlike structure.

**filaria** /fi·lar·ē·ə/ [L, *filum,* thread],   a nematode of the superfamily Filarioidea.

**filariasis** /fil′ərī′əsis/ [L, *filum,* thread; Gk, *osis,* condition],   a disease caused by the presence of filariae or microfilariae in body tissues. Filarial worms are round, long, and threadlike and are common in most tropic and subtropic regions. They tend to infest the lymph nodes, lymphatics, subcutaneous tissues, and skin after entering the body as microscopic larvae through the bite of a mosquito, blackfly, or midge. The infection is characterized by occlusion of the lymphatic vessels, with swelling and pain of the limb distal to the blockage. After many years the limb may become greatly swollen and the skin coarse and tough. Treatment is by oral administration of diethylcarbamazine, ivermectin, albendazole, or mebendazole. Apheresis, antihistimines, and corticosteroid therapy may be performed before the administration of antihelmenthic agents to reduce the risk of reaction associated with heavy worm burden. The most effective means of preventing infestation is flying insect control. See also **elephantiasis,** *Loa loa, Mansonella,* onchocerciasis, *Wuchereria.*

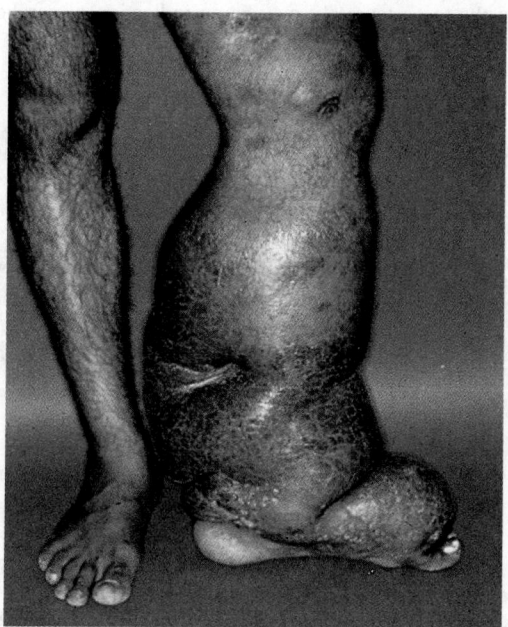

**Filariasis** *(Goldstein and Goldstein, 1997)*

**filariform** /filer′ifôrm/,   pertaining to a structure or organism that is threadlike.

**Filarioidea** /fi·lar′ē·oi′dē·ə/ [L, *filum,* thread + Gk, *eidos,* form],   the filariae, a superfamily or order of nematode parasites, the adults being threadlike worms that invade the tissues and body cavities where the female deposits embryonated eggs (prelarvae) known as microfilariae. These microfilariae are ingested by blood-sucking insects in whom they pass their developmental stage and are returned to humans when the insects bite. Genera infecting humans include *Brugia, Loa, Mansonella, Onchocerca,* and *Wuchereria.*

**-filcon,**   combining form for hydrophilic contact lens material.

**file,**   **1.** (in dentistry) a tool for scaling or removing plaque from the teeth. **2.** a collection of related data or information, assembled for a specified purpose and stored as a unit.

**filial generation** /fil′ē·əl/ [L, *filius,* son, *generare,* to beget],   the offspring produced from a given mating or cross. See also $F_1$, $F_2$.

**filiform bougie** /fil′ifôrm/ [L, *filum,* thread, *forma,* form; Fr, *bougie,* candle],   an extremely thin device for passage through a narrow pathway, such as a sinus tract. See also **bougie.**

**filiform catheter,**   a catheter with a slender, threadlike tip that allows the wider portion of the instrument to be passed through canals that are constricted or irregular because of an obstruction or an angulation in the canal. It may bypass obstructions or dilate strictures.

**filiform papilla.**   See **papilla.**

**filiform warts.**   See **digitate wart.**

**filling,**   a dental restoration consisting of a silver amalgam or other material that is inserted into a prepared tooth cavity to repair a carious lesion.

**filling factor** [AS, *fyllan,* filling; L, *factor,* a maker],   a measure of the geometric relationship between a magnetic resonance (MR) imaging coil and the body. This relationship affects the MR signal-to-noise ratio and, ultimately, image quality. Achieving a high filling factor requires fitting the coil closely to the body, thus potentially decreasing patient comfort.

**filling pressure.**   See **end-diastolic pressure.**

**film** [AS, *filmen,* membrane],   **1.** a thin sheet or layer of any material, such as a coating of oil on a metal part. **2.** (in photography and radiography) a thin, flexible transparent sheet of cellulose acetate or polyester plastic material coated with a light-sensitive emulsion, used to record images, such as organs, structures, and tissues, that may be involved in disease and diagnosis.

**film badge,**   a photographic film packet, sensitive to ionizing radiation, used for estimating the exposure of personnel working with x-rays and other radioactive sources.

**film development,**   the processing of photographic or x-ray films to manifest the latent image resulting from exposure of the chemically treated emulsion to electromagnetic radiation. Development involves wetting the film to loosen the emulsion, followed by a series of chemical baths that reduce the exposed silver ions to black metallic silver. The reducing agents for radiographic films generally contain hydroquinone to produce black tones slowly and phenidone to produce shades of gray rapidly.

**film fault,**   a defect in a photograph or radiograph, usually caused by a chemical, physical, or electrical error in its production. See also **artifact.**

**film on teeth,**   a collection of mucinous deposits that adhere to the teeth by means of acquired pellicle. Plaque, the film on teeth, contains microorganisms, desquamated tissue elements, blood cellular elements, and other debris. See also **plaque.**

**film screen mammography,**   a breast radiographic technique in which a special single-emulsion film and high-detail intensifying screens are used. The technique provides a fine image at radiation exposure levels of less than 1 rad, compared with older methods that generated radiation levels of as much as 16 rad.

**filopressure,** the temporary compression of a blood vessel by a ligature. The ligature is removed when the blood flow has stopped.

*Filovirus,* a genus of single-stranded negative-sense ribonucleic acid viruses in the Filoviridae family. The genus includes the Ebola and Marburg viruses.

**filter** [Fr, *filtrer,* to strain], **1.** a device or material through which a gas or liquid is passed to separate out unwanted matter. **2.** (in radiology) a device added to radiographic equipment that selectively removes low-energy x-rays that have no chance of reaching the film. Examples include bowtie, compensating, and conic filters.

**filtered back projection,** a mathematical technique used in magnetic resonance imaging and computed tomography to create images from a set of multiple projection profiles.

**filtration** /filträ'shən/ [Fr, *filtrer,* to strain], the addition of sheets of metal to a beam of x-rays, for the purpose of altering the energy spectrum and thus the imaging characteristics and penetrating ability of the radiation. Filtration is generally accomplished with aluminum or copper at low to medium energy and with tin, copper, or aluminum at higher energy.

**filtration angle.** See **angle of iris.**

**filum** /fi'ləm/, a threadlike structure, as the filum terminale, which extends from the lower end of the spinal cord.

**fimbria** /fim'brē·ə/ [L, fringe], any structure that forms a border or edge or that resembles a fringe. Kinds of fimbria are **fimbria hippocampi, fimbria ovarica,** and *fimbriae tubae terminale* (**spinal cord**). See also **pilus,** def. 2.

**fimbriae tubae** /fim'brī·ī/, the branched fingerlike projections at the distal end of each of the fallopian tubes. The projections are connected to the ovary and have epithelial cells with cilia that serve to move the ovum toward the uterus.

**fimbria hippocampi,** a band of efferent fibers formed by the alveus hippocampi that is continuous with the posterior pillar of the fornix.

**fimbrial tubal pregnancy** /fim'brē·əl/, a kind of tubal pregnancy in which implantation occurs in the fimbriated distal end of one of the fallopian tubes. See also **tubal pregnancy.**

**fimbria ovarica,** the longest of the fimbriae tubae. It extends from the infundibulum to the ovary. Also called **fimbriated extremity.**

**fimbriated** /fim'brē·ā'tid/ [L, *fimbria,* a fringe], having fimbria, or the fringelike projection of the ovaries or the nerve fibers along the border of the hippocampus.

**fimbriated extremity.** See **fimbria ovarica.**

**financial resource assistance,** a nursing intervention from the Nursing Interventions Classification (NIC) defined as assisting an individual/family to secure and manage finances to meet health care needs. See also **Nursing Interventions Classification.**

**finasteride** /fin'əstrīd, finas'trīd/, a drug used to treat prostatic hypertrophy by reversing the progressive enlargement of the gland.

**finding, 1.** an observation made about a particular disease state, usually in relation to physical examination and laboratory tests. **2.** a conclusion drawn from an examination, study, or experiment.

**fine motor skills** [Fr, *fin,* thin; L, *movere* + ONor, *skilja,* to cut apart], the use of precise coordinated movements in such activities as writing, buttoning, cutting, tracing, or visual tracking.

**fine-needle aspiration,** a diagnostic technique that uses a very thin needle and gentle suction to obtain tissue samples. The needle is thinner than that used for venipuncture, and the procedure is less painful than drawing of blood. Usually the procedure is done on an outpatient basis, and no anesthetic is used. The aspirated tissue is examined by a pathologist.

**fineness** /fīn'nes/ [Fr, *fin,* thin], a means of grading alloys in relation to their gold content. The fineness of an alloy is designated in parts per thousand of pure gold, which is 1000 fine. Gold alloys and pure gold may be used in dental restorations, such as tooth crowns and prepared tooth-cavity fillings.

**fine tremor** [Fr, *fin,* thin; L, *tremor,* to tremble], a vibration that occurs after a voluntary movement or one that results from fatigue in the corresponding muscle group.

**finger** [AS, *fingar*], any of the digits of the hand. The fingers are composed of three bony phalanges. Some anatomists regard the thumb as a finger, since its metacarpal bone ossifies in the same way as a phalanx. Other anatomists regard the thumb as being composed of a metacarpal bone and two phalanges. The digits of the hand are anatomically numbered 1 to 5, starting with the thumb. See also **nail.**

**finger agnosia,** a neurologic disorder in which a patient is unable to distinguish between stimuli applied to two different fingers without visual clues. It is a feature of some types of dementia.

**finger goniometer** [AS, *finger* + Gk, *gonia,* angle, *metron,* meter], an instrument for measuring the angle of a finger joint.

**finger-nose test** [AS, *finger* + *nosu* + L, *testum,* crucible], a test of the coordination of the arms. The patient is asked to draw the tip of the index finger quickly to the nose, first with the eyes open, then with the eyes closed. An inability to perform the test accurately may be an indication of cerebellar disease.

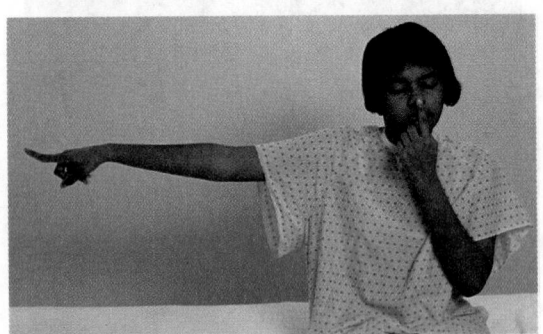

**Finger-nose test** *(Seidel et al, 1999)*

**finger percussion.** See **percussion.**

**finger phenomenon,** a diagnostic test for organic hemiplegia. With the patient's elbow on the table, the examiner grasps the patient's wrist and uses the thumb to put pressure on the radial side of the patient's pisiform bone. If the hemiplegia is organic, the patient's fingers spread fanwise.

**fingerprint,** an image left on a smooth surface by the pattern of the pad of a distal phalanx. The distinctive pattern of loops and whorls represents the fine ridges marking the skin. Because each individual's fingerprints are unique, a classification system of the patterns is useful in identifying individuals.

**finger stick,** the act of puncturing the tip of the finger to obtain a small sample of capillary blood. In some procedures the hand may be first immersed in warm water for 10 minutes to "arterialize" the capillary blood or give it characteristics similar to those of arterial blood.

**finger sweep,** a technique for clearing a mechanical obstruction from the upper airway of an unconscious patient. The rescuer opens the victim's mouth by grasping the lower jaw and tongue between the thumb and fingers. The rescuer then attempts to sweep the foreign object out of the victim's mouth with a finger.

**Finnish bath.** See **Russian bath.**

**FiO₂,** abbreviation for **fraction of inspired oxygen.**

**Fiorinal,** trademark for a group of fixed-combination drugs containing a sedative-hypnotic (butalbital); an analgesic, antipyretic, and antiinflammatory (aspirin); an analgesic (phenacetin); and a central nervous system stimulant (caffeine).

**fire ant sting,** a potentially lethal venomous injection of piperidine alkaloids by a fire ant. The ant attaches itself to the skin with its mandibles and injects venom through a stinger in the posterior part of its abdomen. The ant injects repeatedly as it rotates its body around the attachment site. All victims experience a local wheal and flare reaction that lasts up to an hour, followed by formation of a sterile pustule. The pustule sloughs off after about 48 hours but is followed by itching that may last for days. Fire ant stings are a common cause of anaphylaxis in the southern United States.

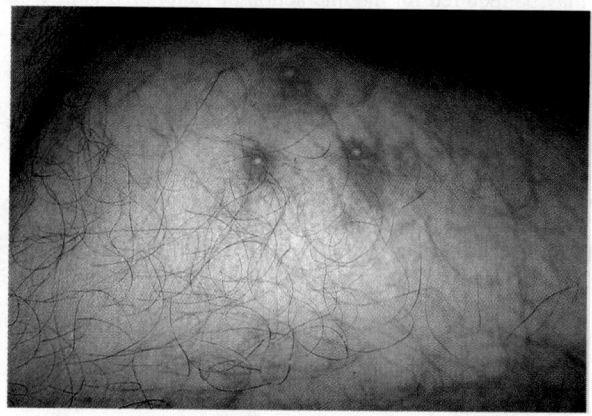

**Fire ant sting** *(Auerbach, 1995/courtesy Cameron Smith)*

**fire damp.** See **damp.**

**fireman's cramp.** See **heat cramp.**

**fire-setting precautions,** a nursing intervention from the Nursing Interventions Classification (NIC) defined as prevention of fire-setting behaviors. See also **Nursing Interventions Classification.**

**first aid**[1] [AS, *fyrst* + Fr, *aider,* to help], the immediate care that is given to an injured or ill person before treatment by medically trained personnel. Attention is directed first to the most critical problems: evaluation of the patency of the airway, the presence of bleeding, and the adequacy of cardiac function. The patient is kept warm and as comfortable as possible. The conscious patient is reassured and queried for significant details of his or her medical history, such as diabetes, a known heart condition, or allergic reactions to drugs; if the patient is unconscious, a medical identification card, bracelet, or necklace is sought. The patient is moved as little as possible, particularly if there is a possibility of fracture. If vomiting occurs, the patient's head is moved to a position for the vomitus to exit easily to prevent aspiration. See also **cardiopulmonary resuscitation, control of hemorrhage, emergency medicine, emergency nursing.**

**first aid**[2], a nursing intervention from the Nursing Interventions Classification (NIC) defined as providing initial care of a minor injury. See also **Nursing Interventions Classification.**

**first cranial nerve.** See **olfactory nerve.**

**first cuneiform.** See **medial cuneiform bone.**

**first dentition.** See **deciduous dentition.**

**first-dollar coverage,** an insurance plan under which the third-party payer assumes liability for covered services as soon as the first dollar of expense for such services is incurred, without requiring the insured to pay a deductible.

**first filial generation (F₁),** the heterozygous offspring produced by the crossing of a homozygous dominant strain with a homozygous recessive strain.

**first-generation scanner,** an early type of computed tomography device that used a finely collimated (pencil) x-ray beam and a single detector moving in a translate-rotate mode. It required 180 translations, each separated by a 1-degree rotation, and up to 5 minutes for one scan.

**first intention.** See **intention.**

**first line therapy.** See **induction therapy.**

**first metacarpal bone,** the metacarpal bone of the thumb.

**first-order change,** a change within a system that itself remains unchanged.

**first-order kinetics,** a chemical reaction in which the rate of decrease in the number of molecules of a substrate is proportional to the concentration of substrate molecules remaining. In first-order reactions involving two substances, only one of the concentrations affects the rate. The rate of metabolism of most drugs follows the rule of first-order kinetics and is independent of the dose. Also called *first-order reaction.* See also **kinetics.**

**first responder,** the first emergency person to arrive at the scene of a traumatic or medical situation. This person is trained according to a national standard curriculum set up by the U.S. Department of Transportation.

**first rib,** the highest rib of the thoracic cage. It moves about the axis of its neck, raising and lowering the sternum. First rib movement during quiet breathing is negligible, but under conditions of stress it can increase the anteroposterior diameter of the chest.

**first stage of labor** [ME, *fyrst* + OFr, *estage* + L, *labor,* work], a period of 8 to 12 hours marked by the onset of regular contractions of the uterus with full dilation of the cervix and the appearance of a small amount of blood-tinged mucus. Danger signs of the first stage include abnormal bleeding, abnormal fetal heart rate, and abnormal fetal presentation and position.

**first-state cementoma.** See **periapical fibroma.**

**fiscal resource management,** a nursing intervention from the Nursing Interventions Classification (NIC) defined as procuring and directing the use of financial resources to ensure the development and continuation of programs and services. See also **Nursing Interventions Classification.**

**fish-handler's disease.** See **erysipeloid.**

**fish poisoning,** toxic effects caused by ingestion of fish that contain substances that may produce symptoms ranging from nausea and vomiting to respiratory paralysis. See also ciguatera poisoning, scombroid poisoning, tetraodon poisoning.

**fish skin disease.** See **ichthyosis.**

**fish tapeworm infection** [AS, *fisc,* fish], an infection caused by the tapeworm *Diphyllobothrium latum* that is transmitted to humans when they eat contaminated raw or undercooked freshwater fish. Fish tapeworm infection is common in temperate zones throughout the world and is found in the Great Lakes region of the United States. Most infections are asymptomatic. However, persons may exhibit abdominal discomfort, vomiting, diarrhea, weight loss, and vitamin $B_{12}$ deficiency. Treatment is praziquantel and vitamin $B_{12}$ if indicated for deficiency. Also called **diphyllobothriasis.** See also *Diphyllobothrium,* tapeworm infection.

**fiss-,** combining form meaning 'split or cleft': *fissile, fissiparous, fissula.*

**fission** /fish′ən/ [L, *fissio,* splitting], **1.** the act or process of splitting or breaking up into two or more parts. **2.** a type of asexual reproduction common in bacteria, protozoa, and other simpler forms of life in which the cell divides into two or more equal components, each of which eventually develops into a complete organism. Kinds of fission are **binary fission** and **multiple fission. 3.** also called **nuclear fission.** (in physics) the splitting of the nucleus of an atom and subsequent release of energy.

**fissiparous** /fisip′ərəs/, reproduced by fission.

**fissura.** See **fissure.**

**fissural angioma** /fish′ərəl/ [L, *fissura,* cleft], a tumor composed of a cluster of dilated blood vessels found on the lip, face, or neck in an embryonal fissure.

**fissure** /fish′ər/ [L, *fissura,* cleft], **1.** a cleft or a groove on the surface of an organ, often marking its division into parts, such as the lobes of the lung. **2.** a cracklike lesion of the skin, such as an anal fissure. **3.** a lineal fault on a bony surface that occurs during the development of a part, such as a fissure in the enamel of a tooth. A fissure is usually deeper than a sulcus, but in the terminology of anatomy *fissure* and *sulcus* are often used interchangeably. Also called **fissura.** Compare **sulcus.** —**fissured,** *adj.*

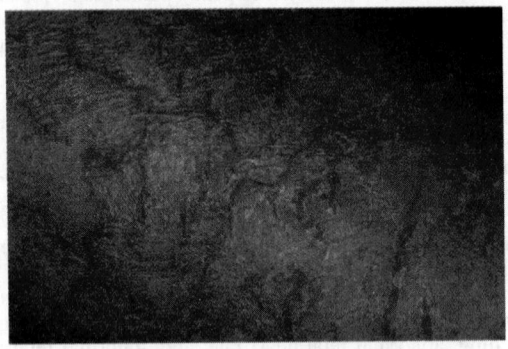

**Fissures** *(Lemmi and Lemmi, 2000)*

**fissured tongue** /fish′ərd/ [L, *fissura,* cleft; AS, *tunge*], a tongue with deep surface furrows that may radiate outward. The condition may be inherited as an autosomal-dominant trait.

**fissure fracture,** any fracture in which a crack extends into the cortex of the bone but not through the entire bone. See also **greenstick fracture.**

**fissure-in-ano.** See **anal fissure.**

**fissure of Bichat.** See **transverse fissure.**

**fissure of Rolando.** See **central sulcus.**

**fissure of Sylvius.** See **lateral cerebral sulcus.**

**fistula** /fis′chŏŏlə, -chələ/, *pl.* **fistulas, fistulae** [L, pipe], an abnormal passage from an internal organ to the body surface or between two internal organs, such as a hepatopleural or pulmonoperitoneal fistula. Fistulas may occur in many sites from the gingiva to the anus. They may be caused by a congenital defect, injury, infection, spreading of a malignant lesion, radiotherapy of a cancerous growth, or trauma during childbirth. They also may be created to achieve therapeutic purposes or obtain body secretions for physiologic studies. An arteriovenous fistula is commonly created to gain access to the patient's bloodstream for hemodialysis. Anal fistulas that result from rupture or drainage of abscesses may be treated by fistulectomy or fistulotomy; fistulas between the vagina and bladder, urethra, ureter, or rectum may be repaired surgically, but the results are not always successful. —**fistulous, fistular, fistulate,** *adj.*

**fistula-in-ano.** See **anal fistula.**

**fistular, fistulate.** See **fistula.**

**fistulectomy** /fis′chəlek′təmē/ [L, *fistula,* pipe; Gk, *ektomē,* excision], the surgical removal of a fistula.

**fistulous.** See **fistula.**

**fit, 1.** (*nontechnical*) a paroxysm or seizure. **2.** the sudden onset of an episode of symptoms such as a fit of coughing. **3.** the manner in which one surface is aligned to another, such as the alignment of a denture with the gingiva and jaw.

**fitness,** a measure of the ability of a person to perform certain tasks. See also **physical fitness.**

**Fitzgerald factor,** a high-molecular-weight kininogen that may be required for the interaction of factors XII and XI in the coagulation process.

**Fitzgerald treatment.** See **zone therapy.**

**Fitz-Hugh−Curtis syndrome** /fitz′hyoo kər′tis/ [Thomas Fitz-Hugh Jr., American physician, 1894−1963; Arthur H. Curtis, American gynecologist, 1881−1955], perihepatitis occurring as a complication of gonorrhea or chlamydial infection in women, marked by fever, upper quadrant pain, tenderness and spasm of the abdominal wall, and occasionally by friction rub over the liver.

**Fitzpatrick, Joyce J.,** a nursing theorist who derived her Life Perspective Rhythm Model from Martha Rogers' conceptualization of unitary man. She began publishing in 1970. Fitzpatrick proposes that the process of human development is characterized by rhythms that occur within the context of continuous person-environment interaction. Nursing activity focuses on enhancing the developmental process toward health. Fitzpatrick believes a central concern of nursing science and the nursing profession is the meaning attributed to life as the basic understanding of human existence. The four major concepts in this model are expressed as nursing, person, health, and environment. The person is viewed as a unified open rhythmic system with temporal patterns, consciousness patterns, and motion and perceptual patterns. Health is a human dimension under continuous development, interacting with the environment. It is seen as a heightened awareness of the meaningfulness of life. See also **Rogers, Martha.**

**5-day fever,** (*informal*) trench fever.

**five-in-one repair.** See **Nicholas procedure.**

**five-step nursing process,** a nursing process comprising five broad categories of nursing behaviors: assessing, analyzing, planning, implementing, and evaluating. The nurse gathers information about the patient, identifies his or her specific needs, develops a plan of care with the patient to answer these needs, implements the plan of care, and evaluates the effects of the implementation. The nurse involves the patient, the patient's family, and significant others in each step of the process to the greatest extent possible and compensates for and acknowledges the factors that may influence the provision of care by the nurse and staff. Implicit in the nursing process is the therapeutic and personal relationship of the nurse, the patient, the patient's family, and significant others. See also **nursing process.**

**fixate, fixated.** See **fixation.**

**fixating eye** /fik′sāting/ [L, *figere*, to fasten; AS, *eage*], (in strabismus) the normal eye that can be focused. Compare **squinting eye.**

**fixation** /fiksā′shən/ [L, *figere*, to fasten, *atio*, process], (in psychoanalysis) an arrest at a particular stage of psychosexual development, such as anal fixation. —**fixate**, *v.*, **fixated**, *adj.*

**fixational ocular movements** /fiksā′shənəl/, rotation of the eyes during voluntary fixation on an object.

**fixation muscle,** a muscle that acts to hold a part of the body in appropriate position. Compare **antagonist, prime mover, synergist.**

**fixative** /fik′sətiv/ [L, *figere*, to fasten], **1.** any substance used to bind, glue, or stabilize. **2.** any substance used to preserve gross or histologic specimens of tissue for later examination.

**fixator,** a device composed of rods and pins designed to provide stabilization of a body part. The external skeletal apparatus may be attached directly to the bone.

**fixed anions** /fikst/, anions that are not part of the body's buffer anions.

**fixed bridgework,** a dental device that incorporates artificial teeth permanently attached to natural teeth or implants in the jaw.

**fixed cantilever.** See **partial denture.**

**fixed cations,** cations that are not part of the body's metabolic buffering system.

**fixed-combination drug** [L, *figere*, to fasten, *combinare*, to combine; Fr, *drogue*], any of a group of multiple-ingredient preparations that provide concomitant administration of specific amounts of two or more medications.

**fixed coupling,** the occurrence of a normal and an ectopic heartbeat with a constant interval between the two each time the ectopic beat occurs.

**fixed delusion** [L, *figere*, to fasten, *deludere*, to deceive], a delusion that is consistent, unaltered, and difficult to interrupt.

**fixed-dose combination.** See **fixed-combination drug.**

**fixed dressing,** a dressing usually made of gauze impregnated with a hardening agent, such as plaster of paris, sodium silicate, starch, or dextrin, applied to support or immobilize a part of the body. The dressing is soaked in water, applied to the part to be immobilized, and allowed to harden. See also **cast, splint.**

**fixed drug eruption,** well-defined red to purple lesions that appear at the same sites on the skin and mucous membranes each time a particular drug is used. The reaction occurs most commonly in patients who are using tetracycline or phenolphthalein.

**fixed fulcrum,** a tomographic fulcrum that remains at a fixed height.

**fixed idea, 1.** a persistent, obsessional thought or notion. **2.** in certain mental disorders, especially obsessive-compulsive disorder, an idea that dominates mental activity and persists despite contrary evidence or rational refutation. Also called **idée fixe.**

**fixed interval (FI) reinforcement,** (in psychiatry) rein-

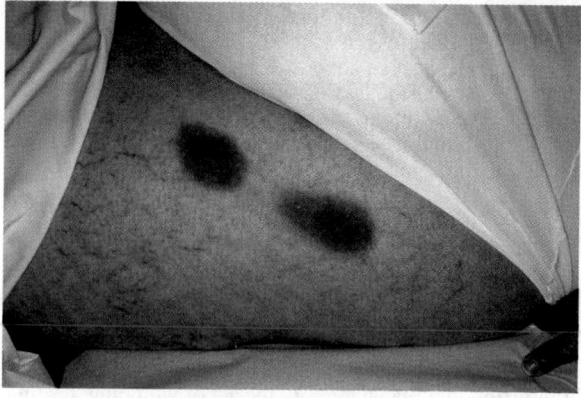

**Fixed drug eruption**
*(Goldstein and Goldstein, 1997/courtesy Department of Dermatology, Medical College of Georgia)*

forcement given after a specific amount of time has elapsed.

**fixed macrophage** [L, *figere*, to fasten; Gk, *makros*, large, *pagein*, to eat], a nonmotile mononuclear phagocyte in the liver sinuses, spleen, lymph glands, and other tissues.

**fixed noncirculating phagocyte.** See **phagocyte.**

**fixed orthodontic appliance,** a prosthetic device cemented to the teeth or attached by adhesive material, for changing the relative positions of the teeth.

**fixed partial denture.** See **partial denture.**

**fixed-performance oxygen delivery system.** See **high-flow oxygen delivery system.**

**fixed phagocyte.** See **phagocyte.**

**fixed pupil** [L, *figere*, to fasten, *pupilla*, little girl], an abnormal condition in which the pupils fail to dilate or contract when stimulated. The cause is commonly adhesions binding the iris to the lens capsule or acute glaucoma causing interference with the nerve supply of the iris.

**fixed rate pacemaker** [L, *figere*, to fasten, *ratum*, calculate, *passus*, step; ME, *maken*], an electronic cardiac stimulator that delivers impulses to the cardiac muscle at a preset rate regardless of the heart's independent activity.

**fixed ratio (FR) reinforcement,** (in psychiatry) reinforcement given after a specific number of responses have occurred.

**fixed torticollis** [L, *figere*, to fasten, *tortus*, twisted, *collum*, neck], a condition in which neck muscles on one side are so short that the head is held continuously in the same position. See also **torticollis.**

**fixed vertebrae.** See **false vertebra.**

**fixer,** a chemical used in processing photographic or x-ray film. Applied after the developing phase, it neutralizes any developer remaining on the film, removes undeveloped silver halides, and hardens the emulsion.

**flaccid** /flak′sid/ [L, *flaccus*, flabby], weak, soft, and flabby; lacking normal muscle tone, such as flaccid muscles associated with peripheral neuritis, poliomyelitis, and early stroke. —**flaccidity, flaccidness**, *n.*

**flaccid bladder,** a form of neurogenic bladder caused by interruption of the neural pathways associated with the voiding reflex, usually as a result of trauma or conditions such as diabetes. It is marked by continual filling and occasional overfilling of the bladder, absence of bladder sensation, and inability to urinate voluntarily. The bladder can be emptied by pressure applied to the area. Also called **atonic bladder, autonomous bladder, nonreflex bladder.** Compare **spastic bladder.**

**flaccid dysarthria.** See **lower motor neuron dysarthria.**
**flaccidity, flaccidness** /flaksid′itē/. See **flaccid.**
**flaccid paralysis,** an abnormal condition characterized by the weakening or the loss of muscle tone. It may be caused by disease or by trauma affecting the nerves associated with the involved muscles. Compare **spastic paralysis.**
**flagell-,** combining form meaning 'whiplike process, tapping': *flagellation, flagelliform, flagellospore.*
**flagella.** See **flagellum.**
**flagellant** /flaj′ələnt/, a person who receives sexual gratification from the practice of flagellation.
**flagellate** /flaj′əlāt′, -lit/ [L, *flagellum,* whip], a protozoon or alga that propels itself with flagella. Examples include *Trypanosoma, Leishmania, Trichomonas,* and *Giardia.* See also **protozoon.**
**flagellation** /flaj′əlā′shən/, 1. the act of whipping, beating, or flogging. 2. a type of massage administered by tapping the body with the fingers. See **massage.** 3. a type of sexual deviation in which a person is erotically gratified by being whipped or by whipping another. See **masochism, sadism.** 4. the arrangement of flagella on an organism; exflagellation.
**flagellum** /flajel′əm/, pl. **flagella** [L, whip], a long, hairlike projection that extends from some unicellular organisms and from the sperm of animals, algae, and some plants. Flagellar motion is a complex, whiplike undulation that propels cells through a fluid environment.
**Flagyl,** trademark for an antibiotic and antiprotozoal (metronidazole).
**flail chest** /flāl/ [ME, *fleyl,* whip; AS, *cest,* box], a thorax in which multiple rib fractures cause instability in part of the chest wall and paradoxic breathing, with the lung underlying the injured area contracting on inspiration and bulging on expiration. If it is uncorrected, hypoxia will result.
■ OBSERVATIONS: Flail chest is characterized by sharp pain; uneven chest expansion; shallow, rapid respirations; and decreased breath sounds. Tachycardia and cyanosis may be present. Potential complications include atelectasis, pneumothorax, hemothorax, cardiac tamponade, shock, and respiratory arrest.
■ INTERVENTIONS: The treatment of choice is internal stabilization of the chest wall through the use of a volume-controlled ventilator with a cuffed tracheostomy tube or endotracheal tube. If the patient breathes against the automatic ventilator, a sedative and muscle relaxant may be ordered to achieve ventilatory control. Chest tubes may be required to remove air or fluid that is preventing expansion of the affected lung, and a nasogastric tube may be ordered to provide food and fluids. The patient's blood pressure, pulse, respirations, and breath sounds are checked every 1 to 2 hours, rectal temperature is measured every 2 to 4 hours, and arterial blood gases are monitored as ordered.
■ NURSING CONSIDERATIONS: The patient with flail chest usually requires a long period of care involving frequent repositioning, scrupulous attention to the patency and cleanliness of the tracheostomy or endotracheal tube, skin care, oral hygiene, and emotional support. The nurse performs passive range-of-motion exercises involving the extremities, explains the various procedures, and provides a pad and pencil or a magic slate with which the patient can communicate.
**flame photometry** [L, *flagrare,* to burn; Gk, *phos,* light, *metron,* measure], measurement of the wavelength of light rays emitted by excited metallic electrons exposed to the heat energy of a flame, used to identify characteristics in clinical specimens of body fluids. The intensity of the emitted light is proportional to the concentration of atoms in the

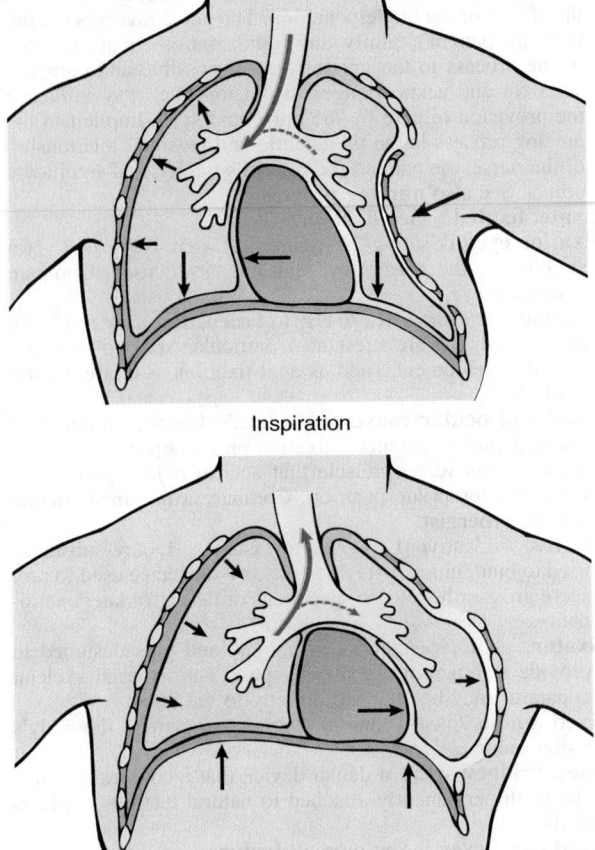

Inspiration

Expiration

**Flail chest** *(Lewis, Heitkemper, and Dirksen, 2000)*

fluid, and a quantitative analysis can be made on that basis. In the clinical laboratory, flame photometry was used to measure sodium, potassium, and lithium levels.
**flammable,** the property of igniting and burning easily and rapidly. Also called **inflammable.**
**flange** /flanj/, 1. the part of a denture base that extends from the cervical ends of the teeth to the border of the denture. 2. a prosthesis with a lateral vertical extension designed to direct a resected mandible into centric occlusion.
**flank,** the posterior portion of the body between the ribs and the ilium. Flank pain is sometimes associated with the kidney.
**flap,** a layer of skin or other tissue surgically separated from deeper structures for transplantation, coverage of an area that has been injured, or examination of deeper tissues.
**flapping tremor.** See **asterixis.**
**flap reconstruction,** an alternative to skin expansion as a method of breast reconstruction after mastectomy. It involves creation of a skin flap using tissue from another part of the body, such as the back or abdomen. The flap is attached to the chest to create a pocket for implantation or to build a breast mound.
**flap surgery,** a type of breast reconstruction that is performed in a single stage, in some cases at the same time as a mastectomy.

**flare** /fler/, **1.** a red blush on the skin at the periphery of an urticarial lesion seen in immediate hypersensitivity reactions. **2.** an expanding skin flush, spreading from an infective lesion or extending from the principal site of a reaction to an irritant. **3.** the sudden intensification of a disease.

**flaring of nostrils,** nasal widening during inspiration, a sign of air hunger or respiratory distress.

**flash,** a sudden or intermittent brief burst of intense heat or light. See also **hot flash, rush.**

**flashback,** a phenomenon experienced by persons who have taken a hallucinogenic drug or had a psychologic trauma and unexpectedly reexperience its effects. This is also suffered by patients with **posttraumatic stress disorder.**

**flash burn,** a lesion caused by exposure to an extremely intense source of radiant energy or heat. Flash burn commonly occurs on the corneas of arc welders.

**flashover phenomenon,** an effect of a lightning strike or other intense electric discharge in which the electric current passes over the body instead of through it. The result is a red, featherlike branching pattern on the skin.

**flask,** **1.** a narrow-neck glass vessel used for heating liquids, distilling chemicals, or culturing fluid media. **2.** a small glass receptacle for holding liquids or powders.

**flask closure** [L, *vasculum,* small vessel, *claudere,* to close], the joining of two halves of a flask that encloses and forms a mold for a denture base.

**flasking** /flask'ing/ /L, *vasculum,* small vessel/, **1.** the act of investing in a flask. **2.** the process of investing the cast and a wax denture in a flask preparatory to molding the denture base material into the form of the denture.

**flat affect,** the absence or near absence of emotional response to a situation that normally elicits emotion. It is observed in schizophrenia and some depressive disorders. Also called **flattened affect.**

**Flatau-Schilder disease.** See **Schilder's disease.**

**flat bone** [AS, *flet,* floor], any of the bones that provide structural contours of the skeleton. Examples include ribs and bones of the cranium.

**flat electroencephalogram,** a graphic chart on which no tracings are recorded during electroencephalography, indicating a lack of brain wave activity. Flat readings are indicative of death except in cases of profound hypothermia and central nervous system depression. Also called **isoelectric electroencephalogram.**

**flatfoot,** an abnormal but relatively common condition characterized by the flattening out of the arch of the foot. Also called **pes planus.** See also **fallen arch.**

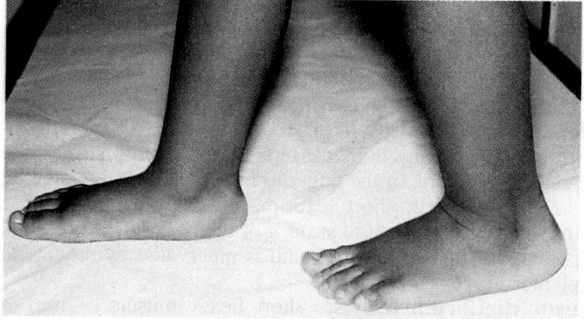

**Flatfoot** *(Zitelli and Davis, 1997)*

**flat spring contraceptive diaphragm,** a kind of contraceptive diaphragm in which the flexible metal spring that forms the rim is a thin, light, flat band made of stainless steel. The rubber dome is approximately 3.8 cm deep, and the diameter of the rubber-covered rim is between 55-100 mm. Seven sizes, in increments of 5 mm, allow the clinician to fit the diaphragm to a particular woman. This kind of diaphragm is prescribed for a woman whose vaginal musculature provides good support, whose uterus is in the normal position and not acutely retroflexed or anteflexed, and whose vagina, neither very long nor very short, has a shallow arch behind the symphysis pubis.

**flattened affect.** See **flat affect.**

**flatulence** /flach'ələns/ [L, *flatus,* a blowing], the presence of an excessive amount of air or gas in the stomach and intestinal tract, causing distension of the organs and in some cases mild to moderate pain.

**flatulence reduction,** a nursing intervention from the Nursing Interventions Classification (NIC) defined as prevention of flatus formation and facilitation of passage of excessive gas. See also **Nursing Interventions Classification.**

**flatulent** /flach'ələnt/ [L, *flatus,* a blowing], pertaining to gas or air in the digestive tract.

**flatus** /flā'təs/ [L, a blowing], air or gas in the intestine that is passed through the rectum. See also **aerophagy.**

**flat wart.** See **verruca plana.**

**flav-,** prefix meaning 'yellow': *flavescens, flavin, flavism.*

*Flavivirus.* a genus of a family of Flaviviridae single-stranded positive-sense ribonucleic acid viruses, including species that cause yellow fever, dengue, and St. Louis encephalitis.

**flavone** /flā'vōn/ [L, *flavus,* yellow], a colorless crystalline flavonoid derivative and component of bioflavonoid.

**flavoprotein,** a group of conjugated proteins that make yellow enzymes essential for cellular respiration. They also are involved in liberation of hydrogen from oxidation of fatty acids and function as electron acceptors in oxidative phosphorylation.

**flavoxate hydrochloride** /flavok'sāt/, a smooth muscle relaxant.

■ INDICATION: It is prescribed for spastic conditions of the urinary tract.

■ CONTRAINDICATIONS: GI hemorrhage or obstruction, urinary tract obstruction, or known hypersensitivity to this drug prohibits its use.

■ ADVERSE EFFECTS: Among the more serious adverse reactions are nervousness, nausea, abdominal pain, fever, and tachycardia.

**flax,** a flowering annual herb found in the United States, Canada, and Europe.

■ USES: This herb is used for constipation and as a source of omega-3 fatty acids.

■ CONTRAINDICATIONS: Flax is contraindicated in people with bowel obstruction and dehydration. It is also not recommended during pregnancy and lactation, in children, or in those with known hypersensitivity to this product. Flax should not be used as a poultice on open wounds.

**fl. dr.,** abbreviation for **fluid dram.**

**flea** [AS], a wingless, bloodsucking insect of the order Siphonaptera, some species of which transmit arboviruses to humans by acting as host or vector to the organism.

**flea bite,** a small puncture wound produced by a bloodsucking flea. Certain species of fleas transmit plague, murine typhus, and probably tularemia.

**flea-borne typhus.** See **murine typhus.**

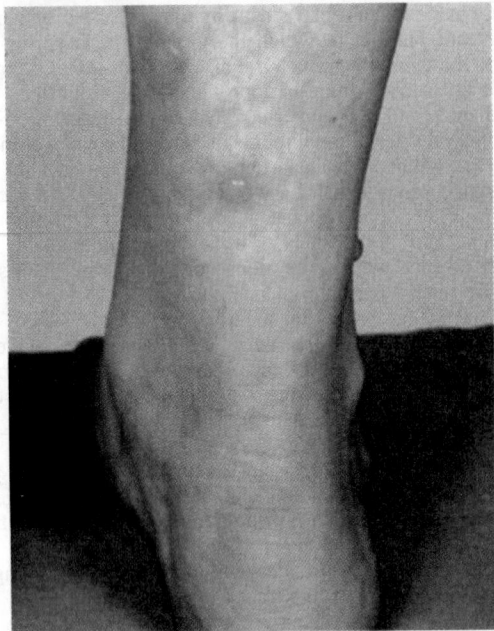

**Flea bite** *(du Vivier, 1993)*

**flecainide acetate** /flekā′nīd/, an oral antiarrhythmic drug.
- INDICATIONS: It is prescribed for the treatment of ventricular arrhythmias.
- CONTRAINDICATIONS: Preexisting second- or third-degree atrioventricular block, right bundle-branch block associated with a left hemiblock in the absence of a pacemaker, or cardiogenic shock prohibits its use. Concurrent therapy with disopyramide and verapamil is not recommended.
- ADVERSE EFFECTS: Among adverse reactions reported are new or increased arrhythmias or congestive heart failure, dizziness, visual disturbances, dyspnea, headache, nausea, fatigue, tremor, constipation, and edema.

**fleck dystrophy of the cornea.** See **speckled dystrophy of the cornea.**

**-flect, -flex,** combining form meaning 'to bend': *anteflect, circumflect.*

**Fleet Enema,** trademark for a manufactured enema formula containing 16 g sodium biphosphate and 6 g sodium phosphate per 100 ml solution. It is available in disposable plastic pouches fitted with prelubricated rectal tubes.

**Fleischner method** /flīsh′nər/ [Felix Fleischner, American radiologist, 1893–1969], a technique for producing lordotic x-ray projections of the lungs. The patient leans backward from the waist to a nearly 45-degree posterior inclination with his or her back against the x-ray film.

**flesh,** the soft, muscular tissues of the body. See also **muscle.**

**Fletcher factor,** a prekallikrein blood coagulation substance that interacts with both factor XII and Fitzgerald factor, activating both and accelerating thrombin formation.

**FLEX,** abbreviation for **Federation Licensing Examination.**

**Flexeril,** trademark for a muscle relaxant (cyclobenzaprine hydrochloride).

**Flex-Foot,** trademark for a stored-energy foot prosthesis. It contains a J-shaped plastic beam that acts like a spring when the wearer walks or runs. See also **stored-energy foot.**

**flexibilitas cerea.** See **cerea flexibilitas.**

**flexibility** /flek′si·bil′i·tē/ [L, *flectere,* to bend], the quality of being readily bent without breaking.

**flexion** /flek′shən/ [L, *flectere,* to bend], **1.** a movement allowed by certain joints of the skeleton that decreases the angle between two adjoining bones, such as bending the elbow, which decreases the angle between the humerus and the ulna. Compare **extension. 2.** a resistance to the descent of the fetus through the birth canal that causes the neck to flex so the chin approaches the chest. Thus the smallest diameter (suboccipitobregmatic) of the vertex presents.

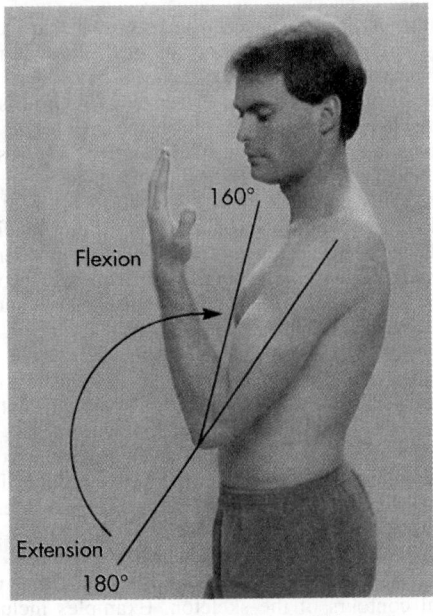

**Flexion and extension of the elbow**
*(Seidel et al, 1995/Patrick Watson)*

**flexion jacket,** a corset designed to provide spinal immobility. It is typically fashioned of a rigid material and, like a Griswald brace, provides three-point fixation in opposite directions.

**flexitime.** See **flextime.**

**flexor** /flek′sər/ [L, bender], a muscle that flexes a joint.

**flexor carpi radialis** [L, *flexor,* bender], a slender, superficial muscle of the forearm that lies on the ulnar side of the pronator teres. It functions to flex and to help abduct the hand. Compare **flexor carpi ulnaris, palmaris longus.**

**flexor carpi ulnaris,** a superficial muscle lying along the ulnar side of the forearm. It functions to flex and adduct the hand. Compare **flexor carpi radialis, palmaris longus.**

**flexor digiti minimi brevis, 1.** short flexor muscle of little finger: a muscle that inserts on the medial side of the proximal phalanx of the finger to flex it and is innervated by the ulnar nerve. **2.** short flexor muscle of little toe: a muscle that inserts on the lateral surface of the base of the proximal phalanx of the toe to flex it and is innervated by the lateral plantar nerve.

**flexor digitorum brevis,** short flexor muscle of toes: a muscle that inserts on the middle phalanges of the four lateral toes and flexes them; it is innervated by the medial plantar nerve.

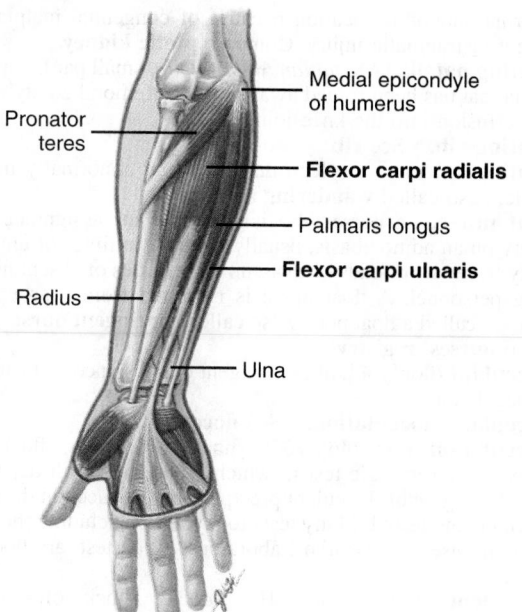

**Flexor carpi radialis and flexor carpi ulnaris**
*(Thibodeau and Patton, 1999/John V. Hagen)*

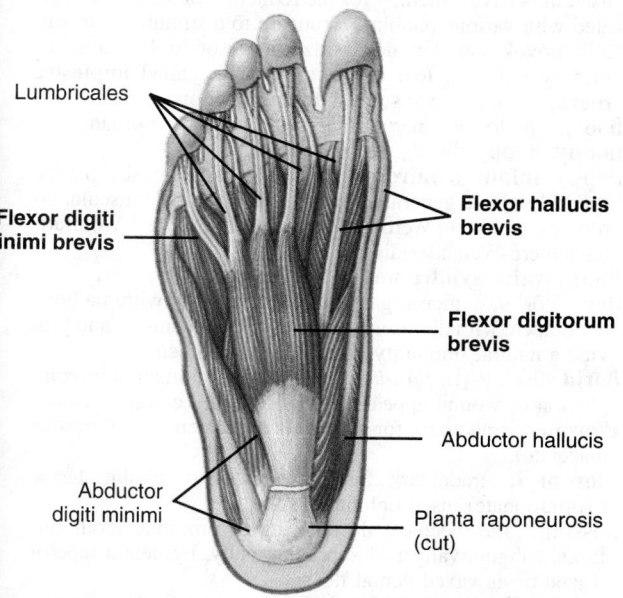

**Flexor digiti minimi brevis, flexor digitorum brevis, and flexor hallucis brevis muscles of the foot**
*(Thibodeau and Patton, 1999/John V. Hagen)*

maris longus. The muscle flexes the second phalanx of each finger and, by continued action, the hand. Also called *flexor digitorum sublimis*. Compare **flexor carpi radialis, flexor carpi ulnaris, palmaris longus, pronator teres.**

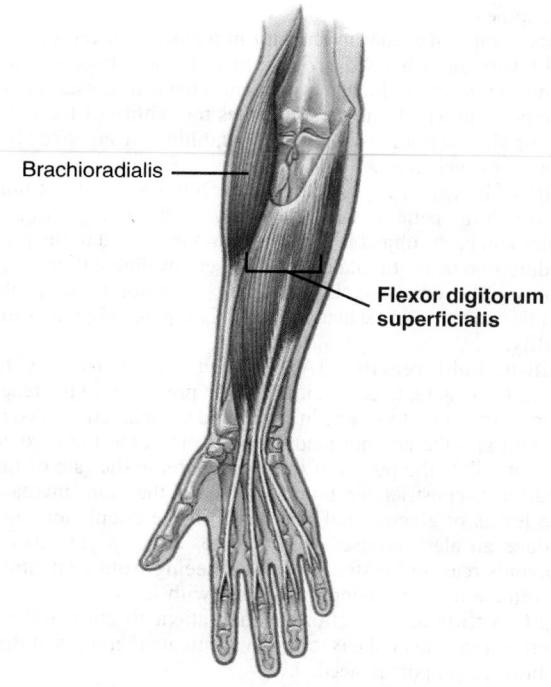

**Flexor digitorum superficialis**
*(Thibodeau and Patton, 1999/John V. Hagen)*

**flexor hallucis brevis,** short flexor muscle of great toe: a muscle that inserts in the base of the proximal phalanx of the great toe and flexes it; it is innervated by the medial plantar nerve.

**flexor retinaculum of ankle** [L, *flexor,* bender, *retinaculum,* halter; AS, *ancleow*], a strong band of fascia from the medial malleolus to the calcaneum, passing over the long flexor tendons and blood vessels and nerves of the posterior tibia.

**flexor retinaculum of hand,** the thick fibrous band of antebrachial fascia that wraps the carpal canal surrounding the tendons of flexor muscles of the forearm at the distal ends of the radius and the ulna. Also called **retinaculum flexorum manus, volar ligament.**

**flexor retinaculum of wrist** [L, *flexor,* bender, *retinaculum,* halter; AS, *wrist*], a strong ligament across the front of the hollow of the carpus and over the flexor tendons of the fingers and median nerve.

**flexor withdrawal reflex,** a common cutaneous reflex consisting of a widespread contraction of physiologic flexor muscles and relaxation of physiologic extensor muscles. It is characterized by abrupt withdrawal of a body part in response to painful or injurious stimuli. A relatively innocuous stimulation of the skin may result in a weak contraction of one or more flexor muscles and a minimal withdrawal reflex.

**flextime** /fleks'tīm/ [L, *flectere,* to bend; AS, *tima*], a system of staffing that allows the individualization of work

**flexor digitorum profundus,** one of two deep flexor muscles of the fingers: a muscle that inserts on the distal phalanges of the fingers and flexes them; it is innervated by the ulnar and anterior interosseous nerves.

**flexor digitorum superficialis,** the largest superficial muscle of the forearm, lying on the ulnar side under the pal-

schedules. A person working days may choose to work from 7:00 to 3:00, 9:00 to 5:00, or other hours. Full staffing must be maintained, but within the group flextime can be arranged. Use of the system tends to improve morale and decrease turnover. Also called **flexitime.**

**flexure** /flek'shər/, a normal bend or curve in a body part, such as the colic flexure of the colon or the dorsal flexure of the spine.

**flicks,** rapid fixation involuntary movements of the eye.

**flight into health** [AS, *fleogan*, to fly], an abnormal but common reaction to an unpleasant physical sensation or symptom in which the person denies the reality of the feeling or observation, insisting there is nothing wrong. See also **illness experience.**

**flight of ideas,** (in psychiatry) a continuous stream of talk in which the patient switches rapidly from one topic to another and each subject is incoherent and unrelated to the preceding one or is stimulated by some environmental circumstance. The condition is frequently a symptom of acute manic states and schizophrenia. Compare **circumstantiality.**

**flight-or-fight reaction** [AS, *fleogan*, to fly, *feohtan*, to fight; L, *reagere*, to act again], **1.** (in physiology) the reaction of the body to stress, in which the sympathetic nervous system and the adrenal medulla act to increase the cardiac output, dilate the pupils of the eyes, increase the rate of the heartbeat, constrict the blood vessels of the skin, increase the levels of glucose and fatty acids in the circulation, and induce an alert, aroused mental state. **2.** (in psychiatry) a person's reaction to stress by either fleeing from a situation or remaining and attempting to deal with it.

**flight to illness,** the effort of the patient to convince the therapist that he or she is too ill to terminate therapy and that continued support is needed.

**flip angle,** in magnetic resonance imaging, the degree of rotation of the macroscopic magnetization vector produced by a radiofrequency pulse with respect to the direction of the static magnetic field.

**floaters** [AS, *flotian*, to float], spots that appear to drift in front of the eye, caused by a shadow cast on the retina by vitreous debris. Most floaters are benign and represent remnants of a network of blood vessels that existed prenatally in the vitreous cavity. The sudden onset of several floaters may indicate serious disease. Hemorrhage into the vitreous humor may cause a large number of big and little shadows and a red discoloration of vision. The cause is often traumatic injury, but spontaneous intraocular hemorrhage is observed in proliferative diabetic retinopathy, hypertension, or increased intracranial pressure. Cancer, detachment of the retina, occlusion of a retinal vein, and other purely ocular diseases may also cause hemorrhage into the vitreous cavity. Inflammation of the retina resulting from chorioretinitis may cause entry of inflammatory cells into the vitreous humor. Inflammatory debris may adhere to the vitreous framework in netlike masses that are very disruptive of normal vision. Retinal detachment also causes a sudden appearance of flashes of light and/or floaters and a diminished field of vision as a shower of red cells and pigment is released into the vitreous humor. Careful ophthalmologic examination through a well-dilated pupil is recommended for all people who experience a sudden occurrence of floaters, because each of the pathologic causes can be treated in the early stages and loss of vision can usually be prevented. Also called **muscae volitantes.**

**floating head** [AS, *flotian*, to float, *heafod*], unengaged fetal head. See also **ballottement, engagement.**

**floating kidney,** a kidney that is not securely fixed in the normal anatomic location because of congenital malplacement or traumatic injury. Compare **ptotic kidney.**

**floating patella** [AS, *flotian* + L, *patella*, small pan], a patella that has been forced away from the femoral condyle by an effusion into the knee joint.

**floating rib.** See **rib.**

**floating spleen,** a spleen displaced and abnormally movable. Also called **wandering spleen.**

**float nurse,** a nurse who is available for assignment to duty on an ad hoc basis, usually to assist in times of unusually heavy workloads or to assume the duties of absent nursing personnel. A float nurse is recruited from a group of nurses called a float pool. Also called **contingent nurse.** See also **nurses' registry.**

**flocculant** /flok'yōōlənt/, an agent or substance that causes flocculation.

**flocculate, flocculation.** See **flocculent.**

**flocculation test** /flok'yōōlā'shən/ [L, *floccus*, flock of wool], a serologic test in which a positive result depends on the degree of flocculent precipitation produced in the material being tested. Many tests for syphilis, including the Venereal Disease Research Laboratories slide test, are flocculation tests.

**flocculent** /flok'yōōlənt/ [L, *floccus*, flock of wool], clumped or tufted, such as a cloud, or covered with a woolly, fuzzy surface. —**flocculate,** *v.,* **flocculation, floccule,** *n.*

**flood fever.** See **typhus.**

**flooding** [AS, *flod*], **1.** profuse bleeding from the uterus especially after childbirth or prolonged menses. **2.** a technique used in behavior therapy for the reduction of anxiety associated with various phobias. Exposure to a stimulus that usually provokes anxiety desensitizes a person to that stimulus, thereby reducing fear and anxiety. Also called **implosive therapy.** Compare **systemic desensitization.**

**floor,** the lower inner surface of any cavity or organ.

**floppy, floppy disk.** See **diskette.**

**floppy infant syndrome** [ME, *flappe,* slap; L, *infans,* speechless], a general term for juvenile spinal muscular atrophies, including Werdnig-Hoffmann disease and Wohlfart-Kugelberg-Welander disease.

**floppy-valve syndrome.** See **Barlow's syndrome.**

**flora** /flôr'ə/, microorganisms that live on or within a body to compete with disease-producing microorganisms and provide a natural immunity against certain infections.

**florid** /flôr'id/ [L, *floridus,* flowery], in human skin complexion or wound appearance, a bright red color.

**Florone,** trademark for a topical corticosteroid (diflorasone diacetate).

**Floropryl,** trademark for an inhibitor of cholinesterase (isoflurophate), used ophthalmically.

**flossing,** the mechanical cleansing of proximal tooth surfaces, subgingivally and supragingivally, by dental tape or waxed or unwaxed dental floss.

**flotation device** /flōtā'shən/ [Fr, *flotter,* to float], a foam mattress with a gellike pad located in its center, designed to protect bony prominences and distribute pressure evenly against the skin's surface.

**flotation therapy,** a state of semiweightlessness produced by various types of hospital equipment and used in the treatment and prevention of pressure ulcers.

**flow,** **1.** the movement of a liquid or gas. **2.** copious menstruation but less profuse than flooding.

**flow chart** [AS, *flowan* + L, *charta,* paper], a graphic representation of a computer program sequence. It is developed before the writing of a computer program.

**flow cytometry,** a technique in which cells suspended in a

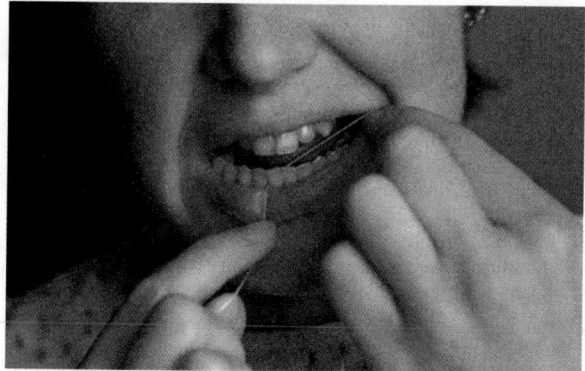

**Flossing** (Potter and Perry, 2001)

fluid flow one at a time through a focus of exciting light, which is scattered in patterns characteristic to the cells and their components; they are often labeled with fluorescent markers so that light is first absorbed and then emitted at altered frequencies. A sensor detecting the scattered or emitted light measures the size and molecular characteristics of individual cells; tens of thousands of cells can be examined per minute and the data gathered are processed by computer.

**flowmeter,** a device operated by a needle valve. In an anesthetic gas machine it is the flowmeter that measures gases by speed of flow, according to their viscosity and density. Also called **rotameter.**

**flow sheet,** (in a patient record) a graphic summary of several changing factors, especially the patient's vital signs or weight and the treatments and medications given. In labor the flow sheet displays the progress of labor, including centimeters of cervical dilation, cervical effacement, position of the baby's head, baby's heart rate, frequency of contractions, mother's temperature and blood pressure, and medications given or procedures performed.

**flow transducer,** a measuring device that calculates volume by dividing flow by time.

**flow-volume curve,** a graphic of the instantaneous rate of air flow during a forced expiration. It is plotted as a function of the volume. It may be a maximum expiratory flow-volume curve or a partial expiratory flow-volume curve.

**flow-volume loop,** a graph of the rate of air flow as a function of lung volume during a complete respiratory cycle consisting of a forced inspiration followed by a forced expiration. The plotted curve appears as a loop and is used in assessing pulmonary function.

**floxuridine** /floksyŏŏr′ədēn/, an antineoplastic agent.
- INDICATIONS: It is prescribed in the treatment of malignant neoplastic disease of the brain, breast, liver, and gallbladder.
- CONTRAINDICATIONS: Bone marrow depression, infection, poor nutritional state, or known hypersensitivity to this drug prohibits its use.
- ADVERSE EFFECTS: Among the more serious adverse reactions are severe depression of the bone marrow and acute GI disturbances, including nausea, vomiting, diarrhea, and stomatitis. Alopecia and dermatitis commonly occur.

**fl. oz.,** abbreviation for **fluid ounce.**

**flu** /flŏŏ/, (informal) 1. influenza. 2. any viral infection, especially of the respiratory or intestinal system.

**fluctuant** /fluk′chŏŏ·ənt/, pertaining to a wavelike motion that is detected when a structure containing a liquid is palpated.

**fluctuation** /fluk·chŏŏ·ā′shən/ [L, fluctuare, to wave], 1. a wavelike motion of fluid in a body cavity that follows a shaking motion. 2. a variation in a fixed value or mass.

**flucytosine** /flŏŏsī′təsēn/, an antifungal.
- INDICATION: It is prescribed in the treatment of certain serious fungal infections.
- CONTRAINDICATIONS: Known hypersensitivity to this drug prohibits its use. Close monitoring is required when administering it to patients with renal disorders or bone marrow depression.
- ADVERSE EFFECTS: Among the more serious adverse reactions are GI disturbances, including enterocolitis, abnormal liver function, hepatomegaly, and bone marrow depression.

**Fludara** trademark for a fluorinated nucleotide analog of vidaribine (fludarabine).

**fludarabine,** a fluorinated nucleotide analog of the antiviral agent vidarabine.
- INDICATIONS: It is prescribed in the treatment of patients with B-cell chronic lymphocyteic leukemia.
- CONTRAINDICATIONS: The drug should not be given to patients who are hypersensitive to this drug or its components. Patients should be closely observed for signs of hematologic and nonhematologic toxicity.
- ADVERSE EFFECTS: Fludarabine is a potent antineoplastic agent with potentially significant side effects. The side effects most often reported include myelosuppression, fever and chills, nausea, and vomiting.

**fluent** /flŏŏ′ənt/ [L. fluens flowing], flowing effortlessly; said of speech.

**-fluent,** suffix meaning 'flowing': diffluent, ossifluent.

**fluent aphasia** /flŏŏ′ənt/ [L, fluere, to flow; Gk, a, not, phasis, speech], form of aphasia in which the patient articulates words easily, although the message may be unintelligible or may not be related to a particular stimulus. Types include **Wernicke's aphasia** and **conduction aphasia.**

**fluid** /flŏŏ′id/ [L, fluere, to flow], 1. a substance, such as a liquid or gas, that is able to flow and to adjust its shape to that of a container because it is composed of molecules that are able to change positions with respect to each other without separating from the total mass. 2. a body fluid, either intracellular or extracellular, involved in the transport of electrolytes and other vital chemicals to, through, and from tissue cells. See also **blood, lymph, cerebrospinal fluid.**

**fluid balance¹,** a state of equilibrium in which the amount of fluid consumed equals the amount lost in urine, feces, perspiration, and exhaled water vapor.

**fluid balance²,** a nursing outcome from the Nursing Outcomes Classification (NOC) defined as balance of water in the intracellular and extracellular compartments of the body. See also **Nursing Outcomes Classification.**

**fluid dram (fl. dr. or ),** a unit of liquid measure equal to 3.696 milliliters (ml), 60 minims, or ⅛ fluid ounce.

**fluid/electrolyte management,** a nursing intervention from the Nursing Interventions Classification (NIC) defined as regulation and prevention of complications from altered fluid and/or electrolyte levels. See also **Nursing Interventions Classification.**

**fluidic ventilator** /flŏŏ·id′ik/, a device used in respiratory therapy that applies the Coanda effect to the movement of the flow of air or gases. As the airstream passes a wall, a pocket of turbulence forms a low-pressure bubble next to the wall, causing the airstream to adhere to the wall. As a gas travels faster over the pocket of turbulence, the surrounding gas molecules not in the stream acquire a higher pressure, holding the stream against the wall. The gas flow tends to remain in that pattern until it is diverted by a different input pressure. See also **Coanda effect.**

**fluid management,** a nursing intervention from the Nursing Interventions Classification (NIC) defined as promotion of fluid balance and prevention of complications resulting from abnormal or undesired fluid levels. See also **Nursing Interventions Classification.**

**fluid monitoring,** a nursing intervention from the Nursing Interventions Classification (NIC) defined as collection and analysis of patient data to regulate fluid balance. See also **Nursing Interventions Classification.**

**fluidotherapy** /floo'idōther'əpē/, a modality of dry heat that uses a suspended air stream with the properties of a liquid. It simultaneously performs the functions of applied heat, massage, sensory stimulation, levitation, and pressure oscillations.

**fluid ounce (fl. oz.),** a measure of liquid volume in the apothecaries' system, which is equal to 8 fluid drams or 29 ml, 480 minims, 1/20 imperial pint, or the volume occupied by 437.5 grains of distilled water at a temperature of 16.7° C. See also **apothecaries' measure, metric system.**

**fluid overload,** an excessive accumulation of fluid in the body caused by excessive parenteral infusion or deficiencies in cardiovascular or renal fluid volume regulation. Compare **circulatory overload, hypervolemia.**

**fluid resuscitation,** a nursing intervention from the Nursing Interventions Classification (NIC) defined as administering prescribed intravenous fluids rapidly. See also **Nursing Interventions Classification.**

**fluid retention,** a failure to excrete excess fluid from the body. Causes may include renal, cardiovascular, or metabolic disorders. In uncomplicated cases the condition can sometimes be corrected with diuretics and a low-salt diet.

**fluid therapy,** the regulation of water balance in patients with impaired renal, cardiovascular, or metabolic function by careful measurement of fluid intake against daily losses.

**fluid volume, deficient,** a nursing diagnosis accepted by the Fourth National Conference on the Classification of Nursing Diagnoses (revised 1996). Fluid volume deficit is the state in which an individual experiences decreased intravascular, interstitial, and/or intracellular fluid. This refers to dehydration, water loss alone without change in sodium.
■ DEFINING CHARACTERISTICS: The defining characteristics are decreased urine output, increased urine concentration, sudden weight loss, decreased venous filling, increased hematocrit, decreased skin/tongue turgor, decreased blood pressure, and dry skin/mucous membranes. Defining characteristics that require further study are thirst, increased pulse rate, decreased pulse volume/pressure, change in mental state, increased body temperature, and weakness.
■ RELATED FACTORS: The related factors are active fluid volume loss and failure of regulatory mechanisms. See also **nursing diagnosis.**

**fluid volume, excess,** a nursing diagnosis accepted by the Fifth National Conference of the Classification of Nursing Diagnoses (revised 1996). Fluid volume excess is defined as a state in which an individual experiences increased isotonic fluid retention.
■ DEFINING CHARACTERISTICS: The defining characteristics are edema, effusion, anasarca, weight gain, shortness of breath, intake greater than output, abnormal breath sounds, rales (crackles), decreased hemoglobin and hematocrit, increased central venous pressure, jugular vein distension, and positive hepatojugular reflex. Both central venous pressure and jugular vein distension have minimal clinical evidence present and need further research. Defining characteristics that require further study: clinical evidence that is lacking in fluid volume excess studies, orthopnea, $S_3$ heart sound, pul-

monary congestion, change in respiratory pattern, change in mental status, blood pressure changes, pulmonary artery pressure changes, oliguria, specific gravity changes, azotemia, altered electrolytes, restlessness, and anxiety.
■ RELATED FACTORS: The related factors are compromised regulatory mechanism, excess fluid intake, and excess sodium intake. See also **nursing diagnosis.**

**fluid volume, imbalanced, risk for,** a nursing diagnosis accepted by the Thirteenth National Conference on the Classification of Nursing Diagnoses. The condition is a risk of a decrease, increase, or rapid shift from one to the other of intravascular, interstitial, and/or intracellular fluid. This refers to the loss or excess of intravascular, interstitial, intracellular body fluids or replacement fluids.
■ RISK FACTORS: Patients scheduled for major invasive procedures are at risk. Other risk factors are being determined. See also **nursing diagnosis.**

**fluid volume, risk for deficient,** a nursing diagnosis accepted by the Fifth National Conference on the Classification of Nursing Diagnoses. Risk for fluid volume deficit is the state in which an individual is at risk of experiencing vascular, cellular, or intracellular dehydration.
■ RISK FACTORS: Risk factors include advanced age; excessive weight; extreme loss of fluid through normal routes, such as diarrhea, or abnormal routes, such as indwelling tubes; lack of fluid intake, as happens during physical immobility; increased fluid needs, as created by hypermetabolic states; and use of diuretics or other medications affecting the retention and excretion of body fluids. See also **nursing diagnosis.**

**fluke** /flook/, a parasitic flatworm of the class Trematoda, including the genus *Schistosoma*. See also **schistosomiasis.**

**flunisolide,** an intranasal (Nasalide, Nasarel) and oral inhalation (Aerobid) steroid antiinflammatory agent.
■ INDICATIONS: It is prescribed in the treatment of seasonal or continuing allergic rhinitis that involves inflammation of the mucous membranes of the nasal passages.
■ CONTRAINDICATIONS: The drug should not be given to patients with allergy to this drug or any of its components or to patients with untreated infection of the mucous membrane.
■ ADVERSE EFFECTS: The side effects most often reported include nasal or throat irritation, stinging, burning, or dryness; nosebleed; sneezing; bloody mucus; congestion; asthma; increased coughing; sore throat; or lesions in the nose or throat.

**fluocinolone acetonide** /floo'ōsin'əlōn/, a topical glucocorticoid.
■ INDICATION: It is prescribed for severe dermatoses.
■ CONTRAINDICATIONS: Impaired circulation, viral and fungal diseases of the skin, or known hypersensitivity to this drug or to other steroid medication prohibits its use.
■ ADVERSE EFFECTS: Among the more serious adverse reactions are systemic side effects that result from prolonged use or excessive application. Various hypersensitivity reactions may occur.

**fluocinonide** /floo'ōsin'ənīd/, a topical corticosteroid.
■ INDICATION: It is prescribed to reduce skin inflammation.
■ CONTRAINDICATIONS: Viral and fungal diseases of the skin, tuberculosis of the skin, or known hypersensitivity to this drug prohibits its use.

**Fluonid,** trademark for a glucocorticoid (fluocinolone acetonide).

**fluorescence** /floores'əns/ [L, *flux,* a discharge], the emission of light of one wavelength by a substance when it is exposed to electromagnetic radiation of a shorter wavelength. Fluorescent substances that emit visible light appear luminous. **—fluoresce,** *v.,* fluorescent, *adj.*

**fluorescent antibody test (FA test)** /flŏōres'ənt/,   a test in which a fluorescent dye is used to stain an antibody for identification of clinical specimens. Fluorescent dyes conjugate with immunoglobulins without altering the antibody-antigen reaction, making the dyed organisms glow visibly when examined under a fluorescent microscope. The fluorescent antibody technique can be used in identification of *Mycobacterium tuberculosis* and in the most common serologic screening test for syphilis. Kinds of fluorescent antibody tests include the **FTA-ABS test.** Also called **immunofluorescence test.**

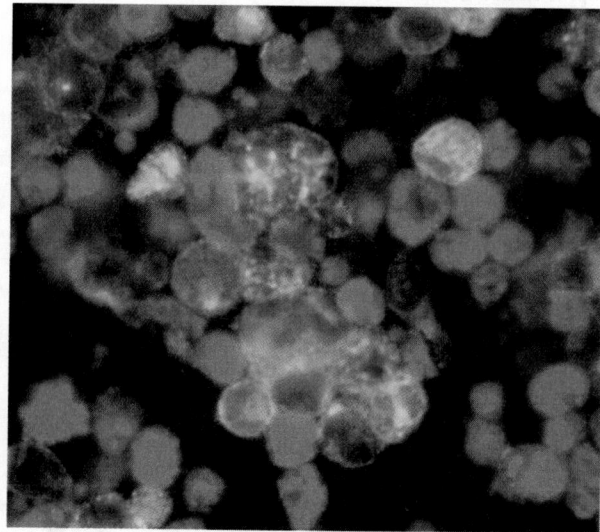

**Fluorescent antibody test**
*(Baron, Peterson, and Finegold, 1994/courtesy Ellena Peterson, University of California–Irvine)*

**fluorescent microscopy,**   examination with a fluorescent microscope equipped with a source of ultraviolet light rays, used to study specimens, such as tissues or microorganisms, that have been stained with fluorescent dye. Also called **ultraviolet microscopy.** See also **fluorescent antibody test.**

**fluorescent treponemal antibody absorption test (FTA-ABS test),**   a serologic test for syphilis. See also **fluorescent antibody test.**

**fluoridation** /flŏōr'idā'shən/ [L, *fluere,* to flow],   the process of adding fluoride, especially to a public water supply, to reduce tooth decay. See also **fluoride.**

**fluoride** /flŏōr'īd/,   an anion of fluorine, fluoride compounds are introduced into drinking water or applied directly to the teeth to prevent tooth decay.

**fluoride dental treatment** [L, *fluere,* to flow, *dens,* tooth; Fr, *traitment*],   the direct oral application of fluoride compounds to reduce the incidence of dental caries.

**fluoride poisoning** [L, *fluere,* to flow, *potio,* drink],   the toxic effects of contact with compounds of fluorine, an intensely poisonous pale yellow gas. Sodium fluoroacetate is a powerful rodent poison; methyl fluoroacetate is regarded as too toxic to use as a pesticide. The fluoroacetate compounds inhibit enzymes of the citric acid cycle. Inhalation of hydrogen fluoride can lead to bronchospasm, laryngospasm, and pulmonary edema.

**fluorination** /flŏōr'inā'shən/,   the addition of fluorine to a compound, such as those commonly found in topical corticosteroids.

**fluorine (F)** /flŏōr'ēn, flŏō'ərēn/ [L, *fluere,* to flow],   an element of the halogen family and the most reactive of the nonmetals. Its atomic number is 9; its atomic mass is 19.00. It occurs in nature only as a component of substances such as fluorspar, cryolite, and phosphate rocks. It can be prepared by the electrolytic decomposition of hydrogen fluoride and in its pure form is a pale yellow toxic gas 1.6 times heavier than air. It is also a component of very stable fluorocarbons used in the manufacture of resins and plastics. As a component of fluorides, it is widely distributed throughout the soils of the earth, enters plants, is ingested by humans, and is absorbed from the GI tract. Fluorides in the atmosphere and industrial dust are absorbed by the lungs and the skin. Relatively soluble compounds, such as sodium fluoride, are almost completely absorbed by humans. The relatively insoluble compounds, such as cryolite, are poorly absorbed. Small amounts of sodium fluoride are added to the water supply of many communities to harden tooth enamel and decrease dental caries. Excessive amounts of fluoride can mottle tooth enamel and cause osteosclerosis. Acute fluoride poisoning and death can result from the accidental ingestion of insecticides and rodenticides containing fluoride salts.

**fluoroacetic acid (CH$_2$FCOOH)** /flŏōr'ō·asē'tik, -aset'ik/,   a colorless water-soluble, highly toxic compound that blocks the citric acid cycle, causing convulsions and ventricular fibrillation. It is derived from a South African tree and is used in some potent pesticides.

**fluorocarbons** /flŏōr'ōkär'bəns/ [L, *fluere,* to flow, *carbo,* coal],   hydrocarbons where some or all of the hydrogens are replaced by fluorine. Fluorocarbons are generally colorless, nonflammable gases, but some are liquids at room temperature. The compounds can produce mild upper respiratory tract irritation, and excessive exposure has been cited as a cause of central nervous system depression.

**fluorometry** /flŏōrom'ətrē/ [L, *fluere* + Gk, *metron,* measure],   measurement of fluorescence emitted by compounds when exposed to ultraviolet or other intense radiant energy. The atoms of certain substances produce fluorescence of a characteristic color and wavelength, allowing identification and quantification of several clinically significant compounds in biologic specimens. Although fluorometry is a highly sensitive method of analysis, test interference by other compounds, especially drugs, may limit its usefulness in some situations. —**fluorometric,** *adj.*

**Fluoroplex,**   trademark for a topical preparation of antineoplastic (fluorouracil).

**fluoroscope** /flŏōr'əskōp'/ [L, *fluere* + Gk, *skopein,* to look],   a device used to project a radiographic image on a fluorescent screen for visual examination. —**fluoroscopic,** *adj.*

**fluoroscopic compression device** /flŏōr'əskop'ik/,   any of several objects that can be placed on a specific area of a patient's abdomen to compress the abdomen and separate loops of bowel during fluoroscopy of the digestive tract.

**fluoroscopy** /flŏōros'kəpē/,   the visual examination of a part of the body or the function of an organ with a fluoroscope. The technique offers continuous imaging of the motion of internal structures and immediate serial images. It is invaluable in many clinical procedures, such as intrauterine fetal transfusion and cardiac catheterization.

**fluorosis** /flŏōrō'sis/ [L, *fluere* + Gk, *osis,* condition],   the condition that results from excessive prolonged ingestion of fluorine. Unusually high concentration of fluorine in the drinking water typically causes mottled discoloration and pitting of the enamel of the secondary and deciduous dentition in children whose teeth developed while maternal intake of fluorinated water was high. Severe chronic fluorine poisoning leads to osteosclerosis and other pathologic bone and joint changes in adults. See also **fluoridation, fluoride.**

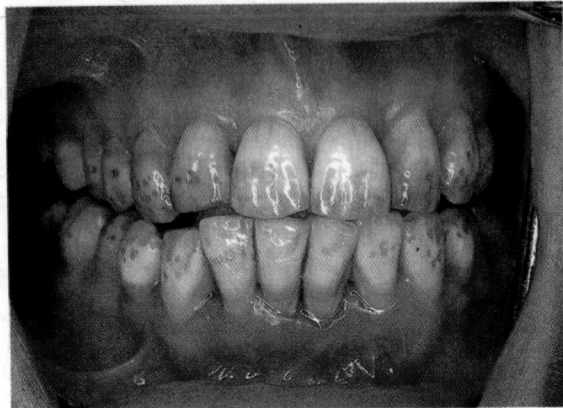

**Fluorosis** (Regezi, Sciubba, and Pogrel, 2000)

**fluorouracil** /floŏr′ōyoŏr′əsil/, an antimetabolite antineoplastic.
- INDICATIONS: It is prescribed in the treatment of malignant neoplastic disease of the skin and internal organs.
- CONTRAINDICATIONS: Bone marrow depression, infection, poor nutritional status, or known hypersensitivity to this drug prohibits its use.
- ADVERSE EFFECTS: Among the more serious adverse reactions are severe depression of the bone marrow and acute GI disturbances, including nausea, vomiting, diarrhea, and stomatitis. Alopecia and dermatitis commonly occur.

**Fluothane,** trademark for an inhalational general anesthetic (halothane).

**fluoxetine hydrochloride** /floŏ·ok′sətēn/, an oral antidepressant that acts by selectively preventing serotonin reuptake.

**fluoxymesterone** /floŏ·ok′simes′tərōn/, an androgenic and anabolic steroid.
- INDICATIONS: It is prescribed in the treatment of testosterone deficiency, breast cancer in females, and delayed puberty in males.
- CONTRAINDICATIONS: Male breast or prostate cancer, liver disease, known or suspected pregnancy, or known hypersensitivity to this drug prohibits its use.
- ADVERSE EFFECTS: Among the more serious adverse reactions are anaphylaxis, hypercalcemia, and jaundice.

**fluphenazine hydrochloride** /floŏfen′əzēn/, a phenothiazine tranquilizer.
- INDICATION: It is prescribed in the treatment of psychotic disorders.
- CONTRAINDICATIONS: Parkinson's disease, concurrent administration of central nervous system depressants, liver or renal dysfunction, severe hypotension, or known hypersensitivity to this drug or to other phenothiazine medication prohibits its use.
- ADVERSE EFFECTS: Among the more serious adverse effects are hypotension, liver toxicity, a variety of extrapyra-

midal reactions, blood dyscrasias, and hypersensitivity reactions.

**flurandrenolide** /floŏ′rəndren′əlīd/, a topical glucocorticoid.
- INDICATION: It is prescribed for the treatment of skin inflammation.
- CONTRAINDICATIONS: Impaired circulation, viral and fungal diseases of the skin, or known hypersensitivity to this drug or to steroid medication prohibits its use.
- ADVERSE EFFECTS: Among the more serious adverse reactions are systemic side effects that result from prolonged use or excessive application and hypersensitivity.

**flurazepam hydrochloride** /floŏraz′əpam/, a benzodiazepine minor tranquilizer.
- INDICATION: It is prescribed in the treatment of insomnia.
- CONTRAINDICATION: Known hypersensitivity to this drug prohibits its use.
- ADVERSE EFFECTS: Among the most serious adverse reactions are possible physical and psychologic dependence. Dizziness and drug hangover may also occur.

**flush** [ME, *fluschen*], **1.** a blush or sudden reddening of the face and neck. **2.** a sudden subjective feeling of heat. **3.** a prolonged reddening of the face such as may be seen with fever, use of certain drugs, or hyperthyroidism. **4.** a sudden rapid flow of water or other liquid.

**flush device,** an apparatus in a hemodynamic monitoring system used to install normal saline to clear blood and assure line patency. This ensures transmission of a clear pressure wave from a catheter to a transducer to provide accurate arterial or venous pressure measures.

**flutamide,** a hormonal (antiandrogen) antineoplastic agent.
- INDICATIONS: It is prescribed in the treatment of recurrent forms of cancer that respond to hormone therapy, such as cancer of the breast, prostate, or kidney. It acts by preventing sex hormones (that aid cancer growth) from getting to cancerous tissue. It may also help other anticancer drugs to reach cancer cells and stop further cancer growth.
- CONTRAINDICATIONS: The drug should not be given to patients who are allergic to the product. Hormonal medications should be avoided or used with extreme caution by women who are breastfeeding or who may be pregnant. Anticoagulants may interact with flutamide.
- ADVERSE EFFECTS: The side effects most often reported include hot flashes, loss of sex drive, impotence, nausea, vomiting, breast enlargement, and stomach upset.

**flutter,** a rapid vibration or pulsation that may interfere with normal function.

**flutter-fibrillation** [AS, *fleotan*, to move quickly; L, *fibrilla*, small fiber], a type of atrial fibrillation (involuntary recurrent contraction) in which the irregular fibrillatory line resembles atrial flutter mixed with atrial fibrillatory waves.

**fluvastatin,** an antilipidemic.
- INDICATIONS: This drug is used as an adjunct treatment in primary hypercholesterolemia (types Ia and Ib) and in coronary atherosclerosis associated with coronary artery disease.
- CONTRAINDICATIONS: Factors that prohibit the use of fluvastatin include known hypersensitivity to this drug, pregnancy, lactation, and active liver disease.
- ADVERSE EFFECTS: Life-threatening effects of this drug are liver dysfunction, myositis, rhabdomyolysis, thrombocytopenia, hemolytic anemia, and leukopenia. Other adverse reactions include rash, pruritus, nausea, constipation, diarrhea, dyspepsia, flatus, pancreatitis, lens opacities, myalgia, headache, dizziness, insomnia, fatigue, influenza, upper respiratory infection, rhinitis, cough, pharyngitis, and sinusitis.

**fluvoxamine maleate,** an antidepressant drug with selective inhibitory action in neuronal serotonin re-uptake.

- INDICATIONS: It is prescribed in the treatment of obsessive-compulsive disorder in adult patients and in depression.
- CONTRAINDICATIONS: The drug should not be given to patients with allergy to fluvoxamine maleate, patients who use monoamine oxidase inhibitors, or patients with a history of seizures, suicide attempts, or mania.
- ADVERSE EFFECTS: The side effects most often reported include rhinitis, increased frequency of urination, painful menstruation, chest pain, back pain, or general body discomfort.

**flux** /fluks/ [L, *fluere*, to flow], **1.** an excessive flow or discharge. **2.** a substance that maintains the cleanliness of metals to be united and facilitates the easy flow and attachment of solder.

**flux gain** /fluks/, the ratio of the number of light photons at the output phosphor of a radiographic image intensifier tube to the number at the input phosphor.

**fly** [AS, *flyge*], a two-winged insect of the order Diptera, some species of which transmit arboviruses to humans.

**fly bites,** bites that may be caused by species of deer flies, horse flies, blackflies, or sand flies. Such bites produce a small painful wound with swelling caused by substances in the insect's saliva that are injected beneath the surface of the skin. Emergency treatment for fly bites includes cleaning the site and placing ice on it. The bite should be monitored for possible infections, as biting flies often transmit diseases.

**Fm,** symbol for the element **fermium.**

**FMD,** abbreviation for **fibromuscular dysplasia.**

**FMET,** abbreviation for **formylmethionine.**

**FMG,** abbreviation for **foreign medical graduate.**

**FML,** trademark for an ophthalmic glucocorticoid agent (fluorometholone).

**FMR-1,** the symbol for a gene associated with a mental retardation disorder of the **fragile X syndrome.** The normal function of the gene has not been determined.

**FMRI,** abbreviation for **functional magnetic resonance imaging.**

**FNP,** abbreviation for **family nurse practitioner.**

**foam** /fōm/ [A.S. *fām*], **1.** *n.* a dispersion of gas in a liquid or solid, such as pumice or whipped cream. **2.** *n.* frothy saliva, produced particularly on exertion or pathologically.

**foam,** *v.* to produce or cause production of such a substance.

**foam bath** [AS, *fam* + *baeth*], a bath taken in water containing a saponin substance that covers the surface of the liquid and through which air or oxygen is blown to form the foam.

**focal** /fō'kəl/ [L, *focus*, hearth], pertaining to a focus.

**focal dermal hypoplasia,** an autosomal dominant X-linked disorder found exclusively in females, characterized by linear areas of dermal hypoplasia with herniation of underlying tissue through the defects; there are also telangi-ectasias, areas of discoloration, localized fatty deposits, papillomas of mucous membranes around orifices, and limb anomalies such as syndactyly, adactyly, and oligodactyly. Also called **Goltz syndrome.**

**focal emphysema,** centriacinar emphysema associated with inhalation of environmental dusts, producing dilation of the terminal and respiratory bronchioles. Also called **focal dust emphysema.**

**focal glomerular sclerosis,** focal sclerosing lesions of renal glomeruli with proteinuria, hematuria, hypertension, and the nephrotic syndrome; it may be idiopathic or secondary to other conditions, including heroin-abuse nephropathy, chronic interstitial nephritis, and malignancies. Exacerbations and remissions may occur, most often in children; progression to renal failure occurs at a variable and unpredictable rate. Also called **focal glomerulosclerosis.**

**focal illumination.** See **illumination.**

**focal lesion** [L, *focus* + *laesio*, hurting], an infection, tumor, or injury that develops at a restricted or circumscribed area of tissue.

**focal plane,** the plane of tissue that is in focus on a tomogram.

**focal point** [L, *focus*, hearth, *punctus*, pricked], a point at which rays of light meet when deflected, either by reflection or refraction.

**focal seizure** [L, *focus*, hearth; OFr, *seisir*], a transitory disturbance in motor, sensory, or autonomic function that results from abnormal neuronal discharges in a localized part of the brain, most frequently motor or sensory areas adjacent to the central sulcus. Focal motor seizures commonly begin as spasmodic movements in the hand, face, or foot. Abnormal neuronal discharges that arise in the motor area that controls mastication and salivation may be manifested by chewing, lip smacking, swallowing movements, and profuse salivation. Abnormal electrical activity in the sensory strip of the cortex may be evident initially as a numb, prickling, tingling, or crawling feeling, and the neuronal discharge may spread to motor areas. Focal seizures may be caused by localized anoxia or a small brain lesion. See also **epilepsy, motor seizure.**

**focal spot,** the area on the anode of an x-ray tube or the target of an accelerator that is struck by electrons and from which the resulting x-rays are emitted. The shape and size of a focal spot influence the resolution of a radiographic image. An increase in focal spot size, which may accompany deterioration of the x-ray tube, reduces the ability to define small structures. Also called **actual focal spot.**

**focal symptom** [L, *focus*, hearth; Gk, *symptoma*, that which happens], a body function disturbance centered on a specific body system or part.

**focal zone,** in ultrasonography, the distance along the beam axis of a focused transducer assembly, from the point where the beam area first becomes equal to four times the focal area to the point beyond the focal surface where the beam area again becomes equal to four times the focal area.

**-focon,** combining form for hydrophobic contact lens material.

**focus** /fō'kəs/ [L, hearth], **1.** a specific location, as the site of an infection or the point at which an electrochemical impulse originates. **2.** The point at which light rays converge after passing through a lens.

**focused activity** /fō'kəst/, a therapeutic technique of actively leading the patient to adaptive coping skills and away from maladaptive ones.

**focused grid,** an x-ray grid that has lead foils placed at an angle so that they all point to a focus at a specific distance.

**foetal.** See **fetus.**

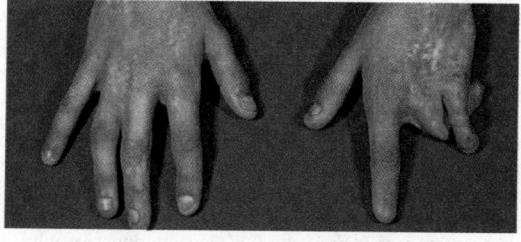

**Focal dermal hypoplasia**
*(Hordinsky, Sawaya, and Scher, 2000)*

**foeti-, foeto-.** See **feti-**.

**foetus.** See **fetus**.

**Fogarty catheter,** a type of balloon-tip catheter used to remove thrombi and emboli from blood vessels.

**fogged film fault** /fogd/ [Dan, *spray* + AS, *filmen*, membrane; L, *fallere*, to deceive], a defect in a photograph or radiograph, that appears as a foggy area. It is usually caused by stray light or radiation, use of expired film, or an unsafe darkroom light. See also **artifact**.

**fogging** [ME, *fogge*], a method of determining refractive error, particularly in cases of astigmatism, by placing excessively convex or concave lenses in front of the eyes. The patient is made artificially hyperopic or myopic by means of the spheres in order to relax all accommodation.

**fog nebulizer** /neb′yəli′zer/, (in respiratory care) a device that humidifies by producing large volumes of particles.

**foil pellet,** a loosely rolled piece of gold foil, used for making various dental restorations, such as permanent tooth cavity fillings and tooth crowns. See also **gold foil**.

**folacin.** See **folic acid, folate**.

**folate** /fō′lāt/, 1. a salt of folic acid. 2. any of a group of substances found in some foods and in mammalian cells that act as coenzymes and promote the chemical transfer of single carbon units from one molecule to another. See also **folic acid**.

**folate deficiency.** See **folic acid**.

**fold.** See **plica**.

**folded cravat sling,** a bandage suspended from the neck, usually for supporting a forearm. It is prepared by placing a broad fold of cloth on the chest vertically with one end over the shoulder of the affected arm. The other end hangs in front of the chest, and the lower end is moved up and over the shoulder and tied.

**Foley catheter** /fō′lē/ [Frederick E.B. Foley, American physician, 1891–1966], a rubber catheter with a balloon tip to be filled with a sterile liquid after it has been placed in the bladder. This kind of catheter is used when continuous drainage of the bladder is desired, such as in surgery, or when repeated urinary catheterization would be necessary if an indwelling catheter were not used. Sterile technique is used in placing the catheter. See also **catheterization**.

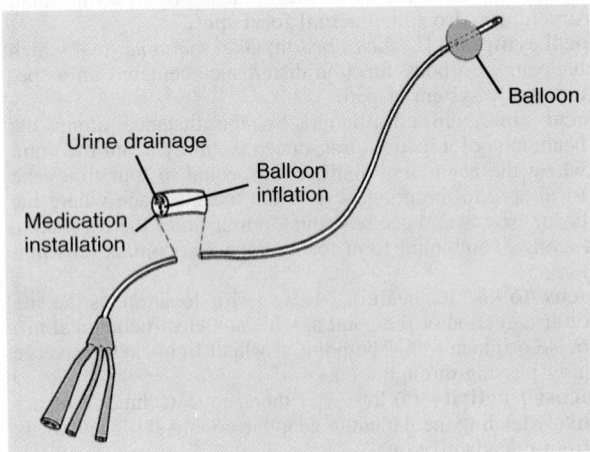

**Foley catheter** *(Potter and Perry, 1993)*

**foliate papillae** /fō′lē·āt/, a series of nipplelike processes that occur in folds along the lateral margins and in the front of the palatoglossus muscle of the tongue.

**folic acid** /fō′lik, fol′ik/, a yellow crystalline water-soluble vitamin essential for cell growth and reproduction. It functions as a coenzyme with vitamins $B_{12}$ and C in the metabolism and use of proteins and in the formation of nucleic acids and heme for hemoglobin. Deficiency results in poor growth, graying of hair, glossitis, stomatitis, GI lesions, and diarrhea, and it may lead to megaloblastic anemia. Deficiency is caused by inadequate dietary intake of the vitamin, malabsorption, metabolic abnormalities, or drug-nutrient interactions. Need for folic acid increases in pregnancy, infancy, and periods of stress. A daily intake of 400 mg before conception and during early pregnancy has been found to lower the risk of fetal neural tube defects. Rich dietary sources include spinach and other green leafy vegetables, liver, kidney, asparagus, lima beans, nuts, orange juice, and whole-grain cereals. It is both heat- and light-labile, and considerable loss of the vitamin occurs during cooking and when it has been stored for a long period. Also called **folacin, pteroylglutamic acid**.

**folic acid deficiency anemia,** a form of megaloblastic (macrocytic) anemia caused by a lack of folic acid in the diet.

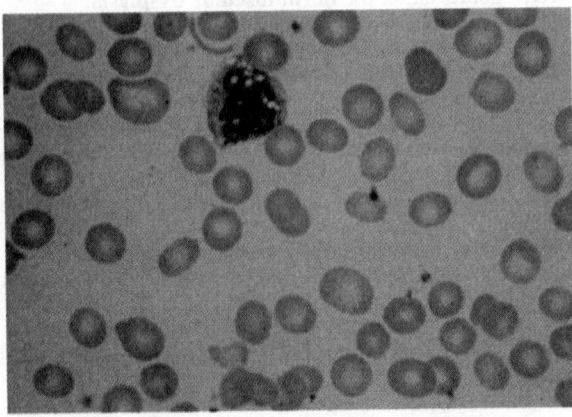

**Folic acid deficiency anemia** *(McLaren, 1992/Dr. A.C. Parker)*

**folic acid test (folate),** a blood test performed to evaluate hemolytic disorders and to detect anemia caused by folic acid deficiency.

**folie** /fōlē′/ [Fr, madness], a psychiatric condition in a person who has previously been in good mental health. Kinds of folie include **folie à deux, folie circulaire, folie du doute, folie du pourquoi, folie gemellaire, folie musculaire,** and **folie raisonnante**.

**folie à deux.** See **shared paranoid disorder**.

**folie circulaire.** See **bipolar disorder**.

**folie du doute** /dYdо̄о̄t′/ [Fr, madness of doubts], an extreme obsessive-compulsive reaction characterized by persistent doubting, vacillation, repetition of a particular act or behavior, and pathologic indecisiveness to the point of being unable to make even the most trifling decision.

**folie du pourquoi** /dYpо̄о̄rkwô·ä′/ [Fr, madness of why], a psychopathologic condition characterized by the persistent tendency to ask questions, usually concerning unrelated topics.

**folie gemellaire** /zhemeler'/ [Fr, madness in twins], a psychotic condition that occurs simultaneously in twins, sometimes in those not living together or closely associated at the time.

**folie musculaire** /mYskYler'/, severe chorea.

**folie raisonnante** /rezônäNt'/ [Fr, deliberating reason], a delusional form of any psychosis marked by an apparent logical thought process but lacking common sense.

**folinic acid** /fōlin'ik/, an active form of folic acid. It is used to treat megaloblastic anemias that are not caused by vitamin $B_{12}$ deficiency and to counteract the toxic effects of antineoplastic folic acid antagonists, such as methotrexate. Also called **citrovorum factor, leucovorin.**

**folk illnesses** /fōk/, health disorders that are attributed to nonscientific causes. The major categories are naturalistic illnesses, caused by impersonal factors such as yin-yang forces, and personalistic illnesses, caused by evil eye or other "magic."

**follicle** /fol'ikəl/ [L, *folliculus,* small bag], **1.** a small, secretory sac, such as the dental follicles that enclose the teeth before eruption or the hair follicles within the epidermis. **2.** a fluid- or colloid-filled ball of cells in some glands such as the thyroid and the ovaries. —**follicular,** *adj.*

**follicles of Lieberkühn.** See **Lieberkühn's glands.**

**follicle-stimulating hormone (FSH),** a gonadotropin that stimulates the growth and maturation of graafian follicles in the ovary and promotes spermatogenesis in the male. It is secreted by the anterior pituitary gland. FSH-releasing factor produced in the median eminence of the hypothalamus controls the release of FSH by the pituitary. Increasing amounts of FSH are secreted in the postmenstrual or resting phase of the menstrual cycle, causing a primordial follicle to develop into a mature graafian follicle containing a mature ovum. The graafian follicle produces estrogen, which reaches a high level before ovulation and suppresses release of FSH. In males FSH maintains the integrity of the seminiferous tubules and influences all the stages of spermatogenesis. It may be used to treat some conditions. One form is derived from the urine of postmenopausal women. Also called **menotropins.**

**follicle stimulating hormone releasing factor (FSH-RF)** [L, *folliculus,* small bag, *stimulare,* to incite; Gk, *horaein,* to set in motion; ME, *relesen* + L, *facere,* to do], the gonadotropin-releasing hormone.

**follicular** /fō·lik'yōō·lər/ [L, *folliculus,* small bag], of or pertaining to a follicle or follicles.

**follicular adenocarcinoma** /fōlik'yələr/, a neoplasm characterized by a follicular arrangement of cells often seen in the thyroid gland. The follicular thyroid carcinoma has a tendency to metastasize distantly to the lungs and bones. Surgery is the preferred treatment; if complete excision of the primary tumor is not feasible, radioiodine therapy is indicated. See also **medullary carcinoma, papillary adenocarcinoma.**

**follicular cyst,** a tooth-forming sac that arises from the epithelium of a tooth bud and dental lamina. The kinds of follicular cysts are dentigerous, multilocular, and primordial.

**follicular goiter,** an enlargement of the thyroid gland characterized by proliferation of the follicles and epithelial tissue.

**follicular phase,** the first part of the menstrual cycle, when ovarian follicles mature to prepare for ovulation.

**follicular tonsillitis** [L, *folliculus,* a small bag, *tonsilla* +

Gk, *itis,* inflammation], inflammation of the tonsils accompanied by a purulent infection of the tonsillar crypts.

**follicular vulvitis** [L, *folliculus,* a small bag, *vulva,* a wrapper; Gk, *itis,* inflammation], an inflammation of the skin follicles of the vulva.

**folliculitis** /fōlik'yōōlī'tis/, inflammation of hair follicles, such as in sycosis barbae.

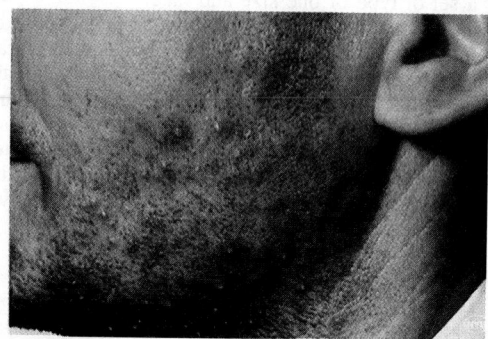

**Folliculitis**
*(Barkauskas et al, 1998/courtesy American Academy of Dermatology and Institute for Dermatologic Communication and Education, Schaumburg, Illinois)*

**folliculitis keloidalis.** See **keloid acne.**

**folliculogenesis** /fōlik'yələjen'əsis/, **1.** the stimulation of follicle development in the ovary by hormones or drugs. **2.** the development of follicles in the ovary, normally under the influence of the follicle stimulating hormone secreted by the anterior pituitary gland.

**folliculoma.** See **granulosa cell tumor.**

**folliculosis** /fōlik'yōōlōsis/, a condition characterized by the development of a large number of lymph follicles, which may or may not be associated with an infection. In conjunctival folliculosis the large number of lymph follicles may give the conjunctival sac a granular appearance.

**follitropin alfa/follitropin beta,** an ovulation stimulant.

- INDICATIONS: This drug is used to induce ovulation during assisted reproductive technologies such as in vitro fertilization.

- CONTRAINDICATIONS: Factors that prohibit the use of follitropin alfa/follitropin beta include known hypersensitivity, pregnancy, undiagnosed vaginal bleeding, intracranial lesion, and ovarian cyst not caused by polycystic ovarian disease.

- ADVERSE EFFECTS: Life-threatening effects of this drug are birth defects and spontaneous abortion. Other adverse reactions include malaise, nausea, vomiting, constipation, increased appetite, abdominal pain, rash, dermatitis, urticaria, alopecia, polyuria, urinary frequency, multiple ovulation, and breast pain.

**follow-up,** an act of renewing contact with sources of information and reviewing data needed to reinforce or evaluate a previous action or report, such as reexamination of an earlier diagnosis or prognosis.

**fomentation** /fō'mentā'shən/ [L, *fomentare,* to apply a poultice], **1.** a topical treatment for pain or inflammation that uses a warm, moist application. **2.** a substance or poultice that is used as a warm, moist application.

**fomite** /fō′mīt/ [L, *fomes,* tinder], nonliving material such as bed linen that may transmit microorganisms.

**Fones' method** /fōnz/ [Alfred C. Fones, American dentist, b. 1869], a toothbrushing technique that uses large, sweeping, scrubbing circles over occluded teeth, with the toothbrush held at right angles to the tooth surfaces. With the jaws parted, the palatal and lingual surfaces of the teeth are scrubbed in smaller circles. Occlusal surfaces of the teeth are scrubbed in an anteroposterior direction.

**font,** a set of type of one size and face.

**fontanel** /fon′tənel′/ [Fr, *fontaine,* fountain], a space covered by tough membranes between the bones of an infant's cranium. The anterior fontanel, roughly diamond-shaped, usually closes at 14 months. The posterior fontanel, triangular in shape, closes about 2 months after birth. Increase in intracranial pressure may cause a fontanel to become tense or bulge, as evidenced in infection such as meningitis. A fontanel may be soft and depressed as a result of dehydration. Also spelled **fontanelle, fonticulus.**

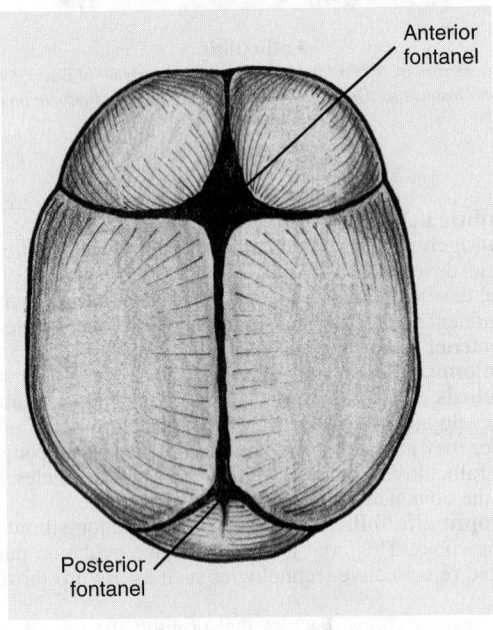

**Fontanels** *(Potter and Perry, 1995)*

**fonticulus.** See **fontanel.**

**food** [AS, *foda*], **1.** any substance, usually of plant or animal origin, consisting of carbohydrates, proteins, fats, and such supplementary elements as minerals and vitamins, that is ingested or otherwise taken into the body and assimilated to provide energy and to promote the growth, repair, and maintenance essential for sustaining life. **2.** nourishment in solid form, as contrasted with liquid form. **3.** a particular kind of solid nourishment, such as breakfast food or snack food.

**food additives,** a large variety of substances that are added to foods to prevent spoilage, improve appearance, enhance flavor or texture, or increase nutritional value. Most food ad-ditives must be approved by the U.S. Food and Drug Administration to determine whether they can cause cancer, birth defects, or other health problems. Examples include butylated hydroxyanisole (BHA) and butylated hydroxytoluene (BHT) in vitro, antioxidants that are added to fats to retard rancidity.

**food allergy,** a hypersensitive state that results from the ingestion, inhalation, or other contact with a specific food antigen. Symptoms of sensitivity to specific foods can include allergic rhinitis, bronchial asthma, urticaria, angioneurotic edema, dermatitis, pruritus, headache, labyrinthitis and conjunctivitis, nausea, vomiting, diarrhea, pylorospasm, colic, spastic constipation, mucous colitis, and perianal eczema. Food allergens are protein in nature and elicit an immunoglobulin response. The most common foods that cause allergic reactions are wheat, milk, eggs, fish and other seafoods, chocolate, corn, nuts (particularly peanuts), strawberries, chicken, pork, legumes, tomatoes, cucumbers, garlic, and citrus fruits. Foods that are rarely allergenic are rice, lamb, gelatin, peaches, pears, lettuce, artichokes, sesame oil, and apples. Diagnosis of a specific food allergy is obtained by a detailed food history, food diary, elimination diet, cutaneous tests, and blood examination for an immunoglobulin response. Compare **gastrointestinal allergy.**

**Food and Drug Administration (FDA),** a U.S. federal agency responsible for the enforcement of federal regulations on the manufacture and distribution of food, drugs, and cosmetics intended to prevent the sale of impure or dangerous substances.

**food and drug interactions,** adverse health effects of certain combinations of foods and medications. Examples include depletion of potassium from body tissues, reduced activity of drug-metabolizing enzymes, and interference with the function of the drug.

**food chain** [AS, *foda + chaine*], an ecologic sequence in which the various organisms within a community subsist on organisms lower in the sequence, as the human eats the fish that eats the worm, and so on. Each level within the chain has a fundamental role, and destruction of any one member affects the rest of the chain negatively.

**food challenge,** a challenge test for determining food allergens; a small amount of a lyophilized preparation of the suspected allergen is administered orally and the patient is monitored for reactions such as rash, rhinorrhea, or diarrhea. Also called **food challenge test.**

**food contaminants** /kəntam′inənts/, substances that make food unfit for human consumption. Examples include bacteria, toxic chemicals, carcinogens, teratogens, and radioactive materials. Also regarded as contaminants are basically harmless substances, such as water, that may be added to food to increase its weight.

**food exchange list.** See **Exchange Lists for Meal Planning.**

**food poisoning,** any of a large group of toxic processes that result from the ingestion of a food contaminated by toxic substances or by bacteria that contain toxins. Kinds of food poisoning include **salmonella food poisoning, ciguatera poisoning, Minamata disease, mushroom poisoning,** and **shellfish poisoning.** See also **botulism, ergot alkaloid, phalloidine, toadstool poisoning.**

**food pyramid,** a diagrammatic proportional representation of human nutritional needs devised in 1992 by the U.S. Department of Agriculture to replace the "four food groups" pie chart used since the 1950s. The USDA "Food Guide Pyramid" features a relatively wide base of 6 to 11 servings

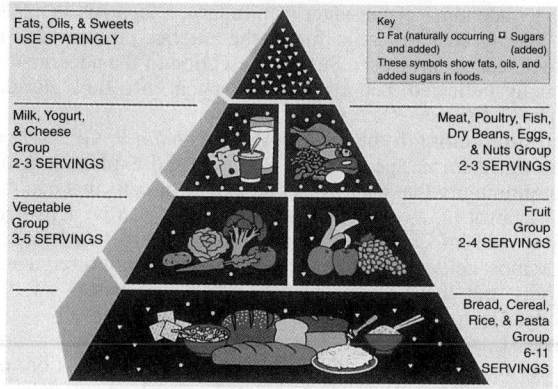

**Food guide pyramid**
*(US Department of Agriculture: USDA Human Nutrition Information, Pub No 249, Washington DC, 1992, US Government Printing Office)*

daily of grains and cereals beneath a layer representing 5 to 9 servings daily of fruits and vegetables. A third tapering level represents 2 to 3 daily servings of meats and 2 to 3 of dairy products. At the peak of the pyramid are fats and sweets, to be eaten sparingly. Other countries use similar diagrammatic depictions to guide the public, for example Canada uses the Rainbow for this purpose.

**food sensitivity/hypersensitivity reaction,** sensitivity to food items that may or may not be protein-aceous in nature. See **food allergy.**

**food service administrator,** a member of a hospital staff who is responsible for the planning and management of the food service system of the facility.

**food service department,** the section of a hospital or similar health facility that is responsible for food preparation and services to patients and personnel. It also provides nutritional care to patients.

**foot** [AS, *fot*], the distal extremity of the leg, consisting of the tarsus, the metatarsus, and the phalanges.

**foot-and-mouth disease,** an acute extremely contagious rhabdovirus, specifically vesicular stomatitis virus, infection of cloven-hooved animals. It is characterized by the development of ulcers on the skin around the mouth, on the mucous membrane in the mouth, and on the udders. Horses are immune. The virus is transmitted to humans by direct contact with infected animals or their secretions or with contaminated milk, although this is uncommon. Symptoms and signs in humans include headache, fever, malaise, and vesicles on the tongue, oral mucous membranes, hands, and feet. Generalized pruritus and painful ulcerations may occur; however, the temperature soon falls, the lesions subside in about a week, and total healing without scars is complete by 2 or 3 weeks. Treatment is symptomatic. Also called **aphthous fever.** See also **picornavirus.**

**footboard,** a board or open box placed at the end of a patient's bed and at a level above the top of the mattress to prevent the weight of the top sheet and blankets from resting on the feet. It is situated so that the soles of the feet are positioned firmly against the board with the legs at right angles to it. Its purposes are to help the bedridden patient retain normal posture and prevent footdrop.

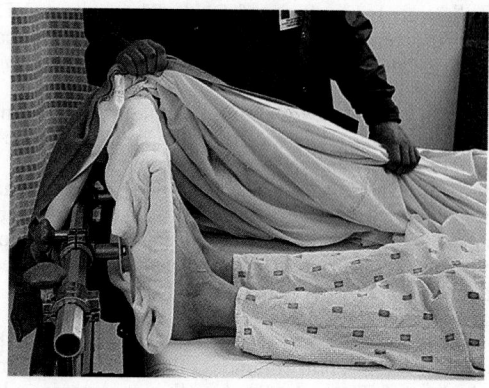

**Footboard** *(Sorrentino, 1996)*

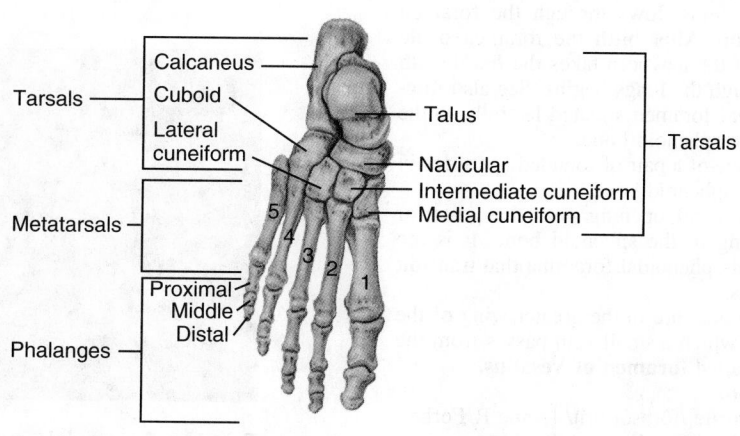

**Bones of the foot** *(Applegate, 2000)*

**foot-candle** /foot'kan·dəl/ [AS, *fot;* L, *candela,* light], a unit of illumination being 1 lumen per square foot or equivalent to 1.0764 milliphots (see **phot**). Compare **lux.**

**foot care,** a nursing intervention from the Nursing Interventions Classification (NIC) defined as cleansing and inspecting the feet for the purposes of relaxation, cleanliness, and healthy skin. See also **Nursing Interventions Classification.**

**footdrop** /foot'drop/ [AS, *fot + dropa*], an abnormal neuromuscular condition of the lower leg and foot, characterized by an inability to dorsiflex, or evert, the foot caused by damage to the common peroneal nerve.

**-footed,** combining form meaning 'having feet' of a specified sort or number: *clubfooted, flatfooted, four-footed.*

**footling breech** [AS, *fot + ME, brech*], an intrauterine position of the fetus in which one or both feet are folded under the buttocks at the inlet of the maternal pelvis; one foot presents in a single footling breech, both in a double footling breech. Compare **frank breech.** See also **breech birth.**

**foot-pound,** a unit for the measurement of work or energy. One foot-pound is the amount of work required to move 1 pound a distance of 1 foot in the same direction as that of the applied force.

**footprinting,** a method for determining the location of binding between a protein and a DNA molecule. The technique involves nuclease digestion of the unbound and therefore unprotected sequences of DNA. The protected DNA fragment that remains can be identified electrophoretically.

**for-,** prefix meaning 'an opening': *foramen, foramina, foration.*

**foramen** /fôrā'mən/, *pl.* **foramina** [L, hole], an opening or aperture in a membranous structure or bone, such as the apical dental foramen and the carotid foramen.

**foramen diaphragmatis.** See **pacchionian foramen.**

**foramen magnum,** a passage in the occipital bone through which the spinal cord enters the spinal column.

**foramen of Monro** /monrō'/, a passage between the lateral and third ventricles of the brain.

**foramen of Vesalius.** See **foramen venosum.**

**foramenotomy,** surgical removal of small pieces of bone around an intervertebral foramen, allowing more room for the spinal nerve. The procedure usually accompanies a laminectomy.

**foramen ovale** /ōvā'lē, ōvä'lā/, **1.** an opening in the septum between the right and the left atria in the fetal heart. This opening provides a bypass for blood that would otherwise flow to the fetal lungs. Most of the blood from the inferior vena cava in the fetus flows through the foramen ovale into the left atrium. After birth the foramen ovale functionally closes when the newborn takes the first breath and full circulation through the lungs begins. See also **ductus arteriosus. 2.** an oval foramen situated laterally to the foramen rotundum of the sphenoid bone.

**foramen rotundum,** one of a pair of rounded apertures in the greater wings of the sphenoid bone.

**foramen spinosum,** a small opening near the posterior angle of the greater wing of the sphenoid bone. It is the smallest of three pairs of sphenoidal foramina that transmit nerves and blood vessels.

**foramen venosum,** an aperture in the greater wing of the sphenoid bone, through which a small vein passes from the cavernous sinus. Also called **foramen of Vesalius.**

**foramina.** See **foramen.**

**Forbes-Albright syndrome** /fôrbsôl'brīt/ [Anne P. Forbes, American physician, 1911–1992; Fuller Albright, American physician, 1900–1969], an endocrine disease characterized by amenorrhea, prolactinemia, and galactorrhea, caused by an adenoma of the anterior pituitary. Diagnosis is made by radiographic examination of the anterior pituitary and a blood test for prolactin. Surgical resection of the adenoma is usually indicated. See also **galactorrhea, pituitary gland.**

**Forbes' disease.** See **Cori's disease.**

**forbidden clone hypothesis** [AS, *forbeodan* + Gk, *klon,* a cutting, *theoria,* speculation], a proposed explanation for autoimmunity that postulates that clones of cells that can react against the body persist after birth and can be activated by a viral infection or by some metabolic change. It holds that most cells of the immune system attack only foreign antigens, but these clones of cells attack the tissues of the body. Compare **sequestered antigens hypothesis.**

**force** [L, *fortis,* strong], **1.** energy applied so that it initiates motion, changes the speed or direction of motion, or alters the size or shape of an object. **2.** a push or pull defined as mass times acceleration. If the force on an object produces movement, it is called dynamic; if the force does not produce movement, it is called static.

**forced expiratory flow (FEF),** the average volumetric flow rate during any stated volume interval while a forced expired vital capacity test is performed. It is usually expressed as a percentage of vital capacity.

**forced expiratory time (FET),** the time required to exhale a given volume of air.

**forced expiratory volume (FEV),** the volume of air that can be forcibly expelled in a fixed period after full inspiration. Compare **vital capacity.** See also **expiratory reserve volume.**

**forced expired vital capacity (FEVC),** the maximum volume of gas that can be forcibly and rapidly exhaled after a full inspiration. Also called **forced vital capacity, timed vital capacity.**

**forced-inhalation abdominal breathing,** a respiratory therapy technique in which the patient inhales through the nose with an effort forceful enough to lift small sandbag weights placed on the abdomen. The technique is said to resemble closely the abdominal effort involved in normal breathing.

**forced vital capacity.** See **forced expired vital capacity.**

**forceps,** *pl.* **forceps** [L, pair of tongs], a pair of any of a large variety and number of surgical instruments, all of which have two handles or sides, each attached to a dull blade. The handles may be joined at one end, such as a pair of tweezers, or the two sides may be separate to be drawn together in use, such as obstetric forceps. Forceps are used

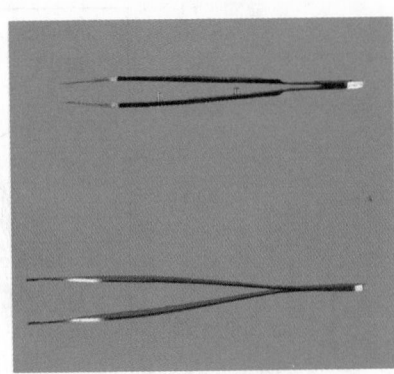

**Forceps: Castroviejo suturing (top) and Brown Adson tissue (bottom)**
*(Tighe, 1999)*

to grasp, handle, compress, pull, or join tissue, equipment, or supplies. See specific forceps.

**forceps delivery,** an obstetric operation in which instruments are used to deliver a baby. It is performed to overcome dystocia, to quickly deliver a baby experiencing fetal distress, or, most often, to shorten normal labor. Local or regional anesthesia is usual, as is episiotomy. Prerequisites to forceps delivery include full dilation of the cervix, engagement of the fetal head, certain knowledge of the position of the head, and ruptured membranes. The blades of the forceps are introduced into the vagina one at a time and applied symmetrically to opposite sides of the baby's head; the handles of the forceps are pulled together so that the head is held firmly between the blades; the head is rotated, if necessary, to the occiput anterior or occiput posterior position; and traction is applied so as to draw the head from the birth passage. When the head has been delivered, the forceps are removed and the delivery is completed manually. Because cesarean section is performed more often now than formerly, traumatic forceps deliveries are uncommon. Kinds of forceps delivery are **high forceps, low forceps,** and **midforceps.** Compare **forceps rotation, trial forceps.** See also **obstetric forceps.**

**forceps rotation,** an obstetric operation in which forceps are used to turn a baby's head that is arrested in transverse or posterior position in the birth canal. It may be performed to facilitate spontaneous birth or to initiate a forceps delivery. Kinds of forceps rotation are **Kielland's rotation** and **Scanzoni's rotation.** Compare **forceps delivery, manual rotation.** See also **obstetric forceps.**

**forceps tenaculum.** See **tenaculum.**

**forcible inspiration** [L, *fortis,* strong, *inspirare*], breathing that is assisted by a mechanical ventilator that forces air into the lungs during inhalation but allows the patient to exhale passively.

**Fordyce-Fox disease** /fôr′disfoks′/ [G. H. Fox, American dermatologist, 1846–1937; John A. Fordyce, American dermatologist, 1858–1925], an apocrine gland disorder that produces symptoms similar to those of miliaria. It is characterized by intensely itchy follicular papules in the axillae, umbilicus, areolae of the breast, and pubic area.

**Fordyce's disease** [John A. Fordyce], the presence of enlarged oil glands in the mucosal membranes of the lips, cheeks, gums, and genitalia. It is a common condition and may be symptomless. The ectopic sebaceous glands of the buccal mucosa appear as tiny, whitish yellow raised lesions (Fordyce spots).

**fore-,** prefix meaning 'front or before': *forearm, foregut, forewaters.*

**forearm,** the portion of the upper extremity between the elbow and the wrist. It contains two long bones, the radius and ulna.

**forebrain.** See **prosencephalon.**

**forefinger,** the first, or index, finger.

**forefoot,** the portion of the foot that includes the metatarsus and toes.

**foregut** /fôr′gut/ [AS, *fore,* in front, *guttas*], the cephalic portion of the embryonic alimentary canal. It consists of endodermal tissue and gives rise to the pharynx, esophagus, stomach, liver, pancreas, most of the small intestine, and respiratory ducts. Compare **hindgut, midgut.**

**forehead** /fÔr′hed/ [AS, *fore,* in front + *heafod,* head], the region of the face superior to the eyes.

**foreign body** /fôr′in/ [Fr, *forain,* alien; AS, *bodig*], any object or substance found in an organ or tissue in which it does not belong under normal circumstances, such as a bolus of food in the trachea or a particle of dust in the eye.

**foreign body granuloma** [OFr, *forain* + AS, *bodig* + L, *granulum,* little grain; Gk, *oma,* tumor], a chronic inflammatory mass of tissue that accumulates around foreign bodies such as gravel, splinters, or bits of sutures.

**foreign body in airway,** anything found in the airway that is not normally present. Examples include food, coins, small pieces of toys, and bones. It is crucial to determine the extent of airway obstruction. The patient may be asymptomatic or may exhibit dyspnea or changes in breathing pattern or color (cyanosis). Removal of the foreign body is generally performed with a fiberoptic laryngoscope and forceps or via bronchoscopy.

**foreign body in ear** [OFr, *forain* + AS, *bodig* + *eare*], any object found in the ear canal that is not normally part of it, such as a bean, insect, or pebble.

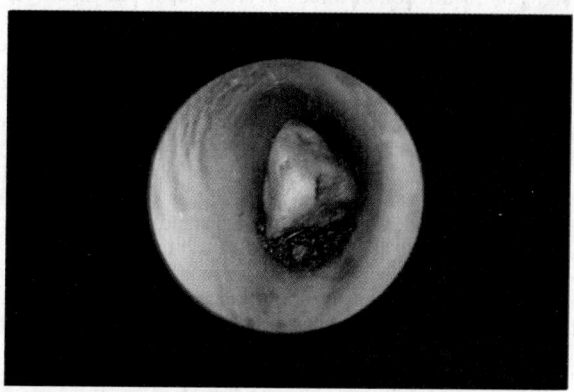

**Foreign body in the ear**
(Bingham, Hawke, and Kwok, 1992/courtesy Dr. Lalitha Shaker, St. Joseph's Health Centre, Toronto)

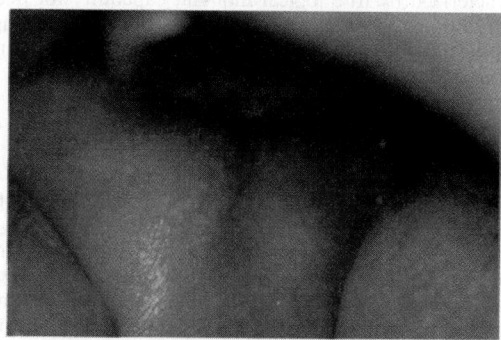

**Fordyce spots** (Lemmi and Lemmi, 2000)

**foreign body in esophagus** [OFr, *forain* + AS, *bodig* + Gk, *oisophagos,* gullet], anything found in the esophagus that is not normally a part of the tissue.

**foreign body in eye** [OFr, *forain* + AS, *bodig* + *eage*], anything found in the eye that is not a normal part of the tissue. Foreign bodies may be superficially embedded in the tissue surfaces or may penetrate the globe.

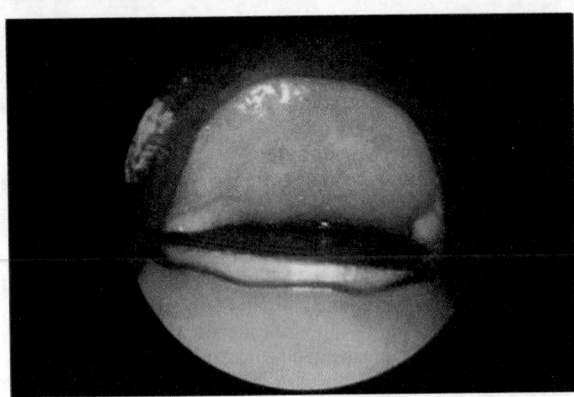

**Foreign body in the esophagus**
*(Bingham, Hawke, and Kwok, 1992/courtesy Dr. Bruce Benjamin)*

**foreign body in throat** [OFr, *forain* + AS, *bodig* + *throte*], anything found in the throat that is not normally present. A common foreign body in the throat is a posteriorly displaced tongue.

**foreign body obstruction,** a disturbance in normal function or a pathologic condition caused by an object lodged in a body orifice, passage, or organ. Most cases occur in children who suddenly inhale or swallow a foreign object or insert it into a body opening. Large boluses of hastily eaten food frequently lodge in the esophagus, causing coughing, choking, and, if the airway is obstructed, asphyxia. Forceful blows to the victim's back between the shoulder blades or the Heimlich maneuver may dislodge the bolus. Esophageal foreign bodies usually produce an immediate reaction but occasionally result in a long asymptomatic period before signs of obstruction or infection are evident. Laryngeal foreign bodies usually cause hoarseness, wheezing, and dyspnea; a sharp object, such as a chicken bone, may perforate the larynx and cause swelling and infection. A foreign body in the trachea may cause wheezing, an audible slap, coughing, and dyspnea; a small object may become lodged in a bronchus, producing coughing, which is often followed by an asymptomatic period before signs of obstruction and inflammation appear. Needles and hairpins ingested by children often pass through the esophagus and stomach without incident but may become lodged at the turn of the duodenum and require removal by a magnetized nasogastric tube or by laparotomy; laxatives are contraindicated, and if tenderness, rigidity, pain, nausea, or vomiting ensues, immediate surgery is necessary. Coins, marbles, and closed safety pins usually pass through the digestive tract without creating problems; but hairballs, vegetable fibers, or shellac concretions sometimes found in the stomach of emotionally disturbed or retarded patients may cause anorexia, nausea, and vomiting. Hairballs may be fragmented by an endoscope and removed by lavage; surgery may be required.

**foreign medical graduate (FMG),** a physician trained in and graduated from a medical school outside the United States and Canada. U.S. citizens graduated from medical schools outside the United States and Canada are also classified as FMGs.

**forensic** /fōren′sik/ [L, *forum*, public place], pertaining to courts of law.

**forensic dentistry,** the branch of dentistry that deals with the legal aspects of professional dental practices and treatment, with particular emphasis on the use of dental records to identify victims of crimes or accidents.

**forensic medicine** [L *forum*, public place, *medicinus*, physician], a branch of medicine that deals with the legal aspects of health care.

**forensic psychiatry** [L, *forum*, public place; Gk, *psyche*, mind, *iatreia*, treament], a branch of psychiatry concerned with the application of psychiatry to law, including criminal responsibility, guardianship, and competence to stand trial.

**foreplay** /fôr′plā/, sexual activities, such as kissing and fondling, that precede coitus.

**foreshortened image.** See **image foreshortening.**

**foreskin** /for′skin/ [AS, *fore* + *skinn*], a loose fold of skin that covers the end of the penis or clitoris. Its removal constitutes circumcision. Also called **prepuce.**

**Forestier's disease** /fō′res·tē·āz′/ [Jacques Forestier, French neurologist, 20th century], hyperostosis of the anterolateral part of the vertebral column, especially in the thoracic region.

**forest yaws** /for′ist/ [L, *foris*, outside; Afr, *yaw*, strawberry], a cutaneous form of American leishmaniasis, common in South and Central America, caused by *Leishmania guyanensis.* The disease is chronic, with multiple deep skin ulcers that occasionally spread to the nasal mucosa. Also called **pian bois.**

**forewaters** /fôr′wôtərs/ [AS, *fore* + *waeter*], the part of the amniotic sac that pouches into the cervix in front of the presenting part of the fetus. It is sometimes called the forebag.

**forgiveness facilitation,** a nursing intervention from the Nursing Interventions Classification (NIC) defined as assisting an individual to forgive and/or experience forgiveness in relationship with self, others, and higher power. See also **Nursing Interventions Classification.**

**fork** /fôrk/ [L, *furca*], **1.** an instrument with prongs. **2.** something resembling such an instrument.

**forked tongue** /fôrkt/ [L, *furca* + AS, *tunge*], a tongue divided by a longitudinal fissure. Also called **bifid tongue, slit tongue.**

**-form, -forme,** suffix meaning 'having a (specified) shape or form': *linguiform, toruliform.*

**formaldehyde (HCHO)** /fərmal′dəhīd/, a toxic, colorless foul-smelling gas that is soluble in water and used in that form as a disinfectant, fixative, or preservative. Also called **methanal.**

**formalin** /fôr′məlin/, a clear solution of formaldehyde in water. A 37% solution is used for fixing and preserving biologic specimens for pathologic and histologic examination.

**formal operations,** a form of thinking following the stage of concrete operations and representing the final, most mature state of thinking; it usually occurs after age 11 and is characterized by true logical thought, capability for deductive reasoning, abstract thinking, formulation and testing of hypotheses, appreciation for multiple perspectives on an issue, and the manipulation of ideas and concepts.

**format** /fôr′mət/, a computer arrangement of data for storage or display. It may involve dividing the space on a disk into marked sectors for storage.

**formation** /fôrmā′shən/, **1.** a cluster of people who occupy and therefore define a quantum of space. **2.** a structure, shape, or figure.

**formative evaluation** /fôr′mətiv/, **1.** judgments made about effectiveness of nursing interventions as they are implemented. **2.** (in nursing education) periodic evaluation of a student during a course, usually a clinical practicum.

**formboard,** equipment used in tactile performance testing. It consists of a board with cutouts of various shapes and sizes and blocks of corresponding geometric characteristics. Subjects are tested on their ability to fit the blocks into the proper cutout spaces.

**forme fruste** /fôrm′ frYst′, fôrm′ fro͞ost′/, *pl.* **formes frustes** [Fr, rough form],    **1.** an incomplete or atypical form of a disease or a disease that is spontaneously arrested before it has run its usual course. **2.** (in genetics) an inherited disorder in which there is minimal expression of an abnormal trait.

**formic acid (HCOOH)** /fôr′mik/,    a colorless pungent liquid found in nature in nettles, in ants, and in other insects. It is prepared commercially from oxalic acid and glycerin and from the oxidation of formaldehyde. Formerly used as a vesicant, it currently has no therapeutic applications. Also called **methanoic acid.**

**formiminoglutamic acid (FIGLU)** /fôrmim′ino͞oglo͞otam′ik/,    a compound formed in the metabolism of histidine, present in urine in elevated levels in folic acid deficiency. Increased excretion of FIGLU may indicate folic acid deficiency.

**-formin,**    combining form for phenformin-type oral hypoglycemics.

**formol.**    See **formaldehyde.**

**formula** /fôr′m(y)ələ/ [L, *forma,* pattern],    a simplified statement, generally using numerals and other symbols, expressing the constituents of a chemical compound, a method for preparing a substance, or a procedure for achieving a desired value or result. —**formulaic,** *adj.*

**formulary** /fôr′myəle′rē/ [L, *forma,* pattern],    a listing of drugs intended to include a large enough range of medications and sufficient information about them to enable health practitioners to prescribe treatment that is medically appropriate. Hospitals maintain formularies that list all drugs commonly stocked in their pharmacy. Third-party organizations such as insurance companies usually maintain formularies that list drugs for which the company will cover under plan benefts. See also **compendium,** *United States Pharmacopeia.*

**formulation** /fôr′myəlā′shən/ [L, *forma,* pattern],    **1.** a pharmacologic substance prepared according to a formula. **2.** a systematic and precise statement of a problem, a theory, or a method of analysis in research.

**formylmethionine (FMET)** /fôr′milməthī′ənēn/,    (in molecular genetics) the first amino acid in a protein sequence.

**fornication** /fôr′nikā′shən/ [L, *fornix,* arch],    (in law) sexual intercourse between two people who are not married to each other. The specific legal definition varies from jurisdiction to jurisdiction. In some, both persons are unmarried; in some, one is unmarried; in some, the charge is adultery rather than fornication if the woman is married, regardless of the man's marital status.

**fornix** /fôr′niks/, *pl.* **fornices** /fôr′nisēz/ [L, arch],    an archlike structure or space, such as the fornix cerebri, the superior or inferior conjunctival fornices, or the vaginal fornices.

**fornix cerebri** /ser′əbrī/,    an archlike body of nerve fibers that lies beneath the corpus callosum of the cranium and serves as the efferent pathway from the hippocampus.

**fornix vaginae.**    See **vaginal fornix.**

**forskolin (FSK),**    an activator of adenylate cyclase. FSK interacts directly with ion channels, increasing glutamate responses and amplitude and decay time of spontaneous excitatory postsynaptic currents.

**Fortaz,**    trademark for a cephalosporin antibiotic (ceftazidime).

**Fort Bragg fever.**    See **pretibial fever.**

**fortified milk** [L, *fortis,* strong; AS, *milc*],    pasturized milk enriched with one or more nutrients, usually vitamins A and D, that has been standardized at 400 International Units per quart (fortified vitamin D milk).

**forward chaining,**    a method of measuring rehabilitation performance: The patient performs the first step independently and the therapist helps the patient perform the rest of the steps. The routine is then repeated with the patient performing the first two steps independently, then the first three steps, and so on.

**forward-leaning posture,**    a respiratory therapy technique intended to reduce or eliminate the involvement of the accessory muscles of respiration in ambulatory patients with breathing difficulty. It involves walking while bent forward in a slightly stooped posture. For patients unable to tolerate functional walking, a special high walker with wheels may be used.

**Foscavir,**    trademark for an antiviral drug used in the treatment of cytomegalovirus retinitis.

**fosfomycin,**    a urinary antiinfective.
- INDICATIONS: This drug is used to treat infections of the urinary tract caused by *Enterococcus faecalis* and *Escherichia coli.*
- CONTRAINDICATIONS: Known hypersensitivity to this drug prohibits its use.
- ADVERSE EFFECTS: Adverse effects of this drug include vaginitis, dysuria, hematuria, menstrual disorder, fever, insomnia, somnolence, migraine, asthenia, nervousness, constipation, dry mouth, flatulence, increased SGPT, dyspepsia, and pruritus. Common side effects are headache, dizziness, nausea, vomiting, anorexia, diarrhea, and rash.

**fosinopril,**    an angiotensin-converting enzyme inhibitor.
- INDICATIONS: It is prescribed in the treatment of high blood pressure. It acts by blocking enzymes involved in body chemisty that results in constriction of blood vessels, increasing blood pressure and causing sodium and fluids to be retained.
- CONTRAINDICATIONS: The drug should not be given to patients with allergy to angiotensin-converting enzyme inhibitors. It should be used with caution in patients with kidney diseases or diabetes or with potassium-containing products.
- ADVERSE EFFECTS: The side effects most often reported include "first-dose effect," including dizziness and fainting caused by lowered blood pressure, persistent dry nonproductive cough, depression, headache, palpitations, breathing difficulty, and fluid retention.

**fosphenytoin,**    an anticonvulsant.
- INDICATIONS: This drug is used to treat generalized tonic-clonic seizures and status epilepticus.
- CONTRAINDICATIONS: Factors that prohibit the use of fosphenytoin include known hypersensitivity to this drug, psychiatric conditions, pregnancy, bradycardia, SA and AV block, and Stokes-Adams syndrome.
- ADVERSE EFFECTS: Life-threatening effects of this drug are ventricular fibrillation, nephritis, agranulocytosis, leukopenia, aplastic anemia, thrombocytopenia, megaloblastic anemia, and Stevens-Johnson syndrome. Other adverse effects include drowsiness, dizziness, insomnia, paresthesias, depression, suicidal tendencies, aggression, headache, confusion, hypotension, nystagmus, diplopia, blurred vision, nausea, vomiting, constipation, anorexia, weight loss, hepatitis, jaundice, gingival hyperplasia, urine discoloration, rash, lupus erythematosus, hirsutism, and hypocalcemia.

**fossa** /fos′ə/, *pl.* **fossae** [L, ditch],    a hollow or depression, especially on the surface of the end of a bone, such as the olecranon fossa or the coronoid fossa.

**Foster bed,**    trademark for a special bed used in the care and treatment of severely injured patients, especially those with spinal injuries. It consists of two Bradford frames mounted on a castered base. The assembly is attached to a rotary bearing mechanism, permitting horizontal turning of the patient without moving the spine. The patient can be rotated to supine and prone positions while maintaining proper immobilization and alignment of injured body structures. A horizontal turning frame permits hyperextension and traction at each end of the frame, and either end of the bed can be elevated to provide countertraction. It can be used in posttraumatic management of patients with spinal instability, with or without cord damage, and in the management of the postoperative patient with multilevel spinal fusion when weight-bearing or ambulation is contraindicated. The Foster bed is also used for halo-femoral traction and maintenance of continuous cervical traction in flexion for patients with unstable cervical neck problems. Compare **CircOlectric (COL) bed, hyperextension bed, Stryker wedge frame.** See also **Bradford frame.**

**Foster Kennedy syndrome** /fos'tər ken'ə·dē/ [Robert Foster Kennedy, American neurologist, 1884−1952], retrobulbar neuritis, central scotoma, optic atrophy on the side of the lesion and papilledema on the opposite side, occurring in tumors of the frontal lobe of the brain which press downward.

**fo-ti,** a climbing perennial herb found in China.
- ■ USES: This herb is used for tiredness, constipation, and elevated cholesterol.
- ■ CONTRAINDICATIONS: Fo-ti is contraindicated during pregnancy and lactation, in children, in those with known hypersensitivity to this product, or diarrhea.

**foulage.** See **pétrissage.**

**foundation** [L, *fundamentum*], (in dentistry) any device or material added to a remaining tooth structure to enhance the stability and retention of an overlying cast restoration, such as a pin retainer, amalgam, or casting.

**foundation model,** a health maintenance organization or other health system that is legally established as a tax-exempt, not-for-profit corporation organized to operate as a charitable institution.

**fourchette** /fōōrshet'/ [Fr, fork], a tense band of mucous membranes at the posterior angle of the vagina that connects the posterior ends of the labia minora.

**four-handed dentistry,** a technique in which a dental assistant or dental hygienist works directly with the dentist on the procedures being done in the mouth of a patient. The technique reduces fatigue and improves the effectiveness of dental procedures.

**Fourier transform (FT)** /fōōryā'/ [Jean B.J. Fourier, French mathematician, 1768–1830; L, *transformare,* to change form], a mathematical procedure that separates out the frequency components of a signal from its amplitudes as a function of time, or vice versa.

**Fourier transform imaging,** [Jean B.J. Fourier], (in medical physics) nuclear magnetic resonance (NMR) imaging techniques in which at least one dimension is phase encoded by applying variable gradient pulses along that dimension before "reading out" the NMR signal with a gradient magnetic field perpendicular to the variable gradient. The Fourier transform is then used to reconstruct an image from the set of encoded NMR signals.

**Fournier's gangrene** /fōōrnyāz'/ [Jean A. Fournier, French syphilographer. 1832–1914], an infective gangrene of the scrotum or vulva caused by an anaerobic hemolytic strain of streptococcus.

**four-poster orthosis,** an orthosis to immobilize the cervical vertebrae. It contains four vertical posts or poles on the anterior and posterior lateral sides of the head and is placed

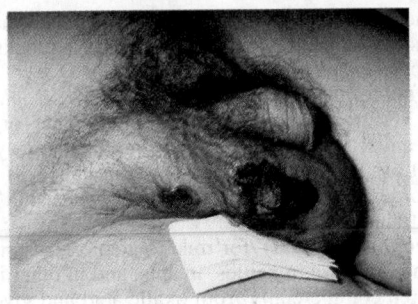

**Fournier's gangrene**
*(Stone and Gorbach, 2000/courtesy Dr. Mark Drapkin, Newton Wellesley Hospital, Newton, Massachusetts)*

over the shoulders. The head is supported under the chin and occiput, and the posts prevent movement.

**four-tailed bandage,** a narrow piece of cloth with two ties on each end for wrapping a joint, such as an elbow or knee, or a prominence, such as the nose or chin.

**fourth cranial nerve.** See **trochlear nerve.**

**fourth-generation scanner,** a computed tomography machine in which the x-ray source rotates but the detector assembly does not. Radiation detection is accomplished through a fixed, circular array of up to 1000 detectors. Fourth generation scanners may have scanning times as short as 1 second.

**fourth stage of labor** [ME, *feower,* four; OFr, *estage* + L, *labor,* work], a postpartum period of about 4 hours after the third stage, or delivery of the placenta. Some complications, especially hemorrhage, occur at this time, necessitating careful observation of the mother.

**fourth ventricle** [ME, *feower,* four; L, *ventriculus,* little belly], a cavity with a diamond-shaped floor in the hindbrain, communicating below with the central canal of the spinal cord and above with the cerebral aqueduct of the midbrain. At the bottom of the ventricle are surfaces of the pons and medulla.

**fovea capitis** /fō'vē·ə/ [L, *fovea,* pit], 1. a depression on the proximal surface of the head of the radius where it meets the capitulum of the humerus. 2. a fovea on the head of the femur, where the ligamentum teres is attached.

**fovea centralis,** an area at the center of the retina where cone cells are concentrated and there are no rod cells. See also **macula lutea.**

**Fowler's position** /fou'lərz/ [George R. Fowler, American surgeon, 1848–1906], the posture assumed by the patient when the head of the bed is raised 45 to 60 degrees and his

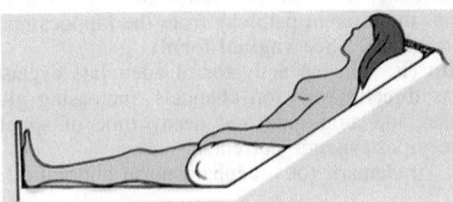

**Fowler's position** *(Potter and Perry, 2001)*

or her knees are elevated slightly. See also **high-Fowler's position.**

**Fox-Fordyce disease** /foks fôr′dīs/ [G. H. Fox, American dermatologist,1846−1937; John Addison Fordyce, American dermatologist, 1858−1925], a chronic skin disease, usually seen in women, characterized by small papular eruptions and other skin changes of apocrine gland−bearing areas, especially the axillae and pubes; the cause is obstruction and rupture of the intraepidermal part of the ducts of the glands. Also called **apocrine miliaria.**

**foxglove** /foks′glov/, the common name for *Digitalis purpura,* the plant that is a source of digitalis.

**Fox's knife.** See **Goldman-Fox knife.**

**Fr,** symbol for the element **francium.**

**fract-,** combining form meaning 'a breaking': *fractional, fractography, fracture.*

**fractional dilation and curettage** /frak′shənəl/, a diagnostic technique in which each section of the uterus is examined and curetted to obtain specimens of the endometrium from all parts of the organ. It is often performed under regional anesthesia in the diagnosis of endometrial cancer.

**fractionation** /frak′shənā′shən/ [L, *frangere,* to break], **1.** (in neurology) a mechanism within the neural arch of the vertebrae whereby only a portion of the efferent nerves innervating a muscle reacts to a stimulus, even when the reflex requirement is maximal, so that a reserve of neurons remains to respond to additional stimuli. Through this phenomenon muscle tension is maintained. **2.** (in chemistry) the separation of a substance into its basic constituents, by using such procedures as fractional distillation or crystallization. **3.** (in bacteriology) the process of isolating a pure culture by successive culturing of a small portion of a colony of bacteria. **4.** (in histology) the process of isolating the different components of living cells by centrifugation. **5.** (in radiology) the process of administering a dose of radiation in smaller units over time to minimize tissue damage rather than in a single large dose. Also called **dose fractionation, fractionation radiation.**

**fractionation radiation.** See **fractionation, def. 5.**

**fraction of inspired oxygen (FiO₂)** [L, *frangere,* to break, *inspirare,* to breathe in; Gk, *oxys,* sharp, *genein,* to produce], the proportion of oxygen in the air that is inspired.

**fracture** /frak′chər/ [L, *frangere,* to break], a traumatic injury to a bone in which the continuity of the bone tissue is broken. A fracture is classified by the bone involved, the part of that bone, and the nature of the break, such as a comminuted fracture of the head of the tibia. See also specific types of fractures.

**fracture-dislocation,** a break in the bony structures of any joint, with associated dislocation of the same joint.

**fracture of clavicle** [L, *frangere + clavicula,* little key], a break in the long bone of the shoulder girdle. It is typically accompanied by pain, swelling, and a protuberance and depression over the site of the injury. The patient usually supports the arm on the injured side at the elbow. Treatment generally involves application of a clavicle strap or a figure-eight bandage.

**fracture of olecranon** [L, *frangere + Gk, olekranon,* point of the elbow], a break in the bony prominence of the ulna at the elbow joint. Different types of olecranon fractures may occur, depending on the articular surfaces involved. The triceps, which normally extends the elbow, may become spastic as a result of the injury.

**fracture of patella** [L, *frangere + patella,* small pan], a break in the sesamoid knee cap. The fracture often occurs in automobile accidents in which the knee strikes the dash-

board. The damage is complicated by reflex bracing of the quadriceps femoris muscle, which pulls the fragments apart. Treatment includes suturing the bone fragments and confining the patient in a long-leg cast.

**fracture of radius** [L, *frangere + ray],* a break in and dislocation of the lower end of the radius, usually with backward and radial displacement of the wrist and hand. The fracture commonly occurs when a falling person extends the arm and hand in an effort to cushion the impact. See also **Colles' fracture.**

**fracture of skull** [L, *frangere +* AS, *skulle,* bowl], a break in one or more of the cranial bones. A fracture in the vault of the skull is usually a compound fracture and is complicated by possible damage to brain tissue, particularly if shards of bone are driven into the brain by the force of the trauma.

**fracture threshold,** a measure of bone density used in predicting osteoporosis risk factors. Various investigators have established different methods of interpreting bone density data. One method predicts that 95% of women will have vertebral fractures if their trabecular bone volume is less than 14% of the mean.

**fragile X syndrome** /fraj′əl/, a reproductive disorder characterized by a nearly broken X chromosome, which has a tip hanging by a flimsy thread. It is the most common inherited cause of mental retardation. Only about 75% of the results of tests for the broken chromosome are accurate. Some healthy individuals may possess fragile X chromosomes without exhibiting symptoms and may transmit the condition to children or grandchildren.

**fragilitas ossium.** See **osteogenesis imperfecta.**

**fragment** /frag′mənt/ [L, *frangere,* to break], one of the small pieces into which a larger entity has been broken.

**fragmented fracture.** See **comminuted fracture.**

**Fragmin,** trademark for a low-molecular-weight heparin (dalteparin sodium).

**frail elder,** an older person (usually above 85 years of age) who has multiple physical or mental disabilities that may interfere with the ability to perform activities of daily living independently.

**fraise** /frāz/ [Fr, strawberry], a smooth hemispheric or conic burr with cutting edges. It is used for enlarging trephine openings or cutting osteopathic flaps.

**frambesia, framboesia.** See **yaws.**

**frame** /frām /, a structure, usually rigid, designed for giving support to or for immobilizing a part.

**frame of reference** [AS, *framian,* to help; L, *referre,* to carry back], the personal guidelines of an individual, taken as a whole. An individual frame of reference reflects the person's social status, cultural norms, and concepts.

**Franceschetti's syndrome** /fran′chesket′ēz/ [Adolphe Franceschetti, Swiss ophthalmologist, 1896–1968], a complete form of mandibulofacial dysostosis. See also **Treacher Collins' syndrome.**

**franchise dentistry** /fran′chīz/ [Fr, exemption; L, *dens,* tooth], the practice of dentistry under a trade name purchased from another dentist or dental practice. Under a franchise license agreement, the franchiser may use the trade name, associated marketing products, and treatment techniques for a sum of money, in accordance with the franchise rules and regulations.

*Francisella,* a genus of nonmotile nonspore-forming pathogenic aerobic bacteria. The organisms cause tularemia in humans.

**francium (Fr)** /fran′sē·əm/ [France], a metallic element of the alkali metal group. Its atomic number is 87; its atomic

## Types and causes of fractures

| Type | Description | Cause |
|------|-------------|-------|
| Avulsed | Fracture that pulls bone and other tissues from usual attachments | Direct energy or force, with resisted extension of bone and joint |
| Bucket-handle | Double vertical fractures of pelvis on same side, resulting in pelvic dislocation | Direct blow or anterior compression force, with or without sacral torsion |
| Butterfly | Butterfly-shaped piece of fractured bone, usually accompanying comminuted fracture | Direct, indirect, or rotational force to bone |
| Comminuted | Fracture with more than two pieces; may have significant associated soft tissue trauma | Direct crushing injury or force to tissues and bone |
| Compound (open) | Skin broken over fracture; possible soft tissue trauma | Moderate to severe energy that is continuous and exceeds tissue tolerances |
| Compression | Fraction is squeezed or wedged together at one side | Compressive, axial energy or force applied directly from above fracture site |
| Displaced | Fracture with one, both, or all fragments out of normal alignment | Direct energy or force to site |
| Greenstick | Break in only one cortex of bone | Minor direct or indirect energy |
| Impacted | Fracture with one end wedged into opposite end or inside fractured fragment | Compressive axial energy or force directly to distal fragment |

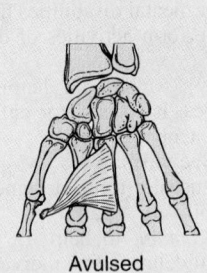

Avulsed

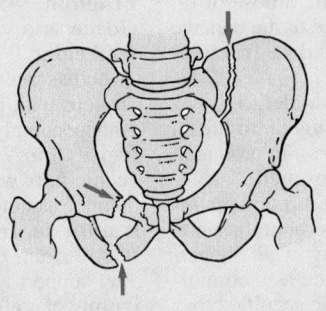

Bucket-handle

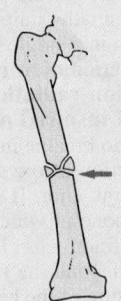

Butterfly

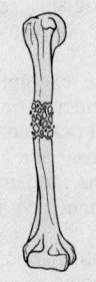

Comminuted

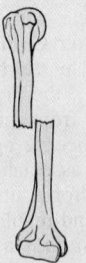

Displaced

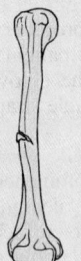

Greenstick

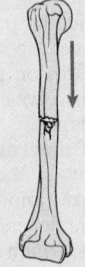

Impacted

Illustrations from Lewis SL, Collier IC, Heitkemper MM: *Medical-surgical nursing: assessment and management of clinical problems,* ed 4, St Louis, 1996, Mosby.

## Types and causes of fractures—cont'd

| Type | Description | Cause |
|---|---|---|
| Intraarticular | Fracture involving bones inside a joint | Direct or indirect energy or force to joint |
| Lead pipe (torus) | Fracture of one cortex of shafts of radius and ulna (one cortex of each bone), shown as wrinkle or buckle | Direct blow to forearm or indirect compressive force, as from a fall |
| Linear | As a line, so can be transverse or oblique | Minor or moderate energy of force directly to bone |
| Neoplastic (pathologic) | Transverse, oblique, or spiral fracture of bone weakened by tumor pressure or presence | Minor energy or force, which may be direct or indirect |
| Oblique | Fracture at oblique angle across both cortices | Direct or indirect energy, with angulation and some compression |
| Occult | Fracture that is hidden or not readily discernible | Minor force or energy |
| Segmental | Fracture with two or more pieces or segments | Direct or indirect moderate to severe force |
| Spiral | Fracture that curves around cortices and may become displaced by twist | Direct or indirect twisting energy or force with distal part held or unable to move |
| Stellate | Central fracture point from which fissures radiate | Direct blow or force of moderate energy |
| Stress | Crack in one cortex of bone | Repetitive direct energy or force, as from jogging, running, or striking a lever, or from osteoporosis |
| Transverse | Horizontal break through bone | Direct or indirect energy toward bone |

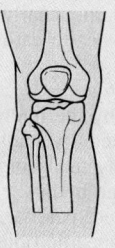

Intraarticular

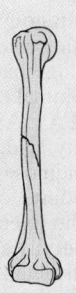

Oblique

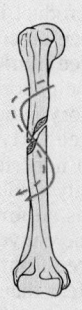

Spiral

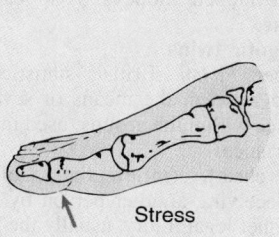

Stress

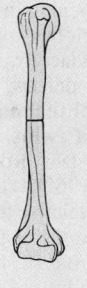

Transverse

mass is 223. Formed from the decay of actinium, all of its 20 isotopes are radioactive and short-lived.

**frank** [L, *francus*, forthright], obvious or clinically evident, such as the unequivocal presence of a condition or a disease. An example is frank bleeding.

**Frank biopsy guide,** trademark for a device consisting of a long needle containing a hooked wire used to obtain biopsy samples of breast tissue. The needle is inserted into the breast until its tip nearly touches the lesion observed by mammography. The needle is withdrawn, but the hooked wire remains to locate the tissue site. The surgeon cuts along the wire or otherwise approaches the hooked end of the wire and removes the tissue. See also **Kopan's needle.**

**frank breech** [L, *francus* + ME, *brec*], an intrauterine position of the fetus in which the buttocks present at the maternal pelvic inlet, the legs are straight up in front of the body, and the feet are at the shoulders. Babies born in this position tend to hold their feet near the head for some days after birth. Compare **complete breech, footling breech.** See also **breech birth.**

**Frankfurt horizontal plane** [Frankfurt-am-Main (anthropologic) Agreement, 1882], (in dentistry) a craniometric surface determined by the inferior borders of the bony orbits and the upper margin of the auditory meatus. It passes through the two orbitales and the two tragions and is commonly used as a reference surface in orthodontic diagnosis and treatment planning.

**Frankfurt line.** See **Reid's base line.**

**Frankfurt-mandibular incisor angle (FMIA),** (in dentistry) the precumbency of the mandibular incisor to the Frankfurt horizontal plane.

**Frank-Starling relationship** [Otto Frank, German physiologist, 1865–1944; Ernest H. Starling, English physiologist, 1866–1927], a mathematical expression stating that stroke volume increases with diastolic volume. The relationship is based on the principle that the force exerted by the myocardial fibers during contraction is directly proportional to their length or degree of stretch at the start of contraction. Because there are no adequate in vivo methods of measuring fiber length or diastolic volume, pulmonary artery obstructive pressure or pulmonary artery end-diastolic pressure is used as an index of diastolic volume. The relationship holds over a range of diastolic volumes. Beyond that range, the myocardial fibers are stretched past the point of maximal overlap between thick and thin filaments, and contractile force and stroke volume decrease. Also called *Frank-Starling mechanism,* **Starling's law of the heart.**

**Fraser syndrome** /frā'zer/ [George Robert Fraser, Czechoslovakian-born American geneticist, b. 1932], an autosomal recessive abnormality, characterized by absence of an opening in the eyelids, disorganization of one or both ocular globes, malformed ears, cleft palate, laryngeal stenosis, syndactyly, meningoencephalocele, imperforate anus, cardiac defects, and maldeveloped kidneys. Also called **cryptophthalmos syndrome.**

**fraternal twins.** See **dizygotic twins.**

**F-ratio** [Sir Ronald Aylmer *Fisher,* British statistician, 1890–1962], the variance between the means of several groups relative to the variance within the groups; used in the *F*-test in the analysis of variance.

**fraud** /frôd/ [L, *fraudare,* to cheat], (in law) the act of intentionally misleading or deceiving another person by any means so as to cause him or her legal injury, usually the loss of something valuable or the surrender of a legal right.

**Fraunhofer zone** /froun'hōfər/ [Joseph von Fraunhofer, German optician, 1787–1826], the zone farthest from the face of an ultrasound transducer. It is characterized by a divergence of the ultrasound beam and a more uniform ultrasound intensity. Also called **far field.** See also **Fresnel zone.**

**FRC,** abbreviation for **functional residual capacity.**

**F.R.C.P.,** abbreviation for *Fellow of the Royal College of Physicians.*

**F.R.C.S.,** abbreviation for *Fellow of the Royal College of Surgeons.*

**freckle** [ME, *freken*], a brown or tan macule on the skin that results from exposure to sunlight. There is an inherited tendency to freckling, and it is most frequently seen in persons with red hair. Freckles are harmless but people who freckle easily should avoid excessive sun exposure or use protective sunscreens because they have a tendency toward development of more serious actinic skin changes. Compare **lentigo.**

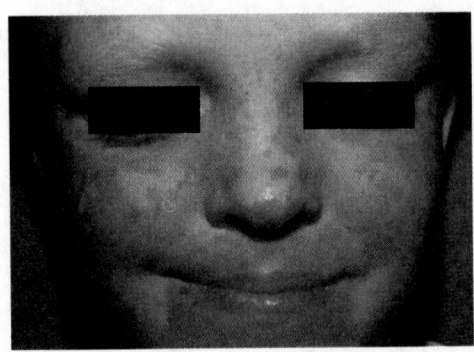

**Freckles** *(Weston, Lane, and Morrelli, 1996)*

**Fredet-Ramstedt operation.** See **pyloromyotomy.**

**free-air chamber** [AS, *freo,* free; Gk, *aer,* air; L, *camera,* vault], a device used throughout the world as a primary standard for calibrating x-ray exposure.

**free association,** 1. spontaneous consciously unrestricted association of ideas, feelings, or mental images. 2. spontaneous verbalization of thoughts and emotions that enter the consciousness during psychoanalysis. It is the basis of classical freudian analysis and also of jungian type analysis.

**free base.** See **crack.**

**free basing,** a chemical process used to increase the stimulating effect of illicit drugs such as cocaine. The resulting product is smoked.

**free circulating phagocyte.** See **phagocyte.**

**free clinic,** a clinic or health program, usually located in a neighborhood setting, that provides health care for ambulatory patients at nominal or no cost.

**free fatty acid (FFA)** [AS, *freo* + *faett* + L, *acidus,* sour], a nonesterified fatty acid, released by the hydrolysis of triglycerides within adipose tissue. Free fatty acids can be used as an immediate source of energy by many organs and can be converted by the liver into ketone bodies.

**free-floating anxiety,** a generalized, persistent, pervasive fear that is not attributable to any specific object, event, or source. See also **anxiety.**

**free-form foot orthosis,** an orthosis that is molded directly to a patient's foot. It requires less material and time to produce than other orthoses but does not provide a positive model for a more exact fabrication of a balanced orthosis.

**free gingiva,** the unattached portion of the gum coronal to the junctional epithelium. It encircles each tooth and forms a gingival sulcus or crevice.

**free gingival groove,** a shallow line or depression on the gum surface at the junction of the free and attached gingivae.

**free graft** [AS, *freo* + Gk, *graphein,* stylus], a graft completely removed from its original site and replaced at a new site in a single one-stage operation.

**free-induction decay (FID),** a signal emitted by the atomic nuclei in a tissue after a radiofrequency pulse has excited the nuclear spins at resonance. The decaying oscillation of the nuclei back to their normal state causes them to emit photons, which provide the signal from which a magnetic resonance image is made.

**free macrophage** [AS, *freo* + Gk, *makros,* large, *phagein,* to eat], a motile macrophage derived from a monocyte. It responds to chemotactic stimuli and migrates from blood vessels to tissue spaces.

**Freeman-Sheldon syndrome** /frē′mən·shel′dən/ [Ernest Arthur Freeman, British orthopedic surgeon, 1900−1975; Joseph Harold Sheldon, British physician, 1920−1964], a congenital anomaly transmitted as an autosomal dominant trait, consisting of characteristic flattened, masklike facies; small mouth, the lips protruding as in whistling; deep-set eyes with hypertelorism; camptodactyly with ulnar deviation of the fingers; and clubfoot. Also called **craniocarpotarsal dystrophy, whistling face syndrome, whistling face−windmill vane hand syndrome.**

**free nerve ending,** a receptor nerve ending that is not enclosed in a capsule. A typical free nerve ending consists of a bare axon that may be myelinated or unmyelinated. It is often found in fibrous capsules, ligaments, or synovial spaces and may be sensitive to mechanical or biochemical stimuli.

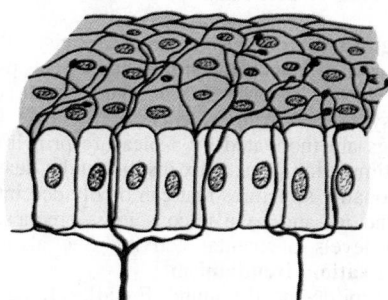

**Free nerve ending** *(Crossman and Neary, 1995)*

**free phagocyte.** See **phagocyte.**

**free radical,** an organic compound with at least one unpaired electron. It is unstable and reacts readily with other molecules.

**free-radical theory of aging,** a concept of aging based on the premise that the main causative factor is an imbalance between the production and elimination of free chemical radicals in the body tissues.

**free-standing tax-exempt clinic,** (in U.S. managed care) an organization that may employ physicians or make arrangements with physicians as independent contractors. It is usually organized as a not-for-profit, tax-exempt corpora-

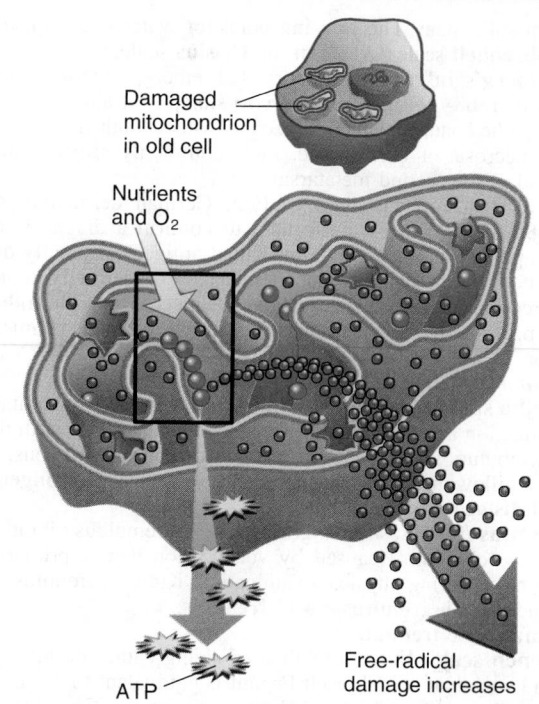

Damaged mitochondrion in old cell

Nutrients and $O_2$

ATP

Free-radical damage increases

**Free-radical theory of aging** *(McCance and Huether, 1998)*

tion. It is the direct provider of health care and holds preferred provider organization and health maintenance organization contracts, bills and collects in its own name, and owns the accounts receivable department.

**free thyroxine,** the amount of the unbound, active thyroid hormone thyroxine ($T_4$) circulating in the blood, measured by specific laboratory procedures. See also **free thyroxine index.**

**free thyroxine index,** the amount of unbound, physiologically active thyroxine ($T_4$) in serum. This amount is determined by direct assay or, more frequently, calculated on the basis of an in vitro uptake test. In this test the uptake (by resin or charcoal) of labeled triiodothyronine ($T_3$) is measured; because $T_3$ is less strongly bound by serum, it is used instead of $T_4$. The free $T_4$ index is then obtained by multiplying the $T_3$ uptake by the total concentration of $T_4$ in serum.

**free thyroxine test (FT$_4$),** a blood test used to determine thyroid function, especially when the patient has concurrent clinical situations that may alter protein blood levels. Abnormal levels indicate either hyper- or hypothyroid states.

**free-water clearance,** the calculated volume of water that must be added to a given volume of urine to make it isotonic to the plasma.

**freeway space** [AS, *freo* + *wegan* + L, *spatiaum*], the separation between the occlusal surfaces of the teeth when the mandible is in its rest position.

**freezing,** a sudden inability to initiate or continue repetitive motor activity of patients with Parkinson's disease. The patient may be unable to take the first step in walking or, if walking, may find a real or imagined obstacle that causes the feet to remain in one spot.

**freezing point** [ME, *fresen,* to be cold; L, *punctus,* pricked], the temperature at which a substance changes from a liquid to a solid state. The freezing point for water is 32° on the **Fahrenheit** scale and 0° on the **Celsius** scale.

**Freiberg's infraction** [Albert H. Freiberg, American surgeon, 1868–1940; L, *infarcire*, to stuff], an abnormal orthopedic condition characterized by osteochondritis or aseptic necrosis of bone tissue, most commonly affecting the head of the second metatarsal.

**Frei's test** /frī/ [William S. Frei, German dermatologist, 1885–1943], a test performed to confirm a diagnosis of lymphogranuloma venereum. Killed antigen, originally derived from infected patients, is injected intradermally in one forearm, and a control material is injected into the other arm. If a red, thickened papule develops at the site of injection of antigen, the test result is positive. See also *Chlamydia.*

**Frejka splint** /frā'kə/, a corrective device used to maintain abduction and articulation of the head of the femur with the acetabulum in a baby born with dislocated hips. It consists of a pillow that is belted between the legs. See also **congenital dislocation of the hip.**

**fremitus** /frem'itəs/ [L, a growling], a tremulous vibration of the chest wall caused by vocalization that is primarily palpated during physical examination. Kinds of fremitus include **tactile fremitus, vocal fremitus.**

**frena.** See **frenum.**

**French scale (Fr),** a method of sizing catheters, tubules, and sounds in which each Fr unit is equivalent to 1.3 mm.

**frenectomy** /frənek'təmē/ [L, *frenum,* bridle; Gk, *ektomē,* excision], a surgical procedure for excising a frenum or frenulum, such as the excision of the lingual frenum from its attachment into the mucoperiosteal covering of the alveolar process to correct ankyloglossia. Compare **frenotomy.**

**Frenkel's exercises** [Heinrich S. Frenkel, Swiss neurologist, 1860–1931], a system of slow repetitious exercises of increasing difficulty developed to treat ataxia in multiple sclerosis and similar disorders.

**frenotomy** /frənot'əmē/ [L, *frenum* + Gk, *temnein,* to cut], a surgical procedure for repairing a defective frenum, such as the cutting or lengthening of the lingual frenum to correct ankyloglossia. Compare **frenectomy.**

**frenulum.** See **frenum.**

**frenulum linguae.** See **frenulum of tongue.**

**frenulum of lips** /fren'yələm/, a fold of movement-limiting mucous membrane running from the gums to the lips or tongue. The frenulum of the lower lip is called the frenulum labii inferioris; that of the upper lip is the frenulum labii superioris.

**frenulum of tongue** [L, *frenum,* bridle; AS, *tunge*], a longitudinal fold of mucous membrane connecting the floor of the mouth to the underside of the tongue in midline. A congenital defect causes an abnormal shortness of the frenulum, causing tongue-tie, which can be surgically corrected. Also called **frenulum linguae, lingual frenum.**

**frenum** /frē'nəm/, *pl.* **frenums, frena** [L, *frenum,* bridle], a restraining portion or structure, a fold of mucous membrane that connects two parts, one more or less movable. Also called **frenulum.**

**frequency (F)** /frē'kwənsē/ [L, *frequens,* frequent], **1.** the number of repetitions of any phenomenon within a fixed period, such as the number of heartbeats per minute. **2.** (in biometry) the proportion of the number of persons having a discrete characteristic to the total number of persons being studied. **3.** (in electronics) the number of cycles of a periodic quantity, such as alternating current, that occur in a period of 1 second. Electromagnetic frequencies, formerly expressed in cycles per second (cps), are now expressed in hertz (Hz).

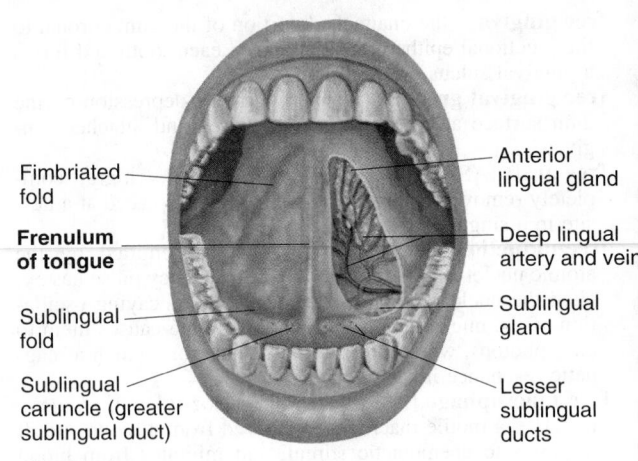

**Frenulum of tongue** *(Seidel et al, 1999)*

**freshening,** a step in the process of wound repair in which fibrin, granulation, and early scar tissue are removed in preparation for secondary closure.

**fresh frozen plasma** [ME, *fresen,* to be cold; Gk, *plassein,* to mold], an unconcentrated form of blood plasma containing all of the clotting factors except platelets. It can be used to supplement red blood cells (RBCs) when whole blood is not available for exchange transfusion or to correct a bleeding problem of unknown cause. It is also used to correct DIC. See also **plasma.**

**Fresnel zone** /freznel'/ [Augustine J. Fresnel, French physicist, 1788–1827], the region nearest the face of an ultrasound transducer. It is characterized by a highly collimated beam with great variation in ultrasound intensity and is generally the area of best image resolution. Also called **near field.**

**Freud, Sigmund** /froid/ [Austrian neurologist, 1856–1939], founder of a complex integrated theory of psychologic causes of mental disorders, some, such as hysteria, with physical symptoms. Among tenets of freudian theory: human beings are motivated by a pleasure principle; receive internal stimulation from a sex instinct and a death instinct; have personality structures that can be divided into ego, superego, and id; and have unconscious, preconscious, and conscious levels of mental activity. See also **freudian, freudian fixation, freudianism.**

**freudian** /froi'dē·ən/ [Sigmund Freud], **1.** pertaining to Sigmund Freud; his theories and doctrines, which stress the formative years of childhood as the basis for later psychoneurotic disorders, primarily through the unconscious repression of instinctual drives and sexual desires; and his system of psychoanalysis, based on free association and dream analysis, for treating such disturbances. **2.** anything that is easily interpreted according to the theories of Freud or in psychoanalytic terms. **3.** pertaining to the school of psychiatry based on Freud's teachings. **4.** one who adheres to Freud's school of psychiatry. See also **psychoanalysis.**

**freudian fixation** [Sigmund Freud], an arrest in psychosexual development characterized by a firm emotional attachment to another person or object. Some kinds of freudian fixation are **father fixation** and **mother fixation.**

**freudianism** /froi'dē·əniz'əm/, the school of psychiatry based on the psychoanalytic theories and psychotherapeutic methods of treating disorders developed by Sigmund Freud and his followers. Also called **freudism.** See also **psychoanalysis.**

**freudian slip,**   (in freudian psychology) a behavioral error in speech or action that is believed to reveal a hidden motive in the unconscious of the perpetrator. Also called *parapraxis.*

**freudism.**   See **freudianism.**

**friable** /frī′əbəl/ [L, *friare,* to crumble],   easily shattered, crumbled, or pulverized, such as tissues of the liver.

**fricative** /frik′ətiv/,   a consonant speech sound such as an /f/ or /s/, made by forcing an air stream through a constricted opening.

**Fricke dosimeter,**   a meter that quantifies radiation dose by measuring the change in the concentration of ferric ions in a solution subject to irradiation.

**friction** /frik′shən/ [L, *fricare,* to rub],   **1.** the act of rubbing one object against another. See also **attrition. 2.** a type of massage in which deeper tissues are stroked or rubbed, usually through strong circular movements of the hand. See also **massage.**

**frictional force** /frik′shənəl/,   the force component parallel to the surfaces at the point of contact between two objects. The frictional component, in contact between curved objects, may be tangential to the surfaces. Frictional force may be increased or decreased by such factors as moisture on a surface.

**friction burn,**   tissue injury caused by abrasion of the skin. See also **abrasion.**

**friction rub,**   a dry, grating sound heard with a stethoscope during auscultation. It is a normal finding when heard over the liver and splenic areas. A friction rub auscultated over the pericardial area is suggestive of pericarditis; a rub over the pleural area may be a sign of lung disease.

**Friedländer's bacillus** /frēd′lendərz/ [Carl Friedländer, German pathologist, 1847–1887],   a bacterium of the species *Klebsiella pneumoniae,* which is associated with infection of the respiratory tract, especially lobar pneumonia.

**Friedländer's pneumonia** [Carl Friedländer; Gk, *pneumon,* lung],   a form of bronchopneumonia with a high mortality rate, particularly among older patients. The pneumonic patches tend to become confluent, and those who survive may experience pulmonary abscesses and necrosis.

**Friedman curve** /frēd′mən/ [Emanuel A. Friedman, American obstetrician, b. 1926],   a graph depicting the progress of labor, prepared by labor attendants to facilitate detection of dysfunctional labor. Observations of cervical dilation and fetal descent are plotted on the vertical axis against time on the horizontal axis. The labor curve is divided into latent and active phases, with the latter subdivided into latent, acceleration, maximum slope, and deceleration.

**Friedman's test** [Maurice H. Friedman, American physiologist, b. 1903],   a modification of the Aschheim-Zondek test. A sample of urine from a woman is injected into a mature unmated female rabbit. If, days later, the rabbit ovaries contain fresh corpora lutea or hemorrhaging corpora, the result is positive, indicating that the woman is pregnant.

**Friedreich's ataxia** /frēd′rīshs/ [Nickolaus Friedreich, German physician, 1825–1882],   an abnormal condition characterized by muscular weakness, loss of muscular control, weakness of the lower extremities, and an abnormal gait. Friedreich's ataxia, which may be hereditary, exhibits both dominant and recessive inheritance patterns. The primary pathologic feature is pronounced sclerosis of the posterior columns of the spinal cord with possible involvement of the spinocerebellar tracts and the corticospinal tracts. Friedreich's ataxia usually affects individuals between 5 and 20 years of age. The highest incidence of onset is at puberty. The characteristically ataxic gait may progress to severe dis-

ability. Over a period of years a child who is affected may also have ataxia of the upper extremities and difficulty in performing simple maneuvers such as writing or handling eating utensils. The characteristic gait of this disease is caused by a cavus deformity, or clawfoot. The gait and the stance of the affected individual are unsteady. A positive Romberg's sign may be evident, and Babinski's sign is present with absent or decreased deep reflexes. The condition may also cause slurred speech, head tremors, tachycardia, and cardiac failure. Thoracic scoliosis is present in approximately 80% to 90% of the patients afflicted. All the signs and symptoms are progressive. There is no curative treatment for Friedreich's ataxia. Orthoses may be useful to varying degrees in prevention of associated deformities and maintenance of an ambulatory status. Correction of the foot deformity allows the patient to remain ambulatory as long as possible and is performed when the disease process does not appear to be progressing, thereby reducing the potential for recurrence. Spinal fusion may correct the associated scoliosis. In progression of this disease death usually results from myocardial failure.

**Friedreich's sign** [Nikolaus Friedreich; L, *signum,* sign],   the diastolic collapse of the jugular veins in adherent pericardium.

**Fried's rule,**   a method of estimating the dose of medicine for a child by multiplying the adult dose by the child's age in months and dividing the product by 150. See also **Clark's rule.**

**frigid** /frij′id/ [L, *frigidus,* cold],   **1.** lacking warmth of feeling; unemotional; unimaginative; without passion or ardor and stiff or formal in manner. **2.** (of a woman) unresponsive to sexual advances or stimuli, abnormally indifferent or averse to sexual intercourse, or unable to have an orgasm during sexual intercourse. Compare **impotence.** See also **orgasm. —frigidity,** *n.*

**fringe field** /frinj′/,   in magnetic resonance imaging, the part of the magnetic field that extends away from the confines of the magnet and cannot be used for imaging. It may affect nearby equipment and personnel.

**frit** /frit, frē/ [Fr, fried],   a partially or wholly fused porcelain that is cracked by plunging into water while hot. It is used to make dental porcelain powders.

**frog leg position.**   See **Lauenstein method.**

**Fröhlich's syndrome.**   See **adiposogenital dystrophy.**

**frôlement** /frôlmäN′/ [Fr, brushing],   **1.** the rustling type of sound often heard on auscultating the chest in diseases of the pericardium. **2.** a kind of massage that uses a light brushing stroke with the hand. See also **massage.**

**Froment's sign.**   See **thumb sign.**

**front-,**   combining form meaning 'forehead or front': *frontad, frontalis, frontonasal.*

**frontal bone** /fron′təl/ [L, *frons,* forehead],   a single cranial bone that forms the front of the skull, from above the orbits, posteriorly to a junction with the parietal bones at the coronal suture.

**frontal lobe,**   the largest of five lobes constituting each of the two cerebral hemispheres. It lies beneath the frontal bone; occupies part of the lateral, medial, and inferior surfaces of each hemisphere; and extends posteriorly to the central sulcus and inferiorly to the lateral fissure. It is responsible for voluntary control over most skeletal muscles. The frontal lobe significantly influences personality and is associated with the higher mental activities, such as planning, judgment, and conceptualization. Compare **central lobe, occipital lobe, parietal lobe, temporal lobe.**

**frontal lobe syndrome,**   behavioral and personality changes usually observed after a neoplastic or traumatic

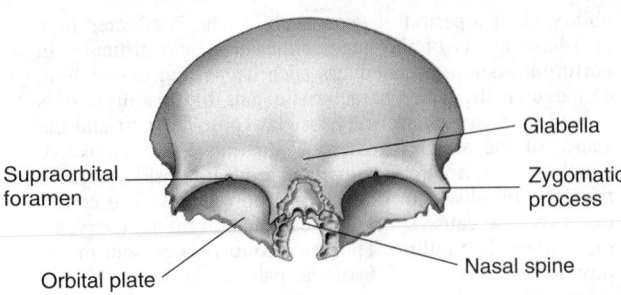

Glabella

Supraorbital foramen

Zygomatic process

Orbital plate

Nasal spine

**Frontal bone**

frontal lobe lesion. The patient may become sociopathic, boastful, hypomanic, uninhibited, exhibitionistic, and subject to outbursts of irritability or violence; in other cases the person may become depressed, apathetic, lacking in initiative, negligent about personal appearance, and inclined to perseverate. Partial frontal lobectomy was formerly performed by some psychosurgeons to reduce drive in extremely disturbed psychotic patients, but the results were highly questionable.

**frontal plane,** any of the vertical planes passing through the body from the head to the feet, perpendicular to the sagittal planes, the plane parallel to the long axis of the body and at right angles to the median sagital plane, dividing the body into front and back portions. Also called **coronal plane.** Compare **median plane, sagittal plane, transverse plane.** See also **frontal section.**

**frontal pole** [L, *frons,* forehead, *polus*], the anterior extremity of the frontal lobe of the cerebrum.

**frontal section** [L, *frons,* forehead, *sectio,* a cutting], a section of the head or other body part cut into anterior and posterior portions. Also called **coronal section.** See also **frontal plane.**

**frontal sinus,** one of a pair of small cavities in the frontal bone of the skull that communicate with the nasal cavity and lie above the orbits. The frontal sinuses are situated behind the superciliary arches and are lined with a mucous membrane that is continuous with that of the nasal cavity. Each sinus opens into the anterior part of the middle meatus

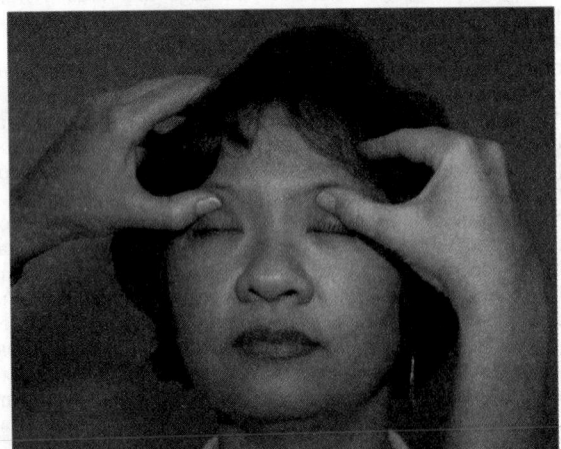

**Assessment of the frontal sinuses** *(Lemmi and Lemmi, 2000)*

through the frontonasal duct. The frontal sinuses are absent at birth, become well developed between the seventh and eighth years, and reach their full size after puberty. Compare **ethmoidal air cell, maxillary sinus, sphenoidal sinus.**

**frontal vein,** one of a pair of superficial veins of the face, arising in the plexus of the forehead. Each frontal vein communicates with the frontal tributaries of the superficial temporal vein and lies near the vein of the opposite side as it courses toward the root of the nose. Compare **angular vein, facial vein.**

**frontocortical aphasia.** See **motor aphasia.**

**frontoethmoidal suture.** See **ethmoidofrontal suture.**

**frontonasal dysplasia,** a hereditary form of defective midline development of the head and face, including ocular hypertelorism, occult cleft nose and maxilla, and sometimes mental retardation or other defects. Also called **median cleft facial syndrome.**

**frostbite** [AS, *frost + bitan*], traumatic effect of extreme cold on skin and subcutaneous tissues that is first recognized by distinct pallor of exposed skin surfaces, particularly the nose, ears, fingers, and toes. Vasoconstriction and damage to blood vessels impair local circulation and cause anoxia, edema, vesiculation, and necrosis. Gentle warming is appropriate first-aid treatment; rubbing of the affected part is avoided. Later therapy is similar to treatment of thermal burns. Iatrogenic frostbite is the result of excessive use of ethyl chloride sprays for local anesthesia for the relief of muscle and tendon strains. Compare **chilblain, immersion foot.**

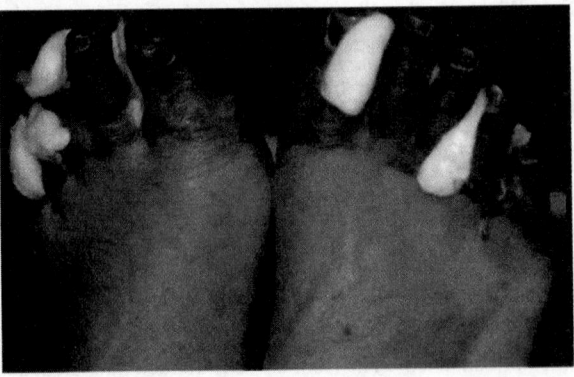

**Frostbite** *(Auerbach, 1995)*

**frottage** /frôtäzh′/ [Fr, rubbing], **1.** sexual gratification obtained by rubbing (especially the genital area) against the clothing of another person, as can occur in a crowd. **2.** a massage technique using rubbing.

**frotteur** /frôtœr′/ [Fr], a person who obtains sexual gratification by the practice of frottage.

**frozen blood.** See **bank blood.**

**frozen section** [ME, *fresen* + L, *sectio*], a histologic section of tissue that has been frozen by exposure to dry ice.

**frozen section method** [AS, *freosan,* to freeze; L, *sectio,* a cutting; Gk *meta* order, *hodos* path], (in surgical pathology) a method used in preparing a selected portion of tissue for pathologic examination. The tissue is moistened and, fixed or unfixed, is rapidly frozen and cut by a microtome ina cryostat. This method is very rapid, allowing the pathologist to examine the specimen during a surgical procedure.

**F.R.S.C.,** abbreviation for *Fellow of the Royal Society of Canada.*

**fructokinase** /fruk'tōkī'nās/, an enzyme that catalyzes the transfer of a high-energy phosphate group from adenosine triphosphate to D-fructose.

**fructosamine test** /frook·tōs'ə·mēn /, determination of the serum fructosamine level by measuring the reduction of nitroblue tetrazolium (NBT) to purple under alkaline conditions; it is used as an index of the average glycemic state over the preceding 2 to 3 weeks.

**fructose** /fruk'tōs, frook'-/, a yellowish-to-white crystalline water-soluble levorotatory ketose monosaccharide that is sweeter than sucrose. It is found in honey and several fruits and combines with glucose to form the disaccharide sucrose. Isomerization of the glucose in corn syrup to fructose allows for the production of high fructose corn syrup that is used to sweeten foods; for example more than 90% of soft drinks in the United States are sweetened with HFCS. Also called **fruit sugar, levulose.**

**fructose intolerance** [L, *fructus,* fruit, *in* + *tolerare,* to bear], an inherited disorder marked by an absence of enzymes needed to metabolize fructose. Symptoms include sweating, tremors, confusion, digestive distress with vomiting, and failure of infants to grow. The condition is transmitted as an autosomal dominant trait.

**fructosemia** /frook'tōsē'mē·ə/ [L, *fructus,* fruit; Gk, *haima,* blood], the presence of fructose in the blood.

**fructose test,** a laboratory fertility examination of the semen of azoospermic men. Fructose comes primarily from the seminal vesicles. The purpose of the test is to rule out possible ejaculatory duct obstruction or agenesis of seminal vesicles.

**fructosuria** /frook'tōsŏŏr'ē·ə/, presence of the sugar fructose in the urine. This usually harmless and asymptomatic condition is caused by the hereditary absence of the enzyme fructokinase, which normally assists fructose metabolism. Essential fructosuria is associated with symptoms of diabetes mellitus. Also called *levulosuria.*

**fruit sugar.** See **fructose.**

**frustration** /frustrā'shən/, a feeling that results from interference with one's ability to attain a desired goal or satisfaction.

**FSH,** abbreviation for **follicle-stimulating hormone.**

**FSH-RF,** abbreviation for **follicle-stimulating hormone releasing factor.**

**FSK,** abbreviation for **forskolin.**

**FT,** abbreviation for *fast-twitch.* See **fast-twitch (FT) fiber.**

**FTA-ABS test.** See **fluorescent treponemal antibody absorption test.**

**FTC,** abbreviation for **Federal Trade Commission.**

**F-test** [Sir Ronald Aylmer *Fisher,* British statistician, 1890−1962], a statistical test comparing the means of more than two groups simultaneously by comparing two different measures of variance of the observations. One statistic measures the variations between the means of the groups (the between-groups variation), the other the variations within the groups (the within-group variation). If the two measures of variance yield similar results and their ratio, the *F*-ratio, approximates 1.0, the null hypothesis that all observations came from the same population cannot be rejected, whereas under the alternative hypothesis, the *F*-ratio is expected to be larger than 1.0. The test is the first step in the analysis of variance.

**FTT,** abbreviation for **failure to thrive.**

**fuchsin bodies.** See **Russell's bodies.**

**fucosidosis** /fyōō'kōsidō'sis/, a hereditary lysosomal storage disorder that results from the absence of the enzyme required to metabolize fucoside moieties. It causes mental retardation, neurologic deterioration, coarse facial features, thickened skin, and hepatosplenomegaly.

**FUDR,** trademark for an antiviral and antineoplastic (floxuridine).

**fugue** /fyōōg/ [L, *fuga,* running away], a state of dissociative reaction characterized by amnesia and physical flight from an intolerable situation. During the episode the person appears normal and seems consciously aware of what may be very complex activities and behavior, but afterward he or she has no recollection of the actions or behavior. The condition may last for only a few days or weeks, or it may continue for several years, during which the person wanders away from the customary environment, enters a new occupation, and undertakes an entirely different way of life. The syndrome appears to be caused by an inability to cope with a severe conflict or with a chronically stressful life situation. A form of fugue also occurs briefly after an epileptic seizure. See also **ambulatory automatism, automatism, dissociative reaction.**

**Fukuhara syndrome.** See **MERRF syndrome.**

**Fukuyama type congenital muscular dystrophy** /fōō'kōō·ya'ma/ [Yukio Fukuyama, Japanese physician, 20th century], an autosomal recessive type of muscular dystrophy evident in infancy; muscle abnormalities resemble those of Duchenne's muscular dystrophy, and patients are mentally retarded with microgyria and other cerebral abnormalities. Also called **Fukuyama's syndrome.** See also **Duchenne's muscular dystrophy.**

**fulcrum** /fŏŏl'krəm, ful'-/ [L, *fulcire,* to support], **1.** the stable point or the position on which a lever, such as the ulna or the femur, turns. Numerous common body movements, such as raising the arm and walking, are combinations of lever actions involving fulcrums. The muscles provide the forces that move the numerous bones acting as levers. **2.** (in radiology) an imaginary pivot point about which the x-ray tube and film move. During computed tomography the fulcrum lies in the focal, or object, plane, and only anatomic areas lying in this plane are focused and imaged.

**fulfillment** [AS, *fullfyllan,* to make full], a perception of harmony in life that results when an individual has found meaning and acts purposefully.

**fulgurate** /ful'gyərāt/ [L, *fulgur,* lightning], **1.** pertaining to sudden, intense, sharp pain. **2.** the use of a movable electrode to destroy superficial tissue.

**fulguration.** See **electrodesiccation.**

**full-arch wire,** a wire that is attached to the teeth and extends from the molar region of one side, across the front of the mouth, to the molar region on the other side. It is used to cause or guide orthodontic tooth movement. A sectional arch wire or shorter version of the full-arch wire may also be used.

**full bath** [AS, *fol* + *baeth*], a bath in which the patient's body is immersed in water up to the neck.

**full denture** [AS, *fol* + L, *dens,* tooth], a removable dental prosthesis that replaces all of the natural teeth in the maxillary or mandibular dental arch. The denture is usually made of methyl methacrylate and is completely supported by the mouth tissues. Also called **complete denture.**

**full hospital diet.** See **regular diet.**

**full-liquid diet,** a diet consisting of only liquids and foods that liquefy at body temperature. It includes milk, milk drinks, carbonated beverages, coffee, tea, strained fruit juices, broth, strained cream soup, eggs cooked to liquid consistency or pasteurized, egg substitutes, cream, melted butter or margarine, strained precooked infant cereals in milk, thin custards, gelatin desserts, ice cream, sherbet, strained vegetables in soup, honey, syrups, sugar, and dry skim milk dissolved in liquids. The diet is prescribed after surgery, in some acute infections of short duration, in the treatment of acute GI disorders, and for patients too ill to chew. See also **liquid diet.**

**full-lung tomography,** a technique for producing general tomographic surveys of both lungs for the purpose of detecting possible occult nodules of metastases. Such lesions usually cannot be visualized with conventional radiologic methods.

**full pulse** [AS, *fol* +, *pulsare,* to beat], a large-volume pulse with a low pulse pressure. Also called **pulsus magnus.**

**full-risk HMO,** (in U.S. managed care) a health maintenance organization in which the hospital receives capitation (money paid) for all facility and hospital-based physician services. The physician group receives capitation and shares the deficit or surplus of the hospital risk pool. The HMO retains premium dollars and assumes risk for out-of-area emergencies, pharmacy benefits, and vision benefits.

**full term** [AS, *fol* + Gk, *terma,* limit], pertaining to the normal period of human gestation, between 38 and 41 weeks.

**full-thickness graft,** a tissue transplant that includes the full thickness of the skin and subcutaneous layers.

**full weight-bearing (FWB)** [AS, *fol* + *gewiht* + ME, *beren*], Relating to a view in radiology that shows the response to stresses of a natural posture. Full weight-bearing views of the foot are useful in studying flatfoot and clawfoot.

**fulminant hepatitis,** a rare and frequently fatal form of acute hepatitis B in which the patient's condition rapidly deteriorates, with hepatic encephalopathy, necrosis of the hepatic parenchyma, coagulopathy, renal failure, and coma.

**fulminating** /ful'minā'ting/ [L, *fulminare,* lightening flash], (of a disease or condition) rapid, sudden, severe, such as an infection, fever, or hemorrhage. Also **fulminant. —fulminate,** *v.*

**Fulvicin,** trademark for an antifungal (griseofulvin).

**fumagillin, fumigacin.** See **helvolic acid.**

**fumigate** /fyo͞o'migāt/, to disinfect by exposing an area or object to pesticidal smoke or fumes.

**fuming,** producing a visible vapor.

**function** /fungk'shən/ [L, *functio,* performance], **1.** an act, process, or series of processes that serve a purpose. **2.** to perform an activity or to work properly and normally.

**functional** /fungk'shənəl/ [L, *functio,* performance], **1.** pertaining to a function. **2.** affecting the functions but not the structure of an organism or organ system.

**functional age,** a combination of the chronologic, physiologic, mental, and emotional ages.

**functional analysis,** (in psychiatry) a type of therapy that traces the sequence of events involved in producing and maintaining undesirable behavior.

**functional antagonism,** (in pharmacology) a situation in which two agonists interact with different receptors and produce opposing effects.

**functional assessment.** See **health history.**

**functional bowel syndrome.** See **irritable bowel syndrome.**

**functional contracture.** See **hypertonic contracture.**

**functional differentiation,** (in embryology) the specialization or diversification that results from the particular function of a cell or tissue.

**functional disease, 1.** a disease that affects function or

performance. **2.** a condition marked by signs or symptoms of an organic disease or disorder although careful examination fails to reveal any evidence of structural or physiologic abnormalities. The symptoms of a functional disorder are as real as those of an organic disease. Headache, impotence, certain heart murmurs, and constipation may be symptoms of organic disease or of functional disease.

**functional dyspepsia,** a condition characterized by impaired digestion caused by an atonic or a neurologic problem. See also **dyspepsia.**

**functional foods,** foods and food supplements marketed for presumed health benefits, such as vitamin supplements and certain herbs.

**functional health history.** See **complete health history.**

**functional hearing loss,** hearing loss that lacks any organic lesion. Also called **nonorganic hearing loss.**

**functional illness,** a physical disorder with no known structural explanation for the symptoms. See also **disorder, functional disease, illness.**

**functional imaging,** a diagnostic procedure in which a sequence of radiographic or scintillation camera images of the distribution of an administered radioactive tracer delineates one or more physiologic processes in the body.

**functional impotence.** See **impotence.**

**functional magnetic resonance imaging (fMRI),** a radiographic technique for imaging brain activity. In fMRI the examiner takes a rapid succession of scans designed to detect increases in oxygen consumption in various regions of the brain, which reflects small changes in blood flow and increased activity in certain cells.

**functional murmur** [L, *functio,* performance], a heart murmur caused by an alteration of function without structural heart disease or damage, as in a murmur related to anemia. Also called **physiologic murmur.**

**functional nursing,** an organizational mode for assigning nursing personnel that is task- and activity-oriented, using auxiliary health workers trained in a variety of skills. Each person is assigned specific functions performed for all patients in a given unit, and all are responsible to the head nurse.

**functional occlusal harmony,** a biting relationship of opposing teeth in all ranges and movements that provides maximum chewing efficiency without pathogenic force on the supporting oral structures.

**functional overlay,** an emotional aspect of an organic disease. It may occur as an overreaction to an illness and is characterized by symptoms that continue long after clinical signs of the disease have ended.

**functional pathology** [L, *functio,* performance; Gk, *pathos,* disease, *logos,* science], a study of the functional changes that result from structural alterations in tissues.

**functional position of the hand,** a position for splinting the hand, including the wrist and fingers. It consists of dorsiflexing both the wrist between 20 and 35 degrees and the proximal interphalangeal joints between 45 and 60 degrees. The thumb is abducted and in opposition and alignment with the pads of the fingers.

**functional progression,** a rehabilitative sequence for a musculoskeletal or similar injury. With variations for individual cases the program usually progresses from immobilization for primary healing through protection of range of motion to endurance and strengthening activities related to the patient's work and play requirements.

**functional psychosis,** a severe emotional disorder characterized by personality derangement and loss of ability to function in reality, but without evidence that the disorder is related to the physical processes of the brain.

**functional residual capacity (FRC),** the volume of gas in the lungs at the end of a normal tidal volume exhalation. The functional residual capacity is equal to the residual volume plus the expiratory reserve volume.

**functional splint** [L, *functio,* performance; ME, *splent*], an orthopedic device that allows or assists a patient's movements. Also called **ambulatory splint, dynamic splint.** See also **splint.**

**functional visual skills,** various normal eye activities such as depth perception, eye aiming and alignment, and oculomotility.

**fundal height** /fun'dəl/ [L, *fundus,* bottom; AS, *heightho*], the height of the fundus, measured in centimeters from the top of the symphysis pubis to the highest point in the midline at the top of the uterus. Fundal height is measured at each prenatal visit with large blunt calipers or with a tape measure. From the twentieth to the thirty-second week of pregnancy the height in centimeters is equal to the gestation in weeks. Two measurements 2 weeks apart showing a deviation of more than 2 cm may indicate that the fetus is large or small for dates, that the estimated gestation is in error, or that the woman is carrying a multiple pregnancy.

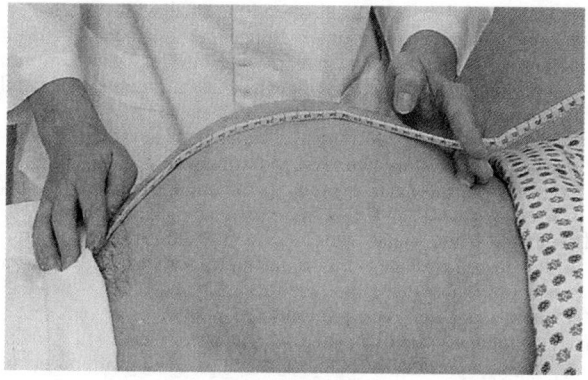

**Measurement of fundal height** *(Seidel et al, 1999)*

**fundal placenta** [L, *fundus,* bottom, *placenta,* flat cake], a placenta that is attached to the fundus of the uterus.

**fundamentals of nursing** /fun'dəmen'təls/, the basic principles and practices of nursing as taught in educational programs for nurses. In a course on the fundamentals of nursing, traditionally required in the first semester of the program, the student attends classes and gives care to selected patients. A fundamentals of nursing course emphasizes the importance of the fundamental needs of humans as well as competence in basic skills as prerequisites to providing comprehensive nursing care.

**fundi.** See **fundus.**

**fundiform ligament of penis** /fun'difôrm/, a band of elastic fibers surrounding the penis. It extends from the linea alba above the pubic symphysis and attaches to the penile fascia.

**fundoplication** /fun'dəplikā'shən/ [L, *fundus,* bottom, *plicare,* to fold], a surgical procedure involving making tucks (plication) in the fundus of the stomach around the lower end of the esophagus. The operation is used in the treatment of gastric acid reflux into the esophagus. See also **plication.**

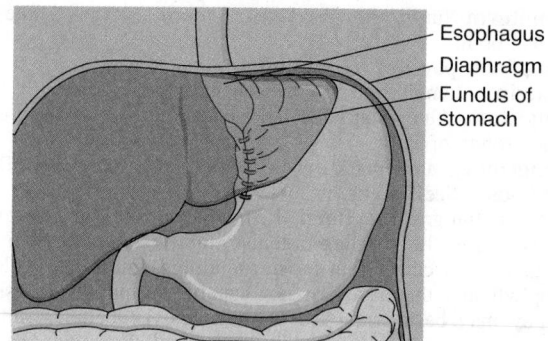

**Nissen fundoplication for hiatal hernia**
*(Beare and Myers, 1998)*

**fundoscopy.** See **funduscopy.**

**fundus** /fun'dəs/, *pl.* **fundi** [L, bottom], the base or the deepest part of an organ; the portion farthest from the mouth of an organ, such as the fundus of the uterus or the fundus of an eye.

**funduscope.** See **ophthalmoscope.**

**funduscopy.** See **ophthalmoscopy.**

**fundus microscopy,** examination of the interior of the eye using an instrument that combines an ophthalmoscope and a lens with high magnifying power for observing minute structures in the cornea, iris, and fundus.

**fundus of the gallbladder,** the closed end of the gallbladder, adjacent to the inferior border of the liver.

**fundus of the stomach,** a cul-de-sac of the stomach that lies above the level of the cardiac orifice, where the esophagus joins the stomach.

**fundus of the urinary bladder,** the bottom of the bladder, formed by the convex posterior wall.

**fungal** /fung'gəl/ [L, *fungus,* mushroom], pertaining to or resembling a fungus or fungi.

**fungal abscess,** a collection of pus produced by a fungal infection.

**fungal infection** [L, *fungus,* mushroom, *inficere,* to stain], any inflammatory condition caused by a fungus. Most fungal infections are superficial and mild, though persistent and difficult to eradicate. Some, particularly in older, debilitated, or immunosuppressed or immunodeficient people, may become systemic and life-threatening. Some kinds of fungal infections are **aspergillosis, blastomycosis, candidiasis, coccidioidomycosis,** and **histoplasmosis.**

**fungal infection of nail,** an infection of the horny cutaneous plates on the dorsal tips of the fingers and toes. The infection is commonly caused by *Tricophyton* organisms and treated with griseofulvin and itraconazole.

**fungal pneumonia,** pneumonia caused by inhaled fungi, usually *Blastomyces dermatitidis, Coccidioides immitis,* or *Histoplasma capsulatum.* Numerous other fungi, such as *Aspergillus* and *Candida,* infect immunocompromised patients. See also **blastomycosis, histoplasmosis.**

**fungal septicemia** [L, *fungus* + Gk, *septikos,* putrid, *haima,* blood], a form of systemic infection in which the causative agent is a fungus in the circulatory bloodstream.

**fungemia** /funjē'mē·ə/ [L, *fungus* + Gk, *haima,* blood], the presence of fungi in the blood. Compare **bacteremia, parasitemia, viremia.**

**fungicide** /fun'jisīd/, a drug that kills fungi. See also **antifungal,** def. 2. **—fungicidal,** *adj.*

**fungiform** /fun′jifôrm/ [L, *funis* + *forma*], shaped like a mushroom.

**fungiform papilla.** See **papilla.**

**-fungin,** combining form for antifungal antibiotics.

**fungistatic** /fun′jēstat′ik/, having an inhibiting effect on the growth of fungi.

**Fungizone,** trademark for an antifungal (amphotericin B).

**fungous.** See **fungus.**

**fungus** /fun′gəs/, *pl.* **fungi,** L, *ungus,* mushroom], a eukaryotic, thallus-forming organism that feeds by absorbing organic molecules from its surroundings. Fungi lack chlorophyll and therefore are not capable of photosynthesis. They may be saprophytes or parasites. Unicellular fungi (yeasts) reproduce by budding; multicellular fungi, such as molds, reproduce by spore formation. Fungi may invade living organisms, including humans, as well as nonliving organic substances. Of the 100,000 identified species of fungi, 100 are common in humans and 10 are pathogenic. See also **fungal infection. —fungal, fungous,** *adj.*

**funic presentation** /fyoo̅′nik/ [L, *funis* + *praesentare,* to show], (in obstetrics) the appearance of the umbilical cord before the main presenting part of the fetus. Also called **cord presentation, funis presentation, presentation.**

**funic souffle** /fyoo̅′nik soo̅′fəl/ [L, *funis,* cord; Fr, *souffle,* breath], a soft, muffled blowing sound produced by blood rushing through the umbilical vessels and synchronous with the fetal heart sound.

**funiculitis** /fənik′yəlī′tis/, any abnormal inflammatory condition of a cordlike structure of the body, such as the spinal cord or spermatic cord.

**funiculopexy** /fənik′yəlōpek′sē/, a surgical procedure for correcting an undescended testicle, in which the spermatic cord is sutured to surrounding tissue.

**funiculus** /fənik′yələs/ [L, little cord], a division of the white matter of the spinal cord, consisting of fasciculi or fiber tracts.

**funiculus umbilicalis.** See **umbilical cord.**

**funis** /fyoo̅′nis, foo̅′nis/, a cordlike structure, such as the umbilical cord.

**funis presentation.** See **funic presentation.**

**funnel chest** [L, *fundere,* to pour], a skeletal abnormality of the chest characterized by a depressed sternum. The deformity may not interfere with breathing, but surgical correction is often recommended for cosmetic reasons. Also called **pectus excavatum.**

**funnel feeding,** a technique in which liquids may be given orally to a patient who cannot move the lips or masticate, such as after surgery at the mouth or lips. A rubber tube attached to a funnel is placed in the mouth, usually at one corner, and a liquid is poured slowly through the funnel and tube into the mouth near the back of the tongue. The patient quickly learns to control the flow with sucking action and tongue position. If the method is used for a weak or young infant, a rubber bulb or a large syringe may be used instead of a funnel. The bulb or syringe is compressed gently, slowly, and continuously to control the rate of flow and prevent choking.

**funny bone,** a popular name for a point at the lower end of the humerus where the ulnar nerve crosses the elbow joint near the surface and, if subjected to external pressure, produces in a tingling sensation.

**FUO,** abbreviation for **fever of unknown origin.**

**Furadantin,** trademark for an antibacterial (nitrofurantoin).

**furazolidone** /foo̅′rəzol′idōn/, an antiinfective and antiprotozoal.

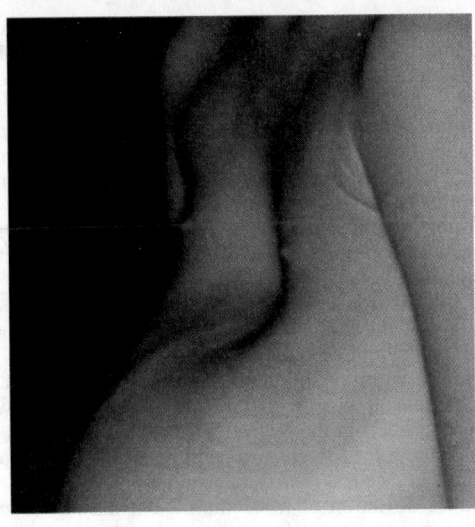

**Funnel chest** *(Zitelli and Davis, 1997)*

■ INDICATIONS: It is prescribed for the treatment of susceptible bacterial or protozoal infections of the GI tract.

■ CONTRAINDICATIONS: Known hypersensitivity to this drug prohibits its use. It is not given to children less than 1 month of age, and it is not used with drugs that are contraindicated with monoamine oxidase inhibitors.

■ ADVERSE EFFECTS: Among the more serious adverse reactions are hemolytic anemia and fever, skin rash, and abdominal pain. Concurrent use with alcohol is contraindicated.

**furcation** /fərkā′shən/ [L, *furca,* fork], the region of division of tooth root. It is a bifurcation if there are two roots or a trifurcation if there are three roots.

**furcation probe** See **periodontal probe.**

**furfuraceous desquamation** /fur′fərā′sē·əs/ [L, *furfur,* bran, *desquamare,* to scale off], the shedding of epidermis in large scales.

**furosemide** /fyoo̅rō′səmīd/, a loop diuretic.

■ INDICATIONS: It is prescribed in the treatment of congestive heart failure, renal failure, and edema.

■ CONTRAINDICATIONS: Anuria, pregnancy, lactation, electrolyte depletion, or known hypersensitivity to this drug prohibits its use.

■ ADVERSE EFFECTS: Among the more serious adverse reactions are fluid and electrolyte imbalances.

**Furoxone,** trademark for an antiinfective antiprotozoal (furazolidone).

**furred tongue.** See **coated tongue.**

**furrow** /fur′ō/ [AS, *furh*], a groove, such as the atrioventricular furrow that separates the atria from the ventricles of the heart.

**furuncle** /fyoo̅r′ungkəl/ [L, *furunculus,* petty thief], a localized suppurative staphylococcal skin infection originating in a gland or hair follicle and characterized by pain, redness, and swelling. Necrosis deep in the center of the inflamed area forms a core of dead tissue that is spontaneously extruded, eventually resorbed, or surgically removed. It is important to avoid irritating or squeezing the lesion to prevent spread of the infection. Treatment may include antibiotics, local moist heat, and, when there is definite fluctuation and the hard white core is evident, incision and drainage. Also called **boil. —furunculous,** *adj.*

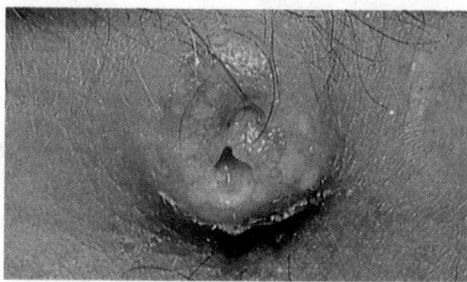

**Furuncle**
*(Seidel et al, 1999/courtesy Jaime A. Tschen, MD, Baylor College of Medicine, Dept. of Dermatology, Houston)*

**furunculosis** /fyŏŏrung'kyŏŏlō'sis/, an acute skin disease characterized by boils or successive crops of boils that are caused by staphylococci or streptococci.

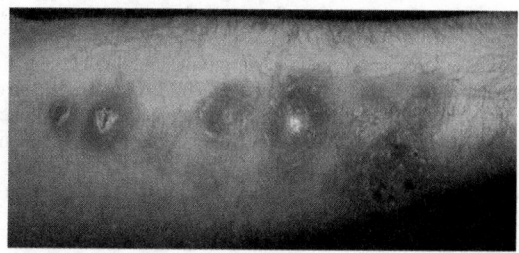

**Furunculosis** *(Weston, Lane, and Morrelli, 1996)*

**furunculous.** See **furuncle.**

**-fuse,** suffix meaning 'to pour or flow': *diffuse, effuse, perfuse.*

**fused teeth** /fyŏŏzd/ [L, *fundere,* to melt], partial or complete fusion of two or more individual teeth.

**fusiform** /fyŏŏ'sifôrm/ [L, *fusus,* spindle, *forma,* form], a structure that is tapered at both ends.

**fusiform aneurysm,** a localized dilation of an artery in which the entire circumference of the vessel is distended. The result is an elongated, tubular or spindlelike swelling. Also called **Richet's aneurysm.** Compare **saccular aneurysm.**

**fusiform gyrus** [L, *fusus,* spindle, *forma,* form; Gk, *gyros,* turn], a convolution of the cerebral hemispheres that lies below the collateral fissures and joins the occipital and temporal lobes.

**fusimotor** /fyŏŏ'zimō'tər/ [L, *fusus* + *motare,* to move about], pertaining to the motor nerve fibers, or gamma efferent fibers, that innervate the intrafusal fibers of the muscle spindle.

**fusion** /fyŏŏ'zhən/ [L, *fusio,* outpouring], **1.** the joining into a single entity, as in optic fusion. **2.** the act of uniting two or more bones of a joint. Also called **ankylosis. 3.** the surgical joining of two or more vertebrae, performed to stabilize a segment of the spinal column after severe trauma, herniation of a disk, or degenerative disease. Under general anesthesia the cartilage pads are removed from between the posterior parts of the involved vertebrae. Bone chips are cut from one of the patient's iliac crests and inserted in place of the cartilage, fusing the articulating surfaces into one segment of bone. **4.** (in psychiatry) the tendency of two people who are experiencing an intense emotion to unite.

**fusional amplitude.** See **amplitude of convergence.**

**fusional movement** /fyŏŏ'zhənəl/, a reflex that moves the visual axes to the point of fixation, producing stereoscopic vision.

**fusion beat,** in an electrocardiogram, a P wave or QRS complex resulting from the concurrent activation of the atria or the ventricles by two stimuli in the same chamber. An atrial fusion beat results when the sinus beat coincides with an atrial ectopic beat, when two atrial ectopic beats coincide, or when an atrial or sinus beat coincides with retrograde conduction from a junctional focus. A ventricular fusion beat results when a ventricular beat coincides with a sinus beat, a ventricular ectopic beat, or a junctional beat.

***Fusobacterium,*** a large cigar-shaped anaerobic bacillus genus with only one species, *Fusobacterium fusiforme,* pathogenic to humans. It is sometimes associated with Vincent's angina.

**fusospirochetal disease** /fyŏŏ'zōspī'rōkē'təl/ [L, *fusus,* spindle; Gk, *speira,* coil, *chaite,* hair], any infection characterized by ulcerative lesions in which both a fusiform bacillus and a spirochete are found, such as trench mouth or Vincent's angina.

**FVIII,** (recombinant blood factor VIII), a large glycoprotein containing more than 2300 amino acids, 24 cysteine residues, and 25 potential glycosylation sites. The factor is used to treat blood-clotting disorders, such as **hemophilia A,** in which the factor is deficient or missing.

**F wave,** a waveform recorded in electroneuromyographic and nerve conduction tests. It appears on supramaximal stimulation of a motor nerve and is caused by antidromic transmission of a stimulus. The F wave is used in studies of motor nerve function in the arms and legs.

**f waves,** in an electrocardiogram, wavy deflections at a rate of 400 or more per minute that represent atrial fibrillation.

**FWB,** abbreviation for **full weight-bearing.**

**-fy,** suffix meaning 'to make into' something specified: *acidify, decalcify, salify.*

**-fying.** See **-factive.**

**-fylline,** combining form for theophylline derivatives.

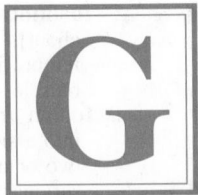

**g,** abbreviation for **gram.**

**G1,** a phase in the cell cycle during which the cell's future can be influenced by various positive and negative signals, such as growth factors. The signals determine whether the cell will advance beyond a certain checkpoint. Once beyond the checkpoint, the cell is committed to entering a phase during which it replicates its DNA in preparation for mitosis.

**G2,** a phase in the cell cycle that follows DNA replication. During G2, the cell checks the accuracy of DNA replication and prepares for mitosis.

**G-6-PD deficiency,** abbreviation for **glucose-6-phosphate dehydrogenase deficiency.**

**Ga,** symbol for the element **gallium.**

**GA,** abbreviation for **general anesthesia.**

**GABA,** abbreviation for **gamma-aminobutyric acid.**

**GABHS,** abbreviation for **group A beta-hemolytic streptococcal skin disease.**

**GAD,** abbreviation for **generalized anxiety disorder.**

**gadolinium (Gd)** /gad′əlin′ē·əm/ [Johan Gadolin, Finnish chemist, 1760–1852], **1.** a rare earth metallic element. Its atomic number is 64; its atomic mass is 157.25. It is now widely used as an MRI contrast agent. **2.** (in radiology) a phosphor used to intensify screens.

**gag** [ME, *gaggen,* to strangle], **1.** a dental device for holding the jaws open during oral surgery or dental restoration. Also called **mouth prop. 2.** to retch or attempt to vomit.

**gag reflex** [ME, *gaggen,* to strangle; L, *reflectere,* to bend back], a normal neural reflex elicited by touching the soft palate or posterior pharynx; the responses are symmetric elevation of the palate, retraction of the tongue, and contraction of the pharyngeal muscles. The reflex is used as a test of the integrity of the vagus and glossopharyngeal nerves. Also called **pharyngeal reflex.**

**gait** [ONorse, *geta,* a way], the manner or style of walking, including rhythm, cadence, and speed.

**Gait Assessment Rating Scale (GARS),** an inventory of 16 abnormal aspects of gait observed by an examiner as a patient walks at a self-selected pace. The abnormalities are commonly seen in elderly people who fall. Each aspect is graded on a scale of 0-1-2-3, with lower numbers indicating less abnormality.

**gait determinant,** one of a number of the kinetic anatomic factors that govern an individual's locomotion in the process of walking. Some authorities have defined pelvic rotation, pelvic tilt, knee and hip flexion, knee and ankle interaction, and lateral pelvic displacement as the main determinants of gait. Such descriptions are often important in analyzing and correcting pathologic gaits of patients afflicted by orthopedic diseases, deformities, or abnormal bone conditions.

**gait disorder,** an abnormality in the manner or style of walking, which usually results from neuromuscular, arthritic, or other body changes. The body's center of gravity may change over the years, causing the degree of knee flexion needed to maintain one's balance when walking to change. Some individuals with neuromuscular disorders may walk with a shuffling gait or move with lurching ac-

tions. At times a gait disorder may be the result of a medication that causes confusion or loss of coordination or an eye or ear disturbance that affects the sense of balance.

**galact-, galacta-. See galacto-.**

**-galactia,** combining form meaning a 'condition involving secretion of milk': *cacogalactia, dysgalactia, oligogalactia.*

**galacto-, galact-, galacta-,** combining form meaning 'milk': *galactochloral, galactogen, galactorrhea.*

**galactocele** /gəlak′təsēl′/, a cyst or hydrocele caused by blockage of a mammary gland milk duct.

**galactokinase** /gəlak′tōkī′nās/ [Gk, *gala,* milk, *kinesis,* movement; Fr, *diastase,* enzyme], an enzyme that functions in the metabolism of glycogen. Galactokinase catalyzes a metabolic step involving the transfer of a high-energy phosphate group from a donor molecule to a molecule of galactose, producing a molecule of D-galactose1-phosphate.

**galactokinase deficiency,** an inherited disorder of carbohydrate metabolism in which the enzyme galactokinase is deficient or absent. As a result, dietary galactose is not metabolized, galactose accumulates in the blood, and cataracts may develop rapidly. Food containing galactose, such as milk and certain milk products, must be eliminated from the diet. Compare **lactase deficiency.**

**galactophorous duct** /-môr′fəs/ [Gk, *gala* + *pherein,* to bear; L, *ducere,* to lead], a passage for milk in the lobes of the breast.

**galactorrhea** /gəlak′tərē′ə/ [Gk, *gala* + *rhoia,* flowing], lactation not associated with childbirth or nursing. The condition is sometimes a symptom of a pituitary gland tumor. See also **Forbes-Albright syndrome.**

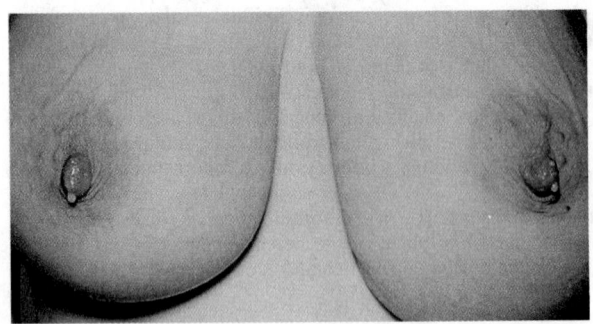

**Galactorrhea** *(Mansel and Bundred, 1995)*

**galactosamine,** galactose that contains an amine group on the second group.

**galactose** /gəlak′tōs/ [Gk, *gala* + *glykys,* sweet], a simple sugar found in the dextrorotatory form in lactose (milk sugar), nerve cell membranes, sugar beets, gums, and seaweed and in the levorotatory form in flaxseed mucilage. Prepared galactose, a white crystalline substance, is less sweet and less soluble in water than glucose but is similar in other properties.

**galactosemia** /gəlak′tōsē′mē·ə/ [Gk, *gala* + *glykys*, sweet, *haima*, blood], an inherited autosomal-recessive disorder of galactose metabolism. It is characterized by a deficiency of the enzyme galactose-1-phosphate uridyl transferase. Shortly after birth an intolerance to milk occurs; it is evidenced by anorexia, nausea, vomiting, and diarrhea and causes failure to thrive. Hepatosplenomegaly, cataracts, and mental retardation develop. Greater than normal amounts of galactose are present in the blood, the galactose tolerance test result indicates an abnormality, and the red cells show deficient galactose-1-phosphate uridyl transferase activity. Because the elimination of galactose from the diet results in the rapid decrease of all symptoms except mental retardation, early diagnosis and prompt therapy are essential. Pregnant women known to be carriers should exclude lactose and galactose from their diet. Compare **diabetes mellitus, glycogen storage disease.** See also **galactose, inborn error of metabolism.**

kodystrophy, Krabbe's disease. Compare **Tay-Sachs disease.**

**galactosyl transferase,** an enzyme in the head of sperm that is required for sperm to bind to eggs.

**galactozymase** /-zī′māz/, an enzyme in milk that is able to hydrolyze starch.

**galacturia** /gal′əkto͞or′ē·ə/ [Gk, *gala*, milk, *ouron*, urine], a condition in which the urine has a milky color caused by the abnormal presence of galactose, a monosaccharide, in the urine.

**galanin** /galan′in, gal′ənin/, a neuropeptide in the small intestine and central and peripheral nervous systems that has a role in bowel motility, pancreas activity, and prolactin and growth hormone release.

**Galant reflex** /gəlant′/, a normal response in the neonate to move the hips toward the stimulated side when the back is stroked along the spinal cord. The reflex disappears by about 4 weeks of age. Absence of the reflex may indicate spinal cord lesion. Also called **trunk incurvation reflex.**

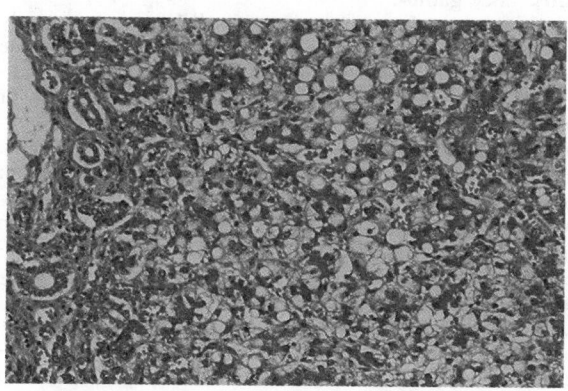

**Galactosemia: fatty changes in the liver**
*(Cotran, Kumar, and Collins, 1999/courtesy Dr. Wesley Tyson, The Children's Hospital, Denver, Colorado)*

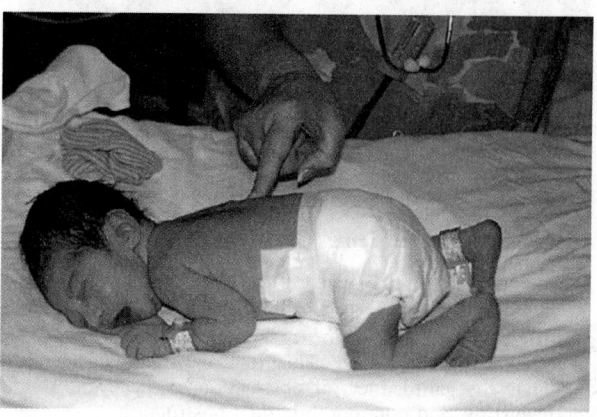

**Elicitation of the Galant reflex**
*(Lowdermilk, Perry, and Bobak, 2000)*

**galactose tolerance test,** a test of the ability of the liver to remove galactose from the blood and convert it to glycogen. The test, which is used to estimate impaired liver function, measures the rate of galactose excretion after ingestion or injection of a measured amount of galactose.

**galactoside** /gəlak′tō′sīd′/, a glycoside containing galactose.

**galactoside permease,** an enzyme that catalyses the transport of lactose into the cell.

**galactosidose,** an enzyme that catalyzes the metabolism of galactosides.

**galactosis** /gal′əktōsis/, lactation; the formation of milk by the lacteal glands.

**galactosuria** /-so͞or′ē·ə/, the presence of galactose, a simple sugar, in the urine.

**galactosyl ceramide lipidosis** /gəlak′təsil/ [Gk, *gala* + *glykys*, sweet; L, *cera*, wax, *lipos*, fat, *osis*, condition], a rare fatal inherited disorder of lipid metabolism, present at birth. Infants become paralyzed, blind, deaf, and increasingly retarded; eventually they die of bulbar paralysis. There is no known treatment for the disorder, but it can be detected in pregnancy by amniocentesis. Also called **globoid leu-**

**galea aponeurotica.** See **epicranial aponeurosis.**

**Galeazzi's fracture** /gal′ē·at′sēz/ [Riccardo Galeazzi, Italian surgeon, 1866–1952], a break in the distal radius accompanied by dislocation of the radioulnar joint. Also called **Dupuytren's fracture.**

**Galen's vein** /gā′lənz/ [Claudius Galen, Greek physician, circa AD 130–200], the large vein formed by the union of the two terminal cerebral veins. It curves around the splenium of the corpus callosum and continues as the straight sinus of the brain. Also called **great cerebral vein of Galen.**

**gall.** See **bile.**

**gallbladder (GB)** /gôl′blad′ər/ [ME, *gal* + AS, *blaedre*], a pear-shaped excretory sac lodged in a fossa on the visceral surface of the right lobe of the liver. It stores and concentrates bile, which it receives from the liver via the hepatic duct. In an adult it holds about 32 mL of bile. During digestion of fats the gallbladder contracts, ejecting bile through the common bile duct into the duodenum. The gallbladder is divided into a fundus, body, and neck and is covered by the peritoneum. Obstruction of the biliary system by gallstones may lead to jaundice and pain; it may require surgical or other intervention. See also **lithotripsy.**

**gallbladder carcinoma,**   a malignant neoplasm of the bile reservoir, characterized by anorexia, nausea, vomiting, weight loss, progressively worsening right upper quadrant pain, and eventually jaundice. Tumors of the gallbladder are predominantly adenocarcinomas; often associated with biliary calculi, they are three to four times more common in women than in men and rarely occur before 40 years of age. Physical examination reveals an enlarged gallbladder in about half of the cases. Ultrasound or radiographic tests may aid in making a diagnosis. Complete removal of the gallbladder may be curative, but partial hepatectomy may be required because the liver is often a site of early metastases. Palliative surgery is often needed. Radiotherapy may be palliative; chemotherapy is usually ineffective.

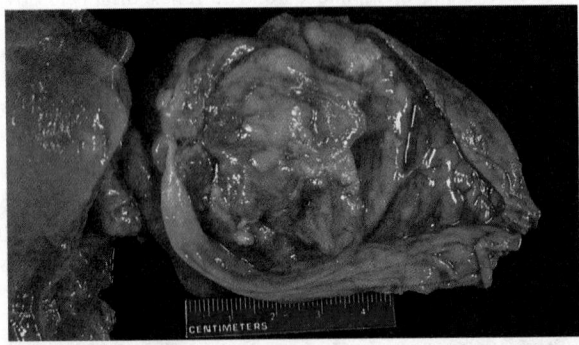

**Gallbladder carcinoma** *(Kumar, Cotran, and Robbins, 1997)*

**gallbladder nuclear scanning,**   a nuclear scan used to evaluate the biliary tract. This test may also be used to evaluate the gallbladder for obstruction of the cystic duct, cholecystitis, and common bile duct obstruction.

**gallium (Ga)** /gal'ē·əm/ [L, *Gallia,* Gaul],   a metallic element. Its atomic number is 31; its atomic mass is 69.72. The melting point of gallium is 29.8° C (88.6° F); it will melt if held in the hand. Because of its high boiling point (1983° C; 3602° F), it is used in high-temperature thermometers. Radioisotopes of gallium are used in total body scanning procedures. Many of its compounds are poisonous.

**gallium scan,**   a nuclear scan of the total body performed after an IV injection of radioactive gallium, a radionuclide that concentrates in areas of inflammation and infection, abscess, and benign and malignant tumor. It is useful in detecting metastatic tumor, especially lymphoma.

**gallop** /gal'əp/ [Fr, *galop*],   a third or fourth heart sound, which at certain heart rates sometimes sounds like the gait of a horse. Also called **gallop rhythm.** See also $S_3$, $S_4$, **summation gallop.**

**gallop rhythm.**   See **gallop.**

**gallstone.**   See **biliary calculus, cholelithiasis.**

**galoche chin** /gəlosh'/ [Fr, *galosh* + AS, *cin*],   a narrow protruding or thrusting chin. It is a congenital condition.

**galvanic** /galvan'ik/ [Luigi Galvani, Italian physician, 1737–1798],   pertaining to or involving electricity.

**galvanic cautery, galvanocautery.**   See **electrocautery.**

**galvanic electric stimulation** [Luigi Galvani],   the use of a high-voltage electric stimulator to treat muscle spasms, edema of acute injury, myofascial pain, and certain other disorders. See also **transcutaneous electric nerve stimulation (TENS).**

**galvanic skin response (GSR)** [Luigi Galvani; AS, *scinn* + L, *respondere,* to reply],   a reaction to certain stimuli as indicated by a change in the electrical resistance of the skin. The effect is related to subconscious activity of the sweat glands and may result from pleasant as well as unpleasant stimuli. The GSR is used in some polygraph examinations.

**galvanoionization.**   See **iontophoresis.**

**galvanometer** /gal'vənom'ətər/ [Luigi Galvani],   an instrument used to measure the strength and direction of flow of an electric current. Its action depends on the deflection of a magnetic needle in the field produced by current passing through a coil. A simple galvanometer is used mainly to detect the presence of an electric current. Galvanometers are used in certain diagnostic instruments, such as electrocardiographs.

**Galveston Orientation and Amnesia Test (GOAT),**   a series of 10 questions asked of a patient to help evaluate posttraumatic amnesia. The test is repeated on a weekly basis and is scored on a scale of 0 to 100. A patient is determined to be out of the amnesic state when the score exceeds 75.

**gam-.**   See **gamo-.**

**Gambian trypanosomiasis** /gam'bē·ən/,   a usually chronic form of African trypanosomiasis, caused by the parasite *Trypanosoma brucei gambiense.* An infected individual may have relatively mild symptoms for months or years before developing the neurologic symptoms of the terminal stage. Also called **West African sleeping sickness.** Compare **Rhodesian trypanosomiasis.** See also **African trypanosomiasis.**

**game knee** [ME, *gamen* + AS, *cneow*],   an informal term for any injury or condition that interferes with normal function of the knee joint.

**gamet-.**   See **gameto-.**

**gamete** /gam'ēt/ [Gk, marriage partner],   **1.** a mature male or female germ cell that is capable of functioning in fertilization or conjugation and contains the haploid number of chromosomes of the organism. **2.** an ovum or a spermatozoon. See also **meiosis. —gametic,** *adj.*

**gamete intrafallopian transfer (GIFT),**   a human fertilization technique in which male and female gametes are injected through a laparoscope into the fimbriated ends of the fallopian tubes.

**gametic** /gəmat'ik/,   pertaining to a reproductive cell such as a spermatozoon or ovum forming the gamete.

**gametic chromosome,**   any of the chromosomes contained in a haploid cell, specifically a spermatozoon or an ovum, as contrasted with those in a diploid, or somatic, cell.

**gameto-, gamet-,**   combining form meaning 'reproductive cell': *gametocyte, gametophore, gametogenesis.*

**gametocide** /gəmē'tōsīd/ [Gk, *gamete* + L, *caedere,* to kill],   any agent that is destructive to gametes or gametocytes. The term is most often used to refer to agents specific for gametocytes of the protozoon *Plasmodium,* which causes malaria. **—gametocidal,** *adj.*

**gametocyte** /gəmē'tōsīt/ [Gk, *gamete* + *kytos,* cell],   any cell capable of dividing into or in the process of developing into a gamete.

**gametogenesis** /gam'itōjen'əsis/ [Gk, *gamete* + *genein,* to produce],   the origin and maturation of gametes, which occurs through meiosis. See also **oogenesis, spermatogenesis. —gametogenic, gametogenous,** *adj.*

**gametophyte** /gəmē'tōfīt/ [Gk, *gamete* + *phyton,* plant],   a cell in the reproductive stage when the nuclei are in a haploid condition.

**gamma** /gam'ə/,   Γ, γ, the third letter of the Greek alphabet. It is a symbol for photon, heavy-chain immunoglobulins, or the third component in a series of certain chemical groups.

**gamma-aminobutyric acid (GABA),** an amino acid that functions as an inhibitory neurotransmitter in the brain and spinal cord. It is also found in the heart, lungs, and kidneys and in certain plants.

**gamma-benzene hexachloride.** See **lindane.**

**gamma camera** [Gk, *gamma,* third letter of Greek alphabet; L, *camera,* vault], a device that uses the emission of light from a crystal struck by gamma rays to produce an image of the distribution of radioactive material in a body organ. The light is detected by an array of light-sensitive electronic components and is converted into electric signals, which are processed to produce the image. The gamma camera is a workhorse of nuclear medicine departments, where it is used to produce scans of patients who have been injected with small amounts of radioactive materials.

**gamma efferent fiber** [Gk, *gamma* + L, *efferre,* to carry out, *fibra,* fiber], any of the motor nerve fibers that transmit impulses from the central nervous system to the intrafusal fibers of the muscle spindle. The gamma efferent fibers are responsible for deep tendon reflexes, spasticity, and rigidity but not for the degree of contractile response. They function in regulating the sensitivity of the spindle and the total tension of the muscle.

**gamma globulin.** See **immune gamma globulin.**

**gamma-glutamyl transpeptidase (GGT),** an enzyme that appears in the serum of patients with several types of liver or gallbladder disorders, including drug hepatotoxicity, biliary tract obstruction, alcohol-induced liver disease, and liver carcinoma. Normal adult (after 45 years of age) GGT blood levels are 8 to 38 U/L.

**gamma-glutamyl transpeptidase test (GGTP),** a blood test used to detect liver cell dysfunction, which accurately indicates cholestasis, biliary obstruction, cholangitis, or cholecystitis. It can also detect chronic alcohol ingestion and therefore is useful in the screening or evaluation of patients with alcoholism. Levels of this enzyme are also elevated after acute myocardial infarction.

**gamma interferon.** See **interferon gamma.**

**gamma knife,** an apparatus for producing intracranial lesions by precisely aimed intersecting beams of gamma rays; used in stereotactic radiosurgery.

**gamma knife stereotaxic radiosurgery,** a method for destroying deep-seated brain tumors with a focused beam of gamma radiation. By using three-dimensional stereoscopic techniques to aim the radiation from several angles, it is possible to concentrate the energy on the tumor while minimizing damage to surrounding tissues.

**gamma radiation** [Gk, *gamma* + L, *radiare,* to emit rays], a very high-frequency form of electromagnetic radiation consisting of photons emitted by radioactive elements in the course of nuclear transition. The wavelength of gamma radiation is characteristic of the radioactive elements involved and ranges from about $4 \times 10^{-10}$ to $5 \times 10^{-13}$ m. Gamma radiation can penetrate thousands of meters of air and several centimeters of soft tissue and bone. It is more penetrating than alpha radiation and beta radiation but has less ionizing power and is not deflected in electric or magnetic fields. Like x radiation, gamma radiation can injure and destroy body cells and tissue, especially cell nuclei. However, controlled application of gamma radiation is important in the diagnosis and treatment of various conditions, including skin cancer and malignancies deep within the body. Also called **gamma rays.** See also **x-rays.**

**gamma ray.** See **gamma radiation.**

**gammopathy** /gamop′əthē/, an abnormal condition characterized by the presence of markedly increased levels of gamma globulin in the blood. Two different types of hypergammaglobulinemia can be distinguished. **Monoclonal gammopathy** is commonly associated with an electrophoretic pattern showing one sharp, homogenous electrophoretic band in the gamma globulin region. This reflects the presence of excessive amounts of one type of immunoglobulin secreted by a single clone of B cells. **Polyclonal gammopathy** reflects the presence of a diffuse hypergammaglobulinemia in which all immunoglobulin classes are proportionally increased. See also **Bence Jones protein, multiple myeloma.**

**gamo-, gam-,** combining form meaning 'marriage or sexual union': *gamobium, gamont, gamophagia.*

**gamogenesis** /gam′ōjen′əsis/ [Gk, *gamos,* marriage, *genein,* to produce], sexual reproduction through the fusion of gametes. **—gamogenetic,** *adj.*

**gamone** /gam′ōn/ [Gk, *gamos,* marriage], a chemical substance secreted by ova and spermatozoa that is believed to attract the gametes of the opposite sex to and facilitate union. Kinds of gamones are **androgamone** and **gynogamone.**

**gampsodactyly.** See **pes cavus.**

**-gamy,** 1. suffix meaning a '(specified) type of marriage': *endogamy, monogamy, pedogamy.* 2. suffix meaning 'possession of organs for reproduction': *cleistogamy, dichogamy, homogamy.* 3. suffix meaning a 'union for propagation': *hologamy, macrogamy, syngamy.*

**ganciclovir** /gansik′lōvir/, an acrylic nucleoside structurally related to acyclovir. It is used to prevent cytomegalovirus disease after allogenic bone marrow transplantation and in persons with acquired immunodeficiency syndrome.

**gangli-.** See **ganglio-.**

**ganglia.** See **ganglion.**

**gangliated.** See **ganglionated.**

**ganglio-, gangli-,** combining form meaning 'ganglion': *gangliocytoma, ganglioneuroma, ganglioplexus.*

**gangliocytoma** /gang′glē-ō′sītō′mə/, a benign tumor involving ganglion cells. These tumors are frequently found in the pituitary gland, where they are associated with hypersecretion of growth hormone–releasing hormone (ganglioneuroma).

**ganglion** /gang′glē-on/, *pl.* **ganglia** [Gk, knot], 1. a knot or knotlike mass of nervous tissue. 2. one of the nerve cell bodies, chiefly collected in groups outside the central nervous system. Very small groups abound in association with alimentary organs. The two types of ganglia in the body are the sensory ganglia on the dorsal roots of spinal nerves and on the sensory roots of the trigeminal, facial, glossopharyngeal, and vagus nerves and the autonomic ganglia of the sympathetic and parasympathetic systems.

**ganglionar neuroma** /gang·glē′ənər/ [Gk, *ganglion* + *neuron,* nerve, *oma,* tumor], a tumor composed of a solid mass of ganglia and nerve fibers. Usually found in abdominal tissues, the tumor occurs most commonly in children. Chemotherapy or surgery is often recommended. Also called **ganglionated neuroma, ganglionic neuroma.**

**ganglionated,** having ganglia. Also **gangliated.**

**ganglionated nerve,** a nerve of the sympathetic nervous system.

**ganglionated neuroma.** See **ganglionar neuroma.**

**ganglionic blockade** /gang′glē-on′ik/, the blocking of nerve impulses at synapses of autonomic ganglia, usually by the administration of ganglionic blocking agents.

**ganglionic blocking agent,** any one of a group of drugs prescribed to produce controlled hypotension, as required in certain surgical procedures or in emergency management of hypertensive crisis. The drugs act by occupying receptor sites on sympathetic and parasympathetic nerve endings of autonomic ganglia, preventing response of these nerves to the action of acetylcholine liberated by the presynaptic nerve endings. Trimethaphan and mecamylamine are the most commonly prescribed ganglionic blocking agents. They are used with great caution in treating patients who are affected with coronary, cerebrovascular, or renal insufficiency or who have a history of severe allergy. Adverse reactions to the drugs include sudden marked hypotension, paralytic ileus, urinary retention, constipation, visual disturbances, heartburn, and nausea.

**ganglionic crest.**    See **neural crest.**

**ganglionic glioma** [Gk, *ganglion* + *glia*, glue, *oma*, tumor], a tumor composed of glial cells and ganglion cells that are nearly mature. See also **neuroblastoma.**

**ganglionic neuroma.**    See **ganglionar neuroma.**

**ganglionic ridge.**    See **neural crest.**

**ganglionitis** /gang′glē·ənī′tis/, an inflammation of a nerve or lymph ganglion.

**ganglioside** /gang′glē·əsīd′/, a glycosphingolipid found in the brain and other nervous system tissues. Gangliosides are members of a group of galactose-containing cerebrosides with a basic composition of ceramide-glucose-galactose-*N*-acetyl neuraminic acid. Accumulation of gangliosides caused by an inborn error of metabolism results in gangliosidosis or Tay-Sachs disease.

**gangliosidosis type I.**    See **Tay-Sachs disease.**

**gangliosidosis type II.**    See **Sandhoff's disease.**

**gang rape,** sexual intercourse against the will of the victim by a group of assailants. Gang sex attacks usually but not always are committed by several males who take turns assaulting a female, but the victim may be another male, as in a prison. See also **rape, statutory rape.**

**gangrene** /gang′grēn/ [Gk, *gangraina*, a gnawing sore], necrosis or death of tissue, usually the result of ischemia (loss of blood supply), bacterial invasion, and subsequent putrefaction. The extremities are most often affected, but it can occur in the intestines and gallbladder. Internally gangrene may be a complication of strangulated hernia, appendicitis, cholecystitis, or thrombosis of the mesenteric arteries to the gut. **Dry gangrene** is a late complication of diabetes mellitus that is already complicated by arteriosclerosis, in which the affected extremity becomes cold, dry, and shriveled and eventually turns black. **Moist gangrene** may

follow a crushing injury or an obstruction of blood flow by an embolism, tight bandages, or a tourniquet. This form of gangrene has an offensive odor, spreads rapidly, and may result in death in a few days. In all types of gangrene surgical debridement is necessary to remove the necrotic tissue before healing can progress. Cleanliness and maintenance of good circulation are nursing considerations essential in preventing this condition. See also **gas gangrene, open amputation. —gangrenous,** *adj.*

**gangrenous appendicitis** /gang′grənəs/ [Gk, *gangraina,* a gnawing sore; L, *appendere,* to hang upon, Gk, *itis,* inflammation], a condition in which the appendix becomes gangrenous because obstruction of its lumen blocks the flow of blood to that body part.

**gangrenous necrosis.**    See **necrosis.**

**gangrenous stomatitis.**    See **noma.**

**gangrenous vulvitis** [Gk, *gaggraina* + L, *vulva,* wrapper; Gk, *itis,* inflammation], the death of tissues in the area of the vulva that results when an inadequate blood supply causes sloughing of cells.

**ganirelix,** a gonadotropin-releasing hormone antagonist.
- ■ INDICATIONS: This drug is used to inhibit premature luteinizing hormone surges in women undergoing controlled ovarian hyperstimulation.
- ■ CONTRAINDICATIONS: Pregnancy, lactation, latex allergy, and known hypersensitivity to this drug prohibit its use.
- ■ ADVERSE EFFECTS: Fetal death is a life-threatening consequence of this drug's use. Other adverse effects of ganirelix include headache, ovarian hyperstimulation syndrome, gynecologic abdominal pain, nausea, and pain on injection. Common side effects include spotting and breakthrough bleeding.

**ganja.**    See **cannabis.**

**Gantanol,** trademark for a sulfa antibiotic (sulfamethoxazole).

**Gantrisin,** trademark for a sulfa antibiotic (sulfisoxazole).

**gantry assembly** /gan′trē/, a subsystem of the computed tomography apparatus consisting of the x-ray tube, the detector array, the high-voltage generator, the patient support and positioning couch, and the mechanical support for each.

**gap** [OE, *gapa,* a hole], a short, missing segment in one strand of a DNA molecule.

**gap junction,** a type of junction between cells; it consists of a narrowed portion of the intercellular space that contains channels or pores composed of hexagonal arrays of membrane-spanning proteins around a central lumen (connexon), through which pass ions and small molecules. In electrically excitable tissues such as myocardial tissue and the central nervous system, gap junctions serve to transmit electrical impulses via movement of ions and are known as **electrotonic synapses.** Also called **nexus.** See also **connexon.**

**gap phenomenon,** a situation in which a premature cardiac stimulus encounters a block where an earlier or later stimulus could be conducted.

**Garamycin,** trademark for an aminoglycoside antiinfective (gentamicin sulfate).

**Gardner-Diamond syndrome** [Frank H. Gardner, American physician, b. 1919; Louis K. Diamond, American physician, b. 1902], a condition resulting from autoerythrocyte sensitization, marked by large, painful transient skin discolorations that appear without apparent cause but often accompany emotional upsets, various collagen disorders, and abnormalities of protein metabolism. Treatment includes topical and systemic corticosteroids. Also called **autoerythrocyte sensitization syndrome.**

*Gardnerella vaginalis* /gärd′nərel′ə/ [Herman L. Gardner,

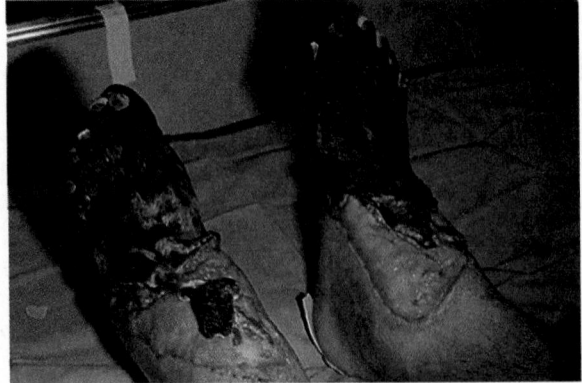

**Gangrene** *(Auerbach, 1995/courtesy Cameron Bangs, MD)*

twentieth-century American bacteriologist; L, *vagina, sheath*], a genus of rod-shaped gram-negative bacteria normally found in the female genital tract. The bacteria, formerly identified as *Haemophilus vaginalis,* may also be a marker for bacterial vaginosis.

**Gardnerella vaginalis vaginitis** [Herman L. Gardner, L, *vagina,* sheath; Gk, *itis,* inflammation], a chronic inflammation of the vagina caused by a bacterium, *Gardnerella vaginalis.* Also called **vulvovaginitis.**

**Gardner, Mary Sewell** (1871–1961), an American public health nurse who wrote the classic *Public Health Nurse.* She directed the Providence, Rhode Island, District Nursing Association and was instrumental in the development of the National Organization for Public Health Nursing and of public health nursing in the American Red Cross.

**Gardner's syndrome** [Eldon J. Gardner, American geneticist, b. 1909], familial polyposis of the large bowel, with fibrous dysplasia of the skull, extra teeth, osteomas, fibromas, and epidermal cysts. The condition is inherited as a dominant trait, and malignancies occur more often than usual in families having this syndrome.

**Gardner-Wells tongs,** pins that are attached to the skull of patients immobilized with cervical injuries. The pins are used to apply traction to reduce a fracture or dislocation while the patient is in a bed with a traction setup.

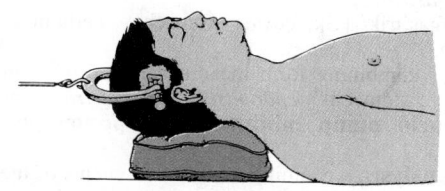

**Gardner-Wells tongs** *(Beare and Myers, 1998)*

**gargle** /gär′gəl/ [Fr, *gargouille,* drainpipe], **1.** to hold and agitate a liquid at the back of the throat by tilting the head backward and forcing air through the solution. The procedure is used for cleansing or medicating the mouth and oropharynx. **2.** a solution used to rinse the mouth and oropharynx.

**gargoylism.** See **Hurler's syndrome.**

**garlic,** an herbal product taken from a perennial bulb grown throughout the world.

■ USES: This herb is used for vascular disease, elevated LDL, elevated triglycerides, low HDL, high blood pressure, poor circulation, risk of cancer, inflammatory disorders, childhood ear infection, and yeast infection.

■ CONTRAINDICATIONS: Garlic should not be used during pregnancy, since it may stimulate labor, or during lactation, since it may cause colic in infants. It is also contraindicated in those with known hypersensitivity, stomach inflammation, gastritis, and hypothyroidism (since garlic may reduce iodine uptake). People who have had or are about to have surgery should also avoid it, since clotting time may be increased.

**GARS,** abbreviation for **Gait Assessment Rating Scale.**

**Gartner's duct** [Hermann T. Gartner, Danish anatomist, 1785–1827], one of two vestigial closed ducts, each parallel to a uterine tube.

**gas** [Gk, *chaos*], an aeriform fluid that possesses complete molecular mobility and the property of indefinite expansion.

A gas has no definite shape, and its volume is determined by its container and by temperature and pressure. Compare **liquid, solid.**

**gas bacillus** [Gk, *chaos* + L, *bacillum,* small rod], any of several species of bacillus that produce a gas as a by-product of their metabolism. Examples include *Escherichia coli,* which ferments lactose and glucose, and the clostridial species that produce gas gangrene.

**gas chromatography,** the separation and analysis of different substances according to their different affinities for a standard absorbent. In the process a gaseous mixture of the substances is passed through a glass cylinder containing the absorbent, which may be dampened with a nonvolatile liquid solvent for one or more of the gaseous components. As the mixture passes through the absorbent, each substance is absorbed to a different extent and leaves a characteristic pigment. The bands of different colors left when all the gaseous mixture has moved through the absorbent constitute a chromatograph for analysis. Compare **column chromatography, ion exchange chromatography.**

**gas distension.** See **flatulence.**

**gas embolism,** an occlusion of one or more small blood vessels, especially in the muscles, tendons, and joints, caused by expanding gas bubbles. Gas emboli can rupture tissue and blood vessels, causing decompression sickness and death. This phenomenon commonly affects deep-sea divers who rise too quickly to the surface without adequate decompression. Gas emboli are most dangerous in the central nervous system because of associated neurologic changes, such as syncope, paralysis, and aphasia. Such emboli are extremely painful. The prevention and treatment of gas emboli involve gradual decompression of atmospheric gases, especially nitrogen, that are dissolved in the blood. See also **air embolism, decompression sickness, embolism.**

**gas endarterectomy.** See **endarterectomy.**

**gaseous** /gas′ē·əs, gash′əs/ [Gk, *chaos*], pertaining to or resembling gas.

**gas exchange, impaired,** a nursing diagnosis accepted by the Fourth National Conference on the Classification of Nursing Diagnoses. Impaired gas exchange is the state in which the individual experiences a decreased passage of oxygen and/or carbon dioxide between the alveoli of the lungs and the vascular system.

■ DEFINING CHARACTERISTICS: The defining characteristics are confusion, restlessness, irritability, somnolence, inability to move secretions, hypercapnia, and hypoxia.

■ RELATED FACTORS: Related factors include altered oxygen supply, alveolar capillary membrane changes, altered blood flow, and altered oxygen-carrying capacity of the blood. See also **nursing diagnosis.**

**gas gangrene,** necrosis accompanied by gas bubbles in soft tissue after surgery or trauma. It is caused by anaerobic organisms, such as various species of *Clostridium,* particularly *C. perfringens.* Symptoms include pain, swelling, and tenderness of the wound area; moderate fever; tachycardia; and hypotension. The skin around the wound becomes necrotic and ruptures, revealing necrotic muscle. A characteristic finding is toxic delirium. If untreated, gas gangrene is rapidly fatal. Prompt treatment, including excision of gangrenous tissue and IV administration of penicillin G, saves 80% of patients. The disease is prevented by proper wound care. Also called **anaerobic myositis.**

**gasoline poisoning.** See **petroleum distillate poisoning.**

**gas pains.** See **flatulence.**

**gas-scavenging system,** the equipment used to prevent waste anesthetic gases from escaping into the atmosphere of the operating room. See also **trace gas.**

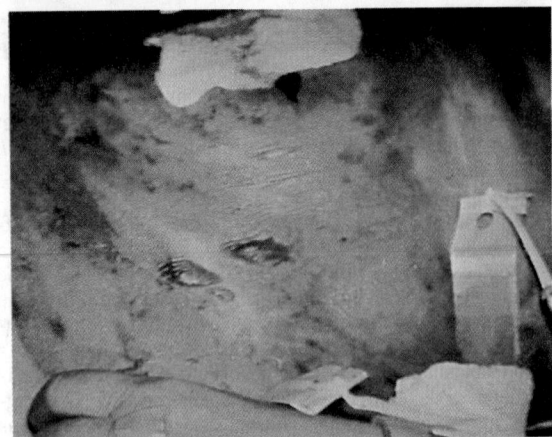

**Gas gangrene** *(Baron, Peterson, and Finegold, 1994)*

**Gasser's syndrome.**   See **hemolytic uremic syndrome.**

**gas sterilization** [Gk, *chaos*, gas; L, *sterilis*, barren],   the use of a gas such as ethylene oxide, $C_2H_4O$, to sterilize medical equipment.

**Gastaut's disease.**   See **Lennox-Gastaut syndrome.**

**gaster-, gastr-.**   See **gastro-.**

**gas therapy,**   the use of medical gases in respiratory therapy. Kinds of gas therapy include **carbon dioxide therapy, controlled oxygen therapy, helium therapy,** and **hyperbaric oxygenation.**

**gastralgia.**   See **stomach ache.**

**gastrectasia** /gas'trektā'zhə/ [Gk, *gaster*, stomach, *ektasis*, stretching],   an abnormal dilation of the stomach. It may be accompanied by pain, vomiting, rapid pulse, and falling body temperature. Causes can include overeating, obstruction of the pyloric valve, or a hernia.

**gastrectomy** /gastrek'təmē/,   surgical excision of all or, more commonly, part of the stomach. It is performed to remove a chronic peptic ulcer, to stop hemorrhage in a perforating ulcer, or to remove a malignancy. Before surgery a GI series is done, and a nasogastric tube is inserted. With the patient under general anesthesia one half to two thirds of the stomach is removed, including the ulcer and a large area of acid-secreting mucosa. A gastroenterostomy is then done, joining the remainder of the stomach to the jejunum or duodenum. After surgery the nurse observes the drainage from the nasogastric suction tube for bright red blood, indicative

of hemorrhage. Blockage of the tube is reported at once, because gastric distension strains the suture lines. Irrigation is done only according to surgeon's orders, gently and with small amounts of fluid, if at all. Adequate medication for pain allows deeper breathing and coughing because the incision is close to the diaphragm. The nurse encourages the patient to breathe deeply and if necessary to cough. With the return of peristalsis water is given orally, and, if tolerated without pain or nausea, the nasogastric tube is removed. The diet gradually progresses to six small bland meals a day with 120 mL of fluid hourly between meals. A temperature elevation or dyspnea may indicate leakage of oral fluids from the incision around the anastomosis. The most common complication of gastrectomy is dumping syndrome, with fullness and discomfort after meals. Other possible complications include marginal peptic ulcer, in which gastric acids come into contact with a suture line; afferent loop syndrome, in which the duodenal loop is blocked and pancreatic juices and bile flow back into the stomach; vitamin $B_{12}$ and folic acid deficiency; reduced absorption of calcium and vitamin D; and functional hyperinsulinism in which carbohydrates now passing directly into the small bowel cause an outpouring of insulin into the bloodstream and a resultant hypoglycemia within 2 hours. See also **dumping syndrome, gastroenterostomy, nasogastric tube, peptic ulcer.**

**-gastria,**   combining form meaning '(condition of) possessing a stomach or stomachs': *atretogastria, macrogastria, megalogastria.*

**gastric** /gas'trik/ [Gk, *gaster*, stomach],   pertaining to the stomach.

**-gastric,**   combining form meaning a 'type of stomach or number of stomachs': *endogastric, paragastric, trigastric.*

**gastric acid pump inhibitor.**   See **proton pump inhibitor.**

**gastric analysis,**   examination of the contents of the stomach, primarily to determine the quantity of acid present and incidentally to ascertain the presence of blood, bile, bacteria, and abnormal cells. It may also be done to detect acid-fast bacillus in a client with undiagnosed tuberculosis. A sample of gastric secretion is obtained via a nasogastric tube. The technique used varies according to the information desired. The total absence of hydrochloric acid is diagnostic of pernicious anemia. Patients with gastric ulcer and gastric cancer may secrete less acid than normal, whereas patients with duodenal ulcers secrete more. The composition and volume of the secretions may also provide diagnostic information. This procedure is rarely performed.

**gastric antacid.**   See **antacid.**

**gastric atrophy.**   See **atrophic gastritis.**

**gastric cancer,**   a malignancy of the stomach. Approximately 97% of stomach tumors are adenocarcinomas, which may be ulcerating, polypoid, diffuse, and fibrous, or superficial spreading lesions; lymphomas and leiomyosarcomas account for less than 3%. Symptoms of gastric cancer are vague epigastric discomfort, dysphagia, anorexia, weight loss, and unexplained iron deficiency anemia; however, many cases are asymptomatic in the early stages, and metastases may cause the first symptoms. Diagnostic measures include a test for occult blood in the stool, a upper GI series, a computed tomographic examination of the gastric mucosa with a flexible endoscope, and biopsy and cytologic studies of exfoliated tumor cells. Surgery is usually recommended for suitable lesions. Radiotherapy and chemotherapy are usually not effective in adenocarcinoma but are often used in gastric lymphoma; chemotherapy is used in treating advanced metastatic gastric adenocarcinoma. Gastric cancer is declining in incidence in North America and Western Eu-

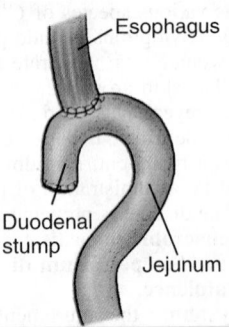

Esophagus

Duodenal
stump

Jejunum

**Total gastrectomy** *(Monahan and Neighbors, 1998)*

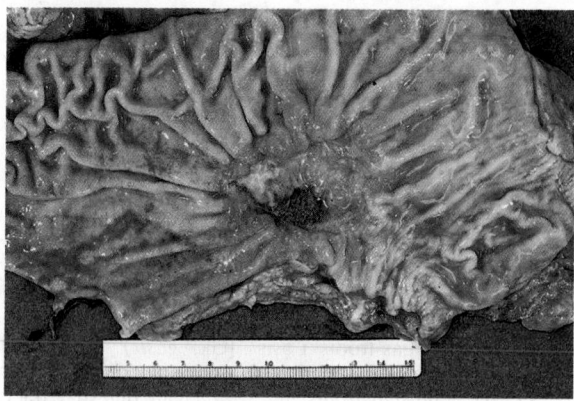

**Gastric cancer** *(Kumar, Cotran, and Robbins, 1997)*

rope but is common in Japan. Dietary factors, such as nitrates, smoked and salted fish and meats, moldy foods containing aflatoxin, and infection with *Helicobacter pylori* are thought to cause gastric cancer, but the cause remains unknown. The incidence is higher in men than in women and peaks in individuals 50 to 59 years of age. The risk increases in workers exposed to asbestos and in patients with pernicious anemia.

**gastric digestion** [Gk, *gaster,* stomach; L, *digere,* to separate], digestion by gastric juice in the stomach.

**gastric dyspepsia,** pain or discomfort localized in the stomach. See also **dyspepsia.**

**gastric emesis** [Gk, *gaster,* stomach, *emesis,* vomiting], vomiting associated with a stomach disorder, such as stomach cancer, stomach ulcer, or severe gastritis.

**gastric fistula,** an abnormal passage into the stomach, communicating most frequently with an opening on the external surface of the abdomen. A gastric fistula may be created surgically to provide tube feeding for patients with severe esophageal disorders. See also **gastrostomy, gastrostomy feeding.**

**gastric glands,** glands in the stomach mucosa that secrete hydrochloric acid, mucin, and pepsinogen.

**gastric inhibitory polypeptide (GIP),** a GI hormone found in the mucosa of the small intestine. Release of the hormone, mediated by the presence of glucose or fatty acids in the duodenum, results in the release of insulin by the pancreas and inhibition of gastric acid secretion.

**gastric intubation,** a procedure in which a Levin tube or other small-caliber catheter is passed through the nose into the esophagus and stomach. It may also be used for the introduction into the stomach of liquid formulas to provide nutrition for unconscious patients or for premature or sick newborns. Medication or a contrast medium may be instilled for treatment or for radiologic examination. See also **gastric lavage, Levin tube.**

**gastric juice,** digestive secretions of the gastric glands in the stomach, consisting chiefly of pepsin, hydrochloric acid, rennin, and mucin. The pH is strongly acid (0.9 to 1.5). Achlorhydria (a deficiency of hydrochloric acid in gastric juice) is present in pernicious anemia and stomach cancer. Excessive secretion of gastric juice may lead to mucosal irritation and peptic ulcer. See also **achlorhydria, gastric analysis, gastric ulcer.**

**gastric lavage,** the washing out of the stomach with sterile water or a saline solution. The procedure is performed before and after surgery to remove irritants or toxic substances and possibly before such examinations as endoscopy or gastroscopy. See also **irrigation.**

**gastric motility,** the spontaneous peristaltic movements of the stomach that aid in digestion, moving food through the stomach and out through the pyloric sphincter into the duodenum. Excess gastric motility causes pain that is usually treated with antispasmodic medication. Below normal motility is common in labor, after general anesthesia, and as a side effect of some sedative hypnotics.

**gastric mucin** [Gk, *gaster,* stomach; L, *mucus*], a viscous secretion of glycoproteins produced from the mucous membrane lining of swine stomachs and formerly used in the treatment of peptic ulcers.

**gastric node,** a node in one of three groups of lymph glands associated with the abdominal and pelvic viscera supplied by branches of the celiac artery. The gastric nodes accompany the left gastric artery and are divided into the superior and inferior gastric nodes. Compare **hepatic node, pancreaticolienal node.**

**gastric resection** [Gk, *gaster,* stomach; L, *re + secare,* to cut], the surgical removal of part or all of the stomach, usually performed in the treatment of stomach cancer or intractable peptic ulcer. See also **gastrectomy, gastroenterostomy.**

**gastric tetany.** See **tetany.**

**gastric ulcer.** See **peptic ulcer.**

**gastrin** /gas′trin/ [Gk, *gaster,* stomach], a polypeptide hormone, secreted by the pylorus, that stimulates the flow of gastric juice and contributes to the stimulus for bile and pancreatic enzyme secretion. Normal findings of blood levels of gastrin are less than 200 pg/mL.

**gastrinoma** /gas′trinō′mə/, a tumor found in the pancreas and in the duodenum. It is associated with the presence of peptic ulcers.

**gastrin-releasing peptide,** a 27-amino acid linear neuropeptide structurally and functionally related to bombesin; it mediates neural release of antral gastrin, causes bronchoconstriction and respiratory tract vasodilation, stimulates growth and mitogenesis of cells in culture, and may act as an excitatory neurotransmitter of enteric interneurons.

**gastrin test,** a blood test used to help identify patients with Zollinger-Ellison (ZE) syndrome and G-cell hyperplasia, who typically have high serum gastrin levels. Test results can help the clinician institute appropriate, aggressive medical and surgical therapy for these patients.

**gastritis** /gastrī′tis/, an inflammation of the lining of the stomach that occurs in two forms. **Acute gastritis** may be caused by severe burns, major surgery, aspirin or other antiinflammatory agents (nonsteroidal antiinflammatory drugs), corticosteroids, drugs, food allergens, or viral, bacterial, or chemical toxins. The symptoms—anorexia, nausea, vomiting, and discomfort after eating—usually abate after the causative agent has been removed. **Chronic gastritis** is usually a sign of underlying disease, such as peptic ulcer, stomach cancer, Zollinger-Ellison syndrome, or pernicious anemia. Differential diagnosis is by endoscopy with biopsy. Kinds of gastritis include **atrophic gastritis, hemorrhagic gastritis,** and **hypertrophic gastritis.** Compare **peptic ulcer.**

**gastro-, gaster-, gastr-,** combining form meaning 'stomach or abdomen': *gastroadynamia, gastrocolitis, gastrophrenic.*

**gastrocamera** /gas′trōkam′ərə/, a small camera that can be lowered into the stomach through the esophagus and retrieved after recording images of the stomach lining.

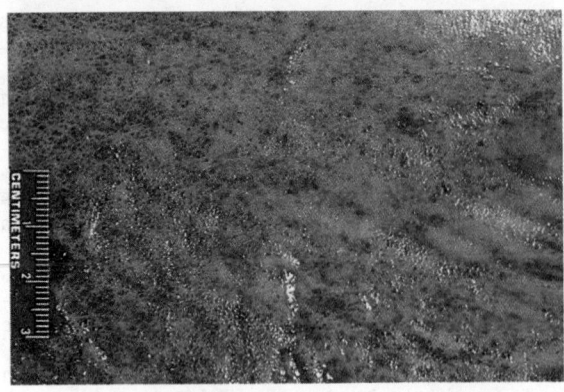

**Acute gastritis** *(Cotran, Kumar, and Collins, 1999)*

**gastrocnemius** /gas'trōnē'me·us/ [Gk, *gastroknemia,* calf of the leg], the most superficial calf muscle in the posterior part of the leg. It joins the tendon of the soleus as part of the tendo calcaneus. Compare **soleus, plantaris.**

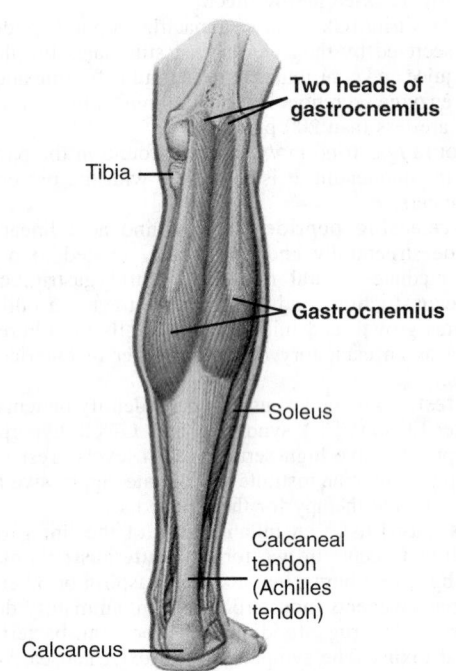

**Gastrocnemius** *(Thibodeau and Patton, 1999/John V. Hagen)*

**gastrocnemius gait,** an abnormal gait associated with a weakness of the gastrocnemius. It is characterized by the dropping of the pelvis on the affected side at the last moment of the stance phase in the walking cycle, accompanied by lagging or slowness in forward pelvic movement.

**gastrocnemius test,** a test of the function of the gastrocnemius muscle by ankle plantar flexion while the patient is in a prone position. The examiner places fingers for palpation on the posterior of the calf while the patient pulls the heel upward, thus plantar flexing the ankle. Flexion of the toes and forefoot before movement of the heel is evidence of muscle substitution.

**gastrocoele.** See **archenteron.**

**gastrocolic omentum.** See **greater omentum.**

**gastrocolic reflex** /-kol'ik/ [Gk, *gaster* + *kolon,* colon; L, *reflectere,* to bend backward], a mass peristaltic movement of the colon that often occurs 15 to 20 minutes after food enters the stomach. When an infant is fed, this reflex may cause bowel movement.

**gastrodidymus** /-did'iməs/ [Gk, *gaster* + *didymos,* twin], conjoined, equally developed twins united at the abdominal region. Also called **omphalodidymus.**

**gastrodisciasis** /gas'trōdiskī'əsis/ [Gk, *gaster* + *diskos,* disk, *eidos,* form, *osis,* condition], an infection of trematodes of the genus *Gastrodiscoides,* which are digestive tract parasites. The species *G. hominis,* a reddish-orange fluke averaging 1 cm in length, is endemic in the hog populations of Southeast Asia and is transmitted to humans.

**gastrodisk.** See **embryonic disk.**

**gastroduodenal** /-dōō'ədē'nəl/ [Gk, *gaster* + L, *duodeni,* 12 fingers], pertaining to the stomach and duodenum.

**gastroduodenitis** /-dōō'ədenī'tis/ [Gk, *gaster,* stomach; L, *duodeni,* 12 fingers; Gk, *itis,* inflammation], inflammation of the stomach and duodenum.

**gastroduodenoscopy** /-dōō'ədenos'kəpē/, inspection of the stomach and duodenum by means of a gastroscope passed through the oral cavity and esophagus or through an incision in the abdominal wall.

**gastroduodenostomy** /-dōō'ədenos'təmē/, surgical establishment of a passageway between the stomach and the duodenum. It may be done, for example, to bypass a pyloric obstruction.

**gastrodynia.** See **stomach ache.**

**gastroenteritis** /gas'trō·en'tərī'tis/ [Gk, *gaster* + *enteron,* intestine, *itis,* inflammation], inflammation of the stomach and intestines accompanying numerous GI disorders. Symptoms are anorexia, nausea, vomiting, fever (depending on causative factor), abdominal discomfort, and diarrhea. The condition may be attributed to bacterial enterotoxins, bacterial or viral invasion, chemical toxins, or miscellaneous conditions, such as lactose intolerance. The onset may be slow, but more often it is abrupt and violent, with rapid loss of fluids and electrolytes caused by persistent vomiting and diarrhea. Hypokalemia and hyponatremia, acidosis, or alkalosis may develop. Treatment is supportive, using bed rest, sedation, IV replacement of electrolytes, and antispasmodic medication to control vomiting and diarrhea. With a precise diagnosis medication and treatment can be specific and curative, such as an antitoxin prescribed for gastroenteritis resulting from a bacterial endotoxin. After the acute phase water may begiven by mouth. If it produces no vomiting or diarrhea, clear fluids may be added, followed, if tolerated, by a diet of foods that appeal to the patient and do not cause symptoms. Also called **enterogastritis.**

**gastroenterologist** /gas'trō·en'tərol'əjist/, a physician who specializes in diseases affecting the GI tract.

**gastroenterology** /gas'trō·en'tərol'əjē/ [Gk, *gaster* + *enteron,* intestine, *logos,* science], the study of diseases affecting the GI tract, including the stomach, intestines, gallbladder, and bile duct.

**gastroenterostomy** /gas'trō·en'təros'təmē/ [Gk, *gaster* + *enteron,* intestine, *stoma,* mouth], surgical formation of an artificial opening between the stomach and the small intestine, usually at the jejunum. The operation is performed with a gastrectomy to route food from the remainder of the stomach into the small intestine or alone to treat a perforating ulcer of the duodenum. A GI series is done before surgery, and a nasogastric tube is inserted. The jejunum is pulled up and anastomosed with the stomach. A new opening is then made for food to pass from the stomach directly into the jejunum. Pancreatic juices and bile are still secreted into the duodenum and pass through its distal end to the jejunum. After surgery complications and care are the same as for gastrectomy. Compare **gastrectomy.**

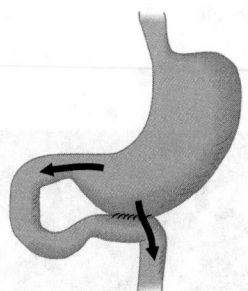

**Gastroenterostomy** *(Black, Hawks, and Keene, 2001)*

**gastroesophageal** /gas′trō·isof′əjē′əl/ [Gk, *gaster* + *oisophagos*, gullet], pertaining to the stomach and esophagus.

**gastroesophageal hemorrhage.** See **Mallory-Weiss syndrome.**

**gastroesophageal reflux,** a backflow of contents of the stomach into the esophagus that is often the result of incompetence of the lower esophageal sphincter. Gastric juices are acid and therefore produce burning pain in the esophagus. Repeated episodes of reflux may cause esophagitis, peptic esophageal stricture, or esophageal ulcer. In uncomplicated cases treatment consists of elevation of the head of the bed, avoidance of acid-stimulating foods, and regular administration of antacids. In complicated cases surgical repair may provide relief. Also called **GERD.** See also **chalasia, esophagitis, heartburn, hiatal hernia, reflux esophagitis.**

**gastroesophageal reflux scan,** a nuclear scan that is used to evaluate patients with symptoms of heartburn, regurgitation, vomiting, and dysphagia, and to evaluate the medical or surgical treatment of patients with gastroesophageal reflux.

**gastroesophagitis** /gas′trō′isof′əjī′tis/, inflammation of the stomach and esophagus.

**gastrofiberscope** /-fī′bərskōp′/, a flexible fiber endoscope for examination of the stomach.

**gastrohepatic omentum.** See **lesser omentum.**

**gastrointestinal (GI)** /gas′trō·intes′tinəl/ [Gk, *gaster* + L, *intestinum,* intestine], pertaining to the organs of the GI tract, from mouth to anus.

**gastrointestinal (GI) allergy,** an immediate reaction of hypersensitivity of the digestive system after the ingestion of certain foods or drugs. GI allergy differs from food allergy, which can affect other organ systems. Characteristic symptoms include itching and swelling of the mouth and oral passages, nausea, vomiting, diarrhea (sometimes containing blood), severe abdominal pain, and, in severe cases, anaphylactic shock. Treatment includes identification and removal of the allergen. In an acute attack epinephrine may be administered as a stimulant, and muscle relaxants may be given to reduce intestinal spasms that cause abdominal pain.

In childhood GI allergy is most often caused by hypersensitivity to cow's milk and is characterized by diarrhea and colicky pain, sometimes with vomiting, eczema, respiratory distress, and thrombocytopenia. Compare **food allergy.** See also **lactose intolerance.**

**gastrointestinal bleeding,** any bleeding from the GI tract. The most common underlying conditions are peptic ulcer, Mallory-Weiss syndrome, esophageal varices, diverticulosis, ulcerative colitis, and carcinoma of the stomach and colon. Vomiting of bright red blood or passage of coffee ground vomitus indicates upper GI bleeding, usually from the esophagus, stomach, or upper duodenum. Aspiration of the gastric contents, lavage, and endoscopy are performed to determine the site and rate of bleeding. Tarry black stools indicate a bleeding source in the upper GI tract; bright red blood from the rectum usually indicates bleeding in the distal colon. GI bleeding is treated as a potential emergency. Patients may require transfusions, fluid replacement, or gastric lavage and are watched carefully so as to prevent shock and hypovolemia. In all patients blood loss is evaluated and ability to coagulate is tested. See also **coffee-ground vomitus, hematochezia, melena.**

**gastrointestinal bleeding scan,** a nuclear scan that is used to localize the site of bleeding in patients who are having active gastrointestinal hemorrhage. It may also be used in patients with suspected intraabdominal (nongastrointestinal) hemorrhage of unknown origin.

**gastrointestinal gas.** See **flatulence.**

**gastrointestinal infection,** any infection of the digestive tract caused by bacteria, viruses, or parasites. All may have common clinical features of nausea, vomiting, diarrhea, and anorexia. Treatment in most cases includes bed rest, ready access to a bathroom, and food and beverages to replenish loss of fluid and electrolytes.

**gastrointestinal intubation,** a nursing intervention from the Nursing Interventions Classification (NIC) defined as insertion of a tube into the gastrointestinal tract. See also **Nursing Interventions Classification.**

**gastrointestinal obstruction,** any obstruction of the passage of intestinal contents, caused by mechanical blockage or failure of motility. Mechanical blockage may be caused by adhesions resulting from surgery or inflammatory bowel disease, an incarcerated hernia, fecal impaction, tumor, intussusception, volvulus, or foreign body ingestion. Failure of motility may follow anesthesia, abdominal surgery, or occlusion of any of the mesenteric arteries to the gut. Symptoms vary with the cause of obstruction but generally include vomiting, abdominal pain, and increasing abdominal distension. Dehydration and prostration may follow. Characteristically bowel sounds are diminished or absent especially distal to the obstruction, and abdominal guarding is prominent. A barium enema may be performed, but barium is never given by mouth because it increases the volume of the obstruction. The objective of therapy is to remove the obstruction as quickly and safely as possible. A tube is inserted into the stomach or small intestine to aspirate contents and relieve distension. During these procedures the patient is monitored for proper fluid and electrolyte balance. Surgical intervention may be necessary. The nurse helps the patient to understand that medication for pain can aggravate the condition by further decreasing motility of the GI tract and that it may not be prescribed in the acute period, before the location and extent of the obstruction are discovered.

**gastrointestinal system assessment,** an evaluation of the patient's digestive system and symptoms.

■ METHOD: Discussion of symptoms is encouraged. The patient is asked whether there is or has been pain or tenderness in the oral cavity, gums, tongue, lips, abdomen, or rectum, and whether there have been instances of dysphagia, belching, heartburn, anorexia, nausea, vomiting, constipation, diarrhea, or painful defecation. Information is elicited about changes in eating; bowel habits; the color, character, and frequency of stools and urine; the use of laxatives or enemas; and the occurrence of fatigue, hemorrhoids, and edema of the extremities. The patient's general appearance, weight, and temperature are noted; the blood pressure, pulse, and respirations are checked in the supine, sitting, and standing positions; and the urinary output and color are determined. The presence of allergies, stomatitis, and halitosis and the condition of the tongue, gums, oral mucosa, and teeth are recorded. The abdomen is examined for distension, rigidity, ascites, symmetry, organomegaly, keloid tissue, visible peristalsis, bowel sounds, masses, and the presence of an ostomy. The perianal area is inspected for its general condition, color, odor, and hemorrhoids; the sclera for signs of jaundice; and the skin for pruritus, spider angioma, purpura, palmar erythema, peripheral edema, jaundice, and distended, tortuous blood vessels. Relevant to the assessment are concurrent endocrine, cardiovascular, and neurologic disorders; severe burns; psychologic problems; carcinoma; alcohol or drug abuse; and previous GI surgery and illnesses such as hepatitis, liver cirrhosis, or pancreatitis. The patient's personality type, attitude toward work, and use of tobacco, antacids, laxatives, anticholinergics, steroids, antidiarrheals, antiemetics, sedatives, tranquilizers, barbiturates, antihypertensives, antibiotics, and aspirin are investigated. The family history, especially of GI disease, carcinoma, and diabetes mellitus, is an important aspect of the evaluation. Diagnostic aids include a complete blood count, stool examination, prothrombin time, and determinations of levels of alkaline phosphatase, serum and urine bilirubin, aspartate aminotransferase, alanine aminotransferase, lactic acid dehydrogenase, blood urea nitrogen, serum lipase, cholinesterase, calcium, albumin, and glucose. Additional laboratory studies for the evaluation are the total protein level, a serum electrolyte profile; serum carotene, delta-xylose tolerance, galactose tolerance, hippuric acid, and bromsulphalein tests; the albumin-globulin ratio, serum flocculation, and thymol turbidity tests; urobilinogen level; the polyvinylpyrrolidone test for protein loss; Sulkowitch's test for calcium in urine; and Schilling's test for GI absorption of vitamin B$_{12}$. Procedures that may be required for the diagnosis include upper GI, small bowel, and gallbladder series; esophageal and gastric endoscopy and biopsy; scans of the liver and pancreas; biopsy of the liver, colon, or rectum; gastric analysis, sigmoidoscopy, abdominal x-ray films, fluoroscopy, percutaneous transhepatic cholangiography, splenoportography, and digital rectal examinations.

■ INTERVENTIONS: The physician or other health care provider conducts the interview, records observations of the patient, and assembles the results of the diagnostic laboratory studies and procedures.

**gastrointestinal tract.** See **digestive tract.**
**gastrojejunostomy.** See **Billroth's operation II.**
**gastrokinetic drugs** /-kinet'ik/, chemicals that stimulate salivation, increase lower esophageal sphincter (LES) pressure, and improve esophageal clearance in the supine but not in the upright position.
**gastromalacia** /-məlā'shə/ [Gk, *gaster,* stomach, *malakia,* softness], an abnormal softening of the walls of the stomach.
**gastromegaly** /-meg'əlē/ [Gk, *gaster* + *megas,* large], an abnormal enlargement of the stomach or abdomen.
**gastroparesis** /-pərē'sis/, failure of the stomach to empty

caused by decreased gastric motility. The major causes are various kinds of abdominal inflammation, scleroderma, diabetic autonomic neuropathy, vagotomy, and use of anticholinergic medications.
**gastroplasty** /gas'troplas'tē/ [Gk, *gaster* + *plassein,* to mold], any surgery performed to reshape or repair any stomach defect or deformity.
**gastropore.** See **blastopore.**
**gastroschisis** /gastros'kəsis/ [Gk, *gaster* + *schisis,* division], a congenital defect characterized by incomplete closure of the abdominal wall with protrusion of the viscera. Compare **omphalocele.**

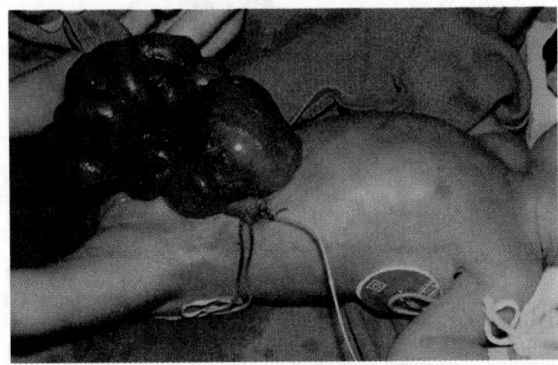

**Neonate with gastroschisis**
*(Moore, Persaud, and Shiota, 2000/courtesy Dr. A.E. Chudley, Department of Pediatrics and Child Health, University of Manitoba, Children's Hospital, Winnipeg, Canada)*

**gastroscope** /gas'trōskōp'/ [Gk, *gaster* + *skopein,* to look], a fiberoptic instrument for examining the interior of the stomach. See also **fiberoptics. gastroscopic,** *adj.*
**gastroscopy** /gastros'kəpē/, the visual inspection of the interior of the stomach by means of a gastroscope inserted through the esophagus. The flexible fiberoptic gastroscope increases the visualization of the prepyloric antrum, but the fundus is still not visible. See also **endoscopy, fiberoptics.** —**gastroscopic,** *adj.*
**gastrostomy** /gastros'təmē/ [Gk, *gaster* + *stoma,* mouth], surgical creation of an artificial opening into the stomach through the abdominal wall. It is performed to feed a patient who has esophageal cancer or tracheoesophageal fistula, who may be unconscious for a prolonged period, or who is unable to swallow as a result of a cerebrovascular accident, Alzheimer's disease, or another disorder. The anterior wall of the stomach is drawn forward and sutured to the abdominal wall. A Foley catheter or other tube or a special prosthesis is then inserted into an incision in the stomach, and the opening is tightly sutured to prevent leakage of the stomach contents. The device is clamped and is opened when liquid food supplement is instilled. After surgery glucose water may be given, followed by a slow continuous feeding of a warm blended formula to increase absorption. The skin is kept clean and dry around the site. Skin irritation indicates leakage of gastric secretions and digestive enzymes. After 2 weeks the tube may be withdrawn after feeding and reinserted before the next meal.

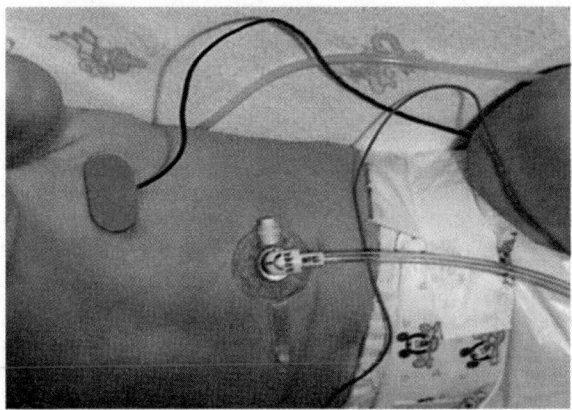

**Gastrostomy device** *(Wong, 1993)*

**gastrostomy feeding,** the introduction of a nutrient solution through a tube that has been surgically inserted into the stomach through the abdominal wall. See also **enteral tube feeding.**

**gastrostomy tube.** See **stomach tube.**

**gastrothoracopagus** /gas'trōthôr'əkop'əgəs/ [Gk, *gaster* + *thorax,* chest, *pagos,* fixture], conjoined twins who are united at the thorax and abdomen.

**gastrula** /gas'trŏŏlə/ [Gk, *gaster,* stomach], the early embryonic stage formed by the invagination of the blastula. The cup-shaped gastrula consists of an outer layer of ectoderm and an inner layer of mesentoderm that subsequently differentiates into the mesoderm and endoderm. See also **blastula, embryonic layer.**

**-gastrula,** combining form meaning an 'embryonic stage after the blastula': *amphigastrula, discogastrula, paragastrula.*

**gastrulation** /gas'trəlā'shən/ [Gk, *gaster,* stomach], the development of the gastrula in lower animals and the formation of the three germ layers in the embryo of humans and higher animals. It is characterized by an extensive series of coordinated morphogenetic movements within the blastula or blastocyst by which the primitive body plan of the organism is established and by which the areas that later differentiate into various structures and organs are in their proper position for development.

**Gatch bed** /gach/ [William D. Gatch, American surgeon, 1878–1961; AS, *bedd*], a bed that has an adjustable joint, allowing the knees to be flexed and the legs supported.

**gatekeeper,** a health care professional, usually a primary care physician or a physician extender, who is the patient's first contact with the health care system and triages the patient's further access to the system.

**gatekeeper effect,** a contraction of the endothelium mediated by immunoglobulin G (IgG). It permits components of the blood to gain access to the extravascular space as a result of the increased vascular permeability.

**gate theory of pain.** See **pain mechanism.**

**gateway drugs,** minor substances of abuse, such as inhalants, used in general by children or young people before they experiment with marijuana or hard drugs; entry drugs.

**gatifloxacin,** a broad-spectrum antiinfective.

■ INDICATIONS: Gatifloxacin is used to treat acute bacterial exacerbation of chronic bronchitis, acute sinusitis, community-acquired pneumonia, gonorrhea, and infections caused by susceptible *Escherichia coli, Staphylococcus au-*

*reus, Haemophilus influenzae, H. parainfluenzae, Klebsiella pneumoniae, Moraxella catarrhalis, Neisseria gonorrhoeae, Proteus mirabilis, Chlamydia pneumoniae, Legionella pneumophila,* and *Mycoplasma pneumoniae.*

■ CONTRAINDICATIONS: Known hypersensitivity to quinolones prohibits the use of gatifloxacin.

■ ADVERSE EFFECTS: Pseudomembranous colitis is a life-threatening effect of this drug. Other adverse effects include dizziness, insomnia, paresthesia, tremor, vasodilation, increased ALT and AST, pruritus, urticaria, photosensitivity, flushing, fever, and chills. Common side effects include headache, nausea, diarrhea, rash, dyspnea, and pharyngitis.

**gating,** the organizing of MRI data so that information used to construct an image originates in the same point in the cycle of a repeating movement, such as a heartbeat. The moving object is thus frozen at that phase of its movement, and image blurring is minimized.

**gating mechanism,** 1. the increasing duration of an action potential from the atrioventricular node to a point in the distal Purkinje system, beyond which it decreases. 2. a process that controls the opening and closing of cell-membrane ion channels.

**Gaucher's disease** /gôshāz'/ [Phillipe C.E. Gaucher, French physician, 1854–1918], a rare familial disorder of fat metabolism caused by an enzyme deficiency, characterized by widespread reticulum cell hyperplasia in the liver, spleen, lymph nodes, and bone marrow. Beginning in infancy or early childhood splenomegaly, hepatomegaly, and abnormal bone growth develop. Diagnosis is made through biopsy of the liver, spleen, or bone marrow. Mortality rate is high, but children who survive adolescence may live for many years. Also called **glucosyl cerebroside lipidosis.**

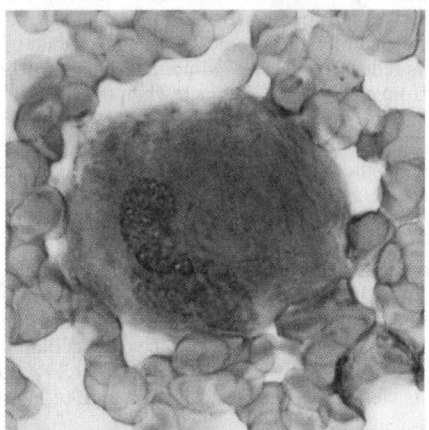

**Bone marrow smear in Gaucher's disease**
*(Carr and Rodak, 1999)*

**gauge** /gāj/ [ME], an instrument for determining physical properties of anything, including caliber, dimensions, or pressure.

**gauntlet bandage** /gônt'lit/ [Fr, *gantlet,* small glove, *bande,* strip], a glovelike bandage covering the hand and the fingers. See also **demigauntlet bandage.**

**gauss** /gôs, gous/ [J.K.F. Gauss, German physicist, 1777–1855], a unit of magnetic field strength. It is equal to $10^{-5}$ tesla.

**gauze** /gôz/ [Fr, *gaze*], a transparent fabric of open weave and differing degrees of fineness, most often cotton muslin, used in surgical procedures and for bandages and dressings. It may be sterilized and permeated by an antiseptic or lotion. Kinds of gauze include **absorbable gauze, absorbent gauze,** and **petrolatum gauze.** See also **bandage.**

**gauze sponge** [Fr, *gaze* + Gk, *spoggia*], a piece of folded gauze used during surgery to wipe up bleeding surfaces and thereby help locate any sources of blood loss.

**gavage** /gäväzh'/ [Fr, *gaver,* to gorge], the process of feeding a patient through a nasogastric tube. Also called **gavage feeding, nasogastric feeding.** See also **drip gavage, enteral tube feeding.**

**gavage feeding.** See **gavage.**

**gavage feeding of the newborn,** a procedure in which a tube passed through the nose or mouth into the stomach is used to feed a newborn with weak sucking, uncoordinated sucking and swallowing, respiratory distress, tachypnea, or repeated apneic spells.

■ METHOD: After the gastric tube is inserted, its placement is checked by radiography or by instillation of air and auscultation of the stomach for air sounds or by immersion of the proximal end of the tube in water. If the amount of residual formula left in the infant's stomach at the time of the next feeding exceeds the quantity specified, the next feeding may be delayed or omitted. Blue food coloring is often added to the gavage to distinguish gastric contents from respiratory secretions to help detect aspiration of gastric contents into the lungs. During feeding the infant is held in a low Fowler's position, preferably by the mother, and is restrained only if necessary. The feeding syringe is held 18 centimeters above the infant's head, and the flow is initiated by pressure on the plunger. As the formula is slowly instilled, the baby is stroked and is offered a pacifier to promote gravity flow, exert a calming effect, and reinforce the relationship between sucking and feeding. If the infant gags, spits, chokes, regurgitates, vomits, or becomes cyanotic, the rate of flow of formula is reduced and the feeding may be stopped. To prevent air from entering the stomach when the feeding is completed, the tube is pinched closed as it is withdrawn. The infant is burped gently by patting or rubbing the back and then positioned on the right side in the crib; postural drainage and percussion are avoided for at least 1 hour after feeding. The time, amount, and kind of feeding and the size of tube used are entered in the nursing care plan.

■ INTERVENTIONS: The nurse administers intermittent gavage feeding to the infant, explains the need for the procedure to the parents and that nipple feedings may be instituted when the infant sucks on the gavage tube or pacifier, actively seeks nourishment, shows good suck and swallow coordination, gains weight, and has a respiratory rate of less than 60 breaths per minute.

■ OUTCOME CRITERIA: Intermittent gavage feedings can enable the high-risk infant to survive.

**gay** [Fr, *gai,* merry], **1.** any person who is homosexual. **2.** pertaining to homosexuality.

**gay bowel syndrome,** a group of GI symptoms that occur most commonly in homosexual males as a consequence of oral-anal sexual practices. It is almost always caused by infection with *Shigella flexneri.* Clinical features include bloating, flatulence, diarrhea, polyps, fissures, and hemorrhoids. Sexually transmitted infections associated with the syndrome include syphilis, gonorrhea, and herpes simplex, as well as diseases caused by human papillomavirus, cytomegalovirus, *Chlamydia trachomatis,* and *Campylobacter* species.

**Gay-Lussac's law** /gä'ləsaks'/ [Joseph L. Gay-Lussac, French scientist, 1778–1850; L, *legu,* a rule], (in physics) a law stating that the volume of a specific mass of a gas increases as the temperature increases if the pressure remains constant. Also called **Charles' law.**

**Gay Nurses' Alliance (GNA),** a national organization of gay and lesbian nurses.

**gaze** /gāz/ [ME, *gazen,* to stare], a state of looking in one direction. A person with normal vision has six basic positions of gaze, each determined by control of different combinations of contractions of extraocular muscles. See also **cardinal position of gaze.**

**gaze palsy.** See **supranuclear gaze disturbance.**

**gaze paresis,** a disturbance of eye conjugate movement in which gaze tends to be tonically deviated in the direction of normal gaze. For example, in left frontal lobe damage the patient cannot voluntarily look to the right and the eyes spontaneously deviate to the left. The patient may be able to return the gaze voluntarily to the midline but cannot move the eyes past the midline into the paretic field of gaze.

**gaze test,** a test of ocular and vestibular functioning; movements of the eye are recorded with the patient gazing straight at an object and at positions off to different sides of it; then with eyes closed for 20 seconds, the patient must perform a small mental exercise. The eyes normally should assume a center gaze while they are closed.

**GB,** abbreviation for **gallbladder.**

**GBIA,** abbreviation for **Guthrie's bacterial inhibition assay.**

**g.c.,** *informal.* abbreviation for **gonococcus.**

**G-CSF,** abbreviation for **granulocyte colony-stimulating factor.**

**Gd,** symbol for the element **gadolinium.**

**GDM,** abbreviation for **gestational diabetes mellitus.**

**GDNF,** abbreviation for **glial-cell-line-derived neurotrophic factor.**

**Ge,** symbol for the element **germanium.**

**gegenhalten** /gā'gənhäl'tən/ [Ger, counterpressure], the involuntary resistance to passive movement of the extremities. It may occur as a symptom of catatonia in which there is passive resistance to stretching movements, even when the patient attempts to cooperate. The effect may be psychogenic in origin or may be a sign of dementia or cerebral deterioration. Also called **paratonia.**

**Geiger-Müller (GM) counter** /gī'gərmil'ər/ [Hans Geiger, German physicist, 1882–1945; Walther Müller, twentieth century German physicist; Fr, *conter,* to tell], an electronic device that indicates the level of radioactivity of a substance by counting the number of ionizing subatomic particles emitted by the substance. As the particles pass through a gas-filled tube inside the counter, they ionize the gas and cause an electric discharge. The tube cannot identify the type or energy of a particle. Also called **Geiger counter.**

**gel** /jel/ [L, *gelare,* to congeal], a colloid that is firm although it contains a large amount of liquid, used in many medicines as a demulcent, a vehicle for other drugs, an antacid, or an astringent, depending on the drug from which it is derived. Also called **jelly.**

**-gel,** suffix meaning 'jellylike substances' formed by cooling a colloid into a semisolid state.

**gelat-,** combining form meaning 'to freeze, congeal': *gelatigenous, gelatinoid, gelatum.*

**gelatin buildup** /jel'ətən/, an x-ray film artifact that may appear as a sharp area of either increased or reduced density.

**gelatin film, absorbable,** a hemostatic.

■ INDICATIONS: It is used to attain hemostasis during surgery, particularly neurologic, thoracic, and ophthalmic procedures.

■ CONTRAINDICATIONS: Infection or gross contamination of the surgical wound prohibits its use.

■ ADVERSE EFFECTS: There are no known adverse reactions.

**gelatiniform carcinoma.** See **mucinous carcinoma.**

**gelatinous** /jəlat'ənəs/ [L, *gelare,* to congeal], pertaining to or resembling a viscous, jellylike substance.

**gelatinous carcinoma,** a former term for **mucinous carcinoma.**

**gelatin sponge,** an absorbable local hemostatic.

■ INDICATIONS: It is prescribed to control surgical bleeding and treat pressure ulcers.

■ CONTRAINDICATIONS: Frank infection, extensive and abnormal bleeding, postpartum bleeding, or menorrhagia prohibits its use.

■ ADVERSE EFFECTS: There are no known adverse reactions.

**gel diffusion.** See **immunodiffusion.**

**gel filtration,** a method of separating molecules by size. A solution containing molecules of various sizes is passed through a filter consisting of a porous material, generally a polyacrylamide or polysaccharide. The larger molecules are excluded from the interior of the filter and thus emerge from it earlier than the smaller molecules.

**Gelfoam,** trademark for an absorbable hemostatic gelatin sponge.

**Gellhorn pessary.** See **pessary.**

**gemcitabine,** a miscellaneous antineoplastic.

■ INDICATIONS: This drug is used to treat adenocarcinoma of the pancreas (nonresectable Stages II and III or metastatic Stage IV) and non-small cell lung cancer (Stage IIIA or B and IV). It is also used in combination with cisplatin to treat inoperable, advanced, or metastatic non-small cell lung cancer.

■ CONTRAINDICATIONS: Known hypersensitivity and pregnancy prohibit this drug's use.

■ ADVERSE EFFECTS: Life-threatening effects of this drug are leukopenia, anemia, neutropenia, thrombocytopenia, and hemorrhage. Other adverse effects include diarrhea, nausea, vomiting, anorexia, constipation, stomatitis, irritation at the site of administration, rash, alopecia, dyspnea, fever, and infection.

**gemellary** /jem'əler'ē/ [L, *gemellus,* twin], pertaining to twins.

**gemellipara** /jem'əlip'ərə/ [L, *gemellus* + *parare,* to give birth], a woman who has given birth to twins.

**gemellology** /jem'əlol'əjē/ [L, *gemellus* + Gk, *logos,* science], the study of twins and the phenomenon of twinning.

**gemellus** /jəmel'əs/, either of a pair of small muscles arising from the ischium. They rotate the thigh laterally.

**gemellus test,** a test of the function of the gemellus superior and gemellus inferior in hip external rotation while the patient is seated with the knees flexed. The examiner places one hand on the lateral aspect of the knee to prevent flexion or abduction of the hip while the patient rotates the thigh outward by moving the foot medially.

**gemfibrozil** /jemfī'brəzil/, an antihyperlipidemic agent.

■ INDICATION: It is prescribed for the treatment of hyperlipidemia.

■ CONTRAINDICATIONS: Renal or hepatic dysfunction, gallbladder disease, or known hypersensitivity to this drug prohibits its use.

■ ADVERSE EFFECTS: Among the adverse reactions are abdominal or epigastric pain, urticaria, dizziness, and anemia.

**gemin-,** combining form meaning 'a twin or double': *geminate, gemini, geminous.*

**gemistocyte** /gemis'təsīt/, an astrocyte with an eccentric nucleus and swollen cytoplasm, as seen in areas of nervous tissue affected by edema, demyelination, or infarction.

**gemma** /jem'ə/, *pl.* **gemmae** [L, bud], **1.** a budlike projection produced by some organisms during budding, a type of asexual reproduction. Also called **gemmule. 2.** any budlike or bulblike structure, such as a taste bud or end bulb. —**gemmaceous,** *adj.*

**gemmate** /jem'āt/ [L, *gemma* + *atus,* function], **1.** having buds or gemmae. **2.** to reproduce by budding.

**gemmation** /jemā'shən/ [L, *gemmare,* to produce buds], the process of reproduction by budding. Also called **gemmulation.**

**gemmiferous** /jemif'ərəs/ [L, *gemma* + *fer,* bearing], having buds or gemmae; gemmiparous.

**gemmiform** /jem'ifôrm'/, resembling a bud or gemma.

**gemmipara** /jemip'ərə/ [L, *gemma* + *parare,* to give birth], an animal that produces gemmae or reproduces by budding, such as a hydra. —**gemmiparous,** *adj.*

**gemmulation.** See **gemmation.**

**gemmule.** See **gemma.**

**Gemonil,** trademark for an anticonvulsant (metharbital).

**gen-, geno-,** combining form meaning 'to become or produce': *generic, genesiology, genophobia, genus.*

**-gen, -gene, 1.** suffix meaning 'that which generates': *aerogen, proteinogen, venogen.* **2.** combining form meaning 'that which is generated': *immunogen, ionogen, nitrogen.*

**Genapax Tampon,** trademark for an antiinfective tampon containing gentian violet.

**gender** /jen'dər/ [L, *genus,* kind], **1.** the classification of the sex of a person into male, female, or ambivalent. **2.** the specific sex of a person. See also **sex.**

**gender identity,** the inner sense of maleness or femaleness. Differentiation of gender identity begins in infancy, continues throughout childhood, and is reinforced during adolescence. Also called **core gender identity.**

**gender identity disorder,** a condition characterized by a persistent feeling of discomfort or inappropriateness concerning one's anatomic sex. The disorder typically begins in childhood with gender identity problems and is manifested in adolescence or adulthood as cross-dressing.

**gender role,** the expression of a person's gender identity; the image that a person presents to both himself or herself and others, demonstrating maleness or femaleness.

**gender testing** [L, *genus,* kind, *testum,* crucible], a procedure for validating the sex of an individual by examining a tissue sample, usually obtained from oral mucous membrane cells, for the presence of a Y chromosome.

**gene** /jēn/ [Gk, *genein,* to produce], the biologic unit of inheritance, consisting of a particular nucleotide sequence within a DNA molecule that occupies a precise locus on a chromosome and codes for a specific polypeptide chain. In diploid organisms, which include humans and other mammals, genes occur as paired alleles. Kinds of genes include **complementary genes, mutant genes, operator genes, pleiotropic genes, regulator genes, structural genes,** and **supplementary genes.** See also **chromosome, cistron, deoxyribonucleic acid, operon.**

**-gene.** See **-gen.**

**gene amplification** [Gk, *genein,* to produce; L, *amplus,* large], a process in which a specific gene or set of genes is duplicated many times in certain cells in response to defined signals or environmental stresses.

**gene expression,** the flow of genetic information from gene to protein. the process, or the regulation of the process, by which the effects of a gene are manifested. the manifestation of a heritable trait in an individual carrying the gene or genes that determine it.

**gene library.** See **DNA library.**

**gene marker.** See **genetic marker.**

## Partial list of single-gene disorders

| Disease | Inheritance | Basic defect | Manifestations | Therapy |
|---|---|---|---|---|
| Achondroplasia | Autosomal dominant, new mutation | Defect in ossification at epiphyseal plate (growth portion of bones) | Very short limbs; large head; lordosis | Supportive |
| Albinism (ocular) | Autosomal recessive | Deficiency of tyrosinase: failure to convert tyrosine to dopa, and hence, lack of melanin synthesis | Lack of pigment in skin, hair, and eyes; eye defects | Symptomatic<br>Avoid exposure to sunlight<br>Ophthalmologic care |
| Cystic fibrosis | Autosomal recessive | Defect in pancreatic enzymes | Abnormal secretions, chronic pulmonary disease, malabsorption | Symptomatic, enzyme therapy |
| Fragile X syndrome | Sex-linked dominant | Unknown | Long face, large ears, large testicles, mental retardation | Symptomatic, folic acid therapy |
| Galactosemia | Autosomal recessive | Defect in galactose metabolism | Hypotonia, vomiting, hepatosplenomegaly, cataracts | Galactose-free diet |
| Hemophilia A | Sex-linked recessive | Defect in factor VIII production | Hemorrhage into tissues, joints after injury | Factor VIII replacement therapy |
| Hypothyroidism (familial) | Autosomal recessive | Deficiency of iodotyrosine deiodinase | Lethargy; stunted growth; mental retardation | Early administration of thyroid hormone |
| Maple syrup urine disease | Autosomal recessive | Defective metabolism of branched-chain amino acids | Onset in early infancy; neurologic disorders; odor of urine similar to that of maple syrup | Diet low in branched-chain amino acids |
| Marfan's syndrome (arachnodactyly) | Autosomal dominant, new mutation | Defect in elastic fibers of connective tissues | Tall and thin, with long tapering fingers; poorly developed musculature; associated defects include aortic aneurysm, dislocation of optic lens, winged scapula | Supportive<br>Surgical correction of deformities |
| Muscular dystrophy (Duchenne) | Sex-linked recessive, new mutation | Protein dystrophin is absent | Muscular atrophy, progressive deterioration of motor function and mental development | Symptomatic |
| Myotonic dystrophy | Autosomal dominant | Defective calcium metabolism in nerve and muscle cells | Hypotonia, characteristic facial features, respiratory distress, poor feeding, high-arched palate, and cataracts; severe neonatal form leads to early death | Symptomatic |
| Neurofibromatosis (von Recklinghausen's disease) | Autosomal dominant, new mutation | Defect in neural cells—exact mechanism unknown | Café-au-lait spots, multiple fibromas, neurologic and ophthalmologic defects, skeletal anomalies | Symptomatic, surgical removal of tumors |
| Noonan's syndrome | Autosomal dominant | Unknown | Small stature, shield-shaped chest, webbed neck, low posterior hair-line, narrow maxilla, low-set ears, ptosis, hypertelorism, cardiac anomalies (pulmonic stenosis) | Correct cardiac anomalies<br>Supportive |
| Osteogenesis imperfecta | Autosomal dominant, new mutation | Defect in production of type 1 procollagen | Fragile, short, bowed bones, blue sclera, hyperextensible joints, hearing loss | Symptomatic, surgical orthopedic procedures |
| Phenylketonuria | Autosomal recessive | Defect in phenylalanine metabolism | Eczema, poor feeding, seizures, musty smell to urine, mental retardation | Low-phenylalanine diet |
| Tay-Sachs disease (amaurotic familial idiocy) | Autosomal recessive | Deficiency of hexosaminidase; defect in synthesis of gangliosides | Predominantly in Ashkenazi Jews; progressive neurologic deterioration; blindness, cherry red spot in macula; early death | Supportive |
| Thalassemias | Autosomal recessive | Defect in synthesis of one or more globin chains of hemoglobin | Anemia, hepatosplenomegaly, thinning of bones | Symptomatic, transfusions |
| Wilson's disease | Autosomal recessive | Failure of biliary excretion of copper, leading to copper toxicity | Liver failure, speech abnormalities, tremors, psychiatric and behavioral problems | Chelation agents, treatment of liver disease |

From Wong DL: *Nursing care of infants and children*, ed 6, St Louis, 1999, Mosby.

**gene pool** [Gk, *genein,* to produce; AS, *pol*],   the total number of genes in a population. If the population reproduces by random sexual selection, there will be a normal (bell-shaped) distribution of genes in the gene pool.

**gene probe,**   a device used in molecular biology for locating a particular gene on a chromosome. It involves pairing a short known segment of deoxyribonucleic acid or ribonucleic acid with a matching sequence of bases on a chromosome.

**genera.**   See **genus.**

**general adaptation syndrome (GAS)** [L, *genus,* kind; L, *adaptare,* to fit; Gk, *syn,* together, *dromos,* course],   the defense response of the body or the psyche to injury or prolonged stress, as described by Hans Selye (1907–1982). It consists of an initial stage of shock or alarm reaction, followed by a phase of increasing resistance or adaptation, using the various defense mechanisms of the body or mind, and culminates in a state of adjustment and healing or of exhaustion and disintegration. Also called **adaptation syndrome.** See also **crisis, posttraumatic stress disorder, stress.**

**general anesthesia,**   the absence of sensation and consciousness as induced by various anesthetic medications, given by inhalation or IV injection. The components of general anesthesia are analgesia, amnesia, muscle relaxation, control of vital signs, and unconsciousness. The depth of anesthesia is planned to allow the surgical procedure to be performed without the patient's experiencing pain, moving, or having any recall of the procedure. Endotracheal intubation and respiratory support are often necessary. General anesthesia may be administered only by an anesthesiologist, anesthesia assistant, or a Certified Registered Nurse Anesthetist. See also **anesthesia, local anesthesia, regional anesthesia.**

**generalization** /jen′(ə)rəlīzā′shən/ [L, *genus,* kind; Gk, *izein,* to cause],   **1.** the reasoning by which a basic conclusion is reached, with application to different items that have a common factor. **2.** the process of reducing or subsuming under a general rule or statement, such as classifying items in general categories. **3.** a principle with general application. **4.** (in occupational therapy) the ability of a patient to apply knowledge and skills learned in therapy to a variety of similar but new situations.

**generalized actinomycosis.**   See **actinomycosis.**

**generalized anaphylaxis** /jen′(ə)rəlīzd′/,   a severe reaction to an allergen characterized by itching, edema, wheezing respirations, apprehension, cyanosis, dyspnea, pupillary dilation, falling blood pressure, and rapid, weak pulse that may quickly produce shock and death. The reaction is mediated by immunoglobulin E antibodies that form in response to an initial sensitizing dose of an allergen and render the individual hypersensitive to the allergen by binding it to mast cells and basophils. A subsequent challenging dose of the allergen causes the cells to release histamine, bradykinin, and other vasoactive amines, producing anaphylaxis. See also **anaphylactic shock, anaphylaxis, reagin-mediated disorder.**

**generalized anxiety disorder (GAD),**   an anxiety reaction characterized by persistent apprehension. The symptoms range from mild, chronic tenseness, with feelings of timidity, fatigue, apprehension, and indecisiveness, to more intense states of restlessness and irritability that may lead to aggressive acts. In extreme cases the overwhelming emotional discomfort is accompanied by physical reactions, including tremor, sustained muscle tension, tachycardia, dyspnea, hypertension, increased respiration, and profuse perspiration. Other physical signs include changes in skin color, nausea, vomiting, diarrhea, restlessness, immobilization, insomnia, and changes in appetite, all occurring without underlying organic cause. The symptoms of anxiety may be controlled with medication, such as tranquilizers, but psychotherapy is the preferred treatment. Also called **anxiety reaction, anxiety state.** See also **anxiety, anxiety attack.**

**generalized emphysema.**   See **panacinar emphysema.**

**generalized peritonitis** [L, *genus,* kind; Gk, *peri,* near, *teinein,* to stretch, *itis,* inflammation],   a bacterial infection of the peritoneum secondary to an infection in another organ, as when an appendix ruptures or an ulcer perforates the gastric wall. The symptoms are usually acute and severe. See also **peritonitis.**

**generally recognized as effective (GRAE),**   one of the statutory criteria that must be met by a drug before it can be approved as a new drug. Meeting these criteria relieves the manufacturer of the necessity of obtaining premarket approval as required by the Federal Food, Drug, and Cosmetic Act. To be recognized as effective, the drug must be, according to the act, considered safe and effective by "experts qualified by scientific training and experience."

**generally recognized as safe (GRAS),**   a 1958 rule established by the U.S. Food and Drug Administration (FDA) to identify foods regarded as safe to use because of lack of evidence that they may be harmful. Originally the rule was applied to all foods that were in use in 1958 and were not then known to be hazardous. Later, because of improved scientific techniques for detecting mutagens and carcinogens, items that had been classified as safe, such as caffeine, were further tested by the FDA to determine whether they should remain on the GRAS list.

**general paresis** [L, *genus,* kind; Gk, paralysis],   a neurological disorder that results from chronic syphilitic infection. It is characterized by degeneration of the cortical neurons; progressive dementia, tremor, and speech disturbances; muscular weakness; and ultimately generalized paralysis. It is often accompanied by periods of exultation and delusions of grandeur. Treatment usually consists of large doses of penicillin, without which the outcomes are almost invariably progressive deterioration and death. Also called **paretic dementia, syphilitic meningoencephalitis.**

**general practitioner (GP)** [L, *genus,* kind; Gk, *praktikos,* practical],   a family practice physician. See also **family medicine, family practice, family practice physician.**

**general relaxation** [L, *genus,* kind, *relaxare,* to ease],   a slackening of strain or tension of the entire body, particularly of the muscles.

**general symptom** [L, *genus* + Gk, *symptoma,* that which happens],   a symptom that affects the entire body rather than a specific organ or location. Also called **constitutional symptom.**

**generation** /jen′ərā′shən/ [L, *generare,* to beget],   **1.** the act or process of reproduction; procreation. **2.** a group of contemporary individuals that have descended through the same number of life cycles from a common ancestor. **3.** the period between the birth of one individual and the birth of its offspring. Kinds of generation include **alternate generation, filial generation,** and **parental generation.**

**generative** /jen′ərā′tiv/ [L, *generare,* to beget],   pertaining to activity that generates new physical or mental growth, such as creative problem solving.

**generic** /jəner′ik/ [L, *genus,* kind],   **1.** pertaining to a genus. **2.** pertaining to a substance, product, or drug that is not protected by trademark. **3.** pertaining to the name of a kind of drug that is also the description of the drug.

**generic equivalent,**   a drug product sold under its generic name whose active ingredients are identical in chemical composition to one or more others sold under trademark. Inactive ingredients may not be the same.

**generic name,** the official established nonproprietary name assigned to a drug. A drug is licensed under its generic name, and all manufacturers of the drug list it by its generic name. However a drug is usually marketed under trademark chosen by the manufacturer. See also **chemical name, established name, trademark.**

**generic nursing program,** a program that prepares people with no professional nursing experience for entry into the field of nursing.

**-genesia,** 1. suffix meaning a '(specified) condition concerning information': *agenesia, morphogenesia, paragenesia.* 2. also **-genesis.** combining form meaning 'the production or procreation of something (specified)': *algogenesia, palingenesia, syngenesia.*

**genesis** /jen′əsis/ [Gk, origin], 1. the origin, generation, or developmental evolution of anything. 2. the act of producing or procreating.

**-genesis.** See **-genesia.**

**gene splicing** /jēn/, a process by which a segment of DNA is attached to or inserted into a strand of DNA from another source. In recombinant DNA technology, DNA from humans or other organisms is spliced into bacterial plasmids.

**gene therapy,** a procedure that involves injection of "healthy genes" into the bloodstream of a patient to cure or treat a hereditary disease or similar illness. Blood is withdrawn from the patient; the white cells are separated and cultured in a laboratory, and inserted into modified viruses. Normal genes from a volunteer are inserted into the viruses, which, in turn, transfer the normal gene into the chromosomes of the patient's white cells. The white cells containing the normal genes are finally injected into the patient's bloodstream. A clinical application of gene therapy may be found in the treatment of thalassemia, a genetically determined disease, in which efforts have been made to increase hemoglobin F production and improve the level of anemia. Research goals include changing the actual hemoglobin genes in red blood cell precursors or transplantation of normal hemoglobin genes into the bone marrow of thalassemia patients. Also called **somatic-cell gene therapy.**

**genetic** /jənet′ik/ [Gk, *genesis,* origin], 1. pertaining to reproduction, birth, or origin. 2. pertaining to genetics or heredity. 3. pertaining to or produced by a gene; inherited.

**-genetic,** 1. suffix meaning 'generation by (specified) agents': *gamogenetic, mitogenetic, spermatogenetic.* 2. suffix meaning 'generating': *glycogenetic, ovigenetic, ureagenetic.* 3. suffix meaning 'something generated by a (specified) agent': *biogenetic, ideogenetic, phylogenetic.*

**genetic affinity,** relationship by direct descent.

**genetically significant dose (GSD)** /jənet′iklē/, an arbitrary measure of the estimated annual gonadal radiation received by the population gene pool. In the United States the estimated GSD is 20 mrad. The figure is not intended to suggest possible genetic effects of exposure to that level of radiation.

**genetic association,** a condition in which specific genotypes are associated with other factors, such as specific diseases.

**genetic carrier,** a person who carries an allele without exhibiting its effects. Such an allele is usually recessive, but it may also be dominant and latent, with symptoms that do not appear until adulthood.

**genetic code,** the information carried by DNA that determines the specific amino acids and their sequence in each protein synthesized by an organism. The code consists of the sequence of nucleotides in the DNA molecule of each chromosome in the nucleus of every cell. During transcription, a specific part of the code is transcribed into a sequence of nucleotides in the messenger RNA (mRNA). The mRNA travels from the nucleus to the cytoplasm, where it is translated into protein by the ribosomes. A codon consisting of three consecutive nucleotides in the mRNA codes for each amino acid in the protein. A change in the code may result in an incorrect sequence of the amino acids in the protein, causing a mutation. See also **anticodon, transcription, translation.**

**genetic colonization,** the process by which a parasite introduces into its host genetic information that induces the host to synthesize products solely for the use of the parasite.

**genetic counseling**[1], the process of determining the occurrence or risk of occurrence of a genetic disorder in a family and of providing information and advice about topics such as care of an affected child, prenatal diagnosis, termination of a pregnancy, sterilization, and artificial insemination. Effective genetic counseling begins with an accurate diagnosis of the condition; because many of the more than 3000 known inherited disorders have similar clinical manifestations, special biochemical cytogenetic or molecular genetic tests may be required. A genetic counselor also must prepare a careful, detailed family history, recorded in the form of a pedigree chart, and must have an understanding of genetic principles, especially a knowledge of the risks related to multifactorial inheritance. The most efficient counseling services consist of a group of specialists, including physicians, geneticists, psychologists, biochemists, cytologists, nurses, and social workers. Nurses must be especially alert to situations in which persons may need genetic counseling, must become familiar with facilities in the area that provide genetic counseling, and must help couples arrive at tentative decisions regarding family planning or the care of a child with a genetic disorder. See also **genetic screening, prenatal diagnosis.**

**genetic counseling**[2] a nursing intervention from the Nursing Interventions Classification (NIC) defined as use of an interactive helping process focusing on assisting an individual, family, or group, manifesting or at risk for developing or transmitting a birth defect or genetic condition, to cope. See also **Nursing Interventions Classification.**

**genetic counselor,** a health professional academically and clinically prepared to communicate genetic, medical, and technical information about the occurrence, or risk of occurrence, of a genetic condition or birth defect. As part of a genetic delivery services team, the genetic counselor consults with individuals, and/or their families, about their birth defects or genetic disorders, their risk for inherited conditions, and their options. A masters' degree in genetic counseling is usually required; the American Board of Genetic Counseling provides certification.

**genetic death,** 1. the failure of an organism to survive as a result of its genetic makeup. 2. the removal of an allele or genotype from the gene pool of a population or from a given familial descent because of the sterility, failure to reproduce, or death before sexual maturity of all individuals bearing that allele or genotype.

**genetic disorder.** See **inherited disorder.**

**genetic drift,** a change in the allelic frequencies within a population as a result of chance. The smaller a population is, the greater is the tendency for variation within each generation so that eventually small, isolated, inbreeding groups become genetically quite different from their ancestors. Also called **random genetic drift.**

**genetic engineering,** the process of producing recombinant DNA for the purposes of altering and controlling the genotype and phenotype of organisms. Enzymes are used to break a DNA molecule into fragments so that genes from another organism can be inserted into the DNA. Genetic engineering has been used to produce a variety of human proteins, including growth hormone, insulin, and interferon, in bacteria. At present, it represents a powerful tool for medical research but is possible only in microorganisms. In the future, genetic engineering may be applicable to more complex organisms, offering the possibility of controlling and eliminating genetic disorders and malformations in humans.

**genetic equilibrium,** the state within a population at which the frequency of alleles and genotypes does not change from generation to generation. It routinely occurs in large, interbreeding populations in which mating is random and there are no or relatively few mutations. See also **Hardy-Weinberg equilibrium principle.**

**genetic homeostasis,** the maintenance of genetic variability within a population through adaptation to varied or changing environments and conditions of life as a result of shifts or resistance to shifts in allelic frequencies.

**genetic immunity.** See **natural immunity.**

**genetic isolate,** a group of individuals that are genetically separated by geographic, racial, social, cultural, or other barriers that prevent them from interbreeding with those outside the group. Depending on the size of the group and the amount of inbreeding that occurs, genetic isolates may show an increased incidence of otherwise rare inherited defects. See also **deme.**

**geneticist** /jənet′isist/, a scientist who specializes in the study or application of genetics.

**genetic load,** the average number of accumulated detrimental genes per individual within a population, including those caused by mutation and selection within a recent generation and those inherited from ancestors. Genetic load is expressed in lethal equivalents.

**genetic map,** the graphic representation of the linear arrangement of genes on a chromosome and the relative distances between them, in map units or morgans. Also called **linkage map.**

**genetic marker,** any specific gene that produces a readily recognizable genetic trait that can be used in family and population studies or in linkage analysis. Also called **gene marker, marker gene.**

**genetic polymorphism,** the recurrence within a population of two or more discontinuous genetic variants of a specific trait in such proportions that they cannot be maintained simply by mutation. Examples include the sickle cell trait, the Rh factor, and the blood groups. Compare **balanced polymorphism.**

**genetic population.** See **deme.**

**genetics** /jənet′iks/, 1. the science that studies the principles and mechanics of heredity, specifically the means by which traits are passed from parents to offspring and the causes of the similarities and differences between related organisms. 2. the total genetic makeup of a particular individual, family, group, or condition. Kinds of genetics are **clinical genetics, molecular genetics,** and **population genetics.** See also **cytogenetics, Mendel's laws.**

**genetic screening,** the process of investigating a specific population of persons for the purpose of detecting the presence of disease, either incipient or overt, such as the generalized screening of all newborns for phenylketonuria. Genetic screening may be used to identify those who possess defective genes, gain information concerning the incidence of a disorder in the population, and provide reproductive information, specifically to those at risk, such as the close relatives of persons affected with inborn errors of metabolism or those in certain ethnic groups who have a high incidence of a particular disease, specifically sickle cell anemia in African-Americans and Tay-Sachs disease in Ashkenazic Jews. When accompanied by education and counseling, mass screening programs can be effective in the management of genetic disorders. See also **genetic counseling.**

**gene transfer** [Gk, *genein,* to produce; L, *transferre,* to bring across], a type of gene therapy in which a gene is transplanted from a donor organism into a recipient organism.

**Genga's bandage.** See **Theden's bandage.**

**-genia,** suffix meaning '(condition or development of the) jaw': *microgenia, opisthogenia, progenia.*

**-genic,** 1. suffix meaning 'causing, forming, producing': *collagenic, hemorrhagenic, phosphagenic.* 2. suffix meaning 'produced by or formed from': *bacillogenic, coccigenic, pituitarigenic.* 3. suffix meaning 'related to a gene': *intragenic, polygenic, trigenic.*

**geniculate neuralgia** /jənik′yəlāt/ [L, *geniculum,* little knee; Gk, *neuron,* nerve, *algos,* pain], a severe debilitating inflammatory condition of the geniculate ganglion of the facial nerve. It is characterized by pain, loss of the sense of taste, facial paralysis, and a decrease in salivation and lacrimation. It sometimes follows herpes zoster infection. See also **Ramsay Hunt's syndrome.**

**geniculate zoster.** See **herpes zoster.**

**genio-,** combining form meaning 'chin': *genion, genioplasty.*

**geniohyoideus** /jē′nē·ōhī·oi′dē·əs/ [Gk, *genion,* chin, *hyoides,* Y-shaped], one of the four suprahyoid muscles that draw the hyoid bone and the tongue forward. Also called **geniohyoid muscle.** Compare **digastricus, mylohyoideus, stylohyoideus.** See also **suprahyoid muscles.**

**genit-,** 1. combining form meaning 'birth or reproduction': *genitalia.* 2. combining form meaning 'generative organs or sexual reproduction': *genitourinary, genitalia.*

**genital.** See **genitals.**

**genital herpes.** See **herpes genitalis, herpes simplex.**

**genitalia.** See **genitals.**

**genital reflex.** See **sexual reflex.**

**genitals** /jen′itəlz/ [L, *genitalis*], the sex, or reproductive, organs visible on the outside of the body. In the female they include the vulva, mons veneris, labia majora, labia minora, clitoris, and vaginal vestibule. The male genitals include the penis, scrotum, and testicles. Also called **genitalia.** —**genital,** *adj.*

**genital self-examination.** See **self-breast examination, testicular self-examination.**

**genital stage** /jen′itəl/ [L, *genitalis* + Fr, *stage,* trial period], (in psychoanalysis) the final period in freudian psychosexual development, beginning with adolescence and continuing through the adult years when the genitals are the predominant source of pleasurable stimulation. The most significant feature of this stage is direction of sexual interest not just toward self-satisfaction but toward establishment of a stable and meaningful relationship. See also **psychosexual development.**

**genital tract.** See **reproductive system.**

**genital wart** [L, *genitalis* + AS, *wearte*], a small soft, moist pink or red swelling of the genitals that becomes pedunculated and may be painless. The growth may be solitary, or a cauliflower-like group may be present in the same area of the genitalia. It is caused by a sexually transmitted disease, human papillomavirus (HPV). Atypical genital warts should be biopsied and examined as possible carcino-

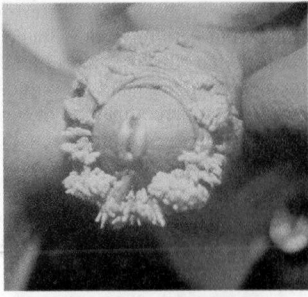

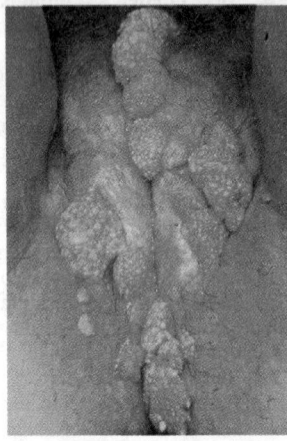

**Genital wart**
*(Monahan and Neighbors, 1998/courtesy New York City Health Department)*

mas because they are associated with cervical cancer. No therapy has been shown to eradicate HPV. One third of lesions disappear without treatment. Treatment may include podofilox, resin, or trichloracetic acid or cryotherapy with liquid nitrogen, laser or surgical removal. Also called **condyloma acuminatum, venereal wart, verruca acuminata.**

**genitourinary (GU)** /jen'itō·yŏŏr'iner'ē/ [L, *genitalis* + Gk, *ouron,* urine], referring to the genital and urinary systems of the body: the organ structures, functions, or both. Also called **urogenital.**

**genitourinary fistula,** an abnormal communication between organs of the urogenital system or between organs of the urogenital system and some other system.

**genitourinary system.** See **urogenital system.**

**genocide** /jen'əsīd/, the systematic extermination of a national, ethnic, political, religious, or other population.

**genogram** /jē'nōgram/, a diagram that depicts family relationships over at least three generations. It is useful as a tool for studying the process of a family system or hereditary disease over time.

**genome** /jē'nōm/ [Gk, *genein,* to produce], the complete set of genes in the chromosomes of each cell of a specific organism. —**genomic,** *adj.*

**genome map,** a graphic representation of the locations of genes in a genome. The human genome map, completed in 1996, locates 5264 markers for genes and has led to the discovery of 223 genes linked to more than 200 diseases. The mouse genome map locates 7377 markers on 20 chromosomes.

**genomic imprinting,** differential expression of a gene or genes as a function of whether they were inherited from the male or the female parent, e.g. a deletion on chromosome 15 that causes Prader-Willi syndrome if inherited from the father causes instead Angelman's syndrome if inherited from the mother.

**genontopia.** See **senopia.**

**genotoxic** /jē'nōtok'sik/, capable of altering DNA, thereby causing cancer or mutation.

**genotoxic carcinogens,** cancer-causing agents that can alter deoxyribonucleic acid (DNA) molecules. Genotoxic carcinogens include organic compounds that induce mutations directly, organic compounds that alter DNA after activating metabolism, and metals or metal salts that can alter DNA.

**genotype** /jē'nōtīp'/ [Gk, *genos,* birth, *typos,* mark], **1.** the complete genetic constitution of an organism or group, as determined by the specific combination and location of the genes on the chromosomes. **2.** the alleles situated at one or more sites on homologous chromosomes. A pair of alleles is usually designated by letters or symbols, such as *AA* when the alleles are identical and *Aa* when they are different. **3.** a group or class of organisms having the same genetic makeup; the type species of a genus. Compare **phenotype.** —**genotypic,** *adj.*

**-genous,** suffix meaning 'to originate from or to contain': *homogenous, hydrogenous.*

**gentamicin sulfate** /jen'təmī'sin/, an aminoglycoside antibiotic.

■ INDICATION: It is prescribed for the treatment of severe infections caused by organisms sensitive to gentamicin.

■ CONTRAINDICATIONS: Concomitant administration of other potentially ototoxic or nephrotoxic drugs or known hypersensitivity to this drug or to other aminoglycoside medications prohibits its use. It is used with caution in patients with impaired renal function.

■ ADVERSE EFFECTS: Among the more serious adverse reactions are nephrotoxicity, auditory or vestibular ototoxicity, impairment of neuromuscular transmission, and hypersensitivity reactions.

**gentian violet** /jen'shən/, a topical antibacterial antiinfective, antifungal, and anthelmintic.

■ INDICATIONS: It is prescribed in the treatment of pinworms, superficial infections of the skin, and vaginal infections.

■ CONTRAINDICATIONS: Known hypersensitivity to this drug prohibits its use. It is not applied to ulcerative lesions of the face.

■ ADVERSE EFFECTS: Among the most serious adverse reactions is permanent discoloration of the skin after topical exposure to the drug. GI distress and purple vomitus may occur after oral administration.

**gentiotannic acid** /jen'shē·ətan'ik/, a form of tannic acid once used as an astringent and in the treatment of burns but no longer recommended because of its hepatotoxicity.

**Gentran 40,** trademark for a plasma volume extender (dextran 40).

**Gentran 75,** trademark for a plasma volume extender (dextran 75).

**genu** /jē'nōo/ [L, knee], the knee or any angular structure resembling the flexed knee.

**genupectoral position** /je'nōopek'tərəl/ [L, *genu,* knee, *pectus,* breast, *positio*], knee-chest position. To assume the genupectoral position the person kneels so that the weight of the body is supported by the knees and chest, with the buttocks raised. The head is turned to one side and the arms are flexed so that the upper part of the body can be supported in part by the elbows.

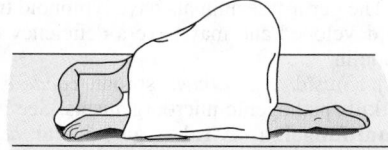

**Genupectoral position** *(Potter and Perry, 2001)*

**genu recurvatum** [L, *genu,* knee, *recurvare,* to bend back], a deformity in which the lower leg is hyperextended at the knee joint. Also called **back knee.**

**genus** /jē′nəs/, *pl.* **genera** /jen′ərə/ [L, kind], a subdivision of a family of organisms. A genus usually is composed of several closely related species. The genus *Homo* has only one species, *Homo sapiens* (humans). See also **family.**

**genu valgum** [L, *genu,* knee, *valgus,* bent inward], a deformity in which the legs are curved inward, so that the knees are close together and strike each other as the person walks, and the ankles are widely separated. Also called **knock-knee.**

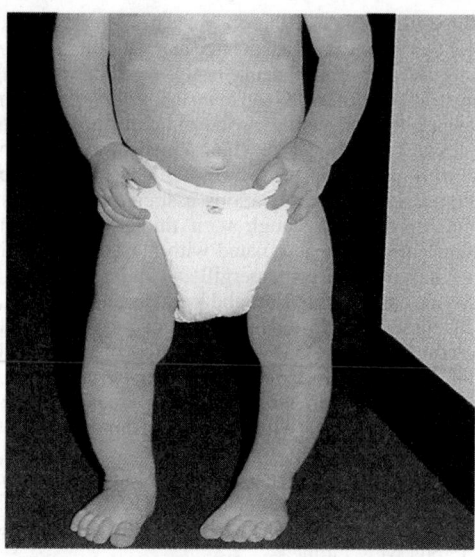

**Genu varum** *(Zitelli and Davis, 1997)*

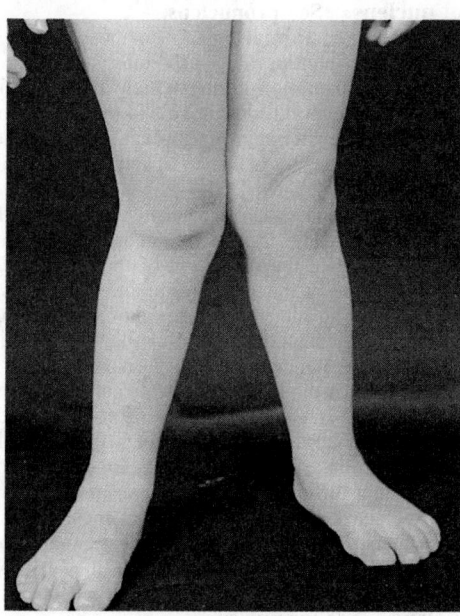

**Genu valgum** *(Zitelli and Davis, 1997)*

surface of the tongue characterized by numerous and continually changing areas of loss and regrowth of the filiform papillae. The wandering shape and outline of the denuded red patches surrounded by thickened white borders present a geographic or maplike appearance. Also called **benign migratory glossitis.**

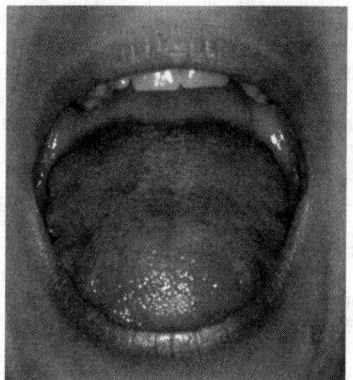

**Geographic tongue** *(Lemmi and Lemmi, 2000)*

**genu varum** [L, knee, *varus,* bent outward], a deformity in which one or both legs are bent outward at the knee. Also called **bowleg.** Compare **genu valgum.**

**-geny,** combining form meaning 'production, generation, origin': *homogeny, hylogeny, morphogeny.*

**geo-,** prefix meaning 'earth or soil': *geobiology, geophagia, geotropism.*

**Geocillin,** trademark for an antibacterial (carbenicillin indanyl sodium).

**geographic tongue** /jē′əgraf′ik/ [Gk, *ge,* earth, *graphein,* to record; AS, *tunge*], an inflammatory disorder on the dorsal

**geometric mean.** See **mean.**

**Geopen,** trademark for an antibacterial (carbenicillin disodium).

**geophagia,** the practice of eating clay or dirt. A form of pica, the compulsion is thought by some to be associated with disorders of mineral balance. Some patients with pica have been found to suffer from an iron deficiency and respond to iron therapy. However, red clay may be so rich in potassium that its ingestion can lead to hyperkalemia in individuals with renal failure.

**geotrichosis** /jē′ōtrikō′sis/ [Gk, *ge,* earth, *thrix,* hair, *osis,* condition], a condition associated with the fungus *Geotrichum candidum* that may cause oral, bronchial, pharyngeal, and intestinal disorders. *Geotrichum candidum* is normally found in healthy individuals, soil, and dairy products and is not necessarily pathogenic. Geotrichosis most commonly occurs in immunosuppressed individuals with diabetes. Bronchopulmonary complications associated with this disorder may produce a cough with thick, bloody sputum. Geotrichosis has been associated with allergic asthmatic reactions similar to allergic aspergillosis and a type of intestinal disorder characterized by abdominal pain, diarrhea, and rectal bleeding. Oral lesions that may occur with this disorder are commonly treated with a solution of gentian violet; associated abdominal lesions are treated with the oral administration of gentian violet capsules; associated pulmonary lesions are treated with the oral administration of potassium iodide.

**Gerbich blood group** /gər′bich /, a blood group consisting of the erythrocytic antigens Ge 1, Ge 2, and Ge 3; although rare in most parts of the world, it has been found often in Papua New Guinea.

**GERD,** abbreviation for *gastroesophageal reflux disease;* see **gastroesophageal reflux.**

**geriatric day care** /jer′ē·at′rik/ [Gk, *geras,* old age; AS, *daeg* + L, *garrire,* chatter], an ambulatory health care facility for elderly people. It usually offers a broad range of professional and community services to maximize functional independence of the patients.

**geriatric dentistry.** See **gerodontics.**

**Geriatric Depression Scale (GDS),** a brief depression screening inventory composed of 30 items that require yes or no answers. A score of 11 or above indicates depressed individuals. There is a 15-item short version. Scores of 5 or more may indicate depression.

**geriatrician** /jer′ē·ətrish′ən/, a physician who has specialized postgraduate education and experience in the medical care of older persons.

**geriatric nurse practitioner,** a registered nurse with additional education obtained through a master's degree program in nursing or a non-degree-granting certificate program that prepares the nurse to deliver primary health care to adults.

**geriatrics** /jer′ē·at′riks/, the branch of medicine dealing with the physiologic characteristics of aging and the diagnosis and treatment of diseases affecting the aged.

**germ** /jurm/ [L, *germen,* sprout], **1.** any microorganism, especially one that is pathogenic. **2.** a unit of living matter able to develop into a self-sufficient organism, such as a seed, spore, or egg. **3.** (in embryology) the first stage in development, such as a spermatozoon or other germ cell.

**German cockroach,** *Blattella germanica,* a small light brown species found as a household pest in North America and Europe.

**germanium (Ge)** /jərmā′nē·əm/ [Germany], a metallic element with some nonmetallic semiconductor properties. Its atomic number is 32; its atomic mass is 72.61.

**German measles.** See **rubella.**

**germ cell, 1.** a sexual reproductive cell in any stage of development, from the primordial embryonic form to the mature gamete. **2.** an ovum or spermatozoon or any of their preceding forms. **3.** any cell undergoing gametogenesis. Also called **gonoblast, gonocyte.** Compare **somatic cell.**

**germ disk.** See **embryonic disk.**

**germ-free animal,** a laboratory animal raised under sterile conditions, free of exposure to microorganisms. The diet is controlled, preventing exposure to microorganisms that may be in food. The germ-free animals have lymphoid tissue that is not fully developed and may have a deficiency of serum immunoglobulin.

**germicide** /jur′misīd/ [L, *germen,* sprout, *caedere,* to kill], a drug that kills pathogenic microorganisms. See also **antibacterial, antifungal, antiviral. —germicidal,** *adj.*

**germinal** /jur′minəl/ [L, *germen,* sprout], pertaining to or characteristic of a germ cell or to the early stages of development.

**germinal center** [L, *germen,* sprout; Gk, *kentron,* center], an antigen-localizing primary follicle with lymphoid tissue, occupying the center of the lymphatic nodules of the spleen, tonsils, and lymph nodes. It reacts to antigens, enlarging and becoming filled with lymphoblasts and macrophages at the center of a ring of small lymphocytes.

**germinal disk.** See **embryonic disk.**

**germinal epithelium, 1.** the epithelial layer covering the genital ridge from which the gonads are derived in early embryonic development. **2.** the epithelial covering of the ovary, formerly thought to be the site of the formation of the oogonia. See also **oogenesis.**

**germinal infection,** an infection transmitted to a child by the ovum or sperm of a parent. Compare **endogenous infection, mixed infection, retrograde infection, secondary infection.**

**germinal membrane.** See **blastoderm.**

**germinal nucleus.** See **pronucleus.**

**germinal pole.** See **animal pole.**

**germinal stage,** (in embryology) the interval of time from fertilization to implantation during which the ovum undergoes cell division several times, travels to the uterus, and, in the form of a blastocyst, begins to implant itself in the endometrium. The germinal stage is over at about 10 days of gestation.

**germination** /jur′minā′shən/ [L, *germen,* sprout], **1.** the initial growth and development of an organism from the time of fertilization to the formation of the embryo. **2.** the sprouting of a spore or the seed of a plant. **—germinate,** *v.*

**germinoma** /jur′minō′mə/, a neoplasm of the germinal tissue of the gonads, the mediastinum, or the pineal region. It is commonly associated with pituitary disorders.

**germ layer,** one of the three primordial cell layers formed during gastrulation in the early stages of embryonic development from which the entire range of body tissue is derived. Each germ layer has the potential for forming different cell types that differentiate into the various structures of the body. See also **ectoderm, endoderm, mesoderm.**

**germ line,** genetic material in a cell lineage that is passed down through the gametes before it is modified by somatic recombination or maturation.

**germ nucleus.** See **pronucleus.**

**germ plasm, 1.** the part of a germ cell that contains the reproductive and hereditary material; the total of the DNA in a specific cell or organism. **2.** *nontechnical.* germ cells in any stage of development together with the tissues from which they originated.

**germ theory** [L, *germen,* sprout; Gk, *theoria,* speculation], the concept that all infectious and contagious diseases are caused by living microorganisms.

**gero-, geronto-,** combining form meaning 'old age or the aged': *gerocomia, gerodontology, geromarasmus.*

**geroderma** /jer′ədur′mə/ [Gk, *geron,* old man, *derma,* skin], **1.** the atrophic skin of aging. **2.** skin that is thin and wrinkled as a result of a defective state of nutrition. **3.** any condition characterized by skin that is thin and wrinkled, resembling the skin of old age.

**gerodontia.** See **gerodontics.**

**gerodontics** /jer′ō·don′tiks/ [Gk, *geron,* old man + *odous,* tooth], the delivery of dental care to aging persons; the diagnosis, prevention, and treatment of problems peculiar to advanced age. Also called **geriatric dentistry, gerodontia, gerodontology.**

**gerodontology.** See **gerodontics.**

**-gerontic, -gerontal,** combining form meaning 'old age': *paragerontic, phylogerontic, ungerontic.*

**gerontic nursing,** nursing care pertaining to an older person, a compromise between geriatric nursing (nursing care primarily for older persons who are ill) and gerontological nursing (a more holistic view of the nursing care of older persons).

**geronto-.** See **gero-.**

**gerontogen** /jeron′təjən/, an environmental agent that contributes to the aging process by accelerating the onset and/or rate of progression of aging. Examples include age-dependent cellular and biochemical responses to oxidant damage (such as from $NO_2$ and ozone); aging of cells that have an intrinsic sensitivity to certain toxins (such as carbon tetrachloride and ethanol); and toxic doses that are more likely to cause adverse effects on aging organisms.

**Gerontological Society of America (GSA),** an organization of scientific and academic professionals interested in studies of the nature of the aging process and the clinical manifestations of disease in the aging organism. GSA members participate with the International Association of Gerontology in periodic seminars at which worldwide research on longevity is presented.

**gerontology** /jer′əntol′əjē/ [Gk, *geras,* old age, *logos,* science], the study of all aspects of the aging process, including the clinical, psychologic, economic, and sociologic issues encountered by older persons and their consequences for both the individual and society.

**gerontoxon.** See **arcus senilis.**

**geropsychiatry** /jer′ōsīkī′ətrē/ [Gk, *geras,* old age, *psyche,* mind], the study and treatment of psychiatric aspects of aging and mental disorders of elderly people.

**-gerous,** suffix meaning 'bearing, producing, or containing' something specified: *calcigerous, ovigerous, setigerous.*

**Gerstmann's syndrome** /gerst′mänz/ [Josef Gerstmann, Austrian neurologist, 1887−1969], a combination of finger agnosia, right-left disorientation, agraphia, acalculia, and often constructional apraxia; it was formerly attributed to a lesion in the angular gyrus of the dominant hemisphere, but now that cause is in doubt.

**Gerstmann-Straussler syndrome.** See **human prion disease.**

**Gesell Developmental Assessment** [Arnold L. Gesell, American pediatrician and psychologist, 1880–1961], an evaluation program that provides information on gross motor, fine motor, language, personal-social, and cognitive development.

**Gestalt** /gəshtält′/, *pl.* **Gestalts, Gestalten** /gəshtäl′tən/ [Ger, form], a single physical, psychologic, or symbolic configuration, pattern, or experience that consists of a number of elements and has an effect as a whole different from that of the sum of its parts.

**Gestalt psychology,** a school of psychology, originating in Germany, that maintains that a psychologic phenomenon is perceived as a total configuration or pattern, rising from the relationships among its constituent elements, rather than as discrete elements possessing attributes of their own, and that the pattern, or Gestalt, cannot be derived from the summation of its constituents. Thus learning is regarded as resulting from insight, defined as a process or reorganization, rather than from association or trial and error, and behavior is seen as an integrated response to a unitary situation rather than as a series of reflexes and sensations. Also called **configurationism, Gestaltism.** See also **Gestalt.**

**Gestalt therapy,** a form of psychotherapy that stresses the unity of self-awareness, behavior, and experience. It incorporates elements of psychoanalytic, behavioristic, and humanistic existential therapy. See **Gestalt psychology.**

**gestant anomaly.** See **odontoma.**

**gestant odontoma.** See **dens in dente.**

**gestate** /jes′tāt/ [L, *gestare,* to bear], **1.** to carry a developing fetus in the womb. **2.** to grow and develop slowly toward maturity, such as a fetus in the womb.

**gestation** /jestā′shən/ [L, *gestare,* to bear], in viviparous animal the period from the fertilization of the ovum until birth. Gestation varies with the species; in humans the average duration is 266 days, or approximately 280 days from the onset of the last menstrual period. A gestation time of less than 37 weeks is regarded as premature; one that continues beyond 42 weeks is considered postmature, regardless of the size of the fetus or other factors. See also **pregnancy.**

**gestational age** /jestā′shənəl/ [L, *gestare* + *aetas,* time of life], the age of a fetus or a newborn, usually expressed in weeks dating from the first day of the mother's last menstrual period.

**gestational assessment** [L, *gestare,* to bear, *assidere,* to sit beside], calculation of the fetal age of the offspring, based on such factors as the menstrual history of the mother, the date when fetal heart sounds are first detected, and the evaluation of ultrasound data. The information is important in planning emergency care in the event of premature birth signs.

**gestational diabetes mellitus (GDM),** a disorder characterized by an impaired ability to metabolize carbohydrate, usually caused by a deficiency of insulin, occurring in pregnancy. It disappears after delivery of the infant but, in a significant number of cases, returns years later as type 2 diabetes mellitus. Evidence suggests that placental lactogen and considerable destruction of insulin by the placenta play a role in precipitating GDM. Treatment consists of self-blood glucose monitoring, insulin administration, a diet that controls the amount of carbohydrate eaten, and an adequate intake of calcium and iron. See also **diabetes mellitus.**

**gestational psychosis** [L, *gestare,* to bear; Gk, *psyche,* mind, *osis,* condition], any mental disorder that can be attributed to a pregnancy and resolves when pregnancy ends.

**gestational sac,** a pouch containing the fetus in extrauterine gestation.

**gestation period** [L, *gestare,* to bear; Gk, *peri,* near, *hodos,* way], the time span between conception and labor. In humans the period is approximately 38 weeks.

**gestures in physical examination** /jes′chərs/, physical appearance clues in diagnosis, such as a patient's pressing a clenched fist against the sternum as a "body language" message of the pain experienced during a myocardial infarction.

**Getman visuomotor theory** [Gerald Getman], a concept that visual perception is based on developmental sequences of physiologic actions in children. The sequence of eight stages begins with innate response systems and advances to cognitive integration of perceptions, abstractions, and higher symbolic activity.

**-geusia, -geustia,** suffix meaning '(condition of the) sense of taste': *glycogeusia, hemiageusia, parageusia.*

**GFP,** abbreviation for **green fluorescent protein.**

**GFR,** abbreviation for **glomerular filtration rate.**

**GH,** abbreviation for **growth hormone.**

**Ghon's complex** [Anton Ghon, Czechoslovakian pathologist, 1866–1936], a combination of pleural surface-healed granulomas or scars on the middle lobe of the lung together with hilar lymph node granulomas. The complex is evidence that a primary tuberculosis case has healed.

**ghost cells** [AS, *gast* + L, *cella,* storeroom], red blood cells that have lost their hemoglobin so that only the plasma membranes are observed in microscopic examinations of urine samples. The hemoglobin is destroyed by the presence of urine. Also called **shadow cells.**

**ghost teeth.** See **odontodysplasia.**

**GHRF,** abbreviation for **growth hormone releasing factor.**

**GHRH,** abbreviation for **growth hormone releasing hormone.**

**GHRIH,** abbreviation for *growth hormone release inhibiting hormone.* See **somatostatin.**

**GI,** abbreviation for **gastrointestinal.**

**Gianotti-Crosti syndrome** /jä·not′ē·kros′tē/ [Fernando Gianotti, Italian dermatologist, 1920−1984; Agostino Crosti, Italian dermatologist, 20th century], a generally benign and self-limited disease of young children representing a primary natural infection with hepatitis B virus, characterized by the appearance of crops of usually nonpruritic, dusky or coppery red, flat-topped, firm papules forming a symmetrical eruption on the face, buttocks, and limbs, including the palms and soles, and associated with malaise, low-grade fever, and few other symptoms. Also called **acrodermatitis papulosa infantum, infantile acrodermatitis, papular acrodermatitis of childhood.**

**giant axonal neuropathy,** an autosomal recessive neuropathy of childhood characterized by enlarged axons made up of masses of tightly woven neurofilaments.

**giant cell** /jī′ənt/ [L, *gigas,* huge, *cella,* storeroom], an abnormally large tissue cell. It often contains more than one nucleus and may appear as a merger of several normal cells.

**giant cell arteritis.** See **temporal arteritis.**

**giant cell carcinoma,** a malignant epithelial neoplasm characteristically containing many large anaplastic cells. A small percentage of adenocarcinomas of the lung and liver also contain such cells. Also called **carcinoma gigantocellulare.**

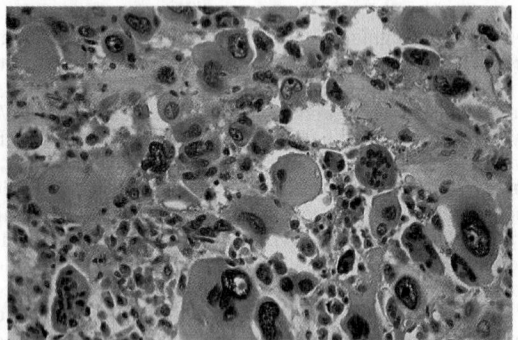

**Giant cell carcinoma of the bladder** *(Fletcher, 2000)*

**giant cell hepatitis.** See **neonatal hepatitis.**

**giant cell interstitial pneumonia.** See **interstitial pneumonia.**

**giant cell myeloma,** a bone tumor of multinucleated giant cells that resembles osteoclasts scattered in a matrix of spindle cells. Myelomas of this kind may be benign or malignant and may cause pain, functional disability, and pathologic fractures. Also called **giant cell tumor of bone.**

**giant cell sarcoma.** See **giant cell myeloma, osteoblastic sarcoma.**

**giant cell thyroiditis.** See **de Quervain's thyroiditis.**

**giant cell tumor of bone.** See **giant cell myeloma.**

**giant chromosome,** any of the excessively large chromosomes found in insects and certain other animals, including the lampbrush and polytene chromosomes.

**giant follicular lymphoma,** a nodular, well-differentiated lymphocytic malignant lymphoma in which nodules distort the normal structure of a lymph node. Also called **Brill-Symmers disease, giant follicular lymphadenopathy, Symmers' disease.**

**giant hypertrophic gastritis,** a rare disease characterized by large folds of nodular gastric rugae that may cover the wall of the stomach, causing anorexia, nausea, vomiting, and abdominal distress. Radiographic or endoscopic examination or surgery may be necessary for diagnosis. The disease is associated with an incidence of stomach cancer that is greater than normal. Also called **Ménétrier disease.**

**giant lymph node hyperplasia.** See **Castleman's disease.**

**giant peristaltic contraction,** a propulsive contraction of the bowel that normally occurs periodically in the distal small intestine and colon. The contractions are 1.5 to 2 times larger than normal in amplitude and 4 to 6 times longer in duration than usual. In certain disease states giant peristaltic contractions may start in the proximal small intestine and proceed uninterrupted. They may also be induced by a variety of stimuli including certain antibiotics, radiation therapy, and parasitic infections.

*Giardia* /jē·är′dē·ə/ [Alfred Giard, French biologist, 1846–1908], a common genus of flagellate protozoans. Many species of *Giardia* normally inhabit the digestive tract and cause inflammation in association with other factors that produce rapid proliferation of the organism. See also **giardiasis.**

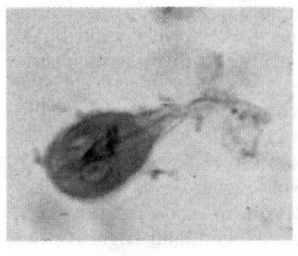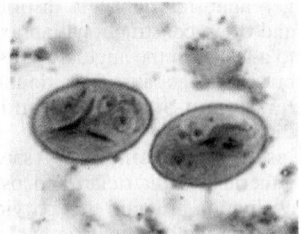

***Giardia lamblia* trophozoite and cyst** *(Murray et al, 1998)*

**giardiasis** /jē·ärdī′əsis/ [Alfred Giard; Gk, *osis,* condition], a diarrheal illness caused by infection with the protozoan *Giardia lamblia.* The source of infection is usually fecally contaminated water. Cases have occurred in day-care facilities with poor hygienic practices. Infection may be asymptomatic or may cause nausea; abdominal cramps; foul-smelling, greasy diarrhea; fatigue; and weight loss. Treatment is metronidazole or tinidazole, furazolidone, or paromomycin. It is treated with flagyl. Also called **traveler's diarrhea.**

**gibbus** /gib′əs, jib′əs/ [L, hump],   **1.** a hump, swelling, or enlargement on a body surface, usually confined to one side. **2.** a convex spinal curvature that may occur after the collapse of a vertebral body as may result from a fracture or tuberculosis of the spine.

**Gibraltar fever.**  See **brucellosis.**

**Gibson's murmur** [George A. Gibson, Scottish physician, 1854–1913],  a heart murmur that is heard continuously throughout the cardiac cycle. It waxes at the end of systole and wanes near the end of diastole and is often described as a "machinery-like" murmur. It is often accompanied by a thrill and occurs in patients with patent ductus arteriosus. Also called **machinery murmur.**

**Gibson walking splint,**  a kind of Thomas splint that enables a patient to be ambulatory.

**Giemsa's stain** /gē·em′səz/ [Gustav Giemsa, German chemist, 1867–1948; Fr, *teindre,* to dye],  an azure dye used as a stain in the microscopic examination of the blood for certain protozoan parasites, viral inclusion bodies, and rickettsia and, more routinely, in the preparation of a smear for a differential white cell count.

**GIFT,**  abbreviation for **gamete intrafallopian transfer.**

**giga-**  prefix meaning 'one billion ($10^9$)': *gigabit, gigabyte, gigahertz.*

**gigantism** /jigan′tizəm/ [L, *gigas,* giant],  an abnormal condition characterized by excessive size and stature. It is caused most frequently by hypersecretion of growth hormone (GH) and occurs to a lesser degree in hypogonadism and in certain genetic disorders. Acromegaly results, with overgrowth of the hands, feet, and face. Gigantism with normal body proportions and normal sexual development usually results from hypersecretion of GH in early childhood. Hypogonadism, by delaying puberty and closure of the epiphyses, may lead to gigantism. Excessive linear growth often occurs in males with more than one Y chromosome, and it may accompany Klinefelter's syndrome, Marfan's syndrome, and some cases of generalized lipodystrophy. Children with cerebral gigantism are mentally retarded and have a large head and extremities and a clumsy gait. Growth is rapid during their first few years and then reverts to a normal rate. Appropriate gonadal hormones may be administered to control abnormal growth of children with hypogonadism. The treatment of acromegalic gigantism is usually irradiation, but hypophysectomy may be indicated. See also **acromegaly, eunuchoidism.**

**giganto-,**  combining form meaning 'huge': *gigantoblast, gigantochromoblast, gigantocyte.*

**Gilbert's syndrome** [Nicolas A. Gilbert, French physician, 1858–1927],  a benign hereditary condition characterized by hyperbilirubinemia and jaundice. No treatment is required. See also **hyperbilirubinemia of the newborn.**

**Gilchrist's disease.**  See **blastomycosis.**

**Gilles de la Tourette's syndrome** /zhēl′dəlätŏŏrets′/ [George Gilles de la Tourette, French neurologist, 1857-1927],  an abnormal condition characterized by facial grimaces, tics, and involuntary arm and shoulder movements. In adolescence the condition worsens; the patient may grunt, snort, and shout involuntarily. Coprolalia often develops, affecting judgment of the condition by the family and society. In adulthood the condition usually lessens and tends to wax and wane. Recently treatment with dopamine antagonists has been found to be very effective, demonstrating an organic cause for this syndrome. Also called **Tourette's syndrome.**

**Gillies' operation** /gil′ēz/ [Harold D. Gillies, English surgeon, 1882–1960],  a surgical procedure for reducing fractures of the zygoma and zygomatic arch by making an incision in the temporal hairline.

**ginger,**  an herb native to the tropics of Asia and now cultivated in the tropics of South America, China, India, Africa, the Caribbean, and parts of the United States.

■ USES: This herb is used for nausea, motion sickness, indigestion, and inflammation.

■ CONTRAINDICATIONS: Ginger is not recommended during pregnancy (it is an abortifacient when taken in large amounts) or lactation, in children, or in those with known hypersensitivity to this product. It should not be used in cholelithiasis unless directed by a physician.

**ginger jake paralysis** /jin′jərjāk′/,  a polyneuropathy that primarily affects motor nerves to the distal parts of the extremities. First observed in Jamaica, it is caused by drinking an alcoholic extract of Jamaican ginger adulterated by a pesticide, tri-ortho-cresyl phosphate.

**gingiva** /jinji′və/, *pl.* **gingivae** [L, gum],  the gum tissues of the mouth, consisting of a mucous membrane with supporting fibrous tissue that overlies the crowns of unerupted teeth and encircles the necks of teeth that have erupted. —**gingival,** *adj.*

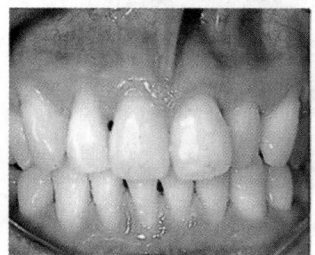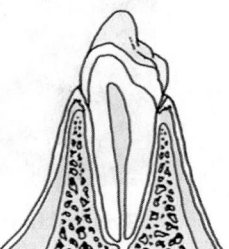

**Normal gingiva** *(Murray et al, 1994)*

**gingival abscess** /jinjī′vəl/,  a pocket of pus that arises under the mucosal covering of the gums and spreads to the neck of a tooth.

**gingival blanching** [L, *gingiva* + Fr, *blanchir,* to whiten],  the lightening of gum color, usually temporary, caused by stretching of gum tissue and decreased blood supply.

**gingival blood supply,**  the vascular supply to the gums. It rises from blood vessels that pass along the outer periosteum of bone and anastomose with vessels of the periodontal membrane as well as intra-alveolar blood vessels.

**gingival cavity,**  a tooth cavity that occurs in the third of the clinical crown nearest to the gum.

**gingival color,**  the color of gum tissues. It is affected by the thickness and degree of keratinization of the epithelium, blood supply, pigmentation, medications, and gingival and systemic diseases.

**gingival consistency,**  the combination of tactile and visual characteristics of healthy gum tissue. The tissue should be firm and resilient and should resemble smooth velvet or a finely or coarsely grained orange peel. Compare **gingival color.**

**gingival corium,**  the most stable connective tissue of the gingiva, which lies between the periosteum and the lamina propria mucosae.

**gingival crater,**  a depression in the gum tissue, especially in the area of the former apex of interdental papilla. It is commonly caused by necrotizing ulcerative gingivitis and food impaction against the tissue subjacent to the contact areas of adjacent teeth.

**gingival crevice,** a normal space located around a tooth between the wall of the unattached gum tissue and the enamel and/or cementum of the tooth. Also called **gingival sulcus.**

**gingival cuff.** See **junctional epithelium.**

**gingival discoloration,** a change in the normal color of the gum tissue, associated with inflammation, reduced blood supply, abnormal pigmentation, and other problems.

**gingival festoon,** the distinct rounding and enlargement of the margins of the gum tissue found in early gingival involvement. Compare **festoon, McCall's festoon.**

**gingival hormonal enlargement,** swelling of the gums associated with hormonal imbalance during pregnancy, puberty, or postmenopausal therapy. Also called **pregnancy epulis.**

**gingival hyperplasia,** overgrowth of the gum tissue, often in patients treated with phenytoin for epileptic seizures.

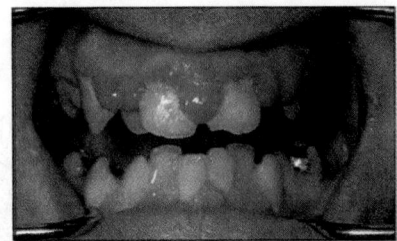

**Gingival hyperplasia** *(Perkin, 1998)*

**gingival hypertrophy,** an overgrowth of gum tissue encircling the teeth. It may be caused by the ingestion of phenytoin, a medication prescribed for the treatment of epilepsy.

**gingival line** [L, *gingiva,* gum, *linea*], the scalloped line formed by the edge of the unattached gum tissue at the margin of the soft tissues beside the teeth. The line is called marginal gingiva when viewed buccally or lingually; between the teeth in the interproximal area, the line is called interdental gingiva. Also called **gum line.**

**gingival massage,** the rubbing of the gum tissues for cleansing purposes, for improvement of tissue tone and blood circulation, and for keratinization of the surface epithelium.

**gingival mat,** the connective tissue of the gum, composed of coarse, broad collagen fibers that attach the gingivae to the teeth and hold the unattached gum close to the teeth.

**gingival papilla.** See **interdental gingiva.**

**gingival physiology,** the function of the gum tissue as supportive and protective investments of the teeth and subjacent tissues. The gingival fiber apparatus serves as a barrier to apical migration of the junctional epithelium and binds the gingival tissues to the teeth. Normal gingival topography permits the free flow of food away from the occlusal surfaces and from the cervical and interproximal areas of the teeth.

**gingival pocket.** See **periodontal pocket.**

**gingival position,** the level of the gum margin in relation to the teeth.

**gingival shrinkage,** the reduction in the size of the gum tissue, especially as a result of the therapeutic elimination of subgingival deposits and curettage of the soft tissue wall of the gingival pocket.

**gingival stippling,** numerous small depressions in the surface of healthy gum tissue, producing an appearance that varies from that of smooth velvet to that of an orange peel. See also **epithelial peg, gingival consistency, rete peg.**

**gingival sulcus.** See **gingival crevice.**

**gingivectomy** /jin'jīvek'təmē/ [L, *gingiva* + Gk, *ektomē,* excision], surgical removal of infected and diseased gum tissue, performed to arrest the progress of periodontal disease. With the patient under local anesthesia and sometimes sedated, the affected tissue is removed, and the accessible root surfaces are debrided of calculus and necrotic cementum. This procedure eliminates periodontal pockets. The healthy gingival tissues are sutured into place, and a periodontal pack may be placed on the surgical site to prevent trauma during eating and to allow new tissue growth to fill in the area. Bleeding, discomfort, and pain are genereally associated with the procedure. After surgery the patient is closely monitored for signs of hemorrhage, frequency in swallowing, or a rise in pulse rate. The periodontal pack is removed after 1 week. Compare **gingivoplasty.**

**gingivitis** /jin'jivī'tis/ [L, *gingiva* + Gk, *itis,* inflammation], inflammation of the gingiva, with symptoms that may include redness, swelling, and bleeding. Gingivitis is generally the result of poor oral hygiene and of the accumulation of bacterial plaque on the teeth, but it may be a sign of other conditions, such as diabetes mellitus, leukemia, hormonal changes, or vitamin deficiency. It is common in pregnancy, is usually painless, and may be acute or chronic. Frequent removal of plaque and regular visits to the dentist or dental hygienist may help in prevention. Compare **acute necrotizing ulcerative gingivitis.**

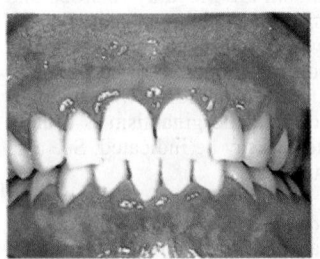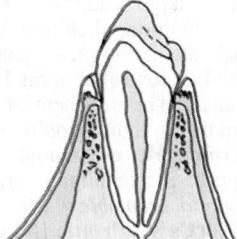

**Gingivitis** *(Murray et al, 1994)*

**gingivo-,** combining form meaning 'gingiva': *gingivoglossitis, gingivolabial, gingivosis.*

**gingivoplasty** /jin'jivōplas'tē/ [L, *gingiva* + Gk, *plassein,* to shape], the surgical contouring of the gum tissues and interdental papillae to restore gingival tissue to more normal form and function. Compare **gingivectomy.**

**gingivostomatitis** /jin'jivōstō'mətī'tis/ [L, *gingiva* + Gk, *stoma,* mouth, *itis,* inflammation], multiple painful ulcers on the gums and mucous membranes of the mouth, the result of a herpesvirus infection. The condition most frequently affects infants and young children. It usually subsides after 1 week, but in rare cases it may progress to a systemic viral infection. See also **herpes simplex.**

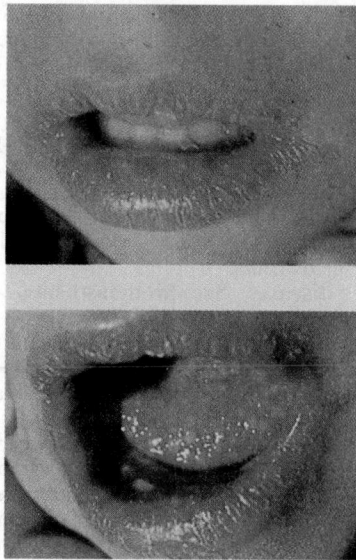

**Gingivostomatitis** *(Doughty and Broadwell, 1993)*

**ginglymus joint.** See **hinge joint.**

**ginkgo,** an herbal product harvested from a tree that is native to China and Japan.

■ USES: This herb is used for poor circulation, diabetes, vascular disease, cancer, inflammatory disorders, impotence, and degenerative nerve conditions. It is also used for age-related declines in cognition and memory.

■ CONTRAINDICATIONS: Ginkgo is contraindicated in people with coagulation or platelet disorders or hemophilia, in children, and in those with known hypersensitivity to this product.

**ginseng,** an herb with red or yellow fruits that is native to the Far East and is now found throughout the world. One species is native to North America.

■ USES: This herb is used for physical and mental exhaustion, stress, viral infections, diabetes, sluggishness, fatigue, weak immunity, and convalescence.

■ CONTRAINDICATIONS: Ginseng should not be used during pregnancy and lactation or in children. It is also contraindicated in those with known hypersensitivity, hypertension, and cardiac disorders.

**Giordano-Giovannetti diet** /jôrdä′nōjō′vənet′ē/, a low-protein, low-fat, high-carbohydrate diet with controlled potassium and sodium intake, used in chronic renal insufficiency and liver failure. Protein is given only in the form of essential amino acids so that the body will use excess blood urea nitrogen to synthesize the nonessential amino acids for the production of tissue protein. The foods included are eggs, small amounts of milk, low-protein bread, and some fruits and vegetables low in potassium, such as green beans, summer squash, cabbage, pears, grapefruit, and fresh or frozen blackberries, blueberries, and boysenberries. There are many modified forms of this diet, depending on patient requirements and tolerance and usually varying in the amount and origin of the protein. Also called **Giovannetti diet.** See also **renal diet.**

**gipoma** /gipō′mə/, a pancreatic tumor that causes changes in secretion of gastric inhibitory polypeptide (GIP).

**girdle** /gur′dəl/, any curved or circular structure, such as

the hipline formed by the bones and related tissues of the pelvis.

**girdle pad,** a covering that fits over the iliac crests and sacrum to protect the hip area in contact sports.

**girdle sensation.** See **zonesthesia.**

**GI tract.** See **digestive tract**.

**Giuliani's sign** [Emilio R. Giuliani, twentieth century American cardiologist], a posterior chest thrill felt between the left scapula and spinal column in mitral insufficiency caused by anterior mitral leaf prolapse.

**glabella** /gləbəl′ə/ [L, *glabrum,* bald], a flat triangular area of bone between the two superciliary ridges of the forehead. It is sometimes used as a baseline for cephalometric measurements.

**glabrous skin** /glā′brəs/ [L, *glaber,* smooth; AS, *scinn*], smooth, hairless skin.

**glacial acetic acid** /glā′shəl/, a clear, colorless liquid or crystalline substance (CH₃COOH) with a pungent odor. It is obtained by the destructive distillation of wood or from acetylene and water or by the oxidation of ethyl alcohol by aerobic bacteria, as in the production of vinegar. Glacial acetic acid is strongly corrosive and potentially flammable, having a low flash point. It is miscible in alcohol, ether, glycerol, and water and is used as a solvent for organic compounds. Also called **vinegar acid.**

**gland** [L, *glans,* acorn], any one of many organs in the body, comprising specialized cells that secrete or excrete materials not related to their ordinary metabolism. Some glands lubricate; others, such as the pituitary gland, produce hormones; hematopoietic glands, such as the spleen and certain lymph nodes, take part in the production of blood components. **Exocrine glands** discharge their secretions into ducts. They may be classified by the shape and complexity of their duct systems. **Endocrine glands** are ductless and

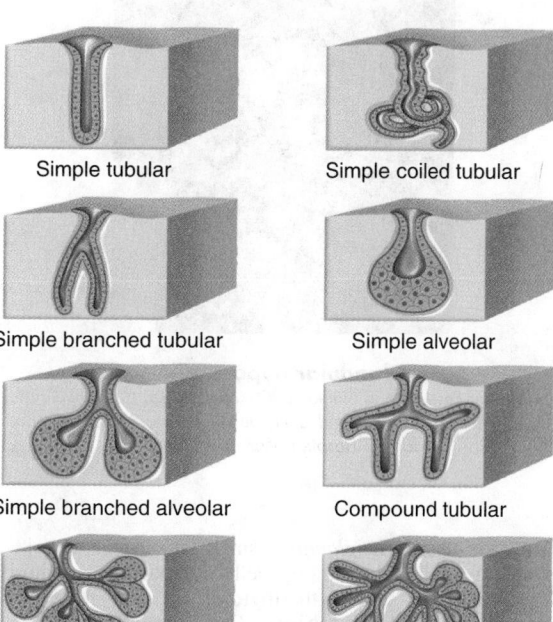

Simple tubular  Simple coiled tubular

Simple branched tubular  Simple alveolar

Simple branched alveolar  Compound tubular

Compound alveolar  Compound tubuloalveolar

**Exocrine glands: structural classification**

discharge their secretions directly into the blood or interstitial fluid.

**glanders** [OFr, *glandres,* neck gland swelling], an infection caused by the bacillus *Burkholderia mallei* (formerly called *Pseudomonas mallei*), transmitted to humans from horses and other domestic animals. It is characterized by purulent inflammation of the mucous membranes and development of skin nodules that ulcerate. If untreated with antibiotics, the infection may spread to the bones, liver, central nervous system, and other tissues and cause death. It is endemic in Africa, Asia, and South America but has been eradicated in Europe and North America.

**glandes.** See **glans.**

**gland of Montgomery.** See **areolar gland.**

**glands of bile duct,** tubuloacinar glands in the mucosa of the bile ducts and the neck of the gallbladder. Also called **biliary glands.**

**glands of Zeis.** See **ciliary gland.**

**glandular** /glan'dyələr/ [L, *glandula,* small gland], pertaining to or resembling a gland.

**glandular carcinoma.** See **adenocarcinoma.**

**glandular epithelium** [L, *glandula,* small gland; Gk, *epi,* above, *thele,* nipple], epithelium that contains glandular cells.

**glandular fever.** See **infectious mononucleosis.**

**glandular hypospadias** [L, *glandula,* small gland *+hypo,* under + *spadōn,* a rent], the most common type of hypospadias, in which the urethral orifice opens at the site of the frenum, which may be rudimentary or absent; the normal site of the urinary meatus is represented on the glans penis as a blind pit. Also called **balanic hypospadias.**

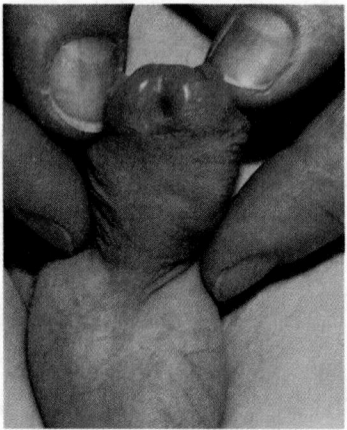

**Glandular hypospadia**
(Moore, Pesaud, and Shiota, 2000/courtesy Dr. A.E. Chudley, Department of Pediatrics and Child Health, University of Manitoba, Children's Hospital, Winnipeg, Canada)

**glandular tissue** [L, *glandula,* small gland; OFr, *tissu*], a group of epithelial secreting cells composing a definitive glandular organ, such as the thyroid.

**glandula vestibularis major.** See **Bartholin's gland.**

**glans** /glanz/, *pl.* **glandes** /glan'dēz/ [L, acorn], **1.** a general term for a small rounded mass or a glandlike body. **2.** erectile tissue, as on the ends of the clitoris and the penis.

**glans of clitoris** [L, *glans* + Gk, *kleitoris*], the erectile tissue at the end of the clitoris. It comprises two corpora cavernosa enclosed in a dense, fibrous membrane and connected to the pubis and ischium. Also called **glans clitoridis.**

**glans penis,** the conical tip of the penis that covers the end of the corpora cavernosa penis and the corpus spongiosum like a cap. The urethral orifice is normally located at the distal tip of the glans penis; the corona glandis, the widest part of the glans penis, is around the base of the proximal portion. A fold of dark, thin, hairless skin forms the foreskin covering the glans penis.

**Glanzmann's disease.** See **thrombasthenia.**

**glare,** a strong, dazzling light that may cause discomfort to the eye. Visual problems that result from glare often involve inadequate lighting conditions; they particularly affect individuals with cataracts or other disease conditions. The condition is relieved somewhat by using incandescent rather than fluorescent lighting, wearing a visor, wearing special antiglare lenses, and using a matte-black cardboard typoscope for reading words on a glaring white paper.

**Glasgow Coma Scale,** a quick, practical standardized system for assessing the degree of conscious impairment in the critically ill and for predicting the duration and ultimate outcome of coma, primarily in patients with head injuries. The system involves three determinants, eye opening, verbal response, and motor response, all of which are evaluated independently according to a rank order that indicates the level of consciousness and degree of dysfunction. The degree of consciousness may vary from determinant to determinant and is assessed numerically by the best response. The results may be plotted on a graph to provide a visual representation of the improvement, stability, or deterioration of a patient's level of consciousness, which is crucial to predicting the eventual outcome of coma. The sum of the numeric values for each parameter can also be used as an overall objective measurement, with 14 indicative of no impairment, 3 compatible with brain death, and 7 usually accepted as a state of coma. The test score can also function as an indicator for certain diagnostic tests or treatments, such as the need for a computed tomography scan, intracranial pressure monitoring, and intubation. The scale has a high degree of consistency even when used by staff with varied experience.

**Glasgow Coma Scale scoring**

**Eyes open**
4 Spontaneously
3 On request
2 To pain stimuli (supraorbital or digital)
1 No opening

**Best verbal response**
5 Oriented to time, place, person
4 Engages in conversation, confused in content
3 Words spoken but conversation not sustained
2 Groans evoked by pain
1 No response

**Best motor response**
5 Obeys a command ("Hold out three fingers.")
4 Localizes a painful stimulus
3 Flexes either arm
2 Extends arm to painful stimulus
1 No response

From Phipps WJ, Sands JK, Marek JE: *Medical-surgical nursing: concepts and clinical practice,* ed 6, St Louis, 1999, Mosby.

**Glasgow Outcome Scale,** a functional assessment inventory based on five global categories: death, persistent vegetative state, severe disability, moderate disability, and good recovery. It measures outcome. It has been criticized as lacking sensitivity to functionally significant changes.

**glass factor.** See **factor XII.**

**glass ionomer cement,** a dental cement used for small restorations on the proximal surfaces of anterior teeth, for restoration of eroded areas at the gingival margin, and as a luting agent for restorations and orthodontic bands.

**glatiramer,** a multiple sclerosis drug.

■ INDICATIONS: This drug is used to reduce the frequency of relapses in patients with relapsing-remitting multiple sclerosis.

■ CONTRAINDICATIONS: Known hypersensitivity to this drug or to mannitol prohibits the use of glatiramer.

■ ADVERSE EFFECTS: Adverse effects of this drug include migraine, palpitations, syncope, tachycardia, vasodilation, nausea, vomiting, diarrhea, anorexia, gastroenteritis, ecchymosis, lymphadenopathy, edema, weight gain, arthralgia, anxiety, hypertonia, tremor, vertigo, speech disorder, agitation, confusion, bronchitis, dyspnea, pruritus, rash, sweating, urticaria, erythema, ear pain, urinary urgency, dysmenorrhea, and vaginal moniliasis.

**glauco-,** combining form meaning 'gray or silver': *glaucoma, glaucomatous.*

**glaucoma** /glôkō′mə, glou-/ [Gk, cataract], an abnormal condition of elevated pressure within an eye caused by obstruction of the outflow of aqueous humor. **Acute (angle-closure, closed-angle,** or **narrow-angle) glaucoma** occurs if the pupil in an eye with a narrow angle between the iris and cornea dilates markedly, causing the folded iris to block the exit of aqueous humor from the anterior chamber. Primary open-angle glaucoma (POAG) is much more common, often bilateral; it develops slowly and is genetically determined. The obstruction is believed to occur within the Schlemm's canal. **—glaucomatous,** *adj.*

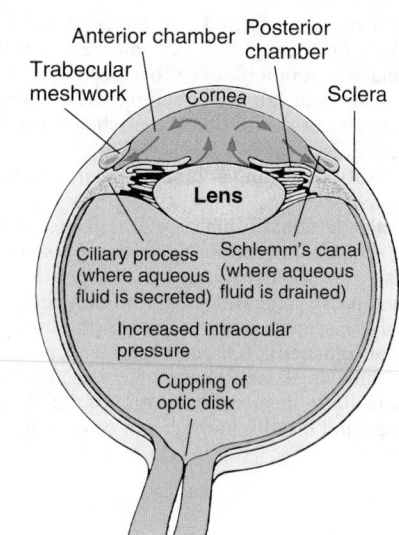

**Open-angle glaucoma** *(Beare and Myers, 1998)*

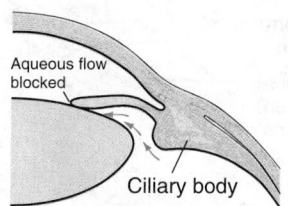

**Closed-angle glaucoma** *(Beare and Myers, 1998)*

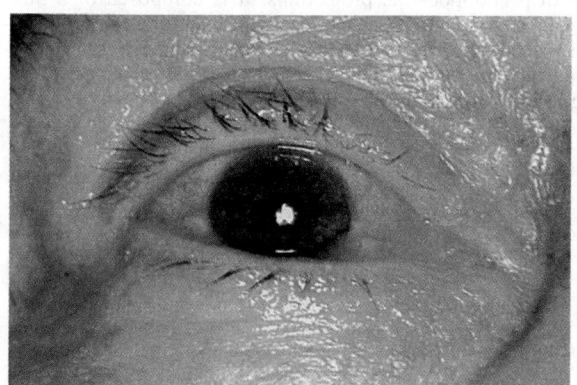

**Ophthamoscopic image of open-angle glaucoma**
*(Apple and Rabb, 1998)*

■ OBSERVATIONS: Acute glaucoma is accompanied by extreme ocular pain, blurred vision, redness of the eye, and dilation of the pupil. Nausea and vomiting may occur. If untreated, acute glaucoma causes complete and permanent blindness within 2 to 5 days. Chronic glaucoma may produce no symptoms except gradual loss of peripheral vision over a period of years. Sometimes present are headaches, blurred vision, and dull pain in the eye. Cupping of the optic discs may be noted on ophthalmoscopic examination. Halos around lights and central blindness are late manifestations. Both types are characterized by elevated intraocular pressure indicated by tonometry.

■ INTERVENTIONS: Acute glaucoma is treated with eyedrops to constrict the pupil and draw the iris away from the cornea; osmotic agents such as urea, mannitol, or glycerol given systemically to lower intraocular pressure; acetazolamide to reduce fluid formation; and surgical iridectomy to produce a filtration pathway for aqueous humor. Chronic glaucoma can usually be controlled with eyedrops such as beta-blockers, topical carbonic anhydrase inhibitors, and prostaglandin analogs. Other treatment includes carbonic anhydrase inhibitors, epinephrine eyedrops, and timolol, a beta-adrenergic blocking agent.

**glaucoma consummatum.** See **absolutum glaucoma.**

**glaucomatocyclitic crisis** /glôkom′ətōsiklit′ik/, a recurrent rise in intraocular pressure in one eye, resembling acute angle-closure glaucoma, associated with minimal signs of uveitis. Also called **Posner-Schlossman syndrome.**

**glaucomatous.** See **glaucoma.**

**glaucomatous halo** /glôkom′ətəs/, **1.** an illusion of a circle of brightness surrounding a light, observed by patients with acute glaucoma, which is caused by edema of the corneal epithelium. **2.** a yellowish white ring surrounding the optic disc, a sign of atrophy of the choroid in glaucoma.

**glaze** /glāz/ [ME, *glasen*], **1.** to cover with a glossy, smooth surface or coating. **2.** a ceramic veneer added to a dental porcelain restoration after it has been fired, to give a completely nonporous, glossy or semiglossy surface. **3.** the final firing (in air) of dental porcelain, when formation of a thin, vitreous, glossy surface takes place.

**-glea, -glia,** suffix meaning a 'binding gelatinous medium': *ooglea, zooglea.*

**glenohumeral** /glē′nōhyōō′mərəl/ [Gk, *glene*, joint socket; L, *humerus*, shoulder], pertaining to the glenoid cavity and the humerus at the shoulder joint.

**glenohumeral joint,** the shoulder joint, formed by the glenoid cavity of the scapula and the head of the humerus.

**glenohumeral ligaments** [Gk, *glene*, joint socket, *humerus*, shoulder], three thickened bands of connective tissue attached proximally to the anterior margin of the glenoid cavity and labrum and distally to the lesser tuberosity and neck of the humerus.

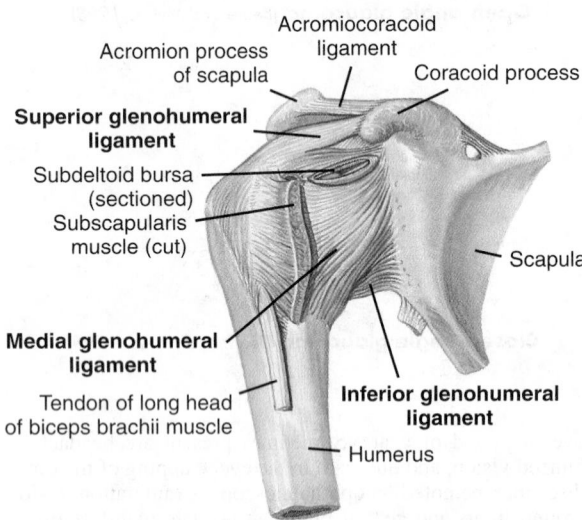

**Glenohumeral ligaments** *(Thibodeau and Patton, 1999)*

**glenoid cavity** /glē′noid/ [Gk, *glene*, joint socket, *eidos*, form; L, *cavum*], a shallow socket with which the head of the humerus articulates below the acromium at the junction of the superior and axillary borders. Also called **glenoid fossa.**

**glenoid fossa.** See **glenoid cavity, mandibular fossa.**

**glia.** See **neuroglia.**

**glia cells** /glī′ə, glē′ə/ [Gk, *glia*, glue; L, *cella*, storeroom], neural cells that have a connective tissue supporting function in the central nervous system. Examples include astrocytes and oligodendroglial cells of ectodermal origin and microglial cells of mesodermal origin.

**gliadin** /glī′ədin/ [Gk, *glia*, glue], a fraction of the gluten protein that is found in wheat and rye and less so from barley and oats. Its solubility in diluted alcohol distinguishes it from another grain protein, glutenin. Those with celiac disease are sensitive to this substance and it is excluded from their diet. See also **celiac disease.**

**glial cell line derived neurotrophic factor (GDNF)** /glī′əl/, a nerve growth drug. It has been used in laboratory animals to reverse the progression of symptoms of Parkinson's disease. GDNF is believed to act as a biologic shield, protecting dopamine nerve cells from damage that normally would destroy them.

**gliding** [AS, *glidan*, to glide], **1.** one of the four basic movements allowed by the various joints of the skeleton. It is common to all movable joints and permits one surface to move smoothly over an adjacent surface, regardless of shape. Gliding is the only motion allowed by most of the wrist and the ankle joints. **2.** a smooth, continuous movement. Compare **angular movement, circumduction, rotation.**

**gliding contusion,** a brain injury caused by displacement of the gray matter of the cerebral cortex during angular acceleration of the head. Most of the damage occurs at the junction between the gray matter and the white matter. Such contusions are associated with diffuse axonal injuries and acute subdural hematomas.

**gliding joint,** a synovial joint in which articulation of contiguous bones allows only gliding movements, as in the wrist and the ankle. The ligaments or the osseous processes around each gliding joint limit movements of apposed plane surfaces or concavoconvex articulations. Also called **arthrodia, articulatio plana.** Compare **hinge joint, pivot joint.**

**gliding zone,** an articular cartilage surface area immediately adjacent to a joint space. It consists of a thin layer of densely packed collagen fibers lying parallel to the surface and covered by a fine acellular, afibrillar membrane. At the periphery the fibrous components merge with the fibrous periosteum of the adjacent bone.

**glio-,** combining form meaning 'neuroglia or a gluey substance': *gliococcus, gliosarcoma, gliosome.*

**glioblastoma.** See **spongioblastoma.**

**glioblastoma multiforme** /glī′ōblastō′mə mul′tifôr′mē/ [Gk, *glia*, glue, *blastos*, germ, *oma*, tumor; L, *multus*, many, *forma*, form], a malignant rapidly growing pulpy or cystic tumor of the cerebrum or the spinal cord. The lesion spreads with pseudopod-like projections. It is composed of a mixture of monocytes, pyriform cells, immature and mature astrocytes, and neural ectodermal cells with fibrous or protoplasmic processes. Also called **anaplastic astrocytoma, glioma multiforme.**

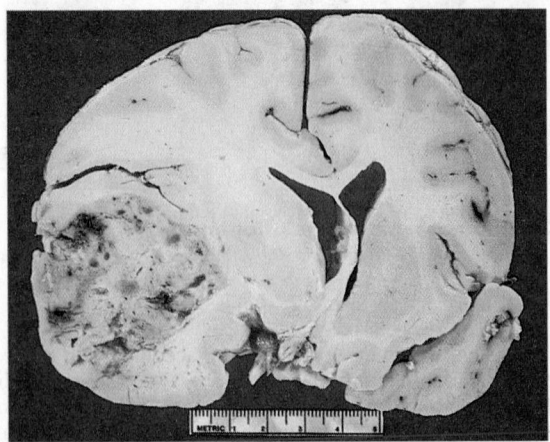

**Glioblastoma multiforme** *(Kumar, Cotran, and Robbins, 1997)*

**glioma** /glī·ō′mə/, *pl.* **gliomas, gliomata** [Gk, *glia* + *oma,* tumor], any of the largest group of primary tumors of the brain, composed of malignant glial cells. Kinds of gliomas are **astrocytoma, ependymoma, glioblastoma multiforme, medulloblastoma,** and **oligodendroglioma.**

**-glioma,** combining form meaning a 'tumor arising from the neuroglia': *angioglioma, fibroglioma, ganglioma.*

**glioma multiforme.** See **glioblastoma multiforme.**

**glioma retinae.** See **retinoblastoma.**

**glioma sarcomatosum.** See **gliosarcoma.**

**gliomata.** See **glioma.**

**glioneuroma** /glī′ōnŏŏrō′mə/, *pl.* **glioneuromas, glioneuromata** [Gk, *glia* + *neuron,* nerve, *oma,* tumor], a neoplasm composed of nerve cells and elements of their supporting connective tissue.

**gliosarcoma** /glī′ōsärkō′mə/, *pl.* **gliosarcomas, gliosarcomata** [Gk, *glia* + *sarx,* flesh, *oma,* tumor], a tumor composed of spindle-shaped cells in the delicate supporting connective tissue of nerve cells. Also called **glioma, glioblastoma, spongioblastoma, spongiocytoma.**

**gliosarcoma retinae.** See **retinoblastoma.**

**gliosis** /glī·ō′sis/, a proliferation of astrocytes that may appear as a sign of healing after a central nervous system injury. See also **fibrogliosis.**

**glipizide** /glip′izīd/, an oral antidiabetic drug.
- ■ INDICATIONS: It is prescribed as an adjunct to diet and exercise to lower blood glucose levels of patients with type 2 diabetes mellitus.
- ■ CONTRAINDICATIONS: The dosage may have to be adjusted for patients who are taking drugs such as diuretics that increase blood glucose levels; elderly, debilitated, or malnourished patients are at risk of development of hypoglycemia.
- ■ ADVERSE EFFECTS: Among the most serious adverse reactions are nausea, heartburn, and skin allergies.

**Glisson's capsule** /glis′ənz/ [Francis Glisson, English physician, 1597–1677; L, *capsula,* little box], the fibrous outer tissue sheath around lobules of the liver that carry branches of the hepatic artery, portal vein, and bile duct. Also called **hepatobiliary capsule.**

**glitter cells** [ME, *gliteren,* to shine], white blood cells in which movement of granules is observed in their cytoplasm. They are seen in microscopic examination of urine samples in cases of pyelonephritis or disorders marked by low osmolality.

**Gln,** abbreviation for **glutamine.**

**global aphasia** /glō′bəl/ [L, *globus,* ball; Gk, *a* + *phasis,* without speech], a loss of ability to use or comprehend any form of written or spoken language. The condition involves both sensory and motor nerve tracts and is a relatively more severe form of aphasia. Communication is attempted through gestures or the use of automatic words and phrases. Also called **mixed aphasia.**

**global price,** (in U.S. managed care) an all-inclusive price for services rendered. It may refer to comprehensive physician services alone or include both hospital and physician services, depending on the contractual agreement.

**global warming,** an ecologic model of world climate changes based on the **greenhouse effect,** exacerbated by burning of fossil fuels, massive deforestation, and conversion of cropland to industrial and other urban uses, all contributing to an increase in the earth's temperature. Major shifts in climate are not unusual in the history of the earth, which has undergone global warming in previous periods of geologic history.

**globin** /glō′bin/ [L, *globus,* ball], a group of four globulin protein molecules that become bound by the iron in heme molecules to form hemoglobin or myoglobin.

**-globin,** suffix meaning 'containing protein': *hemoglobin, myoglobin.*

**-globinuria,** combining form meaning '(condition involving) the presence of complex proteins in the urine': *hemoglobinuria, methemoglobinuria, myoglobinuria.*

**globoid leukodystrophy.** See **galactosyl ceramide lipidosis.**

**globose nucleus,** one of four deeply placed cerebellar nuclei, located medial to the emboliform nucleus. It receives input from the intermediate zone of the cerebellar cortex, and its axons exit via the superior cerebellar peduncle. The globose nucleus is involved in posture control and voluntary movement.

**globule** /glob′yŏŏl/ [L, *globulus,* small ball], a small spheric mass. Kinds of globules are **dentin globule, Dobie's globule, Marchi's globule, milk globule, Morgagni's globule,** and **myelin globule.**

**globulin** /glob′yŏŏlin/, one of a broad category of simple proteins classified by solubility, electrophoretic mobility, and size. Compare **albumin.** See also **euglobulin, plasma protein.**

**globulinuria** /-ŏŏr′ē·ə/ [L, *globulus,* small ball; Gk, *ouron,* urine], the presence of globulin-class proteins in the urine.

**globus hystericus** /glō′bus/ [L, small ball; Gk, *hystera,* womb], a transitory sensation of a lump in the throat that cannot be swallowed or coughed up, often accompanying emotional conflict or acute anxiety. The condition is thought to be caused by a functional disturbance of the ninth cranial nerve and spasm of the inferior constrictor muscle that encircles the lower part of the throat. The physical examination result tends to be normal, as does the result of barium esophagraphy.

**globus pallidus** /pal′idəs/ [L, small ball, pale], the smaller and more medial part of the lentiform nucleus of the brain, separated from the putamen by the lateral medullary lamina and divided into external and internal portions closely connected to the stratum, thalamus, and mesencephalon.

**-gloea.** See **-glea.**

**glomangioma** /glōman′jē·ō′mə/, *pl.,* **glomangiomas, glomangiomata** [L, *glomus,* ball of thread; Gk, *angeion,* vessel, *oma*], a benign tumor that develops from a cluster of blood cells in the skin. Also called **angiomyoneuroma, angioneuroma.**

**glomera.** See **glomus.**

**glomerular** /glōmer′yŏŏlər/ [L, *glomerulus,* small ball], pertaining to a glomerulus, especially a renal glomerulus.

**glomerular capsule.** See **Bowman's capsule.**

**glomerular disease,** any of a group of diseases in which the glomerulus of the kidney is affected. Depending on the particular disease, there may be hyperplasia, atrophy, necrosis, scarring, or deposits in the glomeruli. The symptoms may be abrupt in onset or slowly progressive. Compare **acute tubular necrosis.** See also **glomerulonephritis.**

**glomerular filtration,** the renal process whereby fluid in the blood is filtered across the capillaries of the glomerulus and into the urinary space of Bowman's capsule.

**glomerular filtration rate (GFR)** [L, *glomerulus,* small ball; Fr, *filtre* + L, *ratus*], a kidney function test in which results can be determined from the amount of ultrafiltrate formed by plasma flowing through the glomeruli of the kidney. It may be calculated from inulin and creatinine clearance, serum creatinine, and blood urea nitrogen (BUN).

**glomeruli.** See **glomerulus.**

**glomerulo-,** combining form meaning 'glomerulus', the functional unit of the kidney: *glomerulopathy.*

**glomerulonephritis** /glōmer′yŏŏlōnəfrī′tis/ [L, *glomerulus,* small ball; Gk, *nephros,* kidney, *itis*], an inflammation of the glomerulus of the kidney, characterized by proteinuria, hematuria, decreased urine production, and edema. Kinds of glomerulonephritis are **acute glomerulonephritis, chronic glomerulonephritis,** and **subacute glomerulonephritis.**

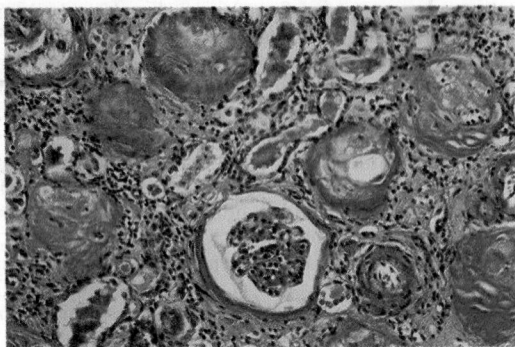

**Chronic glomerulonephritis**
*(Kumar, Cotran, and Robbins, 1997/courtesy Dr. M.A. Venkatachalam, Department of Pathology, University of Texas Health Sciences Center, San Antonio)*

**glomerulosclerosis** /-sklərō′sis/ [L, *glomerulus,* small ball; Gk, *sklerosis,* a hardening, *osis,* condition], a severe kidney disease in which glomerular function of blood filtration is lost as fibrous scar tissue replaces the glomeruli. The disease commonly follows an infection or arteriosclerosis.

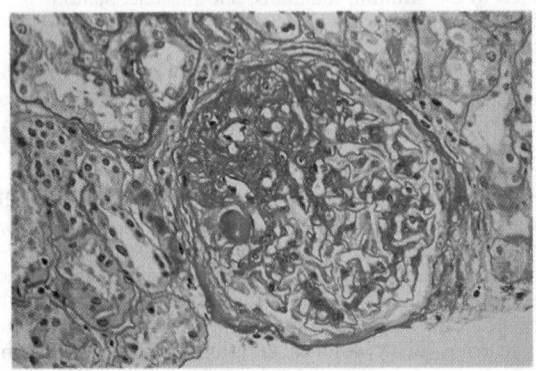

**Glomerulosclerosis**
*(Kumar, Cotran, and Robbins, 1997/courtesy Dr. H. Rennke, Department of Pathology, Brigham and Women's Hospital, Boston)*

**glomerulus** /glōmer′yŏŏləs/, *pl.* **glomeruli** [L, small ball], **1.** a tuft or cluster. **2.** a structure composed of blood vessels or nerve fibers, such as a renal glomerulus.

**glomus** /glō′məs/, *pl.* **glomera** /glom′ərə/ [L, ball of thread], a small group of arterioles connecting directly to veins and having a rich nerve supply.

**glomus cell, 1.** an epithelioid cell surrounding a coiled arteriovenous anastomosis of a glomus body. **2.** a modified smooth muscle cell.

**glomus tumor,** a frequently painful neoplasm involving the arteriovenous anastomoses of the skin. It contains many small vascular channels surrounded by glomus cells.

**gloss-.** See **glosso-.**

**glossa.** See **tongue.**

**glossalgia.** See **glossodynia.**

**glossectomy** /glosek′təmē/ [Gk, *glossa,* tongue, *ektomē,* excision], the surgical removal of all or a part of the tongue.

**-glossia, 1.** suffix meaning 'related to the tongue': *cacoglossia, megaloglossia, schistoglossia.* **2.** suffix meaning the 'possession of a specified number of tongues': *aglossia, diglossia.*

**glossitis** /glosī′tis/ [Gk, *glossa,* tongue, *itis*], inflammation of the tongue. Acute glossitis, characterized by swelling, intense pain that may be referred to the ears, salivation, fever, and enlarged regional lymph nodes, may develop during an infectious disease or after a burn, bite, or other injury. Glossitis in which there is smooth atrophy of the surface and edges of the tongue is seen in pernicious anemia. Glossitis in which irregular, bright red patches appear on the tip or sides of the tongue (**Moeller's glossitis**) occurs in middle-aged people, chiefly women. The condition causes pain or a burning sensation and sensitivity to hot or spicy foods; it often resists treatment. In congenital glossitis there is a flat or slightly elevated patch or plaque anterior to the circumvallate papillae in the midline of the dorsal surface of the tongue.

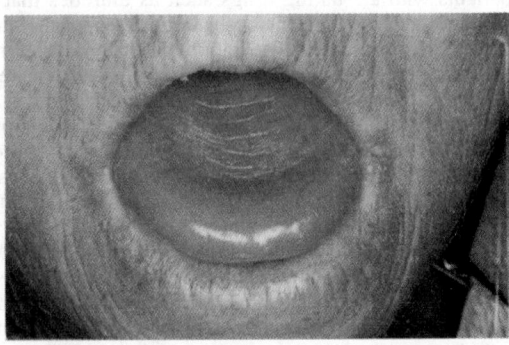

**Severe atrophic glossitis** *(Sleisenger and Fordtran, 1993)*

**glossitis parasitica.** See **parasitic glossitis.**

**glossitis rhomboidea mediana.** See **median rhomboid glossitis.**

**glosso-, gloss-,** combining form meaning 'tongue': *glossocele, glossodynia, glossoplegia.*

**glossodynia** /glos′ōdin′ē·ə/ [Gk, *glossa* + *odyne,* pain], pain in the tongue, caused by acute or chronic inflammation, an abscess, an ulcer, or trauma. Also called **glossalgia.**

**glossodynia exfoliativa.** See **Moeller's glossitis.**

**glossoepiglottic** /glos′ō·ep′iglot′ik/, pertaining to the epiglottis and the tongue.

**glossohyal.** see **hyoglossal.**

**glossolalia** /glos′ōlā′lyə/ [Gk, *glossa* + *lalein,* to babble], speech in an unknown 'language,' as 'speaking in tongues' during a state of religious ecstasy when the message being transmitted through the speaker is believed to be a message from a celestial spirit or from God.

**glossoncus** /glosong′kəs/ [Gk, *glossa* + *onkos,* swelling], a local swelling or general enlargement of the tongue.

**glossopathy** /glosop'əthē/ [Gk, *glossa* + *pathos,* disease], a pathologic condition of the tongue, such as acute inflammation caused by a burn, bite, injury, or infectious disease; enlargement resulting from congenital lymphangioma; or a disorder produced by mycotic infection, a malignant lesion, or a congenital anomaly.

**glossopexy** /glos'əpek'sē/ [Gk, *glossa* + *pexis,* fixation], an adhesion of the tongue to the lip.

**glossopharyngeal** /glos'ōfərin'jē·əl/ [Gk, *glossa* + *pharynx,* throat], pertaining to the tongue and pharynx. See also **glossopharyngeal nerve.**

**glossopharyngeal breathing (GPB),** a technique of forcing air into the lungs with the pharynx and tongue muscles. The technique can be taught to patients whose respiratory muscles are weak.

**glossopharyngeal nerve,** either of a pair of cranial nerves essential to the sense of taste, sensation in some viscera, and secretion from certain glands. The nerve has both sensory and motor fibers that pass from the tongue, parotid gland, and pharynx; communicate with the vagus nerve; and connect with two areas in the brain. Also called **nervus glossopharyngeus, ninth cranial nerve.**

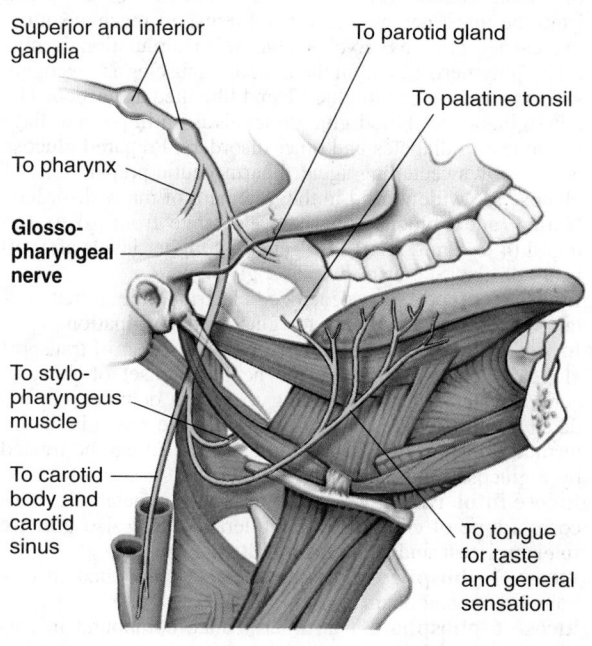

Superior and inferior ganglia
To parotid gland
To palatine tonsil
To pharynx
**Glossopharyngeal nerve**
To stylopharyngeus muscle
To carotid body and carotid sinus
To tongue for taste and general sensation

**Glossopharyngeal nerve**

**glossopharyngeal neuralgia,** a disorder of unknown origin characterized by recurrent attacks of severe pain in the back of the pharynx, the tonsils, the base of the tongue, and the middle ear. It tends to affect more men than women, with an onset after 40 years of age. Attacks lasting from a few seconds to minutes may be triggered by swallowing. The symptoms may be similar to those of trigeminal neuralgia. Treatment is usually pharmaceutical, but surgery may be recommended to sever involved nerve tracts.

**glossophytia** /glos'əfit'ē·ə/ [Gk, *glossa* + *phyton,* plant], a condition of the tongue characterized by a blackish patch on the dorsum on which filiform papillae are greatly elongated

and thickened like bristly hairs. The usually painless condition may be caused by heavy smoking or the extensive use of broad-spectrum antibiotics. See also **parasitic glossitis.**

**glossoplasty** /glos'ōplas'tē/ [Gk, *glossa* + *plassein,* to mold], a surgical procedure or plastic surgery on the tongue performed to correct a congenital anomaly, repair an injury, or restore a measure of function after excision of a malignant lesion.

**glossoptosis** /glos'optō'sis/ [Gk, *glossa* + *ptosis,* falling], the retraction or downward displacement of the tongue.

**glossopyrosis** /glos'ōpīrō'sis/ [Gk, *glossa* + *pyr,* fire, *osis,* condition], a burning sensation in the tongue caused by chronic inflammation, by exposure to extremely hot or spicy food, or by psychogenic glossitis.

**glossorrhaphy** /glosôr'əfē/ [Gk, *glossa* + *rhaphe,* seam], the surgical suturing of a wound in the tongue.

**glossotrichia** /glos'ətrik'ē·ə/ [Gk, *glossa* + *thrix,* hair], a condition of the tongue characterized by a hairlike appearance of the papillae. Also called **hairy tongue.**

**glossy skin** [ONorse, *glosa,* smooth and shiny; AS, *scinn*], a shiny skin that is usually secondary to neuritis and may be associated with other integumentary disorders, including alopecia, skin fissuring, and ulceration. It usually begins as an erythematous area on an extremity.

**glott-,** combining form meaning 'pertaining to the glottis': *glottic, glottidas, glottis.*

**glottal stop** /glot'əl stop /, a speech sound made by closure of the glottis and then an explosive release.

**glottis,** *pl.* **glottises, glottides** [Gk, opening to larynx], **1.** also called **true glottis, rima glottidis.** a slitlike opening between the true vocal cords (plica vocalis). **2.** the phonation apparatus of the larynx, composed of the true vocal cords and the opening between them (rima glottidis). —**glottal, glottic,** *adj.*

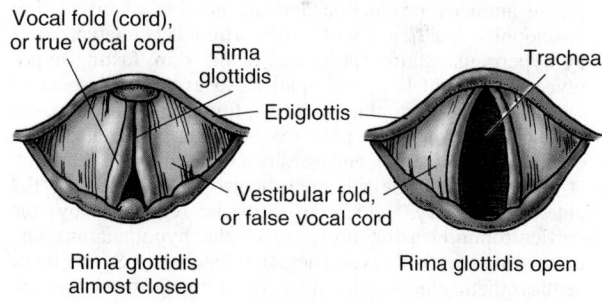

ANTERIOR

Vocal fold (cord), or true vocal cord
Rima glottidis
Trachea
Epiglottis
Vestibular fold, or false vocal cord
Rima glottidis almost closed
Rima glottidis open

POSTERIOR

**Glottis** *(Ignatavicius, Workman, and Mishler, 1999)*

**gloves,** sterile or clean, fitted coverings for the hands, usually with a separate sheath for each finger and thumb. Clean gloves are worn to protect health care personnel from urine, stool, blood, saliva, and drainage from wounds and lesions of patients and to protect patients from health care personnel who may have cuts. Sterile gloves are worn when there is contact with sterile instruments or a patient's sterile part.

**glow curve,** (in thermoluminescence dosimetry) the graphic representation of the emitted light intensity that increases with the increasing phosphor temperature.

**GLP-1,** abbreviation for **glucagon-like peptide 1.**

**Glu,** abbreviation for **glutamic acid.**

**glucagon** /gloo′kəgon/ [Gk, *glykys,* sweet, *agaein,* to lead], a polypeptide hormone, produced by alpha cells in the islets of Langerhans, that stimulates the conversion of glycogen to glucose in the liver. Secretion of glucagon is stimulated by hypoglycemia and by the growth hormone of the anterior pituitary. A preparation of purified crystallized glucagon is used in the treatment of certain hypoglycemic states. Also called **hyperglycemic-glycogenolytic factor.**

**glucagon-like peptide 1 (GLP-1),** an appetite suppressing substance found in the brain and intestine. In the brain GLP-1 acts as a satiety signal. In the intestine it slows emptying of the stomach and stimulates the release of insulin from the pancreas.

**glucagonoma syndrome** /gloo′kəgonō′mə/ [Gk, *glykys* + *agaein* + *oma,* tumor], a disease associated with a glucagon-secreting tumor of the islet cells of the pancreas. It is characterized by hyperglycemia, stomatitis, glossitis, anemia, weight loss, and a characteristic rash. Treatment is surgical removal of the tumor.

**glucagon test,** a blood test used to help diagnose glucagonoma, glucagon deficiency, diabetes mellitus, pancreatic insufficiency, renal failure, and other conditions.

**gluco-, glyco-,** combining form meaning 'sweetness or glucose': *glucofuranose, glucokinetic, glucosuria, glycocholic.*

**glucocorticoid** /gloo′kōkôr′təkoid/ [Gk, *glykys* + L, *cortex,* bark; Gk, *eidos,* form], an adrenocortical steroid hormone that increases gluconeogenesis, exerts an antiinflammatory effect, and influences many body functions. The most important of the three glucocorticoids is cortisol (hydrocortisone); corticosterone is less active, and cortisone is inactive until converted to cortisol. Glucocorticoids promote the release of amino acids from muscle, mobilize fatty acids from fat stores, and increase the ability of skeletal muscles to maintain contractions and avoid fatigue. These hormones are known to stabilize mitochondrial and lysosomal membranes, increase the production of adenosine triphosphate, promote the formation of certain liver enzymes, and decrease antibody production and the number of circulating eosinophils. A deficiency of glucocorticoids is characterized by hyperpigmentation (bronzing) of the skin, fasting hypoglycemia, weight loss, and apathy. An excess is associated with elevated serum glucose levels, thinning of the skin, ecchymosis, osteoporosis, poor wound healing, increased susceptibility to infection, and obesity. Glucocorticoid secretion is stimulated by the adrenocorticotropic hormone of the anterior pituitary, which in turn is regulated by the corticotropin-releasing hormone of the hypothalamus and circulating cortisol levels (negative feedback). Synthetic or semisynthetic glucocorticoids, derived chiefly from cortisol, include prednisone, prednisolone, dexamethasone, methylprednisolone, triamcinolone, and betamethasone. Compare **mineralocorticoid.**

**glucogenesis,** giving rise to or producing glucose.

**Glucometer,** trademark for a battery-powered instrument used to calculate blood glucose from as little as one drop of blood. Also called **blood glucose monitor.**

**gluconeogenesis** /gloo′kōne′ō·jen′əsis/, the formation of glycogen from fatty acids and proteins rather than from carbohydrates. Also called **glyconeogenesis.**

**Glucophage,** trademark for an oral antidiabetic agent (metformin hydrochloride).

**glucosan** /gloo′kəsan/ [Gk, *glykys,* sweet], any of a large group of anhydrous polysaccharides that on hydrolysis yield a hexose, primarily anhydrides of glucose. The glucosans include cellulose, glycogen, starch, and the dextrins.

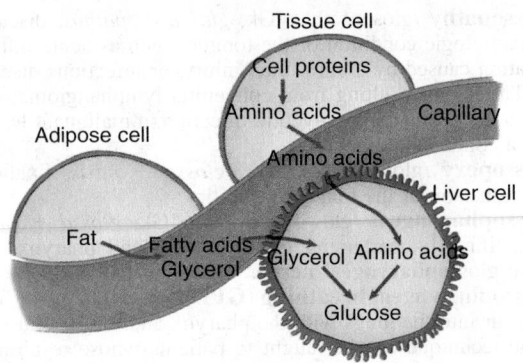

**Gluconeogenesis** *(Thibodeau and Patton, 1999)*

**glucose** /gloo′kōs/ [Gk, *glykys,* sweet], a simple sugar found in certain foods, especially fruits, and a major source of energy present in the blood and animal body fluids. Glucose, when ingested or produced by the digestive hydrolysis of double sugars and starches, is absorbed into the blood from the intestines by a facilitated transport mechanism using carrier proteins. Excess glucose in circulation is normally polymerized within the liver and muscles as glycogen, which is hydrolyzed to glucose and liberated as needed. The determination of blood glucose levels is an important diagnostic test in diabetes and other disorders. Prepared glucose is a syrupy sweetening agent. Pharmaceutic preparations of glucose are widely used in the treatment of many disorders. Normal adult blood glucose levels range from 70 to 115 mg/dl (4 to 6 mmol/L), with generally higher levels after 50 years of age. See also **dextrose, glycogen.**

**glucose electrode,** a specialized electric terminal that contains incorporated enzyme for glucose determination.

**glucose-galactose malabsorption,** a disorder of transport clinically characterized by the neonatal onset of profuse, acidic, watery diarrhea leading to severe dehydration and death if untreated, resulting from a selective defect in the intestinal transport of glucose and galactose; it can be treated by a glucose- and galactose-free diet.

**glucose intolerance,** inability to properly metabolize glucose, a type of carbohydrate intolerance. See also **glucose tolerance test** and **diabetes mellitus.**

**glucose 1-phosphate,** an intermediate compound in carbohydrate metabolism.

**glucose 6-phosphate,** an intermediate compound in carbohydrate metabolism.

**glucose-6-phosphate dehydrogenase (G-6-PD) deficiency,** an inherited disorder characterized by red cells partially or completely deficient in glucose-6-phosphate dehydrogenase, an enzyme critical in aerobic glycolysis. A sex-linked disorder, the defect is fully expressed in affected males despite a heterozygous pattern of inheritance. The disorder is associated with episodes of acute hemolysis under conditions of stress or in response to certain chemicals or drugs. The anemia that results is a kind of nonspherocytic hemolytic anemia. See also **congenital nonspherocytic hemolytic anemia, favism.**

**glucose-6-phosphate dehydrogenase (G-6-PD) test,** a blood test to diagnose G-6-PD deficiency in suspected individuals. Deficiency of this enzyme causes precipitation of hemoglobin and cellular membrane changes, possibly re-

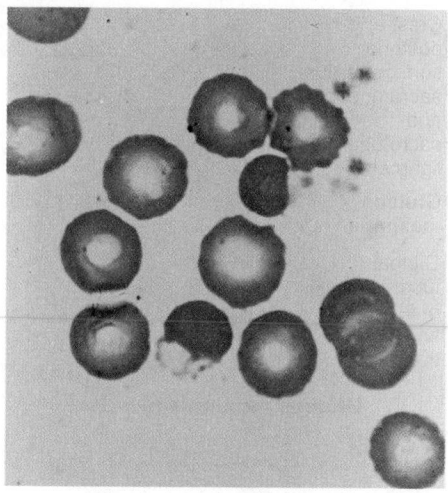

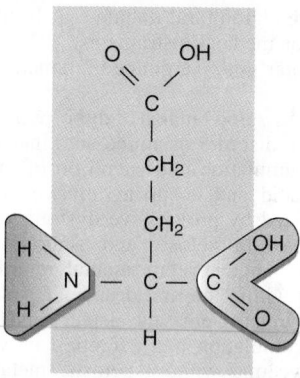

**Chemical structure of glutamic acid**

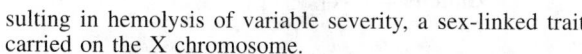

**Glucose-6-phosphate dehydrogenase (G6PD) disease**
*(Zitelli and Davis, 1997)*

sulting in hemolysis of variable severity, a sex-linked trait carried on the X chromosome.

**glucose tolerance test,** a test of the body's ability to metabolize carbohydrates by administering a standard dose of glucose and measuring the blood and urine for glucose level at regular intervals thereafter. The patient usually eats a high-carbohydrate diet for the 3 days before the test and fasts the night before. A fasting blood glucose level is obtained the next morning, and then the patient drinks a 100-g dose of glucose. Blood and urine are collected periodically for up to 6 hours. The glucose tolerance test is most often used to assist in the diagnosis of diabetes or other disorders that affect carbohydrate metabolism.

**glucosuria** /glōō'kōsŏŏr'ē·ə/ [Gk, *glykys* + *ouron*, urine], abnormal presence of glucose in the urine resulting from the ingestion of large amounts of carbohydrate or from a metabolic disease, such as diabetes mellitus. See also **glycosuria.** —**glucosuric,** *adj.*

**glucosyl,** **1.** pertaining to glucose. **2.** a glucose radical.

**glucosyl cerebroside lipidosis.** See **Gaucher's disease.**

**Glucotrol,** trademark for an oral antidiabetic drug (glipizide).

**glue sniffing** [Gk, *gloios* + ME, *sniffen*], the practice of inhaling the vapors of toluene, a volatile organic compound used as a solvent in certain glues. The glue is squeezed into a plastic bag, which is then placed over the nose and mouth. Intoxication and dizziness result. Prolonged accidental or occupational exposure or repeated recreational use may damage a variety of organ systems. Death has resulted from asphyxiation by the plastic bag.

**glutamate** /glōō'təmāt/, a salt of glutamic acid, a major excitatory amino acid of the central nervous system.

**glutamic acid (Glu)** /glōōtam'ik/ [L, *gluten,* glue, *amine,* ammonia; *acidus,* sour], a nonessential amino acid that occurs widely in a number of proteins. Preparations of glutamic acid are used as aids for digestion. See also **amino acid, protein.**

**glutamic acid decarboxylase autoantibody,** an antibody found in patients with insulin-dependent diabetes mellitus. The antibody recognizes glutamic acid decarboxylase, an intracellular enzyme.

**glutamic acidemia** /glōōtam'ikas'idē'mē·ə/, an inherited disorder of amino acid metabolism that causes an excessive level of glutamic acid. The precise enzyme defect is unknown. The condition is characterized by mental and physical retardation, seizures, and fragile hair growth.

**glutamic acid hydrochloride,** a gastric acidifier.
- INDICATION: It is prescribed for the treatment of hypoacidity.
- CONTRAINDICATIONS: Hyperacidity, peptic ulcer, or known hypersensitivity to this drug prohibits its use.
- ADVERSE EFFECTS: The most serious adverse reaction is systemic acidosis that results from overdose.

**glutamic oxaloacetic transaminase.** See **aspartate aminotransferase.**

**glutamic pyruvic transaminase.** See **alanine aminotransferase.**

**glutamine (Gln)** /glōō'təmēn/ [L, *gluten* + *amine,* ammonia], a nonessential amino acid found in the juices of many plants and in many proteins in the body. It functions as an amino donor for many reactions. It is also a nontoxic transport for ammonia because it is readily hydrolyzed to glutamic acid and free ammonia, the latter excreted in the urine. See also **amino acid, protein.**

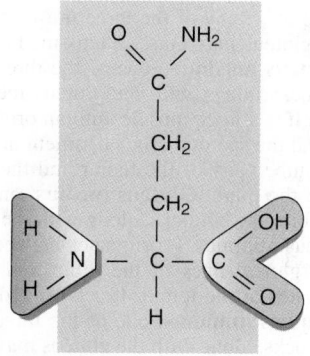

**Chemical structure of glutamine**

**glutaraldehyde** /gloo′tәral′dәhīd/, a histologic fixative and sterilant for medical instruments.

**glutargin** /glootär′gin/, arginine glutamate. See also **arginine.**

**glutaricaciduria** /gloo·tar′ik·as′i·dyoo′rē·ә /, **1.** an autosomal recessive disorder of amino acid metabolism characterized by accumulation and excretion of the dicarboxylic acid glutaric acid and occurring in two types: *Type I* is also characterized by progressive dystonia and dyskinesia, hypoglycemia, mild ketosis and acidosis, opisthotonus, choreoathetosis, motor delay, mental retardation, hypotonia, and death within the first decade. *Type II* is caused by any of several related emzyme defects and is also characterized by accumulation and excretion of various organic acids, hypoglycemia without ketosis, metabolic acidosis, and a spectrum of phenotypic manifestations varying with the particular defect. Increasing age of onset is correlated with decreasing severity; when of neonatal onset it may be accompanied by congenital anomalies and is rapidly fatal. Type II is also called **multiple acyl CoA dehydrogenation deficiency. 2.** excretion of glutaric acid in the urine.

**glutathione** /gloo′tәthī′ōn/ [L, *gluten* + Gk, *theione,* sulfur], a tripeptide of glutamic acid, cysteine, and glycine whose deficiency is commonly associated with hemolytic anemia. It functions by taking up and giving off hydrogen.

**gluteal** /gloo′tē·әl/ [Gk, *gloutos,* buttocks], pertaining to the buttocks or to the muscles that form the buttocks.

**gluteal fold, 1.** a fold of the buttock. **2.** the horizontal lower margin of the buttock at its junction with the thigh.

**gluteal gait.** See **Trendelenburg gait.**

**gluteal reflex,** contraction of the gluteus muscles elicited by stroking the back.

**gluteal region,** the region overlying the gluteal muscles.

**gluteal tuberosity,** a ridge on the lateral posterior surface of the femur to which is attached the gluteus maximus.

**gluten** /gloo′tәn/ [L, glue], the insoluble protein constituent of wheat and other grains. It is obtained from flour by washing out the starch and is used as an adhesive agent, giving to dough its tough, elastic character. See also **celiac disease, food sensitivity.**

**gluten-induced enteropathy.** See **celiac disease.**

**glutethimide** /glooteth′әmīd/, a sedative.

■ INDICATION: It is prescribed in the treatment of anxiety and insomnia.

■ CONTRAINDICATION: Known hypersensitivity to this drug prohibits its use.

■ ADVERSE EFFECTS: Among the most serious adverse reactions are physical and psychologic dependence. Rashes also may occur.

**gluteus** /glootē′әs/, any of the three muscles that form the buttocks: the gluteus maximus, gluteus medius, and gluteus minimus. **Gluteus maximus,** one of the three muscles that form the buttocks, along with the gluteus medius and gluteus minimus. It is a large muscle with an origin in the iliac, the sacrum, and the sacrotuberous ligament and an insertion in the gluteal tuberosity of the femur and the fascia lata. It acts to extend the thigh. **Gluteus medius,** one of the three muscles that form the buttocks, along with the gluteus maximus and gluteus minimus. It originates between the anterior and posterior gluteal lines of the ilium and inserts in the greater trochanter of the femur. It acts to abduct and rotate the thigh. **Gluteus minimus,** one of the three muscles that forms the buttocks, along with the gluteus maximus and gluteus medius. It originates between the inferior and anterior gluteal lines of the ilium and inserts in the greater trochanter of the femur. It acts to abduct the thigh.

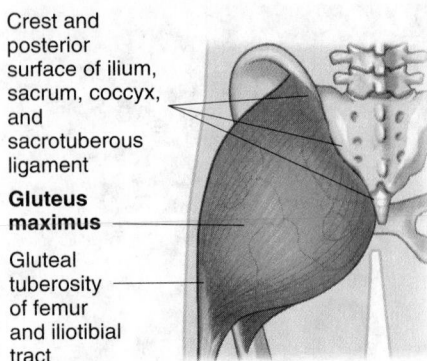

Crest and posterior surface of ilium, sacrum, coccyx, and sacrotuberous ligament

**Gluteus maximus**

Gluteal tuberosity of femur and iliotibial tract

**Gluteus maximus muscle**

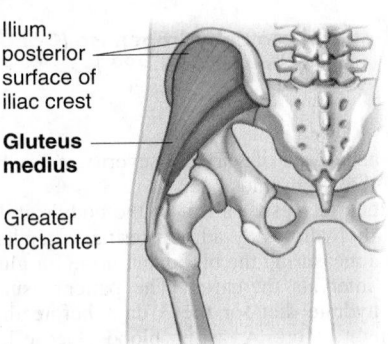

Ilium, posterior surface of iliac crest

**Gluteus medius**

Greater trochanter

**Gluteus medius muscle**

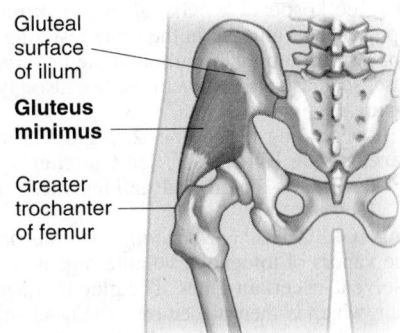

Gluteal surface of ilium

**Gluteus minimus**

Greater trochanter of femur

**Gluteus minimus muscle**

**glutin.** See **gliadin.**

**Gly,** abbreviation for **glycine.**

**glyburide** /glī′bәrīd/, an oral antidiabetic drug.

■ INDICATIONS: It is prescribed as an adjunct to diet and exercise to lower blood glucose levels of patients with type 2 diabetes mellitus.

■ CONTRAINDICATIONS: Because of its long duration of action, glyburide may produce prolonged hypoglycemia; there is also a risk of severe hypoglycemia in elderly, debilitated, or malnourished patients. The dosage may require adjustment for patients taking other drugs that increase blood glucose levels.

■ ADVERSE EFFECTS: Among the more serious adverse reactions are nausea, hypoglycemia, and skin allergies.

**glycate,** the product of a nonenzymic reaction between a sugar and a free amino group of a protein.

**glycated hemoglobin.** See **glycosylated hemoglobin.**

**-glycemia,** combining form meaning a 'condition of sugar in the blood': *dysglycemia, hepatoglycemia, hyperglycemia.*

**glycerin** /glis′ərin/ [Gk, *glykys*, sweet], a sweet, colorless oily fluid that is a pharmaceutic grade of glycerol. Glycerin is used as a moistening agent for chapped skin, as an ingredient of suppositories for constipation, and as a sweetening agent and vehicle for drug preparations. Also spelled **glycerine.**

**glycerol ($C_3H_8O_3$)** /glis′ərôl/ [Gk, *glykys*, sweet], an alcohol that is a component of fats. Glycerol is soluble in ethyl alcohol and water. Also called **1, 2, 3-propanetriol.** See also **glycerin.**

**glycerol kinase,** an enzyme in the liver and kidneys that catalyzes the transfer of a phosphate group from adenosine triphosphate to form adenosine diphosphate and L-glycerol-3-phosphate.

**glyceryl alcohol.** See **glycerin.**

**glyceryl guaiacolate.** See **guaifenesin.**

**glyceryl triacetate.** See **triacetin.**

**glycine (Gly)** /glī′sin/ [Gk, *glykys* + L, *amine*, ammonia], a nonessential amino acid occurring widely as a component of animal and plant proteins. Synthetically produced glycine is used in solutions for irrigation, in the treatment of various muscle diseases, and as an antacid and dietary supplement. See also **amino acid, protein.**

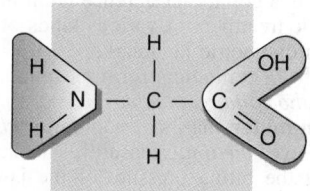

**Chemical structure of glycine**

**glyco-.** See **gluco-.**

**glycocholic acid** /glī′kōkol′ik/ [Gk, *glykys*, sweet; L, *acidus*, sour], a substance in bile, formed by glycine and cholic acid, that aids in digestion and absorption of fats. Glycocholic acid is used as a food additive and an emulsifying agent.

**glycogen** /glī′kəjən/ [Gk, *glykys*, sweet, *genein*, to produce], a polysaccharide that is the major carbohydrate stored in animal cells. It is formed from repeating units of glucose and stored chiefly in the liver and, to a lesser extent, in muscle cells. Glycogen is depolymerized to glucose, which is released into the circulation as needed by the body. Also called **animal starch, hepatin, tissue dextrin.** See also **glucose.**

**glycogenesis** /glī′kōjen′əsis/, the synthesis of glycogen from glucose.

**glycogenolysis** /glī′kōjenol′isis/ [Gk, *glykys* + *genein* + *lysis*, loosening], the breakdown of glycogen to glucose.

**glycogen storage disease** [Gk, *glykys* + *genein* + L, *instaurare,* to renew, *dis,* opposite of; Fr, *aise,* ease], any of a group of inherited disorders of glycogen metabolism. An enzyme deficiency causes glycogen to accumulate in abnormally large amounts in various parts of the body. Biopsy and chemical analysis reveal the missing enzyme. Also called **glycogenosis.**

**glycogen storage disease, type I.** See **von Gierke's disease.**

**glycogen storage disease, type Ib,** a form of glycogen storage disease in which excessive amounts of glycogen are deposited in the liver and leukocytes. Some symptoms are similar to, but less severe than, those of glycogen storage disease, **type Ia** (von Gierke's disease). Additional symptoms include neutropenia and recurrent GI infections. Biopsy of the affected organs reveals the absence of glucose-6-phosphatase translocase, an enzyme necessary for glycogen metabolism. See also **von Gierke's disease.**

**glycogen storage disease, type II.** See **Pompe's disease.**

**glycogen storage disease, type III.** See **Cori's disease.**

**glycogen storage disease, type IV.** See **Andersen's disease.**

**glycogen storage disease, type V.** See **McArdle's disease.**

**glycogen storage disease, type VI.** See **Hers' disease.**

**glycogen storage disease, type VII.** See **Tarui's disease.**

**glycohemoglobin.** See **glycosylated hemoglobin.**

**glycolipid** /glī′kōlip′id/ [Gk, *glykys*, sweet, *lipos*, fat], a compound that consists of a lipid and a carbohydrate, usually galactose, found primarily in the tissue of the nervous system, especially the myelin sheath and the ganglion cells.

**glycolysis** /glīkol′isis/ [Gk, *glykys* + *lysis*, loosening], a series of enzymatically catalyzed reactions by which glucose and other sugars are broken down to yield lactic acid (anaerobic glycolysis) or pyruvic acid (aerobic glycolysis). The breakdown releases energy in the form of adenosine triphosphate. Also called **Embden-Meyerhof pathway.** See also **aldolase, citric acid cycle, lactic acid.**

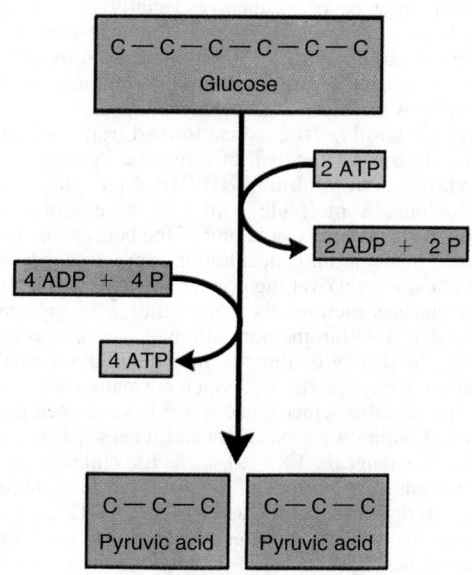

**Aerobic glycolysis** *(Applegate, 2000)*

**glycometabolism** /glī'kōmətab'əl iz'əm/, the metabolism of sugar in the animal body.

**glyconeogenesis.** See **gluconeogenesis.**

**glycopenia** /-pē'nē·ə/, **1.** hypoglycemia. **2.** a deficiency of sugar in the blood or tissues.

**glycopeptides** /-pep'tīdz/, a class of peptides that contain sugars linked with amino acids, as in bacterial cell walls.

**glycophorin** /-fôr'in/, one of a group of proteins that project through the membrane of red blood cells (RBCs). The outside end of glycophorins carries antigen of the MNS blood group. The sialic acid component of glycophorins contributes to the negative charge of the outer erythrocyte plasma membrane. Influenza virus can attach to sialic acid present on all glycophorin A, B, C, D, and E and produce agglutination (does not enter RBC). Malaria virus can attach to glycophorin A and C and infect RBCs. See also **blood group.**

**glycoprotein** /glī'kōprō'tēn/ [Gk, *glykys*, sweet, *proteios*, first rank], any of the large group of conjugated proteins in which the nonprotein substance is a carbohydrate. These include the mucins, the mucoids, and the chondroproteins.

**glycopyrrolate** /glī'kōpir'əlāt/, an anticholinergic.

■ INDICATION: It is prescribed as an adjunct to ulcer therapy and parenterally to reduce secretions before surgery.

■ CONTRAINDICATIONS: Narrow-angle glaucoma, asthma, obstruction of the genitourinary or GI tract, ulcerative colitis, or known hypersensitivity to this drug prohibits its use.

■ ADVERSE EFFECTS: Among the more serious adverse reactions are blurred vision, central nervous system effects, tachycardia, dry mouth, decreased sweating, and hypersensitivity reactions.

**glycoside** /glī'kəsīd/ [Gk, *glykys*, sweet], any of several carbohydrates that yield a sugar and a nonsugar on hydrolysis. The plant *Digitalis purpurea* yields a glycoside used in the treatment of heart disease.

**glycosphingolipids** /glī'kōsfing'gōlip'ids/, compounds formed from carbohydrates and ceramide, a fatty substance, found in tissues of the central nervous system and also in erythrocytes. Deficiency of an enzyme needed to metabolize glycosphingolipids leads to a potentially fatal nervous system disorder.

**glycosuria** /glī'kōsŏŏr'ē·ə/ [Gk, *glykys* + *ouron*, urine], abnormal presence of a sugar, especially glucose, in the urine. Glycosuria can result from the ingestion of large amounts of carbohydrate, or it may be caused by endocrine or renal disorders. It is a finding most routinely associated with diabetes mellitus. —**glycosuric,** *adj.*

**glycosyl** /glī'kō·sil /, the radical formed from a saccharide, such as glucose, by removal of a specific hydroxyl group.

**glycosylated hemoglobin (GHb/Hb A$_{1c}$)** /glīkō'silā'tid/, a hemoglobin A molecule with a glucose group on the *N*-terminal valine amino acid unit of the beta chain. The glycosylated hemoglobin concentration represents the average blood glucose level over the previous several weeks. In controlled diabetes mellitus the concentration of glycosylated hemoglobin is within the normal range, but in uncontrolled cases the level may be three to four times the normal concentration. Assays of Hb A$_{1c}$, which normally has a 4-month life span, reveal whether glucose levels have been properly controlled during a period of several weeks before the test. The normal range is 1.8% to 4.0% for children; 2.2% to 4.8% for adults. Also spelled **glycosylated haemoglobin.**

**glycosylated hemoglobin test (GHb, GHB),** a blood test used to monitor diabetes treatment. It measures the amount of hemoglobin A$_{1c}$ in the blood and provides an accurate long-term index of the patient's average blood glucose level.

**glycosylation** /glī·kə'sə·lā'shən/, the formation of linkages with glycosyl groups, covalently attaching a carbohydrate to another molecule.

**glycyl alcohol.** See **glycerin.**

**glycyrrhizic acid** /glis'iriz'ik/, a sweet compound containing potassium and calcium salts derived from licorice root. It is used as a expectorant and as a flavoring for pharmaceuticals. See also **licorice.**

**gm,** abbreviation for **gram.** The preferred abbreviation is **g.**

**GM-2,** a carbohydrate found in much larger quantities in cancer cells than in normal cells. It is used in some experimental cancer therapy. When it is mixed with bacille Calmette-Guérin (BCG) and injected into melanoma patients, some patients make antibodies against the cancer cells.

**GM-CSF,** abbreviation for **granulocyte-macrophage colony-stimulating factor.**

**GMENAC,** abbreviation for **Graduate Medical Education National Advisory Committee.**

**GMP,** abbreviation for **guanosine monophosphate.**

**GN.** See **graduate nurse.**

**GNA,** abbreviation for **Gay Nurses' Alliance.**

**gnath-.** See **gnatho-.**

**gnathalgia.** See **gnathodynia.**

**-gnathia,** combining form meaning a 'condition of the jaw': *brachygnathia, campylognathia, retrognathia.*

**gnathic** /nath'ik/ [L, *gnathos*, jaw], pertaining to the jaw or cheek.

**gnathic index,** the degree of prominence of the upper jaw, expressed as a percentage of the distance from basion to nasion.

**gnathion** /nā'thē·on/ [L, *gnathos*, jaw], the lowest point in the lower border of the mandible in the median plane. It is found on the bony mandibular border when palpated from below and naturally lies posterior to the tegumental border of the chin. It is a common reference point in the diagnosis and orthodontic treatment of various kinds of malocclusion and is an anthropometric landmark.

**gnatho-, gnath-,** combining form meaning 'jaw': *gnathocephalus, gnathodynia, gnathoplasty.*

**gnathodynamometer** /nā'thōdī'nəmom'ətər/ [Gk, *gnathos* + *dynamis*, force, *metron*, measure], an instrument used for measuring the biting pressure of the jaws of an individual. Also called **occlusometer.**

**gnathodynia** /nā'thōdin'ē·ə/ [Gk, *gnathos* + *odyne*, pain], pain in the jaw, such as that commonly associated with an impacted wisdom tooth. Also called **gnathalgia.**

**gnathology** /nāthol'əjē/, [Gk, *gnathos* + *logos*, science], a field of dental or medical study that deals with the entire chewing apparatus, including its anatomic, histologic, morphologic, physiologic, and pathologic characteristics. Diagnostic, therapeutic, and rehabilitative procedures result from these studies.

**gnathoschisis.** See **cleft palate.**

**gnathostatic cast** /nā'thōstat'ik/ [Gk, *gnathos* + *statike*, weighing; ME, *casten*], a cast of the teeth trimmed so that its occlusal plane is in its normal oral attitude when the cast is set on a plane surface. It is used in orthodontic diagnosis based on gnathostatics.

**gnathostatics** /nā'thōstat'iks/ [Gk, *gnathos* + *statike*, weighing], a technique of orthodontic diagnosis based on an analysis of the relationships between the teeth and certain reference points on the skull. See also **gnathostatic cast.**

*Gnathostoma* /nath·os'to·mə/ [Gk, *gnathos* + *stoma*, mouth], a genus of parasitic nematodes of the family Gnathostomatidae; *G. spini'gerum* is parasitic in cats, dogs, and humans after they eat raw fish containing the larvae, causing gnathostomiasis. See also **gnathostomiasis.**

**gnathostomiasis** /nath′ō·stō·mī′ə·sis/ [Gk, *gnathos* + *stoma,* mouth + *osis,* condition], infection with the nematode *Gnathostoma spinigerum,* occurring when undercooked fish harboring the larvae are eaten. The larvae migrate, often in the subcutaneous tissue, causing a creeping eruption associated with intense eosinophilia (see **cutaneous larva migrans**). Occasionally they migrate to deeper tissues and cause abscesses or to the central nervous system, where they cause eosinophilic myeloencephalitis.

**gno-,** combining form meaning 'to know or discern': *gnosia, gnosis.*

**-gnomonic, -gnomonical,** combining form meaning 'signs or experience in knowing or judging (a condition)': *pathognomonic, physiognomonic, thanatognomonic.*

**-gnomy,** combining form meaning the 'science or means of judging' something specified: *craniognomy, pathognomy, physiognomy.*

**-gnosia,** combining form meaning a '(condition of) perceiving or recognizing': *acognosia, hypergnosia, topognosia.*

**-gnosis,** combining form meaning 'knowledge': *acrognosis, diagnosis, topognosis.*

**gnotobiotic** /nō′tōbī·ot′ik/, pertaining to a germ-free animal or an animal or an environment in which all the microorganisms are known. See also **germ-free animal.**

**GnRH,** abbreviation for **gonadotropin releasing hormone.**

**goal** /gōl/ [ME, *gol,* limit], the purpose toward which an endeavor is directed, such as the outcome of diagnostic, therapeutic, and educational management of a patient's health problem.

**goal-oriented movements,** voluntary movements that are organized around behavioral goals, environmental context, and task specificity, as distinguished from reflexive movements.

**GOAT,** abbreviation for **Galveston Orientation and Amnesia Test.**

**goblet cell** [ME, *gobelet,* small bowl], one of the many specialized epithelial cells that secrete mucus and form glands of the epithelium of the stomach, the intestine, and parts of the respiratory tract. Also called **beaker cell, chalice cell.** See also **gland.**

**goiter** /goi′ter/ [L, *guttur,* throat], an enlarged thyroid gland, usually evident as a pronounced swelling in the neck. The enlargement may be associated with hyperthyroidism, hypothyroidism, or normal levels of thyroid function. It may be cystic or fibrous, containing nodules or an increased

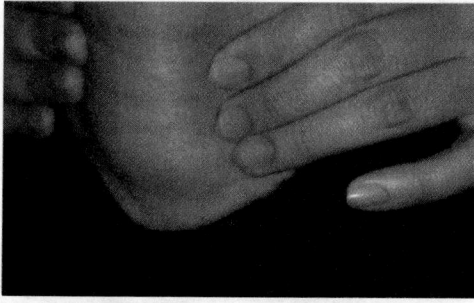

**Palpation of the thyroid gland in goiter**
*(Lemmi and Lemmi, 2000)*

number of follicles. The goiter may surround a large blood vessel, or a part of the enlarged gland may be situated beneath the sternum or in the thoracic cavity. Treatment may include total or subtotal surgical removal, the administration of antithyroid drugs or radioiodine, or use of thyroid hormone to block the pituitary mechanism that releases thyroid-stimulating hormone. After thyroidectomy maintenance therapy with thyroid hormone may be required. Also spelled **goitre.** See specific goiters. **—goitrous,** *adj.*

**goitrogenic glycoside** /goi′trəjen′ik/, a glycoside that may cause hyperthyroidism or a goiter.

**goitrous thyroiditis.** See **Hashimoto's disease.**

**gold (Au)** [AS, *geolu,* yellow], a yellowish soft metallic element that occurs naturally as a free metal and as the telluride $AuAgTe_4$. Its atomic number is 79; its atomic mass is 196.97. Gold has been highly valued since antiquity and has been and is used for currency, for ornamentation, and as a dental restorative material. It is usually hardened by alloying it with small amounts of nickel or copper. It is highly resistive to oxidation but can be dissolved in aqua regia and aqueous potassium cyanide. Gold salts, in which gold is attached to sulfur, are often used in the treatment, or chrysotherapy, of patients with rheumatoid arthritis but cause serious toxicity in about 10% of patients and some toxicity in 25% to 50%. See also **chrysotherapy.**

**gold 198,** a radioactive gold antineoplastic.

■ INDICATIONS: It is prescribed for treatment of cancer of the prostate, cervix, and bladder and for reduction of fluid accumulation secondary to a cancer.

■ CONTRAINDICATIONS: Ulcerative tumors, pregnancy, lactation, or unhealed surgical wounds prohibit its use. It is not prescribed for patients less than 18 years of age.

■ ADVERSE EFFECTS: The most serious adverse reaction is radiation sickness.

**Goldblatt kidney,** an abnormal kidney in which constriction of a renal artery leads to ischemia and release of renin, a pressor substance associated with hypertension.

**gold compound,** a drug containing gold salts, usually administered with other drugs in the treatment of rheumatoid arthritis. Gold is potentially toxic and is administered only under the supervision of a specialist in chrysotherapy. Toxic reactions range from mild dermatoses to lethal poisoning. Various radioisotopes of gold have been used in diagnostic radiology and in radiologic treatment of certain malignant neoplastic diseases.

**Goldenhar's syndrome** /gōl′dən·härz/ [Maurice Goldenhar, Swiss physician, 20th century], a congenital condition in which colobomas of the upper eyelid, dermoids on the eyeball, bilateral accessory auricular appendages anterior to the ears, and vertebral anomalies are frequently associated with characteristic facies, consisting of asymmetry of the skull, prominent frontal bossing, low hairline, mandibular hypoplasia, low-set ears, and sometimes smallness of the mouth on one side. Also called **OAV syndrome, oculoauriculovertebral dysplasia.**

**goldenseal,** a perennial herb found in the Ohio River valley.

■ USES: This herb is used for high blood pressure, poor appetite, infections, menstrual problems, minor sciatic pain, and muscle spasms. It is also used as an eye wash.

■ CONTRAINDICATIONS: Goldenseal is contraindicated in women who are pregnant (it is a uterine stimulant). It also should not be used in people with known hypersensitivity to this herb or who have cardiovascular conditions such as heart block, arrhythmias, or hypertension. It should not be used locally for purulent ear discharge, or in a ruptured ear drum.

**gold foil,** pure gold that has been rolled and beaten into a very thin sheet, used for making foil pellets. The main types of gold foil are cohesive, semicohesive, and noncohesive.

**gold inlay,** an intracoronal cast restoration of gold alloy that restores one or more tooth surfaces. It is held in place by the internal walls of the tooth and dental cements.

**Goldman-Fox knife,** a dental surgical instrument with a sharp cutting edge, designed for the incision and contouring of gingival tissue. Also called **Fox's knife.**

**gold sodium thiomalate,** an antirheumatic.
- INDICATION: It is prescribed for the treatment of rheumatoid arthritis.
- CONTRAINDICATIONS: Severe debilitation, systemic lupus erythematosus, renal or liver disease, blood dyscrasias, Sjögren's syndrome (in rheumatoid arthritis), or known hypersensitivity to this drug or to other gold or heavy metal salts prohibits its use.
- ADVERSE EFFECTS: Among the most serious adverse reactions are various blood dyscrasias, renal damage, and allergic reactions. Dermatitis, stomatitis, and lesions of the mucous membranes also may occur.

**gold standard,** **1.** an accepted test that is assumed to be able to determine the true disease state of a patient regardless of positive or negative test findings or sensitivities or specificities of other diagnostic tests used. **2.** an acknowledged measure of comparison of the superior effectiveness or value of a particular medication or other therapy as compared with that of other drugs or treatments.

**gold therapy.** See **chrysotherapy.**

**golfer's elbow,** an informal term for inflammation of the medial epicondyle of the humerus, associated with repeated use of the wrist flexors.

**Golgi apparatus** /gôl'jē/ [Camillo Golgi, Italian histologist and Nobel laureate, 1843–1926; L, *ad,* toward, *praeparare,* to prepare], one of many small membranous structures found in most cells, composed of various elements associated with the formation of carbohydrate side chains of glycoproteins, mucopolysaccharides, and other substances. Saccules within each structure migrate through the plasma membrane and release substances associated with external and internal secretion. Also called **Golgi body, Golgi complex.**

**Golgi-Mazzoni corpuscles** /gôl'jēmatsō'nē/ [Camillo Golgi; Vittori Mazzoni, Italian physiologist, 1880–1940], a number of thin capsules enveloping terminal nerve fibrils in the subcutaneous tissue of the fingers. They have thicker cores than Pacini's corpuscles but are similar special sensory end organs. Compare **Krause's corpuscles, Pacini's corpuscles, Ruffini's corpuscles.**

**Golgi's cells** [Camillo Golgi; L, *cella,* storeroom], **1. Golgi type I neurons,** nerve cells having long axons that leave the local neurophil area of the parent cell body, traverse the white matter, and project to the rest of the nervous system. **2. Golgi type II neurons,** nerve cells with short trajectory axons, like stellate cells of the cerebral and cerebellar cortex. They generally do not enter white matter but remain within the local neurophil in the cerebral and cerebellar cortices and the retina.

**Golgi tendon organ** [Camillo Golgi], a sensory nerve ending that is sensitive to both tension and excessive passive stretch of a skeletal muscle.

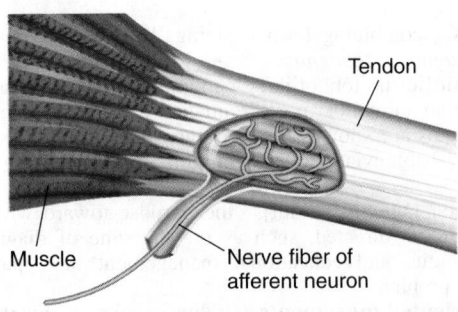

**Golgi tendon organ**

**Golgi type I neurons, Golgi type II neurons.** See **Golgi's cells.**

**Goltz syndrome.** See **focal dermal hypoplasia.**

**gomphosis** /gomfō'sis/, *pl.* **gomphoses** [Gk, *gomphos,* bolt], an articulation by the insertion of a conical process into a socket, such as the insertion of a root of a tooth into an alveolus of the mandible or the maxilla. Gomphosis is not a connection between true bones but is considered a type of fibrous joint. Compare **sutura, syndesmosis.**

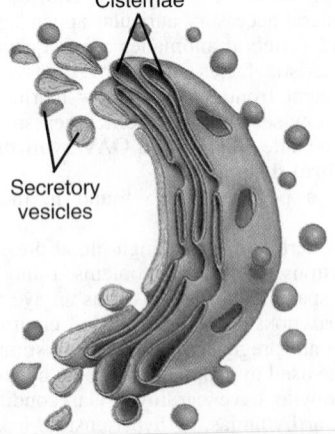

**Golgi apparatus** *(Thibodeau and Patton, 1999/William Ober)*

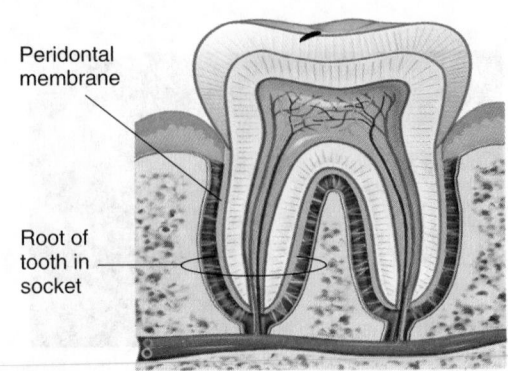

**Gomphosis**

**gon-, gono-, gony-.** **1.** prefix meaning 'semen or seed': *gonococcin, gonophore, gonotome.* **2.** combining form meaning 'knee': *gonycampsis, gonyectyposis, gonyoncus.*

**gonad** /gō′nad/ [Gk, *gone,* seed], a gamete-producing gland, such as an ovary or a testis. —**gonadal,** *adj.*

**gonadal aplasia** /gō′nədəl/, a congenital state in which there is defective development of the germinal tissues of the gonads.

**gonadal dose,** the amount of radiation received by the gonads as a result of a radiographic examination. It may vary from less than 1 mrad for a dental or chest radiograph to 225 mrad for a lumbar spine radiograph and 800 mrad for a fetus during pelvimetry.

**gonadal dysgenesis,** a general designation for a variety of conditions involving anomalies in the development of the gonads, such as Turner's syndrome, hermaphroditism, and gonadal aplasia.

**gonadal shield,** a specially designed contact or shadow shield used to protect the gonadal area of a patient from the primary radiation beam during radiographic procedures. It is generally used for patients who are potentially reproductive, including women less than 40 years of age and all males.

**gonado-** [L. *gonas,* gen. *gonadis* gonad, from Gr. *gonos* procreation], prefix meaning relationship to the gonads.

**gonadoblastoma** /gō′nə·dō·blas·tō′mə/ [Gk, *gone,* seed + *blastos,* germ + *-oma,* tumor], a rare benign type of germ cell tumor, usually occurring in patients with gonadal dysgenesis, and often bilateral. It contains all gonadal elements and is frequently associated with an abnormal chromosomal karyotype. It may give rise to development of a dysgerminoma or other more malignant germ cell tumor. See also **dysgerminoma, gonadal dysgenesis.**

**gonadotropic** /gō′nədōtrof′ik/, acting on or stimulating the gonads. Also called **gonadotrophic.** See also **gonadotropin.**

**gonadotropin** /gō′nədōtrop′in/ [Gk, *gone* + *trophe,* nourishment], a hormonal substance that stimulates the function of the testes and the ovaries. The gonadotropic follicle stimulating hormone and luteinizing hormone are produced and secreted by the anterior pituitary gland. In early pregnancy, human chorionic gonadotropin (HCG) is produced by the placenta. It acts to sustain the function of the corpus luteum of the ovary, forestalling menstruation and thus maintaining pregnancy. Gonadotropins are prescribed to induce ovulation in infertility that is caused by inadequate stimulation of the ovary by endogenous gonadotropic hormones. Excessive stimulation of the ovary may result in vast enlargement of the gland, maturation of many follicles, multiple pregnancy, bleeding into the abdomen, and pain. Also called **gonadotrophin.** —**gonadotropic, gonadotrophic,** *adj.*

**gonadotropin-releasing hormone (GnRH)** [Gk, *gone,* seed, *trope,* a turn; ME, *relesen;* Gk, *hormaein,* to set in motion], a decapeptide hypophysiotropic hormone secreted by the hypothalamus. It stimulates the release of **luteinizing hormone (LH)** and **follicle-stimulating hormone (FSH)** by the anterior pituitary. GnRH may be used in the treatment of endometriosis among conditions.

**gonial angle.** See **angle of mandible.**

**-gonic,** suffix meaning 'work required to facilitate a specified reaction': *dysgonic, endergonic, exergonic.*

**gonio-,** combining form meaning 'angle': *goniocraniometry, goniometer, gonion.*

**goniometer** /gon′ē·om′ətər/, an instrument used to measure angles, particularly range-of-motion angles of a joint.

**goniometry** /gon′ē·om′ətrē/ [Gk, *gonia,* angle, *metron,* measure], a system for measuring angles during testing for

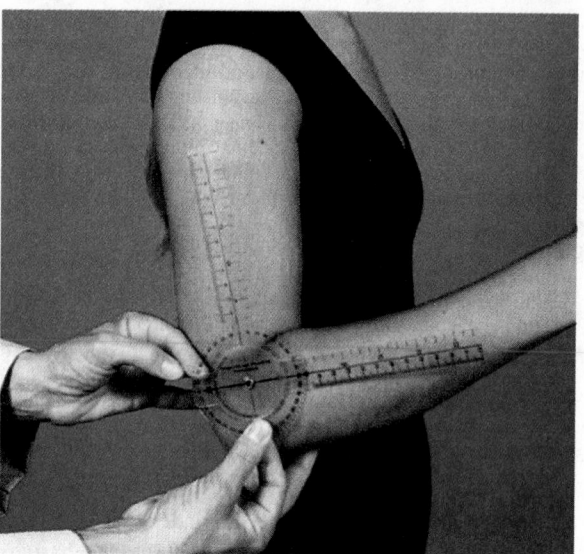

**Goniometer** *(Barkauskas et al, 1998)*

various labyrinthine diseases that affect the sense of balance. One test uses a plank, one end of which may be raised to any desired height. The patient stands on the plank as one end is gradually raised, and the point where he or she can no longer maintain balance is noted. —**goniometric,** *adj.*

**gonion** /gō′nē·on/ *pl.* **gonia** [Gk, *gōnia,* angle], an anthropometric landmark located at the most inferior, posterior, and lateral point on the external angle of the mandible, being the apex of the maximum curvature of the mandible, where the ascending ramus becomes the body of the mandible. See also **mandible.**

**gonioscope** /gō′nē·əskōp′/ [Gk, *gonia* + *skopein,* to look], a mirrored optical instrument used to examine the filtration angle of the anterior chamber of the eye. The mirrors permit visualization of the angle, by means of a reflected image.

**goniotomy** /gon′ē·ot′əmē/, an operation performed to remove any obstruction to the flow of aqueous humor in the front chamber of the eye. The procedure is commonly done in patients with congenital glaucoma.

**gonoblast.** See **germ cell.**

**gonococcal** /gon′əkok′əl/ [Gk, *gone,* seed, *kokkos,* berry], pertaining to or resembling gonococcus.

**gonococcal pyomyositis** [Gk, *gone,* seed, *kokkos,* berry, *pyon,* pus, *mys,* muscle, *itis,* inflammation], an acute inflammatory condition of a muscle caused by infection with *Neisseria gonorrhoeae,* characterized by abscess formation and pain. It is an unusual form of gonorrhea and must be differentiated from sarcoma. Diagnosis is made by the discovery of the gonococcal diplococci within the abscess when a bacterial culture of a specimen is prepared after exploratory surgery. The patient is then usually found to be asymptomatically infected in the urogenital organs. Antibiotic treatment, most often with ceftriaxone, is rapidly effective in curing the infection.

**gonococcal salpingitis** [Gk, *gone,* seed, *kokkos,* berry, *salpigx,* tube, *itis,* inflammation], an inflammation of the fallopian tubes caused by a gonococcal infection. Also called **gonorrheal salpingitis.**

**gonococcal urethritis** [Gk, *gone,* seed, *kokkos,* berry, *ourethra,* urethra, *itis,* inflammation], inflammation of the urethra caused by an infection of *Neisseria gonorrhoeae*. Also called **gonorrheal urethritis.**

**gonococcus** /gon'əkok'əs/, pl. **gonococci** /gon'əkok'sī/ [Gk, *gone + kokkos,* berry], a gram-negative intracellular diplococcus of the species *Neisseria gonorrhoeae,* the cause of gonorrhea. A nonmotile aerobic microorganism of the species *Neisseria gonorrhoeae.* It is a parasite of the mucous membrane and the cause of **gonorrhea.**

**gonocyte.** See **germ cell.**

**gonorrhea** /gon'ərē'ə/ [Gk, *gone + rhoia,* flow], a common sexually transmitted disease that most often affects the genitourinary tract and occasionally the pharynx or rectum. Infection results from contact with an infected person or with secretions containing the causative organism *Neisseria gonorrhoeae.* Infants born to infected women may acquire conjunctival infection from passage through the birth canal. Gonorrheal infections must be reported to local health departments in the United States. Also spelled **gonorrhoea.** —**gonorrheal, gonorrheic,** *adj.*

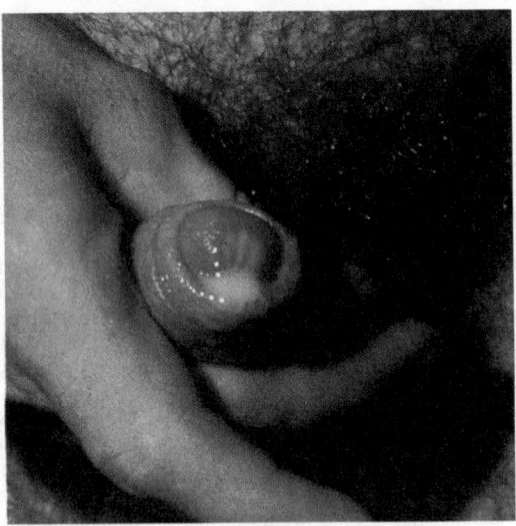

**Gonorrhea in the male patient**
*(Morse, Moreland, and Holmes, 1996)*

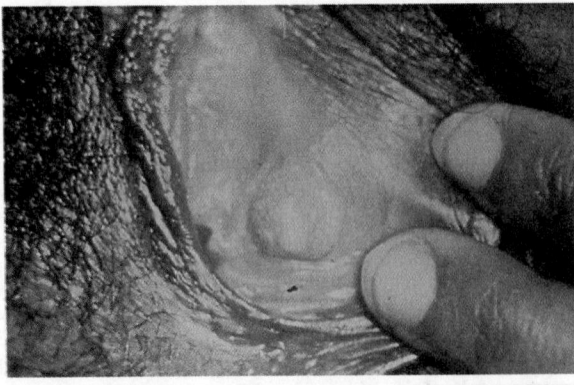

**Gonorrhea in the female patient**
*(Morse, Moreland, and Holmes, 1996)*

■ OBSERVATIONS: Urethritis; dysuria; purulent, greenish-yellow urethral or vaginal discharge; red or edematous urethral meatus; and itching, burning, or pain around the vaginal or urethral orifice are characteristic. The vagina may be massively swollen and red, and the lower abdomen may be tense and very tender. As the infection spreads, as occurs more commonly in women than in men, nausea, vomiting, fever, and tachycardia may occur as salpingitis, oophoritis, or peritonitis develops. Inflammation of the tissues surrounding the liver also may occur, causing pain in the upper right quadrant of the abdomen. Severe disseminated infection is also more common in women than in men and is characterized by signs of septicemia with polyarthritis, tender papillary lesions on the skin of the hands and feet, and inflammation of the tendons of the wrists, knees, and ankles. Gonococcal ophthalmia involves infection of the conjunctiva and may lead to scarring and blindness. Gonorrhea is diagnosed by bacteriologic culture of the organism from a smear obtained from a specimen of exudate. In men a microscopic study of a Gram's-stained specimen of exudate that reveals gram-negative intracellular diplococci is diagnostic of gonorrheal infection, but this finding is not diagnostic in women.

■ INTERVENTIONS: The recommended regimen for uncomplicated gonorrhea is ceftriaxone 125 mg intramuscularly (IM) once or doxycycline, 100 mg, orally twice daily for 7 days. Generally patients with gonorrhea infections should be treated simultaneously for presumptive chlamydial infections. Alternative medications are ciprofloxacin, ofloxacin, cefixime, and azithromycin. Treatment failure of this regimen is rare; therefore a follow-up culture for test of cure is not essential. The routine instillation of 1% solution of silver nitrate or topical ophthalmic antibiotic into the eyes of the newborn provides effective prophylaxis against conjunctival infection in the newborn period that might otherwise result from contact with the infected secretions of an asymptomatic infected mother during vaginal delivery.

■ NURSING CONSIDERATIONS: It is important that the patient's sexual contacts be treated. Before administration of any antibiotic it is ascertained that the patient does not have any known sensitivity to the drug being given and that equipment and drugs are available to treat any hypersensitivity reaction that may occur. Precaution against spread of the disease is recommended through condom use or monogamous sexual relations.

**gonorrheal** /gon'ərē'əl/ [Gk, *gone,* seed, *kokkos*], pertaining to or resembling gonorrhea.

**gonorrheal arthritis** [Gk, *gone,* seed, *kokkos,* berry, *arthron,* joint, *itis,* inflammation], a blood-borne gonococcal infection of the joints. It may affect one or several joints, may occur as a chronic or acute form, and often leads to joint fusion. Infection may result in pus formation in an affected joint.

**gonorrheal conjunctivitis,** a severe, destructive form of purulent conjunctivitis caused by the gonococcus *Neisseria gonorrhoeae.* Prompt treatment by the IV administration of antibiotics is required to prevent scarring of the cornea and blindness. Newborns receive routine prophylaxis of a topical ophthalmic instillation of 1% solution of silver nitrate or an antibiotic ophthalmic ointment; the treatment has largely eradicated the infection in infants. See also **ophthalmia neonatorum.**

**gonorrheal proctitis** [Gk, *gone,* seed, *rhoia,* flow, *proktos,* anus, *itis,* inflammation], an inflammation of the rectum caused by an infection of gonorrhea.

**gonorrheal salpingitis.** See **gonococcal salpingitis.**

**gonorrheal urethritis.** See **gonococcal urethritis.**

**gonorrheic.** See **gonorrhea.**

**-gony,** suffix meaning 'birth, origin, or procreation': *amphigony, merogony, zoogony.*

***Gonyaulax catanella*** /gon′ē·ô′laks/, a species of toxin-producing planktonic protozoa ingested by shellfish along the coasts of North America that causes shellfish poisoning. It colors the sea red in an infected area. The phenomenon is called red tide. See also **shellfish poisoning.**

**Goodell's sign** /go͞odelz′/ [William Goodell, American gynecologist, 1829–1894], softening of the uterine cervix, a probable sign of pregnancy.

**good faith and fair dealing,** actions taken with the best interests of the patient in mind and without harmful intent.

**Goodman's syndrome** /good′mənz/ [Richard M. Goodman, Israeli physician, 20th century], an autosomal recessive form of acrocephalopolysyndactyly characterized also by congenital heart defects, sidewards deviation and abnormal flexion of digits, and ulnar deviation, but with unimpaired intelligence. See also **acrocephalopolysyndactyly.**

**Goodpasture's syndrome** /go͞od′pas·chər/ [Ernest W. Goodpasture, American pathologist, 1886–1960], a chronic relapsing pulmonary hemosiderosis, usually associated with glomerulonephritis and characterized by a cough with hemoptysis, dyspnea, anemia, and progressive renal failure. Mild forms may respond to corticosteroids or immunosuppressive drugs. Severe recurrent cases have a poor prognosis; hemodialysis and kidney transplantation are the only treatments.

**Goodrich, Annie Warburton** (1866–1954), an American nursing educator who was instrumental in advancing nursing from an apprenticeship to a profession. She was superintendent of nurses at several New York hospitals before going to Teachers College, Columbia University, in 1914. In addition to teaching, she was associated with the Henry Street Settlement and the Nursing Department of the U.S. Army. In 1923 she became dean of the newly formed School of Nursing at Yale University, which awarded a degree similar to that awarded in other professions.

**Good Samaritan legislation** /səmar′itən/ [good Samaritan, from New Testament parable; L, *lex,* law, *lator,* proposer], laws enacted in some states to protect physicians, dentists, nurses, and some other health professionals from liability in rendering emergency medical or dental aid, unless there is proven willful wrong or gross negligence.

**gooseflesh.** See **pilomotor reflex.**

**Gopalan's syndrome.** See **burning feet syndrome.**

**Gordon's elementary body** [Mervyn H. Gordon, English physician, 1872–1953], a particle found in tissues containing eosinophils; once thought to be the viral cause of Hodgkin's disease. Also called **Gordon's encephalopathic agent.**

**Gordon's reflex** [Alfred Gordon, American neurologist, 1874–1953], **1.** an abnormal variation of Babinski's reflex, elicited by compressing the calf muscles, characterized by dorsiflexion of the great toe and fanning of the other toes. It is evidence of disease of the pyramidal tract. **2.** an abnormal reflex, elicited by compressing the forearm muscles, characterized by flexion of the fingers or of the thumb and index finger. It is seen in diseases of the pyramidal tract. Compare **Chaddock reflex, Oppenheim reflex.** See also **Babinski's reflex.**

**Gordon's syndrome** /gôr′dənz/ [Richard D. Gordon, Australian physician, 20th century], a type of pseudohypoaldosteronism with hypertension and hyperkalemia but without salt wasting, thought to be caused by abnormally increased absorption of chloride by the renal tubules. See also **pseudohypoaldosteronism.**

**Gorham's disease** /gor′əmz/ [Lemuel Whittington Gorham, American physician, 1885–1968], gradual, but often complete, resorption of a bone or group of bones, which may be associated with multiple hemangiomas; it usually occurs in children or young adults, sometimes following trauma, but its cause is unknown.

**Gosselin's fracture** /gôslaNz′/ [Leon A. Gosselin, French surgeon, 1815–1847], a V-shaped break in the distal tibia, extending to the ankle.

**GOT,** abbreviation for **glutamic-oxaloacetic transaminase.**

**gotu kola,** a creeping herb found in swamps of Africa, Sri Lanka, and Madagascar.

■ USES: This herb is used to treat chronic wounds and psoriasis.

■ CONTRAINDICATIONS: Gotu kola should not be used during pregnancy and lactation or in children until more research is available. Those with known hypersensitivity to this herb or to members of the celery family should not use this product.

**goundou** /go͞on′do͞o/ [West African], a condition characterized by bony exostoses of the nasal and maxillary bones, usually occurring as a late sequela of yaws in people in Africa and Latin America.

**gout** [L, *gutta,* drop], a disease associated with an inborn error of uric acid metabolism that increases production or interferes with excretion of uric acid. Excess uric acid is converted to sodium urate crystals that precipitate from the blood and become deposited in joints and other tissues. Men are more often affected than women. The great toe is a common site for the accumulation of urate crystals. The condition can cause exceedingly painful swelling of a joint, accompanied by chills and fever. The symptoms are recurrent; episodes become longer each year. The disorder is disabling and, if untreated, can progress to the development of destructive joint changes, such as tophi. Treatment usually includes administration of colchicine, phenylbutazone, indomethacin, or glucocorticoid drugs, and a diet that excludes purine-rich foods such as organ meats. It may include surgical removal of ulcerated tophi. Acquired gout is a condition having the signs and symptoms of gout but resulting from another disorder or treatment for a different condition. Diuretic drugs can alter the concentration of uric acid so that uric acid salts precipitate from the blood and are carried to the joints. See also **chondrocalcinosis, Lesch-Nyhan syndrome, tophus.**

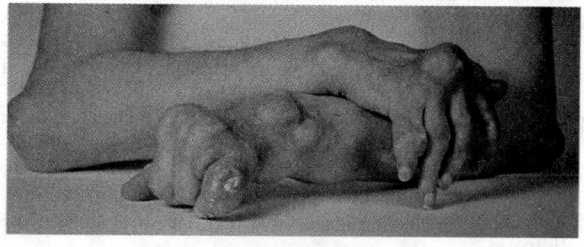

**Gout**
*(Clinical Slide Collection of the Rheumatic Diseases, © 1991, 1995, 1997; used with permission of the American College of Rheumatology)*

**gouty** /gou′tē/ [L, *gutta,* drop], pertaining to or resembling the condition of gout.

**gouty arthritis.** See **gout.**

**Gowers' muscular dystrophy.** See **distal muscular dystrophy.**

**GP,** abbreviation for **general practitioner.**

**gp160,** a glycoprotein found on the outer surface, or envelope, of the human immunodeficiency virus. It is composed of **gp120,** which protrudes from the envelope, and **gp41,** which is embedded in the envelope.

**GPB,** abbreviation for **glossopharyngeal breathing.**

**GPT,** abbreviation for **glutamic pyruvic transaminase.** See **alanine aminotransferase.**

**GPWW,** abbreviation for **group practice without walls.**

**gr,** abbreviation for **grain.**

**graafian follicle** /grä'fē·ən, -grā'-/ [Reijnier de Graaf, Dutch physician, 1641–1673; L, *folliculus,* small bag], a mature ovarian vesicle, measuring about 10 to 12 mm in diameter, that ruptures during ovulation to release the ovum. Many primary ovarian follicles, each containing an immature ovum about 35 μm in diameter, are embedded near the surface of the ovary, just below the tunica albuginea. Under the influence of the follicle stimulating hormone from the adenohypophysis one ovarian follicle ripens into a graafian follicle during the proliferative phase of each menstrual cycle. The cells that form the graafian follicle are arranged in a layer three to four cells thick around a relatively large volume of follicular fluid. Within the follicle the ovum grows to about 100 μm in diameter, ruptures, and is swept into the fimbriated opening of the uterine tube. The cavity of the follicle collapses when the ovum is released, and the remaining follicular cells greatly enlarge to become the corpus luteum. If the ovum is fertilized, the corpus luteum grows and becomes the corpus luteum of pregnancy, which degenerates by the end of 9 months and has a diameter of about 30 mm. As the ovarian follicle ripens into the graafian follicle, it produces estrogen, which stimulates the proliferation of the endometrium and the enlargement of the uterine glands. The growing corpus luteum produces progesterone, which triggers endometrial gland secretion and prepares the uterus to receive the fertilized ovum. If the ovum is not fertilized, the graafian follicle forms the corpus luteum of menstruation, which degenerates before the next menstrual cycle, leaving the small scarred corpus albicans.

**gracile** /gras'il/, long, slender, and graceful.

**gracilis** /gras'ilis/, the most superficial of the five medial femoral muscles. It is a thin, flattened muscle that is broad proximally and narrow distally. It functions to adduct the thigh and flex the leg and to assist in the medial rotation of the leg after it is flexed. Compare **adductor brevis, adductor longus, adductor magnus, pectineus.**

**gradation of activity** /gradā'shən/, therapeutic activities that are appropriately paced and modified to demand maximal capacities at any point in progression or regression of the patient's condition.

**graded exercise test (GXT),** a test given a cardiac patient during rehabilitation to assess prognosis and quantify maximal functional capacity. The test is given before discharge to determine guidelines for activity programs at home and work during convalescence. See also **exercise electrocardiogram.**

**gradient** /grā'dē·ənt/ [L, *gradus,* step], **1.** the rate of increase or decrease of a measurable phenomenon, such as temperature or pressure. **2.** a visual representation of the rate of change of a measurable phenomenon; a curve.

**gradient former,** a device for the preparation of linear density gradient medium in a column for gradient electrophoresis.

**gradient gel electrophoresis,** gel electrophoresis performed in a concentration gradient gel with progressively decreasing pore size.

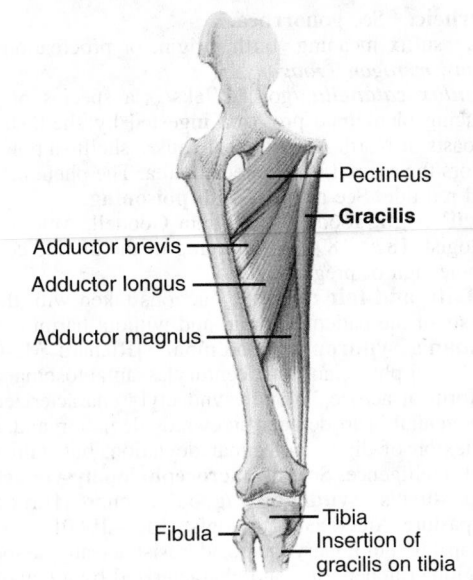

Pectineus
**Gracilis**
Adductor brevis
Adductor longus
Adductor magnus
Tibia
Insertion of gracilis on tibia
Fibula

**Gracilis muscle** *(Thibodeau and Patton, 1999/John V. Hagen)*

**gradient magnetic field,** a magnetic field that changes in strength in a given direction. Such fields are used in magnetic resonance imaging (MRI) to select a region for imaging and to encode the location of MRI signals received from the object being imaged.

**gradient plate technique,** a method for isolating antibiotic-resistant bacteria mutants by exposing an agar plate containing concentration gradient of antibiotic to an inoculation of bacteria to be tested.

**graduated bath** /graj'oo·a'tid/ [L, *gradus,* step; AS, *baeth*], a bath in which the temperature of the water is slowly reduced.

**graduated muscular contractions,** controlled shortening of muscle units in properly timed and adequate response to a stimulus. The contractions may be induced by the central nervous system or by electrical stimulation. Contractile force can be controlled by varying the number of units that contract or by increasing the frequency of contractions.

**graduated resistance exercise.** See **progressive resistance exercise.**

**graduate medical education** /graj'oo·it/, formal medical education pursued after receipt of the doctor of medicine (M.D.) or other professional degree in the medical sciences, usually as an intern, resident, or fellow.

**Graduate Medical Education National Advisory Committee (GMENAC),** a committee established by order of the Secretary of the Department of Health, Education, and Welfare (now the Department of Health and Human Services) to study the personnel issues in medicine. The committee issued its final report in September 1980. Among its conclusions was that the supply of nurses in expanded roles, including nurse practitioners and nurse midwives, should be increased.

**graduate nurse (GN)** [L, *gradus,* step, *nutrix,* nurse], a nurse who is a graduate of an accredited school of nursing but not yet licensed.

**Graduate Record Examination (GRE),** an examination administered to graduates of institutions of higher learning. The scores are used as criteria for admission to master's and doctoral programs in many institutions and areas of specialization, including nursing. The examination tests verbal and mathematical aptitudes and abilities.

**GRAE,** abbreviation for **generally recognized as effective.**

**graft** [Gk, *graphion,* stylus], a tissue or an organ taken from a site or a person and inserted into a new site or person, performed to repair a defect in structure. The graft may be temporary, such as an emergency skin transplant for extensive burns, or permanent with the grafted tissue growing to become a part of the body. Skin, bone, cartilage, blood vessel, nerve, muscle, cornea, and whole organs, such as the kidney or the heart, may be grafted. Preoperative care focuses on a high protein diet and vitamins to ensure optimal physical condition and on freedom from infection. With the patient under general or local anesthesia the tissue is transferred and sutured into place. Rejection is the major complication: fever, pain in the graft area, and evidence of loss of function 4 to 15 days after the procedure are indicative of rejection. Immunosuppressive drugs are given in large doses to suppress antibody production and rejection. Even if an early reaction is prevented, late rejection may occur 1 year or more after the graft is done. Also called **transplant.** See also **allograft, autograft, isograft, skin graft, xenograft.**

**graft facilitation,** a method for extending the survival of a graft by conditioning the recipient with an immunoglobulin-blocking factor, which suppresses graft rejection.

**graft rejection,** the immunologic destruction of transplanted organs or tissues. The rejection may be based on both cell-mediated and antibody-mediated immunity against cells of the graft by a histoincompatible recipient. First-set rejection usually occurs within 10 days. Second-set rejection occurs within 1 week after a second graft with the same antigenic specificity as the first is placed in the same host.

**graft-versus-host disease (GVHD),** a rejection response of certain grafts, especially of bone marrow. It is commonly associated with inadequate immunosuppressive therapy of the donor, which allows immunocompetent cells in the donated tissue to recognize the recipient's tissues as foreign and to attack them. Because the recipient is totally immunosuppressed, the recipients immune system cannot defend against the attack. Characteristic signs may include skin lesions with edema, erythema, ulceration, scaling, loss of hair, lesions of the joints and the heart, and hemolytic anemia with a positive Coombs' test reaction. Also called **graft-versus-host reaction (GVHR), homologous disease.**

**Graham's law** /grā'əmz/ [Thomas Graham, English chemist, 1805–1869], the law stating that the rate of diffusion of a gas through a liquid (or the alveolar-capillary membrane) is directly proportional to its solubility coefficient and inversely proportional to the square root of its density.

**Graham Steell murmur** [Graham Steell, British physician, 1851–1942], an early diastolic murmur heard in the second intercostal space to the left of the sternum. It is associated with pulmonary valve regurgitation in pulmonary hypertension.

**grain (gr)** [L, *granum,* seed], the smallest unit of mass in avoirdupois, troy, and apothecaries' weights, which is the same in all and is equal to 4.79891 mg. The troy and apothecaries' ounces contain 480 grains; the avoirdupois ounce contains 437.5 grains.

**gram (g, gm)** [L, *gramma,* small weight], a unit of mass in the metric system equal to $\frac{1}{1000}$ kilogram, 15.432 grains, and 0.0353 ounce avoirdupois. 453.6 g = 1lb. The preferred abbreviation is **g.**

**-gram, -gramme,** 1. suffix meaning a 'drawing' or a written record: *mammogram, electroencephalogram.* 2. combining form identifying a basic unit of mass: *centigram, kilogram.*

**gram calorie.** See **calorie[1] (cal).**

**gram-equivalent weight (gEq),** an equivalent weight of a substance calculated as the gram mass that contains, replaces, or reacts (directly or indirectly) with the Avogadro number of hydrogen atoms. As 1 atom of sulfur (atomic mass 32) combines with 2 atoms of hydrogen (atomic mass 1), the gram equivalent weight of sulfur is $\frac{32}{2} = 16$.

**gram-molecular weight (gmW),** a mass in grams numerically equal to the molecular weight of a substance, or the sum of all the atomic weights in its molecular formula. In the example of carbon dioxide ($CO_2$), its gram-molecular weight is 12 (atomic mass of carbon) + 2 × 16 (atomic mass of oxygen), or 44 g. See also **mole, molecular weight.**

**gram-negative** [Hans C.J. Gram, Danish physician, 1853–1938; L, *negare,* to say no], having the pink color of the counterstain used in Gram's method of staining microorganisms. This property is a primary method of characterizing organisms in microbiology. Some of the most common gram-negative pathogenic bacteria are *Bacteroides fragilis, Brucella abortus, Escherichia coli, Haemophilus influenzae, Klebsiella pneumoniae, Neisseria gonorrhoeae, Proteus vulgaris, Pseudomonas aeruginosa, Salmonella typhi, Shigella dysenteriae,* and *Yersinia pestis.*

**gram-positive** [Hans C.J. Gram; L, *positivus*], retaining the violet color of the stain used in Gram's method of staining microorganisms. This property is a primary method of characterizing organisms in microbiology. Some of the most common kinds of gram-positive pathogenic bacteria are *Bacillus anthracis, Clostridium* species, *Mycobacterium leprae, Mycobacterium tuberculosis, Staphylococcus aureus, Streptococcus pneumoniae,* and *Streptococcus pyogenes.*

**Gram's method.** See **Gram's stain.**

**Gram's stain** [Hans C.J. Gram], the method of staining microorganisms using a violet stain, followed by an iodine solution; decolorizing with an alcohol or acetone solution; and counterstaining with safranin. The retention of either the violet color of the stain or the pink color of the counterstain serves as a primary means of identifying and classifying bacteria. Also called **Gram's method.** See also **gram-negative, gram-positive.**

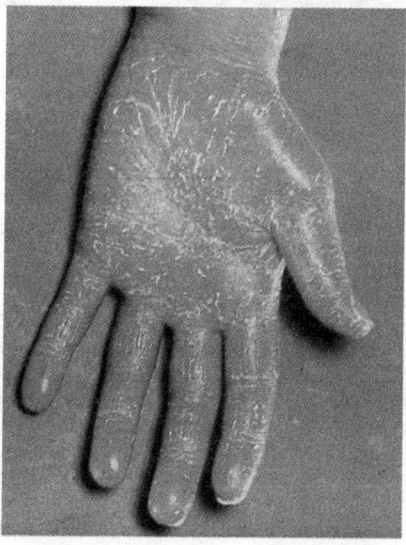

**Graft-versus-host reaction** *(Skarin, 1996)*

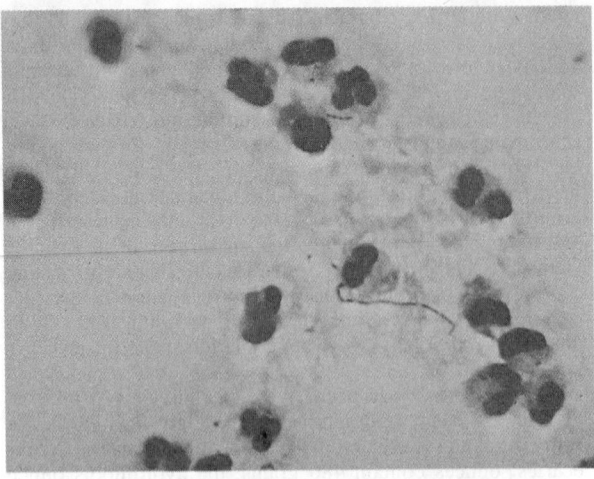

**Gram-negative stain of cerebrospinal fluid containing *Haemophilus influenzae***
*(Baron, Peterson, and Finegold, 1994)*

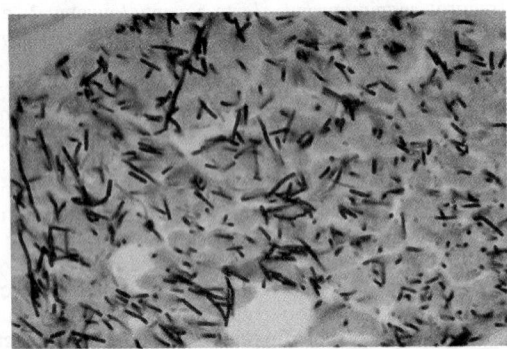

**Gram-positive stain of clostridial infection**
*(Stone and Gorbach, 2000)*

**gram-variable,** gram-positive bacteria that can become gram-negative after culturing.

**grandiose** /gran'dē·ōs'/ [L, *grandis*, great], pertaining to something or somebody imposing, impressive, magnificent, or, also, pompous and showy.

**grandiosity.** See **megalomania.**

**grand mal seizure.** See **tonic-clonic seizure.**

**grand multipara** /grand/ [L, *grandis*, great, *multus*, many, *parere*, to give birth], a woman who has carried six or more pregnancies to a viable stage.

**grand rounds** [L, *grandis* + *rotundus*, wheel], a formal conference in which an expert presents a lecture concerning a clinical issue intended to be educational for the listeners. In some settings grand rounds may be formal teaching rounds conducted by an expert at the bedsides of selected patients.

**grant** [ME, *granten*, to believe a request], a monetary award given to an institution, a project, or an individual, given by a granting agency, the federal government, a foundation, a private business, or an institution to provide financial support for research, service, or training. The applicant usually writes a formal application (proposal) for the grant, which is reviewed by the granting agency and compared with other proposals. The grantee is usually accountable to the grantor for reporting the outcomes as a result of the awarded resources.

**granul-,** prefix meaning 'grains or granules': *granulase, granulocorpuscle, granulocytemia.*

**granular** /gran'yələr/ [L, *granulum*, little grain], **1.** macroscopically resembling or feeling like sand. **2.** microscopically appearing to have a few or many particles within or on its surface, such as a stained granular leukocyte. —**granularity,** *n.*

**granular cast** [L, *granulum*, little grain; ONorse, *kasta*], a mass of pathologic debris composed of cells filled with protein and fatty granules.

**granular conjunctivitis.** See **trachoma.**

**granular endoplasmic reticulum.** See **endoplasmic reticulum.**

**granular induration,** fibrosis of an organ, characterized by the formation of localized granular areas, as seen in cirrhosis of the liver.

**granularity.** See **granular.**

**granulation tissue** /gran'yəlā'shən/ [L, *granulum*, little grain], any soft pink fleshy projections that form during the healing process in a wound that does not heal by first intention. It consists of many capillaries surrounded by fibrous collagen. Overgrowth of granulation tissue causes proud flesh growing above the skin. See also **pyogenic granuloma.**

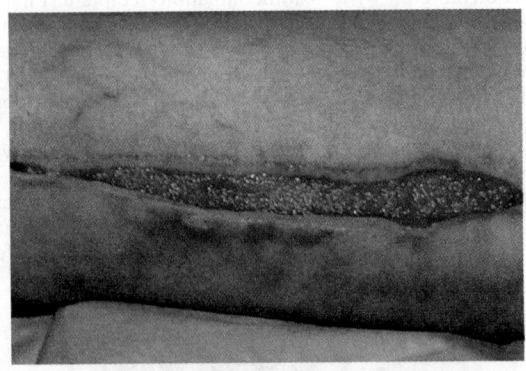

**Granulation tissue**
*(Bryant, 1992/courtesy Abbott Northwestern Hospital, Minneapolis)*

**granule** /gran'yōōl/ [L, *granulum*, little grain], a particle, grain, or other small dry mass capable of free movement. Unlike powders, granules are usually free flowing because of small surface forces involved.

**granulitis** /gran'yəlī'tis/ [L, *granulum*, little grain; Gk, *itis*, inflammation], acute miliary tuberculosis.

**granulocyte** /gran'yōōləsīt'/ [L, *granulum* + Gk, *kytos*, cell], a type of leukocyte characterized by the presence of cytoplasmic granules. Kinds of granulocytes are **basophil, eosinophil,** and **neutrophil.** Compare **agranulocyte.**

**granulocyte colony-stimulating factor (G-CSF),** a glycoprotein secreted by a variety of cells that stimulates the growth of hematopoietic stem cells and their differentiation into granulocytes. It is often used to treat patients who have become severely neutropenic as a result of chemotherapy or irradiation. See also **growth factor.**

**granulocyte-macrophage colony-stimulating factor (GM-CSF),** a glycoprotein secreted by macrophages that stimulates the growth of myeloid progenitor cells and their differentiation into granulocytes and macrophages. See also **growth factor.**

**granulocyte transfusion,** the use of specially prepared leukocytes for the treatment of severe granulocytopenia and for prophylaxis in the prevention of serious infection in patients with leukemia or those receiving cancer chemotherapy. The procedure has the same risks as a blood transfusion. Also called **buffy coat transfusion.**

**granulocytic leukemia.** See **acute myelocytic leukemia, chronic myelocytic leukemia.**

**granulocytic sarcoma.** See **chloroma.**

**granulocytopenia** /gran'yōōlōsī'tōpē'nē-ə/ [L, *granulum* + Gk, *kytos,* cell, *penia,* poverty], an abnormal decrease in the total number of granulocytes in the blood. Also called **granulopenia, neutropenia.** Compare **granulocytosis.** See also **leukopenia.** —**granulocytopenic,** *adj.*

**granulocytosis** /gran'yōōlōsītō'sis/ [L, *granulum* + Gk, *kytos,* cell, *osis,* condition], an abnormal increase in the total number of granulocytes in the blood, for example as occurs in response to infection. Compare **granulocytopenia.**

**granuloma** /gran'yōōlō'mə/, *pl.* granulomas, granulomata [L, *granulum* + Gk, *oma,* tumor], a chronic inflammatory lesion characterized by an accumulation of macrophages; epithelioid macrophages, with or without lymphocytes; and giant cells into a discrete granule. Granulomas may resolve spontaneously, remain static, become gangrenous, spread, or act as a focus of infection. Treatment depends on the cause and probable course of the particular granuloma.

**-granuloma,** combining form meaning a 'tumorlike mass or nodule of granulation tissue': *paragranuloma, ulcerogranuloma, xanthogranuloma.*

**granuloma annulare,** a self-limited chronic skin disease of unknown cause that consists of reddish papules arranged in a ring. It most commonly occurs on the distal portions of the extremities in children.

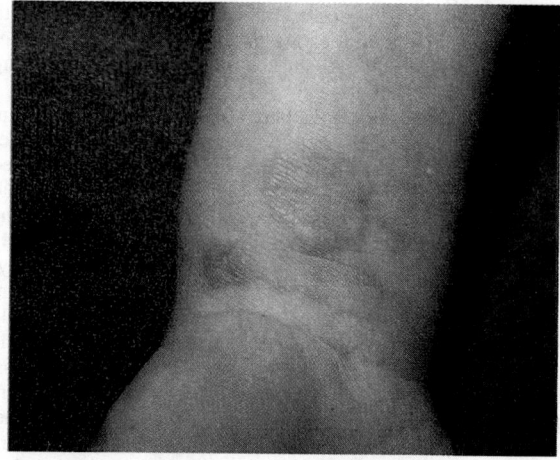

**Granuloma annulare** *(Weston, Lane, and Morrelli, 1996)*

**granuloma gluteale infantum,** a skin condition of the neonate characterized by large elevated bluish or brownish red nodules on the buttocks. It often occurs as a secondary

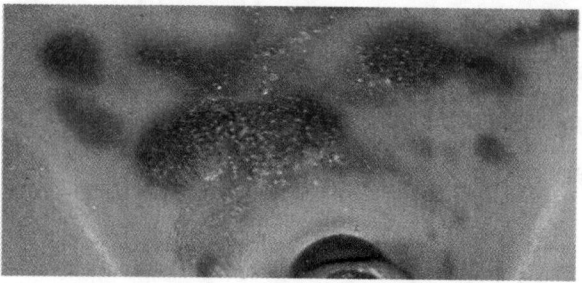

**Granuloma gluteale infantum**
*(du Vivier, 1993/courtesy David Atherton)*

reaction to the application of strong steroid salves over time. The lesions routinely disappear within a couple of months after the use of the preparations is discontinued.

**granuloma inguinale,** a sexually transmitted disease characterized by ulcers of the skin and subcutaneous tissues of the groin and genitalia. It is caused by infection with *Calymmatobacterium granulomatis,* a small gram-negative rod-shaped bacillus. Diagnosis is made by microscopic examination and identification of characteristic "safety-pin"-shaped bodies in the cytoplasm of phagocytes taken from a lesion and dyed with Wright's stain. Untreated, the lesions spread, deepen, multiply, and become secondarily infected. Streptomycin is usually effective in treating the infection. All patients who have or are suspected of having granuloma inguinale are also tested for syphilis, because concurrent infection is common.

**granulomatosis** /gran'yōōlōmətō'sis/ [L, *granulum* + Gk, *oma,* tumor, *osis,* condition], a condition or disease characterized by the development of granulomas, such as **berylliosis, pulmonary Wegener's granulomatosis,** or **Wegener's granulomatosis.**

**granulomatous** /gran'yəlom'ətəs/ [L, *granulum,* little grain], pertaining to or resembling granulomas.

**granulomatous amebic encephalitis,** chronic encephalitis, usually seen in debilitated or immunocompromised patients, caused by infection with species of *Acanthamoeba.* It is marked by the formation of granulomas; headache, seizures, nausea, and vomiting frequently occur.

**granulomatous lipophagia** [L, *granulum,* little grain; Gk, *lipos,* fat, *phagein,* to eat], a disease in which enlarged intestinal and mesenteric lymph spaces become filled with fats and fatty acids.

**granulomatous thyroiditis.** See **de Quervain's thyroiditis.**

**granulopenia.** See **granulocytopenia.**

**granulopoietin** /gran'yōōlō'pō-ē'tin/, a glycoprotein secreted by monocytes that controls the production of granulocytes by bone marrow. See also **granulocyte colony-stimulating factor.**

**granulosa cell carcinoma.** See **granulosa cell tumor.**

**granulosa cell tumor** /gran'yōōlō'sə/ [L, *granulum,* little grain], a fleshy ovarian tumor with yellow streaks that originates in cells of the primordial membrana granulosa and may grow to a large size. Excessive production of estrogen, resulting in endometrial hyperplasia and menorrhagia, may be associated with the tumor.

**granulosa-theca cell tumor,** an ovarian tumor composed of granulosa (follicular) cells or theca cells or both. The tumor is associated with excessive production of estrogen and hyperplasia of the breast and endometrium. See also **luteoma.**

**granulosis** /gran'yŏōlō'sis/, any disorder characterized by an accumulation of granules in an area of body tissue, such as a skin eruption marked by tiny granules beneath the surface.

**grapeseed,** an herb found throughout the world.

■ USES: This herb is used as an antioxidant, as a chronic disease preventative, and as an antiinflammatory.

■ CONTRAINDICATIONS: Use of grapeseed should be avoided during pregnancy and lactation and in children until more research is available.

**-graph,** 1. suffix meaning the 'product of drawing or writing': *hemophotograph, micrograph, retinograph.* 2. combining form meaning a 'machine for making something drawn': *clonograph, pneumograph, scopograph.*

**graphanesthesia** /graf'anəsthē'zhə/, inability to feel writing on the skin, usually caused by a central nervous system lesion. Also called **agraphesthesia.**

**-grapher,** suffix meaning 'one who writes about' something specified: *nosographer, syphilographer.*

**graphesthesia** /graf'esthē'zhə/, ability to feel writing on the skin.

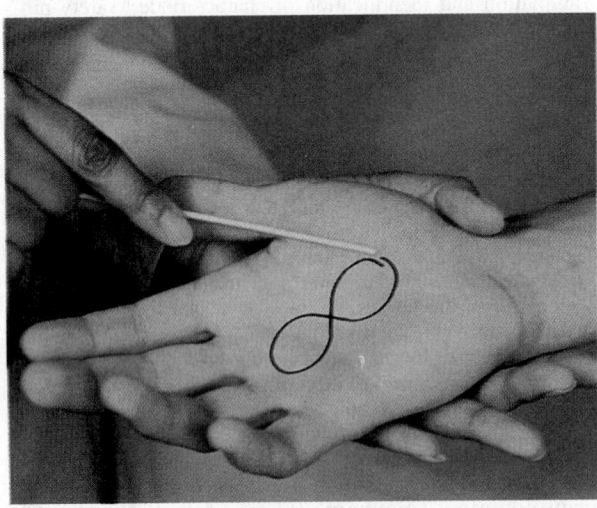

**Testing for graphesthesia** *(Barkauskas et al, 1998)*

**-graphia,** suffix meaning an 'abnormality revealed through handwriting': *dysantigraphia, palingraphia.*

**graphing** /graf'ing/, the organization of data consisting of two or more variables along horizontal and vertical axes of a graph to show relationships between specific quantities or other specific factors.

**graphite** /graf'īt/ [L, *graphites,* from Gk, *graphis* a writing instrument], a form of native mineralized carbon; inhalation of its dust causes a form of pneumoconiosis. See also **pneumoconiosis.**

**graphite pneumoconiosis** /noo'mō·kō'nē·ō'sis /, silicosis resulting from inhalation of graphite dust, which often contains up to 10 per cent silica. Also called **graphite fibrosis** and **graphitosis.**

**graphitosis.** See **graphite pneumoconiosis.**

**grapho-,** combining form meaning 'writing': *graphocatharsis, graphomania, graphophobia.*

**graphospasm.** See **writer's cramp.**

**-graphy,** suffix meaning a 'kind of printing or process of recording': *arteriography, cardiography, dermagraphy.*

**GRAS,** abbreviation for **generally recognized as safe.**

**grasp reflex** [ME, *graspen,* grab; L, *reflectere,* to bend back], a pathologic reflex induced by stroking the palm or sole with the result that the fingers or toes flex in a grasping motion. The reflex occurs in diseases of the premotor cortex. In young infants the tonic grasp reflex is normal: When an examiner strokes the infant's palms, the child grasps the examiner's fingers so firmly that he or she can be lifted into the air. Also called **darwinian reflex.**

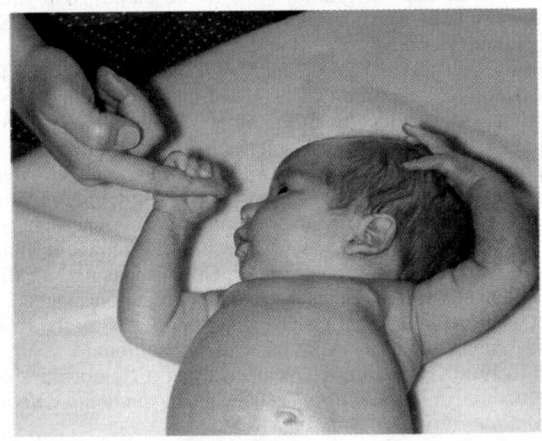

**Grasp reflex in an infant** *(Zitelli and Davis, 1997)*

**grass.** See **cannabis.**

**grass-line ligature** [AS, *graes* + L, *linea,* thread, *ligare,* to bind], a fine cord made from the fibers of a grass-cloth plant, used in orthodontics for minor adjustments or movement of the teeth. The ligature exerts traction by shrinking when wetted by saliva.

**Graves' disease** /grāvz/ [Robert J. Graves, Irish physician, 1796–1853], a multisystem auto immune disorder characterized by pronounced hyperthyroidism usually associated with an enlarged thyroid gland and exophthalmos (abnormal protrusion of the eyeball). The origin is unknown, but the disease is familial and may be caused by thyroid-stimulating autoantibodies that bind to TSH receptors and stimulate thyroid secretion. Graves' disease, which is five times more common in women than in men, occurs most frequently when the individual is between 30 and 60 years of age and can arise after an infection or physical or emotional stress. Typical signs, which are related to hyperthyrpoidism, are nervousness, a fine tremor of the hands, weight loss, fatigue, breathlessness, palpitations, increased heat intolerance, increased metabolic rate, and GI motility. An enlarged thymus, generalized hyperplasia of the lymph nodes, blurred or double vision, localized myxedema, atrial arrhythmias, and osteoporosis may occur. The diagnosis may be established by tests that measure TSH, thyroxine, and triiodothyronine levels in serum. If necessary, radioactive iodine uptake in the gland may be tested. Treatment may include prescription of antithyroid drugs, such as methimazole, propylthiouracil, and iodine preparations. Radioactive iodine may be administered, but hospitalization for a few days is recommended for patients treated with a large dose. Occasionally subtotal thyroidectomy may be an indication. In patients with inadequately controlled disease, infection or stress may precipitate a life-threatening thyroid storm. The exophthalmia may or may not resolve with the treatment of the disease. Also called **exophthalmic goiter, thyrotoxicosis, toxic goiter.**

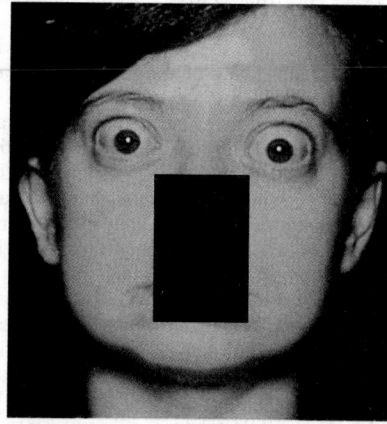

**Graves' disease**
*(Seidel et al, 1999/courtesy Paul W. Ladenson, Maryland)*

**Graves' orbitopathy** /grāvz/ [Robert James *Graves*, Irish physician, 1796–1853; L, *orbita*, wheel track + Gk, *pathos*, disease], the dysthyroid orbitopathy seen in Graves' disease. Also called **Graves' ophthalmopathy.**

**gravid** /grav'id/ [L, *gravidus*, pregnant], pregnant; carrying fertilized eggs or a fetus. —**gravidity, gravidness,** *n.*

**gravid-,** prefix meaning 'pregnancy or pregnant': *gravida, graviditas, gravidocardiac.*

**gravida** /grav'idə/ [L, *gravidus*, pregnant], a woman who is pregnant. The patient may be identified more specifically as **gravida I,** if pregnant for the first time, or **gravida II,** if pregnant a second time.

**-gravida,** suffix meaning 'pregnant woman with (specified) quantity of pregnancies': *nonigravida, plurigravida, unigravida.*

**gravida I or 1.** See **primigravida.**

**gravida II or 2.** See **secundigravida.**

**gravida macromastia,** overdevelopment of the breasts during pregnancy.

**gravidarum chloasma** /grav'ider'əm, gräv'idär'-/ [L, *gravidus*, pregnant; Gk, *chloazein*, to be green], a pigmentary change in the skin that occurs in some women during pregnancy. It usually occurs as patches of hyperpigmentation.

**gravidity, gravidness.** See **gravid.**

**gravidum gingivitis** /grav'idəm/ [L, *gravidus*, pregnant, *gingiva*, gums, *itis*, inflammation], a type of gum inflammation that is associated with plaque formation during pregnancy. It may be associated with hormonal changes. Also called **pregnancy gingivitis.**

**gravid uterus** [L, *gravidus*, pregnant, *uterus*, womb], a pregnant uterus.

**gravimetric analysis.** See **quantitative analysis.**

**gravity** /grav'itē/ [L, *gravis*, heavy], the universal effect of the attraction between any body of matter and any planetary body. The force of the attraction depends on the relative masses of the bodies and on the distance between them.

**gravity-eliminated plane,** a supported position or plane in which the effect of gravity is absorbed or neutralized. In evaluation of muscle strength certain tests are conducted in the gravity-eliminated plane. Other tests may involve movements against the force of gravity.

**gravity gonimeter,** an instrument used for measuring joint angles, consisting of a device that rests on or is strapped to the part to be measured and a dial that rotates behind a weighted pointer that remains vertical by force of gravity.

**gray (Gy),** the SI unit of absorbed radiation dose. One gray equals the energy equivalent of 1 joule/kg of matter; 1 Gy equals 100 rad. See also **rad.**

**gray baby syndrome.** See **gray syndrome.**

**gray column.** any of the three longitudinally oriented thickenings in the spinal cord, composed of the gray substance and containing the nerve cell bodies. They are commonly referred to as *horns* because in transverse sections of the spinal cord they have the appearance of horns. See **anterior horn, latera horn,** and **posterior horn.**

**gray hepatization.** See **hepatization.**

**gray matter.** See **gray substance.**

**gray scale,** the property in which intensity information in ultrasonography is recorded as changes in the brightness of the gray scale display.

**gray scale display,** in ultrasonography, a signal-processing method for selectively amplifying and displaying the level echoes from soft tissues at the expense of the larger echoes. Also called **compression amplification.**

**gray substance** [AS, *graeg* + L, *substantia*], the gray nervous tissue found in the cortex of the cerebrum, cerebellum, and core of the spinal cord. It is predominantly composed of neuron cell bodies and unmyelinated axons. The gray color is produced by cytoplasmic elements seen in all cell bodies and processes not covered by whitish myelin. Nuclei in the gray substance of the spinal cord function as centers for all spinal reflexes. Also called **gray matter.** Compare **white substance.** See also **cerebellum, cerebral cortex, cerebrum, spinal cord, spinal nerves.**

**gray syndrome,** a toxic condition in neonates, especially premature infants, caused by a reaction to chloramphenicol. Because the body's mechanisms for detoxification and excretion of drugs are immature, the infant has limited ability to conjugate and thus eliminate the chloramphenicol. The condition is named for the characteristic ashen-gray cyanosis, which is accompanied by abdominal distension, hypothermia, vomiting, respiratory distress, and vascular collapse. The syndrome, which is fatal if the drug is continued, can be prevented by conservative dosages of the drug and by restriction of its use in women during late pregnancy or labor (because chloramphenicol readily crosses the placental barrier) and in lactating mothers. Also called **gray baby syndrome.**

**GRE,** abbreviation for **Graduate Record Examination.**

**great auricular nerve** [AS, large; L, *auricula*, little ear, *nervus*, nerve], one of a pair of cutaneous branches of the cervical plexus, arising from the second and the third cranial nerves. It is distributed to the skin of the face and the skin of the mastoid process. It also communicates with the smaller occipital nerve, the auricular branch of the vagus nerve, and the posterior auricular branch of the facial nerve.

**great calorie.** See **Calorie² (kcal).**

**great cardiac vein,** one of the five tributaries of the coronary sinus, beginning at the apex of the heart and ascending along the anterior interventricular sulcus to the base of the ventricles. It then curves left in the coronary sulcus, reaches the back of the heart, and opens into the left part of the coronary sinus. It receives various tributaries from the left atrium. The great cardiac vein drains the blood through its tributaries from the capillaries of the myocardium. Also called **vena cordis magna.** Compare **middle cardiac vein, small cardiac vein.**

**great cerebral vein of Galen.** See **Galen's vein.**

**greater circulation.** See **systemic circulation.**

**greater multangular.** See **trapezium.**

**greater omentum** [AS, *great,* large; L, *omentum,* entrails], a filmy, transparent double fold of the peritoneum, draping the transverse colon and coils of the small intestine. It is attached along the greater curvature of the stomach and the first part of the duodenum. It is a readily movable structure that spreads easily into areas of trauma, often sealing hernias and walling off infections that would otherwise cause general peritonitis, as can occur from a ruptured vermiform appendix. It also contains fat and keeps the intestines warm. Also called **gastrocolic omentum.** Compare **lesser omentum.**

**greater sciatic foramen** [AS, *great* + Gk, *ischiadikos,* hip joint; L, *foramen,* hole], an opening between the hip bone, sacrum, and sacrotuberous ligament.

**greater sciatic notch** [AS, *great,* large; Gk, *ischiadikos,* hip joint; OFr, *enochier,* notch], a notch on the posterior border of the hip bone between the posterior inferior iliac spine and the spine of the ischium.

**greater trochanter,** a large projection of the femur, to which are attached various muscles, including the gluteus medius, gluteus maximus, and obturator internus. The greater trochanter projects from the angle formed by the neck and the body of the femur.

**greater vestibular gland.** See **Bartholin's gland.**

**great membrane,** the external components of a membrane, such as the layer of carbohydrate molecules on the outer surface.

**great saphenous vein,** one of a pair of the longest veins in the body, which contains 10 to 20 valves along its course through the leg and the thigh before ending in the femoral vein. It begins in the medial marginal vein of the dorsum of the foot and ascends anterior to the tibial malleolus and up the medial side of the leg in relation to the saphenous nerve. It runs posterior to the medial condyles of the tibia and the femur and passes through the hiatus saphenus immediately before joining the femoral vein. It contains more valves in the leg than in the thigh and receives many cutaneous veins and numerous tributaries, such as those from the sole of the foot. Near the saphenous hiatus it is joined by the superficial epigastric vein, the superficial epigastric circumflex, and the superficial external pudendal veins. Compare **common iliac vein, femoral vein.**

**great vessel,** one of the large arteries and veins entering and leaving the heart. They include the aorta, the pulmonary arteries and veins, and the superior and inferior venae cavae.

**green cancer.** See **chloroma.**

**Greenfield filter** [L. Greenfield, twentieth-century American surgeon], a filter placed in the inferior vena cava under fluoroscopic guidance. Used in patients who are particularly vulnerable to pulmonary embolism, it prevents venous emboli from entering the pulmonary circulation.

**Greenfield's disease** [Joseph G. Greenfield, British pathologist, 1884–1958], a disorder of the white matter of the brain tissue, characterized by an accumulation of sphingolipid in both parenchymal and supportive tissues and a diffuse loss of myelination. An infantile form usually begins by the third year of life, with symptoms that include loss of vision, rigidity, motor disorders, and mental deterioration. A juvenile form usually begins before a child is 10 years of age and an adult form after 16 years of age; the adult form is marked by psychiatric symptoms that progress to dementia. See also **leukodystrophy.**

**green fluorescent protein (GFP),** a protein obtained from the jellyfish *Aequorea victoria* that emits a bright green fluorescence when illuminated. GFP is used to monitor gene expression, gene transfer across plasma membranes, and cell surface activity.

**greenhouse effect,** a theorized change in the earth's climate caused by accumulation of solar heat in the earth's surface and atmosphere. Human activity contributes increasing amounts of the so-called greenhouse gases, such as carbon dioxide, methane, and chlorofluorocarbon, to the atmosphere. Some of the particles and gases in the atmosphere also allow more sunlight to filter through to the earth's surface but reflect back much of the radiant infrared energy that otherwise would escape through the atmosphere back into space. See **global warming.**

**Greenough microscope.** See **stereoscopic microscope.**

**green soap** [AS, *grene* + L, *sapo*], a soft soap made from vegetable oils with sodium or potassium hydroxide in concentrations adjusted to retain glycerol. The soap may be any color, depending on the ingredient oils added.

**green soap tincture** [AS, *grene* + L, *sapo,* soap, *tinctura,* dyeing], an alcoholic solution of green soap with lavender oil added.

**greenstick fracture** [AS, *grene* + *stician*], an incomplete fracture in which the bone is bent but broken only on the outer arc of the bend. Children, especially those with rickets, are particularly likely to have greenstick fractures. Immobilization is usually effective, and healing is rapid. Also called **bent fracture, hickory stick fracture.** See also **fracture.**

**green tea,** an herb that grows as a native shrub in Asia.
■ USES: This herb is used to prevent cancer and heart disease, for hypercholesterolemia, and as an antidiarrheal.
■ CONTRAINDICATIONS: Green tea is contraindicated in those with known hypersensitivity to this product and in those with kidney inflammation, GI ulcers, insomnia, cardiovascular disease, and increased intraocular pressure.

**green tobacco sickness,** a nicotine-induced illness of tobacco harvest workers, characterized by headache, dizziness, vomiting, and prostration. The condition is caused by skin contact with wet tobacco leaves.

**-grel,** combining form for a platelet antiaggregate.

**grenz rays** [Ger, *Grenze,* boundary; L, *radius,* ray], low-energy x-rays used for treatment of skin conditions. They have very little penetrating ability and are frequently applied by dermatologists rather than by radiotherapists.

**Greulich-Pyle method** /groi′lish-pīl′, grōō′lik-/, a technique for evaluating the bone age of children, using a single frontal radiograph of the left hand and wrist.

**Grey Turner's sign** [George Grey Turner, English surgeon, 1877–1951], bruising of the skin of the loin in acute hemorrhagic pancreatitis. Also called **Turner's sign.**

**grid** [ME, *gredire,* grate], a device used during a radiographic examination to absorb radiation that is not heading along a straight line from the x-ray source to the film. Such scattered radiation does not contribute useful information and thus constitutes a source of unwanted density. A **linear grid** consists of alternating parallel strips of radiopaque and radiolucent material. Linear grids may cause variations in image density because of primary-photon attenuation. Den-

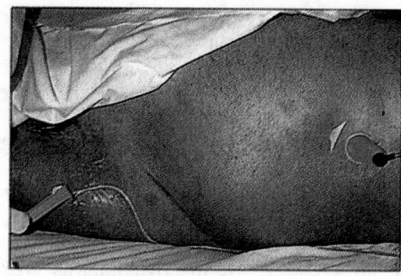

**Grey Turner's sign** *(Grieg and Garden, 1996)*

sity is at a maximum in the center of the film and decreases toward the edges.

**grid cutoff,** an undesirable absorption of primary-beam x-rays by a grid, which prevents useful x-rays from reaching a radiographic film. It is an effect of improper grid positioning and occurs most commonly with linear grids.

**grid ratio,** (in radiology) the ratio of the height of the lead strips to the width of the interspacing of a grid.

**grief** [L, *gravis,* heavy], a nearly universal pattern of physical and emotional responses to bereavement, separation, or loss. It is time linked and must be differentiated from depression. The physical components are similar to those of fear, hunger, rage, and pain. Stimulation of the sympathetic portion of the autonomic nervous system can cause increased heart and respiratory rates, dilated pupils, sweating, bristling of the hair, increased blood flow to the muscles, and increased energy reserves. Digestion slows. The emotional components proceed in stages from alarm to disbelief and denial, to anger and guilt, to a search for a source of comfort, and, finally, to adjustment to the loss. The way in which a grieving person behaves is greatly affected by the culture in which he or she has been raised. See also **bereavement, parental grief.**

**grief reaction,** a complex of somatic and psychologic symptoms associated with extreme sorrow or loss, specifically the death of a loved one. Somatic symptoms include feelings of tightness in the throat and chest with choking and shortness of breath, abdominal distress, lack of muscular power, and extreme tiredness and lethargy. Psychologic reactions involve a generalized awareness of mental anguish and discomfort accompanied by feelings of guilt, anger, hostility, extreme restlessness, inability to concentrate, and lack of capacity to initiate and maintain organized patterns of activities. Such symptoms may appear immediately after a crisis, or they may be delayed, exaggerated, or apparently absent, depending on the degree of involvement of the relationship and the physical and mental status of the person. Although both the somatic and psychologic reactions have the potential for developing into pathologic conditions, appropriate adaptive behavior and normal responses, such as sobbing or talking about the dead person or tragedy, are methods of working through the acute grief and lead to successful resolution of the crisis. Most acute grief reactions are resolved within 4 to 6 weeks, although the period varies and may be much longer, especially in cases of unexpected and sudden death. Intervention by health care professionals, especially nurses, is necessary when individuals exhibit maladaptive behavioral patterns that prevent the resolution of grief and can lead to morbid reactions, including such accepted psychosomatic illnesses as asthma and ulcers. Also called **grief process.** See also **death, parental grief.**

**grief resolution,** a nursing outcome from the Nursing Outcomes Classification (NOC) defined as adjustment to actual or impending loss. See also **Nursing Outcomes Classification.**

**grief work facilitation,** a nursing intervention from the Nursing Interventions Classification (NIC) defined as assistance with the resolution of a significant loss. See also **Nursing Interventions Classification.**

**grief work facilitation: perinatal death,** a nursing intervention from the Nursing Interventions Classification (NIC) defined as assistance with the resolution of a perinatal loss. See also **Nursing Interventions Classification.**

**grieving, anticipatory,** a nursing diagnosis accepted by the Fourth National Conference on the Classification of Nursing Diagnoses (revised 1996). Anticipatory grieving is defined as intellectual and emotional responses and behaviors by which individuals (families, communities) work through the process of modifying self-concept based on the perception of potential loss.
■ DEFINING CHARACTERISTICS: The defining characteristics are potential loss of significant object; expression of distress at potential loss; denial of potential loss; denial of the significance of the loss; guilt, anger, sorrow; bargaining; alteration in: eating habits, sleep patterns, activity level, libido; altered communication patterns; difficulty taking on new or different roles; resolution of grief before the reality of loss.
■ RELATED FACTORS: Related factors are to be developed. See also **nursing diagnosis.**

**grieving, dysfunctional,** a nursing diagnosis accepted by the Fourth National Conference on the Classification of Nursing Diagnoses (revised 1996). Dysfunctional grieving is defined as extended, unsuccessful use of intellectual and emotional responses by which individuals (families, communities) attempt to work through the process of modifying self-concept upon the perception of potential loss.
■ DEFINING CHARACTERISTICS: The defining characteristics are repetitive use of ineffectual behaviors associated with attempts to reinvest in relationships; reliving of past experiences with little or no reduction (diminishment) of intensity of grief; prolonged interference with life functioning; onset of exacerbation of somatic or psychosomatic responses; expression of distress at loss; denial of loss; expression of guilt; expression of unresolved issues; anger; sadness; crying; difficulty in expressing loss; alterations: in eating habits, sleep patterns, dream patterns, activity level, libido, concentration, and/or pursuit of tasks; idealization of lost object; reliving of past experiences; interference with life functioning; developmental regression; and labile affect.
■ RELATED FACTORS: The related factors are an actual or perceived object loss (object loss is used in the broadest sense); objects may include: people, possessions, a job, status, ideals, and parts and processes of the body. See also **nursing diagnosis.**

**griffe des orteils.** See **pes cavus.**

**Grifulvin,** trademark for an antifungal (griseofulvin).

**grinder's asthma** /grīnˈdərz/ [ME, *grinden,* to crush; Gk, panting], a condition characterized by asthmatic symptoms caused by inhalation of fine particles produced by industrial grinding processes. See also **pneumoconiosis.**

**grinder's disease.** See **silicosis.**

**grinding-in,** a clinical corrective grinding of one or more natural or artificial teeth to improve centric and eccentric occlusions. Compare **occlusal adjustment, selective grinding.**

**grip and pinch strength,** the measurable ability to exert pressure with the hand and fingers. It is measured by having a patient forcefully squeeze, grip, or pinch dynamometers;

results are expressed in either pounds or kilograms of pressure.

**gripes** /grīps/ [AS, *gripan,* to grasp], severe and usually spasmodic pain in the abdominal region caused by an intestinal disorder. Also called **gripping.**

**grippe.** See **influenza.**

**gripping.** See **gripes.**

**Grisactin,** trademark for an antifungal (griseofulvin).

**griseofulvin** /gris′ē·ōful′vin/, an antifungal.

■ INDICATIONS: It is prescribed in the treatment of certain fungal infections of the skin, hair, and nails.

■ CONTRAINDICATIONS: Liver dysfunction, porphyria, or known hypersensitivity to this drug prohibits its use.

■ ADVERSE EFFECTS: The most serious adverse reactions are blood dyscrasias. Headache, GI symptoms, and rashes also may occur.

**Griswald brace,** an orthosis for the control of vertebral body compression fractures. It is designed with two anterior forces with each equal to one half the posterior force to extend the spine. Also called **Jewett brace.**

**Grocco's sign, Grocco's triangle.** See **Korányi's sign.**

**grocer's itch** [AS, *gican,* itch], a dermatitis caused by contact with mites found in grain, cheese, or dried foods. Also called *Glycoyphagus domesticus.*

**groin** [ME, *grynde*], each of two areas where the abdomen joins the thighs; inguinal area.

**Grönblad-Strandberg syndrome** /grōn′bladstrand′bərg/ [Ester E. Grönblad, Swedish ophthalmologist, 1898–1942; James V. Strandberg, Swedish dermatologist, 1883–1942], an autosomal-recessive disorder of connective tissue characterized by premature aging and breakdown of the skin, gray or brown streaks on the retina, and hemorrhagic arterial degeneration, including retinal bleeding that causes vision loss. Angina pectoris and hypertension are common; weak pulse, episodic cramplike pains in the calves, and fatigue with exertion may affect the extremities. The prognosis depends on vessel involvement, but life expectancy is shortened. Treatment is symptomatic. Also called **pseudoxanthoma elasticum.**

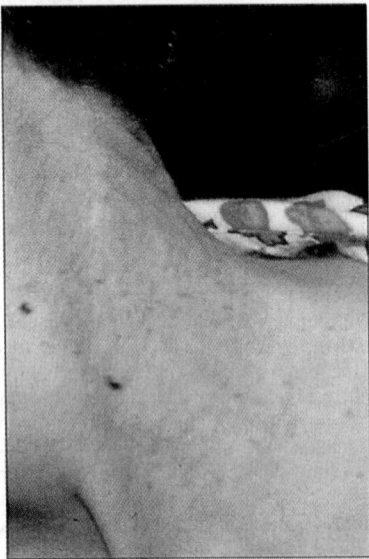

**Grönblad-Strandberg syndrome: skin changes**
*(Michelson and Friedlaender, 1996)*

**groove** [AS, *grafan,* to dig], a shallow, linear depression in various structures throughout the body, as those that form channels for nerves along the bones, those in bones for the insertion of muscles, and those between certain areas of the brain.

**grooved pegboard test,** a method for evaluating psychomotor function by measuring how quickly a subject can insert pegs into grooved holes. The test is reported to be sensitive to the effects of various neurotoxins that can affect perception and dexterity.

**gross** [OFr, *gros,* large], **1.** macroscopic, as *gross pathology,* from the study of tissue changes without magnification by a microscope. **2.** large or obese. Compare **microscopic.**

**gross anatomy,** the study of the organs or parts of the body large enough to be seen with the naked eye. Also called **macroscopic anatomy.**

**Grossman principle,** in tomography, the principle that when the fulcrum or axis of rotation remains at a fixed point, the focal plane is changed by raising or lowering the table top through this point to the desired height.

**gross motor skills** [Fr, *gros,* big; L, *movere,* ONorse, *skilja,* to cut apart], the ability to use large muscle groups that coordinate body movements involved in activities such as walking, running, jumping, throwing, and maintaining balance.

**gross sensory testing,** an evaluation procedure that includes assessment of passive motion sense in the shoulder, elbow, wrist, and fingers and ability to localize touch stimuli to specific fingers. It usually precedes motor evaluation of a patient.

**gross visual skills,** the general ability of a person to track a large, bright object side-to-side or up-to-down without jerkiness, nystagmus, or convergence and to discriminate among various basic shapes and colors.

**ground** [AS, *grund*], **1.** (in electricity) a connection between the electric circuit and the ground, which becomes a part of the circuit. **2.** (in psychology) the background of a visual field that can enhance or inhibit the ability of a patient to focus on an object.

**ground itch,** pruritic papules, urticarial vesiculopustular lesions secondary to penetration of the skin by hookworm larvae. The condition is prevalent in tropic and subtropic climates and may be prevented by wearing shoes and by establishing sanitary disposal of feces. See also **hookworm.**

**ground state,** **1.** the lowest energy level of a physical system. **2.** the stable form of an atom or molecule. See also **fatigue state.**

**ground substance.** See **matrix.**

**group** [Fr, *groupe,* cluster], (in research) any set of items or people under study. See also **control group, experimental group.**

**group dynamics** [Fr, *groupe* + Gk, *dynamis,* force], the interactions and relationships that take place among group members as well as between the group and the rest of society. It includes interdependence of group members, collective problem solving and decision making, and group conformity.

**group function,** (in dentistry) the simultaneous contacting of opposing teeth in a segment or a unit.

**group-model HMO,** a health maintenance organization (HMO) in which a contract is established with multispecialty medical groups for medical services. The HMO is responsible for marketing and developing contracts with enrollees and hospitals. Care is provided at hospitals where the physicians have admitting privileges or at ancillary facilities with which the HMO subcontracts.

**group practice,** two or more physicians, advanced practice nurses, and/or physician's assistants who work together and share facilities. The physicians may practice different specialties. Physicians who are part of a group often are prohibited from becoming independent contractors and earning money by providing medical care outside the group.

**group practice without walls (GPWW),** a medical practice formed to share economic risk, expenses, and marketing efforts. Physicians retain separate offices and finances. Often a central site is established to house administrative services and some or all ancillary services.

**group specificity.** See **specificity.**

**group therapy,** the application of psychotherapeutic techniques within a group of people (usually 10 or fewer) who experience similar difficulties. Generally a group leader directs the discussion of problems in an attempt to promote individual psychologic growth and favorable personality change. The procedure provides opportunities for treating a greater number of people in a shorter time than would be possible with individual therapy, and it is used in clinics, in institutions, and in private practice. Group therapy has been found to be particularly effective in the treatment of various addictions. A kind of group therapy is **psychodrama.** See also **Gestalt therapy, psychotherapy, self-help group, transactional analysis.**

**growing fracture** [AS, *growan* + L, *fractura,* to break], a fracture, usually linear, in which consecutive radiographic images show a gradual separation of the fracture edges over time. The separation is often caused by the pressure of soft tissues, as when arachnoid tissues expand through the edges of a skull fracture.

**growing pains,** 1. rheumatism-like pains that occur in the muscles and joints of children or adolescents as a result of fatigue, emotional problems, postural defects, and other causes that are not related to growth and that may be symptoms of various disorders. 2. emotional and psychologic problems experienced during adolescence.

**growth**[1] [AS, *growan,* to grow], 1. an increase in the size of an organism or any of its parts, as measured in increments of weight, volume, or linear dimensions, that occurs as a result of hyperplasia or hypertrophy. 2. the normal progressive anatomic, physiologic development from infancy to adulthood that is the result of gradual and normal processes of accretion and assimilation. The total of the numerous changes that occur during the lifetime of an individual constitutes a dynamic and complex process that involves many interrelated components, notably heredity, environment, nutrition, hygiene, and disease, all of which are subject to a variety of influences. In childhood growth is categorized according to the approximate age at which distinctive physical changes usually appear and at which specific developmental tasks are achieved. Such stages include the prenatal period, infancy, early childhood (including the toddler and the preschool periods), middle childhood, and adolescence. There are two periods of accelerated growth: the first 12 months, in which the infant triples in weight, increases the height at birth by approximately 50%, and undergoes rapid motor, cognitive, and social development; the second, in the months around puberty, when the child approaches adult height and secondary sexual characteristics emerge. Physical growth may be abnormally accelerated or slowed by a defect in the hypophyseal or pituitary gland. 3. any abnormal localized increase of the size or number of cells, as in a tumor or neoplasm. 4. a proliferation of cells, specifically a bacterial culture or mold. Compare **development, differentiation**[2]**, maturation.**

**growth**[2], a nursing outcome from the Nursing Outcomes Classification (NOC) defined as a normal increase in body size and weight. See also **Nursing Outcomes Classification.**

**growth and development, delayed,** a nursing diagnosis accepted by the Seventh National Conference on the Classification of Nursing Diagnoses. Altered growth and development is defined as the state in which an individual demonstrates deviations in norms from his or her age group.
■ DEFINING CHARACTERISTICS: The defining characteristics are delay or difficulty in performing skills (motor, social, or expressive) typical of the age group; altered physical growth; inability to perform self-care or self-control activities appropriate for the age; flat affect; listlessness; and decreased responses.
■ RELATED FACTORS: Related factors include inadequate caretaking: involving indifference, inconsistent responsiveness, multiple caretakers; separation from significant others; environmental and stimulation deficiencies; effects of physical disability; and prescribed dependence. See **nursing diagnosis.**

**growth charts,** graphic displays of normal progressive changes in height, weight, and head circumference. They consider the range of growth as expressed in percentiles, or as standard deviation from the mean for average height or weight for age. Head circumference measurements are common from birth to 2 years of age.

**growth curve,** a graphic display of data showing proliferation of cell numbers in a culture as a function of time.

**growth, disproportionate, risk for,** a nursing diagnosis accepted by the Thirteenth National Conference on the Classification of Nursing Diagnoses. It is defined as being at risk for growth above the 97th percentile or below the 3rd percentile for age, crossing two percentile channels; disproportionate growth.
■ RISK FACTORS: Prenatal risk factors include congenital or genetic disorders, maternal nutrition, multiple gestation, teratogen exposure, substance use or abuse, and maternal infection. Individual risk factors include infection, prematurity, malnutrition, organic and inorganic factors, caregiver and/or individual maladaptive feeding behaviors, anorexia, insatiable appetite, chronic illness, and substance abuse. Other risk factors include deprivation, teratogens, lead poisoning, poverty, violence, natural disasters, caregiver abuse, caregiver mental illness, caregiver mental retardation, and severe learning disabilities of caregiver. See also **nursing diagnosis.**

**growth factor,** any protein that stimulates the division and differentiation of specific types of cells. Growth factors include platelet-derived growth factor, epidermal growth factor, nerve growth factor, and interleukins, a group of at least 15 proteins produced mainly by T cells but also by mononuclear phagocytes and other cells. Growth factors specifically involved in the division and differentiation of bone marrow stem cells are classified as colony-stimulating factors. Platelets are a rich source of growth factors, some of which may be involved in the cellular proliferation that occurs in diseases such as rheumatoid arthritis and glomerulonephritis. See also **cytokine.**

**growth factor receptor,** a plasma membrane-spanning protein that binds with a specific growth factor on the external surface of a cell and transduces a signal that triggers cell division.

**growth failure,** a lack of normal physical and psychologic development that results from genetic, nutritional, pathologic, or psychosocial factors. See also **failure to thrive, maternal deprivation syndrome.**

**growth hormone (GH),** a single-chain peptide secreted by the anterior pituitary gland in response to growth hormone–releasing hormone (GH-RH). Its secretion is controlled in part by the hypothalamus. GH promotes protein synthesis in all cells, increases fat mobilization and use of fatty acids for energy, and decreases use of carbohydrate. Growth effects depend on the presence of thyroid hormone, insulin, and carbohydrate. Somatomedins, proteins produced chiefly in the liver, play a vital role in GH-induced skeletal growth. GH cannot cause elongation of long bones after the epiphyses close, however, so stature does not increase after puberty. GH accelerates the transport of specific amino acids into cells, stimulates the synthesis of messenger ribonucleic acid (RNA) and ribosomal RNA, influences the activity of several enzymes, increases the storage of phosphorus and potassium, and promotes a moderate retention of sodium. GH secretion, controlled almost exclusively by the central nervous system, occurs in bursts, with more than half of the total daily amount released during early sleep. Somatostatin, an anterior pituitary regulating hormone produced in the hypothalamus, inhibits GH secretion as well as secretion of insulin and gastrin. A deficiency of GH causes dwarfism; an excess results in gigantism in children or acromegaly in adults. Also called **somatotropic hormone, somatotropin.** See also **acromegaly, dwarfism, gigantism, somatostatin.**

**growth hormone release inhibiting hormone.** See **somatostatin.**

**growth hormone–releasing hormone (GH-RH),** somatotropin releasing factor released by the hypothalamus. Also called **somatoliberin.**

**growth hormone (GH) test,** a blood test used to identify growth hormone deficiency in adolescents who have short stature, delayed sexual maturity, or other growth deficiencies. It is also used to document the diagnosis of GH excess in gigantic or acromegalic patients and as a screening test for pituitary hypofunction.

**growth phase,** one of the stages in the growth of a neoplasm.

**growth retardation,** failure of an individual to develop at a normal rate of height and weight for his or her age. See also **intrauterine growth retardation.**

**Grünfelder's reflex** /grYn′feldərz, grēn′-/, an involuntary dorsiflexion of the great toe with a fanlike spreading of the other toes, caused by continued pressure on the posterior lateral fontanel. The reflex occurs in children who have middle-ear disease.

**grunting** [ME, *grunten*], abnormal, short, deep, hoarse sounds in exhalation that often accompany severe chest pain. The grunt occurs because the glottis briefly stops the flow of air, halting the movement of the lungs and their surrounding or supporting structures. Grunting is most often heard in a person who has pneumonia, pulmonary edema, or fractured or bruised ribs. Atelectasis in the newborn also causes grunting, which results from the effort required to fill the lungs.

**GSA,** abbreviation for **Gerontological Society of America.**

**GSR,** abbreviation for **galvanic skin response.**

**G syndrome.** See **Opitz syndrome.**

**gt,** abbreviation for the Latin word *gutta,* 'a drop.'

**GTP,** abbreviation for **guanosine triphosphate.**

**GTPase,** enzyme activity that catalyzes the hydrolysis of guanosine triphosphate to guanosine diphosphate and orthophosphate.

**gtt,** abbreviation for the Latin word *guttae,* 'drops.' Also **gtts, GTTS.**

**G tube.** See **stomach tube.**

**GU,** abbreviation for **genitourinary.**

**guaiac** /gwī′ak/, a wood resin, formerly used as a reagent in laboratory tests for the presence of occult blood.

**guaiacol poisoning.** See **phenol poisoning.**

**guaiac test,** a test, using guaiac as a reagent, performed on feces and urine for detecting occult blood in the intestinal and urinary tracts.

**guaifenesin** /gwī′əfen′əsin/, glyceryl guaiacolate, a white to slightly gray powder with a bitter taste and faint odor, widely used as an expectorant. Guaifenesin increases the flow of fluid in the respiratory tract, reducing the viscosity of bronchial and tracheal secretions and facilitating their removal by the cough reflex and ciliary action. It may increase the risk of hemorrhage in patients taking heparin.

**guanabenz acetate** /gwan′abenz/, a centrally acting antiadrenergic antihypertensive.

■ INDICATION: It is prescribed in the treatment of hypertension.

■ CONTRAINDICATION: Known hypersensitivity to this drug prohibits its use.

■ ADVERSE EFFECTS: Among adverse reactions are dizziness, sedation, and dry mouth.

**guanadrel sulfate** /gwan′ədril/, an antihypertensive agent.

■ INDICATION: It is prescribed in the treatment of hypertension in patients who do not respond to first-step agents.

■ CONTRAINDICATIONS: Pheochromocytoma, administration of monoamine oxidase inhibitors, frank congestive heart failure, or known sensitivity to this drug prohibits its use.

■ ADVERSE EFFECTS: Among the most serious adverse reactions are orthostatic hypotension and syncope.

**guanase.** See **guanine deaminase.**

**guanethidine sulfate** /gwaneth′idēn/, a peripherally acting antiadrenergic antihypertensive.

■ INDICATION: It is prescribed in the treatment of moderate and severe hypertension.

■ CONTRAINDICATIONS: Heart failure, concomitant administration of monoamine oxidase inhibitors, pheochromocytoma, or known hypersensitivity to this drug prohibits its use. It should be avoided in elderly patients.

■ ADVERSE EFFECTS: Among the more serious adverse reactions are orthostatic hypotension, salt and water retention, bradycardia, diarrhea, and inability to ejaculate.

**guanine** /gwan′ēn/, a purine base that is a component of DNA and RNA. In free or uncombined form it occurs in trace amounts in most cells, usually as a product of the enzymatic hydrolysis of nucleic acids and nucleotides. On hydrolysis it is first converted into xanthine and finally into uric acid. See also **adenine.**

**guanine deaminase,** an enzyme that catalyzes the hydrolysis of guanine to xanthine and ammonia. It is present in liver, kidney, spleen, and other tissues. Also called **guanase** /gwan′ās/.

**guanosine** /gwan′ōsēn/, a nucleoside composed of guanine and a sugar, D-ribose. It is a major component of the nucleotides guanosine monophosphate and guanosine triphosphate and of RNA. A related nucleoside, deoxyguanosine, is a major component of DNA.

**guanosine deaminase.** See **deaminase.**

**guanosine monophosphate (GMP),** a nucleotide that plays an important role in various metabolic reactions and in the formation of RNA from DNA templates.

**guanosine triphosphate (GTP),** a high-energy nucleotide, similar to adenosine triphosphate, that functions in various metabolic reactions, such as the activation of fatty acids and the formation of peptide bonds in protein synthesis.

**guaranine** /gwərä′nin/, caffeine.

**guardian ad litem** /ad lī′təm/ [L, *ad litem,* to litigate], (in law) a person who is appointed by a court to prosecute or defend a suit for an infant or an incapacitated person. A guardian ad litem is sometimes appointed when a person's life is in imminent danger and that person refuses treatment.

**guardianship,**  a legal status that places the care and property of an individual in the hands of another person. Implementation of the law varies in different cases and jurisdictions. Some courts have held as legally incompetent mental patients who have jobs and live independently.

**guarding.**  See **abdominal splinting.**

**Guarnieri's bodies** /gōō′ärnyer′ēz/ [Giuseppi Guarnieri, Italian physician, 1856–1918],  acidophilic inclusion bodies that are formed in the cytoplasm of cells infected with cowpox or vaccinia virus.

**Gubbay test of motor proficiency,**  a screening test for the identification of developmental dyspraxia. It consists of eight activities, such as whistling, throwing a tennis ball, and fitting shapes into appropriate slots, the results of which discriminate between impaired motor function and normal development in children.

**Guedel's signs** /gōō′dəlz/ [Arthur E. Guedel, American anesthesiologist, 1883–1956],  a system for describing the stages and planes of anesthesia during an operative procedure. These stages are only applicable to ether anesthesia and are difficult to delineate when combination anesthetics are given. See also **anesthesia.**

**Guérin's fracture** /gāraNz′/ [Alphonse F.M. Guérin, French surgeon, 1816–1895],  a break in the maxilla. Also called **Le Fort I fracture** /ləfôr′/.

**guggul,**  an herb that is native to India.

■ USES: This herb is used for high LDL cholesterol, elevated triglycerides, and weight loss.

■ CONTRAINDICATIONS: Guggul is contraindicated during pregnancy, since it can cause uterine contractions. It also should not be used during lactation, in children, and in those with known hypersensitivity to this product.

**guided imagery** /gī′did/,  a therapeutic technique for relieving pain or anxiety and for promoting relaxation in which a patient is encouraged to concentrate on an image that helps relieve discomfort. See also **visualization.**

**guide dog** [ME, *guiden,* to guard; OE, *docga*],  a dog trained to aid in the mobility of a blind or partially blind person. Guide dogs are usually recruited from certain compatible breeds and tested at 13 weeks of age. If qualified, the dog is then specially trained in private hands for 1 year and retested. Most dogs selected for training pass the final test. Guide dogs also may be trained to serve as "ears" for deaf persons. Also called **companion animals, Seeing Eye dog.**

**guide plane** [ME, *guiden,* to guard; L, *planum,* level ground],  **1.** a part of an orthodontic appliance that has an established inclined plane for changing the occlusal relation of the maxillary and mandibular teeth and for permitting their movement to normal positions. **2.** a plane that is developed on the occlusal surfaces of occlusion rims for positioning the mandible in centric relation. **3.** two or more parallel vertical surfaces of abutment teeth shaped to direct the path of placement and removal of a partial denture.

**guide-shoe marks,**  a radiographic image artifact caused by pressure of the guide shoes, the curved metal lips that guide x-ray film in automatic developing systems. The guide shoes leave scratches called ridge lines in the image.

**guidewire** /gīd′wī·ər/ [ME, *guiden,* to guard; AS, *wir*],  a device used to position an IV catheter, endotracheal tube, central venous line, or gastric feeding tube.

**guiding,**  (in occupational therapy) a method in which therapists assist their patients in perceiving the environment by directing movement of their hands and bodies in functional activities. An example is hand-over-hand guiding in which the therapist's hand is over the patient's hand and assists in performance of a task.

**Guillain-Barré syndrome** /gēyan′bärā′/ [Georges Guillain, French neurologist, 1876–1951; Jean A. Barré, French neurologist, 1880–1967],  an idiopathic, peripheral polyneuritis that occurs 1 to 3 weeks after a mild episode of fever associated with a viral infection or with immunization. Symmetric pain and weakness affect the extremities, and paralysis may develop. The neuritis may spread to the trunk and face. Symptoms vary in intensity from mild to severe enough to require critical nursing care, including ventilator assistance. Treatment consists of supportive care and IV high doses of immunoglobulins. Recovery depends on the extent of neuritis and may take weeks to many months. Also called **acute febrile polyneuritis, acute idiopathic polyneuritis, infectious polyneuritis.**

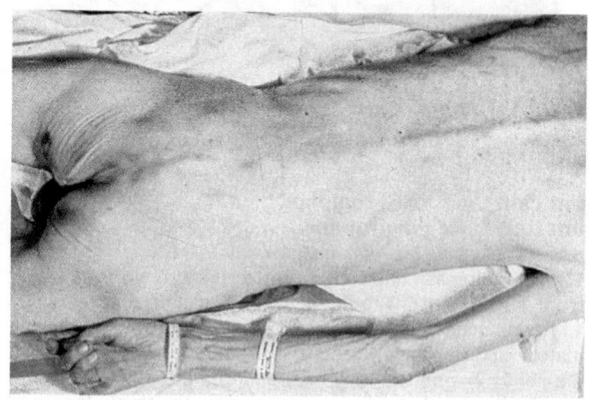

**Limb-wasting in Guillain-Barré syndrome**
*(Perkin et al, 1986/courtesy Dr. P.O. Behen)*

**guilt** [AS, *gylt,* delinquency],  a feeling caused by tension between the ego and superego when one falls below the standards set for oneself, or a remorseful awareness of having done something wrong.

**guilt work facilitation,**  a nursing intervention from the Nursing Interventions Classification (NIC) defined as helping another to cope with painful feelings of responsibility, actual or perceived. See also **Nursing Interventions Classification.**

**guilty,**  (in criminal law) a verdict by the court that to a moral certainty it is beyond reasonable doubt that the defendant committed the crime and is responsible for the offense as charged.

**guinea worm.**  See *Dracunculus medinensis.*

**Guinea worm infection.**  See **dracunculiasis.**

**Gulf War syndrome,**  a group of medical and psychologic complaints, including fatigue, skin rash, memory loss, and headaches experienced by men and women who served in the 1991 Persian Gulf War. Researchers observed similar physical effects in laboratory animals exposed to a mixture of cholinesterase inhibitor insecticides and pyridostigmine; soldiers had been exposed to both agents during the war.

**gullet.**  See **esophagus.**

**gum,**  **1.** a sticky excretion from certain plants. **2.** a firm layer of flesh covering the alveolar processes of the jaws and the base of the teeth. See **gingiva.**

**gumboil** [AS, *goma* + *byl*], an abscess of the gingiva and periosteum resulting from injury, infection, or dental decay. The gum is characteristically red, swollen, and tender. The abscess may rupture spontaneously, or it may require incision. Treatment may include antibiotics and hot mouthwashes. Also called **parulis.**

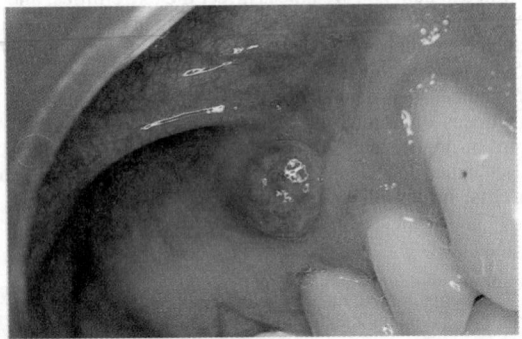

**Gumboil** *(Regezi, Sciubba, and Pogrel, 2000)*

**gum camphor.** See **camphor.**

**gum line.** See **gingival line.**

**gumma** /gum′ə/, *pl.* **gummas, gummata** [AS, *goma,* gum], **1.** a granuloma, characteristic of tertiary syphilis, varying from 1 mm to 1 cm in diameter. It is usually encapsulated and contains a central necrotic mass surrounded by inflammatory and fibrotic zones of tissue. Infectious organisms of the genus *Treponema* may be found in a gumma. The lesion may be localized or diffuse, occurring on the trunk, legs, and face and on various internal organs, especially the liver. Rupture of a gumma produces a shallow ulcer that heals slowly. **2.** a soft granulomatous lesion that sometimes accompanies tuberculosis.

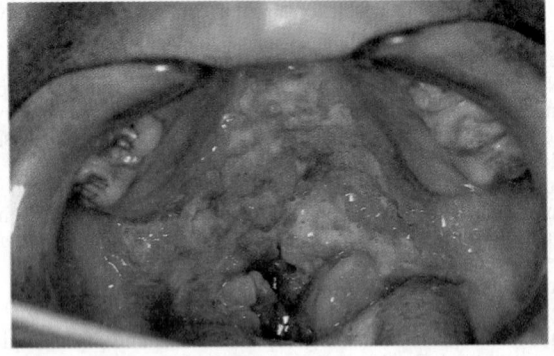

**Gumma on the palate** *(Regezi, Sciubba, and Pogrel, 2000)*

**gun-barrel vision.** See **tunnel vision.**

**Gunning's splint** [Thomas B. Gunning, American dentist, 1813–1889; D, *splinte,* split], a splint used to support the maxilla and the mandible during jaw surgery.

**Gunn's syndrome.** See **jaw-winking.**

**gunshot fracture** [ME, *gunne* + AS, *sceotan,* to shoot; L, *fractura,* break], a fracture caused by a bullet or similar missile.

**gunshot wound (GSW),** penetration of the body by a bullet, commonly marked by a small entrance wound and a larger exit wound. The wound is usually accompanied by damage to blood vessels, bones, and other tissues. There is high risk of infection caused by exposure of the wound to the external environment and debris carried inside the body by the bullet. Additional complications depend on the part of the body wounded.

**Gunson method,** a method of radiographic examination of the pharynx and upper esophagus during swallowing. A dark-colored shoestring is tied around the patient's throat just above the thyroid cartilage. The movement of the larynx is then shown by the elevation of the shoestring as the thyroid cartilage moves anteriorly, followed immediately by displacement of the shoestring as the cartilage passes superiorly.

**Günther's disease** /gun′thərz/ [Hans Gunther, German physician, 1884–1956], a rare congenital disorder of porphyrin metabolism that is associated with sunlight-induced skin lesions. See also **porphyria.**

**gurgle** [Fr, *gargouiller,* to gurgle], an abnormal coarse sound heard during auscultation, especially over large cavities or over a trachea nearly filled with secretions.

**gurney** /gur′nē/, a cot with wheeled legs, used in hospitals to transport patients.

**gurry** /gur′ē/, *(informal)* the detritus incident to physical trauma or surgery, including body fluids, secretions, and tissue.

**Gurvich radiation.** See **mitogenetic radiation.**

**gustation** /gustā′shən/ [L, *gustare,* to taste], the sense and act of tasting foods, beverages, or other substances.

**gustatory** /gus′tətôr′ē/ [L, *gustare,* to taste], pertaining to the act or sense of taste or the organs of taste.

**gustatory hallucination** [L, *gustare,* to taste, *alucinari,* wandering mind], a false taste sensation of either food or beverage on the mucous membrane lining the empty mouth.

**gustatory organ.** See **taste bud.**

**gustatory papilla** [L, *gustare,* to taste, *papilla,* nipple], any of the small tissue elevations in the mouth that contain sense organs of taste such as the circumvallate papilla of the tongue.

**gut** [AS, *guttas*], **1.** intestine. **2.** *informal.* digestive tract. **3.** suture material manufactured from the intestines of sheep.

**gut-associated lymphoid tissue,** lymphoid tissue associated with the gut, including the tonsils, Peyer's patches, lamina propria of the GI tract, and appendix.

**Guthrie's bacterial inhibition assay (GBIA)** /guth′rēz/, a screening for phenylketonuria (PKU) used to detect the abnormal presence of phenylalanine metabolites in the blood. A small amount of blood is obtained and placed in a medium with a strain of *Bacillus subtilis,* a bacterium that cannot grow without phenylalanine. If phenylalanine metabolites are present, the bacteria reproduce, and the test result is positive, indicating that the patient has phenylketonuria. Routine screening of newborns for PKU is now mandatory in most of the United States. The Guthrie blood test has normally been done before discharging the newborn from the hospital. However, it is important to note that this test is not valid until the newborn has ingested an ample amount (for 2 or 3 days) of the amino acid phenylalanine, which is a constituent of both human and cow's milk. Also called **Guthrie's test.** See also **phenylketonuria.**

**gutta (gt)** /gut′ə, gŏŏt′ä/ [L, drop], one drop, or about 1 minim, of a medication.

**guttae (gtt, gtts, GTTS)** [L, drops], the plural of **gutta**, more than one drop, as in **guttae pro auribus**, or eardrops, or **guttae ophthalmicae**, or eyedrops.

**gutta-percha** /gut′əpur′chə/ [Malay, *getah-percha*, latex sap], the coagulated rubbery sap of various tropical trees, used for temporarily sealing the dressings of prepared tooth cavities. When combined with fillers and coloring materials, it may be rolled into sheets and used to make temporary bases for dentures.

**gutta-percha point,** a small cone of gutta-percha, which may be used to fill a root canal. The radiopacity of gutta-percha points permits them to be used also as probes for determining the depth and topographic characteristics of periodontal pockets by means of radiography.

**guttate psoriasis** /gut′āt/ [L, *gutta*, drop; Gk, itch], an acute form of psoriasis that consists of teardrop-shaped red scaly patches measuring 3 to 10 mm all over the body. A beta-hemolytic streptococcal pharyngitis or other upper respiratory infection may precipitate this reaction in susceptible individuals. Treatment is essential to prevent a more severe form of psoriasis. Compare **pustular psoriasis**. See also **psoriasis**.

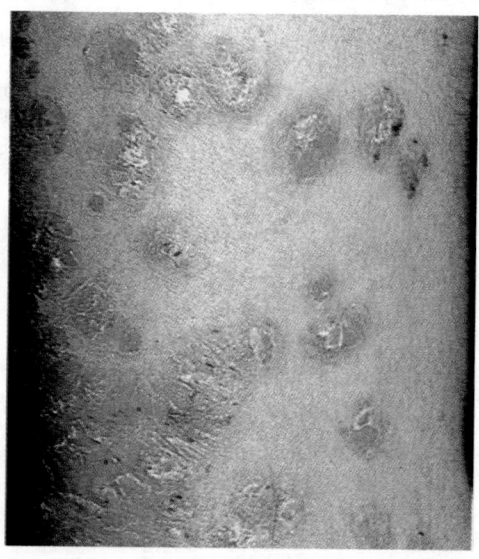

**Guttate psoriasis** (Zitelli and Davis, 1997)

**guttural** /gut′ərəl/ [L, *guttur*, throat], pertaining to or belonging to the throat, including low-pitched, raspy voice quality.

**Guyon tunnel** [Felix J. Guyon, French surgeon, 1831-1920], a fibroosseous tunnel formed in part by the pisohamate ligament of the hand. It contains the ulnar artery and nerve and may be the site of a compression injury.

**GVHD,** abbreviation for **graft-versus-host disease.**

**GVHR,** abbreviation for **graft-versus-host reaction.** See **graft-versus-host disease.**

**G-Well.** See **lindane.**

**Gy,** abbreviation for the SI unit **gray.**

**gymnema,** an herb found in India and Africa.

■ USES: This herb is used to reduce high blood glucose levels.

■ CONTRAINDICATIONS: Gymnema should not be used during pregnancy and lactation, in children, or in those with known hypersensitivity to this product.

**gymno-,** combining form meaning 'nakedness': *gymnocarpus, gymnocyte, gymnospore.*

**gyn,** 1. *informal.* abbreviation for **gynecologist.** 2. abbreviation for **gynecology.**

**gyn-.** See **gyneco-.**

**gynaecoid pelvis.** See **gynecoid pelvis.**

**gynaecology.** See **gynecology.**

**gynaecomastia.** See **gynecomastia.**

**gynandrous** /gīnan′drəs, jī-/ [Gk, *gyne*, woman, *aner*, man], describing a man or a woman who has some of the physical characteristics usually attributed to the other sex, as a female pseudohermaphrodite. Compare **androgynous.** —**gynandry,** *n.*

**gyne-.** See **gyneco-.**

**-gyne, -gyn,** suffix meaning '(specified) female characteristics': *androgyne, epigyne, trichogyne.*

**gyneco-, gyn-, gyne-, gyno-,** combining form meaning 'woman or female gender': *gynecoid, gynecomastia, gynotermon.*

**gynecography** /gī′nə-, jin′əkog′rəfē/, the radiographic examination of the female pelvic organs by means of intraperitoneal gas insufflation.

**gynecoid pelvis** /gī′nəkoid, jin′əkoid/ [Gk, *gyne* + *eidos*, form; L, *pelvis*, basin], a type of pelvis characteristic of the normal female and associated with the smallest incidence of fetopelvic disproportion. The inlet is nearly round, the sacrum is parallel to the posterior aspect of the symphysis pubis, the sidewalls are straight, and the ischial spines are blunt and do not encroach on the space in the true pelvis. It is the ideal pelvic type for childbirth. Also spelled **gynaecoid pelvis.**

**gynecologic** /gī′nə-, jin′əkəloj′ik/ [Gk, *gynaikos*, of a woman], pertaining to gynecology, or the study of diseases of the female reproductive organs and the breasts. Also **gynecological.**

**gynecologic examination,** pelvic examination.

**gynecologic operative procedures** [Gk, *gynaikos*, of a woman; L, *operari*, to work, *procedere*, to proceed], surgical intervention on the female reproductive system. Gynecologic and obstetric problems account for one fifth of all female visits to physicians; many require surgical correction.

**gynecologist** /gī′nəkol′əjist, jī′-, jin′-/, a physician who specializes in the health care of women, including diseases of their reproductive organs and breasts.

**gynecology** /gī′nəkol′əjē, jī′-, jin′-/ [Gk, *gyne* + *logos*, science], the study of diseases of the female reproductive organs, including the breasts. Unlike most specialties in medicine, gynecology encompasses surgical and nonsurgical expertise. It is almost always studied and practiced in conjunction with obstetrics. Also spelled **gynaecology.** —**gynecologic, gynecological,** *adj.*

**gynecomastia** /gī′nəkōmas′tē·ə, jī′-, jin′-/ [Gk, *gyne* + *mastos*, breast], an abnormal enlargement of one or both breasts in men. Milk production may or may not be present. The condition is usually temporary and benign. It may be caused by hormonal imbalance, tumor of the adrenal testis or pituitary, use of medication that contains estrogens or steroidal compounds, or failure of the liver to inactivate circulating estrogen, as in alcoholic cirrhosis. Less commonly the gynecomastia may be caused by a hormone-secreting tumor of the breast, lung, or other organ. It tends to subside spontaneously but, if marked, may be corrected surgically for

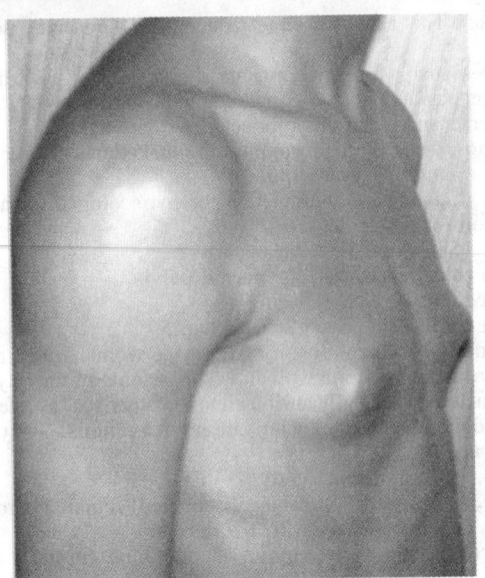

**Prepubertal gynecomastia**
*(Seidel et al, 1999/courtesy Wellington Hurg, MD)*

cosmetic or psychologic reasons. Biopsy may be performed to rule out cancer. Also called **gynecomasty.** Also spelled **gynaecomastia.**

**Gyne-Lotrimin,** trademark for an antifungal (clotrimazole).

**gynephobia** /gī′nəfō′bē·ə, jī′-, jin′-/ [Gk, *gyne* + *phobos*, fear], an anxiety disorder characterized by a morbid fear of women or by a morbid aversion to the society of women. It is an obsessive, phobic phenomenon that occurs almost entirely in men and may usually be traced to some frightening experience involving women that occurred in childhood. Treatment consists of psychotherapy to uncover the causative emotional conflict, followed by behavior therapy, specifically systemic desensitization and flooding to reduce anxiety.

**-gynic, -gynous,** suffix meaning 'human female or female characteristics': *androgynous, hologynic, monogynic, polygynic.*

**gyno-.** See **gyneco-.**

**gynogamone** /gī′nōgam′ōn/ [Gk, *gyne* + *gamos*, marriage], a chemical secreted by female gametes that is believed to attract male gametes.

**-gynous.** See **-gynic.**

**gypsum** /jip′səm/, a mineral composed mainly of crushed calcium sulfate hemihydrate. It is used in making plaster of paris surgical casts and impressions for dentures. Gypsum dust has an irritant action on the mucous membranes of the respiratory tract and the conjunctiva.

**gyrase** /jī′rās/, an enzyme that promotes the unwinding of the closed circular deoxyribonucleic acid helix of bacteria.

**gyri.** See **gyrus.**

**-gyria,** suffix meaning 'spiral or convolution': *oculogyria, polymicrogyria, ulegyria.*

**-gyro,** combining form meaning 'circle or spiral': *gyrus.*

**gyrus** /jī′rəs/, *pl.* **gyri** /jī′rī/ [Gk, *gyro*, circle], one of the winding convolutions of the cerebral hemisphere of the brain. They are caused by infolding of the cortex and are separated by the shallow grooves (sulci) or deeper grooves (fissures).

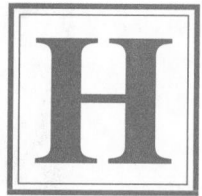

**h,** **1.** abbreviation for **haustus. 2.** symbol for **hecto-. 3.** abbreviation for **height. 4.** symbol for *hora,* the Latin word for hour. **5.** abbreviation for *horizontal.* **6.** abbreviation for **hyperopia.**

**H,** **1.** symbol for the element **hydrogen. 2.** symbol for **henry.**

$^2$**H,** formula for **deuterium,** an isotope of hydrogen.

$^3$**H,** formula for **tritium,** an isotope of hydrogen.

**[H$^+$],** symbol for hydrogen ion molar concentration.

**H$_0$,** symbol for **null hypothesis.**

**HA-1A,** a genetically engineered antibody used in the treatment of certain blood infections. The antibody attacks bacterial toxin rather than attacking the bacteria that produce them. It is relatively free of side effects.

**HAAg,** abbreviation for *hepatitis A antigen.* See also **hepatitis A.**

**Haas method,** a technique for producing radiographic images of the interior of the skull. The patient rests the forehead and nose on the table so that the x-ray beam enters the skull near the base of the occipital bone and emerges on the frontal bone above the nasal bone.

**habeas corpus** /hā′bē·əs kôr′pəs/ [L, you have the body], a right retained by all psychiatric patients that provides for the release of individuals who claim they are being deprived of their liberty and detained illegally. A hearing for this determination takes place in a court of law, where the patient's sanity is at issue.

**Habermann's disease.** See **Mucha-Habermann disease.**

**habilitation** /həbil′itā′shən/, the process of supplying a person with the means to develop maximum independence in activities of daily living through training or treatment.

**habit** [L, *habitus,* condition], **1.** a customary or particular practice, manner, or mode of behavior. **2.** an involuntary pattern of behavior or thought. **3.** the habitual use of drugs or narcotics. See also **habit spasm, habit training, habitus.**

**habitat** /hab′itat/ [L, *habitare,* to dwell], a natural environment where an organism, including a human being, may live and grow normally.

**habit spasm,** an involuntary twitching or tic. It usually involves a small muscle group of the face, neck, or shoulders and causes movements such as spasmodic blinking or rapid jerking of the head to the side. The movements are often generated by emotional conflicts rather than any organic disorder. They may serve as a release for tension or anxiety.

**habit tic** [L, *habitus,* condition; Fr, *tic*], a brief recurrent movement of a muscle group, such as a blink, grimace, or sudden head turning, that is of psychogenic rather than organic origin.

**habit training,** the process of teaching a child how to adjust to the demands of the external world by forming certain habits, primarily those related to eating, sleeping, elimination, and dress.

**habitual abortion** /həbich′ōō·əl/ [L, *habituare,* to become used to], spontaneous termination of three successive pregnancies before the twentieth week of gestation. Habitual abortion can result from chronic infection, abnormalities of the conceptus, maternal hormonal dysfunction, or uterine abnormalities such as cervical incompetence. See also **cerclage, incompetent cervix.**

**habitual dislocation** [L, *habitus,* condition, *dis + locare,* to place], a dislocation that recurs repeatedly after reduction.

**habitual fever.** See **fever, habitual hyperthermia.**

**habitual hyperthermia,** a condition of unknown cause that occurs in young females, characterized by body temperatures of 99° to 100.5° F regularly or intermittently for years, associated with fatigue, malaise, vague aches and pains, insomnia, bowel disturbances, and headaches. No organic cause can be found; the diagnosis is usually made only after a prolonged period of study and observation. No specific treatment is recommended. Reassurance and psychotherapy offer the best relief. Also called **habitual fever.**

**habituation** /həbich′ōō·ā′shən/ [L, *habituare,* to become used to], **1.** an acquired tolerance gained by repeated exposure to a particular stimulus such as alcohol. **2.** a decline and eventual elimination of a conditioned response by repetition of the conditioned stimulus. **3.** psychologic and emotional dependence on a drug, tobacco, or alcohol that results from the repeated use of the substance but without the addictive, physiologic need to increase dosage. Also called **negative adaptation.** Compare **addiction.**

**habitus** /hab′itəs/, a person's appearance or physique, as an athletic habitus. See also **habit.**

**HACEK,** abbreviation for *Hemophilus, Actinobacillus, Cardiobacterium, Eikenella,* and *Kingella,* microorganisms associated with infective endocarditis.

**hacking cough** [AS, *haeccan + cohettan*], a short, weak repeating cough, often caused by irritation of the larynx by a postnasal drip. It can also result from side effects of angiotensin-converting enzyme inhibitor therapy and smoking.

**HAD,** abbreviation for **HIV-associated dementia.**

**Haeckel's law.** See **recapitulation concept.**

**haemangioma.** See **hemangioma.**

**haemarthros.** See **hemarthros.**

**haematemesis.** See **hematemesis.**

**haematocele.** See **hematocele.**

**haematocrit.** See **hematocrit.**

**haematocytoblast.** See **hematocytoblast.**

**haematology.** See **hematology.**

**haematoma.** See **hematoma.**

**haematomyelia.** See **hematomyelia.**

**haematuria.** See **hematuria.**

**haeme.** See **heme.**

**-haemia.** See **-emia.**

**haemochromatosis.** See **hemochromatosis.**

**haemoconcentration.** See **hemoconcentration.**

**haemodialysis.** See **hemodialysis.**

**haemodilution.** See **hemodilution.**

**haemofiltration.** See **hemofiltration.**

**haemoglobin.** See **hemoglobin.**

**haemoglobinometer.** See **hemoglobinometer.**

**haemoglobinopathy.** See **hemoglobinopathy.**

**haemoglobinuria.** See **hemoglobinuria.**

**haemolysin.** See **hemolysin.**

haemolysis.   See hemolysis.
haemolytic anemia.   See hemolytic anemia.
haemoperfusion.   See hemoperfusion.
haemopericardium.   See hemopericardium.
haemoperitoneum.   See hemoperitoneum.
haemophilia.   See hemophilia.
haemophiliac.   See hemophiliac.

*Haemophilus* /hēmof′iləs/ [Gk, *haima,* blood, *philein,* to love], a genus of gram-negative pathogenic bacteria, frequently found in the respiratory tract of humans and other animals. Examples are *Haemophilus influenzae,* which causes respiratory tract infections and one form of meningitis; *H. haemolyticus,* a hemolytic species pathogenic in the upper respiratory tract of humans; and *H. ducreyi,* which causes chancroid. *Haemophilus* species are generally sensitive to cephalosporins, tetracyclines, and sulfonamides.

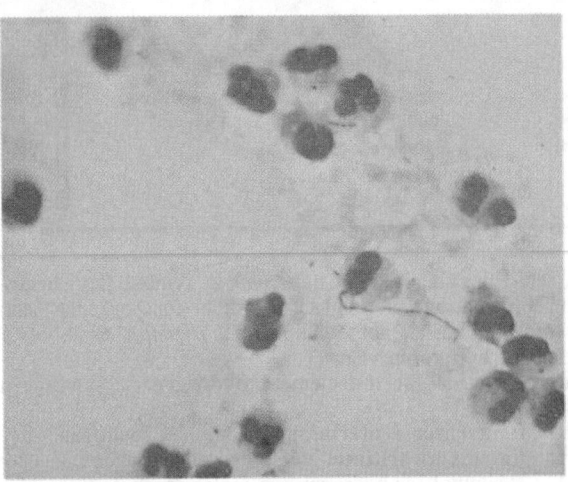

*Haemophilus influenzae* (Baron, Peterson, and Finegold, 1994)

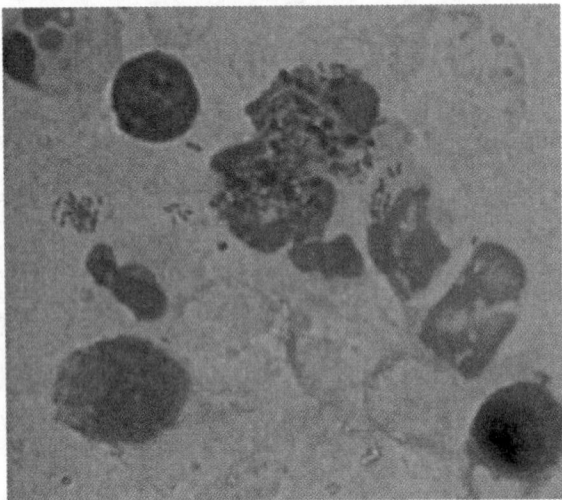

*Haemophilus ducreyi* (Baron, Peterson, and Finegold, 1994)

*Haemophilus influenzae,* a small gram-negative nonmotile parasitic bacterium that occurs in two forms, encapsulated and nonencapsulated, and in six types, a, b, c, d, e, and f. Almost all infections are caused by encapsulated type b organisms. *Haemophilus influenzae* is found in the throats of 30% of healthy, normal people. In children and in debilitated older people, severe destructive inflammation of the larynx, trachea, and bronchi may result from infection. Subacute bacterial endocarditis, purulent meningitis, and pneumonia also may be caused by it. Secondary infection by *H. influenzae* occurs in influenza and in many other respiratory diseases. Immunization is available for pediatric patients.

*Haemophilus influenzae* pneumonia, bacterial pneumonia caused by infection with *Haemophilus influenzae,* seen mainly in young children and debilitated or immunocompromised adults; it sometimes progresses to life-threatening conditions such as meningitis, pericarditis, endocarditis, and epiglottitis that can cause obstruction of the airway.

haemopoietic.   See hemopoietic.
haemoptysis.   See hemoptysis.
haemorrhage.   See hemorrhage.
haemorrhagic disease of newborn.   See hemorrhagic disease of newborn.

haemorrhoid.   See hemorrhoid.
haemorrhoidectomy.   See hemorrhoidectomy.
haemosiderin.   See hemosiderin.
haemostasis.   See hemostasis.
haemostatic.   See hemostatic.
haemothorax.   See hemothorax.

hafnium (Hf) /haf′nē·əm/ [Hafnia, Medieval Latin name of Copenhagen, Denmark], a hard, brittle silver-gray metallic element of the third transition series. Its atomic number is 72; its atomic mass is 178.49. Elements in this group show some nonmetallic chemical characteristics.

Hagedorn needle /hä′gedôrn/ [Werner Hagedorn, German physician, 1831–1894], a flat surgical needle with a cutting edge near its point and a very large eye at the other end.

Hageman factor.   See factor XII.

Haglund's deformity [Sims E.P. Haglund, Swedish orthopedist, 1870–1937], a foot disorder characterized by an enlarged posterior-superior lateral aspect of the calcaneus, often associated with an inverted subtalar joint. It is a common cause of posterior Achilles bursitis.

Hailey-Hailey disease.   See benign familial chronic pemphigus.

hair [AS, *haer*], a filament of keratin consisting of a root and a shaft formed in a specialized follicle in the epidermis. There are three stages of hair development: anagen, the active growing stage; catagen, a short interlude between the growth and resting phases; and telogen, the resting (club) stage before shedding. Scalp hair grows at an average rate of 1 mm every 3 days, body and eyebrow hair at a much slower rate. Hair plucking does not stop hair growth. See also hirsutism, lanugo.

hair analysis [AS, *haer* + Gk, a loosening], chemical analysis of a hair sample to find possible evidence of exposure to a toxic substance. Molecules of lead compounds and other chemicals are absorbed and stored in hair shafts. Hair analysis is also used to determine possible causes of malnutrition. Samples for analysis are taken from areas close to the scalp to eliminate chances that toxic chemicals found in the hair may have been absorbed from air pollutants.

hair care, a nursing intervention from the Nursing Interventions Classification (NIC) defined as promotion of neat, clean, attractive hair. See also Nursing Interventions Classification.

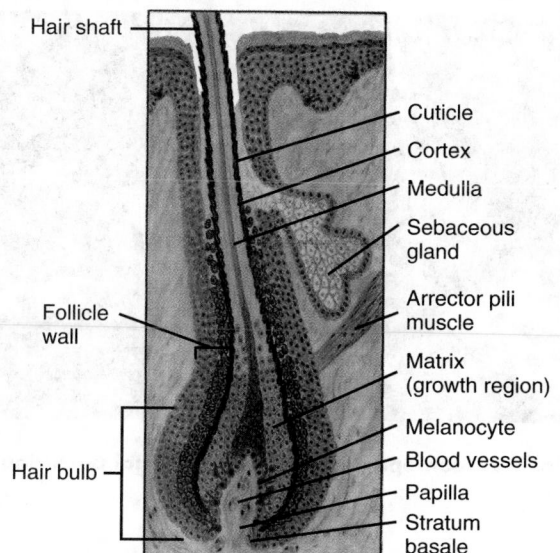

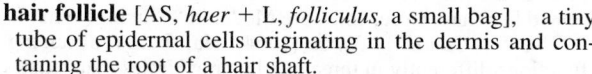

**Structure of hair and hair follicle** *(Applegate, 2000)*

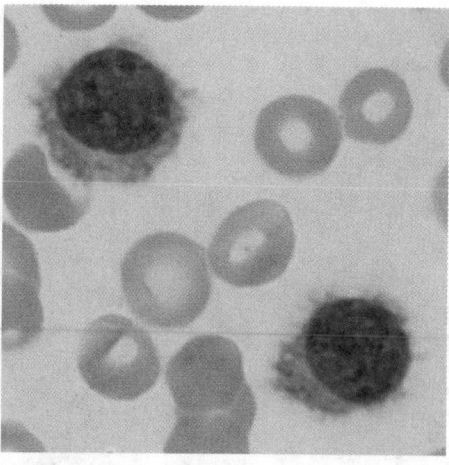

**Hairy-cell leukemia** *(Carr and Rodak, 1999)*

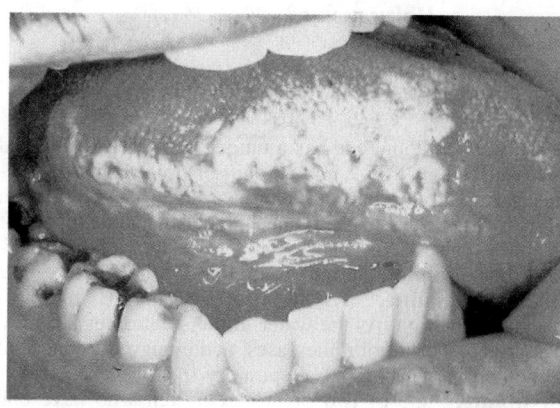

**Hairy leukoplakia caused by Epstein-Barr virus**
*(Murray et al, 1994)*

**hair follicle** [AS, *haer* + L, *folliculus,* a small bag], a tiny tube of epidermal cells originating in the dermis and containing the root of a hair shaft.

**hairline fracture** [AS, *haer* + L, *linea* + *fractura*], a minor fracture that appears on x-ray film as a thin line between two segments of a bone. The segments remain in alignment and the fracture may not extend completely through the bone. A fatigue hairline fracture may develop without apparent injury and in the absence of trauma.

**hair matrix carcinoma.** See **basal cell carcinoma.**

**hair pulling.** See **trichotillomania.**

**hair transplantation,** a form of dermatologic surgery and plastic surgery, performed to correct scalp hair deficiencies caused by hormonal changes, burns, or injuries. The procedure uses existing hair to fill in bald areas. Several sessions are usually required to achieve the level of hair fullness desired by the patient. The sessions consist of grafting the hair-bearing tissue over the bald area directly, or using micrografts of follicles to restore the hairline. It is important that the patient have healthy hair growth on other parts of the head to serve as donor areas and that color, texture, and other aspects of a matching transplant be compatible.

**hairy-cell leukemia** [AS, *haer* + L, *cella,* storeroom; Gk, *leukos,* white, *haima,* blood], an uncommon neoplasm of blood-forming tissues, characterized by pancytopenia, enlargement of the spleen, and many fine projections on the surface of reticulum cells in the blood and bone marrow. The disease occurs six times more frequently in men than in women and usually appears in the fifth decade with an insidious onset and a variable course marked by anemia, thrombocytopenia, and spontaneous bruising. Some cases may achieve long-term remission through alpha-interferon administration or chemotherapy using vincristine and prednisone. Also called **leukemic reticuloendotheliosis.**

**hairy leukoplakia,** a form of leukoplakia characterized by a white plaque that is markedly folded in appearance or smooth and is often visible on one or both lateral borders of the tongue. It is associated with severe immunodeficiency, occurs in human immunodeficiency virus–infected patients, and is believed to result from the Epstein-Barr virus.

**hairy nevus** [AS, *haer* + L, *naevus,* birthmark], a mole, usually pigmented, that has hairs growing from it.

**hairy tongue,** a dark, pigmented overgrowth of the filiform papillae of the tongue that is a benign and frequent side effect of use of some antibiotics. The condition gradually subsides, and no treatment is indicated. See also **glossotrichia.**

**halazone** /hal′əzōn/, a chlorine antiseptic similar to chloramine. It is used for purification of drinking water.

**halcinonide** /həlsin′ənīd/, a topical glucocorticoid.

■ INDICATION: It is prescribed topically for the treatment of inflammation agent.

■ CONTRAINDICATIONS: Viral and fungal diseases of the skin, impaired circulation, or known hypersensitivity to this drug or to steroid medication prohibits its use.

■ ADVERSE EFFECTS: Among the more serious adverse effects are skin reactions and systemic side effects that result from prolonged or excessive application.

**Halcion,** trademark for a hypnotic agent (triazolam).

**Haldol,** trademark for a tranquilizer (haloperidol).

**half-life** (*t-1/2*) [AS, *haelf* + *lif*], **1.** the time required for a radioactive substance to lose 50% of its activity through

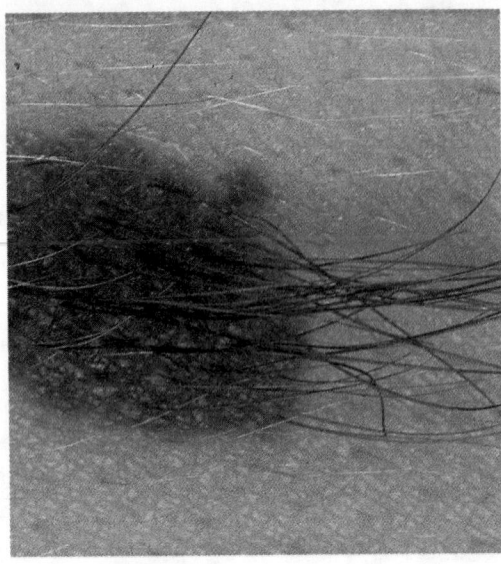

**Hairy nevus** (du Vivier, 1992)

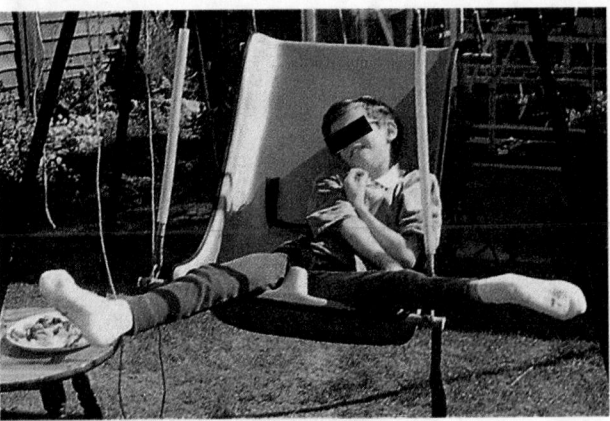

**Hallervorden-Spatz syndrome: abnormal posturing**
(Newton, 1995)

decay. Each radionuclide has a unique half-life. Also called **radioactive half-life. 2.** the amount of time required to reduce a drug level to half of its initial value. Usually the term refers to time necessary to reduce the plasma value to half of its initial value. Drugs commonly have four to five half-lives. See also **biologic half-life, effective half-life.**

**half-normal saline,** a solution of 0.45% NaCl used for mucosal hydration. As the water in the solution evaporates, the saline concentration increases, achieving nearly normal saline concentration in the respiratory tract.

**half-sibling,** one of two or more children who have one parent in common; a half-brother or half-sister. Also called **half-sib.**

**half-value layer (HVL),** the amount of absorbing material required to attenuate a beam of radiation to half its original level. Quantities are indicated by length, as millimeters of aluminum or centimeters of soft tissue.

**halfway house,** a specialized treatment facility, usually for psychiatric patients who no longer require complete hospitalization but who need some care and time to adjust to living independently. Halfway houses are also used for substance abuse recovery.

**halisteresis** /həlis′tərē′sis/ [Gk, *hals,* salt, *steresis,* absence of], a theoretic process of bone resorption in which bone salts are removed by humoral mechanisms and returned to body tissue fluids, leaving behind a decalcified bone matrix. See also **osteolysis.**

**halitosis** /hal′itō′sis/ [L, *halitus,* breath; Gk, *osis,* condition], offensive breath resulting from poor oral hygiene, dental or oral infections, ingestion of certain foods such as garlic or alcohol, use of tobacco, or some systemic diseases such as the odor of acetone in diabetes and ammonia in liver disease.

**Hallervorden-Spatz syndrome** /hol′ərfôr′dən shpots/ [Julius Hallervorden, German neurologist, 1882–1965; H. Spatz, German neurologist, 1888–1969], a progressive neurologic disease of children, with symptoms of parkinsonism. It is characterized by rigidity, athetosis, and dementia. The cause is an accumulation of iron pigments in the globus pallidus and substantia nigra. Treatment is similar to that of Parkinson's disease and Huntington's chorea.

**hallex.** See **hallux.**

**Hall, Lydia E.** (1906–1969), a nursing theorist who presented her Care, Core, and Cure Model in "Nursing: What Is It?" in *The Canadian Nurse* (1964). Hall believed nursing functions differently in three overlapping circles that constitute aspects of patients. She labeled the circles *the body* (the care), *the disease* (the cure), and *the person* (the core). Hall viewed nursing in relation to the core aspect as concerned with the therapeutic use of self in communicating with the patient. Care is the nurturing, comforting component, the "hands-on" care of the patient. Cure is the aspect of nursing involved with treatments and administration of medications. Hall's concept includes adult patients who have passed the acute stage of illness and have rehabilitation and feelings of self-actualization as their goal.

**Hallpike test** See **Dix-Hallpike test.**

**halluces.** See **hallux.**

**hallucination** /həloo′sinā′shən/ [L, *alucinari,* to wander in mind], a sensory perception that does not result from an external stimulus and that occurs in the waking state. It can occur in any of the senses and is classified accordingly as auditory, gustatory, olfactory, tactile, or visual. It is a symptom of psychotic behavior, often noted during schizophrenia, as well as in other mental or organic disorders and conditions. —**hallucinate** /həloo′sənāt/*v.*

**hallucination management,** a nursing intervention from the Nursing Interventions Classification (NIC) defined as promoting the safety, comfort, and reality orientation of a patient experiencing hallucinations. See also **Nursing Interventions Classification.**

**hallucinatory neuralgia** /həloo′sənətôr′ē/, a feeling of localized pain that persists after an episode of severe throbbing pain has subsided.

**hallucinogen** /həloo′sənəjen′, hal′əsin′əjən, hal′yəsin′-əjən/ [L, *alucinari* + Gk, *genein,* to produce], a substance that causes excitation of the central nervous system, characterized by hallucination, mood change, anxiety, sensory distortion, delusion, depersonalization; increased pulse, temperature, and blood pressure; and dilation of the pupils. Psychic dependence may occur, and depressive or suicidal psychotic states may result from the ingestion of hallucinogenic substances. Some kinds of hallucinogens are **lyser-**

gine, **mescaline**, **peyote**, **phencyclidine hydrochloride**, and **psilocybin.**

**hallucinogenesis** /-jen′əsīs/ [L, *alucinari,* to wander in mind; Gk, *genein,* to produce], a cause or source of hallucinations.

**hallucinosis** /halo͞o′sinō′sis/ [L, *alucinari* + Gk, *osis,* condition], a pathologic mental state in which awareness consists primarily or exclusively of hallucinations. A kind of hallucinosis is **alcoholic hallucinosis.**

**hallux** /hal′əks/, *pl.* **halluces** /hal′yo͞osēz/ [L, *hallex,* large toe], the great toe. Also spelled **hallex.**

**hallux rigidus,** a painful deformity of the great toe, limiting motion at the metatarsophalangeal joint.

**hallux valgus,** a deformity in which the great toe is angled away from the midline of the body toward the other toes; in some cases the great toe rides over or under the other toes.

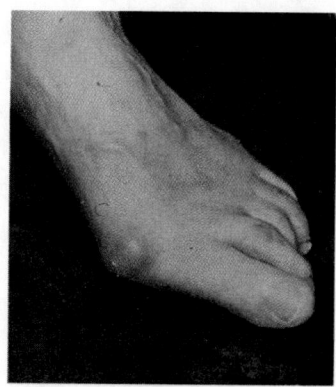

**Hallux valgus**
*(Seidel et al, 1999/courtesy Charles W. Bradley, DPM, MPA, and Caroline Harvey, DPM, California College of Podiatric Medicine)*

**hallux varus,** a deformity in which the great toe is angled away from the other toes.

**halo-** /hal′ō-/, combining form meaning 'salt': *halogen.*

**halo cast.** See **halo vest.**

**haloderma** /hal′ōdur′mə/, skin changes caused by ingestion or injection of halogen, usually a bromide or an iodide.

**halo effect,** the beneficial effect of an interview or other encounter, as may occur in the course of a research project or a health care visit. The halo effect cannot be attributed to the content of the interview or to any specific act or treatment; it is the result of indefinable interpersonal factors present in the interaction.

**halofantrine,** an antimalarial.

■ INDICATIONS: Halofantrine is used to treat mild to moderate malaria.

■ CONTRAINDICATIONS: Known hypersensitivity to halofantrine prohibits its use.

■ ADVERSE EFFECTS: Common side effects of this drug include nausea, vomiting, anorexia, diarrhea, and dysrhythmias.

**Halog,** trademark for a topical glucocorticoid (halcinonide).

**halogen** /hal′ōjən/ [Gk, *hals,* salt, *genein,* to produce], any member of the group 17 elements in the periodic table: fluorine, chlorine, bromine, iodine, and astatine. They are found in sea water as the corresponding halide ion.

**halogenated hydrocarbon** /həloj′ənā′tid/ [Gk, *hals,* salt,

*genein,* to produce, *hydor,* water; L, *carbo,* coal], a volatile liquid used as an inhalation anesthetic, administered in combination with oxygen and/or nitrous oxide. Kinds of halogenated hydrocarbons are **desflurane, enflurane, halothane, isoflurane,** and **sevoflurane.**

**halo nevus,** a benign melanocyte that appears as a central brown mole surrounded by a circle of depigmented skin. Over a period of months the central nevus becomes flat and loses its pigment, leaving a round white macule. Eventually the halo repigments.

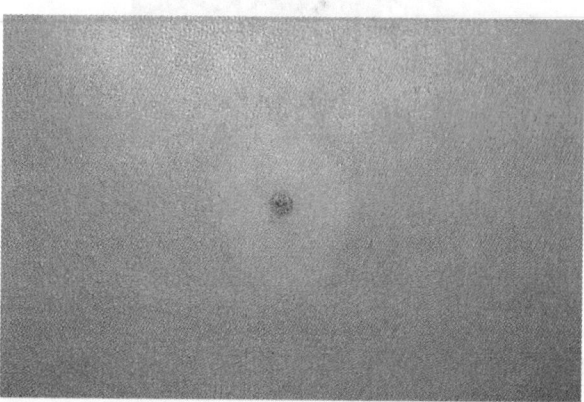

**Halo nevus** *(Lawrence and Cox, 1993)*

**haloperidol** /hal′ōper′ədôl/, a butyrophenone tranquilizer.

■ INDICATIONS: It is prescribed in the treatment of psychotic disorders and in the control of Gilles de la Tourette's syndrome.

■ CONTRAINDICATIONS: Parkinson's disease, concurrent administration of central nervous system depressants, liver or renal dysfunction, severe hypotension, or known hypersensitivity to this drug prohibits its use.

■ ADVERSE EFFECTS: Among the more serious adverse effects are hypotension and a variety of extrapyramidal and hypersensitivity reactions.

**halo sign** [Gk, *halos,* circular floor; L, *signum,* mark], a halo effect produced in the radiograph of the fetal head between the subcutaneous fat and the cranium; said to be indicative of intrauterine death of the fetus.

**Halotestin,** trademark for an androgen (fluoxymesterone).

**halothane** /hal′əthān/, an inhalation anesthetic.

■ INDICATION: It is prescribed for induction and maintenance of general anesthesia.

■ CONTRAINDICATION: It is not recommended for obstetric anesthesia unless uterine relaxation is required.

■ ADVERSE EFFECTS: Among the more serious but rare adverse reactions associated with halothane are hepatic necrosis, cardiac arrest or arrhythmia, hypotension, malignant hyperthermia nausea, and emesis.

**halothane-related hepatitis,** an adverse reaction of some patients to inhalation of halothane, a general anesthetic. The reaction is characterized by hepatitis and a severe fever that develops several days after exposure to the anesthetic. The risk is higher for obese patients, possibly because body fat tends to store the chemical.

**halo vest** [Gk, *halos,* circular floor; AS, *kasta*], an orthopedic device used to help immobilize the neck and head. It incorporates the trunk, usually with shoulder straps, and an outrigger within the cast to secure pins to a band around the skull. The halo vest is used to aid the healing of injuries and cervical dislocations and to position and immobilize a patient after cervical surgery.

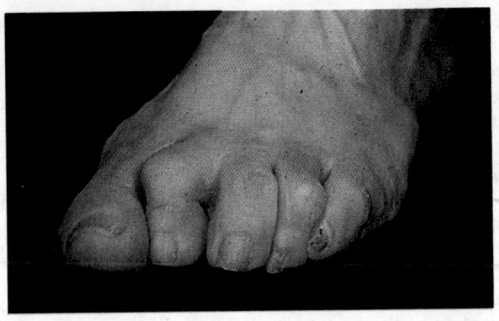

**Hammer toe**
*(Seidel et al, 1999/courtesy Charles W. Bradley, DPM, MPA and Caroline Harvey, DPM, California College of Podiatric Medicine)*

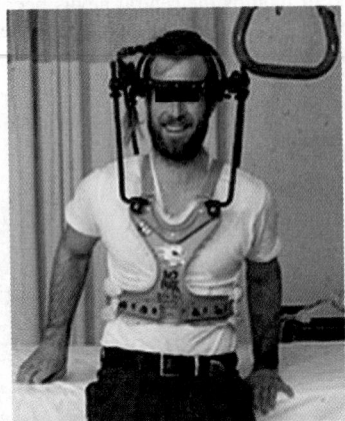

**Halo cast and vest**
*(Phipps, Sands, and Marek, 1999/courtesy Acromed Corp., Cleveland)*

**Halsted's forceps** /hal′stedz/ [William S. Halsted, American surgeon, 1852–1922], **1.** a small pointed hemostatic forceps. **2.** a forceps with slender jaws for grasping arteries and other blood vessels. See also **mosquito forceps.**

**Halsted's suture** [William S. Halsted], the union of two adjoining skin surfaces by a suture placed through the subcuticular fascia.

**HALT,** abbreviation for **Hypertension and Lipid Trial.**

**hamamelis water.** See **witch hazel,** def 2.

**hamartoma,** a new tissue growth resembling a tumor. It results from a defective overgrowth in tissue formation.

**hamartoma syndrome.** See **Cowden's disease.**

**hamate bone** /ham′āt/ [L, *hamatus,* hooked], a carpal (wrist) bone that rests on the fourth and fifth metacarpal bones and projects a hooklike process, the hamulus, from its palmar surface. Its dorsal surface is rough for ligamentous attachment. The hamate bone articulates with the lunate proximally, the fourth and fifth metacarpal distally, the triangular medially, and the capitate laterally. Also called **os hamatum, unciform bone.**

**Hamman-Rich syndrome.** See **interstitial pneumonia.**

**Hamman's disease.** See **pneumomediastinum.**

**hammer finger** [AS, *hamer* + *finger*], a permanently flexed terminal phalanx caused by an injury to the extensor tendon. Also called **mallet finger.**

**hammer toe** [AS, *hamer* + *ta*], a foot digit permanently flexed at the midphalangeal joint, producing a clawlike appearance. The anomaly may be present in more than one digit but is most common in the second toe. It may accompany clawfoot.

**Hampton's hump** [Aubrey O. Hampton, American radiologist, 1900–1955], a soft-tissue image in a radiograph of the lung that is a manifestation of a pulmonary infarction.

**hamstring muscle** [AS, *hamm* + *streng*], any one of three muscles at the back of the thigh: medially the semimembranosus and the semitendinosus and laterally the biceps femoris.

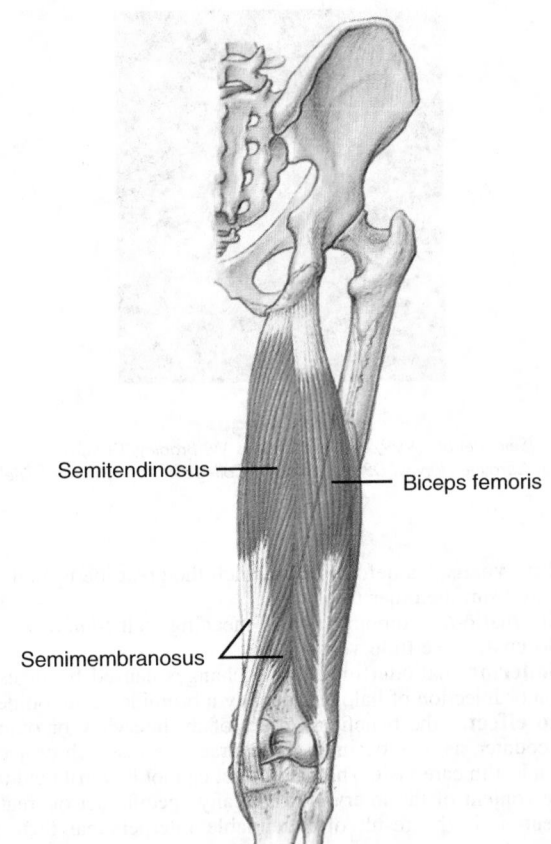

Semitendinosus —     — Biceps femoris

Semimembranosus —

**Hamstring group of muscles: semitendinosus, semimembranosus, and biceps femoris**
*(Seeley and Stephens, 1995/John V. Hagen; used by permission of The McGraw-Hill Companies)*

**hamstring reflex,** a normal deep tendon reflex elicited by tapping one of the hamstring tendons behind the knee, causing contraction of the tendon and flexion of the knee. The patient should be lying in the supine position with the knee and hip partially flexed and the leg supported by the examiner's hand. An accentuated hamstring reflex may result from a lesion of the pyramidal system above the level of the fourth lumbar nerve root. See also **deep tendon reflex.**

**hamstring tendon,**    one of the three tendons from the three hamstring muscles in the back of the thigh. The one lateral and the two medial hamstring tendons connect the hamstring muscles to the knee.

**hamular notch.**    See **pterygomaxillary notch.**

**hamulus** /ham′yoo·ləs/ *pl.* **hamuli** [L, little hook],   a general term denoting a hook-shaped process.

**hand** [AS, *hand*],   the part of the upper limb distal to the forearm. It is the most flexible part of the skeleton and has a total of 27 bones, 8 forming the carpus, 5 forming the metacarpus, and 14 forming the phalangeal section. Also called **manus.**

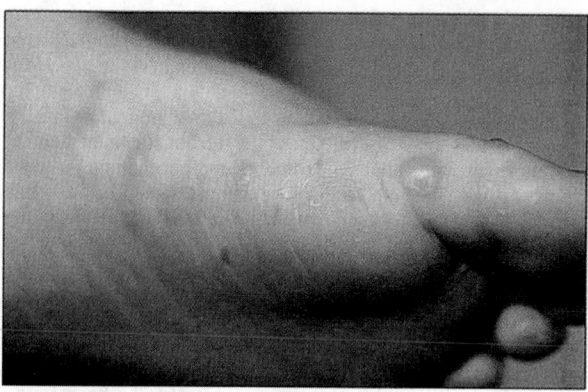

**Hand-foot-and-mouth disease** *(Lawrence and Cox, 1993)*

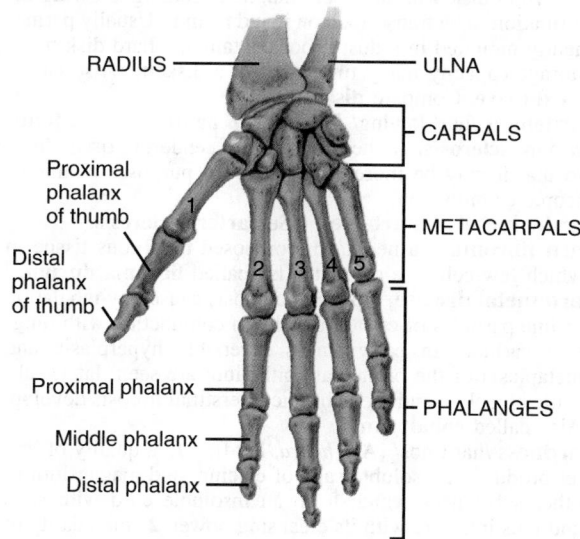

Hand (right, palmar aspect)

**Bones of the hand** *(Applegate, 2000)*

**handblock** [AS, *hand* + Fr, *bloc*],   a device made of a wood block several inches high with a firm handle that can assist a disabled patient in sitting push-ups, which can enhance transfers or mobility in bed. Sometimes called **push-up block.**

**hand condenser,**    (in dentistry) an instrument for compacting amalgams or gold foil using force applied by the operator, with or without supplementary force from a mallet wielded by an assistant.

**handedness** /han′didnes/ [AS, *hand* + *ness,* condition],   voluntary or involuntary preference for use of either the left or right hand. The preference is related to cerebral dominance: left-handedness corresponds to dominance of the right side of the brain, and vice versa. Also called **chirality, laterality.**

**hand-foot-and-mouth disease,**   a viral infection usually caused by coxsackie A virus but also by enterovirus 71. It is characterized by the appearance of painful ulcers and vesicles on the mucous membranes of the mouth and on the hands and feet. The disease is moderately contagious and mainly affects children, including infants. It is spread with oral secretions or stool. There is no specific treatment. Lesions usually resolve in 1 week.

**handicapped** /han′dikapt/ [*hand in cap,* a seventeenth-century game with forfeits],   referring to a person who has a congenital or acquired mental or physical defect that interferes with normal functioning of the body system or the ability to be self-sufficient in modern society. Compare **disability.**

**handpiece** /hand′pēs/,   a device for holding rotary instruments in a dental engine or condensing points in mechanical condensing units. It is connected by an arm, cable, belt, or tube to a power source, such as a motor, or to an air-pressure or water-pressure hose.

**hanging drop preparation** [ME, *hangen,* to hang; AS, *dropa,* to fall; L, *praeparer,* to make ready],   a technique used for the examination and identification of certain microorganisms, such as spirochetes or trichomonads. The technique requires a coverslip, a microscope, and a special slide that has a central concavity. A specimen suspected of containing the microorganism is diluted with a sterile isotonic solution. A drop of this fluid mixture is placed on a glass coverslip, which is then inverted carefully and placed over the slide so that the drop is hanging from the slip into the concavity in the slide. The delicate structures and the method of movement characteristic of the species may then be viewed through the microscope.

**hangman's fracture,**   a break in the posterior elements of the cervical vertebrae with dislocation of C2.

**hangnail** [AS, *angnaegl,* troublesome nail],   a piece of partially disconnected epidermis of the cuticle or nail fold. Tearing the skin fragment causes a red, painful, easily infected sore. Early treatment is to trim the hangnail close with nail clippers. For inflamed cases an antibiotic ointment and protective bandage are used.

**hangover,**   a popular term for a group of symptoms, including nausea, thirst, fatigue, headache, and irritability, resulting from the use of alcohol and certain drugs.

**Hanhart's syndrome** /hän′härts/ [Ernst Hanhart, Swiss physician, 1891−1973],   any of several syndromes of variable inheritance, characterized chiefly by severe micrognathia, high nose root, small eyelid fissures, low-set ears, and variable absence of digits or limbs, usually below the elbow or knee.

**Hanot's disease** /hanōz′/ [Victor C. Hanot, French physician, 1844–1896],   primary biliary cirrhosis. See also **biliary cirrhosis.**

**Hansen's bacillus** [Gerard H.A. Hansen, Norwegian physician, 1841–1912; L, *bacillum,* a small rod],   the acid-fast *Mycobacterium leprae,* which is the cause of leprosy.

**Hansen's disease.** See **leprosy.**

**Hantaan virus,** a virus of the genus *Hantavirus* that causes severe epidemic hemorrhagic fever in Asia; see *Hantavirus.*

**Hantavirus,** a genus of viruses in the *Bunyaviridae* family. *Hantavirus* is the cause of several different forms of hemorrhagic fever with renal syndrome. Some people appear to be more susceptible than others who are presumed to have had similar exposure to the virus. About half of all reported cases have been fatal. A *Hantavirus* infection begins with flulike symptoms and may be mistaken for other diseases. Some patients were diagnosed originally as having hepatitis or inflammation of the pancreas, or both. The disease can be spread by several common rodent species via rodent excreta. Most U.S. cases have been reported in the western United States, but confirmed hantavirus cases have also been found in the New York City suburbs. *Hantavirus* includes the Hantaan, Seoul, Puumala, Prospect Hill, Sin Nombre, and Porogia strains. See also **hemorrhagic fever.**

**hantavirus pulmonary syndrome,** a sometimes fatal febrile illness caused by a virus of the genus *Hantavirus,* characterized by variable respiratory symptoms followed by acute respiratory distress, sometimes progressing to respiratory failure.

**hapadnavirus** /hapad'nəvī'rəs/, a virus similar to that of hepatitis B of the Hepadnaviridae family of microorganisms. It proliferates in the nuclei of liver cells and causes a persistent hepatitis B infection.

**-haphia.** See **-aphia.**

**haplo-,** prefix meaning 'single,' 'simple': *haploderma.*

**haploid** /hap'loid/ [Gk, *haploos,* single, *eidos,* form], having only one complete set of nonhomologous chromosomes. Also called **monoploid, monoploidic. —haploidy,** *n.*

**haploid nucleus** [Gk, *haploos,* single, *eidos,* form; L, *nucleus,* nut], a nucleus possessing only half the normal somatic number of chromosomes. It may occur in a germ cell after meiosis and before fertilization. Also called **hemikaryon.**

**haploidy.** See **haploid.**

**Hapsburg lip,** an overdeveloped, thick lower lip, which often accompanies the Hapsburg jaw (a jaw that projects forward). This kind of lip was characteristic of many members of the royal German-Austrian family that produced several European rulers between 1278 and 1918.

**hapten** /hap'tən/ [Gk, *haptein,* to grasp], a nonproteinaceous substance that acts as an antigen by combining with particular bonding sites on an antibody. Unlike a true antigen, it does not induce the formation of antibodies. A hapten bonded to a carrier protein may cause an immune response. Also called **haptene** /hap'tēn/.

**haptics** /hap'tiks/ [Gk, *haptein,* to grasp], the science concerned with studying the sense of touch. **—haptic,** *adj.*

**haptoglobin** /hap'tōglō'bin/ [Gk, *haptein,* to grasp; L, *globus,* ball], a plasma protein whose only known function is to bind free hemoglobin. The quantity of haptoglobin is increased in certain chronic diseases and inflammatory disorders and is decreased or absent in hemolytic anemia. Normal adult findings range from 100 to 150 mg/dL. Compare **transferrin.** See also **hemoglobinemia, hemoglobinuria.**

**haptoglobin test,** a blood test used to detect hemolysis, the intravascular destruction of red blood cells. Abnormal levels of haptoglobin may indicate hemolytic anemias, primary liver disease, many inflammatory diseases, acute myocardial infarction, and some cancers.

**harborage transmission** /här'bərij/, a mode of infection transmission in which the organism does not undergo morphologic and physiologic changes in the vector.

**hard chancre** [AS, *heard* + Fr, *canker*], a syphilitic chancre or primary lesion that develops at the site of a syphilis infection. The lesion begins as a small red papule that gradually hardens and erodes into an extremely contagious ulcer. A secretion exuded by the sore contains *Treponema pallidum,* the organism that is the causative agent of syphilis in humans.

**hard contact lens** [AS, *heard* + L, *contingere,* to touch, *lentil*], a polymethylmethacrylate, or rigid gas-permeable, contact lens that retains its form without support, in contrast with a soft contact lens, which readily yields to pressure.

**hard data,** information about a patient that is obtained by observation and measurement, including laboratory data, as opposed to information collected by interview of the patient or others.

**hard disk,** a computer data storage medium that consists of a rigid disk with an electromagnetic coating allowing information to be transcribed on it and from it. Usually permanently mounted in a dust-proof container, a hard disk has a storage capacity many times that of a diskette. Also called **hard drive.** Compare **diskette.**

**hardening** /här'dən·ing/ [AS, *heard,* hard], **1.** see **induration, sclerosis. 2.** the procedure of rendering tissue firm, so that it may be more readily cut for purposes of microscopic examination.

**hardening of the arteries.** See **arteriosclerosis.**

**hard fibroma,** a neoplasm composed of fibrous tissue in which few cells are present. Also called **fibroma durum.**

**hard metal disease,** pneumoconiosis caused by inhalation of fine particles of cobalt, usually in conjunction with tungsten carbide. In early stages reversible hyperplasia and metaplasia of the bronchial epithelium are seen; later, subacute alveolitis and then chronic interstitial fibrosis develop. Also called **cobalt lung.**

**hardness** /härd'nəs/ [AS, *heard,* hard], **1.** a quality of water produced by soluble salts of calcium and magnesium or other substances which form an insoluble curd with soap and thus interfere with its cleansing power. **2.** the quality of firmness produced by cohesion of the particles composing a substance, as evidenced by its inflexibility or resistance to indentation, distortion, or scratching. **3.** see **hardness of x-rays.**

**hardness of x-rays,** the relative penetrating power of x-rays. In general, the hardness increases as the wavelength of the x-rays decreases. Also called **hard radiation.** Compare **soft radiation.**

**hard nevus.** See **epidermal nevus.**

**hard palate** [AS, *heard,* hard; L, *palatum*], the bony portion of the roof of the mouth, continuous posteriorly with the soft palate and bounded anteriorly and laterally by the alveolar arches and the gums. The hard palate is covered with stratified squamous epithelium and furnished with numerous palatal glands lying between the mucous membrane and the surface of the bone. Compare **soft palate.**

**hard radiation.** See **hardness of x-rays.**

**hard soap,** a detergent soap made with olive oil and sodium hydroxide.

**HARD syndrome.** See **Walker-Warburg syndrome.**

**hardware,** the tangible parts of a computer, such as chips, boards, wires, transformers, and peripheral devices. See also **software.**

**hardware bug.** See **bug.**

**hard water** [AS, *heard* + *waeter*], water that contains certain cations, particularly calcium and magnesium, that precipitate with soap solutions. The term is generally applied to tap water, and the degree of hardness varies with the source and previous treatment.

**Hardy-Weinberg equilibrium principle** /här′dē wīn′-bərg/ [G. H. Hardy, English mathematician, 1877–1947; Wilhelm Weinberg, German physician, 1862–1937; L, *aequilibris,* equal weight, *principium,* a beginning], a principle stating that the frequency of alleles and genotypes remains relatively unchanged from generation to generation in a large, interbreeding population characterized by random mating, mendelian inheritance, and the absence of migration, mutation, and selection. Under such conditions, the ratio of individuals homozygous for a dominant allele to those heterozygous to those homozygous for a recessive allele is 1:2:1. See also **genetic equilibrium.**

**harelip.** See **cleft lip.**

**hare's eye.** See **lagophthalmos.**

**harlequin color** /här′lək(w)in/ [It, *arlecchino,* goblin; L, *color,* hue], a temporary flushing of the skin on the lower side of the body with pallor on the other side. Commonly seen in normal young infants, it disappears as the child matures.

**harlequin fetus,** an infant whose skin at birth is completely covered with thick, horny scales that resemble armor and are divided by deep red fissures. The condition is the most severe form of lamellar exfoliation of the newborn, and the infant is stillborn or dies within a few days of birth.

**harlequin ichthyosis,** the ichthyosis affecting a harlequin fetus. See also **ichthyosis.**

**Harrington rod** /här′ing·tən/ [Paul R. Harrington, American orthopedic surgeon, b. 1911], one of the rigid, contoured metal rods inserted surgically, along with metal hooks, in the posterior elements of the spine to provide distraction and compression in treatment of scoliosis and other deformities.

**Harrison's groove** [Edward Harrison, English physician, 1776–1838], a deformity of the thorax that develops as a result of the pull of the diaphragm on ribs weakened by rickets or some other calcium deficiency disorder.

**Harris tube** [Franklin Harris, American surgeon, b. 1895], a tube used for gastric and intestinal decompression. It is a mercury-weighted single-lumen tube that is passed through the nose and carried through the digestive tract by gravity. The amount of mercury in the soft bag surrounding the tube varies from 2 to 5 mL according to the age, size, and condition of the patient. The location of the tube and its final placement are checked by fluoroscopy.

sorption of neutral amino acids. Bacterial degradation of unabsorbed amino acids in the gut leads to the absorption of breakdown products and their appearance in urine; the unavailability of tryptophan leads to a deficiency of niacin, the antipellagra vitamin. Common symptoms of the disease are dry, scaly, well-circumscribed skin lesions; glossitis; stomatitis; diarrhea; psychiatric problems; and pronounced photosensitivity. Brief exposure to the sun may cause erythema, edema, and vesiculation. Treatment consists of oral nicotinamide and a diet containing proteins composed of more easily absorbed small peptides.

**Harvard pump,** trademark for a small pump that can be adjusted to deliver small amounts of medication in solution through an IV infusion set. It is commonly used to administer oxytocin in the induction or augmentation of labor. Compare **Abbott pump.**

**harvest fever.** See **leptospirosis.**

**harvest mite.** See **chigger.**

**Hashimoto's disease** /hä′shimō′tōz/ [Hakaru Hashimoto, Japanese surgeon, 1881–1934], an autoimmune thyroid disorder. It is characterized by the production of antibodies in response to thyroid antigens and the replacement of normal thyroid structures with lymphocytes and lymphoid germinal centers. The disease shows a marked hereditary pattern, but it is 20 times more common in women than in men. It occurs most frequently at 30 to 50 years of age but may arise in young children. The thyroid, typically enlarged, pale yellow, and lumpy on the surface, shows dense lymphocytic infiltration, and follicular hyperplasia. The goiter is usually asymptomatic, but occasionally patients have difficulty in swallowing and a feeling of local pressure. The thymus is usually enlarged, and regional lymph nodes often show hyperplasia. A definitive diagnosis can be made if a fluorescent scan shows a decrease or absence of thyroid-stable iodine and if the result of a hemagglutination test for thyroid antigens is positive. Replacement therapy with thyroid hormone is indicated for patients with thyroid deficiency and can prevent further enlargement of the goiter. Also called **Hashimoto's struma, Hashimoto's thyroiditis, lymphocytic thyroiditis, struma lymphomatosa.**

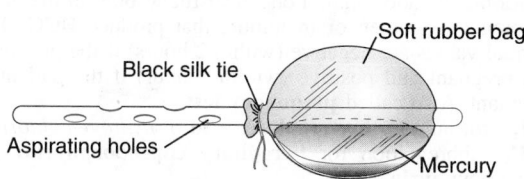

**Harris tube** *(Lewis, Heitkemper, and Dirksen, 2000)*

**Hartmann's curet** [Arthur Hartmann, German physician, 1849–1931], a curet used for the removal of adenoids. See also **curet.**

**Hartmann's solution.** See **Ringer's lactate solution.**

**Hartnup's disease** [Hartnup, family name of first patients diagnosed in England, 1956], a rare recessive genetic metabolic disorder characterized by pellagra-like skin lesions, transient cerebellar ataxia, and hyperaminoaciduria. It is caused by defects in intestinal absorption and renal reab-

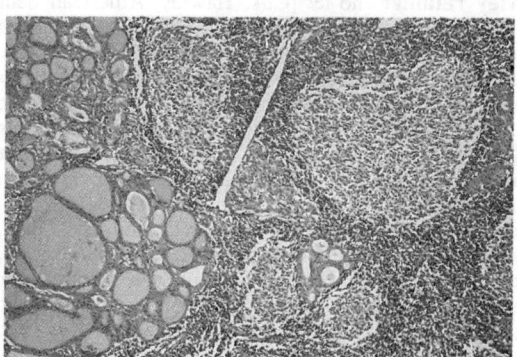

**Hashimoto's disease** *(Kumar, Cotran, and Robbins, 1997)*

**hashish.** See **cannabis.**

**Hasner's fold.** See **lacrimal fold.**

**hatchet** /hach′ət/, a bibeveled or single beveled cutting dental instrument having its cutting edge in line with the axis of its blade; used for breaking down tooth structure undermined by caries, smoothing cavity walls, and sharpening line and point angles. Also called **hatchet excavator.**

**haustrum** /hôs′trəm/ pl. **haustra** [L, *haustor,* drawer], a general term denoting a recess or sacculation.

**haustus (h)** /hôs′təs/, a draught of medicine.

**HAV,** abbreviation for *hepatitis A virus.* See **hepatitis A.**

**Haverhill fever** /hā′vəril/ [Haverhill, Massachusetts, disorder first diagnosed, 1925], a febrile disease, caused by infection with *Streptobacillus moniliformis,* transmitted by the bite of a rat. The spirochete-like bacterium is normally present in rat saliva. Characteristically the wound from the bite heals, but within 10 days fever, chills, vomiting, headache, muscle and joint pain, and a rash appear. Treatment with antibiotics is effective. *S. moniliformis* is identified by laboratory analysis using fluorescent antibody screening. Also called **streptobacillary rat-bite fever.**

**Havers' glands.** See **haversian glands.**

**haversian canal** /havur′shən/ [Clopton Havers, English physician, 1650–1702], one of the many tiny longitudinal canals in bone tissue, averaging about 0.05 mm in diameter. Each contains blood vessels, connective tissue, nerve filaments, and occasionally lymphatic vessels. The canals are interconnected and part of an intricate network. See also **haversian canaliculus, haversian system, Volkmann's canal.**

**haversian canaliculus** /kan′əlik′yələs/ [Clopton Havers], any of the many tiny passages radiating from the lacunae of bone tissue to larger haversian canals. See also **haversian canal, haversian system.**

**haversian glands** [Clopton Havers; L, *glans,* acorn], extrasynovial fat pads that may project into the joint space. Also called **Havers' glands.**

**haversian lamella** [Clopton Havers; L, *lamella,* a small plate], one of a series of lamellae (circular layers) arranged around the central haversian canal of an osteon, or cylindrical unit of bone structure. Also called **Havers' lamella.**

**haversian system** [Clopton Havers], a circular district of bone tissue, consisting of concentric rings of osteocytes and lamellae in the bone around a central blood vessel canal. See also **haversian canal, haversian canaliculus, Volkmann's canal.**

**Haver's lamella.** See **haversian lamella.**

**Hawley retainer** /hô′lē/ [C.A. Hawley, American dentist, early 20th century], an orthodontic appliance consisting of a removable palatal wire and an acrylic biteplate resting against the palate, used to stabilize teeth after their movement or as a basis for tooth movement by providing anchorage for other attachments. Also called **Hawley appliance.**

**hawthorn,** an herbal product taken from a bush or tree found throughout the United States, Canada, Europe, and Asia.

■ USES: This herb is used for poor circulation, chest pain, irregular heartbeat, high blood fats, and high blood pressure.

■ CONTRAINDICATIONS: Hawthorn should not be used during pregnancy and lactation or in children. It is also contraindicated in those with known hypersensitivity to this herb or other members of the Rosaceae family.

**Hawthorne effect** /hô′thôrn/, a general unintentional, but usually beneficial effect on a person, a group of people, or the function of the system being studied. It is the effect of an encounter, as with an investigator or health care provider, or of a change in a program or facility, as by painting of an office or change in the lighting system. The Hawthorne effect is likely to confound the results of a study or investigation, because it is usually present and difficult to identify. It was named for a study in industrial management at the Hawthorne (Illinois) facility of the Western Electric Company.

**hay fever** [AS, *heawan,* to hew; L, *febris,* fever], *informal.* an acute, seasonal, allergic rhinitis stimulated by tree, grass, or weed pollen. Also called **pollen coryza, pollinosis.** See also **allergic rhinitis, organic dust.**

**Hayflick limits** [Leonard Hayflick, American microbiologist, b. 1928; L, *limes,* border], the concept that the life span of living organisms is limited by the number of times that somatic cells will subdivide. On the basis of human cells in cultures, where divisions occur about 50 times, it is estimated the average human life span is limited to around 115 years.

**Hay-Wells syndrome** /hā·welz/ [R.J. Hay, British dermatologist, 20th century; Robert Stuart Wells, British dermatologist, 20th century], an autosomal dominant syndrome of ectodermal dysplasia, cleft lip and palate, and ankyloblepharon; it is also characterized by hypodontia, palmar and plantar keratoderma, partial anhidrosis, sparse wiry hair, and sometimes otologic defects. Also called **AEC syndrome, ankyloblepharon–ectodermal dysplasia–clefting syndrome.**

**hazard** /haz′ərd/ [Fr, *hasard,* chance], a condition or phenomenon that increases the probability of a loss that may result in injury or illness. —**hazardous,** *adj.*

**Hb,** abbreviation for **hemoglobin.**

**HB,** abbreviation for **hepatitis B.**

**Hb A,** abbreviation for **hemoglobin A.**

**Hb A$_2$,** abbreviation for **hemoglobin A$_2$.**

**HBAg,** abbreviation for *hepatitis B antigen.* See also **hepatitis B.**

**Hb C,** abbreviation for **hemoglobin C.**

**HBE,** abbreviation for **His bundle electrogram.**

**Hb F,** abbreviation for **hemoglobin F.**

**HBIG,** abbreviation for **hepatitis B immune globulin.**

**Hb S,** abbreviation for **hemoglobin S.**

**HBsAG,** abbreviation for **hepatitis B surface antigen.** See also **Australia antigen.**

**Hb S-C,** abbreviation for **hemoglobin S-C.**

**HBV,** abbreviation for *hepatitis B virus.* See also **hepatitis B.**

**HCFA.** abbreviation for **Health Care Financing Administration.**

**HCG,** abbreviation for **human chorionic gonadotropin.** See also **chorionic gonadotropin.**

**HCG radioreceptor assay,** a urine test to detect pregnancy or missed abortion, performed by measuring human chorionic gonadotropin, a chemical found only in the urine of pregnant women or in tumors that produce HCG. The normal values are negative (within 2 hours) if the patient is not pregnant and positive (within 1 hour) if the patient is pregnant. Also called **pregnancy test.**

**HCl,** formula for **hydrochloric acid** or *hydrogen chloride.*

**HCP,** abbreviation for **hereditary coproporphyria;** see **coproporphyria.**

**HCV,** abbreviation for *hepatitis C virus.* See also **hepatitis C.**

**HDCV,** abbreviation for **human diploid cell rabies vaccine.**

**H deflection,** a deviation observed on the His bundle electrogram that represents activation of the bundle of His.

**HDI,** abbreviation for **high-definition imaging.**

**HDL,** abbreviation for **high-density lipoprotein.**

**HDV,** abbreviation for *hepatitis D virus.* See also **hepatitis D.**

**He,** symbol for the element **helium.**

**head** [AS, *heafod*], **1.** the uppermost extremity, containing the brain, special sense organs, mouth, nose, and related structures. Most of the tissues are enclosed within the skull, composed of 22 bones. At birth the head is about half the size of an adult head; the greatest changes after infancy involve growth of the facial area. **2.** a rounded, usually proximal portion of some long bones.

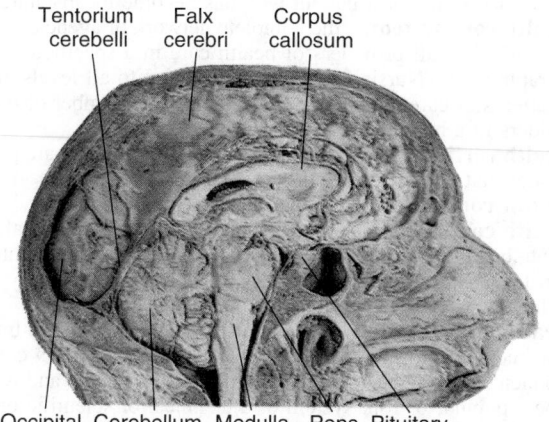

**Cross section of the head** *(Crossman and Neary, 1995)*

**headache** /hed'āk/ [AS, *heafod + acan*, to hurt], a pain in the head from any cause. Kinds of headaches include **cluster headache, functional headache, histamine headache, migraine headache, organic headache, sinus headache,** and **tension headache.** Also called **cephalalgia, cephalgia.**

**head and neck cancer,** any malignant neoplasms of the upper aerodigestive tract, facial features, and structures in the neck, which appear as masses, ulcerations, or flat lesions that usually produce early symptoms. See also specific cancer.

**head banging,** a form of physical exertion observed during some temper tantrums. It usually occurs near the peak of excitement and may be associated with other physical or muscular movements.

**head bobbing,** a sign of respiratory distress in an infant. It occurs when the infant uses the scaleni and sternocleidomastoid muscles to assist ventilation. The contraction of these muscles causes the head to bob because the neck extensor muscles are not strong enough to stabilize the head.

**head box,** a clear plastic chamber that fits over a patient's head with an adjustable seal around the neck for mechanical ventilation. Humidified gas enters the chamber and excess gas is released through an outlet valve. The device may help prevent the need for intubation.

**headcap.** See **headgear.**

**head, eye, ear, nose, and throat (HEENT),** a specialty in medicine concerned with the anatomic, physiologic, and pathologic characteristics of the head, eyes, ears, nose, and throat and with the diagnosis and treatment of disorders of those structures.

**headgear** /hed'gēr/, a harnesslike device fitting over the top and back of the head, serving as a source of resistance for extraoral anchorage for an orthodontic appliance. Also called **headcap.**

**head injury,** any traumatic damage to the head resulting from blunt or penetrating trauma of the skull. Blood vessels, nerves, and meninges can be torn; bleeding, edema, and ischemia may result. See also **concussion.**

**head kidney.** See **pronephros.**

**head louse.** See **lice,** *Pediculus humanus capitis.*

**head nurse.** See **nurse manager.**

**head process,** a strand of cells that extends forward from the primitive node in the early stages of embryonic development in vertebrates. It is the precursor of the notochord and forms the primitive axis around which the embryo develops. Also called **notochordal plate.**

**heads-up tilt table test (HUTT),** a method of evaluating children with neurocardiac syncope. After baseline signs are recorded with the patient in the supine position, the patient is tilted to an 80-degree angle for 30 minutes, or until neurocardiac syncope signs appear.

**head-tilt, chin-lift airway technique,** a method of providing maximum airway opening in an unconscious person. With the victim lying on his or her back, the rescuer pushes down on the victim's forehead with the palm of the hand, tilting the victim's head back. With the other hand, the rescuer lifts the victim's lower jaw near the chin. The technique opens the airway by moving the tongue away from the back of the throat and the epiglottis away from the opening of the trachea. This technique is not recommended if a cervical spine injury is suspected and therefore should not be encouraged. The proper technique for all is chin-lift, jaw-thrust.

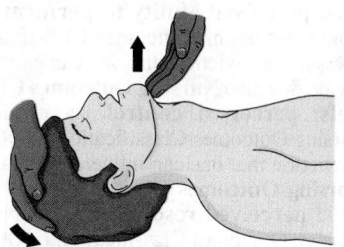

**Head-tilt, chin-lift airway technique**
*(Phipps, Sands, and Marek, 1999)*

**head traction.** See **cervical traction.**

**Heaf test** /hēf/ [Frederick R.G. Heaf, English physician, 1894–1973], a tuberculin skin test that uses a multiple puncture technique. See also **tuberculin test.**

**healing** [AS, *haelan*, to cure], the act or process in which the normal structural and functional characteristics of health are restored to diseased, dysfunctional, or damaged tissues, organs, or systems of the body. See also **intention, wound repair.**

**health** [AS, *haelth*], a condition of physical, mental, and social well-being and the absence of disease or other abnormal condition. It is not a static condition; constant change and adaptation to stress result in homeostasis. René Dubos, often quoted in nursing education, says, "The states of health or disease are the expressions of the success or failure experienced by the organism in its efforts to respond adaptively to environmental challenges." See also **high-level wellness, homeostasis.**

**health assessment,** an evaluation of the health status of an individual by performing a physical examination after obtaining a health history. Various laboratory tests also may be ordered to confirm a clinical impression or to screen for dysfunction. The depth of investigation and the frequency of the assessment vary with the condition and age of the client and the facility in which the assessment is performed. The person's response to any dysfunction present is observed and noted. The techniques of the health assessment include palpation, percussion, auscultation, and inspection, including sight, sound, and smell.

**health behavior,** an action taken by a person to maintain, attain, or regain good health and to prevent illness. Health behavior reflects a person's health beliefs. Some common health behaviors are exercising regularly, eating a balanced diet, and obtaining necessary inoculations.

**health belief model,** a conceptual framework that describes a person's health behavior as an expression of health beliefs. The model was designed to predict a person's health behavior, including the use of health services, and to justify intervention to alter maladaptive health behavior. Components of the model include the person's own perception of susceptibility to a disease or condition, the likelihood of contracting that disease or condition, the person's perception of the severity of the consequences of contracting the condition or the disease, the perceived benefits of care and barriers to preventive behavior, and the internal or external stimuli that result in appropriate health behavior by the person.

**health beliefs,** a nursing outcome from the Nursing Outcomes Classification (NOC) defined as personal convictions that influence health behaviors. See also **Nursing Outcomes Classification.**

**health beliefs: perceived ability to perform,** a nursing outcome from the Nursing Outcomes Classification (NOC) defined as personal conviction that one can carry out a given health behavior. See also **Nursing Outcomes Classification.**

**health beliefs: perceived control,** a nursing outcome from the Nursing Outcomes Classification (NOC) defined as personal conviction that one can influence a health outcome. See also **Nursing Outcomes Classification.**

**health beliefs: perceived resources,** a nursing outcome from the Nursing Outcomes Classification (NOC) defined as personal conviction that one has adequate means to carry out a health behavior. See also **Nursing Outcomes Classification.**

**health beliefs: perceived threat,** a nursing outcome from the Nursing Outcomes Classification (NOC) defined as personal conviction that a health problem is serious and has potential negative consequences for life-style. See also **Nursing Outcomes Classification.**

**health care consumer,** any actual or potential recipient of health care, such as a patient in a hospital, a client in a community mental health center, or a member of a prepaid health maintenance organization.

**Health Care Financing Administration (HCFA)** The branch of the U.S. Department of Health and Human Services responsible for administering the Medicare and Medicaid programs. HCFA sets the coverage policy, payment, and other guidelines and directs the activities of government contractors (e.g., carriers and fiscal intermediaries).

**health care industry,** the complex of preventive, remedial, and therapeutic services provided by hospitals and other institutions, nurses, doctors, dentists, government agencies, voluntary agencies, noninstitutional care facilities, pharmaceutic and medical equipment manufacturers, and health insurance companies.

**health care information exchange,** a nursing intervention from the Nursing Interventions Classification (NIC) defined as providing patient care information to health profes-

sionals in other agencies. See also **Nursing Interventions Classification.**

**health care provider,** any individual, institution, or agency that provides health services to health care consumers.

**health care proxy** [AS, *haelth* + ME, *caru,* sorrow; L, *procuratio,* a deputy], a person designated to make health care decisions for a patient who has become incapacitated.

**health care system,** the complete network of agencies, facilities, and all providers of health care in a specified geographic area. Nursing services are integral to all levels and patterns of care, and nurses form the largest number of providers in a health care system.

**health certificate,** a statement signed by a health care provider that attests to the state of health of a person.

**health consumer.** See **health care consumer.**

**health councils,** *Canada.* organizations that plan and allocate health care facilities. Local participants are represented in the District Health Councils, funded by the Ministry of Health.

**health culture,** a system that attempts to explain and treat sickness and to maintain health. Health cultures are a component of the larger culture or tradition of a people and may be a popular or folk system or a technical or scientific one.

**health economics,** a social system that studies the supply and demand of health care resources and the effect of health services on a population.

**health education$^1$,** an educational program directed to the general public that attempts to improve, maintain, and safeguard the health of the community.

**health education$^2$,** a nursing intervention from the Nursing Interventions Classification (NIC) defined as developing and providing instruction and learning experiences to facilitate voluntary adaptation of behavior conducive to health in individuals, families, groups, or communities. See also **Nursing Interventions Classification.**

**health hazard** [AS, *haelth* + OFr, *hasard*], a danger to health resulting from exposure to environmental pollutants, such as asbestos or ionizing radiation, or to a life-style influence, such as cigarette smoking or chemical abuse.

**health history,** (in nursing and medicine) a collection of information obtained from the patient and from other sources concerning the patient's physical status and psychologic, social, and sexual function. The history provides a data base on which a diagnosis, a plan for management of the diagnosis, treatment, care, and follow-up observation of the patient may be made. The first part of the history describes the chief complaint, the present illness, including its signs and symptoms, onset and character, and any factors or behaviors that aggravate or ameliorate the symptoms. The patient's own words often serve as the best description and may be quoted. The second part of the history comprises an account of previous illnesses and health-promotion behaviors, allergies, transfusions, immunizations, screening tests, and hospitalizations. An occupational history, describing the patient's work and exposure to stress, toxins, radiation, or other occupational hazards, may be included. The effect of the current illness on the patient's work is also noted. A social history is taken in which the patient's social, cultural, environmental, and familial milieu are outlined, focusing on aspects that might have an effect on the current illness. In some instances a sexual history may be relevant. A review of systems may follow or be incorporated into the health history. Kinds of history include **complete health history, episodic health history,** and **interval health history.** Also called **functional assessment.** See also **family history, oc-**

cupational history, past health, personal and social history, present health, review of systems, sexual history.

**health information administrator,** a graduate of a baccalaureate degree program in health information management who contributes to the development or management of computer-based clinical and administrative record systems.

**health information technician,** a graduate of an associate degree program who performs tasks related to computer-based management of health care data.

**health maintenance,** a systematic program or procedure planned to prevent illness, to maintain maximal function, and to promote health. It is central to health care, especially to nursing care at all levels (primary, secondary, and tertiary) and in all patterns (preventive, episodic, acute, chronic, and catastrophic).

**health maintenance, ineffective,** a nursing diagnosis accepted by the Fifth National Conference on the Classification of Nursing Diagnoses. It is defined as an inability to identify, manage, or seek help to maintain health.

■ DEFINING CHARACTERISTICS: The defining characteristics include a demonstrated lack of knowledge regarding basic health practices or the inability to take responsibility for meeting those needs, the inability to adapt to internal or external environmental change, a lack of financial or other resources or support systems, a history of a lack of health-seeking behavior, or an increased interest in improving health behavior.

■ RELATED FACTORS: Related factors include a lack of or significant alteration in communication skills; lack of ability to make deliberate and thoughtful judgments; perceptual or cognitive impairment; ineffective individual coping; dysfunctional grieving; unachieved developmental tasks; ineffective family coping; disabling spiritual distress, and lack of material resources. See also **nursing diagnosis.**

**health maintenance organization (HMO),** a type of group health care practice that provides basic and supplemental health maintenance and treatment services to voluntary enrollees who prepay a fixed periodic fee that is set without regard to the amount or kind of services received. In addition to diagnostic and treatment services, including hospitalization and surgery, an HMO often offers supplemental services, such as dental, mental, and eye care, and prescription drugs. Federal financial support for the establishment of HMOs was provided under Title XIII of the 1973 U.S. Public Health Service Act.

**health nurse,** a community or visiting nurse assigned primarily to promote health maintenance and preventive health measures within the community.

**health orientation,** a nursing outcome from the Nursing Outcomes Classification (NOC) defined as personal view of health and health behaviors as priorities. See also **Nursing Outcomes Classification.**

**health physicist,** a health scientist who directs research, training, and management of programs in which patients and health professionals are exposed to potential hazards associated with the use of diagnostic and therapeutic equipment, such as radioactive materials.

**health physics,** the study of the effects of ionizing radiation on the body and the methods for protecting people from the undesirable effects of the radiation. Health physics is concerned with the development and evaluation of methods, techniques, materials, and procedures to be used to protect people from these untoward effects. Also called **medical physics.**

**health policy,** 1. a statement of a decision regarding a goal in health care and a plan for achieving that goal; for ex-

ample, to prevent an epidemic, a program for inoculating a population is developed and implemented. 2. a field of study and practice in which the priorities and values underlying health resource allocation are determined.

**health policy monitoring,** a nursing intervention from the Nursing Interventions Classification (NIC) defined as surveillance and influence of government and organization regulations, rules, and standards that affect nursing systems and practices to ensure quality care of patients. See also **Nursing Interventions Classification.**

**health professional,** any person who has completed a course of study in a field of health, such as a registered nurse, physical therapist, or physician. The person is usually licensed by a government agency or certified by a professional organization.

**health promoting,** a nursing outcome from the Nursing Outcomes Classification (NOC) defined as actions to sustain or increase wellness. See also **Nursing Outcomes Classification.**

**health-related services,** actions of a health facility other than providing medical care that may contribute directly or indirectly to the physical or mental health and well-being of patients, such as personal or social services.

**health resources,** all materials, personnel, facilities, funds, and anything else that can be used for providing health care and services.

**Health Resources and Services Administration (HRSA),** a U.S. federal agency with responsibilities for the distribution of health information. This includes audiovisual materials relating to a wide range of health subjects such as recruitment of minorities into the health professions, and the role of women in dentistry. The HRSA was involved in establishment of the HIV/AIDS Treatment Information Service.

**health risk,** a disease precursor associated with a higher than average morbidity or mortality rate. The disease precursors may include demographic variables, certain individual behaviors, familial and individual histories, and certain physiologic changes.

**health risk appraisal,** a process of gathering, analyzing, and comparing an individual's characteristics prognostic of health with those of a standard age group, thereby predicting the likelihood that a person may prematurely experience a health problem associated with higher than average morbidity and mortality rates.

**health screening[1],** a program designed to evaluate the health status and potential of an individual. In the process it may be found that a person has a particular disease or condition or is at greater-than-normal risk of its development. Health screening may include taking a personal and family health history and performing a physical examination, tests, laboratory tests, or radiologic examination and may be followed by counseling, education, referral, or further testing.

**health screening[2],** a nursing intervention from the Nursing Interventions Classification (NIC) defined as detecting health risks or problems by means of history, examination, and other procedures. See also **Nursing Interventions Classification.**

**health seeking behavior,** a nursing outcome from the Nursing Outcomes Classification (NOC) defined as actions to promote optimal wellness, recovery, and rehabilitation. See also **Nursing Outcomes Classification.**

**health-seeking behaviors,** a nursing diagnosis accepted by the Eighth National Conference on the Classification of Nursing Diagnoses. This diagnosis describes a state in which a client in stable health is actively seeking ways to alter personal health habits and the environment to move toward optimal health.

■ DEFINING CHARACTERISTICS: The defining characteristics are an expressed or observed desire to seek a higher level of wellness, (stated, demonstrated, or observed) unfamiliarity with wellness community resources, lack of knowledge of health promotion behaviors, desire for increased control of health practice, and concern about environmental conditions or health status.

■ RELATED FACTORS: The related factors are to be developed. See also **nursing diagnosis.**

**health service area,** a geographic region designated under the U.S. National Health Planning and Resources Development Act of 1974, covering such factors as geographic features, political boundaries, population, and health resources, for the effective planning and development of health services.

**health supervision,** health teaching, counseling, or monitoring the status of a patient's health other than for physical care. Such supervision occurs in health care agencies, clinics, physicians' offices, or a patient's home. Compare **care of the sick.**

**health system guidance,** a nursing intervention from the Nursing Interventions Classification (NIC) defined as facilitating a patient's location and use of appropriate health services. See also **Nursing Interventions Classification.**

**health systems agency (HSA),** a body established under the terms of the U.S. National Health Planning and Resources Development Act of 1974. Health planning agencies are intended to provide networks of health planning and resource development services in each of several health service areas established by the Act. Health systems agencies are nonprofit; they may include private organizations, public regional planning bodies, local government agencies, and consumers. See also **health systems plan.**

**health systems plan,** a plan in which the long-range goals of a health services area are specified. Health systems plans are prepared by health systems agencies. See also **health policy.**

**healthy,** a condition of physical, mental, and social well-being and of absence of disease or another abnormal condition.

**hearing** [AS, *hieran*], the sense that enables sound to be perceived. It is a major function of the ear. Any reduction in the ability to perceive sounds results in hearing loss, which can range from mild impairment to complete deafness. See also **deafness.**

**hearing aid,** an electronic device that amplifies sound used by people with impaired hearing. The device consists of a microphone, a battery power supply, an amplifier, and a receiver. The microphone receives sound waves directed to-

ward the person with hearing loss, then converts the sound waves to electrical impulses that are amplified with the aid of the power supply, and the receiver converts the electrical impulses back into sound vibrations. Newer, programmable hearing aids can be customized based on the characteristics of an individual's hearing loss.

**hearing compensation behavior,** a nursing outcome from the Nursing Outcomes Classification (NOC) defined as actions to identify, monitor and compensate for hearing loss. See also **Nursing Outcomes Classification.**

**hearing handicap,** a measure of the impact of a hearing loss on an individual's everyday experiences; the psychosocial impact of a hearing loss.

**hearing impairment,** loss of hearing that adversely affects an individual's ability to communicate.

**hearing loss,** an inability to perceive the normal range of sounds audible to an individual with normal hearing. Hearing loss may be greater at some frequencies than others, or all frequencies may be equally affected. **Conductive hearing loss** is a result of damage to the outer or middle ear, whereas **sensorineural hearing loss** results from damage to the cochlea or auditory nerve. The loss is measured in decibels and may be described as mild, moderate, severe, or profound.

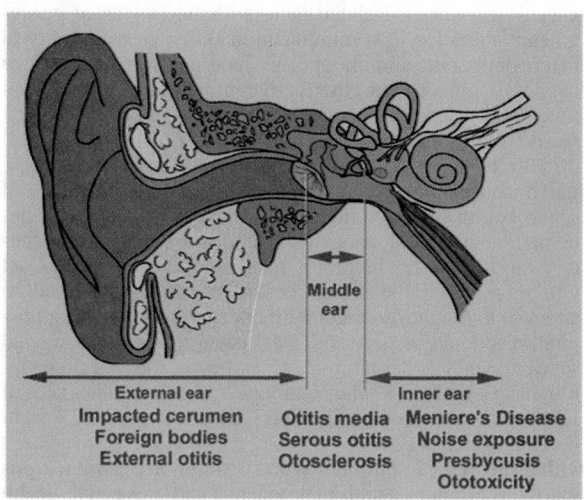

**Causes of hearing loss** *(Lemmi and Lemmi, 2000)*

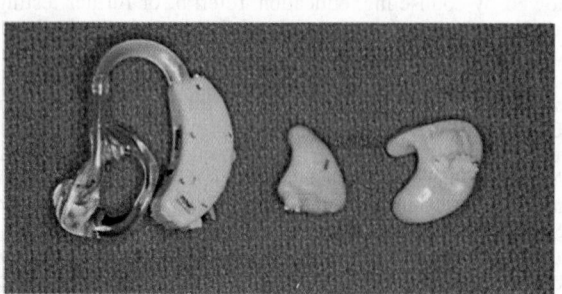

**Hearing aids**
*(Bingham, Hawke, and Kwok, 1992/courtesy Dr. Julain Nedzelski)*

**heart** [AS, *heorte*], the muscular cone-shaped hollow organ, about the size of a clenched fist, that pumps blood throughout the body and beats normally about 70 times per minute by coordinated nerve impulses and muscular contractions. Enclosed in pericardium, it rests on the diaphragm between the lower borders of the lungs, occupying the middle of the mediastinum. It is covered ventrally by the sternum and the adjoining parts of the third to the sixth costal cartilages. The organ is about 12 cm long, 8 cm wide at its broadest part, and 6 cm thick. The weight of the heart in men averages between 280 and 340 g and in women, between 230 and 280 g. The layers of the heart, starting from the outside, are the epicardium, the myocardium, and the endocardium. The chambers include two ventricles with thick muscular walls, making up the bulk of the organ, and two

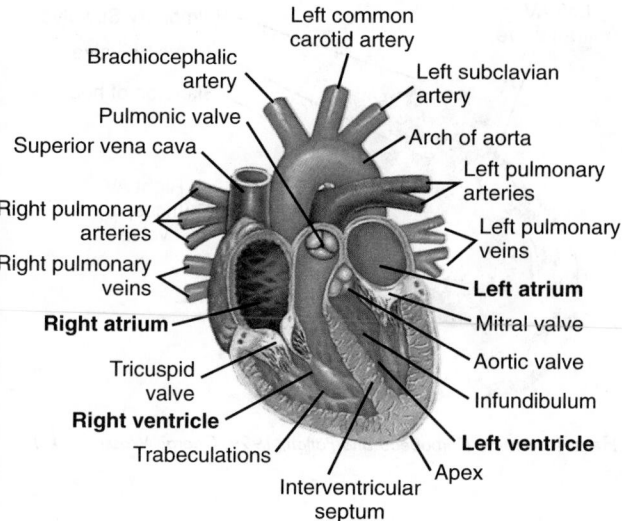

Left common
carotid artery

Brachiocephalic
artery

Left subclavian
artery

Pulmonic valve

Superior vena cava

Arch of aorta

Left pulmonary
arteries

Right pulmonary
arteries

Left pulmonary
veins

Right pulmonary
veins

**Left atrium**

**Right atrium**

Mitral valve

Tricuspid
valve

Aortic valve

Infundibulum

**Right ventricle**

**Left ventricle**

Trabeculations

Apex

Interventricular
septum

**Frontal section of the heart** (Canobbio, 1990)

atria with thin muscular walls. A septum separates the ventricles and extends between the atria (interatrial septum), dividing the heart into the right and the left sides. The left side of the heart pumps oxygenated blood into the aorta and on to all parts of the body. The right side receives deoxygenated blood from the venae cavae and pumps it into the pulmonary arteries. The valves of the heart include the tricuspid valve, the bicuspid (mitral) valve, the semilunar aortic valve, and the semilunar pulmonary valve. The sinoatrial node in the right atrium of the heart (under the control of the medulla oblongata in the brainstem) initiates the cardiac impulse, causing the atria to contract. The atrioventricular (AV) node near the septal wall of the right atrium spreads the impulse over the AV bundle (bundle of His) and its branches, causing the ventricles to contract. Both atria contract simultaneously, followed quickly by the simultaneous contraction of the ventricles. The sinoatrial node of the heartbeat sets the rate. Other factors affecting the heartbeat are emotion, exercise, hormones, temperature, pain, and stress. See also **endocardium, epicardium, heart valve, myocardium.**

**heart attack.** See **myocardial infarction.**

**heartbeat,** a complete cycle of cardiac muscle contraction and relaxation.

**heart block,** an interference with the normal conduction of electrical impulses that control activity of the heart muscle. Heart block is usually specified by the location of the block and the type, such as a first-degree atrioventricular (AV) block, in which atrial impulses are delayed by a fraction of a second before being conducted to the ventricles. Heart block can occur in the sinus node, atria, AV node, AV bundle, fascicles, or a combination of these structures. See also **atrioventricular block, bundle branch block, cardiac conduction defect, infranodal block, intraatrial block, intraventricular block, sinoatrial block.**

**heartburn,** a painful burning sensation in the esophagus just below the sternum. Heartburn is usually caused by the reflux of gastric contents into the esophagus but may result from gastric hyperacidity or peptic ulcer. Antacids relieve the symptoms but do not cure the condition. Also called **pyrosis.** See also **gastroesophageal reflux, hiatal hernia.**

**heart disease risk factor** [AS, *heorte,* heart; L, *dis* + Fr,

*aise,* ease, *risquer,* chance of injury; L, *facere,* to make], one of several hereditary, life-style, and environmental influences that increase one's chance of developing heart disease. Examples include cigarette smoking, high blood pressure, diabetes, obesity, high cholesterol level, lack of routine exercise, and hereditary factors.

**heart failure,** a condition in which the heart cannot pump enough blood to meet the metabolic requirements of body tissues. Many of the symptoms associated with heart failure are caused by the dysfunction of organs other than the heart, especially the lungs, kidneys, and liver. Ventricular dysfunction is usually the basic disorder in congestive heart failure; it often triggers compensatory mechanisms that preserve cardiac output but produce symptoms and signs such as dyspnea, orthopnea, rales, and edema. Heart failure is closely associated with many forms of heart disease, most of which initially affect the left side of the heart. Hence, clinicians commonly divide associated heart failure into left-sided heart failure and right-sided heart failure. Peripheral edema is associated with right-sided heart failure, and dyspnea and other respiratory disorders with left-sided heart failure. Heart failure in infants and children is usually the result of congenital heart disease but also may be caused by myocarditis and ectopic tachycardia. Rheumatic mitral disease and aortic valve disease frequently cause congestive heart failure in young adults. Mitral valve disease, especially mitral stenosis, is the most common cause of heart failure and affects more young women than men. The common causes of heart failure after 40 years of age are coronary atherosclerosis with myocardial infarction, anemia, diastolic hypertension, hypervolemia, valvular heart disease, pulmonary disease, renal disease, and diffuse myocardial disease. Some individuals may suffer heart failure caused by a combination of congenital heart disease and acquired disease. After 50 years of age a common cause of heart failure, especially in men, is calcific aortic stenosis. Some of the extracardiac signs of heart failure are ascites, bronchial wheezing, hydrothorax, edema, liver enlargement, moist rales, and splenomegaly. Cardiac signs associated with heart failure are abnormalities in the jugular venous pulsation, the carotid pulse, and the apex wave on cardiographic tracings. Treatment for heart failure commonly involves reduction of the heart's workload, administration of drugs such as digitalis to increase myocardial contractility and cardiac output, salt-restricted diet, diuretics, angiotensin-converting enzymes to decrease afterload, and surgical intervention. Also called **cardiac failure.** See also **compensated heart failure, congestive heart failure.**

**heart-hand syndrome.** See **Holt-Oram syndrome.**

**heart-lung machine,** an apparatus consisting of a pump and an oxygenator that takes over the functions of the heart and lungs, especially during open heart surgery. The blood is shunted from the venous system through an oxygenator and returned to the arterial circulation.

**heart massage.** See **cardiac massage.**

**heart murmur.** See **cardiac murmur.**

**heart rate,** the frequency with which the heart beats, calculated by counting the number of QRS complexes or ventricular beats per minute. See also **pulse.**

**heart scan,** a radiographic scan of the heart, performed after the injection of a radioactive material into a vein. It is used for determining the size, shape, and location of the heart; for diagnosing pericarditis; and for viewing the chambers of the heart. See also **cardiography, echocardiography.**

**heart sound,** a noise produced within the heart during the cardiac cycle that can be heard over the precordium. It may reveal abnormalities in cardiac structure or function. Cardiac auscultation is performed systematically from the apex to the base of the heart or from base to apex, using a stethoscope to listen, initially with the diaphragm and then with the bell of the instrument. Standard heart sounds include $S_1$, $S_2$, $S_3$, and $S_4$. Additional heart sounds include clicks, gallops, murmurs, rubs, and snaps.

**heart surgery,** any surgical procedure involving the heart, performed to correct acquired or congenital defects, replace diseased valves, open or bypass blocked vessels, or graft a prosthesis or a transplant. Two major types of heart surgery are performed: closed and open. The closed technique is done through a small incision, without using the heart-lung machine. In the open technique the heart chambers are open and fully visible, and blood is detoured around the surgical field by the heart-lung machine. Preoperative care focuses on correcting metabolic imbalances and cardiac and pulmonary ailments and on performing diagnostic and laboratory tests. General anesthesia is used, the chest cavity is opened, and the heart-lung machine is connected. Hypothermia also is used to decrease the metabolic rate and the need of the tissues for oxygen. After surgery constant observation is required in an intensive care unit for signs of hemorrhage, shock, fibrillation, arrhythmia, sudden chest pain, and pulmonary edema. The blood pressure, all pulses, respirations, and venous and pulmonary artery pressures are monitored. If the blood pressure is high enough to ensure cerebral profusion, the head of the patient's bed is elevated to a semi-Fowler's position to encourage chest drainage and lung expansion. The patient is quickly extubated. Oxygen is provided. Chest tube drainage, urinary output, and temperature are noted hourly; IV infusions and sometimes blood transfusions are given. Narcotics help control pain and enable the patient to cough and deep breathe. Antibiotics are given to prevent infection. Mortality rate is highest during the first 48 hours after surgery. Kinds of heart surgery include **Blalock-Taussig procedure, coronary bypass,** and **endarterectomy.** See also **arrhythmia, fibrillation, heart-lung machine, hypothermia, pulmonary edema.**

**heart transplantation** [AS, *hoerte* + L, *transplantare*], the surgical removal of a donor heart and transfer of the organ to a recipient. The donor heart is usually obtained from an accident victim who was healthy before dying, and it is used to replace the severely diseased heart of another person. Most recipients survive for more than 1 year, and nearly three-fourths are able to return to work. Total ischemic time for the transplanted heart is less than 6 hours between donor and recipient. The heart is transplanted with anastomoses of the aorta, pulmonary artery, and pulmonary vein; venous return is provided by an anastomosis between the recipient's right atrium and that of the transplanted organ.

**heart valve,** one of the four structures within the heart that prevent backflow of blood by opening and closing with each heartbeat. The valves include two semilunar valves, the aortic and pulmonary; the mitral or bicuspid valve; and the tricuspid valve. The valves permit blood flow in only one direction, and any of the valves may become defective, permitting the backflow associated with heart murmurs. Also called **cardiac valve.** See also **heart, mitral valve, semilunar valve, tricuspid valve.**

**heat/cold application,** a nursing intervention from the Nursing Interventions Classification (NIC) defined as stimulation of the skin and underlying tissues with heat or cold for the purpose of decreasing pain, muscle spasms, or inflammation. See also **Nursing Interventions Classification.**

**heat cramp** [AS, *haetu* + *crammian,* to fill], any cramp or painful spasm of the voluntary muscles in the arm, leg, or

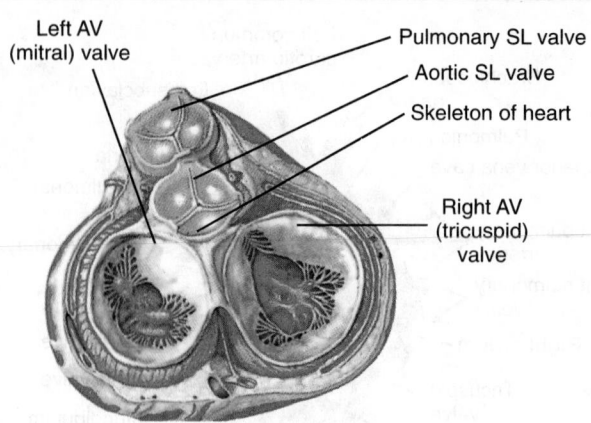

**Heart valves** *(Thibodeau and Patton, 1999/George Wassilchenko)*

abdomen caused by depletion in the body of both water and salt. It usually occurs after vigorous physical exertion in an extremely hot environment or under other conditions that cause profuse sweating and depletion of body fluids and electrolytes. The victim should be moved to a cooler place and given salt-containing fluids. Also called **cane-cutter's cramp, fireman's cramp, miner's cramp, stoker's cramp.** See also **heat exhaustion.**

**heated nebulization,** a method of inhalation therapy that uses a heating device with a nebulizer that produces a spray with a higher water content than that of a cold atomizer. The mist may be administered through a mask or in a tent.

**heat exhaustion,** an abnormal condition characterized by weakness, vertigo, nausea, muscle cramps, and loss of consciousness, caused by depletion of body fluid and electrolytes that results from exposure to intense heat or inability to acclimatize to heat. Body temperature is near normal; blood pressure may drop but usually returns to normal as the person is placed in a recumbent position; the skin is cool, damp, and pale. The person usually recovers with rest and replacement of water and electrolytes. Also called **heat prostration.** Compare **heat hyperpyrexia.** See also **heat cramp.**

**heat exposure treatment,** a nursing intervention from the Nursing Interventions Classification (NIC) defined as management of patient overcome by heat due to excessive environmental heat exposure. See also **Nursing Interventions Classification.**

**heat hyperpyrexia,** a severe and sometimes fatal condition resulting from failure of the temperature regulating capacity of the body, caused by prolonged exposure to sun or to high temperature. Reduction or cessation of sweating is sometimes an early symptom. Body temperature of 105° F or higher, tachycardia, hot and dry skin, headache, altered mental status, and seizures may occur. Treatment includes cooling, sedation, and fluid replacement. Also called **heatstroke, siriasis, sunstroke.** See also **hyperpyrexia.** Compare **heat exhaustion.**

**heat labile** [L, *labilis,* liable to slip], readily destroyed by heat. See also **thermolabile.**

**heat-labile antibody,** an immunoglobulin that loses its ability to interact with antigens when heated above 56°C.

**heat prostration.** See **heat exhaustion.**

**heat rash,** a finely papular or vesicular inflammation of the skin that results from prolonged exposure to heat and high humidity. Tingling and prickling sensations are common.

Prevention and treatment include cool, dry temperatures; ventilation; and absorbent powders. See also **miliaria**.

**heat shock protein (HsP),** an intracellular protein that increases in concentration during metabolic stress, such as exposure to heat. HsPs affect protein assembly, folding, sorting, and uptake into organelles.

**heatstroke.** See **heat hyperpyrexia**.

**heaves** /hēvz/ [AS, *hebban*, to lift], 1. a chronic pulmonary disease of horses, similar to human pulmonary emphysema, characterized by wheezing, coughing, and dyspnea on exertion. The cause of the condition is unknown. 2. *informal.* vomiting and retching.

**heavy chain,** a high-molecular-weight polypeptide that is part of an immunoglobulin molecule. Different types of heavy chains characterize the various categories of immunoglobulins (Igs), such as IgG and IgA.

**heavy chain disease** [AS, *heafig* + L, *catena*, chain; *dis,* opposite of; Fr, *aise*, ease], a plasma cell disorder characterized by a proliferation of immunoglobulin heavy chains. Excessive levels of alpha, gamma, delta, and mu chains are produced, and effects tend to vary according to the predominant type of heavy chain. Alpha heavy chain disease mainly affects children living in the Middle East, causing diffuse abdominal lymphoma and malabsorption disorders. Most gamma heavy chain disease patients are elderly men who have symptoms resembling those of malignant lymphoma: enlarged liver and spleen, fever, anemia, and increased susceptibility to infections. Delta heavy chain disease is rare and marked by symptoms similar to those of multiple myeloma. Mu heavy chain disease presents symptoms of chronic lymphocytic leukemia and treatment is symptomatic.

**heavy function,** increased functional activity of the teeth, which enhances occlusal force.

**heavy hydrogen.** See **deuterium**.

**heavy metal,** a metallic element with a specific gravity five or more times that of water. The heavy metals include antimony, arsenic, bismuth, cadmium, cerium, chromium, cobalt, copper, gallium, gold, iron, lead, manganese, mercury, nickel, platinum, silver, tellurium, thallium, tin, uranium, vanadium, and zinc. Small amounts of many of these elements are common and necessary in the diet. Large amounts of any of them may cause poisoning.

**heavy metal poisoning,** poisoning caused by the ingestion, inhalation, or absorption of various toxic heavy metals. Kinds of heavy metal poisoning include **antimony poisoning, arsenic poisoning, cadmium poisoning, lead poisoning,** and **mercury poisoning**. See also **heavy metal**.

**heavy water,** water in which the hydrogen component is deuterium ($^2$H), or heavy hydrogen. It has properties different from those of ordinary water. Because of its ability to absorb neutrons, heavy water is used as a moderator in nuclear reactions. Also written as $D_2O$.

**hebephrenia, hebephrenic schizophrenia.** See **disorganized schizophrenia**.

**Heberden's node** /hē′bərdənz/ [William Heberden, English physician, 1710–1801; L, *nodus*, knot], an abnormal cartilaginous or bony enlargement of a distal interphalangeal joint of a finger, usually occurring in degenerative diseases of the joints. Compare **Bouchard's node**.

**hebetude** /heb′itōōd′/ [L, *hebeo*, to be blunt], a state of dullness or lethargy, characteristic of some forms of schizophrenia.

**heboid paranoia.** See **paranoid schizophrenia**.

**hectic fever,** a fever that recurs each day, with profound sweating, chills, and facial flushing.

**hecto-** [Gk, *hekaton*, one hundred], prefix in the metric sys-

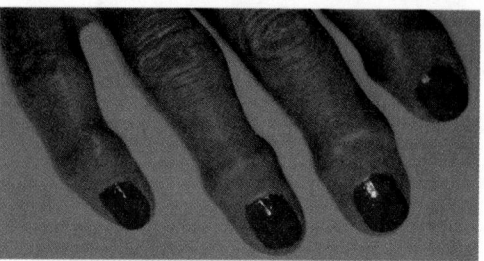

**Heberden's nodes** *(Lemmi and Lemmi, 2000)*

tem indicating 100 units. For example, 1 hectometer equals 100 meters.

**-hedonia,** combining form meaning '(condition of) pleasure, cheerfulness': *anhedonia, hyphedonia, parhedonia*.

**-hedron,** suffix meaning a 'geometric figure with (specified) sides': *decahedron, octahedron, polyhedron*.

**heel** [AS, *hela*], the posterior part of the foot, formed by the largest tarsal bone, the calcaneus.

**heel cup,** a plastic device designed to help relieve pain of a heel spur or contusion by pushing the fat pad of the heel under the calcaneus to increase the cushioning effect.

**heel-knee test** [AS, *hela* + *cneow*, knee; L, *testum*, crucible], a method of assessing coordination of movements of the extremities. In the test the patient, lying supine, is asked to touch the knee of one leg with the heel of the other.

**heel lift,** a foot orthosis, usually made of sheets of cork, to correct a dysfunction that may result from anatomic limb length differences or decreased flexibility.

**heel puncture** [AS, *hela* + L, *punctura*], a method of obtaining a blood sample from a newborn or premature infant by a puncture in the lateral or medial areas of the plantar surface of the heel. Care must be exercised to prevent puncture of the posterior curvature of the heel and to make the puncture as shallow as feasible.

**heel-shin test** [AS, *hela* + *scinu*, shin; L, *testum*, crucible], a method of assessing coordination of movements of the extremities. In the test the patient, lying supine, is asked to pass the heel of one leg slowly down the shin of the other leg from the knee to the ankle.

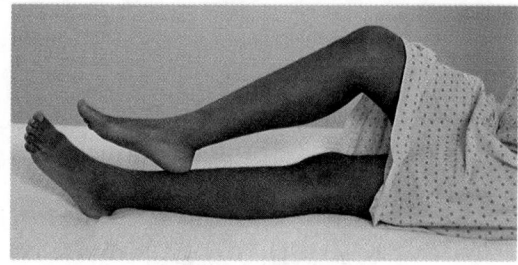

**Heel-shin test** *(Seidel et al, 1999)*

**heel spur.** See **calcaneal spur**.

**HEENT,** abbreviation for **head, eye, ear, nose, and throat**.

**Hegar's dilators** /hā′gərz/ [Alfred Hegar, German gynecologist, 1830–1914], a series of bougies used to dilate the cervical canal. See also **bougie**.

**Hegar's sign** [Alfred Hegar; L, *signum,* sign],   a softening of the isthmus of the uterine cervix that occurs early in gestation. It is a probable sign of pregnancy.

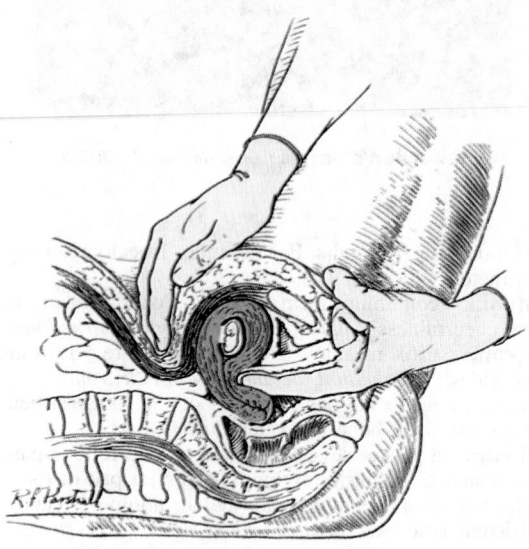

**Assessment for Hegar's sign** (Barkauskas et al, 1998)

**height (ht)** /hīt/ [AS, *hiehtho*],   the vertical measurement of a structure, organ, or other object from bottom to top, when it is placed or projected in an upright position.

**height of contour,**   the greatest convexity of a tooth surface, viewed from a predetermined position.

**Heimlich maneuver** /hīm'lik, -lish/ [H. J. Heimlich, American physician, b. 1920; Fr, *manœuvre,* work done by hand], an emergency procedure for dislodging a bolus of food or other obstruction from the trachea to prevent asphyxiation. The choking person is grasped from behind by the rescuer, whose fist, thumb side in, is placed just below the victim's xiphoid with the other hand placed firmly over the fist. The

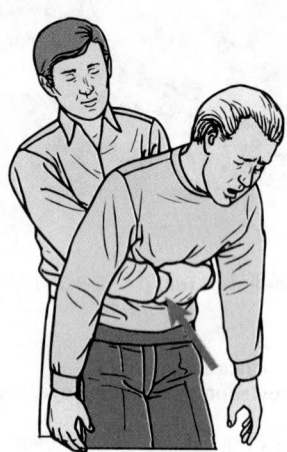

**Heimlich maneuver** (Lewis, Heitkemper, and Dirksen, 2000)

rescuer then pulls the fist firmly and abruptly upward into the epigastrium, forcing the obstruction up the trachea. If repeated attempts do not clear the airway, an emergency cricothyrotomy may be necessary. Also spelled Heimlich manoeuvre. Also known as **abdominal thrust.**

**Heimlich sign** [H. J. Heimlich; L, *signum*],   a universal distress signal that a person is choking and unable to speak, made by grasping the throat with a thumb and index finger, thereby attracting the attention of others nearby. Also called **universal choking signal.**

**Heinz bodies** /hīnts/ [Robert Heinz, German pathologist, 1865–1924],   irregularly shaped bits of altered hemoglobin found in the red blood cells of people who are hypersensitive to certain chemicals, such as aniline, phenylhydrazine, and primaquine.

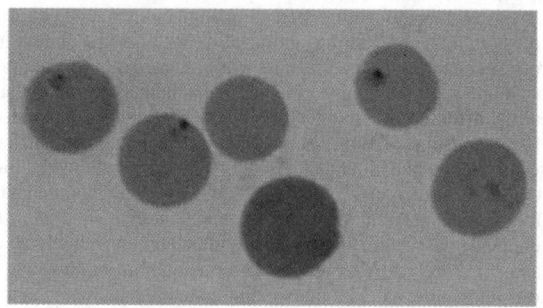

**Heinz bodies** (Carr and Rodak, 1999)

**Helen, Sister (Helen Bowden),**   a nurse who received her education in England and became the first director of the newly formed Bellevue Hospital Training School for Nurses in New York in 1873. Although she had not trained under Florence Nightingale, she set up the Bellevue school according to Nightingale's principles. She was a member of the All Saints Sisterhood. After several years at Bellevue, having established one of the leading nursing schools in the United States, she went to South Africa.

**helical virus** /hel'ikəl/,   a virus in which the protein capsid appears in a coiled pattern.

*Helicobacter* /hel'i·kō·bak'tər/ [Gk, *helix* coil + *bakterion,* small staff],   a genus of gram-negative, microaerophilic bacteria of the family Spirillaceae, consisting of motile, spiral organisms with multiple sheathed flagella; formerly classified in the genus *Campylobacter.*

*Helicobacter pylori*,   a species of spiral or straight gram-negative bacteria with multiple sheathed flagella found in the gastic mucosa of humans and other animals and associated with gastric and peptic ulcers as well as gastric cancers. Formerly called *Campylobacter pylori.*

**helicopod gait** /hel'ikōpod'/ [Gk, *helix,* coil, *pous,* foot],   a manner of walking in which the feet trace half-circles. It is associated with some mental disorders. Also called **helicopodia.**

**heliotherapy.**   See **solar therapy.**

**helium (He)** /hē'lē·əm/ [Gk, *helios,* sun],   a colorless, odorless gaseous element; the second lightest element. Its atomic number is 2; its atomic mass is 4.00. Helium is one of the rare or inert gases and does not combine with other elements. It occurs in the atmosphere at concentrations of five parts per million. Because of its lightness and lack of flam-

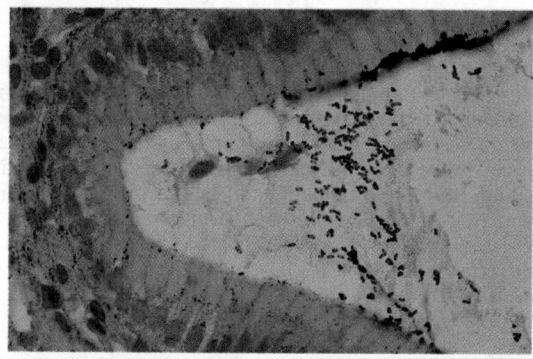

*Helicobacter pylori* (Cotran, Kumar, and Collins, 1999)

mability it is also used to lift airships and balloons. In the liquid state it is used for low-temperature activities. The main physiologic and medical uses of helium are in respiratory therapy and testing and the prevention of nitrogen narcosis and decompression sickness in hyperbaric environments. A mixture of 80% helium and 20% oxygen is commonly breathed by deep-sea divers to prevent gas emboli and by patients undergoing treatment to clear obstruction of the respiratory tract. Problems associated with such uses involve the high velocity of acoustic transmission in helium and the high thermal conductivity of the gas. These characteristics produce voice distortions and hypothermia in persons who inhale it. Helium is one third as soluble in lipids as nitrogen; that characteristic accounts for its preferred use in hyperbaric atmospheres, such as those associated with deep-sea diving. The low density of helium reduces the effort of breathing any gas mixture of which it is a component. Helium is used in pulmonary function testing to calculate the diffusion and residual capacities of the lungs.

**helium therapy,** the use of helium-oxygen gas mixtures to treat patients with airway obstruction. Because of its low density, helium can negotiate an obstruction more easily than nitrogen can, so less driving pressure is required to move the gas mixture in and out of the lungs.

**helix** /hē'liks/ [Gk, coil], a coiled, spirallike formation characteristic of many organic molecules, such as DNA.

**Hellin's law,** a generalized formula for calculating the ratio of multiple births in any population, stating that if twin births occur at the rate of 1:$N$, then the rate of triplet births is approximately 1:$N^2$, the rate of quadruplet births is approximately 1:$N^3$, and so on. The value of $N$ varies greatly but is generally close to 80. Also called **Hellin-Zeleny law.**

**HELLP syndrome** /help/, abbreviation for a form of severe preeclampsia, a hypertensive complication of late pregnancy. The letters stand for *h*emolysis, *e*levated *l*iver function, and *l*ow *p*latelet level.

**helmet cells,** fragmented red blood cells that have been "scooped out" so they resemble helmets. They are found in patients with carcinomatosis, hemolytic anemia, and thrombotic thrombocytopenic purpura. Helmet cells can be seen in blood samples of people with prosthetic heart valves.

**helminth** /hel'minth/ [Gk, *helmins,* worm], a worm, especially one of the pathogenic parasites of the division Metazoa, including flukes, tapeworms, and roundworms.

**-helminth,** suffix meaning 'worm': *nemathelminth, platyhelminth.*

**helminthemesis** /hel'minthem'əsis/ [Gk, *helmins,* worm, *emesis,* vomiting], the vomiting of intestinal worms.

**helminthiasis** /hel'minthī'əsis/ [Gk, *helmins,* worm, *osis,* condition], a parasitic infestation of the body by helminths that may be cutaneous, visceral, or intestinal. Ascariasis, bilharziasis, filariasis, hookworm, and trichinosis are common forms of the disease.

**helminthic** /helmin'thik/ [Gk, *helmins,* worm], pertaining to worms.

**helminthology** /hel'minthol'əjē/, a branch of medicine concerned with parasitic worms.

**helper factor,** a protein produced by helper T lymphocytes that stimulates proliferation of and antibody production by other lymphocytes.

**helper T cell,** a T lymphocyte that promotes the immune response of other lymphocytes to foreign antigens by releasing soluble proteins called helper factors. See also **T cell.**

**helper virus,** a virus that is necessary for the replication of a defective virus. Hepatitis B acts as a helper virus to delta agent, a defective RNA virus.

**helplessness** /help'ləsnəs/, a feeling of a loss of control or ability, usually after repeated failures, or of being immobilized or frozen by circumstances beyond one's control, with the result that one is unable to make autonomous choices.

**Helsinki Accords** /helsing'kē/, a declaration signed by the representatives of 35 member nations of the Conference on Security and Cooperation in Europe in Helsinki, Finland, on August 1, 1975. The declared goals of the nonbinding document comprised four principal aspects of European security: economic cooperation, humanitarian issues, contact between the East and West, and provision for a later follow-up conference (held in Belgrade in 1978). Follow-up conferences were planned in part to allow the member nations to monitor each other's performance on humanitarian issues, such as the right to self-determination of all people and respect for fundamental freedoms, including thought, conscience, and religion or belief, without regard to race, language, sex, or religion. The Helsinki accords grew from the precedent set by the judgments at the Nuremberg tribunals—that crimes against humanity are offenses subject to criminal prosecution. The principle and the practice of informed consent in health care grew from this precedent. Also called **Helsinki Declaration.** See also **Nuremberg tribunal.**

**helvolic acid** /helvol'ik/, an antibiotic, derived from the mold *Aspergillus fumigatus,* formerly used as an amebicide. Also called **fumagillin, fumigacin.**

**hema-** /hē'mə-, hem'ə-/, prefix for terms relating to blood or blood vessels.

**hema-, hemat-,** combining form meaning 'blood': *hematoma, hematophyte.*

**Hemabate,** trademark for a prostaglandin abortifacient (carboprost tromethamine).

**hemacytometer** /-sītom'ətər/ [Gk, *haima,* blood, *kytos,* cell, *metron,* measure], an apparatus for counting the number of cells in a known volume of blood or other fluid. See also **Abbé-Zeiss apparatus.**

**hemadsorption** /hē'madsôrp'shən, hem'-/ [Gk, *haima,* blood; L, *ad* to, *sorbere,* to swallow], a process in which a substance or an agent, such as certain viruses and bacilli, adheres to the surface of an erythrocyte. The process occurs naturally, or it may be induced for laboratory identification of bacteriologic specimens.

**hemagglutination** /hē'məglōō'tinā'shən, hem'-/ [Gk, *haima* + L, *agglutinare,* to glue], the coagulation of erythrocytes. See also **blood clotting.**

**hemagglutination inhibition (HI),** 1. the inhibition of virus-induced hemagglutination as a procedure for identifying hemagglutinating viruses. HI is used in the diagnosis of infections by certain viruses, such as rubella, herpes zoster, and herpes simplex. **2.** a method for measuring the concentration of soluble antigens in biologic specimens in which the specimen is incubated first with homologous antibodies and then with antigen-coated erythrocytes.

**hemagglutinin** [Gk, *haima* + L, *agglutinare*], a type of antibody that agglutinates red blood cells. It is classified according to the source of cells agglutinated as **autologous** (from the same organism), **homologous** (from an organism of the same species), and **heterologous** (from an organism of a different species). Some hemagglutinins clump red cells together as they are suspended in 0.85% sodium chloride solution; others will not agglutinate red cells unless hydrophilic colloids are added or unless the red cells have been treated with a proteolytic enzyme.

**hemangi-,** combining form meaning 'condition of the blood vessel structure or a collection of blood vessels': *hemangioma, hemangiectesis.*

**hemangiectasis,** dilation of a blood vessel.

**hemangioblast** /hēman'jē·ōblast'/, an embryonic mesodermal cell that gives rise to vascular endothelium and blood-forming cells.

**hemangioblastoma** /hēman'jē·ōblastō'mə/, *pl.* **hemangioblastomas, hemangioblastomata** [Gk, *haima* + *angeion,* vessel, *blastos,* germ, *oma,* tumor], a brain tumor composed of a proliferation of capillaries and of disorganized clusters of capillary cells or angioblasts, usually occurring in the cerebellum.

**hemangioendothelioma** /hēman'jē·ō·en'dōthē'lē·ō'mə/, *pl.* **hemangioendotheliomas, hemangioendotheliomata** [Gk, *haima* + *endon,* inside, *thele,* nipple, *oma,* tumor], a tumor, consisting of endothelial cells, that grows around an artery or a vein. The benign form occurs in children and is usually cured by local excision. The tumor rarely becomes malignant. **1.** Also called **angioendothelioma. 2.** malignant hemangioendothelioma. See also **angiosarcoma.**

**hemangiofibroma** /-fībrō'mə/ [Gk, *haima,* blood; L, *fibra,* fiber; Gk, *oma,* tumor], a tumor that has the characteristics of both a hemangioma and a fibroma.

**hemangioma** /hēman'jē·ō'mə/, *pl.* **hemangiomas, hemangiomata** [Gk, *haima* + *angeion,* small vessel, *oma*], a benign tumor consisting of a mass of blood vessels. Also spelled **haemangioma.**

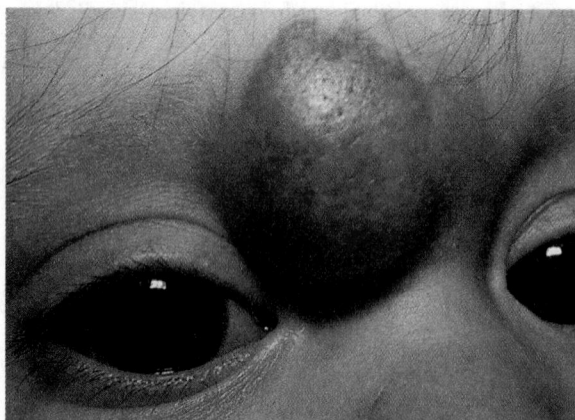

**Hemangioma** *(Zitelli and Davis, 1997)*

**hemangioma simplex.** See **capillary hemangioma.**

**hemangioma-thrombocytopenia syndrome,** a blood disorder usually occurring in the first few months of life in which severe thrombocytopenia and other evidence of intravascular coagulation are accompanied by rapidly expanding hemangiomas of the trunk, extremities, and abdominal viscera, sometimes associated with bleeding and anemia. Bleeding is thought to result from trapping and destruction of platelets within the tumor and depletion of circulating clotting factors. Also called **Kasabach-Merritt syndrome.**

**hemangiosarcoma.** See **angiosarcoma.**

**hemapoiesis** /hem'əpō·ē'sis/ [Gk, *haima,* blood, *poiein,* to make], the formation of blood cells.

**hemarthros** /hem'är'thrəs/ [Gk, *haima,* blood, *arthron,* joint], the extravasation of blood into a joint. Also called **hemarthrosis** /hem'ärthrō'sis/. Also spelled **haemarthros.**

**hematemesis** /hē'mətem'əsis, hem'-/ [Gk, *haima* + *emesis,* vomiting], vomiting of bright red blood, indicating rapid upper GI bleeding, commonly associated with esophageal varices or peptic ulcer. The rate and the source of bleeding are determined by endoscopic examination. Any blood found in the stomach is removed by nasogastric suction. Treatment requires replacement of blood by transfusion and administration of IV fluids for maintenance of fluid and electrolyte balance, and possible gastric lavage. Surgery may be necessary. The patient is usually very anxious and needs quiet, warmth, and reassurance. Also spelled **haematemesis.** See also **gastrointestinal bleeding.**

**hematic.** See **hemic.**

**hematinic** /hem'ətin'ik/, a therapeutic agent that produces an increase in the number of erythrocytes and/or hemoglobin concentration in erythrocytes, such as iron or B complex vitamins.

**hematinuria** /hem'ətinŏŏr'ē·ə/ [Gk, *haima,* blood, *ouron,* urine], a dark-colored urine resulting from the presence of hematin or hemoglobin. See also **hemoglobinuria.**

**hemato-** /hē'mətō-, hem'ətō-/ [Gk, *haima,* blood], prefix for terms relating to blood or blood vessels.

**hematocele** /hem'ətōsēl'/, a cystlike accumulation of blood within the tunica vaginalis of the scrotum. It is usually caused by injury and may require surgery if the blood is not readily resorbed. Also spelled **haematocele.**

**hematochezia** /hem'ətōkē'zhə/ [Gk, *haima* + *chezo,* feces], the passage of red blood through the rectum. The cause is usually bleeding in the colon or rectum, but it may result from the loss of blood higher in the digestive tract. Blood passed from the stomach or small intestine generally loses its red coloration through enzymatic activity on the erythrocytes. Cancer, colitis, and ulcers are among causes of hematochezia. Compare **melena.**

**hematocrit** /hemat'ōkrit/ [Gk, *haima* + *krinein,* to separate], a measure of the packed cell volume of red cells, expressed as a percentage of the total blood volume. The normal range is between 43% and 49% in men, and between 37% and 43% in women. Also spelled **haematocrit.** See also **complete blood count, differential white blood cell count.**

**hematocrit reading.** See **packed cell volume.**

**hematocyte** /hem'ətōsīt/ [Gk, *haima,* blood, *kytos,* cell], a blood cell, particularly a red blood cell. Also called **hemocyte.**

**hematocytoblast** /hem'ətōsī'təblast'/ [Gk, *haima,* blood, *kytos,* cell, *blastos,* germ], a large nucleated reticuloendothelial cell found in bone marrow. It is believed to be a common precursor of various blood elements. Also called **hemocytoblast.**

**hematogenesis** /-jen'əsis/ [Gk, *haima,* blood, *genein,* to produce], pertaining to the formation of blood cells or an increase in the production of blood elements. Also called **hemapoiesis.**

**hematogenic shock.** See **hemorrhagic shock.**

**hematogenous** /hēmətoj'ənəs/ [Gk, *haima + genein,* to produce], originating or transported in the blood.

**hematogenous pigment** [Gk, *haima,* blood, *genein,* to produce; L, *pingere,* to paint], the red color of erythrocytes caused by the presence of hemoglobin.

**hematogenous tuberculosis** [Gk, *haima,* blood, *genein,* to produce; L, *tuberculum,* a small swelling; Gk, *osis,* condition], a form of tuberculosis that is blood-borne.

**hematoid** /hem'ətoid/, bloodlike or resembling blood.

**hematologic, hematological.** See **hematology.**

**hematologic death syndrome** /hem'ətoloj'ik/, a group of clinical signs and symptoms of radiation damage to the blood cells. The condition is characterized by nausea, vomiting, fever, diarrhea, infections, anemia, leukopenia, and hemorrhage. It can result from exposure to a dose of 200 to 1000 rad. The mean survival time for a person with hematologic death syndrome is estimated at between 10 and 60 days.

**hematologic effect,** the response of blood cells to radiation exposure. All types of blood cells are destroyed by radiation, and the degree of cell depletion increases with increasing dose. Lymphocytes are affected first and are reduced in number within minutes or hours after exposure. Erythrocytes are less sensitive than other types of blood cells and may not show radiation effects for several weeks.

**hematologist** /hē'mətol'əjist, hem'-/, a medical specialist in the field of blood and blood-forming tissues.

**hematology** /hē'mətol'əjē, hem'-/ [Gk, *haima + logos,* science], the scientific study of blood and blood-forming tissues. Also spelled **haematology. —hematologic, hematological,** *adj.*

**hematolysis.** See **hemolysis.**

**hematoma** /hē'mətō'mə, hem'-/, *pl.* **hematomas, hematomata** [Gk, *haima + oma,* tumor], a collection of extravasated blood trapped in the tissues of the skin or in an organ, resulting from trauma or incomplete hemostasis after surgery. Initially there is frank bleeding into the space; if the space is limited, pressure slows and eventually stops the flow of blood. The blood clots, serum collects, the clot hardens, and the mass becomes palpable to the examiner and is often painful to the patient. A hematoma may be drained early in the process and bleeding arrested with pressure or, if necessary, with surgical ligation of the bleeding vessel. Considerable blood may be lost, and infection is a serious complication. Also spelled **haematoma.**

**-hematoma,** combining form meaning a 'swelling containing blood': *cephalhematoma, episiohematoma, othematoma.*

**hematometra** /hē'mətōmē'trə/, an accumulation of blood or menstrual fluid in the uterine cavity.

**hematometry** /hem'ətom'ətrē/, an examination of a blood sample to determine the number, type, and properties of blood cells and platelets and the amount of hemoglobin.

**hematomyelia** /hē'mətōmē'lē·ə/ [Gk, *haima + meylos,* marrow], the appearance of frank blood in the fluid of the spinal cord. Also spelled **haematomyelia.**

**hematopathology.** See **hemopathology.**

**hematopericardium.** See **hemopericardium.**

**hematoperitoneum** /-per'itənē'əm/ [Gk, *haima,* blood, *peri,* near, *tenein,* to stretch], the effusion of blood into the peritoneal cavity.

**hematophagous** /hem'ətof'əgəs/, **1.** pertaining to the feeding on blood by insects or other parasites. **2.** the destruction of erythrocytes by phagocytes.

**hematopoiesis** /hē'mətōpō·ē'sis, hem'-/ [Gk, *haima + poiein,* to make], the normal formation and development of blood cells in the bone marrow. In severe anemia and other hematologic disorders, cells may be produced in organs outside the marrow (extramedullary hematopoiesis). See also **erythropoiesis. —hematopoietic,** *adj.*

**hematopoietic growth factor** /-pō·et'ik/, one of a group of proteins, including erythropoietin, interleukins, and colony-stimulating factors, that promote the proliferation of blood cells.

**hematopoietic malignancies,** diseases such as leukemia that arise as a result of unregulated clonal proliferation of stem cells.

**hematopoietic stem cell,** an actively dividing cell that is the source of blood cells.

**hematopoietic syndrome,** a group of clinical features associated with effects of radiation on the blood and lymph tissues. It is characterized by nausea and vomiting, anorexia, lethargy, hemolysis and destruction of the bone marrow, and atrophy of the spleen and lymph nodes.

**hematopoietic system** [Gk, *haima,* blood, *poiein,* to make; L, *systema*], body organs and tissues involved in the formation and functioning of blood elements. It includes the bone marrow and spleen.

**hematoporphyrinuria** /-pôr'firinŏŏr'ē·ə/, the presence of elevated levels of hematoporphyrin in the urine that results from destruction of lysis of erythrocytes. It causes a dark coloration in the urine.

**hematospermia** /-spur'mē·ə/, the presence of blood in the semen. Causes include vascular congestion, infection of the seminal vesicles, coitus interruptus, sexual abstinence, and frequent coitus. The condition is rarely serious and may respond to antibiotic therapy.

**hematothorax.** See **hemothorax.**

**hematoxylin-eosin** /hē'mətok'silin/ [*Haematoxylon campechianum,* logwood; Gk, *eos,* dawn], a stain commonly used to treat tissue sections on microscope slides.

**hematuria** /hē'mətŏŏr'ē·ə, hem'-/ [Gk, *haima + ouron,* urine], abnormal presence of blood in the urine. It is symptomatic of many renal diseases and disorders of the genitourinary system. Microscopic examination of the urine,

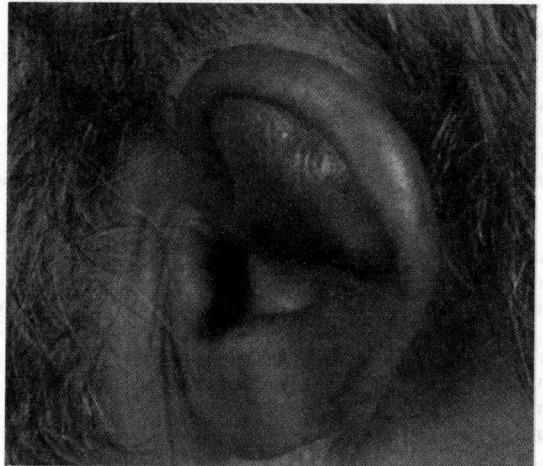

**Hematoma** *(Bingham, Hawke, and Kwok, 1992)*

culture and sensitivity of the urine, and physical examination of the patient are usually performed. Also spelled **haematuria.** **—hematuric,** *adj.*

**heme** /hēm/ [Gk, *haima,* blood], the pigmented iron-containing nonprotein part of the hemoglobin molecule. There are four heme groups in a hemoglobin molecule, each consisting of a cyclic structure of four pyrrole residues, called protoporphyrin, and an atom of iron in the center. Heme binds and carries oxygen in the red blood cells, releasing it to tissues that give off excess amounts of $CO_2$. Also called **haeme.** See also **hemoglobin, porphobilinogen, protoporphyrin.**

**hemeralopia** /hem′ərəlō′pē·ə/ [Gk, *hemera,* day, *alaos,* blind, *ops,* eye], an abnormal visual condition in which bright light causes blurring of vision. Hemeralopia is an unpleasant side effect of certain anticonvulsant medications, including trimethadione, prescribed in treatment of children with petit mal epilepsy. Also called **day blindness, night sight.** **—hemeralopic,** *adj.*

**hemi-,** prefix meaning 'half': *hemiplegia, hemiataxia, hemiopia.*

**-hemia.** See **-emia.**

**hemiacephalus** /hem′ē·āsef′ələs/ [Gk, *hemi,* half, *a,* without, + *kephale,* head], a fetus in which the brain and most of the cranium are lacking. See also **anencephaly.**

**hemiachromatosia** /hem′ē·ak′rōmətō′zhə/, a state of being color-blind in only one half of the visual field.

**hemialgia** /hem′ē·al′jē·ə/, pain that affects one side of the body.

**hemiamblyopia** /hem′ē·am′blē·ō′pē·ə/ [Gk, *hemi,* half, *amblys,* dull, *ops,* eye], blindness in half of the normal visual field. Also called **hemianopia.**

**hemianalgesia** /hem′ē·an′əljē′sē·ə/ [Gk, *hemi,* half, *a,* without, + *algos,* pain], a loss of feeling or sensitivity to pain affecting half of the body or one side of the body.

**hemianesthesia** /hem′ē·an′esthē′zhə/ [Gk, *hemi* + *anaisthesia,* absence of feeling], a loss of feeling on one side of the body.

**hemianopia.** See **hemiamblyopia.**

**hemianopsia.** See **hemiamblyopia.**

**hemiarthroplasty** /hem′ē·är′thrəplas′tē/, a surgical procedure for repair of an injured or diseased hip joint. It involves replacing the head of the femur with a prosthesis without reconstruction of the acetabulum.

**hemiataxia** /hem′ē·ətak′sē·ə/, a loss of muscle control affecting one side of the body, usually as a result of a stroke or cerebellar injury. The condition may be ipsilateral or contralateral.

**hemiazygous vein** /hem′ē·əzī′gəs/ [Gk, *hemi* + *a,* without, + *zygon,* yoke], one of the tributaries of the azygous vein of the thorax. It starts in the left ascending lumbar vein, enters the thorax through the left crus of the diaphragm, ascends on the left side of the vertebral column as high as the ninth thoracic vertebra, and passes dorsal to the aorta to enter the azygous. The hemiazygous vein receives about four of the caudal intercostal veins, the left subcostal vein, and some of the esophageal and mediastinal veins.

**hemiballismus.** See **ballism.**

**hemiblock,** a failure to conduct a cardiac impulse down one division of the left bundle branch, such as an anterior superior or a posterior inferior hemiblock.

**hemic** /hem′ik, hē′mik/, pertaining to blood. Also **hematic.**

**hemicellulose** /hem′ēsel′yo̅o̅lōs/ [Gk, *hemi* + L, *cellula,* little cell], any of a group of polysaccharides that constitute the chief part of the skeletal substances of the cell walls of plants. They resemble cellulose but are soluble and more easily extracted and decomposed. See also **dietary fiber.**

**hemicephalia** /-sefā′lyə/ [Gk, *hemi* + *kephale,* head], a congenital anomaly characterized by the absence of half of the cerebrum, caused by severe arrest of brain development in the fetus. The cerebellum and basal ganglia may be present in rudimentary form.

**hemicephalus** [Gk, *hemi,* half, *kephale,* head], a fetus with congenital absence of half of the cerebrum.

**hemicolectomy** /hem′i·kō·lek′tə·me/ [Gk, *hemi* half + *kolon,* colon + *ektome,* excision], excision of approximately half of the colon.

**hemicrania** /-krā′nē·ə/ [Gk, *hemi* + *kranion,* skull], **1.** a headache, usually migraine, that affects only one side of the head. **2.** a congenital anomaly characterized by the absence of half of the skull in the fetus; incomplete anencephaly.

**hemicraniectomy** /-kran′ē·ek′təmē/ [Gk, *hemi,* half, *kranion,* skull, *ektomē,* excision], a surgical procedure in which part or all of one half of the skull is excised and reflected as a preliminary step to certain types of brain operations.

**hemidiaphragm** /-dī′əfram/, either the left or right functional half of the diaphragm. Although the diaphragm is a single anatomic unit, it is divided by the union of its central tendon and the pericardium into separate leaves, each with its own nerve supply, and each hemidiaphragm can function independently.

**hemidystrophy** /-dis′trəfē/, a condition in which the two sides of the body do not develop equally.

**hemiectromelia** /hem′ē·ek′trōmē′lyə/ [Gk, *hemi* + *ektosis,* miscarriage, *melos,* limb], a congenital anomaly characterized by the incomplete development of the limbs on one side of the body. **—hemiectromelus,** *n.*

**hemiepilepsy** /hem′ē·ep′əlepsē/, a form of epilepsy that affects only one side of the body.

**hemifacial spasm.** See **convulsive tic.**

**hemigastrectomy** /-gastrek′təmē/, surgical removal of one half of the body of the stomach.

**hemiglossal** /-glos′əl/, pertaining to one side of the tongue. Also **hemilingual.**

**hemignathia** /hem′ēnā′thē·ə/ [Gk, *hemi* + *gnathos,* jaw], **1.** a congenital anomaly characterized by incomplete development of the lower jaw on one side of the face. **2.** a condition of having only one jaw. **—hemignathus,** *n.*

**hemihyperplasia** /-hī′pərplā′zhə/ [Gk, *hemi* + *hyper,* excessive, *plassein,* to form], overdevelopment or excessive growth of half of a specific organ or part or all of the organs and parts on one side of the body.

**hemihypertonia** /-hī′pərtō′nē·ə/ [Gk, *hemi* + *hyper* + *tonikos,* stretching], exaggerated tension in the muscles on one side of the body, causing tonic contraction. In one form of the disorder, tonic spasms may occur occasionally in different muscle groups on one side of the body.

**hemihypertrophy** /-hīpur′trəfē/ [Gk, *hemi* + *hyper* + *trophe,* nourishment], an unusual enlargement or overgrowth of half of the body or half of a body part.

**hemihypoplasia** /-hī′pōplā′zhə/ [Gk, *hemi* + *hypo,* under, *plassein,* to form], partial or incomplete development of half of a specific organ or part or all of the organs and parts on one side of the body.

**hemikaryon.** See **diploid nucleus.**

**hemilaminectomy** /hem′i·lam′i·nek′tə·me/ [Gk, *hemi,* half; L, *lamina,* plate; Gk, *ektome,* excision], surgical removal of one side of the vertebral lamina.

**hemilateral** /-lat′ərəl/, pertaining to one side.

**hemilingual.** See **hemiglossal.**

**hemimelia** /-mē′lyə/ [Gk, *hemi* + *melos*], a developmental anomaly characterized by the absence or gross shortening of the lower portion of one or more of the limbs. The condition may involve either or both of the bones of the distal arm or leg and is designated according to which is absent or defective, as fibular, radial, tibial, or ulnar hemimelia. See also **ectromelia, phocomelia.**

**hemiopia** /hem′ē·ō′pē·ə/ [Gk, *hemi,* half, *ops,* eye], a condition involving only one eye or half the visual field.

**hemipagus** /hemip′əgəs/ [Gk, *hemi* + *pagos,* fixture], symmetric twins who are conjoined at the thorax.

**hemiparesis** /-pərē′sis/ [Gk, *hemi* + *paralyein,* to be palsied], muscular weakness of one half of the body.

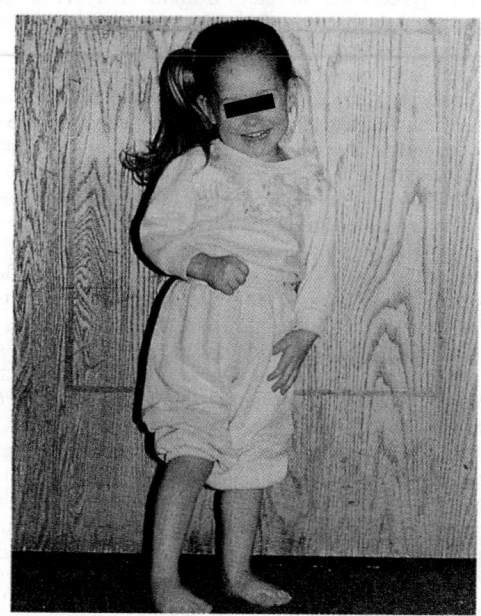

**Posture typical in hemiparesis** *(Zitelli and Davis, 1997)*

**hemiparesthesia** /-per′esthē′zhə/ [Gk, *hemi,* half, *para,* beside, *aisthesis,* sensation], a numbness or other abnormal or impaired sensation that is experienced on only one side of the body.

**hemiplegia** /hem′iplē′jə/ [Gk, *hemi* + *plege,* stroke], paralysis of one side of the body. Kinds of hemiplegia include **cerebral hemiplegia, facial hemiplegia,** and **spastic hemiplegia.** Compare **diplegia, paraplegia, quadriplegia.** —**hemiplegic,** *adj.*

**hemiplegic gait** /-plē′jik/ [Gk, *hemi,* half, *plege,* stroke; ONorse, *gata,* a way], a manner of walking in which an affected limb moves in a semicircle with each step.

**hemisection** /-sek′shən/ [Gk, *hemi,* half; L, *sectare,* to cut], half of a body or other object divided along a longitudinal plane, producing two lateral halves; bisection.

**hemisomus** /hem′isō′məs/ [Gk, *hemi* + *soma,* body], a fetus or individual in whom one side of the body is malformed, defective, or absent.

**hemisphere** /hem′isfir/ [Gk, *hemi* + *sphaira,* sphere], **1.** one half of a sphere or globe. **2.** the lateral half of the cerebrum or of the cerebellum. —**hemispherical,** *adj.*

**hemiteras** /hem′ēter′əs/, *pl.* **hemiterata** [Gk, *hemi* + *teras,* monster], any individual with a congenital malformation that is not so severe or disabling as to be classified as a teratic condition. —**hemiteratic,** *adj.*

**hemithorax** /-thôr′aks/, one side of the chest.

**hemithyroidectomy** /-thī′roidek′təmē/, surgical removal of one lobe of the thyroid gland.

**hemivertebra** /-vur′təbrə/, an abnormal condition characterized by the congenital failure of a vertebra to develop completely. It is possibly caused by the complete failure of the growth center of one vertebral body. Usually half of the vertebra involved is completely or partially developed, and the other half is absent. One or more vertebrae may be involved; the different conditions produce varying degrees of balanced or unbalanced scoliosis. As a result of the developmental abnormality of the spine, a wedge-shaped vertebra develops, and adjacent vertebral bodies expand to fit the deformity or tilt to accommodate wedge-shaped articulation. Hemivertebra may be classified according to the degree of developmental failure of involved vertebral growth centers. When two vertebral bodies are involved and growth centers on the same side fail to develop, moderate to severe unbalanced congenital scoliosis results; when growth centers fail to develop on opposite sides, balanced congenital scoliosis results. Singular hemivertebra may cause few if any signs and symptoms. Depending on the degree of congenital scoliosis involved, any associated deformity may become more apparent with growth. Other types of hemivertebra, especially those involving unbalanced congenital scoliosis, usually progress markedly with growth and have a relatively poor prognosis unless early spinal fusion prevents further spinal curvature. No treatment may be required for the form of the condition associated with balanced congenital scoliosis.

**hemizygote** /-zī′gōt/ [Gk, *hemi* + *zygon,* yoke], an individual, organism, or cell that has only one allele for a specific characteristic. The trait specified by the allele is expressed regardless of whether the allele is dominant or recessive. Such alleles include those on the single X chromosome in males, which have no corresponding alleles on the Y chromosome. —**hemizygosity,** *n.,* **hemizygous, hemizygotic,** *adj.*

**hemlock,** the common name for *Conium maculatum,* a plant indigenous to most of Europe and the source of a poisonous alkaloid, coniine. An extract of the leaves and flowers of conium has been used as a respiratory sedative; its hydrochloride salts have been used as an antispasmodic. Also called **conium.**

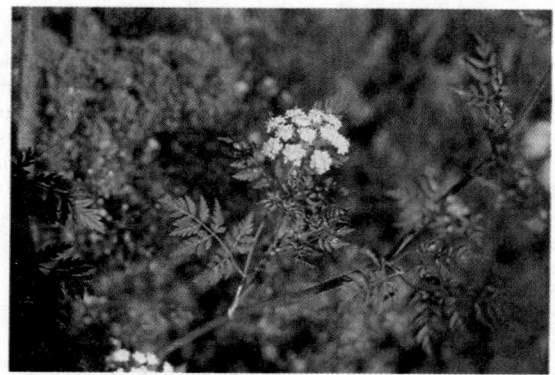

**Poison hemlock** *(Auerbach, 1995)*

**Hemlock Society,** a group who provide information about euthanasia and suicide for terminally ill patients.

**hemo-** /hē′mō-, hem′ō-/, prefix relating to blood or blood vessels.

**hemoagglutination.** See **hemagglutination.**

**hemoagglutinin.** See **hemagglutinin.**

**hemobilinuria** /hē'mōbil'inŏŏr'ē·ə/, the presence of the brown pigment urobilin in the blood and urine.

**hemoblastic leukemia.** See **stem cell leukemia.**

**hemochromatosis** /hē'mōkrō'mətō'sis, hem'-/ [Gk, *haima,* blood, *chroma,* color, *osis,* condition], a rare disease of iron metabolism, characterized by excess iron deposits throughout the body. Hepatomegaly, skin pigmentation, diabetes mellitus, and cardiac failure may occur. The disease most often develops as a complication of a hemolytic anemia such as sickle cell anemia. Multiple blood transfusions are required for treatment. Also spelled **haemochromatosis.** Compare **hemosiderosis.** See also **iron metabolism, siderosis, thalassemia.**

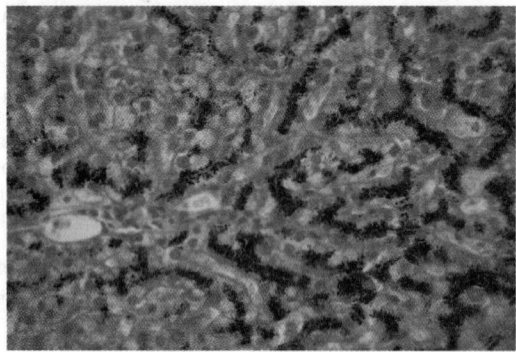

**Genetic hemochromatosis**
*(Kumar, Cotran, and Robbins, 1997)*

**hemoclip,** a malleable metal clip used to ligate small blood vessels during surgery and to mark the location of body structures in radiographic procedures.

**hemoconcentration** /-kon'səntrā'shən/ [Gk, *haima* + L, *cum,* together with, *centrum,* center], an increase in the number of red blood cells resulting from either a decrease in plasma volume or increased production of erythrocytes. Also spelled **haemoconcentration.**

**hemocyanin** /hē'mōsī'ənin/, an oxygen-carrying protein molecule present in certain lower animals, particularly arthropods and mollusks. The molecule is similar to the hemoglobin molecule of human blood but uses copper atoms, rather than iron, and is less efficient than hemoglobin in requiring many more atoms to bind a single molecule of oxygen.

**hemocyte.** See **hematocyte, hematocytoblast.**

**hemocytoblast.** See **hematocytoblast.**

**hemocytoblastic leukemia.** See **stem cell leukemia.**

**hemocytology** /-sītol'əjē/ [Gk, *haima,* blood, *kytos,* cell, *logos,* science], the study of the components of blood.

**hemodiafiltration** /-dī'əfiltrā'shən/, a technique similar to hemofiltration, used to treat uremia by convective transport of the solute rather than diffusion.

**hemodialysis** /hē'mōdī·al'isis, hem'-/ [Gk, *haima* + *dia,* apart, *lysis,* loosening], a procedure in which impurities or wastes are removed from the blood. It is used in treating patients with renal failure and various toxic conditions. The patient's blood is shunted from the body through a machine for diffusion and ultrafiltration and then returned to the pa-

tient's circulation. Hemodialysis requires access to the patient's bloodstream, a mechanism for the transport of the blood to and from the dialyzer, and a dialyzer. Also spelled **haemodialysis.** See **arteriovenous fistula, external shunt.**

■ METHOD: Access may be achieved by an external shunt or an arteriovenous fistula. The external shunt is constructed by inserting two cannulas through the skin into a large vein and a large artery. When dialysis is not being performed, the cannulas are joined, allowing the blood to flow from artery to vein. When dialysis is being performed, the cannulas are separated, allowing the arterial blood to flow to the dialyzer and the dialyzed blood to return from the dialyzer to the circulation through the cannula in the vein. An arteriovenous fistula is created by the anastomosis of a large vein to an artery. Large-bore needles are threaded into superficial vessels enlarged by the increased flow caused by the fistula. Various dialyzers may be used. The procedure takes from 3 to 8 hours depending on patient's condition, weight gain, and laboratory values and may be necessary daily in acute conditions or two or three times a week in chronic renal failure.

■ INTERVENTIONS: A decrease in blood flow through the shunt may cause clotting; therefore any factor that may result in a slowing of the flow is to be avoided. Some of these factors are systemic hypotension, infection of the shunt or fistula, compression of the shunt or fistula, thrombophlebitis, and prolonged inflation of a blood pressure cuff. Infection is prevented in the area around an external shunt by placing a sterile dressing over the shunt and changing the dressing daily. Before the procedure is begun, the patient is told how long it will take, what pain or discomfort may be expected, what will be felt afterward, what food or activity will be allowed during the procedure, and whether family or friends may be present during treatment. Headache, nausea, and muscle cramps are common, especially during the procedure and for a few hours afterward. The patient usually feels best on the day after hemodialysis. Rest, an antiemetic, and a mild analgesic may make the procedure more comfortable. Most patients need emotional support and some physical assistance during hemodialysis. The physical status of the patient is monitored frequently throughout; blood pressure, pulse, and blood tests for electrolyte and acid-base balance are performed. Normal saline solution may be administered to counteract hypotension that results from rapid removal of fluid from the intravascular compartment. The patient is weighed before and after the treatment to determine the amount of fluid lost during the procedure. An anticoagulant is usually given to prevent coagulation of the blood in the dialyzer, cannulas, or catheters; to prevent hemorrhage protamine sulfate may be administered after the procedure to reverse the effect of the anticoagulant. Any treatment that causes tissue trauma, such as dental extraction, venipuncture, or intramuscular injection, is not recommended during or immediately after dialysis.

■ OUTCOME CRITERIA: Infection and clotting of the shunt and erosion of the skin around the shunt are frequent complications with an external shunt; therefore the method that uses an arteriovenous fistula is more common. The discomfort before, during, and just after dialysis; the prolonged time of relative immobility during the procedure; and the dietary restrictions necessary in renal insufficiency all cause considerable stress in the patient. Adjustments in the patterns of daily life are necessary and require the assistance of professionals with experience and training.

**hemodialysis technician,** a registered health professional who has received special training in the operation of hemodialysis equipment and treatment of patients with kidney disorders.

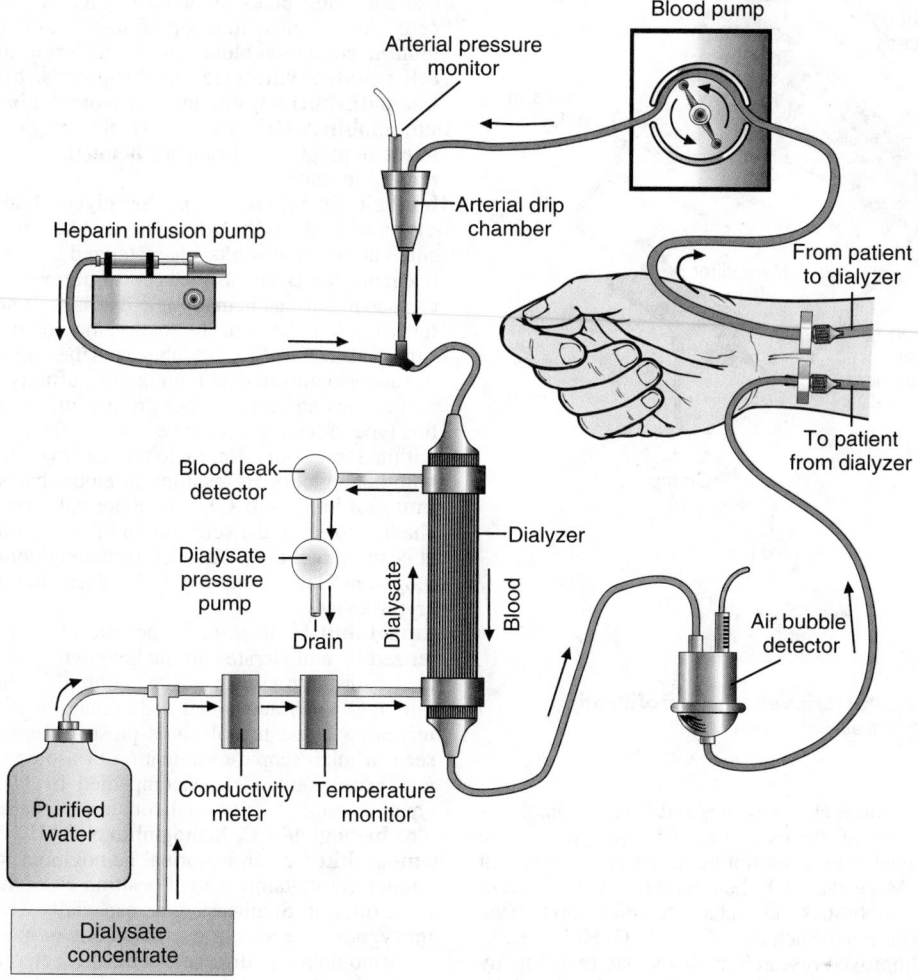

**Hemodialysis** *(Lewis, Heitkemper, and Dirksen, 2000)*

**hemodialysis therapy,** a nursing intervention from the Nursing Interventions Classification (NIC) defined as management of extracorporeal passage of the patient's blood through a dialyzer. See also **Nursing Interventions Classification.**

**hemodialyzer.** See **dialyzer.**

**hemodilution** /-dilōō′shən/ [Gk, *haima,* blood; L, *diluare,* to wash away], a condition in which the concentration of erythrocytes or other blood elements is lowered, usually resulting from an increase in plasma volume. Also spelled **haemodilution.**

**hemodynamic regulation,** a nursing intervention from the Nursing Interventions Classification (NIC) defined as optimization of heart rate, preload, afterload, and contractility. See also **Nursing Interventions Classification.**

**hemodynamics** /-dīnam′iks/ [Gk, *haima* + *dynamis,* force], the study of the physical aspects of blood circulation, including cardiac function and peripheral vascular physiologic characteristics.

**Hemofil M,** trademark for human antihemophilic factor.

**hemofiltration** /-filtrā′shən/, a type of hemodialysis in which there is convective transport of the solute through ul-

trafiltration across the membrane. It is reported to be more effective than diffusion in removing higher-molecular-weight solutes from the blood, particularly in the treatment of uremia. Also spelled **haemofiltration.**

**hemofiltration therapy,** a nursing intervention from the Nursing Interventions Classification (NIC) defined as cleansing of acutely ill patient's blood via a hemofilter controlled by the patient's hydrostatic pressure. See also **Nursing Interventions Classification.**

**hemoglobin (Hb)** /hē′məglō′bən/ [Gk, *haima* + L, *globus,* ball], a complex protein-iron compound in the blood that carries oxygen to the cells from the lungs and carbon dioxide away from the cells to the lungs. Each erythrocyte contains 200 to 300 molecules of hemoglobin, each molecule of hemoglobin contains four groups of heme, and each group of heme can carry one molecule of oxygen. A hemoglobin molecule contains four globin polypeptide chains composed of amino acids. Each polypeptide chain is composed of 141 to 146 amino acids; the absence, replacement, or addition of only one amino acid modifies the properties of the hemoglobin. Different kinds of hemoglobin are identified by their specific combination of polypeptide chains; those found

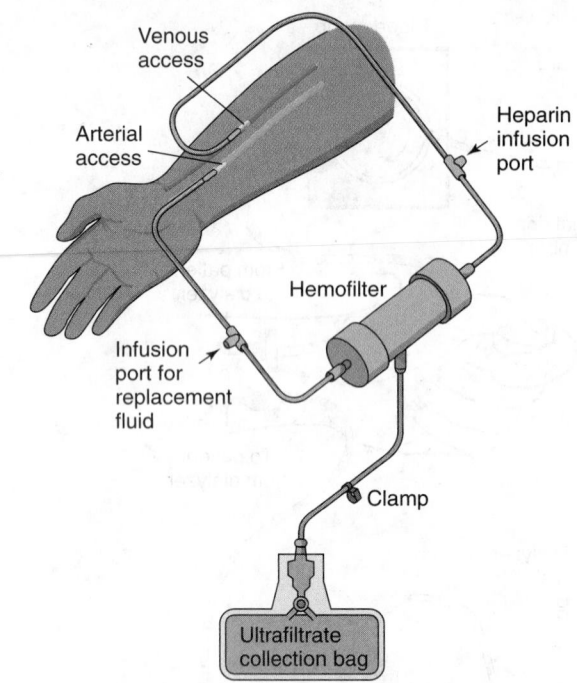

**Continuous arteriovenous hemofiltration**
*(Beare and Myers, 1998)*

most often are α and β chains with γ and δ being found less often. The number of chains of the different types in the molecule is indicated by subscript numerals and superscript capital letters. More than 100 hemoglobins with different electrophoretic mobilities and characteristics have been identified and classified, such as S, C, D, E, G, H, I, J, K, L, M, N, and O. Improved research methods may reveal many more. The normal concentrations of hemoglobin in the blood are 12 to 16 g/dL in women and 13.5 to 18 g/dL in men. In an atmosphere of high oxygen concentration, such as in the lungs, hemoglobin binds with oxygen to form oxyhemoglobin. In an atmosphere of low oxygen concentration, such as in the peripheral tissues of the body, oxygen is replaced by carbon dioxide to form carboxyhemoglobin. Hemoglobin releases the carboxyhemoglobin in the lungs for

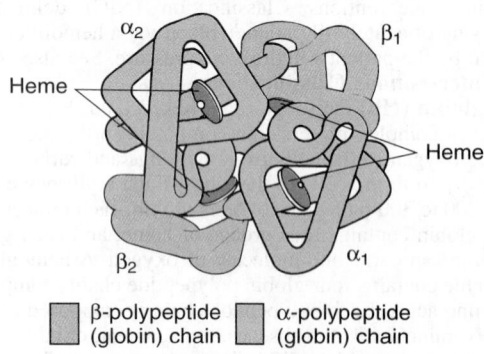

| β-polypeptide (globin) chain | α-polypeptide (globin) chain |

**Molecular structure of hemoglobin**
*(Huether and McCance, 2000)*

excretion and picks up more oxygen for transport to the cells. Also spelled **haemoglobin.** See also **carboxyhemoglobin, complete blood count, differential white blood cell count, erythrocyte, erythropoiesis, heme, hemoglobinopathy, hemolysin,** and **oxyhemoglobin.**

**hemoglobin A (Hb A),** a normal hemoglobin. Also called **adult hemoglobin.** Compare **hemoglobin F.** See also **hemoglobinopathy.**

**Hemoglobin $A_{1e}$ (Hb $A_{1e}$).** See **glycosylated hemoglobin.**

**hemoglobin $A_2$ (Hb $A_2$),** a normal hemoglobin present in small amounts in adults, characterized by the substitution of δ chains for β chains. Its concentration in the blood increases in various hematologic diseases. It normally constitutes 1.5% to 3.5% of the total hemoglobin.

**hemoglobin Bart's,** an abnormal hemoglobin composed of four γ chains having high oxygen affinity, seen in Southeast Asians and a few other groups; infants born with only this type of hemoglobin have hydrops fetalis and usually die within a few hours. Hemoglobin Bart's is often found mixed with hemoglobin H, resulting in alpha-thalassemia.

**hemoglobin C (Hb C),** an abnormal type of hemoglobin characterized by the substitution of lysine for glutamic acid at position 6 of the β chain of the hemoglobin molecule. Hemoglobin C moves slowly and reduces the plasticity of the erythrocytes.

**hemoglobin C disease,** a genetic blood disorder characterized by a moderate chronic hemolytic anemia and associated with the presence of hemoglobin C. Hemoglobin C is inherited as an autosomal codominant gene. No anemia or increased blood hemolysis is present. Target cells may be seen in microscopic examination of a blood smear. Abnormal hemoglobin C is accompanied by an approximately equal amount of its normal counterpart, hemoglobin A. See also **hemoglobin C, hemoglobin S-C (Hb S-C) disease.**

**hemoglobin E,** an abnormal hemoglobin with lysine substituted for glutamic acid at position 26 of the β chain, seen most often in Southeast Asia, especially Thailand. The homozygous state may be asymptomatic or may be manifested as hemoglobin E disease, while the heterozygous state is clinically silent.

**hemoglobin E disease** [Gk, *haima,* blood; L, *globus,* ball; E; Gk, *dis,* not; Fr, *aise,* ease], a mild form of anemia caused by a genetic abnormality of the hemoglobin molecule. Worldwide it is the third most common form of hemoglobin disorder, primarily affecting people of Southeast Asian and African descent.

**hemoglobin electrophoresis,** a test to identify various abnormal hemoglobins in the blood, including certain genetic disorders, such as sickle cell anemia.

**hemoglobinemia** /hē′mōglō′binē′mē·ə, hem′-/, presence of free hemoglobin in the blood plasma.

**hemoglobin F (Hb F),** the normal hemoglobin of the fetus. Most Hb F is replaced by hemoglobin A in the first days after birth. Hb F has an increased capacity to carry oxygen and is present in increased amounts in some pathologic conditions, including sickle cell anemia, aplastic anemia, and leukemia. Small amounts are produced throughout life.

**hemoglobin G,** any of various abnormal hemoglobins with an amino acid substitution on the α chain; the most common one is hemoglobin G Philadelphia, which causes alpha-thalassemia.

**hemoglobin Gower,** a normal hemoglobin present in early embryonic life and disappearing before birth; it occasionally consists entirely of epsilon chains ($\epsilon_4$), but the usual forms are *hemoglobin Gower-1,* consisting of two zeta and two epsilon chains ($\zeta_2\epsilon_2$), and *hemoglobin Gower-2,* consisting of two alpha and two epsilon chains ($\alpha_2\epsilon_2$).

**hemoglobin H,** a rapidly migrating abnormal hemoglobin composed of four β chains, having a high oxygen affinity, found mainly in Southeast Asians, natives of the Mediterranean region, and a few other ethnic groups. Infants may be born with a mixture of hemoglobin H and hemoglobin Bart's.

**hemoglobin H disease,** alpha-thalassemia in individuals heterozygous for hemoglobin H, characterized by chronic hemolytic anemia associated with splenomegaly; red blood cell hypochromia, anisocytosis, and poikilocytosis are accompanied by inclusion bodies detectable by supravital staining.

**hemoglobin Kansas,** an abnormal hemoglobin with threonine substituted for asparagine at position 102 of the β chain, resulting in decreased oxygen affinity and cyanosis.

**hemoglobin Kenya,** an abnormal type of hemoglobin in which the non-α chain has a γ chain portion at the N terminus and a β chain portion at the C terminus, resulting in beta-thalassemia.

**hemoglobin Köln,** an unstable hemoglobin that has methionine substituted for valine at position 95 of the β chain, usually resulting in hemolytic anemia with Heinz bodies in the erythrocytes.

**hemoglobin M,** any of several abnormal hemoglobins having amino acid substitutions in the α or β chains and all associated with methemoglobinemia.

**hemoglobin M disease** [Gk, *haima,* blood; L, *globus,* ball; *M;* Gk, *dis,* not; Fr, *aise,* ease], a type of anemia in which part of the hemoglobin contains iron in the $Fe^{+++}$ state and is unable to combine with oxygen. The patient may experience cyanosis but is able to function because part of the hemoglobin is normal. See **methemoglobin.**

**hemoglobinometer** /-om′ətər/ [Gk, *haima,* blood; L, *globus,* ball; Gk, *metron,* measure], any of several types of instruments designed to measure the percentage of hemoglobin in a blood sample. Some use colorimetric techniques, comparing the color of the blood sample with a standard red color. Also spelled **haemoglobinometer.**

**hemoglobinopathy** /hē′mōglō′binop′əthē, hem′-/ [Gk, *haima* + L, *globus,* ball; Gk, *pathos,* disease], a group of inherited disorders characterized by structural variations of the hemoglobin molecule. An abnormality may occur in the heterozygous or the homozygous form. The alteration appears as the substitution of one or more amino acids in the globin portion of the molecule at selected positions in the two alpha or two beta polypeptide chains. Although more than 100 variants have been described, only hemoglobins S, C, and D are commonly seen. In the heterozygous form the normal adult pigment, hemoglobin A, and the variant both appear in the red cell; little or no clinical manifestation of disease may be present. In the homozygous form only the variant hemoglobin is present, and the characteristic symptoms of that hemoglobinopathy appear. Mixed heterozygous forms are also known to occur. The normal hemoglobin A may be absent, and two or three hemoglobin variants may be present. Kinds of hemoglobinopathies include **hemoglobin C disease, hemoglobin S-C disease,** and **sickle cell anemia.** Compare **thalassemia.** Also spelled **haemoglobinopathy.** See also **hemoglobin, hemoglobin A, sickle cell thalassemia, sickle cell trait.**

**hemoglobin oxygen saturation,** a quantitative measure of volume of oxygen per volume of blood, depending on the grams of hemoglobin per deciliter of blood. For example, two samples of blood, one with hemoglobin at 15 g/dL and the other at 7.5 g/dL, may both be 96% saturated with oxygen, but the hemoglobin oxygen saturation will be greater in the 15 g/dL sample.

**hemoglobin Portland,** a normal hemoglobin present in the fetus late in the first trimester of pregnancy, consisting of zeta and gamma chains ($\zeta_2\gamma_2$); it disappears in utero.

**hemoglobin S (Hb S),** an abnormal type of hemoglobin, characterized by the substitution of the amino acid valine for glutamic acid in the β chain of the hemoglobin molecule. They move more slowly and are much less soluble than hemoglobin A. As the abnormal molecules become deoxygenated, because of decreased oxygen tension in the peripheral circulation, they become sickle-shaped, move slowly, clump together, and hemolyze. If the proportion of Hb S to Hb A is large, as in sickle cell anemia, local thrombosis and infarction may occur. See also **sickle cell anemia, sickle cell crisis, sickle cell trait.**

**hemoglobin saturation,** the amount of oxygen combined with hemoglobin in proportion to the amount of oxygen the hemoglobin is capable of carrying. It is expressed as a percentage of a ratio: content/capacity.

**hemoglobin SC (Hb SC) disease,** a genetic blood disorder in which two different abnormal alleles, one for hemoglobin S and one for hemoglobin C, are inherited. The disorder is characterized by a clinical course considerably less severe than that of sickle cell anemia despite the absence of normal hemoglobin. See also **hemoglobin C disease, sickle cell thalassemia.** Also called **sickle cell-hemoglobin C disease.**

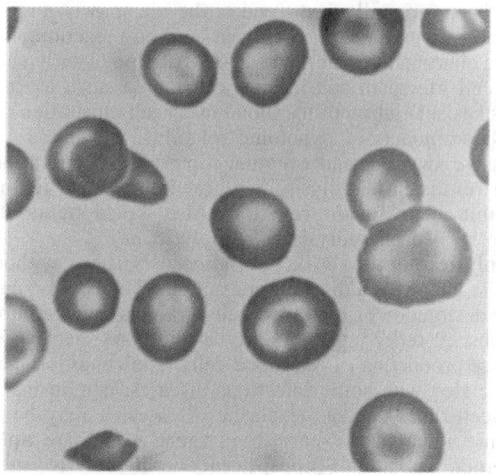

**Hemoglobin SC disease** *(Zitelli and Davis, 1997)*

**hemoglobin SD disease,** a genetically determined anemia in which the erythrocytes contain both hemoglobin S and hemoglobin D, with symptoms like those of mild sickle cell anemia. Also called **sickle cell−hemoglobin D disease.** See also **sickle cell anemia.**

**hemoglobin Seattle,** an abnormal hemoglobin in which glutamic acid replaces alanine at position 76 of the β chain, decreasing the hemoglobin molecule's affinity for oxygen.

**hemoglobin test (Hb, Hgb),** a blood test that measures the total amount of hemoglobin in the peripheral blood, which reflects the number of red blood cells in the blood. The test is normally performed as part of a complete blood count. Abnormal levels indicate anemia, erythrocytosis, and sickle cell disease, among others.

**hemoglobinuria** /-ŏŏr'ē·ə/ [Gk, *haima* + L, *globus,* ball; Gk, *ouron,* urine], abnormal presence in the urine of hemoglobin that is not attached to red blood cells. Hemoglobinuria can result from various autoimmune diseases or episodic hemolytic disorders. It can be diagnosed by using a dipstick reagent that is sensitive to free hemoglobin. Kinds of hemoglobinuria include **cold hemoglobinuria, march hemoglobinuria,** and **nocturnal hemoglobinuria.** Also spelled **haemoglobinuria. —hemoglobinuric,** *adj.*

**hemoglobinuric** /-ŏŏr'ik/ [Gk, *haima,* blood; L, *globus,* ball; Gk, *ouron,* urine], pertaining to the presence of hemoglobin in the urine.

**hemogram** /hē'məgram/ [Gk, *haima* + *gramma,* record], a written or graphic record of a differential blood count that emphasizes the size, shape, special characteristics, and numbers of the solid components of the blood. See also **complete blood count.**

**hemolysin** /himol'əsin/ [Gk, *haima* + *lysis,* loosening], any one of the numerous substances that lyse or dissolve red blood cells. Hemolysins are produced by bacterial strains, including staphylococci and streptococci, and are contained in venoms and vegetables. Bacterial hemolysins are divided into those that are filterable and those that cluster around the bacterial colony on a culture medium containing red blood cells. Hemolysins appear to aid the invasive power of bacteria. Also spelled **haemolysin.** See also **hemoglobin, hemolysis.**

**hemolysis** /himol'isis/ [Gk, *haima* + *lysis,* loosening], the breakdown of red blood cells and the release of hemoglobin that occur normally at the end of the life span of a red cell. Hemolysis may occur in antigen-antibody reactions, metabolic abnormalities of the red cell that significantly shorten red cell life span, and mechanical trauma, such as cardiac prosthesis. Dilution of the blood by IV administration of excessive amounts of hypotonic solutions, which cause progressive swelling and eventual rupture of the erythrocyte, also results in hemolysis. See also **hemolysin, hemolytic anemia, transfusion reaction.** Also called **hematolysis.** Also spelled **haemolysis. —hemolytic,** *adj.*

**hemolytic anemia** /-lit'ik/ [Gk, *haima* + *lysis* + *a,* without, + *haima,* blood], a disorder characterized by chronic premature destruction of red blood cells. Anemia may be minimal or absent, reflecting the ability of the bone marrow to increase production of red blood cells. The condition may be associated with some infectious diseases, certain inherited red-cell disorders, or neoplastic diseases, it may be a response to drugs or other toxic agents. Compare **aplastic anemia, congenital nonspherocytic hemolytic anemia, iron deficiency anemia, myelophthisic anemia.** Also spelled **haemolytic aenemia.** See also **anemia, hemolysis, spherocytosis.**

**hemolytic anemia of newborn.** See **erythroblastosis fetalis.**

**hemolytic antibody,** an antibody capable of dissolving red blood cells in the presence of complement.

**hemolytic jaundice,** a yellowish discoloration of the skin caused by a breakdown of red blood cells, which causes excessive amounts of bilirubin. See also **hyperbilirubinemia.**

**hemolytic jaundice of the newborn.** See **icterus gravis neonatorum.**

**hemolytic uremic syndrome,** a rare kidney disorder marked by renal failure, microangiopathic hemolytic anemia, and platelet deficiency. The syndrome, the cause of which is unknown, usually occurs in infancy. With conservative management including dialysis, most infants and children recover. The prognosis in adults is uncertain.

**hemopathology** /-pəthol'əjē/, the study of diseases of the blood. Also called **hematopathology.**

**hemoperfusion** /-pərfyōō'zhən/, the perfusion of blood through a sorbent device, such as activated charcoal or resin beads, rather than through dialysis equipment. Hemoperfusion may be used in treating uremia, liver failure, and certain forms of drug toxicity. Also spelled **haemoperfusion.**

**hemopericardium** /-per'ikär'dē·əm/ [Gk, *haima* + *peri,* near, *kardia,* heart], an accumulation of blood within the pericardial sac surrounding the heart. Also spelled **haemopericardium.** Also called **hematopericardium** /hē'mətō-per'ikär'dē·əm/.

**hemoperitoneum** /-per'itōnē'əm/ [Gk, *haima* + *peri,* around, *tenein,* to stretch], the presence of extravasated blood in the peritoneal cavity caused by surgical procedures, necrotizing tumors, fistulas, or laparoscopy procedures. Also spelled **haemoperitoneum.**

**hemophil** /hē'mōfil/ [Gk, *haima,* blood, *philein,* to love], bacteria of the genus *Haemophilus,* which thrive in culture media containing blood.

**hemophilia** /hē'mōfē'lyə, hem'-/ [Gk, *haima* + *philein,* to love], a group of hereditary bleeding disorders characterized by a deficiency of one of the factors necessary for coagulation of the blood. The two most common forms of the disorder are hemophilia A and hemophilia B. Hemophilia A (classic hemophilia) is the result of a deficiency or absence of antihemophilic factor VIII. Hemophilia B (Christmas disease) represents a deficiency of plasma thromboplastin component. The clinical severity of the disorder varies with the extent of the deficiency. Greater than usual loss of blood during dental procedures, epistaxis, hematoma, and hemarthrosis are common problems in patients with hemophilia. Severe nonsurgical internal hemorrhage and hematuria are less common. The primary objectives of nursing care are to prevent bleeding and to make the environment as safe as possible. The nurse teaches measures for controlling bleeding and for limiting local joint damage and ways that the patient can be physically active without danger of injury. The nurse also provides assistance in coping with the disorder, refers parents to genetic counselors and parent discussion groups and other available local resources, and provides home care. Also spelled **haemophilia.** See **von Willebrand's disease,** and see specific blood factors. **—hemophiliac,** *n.,* **hemophilic,** *adj.*

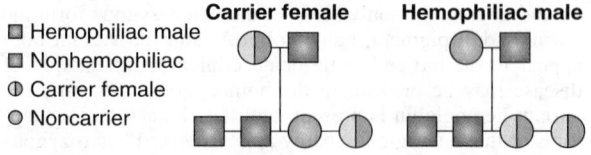

☐ Hemophiliac male
☐ Nonhemophiliac
◑ Carrier female
○ Noncarrier

**Carrier female**  **Hemophiliac male**

**Inheritance patterns in hemophilia**
*(Beare and Myers, 1998)*

**hemophilia A,** a hereditary blood disorder usually expressed in males that is transmitted as an X-linked recessive trait and caused by a deficiency of coagulation factor VIII. Hemophilia A is considered the classic type of hemophilia. See also **coagulation factor, hemophilia.**

**hemophilia B,** a hereditary blood disorder, transmitted as an X-linked recessive trait and caused by a deficiency of factor IX, the plasma thromboplastin component. The condition is clinically similar to but less severe than hemophilia A. Also called **Christmas disease.** See **coagulation factor, hemophilia.**

**hemophilia C,** a hereditary blood disorder, transmitted as an X-linked recessive trait and caused by a deficiency of factor XI, the plasma thromboplastin antecedent. The condition is clinically similar to but may be less severe than hemophilia A. Also called **Rosenthal's syndrome.** See also **coagulation factor, hemophilia.**

**hemophiliac** /-fē′lē·ak/ [Gk, *haima,* blood, *philein,* to love], a person who has inherited the bleeding disease **hemophilia.** Also spelled **haemophiliac.**

**hemophilic.** See **hemophilia.**

**hemopneumopericardium** /hē′mōnōō′mōper′ikär′dē·əm/ [Gk, *haima,* blood, *pneuma,* air, *kardia,* heart], an accumulation of blood and air in the pericardium. Also called **pneumohemopericardium.**

**hemopneumothorax** /hē′mōnōō′mōthôr′aks/ [Gk, *haima,* blood, *pneuma,* air, *thorax,* chest], an accumulation of blood and air in the pleural cavity.

**hemopoietic** /hē′mōpō·et′ik, hem′-/ [Gk, *haima + poiein,* to make], related to the process of formation and development of the various types of blood cells. Also spelled **haemopoietic.**

**hemoptysis** /himop′tisis/ [Gk, *haima + ptyein,* to spit], coughing up of blood from the respiratory tract. Blood-streaked sputum often is present in minor upper respiratory infections or bronchitis. More profuse bleeding may indicate *Aspergillus* infection, lung abscess, tuberculosis, or bronchogenic carcinoma, in which the exsanguination (blood loss) is caused by erosion of the pulmonary vessels by the tumor. The patient should be informed that hemoptysis is normal after some endoscopic procedures to prevent worry. Radiographic examination, endoscopy, and bronchoscopy are often used to diagnose hemoptysis. Also spelled **haemoptysis.**

**hemorheology** /-rē·ol′əjē/ [Gk, *haima,* blood, *rhoia,* flow, *logos,* science], the study of the effects of blood flow on the cellular components of blood and walls of blood vessels. Also spelled **hemorrheology.**

**hemorrhage** /hem′ərij/ [Gk, *haima + rhegnynei,* to gush], a loss of a large amount of blood in a short period, either externally or internally. Hemorrhage may be arterial, venous, or capillary.

■ OBSERVATIONS: Symptoms of massive hemorrhage are related to hypovolemic shock: rapid, thready pulse; thirst; cold, clammy skin; sighing respirations; dizziness; syncope; pallor; apprehension; restlessness; and hypotension. If bleeding is contained within a cavity or joint, pain will develop as the capsule or cavity is stretched by the rapidly expanding volume of blood.

■ INTERVENTIONS: Effort is directed to stopping the hemorrhage. If hemorrhage is external, pressure is applied directly to the wound or to the appropriate pressure points. The part of the body that is wounded may be elevated. Ice, applied directly to the wound, may slow bleeding by causing vasoconstriction. Body temperature may be maintained by keeping the person covered and flat. If an extremity is wounded, and if the bleeding is severe, a tourniquet may be applied proximal to the wound. Also spelled **haemorrhage. —hemorrhagic,** *adj.*

**hemorrhage control,** a nursing intervention from the Nursing Interventions Classification (NIC) defined as reduction or elimination of rapid and excessive blood loss. See also **Nursing Interventions Classification.**

**hemorrhagic diathesis** /-raj′ik/, an inherited predisposition to any of a number of abnormalities characterized by excessive bleeding. See also **Fanconi's syndrome, hemophilia, von Willebrand's disease.**

**hemorrhagic disease of newborn,** a bleeding disorder of neonates that is usually caused by a deficiency of vitamin K. Also spelled **haemorrhagic disease of the newborn.**

**hemorrhagic familial angiomatosis.** See **Osler-Weber-Rendu syndrome.**

**hemorrhagic fever,** a group of viral infections characterized by fever, chills, headache, malaise, and respiratory or GI symptoms, followed by capillary hemorrhages and in severe infection by oliguria, kidney failure, hypotension, and possibly death. Many forms of the disease occur in specific geographic areas. See also **Ebola virus disease, Lassa fever, Marburg virus disease.**

**hemorrhagic gastritis,** a form of acute gastritis usually caused by a toxic agent, such as alcohol, aspirin or other drugs, or bacterial toxins that irritate the lining of the stomach. Nausea, vomiting, and epigastric distress may persist after the irritant is removed. Treatment is symptomatic; the nurse usually includes identification of the irritant and dietary counseling for a patient with hemorrhagic gastritis.

**hemorrhagic infarct** [Gk, *haima,* blood, *rhegnynei,* to gush; L, *infarcire,* to stuff], an area of necrosis that has accumulated so much blood that it resembles a red, swollen bruise.

**hemorrhagic jaundice** [Gk, *haima,* blood, *rhegnynei,* to gush; Fr, *jaune,* yellow], a form of jaundice that occurs in **Weil's syndrome** or other forms of **leptospirosis** in which capillary injury and anemia are present.

**hemorrhagic lung.** See **adult respiratory distress syndrome.**

**hemorrhagic measles** [Gk, *haima,* blood, *rhegnynei,* to gush; ME, *masalas*], a severe form of measles characterized by bleeding into the skin and mucous membranes. See also **black measles.**

**hemorrhagic pericarditis** [Gk, *haima,* blood, *rhegnynei,* to gush, *peri,* near, *kardia,* heart, *itis,* inflammation], inflammation of the pericardium accompanied by a bloody effusion. The condition is frequently caused by tuberculosis or a tumor.

**hemorrhagic plague** [Gk, *haima,* blood, *rhegnynei,* to gush; L, *plaga,* stroke], a severe form of bubonic plague in which bleeding occurs under the skin. Also called **black plague, bubonic plague.**

**hemorrhagic pleurisy** [Gk, *haima,* blood, *rhegnynei,* to gush, *pleuritis*], an inflammation of the pleura in which effusion of blood into the tissues occurs.

**hemorrhagic purpura** [Gk, *haima,* blood, *rhegnynei,* to gush; L, *purpura,* purple], a form of purpura associated with thrombocytopenia and prolonged bleeding time. Also called **thrombopenic purpura, thrombocytopenic purpura.**

**hemorrhagic scurvy.** See **infantile scurvy.**

**hemorrhagic shock,** shock associated with the sudden and rapid loss of significant amounts of blood. Severe traumatic injuries often cause such blood losses. This results in inadequate perfusion to meet the metabolic demands of cellular function. Death occurs within a relatively short time unless transfusion quickly restores normal blood volume. Hemorrhagic shock often accompanies secondary shock. Compare **primary shock.**

**hemorrhagic urticaria** [Gk, *haima,* blood, *rhegnynei,* to gush; L, *urtica,* nettle], a skin eruption characterized by bleeding in the wheals, usually as a complication of another disease such as nephritis. In some cases the bleeding occurs first and the wheals become superimposed. Also called **urticaria hemorrhagica.**

**hemorrheology.** See **hemorheology.**

**hemorrhoid** /hem′əroid/ [Gk, *haima* + *rhoia*, flow], a varicosity in the lower rectum or anus caused by congestion in the veins of the hemorrhoidal plexus.

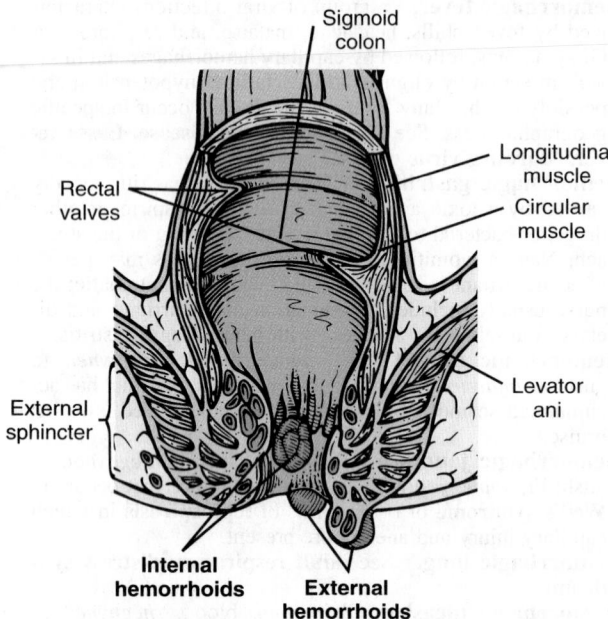

**Hemorrhoids** *(Lewis, Heitkemper, and Dirksen, 2000)*

■ OBSERVATIONS: Internal hemorrhoids originate above the internal sphincter of the anus. If they become large enough to protrude from the anus, they become constricted and painful. Small internal hemorrhoids may bleed with defecation. External hemorrhoids appear outside the anal sphincter. They are usually not painful, and bleeding does not occur unless a hemorrhoidal vein ruptures or thromboses.

■ INTERVENTIONS: Treatment includes local application of a topical medication to lubricate, anesthetize, and shrink the hemorrhoid; sitz baths and cold or hot compresses are also soothing. The hemorrhoids may require sclerosing by injection, ligation, or surgical excision. Ligation is increasingly the preferred treatment because it is simple and effective and does not require anesthesia. The hemorrhoid is grasped with a forceps, and a rubber band is slipped over the varicosity, causing tissue necrosis and sloughing of the hemorrhoid, usually within 1 week.

■ NURSING CONSIDERATIONS: Straining to defecate, constipation, and prolonged sitting contribute to the development of hemorrhoids. The client is counseled about ways to prevent these predisposing factors. Because pregnancy is associated with an increased incidence of hemorrhoids, pregnant women, as well as individuals who have cirrhosis of the liver, are advised to avoid constipation. Also spelled **haemorrhoid.**

**hemorrhoidal** /hem′əroi′dəl/ [Gk, *haimorrhois*, a vein that discharges blood], pertaining to or resembling hemorrhoids.

**hemorrhoidal tag,** an anal skin tag that was originally part of hemorrhoidal tissue.

**hemorrhoidectomy** /hem′əroidek′təmē/ [Gk, *haimorrhois*, a vein that discharges blood, *ektomē*, excision], a surgical procedure performed for excision of a hemorrhoid. Also spelled **haemorrhoidectomy.**

**hemosalpinx** /hē′mōsal′pinks/ [Gk, *haima*, blood, *salpinx*, tube], a collection of blood in a fallopian tube.

**hemosiderin** /hē′mōsid′ərin/ [Gk, *haima* + *sideros*, iron], an iron-rich pigment that is a product of red cell hemolysis. Iron is often stored in this form. Also spelled **haemosiderin.**

**hemosiderosis** /hē′mōsid′ərō′sis, hem′-/ [Gk, *haima* + *sideros*, iron, *osis*, condition], an increased deposition of iron in a variety of tissues, usually in the form of hemosiderin and usually without tissue damage. It is often associated with diseases involving chronic, extensive destruction of red blood cells, such as thalassemia major. Compare **hemochromatosis, sideroblastic anemia.** See also **ferritin, iron transport, siderosis, thalassemia, transferrin.**

**hemostasis** /himos′təsis, hē′məstā′sis/ [Gk, *haima* + *stasis*, halting], the termination of bleeding by mechanical or chemical means or by the complex coagulation process of the body, which consists of vasoconstriction, platelet aggregation, and thrombin and fibrin synthesis. Also spelled **haemostasis.** Compare **blood clotting.** See also **platelet, thrombus, vasoconstriction.**

**hemostat.** See **Halsted's forceps.**

**hemostatic** /-stat′ik/ [Gk, *haima* + *stasis*, halting], pertaining to a procedure, device, or substance that arrests the flow of blood. Direct pressure, tourniquets, and surgical clamps are mechanical hemostatic measures. Cold applications, including the use of an ice bag on the abdomen to halt uterine bleeding and irrigation of the stomach with an iced solution to check gastric bleeding, are hemostatic. Gelatin sponges, solutions of thrombin, and microfibrillar collagen, which causes the aggregation of platelets and the formation of clots, are used to arrest bleeding in surgical procedures. Aminocaproic acid is administered orally or intravenously in the treatment of excessive bleeding caused by systemic hyperfibrinolysis. Phytonadione (vitamin $K_1$) is used in the prevention and treatment of hemorrhagic disease in newborns and the treatment of prothrombin deficiency induced by anticoagulants or other drugs. Also spelled **haemostatic.**

**hemostatic forceps.** See **artery forceps.**

**hemotherapeutics** /-ther′əpyo͞o′tiks/, a form of treatment that involves the use of fresh blood plasma or serum. Also called **hemotherapy.**

**hemothorax** /hē′mōthôr′aks, hem′-/ [Gk, *haima* + *thorax*, chest], an accumulation of blood and fluid in the pleural cavity, between the parietal and visceral pleura, usually the result of trauma. Blood can also accumulate in the thorax cavity as a result of erosion of pulmonary vessels, the rupture of blebs, or granulomas. Hemothorax also may be caused by the rupture of small blood vessels that results from inflammation caused by pneumonia, tuberculosis, or tumors. Shock from hemorrhage, pain, and respiratory failure follow if emergency care is not available. Also spelled **haemothorax.** Also called **hematothorax** /hē′mətōthôr′aks/. Compare **hemopneumothorax.**

**hemotroph** /hē′mətrof/, the total nutritive substances supplied to the embryo from the maternal circulation after the development of the placenta. Also spelled **hemotrophe.** Also called **hemotrophic nutrition.** Compare **embryotroph.** —**hemotrophic,** *adj.*

**Henderson-Hasselbalch equation** [Lawrence J. Henderson, American chemist, 1878–1942; Karl A. Hasselbalch, Danish biochemist, 1874–1962], the relationship among pH, the $pK_a$ of a buffer system, and the ratio of the concentrations of the conjugate base and a weak acid.

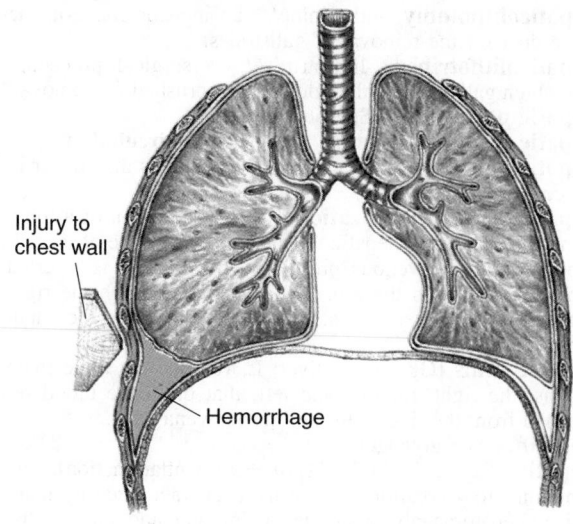

**Hemothorax** *(Wilson and Giddens, 2001)*

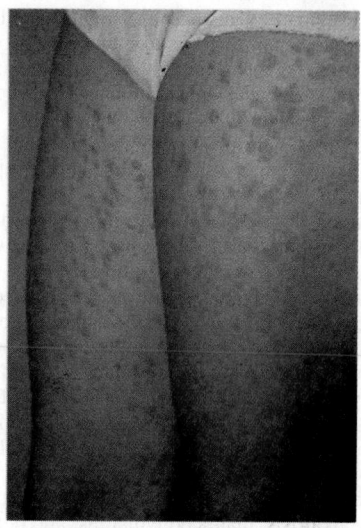

**Henoch-Schönlein purpura** *(Zitelli and Davis, 1997)*

**Henderson, Virginia** (1897–1996), a nursing theorist who introduced a holistic approach to the profession in 1966. The theory is based on the concepts that the body and mind are inseparable, no two individuals are alike, and the role of nursing is independent of the functions of the physician. The Henderson theory proposes that there are 14 components of basic nursing care that contribute to the health of a patient. They relate to (1) breathing, (2) eating and drinking, (3) elimination, (4) movement and posture, (5) sleep and rest, (6) clothing, (7) maintenance of body temperature, (8) cleaning and grooming of the body, (9) avoidance of environmental dangers and injury, (10) communication, (11) worship, (12) work, (13) play and recreation, and (14) learning and discovery.

**Henle's fissure** /hen′lēz/ [Friedrich Gustav Henle, German anatomist, 1809–1885], one of many patches of connective tissue between the muscle fibers of the heart.

**Henle's loop.** See **loop of Henle.**

**Henoch-Schönlein purpura** /hen′ôkhshœn′līn/ [Eduard H. Henoch, German physician, 1820–1910; Johannes L. Schönlein, German physician, 1793–1864], a self-limited hypersensitivity vasculitis, chiefly of children. It is characterized by purpuric skin lesions that appear predominantly on the lower abdomen, buttocks, and legs and are usually associated with pain in the knees and ankles. Other joint involvement, GI bleeding, and hematuria are also common findings. The disease lasts up to 6 weeks and has no sequelae if renal involvement is not severe. Immunosuppressive drugs, such as corticosteroids, may help relieve the nephropathy. Also called **anaphylactoid purpura, Schönlein-Henoch purpura.**

**henry (H)** [Joseph Henry, American physicist, 1797–1878], an International System (SI) unit of electrical inductance equal to 1 volt-second per ampere.

**Henry's law** [William Henry, English chemist, 1774–1836], (in physics) a law stating that the solubility of a gas in a liquid is proportional to the pressure of the gas if the temperature is constant and if the gas does not chemically react with the liquid.

**Henschen method,** a technique for positioning a patient's head in a true lateral position to produce a radiographic image of the mastoid and petrous portions of the head.

**Hensen's knot, Hensen's node.** See **primitive node.**

**hen worker's lung.** See **pigeon breeder's lung.**

**HEP,** abbreviation for **hepatoerythropoietic porphyria.**

**heparin** /hep′ərin/ [Gk, *hēpar,* liver], a naturally occurring mucopolysaccharide that acts in the body as an antithrombin factor to prevent intravascular clotting. The substance is produced by basophils and mast cells, which are found in large numbers in the connective tissue surrounding capillaries, particularly in the lungs and liver. In the form of sodium salt heparin is used therapeutically as an anticoagulant. See also **heparin sodium.**

**heparin lock flush solution (USP)** [Gk, *hēpar,* liver; OE, *loc* + ME, *fluschen* + L, *solutus,* dissolved], a sterile solution of heparin sodium, saline solution, and benzyl alcohol that is intended for use in maintaining patency in IV equipment. It is not used in anticoagulant therapy.

**heparin rebound,** the phenomenon of reactivation of heparin effect that occurs from 5 minutes to 5 hours after neutralization with protamine sulfate.

**heparin sodium,** an anticoagulant.

■ INDICATIONS: It is prescribed in the treatment and prophylaxis of a variety of thromboembolic disorders.

■ CONTRAINDICATIONS: Known hypersensitivity to this drug prohibits its use. It is given only when frequent monitoring of the coagulation status of the patient's blood is possible.

■ ADVERSE EFFECTS: The most serious adverse reaction is hemorrhage. Vasospastic disorders may occur.

**hepat-.** See **hepato-.**

**hepatectomy** /hep′ətek′təmē/ [Gk, *hēpar,* liver, *ektomē,* excision], a surgical procedure performed to remove a portion of the liver.

**-hepatia,** combining meaning '(condition of the) liver or its functioning': *anhepatia, dyshepatia, hypohepatia.*

**hepatic** /hepat′ik/ [Gk, *hēpar,* liver], pertaining to the liver.

**hepatic adenoma,** a rapidly growing tumor of the liver that may become very large and rupture, causing a lethal internal hemorrhage. The incidence is frequently associated with the use of oral contraceptives.

**hepatic amebiasis,** a disorder characterized by enlargement and tenderness of the liver that is often associated with amebic dysentery. The inflammation results from direct infection with *Entamoeba histolytica.* See also **amebiasis, amebic dysentery,** *Entamoeba histolytica.*

**hepatic bile,** a "C" form of bile obtained from a duodenal drainage tube after the gallbladder has been emptied.

**hepatic cells.** See **hepatic cord.**

**hepatic coma,** a neuropsychiatric manifestation of extensive liver damage caused by chronic or acute liver disease. Either endogenous or exogenous waste toxic to the brain is not neutralized in the liver before being shunted back into the peripheral circulation of the blood, or substances required for cerebral function are not synthesized in the liver and therefore are not available to the brain. Commonly, ammonia, a by-product of protein metabolism that is toxic to the brain, is not converted to urea by the liver. The condition is characterized by variable consciousness, including lethargy, stupor, and coma; a tremor of the hands; personality change; memory loss; hyperreflexia; and hyperventilation. Respiratory alkalosis, mania convulsions, and death may occur. The outcome varies according to the pathogenesis of the condition and the treatment. ■ INTERVENTIONS: Treatment in most cases includes cleansing enemas, low-protein diet, parenteral hydration with a balanced electrolyte solution, and specific treatment for the underlying cause. It may also include the use of neomycin orally to kill off bacteria and thus prevent elevated blood urea nitrogen levels. Also called **portal-systemic encephalopathy.** See also **cirrhosis, hepatitis.**

**hepatic cord,** a mass of cells, arranged in irregular radiating columns and plates, spreading outward from the central vein of the hepatic lobule. The cells are many-sided and contain one or sometimes two distinct nuclei. Many such cords join to form the parenchyma of the liver lobule. Each cell usually contains granules, some protoplasmic and others consisting of glycogen, fat, or an iron compound. Also called **hepatic cells.**

**hepatic dyspepsia,** a digestive difficulty caused by a liver disorder.

**hepatic encephalopathy.** See **hepatic coma.**

**hepatic fistula,** an abnormal passage from the liver to another organ or body structure.

**hepatic insufficiency,** a failure or partial failure of normal liver function.

**hepatic keratitis.** See **dendritic keratitis.**

**hepatic lobes** [Gk, *hēpar*, liver, *lobos*, lobes], the large divisions of the liver: caudate, quadrate, left, and right.

**hepatic node,** a node in one of three groups of lymph glands associated with the abdominal and pelvic viscera supplied by branches of the celiac artery. The hepatic nodes are divided into the hepatic and subpyloric groups. The hepatic group, on the stem of the hepatic artery, extends along the common bile duct, between the two layers of the lesser omentum, as far as the porta hepatis. The subpyloric group comprises about five nodes closely relating to the division of the gastroduodenal artery. Both groups receive materials from the stomach, the duodenum, the liver, the gallbladder, and the pancreas. Their efferent vessels join the celiac set of preaortic nodes. Compare **gastric node, pancreaticolienal node.**

**hepatico-.** See **hepato-.**

**hepaticoduodenostomy** /hepat′ikōdo͞o′ōdənos′təmē/, surgical establishment of a passageway between the hepatic duct and the duodenum.

**hepaticoenterostomy** /həpat′ikō·en′teros′təmē/, surgical establishment of a passageway between the hepatic duct and the intestine.

**hepaticolithotomy** /-lithot′əmē/, an incision made in the bile duct for the removal of gallstones.

**hepaticolithotripsy** /-lith′ətrip′sē/, a surgical procedure in which gallstones in the bile duct are crushed for removal.

**hepatic porphyria.** See **porphyria.**

**hepatic portal circulation.** See **portal circulation.**

**hepatic pulse,** pulsation of the liver, such as may occur in tricuspid incompetence.

**hepatic vein catheterization,** the introduction of a long, fine catheter into a hepatic venule for the purpose of recording intrahepatic venous pressure. The catheter is inserted through a vein in the arm and is passed through the right atrium, inferior vena cava, and hepatic vein into the small hepatic vessel.

**hepatic veins** [Gk, *hēpar*, liver; L, *vena*], the three main veins, the right, middle, and left, that drain the blood returned from the liver into the inferior vena cava.

**hepatin.** See **glycogen.**

**hepatitis** /hep′əti′tis/ [Gk, *hēpar* + *itis,* inflammation], an inflammatory condition of the liver, characterized by jaundice, hepatomegaly, anorexia, abdominal and gastric discomfort, abnormal liver function, clay-colored stools, and tea-colored urine. The condition may be caused by bacterial or viral infection, parasitic infestation, alcohol, drugs, toxins, or transfusion of incompatible blood. It may be mild and brief or severe, fulminant, and life-threatening. The liver usually is able to regenerate its tissue, but severe hepatitis may lead to cirrhosis and chronic liver dysfunction. Compare **anicteric hepatitis.** See also **viral hepatitis.**

**hepatitis A,** a viral hepatitis caused by the hepatitis A virus **(HAV),** characterized by slow onset of signs and symptoms. The virus may be spread through fecally contaminated food or water. The infection most often occurs in young adults and is usually followed by complete recovery. Prophylaxis with immune globulin is effective in household and sexual contacts. A vaccine for immunization is available. Also called **acute infective hepatitis.** See **viral hepatitis.**

**hepatitis B,** a viral hepatitis caused by the hepatitis B virus **(HBV).** The virus is transmitted by transfusion of contaminated blood or blood products, by sexual contact with an infected person, or by the use of contaminated needles and instruments. Severe infection may cause prolonged illness, destruction of liver cells, cirrhosis, increased risk of liver cancer, or death. A vaccine is available and recommended for infants, teenagers, and adults at risk for exposure. Treatment may involve transplantation. Also called **serum hepatitis.** See **viral hepatitis.**

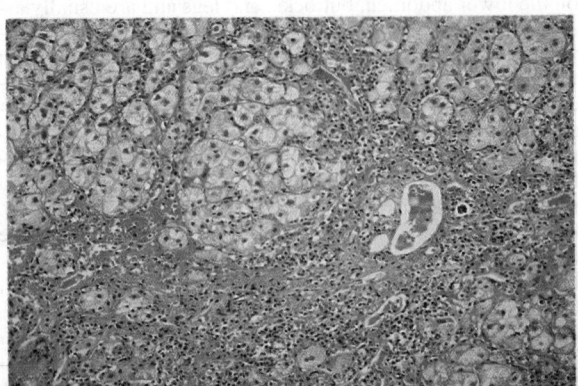

**Chronic hepatitis B infection** *(Damjanov and Linder, 2000)*

## Characteristics of hepatitis viruses

| | Incubation period | Mode of transmission | Sources of infection and spread of disease | Infectivity |
|---|---|---|---|---|
| Hepatitis A (HAV) | 15-50 days (average 28) | Fecal-oral (fecal contamination and oral ingestion) | Crowded conditions; poor personal hygiene; poor sanitation; contaminated food, milk, water, and shellfish; persons with subclinical infections; infected food handlers; sexual contact | Most infectious during 2 wk before onset of symptoms; infectious until 1-2 wk after symptoms start |
| Hepatitis B (HBV) | 45-180 days (average 60-90) | Percutaneous (parenteral)/permucosal exposure to blood or blood products. Sexual contact. Perinatal contact | Contaminated needles, syringes, and blood products; sexual activity with infected partners; asymptomatic carriers | Before and after symptoms appear; infectious for 4-6 mo; in carriers continues for patient's lifetime |
| Hepatitis C (HCV) | 14-180 days (average 56) | Percutaneous (parenteral)/permucosal exposure to blood or blood products | Blood and blood products; needles and syringes; sexual activity with infected partners | 1-2 wk before symptoms; continues during clinical course; indefinitely with carriers |
| Hepatitis D (HDV) | Not firmly established HBV must precede HDV; chronic carriers of HBV are always at risk | Can cause infection only together with HBV; routes of transmission same as for HBV | Same as HBV | Blood is infectious at all stages of HDV infection |
| Hepatitis E (HEV) | 15-64 days (average 26-42 days in different epidemics) | Fecal-oral | Contaminated water; poor sanitation; found in Asia, Africa, and Mexico; not common in the United States and Canada | Not known; may be similar to HAV |

From Lewis SM, Heitkemper MM, Dirksen SR: *Medical-surgical nursing: assessment and management of clinical problems,* ed 5, St Louis, 2000, Mosby.

**hepatitis B immune globulin (HBIG),** a passive immunizing agent.
- INDICATION: It is prescribed for postexposure prophylaxis against infection by the hepatitis B virus.
- CONTRAINDICATIONS: Known hypersensitivity to the drug or to gamma globulin prohibits its use.
- ADVERSE EFFECTS: Among the most serious adverse reactions are severe hypersensitivity reactions. Pain and inflammation at the site of injection also may occur.

**hepatitis B surface antigen.** See **Australia antigen.**

**hepatitis B vaccine,** a vaccine prepared from the blood plasma of asymptomatic human carriers of hepatitis B virus. A series of three doses is recommended to achieve immunity. The vaccine is particularly advised for people who are likely to have contact with blood or fluids of affected people, such as nurses, physicians, dentists, dental hygienists, and laboratory personnel.

**hepatitis B vaccine (recombinant),** a genetically engineered vaccine produced in yeast cells by recombinant deoxyribonucleic acid technology.

**hepatitis C,** a type of hepatitis transmitted most commonly by blood transfusion or percutaneous inoculation, as when IV drug users share needles or when drug users share straws for nasal inhalation of cocaine. It is transmitted less commonly by sexual intercourse. The disease progresses to chronic hepatitis in up to 80% of the patients acutely infected. Diagnosis is made through identification of antibodies of HCV or PCR. Treatment is alpha-interferon and ribavarin.

**hepatitis D,** a form of hepatitis that occurs only in patients co-infected with hepatitis B. HDV relies on HBV replication and cannot replicate independently. The disease usually de-

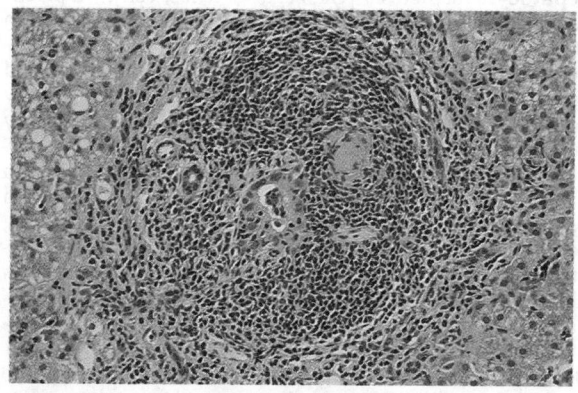

**Chronic hepatitis C infection** *(Damjanov and Linder, 2000)*

velops into a chronic state. Diagnosis is made by detecting serum antibodies to HDV. It is transmitted sexually and through needle sharing. The only treatment is prevention of HBV.

**hepatitis E,** a self-limited type of hepatitis acquired by ingestion of fecally contaminated water or food.

**hepatitis F,** a rare, fulminant form of hepatitis.

**hepatitis G,** a form of hepatitis, caused by the hepatitis G virus (HGV), that is transmitted by contact with blood. Infection is of widespread occurrence and causes generally asymptomatic to mild disease. It is seen in patients after drug transfusions, in patients undergoing hemodialysis, and in IV drug abusers; it is also seen in infants born to infected mothers.

**hepatitis virus studies,** a series of tests used to detect antigens and antibodies to hepatitis B surface antigen (HBsAg), hepatitis B surface antibody (HBsAb), hepatitis B core antibody (HBcAb), hepatitis B e-antigen (HBeAg), hepatitis B e-antibody (HBeAb), and hepatitis C antibodies (HCV IgG).

**hepatization** /hep'ətīzā'shən/ [Gk, *hepatizein,* like the liver], transformation of lung tissue into a solid mass resembling the liver, as in early pneumococcal pneumonia, in which consolidation and effusion of red blood cells in the alveoli produce **red hepatization.** In later stages of pneumococcal pneumonia, when white blood cells fill the alveoli, the consolidation becomes **gray hepatization,** or **yellow hepatization,** when infiltrated by fat deposits.

**hepato-, hepat-, hepatico-,** combining meaning 'liver': *hepatobiliary, hepatocarcinogenic, hepatocellular.*

**hepatobiliary capsule.** See **Glisson's capsule.**

**hepatoblastoma** /hep'ətō'blastō'mə/, a cancer of the liver that tends to occur in children. It is usually detected during examination for causes of failing health and for the presence of a mass in the upper abdomen. Hepatoblastoma also may be associated with precocious puberty.

**hepatocarcinogen** /-kärsin'əjən/, an agent that causes carcinoma of the liver.

**hepatocarcinoma, hepatocellular carcinoma.** See **hepatoma.**

**hepatocele** [Gk, *hēpar,* liver, *kele,* hernia], a hernia of a portion of the liver through the diaphragm or the abdominal wall.

**hepatocellular jaundice** /-sel'yələr/, jaundice resulting from disease or injury to liver cells.

**hepatocholangitis** /hep'ətōkō'lanjī'tis/, an inflammation of both the liver and the bile ducts.

**hepatocyte** /hep'ətōsīt/ [Gk, *hēpar* + *kytos,* cell], a parenchymal liver cell that performs all the functions ascribed to the liver.

**hepatocyte growth factor (HGF),** a potent mitogen and inducer of hepatocyte proliferation, produced in the liver by cells other than hepatic cells and in many other organs by cells of the mesenchyme.

**hepatoduodenal ligament** /hep'ətōdoo'ədē'nəl, -doo·od'in əl/ [Gk, *hēpar* + L, *duodeni,* twelve fingers], the portion of the lesser omentum between the liver and the duodenum, containing the hepatic artery, the common bile duct, the portal vein, the lymphatics, and the hepatic plexus of nerves. These structures are enclosed within a fibrous capsule between the two layers of the ligament. Compare **hepatogastric ligament.**

**hepatoerythropoietic porphyria (HEP)** /hep'ə·tō ə·rith'rōpoi·et'ik/ [Gk, *hēpar,* liver + *erythros,* red + *poiein,* to make], a severe homozygous form of **porphyria cutanea tarda** (PCT) believed to result from an autosomal dominant defect in the same enzyme activity as PCT. It is clinically identical to PCT but onset is in early childhood and activity of the affected enzyme in liver, erythrocytes, and fibroblasts is virtually absent.

**hepatogastric ligament** /hep'ətōgas'trik/ [Gk, *hēpar* + *gaster,* stomach], the portion of the lesser omentum between the liver and the stomach. Compare **hepatoduodenal ligament.**

**hepatogenous jaundice** /hep'ətoj'ənəs/ [Gk, *hēpar,* liver, *genein,* to produce; Fr, *jaune,* yellow], a type of jaundice caused by a condition of the liver.

**hepatogram** /hep'ətōgram'/, **1.** a sphygmographic tracing of the liver pulse. **2.** a radiographic image of the liver.

**hepatography** /hep'ətog'rəfē/, **1.** the recording of the liver pulse. **2.** the radiographic or isotope scintigraphic visualization of the liver.

**hepatojugular** /hep'ətōjug'yŏŏlər/ [Gk, *hēpar,* liver; L, *jugulum,* neck], pertaining to the liver and the jugular vein.

**hepatojugular reflux** [Gk, *hēpar* + L, *jugulum,* neck], an increase in jugular venous pressure when pressure is applied for 30 to 60 seconds over the abdomen, suggestive of right-sided heart failure.

**hepatolenticular degeneration** /həpat'ōlentik'yŏŏlər/ [Gk, *hēpar* + L, *lens,* lentil], an abnormal condition associated with defective copper metabolism in the body, characterized by decreased serum ceruloplasmin and copper levels and increased secretion of urinary copper. In individuals with this condition tissue deposits of copper associated with hepatic cirrhosis, deep marginal pigmentation of the cornea, and extensive degeneration of the central nervous system, especially the basal ganglions, develop. Also called **Wilson's disease.**

**hepatolienal fibrosis.** See **congestive splenomegalia.**

**hepatolithiasis** /lithī'əsis/, the presence of stones in the liver.

**hepatologist** /hep'ətol'əjist/, a physician who specializes in diseases of the liver.

**hepatology** /hep'ətol'əjē/, the branch of medicine that is concerned primarily with diseases of the liver.

**hepatoma** /hep'ətō'mə/, *pl.* **hepatomas, hepatomata** [Gk, *hēpar* + *oma,* tumor], a primary malignant tumor of the liver, which is relatively rare in the United States. It occurs most commonly in the sixth decade, and its incidence is higher in African-Americans than Caucasians. It is characterized by hepatomegaly, pain, hypoglycemia, weight loss, anorexia, ascites, as well as elevated serum alpha-fetoprotein levels, portal hypertension, and jaundice in the plasma. The tumor occurs most frequently in association with hepatitis or cirrhosis of the liver and in those parts of the world where the mycotoxin aflatoxin is found. It is treated with surgical resection when isolated to one lobe of the liver. The prognosis is poor. Chemotherapy and liver transplantation are used in some centers.

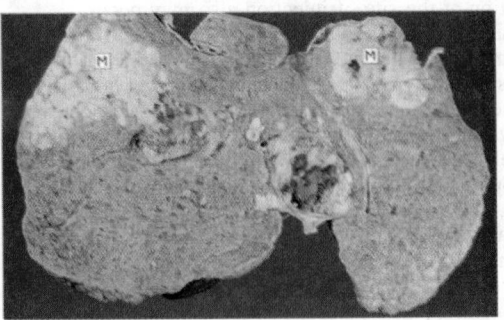

**Hepatoma** *(Stevens and Lowe, 1995)*

**hepatomegaly** /hep'ətōmeg'əlē/ [Gk, *hēpar* + *megas,* large], abnormal enlargement of the liver that is usually a sign of disease. It is often discovered by percussion and palpation as part of a physical examination. In hepatomegaly the liver is easily palpable below the ribs and may be tender to the touch. Hepatomegaly may be caused by hepatitis or other infection, fatty infiltration, as in alcoholism, biliary obstruction, or malignancy.

**hepatonecrosis** /-nekrō'sis/, **1.** the death of liver cells. **2.** gangrene of the liver.

**hepatopancreatic ampulla** /-pan'krē·at'ik/ [Gk, hēpar + pan, all, kreas, flesh], the dilation formed by the junction of the pancreatic and bile ducts as they open into the lumen of the duodenum. Also called **ampulla of the bile duct, ampulla of Vater.**

**hepatorenal** /hep'ətōrē'nəl/, [Gk, hēpar, liver; L, ren, kidney], pertaining to the liver and the kidneys.

**hepatorenal syndrome,** a type of kidney failure characterized by a gradual loss of function without signs of tissue damage. It is associated with hepatitis or cirrhosis of the liver; its exact cause is unknown.

**hepatosplenomegaly** /-splē'nōmeg'əlē/ [Gk, hēpar, liver, splen + megas, large], enlargement of the spleen and liver.

**hepatotoxic** /-tok'sik/, potentially destructive of liver cells.

**hepatotoxicity** /hep'ətōtoksis'itē/ [Gk, hēpar + toxikon, poison], the tendency of an agent, usually a drug or alcohol, to have a destructive effect on the liver.

**hepatotoxin** /-tok'sin/, a poison that damages parenchymal cells of the liver.

**hepta-, hept-,** combining meaning 'seven': heptachromic, heptadactylia, heptavalent.

**heptachlor poisoning** /hep'təklôr'/ [Gk, hepar, seven, chloros, green; L, potio, drink], a form of chlorinated organic insecticide poisoning.

**heptaploid.** See **polyploid.**

**heptavalent.** /hep'tivā'lənt/ pertaining to a chemical that has a valence of 7. Also called **septivalent.**

**herald patch.** See **pityriasis rosea.**

**herb** /(h)urb/ [L, herba, grass], **1.** any plant that is used for culinary or medicinal purposes. **2.** a leafy plant without a wooden stem. **3.** a plant with aerial parts that do not persist from one year to the next.

**herbalist** /hur'bəlist/, **1.** a person who specializes in the study of herbs. **2.** a dealer in medicinal herbs.

**herb bath** [L, herba, grass; AS, baeth], a medicinal bath taken in water containing a decoction of aromatic herbs.

**herbicide poisoning** /hur'bisīd/ [L, herba, grass, caedere, to kill], a poisoning caused by the ingestion, inhalation, or absorption of a substance intended for use as a weed killer or defoliant. Many of the commonly used agricultural herbicides can produce symptoms ranging from skin irritation to hypotension, liver and kidney damage, and coma or convulsions. Estimated fatal doses may be as small as 1 to 10 g. Some herbicides contain extremely toxic substances; poisoning is characterized by dysphagia, burning stomach pain, throat constriction, diarrhea, or other severe symptoms.

**herbivorous** /hərbiv'ərəs/ [L, herba, grass, vorare, to devour], pertaining to feeding on plants or to animals that subsist mostly or entirely on plants. Also called **herbivore** /hur'bivôr/.

**herb tea,** a medicinal beverage prepared by the infusion of a water-soluble extract of leaves, roots, bark, or other parts of an herb. The vegetable matter is commonly macerated and steeped in boiling water, which is strained and served hot. Cold water may be used for herbs containing readily soluble active principles.

**herd immunity** [ME, heord, group; L, immunis, free from], the level of disease resistance of a community or population.

**herd instinct** [ME, heord + L, instinctus, impulse], the basic need of social animals, including humans, for the companionship of peers and a tendency to find compatibility with the behavioral standards of others in the group.

**hereditability** /həred'itəbil'itē/ [L, hereditas, inheritance], the degree to which a specific trait is controlled by inheritance.

**hereditary** /həred'iter'ē/ [L, hereditas, inheritance], transmitted from parent to offspring; inborn; inherited. Compare **acquired, congenital, familial.**

**hereditary angioedema,** an inherited autosomal dominant disorder characterized by the episodic appearance of nonpitting edema involving any part of the body, including mucosal surfaces. The attacks last 48 to 72 hours and can be life-threatening if the edema obstructs the airway.

**hereditary ataxia,** one of a group of inherited degenerative diseases of the spinal cord, cerebellum, and often other parts of the nervous system, characterized by tremor, spasm, muscle wasting, skeletal change, and sensory disturbances resulting in impaired motor activity. Kinds of hereditary ataxia include **ataxia telangiectasia** and **Friedreich's ataxia.**

**hereditary brown enamel.** See **amelogenesis imperfecta.**

**hereditary coproporphyria.** See **coproporphyria.**

**hereditary deforming chondroplasia.** See **diaphyseal aclasis.**

**hereditary disorder.** See **inherited disorder.**

**hereditary elliptocytosis.** See **elliptocytosis.**

**hereditary enamel hypoplasia.** See **amelogenesis imperfecta.**

**hereditary essential tremor.** See **essential tremor.**

**hereditary hemochromatosis,** an autosomal recessive form of hemochromatosis; iron accumulation is lifelong, with symptoms appearing usually in the fifth or sixth decades of life. See also **hemochromatosis.**

**hereditary hemorrhagic telangiectasia.** See **Osler-Weber-Rendu syndrome.**

**hereditary hyperuricemia.** See **Lesch-Nyhan syndrome.**

**hereditary multiple exostoses,** a rare familial dyschondroplastic disease in which bony protuberances form on the shafts of the long bones and eventually develop into caps of cartilage covering the ends of the bones. The affected joints lose their mobility, and the bones stop growing. The disease begins in childhood and has no cure. Very rarely a chondrosarcoma may develop from the cap of an exostosis. See also **Ollier's dyschondroplasia.**

**hereditary opalescent dentin.** See **dentinogenesis imperfecta.**

**hereditary oral disease,** any abnormal condition characterized by genetic defects of structures in or around the mouth, such as deformed dentition, ankyloglossia, hereditary gingivofibromatosis, or cleft palate. Many hereditary oral diseases, including Crouzon's disease, sickle cell anemia, gargoylism, familial amyloidosis, and achondroplasia, are associated with generalized defects.

**hereditary osteo-onychodysplasia.** See **nail-patella syndrome.**

**hereditary protoporphyria.** See **porphyria.**

**hereditary spherocytosis.** See **spherocytic anemia.**

**hereditary tyrosinemia.** See **tyrosinemia.**

**heredity** /həred'itē/ [L, hereditas, inheritance], **1.** the process by which particular traits or conditions are genetically transmitted from parents to offspring, causing resemblance of individuals related by descent. It involves the separation and recombination of genes during meiosis and fertilization and the further interaction of developmental influences and genetic material during embryogenesis. **2.** the total genetic constitution of an individual; the sum of the qualities inherited from ancestors and the potentialities of transmitting these qualities to offspring.

**heredo-,** combining meaning 'hereditary': *heredobiologic, heredosyphilitic, heredotrophedema.*

**Hering-Breuer reflex** /her′ingbroi′ər/ [Heinrich E. Hering, German physiologist, 1866–1948; Joseph Breuer, Austrian physician, 1842–1925], a neural mechanism that terminates inspiration and initiates expiration. The reflex is triggered by impulses that originate in stretch receptors of the bronchi and bronchioles in response to distension of the airway, increased intratracheal pressure, or pulmonary inflation. The impulses travel via afferent fibers of the vagus nerves to the medullary respiratory center. The Hering-Breuer reflex is well developed at birth and is hyperactive in conditions of restrictive ventilatory insufficiency.

**Hermansky-Pudlak syndrome** /hər·män′ske·pŏŏd′läk/ [F. Hermansky, Czechoslovakian internist, 20th century; P. Pudlak, Czechoslovakian internist, 20th century], an autosomal recessive form of oculocutaneous albinism (OCA) with a hemorrhagic diathesis secondary to a platelet defect, and accumulation of a ceroid-like substance in the reticuloendothelial system, oral mucosa, and urine.

**hermaphroditism** /hərmaf′rədītiz′əm/ [Gk, *Hermaphroditos,* son of Hermes and Aphrodite], a rare condition in which both testicular and ovarian tissue exist in the same person; the testicular tissue contains seminiferous tubules or spermatozoa and the ovarian tissue contains follicles or corpora albicantia. The condition results from a chromosomal abnormality. Also called **hermaphrodism.** Compare **pseudohermaphroditism.**

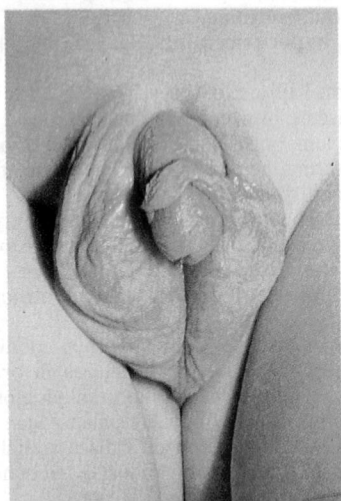

**Hermaphroditism** *(Zitelli and Davis, 1997)*

**hermetic** /hərmet′ik/ [Gk, *Hermes*], from use in alchemy, pertaining to sealing a container so as to make it airtight.

**hernia** /hur′nē·ə/ [L, rupture], protrusion or projection of an organ through an abnormal opening in the muscle wall of the cavity that surrounds it. A hernia may be congenital, may result from the failure of certain structures to close after birth, or may be acquired later in life as a result of obesity, muscular weakness, surgery, or illness. Kinds of hernia include **abdominal, diaphragmatic, femoral, hiatal, inguinal,** and **umbilical.** See also **herniorrhaphy.**

**hernial** /hur′nē·əl/, pertaining to or resembling a hernia.

**hernial sac** [L, *hernia,* rupture; Gk, *sakkos,* sack], a pouch of peritoneum into which organs or other tissues pass to form a hernia.

**herniated** /hur′nē·ā′tid/, pertaining to a tear or abnormal bulge of an organ or organ part through a retaining tissue.

**herniated disk,** a rupture of the fibrocartilage surrounding an intervertebral disk, releasing the nucleus pulposus that cushions the vertebrae above and below. The resultant pressure on spinal nerve roots may cause considerable pain and damage the nerves, resulting in restriction of movement. The condition most frequently occurs in the lumbar region. Also called **herniated intervertebral disk, herniated nucleus pulposus, ruptured intervertebral disk, slipped disk.**

**herniation** /hur′nē·ā′shən/, a protrusion of a body organ or portion of an organ through an abnormal opening in a membrane, muscle, or other tissue. See also **hernia, hiatal hernia.**

**herniography** /hur′nē·og′rəfē/, the radiographic examination of a hernia after it has been injected with a contrast medium.

**herniorrhaphy** /hur′nē·ôr′əfē/, the surgical repair of a hernia.

**herniotomy** /hur′nē·ot′əmē/ [L, *hernia* + Gk, *temnein,* to cut], a surgical procedure to reduce a hernia.

**heroin** /her′ō·in/ [Ger, *heroine,* originally trademark for diacetylmorphine], a morphinelike drug with no currently acceptable medical use in the United States. Heroin is included in Schedule I of the Controlled Substances Act of 1970. Like other opium alkaloids, it can produce analgesia, respiratory depression, GI spasm, and physical dependence. It produces its major effects on the central nervous system and bowel and alters the endocrine and autonomic nervous systems. Heroin, which loses much of its analgesic power when taken orally, is more powerful than morphine and acts more rapidly. Repeated use of this drug produces tolerance to most of the acute opioid effects; physical dependence develops concurrently with tolerance. Withdrawal from heroin after relatively few exposures commonly produces acute abstinence syndrome. Withdrawal signs are usually observed shortly before the next planned dose and commonly include anxiety, restlessness, irritability, and craving for another dose. Other withdrawal signs that may appear 8 to 15 hours after the last dose include lacrimation, perspiration, yawning, and restless sleep. On awakening from such sleep the severely addicted heroin user may experience withdrawal signs, such as vomiting, pain in the bones, diarrhea, convulsions, and cardiovascular collapse. Withdrawal signs usually peak at between 36 and 48 hours and gradually subside during the following 10 days. Methadone is commonly used as a substitute drug in the treatment of heroin addiction (methadone maintenance therapy). Also called **diacetylmorphine.**

**herpangina** /hur′panjī′nə/ [Gk, *herpein,* to creep; L, *angina,* quinsy], a viral infection, usually of young children, characterized by sore throat, headache, anorexia, and pain in the abdomen, neck, and extremities. Febrile convulsions and vomiting may occur in infants. Papules or vesicles may form in the pharynx and on the tongue, the palate, or the tonsils. The lesions evolve into shallow ulcers that heal spontaneously. The disease usually runs its course in less than 1 week. Treatment is symptomatic. The cause is often infection by a strain of coxsackievirus.

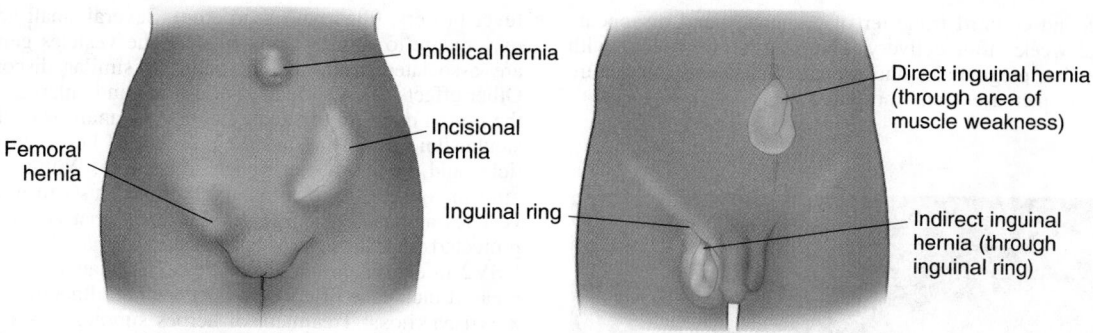

**Common locations of hernias** (Leonard, 2001)

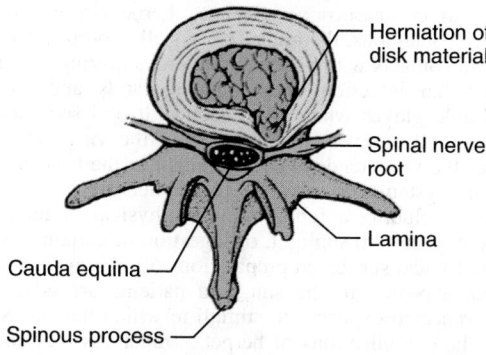

**Herniated disk** (Monahan and Neighbors, 1998)

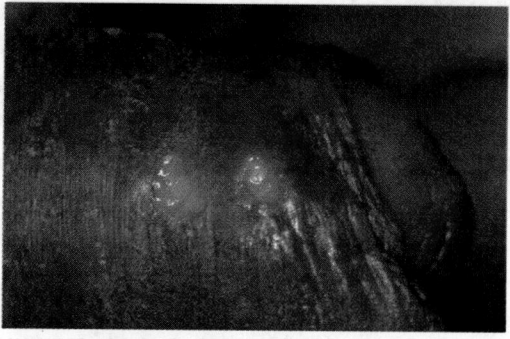

**Herpes genitalis** (Lemmi and Lemmi, 2000)

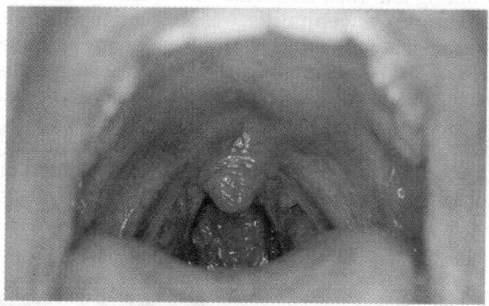

**Herpangina** (Regezi, 2000)

**herpes genitalis** /hur′pēz jen′ital′is/ [Gk, *herpein*, to creep; L, *genitalis*, genitalia], a chronic infection caused by type 2 herpes simplex virus (HSV2), usually transmitted by sexual contact. It causes painful vesicular eruptions on the skin and mucous membranes of the genitalia of males and females. When acquired during pregnancy, HSV2 may be transmitted through the placenta to the fetus and to the newborn by direct contact with infected tissue during birth. It is a precursor of cervical cancer.

■ OBSERVATIONS: In the male herpes genitalis infections may resemble penile ulcers. A small group of vesicular lesions surrounded by erythematous tissue may occur on the glans or prepuce. The lesions erupt into superficial ulcers that often heal in 5 to 7 days, although they also may become the sites of secondary infections. The lesions are painful and are often associated with a burning sensation, urinary dysfunction, fever, malaise, and swelling of the lymph nodes in the inguinal area. The female patient may exhibit the same or similar systemic effects, and members of both sexes may complain of painful sexual intercourse. In the female, herpes genitalis lesions are likely to appear as multiple superficial eruptions on the surfaces of the cervix, vagina, or perineum. There may be a discharge from the cervix. Vaginal lesions may appear as mucous patches with grayish ulcerations. Laboratory tests from smears of fluid taken from the base of lesions show a positive Tzanck reaction with multiple nucleated giant cells, which distinguishes HSV2 infections from other venereal diseases. Infection tends to recur.

■ INTERVENTIONS: Acyclovir taken orally results in partial control of the symptoms and signs of herpes episodes. The drug accelerates healing but does not eradicate the infection. The antiviral agents valacyclovir, penciclovir, and famciclovir may suppress reaction and also may lessen the severity and duration of the outbreak.

■ NURSING CONSIDERATIONS: The nurse teaches patients with genital herpes about the potential for recurrent episodes of lesions and advises them to abstain from sexual activity while the lesions are present. Sexual transmission has been documented during phases when no lesions were present. Women of childbearing age with genital herpes should inform their health care provider if they become pregnant.

**herpes gestationis** [Gk, *herpein* + L, *gestare*, to bear], a generalized pruritic vesicular or bullous rash that appears in the second or third trimester of pregnancy and disappears several weeks after delivery. The lesions often recur with succeeding pregnancies and are associated with premature birth and increased fetal mortality rate.

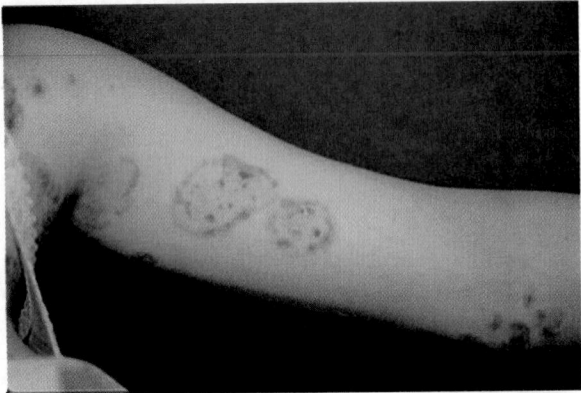

**Herpes gestationis with erythematous, circinate papules and vesicles**
*(Goldstein and Goldstein, 1997/courtesy Beverly Sanders, MD)*

**herpes labialis.**  See **herpes simplex.**

**herpes menstrualis** [Gk, *herpein*, to creep; L, *menstruare*], a form of herpes simplex that tends to erupt during menstrual periods.

**herpes simplex** [Gk, *herpein* + L, *simplex*, uncomplicated], an infection caused by a herpes simplex virus (HSV), which has an affinity for the skin and nervous system and usually produces small transient irritating and sometimes painful fluid-filled blisters on the skin and mucous membranes. HSV1 (oral herpes, herpes labialis) infections tend to occur in the facial area, particularly around the mouth and nose; HSV2 (herpes genitalis) infections are usually limited to the genital region.

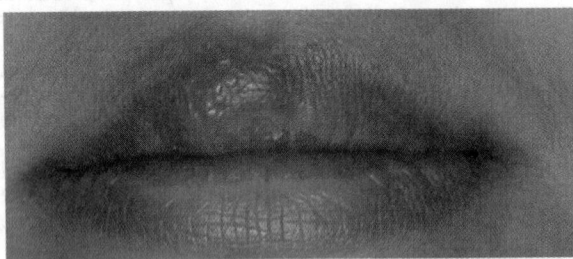

**Herpes simplex I: primary infection**
*(Lemmi and Lemmi, 2000)*

■ OBSERVATIONS: The initial symptoms of an HSV1 infection usually include burning, tingling, or itching sensations about the edges of the lips or nose within 1 or 2 weeks after contact with an infected person. Several hours later small red papules develop in the irritated area; later small vesicles, or

fever blisters, filled with fluid erupt. Several small vesicles may merge to form a larger blister. The vesicles generally are associated with itching, pain, or similar discomfort. Other effects often include a mild fever and enlargement of the lymph nodes in the neck. Laboratory analysis of the vesicular fluid usually shows the presence of herpesvirus particles and the absence of pyogenic bacteria. Within 1 week after the onset of symptoms, thin yellow crusts form on the vesicles as healing begins. In skin areas that are moist or protected and in severe cases, healing may be delayed. HSV2 infections in adolescence are associated with an increased incidence of cervical cancer in adulthood.
■ INTERVENTIONS: Treatment of herpes simplex is symptomatic. The lesions may be washed gently with soap and water to reduce the risk of secondary infection. Topical penciclovir cream may speed healing. Where secondary infections have begun, antibiotics are prescribed. Although there is no cure, treatment includes oral acyclovir or valacyclovir.
■ NURSING CONSIDERATIONS: Because herpesviruses are extremely contagious, the nurse follows all appropriate procedures in contacts with patients to avoid acquiring and transmitting the infection. Washing the hands and wearing disposable gloves when in contact with oral secretions of genitalia help prevent transmission of the virus. Once acquired, the virus tends to remain latent in the tissues of the nervous system and may be reactivated by a variety of stimuli, including a febrile illness, physical or emotional stress, exposure to sunlight, or ingestion of certain foods or drugs. Topical sunscreen preparations offer some protection against exposure to the sun, and patients are advised to avoid repeated exposure to stimuli to which they are sensitive. The complications of herpetic infections may include encephalitis, herpes simplex keratitis, and gingivostomatitis. In cases involving systemic complications, IV acyclovir, blood transfusions, IV solutions, and other therapy may be required. In uncomplicated cases the herpes attack is usually self-limiting and runs its course in 3 weeks or less.

**herpes simplex encephalitis,**  a necrotizing inflammation of the brain that follows an infection with herpes simplex virus (HSV1). It is a common acute form of encephalitis and similar to other viral encephalitis infections. Repeated seizures occur early in the course, and there is severe hemorrhagic necrosis. Affected areas of the brain are usually the orbital portions of the frontal lobes and the inferomedial portions of the temporal lobe. Persons of any age may be in-

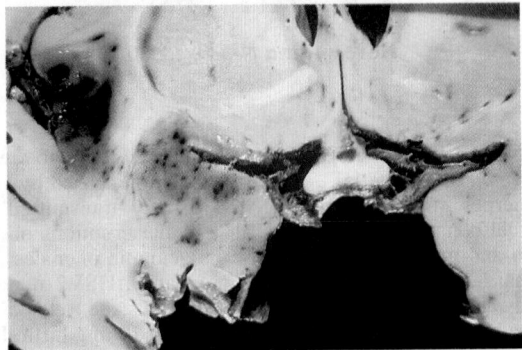

**Herpes simplex encephalitis**
*(Kumar, Cotran, and Robbins, 1997/courtesy Beverly Rogers, MD, and Charles L. White III, MD, Department of Pathology, University of Texas Southwestern Medical Center, Dallas)*

fected, but cerebral sequelae are more likely to occur in infants. The mortality rate varies, but even desperately ill patients may recover completely.

**herpes simplex keratitis.**   See **ocular herpes.**

**herpes simplex test (HSV),**   a blood test or microscopic culture done to detect types 1 and 2 of the herpes simplex virus. HSV 1 is primarily responsible for the oral lesions known as "cold sores," while HSV 2 is a sexually transmitted viral infection of the urogenital tract. Culture is the more accurate of the two types of tests.

**herpesvirus** /hur'pēzvī'rəs/ [Gk, *herpein* + L, *virus,* poison],   any of seven related viruses: herpes simplex viruses 1 and 2, varicella zoster virus, Epstein-Barr virus, cytomegalovirus, human herpesvirus 6, and human herpesvirus 7.

**herpesvirus hominis.**   See **herpes simplex.**

**herpesvirus simiae encephalomyelitis,**   a typically fatal infection of the central nervous system by a B form of herpes simplex virus that usually affects simians. Persons most likely to be infected by the monkey virus are veterinarians and animal laboratory workers.

**herpes zoster** /zos'tər/ [Gk, *herpein* + *zoster,* girdle],   an acute infection caused by reactivation of the latent varicella zoster virus (VZV), which mainly affects adults. It is characterized by the development of painful vesicular skin eruptions that follow the underlying route of cranial or spinal nerves inflamed by the virus. Prompt treatment with antivirals can speed healing and reduce the risk of postherpetic neuralgia. Also called **shingles.** See also **herpes simplex, varicella zoster virus.**

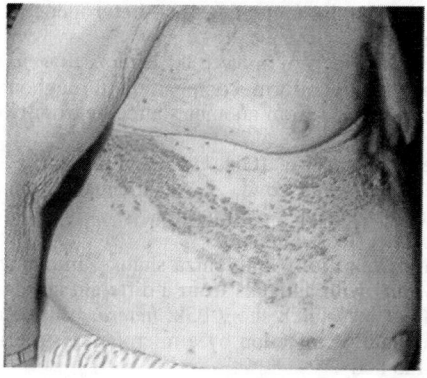

**Herpes zoster**
*(Bryant, 2000/courtesy Mary Brahman, Abbott Northwestern Hospital, Minneapolis)*

**herpes zoster ophthalmicus,**   a form of herpes zoster in which the virus invades the gasserian ganglion, causing pain and skin eruptions along the ophthalmic branch of the fifth cranial nerve. There also may be involvement of the third cranial nerve. The infection frequently leads to corneal ulceration or other ocular complications. Also called **ophthalmic herpes zoster.**

**herpes zoster oticus,**   a herpes zoster infection of the eighth cervical (vestibulocochlear) nerve ganglia and geniculate ganglion, causing severe pain in the external ear structures and pain or paralysis along the facial nerve. The disease also may cause hearing loss and vertigo. The vertigo is usually transient, but the hearing loss and facial paralysis

may be permanent. Vesicular eruptions may occur along the external ear canal and ear pinna. Treatment is generally symptomatic, with diazepam administered for vertigo, analgesics for pain, and corticosteroids for other symptoms. Acyclovir may be prescribed.

**herpes zoster virus.**   See **chickenpox.**

**herpetic encephalitis** /hər·pet'ik/ [Gk, *herpein,* to creep + *enkephalos,* brain + *itis,* inflammation],   the most common form of acute encephalitis, caused by a herpesvirus and characterized by hemorrhagic necrosis of parts of the temporal and frontal lobes. Onset is over several days and involves fever, headache, seizures, stupor, and often coma, frequently with a fatal outcome.

**herpetic keratitis.**   See **dendritic keratitis.**

**herpetic neuralgia** /hərpet'ik/ [Gk, *herpein,* to creep, *neuron,* nerve, *algos,* pain],   a form of neuralgia with intractable pain that develops at the site of a previous eruption of herpes zoster.

**herpetic sore throat,**   a herpes inflammation that develops in the region of the pharynx.

**herpetic stomatitis** [Gk, *herpein,* to creep, *stoma,* mouth, *itis,* inflammation],   a form of inflammation of the mouth caused by a herpesvirus infection.

**herpetiform** /hərpet'ifôrm'/ [Gk, *herpein* + L, *forma,* form],   having clusters of vesicles; resembling the skin lesions of some herpesvirus infections.

**Herplex,**   trademark for a topical antiviral (idoxuridine).

**Hers' disease** /herz, hurz/ [H. G. Hers, 20th-century Belgian physiologist; L, *dis,* opposite of; Fr, *aise,* ease],   an uncommon metabolic disorder of glycogen storage. It is characterized by hepatomegaly and an accumulation of abnormally large amounts of glycogen in the liver as a result of its inability to break down glycogen. The condition is inherited as an autosomal recessive trait. There is no known treatment. Also called **glycogen storage disease, type VI.** See also **glycogen storage disease.**

**hertz (Hz)** /hurts, herts/ [Heinrich R. Hertz, German physicist, 1857–1894],   a unit of measurement of wave frequency equal to 1 cycle per second (cps).

**Herxheimer's reaction** /herks'hī'mərz/ [Karl Herxheimer, German dermatologist, 1861–1944],   an increase in symptoms after administration of a drug. The reaction was originally discovered in penicillin treatment of syphilis, but it has been found to occur with other diseases as well.

**Herzog taping protocol,**   a procedure for immobilizing and balancing a foot with tape after a musculoskeletal injury. The protocol consists of step-by-step instructions for applying tape, beginning with the lateral aspect of the head of the fifth metatarsal and continuing through the lateral plantar aspect of the foot.

**Heschl's gyrus** /hesh'əl/ [Richard L. Heschl, Austrian pathologist, 1824–1881; Gk, *gyros,* turn],   any of several small gyri that run transversely on the upper surface of the temporal operculum of the insula of the cortex.

**hesperidin** /hesper'idin/,   a crystalline flavone glycoside present in most citrus fruits, especially in the spongy casing of oranges and lemons.

**Hesselbach's hernia** /hes'əlbaks, -bäkhs/ [Franz K. Hesselbach, German surgeon, 1759–1816],   a protrusion of diverticula through the femoral sheath, usually associated with direct inguinal hernia.

**hetastarch** /het'əstärch/,   a plasma volume expander.
- INDICATIONS: It is prescribed as an adjunct in shock and leukapheresis.
- CONTRAINDICATIONS: Severe bleeding, severe heart or kidney dysfunction with oliguria or anuria, or known hypersensitivity to this drug prohibits its use.

■ ADVERSE EFFECTS: Among the more serious adverse reactions are influenza-like symptoms, muscle pain, edema, and anaphylaxis.

**heter-.**   See **hetero-.**

**heterauxesis.**   See **allometric growth.**

**hetero-, heter-,** combining meaning 'another or different': *heteroalbumose, heterochronia, heterogamy.*

**heteroallele** /het′ərō-əlēl′/ [Gk, *heteros,* different, *alleolon,* of one another], one of a pair of alleles at a specific locus on homologous chromosomes that differs from the other of the pair. —**heteroallelic,** *adj.*

**heteroantibody** /het′ərō-an′tibod′ē/, an antibody that recognizes an antigen from a species other than that of the antibody producer.

**heteroantigen** /he′tərō-an′təjən/, an antigen that originates in a different species and is foreign to the antibody producer.

**heteroblastic** /het′ərōblas′tik/ [Gk, *heteros* + *blastos,* germ], developing from different germ layers or kinds of tissue rather than from a single type. Compare **homoblastic.**

**heterocellular** /-sel′yələr/, pertaining to a structure formed by more than one kind of cell.

**heterocephalus** /-sef′ələs/ [Gk, *heteros* + *kephale,* head], a malformed fetus that has two heads of unequal size. —**heterocephalous, heterocephalic,** *adj.*

**heterochromatin** /-krō′mətin/ [Gk, *heteros,* different, *chroma,* color], the part of a chromosome that is inactive in gene expression but may function in controlling metabolic activities, transcription, and cell division. It stains most intensely during interphase and usually remains in a condensed state throughout the cell cycle. It consists of two types: constitutive heterochromatin, which is present in all cells and is characteristic of the Y chromosome, and facultative heterochromatin, which is present in the inactivated X chromosome of the mammalian female. Compare **euchromatin.** See also **chromatin.** —**heterochromatic,** *adj.*

**heterochromatinization** /-krō′mətīzā′shən/, the transformation of genetically active euchromatin into genetically inactive heterochromatin. It occurs during the inactivation of one of the X chromosomes in the mammalian female during the early stages of embryogenesis. See also **Lyon hypothesis.**

**heterochromia iridis** /het′ər-ō-krō′mē-ə ī′ri-dis/ [Gk, *heteros,* different + *chroma,* color + *iris,* rainbow], difference of color in the two irides, or in different areas of the same iris.

**heterochromic iridis.** [Gk, *chroma,* color; *iris,* rainbow], a difference in color of the two irides.

**heterochromosome** /-krō′məsōm/, a sex chromosome. See also **heterotypic chromosomes.** —**heterochromosomal,** *adj.*

**heterocytotropic antibody** /-sī′tətrop′ik/, an antibody of immunoglobulin class E that has a greater affinity for antigens when fixed to mast cells of a different species than that of the antibody producer.

**heterodidymus** /het′ərōdid′iməs/ [Gk, *heteros* + *didymos,* twin], a conjoined twin fetus in which the parasitic elements consist of a head, neck, and thorax attached to the thoracic wall of the autosite. Also called **heterodymus.**

**heteroduplex** /-doo′pleks/ [Gk, *heteros* + L, *duoplicare,* to double], a DNA molecule in which the two strands are derived from different individuals, with the result that some base pairs may not be complementary.

**heteroduplex mapping,** a method for determining the location of insertions, deletions, and other heterogeneities in the two strands of a DNA molecule.

**heterodymus.**   See **heterodidymus.**

**heteroenzyme** /het′ərō-en′zīm/, a functionally identical enzyme from a different species.

**heteroeroticism** /het′ərō-irot′isiz′əm/ [Gk, *heteros,* diffrent, *eros,* love], sexual feeling or activity directed toward another individual. Also called **alloeroticism, heteroerotism.** Compare **autoeroticism.**

**heterofermentation** /-fur′məntā′shun/, fermentation that produces major products that are different.

**heterogamete.**   See **anisogamete.**

**heterogametic** /-gamet′ik/, pertaining to the sex that produces gametes of different kinds, in terms of their sex chromosomes. In human beings the male, who possesses X-bearing and Y-bearing sperm, is the heterogametic sex.

**heterogamy** /het′ərog′əmē/ [Gk, *heteros* + *gamos,* marriage], **1.** anisogamy. **2.** heterogenesis. —**heterogamous,** *adj.*

**heterogeneity** /-jənē′itē/, **1.** a quality of being dissimilar in kind. **2.** a state of having different characteristics and qualities.

**heterogeneous** /het′əroj′ənəs/ [Gk, *heteros,* different, *genos,* kind], **1.** consisting of dissimilar elements or parts; unlike; incongruous. **2.** not having a uniform quality throughout. Compare **homogeneous.** —**heterogeneity,** *adj.*

**heterogenesis** /-jen′əsis/ [Gk, *heteros* + *genein,* to produce], **1.** reproduction that differs in successive generations, such as the alternation of sexual and asexual reproduction, so that offspring have characteristics different from those of the parents. In the asexual stage, it often involves one or more parthenogenetic or hermaphroditic generations, often with various hosts, as in the case of many trematode parasites. Also called **heterogamy, heterogeny, heterogony. 2.** asexual reproduction. **3.** abiogenesis. Compare **homogenesis.** See also **metagenesis.** —**heterogenetic, heterogenic,** *adj.*

**heterogenous** /het′əroj′ənəs/ [Gk, *heteros* + *genos,* kind], **1.** Having a nonuniform composition throughout. **2.** derived or developed from another source or from two different sources.

**heterogenous vaccine** [Gk, *heteros,* different, *genein,* to produce; L, *vaccinus,* cow], a vaccine made from a source other than the patient's own tissues.

**heterograft.**   See **xenograft.**

**heteroimmunization** /-im′yənīzā′shun/, immunization of an individual with antigens from a different species.

**heteroinfection** /-infek′shən/ [Gk, *heteros,* different; L, *inficere,* to stain], infection by a microorganism originating outside the body.

**heterolactic acid fermentation** /-lak′tik/, bacterial fermentation that produces a mixture of lactic acid and other products.

**heterologous.**   See **xenogeneic.**

**heterologous anaphylaxis** /het′ərol′əgəs/ [Gk, *heteros,* differen, *logos,* relation, *ana,* again, *phylaxis,* protection], a form of passive anaphylaxis that results from the transfer of serum between two animals of different species.

**heterologous insemination.** See **artificial insemination—donor (AID).**

**heterologous tumor** [Gk, *heteros* + *logos,* relation], a neoplasm consisting of tissue different from that of its site. Compare **homologous tumor, organoid neoplasm.**

**heterologous twins.**   See **dizygotic twins.**

**heterometropia** /-mətrō′pē·ə/ [Gk, *heteros,* different, *metron,* measure, *ops,* eye], a generally mild visual disorder in which one eye refracts differently from the other, causing slightly different images to be perceived by the right and left eyes.

**heteronymous** /het′əron′iməs/ [Gk, *heteros,* different,

*onyma,* name], **1.** having different names; the opposite of synonymous. **2.** an optical phenomenon in which two images are produced by one object. **3.** abnormal.

**heterophil** /het′ərofil′/ [Gk, *heteros* + *philein,* to love], having affinity for something unusual or abnormal, as an antibody that recognizes an antigen other than the one it is expected to challenge. Also spelled **heterophile** /-fīl′/.

**heterophil antibody test** [Gk, *heteros* + *philein,* to love], a test for the presence of heterophil antibodies in the serum of patients suspected of having infectious mononucleosis, based on an agglutination reaction between heterophil antibodies in a person's serum and heterophil antigen, a normal component of sheep erythrocytes. This antibody eventually appears in the serum of more than 80% of the patients with mononucleosis caused by the Epstein-Barr virus; hence it is highly diagnostic of the disease. See also **Epstein-Barr virus.**

**heterophile.** See **heterophil.**

**heterophilic leukocyte** /-fil′ik/ [Gk, *heteros,* different, *philein,* to love, *leukos,* white, *kytos,* cell], a neutrophil of certain animal species that takes an acid stain.

**heteroplastic transplantation** /-plas′tik/ [Gk, *heteros,* different, *plassein,* to mold; L, *transplantare*], the transfer of tissue from one animal to another of a different species. Compare **homoplastic transplantation.**

**heteroploid** /het′ərəploid′/ [Gk, *heteros* + *ploos,* times, *eidos,* form], **1.** an individual, organism, strain, or cell that has a variation in the number of chromosomes characteristic of somatic cells of the species. The change may involve entire sets of chromosomes or single chromosomes. **2.** pertaining to such an individual, organism, strain, or cell. **—heteroploidy,** *n.* See also **aneuploid, euploid.**

**heteroploidy** /het′ərəploi′dē/, the state or condition of having an abnormal number of chromosomes, either more or less than that characteristic of the somatic cell of the species.

**heteropolymer** /-pol′imir/ [Gk, *heteros* + *polys,* many, *meros,* part], a compound formed from subunits that are not all the same, such as a protein composed of various amino acid subunits.

**heterosexual** /-sek′shəl/ [Gk, *heteros,* different; L, *sexus,* male or female], **1.** a person whose sexual desire or preference is for people of the opposite sex. **2.** pertaining to sexual desire or preference for people of the opposite sex. **—heterosexuality,** *n.* See **sexual orientation.**

**heterosexual panic,** an acute attack of anxiety that results in the frantic pursuit of heterosexual activity in response to unconscious or latent homosexual impulses. Compare **homosexual panic.**

**heterosis** /het′ərō′sis/ [Gk, *heteros* + *osis,* condition], the superiority of first-generation hybrid plants and animals with respect to one or more traits when compared with either of the parent strains or with corresponding inbred strains. Also called **hybrid vigor.**

**heterotopic ossification** /-top′ik/ [Gk, *heteros* + *topos,* place], a nonmalignant overgrowth of bone, frequently occurring after a fracture, that is sometimes confused with certain bone tumors when visualized on x-ray film. Also called **exuberant callus, myositis ossificans.**

**heterotopic pain,** pain that appears in the wrong part of the body, as pain originating in the gallbladder that may be felt in the right shoulder. The phenomenon seems to be caused by projection of sensory neurons from different parts of the body into the same regions of the central nervous system. Also called **referred pain.**

**heterotopic pregnancy,** a pregnancy that is both intrauterine and extrauterine.

**heterotopic transplantation** [Gk, *heteros,* different, *topos,* place; L, *transplantare*], the transfer of tissue from one part of a body of a donor to another area of the body of a recipient.

**heterotransplant** /-trans′plant/ [Gk, *heteros,* different; L, *transplantare*], the transfer of tissue from one animal to another of a different species.

**heterotypic** /het′ərōtip′ik/ [Gk, *heteros* + *typos,* pattern], pertaining to or characteristic of a type differing from the usual or the normal, specifically regarding the first meiotic division of germ cells in gametogenesis as distinguished from the second meiotic division or a mitotic division. Also called **heterotypical.** Compare **homeotypic.**

**heterotypic chromosomes,** any unmatched pair of chromosomes, specifically the sex chromosomes.

**heterotypic mitosis,** the division of bivalent chromosomes, as occurs in the first meiotic division of germ cells in gametogenesis; a reduction division. Compare **homeotypic mitosis.**

**heterozygosis** /het′ərōzīgō′sis/ [Gk, *heteros* + *zygotos,* yoked], **1.** the formation of a zygote by the union of two gametes that have dissimilar pairs of alleles. **2.** the production of hybrids through crossbreeding. **—heterozygotic,** *adj.*

**heterozygote** /-zī′gōt/ [Gk, *heteros,* different, *zygotos,* yoked], an organism whose somatic cells have two different allelomorphic genes on the same locus of each pair of chromosomes. It can produce two different types of gametes.

**heterozygote detection,** the use of amniocentesis and other techniques to identify potential inherited X-linked recessive disorders, such as Hunter's syndrome or Duchenne's muscular dystrophy.

**heterozygotic.** See **heterozygosis.**

**heterozygous** /het′ərəzī′gəs/ [Gk, *heteros* + *zygotos,* yoked], having two different alleles at corresponding loci on homologous chromosomes. An individual who is heterozygous for a trait has inherited an allele for that trait from one parent and an alternative allele from the other parent. A person who is heterozygous for a genetic disease caused by a dominant allele, such as Huntington's disease, manifests the disorder. An individual who is heterozygous for a hereditary disorder produced by a recessive allele, such as sickle cell anemia, is asymptomatic or exhibits reduced symptoms of the disease. The offspring of a heterozygous carrier of a genetic disorder have a 50% chance of inheriting the allele associated with the disorder if the other parent does not carry the allele. Compare **homozygous.**

**heuristic** /hyŏŏris′tik/ [Gk, *heuriskein,* to discover], **1.** serving to stimulate interest for further investigation. **2.** a teaching method in which the student is encouraged to learn through independent research and investigation.

**HEV,** abbreviation for *hepatitis E virus.* See **hepatitis E.**

**hex-, hexa-,** combining meaning 'six': *hexabasic, hexavaccine, hexhydric.*

**hexachlorophene** /hek′səklôr′əfēn/, a topical antiinfective and detergent.

■ INDICATIONS: It is used as an antiseptic scrub and as a disinfectant for inanimate objects.

■ CONTRAINDICATIONS: Known hypersensitivity to this drug prohibits its use. Systemic absorption can occur when it is used on burns, broken skin, mucous membranes, and infant skin, with hemotoxic effects.

■ ADVERSE EFFECTS: Among the more serious adverse reactions are skin rash and neurologic abnormalities.

■ NOTE: The skin should be rinsed thoroughly to prevent systemic absorption.

**hexacosanol.** See **ceryl alcohol.**

**hexadactyly** /hek'sə·dak'tə·le/ [Gk, *hex,* six + *daktylos,* finger], the occurrence of six digits on the hand or foot.

**hexadecanoic acid.** See **palmitic acid.**

**hexadecanol.** See **cetyl alcohol.**

**Hexadrol,** trademark for a glucocorticoid (dexamethasone).

**hexamethylenamine.** See **methenamine.**

**hexamethylmelamine** /-meth'ilmel'əmēn/, an antineoplastic that is used to treat persistent or recurrent ovarian carcinomas.

**hexanoic acid.** See **caproic acid.**

**hexaploid.** See **polyploid.**

**hexavalent.** /hek'sivā'lənt/, pertaining to a chemical with a valence of 6. Also called **sexivalent.**

**hexenmilch.** See **witch's milk.**

**hexocyclium methylsulfate** /-sī'klē·əm/, an anticholinergic.

■ INDICATION: It is prescribed as an adjunct to ulcer therapy.

■ CONTRAINDICATIONS: Narrow-angle glaucoma, asthma, obstruction of the genitourinary or GI tract, ulcerative colitis, or known hypersensitivity to this drug prohibits its use.

■ ADVERSE EFFECTS: Among the more serious adverse reactions are blurred vision, central nervous system effects, tachycardia, dry mouth, decreased sweating, and hypersensitivity reactions.

**hexokinase** /hek'səkī'nās/ [Gk, *hex,* six, *glykys,* sweet, *kinein,* to move, *ase,* enzyme], an enzyme present in muscle that catalyzes the transfer of a phosphate group from adenosine triphosphate to glucose 6-phosphate. It is also found in yeast.

**hexosaminidase test,** a blood test used to detect the presence of the enzyme hexosaminidase, which is present in Tay-Sachs disease and Sandhoff's disease, a variant of Tay-Sachs.

**hexose** /hek'sōs/ [Gk, *hex,* six, *glykys,* sweet], a monosaccharide that contains six carbon atoms in the molecule. Glucose, mannose, and fructose are the principal hexoses found in nature, as well as being the principal absorbable end products of carbohydrate digestion.

**hexylcaine hydrochloride** /hek'silkān/, a local anesthetic for use on intact mucous membranes of the respiratory, upper GI, and urinary tracts.

**hexylresorcinol** /hek'ilrəsôr'sənol/, a topical skin anesthetic that is also administered for the treatment of certain types of worm infestations.

**Hf,** symbol for the element **hafnium.**

**HFJV,** abbreviation for *high-frequency jet ventilation.* See **high-frequency ventilation.**

**HFO,** abbreviation for *oscillation.*

**HFV,** abbreviation for **high-frequency ventilation.**

**Hg,** symbol for the element **mercury.**

**Hgb,** abbreviation for **hemoglobin.**

**HGE,** abbreviation for **human granulocytic erlichiosis.**

**HGF,** 1. abbreviation for *human growth factor* 2. abbreviation for *hyperglycemic-glycogenolytic factor.* See also **glucagon.**

**HHS,** abbreviation for **Department of Health and Human Services.**

**HI,** abbreviation for **hemagglutination inhibition.**

**hiatal hernia,** protrusion of a portion of the stomach upward through the diaphragm. The condition occurs in about 40% of the population, and most people display few, if any, symptoms. The major difficulty in symptomatic patients is gastroesophageal reflux, the backflow of the acid contents of the stomach into the esophagus. Diagnosis is made easily on x-ray films and may be an incidental finding of a chest ra-

diogram. Surgical treatment is usually unnecessary, and efforts should be directed to alleviating the discomfort associated with reflux. See also **diaphragmatic hernia, gastroesophageal reflux, heartburn.**

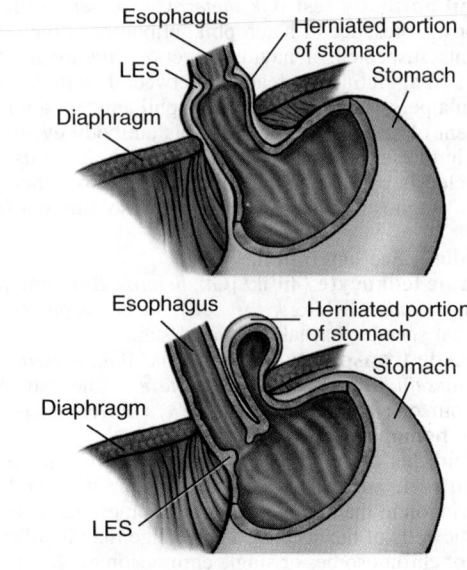

**Hiatal hernia** *(Monahan and Neighbors, 1998)*

**hiatus** /hī·ā'təs/ [L, *hiare,* to stand open], a usually normal opening in a membrane or other body structure. —**hiatal,** *adj.*

**hiatus aorticus** [L, *hiare,* to stand open; Gk, *aerein,* to raise], an opening in the diaphragm for the aorta and thoracic duct.

**hiatus esophagus** [L, *hiare,* to stand open; Gk, *oisophagos,* gullet], the opening in the diaphragm for the esophagus.

**hibakusha** /hē'bäkōō'shä/ [Japanese], people who were exposed to the atomic bomb explosions in Hiroshima and Nagasaki.

**Hib disease,** an infection caused by *Haemophilus influenzae* type b (Hib), which mainly affects children in the first 5 years of life. It is a leading cause of bacterial meningitis, as well as pneumonia, joint or bone infections, and throat inflammations. More than two thirds of the U.S. cases of Hib disease have been attributed to exposure in day-care centers. It is fatal in about 5% of infections. The infection can generally be prevented with a vaccine, given in infancy, usually at 2, 4, 6, and 12-18 months.

**hibernation** /hī'bərnā'shun/ [L, *hibernare,* to winter], a natural physiologic state or process wherein a generalized slowdown in metabolic and body functions produces a somnolescent condition and in which body temperature is maintained at a lower level than normal. It is a survival mechanism used by some species of birds and mammals to cope with periods of low temperature and reduced food supply.

**hibernoma** /hī'bərnō'mə/, *pl.* **hibernomas, hibernomata** [L, *hibernus,* winter; Gk, *oma,* tumor], a benign tumor, usually on the hips or the back, composed of fat cells that are partly or entirely of fetal origin. Also called **fat cell lipoma, fetal lipoma.**

**Hibiclens,** trademark for a topical antiinfective medication for the skin and mucous membranes (chlorhexidine gluconate).

**hiccup** /hik'əp/, a characteristic sound that is produced by the involuntary contraction of the diaphragm, followed by rapid closure of the glottis. Hiccups have various causes, including indigestion, rapid eating, certain types of surgery, and epidemic encephalitis. It can also be caused by or associated with abdominal distension. Most episodes of hiccups do not persist longer than a few minutes, but recurrent and prolonged attacks sometimes occur. The condition is most often seen in men. Sedatives are used in extreme cases. Also spelled **hiccough.** Also called **singultus.**

**Hickman catheter** /hik'mən/ [R. O. Hickman, American surgeon, 20th century], a type of central venous catheter used for the long term administration of substances via the venous system, such as antibiotics, total parenteral nutrition, or chemotherapeutic agents; it can be used for continuous or intermittent administration and may have either a single or a double lumen.

**hickory stick fracture.** See **greenstick fracture.**

**hidradenitis.** See **hydradenitis.**

**hidradenitis suppurativa** /hī'drad·ə·nī'tis·sup'yo͞o·rə·tē'v ə/ [Gk, *hydos,* water + *aden,* gland + *itis,* inflammation; L, *suppurare,* to form pus], a chronic suppurative and cicatricial disease of the apocrine gland−bearing areas, chiefly the axillae (especially in young women) and anogenital region (especially in men), which is caused by occlusion of the pores with secondary bacterial infection of apocrine sweat glands. It is characterized by the development of one or more tender red abscesses that enlarge and eventually break through the skin, yielding purulent or seropurulent drainage. Healing occurs with fibrosis, and recurrences lead to sinus tract formation and progressive scarring. Also called **apocrinitis, hidradenitis axillaris.**

**hidro-,** combining meaning 'sweat or sweat gland': *hidrocystoma, hidrosadenitis.*

**hidrosis** /hidrō'sis, hī-/ [Gk, *hidros,* sweat], sweat production and secretion. Also spelled **hydrosis.** Compare **anhidrosis, hyperhidrosis. —hidrotic,** *adj.*

**hieralgia** /hī'əral'jə/ [Gk, *hieron,* sacrum, *algos,* pain], a painful sacrum.

**hiero-, hier-,** combining meaning 'sacrum or something sacred': *hierolisthesis, hieromania, hierotherapy.*

**high.** See **rush.**

**high-altitude edema** [ME, *heigh* + L, *altitudo* + Gk, *oidema,* swelling], a form of pulmonary edema that occurs in people who move rapidly to higher altitudes. Fluid accumulates in the lungs as atmospheric pressure decreases.

**high blood pressure.** See **hypertension.**

**high-calorie diet,** a diet that provides 1000 or more calories a day beyond what is ordinarily recommended. It may be prescribed for nursing mothers, patients with severe weight loss caused by illness, or people with abnormally high metabolic rates or energy requirements, such as certain athletes or outdoor workers.

**high-copy number,** a large number of repetitive copies of a gene, such as may be produced by cloning.

**high-definition imaging (HDI),** an ultrasound technique used in breast cancer diagnosis to determine without biopsy whether a lump is a solid tumor or a relatively harmless fluid-filled cyst. HDI also provides a clear picture of lumps, revealing such details as irregular colors and edges.

**high-density lipoprotein (HDL)** [ME, *heigh,* high; L, *densus,* thick; Gk, *lipos,* fat, *proteios,* first rank], a plasma protein made mainly in the liver and containing about 50% lipoprotein (apoprotein) along with cholesterol, triglycerides and phospholipid and is involved in transporting cholesterol and other lipids to the liver to be disposed. Higher levels of high-density lipoprotein are associated with decreased cardiac risk profiles. See also **low-density lipoprotein, very-low-density lipoprotein (VLDL).**

**high-dose tolerance,** the absence of an expected immunologic response after repeated injections of large amounts of an antigen.

**high enema** [ME, *heigh* + Gk, *einienai,* to send in], an enema that is inserted into the colon through a long catheter.

**high-energy phosphate compound,** a chemical compound containing an easily hydrolyzed phosphoric anhydride group. The hydrolysis of this group liberates considerable energy, and coupling of this reaction to endothermic reactions provides the energy necessary for the endothermic reaction to proceed. Adenosine triphosphate is the most powerful and ubiquitous of the high-energy phosphate compounds found in the body. All of these compounds liberate energy to fuel muscle contraction, active transport across cell membranes, and synthesis of many substances in the body.

**highest intercostal vein** [ME, *heigh* + L, *inter,* between, *costa,* rib, *vena,* vein], one of a pair of veins that drain the blood from the upper two or three intercostal spaces. The right vein descends and opens into the azygous vein. The left vein crosses the arch of the aorta and opens into the left brachiocephalic vein, usually receiving the left bronchial vein.

**high-flow oxygen delivery system,** a respiratory care apparatus that supplies inspired gases at a consistent preset oxygen concentration. It is generally not affected by changes in the ventilatory pattern. Also called **fixed-performance oxygen delivery system.**

**high forceps,** an obstetric procedure in which forceps are used to deliver a baby whose head is not engaged in the birth canal. No longer considered acceptable or meeting the standard of care. Compare **low forceps, mid forceps.** See also **forceps delivery, obstetric forceps.**

**high-Fowler's position** [ME, *heigh,* high; George R. Fowler, American surgeon, 1848–1906], placement of the patient in a semisitting position by raising the head and trunk 90 degrees. The knees may or may not be flexed.

**high-frequency hearing loss** [ME, *heigh* + L, *frequens;* AS, *deaf*], a loss of ability to hear high-frequency sounds. It is most commonly associated with aging or noise exposure. Hearing loss may begin in early adulthood with a loss of hearing to frequencies in the range of 18 to 20 kHz. At about 60 years of age, loss of hearing may begin to affect lower frequencies, in the range of 4 to 8 kHz, thus interfering with the ability to understand speech. Hearing loss caused by noise exposure is often greatest at or near 4 kHz.

**high-frequency ventilation (HFV),** a technique for providing ventilatory support to patients at a rate of at least 60 breaths per minute with small tidal volumes. It may be used during intraoperative procedures such as laryngoscopy or bronchoscopy, as well as for ventilation in patients with a bronchopleural fistula. Kinds of HFV include high-frequency jet ventilation (HFJV) and high-frequency oscillation (HFO). HFJV uses a high-pressure gas source that can produce short, rapid jets of gas through a small-bore cannula into the airway above the carina at a rate of 100 to 400 per minute. HFO forces small impulses of gas into and out of the airway at a rate of 400 to 4000 per minute.

**high labial arch,** a labial arch wire adapted to lie gingival to the anterior tooth crowns and having auxiliary springs that extend downward in contact with the teeth to be moved.

**high-level wellness,** a concept of optimal health that emphasizes the integration of body, mind, and environment to maximize the function of an individual.

**high lithotomy,** a suprapubic approach for surgical removal of urinary bladder stones that are not easily removed by ultrasonic crushing. Also called **suprapubic lithotomy.**

**high-potassium diet,** a diet that contains foods rich in potassium, including all leafy green vegetables, brussels sprouts, citrus fruits, bananas, dates, raisins, legumes, meats, and whole grains. It is indicated for any condition that causes loss of extracellular fluid such as acute diarrhea, congenital renal alkalosis, aldosteronism, hypokalemia, hypertension, and diabetic coma. It is also indicated for patients who are receiving some diuretics, such as thiazide and furosemide, or corticosteroid therapy.

**high-pressure liquid chromatography,** a method of chromatography to separate and quantitate mixtures of substances in a solution. The procedure uses a high-resolution column, pressure, and gradient elution systems for separation of solutes by absorption, partition, ion exchange, and size exclusion. Also known as **high-performance liquid chromatography.**

**high-protein diet,** a diet that contains large amounts of protein, consisting largely of meats, fish, milk, legumes, and nuts. It may be indicated in protein depletion that results from any cause, as a preoperative preparation, or for patients with severe burns and sepsis, and so on. It may be contraindicated in liver failure or when kidney function is so impaired that added protein could result in azotemia and acidosis.

**high-residue diet** /-rez′idyōō/ [ME, *heigh* + L, *residuum,* remaining; Gk, *diaita,* way of living], a diet that contains a greater than usual proportion of substances the digestive tract will not metabolize and absorb, such as soluble and insoluble dietary fiber.

**high-resolution,** the quality and accuracy of detail presented by a graphics system display, such as on a computer monitor screen or a computer printout. Generally, resolution quality increases as the number of pixels, or image-forming units in the display, increases.

**high-risk infant,** any neonate, regardless of birth weight, size, or gestational age, who has a greater than average chance of morbidity or mortality, especially within the first 28 days of life. Risk factors include preconceptual, prenatal, natal, or postnatal conditions or circumstances that interfere with the normal birth process or impede adjustment to extrauterine growth and development. See also **neonatal period, premature infant.**

**high-risk pregnancy care,** a nursing intervention from the Nursing Interventions Classification (NIC) defined as identification and management of a high-risk pregnancy to promote healthy outcomes for mother and baby. See also **Nursing Interventions Classification.**

**high-speed handpiece,** a dental cutting instrument that rotates at up to 450,000 rpm. Modern high-speed handpieces are powered by miniature turbines driven by compressed air.

**high-vitamin diet,** a dietary regimen that includes a variety of foods that contain therapeutic amounts of all of the vitamins necessary for the metabolic processes of the body. It is often ordered in combination with other therapeutic diets that contain larger than usual amounts of protein or calories, especially when treating severe or chronic infection, malnutrition, or vitamin deficiency.

**hila.** See **hilum.**

**hilar** /hī′lär/ [L, *hilum,* a trifle], pertaining to a hilum.

**Hill-Burton Act,** a 1946 amendment to the U.S. Public Health Service Act authorizing grants to states for surveying their hospital and public health center needs and for planning and constructing additional facilities. Subsequent amendments authorized federal funding for as much as two thirds of the cost of construction projects and broadened the scope of the legislation to include diagnostic and treatment centers, long-term treatment centers, and nursing homes and to aid in modernization of existing hospitals. Also called **Hospital Survey and Construction Act.**

**Hill-Burton programs,** a cluster of programs created by U.S. legislation included in the National Health Planning and Resources Development Act of 1974. The programs allow federal monetary assistance for modernization of health facilities, construction of outpatient health centers, construction of inpatient facilities in underserved areas, and conversion of existing health care facilities for the provision of new health services.

**hilum** /hī′ləm/, *pl.* **hila** [L, *hilum,* a trifle], a depression or recess at that part of an organ where vessels and nerves enter.

**hindbrain** /hīnd′brān/ [ME, *hind* + AS, *bragen*], the division in the brain of an embryo that eventually becomes the pons, the medulla oblongata, and the cerebellum.

**hindgut** /hīnd′gut/ [ME, *hind* + AS, *guttas*], the caudal portion of the embryonic alimentary canal. It is formed by the development of the tail fold and eventually gives rise to part of the small and large intestines, rectum, bladder, and urogenital ducts. Compare **foregut, midgut.** See also **cloaca.**

**hind kidney.** See **metanephros.**

**hinge axis,** a line that passes through the left and right mandibular condyles and coincides with the center of rotation of the mandible. Determining the hinge axis is essential in constructing dental prostheses and in correcting occlusal interferences.

**hinge axis-orbital plane,** a reference plane for the diagnosis of various types of malocclusions and for the development of associated prostheses. It is usually determined by marking three points on a patient's skull. Two of the points, one on each side of the face, are located on the hinge axis. The third point is located on the face at the level of the orbital rim just beneath the eye.

**hinge-bow.** See **kinematic face-bow.**

**hinged knee,** an appliance designed to protect and support the knee during activity. It consists of an elastic sleeve with medial and lateral steel or aluminum bars hinged at the axis of the knee joint. The hinged bars are stabilized with leather or self-adhesive (Velcro) straps.

**hinge joint** [ME, *henge,* hinge; ME, *jointe,* a connection], a synovial joint providing a connection in which articular surfaces are closely molded together in a manner that permits extensive motion in one plane. The distal bone of a hinge joint seldom moves in the same plane as that of the axis of the proximal bone. The interphalangeal joints are hinge joints. Also called **ginglymus joint.** Compare **gliding joint, pivot joint.**

**hip.** See **coxa.**

**hip bath.** See **sitz bath.**

**hipbone.** See **innominate bone.**

**hip joint.** See **coxal articulation.**

**hip-joint disease** [AS, *hype* + L, *jungere,* to join; Gk, *dis,* not; Fr, *aise,* ease], any abnormal condition of the hip joint, such as **Perthes' disease** or congenital dislocation of the hip.

**Hippel's disease** [Eugen von Hippel, German ophthalmologist, 1867–1939], a familial disease, hereditary hemangioma confined mainly to the retina, first described by Hippel. Compare **von Hippel–Lindau disease.**

**hippocampal** /hip'ōkam'pəl/ [Gk, *hippokampos,* seahorse], pertaining to the hippocampus.

**hippocampal commissure** [Gk, *hippokampos,* seahorse; L, *commissura,* a joint], a thin triangular sheet of transverse fibers that connects the medial edges of the posterior pillars of the fornix in the brain.

**hippocampal fissure,** a fissure reaching from the posterior aspect of the corpus callosum to the tip of the temporal lobe.

**hippocampal formation** [Gk, *hippokampos,* seahorse; L, *formatio*], a part of the rhinencephalon, including the dentate gyrus, longitudinal striae, and hippocampus.

**hippocampal gyrus** [Gk, *hippokampos,* seahorse, *gyros,* turn], a convolution on the medial side of the temporal lobe of the cerebral cortex.

**hippocampus** /hip'ōkam'pəs/, *pl.* **hippocampi** [Gk, *hippokampos,* seahorse], a curved convoluted elevation of the floor of the inferior horn of the lateral ventricle of the brain. It is composed of gray substance covered by a layer of white fibers, the alveus, and functions as an important component of the limbic system and of memory processing. Its efferent projections form the fornix of the cerebrum. Also called **Ammon's horn, hippocampus major.**

**hippocampus minor.** See **calcar avis.**

**Hippocrates** /hipok'rətēz/, a Greek physician born about 460 BC on the island of Cos, a center for the worship of Æsculapius. Called the "Father of Medicine," Hippocrates introduced a scientific approach to healing by seeking physical causes of disease rather than magic or mythic relationships used by members of the Æsculapian cults of the time. He also compiled case records of illnesses, including results of treatments administered, and developed the art of ethical bedside care. See **Hippocratic oath.**

**Hippocrates' bandage.** See **capeline bandage.**

**Hippocratic oath** /hip'əkrat'ik/, an oath, attributed to Hippocrates, that serves as an ethical guide for the medical profession. It is traditionally incorporated into the graduation ceremonies of medical colleges and reads as follows: I swear by Apollo the physician, by Æsculapius, Hygeia, and Panacea, and I take to witness all the gods, and all the goddesses, to keep according to my ability and my judgment the following Oath: To consider dear to me as my parents him who taught me this art; to live in common with him and if necessary to share my goods with him; to look upon his children as my own brothers, to teach them this art if they so desire without fee or written promise; to impart to my sons and the sons of the master who taught me and the disciples who have enrolled themselves and have agreed to the rules of the profession, but to these alone, the precepts and the instruction. I will prescribe regimen for the good of my patients according to my ability and my judgment and never do harm to anyone. To please no one will I prescribe a deadly drug, nor give advice which may cause his death. Nor will I give a woman a pessary to procure abortion. But I will preserve the purity of my life and my art. I will not cut for stone, even for patients in whom the disease is manifest; I will leave this operation to be performed by practitioners (specialists in this art). In every house where I come I will enter only for the good of my patients, keeping myself far from all intentional ill-doing and all seduction, and especially from the pleasures of love with women or with men, be they free or slaves. All that may come to my knowledge in the exercise of my profession or outside of my profession or in daily commerce with men, which ought not to be spread abroad, I will keep secret and will never reveal. If I keep this oath faithfully, may I enjoy my life and practice my art, respected by all men and in all times; but if I swerve from it or violate it, may the reverse be my lot. See also **Hippocrates.**

**hippuric acid** [Gk, *hippos,* horse, *ouron,* urine; L, *acidus,* sour], a detoxication product in the urine of some animals. It has been used as a medication in the treatment of arthritic diseases.

**hip replacement** [AS, *hype*], substitution of an artificial ball and socket joint for the hip joint. Hip replacement is performed to relieve a chronically painful and stiff hip in advanced osteoarthritis, an improperly healed fracture, or degeneration of the joint. Antibiotic therapy is begun before surgery, and the patient is taught to walk with crutches or a walker. During surgery the femoral head, neck, and part of the shaft are removed, and the contours of the socket are smoothed. A prosthesis of a durable, hard metal alloy or stainless steel is attached to the femur. A metal or a plastic acetabulum is implanted. After surgery the patient may be placed in traction. The affected leg is kept abducted and in straight alignment with pillows; external rotation of the leg must be prevented. The nurse observes nerve function and circulation in the leg frequently during the first postoperative day. The most frequent complications are infection requiring removal of the new joint and dislocation. Ambulation begins gradually, with frequent short walks. Sitting for more than 1 hour is to be prevented, and hip flexion beyond 60 degrees may cause dislocation of the prosthesis. The patient continues an exercise program after discharge to maintain functional motion of the hip joint and to strengthen the abductor muscles. Weight-bearing may be modified according to the type of prosthesis implanted.

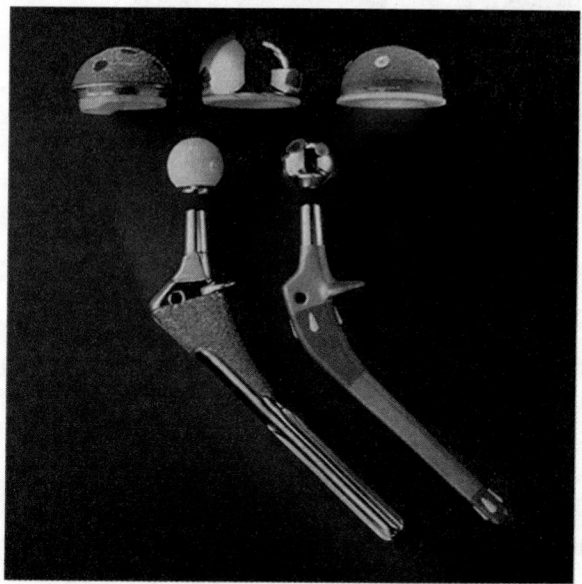

**Hip replacements**
*(Lewis, Collier, and Heitkemper, 1996/courtesy Zimmer, Inc., Warsaw, Indiana)*

**Hiprex,** trademark for a urinary antibacterial (methenamine hippurate).

**Hirschberg's reflex** /hursh'bərgz/, a diagnostic test for pyramidal tract disease. The test result is regarded as positive if inversion of the foot occurs when the sole is stroked at the base of the great toe.

**Hirschfeld's method** [Isador Hirschfeld, American dentist, 1881–1965], a tooth brushing technique in which the bristles are vigorously rotated in very small circles against the gingivae and the axial surfaces of the teeth at a slight incisal or occlusal angle.

**Hirschsprung's disease** /hirsh'sprŏŏngz/ [Harald Hirschsprung, Danish physician, 1830–1916], the congenital absence of autonomic ganglia in the smooth muscle wall of the colon, which causes poor or absent peristalsis in the involved segment of colon, accumulation of feces, and dilation of the bowel (megacolon). Symptoms include intermittent vomiting, diarrhea, and constipation. The abdomen may become distended to several times its normal size. The condition is usually diagnosed in infancy, but it may not be recognized until much later in childhood, when there is anorexia, lack of urge to defecate, distension of the abdomen, and poor health occur. Diagnosis is confirmed by barium enema; biopsy of the affected tissue shows the absence of ganglia. Surgical repair in early childhood is usually successful. A temporary colostomy is performed, and the aganglionic portion of the bowel is resected. The colostomy is almost always reversed a few months later. Also called **aganglionic megacolon, congenital megacolon.**

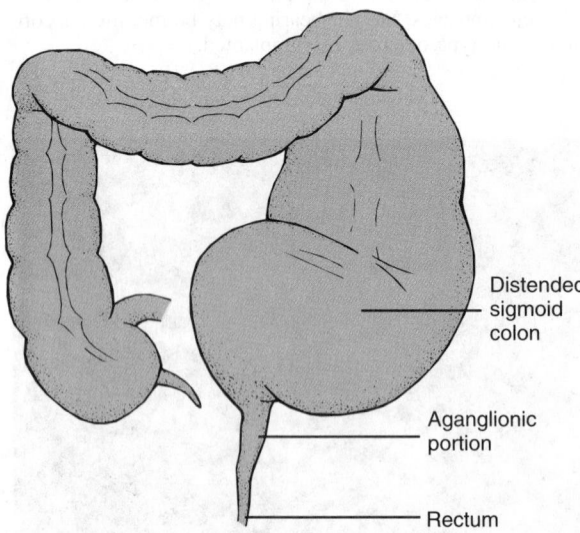

Distended sigmoid colon

Aganglionic portion

Rectum

**Hirschsprung's disease** *(Wong, 1996)*

**hirsutism** /hur'sŏŏtiz'əm/ [L, *hirsutus,* hairy], excessive body hair in a masculine distribution pattern as a result of heredity, hormonal dysfunction, porphyria, or medication. Treatment of the specific cause usually stops growth of more hair. Excess hair may be removed by laser, electrolysis, chemical depilation, shaving, or rubbing with pumice. Fine facial hair may be most effectively minimized by bleaching. Also called **hypertrichosis. —hirsute,** *adj.,* **hirsuteness,** *n.*

**hirsutoid papilloma of the penis** /hur'sŏŏtoid/ [L, *hirsutus,* shaggy; Gk, *eidos,* form], a condition characterized by clusters of small white papules on the coronal edge of the glans penis. Also called **papillomatosis coronae penis, pearly penile papules.**

**His,** abbreviation for **histidine.**

**His bundle.** See **bundle of His.**

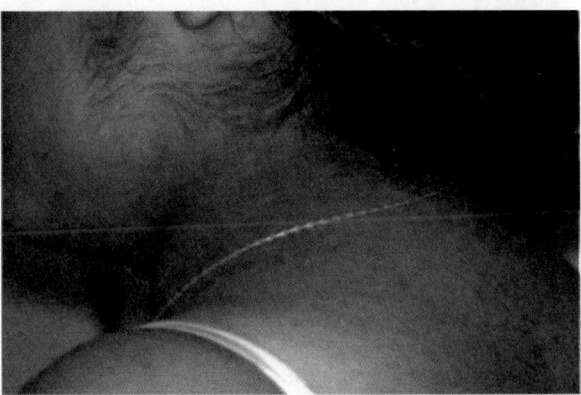

**Hirsutism** *(Lemmi and Lemmi, 2000)*

**His bundle electrogram (HBE)** [Wilhelm His, Jr., German physician, 1863–1934], a direct recording of the electrical activity in the atrioventricular bundle (bundle of His).

**His-Purkinje system** /his'pərkin'jē/ [Wilhelm His, Jr.; Johannes E. Purkinje, Czechoslovakian physiologist, 1787–1869], the conduction system in the heart from the atrioventricular bundle (bundle of His) to the distal Purkinje fibers.

**hist-.** See **histo-.**

**histaminase** /histam'inās/, a soft tissue enzyme found in various body tissues. It catalyzes the decarboxylation of histamine and converts histamine into inactive imidazolacetic acid. Also called **diamine oxidase.**

**histamine** /his'təmēn, -min/ [Gk, *histos,* tissue; L, *amine,* ammonia], a compound, found in all cells, that is produced by the breakdown of histidine. It is released in allergic inflammatory reactions and causes dilation of capillaries, a decrease in blood pressure, an increase in the secretion of gastric juice, and constriction of smooth muscles of the bronchi and uterus.

**histamine blocking agent,** a substance that interferes with stimulation of cells by histamine.

**histamine headache,** a headache associated with the release of histamine from the body tissues and marked by symptoms of dilated carotid arteries, fluid accumulation under the eyes, tearing or lacrimation, and rhinorrhea (runny nose). Symptoms include sudden sharp pain on one side of the head, involving the facial area from the neck to the temple. Treatment includes the use of preparations of antihistamines and ergot that help constrict the arteries. Also called **cluster headache, Horton's histamine cephalalgia.** See also **cephalalgia.**

**-histechia,** combining meaning a 'tissue retaining a (specified) substance': *cholesterohistechia, glycohistechia, uratohistechia.*

**histenzyme** /histen'zīm/, a renal tissue enzyme that splits hippuric acid into glycine and benzoic acid.

**histidine (His)** /his'tidēn/ [Gk, *histos,* tissue], a basic amino acid found in many proteins and a precursor of histamine. It is an essential amino acid in infants. See also **amino acid, protein.**

**histidinemia** /his'tidinē'mē·ə/, an inherited metabolic disorder caused by an enzyme defect involving l-histidine ammonia lyase and affecting the amino acid histidine. The condition leads to retardation and nervous system disorders. It is controlled by diet that limits the intake of histidine.

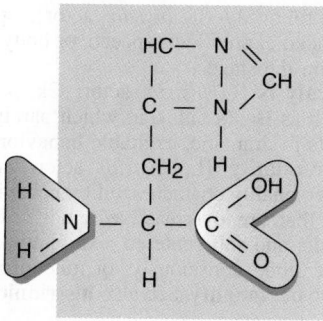

**Chemical structure of histidine**

**histioblast** /his′tē-/, a tissue-forming cell.

**histiocyte.** See **macrophage.**

**histiocytic leukemia.** See **monocytic leukemia.**

**histiocytic malignant lymphoma** /his′tē-ōsit′ik/ [Gk, *histos + kytos,* cell], a lymphoid neoplasm containing undifferentiated primitive cells or differentiated reticulum cells. Also called **reticulum cell sarcoma.**

**histiocytic necrotizing lymphadenitis.** See **Kikuchi's lymphadenitis.**

**histiocytosis X** /his′tē-ōsītō′sis/, *obsolete.* a cluster of conditions encompassing benign eosinophilic granuloma and several malignant lymphomatous diseases.

**histiotypic growth** /his′tē-ōtip′ik/ [Gk, *histos + typos,* mark], the uncontrolled proliferation of cells, as occurs in bacterial cultures and molds. Compare **organotypic growth.**

**histo-, hist-,** combining meaning 'tissue': *histoclastic, histohematin, histonectomy.*

**histocompatibility** /his′tōkəmpat′ibil′itē/ [Gk, *histos,* tissue; L, *compatibilis,* agreeing], a measure of the similarity of the antigens of a donor and a recipient of transplanted tissue.

**histocompatibility antigen** [Gk, *histos* + L, *compatibilis,* agreeable], one of a a group of genetically determined antigens on the surface of many cells. They are the cause of most graft rejections that occur in organ transplantation. See **isoantigen, histocompatibility locus.**

**histocompatibility complex,** a group of genes whose products determine the compatibility of tissues or organs transplanted from one individual to another of the same species or from one species to another. The histocompatibility complex of proteins are found on the plasma membrane cells and help identify tissues as "self" or foreign. In humans the major histocompatibility complex contains 50 genes on the short arm of chromosome number 6. See also **HLA complex.**

**histocompatibility gene** [Gk, *histos,* tissue; L, *compatibilis + genein,* to produce], a gene of the HLA complex that determines an antigen that governs histocompatibility of the donor and recipient of transplanted tissue. See also **human leukocyte antigen (HLA).**

**histocompatibility locus,** one of a set of positions on a chromosome occupied by a complex of genes that govern several tissue antigens. Together the loci and the genes comprise the human leukocyte antigen complex.

**histocyte** /his′təsīt/ [Gk, *histion,* web, *kytos,* cell], a macrophage of connective tissue that plays a role in the body's immune system.

**histogram** /his′təgram′/ [Gk, *histos + gramma,* record], (in research) a graph showing the values of one or more variables plotted against time or against frequency of occurrence. A graph of a patient's temperature, pulse, and respiration is an example of a histogram.

**histography** /histog′rəfē/ [Gk, *histos + graphein,* to record], the process of describing or creating visualizations of tissues and cells. —**histographer,** *n.,* **histographic,** *adj.,* **histographically,** *adv.*

**histoincompatible** /his′tō·in′kəmpat′əbəl/, pertaining to host and donor tissues that have different genotypes and are therefore likely to induce an immune response, leading to rejection of a tissue graft or organ transplant.

**histologic** [Gk, *histos,* tissue, *logos,* science], pertaining to the study of the microscopic anatomic and physiologic characteristics of tissues and the cells found therein.

**histological, histologically.** See **histology.**

**histologic technician,** an allied health professional who prepares tissue specimens of human and animal origin for a pathologist to examine for diagnostic, research, or teaching purposes. Histologic technicians process sections of body tissue by fixation, dehydration, embedding, sectioning, decalcification, microincineration, mounting, and routine and special staining. Educational preparation is usually 12 months for a certificate and 24 months for an associate degree. Also called **histotechnician.** See also **histotechnologist.**

**histologist** /histol′əjist/, a medical scientist who specializes in the study of the structure of organ tissues, including the composition of cells and their organization into various body tissues. See also **histology.**

**histology** /histol′əjē/ [Gk, *histos + logos,* science], **1.** the science dealing with the microscopic identification of cells and tissue. **2.** the structure of organ tissues, including the composition of cells and their organization into various body tissues. —**histologic, histological,** *adj.*

**histolysis** [Gk, *histos,* tissue, *lysis,* loosening], breakdown or dissolution of living organic tissue. —**histolytic,** *adj.*

**histolytic** /his′tōlit′ik/, pertaining to or causing the breakdown or dissolution of living organic tissue. See also **histolysis.**

**histone** /his′tōn/ [Gk, *histos,* tissue], any of a group of strongly basic, low-molecular-weight proteins that are soluble in water and insoluble in dilute ammonia and combine with DNA to form nucleoproteins. They are found in the nucleus of eukaryotic cells, where they form a complex with DNA in the chromatin and function in regulating gene activity. See also **nucleosome.**

**histopathology** /his′tōpathol′əjē/ [Gk, *histos,* tissue, *pathos,* disease, *logos,* science], the study of diseases involving the tissue cells.

**histoplasma agglutinin** /-plaz′mə/ [Gk, *histos + plasma,* a formation], a specific antibody that causes the clumping associated with fungal lung infections when it interacts with antigens.

***Histoplasma capsulatum*** [Gk, *histos + plasma* + L, *capsula,* little box], a dimorphic fungal organism that is a single budding yeast at body temperature and a mold at room temperature. It is the causative organism in histoplasmosis, common in the Mississippi River Valley. The fungus, spread by airborne spores from soil contaminated with excreta from infected birds or bats, acts as a parasite on the cells of the reticuloendothelial system.

**histoplasmin test** /-plaz′min/, a skin test for diagnosis of an infection caused by *Histoplasma capsulatum* fungus.

**histoplasmosis** /his′tōplazmō′sis/ [Gk, *histos + plasma + osis,* condition], an infection caused by inhalation of

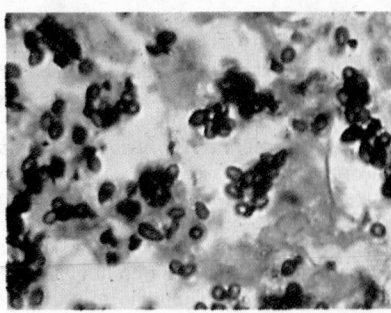

**Histoplasma capsulatum in the lung**
*(Baron, Peterson, and Finegold, 1994)*

spores of the fungus *Histoplasma capsulatum.* **Primary histoplasmosis** is characterized by fever, malaise, cough, and lymphadenopathy. Spontaneous recovery is usual; small calcifications remain in the lungs and affected lymph glands. **Progressive histoplasmosis,** the sometimes fatal disseminated form of the infection, is characterized by ulcerating sores in the mouth and nose; enlargement of the spleen, liver, and lymph nodes; and severe and extensive infiltration of the lungs. The severe form is treated with amphotericin B, and less severe cases may be treated with ketoconazole. Infection confers immunity; a histoplasmin skin test may be performed to identify people who may safely work with contaminated soil. The disease is most common in the Mississippi and Ohio River Valleys. Also called **Darling's disease.**

**history** /his'tərē/ [L, *historia,* inquiry],  **1.** a record of past events. **2.** a systematic account of the medical, emotional, and psychosocial occurrences in a patient's life and of factors in the family, ancestors, and environment that may have a bearing on the patient's condition.

**history of present illness,**  an account obtained during the interview with the patient of the onset, duration, and character of the present illness, as well as of any acts or factors that aggravate or ameliorate the symptoms. The patient is asked what he or she considers to be the cause of the symptoms and whether a similar condition has occurred in the past. See also **health history.**

**histotechnician.**  See **histologic technician.**

**histotechnologist,**  an allied health professional who prepares tissue specimens of human and animal origin for a pathologist to examine for diagnostic, research, or teaching purposes. Histotechnologists perform all functions of the histologic technician as well as identifying tissue structures, cell components, and their staining characteristics and relating them to physiologic functions; implementing and testing new techniques and procedures; making judgments concerning the results of quality control measures; instituting proper procedures to maintain accuracy; and sometimes supervising and teaching. A 4-year baccalaureate degree program is usually required. See also **histologic technician.**

**histotoxin** /-tok'sin/ [Gk, *histos* + *toxikon,* poison],  any substance that is poisonous to body tissues. Histotoxins are usually generated within the body rather than being introduced externally. An example is the tissue-destroying enzymes formed by bacteria such as *Clostridium perfringens.*

**histotroph, histotrophe, histotrophic nutrition.**  See **embryotroph.**

**histrionic** /his'trē·on'ik/ [L, *histrio,* actor],  pertaining to exaggerated facial expressions, speech, or body movements, such as used on the stage.

**histrionic paralysis** [L, *histrio,* actor; Gk, *paralyein*],  a condition, such as **Bell's palsy,** in which paralysis of facial muscles results in dramatic, excitable behavior.

**histrionic personality** [L, *histrio,* actor, *persona,* role played],  a personality characterized by behavioral patterns and attitudes that are overreactive, emotionally unstable, overly dramatic, and self-centered, exhibited as a means of attracting attention, consciously or unconsciously. Also called **hysteric personality.** See also **histrionic personality disorder.**

**histrionic personality disorder,**  a disorder characterized by dramatic, reactive, and intensely exaggerated behavior, which is typically self-centered. It results in severe disturbance in interpersonal relationships that can lead to psychosomatic disorders, depression, alcoholism, and drug dependency. Symptoms include emotional excitability, such as irrational angry outbursts or tantrums; abnormal craving for activity and excitement; overreaction to minor events; manipulative threats and gestures; egocentricity; inconsiderateness; inconsistency; and continuous demand for reassurance generated by feelings of helplessness and dependency. A person having this disorder is perceived by others as vain, demanding, superficial, self-centered, and self-indulgent. The disorder is more prevalent in women than in men and is treated by various psychotherapies, depending on the individual and the severity of the condition. See also **narcissistic personality disorder.**

**His-Werner disease** [Wilhelm His, Jr., German physician, 1863–1934; Heinrich Werner, German physician, 1874–1947; Gk, *dis,* not; Fr, *aise,* ease],  trench fever, an acute louse-borne infection that mainly affected soldiers in World War I.

**HIV,**  abbreviation for **human immunodeficiency virus.**

**HIV-associated dementia (HAD),**  a usually rapidly progressive dementia that is the primary manifestation of encephalopathy caused by human immunodeficiency virus type I infection. It is marked a variety of cognitive, motor, and behavioral abnormalities, including loss of retentive memory, inattentiveness, language disorders, apathy, incoordination, and ataxia. As the disease progresses, paraplegia, incontinence urine and feces, abulia, and mutism may occur. Survival after the onset of dementia is usually three to six months but is occasionally longer.

**HIV-associated nephropathy,**  renal pathology in patients infected with the human immunodeficiency virus, similar to focal glomerular sclerosis, with proteinuria, enlarged kidneys, and dilated tubules containing proteinaceous casts; it may progress to end stage renal disease within weeks.

**HIV-associated retinopathy,**  a usually asymptomatic microangiopathy affecting the retina, seen in human immunodeficiency virus infection; it is manifested by transient cotton-wool exudate, and occasionally hemorrhages, microaneurysms, and other lesions of the microvasculature. Also called **AIDS-associated retinopathy.**

**hives.**  See **urticaria.**

**Hivid,**  trademark for an antiretroviral nucleoside analog (zalcitabine).

**HIVNET,**  an international vaccine test network organized to conduct studies of prospective vaccines for human immunodeficiency virus (HIV) infection. It also supports behavioral and other studies of HIV infections.

**HIV protease inhibitors** /prō'tē·ās in·hib'i·tərz/ [*protein* + *-ase,* enzyme suffix; L, *inhibere,* to restrain],  a group of antiretroviral drugs active against the human immunodeficiency virus; they prevent cleavage of viral polyproteins, causing production of immature viral particles that are noninfective. Examples include indinavir, ritonavir, and saquinavir. Also called **protease inhibitors.**

**H⁺,K⁺-ATPase** /ā·tē·pē′ās /, a membrane-bound enzyme occurring on the secretory surfaces of parietal cells; it uses the energy derived from the hydrolysis of ATP to drive the exchange of ions across the cell membrane, secreting acid into the gastric lumen. Protons and chloride ions are pumped against gradients across the apical membranes of activated parietal cells into the gastric lumen, in exchange for potassium ions. See also **adenosine triphosphatase.**

**HLA,** abbreviation for **human leukocyte antigen.**

**HLA-A,** abbreviation for *human leukocyte antigen A.* See **human leukocyte antigen.**

**HLA-B,** abbreviation for *human leukocyte antigen B.* See **human leukocyte antigen.**

**HLA complex,** human leukocyte antigen group A, the region of chromosome 6 containing genes that code for proteins that enable the immune system to differentiate tissues or proteins between "self" and "nonself." These loci are identified by numbers and letters, such as HLA-B27. Antigens are divided into three classes. Class I antigens (HLA-A, -B, and C) occur on the surface of all nucleated cells and platelets and are important in tissue transplantation. If donor and recipient HLA antigens do not match, the nonself antigens are recognized and destroyed by killer T cells. Class II antigens occur only on immunocompetent cells and normally recognize foreign proteins. Class III antigens are non-histocompatibility antigens, such as some compliment components, that map in the HLA complex. Also called **histocompatibility complex** and **major histocompatibility complex (MHC).**

**HLA-D,** abbreviation for *human leukocyte antigen D.* See **human leukocyte antigen.**

**HLH,** abbreviation for *human luteinizing hormone.*

**HLHS,** abbreviation for **hypoplastic left heart syndrome.**

**HMD,** abbreviation for **hyaline membrane disease.** See **respiratory distress syndrome of the newborn.**

**HME,** abbreviation for **human monocytic erlichiosis.**

**HMG-CoA reductase,** a rate-controlling enzyme of cholesterol synthesis. Activity of the enzyme may be as much as 60 times higher than normal in patients with familial hypercholesterolemia.

**HMO,** abbreviation for **health maintenance organization.**

**HMS Liquifilm,** trademark for an ophthalmic preparation containing a glucocorticoid (medrysone).

**Ho,** symbol for the element **holmium.**

**H₂O,** symbol for **water.**

**hoarseness** /hôrs′nəs/, a condition marked by a rough, harsh, grating voice, indicating an inflammation of the throat and larynx.

**hod-,** prefix meaning 'pathway': *hodology, hodoneuromere.*

**Hodgkin's disease** /hoj′kinz/ [Thomas Hodgkin, English physician, 1798–1866], a malignant disorder characterized by painless, progressive enlargement of lymphoid tissue, usually first evident in cervical lymph nodes; splenomegaly; and the presence of Sternberg-Reed cells, large, atypical macrophages with multiple or hyperlobulated nuclei and prominent nucleoli. Symptoms include anorexia, weight loss, generalized pruritus, low-grade fever, night sweats, anemia, and leukocytosis. The disease is diagnosed in about 7100 Americans annually and causes approximately 1700 deaths a year, affects twice as many males as females, and

usually develops between 15 and 35 years of age, but sometimes as late as 70 years of age. The diagnosis is established by blood studies, x-ray films, lymphangiograms, lymph node biopsies, and ultrasonic and computed tomographic scans. Radiotherapy, using a covering mantle to protect other organs, is the treatment of choice for early stages of the disease; combination chemotherapy is the treatment for advanced disease. Long-term remissions are achieved in more than half of the patients treated, and 60% to 90% of those with localized disease may be cured. There is a threefold increased risk of development of Hodgkin's disease in first-degree relatives, suggesting an unknown genetic mechanism.

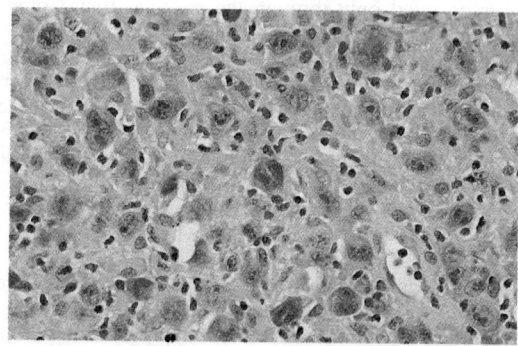

**Hodgkin's disease: lymphocyte depletion type**
*(Kumar, Cotran, and Robbins, 1997/courtesy Dr. Robert W. McKenna, Department of Pathology, University of Texas Southwestern Medical School, Dallas)*

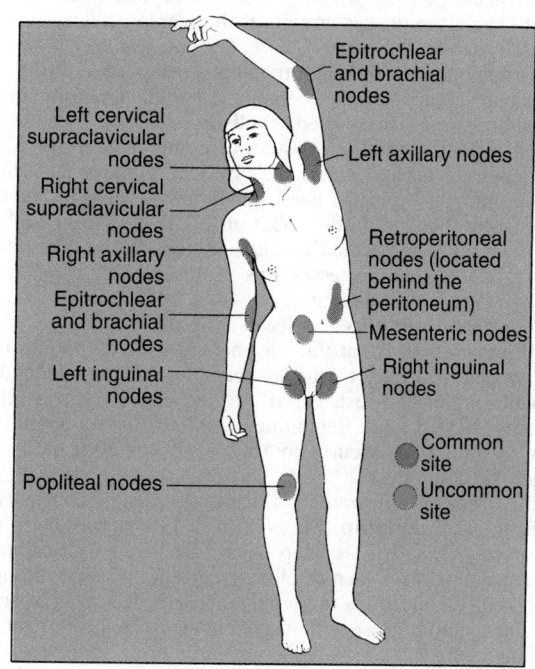

**Lymph node sites for Hodgkin's disease**
*(Huether and McCance, 2000)*

**Hodgson's disease** /hoj'sənz/ [Joseph Hodgson, English physician, 1788–1869; Gk, *dis*, not; Fr, *aise*, ease], an aneurysmal dilation of the aorta.

**Hoffmann's atrophy.** See **Werdnig-Hoffmann disease.**

**Hoffmann's reflex** [Johann Hoffmann, German neurologist, 1857–1919], an abnormal reflex elicited by sudden forceful flicking of the nail of the index, middle, or ring finger, which causes flexion of the thumb and of the middle and distal phalanges of one of the other fingers. It is indicative of pyramidal tract disease above the level of the seventh or eighth cervical and first thoracic vertebrae. Also called **Hoffmann's sign.**

**hol-.** See **holo-.**

**holandric** /holan'drik/ [Gk, *holos*, whole, *aner*, man], **1.** referring to genes located on the nonhomologous portion of the Y chromosome. **2.** pertaining to traits or conditions transmitted only through the paternal line. Compare **hologynic.**

**holandric inheritance,** the acquisition or expression of traits or conditions only through the paternal line, transmitted by genes located on the nonhomologous portion of the Y chromosome. Compare **hologynic inheritance.**

**hold-relax,** a technique of facilitating neuromuscular sensation and awareness. It is used in treating hypertonicity or motor dysfunction. It is often applied when there is muscle tightness on one side of a joint and when immobility is the result of pain.

**holism** /hō'lizəm/ [Gk, *holos*, whole], a philosophic concept in which an entity is seen as more than the sum of its parts. Holism is prominent in current approaches to psychology, biology, nursing, medicine, and other scientific, sociologic, and educational fields of study and practice. Also spelled **wholism.**

**holistic** /hōlis'tik/ [Gk, *holos*], pertaining to the whole; considering all factors, as holistic medicine. Also spelled **wholistic.**

**holistic counseling,** an alternative form of psychotherapy that focuses on the whole person (mind, body, and spirit) and health; the goal is growth of the whole person.

**holistic health** /hōlis'tik/ [AS, *hal*, whole, *haelth*], a concept that concern for health requires a perspective of the individual as an integrated system rather than one or more separate parts. Also spelled **wholistic.**

**holistic health care,** a system of comprehensive or total patient care that considers the physical, emotional, social, economic, and spiritual needs of the person; his or her response to illness; and the effect of the illness on the ability to meet self-care needs. Holistic nursing is the modern nursing practice that expresses this philosophy of care. Also called **comprehensive care.**

**Hollenback condenser.** See **pneumatic condenser.**

**Holliday-Segar formula,** a method of estimating the daily caloric needs of the average hospital patient under conditions of bed rest, based on the body weight in kilograms of the patient. Beginning at 100 kcal/kg for an infant, the formula plots a curve to 1500 kcal plus 20 kcal/kg for each kilogram over 20 kg.

**hollow** /hol'ō/ [OE, *holh*], a depressed area or concavity.

**hollow cathode lamp** [ME, *holwe* + Gk, *kata*, down, *hodos*, way, *lampas*], a lamp consisting of a metal cathode and an inert gas. When an electric current is passed through the cathode, electrons in the metal are excited so as to emit a line spectrum of specific wavelengths related to the metal of the cathode.

**holmium (Ho)** /hōl'mē-əm/ [L, *Holmia*, Stockholm, Sweden], a rare earth metallic element. Its atomic number is 67; its atomic mass is 164.93.

**holo-, hol-,** prefix meaning 'entire or the whole': *holodiastolic, holomastigote, holotonia.*

**holoacardius** /hol'ō-äkär'dē-əs/ [Gk, *holos* + *kardia*, heart], a separate, grossly defective monozygotic twin fetus. It is usually represented by a shapeless, nonformed mass in which the heart is absent and the circulation in utero is accomplished totally by the heart of the viable twin through a vascular shunt.

**holoacardius acephalus,** a grossly defective separate twin fetus that lacks a heart, a head, and most of the upper portion of the body.

**holoacardius acormus,** a grossly defective, separate twin fetus in which the trunk is malformed and little more than the head is recognizable.

**holoacardius amorphus,** a malformed separate twin fetus in which there are no recognizable or formed parts.

**holoarthritis** /-ärthrī'tis/, a form of arthritis that involves all or most of the joints.

**holoblastic** /hol'əblas'tik/ [Gk, *holos* + *blastos*, germ], pertaining to an ovum that contains little or no yolk and undergoes total cleavage. Compare **meroblastic.**

**holocephalic** /hō'lōsifal'ik/ [Gk, *holos* + *kephale*, head], pertaining to a malformed fetus in which several parts are deficient although the head is complete.

**holocrine** /hol'əkrēn/ [Gk, *holos*, whole, *krienein*, to secrete], pertaining to a gland whose only function is to secrete or whose secretion consists of disintegrated cells of the gland itself.

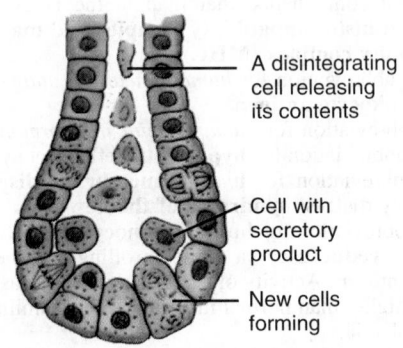

A disintegrating cell releasing its contents

Cell with secretory product

New cells forming

**Holocrine gland** (Applegate, 2000)

**holocrine secretion** [Gk, *holos*, whole, *krienein*, to secrete], a secretion that consists of disintegrated or altered cells of the gland, as in the example of sebaceous glands.

**holodiastolic.** See **pandiastolic.**

**holoendemic** /hol'ō-endem'ik/, pertaining to an intensely endemic disease area.

**holoenzyme** /hol'ō-en'zīm/ [Gk, *holos* + *en*, in, *zymos*, ferment], a complete enzyme-cofactor complex that gives rise to full catalytic activity.

**holographic reconstruction** /-graf'ik/, a method of producing three-dimensional images with diagnostic ultrasound equipment.

**hologynic** /hol'ōjin'ik/ [Gk, *holos* + *gyne*, female], **1.** referring to genes located on attached X chromosomes. **2.** pertaining to traits or conditions transmitted only through the maternal line. Compare **holandric.**

**hologynic inheritance,** the acquisition or expression of traits or conditions only through the maternal line, transmitted by genes located on attached X chromosomes. The phenomenon is not known to occur in humans. Compare **holandric inheritance.**

**holoprosencephaly** /hol′ōpros′ensef′əlē/ [Gk, *holos* + *pro,* before, *enkephalos,* brain], a congenital defect caused by the failure of the prosencephalon to divide into hemispheres during embryonic development. It is characterized by multiple midline facial defects, including cyclopia in severe cases. It can also be caused by an extra chromosome in the 13-15 or D group, manifested as one of many developmental defects. See also **trisomy 13. —holoprosencephalic, holoprosencephalous,** *adj.*

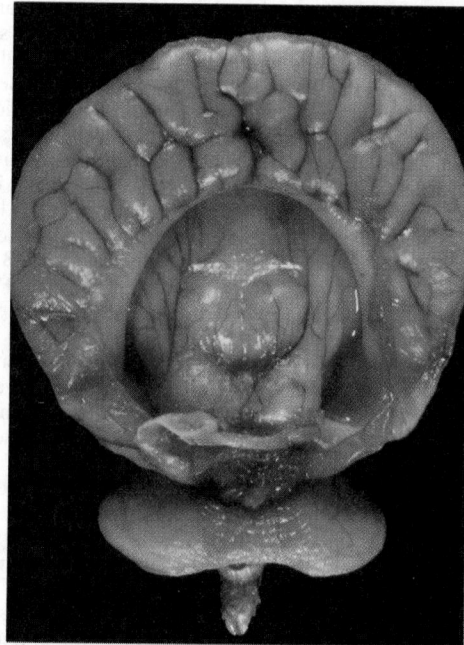

**Holoprosencephaly: view of dorsal surface**
*(Cotran, Kumar, and Collins, 1999)*

**holorachischisis.** See **complete rachischisis.**
**holosystolic.** See **pansystolic.**
**Holter monitor** [Norman J. Holter, American biophysicist, 1914–1983; L, *monere,* to remind], trademark for a device for making prolonged electrocardiograph recordings (usually 24 hours) on a portable tape recorder while the patient conducts normal daily activities. The patient also may keep an activity diary for the purpose of comparing daily events with electrocardiographic tracings. Also called **ambulatory electrocardiograph.**
**Holthouse's hernia.** See **inguinocrural hernia.**
**Holt-Oram syndrome** /hōlt·or′əm/ [Mary Clayton Holt, British cardiologist, 20th century; Samuel Oram, English cardiologist, b. 1913], autosomal dominant heart disease of varying severity, usually an atrial or ventricular septal defect, associated with skeletal malformation (hypoplastic thumb and short forearm). Also called **heart-hand syndrome.**

**Holtzman inkblot technique,** a modification of the Rorschach test in which many more pictures of inkblots are used, the subject is permitted only one response to each design, and the scoring is predominantly objective rather than subjective.
**Homans' sign** [John Homans, American surgeon, 1877-1954; L, *signum,* mark], pain in the calf with dorsiflexion of the foot, indicating thrombophlebitis or thrombosis.
**home assessment** [AS, *ham,* village; L, *assidere,* to sit beside], an examination of the living area of a physically challenged person for the purposes of making recommendations about elimination of safety hazards and suggesting architectural or other modifications that would allow for independent functioning.
**home care** [AS, *ham,* village; L, *garrire,* to chatter], a health service provided in the patient's place of residence for the purpose of promoting, maintaining, or restoring health or minimizing the effects of illness and disability. Service may include such elements as medical, dental, and nursing care; speech and physical therapy; homemaking services of a home health aide; and provision of transportation. The nature and extent of care needed and the ability of the patient's family and friends to assume responsibility for that care are assessed. Nursing may be provided by a registered nurse, licensed practical nurse, or home health aide. Some hospitals have home care services that include regular visits by a nurse and a physician to patients in the home.
**home health agency,** an organization that provides health care in the home. Medicare certification for a home health agency in the United States requires provision of skilled nursing services and at least one additional therapeutic service.
**home health nurse,** a registered nurse who visits patients in the home. The nurse works primarily in the area of secondary or tertiary care, providing hands-on care and educating the patient and family on care and prevention of future episodes.
**homeless person,** an individual who has no permanent home, haven, or domicile. Such individuals usually are indigent and depend on charity or public assistance for temporary lodging and medical care. An estimated 30% of homeless persons suffer from some type of mental disorder. See also **indigence.**
**home maintenance assistance,** a nursing intervention from the Nursing Interventions Classification (NIC) defined as helping the patient/family to maintain the home as a clean, safe, and pleasant place to live. See also **Nursing Interventions Classification.**
**home maintenance, ineffective** a nursing diagnosis accepted by the Fourth National Conference on the Classification of Nursing Diagnoses. Impaired home maintenance management is the inability to independently maintain a safe, growth-promoting immediate environment.
■ DEFINING CHARACTERISTICS: Among the defining characteristics reported by the patient and other members of the household are difficulty in maintaining the home in a comfortable condition, a need for help from the outside in maintaining the home, and the existence of debt or a financial crisis. Among the defining characteristics that may be observed in the home are disorder, an offensive odor, an inappropriate temperature, lack of necessary equipment or supplies, and the presence of rodents or vermin.
■ RELATED FACTORS: Related factors include an individual or family member with a disease or injury; insufficient family organization or planning; insufficient finances; unfamiliarity with neighborhood resources; impaired cognitive or emotional functioning; lack of knowledge; lack of role model-

ing; and inadequate support systems. See also **nursing diagnosis.**

**homeo-, homoeo-, homoio-,** combining meaning 'sameness, similarity': *homeochrome, homeomorphus, homeothermal.*

**homeodynamics** /hō′mē·ədīnam′iks/ [Gk, *homoios,* similar, *dynamis,* force], the constantly changing interrelatedness of body components while maintaining an overall equilibrium.

**homeomorphous** /-môr′fəs/, similar in appearance but different in composition.

**homeopathic.** See **homeopathy.**

***Homeopathic Pharmacopoeia of the United States,*** one of the three official drug compendia specified in the Federal Food, Drug, and Cosmetic Act. See also **compendium,** *National Formulary (NF), United States Pharmacopoeia (USP).*

**homeopathist** /hō′mē·op′əthist/, a physician who practices homeopathy.

**homeopathy** /hō′mē·op′əthē/ [Gk, *homoios,* similar, *pathos,* disease], a system of therapeutics based on the theory that "like cures like." The theory was advanced in the late eighteenth century by Dr. Samuel Hahnemann, who believed that a large amount of a particular drug may cause symptoms of a disease and moderate dosage may reduce those symptoms; thus some disease symptoms could be treated by very small doses of medicine. In practice, homeopathists dilute drugs with milk sugar in ratios of 1 to 10 to achieve the smallest dose of a drug that seems necessary to control the symptoms in a patient and prescribe only one medication at a time. Compare **allopathy. —homeopathic,** *adj.*

**homeostasis** /hō′mē·əstā′sis/ [Gk, *homoios* + *stasis,* standing still], a relative constancy in the internal environment of the body, naturally maintained by adaptive responses that promote healthy survival. Various sensing, feedback, and control mechanisms function to effect this steady state. Some of the key control mechanisms are the reticular formation in the brainstem and the endocrine glands. Some of the functions controlled by homeostatic mechanisms are heartbeat, hematopoiesis, blood pressure, body temperature, electrolytic balance, respiration, and glandular secretion. **—homeostatic,** *adj.*

**homeotherapy** /-ther′əpē/, the treatment or prevention of disease by homeopathic methods.

**homeotic mutation** /hō′mē·ot′ik/, a mutation that causes tissues to alter their normal differentiation pattern, producing integrated structures but in unusual locations. For example, a homeotic mutation in the fruit fly, *Drosphila,* causes legs to develop where antennae normally form.

**homeotypic** /hō′mē·ōtip′ik/ [Gk, *homoios* + *typos,* mark], pertaining to or characteristic of the regular or usual type, specifically regarding the second meiotic division of germ cells in gametogenesis as distinguished from the first meiotic division. Also called **homeotypical.** Compare **heterotypic.**

**homeotypic mitosis,** the separation of sister chromatids, as occurs in the second meiotic division of germ cells in gametogenesis. Compare **heterotypic mitosis.**

**Home's silver precipitation method,** a technique for depositing silver in enamel and dentin by applying ammoniac silver nitrate solution and reducing with formalin or eugenol.

**homicide** /hom′isīd/ [L, *homo,* man, *caedere,* to kill], the death of one human being caused by another.

**hominal physiology** /hom′inəl/ [L, *hominis,* human; Gk, *physis,* nature, *logos,* science], the study of the specific physical and chemical processes involved in the normal functioning of humans; human physiology.

**hominid** /hom′inid/ [L, *homo,* man; Gk, *eidos,* form], pertaining to the primate family Hominidae, which includes humans.

**homo-,** **1.** prefix meaning 'the same': *homocentric, homodont, homolysis.* **2.** prefix meaning 'the addition of one $CH_2$ group to the main compound': *homochelidonine, homocystine, homoquinine.*

**homoblastic** /hō′mōblas′tik/ [Gk, *homos* + *blastos,* germ], developing from the same germ layer or from a single type of tissue. Compare **heteroblastic.**

**homocarnosine** /hō′mō·kär′nō·sēn /, a dipeptide consisting of γ-aminobutyric acid and histidine; in humans it is found in the brain but not in other tissues.

**homochronous inheritance** /hōmok′rənəs/ [Gk, *homos* + *chronos,* time], the appearance of traits or conditions in offspring at the same age when they appeared in the parents.

**homocysteine** /-sis′tēn/, an amino acid containing sulfur and a homolog of cysteine, produced in the demethylation of methionine. It is also an intermediate product in the biosynthesis of cysteine from ʟ-methionine via ʟ-cystathionine in the breakdown of proteins. High levels of homocysteine are associated with an increased risk of collagen cardiovascular disorders, particularly thromboembolic stroke. It is believed the amino acid may have a toxic effect on cells lining the blood vessels. Studies also indicate that low levels of homocysteine are found in people with high intake of B vitamins. See also **homocystine.**

**homocysteine test (HCY),** a blood test used to detect levels of homocysteine, which, if elevated, may act as an independent risk factor for ischemic heart disease, cerebrovascular disease, peripheral arterial disease, and venous thrombosis. This test should be considered for screening in individuals with progressive and unexplained atherosclerosis despite normal lipoproteins and in the absence of other risk factors, and in those with an unusual family history of atherosclerosis.

**homocystine** /sis′tin/, a disulfide analog of homocysteine produced by the oxidation of homocysteine. See also **homocysteine.**

**homocystinemia** /-sis′tinē′mē·ə/, an amino acid disorder that causes an excess of homocystine in the blood. See also **homocystinuria.**

**homocystinuria** /hō′mōsis′tinōŏr′ē·ə/ [Gk, *homos* + (cystine); Gk, *ouron,* urine], a rare biochemical abnormality characterized by the abnormal presence of homocystine, an amino acid, in the blood and urine, which is caused by any of several enzyme deficiencies in the metabolic pathway of methionine to cystine. The disease is inherited as an autosomal-recessive trait; its clinical signs are similar to those of Marfan's syndrome, including mental retardation, osteoporosis leading to skeletal abnormalities, dislocated lenses, and thromboembolism. Treatment may include a diet low in methionine and supplementation with large doses of vitamin $B_6$. Long-term results of treatment are not available. **—homocystinuric,** *adj.*

**homoeo-.** See **homeo-.**

**homogametic** /hō′mōgamet′ik/ [Gk, *homos* + *gamete,* spouse], pertaining to the sex that produces gametes of only one kind, in terms of their sex chromosomes. In human beings, the female is the homogametic sex.

**homogenate** /hōmoj′ənit/, a tissue that is or has been made homogenous, as by grinding cells into a creamy consistency for laboratory studies. A homogenate usually lacks cell structure. Also called **broken cell preparation.**

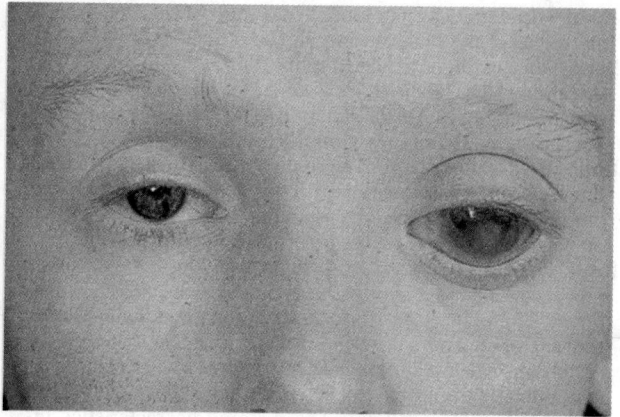

**Homocystinuria: lens dislocation** *(Newton, 1995)*

**homogeneous** /hō'mōjē'nē-əs/ [Gk, *homos* + *genos*, kind], **1.** consisting of similar elements or parts. **2.** having a uniform quality throughout. Compare **heterogeneous.** —**homogeneity,** *adj.*

**homogenesis** /hō'mōjē'nē-əs/ [Gk, *homos* + *genesis*, origin], reproduction by the same process in succeeding generations so that offspring are similar to the parents. Compare **heterogenesis.**

**homogenetic** /-jenet'ik/, **1.** pertaining to homogenesis. **2.** homogenous, def. 2.

**homogenized** /hōmoj'ənīzd/ [Gk, *homos*, same, *genein*, to produce], the state of having undergone homogenization: having a uniform texture or consistency throughout.

**homogenized milk** [Gk, *homos* + *genos*, kind], milk that has been mechanically treated to reduce and emulsify the fat globules so that the cream cannot separate.

**homogenous** /hōmoj'ənəs/ [Gk, *homos* + *genos*, kind], **1.** homogeneous. **2.** having a likeness in form or structure as a result of a common ancestral origin. **3.** homoplasty. Compare **heterogenous.**

**homogenous graft.** See **homologous graft.**

**homogentisic acid,** a compound that is an intermediate product of the metabolism of tyrosine. It forms a melanin-like staining substance in the urine of people who have alkaptonuria.

**homogeny** /hōmoj'ənē/ [Gk, *homos* + *genos*, kind], **1.** homogenesis. **2.** a likeness in structure or form that results from a common ancestral origin. Compare **homoplasty.**

**homograft.** See **allograft.**

**homoio-.** See **homeo-.**

**homoiothermal.** See **warm-blooded.**

**homoiothermic** /hom'ē-əthur'mik/ [Gk, *homos*, same, *therme*, heat], pertaining to the ability of warm-blooded animals to maintain a relatively stable internal temperature regardless of the temperature of the environment. This ability is not fully developed in newborn humans.

**homolateral** /hō'mōlat'ərəl/, pertaining to the same side of the body.

**homolateral limb synkinesis,** a condition of hemiplegia in which there appears to be a mutual dependency between the affected upper and lower limbs. Efforts at flexion of an upper extremity cause flexion of the lower extremity.

**homolog** /hom'əlog/ [Gk, *homos*, same], **1.** any organ corresponding in function, origin, and structure to another organ, as the flippers of a seal that correspond to human hands.

**2.** (in chemistry) one of a series of compounds, each formed by an added common element; for example, CO, carbon monoxide, is followed by $CO_2$, carbon dioxide, with the addition of an oxygen atom. Also spelled **homologue.** Compare **analog.** —**homologous,** *adj.*

**homologous** /hōmol'əgəs/ [Gk, *homos*, same, *logos*, relation], pertaining to corresponding attributes; similar in structure. Compare **analogous.** See also **homolog.**

**homologous anaphylaxis** [Gk, *homos*, same, *logos*, relation, *ana*, back, *phylaxis*, protection], a form of passive anaphylaxis resulting from the transfer of serum between animals of the same species.

**homologous chromosomes** [Gk, *homos*, same, *chroma* color, *soma* body], any two chromosomes in a diploid somatic cell that are identical in size, shape, and gene loci. In humans there are 22 pairs of homologous chromosomes and 1 pair of sex chromosomes, with one member of each pair derived from the mother and the other from the father.

**homologous disease.** See **graft-versus-host disease.**

**homologous graft** [Gk, *homos*, same, *logos*, relation, *graphein*, stylus], a tissue removed from a donor for transplantation to a recipient of the same species. Compare **autograft, heterograft, isograft.** Also called **homogenous graft.**

**homologous insemination.** See **artificial insemination—husband (AIH).**

**homologous organs** [Gk, *homos*, same, *logos*, relation, *organon*, instrument], body parts of different species (or sexes) that are structural equivalents, such as the arms of humans and the forelegs of dogs and cats. Compare **analogous.**

**homologous transplantation.** See **homoplastic transplantation.**

**homologous tumor,** a neoplasm made up of cells resembling those of the tissue in which it is growing. Compare **organoid neoplasm, heterologous tumor.**

**homologue.** See **homolog.**

**homonymous** /hōmon'iməs/ [Gk, *homos*, same, *onyma*, name], having the same name or sound.

**homonymous diplopia** [Gk, *homos*, same, *onyma*, name, *diploos*, double, *opsis*, vision], a type of diplopia in which the image observed by the right eye is located to the right of the image observed by the left eye.

**homonymous hemianopia** [Gk, *homos* + *onyma*, name], blindness or defective vision in the right or left halves of the visual fields of both eyes.

**homophobia** /hō'mōfō'bē-ə/ [Gk, *homos*, same, *phobos*, fear], the fear of or prejudice against homosexuals.

**homoplastic.** See **homoplasty.**

**homoplastic transplantation** [Gk, *homos*, same, *plassein*, to mold; L, *transplantare*, to transplant], the homologous transplantation of tissue from one human to another or from one animal to another of the same species. Also called **homologous transplantation.**

**homoplasty** /hō'məplas'tē/ [Gk, *homos* + *plassein*, to mold], having a likeness in form or structure acquired through similar environmental conditions or parallel evolution rather than resulting from common ancestral origin. Compare **homogeny.** —**homoplastic,** *adj.*

**homopolymer** /hō'mōpol'imir/ [Gk, *homos* + *poly*, many, *meros*, part], a compound formed from subunits that are the same, such as a carbohydrate composed of a series of glucose units.

*Homo sapiens* /hō'mō sā'pē-əns, sä'pē-ens/ [L, *homo*, human, *sapere*, to know or taste], the scientific name of the human species.

**homosexual** /-sek′shəl/ [Gk, *homos* + L, *sexus,* sex, gender], **1.** pertaining to or denoting the same sex. **2.** a person who is sexually attracted to members of the same sex. Compare **heterosexual.** See also **lesbian.**

**homosexuality.** See **sexual orientation.**

**homosexual panic,** an acute attack of anxiety based on unconscious conflicts concerning gender identity and a fear of being homosexual. Compare **heterosexual panic.**

**homosexual sexual intercourse** [Gk, *homos,* same; L, *sexus,* male or female, *intercursus,* interposition], sexual activity of members of the same sex ranging from feelings and fantasies to kissing and genital, oral, or anal contact.

**homothermal.** See **warm-blooded.**

**homotopic pain** /hō′mōtop′ik/, pain experienced at the point of injury.

**homotype** /hō′mōtīp/, any structure or body part, such as a hand or foot, that appears in reversed symmetry with a similar part.

**homovanillic acid** /hō′mōvənil′ik/, an acid that is produced by the normal metabolism of dopamine and may occur at an elevated level in urine in association with tumors of the adrenal gland. Its normal accumulation in a 24-hour collection urine sample is 15 mg.

**homozygosis** /hō′mōzīgō′sis/ [Gk, *homos* + *zygon,* yoke], **1.** the formation of a zygote by the union of two gametes that have one or more pairs of identical alleles. **2.** the production of purebred organisms or strains through inbreeding.

**homozygote** /hō′məzī′gōt/ [Gk, *homos,* same, *zygon,* yoke], an organism whose somatic cells have identical genes on the same locus on one of the chromosome pairs.

**homozygous** /hō′məzī′gəs/ [Gk, *homos* + *zygon,* yoke], having two identical alleles at corresponding loci on homologous chromosomes. An individual who is homozygous for a trait has inherited from each parent one allele for that trait. A person who homozygous for a genetic disease caused by a pair of recessive alleles, such as sickle cell anemia, manifests the disorder, and all of his or her offspring will inherit the allele for the disease. Compare **heterozygous.**

**homunculus** /hōmung′kyələs/, *pl.* **homunculi** [L, little man], **1.** a dwarf in whom all the body parts are proportionally developed and in which there is no deformity or abnormality. **2.** (in early embryologic theories of development, primarily preformation) a minute and complete human being contained in each of the germ cells that after fertilization grows from the microscopic to normal size; by extension, the human fetus. **3.** a small anatomic model of the human form; a manikin, specifically, one believed to have been produced by an alchemist and placed into a flask. **4.** (in psychiatry) a little man created by the imagination who possesses magical powers.

**hook grasp,** a type of prehension in which an object is grasped with the fingers alone, without use of the thumb and palm.

**hookworm** [AS, *hok* + *wyrm*], *nontechnical.* a nematode of the genera *Ancylostoma, Necator,* and *Uncinaria.* Most hookworm infections in the Western Hemisphere are caused by the species *Necator americanus.*

**hookworm disease** [AS, *hok* + *wyrm* + Gk, *dis,* not; Fr, *aise,* ease], a roundworm infestation that may involve either of two important intestinal parasites of humans, *Ancylostoma duodenale* and *Necator americanus.* Both forms of the disease are characterized by abdominal pain and iron deficiency anemia. The worm enters the human body as a larva by penetrating the skin, traveling to the lungs via the circulatory system, and ascending the respiratory tract to the pharynx, where it is swallowed. In the intestinal tract the hookworm attaches its mouth to the mucosa and subsists on the blood of the host.

**hope,** a nursing outcome from the Nursing Outcomes Classification (NOC) defined as presence of internal state of optimism that is personally satisfying and life-supporting. See also **Nursing Outcomes Classification.**

**hope instillation,** a nursing intervention from the Nursing Interventions Classification (NIC) defined as facilitation of the development of a positive outlook in a given situation. See also **Nursing Interventions Classification.**

**hopelessness** [AS, *hopian,* to hope, *laes,* less, *ness,* condition], a nursing diagnosis accepted by the Seventh National Conference on the Classification of Nursing Diagnoses. Hopelessness describes a state in which an individual sees limited or no alternatives or personal choices available and is unable to mobilize energy on his or her own behalf. ■ DEFINING CHARACTERISTICS: The defining characteristics include passivity, decreased verbalization, decreased affect, lack of initiative, decreased response to stimuli, turning away from the speaker, shrugging in response to the speaker, closing eyes, decreased appetite, increased or decreased sleep, and lack of involvement in care. ■ RELATED FACTORS: Related factors include prolonged activity restriction, failing or deteriorating physiologic condition, long-term stress, abandonment, and a loss of belief in transcendent values. See also **nursing diagnosis.**

**hops,** a perennial herb cultivated throughout the world. ■ USES: This herb is used as a mild sedative, diuretic, and weak antibiotic. It is also used to improve appetite and to treat insomnia, hyperactivity, pain, fever, and jaundice. ■ CONTRAINDICATIONS: Hops should not be used in people who are hypersensitive to this product, who have breast, uterine, or cervical cancers, or who suffer from a depressive condition.

**hordeolum** /hôrdē′ələm/ [L, *hordeum,* barley], a furuncle of the margin of the eyelid originating in the sebaceous gland of an eyelash. Treatment includes hot compresses and antibiotic ophthalmic preparations; incision and drainage are occasionally required. Also called **sty.** Compare **chalazion.**

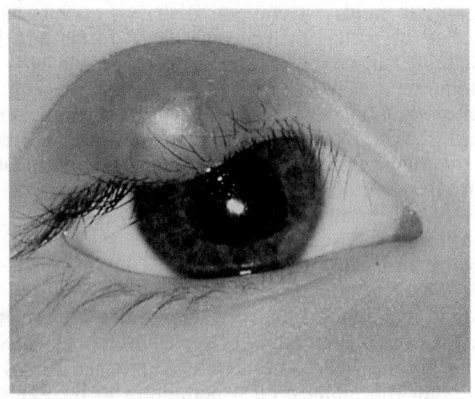

**Hordeolum** *(Zitelli and Davis, 1997)*

**horizon** /hôrī′zən/ [Gk, *horizein,* to encircle], a specific stage of human embryonic development determined by the appearance and ultimate formation of certain anatomic characteristics. The classification comprises 23 stages, each lasting 2 to 3 days, beginning with the fertilization of the ovum and ending 7 to 9 weeks later with the initiation of the fetal period of intrauterine life.

**horizontal abdominal position** /hôr'izon'təl/, prone position.

**horizontal angulation** [Gk, *horizein,* to encircle; L, *angularis,* angle], the angle within the occlusal plane, relative to a reference in the vertical or sagittal plane, at which the central x-ray beam is directed during radiography of oral structures. Compare **vertical angulation.**

**horizontal fissure of the right lung,** a cleft that marks the separation of the upper and middle lobes of the right lung.

**horizontal overlap.** See **overjet.**

**horizontal plane** [Gk, *horizein,* to encircle; L, *planum,* level ground], **1.** any plane of the erect body parallel to the horizon, dividing the body into upper and lower parts. **2.** a plane passing through a tooth at right angles to its long axis.

**horizontal position,** a position in which the patient lies on the back with the legs extended.

**horizontal pursuit,** a visual screening test in which the patient is asked to follow with both eyes a target moving in a horizontal plane while the examiner observes accuracy of alignment and supportive head movements.

**horizontal resorption,** a pattern of bone reduction in marginal periodontitis wherein the marginal crest of the alveolar bone between adjacent teeth remains level and the bases of the periodontal pockets are above the crest. Compare **vertical resorption.** See also **resorption.**

**horizontal transmission,** the spread of an infectious agent from one person or group to another, usually through contact with contaminated material, such as sputum or feces.

**horizontal vertigo,** a giddiness or feeling of instability experienced while lying down, frequently caused by a labyrinthine disorder.

**horm-,** prefix meaning 'an impulse, to urge or stimulate': *hormesis, hormonal, hormothyrin.*

**hormic psychology** /hôr'mic/ [Gk, *hormaien,* to begin action], (in psychology) the school that stresses the purposive, goal-oriented nature of human behavior. Also called **hormism.**

**hormonal** /hôr'mōnəl/ [Gk, *hormaein,* to set in motion], pertaining to or resembling hormones.

**hormone** /hôr'mōn/ [Gk, *hormaein,* to set in motion], a complex chemical substance produced in one part or organ of the body that initiates or regulates the activity of an organ or a group of cells in another part. Hormones secreted by the endocrine glands are carried through the bloodstream to the target organ. Secretion of these hormones is regulated by other hormones, by neurotransmitters, and by a negative feedback system in which an excess of target organ activity or hormone signals a decreased need for the stimulating hormone. Other hormones are released by organs for local effect, most commonly in the digestive tract.

**-hormone, 1.** suffix meaning a 'chemical substance possessing a regulatory effect' classified by source: *necrohormone, phytohormone, zoohormone.* **2.** suffix meaning a 'chemical substance possessing a regulatory effect' classified by activity affected: *cytohormone, neurohormone, parathormone.*

**hormone replacement therapy,** the administration of sex hormones following menopause or hysterectomy or in amenorrhea; there are a number of indications, including the prevention of postmenopausal osteoporosis and coronary artery disease, and the induction of menses in amenorrhea.

**hormone-sensitive lipase** /mō'bilizā'shən/, an enzyme that catalyzes the release of fatty acids from adipose tissues.

**hormone therapy,** the treatment of diseases with hormones obtained from endocrine glands or substances that simulate hormonal effects. Also called **endocrine therapy.**

**horn,** a projection or protuberance on a body structure. Examples include the horn of the hyoid bone and the iliac horn.

**Horner's syndrome** [Johann F. Horner, Swiss ophthalmologist, 1831–1886], a neurologic condition characterized by miotic pupils, ptosis, and facial anhidrosis, which results from a lesion in the spinal cord, with damage to a cervical nerve. In the case of traumatic injury the person is immobilized in the prone or supine position.

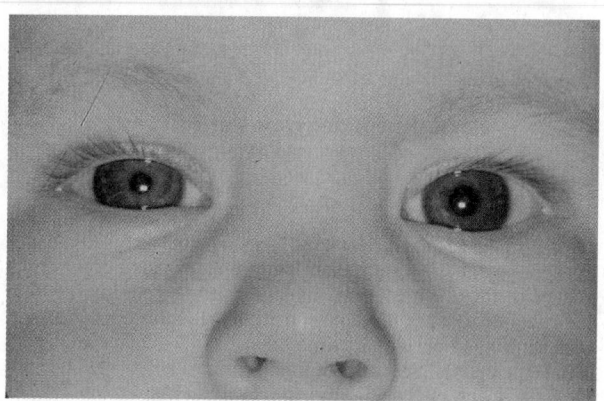

**Horner's syndrome: ptosis of the right eyelid**
*(Zitelli and Davis, 1997)*

**horny** /hôr'nē/, having the nature or appearance of horn. Also called **corneous, keratic.**

**horny layer.** See **stratum corneum.**

**horripilation.** See **pilomotor reflex.**

**horse chestnut,** an herbal product taken from a tree or shrub found worldwide.

■ USES: This herb is used for fever, fluid retention, frostbite, hemorrhoids, inflammation, lower extremity swelling, phlebitis, varicose veins, and wounds.

■ CONTRAINDICATIONS: Horse chestnut is contraindicated during pregnancy and lactation and in children until more research has been completed.

**horse serum** [AS, *hors* + L, *serum,* whey], immune serum prepared from the blood of a horse. Because many people are sensitive to horse serum, a skin test for sensitivity is recommended before immunization. Tetanus immune globulin prepared from human immune serum is preferred.

**horseshoe fistula** /hôrs'shoo/ [AS, *hors* + *scoh,* shoe], an abnormal semicircular passage in the perianal area with both openings on the surface of the skin.

**horseshoe kidney,** a relatively common congenital anomaly characterized by an isthmus of parenchymal tissue connecting the two kidneys at the lower poles. The condition may cause obstruction of the ureters, hydronephrosis, and abdominal pain. It is corrected by surgery to separate and reposition the kidneys.

**horsetail,** a perennial herb known as a pteridophyte, found throughout the world.

■ USES: This herb is used as a diuretic, a genitourinary astringent, and an antihemorrhagic. It is also used for Bell's palsy and for healing broken bones.

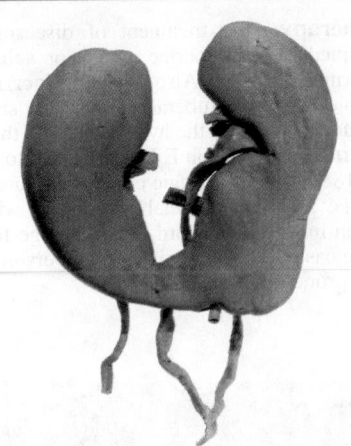

**Horseshoe kidney: posterior view**
*(Moore, Persaud, and Shiota, 2000)*

■ CONTRAINDICATIONS: Horsetail should not be used during pregnancy and lactation or in children. It is also contraindicated in those with known hypersensitivity, edema, cardiac or renal disease, or nicotine sensitivity. It should not be used for prolonged periods of time.

**Hortega cells.** See **microglia.**

**Horton's arteritis.** See **temporal arteritis.**

**Horton's headache.** See **migrainous cranial neuralgia.**

**Horton's histamine cephalalgia.** See **histamine headache.**

**hospice** /hos′pis/ [L, *hospes*, host], a system of family-centered care designed to assist the terminally ill person to be comfortable and to maintain a satisfactory life-style through the phases of dying. Hospice care is multidisciplinary and includes home visits, professional health care available on call, teaching and emotional support of the family, and physical care of the client. Some hospice programs provide care in a center, as well as in the home. See also **emotional care of the dying patient, stages of dying.**

**hospital** /hos′pitəl/ [L, *hospitium*, guesthouse], a health care facility that provides inpatient beds, continuous nursing services, and an organized medical staff.

**hospital-acquired infection.** See **nosocomial infection.**

**hospital clinic,** an ambulatory care site owned by a hospital where persons who do not require hospitalization receive medical care. It may be primary care or subspecialty care.

**hospitalism** /hos′pitəliz′əm/, the physical or mental effects of hospitalization or institutionalization on patients, especially infants and children in whom the condition is characterized by social regression, personality disorders, and stunted growth. See also **anaclitic depression.**

**hospitalist** /hos′pi·təl·ist /, a physician specializing in hospital inpatient care.

**Hospital Survey and Construction Act.** See **Hill-Burton Act.**

**host** /hōst/ [L, *hospes*], **1.** an organism in which another, usually parasitic organism is nourished and harbored. A **primary** or **definitive host** is one in which the adult parasite lives and reproduces. A **secondary** or **intermediate host** is one in which the parasite exists in its nonsexual, larval stage. A **reservoir host** is a primary animal host for organisms that sometimes become parasitic in humans and through which humans may become infected. **2.** the recipient of a transplanted organ or tissue. Compare **donor.**

**host defense mechanisms,** a group of body protective systems, including physical barriers and the immune response, that normally guard against infection.

**hostility** /hostil′itē/ [L, *hostilis*, hostile], an emotional state characterized by enmity toward others and a desire to harm those at whom the antagonism is directed. The hostility may be expressed passively and actively.

**hot bath** [AS, *hat + baeth*], a bath in which the temperature of the water is gradually raised to about 106° F (41.11° C).

**hot compress** [AS, *hat* + L, *comprimere,* to press together], a heated pad of damp, thickly folded cloth applied to an area to reduce pain or inflammation. See also **fomentation.**

**hot flash,** a transient sensation of warmth experienced by some women during or after menopause. Hot flashes result from autonomic vasomotor disturbances that accompany changes in the neurohormonal activity of the ovaries, hypothalamus, and pituitary. The exact causative mechanism is not known. All menopausal women do not experience hot flashes; among those who do, the frequency, duration, and intensity vary widely. Although physically harmless, the symptom may be extremely disturbing or, rarely, disabling. Hot flashes may be alleviated by cyclic or continuous administration of exogenous estrogen. Also called **hot flush.** See **menopause.**

**hot line,** a means of contacting a trained counselor or specific agency for help with a particular problem, such as a rape hot line or a battered child hot line. The person needing help calls a telephone number and speaks to a counselor, who remains anonymous and who offers emotional support, specific recommendations for action, and referral to other medical, social, or community services. Such services are usually maintained by volunteers and are accessible 24 hours a day, 7 days a week.

**hot spot, 1.** a site in a gene sequence at which mutations occur with an unusually high frequency. **2.** an area on a radiographic image that represents an abnormally high absorption of radiation.

**Hounsfield unit** /hounz′fēld/ [Godfrey N. Hounsfield, 20th century English scientist], the numeric information contained in each pixel of a CT image. It is related to the composition and nature of the tissue imaged and is used to represent the density of tissue. Also called **CT number, Hounsfield number.**

**hourglass uterus** [Gk, *hora* + AS, *glaes*], a uterus in which a segment of circular muscle fibers contracts during labor, causing constriction ring dystocia. The condition is marked by lack of progress despite adequate labor contractions and recession of the presenting part during a contraction rather than descent of the presenting part.

**housekeeping department,** a unit of a hospital staff responsible for cleaning the hospital premises and furnishings, including controlling pathogenic organisms. See also **environmental services.**

**housemaid's knee** [AS, *hus + maeden + cneow,* knee], a chronic inflammation of the bursa in front of the kneecap, characterized by redness and swelling. It is caused by prolonged and repetitive pressure of the knee on a hard surface.

**house organ,** a publication designed for distribution to the employees or members of an institution or business. It may be prepared by a staff within the institution or business, or by an outside agency.

**house physician** [AS, *hus* + Gk, *physikos,* natural], a physician on call and immediately available in a hospital or other health care facility.

**house staff,** the interns and residents who are employed at a hospital while receiving additional training after graduation from medical college.

**house surgeon,** a surgeon on call and immediately available on the premises of a hospital.

**housewives' eczema** [AS, *hus* + *wif* + Gk, *ekzein,* to boil over], an informal term for contact dermatitis of the hands caused and exacerbated by their frequent immersion in water and by the use of soaps and detergents.

**Houston's valves.** See **plicae transversales recti.**

**Hovius' plexus.** See **Leber's plexus.**

**Howell-Jolly bodies** /hou′əljol′ē/ [William H. Howell, American physiologist, 1860–1945; Justin M.J. Jolly, French histologist, 1870–1953], spheric and granular inclusions in the erythrocytes observed on microscopic examination of stained blood smears. They are most commonly seen in people who have hemolytic or pernicious anemia, leukemia, thalassemia, or congenital absence of the spleen and in those who have had a splenectomy.

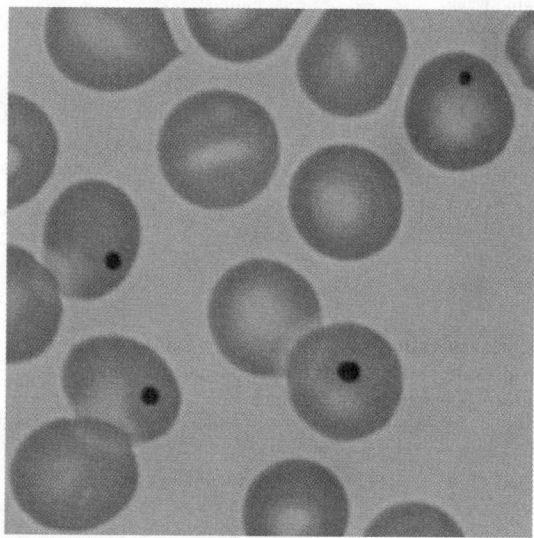

**Howell-Jolly bodies** *(Carr and Rodak, 1999)*

**HPG,** abbreviation for *human pituitary gonadotropin.*

**HPL,** abbreviation for **human placental lactogen.**

**HPV,** 1. abbreviation for **human papillomavirus.** 2. abbreviation for **human parvovirus.**

**hr,** abbreviation for *hour.*

**H$_1$ receptor,** a type of histamine receptor on vascular smooth muscle cells through which histamine mediates vasodilation. See also **histamine blocking agent.**

**H$_2$ receptor,** a type of histamine receptor on various kinds of cells through which histamine mediates bronchial constriction in asthma and GI constriction in diarrhea. See also **histamine blocking agent.**

**HRIG,** abbreviation for *human rabies immune globulin* vaccine.

**HRSA,** abbreviation for **Health Resources and Services Administration.**

**HSA,** abbreviation for **health systems agency.**

**hs, h.s.,** abbreviation for the Latin *hora somni,* at bedtime.

**HsP,** abbreviation for **heat shock protein.**

**HSV,** abbreviation for *herpes simplex virus.* See **herpes genitalis, herpes simplex.**

**HSV1,** abbreviation for *herpes simplex virus type 1.* See **herpes simplex.**

**ht,** abbreviation for **height.**

**HTLV-I,** abbreviation for **human T-cell lymphotropic virus type I.**

**HTLV-I–associated myelopathy.** See **chronic progressive myelopathy.**

**HTLV-II,** abbreviation for **human T-cell lymphotropic virus type II.**

**HTLV-III,** abbreviation for **human T-cell lymphotropic virus type III.**

**Hubbard tank** [Carl P. Hubbard, American engineer, b. 1857; Port, *tanqu*] water tank in which patients can perform underwater exercise. The patient's trunk and extremities are submerged on a stretcher. The water provides buoyancy and heat for the benefit of weakened or painful muscles or joints with limited active range of motion. The tank also may be used for wound debridement. See also **whirlpool bath.**

**huffing,** forced expiration with an open glottis used to clear secretions from the airway when pain limits normal coughing.

**HUGO** /hyo͞o′gō/, abbreviation for **Human Genome Organization.**

**Huhner test** /ho͞o′nər/ [Max Huhner, American urologist, 1873–1947], a test for male fertility in which a semen sample aspirated from the vagina within an hour after coitus is examined for spermatozoal activity.

**human** /h(y)o͞o′mən/ [L, *humanus*], a member of the genus *Homo* and particularly of the species *H. sapiens.*

**human bite** [L, *humanus* + AS, *bitan*], a wound caused by the piercing of skin by human teeth. Bacteria are usually present, and serious infection often follows. The area is thoroughly washed with an antiseptic and rinsed well. The wound is examined frequently, and appropriate antibiotic therapy instituted, if necessary.

**human chorionic gonadotropin.** See **chorionic gonadotropin.**

**human chorionic somatomammotropin (HCS),** a hormone produced by the syncytiotrophoblast during pregnancy. It regulates carbohydrate and protein metabolism of the mother to ensure delivery to the fetus of glucose for energy and protein for fetal growth. HCS also may have a diabetogenic effect in the mother, who therefore may have an increased blood glucose level. Also called placental lactogen (lactogen) and chrionic growth hormone-prolactin.

**human diploid cell rabies vaccine (HDCV),** an inactivated rabies virus vaccine prepared from rabies virus grown in human diploid cell cultures. Active immunization with HDCV begins on the day of exposure, followed by four or five additional injections. Passive immunization with *human rabies immune globulin (HRIG)* may be given concurrently with HDCV.

**human ecology,** the study of the interrelationships between people and their environments, as well as among individuals within an environment.

**Human Genome Organization (HUGO),** an international group established in 1989 to coordinate activities concerned with the human genome project, including the distribution of funding and dissemination of information.

**human granulocytic erlichiosis (HGE).** See **erlichiosis.**

**human growth hormone (synthetic).** See **synthetic human growth hormone.**

**human herpesvirus 6,** a ubiquitous virus belonging to the subfamily Betaherpesvirinae that is the causative agent of exanthema subitum. Most healthy adults carry the virus and are asymptomatic; infection results in lifelong persistence. See also **exanthema subitum, herpesvirus.**

**human herpesvirus 7,** a virus belonging to the subfamily Betaherpesvirinae, closely related to human herpesvirus 6, but not known to be associated with any disease. See also **human herpesvirus 6.**

**human herpesvirus 8,** a virus in the family Herpesviridae that has been implicated as the causative agent of Kaposi's sarcoma and primary effusion lymphoma. Also called **Kaposi's sarcoma—associated herpesvirus.** See also **Kaposi's sarcoma, primary effusion lymphoma.**

**human immunodeficiency virus (HIV)** /im′yōōnō′difish′ ənsē/ [L, *humanus* + *immunis,* free from, *de,* from, *facere,* to make, *virus,* poison], a retrovirus that causes acquired immunodeficiency syndrome (AIDS). Retroviruses produce the enzyme reverse transcriptase, which allows the viral RNA genome to be transcribed into DNA inside the host cell. HIV is transmitted through contact with an infected individual's blood, semen, breast milk, cervical secretions, cerebrospinal fluid, or synovial fluid. It infects CD4-positive helper T cells of the immune system and causes infection with an incubation period that averages 10 years. With the immune system destroyed, AIDS develops as opportunistic infections such as **Kaposi's sarcoma,** *Pneumocystis carinii* pneumonia, candidiasis, and **tuberculosis** attack organ systems throughout the body. Aside from the initial antibody tests (enzyme-linked immunosorbent assay and Western blot) that establish the diagnosis for HIV infection, the most

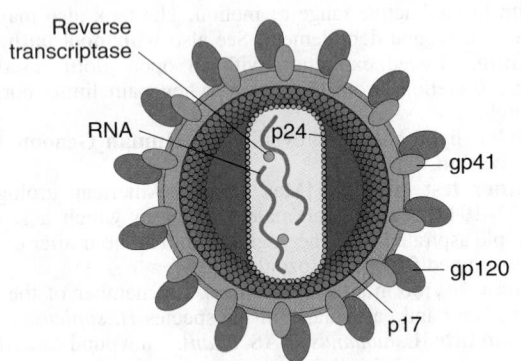

**Reverse transcriptase**

**RNA**

p24

gp41

gp120

p17

**Human immunodeficiency virus**
*(Kumar, Cotran, and Robbins, 1997)*

### Signs and symptoms of HIV infection

| | |
|---|---|
| Chills and fever | Malaise |
| Night sweats | Fatigue |
| Dry productive cough | Oral lesions |
| Dyspnea | Skin rashes |
| Lethargy | Abdominal discomfort |
| Confusion | Diarrhea |
| Stiff neck | Weight loss |
| Seizures | Lymphadenopathy |
| Headache | Progressive generalized edema |

From Phipps WJ, Sands JK, Marek JE: *Medical-surgical nursing: concepts and clinical practice,* ed 6, St Louis, 1999, Mosby.

### CDC classification of HIV infection based on pathophysiology of the disease as immune function progressively worsens

| Class | Criteria |
|---|---|
| Group I | 1. Acute infection with HIV<br>2. Flu-like symptoms; resolve completely<br>3. HIV antibody negative |
| **HIV asymptomatic**<br>Group II | 1. HIV antibody positive<br>2. No laboratory or clinical indicators of immunodeficiency |
| **HIV symptomatic**<br>Group III | 1. HIV antibody positive<br>2. Persistent generalized lymphadenopathy |
| Group IV-A | 1. HIV antibody positive<br>2. Constitutional disease<br>  a. Persistent fever or diarrhea<br>  b. Weight loss >10% of normal body weight |
| Group IV-B | 1. Same as group IV-A, and<br>2. Neurologic disease<br>  a. Dementia<br>  b. Neuropathy<br>  c. Myelopathy |
| Group IV-C | 1. Same as group IV-B, and<br>2. CD4+ T lymphocyte count <200/µl<br>3. Opportunistic infection |
| Group IV-D | 1. Same as group IV-C, and<br>2. Pulmonary tuberculosis, invasive cervical cancer, or other malignancy |

Data from Centers for Disease Control and Prevention, March 1993.
From Price SA, Wilson LM: *Pathophysiology: clinical concepts of disease processes,* ed 5, St Louis, 1997, Mosby.

**Mature form**

**Budding particles**

**Electromicrograph of HIV cultured from a patient with hemophilia**
*(Monahan and Neighbors, 1997/courtesy Jonathan W.M. Gold, MD)*

important laboratory test for monitoring the level of infection is the CD4 lymphocyte test, which determines the percentage of T lymphocytes that are CD4 positive; patients with CD4 cell counts greater than 500/mm$^3$ are considered most likely to respond to treatment with alpha-interferon and/or zidovudine. A significant drop in the CD4 cell count is a signal for therapeutic intervention with antiretroviral therapy. Vaccines based on the HIV envelope glycoproteins gp120 and gp160, intended to boost the immune system of people already infected with HIV, are being investigated. Still in limited trials, Phase III reports are planned for 2001. Formerly called **human T-cell leukemia virus type III, human T-cell lymphotropic virus type III.** See also **acquired immunodeficiency syndrome.**

**human insulin,**   a biosynthetic product manufactured from *Escherichia coli* by recombinant deoxyribonucleic acid technology. The advantage of human insulin is that it eliminates allergic reactions that occur with the use of animal insulins. See also **insulin,** def. 2.

**human investigations committee,**   a group established in a hospital, school, or university to review research proposals involving human subjects to protect the rights of the people to be studied. Also called **human subjects review committee,** and in hospitals, the IRB or Investigational Review Board.

**humanism** /h(y)oo′məniz′əm/,   a system of thought pertaining to the interests, needs, and welfare of human beings; the concept that human needs and values are of utmost importance.

**humanistic existential therapy** /hyoo′mənis′tik/,   a kind of psychotherapy that promotes self-awareness and personal growth by stressing current reality and by analyzing and altering specific patterns of response to help a person realize his or her potential. This process may be facilitated in a group setting, where additional aspects of problems are revealed through interaction with others. Kinds of humanistic existential psychotherapy are **client-centered therapy, existential therapy,** and **Gestalt therapy.** Also called **existential humanistic psychotherapy.**

**humanistic nursing model,**   a conceptual framework in which the nurse-patient relationship is analyzed as a human-to-human event rather than a nurse-to-patient interaction. The nurse makes therapeutic use of herself or himself, understanding the effects of nursing actions. Four phases are recognized in the development of the therapeutic relationship. The encounter phase is followed by the phase in which the identities of the nurse and patient emerge. The nurse empathizes and then sympathizes with the patient. The meaning of the patient's experience is important; hope and suffering are seen as central to that experience. Self-knowledge and self-awareness of the nurse are essential. Nursing intervention proceeds in five steps: observation of the need for intervention; validation of this observation; determination of the ability of the nurse to facilitate any necessary referral; formulation of a plan for meeting the need; and evaluation of the degree to which the need is met.

**humanistic psychology,**   a branch of psychology that emphasizes a person's struggle to develop and maintain an integrated, harmonious personality as the primary motivational force in human behavior. See also **self-actualization.**

**human leukocyte antigen (HLA),**   any one of four significant histocompatibility antigens governed by genes of the HLA complex, specific loci on chromosome 6 designated HLA-A, HLA-B, HLA-C, and HLA-D. Each locus has several genetically determined alleles; each of these is associated with certain diseases or conditions; for example, HLA-B27 is usually present in people who have ankylosing

spondylitis. The HLA system is used to assess tissue compatibility. White blood cells are used for testing. Perfect tissue compatibility exists only between identical twins. See also **histocompatibility gene.**

**human liver fluke.**   See **liver fluke.**

**human lymphocyte antigen B27 test (HLA-B27),**   a blood test done as part of paternity investigations, to indicate tissue compatibility with tissue transplantation, and to assist in the diagnosis of Reiter's syndrome and other conditions.

**human monocytic erlichiosis.**   See **erlichiosis.**

**human natural killer cell,**   a lymphocyte that is able to lyse tumor and virally infected cells as part of the body's natural defense against malignancy and invasion by pathogens.

**human papillomavirus (HPV),**   a virus that is the cause of common warts of the hands and feet, as well as lesions of the mucous membranes of the oral, anal, and genital cavities. More than 50 types of HPV have been identified, some of which are associated with cancerous and precancerous conditions. The virus can be transmitted through sexual contact, and specific types of the virus are a precursor to cancer of the cervix. Transmission has taken place without the presence of warts, indicating that it may occur through body fluids, such as semen or cervical secretions. There is no specific cure for an HPV infection, but the virus often can be controlled by podophyllin or interferon and the warts can be removed by cryosurgery, laser treatment, or conventional surgery.

**human parvovirus (HPV),**   a small single-stranded deoxyribonucleic acid virion that has been associated with several diseases, including erythema infectiosum and aplastic crises of chronic hemolytic anemias. Parvoviruses of various types also infect wild and domestic animals and may replicate in susceptible cells without a helper virus. See also **helper virus, virion.**

**human placental lactogen (HPL),**   a placental hormone that may be deficient in certain abnormalities of pregnancy. The normal concentrations of this hormone in serum after the fifth week of pregnancy are 0.5 μg/mL and increase to approximately 8 μg/mL at the time of delivery. Also called chorionic somatomammotropin.

**human prion diseases**   See **transmissible spongiform encephalopathy.**

**human protein C,**   an anticoagulant that inactivates coagulation cofactors 5 and 8c and mediates clot lysis by tissue plasminogen activator (t-PA).

**human rhinovirus 14,**   the common cold virus. It has a complex protein coat containing "sticky sites" that help attach the virus to cell receptors in the upper respiratory system. Because of the more than 100 strains of the virus that are known, devising a vaccine that would protect against all variations is difficult.

**human subjects review committee.**   See **human investigations committee.**

**human synthetic growth hormone.**   See **Humatrope.**

**human T-cell leukemia virus type I.**   See **human T-cell lymphotropic virus type I.**

**human T-cell leukemia virus type II.**   See **human T-cell lymphotropic virus type II.**

**human T-cell leukemia virus type III.**   See **human immunodeficiency virus.**

**human T-cell lymphotropic virus type I (HTLV-I),**   a type C oncovirus of worldwide distribution but most common in Japan, Africa, and the Caribbean basin, having an affinity for helper/inducer T lymphocytes, that causes chronic infection and is associated with adult T-cell leukemia/lymphoma and tropical spastic paraparesis. Also called **human T-cell leukemia virus type I.**

**human T-cell lymphotropic virus type II (HTLV-II),** a type C oncovirus having extensive serologic cross-reactivity with HTLV-I, isolated from an atypical T-cell variant of hairy cell leukemia; it has also been isolated from patients with other hematologic disorders. Also called **human T-cell leukemia virus type II.**

**human T-cell lymphotropic virus type III (HTLV-III).** See **human immunodeficiency virus.**

**Humatin,** trademark for an amebicde (paromomycin sulfate).

**Humatrope,** trademark for a brand of human synthetic growth hormone produced with recombinant deoxyribonucleic acid techniques. It is a polypeptide hormone with 191 amino acids in the same sequence as **somatotropin,** the human growth hormone produced by the pituitary gland.

**humectant** /hyo͞omek′tənt/, a substance that promotes retention of moisture.

**humer-,** prefix meaning 'the humerus': *humeroradial, humeroulnar.*

**humeral.** See **humerus.**

**humeral articulation.** See **shoulder joint.**

**humerus** /hyo͞o′mərəs/, *pl.* humeri [L, shoulder], the bone of the upper arm, from the elbow to the shoulder joint where it articulates with the scapula. It comprises a body, a head, and a condyle. The body is almost cylindric proximally and prismatic and flattened distally and has two borders and three surfaces. The nearly hemispheric head articulates with the glenoid cavity of the scapula and has a constriction called the surgical neck, frequently the seat of a fracture. The condyle at the distal end has several depressions into which articulate the radius and ulna. Also called **arm bone.** —**humeral,** *adj.*

**humidification** /hyo͞omid′ifikā′shən/ [L, *humidus,* moist, *facere,* to make], the process of increasing the relative humidity of the atmosphere around a patient through the use of aerosol generators or steam inhalers that exert an antitussive effect. Humidification acts by decreasing the viscosity of bronchial secretions, whereas added medications or sodium chloride may stimulate coughing by an irritant effect.

**humidifier** /hyo͞omid′ifī′ər/ [L, *humidus,* moist, *facere,* to make], a machine designed to adjust the amount of moisture in the atmosphere of a room or respiratory device.

**humidifier lung,** hypersensitivity pneumonitis caused by inhalation of air that has been passed through humidifiers, dehumidifiers, or air conditioners contaminated by any variety of fungi, amebas, or thermophilic bacteria.

**humidity** /hyo͞omid′itē/ [L, *humidus,* moist], pertaining to the level of moisture in the atmosphere, which varies with the temperature. The percentage is usually represented in terms of **relative humidity,** with 100% the point of air saturation, or the level at which the air can absorb no additional water.

**humor**[1] /hyo͞o′mər/ [L, *humidus,* moist], any body fluid or semifluid substance such as blood or lymph. The term is often used in reference to the **aqueous humor** or the **vitreous humor** of the eye.

**humor**[2], a nursing intervention from the Nursing Interventions Classification (NIC) defined as facilitating the patient to perceive, appreciate, and express what is funny, amusing, or ludicrous in order to establish relationships, relieve tension, release anger, facilitate learning, or cope with painful feelings. See also **Nursing Interventions Classification.**

**humoral immunity** /hyo͞o′mərəl/ [L, *humor,* liquid, *immunis,* freedom], one of the two forms of immunity that respond to bacteria and other foreign antigens. Humoral im-

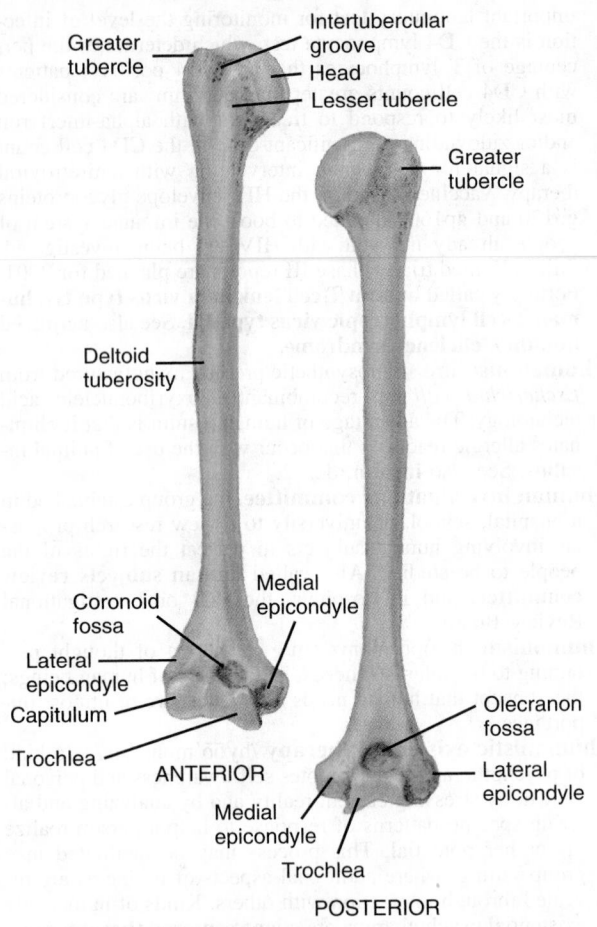

**Humerus** (Applegate, 2000)

munity is mediated by circulating antibodies (immunoglobulins IgA, IgB, and IgM), which coat the antigens and target them for destruction by polymorphonuclear neutrophils. Circulating antibodies are produced by plasma cells of the reticuloendothelial system. The interaction of antibody with antigen also activates the complement system. Compare **cellular immunity.** See also **antigen-antibody reaction.**

**humoral response,** one of a broad category of hypersensitivity reactions. Humoral responses are mediated by B lymphocytes and occur in anaphylactic and immunocomplex hypersensitivities and in cytotoxic anaphylaxis. Compare **cell-mediated immune response.** See also **humoral immunity.**

**Humorsol,** trademark for an ophthalmic anticholinesterase agent (demecarium bromide).

**humpback** /hump′bak/ [Du, *homp,* thick slice; AS, *baec*], a colloquial term for **kyphosis,** an abnormal curvature of the cervicothoracic spine.

**Humulin,** trademark for a brand of human insulin of recombinant deoxyribonucleic acid origin.

**hunger,** a physical sensation usually associated with a craving or desire for food.

**hunger contractions,** strong contractions of the stomach usually associated with a desire for food.

**hunger pain,** epigastric cramps often associated with a desire for food.

**hung-up reflex,** a deep tendon reflex in which, after a stimulus is given and the reflex action takes place, the limb slowly returns to its neutral position. This prolonged relaxation phase is characteristic of reflexes in persons with hypothyroidism. See also **deep tendon reflex.**

**Hunner's ulcer** [Guy LeRoy Hunner, American surgeon, 1868–1957], a deep hemorrhagic lesion in the bladder associated with interstitial cystitis.

**Hunter's canal.** See **adductor canal.**

**Hunter's syndrome** [Charles Hunter, Canadian physician, 1873–1955; Gk, *syn,* together, *dromos,* course], a hereditary defect in mucopolysaccharide metabolism affecting only males, characterized by dwarfism, kyphosis, gargoylism, and mental retardation. It is transmitted as an X-linked recessive trait. Females who carry the gene can be identified by biochemical tests. Also called **MPS II, X-linked mucopolysaccharidosis.** See also **mucopolysaccharidosis.**

**Huntington's chorea.** See **Huntington's disease.**

**Huntington's disease** [George S. Huntington, American physician, 1851–1916], a rare abnormal hereditary condition characterized by chronic progressive chorea and mental deterioration that results in dementia. An individual afflicted with the condition usually shows the first signs in the fourth decade of life and dies within 15 years. It is transmitted as an autosomal trait. There is no known effective treatment, but symptoms can be relieved with medication.

Huntington's disease: dilated lateral ventricle with caudate and lentiform atrophy
*(Perkin, 1998)*

common. The disease process usually results in death during childhood from cardiac complications or pulmonary disorders. Also called **gargoylism, lipochondrodystrophy, MPS I.** See also **mucopolysaccharidosis.**

**Hurter and Driffield curve.** See **characteristic curve.**

**Hürthle cell adenoma** /hirt′lə, hŏŏrth′lē/ [Karl W. Hürthle, German histologist, 1860–1945], a benign tumor of the thyroid gland composed of large cells with granular eosinophilic cytoplasm (Hürthle cells). Compare **Hürthle cell carcinoma.**

**Hürthle cell carcinoma** [Karl W. Hürthle], a malignant neoplasm of the thyroid gland composed of Hürthle cells. These tumors, which occur more often in women than in men, are encapsulated, resemble adenomas, and are locally invasive. Compare **Hürthle cell adenoma.**

**Hürthle cell tumor** [Karl W. Hürthle], a neoplasm of the thyroid gland composed of large cells with granular eosinophilic cytoplasm (Hürthle cells); it may be benign (Hürthle cell adenoma) or malignant (Hürthle cell carcinoma).

**husband-coached childbirth.** See **Bradley method.**

**Hutchinson-Gilford syndrome.** See **progeria.**

**Hutchinson's disease.** See **angioma serpiginosum.**

**Hutchinson's freckle** [Jonathan Hutchinson, English surgeon, 1828–1913], a tan patch on the skin that grows slowly and becomes mottled, dark, thick, and nodular. The lesion is usually seen on one side of the face of an elderly person. Local excision is recommended because it often becomes malignant. Also called **lentigo maligna.** See also **melanoma.**

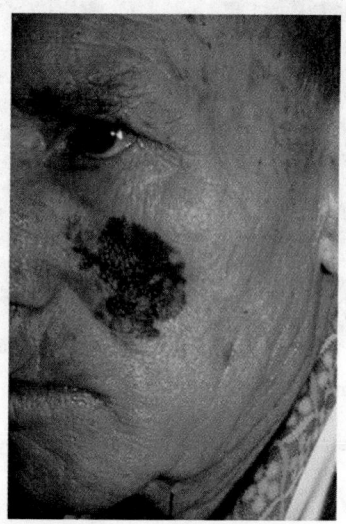

Hutchinson's freckle *(Belcher, 1992)*

**Hurler's syndrome** [Gertrude Hurler, German physician, 1889–1965], a type of mucopolysaccharidosis, transmitted as an autosomal-recessive trait, that produces severe mental retardation. Symptoms appear within the first few months of life. Characteristic signs of the disease are enlargement of the liver and spleen, often with cardiovascular involvement. Facial characteristics include a low forehead and enlargement of the head, sometimes resulting from hydrocephalus. Corneal clouding is common, and the neck is short. Marked kyphosis is apparent at the dorsolumbar level, and the hands and the fingers are short and broad. Flexion contractures are

**Hutchinson's teeth** [Jonathan Hutchinson], a characteristic of congenital syphilis in which the secondary lateral incisors are peg-shaped, widely spaced, and notched at the end, with a central crescent-shaped deformity. See also **syphilis.**

**Hutchinson's triad** [Jonathan Hutchinson], the interstitial keratitis, notched teeth, and deafness characteristic of congenital syphilis. See also **syphilis.**

**Hutchison-type neuroblastoma** [Robert G. Hutchison, English pediatrician, 1871–1960; Gk, *typos,* mark], a neuroblastoma that has metastasized to the cranium.

**HUTT,** abbreviation for **heads-up tilt table test.**

**HVA,** abbreviation for **homovanillic acid.**

**HV interval** /in'tərvəl/, the conduction time of an impulse traveling through the His-Purkinje system. It is measured from the onset of the atrioventricular bundle potential to the onset of ventricular activation as recorded on an electrogram.

**HVL,** abbreviation for **half-value layer.**

**hyal-.** See **hyalo-.**

**hyaline** /hī'əlin/ [Gk, *hyalos,* glass], pertaining to substances that are clear or glasslike.

**hyaline bodies** [Gk, *hyalos* + AS, *bodig*], **1.** the residue of colloidal degeneration found in some cells. **2.** globules of neurosecretory material found in the posterior lobe of the pituitary. **3.** deposits of homogenous eosinophilic material found in renal tubular epithelium and representing excess protein molecules that cannot be metabolized or transported.

**hyaline cartilage** [Gk, *hyalos,* glass; L, *cartilago*], a type of elastic connective tissue composed of specialized cells in a translucent, pearly blue matrix. Hyaline cartilage thinly covers the articulating ends of bones, connects the ribs to the sternum, and supports the nose, the trachea, and part of the larynx. It is covered by a membranous perichondrium, except where it coats the ends of bones, and tends to calcify in advanced age. Compare **yellow cartilage, white fibrocartilage.**

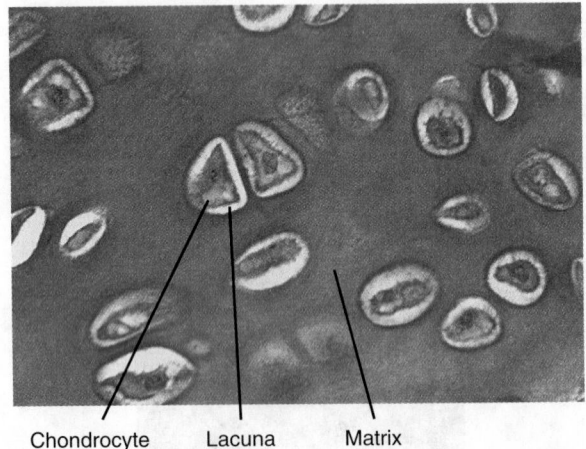

Chondrocyte   Lacuna   Matrix

**Hyaline cartilage** (© Ed Reschke; used with permission)

**hyaline cast,** a transparent cast composed of mucoprotein.

**hyaline membrane** [Gk, *hyalos,* glass; L, *membrana*], a fibrous covering of the alveolar membranes in infants, caused by a lack of pulmonary surfactant associated with prematurity and low-birth-weight delivery. See also **respiratory distress syndrome of the newborn.**

**hyaline membrane disease.** See **respiratory distress syndrome of the newborn.**

**hyaline thrombus,** a transparent mass of hemolyzed erythrocytes.

**hyalinization** /hī'əlin'īzā'shən/ [Gk, *hyalos,* glass], the development of glassy homogenous material within a cell.

**hyalinuria** /-ŏŏr'ē·ə/ [Gk, *hyalos,* glass, *ouron,* urine], the presence of hyaline casts of protein in acidic urine. This condition may occur in glomerulonephrosis.

**hyalo-, hyal-,** prefix meaning 'resembling glass': *hyaloenchondroma, hyaloplasm, hyaloid.*

**hyaloid** /hī'əloid/ [Gk, *hyalos,* glass, *eidos,* form], pertaining to or resembling hyaline.

**hyaloid artery** [Gk, *hyalos* + *eidos,* form], an embryonic blood vessel that branches to supply the vitreous body of the eye and develops part of the blood supply to the capsula vasculosa lentis. The hyaloid artery disappears from the fetus in the ninth month of pregnancy, leaving a vestigial remnant, the hyaloid canal, which persists in the adult as a narrow passage through the vitreous body from the optic disc to the posterior surface of the crystalline lens.

**hyaloid membrane** [Gk, *hyalos,* glass; L, *membrana*], a surface layer of the vitreous body of the eye, at the interface between the primary and secondary vitreous and at the boundaries of the hyaloid canal.

**hyaloplasm** /hī'əlōplaz'əm/ [Gk, *hyalos* + *plasma,* formation], the portion of the cytoplasm that is clear and more fluid than the granular and reticular part. Also called **cytohyaloplasm, cytolymph, enchylema, interfibrillar mass of Flemming, interfilar mass, paramitome.**

**hyaluronic acid** /hī'əlyŏŏron'ik/, a mucopolysaccharide formed by the polymerization of acetylglucosamine and glucuronic acid, which occurs in vitreous humor, synovial fluids, and various tissues. Known as the cement substance of tissues, it forms a gel in intercellular spaces.

**hyaluronidase** /hī'əlyŏŏron'ədās/, an enzyme that hydrolyzes hyaluronic acid.

■ INDICATIONS: It is prescribed to increase the absorption and dispersion of other parenteral drugs, for hypodermoclysis, and for improvement of resorption of radiopaque agents.

■ CONTRAINDICATIONS: Acute inflammation, infection, or known hypersensitivity to this drug prohibits its use.

■ ADVERSE EFFECTS: The most serious adverse reaction is hypersensitivity.

**hybrid** /hī'brid/ [L, *hybrida,* offspring], **1.** an offspring produced by mating organisms from different species, varieties, or genotypes. **2.** pertaining to such an offspring.

**hybrid computer,** a computer that combines the characteristics of a digital computer and an analog computer by its capacity to accept input and provide output in either digital or analog form and to process information digitally. Compare **analog computer, digital computer.**

**hybridization** /hī'bridīzā'shən/, **1.** the process of producing hybrids by crossbreeding. **2.** the process of combining single-stranded nucleic acids from different sources to form stable, double-stranded molecules. The technique involves fragmentation and separation of the source nucleic acids by heating, followed by recombination through cooling. The resulting hybrids can be DNA-DNA, DNA-RNA, or RNA-RNA duplexes.

**hybridoma** /hī'bridō'mə/, a hybrid cell formed by the fusion of a myeloma cell and an antibody-producing cell. Hybridomas are used to produce monoclonal antibodies.

**hybrid subtraction,** a method for producing digitized radiographic images that requires at least four images. It uses both energy and temporal subtraction steps to mitigate patient motion artifacts.

**hybrid vigor.** See **heterosis.**

**Hycodan,** trademark for a fixed-combination drug containing an anticholinergic (homatropine methylbromide) and an antitussive (hydrocodone bitartrate).

**Hycomine,** trademark for a fixed-combination drug containing an adrenergic (phenylpropanolamine hydrochloride) and an antitussive (hydrocodone bitartrate).

**hydantoin** /hīdan'tō·in/, any one of a group of anticonvulsant medications, chemically and pharmacologically similar to the barbiturates, that act to limit seizure activity and reduce the spreading of abnormal electrical excitation from the focus of the seizure. A primary hydantoin in the management of almost all forms of epilepsy is phenytoin, formerly known as diphenylhydantoin. Frequent determination of the blood concentration of hydantoin is necessary.

**hydatid** /hī'dətid/ [Gk, *hydatis,* water drop], a cyst or cyst-like structure that usually is filled with fluid, especially the cyst formed around the developing scolex of the dog tapeworm *Echinococcus granulosus.* Humans and sheep can become hosts to the larval stage by ingesting the eggs. Hydatid cysts may be identified by palpation; they occur most commonly in the liver. An acute anaphylactoid allergic reaction may occur if the cyst ruptures. See also **hydatid cyst, hydatid mole, hydatidosis. —hydatic,** *adj.*

**hydatid cyst,** a cyst in the liver that contains larvae of the tapeworm *Echinococcus granulosus,* whose eggs are carried from the intestinal tract to the liver via the portal circulation. Patients are generally asymptomatic, except for hepatomegaly and a dull ache over the right upper quadrant of the abdomen. Radiologic tests are used in diagnosis, and, because no medical treatment is available, surgical removal of the cyst is indicated. Compare **hydatid mole.**

**hydatid disease.** See **echinococcosis.**

**hydatidiform** /hī'dədid'ifôrm/ [Gk, *hydatis,* water drop; L, *forma*], having the appearance or form of a **hydatid.** Also spelled **hydatiform** /hīdat'ifôrm/.

**hydatid mole,** an intrauterine neoplastic mass of grapelike enlarged chorionic villi that occurs in approximately 1 in 1500 pregnancies in the United States and eight times more frequently in some Asian countries. Molar pregnancies are more common in older and younger women than in those between 20 and 40 years of age. The cause of the degenerative disorder is not known; it may be the result of a primary ovular defect, an intrauterine abnormality, or a nutritional deficiency. Characteristic signs are extreme nausea, uterine bleeding, anemia, hyperthyroidism, an unusually large uterus for the duration of pregnancy, absence of fetal heart sounds, edema, and high blood pressure. Diagnostic measures include ultrasonography, amniography, and measurement of chorionic gonadotropin level in the blood. In most cases the mole is discovered when abortion is threatened or in progress. Oxytocin may be used to stimulate evacuation of a mole that is not spontaneously aborted, and curettage is usually performed several days later to be certain no molar tissue remains in the uterus. It is important that pregnancy be avoided for at least 1 year and that assays for chorionic gonadotropin be performed to monitor for the risk of development of gestational trophoblastic disease. Also called **hydatidiform mole.** See also **trophoblastic cancer.**

**hydatidosis** /hī'dətidō'sis/ [Gk, *hydatis + osis,* condition], infestation with the tapeworm *Echinococcus granulosus.* See also **hydatid cyst.**

**hydatiform.** See **hydatidiform.**

**Hydeltrasol,** trademark for a glucocorticoid (prednisolone sodium phosphate).

**Hydeltra TBA,** trademark for a glucocorticoid (prednisolone tebutate).

**Hydergine,** trademark for a fixed-combination drug containing various ergoloid mesylates.

**hydr-.** See **hydro-.**

**hydradenitis** /hī'dradəni'tis/ [Gk, *hydor,* water, *aden,* gland, *itis,* inflammation], an infection or inflammation of the sweat glands. Also spelled **hidradenitis.**

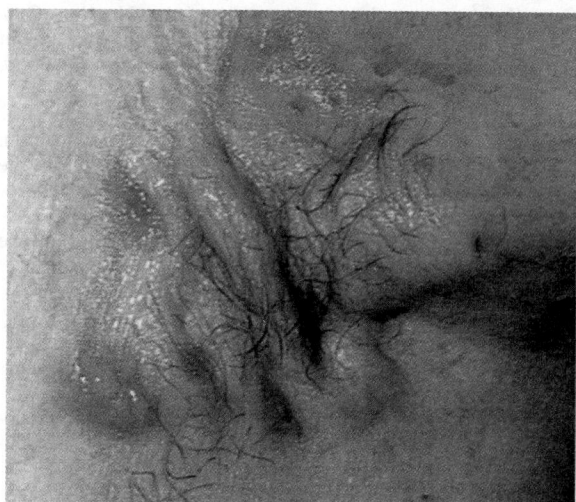

**Hydradenitis suppurativa** *(White, 1994)*

**hydralazine** /hīdral'əzēn/, a vasodilator used in hypertension.

■ INDICATION: It is prescribed in the treatment of hypertension.

■ CONTRAINDICATIONS: Coronary artery disease, mitral valvular rheumatic heart disease, or known sensitivity to this drug prohibits its use.

■ ADVERSE EFFECTS: Among the most serious adverse reactions are angina pectoris, palpitations, tachycardia, hypotension, anorexia, tremors, blood dyscrasias, depression, nausea, and peripheral neuritis.

**hydralazine hydrochloride.** See **hydralazine.**

**hydramnios** /hīdram'nē·əs/ [Gk, *hydor + amnos,* lamb's caul], an abnormal condition of pregnancy characterized by an excess of amniotic fluid. It occurs in less than 1% of pregnancies and is diagnosed by palpation, ultrasound, or radiographic examination. It is associated with maternal disorders, including toxemia of pregnancy and diabetes mellitus. Some fetal disorders, including anomalies of the GI tract, respiratory tract, and cardiovascular system, may interfere with normal exchange of amniotic fluid, causing hydramnios. Fetal hydrops and multiple gestation are also associated with the condition. The incidence of premature

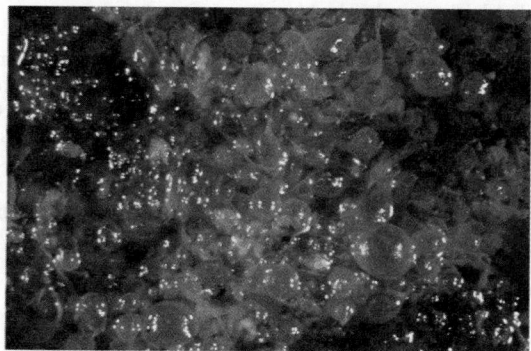

**Hydatid mole** *(Cotran, Kumar, and Collins, 1999)*

rupture of the membranes, premature labor, and perinatal mortality is increased. Periodic amniocentesis may be necessary. Also called **hydramnion, polyhydramnios.** Compare **oligohydramnios.**

**hydranencephaly** /hīdran'ənsef'əlē/, a neurologic disorder in which the cerebral hemispheres are lacking although the cerebellum, brainstem, and other central nervous system tissues may be intact. The newborn with hydranencephaly may have normal neurologic functions but does not develop, and computed tomographic scans indicate an absence of cerebral tissue. Treatment is supportive. See also **anencephaly.**

**hydrargyrism.** See **mercury poisoning.**

**hydrate** /hī'drāt/ [Gk, *hydor,* water], **1.** a combination of a substance with one or more water molecules. **2.** a molecular association of a substance with water.

**hydration**[1] /hīdrā'shən/ [Gk, *hydor,* water], a chemical process in which water is added without disrupting the rest of the molecule.

**hydration**[2], a nursing outcome from the Nursing Outcomes Classification (NOC) defined as amount of water in the intracellular and extracellular compartments of the body. See also **Nursing Outcomes Classification.**

**Hydrea,** trademark for an antineoplastic (hydroxyurea).

**hydremic ascites** /hīdrem'ik/ [Gk, *hydor* + *haima,* blood, *askos,* bag], an abnormal accumulation of fluid within the peritoneal cavity accompanied by hemodilution, as in protein calorie malnutrition. See also **ascites.**

**-hydria,** combining form meaning 'level of fluid in the body': *histohydria, isohydria, oligohydria.*

**hydro-, hydr-,** prefix meaning 'water or hydrogen': *hydroadipsia, hydrocele, hydropexis.*

**hydroa** /hīdrō'ə/ [Gk, *hydor* + *oon,* egg], an unusual vesicular and bullous skin condition of childhood that recurs each summer after exposure to sunlight, sometimes accompanied by itching lichenification, and scars. It usually disappears soon after puberty. Treatment includes use of sunscreen and avoidance of exposure to sunlight.

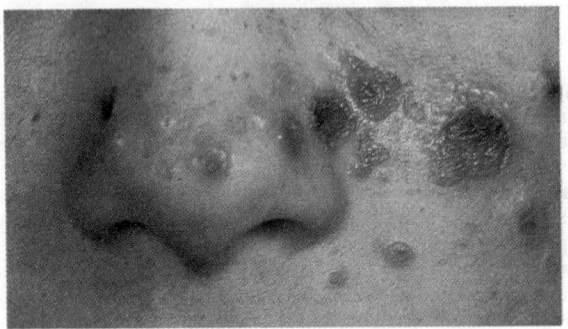

**Hydroa vacciniforme** *(du Vivier, 1993)*

**hydrobilirubin** /hī'drōbil'iroo'bin/ [Gk, *hydor,* water; L, *bilis,* bile, *ruber,* red], a reddish-brown bile pigment produced by the reduction of bilirubin.

**hydrocarbon** /-kär'bən/ [Gk, *hydor* + L, *carbo,* charcoal], any of a large group of organic compounds whose molecules are composed of hydrogen and carbon, many of which are derived from petroleum. Brief incidental exposures to low concentrations of solvent vapors that contain carbon, such as gasoline, lighter fluids, aerosol sprays, and spot removers, may be relatively harmless, but exposures to concentrations of hydrocarbon vapors often found in the home and in manufacturing environments may be dangerous.

**hydrocele** /hī'drōsēl'/ [Gk, *hydor* + *kele,* hernia], an accumulation of fluid in any saclike cavity or duct, specifically in the tunica vaginalis testis or along the spermatic cord. The condition is caused by inflammation of the epididymis or testis or by lymphatic or venous obstruction in the cord. Congenital hydrocele is caused by failure of the canal between the peritoneal cavity and the scrotum to close completely during prenatal development. In some newborns the defect may resolve spontaneously after neonatal obliteration of the communication. Treatment for persistent hydrocele is surgery. Aspiration is only a temporary measure and may induce secondary infection. See also **inguinal hernia.**

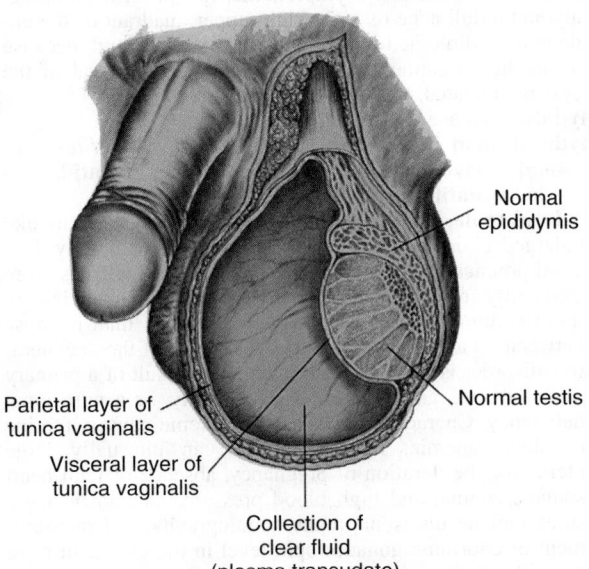

Normal epididymis

Normal testis

Parietal layer of tunica vaginalis

Visceral layer of tunica vaginalis

Collection of clear fluid (plasma transudate)

**Hydrocele** *(Huether and McCance, 2000)*

**hydrocephalic cry** /-səfal'ik/, an involuntary loud nighttime cry of a child who has acquired hydrocephalus.

**hydrocephalocoele,** a hernia consisting of a watery sac of brain tissue protruding through a fissure into the skull. Also called **hydrencephalocoele.**

**hydrocephalus** /-sef'ələs/ [Gk, *hydor* + *kephale,* head], a pathologic condition characterized by an abnormal accumulation of cerebrospinal fluid, usually under increased pressure, within the cranial vault and subsequent dilation of the ventricles. Interference with the normal flow of cerebrospinal fluid may result from increased secretion of the fluid, obstruction within the ventricular system (noncommunicating or intraventricular hydrocephalus), or defective resorption from the cerebral subarachnoid space (communicating or extraventricular hydrocephalus), caused by developmental anomalies, infection, trauma, or brain tumors.

■ OBSERVATIONS: The condition may be congenital, with rapid onset of symptoms, or it may progress slowly so that neurologic manifestations do not appear until early to late childhood or even until early adulthood. In infants the head

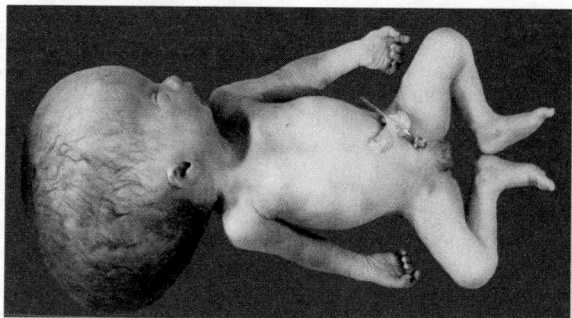

**Fetus with pronounced hydrocephalus**
*(Carlson, 1999/courtesy M. Barr, Ann Arbor, Michigan)*

grows at an abnormal rate with separation of the sutures, bulging fontanels, and dilated scalp veins; the face becomes disproportionately small, and the eyes appear depressed within the sockets. Typical behavior includes irritability with lethargy and vomiting, opisthotonos, lower extremity spasticity, and failure to perform normal reflex actions. If the condition progresses, lower brainstem function is disrupted; the skull becomes enormous; the cortex is destroyed; and the infant displays somnolence, seizures, and cardiopulmonary obstruction and usually does not survive the neonatal period. At later onset, after the cranial sutures have fused and the skull has formed, symptoms are primarily neurologic and include headache, edema of the optic disc, strabismus, and loss of muscular coordination. Hydrocephalus in infants is suspected when head growth is observed to be in excess of the normal rate. In all age groups diagnosis is confirmed by such procedures as cerebrospinal fluid examination, computed tomography, air encephalography, arteriography, and echoencephalography.

■ INTERVENTIONS: Treatment consists almost exclusively of surgical intervention to correct the ventricular obstruction, reduce the production of cerebrospinal fluid, or shunt the excess fluid by ventricular bypass to the right atrium of the heart or to the peritoneal cavity. Surgically treated hydrocephalus with continued neurosurgical and medical management has a survival rate of approximately 80%, although prognosis depends largely on the cause of the condition. Hydrocephalus is frequently associated with myelomeningocele, in which case there is a less favorable prognosis.

■ NURSING CONSIDERATIONS: Primary care of the child with hydrocephalus consists of maintaining adequate nutrition, proper positioning and support to prevent extra strain on the neck, and assistance with diagnostic evaluation and procedures. After surgery, in addition to routine care and observation to prevent complications, especially infection, the nurse gives support to the parents and teaches them how to care for a child with a functioning shunt, specifically how to recognize signs that indicate shunt malfunction or infection and how to pump the shunt. Also called **hydrocephaly.** —**hydrocephalic,** *adj., n.* See **macrocephaly.**

**hydrochloric acid** /-klôr′ik/ [Gk, *hydor* + *chloros*, green], an aqueous solution of hydrogen chloride or hydrogen ions and chloride ions. Hydrochloric acid is secreted in the stomach and is a major component of gastric juice.

**hydrochlorothiazide** /-klôr′ōthī′əzīd/, a thiazide diuretic and antihypertensive.

■ INDICATIONS: It is prescribed in the treatment of hypertension and edema.

■ CONTRAINDICATIONS: Anuria or known hypersensitivity to this drug, to other thiazide medication, or to sulfonamide derivatives prohibits its use.

■ ADVERSE EFFECTS: Among the more serious adverse effects are hypoglycemia, hyperglycemia, hyperuricemia, and hypersensitivity reactions.

**hydrocholeretics** /-kō′ləret′iks/ [Gk, *hydor* + *chloe*, bile, *eresis*, removal], drugs that stimulate the production of bile with a low specific gravity or with a minimal proportion of solid constituents.

**Hydrocil Instant,** trademark for a laxative (psyllium hydrophilic mucilloid).

**hydrocodone bitartrate** /-kō′dōn/, an opioid antitussive and analgesic.

■ INDICATION: It is prescribed in the treatment of cough and pain.

■ CONTRAINDICATIONS: Drug dependence or known hypersensitivity to this drug prohibits its use.

■ ADVERSE EFFECTS: Among the more serious adverse reactions are drug dependence and respiratory and circulatory depression.

**hydrocolloid,** a gelatinous colloid in which water is the dispersion material. It is used in dentistry as an impression material.

**hydrocortisone, hydrocortisone acetate, hydrocortisone cyclopentylpropionate, hydrocortisone sodium succinate.** See **cortisol.**

**hydrocortisone valerate** /- kôr′tisōn/, a topical corticosteroid.

■ INDICATION: It is prescribed for the topical treatment of skin inflammation. Used topically as an antiinflammatory agent.

■ CONTRAINDICATIONS: Viral and fungal diseases of the skin that occur where circulation is impaired or known hypersensitivity to steroids prohibits its use.

■ ADVERSE REACTIONS: Among the more serious adverse reactions are various systemic side effects that may result from prolonged or excessive use. Local irritation of the skin may occur.

**Hydrocortone,** trademark for a glucocorticoid (hydrocortisone acetate).

**HydroDiuril,** trademark for a diuretic (hydrochlorothiazide).

**hydroflumethiazide** /-floo′methī′əzīd/, a diuretic and antihypertensive.

■ INDICATIONS: It is prescribed in the treatment of hypertension and edema.

■ CONTRAINDICATIONS: Anuria or known hypersensitivity to this drug, to other thiazide medication, or to sulfonamide derivatives prohibits its use.

■ ADVERSE EFFECTS: Among the more serious adverse effects are blood disorders, hypotension, hypokalemia, hyperglycemia, hyperuricemia, and hypersensitivity reactions.

**hydrofluoric acid** /hī′drō·floor′ik /, a term applied to aqueous solutions of hydrogen fluoride, an organic acid used in dilute solutions for cleaning and etching. It is extremely poisonous, as well as corrosive to the skin.

**hydrogel,** a gel in which water is the dispersion medium.

**hydrogen (H)** /hī′drəjən/ [Gk, *hydor* + *genein*, to produce], a gaseous monovalent element. Its atomic number is 1; its atomic mass is 1.008. It is the simplest and the lightest of the elements and is a colorless, odorless, highly inflammable diatomic gas. It occurs in pure form only sparsely in the earth and the atmosphere but is plentiful in the sun and in many other stars. Hydrogen is a component of numerous compounds, many of them produced by the body. As a component of water, hydrogen is crucial in the metabolic interaction of acids, bases, and salts within the body and in the fluid balance necessary for the body to survive.

**hydrogenase** /hī′drōjənās′/ [Gk, *hydor,* water, *genein,* to produce, *ase,* suffix indicating an enzyme], an enzyme that catalyzes reduction of molecules by combining them with molecular hydrogen.

**hydrogenation.** See **reduction.**

**hydrogen bonding,** the attractive force of compounds in which a hydrogen atom covalently linked to an electronegative element such as oxygen, nitrogen, or fluorine has a large degree of positive character relative to the electronegative atom, thereby causing the compound to possess a large dipole and to associate strongly with other like molecules.

**hydrogen cyanide (HCN),** a colorless, toxic, volatile liquid or gas with the aroma of bitter almonds. It occurs naturally in almonds and in the stone pits of peaches, plums, and other fruits. When dissolved in water, it is called hydrocyanic acid, prussic acid.

**hydrogen donor,** a compound that gives up hydrogen (usually $H^+$, a proton) to another compound.

**hydrogen ion [$H^+$],** a positively charged hydrogen atom.

**hydrogen ion [$H^+$] concentration of blood,** a measure of blood pH and its effect on the ability of the hemoglobin molecule to hold oxygen. See also **Bohr effect.**

**hydrogen peroxide,** a topical antiinfective.

**hydroglossa.** See **ranula.**

**hydrokinetics** /-kinet′iks/ [Gk, *hydor,* water, *kinesis,* motion], the study of movement of fluids.

**hydrolase** /hī′drōlās/, an enzyme that cleaves ester bonds by the addition of water.

**hydrolysis** /hīdrol′isis/ [Gk, *hydor* + *lysis,* loosening], the chemical alteration or decomposition of a compound with water.

**hydrolytic** /-lit′ik/ [Gk, *hydor,* water, *lysis,* loosening], pertaining to or having the ability to produce hydrolysis.

**hydrolyze** /hī′drōlīz/ [Gk, *hydor,* water, *lysis,* loosening], **1.** to cause or bring about hydrolysis. **2.** to cause a substance to split into component parts by the addition of water.

**hydrometer** /hīdrom′ətər/ [Gk, *hydor* + *metron,* measure], a device that determines the specific gravity or density of a liquid by a comparison of its weight with that of an equal volume of water. A calibrated hollow glass device is placed in the liquid being examined, and the depth to which the device settles in the liquid is noted.

**hydromorphone hydrochloride** /-môr′fōn/, an opioid analgesic.

- INDICATION: It is used to treat moderate to severe pain.
- CONTRAINDICATIONS: It is used with caution in many conditions, including head injuries, asthma, impaired renal or hepatic function, or unstable cardiovascular status. Known hypersensitivity to this drug prohibits its use.
- ADVERSE EFFECTS: Among the most serious adverse reactions are drowsiness, dizziness, nausea, constipation, respiratory and circulatory depression, and drug addiction.

**hydromyelia** /hī′drō·mī·ē′lē·ə/ [Gk, *hydor,* water + *myelos,* marrow], a pathological condition in which there is dilation of the central canal of the spinal cord with increased fluid accumulation. Compare **syringomyelia.**

**hydronephrosis** /hī′drōnefrō′sis/ [Gk, *hydor* + *nephros,* kidney, *osis,* condition], distension of the pelvis and calyces of the kidney by urine that cannot flow past an obstruction in a ureter. Ureteral obstruction may be caused by a tumor, a calculus lodged in the ureter, inflammation of the prostate gland, or edema caused by a urinary tract infection. The person may experience pain in the flank and, in some cases, hematuria, pyuria, and hyperpyrexia. IV pyelography, cytoscopy, or retrograde pyelography may be used in diag-

nosis. Surgical repair or removal of the obstruction may be necessary. Prolonged hydronephrosis causes atrophy and eventual loss of kidney function. See also **urinary calculus.** —**hydronephrotic,** *adj.*

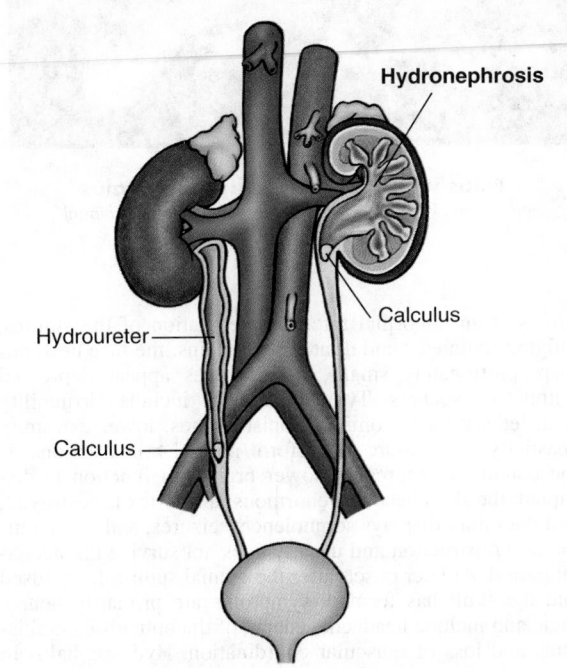

**Hydronephrosis** *(Monahan and Neighbors, 1998)*

**hydropenia** /-pē′nē·ə/, lack of water in the body tissues.

**hydropericarditis,** inflammation of the pericardium accompanied by excessive accumulation of serous fluid.

**hydropericardium,** an excessive accumulation of fluid in the pericardium.

**hydroperitoneum** /-per′itənē′əm/, an accumulation of fluid in the peritoneum.

**hydrophilic** /-fil′ik/ [Gk, *hydor* + *philein,* to love], pertaining to the property of attracting water molecules, possessed by polar radicals or ions. Compare **hydrophobic.**

**hydrophobia** /-fō′bē·ə/ [Gk, *hydor* + *phobos,* fear], **1.** *nontechnical.* rabies. **2.** a morbid, extreme fear of water.

**hydrophobiaphobia,** a morbid fear of hydrophobia, with symptoms that may simulate those of rabies.

**hydrophobic** [Gk, *hydor* + *phobos,* fear], pertaining to the property of repelling water molecules, a quality possessed by nonpolar radicals or molecules that are more soluble in organic solvents than in water. Compare **hydrophilic.**

**hydrophone** /hī′drəfōn/, a small diameter probe with a piezoelectric element, usually about 0.5 mm in diameter, at one end. When placed in an ultrasound beam, the hydrophone produces an electric signal.

**hydrophthalmos.** See **congenital glaucoma.**

**hydropic** /hīdrop′ik/ [Gk, *hydrops*], pertaining to the condition of dropsy.

**Hydropres,** trademark for a fixed-combination drug containing a diuretic (hydrochlorothiazide) and an antihypertensive (reserpine).

**hydrops** /hī'drops/ [Gk, dropsy], an abnormal accumulation of clear watery or serous fluid in a body tissue or cavity, such as a joint, a graafian follicle, a fallopian tube, the abdomen, the middle ear, or the gallbladder. Hydrops in the entire body may occur in infants born with thalassemia or severe Rh sensitization. Formerly called **dropsy.**

**hydrops fetalis,** massive edema in the fetus or newborn, usually in association with severe erythroblastosis fetalis. Severe anemia and effusions of the pericardial, pleural, and peritoneal spaces also occur. The condition usually leads to death, even with immediate exchange transfusions after delivery. Also called **fetal hydrops.**

**hydrops gravidarum** [Gk, hydor, water; L, gravidus, pregnant], edema caused by pregnancy.

**hydrops tubae profluens.** See **intermittent hydrosalpinx.**

**hydroquinone** /hī'drōkwin'ōn/, a dermatologic bleaching agent.

■ INDICATIONS: It is prescribed to reduce pigmentation of the skin in certain conditions in which an excess of melanin causes hyperpigmentation.

■ CONTRAINDICATIONS: Sunburn, prickly heat, other irritation of the skin, or known hypersensitivity to this drug prohibits its use.

■ ADVERSE EFFECTS: Among the more serious adverse reactions are tingling, erythema, burning, and severe inflammation of the skin.

**hydrosalpinx** /hī'drōsal'pingks/ [Gk, hydor + salpinx, tube], an abnormal condition of the fallopian tube in which it is cystically enlarged and filled with clear fluid. It is the result of an infection that has previously occluded the tube at both ends. The purulent material produced by the infection undergoes liquefaction during resolution of the acute phase of the inflammatory process.

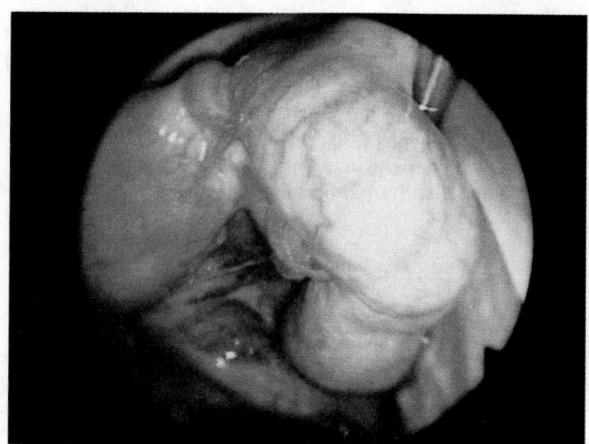

**Hydrosalpinx** (Hunt, 1999/courtesy Robert B. Hunt, Boston)

**hydrosis** [Gk, hydor, water, osis, condition], pertaining to the production of sweat. Also spelled **hidrosis.**

**Hydro-Sphere Nebulizer,** trademark for a type of nebulizer in which a source gas enters a hollow sphere coated with a film of water. The gas exits through slits at the top of the sphere as an aerosol jet, carrying particles of fluid from the sphere's surface.

**hydrostatic** /-stat'ik/ [Gk, hydor, water, statos, standing], pertaining to fluids at rest or in equilibrium and the pressure they exert.

**hydrostatic dosimetry,** the weighing of a person under water to determine the ratio of lean tissue to body fat.

**hydrostatic pressure,** the pressure exerted by a liquid.

**hydrostatics,** the study of pressures in liquids at rest or in equilibrium.

**hydrotherapy** /-ther'əpē/ [Gk, hydor + therapeia, treatment], the use of water in the treatment of various disorders. Hydrotherapy may include continuous tub baths, wet sheet packs, or shower sprays.

**hydrothorax** /-thôr'aks/ [Gk, hydor + thorax, chest], a noninflammatory accumulation of serous fluid in one or both pleural cavities.

**hydrotropism** /-trō'pizəm/ [Gk, hydor + trope, turning], the tendency of a cell or organism to turn or move in a certain direction under the influence of a water stimulus.

**hydrous** /hī'drəs/ [Gk, hydor, water], pertaining to a substance or object that contains water or is moist.

**hydrous wool fat.** See **lanolin.**

**hydroxide** /hīdrok'sīd/, an ion with the formula $OH^-$.

**hydroxyamphetamine hydrobromide** /hīdrok'sē·əmfet'əmēn/, an adrenergic and mydriatic.

■ INDICATIONS: It is prescribed for dilation of the pupil for ophthalmoscopy and as a diagnostic aid in Horner's syndrome.

■ CONTRAINDICATIONS: Narrow-angle glaucoma or known hypersensitivity to this drug prohibits its use.

■ ADVERSE EFFECTS: Among the more serious adverse reactions are increased intraocular pressure and photophobia.

**hydroxyandrosterone** /hīdrok'sē·andros'tərōn/ [Gk hydor + andros, male, stereos, solid], a sex hormone secreted by the testes and adrenal glands. Its normal accumulation in the urine of men after 24-hour collection is 0.1 to 8 mg; in women, 0 to 0.5 mg.

**hydroxyapatite** /hīdrok'sē·ap'ətīt/, an inorganic compound composed of calcium, phosphate, and hydroxide. It is found in the bones and teeth in a crystallized latticelike form that gives these structures rigidity.

**hydroxybenzene.** See **carbolic acid.**

**hydroxychloroquine sulfate** /-klôr'əkwīn/, an antimalarial preparation.

■ INDICATIONS: It is prescribed in the treatment of malaria and the suppression of acute paroxysmal attacks of the disease; in the treatment of extraintestinal, usually hepatic, amebiasis; and in the reduction of symptoms of lupus erythematosus and rheumatoid arthritis.

■ CONTRAINDICATIONS: Concurrent use of other 4-aminoquinolones or of gold salts or a known hypersensitivity to this drug or to other 4-aminoquinolones prohibits its use. It is used with caution in cases of alcoholism, blood dyscrasia, severe neurologic disorder, retinal or visual field damage, psoriasis, or porphyria. The drug is not usually recommended in pregnancy because it has been associated with damage to the central nervous system of the fetus.

■ ADVERSE EFFECTS: Among the many severe adverse reactions are retinopathy, corneal opacity, polyneuritis, seizure, agranulocytosis, and hepatitis. The incidence and severity of these and many other adverse effects increase with the dosage and prolonged duration of treatment.

**17-hydroxycorticosteroid** /-kôr'tikos'təroid/, any steroid hydroxylated at carbon-17 secreted by adrenal glands and occasionally measured in the urine in a test for determining adrenal function and diagnosing hypoadrenalism or hyperadrenalism. The normal accumulation in the urine of men after 24-hour collection is 5.5 to 14.5 μg; in women, 4.9 to

12.9 µg; and in children, slightly less. The levels are normally two to four times higher in all cases after injection of 25 USP units of adrenocorticotropic hormone.

**17-hydroxycorticosteroids test (17-OCHS),** a 24-hour urine test used to detect abnormal levels of 17-OCHS. Elevated levels are seen in hyperfunction of the adrenal gland (Cushing syndrome), while low levels are seen in hypofunction (Addison's disease).

**11-hydroxyetiocholanolone** /hīdrok′sē·ē′tē·ōkolan′əlōn/, a sex hormone secreted by the testes and adrenal glands. The normal accumulation in the urine of men after 24-hour collection is 0.2 to 0.6 mg; in women, 0.1 to 1 mg.

**5-hydroxyindoleacetic acid** /hīdrok′sē·in′dōlē·əset′ik/, an acid produced by serotonin metabolism, measured in the blood and urine to aid in the diagnosis of certain kinds of tumors. It commonly rises above normal levels in whole blood in association with asthma, diarrhea, rapid heartbeat, and other symptoms and is elevated in the urine of patients with carcinoid syndrome. Its normal concentration in whole blood is 0.05 to 0.20 g/mL; its normal accumulation in urine after 24-hour collection is 1 to 5 mg.

**5-hydroxyindoleacetic acid test,** a 24-hour urine test used to detect and follow the clinical course of patients with carcinoid tumors, which may grow in the appendix, intestine, lung, or any tissue derived from the neuroectoderm. The test is also used to reevaluate patients with known tumors for tumor progression or therapeutic response to antineoplastic therapy.

**hydroxyl (OH)** /hīdrok′sil/, a monovalent radical consisting of an oxygen atom and a hydrogen atom.

**hydroxyprogesterone caproate** /-prōjes′tərōn/, a progestation.

- INDICATIONS: It is prescribed in the treatment of advanced adenocarcinoma of the uterine corpus, amenorrhea, and abnormal uterine bleeding caused by hormonal imbalance in the absence of organic disease.
- CONTRAINDICATIONS: Markedly impaired liver function, carcinoma of the breast, undiagnosed abnormal genital bleeding, thromboembolic disorders, or known sensitivity to this drug prohibits its use.
- ADVERSE EFFECTS: Among the most serious adverse reactions are thrombophlebitis, pulmonary embolism, cerebrovascular accident, neuroocular lesions, anorexia, edema, hypertension, cholestatic jaundice, and depression.

**hydroxyproline** /-prō′lēn/, an amino acid whose level in the urine is elevated in diseases of the bone and certain genetic disorders, such as Marfan's syndrome. Its normal accumulation in urine after a 24-hour collection is 10 to 75 mg.

**5-hydroxytryptamine.** See serotonin.

**hydroxyurea** /hīdrok′siyŏŏrē′ə/, an antineoplastic.

- INDICATION: It is prescribed in the treatment of a variety of neoplasms.
- CONTRAINDICATIONS: Bone marrow depression or known hypersensitivity to this drug prohibits its use. It is not to be given to women who are or may become pregnant.
- ADVERSE EFFECTS: The most serious adverse reaction is bone marrow depression. GI disturbances and dermatitis also may occur.

**hydroxyzine hydrochloride** /hīdrok′səzēn/, an antihistamine.

- INDICATIONS: It is prescribed for the relief of anxiety, nervous tension, hyperkinesis, itching, and motion sickness.
- CONTRAINDICATION: Known hypersensitivity to this drug is the only contraindication.
- ADVERSE EFFECTS: No serious adverse reactions have been observed. Decreased mental alertness sometimes occurs.

**hygiene** /hī′jēn/ [Gk, *Hygieia,* the goddess of health], the principles and science of the preservation of health and prevention of disease.

**hygienist** /hī′jənist, hījē′nist/ [Gk, *Hygieia*], one who practices the principles and laws of **hygiene.**

**hygro-** /hī′grō-/ [Gk, *hygros,* moist], prefix for terms relating to moistness or moisture.

**hygroma** /hī·grō′mə/ *pl.* **hygromas, hygromata** [Gk, *hygros,* moist + *-oma,* tumor], a sac, cyst, or bursa distended with a fluid.

**hygrometer** /hīgrom′ətər/ [Gk, *hygros,* moist, *metron,* measure], an instrument that directly measures relative humidity of the atmosphere or the proportion of water in a specific gas or gas mixture, without extracting the moisture.

**hygroscopic humidifier** /-skop′ik/, a humidifying device attached to the tubing circuit of a mechanical ventilator or anesthesia gas machine to maintain a constant rate of humidity in the trachea.

**Hygroton,** trademark for a diuretic (chlorthalidone).

**Hylorel,** trademark for an antihypertensive (guanadrel sulfate).

**hymen** /hī′mən/ [Gk, membrane], a fold of mucous membrane, skin, and fibrous tissue that covers the introitus of the vagina. It may be absent, small, thin and pliant, or rarely tough and dense, completely occluding the introitus. When the hymen is disrupted, small rounded "tags" of tissue remain. See also **carunculae hymenales.**

**hymenal** /hī′mənəl/ [Gk, *hymen,* membrane], pertaining to the hymen.

**hymenal tag,** normal redundant hymenal tissue protruding from the floor of the vagina during the first weeks after birth. It eventually disappears without treatment.

**hymenectomy** /hī′mənek′təmē/ [Gk, *hymen,* membrane, *ektomē,* excision], the surgical excision of a membrane, particularly the hymen.

**hymenolepiasis,** heavy infestation by *Hymenolepis nana* that may cause abdominal pain, bloody stools, and disorders of the nervous system, especially in children. Contaminated food spreads the disease, which is endemic in the United States. Quinacrine hydrochloride or hexylresorcinol is used to treat the infestation.

*Hymenolepis* /hī′mə·nol′ə·pis/ [Gk, *hymen,* membrane + *lepis,* rind], a genus of tapeworms of the family Hymenolepididae, which parasitize birds and mammals, including humans. See also **hymenolepiasis.**

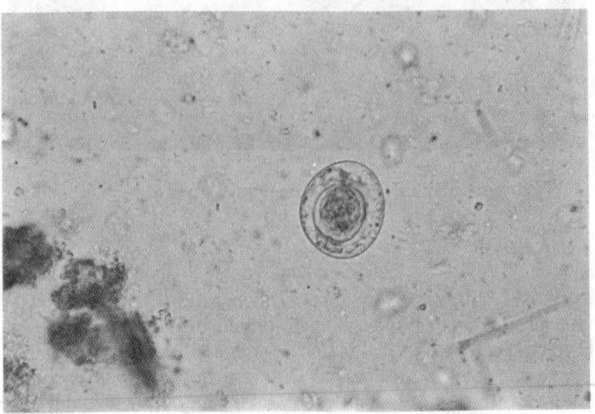

***Hymenolepis nana* egg** *(Mahon and Manuselis, 2000)*

**hymenotomy** /hī'mənot'əmē/ [Gk, *hymen* + *temnein*, to cut], the surgical incision of the hymen.

**hyo-** /hī'ō-/ [Gk, *hyoeides*, upsilon, U-shaped], prefix meaning 'shaped like the letter *u* or pertaining to the hyoid bone': *hyobasioglossus, hyoglossus.*

**hyoglossal** /-glos'əl/ [Gk, *hyoeides* + *glossa*, tongue], pertaining to the tongue and the horseshoe-shaped hyoid bone at the base of the tongue immediately above the thyroid cartilage. Also **glossohyal.**

**hyoglossal membrane,** a widening of the lingual septum connecting the root of tongue to the hyoid bone.

**hyoglossus** /-glos'əs/ [Gk, *hyoeides* + *glossa*, tongue], a depressor muscle of the tongue that arises from the hyoid bone.

**hyoid** /hī'oid/ [Gk, *hyoeides*, upsilon, U-shaped], **1.** the hyoid bone. **2.** pertaining to the hyoid bone.

**hyoid arch** [Gk, *hyoeides* + L, *arcus*, bow], the second pharyngeal or branchial arch. It is present in typical form in the embryo, but the skeletal elements develop into the stapes and styloid process of the temporal bone of the adult.

**hyoid bone** /hī'oid/ [Gk, *hyoeides*, upsilon, U-shaped; AS, *ban*, bone], a single U-shaped bone suspended from the styloid processes of the temporal bones. The body of the hyoid is square and flat, its ventral surface convex and angled cranially. Two greater wings of the bone attach to the lateral thyroid ligaments, and the body of the bone attaches to various muscles, such as the hypoglossus and the sternohyoideus. The hyoid is palpable in the neck. Also called **lingual bone, os hyoideum.**

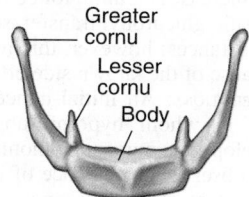

Greater cornu
Lesser cornu
Body

**Hyoid bone**

**hyoscine.** See **scopolamine.**

**hyoscine hydrobromide.** See **scopolamine hydrobromide.**

**hyoscyamine** /hī'əsī'əmēn/, an anticholinergic/antispasmodic.

■ INDICATIONS: It is prescribed in the treatment of hypermotility of the GI and lower urinary tracts.

■ CONTRAINDICATIONS: Narrow-angle glaucoma, asthma, obstruction of the genitourinary or GI tract, severe ulcerative colitis, or known hypersensitivity to this drug prohibits its use.

■ ADVERSE EFFECTS: Among the more serious adverse reactions are blurred vision, central nervous system effects, tachycardia, dry mouth, decreased sweating, and hypersensitivity reactions.

**hyp-.** See **hypo-.**

**hypalgesia** /hī'paljē'zē·ə/ [Gk, *hypo*, below, *algesis*, pain], the perception of a painful stimulus to a degree that varies significantly from a normal perception of the same stimulus.

**hyper-** /hī'pər-/, prefix meaning 'excessive, above, or beyond': *hyperacidaminuria, hyperalkalinity, hyperechema.*

**Hyperab,** trademark for a passive immunizing agent (rabies immune globulin).

**hyperacidity** /-əsid'itē/ [Gk, *hyper*, excess; L, *acidus*, sour], an excessive amount of acidity, as in the stomach. See also **hyperchlorhydria.**

**hyperactive child syndrome.** See **attention deficit hyperactivity disorder.**

**hyperactivity** /-aktiv'itē/ [Gk, *hyper* + L, *activus*, active], any abnormally increased motor activity or function involving either the entire organism or a particular organ, as the heart or thyroid. Compare **hypoactivity.** See also **attention deficit disorder.**

**hyperacuity** /-akyoo'itē/ [Gk, *hyper*, excessive, *akouien*, to hear], excessive sensitivity to sounds.

**hyperadenosis** /-ad'ənō'sis/ [Gk, *hyper*, excessive, *aden*, gland, *osis*, condition], a condition characterized by enlarged glands.

**hyperadrenalism.** See **Cushing's disease.**

**hyperadrenocorticism.** See **Cushing's syndrome.**

**hyperalbuminemia** /-albyoo'minē'mē·ə/, an excessive amount of albumin in the blood.

**hyperaldosteronism.** See **aldosteronism.**

**hyperalgia** /-al'jə/, extreme sensitivity to pain. Also called **hyperalgesia.**

**hyperalimentation** /-al'iməntā'shən/ [Gk, *hyper* + L, *alimentum*, nourishment], **1.** overfeeding or the ingestion or administration of an amount of nutrients that exceeds the demands of the appetite. **2.** See **total parenteral nutrition.**

**hyperalkalinity** /-al'kəlin'itē/, a condition of excessive alkalinity.

**hyperammonemia** /hī'pəram'ōnē'mē·ə/ [Gk, *hyper* + (ammonia), *haima*, blood], abnormally high levels of ammonia in the blood. Ammonia is produced in the intestine, absorbed into the blood, and detoxified in the liver. It is also generated as a by-product of protein metabolism. An increased production of ammonia or a decreased ability to detoxify it increases the blood levels of ammonia. The disorder is controlled by low-protein diets, including essential amino acid mixtures. Untreated, the condition leads to hepatic encephalopathy, characterized by asterixis, vomiting, lethargy, coma, and death.

**hyperbaric chamber** /-ber'ik/ [Gk, *hyper*, excess, *baros*, weight, *kamara*, arched roof], an airtight chamber containing an oxygen atmosphere under high pressure. A patient may be placed in the chamber for the treatment of certain infections, tumors, and cardiovascular diseases in which atmospheric oxygen pressures up to three times normal may have therapeutic value.

**hyperbaric oxygenation** [Gk, *hyper* + *baros*, weight, *oxys*, sharp, *genein*, to produce], the administration of oxygen at greater than normal atmospheric pressure. The procedure is performed in specially designed chambers that permit the delivery of 100% oxygen at atmospheric pressure that is three times normal. The technique is used to overcome the natural limit of oxygen solubility in blood, which is about 0.3 mL of oxygen per 100 mL of blood. In hyperbaric oxygenation, dissolved oxygen can be increased to almost 6 mL per 100 mL and the $PO_2$ in blood may be nearly 2000 mm Hg at 3 atmospheres absolute. Hyperbaric oxygenation has been used to treat carbon monoxide poisoning, air embolism, smoke inhalation, acute cyanide poisoning, decompression sickness, clostridial myonecrosis, and certain cases of blood loss or anemia in which increased oxygen transport may compensate in part for hemoglobin deficiency. Factors limiting the usefulness of hyperbaric oxygenation include the hazards of fire and explosive decompression, pulmonary damage and neurologic toxicity at high atmospheric pressures, cardiovascular debility of the patient, and the need to interrupt treatments repeatedly because exposures at maximum atmospheric pressures must be limited to 90 minutes. Also called **hyperbaric oxygen therapy.**

**hyperbaric oxygen therapy.** See **hyperbaric oxygenation.**

**hyperbaric solution** [Gk, *hyper,* excess, *baros,* weight], a type of spinal anesthetic that has a specific gravity greater than that of cerebrospinal fluid so it will settle into the lowest parts of the spinal canal.

**hyperbarism** /-ber'izəm/, any disorder resulting from exposure to increased ambient pressure, usually caused by sudden exposure to or a significant increase in pressure. See also **barotrauma, decompression sickness.**

**hyperbetalipoproteinemia** /hī′pərbā′təlip′ōprō′tēnē′mē·ə/ [Gk, *hyper + beta,* second letter of Greek alphabet, *lipos,* fat, *proteios,* first rank, *haima,* blood], type II hyperlipoproteinemia, a genetic disorder of lipid metabolism, in which there are abnormally high levels of serum cholesterol, and xanthomas appear on the tendons of the heels, knees, and fingers. There is a marked tendency to development of atherosclerosis and early myocardial infarction, especially among males. Treatment attempts to reduce blood cholesterol levels in the hope of lowering the risk of early death from heart disease. The patient is usually counseled to avoid most meats, eggs, milk products, and all saturated fats and is encouraged to eat fish, grains, fruits, vegetables, lean poultry, and unsaturated fats. Exercise may be recommended, and drugs may be prescribed in some cases. See also **cholesterolemia.**

**hyperbilirubinemia** /hī′pərbil′iroo′binē′mē·ə/ [Gk, *hyper* + L, *bilis,* bile, *ruber,* red; Gk, *haima,* blood], greater than normal amounts of the bile pigment bilirubin in the blood, often characterized by jaundice, anorexia, and malaise. Hyperbilirubinemia is most often associated with liver disease or biliary obstruction, but it also occurs when there is excessive destruction of red blood cells, as in hemolytic anemia. Treatment is specific to the underlying condition. When bilirubin levels are high, treatment includes phototherapy and hydration. Also spelled **hyperbilirubinaemia.** See also **jaundice.**

**hyperbilirubinemia of the newborn,** an excess of bilirubin in the blood of the neonate. It is usually caused by a deficiency of an enzyme that results from physiologic immaturity, or by increased hemolysis, especially that produced by blood group incompatibility, which, in severe cases, can lead to kernicterus. Also called **neonatal hyperbilirubinemia.** See also **breast milk jaundice, cholestasis, Crigler-Najjar syndrome, Dubin-Johnson syndrome, erythroblastosis fetalis, Gilbert's syndrome, kernicterus, phototherapy in the newborn, rotor syndrome.**
■ OBSERVATIONS: Serum bilirubin levels are elevated in the normal newborn; the concentration of circulating erythrocytes is greater and infants have less ability to conjugate and excrete bilirubin because of a lack of the enzyme glucuronyl transferase, a reduced albumin concentration, and a lack of intestinal bacteria. Jaundice appears when blood levels of bilirubin exceed 5 mg/100 mL, usually not before 24 hours in full-term neonates. Clinically observable jaundice or serum bilirubin level exceeding 5 mg/100 mL within the first 24 hours of life is abnormal and indicates a pathologic cause of hyperbilirubinemia. In erythroblastosis fetalis, jaundice is evident shortly after birth, and bilirubin levels rise rapidly. Severely affected infants also show hepatosplenomegaly and signs of anemia, which quickly worsen, causing a decrease in oxygen-carrying capacity that may lead to cardiac failure and shock. Early symptoms of kernicterus are leth-

argy, poor feeding, and vomiting, followed by severe neurologic excitation or depression, including tremors, twitching, convulsion, opisthotonos, a high-pitched cry, hypotonia, diminished deep tendon reflexes, and absence of Moro and sucking reflexes. Brain damage generally does not occur at serum bilirubin levels below 20 mg/100 mL in an otherwise healthy term infant. Factors such as metabolic acidosis, lowered albumin levels, hypoxia, hypothermia, free fatty acids, and certain drugs, especially salicylates and sulfonamides, increase the risk at much lower levels. The mortality rate may reach 50%. Sequelae of kernicterus include mental retardation, minimal brain dysfunction, cerebral palsy, delayed or abnormal motor development, hearing loss, ataxia, athetosis, perceptual problems, and behavioral disorders.
■ INTERVENTIONS: Such preventive measures as frequent feedings during the first 6 to 12 hours of life to increase GI motility have little justification. Infants with mild jaundice require no treatment, only observation. Phototherapy is the usual treatment for severe or increasing hyperbilirubinemia. If hyperbilirubinemia is the result of increased hemolysis caused by blood group incompatibility, exchange transfusion may be done. It is usually indicated if laboratory analysis reveals a positive antiglobulin test result, a hemoglobin concentration of the cord blood below 12 g/100 mL, or a bilirubin level of 20 mg/100 mL or more in a full-term infant or 15 mg/100 mL or more in a premature infant. Phototherapy may be used in conjunction with exchange transfusion, except in cases of Rh incompatibility. If used immediately after the initial exchange transfusion, phototherapy may remove enough bilirubin from the tissues to make subsequent transfusions unnecessary. Pharmacologic management, such as the use of barbiturates to stimulate protein synthesis that in turn increases albumin for conjugating bilirubin and promotes hepatic glucuronyl transferase synthesis, is indicated in some instances; however, this form of therapy is controversial because of the known side effects of the drugs.
■ NURSING CONSIDERATIONS: An initial concern is to identify high-risk infants in whom hyperbilirubinemia and kernicterus may develop. The nurse may monitor the serum bilirubin levels and observe for evidence of jaundice, anemia, central nervous system irritability, and such conditions as acidosis, hypoxia, and hypothermia. In erythroblastosis fetalis exchange transfusion may be necessary. The amounts of blood infused and withdrawn, the vital signs, and any signs of exchange reactions are noted. Resuscitative equipment is kept available. Optimal body temperature is maintained: Hypothermia increases oxygen and glucose consumption, causing metabolic acidosis, and hyperthermia damages the donor's erythrocytes, causing an elevation in the amount of free potassium, which may lead to infant cardiac arrest. After the procedure a sterile dressing is applied to the catheter site.

**hypercalcemia** /hī′pərkalsē′mē·ə/ [Gk, *hyper* + L, *calx,* lime; Gk, *haima,* blood], greater than normal amounts of calcium in the blood, most often resulting from excessive bone resorption and release of calcium, as occurs in hyperparathyroidism, metastatic tumors of bone, Paget's disease, and osteoporosis. Clinically patients with hypercalcemia experience confusion, anorexia, abdominal pain, muscle pain, and weakness. Extremely high levels of blood calcium may result in coma, shock, kidney failure, and death. Hypercalciuria is also found in most patients with elevated blood calcium level. Prednisone, diuretics, isotonic saline solution, and other drugs may be used in treatment. Also spelled **hypercalcaemia. —hypercalcemic,** *adj.*

**hypercalcemic nephropathy** /-kalsē′mik/ [Gk, *hyper,* excessive; L, *calx,* lime, *haima,* blood; Gk, *nephros,* kidney, *pathos,* disease], a progressive disorder of kidney function caused by an excessive level of calcium in the blood. The calcium causes cumulative functional and histologic abnormalities that lead to a decreased glomerular filtration rate and kidney failure.

**hypercalciuria** /hī′pərkal′sēyŏŏr′ē·ə/ [Gk, *hyper* + L, *calx,* lime; Gk, *ouron,* urine], the presence of abnormally great amounts of calcium in the urine, resulting from conditions such as sarcoid, hyperparathyroidism, or certain types of arthritis that are characterized by augmented bone resorption. Immobilized patients are often hypercalciuric. Some people absorb more calcium than is normal and therefore excrete greater than normal amounts into their urine. Concentrated amounts of calcium in the urinary tract may form kidney stones. Treatment is directed to correcting any underlying disease condition and limiting dietary intake of calcium. Also called **hypercalcinuria.** Compare **hypercalcemia.** —**hypercalciuric,** *adj.*

**hypercapnia** /hī′pərkap′nē·ə/ [Gk, *hyper* + *kapnos,* vapor], greater than normal amounts of carbon dioxide in the blood. Also called **hypercarbia.**

**hypercapnic acidosis** /-kap′nik/ [Gk, *hyper,* excessive, *kapnos,* vapor; L, *acidus,* sour, *osis,* condition], an excessive acidity in body fluids caused by an increase in carbon dioxide tension in the blood. The condition may be secondary to pulmonary insufficiency; as carbon dioxide accumulates in the blood its acidity increases.

**hypercarbia.** See **hypercapnia.**

**hyperchloremia** /-klôr′mē·ə/ [Gk, *hyper* + *chloros,* green, *haima,* blood], an excessive level of chloride in the blood that results in acidosis. Also spelled **hyperchloraemia.**

**hyperchlorhydria** /-klôrhid′rē·ə/ [Gk, *hyper* + *chloros* + *hydor,* water], the excessive secretion of hydrochloric acid by cells lining the stomach. Also called **chlorhydria.** See also **hyperacidity.**

**hypercholesterolemia** /-kōles′tərōlē′mē·ə/ [Gk, *hyper* + *chole,* bile, *stereos,* solid, *haima,* blood], a condition in which greater than normal amounts of cholesterol are present in the blood. High levels of cholesterol and other lipids may lead to the development of atherosclerosis. Hypercholesterolemia may be reduced or prevented by avoiding saturated fats, which are found in red meats, eggs, and dairy products, or certain medications. Hypercholesterolemia is sometimes inherited; in such cases diet is a less effective factor. Also spelled **hypercholesterolaemia.**

**hypercholesterolemic xanthomatosis.** See **familial hypercholesterolemia.**

**hyperchromatic.** See **hyperchromic.**

**hyperchromia** /-krō′mē·ə/ [Gk, *hyper,* excessive, *chroma,* color], an increase of hemoglobin in the erythrocytes.

**hyperchromic** /-krō′mik/ [Gk, *hyper* + *chroma,* color], having a greater density of color or pigment. Also **hyperchromatic.**

**hyperchylomicronemia** /-kī′lōmī′krōnē′mē·ə/ [Gk, *hyper* + *chylos,* juice, *mikros,* small, *haima,* blood], type I hyperlipoproteinemia, a rare congenital deficiency of an enzyme essential to fat metabolism. Fat accumulates in the blood as chylomicrons. The condition affects children and young adults, in whom xanthomas (fatty deposits) in the skin, hepatomegaly, and abdominal pain develop. Pancreatitis is the most significant complication. Strict limitation of dietary fat may allow the person to prevent discomfort and complications. Also called **familial lipoprotein lipase deficiency.** See also **chylomicron.**

**hypercoagulability** /-kō·ag′yələbil′itē/ [Gk, *hyper* + L, *coagulare,* to curdle, *habilis,* able], a tendency of the blood to coagulate more rapidly than is normal.

**hyperdactyly.** See **polydactyly.**

**hyperdiploid.** See **hyperploid.**

**hyperdynamic syndrome** /-dīnam′ik/ [Gk, *hyper* + *dynamis,* force], a cluster of symptoms that signal the onset of septic shock, often including a shaking chill, rapid rise in temperature, flushing of the skin, galloping pulse, and alternating rise and fall of the blood pressure. This is a medical emergency treated by keeping the patient warm, elevating the legs to assist venous return, usually ordering IV fluids and antibiotics, and managing blood pressure. Nothing is given by mouth. The patient's head is turned to the side to prevent aspiration if there is vomiting. See also **septic shock.**

**hyperemesis** /hī′per·em′ə·sis/ [Gk, *hyper,* excess + *emesis,* vomit], excessive vomiting.

**hyperemesis gravidarum** /hī′pərem′isis/ [Gk, *hyper* + *emesis,* vomiting; L, *gravida,* pregnant], an abnormal condition of pregnancy characterized by protracted vomiting, weight loss, and fluid and electrolyte imbalance. If the condition is severe and intractable, brain damage, liver and kidney failure, and death may result. The cause of the condition is not known; an increase in levels of chorionic gonadotropins or other hormones, an immunologic sensitivity to products of conception, or aggravation of preexisting emotional conflicts has been suggested, but a causal relationship has not been proved. It occurs in approximately 3 of every 1000 pregnancies; its incidence has diminished in recent years.

■ OBSERVATIONS: Women are frightened of and uncomfortable and embarrassed about their illness. Dry mucous membranes are a sign of dehydration. Other signs include decreased skin elasticity, a rapid pulse, and falling blood pressure. The specific gravity of the urine rises, and the volume of urine excreted falls. The hematocrit is elevated because of hemoconcentration. Loss of electrolytes in vomitus leads to metabolic acidosis with hypokalemia, hypochloremia, and hyponatremia. Severe potassium deficit alters myocardial function; the electrocardiogram may show prolonged P-R and Q-T intervals and inverted T waves. In addition to weight loss, undernourishment causes fever, ketosis, and acetonuria. Severe vitamin B deficiency may result in encephalopathy manifested by confusion and eventually coma. Laboratory analyses of blood indicate increased concentrations of metabolic products normally cleared by the liver and kidneys. Forceful vomiting may cause retinal hemorrhages that impair vision and gastroesophageal tears that bleed, causing hematemesis or melena.

■ INTERVENTIONS: Effective therapy arrests vomiting and achieves rehydration, adequate nutrition, and emotional stabilization. Bed rest is instituted. Antiemetics safe for the fetus are administered. Fluids, electrolytes, nutrients, and vitamins are given parenterally if the woman is unable to retain fluids by mouth. The fetal heart rate is measured frequently. Psychiatric consultation and therapy are sometimes beneficial. Termination of pregnancy is curative but almost never required.

■ NURSING CONSIDERATIONS: Visitors are encouraged; isolation, formerly recommended, is not desirable. Sympathetic listening and supportive, nonjudgmental care are provided. The woman and her family are told often that the prognosis is excellent for both mother and baby. The woman is weighed regularly, and her weight is accurately recorded, for the best evidence of recovery is steady weight gain.

**hyperemesis lactentium,** a condition of excessive vomiting by nursing infants.

**hyperemia** /hī′pərē′mē·ə/ [Gk, *hyper* + *haima,* blood], an excess of blood in part of the body, caused by increased blood flow, as in the inflammatory response, local relaxation of arterioles, or obstruction of the outflow of blood from an area. Skin overlying a hyperemic area usually becomes reddened and warm. —**hyperemic,** *adj.*

**hyperesthesia** /-esthē'zhə/, an extreme sensitivity of one of the body's sense organs, such as pain or touch receptors in the skin.

**hyperextension** /-ikten'shən/ [Gk, *hyper* + L, *extendere,* to stretch out], movement at a joint to a position beyond the joint's normal maximum extension.

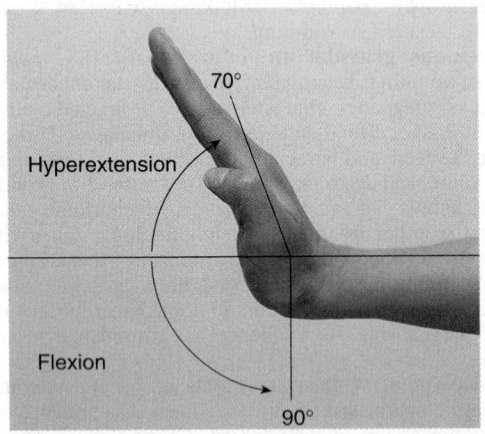

**Hyperextension of the wrist** *(Wilson and Giddens, 2001)*

**hyperextension bed,** a bed used in pediatric orthopedics to maintain any correction achieved by suspension of a body part and to increase the range of motion of the hips after an operative muscle release procedure. The hyperextension bed may be purchased, or a regular hospital bed may be converted. Removal of the mattress from a hospital bed and the addition of three half mattresses allow sufficient height to permit alternating prone and supine positions and the concomitant alternating flexion and extension of the hips. The bilateral extremities of the patient, in casts, are suspended over the lower half of the bed with rings and traction apparatus. The position of the patient's hips is alternated at 2-hour intervals; abduction and adduction can be controlled by the position of the pulleys. Restraints are required to maintain the child in position so that the horizontal, gluteal folds are even with the bottom edge of the stacked mattresses. Also called **Schwartz bed.** Compare **CircOlectric (COL) bed, Foster bed, Stryker wedge frame.**

**hyperflexia** /-flek'shə/ [Gk, *hyper* + L, *flectere,* to bend], the forcible overflexion or bending of a limb.

**hyperfunction** /-fungk'shən/ [Gk, *hyper* + L, *functio,* performance], increased function of any organ or system.

**hypergenesis** /-jen'əsis/ [Gk, *hyper* + *genesis,* origin], excessive growth or overdevelopment. The condition may involve the entire body, as in gigantism, or any part, or it may result in the formation of extra parts, such as additional fingers or toes. —**hypergenetic,** *adj.*

**hypergenetic teratism** /- jənet'ik/ [Gk, *hyper*+ *genesis* + *teras,* monster], a congenital anomaly in which there is excessive growth of a part, an organ, or the entire body, as in gigantism.

**hypergenitalism** /- jen'itəliz'əm/, the presence of abnormally large external genitalia. The condition is usually associated with precocious puberty.

**hyperglobulinemia** /-glob'yəlinē'mē·ə/ [Gk, *hyper,* excessive; L, *globulus,* small globe, *haima,* blood], an excess of globulin in the blood.

**hyperglycemia** /hī'pərglīsē'mē·ə/ [Gk, *hyper* + *glykys,* sweet, *haima,* blood], a greater than normal amount of glucose in the blood. Most frequently associated with diabetes mellitus, the condition may occur in newborns, after the administration of glucocorticoid hormones, and with an excess infusion of IV solutions containing glucose, especially in poorly monitored long-term hyperalimentation. Also spelled **hyperglycaemia.** Also called **hyperglycosemia.** Compare **hypoglycemia.**

**hyperglycemia management,** a nursing intervention from the Nursing Interventions Classification (NIC) defined as preventing and treating above-normal blood glucose levels. See also **Nursing Interventions Classification.**

**hyperglycemic-glycogenolytic factor.** See **glucagon.**

**hyperglycemic-hyperosmolar nonketotic syndrome** /-glīsē'mik/ [Gk, *hyper* + *glykys* + *hyper* + *osmos,* impulse; L, *non,* not, (ketone); Gk, deep sleep], a diabetic syndrome in which the level of ketone bodies is normal; caused by hyperosmolarity of extracellular fluid and resulting in dehydration of intracellular fluid, often a consequence of overtreatment with hyperosmolar solutions. The condition is usually seen in people with type 2 diabetes mellitus.

**hyperglyceridemia** /-glī'səridē'mē·ə/ [Gk, *hyper,* excessive, *glykys* + *haima,* blood], an excess of glycerides, particularly triglycerides, in the blood. It is caused by a congenital defect in the ability to metabolize the amino acid glycine.

**hyperglycogenolysis** /-glī'kōjənol'isis/, excessive breaking down of glycogen to glucose in animal tissue.

**hyperglycosuria** /-glī'kōsŏŏr'ē·ə/, an excess of sugar in the urine.

**hyperglysemia** /-glī'kəsē'mē·ə/, an excess of sugar in the blood. See **hyperglycemia.**

**hypergonadism** /-gō'nədiz'əm/ [Gk, *hyper,* excessive, *gone,* seed], excessive activity of the ovaries or testes.

**HyperHep,** trademark for a hepatitis B immune globulin (human) that is administered intramuscularly to provide passive immunization for people who have been exposed to the hepatitis B virus.

**hyperhidrosis** /hī'pərhīdrō'sis, -hidrō'sis/ [Gk, *hyper* + *hidros,* perspiration], excessive perspiration often caused by heat, hyperthyroidism, strong emotion, menopause, or infection. Symptomatic therapy usually includes topical antiperspirants and other medications.

**hyperhydration.** See **overhydration.**

**hyperimmune** /-imyōon'/ [Gk, *hyper* + L, *immunis,* freedom], having a greater-than-normal immunity because of an unusual abundance of antibodies.

**hyperimmune plasma,** plasma containing extremely high levels of antibodies.

**hyperinsulinism** /-in'səliniz'əm/ [Gk, *hyper* + L, *insula,* island], an excessive amount of insulin in the body. It may be caused by administration of an insulin dose greater than required or the presence of an insulin-secreting tumor in the islets of Langerhans. Symptoms include hunger, shakiness, and diaphoresis caused by hypoglycemia. See also **insulin shock.**

**hyperirritability** /-irit'əbil'itē/ [Gk, *hyper,* excessive; L, *irritare,* to tease], excessive excitability or sensitivity, or exaggerated response to a stimulus.

**hyperkalemia** /hī'pərkəlē'mē·ə/ [Gk, *hyper* + L, *kalium,* potassium; Gk, *haima,* blood], greater than normal amounts of potassium in the blood. This condition is seen frequently in acute renal failure, massive trauma, major burns, and Addison's disease. Early signs are nausea, diarrhea, and muscle weakness. As potassium levels increase, marked cardiac changes are observed in the electrocardiogram. Treatment of severe hyperkalemia includes oral administration of Kayexalate (sodium polystyrene sulfonate) and IV administration of sodium bicarbonate, calcium salts, and dextrose. Hemodialysis is used if these measures fail. Also spelled **hyperkalaemia.**

**hyperkalemic periodic paralysis.** See **adynamia episodica hereditaria.**

**hyperkeratinization** /-ker′ətinīzā′shən/ [Gk, *hyper,* excessive, *keras,* horn], an abnormal horny thickening of the epithelium of the palms and soles.

**hyperkeratosis** /-ker′ətō′sis/ [Gk, *hyper* + *keras,* horn, *osis,* condition], overgrowth of the cornified epithelial layer of the skin. See also **callus, corn.**

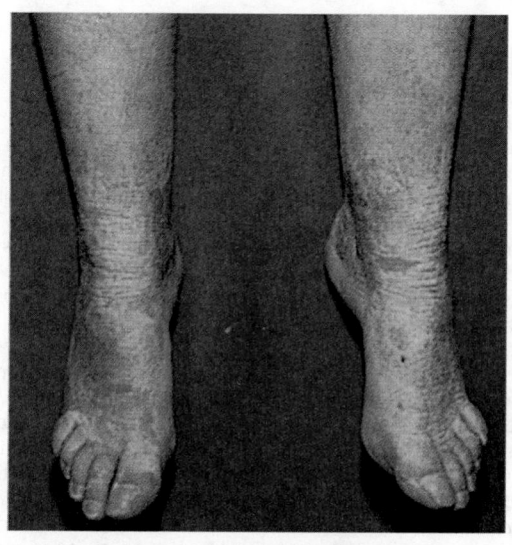

**Epidermolytic hyperkeratosis**
*(Weston, Lane, and Morrelli, 1996)*

**hyperketonemia** /-kē′tōnē′mē·ə/, an abnormally high level of ketone bodies in the blood.

**hyperketonuria** /-kē′tōnŏŏr′ē·ə/, an abnormally high level of ketone bodies in the urine.

**hyperkinesis.** See **attention deficit disorder.**

**hyperlactation** /-laktā′shən/, a condition in which lactation continues beyond the usual period of breastfeeding. Also called *superlactation.*

**hyperlipemia** /-lipē′mē·ə/, an excessive level of blood fats, usually caused by a lipoprotein lipase deficiency or a defect in the conversion of low-density lipoprotein to high-density lipoprotein. The condition occurs in nephrotic syndrome and hypoalbuminemia.

**hyperlipidemia** /-lip′idē′mē·ə/ [Gk, *hyper* + *lipos,* fat, *haima,* blood], an excess of lipids, including glycolipids, lipoproteins, and phospholipids, in the plasma. Also spelled **hyperlipidaemia.** See also **antilipidemic.**

**hyperlipidemia type I,** a condition of elevated blood lipid levels, characterized by an increase in both cholesterol and triglycerides and caused by the presence of chylomicrons. It is inherited as an autosomal-recessive trait with a low risk of atherosclerosis. It results in recurrent bouts of acute pancreatitis. The symptoms begin in childhood. The accumulation of triglycerides is generally proportional to the amount of dietary fat. Treatment is primarily dietary; both saturated and unsaturated fats are restricted to amounts that produce less than 500 mg/dl of blood, evaluated after an overnight fast. Also called **exogenous hypertriglyceridemia, familial hyperglyceridemia, fat-induced hyperlipidemia.**

**hyperlipidemia type IIA, hyperlipidemia type IIB.** See **familial hypercholesterolemia.**

**hyperlipidemia type III.** See **broad beta disease.**

**hyperlipidemia type IV,** a relatively common form of hyperlipoproteinemia characterized by a slight elevation in cholesterol levels, a moderate elevation of triglyceride levels, and an elevation of the triglyceride carrier protein very low-density lipoprotein level. It is sometimes familial and is associated with an increased risk for coronary atherosclerosis. The condition is controlled with weight reduction, a low-carbohydrate diet, drugs, niacin, and avoidance of alcohol. Also called **endogenous hypertriglyceridemia.**

**hyperlipidemia type V,** a condition of elevated blood lipid levels, characterized by slightly increased cholesterol level, greatly increased triglyceride level, elevation of the triglyceride carrier protein very low-density lipoprotein level, and above normal levels of chylomicrons. It is a genetically heterogenous disorder that apparently does not increase the risk of atherosclerosis. Treatment includes weight control, a low-fat diet, drugs, niacin, and abstinence from alcohol. Also called **mixed hypertriglyceridemia, mixed hyperlipemia.**

**hyperlipoproteinemia** /hī′pərlip′ōprō′tēnē′mē·ə/ [Gk, *hyper* + *lipos,* fat, *proteios,* first rank, *haima,* blood], any of a large group of inherited and acquired disorders of lipoprotein metabolism. They are characterized by greater than normal amounts of certain protein-bound lipids and other fatty substances in the blood and usually low levels of HDL cholesterol. Dyslipidemia causes atherosclerosis and pancreatitis. The treatment includes dietary control of obesity; diet may reduce lipoprotein levels in the blood. Medication and other treatment vary according to the specific metabolic defect, its cause, and its prognosis. Previously called hyperlipidemia.

**hypermagnesemia** /hī′pərmag′nisē′mē·ə/ [Gk *hyper* + *magnesia,* magnesium, *haima,* blood], a greater than normal amount of magnesium in the plasma, found in people with kidney failure and in those who use large doses of drugs containing magnesium, such as antacids. Toxic levels of magnesium cause cardiac arrhythmias and depression of deep tendon reflexes and respiration. Treatment often includes IV fluids, a diuretic, and hemodialysis.

**hypermature cataract** /- məchŏŏr′/ [Gk, *hyper,* excessive; L, *maturare,* to make ripe; Gk, *katarrhaktes,* portcullis], an opaque lens that has lost water and has become soft and reduced in size.

**hypermenorrhea.** See **menorrhagia.**

**hypermetabolic state** /-met′əbol′ik/, an abnormally increased rate of metabolism, as in a high fever or hyperthyroidism.

**hypermetabolism** /-mətab′əliz′əm/, increased metabolism, usually accompanied by excessive body heat.

**hypermetaplasia** /-met′əplā′zhə/, an abnormal increase in the rate of transformation of one kind of tissue into another, as in the development of tumors.

**hypermetria** /hī'pərmē'trē·ə/ [Gk, *hyper* + *metron*, measure], an abnormal condition, a form of dysmetria, characterized by a dysfunction of the power to control the range of muscular action and causing movements that overreach the intended goal of the affected individual. Compare **hypometria.**

**hypermetropia, hypermetropy.** See **hyperopia.**

**hypermnesia** /hī'pərm·nē'zhə/, an extraordinarily good state of memory.

**hypermobility** /-mōbil'itē/ [Gk, *hyper,* excessive; L, *mobilis,* movable], an abnormally wide range of movement of the joints. The condition is seen in children and may be associated with **Marfan's syndrome.**

**hypermorph** /hī'pərmôrf'/ [Gk, *hyper* + *morphe,* form], **1.** a person whose arms and legs are disproportionately long in relation to the trunk, and whose sitting height is disproportionately short compared to the standing height. **2.** a mutant allele that has an increased effect on the expression of a trait. Compare **amorph, antimorph, hypomorph.**

**hypermotility** /-motil'itē/, an excessive movement of the involuntary muscles, particularly in the GI tract.

**hypernasality** /hī'pər·nā·zal'i·tē/ [Gk, *hyper,* excess + *nasus,* nose], an excessively nasal quality of voice, which may result in unintelligible speech; the cause is velopharyngeal insufficiency with emission of too much air through the nose. Also called **open rhinolalia.** See also **velopharyngeal insufficiency.**

**hypernatremia** /hī'pərnatrē'mē·ə/ [Gk, *hyper* + L, *natrium,* sodium], a greater than normal concentration of sodium in the blood, caused by excessive loss of water and electrolytes that results from polyuria, diarrhea, excessive sweating, or inadequate water intake. It may also be a result of a large intake of salt, either orally or intravenously. When water loss is caused by kidney dysfunction, urine is profuse and dilute. If water loss is not through the kidneys, such as in diarrhea and excessive sweating, the urine is scanty and highly concentrated. People with hypernatremia may become mentally confused, have seizures, and lapse into coma. The treatment is restoration of fluid and electrolyte balance by mouth or by IV infusion. Care must be taken to restore water balance slowly, because further electrolyte imbalances may occur. Also spelled **hypernatraemia.** See also **diabetes insipidus.**

**hyperopia** /-ō'pē·ə/ [Gk, *hyper* + *ops,* eye], farsightedness, or an inability of the eye to focus on nearby objects. It results from an error of refraction in which rays of light entering the eye are brought into focus behind the retina. Also called **farsightedness, hypermetropia, hypermetropy.** Compare **myopia.**

**hyperorchidism** /-ôr'kidiz'əm/ [Gk, *hyper,* excessive, *orchis,* testis], excessive endocrine activity of the testes.

**hyperornithinemia** /-ôr'nithinē'mē·ə/, a metabolic disorder involving the amino acid ornithine, which tends to accumulate in the tissues, causing seizures and retardation. Treatment is a low-protein diet.

**hyperosmia** /-oz'mē·ə/, an abnormally increased sensitivity to odors. Compare **anosmia.**

**hyperosmolarity** /-oz'məler'itē/ [Gk, *hyper* + *osmos,* impulse], a state or condition of abnormally increased osmolarity. —**hyperosmolar,** *adj.*

**hyperosmotic** /-osmot'ik/, pertaining to a solution that has a higher solute concentration than another solution. Compare **hypoosmotic, isosmotic.**

**hyperostosis.** See **exostosis.**

**hyperostosis frontalis interna,** thickening of the inner table of the frontal bone, which may be associated with hirsutism and obesity; it most commonly affects women near menopause. Also called **Morel's syndrome.**

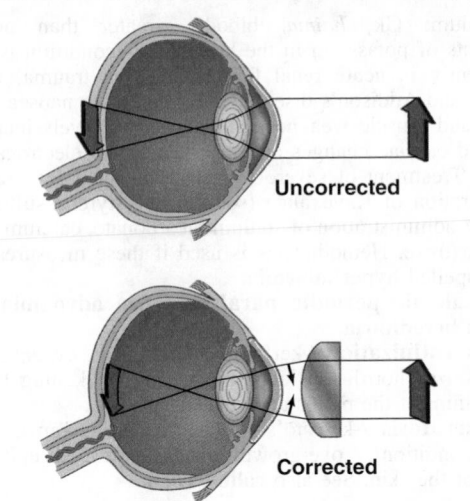

**Hyperopia** *(Thibodeau and Patton, 1999/Network Graphics)*

**hyperoxaluria** /-ok'sələoôr'ē·ə/, an excessive level of oxalic acid or oxalates, primarily calcium oxalate, in the urine. The cause is usually an inherited deficiency of an enzyme needed to metabolize oxalic acid, which is present in many fruits and vegetables, or a disorder of fat absorption in the small intestine. An excess of oxalates may lead to the formation of renal calculi and renal failure. Treatments include pyridoxine, forced fluids, and a low-oxalate diet.

**hyperoxemia** /-oksē'mē·ə/ [Gk, *hyper,* excessive, *oxys,* sharp, *haima,* blood], increased oxygen content of the blood.

**hyperoxia** /-ok'sē·ə/, abnormally high oxygen tension in the blood.

**hyperoxygenation** /-ok'sijənā'shən/ [Gk, *hyper* + *oxys,* sharp, *genein,* to produce], the use of high concentrations of inspired oxygen before and after endotracheal aspiration.

**hyperparathyroidism** /-per'əthī'roidiz'əm/ [Gk, *hyper* + *para,* beside, *thyreos,* shield, *eidos,* form], an abnormal endocrine condition characterized by hyperactivity of any of the four parathyroid glands with excessive secretion of parathyroid hormone (PTH), which causes increased resorption of calcium from the skeletal system, and increased absorption of calcium by the kidneys and GI system. The condition may be primary, originating in one or more of the parathyroid glands and usually caused by an adenoma, or secondary, resulting from an abnormal hypocalcemia-producing condition in another part of the body, which causes a compensatory hyperactivity of the parathyroid glands.

■ OBSERVATIONS: Hypercalcemia in primary hyperparathyroidism results in dysfunction of many body systems. In the kidneys, tissue calcifies, calculi form, and renal failure may ensue. In addition excess phosphorus is excreted and excess 1, 25 (OH)2 D (vitamin D) is synthesized In the bones and joints, osteoporosis develops, causing pain and fragility; fractures, synovitis, and pseudogout often occur. In the GI tract chronic, piercing epigastric pain may develop as a result of pancreatitis and increased gastrin production; anorexia and nausea may occur; and vomiting of blood may result if peptic ulceration occurs. In the neuromuscular system generalized weakness and atrophy develop if the condition is not corrected; and changes in the central nervous system produce alteration of consciousness, coma, psychosis, abnormal behavior, and disturbances of personality. Secondary hyperparathyroidism may result in many of these signs of calcium imbalance and in various abnormalities of the long bones, such as rickets. The diagnosis of primary hyperparathyroidism is made by laboratory findings of increased levels of PTH and calcium in the blood and by the characteristic appearance of the bones on radiographic films. Calcium in the blood and urine and chloride and alkaline phosphatase in the blood are present in excessive amounts; phosphorus is present in the serum in less than normal amounts.

■ INTERVENTIONS: Primary parathyroidism that is the result of an adenoma of one of the glands is treated by excision of the tumor; other causes of primary disease may require excision of up to one half of the glandular tissue. In asymptomatic patients over 50, noninterventional observation may be indicated. Dietary intake of calcium may be limited, and adequate hydration must be maintained. Estrogens may be used in postmenopausal females. Biphosphates may be administered in severe hypercalcemia to lower the serum calcium level. After surgery calcium levels in the blood may drop rapidly to dangerously low levels if frequent laboratory evaluations are not made and supplemental calcium is not given as required. Secondary hyperparathyroidism is managed by treating the underlying cause of hypertrophy of the gland. Vitamin D is frequently given, and peritoneal dialysis may be necessary to remove excess calcium from the circulation.

■ NURSING CONSIDERATIONS: Frequent laboratory evaluations of blood levels of calcium, phosphorus, potassium, and magnesium are necessary throughout the course of treatment. Because fractures occur easily and are common, great care is taken to prevent trauma to the patient. IV hydration is usually performed to dilute the concentration of calcium, and the lungs are assessed regularly to detect pulmonary edema in its earliest stages. Tetany is a warning sign of severe hypoglycemia; calcium gluconate is kept available for immediate use after surgery. Walking and moving about cause pain but accelerate healing of the affected bones and are therefore encouraged.

**hyperperistalis** /-per′istal′is/ [Gk, *hyper,* excessive, *peristellein,* to clasp], a state of excessive motility of the waves of alternate contractions and relaxations that propel contents forward through the digestive tract.

**hyperphagia.** See **polyphagia.**

**hyperphenylalaninemia** /hī′pərfen′ilal′ənine′mē·ə/ [Gk, *hyper* + (phenylalanine), *haima,* blood], an abnormally high concentration of phenylalanine in the blood. This symptom may be the result of one of several defects in the metabolic process of breaking down phenylalanine. See also **phenylketonuria.**

**hyperphoria** /hī′pərfôr′ē·ə/ [Gk, *hyper* + *pherein,* to bear], the tendency of an eye to deviate upward.

**hyperphosphoremia** /-fos′fərē′mē·ə/, an abnormally high level of phosphorus compounds in the blood.

**hyperpigmentation** /-pig′məntā′shən/ [Gk, *hyper* + L, *pigmentum,* paint], darkening of the skin. Causes include heredity, drugs, exposure to the sun, trauma, and adrenal insufficiency. Compare **hypopigmentation.** See also **melasma, melanocyte-stimulating hormone.**

**hyperpituitarism** /-pityŌŌ′itəriz′əm/ [Gk, *hyper,* excessive; L, *pituita,* phlegm], overactivity of the anterior lobe of the pituitary gland, leading to such conditions as **acromegaly** and **Cushing's disease.** See also **gigantism.**

**hyperplasia** /hī′pərplā′zhə/ [Gk, *hyper* + *plassein,* to mold], an increase in the number of cells of a body part that results from an increased rate of cellular division. Types

of hyperplasia include compensatory, hormonal, and pathologic. Compare **hypertrophy, hypoplasia.**

**hyperplastic gingivitis** [Gk, *hyper,* excessive, *plassein,* to mold; L, *gingiva,* gum; Gk, *itis,* inflammation], inflammation and enlargement of the gums caused by an increase in the number of cells, usually because of bacterial plaque accumulation. Compare **hypertrophic gingivitis.**

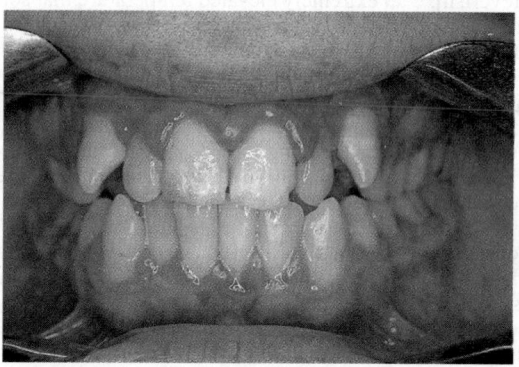

**Hyperplastic gingivitis** *(Regezi, Sciubba, and Pogrel, 2000)*

**hyperplastic obesity.** See **obesity.**

**hyperploid** /hī′pərploid/ [Gk, *hyper* + *eidos,* form], **1.** an individual, organism, strain, or cell that has one or more chromosomes in excess of the haploid number or of an exact multiple of the haploid number characteristic of the species. The result is one or more unbalanced sets of chromosomes, which are referred to as hyperdiploid, hypertriploid, hypertetraploid, and so on, depending on the number of multiples of the haploid number they contain. **2.** pertaining to such an individual, organism, strain, or cell. Compare **hypoploid.** See also **trisomy.** —**hyperploidy,** *adj.*

**hyperploidy** /hī′pərploi′dē/, any increase in chromosome number that involves individual chromosomes rather than entire sets, resulting in more than the normal haploid number characteristic of the species, as in Down syndrome. Compare **hypoploidy.**

**hyperpnea** /hī′pərpnē′ə/ [Gk, *hyper* + *pnoe,* blowing], an exaggerated deep, rapid, or labored respiration. It occurs normally with exercise and abnormally with aspirin overdose, pain, fever, hysteria, or any condition in which the supply of oxygen is inadequate, such as cardiac disease and respiratory disease. Also spelled **hyperpnoea.** Compare **dyspnea, hypopnea, orthopnea, tachypnea.** See also **respiratory rate.** —**hyperpneic, hyperpnoic,** *adj.*

**hyperpolarized helium** /-pō′lərīzd/, a gas used in magnetic resonance imaging studies of respiratory disorders to produce images of the air spaces in the lungs.

**hyperprolactinemia** /-prōlak′tinē′mē·ə/ [Gk, *hyper* + L, *pro,* before, *lac,* milk; Gk, *haima,* blood], an excessive amount of prolactin in the blood. The condition is caused by a hypothalamus-pituitary dysfunction. In women it is usually associated with galactorrhea and secondary amenorrhea; in men it may be a factor in gynecomastia, decreased libido, and impotence. It may be a result of endocrine side effects related to certain antipsychotic medications. Also spelled **hyperprolactinaemia.**

**hyperprolinemia** /hī′pər·prō′li·nē′mē·ə /, an autosomal recessive aminoacidopathy characterized by an excess of proline in the body fluids and occurring as two types, I and II, each of which is caused by deficiency in a different enzyme involved in proline metabolism, and both of which are probably benign.

**hyperproteinemia** /-prō'tēnē'mē·ə/ [Gk, *hyper,* excessive, *proteios,* first rank, *haima,* blood], an abnormally high level of protein elements in the blood.

**hyperptyalism.** See **ptyalism.**

**hyperpyrexia** /hī'pərpīrek'sē·ə/ [Gk, *hyper + pyressein,* to be feverish], an extremely elevated temperature that sometimes occurs in acute infectious diseases, especially in young children. Malignant hyperpyrexia, characterized by a rapid rise in temperature, tachycardia, tachypnea, sweating, rigidity, and blotchy cyanosis, occasionally occurs in patients undergoing general anesthesia. A high temperature may be reduced by sponging the body with tepid water, by giving a tepid tub bath, or by administering antipyretic medication, such as aspirin or acetaminophen. See also **fever. —hyperpyretic,** *adj.*

**hyperreactivity** /-rē'aktiva'itē/ [Gk, *hyper + L, re,* again, *activus,* active], an abnormal condition in which responses to stimuli are exaggerated.

**hyperreflection** /-riflek'shən/, a compulsion to devote excessive attention to oneself.

**hyperreflexia** /-riflek'sē·ə/ [Gk, *hyper + L, reflectere,* to bend back], increased reflex reactions. See also **autonomic hyperreflexia.**

**hypersalivation.** See **sialorrhea.**

**hypersensibility** /-sen'səbil'itē/, excessive ability to perceive or feel, as excessive sensibility to pain.

**hypersensitivity** /-sen'sətiv'itē/ [Gk, *hyper + L, sentire,* to feel], an abnormal condition characterized by an exaggerated response of the immune system to an antigen. See also **allergy. —hypersensitive,** *adj.*

**hypersensitivity pneumonitis,** an inflammatory form of interstitial pneumonia that results from an immunologic reaction in a hypersensitive person. The reaction may be provoked by a variety of inhaled organic dusts, often those containing fungal spores. The disease can be prevented by avoiding contact with the causative agents. Classification of the disease is based solely on the character of the immune response rather than on its clinical manifestations. A wide variety of symptoms may occur, including asthma, fever, chills, malaise, and muscle aches, which usually develop 4 to 6 hours after exposure. Laboratory examination of the blood commonly reveals leukocytosis. Recovery is usually

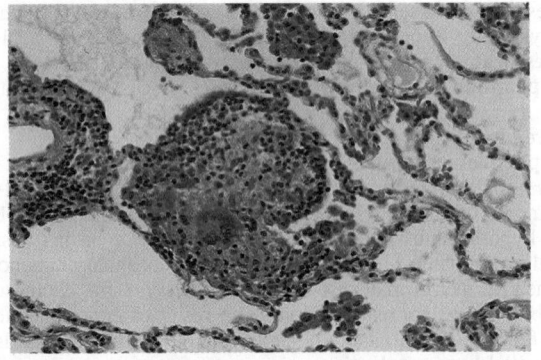

**Hypersensitivity pneumonitis: histologic appearance**
*(Cotran, Kumar, and Collins, 1999)*

spontaneous. In an acute attack corticosteroids may be given to diminish the inflammatory response. Kinds of hypersensitivity pneumonitis include **bagassosis, cork worker's lung, farmer's lung, humidifier lung,** and **mushroom worker's lung.** Also called **extrinsic allergic alveolitis.** See also **Arthus reaction.**

**hypersensitivity reaction,** an inappropriate and excessive response of the immune system to a sensitizing antigen, called an allergen. Several factors determine the degree of the response: the person's genetic predisposition for an exaggerated response, the amount of allergen, the kind of allergen, its route of entrance into the body, the timing of the exposures to the allergen, and the site of the allergen-immune mediator reaction. Hypersensitivity reactions are classified into four types according to the components of the immune system involved in their mediation. A type I or immediate hypersensitivity reaction occurs rapidly, within several minutes, on reexposure to an antigen, and is the result of interaction of immunoglobulin E and the antigen; anaphylaxis is a particularly severe type I hypersensitivity reaction. A type II or cytotoxic hypersensitivity reaction is one of tissue or cell damage resulting from antibody-antigen interactions on cell surfaces. A type III or immune complex-mediated hypersensitivity reaction is a local or general inflammatory response caused by formation of circulating antigen-antibody complexes and their disposition in tissues. A type IV hypersensitivity reaction (also called cell-mediated or T cell-mediated hypersensitivity reaction) is one initiated by antigen-specific T lymphocytes; unlike hypersensitivity reactions mediated by antibodies, this type takes one or more days to develop, and the hypersensitivity can be transferred by lymphocytes but not by serum. The term is often equated with delayed hypersensitivity reactions that are cytokine-mediated (as contrasted with direct cytolysis).

**hypersensitization** /-sen'sitīzā'shən/ [Gk, *hyper,* excessive; L, *sentire,* to feel], a state of increased reactivity or sensitivity to a stimulus.

**hypersomnia** /hī'pərsom'nē·ə/ [Gk, *hyper + L, somnus,* sleep], **1.** sleep of excessive depth or abnormal duration, usually caused by psychologic rather than physical factors and characterized by a state of confusion on awakening. **2.** extreme drowsiness, often associated with lethargy. **3.** a condition characterized by periods of deep, long sleep. Compare **narcolepsy.**

**hyperspadias.** See **epispadias.**

**hypersplenism** /hī'pərsplē'nizəm/ [Gk, *hyper + splen,* spleen], a syndrome consisting of splenomegaly and a deficiency of one or more types of blood cells. The numerous causes of this syndrome include portal hypertension, the lymphomas, the hemolytic anemias, malaria, tuberculosis, and various connective tissue and inflammatory diseases. Patients complain of abdominal pain on the left side and often experience fullness after eating very little, because the greatly enlarged spleen is pressing against the stomach. On physical examination the enlarged spleen is felt and abnormal bruits (vascular sounds) are heard with a stethoscope over the epigastric area. Treatment of the underlying disorder may cure the syndrome. Splenectomy is usually performed only when treating the hemolytic anemias or when splenic enlargement is severe and the danger of vascular accident is significant. See also **splenectomy.**

**Hyperstat,** trademark for an emergency vasodilator (diazoxide).

**hypersthenic** /hī'pərsthen'ik/, **1.** pertaining to a condition of excessive strength or tonicity of the body or a body part. **2.** pertaining to a body type characterized by massive proportions.

**hypersystole** /-sis′tǝlē/,   abnormal force or duration of ventricular contraction.

**hypertaurodontism** /hī′pǝr·tô′rō·don′tiz·ǝm/ [Gk, *hyper,* excess; L, *taurus,* bull; Gk, *odous,* tooth],   taurodontism in which the tooth roots do not branch. See also **mesotaurodontism, taurodontism.**

**hypertelorism** /hī′pǝrtel′ǝriz′ǝm/ [Gk, *hyper* + *tele,* far, *horizo,* separate],   a developmental defect characterized by an abnormally wide space between two organs or parts. A kind of hypertelorism is **ocular hypertelorism.** Compare **hypotelorism.**

**hypertelorism-hypospadias syndrome.**   See **Opitz syndrome.**

**hypertension** /-ten′shǝn/ [Gk, *hyper* + L, *tendere,* to stretch],   a common disorder characterized by elevated blood pressure persistently exceeding 140/90 mm Hg. Essential hypertension, the most common kind, has no single identifiable cause, but risk for the disorder is increased by obesity, a high serum sodium level, hypercholesterolemia, and a family history of high blood pressure. Known causes of secondary hypertension include adrenal disorders such as aldosteronism, Cushing's syndrome, and pheochromocytoma; thyrotoxicosis; preeclampsia; and chronic glomerulonephritis and other renal diseases. The incidence of hypertension is higher in men than in women and is twice as great in African-Americans as in Caucasian. People with mild or moderate hypertension may be asymptomatic or may experience suboccipital headaches, especially on rising; tinnitus; lightheadedness; ready fatigability; and palpitations. With sustained hypertension arterial walls become thickened, inelastic, and resistant to blood flow, and the left ventricle becomes distended and hypertrophied as a result of its efforts to maintain normal circulation against the increased resistance. Inadequate blood supply to the coronary arteries may cause angina or myocardial infarction. Left ventricular hypertrophy may lead to congestive heart failure. Malignant hypertension, characterized by a diastolic pressure higher than 120 mm Hg, severe headaches, blurred vision, and confusion, may result in fatal uremia, myocardial infarction, congestive heart failure, or a cerebrovascular accident. Drugs used to treat hypertension include diuretics such as furosemide and thiazide derivatives, vasodilators such as

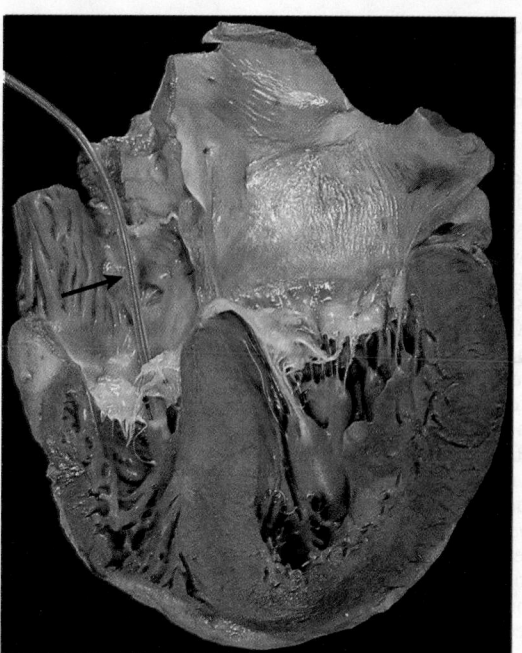

**Hypertrophy of the left ventricle in hypertension**
*(Cotran, Kumar, and Collins, 1999)*

### Classification of hypertension by age group

| Age group | Significant hypertension (mm Hg) | Severe hypertension (mm Hg) |
|---|---|---|
| **Newborns** | | |
| 7 days | Systolic BP ≥ 96 | Systolic BP ≥ 106 |
| 8-30 days | Systolic BP ≥ 104 | Systolic BP ≥ 110 |
| **Infants (<2 yr)** | Systolic BP ≥ 112 | Systolic BP ≥ 118 |
| | Diastolic BP ≥ 74 | Diastolic BP ≥ 82 |
| **Children** | | |
| (3-5 yr) | Systolic BP ≥ 116 | Systolic BP ≥ 124 |
| | Diastolic BP ≥ 76 | Diastolic BP ≥ 84 |
| (6-9 yr) | Systolic BP ≥ 122 | Systolic BP ≥ 130 |
| | Diastolic BP ≥ 78 | Diastolic BP ≥ 86 |
| (10-12 yr) | Systolic BP ≥ 126 | Systolic BP ≥ 134 |
| | Diastolic BP ≥ 82 | Diastolic BP ≥ 90 |
| **Adolescents** | | |
| (13-15 yr) | Systolic BP ≥ 136 | Systolic BP ≥ 144 |
| | Diastolic BP ≥ 86 | Diastolic BP ≥ 92 |
| (16-18 yr) | Systolic BP ≥ 142 | Systolic BP ≥ 150 |
| | Diastolic BP ≥ 92 | Diastolic BP ≥ 98 |
| **Adults** | Systolic BP ≥ 160 | Systolic BP ≥ 240 |
| | Diastolic BP ≥ 90 | Diastolic BP ≥ 115 |

Calculation of systolic blood pressure expected for children over 1 year of age can be estimated with the following formula:

$$80 + (2 \times \text{child's age in years})$$

For example, the calculation of the expected systolic blood pressure of a 5-year-old would be as follows:

$$80 + (2 \times 5) = 90$$

Although this calculation gives a figure below the expected mean, it is still considered within normal limits for a 5-year-old child.

Modified from National Heart, Lung, and Blood Institute: Report of the second task force on blood pressure control in children—1987, *Pediatrics* 79:1, 1987. From Seidel HM, Ball JW, Dains JE, Benedict WG: *Mosby's guide to physical examination,* ed 3, St. Louis, 1995, Mosby.

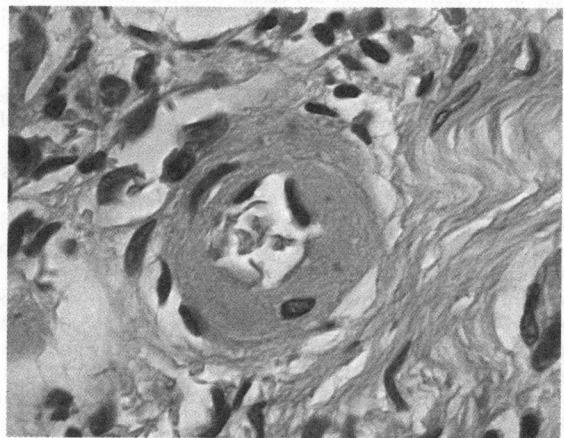

**Vascular pathology in hypertension**
*(Cotran, Kumar, and Collins, 1999/courtesy Helmut Rennke, MD, Brigham and Women's Hospital, Boston)*

hydralazine and prazosin, sympathetic nervous system (SNS) depressants such as rauwolfia alkaloids, SNS inhibitors such as guanethidine and methyldopa, angiotensin converting enzyme inhibitors, calcium channel blockers, and ganglionic blocking agents such as clonidine and propranolol. Patients with high blood pressure are advised to follow a low-sodium, low-saturated-fat diet; to control obesity by reducing caloric intake; to exercise; to avoid stress; and to have adequate rest. Also called **high blood pressure.** See also **blood pressure.**

**Hypertension and Lipid Trial (HALT),** a study to assess the efficacy and safety of alpha-adrenergic blockers in patients with hypertension.

**hypertensive** /-ten′siv/ [Gk, *hyper,* excessive; L, *tendere,* to stretch], pertaining to high blood pressure, its cause, or its effects.

**hypertensive arteriosclerosis,** a form of arteriosclerosis complicated by a buildup of the muscular and elastic tissues of the arterial walls caused by hypertension.

**hypertensive crisis** [Gk, *hyper* + L, *tendere,* to stretch; Gk, *krisi,* turning point], a sudden, severe increase in blood pressure to a level exceeding 200/120 mm Hg, occurring most frequently in individuals who have untreated hypertension or who have stopped taking prescribed antihypertensive medication.
■ OBSERVATIONS: Characteristic signs include severe headache, vertigo, diplopia, tinnitus, photophobia, nosebleed, twitching of muscles, tachycardia or other cardiac arrhythmia, distended neck veins, narrowed pulse pressure, nausea, and vomiting. The patient may be confused, irritable, or stuporous, and the condition may lead to convulsions, coma, myocardial infarction, renal failure, cardiac arrest, or stroke.
■ INTERVENTIONS: Treatment consists of antihypertensive drugs and diuretics; Anticonvulsants, sedatives, and antiemetics may be used if indicated. The patient is usually placed on a cardiac monitor in a bed with the head elevated and is maintained in a quiet environment. The diet is low in calories, and sodium and fluids may be restricted. As the patient's condition improves, the patient is permitted progressive ambulation but is carefully observed for symptoms of orthostatic hypotension, such as pallor, diaphoresis, or faintness, which may be side effects of the antihypertensive drugs.
■ NURSING CONSIDERATIONS: The major concerns of the nurse are to observe and report any sign of hypotension. In preparation for discharge the nurse advises the patient to recognize symptoms of any dramatic increase or decrease in blood pressure, to adhere to the prescribed diet and medication, and to avoid fatigue, heavy lifting, use of tobacco products, and stressful situations. See also **malignant hypertension.**

**hypertensive encephalopathy** [Gk, *hyper* + L, *tendere,* to stretch; Gk, *enkephalos,* brain, *pathos,* disease], a set of symptoms, including headache, convulsions, and coma, associated with glomerulonephritis.

**hypertensive retinopathy** [Gk, *hyper* + L, *tendere,* to stretch, *rete* + *net,* web; Gk, *pathos,* disease], a condition in which retinal changes occur in association with arterial hypertension. The changes may include blood vessel alterations, hemorrhages, exudates, and retinal edema.

**hypertetraploid.** See **hyperploid.**

**hyperthermia¹** /hī′pərthur′mē-ə/ [Gk, *hyper* + *therme,* heat], **1.** a much higher than normal body temperature induced therapeutically or iatrogenically. **2.** *nontechnical.* malignant hyperthermia.

**hyperthermia²,** a nursing diagnosis accepted by the Seventh National Conference on the Classification of Nursing

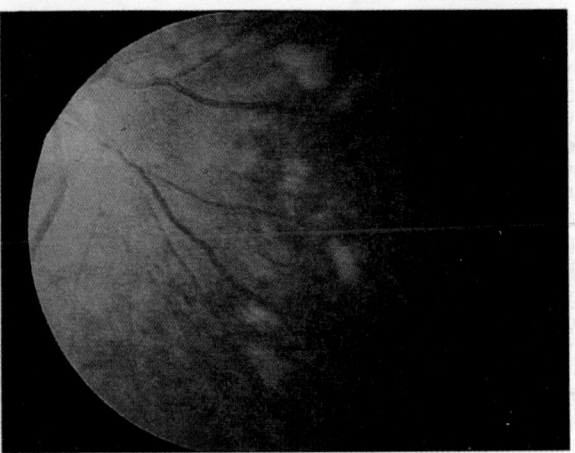

**Hypertensive retinopathy** *(Michelson and Friedlaender, 1996)*

Diagnoses. The condition is defined as a state in which an individual's body temperature is elevated above his or her normal range.
■ DEFINING CHARACTERISTICS: The increase in body temperature is the major defining characteristic. Minor characteristics include flushed skin, skin warm to the touch, increased respiratory rate, tachycardia, and seizures or convulsions.
■ RELATED FACTORS: Related factors include exposure to a hot environment, vigorous activity, medications or anesthesia, inappropriate clothing, increased metabolic rate, illness or trauma, dehydration, and inability or decreased ability to perspire. See also **nursing diagnosis.**

**hyperthyroidism** /-thī′roidiz′əm/ [Gk, *hyper* + *thyreos,* shield, *eidos,* form], a condition characterized by hyperactivity of the thyroid gland. The gland is usually enlarged, secreting greater than normal amounts of thyroid hormones, and the metabolic processes of the body are accelerated. Nervousness, exophthalmos, tremor, constant hunger, weight loss, fatigue, heat intolerance, palpitations, and diarrhea may develop. Antithyroid drugs, as propylthiouracil or methimazole, are usually prescribed. Radioactive iodine may be prescribed in certain cases. Surgical ablation of the gland is sometimes necessary. Untreated hyperthyroidism may lead to death from cardiac failure. See also **Graves' disease, thyroid storm, thyrotoxicosis.**

**hypertonia** /-tō′nē-ə/, **1.** abnormally increased muscle tone or strength. The condition is sometimes associated with genetic disorders, such as trisomy 18, and may be expressed in arm or leg deformities. **2.** a condition of excessive pressure, such as the intraocular pressure of glaucoma.

**hypertonic** /hī′pərton′ik/ [Gk, *hyper* + *tonos,* stretching], pertaining to a solution that causes cells to shrink. Compare **hypotonic, isotonic.**

**hypertonic bladder** [Gk, *hyper,* excessive, *tonos,* tone; AS, *blaedre*], a condition of excessive tension in the detrusor muscle of the bladder, usually caused by an irritant such as a calculus.

**hypertonic contracture,** prolonged muscle contraction that results from continuous nerve stimulation in spastic paralysis. Anesthesia or sleep eliminates this condition. Also called **functional contracture.**

**hypertonicity** /-tənis′itē/ [Gk, *hyper,* excessive, *tonos,* tone], **1.** excessive tone, tension, or activity. **2.** (in ophthalmology) increased intraocular pressure. **3.** excessive tension of the arteries or muscles. **4.** increase in osmotic pressure.

**hypertonic saline,** a saline solution that contains 1% to 15% sodium chloride (compared with normal saline solution at 0.9%). It is used as a bronchial lavage to stimulate sputum production by increasing movement of fluid into the mucosal blanket and causing irritation that promotes coughing.

**hypertonus** /-tō′nəs/, an excessive level of skeletal muscle tension or activity.

**hypertrichosis.** See **hirsutism.**

**hypertriglyceridemia.** See **hyperchylomicronemia.**

**hypertriploid.** See **hyperploid.**

**hypertrophic** /-trof′ik/ [Gk, *hyper,* excessive, *trophe,* nourishment], pertaining to an increase in size, structure, or function.

**hypertrophic angioma.** See **hemangioendothelioma.**

**hypertrophic cardiomyopathy,** an abnormal condition characterized by gross hypertrophy of the interventricular septum and left ventricular free wall of the heart. Ventricular outflow obstruction results in impaired diastolic filling and reduced cardiac output. Signs and symptoms, such as fatigue and syncope, are often associated with exercise when the demand for increased cardiac output cannot be met. Also called **hypertrophic obstructive cardiomyopathy.**

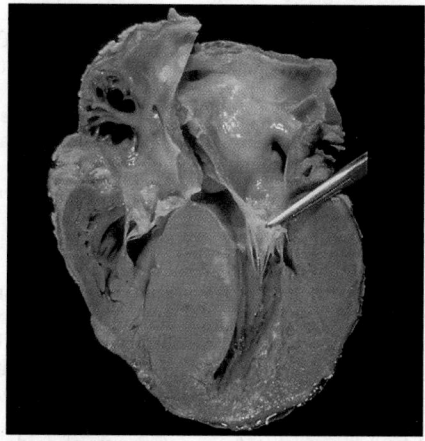

**Hypertrophic cardiomyopathy**
*(Kumar, Cotran, and Robbins, 1997/courtesy Sid Murphree, MD, Department of Pathology, University of Texas Southwestern Medical School, Dallas)*

**hypertrophic catarrh** [Gk, *hyper + trophe,* nourishment, *kata,* down, *rhoia,* flow], a chronic condition characterized by inflammation and discharge from a mucous membrane, accompanied by the thickening of the mucosal and submucosal tissue. Compare **atrophic catarrh.** See also **catarrh.**

**hypertrophic cicatrization.** See **hypertrophic scarring.**

**hypertrophic cirrhosis,** a stage of cirrhosis characterized by an overgrowth of liver tissue.

**hypertrophic gastritis,** an inflammatory condition of the stomach characterized by epigastric pain, nausea, vomiting, and distension. It is differentiated from other forms of gastritis by the presence of prominent rugae (folds), enlarged glands, and nodules on the wall of the stomach. This condition often accompanies peptic ulcer, Zollinger-Ellison syndrome, or gastric hypersecretion.

**hypertrophic gingivitis** [Gk, *hyper,* excessive; *trophe,* nourishment], inflammation and enlargement of the gums resulting from an increase in the size of cells, usually because of an underlying systemic disorder. Compare **hyperplastic gingivitis, gingivitis.**

**hypertrophic obesity.** See **obesity.**

**hypertrophic obstructive cardiomyopathy.** See **hypertrophic cardiomyopathy.**

**hypertrophic pulmonary osteopathy.** See **Marie's hypertrophy.**

**hypertrophic scarring,** scarring caused by excessive formation of new tissue in the healing of a wound. It has the appearance of a hard, tumorlike keloid. Also called **hypertrophic cicatrization.**

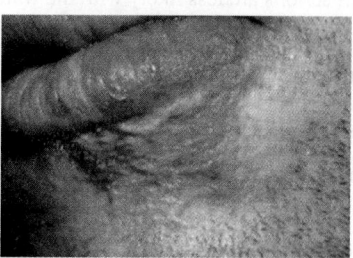

**Hypertrophic scar** *(Goldman and Fitzpatrick, 1994)*

**hypertrophy** /hīpur′trəfē/ [Gk, *hyper + trophe,* nourishment], an increase in the size of an organ caused by an increase in the size of the cells rather than the number of cells. The cells of the heart and kidney are particularly prone to hypertrophy. Kinds of hypertrophy include **adaptive hypertrophy, compensatory hypertrophy, Marie's hypertrophy, physiologic hypertrophy,** and **unilateral hypertrophy.** Also called **overgrowth.** Compare **atrophy, hyperplasia, auxesis.** —**hypertrophic,** *adj.*

**hypertrophy of heart** [Gk, *hyper,* excessive, *trophe,* nourishment; AS, *heorte*], an increase in the size of the heart resulting from enlargement of the heart muscle, but without an increase in the capacity of the heart chambers. It is a compensatory mechanism in heart failure.

**hypertropia.** See **anoopsia.**

**hyperuricaemia, hyperuricemia.** See **gout.**

**hypervalinemia** /hī′pər·val′i·nē′mē·ə /, **1.** an autosomal recessive aminoacidopathy, probably caused by a defect in an enzyme necessary for valine catabolism, characterized by elevated levels of valine in the plasma and urine and by failure to thrive. **2.** elevated levels of valine in the plasma. Also called **valinemia.**

**hyperventilation** /-ven′tilā′shən/ [Gk, *hyper + ventilare,* to fan], pulmonary ventilation rate greater than that metabolically necessary for gas exchange. It is the result of an increased respiration rate, an increased tidal volume, or both. Hyperventilation causes an excessive intake of oxygen and elimination of carbon dioxide. Hypocapnia and respiratory alkalosis then occur, leading to dizziness, faintness, numbness of the fingers and toes, possibly syncope, and psychomotor impairment. Causes of hyperventilation include asthma or early emphysema; increased metabolic rate caused by exercise, fever, hyperthyroidism, or infection; lesions of the central nervous system, as in cerebral thrombosis, encephalitis, head injuries, or meningitis; hypoxia or metabolic acidosis; use of hormones and drugs, such as epinephrine, progesterone, and salicylates; difficulties with mechanical respirators; and psychogenic factors, such as acute anxiety or pain. Compare **hypoventilation.** See also **respiratory center.**

**hyperventilation tetany,** a nervous disorder characterized by muscle twitches, cramps, or spasms caused by abnormally low blood levels of $CO_2$ from forced overbreathing. See also **tetany.**

**hyperviscosity** /-viskos'itē/ [Gk, *hyper,* excessive; L, *viscosus,* sticky], an extremely viscous or thick fluid.

**hypervitaminosis** /-vī'taminō'sis/, an abnormal condition resulting from excessive intake of toxic amounts (self-prescribed, usually from supplements) of one or more vitamins, especially over a long period. Serious effects may result from overdoses of fat-soluble vitamins A, D, E, or K, but adverse reactions are less likely with the water-soluble B and C vitamins, except when taken in megadoses. Compare **avitaminosis.** See also **megadose,** specific vitamins.

**hypervolemia** /-vōlē'mē·ə/ [Gk, *hyper* + L, *volumen,* paper roll; Gk, *haima,* blood], an increase in the amount of intravascular fluid, particularly in the volume of circulating blood or its components. See also **congestive heart failure.**

**hypervolemia management,** a nursing intervention from the Nursing Interventions Classification (NIC) defined as reduction in extracellular and/or intracellular fluid volume and prevention of complications in a patient who is fluid overloaded. See also **Nursing Interventions Classification.**

**hypesthesia** /hī'pisthē'zhə/ [Gk, *hypo,* under, *aisthesis,* feeling], a decrease in sensation in response to stimulation of the sensory nerves or body organs or areas they innervate. Also called **hypoesthesia. —hypesthetic,** *adj.*

**hypha** /hī'fə/, *pl.* **hyphae** [Gk, *hyphe,* web], a threadlike structure in the mycelium in a fungus.

**hyphema** /hīfē'mə/ [Gk, *hypo,* under, *haima,* blood], a hemorrhage into the anterior chamber of the eye, usually caused by a blunt trauma. The patient is treated by an ophthalmologist, who evaluates the need for evacuation of the blood and the use of mydriatic or miotic medications or a carbonic anhydrase inhibitor. Glaucoma may result from recurrent bleeding. Also called **hyphaemia, hyphemia** /hīfē'mē·ə/.

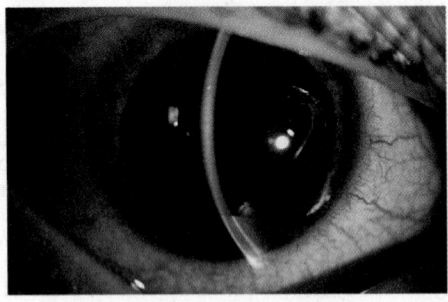

**Hyphema** *(Zitelli and Davis, 1997)*

**hypnagogic.** See **hypnagogue.**

**hypnagogic hallucination** /hip'nəgoj'ik/ [Gk, *hypnos,* sleep, *agogos,* leading], a vivid image that occurs in the period between wakefulness and sleep. Compare **hallucination.**

**hypnagogue** /hip'nəgog/ [Gk, *hypnos* + *agogos,* leading],

an agent or substance that tends to induce sleep or the feeling of dreamy sleepiness, as occurs before falling asleep. See also **hypnotics. —hypnagogic,** *adj.*

**hypno-,** prefix meaning 'sleep': *hypnagogic, hypnalgia.*

**hypnoanalysis** /hip'nə·anal'isis/ [Gk, *hypnos* + *analyein,* to loosen], the use of hypnosis as an adjunct to other techniques in psychoanalysis.

**hypnogenic zone** /hip'nəjen'ik/, a specific area on the body that, when stimulated with pressure, can cause a person to enter a hypnotic state.

**hypnosis**[1] /hipnō'sis/ [Gk, *hypnos,* sleep], a passive, trancelike state that resembles normal sleep during which perception and memory are altered, resulting in increased responsiveness to suggestion. The condition is usually induced by the monotonous repetition of words and gestures while the subject is completely relaxed.

**hypnosis**[2], a nursing intervention from the Nursing Interventions Classification (NIC) defined as assisting a patient to induce an altered state of consciousness to create an acute awareness and a directed focus experience. See also **Nursing Interventions Classification.**

**hypnotherapy** /hip'nəther'əpē/ [Gk, *hypnos* + *therapeia,* treatment], the use of hypnosis as an adjunct to other techniques in psychotherapy.

**-hypnotic,** combining form meaning 'sleep or hypnosis': *anhypnotic, autohypnotic, posthypnotic.*

**hypnotics** /hipnot'iks/ [Gk, *hypnos,* sleep], a class of drugs often used as sedatives. See also **hypnagogue.**

**hypnotic sleep** /hipnot'ik/ [Gk, *hypnos,* sleep; ME, *slep*], sleep induced by hypnosis through the administration of hypnotic medicines.

**hypnotic suggestion** [Gk, *hypnos,* sleep; L, *suggerere,* to suggest], a suggestion implanted in the mind of a person under hypnosis.

**hypnotic trance,** an artificially induced sleeplike state, as in hypnosis.

**hypnotism** /hip'nətiz'əm/ [Gk, *hypnos,* sleep], the study or practice of inducing hypnosis.

**hypnotist** /hip'nətist/, one who practices hypnotism.

**hypnotize** /hip'nətīz/, **1.** to put into a state of hypnosis. **2.** to fascinate, entrance, or control through personal charm.

**hypo-, hyp-,** prefix meaning 'under, below, beneath, deficient,' or, in chemistry, 'lacking oxygen': *hypochlorite, hypodermic, hypodontia.*

**hypoacidity** /hī'pō·əsid'itē/, a deficiency of acid.

**hypoactivity** /-aktiv'itē/ [Gk, *hypo,* under; L, *activus,* active], any abnormally diminished activity of the body or its organs, such as decreased cardiac output, thyroid secretion, or peristalsis. Compare **hyperactivity,** def. 1.

**hypoacusis** /-əkoo̅'sis/ [Gk, *hypo,* under, *akouein,* to hear], a reduced sensitivity to sounds.

**hypoadrenalism.** See **Addison's disease.**

**hypoalbuminemia** /-alboo̅'minē'mē·ə/, a condition of abnormally low levels of albumin in the blood. It may occur in celiac disease, tropical sprue, malnutrition, and some forms of liver or kidney impairment. Also spelled **hypoalbuminaemia.**

**hypoalimentation** /-al'iməntā'shən/ [Gk, *hypo* + L, *alimentum,* nourishment], a condition of insufficient or inadequate nourishment.

**hypoallergenic** /-al'ərjen'ik/ [Gk, *hypo,* under, *allos,* other, *ergein,* to work], having a lowered potential for producing an allergic reaction.

**hypobarism** /-ber'izəm/, air pressure that is significantly less than the sea level normal of 760 mm Hg. See also **barotrauma, decompression sickness.**

**hypobetalipoproteinemia** /hī'pōbā'təlip'ōprō'tēnē'mē·ə/ [Gk, *hypo* + *beta,* second letter of Greek alphabet, *lipos,* fat, *proteios,* first rank, *haima,* blood], an inherited disorder in which there are less than normal amounts of beta-lipoprotein in the serum. Blood lipids and cholesterol are present at less than the expected levels regardless of dietary intake of fats. There are no clinical signs, and treatment is unnecessary. Compare **hyperbetalipoproteinemia.**

**hypoblast** /hī′pōblăst/ [Gk, *blastos,* germ], the lower layer of the bilaminar embryonic disk in a human embryo, present during the second week. It gives rise to the endoderm.

**hypocalcemia** /hī′pōkalsē′mē·ə/ [Gk, *hypo* + L, *calx,* lime; Gk, *haima,* blood], a deficiency of calcium in the serum that may be caused by hypoparathyroidism, vitamin D deficiency, kidney failure, acute pancreatitis, or inadequate amounts of plasma magnesium and protein. Normal serum calcium levels range from 8.5 to 10.5 mg/dL. Mild hypocalcemia is asymptomatic. Severe hypocalcemia is characterized by cardiac arrhythmias and tetany with hyperparesthesia of the hands, feet, lips, and tongue. The underlying disorder is diagnosed and treated, and calcium is given by mouth or IV infusion. Hypocalcemia is also seen in dysmature newborns, in infants born of mothers with diabetes, or in normal babies of normal mothers delivered after a long or stressful labor and delivery. The condition is signaled by vomiting, twitching of extremities, poor muscle tone, high-pitched crying, and difficulty in breathing. Also spelled **hypocalcaemia.** See also **Chvostek's sign, tetany. —hypocalcemic,** *adj.*

**hypocalcemic tetany** /-kalsē′mik/ [Gk, *hypo,* under, L, *calx,* calcium, *haima,* blood, *tetanos,* convulsive tension], a disease caused by an abnormally low level of calcium in the blood. It is characterized by hyperexcitability of the neuromuscular system and results in carpopedal spasms. A common cause is a deficiency of parathyroid hormone secretion.

**hypocalciuria** /-kal′siuŏŏr′ē·ə/ [Gk, *hypo,* under; L, *calx,* lime; Gk, *ouron,* urine], a diminished level of calcium in the urine.

**hypocapnia** /-kap′nē·ə/, an abnormally low arterial carbon dioxide level. Also called **hypocarbia.**

**hypochloremia** /-klôrē′mē·ə/ [Gk, *hypo* + *chloros,* green, *haima,* blood], a decrease in the chloride level in the blood serum, below 95 mEq/L. The condition may result from prolonged gastric suctioning. Also spelled **hypochloraemia.**

**hypochloremic alkalosis** /-klôrē′mik/, a metabolic disorder resulting from an increase in blood bicarbonate level secondary to loss of chloride from the body.

**hypochlorhydria** /-klôrhid′rē·ə/ [Gk, *hypo* + *chloros,* green, *hydor,* water], a deficiency of hydrochloric acid in the stomach's gastric juice.

**hypochlorite poisoning** /-klôr′īt/, toxic effects of ingestion of or skin contact with household or commercial bleaches or similar chlorinated products. Symptoms include pain and inflammation of the mouth and digestive tract, vomiting, and breathing difficulty. Skin contact may produce blisters.

**hypochlorous acid** /-klôr′əs/ [Gk, *hypo* + *chloros,* green; L, *acidus,* sour], a compound that is stable only in the form of a dilute aqueous solution formed by dissolving chlorine gas in water to yield a greenish-yellow solution. An unstable compound that decomposes to hydrochloric acid and water, it is used as a bleaching agent and disinfectant.

**hypocholesteremia** /-kəles′tərē′mē·ə/, an abnormally low level of cholesterol in the blood. Also called **hypocholesterolemia.**

**hypochondria.** See **hypochondriasis.**

**hypochondriac** /-kon′drē·ak/ [Gk, *hypo,* under, *chondros,* cartilage], **1.** pertaining to the regions of the upper abdomen beneath the lower ribs and lateral to the epigastric region. See **hypochondriac region. 2.** pertaining to a person who is so preoccupied with matters of ill health that the state of mind itself becomes a disability. **—hypochondriacal,** *adj.*

**hypochondriac region** [Gk, *hypo* + *chondros,* cartilage; L, *regio,* direction], the part of the abdomen in the upper zone on both sides of the epigastric region and beneath the cartilages of the lower ribs. Also called **hypochondrium.** See also **abdominal regions.**

**hypochondriasis** /hī′pōkəndrī′əsis/ [Gk, *hypo* + *chondros,* cartilage, *osis,* condition], a chronic abnormal concern about the health of the body. It is characterized by extreme anxiety, depression, and an unrealistic interpretation of real or imagined physical symptoms as indications of a serious illness or disease despite rational medical evidence that no disorder is present. The condition is caused by some unresolved intrapsychic conflict and may involve a specific organ, such as the heart, lungs, or eyes, or several body systems at various times or simultaneously. In severe cases the distorted body-mind relationship is so strong that actual symptoms and disease may develop. Treatment usually consists of psychotherapy to uncover the underlying emotional conflict. Also called **hypochondria.**

**hypochondrium.** See **hypochondriac region.**

**hypochondroplasia** /-kon′drōplā′zhə/, an inherited form of dwarfism that resembles a mild form of achondroplasia. It is relatively uncommon and is transmitted as an autosomal dominant trait.

**hypochromic** /hī′pōkrō′mik/ [Gk, *hypo* + *chroma,* color], pertaining to less than normal color. The term usually describes a red blood cell and characterizes anemias associated with decreased synthesis of hemoglobin. Compare **normochromic.** See also **hypochromic anemia, red cell indexes.**

**hypochromic anemia, 1.** a group of anemias characterized by a decreased concentration of hemoglobin in the red blood cells. **2.** a form of anemia in which the hemoglobin is deficient in proportion to the size of erythrocytes or the individual erythrocyte has the capacity to contain more hemoglobin in, for example, iron deficiency anemia. See also **anemia, red cell indexes.**

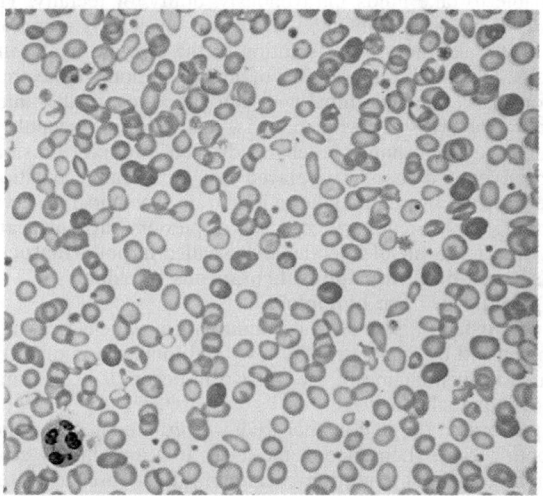

**Hypochromic microcytic anemia**
*(Kumar, Cotran, and Robbins, 1997/courtesy Dr. Robert W. McKenna, Department of Pathology, University of Texas Southwestern Medical School, Dallas)*

**hypocycloidal motion** /-sī′kloidəl/, a complex circular movement of the x-ray tube and film during the acquisition of CT images. It is used to blur structures outside the focal plane and eliminate ghost images.

**hypocytic leukemia.** See **aleukemic leukemia.**

**hypodermatoclysis.** See **hypodermoclysis.**

**hypodermic** /-durmik/ [Gk, *hypo* + *derma*, skin], pertaining to the area below the skin, such as a hypodermic injection.

**hypodermic implantation** [Gk, *hypo*, under, *derma*, skin; L, *implantare*, to set into], the introduction of a solid medicine under the skin, usually on the chest or abdominal wall, to ensure local action or slow absorption.

**hypodermic needle,** a short, thin hollow needle that attaches to a syringe for injecting a drug or medication under the skin or into vessels and for withdrawing a fluid, such as blood, for examination.

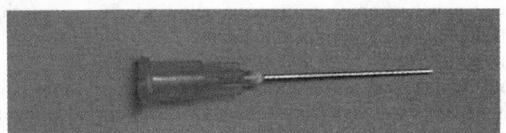

**Hypodermic needle** *(Potter and Perry, 2001)*

**hypodermic syringe** [Gk, *hypo*, under, *derma*, skin, *syrigx*, tube], an instrument designed to direct fluid under the skin through a fine hollow needle.

**hypodermic tablet,** a compressed or molded dosage form of a medication that can be dissolved for IV administration.

**hypodermoclysis** /hī′pōdərmok′lisis/ [Gk, *hypo* + *derma*, skin, *klysis*, flushing out], the injection of an isotonic or hypotonic solution into subcutaneous tissue to supply a continuous and large amount of fluid, electrolytes, and nutrients. The procedure is used to replace the loss or inadequate intake of water and salt during illness or surgery or after shock or hemorrhage. It is performed only when a patient is unable to take fluids intravenously, orally, or rectally. The rate of absorption into the circulatory system is increased with the addition to the solution of the enzyme hyaluronidase. The most common sites of administration are the anterior thighs, the abdominal wall along the crest of the ilium, below the breasts in women, and directly over the scapula in children; sites should be changed when multiple infusions are given. The patient is placed in a comfortable position, because the procedure takes a long time. The nurse observes for signs of circulatory collapse, respiratory difficulty, and edema at the site of injection. Also called **hypodermatoclysis, interstitial infusion, subcutaneous infusion.**

**hypodiploid.** See **hypoploid.**

**hypodipsia** /-dip′sē·ə/, a condition in which health is threatened by an abnormally low fluid intake. It is often related to dysfunction of the thirst osmoreceptor in the anterior hypothalamus.

**hypodontia** /hī′pō·don′shə/ [Gk, *hypo*, under + *odous*, tooth], partial absence of the teeth. It is a relatively common congenital condition characterized by absence of one or more teeth because of absence of their anlage, which is seldom associated with other anomalies. Also called **partial anodontia.**

**hypoesthesia.** See **hypesthesia.**

**hypofibrinogenemia** /-fī′brinōjənē′mē·ə/ [Gk, *hypo* + L, *fibra*, fiber; Gk, *genein*, to produce, *haima*, blood], a deficiency of fibrinogen, a blood clotting factor, in the blood. The condition may result from DIC as a complication of abruptio placentae. Also spelled **hypofibrinogenaemia.**

**hypofunction** /-fungk′shən/ [Gk, *hypo*, under; L, *functio*, performance], a diminished or inadequate level of activity of an organ system or its parts.

**hypogammaglobulinemia** /- gam′əglō′byəlinē′mē·ə/ [Gk, *hypo* + *gamma*, third letter in Greek alphabet; L, *globus*, small sphere; Gk, *haima*, blood], a less than normal concentration of gamma globulin in the blood, usually the result of increased protein catabolism or loss of protein in the urine. The condition is associated with a decreased resistance to infection. Also spelled **hypogammaglobulinaemia.** Compare **agammaglobulinemia.**

**hypogastric** /-gas′trik/ [Gk, *hypo*, under, *gaster*, stomach], pertaining to the hypogastrium, or the lower abdominal region below the umbilical region and between the right and left iliac regions.

**hypogastric artery.** See **internal iliac artery.**

**hypogastric pain,** pain in the lower abdomen.

**hypogastric plexus,** a complex of nerve fibers in the pelvic area near the termination of the aorta and the beginning of the common iliac artery.

**hypogastric region.** See **pubic region.**

**hypogastrium.** See **pubic region.**

**hypogenitalism** /- jen′itəliz′əm/ [Gk, *hypo* + L, *genitalis*, fruitful], a condition of retarded sexual development caused by a defect in male or female hormonal production in the testis or ovary.

**hypogeusia** /-gōō′zē·ə/, reduced taste.

**hypoglossal** /-glos′əl/ [Gk, *hypo*, under, *glossa*, tongue], pertaining to nerves or other structures under the tongue.

**hypoglossal nerve** [Gk, *hypo* + *glossa*, tongue], either of a pair of cranial nerves essential for swallowing and for moving the tongue. Each nerve has four major branches, communicates with the vagus nerve, and arises from nucleus XII in the brain. Also called **nervus hypoglossus, twelfth cranial nerve.**

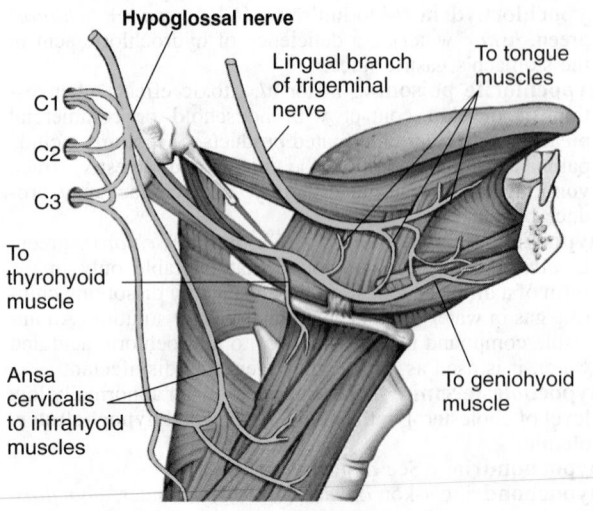

**Hypoglossal nerve**

**hypoglossus** /-glos′əs/, **1.** a muscle that retracts and pulls down the side of the tongue. **2.** the hypoglossal nerve.

**hypoglycemia** /hī′pōglīsē′mē·ə/ [Gk, *hypo* + *glykys,* sweet, *haima,* blood], a less than normal amount of glucose in the blood, usually caused by administration of too much insulin, excessive secretion of insulin by the islet cells of the pancreas, or dietary deficiency. The condition may cause weakness, headache, hunger, visual disturbances, ataxia, anxiety, personality changes, and, if untreated, delirium, coma, and death. The treatment is the administration of glucose in orange juice (or other fluids) by mouth if the person is conscious or in an IV glucose solution if the person is unconscious. Glycogen or complex carbohydrates may also be given. Also spelled **hypoglycaemia.** Compare **diabetic coma.**

**hypoglycemia management,** a nursing intervention from the Nursing Interventions Classification (NIC) is defined as preventing and treating low blood glucose levels. See also **Nursing Interventions Classification.**

**hypoglycemic** /-glīsē′mik/ [Gk, *hypo,* under, *glykys,* sweet, *haima,* blood], pertaining to or resembling a state of low blood glucose level. Also spelled **hypoglycaemic.**

**hypoglycemic agent,** any of a large heterogeneous group of drugs prescribed to decrease the amount of glucose circulating in the blood.

**hypoglycemic coma** [Gk, *hypo,* under, *glykys,* sweet, *koma,* deep sleep], a loss of consciousness that results from abnormally low blood glucose levels.

**hypoglycogenolysis** /-glī′kōjənol′isis/, a metabolic disorder in which defective splitting of glycogen molecules results in a decreased formation of glucose.

**hypogonadism** /-gō′nədiz′əm/, a deficiency in the secretory activity of the ovary or testis. The condition may be primary or caused by a gonadal dysfunction involving the Leydig's cells in the male, or it may occur secondary to a hypothalamus-pituitary disorder. Secondary hypogonadism is sometimes further differentiated into pituitary hypogonadism and hypothalamic hypogonadism.

**hypohidrotic ectodermal dysplasia.** See **anhidrotic ectodermal dysplasia.**

**hypoinsulinism** /-in′səliniz′əm/ [Gk, *hypo,* under; L, *insula,* island (of Langerhans)], a deficiency of insulin secretion by cells of the pancreas and associated signs and symptoms of diabetes.

**hypokalemia** /hī′pōkəlē′mē·ə/ [Gk, *hypo* + L, *kalium,* potassium; Gk, *haima,* blood], a condition in which an inadequate amount of potassium, the major intracellular cation,

is found in the circulating bloodstream. Hypokalemia is characterized by abnormal electrocardiographic findings, weakness, confusion, mental depression, and flaccid paralysis. The cause may be starvation, treatment of diabetic acidosis, adrenal tumor, or diuretic therapy. Mild hypokalemia may resolve itself when the underlying disorder is corrected. Severe hypokalemia may be treated by the administration of potassium chloride, orally or parenterally, and by a diet high in potassium. Also spelled **hypokalaemia.** Also called **kaliopenia.** Compare **hyperkalemia.** See also **electrolyte balance. —hypokalemic,** *adj.*

**hypokalemic alkalosis** /-kalē′mik/, a pathologic condition resulting from the accumulation of base or the loss of acid from the body associated with a low level of serum potassium. The retention of alkali or the loss of acid occurs primarily in extracellular fluid, but the pH of intracellular fluid may also be subnormal. See also **hypokalemia.**

**hypokalemic periodic paralysis** [Gk, *hypo,* under; L, *kalium,* potassium; Gk, *peri,* near, *hodos,* way, *paralyein,* to be palsied], a state of recurring attacks of muscular weakness associated with low blood levels of potassium.

**hypokinesia.** See **hypomotility.**

**hypokinetic** /-kinet′ik/ [Gk, *hypo,* under, *kinesis,* movement], pertaining to diminished power of movement or motor function, which may or may not be accompanied by a mild form of paralysis.

**hypolipoproteinemia** /hī′pōlip′ōprō′tēnē′mē·ə/ [Gk, *hypo* + *lipos,* fat, *proteios,* first rank, *haima,* blood], a group of defects of lipoprotein metabolism that cause varying complexes of signs. Primary, or hereditary, hypolipoproteinemia factors include abnormal transport of triglycerides in the blood, low levels of high-density lipoproteins, high levels of low-density lipoproteins, and abnormal fat deposits in the body, especially in the kidneys and the liver. In some of the syndromes ocular, cardiovascular intestinal, and neurologic effects are also present. The condition also may be secondary to anemia, malabsorption syndromes, or malnutrition. Kinds of hypolipoproteinemia are **abetalipoproteinemia, hypobetalipoproteinemia, familial hypocalphalipoproteinemia, lecithin-cholesterol acyltransferase deficiency,** and **Tangier disease.** Also called hypolipidemia

**hypomagnesemia** /hī′pōmag′nisē′mē·ə/, an abnormally low concentration of magnesium in the blood plasma, which causes nausea, vomiting, muscle weakness, tremors, tetany, and lethargy. Tachycardia and arrhythmia may also occur. Mild hypomagnesemia is usually the result of inadequate absorption of magnesium in the kidney or intestine, although it is also seen after prolonged parenteral feeding and during lactation. A more severe form is associated with malabsorption syndrome, protein malnutrition, and parathyroid disease. Magnesium salts to correct the deficiency may be given orally or intravenously.

**hypomania** /-mā′nē·ə/ [Gk, *hypo* + *mania,* madness], a mild degree of mania characterized by optimism; excitability; energetic, productive behavior; marked hyperactivity and talkativeness; heightened sexual interest; quick anger and irritability; and a decreased need for sleep. It may be observed before a full-blown manic episode. **—hypomaniac,** *n.,* **hypomanic,** *adj.*

**hypomelanosis of Ito.** See **incontinentia pigmenti achromians.**

**hypometria** /hī′pōmē′trē·ə/ [Gk, *hypo* + *metron,* measure], an abnormal condition, a form of dysmetria, characterized by a dysfunction of the power to control the range of muscular action, resulting in movements that fall short of the intended goals of the affected individual. Compare **hypermetria.**

### Signs and symptoms of hypoglycemia

| Sympathetic nervous system activity | | |
|---|---|---|
| Pallor | Palpitation | Weakness* |
| Perspiration* | Nervousness* | Trembling |
| Piloerection | Irritability | Hunger |
| Tachycardia | | |

| Central nervous system activity | |
|---|---|
| Headache | Fatigue |
| Blurred vision | Numbness of lips, tongue |
| Diplopia | Mental confusion* |
| Incoherent speech | Convulsions* |
| Emotional changes | Coma |

From Phipps WJ, Sands JK, Marek JE: *Medical-surgical nursing: concepts and clinical practice,* ed 6, St Louis, 1999, Mosby.
*Signs most commonly reported by patients.

**hypomobility** /-mōbil′itē/, a lack of normal movement of a joint or body part, as may result from an articular surface dysfunction or from disease or injury that affects a bone or muscle.

**hypomorph** /hī′pōmôrf/ [Gk, *hypo* + *morphe*, form], **1.** a person whose arms and legs are disproportionately short in relation to the trunk and whose sitting height is disproportionately tall compared to the standing height. **2.** a mutant allele that has a reduced effect on the expression of a trait but does not cause abnormal development. Also called **leaky gene.** Compare **amorph, antimorph, hypermorph.**

**hypomotility** /-mōtil′itē/ [Gk, *hypo,* under; L, *motare,* to move frequently], a state of diminished motility or loss of power to move about. Also called **hypokinesia.**

**hyponasality** /hī′pō·nā·zal′i·tē/ [Gk, *hypo,* under + *nasus,* nose], a quality of voice in which there is a complete lack of nasal emission of air and nasal resonance, so that speakers sound as if they have a cold. Also called **denasality.**

**hyponatremia** /hī′pōnatrē′mē·ə/ [Gk, *hypo* + L, *natrium,* sodium; Gk, *haima,* blood], a lower than normal concentration of sodium in the blood, caused by inadequate excretion of water or by excessive water in the circulating bloodstream. In a severe case the person may experience water intoxication, with confusion and lethargy, leading to muscle excitability, convulsions, and coma. Fluid and electrolyte balance may be restored by IV infusion of a balanced solution or a fluid-restricted diet. Also spelled **hyponatraemia.**

**hypoosmolality** [Gk, *hypo* + *osmos,* impulse], a state or condition of abnormally reduced osmolality. The normal serum concentration (millimoles per liter) is 0.43-0.50 times the serum osmolality (milliosmoles per kilogram). A decrease in this ratio is caused by an increase in other osmolutes such as glucose or ketone bodies in diabetes mellitus, urea in uremia, or salicylate in salicylic poisoning. See also **osmolality.**

**hypoosmotic** /hī′po·ozmot′ik/, pertaining to a solution that has a lower solute concentration than another solution. Compare **hyperosmotic, isosmotic.**

**hypoparathyroidism** /-per′əthī′roidiz′əm/ [Gk, *hypo* + *para,* beside, *thyreos,* shield, *eidos,* form], a condition of insufficient secretion of the parathyroid glands. It can be caused by primary parathyroid dysfunction or by elevated serum calcium level.

**hypoperistalsis** /-per′istal′sis/ [Gk, *hypo,* under, *peristellein,* to clasp], a state of abnormally slow motility of waves of alternate contraction and relaxation that impel contents forward through the digestive tract.

**hypopharyngeal** /-fərin′jē·əl/ [Gk, *hypo* + *pharynx,* throat], **1.** pertaining to the hypopharynx. **2.** situated below the pharynx.

**hypopharynx** /-fer′ingks/, the inferior portion of the pharynx, between the epiglottis and the larynx. It corresponds to the height of the epiglottis and is a critical dividing point in separating solids and fluids from air entering the region.

**hypophonia** /-fō′nē·ə/ [Gk, *hypo,* under, *phone,* voice], a weak or whispered voice.

**hypophoria** /-fôr′ē·ə/, a type of strabismus in which the patient may not show signs of ocular muscle imbalance until the affected eye is covered, resulting in a downward deviation. Otherwise the central nervous system may attempt to compensate for the defect through a fusion of the images received from both of the eyes.

**hypophosphatasia** /hī′pōfos′fətā′zhə/ [Gk, *hypo* + *phosphoros,* lightbearing], congenital absence of alkaline phosphatase, an enzyme essential to the calcification of bone tissue. Affected newborns vomit, grow slowly, and often die in infancy. Children who survive have numerous skeletal abnormalities and are dwarfs. There is no known treatment.

**hypophosphatemic rickets** /hī′pōfos′fətē′mik/, a rare familial disorder characterized by impaired resorption of phosphate in the kidneys and poor absorption of calcium in the small intestine, which result in osteomalacia, retarded growth, skeletal deformities, and pain. Treatment includes the prescription of phosphate and vitamin D, to be taken by mouth.

**hypophyseal** /-fizē′əl, -fiz′ē·əl/ [Gk, *hypo,* under, *phyein,* to grow], pertaining to the hypophysis or pituitary body.

**hypophyseal cachexia.** See **panhypopituitarism.**

**hypophyseal dwarf.** See **pituitary dwarf.**

**hypophyseal hormones,** pituitary hormones that are associated with body growth and exercise effects, such as luteinizing hormone, which stimulates testosterone production and muscular hypertrophy; growth hormone; and antidiuretic hormone.

**hypophyseal portal system,** a set of veins that carry blood and regulatory hormones from the hypothalamus to the adenohypophysis, where the target cells of the releasing hormones are located.

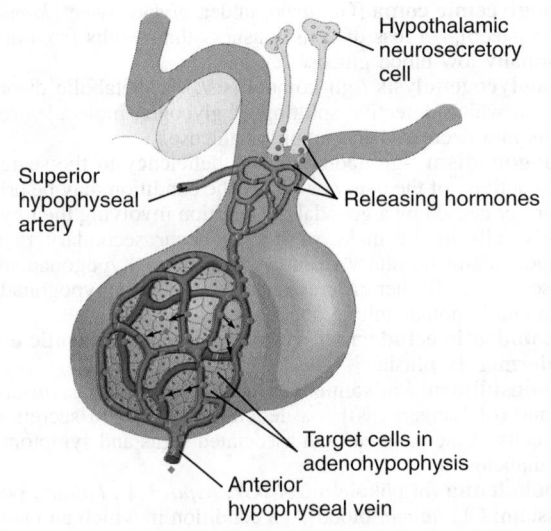

**Hypophyseal portal system**
*(Thibodeau and Patton, 1999/Network Graphics)*

**hypophysectomy** /hīpof′əsek′təmē/ [Gk, *hypo* + *phyein,* to grow, *ektomē,* excision], surgical removal of the pituitary gland. It may be performed to slow the growth and spread of endocrine-dependent malignant tumors or to excise a pituitary tumor. The gland is removed only if other treatment, such as x-ray therapy, radioactive implants, or cryosurgery, fails to destroy all pituitary tissue. General anesthesia is given and the gland is completely removed. Postoperative nursing care is as for a craniotomy. Levels of hormones, including thyroid-stimulating hormone, adrenocorticotropic hormone, and antidiuretic hormone, are monitored, and replacement therapy is begun as needed. Urinary output is measured every 2 hours for several days, and an amount in excess of 300 mL in any 2-hour period is reported. The patient is closely monitored for early signs of thyroid crisis, addisonian crisis, electrolyte imbalance, hemorrhage, hypothermia, and meningitis. **—hypophysectomize,** *v.*

**hypophyseoprivic** /-fiz'ē-ōpriv'ik/ [L, *privus,* deprived], pertaining to a deficiency of hormone secretions by the pituitary gland (hypophysis). The condition may be caused by functional inactivity or surgical removal of the gland.

**hypophysis** /hīpof'isis/ [Gk, *hypo,* under, *phyein,* to grow], the pituitary body (gland). The anterior lobe is sometimes identified as the **adenohypophysis** and the posterior lobe as the **neurohypophysis.**

**hypophysis cerebri.** See **pituitary gland.**

**hypopigmentation** /-pig'məntā'shən/ [Gk, *hypo* + L, *pigmentum,* paint], unusual lack of skin color, but not complete lack of pigment as seen in albinism. Compare **hyperpigmentation.**

**hypopituitarism** /-pityo͞o'iteriz'əm/ [Gk, *hypo* + L, *pituita,* phlegm], an abnormal condition caused by diminished activity of the pituitary gland and marked by excessive deposits of fat and persistence or acquisition of adolescent characteristics. Serum levels of pituitary hormones are lower than normal.

**hypoplasia** /hī'pōplā'zhə/ [Gk, *hypo* + *plassein,* to mold], underdevelopment of an organ or a tissue, usually resulting from the presence of a smaller-than-normal number of cells. Kinds of hypoplasia are **cartilage-hair hypoplasia** and **enamel hypoplasia.** Also called **hypoplasty.** Compare **aplasia, hyperplasia.** See also **oligomeganephronia, osteogenesis imperfecta. —hypoplastic,** *adj.*

**hypoplasia of the mesenchyme.** See **osteogenesis imperfecta.**

**hypoplastic.** See **hypoplasia.**

**hypoplastic anemia** /-plas'tik/, a broad category of anemias characterized by decreased production of red blood cells. Compare **aplastic anemia, polycythemia.** See also **anemia.**

**hypoplastic dwarf.** See **primordial dwarf.**

**hypoplastic left heart syndrome (HLHS),** any of a group of congenital anomalies consisting of hypoplasia or atresia of the left ventricle and of the aortic or mitral valve or both and hypoplasia of the ascending aorta; it is characterized by respiratory distress and extreme cyanosis, with cardiac failure and death in early infancy.

**hypoplasty.** See **hypoplasia.**

**hypoploid** /hī'pəploid/ [Gk, *hypo* + *eidos,* form], **1.** an individual, organism, strain, or cell that has fewer than the haploid number or than an exact multiple of the haploid number of chromosomes characteristic of the species. The result is one or more unbalanced sets of chromosomes, which are referred to as hypodiploid, hypotriploid, hypotetraploid, and so on, depending on the number of multiples of the haploid chromosomes they contain. **2.** pertaining to such an individual, organism, strain, or cell. Also called **hypoploidic.** Compare **hyperploid.** See also **monosomy. —hypoploidy,** *n.*

**hypoploidy** /hī'pōploi'dē/, any decrease in chromosome number that involves individual chromosomes rather than entire sets, so that fewer than the normal haploid number of chromosomes characteristic of the species are present, as in Turner's syndrome. Compare **hyperploidy.**

**hypopnea** /hīpop'nē-ə, hī'pōnē'ə/ [Gk, *hypo* + *pnoe,* breath], abnormally shallow and slow respiration. In well-conditioned athletes it may be appropriate and is often accompanied by a slow pulse; otherwise it is apparent when pleuritic pain limits excursion and is characteristic of damage to the brainstem. Accompanied by a rapid, weak pulse, it is a grave sign. See also **respiratory rate.**

**hypopotassemia** /-pot'əsē'mē-ə/ [Gk, *hypo* + D, *potasch,*

potash; Gk, *haima,* blood], a deficiency of potassium in the blood. See also **hypokalemia.**

**hypoproliferative anemias** /- prolif'ərətiv'/, a group of anemias caused by inadequate production of erythrocytes. The condition is associated with protein deficiencies, renal disease, and myxedema.

**hypoproteinemia** /hī'pōprō'tēnē'mē-ə/ [Gk, *hypo* + *proteios,* first rank, *haima,* blood], a disorder characterized by a decrease in the amount of protein in the blood to an abnormally low level, accompanied by edema, nausea, vomiting, diarrhea, and abdominal pain. It may be caused by an inadequate dietary supply of protein, by intestinal lymphangiectasia, or by renal failure. It can also result from burns. Also spelled **hypoproteinaemia.** Also called **intestinal lymphangiectasia.**

**hypoprothrombinemia** /hī'pōprōthrom'binē'mē-ə/ [Gk, *hypo* + L, *pro,* before; Gk, *thrombos,* lump, *haima,* blood], an abnormal reduction in the amount of prothrombin (factor II) in the circulating blood, characterized by poor clot formation, longer bleeding time, and possible hemorrhage. The condition is usually produced by inadequate synthesis of prothrombin in the liver, most often the result of a deficiency of vitamin K caused by severe liver disease, or by anticoagulant therapy with the drug dicumarol, or in newborns. Also spelled **hypoprothrombinaemia.** See also **blood clotting.**

**hypoptyalism.** See **hyposalivation.**

**hypopyon** /hīpō'pē-on/ [Gk, *hypo* + *pyon,* pus], an accumulation of pus in the anterior chamber of an eye, which appears as a gray fluid between the cornea and the iris. It may occur as a complication of conjunctivitis, herpetic keratitis, or corneal ulcer.

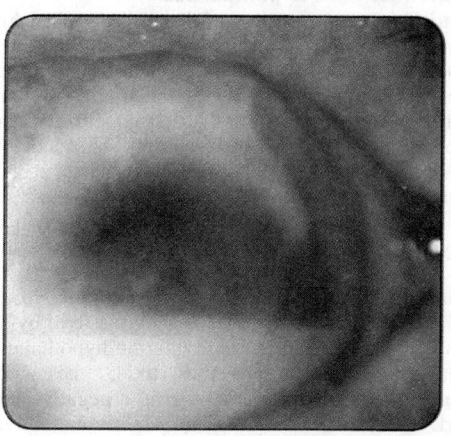

**Hypopyon** *(Kanski and Nischal, 1999)*

**hyporeflexia** /-riflek'sē·ə/ [Gk, *hypo* + L, *reflectere,* to bend back], decreased reflex reactions.

**hyposalivation** /-sal'ivā'shən/ [Gk, *hypo* + L, *saliva,* spittle], a decreased flow of saliva. It may be associated with dehydration, radiation therapy of the salivary gland regions, anxiety, the use of drugs such as atropine and antihistamines, vitamin deficiency, inflammation or infection of the salivary glands, or various syndromes, such as Plummer-Vinson syndrome. Also called **asialorrhea.** See also **xerostomia.**

**hyposensitization.** See **immunotherapy.**

**hypospadias** /hī'pō·spā'dē·əs/ [Gk, *hypo,* under + *spadōn,* a rent], a developmental anomaly in the male in which the urethra opens on the underside of the penis or on the perineum.

**hypostatic** /-stat'ik/ [Gk, *hypo* + *stasis,* standing still], pertaining to an accumulation of deposits of substances or congestion in a body area that results from a lack of activity.

**hypostatic lung collapse** [Gk, *hypo,* under, *stasis,* standing still; AS, *lungen* + L, *collabi,* to fall together], a disorder in which fluids or suspended solids pool or settle in a part of the lung, resulting in congestion.

**hypostatic pneumonia,** a type of pneumonia associated with elderly or debilitated people who remain in the same position for long periods. Fluids tend to settle in one area of the lungs, increasing the susceptibility to infection.

**hyposthenic** /hī'pōsthen'ik/, **1.** pertaining to a lack of strength or muscle tone. **2.** a body type characterized by a slender build.

**hypotelorism** /hī'pōtel'əriz'əm/ [Gk, *hypo* + *tele,* far, *horizo,* separate], a developmental defect characterized by an abnormally decreased distance between two organs or parts. A kind of hypotelorism is **ocular hypotelorism.** Compare **hypertelorism.**

**hypotension** /-ten'shən/ [Gk, *hypo* + L, *tendere,* to stretch], an abnormal condition in which the blood pressure is not adequate for normal perfusion and oxygenation of the tissues. An expanded intravascular space, hypovolemia, or diminished cardiac output may be the cause.

**hypotensive** /-ten'siv/ [Gk, *hypo,* under; L, *tendere,* to stretch], pertaining to abnormally low blood pressure.

**hypotensive anesthesia.** See **deliberate hypotension.**

**hypotetraploid.** See **hypoploid.**

**hypothalamic.** See **hypothalamus.**

**hypothalamic amenorrhea** /-thalam'ik/ [Gk, *hypo* + *thalamos,* chamber], cessation of menses caused by disorders that inhibit the hypothalamus from initiating the cycle of neurohormonal interactions of the brain, pituitary, and ovary necessary for ovulation and subsequent menstruation. Examples of causes are stress, anxiety, and acute weight loss. See **amenorrhea.**

**hypothalamic hormones,** a group of hormones secreted by the hypothalamus, including vasopressin, oxytocin, and the thyrotropin-releasing and gonadotropin-releasing hormones.

**hypothalamic obesity** [Gk, *hypo,* under, *thalamos,* chamber; L, *obesitas,* fatness], obesity that is caused by damage or a functional disturbance involving the hypothalamus.

**hypothalamic-pituitary-adrenal axis,** the combined system of neuroendocrine units that in a negative feedback network regulate the adrenal gland's hormonal activities.

**hypothalamus** /hī'pōthal'əməs/ [Gk, *hypo* + *thalamos,* chamber], a portion of the diencephalon of the brain, forming the floor and part of the lateral wall of the third ventricle. It activates, controls, and integrates the peripheral autonomic nervous system, endocrine processes, and many somatic functions, such as body temperature, sleep, and appetite. Compare **epithalamus, metathalamus, subthalamus, thalamus. —hypothalamic,** *adj.*

**hypothenar eminence** /hīpoth'ənär, hī'pōthē'när/ [Gk, *hypo* + *thenar,* palm], a fleshy pad on the ulnar side of the palm of the hand.

**hypothermal** /-thur'məl/ [Gk, *hypo,* under, *therme,* heat], **1.** pertaining to a condition in which the body temperature is significantly below normal as a result of external exposure to cold or has been reduced markedly for surgical or thera-

peutic purposes. **2.** pertaining to temperatures that are tepid to slightly warm.

**hypothermia**[1] /hī'pōthur'mē·ə/ [Gk *hypo* + *therme,* heat], **1.** an abnormal and dangerous condition in which the oral temperature is below 95° F (35° C) or the rectal temperature is below 96° F (35.5° C), usually caused by prolonged exposure to cold and/or damp conditions. Respiration is shallow and slow, and the heart rate is faint and slow. The person may appear to be dead. People who are very old or very young, people who have cardiovascular problems, and people who are hungry, tired, or under the influence of alcohol are most susceptible to hypothermia. Hospitalization is necessary for evaluating and treating any metabolic abnormalities that may result from hypothermia. Hypothermic patients in cardiac arrest should be rewarmed to 32° C (92° F) before resuscitation efforts are abandoned. **2.** the deliberate and controlled reduction of body temperature with cooling mattresses or ice as preparation for some surgical procedures.

**hypothermia**[2], a nursing diagnosis accepted by the Eighth National Conference on the Classification of Nursing Diagnoses. This diagnosis is defined as the state in which an individual's body temperature is reduced below his or her normal range but not below 96° F (rectal) or 97.5° F (rectal newborn).

■ DEFINING CHARACTERISTICS: Defining characteristics are mild shivering, cool skin, moderate pallor, slow capillary refill, tachycardia, cyanotic nailbeds, hypertension, and piloerection.

■ RELATED FACTORS: Related factors include exposure to a cool or cold environment, illness or trauma, inability or decreased ability to shiver, malnutrition, inadequate clothing, consumption of alcohol, medications causing vasodilation, evaporation from skin in cool environment, decreased metabolic rate, inactivity, and aging. See also **nursing diagnosis.**

**hypothermia blanket,** a covering used to conserve heat in the body of a patient suffering from hypothermia.

**hypothermia therapy,** the reduction of a patient's body temperature to counteract high prolonged fever caused by an infectious or neurologic disease or less frequently as an adjunct to anesthesia in heart or brain surgery.

■ METHOD: Hypothermia may be produced by placing crushed ice around the patient, by immersing the body in ice water, by autotransfusing blood after it is circulated through coils submerged in a refrigerant, or most commonly by applying cooling blankets or vinyl pads containing coils through which cold water and alcohol are circulated by a pump. The cooling unit is placed in an open area; any kinks or twists in the tubing are removed, and the blanket is checked for leaks. The patient is wrapped in bath blankets and then covered with the cooling blanket; the patient's temperature, registered by means of a probe inserted into the rectum, is read and recorded before hypothermia is initiated, every 5 minutes until the desired reduction is achieved, and then every 15 minutes. The blood pressure, pulse, respirations, and neurologic status are checked every 5 to 10 minutes until the temperature is stabilized, then every 30 minutes for 2 hours, every 4 hours in the next 24 hours, and subsequently as required. Every 1 to 2 hours the patient is assisted in turning, coughing, and deep breathing. At similar intervals the chest is auscultated for breath sounds, and oral, nose, and skin care are administered; the skin is lubricated with oil or lotion before and during the procedure. An indwelling catheter is connected to a closed gravity drainage system, as ordered, and fluid intake and output are measured; if less than 30 mL of urine per hour is excreted, the physician is notified. If the patient's oral temperature is less than 90° F (32.2° C), the gag reflex is tested before any oral fluids

or foods are administered. Nasooral suction is performed as indicated, body alignment is maintained, and passive or active range-of-motion exercises are performed every 4 hours. Because shivering increases body heat, medication for its prevention, such as chlorpromazine hydrochloride, may be ordered. The patient is observed for medication reactions, decrease in blood pressure, bradycardia, arrhythmias, bradypnea, respiratory failure, unequal pupils, increase in intracranial pressure, changes in consciousness, intestinal ileus, and frostbite. Any changes in skin color or signs of edema and induration are reported to the physician immediately. At the termination of therapy, the cooling blanket is replaced by regular blankets and the patient usually warms at his or her own rate. As the patient's temperature approaches normal, the warming blankets are removed, but the temperature probe remains in place until the body temperature is stable. ■ INTERVENTIONS: The nurse administers hypothermia, carefully monitoring the patient's vital signs and any evidence of complications.
■ OUTCOME CRITERIA: Hypothermia therapy used in the treatment of high fever associated with generalized severe infections reduces body heat by decreasing metabolism and inhibits the multiplication of the causative pathogenic organisms. Patients with a high temperature caused by a neurologic disease may be maintained in a state of mild hypothermia (87° to 95° F or 30.6° to 35° C) for as long as 5 days. The procedure is successful if the fever is broken and complications do not occur.

**hypothermia treatment,** a nursing intervention from the Nursing Interventions Classification (NIC) defined as rewarming and surveillance of a patient whose core body temperature is below 35° C. See also **Nursing Interventions Classification.**

**hypothesis** /hīpoth′isis/ [Gk, groundwork], (in research) a statement derived from a theory that predicts the relationship among variables representing concepts, constructs, or events. Kinds of hypotheses include **causal hypothesis, null hypothesis,** and **predictive hypothesis.**

**hypothrombinemia** /-throm′binē′mē-ə/, a deficiency of the clotting factor thrombin in the blood.

**hypothyroid** /-thī′roid/ [Gk, *hypo,* under, *thyreos,* shield, *eidos,* form], pertaining to or resembling thyroid deficiency.

**hypothyroid dwarf.** See **cretin dwarf.**

**hypothyroidism** /-thī′roidiz′əm/ [Gk, *hypo* + *thyreos,* shield, *eidos,* form], a condition characterized by decreased activity of the thyroid gland. It may be caused by surgical removal of all or part of the gland, overdosage with antithyroid medication, decreased effect of thyroid releasing hormone secreted by the hypothalamus, decreased secretion of thyroid stimulating hormone by the pituitary gland, atrophy of the thyroid gland itself, or peripheral resistance to thyroid hormone. Weight gain, mental and physical lethargy, dryness of the skin, constipation, arthritis, and slowing of the body's metabolic processes may occur. Untreated, hypothyroidism leads to myxedema coma, and death. Treatment is by administration of the deficient hormone. Dosage is adjusted to maintain normal serum levels of thyroid hormones. See **Hashimoto's disease, myxedema.**

**hypotonia** /-tō′nē·ə/ [Gk, *hypo,* under, *tonos,* stretching], a condition of diminished tone or tension that may involve any body structure.

**hypotonic** /hī′pōton′ik/ [Gk, *hypo,* under, *tonos,* stretching], **1.** pertaining to a lower or lessened tone or tension in any body structure, as in paralysis. **2.** pertaining to a solution that causes cells to swell. Compare **hypertonic, isotonic.**

**hypotonic saline** [Gk, *hypo,* under, *tonos,* tone; L, *sal,* salt], a saline solution that is less than isotonic in strength.

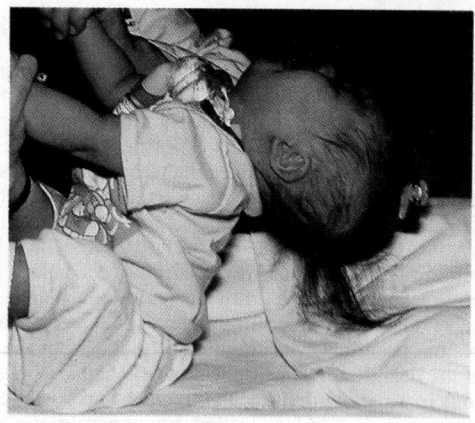

**Hypotonic infant** *(Zitelli and Davis, 1997)*

**hypotriploid.** See **hypoploid.**

**hypoventilation** /-ven′tilā′shən/ [Gk, *hypo* + L, *ventilare,* to fan], an abnormal condition of the respiratory system that occurs when the volume of air that enters the alveoli and takes part in gas exchange is not adequate for the body's metabolic needs. It is characterized by cyanosis, polycythemia, increased $PaCO_2$, and generalized decreased respiratory function. Hypoventilation may be caused by an uneven distribution of inspired air (as in bronchitis), obesity, neuromuscular or skeletal disease affecting the thorax, decreased response of the respiratory center to carbon dioxide, or a reduced amount of functional lung tissue, as in atelectasis, emphysema, and pleural effusion. The results of hypoventilation are hypoxia, hypercapnia, pulmonary hypertension with cor pulmonale, and respiratory acidosis. Treatment includes weight reduction in cases of obesity, artificial respiration, and possibly tracheostomy. Compare **hyperventilation.** See also **respiratory center.**

**hypovitaminosis.** See **avitaminosis.**

**hypovolemia** /-vōlē′mē·ə/ [Gk, *hypo* + L, *volumen,* whirl; Gk, *haima,* blood], an abnormally low circulating blood volume. Also spelled **hypovolaemia.**

**hypovolemia management,** a nursing intervention from the Nursing Interventions Classification (NIC) defined as expansion of intravascular fluid volume in a patient who is volume depleted. See also **Nursing Interventions Classification.**

**hypovolemic shock** /-vōlē′mik/, a state of physical collapse and prostration caused by massive blood loss, about one fifth or more of total blood volume. The common signs include low blood pressure, thready pulse, clammy skin, tachycardia, rapid breathing, and reduced urinary output. The associated blood losses may stem from GI bleeding, internal or external hemorrhage, or excessive reduction of intravascular plasma volume and body fluids. Disorders that may cause hypovolemic shock are dehydration from excessive perspiration, severe diarrhea, protracted vomiting, intestinal obstruction, peritonitis, acute pancreatitis, and severe burns, which deplete body fluids. Associated effects may include metabolic acidosis with the accumulation of lactic acid, irreversible cerebral and renal damage, and disseminated intravascular coagulation. Treatment of hypovolemic shock focuses on prompt replacement of blood and fluid volumes, identification of bleeding sites, and control of bleeding. Without fast, aggressive treatment, further collapse that can cause death ensues. Compare **cardiogenic shock.** See also **electric shock, shock.**

**hypoxemia** /hī′poksē′mē·ə/ [Gk, *hypo + oxys,* sharp, *genein,* to produce, *haima,* blood], an abnormal deficiency in the concentration of oxygen in arterial blood. Symptoms of acute hypoxemia are cyanosis, restlessness, stupor, coma, Cheyne-Stokes respiration, apnea, increased blood pressure, tachycardia, and an initial increase in cardiac output that later falls, producing hypotension and ventricular fibrillation or asystole. Chronic hypoxemia stimulates red blood cell production by the bone marrow, leading to secondary polycythemia. Hypoxemia caused by decreased alveolar oxygen tension or underventilation improves with oxygen therapy. Hypoxemia resulting from shunting of blood from the right side of the heart to the left side without exchange of gases in the lungs is treated with bronchial hygiene and positive endexpiratory pressure. Also spelled **hypoxaemia.** Compare **hypoxia.** See also **anoxia, asphyxia.**

**hypoxia** /hīpok′sē·ə/ [Gk, *hypo + oxys,* sharp, *genein,* to produce], inadequate oxygen tension at the cellular level, characterized by tachycardia, hypertension, peripheral vasoconstriction, dizziness, and mental confusion. Mild hypoxia stimulates peripheral chemoreceptors to increase heart and respiration rates. The central mechanisms that regulate breathing fail in severe hypoxia, leading to irregular respiration, Cheyne-Stokes respiration, apnea, and respiratory and cardiac failure. Increased sensitivity to the depressant effect of opiates on the respiratory system is common in chronic hypoxia, causing severe depression of respiration or apnea from relatively small doses. If the availability of oxygen is inadequate for aerobic cellular metabolism, energy is provided by less efficient anaerobic pathways that produce metabolites other than carbon dioxide and water. The tissues most sensitive to hypoxia are the brain, heart, pulmonary vessels, and liver. Treatment may include cardiotonic and respiratory stimulant drugs, oxygen therapy, mechanical ventilation, and frequent analysis of blood gases. Compare **hypoxemia.** See also **anoxia, chemoreceptor, hyperventilation, respiratory center.**

**hypoxic drive** /-hīpok′sik/, stimulation of respiration by low $PaO_2$, mediated through the carotid and aortic bodies.

**hypsi-,** prefix meaning 'high': *hypsicephalia, hypsiconchous, hypsistaphylie.*

**hypsibrachycephaly** /hips′ibrakisef′əlē/ [Gk, *hypsi,* high, *brachys,* short, *kephale,* head], the condition of having a skull that is high with a broad forehead. See also **brachycephaly, oxycephaly. —hypsibrachycephalic,** *adj., n.*

**hypsicephaly.** See **oxycephaly.**

**hypso-,** prefix meaning 'height': *hypsonosus, hypsophobia, hypsotherapy.*

**hyster-.** See **hystero-.**

**hysteralgia.** See **metralgia.**

**hysterectomy** /his′tərek′təmē/ [Gk, *hystera,* womb, *ektomē,* excision], surgical removal of the uterus. It is performed to remove fibroid tumors of the uterus or to treat chronic pelvic inflammatory disease, severe recurrent endometrial hyperplasia, uterine hemorrhage, and precancerous and cancerous conditions of the uterus. Types of hysterectomy include **total hysterectomy,** in which the uterus and cervix are removed, and **radical hysterectomy,** in which ovaries, oviducts, lymph nodes, and lymph channels are removed with the uterus and cervix. Menstruation ceases after either type is performed. A vaginal irrigation may be given preoperatively. During surgery the uterus is excised and removed, either through the abdominal wall or through the vagina. In some cases it may be removed laparoscopically. One or both ovaries and oviducts may be removed at the same time. Af-

ter surgery the nurse frequently observes the abdominal dressing, if present, and vaginal pad for bleeding. Food and oral fluids are restricted to prevent abdominal distension. The lower half of the bed is kept flat, and the patient is instructed to avoid sharply flexing the thighs or knees, because thrombophlebitis of the blood vessels of the pelvis and upper thigh is a frequent complication. Leg exercises are encouraged. Low back pain or scanty urine may indicate a ligated ureter. A kind of hysterectomy is **cesarean hysterectomy.** Compare **hysterosalpingo-oophorectomy. —hysterectomize,** *v.*

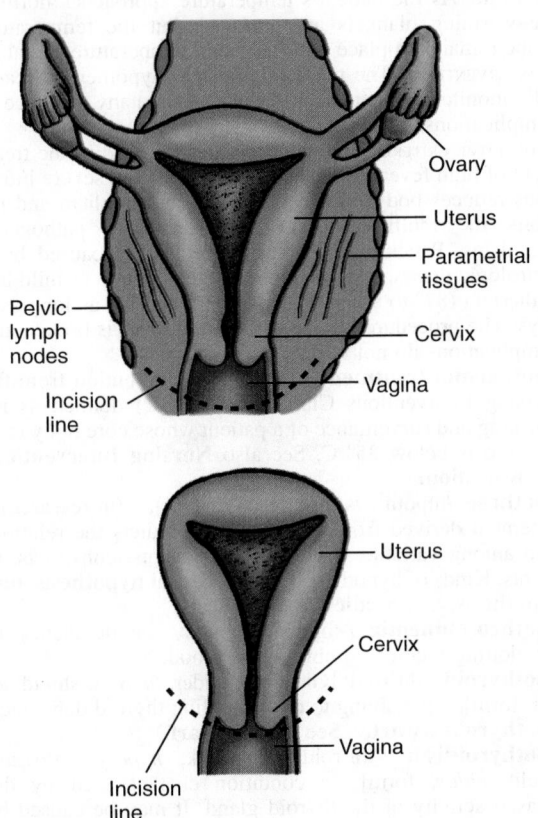

**Hysterectomy** *(Monahan and Neighbors, 1998)*

**hysteresis** /his′tərē′sis/ [Gk, *hysterein,* to be late], **1.** a lagging or retardation of one of two associated phenomena or a failure to act in unison. **2.** the influence of the previous condition or treatment of the body on its subsequent response to a given force, as in the example of the elastic property of a lung. At any given lung volume the elastic recoil pressure within the airways during expiration is less than that which exists at the same lung volume during inspiration.

**hysteria** /histir′ē·ə/ [Gk, *hystera,* womb], a general state of tension or excitement in a person or a group, characterized by unmanageable fear and temporary loss of control over the emotions.

**hysteric** /hister′ik/ [Gk, *hystera,* womb], pertaining to or resembling hysteria. Also **hysterical.**

**hysteric amaurosis** [Gk, *hystera + amauroein,* to darken], monocular or, more rarely, binocular blindness that follows an emotional shock. It may last for hours, days, or months.

**hysteric aphonia.**  See **conversion dysphonia.**

**hysteric ataxia** [Gk, *hystera*, womb, *ataxia*, without order], a loss of control over voluntary movements in walking or standing although the involved muscles function normally when the person is lying or sitting. See also **astasia-abasia.**

**hysteric blindness.**  See **psychic blindness.**

**hysteric chorea** [Gk, *hystera*, womb, *choreia*, dance], a condition in which an individual has choreiform movements, usually associated with his or her occupation, although the actions are the result of hysteria rather than true chorea.

**hysteric convulsion,**  a violent involuntary contraction and relaxation of the skeletal muscles marked by spasmodic muscular contractions with no organic cause.

**hysteric dyspepsia,**  difficulty in digestion caused by emotional disturbances.

**hysteric lethargy** [Gk, *hystera* + *lethargia*, drowsiness], a sleep induced by hypnosis. See also **hypnosis, lethargy.**

**hysteric paralysis** [Gk, *hystera*, womb, *paralyein*, to be palsied], a loss of movement or muscular weakness that is caused by hysteria rather than an identifiable organic defect.

**hysteric personality.**  See **histrionic personality.**

**hysteric syncope,**  a temporary loss of consciousness or a fainting spell caused by emotional agitation.

**hysteric tremor** [Gk, *hystera*, womb; L, *tremere*, to tremble], **1.** a fine rhythmic shaking in one extremity or of a generalized nature that may be an expression of fear, anxiety, or hysteria. **2.** a coarse irregular shaking that increases with voluntary movements. **3.** a shaking that is transient and is caused by exposure to drugs or toxic substances rather than an organic disorder.

**hysteric vertigo,**  a giddiness or loss of stability, often with a sensation of rotation, with no organic cause.

**hystero-, hyster-,**  combining form meaning 'uterus': *hysterocarcinoma, hysterocleisis, hysterolith.*

**hysterodynia.**  See **metralgia.**

**hysterogram** /his'tərōgram'/ [Gk, *hystera* + *gramma*, record], a radiographic image of a uterus made after the injection of a contrast medium into the uterine cavity. See also **hysterosalpingogram.**

**hysterography** /his'tərog'rəfē/ [Gk, *hystera*, womb, *graphein*, to record], the use of x-ray film and other instruments to make a medical assessment of the condition of the uterus.

**hysterolaparotomy** /his'tərōlap'ərot'əmē/ [Gk, *hystera* + *lapara*, loin, *temnein*, to cut], abdominal hysterectomy or hysterotomy.

**hystero-oophorectomy** /-ō'əfərek'təmē/ [Gk, *hystera*, womb, *oophoron*, ovary, *ektomē*, excision], the surgical removal of the uterus and both ovaries.

**hysterosalpingogram** /his'tərō'salping'gōgram'/ [Gk, *hystera* + *salpinx*, tube, *gramma*, record], an x-ray film of the uterus and the fallopian tubes using gas or a radiopaque substance introduced through the cervix to allow visualization of the cavity of the uterus and the passageway of the tubes. A blockage of a structure is demonstrated on the film because the radiopaque substance cannot pass to the more distal structures and escape from the ends of the tubes into the peritoneal cavity. Serial hysterosalpingography is useful in the diagnosis of the cause of infertility.

**hysterosalpingography** /his'tərōsal'ping·gog'rəfē/, a method of producing radiographic images of the uterus and

fallopian tubes as part of the diagnosis of abnormalities in the reproductive tract of a nonpregnant woman. The technique outlines the size, shape, and position of the organs, including any tumors, fistulas, or polyps. It also reveals any obstructions in the fallopian tubes.

**hysterosalpingo-oophorectomy** /-salping'gō·ō'əfərek't əmē/ [Gk, *hystera* + *salpinx*, tube, *oophoron*, ovary, *ektomē*, excision], surgical removal of one or both ovaries and oviducts along with the uterus, performed commonly to treat malignant neoplastic disease of the reproductive tract and chronic endometriosis. Removal of the ovaries and oviducts is routinely done with a hysterectomy on menopausal or postmenopausal women. To prevent the severe symptoms of sudden menopause in premenopausal women, a portion of one ovary is left, unless a malignancy is present. If both ovaries are removed and no malignancy is present, estrogen replacement therapy is often begun immediately. Elastic stockings or bandages may be applied to the legs to prevent circulatory stasis because thrombophlebitis of the blood vessels of the pelvis or thigh is a frequent complication. The lower half of the bed is kept flat, and the patient is instructed not to flex the thighs or knees. Low back pain or scanty urine may indicate a ligated ureter. Compare **hysterectomy.**

**hysteroscope** /his'tər·ō·skōp'/ [Gk, *hystera*, womb + *skopein*, to view], an endoscope used in direct visual examination of the canal of the uterine cervix and the cavity of the uterus.

**hysteroscopy** /his'təros'kepē/ [Gk, *hystera* + *skopein*, to look], direct visual inspection of the cervical canal and uterine cavity through a hysteroscope. Hysteroscopy is performed to examine the endometrium, to secure a specimen for biopsy, to remove an intrauterine device, or to excise cervical polyps. The endoscope is passed through the vagina and into the uterus, and the surrounding tissues are examined. The procedure is contraindicated in pregnancy, acute pelvic inflammatory disease, chronic upper genital tract infection, recent uterine perforation, and known or suspected cervical malignancy. —**hysteroscope,** *n.,* **hysteroscopic,** *adj.*

**hysterotome** /his'tərotōm'/ [Gk, *hystera*, womb, *temnein*, to cut], a surgical knife used for certain procedures involving the uterus.

**hysterotomy** /his'tərot'əmē/ [Gk, *hystera* + *temnein*, to cut], surgical incision of the uterus, performed as a method of abortion in a pregnancy beyond the first trimester of gestation in which a saline injection abortion was incomplete or in which a tubal sterilization is to be done with the abortion. During surgery the lower segment of the uterus is incised, and the products of conception are withdrawn. Postoperative care includes close observation for excessive vaginal bleeding.

**hysterovaginoenterocele** /-vaj'inō·en'tərōsēl'/ [Gk, *hystera*, womb; L, *vagina*, sheath; Gk, *enteron*, bowel, *kele*, hernia], a hernia involving the uterus, vagina, and intestines. Prolapse of the pelvic organs may be caused by pregnancy or an inherent weakness of the supporting structures. It is also common after menopause. Surgical repair or the use of a pessary may help.

**Hytone,**  trademark for a glucocorticoid (hydrocortisone).

**Hz,**  abbreviation for **hertz.**

**HZV,**  abbreviation for *herpes zoster virus.* See **chickenpox, herpes zoster.**

**I, 1.** symbol for *inspired gas.* **2.** symbol for the element **iodine.**

**-i,** plural-forming suffix used in native and later scientific Latin words: *bacilli, bronchi, plumbi,* and in scientific terms derived through Latin from Greek: *encephali, pylori, tympani.*

**$^{131}$I,** symbol for *radioactive iodine, isotopic mass (atomic weight) 131.*

**$^{132}$I,** symbol for *radioactive iodine, isotopic mass (atomic weight) 132.*

**-ia,** suffix meaning a 'specified condition of a disease or process': *athrombia, phrenoblabia, pontobulbia.*

**IABC,** abbreviation for *intraaortic balloon counterpulsation.* See **intraaortic balloon pump.**

**IABP,** abbreviation for **intraaortic balloon pump.**

**IADL,** abbreviation for **instrumental activities of daily living.**

**I.A.D.R.,** abbreviation for **International Association for Dental Research.**

**IAH,** abbreviation for **idiopathic diffuse alveolar hemorrhage.**

**I and O,** abbreviation for *intake and output.*

**-iasis,** suffix meaning 'the formation or presence of an abnormal condition or disease': *dicrocoeliasis, elephantiasis.*

**-iatria.** See **-iatry.**

**-iatric, -iatrical,** combining form meaning 'relating to medicine, physicians, or medical treatment': *neuropsychiatric, orthopsychiatric, pithiatric.*

**-iatrist, -iatrician,** combining form meaning 'one who treats or a physician': *hydriatrist, pediatrician, podiatrist.*

**iatro-,** combining form meaning 'physician or treatment': *iatrogenic, iatrophysics, iatrotechnics.*

**iatrogenic** /ī′atrōjen′ik, yat-/ [Gk, *iatros,* physician, *genein,* to produce], caused by treatment or diagnostic procedures. An iatrogenic disorder is a condition caused by medical personnel or procedures or through exposure to the environment of a health care facility. See also **nosocomial. —iatrogenesis, iatrogeny,** *n.*

**iatrogenic diabetes mellitus,** a form of diabetes that develops as an adverse effect of treatment for a different medical problem. Patients who are presented high doses of corticoteroids usually develop iatrogenic diabetes mellitus. Also called **secondary diabetes.**

**iatrogenic pneumothorax,** a condition in which air or gas is present in the pleural cavity as a result of mechanical ventilation, tracheostomy tube placement, or other therapeutic intervention.

**iatrology,** the science of medicine.

**iatropic** /ī′atrop′ik/ [Gk, *iatros,* physician, *trepein,* to turn], describing a need to see a physician.

**iatropic stimulus,** the symptoms that induce a patient to seek professional health care. See also **chief complaint.**

**-iatry, -iatria,** combining form meaning a '(specified) type of medical treatment, the medical profession, or physicians': *andriatry, pediatry, pithiatry.*

**I band** [ME, *band,* flat strip], an isotropic band within a striated muscle fiber that appears dark in polarized light but light when stained. See also **sarcomere.**

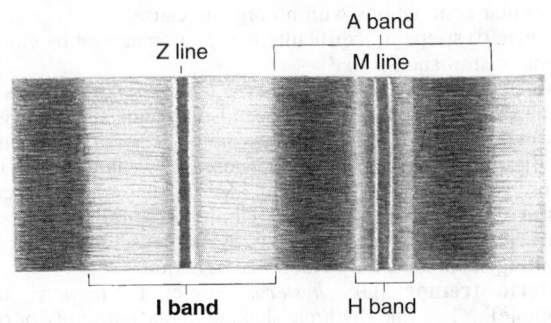

**I band** *(Thompson et al, 1997)*

**IBC,** abbreviation for *iron-binding capacity.*

**IBD,** abbreviation for **inflammatory bowel disease.** See **Crohn's disease, ulcerative colitis.**

**-ible.** See **-able.**

**IBS,** abbreviation for **irritable bowel syndrome.**

**ibuprofen** /ī′byoō′prōfin/, a nonsteroidal antiinflammatory agent.

■ INDICATIONS: It is prescribed in the treatment of rheumatoid arthritis and osteoarthritis, muscle aches, and menstrual cramps.

■ CONTRAINDICATIONS: Renal dysfunction, disorders of the GI tract, or known hypersensitivity to this drug, to other nonsteroidal antiinflammatory drugs, or to aspirin prohibits its use.

■ ADVERSE EFFECTS: Among the more serious adverse reactions are GI disturbances, gastric or duodenal ulceration, dizziness, skin rash, and tinnitus.

**ibutilide fumarate,** a drug that controls atrial fibrillation and atrial flutter.

■ INDICATIONS: It is prescribed in the treatment of heart arrhythmias by converting atrial fibrillation and atrial flutter of recent onset to normal sinus rhythm.

■ CONTRAINDICATIONS: If the drug does not result in conversion after an initial 10-minute infusion, a second 10-minute infusion may be given, but not sooner than 10 minutes after the first dose has been completed.

■ ADVERSE EFFECTS: The side effects most often reported include life-threatening arrhythmias, including ventricular tachycardia.

**IBW,** abbreviation for *ideal body weight.*

**IC,** abbreviation for **inspiratory capacity.**

**-ic, -ac,** suffix meaning 'pertaining to, similar to': *allelic, cadaveric, hypochondriac.*

**ICA,** abbreviation for **islet cell antibody.**

**-icam,** suffix for antiinflammatory agents of the isoxicam group.

**ICD,** abbreviation for **implantable cardioverter-defibrillator.**

**ICD**, abbreviation for *International Classification of Diseases.*

**ice burn,** partial-thickness thermal necrosis of the skin caused by prolonged therapy entailing applications of ice.

**Iceland disease** /īs′land/, a group of symptoms associated with effects of a viral infection of the nervous system, including muscular pain and weakness, depression, and sensory changes. It mainly affects young adults; its exact cause is unknown. Also called **benign myalgic encephalomyelitis, chronic fatigue syndrome, royal free disease.**

**I cell disease,** a form of lysosomal disease characterized by progressive mental deterioration, heart disease, and respiratory failure in the first 10 years of life. A number of lysosomal enzymes are lacking, and fibroblasts display numerous coarse inclusions. Also called **inclusion cell disease, mucolipidosis II.**

**ice pack** [ME, *is* + *pakke*], a container of crushed ice placed on the body to reduce tissue temperature, relieve pain, soothe inflamed tissue, or control bleeding.

**ICF,** abbreviation for **intermediate care facility.**

**ICF/MR,** abbreviation for *intermediate care facility for the mentally retarded.* See **intermediate care facility.**

**ICH,** abbreviation for **intracerebral hemorrhage.**

**ichor** /ī′kôr/, a thin watery fluid discharged from a sore.

**ichthyo-,** combining form meaning 'fish': *ichthyocolla, ichthyophagy, ichthyotoxic.*

**ichthyoid** /ik′thē·oid/ [Gk, *ichthys,* fish, *eidos,* form], pertaining to objects or structures that are fish-shaped or fish-like.

**ichthyosis** /ik′thē·ō′sis/ [Gk, *ichthys,* fish, *osis,* condition], any of several inherited dermatologic conditions in which the skin is dry and hyperkeratotic, resembling fish scales. It usually appears at or shortly after birth and may be part of one of several rare syndromes. Some types respond temporarily to bath oils or lactic acid. A rare, acquired variety accompanying a lymphoma or multiple myeloma occurs in adults. Also called **fish skin disease, xeroderma.** —**ichthyotic,** *adj.*

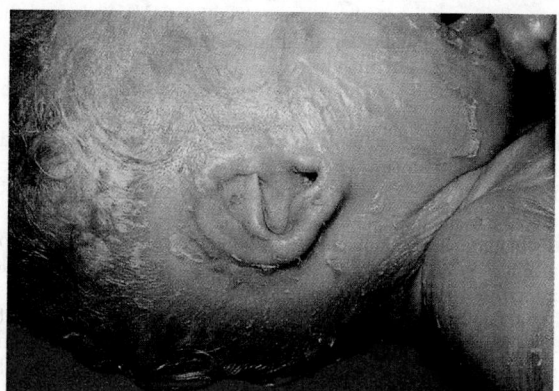

**Lamellar ichthyosis** *(Weston, Lane, and Morelli, 1996)*

**ichthyosis congenita, ichthyosis fetalis.** See **lamellar exfoliation of the newborn.**

**ichthyosis fetus.** See **harlequin fetus.**

**ichthyosis hystrix** [Gk, *ichthys,* fish + *-osis,* condition + *hystrix,* porcupine], a localized form of epidermolytic hy-

perkeratosis having the appearance of linear epidermal nevi. See also **epidermolytic hyperkeratosis.**

**ichthyosis vulgaris** [Gk, *ichthys* + *osis* + L, *vulgaris,* common], a hereditary skin disorder characterized by large, dry, dark scales that cover the face, neck, scalp, ears, back, and extensor surfaces but not the flexor surfaces of the body. The condition is transmitted as an autosomal dominant trait; it appears several months to 1 year after birth. Management consists of topical application of emollients and use of keratolytic agents to facilitate removal of the scales. Also called **ichthyosis simplex.** See also **sex-linked ichthyosis.**

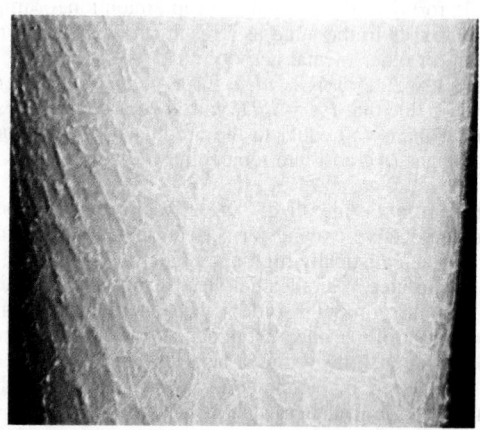

**Ichthyosis vulgaris** *(Zitelli and Davis, 1997)*

**ichthyotic.** See **ichthyosis.**

**-ician,** suffix meaning a 'specialist in a field': *clinician, pediatrician, technician.*

**ICN,** abbreviation for **International Council of Nurses.**

**icon** /ī′kən/, an image on the screen of a computer terminal representing a specific command.

**ICP,** abbreviation for **intracranial pressure.**

**-ics,** combining form meaning the 'systematic formulation of a body of knowledge': *bionomics, osmics, psychics.*

**I.C.S.,** abbreviation for **International Congress of Surgeons.**

**ICSH,** abbreviation for **interstitial cell-stimulating hormone.** See **luteinizing hormone.**

**ictal** /ik′təl/ [Gk, *ikteros,* jaundice], pertaining to a sudden acute onset, as convulsions of an epileptic seizure.

**-ictal,** combining form meaning 'to be caused by a sudden attack or stroke': *postictal.*

**icter-,** combining form meaning 'jaundice': *icterohepatitis.*

**icteric** /ikter′ik/ [Gk, *ikteros,* jaundice], pertaining to or resembling jaundice.

**icterogenic** /ik′tərōjen′ik/, causing jaundice.

**icterus.** See **jaundice.**

**icterus gravis neonatorum** /ik′tərəs/ [Gk, *ikteros,* jaundice; L, *gravis,* weight, *neonatus,* newborn], a hemolytic jaundice of the newborn caused by incompatibility between the mother's serum and infant's red corpuscles.

**icterus neonatorum,** a jaundiced condition in a newborn.

**ictus** /ik′təs/, *pl.* **ictuses, ictus** [L, stroke], **1.** a seizure. **2.** a cerebrovascular accident. —**ictal, ictic,** *adj.*

**ICU,** abbreviation for **intensive care unit.**

**id** [L, it], **1.** (in freudian psychoanalysis) the part of the psyche functioning in the unconscious that is the source of instinctive energy, impulses, and drives. It is based on the pleasure principle and has strong tendencies toward self-preservation. Compare **ego, superego. 2.** the true unconscious.

**ID,** abbreviation for *infectious disease.*

**-id, 1.** suffix meaning 'structure or body': *plasmid, protoconid, talonid, trigonid.* **2.** suffix meaning 'a member of a group': *tuberculid.*

**IDDM,** abbreviation for **insulin-dependent diabetes mellitus.** See **type 1 diabetes mellitus.**

**-ide,** suffix meaning 'a compound of': *chloride, monoxide, sulfide.*

**idea** [Gk, form], any thought, concept, intention, or impression that exists in the mind as a result of awareness, understanding, or other mental activity.

**ideal gas law** /īdē′əl/ [Gk, *idea,* form, *chaos,* gas; AS, *lagu,* law], the rule that $PV = nRT$, with the product of pressure *(P)* and volume *(V)* equal to the product of the number of moles of gas *(n),* absolute temperature *(T),* and a gas constant *(R).*

**idealized image** /īdē′əlīzd/, a self-concept of a person with a compulsive craving for perfection and admiration. It results in unrealistically high and unattainable goals.

**idea of influence,** an idea held less firmly than a delusion, often seen in paranoid disorders, that external forces or persons are controlling one's thoughts, actions, and feelings.

**idea of persecution,** an idea held less firmly than a delusion, often seen in paranoid disorders, that one is being threatened, discriminated against, or mistreated by other persons or by external forces.

**idea of reference,** a delusion that the statements or actions of others, usually interpreted as deprecatory, refer to oneself. It is often seen in paranoid disorders. Also called **delusion of reference, referential idea.**

**ideational apraxia** /ī′dē·ā′shənəl/ [Gk, *idea,* form, *a + prassein,* not to do], a condition in which the conceptual process is lost, often because of a lesion in the submarginal gyrus of the parietal lobe. The individual is unable to formulate a plan of movement and does not know the proper use of an object because of a lack of perception of its purpose. There is no loss of motor movement, but the reason for the movement is confused. Also called **sensory apraxia.** See also **apraxia.**

**idée fixe.** See **fixed idea.**

**identical twins.** See **monozygotic twins.**

**identification** /īden′tifikā′shən/ [L, *idem,* the same, *facere,* to make], an unconscious defense mechanism by which a person patterns his or her personality on that of another person, assuming the person's qualities, characteristics, and actions. The process is a normal function of personality development and learning, specifically of the superego, and it contributes to the acquisition of interests and ideals. Identification first occurs in early childhood when 3- to 5-year-olds first identify with parental same-sex figures; it resurges in adolescence as a major task of identifying with peers.

**identity**[1] /īden′titē/, a component of self-concept characterized by one's persisting consciousness of being oneself, separate and distinct from others. **Identity diffusion,** or identity confusion, is a lack of clarity and consistency in one's perception of the self, which produces a high degree of anxiety.

**identity**[2], a nursing outcome from the Nursing Outcomes Classification (NOC) defined as ability to distinguish between self and non-self and to characterize one's essence. See also **Nursing Outcomes Classification.**

**identity crisis** [L, *idem,* the same; Gk, *krisis,* turning point], a period of confusion concerning an individual's sense of self and role in society, which occurs most frequently in the transition from one stage of life to the next. It is often expressed by isolation, negativism, extremism, and rebelliousness.

**identity diffusion.** See **identity.**

**identity disorder.** See **spiritual therapy.**

**identity disorder of childhood,** a mental disturbance of childhood in which the person is abnormally uncertain and concerned about long-term goals such as career choice or sexual preference to the point that the concerns interfere with educational and social functions. See also **identity crisis.**

**ideo-** [Gr, *idea*], prefix meaning 'idea': *ideogram.*

**ideokinetic apraxia.** See **ideomotor apraxia.**

**ideology** /ī′de·ol′əjē/ [Gk, *idea*], a scheme of ideas or systematic organization of ideas associated with doctrine and philosophy.

**ideomotor apraxia** /īdē′əmō′tor/ [Gk, *idea* + L, *motare,* to move about; Gk *a* + *prassein,* not to do], the inability to translate an idea into motion, resulting from some interference with the transmission of the appropriate impulses from the brain to the motor centers. There is no loss of the ability to perform an action automatically, such as tying the shoelaces, but the action cannot be performed on request. The condition is often caused by diffuse cortical disease. Also called **ideokinetic apraxia, limb-kinetic apraxia, transcortical apraxia.** See also **apraxia.**

**ideophobia** /-fō′bē·ə/ [Gk, *idea* + *phobos,* fear], an anxiety disorder characterized by the irrational fear or distrust of ideas or reason. See also **phobia.**

**idio-,** prefix meaning 'private, distinctive, peculiar': *idiopathic.*

**idiocrasy.** See **idiosyncrasy.**

**idiogram** /id′ē·əgram′/, a diagram or graphic representation of a karyotype, showing the number, relative sizes, and morphologic characteristics of the chromosomes of a species, individual, or cell.

**idiojunctional rhythm** /-jungk′shənəl/ [Gk, *idios,* own; L, *jungere,* to join; Gk, *rhythmos*], a heart rhythm emanating from the junction of the atrioventricular (AV) node and the AV bundle but without retrograde conduction to the atria.

**idiomere.** See **chromomere.**

**idiopathic** /-path′ik/ [Gk, *idios* + *pathos,* disease], without a known cause.

**idiopathic diffuse alveolar hemorrhage (IAH),** bleeding into the alveoli of the lungs caused by any of a number of disorders, including Goodpasture's syndrome, Wegener's granulomatosis, and collagen vascular disease.

**idiopathic disease,** a disease that develops without an apparent or known cause, although it may have a recognizable pattern of signs and symptoms and may be curable.

**idiopathic edema,** edema of unknown cause, usually affecting women, occurring intermittently over a period of years, and usually worse during the premenstrual phase; it is associated with increased aldosterone secretion.

**idiopathic gangrene** [Gk, *idios,* own, *pathos,* disease, *gangraina*], a gangrenous condition of unknown cause.

**idiopathic guttate hypomelanosis** /hī′pōmel′ənō′sis/, a drop-shaped hypopigmented skin lesion of unknown origin. It is fairly common, occurring in approximately half of all normal adults.

**idiopathic hemosiderosis,** the accumulation of iron-containing deposits in cells of the lungs as a result of bleeding in the lungs.

**idiopathic hypoventilation,** a disorder of unknown cause

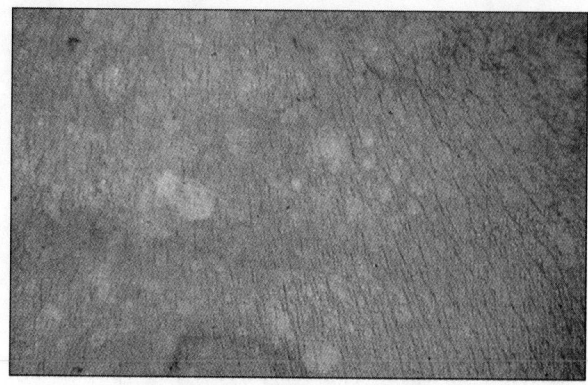

**Idiopathic guttate hypomelanosis**
*(Lawrence and Cox, 1993)*

sis and up to 80% of those with structural scoliosis. It may occur at any age, but three types are commonly associated with certain age groups. The infantile type affects 1- to 3-year-olds. The juvenile type affects 3- to 10-year-olds. The adolescent type affects preadolescents and adolescents. The main factors in diagnosing idiopathic scoliosis are the degree, balance, and rotational component of the curvature. The rotational component may contribute to rib cage deformities and impingement on the pulmonary and cardiac systems.

associated with deficient ventilation of the alveoli of the lungs.

**idiopathic midline destructive disease (IMDD),**  a disorder of unknown cause characterized by ulceration and necrosis of the midline facial tissues and obstruction of the upper airways. IMDD develops without systemic involvement.

**idiopathic multiple pigmented hemorrhagic sarcoma.** See **Kaposi's sarcoma.**

**idiopathic necrotizing crescentic glomerulonephritis,** an autoimmune disorder that causes intracapsular hemorrhage and cellular crescent formation in the renal glomerulus. See also **glomerulonephritis.**

**idiopathic nephrotic syndrome** [Gk, *idios,* own, *pathos,* disease, *nephros,* kidney],  a kidney disease of unknown origin characterized by hematuria, albuminuria, edema, and hypertension resulting from damaged glomerular capillaries.

**idiopathic neuralgia** [Gk, *idios,* own, *pathos,* disease, *neuron,* nerve, *algos,* pain],  a form of neuralgia that occurs without any identifiable structural nerve lesion.

**idiopathic pericarditis** [Gk, *idios,* own, *pathos,* disease, *peri,* near, *kardia,* heart, *itis,* inflammation],  inflammation of the pericardium of unknown cause.

**idiopathic postpartum renal failure,**  kidney failure that begins 1 day to several weeks after delivery following an uneventful gestation. Symptoms include oliguria or anuria, which progresses to azotemia, with complications of hemolytic anemia or coagulopathy. Treatment is supportive but aimed primarily at reducing blood pressure.

**idiopathic pulmonary fibrosis** [Gk, *idios,* own, *pathos,* disease; L, *pulmoneous,* the lungs, *fibra,* fiber],  a disorder of unknown cause characterized by fibrosis of the lungs. It may follow an earlier inflammation or disease, such as tuberculosis or pneumoconiosis.

**idiopathic pulmonary hemorrhage,**  bleeding in the lungs without a known cause. It may be a cause of secondary spontaneous pneumothorax.

**idiopathic reactive hypoglycemia,**  a condition of diminished blood glucose level that occurs after the ingestion of carbohydrates and has no known cause. It may be related to increased insulin sensitivity or excess counterregulatory hormone secretion or action.

**idiopathic respiratory distress syndrome.**  See **respiratory distress syndrome of the newborn.**

**idiopathic scoliosis,**  an abnormal condition characterized by a lateral curvature of the spine. It is the most common type of scoliosis, evident in 70% of all patients with scolio-

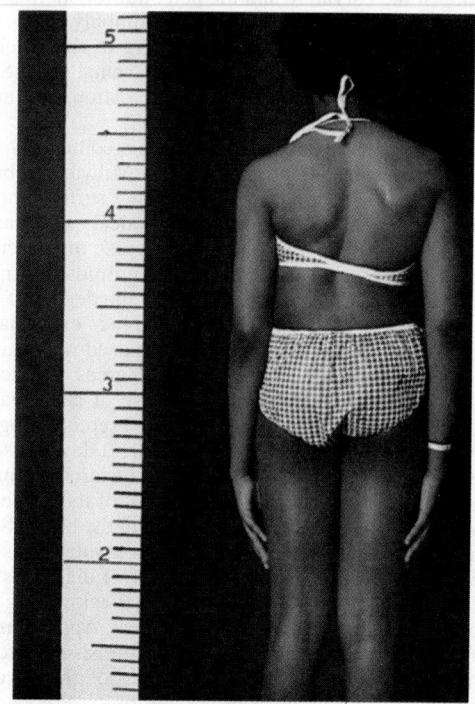

**Idiopathic scoliosis: scapular asymmetry**
*(Zitelli and Davis, 1997)*

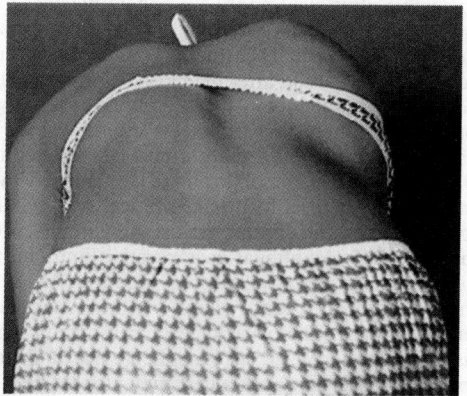

**Idiopathic scoliosis: rib hump deformity**
*(Zitelli and Davis, 1997)*

■ OBSERVATIONS: The most common type is the adolescent type. Early diagnosis is difficult because the associated curvature is often hidden by clothing. Preadolescent screening is encouraged in schools. The signs commonly associated with scoliosis include unlevel shoulders, a prominent scapula, a prominent breast, a prominent flank area, an unlevel or prominent hip, poor posture, and an obvious curvature. During diagnosis it is necessary to view the patient from the front and from the back and while the patient is bending. Other signs that may be associated with idiopathic scoliosis are occasional transient pain and fatigue and decreased pulmonary function. Radiographic films of the spine in the bending position are important in ascertaining the flexibility of the curvature and the potential for spontaneous correction. Neurologic deficits are commonly associated with severe curvature and vary according to the extent to which the curvature has impinged on the spinal cord. Some signs of such impingement are reflex, sensation, and motor alterations of the lower extremities.

■ INTERVENTIONS: Nonsurgical intervention commonly uses observation, an exercise program, and a Milwaukee brace. Observation and an exercise program often suffice; the observation is implemented by frequent physical examinations and radiographic monitoring of the progress of the curvature. Exercise programs are designed to promote the maximum correction possible, as indicated by the degree of flexibility shown in the initial radiographic examination. Observation and the exercise program are used with patients who have a curvature less than 15 to 20 degrees. Greater degrees of curvature usually require the use of a Milwaukee brace in addition to observation and an exercise program. The brace, which is usually worn 23 hours a day, is used to control the progress of the curvature. The exercise program is implemented when the adolescent is out of the brace, and additional exercises are performed while in the brace. Surgical intervention may be required if the curvature has progressed to 40 degrees or more at the time of diagnosis or if a slightly lesser degree of curvature exists with a high degree of rotational component or imbalance. Approximately 5% to 10% of patients with idiopathic scoliosis require surgical intervention, which involves fusing of the involved vertebrae to prevent progress of the deformity. Preoperative traction such as Cotrel traction and halo-femoral traction may also be used to encourage gradual tissue alterations and to decrease postoperative complications. The patient involved may be placed in Cotrel traction for a period of 5 to 10 days before surgery. If halo-femoral traction is used, the patient may be placed in traction 1 to 3 weeks before surgery. Some physicians apply a preoperative cast to their patients with idiopathic scoliosis to achieve immobilization and adjustment, especially if surgery must be postponed for a considerable period after diagnosis. Common surgical intervention techniques for this condition are the Harrington rod instrumentation technique and the Dwyer cable instrumentation technique; the former is more common. Initial postoperative immobilization is achieved with a posterior plaster shell, a Milwaukee brace, or a windowed cast. A Stryker frame, Foster frame, or CircOlectric bed may also be used. Additional postoperative immobilization by means of cast therapy is often required for 8 to 12 months or until the bony union of the fused area is absolutely ensured. The usual type of cast in this application is a Risser localizer cast, applied with a degree of traction. The Risser turnbuckle cast may also be used when instrumentation has not been used. A Milwaukee brace or a plastic body jacket may be used when less immobilization is desired.

**idiopathic steatorrhea** [Gk, *idios,* own, *pathos,* disease, *stear,* fat, *rhoia,* flow],   excess fat in the stools, particularly as in celiac disease in adults.

**idiopathic tetanus** [Gk, *idios,* own, *pathos,* disease, *tetanos,* convulsive tension],   a tetanus infection of unknown cause.

**idiopathic thrombocytopenic purpura (ITP),**   a deficiency of platelets that results in bleeding into the skin and other organs. **Acute ITP** is a disease of children that may follow a viral infection, lasts a few weeks to a few months, and usually has no residual effects. **Chronic ITP** is more common in adolescents and adults, begins more insidiously, and lasts longer. Antibodies to platelets are found in patients with ITP; the condition may be transmitted to the fetus if the mother is affected. Treatment includes hemophoresis, corticosteroids, therapeutic plasmapheresis, and splenectomy. See also **thrombocytopenia, thrombocytopenic purpura.**

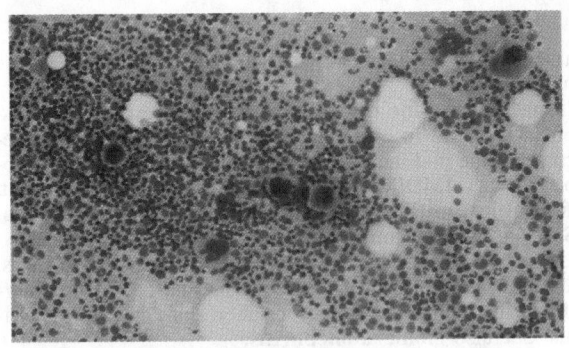

**Idiopathic thrombocytopenia purpura: bone marrow aspirate**
*(Zitelli and Davis, 1997)*

**idiopathic ventricular tachycardia,**   an accelerated heart rhythm (greater than 100/min) that originates in a focus within a ventricle but is of unknown cause.

**idiopathy** /id′ē·op′əthē/,   any primary disease that arises without an apparent cause. —**idiopathic,** *adj.*

**idiosyncrasy** /-sin′krəsē/ [Gk, *idios* + *synkrasis,* mixing together],   **1.** a physical or behavioral characteristic or manner that is unique to an individual or to a group. **2.** an individual's unique hypersensitivity to a particular drug, food, or other substance. Also called **idiocrasy** /id′ē·ok′rəsē/. See also **allergy. —idiosyncratic,** *adj.*

**idiosyncratic** /-sinkrat′ik/ [Gk, *idios,* own, *synkrasis,* mixing together],   pertaining to personal peculiarities or mannerisms.

**idiosyncratic drug** [Gk, *idios,* own, *sygkrasis,* mixing together; Fr, *drogue*],   an individual sensitivity to effects of a drug caused by inherited or other body constitution factors. In some cases a drug may have idiosyncratic effects that are contrary to the expected results.

**idiotope** /id′ē·ətōp′/,   an antigenic determinant on a variable region of an immunoglobulin molecule.

**idiotrophic** /-trof′ik/,   describing an organism capable of choosing its own food.

**idiot savant** /idē·ō′ savänt′/,   an individual with mental retardation who is nonetheless capable of performing certain unusual mental feats, primarily those involving music, puzzle solving, or manipulation of numbers.

**idiotype** /id′ē·ətīp′/ [Gk, *idios* + *typos,* mark],   the portion of an immunoglobulin molecule that confers the molecule's unique character, most often including its antigen-binding site.

**idioventricular** /-ventrik′yələr/ [Gk, *idios* + L, *ventriculus,* little belly],   originating in a ventricle.

**idioventricular rhythm** [Gk, *idios,* own; L, *ventriculus,* little belly; Gk, *rhythmos*],   an independent cardiac rhythm caused by a repeated discharge of impulses at a rate of less than 100/min from a focus within a ventricle.

**-idium,**   noun-forming suffix: *coracidium, parorchidium, thrombidium.*

**IDL,**   abbreviation for **intermediate-density lipoprotein.**

**IDM,**   abbreviation for *infant of a diabetic mother.*

**idoxuridine** /ī′doksyŏŏr′ədēn/,   an ophthalmic antiviral.

■ INDICATION: It is prescribed for the treatment of herpes simplex keratitis.

■ CONTRAINDICATIONS: Deep ulceration of the cornea or known hypersensitivity to this drug prohibits its use.

■ ADVERSE EFFECTS: Among the more serious adverse reactions are visual disturbances and eye discomfort.

**id reaction,**   the autosensitization resulting from any inflammatory condition that causes pruritus and vesicular lesions. These secondary lesions are caused by circulating antigens and are usually distant from the primary infection.

**I:E ratio,**   the ratio of the duration of inspiration to the duration of expiration. A range of 1:1.5 to 1:2 for an adult is considered acceptable for mechanical ventilation. Ratios of 1:1 or higher may cause hemodynamic complications, whereas ratios lower than 1:2 indicate lower mean airway pressure and fewer associated hazards.

**-ifene,**   combining form for antiestrogen products of the clomiphene and tamoxifen groups.

**-iform,**   suffix meaning 'in the form of': *amebiform, bulbiform, nucleiform.*

**Ig,**   abbreviation for **immunoglobulin.**

**IgA, IgD, IgE, IgG, IgM,**   abbreviations for **immunoglobulins A, D, E, G, and M.**

**IgA deficiency,**   a selective lack of immunoglobulin A, (IgA). The most common type of immunoglobulin deficiency, it occurs in about 1 in 400 individuals. IgA is a major antibody in the saliva and in the mucous membranes of the intestines and the bronchi. It protects against bacterial and viral infections. IgA deficiency is inheritied as  an autosomal-dominant or autosomal-recessive trait and is associated with autoimmune abnormalities. It is common in patients with rheumatoid arthritis and in those with systemic lupus erythematosus. Many individuals with this deficiency have normal numbers of peripheral blood lymphocytes with IgA receptors and normal amounts of other immunoglobulins. Normality accompanied by IgA deficiency suggests that the B lymphocytes of the patient may not secrete IgA. In some patients with this deficiency, T cells seem to depress the synthesis of IgA.

■ OBSERVATIONS: Common symptoms are respiratory allergies associated with chronic sinopulmonary infection; GI diseases, such as celiac disease and regional enteritis; autoimmune diseases, such as rheumatoid arthritis, systemic lupus erythematosus, and chronic hepatitis; and malignant tumors, such as squamous cell carcinoma of the lungs, reticulum cell sarcoma, and thymoma. However, symptoms of IgA deficiency are often lacking in patients whose immune system may compensate for low IgA levels with extra amounts of IgM. The age of onset varies. Some children with IgA deficiency may begin to synthesize IgA spontaneously when a recurrent infection wanes and their condition

improves. Diagnoses of IgA-deficient patients depend on the results of tests that commonly show normal IgE and IgM levels while IgA levels are below 5 mg/dL in serum. The cell-mediated immune response and circulating B cell levels often appear normal, although tests may indicate autoantibodies and antibodies against IgG, IgM, and cow's milk. T cell interferon production may be decreased in some patients with IgA deficiency, increasing the chances of infection.

■ INTERVENTIONS: There is no known cure for selective IgA deficiency. Treatment usually involves efforts to control associated diseases, such as respiratory and GI infections.

■ NURSING CONSIDERATIONS: The patient with IgA deficiency should not receive gamma globulin, because associated sensitization may cause anaphylaxis during administration of blood products. If patient requires a blood transfusion, the risk of any harmful reaction can be reduced by using washed red blood cells. Using the crossmatched blood of an IgA-deficient donor in such a transfusion is considered safer, since it completely eliminates the risk of an adverse reaction. IgA deficiency is a lifelong condition, and patients with this disorder are commonly instructed to identify its symptoms and to seek treatment promptly when the symptoms appear.

**IgD,**   abbreviation for **immunoglobulin D.**

**IgE,**   abbreviation for **immunoglobulin E.**

**IGF,**   abbreviation for **insulin-like growth factors.**

**IgG,**   abbreviation for **immunoglobulin G.**

**IgM,**   abbreviation for **immunoglobulin M.**

**ignipeditis** /ig′nēpedī′tis/ [L, *ignis,* fire, *pes,* foot],   a burning pain in the soles of the feet caused by peripheral neuritis.

**IGT,**   abbreviation for **impaired glucose tolerance.**

**I.H.,**   an abbreviation for *infectious hepatitis.* See **hepatitis A.**

**Ikwa fever.**   See **trench fever.**

**IL-1,**   abbreviation for **interleukin-1.**

**IL-2,**   abbreviation for **interleukin-2.**

**IL-3,**   abbreviation for **interleukin-3.**

**IL-4,**   abbreviation for **interleukin-4.**

**IL-5,**   abbreviation for **interleukin-5.**

**IL-6,**   abbreviation for **interleukin-6.**

**IL-7,**   abbreviation for **interleukin-7.**

**IL-8,**   abbreviation for **interleukin-8.**

**IL-9,**   abbreviation for **interleukin-9.**

**IL-10,**   abbreviation for **interleukin-10.**

**IL-11,**   abbreviation for **interleukin-11.**

**IL-12,**   abbreviation for **interleukin-12.**

**IL-13,**   abbreviation for **interleukin-13.**

**IL-14,**   abbreviation for **interleukin-14.**

**IL-15,**   abbreviation for **interleukin-15.**

**ILD,**   abbreviation for **interstitial lung disease.**

**Ile,**   abbreviation for **isoleucine.**

**ilea.**   See **ileum.**

**ileac, ileal.**   See **ileum.**

**ileal bypass** /il′ē·əl/ [L, *ileum,* intestine; AS, *bi,* near; Fr, *passer*],   a surgical procedure for treating obesity by anastomosing the upper portion of the small intestine to a part closer to the end of the small intestine, thereby bypassing much of the length of the ileum that normally absorbs nutrients. See also **intestinal bypass.**

**ileal conduit** [Fr, *conduire,* to guide],   a method of urinary diversion through intestinal tissue. The ureters are implanted in a section of dissected ileum. This section is sutured closed on one end; the other end is drawn through the abdominal wall (right lower quadrant) to create a stoma. The patient wears a pouch to collect the urine.

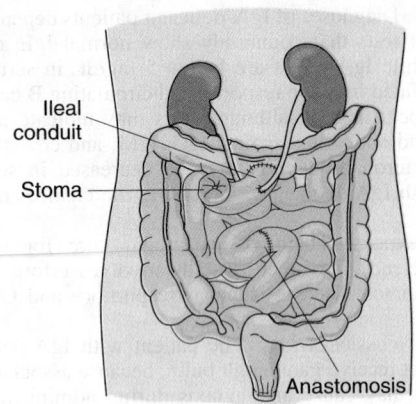

**Ileal conduit** *(Phipps, Sands, and Marek, 1999)*

**ileectomy** /il′ē-ek′təmē/, surgical removal of the ileum.

**ileitis** /il′ē-ī′tis/ [L, *ileum*, intestine; Gk, *itis*], inflammation of the ileum. See also **Crohn's disease.**

**ileo-**, prefix meaning 'the ileum': *ileocecum, ileorectostomy, ileotomy.*

**ileoanal anastomosis** /il′ē-ō-ā′nəl/, a surgical procedure in which the colon and rectum are removed but the anus and anal sphincter are left intact. An anastomosis is formed between the lower end of the small intestine and the anus. The operation is an alternative to proctocolectomy for the treatment of ulcerative colitis.

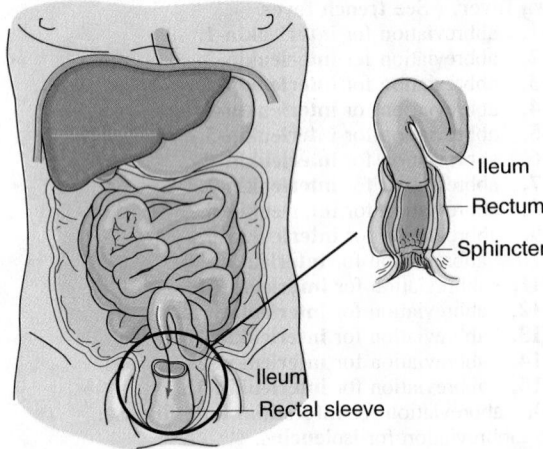

**Ileoanal anastomosis** *(Phipps, Sands, and Marek, 1999)*

**ileocecal** /il′ē-ōsē′kəl/ [L, *ileum*, intestine, *caecus*, blind], pertaining to both the ileum and the cecum and the region where they are joined. Also spelled **ileocaecal.**

**ileocecal incompetence.** See **incompetence.**

**ileocecal insufficiency.** See **insufficiency.**

**ileocecal syndrome,** appendicitis.

**ileocecal valve** [L, *ileum*, intestine, *caecus*, blind, *valvarum*, folding door], the sphincter muscle between the ileum of the small intestine and the cecum of the large intestine. It consists of two flaps that project into the lumen of the large intestine, immediately above the vermiform appendix, preventing food from reentering the small intestine.

**ileocecostomy.** See **cecoileostomy.**

**ileocolic node** /il′ē-ōkol′ik/ [L, *ileum* + Gk, *kolon,* colon; L, *nodus,* knot], a node in one of three groups of superior mesenteric lymph glands, forming a chain of approximately 15 nodes around the ileocolic (mesenteric) artery. They tend to form in two main groups, one near the duodenum, the other on the lower part of the ileocolic artery. The chain breaks into several groups where the artery divides into its terminal branches. The ileocolic nodes receive materials from the jejunum, ileum, cecum, vermiform appendix, ascending colon, and transverse colon. Their efferent vessels pass to the preaortic nodes. Compare **mesenteric node, mesocolic node.**

**ileocolitis** /-kōlī′tis/, an inflammation of the ileum and colon.

**ileocystoplasty** /-sis′təplas′tē/ [L, *ileum* + Gk, *kystis,* bag, *plassein,* to mold], a surgical procedure in which the bladder is reconstructed by using a segment of the ileum for the bladder wall.

**ileocystostomy** /-sistos′təmē/ [L, *ileum* + intestines; Gk, *kystis,* bag, *stoma, mouth],* a surgical procedure to form a passage to direct urine through the abdominal wall by using a segment of small intestine as a tube from the bladder.

**ileorectal** /-rek′təl/, pertaining to the ileum and rectum.

**ileosigmoidostomy** /-sig′moidos′təmē/, surgical formation of a passageway between the ileum and the colon.

**ileostomate** /il′ē-os′təmāt/, a person who has undergone an ileostomy.

**ileostomy** /il′ē-os′təmē/ [L, *ileum* + Gk, *stoma,* mouth, *temnein,* to cut], surgical formation of an opening of the ileum onto the surface of the abdomen, through which fecal matter is emptied. The operation is performed in advanced or recurrent ulcerative colitis, Crohn's disease, or cancer of the large bowel. A low-residue diet is given before surgery and is reduced to fluids 24 hours before surgery to decrease intestinal residue. Intestinal antibiotics are given to decrease the bacterial count. A nasogastric or intestinal tube is passed. The diseased portion of the large bowel is removed in a permanent ileostomy; occasionally the distal and proximal segments of bowel may be reconnected after ulcerated areas have healed. A loop of the proximal ileum is then drawn out onto the abdomen and sutured in place, and a stoma is formed. A pouch may be made with part of the terminal ileum, in which the open end is woven through the rectus

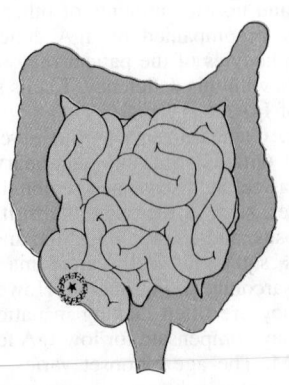

**Ileostomy** *(Potter and Perry, 2001)*

muscles to form a valve and then opens onto the abdomen. After surgery the patient wears a disposable bag to collect the semiliquid fecal matter, which begins to drain once peristalsis is restored and the nasogastric tube is removed. Since the secretions contain digestive enzymes that can ulcerate the skin around the stoma, the nurse ensures that nothing leaks from the bag. The nurse instructs the patient in how to apply and care for the stoma and the ileostomy bag. If a pouch is present, it is drained three or four times a day through a small irrigating catheter through the valve. Compare **colostomy**. See also **enterostomy, ostomy irrigation, stoma.**

**ileum** /il′ē·əm/, *pl.* **ilea** [L, intestine], the lower-third distal portion of the small intestine, extending from the jejunum to the cecum. Internally it has a few small circular folds and numerous clusters of lymphatic tissues. It ends in the right iliac fossa, opening into the medial side of the large intestine. See **ileocecal valve.** —**ileac, ileal,** *adj.*

**ileus** /il′ē·əs/ [L; Gk, *eilein,* to pack close together], an obstruction of the intestines, such as an adynamic ileus caused by immobility of the bowel or a mechanical ileus in which the intestine is blocked by mechanical means. See also **paralytic ileus.**

**ilia.** See **ilium.**

**-iliac,** suffix meaning 'the ilium': *occipitoiliac, subiliac, vertebroiliac.*

**iliac circumflex node** /il′ē·ak/ [L, *ilium* + flank; *circum,* around, *flectere,* to bend, *nodus,* knot], a node in one of the seven clusters of parietal lymph nodes of the abdomen. This node is one of a group found along the course of the deep iliac circumflex vessels. Compare **common iliac node, external iliac node, internal iliac node.** See also **lymph, lymphatic system, lymph node.**

**iliac crest** [L, *ilia,* intestines; ME, *creste*], the upper elevated margins of the ilium.

**iliac fascia,** the portion of the endoabdominal fascia that is attached with the iliacus to the crest of the ilium and passes under the inguinal ligament into the thigh.

**iliac horns,** accessory bony spurs on the posterior of the ilium, one of the symptoms of nail-patella syndrome.

**iliac region.** See **inguinal region.**

**iliacus** /ilī′əkəs/ [L, *ilium,* flank], a flat triangular muscle that covers the inner curved surface of the iliac fossa. It arises from the inner aspect of the superior iliac crest, from the anterior and the iliolumbar ligaments, and from the sacrum. It joins the psoas major to form the iliopsoas at the inguinal ligament. The iliacus is innervated by branches of the femoral nerve that contain fibers from the second and third lumbar nerves. It acts to flex and laterally rotate the thigh. Compare **psoas major, psoas minor.**

**ilio-,** combining form meaning 'ilium or flank': *iliocostal, iliolumbar, iliometer.*

**iliofemoral** /il′ē·ōfem′ərəl/, pertaining to the ilium and femur.

**iliofemoral ligament** [L, *ilium* + flank, *femur,* thigh, *ligamentum*], a triangular band of connective tissue attached by its apex to the anterior inferior spine of the ilium and acetabular margin and by its base to the intertrochanteric line of the femur.

**iliofemoral thrombosis,** an abnormal vascular condition in which a clot develops in the iliofemoral circulation.

**ilioinguinal** /il′ē·ō·ing′gwinəl/ [L, *ilium* + *inguen,* groin], pertaining to the hip and inguinal regions.

**iliolumbar ligament** /-lum′bər/ [L, *ilium* + *lumbus,* loin, *ligare,* to bind], one of a pair of ligaments forming part of the connection between the vertebral column and the pelvis. Each iliolumbar ligament attaches to a transverse process of

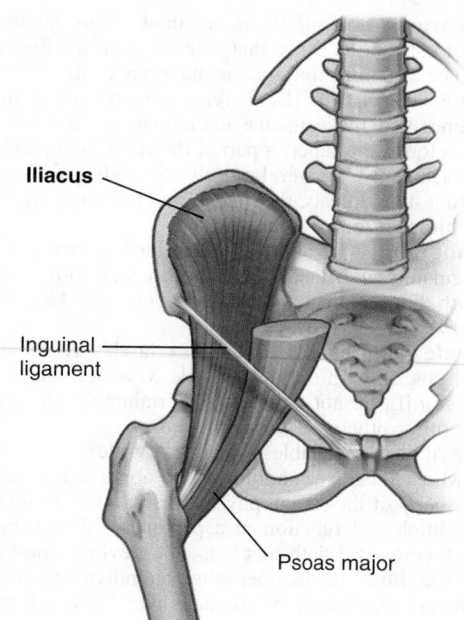

**Iliacus muscle**

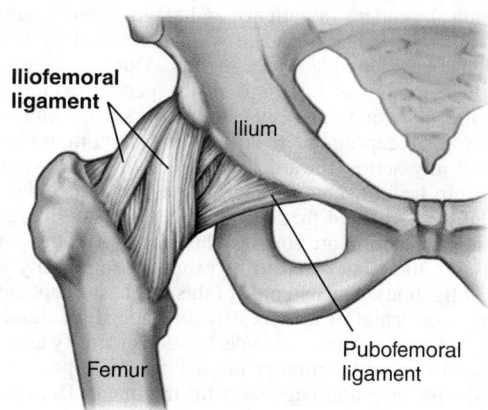

**Iliofemoral ligament**

the fifth lumbar vertebra and laterally to the ileum and inferiorly passes to the base of the sacrum, where it blends with the sacroiliac ligament.

**iliopectineal line** /- pek′tənəl/ [L, *ilium* + *pectus,* breast, *linea*], a bony ridge on the inner surface of the ilium and pubic bones that divides the true and false pelves. Also called **brim of true pelvic cavity, inlet.**

**iliopsoas** /il′ē·ōsō′əs/ [L, *ilium* + Gk, *psoa,* loin muscle], one of the pair of muscle complexes that flex the thigh and the lumbar vertebral column, consisting of the psoas major, the psoas minor, and the iliacus; the psoas minor is often absent.

**iliopsoas abscess** [L, *ilium,* intestine], an abscess, possibly tuberculous in origin, that spreads from the thoracic or lumbar spine to the upper leg muscles.

**iliotibial tract** /-tib′ē·əl/ [L, *ilium,* flank, *tibia,* shinbone], a band of connective tissue that extends from the iliac crest to the knee and links the gluteus maximus to the tibia.

**ilium** /il′ē·əm/, *pl.* **ilia** [L, flank], the uppermost of the three bones that make up the innominate bone (hipbone). The ilium forms the superior part of the acetabulum and provides attachment for several muscles, including the obturator internus, the gluteals, the iliacus, and the sartorius. Compare **ischium, pubis. —iliac,** *adj.*

**illegal abortion,** an abortion performed contrary to the laws regulating abortion. Illegal abortions are often associated with life-threatening complications. See also **septic abortion.**

**illegitimate** /il′ejit′imit/ [L, *in,* not, *lex,* law], **1.** not authorized by law. **2.** born out of wedlock. **3.** abnormal.

**illicit** /ilis′it/ [L, *in,* not, *lex,* law], pertaining to an act that is unlawful or otherwise not permitted.

**illiterate** /ilit′ərit/, unable to read and write.

**illness** [ME, unhealthy condition], an abnormal process in which aspects of the social, physical, emotional, or intellectual condition and function of a person are diminished or impaired, compared with that person's previous condition.

**illness behavior,** the manner in which individuals monitor the structure and functions of their own bodies, interpret symptoms, take remedial action, and make use of health care facilities.

**illness experience,** the process of being ill. A commonly used model is Suchman's stages of illness, comprising five stages: stage I, experiencing a symptom; stage II, assuming a sick role; stage III, making contact for health care; stage IV, being dependent (a patient); and stage V, recovering or being rehabilitated. Each stage is characterized by certain decisions, behaviors, and end points. During stage I, in which a symptom is experienced, the person decides that something is wrong and seeks a remedy. Stage I ends with the person's accepting the reality of the symptom, no longer delaying any action toward help or denying the symptom (flight into health). During stage II the person decides that the illness is real and that care is necessary. Advice, guidance, and validation are sought. This stage gives the person permission to act sick and to be excused temporarily from usual obligations. The outcome of this stage is acceptance of the role—or denial of its necessity. In stage III professional advice is sought; authoritative declarations identify and validate the illness and legitimize the sick role. The person usually asks for help and negotiates for treatment. Denial may still occur, and the patient may "shop" further for medical care or may accept the illness, the medical authority, and the plan for treatment. In stage IV, professional treatment is performed and accepted by the person, who is now perceived as a patient. At any time during this stage the dependent patient may experience ambivalent feelings and may decide to reject the treatment, the caregiver, and the illness. More often care is accepted with ambivalence. The patient has a particular need to be informed and to be given emotional support during this stage. During stage V the patient relinquishes the sick role. The usual tasks and roles are reassumed to the greatest degree possible. Some people do not willingly give up the sick role, becoming in their own eyes chronically ill, or they may, for secondary gain, malinger, acting sick. Most people accept recovery and work toward rehabilitation.

**illness prevention,** a system of health education programs and activities directed to protecting patients from real or potential health threats, minimizing risk factors, and promoting healthy behavior.

**illumination** /iloo′minā′shən/ [L, *illuminare,* to make light], the lighting up of a part of the body or of an object under a microscope for the purpose of examination. **—illuminate,** *v.*

**illusion** /iloo′zhən/ [L, *illudere,* to mock], a false interpretation of an external sensory stimulus, usually visual or auditory, such as a mirage in the desert or voices on the wind. Compare **delusion, hallucination.**

**Ilopan,** trademark for a precursor of coenzyme A (dexpanthenol).

**Ilosone,** trademark for an antibacterial (erythromycin estolate).

**im-,** prefix in chemistry indicating the bivalent group NH: *imadyl, imide, imperialine.*

**IM,** abbreviation for *intramuscular.*

**I.M.A.,** abbreviation for **Industrial Medical Association.**

**image** /im′ij/ [L, *imago,* likeness], **1.** a representation or visual reproduction of the likeness of someone or something, such as a painting, photograph, or sculpture. **2.** an optic representation of an object, such as that produced by refraction or reflection. **3.** a person or thing that closely resembles another; semblance. **4.** a mental picture, representation, idea, or concept of an objective reality. **5.** (in psychology) a mental representation of something previously perceived and subsequently modified by other experiences, resulting from intrapsychic or extrapsychic stimuli, or both.

**image acquisition time,** the time required to acquire the data used in producing a magnetic resonance image. It does not include the time involved in constructing the image from the data. In comparing sequential plane imaging and volume imaging techniques, the equivalent image acquisition time per slice must be considered, as well as the actual image acquisition time.

**image foreshortening,** a type of shape distortion in which a radiographic image appears shorter and wider than the actual structure it represents. It results from misalignment of the x-ray tube relative to the patient, of the patient relative to the film, or of the tube relative to the film.

**image format,** the manner in which a CT image is stored, such as on a computer disk, magnetic tape, or film.

**image intensifier,** an electronic device used to produce a fluoroscopic image with a low-radiation exposure. A beam of x-rays passing through the patient is converted into a pattern of electrons in a vacuum tube. The electrons are accelerated and concentrated onto a small fluorescent screen, where they present a bright image, which is generally displayed on a video monitor.

**image matrix,** an arrangement of columns or rows of cells, or pixels, forming a digital image.

**imagery** /im′ijrē/ [L, *imago*], (in psychiatry) the formation of mental concepts, figures, ideas; any product of the imagination. An imagery technique is applied therapeutically to decrease anxiety. See also **guided imagery.**

**imagination** /imaj′inā′shən/ [L, *imaginare,* picture to oneself], **1.** the ability to form, or the act or process of forming, mental images or conscious concepts of things that are not immediately available to the senses. **2.** (in psychology) the ability to reproduce images or ideas stored in the memory by the stimulation or suggestion of associated ideas or to regroup former ideas and concepts to form new images and ideas concerned with a particular goal or problem. See also **fantasy.**

**imaging** /im′ijing/ [L, *imago*], the formation of a mental picture or representation of someone or something using the imagination. See also **fantasy.**

**imago** /imā′gō/ [L, likeness], (in analytic psychology) an unconscious, usually idealized mental image of a significant individual, such as one's mother, in a person's early formative years. See also **identification.**

**imbalance** /imbal'əns/ [L, *im*, not, *bilanx*, having two scales], **1.** lack of balance between opposing muscle groups, such as in the imbalance of extraocular muscles leading to strabismus. **2.** abnormal balance of fluid and electrolytes in the body tissues. **3.** unequal distribution of subjects in a population group, such as the only girl in a large family of boys. **4.** pertaining to a person with mental abilities that are remarkable in one area but deficient in others, as an idiot savant.

**imbedded tooth.** See **embedded tooth.**

**imbricate** /im'brikāt/ [L, *imbrex*, roofing tile], to build a surface with overlapping layers of material. Surgeons may imbricate with layers of tissue when closing a wound or other opening in a body part. —**imbrication**, *n.*

**IMDD,** abbreviation for **idiopathic midline destructive disease.**

**Imferon,** trademark for an injectable hematinic (iron dextran).

**imide-, imido-,** combining form indicating the presence in a chemical compound of the bivalent group NH: *imidogen.*

**imiglucerase,** an analog of a human enzyme produced by recombinant deoxyribonuclease technology.
■ INDICATIONS: It is prescribed as enzyme replacement therapy for patients with type I Gaucher disease.
■ CONTRAINDICATIONS: There are no known contraindications to the use of imiglucerase by injection.
■ ADVERSE EFFECTS: The side effects most often reported include headache, nausea, abdominal discomfort, dizziness, and rash.

**imino-,** combining form indicating the presence of the bivalent group NH attached to a nonacid radical: *iminourea.*

**iminoglycinuria** /im'inōglī'sinŏŏr'ē-ə/, a benign familial condition characterized by the abnormal urinary excretion of the imino acids glycine, proline, and hydroxyproline.

**imipenem-cilastatin sodium** /im'ipē'nəm sil'əstat'in/, a broad-spectrum parenteral antibiotic.
■ INDICATIONS: It is prescribed for the treatment of infections caused by susceptible organisms in the lower respiratory or urinary tracts, skin, abdomen, reproductive organs, bones, or joints. It is also used in the treatment of endocarditis and septicemia.
■ CONTRAINDICATIONS: This product is not recommended for children. Caution should be used in administering the drug to patients with pseudomembranous colitis, hypersensitivity reactions, or a history of seizures.
■ ADVERSE EFFECTS: The most common adverse reactions are phlebitis, thrombophlebitis, nausea, vomiting, diarrhea, rash, fever, and central nervous system symptoms.

**imipramine hydrochloride** /imip'rəmēn/, a tricyclic antidepressant.
■ INDICATION: It is prescribed in the treatment of mental depression.
■ CONTRAINDICATIONS: Concomitant administration of monoamine oxidase inhibitors, recent myocardial infarction, cardiovascular disease or seizure disorder, or known hypersensitivity to this drug or to other tricyclic medication prohibits its use.
■ ADVERSE EFFECTS: Among the more serious adverse reactions are sedation, GI disturbances, and cardiovascular and neurologic reactions. It should not be withdrawn abruptly. This drug interacts with many other drugs.

**immature baby** /iməchŏŏr'/ [L, *im*, not, *maturus*, ripe], a term sometimes applied to an infant who weighs less than 1134 g (2.5 lb) and who is significantly underdeveloped at birth.

**immature cataract** [L, *im* + *maturus*, ripe; Gk, *katarrhaktes*], a cataract at an early stage of development when the lens, partially opaque, absorbs fluid and increases by swelling. Only part of the lens is opaque.

**immature erythrocyte** [L, *im* + *maturus*, ripe; Gk, *erythros*, red, *kytos*, cell], any of the intermediate blood cells between the hemocytoblasts and nonnucleated red blood cells. They may be found in the blood circulation after birth of the fetus.

**immediate auscultation** /imē'dē·it/ [L, *im* + *medius*, middle, *auscultare*, to listen], a method of examining a patient by placing an ear or stethoscope on the skin directly over the body part being studied.

**immediate automatism,** a state in which a person acts spontaneously and automatically and later has no recollection of the behavior.

**immediate denture** [L, *im* + *medius* + *dens*, tooth], a removable artificial denture that is placed in the mouth to maintain normal appearance and the ability to chew food. It may be complete or partial.

**immediate hypersensitivity,** an allergic reaction that occurs within minutes after exposure to an allergen and is mediated by antibodies. Compared **delayed hypersensitivity.**

**immediate hypersensitivity reaction,** type I hypersensitivity reaction; see **hypersensitivity reaction.**

**immediate percussion.** See **percussion.**

**immediate postoperative fit prosthesis (IPOF),** a temporary or preparatory prosthesis, such as a pylon.

**immediate posttraumatic automatism,** a posttraumatic state in which a person acts spontaneously and automatically and later has no recollection of the behavior.

**immersion** /imur'zhən/ [L, *im* + *mergere*, to dip], the placing of a body or an object into water or other liquid so that it is completely covered by the liquid. —**immerse**, *v.*

**immersion foot,** an abnormal condition of the feet characterized by damage to the muscles, nerves, skin, and blood vessels, caused by prolonged exposure to dampness or by prolonged immersion in cold water. See also **frostbite, trench foot.**

**Immerslund-Gräsbeck syndrome,** a familial form of megaloblastic anemia and cobalamin deficiency. It is characterized by selective intestinal malabsorption of vitamin $B_{12}$, uninfluenced by intrinsic factor. About 90% of the cases are associated with a mild, nonspecific form of proteinuria.

**imminent abortion.** See **inevitable abortion.**

**immiscible** /imis'əbəl/ [L, *im* + *miscere*, to mix], not capable of being mixed, such as oil and water. Compare **miscible.**

**immobility consequences: physiological,** a nursing outcome from the Nursing Outcomes Classification (NOC) defined as extent of compromise in physiological functioning due to impaired physical mobility. See also **Nursing Outcomes Classification.**

**immobility consequences: psycho-cognitive,** a nursing outcome from the Nursing Outcomes Classification (NOC) defined as extent of compromise in psycho-cognitive functioning due to impaired physical mobility. See also **Nursing Outcomes Classification.**

**immobilization** /imō'bəlīzā'shən/, **1.** fixation of a body part so that it cannot move during surgery or after setting of a fracture. **2.** prolonged inactivity of an individual.

**immobilization test,** a procedure for identifying antibodies to motile microorganisms by measuring the ability of the antibodies to restrict the motility of the microorganisms.

**immotile cilia syndrome** /imō'til/ [L, *im*, *motilis*, movable, *cilia*, eyelashes; Gk, *syn*, together, *dromos*, course], a condition in which cilia, the hairlike processes of epithelial cells, fail to function normally. As a result, the patient has difficulty in filtering dust and other airborne debris from the respiratory system. See also **Kartagener's syndrome.**

**immune** /imyo͞on'/ [L, *immunis,* free from], being protected against infective or allergic diseases by a system of antibody molecules and related resistance factors.

**immune body.** See **antibody.**

**immune cytolysis,** cell destruction mediated by a specific antibody, which activate the complement system, resulting in rupture of the cell membrane.

**immune deviation,** modification of an immune response to an antigen caused by a previous exposure to the same antigen.

**immune elimination,** 1. a method for determining antibody response by measuring the rate of removal of labeled antigens from the circulation. 2. an accelerated removal of antigens as a result of their binding to antibodies.

**immune exclusion,** the prevention of an antigen from entering the body by a specific immune response.

**immune gamma globulin,** passive immunizing agent obtained from pooled human plasma. Also called **immune globulin.** See also **immunoglobulin G.**

■ INDICATIONS: It is prescribed for immunization against measles, poliomyelitis, chickenpox, serum hepatitis after transfusion, hepatitis A, agammaglobulinemia, and hypogammaglobulinemia.

■ CONTRAINDICATION: Known hypersensitivity to gamma globulins prohibits its use.

■ ADVERSE EFFECTS: Among the more serious adverse reactions are pain and inflammation at the site of injection, allergic reactions, and headache.

**immune globulin.** See **immune gamma globulin.**

**immune hemolysis,** the destruction of red blood cells caused by the formation of specific antigen-antibody complexes in the presence of complement.

**immune human globulin,** a sterile solution of globulins that is used as a passive immunizing agent and derived from adult human blood.

**immune hypersensitivity control,** a nursing outcome from the Nursing Outcomes Classification (NOC) defined as extent to which inappropriate immune responses are suppressed. See also **Nursing Outcomes Classification.**

**immune neutropenia,** neutrophil destruction caused by antibodies specific for neutrophil antigenic determinants, as often occurs in autoimmune diseases.

**immune protein** [L, *immunis,* free from; Gk, *proteios,* first rank], a protein, such as an antibody or antitoxin, that contributes to the immunity of a host.

**immune reaction.** See **immune response.**

**immune recognition,** the activation of a T or B cell by an antigen.

**immune response,** a defense function of the body that protects the body against invading pathogensm foreign tissuesm and malignancies. It consists of the humoral immune response and the cell-mediated immune response. In the humoral immune response, B lymphocytes produce antibodies that react with specific antigens. The antigen-antibody reactions activate the complement cascade, which causes the lysis of cells bearing those antigens. The humoral response may begin immediately on invasion by an antigen or up to 48 hours later. In the cell-mediated immune response, T lymphocytes mobilize tissue macrophages in the presence of foreign antigens. Also called **immune reaction.** See also **cell-mediated immune response, humoral immunity, immune system.**

**immune serum.** See **antiserum.**

**immune serum globulin.** See **immunoglobulin.**

**immune status,** a nursing outcome from the Nursing Outcomes Classification (NOC) defined as adequacy of natural and acquired appropriately targeted resistance to internal and external antigens. See also **Nursing Outcomes Classification.**

**immune surveillance.** See **immunologic surveillance.**

**immune system,** a system of tissues and organs that protects the body against pathogenic organisms and other foreign bodies. The principal components of the immune system include the bone marrow, the thymus, and the lymphoid tissues. The system also uses peripheral organs, such as the lymph nodes, the spleen, and the lymphatic vessels. The immune system protects the body initially by creating local barriers and inflammation. The local barriers provide chemical and mechanical defenses through the skin, the mucous membranes, and the conjunctiva. Inflammation draws polymorphonuclear leukocytes and neutrophils to the site of injury, where these phagocytes engulf the invading pathogens. If these first-line defenses fail or are inadequate to protect the body, the humoral immune response and the cell-mediated immune response are activated. See also **immune response.**

**immunity** /imyo͞o'nitē/ [L, *immunis,* free], 1. (in civil law) exemption from a duty or an obligation generally required by law, as an exemption from taxation or from penalty for wrongdoing or protection against liability. 2. the quality of being insusceptible to or unaffected by a particular disease or condition. Kinds of immunity are **active immunity** and **passive immunity. —immune,** *adj.*

**immunization** /im'yənīzā'shən/ [L, *immunis,* free], a process by which resistance to an infectious disease is induced or augmented.

**immunization behavior,** a nursing outcome from the Nursing Outcomes Classification (NOC) defined as actions to obtain immunization to prevent a communicable disease. See also **Nursing Outcomes Classification.**

**immunization/vaccination management,** a nursing intervention from the Nursing Interventions Classification

**Comparison of humoral immunity and cell-mediated immunity**

| Characteristics | Humoral immunity | Cell-mediated immunity |
|---|---|---|
| Cells involved | B lymphocytes | T lymphocytes, macrophages |
| Products | Antibodies | Sensitized T cells, lymphokines |
| Memory cells | Present | Present |
| Reaction | Immediate | Delayed |
| Protection | Bacteria | Fungus |
| | Viruses (extracellular) | Viruses (intracellular) |
| | | Tumor cells |
| | Respiratory and gastrointestinal pathogens | |
| Examples | Anaphylactic shock | Tuberculosis |
| | Atopic diseases | Fungal infections |
| | Transfusion reaction | Contact dermatitis |
| | Neutralization of exotoxins | Graft rejection |
| | Bacterial infections | Destruction of cancer cells |

From Lewis SM, Heitkemper MM, Dirksen SR: *Medical-surgical nursing: assessment and management of clinical problems,* ed 5, St Louis, 2000, Mosby.

(NIC) defined as monitoring immunization status, facilitating access to immunizations, and provision of immunizations to prevent communicable disease. See also **Nursing Interventions Classification.**

**immunoabsorbent** /im′yənō′absôr′bənt/, a gel or other inert substance used to absorb antibodies from a solution or to purify them.

**immunoabsorption** /im′yənō′absôrp′shən/, **1.** removal of a specific group of antibodies by antigens. **2.** removal of antigen by interaction with specific antibodies.

**immunoadsorbent** /im′yənō′adsôr′bənt/, an insoluble preparation of antigens or antibodies used to bind homologous antibodies or antigens and remove them from a mixture of substances.

**immunoassay** /im′yənō·as′ā/ [L, *immunis* + Fr, *essayer,* to try], a competitive-binding assay in which the binding protein is an antibody.

**immunobead** /im′yənōbēd′/, a tiny, inert plastic sphere coated with antigens or antibody, used for immunoassays, such as the isolation of B cells from T cells.

**immunoblastic lymphoma** /-blas′tik/, a proliferation of immunoblasts involving the lymph nodes.

**immunoblotting** /-blot′ing/, a method for identifying antigens. The antigens are allowed to adhere to cellulose sheets where they bond nonspecifically, and are identified by staining with labeled antibodies. The method is also used to detect monoclonal proteins. See also **Western blot test.**

**immunochemistry,** the study of the chemical properties of antigens and antibodies, complement, and T cell receptors.

**immunochemotherapy** /-kem′ōther′əpē/, a combination of biotherapy and chemotherapy. See also **chemotherapy, immunotherapy.**

**immunocompetence** /-kom′pətəns/, the ability of an immune system to mobilize and deploy its antibodies and other responses to stimulation by an antigen. Immunocompetence may be weakened in older individuals as a result of age-related attenuation in T cell function. It may also be diminished by viruses, radiation, and chemotherapeutic drugs.

**immunocomplex,** a multimolecular complex formed when an antibody binds to a specific antigen. The complex is capable of activating complements and is a factor in diseases such as arthritis, vasculitis, serum sickness, and glomerulonephritis.

**immunocomplex assay,** a laboratory assessment of the amounts of components in multimolecular antigen-antibody complexes. The assay is used in various diagnostic tests for collagen-vascular disorders, glomerulonephritis, vasculitis, hepatitis, and neoplastic diseases.

**immunocomplex hypersensitivity** [L, *immunis,* free; *complexus,* embrace; Gk, *hyper,* excess; L, *sentire,* to feel], a complement-dependent, immediate-acting, humoral hypersensitivity to certain soluble antigens. It occurs when antibodies (immunoglobulins G or M) bind to circulating antigens, forming immune complexes. These complexes are deposited in tissues, such as blood vessels and renal glomeruli. Augmented by complement activation, they induce injury or dysfunctional responses in those tissues. Immune complex hypersensitivity is a dynamic, ever-changing process. Also called **type III hypersensitivity.** Compare **anaphylactic hypersensitivity, cell-mediated immune response, cytotoxic anaphylaxis.**

**immunocomplex−mediated hypersensitivity reaction,** type III hypersensitivity reaction; see **hypersensitivity reaction.**

**immunocompromised** /-kom′prəmīzd′/ [L, *immunis,* free from, *compromittere,* to promise mutually], pertaining to

an immune response that has been weakened by a disease or an immunosuppressive agent.

**immunocompromised host,** an individual whose immune response is weakened as a result of an immunodeficiency disorder or exposure to immunosuppressive drugs or irradiation.

**immunodeficiency.** See **dysgammaglobulinemia.**

**immunodeficiency disease** /-difish′ənsē/, any of a group of diseases caused by a defect in the immune system and generally characterized by susceptibility to infections and chronic diseases. Such diseases are sometimes classified as B cell (antibody) deficiencies, T cell (cellular) deficiencies, combined T and B cell deficiencies, defects of cell movement, and defects of microbicidal activity. See also **severe combined immunodeficiency disease (SCID).**

**immunodeficient** /-difish′ənt/ [L, *immunis* + *de,* from, *facere,* to make], pertaining to an abnormal condition of the immune system in which cellular or humoral immunity is inadequate and resistance to infection is decreased. Kinds of immunodeficient conditions include **hypogammaglobulinemia** and **lymphoid aplasia.**

**immunodiagnosis.** See **serologic diagnosis.**

**immunodiagnostic** /-dī′əgnos′tik/ [L, *immunis* + Gk, *dia,* through, *gnosis* knowledge], pertaining to or characterizing a diagnosis based on an antigen-antibody reaction. In many cases a tumor releases a discrete antigenic substance into the blood; detection of a particular antigen can provide an immunodiagnostic sign of the presence of the tumor associated with that antigen.

**immunodiffusion** /-difyo͞o′zhən/ [L, *immunis* + *diffundere,* to spread], a technique for the identification and quantification of any of the immunoglobulins. It is based on the presence of a visible precipitate that results from an antigen-antibody combination under certain circumstances. **Gel diffusion** is a technique that involves evaluation of the precipitin reaction in a clear gel, seen when an antigen placed in a hole in the agarose diffuses evenly into the medium. An obvious ring forms where the antigen meets the antibody. **Electroimmunodiffusion** is a gel diffusion to which an electrical field is applied, accelerating the reaction. **Double gel diffusion** is a technique that permits identification of antibodies in mixed specimens. In an agar plate antigen is placed in one well, antibody in another. Antigen and antibody diffuse out of their wells. In mixed antigen specimens each antigen-antibody combination forms a separate line;

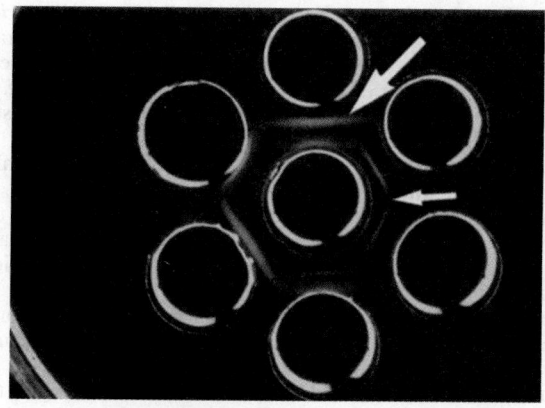

**Immunodiffusion** *(Murray et al, 1998)*

observation of the location, shape, and thickness of a line permits identification and quantification of the antibody.

**immunoelectroadsorption** /im'yənō'ilek'trō·adsôrp'shən/, an antibody assay technique in which antigens are adsorbed onto a metal-coated glass slide with an electric current. Serum containing antibodies is then applied to the slide.

**immunoelectrodiffusion.** See **immunodiffusion.**

**immunoelectron microscopy** /im'yənō'ilek'tron/, electron microscopy of specimens labeled with antibodies that have been conjugated with gold. The gold makes the antibody labels electron-dense.

**immunoelectrophoresis** /-ilek'trōfôrē'sis/ [L, *immunis* + Gk, *elektron,* amber, *pherein,* to bear], a technique that combines electrophoresis and immunodiffusion to separate and allow identification of complex proteins. The proteins in the test serum are spread out in agar and separated by electrophoresis. Wells or troughs are then cut into the agar, and parts of antibody are placed in the troughs and allowed to diffuse toward the separated proteins. A visible precipitin will form in a series of arcs in the agar when an antigen-antibody reaction occurs. The shape and location of each arc are specific for known proteins. Unusual arcs are representative of abnormal or unknown protein. Although the density of the precipitation corresponds to the concentration of protein in each electrophoretic band, immunoelectrophoresis does not accurately quantify the amount of protein in the test serum. —**immunoelectrophoretic,** *adj.*

**immunoenhancement** /im'yənō'enhans'mənt/, the augmentation of immune responsiveness by immunization or other means.

**immunoferritin** /-fer'itin/, an antibody labeled with ferritin used to identify specific antigens in electron microscopy.

**immunoferritin technique,** a method of labeling antibody molecules with ferritin, an electron-dense material. The ferritin renders the sites of antibody attachment visible in electron microscopy.

**immunofixation** /-fiksā'shən/, a process by which antigens in a protein mixture are separated on an electrophoretic gel and identified by the application of labeled antibodies.

**immunofluorescence** /- flōōres'əns/ [L, *immunis* + *fluere,* to flow], a technique used for the rapid identification of an antigen by exposing it to known antibodies tagged with the fluorescent dye fluorescein and observing the characteristic antigen-antibody reaction of precipitation. As the fluorescent antibody reacts with its specific antigen, the precipitate appears luminous in the ultraviolet light projected by a fluorescent microscope. Many of the most common infectious organisms can be identified by this technique. Among them are *Candida albicans, Haemophilus influenzae, Neisseria gonorrhoeae, Shigella, Staphylococcus aureus,* and several viruses, including rabies virus and many enteroviruses. See also **fluorescent microscopy.** —**immunofluorescent,** *adj.*

**immunofluorescence test.** See **fluorescent antibody test.**

**immunofluorescent.** See **immunofluorescence.**

**immunofluorescent microscopy.** See **fluorescent microscopy, immunofluorescence.**

**immunogen** /imyōō'nəjən/ [L, *immunis* + Gk, *genein,* to produce], any agent or substance capable of provoking an immune response or producing immunity. —**immunogenic,** *adj.*

**immunogenetics** /-jənet'iks/, a branch of medicine concerned with the role of genetics in tissue transplantation and immunologic response.

**immunogenicity** /-jənis'itē/, the ability of an antigen to induce a specific immune response. —**immunogenic,** *adj.*

**immunoglobulin (Ig)** /-glob'yəlin/ [L, *immunis* + *globus,*

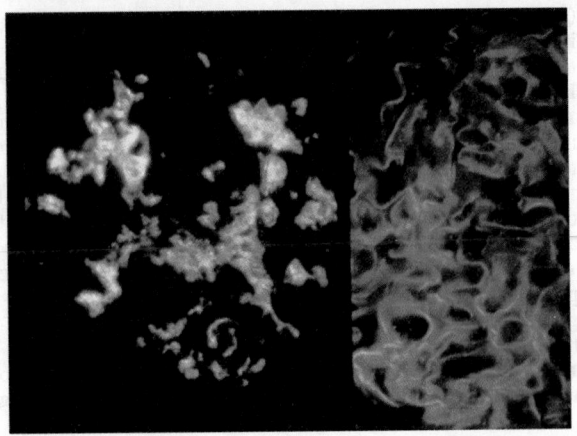

**Immunofluorescence** *(Mudge-Grout, 1992)*

small sphere], any of five structurally distinct classes of proteins that function as antibodies in the serum and external secretions of the body. In response to specific antigens, immunoglobulins are formed in the bone marrow, spleen, and all lymphoid tissues except the thymus. Classes of immunoglobulins are **IgA, IgD, IgE, IgG,** and **IgM.** Also called **immune serum globulin.** See also **antibody, antigen, immunity.**

**immunoglobulin A (IgA),** one of the most prevalent of the five classes of antibodies produced by the body. It is found in all secretions of the body and is the major antibody in the tears, and saliva, mucous membranes lining the intestines and bronchi. IgA combines with a protein in the mucosa and defends body surfaces by seeking out foreign microorganisms and triggering an antigen-antibody reaction. The normal concentration of IgA in serum is 50 to 250 mg/dL. Compare **immunoglobulin D, immunoglobulin E, immunoglobulin G, immunoglobulin M.** See also **IgA deficiency.**

**immunoglobulin D (IgD),** one of the five classes of antibodies produced by the body. It is a found in small amounts in serum tissue. Although its precise function is not known,

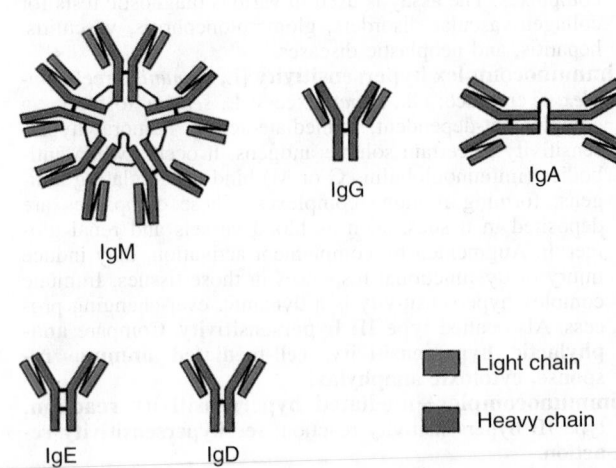

**Immunoglobulins** *(Thibodeau and Patton, 1999/Rolin Graphics)*

**Properties of immunoglobulin classes**

| Property | Immunoglobulin class | | | | |
|---|---|---|---|---|---|
| | IgG | IgM | IgA | IgE | IgD |
| Physiochemical Principal site found | Internal body fluids | Serum | Serum and exocrine secretions | Tissue bound | Bound to lymphocyte surface |
| Fixed complement | Yes | Yes | No | No | No |
| Crosses placenta | Yes | No | No | No | No |
| Principal functions | Agglutination, detoxification, virus neutralization; enhancement of phagocytosis | Agglutination, cytolysis; enhancement of phagocytosis | Protection of mucosal surfaces | Mediation of immediate type of hypersensitivity | Control of lymphocytic activation and suppression |

IgD increases in quantity during allergic reactions to milk, insulin, penicillin, and various toxins. The normal concentration of IgD in serum is 0.5 to 3 mg/dL. Compare **immunoglobulin A, immunoglobulin E, immunoglobulin G, immunoglobulin M.**

**immunoglobulin E (IgE),** one of the five classes of antibodies produced by the body. It is concentrated in the lungs, skin, and mucous membranes. It provides the primary defense against environmental antigens and is believed to be responsive to immunoglobulin A. IgE reacts with certain antigens to trigger the release of chemical mediators that cause anaphylactic hypersensitivity reactions characterized by wheal and flare. The normal concentration of IgE in serum is 0.01 to 0.04 mg/dL. Compare **immunoglobulin A, immunoglobulin D, immunoglobulin G, immunoglobulin M.**

**immunoglobulin electrophoresis,** a blood test done to detect and identify the various immunoglobulins (antibodies), such as IgG, IgA, IgM, IgE, and IgD. Serum immunoelectrophoresis is used to detect and monitor the course of diseases such as hypersensitivity diseases, immune deficiencies, autoimmune diseases, chronic infections, multiple myeloma, chronic viral infections, and intrauterine fetal infections.

**immunoglobulin G (IgG),** one of the five classes of antibodies produced by the body. It is synthesized in response to invasions by bacteria, fungi, and viruses. IgG crosses the placenta and protects the fetus against red cell antigens and white cell antigens. The normal concentration of IgG in serum is 800 to 1600 mg/dL. Compare **immunoglobulin A, immunoglobulin D, immunoglobulin E, immunoglobulin M.**

**immunoglobulin M (IgM),** one of the five classes of antibodies produced by the body and the largest in molecular structure. It is found in circulating fluids and is the first immunoglobulin produced when the body is challenged by antigens. IgM triggers the increased production of immunoglobulin G and the complement fixation required for effective immune response. It is the dominant antibody in ABO blood group incompatibilities. The normal concentration of IgM in serum is 40 to 120 mg/dL. Compare **immunoglobulin A, immunoglobulin D, immunoglobulin E, immunoglobulin G.**

**immunohematology** /-hem′ətol′əjē/ [L, *immunis* + Gk, *haima,* blood, *logos,* science], the study of antigen-antibody reactions and their effects on blood.

**immunoincompetence** /im′yənō′inkom′pətəns/, inability to develop an immune reaction. See also **immunocompromised host. —immunoincompetent,** *adj*

**immunoincompetent** /im′yənō′inkom′pətənt/, an inability to develop an immune response to the challenge of antigens.

**immunologic barrier** /-loj′ik/, an apparent protection against an immune response afforded by certain areas of the body as demonstrated by the prolonged survival of foreign grafts in those areas. The barrier may be related to the nature of lymphatic drainage in those areas.

**immunologic disease** [L, *immunis,* free from; Gk, *logos,* science; L, *dis* + Fr, *aise,* ease], any condition caused by the reactions of antibodies to antigens, as in anaphylaxis.

**immunologic granuloma,** a small, organized, compact collection of mononuclear phagocytes that develops within 2 or 3 weeks after the introduction of a foreign material, provoking an inflammatory response. Such materials include sea urchin toxin, chemicals used in making tattoos, and antigens associated with leprosy, tuberculosis, and cat-scratch fever.

**immunologic model of aging,** an idea that a decline in the function of T cells and B cells causes normal cells to be unrecognized as such, thereby triggering immune reactions against an individual's own tissues.

**immunologic pregnancy test,** a method of detecting pregnancy through an increase in the concentration of human chorionic gonadotropin (HCG) in the plasma or urine, as determined by the reaction of HCG with a specific antiserum.

**immunologic surveillance** [L, *immunis,* free from; Gk, *logos,* science; Fr, *surveiller,* to watch over], the constant monitoring by the immune system of microorganisms, foreign tissue, and diseases caused by altered cells, especially cancer cells. Also called **immune surveillance, immunosurveillance.**

**immunologic test** [L, *immunis* + *testum,* crucible], a test based on the principles of antigen-antibody reactions.

**immunologist** /im′yənol′əjist/, a specialist in immunology.

**immunology** /im′yənol′əjē/ [L, *immunis* + Gk, *logos,* science], the study of the reaction of tissues of the immune system of the body to antigenic stimulation.

**immunomodulator** /-mod′yəlā′tər/ [L, *immunis* + *modulus,* little measure], a substance that alters the immune response by augmenting or reducing the ability of the immune system to produce antibodies or sensitized cells that recognize and react with the antigen that initiated their production. Immunomodulators include corticosteroids, cytotoxic agents, thymosin, and immunoglobulins. Some immunomodulators are naturally present in the body, and certain of these are available in pharmacologic preparations. —**immunomodulation,** *n.*

**immunopathology** /-pəthol′əjē/, **1.** the study of disease processes that have an immunologic cause. **2.** injury induced by antibodies or other products of an immune response.

**immunophenotypic analysis** /-fē′nōtip′ik/, a method for dividing lymphomas and leukemias into clonal subgroups on the basis of differences in cell surfaces and cytoplasmic antigens. The antigenic differences are detected with monoclonal antibodies and flow cytometry.

**immunopotency** /-pō′tənsē/ [L, *immunis* + *potentia*, power], the ability of an antigen to elicit an immune response.

**immunoprecipitation** /-prisip′itā′shən/, a procedure used to isolate target molecules with which antibodies react. Precipitation results when insoluble antigen-antibody complexes are formed by the reaction between soluble antigens and antibodies.

**immunoproliferative disorder,** a condition characterized by the continuous proliferation of a subset of immune cells, such as lymphocytes or plasma cells, that is associated with autoimmune and immunoglobulin disorders.

**immunoproliferative small intestine disease (IPSID),** a disorder characterized by a small, diffuse lesion with cells that have features of plasma cells, histiocytes, and atypical lymphocytes. The disease mainly affects the duodenum and proximal jejunum. Patients experience diarrhea, weight loss, abdominal pain, and clubbing of the fingers and toes. Also called **alpha chain disease, Mediterranean lymphoma.**

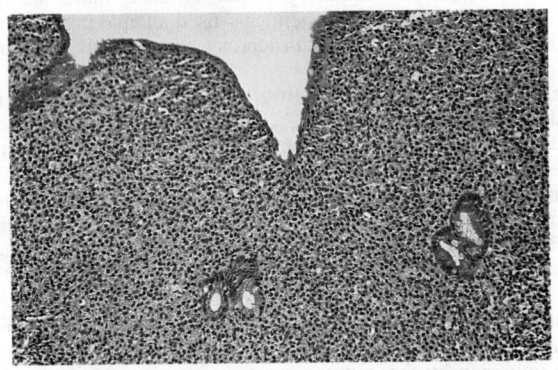

**Immunoproliferative small intestine disease**
*(Fletcher, 2000)*

**immunoprophylaxis** /-prō′filak′sis/, the introduction of active immunization through vaccines or passive immunization through antisera.

**immunoradiometric assay** /-rā′dē·ō·met′rik/, a method for measuring certain plasma proteins by using radiolabeled antibodies.

**immunoregulation** /-reg′yəlā′shən/, control of the immune response, as by manipulation of pathways involving suppressor and contrasuppressor T cells.

**immunoregulatory hormones** /-reg′yələtôr′ē/, chemical substances secreted by endocrine glands and lymphocytes that influence activities of the immune system.

**immunoselection** /-silek′shən/ [L, *immunis* + *seligere*, to select], the survival of certain cells as a result of their lack of surface antigens that would otherwise make them vulner-able to attack and destruction by antibodies. See also **erythroblastosis fetalis, Rh factor.**

**immunosorbent** /-sôr′bənt/, a substance containing attached antigens used to remove homologous antibodies from a solution. See also **enzyme-linked immunosorbent assay.**

**immunostimulant** /-stim′yələnt/, an agent, such as bacille Calmette-Guérin vaccine, that induces an immune response.

**immunosuppression** /-səpresh′ən/ [L, *immunis* + *supprimere,* to press down], **1.** the administration of agents that significantly interfere with the ability of the immune system to respond to antigenic stimulation by inhibiting cellular and humoral immunity. Corticosteroids; cytotoxic drugs, including antimetabolites and alkylating agents; antilymphocytic antibodies; and irradiation may produce immunosuppression. Immunosuppression may be deliberate, such as in preparation for bone marrow or other transplantation to prevent rejection by the host of the donor tissue, or incidental, such as often results from chemotherapy for the treatment of cancer. **2.** an abnormal condition of the immune system characterized by markedly inhibited ability to respond to antigenic stimuli. —**immunosuppressed,** *adj.*

**immunosuppressive** /-səpres′iv/, **1.** pertaining to a substance or procedure that lessens or prevents an immune response. **2.** an immunosuppressive agent. The immunosuppressive drugs used most frequently to prevent homograft rejection are the cytotoxic purine antimetabolite azathioprine, the alkylating agent cyclophosphamide, and the adrenocorticosteroid prednisone. Methotrexate, cytarabine, dactinomycin, thioguanine, and antilymphocyte globulin are also potent immunosuppressives. The use of some of these agents is being explored for the treatment of autoimmune diseases such as systemic lupus erythematosus and many other disorders.

**immunosurveillance.** See **immunologic surveillance.**

**immunotherapy** /-ther′əpē/ [L, *immunis* + Gk, *therapeia,* treatment], the application of immunologic knowledge and techniques to prevent and treat disease. Examples include the administration of increasing doses of allergens in the treatment of allergies, the use of immunostimulants and immunosuppressants, the transfer of immunocompetent cells and tissues from one person to another, and the use of interferon for its antiviral and antitumor properties. —**immunotherapeutic,** *adj.*

**immunotoxin (IT)** /-tok′sin/, a toxin that is attached to a monoclonal antibody and used to destroy a specific type of target cell. An example is the plant toxin ricin, which inhibits protein synthesis in tumor cells that are recognized by the antibodies to which ricin is attached.

**Imodium,** trademark for an antidiarrheal (loperamide hydrochloride).

**Imovax,** trademark for a rabies virus vaccine (rabies human diploid cell vaccine).

**impacted** /impak′tid/ [L, *impingere,* to drive against], tightly or firmly wedged in a limited amount of space. —**impact,** *v.,* **impaction,** *n.*

**impacted cerumen,** accumulated cerumen forming a solid mass that adheres to the wall of the external auditory canal.

**impacted fracture,** a bone break in which the adjacent fragmented ends of the fractured bone are wedged together.

**impacted tooth,** a tooth so positioned against another tooth, bone, or soft tissue that its complete and normal eruption is impossible or unlikely. An impacted third molar tooth may be further described according to its position, such as buccoangular, distoangular, or vertical. Compare **embedded tooth.**

**impaction** /impak′shən/, **1.** an obstacle or malposition that prevents a tooth from erupting. **2.** the presence of a large or hard fecal mass in the rectum or colon.

**impact printer** /im′pakt/, a mechanical printer that imprints computer characters on paper by striking it as a typewriter does, usually through an inked ribbon. Compare **nonimpact printer.** See also **dot-matrix printer.**

**impaired glucose tolerance (IGT)** /imperd′/ [L, *impejorare,* to make worse; Gk, *glykys,* sweet; L, *tolerare,* to endure], a condition in which fasting plasma glucose levels are higher than normal but lower than those diagnostic of diabetes mellitus. In some patients this represents a stage in the natural history of diabetes, but in a substantial number of persons IGT either does not progress or ends, and glucose tolerance reverts to normal. Also called impaired fasting glucose (IFG). See also **diabetes mellitus.**

**impairment** [L, *impejorare,* to make worse], any disorder in structure or function resulting from anatomic, physiologic, or psychologic abnormalities that interfere with normal activities.

**impedance** /impē′dəns/ [L, *impedire,* to entangle], a form of electrical resistance observed in an alternating current that is analogous to the classic electric resistance that occurs in a direct current circuit. It is expressed as a ratio of voltage applied to a circuit to the current it produces, as an alternating current oscillates ahead of or behind the voltage.

**impedance audiometry.** See **audiometry.**

**impedance plethysmography,** a technique for detecting blood vessel occlusion that determines volumetric changes in the limb by measuring changes in its girth as indicated by changes in the electrical impedance of mercury-containing polymeric silicone (Silastic) tubes in a pressure cuff. The method is based on the principle that any circumferential rate of change in a limb segment is directly proportional to the volumetric rate of change, which in turn reflects occlusion of venous and arterial blood flow. However, the technique does not accurately indicate the presence or absence of partially obstructing thrombi in major vessels.

**imperative conception** /imper′ətiv/ [L, *imperare,* to command], a thought or impression that appears spontaneously in the mind and cannot be eliminated, such as an obsession.

**imperative idea.** See **compulsive idea.**

**imperforate** /impur′fərit/ [L, *im,* not, *perforare,* to pierce], lacking a normal opening in a body organ or passageway. An infant may be born with an imperforate anus. Compare **perforate.**

**imperforate anus,** any of several congenital developmental malformations of the anorectal portion of the GI tract.

■ OBSERVATION: The most common form is anal agenesis, in which the rectal pouch ends blindly above the surface of the perineum. An anal fistula is present in 80% to 90% of cases. Other forms include anal stenosis, in which the anal aperture is small, and anal membrane atresia, in which the anal membrane covers the aperture, creating an obstruction.

■ INTERVENTIONS: The defect is usually discovered at birth; inspection reveals absence of the anus or the presence of a thin translucent membrane covering it. Digital and endoscopic examination allows identification of the anatomic character of the malformation. Radiographic examination is performed to outline the rectal pouch. A radiopaque marker is placed at the usual site of the anus, and the infant is held upside down. Air moving through the intestines into the distal portion of the bowel or the rectum is visible on the x-ray film. Anal stenosis is treated with daily digital dilation begun in the hospital and continued at home by the parents. An

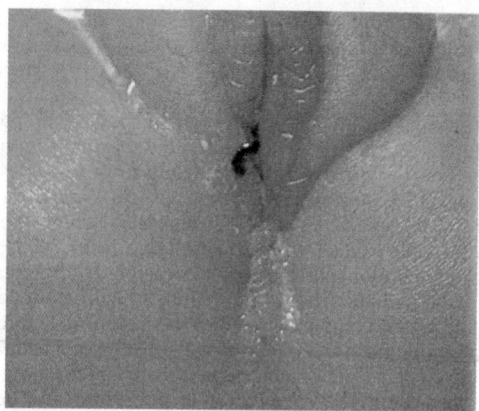

**Imperforate anus**
*(Zitelli and Davis, 1997/courtesy Dr. Christine L. Williams, New York Medical College)*

imperforate anal membrane is excised, and digital dilation is performed daily as the skin heals. Surgical reconstruction is performed to treat anal agenesis in infants in whom the pouch is below the puborectalis of the levator ani; an anus is created surgically by an anoplasty. Anal atresia in which the pouch at the end of the bowel is high above the perineum may require a colostomy.

■ NURSING CONSIDERATIONS: Often it is the nurse who identifies the anal malformation during the routine newborn assessment. A newborn who does not pass any stool in the first 24 hours requires further evaluation for the possibility of the defect. The passage of meconium from the vagina or urinary meatus clearly indicates the presence of anal fistula and usually occurs in association with an imperforate anus. Postoperative care in the newborn treated surgically for any of these conditions requires scrupulous attention to the perineal area.

**imperforate hymen** [L, *im* + *perforare,* to pierce through; Gk, *hymen,* membrane], a hymen that completely encloses the external orifice of the vagina.

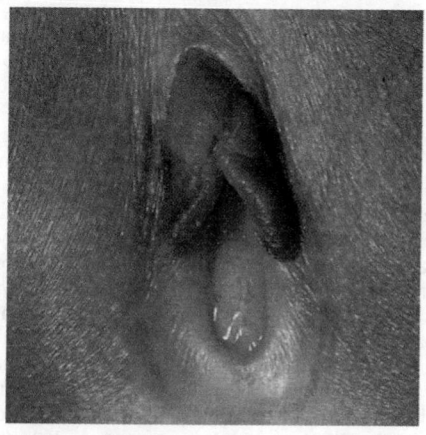

**Imperforate hymen** *(Zitelli and Davis, 1997)*

**impermeable** /impur′mē·əbəl/ [L, *im,* not, *permeare,* to pass through],   (of a tissue, membrane, or film) preventing the passage of a substance through it. Also called **impervious** /impur′vē·əs/.

**impetigo** /im′pətī′gō/ [L, *impetus,* an attack],   a streptococcal, staphylococcal, or combined infection of the skin beginning as focal erythema and progressing to pruritic vesicles, erosions, and honey-colored crusts. Lesions usually form on the face and spread locally. The disorder is highly contagious through contact with the discharge from the lesions. Acute glomerulonephritis is an occasional complication. Treatment includes thorough cleansing with antibacterial soap and water, compresses of Burow's solution, and topical or oral antibiotics. Treatment of the sores, use of individual washcloths and linens, and scrupulous handwashing help prevent spread of the infection. —**impetiginous** /im′petij′in əs/, *adj.*

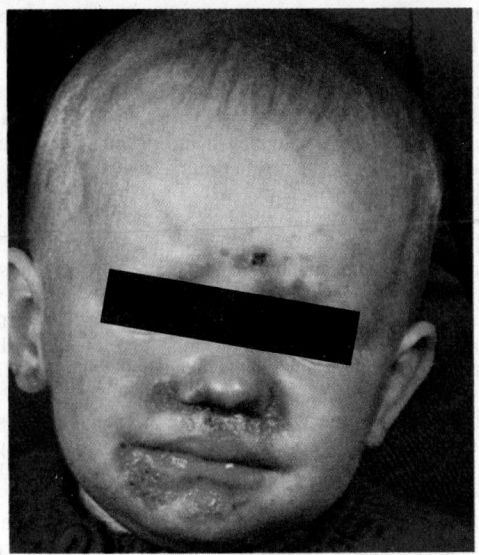

**Impetigo contagiosa** *(du Vivier, 1993)*

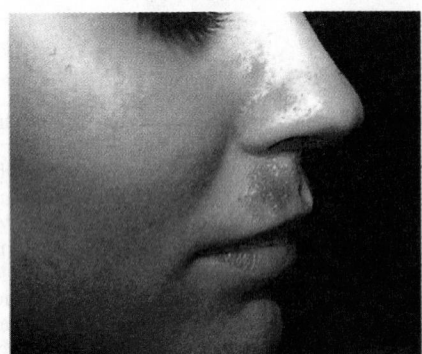

**Impetigo** *(Weston, Lane, and Morelli, 1996)*

**impetigo contagiosa** [L, *impetus,* attack; *contingere,* to touch],   an acute contagious superficial infection of the skin. It is characterized by vesicles that rupture, leaving a purulent exudate that dries into golden crusts.

**impetigo herpetiformis** [L, *impetus,* attack; Gk, *herpein,* to creep; L, *forma*],   a rare skin disorder that mainly affects pregnant women, beginning as an eruption in the genitofemoral area and spreading to other areas. The eruptions are usually irregular or circular groups of pustules that tend to coalesce.

**impingement injection test** /impinj′mənt/,   an appraisal of shoulder injury in which the injection of 10 mL of lidocaine into the subacromial space reduces the painful arc of abduction by more than half.

**impingement sign,**   a painful arc produced by forceful abduction of the internally rotated arm against the acromion in evaluation of a shoulder injury.

**impingement syndrome,**   a progressive condition of shoulder pain and dysfunction, usually caused by repetitive placement of the arm in overhead positions. The disorder is a common sports injury, particularly among persons who participate in baseball, tennis, swimming, and volleyball.

**implant** /im′plant, implant′/ [L, *implantare,* to set into],   **1.** (in radiotherapy) an encapsulated radioactive substance embedded in tissue for therapy. Seeds containing iodine-125 may be implanted permanently in prostate and chest tumors, and seeds of iridium-192 in ribbons or wire may be embed-

ded temporarily in head and neck cancers. Sealed sources of cesium-137 or radium-226 may be implanted in the body cavity temporarily in the treatment of gynecologic malignancies; strontium-90 in sealed sources may be embedded for a brief period (usually less than 2 minutes) in the treatment of eye tumors; needles containing radium-226 may be used as temporary interstitial implants. Patients with radioactive implants are isolated from other patients whenever possible. **2.** (in surgery) material inserted or grafted into an organ or structure of the body. The implant may be of tissue, such as in a blood vessel graft, or of an artificial substance, such as in a hip prosthesis, a cardiac pacemaker, or a container of radioactive material.

**implantable cardioverter-defibrillator (ICD),**   a surgically implanted electric device that automatically terminates lethal ventricular arrhythmias by delivering low-energy shocks to the heart, restoring proper rhythm when the heart begins beating rapidly or erratically. About the size of an audiotape cassette, the device can be implanted without thoracotomy in many cases. It is attached to the abdomen or chest wall with a wire link to the heart.

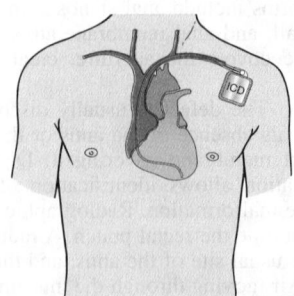

**Implantable cardioverter-defibrillator**
*(Lewis, Heitkemper, and Dirksen, 2000)*

**implantation,** (in embryology) the process involving the attachment, penetration, and embedding of the blastocyst in the lining of the uterine wall during the early stages of prenatal development. It may be artificial or natural. Kinds of implantation include **eccentric implantation, interstitial implantation,** and **superficial implantation.** Also called **nidation.**

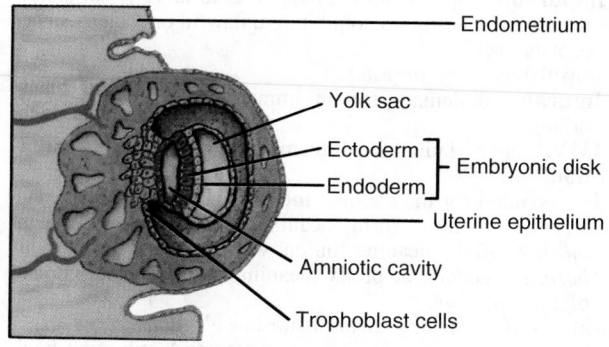

**Implantation** *(Applegate, 2000)*

Labels: Endometrium, Yolk sac, Ectoderm, Endoderm, Embryonic disk, Uterine epithelium, Amniotic cavity, Trophoblast cells

**implantation dermoid cyst,** a tumor derived from embryonal tissues, caused by an injury that forces part of the ectoderm into the body.

**implantation endometriosis** [L, *implantare,* to set into; Gk, *endon,* within, *metra,* womb, *osis,* condition], ectopic endometrial tissue prevalent throughout the peritoneal cavity. Also called **peritoneal endometriosis.**

**implant denture,** complete or partial denture that includes a subperiosteally or intraperiosteally implanted framework in contact with alveolar bone. The denture attaches to one or more posts that project from the framework through the connective tissues and mucous membranes. A variety of designs are available. This type of solution to the loss of natural teeth requires a strong commitment by the patient to practice effective oral hygiene measures.

**implanted infusion port,** a self-sealing silicone septum encased in a metal or plastic case with an attached silicone catheter that is threaded intravenously. It is implanted subcutaneously and used for long-term venous access for infusion of medications, parenteral nutrition, or IV solutions.

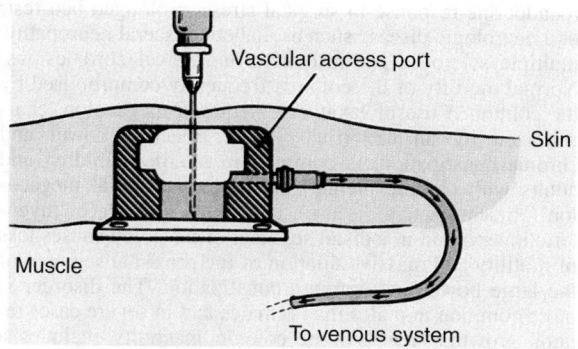

**Implanted infusion port** *(Potter and Perry, 2001)*

Labels: Vascular access port, Skin, Muscle, To venous system

**implanted suture** [L, *implantare,* to set into, *sutura*], a suture formed by inserting pins on opposite sides of a wound and drawing the edges of the wound together by winding thread tightly around the pins.

**implant restoration,** a single- or multiple-tooth implant crown or bridge that replaces a missing tooth or teeth.

**implementation** /im′pləməntā′shən/ [L, *implere,* to fill], a deliberate action performed to achieve a goal, such as carrying out a plan in caring for a patient.

**implementation mechanism,** the means by which innovations are transferred from the planners to the units of service.

**implementing** /im′pləmen′ting/ [L, *implere,* to fill], (in five-step nursing process) a category of nursing behavior in which the actions necessary for accomplishing the health care plan are initiated and completed. Implementing includes performing or assisting in the performance of the patient's activities of daily living, if necessary; counseling and teaching the patient or the patient's family; giving care to achieve patient comfort and therapeutic goals and to optimize the patient's achievement of health goals; supervising and evaluating the work of staff members; and recording and exchanging information relevant to the patient's continued health care. The nurse helps the patient and the patient's family to recognize and manage the emotional and psychologic stress attendant on the patient's condition and facilitates the relationships of the patient, patient's family, staff, and other significant people. Correct principles, procedures, and techniques of health care are taught, and the patient is informed about the current status of his or her health. If necessary, the patient or the patient's family is referred to a health or social resource in the community. Care is given to achieve therapeutic goals, including acting to compensate for adverse reactions; using preventive and precautionary measures and correct technique in administering care; preparing the patient for surgery, delivery, or other procedure; or initiating lifesaving measures in emergencies. Care is given to the patient in a manner and to a degree that best promotes the patient's attainment of the goals by providing an environment that is conducive to attaining them; by adjusting the care given according to the patient's needs; by stimulating and motivating the patient to achieve independence; by encouraging the patient to comply with and accept the regimen of care; and by compensating for the staff reactions to factors that influence the relationship with the patient and the therapy planned. Implementing follows planning and precedes evaluating in the five-step nursing process. See also **analyzing, assessing, evaluating, nursing process, planning.**

**implied consent** /implīd′/ [L, *implicare,* to involve, *consentire,* to feel], the granting of permission for health care without a formal agreement between the patient and health care provider. An example is an appointment made with a physician by a patient with a physical complaint; it is implied that by making the appointment the patient gives consent to the physician to make a diagnosis and offer treatment.

**implosion** /implō′zhən/ [L, *im + plaudere,* to strike], **1.** a bursting inward. **2.** a psychiatric treatment for people disabled by phobias and anxiety in which the person is desensitized to anxiety-producing stimuli by repeated intense exposure in imagination or reality, until the stimuli are no longer stressful. Also called **flooding. —implode,** *v.*

**implosive therapy.** See **flooding.**

**impotence** /im′pətəns/ [L, *im,* not, *potentia,* power], **1.** weakness. **2.** inability of the adult male to achieve penile erection or, less commonly, to ejaculate after achieving an erection. Several forms are recognized. **Functional impotence** has a psychologic basis. **Anatomic impotence** results from physically defective genitalia. **Atonic impotence** involves disturbed neuromuscular function. Poor health, old or advancing age, drugs, and fatigue can induce impotence. Also called **impotency, erectile dysfunction. —impotent, erectile dysfunction,** *adj.*

**impregnate** /impreg'nāt/ [L, *impregnare,* to make pregnant], **1.** to inseminate and make pregnant; to fertilize. **2.** to saturate or mix with another substance. **—impregnable,** *adj.,* **impregnation,** *n.*

**impression** /impresh'ən/ [L, *imprimere,* to press into], **1.** (in dentistry and prosthetic medicine) a mold of a part of the mouth or other part of the body from which a replacement or prosthesis may be formed. **2.** (in the medical record) the examiner's diagnosis or assessment of a problem, disease, or condition. **3.** a strong sensation or effect on the mind, intellect, or feelings.

**impression material** [L, *imprimere,* to press into, *materia,* stuff], any substance used for making impressions of teeth and oral structures to produce dental restorations.

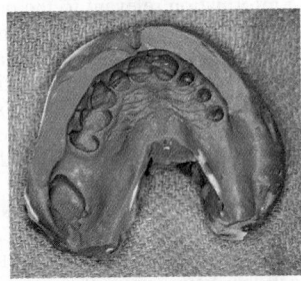

**Polyether impression material** *(Cranin, 1999)*

**imprinting** [Fr, *empreindre,* to impress], (in ethology) a special type of learning that occurs at critical points during the early stages of development in animals. It involves behavioral patterning and social attachment, is characterized by rapid acquisition and irreversibility, and is usually species-specific, although animals exposed to members of a different species during this short period may become attached to and identify with that particular species instead of their own. The degree to which imprinting occurs in human development has not been determined. See also **bonding.**

**imprisonment** /impriz'ənment/ [Fr, *emprisonner,* to confine], (in law) the act of confining, detaining, or arresting a person or in any way restraining personal liberty and preventing free exercise of movement.

**impulse** /im'puls/ [L, *impellere,* to drive], **1.** (in psychology) a sudden irresistible, often irrational inclination, urge, desire, or action resulting from a particular feeling or mental state. **2.** also called **nerve impulse, neural impulse.** (in physiology) the electrochemical process involved in neural transmission. **—impulsive,** *adj.*

**impulse-conducting system** [L, *impellere,* to drive before, *conducere,* to conduct; Gk, *systema*], the Purkinje fibers within the heart muscle that conduct impulses controlling the contractions of the atria and ventricles.

**impulse control,** a nursing outcome from the Nursing Outcomes Classification (NOC) defined as self-restraint of compulsive or impulsive behaviors. See also **Nursing Outcomes Classification.**

**impulse control disorder,** a behavior in which the individual fails to resist performing a potentially harmful act.

The individual usually has a sense of tension or arousal before committing the act and a sense of relief or pleasure when it is committed.

**impulse control training,** a nursing intervention from the Nursing Interventions Classification (NIC) defined as assisting the patient to mediate impulsive behavior through application of problem-solving strategies to social and interpersonal situations. See also **Nursing Interventions Classification.**

**impulsion** /impul'shən/ [L, *impellere,* to drive], an abnormal, irrational urge to commit an unlawful or socially unacceptable act.

**impulsive.** See **impulse.**

**Imuran,** trademark for an immunosuppressive (azathioprine).

**IMV,** abbreviation for **intermittent mandatory ventilation.**

**In,** symbol for the element **indium.**

**in-,** **1.** combining form meaning 'fiber': *inaxon, inemia, initis.* **2.** prefix meaning 'in, on, within, into or toward': *inborn, inbreeding.* **3.** prefix meaning 'not, lack of, opposite of': *inarticulate.*

**-in,** suffix meaning 'neutral substance': *albumin, gelatin.*

**-in, -ine,** **1.** combining form meaning an 'antibiotic': *bacitracin, penicillin, streptomycin.* **2.** combining form meaning a 'pharmaceutic product': *aspirin, niacin.* **3.** combining form meaning a 'chemical compound': *albumin, gelatin, palmitin.* **4.** combining form meaning an 'enzyme': *emulsin, pepsin, myrosin.*

**inactivated measles virus vaccine** /inak'tivā'tid/ [L, *in,* not, *activus* + OE, *masala,* blister; L, *virus,* poison, *vaccinus,* of a cow], a measles vaccine virus that has been treated so that it is no longer capable of replication. It is an alternative to live attenuated measles vaccine, which may be contraindicated for some individuals, such as those who are immunodeficient.

**inactivation** /inak'tivā'shən/ [L, *in,* not, *activus,* active], a reversible denaturation of a protein. See also **deactivation.**

**inactivation of complement** [L, *in* + *activus, complere,* to complete], the loss of activity of the enzymatic proteins in blood, achieved by heating the serum to about 122° F (50° C). Inactivation of complement is a step in the process of **complement fixation.**

**inactive colon** /inak'tiv/ [L, *in,* not, *activus,* active; Gk, *kolon,* colon], hypotonicity of the bowel that results in decreased contractions and propulsive movements and a delay in the normal 12-hour transit time of luminal contents from the cecum to the anus. Colonic inactivity may be caused by acquired or congenital megacolon, anticholinergic drugs, depression, faulty habits of elimination, inadequate fluid intake, lack of exercise, a low-residue or starvation diet, neuroendocrine response to surgical stress, prolonged bed rest, or a neurologic disease such as diabetic visceral neuropathy, multiple sclerosis, parkinsonism, and spinal cord lesions. Normal motility of the colon is frequently compromised by the continued use of laxatives. Acquired megacolon, characterized by an abnormally large, inactive bowel and chronic constipation, is common in retarded children and adults with chronic mental illness. In congenital megacolon (Hirschsprung's disease), congenital absence of myenteric innervation in a distal segment of the colon causes loss of motility and massive dilation of the proximal segment of the large bowel and extreme constipation. The disorder is more common in males than females and in severe cases retards growth. Treatment of colonic inactivity includes a stimulus-response training program to establish regular bowel habits, the use of stool softeners and hydrophilic colloids to increase fecal bulk, and a diet containing adequate roughage.

**inadequate personality** /inad′əkwit/ [L, *in*, not, *adaequare*, to equal, *personalis*, of a person], a personality characterized by a lack of physical stamina, emotional immaturity, social instability, poor judgment, reduced motivation, ineptness—especially in interpersonal relationships—and an inability to adapt or react effectively to new or stressful situations.

**inamrinone lactate** /am′rinōn/, an IV cardiac inotropic drug.

■ INDICATIONS: It is prescribed in the short-term management of congestive heart failure in patients who do not respond to therapy with digitalis, diuretics, and vasodilators.

■ CONTRAINDICATIONS: Concomitant use with disopyramide and any combination therapy should be closely monitored for potential interactions.

■ ADVERSE EFFECTS: Among the more serious adverse reactions are thrombocytopenia, arrhythmias, hypotension, nausea, vomiting, liver impairment, and hypersensitivity effects.

**inanimate** /inan′imit/ [L, *in*, not, *animus*, life spirit], not alive; lacking signs of life.

**inanition** /in′ənish′ən/ [L, *inanis*, empty], **1.** an exhausted condition resulting from lack of food and water or a defect in assimilation; starvation. **2.** a state of lethargy characterized by a loss of vitality or vigor in all aspects of social, moral, and intellectual life.

**inanition fever,** a temporary mild febrile condition of the newborn in the first few days after birth, usually caused by dehydration.

**inborn** /in′bôrn/ [L, *in*, within; AS, *beran*, to bear], innate; acquired or occurring during intrauterine life, with reference to both normally inherited traits and developmental or genetically transmitted anomalies. See also **congenital, hereditary, inborn error of metabolism.**

**inborn error of metabolism,** one of many abnormal metabolic conditions caused by an inherited defect of a single enzyme or other protein. Although people with such diseases are defective in only protein, they generally display a large number of physical signs that are characteristic of the genetic trait. The diseases are rare. Kinds of inborn errors of metabolism include **phenylketonuria, Tay-Sachs disease, Lesch-Nyhan syndrome, galactosemia,** and **glucose-6-phosphate dehydrogenase deficiency.**

■ OBSERVATIONS: Inborn errors of metabolism may be detected in the fetus in utero by the examination of squamous and blood cells obtained by amniocentesis and fetoscopy. Laboratory tests after birth often show higher than normal levels of particular metabolites in the blood and urine, such as phenylpyruvic acid and phenylalanine in phenylketonuria (PKU) and galactose in galactosemia. The values are higher in homozygous than in heterozygous carriers. Signs of the various defects are usually seen only in homozygous carriers.

■ INTERVENTIONS: Treatment for some pathologic inborn errors may be removal of food in the diet containing the nondegradable metabolite to prevent its accumulation. Removal of dietary phenylalanine in PKU and galactose in galactosemia is effective in preventing the development of symptoms if treatment is begun early. In those cases of inborn errors of metabolism in which the nondegradable metabolite is endogenous, such as in the mucopolysaccharidoses, no treatment is available.

**inborn lysosomal disease,** one of many inherited disorders of metabolism involving degradative enzymes normally located in lysosomes. The condition leads to storage of ab-normal amounts of lysosomal agents. Also called **lysosomal storage disease.**

**inborn reflex.** See **unconditioned response.**

**inbreeding** /in′brēding/ [L, *in*, within; AS, *bredan*, to reproduce], the production of offspring by the mating of closely related organisms; the most extreme form is self-fertilization, which occurs in certain plants and animals. Inbreeding increases the chance that recessive alleles for both desirable and undesirable traits will become homozygous and be expressed phenotypically. In humans the amount of inbreeding in a specific population is largely controlled by tradition and cultural practices. Inbreeding is a standard agricultural method for developing desirable genotypes and pure lines in plants and animals. Compare **outbreeding.**

**incandescent** [L, *incandescere*, to begin to glow], hot to the point of glowing or emitting intense light rays, as an incandescent light bulb.

**incarcerate** /inkar′sərāt/ [L, *in*, within, *carcerare*, to imprison], to trap, imprison, or confine, such as a loop of intestine in an inguinal hernia. See also **hernia.**

**incarcerated hernia** [L, *in* + *carcerare*, to imprison, *hernia*, rupture], a loop of bowel with ends occluded so that solids cannot pass; the herniated bowel will not return to its normal position without manipulation or surgery. It is essential to correct the condition before the bowel becomes strangulated. Also called **irreducible hernia.**

**incentive spirometry** /insen′tiv/, a method of encouraging voluntary deep breathing by providing visual feedback about inspiratory volume. Using a specially designed spirometer, the patient inhales until a preset volume is reached, then sustains the inspiratory volume by holding his or her breath for 3 to 5 seconds. Incentive spirometry reduces the risk of atelectasis and pulmonary consolidation.

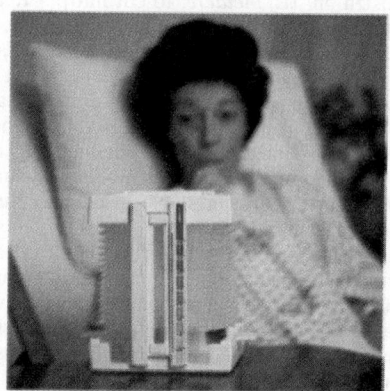

**Incentive spirometry** *(Potter and Perry, 2001)*

**inception** /insep′shən/ [L, *incipere*, to begin], the origin or beginning of anything.

**incest** /in′sest/ [L, *incestum*, defiled], sexual intercourse between persons too closely related to marry legally. **—incestuous,** *adj.*

**incidence** /in′sidəns/ [L, *incidere*, to happen], **1.** the number of times an event occurs. **2.** (in epidemiology) the number of new cases in a particular period. Incidence is often expressed as a ratio, in which the number of cases is the numerator and the population at risk is the denominator. See also **rate.**

**incidence rate,** the rate of new cases of a disease in a specified population over a defined period.

**incidental additives** /in'siden'təl/ [L, *incidere,* to happen, *additio,* something added], material added to food by the use of pesticides, herbicides, or chemicals used in food processing.

**incident report,** a document, usually confidential, describing any accident or deviation from policies or orders involving a patient, employee, visitor, or student on the premises of a health care facility.

**incident reporting,** a nursing intervention from the Nursing Interventions Classification (NIC) defined as written and verbal reporting of any event in the process of patient care that is inconsistent with desired patient outcomes or routine operations of the health care facility. See also **Nursing Interventions Classification.**

**incineration** /insin'ərā'shən/ [L, *incinerare,* to burn to ashes], the removal or reduction of waste materials by burning.

**incipient** /insip'ē·ənt/ [L, *incipire,* to commence], coming into existence; at an initial stage; beginning to appear, such as a symptom or disease.

**incipient carious lesion.** See **primary dental caries.**

**incipient dental caries,** the earliest detectable signs of tooth decay. At this stage, the lesion has not penetrated the dentin.

**incisal** /in·sī'zəl/ [L, *incidere,* to cut into], **1.** cutting. **2.** pertaining to the cutting edge of an anterior tooth.

**incisal angle** /insī'səl/ [L, *incidere,* to cut into, *angulus,* corner], the angle between the hinge axis-orbital plane and the discluding surface of the maxillary incisors.

**incisal guide.** See **anterior guide.**

**incisal guide pin,** a metal rod, attached to the upper member of a dental articulator, that touches the incisal guide table to maintain the established vertical separation of the upper and lower members of the articulator.

**incision** /insizh'ən/ [L, *incidere,* to cut into], **1.** a cut produced surgically by a sharp instrument that creates an opening into an organ or space in the body. **2.** to incise.

**incisional hernia** /insish'ənəl/ [L, *incidere,* to cut into, *hernia,* rupture], a herniation through a surgical scar.

**incision site care,** a nursing intervention from the Nursing Interventions Classification (NIC) defined as cleansing, monitoring, and promotion of healing in a wound that is closed with sutures, clips, or staples. See also **Nursing Interventions Classification.**

**incisor** /insī'zər/, one of the four front teeth in each dental arch. Deciduous incisors appear during infancy and are replaced during childhood by secondary incisors, which last until old age. The crown of each incisor is chisel shaped and has a sharp cutting edge. Its labial surface is convex, smooth, and highly polished; its lingual surface is concave and, in many individuals, is marked by an inverted V-shaped basal ridge near the gingiva of the maxillary arch. The neck of an incisor is constricted, and the root is single, long, and conic. The upper incisors are larger and stronger than the lower and are directed downward and forward. Compare **canine tooth, molar, premolar.**

**incisura** /in'sisyoo'rə/ [L, *incidere,* to cut into], a notch or incision on an organ or body part.

**inciting eye.** See **exciting eye.**

**inclusion** /inkloo'zhən/ [L, *in,* within, *claudere,* to shut], **1.** the act of enclosing or the condition of being enclosed. **2.** a structure within another, such as an inclusion in the cytoplasm of the cells.

**inclusion bodies,** microscopic objects of various shapes and sizes observed in the nucleus or cytoplasm of blood cells or other tissue cells, depending on the type of disease.

**inclusion body myositis,** a progressive inflammatory myopathy primarily involving muscles of the pelvic region and legs, usually seen in older people; the muscles are infiltrated by mononuclear inflammatory cells, sarcoplasmic vacuoles, masses of filaments and filamentous microtubules, and sometimes eosinophilic bodies.

**inclusion cell disease.** See **I cell disease.**

**inclusion conjunctivitis,** an acute purulent conjunctival infection caused by *Chlamydia* organisms. It occurs in two forms: the infection in infants is characterized by bilateral chemosis, redness, and purulent discharge; the adult variety is unilateral, less severe, and less purulent, and is associated with preauricular lymphadenopathy. Local instillation of antibiotics is effective treatment.

**inclusion dermoid cyst,** a tumor derived from embryonal tissues, caused by the inclusion of foreign tissue when a developmental cleft closes.

**inclusiveness principle** /inkloo'sivnəs/ [L, *in,* within, *claudere,* to shut, *principium,* a beginning], a rule that response to various objects in the environment is proportional to the amount of stimulus provided by each object.

**inclusive rate** /inkloo'siv/, a method of calculating inpatient hospital charges in which a fixed amount covers all services, regardless of the number or intensity of services provided.

**incoercible** /in'kō·ur'sibəl/, pertaining to something that cannot be restrained or willfully terminated, as a siege of hiccups.

**incoercible vomiting,** vomiting that is intractable or out of control. See also **pernicious vomiting.**

**incoherent** /in'kōhir'ənt/ [L, *in,* not, *cohaere,* to hold together], **1.** disordered; without logical connection; disjointed; lacking orderly continuity or relevance. **2.** unable to express one's thoughts or ideas in an orderly, intelligible manner, usually as a result of emotional stress.

**incompatibility** /in'kəmpat'ibil'itē/ [L, *in* + *compatibilus,* agreeing], a state of not being able to exist in harmony, as when transfused blood produces adverse effects because the donor and recipient blood groups conflict.

**incompatible** /in'kəmpat'əbəl/ [L, *in,* not, *compatibilus,* agreeing], unable to coexist. A tissue transplantation may be rejected because recipient and donor antibody factors are incompatible.

**incompetence** /inkom'pətəns/ [L, *in,* not, *competentia,* capable], lack of ability to function. Kinds of incompetence include **aortic incompetence, ileocecal incompetence,** and **valvular incompetence.** See also **incompetency. —incompetent,** *adj.*

**incompetency** /inkomp'ətənsē/, legal status of a person declared to be unable to provide for his or her own needs and protection proved in a court hearing.

**incompetent.** See **incompetence.**

**incompetent cervix** [L, *in,* not, *competentia,* capable, *cervix,* neck], (in obstetrics) a condition characterized by painless dilation of the cervical os of the uterus before term without labor or contractions of the uterus. Miscarriage or premature delivery may result. Incompetent cervix is treated prophylactically by a Shirodkar or other procedure in which the cervix is held closed by a surgically implanted suture.

**incomplete abortion** /in'kəmplēt'/ [L, *in,* not, *complere,* to fill, *ab,* away from, *oriri,* to be born], termination of pregnancy in which the products of conception are not entirely expelled or removed. It often causes hemorrhage that may require surgical evacuation by curettage, oxytocics, and blood replacement. Infection is also a frequent complication of incomplete abortion. Compare **complete abortion.**

**incomplete dislocation** [L, *in* + *complere,* to fill up, *dis* + *locare,* to place], a partial abnormal separation of the articular surfaces of a joint. Also called **subluxation.**

**incomplete fistula.** See **blind fistula.**

**incomplete fracture,** a bone break in which the crack in the osseous tissue does not completely traverse the width of the affected bone but may angle off in one or more directions.

**incomplete hemianopia,** loss of only a part of the half of the visual field. See also **hemianopia.**

**incomplete hernia** [L, *in* + *complere,* to fill up, *hernia,* rupture], a hernia that has not yet protruded through a weak spot or opening.

**incomplete protein,** a food that is inadequate in one or more of the nine amino acids essential for normal growth and maintenance of tissue when used as the sole source of protein and adequate energy is available.

**incongruent communication** /inkong′grōō·ənt/, a communication pattern in which the sender gives conflicting messages on verbal and nonverbal levels and the listener does not know which message to accept. See also **double bind.**

**incontinence** /inkon′tinəns/ [L, *incontinentia,* inability to retain], the inability to control urination or defecation. Urinary incontinence may be caused by anatomic, physiologic, or pathologic factors. Treatment depends on the diagnosed cause. Fecal incontinence may result from relaxation of the anal sphincter or disorders of the central nervous system or spinal cord and may be treated by a program of bowel training. A Bradford frame with an opening for a bedpan or urinal may be used for bedridden incontinent patients. See also **bowel training, urinary incontinence. —incontinent,** *adj.*

**incontinence, bowel,** a nursing diagnosis accepted by the Fourth National Conference on the Classification of Nursing Diagnoses. The condition is defined as a state in which an individual experiences a change in normal bowel habits characterized by involuntary passage of stool. The cause of the condition, developed at the Fifth National Conference, is neuromuscular or musculoskeletal impairment; depression, severe anxiety, or perceptive or cognitive impairment; multiple life changes; inadequate relaxation; little or no exercise; poor nutrition; work-related tensions; no vacations; unmet expectations; unrealistic perceptions; and inadequate support systems or coping methods.

■ DEFINING CHARACTERISTICS: The defining characteristic is an involuntary passage of stool.

■ RELATED FACTORS: Related factors include gastrointestinal disorders, neuromuscular disorders, colostomy, loss of rectal sphincter control, and impaired cognition. See also **nursing diagnosis.**

**incontinence, functional,** a nursing diagnosis accepted by the Seventh National Conference on the Classification of Nursing Diagnoses. The condition is defined as the state in which an individual experiences an involuntary, unpredictable passage of urine.

■ DEFINING CHARACTERISTICS: The defining characteristics are the urge to void or bladder contractions sufficiently strong to result in loss of urine before reaching an appropriate receptacle.

■ RELATED FACTORS: Related factors include altered environment and sensory, cognitive, or mobility deficits. See also **nursing diagnosis.**

**incontinence, reflex,** a nursing diagnosis accepted by the Seventh National Conference on the Classification of Nursing Diagnoses. The diagnosis describes the state in which an individual experiences an involuntary loss of urine occurring at somewhat predictable intervals when a specific bladder volume is reached.

■ DEFINING CHARACTERISTICS: Defining characteristics include lack of awareness of bladder filling; lack of urge to void or feeling of bladder fullness; or uninhibited bladder contractions/spasms at regular intervals.

■ RELATED FACTORS: Related factors include neurologic impairment, as a spinal cord lesion that interferes with conduction of cerebral messages above the level of the reflex arc. See also **nursing diagnosis.**

**incontinence, urinary, stress,** a nursing diagnosis accepted by the Seventh National Conference on the Classification of Nursing Diagnoses. The condition is defined as the state in which an individual experiences a loss of urine of less than 50 mL occurring with increased abdominal pressure, such as experienced during coughing, sneezing, laughing, and lifting.

■ DEFINING CHARACTERISTICS: The defining characteristics are reported or observed dribbling with increased abdominal pressure and urinary urgency or urinary frequency (more often than every 2 hours).

■ RELATED FACTORS: Related factors are degenerative changes in pelvic muscles and structural supports associated with increased age; high intraabdominal pressure such as obesity, or gravid uterus; incompetent bladder outlet; overdistension between voidings; and weak pelvic muscles and structural supports. See also **nursing diagnosis.**

**incontinence, urinary, total,** a nursing diagnosis accepted by the Seventh National Conference on the Classification of Nursing Diagnoses. The condition is defined as the state in which an individual experiences a continuous and unpredictable loss of urine.

■ DEFINING CHARACTERISTICS: Defining characteristics include a constant flow of urine that occurs at unpredictable times without distension or uninhibited bladder contractions or spasms, unsuccessful incontinence refractory to treatments, nocturia (urination more than two times per night), lack of perineal or bladder awareness, and unawareness of incontinence.

■ RELATED FACTORS: Related factors include neuropathy preventing transmission of a reflex indicating bladder fullness; neurologic dysfunction causing triggering of micturition at unpredictable times; independent contraction of detrusor reflex caused by surgery; trauma or disease that affects spinal cord nerves; or anatomic factors such as a fistula. See also **nursing diagnosis.**

**incontinence, urinary, urge,** a nursing diagnosis accepted by the Seventh National Conference on the Classification of Nursing Diagnoses. Urge incontinence is defined as the state in which an individual experiences involuntary passage of urine occurring soon after a strong sense of urgency to void.

■ DEFINING CHARACTERISTICS: Defining characteristics are urinary urgency, frequency (voiding more often than every 2 hours), bladder contractions or spasms, nocturia (urination more than two times per night), voiding in small amounts (less than 100 mL) or in large amounts (500 mL), and an inability to reach a toilet in time.

■ RELATED FACTORS: Related factors include decreased bladder capacity, as with a history of pelvic inflammatory disease, abdominal surgery, or an indwelling urinary catheter; irritation of bladder stretch receptors, which causes spasm, as with a bladder infection; alcohol; caffeine; increased fluids; increased urine concentration; and overdistension of the bladder. See also **nursing diagnosis.**

**incontinence, urinary, urge, risk for,**   a nursing diagnosis accepted by the Thirteenth National Conference on the Classification of Nursing Diagnoses. The condition is a risk for involuntary loss of urine associated with a sudden, strong sensation of urinary urgency.
■ RISK FACTORS: Risk factors include effects of medications, caffeine, alcohol; detrusor hyperreflexia from cystitis, urethritis, tumors, renal calculi, central nervous system disorders above the pontine micturition center, detrusor muscle instability with impaired contractility, involuntary sphincter relaxation, ineffective toileting habits, and small bladder capacity. See also **nursing diagnosis.**

**incontinent.**   See **incontinence.**

**incontinentia pigmenti** /in·kon′ti·nen′shə pig·men′tī /,   a male-lethal X-linked dominant syndrome with onset at birth or shortly thereafter, characterized by the presence of brown or slate-brown bands, whorls, swirls, or splatter-like hyperpigmented cutaneous lesions, preceded by vesiculobullous and verrucous inflammatory changes, often associated with developmental anomalies involving other structures, such as the hair, eyes, and skeletal and central nervous systems. Also called **Bloch-Sulzberger incontinentia pigmenti, Bloch-Sulzberger syndrome.**

**incontinentia pigmenti achromians,**   a congenital neurocutaneous syndrome, not present at birth but appearing in early life, characterized by the presence of peculiar whorled, linear, and splatter-like patterns of hypopigmentation, and often associated with other abnormalities, including hair loss and ocular, musculoskeletal, and mental disturbances. It is unrelated to incontinentia pigmenti. Also called **hypomelanosis of Ito.** Compare **incontinentia pigmenti.**

**increment** /ing′krəmənt/ [L, *incresere,* to grow],   1. an increase or gain. 2. the act of growing or increasing. 3. the amount of an increase or gain in intrauterine pressure as uterine contractions begin in labor. —**incremental,** *adj.*

**incremental line** /ing′krəmen′təl/,   1. one of a series of lines showing successive layers deposited in a tissue. 2. a very fine line of cementum that follows the contours of a tooth.

**incremental lines of Ebner** [Victor von Ebner, Austrian histologist, 1842–1925],   delicate lines seen on ground sections of a tooth, demarking increments of dentin.

**incrustation,**   hardened exudate, scale, or scab.

**incubation period** /in′kyəbā′shən/ [L, *incubare,* to lie on; Gk, *peri,* around, *hodos,* way],   1. the time between exposure to a pathogenic organism and the onset of symptoms of a disease. 2. the time required to induce the development of an embryo in an egg or to induce the development and replication of tissue cells or microorganisms being grown in culture media or other special laboratory environment. 3. the time allowed for a chemical reaction or process to proceed.

**incubator** /in′kyəbā′tər/,   an apparatus used to provide a controlled environment, especially temperature. Other environmental components, such as darkness, light, oxygen, moisture, or dryness, may also be controlled, as in an incubator for the cultivation of eggs or microorganisms in a laboratory or an incubator for premature infants.

**incud-,**   combining form meaning 'an anvil (the incus)': *incudectomy, incudiform, incudomalleal.*

**incudectomy** /in′kyo͞odek′təmē/ [L, *incus,* anvil, *ektomē,* excision],   surgical removal of the incus, performed to treat conductive hearing loss that results from necrosis of the tip of the incus. Local or general anesthesia is used. The defective incus is excised and replaced with a bone chip graft so that sound vibrations are again transmitted. After surgery the nurse instructs the patient to change position slowly to avoid dizziness, to prevent blowing the nose and sneezing, and to report any fever, headache, dizziness, or ear pain.

**incurable** /inkyo͞o′rəbəl/,   not responding to medical or surgical treatment.

**incus** /ing′kəs/, *pl.* **incudes** /inko͞o′dēz/ [L, anvil],   one of the three ossicles in the middle ear, resembling an anvil. It transmits sound vibrations from the malleus to the stapes. Compare **malleus, stapes.** See also **middle ear.**

**IND,**   abbreviation for **investigational new drug.**

**indanedione derivative** /indane′dē·ōn/,   one of a small group of oral anticoagulants designed for long-term therapeutic use in patients who cannot tolerate other oral anticoagulants. Anticoagulation using indanediones is difficult to control, and these agents may cause grave adverse effects, including severe renal and hepatic toxicity, agranulocytosis, and leukopenia; for this reason coumarin derivatives are preferred. Regular evaluations of prothrombin time are necessary. Extreme fatigue, sore throat, chills, and fever are signs of impending toxicity and require discontinuation of the drug. Compare **coumarin.**

**indemnify** /indem′nifī/,   to protect against loss or injury by compensating for the loss or injury.

**indentation** /in′dəntā′shən/ [L, *in,* within, *dens,* tooth],   a notch, pit, or depression in the surface of an object, such as toothmarks on the tongue or skin. —**indent,** *v.*

**independence** /in′dəpen′dəns/ [L, *in,* not, *de,* from, *pendere,* to hang],   1. the state or quality of being independent; autonomy; free of the influence, guidance, or control of a person or a group. 2. a lack of requirement or reliance on another for physical existence or emotional needs. —**independent,** *adj.*

**independent assortment.**   See **Mendel's laws.**

**independent intervention.**   See **intervention.**

**independent living center,**   rehabilitation facility in which disabled persons can receive special education and training in the performance of all or most activities of daily living with a particular handicap. A typical independent living center may contain a completely furnished multi-room apartment, including a kitchen with cabinets and cooking facilities that can be reached easily by a person in a wheelchair, designed for training patients in homemaking skills.

**independent practice,**   (in nursing) the practice of certain aspects of professional nursing that are encompassed by applicable licensure and law and require no supervision or direction from others. Nurses in independent practice may have an office in which they see patients and charge fees for service. In all nursing settings, state practice acts define certain aspects of nursing practice that are independent and may define those that must be done only under supervision or direction of another individual, usually a physician.

**Independent Practice Association (IPA),**   a U.S. type of physician alliance in which the physicians own the practice, as opposed to physicians employed by an entity such as a health maintenance organization. Physicians in the IPA are legally organized as a corporation, partnership, professional corporation, or foundation to contract as a group to provide services. Economic risk is shared, but overhead is not. See also **health maintenance organization.**

**independent variable,**   (in research) a variable that is manipulated by the researcher and evaluated by its measurable effect on the dependent variable or variables; for example, in a study of the effect of nursing intervention on postoperative vomiting, nursing intervention is the independent variable evaluated by its effect on the incidence of postoperative vomiting. Also called **experimental variable, predictor variable.** Compare **dependent variable.**

**Inderal,** trademark for a nonselective beta-adrenergic blocking agent (propranolol).

**indeterminate cleavage** /in′ditur′minit/ [L, *in*, not, *determinare*, to fix limits; AS, *cleofan*, to split], mitotic division of the fertilized ovum into blastomeres that have similar developmental potential and, if isolated, can give rise to a complete individual embryo. Also called **regulative cleavage.** Compare **determinate cleavage.** See also **regulative development.**

**index** /in′deks/ *pl.* **indexes, indices** [L, that which points out], **1.** also called **forefinger, index finger.** the second digit of the hand, the finger adjacent to the thumb. **2.** a unitless quantity, usually a ratio of two measurable quantities having the same dimensions, or such a ratio multiplied by 100. **3.** a core or mold used in dentistry to record or maintain the relative position of a tooth or teeth to one another and/or to a cast, to ensure reproduction in the dental prosthesis of their original position. **4.** a directory, in particular an alphabetized list of terms, each term accompanied by page numbers or other notations telling where it appears in a given work or set of works.

**index astigmatism** [L, *indicare*, to make known, *a + stigma*, point], an astigmatism caused by unequal refractive indices in different parts of the lens.

**index case** [L, *indicare*, to make known], (in epidemiology) the first case of a disease, as contrasted with subsequent cases. See also **propositus.**

*Index Medicus,* an index published monthly by the National Library of Medicine, which lists articles from the medical, nursing, and allied health literature from throughout the world by subject and by author. The *Cumulative Index Medicus* is published yearly; it contains the citations in all 12 issues of the *Index Medicus,* which can be accessed electronically.

**index myopia,** a kind of nearsightedness caused by a variation in the index of refraction of the eye media.

**Indian Health Service,** a bureau of the Department of Health and Human Services for providing public health and medical services to Native Americans in the United States. In Canada the services are provided by the **Ministry of Indian Affairs.**

**Indian tick fever.** See **Marseilles fever.**

**indican** /in′dikən/ [Gk, *indikon*, indigo], a substance (potassium indoxyl sulfate) produced in the intestine by the decomposition of tryptophan, absorbed by the intestinal wall, and excreted in the urine. Its level may be elevated in the urine of patients on high-protein diets or those suffering from GI disease. The normal accumulation of indican in urine is 10 to 20 mg/24 hr.

**indication** /in′dikā′shən/ [L, *indicare*, to make known], a reason to prescribe a medication or perform a treatment. A bacterial infection may be an indication for the prescription of a specific antibiotic; appendicitis is an indication for appendectomy. —**indicate,** *v.*

**indicator** /in′dikā′tər/, a tape, paper, tablet, or other substance that is used to test for a specific reaction because it changes in a predictable visible way. Some kinds of indicators are **autoclave indicator, dipsticks,** and **litmus paper.** Also called **reagent.**

**indicator-dilution method,** a method for measuring blood volume. A known amount of a substance that dissolves freely in blood but does not leave the capillaries is injected intravenously. After a few minutes a sample of blood is withdrawn, and the volume of blood in the body is calculated from the concentration of the substance in the sample, the sample's volume, and the hematocrit.

**indifference-to-pain syndrome** /indif′ərəns/, a congenital lack of pain sensitivity caused by defective development of sensory nerve endings in the skin.

**indigence** /in′dijəns/ [L, *indigere*, to need], a condition of having insufficient income to pay for adequate medical care without depriving oneself or one's dependents of food, clothing, shelter, or other living essentials.

**indigenous** /indij′ənəs/ [L, *indigena*, a native], native to or occurring naturally in a specified area or environment, as certain species of bacteria in the human digestive tract.

**indigestible** /in′dijes′təbəl/ [L, *in*, not, *digerere*, to separate], pertaining to a food substance that cannot be broken down within the digestive tract and converted into an absorbable nutrient.

**indigestion.** See **dyspepsia.**

**indinavir,** an antiretroviral protease inhibitor.

■ INDICATIONS: It is prescribed in the treatment of human immunodeficiency virus infection.

■ CONTRAINDICATIONS: The drug should not be given to patients with a risk of kidney stones. It should be administered with other medications to reduce the risk of resistance development.

■ ADVERSE EFFECTS: The side effects most often reported include nephrolithiasis and hyperbilirubinemia.

**indirect anaphylaxis** [L, *in*, not, *directus,* straight; Gk, *ana,* again, *phylaxis,* protection], an exaggerated reaction of hypersensitivity to one of a person's own antigens that occurs because the antigen has been altered in some way.

**indirect calorimetry,** the measurement of the amount of heat generated in an oxidation reaction by determining the intake or consumption of oxygen or by measuring the amount of carbon dioxide or nitrogen released and translating these quantities into a heat equivalent. Compare **direct calorimetry.**

**indirect Coombs' test,** a blood test used during blood compatibility crossmatching to detect the presence of circulating antibodies against red blood cells. The major purpose of this test is to determine whether the patient has minor serum antibodies (besides the major ABO/Rh system) to red blood cells that he or she is about to receive by blood transfusion.

**indirect division.** See **mitosis.**

**indirect laryngoscopy** [L, *in*, not, *directus,* straight; Gk, *larynx + skopein,* to view], a method of examining the larynx with a mirror.

**indirect nursing care functions,** liaison nurse activities used to solve problems with a consultee who is responsible and accountable for implementing and evaluating any recommended changes.

**indirect ophthalmoscope,** an ophthalmoscope with a biconvex lens that produces a reversed direct stereoscopic image.

**indirect percussion.** See **percussion.**

**indirect provider reimbursement,** a method of payment to an agency for health services delivered by providers, such as nurses.

**indirect restorative method,** a technique for fabricating a restoration on a cast of the original tooth, such as the indirect construction of an inlay. After a die is made from an impression of the prepared tooth, a wax pattern is formed and the inlay is cast. The cast inlay is then fitted and finished on the die and then cemented into the tooth.

**indirect retainer,** that part of a removable partial denture which resists movement of a free end denture base away from its tissue support by means of lever action on the opposite side of the the fulcrum line.

**indirect transfusion** [L, *in + directus,* straight, *transfundere,* to pour through], the transfusion of blood to a recipi-

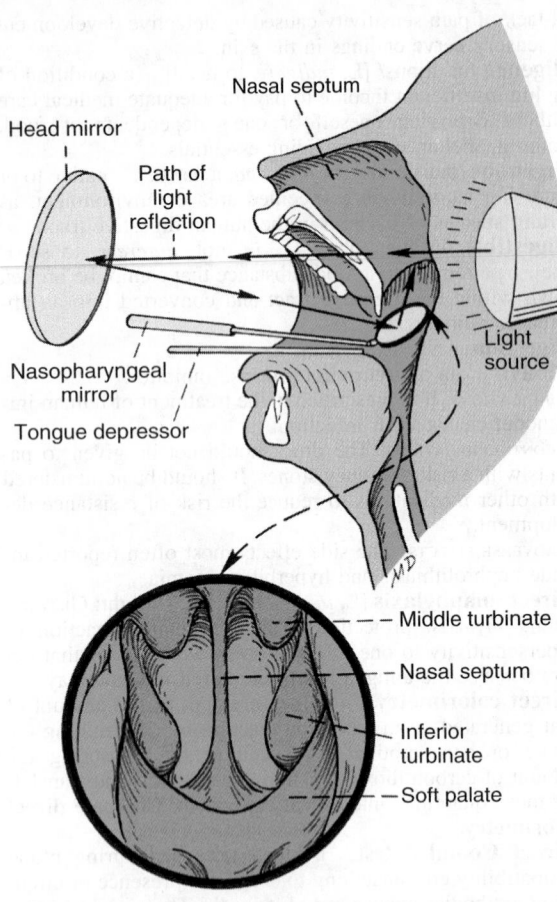

Head mirror

Nasal septum

Path of light reflection

Nasopharyngeal mirror

Tongue depressor

Light source

Middle turbinate

Nasal septum

Inferior turbinate

Soft palate

**Indirect laryngoscopy** (Black, Hawks, and Keene, 2001)

ent after the donor blood has been prepared with anticoagulants, defibrinating agents, or other substances, as opposed to direct transfusion of blood from donor to recipient.

**indirect vision** [L, *in* + *directus,* straight, *visio,* seeing], a visual sensation caused by stimulation of the extramacular portion of the retina. Also called **peripheral vision.**

**indium (In)** [L, *indicum,* indigo], a silvery metallic element with some nonmetallic chemical properties. Its atomic number is 49; its atomic mass is 114.82. It is used in electronic semiconductors.

**individual immunity** /in'divij'ōō·əl/ [L, *individuus,* indivisible, *immunis,* free], a form of natural immunity not shared by most other members of the race and species. It is rare and probably occurs as the result of an infection that was not recognized when it occurred. Compare **racial immunity, species immunity.**

**individual-model HMO,** a health maintenance organization (HMO) in which individual physicians contract directly and independently with the HMO.

**individual psychology,** a modified system of psychoanalysis, developed by Alfred Adler, that views maladaptive behavior and personality disorders as resulting from a conflict between the desire to dominate and feelings of inferiority. See also **inferiority complex.**

**Indocin,** trademark for an antiinflammatory agent (indomethacin).

**indocyanine green** /in'dō·sī'ə·nēn /, a dye occurring as an olive-brown, dark green, dark blue, or black powder; used intravenously as a diagnostic aid in the determination of blood volume, cardiac output, and hepatic function.

**indole** /in'dōl/, a volatile chemical produced during tryptophan metabolism. It is partly responsible for the odor of the feces.

**indoleacetic acid** /in'dōləsē'tik, -əset'ik/, a major terminal metabolite of tryptophan that is present in very small amounts in normal urine and excreted in elevated quantities by patients with carcinoid tumors. It is measured as 5-hydroxyindoleacetic acid (5-HIAA).

**indolent** /in'dələnt/ [L, *in* + *dolere,* to suffer pain], pertaining to an organic disorder that is accompanied by little or no pain.

**indomethacin** /in'dōmeth'əsin/, a nonsteroidal antiinflammatory agent.

■ INDICATIONS: It is prescribed in the treatment of arthritis, gout attacks, and certain other inflammatory conditions.

■ CONTRAINDICATIONS: Upper GI disease or known hypersensitivity to this drug or to aspirin prohibits its use. It is not given to children less than 15 years of age or to pregnant or lactating women.

■ ADVERSE EFFECTS: The most serious adverse reaction is peptic ulcers. GI upset, dizziness, tinnitus, and rashes also may occur.

**induce** /ind(y)ōōs'/ [L, *inducere,* to lead in], to cause or stimulate the start of an activity, as an enzyme induces a metabolic activity. See also **induced fever. —inducer, induction,** *n.*

**induced abortion,** an intentional termination of pregnancy before the fetus has developed enough to live if born. From 20% to 50% of pregnancies are terminated deliberately, at the request of the mother or for medical indications—during the first trimester by vacuum aspiration and/or curettage, or during the second trimester by dilation and evacuation, induction of labor or hysterotomy. Termination of pregnancy by a trained person under proper conditions is safe. Compare **spontaneous abortion.** See also **septic abortion, therapeutic abortion.**

**induced fever,** a deliberate elevation of body temperature by application of heat or by inoculation with a fever-producing organism to kill heat-sensitive pathogens.

**induced lethargy,** a trancelike state produced during hypnosis. See also **hypnosis, lethargy.**

**induced mutation** [L, *inducere,* to lead in, *mutare,* to change], a mutation that has been produced by treatment with a physical or chemical agent that affects the deoxyribonucleic acid molecules of a living organism.

**induced phagocytosis** [L, *inducere,* to lead in; Gk, *phagein,* to eat, *kytos,* cell], the ingestion of microorganisms and other foreign particles by cells of the reticuloendothelial system.

**induced psychotic disorder,** a severe mental disturbance in which there is a withdrawal from reality, resulting from exposure to a toxic agent such as a drug or hallucinogen.

**induced trance,** a somnambulistic state resulting from hypnotism.

**induced vomiting** [L, *inducere,* to lead in; *vomere,* to vomit], vomiting produced by administration of ipecac syrup, soapy water, or handwashing liquid detergent or by insertion of a finger or blunt instrument into the throat. Vomiting may be medically indicated in cases of ingestion of noncaustic poisons but may also be self-induced by patients afflicted with **bulimia.**

**inducer** /indōō'sər/, a substance, usually a substrate of a specific enzyme, that combines with and inactivates the repressor produced by a regulator gene in bacteria. This combination prevents the repressor from blocking activation of the operator gene, allowing one or more structural genes to be transcribed.

**induction** /induk′shən/ [L, *inducere,* to lead in],   the process of stimulating and determining morphogenetic differentiation in a developing embryo through the action of chemical substances transmitted from one embryonic part to another. See also **evocation.**

**induction chemotherapy,**   chemotherapy as the initial treatment for cancer, especially as part of combined modality therapy.

**induction of anesthesia,**   the administration of a drug or combination of drugs that results in a state of general anesthesia; the process of causing general anesthesia by the administration of pharmaceuticals.

**induction of labor,**   an obstetric procedure in which labor is initiated artificially by means of amniotomy or administration of oxytocics. It is performed electively or for fetal or maternal indications. Elective induction is carried out for the convenience of the mother or the obstetrician, often to avert the possibility of delivery outside the hospital when labor is judged to be imminent and the mother is expected to have an unusually rapid birth. Elective inductions are performed less often now than in the past. Prerequisites for elective induction are a term gestation, a fetal weight of at least 2500 g, a cervix judged ready to dilate, a vertex presentation, and engagement of the presenting part of the fetus in the pelvis. Errors in the estimation of gestational age and fetal weight may result in the delivery of an unexpectedly immature or low–birth weight infant. Indicated induction is performed when its risk is judged to be less than that of continuing the pregnancy in such conditions as premature rupture of the membranes, severe maternal diabetes, and intractable preeclampsia. Surgical induction is effected by amniotomy, often with stripping of the membranes and digital stretching of the cervix; it is very often carried out in conjunction with medical induction. Medical induction is achieved through the administration of oxytocin, almost always by IV infusion, in a carefully controlled manner using microdrip equipment or an infusion pump. Beginning with very small amounts of oxytocin in an IV solution, the dosage is increased by gradual increments of the rate or concentration of infusion until effective labor is established. With IV oxytocin inductions a secondary, piggyback infusion without medication is always attached to the tubing so that an unmedicated infusion can be maintained if oxytocin is stopped. Prostaglandins are more commonly used to induce labor in the second trimester, particularly for therapeutic abortions. Electronic fetal and uterine monitoring is usually instituted during induction of labor to prevent hyperstimulation of the uterus and fetal distress. Ideally induced labor mimics natural labor, but in practice it usually does not. Longer and harder contractions commonly occur. In addition to unexpected fetal immaturity, complications of induction of labor include umbilical cord prolapse after amniotomy, tumultuous labor, tetanic uterine contractions, rupture of the uterus, placental abruption, fetal maternal hypotension, water intoxication, postpartum uterine atony and hemorrhage, and fetal asphyxia, hypoxia, or death. If the induction fails to produce effective labor, cesarean section is often required to prevent the adverse sequelae of the procedures used in the induction. For this reason it is usually recommended that induction of labor not be attempted unless delivery must be accomplished to prevent severe fetal or maternal morbidity.

**induction phase,**   the period during which a normal cell becomes transformed into a cancerous cell.

**induction therapy,**   the first therapeutic measure used to treat a disease, especially when combined modality therapy is planned. Also called **first line therapy.**

**inductive approach** /induk′tiv/,   the analysis of data and examination of practice problems within their own context rather than from a predetermined theoretical basis.

**inductor** /induk′tər/ [L, *inducere,* to lead in],   (in embryology) a tissue or cell that emits a chemical substance that stimulates some morphogenetic effect in the developing embryo. See also **evocator, organizer.**

**induration** /in′dyərā′shən/ [L, *indurare,* to make hard],   hardening of a tissue, particularly the skin, caused by edema, inflammation, or infiltration by a neoplasm. —**indurated,** *adj.*

**indurative myocarditis** /in′dyərā′tiv/ [L, *indurare,* to make hard; Gk, *mys,* muscle, *kardia,* heart, *itis,* inflammation], inflammation of the myocardium that leads to a hardening of the muscles of the heart walls.

**industrial health** [L, *industria,* diligence; ME, *helthe*],   the health concerns associated with the workplace, such as exposure to asbestos, mining and milling dusts, metal and acid vapors, lighting, and ergonomic factors.

**Industrial Medical Association (I.M.A.),**   a professional organization whose members are concerned with the identification, prevention, diagnosis, and treatment of disorders associated with technology and industry.

**industrial psychology** [L, *industria,* diligence],   the application of psychologic principles and techniques to the problems of business and industry, including the selection of personnel, the motivation of workers, and the development of training programs.

**indwelling catheter** /in′dweling/ [L, *in,* within; AS, *dwellan,* to remain],   any catheter designed to be left in place for a prolonged period. See also **self-retaining catheter.**

**-ine,**   suffix meaning a 'chemical substance': *chlorine, pyrrolidine, strychnine.*

**inebriant** /inē′brē·ənt/ [L, *inebriare,* to make drunk],   a substance that induces inebriation or intoxication, as does ethanol.

**inebriate** /inē′brē·āt/,   to make drunk.

**inert** /inurt′/ [L, *iners,* idle],   **1.** not moving or acting, such as inert matter. **2.** (of a chemical substance) not taking part in a chemical reaction. **3.** (of a medical ingredient) not active pharmacologically; serving only as a bulking, binding, or sweetening agent or other excipient in a medication.

**inert gas,**   neutral monotomic elements with completely filled outer electron shells. These elements are all gaseous and extremely nonreactive. The inert gases are argon, helium, and neon. Also called **noble gas.**

**inertia** /inur′shə/ [L, idleness],   **1.** the tendency of a body at rest to remain at rest unless acted on by an outside force, and the tendency of a body in motion to remain at motion in the direction in which it is moving unless acted on by an outside force. **2.** an abnormal condition characterized by a general inactivity or sluggishness, such as colonic inertia or uterine inertia.

**inertial impaction** /inur′shəl/,   the deposition of large aerosol particles on the walls of an airway conduit. The impaction tends to occur where the airway direction changes. Small particles have less inertia and are more likely to be carried around corners and continue in the path of the airflow.

**inevitable abortion** /inev′itəbəl/ [L, *inevitabilis,* unavoidable],   a condition of pregnancy in which spontaneous termination is imminent and cannot be prevented. It is characterized by bleeding, uterine cramping, dilation of the cervix, and presentation of the conceptus in the cervical os. If heavy bleeding supervenes, immediate evacuation of the uterus may be required. Transvaginal ultrasound makes it possible to determine presence or absence of fetal heart movement at 5 weeks gestation. Compare **incomplete abortion, threatened abortion.**

**in extremis,** in the extremity, or at the point of death.

**infant** /in′fənt/ [L, *infans*, unable to speak], **1.** a child who is in the earliest stage of extrauterine life, a time extending from the first month after birth to approximately 12 months of age, when the baby is able to assume an erect posture. **2.** (in law) a person not of full legal age; a minor. **3.** pertaining to infancy; in an early stage of development. —**infantile,** *adj.*

**infant behavior, disorganized,** a nursing diagnosis accepted by the Eleventh National Conference on the Classification of Nursing Diagnoses. It is defined as an alteration in integration and modulation of the physiologic and behavioral systems of functioning (i.e., the autonomic, motor, state, organizational, self-regulatory, and attentional-interactional systems).

■ DEFINING CHARACTERISTICS: Major defining characteristics are change from baseline physiologic measures; tremors, startles, and twitches; hyperextension of arms and legs; diffuse/unclear sleep; deficient self-regulatory behaviors; and deficient response to visual/auditory stimuli. Minor defining characteristics are yawning and apnea.

■ RELATED FACTORS: The related factors are pain, oral motor problems, feeding intolerance, environmental overstimulation, lack of containment or boundaries, prematurity, and invasive or painful procedures. See also **nursing diagnosis.**

**infant behavior, disorganized: risk for,** a nursing diagnosis accepted by the Eleventh National Conference on the Classification of Nursing Diagnoses. It is defined as a risk for alteration in integration and modulation of the physiologic and behavioral systems of functioning (i.e., autonomic, motor, state, organizational, self-regulatory, and attentional-interactional systems).

■ RISK FACTORS: The risk factors are pain, oral motor problems, environmental overstimulation, lack of containment or boundaries, prematurity, and invasive or painful procedures. See also **nursing diagnosis.**

**infant behavior, organized, readiness for enhanced,** a nursing diagnosis accepted by the Eleventh National Conference on the Classification of Nursing Diagnoses. It is defined as a pattern of modulation of the physiologic and behavioral systems of functioning of an infant (i.e., autonomic, motor, state, organizational, self-regulatory, and attentional-interactional systems) that is satisfactory but can be improved, producing higher levels of integration in response to environmental stimuli.

■ DEFINING CHARACTERISTICS: The defining characteristics are stable physiologic measures, definite sleep/wake states, use of some self-regulatory behaviors, and response to visual or auditory stimuli.

■ RELATED FACTORS: The related factors are prematurity and pain. See also **nursing diagnosis.**

**infant botulism,** an intoxication by neurotoxins produced by *Clostridium botulinum* that occurs in children less than 6 months of age. The condition is characterized by severe hypotonicity of all muscles, constipation, lethargy, and feeding difficulties, and it may lead to respiratory insufficiency. The botulism neurotoxin is usually found in the GI tract rather than in the blood, indicating that it is probably produced in the gut rather than ingested; the epidemiologic and pathophysiologic characteristics of the syndrome are not clearly understood. Treatment is supportive, including optimal

management of fluids, electrolytes, and nutrition. Ventilatory support may also be necessary. There is no evidence that antitoxin therapy is helpful, and it is usually not recommended.

**infant care,** a nursing intervention from the Nursing Interventions Classification (NIC) defined as provision of developmentally appropriate family-centered care to the child under 1 year of age. See also **Nursing Interventions Classification.**

**infant death,** the death of a live-born infant before 1 year of age.

**infant feeder,** a device for nourishing small or weak babies who cannot suck hard enough to get milk from the breast or a bottle. The feeder resembles a bulb syringe with a long soft nipple on the end. The bulb is squeezed slowly and gently, permitting the baby to suck and swallow without great effort and preventing the escape of fluid into the infant's trachea, where it may cause asphyxiation or aspiration pneumonia.

**infant feeding.** See **bottle feeding, breastfeeding.**

**infant feeding pattern, ineffective,** a nursing diagnosis accepted by the Tenth National Conference on the Classification of Nursing Diagnoses. It is defined as a state in which an infant demonstrates an impaired ability to suck or coordinate the suck-swallow response.

■ DEFINING CHARACTERISTICS: The defining characteristics are an inability to initiate or sustain an effective suck and inability to coordinate sucking, swallowing, and breathing.

■ RELATED FACTORS: Related factors are prematurity, neurologic impairment or delay, oral hypersensitivity, prolonged NPO status, and anatomic abnormalities. See also **nursing diagnosis.**

**infanticide** /infan′tisīd/ [L, *infans*, unable to speak, *caedere,* to kill], **1.** the killing of an infant or young child. The act is usually a psychotic reaction often associated with severe depression, such as occurs in bipolar disorder and occasionally in extreme postpartum disturbances. Infanticide may become a neurotic obsession among mothers who do not want the baby or who do not feel physically, mentally, or emotionally capable of caring for or coping with the infant. **2.** one who takes the life of an infant or young child. —**infanticidal,** *adj.*

**infantile** /in′fəntīl/ [L, *infans*, unable to speak], **1.** of, relating to, or characteristic of infants or infancy. **2.** lacking maturity, sophistication, or reasonableness. **3.** affected with infantilism. **4.** being in a very early stage of development.

**infantile acrodermatitis.** See **Gianotti-Crosti syndrome.**

**infantile amnesia,** (in psychology) the inability to remember events from early childhood. It is explained by a theory that a memory for skills develops earlier than a fact-memory system, which may not develop until the third year. Thus a person may learn skills without remembering how the skills were acquired.

**infantile arteritis,** a disorder in infants and young children characterized by inflammation of many arteries in which atherosclerotic lesions are rarely present.

**infantile autism,** a pervasive developmental disorder characterized by abnormal emotional, social, and linguistic development in a child. Symptoms include abnormal ways of relating to people, objects, and situations. It may result from organic brain dysfunction, in which case it occurs before 3 years of age. See also **autistic disorder.**

**infantile celiac disease.** See **celiac disease.**

**infantile cerebral ataxic paralysis** [L, *infans*, unable to speak, *cerebrum*, the brain; Gk, *ataxia*, without order, *paralyein,* to be palsied], a form of congenital diplegia, characterized by cerebral maldevelopment, ataxia, spasticity of the legs, and possibly mental deficiency.

**infantile cerebral sphingolipidosis.** See **Tay-Sachs disease.**

**infantile cirrhosis,** a progressive fibrous liver disorder caused by protein malnutrition.

**infantile colic** [L, *infans,* unable to speak; Gk, *kolikos,* pain in the colon], a descriptive term for a suggested intestinal cause of discomfort in a newborn; specific causes and mechanisms have not been defined. The typical infantile colic patient eats and gains weight but may also appear excessively hungry. Aerophagia caused by crying may lead to flatulence and abdominal distension.

**infantile cortical hyperostosis,** a familial disorder characterized in an infant by bony swellings and tenderness in the affected areas. The child also tends to be feverish and irritable. The mandible is most commonly involved. Radiographs indicate areas of new bone growth beneath the periosteum. Also called **Caffey's disease.**

**infantile dwarf,** a person whose mental and physical development is greatly retarded as a result of various causes, such as genetic or developmental defects.

**infantile eczema.** See **atopic dermatitis.**

**infantile encephalitis** [L, *infans,* unable to speak; Gk, *enkephalos,* brain, *itis,* inflammation], any of a group of brain inflammation conditions affecting infants. The cause may be a direct viral infection or a secondary encephalitis that is a complication of measles, chickenpox, rubella, or other diseases.

**infantile hemiplegia,** paralysis of one side of the body that may occur at birth as a result of a cerebral hemorrhage, in utero as a result of lack of oxygen, or during a febrile illness in infancy.

**infantile hydrocele** [L, *infans* + Gk, *hydor,* water, *kele,* hernia], an accumulation of fluid in the tunica vaginalis. It may be present at birth or acquired.

**infantile neuroaxonal dystrophy,** progressive hereditary degenerative encephalopathy transmitted as an autosomal recessive trait, beginning in infancy with muscular hypotonia and arrest of development in late infancy, followed by dementia, blindness, spasticity, and ataxia. Pathologically it is characterized by widespread focal swellings and degeneration of the axons with scattered globular bodies in the brain. Also called **Seitelberger's disease.**

**infantile paralysis.** See **poliomyelitis.**

**infantile pellagra.** See **kwashiorkor.**

**infantile poliomyelitis.** See **acute atrophic paralysis.**

**infantile scurvy,** a nutritional disease caused by an inadequate dietary supply of vitamin C, which may occur because cow's milk unfortified with vitamin C is the principal food in an infant's diet. Families are counseled to feed their children foods rich in vitamin C or to use a formula supplemented with this vitamin. Also called **Barlow's disease, hemorrhagic scurvy.** See also **ascorbic acid, scurvy.**

**infantile spinal muscular atrophy.** See **Werdnig-Hoffmann disease.**

**infantile spinal paralysis** [L, *infans,* unable to speak, *spina* + Gk, *paralyein,* to be palsied], acute anterior poliomyelitis, a viral infection characterized by nonspecific illnesses, aseptic meningitis, and flaccid weakness of muscle groups.

**infantile uterus,** a uterus that has failed to attain adult characteristics.

**infantilism** /infan'tiliz'əm/ [L, *infans,* unable to speak], **1.** a condition in which various anatomic, physiologic, and psychologic characteristics of childhood persist in the adult. It is characterized by mental retardation, underdeveloped sexual organs, and usually small stature. Compare **progeria.**

**2.** a condition, usually of psychologic rather than organic origin, characterized by speech and voice patterns in an older child or adult that are typical of very young children.

**infant mortality,** the statistical rate of infant death during the first year after live birth, expressed as the number of such deaths per 1000 live births in a specific geographic area or institution in a given period. Neonatal mortality (death within 28 days of birth) accounts for 70% of infant mortality.

**infant of chemically dependent mother,** a newborn who shows withdrawal symptoms, usually within the first 24 hours of life, most commonly caused by maternal antepartum dependence on heroin, methadone, diazepam, phenobarbital, or alcohol. See also **fetal alcohol syndrome.**

■ OBSERVATIONS: Characteristic symptoms include tremors, irritability, hyperactive reflexes, increased muscle tone, twitching, increased mucus production, nasal congestion, respiratory distress, excessive sweating, elevated temperature, vomiting, diarrhea, and dehydration. The infants cry shrilly, often sneeze, frantically suck their fists but feed poorly, and frequently yawn but have difficulty falling asleep. They are usually pale, are often born with nose and knee abrasions, and are subject to convulsions.

■ INTERVENTIONS: The infant is kept warm, snugly swaddled in a padded crib, and exposed to minimal visual, auditory, and tactile stimulation. The baby is handled only when necessary and is then held firmly, close to the body.

■ NURSING CONSIDERATIONS: These high-risk infants require special attention, and it is important for the mother to be encouraged to participate in her baby's care as soon as possible. The nurse may help promote parent-child bonding.

**infarct** /infärkt'/ [L, *infarcire,* to stuff], a localized area of necrosis in a tissue resulting from anoxia. It is caused by an interruption in the blood supply to the area or, less frequently, by circulatory stasis produced by the occlusion of a vein that ordinarily carries blood away from the area. Some infarcts are pale and white because of the lack of circulation. Others may resemble a red, swollen bruise because of hemorrhage and an accumulation of blood in the area. Also called **infarction.**

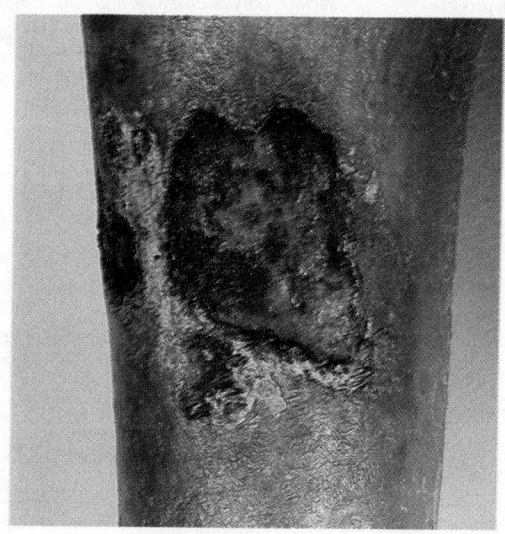

**Infarct** (du Vivier, 1993)

**infarct extension,** a myocardial infarction that has spread beyond the original area, usually as a result of the death of cells in the ischemic margin of the infarct zone.

**infarction** /infärk'shən/ [L, *infarcire,* to stuff], **1.** an infarct. **2.** the development and formation of an infarct. Kinds of infarction include **myocardial infarction** and **pulmonary infarction.**

**infect** [L, *inficere,* to stain], to transmit a pathogen that may induce development of an infectious disease in another person.

**infected abortion,** a spontaneous or induced termination of an immature pregnancy in which the products of conception have become infected, causing fever and requiring antibiotic therapy and evacuation of the uterus. Compare **septic abortion.**

**infection** /infek'shən/ [L, *inficere,* to stain], **1.** the invasion of the body by pathogenic microorganisms that reproduce and multiply, causing disease by local cellular injury, secretion of a toxin, or antigen-antibody reaction in the host. **2.** a disease caused by the invasion of the body by pathogenic microorganisms. Compare **infestation. —infectious,** *adj.*

**infection control[1],** the policies and procedures of a hospital or other health facility to minimize the risk of spreading of nosocomial or community-acquired infections to patients or members of the staff.

**infection control[2],** a nursing intervention from the Nursing Interventions Classification (NIC) defined as minimizing the acquisition and transmission of infectious agents. See also **Nursing Interventions Classification.**

**infection control committee,** a group of hospital health professionals composed of infection control personnel, with medical, nursing, administrative, and occasionally dietary and housekeeping department representatives, who plan and supervise infection control activities.

**infection control: intraoperative,** a nursing intervention from the Nursing Interventions Classification (NIC) defined as preventing nosocomial infection in the operating room. See also **Nursing Interventions Classification.**

**infection control nurse,** a registered nurse who is assigned responsibility for surveillance and infection prevention, education, and control activities.

**infection protection,** a nursing intervention from the Nursing Interventions Classification (NIC) defined as prevention and early detection of infection in a patient at risk. See also **Nursing Interventions Classification.**

**infection, risk for,** a nursing diagnosis accepted by the Seventh National Conference on the Classification of Nursing Diagnoses. Risk for infection is defined as the state in which an individual is at increased risk for being invaded by pathogenic organisms.

■ RISK FACTORS: Risk factors include inadequate primary defenses, such as broken skin, traumatized tissue, decrease in ciliary action, stasis of body fluids, change in pH secretions, and altered peristalsis; inadequate secondary defenses, such as decreased hemoglobin, leukopenia, suppressed inflammatory response, and immunosuppression; inadequate acquired immunity; tissue destruction and increased environmental exposure; chronic disease; invasive procedures; malnutrition; pharmaceutic agents; trauma; rupture of amniotic membranes; and insufficient knowledge to avoid exposure to pathogens. See also **nursing diagnosis.**

**infection status,** a nursing outcome from the Nursing Outcomes Classification (NOC) defined as presence and extent of infection. See also **Nursing Outcomes Classification.**

**infectious** /infek'chəs/, **1.** capable of causing an infection. **2.** caused by an infection.

**infectious arthritis** [L, *inficere,* to stain; Gk, *arthron,* joint + *-itis,* inflammation], arthritis caused by bacteria, rickettsiae, mycoplasmas, viruses, fungi, or parasites.

**infectious bulbar paralysis** [L, *inficere,* to stain, *bulbus,* swollen root; Gk, *paralyein,* to be palsied], a herpesvirus disease of animals that may cause a mild pruritus when transmitted to humans. Also called **pseudorabies.**

**infectious disease** [L, *inficere,* to stain, *dis* + Fr, *aise,* ease], any communicable disease, or one that can be transmitted from one human being to another or from animal to human by direct or indirect contact.

**infectious endocarditis,** endocarditis caused by infection with microorganisms, especially bacteria and fungi. It has been classified according to course as acute and subacute: the *acute* form is usually due to staphylococci, pneumococci, gonococci, or streptococci, involves a normal heart valve, and has a short history and rapid course; the *subacute* form usually is due to viridans or fecal streptococci or to fungi, affects damaged heart valves, and has a prolonged course. Because underlying causes and available therapies have changed, this division has little current clinical validity and has been largely replaced by classification on the basis of cause or underlying anatomy.

## Defenses against infection

| Types of defense | Specific mechanism |
| --- | --- |
| Surface defenses | Physical barriers: skin, conjunctivae, mucous membranes |
| | Mechanical removal: desquamation of skin, tears, mucus, ciliary action, coughing, salivation, swallowing, urination, defecation |
| | Normal bacterial flora: antibacterial factors |
| | Chemical inhibitors: gastric acid, lactic acid, fatty acids, spermine, lactoperoxidase, bile salts |
| | Antimicrobial substances: lysozyme, secretory IgA |
| Nonspecific resistance factors | Fever, interferons, complement, lysozyme, C-reactive protein (reacts with bacterial surface polysaccharides and activates complement), lactoferrin (binds and removes iron as a bacterial nutrient), α-l-antitrypsin (inhibits bacterial enzymes) |
| Inflammation | Soluble factors: |
| | Clotting system: Hageman factor (factor XII) |
| | Complement system: chemotactic factors, anaphylatoxins |
| | Kinin system: bradykinin |
| | Phagocytes |
| | Circulating neutrophils, eosinophils, monocytes, macrophages |
| | Fixed cells (of mononuclear phagocyte system) in alveoli, spleen, liver, bone marrow |
| Immune response | Humoral immune response: B cells, plasma cells, immunoglobulins |
| | Cell-mediated immune response: T cells, lymphokines |

From McCance KL, Huether SE: *Pathophysiology: the biological basis for disease in adults and children,* ed 2, St Louis, 1994, Mosby.

**infectious-exhaustive syndrome.** See **postinfectious psychosis.**

**infectious granuloma** [L, *inficere,* to stain, *granulum,* little grain; Gk, *oma,* tumor], a lumpy lesion of granuloma tissue that may develop in diseases such as tuberculosis, syphilis, and actinomycosis.

**infectious hepatitis.** See **hepatitis A.**

**infectious isolation** [L, *inficere,* to stain; It, *isolare,* to detach], a practice of confining a patient with a particularly virulent disease to an isolated room or other area so as to reduce the risk of contact and spread of the disease among hospital personnel.

**infectious mononucleosis** [L, *inficere,* to stain; Gk, *monos,* single; L, *nucleus,* nut; Gk, *osis,* condition], an acute herpesvirus infection caused by the Epstein-Barr virus. It is characterized by fever, sore throat, swollen lymph glands, atypical lymphocytes, splenomegaly, hepatomegaly, abnormal liver function, and bruising. The disease is usually transmitted by droplet infection but is not highly or predictably contagious. Young people are most often affected. In childhood the disease is mild and usually unnoticed; the older the person, the more severe the symptoms are likely to be. Infection confers permanent immunity, although the virus continues to replicate and can be transmitted. Treatment is primarily symptomatic, with enforced bed rest to prevent serious complications of the liver or spleen, analgesics to control pain, and saline gargles for throat discomfort. Rupture of the spleen may occur, requiring immediate surgery and blood transfusion. See also **Epstein-Barr virus, viral infection.**

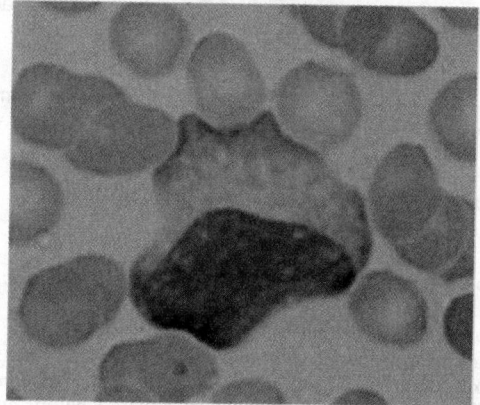

**Infectious mononucleosis** *(Zitelli and Davis, 1997)*

**infectious myringitis,** an inflammatory contagious condition of the eardrum caused by viral or bacterial infection. It is characterized by the development of painful vesicles on the drum. Also called **bullous myringitis.**

**infectious nucleic acid,** deoxyribonucleic acid or, more commonly, viral ribonucleic acid that is able to infect the nucleic acid of a cell and to induce the host to produce viruses.

**infectious parotitis.** See **mumps.**

**infectious polyneuritis.** See **Guillain-Barré syndrome.**

**infective endocarditis.** See **bacterial endocarditis.**

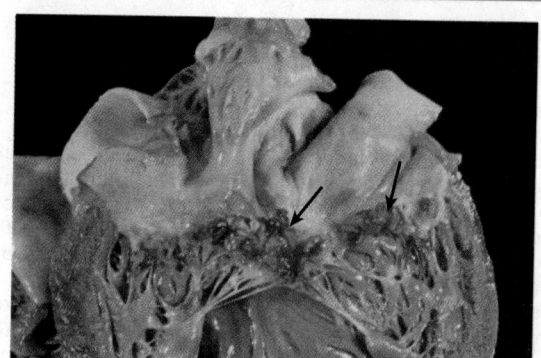

**Bacterial infective endocarditis**
*(Cotran, Kumar, and Collins, 1999)*

**infective tubulointerstitial nephritis** [L, *inficere,* to stain, *tubulus,* tubule, *interstitium,* space between], an acute inflammation of the kidneys caused by an infection by *Escherichia coli* or another pyogenic pathogen. The condition is characterized by chills, fever, nausea and vomiting, flank pain, dysuria, proteinuria, and hematuria. The kidney may become enlarged, and portions of the renal cortex may be destroyed. Infection is usually the result of bacterial contamination of a urinary catheter, but it may occur in any condition characterized by urinary stasis.

**infectivity** /infektiv′itē/ [L, *inficere,* to stain], the ability of a pathogen to spread rapidly from one host to another.

**inferior** /infir′ē·ər/ [L, *inferus,* lower], **1.** situated below or lower than a given point of reference, as the feet are inferior to the legs. **2.** of poorer quality or value. Compare **superior.**

**inferior alveolar artery,** an artery that descends with the inferior alveolar nerve from the first or mandibular portion of the maxillary artery to the mandibular foramen on the medial surface of the ramus of the mandible. It enters the mandibular canal and runs through to the first premolar tooth, where it divides into the mental and incisor branches. Also called **arteria alveolaris inferior.**

**inferior aperture of minor pelvis,** an irregular aperture bounded by the coccyx, the sacrotuberous ligaments, part of the ischium, the sides of the pubic arch, and the pubic symphysis.

**inferior aperture of thorax,** an irregular opening bounded by the twelfth thoracic vertebra, the eleventh and twelfth ribs, and the edge of the costal cartilages as they meet the sternum.

**inferior carotid triangle** [L, *inferior,* lower; Gk, *karos,* heavy sleep; L, *triangulus,* three-cornered], a triangular area bounded by the midline of the neck, the superior belly of the omohyoid muscle above, and the sternocleidomastoid muscle behind. Also called **muscular triangle.**

**inferior conjunctival fornix,** the space in the fold of conjunctiva created by the reflection of the conjunctiva covering the eyeball and the lining of the lower eyelid. Compare **superior conjunctival fornix.**

**inferior gastric node,** a node in one of two groups of gastric lymph glands, lying between the two layers of the lesser omentum along the pyloric half of the greater curvature of the stomach. Compare **hepatic node, superior gastric node.**

**inferiority complex** /infir′ē·ôr′itē/, **1.** a personal feeling or sense of being inadequate. It is largely unconscious and influences attitudes and behaviors. **2.** (in psychoanalysis) a complex characterized by striving for unrealistic goals motivated by an unresolved Oedipus complex. **3.** *informal.* a feeling of being inferior.

**inferior maxillary bone.** See **mandible.**

**inferior mesenteric artery,** a visceral branch of the abdominal aorta, arising just above the division into the common iliacs and supplying the left half of the transverse colon, all of the descending and iliac colons, and most of the rectum. It has left colic, sigmoid, and superior rectal branches.

**inferior mesenteric node,** a node in one of the three groups of visceral lymph glands serving the viscera of the abdomen and the pelvis. The inferior mesenteric nodes are associated with the branches of the inferior mesenteric artery. The inferior mesenteric nodes drain the descending colon, the iliac and sigmoid parts of the colon, and the upper part of the rectum. Their efferent vessels pass to the preaortic nodes. Compare **gastric node, superior mesenteric node.**

**inferior mesenteric vein,** the vein in the lower body that returns the blood from the rectum, the sigmoid and descending colons, and part of the transverse colon. It receives the sigmoid veins from the sigmoid colon and the iliac colon and the left colic vein from the descending colon and the left colic flexure. Compare **superior mesenteric vein.**

**inferior olivary nucleus** [L, *inferior,* lower, *oliva,* olive, *nucleus,* nut kernel], a small purse-shaped collection of nerve cells lying posterolateral to the pyramid, just below the level of the pons. It is a source of cerebellar climbing fibers.

**inferior orbital fissure,** a groove in the inferolateral wall of the orbit that contains the infraorbital and zygomatic nerves and the infraorbital vessels.

**inferior phrenic artery,** a small visceral branch of the abdominal aorta that arises from the aorta itself, the renal artery, or the celiac artery. It divides into the medial and lateral branches and supplies the diaphragm. A few vessels of the inferior vena cava stem from the lateral branch of the right phrenic artery. Some branches of the left phrenic artery supply the esophagus.

**inferior pole of kidney.** See **poles of kidney.**

**inferior radioulnar joint.** See **distal radioulnar articulation.**

**inferior sagittal sinus,** one of the six venous channels of the posterior dura mater, draining blood from the brain into the internal jugular vein. It receives deoxygenated blood from several veins from the falx cerebri and in some individuals from a few veins from the cerebral hemispheres. Compare **straight sinus, superior sagittal sinus, transverse sinus.**

**inferior subscapular nerve** /subskap′yo͞olər/, one of two small nerves on opposite sides of the back that arise from the posterior cord of the brachial plexus. It supplies the distal part of the subscapularis and ends in the teres major. Compare **superior subscapular nerve.**

**inferior thyroid vein,** one of the few veins that arise in the venous plexus on the thyroid gland and form a plexus ventral to the trachea, under the sternothyroideus muscle. A left vein descends from this plexus to join the left brachiocephalic trunk; a right vein descends obliquely to open into the right brachiocephalic vein at its junction with the superior vena cava.

**inferior ulnar collateral artery,** one of a pair of branches of the deep brachial arteries, arising about 5 cm from the elbow, passing inward to form an arch with the deep brachial artery, and carrying blood to the muscles of the forearm. Compare **superior ulnar collateral artery.**

**inferior vena cava,** the large vein that returns deoxygenated blood to the heart from parts of the body below the diaphragm. It is formed by the junction of the two common iliac veins to the right of the fifth lumbar vertebra and ascends along the vertebral column, pierces the diaphragm, and opens into the right atrium of the heart. As it passes through the diaphragm it receives a covering of serous pericardium. The inferior vena cava contains a semilunar valve that is rudimentary in the adult but very large and important in the fetus. The vessel receives blood from the two common iliacs, the lumbar veins, and the testicular veins. Compare **superior vena cava.**

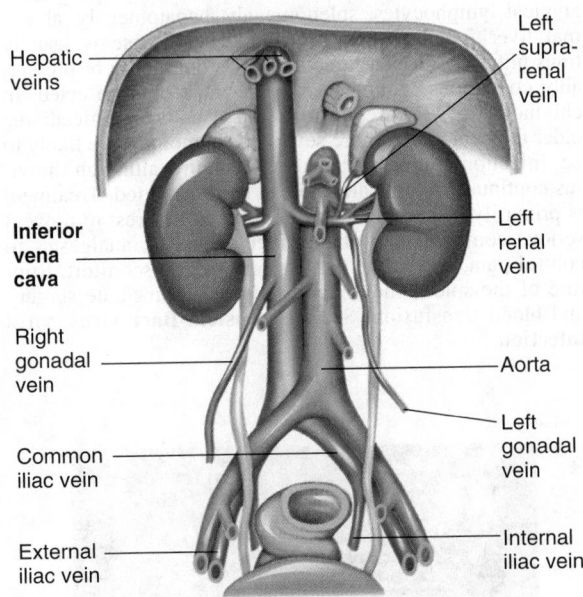

Hepatic veins
Left suprarenal vein
Inferior vena cava
Left renal vein
Right gonadal vein
Aorta
Left gonadal vein
Common iliac vein
External iliac vein
Internal iliac vein

**Inferior vena cava and its tributaries**

**infero-,** prefix meaning 'low': *inferolateral, inferomedial, inferoposterior.*

**inferolateral** /in′fərōlat′ərəl/ [L, *inferus,* lower, *latus,* side], pertaining to a location situated below and to the side.

**inferomedial** /in′fərōmē′dē·əl/ [L, *inferus,* lower, *medius,* middle], pertaining to a location situated below and toward the center.

**infertile** /infur′təl/ [L, *in,* not, *fertilis,* fruitful], denoting the inability to produce offspring. This condition may be present in one or both sex partners and may be temporary and reversible. The cause may be physical, including immature sexual organs, abnormalities of the reproductive system, hormonal imbalance, and dysfunction or anomalies in other organ systems, or it may result from psychologic or emotional problems. The condition is classified as primary, in which pregnancy has never occurred, and secondary, when there have been one or more pregnancies. Compare **sterile.**

**infertility** /in′furtil′itē/, the condition of being unable to produce offspring. Compare **sterility.**

**infest** /infest′/, to attack, invade, and subsist on the skin or in the internal organs of a host. Compare **infect.**

**infestation** /in'festā'shən/ [L, *infestare,* to attack], the presence of animal parasites in the environment, on the skin, or in the hair of a host.

**infiltrate** /infil'trāt/ **1.** *v.* to penetrate the interstices of a tissue or substance. **2.** *n.* the material or solution so deposited.

**infiltration** /in'filtrās'hən/ [L, *in,* within, *filtare,* to strain through], the process whereby a fluid passes into the tissues, such as when a local anesthetic is administered or an IV infusion infiltrates.

**infiltrative disorder** /infil'trətiv/, a condition caused by the diffusion or accumulation in cells or tissues of substances not normally found in those cells or tissues, as in granulomatous diseases.

**infirmary** /infur'mərē/ [L, *infirmus,* weak], a hospital, originally a part of a monastery, that provides care for sick or infirm persons, particularly indigent patients.

**inflammable.** See **flammable.**

**inflammation** [L, *inflammare,* to set afire], the protective response of body tissues to irritation or injury. Inflammation may be acute or chronic; its cardinal signs are redness (rubor), heat (calor), swelling (tumor), and pain (dolor), often accompanied by loss of function. The process begins with a transitory vasoconstriction, then is followed by a brief increase in vascular permeability. The second stage is prolonged and consists of sustained increase in vascular permeability, exudation of fluids from the vessels, clustering of leukocytes along the vessel walls, phagocytosis of microorganisms, deposition of fibrin in the vessel, disposal of the accumulated debris by macrophages, and finally migration of fibroblasts to the area and development of new, normal cells. The severity, timing, and local character of any particular inflammatory response depend on the cause, the area affected, and the condition of the host. Histamine, kinins, and various other substances mediate the inflammatory process.

**inflammation of the liver.** See **hepatitis.**

**inflammatory** /inflam'ətôr'ē/ [L, *inflammare,* to set afire], pertaining to or resembling inflammation.

**inflammatory autobullectomy,** spontaneous regression of a bulla caused by inflammation in patients with bullous emphysema.

**inflammatory bowel disease.** See **Crohn's disease, ulcerative colitis.**

**inflammatory cell,** a cell (neutrophil, macrophage, etc.) participating in the inflammatory response to a foreign substance.

**inflammatory dysmenorrhea** [L, *inflammare* + Gk, *dys* + *men,* month, *rhein,* to flow], menstrual pain that accompanies pelvic infection, fibroids, or endometritis. Also called **secondary dysmenorrhea.**

**inflammatory fracture** [L, *inflammare,* to set afire, *fractura,* break], a break in bone tissue weakened by inflammation.

**inflammatory response,** a tissue reaction to injury or an antigen that may include pain, swelling, itching, redness, heat, and loss of function. The response may involve dilation of blood vessels and consequent leakage of fluid, causing edema; leukocytic exudation; and release of plasma proteases and vasoactive amines such as histamine.

**inflammatory scoliosis** [L, *inflammare* + Gk, *skoliosis,* curvature], a form of scoliosis caused by muscle spasms associated with acute inflammation.

**inflatable pessary.** See **pessary.**

**inflatable splint** /inflā'təbəl/ [L, *in,* within, *flare,* to blow;

ME, *splente*], a tubular device that is placed around a patient's extremity and inflated with air to maintain rigidity. Also called **pneumatic splint.**

**infliximab,** a monoclonal antibody.

■ INDICATIONS: Infliximab is used to treat moderate to severe fistulizing Crohn's disease.

■ CONTRAINDICATIONS: Known hypersensitivity to murines prohibits the use of infliximab.

■ ADVERSE EFFECTS: Life-threatening effects of this drug are anaphylaxis, anemia, and tachycardia. Other adverse reactions include dry skin, sweating, flushing, hematoma, pruritus, upper respiratory infection, pharyngitis, bronchitis, cough, dyspnea, sinusitis, myalgia, back pain, arthralgia, dysuria, urinary frequency, chest pain, hypertension, and hypotension. Common side effects include nausea, vomiting, abdominal pain, stomatitis, constipation, dyspepsia, flatulence, headache, dizziness, depression, vertigo, fatigue, anxiety, fever, rash, dermatitis, and urticaria.

**influenza** /in'floo·en'zə/ [It, influence], a highly contagious infection of the respiratory tract caused by a myxovirus and transmitted by airborne droplet infection. It occurs in isolated cases, epidemics, and pandemics. Symptoms include sore throat, cough, fever, muscular pains, and weakness. The incubation period is brief (from 1 to 3 days), and the onset is usually sudden, with chills, fever, respiratory symptoms, headache, myalgia, and extreme fatigue. Treatment is symptomatic and usually involves bed rest, acetaminophen, and drinking of fluids. Fever and constitutional symptoms distinguish influenza from the common cold. Complete recovery in from 3 to 10 days is the rule, but bacterial pneumonia may occur among high-risk patients, such as the elderly, the very young, and people who have chronic pulmonary disease. Three main strains of influenza virus have been recognized: type A, type B, and type C. New strains of the virus emerge at regular intervals and are named according to their geographic origin, for example, **Asian flu.** Yearly vaccination with the currently prevalent strain of influenza virus is recommended for elderly or debilitated persons and health care personnel. Treatment or prophylaxis in high-risk patients may be achieved with rimantadine. Oseltamivir (oral) and Zanamivir (aerosol), when administered within 48 hours of onset, can lessen the severity and duration of symptoms. Also called **grippe, la grippe,** *(informal)* **flu.**

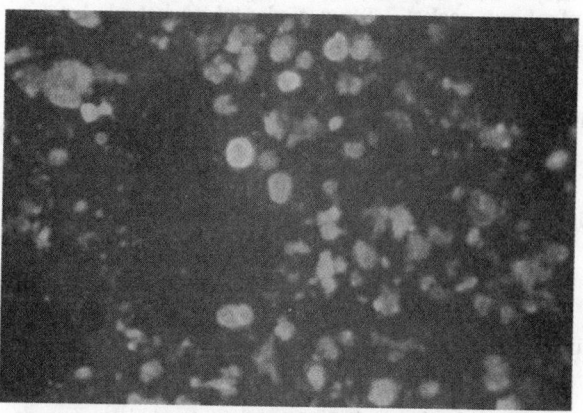

**Respiratory secretion showing influenza A virus**
*(Murray et al, 1990/courtesy Richard Thomson, Akron, Ohio)*

**Influenzavirus A,** a genus of viruses of the family Orthomyxoviridae, containing the agent of influenza A. See also **influenza.**

**Influenzavirus B,** a genus of viruses of the family Orthomyxoviridae containing the agent of influenza B. See **influenza.**

**Influenzavirus C,** a genus of viruses of the family Orthomyxoviridae containing the agent of influenza C. See **influenza.**

**influenza-virus vaccine,** an active immunizing agent.
- INDICATION: It is prescribed for immunization against influenza.
- CONTRAINDICATIONS: Acute infection or allergy to eggs prohibits its use.
- ADVERSE EFFECTS: Among the more serious adverse reactions are anaphylaxis and Guillain-Barré syndrome.

**informal admission,** a type of admission to a psychiatric hospital in which there is no formal or written application and the patient is free to leave at any time. See also **involuntary patient.**

**information processing,** a nursing outcome from the Nursing Outcomes Classification (NOC) defined as the ability to acquire, organize, and use information. See also **Nursing Outcomes Classification.**

**information systems director** [L, *informatio,* idea], a person who directs and administers a data processing facility. Also called **chief information officer (CIO).**

**informed consent** [L, *informare,* to give form, *consentire,* to sense], permission obtained from a patient to perform a specific test or procedure. Informed consent is required before performing most invasive procedures and before admitting a patient to a research study. The document used must be written in a language understood by the patient and be dated and signed by the patient and at least one witness. Signed consent should be obtained by the person performing the procedure. Included in the document are clear, rational statements that describe the procedure or test. Also required is a statement that care will not be withheld if the patient does not consent; informed consent is voluntary. By law, informed consent must be obtained more than a given number of days or hours before certain procedures, including therapeutic abortion and sterilization, and must always be obtained when the patient is fully competent. An individual must be of a certain legal age to give consent; laws vary from state to state.

**infra-,** prefix meaning 'situated, formed, or occurring beneath': *infraclavicular, infracortical, infratemporal.*

**infrabony pocket.** See **periodontal pocket.**

**infraclavicular fossa** /in′frəkləvik′yələr/, a small pocket or indentation just below the clavicle on both sides of the body.

**infraclusion** /in′frə·kloo′zhən/ [L, *infra,* below + *occludere,* to close up], malocclusion in which a tooth has failed to erupt fully and reach the line of occlusion and is out of contact with the opposing tooth. Also called **infraversion.**

**infraction fracture** /infrak′shən/ [L, *infractio,* a breaking, *fractura,* break], a neoplastic fracture characterized by a small radiolucent line in radiographs and most commonly associated with a disorder of metabolism. See also **greenstick fracture.**

**infradentale** /in′frə·den·tā′lē /, a bone measurement landmark, being the highest anterior point on the gingiva between the mandibular central incisors.

**infradian rhythm** /in′frā′dē·ən/ [L, *infra,* below, *dies,* day; Gk, *rhythmos*], a biorhythm that has a period shorter than 24 hours.

**infraglottic.** See **subglottic.**

**infrahyoid** /in′frəhī′oid/, pertaining to the area below the hyoid bone, particularly the group of muscles attached to it.

**inframandibular.** See **submandibular.**

**inframaxillary, 1.** pertaining to the mandible, or lower jaw. **2.** lying below the maxilla, or upper jaw.

**infranodal block** /in′frəno′dəl/ [L, *infra,* below, *nodus,* knot; Fr, *bloc*], a type of atrioventricular (AV) block caused by an abnormality below the AV node, either in the AV bundle or in both bundle branches. An infranodal block has more serious clinical implications than a block at the level of the AV node. The condition is often the result of arteriosclerosis, degenerative diseases, a defect in the conduction system, or a tumor. It most often occurs in older persons. Symptoms include frequent episodes of fainting and a pulse rate of 20 to 40/min. Diagnosis is made by an electrocardiogram, which shows intraventricular conduction disturbances during sinus rhythm and distinguishes nodal from infranodal block. The usual therapy is implantation of a demand pacemaker. Compare **bundle branch block, intraventricular block.** See also **Adams-Stokes syndrome, atrioventricular block, cardiac conduction defect, heart block, intraatrial block, sinoatrial block.**

**infranodal disease,** a cardiac disorder involving the electrical conduction system of the heart below the atrioventricular node. Examples include bundle branch block.

**infraorbital** /in′frə·ô′bitəl/ [L, *infra,* below, *orbita,* wheeltrack], pertaining to the area beneath the floor of the bony cavity in which the eyeball is located.

**infraorbital foramen** [L, *infra,* below, *orbita,* wheeltrack, *foramen,* hole], an opening on the anterior aspect of the maxilla. Through it pass the inferior orbital nerves and blood vessels.

**infrapatellar fat pad** /in′frəpatel′ər/, an area of palpable soft tissue in front of the joint space on either side of the patellar tendon.

**infrared radiation** /in′frəred′/ [L, *infra* + AS, *read,* red; L, *radiare,* to emit rays], electromagnetic radiation with wavelengths between about 700 nm and 1 mm, or longer than those of visible light but shorter than those of microwaves and radio waves. Infrared radiation that strikes the body surface is perceived as heat.

**infrared therapy,** treatment by exposure to various wavelengths of infrared radiation. Hot water bottles and heating pads of all kinds emit longwave infrared radiation; incandescent lights emit shortwave infrared radiation. Infrared treatment is performed to relieve pain and to stimulate circulation of blood.

**infrared thermography,** measurement of temperature through the detection of infrared radiation emitted by heated tissue. Temperature measurement from multiple body areas can be used to generate an image of the body in real time.

**infrasonics** /in′frəson′iks/, sound frequencies that are below the range of human hearing.

**infraspinous fossa.** See **supraspinous fossa.**

**infraspinous muscle** /in′frə·spī′nəs/ [L, *infra,* below + *spina,* spine], the muscle arising from the infraspinous fossa and inserting in the greater tubercle of the humerus. It functions to rotate the humerus laterally.

**infraversion** /in′frə·ver′zhən/ [L, *infra,* below + **vertere,** to turn], **1.** see **infraclusion. 2.** the downward deviation of one eye. **3.** conjugate downward rotation of both eyes. Also called **deorsumversion.**

**infundibula.** See **infundibulum.**

**infundibular stalk** /in′fundib′yələr/ [L, *infundibulum,* funnel; ME, *stalke*], an elongated funnel-shaped structure that connects the hypothalamus with the pituitary gland.

**infundibulum** /in′fundib′yələm/ *pl.* **infundibula** [L, funnel], a funnel-shaped structure or passage, such as the cavity formed by the fimbriae tubae at the distal end of the fallopian tubes, the stalk that extends from the hypothalamus to the posterior lobe of the pituitary gland, or the passage connecting the middle meatus of the nose with the frontal sinus.

**infusate** /infyōō′sāt/, a parenteral fluid slowly introduced into a patient over a specific period.

**infusate contamination,** nosocomial infections transmitted through intravascular devices such as catheters, cannulas, or needles during surgery or other procedures.

**infusion** /infyōō′zhən/ [L, *in,* within, *fundere,* to pour], **1.** the introduction of a substance, such as a fluid, electrolyte, nutrient, or drug, directly into a vein or interstitially by means of gravity flow. Sterile techniques are maintained, the equipment is periodically checked for mechanical difficulties, and the patient is observed for swelling at the site of injection and for cardiac or respiratory difficulties. Compare **injection, instillation, insufflate. 2.** the substance introduced into the body by infusion. **3.** the steeping of a substance, such as an herb, to extract its medicinal properties. **4.** the extract obtained by the steeping process. —**infuse,** *v.*

**infusion pump,** an apparatus designed to deliver measured amounts of a drug or IV solution through IV injection over time. Some kinds of infusion pumps can be implanted surgically.

**ingestion** /injes′chən/ [L, *in,* within, *gerere,* to carry], the oral taking of substances into the body. The term is generally applied to both nutrients and medications.

**ingrown hair** [L, *in,* within; AS, *growen,* to grow, *haer*], a hair that fails to follow the normal follicle channel to the surface, with the free end becoming embedded in the skin. The hair then acts like a foreign body, and inflammation and suppuration follow.

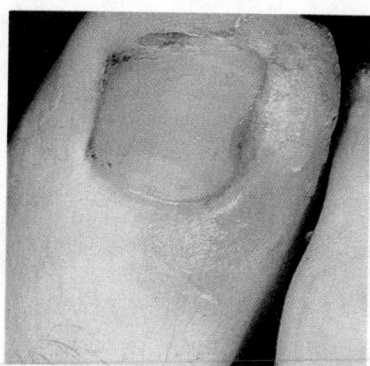

**Ingrown toenail** *(Habif, 1994)*

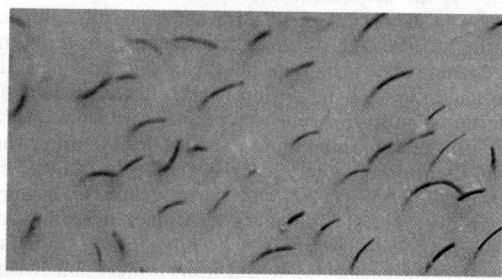

**Ingrown hair** *(du Vivier, 1993/courtesy Institute of Dermatology)*

**ingrown toenail,** a toenail whose distal lateral margin grows or is pressed into the skin of the toe, causing an inflammatory reaction. Granulation tissue may develop, and secondary infection is common. Treatment includes use of wider shoes, proper trimming of the nail, and various surgical procedures to narrow the nail or to reduce the size of the lateral nail fold.

**inguinal** /ing′gwinəl/ [L, *inguen,* groin], pertaining to the groin.

**inguinal canal,** the tubular passage through the lower muscular layers of the abdominal wall that contains the spermatic cord in the male and the round ligament in the female. It is a common site for hernias.

**inguinal falx,** the inferior terminal portion of the common aponeurosis of the internal abdominal oblique and the trans-

verse abdominis. It is inserted into the crest of the pubis, just below the superficial inguinal ring, and strengthens that part of the anterior abdominal wall. The width and the strength of the inguinal falx vary. Also called **conjoined tendon.**

**inguinal hernia,** a hernia in which a loop of intestine enters the inguinal canal; in a male it sometimes fills the entire scrotal sac. An inguinal hernia is usually repaired surgically to prevent the herniated segment from becoming strangulated, gangrenous, or obstructive, thereby blocking passage of waste through the bowel. Of all hernias, 75% to 80% are inguinal hernias. See also **hernia.**

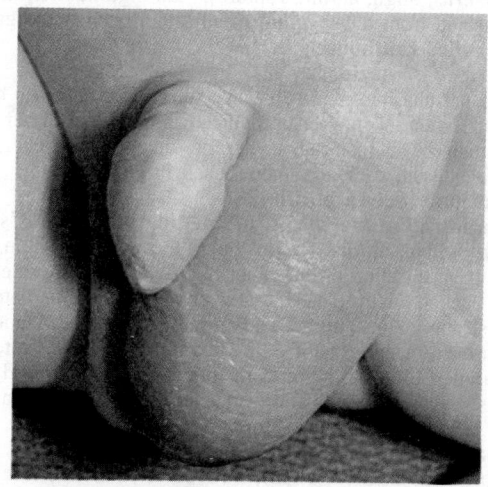

**Inguinal hernia** *(Zitelli and Davis, 1997)*

**inguinal node,** any of the approximately 18 nodes in the group of lymph glands in the upper femoral triangle of the thigh. These nodes are divided into the superficial inguinal nodes and the subinguinal nodes. Compare **anterior tibial node, popliteal node.**

**inguinal region,** the part of the abdomen surrounding the inguinal canal, in the lower zone on both sides of the pubic region. Also called **iliac region.** See also **abdominal regions.**

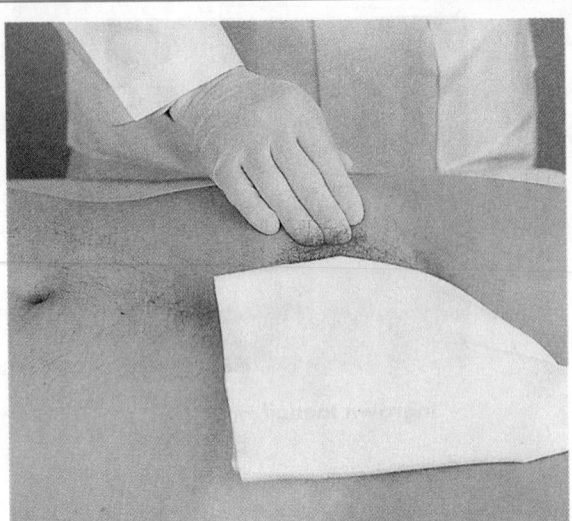

**Palpation of inguinal nodes** (Seidel et al, 1999)

**inguinal ring,** either of the two apertures of the inguinal canal, the internal end opening into the abdominal wall and the external end opening into the aponeurosis of the obliquus externus abdominis above the pubis.

**inguino-,** combining form meaning 'groin': *inguinocrural, inguinodynia, inguinoscrotal.*

**inguinocrural hernia** /ing′gwinōlkrōō′rəl/ [L, *inguen,* groin, *crus,* thigh, *hernia,* rupture], an inguinal hernia that has turned from the inguinal canal laterally over the groin. Also called **Holthouse's hernia.**

**INH.** See **isoniazid.**

**inhalant** /inhā′lənt/, a substance introduced into the body by inhalation. It may be a medication, such as an aerosol, administered in respiratory therapy, or a volatile chemical that is abused, such as toluene, used in glue sniffing.

**inhalation.** See **inspiration.**

**inhalation administration of medication** /in′həlā′shən/ [L, *in,* within, *halare,* to breathe], the administration of a drug by inspiration of the vapor released from a fragile ampule packed in a fine mesh that is crushed for immediate administration. Amyl nitrate and ammonia act quickly and are often used in this way. The medication is absorbed into the circulation through the mucous membrane of the nasal passages. Vaporized medication is also given by inhalation. See also **inhalation therapy, respiratory therapy.**

**inhalational anesthesia.** See **dental anesthesia.**

**inhalational challenge test,** a type of challenge test done to determine reactivity to drugs or causative allergens in allergic asthma; a dilute concentrate of the suspected substance is inhaled and the patient is assessed for bronchial reactivity, which may be either early or late. Also called **inhalational challenge** and **inhalational provocation.**

**inhalation anesthesia,** surgical narcosis achieved by the inhalation of an anesthetic gas or a vapor. Although general anesthesia by inhalation has been used to permit surgical operations for over a century, the mechanism by which these anesthetics dull the pain centers of the brain is not completely understood. Administration of an inhalation anesthetic is usually in conjunction with IV administration of a short-acting hypnotic drug, such as sodium pentothal or propofol. The procedure may require endotracheal intuba-tion. Among the principal inhalation anesthetics are nitrous oxide, desflurane, sevoflurane, enflurane, and isoflurane.

**inhalation injury,** damage to the pulmonary parenchyma caused by inhalation of substances such as very hot air, toxic gas, asbestos, and chemical products of plastic manufacture.

**inhalation therapy,** a treatment in which a substance is introduced into the respiratory tract with inspired air. Oxygen, water, and various drugs may be administered by techniques of inhalation therapy. The goals of treatment are varied, such as improved strength of respiratory function in a bedridden patient, bronchodilation in an asthmatic patient, or liquefaction of mucus in a person with chronic obstructive lung disease.

**inhalation toxicity,** a severe neuromuscular disorder with symptoms like those of Parkinson's disease, caused by prolonged inhalation of manganese dust.

**inhale** /inhāl′/ [L, *in,* within, *halare,* to breathe], to breathe in or to draw in with the breath. Also called **inspire.**

**inhaler** [L, *in* + *halare;* to breathe], a device for administering medications to be inhaled, such as vapors, fine powders, or volatile substances. An inhaler also may be designed to administer anesthetic gases.

**inherent** /inhir′ənt/ [L, *inhaerere,* to cling to], inborn, innate; natural to an environment. Compare **indigenous.**

**inherent rate,** the frequency of impulse formation attributed to a given pacemaker location within the heart. The following rates are representative of the adult heart: sinus node, 60 to 100/min; atrioventricular junction; 40 to 60/min; ventricle: 15 to 40/min. In adults a rate above 100/min is normal during exercise, exertion, strong emotion, or pain. Most clinicians are alert to possible problems when the sinus rate is greater than 90/min and are not concerned unless drops to less than 50/min. In children the normal sinus rate is higher, decreasing as the age of the child increases.

**inheritance** /inher′itəns/ [L, *in,* within, *hereditare,* to inherit], **1.** the acquisition or expression of traits or conditions by transmission of genetic material from parents to offspring. **2.** the sum of the genetic qualities or traits transmitted from parents to offspring; the total genetic makeup of a fertilized ovum. Kinds of inheritance include **alternative inheritance, amphigenous inheritance, autosomal inheritance, blending inheritance, codominant inheritance, complemental inheritance, crisscross inheritance, cytoplasmic inheritance, holandric inheritance, hologynic inheritance, homochronous inheritance, maternal inheritance mendelism, monofactorial inheritance, multifactorial inheritance, supplemental inheritance,** and **X-linked inheritance.** —**inherited,** *adj.* **inherit,** *v.*

**inherited disorder** /inher′itid/, any disease or condition that is genetically determined and involves either a single gene mutation, multifactorial inheritance, or a chromosomal aberration. Also called **genetic disorder, hereditary disorder.**

**inherited trait** [L, *in,* within, *hereditare,* to inherit; Fr, *trait,* a draft], a distinguishing quality or characteristic that is transmitted genetically from one generation to the next.

**inhibin** /inhib′in/, a gonadal hormone that inhibits activity of the follicle stimulating hormone secreted by the anterior pituitary gland.

**inhibiting gene** /inhib′iting/ [L, *inhibere,* to restrain; Gk, *genein,* to produce], a gene that prevents the expression of another gene. See also **epistasis.**

**inhibiting hormone.** See **hormone.**

**inhibition** /in′hibish′ən/ [L, *inhibere,* to restrain], **1.** (in psychology) the unconscious restraint of a behavioral process, usually resulting from the social or cultural forces of the environment; the condition inducing such restraint.

**2.** (in psychoanalysis) the process in which the superego prevents the conscious expression of an unconscious instinctual drive, thought, or urge. **3.** (in physiology) restraining, checking, or arresting the action of an organ or cell or reducing a physiologic activity by antagonistic stimulation. **4.** (in chemistry) the stopping or slowing of the rate of a chemical reaction.

**inhibition assay,** an immunoassay in which an excess of antigens prevents or inhibits the completion of either the initial or the indicator phase of the reaction.

**inhibition of reflexes** [L, *inhibere,* to restrain, *reflectere,* to bend back], **1.** the prevention of a reflex action, requiring a series of biochemical mechanisms to restrict the flow of excitatory impulses at presynaptic and postsynaptic points in the system. **2.** a negative reflex effect that may become established during differential conditioning. The negative conditioned reflex represents an inhibition of a conditioned reflex.

**inhibitor** /inhib′itər/, a drug or other agent that prevents or restricts a certain action.

**inhibitory** /inhib′itôr′ē/ [L, *inhibere,* to restrain], tending to stop or slow a process, such as a neuron that suppresses the intensity of a nerve impulse. Compare **induce.**

**inhibitory enzyme** [L, *inhibere,* to restrain; Gk, *en,* within; *zyme,* ferment], an enzyme that blocks rather than catalyzes a chemical reaction.

**inio-,** combining form meaning 'the occiput': *iniodymus, iniopagus, iniops.*

**inion** /in′ē·on/ [Gk], the most prominent point of the back of the head, where the occipital bone protrudes farthest.

**initial contact stance stage** /inish′əl/ [L, *initium,* beginning, *contigere,* to touch], one of the five stages in the stance phase of walking or gait, specifically associated with the moment when the foot touches the ground or floor and the leg prepares to accept the weight of the body. The initial contact stance stage figures in the diagnoses of many abnormal orthopedic conditions and is often correlated with electromyographic studies of the muscles used in walking, such as the pretibial muscle and the gluteus maximus. Compare **loading response stance stage, midstance, preswing stance stage, terminal stance.** See also **swing phase of gait.**

**initial lesion.** See **primary lesion.**

**initiation codon** /inish′ē·ā′shən kō′don/ [L, *initium,* beginning, *caudex,* book], the triplet of nucleotides, usually adenine-uracil-guanine (AUG) or, in some cases, guanine-uracil-guanine (GUG), that code for formylmethionine, the first amino acid in all protein sequences. Also called **initiator codon, start codon.**

**initiator** /inish′ē·ā′tər/, a cocarcinogenic factor that causes a usually irreversible genetic mutation in a normal cell and primes it for uncontrolled growth. Examples include radiation, aflatoxins, urethane, and nitrosamines.

**inject.** See **injection.**

**injectable contraceptive,** medroxyprogesterone acetate, a progestin, administered intramuscularly at a dose sufficient to prevent ovulation and used as a contraceptive. The muscle into which the hormone is injected serves as a depot from which the hormone is slowly released, so that injections need to be given only every three months. This is a very convenient and highly effective method of contraception.

**injectable silicone** /injek′təbəl/ [L, *in* + *jacere,* to throw, *silex,* silicon], polymeric organic compounds of silicone that are used in plastic surgery. The silicones are injected beneath the skin for cosmetic benefits. Foreign body reactions to silicone injections for breast augmentation may cause an appearance of tender hard nodules.

**injection** /injek′shən/ [L, *in,* within, *jacere,* to throw], **1.** the act of forcing a liquid into the body by means of a needle and syringe. Injections are designated according to the anatomic site involved; the most common are intraarterial, intradermal, intramuscular, intravenous, and subcutaneous. Parenteral injections are usually given for therapeutic reasons, although they may be used diagnostically. Sterile technique is maintained. Compare **infusion, instillation, insufflate. 2.** the substance injected. **3.** redness and swelling observed in the physical examination of a part of the body, caused by dilation of the blood vessels secondary to an inflammatory or infectious process. —**inject,** *v.*

**injection cap,** a rubber diaphragm under a plastic cap. It permits needle insertion into a catheter or vial.

**injection technique.** See **intradermal injection, intramuscular injection, intrathecal injection, intravenous injection, subcutaneous injection,** and see other specific injection techniques.

**injunction** /injungk′shən/ [L, *injungere,* to enjoin], a court order that prevents a party from performing a specified act.

**injury, perioperative positioning: risk for,** a nursing diagnosis accepted by the Eleventh National Conference on the Classification of Nursing Diagnoses. It is defined as a state in which the client is at risk for injury as a result of the environmental conditions found in the perioperative setting. ■ RISK FACTORS: The risk factors are disorientation, immobilization, muscle weakness, sensory or perceptual disturbances resulting from anesthesia, obesity, emaciation, and edema. See also **nursing diagnosis.**

**injury, risk for** /in′jərē/, a nursing diagnosis accepted by the Fourth National Conference on the Classification of Nursing Diagnoses. It is defined as a state in which an individual is at risk of injury as a result of environmental conditions interacting with the individual's adaptive and defensive resources. ■ RISK FACTORS: A somatic risk for injury includes abnormal sensory function, autoimmune condition, malnutrition, hemoglobinopathy or other abnormal hematologic condition, broken skin, developmental abnormality, and psychologic dysfunction. An environmental risk for injury includes lack of immunization; presence of pathogenic microorganisms, chemical pollutants, poisons, alcohol, nicotine, or food additives; modes of transportation; physical aspects of the community, buildings, equipment, or facilities; nosocomial agents; nonavailability of assistance; and various psychologic factors. See also **nursing diagnosis.**

**injury severity score (ISS),** an evaluation system developed to predict the outcomes of traumas, including mortality and length of hospital stay. See also **Glasgow Coma Scale.**

**inlay** /in′lā/ [L, *in,* within; AS, *lecan,* lay], **1.** material, such as bone or skin, inserted into a tissue defect. **2.** (in dentistry) a restoration made outside of a tooth to correspond with the form of a prepared cavity and then cemented into the tooth.

**inlay splint** [L, *in,* within; AS, *lecan,* lay], a casting for fixing or supporting one or more approximating teeth. It is composed of either a single casting or two or more inlays soldered together.

**inlet** [L, *in,* within; ME, *leten*], a passage leading into a cavity, such as the pelvic inlet that marks the brim of the pelvic cavity.

**inlet contraction.** See **contraction.**

**in loco parentis** /in lō′kō pəren′tis/ [L, in the parents' place], the assumption by a person or institution of the parental obligations of caring for a child without adoption.

**innate** /in′āt, ināt′/ [L, *innatus,* inborn], **1.** existing in or belonging to a person from birth; inborn; hereditary; congenital. **2.** a natural and essential characteristic of something or someone; inherent. **3.** originating in or produced by the intellect or the mind.

**innate immunity.** See **natural immunity.**

**inner cell mass** [AS, *innera,* within; L, *cella,* storeroom, *massa,* lump], a cluster of cells localized around the animal pole of the blastocyst of placental mammals from which the embryo develops. See also **trophoblast.**

**inner ear.** See **internal ear.**

**innervate** /in′ərvāt/ [L, *in* + *nervus*], to supply a body part or organ with nerves or nervous stimuli.

**innervation** /in′ərvā′shən/ [L, *in,* within, *nervus,* nerve], the distribution or supply of nerve fibers or nerve impulses to a body part.

**innervation apraxia.** See **motor apraxia.**

**innidation.** See **nidation.**

**innocent** /in′əsənt/ [L, *innocens,* harmless], benign, innocuous, or functional; not malignant, such as an innocent heart murmur.

**innocuous** /inok′yoo·əs/ [L, *innocuus,* harmless], pertaining to use of a substance or procedure that causes no ill effects.

**innominate** /inom′ināt/ [L, *innominatum,* nameless], without a name; unnamed. The term is traditionally applied to certain anatomic structures, often identified by their descriptive name, such as the hipbone, brachiocephalic artery, and brachiocephalic vein.

**innominate artery,** one of the three arteries branching from the arch of the aorta, running about 5 cm from the level of the cranial border of the second right costal cartilage; ascending cranially, dorsally, and obliquely to the right; and dividing into the right common carotid and the right subclavian arteries. Also called **brachiocephalic artery, brachiocephalic trunk.**

**innominate bone,** the hipbone. It consists of the ilium, ischium, and pubis and unites with the sacrum and coccyx to form the pelvis. Also called **os coxae.**

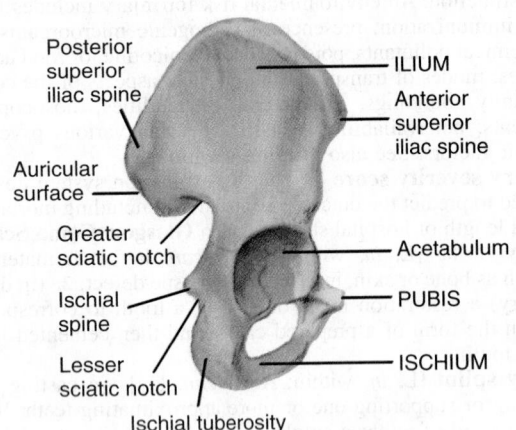

Posterior superior iliac spine
ILIUM
Anterior superior iliac spine
Auricular surface
Greater sciatic notch
Acetabulum
Ischial spine
PUBIS
Lesser sciatic notch
ISCHIUM
Ischial tuberosity

**Innominate bone** *(Applegate, 2000)*

**innominate vein,** a large vein on either side of the neck that is formed by the union of the internal jugular and subclavian veins. The two veins drain blood from the head, neck, and upper extremities and unite to form the superior vena cava. Also called **brachiocephalic vein.**

**Inocor,** trademark for a cardiac inotropic drug (amrinone lactate).

**inocula.** See **inoculum.**

**inoculate** /inok′yəlāt/ [L, *inoculare,* to graft], to introduce a substance (inoculum) into the body to produce or to increase immunity to the disease or condition associated with the substance. It is introduced by multiple scratches in the skin after placement of a drop of the substance on the skin, by puncture of the skin with an implement bearing multiple short tines, or by intradermal, subcutaneous, or intramuscular injection.

**inoculum** /inok′yōoləm/, *pl.* **inocula** [L, *inoculare,* to graft a bud], a substance introduced into the body to cause or to increase immunity to a specific disease or condition. It may be a toxin; a live, attenuated, or killed virus or bacterium; or an immune serum. Also called **inoculant.** See also **immune system.**

**inoperable** /inop′ərəbəl/ [L, *in* + *operari,* to work], pertaining to a medical condition that would not benefit from surgical intervention or for which the risk outweighs the benefits.

**inorganic** /in′ôrgan′ik/ [L, *in,* not; Gk, *organikos,* natural], (in chemistry) a chemical compound that does not contain hydrocarbon or other derivatives.

**inorganic acid,** a compound containing no carbon that is composed of hydrogen and one or more electronegative element, such as chlorine. An example is hydrochloric acid.

**inorganic chemistry,** the study of the properties and reactions of all chemical elements and compounds other than hydrocarbons or their derivatives.

**inorganic dust,** dry, finely powdered particles of an inorganic substance, especially dust, which, when inhaled, can cause abnormal conditions of the lungs. See also **anthracosis, asbestosis, berylliosis, pneumoconiosis, silicosis.**

**inorganic phosphorus,** phosphorus that may be measured in the blood as phosphate ions. Its increased concentration may indicate bone, kidney, or glandular disease; decreased concentration may be associated with alcoholism, vitamin deficiency, and other problems. Normal concentrations in the serum of adults are 1.8 to 2.6 mEq/L. See also **phosphorus.**

**inosine** /in′əsēn, -sīn/, a nucleoside, derived from animal tissue, especially intestines, originally used in food processing and flavoring. It has been used in the treatment of cardiac disorders and now is under investigation in studies of cancer and virus chemotherapy. See also **inosiplex.**

**inosiplex** /inō′sipleks/, a form of inosine that acts as a stimulator of the immune system. It is currently under investigation for use in cancer therapy, in the treatment of herpesvirus and rhinovirus infections, and in immune restoration in pre-AIDS patients. Also called **methisoprinol.**

**inositol** /inō′sətol, inos′-/, an isomer of glucose that occurs widely in plant and animal cells. Although inositol has no current therapeutic use, it may be an essential cell constituent.

**inotropic** /in′ōtrop′ik/ [Gk, *inos,* fiber, *trope,* turning], pertaining to the force or energy of muscular contractions, particularly those of the heart. An inotropic agent increases myocardial contractility.

**inotropic agent,** a substance that influences the force of muscular contractions; *inotropic* is often used to describe an agent that increases muscular contractions of the heart.

**inpatient** /in′pāshənt/ [L, *in,* within, *patior,* to suffer], **1.** a patient who has been admitted to a hospital or other health care facility for at least an overnight stay. **2.** pertaining to the treatment or care of such a patient or to a health care facility to which a patient may be admitted for 24-hour care. Compare **outpatient.**

**inpatient care unit,** a unit of a hospital organized for medical and continuous nursing services for a group of inpatients who are usually grouped according to diagnosis or other common characteristics, such as maternity or surgical patients.

**input,** the information or material that enters a system.

**input device** [L, *in,* within; ME, *putten,* to place], an implement that allows for the entry of commands or information for processing in a form acceptable to a computer, such as a mouse, keyboard, tape drive, disk drive, microphone, or light pen.

**inquest** /in′kwest/ [L, *in* + *quaerere,* to seek], a legal inquiry into the cause, manner, and circumstances of a sudden, unexpected, or violent death.

**INR,** abbreviation for *International Normalized Ratio.*

**insane** /insān′/ [L, *in,* not, *sanus,* sound], a legal term for unsound, diseased, or deranged mental functioning, particularly pertaining to a person who is unable to provide adequate self-care if there is a need to protect the patient and the public from each other. In the United States the precise definition of this legal term varies from state to state.

**insanity** /insan′itē/ [L, *in,* not, *sanus,* sound], *informal.* a term used more in legal and social than in medical terminology. It refers to those mental illnesses that are of such a serious or debilitating nature as to interfere with one's capability of functioning within the legal limits of society and performing the normal activities of daily living.

**insatiable** /insā′sh(ē)əbəl/ [L, *insatiatus,* not satisfied], pertaining to an appetite for food or other needs that cannot be satisfied.

**insect bite** [L, *in,* within, *secare,* to cut], the bite of any parasitic or venomous arthropod such as a louse, flea, mite, tick, or arachnid. Many arthropods inject venom that produces poisoning or severe local reaction, saliva that may contain viruses, or substances that produce mild irritation. The degree of irritation of an insect's bite is affected by the design and shape of its mouth parts: A horsefly, for example, makes a short lateral and coarse wound, whereas a tick takes hold with its backward curved teeth, making its removal difficult. Spiders inflict a sharp pinprick bite that may remain unnoticed until the injected venom has begun to produce a painful reaction. Treatment of a bite depends on the species of insect, the reaction to the bite, and the risk of sequelae from it. First aid treatment is generally symptomatic and includes ice or cold packs, careful cleaning of the wound, and antihistamines or specific antivenin as necessary.

**insecticide** /insek′tisīd/, a chemical agent that kills insects.

**insecticide poisoning.** See **chlorinated organic insecticide poisoning.**

**insemination** /insem′inā′shən/, the injection of semen into the vagina. It may involve an artificial process unrelated to sexual intercourse.

**insenescence** /in′sines′əns/ [L, *insenescere,* to begin to grow old], **1.** the process of aging. **2.** the state of being chronologically old but retaining the vitality of a young person.

**insensible** /insen′sibəl/ [L, *in* + *sentire,* to feel], **1.** pertaining to a person who is unconscious for any reason. **2.** pertaining to a person who is apathetic or deprived of normal sense perceptions.

**insensible perspiration** [L, *in,* not, *sentire,* to feel, *per,* through, *spirare,* to breath], the loss of body fluid by evaporation, such as normally occurs during respiration. A small amount of perspiration is continually excreted by the sweat glands in the skin; the portion that evaporates before

it may be observed also contributes to insensible perspiration. Also called **insensible water loss.**

**insertion** /insur′shən/ [L, *inserere,* to introduce], (in anatomy) the place of attachment, such as that of a muscle to the bone it moves.

**insertion forceps.** See **point forceps.**

**insertion site,** the point in a vein where a needle or catheter is inserted.

**in-service education** [L, *in,* within, *servus,* a slave, *educare,* to rear], a program of instruction or training that is provided by an agency or institution for its employees. The program is held in the institution or agency and is intended to increase the skills and competence of the employees in a specific area. In-service education may be a part of any program of staff development. See also **staff development.**

**insheathed** /in·shēthd′/ [L, *in,* within; AS, *scaeth,* sheath], enclosed within a sheath.

**insidious** /insid′ē·əs/ [L, *insidiosus,* cunning], describing a development that is gradual, subtle, or imperceptible. Certain chronic diseases, such as glaucoma, can develop insidiously with symptoms that are not detected by the patient until the disorder is established. Compare **acute.**

**insight** /in′sīt/ [L, *in,* within; AS, *gesihth,* sight], **1.** the capacity of comprehending the true nature of a situation or of penetrating an underlying truth. **2.** an instance of penetrating or comprehending an underlying truth, primarily through intuitive understanding. **3.** (in psychology) a type of self-understanding encompassing both intellectual and emotional awareness of the unconscious nature, origin, and mechanisms of one's attitudes, feelings, and behavior. It is one of the most important goals of psychotherapy and, with integration, leads to modification of maladaptive behavioral patterns. See also **integration.**

**insipid** /insip′id/ [L, *in* + *sapidus,* savory], dull, tasteless, or lifeless.

**in situ** /in sī′tōō, sit′ōō/ [L, *in,* within, *situs,* position], **1.** in the natural or usual place. **2.** describing a cancer that has not metastasized or invaded neighboring tissues, such as carcinoma in situ.

**insoluble** /insol′yəbəl/ [L, *in,* not, *solubilis,* soluble], unable to be dissolved, usually in a specific solvent, such as a substance that is insoluble in water.

**insoluble fiber,** fiber that is not soluble in water, composed mainly of lignin, cellulose, and hemicelluloses and primarily found in the bran layers of cereal grains; its actions include increasing fecal bulk and decreasing free radicals in the GI tract.

**insomnia** /insom′nē·ə/ [L, *in,* not, *somnus,* sleep], chronic inability to sleep or to remain asleep throughout the night; wakefulness; sleeplessness. Insomnia may be the symptom of a psychiatric disorder. Formerly called **agrypnia.**

**insomniac** /insom′nē·ak/, **1.** a person with insomnia. **2.** pertaining to, causing, or associated with insomnia. **3.** characteristic of or occurring during a period of sleeplessness.

**inspiration** /in′spirā′shən/ [L, *inspirare,* to breathe in], the act of drawing air into the lungs. The major muscle of inspiration is the diaphragm, the contraction of which creates a reduced pressure in the chest, causing the lungs to expand and air to flow inward. Accessory inspiratory muscles include the external intercostals, scaleni, scapular elevators, and sternocleidomastoids. Since expiration is usually a passive process, these muscles of inspiration alone produce normal respiration. Lungs at maximal inspiration have an average total capacity of 5.5 to 6 L of air. Also called **inhalation.** Compare **expiration.** See also **inspiratory reserve volume.** —**inspiratory,** *adj.*

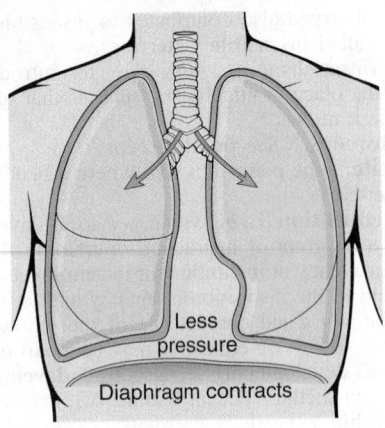

**Inspiration** *(Chabner, 2001)*

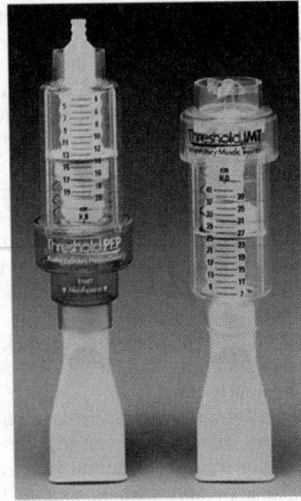

**Inspiratory muscle trainer**
*(Beare and Myers, 1998/courtesy HealthScan Products, Inc., Cedar Grove, New Jersey)*

**inspiratory** /inspī′rətôr′ē/ [L, *inspirare*, to breathe in], pertaining to inspiration.

**inspiratory capacity (IC),** the maximum volume of gas that can be inhaled from the end of a resting exhalation. Equal to the sum of the tidal volume and the inspiratory reserve volume, it is measured with a spirometer.

**inspiratory dyspnea** [L, *inspirare*, to breathe in; Gk, *dys,* without, *pnoia,* breath], a form of breathing difficulty caused by an obstruction in the larynx, trachea, or bronchi. The patient attempts to compensate for this deficiency with prolonged, deep inspirations.

**inspiratory gas flow rate,** the amount of gas delivered per minute to a patient's lungs by mechanical ventilation.

**inspiratory hold,** either of two kinds of modification in an inhalation produced by intermittent positive-pressure breathing: (1) a pressure hold, in which a preset pressure is reached and held for a designated period, or (2) a volume hold, in which a predetermined volume is delivered and then held for a designated period.

**inspiratory muscle fatigue,** weakness or exhaustion of the muscles that produce inspiration, resulting in a condition of threatened acute respiratory failure.

**inspiratory reserve volume,** the maximum volume of gas that can be inhaled beyond a normal resting inspiration.

**inspiratory resistance muscle training,** exercises that require inhalation against some type of resisting force. An example of such training is abdominal breathing practice with the Pflex or threshold inspiratory muscle trainer. The amount of resistance is gradually increased over several weeks of abdominal muscle training. Resistance may also be used against expansion of the rib cage by the intercostal musculature during inspiration. The resistance may be provided by a therapist pushing against the ribs or by applying a belt or swathe tightly about the costal margin.

**inspiratory waveform,** one of several flow patterns during inspiration associated with mechanical ventilation. These patterns include a square wave, in which the inspiratory flow rises rapidly to a preset level and stays at that level until expiration begins; a sinusoidal wave, in which the flow gradually increases and decreases throughout inspiration; and a descending ramp wave, in which the flow increases very rapidly and then decreases gradually until the end of inspiration. The last pattern is most similar to normal breathing.

**inspire.** See **inhale.**

**inspirometer** /in′spirom′ətər/ [L, *inspirare,* to breathe in; Gk, *metron,* measure], an apparatus used to measure the volume, force, and frequency of a patient's inspirations.

**inspissate** /inspis′āt/ [L, *inspissare,* to thicken], (of a fluid) to thicken or harden through the absorption or evaporation of the liquid portion, such as milk in an inspissated milk duct. —**inspissation,** *n.*

**instillation** /in′stilā′shən/ [L, *instillare,* to drip], 1. a procedure in which a fluid is slowly introduced into a cavity or passage of the body and allowed to remain for a specific length of time before being drained or withdrawn. It is performed to expose the tissues of the area to the solution, to warmth or cold, or to a drug or substance in the solution. 2. a solution so introduced. Compare **infusion, injection, insufflate.** —**instill,** *v.*

**instinct** /in′stingkt/ [L, *instinctus,* impulse], an inborn psychologic representation of a need, such as life instincts of hunger, thirst, and sex, as well as the destructive and aggressive death instincts.

**instinctive reflex.** See **unconditioned response.**

**institutionalism syndrome** /in′stityōō′shənəliz′əm/, a condition characterized by apathy, withdrawal, submissiveness, and lack of initiative. The person may resist leaving a hospital, even when the surroundings are barely adequate, because it is familiar and predictable and demands are minimal.

**institutionalize** /in′stityōō′shənəlīz′/ [L, *instituere,* to put in place], to place a person in an institution for psychologic or physical treatment or for the protection of the person or society. —**institutionalization,** *n.,* **institutionalized,** *adj.*

**institutional licensure** /in′stityōō′shənəl/ [L, *instituere,* to put in place, *licere,* to be permitted], a proposed procedure in which licensure for almost all health professions would be abandoned and the responsibility for assessing professional competence would fall to the health care facility where the health professional is used. Proponents of the procedure maintain that health needs would be better and more flexibly served. Opponents maintain that knowledge, judgment, and competency are the products of a good basic education in the profession and that educators cannot teach the profession without a set of standardized expectations, as are now provided by government-controlled licensing procedures and certifying examinations. In addition, health care facilities may not have the expertise or resources necessary to evaluate the various kinds of health care providers.

**institutional review board (IRB),** an organizational committee that reviews and approves biomedical research that involves using humans as subjects.

**instrument** /in′strəmənt/ [L, *instrumentum,* tool], a surgical tool or device designed to perform a specific function, such as cutting, dissecting, grasping, holding, retracting, or suturing. Surgical instruments are usually made of steel and are specially treated to be durable, heat-resistant, rust-resistant, and stain-proof. Some kinds of instruments are **clamp, needle holder, retractor,** and **speculum.**

**instrumental activities of daily living (IADL)** /in′strəmen′təl/, the activities often performed by a person who is living independently in a community setting during the course of a normal day, such as managing money, shopping, housekeeping, preparing meals, and taking medications correctly. See also **activities of daily living.**

**instrumental conditioning.** See **operant conditioning.**

**instrumental labor** [L, *instrumentum,* tool, *labor,* work], child delivery in which the use of instruments, such as forceps or perforators, is required.

**instrumentation** /in′strəməntā′shən/, the use of instruments for treatment and diagnosis.

**insufficiency** /in′səfish′ənsē/ [L, *in,* not, *sufficere,* to be adequate], inability to perform a necessary function adequately. Some kinds of insufficiency are **adrenal insufficiency, aortic insufficiency, ileocecal insufficiency, pulmonary insufficiency,** and **valvular insufficiency.**

**insufficient sleep syndrome** /in′səfish′ənt/, a neurologic disorder in which individuals persistently fail to obtain enough sleep to support normal wakefulness.

**insufflate** /in′səflāt, insuf′lāt/ [L, *insufflare,* to blow into], to blow a gas or powder into a tube, cavity, or organ to allow visual examination, to remove an obstruction, or to apply medication. See also **Rubin's test. —insufflation,** *n.*

**insufflator** /in′səflā′tər/ [L, *insufflare,* to blow into], an apparatus used to blow air or gas into a body cavity.

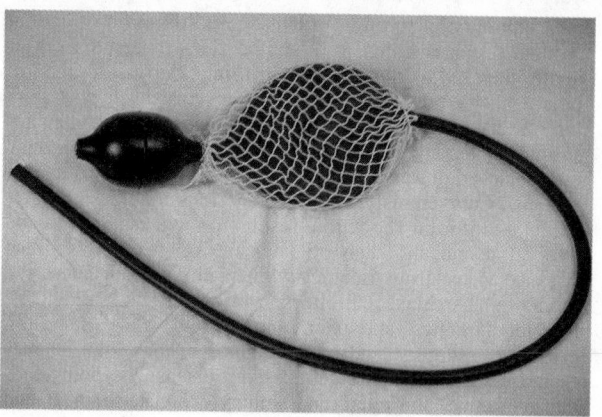

**Insufflator** *(Zakus, 1995)*

**insul-,** combining form meaning 'island or island-shaped': *insula, insulin, insuloma.*

**insulation** /in′səlā′shən/, a nonconducting substance that offers a barrier to the passage of heat or electricity.

**insulin** /in′səlin/ [L, *insula,* island], **1.** a naturally occurring polypeptide hormone secreted by the beta cells of the islets of Langerhans in the pancreas in response to increased levels of glucose in the blood as well as the parasympathetic nervous system. The hormone acts to regulate the metabolism of glucose and the processes necessary for the intermediary metabolism of fats, carbohydrates, and proteins. Insulin lowers blood glucose level and promotes transport and entry of glucose into the muscle cells and other tissues. Inadequate secretion of insulin causes elevated blood glucose and lipid levels, and ketonemia, as well as the characteristic signs of diabetes mellitus, including increased desire to eat, excessive thirst, increased urination, and eventually lethargy and weight loss. Uncorrected severe deficiency of insulin is incompatible with life. Normal findings of insulin assay in adults are levels of 5 to 24 μmU/ml. **2.** a pharmacologic preparation of the hormone administered in treating diabetes mellitus. The various preparations of insulin available for

## Insulins

| Type | Description | Effect on blood glucose (hours after administration) | | |
|------|-------------|------|------|------|
| | | Onset | Peak | Termination |
| **Short acting** | | | | |
| Regulate (crystalline zinc) | Clear | Immediate | 2 to 4 | 6 to 8 |
| Semilente (SL) | Cloudy: amorphous insulin zinc suspension, no protamine | 1 | 4 to 6 | 12 to 16 |
| **Intermediate acting** | | | | |
| NPH | Cloudy: crystalline zinc insulin suspension, 50% saturated with protamine | 2 to 3 | 8 to 12 | 18 to 24 |
| Lente | Cloudy: mixture 30% SL + 70% UL, no protamine | 2 to 3 | 8 to 12 | 18 to 24 |
| **Long acting** | | | | |
| PZI | Cloudy: excess protamine | 6 | 14 to 20 | 24 to 36 |
| Ultralente (UL) | Cloudy: crystalline insulin suspension, high zinc content, no protamine | 6 | 16 to 18 | 30 to 36 |

prescription vary in onset, intensity, and duration of action. Animal source insulins, pork and beef, have been discontinued in the U.S. market. Human insulin is derived by recombinant DNA technology. They are termed quick-acting, intermediate-acting, and long-acting. Most replacement insulin is given by subcutaneous injection in individualized dosage schedules and insulin pumps, but insulin also can be replaced intravenously. Adverse reactions include hypoglycemia and insulin shock that result from excess dosage and hyperglycemia and diabetic ketoacidosis from inadequate dosage. Many drugs interact with insulin, among them the monoamine oxidase inhibitors, corticosteroids, salicylates, thiazide diuretics, and phenytoin. Fever, stress, infection, pregnancy, surgery, and hyperthyroidism may significantly increase insulin requirements; liver disease, hypothyroidism, vomiting, and renal disease may decrease them. Blood tests for glucose and ketones are performed to determine the need for adjustment of the dosage or of the schedule of administration. See also **human insulin.**

**insulin antibody test,** a blood test used to detect the presence of insulin antibodies, which develop in nearly all patients treated with exogenous insulin. These antibodies may reduce the amount of insulin available for glucose metabolism and may contribute to insulin resistance.

**insulinase,** an enzyme that inactivates insulin.

**insulin assay,** a blood test used to diagnose insulinoma (tumor of the islets of Langerhans) and to evaluate patients with fasting hypoglycemia. It is often combined with a fasting plasma glucose test to increase its accuracy.

**insulin-dependent diabetes mellitus (IDDM),** See **type 1 diabetes mellitus.**

**insulinemia** /in′səlinēmē·ə/ [L, *insula,* island; Gk, *haima,* blood], an abnormally high level of insulin in the blood.

**insulin hypoglycemic test,** a postoperative procedure for determining the completeness of vagotomy for peptic ulcer disease. Insulin is administered to cause hypoglycemia. If vagotomy is complete, the acid output from the stomach should be less than before the surgery.

**insulin injection sites,** body tissue areas that allow optimal use of subcutaneous injections of insulin. The choice of sites can affect the rate of absorption and peak action times, but repeated use of the same injection site can lead to localized tissue damage, resulting in malabsorption of insulin. These problems are minimized by systematic rotation of injection sites within the selected anatomic area.

**insulin kinase,** an enzyme, assumed to be present in the liver, that activates insulin.

**insulin-like growth factor (IGF),** hormones that stimulates protein synthesis and sulfation. IGF I and II play a role in uterine and placental growth and early fetal growth during pregnancy. IGF I is also called **somatomedin C.**

**insulin lipodystrophy** [L, *insula,* island; Gk, *lipos,* fat; *dys,* bad, *trophe,* nourishment], the loss of local fat deposits in patients with diabetes, as a complication of repeated insulin injections into the same area.

**insulin lispro,** a pancreatic hormone.
- ■ INDICATIONS: Insulin lispro is used to treat ketoacidosis types I and II and types 1 and 2 diabetes mellitus.
- ■ CONTRAINDICATIONS: Known hypersensitivity to this drug or to protamine prohibits its use.
- ■ ADVERSE EFFECTS: Anaphylaxis is a life-threatening effect of this drug. Other adverse reactions include blurred vision, dry mouth, flushing, rash, urticaria, warmth, lipohypertrophy, swelling, redness, rebound hyperglycemia (the Somogyi effect). Lipodystrophy and hypoglycemia are common side effects.

**insulinogenic** /in′səlin′ōjen′ik/ [L, *insula* + Gk, *genein,* to

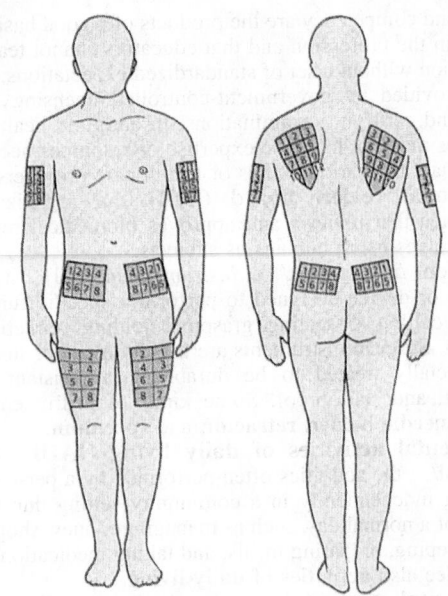

**Insulin injection sites** *(Potter and Perry, 1997)*

produce], promoting the production and release of insulin by the islets of Langerhans in the pancreas.

**insulinoma** /in′səlinō′mə/ *pl.* **insulinomas, insulinomata** [L, *insula* + Gk, *oma,* tumor], a tumor of the insulin-secreting cells of the islets of Langerhans. The majority are benign. Surgical resection of the tumor may be possible, thus limiting the development of hypoglycemia. Also called **insuloma, islet cell adenoma.** Compare **islet cell tumor.**

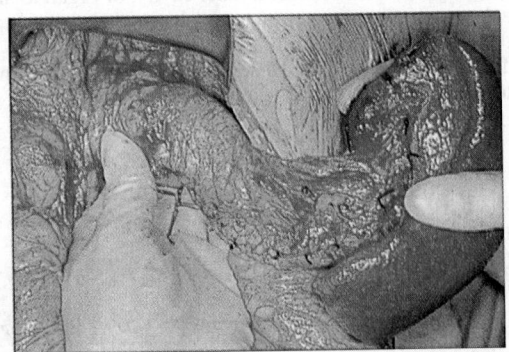

**Insulinoma** *(Greig and Garden, 1996)*

**insulin pump** [L, *insula,* island; ME, *pumpe*], a portable battery-powered instrument that delivers a measured amount of insulin through the abdominal wall. It can be programmed to deliver varied doses of insulin according to the body's needs at the time.

**insulin reaction,** the adverse effects caused by excessive levels of circulating insulin. See **hyperinsulinism.**

**insulin resistance,** a complication of diabetes mellitus characterized by a need for an increased amount of insulin

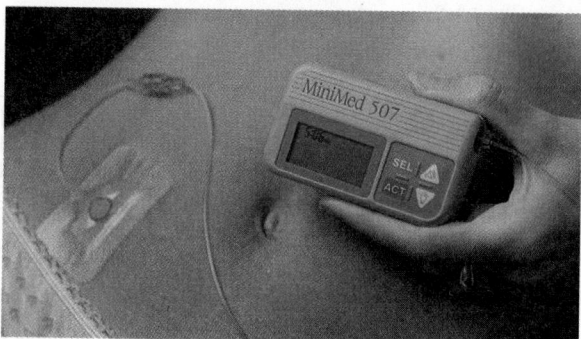

**External insulin pump**
*(Monahan and Neighbors, 1998/courtesy MiniMed Technologies, Sylmar, California)*

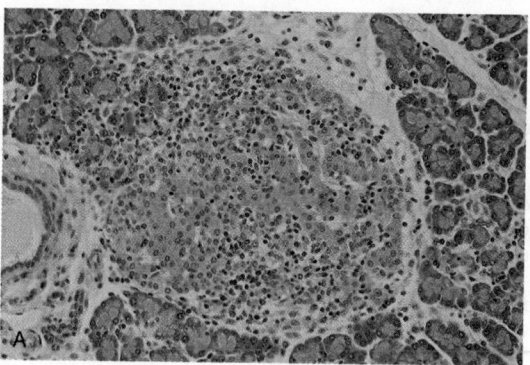

**Insulitis** *(Cotran, Kumar, and Collins, 1999)*

per day to control hyperglycemia and ketosis. The cause is associated with insulin binding by high levels of antibody. Insulin-resistant states also may occur with acanthosis nigrans, Werner's syndrome, ataxia telangiectasia, Alström syndrome, pineal hyperplasia syndrome, and various lipodystrophic disorders.

**insulin shock,** a condition of hypoglycemic shock caused by an overdose of insulin, decreased intake of food, or excessive exercise. It is characterized by sweating, trembling, chilliness, nervousness, irritability, hunger, hallucination, numbness, and pallor. Uncorrected, it progresses to convulsions, coma, and death. Treatment requires an immediate dose of glucose orally or parenterally or glucagon IM or IV. Persons with insulin-treated diabetes mellitus should wear a bracelet (Medic-Alert) that indicates that they have the disease. Compare **diabetic coma, ketoacidosis.**

**insulin tolerance test,** a test of the body's ability to use insulin, in which insulin is given and blood glucose is measured at regular intervals. Thirty minutes after the insulin is administered, blood glucose level is usually lower but not less than half of the fasting glucose level. Glucose levels usually return to normal after about 90 minutes. In people who have hypoglycemia, the glucose levels may drop lower and be slower to return to normal.

**insulintropin** /in'səlintrop'in/ [L, *insula,* island], a naturally occurring hormone produced in the intestines when food is ingested. It causes the release of insulin from the pancreas, which in turn regulates blood glucose levels. It has been administered to type 2 diabetes patients but is not useful in its present form in the treatment of type 1 diabetes patients, in whom the pancreas does not secrete insulin.

**insulitis** /in'səlī'tis/, a lymphocytic infiltration of the pancreatic beta cells in the islets of Langerhans. The condition is associated with the development of type 1 diabetes mellitus. Also called **isletitis.**

**insuloma.** See **insulinoma.**

**insurance authorization,** a nursing intervention from the Nursing Interventions Classification (NIC) defined as assisting the patient and provider to secure payment for health services or equipment from a third party. See also **Nursing Interventions Classification.**

**intake** [L, *in,* within; AS, *tacan,* to take], **1.** the process in which a person is admitted to a clinic or hospital or is signed in for an office visit. The reason for the visit and various identifying data about the patient are noted. Certain routine preliminary procedures may be performed, such as obtaining a blood pressure reading or a urine specimen. In some clinical settings the intake may also include obtaining such additional information as the patient's basic health history and previous source of care. **2.** (in nursing) the amount of food or fluid ingested in a given period. Intake is measured and noted in milliliters or grams per 8-, 12-, or 24-hour period.

**Intal,** trademark for an antiasthmatic mast cell inhibitor agent (cromolyn sodium).

**integral dose** /in'təgrəl/ [L, *integrare,* to make whole; Gk, *dosis,* giving], the total amount of energy absorbed by a patient or object during exposure to radiation. Also called **volume dose.**

**integrate.** See **integration.**

**Integrated Group Without Walls** /in'təgrā'tid/, a network of physicians who have merged legally but continue to practice individually. Selected functions, such as information management, are centralized.

**Integrated Health Care Delivery System,** a managed care system in the United States that includes a hospital organization that provides acute patient care, a multispecialty medical care delivery system, the capability of contracting for any other needed services, and a payer. Services are provided to enrollees of the health plan.

**Integrated Multispecialty Group,** a managed care system similar to a single-specialty medical group, except that various specialties and usually primary care are also provided. Also called **Multispecialty Medical Group.**

**integrated system,** **1.** (in managed care) a legal partnership between groups of physicians and hospitals that contract and share risk while working together. It may include foundations, management service organizations, and physician-hospital organizations. **2.** a group of interconnected units that form a functioning computer system.

**integrating dose meter** /in'təgrā'ting/, a device that measures the total amount of radiation administered to a patient during a radiotherapy exposure. It is usually placed on the patient's skin and may terminate the exposure when the desired amount is reached.

**integration** /in'təgrā'shən/ [L, *integrare,* to make whole], **1.** the act or process of unifying or bringing together. **2.** (in psychology) the organization of all elements of the personality into a coordinated functional whole that is in harmony with the environment, one of the primary goals in psychotherapy. It involves the assimilation of insight and the coordination of new and old data, experiences, and emotional reactions so that an effective change can occur in behavior, thinking, or feeling. See also **insight. —integrate,** *v.*

**integration of self,** one of the components of high-level wellness. It is a prerequisite for the achievement of maturity and is characterized by the integration of mind, body, and spirit into one harmoniously functioning unit.

**integrin** /integ′rin/, **1.** a protein that links the outside of a cell with its interior. **2.** a heterodimeric molecule involved in cell-substate and cell-cell adhesion.

**integument** /integ′yōōmənt/ [L, *integumentum,* a covering], a covering or skin. —**integumentary,** *adj.*

**integumentary system** /integ′yəmen′tərē/, the skin and its appendages, hair, nails, and sweat and sebaceous glands. See also the Color Atlas of Human Anatomy.

**integumentary system assessment,** an evaluation of the general condition of a patient's integument and of factors or abnormalities that may contribute to the presence of a dermatologic disorder.

■ METHOD: The patient is asked about itching, pain, rashes, blisters, or boils; whether the skin usually is dry, oily, thin, rough, bumpy, or puffy; or whether it feels hot or cold, peels, changes in color, or is marked with dark liver (aging) spots. Observations are made of the intactness, turgor, elasticity, temperature, cleanliness, odor, wetness or dryness, and color of the skin. Cyanosis of the lips, circumoral area, or mucous membranes, ear lobes, or nailbeds; jaundice of the sclera; paleness of conjunctivae; and distribution of pigment are noted. Evidence of rashes, edema, needle marks, insect bites, scabies, acne, sclerema, decubiti, uremic frost on the beard or eyebrows, or pressure areas over bony prominences is recorded. The nails are examined for brittleness, lines, a convex ram's horn or concave spoon shape, and the condition of surrounding tissue, including clubbing of the fingers and toes. The existence and characteristics of lesions such as maculae, papules, vesicles, pustules, bullae, hives, warts, moles, ulcers, scars, keloids, petechiae, lipomas, crusts of dried exudate, flakes of dead epidermis, excoriations, blackheads, and chancres are noted. The patient's exposure to parasites, to internal allergens in food and drugs, and to external allergens in cosmetics, soaps, topical medication, and plants, as well as a family history of allergies, is investigated, as well as currently used medication, creams, lotions, ointments, hygienic measures, and sexual practices. Diagnostic aids contributing to the evaluation are skin and lesion cultures, punch biopsies, skin tests for allergies, a lupus erythematosus preparation, and a blood culture.

■ NURSING INTERVENTIONS: The nurse conducts the interview to obtain subjective data on the patient's condition, makes the necessary observations, and assembles the background information and results of the diagnostic tests.

■ OUTCOME CRITERIA: A well-conducted assessment of the patient's integument is a valuable aid in diagnosing a dermatologic disorder.

**intellect** /in′təlekt/ [L, *intellectus,* perception], **1.** the power and ability of the mind for knowing and understanding, as contrasted with feeling or with willing. **2.** a person possessing a great capacity for thought and knowledge. —**intellectual,** *adj., n.*

**intellectualization** /in′təlek′chōō·əlīzā′shən/ [L, *intellectus* + Gk, *izein,* to cause], **1.** (in psychiatry) a defense mechanism in which reasoning is used as a means of blocking a confrontation with an unconscious conflict and the emotional stress associated with it. **2.** the overuse of abstract thinking or generalizations to control or minimize painful feelings.

**intelligence** /intel′ijəns/ [L, *intelligentia,* perception], **1.** the potential ability and capacity to acquire, retain, and apply experience, understanding, knowledge, reasoning, and judgment in coping with new experiences and in solving problems. **2.** the manifestation of such ability. See also **intelligence quotient.** —**intelligent,** *adj.*

**intelligence quotient (IQ),** a numeric expression of a person's intellectual level as measured against the statistical average of his or her age group. On several of the traditional scales, it is determined by dividing the mental age, derived through psychologic testing, by the chronologic age and multiplying the result by 100. Average IQ is considered to be 100.

**intelligence test,** any of a variety of standardized tests designed to determine the mental age of an individual by measuring the relative capacity to absorb information and to solve problems.

**intelligent.** See **intelligence.**

**intelligent terminal,** a computer terminal that can function as a processing device in addition to providing input/output facilities, whether operated independently or connected to a main computer.

**intemperance** /intem′pərəns/ [L, *in,* not, *temperare,* to moderate], excessive indulgence in eating, drinking, or other life-style functions.

**intensifying screen** /inten′sifī′ing/ [L, *intensus,* tighten, *facere,* to make; ME, *screne*], a device consisting of fluorescent material, which is placed in contact with the film in a radiographic cassette. Radiation interacts with the fluorescent phosphor, releasing light photons. These photons expose the film with greater efficiency than would the radiation alone; thus, patient exposure to radiation can be reduced.

**intensive care** /inten′siv/ [L, *intensus,* tighten, *garrire,* to chatter], constant complex health care as provided in various acute life-threatening conditions such as multiple trauma, severe burns, or myocardial infarction or after certain kinds of surgery. Care is most frequently given in a unit equipped with various technologically sophisticated machines and devices for treating and monitoring the condition of the patient and given by specially trained personnel. Also called **critical care.**

**intensive care unit (ICU),** a hospital unit in which patients requiring close monitoring and intensive care are kept. An ICU contains highly technical and sophisticated monitoring devices and equipment, and is staffed by personnel to deliver critical care. A large tertiary care facility usually has separate units specifically designed for the intensive care of adults, infants, children, or newborns or for other groups of patients requiring a certain kind of treatment. See also **coronary care unit.**

**intention** /inten′shən/ [L, *intendere,* to aim], a kind of healing process. Healing by **primary intention** is the initial union of the edges of a wound, progressing to complete healing without granulation. Healing by **secondary intention** is wound closure in which the edges are separated, granulation tissue develops to fill the gap, and epithelium grows in over the granulations, producing a scar. Healing by **tertiary intention** is wound closure in which granulation tissue fills the gap between the edges of the wound, with epithelium growing over the granulation at a slower rate and producing a larger scar than results from healing from secondary intention. Suppuration is also usually found.

**intentional additives,** substances that are deliberately added in the manufacture of food or pharmaceutical products to improve or maintain flavor, color, texture, or consistency or to enhance or conserve nutritional value. Compare **incidental additives.**

**intention tremor,** fine, rhythmic purposeless movements that tend to increase during voluntary movements. Compare **resting tremor.** See also **tremor.**

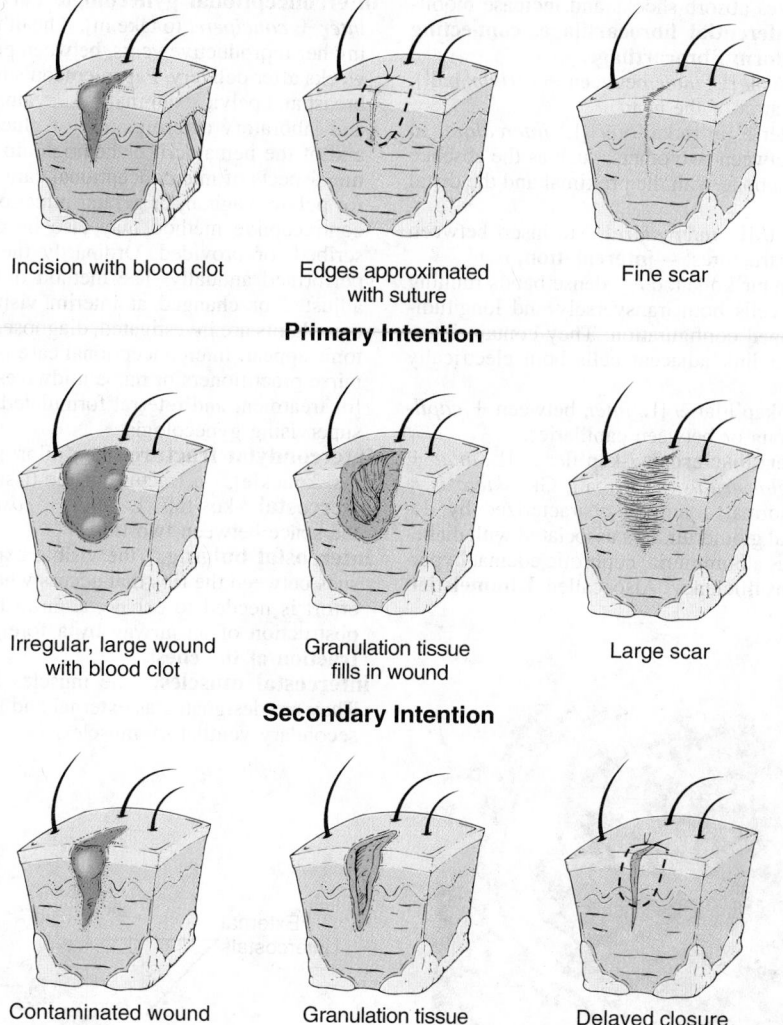

Incision with blood clot     Edges approximated with suture     Fine scar

**Primary Intention**

Irregular, large wound with blood clot     Granulation tissue fills in wound     Large scar

**Secondary Intention**

Contaminated wound     Granulation tissue     Delayed closure with suture

**Tertiary Intention**

**Intention** *(Lewis, Heitkemper, and Dirksen, 2000)*

**inter-** prefix meaning 'situated, formed, or occurring between': *interacinar, intercalary, intercartilaginous.*

**interactional model** /-ak′shənəl/ [L, *inter,* between, *agere,* to do], a therapy model that views the family as a communication system comprising interlocking subsystems of family members. Family dysfunction occurs when the rules governing family interaction become vague and ambiguous. The therapeutic goal is to help the family clarify the rules governing their relationships.

**interactionist theory** /-ak′shənist/, an aging theory that views age-related changes as resulting from the interactions among the individual characteristics of the person, the circumstances in society, and the history of social interaction patterns of the person.

**interaction processes,** a component of the theory of effective practice. The processes consist of a series of interactions between a nurse and a patient. The series occurs in a sequence of actions and reactions until the patient and the nurse both understand what is wanted and the desired behavior or act is achieved.

**interaction theme.** See **communication theme.**

**interactive terminal** /-ak′tiv/, a data processing terminal that is integrated into a system to allow two-way communication between the user and the system. Also called **interactive system, user interaction.**

**interalveolar** /-alvē′ələr/ [L, *inter,* between, *alveolus,* little hollow], pertaining to the area between alveoli.

**interarticular** /-ärtik′yələr/ [L, *inter,* between, *articulus,* joint], pertaining to the areas between two joints or between facing surfaces of a joint.

**interarticular fibrocartilage** [L, *inter + articulus,* joint], one of four kinds of fibrocartilage, consisting of flattened fibrocartilaginous plates between the articular cartilage of the most active joints, such as the sternoclavicular, wrist, and knee joints. The synovial surfaces extend over the fibrocartilaginous plates and attach to surrounding ligaments. The fibrocartilaginous plates absorb shocks and increase mobility. Compare **circumferential fibrocartilage, connecting fibrocartilage, stratiform fibrocartilage.**

**interatrial** /in′tər·ā′trē·əl/ [L, *inter,* between + *atrium,* hall], situated between the atria of the heart.

**intercalary** /intur′kəler′ē, in′tərkal′ərē/ [L, *intercalare,* to insert], occurring between two others, such as the absence of the middle part of a bone with the proximal and the distal parts present.

**intercalate** /intur′kəlāt/ [L, *intercalare*], to insert between adjacent surfaces or structures. —**intercalation,** *n.*

**intercalated disks** /in·tur′kə·lā·təd /, dense bands running between myocardial cells both transversely and longitudinally, forming a stepped configuration. They contain intercellular junctions that link adjacent cells both electrically and mechanically.

**intercapillary** /in′tər·kap′i·lar·ē/ [L, *inter,* between + *capillaris,* hairlike], among or between capillaries.

**intercapillary glomerulosclerosis** /-kap′iler′ē/ [L, *inter* + *capillaris,* hairlike, *glomerulus,* small ball; Gk, *sklerosis,* a hardening], an abnormal condition characterized by degeneration of the renal glomeruli. It is associated with diabetes and often produces albuminuria, nephrotic edema, hypertension, and renal insufficiency. Also called **Kimmelstiel-Wilson syndrome.**

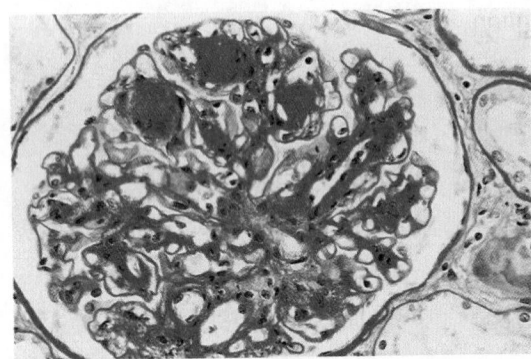

**Intercapillary glomerulosclerosis**
*(Cotran, Kumar, and Collins, 1999)*

**intercavernous sinuses** /-kav′ərnəs/ [L, *inter,* between, *caverna,* cavity, *sinus,* curve], the cavities through which the cavernous sinuses of the dura mater communicate.

**intercellular** /-sel′yələr/ [L, *inter* + *cella,* storeroom], pertaining to the area between or among cells.

**intercellular bridge,** a structure that connects adjacent cells, occurring primarily in the epithelium and other stratified squamous epithelia. It consists of slender strands of cytoplasm that project from the surfaces of adjacent cells and merge at the desmosome. Also called **cytoplasmic bridge.**

**interceptive orthodontics** /in′tər·sep′tiv/, that phase of orthodontics concerned with elimination of a condition that might lead to the development of malocclusion.

**intercerebral** /-ser′əbrəl/ [L, *inter,* between, *cerebrum,* brain], pertaining to the area between the left and right cerebral hemispheres.

**interchange.** See **reciprocal translocation.**

**interclavicular** /-kləvik′yələr/ [L, *inter,* between, *clavicula,* little key], pertaining to the area between the clavicles.

**interconceptional gynecologic care** /-kənsep′shənəl/ [L, *inter* + *concipere,* to take in], health care of a woman during her reproductive years, between pregnancies, and after 6 weeks after delivery. Papanicolaou's test for cervical cancer, breast and pelvic examinations, evaluation of general health, and laboratory determination of glucosuria and proteinuria and of the hematocrit or hemoglobin are common and routine aspects of interconceptional care. Testing and treatment for pelvic, vaginal, or genital infections may be required. A contraceptive method may also be discussed, taught, prescribed, or provided. Ordinarily the basic examination is performed annually. The method of contraception may be adjusted or changed at interim visits; infections or other complaints are investigated, diagnosed, and treated as symptoms appear. Interconceptional care is increasingly given by nurse practitioners or nurse midwives who follow protocols for treatment and referral formulated in consultation with a supervising gynecologist.

**intercondylar fracture** /-kon′dilər/ [L, *inter* + Gk, *kondylos,* knuckle], a fracture of the tissue between condyles.

**intercostal** /-kos′təl/ [L, *inter* + *costa,* rib], pertaining to the space between two ribs.

**intercostal bulging,** the visible expansion of the soft tissues between the ribs that occurs when increased expiratory effort is needed to exhale, as in asthma, cystic fibrosis, or obstruction of an airway by a foreign body. Compare **retraction of the chest.**

**intercostal muscles,** the muscles between adjacent ribs. They are designated as external and internal and function as secondary ventilatory muscles.

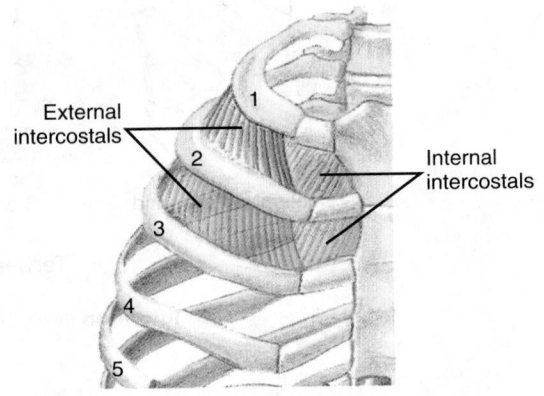

**Intercostal muscles**
*(Thibodeau and Patton, 1999/John V. Hagen)*

**intercostal neuralgia,** pain in the intercostal spaces of the chest wall, involving intercostal nerves.

**intercostal node,** a node in one of three groups of thoracic parietal lymph nodes situated near the dorsal parts of the intercostal spaces. The nodes are associated with lymphatic vessels that drain the posterolateral area of the chest. The efferent vessels from the nodes in the caudal four or five spaces form a descending trunk that opens into the dilated origin of the thoracic duct. The efferent vessels from the nodes in the upper intercostal spaces on the left side connect with the thoracic duct; those on the right side end in the right lymphatic duct. Compare **diaphragmatic node, sternal node.** See also **lymphatic system, lymph node.**

**intercostal space** [L, *inter,* between, *costa,* rib, *spatium*], the region between the ribs.

**intercourse** /in'tərkôrs'/ [L, *intercursus,* running between], *informal.* sexual intercourse between individuals. See **coitus.**

**intercristal** /-kris'təl/ [L, *inter* + *crista,* ridge], pertaining to the space between two crests.

**intercurrent disease** /-kur'ənt/ [L, *intercurrere,* to run between], a disease that develops in and may alter the course of another disease.

**interdental canal** /-den'təl/ [L, *inter* + *dens,* tooth], any one of the nutrient channels that pass upward to the teeth through the body of the mandible. Also called **nutrient canal.**

**interdental canals,** channels in the alveolar process of the mandible, between the roots of the medial and lateral incisors, for the passage of anastomosing blood vessels between the sublingual and inferior dental arteries. Also called **nutrient canals.**

**interdental gingiva,** the supporting gingival tissues, containing prominent horizontal collagen fibers, that normally fill the space between two approximating teeth. Also called **gingival papilla.**

**interdental groove,** a linear vertical depression on the surface of the interdental papillae, which functions as a channel for the egress of food from the interproximal areas.

**interdental spillway,** a channel formed by the interproximal contours of adjoining teeth and their investing tissues.

**interdependent intervention.** See **intervention.**

**interdigestive migrating motor complex** /-dijes'tiv/, a pattern of small bowel cyclic motor activity that follows completion of food digestion and absorption. It consists of periods of inactivity alternating with segmental or propulsive contractions.

**interest tests,** psychologic tests designed to clarify an individual's vocational potential or to compare an individual's performance with the average scores of a specific population.

**interface** /in'tərfās/ [L, *inter* + *facies,* face], **1.** the connection between different elements of a computer system or between different computers. **2.** The method by which a computer user interacts with a computer system as displayed on a monitor screen, such as a graphical user interface.

**interfemoral** /in'tər·fem'ə·rəl/ [L, *inter,* between + *femur,* thigh], between the thighs.

**interference** /-fir'əns/ [L, *inter* + *ferire,* to strike], the effect of a component on the accuracy of measurement of the desired analyte.

**interferent** /-fir'ənt/ [L, *inter* + *ferire,* to strike], any chemical or physical phenomenon that can interfere with or disrupt a reaction or process.

**interferential current therapy** /-fərən'shəl/, a form of electrical stimulation therapy using two or three distinctly different currents that are passed through a tissue from surface electrodes. Portions of each current are canceled by the other, with the result that a different net current is applied to the target tissue.

**interferon** /-fir'on/ [L, *inter* + *ferire,* to strike], a natural glycoprotein formed by cells exposed to a virus or another foreign particle of nucleic acid. It induces the production of translation inhibitory protein (TIP) in noninfected cells. TIP blocks translation of viral RNA, thus giving other cells protection against both the original and other viruses. Interferon is species specific.

**interferon alfacon-1,** a recombinant type 1 interferon.

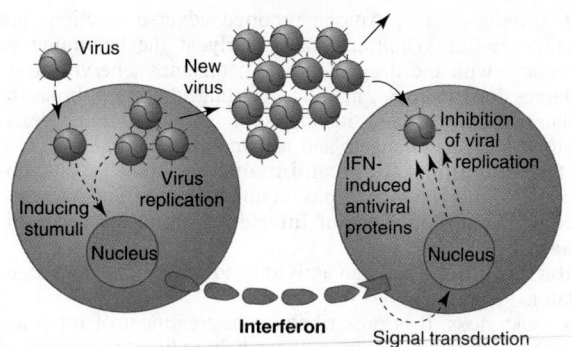

**Mechanisms of action of interferon**
*(Lewis, Heitkemper, and Dirksen, 2000)*

■ INDICATIONS: This drug is used to treat chronic hepatitis C infections. It is being used investigationally to treat hairy cell leukemia in combination with G-CSF.

■ CONTRAINDICATIONS: Hypersensitivity to alpha interferons or to products derived from *Escherichia coli* prohibit the use of this drug.

■ ADVERSE EFFECTS: Life-threatening effects of interferon alfacon-1 include granulocytopenia, thrombocytopenia, and leukopenia. Other adverse effects include headache, rigors, insomnia, dizziness, nausea, diarrhea, anorexia, vomiting, constipation, hemorrhoids, decreased salivation, musculoskeletal pain, dysmenorrhea, vaginitis, menstrual disorders, alopecia, pruritus, rash, erythema, tinnitus, earache, conjunctivitis, eye pain, granulocytopenia, ecchymosis, hypertension, palpitations, nervousness, depression, anxiety, emotional lability, abnormal thinking, upper respiratory infection, respiratory tract congestion, and bronchitis.

**interferon alfa-n 1 lymphoblastoid,** a recombinant type 1 interferon.

■ INDICATIONS: This drug is used to treat chronic hepatitis C infections.

■ CONTRAINDICATIONS: Factors that prohibit the use of this drug include known hypersensitivity to alpha interferons and a history of anaphylactic reactions to bovine or ovine immunoglobulins, egg protein, polymyxin B, or neomycin sulfate.

■ ADVERSE EFFECTS: Life-threatening effects of this drug are granulocytopenia, thrombocytopenia, and leukopenia. Other adverse effects include ecchymosis and epistaxis. Common side effects include headache, fever, insomnia, dizziness, anxiety, hostility, lability, nervousness, depression, confusion, abnormal thinking, amnesia, abdominal pain, nausea, diarrhea, anorexia, vomiting, back pain, alopecia, pruritus, rash, erythema, dry skin, pharyngitis, upper respiratory infection, cough, dyspnea, and bronchitis.

**interferon-alpha,** the major interferon produced by virus-induced leukocyte cultures; the primary producer cells are null lymphocytes, and the major activities are antiviral activity and activation of NK cells. It is used in the experimental treatment of hairy cell leukemia and other selected neoplasias. Also spelled *interferon-alfa.*

**interferon alpha-2a, recombinant,** a parenteral antineoplastic drug.

■ INDICATIONS: It is administered in the treatment of AIDS-related Kaposi's sarcoma.

■ CONTRAINDICATIONS: Caution is recommended in prescribing this product for patients with severe cardiovascular disease.

■ ADVERSE EFFECTS: Among reported adverse reactions are influenza-like symptoms, particularly at the beginning of therapy with the drug; confusion; dizziness; nervousness; depression; anorexia; nausea; vomiting; diarrhea; throat inflammation; dry and itching skin; alopecia; diaphoresis; blood pressure changes; and tachycardia.

**interferon alpha-2b, recombinant,** a parenteral antineoplastic drug with indications, contraindications, and adverse effects similar to those of **interferon alpha-2a, recombinant.**

**interferon beta-1a,** an antiviral and immune system regulator.

■ INDICATIONS: It is prescribed in the treatment of relapsing forms of multiple sclerosis. It can help reduce the number of neurologic attacks and slow the progress toward physical disability.

■ CONTRAINDICATIONS: The drug should not be given to patients with allergy or sensitivity to interferon beta-1a or components of its formulation.

■ ADVERSE EFFECTS: The side effects most often reported include muscle aches, chills, fever, weakness, and influenza-like symptoms.

**interferon beta-2,** a cytokine derived from T cells that stimulate B cells to proliferate in vitro but (unlike B cell differentiation factors) do not stimulate antibody secretion.

**interferon gamma,** a small, species-specific glycoprotein produced by mitogen-stimulated T cells. It possesses antiviral activity and plays a central role in the immunoregulatory processes.

**interferon nomenclature,** a system recommended by the International Interferon Nomenclature Committee for identifying interferon compounds. For a specific interferon, the name consists of "interferon" followed by a Greek letter (spelled out), a dash, and an arabic number, and a lowercase letter, as in the example, *interferon alpha-2a.*

**interfibrillar mass of Flemming, interfilar mass.** See **hyaloplasm.**

**interim rate** /in'tərim/ [L, meanwhile, *ratum,* calculate], a method of third-party payment for costs of hospital services in which an amount is paid periodically pending an accounting of actual costs at the end of a designated period.

**interior** /in·tēr'ē·ər/ [L, inner], **1.** situated inside; inward. **2.** an inner part or cavity.

**interiorization** /intir'ə·ərīzā'shən/ [L, *interior,* inner; Gk, *izein,* to cause], the merging of reflex and cognitive processes as a response to the environment.

**interior mesenteric artery** [L, inner; Gk, *mesos,* middle, *enteron,* intestine, *arteria,* airpipe], a visceral branch of the abdominal aorta, arising just above the division into the common iliacs and supplying the left half of the transverse colon, all of the descending and iliac colons, and most of the rectum. It has left colic, sigmoid, and superior rectal branches.

**interkinesis** /in'tərkinē'sis, -kīnē'sis/ [L, *inter* + Gk, *kinein,* to move], the interval between the first and second nuclear divisions in meiosis. See also **interphase.**

**interlace mode** /-lās'/, a process whereby a conventional video camera tube produces two fields of 262.5 lines each in 17 ms to form a 525-line video frame in 33 ms. Each field represents repeated adjacent active traces and horizontal retraces of the electron beam across a video screen.

**interleukin** /-lōō'kin/, one of a large group of proteins produced mainly by T cells and in some cases by mononuclear phagocytes or other cells. Interleukins participate in communication among leukocytes and are important in the inflammatory response. Most interleukins direct other cells to divide and differentiate. Each acts on a particular group of cells that have receptors specific for that interleukin.

**interleukin-1 (IL-1),** a protein with numerous immune system functions, including activation of resting T cells, endothelial cells, and macrophage; mediation of inflammation, and stimulation of the synthesis of lymphokines, collagen, and collagenases. IL-1 can also induce fever, sleep, adrenocorticotropic hormone release, and nonspecific resistance to infection.

**interleukin-2 (IL-2),** a protein with various immunologic functions, including the ability to initiate proliferation of activated T cells. IL-2 is used in the laboratory to grow T cell clones with specific helper, cytotoxic, and suppressor functions.

**interleukin-3 (IL-3),** an immune-response protein that supports the growth of pluripotent bone marrow stem cells and is a growth factor for mast cells.

**interleukin-4 (IL-4),** an immune-response protein that is a growth factor for activated B cells, resting T cells, and mast cells. Also called **B cell stimulating factor-1.**

**interleukin-5 (IL-5),** a cytokine produced by helper T cells. It stimulates B cells and eosinophils and facilitates the differentiation of B cells that secrete immunoglobulin A.

**interleukin-6 (IL-6),** a cytokine derived from fibroblasts, macrophages, and tumor cells. It is an antiviral protein that is also used in the treatment of some types of cancer. Also called **beta$_2$-interferon.**

**interleukin-7 (IL-7),** a cytokine produced by bone marrow stromal cells that causes lymphoid stem cells to differentiate into progenitor B and T cells and stimulates the killing of foreign cells by T cells and monocytes.

**interleukin-8 (IL-8),** a cytokine produced by various cell types involved in inflammation that attracts and activates neutrophils.

**interleukin-9 (IL-9),** a glycoprotein that helps induce the growth of some helper T cell clones but not cytotoxic T cell clones.

**interleukin-10 (IL-10),** a protein expressed by CD4 and CD8 T cells, monocytes, macrophages, and activated B cells. It inhibits cytokine synthesis and suppresses the functions of macrophages and natural killer T cells.

**interleukin-11 (IL-11),** a cytokine produced by bone marrow stromal cells. It induces IL-6-dependent murine plasmacytoma cells to proliferate and plays an important role in early platelet hematopoiesis.

**interleukin-12 (IL-12),** a protein produced by activated T cells that stimulates cell-mediated killing by natural killer cells and lymphocytes. It promotes the maturation of cytotoxic T cells.

**interleukin-13 (IL-13),** a protein produced by activated T cells that inhibits inflammatory cytokine production by peripheral blood monocytes. It suppresses cell-mediated immune responses and promotes B cell differentiation.

**interleukin-14 (IL-14),** a protein produced by follicular dendritic cells, germinal T cells, and some malignant B cells. It enhances the proliferation of B cells and induces memory B cell production and maintenance.

**interleukin-15 (IL-15),** a growth factor that enhances peripheral blood T cell production.

**interlobular duct** /-lob'yələr/ [L, *inter* + *lobulus,* small lobe], any duct connecting or draining the lobules of a gland.

**interlobular emphysema.** See **distal acinar emphysema.**

**interlocked twins** [L, *inter* + AS, *loc,* a fastening], monozygotic twins so positioned in the uterus that the neck of one becomes entwined with that of the other during presentation so that vaginal delivery is not possible. Such interlocking occurs when one fetus is a breech presentation and the other a vertex presentation. Also called *interlocking twins.*

**intermediary** /-mē′dē·er′ē/ [L, *inter* + *mediare,* to divide], a private insurance company or public or private agency selected by health care providers to pay claims under the Medicare program.

**intermediary metabolism** [L, *inter,* between, *mediary,* to divide; Gk, *metabole,* change], the metabolic processes involved in the synthesis of cellular components between digestion of food and excretion of waste products.

**intermediate-acting insulin** [L, *inter* + *mediare,* to divide, *activus,* active], a preparation of the synthetic human or pork insulin to which zinc has been added under specific chemical conditions and having an intermediate range of action. Neutral protamine Hagedorn (NNPH) insulin starts to work about 60 to 90 minutes after injection, peaks 4 to 12 hours after injection, and lasts about 18 hours. Lente insulin has a simular time course of action. See also **insulin.** Compare **long-acting insulin, rapid-acting insulin, short-acting insulin.**

**intermediate care** /-mē′dē·it/, **1.** a level of medical care for certain chronically ill or disabled individuals in which room and board are provided but skilled nursing care is not. Title XI of U.S. Medicaid legislation mandates standards and federal subsidies for intermediate care of the recipients of public assistance. **2.** A unit where patients are kept who do not require intensive care but who are not yet ready to be kept in a regular medical-surgical unit.

**intermediate care facility (ICF),** a health facility that provides medically related services to persons with a variety of physical or emotional conditions requiring institutional facilities but without the degree of care provided by a hospital or skilled nursing facility. An example is a health care facility for mentally retarded or other developmentally disabled persons.

**intermediate care unit,** a transitional unit for patients from critical care units that provides close monitoring before discharge.

**intermediate cell mass.** See **nephrotome.**

**intermediate column.** See **lateral horn.**

**intermediate cuneiform bone,** the smallest of the three cuneiform bones of the foot, located between the medial and the lateral cuneiform bones. Also called **middle cuneiform bone, second cuneiform bone.**

**intermediate-density lipoprotein (IDL),** a lipid-protein complex with a density between those of very low–density lipoprotein and low-density lipoprotein. The product has a relatively short half-life and is normally in the blood in very low concentrations. In a type III hyperlipoproteinemic state the IDL concentration in the blood is elevated.

**intermediate disk.** See **Z line.**

**intermediate host,** any animal in which the larval or intermediate stage of a parasite develops. Certain snails are intermediate hosts for liver flukes and schistosomes. Humans are intermediate hosts for malaria parasites. Also called **secondary host.** Compare **dead-end host, definitive host, reservoir host.** See also **host,** def. 1.

**intermediate mass,** the connecting mass of nervous tissue between two lobes of the diencephalon.

**intermediate mesoderm.** See **nephrotome.**

**intermenstrual** /-men′stroo͞·əl/ [L, *inter* + *menstruum,* menstrual fluid], pertaining to the time between menstrual periods.

**intermenstrual fever,** the normal slight elevation of temperature that marks ovulation, usually occurring about 14 days before the onset of menses.

**intermenstrual pain.** See **mittelschmerz.**

**intermittent** /-mit′ənt/ [L, *inter* + *mittere,* to send], occurring at intervals; alternating between periods of activity and inactivity, such as rheumatoid arthritis, which is marked by periods of signs and symptoms followed by periods of remission.

**intermittent assisted ventilation (IAV),** a system of respiratory therapy in which assisted ventilation is combined with spontaneous breathing. Also called **intermittent demand ventilation (IDV).**

**intermittent claudication.** See **claudication.**

**intermittent compression,** external compression used to control and reduce accumulation of lymph in body tissues. Devices to provide intermittent compression in an on-off timing sequence include inflated pressure sleeves and linear compression pumps. Some devices provide cold temperatures with compression to assist in controlling edema. Intermittent compression is also used to decrease acute bleeding.

**intermittent demand ventilation (IDV).** See **intermittent assisted ventilation.**

**intermittent explosive disorder,** a mental disturbance beginning in childhood and characterized by discrete episodes of violence and aggressive behavior or destruction of property in otherwise normal individuals. The acts may occur as an overreaction to an ordinarily minor event.

**intermittent fever,** a fever that recurs in cycles of paroxysms and remissions, such as in malaria. Kinds of intermittent fever include **biduotertian malaria, double quartan malaria,** and **quartan malaria.**

**intermittent hydrosalpinx** [L, *inter,* between, *mittere,* to send; Gk, *hydor,* water, *salpinx,* tube], a fluid accumulation in a fallopian tube. The fluid is released periodically through the uterine cavity. Also called **hydrops tubae profluens.**

**intermittent incontinence** [L, *inter,* between, *mittere,* to send, *incontinentia,* inability to retain], urinary incontinence that occurs only when there is pressure on the bladder or exertion of muscular effort. See also **incontinence.**

**intermittent mandatory ventilation (IMV),** a mode of mechanical ventilation in which the patient is allowed to breathe independently except during certain prescribed intervals, when a ventilator delivers a breath either under positive pressure or in a measured volume. Compare **intermittent positive-pressure breathing.** See also **respiratory therapy.**

**intermittent positive-pressure breathing,** a form of assisted or controlled respiration produced by a ventilatory apparatus in which compressed gas is delivered under positive pressure into a person's airways until a preset pressure is reached. Passive exhalation is allowed through a valve, and the cycle begins again as the flow of gas is triggered by inhalation. Also called **IPPV (intermittent positive-pressure ventilation).**

■ METHOD: The use of the IPPB unit involves the combined efforts of the physician, the respiratory therapist or technician, and the nurse. The specific pressure and volume and the use of nebulizing or other attachments are ordered individually. The equipment is tested and is introduced to the patient by the inhalation therapist. The nurse observes that the patient closes the lips around the mouthpiece and does not allow air to escape from the nose or mouth during inspiration and determines whether the therapy is effective.

■ INTERVENTIONS: The patient may require reassurance that the machine will automatically shut off airflow at the end of inspiration and encouragement to relax and allow the lungs to be completely filled by the machine. The patient is cautioned not to manipulate any of the controls.

■ OUTCOME CRITERIA: Ventilation may be greatly improved by the use of the IPPB unit. Secretions may be thinned and cleared, and the passages may be humidified, allowing greater comfort and a better exchange of gases.

**intermittent positive-pressure breathing unit.** See **IPPB unit.**

**intermittent positive-pressure ventilation.** See **intermittent positive-pressure breathing.**

**intermittent pulse** [L, *inter,* between, *mittere,* to send, *pulsare,* to beat], a pulse in which an occasional beat is absent. It tends to occur with second-degree heart block or extrasystole. Also called **dropped-beat pulse.**

**intermittent torticollis** [L, *inter,* between, *mittere,* to send, *tortus,* twisted, *collum,* neck], intermittent, powerful spasms of the neck muscles, drawing the head to one side. The spasms usually occur in the sternocleidomastoid muscle.

**intermittent tremor** [L, *inter,* between, *mittere,* to send, *tremere,* to tremble], a rhythmic involuntary shaking that occurs intermittently or a tremor that occurs after a voluntary movement is attempted.

**intern** /in'turn/ [L, *internus,* inward], **1.** a physician in the first postgraduate year, learning medical practice under supervision before beginning a residency program. **2.** any immediate postgraduate trainee in a clinical program. **3.** to work as an intern. Also spelled *interne.*

**internal** /intur'nəl/ [L, *internus,* inward], within or inside. —**internally,** *adv.*

**internal abdominal oblique muscle,** one of a pair of anterolateral muscles of the abdomen, lying under the external oblique muscle in the lateral and ventral part of the abdominal wall. It is smaller and thinner than the external oblique muscle. It functions to compress the abdominal contents and assists in micturition, defecation, emesis, parturition, and forced expiration. Both sides acting together serve to flex the vertebral column, drawing the costal cartilages toward the pubis. One side acting alone bends the vertebral column laterally and rotates it, drawing the shoulder of the opposite side downward. Also called **obliquus internus abdominis.** Compare **external abdominal oblique muscle.**

**internal acoustic meatus,** an opening in the petrous portion of the temporal bone through which the facial, intermediate, and vestibulocochlear nerves and the labyrinthine artery pass. Also called **meatus acusticus internus.**

**internal aperture of tympanic canaliculus,** the upper opening of the tympanic channel in the temporal bone, leading to the tympanum.

**internal bleeding** [L, *internus,* inward; AS, *blod*], any hemorrhage from an internal organ or tissue, such as intraperitoneal bleeding into the peritoneal cavity or intestinal bleeding into the bowel.

**internal carotid artery,** each of two arteries starting at the bifurcation of the common carotid arteries, opposite the cranial border of the thyroid cartilage, through which blood circulates to many structures and organs in the head.

**internal carotid plexus,** a network of nerves on the internal carotid artery, formed by the internal carotid nerve. The internal carotid plexus supplies sympathetic fibers to the branches of the internal carotid artery, the tympanic plexus, the nerves of the cavernous sinus, and the cranial parasympathetic ganglia through which the fibers pass. Compare **common carotid plexus, external carotid plexus.**

**internal cervical os,** an internal opening of the uterus that corresponds to the slight constriction or isthmus of that organ about midway in its length. The internal cervical os separates the body of the uterus from the cervix. Compare **external cervical os.**

**internal cuneiform bone.** See **medial cuneiform bone.**

**internal ear,** the complex inner structure of the ear, containing receptors for hearing and balance. The maculae and crystae cells help maintain equilibrium; the organ of Corti cells translate sound vibrations into impulses for the sense of hearing. The auditory receptor cells are innervated by the cochlear nerve. Also called **inner ear, labyrinth.** Compare **external ear, middle ear.**

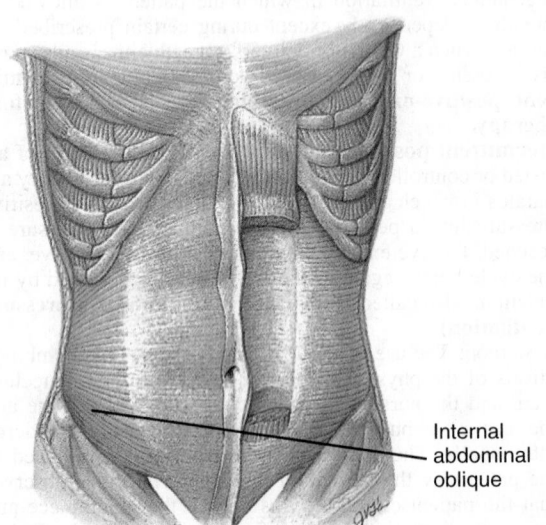

**Internal oblique muscle**
*(Thibodeau and Patton, 1999/John V. Hagen)*

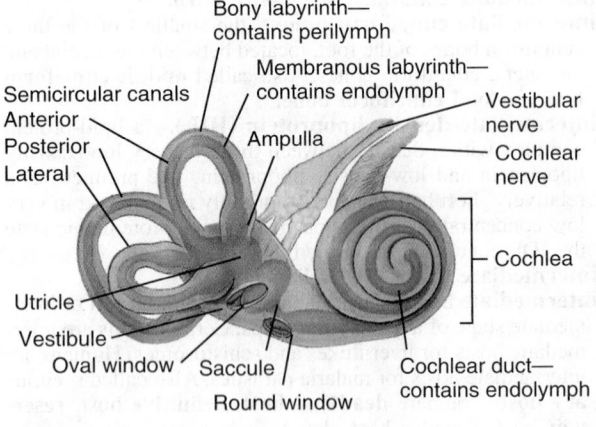

**Internal ear** *(Applegate, 2000)*

**internal fertilization,** the union of gametes within the body of the female after insemination. See also **artificial insemination.**

**internal fistula,** an abnormal passage between two internal organs or structures.

**internal fixation,** any method of holding together the fragments of a fractured bone without the use of appliances external to the skin. After open reduction of the fracture, through an appropriate incision smooth or threaded pins, Kirschner wires, screws, plates attached by screws, or medullary nails may be used to stabilize the fragments. In some instances the device is removed at a later operation, but it may remain in the body permanently. Compare **external pin fixation.**

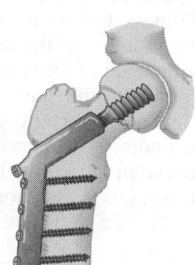

**Internal fixation** *(Black and Matassarin-Jacobs, 1997)*

**internal hemorrhage,** bleeding into a serous cavity, a hollow viscus, or tissues.

**internal hemorrhoid,** a fold of mucous membrane at the anorectal junction, caused by edema or dilation of the interior rectal vein.

**internal hernia,** a protrusion of an intraperitoneal viscus into a recess or compartment within the peritoneal cavity.

**internal iliac artery,** a division of the common iliac artery, supplying the walls of the pelvis, the pelvic viscera, the genital organs, and part of the medial thigh. In the fetus the internal iliac artery is twice as large as the external iliac and is the direct continuation of the common iliac artery. After birth the internal iliac becomes smaller than the external iliac. Also called **hypogastric artery.** Compare **external iliac artery.**

**internal iliac node,** a node in one of seven groups of parietal lymph nodes serving the abdomen and the pelvis. The internal iliac nodes surround the internal iliac vessels and receive lymphatic vessels corresponding to the branches of the internal iliac artery. Their afferent vessels drain lymph from the pelvic viscera, the buttocks, and the dorsal portions of the thighs. Their efferent vessels end in the common iliac nodes. Compare **external iliac node, iliac circumflex node.** See also **lymph, lymphatic system, lymph node.**

**internal iliac vein,** one of the pair of veins in the lower body that join the external iliac vein to form the two common iliac veins. Each vein begins at the greater sciatic foramen and at the pelvic brim joins the external iliac vein. Compare **external iliac vein.**

**internal injury** [L, *internus,* inward, *injuria*], any hurt, wound, or damage to the viscera.

**internalization** /intur'nəlīzā'shən/ [L, *internus* + Gk, *izein,* to cause], the process of adopting within the self, either unconsciously or consciously through learning and socialization, the attitudes, beliefs, values, and standards of another person or more generally of the society or group to which one belongs. See also **socialization.**

**internal jugular vein,** one of a pair of veins in the neck. Each vein collects blood from one side of the brain, the face, and the neck, and both unite with the subclavian vein to form the brachiocephalic vein. Each internal jugular vein is continuous with the transverse sinus in the posterior part of the jugular foramen at the base of the skull. Compare **external jugular vein.**

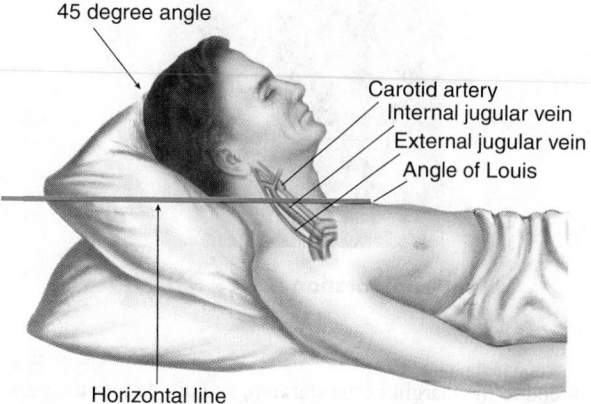

**Internal jugular vein** *(Thompson, 1997)*

**internal locus of control.** See **locus of control.**

**internally.** See **internal.**

**internal malleolus.** See **medial malleolus.**

**internal mammary artery bypass,** a surgical procedure to correct a coronary artery obstruction. The internal mammary artery in situ and still attached to the subclavian artery is anastomosed to the coronary artery beyond the obstruction.

**internal mammary node.** See **sternal node.**

**internal medicine,** the branch of medicine concerned with the study of the physiologic and pathologic characteristics of the internal organs and with the medical diagnosis and treatment of disorders of these organs.

**internal os,** the internal opening of the cervical canal.

**internal podalic version and total breech extraction.** See **version and extraction.**

**internal pterygoid muscle,** one of the four muscles of mastication. It acts to close the jaws. Also called **pterygoideus medialis.** See also **external pterygoid muscle.**

**internal respiratory nerve of Bell.** See **phrenic nerve.**

**internal rotation,** the turning of a limb about its axis of rotation toward the midline of the body.

**internal secretion** [L, *internus,* inward, *secernere,* to separate], a type of secretion in which substances pass directly from a gland into the bloodstream.

**internal standard,** an element or compound added in a known amount to yield a signal against which an instrument or an analyte to be measured can be calibrated.

**internal strabismus.** See **esotropia.**

**internal strangulation** [L, *internus,* inward, *strangulare,* to choke], a state of extreme constriction of an organ, such as a loop of intestine trapped in an opening, resulting in an interruption in the blood supply and ischemia. See also **inguinal hernia, intestinal strangulation.**

**internal thoracic artery,** one of a pair of arteries that arise from the first portions of the subclavian arteries, de-

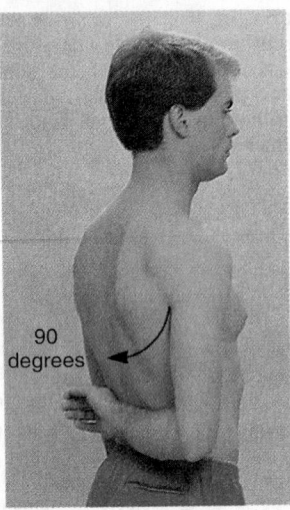

**Internal rotation** *(Seidel et al, 1999)*

scend to the margin of the sternum, and divide into the musculophrenic and superior gastric arteries at the level of the sixth intercostal space. The artery supplies the pectoral muscles, the breasts, the pericardium, and the abdominal muscles.

**internal thoracic vein,** one of a pair of veins that accompany the internal thoracic artery, receiving tributaries that correspond to those of the artery. It forms a single trunk that runs up on the medial side of the artery and ends in the corresponding brachiocephalic vein. The superior phrenic vein usually opens into the internal thoracic vein.

**International Association for Dental Research (IADR),** an international organization concerned with research in dentistry and the exchange of information regarding such research.

*International Classification of Diseases (ICD),* an official list of categories of diseases, physical and mental, issued by the World Health Organization (WHO). It is used primarily for statistical purposes in the classification of morbidity and mortality data. Any nation belonging to WHO may adjust the classification to meet specific needs. See also *Diagnostic and Statistical Manual of Mental Disorders.*

**International Commission on Radiation Protection (ICRP),** a nongovernmental organization founded in England in 1928 to provide general guidance on the safe use of radiation sources, including appropriate protective measures and codes of practice for medical radiology. The ICRP was originally established as a source of information about the hazards of x-rays and radium in medicine but was reorganized in 1950 to include effects of nuclear energy.

**International Congress of Surgeons (I.C.S.),** an international professional organization of surgeons.

**International Council of Nurses (ICN),** the oldest international health organization. It is a federation of nurses' associations from 112 countries and was one of the first health organizations to develop strict policies of nondiscrimination based on nationality, race, creed, color, politics, sex, or social status. The objectives of the ICN include promotion of national associations of nurses, improvement of standards of nursing and competence of nurses, improvement of the status of nurses within their countries, and provision of an authoritative international voice for nurses. The following ICN

definition of the nurse is accepted internationally and serves as a pattern in developing nursing practice and nursing education throughout the world: "A nurse is a person who has completed a program of basic education and is qualified and authorized in her/his country to practice nursing. Basic nursing education is a formally recognized program of study that provides a broad and sound foundation for the practice of nursing, and for postbasic education, which develops specific competency. At the first level, the educational program prepares the nurse, through study of behavior, life, and nursing sciences and clinical experience, for effective practice and direction of nursing care and for the leadership role. The first level nurse is responsible for planning, providing, and evaluating nursing care in all settings for the promotion of health, prevention of illness, care of the sick, and rehabilitation; and functions as a member of the health team. In countries with more than one level of nursing personnel, the second level program prepares the nurse, through study of nursing theory and clinical practice, to give nursing care in cooperation with and under the supervision of a first level nurse." The ICN is active in the World Health Organization (WHO), the United Nations Educational, Scientific, and Cultural Organization (UNESCO), and other international organizations.

**International Normalized Ratio (INR),** a comparative rating of a patient's prothrombin time (PT) ratio, used as a standard for monitoring the effects of warfarin. The INR indicates what the patient's PT ratio would have been if measured by using the primary World Health Organization International Reference reagent.

**International Red Cross Society,** an international philanthropic organization, based in Geneva, Switzerland, concerned primarily with the humane treatment and welfare of the victims of war and calamity and with the neutrality of hospitals and medical personnel in times of war. See also **American Red Cross.**

**International System of Units (SI),** an internationally accepted scientific system of expressing length, mass, and time in base units (IU) of meters, kilograms, and seconds, replacing the old centimeter-gram-second system (**CGS**). The SI system includes as standard measurements the **ampere, kelvin, candela,** and **mole.**

**International Unit (IU, I.U.),** a unit of measure in the International System of Units. See also **SI units.**

**interneuron** /-nŏŏr′on/, a nerve cell whose axon and dendrite lie entirely within the central nervous system and whose function is to relay impulses within the central nervous system.

**internist** /intur′nist, in′turnist/ [L, *internus,* inward], a physician who specializes in internal medicine.

**internship** /in′turnship′/, a period of apprenticeship for a medical school graduate who serves in a hospital for a specified period before beginning a professional practice. Some hospitals offer internships for new graduates in nursing.

**internuncial neuron** /-nun′sē·əl/ [L, *inter + nuntius,* messenger], a connecting neuron in a neural pathway, usually serving as a link between two other neurons.

**interocclusal record** /-əklōō′səl/, an imprint of the positional relation of opposing teeth or jaws to each other, made on the surfaces of occlusal rims or teeth with a material such as plaster of paris, wax, zinc oxide-eugenol paste, or acrylic resin.

**interoceptive** /in′tərōsep′tiv/ [L, *internus,* inward, *capere,* to take], pertaining to stimuli originating from within the body that are related to the functioning of the internal organs or the receptors they activate. Compare **exteroceptive, proprioception.**

**interoceptor** /-sep'tər/ [L, *internus* + *capere*, to take], any sensory nerve ending located in cells in the viscera that responds to stimuli originating from within the body in relation to the function of the internal organs, such as digestion, excretion, and blood pressure. Compare **exteroceptor, proprioceptor.**

**interosseous** /-os'ē·əs/ [L, *inter*, between, *os*, bone], pertaining to an area between bones or a structure, such as a ligament, connecting two bones.

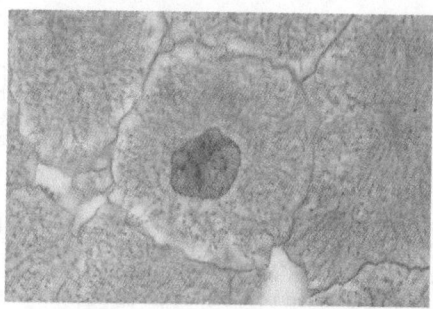

**Interphase** (© *Ed Reschke; used with permission*)

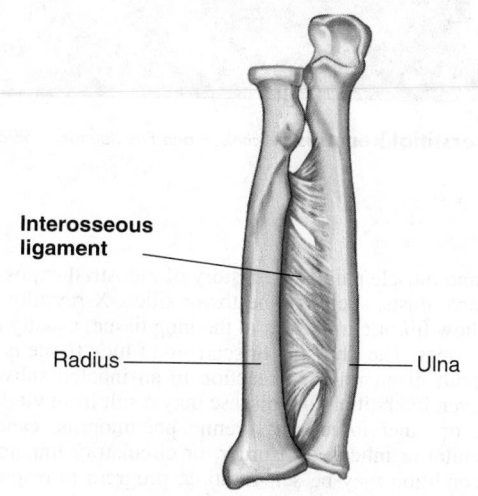

Interosseous ligament

Radius — Ulna

**Interosseus ligament**

**interparietal fissure.** See **intraparietal sulcus.**

**interparoxysmal** /-per'əksis'məl/ [L, *inter*, between, *paroxysmos*, irritation], pertaining to something that happens between paroxysms.

**interperiosteal fracture** /in'tərper'ē·os'tē·əl/ [L, *inter* + Gk, *peri*, around, *osteon*, bone], an incomplete fracture in which the periosteum is not disrupted.

**interpersonal** /-pur'sənəl/ [L, *inter*, between, *personalis*], pertaining to the interactions of individuals.

**interpersonal psychiatry** [L, *inter* + *persona*, mask], a theory of psychiatry introduced by Harry Stack Sullivan [1892–1949] that stresses the nature and quality of relationships with significant others as the most critical factor in personality development.

**interpersonal therapy,** a kind of psychotherapy that views faulty communications, interactions, and interrelationships as basic factors in maladaptive behavior. A kind of interpersonal therapy is **transactional analysis.**

**interphase** /in'tərfās'/ [L, *inter* + Gk, *phasis*, phase], the stage in the cell cycle during which the cell is not dividing, the chromosomes are not individually distinguishable, and such biochemical and physiologic activities as DNA synthesis occur. Interphase follows telophase of one cell division and extends to the beginning of prophase of the next division. See also **anaphase, interkinesis, metaphase, mitosis, prophase, telophase.**

**interpleural space** /-plŏŏr'əl/ [L, *inter*, between; Gk, *pleura*, rib; L, *spatium*], the potential space of the mediastinum between the two pleural linings, which contains serous fluid. Also called **pleural cavity.**

**interpolated premature ventricular contraction** /intur'pəlā'tid/ [L, *interpolare*, to refurbish], a ventricular extrasystole that occurs between two consecutive sinus-

conducted beats. It is not followed by a compensatory pause.

**interpolation** /intur'pəlā'shən/, **1.** the transfer of tissues, as in plastic surgery or transplantation. **2.** (in statistics) the introduction of an estimated intermediate value of a variable between known values.

**interpreter** /intur'prətər/ [Fr, *interpreter*, to translate], a computer program that remains in the memory and translates or executes higher-level language.

**interproximal film.** See **bite wing film.**

**interpubic disk** /-pyŏŏ'bik/ [L, *inter* + *os pubis*, pubic bone; Gk, *diskos*, flat plate], the fibrocartilaginous plate connecting the opposed surfaces of the pubic bones at the pubic symphysis. Varying in thickness, it is strengthened by interlacing fibers and often contains a cavity that usually appears after the tenth year of life. Also called **discus interpubicus.**

**interpulse interval** /-puls'/, the time elapsed between successive nerve impulses; the reciprocal of impulse frequency.

**interradicular space** /-radik'yələr/ [L, *inter* + *radix*, root, *spatium*], the area between the roots of a multirooted tooth, normally occupied by a bony septum and the periodontal membrane.

**interrogatories** /in'tərog'ətôr'ēz/ [L, *inter* + *rogare*, to ask], (in law) a series of written questions submitted to a witness or other person having information of interest to the court. The answers are transcribed and are sworn to under oath. Interrogatories are used during the pretrial period as a means of discovery. They differ from depositions in that there is no opportunity for cross-examination. Compare **discovery, deposition.**

**interrupted suture** /in'tərup'tid/ [L, *interrumpere*, to sever, *sutura*], a single suture tied separately, as distinguished from a continuous suture.

**intersection syndrome,** a condition of pain, crepitus, and a squeaky sensation in the dorsal radial forearm. It occurs most commonly among weight lifters and rowers and is treated with splinting, analgesics, and steroid injection as needed.

**intersex** /in'tərseks'/ [L, *inter* + *sexus*, sex, gender], any individual who has anatomic characteristics of both sexes or whose external genitalia are ambiguous or inappropriate for either the normal male or female. See also **intersexuality, pseudohermaphroditism.**

**intersexuality** /-sek'shŏŏ·al'itē/ [L, *inter* + *sexus*, male or female], the condition in which an individual has both male and female anatomic characteristics to varying degrees or in which the appearance of the external genitalia is ambiguous or differs from that characteristic of the gonadal or genetic sex. See also **hermaphroditism, pseudohermaph-roditism. —intersexual,** *adj.*

**interspinal ligament** /-spī'nəl/ [L, *inter* + *spina,* spine, *ligare,* to bind], one of many thin, narrow membranous ligaments that connect adjoining spinous processes of the vertebrae and extend from the root of each process to the apex. The interspinal ligaments are only slightly developed in the neck.

**interspinous** /-spī'nəs/ [L, *inter* + *spina,* spine], pertaining to the space between any spinous processes.

**interstitial** /in'tərstish'əl/ [L, *inter* + *sistere,* to stand], pertaining to the space between cells, as interstitial fluid, or between organs. Also called **intercellular.**

**interstitial cell-stimulating hormone (ICSH),** a hormone secreted by the anterior pituitary gland that stimulates the production of testosterone by the Leydig, or interstitial, cells of the testis. Also called **luteinizing hormone** for its effects on the female reproductive system.

**interstitial cystitis,** an inflammation of the bladder, believed to be associated with an autoimmune or allergic response. The bladder wall becomes inflamed, ulcerated, and scarred, causing frequent painful urination. Hematuria often occurs. Treatment may include distension of the bladder and cauterization of the ulcers (if present), dietary modification, oral or intravesical medication, pain management, and alternative therapies such as acupuncture. Cystectomy with urinary diversion is rarely indicated. The condition occurs most often in women and may resemble the early stages of bladder cancer. Diagnosis is often by exclusion and may require cystoscopy and biopsy. See also **Hunner's ulcer.**

**interstitial emphysema,** a form of emphysema in which air or gas escapes into the interstitial tissues of the lung after a penetrating injury or a rupture in an alveolar wall. Since the alveoli must be decompressed, there is danger that the pleura will be torn, causing a pneumothorax. The condition is diagnosed by chest x-ray films. See also **pneumothorax.**

**interstitial fibroid** [L, *interstitium,* space between, *fibra,* fiber; Gk, *eidos,* form], a fibrous tumor that develops in the muscular wall of the uterus and tends to grow inward.

**interstitial fluid,** an extracellular fluid that fills the spaces between most of the cells of the body and provides a substantial portion of the liquid environment of the body. Formed by filtration through the blood capillaries, it is drained away as lymph. It closely resembles blood plasma in composition but contains less protein. Compare **intracellular fluid, lymph, plasma.**

**interstitial growth,** an increase in size by hyperplasia or hypertrophy within the interior of a part or structure that is already formed. Compare **appositional growth.**

**interstitial hypertrophic neuropathy.** See **Déjérine-Sottas disease.**

**interstitial implantation,** (in embryology) the complete embedding of the blastocyst within the endometrium of the uterine wall.

**interstitial inflammation** [L, *interstitium,* space between, *inflammare,* to set afire], an inflammation in an area of connective tissues.

**interstitial infusion.** See **hypodermoclysis.**

**interstitial keratitis,** an uncommon inflammation within the layers of the cornea. The first symptom is a diffuse haziness. Blood vessels may grow into the area and cause permanent opacities. The causes are syphilis, tuberculosis, leprosy, and vascular hypersensitivity. Treatment is specific to the infection or condition.

**interstitial lung disease (ILD),** a respiratory disorder characterized by a dry, unproductive cough and dyspnea on exertion. The patient may have swallowing disorders or

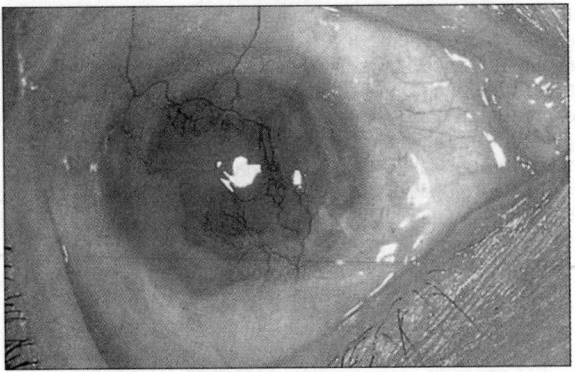

**Interstitial keratitis** *(Michelson and Friedlaender, 1996)*

joint and muscle pain and a history of industrial exposure to inorganic dusts, such as asbestos or silica. X-ray films usually show fibrotic infiltrates in the lung tissue, usually in the lower lobes. The fibrosing or scarring of lung tissue is often the result of an immune reaction to an inhaled substance. However, interstitial lung disease may result from viral, bacterial, or other infections; uremic pneumonitis; cancer; a congenital or inherited disorder; or circulatory impairment. The condition may be self-limiting, progress to respiratory or cardiac failure, or undergo spontaneous recovery.

**interstitial mastitis** [L, *interstitium,* space between; Gk, *mastos,* breast], an inflammation of the connective tissue between ducts of the breast.

**interstitial myositis.** See **myositis fibrosa.**

**interstitial nephritis,** inflammation of the interstitial tissue of the kidney, including the tubules. The condition may be acute or chronic. **Acute interstitial nephritis** is an immunologic adverse reaction to certain drugs, often sulfonamide or methicillin. Acute renal failure, fever, rash, and proteinuria are characteristic of this condition. Most people regain normal kidney function when the offending drug is discontinued. **Chronic interstitial nephritis** is a syndrome of interstitial inflammation and structural changes, sometimes associated with such conditions as ureteral obstruction, pyelonephritis, exposure of the kidney to a toxin, rejection of a transplant, and certain systemic diseases. Gradually renal failure, nausea, vomiting, weight loss, fatigue, and anemia develop. Acidosis and hyperkalemia may follow. The nurse watches carefully for signs of electrolyte imbalance, dehydration, and hypovolemia, especially if there is frequent vomiting. Fluids and electrolytes may be replaced intravenously. Treatment includes correction of the underlying cause. If the cause is an obstruction of the urinary tract, rapid recovery may follow removal of the obstruction; in other cases, hemodialysis and kidney transplantation may be necessary.

**interstitial plasma cell pneumonia.** See **pneumocystosis.**

**interstitial pneumonia,** a condition of diffuse, chronic inflammation of the lungs beyond the terminal bronchioles, characterized by fibrosis and collagen formation in the alveolar walls and by the presence of large mononuclear cells in the alveolar spaces. The symptoms are progressive dyspnea, clubbing of the fingers, cyanosis, and fever. The disease may result from a hypersensitive reaction to busulfan, chlorambucil, hexamethonium, or methotrexate. It may also be an autoimmune reaction because it often accompanies celiac disease, rheumatoid arthritis, Sjögren's syndrome, and systemic sclerosis. X-ray films of the lungs show patchy shadows and mottling, as in bronchopneumonia. Later stages of the disease reveal bronchiectasis, dilation of the bronchi, and shrinkage of the lungs. Treatment includes bed rest, oxygen therapy, and corticosteroids. Most patients die within 6 months to a few years, usually as a result of cardiac or respiratory failure. Also called **diffuse fibrosing alveolitis, giant cell interstitial pneumonia, Hamman-Rich syndrome.** Compare **bronchopneumonia.**

**interstitial pregnancy.**   See **ectopic pregnancy.**

**interstitial therapy,**   radiotherapy in which needles or wires that contain radioactive material are implanted directly into tumor areas. See **brachytherapy.**

**interstitial tissue** [L, *interstitium,* space between; OFr, *tissu*],   the connective and supporting tissue within and surrounding major functional elements of an organ.

**interstitial tubal pregnancy,**   a kind of tubal pregnancy in which implantation occurs in the proximal interstitial portion of one of the fallopian tubes. See also **tubal pregnancy.**

**interstitium** /-stish′ē·əm/,   the space between cells in a tissue.

**intertransverse ligament** /-transvurz′/ [L, *inter* + *transversus,* cross-direction],   one of many fibrous bands connecting the transverse processes of vertebrae. In the cervical region intertransverse ligaments consist of a few scattered fibers; in the thoracic region they are rounded cords intimately connected with the deep muscles of the back; in the lumbar region they are thin and membranous.

**intertrigo** /in′tərtrī′gō/ [L, *inter* + *terere,* to scour],   an erythematous irritation of opposing skin surfaces caused by friction. Common sites are the axillae, the folds beneath large or pendulous breasts, and the inner aspects of the thighs. Maceration and candidal infection may be complications if the area is also warm and moist. Prevention is by weight reduction, powdering, cleansing, and use of antifungal topical medication when necessary. **—intertriginous,** *adj.*

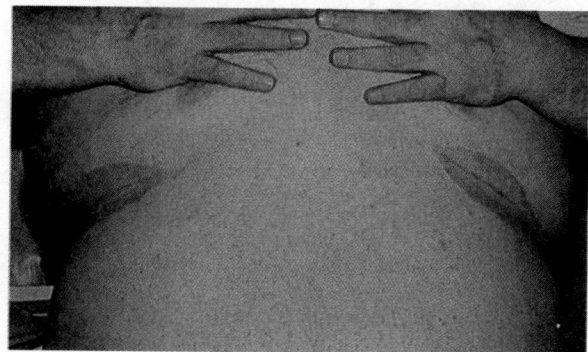

**Intertrigo** *(White, 1994)*

**intertrochanteric crest** /in′tərtrō′kanter′ik/ [L, *inter* + *trochanter,* runner, *crista,* ridge],   one of a pair of ridges along the thigh bones, curving obliquely from the greater to the lesser trochanter.

**intertrochanteric fracture,**   a crack in the proximal femur between the greater and the lesser trochanters.

**intertrochanteric line,**   a line that runs across the anterior surface of the thigh bone from the greater to the lesser trochanter, winding around the medial surface and ending in the linea aspera. The proximal half of the intertrochanteric line is the attachment for the iliofemoral ligament; the distal half holds the vastus medialis muscle.

**intertuberous diameter** /-too′bərəs/ [L, *inter* + *tuber,* swelling; Gk, *dia,* across, *metron,* measure],   the distance between the ischial tuberosities, a factor used in determining the dimensions, including the narrowest diameter, of the pelvic outlet.

**interval** /in′tərval/ [L, *intervallum,* space between],   a space between things or events, or a break or interruption in an otherwise continuous flow.

**interval health history** [L, *intervallum,* space between],   a kind of health history that notes the general condition of a client during the period between visits and is not limited to facts relevant to a particular condition. The interval health history provides an ongoing account of a person's health, serving to bring the data base up to date.

**intervention** /in′tərven′shən/ [L, *inter* + *venire,* to come],   any act performed to prevent harming of a patient or to improve the mental, emotional, or physical function of a patient. A physiologic process may be monitored or enhanced, or a pathologic process may be arrested or controlled. **Independent intervention** is any health care activity pertaining to certain aspects of professional practice that are encompassed by applicable licensure and law and require no supervision or direction from others. **Interdependent intervention** refers to any health care activity carried out by one health care professional in collaboration with another. See also **nursing intervention.**

**interventricular** /-ventrik′yələr/ [L, *inter,* between, *ventriculus,* little belly],   pertaining to the location between the ventricles, as the septum of the heart.

**interventricular septum** [L, *inter,* between, *ventriculus,* little belly, *saeptum,* fence],   the wall between the ventricles of the heart. Also called **ventricular septum.**

**intervertebral** /in′tərvur′təbrəl/ [L, *inter* + *vertebra,* back joint],   pertaining to the space between any two vertebrae, such as the fibrocartilaginous disks.

**intervertebral disk,**   one of the fibrous, broad, and flattened disks found between adjacent spinal vertebrae, except the axis and the atlas. The disks vary in size, shape, thickness, and number, depending on the location in the back and on the particular vertebrae they separate.

**intervertebral fibrocartilage.**   See **intervertebral disk.**

**intervertebral foramen,**   any of the passages between adjacent vertebrae through which the spinal nerves and vessels pass.

**intervertebral ganglion** [L, *inter,* between, *vertebra,* back joint; Gk, *ganglion,* knot],   the ganglionic enlargement of a spinal nerve root between adjacent vertebrae.

**interview** /in′tərvyoo/,   a verbal interaction with a patient initiated for a specific purpose and focused on a specific content area. A **problem-seeking interview** is an inquiry that focuses on gathering data to identify problems the patient needs to resolve. A **problem-solving interview** focuses on problems that have been identified by the patient or health care professional.

**intervillous space** /in′tərvil′əs/ [L, *inter* + *villus,* hair, *spatium*],   one of many spaces between the chorionic villi of the endometrium of the gravid uterus, beneath the placenta. The intervillous spaces act as small reservoirs for oxygenated maternal blood from which the fetal circulation may take up the nutrients and gases by osmosis, hydrostatic pressure, and diffusion.

**intestinal** /intes′tinəl/ [L, *intestinum*], pertaining to the intestines.

**intestinal absorption** [L, *intestinum*, intestine, *absorbare*, to swallow], the passage of the products of digestion from the lumen of the small intestine into the blood and lymphatic vessels in the wall of the gut. The surface area of the intestine is greatly increased by the presence of fingerlike projections, called *villi*, each of which contains capillaries and a lymphatic vessel, or lacteal. Most dissolved nutrients pass quickly into the capillary bed for transport through the portal circulation to the liver. Lipids enter the lymphatic channels, which eventually rejoin the venous circulation at the thoracic duct in the neck.

**intestinal amebiasis.** See **amebic dysentery.**

**intestinal angina,** chronic vascular insufficiency of the mesentery caused by atherosclerosis and resulting ischemia of the smooth muscle of the small bowel. Also called **chronic intestinal ischemia.**

**intestinal apoplexy,** the sudden occlusion of one of the three principal arteries to the intestine by an embolism or a thrombus. This condition leads rapidly to necrosis of intestinal tissue and is often fatal. Treatment is usually surgical. The occlusion is removed, and often the affected portion of the bowel is resected. See also **atherosclerosis.**

**intestinal atresia** [L, *intestinum* + Gk, *a* + *tresis*, boring], a pathologic obstruction of the continuous lumen of the intestinal tract caused by a defect of development in utero.

**intestinal bypass** [L, *intestinum* + AS, *bi* + Fr, *passer* + Gk, *cheirourgos*], a surgical procedure to shorten the digestive tract. It is performed so that less intestinal surface will be available to absorb nutrients from the digested food passing through, as in morbid obesity, or to bypass a blocked or diseased portion of the intestine. The technique usually involves anastomosing the jejunum to the ileum. See also **ileal bypass.**

**intestinal colic** [L, *intestinum* + Gk, *kolikos,* colonic pain], spasmodic pain in intestinal disorders.

**intestinal dyspepsia,** an abnormal condition characterized by impaired digestion associated with a disorder that originates in the intestines. See also **dyspepsia.**

**intestinal fistula,** an abnormal passage from the intestine to an external abdominal opening or stoma, usually created surgically for the exit of feces after removal of a malignant or severely ulcerated segment of the bowel. See also **colostomy.**

**intestinal flora** [L, *intestinum* + *flos,* flowers], the natural bacterial content of the inside of the digestive tract.

**intestinal flu,** a viral gastroenteritis, usually caused by infection by an enterovirus. It is characterized by abdominal cramps, diarrhea, nausea, and vomiting. Outbreaks may be sporadic or epidemic, and the disease usually is mild and self-limited. Treatment is symptomatic. Control of diarrhea may be achieved with antidiarrheal medication and a diet limited to clear fluids. See also **enteric infection, gastroenteritis.**

**intestinal fluke** [L, *intestinum* + AS, *floc*], any internal parasite of the genera *Fasciolopsis, Heterophyes,* and *Metagonimus* in North America and of other genera in Asia and in tropical countries. They enter the body through the mouth as encysted larvae in aquatic vegetation or freshwater fish. Symptoms of intestinal fluke infestation usually include abdominal pain and obstruction and diarrhea.

**intestinal gas** [L, *intestinum*], gas in the digestive tract arising from three sources—swallowed air, gas produced by digestive processes, and blood gases diffused into the intestinal lumen. Gases produced in the intestine and diffused from blood are mainly hydrogen ($H_2$), most of which is a bacterial fermentation product of ingested carbohydrates; carbon dioxide ($CO_2$); and methane ($CH_4$).

**intestinal glands.** See **Lieberkühn's glands.**

**intestinal infarction.** See **intestinal strangulation.**

**intestinal juices,** the secretions of glands lining the intestine.

**intestinal lipodystrophy.** See **lipodystrophy.**

**intestinal lymphangiectasia.** See **hypoproteinemia.**

**intestinal obstruction,** any obstruction that results in failure of the contents of the intestine to progress through the lumen of the bowel. The most common cause is a mechanical blockage resulting from adhesions, impacted feces, tumor of the bowel, hernia, intussusception, volvulus, or the strictures of inflammatory bowel disease. Obstruction may also be the result of paralytic ileus. Obstruction of the small bowel may cause severe pain, vomiting of fecal matter, dehydration, and eventually a drop in blood pressure. Obstruction of the colon causes less severe pain, marked abdominal distension, and constipation. Radiographic examination reveals the level of obstruction and its cause. Treatment includes the evacuation of intestinal contents by means of an intestinal tube. Surgical repair is sometimes necessary. Fluid balance and electrolyte balance are restored by carefully monitored IV infusion. Nonnarcotic analgesics are usually prescribed to prevent the decrease in intestinal motility that often accompanies the administration of narcotic analgesics. Also called *(informal)* **ileus.** See also **hernia, intussusception, volvulus.**

**intestinal perforation** [L, *intestinum* + *perforare,* to pierce], the escape of digestive tract contents into the peritoneal cavity that results from trauma or a disease condition such as a ruptured appendix or perforated ulcer. The condition inevitably leads to peritonitis.

**intestinal pseudo-obstruction** [L, *intestinum,* intestine; Gk, *pseudes,* false; L, *obstruere,* to build against ], a condition characterized by constipation, colicky pain, and vomiting, but without evidence of organic obstruction apparent at laparotomy.

**intestinal strangulation,** the arrest of blood flow to the bowel, causing edema, cyanosis, and gangrene of the affected loop of bowel. This condition is usually caused by a hernia, intussusception, or volvulus. Early signs of intestinal strangulation resemble those of intestinal obstruction, but peritonitis, shock, and presence of a tender mass in the abdomen are important findings in making a differential diagnosis. In addition to surgery, treatment includes the immediate correction of fluid and electrolyte imbalance. Also called **intestinal infarction.**

**intestinal tonsil,** one of a group of lymphatic nodules forming a single layer in the mucous membrane of the ileum opposite the mesenteric attachment. They are oval patches about 1 cm wide and extend for about 4 cm along the intestine. In most individuals they appear in the distal ileum, but they also appear in the jejunum of a few individuals. Also called **Peyer's patches.** Compare **lingual tonsil, palatine tonsil, pharyngeal tonsil.**

**intestinal tract** [L, *intestinum* + *tractus*], the segments of the small and large intestines between the pyloric valve and the rectum. It forms part of the digestive tract.

**intestinal tubes** [L, *intestinum* + *tubus*], the alimentary canal or digestive tract.

**intestine** /intes′tin/ [L, *intestinum*], the portion of the alimentary canal extending from the pyloric opening of the stomach to the anus. It includes the small and large intestines. —**intestinal,** *adj.*

**intima** /in′timə/, *pl.* **intimae** [L, *intimus,* innermost], the innermost layer of a structure, such as the lining membrane of an artery, vein, lymphatic vessel, or organ. —**intimal,** *adj.*

**intimal sclerosis** [L, *intimus,* innermost; Gk, *sklerosis,* hardening], a hardening of the innermost layer of a blood vessel wall. See also **atherosclerosis**.

**intoe.** See **metatarsus varus**.

**intolerance** /intol'ərəns/ [L, *in*, not, *tolerare*, to bear], a condition characterized by inability to absorb or metabolize a nutrient or medication. Exposure to the substance may cause an adverse reaction, as in lactose intolerance. Compare **allergy, atopic**.

**intoxicant** /intok'sikənt/ [L, *in* + Gk, *toxikon*, poison], any agent that can cause intoxication or poisoning.

**intoxication** /intok'sikā'shən/ [L, *in*, within; Gk, *toxikon*, poison], **1.** the state of being poisoned by a drug or other toxic substance. **2.** the state of being inebriated as a result of an excessive consumption of alcohol. **3.** a state of mental or emotional hyperexcitability, usually euphoric.

**intra-** prefix meaning 'situated, formed, or occurring within': *intrabronchial, intracutaneous, intramatrical*.

**intraabdominal infections** /in'trə·abdom'inəl/, diseases caused by organisms, usually bacterial or fungal, situated within the cavity of the abdomen. The infection may be in the retroperitoneal space or the peritoneal cavity. Intraperitoneal infections may be diffuse or localized in one or more abscesses in recesses such as the pelvic space or perihepatic spaces. Abscesses also form about diseased viscera. Treatment depends on the type of infectious organism and the site of the infection.

**intraabdominal pressure** [L, *intra*, within, *abdomen*, belly], the degree of pressure within the abdominal cavity.

**intraalveolar pocket.** See **periodontal pocket**.

**intraaortic balloon pump** /in'trə·ā·ôr'tik/ [L, *intra* + *aeirein*, to rise], a counterpulsation device that provides temporary cardiac assist in the management of refractory left ventricular failure that may follow myocardial infarction or occur in preinfarction angina. The balloon is attached to a catheter inserted into the aorta and is automatically inflated during diastole and deflated during systole. Also called **intraaortic balloon counterpulsation (IABC)**. See also **counterpulsation**.

**intraarterial** /in'trə·ärtir'ē·əl/, pertaining to a structure or action inside an artery.

**intraarticular** /in'trə·ärtik'yələr/ [L, *intra* + *articulus*, joint], within a joint.

**intraarticular fracture**, a fracture involving the articular surfaces of a joint.

**intraarticular injection**, the injection of a medication into a joint space, usually to reduce inflammation, such as in bursitis or fibromyositis. With the same technique abnormally excessive fluid may be withdrawn from the joint space. The fluid may be a result of trauma or inflammation.

**intraarticular ligament**, a ligament that forms part of the joints between 16 of the 24 ribs, dividing the joints into two cavities, each containing a synovial membrane. Each intraarticular ligament consists of a short, flattened band of fibers inside the joint, attached by one extremity to the rib and by the other to the intervertebral disk. Intraarticular ligaments are not present in the joints of the first, tenth, eleventh, and twelfth ribs, each of which has only one synovial cavity. Compare **radiate ligament**.

**intraatrial** /in'trə·ā'trē·əl/ [L, *intra* + *atrium*, hall], pertaining to the space or substance within an atrium of the heart.

**intraatrial block**, delayed or abnormal conduction of the cardiac impulse within the atria. It is identified on an electrocardiogram by a prolonged and often a notched P wave. See also **atrioventricular block, heart block, intraventricular block, sinoatrial block**.

**intrabony pocket.** See **periodontal pocket**.

**intracanalicular fibroma** /-kan'əlik'yələr/ [L, *intra* + *canaliculus*, small channel], a tumor containing glandular epithelium and fibrous tissue, occurring in the breast.

**intracanicular papilloma** /-kənik'yələr/, a benign warty growth in certain glands, especially the breast.

**intracapsular fracture** /-kap'syələr/ [L, *intra* + *capsula*, little box], a fracture within the capsule of a joint.

**intracardiac** /-kär'dē·ak/ [L, *intra*, within; Gk, *kardia*, heart], pertaining to the interior of the heart chambers.

**intracardiac catheter.** See **cardiac catheter**.

**intracardiac lead** /lēd/ [L, *intra* + Gk, *kardia*, heart; AS, *laedan*, lead], **1.** an electrocardiographic conductor in which the exploring electrode is placed within one of the cardiac chambers, usually by means of cardiac catheterization. **2.** *informal*. a tracing produced by such a lead on an electrocardiograph.

**intracartilaginous ossification.** See **ossification**.

**intracatheter** /-kath'ətər/ [L, *intra* + Gk, *katheter*, something lowered], a thin, flexible plastic catheter introduced through a stainless steel needle and threaded into a blood vessel to infuse blood, fluid, or medication. Also called *(informal)* **intracath**.

**intracavitary** /in'trəkav'itər'ē/ [L, *intra* + *cavum*, cave], pertaining to the space within a body cavity.

**intracavitary therapy**, a kind of radiotherapy in which one or more radioactive sources are placed, usually with the help of an applicator or holding device, within a body cavity to irradiate the walls of the cavity or adjacent tissues.

**intracellular** /-sel'yələr/ [L, *intra*, within, *cella*, storeroom], pertaining to the interior of a cell; within a cell.

**intracellular fluid (ICF)** [L, *intra* + *cella*, storeroom, *fluere*, to flow], a fluid within cell membranes throughout most of the body, containing dissolved solutes that are es-

Left common carotid artery

Left subclavian artery

Brachiocephalic trunk

Arch of aorta

Coronary artery

Left ventricle

Balloon

**Systole**

**Early Diastole**

**Late Diastole**

**Intraaortic balloon pump**
*(Lewis, Heitkemper, and Dirksen, 2000)*

sential to electrolytic balance and to healthy metabolism. Also called **intracellular water (ICW).** Compare **extracellular fluid, interstitial fluid, lymph, plasma.**

**intracerebral** /-ser′əbrəl/ [L, *intra* + *cerebrum,* brain], pertaining to the area or substance within the cerebrum.

**intracerebral hematoma,** a localized collection of extravasated blood within the cerebrum, associated with a cerebral laceration resulting from a contusion. See also **intracerebral hemorrhage.**

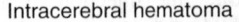
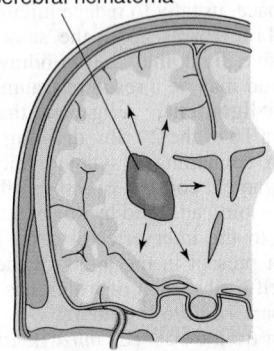

**Intracerebral hematoma (arrows indicate direction of pressure)**
*(Phipps, Sands, and Marek, 1999)*

**intracerebral hemorrhage (ICH),** a type of hemorrhagic stroke in which bleeding directly into the brain occurs. It is most often caused by hypertension and is associated with increased intracranial pressure. ICH usually occurs in the basal ganglia, thalamus, pons, and cerebral and cerebellar white matter.

**intracervical.** See **endocervical.**

**intracistronic** /in′trəsistron′ik/ [L, *intra* + *cis,* this side, *trans,* across], within a cistron.

**intracoronal retainer** /-kôr′ənəl/ [L, *intra* + *corona,* crown], **1.** a cast restoration, such as an inlay, that lies largely within the contour of the tooth crown. The retention to displacement is developed between the restoration and the walls of the prepared tooth cavity. **2.** a direct retainer used in the construction of removable partial dentures. It consists of a female portion within the coronal segment of the crown of an abutment and a male portion attached to the denture proper.

**intracostal** /-kos′təl/, pertaining to the inner surface of a rib.

**intracranial** /-krā′nē·əl/ [L, *intra,* within; Gk, *kranion,* skull], pertaining to the area within the cranium (the bony skull).

**intracranial abscess.** See **brain abscess.**

**intracranial aneurysm,** localized dilation of any of the cerebral arteries. Characteristics of the condition include sudden severe headache, stiff neck, photophobia, nausea, vomiting, and sometimes loss of consciousness. Rupture of an intracranial aneurysm produces a mortality rate approaching 50%, and survivors face a high risk of recurrence. Some forms of intracranial aneurysm may be treated surgically. Kinds of intracranial aneurysms include **berry aneurysm, fusiform aneurysm,** and **mycotic aneurysm.**

**intracranial hemorrhage** [L, *intra,* within; Gk, *kranion,* skull, *haima,* blood], a hemorrhage within the cranium.

**intracranial pneumatocele.** See **pneumocephalus.**

**intracranial pressure (ICP),** pressure that occurs within the cranium.

**intracranial pressure (ICP) monitoring,** a nursing intervention from the Nursing Interventions Classification (NIC) defined as measurement and interpretation of patient data to regulate intracranial pressure. See also **Nursing Interventions Classification.**

**intractable** /intrak′təbəl/ [L, *intractabilis,* hard to manage], having no relief, such as a symptom or a disease that is not relieved by the therapeutic measures used.

**intractable pain** [L, *intractabilis,* hard to manage, *poena,* penalty], pain that is not relieved by ordinary medical, surgical, and nursing measures. The pain is often chronic, persistent, and psychogenic in nature.

**intracutaneous** /-kyo͞otā′nē·əs/ [L, *intra* + *cutis,* skin], within the skin.

**intracystic papilloma** /-sis′tik/ [L, *intra* + Gk, *kystis,* bag], a benign epithelial tumor formed within a cystic adenoma.

**intradermal** /-dur′məl/ [L, *intra,* within; Gk, *derma,* skin], within the dermis.

**intradermal injection,** the introduction of a hypodermic needle into the dermis for the purpose of instilling a substance, such as a serum or vaccine.

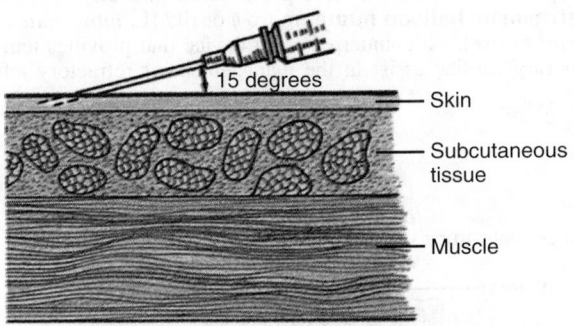

**Intradermal injection showing angle of needle placement in skin**
*(Potter and Perry, 2001)*

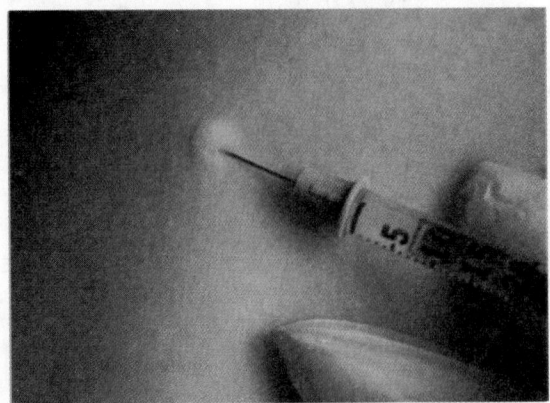

**Formation of bleb following intradermal injection**
*(Potter and Perry, 2001)*

**intradermal test** [L, *intra* + Gk, *derma,* skin], a procedure used to identify suspected allergens by subcutaneously injecting the patient with small amounts of extracts of the suspected allergens. The injections are made at spaced intervals, usually in the forearm or the scapular region. The patient is concurrently injected with the diluent alone as a control procedure. The test result is positive if within 15 to 30 minutes the injection of extract produces a wheal surrounded by erythema and the control injection produces no symptoms. The intradermal test is started with highly diluted solutions; if the initial test result is negative, the procedure is repeated with stronger solutions. This gradual method is used to prevent a systemic reaction, which is more of a risk with intradermal testing than with other kinds of allergy testing, such as the scratch test. The intradermal test tends to be more accurate than the scratch test and is often performed if scratch test results are negative or unclear. Intradermal testing also limits to between 20 and 30 the number of suspected allergens that can be examined simultaneously in the skin of one patient. Also called **subcutaneous test.** Compare **patch test, scratch test.** See also **conjunctival test, use test.**

**intraductal** /-duk′təl/, within a duct.

**intraductal carcinoma** [L, *intra* + *ductus,* duct], a neoplasm that occurs most often in the breast but can occur elsewhere, as in the salivary glands. The lesion on cross section usually shows well-differentiated tumor cells in calcified and dilated ducts.

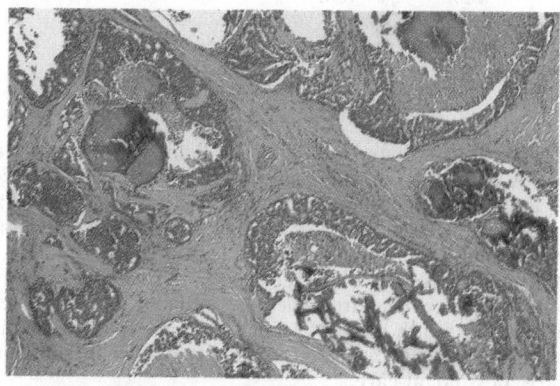

**Intraductal carcinoma of the salivary gland**
*(Fletcher, 2000)*

**intraductal papilloma,** a small benign epithelial tumor in a milk duct of the breast, occasionally marked by bleeding from the nipple. See also **papilloma.**

**intradural lipoma** [L, *intra* + *dura,* hard], a fatty tumor in or beneath the dura mater of the spine or sacrum that tends to infiltrate the dorsal column and roots of spinal nerves, causing pain and dysfunction.

**intraepidermal carcinoma** /in′trə·ep′idur′məl/ [L, *intra* + Gk, *epi,* above, *derma,* skin], a neoplasm of squamous epidermal cells that does not proliferate into the basal area and often occurs in many sites simultaneously. The lesions, which enlarge slowly, are resistant to chemotherapy and to radiation. Also called **precancerous dermatitis.** See also **Bowen's disease.**

**intraepidermal vesicle,** a fluid-filled blisterlike cavity within the epidermis. It is usually less than 1 cm in diameter.

**intraepithelial carcinoma.** See **carcinoma in situ.**

**intrafusal muscle fiber** /-fyo͞o′zəl/, the striated muscle fiber within a muscle spindle.

**intraluminal** /-lo͞o′minəl/, **1.** within the lumen of any tubular structure or organ. **2.** between or among tubes.

**intraluminal coronary artery stent,** a device permanently inserted into a coronary artery to maintain patency of the lumen of the vessel.

**intramammary abscess** /-mam′ərē/, a collection of pus within a mammary gland.

**intramembranous ossification.** See **ossification.**

**intramenstrual pain** /-men′stro͞o·əl/ [L, *intra,* within, *menstrualis,* monthly, *poena,* penalty], pelvic or lower abdominal pain that occurs about midway between menstrual periods and may be associated with ovulation. See also **mittelschmerz.**

**intramural** /-myo͞o′rəl/ [L, *intra,* within, *murus,* wall], pertaining to events or structures within the walls of an organ or body part or cavity.

**intramuscular** /-mus′kyələr/ [L, *intra,* within, *musculus*], pertaining to the interior of muscle tissue.

**intramuscular injection** [L, *intra* + *musculus,* muscle], the introduction of a hypodermic needle into a muscle to administer a medication.

■ METHOD: The equipment is selected, and the medication drawn up into the syringe. The selected site is prepared by cleansing with alcohol. The sites most commonly used are the upper outer quadrant of the gluteal area, the ventrogluteal area, the vastus lateralis of the thigh, or the deltoid muscle. Care must be taken to identify landmarks and select sites to prevent damage to nerves and adjacent structures. The skin is stretched between the thumb and forefinger. The needle is introduced at a 90-degree angle to the muscle with a quick thrust and advanced as necessary—not as far as the hub of the needle, but deep into the muscle. The plunger is withdrawn slightly to be sure that the needle has not been placed in a blood vessel. The solution is injected slowly, the needle is withdrawn, and the injection site is massaged unless contraindicated.

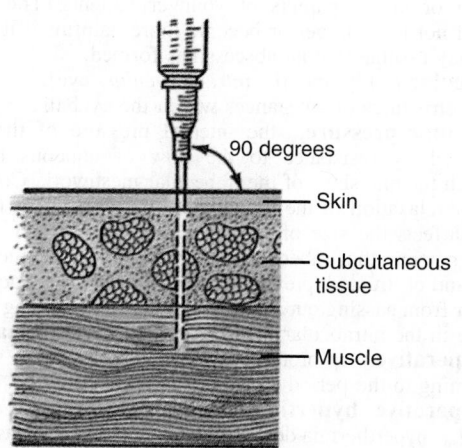

**Intramuscular injection showing angle of needle and placement in the skin**
*(Potter and Perry, 2001)*

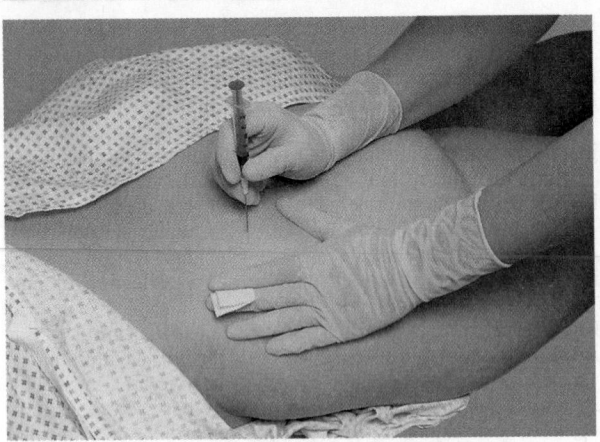

**Hand position for intramuscular injection**
*(Potter and Perry, 1997)*

■ INTERVENTIONS: If the gluteal area is chosen, the patient is asked to lie prone with ankles bent and feet curved in, so that the toes of each foot are directed toward the opposite foot to relax the gluteal muscles, thus making the injection less painful. Injection into deltoid muscles is more painful than in other sites and is avoided if possible. The ventrogluteal area and the vastus lateralis are the preferred injection sites in infants. Care is taken not to hit the femur with the tip of the needle when injecting into the vastus lateralis. Needles and syringes are always disposed of safely in a puncture-resistant container without recapping.

■ OUTCOME CRITERIA: Infection may result from nonaseptic technique; care is taken not to contaminate the needle before injection or to suffer a needlestick. Certain medications can cause tissue necrosis if injected into the subcutaneous tissues. Many medications may be given intravenously or intramuscularly, but the intravenous dose may be much smaller; inadvertent injection into a blood vessel can cause severe systemic reactions or an overdose. Often biologics, such as antigens, serums, or vaccines, may leave a knot in the muscle that is not painful and that subsides slowly over several weeks or months, though it may cause concern in the patient or in the parents of younger patients. The lump should not grow larger or become more painful; if it does, one may assume that an abscess has formed.

**intraocular** /-ok'yələr/ [L, *intra* + *oculus*, eye], pertaining to structures or substances within the eyeball.

**intraocular pressure,** the internal pressure of the eye, regulated by resistance to the flow of aqueous humor through the fine sieve of the trabecular meshwork. Contraction or relaxation of the longitudinal muscles of the ciliary body affects the size of the opening in the meshwork. In older persons the trabecular meshwork may become sclerotic and obstructed, preventing the normal flow of aqueous humor from passing out at the proper rate and causing an increase in the intraocular pressure. See also **glaucoma.**

**intraoperative** /-op'ərətiv'/ [L, *intra* + *operari*, to work], pertaining to the period during a surgical procedure.

**intraoperative hyperthermia** [L, *intra* + *operari*, to work], hyperthermia delivered as a therapeutic measure to internal sites that have been exposed by a surgical procedure. After heating the incision is "closed."

**intraoperative ultrasound,** a diagnostic technique that uses a portable ultrasound device to scan the spinal cord

during spinal surgery. The method enables surgeons to locate and identify tumors of the central nervous system that may not be detected by computed tomography or other techniques. Intraoperative ultrasound can distinguish between syrinxes, or fluid-filled cysts, and neoplastic growths in nervous system tissue.

**intraoral examination.** See **dental examination.**

**intraoral orthodontic appliance** /in'trə·ôr'əl/ [L, *intra* + *oralis*, mouth], a device placed inside the mouth to correct or alleviate malocclusion.

**intraosseous** /in'trə·os'ē·əs/ [L, *intra,* within, *os,* bone], pertaining to the interior of bone.

**intraosseous infusion,** the injection of blood, medications, or fluids into bone marrow rather than into a vein. The technique may be performed in emergency treatment of a child when IV infusion is not feasible.

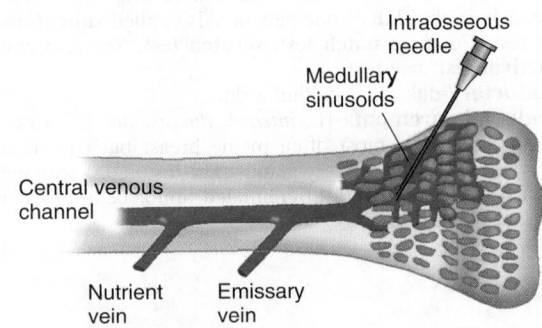

**Intraosseous infusion** *(Sanders et al, 2000)*

**intraparietal sulcus** /-perī'ətəl/ [L, *intra* + *paries,* wall, *sulcus,* groove], an irregular groove on the convex surface of the parietal lobe that marks the division of the inferior and superior parietal lobules of the cerebrum. Also called **interparietal fissure.**

**intrapartal care**[1] /-pär'təl/ [L, *intra* + *partus,* birth], care of a pregnant woman from the onset of labor to the completion of the fourth stage of labor with the expulsion of the placenta. See also **antepartal care, newborn intrapartal care, postpartal care.**

■ METHOD: The signs and symptoms of true labor are observed. Uterine contractions increase in frequency, duration, and strength. Pressure of the presenting part of the fetus causes dilation and effacement of the cervix and contractions of the amniotic sac, producing a bloody discharge called "bloody show." A physical examination of the mother is performed. Urine is measured regularly through labor and may be tested for levels of ketones, protein, and glucose for specific gravity. A microhematocrit is often done. The position, attitude, and presentation of the fetus are ascertained by abdominal palpation. The cervical effacement and dilation and the station of the presenting part of the fetus are determined periodically by vaginal examination, using careful aseptic technique. If the amniotic sac has broken, the color, character, and quantity of the amniotic fluid are noted. The fetal heart rate is counted, and variations are noted in relation to the timing and intensity of contractions. See also **emergency childbirth.**

**intrapartal care**[2], a nursing intervention from the Nursing Interventions Classification (NIC) defined as monitoring and management of stages one and two of the birth process. See also **Nursing Interventions Classification.**

**intrapartal care: high-risk delivery,** a nursing intervention from the Nursing Interventions Classification (NIC) defined as assisting vaginal birth of multiple or malpositioned fetuses. See also **Nursing Interventions Classification.**

**intrapartal period,** the period spanning labor and birth.

**intrapartum** /-pär′təm/, pertaining to the period of labor and birth.

**intrapartum hemorrhage,** copious bleeding, usually caused by abruptio placentae or placenta previa during labor. See also **hemorrhage.**

**intraperiosteal fracture** /in′trəper′ē·os′tē·əl/ [L, *intra* + Gk, *peri*, around, *osteon*, bone], a fracture that does not rupture the periosteum.

**intrapleural space** /-plŏōr′əl/ [L, *intra*, within; Gk, *pleura*, rib; L, *spatium*], within pertaining to the cavity of the pleura.

**intrapsychic conflict** /-sī′kik/ [L, *intra* + Gk, *psyche*, mind], an emotional clash of opposing impulses within oneself, for example, of the id versus the ego or the ego versus the superego. See also **conflict.**

**intrapulmonary** /-pul′məner′ē/ [L, *intra*, within, *pulma*, lung], pertaining to the interior of the lungs.

**intrapulmonary shunt** [L, *intra* + *pulmoneus*, relating to the lung], (in respiratory therapy) a condition in which a region of the lungs is perfused with little or no ventilation. It is indicated by a low ratio of QS/QT, in which QS represents the difference between end capillary oxygen content and mixed venous oxygen content and QT represents cardiac output. The condition may occur in atelectasis, pneumonia, pulmonary edema, and adult respiratory distress syndrome.

**intrarenal hemodynamics** /-rē′nəl/ [L, *intra* + *ren*, kidney], the pattern of blood flow or distribution in the various parts of the kidney. Normally the renal cortex and outer medulla receive the major portion of renal blood flow.

**intraspinal hypodermic** /-spī′nəl/ [L, *intra*, within, *spina*, spine, *hypo*, under, *derma*, skin], pertaining to the injection of a substance into the spinal canal.

**intrathecal** /in′trəthē′kəl/ [L, *intra* + *theca*, sheath], pertaining to a structure, process, or substance within a sheath, such as within the spinal canal.

**intrathecal injection,** the introduction of a hypodermic needle into the subarachnoid space for the purpose of instilling a material for diffusion throughout the spinal fluid.

**intrathoracic goiter** /-thôras′ik/ [L, *intra* + Gk, *thorax*, chest; L, *guttur*, throat], an enlargement of the thyroid gland that protrudes into the thoracic cavity.

**intrauterine** /in′trəyōō′tərin/ [L, *intra*, within, *uterus*, womb], pertaining to the inside of the uterus.

**intrauterine catheter.** See **catheter.**

**intrauterine device (IUD)** [L, *intra* + *uterus*, womb; Fr, *devise*], a contraceptive device. It consists of a bent strip of radiopaque plastic with a fine monofilament tail. The addition of copper wire and/or bands increases the effectiveness. Progesterone-filled IUDs are also available. The mechanism of action is not known. Insertion is performed during or just after menstruation when the cervix is slightly open and menstruation assures that a pregnancy does not exist. The tail string of the IUD is left projecting a few centimeters from the cervix. By feeling the string with her finger at least once each menstrual cycle the wearer can be sure the device is in place. The string also provides a hold for removing the IUD. The rate of failure for the IUD method of contraception is approximately one to five unplanned pregnancies in 100 women using the device for 1 year. IUDs can cause complications; the most serious is pelvic inflamma-

tory disease. When such infections occur in pregnancy, they may be overwhelming and lethal; therefore the IUD is removed if pregnancy is suspected. Some other complications are cervicitis, perforation of the uterus, salpingitis that causes sterility, ectopic pregnancy, abortion, embedding of the device in the wall of the uterus, endometritis, bleeding, pain, cramping, undetected expulsion, and irritation of the penis. Also called **intrauterine contraceptive device (IUCD),** *(informal)* **coil,** *(informal)* **loop.**

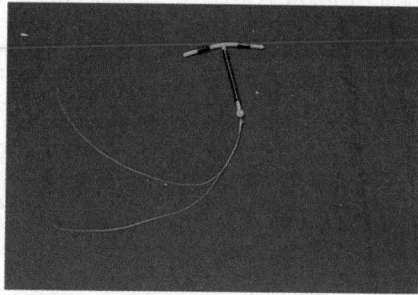

**Intrauterine device** *(Edge and Miller, 1994)*

**intrauterine fracture,** a fracture that occurs during fetal life.

**intrauterine growth curve,** a line on a standardized graph representing the mean weight for gestational age through pregnancy to term. It provides a method for classifying infants according to their state of maturity and fetal development.

**intrauterine growth retardation,** an abnormal process in which the development and maturation of the fetus are impeded or delayed more than two deviations below themean for gestational age, sex, and ethnicity. It may be caused by genetic factors, maternal disease, or fetal malnutrition that results from placental insufficiency. See also **growth retardation, small for gestational age (SGA) infant.**

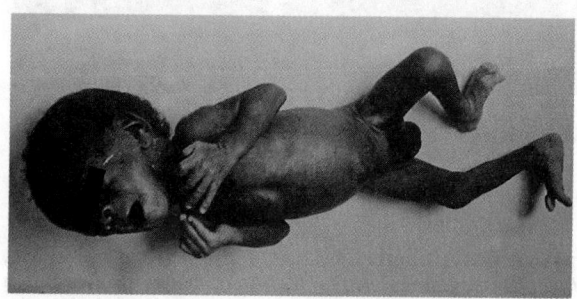

**Intrauterine growth retardation**
*(Zitelli and Davis, 1997/courtesy TALC, Institute of Child Health)*

**intravascular** /-vas′kyələr/ [L, *intra* + *vasculum*, little vessel], pertaining to the inside of a blood vessel.

**intravascular coagulation test,** a test for detecting coagulation of blood within the blood vessels.

**intravenous (IV)** /-vē′nəs/ [L, *intra* + *vena,* vein], pertaining to the inside of a vein, as of a thrombus or an injection, infusion, or catheter.

**intravenous alimentation.** See **total parenteral nutrition.**

**intravenous bolus,** a relatively large dose of medication administered into a vein in a short period, usually within 1 to 30 minutes. The IV bolus is commonly used when rapid administration of a medication is needed, such as in an emergency; when drugs that cannot be diluted, such as many cancer chemotherapeutic drugs, are administered; and when the therapeutic purpose is to achieve a peak drug level in the bloodstream of the patient. The IV bolus is not used when the medication must be diluted in a large-volume parenteral fluid before entering the bloodstream or when the rapid administration of a medication, such as potassium chloride, may be life-threatening. The IV bolus is normally not used for patients who have decreased cardiac output, decreased urinary output, pulmonary congestion, or systemic edema. Such patients have decreased tolerance to medications, which therefore must be diluted more than usual and administered at slower rates. A wristwatch with a second hand is recommended for the timing of all IV bolus injections. The amount of medication to be delivered per minute is determined by dividing the total amount to be injected by the prescribed time for delivery. The IV bolus site is prepared with an appropriate antiseptic, and the site is entered with a venipuncture needle, using sterile technique. A winged-tip needle is used for administering an IV bolus because it is small enough to lessen the risk of collapsing the vein and causing trauma and is more stable than a syringe needle. If a primary IV line is already established, the IV bolus is administered by mixing the prescribed drug with the appropriate amount of diluent and then administering the drug into the primary line, after first determining whether it is compatible with the primary IV solution. Also called **intravenous push.**

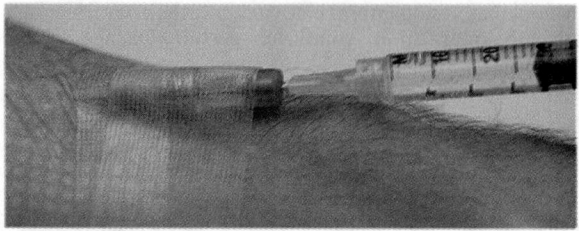

**Administration of medication by intravenous bolus**
*(Potter and Perry, 2001)*

**intravenous catheter** [L, *intra,* within, *vena,* vein; Gk, *katheter,* a thing inserted], a catheter that is inserted into a vein for supplying medications or nutrients directly into the bloodstream, or for diagnostic purposes such as studying blood pressure.

**intravenous cholangiography (IVC),** (in diagnostic radiology) a procedure for outlining the major bile ducts. A radiopaque contrast material is injected intravenously, and serial radiographic films are taken. See also **cholangiography.**

**intravenous controller,** any of several devices that automatically deliver IV fluid at selectable flow rates. The controller is commonly equipped with a rate selector, drop sensor, and alarm. When the infusion does not flow at the prescribed rate, the drop alarm emits a visual and an audible signal. The IV controller works by gravity so that the IV container must be placed at least 30 inches (76.20 centimeters) above the venipuncture site. The controller cannot exert the positive pressure of a true pump and is not recommended for the delivery of highly viscous fluid or for maintenance of an open arterial line. Compare **intravenous peristaltic pump, intravenous piston pump, intravenous syringe pump.**

**intravenous digital subtraction angiography (IV-DSA),** a procedure for the radiographic visualization of arteries following injection of a radiopaque contrast medium is injected into a vein.

**intravenous fat emulsion,** a preparation of 10% fat administered into a vein to help maintain the weight of an adult patient or the weight and growth of a younger patient. Such fat emulsions are prepared from refined soybean oil and egg-yolk phospholipids and may contain such major fatty acids as linoleic, oleic, palmitic, and linolenic acids. The IV fat emulsion is isotonic and may be administered into a peripheral vein, but it is not mixed with other solutions used in parenteral alimentation. IV fat emulsions are often administered when hyperalimentation is not sufficient to maintain adequate treatment of a patient or when the patient needs calories but cannot tolerate the high percentage of dextrose contained in hyperalimentation solutions. Such emulsions may also be administered to patients who need more essential fatty acids than are contained in hyperalimentation solutions or to patients who need general nutritional improvement, especially postoperative patients. IV emulsions are not administered to patients suffering from disturbances of normal fat metabolism (such as hyperlipemia), severe hepatic diseases, blood coagulation defects caused by decreased blood-platelet counts, pulmonary diseases, lipoid nephrosis, hepatocellular damage, or bone marrow dyscrasia, or to those being treated with anabolic inhibitory drugs. If possible, the IV fat emulsion is usually administered during the day so that the patient may follow a normal eating pattern with rest during the night and lower nocturnal urinary flow. Once the primary IV line has been established, IV fat emulsions are usually administered with the aid of an electronic control device to maintain an even flow rate and prevent fatty-acid overload. The patient's fluid intake and output are regularly measured during the delivery of such an emulsion, and daily blood studies are conducted to determine the level of free-floating triglycerides. Hepatic function tests are performed if the patient receives consecutive IV fat emulsion infusions over a long period. Immediate adverse reactions or those that may occur up to 2½ hours after the onset of the infusion may include temperature rise, flushing, sweating, pressure sensations over the eyes, nausea, vomiting, headache, chest and back pain, dyspnea, and cyanosis. Delayed adverse reactions or those that may occur within 10 days of the onset of such infusions may include hepatomegaly, splenomegaly, thrombocytopenia, focal seizures, hyperlipemia, hepatic damage, jaundice, hemorrhagic diathesis, and gastroduodenal ulcer.

**intravenous feeding,** the administration of nutrients through a vein or veins.

**intravenous infusion,** 1. a solution administered into a vein through an infusion set that includes a plastic or glass vacuum bottle or bag containing the solution and tubing connecting the bottle to a catheter or a needle in the patient's vein. 2. the process of administering a solution intravenously. Swelling of the limb around and distal to the site of injection may indicate that the tip of the catheter or needle is

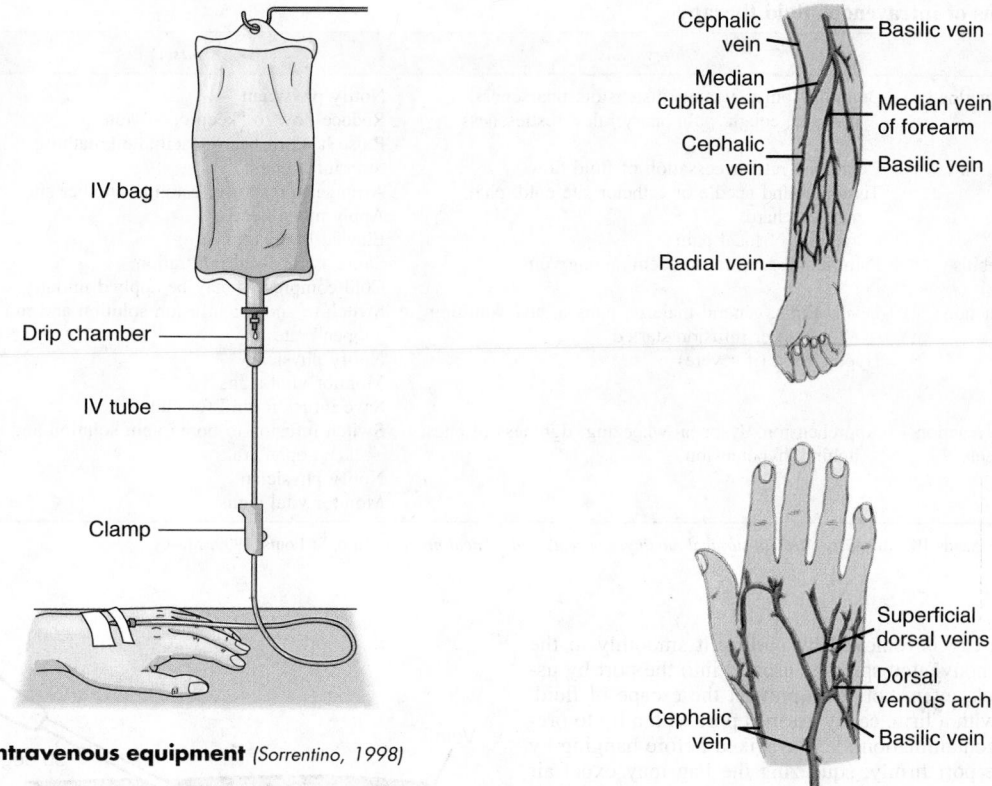

**Intravenous equipment** *(Sorrentino, 1998)*

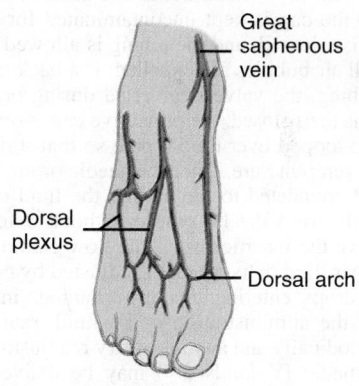

**Common intravenous infusion sites**
*(Potter and Perry, 2001)*

in the subcutaneous tissue and not in the vein. The fluid may be infiltrating the tissue spaces. It should be withdrawn and the limb elevated. Redness, swelling, heat, and pain around the vein at the site of injection or proximal to it may indicate thrombophlebitis. The infusion should be discontinued and the inflammatory condition treated. The infusion is usually begun again at another site. See also **venipuncture.**

**intravenous infusion filter,** any of the numerous devices used in helping to ensure the purity of an IV solution. IV filters strain the solution to remove such contaminants as dissolved impurities (detergents, proteins, and polysaccharides), extraneous salts, microorganisms, particles, precipitates, and undissolved drug powders. Any such contaminants may complicate the IV therapy and patient recovery. Some filters are built into the primary IV tubing; others must be attached. One of the main criteria for selecting a filter is the assurance that the filter is not too fine for the IV solution to be strained; filters that are too fine clog. The size of filter membranes varies from 5 μm to 0.22 μm. Filters of 1 to 5 μm will remove most particulate debris but not most fungi or bacteria. Filters that are 0.45 μm or less remove fungi and most bacteria; filters that are 0.22 μm remove all fungi and bacteria but also reduce the flow rate of the IV solution, which is crucial when rapid delivery is required. See also **needle filter.**

**intravenous infusion technique,** the calculations for determining the delivery rate of IV fluid for the individual patient and the necessary spiking of the container and priming of the tubing before venipuncture and fluid administration.

■ METHOD: The rate at which solution is to be administered by IV infusion can be determined from the procedure formula. The hands are washed thoroughly before assembling the container of IV solution, the IV pole, and the proper tub-

ing with the flow clamp placed in a position directly beneath the drip chamber and clamped. If a bottle with a rubber stopper is used, the protective metal cap is removed, and, with the bottle held securely on a stable surface, the spike of the tubing is pushed firmly into the stopper. To spike an IV bottle with an indwelling vent and latex diaphragm, the metal cap and diaphragm are removed and the spike is inserted into the nonvented hole; if a hiss, indicating a vacuum, does not follow, the bottle is contaminated and should be discarded. Nonvented tubing is used with this kind of bottle. A plastic bag of IV fluid is hung on a hook for

## Complications of intravenous fluid therapy

| Complication | Observations | Nursing actions |
|---|---|---|
| Circulatory overload | Bounding pulse, venous distension, hoarseness, dyspnea, cough, pulmonary rales, restlessness | Notify physician<br>Reduce flow to "keep open" rate<br>Raise head of bed to facilitate breathing |
| Local infiltration | Decreased rate or cessation of fluid flow<br>Tissue around needle or catheter site cold, pale, swollen, hard<br>Complaint of local pain | Stop infusion<br>Arrange to restart infusion at another site<br>Apply moist heat<br>Elevate lower arm |
| Thrombophlebitis | Pain, redness, warmth, edema along vein | Same as for local infiltration<br>Cold compresses may be applied initially |
| Pyrogenic reaction | Fever, chills, general malaise, nausea, and vomiting 30 min after infusion started<br>Hypotension (if severe) | Switch to another infusion solution and run at "keep open" rate<br>Notify physician<br>Monitor vital signs<br>Save infusion fluid for culture |
| Anaphylactic reaction (with proteins) | Apprehension, dyspnea, wheezing, tightness of chest, itching, hypotension | Switch infusion to nonprotein solution and run at "keep open" rate<br>Notify physician<br>Monitor vital signs |

From Phipps WJ, Sands JK, Marek JE: *Medical-surgical nursing: concepts and clinical practice,* ed 6, St Louis, 1999, Mosby.

spiking; the cap is removed by pulling it smoothly to the right, and a nonvented spike is inserted into the port by using one quick, even motion to prevent the escape of fluid. An IV bag with a firm, easily grasped port with a lip to prevent touch contamination may be spiked before hanging by grasping the port firmly; squeezing the bag may expel air and is carefully prevented. After the hanging bag or bottle is spiked, the drip chamber is gently squeezed until it is half full before the tubing is primed. The end of the tubing is held over a sink or wastebasket as the protective cap is removed, and the cap is kept uncontaminated for reuse. The flow clamp is released, and the tubing is allowed to fill with fluid until all air bubbles are expelled; if a back check valve is on the tubing, the valve is inverted during priming. The flow clamp is then closed, the protective cap is replaced, and the tubing is looped over the IV pole so that it does not interfere with venipuncture. Once the needle or intracatheter is inserted and connected to the tubing, the fluid container is hung securely from the IV pole or a hook 3 feet (0.0762 meters) above the insertion site. The flow clamp is opened, and the proper fluid delivery rate is adjusted by counting the number of drops entering the drip chamber in a minute. Throughout the administration of IV fluid, rate of flow is checked periodically and any necessary readjustments of the clamp are made. IV fluids also may be delivered via IV pump. IV pump tubing is then used, and the flow rate is calculated in mL/hr.

■ INTERVENTIONS: The nurse assembles the apparatus for the IV infusion, spikes the fluid container, primes the tubing, calculates the proper rate for the patient, and ensures that the rate of delivery and asepsis are maintained. The nurse carefully observes the patient for signs of circulatory overload, such as a bounding pulse, engorged peripheral veins, dyspnea, cough, and pulmonary edema, indicating that the infusion rate is too rapid and requires adjustment.

■ OUTCOME CRITERIA: IV solutions administered to maintain normal body fluid levels and electrolyte balance do not overload the circulation when delivered at the flow rate required by the individual patient.

**intravenous injection,** a hypodermic injection into a vein for the purpose of instilling a single dose of medication, injecting a contrast medium, or beginning an IV infusion of

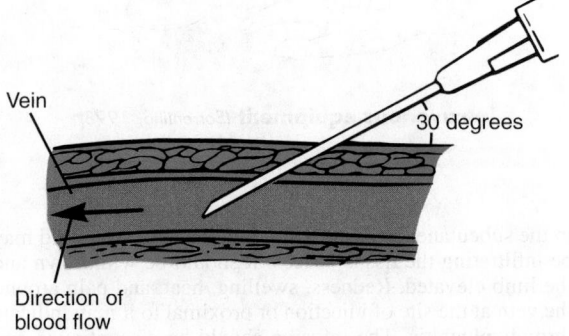

**Intravenous injection showing angle of needle and bevel direction**

blood, medication, or a fluid solution, such as saline or dextrose in water. See also **venipuncture.**

**intravenous (IV) insertion,** a nursing intervention from the Nursing Interventions Classification (NIC) defined as insertion of a needle into a peripheral vein for the purpose of administering fluids, blood, or medications. See also **Nursing Interventions Classification.**

**intravenously (IV),** through a vein.

**intravenous medication** [L, *intra,* within, *vena,* vein, *medicare,* medicine], pharmaceutical delivered directly into the bloodstream via a vein.

**intravenous peristaltic pump,** any one of several devices for administering IV fluids by exerting pressure on the IV tubing rather than on the fluid itself. Most peristaltic pumps operate with normal IV tubing and deliver fluid at a selectable cubic centimeter per hour rate. This device is equipped with a drop sensor, rate selector, power switch indicator lamp, and drop indicator and alarm. The alarm sounds when the infusion does not flow at the prescribed rate. Compare **intravenous controller, intravenous piston pump, intravenous syringe pump.**

**intravenous piston pump,** any of several devices that accurately control the infusion of IV fluids by piston action. Most IV piston pumps can be operated by battery, as well as by electric current, and require special tubing. Some models are portable. IV piston pumps are commonly equipped with controls that allow selectable flow rates and indicators that display flow rates, dose limits, and cumulative fluid volumes. Such pumps commonly monitor the patient's skin for infiltration by IV fluid and are equipped with infiltration and flow alarms. The IV piston pump monitors the actual volume of IV fluid administered instead of counting drops of fluid. Hence its accuracy is not affected by drop size, temperature, or fluid viscosity. The pump is designed to reduce the delivery rate to a keep-vein-open rate if the proper flow rate or the dose limit is exceeded. The pump also stops delivery of the IV fluid if the line is clogged or if infiltration is detected. Compare **intravenous controller, intravenous peristaltic pump, intravenous syringe pump.**

**intravenous pump,** a pump designed to regulate the rate of flow of a fluid administered through an IV catheter. See also **Abbott pump, Harvard pump.**

**intravenous push.** See **intravenous bolus.**

**intravenous pyelography (IVP),** a radiographic technique for examining the structure function of the urinary system. A contrast medium is injected intravenously, and serial x-ray films are taken as the medium is cleared from the blood by the kidneys. The renal calyces, renal pelvis, ureters, and urinary bladder are all visible on the radiographs. Tumors, cysts, stones, and many structural and functional abnormalities may be diagnosed with this technique. Fasting and bowel cleansing with a cathartic or an enema before the procedure improve visualization of the urinary tract. The patient may also be asked to void immediately before injection of the contrast medium to prevent dilution of the medium in the bladder and immediately afterward to check residual urine in the bladder. Also called **descending urography, excretory urography, intravenous urography.**

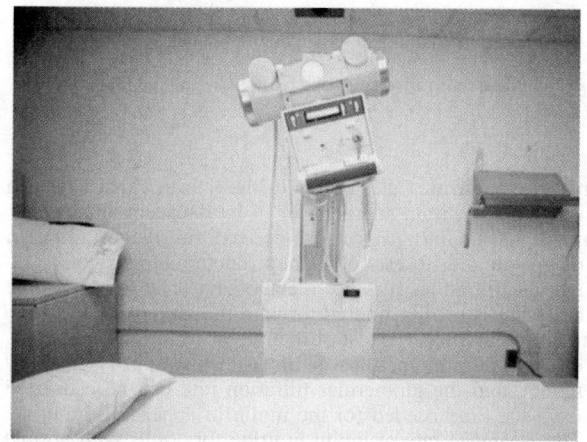

**Equipment for intravenous pyelography** (Gray, 1992)

**intravenous syringe pump,** any one of several devices that automatically compress a syringe plunger at a controlled rate. Such devices are used with disposable syringes that can deliver blood, medications, or nutrients by IV, arte-

rial, or subcutaneous routes. IV syringe pumps can deliver small volumes of fluid at rates as low as 0.01 mL/hour and are often used in the treatment of infants and are especially useful in the care of ambulatory patients. They are ideal for keeping arterial lines open and are usually battery-operated and portable. Compare **intravenous controller, intravenous peristaltic pump, intravenous piston pump.**

**intravenous team,** a group of registered nurses and licensed practical nurses with special training who administer IV therapy under the direction of a physician. State laws may restrict practice of IV therapy to specific categories of health professionals.

**intravenous (IV) therapy[1],** the administration of fluids or drugs, or both, into the general circulation through a venipuncture.

**intravenous (IV) therapy[2],** a nursing intervention from the Nursing Interventions Classification (NIC) defined as administration and monitoring of intravenous fluids and medications. See also **Nursing Interventions Classification.**

**intravenous urography.** See **intravenous pyelography.**

**intraventricular** /-ventrik′yələr/ [L, *intra* + *ventriculus,* little belly], pertaining to the space within a ventricle or to the conduction system within the walls of a ventricle.

**intraventricular block,** altered conduction of the cardiac impulse within the ventricles. The block can occur as a right bundle branch block, left bundle branch block, hemiblock, left anterior or posterior fascicular block, or bifascicular block. Intraventricular blocks are identified on an electrocardiogram when the QRS duration is greater than normal. They can be caused by coronary artery disease, valvular heart disease, ventricular hypertrophy and fibrosis, cardiomyopathy, or degeneration of the conduction system. Prognosis is based on the underlying cardiac condition. See also **bundle branch block, heart block, hemiblock, intraatrial block, sinoatrial block.**

**intraventricular conduction defect,** a delay in conduction of a ventricular impulse within the ventricles.

**intraventricular hydrocephalus.** See **hydrocephalus.**

**intraventricular pressure** [L, *intra,* within, *ventriculus,* little belly], the pressure of the blood within the heart's ventricles. It varies with the phase of the cardiac cycle.

**intrinsic** /intrin′sik/ [L, *intrinsecus,* inside], **1.** denoting a natural or inherent part or quality. **2.** originating from or situated within an organ or tissue.

**intrinsic asthma,** a nonseasonal, nonallergic form of asthma, which usually first occurs later in life than allergic asthma and tends to be chronic and persistent rather than episodic. Precipitating factors include inhalation of irritating pollutants, such as dust particles, smoke, aerosols, strong cooking odors, paint fumes, and other volatile substances. Intrinsic asthma may also be triggered by exposure to cold, damp weather; sudden inhalation of cold, dry air; physical exercise; violent coughing or laughing; respiratory infections, such as the common cold; or psychologic factors, such as anxiety. Compare **allergic asthma.** See also **asthma.**

**intrinsic factor,** a substance secreted by the gastric mucosa that is essential for the intestinal absorption of cyanocobalamin. Intrinsic factor forms a bond with molecules of cyanocobalamin and transports them across the membranes of the ileum. A deficiency of intrinsic factor, caused by gastrectomy, myxedema, or atrophy of the gastric mucosa, causes pernicious anemia. See also **pernicious anemia.**

**intrinsic minus hand deformity,** an abnormality that results from interruption of the ulnar and median nerves at the wrist. It causes metacarpophalangeal joint hyperextension and interphalangeal joint flexion.

**intrinsic muscles,** muscles that are entirely within the body part or segment moved by them, as the tongue muscles.

**intrinsic pathway of coagulation,** a sequence of reactions leading to fibrin formation, beginning with the contact activation of factor XII, followed by the sequential activation of factors XI and IX and resulting in the activation of factor X, which in activated form initiates the common pathway of coagulation. Compare **extrinsic pathway of coagulation.** See also **coagulation cascade, common pathway of coagulation.**

**intro-,** prefix meaning 'into or within': *introgastric, introjection, introspection.*

**introitus** /intrō′itəs/ [L, *intro,* inside, *ire,* to go], an entrance or orifice in a cavity or a hollow tubular structure of the body, such as the vaginal introitus.

**introjection** /-jek′shən/ [L, *intro + jacere,* to throw], an ego defense mechanism whereby an individual unconsciously incorporates into his own ego structure the qualities of another person, usually a significant other. It happens early in life and continues less intensely throughout.

**intromission** /-mish′ən/, the insertion of one object into another, such as the introduction of the penis into the vagina.

**intron** /in′tron/ [L, *intra,* within, *regin,* region], a sequence of nucleotides in eukaryotic DNA that does not code for amino acids and interrupts the coding sequence of a gene. Some genes contain a number of long introns.

**Intron A,** trademark for a parenteral antineoplastic (interferon alpha-2b, recombinant).

**Intropin,** trademark for an adrenergic (dopamine hydrochloride).

**introspection** /-spek′shən/ [L, *introspicere,* to look into], **1.** the act of examining one's own thoughts and emotions by concentrating on the inner self. **2.** a tendency to look inward and view the inner self. —**introspective,** *adj.*

**introsusception** /-susep′shən/ [L, *intro,* inside, *suscipere,* to receive], the telescoping or invagination of one segment of the digestive tract into another segment, usually a lower segment. The process can cause obstruction and strangulation of the bowel.

**introversion** /-vur′zhən/ [L, *intro + vertere,* to turn], **1.** the tendency to direct one's interests, thoughts, and energies inward or toward things concerned with the self. **2.** the state of being totally or primarily concerned with one's own intrapsychic experience. Also spelled **intraversion.** Compare **extroversion.**

**introvert** /in′trəvurt/ [L, *intro + vertere,* to turn], **1.** a person whose interests are directed inward and who is shy, withdrawn, emotionally reserved, and self-absorbed. **2.** to turn inward or to direct one's interests and thoughts toward oneself. Compare **ambivert, extrovert.** See also **egocentric.**

**introverted personality** /-vur′tid/ [L, *intro,* inside, *vertere,* to turn, *personalis*], a personality that is preoccupied with inner thoughts and fantasies rather than with the outer world of people and things.

**intrusion** /in·trōō′zhən/ [L, *intrudere,* to push or force in], an orthodontic technique of depressing a tooth back into the occlusal plane or attempting to prevent its eruption or elongation during correction of an excessive overbite. Compare **extrusion** (def. 3).

**intubate** /in′tyōōbāt/ [L, *in,* within, *tubus,* tube], to catheterize or insert a tube into an organ or body part.

**intubation** [L, *in,* within, *tubus,* tube, *atio,* process], passage of a tube into a body aperture, specifically the insertion of a breathing tube through the mouth or nose into the trachea to ensure a patent airway for the delivery of anesthetic gases and oxygen or both. **Blind intubation** is the insertion of a breathing tube without the use of a laryngoscope. Kinds of intubation include **endotracheal intubation** and **nasotracheal intubation.**

**intussusception** /in′təsəsep′shən/ [L, *intus,* within, *suscipere,* to receive], prolapse of one segment of bowel into the lumen of another segment. This kind of intestinal obstruction may involve segments of the small intestine, the colon, or the terminal ileum and cecum. Intussusception occurs most often in infants and small children and is characterized by abdominal pain, vomiting, and presence of bloody mucus in the stool (currant jelly stool). Barium enema is used to confirm the diagnosis, and surgery is usually necessary to correct the obstruction. See also **intestinal obstruction.**

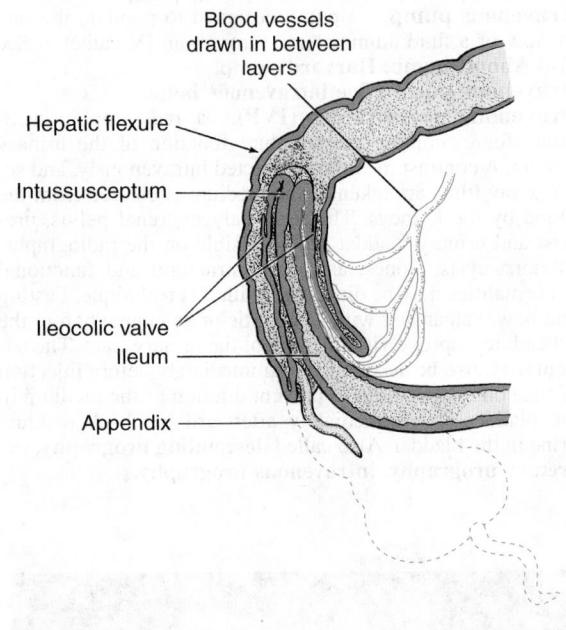

**Ileocolic intussusception** *(Wong et al, 1999)*

**intussusceptum,** the portion of the intestine that has been invaginated within another part in intussusception.

**inulin** /in′yōōlin/, a fructose-derived substance used as a diagnostic aid in tests of kidney function, specifically glomerular filtration. It is not metabolized or absorbed by the body but is readily filtered through the kidney.

**inulin clearance,** a test of the rate of filtration of a starch, inulin, in the glomerulus of the kidney. Inulin is given by mouth, and the glomerular filtration rate can be estimated from the time needed for the inulin to appear in the urine. The clearance rate of inulin in urine for adults with normal renal function is 100 to 150 mL/minute.

**inunction** /inungk′shən/ [L, *in,* within, *ungere,* to smear], **1.** the rubbing of a drug mixed with an oil or fatty substance into the skin, with absorption of the active ingredient. **2.** any compound so applied.

**inundation fever.** See **scrub typhus.**

**in utero** /inyōō′tərō/, inside the uterus.

**invagination** /invaj′ənā′shən/ [L, *in,* within, *vagina,* sheath], **1.** a condition in which one part of a structure telescopes into another, as the intestine during peristalsis. If the invagination is extensive or involves a tumor or polyp, it may cause an intestinal obstruction, necessitating surgery. **2.** surgery for repair of a hernia by replacement of the contents of the hernial sac in the abdominal cavity. General or spinal anesthesia may be used. See also **hernia, intestinal obstruction, peristalsis. —invaginate,** *v.*

**invariable behavior** /inver′ē·əbəl/ [L, *in,* not, *variare,* to vary], behavior that results from physiologic response to a stimulus and is not modified by individual experience, such as a reflex. Compare **variable behavior.**

**invasion** /invā′zhən/ [L, *in,* within, *vadere,* to go], the process by which malignant cells move through the basement membrane and gain access to blood vessels and lymphatic channels.

**invasion of privacy,** (in law) the violation of another person's right to be left alone and free of unwarranted publicity and intrusion.

**invasive** /invā′siv/ [L, *in,* within, *vadere,* to go], characterized by a tendency to spread, infiltrate, and intrude.

**invasive carcinoma,** a malignant neoplasm composed of epithelial cells that infiltrate and destroy surrounding tissues and may metastasize.

**invasive hemodynamic monitoring,** a nursing intervention from the Nursing Interventions Classification (NIC) defined as measurement and interpretation of invasive hemodynamic parameters to determine cardiovascular function and regulate therapy as appropriate. See also **Nursing Interventions Classification.**

**invasive mole.** See **chorioadenoma destruens.**

**invasive procedure** [L, *in + vadere,* to go, *procedere,* to proceed], a diagnostic or therapeutic technique that requires entry of a body cavity or interruption of normal body functions. Examples include the Pap test and colonoscopy.

**invasive thermometry,** measurement of tissue temperature using probes placed directly into the tissue.

**inverse anaphylaxis** /invurs′, in′vurs/, an exaggerated reaction of hypersensitivity induced by an antibody rather than by an antigen. Also called **reverse anaphylaxis.**

**inverse I:E ratio,** an inspiratory/expiratory ratio in mechanical ventilation in which the duration of inspiration is prolonged relative to that of expiration. This condition is sometimes instituted to improve oxygenation, as in the care of infants with idiopathic respiratory distress syndrome and of adults in whom conventional ventilator techniques fail. I:E ratios in such cases may be approximately 2:1 or 3:1. Also called **reversed I:E ratio.** See also **I:E ratio.**

**inverse Marcus Gunn syndrome.** See **Marin Amat's syndrome.**

**inverse relationship.** See **negative relationship.**

**inverse square law,** a law stating that the amount of radiation reaching a surface is inversely proportional to the square of the distance between the source and the surface. For example, a person standing 1 m from a patient being treated with radium is exposed to four times more radiation than a person standing 2 m from the patient.

**Inversine,** trademark for a ganglionic blocking agent (mecamylamine hydrochloride).

**inversion** /invur′zhən/ [L, *invertere,* to turn over], **1.** an abnormal condition in which an organ is turned inside out, such as a uterine inversion. **2.** a chromosomal defect in which a segment of a chromosome breaks off and then reattaches to the chromosome in the reverse orientation, causing the genes carried on that part of the chromosome to be in an abnormal position and sequence.

**inversion traction,** a positional form of traction for the prevention and treatment of back disorders. Special equip-

ment is used to lengthen the spinal column while the patient is in an inverted position. A similar effect is achieved by hanging upside down from a chinning bar.

**invert** /in′vurt/ [L, *invertere,* to turn over], to turn something upside down or inside out.

**invertebrate** /invur′təbrit/, an animal that lacks a vertebral column. Invertebrates comprise more than 95% of all species of animals.

**invert sugar** [L, *invertere,* to turn over; Gk, *sakcharon*], a mixture of glucose and fructose produced by the hydrolysis of sucrose. The process results in an inversion of optical rotation from dextrorotation of sucrose to levorotation of the mixture.

**investigational device exemption (IDE)** /inves′tigā′shən əl/ [L, *investigare,* to search for], an agreement through which the federal government permits the testing of new medical devices.

**investigational new drug (IND),** a drug not yet approved for marketing by the Food and Drug Administration and available only for use in experiments to determine its safety and effectiveness. The use of an investigational new drug in human subjects requires approval by the Food and Drug Administration of an application that includes reports of animal toxicity tests, descriptions of proposed clinical trials, and a list of the investigators and their qualifications.

**Invirase,** trademark for an antiretroviral protease inhibitor (saquinavir).

**invisible differentiation** /inviz′ibəl/ [L, *in,* not, *visibilis,* visible, *differentia,* difference], (in embryology) a fixed determination for specialization and diversification that exists in embryonic cells but is not yet visibly apparent. See also **chemodifferentiation.**

**in vitro** /invē′trō/ [L, *in,* within, *vitreus,* glassware], occurring in a laboratory apparatus. Compare **in vivo.**

**in vitro fertilization (IVF),** a method of fertilizing human ova outside the body by collecting the mature ova and placing them in a dish with a sample of spermatozoa. After an incubation period of 48 to 72 hours, the fertilized ova are injected into the uterus through the cervix. The procedure takes from 2 to 3 days. See also **gamete intrafallopian transfer.**

**in vitro susceptibility testing,** a laboratory trial of the sensitivity of microorganisms, particularly fungi, to potential therapeutic chemicals.

**in vivo** /invē′vō/ [L, *in,* within, *vivo,* alive], occurring in an organism. Compare **in vitro.**

**in vivo fertilization,** a method of fertilization of an ovum within a fallopian tube of a fertile female donor for transplantation into an infertile recipient.

**in vivo tracer study,** a diagnostic procedure in which a series of images of an administered radioactive tracer demonstrates normal or abnormal structures or processes as the tracer passes through a patient's body. A strip-chart recording of the procedure, such as a radionuclide angiocardiogram, shows the passage of the tracer through body.

**involucrum** /in′vəl̅o̅o̅′krəm/, *pl.* **involucra** [L, *involvere,* to wrap up], a sheath or coating, such as that encasing a sequestrum of necrotic bone.

**involuntary** /invol′ənter′ē/ [L, *in,* not, *voluntas,* will], occurring without conscious control or direction. See also **autonomy.**

**involuntary muscle.** See **smooth muscle.**

**involuntary nervous system.** See **visceral nervous system.**

**involuntary patient,** a person admitted to a psychiatric facility against his or her will. See also **informal admission.**

**involution** /in′vəloo′shən/ [L, *involvere,* to wrap up], **1.** a normal process of turning or rolling inward characterized by a decrease in the size of an organ caused by a decrease in the size of its cells, such as postpartum involution of the uterus. **2.** (in embryology) a developmental process in which a group of cells grows over the rim at the border of the organ or part and, rolling inward, rejoins the organ or part to form a tube, such as in the heart or bladder.

**involutional melancholia,** a former term for a state of depression that occurs during the climacteric (menopause of women). It is now treated as a form of a major depressive episode. See also **depression.**

**inward aggression** /in′wərd/ [AS, *inweard*], destructive behavior that is directed against oneself. See also **aggression, masochism.**

**-io,** **1.** noun-forming combining form: *abrasio, evulsio, injectio.* **2.** combining form for iodine-containing contrast medium.

**iodide** /ī′ədīd/ [Gk, *ioeides,* violet], an anion of iodine. Sodium and potassium iodide are the salts most commonly used in medicine.

**iodinated serum albumin** /ī′ədinā′tid/, a sterile, buffered, isotonic solution containing radioiodinated normal human serum used in diagnostic tests of blood volume and cardiac output. It is adjusted to provide not more than 1 mCi of radioactivity per milliliter.

**iodine (I)** /ī′ədīn/ [Gk, *ioeides,* violet], a nonmetallic element of the halogen group. Its atomic number is 53; its atomic mass is 126.90. Iodine is a bluish black solid that becomes a violet vapor on heating without going through a liquid phase. Iodine is an essential micronutrient or trace element; almost 80% of the iodine present in the body is in the thyroid gland, mostly in the form of thyroglobulin. Iodine deficiency can result in goiter or cretinism. Iodine is found in seafood, iodized salt, and some dairy products. It is used as a contrast agent for blood vessels in computed tomography scans. Radioisotopes of iodine are used in radioisotope scanning procedures and in palliative treatment of cancer of the thyroid.

**iodine poisoning** [Gk, *ioeides,* violet; L, *potio,* drink], toxic effects of ingesting iodine, a potent antiseptic with low tissue toxicity. Symptoms include burning pain in the mouth and esophagus, abdominal pain, vomiting, diarrhea, shock, nephritis, laryngeal edema, and circulatory collapse. The mucous membranes are stained brown by the iodine.

**iodism** /ī′ədiz′əm/ [Gk, *ioeides* + *ismos,* process], a condition produced by excessive amounts of iodine in the body. It is characterized by increased lacrimation and salivation, rhinitis, weakness, and a characteristic skin eruption.

**iodize** /ī′ədīz/ [Gk, *ioeides* + *izein,* to cause], to treat or impregnate with iodine or an iodide. Table salt is iodized to prevent the occurrence of goiter in areas with insufficient iodine in the drinking water or food. Iodized oil, a viscous liquid with the odor of garlic, has been used as a contrast medium in radiology.

**iodized salt** [Gk, *ioeides,* violet; AS, *sealt*], table salt to which potassium or sodium iodide has been added to protect against goiter, particularly in regions where soil and drinking water have low iodine content. The iodides are added to achieve approximately 100 ppm.

**iodo-,** combining form meaning 'iodine': *iododerma, iodogenic, iodolography.*

**iodochlorhydroxyquin** /ī·ō′dōklôr′hīdrok′səkwin/, an antibacterial and antifungal.

■ INDICATIONS: It is prescribed in the treatment of eczema, athlete's foot, and other fungal infections.

■ CONTRAINDICATIONS: The presence of tuberculosis or viral skin conditions or known hypersensitivity to this drug or to iodine prohibits its use.

■ ADVERSE EFFECTS: The most serious adverse reaction is irritation to sensitive skin.

**iododerma** /ī·ō′dōdur′mə/ [Gk, *ioeides* + *derma,* skin], a skin rash caused by a hypersensitivity to ingested iodides. The lesions may be acneiform, bullous, or fungating. Treatment requires removal of iodides.

**iodoform** /ī·ō′dəfôrm/ [Gk, *ioeides* + formyl], a topical antiinfective used as an antiseptic.

**iodophor** /ī·ōdəfôr/ [Gk, *ioeides* + *phoros,* bearer], an antiseptic or disinfectant that combines iodine with another agent, such as a detergent.

**iodopsin** /ī′ōdop′sin/ [Gk, *ioeides* + *optikos,* vision], a photosensitive chemical in the cones of the retina that reacts in association with other chemicals and plays a part in color vision. Iodopsin is more stable when exposed to bright light than rhodopsin, which is found in the rods of the retina. Color vision, a synthesis of red, green, and blue light, is induced by changes within the pigments of different types of cones during a photochemical process in which coded nerve impulses are sent to the brain. Research on the exact role of iodopsin in color vision, which is still unknown, is ongoing.

**iodoquinol** /ī′ōdō′kwinol/, an amebicide.

■ INDICATION: It is prescribed in the treatment of intestinal amebiasis. It is also used as a preventive in high-risk people.

■ CONTRAINDICATIONS: Hepatic disease and known hypersensitivity to iodine or 8-hydroxyquinoline prohibit its use.

■ ADVERSE EFFECTS: Among the most serious adverse reactions are dizziness, thyroid enlargement, optic neuropathy, optic atrophy, and peripheral neuropathy.

**iodotherapy** /ī·ō′dōther′əpē/, a treatment that uses iodine or an iodide.

**ion** /ī′ən, ī′on/ [Gk, *ienai,* to go], an atom or group of atoms that has acquired an electrical charge through the gain or loss of an electron or electrons.

**-ion,** **1.** suffix meaning an 'electrically charged particle': *anion, cation, ion.* **2.** noun-forming combining form: *endognathion, osteopedion, parhelion.*

**ion exchange chromatography,** the process of separating and analyzing different substances according to their affinities for chemically stable but very reactive synthetic exchangers, which are composed largely of polystyrene and cellulose. The process uses an absorbent containing ionizing groups and accommodates the exchange of ions between a solution of substances to be analyzed and the absorbent. Ion exchange chromatography is often used to separate components of nucleic acids and proteins elaborated by various structures throughout the body. Different ions deposited in the absorbent during the exchange produce bands of different colors, which constitute a chromatograph. Compare **column chromatography, gas chromatography.**

**ionic bonding** /ī·on′ik/ [Gk, *ienai* + ME, *band,* to bind], an electrostatic force between ions. Ionic compounds do not form true molecules; in aqueous solution they separate into their hydrated constituent ions.

**ionic dissociation,** a phenomenon whereby ions in ionic compounds in an aqueous solution are freed from their mutual attractions and distribute themselves uniformly throughout the solvent.

**ionic strength,** the sum of the concentrations of all ions in a solution, multiplied by the square of their charge.

**ionization** /ī′ənīzā′shən/ [Gk, *ienai* + *izein,* to cause], the process in which a neutral atom or molecule gains or loses electrons and thus acquires a negative or positive electrical charge. Ionizing radiation produces ionization in its passage

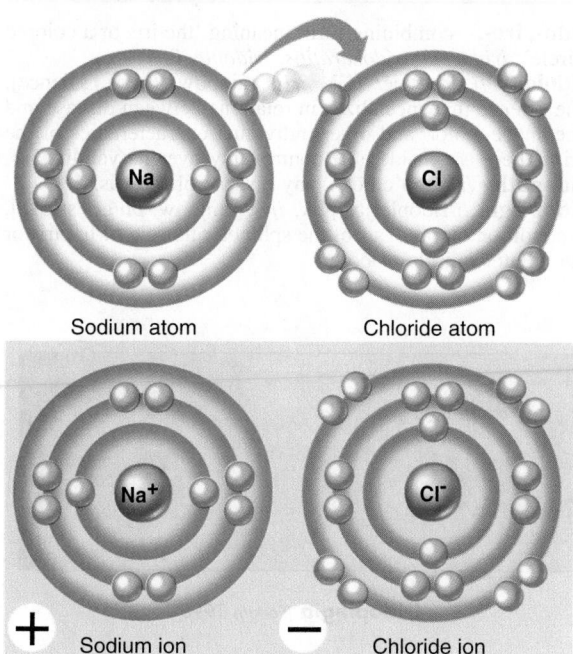

Sodium atom      Chloride atom

Sodium ion      Chloride ion

**Ionization**

through body tissue or other matter. Ionization can also cause cell death or mutation.

**ionization chamber,** a small cavity filled with air that collects the ionic charge liberated during irradiation. The exposure and dose of radiation can be calculated from the amount of change liberated and the mass of air in the chamber.

**ionization constant (K),** after establishment of ionic equilibrium, the product of the molar concentration of the ions divided by the molar concentration of the nonionized molecules.

**ionize** /ī′ənīz/ [Gk, *ienai* + *izein,* to cause], to separate or change into ions. See also **ion.**

**ionized calcium,** the ionized, unbound, noncomplexed fraction of serum calcium that is biologically active.

**ionizing energy** /ī′əni′zing/, the average energy lost by ionizing radiation in producing an ion pair in a gas. In air the value is approximately 33.73 electron-volts.

**ionizing radiation,** high-energy electromagnetic waves (such as x-rays and gamma rays) and particles (such as alpha and beta particles, neutrons, protons, and heavy nuclei) that cause substances in their paths to dissociate into ions. The spatial distribution of the ionization depends on the kind of radiation, its penetrating power, the location of the source, and the nature of the irradiated material. High-energy x-rays penetrate deeply, most beta particles penetrate only a few millimeters, and alpha particles penetrate only a fraction of a millimeter. However, all three produce intense ionization along their tracks. Ionizing radiation directly affects living organisms by killing cells or retarding their development; and by producing gene mutations and chromosome breaks. Tissues containing elements with relatively high atomic weights, such as calcium in bones and teeth, absorb much higher doses of ionizing radiation than do soft tissues.

**ionizing radiation injury** [Gk, *ion,* going; L, *radiare,* to shine, *injuria*], damage or ill effects suffered by exposure to ionizing radiation, including cellular harm resulting from radiation for diagnostic or therapeutic application. The risk of cell death or injury from radiation depends on the type of tissue cells, the stage of cell division at the time of exposure, the intensity and time span of exposure, and the type of radiation administered. See also **radiation burn.**

**ion-selective electrode,** a potentiometric electrode that develops a potential in the presence of one ion (or class of ions) but not in the presence of a similar concentration of other ions.

**iontophoresis** /ī·on′tōfôrē′·sis/ [Gk, *ion,* going, *pherein,* to carry], the introduction of ions of soluble salts into the tissues by direct current. Also called **galvanoionization, ionophoresis** /ī·ō′nō-/, **medical ionization.**

**iontophoretic pilocarpine test** [Gk, *ienai* + *pherein,* to carry], a sweat test used in the diagnosis of cystic fibrosis. Pilocarpine iontophoresis is used to stimulate production of sweat, which is absorbed from the forearm in a previously weighed gauze pad. The sweat sample is then analyzed for concentrations of sodium and chloride electrolytes.

**ion transfer,** a method of transporting chemicals across a membrane, using an electric current as a driving force.

**iota** /ī·ō′tə/, I, ι, the ninth letter of the Greek alphabet. Iota is also used to refer to something tiny, such as one iota.

**Iowa trumpet** /ī′əwə/, trademark for a kind of needle guide used in performing a pudendal block. It consists of a long thin cylinder through which a needle may be passed. A ring is attached to the proximal end of the guide, allowing the operator to hold it securely.

**IPA,** abbreviation for **independent practice association.**

**IPAA,** abbreviation for *International Psychoanalytical Association.*

**IPA-Model HMO,** a health maintenance organization (HMO) that contracts with an independent practice association (IPA) for physician services. The IPA processes and adjudicates claims. The HMO provides enrollees and hospital contracts.

**IPA paradigm shift,** an independent practice association that takes on the role of the health maintenance organization and contracts with its participating providers, but is neither a payer nor a provider.

**ipecac** /ip′əkak/, an emetic.

■ INDICATIONS: It is prescribed to cause emesis in certain types of recent poisonings and drug overdoses.

■ CONTRAINDICATIONS: Known hypersensitivity to this drug prohibits its use. It is not used in unconscious patients or for poisoning by petroleum distillates, strong alkalis, acids, or strychnine.

■ ADVERSE EFFECT: The most serious adverse reaction is cardiotoxicity if vomiting does not occur and the substance is retained.

■ NOTE: If vomiting does not occur, the ipecac can be recovered by gastric lavage.

**IPOF,** abbreviation for **immediate postoperative fit prosthesis.**

**ipomea** /ipəmē′ə/, a resin prepared from the dried root of *Ipomoea orizabensis,* formerly used as a cathartic.

**IPPB,** Abbreviation for **intermittent positive-pressure breathing.**

**IPPB unit,** a pressure-cycled ventilator providing a flow of air into the lungs at a predetermined pressure. As the pressure is attained, the flow is stopped, pressure is released, and the patient exhales. The intermittent positive-pressure breathing device is used to prevent postoperative atelectasis, to promote full expansion of the lungs, to improve oxygenation, and to administer nebulized medications into the respiratory passages.

**IPPV,** abbreviation for **intermittent positive pressure ventilation.** See **IPPB.**

**ipsi-,** prefix meaning 'the same, or self': *ipsilateral.*

**IPSID,** abbreviation for **immunoproliferative small intestine disease.**

**ipsilateral** [L, *ipse,* same, *latus,* side], affecting the same side of the body. Compare **contralateral.**

**IPSP,** abbreviation for *inhibitory postsynaptic potential.*

**IQ,** abbreviation for **intelligence quotient.**

**Ir,** symbol for the element **iridium.**

**IRB,** abbreviation for **institutional review board.**

**irbesartan,** an antihypertensive.

■ INDICATIONS: Irbesartan is used to treat hypertension, either alone or in combination with other drugs. It is also used investigationally to treat heart failure and hypertensive patients with diabetic nephropathy caused by type 2 diabetes mellitus.

■ CONTRAINDICATIONS: Known hypersensitivity and 2nd- and 3rd-trimester pregnancy prohibit the use of this drug.

■ ADVERSE EFFECTS: Anxiety, headache, fatigue, diarrhea, and dyspepsia are among the adverse effects of this drug. Common side effects include dizziness, cough, and upper respiratory infection.

**Ir g,** abbreviation for *immune response function gene.* See **immune response.**

**irid-,** prefix for terms pertaining to the iris.

**iridectomy** /ī′ridek′təmē/ [Gk, *iris,* rainbow, *ektomē,* excision], surgical removal of part of the iris of the eye. It is performed most often to restore drainage of the aqueous humor in glaucoma or to remove a foreign body or a malignant tumor. An incision is made through the cornea, and the iris is grasped with forceps or a hook and drawn out through the incision. The affected area is cut away, and the elastic iris is allowed to slip back into place. Atropine and an antibiotic are instilled, and a dressing and a shield are applied. After surgery, the patient is observed for signs of local hemorrhage or excessive pain.

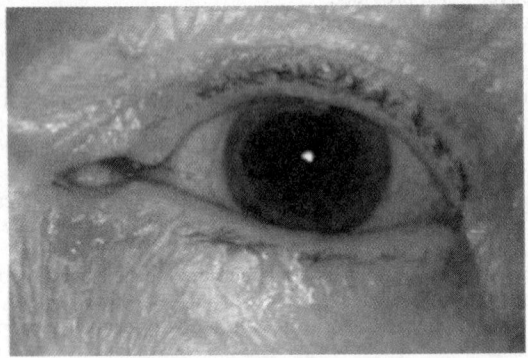

**Irregular pupil caused by iridectomy**
*(Lemmi and Lemmi, 2000)*

**iridemia** /ī′ridē′mə/, hemorrhage from the iris.

**iridescence** /ir′ides′əns/ [L, *iridescere,* to shine like a rainbow], the property of light interference or ability to break up light waves into colors of the spectrum.

**iridic.** See **iris.**

**iridium (Ir)** /irid′ē·əm/ [Gk, *iris,* rainbow], a silvery-bluish metallic element. Its atomic number is 77; its atomic mass is 192.22.

**irido-, iro-,** combining form meaning 'the iris or a colored circle': *iridocele, iridokeratitis, iridoplegia.*

**iridology** /ī′ridol′əjē/ [Gk, *iris,* rainbow, *logos,* science], the science that specializes in relations between disease and the shape, color, and other individual characteristics of the iris. There is considerable controversy over its validity.

**iridopathy** /ī′ridop′əthē/, any disease of the iris.

**iridoplegia** /ī′ridōplē′jə/ [Gk, *iris,* rainbow, *plege,* stroke], a condition of paralysis of the sphincter muscle of the iris or the dilator muscle or both.

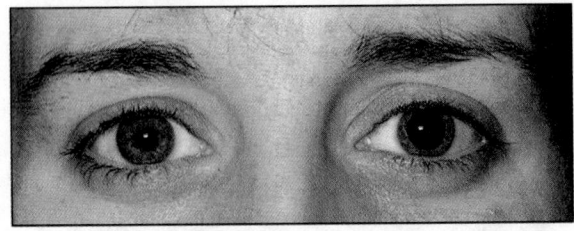

**Iridoplegia** *(Perkin, 1998)*

**iridotomy** /ī′ridot′əmē/ [Gk, *iris* + *temnein,* to cut], a surgical incision into the iris of the eye. It is performed to relieve occlusion of the pupil, to enlarge the pupil in cataract extraction, or to treat postoperative glaucoma. Local or general anesthesia is used. An incision is made through the cornea, and a cut is made transversely across the sphincter fibers of the iris. Atropine and an antibiotic are instilled, and a dressing and shield are applied. After surgery the dressing is observed for signs of drainage. Excessive pain is abnormal. See also **iridectomy, iris.**

**irinotecan,** an antineoplastic hormone.

■ INDICATIONS: This drug is used to treat metastatic carcinoma of the colon or rectum.

■ CONTRAINDICATIONS: Pregnancy and known hypersensitivity to this drug prohibit its use.

■ ADVERSE EFFECTS: Life-threatening effects of irinotecan include leukopenia, anemia, and neutropenia. Other adverse effects include fever, headache, chills, dizziness, diarrhea, nausea, vomiting, anorexia, constipation, cramps, flatus, stomatitis, dyspepsia, site irritation, rash, sweating, dyspnea, increased cough, rhinitis, vasodilation, edema, asthenia, and weight loss.

**iris** /ī′ris/ [Gk, rainbow], an annular, colored membrane shaped like a disc and suspended in aqueous humor between the cornea and the crystalline lens of the eye enclosing a circular pupil. Smooth muscle fibers of the iris contract and relax to allow more or less light to enter the eye through the pupil. The periphery of the iris is continuous with the ciliary body and is connected to the cornea by the pectinate ligament. The iris divides the space between the lens and the cornea into an anterior and a posterior chamber. The involuntary muscle of the iris is composed of circular fibers and radiating fibers. Dark pigment cells under the translucent tissue of the iris are variously arranged in different people to produce different colored irises. The pigment is absent in albinos. In blue eyes the pigment cells are confined to the posterior surface of the iris, but in gray eyes, brown eyes, and black eyes the pigment cells appear in the anterior layer of epithelium and in the stroma. See also **dilator pupillae, sphincter pupillae. —iridic,** *adj.*

**iritis** /īrī'tis/ [Gk, *iris* + *itis*], an inflammatory condition of the iris of the eye characterized by pain, lacrimation, photophobia, and, if severe, diminished visual acuity. On ophthalmic examination the eye looks cloudy, the iris bulges, and the pupil is contracted. The underlying cause is treated if identified, but the condition is most often idiopathic. The pupil is dilated, usually with atropine, and a corticosteroid may be prescribed to reduce inflammation. If the inflammation is allowed to continue and the pupil is left constricted, permanent scarring may occur, causing an opacity over the lens and diminished vision.

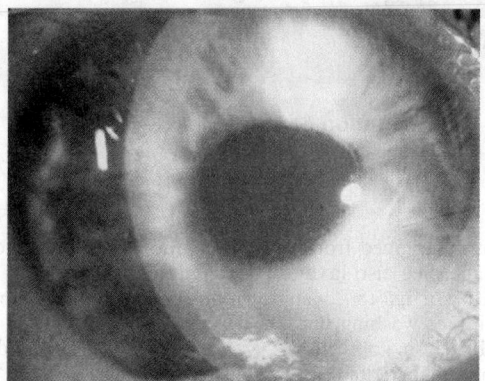

**Iritis** *(Zitelli and Davis, 1997)*

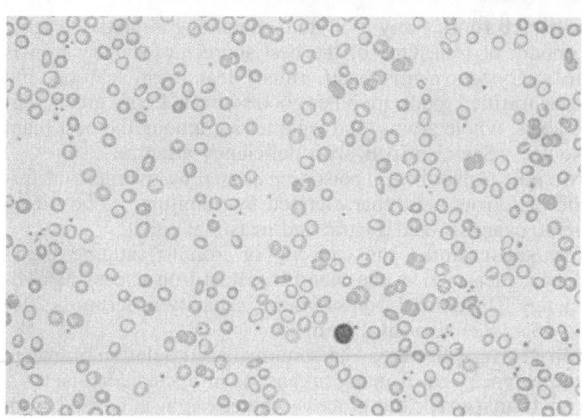

**Iron deficiency anemia** *(Zitelli and Davis, 1997)*

**iro-.** See **irido-.**

**iron (Fe)** /ī'ərn/ [AS, *iren*], a common metallic element essential for the synthesis of hemoglobin. Its atomic number is 26; its atomic mass (weight) is 55.85. It is used as a hematinic in the form of its salts and complexes, as ferrocholinate, ferrous fumarate, ferrous gluconate, ferrous sulfate, and iron dextran.

**iron-binding capacity (IBC),** the extent to which transferrin in the serum of a given patient can bind serum iron.

**iron deficiency anemia,** a microcytic hypochromic anemia caused by inadequate supplies of iron needed to synthesize hemoglobin, characterized by pallor, fatigue, and weakness. Laboratory diagnosis includes hemoglobin, hematocrit, transferrin, and serum iron evaluation. Iron deficiency may be the result of an inadequate dietary supply of iron, of poor absorption of iron in the digestive system, or of chronic bleeding. Replacement iron can be supplied by ferrous sulfate, preferably the oral form. The anemia should be corrected in 2 months, but therapy is continued for another 4 months to replace tissue stores. Compare **hemolytic anemia, hypoplastic anemia.** See also **anemia, iron metabolism, nutritional anemia, red cell indexes.**

**iron dextran,** an injectable hematinic.

■ INDICATION: It is prescribed in the treatment of iron deficiency anemia that is not responsive to oral iron therapy.

■ CONTRAINDICATIONS: Early pregnancy, anemias other than iron deficiency anemia, or known hypersensitivity to this drug prohibits its use.

■ ADVERSE EFFECTS: Among the more serious adverse effects are severe hypersensitivity reactions, including fatal anaphylaxis. Inflammation or phlebitis at the site of injection, arthralgia, headache, GI distress, fever, and lesser hypersensitivity reactions may occur.

**iron level and total iron-binding capacity test,** a blood test used to diagnose iron deficiency anemia and hemochromatosis (iron overload or poisoning), among other conditions.

**iron lung.** See **Drinker respirator.**

**iron metabolism,** a series of processes involved in the entry of iron into the body and its absorption, transport, storage, use in the formation of hemoglobin and other iron compounds, and eventual excretion. Iron normally enters through the epithelium of the intestinal mucosa and is oxidized from ferrous to ferric iron in the process. The rate at which iron enters is modulated by this absorption mechanism. When iron stores are high, iron no longer passes through but is trapped by the mucosal cells of the intestine to be eliminated. Once in the blood, iron cycles between the plasma and the reticuloendothelial or erythropoietic system. For hemoglobin synthesis plasma iron is delivered to the normoblast, where it remains up to 4 months, trapped in the hemoglobin molecules of a mature red cell. Senescent red cells then deteriorate and break down. The iron is released from the hemoglobin by the reticuloendothelial system to reenter the transport pool for recycling. The normal iron distribution in a 70-kg adult (male) totals approximately 3.7 g, more than 65% in circulating hemoglobin. Another 27% is found in the storage pool as hemosiderin or ferritin. The body normally conserves iron so well that loss, usually only through the feces, is normally limited to about 1 mg/day. This amount is easily provided by a dietary intake of only 10 mg/day. Iron deficiency may follow extended intervals of inadequate iron intake (especially in women), in pregnancy when higher levels of iron are needed, or with excessive blood loss. Iron overload sometimes occurs in disorders in which normal regulation of iron absorption is impaired. It is most commonly produced iatrogenically through the parenteral administration of large amounts of iron or blood for therapeutic purposes. See also **anemia, hemochromatosis, iron deficiency anemia, iron transport.**

**iron poisoning** [AS, *iren* + L, *potio,* drink], toxic effects of ingesting iron salts, particularly ferrous sulfate and ferrous chloride. Ferrous sulfate tablets, sometimes mistaken for candy, can cause vomiting, collapse, and liver necrosis. Ferrous chloride, a corrosive substance, causes vomiting, diarrhea, and hemorrhage when taken internally. Iron encephalopathy has resulted from excessive use of iron preparations.

**iron-rich food,** any food item containing a relatively large amount of iron. One of the best sources of dietary iron is liver. Oysters, clams, heart, kidney, lean meat, seafood, and iron-fortified foods are other good sources. Leafy green vegetables, whole grains, and legumes are among the best plant sources. See also **iron, iron deficiency anemia.**

**iron salt poisoning,** poisoning caused by overdose of ferric or ferrous salt, characterized by vomiting, bloody diarrhea, cyanosis, and gastric and intestinal pain.

**iron saturation,** the capacity of iron to saturate transferrin, measured in the blood to detect iron excess or deficiency. The normal iron saturation capacity in serum is 20% to 55%. See also **total iron.**

**iron-storage disease,** an abnormal accumulation of iron in the parenchyma of many organs, as in hemosiderosis.

**iron transport,** the process whereby iron is carried from the intestinal mucosa to sites of use and storage. Iron binds with transferrin and shuttles to storage and utilization sites. Transferrin becomes attached to exogenous iron that enters through the intestinal villi or that reenters the plasma from the sinusoids of the spleen. The iron is then released to the normoblasts, and the transferrin is freed for additional transport functions that may involve iron stored as ferritin or hemosiderin. See also **hemosiderosis, iron metabolism, transferrin.**

**irradiation** /irā′dē·ā′shən/ [L, *irradiare,* to beam upon], exposure to any form of radiant energy, such as heat, light, or x-rays. Radioactive sources of radiant energy, such as x-rays or isotopes of iodine or cobalt, are used diagnostically to examine internal body structures. The same or similar sources of radioactivity in larger amounts are used to destroy microorganisms or tissue cells that have become cancerous. Infrared or ultraviolet light may be used to produce heat in body tissues for pain relief or to treat acne, psoriasis, or other skin ailments. Ultraviolet light is also used to identify certain bacteria and toxic molds. See also **radiation sickness, radioactivity, ultraviolet. —irradiate,** *v.*

**irrational** /irash′ənəl/ [L, *irrationalis,* contrary to reason], pertaining to events, conditions, or behavior that may be considered unreasonable.

**irreducible** /ir′əd(y)oo͞′sibəl/ [L, *in,* not, *reducere,* to bring back], unable to be returned to the normal position or condition, as an irreducible hernia. See also **incarcerate.**

**irreducible hernia.** See **incarcerated hernia.**

**irregular pulse** /ireg′yələr/ [L, *in,* not, *regula,* rule, *pulsare,* to beat], a variation in the force or rhythm of impulses in an artery caused by cardiac arrhythmia.

**irreversible** /ir′əvur′sibəl/ [L, *irrevertere,* to not turn back], pertaining to a situation or condition that cannot be reversed.

**irreversible coma.** See **brain death.**

**irreversible shock,** a condition in which shock does not respond to available forms of treatment and in which recovery is impossible as a result of massive cellular damage.

**irrigate** /ir′igāt/ [L, *irrigare,* to supply water], to flush with a fluid, usually with a slow steady pressure on a syringe plunger. It may be done to cleanse a wound or to clear tubing.

**irrigation** /ir′igā′shən/, the process of washing out a body cavity or wounded area with a stream of water or other fluid. It is also used to cleanse a tube or drain inserted into the body, such as an indwelling catheter. The procedure is most commonly performed with water, saline, aminoacetic acid, or antiseptic solution on the eye, ear, throat, vagina, and urinary tract. Gentle pressure is applied in the introduction of the fluid, except in the debridement of wounds, and the so-

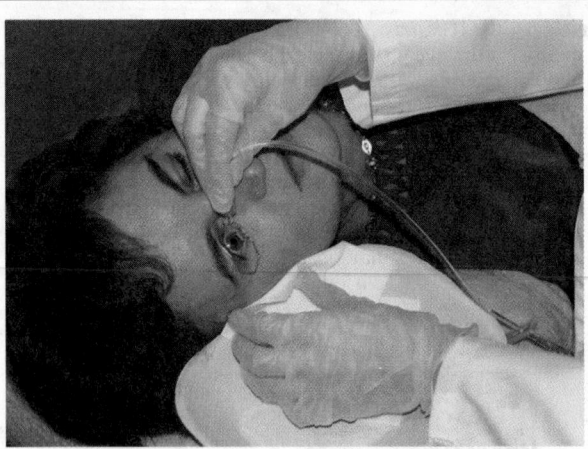

**Eye irrigation** *(Phipps, Sands, and Marek, 1999)*

lution is removed from internal cavities through suction or drainage. See also **lavage. —irrigate,** *v.*

**irrigator** /ir′igā′tər/, an apparatus with a flexible tube for flushing or washing out a body cavity.

**irritability** /ir′itəbil′itē/ [L, *irritare,* to tease], a condition of abnormal excitability or sensitivity.

**irritable bladder** /ir′itəbəl/ [L, *irritare,* to tease; AS, *blaedre*], a condition characterized by a nearly constant urge to urinate. See also **urgency, urinary incontinence.**

**irritable bowel syndrome (IBS)** [L, *irritare,* to tease; OFr, *boel* + Gk, *syn,* together, *dromos,* course], abnormally increased motility of the small and large intestines, of unknown origins. Most of those affected are young adults, who complain of diarrhea and occasionally pain in the lower abdomen. The pain is usually relieved by passing flatus or stool. In diagnosing irritable bowel syndrome other more serious conditions, such as dysentery, lactose intolerance, and the inflammatory bowel diseases, must be ruled out. Because there is no organic disease present in irritable bowel syndrome, no specific treatment is necessary. Many persons benefit from the use of bulk-producing agents in the diet, because bulk tends to stabilize the water content of the stool. Antidiarrheal drugs are helpful in decreasing the frequency of stool. Although this is a functional disorder, patients experience pain and discomfort and need emotional support. Mild tranquilizers or antidepressants are sometimes given to relieve anxiety or depression. Also called **functional bowel syndrome, mucous colitis, spastic colon.**

**irritant** /ir′itənt/ [L, *irritare,* to tease], an agent that produces inflammation or irritation.

**irritant poison** [L, *irritare,* to tease, *potio,* drink], any of a large number of toxic substances in the environment that can cause pain in the digestive tract, diarrhea, vomiting, abdominal cramps, and urinary tract disorders. Some irritant chemicals are industrial gases, such as ammonia, chlorine, phosgene, sulfur dioxide, hydrogen sulfide, and nitrogen dioxide, which may leak into the atmosphere.

**irritation fibroma** /ir′itā′shən/, a localized, peripheral, tumorlike enlargement of connective tissue caused by prolonged irritation. It commonly develops on the gums or the buccal mucosa.

**IRV,** abbreviation for **inspiratory reserve volume.** See also **pulmonary function test.**

**Isaacs' syndrome** /ī'zəks/ [H. Isaacs, American neurologist, 20th century], progressive muscle stiffness and spasms, with continuous muscle fiber activity similar to that seen with neuromyotonia.

**ischaemic contracture.** See **Volkmann's contracture.**

**ischemia** /iskē'mē·ə/ [Gk, *ischein,* to hold back, *haima,* blood], a decreased supply of oxygenated blood to a body part. The condition is often marked by pain and organ dysfunction, as in ischemic heart disease. Some causes of ischemia are arterial embolism, atherosclerosis, thrombosis, and vasoconstriction. Also spelled **ischaemia.** Compare **infarction. —ischemic,** *adj.*

**ischemic contracture.** See **Volkmann's contracture.**

**ischemic heart disease** /iskē'mik/, a pathologic condition caused by lack of oxygen in cells of the myocardium.

**ischemic lumbago,** a pain in the lower back and buttocks caused by vascular insufficiency, as in occlusion of the abdominal aorta.

**ischemic necrosis.** See **coagulation necrosis.**

**ischemic pain,** unpleasant, often excruciating pain associated with decreased blood flow caused by mechanical obstruction, constricting orthopedic casts, or insufficient blood flow that results from injury or surgical trauma. Ischemic pain caused by occlusive arterial disease is often severe and may not be relieved, even with narcotics. The individual with peripheral vascular disease may experience ischemic pain only while exercising because the metabolic demands for oxygen cannot be met as a result of occluded blood flow. The ischemic pain of partial arterial occlusion is not as severe as the abrupt, excruciating pain associated with complete occlusion, such as by an embolus or thrombus. See also **pain intervention.**

**ischemic paralysis,** loss of motor control in a body area caused by an interruption in the blood supply to the area's muscles or nerves.

**ischemic penumbra,** an area of moderately ischemic brain tissue surrounding an area of more severe ischemia; blood flow to this area may be enhanced in order to prevent the spread of a cerebral infarction.

**ischemic pericarditis** [Gk, *ischein,* to hold back, *haima,* blood, *peri,* near, *kardia,* heart, *itis,* inflammation], inflammation of the pericardium caused by interruption of its blood supply during myocardial infarction.

**ischemic stroke,** a cerebrovascular disorder caused by deprivation of blood flow to an area of the brain, generally as a result of thrombosis, embolism, or reduced blood pressure.

**ischia.** See **ischium.**

**ischial spines** /is'kē·əl/ [Gk, *ischion,* hip joint; L, *spina,* thorn], two relatively sharp posterior bony projections into the pelvic outlet from the ischial bones that form the lower border of the pelvis.

**ischial tuberosity** [Gk, *ischion,* hip joint; L, *tuber,* swelling], a rounded protuberance of the lower part of the ischium. It forms a bony area on which the human body rests when in a sitting position.

**ischio-,** combining form meaning 'the ischium or the hip': *ischioanal, ischiodidymus, ischiopagus.*

**ischiocele.** See **sciatic hernia.**

**ischium** /is'kē·əm/, *pl.* **ischia** [L; Gk, *ischion,* hip joint], one of the three parts of the hip bone, which joins the ilium and the pubis to form the acetabulum. The ischium comprises the dorsal part of the hip bone and is divided into the body of the ischium, which forms the posteroinferior two fifths of the acetabulum, and the ramus, which joins the inferior ramus of the pubis. The spine of the ischium provides attachment for various muscles, such as the gemellus superior, the coccygeus, and the levator ani. The greater sciatic notch above the spine transmits the superior and inferior gluteal vessels and various nerves, such as gluteal nerves and the sciatic nerve. A notch below the spine of the ischium transmits various ligaments, vessels, and nerves for other parts. The large dorsal tuberosity of the ischium provides attachment for various muscles, such as the adductor longus, the semimembranosus, the biceps femoris, and the semitendinosus. Compare **ilium, pubis.**

**ischo-,** prefix meaning 'restraint or suppression': *ischemia, ischesis.*

**ISCLT,** abbreviation for *International Society of Clinical Laboratory Technologists.*

**ISG,** abbreviation for **immune serum globulin.**

**ISH,** abbreviation for **isolated systolic hypertension.**

**Ishihara color test** /ish'ēhä'rə/ [Shinobu Ishihara, Japanese ophthalmologist, 1879–1963], a test of color vision that uses a series of plates on which are printed round dots in a variety of colors and patterns. People with normal color vision are able to discern specific numbers or patterns on the plates; the inability to pick out a given number or shape is symptomatic of a specific deficiency in color perception.

**ISIS,** abbreviation for *International Study of Infarct Survival.*

**island** /i'lənd/ [OE, *īegland,* island], a cluster of cells or an isolated piece of tissue. See also **islet.**

**island fever.** See **scrub typhus.**

**island of Reil.** See **central lobe.**

**islands of Langerhans** /lang'gərhanz/ [L, *insula,* island; Paul Langerhans, German pathologist, 1847–1888], clusters of cells within the pancreas that produce insulin, glucagon, and pancreatic polypeptide. They form the endocrine portion of the gland, and their hormonal secretions released into the bloodstream are balanced, important regulators of carbohydrate metabolism. The islands of Langerhans are scattered throughout the pancreas; the beta cells, which secrete insulin, usually appear in the center of each of the lobules. Alpha cells secrete glucagon, and pancreatic peptide cells secrete pancreatic peptide. The cells the islands comprise are arranged in plates interspersed by capillaries. Also called **islets of Langerhans.**

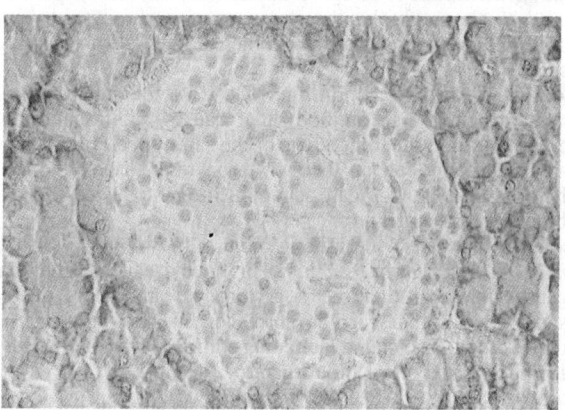

**Island of Langerhans: normal islet**
*(Bodansky, 1989/ Professor K.D. Buchanan)*

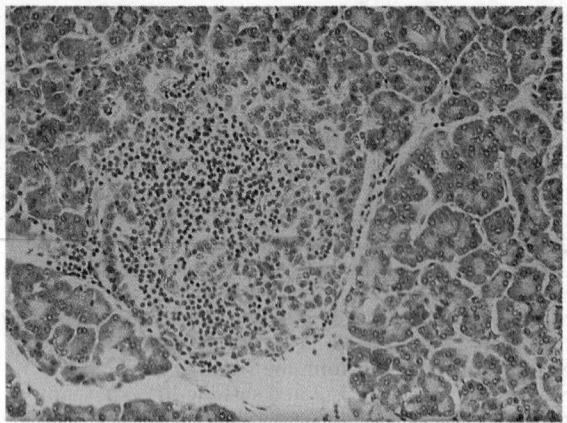

**Island of Langerhans in type I diabetes mellitus**
(Bodansky, 1989/Professor W. Gepts, Brussels)

**islet** /ī'lət/ [MFr, *islette,* little island], a cluster of cells or an isolated piece of tissue. See also **island.**

**islet cell adenoma.** See **insulinoma.**

**islet cell antibody (ICA)** /ī'lit/ [MFr, *islette,* little island], an immunoglobulin that reacts with cytoplasmic components of all of the cells in the pancreatic islets. These antibodies occur in about 60% to 70% of newly diagnosed patients with insulin-dependent diabetes mellitus, providing strong evidence for an autoimmune origin and pathogenesis of the disease. The presence of ICA can be demonstrated for years before the occurrence of symptoms. The antibody tends to disappear with time.

**islet cell tumor,** any tumor of the islands of Langerhans. Kinds of islet cell tumors include insuloma, gastrinoma, glucagonoma, and somatostatinoma.

**isletitis.** See **insulitis.**

**islets of Langerhans.** See **islands of Langerhans.**

**-ism, -simus,** suffix meaning 'condition of, practice of, theory of': *hyperthyroidism, hypopituitarism, strabismus.*

**Ismelin,** trademark for an antihypertensive (guanethidine sulfate).

**iso-** /ī'sō-/, prefix meaning 'equal': *isobar, isochromatic, isohydric.*

**isoagglutination** /ī'sō·əgloo̅'tinā'shən/ [Gk, *isos,* equal; L, *agglutinate,* to glue], the clumping of erythrocytes by agglutinins from the blood of another individual of the same species.

**isoagglutinin** /ī'sō·əgloo̅'tinin/ [Gk, *isos,* equal; L, *agglutinate,* to glue], an antibody that causes agglutination of erythrocytes in other members of the same species that carry an isoagglutinogen on their erythrocytes. Also called **isohemagglutinin.** Compare **isoagglutinogen.** See also **ABO blood group, antibody.**

**isoagglutinogen** /ī'sō·əgloo̅otin'əjən/ [Gk, *isos* + L, *agglutinate,* to glue; Gk, *Geenen,* to produce], an antigen that causes the agglutination of erythrocytes in others of the same species that carry a corresponding isoagglutinin in their serum. Also called **isohemagglutinin.** Compare **agglutinin.** See also **ABO blood group.**

**isoamyl alcohol.** See **amyl alcohol.**

**isoantibody** /ī'sō·an'tibod'ē/ [Gk, *isos* + *anti,* against; AS, *boding,* body], an antibody to isoantigens found in other members of the same species. See also **autoimmune disease, tissue typing.**

**isoantigen** /ī'sō·an'tijən/ [Gk, *isos* + *anti,* against; AS, *boding,* body; Gk, *Geenen,* to produce], a substance that interacts with isoantibodies in other members of the same species. Compare **autoantigen, autoimmune disease.** See also **antigen, isoagglutinogen.**

**isobar** /ī'səbär/ [Gk, *isos* + *barrios,* weight], **1.** a line connecting points of equal pressure on a graph, as lines connecting points of equal carbon dioxide tension on a pH-bicarbonate diagram. **2.** (in nuclear medicine) one of a group of nuclides having the same total number of neutrons and protons in the nucleus but so proportioned that their atomic numbers have different values.

**isobaric** /-bär'ik/ [Gk, *isos,* equal, *barrios,* weight], **1.** pertaining to two substances or solutions of the same specific gravity. **2.** pertaining to two isotopes that have the same mass number but different atomic numbers. **3.** having the same barometric pressure.

**isobutyl alcohol (C₄H₁₀O)** $(C_4H_{10}O)$ /ī'sobyoo̅'til/ [Gk, *isos* + *butyrin,* butter, *hyl,* matter; AR, *alcohol,* essence], a clear colorless liquid that is miscible with ethyl alcohol or ether. Also called **2-methyl-1-propanol.**

**isocapnic** /-kap'ink/, pertaining to a level of carbon dioxide in the tissues that remains steady despite changing levels of ventilation.

**isocarboxazid** /-kärbok'səzid/, a monoamine oxidase inhibitor.

■ INDICATION: It is prescribed in the treatment of mental depression.

■ CONTRAINDICATIONS: Liver or kidney dysfunction, congestive heart failure, pheochromocytoma, concomitant use of a sympathomimetic drug or foods high in tryptophan or tyramine, or known hypersensitivity to the drug prohibits its use.

■ ADVERSE EFFECTS: Among the more serious adverse reactions are hyperactivity, cardiac arrhythmia, hypotension, vertigo, dryness of mouth, constipation, and blurred vision. Monoamine oxidase inhibitors produce many adverse drug interactions.

**isochromosome** /-krō'məsōm/, a chromosome whose arms are of equal length.

**isocrotic,** describing the separation of a mixture by chromatography using a single solvent or solvent mixture.

**isodose chart** /ī'sədōs/ [Gk, *isos* + *doss,* giving, *charta,* paper], a graphic representation of the distribution of radiation in a medium; lines are drawn through points receiving equal doses. Isodose charts are determined for x-rays traversing the body, for radium applicators used in intracavitary or interstitial treatment, and for working areas where x-rays or radionuclides are used.

**isodynamic law** /ī'sōdīnam'ik/, the rule that for energy purposes different foods may replace one another in accordance with their caloric values, as determined when burned in a calorimeter.

**isoeffect lines** /ī'sō·ifekt'/, lines on a graph representing doses of radiation that have tumoricidal effects in normal tissues.

**isoelectric** /ī'sō·ilek'trik/ [Gk, *isos* + *electron,* amber], pertaining to the electric baseline of an electrocardiogram.

**isoelectric electroencephalogram.** See **flat electroencephalogram.**

**isoelectric focusing,** the ordering and concentration of substances according to their isoelectric points.

**isoelectric period,** a period in physiologic activity, such as nerve conduction or muscle contraction, when there is no variation in electric potential.

**isoelectric point,** the pH at which a molecule containing two or more ionizable groups is electrically neutral. The average number of positive charges equals the average number of negative charges.

**isoenzyme** /ī'sō·en'zīm/ [Gk, *isos* + *en,* in, *syme,* ferment], a chemically distinct form of an enzyme. The various forms are distinguishable in analysis of blood samples, which aids in the diagnosis of disease. Different enzymes that catalyze the same physiologic reaction may also exist as isoenzymes in different animal species. Also called **isozyme.**

**isoetharine, isoetharine hydrochloride.** See **isoetharine mesylate.**

**isoetharine mesylate** /ī'sō·eth'ərēn/, a beta-adrenergic bronchodilator.

■ INDICATIONS: It is prescribed in the treatment of bronchial asthma, bronchitis, and emphysema.

■ CONTRAINDICATIONS: A history of cardiac arrhythmia or known hypersensitivity to this drug or to sympathomimetic medications prohibits its use.

■ ADVERSE EFFECTS: Among the more serious adverse reactions are palpitations, tachycardia, arrhythmias, vertigo, nervousness, and headache.

**isoexposure line** /ī'sō·ikspō'zhər/, an imaginary line representing positions of equal exposure to radiation around a fluoroscopic instrument.

**isoflows** /ī'sōflōz/, a measure of early small airway dysfunction in a patient made by comparing forced expiratory flow rates of air and of helium at fixed points in time.

**isofosfamide.** See isophosphamide.

**isogamete** /ī'sōgam'ēt/ [Gk, *isos* + *gamete,* wife], a reproductive cell of the same size and structure as the one with which it unites. Compare **anisogamete. —isogametic,** *adj.*

**isogamy** /īsog'əmē/ [Gk, *isos* + *gamos,* marriage], sexual reproduction in which there is fusion of gametes of the same size and structure, such as in certain algae, fungi, and protists. Compare **anisogamy. —isogamous,** *adj.*

**isogeneic.** See **syngeneic.**

**isogenesis** /-jen'əsis/ [Gk, *isos* + *genein,* to produce], development from a common origin and according to similar processes. Also called **isogeny** /īsoj'ənē/. **—isogenetic, isogenic,** *adj.*

**isograft** /ī'səgraft'/ [Gk, *isos* + *graphion,* stylus], surgical transplantation of histocompatible tissue between genetically identical individuals, such as identical twins. Compare **allograft, autograft, xenograft.** See also **graft.**

**isohemagglutinin.** See **isoagglutinin.**

**isohydric shift** [Gk, *isos* + *hydor,* water; AS, *sciftan,* to divide], the series of reactions in red blood cells in which $CO_2$ is taken up and oxygen is released without the production of excess hydrogen ions.

**isoimmunization** /ī'sō·im'yənīzā'shən/, the development of antibodies against antigens from the same species, such as anti-Rh antibodies in an Rh-negative person. See also **erythroblastosis fetalis.**

**isokinetic** /-kinet'ik/, pertaining to a concentric or eccentric contraction that occurs at a set speed against a force of maximal resistance produced at all points in the range of motion.

**isokinetic exercise** [Gk, *isos,* equal, *kinesis,* motion; L, *exercere,* to keep at work], a form of exercise in which maximum force is exerted by a muscle at each point throughout the active range of motion as the muscle contracts. The effort of the patient to resist the movement is measured.

**isolate** /ī'səlāt/ [It, *isolare,* to detach], **1.** to separate a pure chemical substance from contamination by foreign matter. **2.** to derive from any source a pure culture of a microorganism. **3.** to prevent an individual from having contact with the rest of a population.

**isolated systolic hypertension (ISH),** a type of hypertension in which only the systolic blood pressure is elevated. The condition, which usually affects the elderly, increases the risk of stroke or heart attack.

**isolation** /-lā'shən/ [L, *insula,* island], the separation of a seriously ill patient from others to prevent the spread of an infection or to protect the patient from irritating environmental factors. A patient undergoing radiation therapy may also be isolated to reduce the exposure of hospital personnel to effects of radioactive materials.

**isolation incubator,** an incubator bed regularly maintained for premature or other infants who require isolation.

**isolation ward** [It, *isolare,* to detach; ME, *warden*], a room or section of a hospital in which certain categories of patients, particularly those infected with acute contagious diseases, can be treated with a minimum of contact with the rest of the patients and hospital personnel.

**Isolette,** trademark for a self-contained incubator unit that provides a controlled heat, humidity, and oxygen microenvironment for the isolation and care of premature and low–birth weight neonates. The apparatus is made of a clear plastic material and has a large door and portholes for easy access to the infant with a minimum of heat and oxygen loss. A servocontrol mechanism constantly monitors the infant's temperature and controls the heat within the unit.

**isoleucine (Ile)** /ī'sōloo'sēn/ [Gk, *isos* + *leukos,* white], an amino acid that occurs in most dietary proteins and is essential for proper growth in infants and for nitrogen balance in adults. Also spelled **isoleuceine.** See also **amino acid, maple syrup urine disease, protein.**

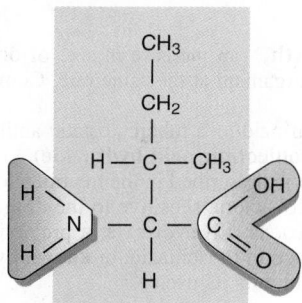

**Chemical structure of isoleucine**

**isologous graft** /īsol'əgəs/ [Gk, *isos,* equal, *logos,* relation, *graphion,* stylus], a tissue transplant between two individuals who are genetically identical, as identical twins.

**isomeric** /-mer'ik/ [Gk, *isos,* equal, *meros,* part], pertaining to a chemical phenomenon in which two compounds of the same chemical formula may differ in chemical and physical properties. The difference is the result of the arrangement of atoms in the respective molecules, either the connections between the atoms or their arrangements in three-dimensional space.

**isomers** /ī'səmərz/, molecules that have the same molecular mass and formula but different structures, resulting in different properties.

**isometheptene hydrochloride** /-məthep'tēn/, an antispasmodic and vasoconstrictor drug that is a component in some fixed-combination drugs used to treat migraine.

**isometric** /ī'səmet'rik/ [Gk, *isos* + *metron,* measure], maintaining the same length or dimension.

**isometric contraction** [Gk, *isos,* equal, *metron,* measure; L, *contractio,* a drawing together], muscular contraction not accompanied by movement of the joint. Resistance applied to the contraction increases muscle tension without producing movement of the joint. Sometimes called *muscle setting exercises.*

**isometric exercise,** a form of active exercise in which muscle tension is increased while pressure is applied against stable resistance. This exercise may be accomplished by pushing or pulling against an immovable object or by simultaneously contracting opposing muscles, such as by pressing the hands together. There is no joint movement, and muscle length remains unchanged, but muscle strength and tone are maintained or improved. Compare **isotonic exercise.** See also **exercise.**

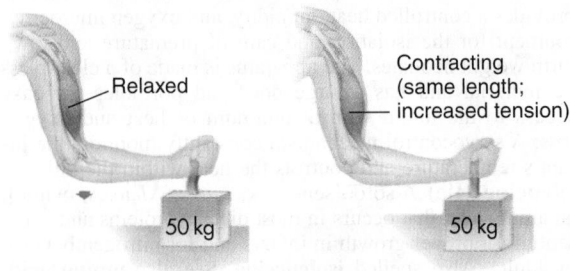

**Isometric exercise** *(Thibodeau and Patton, 1999/Rolin Graphics)*

**isometric growth,** an increase in size of different organs or parts of an organism at the same rate. Compare **allometric growth.**

**isoniazid** /ī′sənī′əzid/, a tuberculostatic antibacterial. Also called **INH (isonicotinic acid hydrazide).**
- INDICATION: It is prescribed in the treatment of tuberculosis caused by mycobacteria sensitive to the drug.
- CONTRAINDICATIONS: Liver disease, a previous history of a hepatotoxic reaction to isoniazid, or known hypersensitivity to this drug prohibits its use.
- ADVERSE EFFECTS: Among the more serious adverse reactions in long-term treatment are hepatotoxicity and peripheral neuropathy. Rashes, fever, and central nervous system effects commonly occur.

**isoosmotic** See **isosmotic.**

**isopentoic acid.** See **isovaleric acid.**

**isophane insulin suspension** /ī′səfān/ [Gk, *isos* + *phanein,* to show; L, *insula,* island; *suspendere,* to hang up], a modified form of protamine zinc insulin suspension. It is an intermediate-acting insulin that is a stable commonly prescribed preparation. Also spelled **NPH insulin.**

**isophosphamide** /-fos′fəmīd/, an antineoplastic that is a derivative of cyclophosphamide; its use is similarly to that of cyclophosphamide. Also called **isofosfamide.** See also **cyclophosphamide.**

**isoprenaline.** See **isoproterenol hydrochloride.**

**isopropamide iodide** /-prō′pəmīd/, an anticholinergic.
- INDICATION: It is prescribed as an adjunct to ulcer therapy.
- CONTRAINDICATIONS: Narrow-angle glaucoma, asthma, obstruction of the genitourinary or GI tract, ulcerative colitis, or known hypersensitivity to this drug prohibits its use.
- ADVERSE EFFECTS: Among the more serious adverse reactions are blurred vision, central nervous system effects,

tachycardia, dry mouth, decreased sweating, and hypersensitivity reactions.

**isopropanol.** See **isopropyl alcohol.**

**isopropylacetic acid.** See **isovaleric acid.**

**isopropyl alcohol (C₃H₈O)** /ī′sōprō′pil/, a clear, colorless bitter aromatic liquid that is miscible with water, ether, chloroform, and ethyl alcohol. A solution of approximately 70% isopropyl alcohol in water is used as a rubbing compound. Also called **avantin, dimethyl carbinol, isopropanol, 2-propanol.** See also **alcohol.**

**isopropylaminoacetic acid.** See **valine.**

**isoproterenol hydrochloride** /ī′sōprəter′ənol/, a beta-adrenergic stimulant.
- INDICATIONS: It is used as a bronchodilator and as a cardiac stimulant.
- CONTRAINDICATIONS: Cardiac arrhythmia or known hypersensitivity to this drug prohibits its use.
- ADVERSE EFFECTS: Among the more serious adverse reactions are arrhythmias, tachycardia, hypotension, and intensification of angina.

**Isoptin,** trademark for a calcium channel blocker or calcium ion antagonist (verapamil).

**Isopto Atropine,** trademark for an anticholinergic (atropine sulfate).

**Isopto Carbachol,** trademark for a cholinergic (carbachol).

**Isopto Carpine,** trademark for a cholinergic (pilocarpine hydrochloride).

**Isopto Cetamide,** trademark for an antibacterial (sulfacetamide sodium).

**Isopto Homatropine,** trademark for an anticholinergic (homatropine hydrobromide).

**Isopto Hyoscine,** trademark for an anticholinergic (scopolamine hydrobromide).

**Isordil,** trademark for an antianginal agent (isosorbide dinitrate).

**isosmotic** /ī′sozmot′ik/, pertaining to a solution that has the same solute concentration as another solution. Also called **isoosmotic.** Compare **hyperosmotic, hypoosmotic**

**isosorbide dinitrate** /-sôr′bīd/, an antianginal agent.
- INDICATION: It is prescribed as a coronary vasodilator in the treatment of angina pectoris and congestive heart failure.
- CONTRAINDICATION: Known hypersensitivity to this drug prohibits its use.
- ADVERSE EFFECTS: The most serious reaction is occasional marked hypotension. Flushing, headache, and dizziness also may occur.

***Isospora*** /ī·sos′pə·rə/ [Gk, *isos,* equal + *sporos,* seed], a genus of coccidian protozoa found in birds, amphibians, reptiles, and mammals, including humans. It includes the species *I. belli* and *I. hominis.* See also **isosporiasis.**

**isosporiasis** /ī·sos′pə·rī′ə·sis/, infection with *Isospora.* See **coccidiosis.**

**isotachophoresis** /-tak′ōfôrē′sis/ [Gk, *isos* + *tachos,* speed, *pherein,* to bear], the ordering and concentration of substances of intermediate effective mobilities between an ion of high effective mobility and one of much lower effective mobility, followed by their migration at a uniform speed.

**isothermal** /-thur′məl/ [Gk, *isos,* equal, *therme,* heat], having the same temperature. See **synthermal.**

**isotones** /ī′sətōnz′/, atoms that have the same number of neutrons but different numbers of protons.

**isotonic** /ī′səton′ik/ [Gk, *isos* + *tonikos,* stretching], pertaining to a solution that causes no change in cell volume.

**isotonic exercise,** a form of active exercise in which muscles contract and cause movement. There is no significant change in resistance throughout the movement, so the force of contraction remains constant. Such exercise greatly enhances joint mobility and helps improve muscle strength and tone. Two examples of isotonic exercise are rising on tiptoes and stretching arms overhead. Compare **isometric exercise**. See also **exercise.**

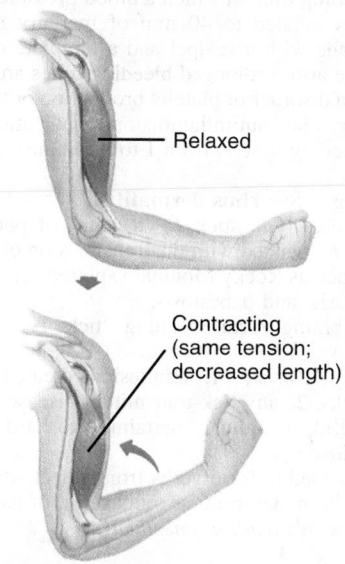

Relaxed

Contracting (same tension; decreased length)

**Isotonic muscle contraction**
*(Thibodeau and Patton, 1999/Rolin Graphics)*

**isotonicity law** /ī′sətonis′itē/, a law that describes a state of equal osmotic pressure in extracellular body fluids that results from equal concentrations of electrolytes and other solute particles in the fluid. If a hypertonic solution is ingested, additional water will be drawn from surrounding blood plasma to dilute the intestinal contents and maintain tonicity.

**isotope** /ī′sətōp/ [Gk, *isos* + *topos,* place], one of two or more forms of a chemical element having the same number of protons in the atomic nucleus but different numbers of neutrons and thus a different atomic mass. For example, two common isotopes of carbon are ($^{12}$C), which has six neutrons, and ($^{14}$C), which has eight. Many isotopes are used in diagnostic and therapeutic procedures.

**isotopic tracer** /ī′sətop′ik/ [Gk, *isos* + *topos,* place; Fr, *tracer,* to track], an isotope or mixture of isotopes of an element incorporated into a sample to permit observation of the course of the element through a chemical, physical, or biologic process. The observations may be made by measuring the radioactivity or the abundance of the isotope.

**isotretinoin** /-trətin′ō·in/, an antiacne agent.

■ INDICATION: It is prescribed for the treatment of cystic acne.

■ CONTRAINDICATIONS: Pregnancy or sensitivity to hydroxybenzoic acid esters prohibits its use.

■ ADVERSE EFFECTS: The most serious adverse reactions are epistaxis, cheilitis, conjunctivitis, paresthesia, dizziness, and serum lipid and hematologic disturbances.

**isotype** /ī′sətīp/, an antigenic determinant that occurs in all members of a subclass of an immunoglobulin class. An antigenic determinant that is isotypic in one subclass may appear as an allotypic marker in another class.

**isovaleric acid** /-vəler′ik/ [Gk, *isos* + L, *valeriana,* herb, *acidus,* sour], a fatty acid with a pungent taste and dis-

agreeable odor that is found in valerian and other plant products, as well as in cheese. It also occurs as a metabolite of the amino acid leucine and is found in the sweat of feet and in the urine of patients with smallpox, hepatitis, and typhus. It has been used commercially in a variety of drugs, perfumes, and flavorings. Isovaleric acidemia occurs in patients who have abnormally high levels of isovaleric acid in the blood and urine as a result of an inherited deficiency of the enzyme isovaleryl coenzyme A dehydrogenase. The condition is treated with diets that contain low-leucine foods. Also called **isopentoic acid, isopropylacetic acid.**

**isovolume pressure-flow curve** /-vol′yəm/, a curve on a graph describing the relationship of driving pressure to the resulting volumetric flow rate in the airways at any given lung inflation.

**isovolumic contraction** /-vəloo′mik/ [Gk, *isos* + L, *volumen,* paper roll, *contractio,* drawing together], the early phase of systole, in which the myocardial muscle fibers have begun to shorten but have not developed enough pressure in the ventricles to overcome the aortic and pulmonary end-diastolic pressures and open the aortic and pulmonary valves. During this period of muscle fiber contraction, the ventricular volumes do not change. See also **afterload.**

**isoxsuprine hydrochloride** /ī′sok′səprēn/, a peripheral vasodilator.

■ INDICATIONS: It is prescribed for the symptomatic relief of cerebrovascular insufficiency and improvement of circulation in arteriosclerosis, Raynaud's disease, and Buerger's disease.

■ CONTRAINDICATION: Known hypersensitivity to this drug is the only contraindication.

■ ADVERSE EFFECTS: Among the more serious adverse reactions are tachycardia, hypotension, and dermatitis.

**isozyme.** See **isoenzyme.**

**ISS,** abbreviation for **injury severity score.**

**-ist,** suffix meaning a 'practitioner of a science': *audiologist, pharmacist, psychosomaticist.*

**isthmus** /is′məs/, *pl.* **isthmuses, isthmi** [Gk, *isthmos,* a narrow, connection, passage, or constriction], a constriction between two larger parts of an organ or anatomic structure, such as the isthmus of the thyroid.

**isthmus of thyroid** [Gk, *isthmos* + *thyreos* + *eidos,* form], a part of the thyroid gland, anterior to the trachea, which joins the two lateral lobes of the gland.

**Isuprel,** trademark for a beta-adrenergic stimulant (isoproterenol).

**IT,** abbreviation for **immunotoxin.**

**itch** [AS, *giccan*], **1.** to feel a sensation, usually on the skin, that makes one want to scratch. **2.** a tingling, annoying sensation on an area of the skin that makes one want to scratch it, caused in some people, for example, by rhus dermatitis, a mosquito bite, or an allergic reaction. **3.** the pruritic condition of the skin caused by infestation with the parasitic mite *Sarcoptes scabiei.* See also **pruritus. —itchy,** *adj.*

**itch mite** [AS, *giccan* + *mite*], a tiny arachnid with piercing and sucking mouthparts. At least three genera of itch mites are recognized: *Chorioptes, Notoedres,* and *Sarcoptes.*

**itchy.** See **itch.**

**-ite,** **1.** suffix meaning 'compounds': *nitrite, phosphite, sulfite.* **2.** combining form meaning a 'body part': *chondriomite, osteite, zygoite.*

**ithy-,** combining form meaning 'erect or straight': *ithylordosis, ithyokyphosis.*

**-itic,** suffix meaning 'related to something specified': *encephalitic, nephritic, syphilitic.*

**-itis,** suffix meaning an 'inflammation of a (specified) organ': *carditis, cecitis, sarcitis.*

**ITP,** abbreviation for **idiopathic thrombocytopenic purpura.**

**IU, I.U.,** abbreviation for **International Unit.**

**IUD,** abbreviation for **intrauterine device.**

**-ium,** **1.** suffix used to name metallic elements: *radium, sodium.* **2.** suffix for quaternary ammonium derivatives.

**IUPC,** abbreviation for *intrauterine pressure catheter.*

**IV,** **1.** abbreviation for **intravenous** or **intravenously.** **2.** *informal.* equipment consisting of a bottle or bag of fluid, infusion set with tubing, and intravenous catheter, used in intravenous therapy. **3.** intravenous administration of fluids or medication by injection into a vein.

**IVAC pump,** trademark for a portable IV pump that electronically regulates and monitors the flow of IV fluid. It is usually attached to the IV stand. See also **intravenous pump.**

**IVC,** abbreviation for **intravenous cholangiography.**

**Ivemark's syndrome** /ē′vəmärks, ī′v′märks/, a congenital defect in which organs on the left side of the body are a mirror image of their counterparts on the right side.

**IVF,** abbreviation for **in vitro fertilization.**

**ivory bones.** See **osteopetrosis.**

**IVP,** abbreviation for **intravenous pyelography.**

**IV push.** See **intravenous bolus.**

**IVT,** abbreviation for *intravenous transfusion.*

**IV-type traction frame,** a metal structure for holding traction equipment. It consists of two metal uprights, one at each end of the bed, which support an overhead metal bar. The base of each upright is clamped to a horizontal bar that fits into holders inserted at the corners of the bed. Compare **claw-type traction frame.** See also **traction frame.**

**Ivy method** [Robert H. Ivy, American surgeon, 1881–1947], a test of bleeding time in which a blood pressure cuff on the upper arm is inflated to 40 mm of mercury and a small wound is made with a scalpel and a template on the volar surface of the arm. Prolonged bleeding times are most often the result of a disorder of platelet production or the ingestion of aspirin or other antiinflammatory medications. Normal adult Ivy bleeding time is from 1 to 9 minutes. See also **hemostasis.**

**ivy poisoning.** See **rhus dermatitis.**

***Ixodes*** /iksō′dēz/ [Gk, sticky], a genus of parasitic hard-shelled ticks associated with the transmission of a variety of infections, such as Rocky Mountain spotted fever, Lyme disease, erlichiosis, and babesiosis.

**ixodi-,** combining form meaning 'ticks': *ixodiasis, ixodism.*

**ixodiasis** /ik′sōdī′əsis/, **1.** skin lesions created by the bites of ixodid ticks. **2.** any tick-transmitted disease.

**ixodid** /iksod′id, iksō′did/, pertaining to hard ticks of the family Ixodidae.

**-ize,** suffix added to form verbs from adjectives and nouns. Verbs mean 'to make, become, engage in, or use, or to treat or combine with': *oxidize, anesthetize.*

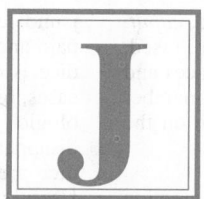

**J,** abbreviation for **joule.**

**Jaccoud's dissociated fever** /zhäkooz'/ [Sigismond Jaccoud, French physician, 1830–1913], a form of meningitic fever accompanied by a paradoxical slow pulse rate.

**jacket** [Fr, *jaquette*], a supportive or confining therapeutic casing or garment for the torso. It is also used to prevent edema in the extremities. See also **Minerva cast, Sayre's jacket.**

**jacket restraint,** an orthopedic device used to help immobilize the trunk of a patient in traction and to discourage the patient from sitting up in bed. The jacket restraint is attached to both sides of the bedspring frame by means of buckled webbing straps that are sewn into the side seams of the restraint. The jacket restraint may be used with most kinds of traction but is not usually used with Dunlop skin traction, Dunlop skeletal traction, Bryant traction, halo-femoral traction, or halo-pelvic traction. Compare **diaper restraint, sling restraint.**

**jackknife position** /jak'nīf/, an anatomic position in which the patient is placed on the stomach with the hips flexed and the knees bent at a 90-degree angle and the arms outstretched in front of the patient. Examination and instrumentation of the rectum are facilitated by this position.

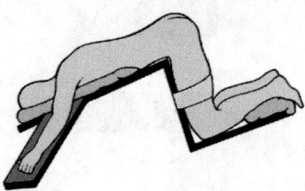

**Jackknife position** (Monahan and Neighbors, 1997)

**jackscrew** /jak'skroo /, a threaded device used in orthodontic appliances for the separation or approximation of teeth or jaw segments.

**Jackson crib,** a removable orthodontic appliance retained in position by crib-shaped wires.

**jacksonian epilepsy** /jak·sō'nē·ən/, epilepsy characterized by focal motor seizures with unilateral clonic movements that start in one group of muscles and spread systematically to adjacent groups, reflecting the march of the epileptic activity through the motor cortex (**jacksonian march**). The seizures are due to a discharging focus in the contralateral motor cortex.

**jacksonian march,** the spread of abnormal electrical activity from one area of the cerebral cortex to adjacent areas, characteristic of **jacksonian epilepsy.** Also called **cortical march, epileptic march.**

**jacksonian seizure,** a series of focal seizures with unilateral clonic movements that start in one group of muscles and spread systematically to adjacent groups, reflecting the march of the epileptic activity through the motor cortex.

**Jackson's sign** [John H. Jackson, English neurologist, 1835–1911], (in hemiparesis) an observation that during quiet respiration the movement of the paralyzed side of the chest may be greater than that of the opposite side. However, the paralyzed side moves less under forced respiration.

**Jackson tracheostomy tube,** trademark for a silver tracheostomy tube with a rubber cuff built onto the tube. The design is intended to prevent accidental migration of the cuff off the end of the tube, causing interference with airflow to the patient.

**Jacob x membrane.** See **retina.**

**Jacquemier's sign** /zhäkmē·āz'/ [Jean M. Jacquemier, French obstetrician, 1806–1879], a deepening of the color of the vaginal mucosa just below the urethral orifice. It may sometimes be noted after the fourth week of pregnancy, but it is not a reliable sign of pregnancy.

**jactitation** /jak'titā'shən/ [L, *jactare*, show off, display], twitchings or spasms of muscles or muscle groups, as observed in the restless body movements of a patient with a severe fever.

*JADA,* abbreviation for *Journal of the American Dental Association.*

**jail fever.** See **epidemic typhus.**

**Jakob-Creutzfeldt disease.** See **Creutzfeldt-Jakob disease.**

*JAMA* /jä'mä, jam'ə, jā'ā'em'ā'/, abbreviation for *Journal of the American Medical Association.*

**jamais vu** /zhämävY', -vē', -voo'/ [Fr, never seen], the sensation of being a stranger when with a person one knows or when in a familiar place. The phenomenon occurs occasionally in normal people but more frequently in those who have temporal lobe epilepsy. Compare **déjà vu.**

**Janeway lesion** /jān'wā/ [Edward G. Janeway, American physician, 1841–1911; L, *laedere*, to injure], a small erythematous or hemorrhagic macule on the palms or soles. It is diagnostic of subacute bacterial endocarditis.

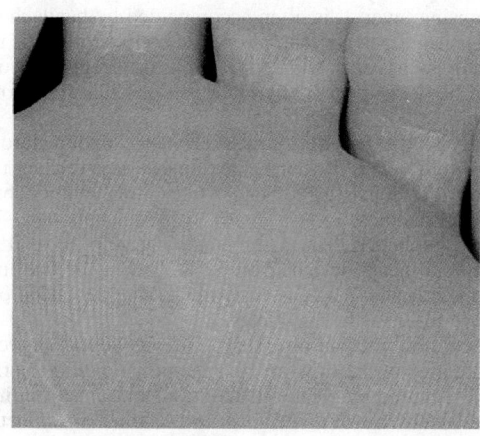

**Janeway lesion** (Zitelli and Davis, 1997)

**janiceps** /jan′əseps/ [L, *Janus*, two-faced Roman god, *caput*, head], a conjoined twin fetus in which the heads are fused, with the faces looking in opposite directions. The faces and bodies of both twins may be fully formed, or one member may be only partially formed and act as a parasite on the more fully developed fetus.

**Jansen's disease.** See **metaphyseal dysostosis.**

**Japanese encephalitis (JE),** a severe epidemic infection of brain tissue seen in East and Southeast Asia and the South Pacific, including Australia and New Zealand. The virus is carried by domestic pigs and wild birds. The disease is characterized by shaking chills, paralysis, and weight loss and is caused by *Flavivirus* transmitted by mosquitoes. Symptoms include headache, fever, neck stiffness, tremors, seizures, spastic paralysis, and coma. Mortality rate ranges widely from 0.3% to 60%. Various neurologic and psychiatric sequelae are common. An inactivated JE vaccine is available and recommended for travel to endemic areas. Treatment is supportive. Also called **Japanese B encephalitis.**

**Japanese flood fever, Japanese river fever.** See **scrub typhus.**

*JAPHA* /jaf′ə, jā′ā′pē′āch′ā′/, abbreviation for *Journal of the American Public Health Association.*

**jar¹,** to shake or jolt.

**jar²,** a cylindrical container.

**Jarcho-Levin syndrome** /jär′kō·lev′in/ [Saul Wallenstein Jarcho, American physician, b. 1906; Paul M. Levin, American physician, 20th century], an autosomal recessive disorder consisting of multiple vertebral defects, short thorax, rib abnormalities, camptodactyly, and syndactyly; urogenital abnormalities are sometimes present. Death, from respiratory insufficiency, usually occurs in infancy. Also called **spondylothoracic dysplasia.**

**jargon (jar.)** /jär′gən/ [Fr, *jargonner,* to speak indistinctly], **1.** incoherent speech or gibberish. **2.** a terminology used by scientists, artists, or others of a professional subculture that is not understood by the general population.

**jargon aphasia** [Fr, *jargonner* + Gk, *a* + *phasis,* speech], a form of speech in which several words are combined in a single word but in a jumbled manner with incorrect accents or words mixed with neologisms. Although outwardly incomprehensible, the speech may be meaningful when analyzed by a psychotherapist. It is noted in schizophrenia, especially the disorganized type. Also called **word salad.**

**Jarisch-Herxheimer reaction** /jä′risherks′hīmər/ [Adolph Jarisch, Austrian dermatologist, 1850–1902; Karl Herxheimer, German dermatologist, 1861–1944], an acute febrile reaction that may follow therapy for syphilis, leptospirosis, or relapsing fever. It is often accompanied by headache and myalgia, rigors, hyperventilation, and confusion and is more common in patients with early syphilis. Pregnant women should be warned that early labor is a possible result of the reaction.

**Jarotzky's treatment** /jərot′skēz/ [Alexander Jarotsky, Russian physician, b. 1866], therapy of gastric ulcer using a bland diet consisting of egg whites, fresh butter, bread, milk, and noodles.

**Jarvik-7** [Robert K. Jarvik, American cardiologist, b. 1946], an artificial heart designed by R. K. Jarvik for use in humans. The Jarvik-7 was an early model that depended on air pressure to drive the ventricles.

**jaundice** /jôn′dis, jän′dis/ [Fr, *jaune,* yellow], a yellow discoloration of the skin, mucous membranes, and sclerae of the eyes, caused by greater than normal amounts of bilirubin in the blood. Because persons with dark skin sometimes have yellow-tinged sclerae, the hard palate of the mouth is often the best place to assess for jaundice. Persons with jaundice may experience nausea, vomiting, and abdominal pain and may pass dark urine and clay-colored stools. Jaundice is a symptom of many disorders, including liver diseases, biliary obstruction, and the hemolytic anemias. Physiologic jaundice commonly develops in newborns and disappears after a few days. Rarer disorders causing jaundice are Crigler-Najjar syndrome and Gilbert's syndrome. Useful diagnostic procedures include a clinical evaluation of the signs and symptoms, tests of liver function, and techniques for direct or indirect visualization such as x-ray film, computed tomographic scan, ultrasound, endoscopy or exploratory surgery, and biopsy. Also called **icterus** /ik′tərəs/. See also **anicteric hepatitis, hyperbilirubinemia. —jaundiced,** *adj.*

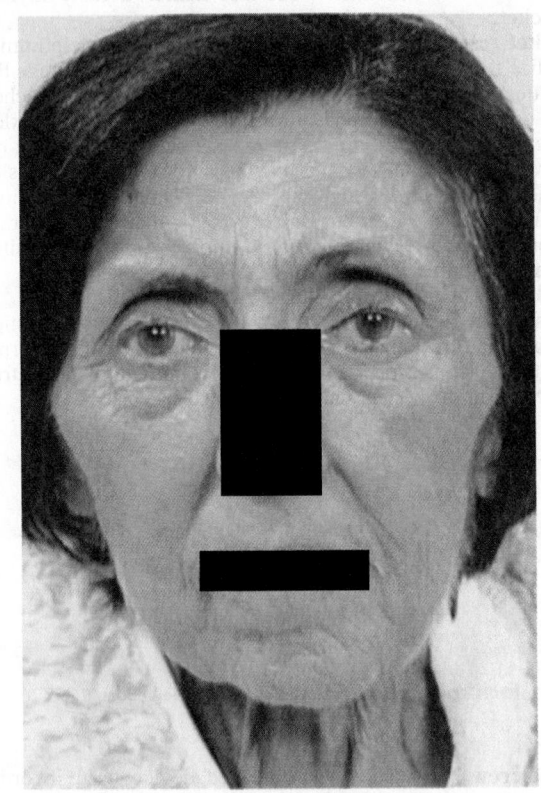

**Severe jaundice** *(Kamal and Brockelhurst, 1991)*

**jaw** [AS, *ceowan,* to chew], a common term used to describe the maxillae and the mandible and the soft tissue that covers these structures, which contain the teeth and form the framework for the mouth. See also **jaw relation.**

**jaw reflex,** an abnormal reflex elicited by tapping the chin with a rubber hammer while the mouth is half open and the jaw muscles are relaxed. A quick snapping shut of the jaw implies damage to the area of cerebral cortex governing motor activity of the fifth cranial nerve. Also called **chin reflex, jaw jerk, mandibular reflex.**

**jaw relation,** any relation of the mandible to the maxilla.

**jaw-winking,** an involuntary facial movement phenomenon in which the eyelid droops, usually on one side of the face, when the jaw is closed but raises when the jaw is opened or when the jaw is moved from side to side. The raising of the eyelid often appears exaggerated. Also called **Gunn's syndrome, Marcus Gunn's syndrome.** See also **Marin Amat's syndrome.**

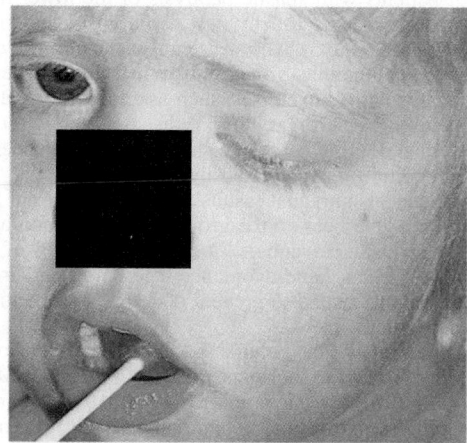

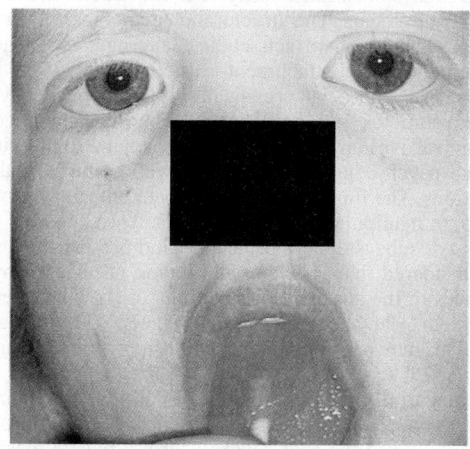

**Jaw-winking** *(Zitelli and Davis, 1997)*

**JCAHO,** abbreviation for **Joint Commission on Accreditation of Healthcare Organizations.**

**J chain,** a polypeptide chain that holds immunoglobulin A (IgA) dimers and IgM pentamers together.

**J/deg,** abbreviation for *joules per degree.*

**Jefferson fracture,** a fracture characterized by bursting of the ring of the first cervical vertebra.

**jejuna.** See **jejunum.**

**jejunal** /jijōō'nəl/ [L, *jejunus*, empty], pertaining to the **jejunum,** the length of intestine between the duodenum and the ileum.

**jejunal feeding tube,** a hollow tube inserted into the jejunum through the abdominal wall for administration of liquefied foods to patients who have a high risk of aspiration. See also **enteral tube feeding, tube feeding.**

**jejunectomy** /jij'ōōnek'təmē/, the surgical removal of all or part of the jejunum.

**jejuno-,** combining form meaning 'the jejunum': *jejunocecostomy, jejunocolostomy, jejunotomy.*

**jejunocolostomy** /jijōō'nōkəlos'təmē/, the surgical creation of an anastomosis between the jejunum and colon.

**jejunoileitis.** See **Crohn's disease.**

**jejunostomy** /jij'ōōnos'təmē/, a surgical procedure to create an artificial opening to the jejunum through the abdominal wall. It may be a permanent or a temporary opening.

**jejunostomy feeding.** See **tube feeding.**

**jejunotomy** /jij'ōōnot'əmē/, a surgical incision in the jejunum.

**jejunum** /jijōō'nəm/, *pl.* jejuna [L, *jejunus*, empty], the intermediate or middle of the three portions of the small intestine, connecting proximally with the duodenum and distally with the ileum. The jejunum has a slightly larger diameter, a deeper color, and a thicker wall than the ileum and contains heavy, circular folds that are absent in the lower part of the ileum. The jejunum also has larger villi than the ileum. Compare **ileum.** —**jejunal,** *adj.*

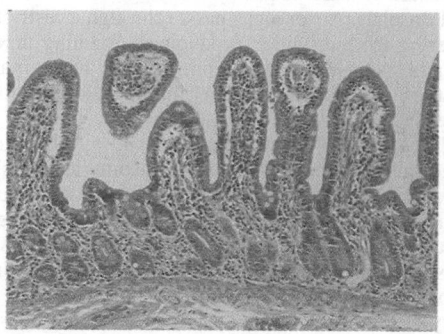

**Jejunum** *(Cotran, Kumar, and Collins, 1999)*

**jelly,** a semisolid nonliquid colloidal solution. See also **gel.**

**jellyfish sting** [L, *gelare*, to congeal; AS, *fisc + stingan*], a wound caused by skin contact with a jellyfish, a sea animal with a bell-shaped gelatinous body and numerous suspended long tentacles containing stinging structures. In most cases a tender, red welt develops on the affected skin. In some cases, depending on the sensitivity of the person and the

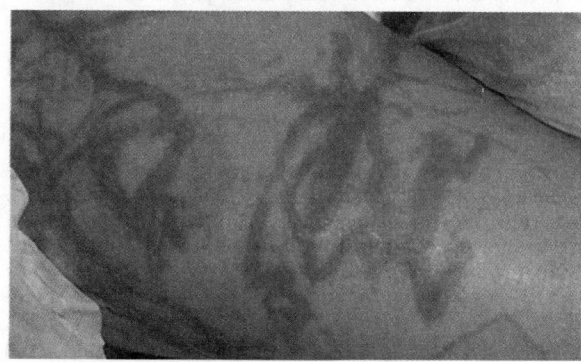

**Tissue necrosis caused by a jellyfish sting**
*(Auerbach, 1995/courtesy John Williamson, MD)*

species of jellyfish, severe localized pain and nausea, weakness, excessive lacrimation, nasal discharge, muscle spasm, perspiration, and dyspnea may occur.

**Jendrassik's maneuver** /yendrä′shiks/ [Ernst Jendrassik, Hungarian physician, 1858–1921; Fr, *manoeuvre*, action], (in neurology) a diagnostic procedure in which the patient hooks the flexed fingers of the two hands together and forcibly tries to pull them apart. While this tension is being exerted, the lower extremity reflexes, particularly the patellar reflex, are tested.

**jerk,** **1.** a sudden abrupt motion such as a thrust, yank, push, or pull. **2.** a quick muscular contraction induced when a tendon over a bone is tapped. See also **spasm.**

**jerk finger.** See **trigger finger.**

**jerk nystagmus,** a slow drift of the eyes in one direction, followed by a rapid recovery movement in the other direction.

**jerks,** a form of choromania, or morbid desire to make rhythmic movements, sometimes associated with emotional fervor.

**jet humidifier,** a humidifier that increases the surface area for exposure of water to gas by breaking the water into small aerosol droplets. Air or a gas passes through a restriction after entering the humidifier, producing a foaming mixture of liquid and gas. Gas issuing from the unit has a maximum amount of water vapor and a minimum of liquid water particles.

**jet lag** [L, *jacere*, to throw; Scand, *lagga*, to fall behind], a condition characterized by fatigue, insomnia, and sluggish body functions caused by disruption of the normal circadian rhythm resulting from rapid travel across several time zones.

**jet nebulizer** [L, *nebula*, mist], a humidifier that uses Bernoulli's principle to convert a pool of liquid into a fine mist of aerosol particles. A jet stream of gas is projected at high velocity across the end of a capillary tube. The gas jet reduces the pressure at the top of the tube, causing the liquid to move to the top, where it is continuously drawn off as aerosol particles that enter the outflow passage of the humidifier.

**Jeune's syndrome** /zhœnz, zhōōnz/ [Mathis Jeune, French pediatrician, b. 1910], a form of lethal short-limbed dwarfism characterized by constriction of the upper thorax and occasionally by polydactylism. It is inherited as an autosomal recessive trait. Also called **asphyxiating thoracic dysplasia.**

**Jewett brace.** See **Griswald brace.**

**jigger.** See **chigoe.**

**jimson weed** /jim′sən/, a common name for *Datura stramonium*, a poisonous plant with large trumpet-shaped flowers. It is a member of solanaceous plants and a natural source of cholinergic blockers. Its chief components are the anticholinergics hyoscyamine and scopolamine.

**jitters,** **1.** irregularities in ultrasound echo locations caused by mechanical or electronic disturbances. **2.** a very uneasy, nervous feeling.

**J/kg,** abbreviation for *joules per kilogram.*

**Jobst garment,** trademark for a type of pressure wrap applied to control hypertrophic scar formation or lymphedema.

**jock itch.** See **tinea cruris.**

**JOD.** abbreviation for **juvenile-onset diabetes.** See **type 1 diabetes mellitus.**

**Jod-Basedow phenomenon** /jod′bä′zədō′/ [Ger, *Jod*, iodine; Karl A. von Basedow, German physician, 1799–1854], thyrotoxicosis that may occur when dietary iodine is given to a patient with endemic goiter in an area of environmental iodine deficiency. It is presumed that iodine deficiency protects some patients with endemic goiter from development

of thyrotoxicosis. The phenomenon may also occur when large doses of iodine are given to patients with nontoxic multinodular goiter in areas with sufficient environmental iodine. Also called iodine-induced hyperthyroidism.

**Joffroy's reflex** /zhôfrô·äz′, jof′roiz/ [Alexis Joffroy, French physician, 1844–1908], a reflex contraction of the gluteus muscles produced when firm pressure is applied to the buttocks of patients with spastic paralysis of the lower limbs.

**Joffroy's sign** [Alexis Joffroy], **1.** an upward direction of a patient's gaze, caused by the absence of facial muscle contraction in ophthalmic goiter. **2.** an inability to perform simple mathematical exercises, such as addition or multiplication, caused by an organic brain disease.

**jogger's heel** [ME, *joggen*, to shake; AS, *hela*, heel], a painful condition characterized by bruising, bursitis, fasciitis, or calcaneal spurs that results from repetitive and forceful striking of the heel on the ground. It is common among joggers and distance runners. Judicious selection of well-fitting running shoes and avoidance of running on hard surfaces are recommended to prevent occurrence or recurrence of the condition.

**Johnson, Dorothy E.,** a nursing theorist who developed a behavioral systems model presented in *Conceptual Models for Nursing Practice* (Riehl and Roy, eds., 1973). Johnson's theory addresses two major components: the patient and nursing. The patient is a behavioral system with seven interrelated subsystems. Each subsystem has structural and functional requirements. The structural elements include drive or goal; predisposition to act; choice, alternatives for action; and behavior. The attachment-affiliative subsystem forms the basis for all social organization. The dependency subsystem promotes helping behavior. The biologic (ingestive and eliminative) and sexual subsystems have to do with social and psychological functions as well as biological considerations. The function of the achievement subsystem is to attempt to manipulate the environment. The functions of the aggressive subsystem are protection and preservation. Johnson considered that problems in nursing are caused by disturbances in the structure or functions of the subsystems or the system. Her behavioral systems theory provides a conceptual framework for nursing education, practice, and research.

**Johnson's method,** a technique for filling root canals, in which gutta-percha cones are dissolved in a chloroform-rosin solution in the root canal to form a plastic mass. The plastic material is forced into the apex of the root canal, and more is added until the canal is sealed. Compare **lateral condensation method.**

**joint** [L, *jungere*, to join], any one of the articulations between bones. Each is classified according to structure and movability as fibrous, cartilaginous, or synovial. Fibrous joints are immovable, cartilaginous joints slightly movable, and synovial joints freely movable. Typical immovable joints are those connecting most of the bones of the skull with a sutural ligament. Typical slightly movable joints are those connecting the vertebrae and the pubic bones. Most of the joints in the body are freely movable and allow gliding, circumduction, rotation, and angular movement. Also called **articulation.** See also **cartilaginous joint, fibrous joint, synovial joint.**

**joint and several liability,** (in law) a condition in which several persons share the liability for a plaintiff's injury and may be found liable individually or as a group.

**joint appointment,** **1.** a faculty appointment to two institutions within a university or system, as to the schools of nursing and medicine of the same university. **2.** (in academic nursing) the appointment of a member of the faculty

## Classification of joints

| Type of joint | Example | Description |
|---|---|---|
| **Fibroid (synarthrosis)** | | No movement is permitted |
| Suture | Cranial sutures | United by thin layer of fibrous tissue |
| Synchondrosis | Joint between the epiphysis and diaphysis of long bones | Temporary joint in which the cartilage is replaced by bone later in life |
| **Cartilaginous (amphiarthrosis)** | | Slightly movable joint |
| Symphysis | Symphysis pubis | Bones are connected by a fibrocartilage disk |
| Syndesmosis | Radius-ulna articulation | Bones are connected by ligaments |
| **Synovial (diarthrosis)** | | Freely movable; enclosed by joint capsule, synovial membrane |
| Ball and socket | Shoulder | Widest range of motion, movement in all planes |
| Hinge | Elbow | Motion limited to flexion and extension in a single plane |
| Pivot | Atlantoaxis | Motion limited to rotation |
| Condyloid | Wrist between radius and carpals | Motion in two planes at right angles to each other, but no radial rotation |
| Saddle | Thumb at carpal-metacarpal joint | Motion in two planes at right angles to each other, but no axial rotation |
| Gliding | Intervertebral: between the articular surfaces of successive vertebrae | Motion limited to gliding |

Adapted from Seidel HM, Ball JW, Dains JE, Benedict GW: *Mosby's guide to physical examination,* ed 4, St Louis, 1999, Mosby. Illustrations from Thibodeau and Patton, 1996/Rolin Graphics.

of a university to a clinical service of an associated service institution. A psychiatric nurse might hold appointment in a university as an assistant professor and might also be a clinical nurse specialist in a service institution. The practice of joint appointments is said to have begun at Case Western Reserve University, University Hospital, Cleveland. See also **unification model.**

**joint audit.** See **nursing audit.**

**joint capsule** [L, *jungere*, to join, *capsula*, little box], a fibrous saclike structure of connective tissue that envelops the end of bones in a diarthroidal joint and contains synovial fluid.

**joint chondroma,** a cartilaginous mass that develops in the synovial membrane of a joint.

**Joint Commission on Accreditation of Healthcare Organizations (JCAHO),** a private nongovernmental agency that establishes guidelines for the operation of hospitals and other health care facilities, conducts accreditation programs and surveys, and encourages the attainment of high standards of institutional medical care in the United States. Members of the JCAHO include representatives from the American Medical Association, American College of Physicians, American College of Surgeons, American Dental Association, and American Hospital Association.

**joint conference committee,** a hospital organization composed of the governing board, administration, and medical staff representatives whose purpose is to facilitate communication between the groups.

**joint fracture.** See **intraarticular fracture.**

**joint instability,** an abnormal increase in joint mobility. See also **hypermobility.**

**joint mouse,** a small movable stone formed in or near a joint, usually a knee.

**joint movement: active,** a nursing outcome from the Nursing Outcomes Classification (NOC) defined as the range of motion of joints with self-initiated movement. See also **Nursing Outcomes Classification.**

**joint movement: passive,** a nursing outcome from the Nursing Outcomes Classification (NOC) defined as the range of motion of joints with assisted movement. See also **Nursing Outcomes Classification.**

**joint planning,** the development by two or more health care providers of a strategic plan to serve the health care needs of an area while sharing clinical or administrative services or data but not assets.

**joint practice,** **1.** the practice of one or more physicians, nurses, and other health professionals, usually private, who work as a team, sharing responsibility for a group of patients. **2.** (in inpatient nursing) the practice of making joint decisions about patient care by committees of the physicians and nurses working on a division.

**joint protection,** the use of orthotics with therapeutic exercise to prevent damage or deformity of a joint during rehabilitation to restore power and range of motion. An example is a metal ankle-foot orthosis that allows weight-bearing on an extended knee.

**Jones criteria** /jōnz/, a standardized set of guidelines for the diagnosis of rheumatic fever, as recommended by the American Heart Association. See also **rheumatic fever.**

**Joseph disease.** See **Machado-Joseph disease.**

**Joubert's syndrome** /zhoo·bārz'/ [Marie Joubert, Canadian neurologist, 20th century], an autosomal recessive syndrome consisting of partial or complete agenesis of the cerebellar vermis, with hypotonia, episodic hyperpnea, mental retardation, and abnormal eye movements; most patients die in infancy.

**joule** /jool/ [James P. Joule, English physicist, 1818–1889], a unit of energy or work in the meter-kilogram-second system and the SI system. It is equivalent to $10^7$ ergs or 1 watt second.

**joystick,** a vertical stick or lever that can be manipulated in various directions to control cursor or other movements on a computer screen. It is used mainly in playing computer games. See also **mouse, trackball.**

**J-pouch,** a fecal reservoir formed surgically by folding over the lower end of the ileum in an ileoanal anastomosis.

**JRA,** abbreviation for **juvenile rheumatoid arthritis.**

**Judd method,** a technique for positioning a patient for radiographic examination of the atlas and odontoid process.

**judgment** /juj'mənt/ [L, judicare, to judge], **1.** (in law) the final decision of the court regarding the case before it. **2.** the reason given by the court for its decision; an opinion. **3.** an award, penalty, or other sentence of law given by the court. **4.** the ability to recognize the relationships of ideas and to form correct conclusions from those data as well as from those acquired from experience.

**judgment call,** slang. a decision based on experience, especially a judgment that resolves a serious problem in which the data are inconclusive or equivocal.

**jug-,** **1.** combining form meaning 'a yoke type of connection': jugal, jugum, conjugal. **2.** a combining form meaning 'collarbone, throat, neck': jugular, jugate.

**jugal** /joo'gəl/ [L, jugum, yoke], pertaining to structures attached or yoked, as the zygomatic bone or malar bone.

**jugu-,** a combining form meaning 'to kill': jugulate, jugulation.

**jugular** /jug'yələr/ [L, jugulum, neck], **1.** pertaining to or involving the throat. **2.** informal. the jugular vein.

**jugular foramen** [L, jugulum, neck, foramen, hole], one of a pair of openings between the lateral part of the occipital bone and the petrous part of the temporal bones in the skull. The foramen contains the inferior petrosal sinus, the transverse sinus, some meningeal branches of the occipital and ascending pharyngeal arteries, and the glossopharyngeal, vagus, and accessory nerves.

**jugular foramen syndrome.** See **Vernet's syndrome.**

**jugular fossa,** a deep depression adjacent to the interior surface of the petrosa of the temporal bone of the skull.

**jugular process,** a portion of the occipital bone that projects laterally from the squamous part to the temporal bone. On its anterior border a deep notch forms the posterior and medial boundary of the jugular foramen.

**jugular pulse,** a pulsation in the jugular vein caused by conditions that inhibit diastolic filling of the right side of the heart.

**jugular venous pressure (JVP),** blood pressure in the **jugular vein,** which reflects the volume and pressure of venous blood. JVP is estimated by positioning the head of a supine patient at a 45-degree angle and observing the neck veins. If the neck veins are filled only to a point a few millimeters above the clavicle at the end of exhalation, JVP is usually normal. With an elevated JVP the neck veins may be distended as high as the angle of the jaw.

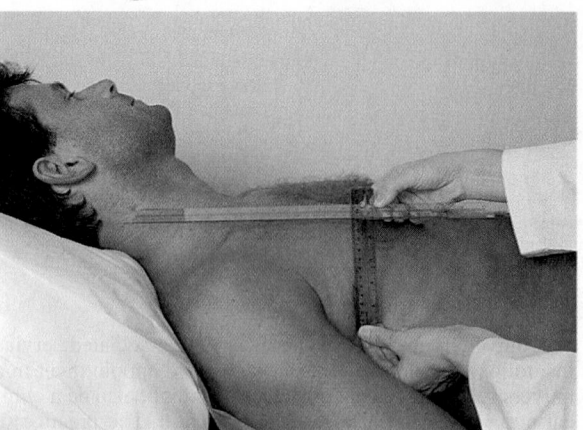

**Measurement of jugular venous pressure**
(Seidel et al, 1999)

**jugum** /jōō′gəm/ [L, yoke], a ridge or furrow joining to points.

**juice** /jōōs/ [L, *jus*, broth], any fluid secreted by the tissues of animals or plants. In humans it usually refers to the secretions of the digestive glands. Kinds of juices include **gastric juice, intestinal juice,** and **pancreatic juice.**

**jumentous** /jōōmen′təs/ [L, *jumentum*, beast of burden], having a strong animal odor, especially that of a horse. The term is used to describe the odor of urine during certain disease conditions.

**jumping disease,** any of several culture-specific disorders characterized by exaggerated responses to small stimuli, muscle tics including jumping, automatic obedience even to dangerous suggestions, and sometimes coprolalia or echolalia. It is unclear whether they are neurogenic or psychogenic in origin. Examples include **jumping Frenchmen of Maine syndrome** and **Gilles de la Tourette's syndrome.**

**jumping Frenchmen of Maine syndrome,** a form of jumping disease observed in a group of lumbermen of French-Canadian descent working in a remote area of Maine; affected individuals had exaggerated startle responses, automatic obedience, and often echolalia. It is believed to have represented a form of operant conditioning rather than a true disease. See also **jumping disease.**

**jumping gene.** See **transposon.**

**junction** /jungk′shən/ [L, *jungere*, to join], an interface or meeting place for tissues or structures.

**junctional bigeminy** /jungk′shənəl/ [L, *jungere*, to join, *bis*, twice, *geminus*, twin], cardiac arrhythmia in which each sinus beat is followed by a junctional beat after a constant delay.

**junctional epithelium** [L, *jungere*, to join; Gk, *epi + thele*, nipple], an area of epithelial soft tissue surrounding the abutment post of a tooth. Also called **attached epithelial cuff, epithelial cuff, gingival cuff.**

**junctional extrasystole** [L, *jungere*, to join, *extra*, beyond; Gk, *systole*, contraction], a premature heartbeat that usually arises from the junction of the atrioventricular (AV) node and the AV bundle, the primary junctional pacing site, but may also arise from within the AV bundle.

**junctional rhythm,** a cardiac rhythm usually originating at the junction of the atrioventricular (AV) node and the AV bundle. It may be a normal escape rhythm (rate less than 60/min) or an active focus (rate 60/min or greater).

**junctional tachycardia,** a junctional rhythm with a rate greater than 100/min. The mechanism may be enhanced normal automaticity, abnormal automaticity, or triggered activity caused by digitalis toxicity.

**junction lines,** vertical lines that appear in the mediastinum on a posterior-anterior (P-A) projection radiographic image of the chest.

**junction nevus** [L, *jungere*, to join, *naevus*, birthmark], a hairless flat or slightly raised brown skin blemish arising from pigment cells at the epidermal-dermal junction. A junction nevus may be found anywhere on the surface of the body. Malignant change may be signaled by increase in size, hardness or darkening, bleeding, or appearance of satellite discoloration around the nevus. Junction nevi undergoing these changes and lesions found in areas subject to trauma should be evaluated by a dermatologist.

**junctura cartilaginea.** See **cartilaginous joint.**

**junctura fibrosa.** See **fibrous joint.**

**junctura synovialis.** See **synovial joint.**

**juncture,** a joint or union of two parts.

**Jungian psychology.** See **analytic psychology.**

**Junin fever.** See **Argentine hemorrhagic fever.**

**juniper tar** /jōō′nipər/ [L, *juniperus* + AS, *teoru*], a dark

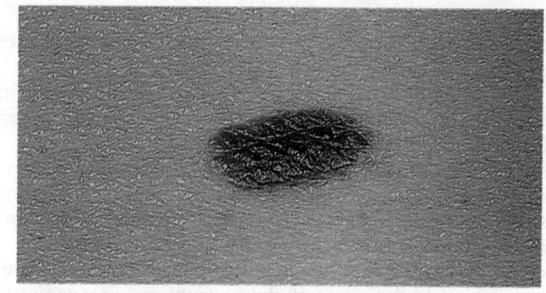

**Junction nevus** *(Habif, 1996)*

oily liquid obtained by the destructive distillation of the wood of *Juniperus oxycedrus* trees. It is used as an antiseptic stimulant in ointments for skin disorders such as psoriasis and eczema. Also called **Cade oil.**

**junk,** *slang.* **heroin.**

**jurisprudence** /jōō′risprōō′dəns/ [L, *jus*, law, *prudentia*, knowledge], the science and philosophy of law. **Medical jurisprudence** relates to the interfacing of medicine with criminal and civil law.

**justice** [L, *justus*, sufficient], a principle of fair and equal treatment for all, with due reward and honor.

**juvenile** /jōō′vənəl, -vənīl/ [L, *juvenus*, youthful], **1.** a young person; youth; child; youngster. **2.** pertaining to, characteristic of, or suitable for a young person; youthful. **3.** physiologically underdeveloped or immature. **4.** denoting psychologic or intellectual immaturity; childish.

**juvenile alveolar rhabdomyosarcoma,** a rapidly growing tumor of striated muscle occurring in children and adolescents, chiefly in the extremities. The prognosis is grave.

**juvenile angiofibroma.** See **nasopharyngeal angiofibroma.**

**juvenile delinquency,** persistent antisocial, illegal, or criminal behavior by children or adolescents to the degree that it cannot be controlled or corrected by the parents, it endangers others in the community, and it becomes the concern of a law enforcement agency.

**juvenile delinquent,** a person who performs illegal acts and who has not reached an age at which treatment as an adult can be accorded under the laws of the community having jurisdiction. Also called **juvenile offender, young offender.**

**juvenile diabetes.** See **type 1 diabetes mellitus.**

**juvenile glaucoma** [L, *juvenus*, young; Gk, *glaukcos*, bluish-gray], increased intraocular tension in a young adult caused by developing structural defects that restrict the outflow of fluid.

**juvenile kyphosis.** See **Scheuermann's disease.**

**juvenile laryngeal respiratory papillomatosis,** multiple squamous cell tumors that develop in the larynx, usually in young children. The growths are transmitted by a papilloma virus and may be acquired from the mother. The laryngeal papillomas tend to undergo periods of remission and recurrence over a period of several years.

**juvenile lentigo.** See **lentigo.**

**juvenile myoclonic syndrome,** a condition in which myoclonic seizures begin to appear around the time of puberty. The myoclonic jerks are more likely to occur immediately after awakening and are often associated with sleep deprivation and photosensitivity.

**juvenile myxedema.** See **childhood myxedema.**

**juvenile offender.** See **juvenile delinquent.**

**juvenile-onset diabetes, juvenile onset–type diabetes.** See **type 1 diabetes mellitus.**

**juvenile periodontitis,** an abnormal condition characterized by severe localized pocketing and bone loss in the dental alveoli of children and adolescents.

**juvenile rheumatoid arthritis (JRA),** a form of rheumatoid arthritis, usually affecting the larger joints of children less than 16 years of age and often accompanied by systemic manifestations. As bone growth in children is dependent on the epiphyseal plates of the distal epiphyses, skeletal development may be impaired if these structures are damaged. Treatment is supportive and includes analgesia, antiinflammatory medication, and rest. Also called **Still's disease.**

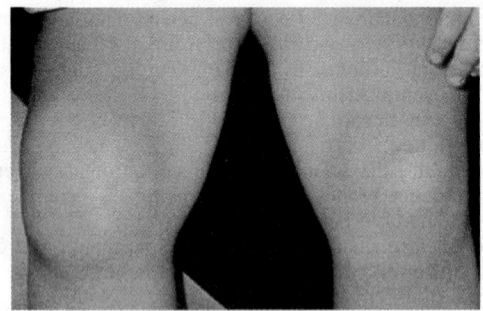

**Juvenile rheumatoid arthritis: swelling and inflammation of the knees**
*(Zitelli and Davis, 1997)*

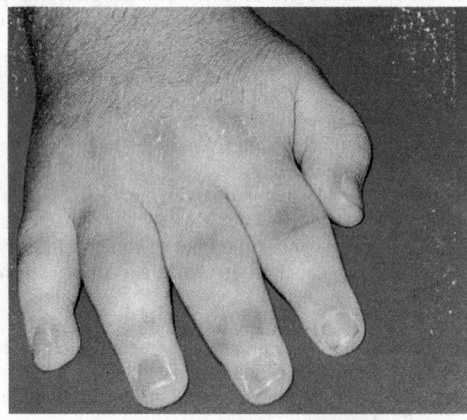

**Juvenile rheumatoid arthritis: deformity of the fingers**
*(Zitelli and Davis, 1997)*

**juvenile spinal muscular atrophy,** a disorder beginning in childhood in which progressive degeneration of anterior horn and medullary nerve cells leads to skeletal muscle wasting. The condition usually begins in the legs and pelvis. Also called **Wohlfart-Kugelberg-Welander disease.**

**juvenile xanthogranuloma,** a skin disorder characterized by groups of yellow, red, or brown papules or nodules on the extensor surfaces of the arms and legs, and in some cases on the eyeball, meninges, and testes. The lesions typically appear in infancy or early childhood and usually disappear in a few years.

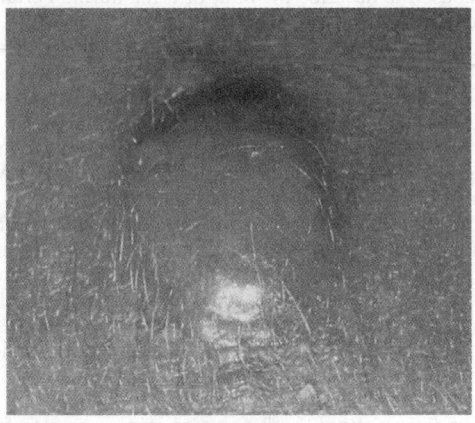

**Juvenile xanthogranuloma** *(Zitelli and Davis, 1997)*

**juxta-,** prefix meaning 'near': *juxtaglomerular, juxtangina, juxtaposition.*

**juxtaarticular** /juk′stə·ärtik′yələr/ [L, *juxta,* near, *articulus,* joint], pertaining to a location near a joint.

**juxtacrine** /juks′təkrin/, describing a hormonal relationship in which the secretory cell is adjacent to an effector cell.

**juxtaglomerular** /-glōmer′ələr/ [L, *juxta,* near, *glomerulus,* small ball], pertaining to an area near or adjacent to the afferent and efferent arterioles of the kidney glomerulus.

**juxtaglomerular apparatus,** a collection of cells located beside each renal glomerulus, consisting of a portion of the distal convoluted tubule arising from that glomerulus, segments of the afferent and efferent arterioles closest to the glomerulus, and cells lying between these structures. It is involved in the secretion of renin in response to blood pressure changes and is important in autoregulation of certain kidney functions. Also called **juxtaglomerular complex.**

**juxtaglomerular cells** [L, *juxta,* near, *glomerulus,* small ball, *cella,* storeroom], smooth myoepitheloid cells lining the glomerular end of the afferent arterioles in the kidney that are in opposition to the macula densa region of the early distal tubule. These cells synthesize and store renin and release it in response to decreased renal perfusion pressure, increased sympathetic nerve stimulation of the kidneys, or decreased sodium concentration in fluid in the distal tubule.

**juxtaglomerular complex.** See **juxtaglomerular apparatus.**

**juxtamedullary** /-med′ələr′ē/, near the border of a medulla.

**juxtaposition** /-pəzish′ən/, the placement of objects side by side or end to end.

**JVP,** abbreviation for **jugular venous pressure.**

**J wave.** See **Osborn wave.**

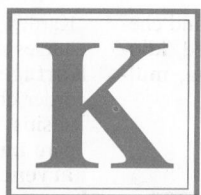

**k,** abbreviation for **kilo,** 1000, or $10^3$.

**K, 1.** symbol for **ionization constant. 2.** symbol for **Kelvin scale. 3.** symbol for the element **potassium** (kalium). **4.** abbreviation for **kilobyte. 5.** symbol in electronics for 1024 ($2^{10}$). **6.** abbreviation for **katal.**

**K$_m$,** symbol for *Michaelis-Menten constant.* See **Michaelis-Menten kinetics.**

**kA,** abbreviation for *kiloampere.*

**-kacin,** suffix for antibiotics derived from *Streptomyces kanamyceticus.*

**kainate** /kī′nāt/, a non-NMDA (*N*-methyl-D-aspartate) receptor agonist. The natural mineral is used as a fertilizer.

**kak-,** combining form meaning 'bad': *kakidrosis, kakosmia.*

**kakosmia.** See **cacosmia.**

**kala-azar** /kä′lə·äzär′/ [Hindi, *kala,* black; Assamese, *azar,* fever], a disease caused by the protozoan *Leishmania donovani,* transmitted to humans, particularly to children, by the bite of the sand fly. Kala-azar occurs primarily in Asia, parts of Africa, several South and Central American countries, and the Mediterranean region. The liver and spleen are the main sites of infection; signs and symptoms include anemia, hepatomegaly, splenomegaly, irregular fever, and emaciation. Patients with kala-azar are also susceptible to secondary bacterial infections. Untreated, the disease has an extremely high mortality. Treatment includes sodium antimony gluconate, blood transfusions (for anemia), bed rest, and adequate nutrition. Also called **Assam fever, black fever, dumdum fever, ponos, visceral leishmaniasis.** See also **leishmaniasis.**

**kalak** /kal′ak/, a pustular skin disease observed among Eskimos.

**kalemia** /kəlē′mē·ə/, the presence of potassium in the blood.

**kali-,** combining form meaning 'potassium': *kaligenous, kalinite, kalium.*

**kaliopenia.** See **hypokalemia.**

**kalium (K)** /kā′lē·əm/ [Ar, *quali,* potash], potassium.

**kaliuresis** /kal′iyŏŏrē′sis/, the excretion of potassium in the urine.

**kallikrein-kinin system** /kalik′rē·in-/, a proposed hormonal system that functions within the kidney, with the enzyme kallikrein in the renal cortex mediating production of bradykinin, which acts as a vasodilator peptide. Kallikrein is present in blood plasma, urine, and tissues in an inactive state. Also spelled **kallikren-kinin system.**

**Kallmann's syndrome** [Franz J. Kallmann, American psychiatrist, 1897–1965], a condition characterized by the absence of the sense of smell. It is caused by agenesis of the olfactory bulbs and secondary hypogonadism related to a decrease of luteinizing hormone-releasing hormone.

**kanamycin** /kan′əmī′sin/, an antibacterial substance derived from *Streptomyces kanamyceticus.*

**kanamycin sulfate,** an aminoglycoside antibiotic.

■ INDICATIONS: It is prescribed in the treatment of certain severe infections and those resistant to other antibiotics.

■ CONTRAINDICATIONS: Concomitant administration of ototoxic drugs or known hypersensitivity to this drug or to other aminoglycoside antibiotics prohibits its use. It is used with caution in patients having impaired renal function and in the elderly.

■ ADVERSE EFFECTS: Among the more serious adverse reactions are nephrotoxicity, vestibular and auditory ototoxicity, neuromuscular blockade, and hypersensitivity reactions.

**kangaroo care,** a nursing intervention from the Nursing Interventions Classification (NIC) defined as promoting closeness between parent and physiologically stable preterm infant by preparing the parent and providing the environment for skin-to-skin contact. See also **Nursing Interventions Classification.**

**Kanner's syndrome** [Leo Kanner, Austrian-born American child psychiatrist, b. 1894], a form of infantile psychosis with an onset in the first 30 months of life. It is characterized by infantile autism, with signs of lack of attachment, avoidance of eye contact, and general failure to develop social relationships; rituals and compulsive behavior manifested by a resistance to change and repetitive acts; general intellectual retardation; and language disorders, which may range from muteness to echolalia. Treatment may include psychotherapy and special education, depending on the child's intelligence level.

**Kantrex,** trademark for an antibacterial (kanamycin sulfate).

**Kaochlor,** trademark for an electrolyte-replacement solution (potassium chloride).

**kaodzera.** See **Rhodesian trypanosomiasis.**

**kaolin** /kā′əlin/ [Chin, *kao-ling,* high ridge], an adsorbent used internally to treat diarrhea, often in combination with pectin. Kaolin in an ointment base is also used topically as an absorbent and a protective emollient.

**kaolinosis** /kā′əlinō′sis/, a form of pneumoconiosis acquired by inhaling clay dust (kaolin). Kaolin is used in the manufacture of paper, ceramics, heat-resistant wood, soaps, toothpaste, and some medicines.

**Kaon Cl,** trademark for an electrolyte-replacement (potassium chloride).

**Kaopectate,** trademark for an antidiarrheal fixed-combination drug containing an adsorbent (kaolin) and an emollient (pectin).

**Kaposi's disease** /kap′əsēz/ [Moritz K. Kaposi, Austrian dermatologist, 1837–1902; L, *dis* + Fr, *aise,* ease], a rare inherited skin disorder that begins in childhood and involves mainly exposed skin areas. Exposure to sunlight results in erythema and vesiculation, followed by increased pigmentation and telangiectasia, skin ulcers, warts, and malignant epitheliomas. Also called **xeroderma pigmentosum.**

**Kaposi's sarcoma (KS, ks)** [Moritz K. Kaposi], a malignant, multifocal neoplasm of reticuloendothelial cells that begins as soft brownish or purple papules on the feet and slowly spreads in the skin, metastasizing to the lymph nodes and viscera. It occurs most often in men and is associated with diabetes, malignant lymphoma, acquired immunodeficiency syndrome, or other disorders. Radiotherapy and chemotherapy are usually recommended. Also called **idiopathic multiple pigmented hemorrhagic sarcoma, multiple idiopathic hemorrhagic sarcoma.**

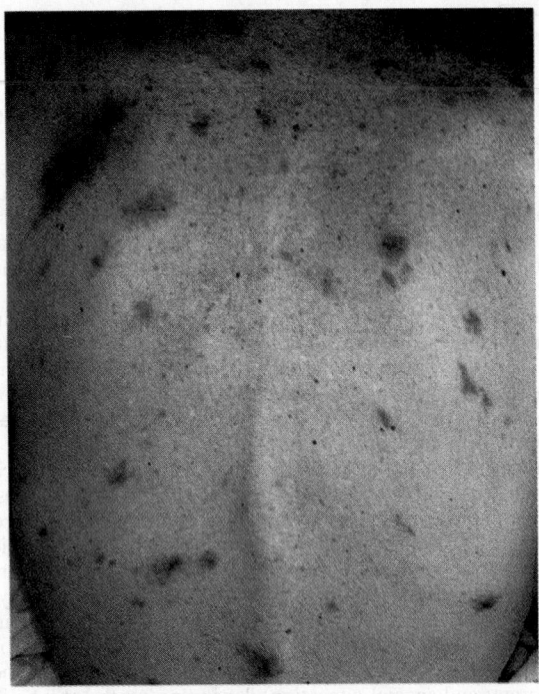

**Kaposi's sarcoma** *(Callen et al, 1993)*

**Kaposi's sarcoma—associated herpesvirus.** See **human herpesvirus 8.**

**Kaposi's varicelliform eruption.** See **eczema herpeticum.**

**kappa** /kap′ə/, K, κ, the tenth letter of the Greek alphabet, used to denote (in chemistry) the tenth carbon atom in a chain; one of two light chains in an immunoglobulin molecule; a type of killer particle present in certain strains of *Paramecium;* and a visual axis angle.

**kappa** (κ) **light chain,** one of two kinds of smaller peptide chains present in an immunoglobulin molecule. See also **lambda** (λ) **light chain.**

**kaps-.** See **caps-.**

**karaya powder** /kär′äyä/ [Hindi, *karayal,* resin; L, *pulvis,* dust], a dried form of *Sterculia urens* or other species of *Sterculia,* used as a bulk cathartic. The use of such a bulk-forming cathartic may also increase the loss of sodium, potassium, and water. With some individuals the use of karaya powder may cause allergic reactions such as urticaria, rhinitis, dermatitis, and asthma. Methylcellulose has largely replaced this drug in modern use. Externally it is used as a drying agent for stage I and stage II pressure ulcers.

**Kardex,** trademark for a card-filing system that allows quick reference to the particular needs of each patient for certain aspects of nursing care. Included on the card may be a schedule of medications, level of activity allowed, ability to perform basic self-care, diet, any special problems, a schedule of treatments and procedures, and a care plan. The Kardex is updated as necessary and is usually kept at the nurses' station.

**Kartagener's syndrome** /kärtag′ənərz/, an inherited disorder characterized by bronchiectasis, chronic paranasal sinusitis, and transposed viscera, usually dextrocardia. Compare **immotile cilia syndrome.**

**karyenchyma.** See **karyolymph.**

**karyo-** /ker′ē·ō-/, combining form meaning 'nucleus': *karyochrome, karyokinesis, karyolymph.*

**karyoclasis, karyoclastic.** See **karyoklasis.**

**karyocyte** /ker′ē·əsīt′/ [Gk, *karyon,* nut + *kytos,* cell], a normoblast, or developing red blood cell with a nucleus condensed into a homogenous staining body. It is normally found in the red bone marrow.

**karyogamy** /ker′ē·og′əmē/ [Gk, *karyon,* nut + *gamos,* marriage], the fusion of cell nuclei, as in conjugation and zygosis. —**karyogamic,** *adj.*

**karyogenesis** /ker′ē·ōjen′əsis/ [Gk, *karyon* + *genein,* to produce], the formation and development of the nucleus of a cell. —**karyogenetic,** *adj.*

**karyokinesis** /ker′ē·ōkinē′sis, -kīnē′sis/ [Gk, *karyon* + *kinesis,* motion], the division of the nucleus and equal distribution of nuclear material during mitosis and meiosis. The process involves the four stages of prophase, metaphase, anaphase, and telophase; it precedes the division of the cytoplasm. Also called **karyomitosis.** See also **cytokinesis.** —**karyokinetic,** *adj.*

**karyoklasis** /ker′ē·ok′ləsis/ [Gk, *karyon* + *klasis,* breaking], **1.** the disintegration of a cell nucleus or nuclear membrane. **2.** the interruption of mitosis. Also spelled **karyoclasis.** —**karyoclastic, karyoklastic,** *adj.*

**karyology** /ker′ē·ol′əjē/ [Gk, *karyon* + *logos,* science], the branch of cytology that concentrates on the study of the cell nucleus, especially the structure and function of the chromosomes. —**karyologic, karyological,** *adj.,* **karyologist,** *n.*

**karyolymph** /ker′ē·əlimf′/ [Gk, *karyon* + *lympha,* water], the clear, usually nonstaining, fluid substance of a cell nucleus. It consists primarily of proteinaceous, colloidal material in which the nucleolus, chromatin, linin, and various submicroscopic particles are dispersed. Also called **karyenchyma, nuclear hyaloplasm, nuclear sap, nucleochyme.** —**karyolymphatic,** *adj.*

**karyolysis** /ker′ē·ol′isis/ [Gk, *karyon* + *lysis,* loosening], the dissolution of a cell nucleus. It occurs normally, both as a form of necrobiosis and during the generation of new cells through mitosis and meiosis.

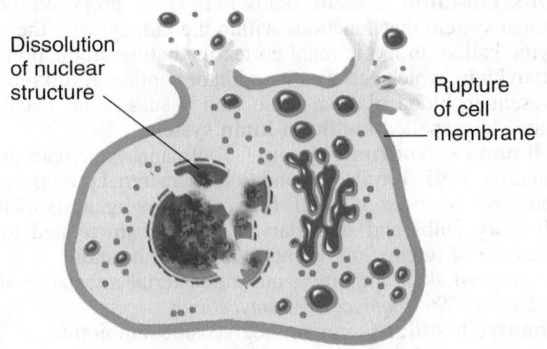

**Karyolysis** *(Huether and McCance, 2000)*

**karyolytic** /ker′ē·əlit′ik/, **1.** pertaining to karyolysis. **2.** something that causes the destruction of a cell nucleus.

**karyomegaly** /ker′ē·ōmeg′əlē/ [Gk, *karyon,* nut + *megas,* large], an increase in the nuclear size of tissue cells.

**karyomere** /ker′ē·əmir′/ [Gk, *karyon* + *meros,* part], **1.** a saclike structure containing an unequal portion of the nuclear material after atypical mitosis. **2.** a segment of a chromosome. See also **chromomere.**

**karyometry** /ker′ē·om′ətrē/, the measurement of the nucleus of a cell. —**karyometric,** *adj.*

**karyomit** /ker′ē·əmit′/ [Gk, *karyon* + *mitos,* thread], **1.** a single chromatin fibril of the network within the nucleus of a cell. **2.** a chromosome.

**karyomitome** /ker′ē·om′itōm/ [Gk, *karyon* + *mitos,* thread], the fibrillar chromatin network within the nucleus of a cell. Also called **karyoreticulum.**

**karyomitosis.** See **karyokinesis.**

**karyomorphism** /-môr′fizəm/ [Gk, *karyon* + *morphe,* form], the shape or form of a cell nucleus, especially that of a leukocyte. —**karyomorphic,** *adj.*

**karyon** /ker′ē·on/ [Gk, nut], the nucleus of a cell. —**karyontic,** *adj.*

**karyophage** /ker′ē·ōfāj′/ [Gk, *karyon* + *phagein,* to eat], an intracellular protozoan parasite that destroys the nucleus of the cell it infects. —**karyophagic, karyophagous,** *adj.*

**karyoplasm.** See **nucleoplasm.**

**karyoplasmic ratio.** See **nucleocytoplasmic ratio.**

**karyopyknosis** /-piknō′sis/ [Gk, *karyon* + *pyknos,* thick], the state of a cell in which the nucleus has shrunk and the chromatin has condensed into solid masses, as in cornified cells of stratified squamous epithelium. —**karyopyknotic,** *adj.*

**karyoreticulum.** See **karyomitome.**

**karyorrhexis** /-rek′sis/ [Gk, *karyon* + *rhexis,* rupture], the fragmentation of chromatin and distribution of it throughout the cytoplasm as a result of nuclear disintegration. —**karyorrhectic,** *adj.*

**karyosome** /ker′ē·əsōm′/ [Gk, *karyon* + *soma,* body], a dense, irregular mass of chromatin filaments in a cell nucleus. It is often seen during interphase and may be confused with the nucleolus because of similar staining properties. Also called **chromatin nucleolus, chromocenter, false nucleolus, prochromosome.**

**karyospheric** /-sfer′ik/ [Gk, *karyon* + *sphaira,* ball], **1.** a spheric nucleus. **2.** pertaining to such a nucleus.

**karyostasis** /ker′ē·os′təsis/ [Gk, *karyon* + *stasis,* standing], the resting stage of the nucleus between cell division. See also **interphase.** —**karyostatic,** *adj.*

**karyotheca.** See **nuclear envelope.**

**karyotin.** See **chromatin.**

**karyotype** /ker′ē·ətīp′/ [Gk, *karyon* + *typos,* mark], **1.** the number, form, size, and arrangement within the nucleus of the somatic chromosomes of an individual or species, as determined by a microphotograph taken during metaphase of mitosis. **2.** a diagrammatic representation of the chromosome complement of an individual or species, in which the chromosomes are arranged in pairs in descending order of size and according to the position of the centromere. See also **chromosome, Denver classification.** —**karyotypic,** *adj.*

**Kasabach-Merritt syndrome.** See **hemangioma-thrombocytopenia syndrome.**

**Kasabach method** /kas′əbak/, (in radiology) a technique for positioning a patient for radiographic examination of the odontoid process.

**Kasai operation.** See **portoenterostomy.**

**Kashin-Bek disease** [Nikolai I. Kashin, Russian orthopedist, 1825–1872; E.V. Bek; L, *dis* + Fr, *aise,* ease], a form of osteoarthrosis afflicting mainly children living in China, Korea, and eastern Siberia. It is believed to be caused by eating foods made with wheat contaminated by a fungus, *Fusarium sporotrichiella.* Also spelled **Kaschin-Beck disease.** Also called **osteoarthritis deformans edemica.**

**kat,** abbreviation for **katal.**

**kat-, kata-, cat-, cata-,** prefix meaning 'to go down, to go against, or to reverse': *katadidymus, katakinetomeric, katolysis.*

**katadidymus** /kat′ədid′əməs/ [Gk, *kata,* down + *didymos,* twin], conjoined twins united in the lower portion of the body and separated at the top.

**katal (K, kat)** /kat′al/ [Gk, *kata,* down], an enzyme unit in moles per second defined by the SI system: $1 K = 6.6 \times 10^9$ U.

**kava,** an herb that is harvested from a shrub that grows in the South Sea islands.

■ USES: This herb is used for nervous anxiety, restlessness, sleep disturbances, and stress.

■ CONTRAINDICATIONS: Kava should not be used during pregnancy and lactation, in children less than 12 years of age, or in those with known hypersensitivity, major depressive disorder, or Parkinson's disease.

**Kawasaki disease.** See **mucocutaneous lymph node syndrome.**

**Kay Ciel,** trademark for an electrolyte replacement solution (potassium chloride).

**Kayser-Fleischer ring** /kī′zər flī′shər/ [Bernhard Kayser, German ophthalmologist, 1869–1954; Bruno Fleischer, German ophthalmologist, 1874–1904], a gray-green to red-gold pigmented ring at the outer margin of the cornea, pathognomonic of hepatolenticular degeneration, a rare progressive disease caused by a defect in copper metabolism and transmitted as an autosomal-recessive trait. The disease is characterized by cerebral degenerative changes, liver cirrhosis, splenomegaly, involuntary movements, muscle rigidity, psychic disturbances, and dysphagia. See also **Wilson's disease.**

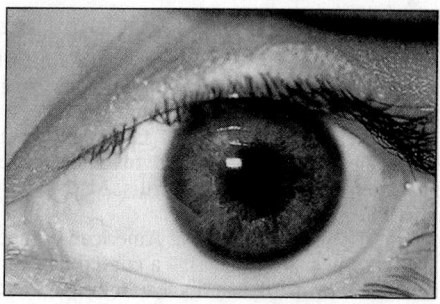

**Kayser-Fleischer ring as seen in Wilson's disease**
*(Perkin, 1998)*

**Kazanjian's operation** /kasan′jē·ənz/ [Varaztad J. Kazanjian, Armenian-born maxillofacial surgeon in U.S., 1879–1974], a surgical procedure for extending the vestibular sulcus to improve the prosthetic foundation of toothless dental ridges.

**kb,** **1.** abbreviation for **kilobase.** **2.** abbreviation for **kilobyte.**

**kbe,** abbreviation for *keyboard entry.*

**kbp,** abbreviation for **kilobase pair.**

**kbs,** abbreviation for *kilobits per second.* Also *kpps.*

**kcal,** abbreviation for **kilocalorie.**

**kcalorie.** See **Calorie (Cal).**

**K cell.** See **null cell.**

**kCi,** abbreviation for *kiloCurie.*

**KE,** abbreviation for **kinetic energy.**

**Kearns-Sayre syndrome** /kernz·sār/ [Thomas P. Kearns, American ophthalmologist, b. 1922; George P. Sayre, American pathologist, b. 1911], progressive ophthalmoplegia, pigmentary degeneration of the retina, myopathy, ataxia, and cardiac conduction defect; onset is before age 20. Almost all patients have large mitochondrial DNA deletions, and ragged red fibers are seen on muscle biopsy. Also called **ophthalmoplegia plus.**

**Kedani fever.** See **scrub typhus.**

**keel,** (in prosthetics) a device in a stored-energy foot prosthesis that bends the foot upward when weight is applied to the toe. See also **carina, Seattle Foot, stored-energy foot.**

**kefir** /kef′ər/ [Russ, fermented milk], a slightly effervescent, acidulous beverage prepared from the milk of cows, sheep, or goats through fermentation by kefir grains, which contain yeasts and lactobacilli. It is an important source of the bacteria necessary in the GI tract to synthesize vitamin K. Also spelled **kephir.**

**Keflex,** trademark for an antibacterial (cephalexin).

**Kefzol,** trademark for an antibacterial (cefazolin sodium).

**Kegel exercises.** See **pubococcygeus exercises.**

**Keith-Flack node.** See **sinoatrial (SA) node.**

**Keith's bundle.** See **sinoatrial (SA) node.**

**Keith-Wagener-Barker classification system** [Norman M. Keith, Canadian physician, b. 1885; Henry P. Wagener, American physician, b. 1890; N. W. Barker, 20th century American physician], a method of classifying the degree of hypertension in a patient on the basis of retinal changes. The stages are group 1, identified by constriction of the retinal arterioles; group 2, constriction and sclerosis of the retinal arterioles; group 3, characterized by hemorrhages and exudates in addition to group 2 conditions; and group 4, papilledema of the retinal arterioles.

**kel-,** combining form meaning 'tumor or fibrous growth': *kelectome, keloid, keloplasty.*

**Kellgren's syndrome** /kel′grinz/ [Henry Kellgren, Swedish physician, b. 1827], a form of osteoarthritis affecting the proximal and distal interphalangeal joints, the first metatarsophalangeal and carpometacarpal joints, the knees, and the spine. The absence of rheumatoid factor and rheumatoid nodules and the lack of systemic involvement differentiate this syndrome from rheumatoid arthritis. Also called **erosive osteoarthritis.**

**Kelly clamp** [Howard A. Kelly, American gynecologist, 1858–1943; AS, *clam,* to fasten], a curved hemostat without teeth, used primarily in gynecologic procedures for grasping vascular tissue.

**Kelly's pad,** a horseshoe-shaped inflatable rubber drainage pad used in a bed or on the operating table.

**keloid** /kē′loid/ [Gk, *kelis,* spot + *eidos,* form], an overgrowth of collagenous scar tissue at the site of a skin injury, particularly a wound or a surgical incision. The new tissue is elevated, rounded, and firm. Young women and African-Americans are particularly susceptible to keloid formation. Types of therapy include solid carbon dioxide, liquid nitrogen, intralesional corticosteroid injections, radiation, silicon gel, and surgery. Treatment may worsen the condition and should be performed only by skilled professionals. Also spelled **cheloid.** —**keloidal, cheloidal,** *adj.*

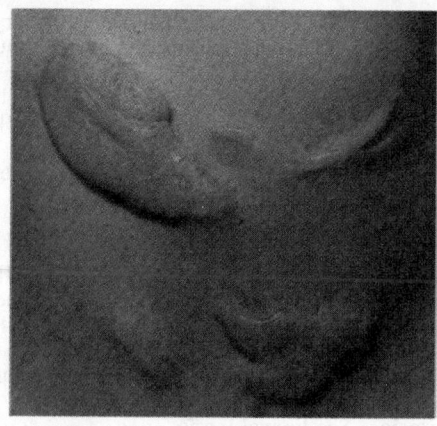

**Keloids** *(Zitelli and Davis, 1997)*

**keloid acne** [Gk, *kelis,* spot + *eidos,* form + *akme,* point], pyoderma in and around the pilosebaceous structures, resulting in keloid scarring. African-Americans are highly susceptible. Also called **dermatitis papillaris capillitii, folliculitis keloidalis.**

**keloidal.** See **keloid.**

**keloidal scar.** See **keloid.**

**keloidosis** /kē′loidō′sis/ [Gk, *kelis* + *eidos,* form + *osis,* condition], habitual or multiple formation of keloids. Also spelled **cheloidosis.**

**keloid scar** [Gk, *kelis,* spot + *eidos,* form *eschara,* scab], an overgrowth of tissue in a scar at the site of skin injury, particularly a wound or a surgical incision. The amount of tissue growth is in excess of that necessary to repair the wound and is partially caused by an accumulation of collagen at the site. Also called **keloidal scar.**

**kelp** [ME, *culp*], **1.** any of the brown seaweed species of *Laminaria* found on the Atlantic coast of Europe. **2.** the ashes of *Laminaria* seaweed burned in a process of extracting iodine and potassium salts.

**Kelvin scale (K)** [Lord Kelvin (William Thomson), British physicist, 1824–1907], an absolute temperature scale calculated in Celsius units from the point at which molecular activity apparently ceases, −273.15° C. To convert Celsius degrees to Kelvin, add 273.15.

**Kemadrin,** trademark for an antiparkinsonian skeletal muscle relaxant (procyclidine hydrochloride).

**Kempner rice-fruit diet.** See **rice diet.**

**Kenalog,** trademark for a glucocorticoid (triamcinolone acetonide).

**Kennedy classification** [Edward Kennedy, American dentist, b. 1883], a method of classifying partial edentulous conditions and partial dentures, based on the position of the spaces once occupied by the missing teeth in relation to the remaining teeth.

**Kenny treatment.** See **Sister Kenny's treatment.**

**keno-,** combining form meaning 'empty': *kenophobia, kenotoxin, kenotron.*

**kenogenesis.** See **cenogenesis.**

**kenophobia** /kē′nōfō′bē·ə/ [Gk, *kenos,* empty + *phobos,* fear], the morbid fear of large and open spaces; agoraphobia. Also called **cenophobia.**

**Kent bundle** [Albert F. S. Kent, English physiologist, 1863–1958; AS, *byndel,* to bind], an accessory pathway between an atrium and a ventricle outside of the conduction system.

This congenital anomaly causes Wolff-Parkinson-White syndrome. The term "accessory pathway" is preferred because the one Kent described had a precise location (anterior and near the fibrous ring of the tricuspid valve).

**Kenya fever.** See **Marseilles fever.**

**kephal-.** See **cephalo-.**

**kephir.** See **kefir.**

**kera-,** combining form meaning 'horn': *keracele, keraphyllocele, keratosis, keratin.*

**kerasin** /ker′əsin/ [L, *cera,* wax], a cerebroside, found in brain tissue, that consists of a fatty acid, galactose, and sphingosine.

**kerat-, kerato-,** 1. combining form meaning 'horny, cornified': *keratolysis, keratoma, keratonosis.* 2. combining form meaning 'cornea, corneal': *keratoiritis, keratoleukoma, keratome.*

**keratectomy** /ker′ətek′təmē/ [Gk, *keras,* horn + *ektomē,* excision], surgical removal of a part of the cornea performed to excise a small, superficial lesion that does not warrant a corneal graft. Local anesthesia is used. The scar is excised, and an antibiotic is injected under the conjunctiva. A topical steroid is given and a light pressure dressing applied. After surgery, the dressings are changed daily. Corneal epithelium grows rapidly, filling a small surgical area in about 60 hours.

**keratic** /kərat′ik/ [Gk, *keras,* horn + L, *icus,* like], 1. pertaining to keratin. 2. pertaining to the cornea.

**keratic precipitate,** a group of inflammatory cells deposited on the endothelial surface of the cornea after trauma or inflammation, sometimes obscuring vision.

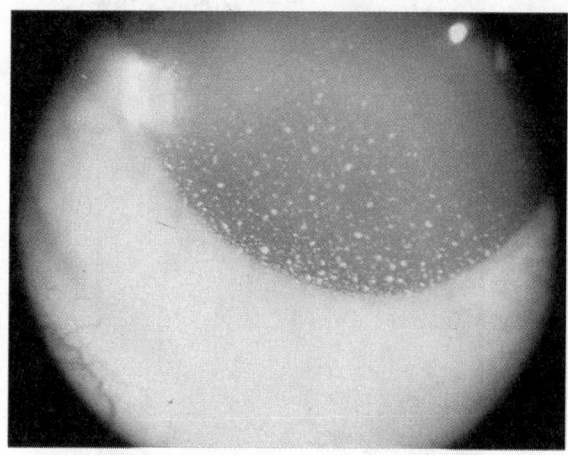

**Keratic precipitate** *(Michelson and Friedlaender, 1996)*

**keratin** /ker′ətin/ [Gk, *keras,* horn], a fibrous sulfur-containing protein that is the primary component of the epidermis, hair, nails, enamel of the teeth, and horny tissue of animals. The protein is insoluble in most solvents, including gastric juice. For this reason, it is often used as a coating for pills that must pass through the stomach unchanged to be dissolved in the intestines.

**keratin cyst,** an epithelial cyst containing keratin.

**keratinization** /-īzā′shən/ [Gk, *keras* + L, *izein,* to cause], a process by which epithelial cells lose their moisture and are replaced by horny tissue.

**keratinize** /ker′ətinīz/, to make or become horny tissue.

**keratinocyte** /kerat′inōsīt′/ [Gk, *keras* + *kytos,* cell], an epidermal cell that synthesizes keratin and other proteins and sterols. These cells constitute 95% of the epidermis, being formed from undifferentiated, or basal, cells at the dermal-epidermal junction. In its various successive stages, keratin forms the prickle cell layer and the granular cell layer, in which the cells become flattened and slowly die to form the final layer, the stratum corneum, which gradually exfoliates.

**keratinophilic** /kerat′inōfil′ik/, describing a type of fungi that uses keratin as a substrate.

**keratitis** /ker′ətī′tis/, any inflammation of the cornea. Kinds of keratitis include **dendritic keratitis, interstitial keratitis, keratoconjunctivitis sicca,** and **trachoma.** Compare **keratopathy. —keratic,** *adj.*

**keratoacanthoma** /ker′ətō·ak′anthō′mə/, *pl.* **keratoacanthomas, keratoacanthomata** [Gk, *keras* + *akantha,* thorn + *oma,* tumor], a benign, rapidly growing, flesh-colored papule or nodule of the skin with a central plug of keratin. The lesion is most common on the face or the back of the hands and arms. It disappears spontaneously in 4 to 6 months, leaving a slightly depressed scar. Biopsy is often necessary to differentiate it from a squamous carcinoma.

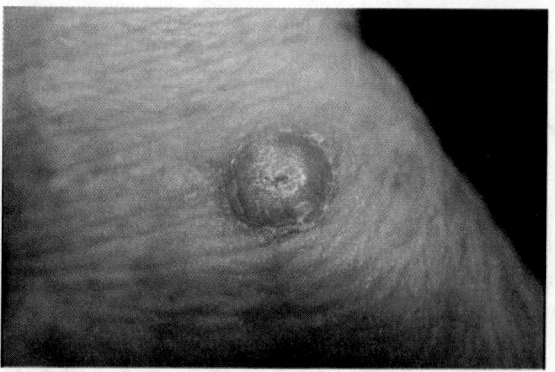

**Keratoacanthoma**
*(McCance and Huether, 1998/courtesy Department of Dermatology, School of Medicine, University of Utah)*

**keratocele** /ker′ətōsēl′/, a hernia of Descemet's membrane through an ulcer in the outer layers of the cornea.

**keratoconjunctivitis** /ker′ətōkənjungk′tivī′tis/ [Gk, *keras* + L, *conjunctivus,* connecting + Gk, *itis,* inflammation], inflammation of the cornea and the conjunctiva. Kinds of keratoconjunctivitis include **eczematous conjunctivitis, epidemic keratoconjunctivitis,** and **keratoconjunctivitis sicca.**

**keratoconjunctivitis sicca,** dryness of the cornea caused by a deficiency of tear secretion in which the corneal surface appears dull and rough and the eye feels gritty and irritated. The condition may be associated with erythema multiforme, Sjögren's syndrome, trachoma, and vitamin A deficiency. Methylcellulose artificial tears may give some relief.

**keratoconus** /ker′ətōkō′nəs/ [Gk, *keras* + *konos,* cone], a noninflammatory protrusion of the central part of the cornea. It is more common in females and may cause marked astigmatism; contact lenses usually restore visual acuity. The cause of the condition is unknown.

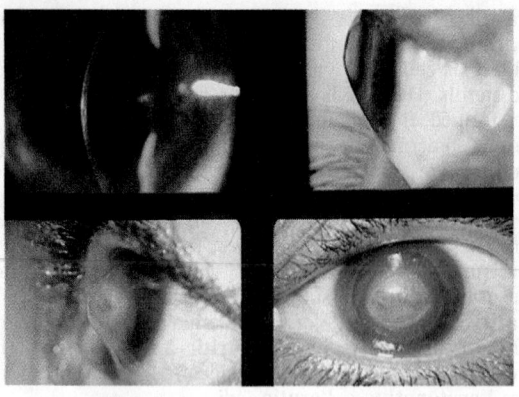

**Keratoconus** *(Apple and Rabb, 1998)*

**keratocyst** /ker′ətōsist′/, a thin-walled, tooth-forming cyst lined by keratinizing epithelium. It may be solitary or part of a multiple lesion, most frequently in the posterior body or ramus of the mandible, and may or may not be associated with teeth.

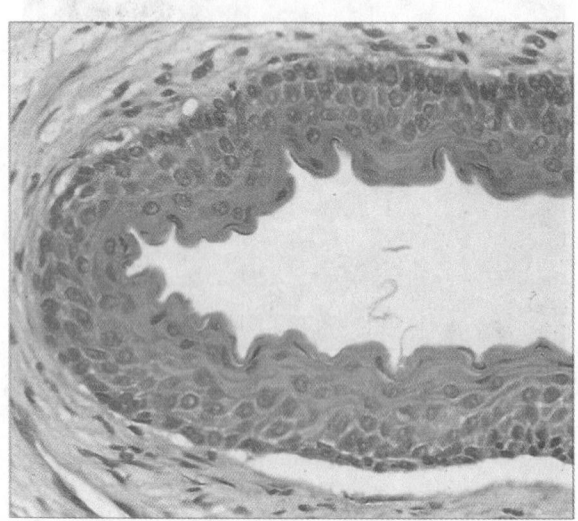

**Keratocyst** *(Eveson and Skully, 1995)*

**keratocyte.** See **corneal corpuscle.**

**keratoderma** /ker′ə·tō·dur′mə/ [Gk, *keras,* horn + *derma,* skin], **1.** a horny skin or covering. **2.** hypertrophy of the horny layer of the skin; see also **callus, hyperkeratosis.**

**keratoderma blennorrhagica** /-durmə/, the development of hyperkeratotic skin lesions of the palms, soles, and nails. The condition tends to occur in some patients with Reiter's syndrome.

**keratodermatitis** /-dur′mətī′tis/, an inflammation and proliferation of the cells of the horny layer of the skin.

**keratoectasia** /ker′ətō·ektā′zha/, a forward bulging or protrusion of the cornea. Also called **kerectasis.**

**keratoepithelioplasty** /-ep′ithē′lē·əplas′tē/, a surgical procedure for the repair of corneal epithelial defects. The defective cornea is removed and replaced with small pieces of donor cornea, which proliferate and replace the original tissue.

**keratogenesis** /-jen′əsis/, the formation of horny tissue caused by the growth of keratin-producing cells.

**keratogenic** /-jen′ik/, pertaining to an agent that induces a growth of horny tissue.

**keratogenous** /ker′ətoj′ənəs/, pertaining to development of the horny layer of the skin or its growth.

**keratoglobus** /-glō′bəs/, a congenital anomaly characterized by distension of the eyeball or the anterior segment of the eye. Also called **megalocornea.**

**keratohyalin** /-hī′əlin/ [Gk, *keras* + *hyalos,* glass], a substance in the granules found in keratinocytes of the epidermis. The keratohyalin granule develops within and around the fibrillar protein, contributing in an unknown manner to the functional maturity of keratin.

**keratoid** /ker′ətoid/ [Gk, *keras,* horn, *eidos,* form], resembling horny or corneal tissue.

**keratoiritis** /ker′ətō·īrī′tis/, an inflammation of the cornea in association with iritis.

**keratolysis** /ker′ətol′ə-sis/ [Gk, *keras* + *lysis,* loosening], the loosening and shedding of the outer layer of the skin, which may occur normally by exfoliation or as a congenital condition in which the skin is shed at periodic intervals. —**keratolytic,** *adj.*

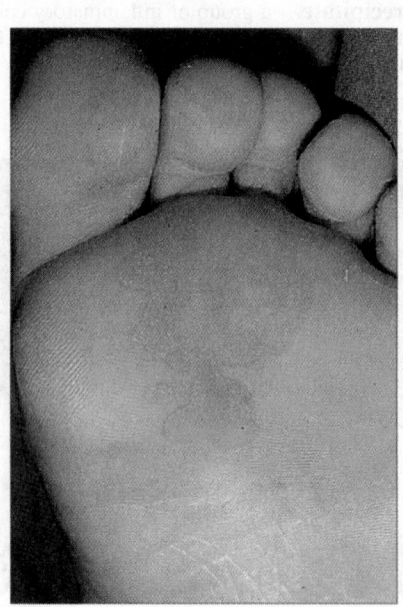

**Keratolysis** *(Lawrence and Cox, 1993)*

**keratoma** /ker′ətō′mə/, a hard, thick epidermal growth caused by hypertrophy of the horny layer of the skin. See also **callus.**

**keratomalacia** /-məlā′shə/ [Gk, *keras* + *malakia,* softness], a condition characterized by xerosis and ulceration of the cornea, resulting from severe vitamin A deficiency. It commonly occurs as a secondary result of diseases that affect vitamin A absorption or storage such as ulcerative colitis, celiac syndrome, cystic fibrosis, or sprue. Also at risk are infants and children who are given dilute formula, who are malnourished, or who are allergic to whole milk and fed skimmed milk, which is a poor source of vitamin A. Early symptoms include night blindness; photophobia; swelling and redness of the eyelids; and drying, roughness, pain, and wrinkling of the conjunctiva. In advanced deficiency, Bitot's spots appear; the cornea becomes dull, lusterless, and hazy, and without adequate therapy it eventually softens and perforates, resulting in blindness. Treatment consists of vitamin A supplements determined by the severity of the condition, although prolonged daily administration of large doses, especially to infants, may result in hypervitaminosis. An adequate diet containing whole milk and foods high in vitamin A or carotenes prevents the condition. See also **vitamin A.**

**keratosis** /ker′ətō′sis/ [Gk, *keras* + *osis,* condition], any skin lesion in which there is overgrowth and thickening of the cornified epithelium. Kinds of keratosis include **actinic keratosis, keratosis senilis,** and **seborrheic keratosis.** —**keratotic,** *adj.*

**keratosis follicularis,** a group of several skin disorders characterized by keratotic papules that coalesce to form brown or black, crusted, wartlike patches. These vegetations may spread widely, ulcerate, and become covered with a purulent exudate. Treatment includes large doses of topical or oral retinoids and oral or topical corticosteroids. Also called **Darier's disease.**

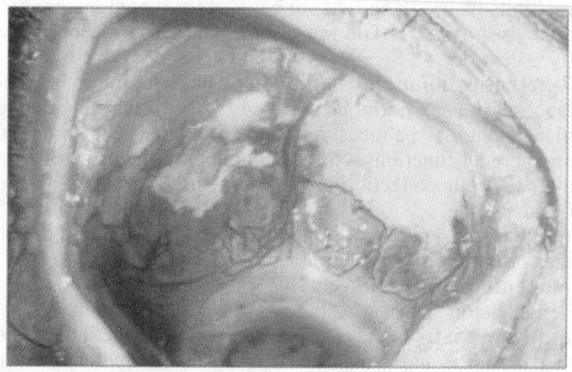

**Keratomalacia**
*(Michelson and Friedlaender, 1996/by permission of Wills Eye Hospital, Residents Teaching Collection)*

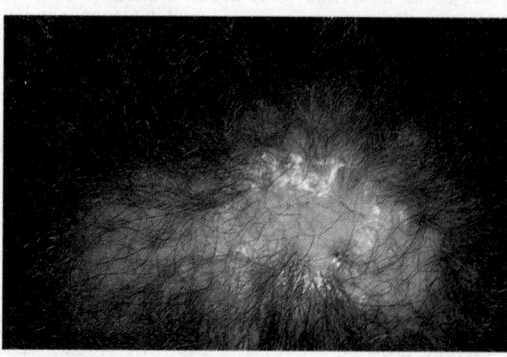

**Keratosis follicularis** *(Hordinsky, Sawaya, and Scher, 2000)*

**keratomycosis** /-mīkō′sis/, a fungal disease of the cornea.
**keratopathy** /ker′ətop′əthē/ [Gk, *keras* + *pathos,* disease], any noninflammatory disease of the cornea. Compare **keratitis.**
**keratophakia** /-fā′kē·ə/, the surgical implantation of donor cornea to the anterior cornea to modify a refractive error.
**keratoplasty.** See **corneal grafting.**

**keratosis seborrheica.** See **seborrheic keratosis.**
**keratosis senilis, keratotic.** See **keratosis.**
**kerauno-,** combining form meaning 'lightning': *keraunoneurosis, keraunophobia.*
**kerectasis.** See **keratoectasia.**
**kerion** /kir′ē·on/ [Gk, honeycomb], an inflamed, boggy granuloma that develops as an immune reaction to a superficial fungus infection, generally in association with *Tinea*

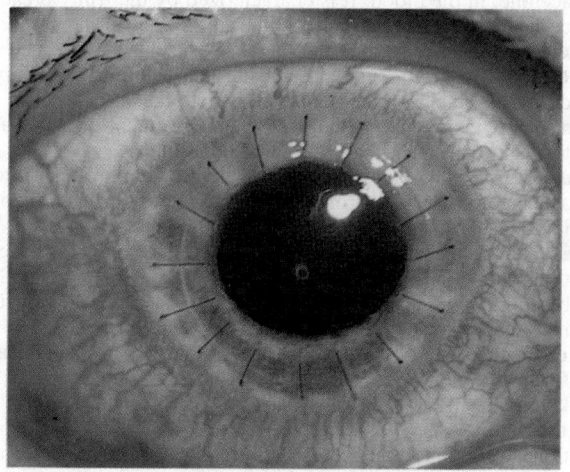

**Clinical appearance of the eye after keratoplasty**
*(Black, Hawks, and Keene, 2001/courtesy Ophthalmic Photography, University of Michigan W.K. Kellogg Eye Center, Ann Arbor)*

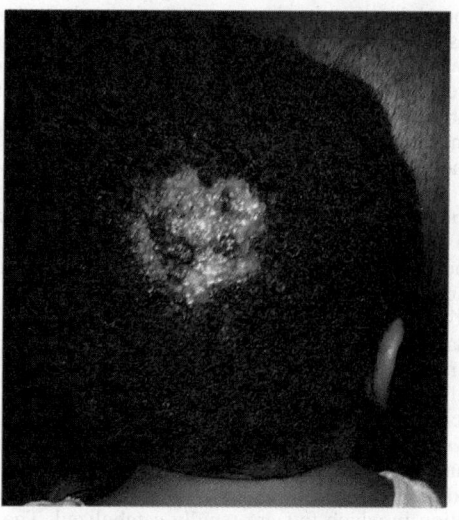

**Kerion** *(Shah, 2000)*

*capitis* of the scalp. The lesion heals within a short time without treatment.

**Kerley lines** /kur′lē/ [Peter J. Kerley, English radiologist, b. 1900], lines resembling interstitial infiltrate that appear on chest x-ray images and are associated with certain disease conditions, such as congestive heart failure and pleural lymphatic engorgement.. They are several centimeters long and may be oriented in many directions. Also called **everywhere lines.**

**KERMA,** abbreviation for *kinetic energy released in the medium,* a quantity that describes the transfer of energy from a photon to a medium as the ratio of energy transferred per unit mass at each point of interaction.

**kernicterus** /kərnik′tərəs/ [Ger, *kern,* kernel; Gk, *ikteros,* jaundice], an abnormal toxic accumulation of bilirubin in central nervous system tissues caused by hyperbilirubinemia. See also **hyperbilirubinemia of the newborn.**

**Kernig's sign** /ker′niks/ [Vladimir M. Kernig, Russian physician, 1840–1917], a diagnostic sign for meningitis marked by a loss of the ability of a supine patient to completely straighten the leg when it is fully flexed at the knee and hip. Pain in the lower back and resistance to straightening the leg constitutes a positive Kernig's sign. Usually the patient can extend the leg completely when the thigh is not flexed on the abdomen.

**kerosene poisoning** /ker′əsen/ [Gk, *keros,* wax; L, *potio,* drink], a toxic condition caused by the ingestion of kerosene or the inhalation of its fumes. Symptoms after ingestion include drowsiness, fever, a rapid heartbeat, tremors, and severe pneumonitis if the fluid is aspirated. Vomiting is not induced. See also **petroleum distillate poisoning.**

**Ketalar,** trademark for a general anesthetic (ketamine hydrochloride).

**ketamine hydrochloride** /kē′təmēn/, a potent nonbarbiturate general anesthetic induction agent administered parenterally to achieve dissociative anesthesia. Ketamine hydrochloride does not cause muscle relaxation. It is a potent somatic analgesic and is particularly useful for brief, minor surgical procedures. Hallucinations, confusion, and disorientation may occur on emergence from anesthesia can occur regardless. See also **dissociative anesthesia.**

**keto-** /kē′tō-/, combining form indicating possession of the carbonyl (=CO) group: *ketoheptose, ketolysis, ketonuria.*

**ketoacidosis** /-as′idō′sis/ [Gk, *keton,* form of acetone; L, *acidus,* sour, *osis,* condition], acidosis accompanied by an accumulation of ketones in the body, resulting from extensive breakdown of fats because of faulty carbohydrate metabolism. It occurs primarily as a complication of diabetes mellitus and is characterized by a fruity odor of acetone on the breath, mental confusion, dyspnea, nausea, vomiting, dehydration, weight loss, and, if untreated, coma. Emergency treatment includes the administration of insulin and IV fluids and the evaluation and correction of electrolyte imbalance. Nasogastric intubation and bladder catheterization may be required if the patient is comatose. Before discharge of the patient from the hospital, the nurse carefully reviews the diet, activity, blood glucose and urine ketone monitoring, and insulin schedule prescribed, emphasizing to the patient that ketoacidosis may be life-threatening and is largely avoidable by strict adherence to the patient's diabetic regimen, monitoring, and appropriate action for illness or stress. See also **diabetes mellitus, ketosis. —ketoacidotic,** *adj.*

**ketoaciduria** /-as′idoor′ē·ə/ [Gk, *keton* + L, *acidus,* sour; Gk, *ouron,* urine], presence in the urine of excessive amounts of ketone bodies, occurring as a result of uncontrolled diabetes mellitus, starvation, or any other metabolic condition in which fats are rapidly catabolized. The condi-

tion can be diagnosed with a dipstick reagent or acetone test tablet. Also called **ketonuria.** See also **Acetest, ketosis. —ketoaciduric,** *adj.*

**17-ketoandrosterone** /-andros′tərōn/, a metabolite of a sex hormone secreted by the testes and adrenal glands that may be measured in the urine to assess hormonal and adrenal functions. Normal amounts in the urine of men after 24-hour collection are 0.2 to 1 mg; in women, 0.2 to 0.8 mg.

**ketoconazole** /-kō′nəzōl/, an antifungal agent.

■ INDICATIONS: It is prescribed for the treatment of candidiasis, coccidioidomycosis, histoplasmosis, and other fungal diseases.

■ CONTRAINDICATIONS: Known hypersensitivity to this drug prohibits its use. It should not be used for fungal meningitis.

■ ADVERSE EFFECTS: The most serious adverse reactions are liver disorders.

**17-ketoetiocholanolone** /-kē′tō·ē′tē·ōkələn′əlōn/, a metabolite of a sex hormone secreted by the testes and adrenal glands that may be measured in the urine to assess hormonal and adrenal functions. Normal amounts in the urine of men after 24-hour collection are 0.2 to 1 mg; in women, 0.2 to 0.8 mg.

**ketogenesis** /-jen′əsis/ [Fr, *keton* + Gk, *genein,* to produce], the formation or production of ketone bodies.

**ketogenic amino acid** /-jen′ik/, an amino acid whose carbon skeleton serves as a precursor for ketone bodies.

**ketogenic diet,** a diet high in fats (often as medium chain triglycerides) and proteins and low in carbohydrates, often indicated in the treatment of epilepsy.

**ketonaemia.** See **ketonemia.**

**ketone** /kē′tōn/ [Fr, *acetone*], an organic chemical compound characterized by having in its structure a carbonyl, or keto, group, =CO, attached to two alkyl groups. It is produced by oxidation of secondary alcohols.

**ketone alcohol** [Gk, *keton* + Ar, *alkohl,* essence], an alcohol containing the ketone group.

**ketone bodies,** two products of lipid pyruvate metabolism, beta-hydroxybutyric acid and aminoacetic acid, from which acetone may arise spontaneously. Ketone bodies are produced via acetyl-CoA in the liver and are oxidized by the muscles. Excessive production leads to their excretion in urine, as in diabetes mellitus. Also called **acetone bodies.**

**ketone group,** the chemical carbonyl group with attached hydrocarbons. See also **ketone.**

**ketonemia** /kē′tōnē′mē·ə/, the presence of ketones, mainly acetone, in the blood. It is characterized by the fruity breath odor of ketoacidosis. Also spelled **ketonaemia.**

**ketonuria.** See **ketoaciduria.**

**ketoprofen** /-prō′fən/, a nonsteroidal antiinflammatory drug with analgesic and antipyretic actions.

■ INDICATIONS: It is prescribed for the treatment of rheumatoid and osteoarthritis and related conditions.

■ CONTRAINDICATIONS: Hypersensitivity to ketoprofen or to aspirin or other nonsteroidal antiinflammatory drugs prohibits its use.

■ ADVERSE EFFECTS: Among the more serious adverse reactions are GI disturbances, including peptic ulcer and GI bleeding; central nervous system effects of headache, dizziness, and drowsiness; and skin rash.

**ketose** /kē′tōs/ [Gk, *keton* + *glykys,* sweet], the chemical form of a monosaccharide in which the carbonyl group is a ketone.

**ketosis** /kitō′sis/ [Gk, *keton* + *glykys,* sweet + *osis,* condition], the abnormal accumulation of ketones in the body as a result of excessive breakdown of fats caused by a deficiency or inadequate use of carbohydrates. Fatty acids are metabolized instead, and the end products, ketones, begin to accumulate. This condition is seen in starvation, occasionally in pregnancy if the intake of protein and carbohydrates is inadequate, and most frequently in diabetes mellitus. It is characterized by ketonuria, loss of potassium in the urine, and a fruity odor of acetone on the breath. Untreated, ketosis may progress to ketoacidosis, coma, and death. See also **diabetes mellitus, ketoacidosis, starvation. —ketotic,** *adj.*

**ketosis-prone diabetes.** See **type 1 diabetes mellitus.**

**ketosis-resistant diabetes.** See **type 2 diabetes mellitus.**

**17-ketosteroid** /kē′tōstir′oid, kētō′stəroid/, any of the adrenal cortical hormones, or ketosteroids, that has a ketone group attached to its seventeenth carbon atom. They are commonly measured in the blood and urine to aid the diagnoses of Addison's disease; Cushing's syndrome; stress; and endocrine problems associated with precocious puberty, feminization in men, and excessive hair growth. Measured in patients in the morning, the normal concentration in plasma is less than 30 µg/dl; in the evening, less than 10 µg/dl. The normal amounts in the urine of men after 24-hour collection are 8 to 15 mg; in women, 6 to 11.5 mg; in children 12 to 15 years of age, 5 to 12 mg; in children younger than 12 years of age, less than 5 mg. Levels of 17-ketosteroids increase 50% to 100% after an injection of ACTH.

**17-ketosteroids test (17-KS),** a 24-hour urine test that is useful in diagnosing adrenocortical dysfunction. It is used to detect levels of 17-KS, which are metabolites of the testosterone and nontestosterone androgenic sex hormones secreted from the adrenal cortex and the testes.

**ketotic** /kētot′ik/ [Fr, *acetone*], **1.** pertaining to the presence of ketone in the body. **2.** denoting the presence of a carbonyl group in a chemical compound.

**keV,** an abbreviation for *kiloelectron volts,* an energy unit equivalent to 1000 electron volts. Also abbreviated *kev.*

**Kew Gardens spotted fever.** See **rickettsialpox.**

**keyboard,** a computer input device consisting of rows of switches with keytops marked as letters or numbers. Manual pressure on a series or combination of the keys generates an electronic code representing words, data, commands, or other input.

**keypad,** a numeric keyboard consisting of the numerals 1 to 9 arranged in three ranks of three keys each and an additional key for zero, as on some calculators.

**key pinch.** See **lateral pinch.**

**key points of control,** areas of the body that can be handled by a therapist in a specific manner to change an abnormal pattern, to reduce spasticity throughout the body, and to guide the patient's active movements. The key points are the shoulder and pelvic girdles.

**key ridge,** the lowest point of the zygomaticomaxillary ridge. Also called **zygomaxillare.**

**kg,** abbreviation for **kilogram.**

**kG,** abbreviation for *kilogauss.*

**kg cal,** abbreviation for *kilogram calorie.* See **calorie.**

**khat,** an herbal product taken from a tree found in Africa and the Arabian peninsula.

■ USES: This herb is used for obesity and gastric ulcers, and as a stimulant.

■ CONTRAINDICATIONS: Khat should not be used during pregnancy and lactation, in children, or in those with known hypersensitivity. People with renal, cardiac, or hepatic disease also should avoid its use.

**kHz,** abbreviation for **kilohertz.**

**kidney** [ME, *kidnere*], one of a pair of bean-shaped, purplish brown urinary organs in the dorsal part of the abdomen; one is located on each side of the vertebral column between the twelfth thoracic and third lumbar vertebrae. In

most individuals the right kidney is slightly lower than the left. Each kidney is about 11 cm long, 6 cm wide, and 2.5 cm thick. In the newborn the kidneys are about three times as large in proportion to the body weight as in the adult. The kidneys filter the blood and eliminate wastes in the urine through a complex filtration network and resorption system comprising more than 2 million nephrons. The nephrons are composed of glomeruli and renal tubules that filter blood under high pressure, removing urea, salts, and other soluble wastes from blood plasma and returning the purified filtrate to the blood. More than 1183 L of blood passes through the kidneys every day, entering the kidneys through the renal arteries and leaving through the renal veins. All the blood in the body passes through the kidneys about 20 times every hour, but only about one fifth of the blood volume is routed through the nephrons. The kidneys remove water as urine and return water that has been filtered to the blood plasma, thus helping to maintain the water balance of the body. Hormones, especially the antidiuretic hormone, produced by the pituitary gland, control the function of the kidneys in regulating the water-electrolyte balance of the body.

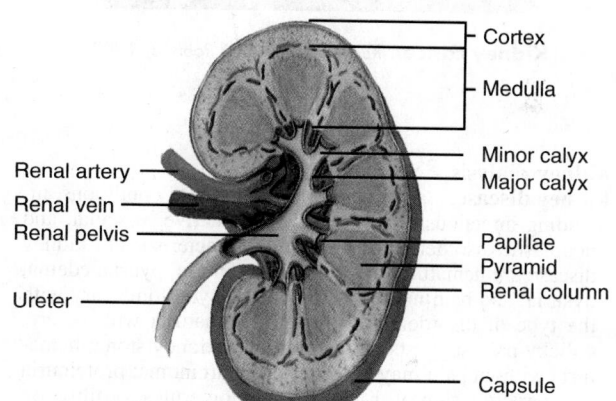

Renal artery
Renal vein
Renal pelvis
Ureter

Cortex
Medulla
Minor calyx
Major calyx
Papillae
Pyramid
Renal column
Capsule

**Kidney: coronal section** *(Applegate, 2000)*

**kidney cancer,** a malignant neoplasm of the renal parenchyma or renal pelvis. Factors associated with an increased incidence of disease are exposure to aromatic hydrocarbons or tobacco smoke and the use of drugs containing phenacetin. A long asymptomatic period may precede the onset of the characteristic symptoms, which include hematuria, flank pain, fever, and a palpable mass. Diagnostic measures include urinalysis, excretory urography, nephrotomography, ultrasonography, renal arteriography, and microscopic and cytologic studies of cells from the renal pelvis. Adenocarcinoma of the renal parenchyma accounts for 80% of kidney tumors, occurring twice as frequently in men as in women; transitional cell or squamous cell carcinomas in the renal pelvis account for approximately 15% and are equally frequent in men and women. Radical nephrectomy with lymph node dissection is usually recommended for tumors of the parenchyma; nephroureterectomy is usually recommended for operable tumors of the renal pelvis. Radiotherapy may be used before or after surgery and as palliation for inoperable tumors. Chemotherapeutic agents may induce temporary remission. See also **Wilms' tumor.**

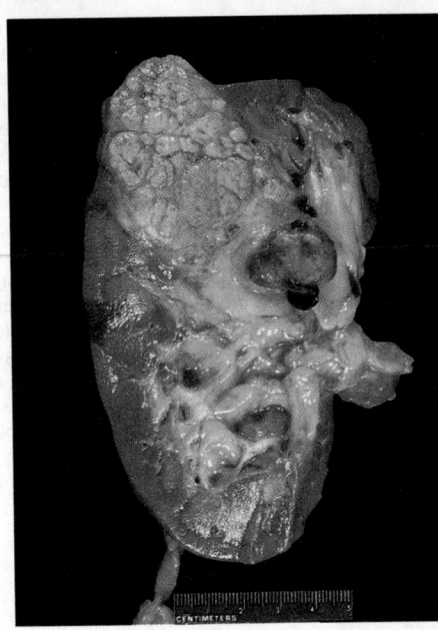

**Kidney cancer** *(Kumar, Cotran, and Robbins, 1997)*

**kidney dialysis.** See **hemodialysis.**

**kidney disease,** any one of a large group of conditions, including infectious, inflammatory, obstructive, vascular, and neoplastic disorders of the kidney. Characteristics of kidney disease are hematuria, persistent proteinuria, pyuria, edema, dysuria, and pain in the flank. Specific symptoms vary with the type of disorder. For example, hematuria with severe, colicky pain suggests obstruction by a kidney stone; hematuria without pain may indicate renal carcinoma; proteinuria is generally a sign of disease in the glomerulus, or filtration unit, of the kidney; pyuria indicates infectious disease; and edema is characteristic of the nephrotic syndrome. Diagnosis of kidney disease is made after laboratory tests and other procedures have been performed. Among the special tests for kidney disorders are excretory urography, IV pyelography, tests of the glomerular filtration rate, biopsy, and ultrasound examination. Treatment depends on the type of disease diagnosed. Some forms of advanced kidney disease may lead to renal failure, coma, and death unless hemodialysis is started. See also **glomerulonephritis, nephrotic syndrome, renal failure, urinary calculus.**

**kidney failure.** See **renal failure.**

**kidney machine.** See **artificial kidney, dialyzer,** def. 1.

**kidney stone.** See **renal calculus.**

**Kielland's forceps.** See **obstetric forceps.**

**Kielland's rotation** /kē'land/ [Christian Kielland, Norwegian obstetrician, 1871–1941], an obstetric procedure in which Kielland's forceps are used in turning the head of the fetus from an occiput posterior or occiput transverse position to an occiput anterior position. It is performed most commonly to correct an arrest in the active stage of labor. The rotation is done at the midplane of the pelvis. As it is associated with increased harm to the mother and to the baby, cesarean section is often preferred instead. See also **forceps delivery, obstetric forceps.**

**Kiesselbach's plexus** /kē'səlbäkhs', -bäks'/ [Wilhelm Kiesselbach, German laryngologist, 1839–1902], a conver-

gence of small fragile arteries and veins located superficially on the anterosuperior part of the nasal septum. It is the most common site for septal bleeding.

**Kikuchi's lymphadenitis** /kē·kōō'chēz/ [M. Kikuchi, Japanese pathologist, 20th century], a benign, self-limited syndrome of lymphadenopathy, usually in the neck, with a female predominance; characteristics include patchy necrotizing lesions of the paracortex and proliferation of distinctive histiocytes, plasmacytoid monocytes, and lymphoblasts surrounded by karyorrhectic debris. Some consider it a self-limited form of systemic lupus erythematosus. Also called **histiocytic necrotizing lymphadenitis, Kikuchi's disease, subacute necrotizing lymphadenitis.** See also **systemic lupus erythematosus.**

**killed vaccine** [ME, *killen* + L, *vaccinus,* of a cow], a vaccine prepared from dead microorganisms. Killed vaccines are generally used to provide immunization from organisms that are too virulent to be used in the living attenuated state. The immune system reacts to the presence of the pathogen in the same manner, whether the organism is live or dead. However, when possible, immunity produced by a live, attenuated vaccine is usually more effective.

**killer cell,** a small lymphocyte without B or T cell markers. It is the effector cell of antibody-dependent cell-mediated cytotoxicity, recognizes antibodies on target cells, and lyses those cells through a cell-cell interaction that does not require complement. Compare **killer T cell, natural killer (NK) cell.** See also **null cell.**

**killer T cells,** antigen-stimulated T lymphocytes or cytotoxic T cells that attack foreign antigens directly and destroy cells that bear those antigens. Compare **killer cell, natural killer (NK) cell.**

**killer yeast,** a strain of yeast cells contains a toxic protein that destroys other yeast strains.

**kilo-** /kil'ə-/, prefix meaning 'one thousand': *kilocalorie, kilogram, kilometer.*

**kilobase (kb),** a length of nucleic acid equal to 1000 bases or nucleotides.

**kilobase pair (kbp),** a length of DNA or double-stranded RNA equal to 1000 base pairs.

**kilobyte (K, kb)** /-bīt/, one thousand (or, more precisely, 1024) bytes.

**kilocalorie (kcal)** /-kəl'ərē/ [Gk, *chilioi,* thousand; L, *calor,* heat], a unit of heat equal to 1000 small calories (cal) or 4,186 joules. Also called **large calorie (Cal).**

**kilogram (kg)** /-gram/ [Gk, *chilioi,* thousand; Fr, *gramme*], a unit for the measurement of mass in the metric system. One kilogram is equal to 1000 grams or to 2.2046 pounds avoirdupois.

**kilogram calorie.** See **calorie.**

**kilohertz (kHz)** /-hurts/ [Gk, *chilioi,* thousand; *hertz,* Heinrich R. Hertz, German physicist, 1857–1894], unit of frequency equal to 1000 ($10^3$) hertz. See also **hertz.**

**kiloliter (kL)** /-lē'tər/ [Gk, *chilioi,* thousand; Fr, *litre*], unit of volume equivalent to 1057 quarts, 1000 liters. Also spelled **kilolitre.**

**kilometer (km)** /-mē'tər/ [Gk, *chilioi,* thousand, *metron*], measure equivalent to 1000 meters (about 0.62 miles).

**kilovolt (kV)** /-volt/ [Gk, *chilioi,* thousand; volt, Count Alessandro Volta, Italian scientist, 1745–1827], measure of electrical potential, 1000 volts.

**kilovolt peak (kVp),** a measure of the maximum electrical potential in kilovolts across an x-ray tube. Most diagnostic x-ray machines have a kVp of 40 to 150. However, x-ray equipment is usually operated at the minimum potential necessary for an examination.

**Kimmelstiel-Wilson syndrome** [Paul Kimmelstiel, German pathologist in the U.S., 1900–1970; Clifford Wilson, English physician, b. 1906]. See **intercapillary glomerulosclerosis.**

**kinaesthesia.** See **kinesthesia.**

**kinanesthesia** /kin'anesthē'zhə/, **1.** an inability to perceive the movement or position of one's body parts. The condition is observed as a sign of ataxia. **2.** loss of movement sense.

**kinase** /kī'nās/ [Gk, *kinesis,* motion; *ase,* enzyme], **1.** an enzyme that catalyzes the transfer of a phosphate group or another high-energy molecular group to an acceptor molecule. Each of these kinases is named for its receptor, such as acetate kinase, fructokinase, or hexokinase. **2.** an enzyme that activates a preenzyme (zymogen). Each of these kinases is named for its source, such as bacterial kinase, enterokinase, fibrinokinase, insulin kinase, staphylokinase, streptokinase, streptokinase-streptodornase, or urokinase.

**kind firmness,** (in psychology) a direct, clear, and confident approach to a patient in which rules and regulations are calmly cited in response to infractions and requests.

**kindred** /kin'drid/, a group of genetically related individuals.

**kine-.** See **kinesio-.**

**kinematic face-bow** /kin'əmat'ik/, an adjustable caliperlike device used for precisely locating the axis of rotation of a mandible through the sagittal plane. Also called **adjustable axis face-bow and hinge-bow.**

**kinematics** /kin'əmat'iks, kī-'/ [Gk, *kinema,* motion], the description, measurement, and recording of body motion without regard to the forces acting to produce the motion. Recordings of body motions are defined in one-plane relationships, although natural motions of the body often occur in more than one plane. Kinematics considers the motions of all body parts relative to the segments of the part involved in the motion and not necessarily in relation to the standard anatomic position; for example, the movements of the fingers are considered in relation to the midline of the hand, not the midline of the body. The most common types of motions studied in kinematics are flexion, extension, adduction, abduction, internal rotation, and external rotation. Kinematics is especially important in orthopedics, rehabilitation medicine, and physical therapy. Also called **cinematics.** Compare **kinetics.**

**kinesia** /kīnē'zhə/ [Gk, *kinein,* to move], a condition caused by erratic or rhythmic motions in any combination of directions, such as in a boat or a car. Severe cases are characterized by nausea, vomiting, vertigo, and headache; mild cases by headache and general discomfort. Various antihistamines are used prophylactically. Motion sickness includes air sickness, car sickness, and seasickness (mal de mer). Also spelled **cinesia.** Also called **kinetosis,** (informal) **motion sickness.**

**-kinesia,** suffix meaning 'movement': *hyperkinesia.*

**kinesic behavior** /kīnē'sik/, nonverbal cues of communication that function to achieve and maintain bonds of attachments between people.

**kinesics** /kīnē'siks/ [Gk, *kinesis,* motion], the study of body position, posture, movement, and facial expression in relation to communication. The observance of nonverbal interactional behavior is an integral part of health assessment and is used especially in mental health assessment as an objective and measurable tool for diagnosing disturbances of communication and behavioral disorders. See also **body language, communication.**

**kinesio-, kine-,** combining form meaning 'movement': *kinesiology, kinesioneurosis, kinesiotherapy.*

**kinesiologic electromyography** /kinē'sē·əloj'ik/, the study of muscle activity involved in body movements.

**kinesiology** /-ol'əjē/ [Gk, *kinesis + logos,* science], the scientific study of muscular activity and the anatomy, physiology, and mechanics of the movement of body parts.

**kinesiotherapist,** a health care professional who, under the direction of a physician, treats the effects of disease, injury, and congenital disorders through the use of rehabilitative exercise and education alone. See also **kinesiotherapy.**

**kinesiotherapy,** a specialized area of medicine in which exercise and movement are used as the primary form of rehabilitation. It is typically used in the treatment of amputees. See also **kinesiotherapist.**

**kinesis** /kīnē'sis, kinē'sis/, physical movement or force, particularly when induced by a stimulus.

**-kinesis, -kinesia,** suffix meaning an 'activation': *angiokinesis, lymphokinesis, thrombokinesis.*

**kinesthesia** /kin'esthē'zhə/ [Gk, *kinesis,* motion, *aisthesis,* feeling], the perception of one's own body parts, weight, and movement. Also spelled **kinaesthesia.**

**kinesthetic memory** /kin'esthet'ik/, the recollection of movement, weight, resistance, and position of the body or parts of the body.

**kinesthetic sense** [Gk, *kinesis,* motion; L, *sentire,* to feel], an ability to be aware of muscular movement and position. By providing information through receptors about muscles, tendons, joints, and other body parts, the kinesthetic sense helps control and coordinate activities such as walking and talking.

**-kinetic, -cinetic, -cinetical,** suffix meaning 'movement': *akinetic, parakinetic, synkinetic.*

**kinetic analysis** /kinet'ik/, analysis in which the change of the monitored parameter with time is related to concentration, such as change of absorbance per minute, to determine the rate of a reaction.

**kinetic ataxia.** See **motor ataxia.**

**kinetic energy (KE)** [Gk, *kinesis,* motion, *energeia*], the energy possessed by an object by virtue of its motion. It is expressed by the formula $E = (1/2)mv^2$, where $m$ represents the mass of the object and $v$ is its velocity.

**kinetic hallucination** [Gk, *kinesis,* motion + L, *allucinari,* wandering mind], a false perception of body movement.

**kinetic proofreading, 1.** a molecular activity in which an enzyme distinguishes correct substrates. **2.** a mechanism that permits a ribosome to make correct codon-anticodon interactions.

**kinetic reflex** [Gk, *kinesis,* motion + L, *reflectere,* to bend back], a postural response resulting from stimulation of the vestibular apparatus. Also called **labyrinthine reflex.**

**kinetics** /kinet'iks/ [Gk, *kinesis* + L, *icus,* like], the study of the forces that produce, arrest, or modify the motions of the body. Newton's first and third laws of motion are especially applicable to kinetics. Newton's first law states that bodies at rest stay at rest and bodies in motion keep moving unless they are acted on by an unbalancing force. Newton's third law states that every action force has a reaction force that is equal in magnitude but opposite in direction. These two laws apply to the forces produced by muscles that act on joints. The reaction forces of the muscles contribute to equilibrium and the motion of the body. Compare **kinematics.**

**kineto-,** combining form meaning 'movable': *kinetochore, kinetogenic, kinetoplasm.*

**kinetochore.** See **centromere.**

**kinetoplasm** /kīnet'ōplaz'əm/, the most highly contractile part of a cell.

**kinetosis.** See **kinesia.**

**kinetotherapeutic bath** /kinet′ōthur′əpyo͞o′tik/ [Gk, *kinesis* + *therapeutike,* medical practice + AS, *baeth*], a bath in which underwater exercises are performed to strengthen weak or partially paralyzed muscles.

**King, Imogene,** a nursing theorist who introduced her theory of goal attainment in her book, *Toward a Theory of Nursing* (1971). King's conceptual framework specifies three interacting systems: personal system, interpersonal system, and social system. King defined nursing as a process of human interactions between nurse and clients who communicate to set goals and then agree to meet the goals. She believes that the patient is a personal system within a social system, co-existing through interpersonal processes with other personal systems. The nurse and patient perceive each other and the situation, act and react, interact, and transact. From her major concepts (interaction, perception, communication, transaction, role, stress, growth and development, and time and space), she derived her theory of goal attainment. King describes nursing as a discipline and an applied science, with emphasis on the derivation of nursing knowledge from other disciplines. She suggests that the patient's and nurse's perceptions, judgments, and actions lead to reaction, interaction, and transaction, which she calls the process of nursing.

**kin group,** family members who are related genetically or by marriage.

**kinin** /kī′nin/, any of a group of polypeptides with varying physiologic activity such as contraction of visceral smooth muscle, vascular permeability, and vasodilation. Two principal kinins, bradykinin and lysylbradykinin, are formed in the blood from precursor kininogens by the action of kallikreins and kinases.

**kinky hair disease** [Du, *kink,* short twist + AS, *haer* + L, *dis* + Fr, *aise,* ease], an inherited condition characterized by short, sparse, poorly pigmented hair with shafts that are twisted and broken. Other mental and physical disorders are usually associated with the disease.

**kino-, kinesi-, kinesio-,** combining form meaning 'movement': *kinematics, kinesiology, hyperkinesia.*

**kinomere.** See **centromere.**

**Kinsbourne syndrome** /kinz′born /, a neurologic disorder of unknown cause with onset between ages 1 and 3 years, characterized by myoclonus of trunk and limbs and by non-rhythmic horizontal and vertical oscillations of the eyes, with ataxia of gait and intention tremor; some cases have been associated with occult neuroblastoma. Also called **myoclonic encephalopathy of childhood.**

**kinship model family group,** a family unit comprising the biologic parents and their offspring. It is like a nuclear family but more closely tied to an extended family. Characteristics of this family group include dominance by the maternal grandmother, who raises the children and makes most of the decisions; clearly delineated sex roles; and resistance to change.

**Kirkland knife** [Olin Kirkland, American periodontist, 1876–1969; AS, *cnif*], a surgical knife with a heart-shaped blade that is sharp on all edges. It is used for a primary gingivectomy incision.

**Kirklin staging system,** a system for determining the prognosis of colon cancer, based on the extent to which the tumor has penetrated the bowel area. See also **cancer staging, Dukes' classification, TNM.**

**Kirschner's wire** /kursh′nərz/ [Martin Kirschner, German surgeon, 1879–1942; AS, *wir*], a threaded or smooth metallic wire available in three diameters and 22.86 cm long. The wire is used in internal fixation of fractures or for skeletal traction.

**Kite method,** a technique for positioning a patient for radiographic examination of congenital clubfoot. The foot is imaged in two planes and is placed on the film holder without altering the foot's abnormal alignment.

**kiting** /kī′ting/, *informal.* the improper and illegal practice of altering a drug prescription to indicate that more of a drug was prescribed than was actually ordered by the physician. Kiting may be done by a patient seeking greater quantities of drugs, especially opioids, than the physician prescribed, or by the pharmacist to increase reimbursement from a third party, such as an insurance company.

**KJ,** abbreviation for *knee jerk.*

**kL,** abbreviation for **kiloliter.**

**klang association.** See **clang association.**

*Klebsiella* /kleb′zē·el′ə/ [Theodore A.E. Klebs, German bacteriologist, 1834–1913], a genus of diplococcal bacteria that appear as small, plump rods with rounded ends. Several respiratory diseases, including bronchitis, sinusitis, and some forms of pneumonia, are caused by infection by species of *Klebsiella.*

*Klebsiella pneumoniae* [Theodore A.E. Klebs; Gk, *pneumon,* lung], a species of bacteria found in soil, water, cereal grains, and the intestinal tract of humans and other animals. It is associated with several pathologic conditions, including pneumonia. See also **Friedländer's bacillus.**

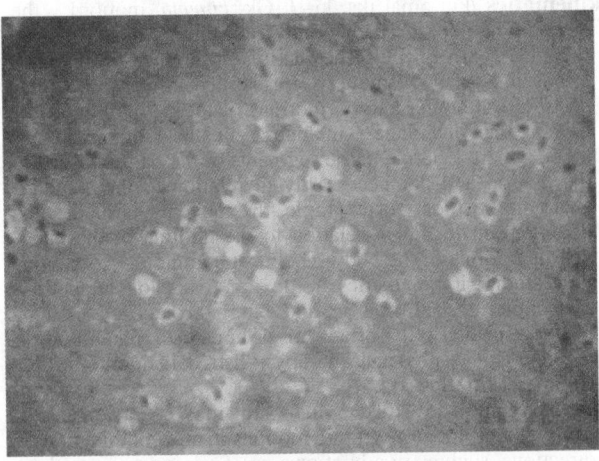

***Klebsiella pneumoniae***
*(Farrar et al, 1993/courtesy Dr. V.E. Del Bene)*

**Klebs-Loeffler bacillus** /klebz′lef′lər/ [Theodore A.E. Klebs; Friederich A.J. Loeffler, German bacteriologist, 1852–1915; L, *bacillum,* small rod], *Corynebacterium diphtheriae.* See also *Corynebacterium.*

**kleeblattschädel deformity syndrome.** See **cloverleaf skull deformity.**

**Kleine-Levin syndrome** /klīn′lev′in/ [Willi Kleine, 20th century German psychiatrist; Max Levin, Russian-born American neurologist, b. 1901], a disorder of unknown cause often associated with psychotic conditions that is characterized by episodic sleep, abnormal hunger, and hyperactivity. The episodes of sleep may last for several hours or days and are followed by confusion on awakening. There is no specific treatment. Compare **narcolepsy.**

**Klein-Waardenburg syndrome.** See **Waardenburg's syndrome** (def. 2).

**klepto-,** prefix meaning 'theft or stealing': *kleptolagnia, kleptomania.*

**kleptolagnia** /klep'tōlag'nē·ə/ [Gk, *kleptein,* to steal, *lagneia,* lust], sexual excitement or gratification produced by stealing.

**kleptomania** /-mā'nē·ə/ [Gk, *kleptein,* to steal, *mania,* madness], an anxiety disorder characterized by an abnormal, uncontrollable, and recurrent urge to steal. The objects are taken not for their monetary value, immediate need, or utility but because of a symbolic meaning usually associated with some unconscious emotional conflict; they are usually given away, returned surreptitiously, or kept and hidden. People who have the condition experience an increased sense of tension before committing the theft and intense gratification during the act. Afterward they display signs of depression, guilt, and anxiety over the possibility of being apprehended and losing status in society. In less severe cases the impulse is expressed by continuously borrowing objects and not returning them. Treatment consists of psychotherapy to uncover the underlying emotional problems. See also **impulse control disorder. —kleptomaniac,** *n.*

**Klinefelter's syndrome** /klīn'feltərz/ [Harry F. Klinefelter, American physician, b. 1912], a condition of gonadal defects appearing in males after puberty, with an extra X chromosome in at least one cell line. Characteristics are small firm testes, long legs, gynecomastia, poor social adaptation, subnormal intelligence, chronic pulmonary disease, and varicose veins. The severity of the abnormalities increases with greater numbers of X chromosomes. The most common abnormality is a 47 XXY karyotype. Men with the karyotype XXXXY have marked congenital malformations and mental retardation.

**Klippel-Feil syndrome** /klipel'fel', klip'əlfīl'/ [Maurice Klippel, French neurologist, 1858–1942; Andre Feil, French neurologist, b. 1884], a condition of short neck and limited neck movements because of congenital fusion of the cervical vertebrae or reduction in the number of cervical vertebrae. Also called **Klippel's disease, Klippel-Feil disease, Klippel-Feil malformation.** See **congenital short neck syndrome.**

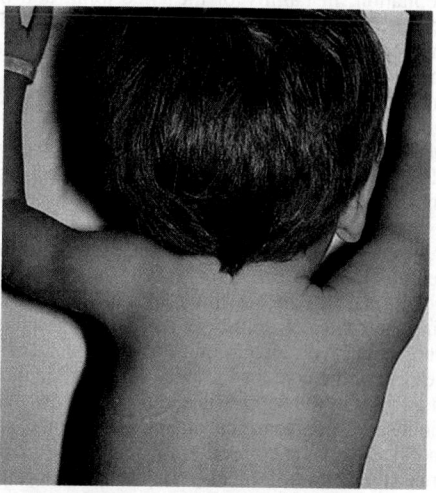

**Klippel-Feil syndrome** *(Zitelli and Davis, 1997)*

**Klippel-Trénaunay syndrome** /kli·pel'trā·nō·nā'/ [Maurice Klippel, French neurologist, 1858−1942; Paul Trénaunay, French physician, 20th century], a rare condition usually affecting one extremity, characterized by hypertrophy of the bone and related soft tissues, large cutaneous hemangiomas, persistent nevus flammeus, and skin varices.

**Kloehn headgear,** an extraoral orthodontic appliance consisting of a cervical strap and a long outer bow. It is used to retract maxillary teeth or to reinforce tooth anchorage during retraction,

**Klonopin,** trademark for an anticonvulsant (clonazepam).

**Klor,** trademark for an electrolyte replacement solution (potassium chloride).

**Klorvess,** trademark for an electrolyte replacement solution (potassium chloride).

**Klumpke's palsy** /kloomp'kēz/ [Augusta Dejerine-Klumpke, French neurologist, 1859–1927], atrophic paralysis of the forearm. It is present at birth and involves the seventh and eighth cervical nerves and the first thoracic nerve. The condition may be accompanied by Horner's syndrome, ptosis, and miosis because of involvement of sympathetic nerves. Also called **Dejerine-Klumpke's paralysis.**

**K-Lyte/Cl,** trademark for an electrolyte replacement solution (potassium chloride).

**km,** abbreviation for **kilometer.**

**kneading** /nē'ding/ [AS, *cnedan*], a grasping, rolling, and pressing movement, as is used in massaging the muscles. See also **massage.**

**knee** /nē/ [AS, *cneow*], a joint complex that connects the thigh with the lower leg. It consists of three condyloid

**Klinefelter's syndrome**
*(Thibodeau and Patton, 1999/Nancy S. Wexler)*

joints, 12 ligaments, 13 bursae, and the patella. The motion of this joint is not a simple gliding motion, because the articular surfaces of the bones involved are not mutually adapted to each other. Various orthopedic conditions such as arthritis commonly affect the knee, especially in elderly individuals. The knee is relatively unprotected by surrounding muscles and is often injured by blows, sudden stops, and turns, especially those associated with sports. Ligamental tears of the knee joint are extremely common in athletes and produce a variety of signs and symptoms, such as effusion surrounding the knee joint, varying degrees of edema, differences in the shape of the knee joint, tenderness on palpation, crepitation, instability of the knee joint, and possible ecchymosis. Torn menisci are very common sports injuries and can cause severe pain, limping, edema, and greatly reduced motion.

**knee-ankle interaction,** one of the five major kinetic determinants of gait, which helps to minimize the displacement of the body's center of gravity during the walking cycle. The knee and the foot work simultaneously to lower the body's center of gravity. When the heel of the foot is in contact with the ground, the foot is dorsiflexed, and the knee is fully extended so that the associated limb is at its maximum length with the center of gravity at its lower point. Plantar flexion of the foot with the initiation of knee flexion maintains the center of gravity in its forward progression at about the same level, also helping to minimize the vertical displacement of the center of gravity. Knee-ankle interaction is often a factor in the diagnosis and treatment of various orthopedic diseases, deformities, and abnormal conditions and in the analysis and the correction of pathologic gaits. Compare **knee-hip flexion, lateral pelvic displacement, pelvic rotation, pelvic tilt.**

**kneecap.** See **patella.**

**knee-chest position.** See **genupectoral position.**

**knee-elbow position** [AS, *cneow + elboga*], a position in which a patient being examined rests on the knees and elbows with the head supported on the hands.

**knee-hip flexion,** one of the five major kinetic determinants of gait, which allows the passage of body weight over the supporting extremity during the walking cycle. Knee-hip flexion occurs during the stance and swing phases of the cycle. The knee first locks into extension as the heel of the weight-bearing limb strikes the ground and is unlocked by final flexion and initiation of the swing phase in the walking cycle. Hip flexion is synchronized with these movements, which help minimize the vertical displacement of the body's center of gravity in the act of walking. Knee-hip flexion is often a factor in the diagnosis and treatment of various orthopedic diseases, deformities, and abnormal conditions and in the analysis and correction of pathologic gaits. Compare **knee-ankle interaction, lateral pelvic displacement, pelvic rotation, pelvic tilt.**

**knee-jerk reflex.** See **patellar reflex.**

**knee joint,** the complex, hinged joint at the knee, regarded as three articulations in one, comprising condyloid joints connecting the femur and the tibia and a partly arthrodial joint connecting the patella and the femur. The knee joint and its ligaments permit flexion, extension, and, in certain positions, medial and lateral rotation. It is a common site for sprain and dislocation. Also called **articulatio genus.**

**knee replacement,** the surgical insertion of a hinged prosthesis performed to relieve pain and restore motion to a knee severely affected by osteoarthritis, rheumatoid arthritis, or trauma. With the patient under general or spinal anesthesia, the diseased surfaces are removed, and a two-piece metallic hinge is inserted into the medullary cavities of the femur and

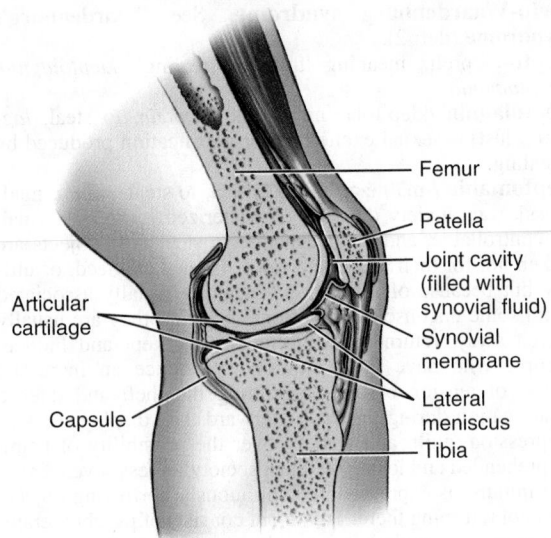

**Knee joint** *(Herlihy and Maebius, 2000)*

tibia. After surgery progressive exercise and whirlpool baths are prescribed through physical therapy. Possible complications include infection, fat embolism, thrombophlebitis, peroneal nerve palsy, loosening of the prosthesis, and flexion contractures. To prevent contractures the patient is cautioned to keep the leg extended in bed; a blanket roll along the femur prevents external rotation. The mobility and range of motion of the joint increase slowly. See also **arthroplasty, hip replacement, osteoarthritis, plastic surgery.**

**knee sling,** a leg support in sling form used under the knee for Russell traction. See also **Russell traction.**

**knife needle** /nīf/ [AS, *cnif + neal*], a slender surgical knife with a needle point, used in the discission of a cataract and other ophthalmic procedures such as goniotomy and goniopuncture.

**knock-knee.** See **genu valgum.**

**Knoop hardness test** /noop/ [Frederick Knoop, 20th century American metallurgist], a method of assessing surface hardness by measuring resistance to the penetration of an indenting tool made of diamond. The test is commonly used for testing the hardness of teeth.

**knot** /not/ [AS, *cnotta*], (in surgery) the interlacing of the ends of a ligature or suture so they remain in place without slipping or becoming detached. The ends of the suture are passed twice around each other before being pulled taut to form a simple surgeon's knot. For additional stability the ends may be recrossed, and a second simple knot made over the first.

**knowledge: breastfeeding,** a nursing outcome from the Nursing Outcomes Classification (NOC) defined as the extent of understanding conveyed about lactation and nourishment of infant through breastfeeding. See also **Nursing Outcomes Classification.**

**knowledge: child safety,** a nursing outcome from the Nursing Outcomes Classification (NOC) defined as the extent of understanding conveyed about safely caring for a child. See also **Nursing Outcomes Classification.**

**knowledge: conception prevention,** a nursing outcome from the Nursing Outcomes Classification (NOC) defined as the extent of understanding conveyed about pregnancy prevention. See also **nursing outcomes classification.**

**knowledge deficient** /nol'ij/,    a nursing diagnosis accepted by the Fourth National Conference on the Classification of Nursing Diagnoses (revised). It is defined as an absence or deficiency of cognitive information related to specific topics. The nature of the knowledge is to be specified.

■ DEFINING CHARACTERISTICS: The defining characteristics are verbalization of the problem; inaccurate follow-through of instruction; inaccurate performance of test; and inappropriate or exaggerated behaviors, e.g., hysterical, hostile, agitated, apathetic.

■ RELATED FACTORS: Related factors are lack of exposure; lack of recall; information misinterpretation; cognitive limitation; lack of interest in learning; and unfamiliarity with information resources. See also **nursing diagnosis.**

**knowledge: diabetes management,**    a nursing outcome from the Nursing Outcomes Classification (NOC) defined as the extent of understanding conveyed about diabetes mellitus and its control. See also **Nursing Outcomess Classification.**

**knowledge: diet,**    a nursing outcome from the Nursing Outcomes Classification (NOC) defined as the extent of understanding conveyed about diet. See also **Nursing Outcomes Classification.**

**knowledge: disease process,**    a nursing outcome from the Nursing Outcomes Classification (NOC) defined as the extent of understanding conveyed about a specific disease process. See also **Nursing Outcomes Classification.**

**knowledge: energy conservation,**    a nursing outcome from the Nursing Outcomes Classification (NOC) defined as the extent of understanding conveyed about energy conservation techniques. See also **Nursing Outcomes Classification.**

**knowledge: fertility promotion,**    a nursing outcome from the Nursing Outcomes Classification (NOC) defined as the extent of understanding conveyed about fertility testing and the conditions that affect conception. See also **Nursing Outcomes Classification.**

**knowledge: health behaviors,**    a nursing outcome from the Nursing Outcomes Classification (NOC) defined as the extent of understanding conveyed about the promotion and protection of health. See also **Nursing Outcomes Classification.**

**knowledge: health promotion,**    a nursing outcome from the Nursing Outcomes Classification (NOC) defined as the extent of understanding of information needed to obtain and maintain optimal health. See also **Nursing Outcomes Classification.**

**knowledge: health resources,**    a nursing outcome from the Nursing Outcomes Classification (NOC) defined as the extent of understanding conveyed about health care resources. See also **Nursing Outcomes Classification.**

**knowledge: illness care,**    a nursing outcome from the Nursing Outcomes Classification (NOC) defined as the extent of understanding of illness-related information needed to achieve and maintain optimal health. See also **Nursing Outcomes Classification.**

**knowledge: infant care,**    a nursing outcome from the Nursing Outcomes Classification (NOC) defined as the extent of understanding conveyed about caring for a baby up to 12 months. See also **Nursing Outcomes Classification.**

**knowledge: infection control,**    a nursing outcome from the Nursing Outcomes Classification (NOC) defined as the extent of understanding conveyed about prevention and control of infection. See also **Nursing Outcomes Classification.**

**knowledge: labor and delivery,**    a nursing outcome from the Nursing Outcomes Classification (NOC) defined as the extent of understanding conveyed about labor and delivery. See also **Nursing Outcomes Classification.**

**knowledge: maternal-child health,**    a nursing outcome from the Nursing Outcomes Classification (NOC) defined as the extent of understanding of information needed to achieve and maintain optimal health of a mother and child. See also **Nursing Outcomes Classification.**

**knowledge: medication,**    a nursing outcome from the Nursing Outcomes Classification (NOC) defined as the extent of understanding conveyed about the safe use of medication. See also **Nursing Outcomes Classification.**

**knowledge: personal safety,**    a nursing outcome from the Nursing Outcomes Classification (NOC) defined as the extent of understanding conveyed about preventing unintentional injuries. See also **Nursing Outcomes Classification.**

**knowledge: postpartum,**    a nursing outcome from the Nursing Outcomes Classification (NOC) defined as the extent of understanding conveyed about maternal health following delivery. See also **Nursing Outcomes Classification.**

**knowledge: preconception,**    a nursing outcome from the Nursing Outcomes Classification (NOC) defined as the extent of understanding conveyed about maternal health prior to conception to ensure a healthy pregnancy. See also **Nursing Outcomes Classification.**

**knowledge: pregnancy,**    a nursing outcome from the Nursing Outcomes Classification (NOC) defined as the extent of understanding conveyed about maintenance of a health pregnancy and prevention of complications. See also **Nursing Outcomes Classification.**

**knowledge: prescribed activity,**    a nursing outcome from the Nursing Outcomes Classification (NOC) defined as the extent of understanding conveyed about prescribed activity and exercise. See also **Nursing Outcomes Classification.**

**knowledge: sexual functioning,**    a nursing outcome from the Nursing Outcomes Classification (NOC) is defined as the extent of understanding conveyed about sexual development and responsible sexual practices. See also **Nursing Outcomes Classification.**

**knowledge: substance abuse control,**    a nursing outcome from the Nursing Outcomes Classification (NOC) defined as the extent of understanding conveyed about managing substance use safely. See also **Nursing Outcomes Classification.**

**knowledge: treatment procedures,**    a nursing outcome from the Nursing Outcomes Classification (NOC) defined as the extent of understanding conveyed about procedure(s) required as part of a treatment regimen. See also **Nursing Outcomes Classification.**

**knowledge: treatment regimen,**    a nursing outcome from the Nursing Outcomes Classification (NOC) defined as the extent of understanding conveyed about a specific treatment regimen. See also **Nursing Outcomes Classification.**

**knuckle** /nuk'əl/,    the dorsal aspect of any phalangeal joint, especially of the metacarpophalangeal joints of the flexed fingers. By extension sometimes applied to any anatomical structure of similar appearance, such as an extruded loop of intestine in hernia.

**Kocher's forceps** /kō'kərz/ [Emil T. Kocher, Swiss surgeon, 1841–1917],    a kind of surgical forceps that has notched jaws, interlocking teeth, and thick curved or straight powerful handles.

**Koch's bacillus** /kōks/ [Robert Koch, German bacteriologist, 1843–1910; L, *bacillum*, small rod],    the *Mycobacterium tuberculosis* microorganism.

**Koch's phenomenon** [Robert Koch; Gk, *phainomenon*, anything seen], a tuberculin reaction that occurs when a culture of tubercle bacilli is injected into the skin of subjects already infected with the disease. In humans a positive tuberculin reaction indicates sensitization resulting from a tuberculosis infection. Also called **Koch's reaction.**

**Koch's postulates** [Robert Koch; L, *postulare*, to demand], the prerequisites for experimentally establishing that a specific microorganism causes a particular disease. The conditions are the following: (1) the microorganism must be observed in all cases of the disease; (2) the microorganism must be isolated and grown in pure culture; (3) microorganisms from the pure culture, when inoculated into a susceptible animal, must reproduce the disease; and (4) the microorganism must be observed in and recovered from the experimentally diseased animal.

**Koch's reaction.** See **Koch's phenomenon.**

**Kock's pouch.** See **continent ileostomy.**

**Koebner phenomenon** /kōb'nər/ [Heinrich Koebner, Polish dermatologist, 1838–1904; Gk, *phainomenon*, something observed], the development of isomorphic lesions at the site of an injury occurring in psoriasis, lichen nitidus, lichen planus, and verruca plana.

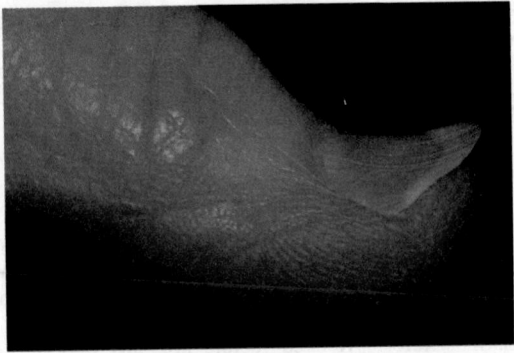

**Koilonychia** *(Hordinsky, Sawaya, and Scher, 2000)*

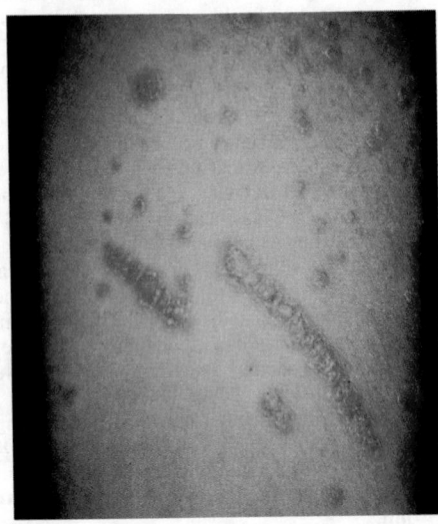

**Koebner phenomenon** *(Zitelli and Davis, 1997)*

**KOH,** chemical formula for **potassium hydroxide.**

**Kohnstamm's phenomenon.** See **aftermovement.**

**koilo-,** combining form meaning 'hollow or concave': *koilonychia, koilorrhachic, koilosternia.*

**koilonychia** /koi'lōnik'ē·ə/ [Gk, *koilos*, hollow, *onyx*, nail], spoon nails; a condition in which nails are thin and concave from side to side. It is usually familial but may occur with trauma and iron deficiency anemia.

**koinoni-,** combining form meaning 'community': *koinonia, koinoniphobia.*

**kolpo-.** See **colpo-.**

**koly-,** combining form meaning 'to hinder': *kolypeptic, kolyphrenia, kolyseptic.*

**kon-,** combining form meaning 'dust': *konometer, koniocortex.*

**Konakion,** trademark for a vitamin K formulation (phytonadione).

**Kopan's needle** /kō'pənz/, a long biopsy needle used to locate the position of a breast tumor on x-ray film. The needle is inserted into the approximate location of the tumor and is left in place during radiography so that it can be repositioned if necessary. In some cases the site is further identified for the surgeon by injecting a colored dye such as methylene blue.

**Koplik's spots** /kop'liks/ [Henry Koplik, American pediatrician, 1858–1927], small red spots with bluish-white centers on the lingual and buccal mucosa, characteristic of measles. The rash of measles usually erupts a day or two after the appearance of Koplik's spots.

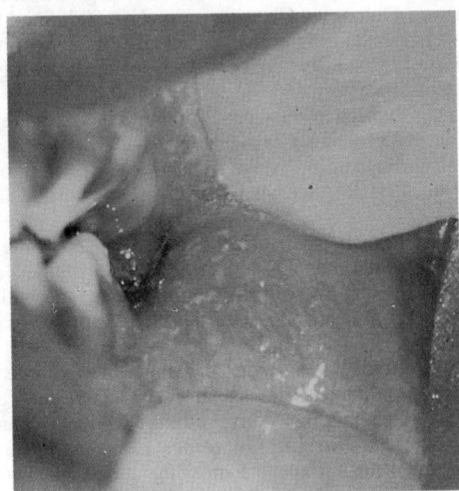

**Koplik's spots** *(Zitelli and Davis, 1997)*

**kopr-, kopra-.** See **copro-.**

**Korányi's sign** /kôr'ənyēz/ [Friedrich von Korányi, Hungarian physician, 1828–1913; L, *signum*], a paravertebral area of dullness found posteriorly on the side opposite a pleural effusion. Also called **Grocco's sign, Korányi-Grocco triangle, triangular dullness.**

**Korean hemorrhagic fever.** See **epidemic hemorrhagic fever.**

**Korotkoff sounds** /kôrot′kôf/ [Nickolai Korotkoff, Russian physician, 1874–1920], sounds heard during the taking of a blood pressure reading using a sphygmomanometer and stethoscope. As air is released from the cuff, pressure on the artery is reduced, and the blood is heard pulsing through the vessel. See also **blood pressure, diastole, sphygmomanometer, systole.**

**Korsakoff's psychosis** /kôr′səkôfs/ [Sergei S. Korsakoff, Russian psychiatrist, 1854–1900], a form of amnesia often seen in chronic alcoholics that is characterized by a loss of short-term memory and an inability to learn new skills. The person is usually disoriented, may present with delirium and hallucinations, and confabulates to conceal the condition. The cause of the condition can often be traced to degenerative changes in the thalamus as a result of a deficiency of B complex vitamins, especially thiamine and $B_{12}$. Compare **Wernicke's encephalopathy.**

**kosher** [Heb, *kasher,* fit or proper], pertaining to the preparation and serving of foods according to Jewish dietary laws. Inherently kosher foods include common fruits, vegetables, and cereals, as well as tea and coffee. Foods that are not kosher include pork, birds of prey, and seafood that lacks fins and scales such as lobster and eels. Most poultry and meat products, excluding pork, are kosher if properly processed.

**$K^+$ pump.** See **potassium pump.**

**Kr,** symbol for the element **krypton.**

**Krabbe's disease.** See **galactosyl ceramide lipidosis.**

**Kraske position** /kras′kə/ [Paul Kraske, Swiss surgeon, 1851–1930], an anatomic position in which the patient is prone, with hips flexed and elevated, head and feet down. The position is used for renal surgery, as it enlarges the costovertebral angle, allowing the surgeon to have optimal access to the kidneys.

**kraurosis** /krôrō′sis/ [Gk, *krauros,* dry, *osis,* condition], a thickening and shriveling of the mucous membranes, particularly female genitalia. See also **kraurosis vulvae.**

**kraurosis vulvae,** a skin disease of aged women characterized by dryness, itching, and atrophy of the external genitalia. It is a condition that exhibits a predisposition to leukoplakia and carcinoma of the vulva. See also **lichen sclerosis et atrophicus.**

**Krause's corpuscles** [Wilhelm J. F. Krause, German anatomist, 1833–1910; L, *corpusculum,* little body], any of a number of sensory end organs in the conjunctiva of the eye; mucous membranes of the lips and tongue; epineurium of nerve trunks, the penis, and the clitoris; and synovial membranes of certain joints. Krause's corpuscles are tiny cylindric oval bodies with a capsule formed by the expansion of the connective tissue sheath of a medullated fiber. They contain a soft, semifluid core in which the axon terminates either in a bulbous extremity or in a coiled mass. Also called **end bulbs of Krause.** Compare **Golgi-Mazzoni corpuscles, Pacini's corpuscles.**

**Krebs cycle.** See **citric acid cycle.**

**Krebs-Henseleit cycle.** See **urea cycle.**

**Krukenberg's tumor** /krōō′kənbərgz/ [Friedrich E. Krukenberg, German pathologist, 1871–1946], a neoplasm of the ovary that is a metastasis of a GI malignancy, usually stomach cancer. Cytologic examination often reveals mucoid degeneration and many large cells shaped like signet rings. Also called **carcinoma mucocellulare.**

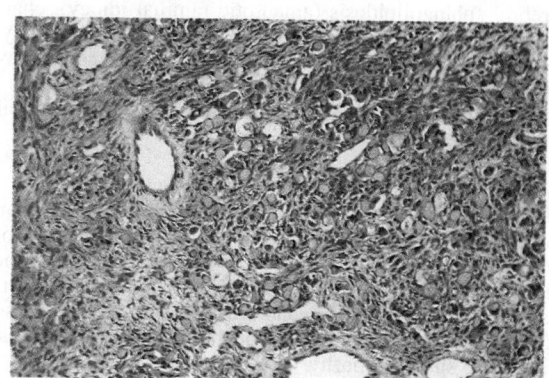

**Krukenberg's tumor** *(Fletcher, 2000)*

**krypto-.** See **crypto-.**

**krypton (Kr)** /krip′ton/, a generally inert rare gaseous element present in air. Its atomic number is 36; its atomic mass is 83.80.

**KS, ks,** abbreviation for **Kaposi's sarcoma.**

**KUB,** abbreviation for *kidney, ureter, and bladder;* a term used in a radiographic examination to determine the location, size, shape, and malformation of the kidneys, ureters, and bladder. Stones and calcified areas may be detected.

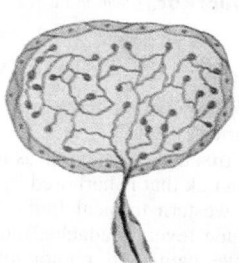

**Krause's corpuscles**
*(Thibodeau and Patton, 1993/Rolin Graphics)*

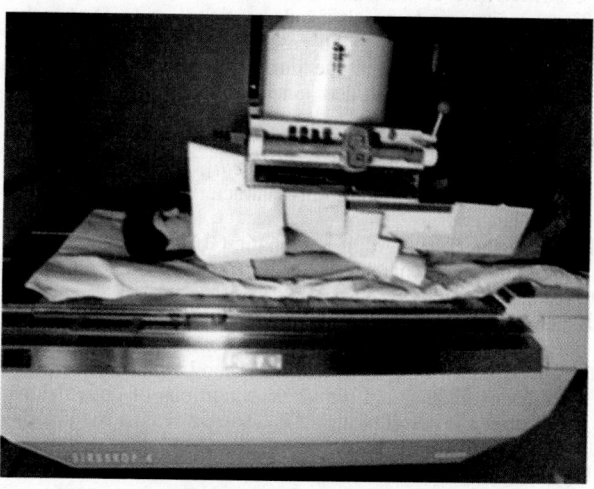

**KUB equipment** *(Brundage, 1992)*

**Kuchendorf method** /koo'kəndôrf/, (in radiology) a technique for positioning a patient for radiographic examination of the patella. The patella is placed against the image receptor and is moved laterally to reduce superimposition.

**kudzu,** an herb that grows in vine form, native to China and Japan and introduced to the United States.

■ USES: This herb is used to reduce alcohol cravings and menopausal symptoms.

■ CONTRAINDICATIONS: Kudzu should not be used during pregnancy and lactation, in children, or in those with known hypersensitivity. It should be used with caution by people who have heart disease.

**Kufs' disease** /koofs/ [H. Kufs, German psychiatrist, 1871–1955; L, *dis* + Fr, *aise*, ease], an adult form of hereditary cerebral sphingolipidosis (amaurotic familial idiocy), characterized by cerebromacular degeneration, hypertonicity, and progressive spastic paralysis. Also called **adult ceroidlipofuscinosis.**

**Kugelberg-Welander syndrome.** See **juvenile spinal muscular atrophy.**

**Kulchitsky's cell.** See **argentaffin cell.**

**Kulchitsky cell carcinoma.** See **carcinoid.**

**Kümmell's disease** /kim'əlz/ [Hermann Kümmell, German surgeon, 1852–1937; L, *dis* + Fr, *aise*, ease], a set of symptoms that develop after a compression fracture of the vertebrae with spinal injury. They include spinal pain, intercostal neuralgia, kyphosis, and weakness in the legs. Also called **Kümmell's spondylitis, posttraumatic spondylitis, traumatic spondylopathy.**

**kunitz inhibitor.** See **trypsin inhibitor.**

**Küntscher nail** /koon'chər, kin'chər/ [Gerhard Küntscher, German surgeon, 1902–1972; AS, *naegel*], a stainless steel nail used in orthopedic surgery for the fixation of fractures of the long bones, especially the femur. Also called **Küntscher intramedullary nail.**

**Kupffer's cells** /koop'fərz/ [Karl W. von Kupffer, German anatomist, 1829–1902], specialized cells of the reticuloendothelial system lining the sinusoids of the liver. The function of Kupffer's cells is to filter bacteria and other small foreign proteins out of the blood.

**kuru** /koo'roo/ [New Guinea, trembling], a slow, progressive, fatal infection of the central nervous system that was endemic to natives of the New Guinea highlands. The incubation period could be 30 or more years, but death usually occurred within months of the onset of symptoms. Characteristic of kuru are ataxia and decreased coordination progressing to paralysis, dementia, slurring of speech, and visual disturbances. Disease was transmitted by ritual cannibalism of brain tissue during funeral rites. No new cases have been recorded since cessation of the cannibalism.

**Kussmaul breathing** /koos'moul/ [Adolf Kussmaul, German physician, 1822–1902; AS, *braeth*], abnormally deep, very rapid sighing respirations characteristic of diabetic ketoacidosis.

**Kussmaul's coma** [Adolf Kussmaul; Gk, *koma*, deep sleep], a diabetic coma characterized by acidosis and deep breathing or extreme hyperpnea.

**Kussmaul's sign** [Adolf Kussmaul; L, *signum,* mark], **1.** a paradoxic rise in venous pressure with distension of the jugular veins during inspiration, as seen in constrictive pericarditis or mediastinal tumor. **2.** conditions of convulsions and coma associated with a GI disorder caused by absorption of a toxic substance.

**kV,** abbreviation for **kilovolt.**

**Kveim reaction** [Morton A. Kveim, Norwegian physician, b. 1892; L, *re*, again, *agere,* to act], a reaction used in a diagnostic test for sarcoidosis, based on an intradermal injection of antigen derived from a lymph node known to be sarcoid. If a noncaseating granuloma appears on the skin at the test site in 4 to 8 weeks, the reaction is said to be positive evidence that the patient has sarcoidosis.

**kVp,** abbreviation for **kilovolt peak.**

**kVp test cassette,** (in radiology) a lightproof box containing a copper filter, a series of stepwedges, and an optical attenuator, used to test the accuracy of kVp settings for peak electrical potential across an x-ray tube.

**kwashiorkor** /kwä'shē·ôr'kôr/ [Afr], a malnutrition disease, primarily of children, caused by severe protein deficiency that usually occurs when the child is weaned from the breast. The child does not lose weight as dramatically and does not look as sick as a marasmic child, who lacks protein and calories. Some now believe Kwashiorkor may relate to bacterial grain contamination and occur when the newly weaned child begins to ingest grain products. Eventually the following symptoms occur: retarded growth, changes in skin and hair pigmentation, diarrhea, loss of appetite, nervous irritability, lethargy, edema, anemia, fatty degeneration of the liver, necrosis, dermatoses, and fibrosis, often accompanied by infection and multivitamin deficiencies. Because dietary fats are poorly tolerated in kwashiorkor, a skimmed milk formula is used in initial feedings, followed by additional foods until a full, well-balanced diet is achieved. See also **marasmic kwashiorkor, marasmus, protein-energy malnutrition.**

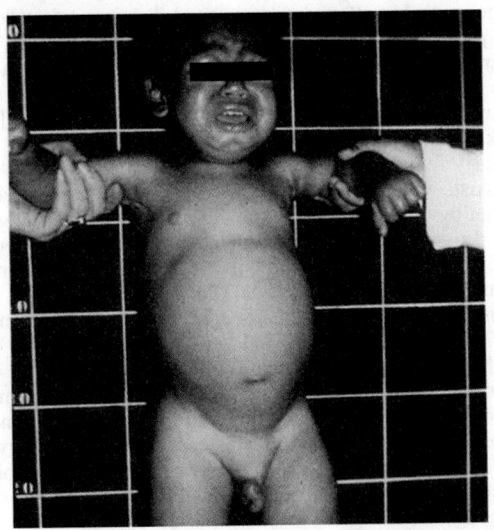

**Kwashiorkor** *(Zitelli and Davis, 1997)*

**Kwell,** trademark for a pediculicide and scabicide (gamma benzene hexachloride).

**Kyasanur Forest disease,** a flavivirus infection transmitted by the bite of a tick that is harbored by shrews and other forest animals in western tropical India. Characteristics of the infection include fever, headache, muscle ache, cough, abdominal and eye pain, and photophobia. Treatment is symptomatic. A vaccine is used in India.

**kymo-,** combining form meaning 'waves': *kymograph, kymoscope, kymotrichous.*

**kymography** /kēmog′rəfē/ [Gk, *kyma*, wave + *graphein*, to record], a technique for graphically recording motions of body organs, such as the heart and the blood vessels.

**kyno-,** combining form meaning 'dogs': *kynocephalus, kynophobia.*

**kypho-,** combining form meaning 'hump': *kyphoscoliosis, kyphosis, kyphotone.*

**kyphos** /kī′fəs/ [Gk, *kyphos,* hunchbacked], the exaggeration or angulation from the normal position of the thoracic vertebral column that is associated with kyphosis. See also **kyphosis.**

**kyphoscoliosis** /kī′fōskō′lē·ō′sis/ [Gk, *kyphos,* hunchbacked + *skolios* curved + *osis,* condition], an abnormal condition characterized by an anteroposterior and a lateral curvature of the spine. It occurs in children and adults and is often associated with cor pulmonale. Compare **kyphosis, scoliosis. —kyphoscoliotic,** *adj.*

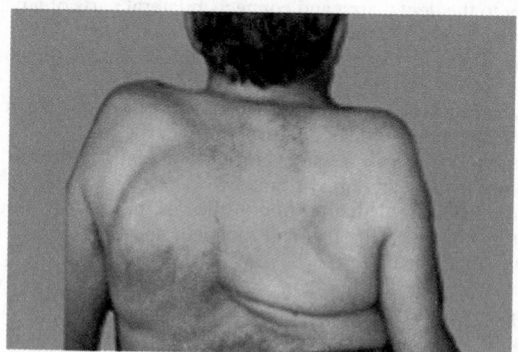

**Kyphoscoliosis** *(Lemmi and Lemmi, 2000)*

**kyphosis** /kīfō′sis/ [Gk, *kyphos,* hunchbacked], an abnormal condition of the vertebral column, characterized by increased convexity in the curvature of the thoracic spine as viewed from the side. The spinal sagittal contour ordinarily consists of a lordosis in the lumbar and cervical spinal seg-

ments that balances the rounding, or the kyphosis, in the thoracic segment. Kyphosis describes this expected rounding but also is used to describe the abnormal condition of the vertebral column. It may be caused by rickets or tuberculosis of the spine. Adolescent kyphosis is usually self-limiting and often undiagnosed; but, if the curvature progresses, there may be moderate back pain. Conservative treatment consists of spine-stretching exercises and sleeping without a pillow with a board under the mattress. A modified Milwaukee brace may be used for severe kyphosis, and, rarely, spinal fusion may be required. Also called **humpback,** roundback. **—kyphotic,** *adj.*

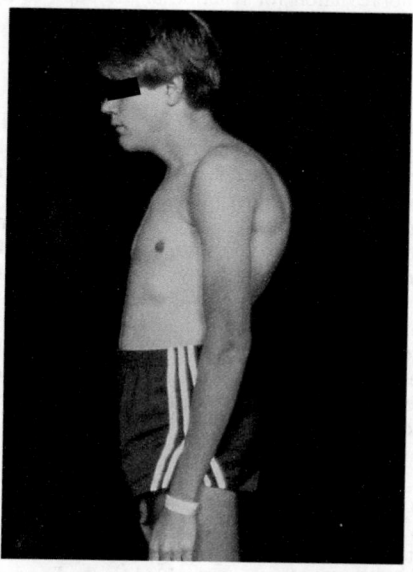

**Severe kyphosis of the thoracic spine**
*(Zitelli and Davis, 1997)*

**kysth-, kystho-.** See **colpo-.**
**kyto-.** See **cyt-.**

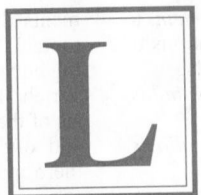

L, **1.** symbol for *kinetic potential*. **2.** abbreviation for *Lactobacillus*. **3.** abbreviation for **lambert**. **4.** abbreviation for *Latin*. **5.** symbol for **liter**. **6.** abbreviation for **lung**.

**L & A,** abbreviation for reaction of the pupil to *light and accommodation*.

**La,** symbol for the element **lanthanum**.

**LA,** abbreviation for **left atrium**.

**lab,** abbreviation for **laboratory**.

**label** [ME, band], *n.* **1.** a substance with a special affinity for an organ, tissue, cell, or microorganism in which it may become deposited and fixed. **2.** an atom or molecule attached to either a ligand or binding protein and capable of generating a signal for monitoring in the binding reaction. **3.** the process of attaching a radioisotope to a compound for the purpose of tracing it during a physiologic action in the body.

**label** *v.* the process of depositing and fixing a substance in an organ, tissue, cell, or microorganism.

**labeled compound,** a chemical substance in which part of the molecules are labeled with a radionuclide or isotope so that observations of the radioactivity or isotopic composition make it possible to follow the compound or its fragments through physical, chemical, or biologic processes.

**labeling,** **1.** the providing of information on a drug, food, device, or cosmetic to the purchaser or user. The information may be in any one of various forms, including printing on a carton, adhesive label, package insert, and monograph. Regulations for labeling are provided by the Food and Drug Administration. The label must contain directions for use, unless such directions are exempted by regulation, as well as warnings or contraindications. It must not contain false or misleading information. **2.** the assignment of a word or term to a form of behavior. **3.** the act of classifying a patient according to a diagnostic category. Labeling can be misleading because not all patients conform to defined characteristics of standard diagnostic categories. Also spelled **labelling**.

**la belle indifference** /lä bel eNdifärä Ns'/ [Fr, nice indifference], an air of unconcern displayed by some patients toward their physical symptoms. It is believed the physical symptoms may relieve anxiety and result in secondary gains in the form of sympathy and attention given by others.

**labetalol hydrochloride** /ləbet'əlol/, an antihypertensive drug with beta and alpha blocking properties.

■ INDICATIONS: It is prescribed for the treatment of hypertension.

■ CONTRAINDICATIONS: The presence of asthma or emphysema prohibits its use. It should be used with caution in patients with diabetes as it may mask symptoms of hypoglycemia, particularly tachycardia.

■ ADVERSE EFFECTS: Among the most serious adverse reactions are orthostatic hypotension, fatigue, headache, skin rashes, scalp paresthesia, nausea, vomiting, and constipation.

**labia** /lā'bē·ə/ *sing.* **labium** [L, lip], **1.** the lips; the fleshy liplike edges of an organ or tissue. **2.** the folds of skin at the opening of the vagina.

**labial** /lā'bē·əl /, pertaining to the lips. See **bilabial**.

**-labial,** combining form meaning 'lips': *alveololabial, glossolabial, maxillolabial.*

**labial arch wire,** a stainless steel arch wire of high tensile strength whose arms come through the embrasure between the canine and lateral incisors in the maxillary arch, and between the canines and first premolar in the mandibular arch. It is used primarily for moving teeth in the lingual direction and for retruding the anterior teeth and closing spaces.

**labial bar** /lā'bē·əl/, a bar that is installed labially or buccally to the dental arch and connects bilateral parts of a mandibular removable partial denture.

**labial flange,** the part of a denture that occupies the outer vestibule of the mouth.

**labial glands** [L, *labium*, lip, *glans*, acorn], small mucous or serous glands embedded in the lips.

**labial notch,** a depression in the border of a denture that accommodates the labial frenum.

**labial vestibule,** that portion of the vestibule of the mouth that lies between the lips and the teeth and gingivae, or residual alveolar ridges.

**labia majora** /major'ə/, *sing.* **labium majus** /mā'jəs/, two long lips of skin, one on each side of the vaginal orifice outside the labia minora. They extend from the anterior labial commissure to the posterior labial commissure and form the lateral boundaries of the pudendal cleft. Each labium contains areolar tissue, fat, and a thin layer of nonstriated muscle. In some women the outer surface of each lip may be covered with coarse pubic hair. The embryonic derivations of the labia majora and the scrotum are homologous.

**labia minora** /minôr'ə/, *sing.* **labium minus** /mē'nəs/, two thin folds of skin between the labia majora, extending from the clitoris backward on both sides of the vaginal orifice, ending between it and the labia majora. Anteriorly each labium divides into an upper and a lower division. The upper divisions pass above the clitoris and meet to form the preputium clitoridis; the lower divisions pass beneath the clitoris and unite to form the frenulum of the clitoris. Opposed surfaces of the labia minora contain sebaceous follicles.

**labile** /lā'bil/ [L, *labilis*, slipping], **1.** unstable; characterized by a tendency to change or be altered or modified. **2.** (in psychiatry) characterized by rapidly shifting or changing emotions, as in bipolar disorder and certain types of schizophrenia; emotionally unstable. **—lability,** *n.*

**-labile,** combining form meaning 'unstable, subject to change': *frigolabile, siccolabile, thixolabile.*

**lability.** See **labile**.

**labio-,** combining form meaning 'lips, particularly the lips of the mouth': *labiocervical, labiodental, labiomental.*

**labiodental** /lā'bē·ōden'təl/ [L, *labium*, lip, *dens*, tooth], **1.** pertaining to the labial, or lip-facing, surfaces of the 12 anterior teeth. **2.** pertaining to the sounds of speech that require a special coordination of teeth and lips.

**labioglossolaryngeal paralysis.** See **bulbar paralysis**.

**labiolingual fixed orthodontic appliance** /lā'bē·ōling'gwəl/ [L, *labium*, lip, *lingua*, tongue], an appliance for correcting or improving malocclusion that is anchored to the maxillary and mandibular first permanent molars. The appliance has labial arches that fit into horizontal buccal tubes attached to anchor bands and lingual arches that are fastened to the lingual side of the anchor bands.

**labioversion** /lā′bē·ō·ver′zhən/ [L, *labium,* lip + vertere, to turn], displacement of a tooth labially from the line of occlusion.

**labium.** See **labia.**

**labium majus.** See **labia majora.**

**labium minus.** See **labia minora.**

**labor** [L, work], the time and the processes that occur during parturition from the beginning of cervical dilation to the delivery of the placenta. Also spelled **labour.** See also **birth, cardinal movements of labor, station.**

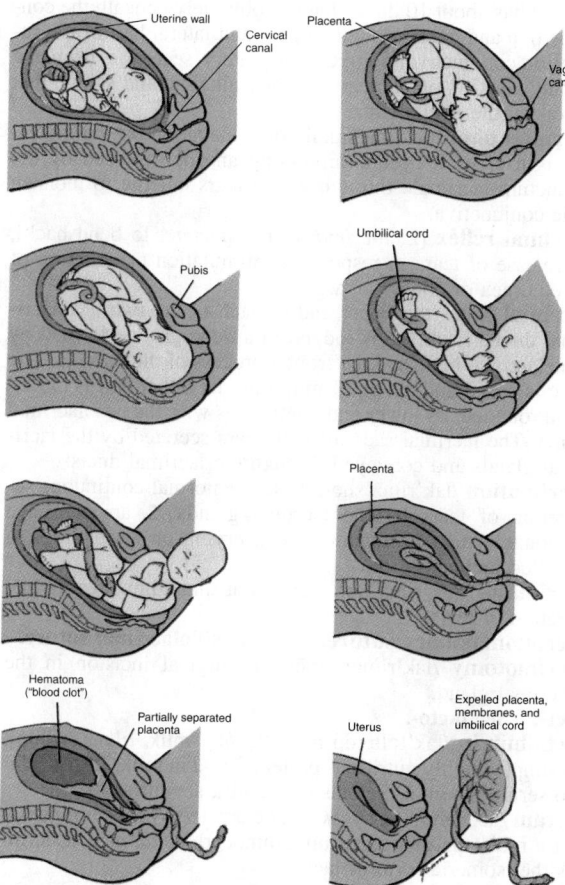

**Mechanisms of labor** *(Moore, 2000)*

**labor, abnormal.** See **dystocia.**

**laboratory (lab)** /lab′(ə)rətôr′e/ [L, *laborare,* to labor], **1.** a facility, room, building, or part of a building in which scientific research, experimentation, testing, or other investigative activities are carried out. **2.** pertaining to a laboratory.

**laboratory core.** See **core.**

**laboratory data interpretation,** a nursing intervention from the Nursing Interventions Classification (NIC) defined as critical analysis of patient laboratory data in order to assist with clinical decision making. See also **Nursing Interventions Classification.**

**laboratory diagnosis,** a diagnosis arrived at after study of secretions, excretions, or tissue through chemical, microscopic, or bacteriologic means or by biopsy. See also **diagnosis.**

**laboratory error,** any error made by the personnel in a clinical laboratory in performing a test, interpreting data, or reporting or recording the results. Laboratory error must always be considered a possible explanation for findings that are at variance with the composite clinical condition of the patient or are widely divergent from previous laboratory tests. General procedure is to repeat the test when an abnormal result is found.

**laboratory medicine,** the branch of medicine in which specimens of tissue, fluid, or other body substance are examined outside of the person, usually in the laboratory. Some fields of laboratory medicine are **chemistry, cytology, hematology, histology,** and **pathology.**

**laboratory test,** a procedure, usually conducted in a laboratory, that is intended to detect, identify, or quantify one or more significant substances, evaluate organ functions, or establish the nature of a condition or disease. Laboratory tests range from quite simple to extremely sophisticated. In modern medical practice they are commonly used to help establish or confirm a diagnosis and often aid in the management of disease.

**labor coach,** a person who assists a woman in labor and delivery by closely attending to her emotional needs and encouraging her to use properly the breathing patterns, concentration techniques, body positions, and massage techniques that were taught in a program of psychophysical preparation for childbirth. The task of a labor coach is to minimize the need for pharmacologic pain relief and to decrease or eliminate the use of analgesia or anesthesia. Usually the coach is the father of the baby or a close friend of the mother, but a professional labor coach, often a registered nurse specially trained in a method, may fill the role. Also called **doula, labor support person.** See also **monitrice.**

**labored breathing,** abnormal respiration characterized by evidence of increased effort, including the use of accessory muscles of respiration in the chest wall, stridor, grunting, or nasal flaring.

**labor induction,** a nursing intervention from the Nursing Interventions Classification (NIC) defined as initiation or augmentation of labor by mechanical or pharmacological methods. See also **Nursing Interventions Classification.**

**labor pains** [L, *labor,* work, *poena,* penalty], pain associated with contraction of the uterus in labor.

**labor support person.** See **labor coach.**

**labor suppression,** a nursing intervention from the Nursing Interventions Classification (NIC) defined as controlling uterine contractions prior to 37 weeks of gestation to prevent preterm birth. See also **Nursing Interventions Classification.**

**labour.** See **labor.**

**labyrinth.** See **internal ear.**

**labyrinth-,** combining form meaning 'labyrinth or inner ear': *labyrinthitis, labyrinthectomy.*

**labyrinthectomy** /lab′ərinthek′təme/, the surgical excision of the aural labyrinth.

**labyrinthine** /lab′ərin′thin/ [Gk, *labyrinthos,* maze], pertaining to or resembling a labyrinth or maze, such as the structure of the inner ear.

**labyrinthine reflex.** See **kinetic reflex.**

**labyrinthine righting,** one of the five basic neuromuscular reactions involved in a change of body positions. The change stimulates cells in the semicircular canals of the inner ear, causing neck muscles to respond by automatically adjusting the head to the new position.

**labyrinthine vertigo.** See **Ménière's disease.**

**labyrinthitis** /lab′ərinthī′tis/ [Gk, *labyrinthos,* maze, *itis*], inflammation of the labyrinthine canals of the inner ear, resulting in vertigo.

**labyrinthus osseus.** See **osseous labyrinth.**

**laceration** /las′ərā′shən/ [L, *lacerare,* to tear], **1.** the act of tearing or slashing. **2.** a torn, jagged wound. —**lacerate,** *v.,* **lacerated,** *adj.*

**laceration of cervix** [L, *lacerare,* to tear, *cervix,* neck], a wound or irregular tear of the cervix uteri during childbirth.

**laceration of the perineum** [L, *lacerare,* to tear; Gk, *perineos*], a wound or irregular tear of the perineal tissues during childbirth.

**lacertus** /lə·ser′təs/ [L, lizard, because of a fancied resemblance], a general term for certain fibrous attachments of muscles.

**lachrymal.** See **lacrimal.**

**lachrymation.** See **lacrimation.**

**lacri-, lachry-,** combining form meaning 'tears': *lacrimalin, lacrimator, lacrimotomy.*

**lacrimal** /lak′riməl/ [L, *lacrima,* tear], pertaining to tears. Also spelled **lachrymal.**

**lacrimal apparatus,** a network of structures of the eye that secrete tears and drain them from the surface of the eyeball. These parts include the lacrimal glands, the lacrimal ducts, the lacrimal canals, the lacrimal sacs, and the nasolacrimal ducts.

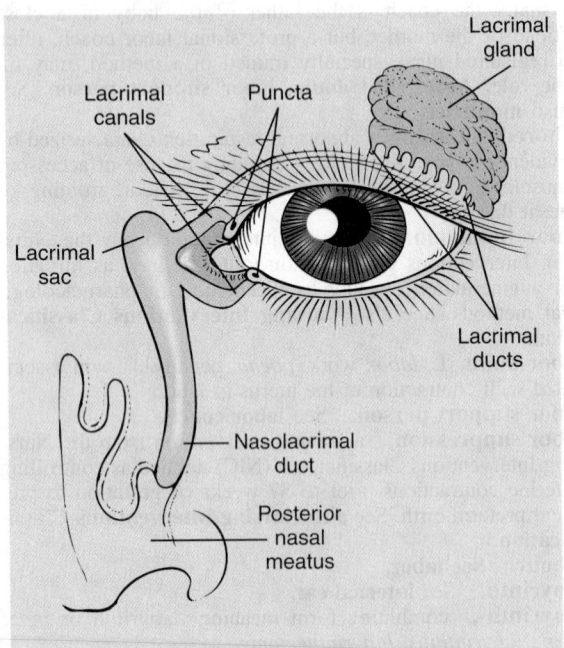

**Lacrimal apparatus** *(Lewis, Heitkemper, and Dirksen, 2000)*

**lacrimal bone,** one of the smallest and most fragile bones of the face, located at the anterior part of the medial wall of the orbit. It unites with the maxilla to form the groove for the lacrimal sac.

**lacrimal canaliculus.** See **lacrimal duct.**

**lacrimal caruncle,** the small, reddish, fleshy protuberance that fills the triangular space between the medial margins of the upper and lower eyelids. It contains sebaceous and sudoriferous glands and secretes a whitish substance that collects and often dries in the corner of the eye.

**lacrimal duct,** one of a pair of channels through which tears pass from the lacrimal lake to the lacrimal sac of each eye. Also called **lacrimal canaliculus.**

**lacrimal fold** [L, *lacrima,* tear; AS, *fealdan*], a valvelike fold of mucous membrane at the lower part of the nasolacrimal duct. Also called **Hasner's fold.**

**lacrimal gland,** one of a pair of glands situated superior and lateral to the eye bulb in the lacrimal fossa of the frontal bone. It is an oval structure about the size of an almond. The gland has about 10 ducts that run obliquely beneath the conjunctiva and open along the upper and lateral half of the superior conjunctival fornix. The watery secretion from the gland consists of the tears, slightly alkaline and saline, that moisten the conjunctiva.

**lacrimal papilla,** the small conic elevation on the medial margin of each eyelid, supporting an apex pierced by the punctum lacrimale through which tears emerge to moisten the conjunctiva.

**lacrimal reflex** [L, *lacrima,* tear, *reflectere,* to bend back], a release of tears in response to stimulation or irritation of the cornea or conjunctiva.

**lacrimal sac,** the upper end of each of the two nasolacrimal ducts. Each sac is lodged in a deep groove formed by the lacrimal bone and the frontal process of the maxilla. The sac is ovoid and about 13 mm long. Its upper end is closed and rounded, its lower end continuous with the nasolacrimal duct. The lacrimal sacs fill with tears secreted by the lacrimal glands and conveyed through the lacrimal ducts.

**lacrimation** /lak′rimā′shən/, **1.** the normal continuous secretion of tears by the lacrimal glands. **2.** an excessive amount of tear production, as in crying or weeping. Also spelled **lachrymation.**

**lacrimator** /lak′rimā′tər/, an agent that stimulates the secretion of tears.

**lacrimomaxillary suture.** See **maxillolacrimal suture.**

**lacrimotomy** /lak′rimot′əmē/, a surgical incision in the lacrimal gland.

**lact-.** See **lacto-.**

**lactalbumin** /lak′təlbyo͞o′min/ [L, *lac,* milk, *albus,* white], a simple, highly nutritious protein found in milk. It is similar to serum albumin. See also **albumin, serum albumin.**

**lactam** /lak′təm/, a cyclic amide created by the elimination of a molecule of water from aminocarboxylic acid. **Lactim** is the isomeric form of lactam.

**lactase** /lak′tās/ [L, *lac* + Fr, *diastase,* enzyme], an enzyme that catalyzes the hydrolysis of lactose to glucose and galactose. Lactase is concentrated in the kidney, liver, and intestinal mucosa. Also called **beta-galactosidase.**

**lactase deficiency,** an inherited abnormality in which the amount of the digestive enzyme lactase is inadequate for the normal digestion of milk products, resulting in the inability to digest lactose (except for the bacterial breakdown of lactose in the large intestine). Lactose intolerance usually doesn't appear until 4 or 5 years of age, begins gradually, and persists throughout life. In adults a relative deficiency may appear as a natural process of aging; it occurs more frequently in persons of Asiatic and African heritage. A lactase inadequacy also may result from subtotal gastrectomy and may be secondary to any disease of the small intestine in which structural changes occur such as tropical sprue, ulcerative colitis, infectious hepatitis, and kwashiorkor; severe malnutrition; or from some types of antibiotic therapy. See also **lactose intolerance.**

**lactate** /lak'tāt/, an anion of lactic acid.

**lactate dehydrogenase (LD),** an enzyme that is found in the cytoplasm of almost all body tissues, where its main function is to catalyze the oxidation of L-lactate to pyruvate. It is assayed as a measure of anaerobic carbohydrate metabolism and as one of several serum indicators of myocardial infarction and muscular dystrophies. Serum levels of LD usually rise 12 to 18 hours after myocardial cell necrosis. See also **CK isoenzyme fraction, Duchenne's muscular dystrophy, aspartate aminotransferase.**

**lactate dehydrogenase test (LDH),** a blood test used to detect levels of LDH, which is widely distributed throughout the body. Disease or injury to body tissues such as the heart, liver, red blood cells, kidneys, skeletal muscles, brain, and lungs will result in higher-than-normal blood levels. Five separate isoenzymes make up the total LDH, with each body tissue containing a predominance of one or more of these fractions.

**lactation** /laktā'shən/ [L, *lac*, milk, *atio*, process], the process of synthesis and secretion of milk from the breasts in the nourishment of an infant or child. See also **breastfeeding.**

**lactation counseling,** a nursing intervention from the Nursing Interventions Classification (NIC) defined as use of an interactive helping process to assist in maintenance of successful breastfeeding. See also **Nursing Interventions Classification.**

**lactation mastitis.** See **caked breast.**

**lactation suppression,** a nursing intervention from the Nursing Interventions Classification (NIC) defined as facilitating the cessation of milk production and minimizing breast engorgement after giving birth. See also **Nursing Interventions Classification.**

**lacteal** /lak'tē·əl/, referring to the tiny vessels in the villi of the wall of the small intestine through which chylomicrons are absorbed and released into the lymphatic system.

**lacteal fistula,** an abnormal passage opening into a lacteal duct.

**lacteal vessel,** one of the many central intestinal capillaries in the villi of the small intestine. They open into the lymphatic vessels in the submucosa. The capillary is filled with milky-white chyle caused by the absorption of fat from the lumen (chylomicrons) and passes chyle to the lymph circulation via the thoracic duct to the blood vascular system.

**lactic** /lak'tik/ [L, *lac* + *icus*, like], referring to milk and milk products. See also **lactic acid, lactose.**

**lactic acid,** a three-carbon organic acid produced by anaerobic respiration. L-lactic acid in muscle and blood is a product of glucose and glycogen metabolism; D-lactic acid is produced by the fermentation of dextrose by a species of micrococcus; a mixture of both D- and L-isomers is found in the stomach, in sour milk, and in certain foods prepared by bacterial fermentation, such as sauerkraut. Also called **alpha-hydroxypropionic acid.** See also **glycolysis.**

**lactic acid fermentation,** 1. the anaerobic production of lactic acid from glucose. 2. the souring of milk.

**lactic acidosis,** a disorder characterized by an accumulation of lactic acid in the blood, resulting in a lowered pH in muscle and serum. The condition occurs most commonly in tissue hypoxia, but may also result from liver impairment,

respiratory failure, burn trauma, neoplasms, and cardiovascular disease.

**lactic acid test (lactate),** a blood test that measures lactate levels, which are a fairly sensitive and reliable indicator of tissue hypoxia. Lactic acid blood levels are used to document the presence of tissue hypoxia, determine the degree of hypoxia, and monitor the effect of therapy.

**lactiferous** /laktif'ərəs/ [L, *lac* + *ferre*, to carry], pertaining to a structure that produces or conveys milk, such as the tubules of the breasts.

**lactiferous duct,** one of many channels that carry milk from the lobes of each breast to the nipple.

**lactiferous glands** [L, *lac*, milk, *ferre,* to carry, *glans,* acorn], glands that secrete or convey milk such as mammary glands.

**lactim.** See **lactam.**

**lactin.** See **lactose.**

**Lactinex,** trademark for a GI, fixed-combination drug containing *Lactobacillus acidophilus* and *Lactobacillus bulgaricus.*

**lacto-, lact-,** combining form meaning 'milk or lactic acid': *Lactobacillus, lactopeptin, lactotoxin.*

***Lactobacillus*** /lak'tōbəsil'əs/ [L, *lac* + *bacillum*, small rod], any one of a group of nonpathogenic gram-positive rod-shaped bacteria that produce lactic acid from carbohydrates. Many species are normally found in the human intestinal tract and vagina.

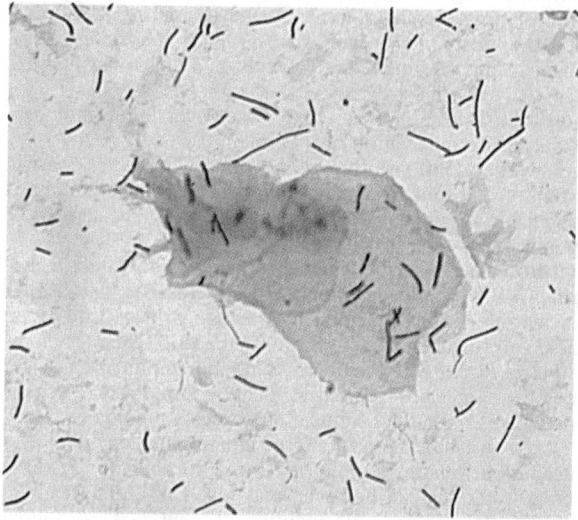

***Lactobacillus*** (Morse, Moreland, and Holmes, 1996)

***Lactobacillus acidophilus*** [L, *lac*, milk, *bacillum*, small rod, *acidus*, sour; Gk, *philein*, to love], a bacterium found in milk and dairy products and feces of bottlefed babies and adults. The strain is used to manufacture a fermented milk product. See also **acidophilus milk.**

***Lactobacillus bulgaricus***, a genus of bacteria used in the production of yogurt.

***Lactodectus mactans.*** See **black widow spider.**

**lactoferrin** /lak'tō·fer'in/, an iron-binding protein present in neurophil granules. By combining with iron, lactoferrin prevents microorganisms from combining with and using iron for their growth and development.

**lactogen** /lak'təjən/ [L, *lac* + Gk, *genein*, to produce], a drug or other substance that enhances the production and secretion of milk. —**lactogenic,** *adj.*

**lactogenic hormone.** See **prolactin.**

**lacto-ovo-vegetarian** /lak'tō·ōv'ōvej'əter'ē·ən/, one whose diet consists primarily of foods of vegetable origin but also includes some animal products such as eggs *(ovo),* milk, and cheese *(lacto),* but no meat, fish, or poultry. Also called **ovo-lacto-vegetarian.**

**lactoperoxidase** /-pərok'sidās/, an enzyme found in milk and saliva. It is believed to inhibit a number of microorganisms, functioning in a nonspecific immunity role.

**lactose** /lak'tos/ [L, *lac* + Gk, *glykys*, sweet], a disaccharide found in the milk of all mammals. On hydrolysis, lactose yields the monosaccharides glucose and galactose. Lactose is used as a laxative, a diuretic, and a component of formulas for infants. Also called **lactin, milk sugar.** See also **lactase deficiency, lactose intolerance, sugar.**

**lactose intolerance,** a sensitivity disorder resulting in the inability to digest lactose from milk products because of a inadequate production of or defect in the enzyme lactase. Symptoms of the disorder are bloating, flatus, nausea, diarrhea, and abdominal cramps. The diet is adjusted according to the tolerance level; milk-derived foods as milk, cheese, butter, margarine, and any products containing milk such as cakes, ice cream, cream soups, and sauces are restricted. Also called **milk intolerance.** See also **lactase deficiency.**

**lactosuria** /lak'təsŏŏr'ē·ə/ [L, *lac* + Gk, *glykys*, sweet, *ouron*, urine], the presence of lactose in the urine, a condition that may occur in late pregnancy or during lactation.

**lactotherapy** /-ther'əpē/ [L, *lac*, milk; Gk, *therapeia*, treatment], any treatment that depends on a diet consisting exclusively or almost exclusively of milk.

**lactotoxin** /-tok'sin/, any toxic base occurring in milk as a result of decomposition of its proteins.

**lacto-vegetarian** /-vej'əter'ē·ən/, one whose diet consists of milk and milk products *(lacto)* in addition to foods of vegetable origin but does not include eggs, meat, fish, or poultry.

**lactulose** /lak'tyəlōs/, a nonabsorbable synthetic disaccharide, 4-0-[β]-D-galactopyranosyl-D-fructose, $C_{12}H_{22}O_{11}$. It is hydrolyzed in the colon by bacteria primarily to lactic acid and small amounts of formic and acetic acids, which results in increased osmotic pressure and acidification of the colonic contents. It is used as a cathartic in chronic constipation. Because the acidification causes ammonia to be removed from the blood to form ammonium ion, it is also used in the treatment of hepatic coma. Its ability to increase fecal water content, however, may also cause diarrhea.

**lacuna** /ləkyōō'nə/, *pl.* **lacunae** [L, pit], **1.** a hollow within a structure, especially bony tissue, in which lie osteoblasts. **2.** a gap, as in the field of vision.

**lacunar** /lakyōō'nər/ [L, *lacuna*, pit], pertaining to or characterized by the presence of pits, depressions, hollows, or spaces.

**lacunar state,** a pseudobulbar disorder characterized by the appearance of small, smooth-walled cavities in the brain tissue. The condition usually follows a series of small strokes, particularly in older adults with arterial hypertension and arteriosclerosis. Also called **status lacunaris.**

**lacus lacrimalis** /lā'kəs lak'rimā'ləs/ [L, *lacus*, lake, *lacrimalis*, tears], a triangular space separating the medial ends of the upper and the lower eyelids at the inner canthus where the tears collect. It is an extension of the medial canthus and contains the lacrimal caruncle.

**LAD,** **1.** abbreviation for *left anterior descending.* **2.** abbreviation for **leukocyte adhesion deficiency.**

**LADME** /lad'mē/, an abbreviation for the time course of drug distribution, representing the terms *liberation, absorption, distribution, metabolism,* and *elimination.*

**Laënnec's catarrh** /lā'əneks'/ [René T. H. Laënnec, French physician, 1781–1826; Gk, *kata,* down, *rhoia,* flow], a form of bronchial asthma characterized by the expectoration of small, viscous, beadlike bodies of sputum. These bodies, called **Laënnec's pearls,** are formed in the bronchioles.

**Laënnec's cirrhosis** [René T. H. Laënnec; Gk, *kirrhos,* yellow-orange, *osis,* condition], a fibrotic form of cirrhosis precipitated by alcohol abuse. Also called **alcoholic cirrhosis.** See **cirrhosis.**

**Laënnec's pearls.** See **Laënnec's catarrh.**

**Laetrile** /lā'ətril/, a substance composed primarily of amygdalin, a cyanogenic glycoside derived from apricot pits. Laetrile has been offered as a cancer medication despite clinical studies by the National Cancer Institute that failed to show benefits from its use. It is claimed that amygdalin is hydrolyzed by enzymes in cancer cells to produce benzaldehyde and hydrogen cyanide, which kill the cancer cells. It is not FDA approved. Also called **vitamin $B_{17}$.**

**laevo-.** See **levo-.**

**laf,** abbreviation for **laminar air flow.**

**lagen-,** combining form meaning 'flasklike': *lageniform.*

**-lagnia, -lagny,** suffix meaning 'lust or a sexual predilection': *osmolagnia, pyrolagnia, scoptolagnia.*

**lagophthalmos** /lag'əfthal'məs/ [Gk, *lagos,* hare, *ophthalmos,* eye], an abnormal condition in which an eye may not be fully closed because of a neurologic or muscular disorder.

**lag phase** [Dan, *lakke,* go slowly; Gk, *phasis,* appearance], a time span during which bacteria injected into a fresh medium have not begun to multiply, although they may enlarge.

**la grippe.** See **influenza.**

**laity** /lā'itē/ [Gk, *laikos,* of the people], a nonprofessional segment of the population, as viewed from the perspective of a member of a particular profession. A clergyman may regard a physician as a member of the laity and vice versa.

**LAK,** abbreviation for **lymphokine-activated killer cells.**

**laked blood** /lākt/ [Fr, *laque,* a deep red color], blood that is clear, red, and homogenous because of hemolysis of the red blood cells, as may occur in poisoning and severe extensive burns.

**Laki-Lorand factor.** See **factor XIII.**

**lal-, lalio-, lalo-,** prefix meaning 'talk, babble': *laliatry, lalognosis, lalopathology.*

**La Leche League International** /lä lech'ā/ [Sp, *la leche,* the milk], an organization that promotes and provides education about breastfeeding.

**-lalia,** suffix meaning a 'disorder of speech': *agitolalia, echolalia, oxylalia.*

**lalio-.** See **lal-.**

**lallation** /lalā'shən/ [L, *lallare,* to babble], **1.** babbling, repetitive, unintelligible utterances, such as the babbling of an infant and the mumbled speech of schizophrenics, alcoholics, and the severely mentally retarded. **2.** a speech disorder characterized by a defective pronunciation of words containing the sound /l/ or by the use of the sound /l/ in place of the sound /r/. Compare **rhotacism.**

**lalo-.** See **lal-.**

**lalophobia** /lal'ōfō'bē·ə/ [Gk, *lalia,* speech, *phobos,* fear], a morbid dread of talking caused by fear and anxiety that one will stammer or stutter.

**lamarckism** /ləmär'kizəm/ [Jean B. P. de Lamarck, French naturalist, 1744–1829; Gk, *ismos,* practice], the theory postulated that organic evolution results from structural changes in plants and animals caused by adaptation to environmental conditions and that these acquired characteristics are transmitted to offspring. Also called **lamarckianism, Lamarck's theory.** Compare **darwinism.** —**lamarckian,** *adj., n.*

**Lamaze method** /ləmäz′/ [Fernand Lamaze, French obstetrician, 1890–1957],  a method of psychophysical preparation for childbirth developed in the 1950s. It requires classes, practice at home, and coaching during labor and delivery, often by a trained coach called a 'monitrice.' The classes, given during pregnancy, teach the physiology of pregnancy and childbirth, exercises to develop strength in the abdominal muscles and control of isolated muscles of the vagina and perineum, and techniques of breathing and relaxation to promote control and relaxation during labor. The woman is conditioned by repetition and practice to dissociate herself from the source of a stimulus by concentration on a focal point, by consciously relaxing all muscles, and by breathing in a special way at a particular rate—thereby training herself not to pay attention to the stimuli associated with labor. The kind and rate of breathing change with the advancing stages of labor. During the early part of the first stage of labor, when the uterine cervix is dilated less than 5 cm and the contractions occur every 2 to 4 minutes, last 40 to 60 seconds, and are of mild to moderate strength, the mother does slow chest breathing during contractions. Her fingers may rest lightly on her lower ribs to feel them rise and fall. The abdominal wall does not move with respiration. She may perform an effleurage, or rhythmic fingertip massage, of her lower abdomen during the contractions. The rate of respiration is 10 or fewer breaths a minute, increasing to 12 per minute as labor intensifies. A deep 'cleansing breath' is taken before and after each contraction. During the active part of the first stage of labor up to the transition to the second stage, the cervix is from 5 cm to nearly fully dilated, the interval between contractions is from 1-1/2 to 4 minutes, and the duration of contractions is from 45 to 90 seconds. (The interval decreases, and the intensity and duration increase as labor progresses.) During contractions the mother breathes quietly and shallowly in her chest. The rate of her breathing varies with the strength of the contractions, increasing during a contraction to as fast as once a second at the peak and slowing to every 6 seconds as the uterus relaxes. She is coached to concentrate on the focal point she has selected, to perform the effleurage of her abdomen, to relax her perineal and vaginal muscles, and to take a cleansing breath at the beginning and end of each contraction. At the end of the first stage of labor, when the cervix is almost completely dilated and the contractions are strong, occurring every 1-1/2 to 2 minutes and lasting 60 to 90 seconds, the mother begins to feel the urge to bear down and push during contractions. She avoids pushing before full dilation by combining several light, shallow breaths in the chest with short puffing exhalations as the urge increases during the contractions. During the second stage of labor the cervix is fully dilated and contractions are strong, frequent, and expulsive. The mother's head and shoulders are supported on pillows. During contractions she is helped to draw her legs back, flexing the thighs against the abdomen, holding them behind the lower thigh with her hands. Her chin is tucked on her chest, the air is blocked from escaping from her lungs, her perineum is relaxed, and she bears down forcibly. Depending on the length of the contraction, several pushes of 10 to 15 or more seconds may be possible during the contraction. As the baby's head crowns, she is asked to pant lightly so that the head may be delivered slowly. The advantages of the method include the need for little or no analgesia for relief of pain and participation in the labor by the mother, giving her a great sense of self-satisfaction at delivery. The father of the baby also benefits by participating in the birth of his child. Compare **Bradley method, Read method.**

**lambda** /lam′də/,  **1.** Λ, λ, the eleventh letter of the Greek alphabet. **2.** a posterior fontanel of the skull marking the point where the sagittal and lambdoidal sutures meet.

**lambda (λ) light chain,**  one of two kinds of smaller polypeptide chains present in an immunoglobulin molecule. See also **kappa (κ) light chain.**

**lambda wave,**  a low-voltage occipital wave recorded by electroencephalography during visual activity.

**lambdoid** /lam′doid/,  having the shape of the Greek letter lambda. See also **lambdoidal suture.**

**lambdoidal suture** /lamdoi′dəl/,  the interdigitating connection between the occipital bone and the parietal bones of the skull. It is continuous with the occipitomastoid suture between the occipital and the mastoid portions of the temporal bones.

**lambert (L)** /lom′bert, lam′bərt/ [J.H. Lambert, German physicist, 1728–1777],  a unit of luminance or brightness of a perfectly diffusing surface, whether emitting or reflecting, equal to a total luminous flux of one lumen per square centimeter.

**lamella** /ləmel′ə/, *pl.* **lamellae** [L, small plate],  **1.** a thin leaf or plate, as of bone. **2.** a medicated disk of glycerin and an alkaloid, for insertion under the eyelid, where it dissolves and is absorbed for local application.

**lamellar** /ləmel′ər/ [L, *lamella,* small plate],  pertaining to or characterized by lamellae.

**lamellar exfoliation** [L, *lamella* + *ex,* without, *folium,* leaf; AS, *niwe,* new, *boren,* born],  a congenital skin disorder transmitted as an autosomal-recessive trait in which a parchmentlike scaly membrane that covers the infant peels off within 24 hours of birth. Complete healing or a progressively less severe process of reforming and shedding of the scales then occurs. Also called **ichthyosis congenita, ichthyosis fetalis, lamellar desquamation of the newborn, lamellar ichthyosis of the newborn.** See also **collodion baby.**

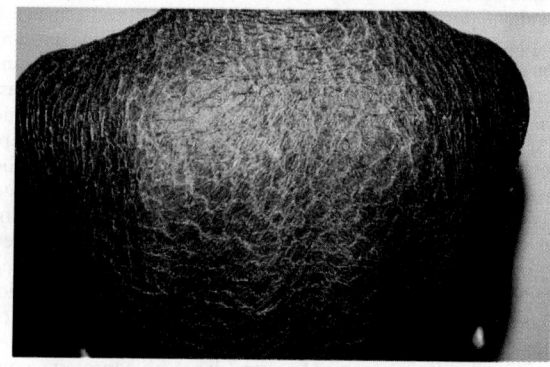

**Lamellar exfoliation in an adult**
*(Zitelli and Davis, 1997)*

**lameness** /lām′nəs/ [ME, *lama,* to break],  a condition of diminished function, particularly because of a foot or leg injury. The term may also be applied to a stiff or painful back that makes walking difficult.

**Lamictal,** trademark for an anticonvulsant drug (lamotrigine).

**lamin-,** combining form meaning 'layer or lamina': *laminagram, laminated, laminotomy.*

**lamina** /lam'inə/, *pl.* **laminae** [L, thin plate], any thin, flat layer of membrane or other bulkier tissue. It may be structureless or part of a structure, as the laminae of the vertebral arch.

**lamina densa,** a layer of epithelial basal lamina that appears dark in electron micrographs.

**lamina dura,** 1. a sheet of compact alveolar bone that lies adjacent to the periodontal membrane, the lining of the tooth socket. 2. a radiographic term used to identify the radiopaque lining of a tooth socket.

**lamina lucida,** a layer of epithelial basal lamina that appears light or clear in electron micrographs.

**lamin antibody** /lam'in/, a type of immunoglobulin found in the serum of some patients with autoimmune diseases, including systemic lupus erythematosus.

**lamina propria,** a layer of connective tissue that lies just under the epithelium of a mucous membrane.

**laminar air flow (laf)** /lam'inər/ [L, *lamina*, plate; Gk, *aer*; AS, *flowan*], a system of circulating filtered air in parallel-flowing planes in hospitals or other health care facilities. The system reduces the risk of airborne contamination and exposure to chemical pollutants in surgical theaters, food preparation areas, hospital pharmacies, and laboratories.

**laminar flow.** See **laminar air flow.**

**laminaria** /lam'iner'ē·ə/ [L, *lamina*, plate], a type of seaweed that swells on absorption of water.

**laminaria tent,** a cone of dried seaweed that swells as it absorbs water and therefore is used to dilate the cervix nontraumatically in preparation for induced abortion or induced labor.

**laminated thrombus** /lam'inā'tid/, a blood clot composed of blood platelets, fibrin, clotting factors, and cellular elements arranged in layers, apparently formed at different times.

**laminectomy** /lam'inek'təmē/ [L, *lamina* + Gk, *ektomē*, excision], surgical removal of the bony arches of one or more vertebrae. It is performed to relieve compression of the spinal cord as caused by a bone displaced in an injury, as the result of degeneration of a disk, or to reach and remove a displaced intervertebral disk. With the patient prone and under general anesthesia, the laminae are removed, and the underlying problem is corrected. Spinal fusion with cages, rods, screws, and/or bone graft is used to stabilize the spine if several laminae are removed. After surgery the bed is kept flat to hold the patient's spine in correct alignment. If the procedure is a cervical laminectomy, the patient is observed for signs of respiratory distress caused by cord edema. Motor function and sensation in the extremities are evaluated every 2 to 4 hours for 48 hours. The dressing is examined frequently for hemorrhage or leakage of cerebrospinal fluid. The patient is taught to logroll without twisting the spine or hips. —**laminectomize,** *v.*

**laminin** /lam'inin/, any of several large glycoproteins consisting of three polypeptide subunits and found in basement membranes. It facilitates linkage with collagen and other basement membrane components and is involved in neurite regeneration.

**laminotomy** /-ot'əmē/, the surgical division of the lamina of a vertebral arch. Also called **rachiotomy.**

**laminotrigine,** an anticonvulsant drug.
■ INDICATIONS: It is prescribed as adjunctive therapy in the treatment of partial seizures in epilepsy patients over the age of 16.

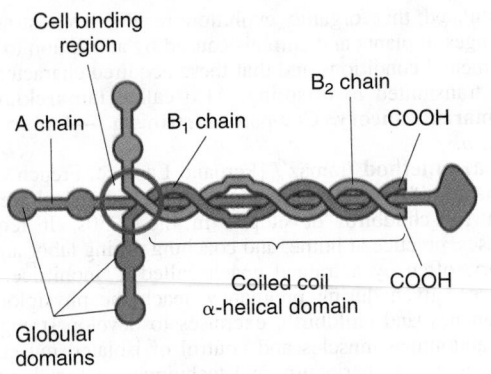

**Laminin** *(Carlson, 1999)*

■ CONTRAINDICATIONS: The drug should not be given to patients with an allergy to laminotrigine or the components of its formulation. Caution is advised in the use of the drug in patients with heart, kidney, or liver disease or skin rash.
■ ADVERSE EFFECTS: The side effects most often reported include headache, bruising, bleeding, flulike symptoms, stomach ache, hot flashes, sore throat, and dermatitis.

**lamivudine (3TC),** an antiviral.
■ INDICATIONS: The Epivir brand name form of this drug is used to treat HIV infection in combination with zidovudine. The Epivir-HBV brand name form is used to treat hepatitis B.
■ CONTRAINDICATIONS: Known hypersensitivity to this drug prohibits its use.
■ ADVERSE EFFECTS: Life-threatening effects of this drug are neutropenia, anemia, thrombocytopenia, and pediatric pancreatitis. Other adverse effects are anorexia, cramps, dyspepsia, taste change, hearing loss, and photophobia. Common side effects are fever, headache, malaise, dizziness, insomnia, depression, fatigue, chills, nausea, vomiting, diarrhea, cough, rash, myalgia, arthralgia, and musculoskeletal pain.

**lampbrush chromosome** [Gk, *lampas*, torch; AS, *bryst*, bristle], an excessively large type of chromosome found in the oocytes of many animals. It has long, threadlike, projecting loops, giving it a hairy, brushlike appearance. See also **giant chromosome.**

**lampro-,** combining form meaning 'clear': *lamprophonia, lamprophonic.*

**LAN,** an abbreviation for **local area network.**

**lance** [L, *lancea*, spear], to incise a furuncle or an abscess to release accumulated pus. A topical anesthetic is applied, the lesion is incised, and the pus is drained. A drain is inserted if the infection is deep. The bacteria involved are most often staphylococci. An antibiotic is given systemically if the boil is facial to prevent infection from spreading into the cranial sinuses. Infected drainage is kept off surrounding skin to prevent a recurrence. Careful handwashing is essential to prevent infection.

**Lancefield's classification** [Rebecca C. Lancefield, American bacteriologist, 1895–1981], a serologic classification of streptococci based on their antigenic characteristics. The bacteria are divided into 13 groups by the identification of their pathologic action. Group A contains most of the streptococci that cause infection in humans. Groups B to T are less pathogenic and are often present without causing disease. Most are hemolytic; of those, the beta subgroup is the most likely to be the cause of infection.

**lancet** /lan'sit/ [L, *lancea,* lance], a short pointed blade used to obtain a drop of blood for a capillary sample. It has a guard above the blade that prevents deep incision, and it is usually disposable.

**lancinating** /lan'sinā'ting/ [L, *lancea,* lance], sharply cutting or tearing, such as lancinating pain.

**Landau-Kleffner syndrome** /län'dou klef'nər/ [William M. Landau, American neurologist, 20th century; F.R. Kleffner, American neurologist, 20th century], an epileptic syndrome of childhood characterized by partial or generalized seizures, psychomotor abnormalities, and aphasia progressing to mutism. The electroencephalogram from bilateral temporal regions is abnormal. Also called **acquired epileptic aphasia.**

**Landau reflex** /lan'dou/, a normal response of infants when held in a horizontal prone position to maintain a convex arc with the head raised and the legs slightly flexed. The reflex is poor in those with floppy infant syndrome and exaggerated in hypertonic and opisthotonic infants.

**landmark** /land'märk/ [AS *land,* + *meark,* mark], a readily recognizable anatomical structure used as a point of reference in establishing the location of another structure or in determining certain measurements.

**landmark position** [AS, *land* + *meark,* mark; L, *positio*], the correct placement of the hands on the chest in cardiopulmonary resuscitation. See also **cardiopulmonary resuscitation.**

**Landouzy-Dejerine muscular dystrophy.** See **fascioscapulohumeral muscular dystrophy.**

**Landsteiner's classification** /land'stī'nərz/ [Karl Landsteiner, American pathologist and Nobel laureate, 1868–1943], the classification of blood groups A, B, AB, and O on the basis of the presence or absence of the two agglutinogens A and B on the erythrocytes in human blood.

**Langer-Giedion syndrome** /lang'ər zhē-dē-ôN'/ [Leonard O. Langer, Jr. American physician, 20th century; A. Giedion, Swiss physician, 20th century], an inherited disorder characterized by mental retardation, microcephaly, multiple exostoses, characteristic facies with bulbous nose, sparse hair, cone shaped epiphyses, loose redundant skin, joint laxity, and other anomalies.

**Langerhans' cells** /lung'ərhuns, lang'ərhans/ [Paul Langerhans, German pathologist, 1847–1888], a stellate dendritic cell found mostly in the stratum spinosum of the epidermis. It is believed to have an immune function with surface markers characteristic of macrophages and monocytes.

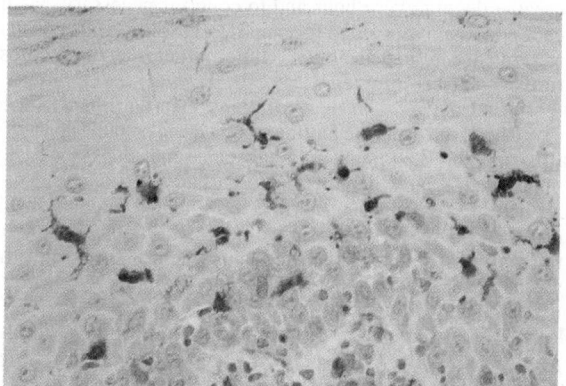

**Normal Langerhans' cells**
*(Regezi, Sciubba, and Pogrel, 2000)*

**Langer's line.** See **cleavage line.**

**Langer's muscle** /läng'ərz/ [Carl Ritter von Edenberg von Langer, Austrian anatomist, 1819–1887], muscular fibers from the insertion of the pectoralis major muscle over the bicipital groove to the insertion of the latissimus dorsi.

**Langhans' layer.** See **cytotrophoblast.**

**language** /lang'gwij/ [L, *lingua,* tongue], **1.** a defined set of characters that, when used alone or in combinations, form a meaningful set of words and symbols that are used for communication. **2.** a unified, related set of commands or instructions that a computer can accept.

**language disorder,** a partial or complete disruption in the ability to understand and produce the conventional symbols or words that comprise one's native language.

**lano-,** combining form meaning 'wool': *lanolin, lanonol, lanosterol.*

**lanolin** /lan'əlin/ [L, *lana,* wool, *oleum,* oil], a fatlike substance from the wool of sheep. It contains about 25% water as a water-in-oil emulsion and is used as an ointment base and an emollient for the skin. Also called **hydrous wool fat.**

**Lanoxin,** trademark for a cardiac glycoside (digoxin).

**lansoprazole,** an antiulcer agent and proton pump inhibitor.

■ INDICATIONS: This drug is used to treat gastroesophageal reflux disease (GERD), severe erosive esophagitis, poorly responsive systemic GERD, and pathologic hypersecretory conditions (Zollinger-Ellison syndrome, systemic mastocytosis, multiple endocrine adenomas). It is also a potentially effective treatment for duodenal and gastric ulcers and for maintenance of healed duodenal ulcers.

■ CONTRAINDICATIONS: Known hypersensitivity to this drug prohibits its use.

■ ADVERSE EFFECTS: Life-threatening effects of this drug are cerebrovascular accident, myocardial infarction, shock, hematuria, and hemolysis. Other adverse effects include confusion, agitation, amnesia, depression, diarrhea, vomiting, nausea, acid regurgitation, anorexia, irritable colon, upper respiratory infections, asthma, bronchitis, dyspnea, alopecia, weight gain or loss, gout, deafness, eye pain, otitis media, chest pain, angina, tachycardia, bradycardia, palpitations, hypertension or hypotension, vasodilation, glycosuria, impotence, kidney calculus, breast enlargement, and anemia.

**lanthanum (La)** /lan'thənəm/ [Gk, *lanthanein,* to escape notice], a rare earth metallic element. Its atomic number is 57; its atomic mass is 138.91.

**lanuginous** /lənⁿōō'jinəs/ [L, *lanugo,* down], pertaining to lanugo.

**lanugo** /lanyōō'gō/ [L, down], **1.** the soft, downy hair covering a normal fetus beginning in the fifth month of gestation and almost entirely shed by the ninth month. **2.** the fine, soft hair covering all parts of the body except palms, soles, and areas where other types of hair are normally found. Also called **vellus hair.**

**lanulous** /lan'yŏōləs/ [L, *lana,* wool, *osus,* filled with], downy or covered with short, fine wooly hair, such as the skin of a fetus. See also **lanugo.**

**lap,** abbreviation for **laparotomy.**

**LAP, 1.** abbreviation for *left atrial pressure.* **2.** abbreviation for **leukocyte alkaline phosphatase.**

**laparectomy** /lap'ərek'təmē/, the surgical excision of tissue from the abdomen wall, usually performed to correct muscle laxity.

**laparo-** /lap'ərō/, combining form meaning 'abdomen or abdominal wall': *laparectomy, laparotomy, laparorrhaphy.*

**laparoenterostomy** /lap'ərō-en'təros'təmē/ [Gk, *lapara,* loin, *enteron,* bowel, *stoma,* mouth], the surgical installation of a tube through an external opening in the abdomen to drain the bowel. A similar procedure may be used to supply

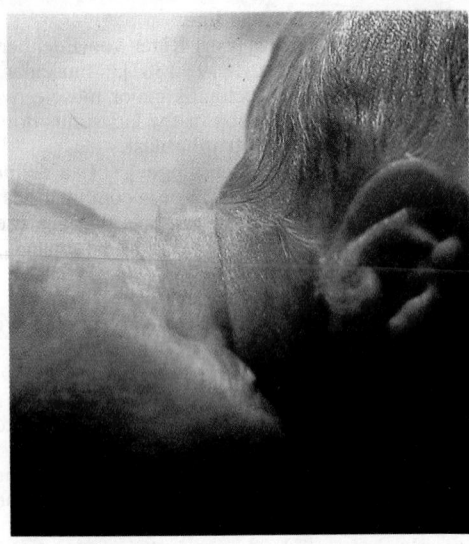

**Lanugo** *(Zitelli and Davis, 1997)*

nutrients to a patient with an upper digestive tract obstruction.

**laparoenterotomy** /lap′ərō·en′tərot′əmē/ [Gk, *lapara*, loin, *enteron*, bowel, *temnein*, to cut], a surgical incision in the intestine through the abdominal wall.

**laparohysterectomy** /-his′tərek′təmē/ [Gk, *lapara*, loin, *hystera*, womb, *ektomē*, excision], a hysterectomy performed by making an excision through the abdominal wall.

**laparohystero-oophorectomy** /-his′tərō-/, the surgical removal of the uterus and ovaries through a small incision in the abdominal wall.

**laparohysterosalpingo-oophorectomy** /-his′tərō′salping′gō-/, the surgical removal of the uterus, ovaries, and fallopian tubes through a small incision in the abdominal wall.

**laparomyitis** /-mī·ī′tis/, an inflammation of the abdominal or lumbar muscles.

**laparosalpingo-oophorectomy** /-salping′gō-/, the surgical removal of the ovaries and fallopian tubes through a small incision in the abdominal wall.

**laparoscope** /lap′ərəskōp′/ [Gk, *lapara*, loin, *skopein*, to look], a type of endoscope consisting of an illuminated tube with an optical system. It is inserted through the abdominal wall for examining the peritoneal cavity. Also called **celioscope, peritoneoscope.** —**laparoscopic,** *adj.,* **laparoscopy,** *n.*

**laparoscopic-assisted vaginal hysteroscopy** /-skop′ik/, a procedure for viewing the inner surface of the uterus with a specially designed endoscope inserted through the cervix. Before insertion the uterus is inflated with carbon dioxide or a glucose solution administered through the cervix. See also **laparoscopy, hysteroscopy.**

**laparoscopic cholecystectomy.** See **cholecystectomy.**

**laparoscopic sterilization** [Gk, *lapara*, loin, *skopein*, to view; L, *sterilis*, barren], the process of rendering a woman incapable of reproduction by inserting a specialized endoscope through a small incision in the abdominal wall. Sterilization may be performed through the incision with clips to occlude the fallopian tubes or by electrocoagulation and severance.

**laparoscopy** /lap′əros′kəpē/, the examination of the abdominal cavity with a laparoscope through one or more small incisions in the abdominal wall, usually at the umbilicus. The procedure is used for inspection of the ovaries and fallopian tubes, diagnosis of endometriosis, destruction of uterine leiomyomas, and myomectomy. Gynecologic sterilization also can be accomplished by fulguration of the oviducts or by tubal ligation. A general anesthetic is used, but the patient does not require overnight hospitalization. Also called **abdominoscopy.** See also **endoscopy, laparoscope.**

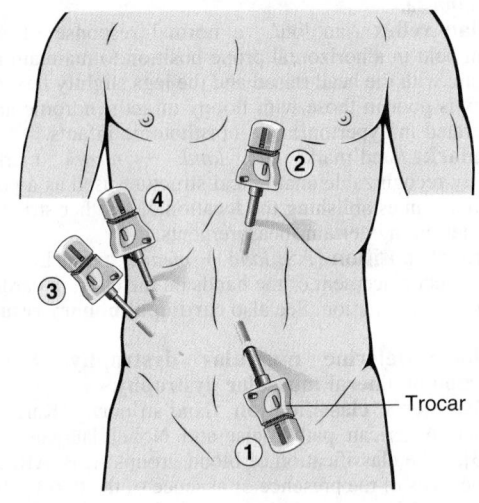

— Trocar

**Laparoscopy: placement of trocars** *(Chabner, 2001)*

**laparotomy (lap)** /lap′ərot′əmē/ [Gk, *lapara* + *temnein*, to cut], any surgical incision into the peritoneal cavity, usually performed under general or regional anesthesia, often on an exploratory basis. Before surgery a complete blood count and urinalysis are done; immediately before surgery the skin may be shaved and cleansed from the nipple line to the pubis. Food and fluids by mouth are withheld for several hours before surgery. If the intestine is to be opened, a nasogastric tube is inserted. Frequent observation of vital signs and drainage systems is essential. Fluid intake and output are recorded. The patient is turned and encouraged to breathe deeply every hour and to cough if necessary. Medication is given as needed for pain relief. Some kinds of laparotomy are **appendectomy, cholecystectomy,** and **colostomy.** —**laparotomize,** *v.*

**lap-board** [ME, *lappa* + *bord*, plank], a flat board placed over the lap to serve as a temporary desk or table.

**lapis** /lap′is/ [L, stone], any substance that does not easily volatilize, as lapis dentalis, or tooth tartar.

**Laplace's law** /läpläs′/ [Pierre S. de Laplace, French physicist, 1749–1827], a principle of physics that the tension on the wall of a sphere is the product of the pressure times the radius of the chamber and the tension is inversely related to the thickness of the wall.

**-lapse,** suffix meaning 'a slip or fall backward': *collapse, prolapse, relapse.*

**large calorie.** See **Calorie.**

**large for gestational age (LGA) infant,** an infant whose fetal growth was accelerated and whose size and weight at birth fall above the ninetieth percentile of appropriate for gestational age infants, whether delivered prematurely, at term, or later than term. Factors other than genetic influences that cause accelerated intrauterine growth include maternal diabetes mellitus and Beckwith's syndrome. LGA infants born of diabetic mothers are generally obese and plethoric, with very pink skin and red, shiny cheeks. They are often listless and limp, feed poorly, and become hypoglycemic within the first few hours. A major problem is that preterm LGA infants, because of their size, are not recognized as high-risk neonates with immature organ system development. Often these infants develop respiratory distress syndrome because pulmonary maturation occurs later in gestation. In cases of Beckwith's syndrome the infant is characterized by gigantism, macroglossia, omphalocele or umbilical hernia, and visceromegaly. Compare **small for gestational age (SGA) infant.**

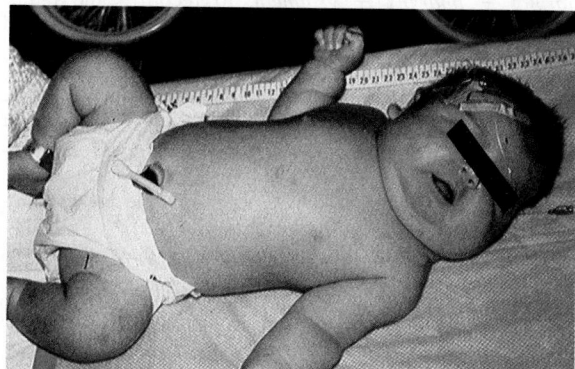

**Large for gestational age infant** (Zitelli and Davis, 1997)

**large intestine** [L, *largus,* abundant, *intestinum*], the part of the digestive tract comprising the cecum; appendix; ascending, transverse, descending, and sigmoid colons; and rectum. The ileocecal valve separates the cecum from the ileum.

**lariat structure** /ler′ē·ət/, a ring of intron segments that have been spliced out of a messenger ribonucleic acid molecule by enzymes. Some introns form a long tail attached to the ring, giving the structure the appearance of a microscopic cowboy lariat.

**Larmor frequency** [Joseph Larmor, Irish physicist, 1857–1942], the frequency of the precession of a charged particle when its motion comes under the influence of an applied magnetic field and a central force.

**Larodopa,** trademark for an antiparkinsonian (levodopa).

**Laron dwarfism** /lä·rôN′/ [Zvi Laron, Israeli endocrinologist, b. 1927], an autosomal recessive syndrome of skeletal growth retardation resulting from impaired inability to synthesize insulin-like growth factor I, usually because of growth hormone receptor defects. Also called **Laron syndrome.**

**Larsen's syndrome** /lär′sənz/ [Loren Joseph Larsen, American orthopedic surgeon, b. 1914], cleft palate, flattened facies, multiple congenital dislocations, and foot deformities.

**larva** /lär′və/ [L, specter], the early immature form of an animal, which undergoes metamorphosis to an adult form. **—larval,** *adj.*

**larval** /lär′vəl/, pertaining to an organism in the preadult stage of a larva.

**larva migrans.** See **cutaneous larva migrans, visceral larva migrans.**

**laryng-.** See **laryngo-.**

**laryngeal** /lerin′jē·əl/ [Gk, *larynx*], pertaining to the larynx.

**laryngeal cancer** [Gk, *larynx* + L, *cancer,* crab], a malignant neoplastic disease characterized by a tumor arising from the epithelium of the structures of the larynx. Laryngeal tumors are more common in men than in women and occur most frequently between 50 and 70 years of age. Chronic alcoholism and heavy use of tobacco increase the risk of developing the cancer. Persistent hoarseness is usually the first sign; advanced lesions may cause a sore throat, dyspnea, dysphagia, and cervical adenopathy. Diagnostic measures include direct laryngoscopy, biopsy, and radiologic examination, including tomographic studies and chest films. Malignant tumors of the larynx are usually epidermoid carcinomas. Radiation is generally recommended for small lesions; total laryngectomy, often combined with radiotherapy, is indicated for extensive lesions. Chemotherapy may be used to try to spare the larynx. After the operation many persons with laryngectomies learn esophageal speech; some use an electric larynx, and a few undergo surgical reconstruction. See also **laryngectomy.**

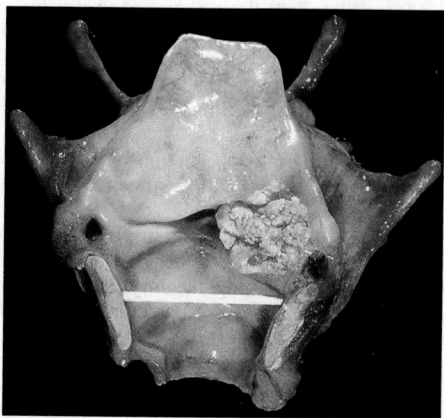

**Squamous cell carcinoma of the larynx** (Fletcher, 2000)

**laryngeal catheterization,** the insertion of a catheter into the larynx for the purpose of removing secretions or introducing gases.

**laryngeal diphtheria.** See **diphtheritic laryngitis.**

**laryngeal edema.** See **edema of glottis.**

**laryngeal mask airway,** a device for maintaining a patent airway without tracheal intubation, consisting of a tube connected to an oval inflatable cuff that seals the larynx. Also called **Brain airway.**

**laryngeal polyp** [Gk, *larynx* + *poly,* many, *pous,* foot], a polyp on the vocal cords that causes hoarseness as a result of vocal abuse or smoking.

**laryngeal pouch.** See **laryngocele.**

**laryngeal prominence.** See **Adam's apple.**

**laryngeal reflex** [Gk, *larynx* + L, *reflectere,* to bend back], a cough reflex caused by irritation of the fauces and larynx.

**laryngeal vertigo** [Gk, *larynx* + L, *vertere,* to turn], a short episode of dizziness or unconsciousness following a paroxysmal attack of coughing or laryngeal spasm. Also called **cough syncope.**

**laryngeal web,** a common congenital malformation of the larynx that may be thin and translucent or thicker and more fibrotic; it is spread between the vocal folds near the anterior commissure and may cause hoarseness, aphonia, and other symptoms.

**laryngectomy** /ler'injek'təmē/ [Gk, *larynx* + *ektomē,* excision], surgical removal of the larynx performed to treat cancer of the larynx. Before surgery the patient is referred to a speech pathologist to discuss esophageal speech and prostheses. Antibiotics are usually administered to reduce the risk of infection. With the patient under regional or general anesthesia, the trachea is sutured to the skin, as in a tracheostomy, to ensure an adequate airway. In a partial laryngectomy only the vocal cords are removed, and the tracheostomy is closed within several days. If the malignancy is extensive, the entire larynx is removed, along with the hyoid, epiglottis, false chords, true chords, cricoid cartilage, and two or three rings of the trachea; the tracheostomy is permanent; and a laryngectomy tube is left in place. After surgery the patient is observed for excessive coughing or any vomiting of blood, and the laryngectomy tube is kept free of mucus. A humidifier or vaporizer is useful to decrease coughing and mucus production. IV fluids are given, and liquid feedings may be given via nasogastric tube. After surgery the patient cannot smell, sniff, or blow his or her nose. A Magic Slate and flash cards are useful for communication between patient, staff, and family. The laryngectomy tube is removed 3 to 6 weeks after surgery. There is permanent speech loss with the total laryngectomy. Compare **neck dissection, radical neck dissection. —laryngectomize,** *v.*

**laryngismus** /ler'injiz'məs/ [Gk, *laryngismos,* whooping], spasm of the larynx. Also called **spasmatic croup, spasmodic croup.**

**laryngismus stridulus.** See **crowing inspiration.**

**laryngitis** /ler'injī'tis/ [Gk, *larynx* + *itis*], inflammation of the mucous membrane lining the larynx, accompanied by edema of the vocal cords with hoarseness or loss of voice, occurring as an acute disorder caused by a cold, by irritating fumes, by sudden temperature changes, or as a chronic condition resulting from excessive use of the voice, heavy smoking, or exposure to irritating fumes. In acute laryngitis there may be a cough, and the throat usually feels scratchy and painful. The patient is advised to remain in an environment with an even temperature, to avoid talking and exposure to tobacco smoke, and to inhale steam containing aromatic vapors such as tincture of benzoin, oil of pine, or menthol. Acute laryngitis may cause severe respiratory distress in children under 5 years of age because the relatively small larynx of the young child is subject to spasm when irritated or infected and readily becomes partially or totally obstructed. The youngster may develop a hoarse, barking cough and an inspiratory stridor and may become restless, gasping for air. Treatment consists of the administration of copious amounts of vaporized cool mist. Chronic laryngitis may be treated by removal of irritants, avoidance of smoking, voice rest, correction of stressful voice habits, cough medication, steam inhalations, and spraying the throat with an astringent antiseptic, such as hexylresorcinol.

**laryngo-, laryng-,** combining form meaning 'larynx': *laryngocentesis, laryngograph.*

**laryngocele** /ləring'gōsēl'/, an abnormal air-containing cavity connected to the laryngeal ventricle. It is caused by an evagination of the mucous membrane of the ventricle and may displace and enlarge the false vocal cord, resulting in hoarseness and airway obstruction. Because a laryngocele is also a potential reservoir of infection, it is usually excised. Also called **laryngeal pouch, saccule of larynx.**

**laryngography.** See **laryngopharyngography.**

**laryngologist** /ler'ing·gol'əjist/, a physician who specializes in the diagnosis and treatment of disorders of the larynx.

**laryngology** /ler'ing·gol'əjē/, [Gk, *larynx* + *logos,* science], the branch of medicine that specializes in the causes and treatments of disorders of the larynx.

**laryngopharyngeal** /-ferin'jē·əl/, pertaining to the larynx and pharynx. See also **laryngopharynx.**

**laryngopharyngitis** /ləring'gōfer'injī'tis/ [Gk, *larynx* + *pharynx,* throat, *itis*], inflammation of the larynx and pharynx. See also **laryngitis, pharyngitis.**

**laryngopharyngography** /lering'gōfer'ing·gog'rəfē/ [Gk, *larynx* + *pharynx* + *graphein,* to record], the radiographic examination of the larynx and pharynx. Also called **laryngography.**

**laryngopharynx** /lering'gōfer'ingks/ [Gk, *larynx* + *pharynx,* throat], one of the three regions of the throat, extending from the hyoid bone to the esophagus. Compare **nasopharynx, oropharynx. —laryngopharyngeal** /lering'-gōferin'jē·əl/, *adj.*

**laryngoscope** /ləring'gəskōp/, an endoscope for examining the larynx.

**laryngoscopic** /-skop'ik/ [Gk, *larynx* + *skopein,* to view], pertaining to the use of a laryngoscope.

**laryngoscopy** /ler'ing·gos'kəpē/ [Gk, *larynx* + *skopein,* to view], the use of a laryngoscope to view the larynx.

**laryngospasm** /ləring'gōspaz'əm/ [Gk, *larynx* + *spasmos,* spasm], a spasmodic closure of the larynx.

**laryngostasis.** See **croup.**

**laryngotomy** /ler'ing·got'əmē/ [Gk, *larynx* + *temnein,* to cut], a surgical incision into the larynx through the cricovocal membrane. It is usually an emergency procedure that is performed when a standard tracheotomy cannot be done.

**laryngotracheitis** /-trā'kē·ī'tis/, an inflammation of the larynx and trachea.

**laryngotracheobronchitis (LTB)** /lering'gōtrā'kē·ō'brongkī'tis/ [Gk, *larynx* + L, *trachea;* Gk, *bronchos,* windpipe, *itis*], an inflammation of the major respiratory passages, usually causing hoarseness, nonproductive cough, and dyspnea. Among the causes are infections by coxsackieviruses, echoviruses, *Haemophilus influenzae,* and *Corynebacterium diphtheriae.* Treatment usually includes steam inhalations, cough suppressants, and, for bacterial infections, appropriate antibiotics. See also **croup.**

**laryngotracheotomy** /-trā'kē·ot'əmē/, a surgical incision into the larynx and trachea.

**larynx** /ler'ingks/ [Gk], the organ of voice that is part of the upper air passage connecting the pharynx with the trachea. It accounts for a large bump in the neck called the Adam's apple and is larger in men than in women, although it remains the same size in men and women until puberty. The larynx forms the caudal portion of the anterior wall of the pharynx and is lined with mucous membrane that is continuous with that of the pharynx and the trachea. The larynx extends vertically to the fourth, fifth, and sixth cervical vertebrae and is somewhat higher in the female and during childhood. It is composed of three single cartilages and three paired cartilages, all connected together by ligaments and moved by various muscles. The single cartilages are the thy-

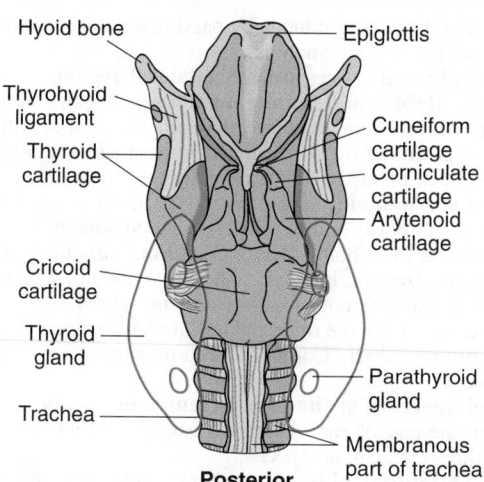

Labels: Hyoid bone, Epiglottis, Thyrohyoid ligament, Cuneiform cartilage, Thyroid cartilage, Corniculate cartilage, Arytenoid cartilage, Cricoid cartilage, Thyroid gland, Parathyroid gland, Trachea, Membranous part of trachea, Posterior

**Larynx: posterior view** *(Phipps, Sands, and Marek, 1999)*

roid, cricoid, and epiglottis. The paired cartilages are the arytenoid, corniculate, and cuneiform, which support the vocal folds. —**laryngeal**, *adj.*

**LAS,** abbreviation for **lymphadenopathy syndrome.**

**Lasan,** trademark for an antipsoriatic (anthralin).

**laser** /lā'zər/, abbreviation for *light amplification by stimulated emission of radiation,* a source of intense monochromatic radiation of the visible, ultraviolet, or infrared portions of the spectrum. Lasers are used in surgery to divide or cause adhesions or to destroy or fix tissue in place. Also called **optic laser.**

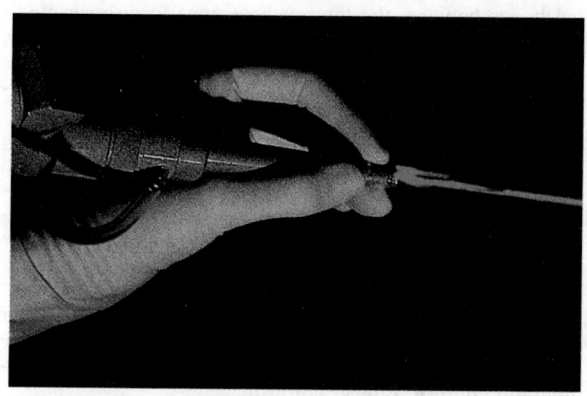

**Carbon dioxide laser handpiece** *(Ball, 1995)*

**laser angioplasty,** the opening of an occluded artery with laser energy delivered to the site through a fiberoptic probe.

**laser bronchoscopy,** bronchoscopy that is performed with the aid of a laser beam directed through fiberoptic equipment. It is used in the diagnosis and treatment of bronchial disorders, tracheobronchial tumors, and subglottic stenosis.

**laser disk,** a plastic disk that stores computer data as tiny pits etched in the surface. A laser beam scanning the pits

translates the data into a computer language. They are frequently used for computer-assisted instruction.

**laser iridotomy,** a procedure for the treatment of closed-angle glaucoma in which the patient has intermittent periods of increased intraocular pressure. The iris gradually occludes the trabecular meshwork. Symptoms may be absent, but there is increased intraocular pressure. The angle-closure mechanism is controlled by creating an opening in the iris. It is usually performed after control of an acute attack when signs of ocular congestion have disappeared. Laser iridotomy can be performed by several kinds of lasers. A topical anesthetic is applied, and a contact lens with a small condensing lens is used to focus the beam on the iris. Iridotomy is made in the mid-iris on the nasal or temporal superior side. Specific techniques vary with the type of laser used.

**laser pain management,** the use of lasers to relieve pain. This treatment has been applied effectively to specific acupuncture points where there is no anatomic dysfunction at the base of the pain.

**laser precautions,** a nursing intervention from the Nursing Interventions Classification (NIC) defined as limiting the risk of injury to the patient related to use of a laser. See also **Nursing Interventions Classification.**

**laser printer,** a high-speed output device for computers using a technique in which laser beams focus images on photosensitive drums. Compare **dot-matrix printer, impact printer.**

**laser trabeculoplasty,** an application of laser energy in the treatment of primary open-angle glaucoma. The procedure may be recommended when intraocular pressure increases despite administration of topical agents. Laser trabeculoplasty increases aqueous outflow facility. An argon laser is commonly used. The eye is anesthetized with a topical anesthetic. The trabecular network is viewed through an antireflective-coated four-mirror gonioprism. A power setting and exposure time are selected to blanch the anterior trabecular meshwork with laser energy without causing bubble formation. A potential complication is a temporary increase in intraocular pressure, which is treated with drugs. The effects of laser trabeculoplasty are not always long lasting. Episcleral fibrosis and scarring are main causes of failure of the therapy. The procedure is usually not effective with additional application, and many patients eventually require antiglaucoma medications again.

**LASIK** /lā'sik/, plastic surgery on the cornea in which the excimer laser and microkeratome are combined for vision correction; the microkeratome is used to shave a thin slice and create a hinged flap in the cornea, the flap is reflected back, the exposed cornea is reshaped by the laser, and the flap is replaced, without sutures, to heal back into position.

**Lasix,** trademark for a diuretic (furosemide).

**Lassa fever** /lä'sə/ [Lassa, Nigeria; L, *febris,* fever], a highly contagious disease of West Africa caused by an arenavirus. It is transmitted by contact with or inhalation of excreta of infected rodents. Person-to-person transmission occurs through contact with infected blood, secretions, or excreta, or transmission may be airborne. Lassa fever is characterized by fever, pharyngitis, dysphagia, and ecchymoses. Varying degrees of deafness occur in one third of cases. Pleural effusion, edema and renal involvement, mental disorientation, confusion, and death from cardiac failure often ensue. Stringent precautions are taken against the spread of infection. Early treatment with ribovirin and supportive symptomatic care are essential. See also **arenavirus, Argentine hemorrhagic fever, Bolivian hemorrhagic fever.**

**last sacraments** [ME, *laste* + L, *sacramentum,* solemn oath], a religious ceremony performed by a member of the clergy in behalf of a person about to die. Also called **last rites.**

**latchkey children,** minors who are often at home alone because their parents are at work.

**late dyspituitary eunuchism.** See **acromegalic eunuchoidism.**

**latency period** /lā′tənsē/ [L, *latere,* to be concealed; Gk, *peri* + *hodos,* way], **1.** also called **incubation period.** The period between contact with a pathogen and development of symptoms. **2.** also called **latency of response.** The time between stimulus and response. **3.** also called **latency stage.** A period between early childhood and puberty when there is little overt interest in the opposite sex.

**latency stage** [L, *latere,* to be concealed; Fr, *estage,* stage], (in psychoanalysis) a period in psychosexual development occurring between early childhood and puberty when sexual motivation and expression are repressed or transferred, through sublimation, to the feelings and behavioral patterns expected as typical of the age.

**latent** /lā′tənt/ [L, *latere,* to be concealed], dormant; existing as a potential; for example, tuberculosis may be latent for extended periods of time and become active under certain conditions.

**latent carcinoma.** See **occult carcinoma.**

**latent diabetes.** See **impaired glucose tolerance.**

**latent energy** [L, *latere,* to be concealed; Gk, *energeia*], the energy contained in an object as a result of its position in space, its internal structure, and stresses imposed on it. Also called **potential energy.**

**latent heat** [L, *latere,* to be concealed; AS, *haetu*], the heat absorbed by a substance when it changes from a solid to a liquid or from a liquid to a gas without an accompanying rise in temperature.

**latent image,** an invisible image produced in a film emulsion by x-rays or visible light that can be converted into a visible image by development.

**latent learning** [L, *latere,* to be concealed; ME, *lernen*], learning acquired unintentionally. It may remain in the subconscious, or be latent, until a need for the knowledge arises.

**latent malaria** [L, *latere,* to be concealed; It, *mal* + *aria,* bad air], a continuing infection without clinical symptoms, resulting from a balance established between the parasite and the body's immune system. See also **malaria.**

**latent period,** the interval between the time of exposure to an injurious dose of radiation and the response.

**latent phase,** the early stage of labor that is characterized by irregular, infrequent, and mild contractions and little or no dilation of the cervix or descent of the fetus. Also called **prodromal labor.** See also **Friedman curve.**

**latent syphilis** [L, *latere,* to be concealed; Gk, *syn,* together, *philein,* to love], a stage of syphilis infection that occurs after 1 year of infection in which no clinical symptoms appear but serologic tests indicate the presence of the syphilis spirochete.

**latent tetany** [L, *latere,* to be concealed; Gk, *tetanos,* convulsive tension], a form of tetany that is elicited only by mechanical or electrical stimuli.

**late-phase hypersensitivity reaction,** an inflammatory response in IgE allergic diseases. It begins 2 to 4 hours after exposure to an antigen, peaks at 6 to 12 hours, and disappears after 24 hours.

**lateral** /lat′ərəl/ [L, *latus,* side], **1.** pertaining to the side. **2.** away from the midsagittal plane. **3.** farther from the midsagittal plane. **4.** to the right or left of the midsagittal plane.

**5.** a speech sound produced by passing air along one or both sides of the tongue, such as *l.*

**lateral abdominal region.** See **lateral region.**

**lateral antebrachial cutaneous nerve,** a continuation of the musculocutaneous nerve that innervates the skin over the radial side of the forearm and sometimes an area of skin of the back of the hand; its modality is sensory.

**lateral aortic node,** a lumbar lymph node in any of three clusters of nodes serving the pelvis and abdomen. The afferent vessels from both sides drain various structures such as the testes, ovaries, kidneys, and lateral abdominal muscles. Most of the efferent vessels from the lateral aortic nodes converge to form the right and left lumbar trunks, which join the cisterna chyli. Compare **preaortic node, retroaortic node.**

**lateral aperture of the fourth ventricle,** an opening between the end of each lateral recess of the fourth ventricle and the subarachnoid space.

**lateral atlantoaxial joint,** either of a pair of joints, one on each side of the body, formed by the inferior articular surface of the atlas and the superior surface of the axis.

**lateral cerebellar nucleus.** See **dentate nucleus.** This term is more commonly used to refer to animals other than primates.

**lateral cerebral sulcus,** a deep cleft marking the division of the temporal from the frontal and parietal lobes of brain. Also called **fissure of Sylvius, lateral cerebral fissure.**

**lateral column.** See **lateral horn.**

**lateral condensation method,** a technique for filling root canals, in which a preselected gutta-percha cone is sealed into the apex of the root and other cones are forced laterally with a spreader until the canal is filled. Compare **Johnson's method.**

**lateral corticospinal tract,** a group of nerve fibers in the lateral funiculus of the spinal cord, originating in the cerebral cortex.

**lateral cuneiform bone,** one of the three cuneiform bones of the foot. It is located in the center of the front row of tarsal bones between the intermediate cuneiform bone medially, the cuboid bone laterally, the scaphoid bone posteriorly, and the third metatarsal anteriorly. It also articulates with the second and fourth metatarsals. Also called **external cuneiform bone, third cuneiform bone.**

**lateral decentering,** in radiology, an error in positioning of the tube head or a focused grid, resulting in partial grid cutoff over the entire film.

**lateral geniculate body,** one of two elevations of the lateral posterior thalamus receiving visual impulses from the retina via the optic nerves and tracts and relaying the impulses to the calcarine (visual) cortex.

**lateral horn,** a small hornlike projection of gray matter into the white matter of the spinal cord, located between the anterior and posterior horns or columns. Also called **intermediate column, lateral column.**

**lateral humeral epicondylitis,** inflammation of the tissue at the lower end of the humerus at the elbow joint, caused by the repetitive flexing of the wrist against resistance. It may result from athletic activity or manual manipulation of tools or other equipment. Pain radiates from the elbow joint. Also called **tennis elbow.** See also **epicondylitis.**

**lateral incisal guide angle,** the inclination of the incisal guide of a dental articulator in the frontal plane.

**lateralis, lateral,** a term denoting a structure situated farther from the median plane of the body or the midline of an organ.

**laterality.** See **handedness.**

**lateralization** /lat′ərəl·īzā′shən/, the tendency for certain processes to be more highly developed on one side of the brain than the other, such as development of spatial and musical thoughts in the right hemisphere and verbal and logical processes in the left hemisphere in most persons.

**lateral lobes of thyroid gland** [L, *latus*, side; Gk, *lobos* + *thyreos*, shield; L, *glans*, acorn], the left and right lobes of a highly vascular thyroid gland situated in front of the neck. The two conical lobes lying on either side of and attached to the larynx are connected by a narrow isthmus.

**lateral medullary syndrome.** See **Wallenberg's syndrome.**

**lateral nystagmus** [L, *latus*, side; Gk, *nystagmos*, nodding], an involuntary jerky movement in which the eyes move from side to side.

**lateral pectoral nerve,** one of a pair of branches from the brachial plexus that, with the medial pectoral nerve, supplies the pectoral muscles. It lies lateral to the axillary artery, arises from the lateral cord of the plexus or from the anterior divisions of the superior and middle trunks just before they unite into the cord, and ends on the deep surface of the clavicular and the cranial sternocostal parts of the pectoralis major. Compare **medial pectoral nerve.**

**lateral pelvic displacement,** one of the five major kinetic determinants of gait. It helps to synchronize the rhythmic movements of walking and is produced by the horizontal shift of the pelvis or relative hip abduction. It is often a factor in the diagnosis and treatment of various orthopedic diseases, deformities, and abnormal conditions and in the analysis and correction of dysfunctional gaits. Compare **knee-ankle interaction, knee-hip flexion, pelvic rotation, pelvic tilt.**

**lateral pinch,** a grasp in which the thumb is opposed to the middle phalanx of the index finger. Also called **key pinch.** See also **palmar pinch, pinch, tip pinch.**

**lateral projection,** a radiographic representation of the body produced by an x-ray beam that travels from the left to the right side of the body, or vice versa. It is a right lateral projection if the right side of the body is adjacent to the cassette and a left lateral projection if the left side is adjacent to it.

**lateral recumbent position,** the posture assumed by the patient lying on the left side with the right thigh and knee drawn up. Also called **English position, obstetric position, Sims' position.**

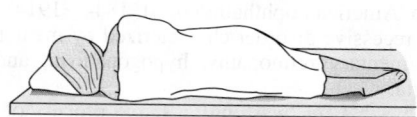

**lateral recumbent position** *(Potter and Perry, 2001)*

**lateral region,** the part of the abdomen in the middle zone on both sides of the umbilical region. Also called **external abdominal region, lateral abdominal region, lumbar region.** See also **abdominal regions.**

**lateral resolution,** the resolution of objects in a plane perpendicular to the axis of an ultrasound beam. It is a measure of the ability of the system to detect closely separated objects, such as adjacent blood vessels.

**lateral rocking,** a sideways rocking of the body used to move the body forward or backward when normal muscle action is not possible. The technique is used by some handicapped patients to move the body to or from the edge of a chair or to a different sitting position on a bed. The rocking is performed while leaning the trunk forward with the arms in front and the head in line above the knees and feet, which are pulled back.

**lateral rotation,** a turning away from the midline of the body. Compare **medial rotation.** See also **rotation.**

**lateral sinus** [L, *latus*, side, *sinus*, hollow], one of the transverse bilateral sinuses of the dura mater that lie along the attached margin of the tentorium cerebelli. They receive the superior sagittal and straight sinuses and drain into the internal jugular veins.

**lateral spinal curvature** [L, *latus*, side, *spina*, backbone, *curvatura*, bend], a bending or abnormal curve of the vertebral column to the right or left side. See also **scoliosis.**

**lateral umbilical fold,** a fold in the peritoneum produced by a slight protrusion of the inferior epigastric artery and the interfoveolar ligament. The lateral umbilical fold is about 3 cm lateral to the middle umbilical fold. Also called **plica umbilicalis lateralis.**

**lateral ventricle** [L, *latus*, side, *ventriculus*, little belly], a cavity in each cerebral hemisphere that communicates with the third ventricle through the interventricular foramen.

**late rickets** [Gk, *rhachis*, backbone], a form of rickets in which bone changes because of a kidney defect that results in a vitamin D or calcium deficiency. The disorder tends to affect older children.

**latero-,** prefix meaning 'side': *laterodeviation, lateroduction, laterotorsion.*

**lateroduction** /lat'ərōduk'shən/, **1.** muscular action in movement to one side or the other. **2.** a turning away from the midline.

**laterognathism** /lat'ərōnath'izəm/, an asymmetric mandible resulting from irregular growth and development, fractures, tumors, or soft tissue atrophy or hypertrophy.

**laterotorsion** /-tôr'shən/, displacement of the uterus to one side.

**lateroversion** /-vur'zhən/, the act of turning over or being deflected from one side to the other.

**latex** /lā'teks/ [L, liquid], an emulsion or fluidlike sap produced in special cells or vessels of certain plants. Latex contains resins, proteins, and other substances and is a source of rubber. It can cause allergic reactions in some individuals.

**latex allergy,** anaphylactic hypersensitivity to soluble proteins in latex, seen most often in patients sensitized by repeated exposure to latex.

**latex allergy response,** a nursing diagnosis accepted by the Thirteenth National Conference on the Classification of Nursing Diagnoses. The condition is an allergic response to natural latex rubber products.
■ DEFINING CHARACTERISTICS: The defining characteristics can be described as Type I, or immediate, reactions, or Type IV, delayed onset, reactions which include eczema, irritation, discomfort caused by reaction to additives, and redness. Irritant reactions include erythema, chapped or cracked skin, and blisters.
■ RELATED FACTORS: Related factors include a lack of immune mechanism response. See also **nursing diagnosis.**

**latex allergy response, risk for,** a nursing diagnosis accepted by the Thirteenth National Conference on the Classification of Nursing Diagnoses. The condition is a risk for allergic response to natural latex rubber products.
■ RISK FACTORS: Risk factors include multiple surgical procedures, especially from infancy; allergies to bananas, avocados, tropical fruits, kiwi, and chestnuts; professions with daily exposure to latex; conditions needing continuous or in-

termittent catheterization; history of reactions to latex; allergies to poinsettia plants, and a history of allergies and asthma. See also **nursing diagnosis.**

**latex fixation test** [L, *latex,* fluid, *figere,* to fasten], a serologic test used in the diagnosis of rheumatoid arthritis in which antigen-coated latex particles agglutinate with rheumatoid factors in a slide specimen of serum or synovial fluid. If positive, the screening slide test is followed by titration. Also called **RA latex test, RF test.** See also **rheumatoid factor.**

**latex precautions,** a nursing intervention from the Nursing Interventions Classification (NIC) defined as reducing the risk of a systemic reaction to latex. See also **Nursing Interventions Classification.**

**Lathrop, Rose Hawthorne** (1851–1926), an American nurse who was a daughter of Nathaniel Hawthorne. She established a home in New York for incurable cancer patients, mostly those who were poor and not accepted in hospitals because of the nature of their disease. Later she became a member of the Third Order of St. Dominic and founded the order of sisters called Servants of Relief for Incurable Cancer, which was received into the Third Order of St. Dominic in 1899. The order founded hospitals wherever there was sufficient need and offered quality care to their patients.

**latissimus dorsi** /latis′iməs dôr′sī/ [L, widest, *dorsum,* the back], one of a pair of large triangular muscles on the thoracic and lumbar areas of the back. The base of the triangle

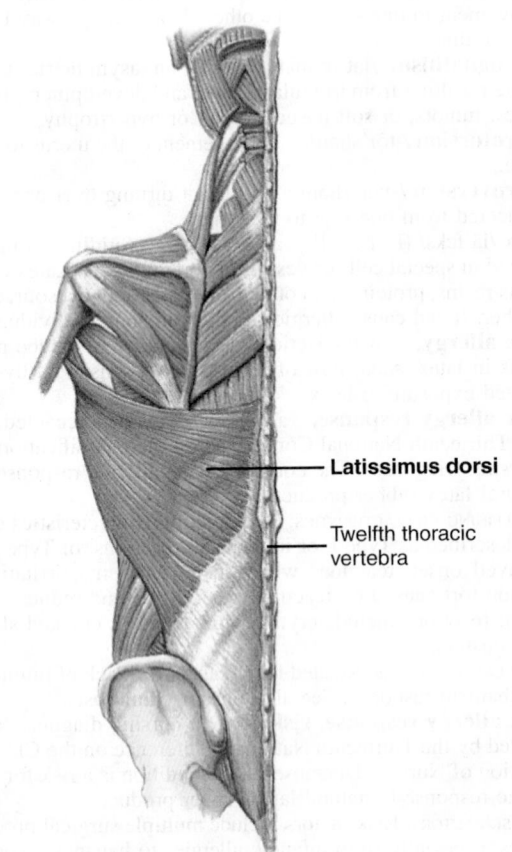

— **Latissimus dorsi**

Twelfth thoracic vertebra

**Latissimus dorsi** *(Thibodeau and Patton, 1999/John V. Hagen)*

inserts through lumbar aponeuroses to the spines of lumbar and sacral vertebrae and in the supraspinous ligaments, posterior iliac crest, and the lower four ribs. The fibers of the muscle twist as they pass the scapula and converge at the base of the intertubercular groove of the humerus. The latissimus dorsi extends, adducts, and rotates the arm medially, draws the shoulder back and down, and, with the pectoralis major, draws the body up when climbing. It is innervated by the thoracodorsal nerve. Compare **levator scapulae, rhomboideus major, rhomboideus minor, trapezius.**

**latitude** [L, *latitudio,* breadth], the ability of an x-ray imaging system to produce acceptable images over a range of exposures. If a system has wide latitude, it is possible to image parts of the body that vary in thickness or density with only one exposure. A system of lesser latitude would require a lower exposure over the thin section and a greater exposure where the absorption was greater.

**LATS,** abbreviation for **long-acting thyroid stimulator.**

**LATS-P,** abbreviation for **long-acting thyroid stimulator protector.**

**lattice formation** [OFr, *lattis,* geometric design], a three-dimensional cross-linked structure formed by the reaction of polyvalent antigens with antibodies.

**latus** /lā′təs/ [L], broad, wide.

**laudanum** /lôd′(ə)nəm/ [Gk, *landanon,* gum resin], a tincture of opium made from a solution of macerated raw opium and 50% alcohol. It is believed to have originated as a secret remedy of Paracelsus, sixteenth century Swiss alchemist and physician.

**Lauenstein method,** a technique for positioning a patient for radiographic examination of the hip joint. It emphasizes the relationship of the femur to the acetabulum. The knee of the affected leg is flexed, and the thigh is drawn up to nearly a right angle. Also called **frog leg position.**

**laughing gas** /laf′ing/, *informal.* nitrous oxide, a side effect of which is laughter or giggling when administered in less than anesthetizing amounts.

**Laurence-Moon-Bardet-Biedl syndrome** /lôr′əns mōōn′ bärdā′ bē′dəl/ [John Z. Laurence, English ophthalmologist, 1829–1870; Robert C. Moon, American ophthalmologist, 1844–1933; Georges Bardet, French physician, b. 1885; Artur Biedl, Czechoslovakian physician, 1869–1933], a hereditary condition characterized by obesity, hypogenitalism, mental deficiency, polydactylism, and retinitis pigmentosa. It is transmitted as an autosomal-recessive trait.

**Laurence-Moon syndrome** /lô′rəns·mōōn/ [John Zachariah Laurence, British ophthalmologist, 1830–1874; Robert C. Moon, American ophthalmologist, 1844–1914], an autosomal recessive disorder characterized by mental retardation, pigmentary retinopathy, hypogonadism, and spastic paraplegia.

**lavage** /ləväzh′/ [Fr, washing], **1.** the process of washing out an organ, usually the bladder, bowel, paranasal sinuses, or stomach for therapeutic purposes. **2.** to perform a lavage. Kinds of lavage are **blood lavage, gastric lavage,** and **peritoneal dialysis.** See also **irrigation.**

**law** [AS, *lagu*], **1.** (in a field of study) a rule, standard, or principle that states a fact or a relationship between factors, such as Dalton's law regarding partial pressures of gas or Koch's law regarding the specificity of a pathogen. **2.** a rule, principle, or regulation established and promulgated by a government to protect or restrict the people affected; the field of study concerned with such laws; or the collected body of the laws of a people, derived from custom and from legislation.

**Law method,** (in radiology) any of several techniques for positioning a patient for radiographic examination of the facial bones, mastoid process, and relationship of the teeth to the maxillary sinuses.

**law of definite composition,** (in chemistry) a law stating that a given compound is always made of the same elements present in the same proportion.

**law of dominance,** formerly considered as a separate principle of Mendel's laws of inheritance, but in modern genetics it is incorporated as part of the first mendelian law, the law of segregation. See also **Mendel's laws.**

**law of independent assortment.** See **Mendel's laws.**

**law of initial value,** the physiologic and psychologic principle that states that, with a given intensity of stimulation, the degree of change produced tends to be greater when the initial value of that variable is low; or the higher the initial level of functioning, the smaller is the change that can be produced.

**law of segregation.** See **Mendel's laws.**

**law of specific nerve energies.** See **Müller's law.**

**law of universal gravitation,** (in physics) the law stating that the force with which bodies are attracted to each other is directly proportional to the masses of the objects and inversely proportional to the square of the distance by which they are separated. See also **gravity, mass.**

**lawrencium (Lr)** /lôren′sē·əm/ [Ernest O. Lawrence, American physicist, 1901–1958], a synthetic transuranic metallic element. Its atomic number is 103; its atomic mass is 257.

**lax,** 1. abbreviation for **laxative.** 2. a condition of relaxation or looseness.

**laxative (lax)** /lak′sətiv/ [L, *laxare*, to loosen], 1. pertaining to a substance that causes evacuation of the bowel by a mild action. 2. a laxative agent that promotes bowel evacuation by increasing the bulk of the feces, softening the stool, or lubricating the intestinal wall. Compare **cathartic.**

**laxative regimen,** a diet that ensures an adequate intake of high-fiber bulk foods, including fruits and vegetables, to avoid chronic constipation. The regimen is supplemented with fluids and physical exercise.

**lay referral system,** an illness referral system through which a person passes from the first recognition of an abnormality to an announcement to the family, to members of the community, to traditional or culturally recognized healers, and then to the regular medical system that includes nurses and physicians. Depending on the culture and the medical care available, some steps may be omitted.

**lazy colon.** See **atonic constipation.**

**lazy leukocyte syndrome,** an immunodeficiency disease of children characterized by recurrent stomatitis, gingivitis, otitis media, and low-grade fever with severe neutropenia. The condition has been associated with abnormal chemotaxis by leukocytes. It is treated with normal human serum transfusions.

**lb** [L, *libra*], abbreviation for **pound.**

**lb ap,** abbreviation for *apothecary pound.*

**lb avdp,** abbreviation for *avoirdupois pound.*

**LBBB,** abbreviation for *left bundle branch block.*

**lbd,** abbreviation for *lower back disorder.*

**lbf,** abbreviation for *pound-force.*

**lbf/ft²,** abbreviation for *pound-force per square foot.*

**lbf/in²,** abbreviation for *pound-force per square inch.*

**lbm,** abbreviation for **lean body mass.**

**lbp,** 1. abbreviation for **low back pain.** 2. abbreviation for *low blood pressure.*

**LBW,** abbreviation for *low birth weight.* See **low-birth weight (LBW) infant.**

**LCAT,** abbreviation for **lecithin-cholesterol acyltransferase.**

**LCBF,** abbreviation for **local cerebral blood flow.**

**LCMRG,** abbreviation for **local cerebral metabolic rate of glucose utilization.**

**LD,** abbreviation for **lethal dose.**

**LD$_{50}$,** symbol for *lethal dose in 50% of population.*

**LDH,** abbreviation for **lactate dehydrogenase.**

**LDL,** abbreviation for **low-density lipoprotein.**

**L-dopa.** See **levodopa.**

**le,** abbreviation for *left eye.*

**LE,** abbreviation for *lupus erythematosus.* See **systemic lupus erythematosus.**

**leaching** /lē′ching/, removal of the soluble contents of a substance by running water or another liquid through it, leaving the insoluble portion behind.

**lead** /lēd/ [As, *laedan*, to lead], an electrical connection attached to the body to record electrical activity, especially of the heart or brain. See also **electrocardiograph, electroencephalograph.**

**lead (Pb)** /led/ [ME, *leed*], a common soft blue-gray metallic element. Its atomic number is 82; its atomic mass (weight) is 207.19. In its metallic form, lead is used as a protective shielding against x-rays. Lead is poisonous, a characteristic that has led to a reduction in the use of lead compounds as pigments for paints and inks. Normal concentrations in whole blood are 0 to 5 μg/dl. The normal amount in urine after 24-hour collection is less the 100 μg.

**lead apron** /led/ [AS, *led* + Fr, *napperon*], a protective shield of lead and rubber that may be worn by a patient, radiologic technologist or radiologist, or both during exposure to x-rays or other diagnostic radiation. It is intended to guard against excessive exposure of the reproductive and other vital body organs to ionizing radiation. Also called **protective apron.**

**lead-containing eyeglasses** /led/, glasses that provide radiation shielding for the eyes of radiographic personnel. They are particularly useful during fluoroscopic procedures or angiographic examinations.

**lead encephalopathy** /led/ [AS, *led* + Gk, *enkephalos*, brain, *pathos*, disease], a condition of brain structure and function as a result of lead poisoning, including exposure to tetraethyl lead. Children are commonly afflicted after eating chips of lead-based paints. The untreated disorder is characterized by delirium, convulsions, mania, cortical blindness, and coma.

**lead equivalent** /led/, the thickness of lead required to achieve the same shielding effect against radiation, under specified conditions, as that provided by a given material.

**leadership** [AS, *leadan*, to lead, *scieppan*, to shape], the ability to influence others to the attainment of goals. Kinds of leadership include authoritarian, democratic, participative, and permissive.

**lead pipe fracture** /led/, a linear fracture that is produced on the side of a bone opposite from the side of impact with a hard object. The point of impact is marked by a compression of bony tissue.

**lead-pipe rigidity** /led/, a state of stiffness and inflexibility that remains uniform throughout the range of passive movement. It is associated with diseases of the basal ganglia.

**lead poisoning** /led/, a toxic condition caused by the ingestion or inhalation of lead or lead compounds. Many children have developed the condition as a result of eating flaked lead paint. Poisoning also occurs from the ingestion of water from lead pipes and lead salts in certain foods and wines, the use of pewter or earthenware glazed with a lead glaze, and the use of leaded gasoline. Inhalation of lead fumes is common in industry. The acute form of intoxication is characterized by a burning sensation in the mouth and esophagus, colic, constipation or diarrhea, mental disturbances, and paralysis of the extremities, followed in severe cases by convulsions and muscular collapse. Chronic lead poisoning, which is characterized by extreme irritability, anorexia, and anemia, may progress to the acute form. Encephalopathy must be anticipated in children with lead poisoning.

**lead shielding** /led/, the use of aprons and other devices containing lead as protective measures against radiation. A layer of lead 1 mm thick can attenuate 99% of x-rays of 50 kVp and 94% of x-rays of 100 kVp.

**leakage radiation** /lē′kij/ [ONorse, *leka,* to drip; L, *radiare,* to emit rays], radiation, exclusive of the primary beam, that is emitted through the housing of equipment used in radiation therapy and radiography.

**leaky gene.** See **hypomorph.**

**lean body mass (lbm)** [ME, *lenen,* slender; AS, *bodig* + ME, *massa,* lump], the combination of cell solids, extracellular and intracellular water, and mineral mass of the body.

**learned helplessness** /lurnd/, a behavioral state and personality trait of a person who believes that he or she is ineffectual, responses are futile, and control over reinforcers in the environment has been lost.

**learning** [AS, *leornian,* to learn], **1.** the act or process of acquiring knowledge or some skill by means of study, practice, or experience. **2.** knowledge, wisdom, or a skill acquired through systematic study or instruction. **3.** (in psychology) the modification of behavior through practice, experience, or training. See also **conditioning.**

**learning curve,** a graphic presentation of the effects of a specified method of teaching or training on the ability of a subject to learn, as shown by improved performance in a particular task.

**learning disability,** an abnormal condition often affecting children of normal or above-average intelligence, characterized by difficulty in learning such fundamental procedures as reading, writing, and numeric calculation. The condition may result from psychologic or organic causes and is usually related to slow development of perceptual motor skills. See also **attention deficit disorder, dysgraphia, dyslexia.**

**learning-disabled adult,** a nonspecific difficulty in the learning process, commonly resulting from developmental lag rather than brain damage or demonstrable illness. Research into adult learning disabilities indicates that, as among children, the disability may be expressed throughout the total personality: cognitively, perceptually, and emotionally. Functional difficulties persist, but in adulthood they are expressed in vocational adjustment, work management, and social and family interactions.

**learning environment,** the sum of the internal and external circumstances and influences surrounding and affecting a person's learning.

**learning facilitation,** a nursing intervention from the Nursing Interventions Classification (NIC) defined as promoting the ability to process and comprehend information. See also **Nursing Interventions Classification.**

**learning readiness enhancement,** a nursing intervention from the Nursing Interventions Classification (NIC) defined as improving the ability and willingness to receive information. See also **Nursing Interventions Classification.**

**learning theory** [AS, *leornian,* to learn; Gk, *theoria,* speculation], a group of concepts and principles that attempts to explain the learning process. One concept, Guthrie's contiguous conditioning premise, postulates that each response becomes permanently linked with stimuli present at the time so that contiguity rather than reinforcement is a part of the learning process.

**leather-bottle stomach.** See **linitis plastica.**

**Leber's congenital amaurosis** /lā′bərz/ [Theodor von Leber, German ophthalmologist, 1840–1917; L, *congenitus,* born with; Gk, *amauroein,* to darken], a rare kind of blindness or severely impaired vision caused by a defect transmitted as an autosomal-recessive trait and occurring at birth or shortly thereafter. The eyes appear normal externally, but pupillary constriction to light is sluggish or absent, and electroretinographic responses are decreased or absent. Pendular nystagmus, photophobia, cataract, and keratoconus may be present; and the ophthalmic disorder may be associated with mental retardation and epilepsy. One type of Leber's amaurosis results in complete blindness; in a second kind the pathology does not progress, and the patient has very mild vision loss.

**Leber's plexus** /lā′bərz/ [Theodor Leber, German ophthalmologist, 1840−1917], a venous plexus in the ciliary region connected with the **canal of Schlemm.** Also called **Hovius' plexus.**

**Leboyer method of delivery** /ləboiyā′/ [Frederick LeBoyer, French obstetrician, b. 1918], a psychophysical approach to delivery with the goal of minimizing the trauma of birth by gently and pleasantly introducing the newborn to life outside the womb. It has four aspects: a gentle controlled delivery in a quiet dimly lit room, avoidance of pulling on the head, avoidance of overstimulation of the infant's sensorium, and encouragement of maternal-infant bonding. Unnecessary intervention in the process of birth is eschewed. After delivery, the baby is gently laid on the mother's abdomen, the back is massaged as the cord stops pulsating, and, when regular spontaneous respirations are established, the baby is gently supported in a warm tub of water by the father. Many birth centers and obstetric services in the United States have found that no adverse effects result from this method. Some studies in France have suggested superior psychologic, social, and intellectual development in young children delivered by this method. Compare **Bradley method, Lamaze method, Read method.**

**LE cell (lupus erythematosus cell),** a neutrophil that has phagocytosed the nucleus of another leukocyte that has already been altered by interacting with the LE factor in the bloodstream.

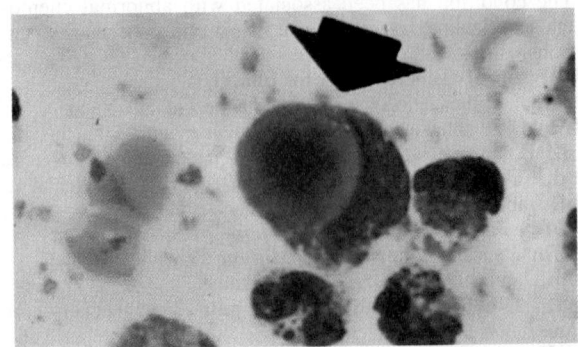

**Lupus erythematosus preparation**
*(Tilton, Ballows, and Hohnadel, 1992)*

**lecithin** /les′ithin/ [Gk, *lekithos,* yolk], phosphatidylcholine, a phospholipid common in plants and animals. Lecithin is found in the liver, nerve tissue, semen and in smaller amounts in bile and blood. It is an essential component of all cell membranes and for fat metabolism and is used in the processing of foods, pharmaceutical products, cosmetics, and inks. Rich dietary sources are soybeans, egg yolk, and corn. See also **choline, inositol.**

**lecithin-cholesterol acyltransferase (LCAT) deficiency,** an autosomal-recessive disorder characterized by an accumulation of unesterified cholesterol in the tissues, corneal opacity, hemolytic anemia, proteinuria, renal insufficiency, and premature atherosclerosis. It is caused by a deficiency of LCAT activity.

**lecithin/sphingomyelin (LS) ratio,** the ratio of two components of amniotic fluid, used for predicting fetal lung maturity. The normal ratio in amniotic fluid is 2:1 or greater when fetal lungs are mature.

**lecitho-,** combining form meaning 'yolk of an egg or ovum': *lecithoblast, lecithoprotein, lecithovitellin.*

**lecithoblast** /les′ithəblast′/, an embryonic cell, the primitive entoderm of a two-layered blastodisc.

**lecithoprotein** /les′ithəprō′tēn/, a compound formed by a combination of lecithin and a protein.

**lectin** /lek′tin/, a protein in seeds and other parts of certain plants that binds with glycoproteins and glycolipids on the surface of animal cells, causing agglutination. Some lectins agglutinate erythrocytes in specific blood groups, and others stimulate the production of T lymphocytes.

**Ledercillin VK,** trademark for a bacterial antibiotic (penicillin V potassium).

**leech therapy,** a nursing intervention from the Nursing Interventions Classification (NIC) defined as application of medicinal leeches to help drain replanted or transplanted tissue engorged with venous blood. See also **Nursing Interventions Classification.**

***Leeuwenhoekia australiensis*** [Anton van Leeuwenhoek, Dutch microscopist, 1632–1723; Australia], a mite indigenous to New South Wales that burrows into the skin, producing severe irritation. Also called **scrub itch.**

**leeway space,** the amount by which the space occupied by the deciduous canine and first and second deciduous molars exceeds that occupied by the canine and premolar teeth of the secondary dentition, usually averaging 1.7 mm on each side of the dental arch.

**Lee-White method** [Roger I. Lee, American physician, b. 1881; Paul D. White, American physician, 1886–1973; Gk, *meta,* beyond, *hodos,* way], a method of determining the length of time required for a clot to form in a test tube of venous blood. It is not specific for any coagulation disorder but is often used to monitor coagulation during heparin therapy. Because normal values and precise methodology vary, instructions are provided by most laboratories. See also **clotting time.**

**leflunomide,** a pyrimidine synthesis inhibitor.
■ INDICATIONS: Leflunomide is used to treat rheumatoid arthritis.
■ CONTRAINDICATIONS: Pregnancy, lactation, and known hypersensitivity to leflunomide prohibit its use.
■ ADVERSE EFFECTS: Adverse reactions to this drug include chest pain, angina pectoris, migraine, bronchitis, cough, respiratory infection, pneumonia, and sinusitis. Common side effects include nausea, anorexia, vomiting, constipation, flatulence, dizziness, insomnia, depression, paresthesia, palpitations, hypertension, rash, pruritus, pharyngitis, and rhinitis.

**LeFort I fracture.** See **Guérin's fracture.**

**left atrioventricular valve.** See **mitral valve.**

**left atrium (LA),** the uppermost chamber on the left side of the heart. It receives blood from the pulmonary veins.

**left brachiocephalic vein** [ME, *left,* weak; Gk, *brachys,* short, *kephale,* head], a vessel about 6 cm long that starts in the root of the neck at the junction of the internal jugular and the subclavian veins on the left side and runs obliquely across the thorax to join the right brachiocephalic vein and form the superior vena cava. Also called **left innominate vein.** Compare **right brachiocephalic vein.**

**left bundle branch block (LBBB),** the failure of the cardiac impulse to propagate down the left bundle branch from the bundle of His, resulting in early activation of the right side of the septum and the right ventricular myocardium. See also **bundle branch block (BBB).**

**left common carotid artery,** the longer of the two common carotid arteries, arising from the aortic arch and having cervical and thoracic parts. The cervical part passes obliquely from the level of the sternoclavicular articulation to the cranial border of the thyroid cartilage, dividing into the left internal and the left external carotid arteries. Compare **right common carotid artery.**

**left coronary artery,** one of a pair of branches from the ascending aorta, arising in the left posterior aortic sinus, dividing into the left interventricular artery and the circumflex branch, and supplying both ventricles and the left atrium. Compare **right coronary artery.**

**left-handedness** /left′han′didnes/, a natural tendency by some persons to favor the use of the left hand in performing certain tasks. Also called **sinistrality.** See also **cerebral dominance, handedness.**

**left-heart failure,** an abnormal cardiac condition characterized by the impairment of the left side of the heart and elevated pressure and congestion in the pulmonary veins and capillaries. Left-heart failure may be related to right-heart failure, because both sides of the heart are part of a circuit and the impairment of one side will eventually affect the other. Experimentally produced failure of one ventricle may produce significant hemodynamic and biochemical abnormalities of the opposite ventricle, even without the usual signs of failure. In "pure" left-heart failure, the body retains significant amounts of sodium and water and consequently develops peripheral edema without clinical evidence of right-heart failure. Also called **left-sided failure.** Compare **right-heart failure.** See also **heart failure.**

**left hepatic duct,** the duct that drains the bile from the left lobe of the liver into the common bile duct.

**left innominate vein.** See **left brachiocephalic vein.**

**left lateral recumbent position** [ME, *left* + L, *latus,* side, *recumbere,* to lie down, *positio*], a position in which the patient lies on the left side with the upper knee and thigh drawn upward. See also **Sims' position.**

**left lymphatic duct.** See **thoracic duct.**

**left pulmonary artery,** the shorter and smaller of two arteries conveying venous blood from the heart to the lungs, rising from the pulmonary trunk, connecting to the left lung, and tending to have more separate branches than the right pulmonary artery. In the fetus, it is larger and more important than the right pulmonary artery because it provides the ductus arteriosus that degenerates to become a ligament after birth. Compare **right pulmonary artery.**

**left-sided failure.** See **left-heart failure.**

**left subclavian artery,** an artery, divided into three parts, that arises from the aortic arch to supply the vertebral column, spinal cord, ear, and brain. The short second part lies dorsal to the scalenus anterior and forms the arch described by the vessel. The third part runs from the scalenus anterior to the first rib, where it becomes the axillary artery. See also **subclavian artery.** Compare **right subclavian artery.**

**left-to-right shunt,** **1.** a diversion of blood from the left side of the heart to the right, such as through a septal defect. **2.** a diversion of blood from the systemic to the pulmonary circulation, such as from a patent ductus arteriosus.

**left ventricle (LV),** the thick-walled chamber of the heart that pumps blood through the aorta and the systemic arteries, the capillaries, and back through the veins to the right atrium. It has walls about three times thicker than those of the right ventricle and contains a mitral valve with two flaps that controls the flow of blood from the left atrium. The left ventricle occupies about half the diaphragmatic surface of the heart and is longer and more conical than the right ventricle, narrowing caudally to form the apex. The chordae tendineae of the left ventricle are thicker, stronger, and less numerous than those in the right ventricle. See also **chordae tendineae.**

**left ventricular assist device (LVAD),** a mechanical pump that temporarily and artificially aids the natural pumping action of the left ventricle.

**left ventricular failure,** heart failure in which the left ventricle fails to contract forcefully enough to maintain a normal cardiac output and peripheral perfusion. Pulmonary congestion and edema develop from back pressure of accumulated blood in the left ventricle. Signs include breathlessness, crackles, dyspnea, orthopnea, pallor, sweating, and peripheral vasoconstriction. The heart is usually enlarged, resulting in a displaced point of maximum impulse. A prominent third heart sound (gallop), normal in children and young adults, is a sign of left ventricular failure in older adults with heart disease. Hypertension is common and may be a causative factor or a result of pulmonary edema. Treatment includes meperidine or morphine for sedation, angiotensin-converting enzyme inhibitors or calcium channel blockers to reduce afterload, diuretics, digitalis, and rest. See also **congestive heart failure.**

**left ventricular thrust.** See **precordial movement.**

**leg** /leg/ [ONor, *leggr*], **1.** that section of the lower limb between the knee and ankle. **2.** in common usage, the entire lower limb (in which case, the part below the knee is called the lower leg).

**legacy** /leg'əsē/ [L, *legatum,* bequest], something that is handed down from the past or intended to be bestowed on future generations.

**legal** [L, *lex,* law], actions or conditions that are permitted or authorized by law.

**legal blindness** [L, *lex,* law; ME, *blend,* sightless], a state of visual acuity in which no better than 20/200 is measured in the better eye with corrective lenses or a visual field of not more than 20 degrees is obtained.

**legal death.** See **death.**

**leg cylinder cast** [ONor, *leggr* + Gk, *kylindros* + ONorse, *kasta*], an orthopedic device of plaster of paris or fiberglass used to immobilize the leg in treating fractures from the ankle to the upper thigh. It is used especially for repairing knee fractures and dislocations, for treating soft tissue trauma around the knee, for maintaining postoperative positioning and immobilization of the knee, and for correcting or maintaining correction of knee deformities. The long-leg cast may also be used for these purposes because it encases the foot and ensures greater immobilization.

**Legg-Calvé-Perthes disease** [Arthur T. Legg, American surgeon, 1874–1939; Jacque Calvé, French orthopedist, 1875–1954; Georg C. Perthes, German surgeon, 1869–

1927], osteochondrosis of the head of the femur in children. It is characterized initially by epiphyseal necrosis or degeneration, followed by regeneration or recalcification. Also called **coxa plana, Perthes disease, pseudocoxalgia.**

**Legionella pneumonia** /lē'jənel'ə/ [American Legion; Gk, *pneumon,* lung], a form of pneumonia caused by a gram-negative bacillus identified as *Legionella pneumophila.* It was discovered after an outbreak of the disease among veterans attending a 1976 convention of the American Legion. See also *Legionella pneumophila,* **Legionnaires' disease.**

***Legionella pneumophila*** /noomof'ələ/, a small gram-negative rod-shaped bacterium that is the causative agent in **Legionnaires' disease.**

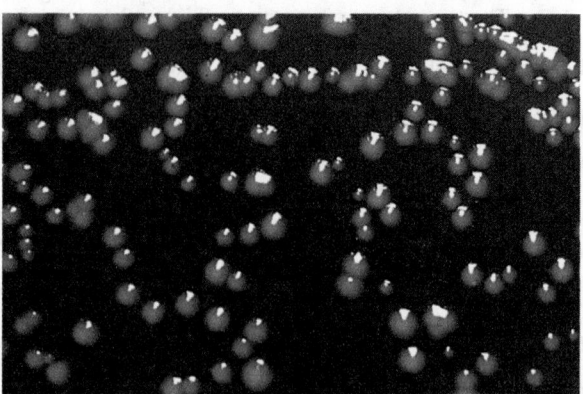

***Legionella pneumophila***
*(Baron, Peterson, and Finegold, 1994/courtesy Dr. Clifford Mintz)*

**legionellosis** /lē'jə·nel·ō'sis /, infection with species of *Legionella,* which may cause any of several illnesses, including **Legionnaires' disease** and **Pontiac fever.**

**Legionnaires' disease** /lē'jənerz'/ [American Legion], an acute bacterial pneumonia caused by infection with *Legionella pneumophila.* It is characterized by an influenza-like illness followed within a week by high fever, chills, muscle aches, and headache. The symptoms may progress to dry cough, pleurisy, and sometimes diarrhea. Usually the disease is self-limited, but mortality has been 15% to 20% in a few localized epidemics. Contaminated air conditioning cooling towers and warm stagnant water supplies, including water vaporizers, water sonicators, whirlpool spas, and showers, may be sources of organisms. Person-to-person contagion has not occurred. Risk of infection is increased by the presence of other conditions such as cardiopulmonary diseases. Treatment includes supportive care and erythromycin. Also called **legionellosis.**

**legume** /leg'yoom/ [L, *legumen,* pulse], any of the members of the Fabales order of dicotyledenous plants, including dried peas, beans, and lentils.

**Leigh disease** /lē/ [Archibald Denis Leigh, British neuropathologist, b. 1915], an encephalopathy of unclear clinical and pathological criteria, causing neuropathologic damage like that of the Wernicke-Korsakoff syndrome. It occurs in two forms: the *infantile form,* which may be the same as **pyruvate carboxylase deficiency,** is characterized by degeneration of gray matter with necrosis and capillary proliferation in the brainstem; hypotonia, seizures, and dementia;

anorexia and vomiting; slow or arrested development; and ocular and respiratory disorders. Death usually occurs before age 3. The *adult* form usually first manifests as bilateral optic atrophy with central scotoma and colorblindness; then there is a quiescent period of up to 30 years; and then late symptoms appear such as ataxia, spastic paresis, clonic jerks, grand mal seizures, psychic lability, and mild dementia. Also called **subacute necrotizing encephalomyelopathy, subacute necrotizing encephalopathy.** See also **Wernicke-Korsakoff syndrome.**

**Leiner's disease** /lī'nərz/ [Karl Leiner, Austrian pediatrician, 1871–1930], an infant condition of generalized dermatitis, with scaling and erythema, as well as seborrheic dermatitis of the scalp. Also called **erythroderma desquamativum.**

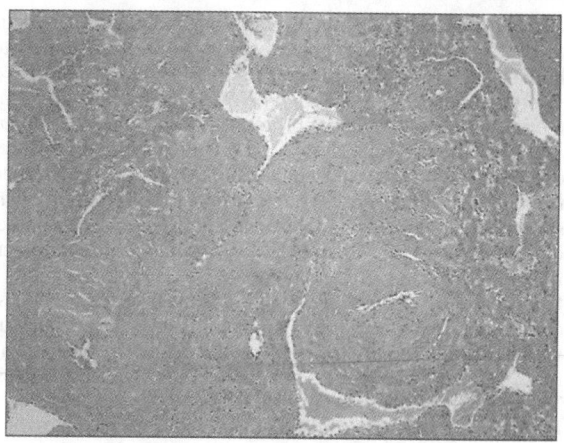
**Leiomyoma** *(Eveson and Scully, 1995)*

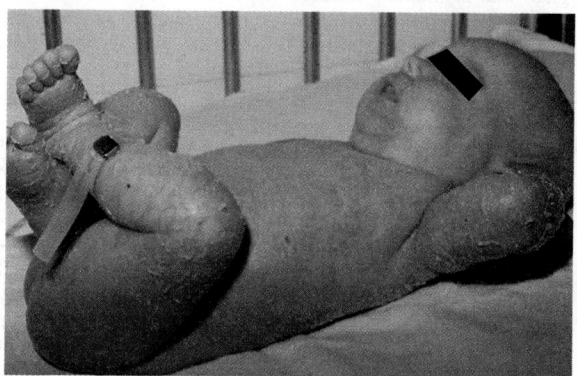
**Leiner's disease: characteristic exfoliative dermatitis**
*(Zitelli and Davis, 1997)*

**Leininger, Madeleine,** a nursing theorist who is credited with the foundation of transcultural nursing and the resultant nursing research, education, and practice in this subfield of nursing. The most complete account of transcultural care theory is found in her book, *Care: The Essence of Nursing and Health* (1984). Some of the major concepts are care, caring, culture, cultural values, and cultural variations. A basic tenet of Leininger's theory is that human beings are inseparable from their cultural background and social structure. She advocates caring as the central theme in nursing care, nursing knowledge, and practice. Caring includes assistive, supportive, or facilitative acts toward an individual or group with evident or anticipated needs. Caring serves to ameliorate or improve human conditions and life ways (life process). Her methodology is borrowed from anthropology, but the concept of caring is an essential characteristic of nursing practice.

**leio-, lio-,** prefix meaning 'smooth': *leiodermia, leiodystonia, leiomyofibroma.*

**leiomyoblastoma.** See **epithelioid leiomyoma.**

**leiomyofibroma** /lī'ōmī'ōfībrō'mə/, *pl.* **leiomyofibromas, leiomyofibromata** [Gk, *leios,* smooth, *mys,* muscle; L, *fibra,* fiber; Gk, *oma,* tumor], a tumor consisting of smooth muscle cells and fibrous connective tissue, commonly occurring in the uterus in middle-aged women. See also **fibroid.**

**leiomyoma** /lī'ōmī·ō'mə/, *pl.* **leiomyomas, leiomyomata,** a benign smooth-muscle tumor occurring most commonly in

the uterus, stomach, esophagus, or small intestine. Surgical resection is usually indicated.

**leiomyoma cutis,** a neoplasm of the smooth muscles of the skin. The lesion is characterized by many small tender red nodules.

**leiomyoma uteri,** a benign neoplasm of the smooth muscle of the uterus. The tumor is characteristically firm, well circumscribed, round, and gray-white. Histologically a pattern of whorls is present. Tumors of this kind develop in the myometrium and occur in women between 30 and 50 years of age. Also called **fibromyoma uteri, myoma previum,** and *(informal)* **fibroid.**

**leiomyosarcoma** /-särkō'mə/ [Gk, *leios,* smooth, *mys,* muscle, *sarx,* flesh, *oma,* tumor], a sarcoma that contains large spindle cells of unstriated muscle.

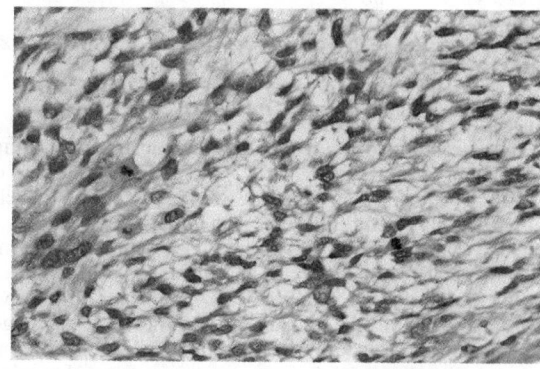
**Leiomyosarcoma** *(Fletcher, 2000)*

**leipo-.** See **lip-.**

**Leishman-Donovan body** /lēsh'məndon'əvən/ [William B. Leishman, English pathologist, 1865–1926; Charles Donovan, Irish physician, 1863–1951], the resting stage of an intracellular nonflagellated protozoan parasite *(Leishmania donovani)* that causes kala-azar, or visceral leishmaniasis, as it appears in infected tissue specimens.

**Leishmania** /lēshmā'nē·ə/ [William B. Leishman], a genus of protozoan parasites. These organisms are transmitted to humans by any of several species of sand flies.

**leishmaniasis** /lēsh'mənī'əsis/ [William B. Leishman], infection with any species of protozoan of the genus *Leishmania*. The diseases caused by these organisms may be cutaneous/mucocutaneous or visceral. The infection is transmitted to humans by several species of nocturnal *Phlebotomus* sandflies. Other species of the blood-sucking insects infect other animals. Diagnosis is made by microscopic identification of the intracellular nonflagellated protozoan on a Giemsa-stained smear taken from a cutaneous lesion or visceral biopsy. A typical infection may begin with a cutaneous sore and progress to ulceration of the mouth, palate, and nose. Some cases are accompanied by a febrile illness. There are three major types of leishmaniasis: **visceral leishmaniasis** or **kala-azar, cutaneous leishmaniasis** or **oriental sore,** and **American leishmaniasis,** the form found in Central America and South America. Visceral leishmaniasis occurs mainly in the tropical areas of Asia; cutaneous leishmaniasis is encountered most frequently in the Middle East. See also *Leishmania.* —**leishmanial,** *adj.*

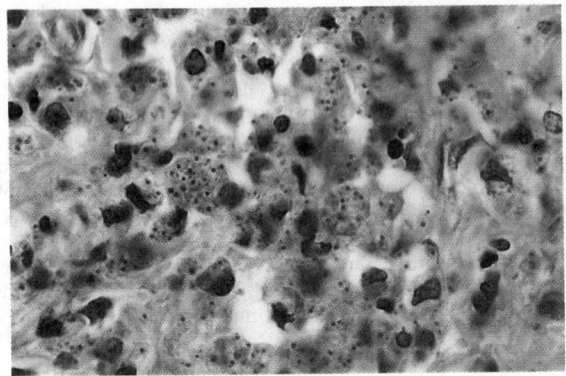

**Visceral leishmaniasis** *(Cotran, Kumar, and Collins, 1999)*

**leishmanin test.** See **Montenegro test.**

**leisure participation,** a nursing outcome from the Nursing Outcomes Classification (NOC) defined as the use of restful or relaxing activities as needed to promote well-being. See also **Nursing Outcomes Classification.**

**-lemma,** combining form meaning a 'confining membrane': *axiolemma, epilemma, neurolemma.*

**lemniscal system** /lemnis'kəl/ [Gk, *lemniskos,* fillet, *systema*], a part of the somatosensory network of large-diameter myelinated A fibers. It includes the dorsal columns and the neospinothalamic tract extending from the spinal cord to the thalamus and cortex.

**lemniscus** /lemnis'kəs/ [Gk, *lemniskos,* fillet], a band or tract of central nervous system fibers, particularly the ascending axons of secondary sensory neurons leading to the thalamus.

**lemon balm,** a perennial herb found in the Mediterranean, Asia, Europe, and North America.

■ USES: This herb is used for abdominal gas and cramping, and for cold sores.

■ CONTRAINDICATIONS: Use of lemon balm is not recommended during pregnancy and lactation, in children, or in those with known hypersensitivity to this herb. It should not be used in people with hypothyroidism.

**Lenègre's disease** /lenāgrāz/, [Jean Lenègre, 20th century French cardiologist, b. 1904], sclerodegeneration of the conduction system of the heart that eventually results in complete heart block.

**length of stay (LOS),** the period of time a patient remains in a hospital or other health care facility as an inpatient.

**Lennox-Gastaut syndrome** /len'oks-gästō'/ [William G. Lennox, American neurologist, 1884–1960; Henri Gastaut, French biologist, b. 1914], a condition in which a variety of generalized seizures, such as tonic, tonic-clonic, akinetic, and myoclonic, begin to appear in the first 5 years of life. Mental retardation is often present. Among suggested causes are inherited metabolic abnormalities and perinatal or postnatal disorders. Also called **Gastaut's disease.**

**lens** [L, lentil], **1.** a curved transparent piece of plastic or glass that is shaped, molded, or ground to refract light in a specific way, as in eyeglasses, microscopes, or cameras. **2.** *informal.* the crystalline lens of the eye. —**lenticular,** *adj.*

**lens capsule,** the clear thin elastic capsule that surrounds the lens of the eye. Also called **capsule of the lens.**

**lens implant,** an artificial lens that is usually implanted at the time of cataract extraction but may also be used for patients with extreme myopia, diplopia, ocular albinism, and certain other abnormalities. The operation is usually performed with a local anesthetic in an outpatient center. Eyedrops containing an antibiotic such as neomycin are instilled before surgery to prevent infection and several times a day for a number of weeks after surgery. After extraction of the cataract, the lens is inserted through a corneal incision. It may be held in place in the anterior chamber by extremely fine sutures to the iris, or, if the lens is implanted into the capsular sac, a miotic agent such as pilocarpine is used to prevent the iris from dilating too widely, which would allow the implant to slip. The implanted lens does not cause the problems with abnormal peripheral vision that are associated with cataract spectacles.

**Lente Insulin,** trademark for an intermediate-acting insulin. See **intermediate-acting insulin.**

**lenticonus** /len'tikō'nəs/, an abnormal spheric or conic protrusion on the lens of the eye. It is a congenital defect found in Alport's syndrome.

**lenticular.** See **lens.**

**lenticular nucleus** /lentik'yələr/ [L, *lens,* lentil, *nucleus,* nut], biconvex basal ganglia of the cerebrum, composed of lateral putamen and medial globus pallidus tissue as part of the corpus striatum.

**lentiform** /len'tifôrm/ [L, *lens* + *forma*], pertaining to or resembling a lentil shape, such as the lens of the eye.

**lentigo** /lentī'gō/, *pl.* **lentigines** /lentij'ənēz/ [L, freckle], a tan or brown macule on the skin brought on by sun exposure, usually in a middle-aged or older person. It is benign, and no treatment is necessary. Compare **freckle.**

**lentigo maligna.** See **Hutchinson's freckle.**

**lentigo maligna melanoma,** a neoplasm developing from Hutchinson's freckle on the face or other exposed surfaces of the skin in elderly patients. It is asymptomatic, flat, and tan or brown, with irregular darker spots and frequent hypopigmentation. It is one of the major clinical types of melanoma and occurs in 10% to 15% of melanoma patients. See also **nodular melanoma, superficial spreading melanoma.**

**lentivirus** /len'tivī'rəs/, a member of a subfamily of retroviruses that includes human immunodeficiency virus. Lentiviruses are usually slow viruses, with long incubation peri-

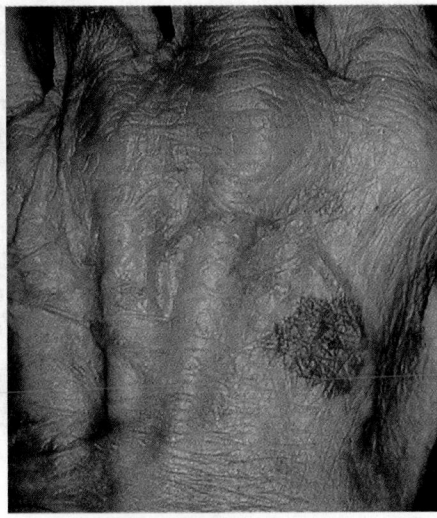

**Lentigo** *(Habif, 1995)*

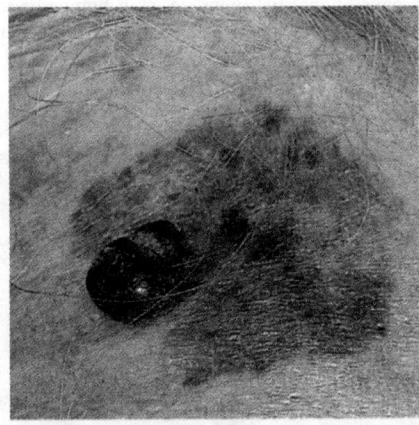

**Lentigo maligna melanoma** *(du Vivier, 1986)*

■ CONTRAINDICATIONS: Known hypersensitivity to hirudins prohibits this drug's use.

■ ADVERSE EFFECTS: Life-threatening effects of lepirudin include heart failure, pericardial effusion, ventricular fibrillation, multiorgan failure, sepsis, hematuria, hemorrhage, and thrombocytopenia. Other adverse reactions include GI bleeding, abnormal liver function tests, abnormal kidney function, pneumonia, and allergic skin reactions. Fever is a common side effect.

**leprechaunism** /lep′rə·kän′izəm /, a rare lethal familial condition marked by slow physical and mental development, the elfin facies suggested by the name (wide-set eyes, low-set ears, and hirsutism), and severe endocrine disorders such as enlargement of the clitoris and breasts in females and of the phallus in males. Also called **Donohue's syndrome.**

**lepro-,** prefix meaning 'leprosy': *leprologist, lepromatous, leprosarium.*

**lepromatous, lepromatous leprosy.** See **leprosy.**

**lepromin test** /leprō′min/, a skin sensitivity test used to distinguish between the lepromatous and tuberculoid forms of leprosy. The test consists of an intradermal injection of lepromin, which is prepared from heat-sterilized *Mycobacterium leprae.* The appearance of a palpable nodule in 8 to 10 days is indicative of the tuberculoid form of leprosy. As no nodule appears in the lepromatous form, the test is not diagnostic of leprosy. The test is used only to follow the course of the disease. See also **leprosy.**

**leprosarium** /lep′rōser′ē·əm/ [Gk, *lepra,* leprosy], a hospital for persons who have Hansen's disease.

**leprosy** /lep′rəsē/ [Gk, *lepra*], a chronic communicable disease caused by *Mycobacterium leprae* that may take either of two forms, depending on the degree of immunity of the host. **Tuberculoid leprosy,** seen in those with high resistance, presents as thickening of cutaneous nerves and anesthetic, saucer-shaped skin lesions. **Lepromatous leprosy,** seen in those with little resistance, involves many body systems, with widespread plaques and nodules in the skin, iritis, keratitis, destruction of nasal cartilage and bone, testicular atrophy, peripheral edema, and involvement of the reticuloendothelial system. Blindness may result. Death is rare unless amyloidosis or tuberculosis occurs concurrently. Contrary to traditional belief, leprosy is not very contagious, and prolonged intimate contact is required for it to be spread between individuals. Children are more susceptible than

ods that may delay the onset of symptoms until several years after exposure.

**LEOPARD syndrome,** a hereditary syndrome transmitted as an autosomal dominant trait, consisting of multiple lentigines, asymptomatic cardiac defects, and typical coarse facies; it may also be associated with pulmonary stenosis, sensorineural hearing loss, skeletal changes, ocular hypertelorism, and abnormalities of the genitalia. Also called **multiple lentigines syndrome.**

**Leopold's maneuver** [Christian G. Leopold, German physician, 1846–1911], a series of four steps used in palpating the abdomen of a pregnant woman to determine position and presentation of the fetus.

**leper** /lep′ər/ [Gk, *lepis,* scaly], an outdated term for a person afflicted with leprosy (Hansen's disease).

**lepido-,** prefix meaning 'flake or scale': *lepidoma, lepidosis.*

**lepirudin,** an anticoagulant.

■ INDICATIONS: Lepirudin is used to treat heparin-induced thrombocytopenia and other thromboembolic conditions.

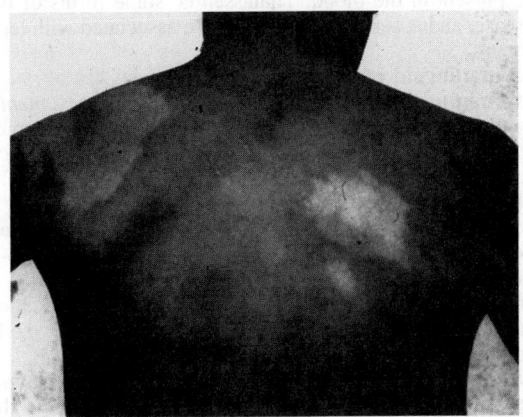

**Borderline tuberculoid leprosy** *(Stone and Gorbach, 2000)*

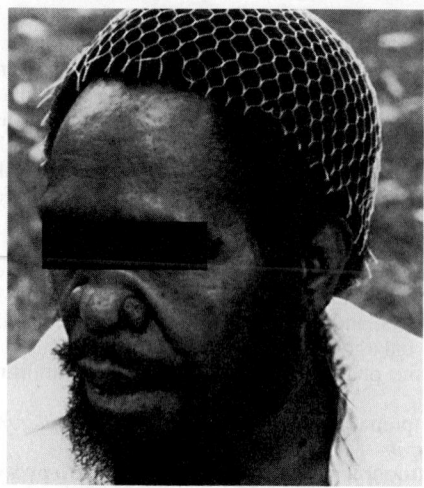

**Advanced lepromatous leprosy** *(Stone and Gorbach, 2000)*

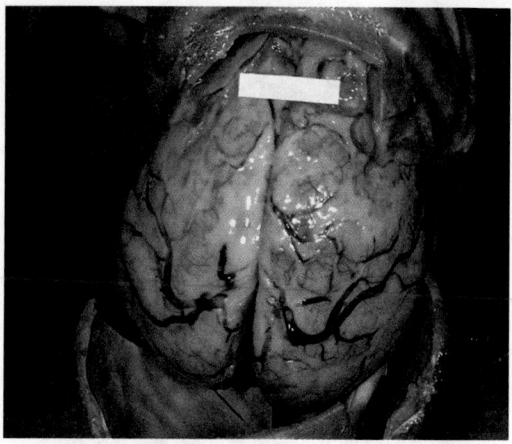

**Acute leptomeningitis** *(Kumar, Cotran, and Robbins, 1997)*

adults. Plastic surgery, physical therapy, and psychotherapy are often necessary. Treatment with sulfones such as dapsone continued for several years usually results in improvement of skin lesions, but recovery from nerve impairment is limited. The disease is found mostly in underdeveloped tropic and subtropic countries. In the United States patients may be referred to the U.S. Public Health Service leprosarium in Carville, Louisiana. Bacille Calmette-Guérin vaccine may be at least partially protective against leprosy. Also called **Hansen's disease.** See also *Mycobacterium.* **—lepromatous, leprotic, leprous,** *adj.*

**-lepsy, -lepsia, -lepsis,** suffix meaning a 'seizure': *deolepsy, electrolepsy, pyknolepsy.*

**-leptic,** suffix meaning 'a (specified) type of seizure': *cataleptic, epileptic, hypnoleptic.*

**leptin** /lep'tin/ [Gk, thin], a peptide associated with obesity. Leptin inhibits neuropeptide Y and is thought to be an appetite suppressant. Excess leptin in obese humans suggests they may be insensitive to leptin.

**lepto-** /lep'tō-/, combining form meaning 'slender, small, thin, or delicate': *leptodermic, leptodactylosis.*

**leptocyte.** See **target cell.**

**leptocytosis** /lep'tōsītō'sis/ [Gk, *leptos,* thin, *kytos,* cell, *osis,* condition], a hematologic condition in which target cells are present in the blood. Thalassemia, some forms of liver disease, and absence of the spleen are associated with leptocytosis.

**leptomeningeal cyst.** See **arachnoid cyst.**

**leptomeninges** /lep'tōminin'jēz/ [Gk, *leptos* + *meninx,* membrane], the arachnoid membrane and the pia mater, two of the three layers covering the brain and spinal cord. Compare **meninges.**

**leptomeningitis** /-men'inji'tis/, an inflammation of the arachnoid and pia mater layers of the meninges. See also **meningitis.**

**leptonema** /lep'tənē'mə/ [Gk, *leptos* + *nema,* thread], the threadlike chromosome formation in the leptotene stage in the first meiotic prophase of gametogenesis, before the beginning of synapsis.

***Leptospira*** /-spī'rə/ [Gk, *leptos* + *speira,* coil], a genus of the family Treponemataceae, order Spirochaetales; tightly coiled microorganisms having spirals with hooked ends. The spirochete thrives in the urine of infected animals, espe-

cially rodents; is pathogenic to humans and other mammals; and may cause hepatitis, jaundice, skin hemorrhages, fever, renal failure, mental status changes, and muscular illness. See also **leptospirosis.**

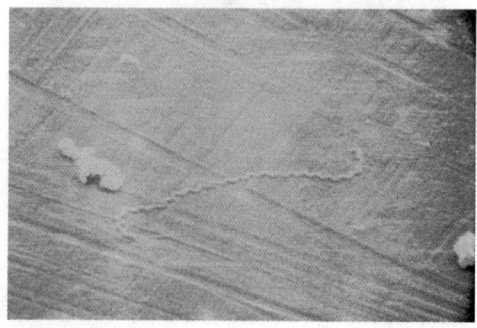

***Leptospira interrogans*** *(Mahon and Manuselis, 2000)*

***Leptospira* agglutinin,** an agglutinin found in the blood of patients with leptospirosis.

**leptospirosis** /lep'tōspīrō'sis/ [Gk, *leptos* + *speira* + *osis,* condition], an acute infectious disease caused by several serotypes of the spirochete *Leptospira interrogans.* It is transmitted in the urine of infected cattle, horses, pigs, dogs, rodents, or wild animals. Human infections arise directly from contact with an infected animal's urine or tissues or indirectly from contact with contaminated water, food, or soil. Clinical symptoms may include hepatitis, jaundice, hemorrhage into the skin, fever, chills, renal failure, meningitis with mental status changes, and muscular pain. The spirochete can be isolated from the urine or blood during the acute stage of the disease, and antibodies can be found in the patient's blood during convalescence. Treatment with antibiotics, usually penicillin or doxycycline, may be effective if they are administered during the first few days of the disease. Fluid and electrolyte replacement is essential if jaun dice or other signs of severe illness are present. The disease is usually short-lived and mild, but severe infections can damage the kidneys and the liver. Blood pressure and vital signs should be monitored, and the patient's urine should be disposed of carefully to prevent spread of the organism. The most serious form of the disease is called **Weil's disease.** Also called **autumn fever.** See also **nanukayami.**

**leptotene** /lep′tətēn/ [Gk, *leptos* + *tainia,* ribbon], the initial stage in the first meiotic prophase in gametogenesis, in which the chromosomes consense and become visible as single, thin filaments. See also **diakinesis, diplotene, pachytene, zygotene.**

**Leriche's syndrome** /lərēshs′/ [René Leriche, French surgeon, 1879–1955], a vascular disorder marked by gradual occlusion of the terminal aorta; intermittent claudication in the buttocks, thighs, or calves; absence of pulsation in femoral arteries; pallor and coldness of the legs; gangrene of the toes; and, in men, impotence. Symptoms are the result of chronic tissue hypoxia caused by inadequate arterial perfusion of the affected areas. Treatment may include endarterectomy, embolectomy, or synthetic bypass graft at the aortic bifurcation.

**lesbian** /lez′bē·ən/ [Gk, island of Lesbos, home of Sappho], **1.** a female homosexual. **2.** pertaining to the sexual preference or desire of one woman for another. —**lesbianism,** *n.*

**Lesch-Nyhan syndrome** /lesh′nī′han/ [Michael Lesch, American pediatrician, b. 1939; William L. Nyhan, Jr., American pediatrician, b. 1926], a hereditary disorder of purine metabolism, characterized by mental retardation, self-mutilation of the fingers and lips by biting, impaired renal function, and abnormal physical development. It is transmitted as a recessive, sex-linked trait.

**Leser-Trélat sign** /lā′zər-trālä′/ [Edmund Leser, German surgeon, 1828–1916; Ulysse Trélat, French surgeon, 1828–1890], a condition of malignant cells present in the skin. It is characterized by the sudden onset of seborrheic keratoses with pruritus or enlargement of preexisting keratosis in older adults. It is associated with adenoma carcinoma of the stomach, breast cancer, and lung cancer.

**lesion** /lē′zhen/ [L, *laesus,* an injury], **1.** a wound, injury, or pathologic change in body tissue. **2.** any visible, local abnormality of the tissues of the skin, such as a wound, sore, rash, or boil. A lesion may be described as benign, cancerous, gross, occult, or primary.

**lesser circulation.** See **pulmonary circulation.**

**lesser multangular bone.** See **trapezoid bone.**

**lesser occipital nerve** [AS, *losian,* to lose; L, *occiput,* back of the head, *nervus,* nerve], one of a pair of cutaneous branches of the cervical plexus, arising from the second cervical nerve, and ascending along the side of the head behind the ear to supply the skin. It communicates with the posterior auricular branch of the facial nerve.

**lesser omentum** [AS, *losian,* to lose; L, *omentum,* entrails], a membranous extension of the peritoneum from the peritoneal layers covering the ventral and the dorsal surfaces of the stomach and the first part of the duodenum. The lesser omentum extends from the portal fissure of the liver to the diaphragm, where the layers separate to enclose the end of the esophagus. It also forms two ligaments, one associated with the liver, the ligamentum hepatogastricum, and the other, the ligamentum hepatoduodenale, with the duodenum. Also called **gastrohepatic omentum, small omentum.**

**lesser sciatic notch** [AS, *losian,* to lose; Gk, *ischiadikos,* hip joint; OFr, *enochier*], a notch on the posterior border of the ischium of the hip bone. It is smooth, is coated with cartilage, and has several ridges corresponding to subdivisions of the obturator internus tendon.

**lesser trochanter,** one of a pair of conic projections on the shaft of the femur, just below the neck. It is the site of insertion of the psoas major muscle. Also called **trochanter minor.** Compare **greater trochanter.**

**let-down,** a sensation in the breasts of lactating women that often occurs as the milk flows into the ducts. It may occur when the infant begins to suck or when the mother hears the baby cry or even thinks of nursing the child.

**let-down reflex.** See **milk ejection reflex.**

**lethal** /lē′thəl/, deadly, capable of causing death.

**lethal allele,** an allele that produces a phenotypic effect that causes the death of the organism at any stage of life. The allele may be dominant, incompletely dominant, or recessive. Human diseases caused by lethal genes include Huntington's disease, which is transmitted as an autosomal dominant trait, and sickle cell anemia, which shows recessive lethality. Compare **sublethal allele.** See also **lethal equivalent.**

**lethal dose (LD),** the amount of toxin that produces death in all members of a species population within a specified period of time. See also **LD$_{50}$.**

**lethal equivalent** [L, *letum,* death, *aequus,* equal, *valere,* to be strong], a recessive allele carried in the heterozygous state that would be lethal in the homozygous state, or any combination of alleles, each with slightly deleterious effects, that are equivalent to such an allele. It is estimated that a person carries an average of 3 to 8 lethal equivalents.

**lethality** /lēthal′itē/, the probability that a person threatening suicide will succeed, based on the method described, the specificity of the plan, and the availability of the means.

**lethargic.** See **lethargy.**

**lethargic encephalitis.** See **epidemic encephalitis.**

**lethargy** /leth′ərjē/ [Gk, *lethargos,* forgetful], the state or quality of dullness, prolonged sleepiness, sluggishness, or serious drowsiness. Compare **stupor.** —**lethargic,** *adj.*

**letrozole,** an antineoplastic nonsteroidal aromatase inhibitor.

■ INDICATIONS: Letrozole is used to treat metastatic breast cancer in postmenopausal women.

■ CONTRAINDICATIONS: Known hypersensitivity and pregnancy prohibit the use of this drug.

■ ADVERSE EFFECTS: Hepatotoxicity is a life-threatening effect of this drug. Other adverse effects include dyspnea, cough, constipation, heartburn, diarrhea, alopecia, sweating, hot flashes, hypertension, somnolence, dizziness, depression, and anxiety. Common side effects include nausea, vomiting, anorexia, rash, pruritus, headache, and lethargy.

**Letterer-Siwe syndrome** /let′ərərzē′və/ [Erich Letterer, German pathologist, b. 1895; Sture A. Siwe, Swedish physician, 1897–1966], any of a group of malignant neoplastic diseases of unknown origin, characterized by histiocytic elements. The syndrome, which is fatal, occurs in infancy and is not familial. Anemia, hemorrhage, splenomegaly, lymphadenopathy, and localized tumefactions over bones are usually present.

**letter quality printer,** an electronic printer that produces characters resembling those of a typewriter in production quality. Laser printers and daisywheel printers produce letter-quality copy as do some inkjet and dot matrix printers.

**leucine** (Leu) /lōō′sēn/ [Gk, *leukos,* white], a white crystalline essential amino acid required for optimal growth in infants and nitrogen equilibrium in adults. It cannot be synthesized by the body and is obtained by the hydrolysis of food protein during digestion. An inherited defect in one of the enzymes involved in the process results in a rare disorder called maple syrup urine disease. See also **amino acid, leucinosis, maple syrup urine disease.**

## Primary skin lesions

| Description | Examples | | |
|---|---|---|---|
| **Macule**<br>A flat, circumscribed area that is a change in the color of the skin; less than 1 cm in diameter | Freckles, flat moles (nevi), petechiae, measles, scarlet fever | 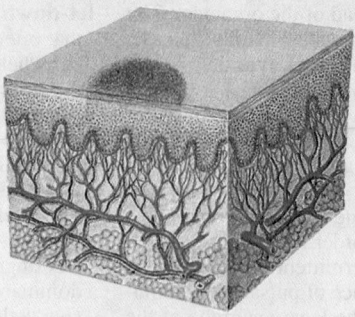 | 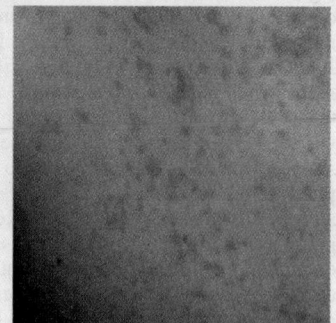<br>**Measles** *(Habif, 1996)* |
| **Papule**<br>An elevated, firm, circumscribed area less than 1 cm in diameter | Wart (verruca), elevated moles, lichen planus | 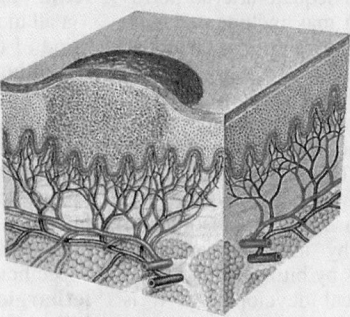 | **Lichen planus**<br>*(Weston, Lane, Morelli, 1996)* |
| **Patch**<br>A flat, nonpalpable, irregular-shaped macule more than 1 cm in diameter | Vitiligo, port-wine stains, mongolian spots, café-au-lait spot | 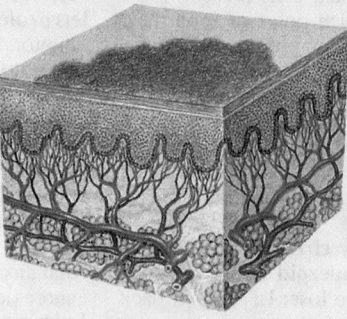 | 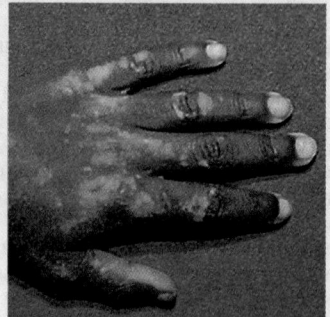<br>**Vitiligo**<br>*(Weston, Lane, Morelli, 1991)* |
| **Plaque**<br>Elevated, firm, and rough lesion with flat top surface greater than 1 cm in diameter | Psoriasis, seborrheic and actinic keratoses | 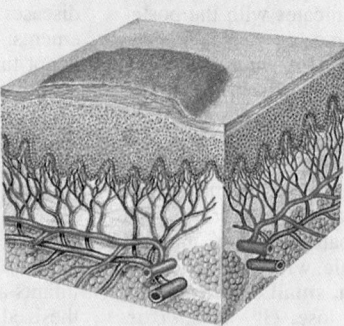 | 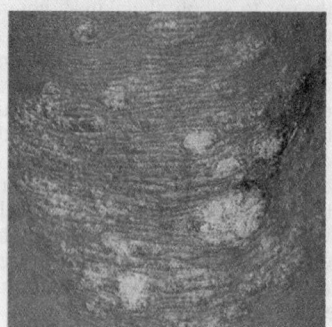<br>**Plaque** *(Habif, 1996)* |

From Seidel HM, Ball JW, Dains JE, Benedict GW: *Mosby's guide to physical examination,* ed 4, St Louis, 1999, Mosby. Modified from Thompson JM, Wilson SF: *Health assessment for nursing practice,* St Louis, 1996, Mosby.

## Primary skin lesions—cont'd

| Description | Examples | | |
|---|---|---|---|
| **Wheal**<br>Elevated irregular-shaped area of cutaneous edema; solid, transient; variable diameter | Insect bites, urticaria, allergic reaction | 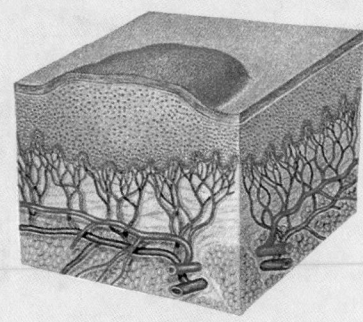 | <br>**Wheal** *(Farrar et al, 1992)* |
| **Nodule**<br>Elevated, firm, circumscribed lesion; deeper in dermis than a papule; 1 to 2 cm in diameter | Erythema nodosum, lipomas | 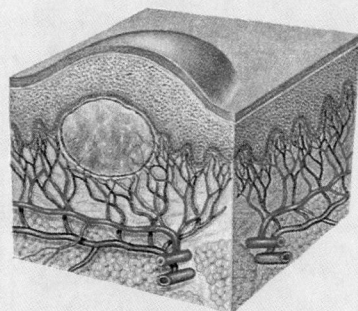 | 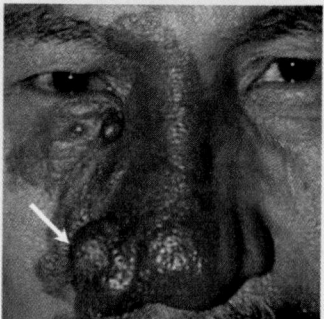<br>**Hypertrophic nodule**<br>*(Goldman and Fitzpatrick, 1994)* |
| **Tumor**<br>Elevated and solid lesion; may or may not be clearly demarcated; deeper in dermis; greater than 2 cm in diameter | Neoplasms, benign tumor, lipoma, hemangioma | 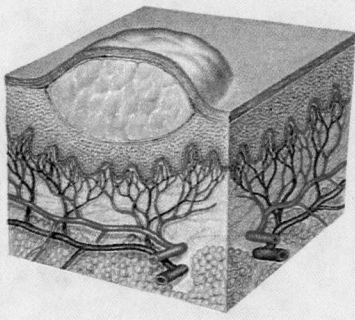 | 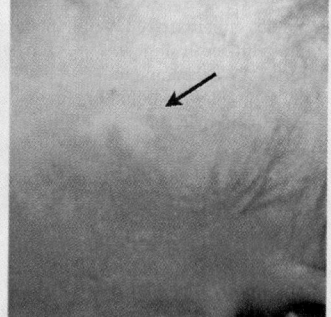<br>**Hemangioma**<br>*(Weston, Lane, Morelli, 1996)* |
| **Vesicle**<br>Elevated, circumscribed, superficial, not into dermis; filled with serous fluid; less than 1 cm in diameter | Varicella (chickenpox), herpes zoster (shingles) | 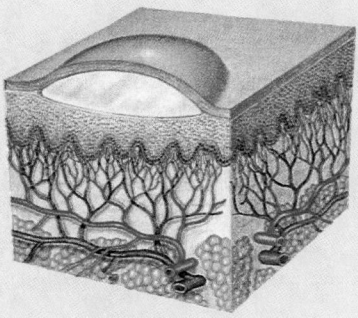 | 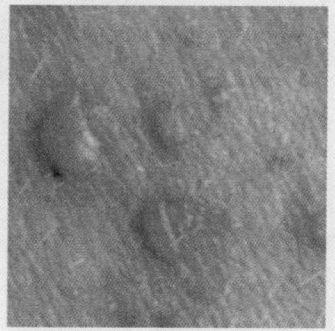<br>**Vesicles caused by Varicella**<br>*(Farrar et al, 1992)* |

*Continued*

## Primary skin lesions—cont'd

| Description | Examples |
|---|---|

**Bulla**
Vesicle greater than 1 cm in diameter

Blister, pemphigus vulgaris

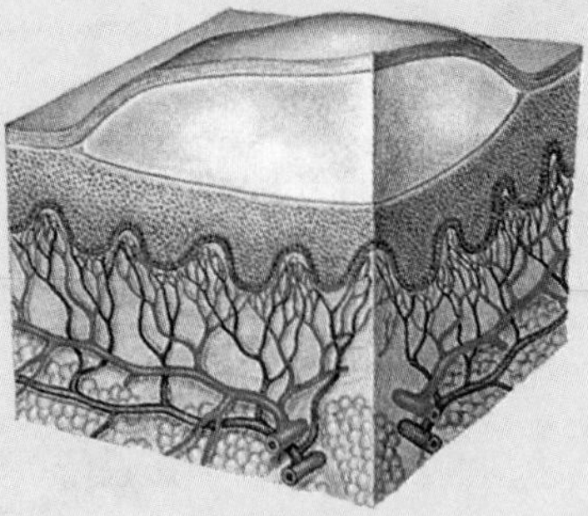

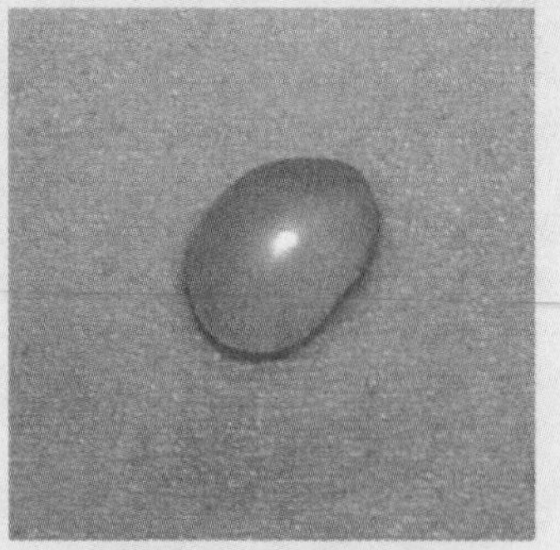

**Blister** *(White, 1994)*

**Pustule**
Elevated, superficial lesion; similar to a vesicle but filled with purulent fluid

Impetigo, acne

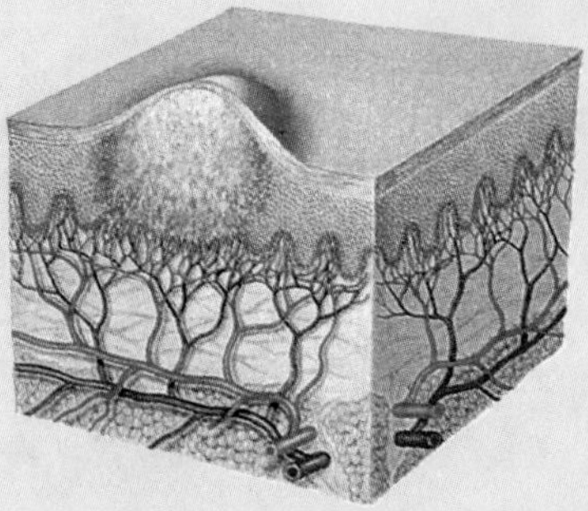

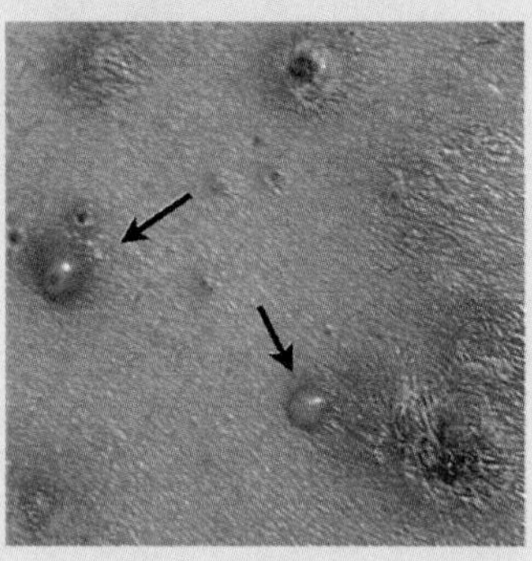

**Acne**
*(Weston, Lane, Morelli, 1996)*

**Cyst**
Elevated, circumscribed, encapsulated lesion; in dermis or subcutaneous layer; filled with liquid or semi-solid material

Sebaceous cyst, cystic acne

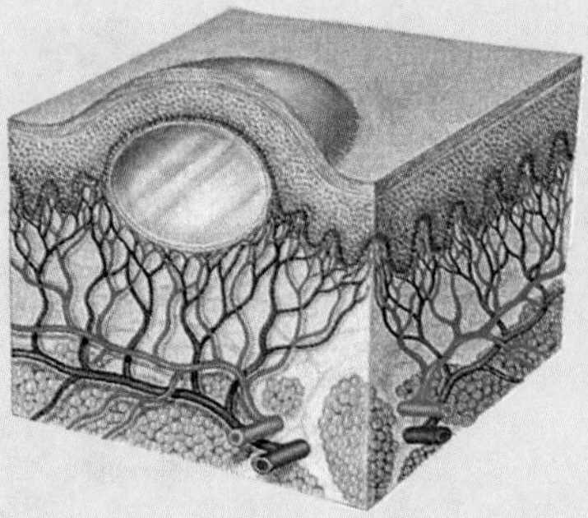

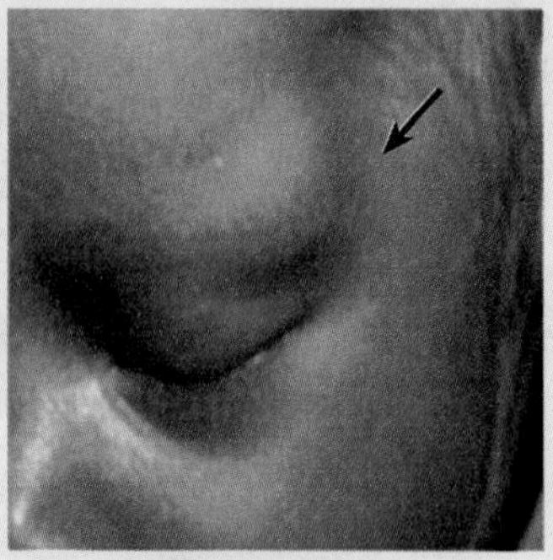

**Sebaceous cyst**
*(Weston, Lane, Morelli, 1996)*

**Telangiectasia**
Fine, irregular red lines produced by capillary dilation

Telangiectasia in rosacea

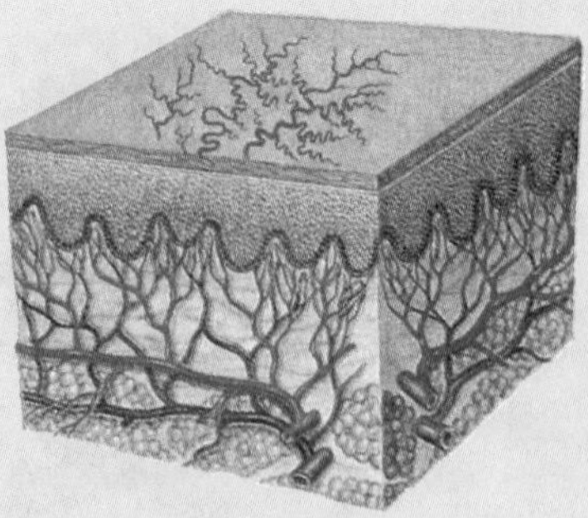

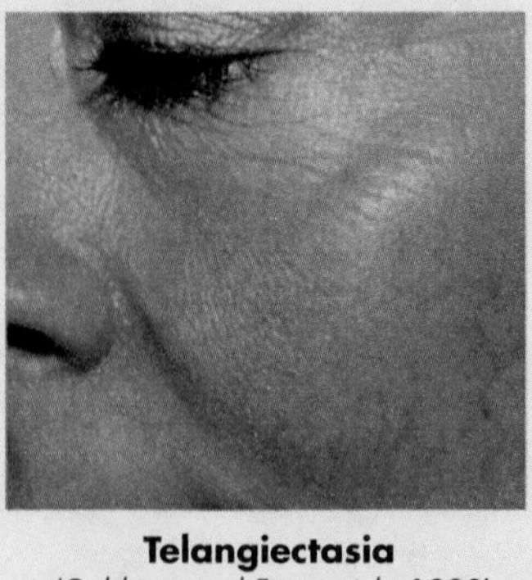

**Telangiectasia**
*(Goldman and Fitzpatrick, 1999)*

From Seidel HM, Ball JW, Dains JE, Benedict GW: *Mosby's guide to physical examination,* ed 4, St Louis, 1999, Mosby. Modified from Thompson JM, Wilson SF: *Health assessment for nursing practice,* St Louis, 1996, Mosby.

## Secondary skin lesions

| Description | Examples | | |
| --- | --- | --- | --- |

**Scale**
Heaped-up keratinized cells; flaky skin; irregular; thick or thin; dry or oily; variation in size

Flaking of skin with seborrheic dermatitis after scarlet fever, or flaking of skin after a drug reaction; dry skin

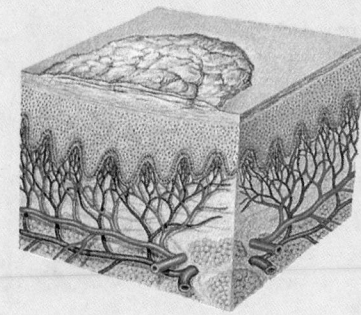

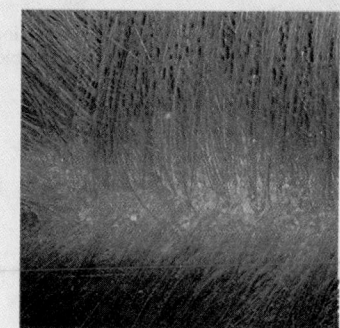

**Fine scaling**
*(Baran et al, 1991)*

**Lichenification**
Rough, thickened epidermis secondary to persistent rubbing, itching, or skin irritation; often involves flexor surface of extremity

Chronic dermatitis

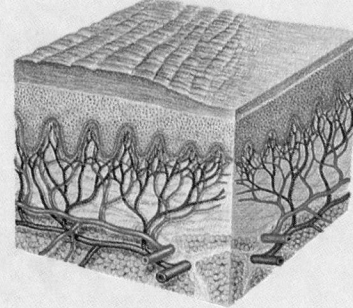

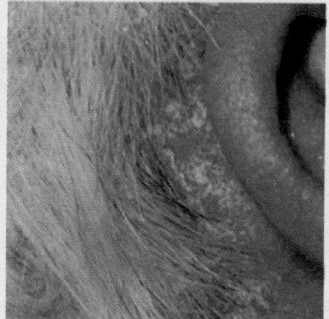

**Statis dermatitis in an early stage**
*(Seidel et al, 1999)*

**Keloid**
Irregular-shaped, elevated, progressively enlarging scar; grows beyond the boundaries of the wound; caused by excessive collagen formation during healing

Keloid formation after surgery

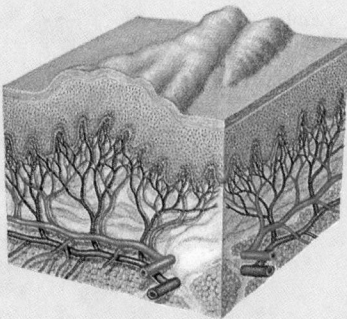

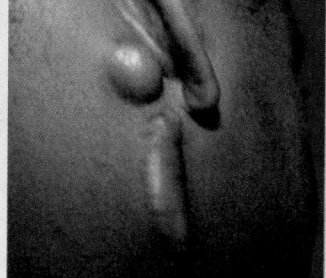

**Keloid**
*(Weston, Lane, Morelli, 1996)*

**Scar**
Thin to thick fibrous tissue that replaces normal skin following injury or laceration to the dermis

Healed wound or surgical incision

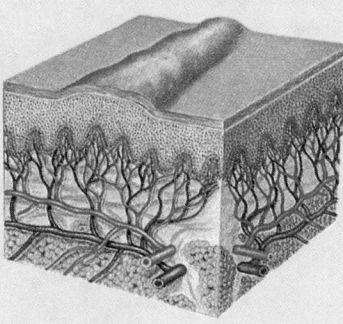

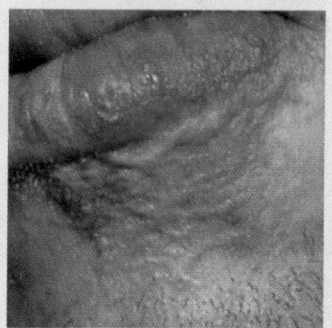

**Hypertrophic scar**
*(Goldman and Fitzpatrick, 1994)*

*Continued*

## Secondary skin lesions—cont'd

| Description | Examples | | |
|---|---|---|---|

**Excoriation**

Loss of the epidermis; linear hollowed-out crusted area

Abrasion or scratch, scabies

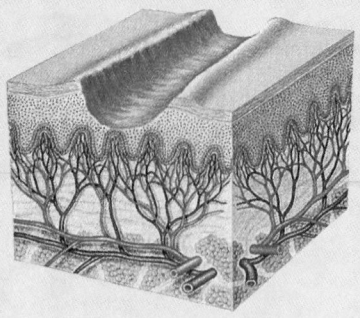 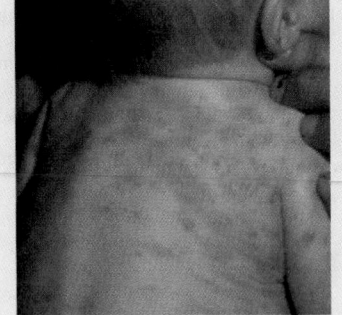

**Scabies**
*(Weston and Lane, 1991)*

**Fissure**

Linear crack or break from the epidermis to the dermis; may be moist or dry

Athlete's foot, cracks at the corner of the mouth

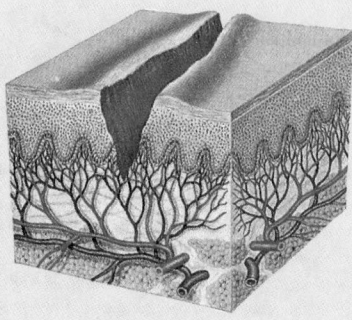 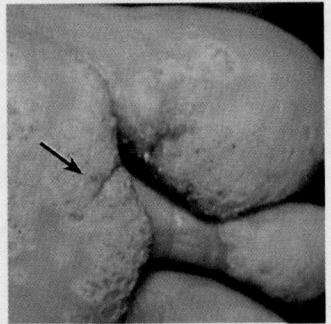

**Fissures**
*(Goldman and Fitzpatrick, 1994)*

**Erosion**

Loss of part of the epidermis; depressed, moist, glistening; follows rupture of a vesicle or bulla

Varicella, variola after rupture

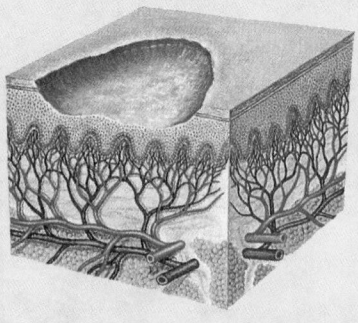 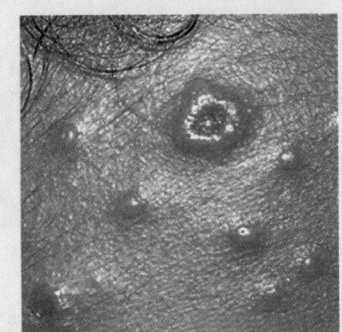

**Erosion**
*(Cohen, 1993)*

**Ulcer**

Loss of epidermis and dermis; concave; varies in size

Decubiti, stasis ulcers

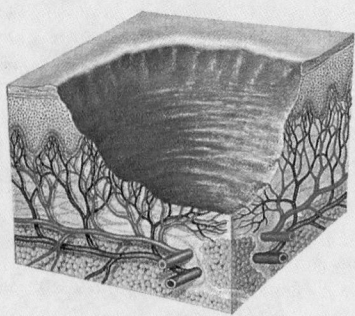 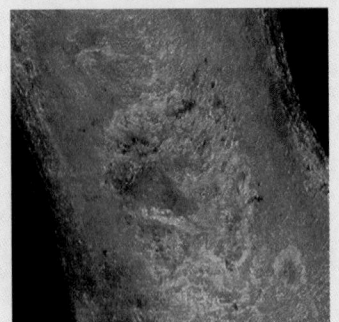

**Statis ulcer** *(Habif, 1996)*

From Seidel HM, Ball JW, Dains JE, Benedict GW: *Mosby's guide to physical examination,* ed 4, St Louis, 1999, Mosby. Modified from Thompson JM, Wilson SF: *Health assessment for nursing practice,* St Louis, 1996, Mosby.

## Secondary skin lesions—cont'd

| Description | Examples | |
|---|---|---|
| **Crust**<br>Dried serum, blood, or purulent exudate; slightly elevated; size varies; brown, red, black, tan, or straw. Scab on abrasion; eczema | Scab on abrasion, eczema | |

**Scab**
*(Seidel et al, 1999)*

| Description | Examples | |
|---|---|---|
| **Atrophy**<br>Thinning of skin surface and loss of skin markings; skin translucent and paperlike | Striae; aged skin | |

**Striae**
*(Seidel et al, 1999)*

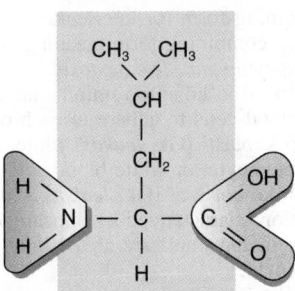

**Chemical structure of leucine**

**leucine aminopeptidase test (LAP),** a blood or 24-hour urine test that detects levels of LAP, used primarily in diagnosing liver disorders and in the differential diagnosis of increased levels of alkaline phosphatase (ALP).

**leucinosis** /lo͞o'sinō'sis/ [Gk, *leukos + osis,* condition], a condition in which the pathways for the degradation of leucine are blocked and large amounts of the amino acid accumulate in body tissue. See also **leucine.**

**leuco-.** See **leuko-.**

**leucocyte.** See **leukocyte.**

**leucocyte migration inhibition factor.** See **macrophage migration inhibiting factor.**

**leucocytopenia.** See **leukopenia.**

**leucocytosis.** See **leukocytosis.**

**leucoderma.** See **leukoderma.**

**leuconychia.** See **leukonychia.**

**leucopenia.** See **leukopenia.**

**leucophoresis.** See **leukophoresis.**

**leucopoiesis.** See **leukopoiesis.**

**leucorrhoea.** See **leukorrhea.**

**leucovorin.** See **folinic acid.**

**leucovorin calcium** /lo͞o'kəvôr'in/, an antianemic.

■ INDICATIONS: It is prescribed in the treatment of an overdose of a folic acid antagonist and certain cases of megaloblastic anemia. It is also used for leucovorin "rescue" after high-dose methotrexate therapy in osteosarcoma to diminish the toxicity of the methotrexate.

■ CONTRAINDICATIONS: Anemia caused by vitamin $B_{12}$ deficiency or known hypersensitivity to this drug prohibits its use.

■ ADVERSE EFFECTS: Hypersensitivity reactions may occur.

**leukaemia.** See **leukemia.**

**leukapheresis** /lo͞o'kəfərē'sis/ [Gk, *leukos + aphairesis,* removal], a process by which blood is withdrawn from a vein, white blood cells are selectively removed, and the remaining blood is reinfused in the donor. It is a treatment/supportive care measure in patients with leukosytosis R/T leukemia. The white blood cells may be used for treating patients with blood deficiencies or for research. Compare **plasmapheresis, plateletpheresis.** See also **apheresis.**

**leukemia** /lōōkē′mē·ə/ [Gk, *leukos* + *haima*, blood], a broad term given to a group of malignant diseases characterized by diffuse replacement of bone marrow with proliferating leukocyte precursors; abnormal numbers and forms of immature white cells in circulation; and infiltration of lymph nodes, spleen, and liver. The incidence of leukemia is about 15 per 100,000 for all age groups but increases around the age of 40 and reaches 160 per 100,000 by age 80. The disease causes about 15,900 deaths a year. Males are affected twice as often as females. The origin of leukemia is not clear, but it may result from genetic predisposition plus exposure to ionizing radiation, benzene, or other chemicals that are toxic to bone marrow. The risk of the disease increases in individuals with Down syndrome, Fanconi's syndrome, ataxia-telangiectasia, Bloom's syndrome, or some other forms of congenital aneuploidy, and in an identical twin of a leukemia victim. Classification has become increasingly complex, sophisticated, and essential since identification of the subtype has therapeutic and prognostic implications. Leukemia is classified according to the predominant proliferating cells. Acute leukemia usually has a sudden onset and rapidly progresses from early signs such as fatigue, pallor, weight loss, and easy bruising to fever, hemorrhages, extreme weakness, bone or joint pain, and repeated infections. Chronic leukemia develops slowly, and signs similar to those of the acute forms of the disease may not appear for years. Diagnoses of acute and chronic forms are made by blood tests and bone marrow biopsies. Involved marrow may range in color from muddy red-brown to pale gray, and changes are usually first evident in the vertebrae, ribs, sternum, and pelvis. The most effective treatment includes intensive combination chemotherapy, antibiotics to prevent infections, and blood transfusions to replace red cells and platelets. Also spelled **leukaemia.** See also **acute childhood leukemia, acute lymphocytic leukemia, acute myelocytic leukemia. —leukemic,** *adj.*

**-leukemia,** combining form meaning an 'increased number of leukocytes in the tissues and/or in the blood': *chloroleukemia, erythroleukemia, hypoleukemia.*

**leukemia cutis,** a condition of the skin in which yellow-brown, red, or purple nodular lesions form localized or general diffuse infiltrations. Also called **lymphoderma perniciosa.**

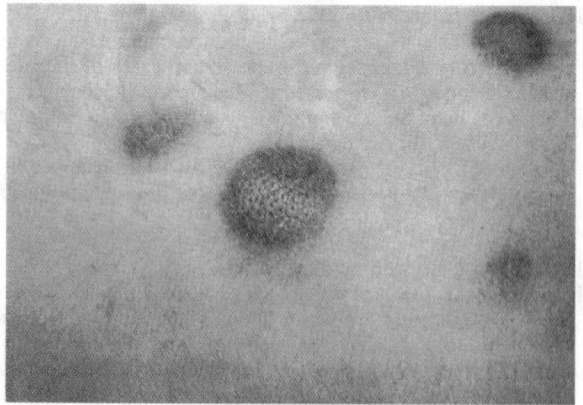

**Leukemia cutis** *(Weston, Lane, and Morrelli, 1996)*

**leukemia inhibitory factor (LIF),** a cytokine named for its ability to suppress the spontaneous proliferation of lymphoid stem cells.

**leukemic.** See **leukemia.**

**leukemic reticuloendotheliosis.** See **hairy-cell leukemia.**

**leukemogenesis** /lōōkē′mōjen′əsis/, the onset, development, or progression of leukemia.

**leukemoid** /lōōkē′moid/, resembling leukemia.

**leukemoid reaction** [Gk, *leukos* + *eidos*, form; L, *re*, again, *agere*, to act], a clinical syndrome resembling leukemia in which the white blood cell count is elevated in response to an allergy, inflammatory disease, infection, poison, hemorrhage, burn, or severe physical stress. Compare **leukemia.**

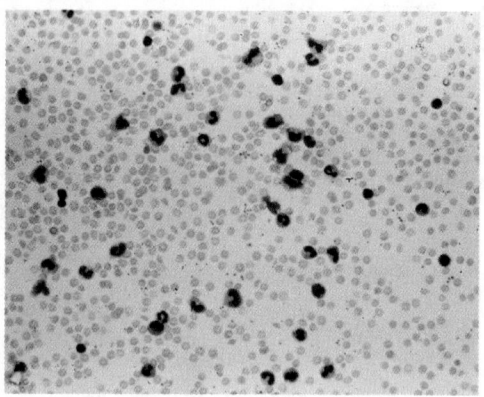

**Leukemoid reaction** *(Zitelli and Davis, 1997)*

**Leukeran,** trademark for an antineoplastic (chlorambucil).

**-leukin,** combining form for interleukin-2-type products.

**leuko-, leuco-,** combining form meaning 'white corpuscle or white': *leukocytopenia, leukocytosis.*

**leukoagglutinin** /lōō′kō·aglōō′tinin/, an antibody that causes white blood cells to adhere to each other.

**leukoblast** /lōō′kəblast/ [Gk, *leukos,* white, *blastos,* germ], an immature leukocyte, or white blood cell.

**leukocoria** /lōō′kō·kor′ē·ə/ [Gk, *leukos,* white + *korē,* pupil], a condition characterized by appearance of a whitish reflex or mass in the pupillary area behind the lens; also spelled **leukokoria.**

**leukocyte** /lōō′kəsīt/ [Gk, *leukos* + *kytos,* cell], a white blood cell, one of the formed elements of the circulating blood system. Five types of leukocytes are classified by the presence or absence of granules in the cytoplasm of the cell. The agranulocytes are **lymphocytes** and **monocytes.** The granulocytes are **neutrophils, basophils,** and **eosinophils.** White cells are able to squeeze through intracellular spaces by diapedesis and migrate by ameboid movements. Leukocytes measure 8 to 20 μm in diameter. Normal blood values vary from 5000 to 10,000 leukocytes per cubic millimeter. Leukocytes function as phagocytes of bacteria, fungi, and viruses, detoxifiers of toxic proteins that may result from allergic reactions and cellular injury, and immune system cells. Also called **leucocyte, white blood cell, white corpuscle.** Also spelled **leucocyte.** Compare **erythrocyte, platelet.** See also **complete blood count, differential white**

blood cell count, **leukocytosis, leukopenia,** and specific types of leukocytes. —**leukocytic,** *adj.*

**leukocyte adhesion deficiency (LAD),** an autosomal inherited disorder caused by a defective integrin molecule (CD18) that is important for cellular adhesion. This defect causes neutrophils to be immotile and unable to phagocytose. Patients with LAD have recurring bacterial infections and impaired wound healing, which may lead to necrosis and gangrene.

**leukocyte alkaline phosphatase (LAP),** an enzyme present in lymphocytes that is elevated in various diseases such as cirrhosis and polycythemia and in certain infections. It may be measured in the blood to detect these disorders and to differentiate chronic myelogenous (myelocytic) leukemia from leukemoid reactions. Normal amounts of this enzyme in a smear of fresh venous blood are 50 to 150 units. Also called **neutrophil alkaline phosphatase.**

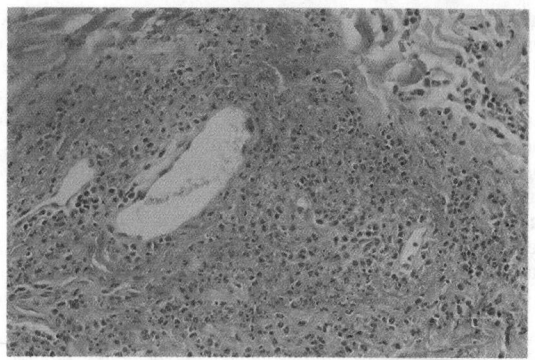

**Leukocytoclastic vasculitis**
*(Cotran, Kumar, and Collins, 1999/courtesy Scott Granter, MD, Brigham and Women's Hospital, Boston)*

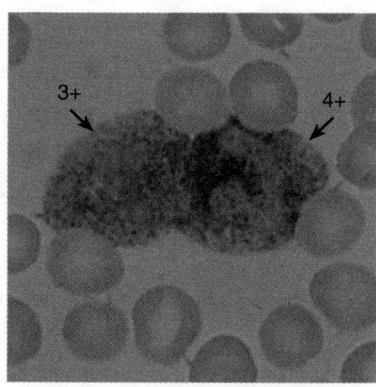

**Leukocyte alkaline phosphatase reaction**
*(Carr and Rodak, 1999)*

**leukocyte migration inhibition factor.** See **macrophage migration inhibiting factor.**

**leukocytic.** See **leukocyte.**

**leukocytic crystal.** See **Charcot-Leyden crystal.**

**leukocytoclastic vasculitis** /loo'kəsī'təklas'tik/, an allergic inflammation of blood vessels, characterized by deposits of fragmented cells, nuclear dust, necrotic debris, and fibrin staining in the vessels. Many patients develop skin lesions, particularly on the legs, accompanied by arthralgia and fever. The disorder is seen in rheumatoid arthritis and other diseases.

**leukocytogenesis** /-jen'əsis/, the origin and development of leukocytes.

**leukocytopenia.** See **leukopenia.**

**leukocytopoiesis.** See **leukopoiesis.**

**leukocytosis** /loo'kōsītō'sis/ [Gk, *leukos* + *kytos,* cell, *osis,* condition], an abnormal increase in the number of circulating white blood cells. An increase often accompanies bacterial, but not usually viral, infections. The normal range is 5000 to 10,000 white cells per cubic millimeter of blood. Leukemia may be associated with a white blood cell count as high as 500,000 to 1 million per cubic millimeter of blood, the increase being either equally or disproportionately distributed among all types. Kinds of leukocytosis include **basophilia, eosinophilia,** and **neutrophilia.** Also

spelled **leucocytosis.** Compare **leukemia, leukemoid reaction, leukopenia.** See also **leukocyte.**

**leukocyturia** /loo'kəsītoor'ē·ə/, the presence of white blood cells in the urine.

**leukoderma** /loo'kōdur'mə/ [Gk, *leukos* + *derma,* skin], localized loss of skin pigment caused by several specific causes. Compare **vitiligo.** Also spelled **leucoderma.**

**leukodystrophy** /-dis'trəfē/ [Gk, *leukos,* white, *dys* + *trophe,* nourishment], a disease of the white matter of the brain, characterized by demyelination. See also **leukoencephalopathy.**

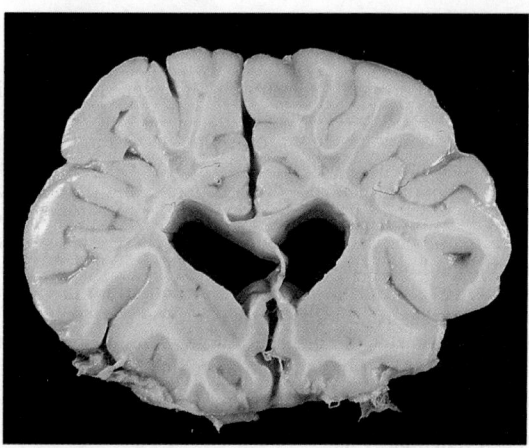

**Leukodystrophy** *(Kumar, Cotran, and Robbins, 1997)*

**leukoencephalopathy** /loo'kō·ən·sef'ə·lop'ə·thē/ [Gk, *leukos,* white + *enkephalos,* brain + *pathos,* disease], any of a group of diseases affecting the white matter of the brain, especially of the cerebral hemispheres, and occurring as a rule in infants and children. The term **leukodystrophy** is used to denote such disorders resulting from a defect in the formation and the maintenance of myelin in infants and children.

**leukoerythroblastic anemia** /loo'kō·erith'rōblas'tik/ [Gk, *leukos* + *erythros*, red, *blastos*, germ, *a* + *haima*, not blood], an abnormal condition in which large numbers of immature white and red blood cells are present. It is characteristic of some anemias that occur as a result of the replacement of normal bone marrow with malignant tumor. See also **myeloid metaplasia, myelophthisic anemia.**

**leukokoria.** See **leukocoria.**

**leukonychia** /loo'kōnik'ē·ə/ [Gk, *leukos* + *onyx*, nail], a benign condition in which white patches appear under the nails. Trauma, infection, and many disorders can cause white spots or streaks on nails. Also spelled **leuconychia.**

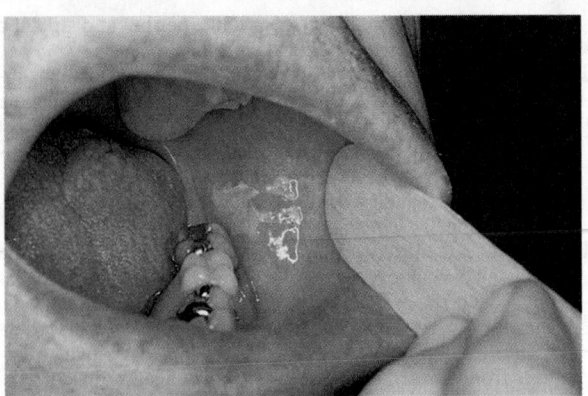

**Leukoplakia** *(Callen, Greer, and Hood, 1993)*

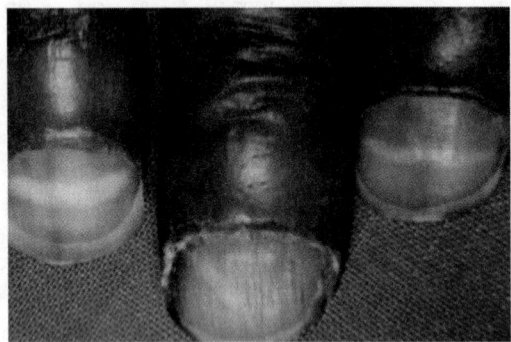

**Leukonychia** *(Hordinsky, Sawaya, and Scher, 2000)*

**leukopenia** /loo'kōpē'nē·ə/ [Gk, *leukos* + *penes*, poor], an abnormal decrease in the number of white blood cells to fewer than 5000 cells per cubic millimeter. The condition may be caused by an adverse drug reaction, radiation poisoning, or pathologic conditions. One or all kinds of white blood cells may be affected. The two most common forms of leukopenia are neutrophilic leukopenia and lymphocytic leukopenia. Also called **leucocytopenia.** Also spelled **leucopenia.** Compare **aleukia, leukocytosis.** See also **aplastic anemia, leukocyte.** —**leukopenic,** *adj.*

**leukopenic leukemia.** See **aleukemic leukemia.**

**leukophlegmasia.** See **phlegmasia alba dolens.**

**leukophoresis** /loo'kōfərē'sis/ [Gk, *leukos* + *phoresis*, being transmitted], a laboratory procedure in which blood is drawn and white blood cells are separated from the blood and the red blood cells are returned to the patient. Also spelled **leucophoresis.**

**leukoplakia** /loo'kōplā'kē·ə/ [Gk, *leukos* + *plakos*, plate], a precancerous, slowly developing change in a mucous membrane characterized by thickened, white, firmly attached patches that are slightly raised and sharply circumscribed. They may occur on the penis or vulva; those appearing on the lips and buccal mucosa are associated with pipe smoking. Malignant potential is evaluated by microscopic study of biopsied tissue. Compare **lichen planus.** See also **lichen sclerosis et atrophicus.**

**leukoplakic vulvitis** /-plā'kik/ [Gk, *leukos*, white, *plakos*, plate, *vulva* + *itis*, inflammation], a condition in which the skin of the vulva becomes thick and white, develops bleeding fissures, and later becomes atrophic. The condition may progress to cancer.

**leukopoiesis** /loo'kōpō·ē'sis/ [Gk, *leukos* + *poiein*, to make], the process by which white blood cells form and develop. Neutrophils, basophils, and eosinophils are produced in myeloid tissue in the bone marrow. Lymphocytes and monocytes are normally derived from hemocytoblasts in lymphoid tissue, but a few develop in the marrow. Also called **leukocytopoiesis.** Also spelled **leucopoiesis.** —**leukopoietic,** *adj.*

**leukorrhea** /loo'kôrē'ə/ [Gk, *leukos* + *rhoia*, flow], a white discharge from the vagina. Normally, vaginal discharge occurs in regular variations of amount and consistency during the course of the menstrual cycle. A greater than usual amount is normal in pregnancy, and a decrease is to be expected after delivery, during lactation, and after menopause. Leukorrhea is the most common reason for women to seek gynecologic care. Also spelled **leucorrhoea.** See also **vaginal discharge.**

**leukosarcoma.** See **lymphoma.**

**leukotomy.** See **lobotomy.**

**leukotoxin** /loo'kətok'sin/ [Gk, *leukos* + *toxikon*, poison], a substance that can inactivate or destroy leukocytes. —**leukotoxic,** *adj.*

**leukotrienes** /-trī'ēnz/, a class of biologically active compounds that occur naturally in leukocytes and produce allergic and inflammatory reactions similar to those of histamine. They are thought to play a role in the development of allergic and autoallergic diseases such as asthma, rheumatoid arthritis, inflammatory bowel disease, and psoriasis.

**leukovirus** /-vī'rus/ [Gk, *leukos*, white; L, *virus*, poison], any of a group of ribonucleic acid viruses that cause disease in animals. The diseases include Rous sarcoma and murine leukemia.

**leuprolide acetate** /loo'prōlīd/, a parenteral antineoplastic drug.

■ INDICATIONS: It is prescribed for the palliative treatment of advanced prostatic cancer, in the management of endometriosis, and for the treatment of children with central precocious puberty.

■ CONTRAINDICATIONS: Caution should be exercised during the beginning of leuprolide acetate therapy when symptoms of bone pain, urinary obstruction, and neurologic problems may increase.

■ ADVERSE EFFECTS: Among adverse reactions reported are hot flashes, transient increases in testosterone levels, dizziness, pain, headache, decreased libido, impotence, and injection site irritation.

**levalbuterol,** an adrenergic β₂-agonist.

- INDICATIONS: Levalbuterol is used in the treatment and prevention of bronchospasm (reversible obstructive airway disease).

- CONTRAINDICATIONS: Tachydysrhythmias, severe cardiac disease, and known hypersensitivity to sympathomimetics prohibit the use of this drug.

- ADVERSE EFFECTS: Among this drug's adverse effects are insomnia, headache, dizziness, stimulation, hallucinations, flushing, irritability, dry nose, irritation of the nose and throat, palpitations, tachycardia, hypertension, angina, hypotension, dysrhythmias, heartburn, nausea, vomiting, and muscle cramps. Common side effects include tremors, anxiety, and restlessness.

**levamfetamine.** See **levamphetamine.**

**levamisole,** an immunomodulator used as an adjuvant treatment in combination with fluorouracil after surgical resection in patients with Dukes' stage C colon cancer.

**levamphetamine** /lev′əmfet′əmēn/, an isomer of amphetamine, formerly used as an anorexiant. Also spelled **levamfetamine.**

**levarterenol bitartrate.** See **norepinephrine bitartrate.**

**levator** /livā′tər/, pl. **levatores** /lev′ətôr′ēz/ [L, *levare,* to lift up], **1.** a muscle that raises a structure of the body, as the levator ani raises parts of the pelvic diaphragm. **2.** a surgical instrument used to lift depressed bony fragments in fractures of the skull and other bones.

**levator ani,** one of a pair of muscles of the pelvic diaphragm that stretches across the bottom of the pelvic cavity like a hammock, supporting the pelvic organs. It is a broad thin muscle that separates into the pubococcygeus and the iliococcygeus. It originates from the ramus of the pubic bone, the spine of the ischium, and a band of fascia between the pubis and the ischium; it inserts into the last two segments of the coccyx, the anococcygeal raphe, the sphincter ani externus, and the central tendinous point of the perineum. The left and right levator ani muscles are divided ventrally but converge as a single sheet across the midline dorsally, forming most of the pelvic diaphragm. The levator ani is innervated by branches of the pudendal plexus, which contains fibers from the fourth sacral nerve. It functions to support and slightly raise the pelvic floor. The pubococcygeus draws the anus toward the pubis and constricts it. Compare **coccygeus.**

**levatores.** See **levator.**

**levator palpebrae superioris,** one of the three muscles of the eyelid, also considered an extrinsic muscle of the eye. It is thin and flat and rises from the small wing of the sphenoid. It is innervated by the oculomotor nerve. It elevates the upper eyelid and is the antagonist of the orbicularis oculi. Compare **corrugator supercilii, orbicularis oculi.**

**levator scapulae,** a muscle of the dorsal and lateral aspects of the neck. It arises from the axis and the atlas, and it inserts into the transverse processes of the four upper cervical vertebrae. It is innervated by the third and fourth cervical nerves and acts to raise the scapula and pull it toward the midline.

**LeVeen shunt** [Harry H. LeVeen, American surgeon, b. 1914], a tube that is surgically implanted to connect the peritoneal cavity and the superior vena cava to drain accumulated fluid from the peritoneal cavity. It is used in cirrhosis of the liver, right-sided heart failure, or abdominal cancer. Before surgery a sodium-restricted diet and diuretics are used to decrease sodium and water retention. With the patient under general anesthesia, a silicone rubber tube is inserted under the subcutaneous tissue from the peritoneal cavity to the superior vena cava. As the patient inhales, the fluid pressure in the peritoneal cavity increases, and that in

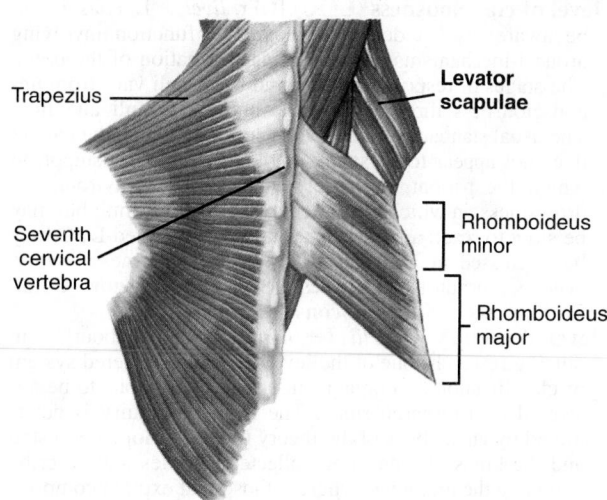

**Levator scapulae** *(Thibodeau and Patton, 1999/John V. Hagen)*

the blood vessel falls, allowing peritoneal fluid to enter the shunt valve. After surgery the patient is closely observed for signs of occlusion of the shunt, GI bleeding, or leakage of peritoneal fluid from the incision. Excessive dilution of the blood may lead to coagulation abnormalities.

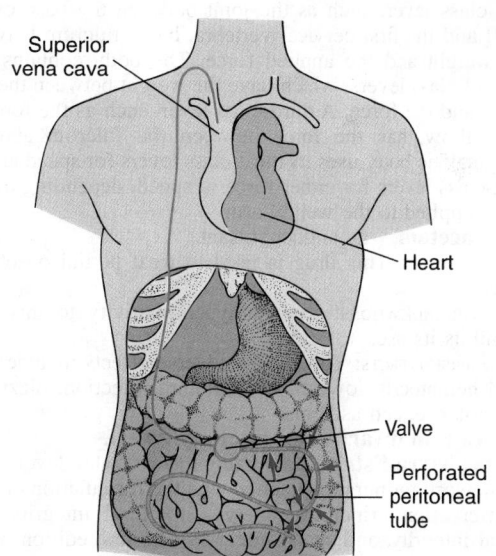

**LeVeen shunt** *(Beare and Myers, 1998)*

**level of activities** [OFr, *livel* + L, *activus*], pertaining to the hierarchy of nervous system activity that determines the level responsible for certain functions while also being controlled by a higher level above it, as in the sequence of events in a reflex action.

**level of consciousness (LOC)** [OFr, *livel* + L, *conscire,* to be aware of], a degree of cognitive function involving arousal mechanisms of the reticular formation of the brain. The stages of response of the mind to stimuli vary from unconsciousness through vague awareness to full attention. The usual standard levels include coma, in which the patient does not appear to be aware of the environment; stupor, in which the patient is vaguely aware of the environment; drowsiness, in which the patient responds to stimuli but may be slow to react, and alert wakefulness. Impaired LOC may be expressed in obtundation or reduced alertness, stupor, syncope, or unresponsiveness. See also **Glasgow Coma Scale, preconscious, subconscious.**

**level of inquiry** [OFr, *livel* + *inquirere,* to ask about], (in nursing research) one of the levels in a rank-ordered system of classification and organization of the questions to be answered in a research study. The level of inquiry is determined by an analysis of the theory to be developed or tested and the kinds of data to be collected. Studies that describe comprise the first level, whereas those that explain comprise the second level. Those that prescribe or predict are the most difficult to answer or to support.

**levels of care,** a classification of health care service levels by the kind of care given, the number of people served, and the people providing the care. Kinds of health care service levels are **primary health care, secondary health care,** and **tertiary health care.**

**lever** /lē′vər, lev′ər/ [L, *levare,* to lift up], any one of the numerous bones and associated joints of the body that act as a simple machine so that force applied to one end of the bone tends to rotate the bone in the direction opposite from that of the applied force. The muscles of the body produce the forces that move the levers. The basic components of a lever are the fulcrum, the force arm, and the weight arm. A first-class lever, such as the joint between the base of the skull and the first cervical vertebra, has a fulcrum between the weight and the applied force. The body contains few second-class levers, which have the weight between the fulcrum and the force. A third-class lever, such as the forearm and elbow, has the force between the fulcrum and the weight. The body uses its third-class levers for speed and its first-class levers for either force or speed, depending on the force applied to the weight arm.

**levetiracetam,** an anticonvulsant.
- INDICATIONS: This drug is used to treat partial onset seizures.
- CONTRAINDICATIONS: Known hypersensitivity to this drug prohibits its use.
- ADVERSE EFFECTS: This drug's adverse effects include lowered hematocrit, lowered hemoglobin, infection, dizziness, somnolence, and asthenia.

**Lévi-Lorain dwarf.** See **pituitary dwarf.**

**Levine, Myra Estrin,** a nursing theorist who developed a framework for nursing practice with the formulation of Four Conservation Principles: energy, structural integrity, personal integrity, and social integrity. The first edition of her book using the conservation principles, *Introduction to Clinical Nursing,* was published in 1969. Levine's emphasis on the ill person in the health care setting reflects the history of health care in the 1960s. Levine's model stresses nursing interventions and interactions based on the scientific background of these principles. Levine viewed people in a holistic manner, having their own environment, both internal and external. She identified four levels of integration that help a person maintain his integrity or wholeness: fight or flight, inflammatory response, response to stress, and perceptual response. The individual's stability is organized by his or her availability of responses and adaptation processes. It is the nurse's task to bring a body of scientific principles on which decisions are based into the situation shared with the patient.

**Levin tube** /lev′in/ [Abraham L. Levin, American physician, 1880–1940], a plastic catheter introduced through the nose and used in gastric intubation for gastric decompression or gavage feeding. Compare **Miller-Abbott tube.** See also **gastric intubation.**

**levitation** /lev′itā′shən/ [L, *levitas,* lightness, *atus,* process], (in psychiatry) a hallucinatory sensation of floating or rising in the air. —**levitate,** *v.*

**levo-** /lē′vō-/, prefix meaning 'left': *levocardia, levoclination, levotorsion.*

**levobunolol hydrochloride** /-bun′əlol/, a topical ophthalmic beta-adrenergic blocker drug for glaucoma.
- INDICATIONS: It is prescribed for the treatment of chronic open-angle glaucoma and ocular hypertension.
- CONTRAINDICATIONS: Levobunolol hydrochloride is contraindicated for patients with bronchial asthma, severe chronic obstructive pulmonary disease, sinus bradycardia, second- or third-degree atrioventricular block, overt cardiac failure, or cardiogenic shock.
- ADVERSE EFFECTS: Adverse reactions may include transient ocular burning or stinging, bradycardia, pulmonary edema, and blepharoconjunctivitis.

**levobupivacaine,** a local anesthetic.
- INDICATIONS: This drug is used to produce local and regional anesthesia, for pain management, and for continuous epidural analgesia.
- CONTRAINDICATIONS: Severe liver disease and known hypersensitivity to this drug contraindicate its use. Levobupivacaine is also contraindicated in children less than 12 years of age and in the elderly.
- ADVERSE EFFECTS: Life-threatening effects of this drug are convulsions, loss of consciousness, myocardial depression, cardiac arrest, dysrhythmias, fetal bradycardia, status asthmaticus, respiratory arrest, and anaphylaxis. Other adverse effects include anxiety, restlessness, drowsiness, disorientation, tremors, shivering, bradycardia, hypotension, hypertension, nausea, vomiting, blurred vision, tinnitus, pupil constriction, rash, urticaria, allergic reactions, edema, burning, skin discoloration at the injection site, and tissue necrosis.

**levocardia** /-kär′dē·ə/, a congenital anomaly in which the viscera are transposed to the opposite side of the body, except for the heart, which is in its normal position.

**levocarnitine** /elkär′nitēn/, an oral drug for carnitine deficiency.
- INDICATIONS: The product is prescribed for the treatment of primary systemic carnitine deficiency.
- CONTRAINDICATIONS: It should not be given to patients with a known hypersensitivity to carnitine.
- ADVERSE EFFECTS: Adverse reactions include nausea, vomiting, abdominal cramps, diarrhea, and body odor.

**levoclination.** See **levotorsion.**

**levodopa** /lē′vōdō′pə/, an antiparkinsonian.
- INDICATIONS: It is prescribed in the treatment of Parkinson's disease, juvenile forms of Huntington's disease, and chronic manganese poisoning.
- CONTRAINDICATIONS: Narrow-angle glaucoma, concomitant use of a monoamine oxidase inhibitor, suspected melanoma, or known hypersensitivity to this drug prohibits its use.
- ADVERSE EFFECTS: Among the more serious adverse reactions are severe GI disturbances, hypotension, various movement disorders, emotional changes, cardiac arrhythmia, and anorexia.

**Levo-Dromoran,** trademark for an opioid analgesic (levorphanol tartrate).

**levofloxacin,** an antiinfective.

■ INDICATIONS: This drug is used to treat acute sinusitis, acute chronic bronchitis, community-acquired pneumonia, uncomplicated skin infections, complicated urinary tract infections, and acute pyelonephritis caused by *Streptococcus pneumoniae, Haemophilus influenzae, H. parainfluenzae,* and *Moraxella catarrhalis.*

■ CONTRAINDICATIONS: Known hypersensitivity to quinolones and photosensitivity prohibit the use of this drug.

■ ADVERSE EFFECTS: Life-threatening effects of this drug are anaphylaxis, multisystem organ failure, hemolytic anemia, pseudomembranous colitis, and Stevens-Johnson syndrome. Other adverse effects include hypoglycemia, hypersensitivity, dizziness, anxiety, encephalopathy, paresthesia, chest pain, palpitations, vasodilation, eosinophilia, lymphopenia, pneumonitis, flatulence, diarrhea, abdominal pain, vaginitis, crystalluria, rash, and pruritus. Common side effects are headache, insomnia, nausea, vomiting, and photosensitivity.

**levonorgestral implant.** See **Norplant System.**

**Levophed Bitartrate,** trademark for an adrenergic (norepinephrine bitartrate).

**levorphanol tartrate** /lē′vôrfā′nol/, an opioid analgesic.

■ INDICATIONS: It is prescribed for the treatment of pain and preoperative analgesia.

■ CONTRAINDICATIONS: Alcoholism, asthma, increased intracranial pressure, respiratory depression, anoxia, or known hypersensitivity to this drug prohibits its use.

■ ADVERSE EFFECTS: Among the more serious adverse reactions are drug dependence, orthostatic hypotension, cardiac arrhythmia, and retention of urine.

**levothyroxine sodium** /-thī′rəksēn/, a thyroid hormone. Also called **ʟ-thyroxine.**

■ INDICATION: It is prescribed in the treatment of hypothyroidism.

■ CONTRAINDICATIONS: Recent myocardial infarction or known hypersensitivity to this drug prohibits its use.

■ ADVERSE EFFECTS: The most serious adverse reactions are angina, tachycardia, arrhythmias, and tremors.

**levotorsion** /lev′itôr′shən/, the rotation to the left of the upper pole of the cornea of one or both eyes. Also called **levoclination.**

**Lev's disease** [Maurice Lev, American pathologist, 1908–1994], fibrosis or calcification of the conduction system of the heart that results in varying degrees of heart block in patients with normal a myocardium and coronary arteries.

**Levsinex,** trademark for an anticholinergic (hyoscyamine sulfate).

**levulose.** See **fructose.**

**levulosuria.** See **fructosuria.**

**Lewis Blood Group System,** a blood-group system based on antigens present in soluble forms in blood and secretions. The antigens are adsorbed from the plasma onto the red cell membrane. The expressed Lewis phenotype is based on whether the patient is a secretor or nonsecretor of the Lewis gene product.

**lewisite** /loo′isīt/ [Winford L. Lewis, American chemist, 1878–1943], 2-chlorovinyl arsine; a poisonous blister gas, used in World War I, that causes irritation of the lungs, dyspnea, damage to the tissues of the respiratory tract, tears, and pain.

**Lewy bodies** /lā′wē, loo′ē/ [Frederick H. Lewy, German neurologist, 1885–1950], concentric spheres found inside vacuoles in midbrain and brainstem neurons in patients with idiopathic parkinsonism, Alzheimer's disease, and other neurodegenerative conditions.

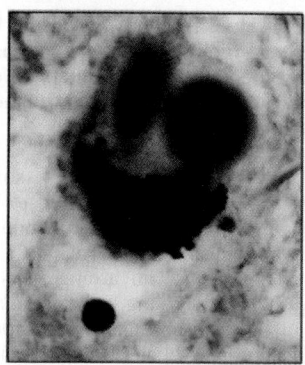

**Lewy body in the substantia nigra** *(Perkin, 1998)*

**-lexia,** suffix meaning 'reading': *alexia, bradylexia, dyslexia.*

**Leyden-Möbius muscular dystrophy** /lī′dən-mœ′bē·əs, -mē′bē·əs/, a form of limb-girdle muscular dystrophy that begins in the pelvic girdle. Also called **pelvifemoral muscular dystrophy.**

**Leydig cells** /lī′dig/ [Franz von Leydig, German anatomist, 1821–1908], **1.** cells of the interstitial tissue of the testes that secrete testosterone. **2.** mucous cells that do not pour their secretions out over the surface of the epithelium.

**Leydig cell tumor,** a generally benign neoplasm of interstitial cells of a testis that may cause gynecomastia in adults and precocious sexual development if the lesion occurs before puberty. The tumor is usually a circumscribed lobulated palpable mass.

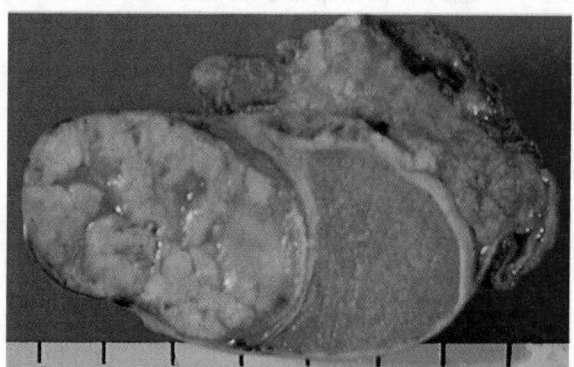

**Leydig cell tumor** *(Fletcher, 2000)*

**LF,** abbreviation for *low frequency.*

**LFA,** abbreviation for *left frontoanterior fetal position.*

**LFP,** abbreviation for *left frontoposterior fetal position.*

**LFT,** abbreviation for **liver function test.**

**LGA,** abbreviation for *large for gestational age.* See **large for gestational age (LGA) infant.**

**LGV,** abbreviation for **lymphogranuloma venereum.**

**LH,** abbreviation for **luteinizing hormone.**

**Lhermitte's sign** /ler′mits/ [Jacques J. Lhermitte, French neurologist, 1877–1959], sudden, transient, electric-like shocks spreading down the body when the head is flexed forward, occurring chiefly in multiple sclerosis but also in compression disorders of the cervical spinal cord.

**LHRH,** abbreviation for **luteinizing hormone-releasing hormone.**

**Li,** symbol for the element **lithium.**

**liability** /lī′əbil′itē/ [L, *ligare,* to bind], **1.** something one is obligated to do or an obligation required to be fulfilled by law, usually financial in nature. **2.** the amount of money required to fulfill a financial obligation.

**liaison nursing** /lē·ā′zən/, an arrangement with clinical specialists in psychiatric nursing whereby nurses and health professionals in other disciplines obtain consultation services in medical-surgical, parent-child, and geriatric settings.

**libel** /lī′bəl/ [L, *libellus,* little book], a false accusation written, printed, or typewritten, or presented in a picture or a sign that is made with malicious intent to defame the reputation of a person who is living or the memory of a person who is dead, resulting in public embarrassment, contempt, ridicule, or hatred.

**liberation** /lib′ərā′shən/ [L, *liber,* free], the process of drug release from the dosage form.

**libidinal.** See **libidinous.**

**libidinal development.** See **psychosexual development.**

**libidinous** /libid′inəs/ [L, *libidinosus,* lustful], **1.** pertaining to or belonging to the libido. **2.** having or characterized by sexual desire. Also **libidinal.** —**libidinize,** *v.*

**libido** /libē′dō, libī′dō/, **1.** the psychic energy or instinctual drive associated with sexual desire, pleasure, or creativity. **2.** (in psychoanalysis) the instinctual drives of the id. **3.** lustful desire or striving.

**Libman-Sacks endocarditis** /lib′mənsaks′/ [Emanuel Libman, American physician, 1872–1946; Benjamin Sacks, American physician, 1896–1939], the most common manifestation of lupus erythematosus, characterized by warty lesions that develop near the heart valves but rarely affect valvular action. The lesions usually are dry and granular, with a pink or tawny color; they contain basophilic cellular debris and develop in the angle of the atrioventricular

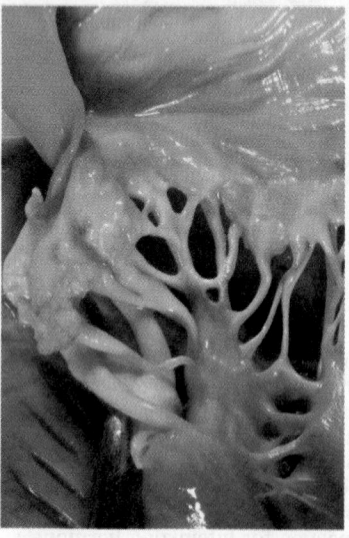

**Libman-Sacks endocarditis**
*(Cotran, Kumar, and Collins, 1999/courtesy Dr. Fred Schoen, Department of Pathology, Brigham and Women's Hospital, Boston)*

valves and at the base of the mitral valve. Also called **Libman-Sacks disease, Libman-Sacks syndrome.**

**Librax,** trademark for a GI, fixed-combination drug containing an anticholinergic (clidinium bromide) and a sedative (chlordiazepoxide hydrochloride).

**Libritabs,** trademark for an antianxiety agent (chlordiazepoxide hydrochloride).

**Librium,** trademark for an antianxiety agent (chlordiazepoxide hydrochloride).

**lice,** *sing.* **louse** [AS, *lus*], any of the small wingless insect order of Anoplura. Lice are ectoparasites of birds and mammals and may spend their entire life cycle on a single host, attaching eggs to the hair shafts or feathers. They transfer to humans by direct contact. Three forms that infect humans are the **head louse,** *Pediculus humanus capitis;* the **body louse,** *Pediculus humanus corporis;* and the **crab louse,** *Phthirus pubis.* See also **pediculosis.**

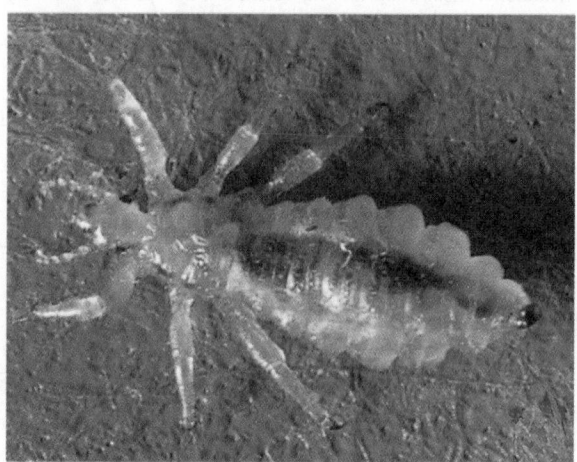

**Human body louse**
*(Habif, 1996/courtesy Ken Gray, Oregon State University Extension Services)*

**license,** an agency- or government-granted permission issued to a health care professional to engage in a given occupation on finding that the applicant has attained the degree of competency necessary to ensure that the public health, safety, and welfare are reasonably well-protected.

**licensed practical nurse (LPN)** /lī′sənst/ [L, *licere,* to be allowed; Gk, *praktikos,* fit for action; L, *nutrix,* nurse], *U.S.* a person educated in basic nursing techniques and direct patient care who practices under the supervision of a registered nurse. The course of education usually lasts 1 year. In Canada an LPN is called a certified nursing assistant. Also called *(U.S.)* **licensed vocational nurse.**

**licensed psychologist,** a person who has earned a PhD in psychology from an accredited graduate school and who has completed 2 to 3 years of postgraduate training with special emphasis on the diagnosis and treatment of psychologic disorders. Also called **clinical psychologist.** See also **psychotherapist.**

**licensed vocational nurse.** See **licensed practical nurse.**

**licensure** /lī′sənshŏŏr/ [L, *licere,* to be allowed], the granting of permission by a competent authority (usually a government agency) to an organization or individual to engage in a practice or activity that would otherwise be illegal.

Kinds of licensure include the issuing of licenses for general hospitals or nursing homes, for health professionals such as physicians, and for the production or distribution of biologic products. Licensure is usually granted on the basis of education and examination rather than performance. It is usually permanent, but a periodic fee, demonstration of competence, or continuing education may be required. Licensure may be revoked by the granting agency for incompetence, criminal acts, or other reasons stipulated in the rules governing the specific area of licensure.

**lichen amyloidosis** /lī′kən/, a common form of amyloidosis. The condition is characterized by symmetric distribution over the skin of translucent yellowish-brown dome-shaped pruritic papules.

**lichenification** /līken′ifikā′shən/ [Gk, *leichen,* lichen, *facere,* to make], thickening and hardening of the skin, often resulting from the irritation caused by repeated scratching of a pruritic lesion. **—lichenified,** *adj.*

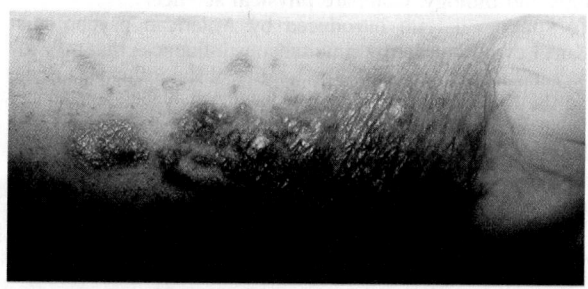

**Lichenification** *(Zitelli and Davis, 1997)*

**lichen nitidus** [Gk, *leichen* + L, *nitidus,* bright], a rare skin disorder characterized by numerous flat, glistening, pale, discrete papules measuring 2 to 3 mm in diameter.

**lichenoid eczema** /lī′kənoid/, a chronic inflammatory cutaneous condition characterized by skin thickening and accentuated skin lesions.

**lichen planus,** a nonmalignant, chronic, pruritic skin disease of unknown cause that is characterized by small flat purplish polygonal papules or plaques with fine gray lines on the surface. Common sites are flexor surfaces of wrists, forearms, ankles, abdomen, and sacrum. On mucous membranes the lesions appear gray and lacy. Nails may have longitudinal ridges. Episodes of disease activity vary but may last for months and may recur.

**lichen sclerosus et atrophicus,** a chronic skin disease characterized by white flat papules and black hard follicular plugs. In advanced cases the papules tend to coalesce into large white patches of thin pruritic skin. Lesions often occur on the torso and in the anogenital regions.

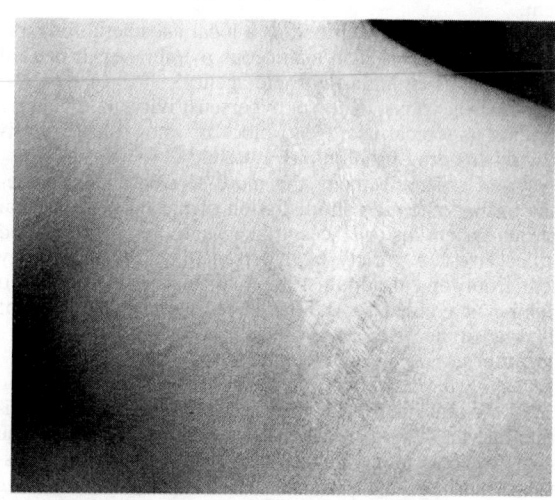

**Lichen sclerosus et atrophicus on the neck** *(Weston, Lane, and Morrelli, 1996)*

**lichen simplex chronicus,** a form of dermatitis characterized by a patch of pruritic confluent papules. Factors such as scratching contribute to its chronicity. Treatment may include topical or intralesional application of corticosteroids to relieve the pruritus.

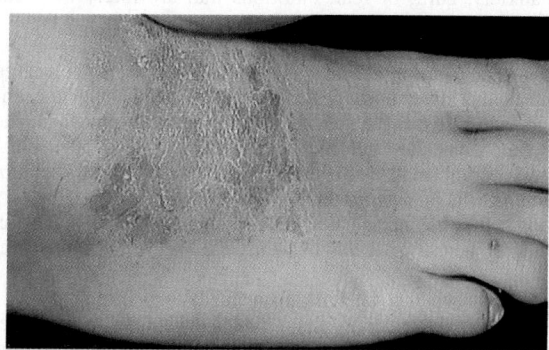

**Lichen simplex chronicus on the foot** *(Habif, 1996)*

**lichen urticatus.** See **papular urticaria.**

**licorice,** an herb that grows in shrub form in many subtropical areas.

■ USES: This herb is used for allergies, arthritis, asthma, constipation, esophagitis, gastritis, hepatitis, inflammatory con-

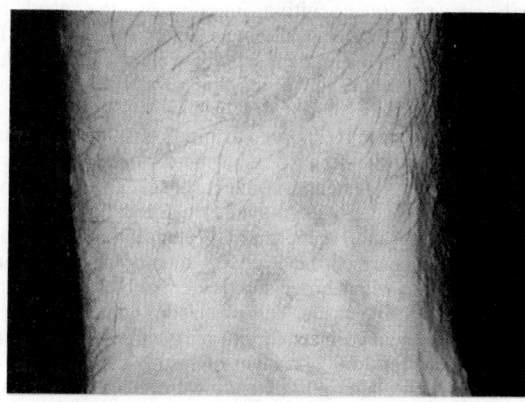

**Lichen planus on the forearm** *(Habif, 1996)*

ditions, peptic ulcers, poor adrenal function, and poor appetite.

■ CONTRAINDICATIONS: Licorice should not be used during pregnancy and lactation, in children, or in those with known hypersensitivity. It is also contraindicated in people with liver disease, renal disease, hypokalemia, hypertension, arrhythmias, and congestive heart failure.

**lid.** See **eyelid.**

**Lidex,** trademark for a glucocorticoid (fluocinonide).

**lidocaine hydrochloride** /lī′dəkān/, a local anesthetic agent.

■ INDICATIONS: It is prescribed as a local anesthetic for topical administration to skin or mucous membranes. It is used parenterally as an antiarrhythmic agent.

■ CONTRAINDICATIONS: Known hypersensitivity to this drug prohibits its topical use. Heart block or known hypersensitivity to this drug prohibits its systemic use.

■ ADVERSE EFFECTS: Among the more serious adverse reactions to the systemic administration of the drug are central nervous system disturbances, hypotension, bradycardia, and cardiac arrest. A variety of hypersensitivity reactions may occur from topical administration of this drug. Eating and drinking is avoided for 1 hour after topical application of this drug to the pharynx or the esophagus.

**lid poppers,** *slang.* amphetamines.

**lie** [AS, *licgan,* position], the relationship between the long axis of the fetus and the long axis of the mother. In a longitudinal lie the fetus is lying lengthwise, or vertically, in the uterus, whereas in a transverse lie the fetus is lying crosswise, or horizontally.

**Lieberkühn's glands** /lē′bərkēnz/ [Johann N. Lieberkühn, German anatomist, 1711–1756; L, *glans,* acorn], tubular glands between the bases of the villi of the small intestine and on the surface of the epithelium of the large intestine. They do not secrete digestive enzymes but a watery fluid. Also called **intestinal glands, crypts of Lieberkühn, follicles of Lieberkühn.**

**lie detector** [AS, *leogan,* untruth; L, *detegere,* to uncover], an electronic device or instrument used to detect lying or anxiety in regard to specific questions. A commonly used lie detector is the polygraph recorder that senses and records pulse, respiratory rate, blood pressure, and perspiration. Some experts hold that certain patterns indicate the presence of anxiety, guilt, or fear, emotions that are likely to occur when the subject is lying.

**lien.** See **spleen.**

**lienal vein** /lī′ənəl, lē-ē′nəl/ [L, *lien,* spleen, *vena*], a large vein of the lower body that unites with the superior mesenteric vein to form the portal vein. It returns blood from the spleen. Also called **splenic vein.**

**lieno-,** combining form meaning 'spleen': *lienomalacia, lienomedullary, lienopathy.*

**lienography** /lē′ənog′rəfē/, the radiographic examination of the spleen after it has been injected with a contrast medium.

**LIF,** abbreviation for **leukemia inhibitory factor.**

**life** [AS, *lif*], the energy that enables organisms to grow, reproduce, absorb and use nutrients, evolve, and in some organisms achieve mobility, express consciousness, and demonstrate a voluntary use of the senses.

**life costs** [AS, *lif* + L, *constare,* constant], the mortality, morbidity, and suffering associated with a given disease or medical procedure.

**life cycle,** **1.** the interval of time from conception to natural death. **2.** the series of stages from any stage of one generation to the same stage of the next generation.

**life expectancy,** the probable number of years a person

will live after a given age, as determined by mortality in a specific geographic area. It may be individually qualified by the person's condition or race, sex, age, or other demographic factors. Also called **expectation of life.**

**life extension** [AS, *lif,* life; L, *extenere,* to stretch out], the process of extending the life span of an individual or population by intervention that promotes better use of preventive medicine and use of established diagnostic and therapeutic facilities.

**life island,** a plastic bubble enclosing a bed, used to provide a germ-free environment for patients with a specific kind of immune deficit.

**life review,** **1.** (in psychiatry) a progressive return to consciousness of past experiences. **2.** reminiscences that occur in old age as a consequence of the realization of the inevitability of death. Also called **reminiscence therapy.**

**lifesaving measure,** any medical intervention that is implemented when a patient's life is threatened.

**life science,** the study of the laws and properties of living matter. Some kinds of life science are **anatomy, bacteriology,** and **biology.** Compare **physical science.**

**life space,** a term introduced by American psychologist Kurt Lewin to describe simultaneous influences that may affect individual behavior. The totality of the influences make up the life space.

**life span,** the length of life of an individual or the average length of life in a population or species.

**life-style–induced health problems,** diseases with natural histories that include conscious exposure to certain health-compromising or risk factors. An example is heart disease associated with cigarette smoking, poor dietary habits, lack of exercise, and sustaining unbuffered stress.

**life support** [AS, *lif,* life; L, *supportare,* to bring up to], the use of any therapeutic technique or device to maintain life functions.

**lifetime reserve** [AS, *lif* + *tid,* time; L, *re,* again, *servare,* to keep], a lifetime total of days of inpatient hospitalization benefits that may be drawn on by a patient who has exhausted the maximum benefits allowed under Medicare for a single spell of illness.

**Li-Fraumeni cancer syndrome** /lē′frômen′ē/ [Frederick P. Li; Joseph F. Fraumeni, Jr.; 20th century American epidemiologists], a type of familial breast carcinoma affecting young women and associated with soft-tissue sarcomas and other cancers in close relatives.

**lift assessment** [AS, *lyft,* loft; L, *assidere,* to sit beside], the selection of the most appropriate lift method to use when moving a patient, as from the bed to a chair. The assessment involves consideration of such factors as whether the patient is conscious or unconscious, whether the patient has a visual, hearing, or cognitive impairment, the need for special care in handling patient attachments such as IV lines or monitors, the patient's body weight, and whether the patient has full range of motion or flaccid or spastic limbs.

**ligament** /lig′əmənt/ [L, *ligare,* to bind], **1.** one of many predominantly white shiny flexible bands of fibrous tissue binding joints together and connecting the articular bones and cartilages to facilitate movement. Such ligaments are slightly elastic and composed of parallel collagenous bundles. When part of the synovial membrane of a joint, they are covered with fibroelastic tissue that blends with surrounding connective tissue. Yellow elastic ligaments such as the ligamenta flava connect certain parts of adjoining vertebrae. Compare **tendon.** **2.** a layer of serous membrane with little or no tensile strength, extending from one visceral organ to another, such as the ligaments of the peritoneum. See

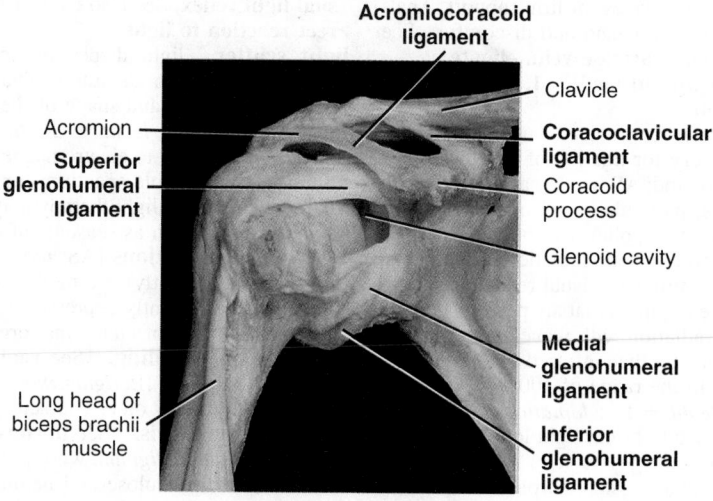

**Ligaments of the shoulder** *(Thibodeau, Patton, 1999)*

also **broad ligament.** Also called **ligamentum.** —**ligamentous,** *adj.*

**ligamenta flava** [L, *ligare* + *flavus,* yellow], the bands of yellow elastic tissue connecting the laminae of adjacent vertebrae from the axis to the first segment of the sacrum. They are thin, broad, and long in the cervical region, thicker in the thoracic region, and thickest in the lumbar region. They help hold the body erect.

**ligamental tear** /lig′əmen′təl/ [L, *ligare,* to bind; AS, *teran,* to destroy], a complete or partial rupture of a ligament caused by an injury to a joint, as by a sudden twisting motion or a forceful blow.

■ OBSERVATIONS: Ligamental tears may occur at any joint but are most common in the knees, where they typically involve the medial, lateral, and posterior ligaments and the anterior and posterior cruciate ligaments. Usually more than one structure is injured because of the way the structures connect with and support each other. The pathologic features of knee ligamental tears depend on the location and severity of the injury. A mild tear may cause little damage, with tenderness, swelling, and pain with stress.

■ INTERVENTIONS: Treatment depends on the severity of the injury. Rest, compression, applications of heat and cold, elevation, and early use are usually recommended for mild tears. Injection of an antiinflammatory agent may be desirable. Treatment for a moderate tear in which few fibers have been completely severed is protective. In addition to the above measures, the joint is aspirated and supported. Treatment for a severe, complete tear is restorative and may include immobilization followed by physical therapy or, if necessary, by surgical repair.

■ NURSING CONSIDERATIONS: Ligamental tears of the knee joint are extremely common in young adults and are associated with sports injuries. Good physical condition may help prevent many injuries, and proper care during healing is necessary to prevent permanent disability, which is often accompanied by joint instability, stiffness, or pain.

**ligament of the neck of the rib,** one of five ligaments of each costotransverse joint, consisting of short, strong fibers passing from the neck of the rib to the transverse process of the adjacent vertebra. Also called **middle costotransverse ligament.**

**ligament of the tubercle of the rib,** one of the five ligaments of each costotransverse joint, comprising a short thick fasciculus passing obliquely from the transverse process of a vertebra to the tubercle of the associated rib. Compare **ligament of the neck of the rib.**

**ligamentous** /lig′əmen′təs/ [L, *ligare,* to bind], pertaining to or having the characteristics of a ligament.

**ligamentum.** See **ligament.**

**ligamentum falciforme** See **broad ligament of liver.**

**ligamentum latum uteri.** See **broad ligament.**

**ligamentum nuchae** /lig′əmen′təm/, the fibrous membrane that reaches from the external occipital protuberance and median nuchal line to the spinous process of the seventh vertebra. A fibrous lamina from the ligament attaches to the posterior tubercle of the atlas and the spinous processes of the cervical vertebrae, forming a septum between muscles on either side of the neck.

**ligand** /lig′ənd, lī′gənd/ [L, *ligare,* to bind], **1.** a molecule, ion, or group bound to the central atom of a chemical compound, such as the oxygen molecule in hemoglobin, which is bound to the central iron atom. **2.** an organic molecule attached to a specific site on a cell surface or to a tracer element. The binding is reversible in a competitive binding assay. It may be the analyte or a cross-reactant. Examples include vitamin $B_{12}$, a ligand with intrinsic factor as the binding protein, and various antigens, which are ligands with antibody-binding proteins.

**ligases** /lī′gāsəz/ [L, *ligare* + Fr, *diastase,* enzyme], a group of enzymes that catalyze the formation of a bond between substrate molecules coupled with the breakdown of a pyrophosphate bond in ATP or a similar donor molecule. Examples of ligases include the synthetase enzymes.

**ligation** /līgā′shən/ [L, *ligare,* to bind], the procedure of tying off a blood vessel or duct with a suture or wire ligature. It may be performed to stop or prevent bleeding during surgery, to stop spontaneous or traumatic hemorrhage, to prevent passage of material through a duct as in tubal ligation, or to treat varicosities. In venous ligation the saphenous vein is tied above the varicosed part, and the distal parts are removed. After surgery the nurse observes the patient's feet and legs for circulatory impairment; the foot of the bed is raised to encourage venous return. Ambulation is begun the day of surgery, with elastic bandages for firm support. Analgesics are given as necessary for pain and discomfort. See also **ligature, tubal ligation, varicose vein.** –**ligate,** *v.*

**ligature** /lig′əchər/ [L, *ligare,* to bind], **1.** a suture. **2.** a wire, as used in orthodontia.

**ligature needle,** a long thin curved needle used for passing a suture underneath an artery for ligation of the vessel.

**ligature wire** [L, *ligare,* to bind; AS, *wir*], a soft, thin wire used in dental procedures, particularly to connect brackets or attachments on orthodontic appliances.

**light** [AS, *leoht*], **1.** electromagnetic radiation of the wavelength and frequency that stimulate visual receptor cells in the retina to produce nerve impulses that are perceived as vision. **2.** electromagnetic radiation with wavelengths shorter than ultraviolet light and longer than infrared light, the range of visible light generally in the range of 400 to 800 nm.

**light-adapted eye** [AS, *leoht* + L, *adaptatio* + AS, *eage*], an eye that has been exposed to bright light long enough for chemical and physiologic changes to take place, such as bleaching of the rhodopsin or visual purple. The loss of cone sensitivity to light may require increased light intensity to obtain the same degree of visual acuity. Also called **photopic eye.**

**light bath,** the exposure of the patient's uncovered skin to the sun or to actinic light rays from an artificial source for therapeutic purposes.

**light chain,** a subunit of an immunoglobulin molecule composed of a polypeptide chain of about 22,000 daltons, or atomic mass units. An example of a light chain is a Bence Jones protein molecule associated with multiple myeloma.

**light chain deficiency,** an immunodeficiency disease, such as megaloblastic anemia, that is associated with an alteration in the kappa or lambda light chains of immunoglobulins.

**light chain disease,** a type of multiple myeloma in which plasma cell tumors produce only monoclonal light chain proteins. Persons with light chain disease may develop lytic bone lesions, hypercalcemia, impaired kidney function, and amyloidosis. See also **gammopathy, heavy chain disease, multiple myeloma.**

**lightening** /lī′tӘning/ [AS, *leoht,* light], a subjective sensation reported by many women late in pregnancy as the fetus settles lower in the true pelvis, leaving more space in the upper abdomen. The diaphragm, no longer restricted by the fundus of the uterus beneath it, can move down more fully during inspiration, allowing deeper breaths. The stomach, too, is less compressed, so the woman can comfortably eat more food at each meal. Urinary frequency occurs as the fetus drops. The profile of the abdomen changes with lightening, because the round, full uterus is visibly lower. The baby is then said to have "dropped."

**light film fault** [AS, *leoht,* light, *filmen,* membrane; L, *fallere,* to deceive], a defect in a radiograph photograph that appears as a barely distinct and inadequate image. It is caused by underexposure, underdevelopment, or use of the wrong film speed or film/screen combination.

**light-headedness,** a condition of feeling giddy, faint, delirious, or slightly dizzy.

**light microscope** [AS, *leoht* + Gk, *mikros,* small, *skopein,* to view], a microscope that uses visible light to view objects too small for the naked eye to see.

**light pen,** an electrical device, resembling a pen, that may be used with a computer terminal to enter or modify information displayed on the screen.

**light reflex,** the mechanism by which the pupil of the eye constricts in response to direct or consensual stimulation with light. Also called **pupillary reflex.** Compare **consen-**sual light reflex. See also **consensual reaction to light, direct reaction to light.**

**light scatter,** light dispersion in any direction by suspended particles in a solution. The degree of scattering depends on the size and shape of the particles.

**light therapy** [AS, *leoht* + Gk, *therapeia,* treatment], exposure of the body to electromagnetic waves of the infrared, ultraviolet, or visible spectrum for therapeutic purposes. In the winter months light therapy may be used to treat depressive disorders such as seasonal affective disorder.

**light-touch palpations** [AS, *leoht* + Fr, *toucher* + L, *palpare,* to touch gently], a method of examination in which the abdomen is gently depressed 1 to 2 cm to determine the size and position of abdominal organs.

**light vaginal bleeding.** See **vaginal bleeding.**

**ligneous** /lig′nē·әs/ [L, *ligum,* wood], woody or resembling wood in texture or other characteristics.

**ligneous thyroiditis.** See **fibrous thyroiditis.**

**lignin** /lig′nin/ [L, *lignum,* wood], an insoluble polysaccharide that with cellulose and hemicellulose forms the chief part of the skeletal substances of the cell walls of plants. It provides bulk in the diet necessary for proper GI functioning. See also **dietary fiber.**

**lignocaine.** See **lidocaine hydrochloride.**

**lilliputian hallucination** /lil′ipyo͞o′shәn/ [Lilliput, mythic island in Swift's *Gulliver's Travels*], a hallucination in which things seem smaller than they actually are. See also **hallucination.**

**limb** /lim/ [AS, *lim*], **1.** an appendage or extremity of the body, such as an arm or leg. **2.** a branch of an internal organ, such as a loop of a nephron.

**limb-girdle muscular dystrophy** [AS, *lim,* limb, *gyrdel*], a form of muscular dystrophy transmitted as an autosomal-recessive trait. The characteristic weakness and degeneration of the muscles begins in the shoulder girdle or in the pelvic girdle. The condition is progressive, regardless of the area in which it is first manifest. Kinds of limb-girdle muscular dystrophy are **Erb muscular dystrophy, Leyden-Möbius muscular dystrophy.**

**limbic** /lim′bik/ [L, *limbus,* edge], pertaining to something that is marginal or at a junction between structures.

**limbic lobe** [L, *limbus,* edge; Gk, *lobos,* lobe], the marginal section of the cerebral hemispheres on the medial aspects. It forms a ring of neural tissue around the hypothalamus and some nuclei.

**limbic system** [L, *limbus,* edge], a group of structures within the rhinencephalon of the brain that are associated with various emotions and feelings such as anger, fear, sexual arousal, pleasure, and sadness. The structures of the limbic system include the cingulate gyrus, the isthmus, the hippocampal gyrus, the uncus, and the amygdala. The structures connect with various other parts of the brain such as the septum and the hypothalamus. Unless the limbic system is modulated by other cortical areas, periodic attacks of uncontrollable rage may occur in some individuals. The function of the system is incompletely understood.

**limb kinetic apraxia.** See **ideomotor apraxia.**

**limb lead** /lēd/ [AS, *lim,* limb, *laeden,* lead], an electrocardiographic electrode that is attached to an arm or a leg.

**limbus** /lim′bәs/, an edge or border, such as the corneal limbus at the edge of the cornea bordering the sclera.

**lime** [AS, *lim*], **1.** any of several oxides and hydroxides of calcium. The various kinds of lime have many uses, including the treatment of sewage, the purification of water and refining of sugar, and the manufacture of materials such as plaster and fertilizers. **2.** a citrus fruit yielding a juice with a high ascorbic acid content. Lime juice was one of the first

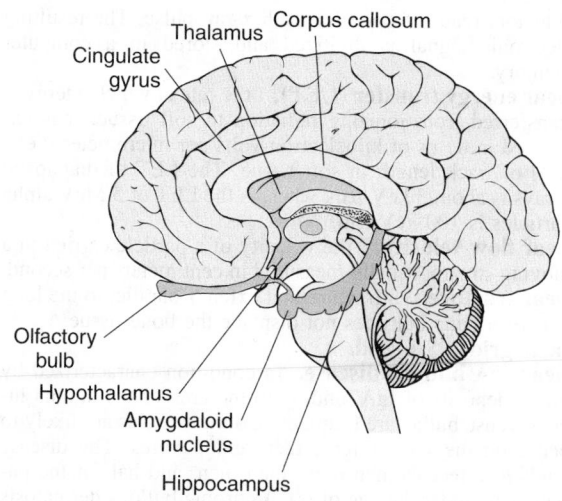

**Limbic system** *(McKenry and Salerno, 1998)*

effective agents to be used in the treatment of scurvy. See also **ascorbic acid, scurvy.**

**limen.** See **threshold stimulus.**

**lime water.** See **calcium hydroxide solution.**

**liminal stimulus.** See **threshold stimulus.**

**limitation of motion** /lim′itā′shən/ [L, *limes,* limit], the restriction of or reduction to a normal range of motion of a body part, caused by disease or injury.

**limited fluctuation method of dosing** [L, *limes,* limit, *fluctuare,* to wave], a method of drug administration in which the dose is not allowed to rise or fall beyond specified maximum and minimum limits.

**limiting charge,** the maximum amount that can be charged in the United States for the services of a physician who does not accept the restrictions on fees established by Medicare laws. Also called **billing limit.**

**limiting resolution,** in computed tomography, the spatial frequency at a modulation transfer function equal to 0.1. The absolute object size that can be resolved by a scanner is equal to the reciprocal of the spatial frequency.

**limit of stability,** the greatest distance in any direction a person can lean away from a midline vertical position without falling, stepping, or reaching for support.

**limit setting,** a nursing intervention from the Nursing Interventions Classification (NIC) defined as establishing the parameters of desirable and acceptable patient behavior. See also **Nursing Interventions Classification.**

**limo-,** combining form meaning 'hunger': *limophthisis, limosis, limotherapy.*

**limp** [ME, not firm], an abnormal pattern of ambulation in which the two phases of gait are markedly asymmetric. See also **stance phase of gait, swing phase of gait.**

**LINAC,** abbreviation for **linear accelerator.**

**Lincocin,** trademark for an antibacterial (lincomycin hydrochloride).

**lincomycin hydrochloride** /lin′kəmī′sin/, an antibiotic.

■ INDICATIONS: It is prescribed in the treatment of certain infections caused by susceptible bacteria.

■ CONTRAINDICATIONS: Known hypersensitivity to this drug or to clindamycin prohibits its use.

■ ADVERSE EFFECTS: Among the more serious adverse reactions are blood disorders, diarrhea, and the development of

life-threatening pseudomembranous colitis caused by superinfection.

**lindane** /lin′dān/, gamma-benzene hexachloride. Also known as G-Well.

■ INDICATIONS: It is prescribed in the treatment of pediculosis and scabies.

■ CONTRAINDICATIONS: It is not usually given to infants or pregnant women and is not applied to the face. Known hypersensitivity to this drug prohibits its use.

■ ADVERSE EFFECTS: Among the most serious adverse reactions are neurologic damage and aplastic anemia. Given topically, irritation of eyes, skin, and mucosa may occur.

**Lindau–von Hippel disease.** See **von Hippel–Lindau disease.**

**Lindbergh pump** [Charles A. Lindbergh, American technician, 1902–1974; ME, *pumpe*], a pump used to preserve an organ of the body by perfusing its tissues with oxygen and other essential nutrients, usually during the transport of an organ from a donor to a recipient. Also called **Carrel-Lindbergh pump.**

**line** [L, *linea*], 1. a connection between two points. 2. a stripe, streak, or narrow ridge, often imaginary, that serves to connect reference points or to separate various parts of the body, as the hairline or nipple line. 3. a black absorption line in a continuous spectrum passing through a medium. 4. an accretion line in the enamel of a tooth marking successive layers of calcification. 5. a catheter or wire that may be inserted in a vein, as an IV line. 6. the base line of an electrocardiogram when neither positive nor negative potentials are recorded. 7. line of sight. Also called **linea.** See also **Frankfurt horizontal plane.**

**linea** /lin′ē·ə/ [L, line], a line defining anatomic features such as the **linea alba** of the abdomen, the **linea albicantes** or **linea nigra** seen on the abdomen during pregnancy, or the **linea vitalis** curving across the palm at the base of the thumb.

**linea alba** [L, *linea,* line, *albus,* white], the white part of the anterior abdominal aponeurosis in the middle line of the abdomen, made of connective tissue representing the fusion of three aponeuroses into a single tendinous band extending

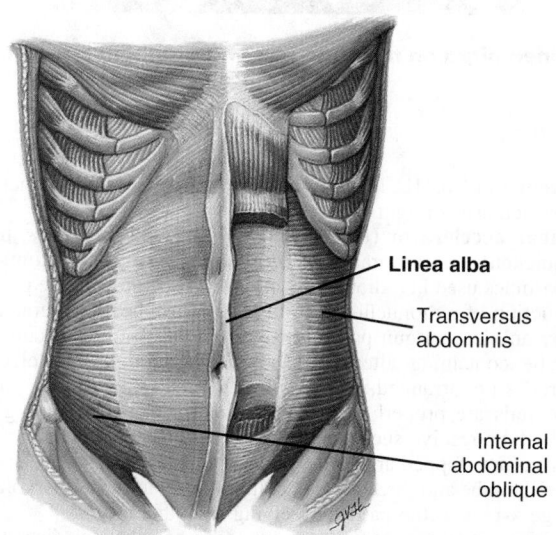

— Linea alba

Transversus abdominis

Internal abdominal oblique

**Linea alba** *(Thibodeau and Patton, 1999/John V. Hagen)*

from the xiphoid process to the symphysis pubis. It contains the umbilicus. Also called **Hunter's line, white line.** Compare **linea semilunaris.**

**linea arcuata,** the curved tendinous band in the sheath of the rectus abdominis below the umbilicus. It is usually derived from the aponeurosis of the transversus abdominis or the obliquus internus, sometimes from both of those muscles. It inserts into the linea alba. Compare **linea semilunaris.**

**linea aspera,** the posterior crest of the femur (thigh bone) that extends proximally into three ridges to which are attached various muscles, including the gluteus maximus, pectineus, and iliacus.

**lineae albicantes,** lines, white to pink or gray, that occur on the abdomen, buttocks, breasts, and thighs and are caused by the stretching of the skin and weakening or rupturing of the underlying elastic tissue. The condition is usually associated with pregnancy, excessive obesity, rapid growth during adolescence, Cushing's syndrome, or prolonged adrenocortical hormone therapy. Also called **stretch marks.**

**linea nigra,** /lin′ē′ənī′guə/ a dark line appearing longitudinally on the abdomen of a pregnant woman during the latter 24 weeks of term. It usually extends from the symphysis pubis midline to the umbilicus and sometimes as far as the sternum.

detectors read off once for each x-ray pulse. The resulting electronic signal is digitized and stored in a computer memory.

**linear energy transfer (LET),** the rate at which energy is transferred from ionizing radiation to soft tissue. It is expressed in terms of kiloelectron volts per micrometer (keV/μm) of track length in soft tissue. The LET of diagnostic x-rays is about 3 keV/μm, whereas the LET of 5 MeV alpha particles is 100 keV/μm.

**linear flow velocity,** the velocity of a particle carried in a moving stream, usually measured in centimeters per second.

**linear fracture,** a fracture that extends parallel to the long axis of a bone but does not displace the bone tissue.

**linear grid.** See grid.

**linear IgA bullous disease,** a condition characterized by linear deposits of IgA binding to the area of the lamina lucida. Tense bullae are frequent, and the vesicles are likely to occur on the face, thighs, feet, and flexures. The disease tends to affect women more than men, and half of the patients are under the age of 60. A chronic bullous dermatosis disease of childhood begins in the first 10 years of life with bullae on the trunk, perioral, and pelvic areas but undergoes total remission at adolescence.

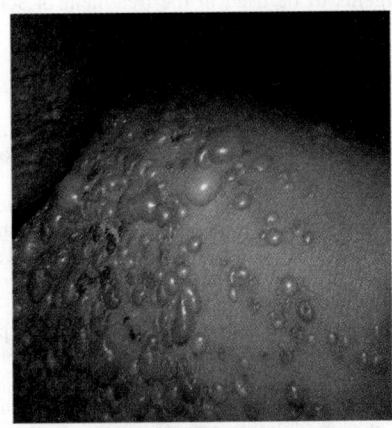

**Linear IgA bullous disease** *(Shah and Laude, 2000)*

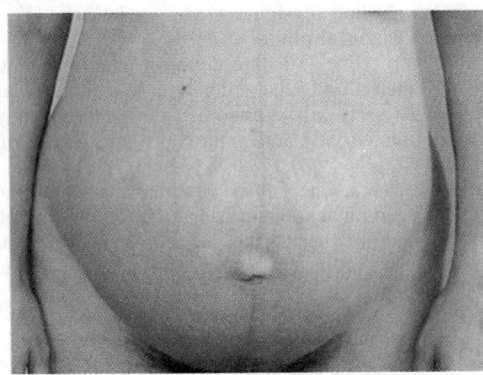

**Linea nigra on the abdomen of a pregnant woman**
*(Seidel et al, 1999)*

**linear** /lin′ē·ər/ [L, *linea,* line], pertaining to a line or lines, particularly straight lines.

**linear accelerator (LINAC)** [L, *linea,* line, *accelerare,* to quicken], an apparatus for accelerating charged subatomic particles used in radiotherapy, physics research, and the production of radionuclides. A pulsed electron beam generated by an electron gun passes through a long, straight vacuum tube containing alternating hollow electrodes. The electrodes are arranged so that, when their high-frequency potentials are properly varied, the electrons passing through the tube receive successive increments of energy. The electrons are stopped abruptly by a heavy metal target at the end of the tube and directed by a collimator to deliver supervoltage x-rays to the patient receiving radiotherapy.

**linear array,** a contiguous sequence of identical discrete detectors, either gas-filled ionization chambers or solid-state semiconductors, used with a fan beam x-ray generator. The

**linearity** /lin′ē·er′itē/, the principle that the density of a radiographic exposure is determined by the product of the current and the exposure time.

**linear regression,** a statistical procedure in which a straight line is established through a data set that best represents a relationship between two subsets or two methods.

**linear scan,** an ultrasound scan in which the transducer moves at a constant speed along a straight line at right angles to the ultrasound beam.

**linear staining,** the use of fluorescein-labeled goat or rabbit antiimmunoglobulins to produce smooth-staining patterns for study by immunofluorescence microscopy.

**linear tomography,** tomography that produces a blurring pattern consisting of indistinguishable linear streaks or blurs over the focal-plane image. The pattern is caused by elongation of structures outside the focal plane.

**linea semilunaris,** the slightly curved line on the ventral abdominal wall, approximately parallel to the median line and lying about halfway between the median line and the side of the body. It marks the lateral border of the rectus abdominis and is visible as a shallow groove when that muscle is tensed. Compare **linea alba.**

**linea terminalis,** a hypothetic line dividing the upper, or false, pelvis, from the lower, or true, pelvis.

**linea vitalis.** See **linea.**

**line compensator,** a device that monitors electric power for medical devices such as x-ray equipment and adjust for voltage fluctuations.

**line of demarcation** [L, *linea* + *de* + *marcare,* to mark], a line that indicates a change in the condition of tissues, such as the boundary between gangrenous and healthy tissues.

**line of gravity,** an imaginary line that extends from the center of gravity to the base of support.

**line pair (lp),** a factor that determines the spatial frequency of CT and radiographic images. It consists of two parallel lines or bars separated by a space. As the number of line pairs per centimeter increases, the fidelity of the image decreases.

**Lineweaver-Burk transformation** /lī′nwēvərburk′/ [Hans Lineweaver, American chemist, b. 1907; Dean Burk, American scientist, 1904–1988; L, *transformare,* to change shape], a method of converting experimental data from studies of enzyme activity so that they can be displayed on a linear plot. The linear form is derived by using reciprocals of both sides of the equation.

**lingu-, linguo-,** combining form meaning 'tongue': *linguiform, lingulectomy, linguodental.*

**lingua.** See **tongue.**

**lingual** /ling′gwəl/ [L, *lingua,* tongue], pertaining to or resembling the tongue.

**lingual artery** [L, *lingua,* tongue], one of a pair of arteries that arises from the external carotid arteries and supplies the tongue and surrounding muscles.

**lingual bar,** a bar that is installed on the tongue side of the dental arch and connects bilateral parts of a mandibular removable partial denture.

**lingual bone.** See **hyoid bone.**

**lingual crib,** an orthodontic appliance consisting of a wire frame suspended behind the maxillary incisors. It is used to obstruct undesirable thumb and tongue habits that can produce malocclusions, especially in children.

**lingual flange,** the part of a mandibular denture that occupies the space adjacent to the residual ridge and next to the tongue.

**lingual frenum.** See **frenulum of tongue.**

**lingual gingiva** [L, *lingua,* tongue, *gingiva,* gum], the gum tissue covering the teeth on the surfaces facing the tongue.

**lingual goiter,** a tumor at the back of the tongue formed by an enlargement of the primordial thyrolingual duct.

**lingualis leukoplakia** [L, *lingua,* tongue; Gk, *leukos,* white, *plax,* plate], a chronic inflammatory lesion characterized by smooth thick white patches on the surface of the tongue, generally attributed to excessive use of alcohol and tobacco. The lesions may be a precursor of epithelioma.

**lingual occlusion.** See **linguoclusion.**

**lingual pain,** a pain in the tongue, which may be caused by biting the tongue, heavy metal poisoning, Vincent's stomatitis, or infiltration of the lingual muscles by a neoplasm.

**lingual papilla.** See **papilla.**

**lingual rest,** a metallic extension attached to the tongue side of an anterior tooth to provide support or indirect retention for a removable partial denture.

**lingual thyroid,** residual thyroid tissue at the base of the tongue that failed to descend into the neck during embryologic development.

**lingual tonsil,** a mass of lymphoid follicles near the root of the tongue. Each follicle forms a rounded eminence containing a small opening leading into a funnel-shaped cavity surrounded by lymphoid tissue.

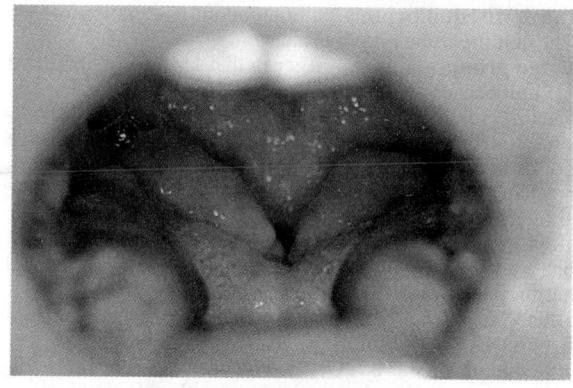

**Lingual tonsil** *(Bingham, 1992)*

**lingula** /ling′gyələ/ [L, small tongue], any anatomic structure that resembles a tongue.

**lingula of the lung** [L, *lingula,* small tongue; AS, *lungen*], a tonguelike projection from the costal surface of the upper lobe of the left lung.

**lingulectomy** /ling′gyəlek′təmē/, a surgical excision of the tongue-shaped lingula part of the left upper lobe of the lung.

**linguoclusion** /ling′gwō·klō′zhən/ [L, *lingua,* tongue + *occludere,* to close up], malocclusion in which the tooth is lingual to the line of the normal dental arch. Also called **lingual occlusion.**

**linguoversion** /ling′gwō·ver′zhən/ [L, *lingua,* tongue + *vertere,* to turn], displacement of a tooth lingually from the line of occlusion.

**liniment** /lin′imənt/ [L, *linere,* to smear], a preparation, usually containing an alcoholic, oily, or soapy vehicle, that is rubbed on the skin as a counterirritant.

**linin** /li′nin/ [Gk, *linon,* flax], the faintly staining threads seen in the nuclei of cells, with granules of chromatin attached to the threads. See also **karyolymph.**

**linitis** /linī′tis/ [Gk, *linon,* flax, *itis,* inflammation], inflammation of cellular tissue of the stomach as in linitis plastica, seen frequently in adenocarcinoma of the stomach.

**linitis plastica,** a diffuse fibrosis and thickening of the wall of the stomach, resulting in a rigid, inelastic organ. The layer of connective tissue of the stomach becomes fibrotic and thick, and the stomach wall becomes shrunken and rigid. Causes of this condition include infiltrating undifferentiated carcinoma, syphilis, and Crohn's disease involving the stomach. Also called **leather bottle stomach.**

**linkage** /ling′kij/ [Gk, *linke,* connection], **1.** (in genetics) the location of two or more genes on the same chromosome so that they do not segregate independently during meiosis but tend to be transmitted together as a unit. The closer the loci of the genes, the more likely they are to be inherited as a group and associated with a specific trait, whereas the farther apart they are, the greater the chance that they will be separated by crossing over and carried on homologous chromosomes. The concept of linkage, which opposes the independent assortment theory of mendelian genetics, led to the foundation of the modern chromosome theory of genetics. See also **synteny. 2.** (in psychology) the association between a stimulus and the response it elicits. **3.** (in chemistry) the bond between two atoms or radicals in a chemical compound or the lines used to designate valency connections between the atoms in structural formulas.

**linkage disequilibrium,** a nonrandom association of two genes on the same chromosome.

**linkage group,** a group of genes that tend to be inherited as a unit because they are located on the same chromosome. Without crossing over, all of the genes on a given chromosome constitute a linkage group, and the number of linkage groups in an organism is equal to the number of autosomes in a haploid cell.

**linkage map.** See **genetic map.**

**linked genes** [ME, *linke* + Gk, *genein,* to produce], genes that are located so close together on the same chromosome that they tend to be transmitted as a linkage group.

**linker** [ME, *linke,* connection], a small segment of synthetic DNA used to join DNA fragments in cloning.

**linoleic acid** /lin′əlē′ik/ [Gk, *linon,* flax, *oleum,* oil], a colorless to straw-colored essential fatty acid with two unsaturated bonds, occurring in many vegetable oils such as corn, soy, and safflower oils. Commercially produced linoleic acid is used in margarine and animal feeds.

**linolenic acid** /lin′ōlen′ik/ [Gk, *linon,* flax, *oleum,* oil], an unsaturated essential fatty acid. It occurs in triglycerides of canola, soy, linseed, and other vegetable oils.

**lio-.** See **leio-.**

**Lioresal,** trademark for an antispastic agent (baclofen).

**liothyronine sodium** /lī′ōthī′rənēn/, a synthetic thyroid hormone. Also known as **triiodothyronine.**

■ INDICATIONS: It is prescribed in the treatment of primary hypothyroidism, myxedema, simple goiter, cretinism, and secondary hypothyroidism.

■ CONTRAINDICATIONS: Hyperthyroidism, thyrotoxicosis, acute myocardial infarction, or known hypersensitivity to this drug prohibits its use. It is used with caution in patients with diabetes mellitus or cardiovascular disease.

■ ADVERSE EFFECTS: Among the serious adverse reactions, usually caused by overdosage, are tachycardia, arrhythmias, thyrotoxicosis, nausea, vomiting, hypertension, nervousness, and loss of weight.

**liotrix** /lī′ətriks/, a uniform mixture of the thyroid hormones $T_3$ and $T_4$.

■ INDICATION: It is prescribed in the treatment of hypothyroid conditions.

■ CONTRAINDICATIONS: Most diseases and abnormal conditions of the myocardium or known hypersensitivity to this drug prohibits its use.

■ ADVERSE EFFECTS: Among the more serious adverse reactions are symptoms of thyrotoxicosis, including tachycardia, nervousness, insomnia, and fever.

**lip** [AS, *lippa*], **1.** either the upper or lower fleshy structure surrounding the opening of the oral cavity. **2.** any rimlike structure bordering a cavity or groove; labium.

**LIP,** abbreviation for **lymphocytic interstitial pneumonia.**

**lip-,** See **lipo-.**

**lipase** /lī′pās, lip′ās/ [Gk, *lipos,* fat; Fr, *diastase,* enzyme], any of several enzymes produced by the organs of the digestive system that catalyze the breakdown of lipids through the hydrolysis of the linkages between fatty acids and glycerol in triglycerides and phospholipids. Normal blood levels of lipase range from 0 to 110 U/L. See also **fat, fatty acid, glycerol, phospholipid, triglyceride.**

**lipase test,** a blood test whose results are used most often to diagnose acute pancreatitis, but also are useful in helping to diagnose renal failure, intestinal infarction or obstruction, and several other conditions.

**lipectomy** /lipek′təmē/ [Gk, *lipos* + *ektomē,* excision], an excision of subcutaneous fat, as from the abdominal wall. Also called **adipectomy.**

**lipedema** /lip′ədē′mə/, a condition in which fat deposits accumulate in the lower extremities from the hips to the ankles, accompanied by symptoms of tenderness in the affected areas. Treatment is dietary.

**lipemia** /lipē′mē·ə/ [Gk, *lipos* + *haima,* blood], a condition in which increased amounts of lipids are present in the blood, a normal occurrence after eating.

**lipid** /lip′id, lī′pid/ [Gk, *lipos,* fat, *eidos,* form], any of a structurally diverse group of organic compounds that are insoluble in water but soluble in alcohol, chloroform, ether, and other solvents. Some lipids are stored in the body and serve as an energy reserve, but are elevated in various diseases such as atherosclerosis. Kinds of lipids include **cholesterol, fatty acids, phospholipids,** and **triglycerides.** The normal concentrations of lipids in serum are total, 400 to 800 mg/dL; cholesterol, 150 to 250 mg/dL; fatty acids, 9 to 15 mM/L; phospholipids, 150 to 380 mg/dL; phospholipid as phosphorus, 9 to 16 mg/dL; and triglycerides, 10 to 190 mg/dL.

**lipidosis** /lip′idō′sis/ [Gk, *lipos* + *osis,* condition], a general term that includes several rare familial disorders of fat metabolism. The chief characteristic of these disorders is the accumulation of abnormal levels of certain lipids in the body. Kinds of lipidoses are **Gaucher's disease, Krabbe's disease, Niemann-Pick disease,** and **Tay-Sachs disease.**

**lipid pneumonia,** an inflammation of the spongy tissue of the lung caused by inhalation of oil droplets into the alveoli. The condition may result from accidentally inhaling oily medications, milk, or other fatty foods or from swimming in petroleum-contaminated water.

**lipiduria** /lip′idoor′ē·ə/, the presence of lipids (fatty bodies) in the urine.

**lipo-, lip-** prefix meaning 'fat': *lipase, lipodystrohy, lipoma.*

**lipoatrophic diabetes** /lip′ō·atrof′ik/, an inherited disease characterized by insulin-resistant diabetes mellitus, loss of body fat, acanthosis nigricans, hypermetabolism, hepatomegaly, and hypertrophied musculature. It is associated with a disorder of the hypothalamus resulting in excessive blood levels of growth hormone and adrenocorticotropic-releasing hormones.

**lipoatrophy** /lip′ō·at′rəfē/, a breakdown of subcutaneous fat at the site of an insulin injection. It usually occurs after several injections at the same site. Compare **lipohypertrophy.**

**lipocele.** See **adipocele.**

**lipochondrodystrophy.** See **Hurler's syndrome.**

**lipochrome** /lip′əkrōm/ [Gk, *lipos* + *chroma,* color], any of the naturally occurring pigments that contain a lipid and give a yellow color to fats, such as carotene.

**lipodystrophia progressiva** /-distrō′fē·ə/ [Gk, *lipos* + *dys,* bad, *trophe,* nourishment; L, *progredior,* to go forth], an abnormal accumulation of fat around the buttocks and thighs and a progressive, symmetric disappearance of subcutaneous fat from areas above the pelvis and on the face. Also called **lipomatosis atrophicans.**

**lipodystrophy** /lip′ōdis′trəfē/ [Gk, *lipos* + *dys,* bad, *trophe,* nourishment], any abnormality in the metabolism or deposition of fats. Kinds of lipodystrophy are **bitrochanteric lipodystrophy, insulin lipodystrophy,** and **intestinal lipodystrophy.**

**lip of hip fracture,** a break in the posterior lip of the acetabulum, often associated with displacement of the hip.

**lipofibroma.** See **fibrolipoma.**

**lipofuscin** /lip′əfus′in/, a class of fatty pigments consisting mostly of oxidized fats that are found in abundance in the cells of adults. Lipofuscins accumulate in lysosomes with age.

**lipogenesis** /-jen′əsis/ [Gk, *lipos,* fat, *genein,* to produce], the production and accumulation of fat.

**lipogranuloma** /lip′ōgran′yŏŏlō′mə/, *pl.* **lipogranulomas, lipogranulomata** [Gk, *lipos* + L, *granulum,* little grain; Gk, *oma,* tumor], a nodule of necrotic, fatty tissue associated with granulomatous inflammation or a foreign-body reaction around a deposit of injected material containing an oily substance.

**lipohypertrophy** /lip′ōhīpur′trəfē/, a build-up of subcutaneous fat tissue at a site where insulin has been injected continuously. Compare **lipoatrophy.**

**lipoic acid** /lipō′ik/, a bacterial growth factor found in liver and yeast.

**lipoid** /lip′oid/, resembling a lipid.

**lipoid nephrosis.** See **minimal change disease.**

**lipolysis** /lipol′isis/, the breakdown or destruction of fats.

**lipolytic** /-lit′ik/ [Gk, *lipos,* fat, *lysis,* loosening], the chemical breakdown of fat.

**lipolytic digestion,** a phase of food digestion in which fat molecules are split into glycerol and fatty acids.

**lipoma** /lipō′mə/, *pl.* **lipomas, lipomata** [Gk, *lipos* + *oma,* tumor], a benign tumor consisting of mature fat cells. Also called **adipose tumor.** See also **multiple lipomatosis. —lipomatous,** *adj.*

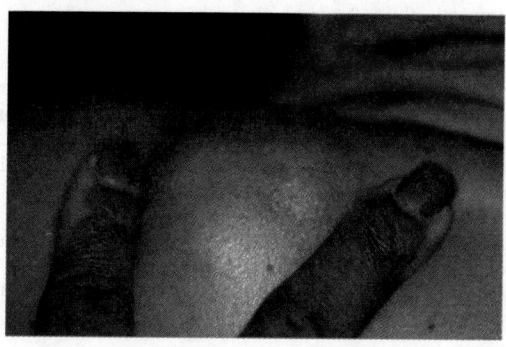

**Lipoma** *(Lemmi and Lemmi, 2000)*

**-lipoma,** combining form meaning a 'tumor made up of fatty tissue': *angiolipoma, fibrolipoma, osteolipoma.*

**lipoma annulare colli,** a diffuse, symmetric accumulation of fat around the neck, not a true lipoma. Also called **Madelung's neck.**

**lipoma arborescens,** a fatty tumor of a joint, characterized by a treelike distribution of fat cells.

**lipoma capsulare,** a benign neoplasm characterized by the abnormal presence of fat cells in the capsule of an organ.

**lipoma cavernosum.** See **angiolipoma.**

**lipoma diffusum renis.** See **lipomatous nephritis.**

**lipoma dolorosa.** See **lipomatosis dolorosa.**

**lipoma fibrosum,** a fatty tumor containing masses of fibrous tissue.

**lipoma myxomatodes.** See **lipomyxoma.**

**lipoma sarcomatodes.** See **liposarcoma.**

**lipomata.** See **lipoma.**

**lipomatosis** /lip′ōmətō′sis/ [Gk, *lipos* + *oma,* tumor, *osis,* condition], a disorder characterized by abnormal tumorlike accumulations of fat in body tissues.

**lipomatosis atrophicans.** See **lipodystrophia progressiva, lipomatosis.**

**lipomatosis dolorosa,** a disorder characterized by the abnormal accumulation of painful or tender fat deposits. Also called **lipoma dolorosa.**

**lipomatosis gigantea,** a condition characterized by massive deposits of fat.

**lipomatosis renis.** See **lipomatous nephritis.**

**lipomatous** /lipō′mətəs/ [Gk, *lipos,* fat, *oma,* tumor], pertaining to or resembling a benign tumor made up of mature fat cells.

**lipomatous myxoma,** a tumor containing fatty tissue that arises in connective tissue.

**lipomatous nephritis,** a rare condition in which the renal nephrons are replaced by fatty tissue. Kidney failure may result. Also called **lipoma diffusum renis, lipomatosis renis.**

**lipometabolism** /-metab′əliz′əm/ [Gk, *lipos,* fat, *metabole,* change], the chemical processes involved in building up or breaking down fat molecules.

**lipomyoma** /-mī·ō′mə/ [Gk, *lipos,* fat; *mys,* muscle, *oma,* tumor], a tumor that combines characteristics of a lipoma and myoma.

**lipomyxoma** /lip′ōmiksō′mə/, *pl.* **lipomyxomas, lipomyxomata** [Gk, *lipos* + *myxa,* mucus, *oma,* tumor], a myxoma that contains fat cells. Also called **lipoma myxomatodes.**

**lipophilia** /-fil′yə/ [Gk, *lipos,* fat, *philein,* to love], a tendency to attract or absorb fat.

**lipoprotein** /lip′ōprō′tēn/ [Gk, *lipos* + *proteios,* first rank], a conjugated protein in which lipids form an integral part of the molecule. They are synthesized primarily in the liver; contain varying amounts of triglycerides, cholesterol, phospholipids, fat-soluble vitamins, and protein; and are classified according to their composition and density. Practically all of the plasma lipids are present as lipoprotein complexes. The elevation of low-density lipoproteins (LDLs) in plasma is associated with an increased risk of atherosclerosis. Normal adult levels of lipoproteins include: high-density lipoproteins, greater than 35 mg/dL; LDL, 60 to 180 mg/dL; very low–density lipoproteins, 25% to 50%. Kinds of lipoproteins are **chylomicrons, high-density lipoproteins, low-density lipoproteins,** and **very low–density lipoproteins.**

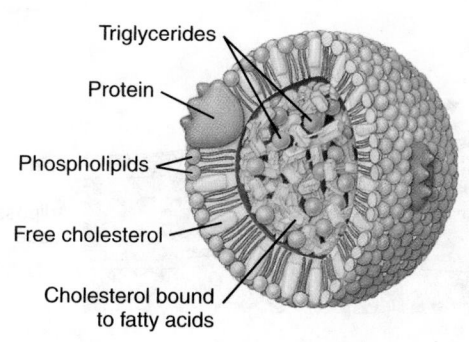

Triglycerides
Protein
Phospholipids
Free cholesterol
Cholesterol bound to fatty acids

**Lipoprotein** *(Thibodeau and Patton, 1999)*

**lipoprotein lipase (LPL),**   an enzyme that plays a key role in breaking down triglycerides present in chylomicrons and very low–density lipoprotein particles, releasing their fatty acids for entry into tissue cells.

**lipoproteins test (HDL, LDL, and VLDL),**   a blood test performed as part of a lipid profile, to identify persons who are at risk for developing heart disease and to monitor therapy if abnormalities are found. Lipoproteins are considered to be an accurate predictor of coronary heart disease.

**liposarcoma** /lip′ōsärkō′mə/, *pl.* **liposarcomas, liposarcomata** [Gk, *lipos* + *sarx,* flesh, *oma,* tumor],   a malignant growth of primitive fat cells. Also called **lipoma sarcomatodes.**

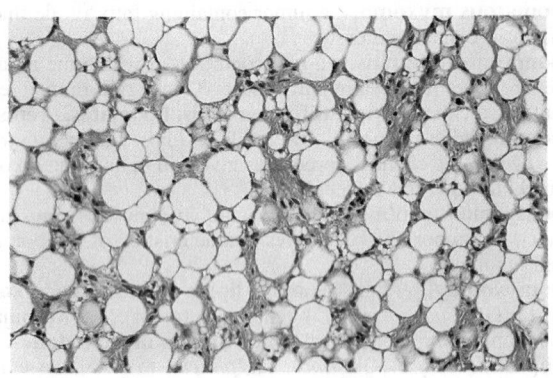

**Liposarcoma** *(Fletcher, 2000)*

**liposis.**   See **lipomatosis.**

**liposoluble** /-sol′yəbəl/ [Gk, *lipos,* fat; L, *solubilis*],   fat soluble.

**liposome** /lip′əsōm/ [Gk, *lipos,* fat, *soma,* body],   a small, spheric particle consisting of a bilayer of phospholipid molecules surrounding an aqueous solution.

**liposuction** /-suk′shən/,   a technique for removing adipose tissue with a suction pump device. It is used primarily to remove or reduce localized areas of fat around the abdomen, breasts, legs, face, and upper arms where the skin is contractile enough to redrape in a normal manner. Also called **suction lipectomy.**

**lip reading,**   a former name for **speech reading.**

**-lipsis, -lipse,**   combining form meaning 'to leave out, fail, omit': *eclipsis, ellipsis, menolipsis.*

**Liquaemin Sodium,**   trademark for an anticoagulant (heparin sodium).

**liquefaction** /lik′wəfak′shən/ [L, *liquere,* to flow, *facere,* to make],   the process in which a solid or a gas is made liquid.

**liquefactive degeneration** /lik′wəfak′tiv/,   dissolution of tissues resulting from hydrolytic enzymes released by leukocytes and tissue cells. It occurs in the skin of patients with lichen planus and lupus erythematosus.

**liquid** /lik′wid/ [L, *liquere,* to flow],   a state of matter, intermediate between solid and gas, in which the molecules move freely among themselves and the substance flows freely with little application of force and assumes the shape of the vessel in which it is contained. Compare **fluid.** See also **gas, solid.**

**liquid diet,**   a diet consisting of foods that can be served in liquid or strained form but that may include custard, ice cream, pudding, tapioca, and soft-cooked eggs. It is prescribed in acute infections, in acute inflammatory conditions of the GI tract, and for patients unable to consume other soft or semifluid foods, usually after surgery. See also **full-liquid diet.**

**liquid glucose,**   a thick, syrupy odorless and colorless or yellowish liquid obtained by the incomplete hydrolysis of starch, primarily consisting of dextrose with dextrins, maltose, and water. It is used as a flavoring agent and may be used as a calorie source, chiefly in treating dehydration.

**liquid nitrogen.**   See **cryogen.**

**liquid scintillation counter,**   a device for measuring radioactivity, usually beta particles, emitted from a sample dispersed in a liquid scintillation cocktail.

**liquor** /lik′ər/,   **1.** any fluid or liquid, such as liquor amnii, the amniotic fluid. **2.** an alcoholic beverage.

**liquor amnii.**   See **amniotic fluid.**

**liquorice.**   See **licorice.**

**Lisfranc's fracture** /lisfrangks′/ [Jacques Lisfranc, French surgeon, 1790–1847],   a fracture dislocation of the foot in which one or all of the proximal metatarsals are displaced.

**lisping,**   the mispronunciation of one or more of the sibilant consonant sounds, usually /s/ and /z/.

**lissencephaly.**   See **agyria** (def. 2).

***Listeria monocytogenes*** /lister′ē·ə mon′ōsītoj′inēz/ [Joseph Lister; Gk, *mono,* single, *kytos,* cell, *genein,* to produce],   a common species of gram-positive, motile bacillus that causes listeriosis.

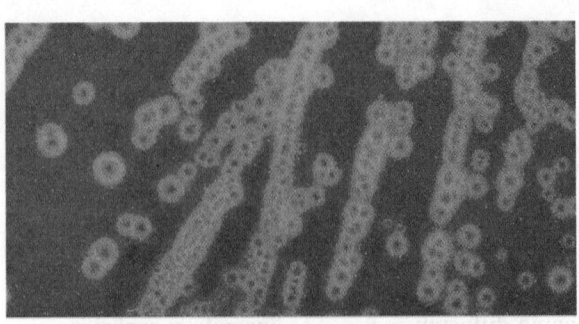

**Colonies of *Listeria monocytogenes***
*(Baron, Peterson, and Finegold, 1994)*

**Liposuction** *(Beare and Myers, 1998)*

**listeriosis** /listir′ē·ō′sis/ [Joseph Lister; Gk, *osis,* condition], an infectious disease caused by a genus of gram-positive motile bacteria that are nonsporulating. *Listeria monocytogenes* infects shellfish, birds, spiders, and mammals in all areas of the world; but infection in humans is uncommon. It is transmitted by direct contact from infected animals to humans; through ingesting contaminated meat and dairy products; by inhalation of dust; or by contact with mud, sewage, or soil contaminated with the organism. The disorder is characterized in mild cases by fever, myalgia, nausea, and diarrhea and in severe cases by circulatory collapse, shock, endocarditis, hepatosplenomegaly, and a dark red rash over the trunk and legs. Fever, bacteremia, malaise, and lethargy are commonly seen. Newborns and immunosuppressed debilitated older people are more vulnerable to infection than are immunocompetent children and young or middle-aged adults. The signs of infection and the severity of the disease vary according to the site of infection and the age and condition of the person. Pregnant women characteristically experience a mild brief episode of illness, but fetal infection acquired through the placental circulation in utero is usually fatal. Infection in the newborn apparently results from exposure to the organism in the birth canal of an infected mother. Meningitis and encephalitis occur in 75% of cases. Treatment may include ampicillin, penicillin, tetracycline, or erythromycin given intramuscularly or intravenously. If infection is suspected in a pregnant woman, treatment is begun immediately, even before bacteriologic culture of the blood, spinal fluid, or vaginal secretions can confirm the diagnosis. All secretions from the patient may contain the organism. Also called **listerosis.**

**Lister, Joseph** (Scottish surgeon, 1827–1912), introduced the use of antiseptic surgery in London hospitals in 1867. Lister operations were performed under a spray of diluted carbolic acid, instruments were dipped in carbolic acid, and wounds were dressed with gauze similarly treated.

**Liston's forceps** [Robert Liston, Scottish surgeon, 1794–1847], a kind of bone-cutting forceps.

**liter (L)** /lē′tər/ [Fr], a derived unit of volume equivalent to 1.057 quarts and defined as the volume occupied by a mass of 1 kg of water at standard temperature and pressure.

**lith-.** See **litho-.**

**-lith,** suffix meaning 'a calculus' or 'a stone': *pneumolith, ptyalith, tonsillolith.*

**Lithane,** trademark for an antimanic drug (lithium carbonate).

**lithiasis** /lithī′əsis/ [Gk, *lithos,* stone, *osis,* condition], the formation of calculi in the hollow organs or ducts of the body. Calculi are formed of mineral salts and may irritate, inflame, or obstruct the organ in which they form or lodge. Lithiasis occurs most commonly in the gallbladder, kidney, and lower urinary tract. Lithiasis may be asymptomatic, but more often the condition is extremely painful. Surgery may be necessary if the stones cannot be excreted spontaneously. Lower urinary tract calculi often can be dissolved. See also **biliary calculus, cholelithiasis, renal calculus, urinary calculus.**

**-lithiasis,** suffix meaning 'the presence, condition, or formation of stones': *cholelithiasis, uterolithiasis.*

**lithium (Li)** /lith′ē·əm/ [Gk, *lithos,* stone], a silver-white alkali metal occurring in various compounds such as petalite and spodumene. Its atomic number is 3; its atomic mass is 6.94. Lithium is the lightest known metal and one of the most reactive elements. Traces of lithium ion occur in animal tissue, and it abounds in many alkaline mineral spring waters. Its salts are used in the treatment of manias, but the mechanisms by which these compounds help to stabilize psychologic moods are not understood. Lithium carbonate is a salt commonly used for psychiatric purposes in the United States; it has been effective in the prevention of recurrent attacks of manic-depressive illnesses. It has helped correct sleep disorders in manic patients, apparently by suppressing the rapid eye movement phases of sleep. Therapeutic concentrations of lithium have no observable psychotropic effects on normal individuals. In manic patients lithium salts also produce high-voltage slow waves in the electroencephalograph, often with superimposed beta waves. An important feature of the lithium ion is its relatively small gradient of distribution across biologic membranes. Patients suffering severe manic attacks are hospitalized so that they can receive proper medical maintenance; treatments start with large doses of antipsychotic drugs, which are followed by the gradual and safe introduction of lithium therapy. Ideally lithium treatment is prescribed only for patients with normal sodium intake and normal heart and kidney function.

**lithium carbonate,** an antimanic agent.

■ INDICATION: It is prescribed in the treatment of manic episodes of manic-depressive disorder.

■ CONTRAINDICATIONS: It is used with caution in the presence of renal or cardiovascular disease and is not recommended for children under 12 years of age. Known hypersensitivity to this drug and pregnancy prohibit its use.

■ ADVERSE EFFECTS: Among the most serious adverse reactions are renal damage, polydipsia and polyuria, and impairment of mental and physical abilities. Retention of sodium and fluid may occur.

**lithium fluoride (LiF),** a compound commonly used for thermoluminescent dosimetry.

**litho-, lith-,** combining form meaning 'stone or calculus': *litholysis, lithomyl, lithophone.*

**Lithobid,** trademark for an antimanic drug (lithium carbonate).

**lithogenesis** /lith′əjen′əsis/ [Gk, *lithos,* stone, *genein,* to produce], the origin of the formation of a calculus.

**lithopedion** /lith′əpē′dē·ən/ [Gk, *lithos* + *paidion,* child], a fetus that has died in utero and has become calcified or ossified. Also called **lithopedium, calcified fetus, ostembryon, osteopedion.**

**lithoscope** /lith′əskōp′/, a device used to inspect calculi in the bladder. See also **cystoscope.**

**Lithotabs,** trademark for an antimanic drug (lithium carbonate).

**lithotomy** /lithot′əmē/ [Gk, *lithos* + *temnein,* to cut], **1.** the surgical excision of a calculus, especially one from the urinary tract. **2.** a position in operating room.

**lithotomy forceps,** a forceps for the extraction of a calculus, usually from the urinary tract.

**lithotomy position,** the posture assumed by the patient lying supine with the hips and the knees flexed and the thighs abducted and rotated externally. Also called **dorsosacral position.**

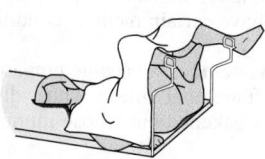

**Lithotomy position** *(Potter and Perry, 2001)*

**lithotripsy** /lith'ətrip'sē/ [Gk, *lithos,* stone, *tribein,* to wear away], a procedure for eliminating a calculus in the renal pelvis, ureter, bladder, or gallbladder. It may be crushed surgically or by using a noninvasive method such as a hydraulic, or high-energy, shock wave or a pulsed dye laser. The fragments may then be expelled or washed out.

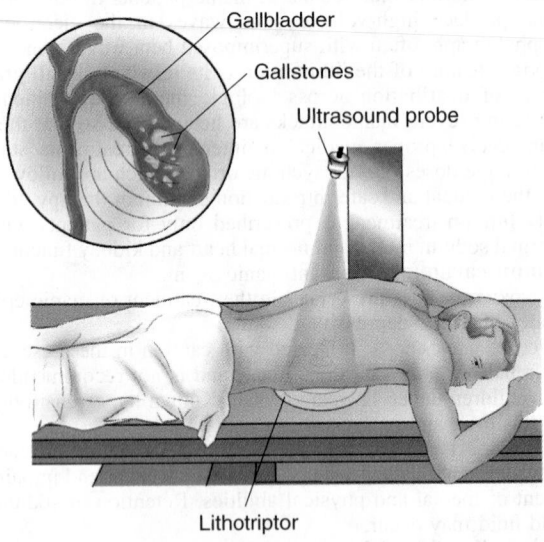

Gallbladder

Gallstones

Ultrasound probe

Lithotriptor

**Lithotripsy** *(Leonard, 2001)*

**lithotrite** /lith'ətrīt/ [Gk, *lithos* + L, *terere,* to rub], an instrument for crushing a stone in the urinary bladder. Also called **lithotriptor. —lithotrity,** *n.*

**litigant** /lit'əgənt/ [L, *litigare,* to go to law], (in law) a party to a lawsuit. See also **defendant, plaintiff.**

**litigate** /lit'əgāt/, (in law) to carry on a suit or to contest.

**litigious paranoia** [L, *litigare,* to go to law; Gk, *paranous,* madness], a form of paranoia in which the person seeks legal proof or justification for systematized delusions.

**litmus paper** /lit'məs/ [ONorse, *litmosi,* coloring herb; L, *papyrus,* paper], absorbent paper coated with litmus, a blue dye, that is used to determine pH. Acid substances or solutions turn blue litmus to red. Alkaline substances or solutions do not cause a color change in blue litmus. The pH range is 4.5 (red) to 8.5 (blue).

**litter** [Fr, *lit,* bed], a stretcher.

**Little's disease.** See **cerebral palsy.**

**Litzmann obliquity.** See **asynclitism.**

**live attenuated measles virus vaccine** /əten'yōō·ā'tid/, a vaccine prepared from live strains of measles virus that have been cultured under conditions that cause them to lose their virulence without losing their ability to induce immunity. The vaccine is not recommended for pregnant women or others who may have certain medical conditions that tend to diminish immunity.

**live attenuated vaccine,** a vaccine prepared from live microorganisms or functional viruses whose disease-producing ability has been weakened but whose immunogenic properties have not.

**live birth** [AS, *libben,* to be alive; ONorse, *byrth*], the birth of an infant, irrespective of the duration of gestation, that exhibits any sign of life, such as respiration, heartbeat, umbilical pulsation, or movement of voluntary muscles. A live birth is not always a viable birth.

**livedo** /livē'dō/ [L, *liveo,* bluish spot], a blue or reddish mottling of the skin that worsens in cold weather and is probably caused by arteriolar spasm. **Cutis marmorata** is a transient form of livedo. See also **livedo reticularis.**

**livedo reticularis,** a disorder accentuated by exposure to cold and presenting with a characteristic reddish-blue mottling with a typical 'fishnet' appearance. The condition involves the entire leg and, less often, the arms. See also **livedo.**

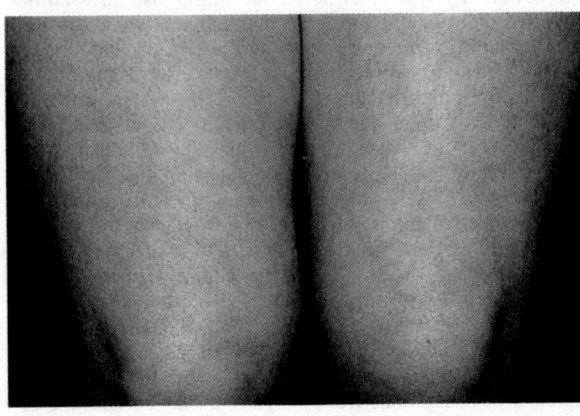

**Livedo reticularis** *(Lawrence and Cox, 1993)*

**livedo vasculitis.** See **segmented hyalinizing vasculitis.**

**live measles and mumps virus vaccine,** a vaccine prepared from live strains of measles and mumps viruses. The vaccine is commonly combined with live rubella viruses as **MMR vaccine** and administered to normal infants at the age of 15 months.

**live oral poliovirus vaccine,** a vaccine prepared from three strains (trivalent) of live polioviruses. Primary immunization with the vaccine usually begins at the age of 2 months.

**liver** [AS, *lifer*], the largest gland of the body and one of its most complex organs. It is located in the upper cranial, right part of the abdominal cavity, occupying almost the entire right hypochondrium and the greater part of the epigastrium. In many individuals it extends into the left hypochondrium as far as the mammary line. It has a soft solid consistency, is shaped like an irregular hemisphere, and is dark reddish-brown. The ventral part of the liver is separated by the diaphragm from the sixth to the tenth ribs on the right side and from the seventh and eighth costal cartilages on the left side. The central section has a deep concavity that fits the vertebral column and the crura of the diaphragm. The liver is divided into four lobes, contains as many as 100,000 lobules, and is served by two distinct blood supplies. The hepatic artery conveys oxygenated blood to the liver, and the hepatic portal vein conveys nutrient-filled blood from the stomach and the intestines. At any given moment the liver holds about 1 pint of blood, or approximately 13% of the total blood supply of the body. The tiny lobules of the organ are composed of polyhedral hepatic cells. These cells communicate with small ducts that connect with larger ducts to form the left and right hepatic ducts that emerge on the caudal

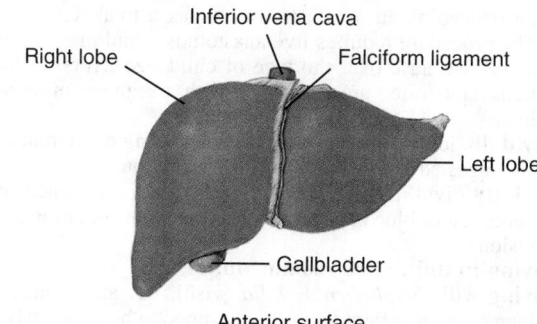

Inferior vena cava

Right lobe

Falciform ligament

Left lobe

Gallbladder

Anterior surface

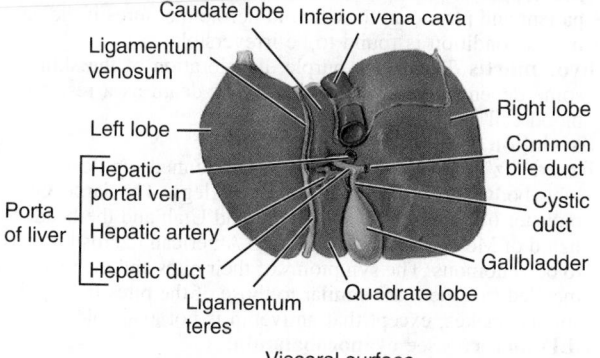

Caudate lobe   Inferior vena cava

Ligamentum venosum

Left lobe

Porta of liver
- Hepatic portal vein
- Hepatic artery
- Hepatic duct

Ligamentum teres

Right lobe

Common bile duct

Cystic duct

Gallbladder

Quadrate lobe

Visceral surface

**Liver** *(Applegate, 2000)*

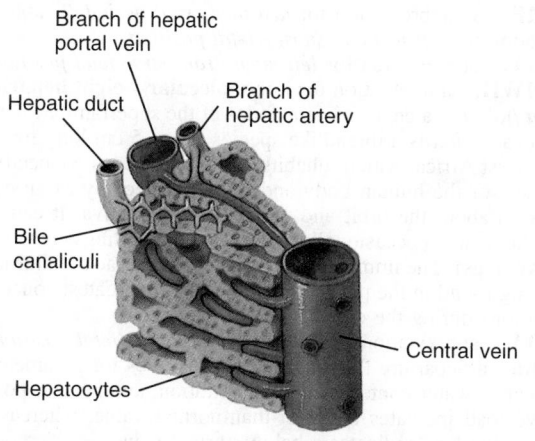

Branch of hepatic portal vein

Hepatic duct

Branch of hepatic artery

Bile canaliculi

Central vein

Hepatocytes

**Cross section of a liver lobule** *(Applegate, 2000)*

surface of the liver. The left and right hepatic ducts converge to form the single hepatic duct, which conveys the bile to the duodenum and gallbladder for storage. More than 500 functions of the liver have been identified. Some of the major functions are the production of bile by hepatic cells; the secretion of glucose, proteins, vitamins, fats, and most of the other compounds used by the body; the processing of hemoglobin for vital use of its iron content; and the conversion of poisonous ammonia to urea. Bile from the liver is stored in

the hepatic duct, in numerous blood vessels, and in the gallbladder, which is connected to the liver by connective tissue. The liver cells produce about 1 pint of bile daily. The hepatic cells also detoxify numerous ingested substances such as alcohol, nicotine, and other poisons, as well as various toxic substances produced by the intestine. See also **gallbladder.**

**liver abscess** [L, *abscedere*, to go away; AS, *lifer*], an abscess in the liver cells, usually caused by an amebic infection, bacterial infection, or trauma. It is characterized by sweats and chills, pain, nausea, and vomiting.

**liver biopsy,** a diagnostic procedure in which a special needle is introduced into the liver under local anesthesia to obtain a specimen for pathologic examination.

■ METHOD: Before a liver biopsy is performed by a physician, the procedure is explained to the patient, whose baseline vital signs are recorded and who is taught how to inhale and hold the breath during needle insertion. After the patient's possible allergy to the local anesthetic is checked and results of bleeding, clotting, and prothrombin tests are obtained, an analgesic or sedative is administered as ordered. On completion of the biopsy, pressure is applied to the site for 15 minutes; the patient is positioned on the right side for the first 2 hours and remains in a supine position in bed for the next 22 hours. The blood pressure, pulse, and respirations are checked every 15 minutes for the first hour, then every 30 minutes for the next 2 hours, and subsequently every 4 hours or as ordered. The biopsy site is observed every 30 minutes for bleeding, swelling, or increased pain; epigastric or referred shoulder pain may occur. Analgesia and vitamin K may be given as ordered, and the recumbent patient is assisted with eating and other activities as needed.

■ INTERVENTIONS: The health care provider reinforces explanations of the biopsy and its purpose, provides care before and after the procedure, and closely observes the patient for postbiopsy complications such as intraperitoneal hemorrhage, shock, and pneumothorax.

■ OUTCOME CRITERIA: An uneventful liver biopsy is a valuable aid in establishing a diagnosis of hepatic disease, including primary and metastatic malignant neoplastic disease.

**liver breath.** See **fetor hepaticus.**

**liver cancer,** a malignant neoplastic disease of the liver, occurring most frequently as a metastasis from another malignancy. Primary liver cancer is common in Africa and Southeast Asia but relatively uncommon in the United States. Primary tumors are six to 10 times more prevalent in men than in women, develop most often in the sixth decade of life, and are associated with cirrhosis of the liver in 70% of the cases. Other risk factors include hemochromatosis, hepatitis, schistosomiasis, exposure to vinyl chloride or arsenic, and possibly nutritional deficiencies. Alcoholism may be a predisposing factor, but nonalcoholic cirrhosis is a greater risk than alcoholic cirrhosis. Aflatoxins in moldy grain and peanuts appear to be linked to high rates of hepatocellular carcinoma in parts of Africa. Characteristics of liver cancer are abdominal bloating, anorexia, weakness, dull upper abdominal pain, ascites, mild jaundice, and a tender enlarged liver; in some cases tumor nodules are palpable on the liver surface. Diagnostic procedures include radioisotope scan, biopsy, and various laboratory studies of liver function. An elevated level of alkaline phosphatase, increased retention of sulfobromophthalein, and the presence of alpha-fetoprotein in the blood suggest liver cancer. Most primary liver tumors are adenocarcinomas, classified as hepatomas when derived from hepatic cells and cholangiomas if they originate in cells of the bile duct. Systemic chemotherapy may result in temporary tumor regression. Irra-

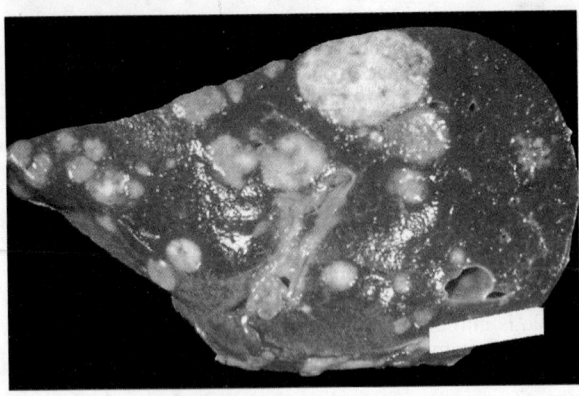

**Metastatic liver cancer** *(Kumar, Cotran, and Robbins, 1997)*

diation is very destructive to liver cells and not very toxic to tumor cells in the liver. See also **hepatoma.**

**liver cell carcinoma.** See **hepatoma.**

**liver disease,** any one of a group of disorders of the liver. Characteristics of liver disease are jaundice, anorexia, hepatomegaly, ascites, and impaired consciousness. The exact diagnosis of liver disease is made through a combination of laboratory tests and clinical findings. See also **cholestasis, cirrhosis, hepatitis.**

**liver failure** [AS, *lifer* + L, *fallere,* to deceive], a condition in which the liver fails to fulfill its function or is unable to meet the demands made on it. Anorexia, fatigue, and weakness are common symptoms of liver cell failure, whereas jaundice indicates a biliary obstruction and fever may accompany viral or alcoholic liver diseases.

**liver flap.** See **asterixis.**

**liver fluke** [AS, *lifer* + *floc*], a parasitic trematode belonging to the class Trematoda with six genera that may infest the liver. The most important species affecting humans in industrialized countries is *Clonorchis sinensis,* which is usually acquired by eating freshwater fish containing the encysted larvae. The larvae are released in the duodenum, enter the common bile duct, and migrate to other bile ducts, the gallbladder, and pancreatic ducts. The liver fluke may survive for many years in the human biliary tree, releasing eggs into the feces. Infestations are most likely to result from ingestion of raw, dried, salted, or pickled freshwater fish and can be prevented by thorough cooking of such fish.

**liver function test (LFT),** one of several tests used to evaluate various functions of the liver—for example, metabolism, storage, filtration, and excretion. Kinds of liver function tests include **alkaline phosphatase, prothrombin time, serum bilirubin,** and **alanine aminotransferase.**

**liver scan,** a noninvasive technique of visualizing the size, shape, and consistency of the liver and for assessing the liver's functional status. It involves IV injection of a radioactively labeled compound that is readily taken up and trapped in the Kupffer cells of the liver. The radiation emitted by the compound is recorded by a radiation detector and can be photographed with a scintillation camera or x-ray film. Liver scans are useful for diagnosing three-dimensional lesions such as abscesses and tumors; for performing biopsies; and for evaluating hepatomegaly, jaundice, and ascites.

**liver spot,** *nontechnical.* a senile lentigo or actinic keratosis.

**liver transplantation,** a treatment for end-stage hepatic dysfunction in which a donor liver is matched in size and blood group to the recipient. The transplanted organ may be introduced as an auxiliary liver or as a total replacement. The procedure requires five anastomoses and many units of blood. Because of a shortage of child-size livers, pediatric transplants often are performed with a segment of an adult liver.

**livid** /liv′id/ [L, *lividus,* bluish], pertaining to an injury that is congested and has a bluish discoloration.

**lividity** /livid′itē/ [L, *lividus,* bluish], a tissue condition of being red or blue because of venous congestion, as in a contusion.

**living-in unit.** See **rooming-in.**

**living will** [AS, *libben* + *willa,* wish], **1.** an advance declaration by a patient that, if determined to be hopelessly and terminally ill, the person does not want to be connected to life support equipment. **2.** a written agreement between a patient and physician to withhold heroic measures if the patient's condition is found to be irreversible.

**livor mortis** /lī′vər/, a purple discoloration of the skin in some dependent body areas following death as a result of blood cell destruction.

**lixiviation,** See **leaching.**

**lizard** /liz′ərd/ [L, *lacerta*], a scaly-skinned reptile with a long body and tail and two pairs of legs. The large Gila monster of Arizona, New Mexico, and Utah and the beaded lizard of Mexico are the only North American lizards known to be venomous. The symptoms of their bites and the recommended treatment are similar to those of the bites from poisonous snakes, except that antivenin is not available.

**LLD factor.** See **cyanocobalamin.**

**LLE,** abbreviation for *left lower extremity.*

**LLQ,** abbreviation for *left lower quadrant of abdomen.*

**LMA,** abbreviation for *left mentoanterior fetal position.*

**LMD.** See **dextran preparation.**

**L.M.D.,** abbreviation for *licensed medical doctor.* Also called **P.M.D.**

**LMP,** **1.** abbreviation for *last menstrual period.* **2.** abbreviation for *left mentoposterior fetal position.*

**LMT,** abbreviation for *left mentotransverse fetal position.*

**LMWH,** abbreviation for **low-molecular-weight heparin.**

*Loa* /lo′ə /, a genus of nematodes of the superfamily Filarioidea. *L. loa* is a threadlike species 2.5 to 5 cm long found in West Africa, which inhabits the subcutaneous connective tissue of the human body and is seen especially as an eye worm about the orbit and under the conjunctiva. It causes itching and occasionally edematous swellings (calabar swellings). The immature forms or microfilariae are diurnal, being found in the peripheral circulation in greatest concentrations during the day.

**LOA,** abbreviation for *left occipitoanterior fetal position.*

**load,** a departure from normal body values for parameters such as water content, salt concentration, and heat. A positive load indicates a higher-than-normal value, whereas a negative load indicates a below-normal value.

**loading,** **1.** the administration of a substance in sufficient quantity to test a patient's ability to metabolize or absorb it. **2.** the exertion of force on a muscle or ligament to increase its strength.

**loading response stance stage** [AS, *lad,* support; L, *responsum,* reply], one of the five stages of the stance phase of walking or gait, specifically associated with the moment when the leg reacts to and accepts the weight of the body. The loading response stance stage is one of the factors in the diagnoses of many abnormal orthopedic conditions and is often studied in conjunction with analyses of the electromyographic activity of the muscles used in walking. Compare **initial contact stance stage, midstance, preswing stance stage, terminal stance.**

**loads** [AS, *lad,* support],   *slang.* a fixed combination of a sedative hypnotic (glutethimide) and a major opioid analgesic (codeine). The medications are taken orally by drug abusers for a euphoric effect reported to be similar to that produced by heroin, but longer lasting. Toxicity may develop, characterized by nystagmus, slurred speech, seizures, coma, pulmonary edema, or sudden apnea and death. Detoxification of an addicted person is managed under close medical supervision with methadone and phenobarbital, as sudden withdrawal can cause death.

***Loa loa*** /lō′älō′ä/,   a parasitic worm of western and central Africa that causes loiasis. Also called **eye worm.**

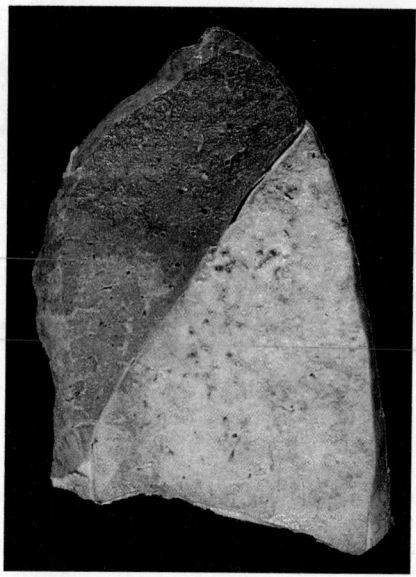

**Lobar pneumonia** *(Kumar, Cotran, and Robbins, 1997)*

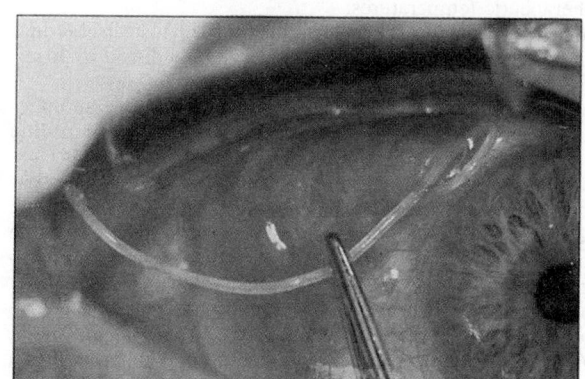

***Loa loa* being extracted from under the conjunctiva**
*(Michelson and Friedlaender, 1996/courtesy Jonathan Belmont, MD)*

**lobar.**   See **lobe.**

**lobar bronchus** /lō′bär/ [Gk, *lobos,* lobe, *bronchos,* windpipe],   a bronchus extending from a primary bronchus to a segmental bronchus into one of the lobes of the right or left lung.

**lobar pneumonia,**   a severe infection of one or more of the five major lobes of the lungs that, if untreated, eventually results in consolidation of lung tissue. The disease is characterized by fever, chills, cough, rusty sputum, rapid shallow breathing, cyanosis, nausea, vomiting, and pleurisy. *Streptococcus pneumoniae* is the usual cause; but *Klebsiella pneumoniae, Haemophilus influenzae,* and other streptococci can produce the disease. If the diagnosis is made early, appropriate antibiotic therapy is highly successful. Complications include lung abscess, atelectasis, empyema, pericarditis, and pleural effusion. Precautions against spread of the contagious disease are important. Because the fatality rate in the elderly and those with underlying systemic illness is high, prophylactic polyvalent pneumococcal vaccine is recommended for them. Compare **bronchopneumonia.**

**lobate** /lō′bāt/,   organized in lobes or rounded divisions. Also **lobular.**

**lobe** /lōb/ [Gk, *lobos*],   **1.** a roundish projection of any structure. **2.** a part of any organ, demarcated by sulci, fissures, or connective tissue, as the lobes of the brain, liver, and lungs. —**lobar, lobular,** *adj.*

**lobe-, -lobe,**   combining form meaning a 'rounded prominence', a lobe: *lobotany gonilobe, multilobe.*

**lobectomy** /lōbek′təmē/ [Gk, *lobos* + *ektomē,* excision],   the surgical excision of one or more lobes of a lung. It is performed to remove a malignant tumor or large benign tumor and to treat uncontrolled bronchiectasis, trauma with hemorrhage, congenital anomalies, or intractable tuberculosis. Any respiratory infection is cleared before surgery. Administration of antibiotics is begun. General anesthesia is administered. The chest cavity is entered through a long back-to-front incision, and the diseased lobe is removed. A large-caliber tube remains in the wound and is connected to a water-sealed drainage system. Oxygen is given after surgery. Vital signs are closely monitored, and deep breathing is encouraged hourly. Blood transfusion may be given, and IV fluids are continued. Pain medication is given. Care is taken that the chest tube remain patent and that the drainage system is sealed and functional. The chest tube is removed 2 to 3 days after surgery. Some compensatory emphysema is expected as the remaining lung tissue overexpands to fill the new space. —**lobectomize,** *v.*

**lobe of ear** [Gk, *lobos,* lobe; AS, *eare*],   the lower part of the auricle that contains no cartilage.

**lobotomy** /lōbot′əmē/ [Gk, *lobos* + *temnein,* to cut],   a neurosurgical procedure in which the nerve fibers in the bundle of white matter in the frontal lobe of the brain are severed to interrupt the transmission of various affective responses. Severe intractable depression and pain are among the indications for the operation. It is seldom performed, because it has many unpredictable and undesirable effects, including personality change, aggression, socially unacceptable behavior, incontinence, apathy, and lack of consideration for others. Because lobotomy is simple to perform, it was overused in the treatment of mentally ill patients in the past. A cannula is passed through the bony orbit of the eye, and a wire loop is inserted through the cannula to the cingulum. The nerve fibers are severed with the wire loop. Also called **leukotomy.**

**lobster claw deformity.**   See **bidactyly.**

**lobular.**   See **lobate, lobe, lobule.**

**lobular carcinoma** /lob′yələr/ [Gk, *lobos* + *karkinos,* crab, *oma,* tumor],   a neoplasm that often forms a diffuse mass and accounts for a small percentage of breast tumors.

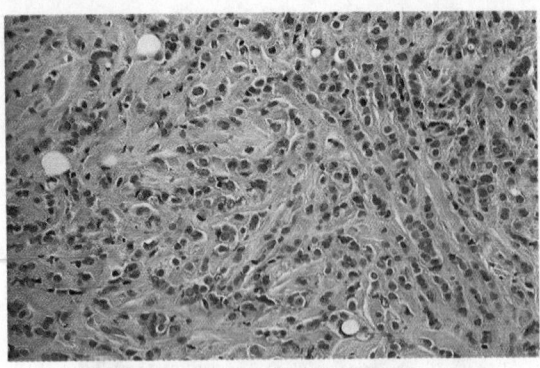

**Lobular carcinoma** *(Fletcher, 2000)*

**lobule** /lob'yōōl/, a small lobe, such as the soft lower pendulous part of the external ear. **—lobular,** *adj.*

**loc-,** prefix meaning 'from a place': *locomotor, locum, locus.*

**LOC,** abbreviation for **level of consciousness.**

**local** [L, *locus,* place], **1.** pertaining to a small circumscribed area of the body. **2.** pertaining to a treatment or drug applied locally. **3.** *informal.* a local anesthetic.

**local adaptation syndrome (LAS),** the localized response of a tissue, organ, or system that occurs as a reaction to stress. See also **general adaptation syndrome.**

**local anaphylaxis** [L, *locus,* place; Gk, *ana + phylaxis*], a hypersensitivity reaction in which injections of an antigen result in localized swellings and necrosis of the skin and subcutaneous tissues.

**local anesthesia,** the infiltration of a local anesthetic medication into to induce the absence of sensation a small area of the body. Brief surgical or dental procedures are the most common indications to avoid general anesthesia. The anesthetic may be applied topically to the surface of the skin or membrane or injected subcutaneously or intradermally. The principal drawback to the use of local anesthesia is the occasional difficulty in achieving adequate anesthesia. Advantages include low cost, ease of administration, low toxicity, and rapid recovery. A conscious patient can cooperate and does not require respiratory support or intubation. In all cases, the recommended dosage of any agent is the smallest possible to achieve the desired effect, because toxicity is directly related to the total amount of drug given rather than to the initial amount or the concentration of the agent used. Each local anesthetic agent also has a recommended maximum allowable dose that is not safely exceeded. Compare **general anesthesia, regional anesthesia, topical anesthesia.**

**local anesthetic,** a medication used to prevent the transmission of impulses through nerves to eliminate sensation in a defined area of the body. It can also prevent motor and atonomic function in this area. The effect is transient (time limited). Drugs available for local anesthesia are classified as members of the ester or the amide family. Specific preparations are available for topical administration; infiltration; and various kinds of regional administration, including field block, regional block, epidural block, and spinal block. People who are sensitive to local anesthetics of one group often can tolerate those of the other group. The vascularity of the injection site, the speed with which the drug is given, the rapidity of action of the drug, and the presence of epinephrine in the solution may affect adverse response.

**local area network (LAN),** a system of linking together computers and other electronic office equipment within an office or building, permitting shared use of software and/or peripherals. Compare **wide area network (WAN).**

**local cerebral blood flow (LCBF),** in positron emission tomography, a parametric image of blood flow through the brain expressed as milliliters per minute per 100 g of brain tissue.

**local cerebral metabolic rate of glucose utilization (LCMRG),** in positron emission tomography, a parametric image of brain activity expressed as milligrams of glucose used per minute per 100 g of brain tissue.

**local control,** the arrest of cancer growth at the site of origin.

**local hypothermia,** the heating of a local area of tissue to therapeutic temperatures.

**local immunity,** a state of protection against disease in a particular organ, tissue, or anatomic site mediated by localized antibodies or lymphoid cells.

**local infection** [L, *locus,* place, *inficere,* to stain], an infection involving bacteria that invade the body at a specific point and remain there, multiplying, until eliminated.

**localization** /lō'kəlīzā'shən/ [L, *locus,* place], **1.** the designation of a particular site for a lesion or organ function. **2.** the determination of the site of a biologic function. **3.** the assignment of a position to an object detected by radiography.

**localization audiometry.** See **audiometry.**

**localization film** [L, *locus,* place; Gk, *izein,* to cause; AS, *filmen,* membrane], a radiographic film taken to confirm a treatment effect or to view the position of an intracavitary or interstitial implant, especially for the purpose of computing the dose delivered.

**localized scleroderma.** See **morphea.**

**localizer image,** an image used to localize a specific body part in computed tomography.

**localizing symptom.** See **symptom.**

**local lesion** [L, *locus,* place, *laesio,* hurting], **1.** a lesion anywhere on the body that does not spread. **2.** a lesion of the central nervous system characterized by distinctive local symptoms.

**local osteolytic hypercalcemia (LOH),** a syndrome of malignancy-associated hypercalcemia resulting from the action of locally acting osteolytic factors released in conjunction with tumor deposits adjacent to bone. LOH is frequently produced by multiple myeloma and lung and breast cancer.

**local paralysis,** a loss of motor control that is confined to a single muscle, muscle group, or part of the body.

**local reaction** [L, *locus,* place, *re + agere,* to act], a reaction to treatment that occurs at the site where it was administered.

**locant** /lō'kənt/, a number or letter code that locates the position of an atom, radical, or compound in the structure of a more complex molecule.

**location** [L, *locus,* place, *atus,* process], a specific place in the memory of a computer where a unit of information is stored.

**lochia** /lō'kē·ə/ [Gk, *lochos,* childbirth], the discharge that flows from the vagina after childbirth. During the first 2 to 4 days after delivery, the lochia is red or brownish red (called **lochia rubra**) and is made up of blood, endometrial decidua, fetal lanugo, vernix, and sometimes meconium, and it has a fleshy odor. About the third day the amount of blood diminishes; the placental site exudes serous material, erythrocytes, lymph, cervical mucus, and microorganisms from the superficial layer called lochia serosa. During the next 10 to 14 days bacteria appear in large numbers along with mucinous decidual material and epithelial cells, causing the lochia to appear whitish yellow (**lochia alba**). This may continue for 3 to 6 weeks into the postpartum period. —**lochial**, *adj.*

**loci.** See **locus.**

**locked-in syndrome** [ME, *loc* + Gk, *syn,* together, *dromos,* course], a paralytic condition in which a person may be conscious and alert but unable to communicate except by eye movements or blinking (e.g., pseudocoma). Bilateral destruction of the medulla oblongata or pons has rendered the individual unable to speak or move any of the limbs.

**locked knee** [AS, *loc* + *cneow*], a condition in which the knee is fixed in either a flexed or an extended position, often caused by longitudinal splitting of the medial meniscus. Also called **trick knee.**

**locked twins.** See **interlocked twins.**

**lock forceps.** See **point forceps.**

**locking point** [AS, *loc,* lock; L, *punctum,* puncture], a point on the body at which light pressure can be applied to help a weak or debilitated patient maintain a desired posture or position. A basic locking point is the body's center of gravity, at the level of the second sacral vertebra, where mild pressure can assist a patient in standing or walking erect.

**lockjaw.** See **tetanus, trismus.**

**locomotion** [L, *locus,* place, *motio,* movement], movement or the ability to move from one place or position to another.

**locomotor** [L, *locus* + *motio*], pertaining to locomotion.

**locomotor ataxia.** See **tabes dorsalis.**

**loculate** /lok′yŏŏlāt/ [L, *loculus,* little place], divided into small spaces or cavities.

**loculation** /lok′yəlā′shən/, the presence of numerous small spaces or cavities.

**loculus** /lok′yŏŏləs/ [L, little place], a small chamber, pocket, or cavity, such as the interior of a polyp.

**locum tenens** /lō′kəm ten′ənz/ [L, *locus,* place, *tenere,* to hold], a physician who is contacted to work on a temporary basis to fill in for a vacancy, vacation, or extended leave.

**locus,** *pl.* **loci** /lō′sī, lō′kē/ [L, place], a specific place or position, such as the locus of a particular gene on a chromosome.

**locus ceruleus** [L, *locus,* place, *caeruleus,* sky-blue], a deeply pigmented group of several thousand neurons in the floor of the fourth ventricle. It is part of a major norepinephrine pathway of the central nervous system.

**locus of control** [L, *locus,* place; Fr, *controle*], a center of responsibility for one's behavior. Individuals with an **internal locus of control** believe they can control events related to their life, whereas those with an **external locus of control** tend to believe that real power resides in forces outside themselves and determines their life.

**locus of infection,** a site in the body where an infection originates.

**Loeffler's syndrome.** See **Löffler's syndrome.**

**Loestrin,** trademark for an oral contraceptive containing an estrogen (ethinyl estradiol) and a progestin (norethindrone acetate).

**Lofenalac,** trademark for a commercial milk-substitute formula that is low in phenylalanine and used for infants with phenylketonuria. It is made from hydrolyzed casein, supplemented with tyrosine, and fortified with added fat, carbohydrate, minerals, and vitamins to balance the formula. A common problem with the formula is diarrhea, which may appear after the first few feedings but generally disappears in a few days.

**Löffler's syndrome** /lef′lərz/ [Wilhelm Löffler, Swiss physician, 1887–1972], a benign, idiopathic disorder marked by episodes of pulmonary eosinophilia, transient opacities in the lungs, anorexia, breathlessness, fever, and weight loss. Recovery is spontaneous and prompt. Also spelled **Loeffler's syndrome.** See also **pulmonary infiltrate with eosinophilia.**

**log-, logo-, -log, -logue,** combining form meaning 'word, speech, thought': *logagnosia, logorrhea, dialog, dialogue.*

**logad-,** combining form meaning 'whites of the eyes': *logadectomy, logaditis, logadoblennorrhea.*

**-logia.** See **-logy.**

**login,** a procedure for initiating interaction between a user and a computer.

**logo-.** See **log-.**

**logoff,** a procedure for terminating interaction between a user and a computer.

**logotherapy** /log′ōther′əpē/ [Gk, *logos,* word, *therapeia,* treatment], a treatment modality based on the application of humanistic and existential psychology to assist a patient in finding meaning and purpose in life and unique life experiences.

**log roll** [ME, *logge* + L, *roto,* turn around], a maneuver used to turn a reclining patient from one side to the other or completely over without flexing the spinal column. The arms of the patient are folded across the chest, and the legs extended. A draw sheet under the patient is manipulated by attending health care team members nursing personnel to facilitate the procedure.

**-logue.** See **-log.**

**-logy, -logia,** suffix meaning 'a science or study of': *mammalogy, metabology, neonatology.*

**LOH,** abbreviation for **local osteolytic hypercalcemia.**

**loiasis** /lō·ī′əsis/, a form of filariasis caused by the worm *Loa loa.* The worms may migrate for 10 to 15 years in subcutaneous tissue, producing localized inflammation known as Calabar swellings. Occasionally, the migrating worms may be visible beneath the conjunctiva. The disease is acquired through the bite of an infected African deer fly. Treatment with diethylcarbamazine usually results in cure and may also be successful as prophylaxis. See also **filariasis, onchocerciasis.**

**loin** [ME, *loyn,* flank], a part of the body on each side of the spinal column between the false ribs and the hip bones.

**Lomotil,** trademark for an antidiarrheal fixed-combination drug containing an antiperistaltic (diphenoxylate hydrochloride) and an anticholinergic (atropine sulfate).

**lomustine** /lōmus′tēn/, an antineoplastic alkylating agent.

■ INDICATIONS: It is prescribed in the treatment of a variety of malignant neoplastic diseases, including brain tumors and Hodgkin's disease.

■ CONTRAINDICATION: Known hypersensitivity to this drug prohibits its use.

■ ADVERSE EFFECTS: Among the more serious adverse reactions are bone marrow depression, nausea, and vomiting.

**Lonalac,** trademark for a low-sodium, nutritional supplement.

**loneliness,** a nursing outcome from the Nursing Outcomes Classification (NOC) defined as the extent of emotional, social, or existential isolation response. See also **Nursing Outcomes Classification.**

**loneliness, risk for,** a nursing diagnosis accepted by the Eleventh National Conference on the Classification of Nursing Diagnoses. It is defined as a subjective state in which an individual is at risk of experiencing vague dysphonia.

■ RISK FACTORS: The risk factors are affectional deprivation, physical isolation, cathectic deprivation, and social isolation. See also **nursing diagnosis.**

**long-acting drug** [AS, *lang* + L, *agere,* to do; Fr, *drogue,* drug], a pharmacologic agent with a prolonged effect because of a formulation resulting in the slow release of the active principle or the continued absorption of small amounts of the dosage of the drug over an extended period.

**long-acting insulin,** a preparation of insulin modified by an interaction with zinc under specific chemical conditions and supplied as a suspension with a prolonged action. An injection of the preparation takes effect within 8 hours, reaches a peak of action in 16 to 24 hours, and has a duration of action of more than 36 hours. Also called **slow-acting insulin, ultralente insulin.** See also **insulin.** Compare **intermediate-acting insulin, short-acting insulin.**

**long-acting thyroid stimulator (LATS),** an immunoglobulin, probably an autoantibody, that exerts a prolonged stimulatory effect on the thyroid gland, causing rapid growth of the gland and excess activity of thyroid function, resulting in hyperthyroidism. It is found circulating in the blood of 50% of people with Graves' disease.

**long-acting thyroid stimulator protector (LATS-P),** an antibody that inhibits the neutralization of long-acting thyroid stimulator and is found in the serum of persons with Graves' disease. LATS-P interferes with the binding of thyroid-stimulating hormone to its receptor on the plasma membrane of thyroid cells. See also **long-acting thyroid stimulator.**

**long-arm cast** [As, *lang* + *earm,* arm; ONorse, *kasta*], an orthopedic cast applied to immobilize the arm from the hand to the upper arm. It is used in treating fractures of the forearm, elbow, and humerus; for maintaining postoperative positioning of the distal arm, elbow, or upper arm; and for correcting or maintaining the correction of deformities of the distal arm, wrist, or elbow. See also **cast.** Compare **short-arm cast.**

**long bones,** the bones that contribute to the height or length of an extremity, particularly the bones of the legs and arms.

**longevity** /lonjev′itē/ [L, *longus,* long, *aveum,* age], the number of years an average person of a particular age is expected to continue living. It is determined by statistical tables based on mortality rates of various population groups.

**longissimus** /lon·jis′i·məs/ [L, longest, very long], a general term denoting a long structure, as a muscle.

**longitudinal** /lon′jətoo̅′dənəl/ [L, *longitudo,* length], **1.** pertaining to a measurement in the direction of the long axis of an object, body, or organ, such as the longitudinal arch of the foot. **2.** pertaining to a scientific study that is conducted over a long period of time, such as the Framingham (Massachusetts) Study of heart disease.

**longitudinal diffusion,** the diffusion of solute molecules in the direction of flow of the mobile phase.

**longitudinal dissociation,** the insulation of parallel pathways of cardiac impulses from each other, usually in the atrioventricular junction.

**longitudinal fissure** [L, *longitudo,* length, *fissura,* cleft], the largest and deepest groove between the medial surfaces of the cerebral hemispheres.

**longitudinal presentation** [L, *longitudo,* length, *praesentare,* to show], the normal presentation of a fetus, with the long axis of the infant body parallel to that of the mother.

**longitudinal sound waves,** pressure waves formed by the oscillation of particles or molecules parallel to the axis of wave propagation. The compression and expansion of such waves at high frequencies is the principle on which ultrasonography is based.

**long-leg cast,** an orthopedic cast applied to immobilize the leg from the toes to the upper thigh. It is used in treating fractures and dislocations of the knee; for maintaining postoperative positioning and immobilization of the knee, distal leg, and ankle; and for correcting or maintaining the correction of the foot, distal leg, and knee. See also **cast.** Compare **short-leg cast.**

**long-leg cast with walker,** an orthopedic cast applied to immobilize the leg from the toes to the upper thigh in treating certain leg fractures. This type of cast is the same as the long-leg cast but incorporates a rubber walker, enabling the patient to walk while the leg is encased in the cast and when weight-bearing ambulation is allowed. See also **cast.**

**long QT syndrome,** an inherited cardiac disorder characterized by prolongation of the Q-T interval. The disorder is associated with ventricular tachycardia, cardiac arrhythmias, syncope, and sudden death. Syncopal episodes often occur during physical exercise in young, otherwise healthy persons.

**long-scale contrast,** a high-kilovolt radiographic image containing a wide range and great number of shades of gray with little difference in the adjacent tones.

**long-term care (LTC),** the provision of medical, social, and personal care services on a recurring or continuing basis to persons with chronic physical or mental disorders. The care may be provided in environments ranging from institutions to private homes. Long-term care services usually include symptomatic treatment, maintenance, and rehabilitation for patients of all age groups.

**long-term memory,** the ability to recall sensations, events, ideas, and other information for long periods of time without apparent effort. It is generally the last memory store to be destroyed in patients with Alzheimer's disease. Compare **short-term memory.**

**long thoracic nerve,** one of a pair of supraclavicular branches from the roots of the brachial plexus. It arises by three roots, from the fifth, the sixth, and the seventh cervical nerves. The fibers from the fifth and the sixth cervical nerves join just after they pierce the scalenus medius and are united with the fibers from the seventh cervical nerve at the level of the first rib. Compare **phrenic nerve.**

**long thoracic nerve injury,** damage to the nerve (C5-7) that innervates the serratus muscle, which anchors the apex of the scapula to the posterior of the rib cage. Symptoms include an abnormally prominent scapula and difficulty in flexing the outstretched arm above the shoulder level, protracting the shoulder, or performing scapula abduction and adduction.

**long tract signs,** neurologic signs such as clonus, muscle spasticity, or bladder involvement that usually indicate a lesion in the middle or upper parts of the spinal cord or in the brain.

**Loniten,** trademark for an antihypertensive (minoxidil).

**loop** [ME, *loupe*], a set of instructions in a computer program that causes certain commands to be executed repeatedly if specified criteria are met.

**loop colostomy** [ME, *loupe* + Gk, *kolon,* colon, *stoma,* mouth], a type of temporary colostomy performed as part of the surgical treatment for repair of some colon diseases. The procedure involves bringing an intact segment of colon anterior to the repair through an abdominal incision and suturing it onto the abdomen. A loop is formed and held in position by placing a piece of glass rod between the segment and the abdomen. The two ends of the rod are connected with a piece of rubber tubing to prevent the rod from slipping. The stomal opening is made on the exterior surface of the segment. The colostomy is reversed after resolution of the original pathology. Also called **double-barrel colostomy.** See also **colostomy irrigation, Hirschsprung's disease.**

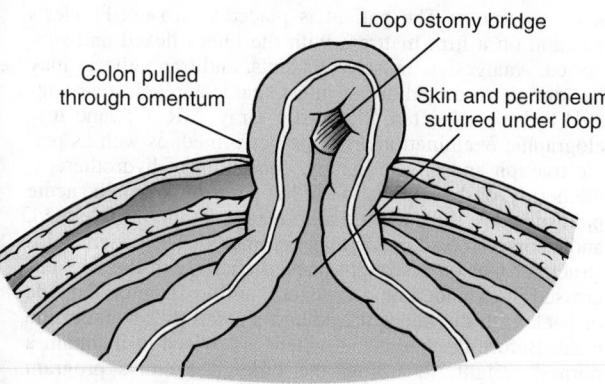

**Loop colostomy** *(Lewis, Heitkemper, and Dirksen, 2000)*

Labels on diagram:
- Loop ostomy bridge
- Colon pulled through omentum
- Skin and peritoneum sutured under loop

**loop diuretic.** See **diuretic.**

**loop excision,** the surgical removal of dysplastic tissue cells with a small wire loop. The technique is used in gynecologic diagnosis and therapy to remove intraepithelial neoplasms from the uterine cervix. Also called *loop electrical excision procedure.*

**loop of Henle** /hen'lē/ [ME, *loupe;* [Friedrich Gustave Henle, German anatomist, 1809–1885], the U-shaped part of a renal tubule, consisting of a thin descending limb and a thick ascending limb. Also called **Henle's loop.**

**loose association** [ME, *lous,* not fastened], (in psychiatry) a disturbance of thinking in which the association of ideas and thought patterns becomes so vague, fragmented, diffuse, and unfocused as to lack any logical sequences or relationship to any preceding concepts or themes. It is a symptom of schizophrenia. When severe, speech may be incoherent. Also called **loosening.**

**loose body,** a fragment of solid tissue in a body cavity or joint. A kind of loose body is a **joint mouse.**

**loose connective tissue.** See **connective tissue.**

**loose fibrous tissue** [ME, *lous,* not fastened], a constrictive, pliable fibrous connective tissue consisting of interwoven elastic and collagenous fibers, interspersed with fluid-filled areolae. It is found in adipose tissue, areolar tissue, reticular tissue, and fibroelastic tissue. Compare **dense fibrous tissue.**

**loosening.** See **loose association.**

**loose-pack joint position,** a point in the range of motion of a joint at which articulating surfaces are the least congruent and the supporting structures are the most lax.

**Looser's zones** /lō'zərz/ [Emil Looser, Swiss physician, 1877–1936], transverse translucent bands, sometimes symmetric, seen radiographically in the cortex of bones affected with osteomalacia or certain other deficiency diseases.

**Lo/Ovral,** trademark for an oral contraceptive containing an estrogen (ethinyl estradiol) and a progestin (norgestrel).

**LOP,** abbreviation for *left occipitoposterior fetal position.*

**loperamide hydrochloride** /lōper'əmīd/, an antiperistaltic.

■ INDICATION: It is prescribed in the treatment of diarrhea.

■ CONTRAINDICATIONS: Known hypersensitivity to this drug prohibits its use. It is not given to patients in whom constipation must be avoided.

■ ADVERSE EFFECTS: Among the most serious reactions are abdominal pain, constipation, nausea, and vomiting.

**loph-,** combining form meaning 'ridge': *lophius, lophodont, lophotrichous.*

**Lopid,** trademark for a lipid-regulating agent (gemfibrozil).

**Lopressor,** trademark for a beta-adrenergic receptor blocking agent (metoprolol tartrate) used in the treatment of hypertension.

**Loprox,** trademark for an antifungal (ciclopirox olamine).

**lorazepam** /lôrā'zəpam/, a benzodiazepine tranquilizer.

■ INDICATIONS: It is prescribed in the treatment of anxiety, nervous tension, and insomnia.

■ CONTRAINDICATIONS: Acute glaucoma, psychosis, pregnancy, or known hypersensitivity to this drug or to any benzodiazepine prohibits its use.

■ ADVERSE EFFECTS: Among the more serious adverse reactions are drowsiness and fatigue. Withdrawal symptoms may occur on discontinuation of the drug, especially after prolonged use or high dosage.

**lordoscoliosis** /lôr'dōskō'lē·ō'sis/ [Gk, *lordos,* bent, *skoliosis,* curvature], a combination of lordosis and scoliosis.

**lordosis** /lôrdō'sis/ [Gk, *lordos,* bent forward, *osis,* condition], an abnormal anterior concavity of the lumbar part of the back.

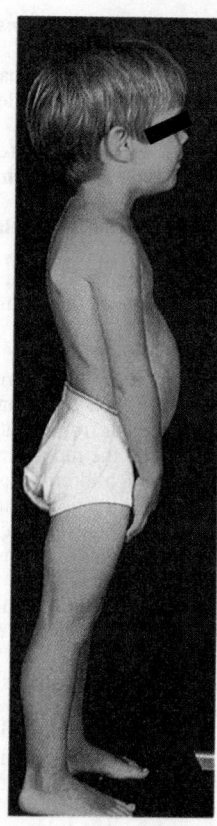

**Lordosis** *(Zitelli and Davis, 1997)*

**lordotic pelvis** /lôrdot'ik/ [Gk, *lordos,* bent forward; L, *pelvis,* basin], a deformed pelvis that bends forward in the lumbar region and is associated with lordosis.

**LOS,** abbreviation for *length of stay.*

**losartan,** an antihypertensive.

■ INDICATIONS: This drug is used to treat hypertension, either alone or in combination with other drugs.

■ CONTRAINDICATIONS: Factors that prohibit the use of this drug are known hypersensitivity to tramadol and 2nd- and 3rd-trimester pregnancy.

■ ADVERSE EFFECTS: Life-threatening effects of this drug are cerebrovascular accident and myocardial infarction. Other adverse effects are anxiety, confusion, abnormal dreams, migraine, tremor, vertigo, task perversion, angina pectoris, 2nd-degree atrioventricular block, hypotension, blurred vision, burning eyes, conjunctivitis, anorexia, constipation, dry mouth, flatulence, gastritis, vomiting, impotence, nocturia, urinary frequency, urinary tract infection, anemia, alopecia, dermatitis, dry skin, flushing, photosensitivity, rash, pruritus, sweating, gout, cramps, myalgia, pain, stiffness, congestion, dyspnea, and bronchitis. Common side effects are dizziness, insomnia, dysrhythmias, diarrhea, dyspepsia, cough, and upper respiratory infection.

**loss of consortium** [ME, *lossen,* to lose; L, *consortionis,* companionship], (in law) a claim for damages sought in recompense for the loss of conjugal relations, including society, affection, and assistance, and impairment or loss of sexual relations. Loss of consortium may be charged against a person whose negligence or malfeasance caused injury to the spouse or against a person who caused a marriage to break up.

**LOT,** abbreviation for *left occipitotransverse fetal position.*

**lotion** [L, *lotio,* a washing], a liquid preparation applied externally to protect the skin or to treat a dermatologic disorder.

**Lotrimin,** trademark for an antifungal (clotrimazole).

**Lou Gehrig's disease.** See **amyotrophic lateral sclerosis.**

**Louis-Bar syndrome.** See **ataxia-telangiectasia syndrome.**

**loupe** /lo͞op/ [Fr, magnifying glass], a magnifying lens mounted in a frame worn on the head, as used to examine the eyes.

**louse.** See **lice.**

**louse bite,** a minute puncture wound produced by a louse that may transmit typhus, trench fever, and relapsing fever. Secondary infection may result from scratching the affected area. Head and body lice are the most common and are frequently found among schoolchildren. Washing and bathing, application of an approved insecticide, and the washing or cleaning of clothes and bed linens are recommended procedures for treatment and prophylaxis against spread of the infestation. See also **pediculosis.**

**louse-borne typhus.** See **epidemic typhus.**

**low back pain (lbp)** [ME, *low* + AS, *baec* + L, *poena,* penalty], local or referred pain at the base of the spine caused by a sprain, a strain, osteoarthritis, ankylosing spondylitis, a neoplasm, or a herniated intervertebral disk. Low back pain is a common complaint and is often associated with poor posture, obesity, sagging abdominal muscles, sitting for prolonged periods of time, or improper body mechanics.

■ OBSERVATIONS: Pain may be localized and static; it may be accompanied by muscle weakness or spasms; or it may radiate down one or both legs, as in sciatica. Pain may be initiated or increased by coughing, sneezing, rising from a seated position, lifting, stretching, bending, or turning. To guard against the pain, the person may decrease the range of motion of the spine. If an intervertebral disk is herniated, deep pressure over the interspace generally causes pain, and flexion of the hip elicits sciatic pain when the knee is extended but not when the knee is flexed (Lasègue's sign).

■ INTERVENTIONS: The patient is placed in a semi-Fowler's position on a firm mattress with the knees flexed and supported. Analgesics, muscle relaxants, and tranquilizers may be administered; and dry or moist heat is applied. If a herniated disk is suspected, diagnostic x-ray, MR, CT, and myelographic examinations may be performed, as well as pelvic traction and physiotherapy, consisting of hydrotherapy, diathermy, or the application of hot paraffin. When the acute pain subsides, the patient may increase activity as tolerated, and a corset or back brace may be ordered. The patient is instructed to sit on a straight-backed chair, with the legs uncrossed or extended on a footstool, and to sleep on the side or back with the knees flexed and a small pillow under the head. Before discharge the patient is advised to maintain a normal weight, to follow the ordered exercise program while avoiding fatigue, to wear flat-heeled shoes, and to avoid constipation by using natural laxatives, if required.

■ NURSING CONSIDERATIONS: The nurse encourages the patient to follow the recommended regimen. Correct body mechanics, adequate and appropriate exercise, and the elimination of excess weight are emphasized.

**low-birth weight (LBW) infant,** an infant whose weight at birth is less than 2500 g, regardless of gestational age.

**low blood,** *informal.* anemia.

**low-calcium diet,** a diet that restricts the use of calcium and eliminates most of the dairy foods, all breads made with milk or dry skimmed milk, and deep-green leafy vegetables. It is prescribed for patients who form renal calculi or with absorptive hypercalciuria. Meats, including beef, lamb, pork, veal, and poultry, fish, vegetables, legumes, and fruits, are recommended.

**low-caloric diet,** a diet that is prescribed to limit calorie intake, usually to cause a reduction in body weight. Such diets may be designated as actually a very low-calorie diet (VLCD), 1000 calorie, or other specific numbers of calories. Exchange lists may be used to allow the patient to select preferred foods from groups of foods categorized as carbohydrate, meat and meat substitutes, and fat.

**low cervical cesarean section,** a surgical procedure to deliver a baby through a transverse incision in the thin supracervical part of the lower uterine segment, behind the bladder and the bladder flap. This incision bleeds less during surgery and heals with a stronger scar than the higher vertical scar of the classic cesarean section. Compare **extraperitoneal cesarean section.** See also **cesarean section.**

**low-cholesterol diet,** a diet that restricts foods containing animal fats and saturated fatty acids, egg yolk, cream, butter, milk, muscle and organ meats, and shellfish. It concentrates instead on poultry, fish, vegetables, fruits, low-fat dairy products, and polyunsaturated fats. The diet is indicated for persons with high serum cholesterol levels, cardiovascular disorders, obesity, hyperlipidemia, hypercholesterolemia, or hyperlipoproteinemia. Also called **cholesterol-restricted diet** or **low-saturated-fat diet.**

**low-density lipoprotein (LDL),** a plasma protein provided from very low–density lipoproteins or by the liver, containing relatively more cholesterol and triglycerides than protein. It is derived in part, if not completely, from the intravascular breakdown of the very low–density lipoproteins and delivers lipids and cholesterol to the body tissues. The high cholesterol content may account for its greater atherogenic potential as compared with the VLDLs.

**low-density lipoprotein (LDL) receptor disorder,** an inherited autosomal-dominant trait characterized by an abnormality in clearance of low-density lipoprotein. It is caused by a defect in LDL receptor activity and is also called familial hypercholesterolemia.

**low-dose tolerance,** a temporary and incomplete immunosuppression induced by the administration of subimmunogenic doses of soluble antigen. The tolerance is achieved in the neonatal period, when lymphoid cells have not matured enough to activate a response.

**lower extremity suspension** [ME, *low* + L, *extremitas* + *suspendere,* to hang], an orthopedic procedure used in the treatment of bone fractures and the correction of orthopedic abnormalities of the lower limbs. Traction equipment, including metal frames, ropes, and pulleys, is applied to relieve the weight of the involved lower limb rather than to exert traction pull. Lower extremity suspension may be either unilateral or bilateral and is used in the postoperative, posttraumatic, or postreduction control of edema. Compare **balanced suspension, upper extremity suspension.**

**lower level discriminator (LLD),** an electronic device used in nuclear medicine to discriminate against all radionuclide pulses whose heights are below a given level.

**lower motor neuron dysarthria,** a disorder of articulation caused by weakness or paralysis of the articulatory muscles and marked by a rasping, monotonous voice and, in advanced forms, shriveling and flaccidity of the tongue and laxness and tremulousness of the lips, seen in advanced cases of lesions of motor nuclei in the lower pons or medulla oblongata. Also called **flaccid dysarthria.**

**lower motor neuron paralysis,** an injury to or lesion that damages the cell bodies or axons, or both, of the lower motor neurons, which are located in the anterior horn cells of the spinal cord and the spinal and peripheral nerves. If complete transection of the spinal cord occurs, voluntary muscle control is totally lost. In partial transection, function is altered in varying degrees, depending on the areas innervated by the nerves involved. In lower motor neuron paralysis the reflex arcs are permanently damaged, causing decreased muscle tone and flaccidity, diminished or absent reflexes, absence of pathologic reflexes, local twitching of muscle groups (fasciculations), and progressive atrophy of the atonic muscles. Compare **upper motor neuron paralysis.**

**lower respiratory infection.** See **respiratory tract infection.**

**lower respiratory tract,** one of the two divisions of the respiratory system. The lower respiratory tract includes the left and right bronchi and the alveoli where the exchange of oxygen and carbon dioxide occurs during the respiratory cycle. The bronchi divide into smaller bronchioles in the lungs, the bronchioles into alveolar ducts, the ducts into alveolar sacs, and the sacs into alveoli. The alveolar sacs and the alveoli present a total lung surface of about 850 square feet (79 square meters) for the exchange of oxygen and carbon dioxide, which occurs between the most internal alveolar surface and the tiny capillaries surrounding the external alveolar wall. The lower respiratory tract is a continuation of the upper respiratory tract and is a common site of infections, obstructive conditions, and neoplastic disease. Compare **upper respiratory tract.** See also **lung.**

**Lowe's syndrome** [Charles U. Lowe, American pediatrician, b. 1921], a sex-linked condition in males characterized by progressive mental deterioration, renal tubular dysfunction, and cortical cataracts with or without glaucoma.

**low-fat diet** [ME, *low;* AS, *faett;* Gk, *diaita,* life-style], a diet containing limited amounts of fat and consisting chiefly of easily digestible foods of high carbohydrate content. It includes all vegetables, lean meats, fish, fowl, pasta, cereals, and whole wheat or enriched bread. Egg yolk and fatty meats are restricted. Cream, fried foods, foods prepared in fats, oils, gravy, cheese, peanut butter, nuts, and olives are among the foods omitted or consumed in small amounts. Experts recommend that no more than 30% of one's daily calories should come from fatty foods and no more than 10% should come from saturated fats. A typical low-fat diet providing approximately 1700 calories per day would contain 85 grams of protein, 220 grams of carbohydrate, and 50 grams of fat. Meat, eggs, butter and margarine are omitted or restricted. Low-fat diets supply 10% to 15% of total energy as fat and may be indicated in gallbladder disease, obesity, heart diseases, malabsorption syndromes, and hyperlipidemia.

**low-fat milk,** milk containing 1% to 2% fat, making it an intermediate in fat content between whole and skimmed milk.

**low-fiber diet.** See **low-residue diet.**

**low-flow oxygen delivery system,** respiratory care equipment that allows the patient to inhale some ambient air along with the delivered oxygen. As the patient's ventilatory pattern changes, different amounts of air are mixed with the constant flow of oxygen, thus causing the inspired oxygen concentration to vary. Also called **variable-performance oxygen delivery system.**

**low forceps** [ME, *low* + L, *forceps,* pair of tongs], an obstetric operation in which forceps are used to deliver a baby whose head is on the pelvic floor. The procedure is performed most often as an elective procedure to shorten normal labor and to control delivery, usually in conjunction with anesthesia and episiotomy. It is commonly required for the delivery of mothers whose expulsive powers have been weakened by analgesia, anesthesia, or fatigue. Also called **outlet forceps, prophylactic forceps.** Compare **high forceps, mid forceps, natural childbirth, spontaneous delivery.** See also **forceps delivery, obstetric forceps.**

**low-grade fever,** an oral temperature that is above 98.6° F (37° C) but lower than 100.4° F (38° C) for 24 hours.

**low-grade infection** [ME, *lah* + L, *gradus,* degree, *inficere,* to stain], a subacute or chronic infection with mild fever and no pus production.

**low-level language,** a computer language using mathematical logic but requiring precise manipulation of binary numbers.

**low-lying placenta.** See **placenta previa.**

**low-molecular weight heparin (LMWH),** a drug used to prevent potentially fatal blood clots in patients undergoing surgery or other patients at risk for blood clots. It has been used to prevent deep vein thrombosis in patients undergoing hip and knee replacements.

**Lown-Ganong-Levine syndrome (LGL)** /loun'gənong' ləvēn'/ [Bernard Lown, American physician, b. 1921; William F. Ganong, American physiologist, b. 1924; S. A. Levine, American physician, 1891–1966], a disorder of the atrioventricular (AV) conduction system marked by ventricular preexcitation. Part or all of the AV nodal connection is bypassed by an abnormal connection between the atria and the AV bundle. The condition may be discovered by routine electrocardiogram or may be seen in association with paroxysmal atrial arrhythmias, supraventricular tachycardia, atrial flutter, and fibrillation. Treatments include the use of antiarrhythmic drugs such as quinidine sulfate, procainamide, and propranolol; surgical interruption of the abnormal pathway; and implantation of a pacemaker. Also called **short-PR-normal-QRS syndrome.** Compare **Wolff-Parkinson-White syndrome.**

**low-power field,** the low magnification field of vision under a light microscope.

**low-protein diet** [ME, *lah,* low; Gk, *proteios,* first rank, *diaita,* way of living], a diet proportionally low in protein, usually designed for persons who must restrict protein intake because of a metabolic abnormality associated with kidney failure or a liver disease.

**low-purine diet,** a diet used as adjunct therapy for gout patients who suffer from a painful accumulation of salts of uric acid in the joints. Purine-rich foods are primary sources of uric acid. They include meat, poultry, fish, and particularly organ meats such as liver, kidney, and sweetbreads. Purine-rich foods are replaced in the diet by dairy products, eggs, and some vegetable sources of proteins. Also called **purine-restricted diet.**

**low-residue diet,** a diet that will leave a minimal residue in the lower intestinal tract after digestion and absorption. It consists of tender meats, poultry, fish, eggs, white bread, pasta, simple desserts, clear soups, tea, and coffee. Omitted are highly seasoned or fried foods, all fruits and fruit juices, raw vegetables, whole grain cereals and bread, nuts, jams, and usually milk. The diet is prescribed in cases of diverticulitis, GI irritability or inflammation, and before and after GI surgery. Because it is lacking in calcium, iron, and vitamins, it should be used only for a limited time or with nutrient supplementation. Physician's orders must read low fiber/low residue as low fiber may not always indicate low residue. Also called **low-fiber diet.**

**low-salt diet.** See **low-sodium diet.**

**low-saturated-fat diet.** See **low-cholesterol diet.**

**low-sodium diet,** a diet that restricts the use of sodium chloride plus other compounds containing sodium such as baking powder or soda, monosodium glutamate, sodium citrate, sodium propionate, and sodium sulfate. It is indicated in hypertension, edematous states (especially when associated with cardiovascular disease), renal or liver disease, and therapy with corticosteroids. The degree of sodium restriction depends on the severity of the condition. Foods included in the diet are eggs, skimmed milk, beef, poultry, lamb, pork, veal, fish, potatoes, green beans, broccoli, asparagus, peas, salad ingredients, and fresh fruits. Many flavoring extracts, spices, and herbs can be used to add taste to the diet. Foods to be avoided include fresh or canned shellfish, ham, bacon, frankfurters, luncheon meats, sausage, cheese, salted butter or margarine, any breads or cereals made with salt, beets, carrots, celery, sauerkraut, spinach, and most canned or frozen foods—unless prepared without sodium, for example, frozen fruits and vegetables. Also to be avoided are many drugs such as laxatives, sedatives, and alkalizers, which contain sodium, and drinking water from a source using a water softener that adds sodium. Also called **low-salt diet, salt-free diet, sodium-restricted diet.**

**loxapine** /lok′səpēn/, a tranquilizer.

■ INDICATION: It is prescribed in the treatment of schizophrenia.

■ CONTRAINDICATIONS: Parkinson's disease, concurrent administration of central nervous system depressants, liver or kidney dysfunction, severe hypotension, or known hypersensitivity to this drug prohibits its use.

■ ADVERSE EFFECTS: Among the more serious adverse effects are hypotension, liver toxicity, a variety of extrapyramidal reactions, and hypersensitivity reactions.

**Loxitane,** trademark for an antipsychotic (loxapine succinate).

**loxo-,** combining form meaning 'oblique, slanting': loxophthalmus, loxotic, loxotomy.

**lozenge.** See **troche.**

**LPL,** abbreviation for **lipoprotein lipase.**

**Lpm,** abbreviation for liters per minute.

**LPN,** abbreviation for **licensed practical nurse.**

**LPS Act,** a California law named for sponsors of the legislation (Lanterman, Petris, and Short) that provides for the protection and treatment of persons judged to be 'gravely disabled' and thus unable to provide food, clothing, or shelter for themselves. The legislation was designed to safeguard the constitutional rights of persons threatened with involuntary commitment on the basis of a psychiatric diagnosis. Some other states have similar laws.

**Lr,** symbol for the element **lawrencium.**

**LSD,** abbreviation for lysergic acid diethylamide. See **lysergide.**

**L/S ratio,** the lecithin/sphingomyelin ratio, used in a test for fetal lung maturity.

**LTB,** abbreviation for **laryngotracheobronchitis.**

**LTC,** abbreviation for **long-term care.**

**LTH,** abbreviation for luteotropic hormone.

**L-thyroxine.** See **levothyroxine sodium.**

**L-Trp,** abbreviation for L-tryptophan. See **tryptophan.**

**Lu,** symbol for the element **lutetium.**

**lubb** /lub/, a syllable used to represent the first heart sound in auscultation; it is longer and lower pitched than the second heart sound. See **heart sounds.**

**lubb-dupp,** an imitation of the two basic sounds heard in the cardiac cycle. Lubb represents the first sound ($S_1$) and is made by the closure of the mitral and tricuspid valves. It is lower in pitch and lasts slightly longer than the second sound, dupp ($S_2$), which is made by the closure of the aortic valve.

**lubricant** /loo′brikənt/ [L, lubricans, making slippery], a fluid, ointment, or other agent capable of diminishing friction and making a surface slippery.

**lubricating enema** /loo′brəkā′ting/ [L, lubricans, making slippery; Gk, enienai, to send in], an enema used to lubricate the anal canal after surgery for hemorrhoids or to prevent fecal impaction. The enema solution may be made with warm olive or mineral oil. See also **oil retention enema.**

**luc-,** combining form meaning 'light': lucifugal, lucipetal, lucotherapy.

**-lucent,** suffix meaning 'light-admitting': radiolucent, translucent.

**lucid** /loo′sid/ [L, lucidus, clear], clear, rational, and able to be understood. See also **lucid interval.**

**lucid interval,** a period of relative mental clarity between periods of irrationality, especially in organic mental disorders, such as delirium and dementia.

**lucidity** /loosid′itē/ [L, lucidus, clear], pertaining to clarity of mind, perception, or intelligibility.

**lucid lethargy,** a mental state characterized by a loss of will; hence an inability to act, even though the person is conscious and intellectual function is normal. See also **lethargy.**

**lucifugal** /loosif′yəgəl/, repelled by bright light.

**Lucio's leprosy phenomenon** [R. Lucio, Mexican physician, 1819–1866], an acute form of diffuse lepromatous infection of the skin, characterized by intensely red, tender plaques, particularly on the legs. The plaques tend to progress to obstructive vasculitis, ulcers, necrosis, and scarring.

**lucipetal** /loosip′ətəl/, attracted to bright light.

**lucotherapy.** See **phototherapy.**

**Ludiomil,** trademark for an antidepressant (maprotiline hydrochloride).

**Ludwig's angina** /lood′vigz/ [Wilhelm F. von Ludwig, German surgeon, 1790–1865; L, angina, quinsy], a severe form of cellulitis in the region of the submandibular gland. Inflammatory edema may distort the floor of the mouth and make swallowing difficult. The glottis may swell suddenly, causing respiratory obstruction. Penicillin is the usual treatment.

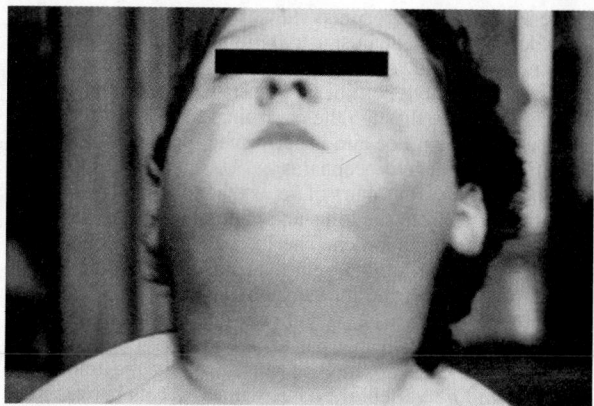

**Ludwig's angina** *(Farrar, 1992)*

**lue-**, combining form meaning 'syphilis': *luetic, luetin, luetism.*

**LUE**, abbreviation for *left upper extremity.*

**Luer-Lok syringe** /lo͞o′ərlōk′/, a glass or plastic syringe for injection having a simple screw lock mechanism that securely holds the needle in place. Also called **Luer's syringe.**

**lues.** See **syphilis.**

**-luetic, -luic**, suffix meaning 'syphilis': *antiluetic, heredoluetic, paraluetic.*

**luetic aortitis.** See **syphilitic aortitis.**

**Lufyllin,** trademark for a smooth muscle relaxant (dyphylline).

**Lugol's solution** [Jean G. A. Lugol, French physician, 1786–1851; L, *solutus,* unbound], an aqueous solution of iodine (5%) and potassium iodide (10%).

**-luic.** See **-luetic.**

**Lukes-Collins classification** [L. J. Lukes; R. D. Collins, 20th century American pathologists], a system of identifying non-Hodgkin's lymphomas according to B cell, T cell, true, and unclassifiable types. B-cell types include lymphocytic, plasmacytic, follicular cell lymphomas, and B cell–derived immunoblastic lymphoma. T-cell types include T cell–derived immunoblastic lymphoma and convoluted cell lymphoma. True types are of histiocytic origin.

**lukewarm bath** [ME, *luke* + AS, *wearm, baeth*], a bath in which the temperature of the water is between 90° and 96° F.

**LUL**, abbreviaion for *left upper lobe* of lung.

**lumbago** /lumbā′gō/ [L, *lumbus,* loin], pain in the lumbar region caused by a muscle strain, rheumatoid arthritis, osteoarthritis, or a herniated intervertebral disk. Ischemic lumbago, characterized by pain in the lower back and buttocks, is caused by vascular insufficiency, as in terminal aortic occlusion. See also **low back pain.**

**lumbar** /lum′bər, lum′bär/ [L, *lumbus,* loin], pertaining to the part of the body between the thorax and the pelvis.

**lumbar nerves,** the five pairs of spinal nerves rising in the lumbar region of the vertebral column. They become increasingly large the more caudal their origin and pass laterally and downward under the cover of the psoas major or between its fasciculi and form part of the lumbar plexus. The lumbar sympathetic ganglia follow no fixed pattern, and fusions of adjacent ganglia are common. When occurring separately, lumbar ganglia lie on the corresponding vertebra or the intervertebral disk caudally. The ganglion of the second lumbar segment is the largest, and the most constant.

**lumbar node,** a node in one of the seven groups of parietal lymph nodes serving the abdomen and the pelvis. The lumbar nodes are numerous and are divided into the lateral aortic nodes, preaortic nodes, and retroaortic nodes. They receive the afferent vessels from many different structures, such as the kidneys, the internal reproductive organs, the lateral abdominal muscles, and certain vertebrae, and pass efferents that form lymphatic trunks. Compare **sacral node.** See also **lymph, lymphatic system, lymph node.**

**lumbar plexus,** a network of nerves formed by the ventral anterior primary divisions of the first three and the greater part of the fourth lumbar nerves. It is located on the inside of the posterior abdominal wall, either dorsal to the psoas major or among its fibers and ventral to the transverse processes of the lumbar vertebrae. The branches of the lumbar plexus are the iliohypogastric, ilioinguinal, genitofemoral, lateral femoral cutaneous, obturator, accessory obturator, and femoral nerves. The iliohypogastric, ilioinguinal, and genitofemoral nerves supply the caudal part of the abdominal wall. The lateral femoral cutaneous, obturator, accessory obturator, and femoral nerves supply the anterior thigh and the middle of the leg. Only 20% of people have the accessory obturator nerve, which comes from the third and the fourth lumbar nerves. Compare **sacral plexus.** See also **lumbosacral plexus.**

**lumbar puncture (LP),** the introduction of a hollow needle and stylet into the subarachnoid space of the lumbar part of the spinal canal. It is performed in various therapeutic and diagnostic procedures. Strict aseptic technique is

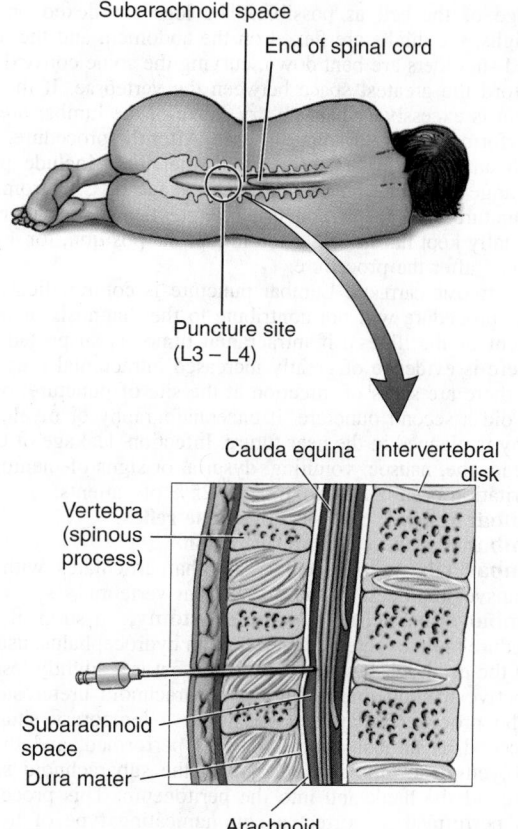

**Lumbar puncture** *(Herlihy and Maebius, 2000)*

used. Diagnostic indications include measuring of cerebrospinal fluid (CSF) pressure; obtaining CSF for laboratory analysis; evaluating the canal for the pressure of a tumor; and injecting air, oxygen, or a radiopaque substance for radiographic visualization of the structures of the nervous system of spinal canal and meninges and brain. Therapeutic indications for lumbar puncture include removing blood or pus from the subarachnoid space, injecting sera or drugs, withdrawing CSF to reduce intracranial pressure, introducing a local anesthetic to induce spinal anesthesia, and placing a small amount of the patient's blood in the subarachnoid space to form a clot to patch a rent or hole in the dura to prevent leak of CSF into the epidural space.

■ METHOD: The skin over the interspace of the third and fourth lumbar vertebrae is cleansed. A fenestrated sterile drape is placed over the back, the window over the puncture site. The needle is inserted through the interspace to the subarachnoid space, and the stylet is withdrawn. If the needle is in the proper place, clear, straw-colored CSF will begin to drip out through the needle. Depending on the indication for the procedure, various techniques follow. The pressure of the CSF may be measured using a manometer attached to a catheter and stopcock, or fluid may be withdrawn, visually examined, and sent to the laboratory for chemical or bacteriologic analysis.

■ INTERVENTIONS: The nurse is often responsible for obtaining the patient's written permission for the physician to perform a lumbar puncture. If the patient is apprehensive, he or she is given a sedative one-half hour before the procedure. The techniques to be used and the treatments to be given or the information to be obtained are explained. The patient is placed in a lateral recumbent position, the back as near the edge of the bed as possible. The legs are flexed on the thighs, the thighs are flexed on the abdomen, and the head and shoulders are bent down, curving the spine convexly to afford the greatest space between the vertebrae. If the patient is excessively hairy, a dry shave of the lumbar area is performed before draping the area. After the procedure, significant signs to be observed by the nurse include pain, change in mentation or alertness, leakage of CSF from the puncture site, fever, and urinary retention. The patient is usually kept flat in bed, often in a prone position, for 4 to 6 hours after the procedure.

■ OUTCOME CRITERIA: Lumbar puncture is contraindicated if the procedure will not contribute to the diagnosis or treatment of the illness, if intracranial tumor is suspected and there is evidence of greatly increased intracranial pressure, if there are signs of infection at the site of puncture, or, to avoid a second puncture, if encephalography or myelography is planned in the near future. Infection, leakage of CSF, headache, nausea, vomiting, dysuria, or signs of meningeal irritation occur in approximately 25% of patients.

**lumbar reflex.** See **erector spinae reflex.**

**lumbar region.** See **lateral region.**

**lumbar rib,** a rudimentary rib that articulates with the transverse process of the first lumbar vertebra.

**lumbar subarachnoid peritoneostomy,** a surgical procedure to drain cerebrospinal fluid in hydrocephalus, usually in the newborn. It spares the kidney but is a slightly less effective method than a lumbar subarachnoid ureterostomy. The procedure may be used when a temporary shunt is needed. A lumbar laminectomy is performed, and then a polyethylene tube is passed from the subarachnoid space around the flank and into the peritoneum. This procedure is performed to correct a communicating type of hydrocephalus.

**lumbar subarachnoid ureterostomy,** a surgical procedure to drain cerebrospinal fluid through the ureter to the bladder in hydrocephalus, usually in the newborn. A lumbar laminectomy and a left nephrectomy are performed, after which a polyethylene tube is passed from the lumbar subarachnoid space through the paraspinal muscles and into the free ureter. The procedure is performed to correct a communicating type of hydrocephalus.

**lumbar veins,** four pairs of veins that collect blood by dorsal tributaries from the loins and abdominal tributaries from the walls of the abdomen. The lumbar veins are connected by the ascending lumbar vein that runs ventral to the transverse processes of the lumbar vertebrae.

**lumbar vertebra,** *pl.* **vertebrae,** one of the five largest segments of the movable part of the vertebral column, distinguished by the absence of a foramen in the transverse process and by vertebral bodies without facets between the sacrum and thoracic vertebrae. The body of each lumbar vertebra is flattened or slightly concave superiorly and inferiorly and is deeply constricted ventrally at the sides. The spinous process of each is thick, broad, and somewhat quadrilateral. The body of the fifth lumbar vertebra is much deeper ventrally than dorsally and in some individuals is defective, tending to weaken the spinal column. Compare **cervical vertebra, coccygeal vertebra, sacral vertebra, thoracic vertebra.**

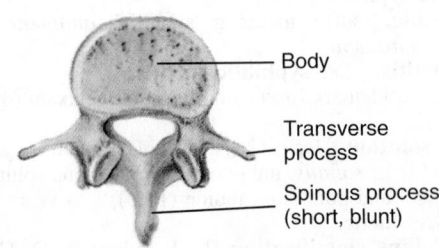

— Body

— Transverse process

— Spinous process (short, blunt)

**Lumbar vertebra** *(Applegate, 2000)*

**lumbo-,** combining form meaning 'loins': *lumbocolostomy, lumbocostal, lumbosacral.*

**lumbocostal** /lum'bōkos'təl/, pertaining to the lumbar region and ribs.

**lumbodorsal fascia.** See **fascia thoracolumbalis.**

**lumbosacral** /lum'bōsā'krəl/ [L, *lumbus,* loin, *sacrum,* sacred], pertaining to the lumbar vertebrae and the sacrum. Also called **sacrolumbar.**

**lumbosacral plexus** [L, *lumbus,* loin, *sacrum,* sacred, *plexus,* braided], the combination of all the ventral anterior primary divisions of the lumbar, the sacral, and the coccygeal nerves. The lumbar and sacral plexuses supply the lower limb. The sacral nerves also supply the perineum through the pudendal plexus and the coccygeal area through the coccygeal plexus. See also **lumbar plexus, sacral plexus.**

**lumbrical.** See **vermiform.**

**lumbrical plus deformity** /lum'brikəl/, a complication of rheumatoid arthritis in which the lumbricals (muscles in the hands and feet) become contracted. A main effect of the dysfunction is metacarpophalangeal joint flexion and interphalangeal joint extension. Compare **boutonnière deformity.**

**lumen** /loo'mən/, *pl.* **lumina, lumens** [L, light], **1.** a tubular space or the channel within any organ or structure of the

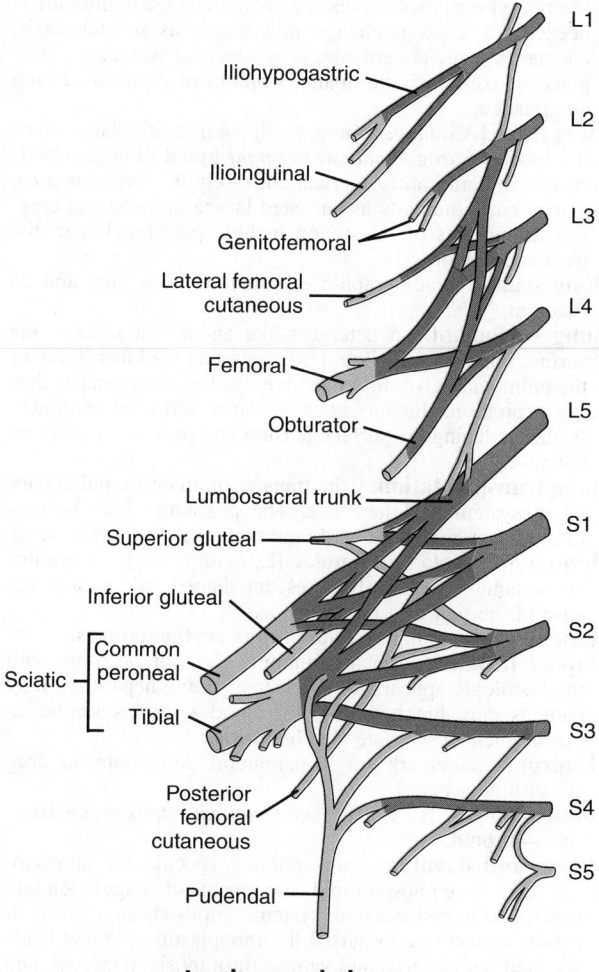

L1
L2
L3
L4
L5
S1
S2
S3
S4
S5

Iliohypogastric
Ilioinguinal
Genitofemoral
Lateral femoral cutaneous
Femoral
Obturator
Lumbosacral trunk
Superior gluteal
Inferior gluteal
Common peroneal
Sciatic
Tibial
Posterior femoral cutaneous
Pudendal

**Lumbosacral plexus**
*(Thibodeau and Patton, 1999/Network Graphics)*

body. **2.** a unit of luminous flux that equals the flux emitted in a unit solid angle by a point source of one candle intensity. —**lumenal, luminal,** *adj.*

**lumin-,** combining form meaning 'light': *luminescence, luminiferous, luminophore.*

**luminal.** See **lumen.**

**luminescence** /loo'mines'əns/ [L, *lumen,* light, *escens,* beginning], **1.** the emission of light by a material after excitation by some stimulus. **2.** the emission of light by intensifying-screen phosphors after x-ray interaction. See also **thermoluminescent dosimetry.**

**luminiferous** /loo'minif'ərəs/ [L, *lumen,* light, *ferre,* to bear], pertaining to a medium that will transmit light.

**luminophore** /loomin'əfôr/, **1.** an organic compound or chemical grouping that emits light. **2.** a substance that emits light when illuminated.

**lumpectomy** /lumpek'təmē/ [ME, *lump,* mass, *ektomē,* excision], surgical excision of a tumor without removing large amounts of surrounding tissue. See also **breast cancer.**

**lumpy jaw** [ME, *lump,* mass, *ceowan,* to chew], *nontechnical.* actinomycosis of cows, caused by infection with *Actinomyces bovis* and not communicable to humans.

**lun-,** combining form meaning 'moon': *lunacy, lunate, lunatism.*

**lunar month** /loo'nər/ [L, *luna,* moon; AS, *monath,* month], a period of 4 weeks or 28 days, approximately the time required for the moon to revolve about the earth.

**lunate bone** /loo'nāt/ [L, *luna,* moon; AS, *ban*], the carpal bone in the center of the proximal row of carpal bones between the scaphoid and triangular bones. It articulates with five bones, the radius proximally, the capitate and the hamate distally, the scaphoid laterally, and the triangular medially. Also called **os lunatum, semilunar bone.**

**lung (L)** [AS, *lungen*], one of a pair of light, spongy organs in the thorax, constituting the main component of the respiratory system. The two highly elastic lungs are the main mechanisms in the body for inhaling (inspiring) air from which oxygen is extracted for the arterial blood system and for exhaling carbon dioxide dispersed from the venous system. The right lung is divided into three lobes; the left lung, two lobes. Each lung is conical and has an apex, a base, three borders, and two surfaces. The apex is rounded and extends into the root of the neck about 4 cm above the first rib. The base of the lung is broad and concave, rests on the convex surface of the diaphragm, and with the diaphragm moves up during expiration and down during inspiration. Each lung is composed of an external serous coat, a subserous layer of areolar tissue, and the parenchyma. The serous coat comprises the thin, visceral pleura. The subserous areolar tissue contains many elastic fibers and invests the entire surface of the organ. The parenchyma is composed of secondary lobules divided into primary lobules, each of which consists of blood vessels, lymphatics, nerves, and an alveolar duct connecting with air spaces. The surfaces of the lungs are partially concave, with a cardiac impression that cradles the heart. The bronchial arteries supply blood to nourish the lungs and are derived from the ventral side of the thoracic aorta or from the aortic intercostal arteries. The bronchial vein is formed at the root of the lung. Most of the blood supplied by the bronchial arteries are returned by the pulmonary veins to the left atrium of the heart. The lungs are pinkish white at birth, and darken in later life. The coloring is from carbon granules deposited in the areolar tissue near the surface of the lung. The carbon deposits increase with age. The lungs of men are usually heavier than those of women and usually have a greater capacity. The quantity of air that can be exhaled from the lungs after the deepest inspiration, the vital capacity, averages 3700 cc.

**lung abscess** [AS, *lungen* + L, *abscedere,* to go away], a complication of an inflammation and infection of the lung, often caused by aspiration of infected material from the mouth.

**lung cancer,** a pulmonary malignancy attributable in the majority of cases to cigarette smoking. Other predisposing factors are exposure to acronitrile, arsenic, asbestos, beryllium, chloromethyl ether, chromium, coal products, ionizing radiation, iron oxide, mustard gas, nickel, petroleum, uranium, and vinyl chloride. Lung cancer develops most often in scarred or chronically diseased lungs. It is usually far advanced when detected, because metastases may precede detection of the primary lesion in the lung. Symptoms of lung cancer include persistent cough, dyspnea, purulent or blood-streaked sputum, chest pain, and repeated attacks of bronchitis or pneumonia. Diagnostic measures include x-ray films, fluoroscopy, tomography, bronchography, angiography, cytologic studies of sputum, bronchial washings or brushings, and needle biopsy. Epidermoid cancers and adenocarcinomas each account for approximately 30% of lung tumors, about 25% are small or oat cell carcinomas, and

15% are large-cell anaplastic cancers. Small cell carcinomas frequently metastasize widely before diagnosis. Surgery is the most effective treatment, but only about 20% are resectable. Lung cancer is essentially incurable unless surgical resection can be accomplished. Thoracotomy is contraindicated if metastases are found in contralateral or scalene lymph nodes. Irradiation is used to treat localized lesions and unresectable intrathoracic tumors and as palliative therapy for metastatic lesions. Radiotherapy may also be administered after surgery to destroy remaining tumor cells and may be combined with chemotherapy. Remissions are obtained in some cases treated with chemotherapeutic agents such as cyclophosphamide, procarbazine, cisplatin, VP-16, doxorubicin hydrochloride, and bleomycin. Chemotherapy is especially indicated for small-cell carcinoma.

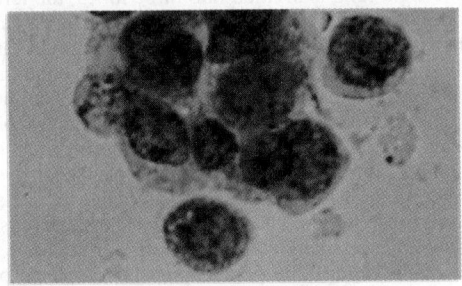

**Lung cancer cells**
*(McCance and Huether, 1998/courtesy American Cancer Society, Atlanta)*

**lung capacity,** a lung volume that is the sum of two or more of the four primary, nonoverlapping lung volumes. Lung capacities are **functional residual capacity, inspiratory capacity, total lung capacity,** and **vital capacity.**

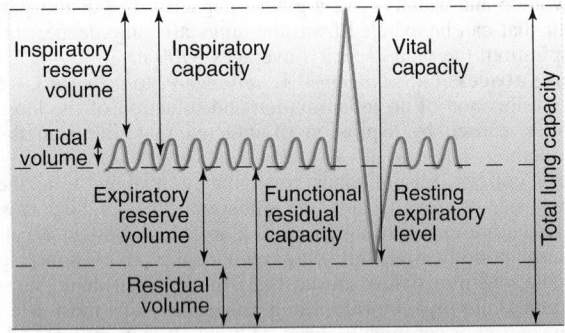

**Lung volumes and capacities**
*(Phipps, Sands, and Marek, 1999)*

**lung compliance,** a measure of the ease of expansion of the lungs and thorax. It is determined by pulmonary volume and elasticity. A high degree of compliance indicates a loss of elastic recoil of the lungs, as in old age or emphysema.

Decreased compliance means a greater change in pressure is needed for a given change in volume, as in atelectasis, edema, fibrosis, pneumonia, or absence of surfactant. Dyspnea on exertion is the main symptom of diminished lung compliance.

**lung fluke** [AS, *lungen,* lung, *floc*], a parasitic flatworm of the species *Paragonimus westermani* found throughout Africa, Asia, and Latin America, but rarely in North America. It may enter the body as encysted larvae in crabs and crayfish. Symptoms of infestation include peribronchiolar distress and hemoptysis.

**lung scan,** a radiographic examination of a lung and its function.

**lung surfactant,** a detergent-like agent that reduces the surface tension of the liquid film covering the inner lining of the pulmonary alveoli. As an alveolus becomes smaller during expiration, the surfactant becomes more concentrated, further reducing the surface tension and preventing alveolar collapse.

**lung transplantation,** the transfer of an entire pulmonary organ system to a new site. The procedure may be performed as a combined cardiopulmonary transplantation.

**lunula** /lōōn′yələ/, *pl.* **lunulae** [L, *luna,* moon], a semilunar structure, such as the crescent-shaped pale area at the base of the nail of a finger or toe.

**lupoid,** resembling **systemic lupus erythematosus.**

**lupoid hepatitis,** an autoimmune form of hepatitis with the histologic appearance of chronic active hepatitis. Many patients show lupoid cells in the blood without systemic lupus erythematosus. See also **hepatitis.**

**Lupron,** trademark for a parenteral antineoplastic drug (leuprolide acetate).

**lupus** /lōō′pəs/ [L, wolf], *nontechnical.* lupus erythematosus. **—lupoid,** *adj.*

**lupus anticoagulant,** an antibody specific for phospholipoproteins or phospholipid components of coagulation factors found in patients with systemic lupus erythematosus. It causes an increase in partial thromboplastin time and is associated with arterial and venous thrombosis, fetal loss, and thrombocytopenia.

**lupus band test,** a direct immunofluorescent method of visualizing a band of immunoglobulins and complement at the dermal-epidermal junction of involved skin in patients with systemic lupus erythematosus.

**lupus erythematosus.** See **systemic lupus erythematosus.**

**lupus erythematosus cell.** See **LE cell.**

**lupus pernio,** a cutaneous form of sarcoidosis, characterized by smooth, shiny plaques on the face, fingers, and toes, clinically resembling frostbite.

**lupus vulgaris,** a rare cutaneous form of tuberculosis in which areas of the skin become ulcerated and heal slowly, leaving deeply scarred tissue. The disease is not related to systemic lupus erythematosus.

**LUQ,** abbreviation for *left upper quadrant of abdomen.*

**Luride,** trademark for a chemical prophylactic (sodium fluoride) that reduces dental caries.

**lusus naturae** /lōō′səs/ [L, *lusus,* sport, *natura,* nature], a congenital anomaly; teratism.

**lute** /lōōt/ [L, *lutum,* mud], **1.** also called **luting agent.** a substance such as cement, wax, or clay that coats a surface or joint area to make a tight seal. **2.** to coat or seal with such a substance.

**lute-,** combining form meaning 'yellow': *luteinizing.*

**luteal** /lōō′tē-əl/, pertaining to the corpus luteum or its functions or effects.

**luteal hormone** [L, *luteus,* yellow; Gk, *hormaein,* to set in motion], a hormone produced by the **corpus luteum.** See also **progesterone.**

**luteal phase.** See **secretory phase.**

**luteal phase deficiency,** female infertility caused by inadequate secretion of progesterone during the luteal phase of the menstrual cycle. It is associated with an abnormality in pituitary gland function.

**lutein** /l$\overline{oo}$′tē·in/ [L, *luteus,* yellow], a yellow-red crystalline carotenoid pigment found in plants with carotenes and chlorophylls.

**luteinization** /l$\overline{oo}$′tē·in′īzā′shən/ [L, *luteus,* yellow], the formation of the corpus luteum from an ovarian follicle that had recently discharged an ovum. The process involves the hypertrophy of the follicular lutein cells and the development of blood vessels and connective tissue at the site.

**luteinizing hormone (LH)** /l$\overline{oo}$′tē·inī′zing/ [L, *luteus,* yellow; Gk, *izein,* to cause, *hormein,* to begin activity], a glycoprotein hormone produced by the anterior pituitary gland. It stimulates the secretion of sex hormones by the ovary and the testes and is involved in the maturation of spermatozoa and ova. In men, it induces the secretion of testosterone by the interstitial cells of the testes. Testosterone, together with follicle-stimulating hormone (FSH), induces the maturation of seminiferous tubules and stimulates them to produce sperm. In females, LH, working together with FSH, stimulates the growing follicle in the ovary to secrete estrogen. High concentrations of estrogen stimulate the release of a surge of LH, which stimulates ovulation. LH then induces the development of the ruptured follicle into the corpus luteum, which continues to secrete estrogen and progesterone. The normal LH concentration in the plasma of men is less than 11 mIU/mL. In premenopausal women it is less than 25 mIU/mL; at midcycle peak it is greater than three times the baseline concentration; in postmenopausal women it is more than 25 mIU/mL. See also **interstitial cell-stimulating hormone (ICSH), menstrual cycle.**

**luteinizing hormone assay and follicle-stimulating hormone test (LH and FSH),** a blood test used in the evaluation of infertility. An LH assay is an easy way to determine if ovulation has occurred. The LH assay and FSH test also are used to determine whether a gonadal insufficiency is primary (a problem with the ovary or testicle) or secondary (caused by pituitary insufficiency resulting in reduced levels of FSH and LH).

**luteinizing hormone–releasing hormone (LHRH),** a neurohormone of the hypothalamus that stimulates and regulates the pituitary gland's release of the luteinizing hormone.

**luteoma** /l$\overline{oo}$′tē·ō′mə/, *pl,* **luteomas, luteomata** [L, *luteus* + Gk, *oma,* tumor], **1.** a granulosa or theca cell tumor whose cells resemble those of the corpus luteum. **2.** also called **pregnancy luteoma.** A unilateral or bilateral nodular hyperplasia of ovarian lutein cells, occasionally developing during the last trimester of pregnancy.

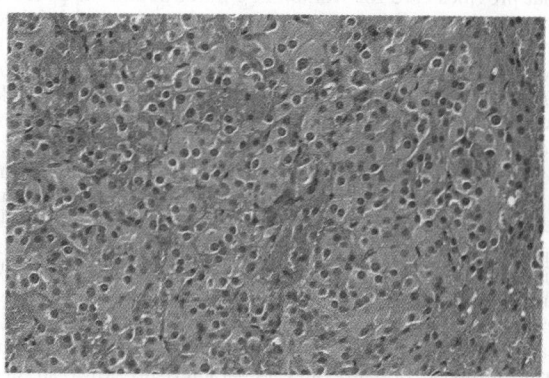

**Luteoma of pregnancy** *(Fletcher, 2000)*

**luteotropin.** See **prolactin.**

**lutetium (Lu)** /l$\overline{oo}$tē′shē·əm/ [L, *Lutetia,* Paris], a rare earth metallic element. Its atomic number is 71; and its atomic mass is 174.97.

**luting agent.** See **lute** (def. 1).

**Luvox,** trademark for an antidepressant drug (fluvoxamine maleate).

**lux (lx),** a unit of illumination equivalent to one lumen per square meter of surface when measured at right angles to the direction of the light.

**luxated joint** /luk′sātid/, a dislocated joint in which there is no contact between articular surfaces.

**luxation** /luksā′shən/ [L, *luxare,* to dislocate], dislocation.

**LV,** abbreviation for **left ventricle.**

**LVAD,** abbreviation for **left ventricular assist device.**

**LVN,** abbreviation for **licensed vocational nurse.** See **licensed practical nurse.**

**LWD,** abbreviation for *living with disease.*

**lx,** abbreviation for **lux.**

**lyases** /lē′āsez/ [Gk, *lyein,* to loosen; Fr, *disastase,* enzyme], a group of enzymes that reversibly split carbon bonds with carbon, nitrogen, or oxygen without hydrolysis or oxygen reduction reactions. The activity results in two subunits in

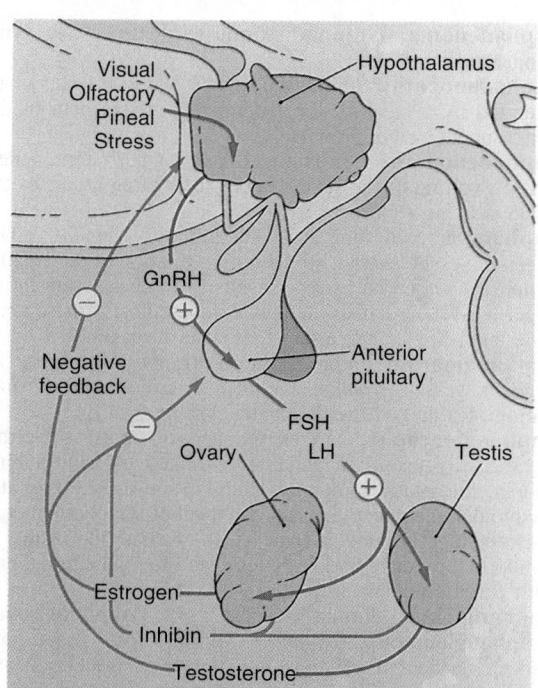

**Feedback regulation of luteinizing hormone**
*(Zitelli and Davis, 1997)*

which one or both may contain a double-bonded carbon. An example of a lyase is deaminase.

**lyco-,** combining form meaning 'wolf': *lycomania, lycorexia.*

**lycopene** /lī′kəpēn/ [Gk, *lykopersikon*, tomato], a red crystalline unsaturated hydrocarbon that is the carotenoid pigment in tomatoes and various berries and fruits. It is considered the primary substance from which all natural carotenoid pigments are derived.

**lycopenemia** /lī′kōpēnē′mē·ə/, a condition characterized by a high concentration of the carotenoid pigment lycopene in the blood, the result of ingesting large amounts of tomato products and other lycopene-rich fruits. Lycopenemia patients may develop a yellowish skin color.

**lye poisoning** /lī/ [AS, *leah*, lye; L, *potio*, drink], toxic effects of ingesting caustic soda or sodium hydroxide (NaOH), a powerful alkali. If the chemical has a pH above 11.5, the chemical burn damage to the mouth and throat is usually irreversible. An alkali burn can be more serious than an acid burn because an acid is usually neutralized by the tissues it contacts. See also **alkali poisoning.**

**lying-in** [AS, *licgan*, lying; L, *in*], **1.** designating the time before, during, and after childbirth. **2.** designating a hospital that provides care for women in childbirth and the puerperium. **3.** the condition of being in confinement, or childbed.

**Lyme disease** /līm/ [Lyme, Connecticut, where originally described], an infection caused by the spirochete, *Borrelia burgdorferi,* transmitted by the bite of infected *Ixodes* ticks (which are far smaller than dog ticks). In the northeast and north-central United States, the ticks normally feed on the white-footed mouse, the white-tailed deer, or other mammals and birds. Ticks are most likely to spread infection after 2 or more days of feeding. Most commonly, nymph ticks spread the disease because they are smaller than 2 mm in size and are rarely noticed. In contrast, the larger adult ticks are more likely to be found and removed before they have transmitted infection. Early stage symptoms of Lyme disease are fatigue, fever, chills, headache, muscle and joint pain, lymphadenopathy, and a characteristic skin rash, erythema migrans. Untreated infection in a small percentage of people can eventually result in arthritis, nervous system abnormalities, and cardiac dysrhythmias. Laboratory tests for infection and disease have not been fully standardized. Treatment consists of oral or IV antibiotics. A licensed vaccine is available but is only partially effective in preventing disease. See also **bullseye rash, erythema migrans.**

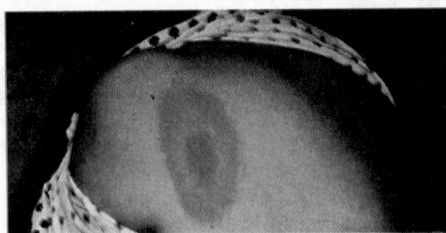

**Lyme disease** *(Stone and Gorbach, 2000)*

**lymph** /limf/ [L, *lympha*, water], a thin watery fluid originating in organs and tissues of the body that circulates through the lymphatic vessels and is filtered by the lymph nodes. Lymph enters the bloodstream at the junction of the internal jugular and subclavian veins. Lymph contains chyle, erythrocytes, and leukocytes, most of which are lymphocytes. See also **chyle, lymphatic system, lymphatic vessels.**

**lymph-, lympho-, -lymph,** combining meaning 'the lymph': *lymphoduct, neurolymph, perilymph.*

**lymphadenectomy,** surgical removal of a lymph node or nodes. Also called **lymph node dissection.**

**lymphadenitis** /limfad′inī′tis, lim′fəd-/ [L, *lympha* + Gk, *aden*, gland, *itis*, inflammation], an inflammatory condition of the lymph nodes, usually the result of systemic neoplastic disease, bacterial infection, or other inflammatory condition. The nodes may be enlarged, hard, smooth or irregular, and red and may feel hot. The location of the affected node is indicative of the site or origin of disease.

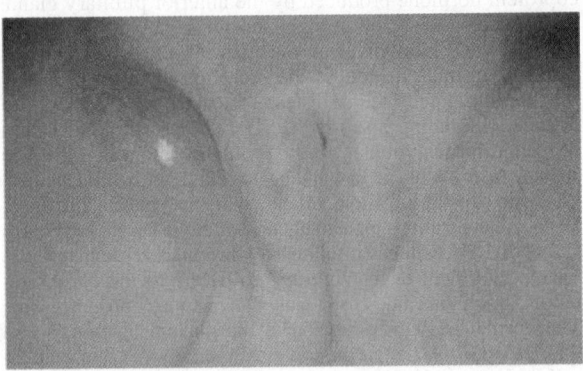

**Lymphadenitis** *(Zitelli and Davis, 1997)*

**lymphadenoma, lymphadenoma venerum.** See **lymphogranulomatosis.**

**lymphadenopathy** /limfad′inop′əthē/, any disorder characterized by a localized or generalized enlargement of the lymph nodes or lymph vessels.

**lymphadenopathy syndrome (LAS),** a persistent, generalized swelling of the lymph nodes. It is often a part of the AIDS-wasting syndrome.

**lymphangiectasia** /limfan′jē·ektā′zhə/ [L, *lympha* + Gk, *angeion,* vessel, *ektasis,* stretching], dilation of the smaller lymphatic vessels. It usually results from obstruction in the larger vessels, such as in pelvic tuberculosis, mesenteric node metastases, and certain protozoan diseases.

**lymphangiogram** /limfan′jē·əgram′/ [L, *lympha,* water; Gk, *angeion,* vessel, *gramma,* record], a radiographic visualization of a part of the lymphatic system.

**lymphangiography,** an x-ray done with contrast dye that is especially useful in patients suspected of having lymphoma, metastatic tumor, or Hodgkin's disease. It is also used to demonstrate the extent and level of lymphatic metastasis, to stage lymphoma patients, to evaluate the results of chemotherapy or radiation therapy, and to evaluate patients with chronic leg swelling.

**lymphangioma** /limfan′jē·ō′mə/, *pl.* **lymphangiomas, lymphangiomata** [L, *lympha* + Gk, *angeion,* vessel, *oma,* tumor], a benign yellowish-tan tumor on the skin, composed of a mass of dilated lymph vessels. The tumor is removed by excision or electrocoagulation for cosmetic reasons. Also called **angioma lymphaticum.** Compare **hemangioma.**

**lymphangioma cavernosum,** a tumor formed by dilated lymphatic vessels and filled with lymph mixed with coagulated blood. The lesion, which is often congenital, may cause extensive enlargement of the affected tissue, especially of the tongue and lips. Also called **cavernous lymphangioma.**

**lymphangioma circumscriptum,** a benign skin lesion that develops from superficial hypertrophic lymph vessels. Most often occurring in children, the lesion is characteristically pigmented and may grow to several centimeters in diameter.

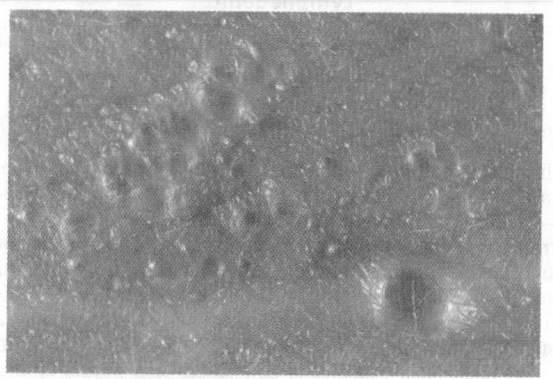

**Lymphangioma circumscriptum** *(Habif, 1996)*

**lymphangioma cysticum.** See **cystic lymphangioma.**
**lymphangioma simplex,** a growth formed by moderately dilated lymph vessels in a circumscribed area, on the skin.
**lymphangiomata.** See **lymphangioma.**
**lymphangiosarcoma** /limfan′jē·ō′särkō′mə/ [L, *lympha,* water; Gk, *angeion,* vessel, *sarx,* flesh, *oma,* tumor], a tumor arising from the lymphatic vessels.
**lymphangitis** /lim′fanjī′tis/ [L, *lympha* + Gk, *angeion,* vessel, *itis*], an inflammation of one or more lymphatic vessels, usually resulting from an acute streptococcal infection of one of the extremities. It is characterized by fine red streaks extending from the infected area to the axilla or groin and by fever, chills, headache, and myalgia. The infection may spread to the bloodstream. Penicillin and hot soaks are usually prescribed; aseptic technique is important to avoid contagion.

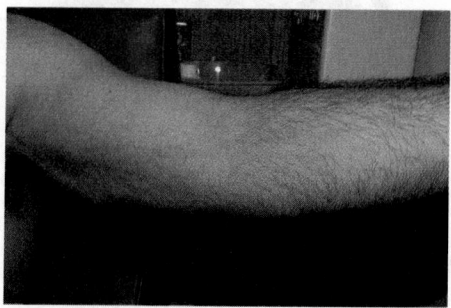

**Streptococcal lymphangitis** *(Stone and Gorbach, 2000)*

**lymphatic** /limfat′ik/ [L, *lympha* + *icus,* form], **1.** pertaining to the lymphatic system of the body, consisting of a vast network of tubes transporting lymph. **2.** any of the vessels associated with the lymphatic network.
**lymphatic capillary plexus,** one of the numerous networks of lymphatic capillaries that collect lymph from the intercellular fluid and constitute the beginning of the lymphatic system. The lymphatic vessels arise from the capillary plexuses, which vary in size and number in different regions and organs of the body. The capillary networks do not contain lymphatic valves as do the vessels. The plexuses are especially abundant in the dermis of the skin but also lace many other areas such as the mucous membranes of the respiratory and digestive systems, testes, ovaries, liver, kidneys, and heart. See also **lymphatic system.**

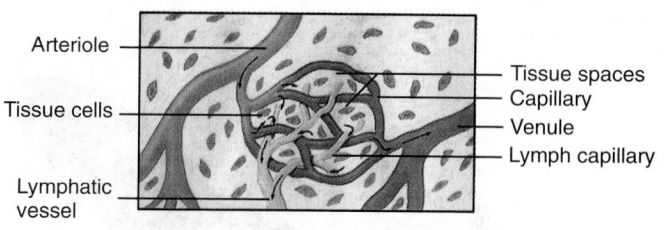

Arteriole
Tissue cells
Lymphatic vessel
Tissue spaces
Capillary
Venule
Lymph capillary

**Lymphatic capillary plexus** *(Applegate, 2000)*

**lymphatic leukemia.** See **acute lymphocytic leukemia, chronic lymphocytic leukemia.**
**lymphatic nodule.** See **malpighian body.**
**lymphatic organ** [L, *lympha,* water; Gk, *organon,* instrument], any body structure composed of lymphatic tissue, such as the thymus, spleen, tonsils, and lymph nodes.
**lymphatic system,** a vast, complex network of capillaries, thin vessels, valves, ducts, nodes, and organs that helps protect and maintain the internal fluid environment of the entire body by producing, filtering, and conveying lymph and producing various blood cells. The lymphatic network also transports fats, proteins, and other substances to the blood system and restores 60% of the fluid that filters out of the blood capillaries into interstitial spaces during normal metabolism. Small semilunar valves throughout the lymphatic network help to control the flow of lymph and, at the junction with the venous system, prevent venous blood from flowing into the lymphatic vessels. The lymph collected throughout the body drains into the blood through two ducts situated in the neck. The thoracic duct that rises into the left side of the neck is the major vessel of the lymphatic system and conveys lymph from the whole body, except for the right quadrant, which is served by the right lymphatic duct. Lymph flows into the general circulation through the thoracic duct at a rate of about 125 ml per hour during routine exertion. Various body dynamics such as respiratory pressure changes, muscular contractions, and movements of organs surrounding lymphatic vessels combine to pump the lymph through the lymphatic system. The lymphatic capillaries, which are the beginning of the system, abound in the dermis of the skin, forming a continuous network over the entire body, except for the cornea. The system also includes specialized lymphatic organs such as the tonsils, the thymus, and the spleen. See also **lymph, lymph node, lymph ves-**

**sels, spleen, thymus,** and the Color Atlas of Human Anatomy.

**lymphatic vasculitis,** a condition of blood vessel necrosis in which the vessels acquire fibrinoid deposits and are infiltrated by lymphocytes. It is associated with graft-versus-host disease.

**lymphatic vessels** [L, *lympha,* water, *vascellum,* little vase], fine, thin-walled, transparent valved channels distributed through most tissues. They are often distinguished by their beaded appearance, which is caused by an irregular lumen. The collecting branches form two systems, one generally running with the superficial veins and the other below the deep fascia and including the intestinal lacteals. Lymphatics resemble veins but have more valves, thinner walls, and contain lymph nodes. They drain through a thoracic duct and a right lymphatic duct into the venous system near the base of the neck. They include three layers: intima, media, adventitia.

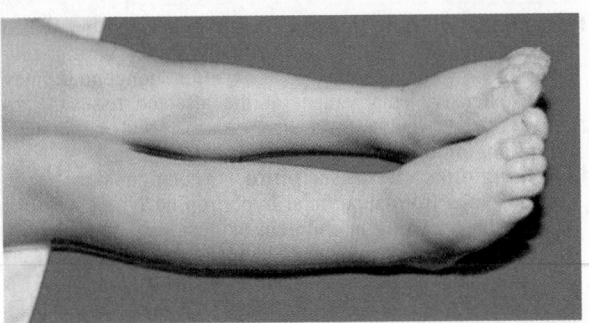

**Lymphedema**
(Seidel et al, 1995/courtesy Walter Tunnessen, MD, University of Penn, School of Medicine, Philadelphia)

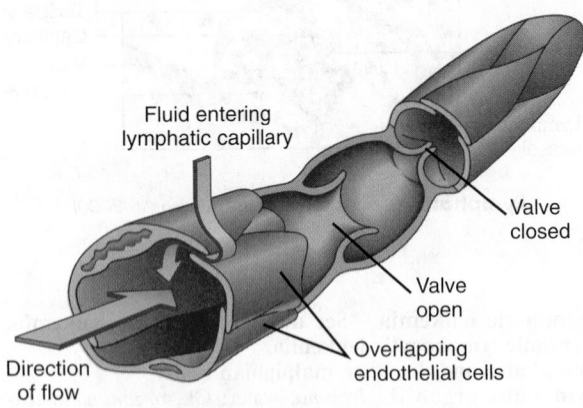

**Lymphatic vessel**
(Thibodeau and Patton, 1999/Network Graphics)

thirst are contraindicated. Surgery may be performed to remove hypertrophied lymph channels and disfiguring tissue. —**lymphedematous, lymphedematose,** *adj.*

**lymph node** [L, *lympha* + *nodus,* knot], one of the many small oval structures that filter the lymph and fight infection and in which lymphocytes, monocytes, and plasma cells are formed. The lymph nodes are of different sizes, some as small as pinheads, others as large as lima beans. Each node is enclosed in a capsule; is composed of a lighter-colored cortical part and a darker medullary part; and consists of closely packed lymphocytes, reticular connective tissue laced by trabeculae, and three kinds of sinuses: subcapsular, cortical, and medullary. Lymph flows into the node through afferent lymphatic vessels that open into the subcapsular sinuses. Most lymph nodes are clustered in areas such as the mouth, the neck, the lower arm, the axilla, and the groin. The lymphatic network and nodes of the breast are especially crucial in the diagnosis and treatment of breast cancer. Also called **lymph gland.**

**lymph cell** See **lymphocyte.**

**lymphedema** /lim′fidē′mə/ [L, *lympha* + Gk, *oidema,* swelling], a primary or secondary condition characterized by the accumulation of lymph in soft tissue and the resultant swelling caused by inflammation, obstruction, or removal of lymph channels. Congenital lymphedema (Milroy's disease) is a hereditary disorder characterized by chronic lymphatic obstruction. Lymphedema praecox occurs in adolescence, chiefly in females, and causes puffiness and swelling of the lower limbs, apparently because of hyperplastic development of lymph vessels. Secondary lymphedema may follow surgical removal of lymph channels in mastectomy, obstruction of lymph drainage caused by malignant tumors, or the infestation of lymph vessels with adult filarial parasites. Lymphedema of the lower extremities begins with mild swelling of the foot; gradually extends to the entire limb; and is aggravated by prolonged standing, pregnancy, obesity, warm weather, and the menstrual period. The disorder has no cure, but lymph drainage from the extremity can be improved if the patient sleeps with the foot of the bed elevated 4 to 8 inches, wears elastic stockings, and takes moderate exercise regularly. Light massage in the direction of the lymph flow and thiazide diuretics may be prescribed; constricting clothing and salty or spicy foods that increase

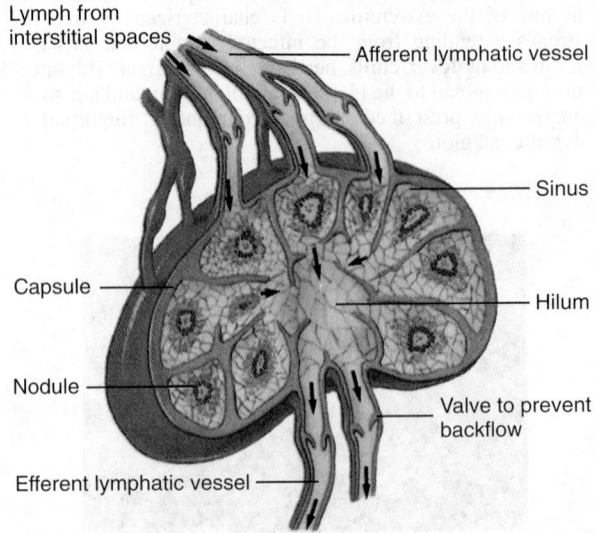

**Lymph node** (Applegate, 2000)

**lymph node dissection.** See **lymphadenectomy.**

**lymph nodule** [L, *lympha,* water, *nodulus,* small knot], any of the small densely packed spheric nodes or aggregations of lymph cells embedded in the reticular meshwork of the lymphatic system, mainly in the tonsils, spleen, and thymus.

**lympho-** See **lymph-.**

**lymphoblast** /lim'fəblast'/, a large, immature cell that develops into a lymphocyte after an antigenic or mitogenic challenge.

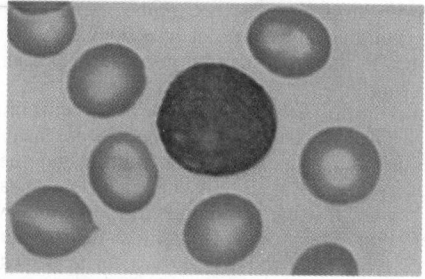

**Lymphoblast** *(Carr and Rodak, 1999)*

**lymphoblastic lymphoma, lymphoblastic lymphosarcoma, lymphoblastoma.** See **poorly differentiated lymphocytic malignant lymphoma.**

**lymphocele** /lim'fəsēl/, a tumor that contains lymph from injured lymph vessels. Also called **lymphocyst.**

**lymphocyte** /lim'fəsīt/ [L, *lympha* + Gk, *kytos,* cell], small agranulocytic leukocytes originating from fetal stem cells and developing in the bone marrow. Lymphocytes normally comprise 25% of the total white blood cell count but increase in number in response to infection. Two forms occur: B cells and T cells. B cells circulate in an immature form and synthesize antibodies for insertion into their own cytoplasmic membranes. Both reproduce mitotically, each of the clones displaying identical antibodies on their surface membranes. When an immature B cell is exposed to a specific antigen, the cell is activated, traveling to the spleen or to the lymph nodes, differentiating, and rapidly producing **plasma cells** and **memory cells.** Plasma cells synthesize and secrete antibody. Memory cells do not secrete antibody but, on reexposure to the specific antigen, develop into antibody-secreting plasma cells. T cells are lymphocytes that have cir-

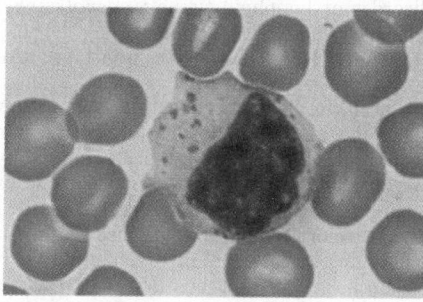

**Lymphocyte** *(Carr and Rodak, 1999)*

culated through the thymus gland and have differentiated to become thymocytes. When exposed to an antigen they divide rapidly and produce large numbers of new T cells sensitized to that antigen. Some T cells are often called 'killer cells' because they secrete immunologically essential chemical compounds and assist B cells in destroying foreign protein. T cells also appear to play a significant role in the body's resistance to the proliferation of cancer cells. Also called **lymph cell, lymphocyst.** See also **lymphokine.**

**lymphocyte activation,** the stimulation of lymphocytes by antigens or mitogens, rendering them metabolically active and causing them to differentiate into effector cells.

**lymphocyte immune globulin (anti-thymocyte),** an immunosuppressant.

■ INDICATIONS: This drug is used to prevent rejection of organ transplants and to treat aplastic anemia.

■ CONTRAINDICATIONS: Known hypersensitivity to this drug prohibits its use.

■ ADVERSE EFFECTS: When this drug is used in renal transplants, life-threatening effects include seizures and anaphylaxis. Other adverse effects include fever, headache, dizziness, weakness, faintness, rash, pruritus, urticaria, wheals, diarrhea, nausea, vomiting, epigastric pain, chest pain, hypertension, and tachycardia. When the drug is used to treat aplastic anemia, seizures are a life-threatening effect. Other adverse effects include fever, chills, headache, lightheadedness, encephalitis, postviral encephalopathy, bradycardia, myocarditis, irregularity, nausea, and abnormal liver function tests.

**lymphocyte immunophenotyping,** a blood test used to detect the progressive depletion of CD4 T lymphocytes, which is associated with an increased likelihood of clinical complications from AIDS. Test results can also indicate if an AIDS patient is at risk for developing opportunistic infections.

**lymphocyte transformation,** an in vitro immunity test process in which a patient's lymphocytes are placed in a culture with an antigen. The rate of transformation, in terms of proliferation and enlargement of T memory cells, is measured by the uptake of radioactive thymidine by the lymphocytes, indicating protein synthesis.

**lymphocytic choriomeningitis** /lim'fəsit'ik/ [L, *lympha* + Gk, *kytos,* cell, *chorion,* skin, *meninx,* membrane, *itis,* inflammation], an arenavirus infection of the meninges and the cerebrospinal fluid. It is caused by the lymphocytic choriomeningitis virus and characterized by fever, headache, and stiff neck. The infection occurs primarily in young adults, most often in the fall and winter months. Recovery usually takes place within 2 weeks.

**lymphocytic hypophysitis,** the massive infiltration of the pituitary gland by lymphocytes and plasma cells, with destruction of the normal parenchyma. The disorder is believed to have an autoimmune basis.

**lymphocytic interstitial pneumonia (LIP),** a diffuse respiratory disorder characterized by fibrosis and accumulation of lymphocytes in the lungs. It is commonly associated with lymphoma and may progress to lymphoma.

**lymphocytic leukemia.** See **acute lymphocytic leukemia, chronic lymphocytic leukemia.**

**lymphocytic lymphoma, lymphocytic lymphosarcoma.** See **well-differentiated lymphocytic malignant lymphoma.**

**lymphocytic thyroiditis.** See **Hashimoto's disease.**

**lymphocytoma.** See **well-differentiated lymphocytic malignant lymphoma.**

**lymphocytopenia** /lim'fōsī'təpē'nē·ə/ [L, *lympha* + Gk, *kytos,* cell, *penes,* poor], a decreased number of lymphocytes in the peripheral circulation, occurring as a primary hematologic disorder or in association with nutritional deficiency, malignancy, or infectious mononucleosis. Compare **alymphocytosis.** See also **agranulocyte.**

**lymphocytosis** /lim′fōsītō′sis/,   a proliferation of lymphocytes, as occurs in certain chronic diseases and during convalescence from acute infections.

**lymphocytotoxic antibody** /lim′fōsītotok′sik/,   an antibody that induces the cell-killing activity of killer lymphocytes on combining with a certain antigen.

**lymphocytotrophic** /-trof′ik/,   having an affinity for lymphocytes.

**lymphoderma perniciosa.**   See **leukemia cutis.**

**lymphoepithelioma** /lim′fō·ep′ithē′lē·ō′mə/ [L, *lympha* + Gk, *epi,* above, *thele,* nipple, *oma,* tumor],   a poorly differentiated neoplasm developing from the epithelium overlying lymphoid tissue in the nasopharynx. It occurs most frequently in young people of Asian origin. Also called **lymphoepithelial carcinoma.**

**lymphogenesis** /-jen′əsis/,   the formation of lymph.

**lymphogenous leukemia.**   See **acute lymphocytic leukemia, chronic lymphocytic leukemia.**

**lymphogranulomatosis** /-gran′yəlō′mətō′sis/ [L, *lympha,* water, *granulum,* small grain + Gk, *oma,* tumor, *osis,* condition],   an infectious granuloma of the lymphatic system. The term is used to identify several inflammatory, granulomatous or sarcomatous disorders, such as **Hodgkin's disease, sarcoidosis, lymphadenoma,** and **lymphadenoma venereum.**

**lymphogranuloma venereum (LGV)** /-gran′yəlō′mə/ [L, *lympha* + *granulum,* small grain; Gk, *oma,* tumor; L, *Venus,* goddess of love],   a sexually transmitted disease caused by a strain of the bacterium *Chlamydia trachomatis.* It is characterized by ulcerative genital lesions, marked swelling of the lymph nodes in the groin, headache, fever, and malaise. Ulcerations of the rectal wall occur less commonly. The disease is diagnosed by isolating the organism from an infected node, demonstrating LGV antibodies by serologic blood test. Doxycycline is usually prescribed for the patient and any person with whom there has been sexual contact. When changing dressings, aseptic technique is used. Also called **lymphopathia venereum.** See also *Chlamydia.*

**lymphography.**   See **lymphangiography.**

**lymphoid** /lim′foid/ [L, *lympha,* water; Gk, *eidos,* form],   pertaining to lymph or lymphatics.

**lymphoid aplasia,**   failure of development of lymphoid tissue, as in severe combined immunodeficiency.

**lymphoid interstitial pneumonia (LIP),**   a form of pneumonia that involves the lower lobes with extensive alveolar infiltration by mature lymphocytes, plasma cells, and histiocytes. It is associated with human immunodeficiency virus infection, especially in children; dysproteinemia; and Sjögren's syndrome. This is an AIDS-defining illness in children.

**lymphoid leukemia.**   See **acute lymphocytic leukemia, chronic lymphocytic leukemia.**

**lymphoidocytic leukemia.**   See **stem cell leukemia.**

**lymphoid ring.**   See **Waldeyer's throat ring.**

**lymphoid system,**   the lymphoid tissue of the body considered collectively; it can be divided into primary (or central) lymphoid tissues, the thymus and bone marrow where lymphocytes differentiate from stem cells, and secondary (or peripheral) tissues, the lymph nodes, spleen, and gut-associated lymphoid tissue (tonsils, Peyer's patches) where lymphocytes take part in immune responses.

**lymphoid tissue** [L, *lympha,* water; Gk, *eidos,* form; OFr, *tissu*],   tissue that consists of lymphocytes on a framework of reticular cells and fibers, as the tonsils and adenoids.

**lymphokine** /lim′fōkīn/ [L, *lympha* + Gk, *kinesis,* motion],   one of the chemical factors produced and released by T lymphocytes that attract macrophages to the site of infection or inflammation and prepare them for attack. Kinds of lymphokines include **chemotactic factor, cytokine, lymphotoxin, migration inhibiting factor,** and **mitogenic factor.**

**lymphokine-activated killer (LAK) cells,**   nonspecific cytotoxic cells that are generated in the presence of interleukin-2 and the absence of antigen. They are distinct from human natural killer cells, peripheral T lymphocytes, or memory cytotoxic thymus-derived lymphocytes. LAK cell infusions have been used investigationally for the treatment of cancer.

**lympholysis** /limfol′əsis/ [L, *lympha* + Gk, *lysein,* to loosen],   cellular destruction of lymphocytes, especially of certain ones in the process of an immune response. —**lympholytic,** *adj.*

**lymphoma** /limfō′mə/, *pl.* **lymphomas, lymphomata** [L, *lympha* + Gk, *oma,* tumor],   a type of neoplasm of lymphoid tissue that originates in the reticuloendothelial and lymphatic systems. It is usually malignant but in rare cases may be benign. It usually responds to treatment. Two main kinds of lymphomas are Hodgkin's disease and non-Hodgkin's lymphoma (NHL). A third form, Burkitt's lymphoma, is rare in North America but relatively common in Central Africa. A rare form of lymphoma is mycosis fungoides, a chronic T-cell variation of the disease affecting the skin and internal organs. It is an insidious disorder, beginning as a plaquelike pruritic rash that spreads through the skin and becomes nodular and systemic. The various lymphomas differ in degree of cellular differentiation and content, but the manifestations are similar in all types. Hodgkin's disease lymphomas tend to affect young adults but usually respond to recently developed types of therapy. The NHL type usually strikes patients around middle age and can be more difficult to treat. Characteristically the appearance of a painless enlarged lymph node or nodes is followed by weakness, fever, weight loss, and anemia. With widespread involvement of lymphoid tissue, the spleen and liver usually enlarge; and GI disturbances, malabsorption, and bone lesions frequently develop. Men are more likely than women to develop lymphoid tumors. There has been a dramatic increase in the incidence of acquired immunodeficiency syndrome–related NHL, which is attributed to prolonged survival of such patients related to the availability of antiretroviral agents. Treatment for lymphoma includes intensive radiotherapy, chemotherapy, and biologic therapies, including interferon and monoclonal antibodies. Kinds of lymphoma include **Burkitt's lymphoma, giant follicular lymphoma, histiocytic malignant lymphoma, Hodgkin's disease,** and **mixed cell malignant lymphoma.** Formerly called **leukosarcoma.** —**lymphomatoid,** *adj.*

**-lymphoma,**   combining form meaning a 'tumor or neoplastic disorder of lymphoid tissue': *adenolymphoma, angiolymphoma, cystadenolymphoma.*

**lymphoma, non-Hodgkin's.**   See **non-Hodgkin's lymphoma.**

**lymphoma staging,**   a system for classifying lymphomas according to the extent of the disease for the purpose of treatment and prognosis. Stage I is characterized by the involvement of a single lymph node region or one extralymphatic organ or site. Stage II is characterized by the involvement of two or more lymph node regions on the same side of the diaphragm or a localized involvement of an extralymphatic organ or site plus one or more node regions on the same side of the diaphragm. In stage III, lymph nodes on both sides of the diaphragm are affected, and there may be involvement of the spleen or localized involvement of an extralymphatic organ or site. Stage IV is typified by diffuse or disseminated involvement of one or more extralymphatic organs or sites with or without associated lymph node involvement.

**lymphomata, lymphomatoid.** See **lymphoma.**

**lymphomatoid granulomatosis** /limfō'mətoid/, a condition of unknown cause in which lymphocytes and plasma cells infiltrate the blood vessels, producing an angiocentric lesion. It most often affects the lungs, causing chest pains, cough, and shortness of breath. See also **Wegener's granulomatosis.**

**lymphopathia venereum.** See **lymphogranuloma venereum.**

**lymphopenia.** See **lymphocytopenia.**

**lymphopoiesis** /-pō·ē'sis/ [L, *lympha,* water; Gk, *poien,* to make], the formation of lymphocytes. —**lymphopoietic** /-pō·et'ik/, *adj.*

**lymphoproliferative** /-prōlif'ərətiv'/ [L, *lympha,* water, *prolles,* offspring, *ferre,* to bear], pertaining to the proliferation of lymphoid tissue.

**lymphoproliferative syndrome, induced,** a group of malignant neoplasms associated with infections by human T-cell lymphotropic virus type I (HTLV-I). The neoplasms arise from the clonal proliferation of lymphoid cells. They may originate in the bone marrow, as lymphoid leukemias, or in extramedullary sites as lymphomas. The most common lymphoid leukemias include lymphoblastic leukemia, which can be rapidly fatal if untreated.

**lymphoreticular malignancy** /-retik'yələr/, a disease of the lymphoreticular system commonly associated with cell-mediated immune deficiencies in which patients have a scarcity of normal white blood cells. It is one cause of hypogammaglobulinemia.

**lymphoreticular system,** the tissues of the lymphoid and reticuloendothelial systems considered together as one system.

**lymphoreticulosis** /-retik'yəlō'sis/ [L, *lympha* + *reticulum,* little net; Gk, *osis,* condition], subacute granulomatous inflammation of lymphoid tissue with proliferation of reticuloendothelial cells, occurring most commonly as the result of a cat scratch. No causative agent is known. The disorder is characterized by the formation of an ulcerated papule at the site of the scratch, fever, and tender lymphadenopathy, sometimes progressing to suppuration. Also called **cat scratch fever.**

**lymphorrhagia,** an escape of lymph from a damaged vessel.

**lymphorrhoid** /limfôr'oid/, a dilated lymph vessel.

**lymphosarcoma.** See **non-Hodgkin's lymphoma.**

**lymphosarcoma cell leukemia** /-särkō'mə/ [L, *lympha* + Gk, *sarx,* flesh, *oma,* tumor], a malignancy of blood-forming tissues characterized by many lymphosarcoma cells in the peripheral circulation that tend to infiltrate surrounding tissues. These cells are extremely immature and larger and more reticulated than lymphocytes. The disease may accompany lymphoma or exist as a separate entity with bone marrow involvement. Also called **lymphoblastic lymphoma.**

**lymphoscintigraphy** /-sintig'rəfē/, a diagnostic technique using scintillation scanning of technetium-99m antimony trisulfide colloid in a noninvasive test for primary and secondary lymphedema. The radiopharmaceutical is injected subcutaneously in the interdigital space of the hands and feet.

**lymphotrophy** /limfot'rəfē/, the nourishment of cells by lymph, particularly in areas lacking adequate blood vessels.

**lymph sinuses** [L, *lympha,* water, *sinus,* hollow], continuous small endothelial-lined spaces just below the capsule of the lymph node. The sinuses slow the flow of lymph through the nodes.

**lymph vessels.** See **lymphatic system.**

**lyo-,** combining form meaning 'to loosen or dissolve': *lyogel, lyophobe, lyotropic.*

**Lyon hypothesis** /lī'ən/ [Mary L. Lyon, English geneticist, b. 1925], a hypothesis stating that only one of the two X chromosomes in a female is functional, the other having become inactive early in development. Either the maternal or the paternal X chromosome may be inactivated in any given cell. Therefore an X-linked trait may be expressed by some cells and not by others.

**lyonization** /lī'ənīzā'shən/ [Mary L. Lyon; Gk, *izein,* to cause], the process of random inactivation of one of the X chromosomes in the cells of females to compensate for the presence of the double X gene dose. See also **Lyon hypothesis.**

**Lyon's ring** [Mary L. Lyon], a type of congenital uropathy in females in which submeatal or distal urethral stenosis causes enuresis, dysuria, and recurring infections. The disorder is treated surgically.

**lyophilic** /lī'ōfil'ik/ [Gk, *lyein,* to dissolve, *philein,* to love], pertaining to substances having an affinity for stability, in solution. Lyophilic substances are used to stabilize colloids.

**lyophilize,** to freeze-dry a substance under vacuum conditions.

**lypressin** /līpres'in/, an antidiuretic and vasoconstrictor.

■ INDICATION: It is prescribed in diabetes insipidus to decrease urinary water loss.

■ CONTRAINDICATIONS: Vascular disease or known hypersensitivity to this drug prohibits its use.

■ ADVERSE EFFECTS: Among the most serious adverse reactions are angina in people with cardiovascular disease, nausea, cramping, and marked facial pallor.

**Lys,** abbreviation for **lysine.**

**lysate** /lī'sāt/, a product of dissolution of matter by lysis, as in the destruction of proteins by hydrolysis.

**-lyse.** See **-lyze.**

**lysemia** /līsē'mē·ə/, the disintegration of red blood cells, accompanied by the release of hemoglobin in the plasma.

**lysergide** /līsur'jīd/, a psychotomimetic, semisynthetic derivative of ergot that acts at multiple sites in the central nervous system from the cortex to the spinal cord. In susceptible individuals, as little as 20 to 25 μg of the potent drug may cause pupillary dilation, increased blood pressure, hyperreflexia, tremor, muscle weakness, piloerection, and increased body temperature. Larger doses also produce dizziness, drowsiness, paresthesia, euphoria or dysphoria, and synesthesias; colors may be heard, sounds visualized, and time is felt to pass slowly. Psychologic dependence may develop; and use of lysergide is associated with significant hazards such as panic, serious depression, paranoid behavior, and prolonged psychotic episodes. Also called **LSD** (an abbreviation of the original German name, **Lyserg-Säure-Diäthylamid, lysergic acid diethylamide**), *(slang)* **acid.** See also **hallucinogen.**

**Lysholm method,** any of several techniques for positioning a patient for radiographic examination of the cranial base, the mastoid and petrous regions of the temporal bone, the optic foramen, and the orbital fissure.

**lysin** /lī'sin/, a specific complement-fixing antibody that initiates the lysis of cells.

**-lysin,** suffix meaning a 'cell-dissolving antibody': *antilysin, betalysin, paralysin.*

**lysine (Lys)** /lī'sēn, lī'sin/,   an essential amino acid needed for proper growth in infants and for maintenance of nitrogen balance in adults. See also **amino acid, protein.**

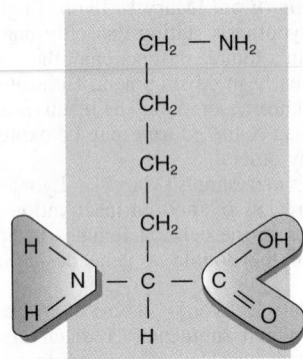

**Chemical structure of lysine**

**lysine intolerance,**   a congenital disorder resulting in the inability to hydrolyse the essential amino acid lysine because of an enzyme deficiency or defect. The disorder is characterized by weakness, vomiting, and coma. It is treated by adjusting the protein content of the diet, restricting foods especially high in lysine. See also **lysinemia.**

**lysinemia** /lī'sinē'mē-ə/,   a condition caused by an inborn error of metabolism and resulting in the inability to hydrolyse the essential amino acid lysine because of an enzyme defect or deficiency. It is characterized by muscle weakness and mental retardation. See also **lysine intolerance.**

**lysine monohydrochloride,**   a salt of the amino acid lysine, used as a dietary supplement to increase the use of vegetable proteins such as corn, rice, and wheat.

**lysinogen** /līsin'əjən/,   an antigen that stimulates the production of a specific lysin.

**lysinurea** /lī'sinŏŏr'ē-ə/,   the presence of lysine in the urine.

**lysis** /lī'sis/ [Gk, *lysein*, to loosen],   **1.** destruction or dissolution of a cell or molecule through the action of a specific agent. Cell lysis is frequently caused by a lysin. **2.** gradual diminution in the symptoms of a disease. Compare **crisis.**

**-lysis,**   suffix meaning a 'breaking down or detachment': *cytolysis, dialysis, osteolysis.*

**lysis of adhesions,**   surgery performed to free adhesions of tissues. See also **adhesiotomy.**

**lyso-,**   combining form meaning 'dissolution': *lysocephalin, lysotype, lysozyme.*

**Lysodren,**   trademark for an antineoplastic (mitotane).

**lysogenesis** /lī'səjen'əsis/ [Gk, *lysein*, loosening, *genein*, to produce],   the formation of lysins, or antibodies that cause partial or complete dissolution of the target cell.

**lysokinase** /lī'sōkī'nās/,   an enzyme that serves as an activating agent for the production of plasmin.

**lysosomal storage disease.**   See **inborn lysosomal disease.**

**lysosome** /lī'səsōm/ [Gk, *lysein* + *soma*, body],   a cytoplasmic, membrane-bound particle that contains hydrolytic enzymes that function in intracellular digestive processes. The organelles are found in most cells but are particularly prominent in leukocytes and the cells of the liver and kidney. If the hydrolytic enzymes are released into the cytoplasm, they cause self-digestion of the cell so that lysosomes may play an important role in certain self-destructive diseases characterized by the wasting of tissue, such as muscular dystrophy.

**lysotype** /lī'sətīp/,   a bacterial species type determined by its reaction to certain phages.

**lysozyme** /lī'səzīm/ [Gk, *lysein* + *en*, within, *zyme*, ferment],   an enzyme with antiseptic actions that destroys some foreign organisms. It is found in granulocytic and monocytic blood cells and is normally present in saliva, sweat, breast milk, and tears.

**lysso-,**   combining form meaning 'rabies or hydrophobia': *lyssodexis, lyssoid, lyssophobia.*

**-lyte,**   **1.** suffix meaning 'electrolyte': *ampholyte.* **2.** suffix meaning a 'substance capable of or resulting from decomposition': *cytolyte, sarcolyte.*

**lytes** /līts/,   an informal abbreviation of *electrolytes,* especially the levels of potassium, sodium, phosphorus, magnesium, and calcium in the blood, as determined by laboratory testing.

**-lytic,**   suffix meaning 'to produce decomposition': *fibrillolytic, leukolytic, myelolytic.*

**Lytren,**   trademark for a nutritional supplement containing various electrolytes.

**-lyze, -lyse,**   suffix meaning 'to produce decomposition': *bacteriolyze, hemolyze, paralyze.*

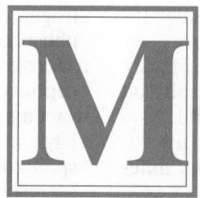

**m,** 1. abbreviation **meter.** 2. abbreviation for **milli-.**

**M,** 1. abbreviation for **mega-.** 2. abbreviation for **molar.** 3. abbreviation for *metastasis* in the tumor, node, metastasis (TNM) system for staging malignant neoplastic disease. See also **cancer staging.**

**M$_r$,** symbol for **relative molecular mass.** See **molecular mass.**

**ma,** abbreviation for **milliampere.**

**MA,** 1. abbreviation for **milliampere.** 2. abbreviation for **mental age.**

**M.A.,** abbreviation for *Master of Arts* degree.

**MAA,** abbreviation for **methacrylic acid.**

**Maass, Clara** an American nurse (1876–1901) who volunteered for military service at the outbreak of the Spanish-American War, after training and working at the Newark German Hospital, which has since been renamed for her. She worked at army camps where soldiers were dying of yellow fever, and then volunteered to go to Havana to participate in experiments to determine the cause of that disease. She was bitten by a mosquito and died 10 days later of yellow fever. She was one of the first nurses to be inducted into the Hall of Fame of the American Nurses Association.

**MAB,** abbreviation for **monoclonal antibodies.**

**mabp,** abbreviation for *mean arterial blood pressure.* See **mean arterial pressure.**

**MAC,** 1. abbreviation for **membrane attack complex.** 2. abbreviation for **microcystic adnexal carcinoma.** 3. abbreviation for **midupper arm circumference.** 4. abbreviation for **minimum alveolar concentration.**

**MAC awake,** endtidal concentration of an anesthetic agent at which 50% of patients appropriately respond to verbal commands (like "open your eyes"). It applies only to inhalation agents and is affected by the adjunctive needs, age, hypothermia, and sedatives.

**MAC disease.** See *Mycobacterium avium* **complex disease.**

**mace** /mās/, the oil-containing, red, fibrous wrapping of the nutmeg kernel. Dried and ground, it is used as an aromatic spice and flavoring. Compare **Mace.**

**Mace,** trademark for a chemical lacrimator. The name is an abbreviation formed by letters in *m*ethylchloroform-2-chloro*ace*tophenone, which is dispersed from a pressurized container to immobilize an attacker.

**macerate** /mas′ərāt/ [L, *macerare,* to soften], to soften something solid by soaking.

**maceration** /-ā′shən/, the softening and breaking down of skin resulting from prolonged exposure to moisture. Prolonged exposure to wetness causes softening of the keratin, redness, oozing, and scaling. In a postterm infant or dead fetus maceration may result from prolonged exposure to amniotic fluid.

**Machado-Joseph disease** /mä·chä′dō· jō′səf/ [Machado and Joseph, afflicted families], a progressive degenerative disease of the central nervous system occurring in families of Portuguese-Azorean descent, having a variety of forms and inherited as an autosomal dominant trait. There are four major types: *Type I,* with pyramidal and extrapyramidal

deficits; *Type II,* with cerebellar, pyramidal, and extrapyramidal deficits; *Type III,* with cerebellar deficits and distal sensorimotor neuropathy; *Type IV,* with parkinsonism and distal sensory neuropathy. Also called **Azorean disease, Joseph disease, Portuguese-Azorean disease.**

**machinery murmur.** See **Gibson's murmur.**

**machismo** /mächis′mō/, (in psychology) a concept of the male that includes both desirable traits of courage and fearlessness and the dysfunctional behaviors of heavy drinking, seduction of women, and domineering and abusive spouse behavior.

**Machover Draw-A-Person Test.** See **Draw-A-Person Test.**

**Machupo.** See **Bolivian hemorrhagic fever.**

**Macleod, John J.** (1876–1935) Scottish physiologist, cowinner, with Sir Frederick G. Banting, of the 1923 Nobel prize for medicine and physiology, for their discovery of insulin. See also **Banting, Sir Frederick G.**

**macrencephaly** /mak′rənsef′əlē/ [Gk, *makros,* large, *enkephalos,* brain], a congenital anomaly characterized by abnormal largeness of the brain. See also **macrocephaly.** —**macrencephalic,** *adj.*

**macro-, makro-** /mak′rō-/, prefix meaning 'large, or abnormal size': *macrobiosis, macrocardius, macrophage.*

**macroadenoma** /-ad′ənō′mə/, a glandular tumor more than 10 mm in diameter.

**macroamylase** /-am′ilās/, a form of serum amylase in which the enzyme is bound to a globulin. Because the resulting complex is too large for renal clearance, plasma amylase levels are increased. The elevated amylase level may not be harmful but may be diagnostic of other disorders, such as pancreatitis or biliary tract disease.

**macroamylasemia** /mak′rō-am′ilāsē′mē-ə/, the presence of macroamylase in the blood.

**macrobiosis** /-bī-ō′sis/ [Gk, *makros,* long, *bios,* life], a long life.

**macrobiotic diet** /-bī-ot′ik/, a restrictive dietary regimen consisting of grains and unprocessed foods. Also called **zen macrobiotic diet.**

**macroblepharia** /mak′rōblifer′ē-ə/ [Gk, *makros* + *blepharon,* eyelid], the condition of having abnormally large eyelids.

**macrocephaly** /mak′rōsef′əlē/ [Gk, *makros* + *kephale,* head], a congenital anomaly characterized by abnormal largeness of the head and brain in relation to the rest of the body, resulting in some degree of mental and growth retardation. The head is more than two standard deviations above the average circumference size for age, sex, race, and period of gestation, with excessively wide fontanels; the facial features are usually normal. The condition may be caused by some defect in formation during embryonic development, or it may be the result of progressive degeneration processes, such as Schilder's disease, Greenfield's disease, or congenital lipoidosis. In macrocephaly the head experiences symmetric overgrowth at the head without increased intracranial pressure, as differentiated from hydrocephalus, in which the lateral, asymmetric growth of the head is caused by excessive accumulation of cerebrospinal fluid, usually under increased pressure. Specific diagnostic tests may be necessary to differentiate the two conditions. Treatment is primarily symptomatic, with nursing care concentrated specifically on helping parents learn to care for a brain-damaged child. Also called **macrocephalia, megalocephaly.** Compare **microcephaly.** See also **hydrocephalus. —macrocephalic, macrocephalous,** *adj.,* **macrocephalus,** *n.*

**macrocyte** /mak′rəsīt/ [Gk, *makros* + *kytos,* cell], an abnormally large mature erythrocyte usually exceeding 9 μm in diameter that is commonly seen in megaloblastic anemias, for example vitamin B$_{12}$ deficiency. Compare **microcyte.** See also **macrocytic anemia.**

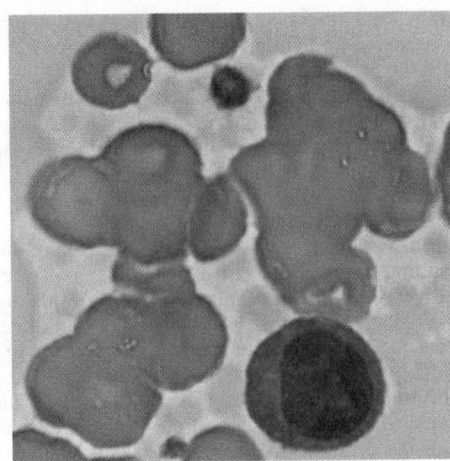

**Macrocyte** *(Carr and Rodak, 1999)*

**macrocytic** /mak′rōsit′ik/ [Gk, *makros* + *kytos* + L, *icus,* form], (of a cell) larger than normal, such as the erythrocytes in macrocytic anemia.

**macrocytic anemia,** a disorder of the blood characterized by impaired erythropoiesis and the presence of large red blood cells in the circulation. Macrocytic anemia is most often the result of a deficiency of folic acid or vitamin B$_{12}$. Compare **microcytic anemia.**

**macrocytosis** /mak′rōsītō′sis/ [Gk, *makros* + *kytos* + *osis,* condition], an abnormal proliferation of macrocytes in the peripheral blood. Compare **poikilocytosis.** See also **anisocytosis.**

**Macrodantin,** trademark for a urinary antibacterial (nitrofurantoin).

**Macrodex,** trademark for a plasma expander (dextran).

**macrodrip** /mak′rōdrip/ [Gk, *makros* + AS, *drypan,* to fall in drops], (in IV therapy) an apparatus that is used to deliver measured amounts of IV solutions at specific flow rates based on the size of drops of the solution. The size of the drops is controlled by the fixed diameter of a plastic delivery tube. Different macrodrips deliver 10, 15, or 20 drops per milliliter of solution. Macrodrips are not usually used to deliver a small amount of IV solution or to keep a vein open, because the interval between drips is so long that a clot may form at the tip of the IV catheter. Compare **microdrip.**

**macroelement,** a chemical element required in relatively large quantities for the normal physiologic processes of the body. Macroelements include carbon, hydrogen, oxygen, nitrogen, potassium, sodium, calcium, chloride, magnesium, phosphorus, and sulfur. See also **macronutrient.**

**macroencephalic, macroencephaly.** See **macrencephaly.**

**macrogamete** /-gam′ēt/ [Gk, *makros* + *gamete,* spouse], a large nonmotile female gamete of certain thallophytes and sporozoa, specifically the malarial parasite *Plasmodium.* It corresponds to the ovum of the higher animals and is fertilized by the smaller, motile male gamete. See also **microgamete.**

**macrogametocyte** /-gamē′təsīt/ [Gk, *makros* + *gamete* + *kytos,* cell], an enlarged merozoite that undergoes meiosis to form the mature female gamete during the sexual phase of the life cycle of certain thallophytes and sporozoa, specifically the malarial parasite *Plasmodium.* Macrogametocytes are found in the red blood cells of a person infected with the malarial parasite, but they must be ingested by a female *Anopheles* mosquito to complete the maturation process and develop into macrogametes.

**macrogenitosomia** /mak′rōjen′itōsō′mē·ə/ [Gk, *makros* + L, *genitalis,* genitalia; Gk, *soma,* body], a congenital condition in which the genitalia are abnormal because of an excess of androgen during fetal development. It is characterized in boys by enlarged external genitalia and in girls by pseudohermaphroditism.

**macroglobulin** /-glob′yəlin/, a globular serum protein with a molecular mass above 400 kilodaltons, such as the proteinase inhibitor alpha$_2$-macroglobulin. See also **immunoglobulin M.**

**macroglobulinemia** /mak′rōglob′yŏŏlinē′mē·ə/ [Gk, *makros* + L, *globulus,* small ball; Gk, *haima,* blood], a form of monoclonal gammopathy in which immunoglobulin (IgM) is overproduced by the clones of a plasma B cell in response to an antigenic signal. Increased viscosity of the blood may result in circulatory impairment, weakness, neurologic disorders, and fatigue. Normal immunoglobulin synthesis is decreased, and the person is susceptible to infection, particularly bacterial pneumonia and septicemia. Treatment may include therapeutic plasma exchange to lower the viscosity. Also spelled **macroglobulinaemia.** Also called **Waldenström's macroglobulinemia.** See also **multiple myeloma.**

**Macroglobulinemia** *(Carr and Rodak, 1999)*

**macroglossia** /mak′rōglos′ē·ə/ [Gk, *makros* + *glossa*, tongue], an excessively large tongue. It is seen in certain syndromes of congenital defects, including Down syndrome.

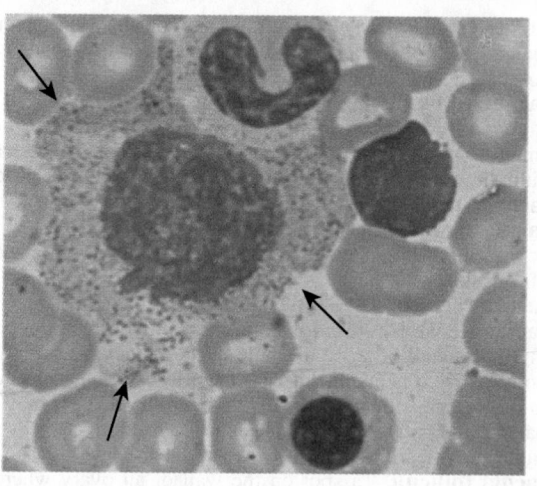

**Macrophage** *(Carr and Rodak, 1999)*

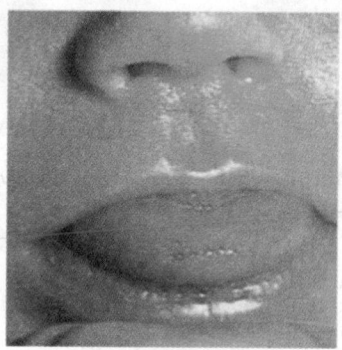

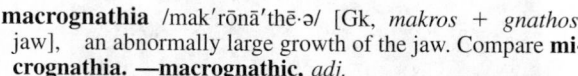

**Macroglossia**
*(Zitelli and Davis, 1992/courtesy Dr. Christine L. Williams, New York Medical College)*

**macrognathia** /mak′rōnā′thē·ə/ [Gk, *makros* + *gnathos*, jaw], an abnormally large growth of the jaw. Compare **micrognathia.** —**macrognathic,** *adj.*

**macrolide** /ma′krōlīd/, any of a group of antibiotics produced by actinomycetes. They include erythromycin, azithromycin, and clarithromycin. Macrolides are generally used against gram-positive bacteria and in patients allergic to penicillins.

**macromolecule** /-mol′əkyōōl/ [Gk, *makros* + L, *moles,* mass], a molecule of colloidal size, such as a protein, nucleic acid, or polysaccharide.

**macronodular adrenal disease** /-nod′yələr/, a form of Cushing's syndrome characterized by massively enlarged adrenal glands.

**macronucleus** /-nōō′klē·əs/ [Gk, *makros* + L, *nucleus,* nut], **1.** a large nucleus that occupies a relatively large portion of the cell. **2.** (in protozoa) the larger of two nuclei in each cell; it governs cell metabolism and growth as opposed to the micronucleus, which functions in sexual reproduction.

**macronutrient** /-nōō′triənt/ [Gk, *makros* + L, *nutriens,* food that nourishes], nutrient required in the greatest amounts: carbohydrate, protein, fat or lipid, and water. See also **macroelement.**

**macrophage** /mak′rəfāj/ [Gk, *makros* + *phagein,* to eat], any phagocytic cell of the reticuloendothelial system, including specialized Kupffer's cells in the liver and spleen, and histocyte in loose connective tissue. See also **Kupffer's cells, phagocyte, reticuloendothelial system.**

**macrophage activating factor (MAF)** [Gk. *makros,* large, *phagein,* to eat; L, *activus,* active, *facere,* to make], a lymphokine released from a sensitized leukocyte that induces changes in the appearance and function of macrophages, which make macrophages active against certain antigens.

**macrophage colony-stimulating factor (M-CSF),** a glycoprotein growth factor that induces committed bone marrow stem cells to differentiate and mature into mononuclear phagocytes.

**macrophage migration inhibiting factor** [Gk, *makros,* large; *phagein,* to eat; L, *migrare,* to wander, *inhibere,* to restrain, *facere,* to make], a lymphokine produced by leukocytes that immobilizes macrophages after contact with an antigen. Also called **leukocyte (or leucocyte) migration inhibition factor, macrophage inhibition factor (MIF).**

**macroprolactinoma** /-prōlak′tinō′mə/, a pituitary tumor more than 10 mm in diameter that causes serum prolactin levels higher than 200 ng/mL. Bromocriptine is used with some success to shrink tumor size before surgery. Frequent monitoring of endocrine status is indicated for the remainder of the patient's life after therapy.

**macropsia** /makrop′sē·ə/ [Gk, *makros,* large, *opsis,* vision], a visual abnormality in which objects appear larger than they actually are.

**macroreentry circuit** /mak′rōrē·en′trē/ [Gk, *makros* + L, *re,* again; Fr, *entree,* entry], a relatively large pathway for the reactivation of myocardial tissue by the same impulse. Examples include a reentry circuit that uses one bundle branch for anterograde conduction and another for retrograde conduction to produce the highly malignant bundle branch reentry ventricular tachycardia. Another circuit runs between the top and bottom of the right atrium and produces atrial flutter.

**macroscopic** /-skop′ik/ [Gk, *makros,* large, *skopein,* to view], large enough to be examined with the naked eye.

**macroscopic anatomy.** See **gross anatomy.**

**macroshock,** shock from an electric current of 1 milliampere (mA) or greater. Currents from 1 to 15 mA produce a tingling sensation and some muscle contraction, those from 15 to 100 mA can cause a painful shock, those from 100 to 200 mA can cause cardiac fibrillation or respiratory arrest, and those above 200 mA may produce rapid burning and destruction of tissue.

**macrosis** /makrō′sis/ [Gk, *makros,* large, *osis,* condition], an increase in the size or volume of an object.

**macrosomia.** See **gigantism.**

**macrostomia.** See **cleft cheek.**

**macrotear** /-ter/, a significant damage to soft tissues caused by acute trauma.

**macula** /mak'yələ/, *pl.* **maculae** [L, spot], a small pigmented area or a spot that appears separate or different in color from the surrounding tissue.

**macula adherens.** See **desmosome.**

**macula albida** [L, *macula*, spot, *albidare*, to make white], small white areas in the serous membranes of the pericardium or in the peritoneum or pleura. Also called **milk patch, tache laiteuse** /täsh'latœs'/.

**macula atrophica,** a condition of cutaneous atrophy characterized by the appearance of small glistening white spots on the skin.

**macula cerulea.** See **blue spot,** def. 1.

**macula densa** [L, *macula*, spot, *densus*, thick], a thickening in the wall of a distal tubule of the kidney nephron at a point where it is in contact with the afferent glomerulus and in direct opposition to the juxtaglomerular cells. It may be part of a negative-feedback system for sodium.

**maculae.** See **macula.**

**macula folliculi,** a spot on the wall of an ovary where a mature follicle will rupture to release an ovum.

**macula lutea,** an oval yellow spot at the optical "center" of the retina 2 mm from the optic nerve. It contains a pit, no blood vessels, and the fovea centralis which contains only retinal cones. Central high-acuity vision occurs when an image is focused directly on the fovea centralis of the macula lutea. Also called *(informal)* **macula.**

**macular.** See **macule.**

**macular degeneration** /mak'yələr/ [L, *macula*, spot, *degenerare*, to deviate], a progressive deterioration of the maculae of the retina. The condition may occur as a primary disorder or may be an effect of several diseases, such as **retinitis pigmentosa.**

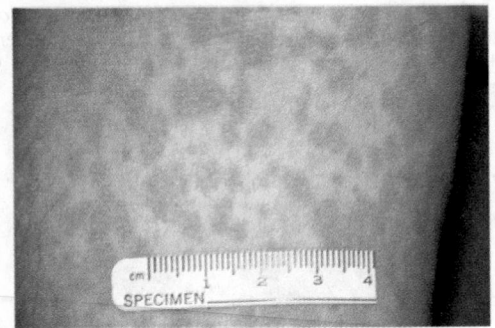

**Macular rash** *(Lemmi and Lemmi, 2000)*

**macula solaris** [L, *macula*, spot, *solaris*, sun], a freckle.

**macule** /mak'yo͞ol/ [L, *macula*, spot], **1.** a small flat blemish or discoloration that is level with the skin surface. Examples are freckles and some rashes. Compare **papule. 2.** a gray scar on the cornea that is visible without magnification. —**macular,** *adj.*

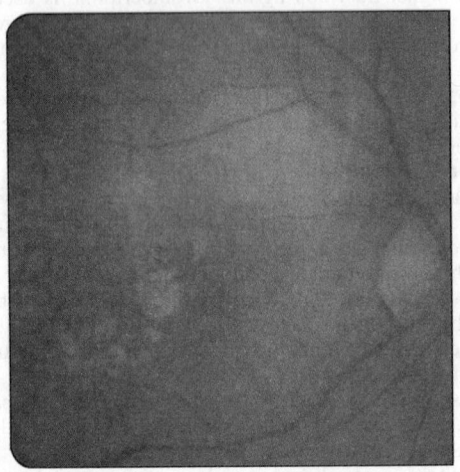

**Macular degeneration** *(Kanski and Nischal, 1999)*

**macular dystrophy,** any of a variety of eye disorders that damage the central part of the retina. Several of the disorders are related to gene mutations that affect older adults, including Sorsby's fundus dystrophy, caused by an excessive growth of blood vessels through the basal membrane, which thickens and bleeds. See also **macular degeneration.**

**macular rash** [L, *macula*, spot; OFr, *rasche*], a skin eruption in which the lesions are flat and less than 1 cm in diameter.

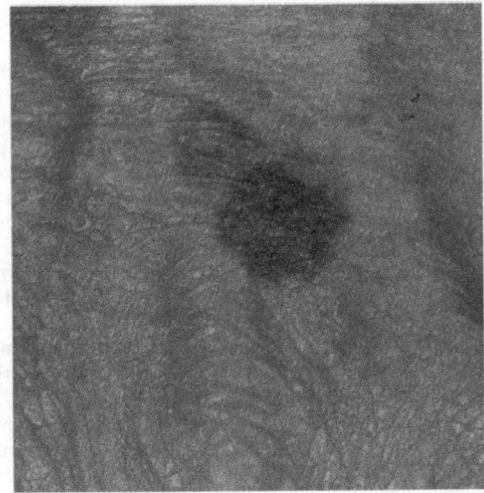

**Macule** *(du Vivier, 1993)*

**maculopapular rash** /mak'yələpap'yələr/ [L, *macula*, spot, *papula*, pimple; OFr, *rasche*], a skin eruption characterized by distinctive macules or papules.

**maculopathy** /mak'yələp'əthē/ [L, *macula*, spot; Gk, *pathos*, disease], a form of macular degeneration primarily involving the macula lutea.

**MAD,** abbreviation for **multiple autoimmune disorder.**

**mad cow disease.** See **bovine spongiform encephalopathy.**

**Madelung's neck.** See **lipoma annulare colli.**

**mad hatter's disease.** See **mercury poisoning.**

**Madura foot** /maj'o͞or'e/ [Madura, India; AS, *fot*, foot], a progressive destructive tropical fungal infection of the foot. Also called **maduromycosis.** See also **mycetoma.**

**MAF,** abbreviation for **macrophage activating factor.**

**mafenide acetate** /maf'ənīd/, a topical antiinfective.

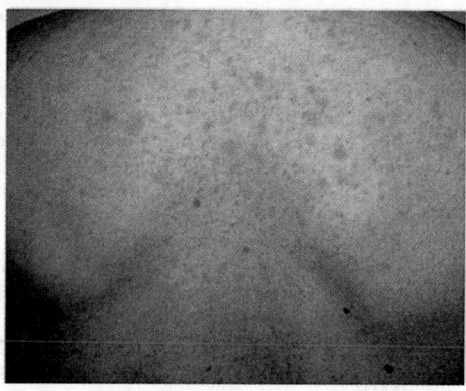

**Maculopapular rash** *(Farrar, 1993/courtesy Dr. B.K. Fisher)*

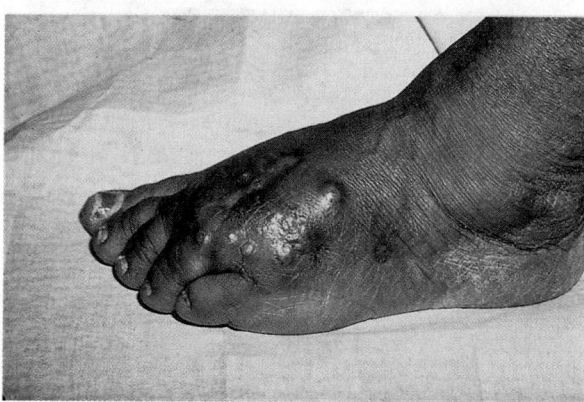

**Madura foot** *(du Vivier, 1993/courtesy Dr. Rod Hay)*

■ INDICATION: It is prescribed in the treatment of burns.

■ CONTRAINDICATIONS: Known hypersensitivity to this drug or to sulfonamide prohibits its use.

■ ADVERSE EFFECTS: Among the more serious adverse effects are hypersensitivity reactions and superinfections, particularly by *Candida albicans.*

**Maffucci's syndrome,** a congenital disorder characterized by the proliferation of cartilage at the ends of long bones and by benign, blood-filled tumors of the skin or viscera. See also **enchondromatosis, cavernous hemangioma.**

**magaldrate** /mag′əldrāte/, an antacid containing a combination of magnesium and aluminum compounds.

■ INDICATIONS: It is prescribed in the treatment of hypersensitivity and stomach upset associated with heartburn, sour stomach, or acid indigestion.

■ CONTRAINDICATIONS: It may alter the absorption of several drugs, such as tetracycline.

■ ADVERSE EFFECTS: A change in bowel function may occur.

**Magendie's law.** See **Bell's law.**

**magical thinking** /maj′ikəl/, (in psychology) a belief that merely thinking about an event in the external world can cause it to occur. It is regarded as a form of regression to an early phase of development. It may be part of ideas of reference, considered normal in those instances, or may reach delusional proportions when the individual maintains a firm conviction about the belief, despite evidence to the contrary. It is a symptom associated with certain stages of schizophrenia.

**magic-bullet approach** [Gk, *magikos,* sorcerer; Fr, *boulette,* small ball; L, *ad,* toward, *prope,* near], **1.** a therapeutic or diagnostic method that makes use of a specific relationship between a drug and a disease or organ. **2.** (in clinical medicine) the administration of a specific drug to cure or ameliorate a given disease or condition. **3.** (in traditional diagnostic radiology) the administration of a specific dye to facilitate the radiographic visualization of a given organ, such as the IV injection of a specific dye for renal studies. **4.** (in nuclear medicine) the administration of a specific radionuclide tagged to an appropriate carrier to provide a scintillation camera image of a given organ or structure, such as the use of a substance containing phosphate and technetium for bone scanning.

**Magill forceps,** an intubation forceps used to guide a tracheal tube into the larynx or to remove a foreign body from an obstructed airway.

**magnesemia** /mag′nəsē′mē·ə/, the presence of magnesium in the blood.

**magnesia magma.** See **milk of magnesia.**

**magnesium (Mg)** /magnē′sē·əm, magnē′zhəm/ [Gr, magnesia; L, lodestone], a silver-white mineral element. Its atomic number is 12; its atomic mass (weight) is 24.32. Magnesium occurs abundantly in nature, always in combination with other elements. It is obtained chiefly by the electrolysis of fused salts containing magnesium chloride or by the thermal reduction of magnesia and is used in photography, metallurgy, and various pharmaceuticals such as magnesium sulfate. Magnesium is the second most abundant cation of the intracellular fluids in the body. It is essential for many enzyme activities and the interaction of intracellular particles and binding of macromolecules to subcellular organelles, such as the binding of messenger ribonucleic acid to ribosomes. It also is important to neurochemical transmissions and muscular excitability. The body of the average 145-pound adult contains about 2000 mEq of magnesium, about 50% of which is in the bones, 45% existing as intracellular cations, and about 5% in the extracellular fluid. Absorption of magnesium occurs in the upper small bowel by means of an active process closely related to the transport system for calcium. Magnesium is excreted mainly by the kidney. Renal excretion of magnesium increases during diuresis induced by ammonium chloride, glucose, and organic mercurials. Magnesium affects the central nervous, neuromuscular, and cardiovascular systems. Insufficient magnesium (hypomagnesemia) in extracellular fluid increases the release of acetylcholine and can cause changes in cardiac and skeletal muscle. Some of the conditions that can produce hypomagnesemia are diarrhea, steatorrhea, chronic alcoholism, and diabetes mellitus. Hypomagnesemia may occur in newborns and infants who are fed cow's milk or artificial formulas, apparently because of the high phosphate/magnesium ratio in such diets. Hypomagnesemia is often treated with parenteral fluids containing magnesium sulfate or magnesium chloride. Excess magnesium (hypermagnesemia) in the body can slow the heartbeat, and concentrations greater than 15 mEq/L can produce cardiac arrest in diastole. Excess magnesium also causes vasodilation by direct effects on the blood vessels and by ganglionic blockade. Hypermagnesemia is usually caused by renal insufficiency and is manifested by hypotension, electrocardiographic changes, muscle weakness, sedation, and a confused mental state.

**magnesium sulfate,** a salt of magnesium.

■ INDICATIONS: It is prescribed parenterally to prevent seizures, especially in preeclampsia, and acute nephritis in children and orally to treat constipation and heartburn and to correct magnesium deficiency.

■ CONTRAINDICATIONS: It is used with caution in patients with renal impairment or hypersensitivity to the drug. Respiratory depression, severe cardiac myopathy, heart block, or symptoms of appendicitis or fecal impaction prohibit its use. It is also prohibited in patients in toxemia of pregnancy during the 2 hours before labor.

■ ADVERSE EFFECTS: The most serious adverse reaction is circulatory collapse from excessive serum concentrations of magnesium. Respiratory depression, confusion, and muscle weakness also may occur.

**magnesium test,** a blood test used to measure levels of magnesium, an electrolyte that is critical in nearly all metabolic processes. Abnormal levels may indicate renal insufficiency, chronic renal disease, uncontrolled diabetes, diabetic acidosis, Addison's disease, hypothyroidism, malnutrition, malabsorption, hypoparathyroidism, and alcoholism.

**magnetic field** /magnet´ik/ [Gk, *magnesia,* lodestone; AS, *feld*], the region around any magnet in which its effects can be detected.

**magnetic lines of force** [Gk, *magnesia,* lodestone; L, *linea,* line, *fortis,* strong], theoretical lines of magnetism that surround a magnet or fill a magnetic field. The presence of the magnetic force along the imaginary lines can be demonstrated by inserting a sensitive material such as iron filings into the lines of magnetic effect.

**magnetic moment** [Gk, *magnesia,* lodestone, *momentum,* movement], a measure of the net magnetic field produced by an elementary particle or an atomic nucleus spinning about its own axis. Such fields are similar to the field surrounding a bar magnet and are the basis for magnetic resonance imaging.

**magnetic permeability,** the ratio of the magnetism induced in a body to the strength of the magnetic field of induction. See also **permeability.**

**magnetic resonance (MR),** a phenomenon in which the atomic nuclei of certain materials placed in a strong, static magnetic field absorb radio waves supplied by a transmitter at particular frequencies. The energy of the radio waves promotes the nuclei from a low-energy state, in which the nuclear spin is aligned parallel to the magnetic field, to a higher-energy state, in which the nuclear spin has a component transverse or opposed to the field. These nuclei occasionally revert to the lower-energy state by emitting photons at characteristic (resonance) frequencies, providing information about the local magnetic field at the nuclei. The rate at which the nuclei revert, or relax, to the lower-energy state when the source of radio waves is turned off is another important factor. See also **relaxation time.**

**magnetic resonance imaging (MRI)** [Gk, *magnesia,* lodestone, *resonare,* to sound again, *imago,* image], medical imaging based on the resonance of atomic nuclei in a strong magnetic field. The field causes those nuclei with an odd number of protons to align and rotate around the axis of the field. Application of a radiofrequency pulse causes the protons to resonate. When the pulse is terminated, the protons "relax" back toward equilibrium. As they do so, they release energy that is detected as a radio signal. Analysis of the amplitude and frequency of the signal yields information about the number and position of nuclei in the tissue, from which the image is produced. MRI is the method of choice for a growing number of disease processes. Among its advantages are its superior soft-tissue contrast resolution, ability to im-

age in multiple planes, and lack of ionizing radiation hazards. MRI is regarded as superior to computed tomography for most central nervous system abnormalities, particularly those of the posterior fossa, brainstem, and spinal cord. It has also become an important tool in musculoskeletal and pelvic imaging. The procedure usually does not require a contrast medium but may use an IV injection of gadolinium. About 15% of patients require an anxiolytic to overcome claustrophobia during MRI, and children may need a sedative as well. Patients must remain motionless for high-quality imaging. Images also may be degraded by motions related to heart contractions, respiration, and bowel peristalsis. Contraindications to MRI are pacemakers, metallic aneurysm clips, and some metallic prostheses and foreign objects. Also called **zeugmatography.** See also **magnetic resonance (MR).**

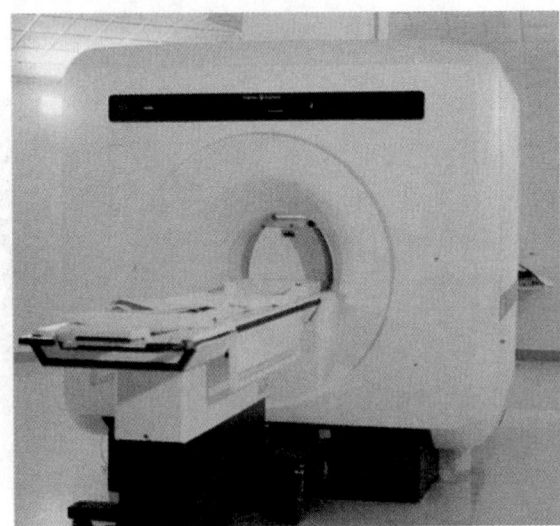

**Clinical setting for magnetic resonance imaging**
*(Mourad, 1991)*

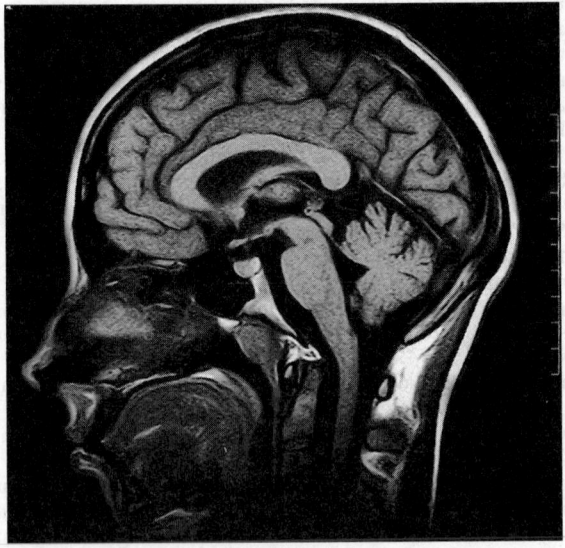

**Magnetic resonance image** *(Crossman and Neary, 1995)*

**magnetic susceptibility,** a measure of the ability of a substance to become magnetized.

**magnetization** /mag'nətīzā'shən/ [Gk, *magnesia,* lodestone; Gk, *izein,* to cause], the magnetic polarization of a material produced by a magnetic field (magnetic moment per unit volume).

**magnetron** /mag'nətron/ [Gk, *magnesia,* lodestone, *trum,* device], a source of microwave energy used in medical linear accelerators to accelerate electrons to the therapeutic energies.

**magnification** /mag'nifikā'shən/, (in psychology) cognitive distortion in which the effects of one's behavior are magnified. See also **minimization.**

**magnification factor,** the size of a radiographic, photographic, or microscopic image divided by the object size. In radiography, it is equal to the source-to-image receptor distance divided by the source-to-object distance.

**MAHA,** abbreviation for **microangiopathic hemolytic anemia.**

**Mahaim fiber** [I. Mahaim, twentieth century French physician, 1897–1965], one of the conductive tracts in cardiac tissue running between the atrioventricular (AV) node or the AV bundle and the muscle of the ventricular septum. The fibers conduct early excitation impulses.

**Mahoney, Mary Eliza** (1845–1926), the first African-American American nurse, Mahoney did private nursing in the Boston area and was active in furthering intergroup relationships and improving the role of the African-American nurse in the community. A medal in her name, established after her death, was first presented in 1936. It is given to an African-American nurse in recognition of an outstanding contribution to the nursing profession.

**main en griffe.** See **clawhand.**

**mainframe computer** [OE, *maegen,* strength, *framian,* to progress; L, *computare,* to count], a large general-purpose computer system for high-volume data processing tasks. It may support large numbers of users simultaneously. Compare **microcomputer, minicomputer, personal computer.**

**mainstreaming** /mān'strēming/ [OE, *maegan,* strength; ME, *strem*], **1.** the system of educating children with disabilities in regular classrooms, with special assistance as needed. **2.** the return of persons recovering from mental illness to the community.

**maintenance dose** /mān'tənəns/ [Fr, *maintenir,* to uphold; Gk, *dosis,* giving], the amount of drug required to keep a desired mean steady-state concentration in the tissues.

**maitake,** an herbal product derived from a mushroom that is native to Japan.

■ USES: This herb is used as an immunostimulant and as a treatment for diabetes, hypertension, high cholesterol, and obesity.

■ CONTRAINDICATIONS: Maitake is not recommended during pregnancy and lactation, in children, or in those with known hypersensitivity until more information is available.

**Majocchi's granuloma** /mäjok'ēz/ [Domenico Majocchi, Italian dermatologist, 1849–1929; L, *granulum,* small grain; Gk, *oma,* tumor], a rare type of tinea corporis that mainly affects the lower legs. It is caused by the fungus *Trichophyton,* which infects the hairs of the affected site and raises spongy granulomas. The lesions persist for 3 to 4 months and are gradually absorbed, or they necrose, often leaving deep scars. Also called **trichophytic granuloma.**

**major affective disorder.** See **major depressive disorder.**

**major connector,** a metal plate or bar used for joining the two halves of a removable partial denture.

**major depressive disorder,** a major disorder of mood

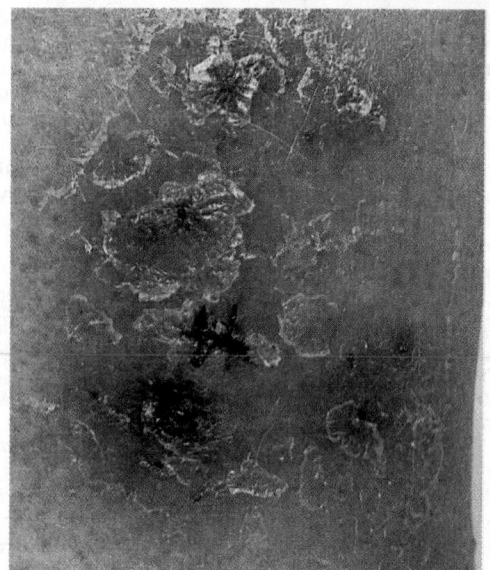

**Majocchi's granuloma** *(du Vivier, 1993)*

characterized by a persistent dysphoric mood, anxiety, irritability, fear, brooding, appetite and sleep disturbances, weight loss, psychomotor agitation or retardation, decreased energy, feelings of worthlessness or guilt, difficulty in concentrating or thinking, possible delusions and hallucinations, and thoughts of death or suicide. The disorder, which occurs in children, adolescents, and adults, may develop over a period of days, weeks, or months; episodes may occur in clusters or singly, separated by several years of normality. The causes of the disorder are multiple and complex and may involve biologic, psychologic, interpersonal, and sociocultural factors that lead to an unidentifiable intrapsychic conflict. Treatment includes use of antidepressants and electroconvulsive therapy, followed by long-term psychotherapy. Nursing care is needed to ensure adequate nutrition, appropriate balance of fluid intake and output, good personal hygiene, and protection of the patient from self-injury. Also called **unipolar disorder.** See also **bipolar disorder, depression, dysthymic disorder.** Also called **major affective disorder.**

**major histocompatibility antigen,** one of a group of proteins encoded by genes of the major histocompatibility complex on chromosome 6.

**major histocompatibility complex (MHC).** See **HLA complex.**

**major hysteria** [ME, *maiour,* great; Gk, *hystera,* womb], an episode of psychogenic illness affecting a large group of individuals at the same time. Examples include the witchcraft trials of the seventeenth century and the irrational mass reaction to the 1938 radio show based on H.G. Wells' science-fiction novel, *War of the Worlds.* Also called **collective hysteria, epidemic hysteria, mass hysteria, mass panic, mass psychogenic illness.**

**major medical insurance,** insurance coverage designed to offset the costs of prolonged or catastrophic illness and injury. Most major medical insurance policies are written to pay a certain percentage of costs up to a predetermined figure, beyond which payment is in full up to a maximum amount, at which point payment ceases. Many require the insured to pay a specified initial, or deductible, amount.

**major renal calyx.** See **renal calyx.**

**major surgery,** a surgical procedure that is extensive and/or life-threatening. It can be and often is done under other than general anesthesia. For example, carotid endarterectomy uses local anesthesia, amputation uses regional anesthesia, and a multitude of other types of major surgery use epidural anesthesia. Compare **minor surgery.** See also **anesthesia, surgery.**

**making weight,** (in sports medicine) the practice of rapid weight loss based on the belief that training at a heavier body weight, then dropping weight shortly before competition, gives an athlete an advantage.

**makro-.** See **macro-.**

**mal** /mal, mäl/ [L, *malus,* bad], an illness or disease, such as grand mal or petit mal.

**mal-,** prefix meaning 'bad, poor, or abnormal': *maladjustment, malalignment, malignant.*

**malabsorption** /mal′əbsôrp′shən/ [L, *malus* + *absorbere,* to swallow], impaired absorption of nutrients from the GI tract. It occurs in celiac disease, sprue, dysentery, diarrhea, inflammatory bowel disease, and other disorders. It may result from an inborn error of metabolism, malnutrition, or any chemical or anatomic condition of the digestive system that prevents normal absorption. See **inborn error of metabolism, malnutrition.**

**malabsorption syndrome,** a complex of symptoms resulting from disorders in the intestinal absorption of nutrients, characterized by anorexia, weight loss, abdominal bloating, muscle cramps, bone pain, and steatorrhea. Anemia, weakness, and fatigue occur because iron, folic acid, and vitamin $B_{12}$ are not absorbed in sufficient amounts. Among the many conditions causing this syndrome are gastric or small bowel resection, celiac disease, tropical sprue, Whipple's disease, intestinal lymphangiectasia, and cystic fibrosis. Treatment and prognosis are determined by the underlying condition. See also **celiac disease, cystic fibrosis, hypoproteinemia, tropical sprue.**

**malacia** /məlā′shə/ [Gk, *malakia,* softness], **1.** a morbid softening or sponginess in any part or any tissue of the body. **2.** a craving for spicy foods, such as mustard, hot peppers, or pickles. —**malacic,** *adj.*

**-malacia,** suffix meaning the 'softening of tissue': *cardiomalacia, esophagomalacia, tracheomalacia.*

**malacic.** See **malacia.**

**malaco-,** combining form meaning 'a condition of abnormal softness': *malacoplakia, malacosarcosis.*

**maladaptation** /mal′adəptā′shən/ [L, *malus* + *adaptatio*], faulty intrapersonal adjustment to stress or change. It may involve a failure to make necessary changes in the desires, values, needs, and attitudes or an inability to make necessary adjustments in the external world. Illness often provokes maladaptive behavior that worsens the problems accompanying the illness.

**maladjusted** /mal′adjus′tid/ [L, *malus,* bad, *adjuxtare,* to bring together], appearing unable to maintain effective relationships needed to fit into the environment and showing irritability, depression, and other psychogenic influences.

**malady** /mal′ədē/ [ME, *maladie,* sick], a disease or illness.

**malaise** /malāz′/ [Fr, discomfort], a vague uneasy feeling of body weakness, distress, or discomfort, often marking the onset of and persisting throughout a disease.

**malalignment** /mal′əlīn′mənt/ [L, *malus* + *ad,* to, *linea,* line], a failure of parts of the body to align normally, such as the teeth in the dental arch.

**malar** /mā′lər/ [L, *mala,* cheek], pertaining to the cheek or the cheekbone.

**malaria** /məler′ē·ə/ [It, *mal,* bad, *aria,* air], a severe infectious illness caused by one or more of at least four species of the protozoan genus *Plasmodium.* The disease is transmitted from human to human by a bite from an infected *Anopheles* mosquito. Malarial infection can also be spread by blood transfusion from an infected patient or by the use of a contaminated or an infected hypodermic needle. Although the endemic disease is limited largely to tropical areas of South and Central America, Africa, and Asia, a number of new cases are introduced into the United States by refugees, military personnel, and travelers returning from malarial areas.
■ OBSERVATIONS: Malaria is characterized by chills and fever, anemia, an enlarged spleen, myalgia, arthralgia, weakness, and vomiting. Splenomegaly, anemia, thrombocytopenia, hypoglycemia, pulmonary or renal dysfunction, and neurosis may also occur. *P. falciparum, P. ovale,* or *P. vivax* parasites penetrate the erythrocytes of the human host, where they mature, reproduce, and burst out periodically. Malarial paroxysms occur at regular intervals, coinciding with the development of a new generation of parasites in the body. Because the life cycle of the infecting parasite varies according to species, the clinical patterns of chills and fever vary, as do the course and severity of the disease. Bouts of malaria usually last from 1 to 4 weeks, with attacks occurring less frequently as the disease progresses. Relapse is common, and the disease can persist for years.
■ INTERVENTIONS: Malaria prophylaxis involves the administration of chloroquine, tetracycline, doxycycline, or mefloquine. Treatment for active malaria includes the administration of chloroquine, quinine, tetracycline, clindamycin, doxycycline, mefloquine, primaquine, sulfonamides, or pyrimethamine. See also **antimalarial, biduotertian fever, blackwater fever, falciparum malaria,** *Plasmodium,* quartan malaria, tertian malaria. —**malarial,** *adj.*

**malarial hemoglobinuria.** See **blackwater fever.**

**malarial parasite** /məler′ē·əl/ [It, *mal aria,* bad air; Gk, *parasitos,* guest], one of four known species of *Plasmodium* that may be injected into the human bloodstream by an anopheline mosquito to begin the cycle of malarial disease.

*Malassezia* /mal′əsē′zē·ə/ [Louis C. Malassez, French physiologist, 1842–1910], a genus of fungi. *Malassezia furfur* causes tinea versicolor (previous name: *Pityrosporum oviculare*). *M. ovalis* is a nonpathogenic organism found in sebaceous areas. Formerly called *Pityrosporum ovale.*

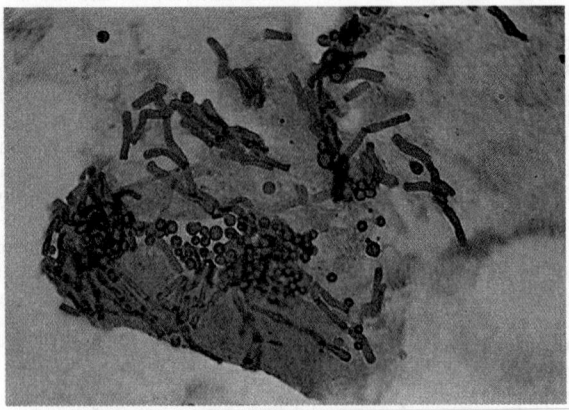

***Malassezia furfur*** (Murray et al, 1998)

**malathion poisoning** /malā′thē·on, məl′əthī′on/, a toxic condition caused by the ingestion or absorption through the skin of malathion, an organophosphorus insecticide. Symptoms include vomiting, nausea, abdominal cramps, headache, dizziness, weakness, confusion, convulsions, and respiratory difficulties. Malathion is much less toxic than parathion and is the only organophosphorus insecticide approved for household use.

**malaxation.** See **pétrissage.**

**Malayan pit viper venom.** See **ancrod.**

**mal del pinto.** See **pinta.**

**mal de Meleda** /mal·də mel′ədä/ [Fr, Meleda sickness], a chronic, autosomal recessive form of keratoderma of the palms and the soles of the feet in which the hyperkeratosis spreads to involve the dorsal aspects of the hands and feet and other areas of the body, with erythematous, scaling, malodorous cutaneous lesions that may cause deep fissuring. Also called **Meleda disease.**

**mal de mer.** See **motion sickness.**

**male** [L, *mas*], **1.** pertaining to the sex that produces sperm cells and fertilizes the female egg to beget offspring; masculine. **2.** a male person.

**male catheterization,** the passage of a catheter through the male urethra for the purpose of draining the urinary bladder. A French size 16-18 catheter is usually determined for adult men unless the physician orders a larger size. The male patient is placed in a supine position with the legs extended. The catheter is inserted 17.5 to 22.5 cm, or until urine flows. Sterile technique is important throughout the procedure to prevent the introduction of infectious organisms into the bladder.

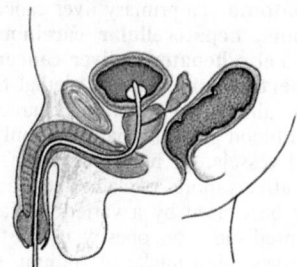

**Male catheterization** *(Potter and Perry, 2001)*

**male menopause** [L, *mas,* male, *men,* month; Gk, *pauein,* to cease], a late middle-age psychogenic condition affecting some men, who experience anxiety over diminished potency, increased fatigue, thinning and graying hair, and other signs of aging. Also called **male climacterium.**

**male pattern alopecia** [L, *mas,* male; ME, *patron* + Gk, *alopex,* fox mange], a common form of baldness in males, beginning at the front and spreading gradually until a fringe remains around the back and temples. Individual differences are determined by heredity, androgenic stimulation, and aging. Also called **male pattern baldness.**

**male reproductive system assessment,** an evaluation of the condition of the patient's genitalia, reproductive history, and past and present genitourinary infections and disorders.

■ METHOD: In a relaxed professional interview the procedures to be conducted are explained and the patient is reassured that his privacy will be scrupulously maintained. He is

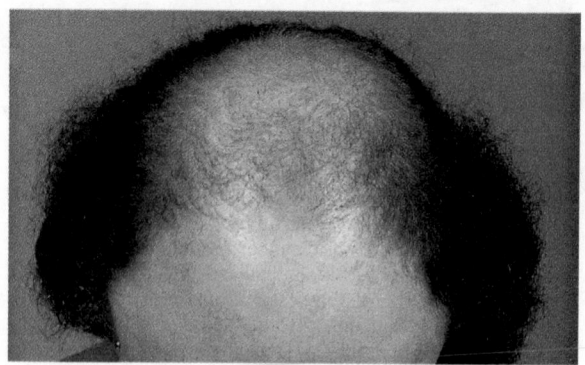

**Male pattern alopecia** *(du Vivier, 1993)*

questioned about his offspring; sexual activity; the existence of nocturia, urgency, frequency, dysuria, urethral discharge, hernia, genital sores; discomfort or pain in the groin, lower back, or legs; and past treatment for epididymitis, gonorrhea, herpes genitalis, hydrocele, nonspecific urethritis, orchitis, prostatitis, syphilis, and varicocele. The examiner, while inspecting the genitalia, observes universal precautions as indicated by the condition. The penis is examined for swelling, inflammation, and lesions such as herpes vesicles or syphilitic sores, chancres, or scars. Anomalies that may be noted include hypospadias or epispadias, resulting from failed closure of the urethra; elongation of the foreskin constricting the urinary meatus; or swelling of the glans caused by a retracted, tight foreskin. The urethral orifice is inspected for a purulent or bloody discharge, and the scrotum is observed for symmetry and shape; in elderly or debilitated men the scrotum may be elongated and flat. The normally smooth testes, epididymis, and spermatic cords are palpated for the presence of beading and varicosities and the size, location, and consistency of any scrotal mass; fluid felt around the testes may be seen by darkening the room and illuminating the scrotum with a flashlight. Wrapping the flashlight with clear plastic wrap, which is changed between patients, decreases the risk of bacteria transfer. The patient is asked to cough or bear down to reveal a hernia, and the abdomen is palpated above the symphysis pubis to determine whether the bladder is distended. The inguinal lymph nodes are palpated, and the amount and distribution of pubic hair are observed. The prostate may be examined with the patient in the Sims' knee-chest position or lithotomy position, but, when possible, it is preferable for the patient to

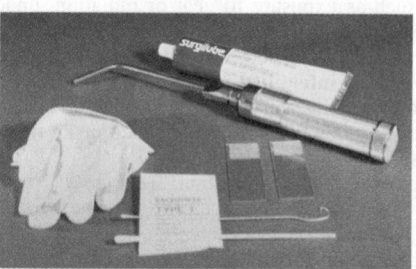

**Equipment for male reproductive system assessment**
*(Lemmi and Lemmi, 2000)*

stand bent at a right angle over a table as the examiner's well-lubricated gloved forefinger sweeps the rectal circumference and palpates the lobes and medial sulcus of the gland. The size, consistency, and any localized nodule suggesting a neoplasm of the normally smooth, firm prostate are carefully noted, and the findings are recorded as on a clock dial with the symphysis pubis representing 12 o'clock. When additional studies are indicated, a smear is prepared from the first urine voided after massage of the prostate. Primary screening for prostatic cancer includes the digital rectal examination and a blood test for PSA. Prostatic acid phosphatase (PAP) is also assessed if prostatic cancer is suspected. Diagnosis is usually established by a biopsy. The assessment includes laboratory studies of any discharge from the penis. A Gram-stained smear usually confirms or rules out a diagnosis of gonorrhea, and a fluorescent-tagged antibody method may be required if the result is equivocal. Cultures may be needed to determine whether nonspecific urethritis is caused by *Escherichia coli, Pseudomonas, Staphylococcus, Streptococcus,* or organisms of other pathogenic genera. Syphilis may be diagnosed by the Venereal Disease Research Laboratories serologic test, but the fluorescent treponemal antibody-absorption test is the most sensitive and specific diagnostic measure. If infertility is a problem, examinations of multiple semen samples are conducted; each specimen collected after 3 days of abstinence is inspected in the laboratory to determine whether the volume of the ejaculate approximates the normal 2 to 5 ml average and whether the semen has a pH of 7.7 and a sperm count of 60 to 150 million per milliliter.

■ INTERVENTIONS: The health care provider conducts the interview and examination, assembles the results of laboratory studies, and urges the patient to inform his sex partner, or partners, if an infectious disease is diagnosed. Throughout the assessment the health care provider recognizes that the patient may be reluctant to discuss his symptoms and activities and may be sensitive about the necessary procedures.

■ OUTCOME CRITERIA: A careful, understanding evaluation of the male patient's reproductive system helps to establish the diagnosis and plan the treatment and aids in allaying the patient's anxiety. The assessment also serves as a public health measure by encouraging the reporting of a sexually transmitted disease to the patient's contacts and proper authorities.

**male sexual dysfunction,** impaired or inadequate ability of a man to carry on his sex life to his own satisfaction. Symptoms include difficulties in starting and maintaining an erection, premature ejaculation, inability to ejaculate, and loss of desire. Compare **female sexual dysfunction. See** also **erectile dysfunction, impotence, premature ejaculation, sexual dysfunction.**

**male sterility** [L, *mas + sterilis,* barren], the inability of a man to produce sperm. Causes may include environmental factors such as exposure to heat or radiation, undescended testes, varicocele, prolonged fever, endocrine disorders, cancer chemotherapy, vasectomy, and abuse of alcohol or marijuana. See also **infertility.**

**malfeasance** /malfē′zəns/ [Fr, *malfaire,* to do evil], performance of an unlawful, wrongful act. Compare **misfeasance, nonfeasance.**

**malformation** /mal′fôrmā′shən/ [L, *malus,* bad, *forma,* shape], an anomalous structure in the body. See also **congenital anomaly.**

**malfunction** /mal′fungk′shən/ [L, *malus,* bad, *functio,* performance], **1.** the inability to function normally. **2.** not to function normally.

**Malgaigne's fracture of pelvis** /malgā′nyəz/ [Joseph F.

Malgaigne, French surgeon, 1806–1865], breaks in multiple pelvic bones, including the pubic rami and the wing of the ipsilateral ilium or the sacrum with associated upper displacement of the hemipelvis.

**malicious prosecution** /məlish′əs/ [L, *malitia,* wickedness, *prosequi,* to pursue], (in law) a suit begun in malice and pursued without sufficient cause. It is usually an action for damages. Malicious prosecution is a wrongful civil proceeding, and a person who takes an active part in initiating or continuing it is subject to liability.

**malign** /məlīn′/ [ME, *malignen,* deceptive], to show ill will or maliciousness; to act viciously; to harm.

**malignant** /məlig′nənt/ [L, *malignus,* bad disposition], **1.** also **virulent.** Tending to become worse and to cause death. **2.** (describing a cancer) anaplastic, invasive, and metastatic. **—malignancy,** *n.*

**malignant astrocytoma,** a high grade astrocytoma, such as **glioblastoma multiforme.**

**malignant atrophic papulosis,** a form of cutaneous lymphocytic vasculitis. The skin disease shows erythematous papules with characteristic porcelain-white centers and elevated borders. The early signs are followed by perforated intestinal ulcers, leading to peritonitis, occluded arterioles, and progressive neurologic disability. Also called **Degos′ disease.**

**malignant dysentery** [L, *malignus,* bad disposition; Gk, *dys,* bad, *enteron,* bowel], a potentially fatal form of dysentery in which symptoms are severe.

**malignant endocarditis.** See **bacterial endocarditis.**

**malignant ependymoma.** See **ependymoblastoma.**

**malignant granuloma** [L, *malignus,* bad disposition, *granulum,* little grain, *oma,* tumor], a malignant lymphoma, such as Hodgkin's disease, or a lymphosarcoma.

**malignant hemangioendothelioma.** See **angiosarcoma.**

**malignant hepatoma,** a primary liver cancer. Also called **hepatocarcinoma, hepatocellular carcinoma, liver cell carcinoma.** See also **hepatoma, liver cancer.**

**malignant hypertension,** the most lethal form of hypertension. It is a fulminating condition, characterized by severely elevated blood pressure that commonly damages the intima of small vessels, the brain, the retina, the heart, and the kidneys. It affects more African-Americans than Caucasians and may be caused by a variety of factors, such as stress, genetic predisposition, obesity, use of tobacco, use of oral contraceptives, high intake of sodium, sedentary life-

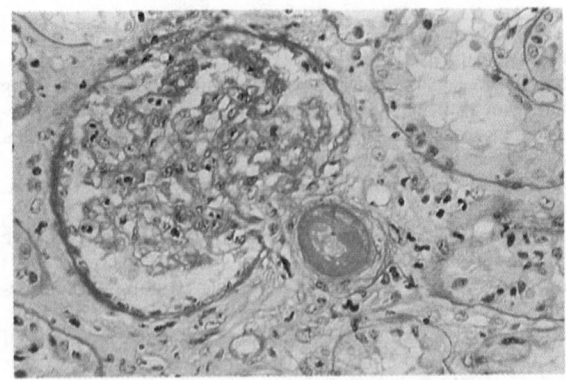

**Malignant hypertension: kidney damage**
*(Cotran, Kumar, and Collins, 1999/courtesy Dr. H. Rennke, Brigham and Women's Hospital, Boston)*

style, renal disease, and aging. Many patients with this condition exhibit signs of hypokalemia and alkalosis and have aldosterone secretion rates even higher than those associated with primary aldosteronism. Also called **accelerated hypertension.** See also **essential hypertension.**

**malignant hyperthermia (MH),** a rare genetic hypermetabolic condition characterized by severe hyperthermia and rigidity of the skeletal muscles occurring in affected people exposed to inhalation anesthetics and succinylcholine, a nondepolarizing muscle relaxant. Treatment includes the administration of large quantities of Dantrolene sodium, administration of 100% oxygen, immediate cooling, cessation of surgery; and correction of acidosis and hyperkalemia. Patients susceptible to malignant hyperthermia must be informed of the condition and susceptible relatives screened. The family is referred to the Malignant Hyperthermia Registry MHAUS.

**malignant hyperthermia precautions,** a nursing intervention from the Nursing Interventions Classification (NIC) defined as prevention or reduction of hypermetabolic response to pharmacological agents used during surgery. See also **Nursing Interventions Classification.**

**malignant malnutrition.** See **kwashiorkor.**

**malignant melanoma.** See **melanoma.**

**malignant mesenchymoma,** a sarcoma that contains mesenchymal elements.

**malignant mole.** See **melanoma.**

**malignant neoplasm,** a tumor that tends to grow, invade, and metastasize. The tumor usually has an irregular shape and is composed of poorly differentiated cells. If untreated, it may result in death.

**malignant neuroma.** See **neurosarcoma.**

**malignant pustule.** See **anthrax.**

**malignant transformation,** the changes that a normal cell undergoes as it becomes a cancerous cell.

**malignant tumor,** a neoplasm that characteristically invades surrounding tissue, metastasizes to distant sites, and contains anaplastic cells. A malignant tumor may cause death if treatment does not intervene.

**malingering** /məling'gəring/ [Fr, *malingre,* puny, weak], a willful and deliberate feigning of the symptoms of a disease or injury to gain some consciously desired end. **—malinger,** *v.,* **malingerer,** *n.*

**malleable** /mal'ē·əbəl/ [L, *malleare,* to beat], able to be pressed, hammered, or otherwise forced into a shape without breaking.

**mallei.** See **malleus.**

**malleolus** /məlē'ələs/, *pl.* **malleoli** [L, little hammer], a rounded bony process, such as the protuberance on each side of the ankle.

**malleolus fibulae.** See **external malleolus.**

**mallet deformity** [ME, *maillet,* maul], a loss of the ability to extend the distal joint of a finger or toe. It may be caused by severe damage, such as rupture of the terminal tendon. See also **hammer finger, hammer toe.**

**mallet finger.** See **hammer finger.**

**mallet fracture,** a fracture in which the dorsal base of a distal phalanx of the hand or foot is torn away. The fracture disrupts the associated extensor apparatus and causes dropped flexion of the distal segment.

**malleus** /mal'ē·əs/, *pl.* **mallei** [L, hammer], one of the three ossicles in the middle ear, resembling a hammer with a head, neck, and three processes. It is connected to the tympanic membrane and transmits sound vibrations to the incus, which communicates with the stapes. Compare **incus, stapes.** See also **middle ear.**

**Mallory body** /mal'ərē/ [Frank B. Mallory, American pathologist, 1862–1941; AS, *bodig,* body], an eosinophilic cytoplasmic inclusion, alcoholic hyalin, found in the liver cells. It is typically, but not always, associated with acute alcoholic liver injury. See also **cirrhosis.**

**Mallory-Weiss syndrome** [G. Kenneth Mallory, American pathologist, b. 1926; Soma Weiss, American physician, 1899–1942], a condition characterized by massive bleeding after a tear in the mucous membrane at the junction of the esophagus and the stomach. The laceration is usually caused by protracted vomiting, most commonly in alcoholics or in people whose pylorus is obstructed. The esophageal tear is located by esophagoscopy or arteriography. Surgery is usually necessary to stop the bleeding. After repair the prognosis is excellent.

**malnutrition** /mal'nōōtrish'ən/ [L, *malus,* bad, *nutrire,* to nourish], any disorder of nutrition. It may result from an unbalanced, insufficient, or excessive diet or from impaired absorption, assimilation, or use of foods. Compare **deficiency disease.**

**malocclusion** /mal'əklōō'zhən/ [L, *malus* + *occludere,* to shut up], abnormal contact between the teeth of the upper jaw and those of the lower jaw. See also **Angle's Classification of Malocclusion, occlusion.**

**malonic acid (CH$_2$(COOH)$_2$)** /məlō'nik/, a white crystalline highly toxic substance used as an intermediate compound in the production of barbiturates. A dicarboxylic acid, also called **propanedioic acid.**

**malpighian body** /malpig'ē·ən/ [Marcello Malpighi, Italian physician, 1628–1694; AS, *bodig,* body], **1.** the renal corpuscle, which includes a glomerulus with Bowman's capsule. **2.** lymphoid tissue surrounding the arteries of the spleen. Also called **lymphatic nodule.**

**malpighian corpuscle** [Marcello Malpighi; L, *corpusculum,* little body], one of a number of small, round, deep-red bodies in the cortex of the kidney, each communicating with a renal tubule. Malpighian corpuscles average about 0.2 mm in diameter, with each capsule composed of two parts: a central glomerulus and a glomerular capsule. The corpuscles are part of a filtering system through which nonprotein components of blood plasma enter the tubules for urinary excretion. Also called **malpighian body, renal corpuscle.**

**malposition** /mal'pəzish'ən/, a wrong or faulty placement of a body part, such as in an untreated fracture.

**malpractice** /malprak'tis/ [L, *malus* + Gk, *praktikos,* practical], (in law) professional negligence that is the proximate cause of injury or harm to a patient, resulting from a lack of professional knowledge, experience, or skill that can be expected in others in the profession or from a failure to exercise reasonable care or judgment in the application of professional knowledge, experience, or skill.

**malpresentation** /malpres'əntā'shən/ [L, *malus,* bad, *praesentare,* to show], an abnormal position of the fetus in the birth canal.

**malrotation** /mal'rōtā'shən/, **1.** any abnormal rotation of an organ or body part, such as the vertebral column or a tooth. **2.** a failure of the intestinal tract or other viscera to undergo normal rotation during embryonic development.

**malt** /môlt/ [AS, *mealt*], a preparation obtained from germinated grain, such as barley, that contains partially degraded starch and protein with nutritive and digestive properties.

**Malta fever.** See **brucellosis.**

**malunion** /malyōō'nyən/ [L, *malus* + *unus,* one], an imperfect union of previously fragmented bone or other tissue. Causes of bone malunion include osteomyelitis and improper immobilization of a fracture.

**mamillary body** /mam′iler′ē/ [L, *mammilla*, nipple; AS, *bodig*, body], either of the two small round masses of gray matter in the hypothalamus located close to one another in the interpeduncular space. They may be involved with olfactory reflexes.

**mamm-,** a combining form meaning 'mammary gland or the breast': *mammectomy, mammogram, mammotropic.*

**mamma.** See **mammary gland.**

**mammary** /mam′ərē/ [L, *mamma*, breast], pertaining to the breast.

**mammary duct.** See **lactiferous duct.**

**mammary glands** [L, *mamma*, breast, *glans,* acorn], lactiferous glands within the breasts. Glandular tissue forms a radius of lobes containing alveoli, each lobe having a system of ducts for the passage of milk from the alveoli to the nipple. The central part of the breast is filled with glandular tissue. Also called **breast, mamma.** See also **lactation.**

**mammary papilla.** See **nipple.**

**mammogram** /mam′əgram/ [L, *mamma* + Gk, *gramma,* record], an x-ray film of the soft tissues of the breast.

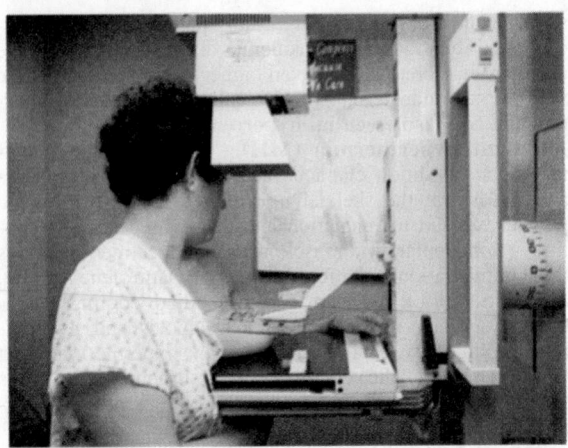

**Clinical setting for mammography** *(Belcher, 1992)*

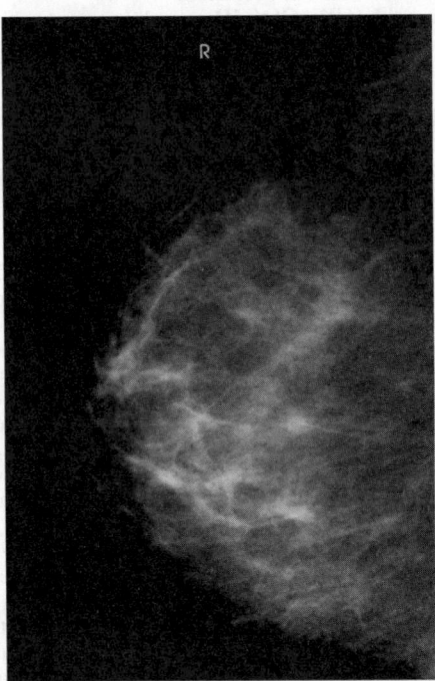

**Mammogram**

**mammography** /mamog′rəfē/, the radiographic examination of the soft tissues of the breast. It is used to identify various benign and malignant neoplastic processes and may show conclusively that a lesion is malignant. Routine mammography reduces the breast cancer mortality rate by 25% to 35% in asymptomatic women in middle age. The baseline mammographic examination is recommended at 35 years of age. The National Cancer Institute recommends a yearly mammogram for women between 50 and 75 years of age. After 75 years of age, routine mammography screening depends on a woman's overall health. Because of newer techniques using lower doses of radiation, the advantage of having regular mammograms greatly outweighs the risk of radiation exposure.

**mammoplasty** /mam′əplas′tē/ [L, *mamma* + Gk, *plassein,* to mold], plastic reshaping of the breasts, performed to reduce or lift large or sagging breasts, to enlarge small breasts, or to reconstruct a breast after removal of a tumor. To reduce the size of the breasts and raise them, excess tissue is removed from the underside of the breasts; the breast is then lifted, and the nipple drawn through an opening in an overhanging skin flap. To enlarge a breast, a saline-filled or silicone gel prosthesis is inserted in a pocket formed beneath the breast on the chest wall. The complications after surgery are infection and, with the use of implants, rejection of tissues to the foreign body. The nurse observes the nipples for signs of vascular insufficiency or congestion, applies a firm supporting breast binder or brassiere, and instructs the patient not to use her arms to lift herself.

**mammothermography** /mam′ōthərmog′rəfē/ [L, *mamma* + Gk, *therme,* heat, *graphein,* to record], a diagnostic procedure in which the breast is examined for abnormal growths by means of a heart-sensitive probe that detects regional differences in blood flow. Compare **mammography.** See also **thermography.**

**man-,** combining form meaning 'hand': *manoptoscope, manual, manudynamometer.*

**managed care,** a health care system in which there is administrative control over primary health care services in a medical group practice. The intention is to eliminate redundant facilities and services and to reduce costs. Health education and preventive medicine are emphasized. Patients may pay a flat fee for basic family care but may be charged additional fees for secondary care services. The system of managed care evolved following World War II from the traditional fee for service, in which the patient paid the physician directly for services performed; through a shift toward health insurance organizations, which paid physicians and hospitals from premiums paid by the patients to the insurers; to the advent in the 1960s of government programs, such as Medicare and Medicaid. In the 1980s another economic shift, originating in California, led to the concept of health maintenance organizations (HMOs), with large corporations initially negotiating with groups of health care workers for financing of medical and hospital expenses of the corporation employees. HMOs also began enrolling individual patients and by the mid-1990s challenged the survival of the traditional insurance systems. See also **health maintenance organization.**

**managed care organization (MCO),** an organization that combines the functions of health insurance, delivery of care, and administration. Examples include the independent practice association, third-party administrator, management service organization, and physician-hospital organization.

**management service organization (MSO),** an entity that under contract provides services such as a facility, equipment, staffing, contract negotiation, administration, and marketing. Services may be provided to solo practitioners or groups. Approaches to establishment of the MSO include the hospital-related MSO; the provider-of-care, hospital-related, tax-exempt clinic MSO; and the nonprofit, hospital-sponsored equity MSO.

**Mandelamine,** trademark for an antibacterial (methenamine mandelate).

**mandible** /man′dibəl/ [L, *mandere,* to chew], a large U-shaped bone constituting the lower jaw. It contains the lower teeth and consists of a horizontal part, a body, and two perpendicular rami that join the body at almost right angles. The body of the mandible is curved, somewhat resembling a horseshoe, and has two surfaces and two borders. The superior border of the mandible contains sockets for the 16 lower teeth. The inferior border provides a groove for the facial artery. Compare **maxilla.** —**mandibular,** *adj.*

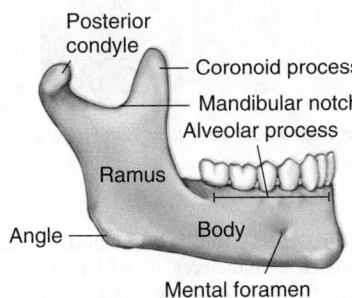

Posterior condyle
Coronoid process
Mandibular notch
Alveolar process
Ramus
Angle
Body
Mental foramen

**Mandible**

**mandibular,** pertaining to the mandible.

**mandibular arch** /mandib′yələr/ [L, *mandere,* to chew, *arcus,* bow], the first visceral arch from which the lower jawbone develops.

**mandibular block,** regional anesthesia of the lower jaw produced by injection of a local analgesic near the third division of the trigeminal nerve.

**mandibular canal** [L, *mandere,* to chew + *canalis,* channel], a passage or channel that extends from the mandibular foramen on the medial surface of the ramus of the mandible to the mental foramen. It holds mandibular blood vessels and a part of the mandibular branch of the trigeminal nerve.

**mandibular fossa** [L, *mandere,* to chew, *fossa,* ditch], a prominent depression in the inferior surface of the squamous part of the temporal bone at the base of the zygomatic process, in which the condyle of the mandible rests. Also called **glenoid cavity, glenoid fossa.**

**mandibular notch,** a depression in the inferior border of the mandible, anterior to the attachments of the masseter muscle, where the external facial muscles cross the inferior

border of the mandible. It is a landmark that may be accentuated by arrested condylar growth and other developmental disturbances of the mandible.

**mandibular process** [L, *mandere,* to chew, *processus*], **1.** the upper alveolar part of the mandible. **2.** the projection of the upper posterior part of the ramus of the mandible bearing the condyle.

**mandibular ramus** [L, *mandere,* to chew, *ramus,* branch], a broad quadrilateral part of the mandible projecting upward from the posterior end of the body behind the lower teeth. It has two surfaces, four borders, and two processes.

**mandibular reflex** [L, *mandere,* to chew, *reflectere,* to bend back], a reflex contraction of the masseter muscle after a downward tap on the point of the jaw while the mouth is open. Also called **chin reflex, chin-jerk reflex, jaw jerk.**

**mandibular retrusion, mandibular retroposition.** See **retrognathia.**

**mandibular sling,** the connection between the mandible and the maxilla, formed by the masseter and the pterygoideus at the angle of the mandible. When the mouth is opened and closed, the mandible moves around a center of rotation formed by the mandibular sling and the sphenomandibular ligament.

**mandibular spine,** a protuberance on the mandibular ramus to which the sphenomandibular ligament is attached.

**mandibulofacial dysostosis** /mandib′yəlofā′shəl/ [L, *mandere* + *facies,* face; Gk, *dys,* bad, *osteon,* bone], an abnormal hereditary condition characterized by an antimongoloid slant of the palpebral fissures, coloboma of the lower lid, micrognathia and hypoplasia of the zygomatic arches, and microtia. Evidence indicates that this disorder is transmitted as an autosomal dominant trait. The condition occurs in the complete form as Franceschetti's syndrome and in the incomplete form as Treacher Collins' syndrome. See also **dysostosis.**

**Mandol,** trademark for a cephalosporin antibiotic (cefamandole nafate).

**mandrel** /man′drəl/ [Fr, *mandrin,* boring tool], the shaft of an object, such as a dental polishing disk, cutting device, or sharpening stone, which is inserted into a handpiece or lathe and supports the object while it rotates.

**maneuver** /mənoo′vər/ [Fr, *manœuvre,* action], **1.** an adroit or skillful manipulation or procedure. **2.** (in obstetrics) a manipulation of the fetus performed to aid in delivery. Also spelled **manoeuvre.**

**manganese (Mn)** /mang′gənēs/ [L, *manganesium,* associated with magnesium], a common metallic element found in trace amounts in tissues of the body, where it aids in the functions of various enzymes. Its atomic number is 25; its atomic mass is 54.938.

**manganese nodule,** a small node produced by microbial reduction of manganese oxides.

**mange** /mānj/, a cutaneous disease of domestic and wild animals caused by skin-burrowing mites. See also **scabies.**

**mani-,** prefix meaning 'mental aberration or madness': *mania, maniaphobia.*

**mania** /mā′nē·ə/ [Gk, madness], a mood characterized by an unstable expansive emotional state, extreme excitement, excessive elation, hyperactivity, agitation, overtalkativeness, flight of ideas, increased psychomotor activity, fleeting attention, and sometimes violent, destructive, and self-destructive behavior.

**-mania, -manic 1.** suffix meaning a 'state of mental disorder'. **2.** suffix meaning 'a state of psychosis': *hypermania, melanomanic.*

**-maniac, 1.** suffix meaning a 'person exhibiting a type of psychosis': *kleptomaniac, narcomaniac, toxicomaniac.*

**2.** suffix meaning a 'person revealing an inordinate interest in something': *ergomaniac, nymphomaniac, opiomaniac.*

**manic depressive.** See **bipolar disorder.**

**manifest deviation.** See **eye deviation.**

**manipulation** /mənip′yəlā′shən/ [L, *manipulare,* to work with the hands], the skillful use of the hands in therapeutic or diagnostic procedures, such as palpation, reduction of a dislocation, turning a fetus, or various treatments in physical therapy and osteopathy. A kind of manipulation is **conjoined manipulation.** See also **massage.**

**mannitol** /man′itol/, a poorly metabolized sugar used as an osmotic diuretic and in kidney function tests.

■ INDICATIONS: It is prescribed to promote diuresis, to decrease intraocular and intracranial pressure, to promote the excretion of poisons and other toxic wastes, and to evaluate renal function.

■ CONTRAINDICATIONS: Pulmonary edema, dehydration, or known hypersensitivity to this drug prohibits its use.

■ ADVERSE EFFECTS: Among the more serious adverse reactions are pulmonary edema, heart failure, hyponatremia, headache, vomiting, and confusion.

**mannose** /man′ōs/, a six-carbon sugar epimeric with glucose, occurring in oligosaccharides of many glycoproteins and glycolipids.

**mannosidosis** /man′ō·si·dō′sis/, a lysosomal storage disease caused by an enzymatic defect in the metabolism of mannose-containing glycoproteins, resulting in accumulation of oligosaccharides. Characteristics include coarse facies, upper respiratory congestion and infections, profound mental retardation, hepatosplenomegaly, cataracts, radiographic signs of skeletal abnormalities, and gibbus deformity. Mannosidosis is divided into type I (infantile onset) and type II (juvenile-adult onset).

**Mann-Whitney test, Mann-Whitney** *U* **test.** See **rank sum test.**

**manoeuvre.** See **maneuver.**

**manometer** /mənom′ətər/ [Gk, *manos,* thin, *metron,* measure], a device for measuring the pressure of a fluid, consisting of a tube marked with a scale and containing a relatively incompressible fluid, such as mercury. The level of the fluid in the tube varies with the pressure of the fluid being measured. Kinds of manometers are **aneroid manometer** and **sphygmomanometer.**

**-manometer,** combining form meaning 'an instrument to measure pressure': *sphygmomanometer.*

**manometry** /mənom′ətrē/ [Gk, *manos,* thin, *metron,* measure], **1.** the science of pressure movements of liquids or gases. **2.** a technique for measuring changes in the pressure of a gas or liquid that result from a biologic or chemical action.

**Mansonella** /man′sə·nel′ə/, a genus of nematodes of the superfamily Filarioidea, found in Central and South America and Africa. *M. ozzardi* and *M. perstans* are two species that parasitize humans and cause mild symptoms. See also **mansonellosis.**

**Mansonella ozzardi** /man′sənel′ə/, a parasitic worm that is indigenous to much of Latin America and the Caribbean islands. It is a relatively benign nematode that infects humans, sometimes causing hydrocele or lymphadenopathy. The larvae live in the bloodstream, and adult worms are found in the visceral mesenteries. The intermediate hosts are biting flies of the genus *Culicoides.*

**mansonellosis** /man′sə·nel·ō′sis/, infection with nematodes of the genus *Mansonella,* an ill-defined syndrome of headache, coldness of the legs, pruritis, and articular swelling. Also called **acanthocheilonemiasis.**

**Mantadil,** trademark for a fixed-combination topical drug

containing a glucocorticoid (hydrocortisone acetate) and an antihistamine (chlorcyclizine hydrochloride).

**mantle cell lymphoma** /man′təl/, a rare form of non-Hodgkin's lymphoma having a usually diffuse pattern; it mainly affects people over 50 years of age and runs an indolent course although it may metastasize to the spleen or liver. See also **non-Hodgkin's lymphoma.**

**Mantoux test** /mantoo′/ [Charles Mantoux, French physician, 1877–1947], a tuberculin skin test that consists of intradermal injection of a purified protein derivative of the tubercle bacillus. A hardened, raised red area of 8 to 10 mm, appearing 24 to 72 hours after injection, is a positive reaction. This method is the most reliable means of testing tuberculin sensitivity. See also **tuberculin test.**

**Positive Mantoux test** *(Hart and Broadhead, 1992)*

**manual rotation** /man′yoo·əl/ [L, *manualis,* hand, *rotare,* to turn], an obstetric maneuver in which a baby's head is turned by hand from a transverse to an anteroposterior position in the birth canal to facilitate delivery. Compare **forceps rotation.**

**manubrial.** See **manubrium.**

**manubriosternal articulation** /mənoo′brē·ōstur′nəl/ [L, *manubrium,* handle; Gk, *sternum,* chest; L, *articularis,* joints], the fibrocartilaginous connection between the manubrium and the body of the sternum. This joint usually closes by 25 years of age. Compare **xiphisternal articulation.**

**manubrium** /mənoo′brē·əm/ [L, handle], the most anterior of the three bones of the sternum, presenting a broad quadrangular shape that narrows caudally at its articulation with the superior end of the body of the sternum. The pectoralis major and the sternocleidomastoideus are attached to the manubrium. Compare **xiphoid process. —manubrial,** *adj.*

**manudynamometer** /man′oodī′nəmom′ətər/ [L, *manus,* hand; Gk, *dynamis,* force, *metron,* measure], a device for measuring the force or extent of thrust.

**manus.** See **hand.**

**many-tailed bandage** [AS, *manig,* many, *taegel,* tail; Fr, *bande,* strip], **1.** a broad evenly shaped bandage with both ends split into strips of equal size and number. As the bandage is placed on the abdomen, chest, or limb, the ends may be overlapped and secured. **2.** an irregularly shaped bandage with torn or cut ends that are secured together. See also **Scultetus bandage.**

**MAO,** abbreviation for **monoamine oxidase.**

**MAOI,** abbreviation for **monoamine oxidase inhibitor.**

**Maolate,** trademark for a skeletal muscle relaxant (chlorphenesin carbamate).

**MAP,** 1. abbreviation for *medical aid post.* 2. abbreviation for **mean arterial pressure.**

**map distance.** See **map unit.**

**maple bark disease** [AS, *mapul* + ONorse, *bark* + L, *dis,* opposite of; Fr, *aise,* ease], a hypersensitivity pneumonitis caused by exposure to the mold *Cryptostroma corticale,* found in the bark of maple trees. In the susceptible person the condition may be acute, accompanied by fever, cough, dyspnea, and vomiting, or chronic, characterized by fatigue, weight loss, dyspnea on exertion, and a productive cough. Although differential diagnosis may be difficult, a thorough occupational history may reveal the cause and source of exposure. In an acute or severe case a short course of prednisone may be used to control the symptoms; avoiding exposure to the bark prevents further reaction.

**maple syrup urine disease** [AS, *mapul* + Ar, *sharab* + Gk, *ouron,* urine], an inherited metabolic disorder in which an enzyme necessary for the breakdown of the amino acids valine, leucine, and isoleucine is lacking. The disease is usually diagnosed in infancy; it is recognized by the characteristic maple syrup odor of the urine and by hyperreflexia. Stress, fever, and infection aggravate the condition. Treatment includes a diet avoiding these amino acids and rarely dialysis or transfusion. Also called **branched chain ketoaciduria.**

**mapping** [L, *mappa,* napkin], the process of locating the relative position of genes on a chromosome through the analysis of genetic recombination. Distances between genes in a linkage group are expressed in map units or morgans. Also called **chromosome mapping.**

**maprotiline hydrochloride** /maprō′tilēn/, an antidepressant similar to the tricyclics.

■ INDICATION: It is prescribed for the treatment of depression.

■ CONTRAINDICATIONS: It is used with caution in conditions in which anticholinergics are contraindicated, in seizure disorders, and in cardiovascular disorders. Concomitant administration of monoamine oxidase inhibitors, recent myocardial infarction, or known hypersensitivity to this drug prohibits its use.

■ ADVERSE EFFECTS: Among the more serious adverse reactions are sedation and anticholinergic side effects. A variety of GI, cardiovascular, and neurologic reactions (including convulsions) may occur. The drug, like the tricyclics, is involved in many potential drug interactions.

**map unit** [L, *mappa,* napkin, *unus,* one], an arbitrary unit of measure used to express the distance between genes on a chromosome. It is calculated from the percentage of recombinations that occur between specific genes so that 1% of crossing over represents one unit on a genetic map, or approximately the number of new combinations that can be detected. The measurement is accurate only for small distances, because double cross-overs do not appear as new recombinations. Also called **map distance.** See also **morgan.**

**marasmic kwashiorkor** /məraz′mik/ [Gk, *marasmos,* a wasting; Afr], a malnutrition disease, primarily of children, resulting from the deficiency of both calories and protein. The condition is characterized by severe tissue wasting, dehydration, loss of subcutaneous fat, lethargy, and growth retardation. See also **kwashiorkor, marasmus.**

**marasmoid** /mərasˈmoid/, resembling marasmus.

**marasmus** /mərazˈməs/ [Gk, *marasmos,* a wasting], a

condition of extreme malnutrition and emaciation, occurring chiefly in young children. It is characterized by progressive wasting of subcutaneous tissue and muscle. Marasmus results from a lack of adequate calories and proteins and is seen in children with failure to thrive and in individuals in a state of starvation. Less commonly it results from an inability to assimilate or use protein because of a defect in metabolism. Care of the marasmic child involves the reestablishment of fluid and electrolyte balance, followed by the slow and gradual addition of foods as they are tolerated. See also **kwashiorkor.**

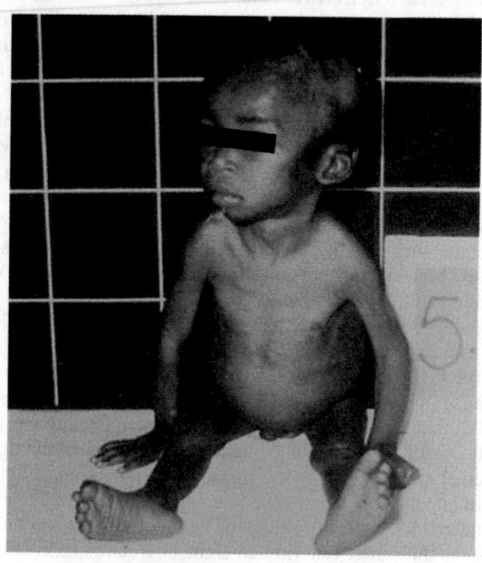

**Marasmus** *(Zitelli and Davis, 1997)*

**marathon encounter group** /merˈəthon/ [Marathon, Greece; L, *in,* in, *contra,* against; Fr, *groupe*], an intensive group experience that accelerates self-awareness and promotes personal growth and behavioral change through the continuous interaction of group members for a period ranging from 16 to more than 40 hours. See also **encounter group.**

**Marax,** trademark for a fixed-combination respiratory drug containing a smooth muscle relaxant (theophylline), an adrenergic (ephedrine sulfate), and an antihistamine (hydroxyzine hydrochloride).

**marble bones.** See **osteopetrosis.**

**Marburg virus disease** /märˈbərg/, a severe febrile viral disease characterized by rash, hepatitis, pancreatitis, and severe GI hemorrhages. The disease is caused by the Marburg virus, a member of the Filoviridae family, which also includes the Ebola virus. An epidemic in Marburg, Germany, in 1967 was apparently contracted from infected imported African green monkeys. The disease may be transmitted to hospital personnel by improper handling of contaminated needles or from hemorrhagic lesions of patients. The diagnosis is made through serologic abnormalities. There is no effective treatment. Also called **hemorrhagic fever.** See also **Ebola virus disease.**

**Marcaine Hydrochloride,** trademark for a local anesthetic (bupivacaine hydrochloride).

**Marchesani's syndrome** /mär·kəsä′nēz/. See **Weill-Marchesani syndrome.**

**march foot** [Fr, *marcher,* to walk; AS, *fot*], an abnormal condition of the foot caused by excessive use, such as in a long march. The forefoot is swollen and painful, and one or more of the metatarsal bones may be broken. See also **stress fracture.**

**march fracture.** See **metatarsal stress fracture.**

**march hemoglobinuria,** a rare abnormal condition, characterized by the presence of hemoglobin in the urine, that occurs after strenuous physical exertion or prolonged exercise, such as marching or distance running. See also **hemolysis.**

**Marchiafava-Micheli disease** /mär′kyəfä′və mikä′lē/ [Ettore Marchiafava, Italian physician, 1847–1935; F. Micheli, Italian physician, 1872–1929], a rare disorder of unknown origin characterized by episodic hemoglobinuria, which occurs usually, but not always, at night.

**Marchi's globule** /mär′kēz/ [Vittoria Marchi, Italian physician, 1851–1908], fragments and particles of broken-up myelin that stain by Marchi's method, seen in degeneration of the spinal cord.

**Marchi's method,** a laboratory staining procedure for demonstrating degenerated nerve fibers. The tissue specimen is first fixed in a solution of potassium bichromate (Müller's fluid), which prevents normal nerve fibers from being stained with osmic acid; osmic acid is then applied as a definitive black stain for abnormal nerve fibers.

**Marcus Gunn pupil sign** [Robert Marcus Gunn, English ophthalmologist, 1850–1909], paradoxical dilation of the pupils in an ophthalmologic examination in response to afferent visual stimuli. In a dark room a beam of light is moved from one eye to the other. Normal miosis is caused by the consensual pupil reaction when the normal eye is illuminated, but as the light is moved to the opposite, abnormal eye, the direct reaction to light is weaker than the consensual reaction; hence both pupils dilate.

**Marcus Gunn's syndrome.** See **jaw-winking.**

**Marezine,** trademark for an antiemetic (cyclizine hydrochloride).

**Marfan's syndrome** /märfäNz′/ [Bernard-Jean A. Marfan, French pediatrician, 1858–1942], a hereditary condition that affects the musculoskeletal system and is often associated with abnormalities of the cardiovascular system and of the eyes. Inherited as an autosomal dominant trait, Marfan's syndrome affects men and women equally. Its major musculoskeletal effects include muscular underdevelopment, ligamentous laxity, joint hypermobility, and bone elongation. The extremities of individuals with Marfan's syndrome are very long and spiderlike, with greatly extended hands, feet, and fingers. Most adult patients are over 6 feet (1.8 meters) tall and have asymmetric skulls. Funnel chest is common, and a lateral curvature of the spine may develop and increase during years of rapid vertebral growth, with kyphoscoliosis developing to varying degrees. The severe ligamental laxity and joint hypermobility associated with Marfan's syndrome may be seen by radiographic examination and often result in pes valgus and back knee. Pathologic alterations of the cardiovascular system appear to produce fragmentation of the elastic fibers in the media of the aorta, which may lead to aneurysm. Ocular changes include a variety of disorders, including dislocation of the lens. No specific treatment is available, and symptomatic management of the associated problems is the usual alternative. Resulting deformities, such as kyphoscoliosis, may be treated with orthoses or surgery, as indicated.

**margin.** See **border.**

**marginal gingiva** /mär′jənəl/ [L, *margo,* margin, *gingiva,* gum], the uppermost part of the free gingiva. It overlaps the neck and base of the crown of the tooth.

**marginal gyrus** [L, *margo,* margin; Gk, *gyros,* turn], the superior frontal convolution on the surface of the cerebral hemispheres.

**marginal peptic ulcer** [L, *margo,* margin; Gk, *peptein,* to digest; L, *ulcus,* ulcer], an ulcer that develops postoperatively at the surgical anastomosis of the stomach and jejunum. See also **peptic ulcer.**

**marginal placenta previa,** placenta previa in which the placenta is implanted in the lower uterine segment, with its margin touching or spreading to some degree over the internal os of the uterine cervix. During labor as the cervix dilates, bleeding may occur from the separation of the edge of the placenta from the uterus beneath it. Bleeding may be so scant as to pose no clinical problem. In some cases frank severe hemorrhage may occur, but the pressure of the presenting part of the baby is often sufficient to act as a tamponade, arresting the hemorrhage. Diagnosis of marginal placenta previa may be suggested by the apparent location of the placenta on ultrasonic visualization. Cesarean section is not usually necessary. See also **placenta previa.**

**marginal ridge,** an elevation of enamel that forms the proximal boundary of the occlusal surface of a tooth.

**marginal sinus** [L, *margo* + *sinus,* hollow], a sinus that may encircle the placenta. Also called **placental sinus.**

**marginal sinus rupture,** a detachment of the placenta from the implantation site. It may be complete, partial, or marginal in abruptio placentae.

**Marie's hypertrophy** [Pierre Marie, French neurologist, 1853–1940; Gk, *hyper,* excess, *trophe,* nourishment], chronic enlargement of the joints caused by periostitis. Also called **hypertrophic pulmonary osteopathy.**

**Marie-Strümpell arthritis, Marie-Strümpell disease.** See **ankylosing spondylitis.**

**marijuana.** See **cannabis.**

**Marin Amat's syndrome** [Manuel Marin Amat, Spanish ophthalmologist, b. 1879] an involuntary facial movement phenomenon in which the eyes close when the mouth opens or when the jaws move in mastication. The effect results from a facial nerve paralysis. Also called **inverse Marcus Gunn's syndrome.**

**Marinesco-Sjögren syndrome** /mä·rē·nes′kō shur′gren/ [Georges Marinesco, Romanian neurologist, 1863–1938; Karl Gustav Torsten Sjögren, Swedish physician, b. 1896], a hereditary syndrome transmitted as an autosomal recessive trait, consisting of cerebellar ataxia, mental and somatic growth retardation, congenital cataracts, inability to chew, thin brittle fingernails, and sparse, incompletely keratinized hair.

**Marinol,** trademark for an oral antiemetic (dronabinol).

**marital rape** [L, *rapere,* to seize], forcible sexual intercourse by a man with his wife.

**marital therapy,** a type of family therapy aimed at understanding and treating one or both members of a couple in the context of a distressed relationship, but not necessarily addressing the discordant relationship itself. In the past the term has also been used more restrictively as synonymous with marriage therapy, but that is increasingly considered a subset of marital therapy. Also called **couples therapy.**

**mark** [AS, *mearc*], any nevus or birthmark.

**marker gene.** See **genetic marker.**

**markers** [AS, *mearc*], body language movements that serve as indicators and punctuation marks in interpersonal communication.

**mark:space ratio.** See **duty cycle.**

**Maroteaux-Lamy syndrome** /mä·rō·tō′ lä·mē′/ [Pierre Maroteaux, French physician, b. 1926; Maurice Emile Joseph Lamy, French physician, 1895−1975], a mucopolysaccharidosis characterized biochemically by the predominance of the mucopolysaccharide dermatan sulfate in the urine and the presence of coarse granules in the leukocytes, and clinically by Hurler-like signs with normal intelligence. There are three clinical forms: the severe or classic form shows Hurler-like symptoms (see **Hurler's syndrome**); the intermediate form has the same phenotype as **pseudo-Hurler polydystrophy;** the mild form is difficult to distinguish from the **Scheie syndrome.** Also called **mucopolysaccharidosis VI** (see **mucopolysaccharidosis**).

**Marplan,** trademark for an antidepressant (isocarboxazid).

**marriage therapy,** a subset of marital therapy that focuses specifically on the bond of marriage between two people, enhancing and preserving it.

**marrow.** See **bone marrow.**

**Marseilles fever** /märsälz′, märsä′/ [Marseille, France; L, *febris,* fever], a disease endemic around the Mediterranean, in Africa, in the Crimea, and in India, caused by *Rickettsia conorii* transmitted by the brown dog tick *(Rhipicephalus sanguineus).* Characteristic symptoms are chills, fever, an ulcer covered with a black crust at the site of the tick bite, and a rash appearing on the second to fourth day. Also called **boutonneuse fever, Bruch's disease, Conor's disease, escharonodulaire, Indian tick fever, Kenya fever.**

**Marshall-Marchetti operation** [Victor F. Marshall, American urologist, b. 1913; Andrew A. Marchetti, American obstetrician, 1901–1970], a surgical procedure performed to correct stress incontinence. The vesicourethropexy involves a retropubic incision and suturing of the urethra, vesicle neck, and bladder to the posterior surface of the pubic bone. Also called **Marshall-Marchetti-Krantz operation.**

**marsupialize** /märsoo′pē·əlīz/ [L, *marsupium,* pouch; Gk, *izein,* to cause], to form a pouch surgically to treat a cyst when simple removal would not be effective, such as in a pancreatic or a pilonidal cyst. With the patient under general or local anesthesia, the cyst sac is opened and emptied. Its edges are sutured to adjacent tissues, and a drain is left in place. Secretions decrease over a period of several months and may eventually cease.

**Martorell's syndrome.** See **Takayasu's arteritis.**

**MAS,** abbreviation for **mobile arm support.**

**masculine** /mas′kyəlin/ [L, *masculinus,* male], having the characteristics of a male.

**masculinization** /mas′kyəlin′īzā′shən/ [L, *masculinus* + Gk, *izein,* to cause], the normal development or induction of male sex characteristics. See also **virilization.** —**masculinize,** *v.*

**MASER** /mā′sər/, abbreviation for *microwave amplification by stimulated emission of radiation.*

**MASH** /mash/, abbreviation for *mobile army surgical hospital.*

**mask** [Fr, *masque*], **1.** to obscure, as in symptomatic treatment that may conceal the development of a disease. **2.** to cover, as does a skin-toned cosmetic that may hide a pigmented nevus. **3.** a cover worn over the nose and mouth to prevent inhalation of toxic or irritating materials, to control delivery of oxygen or anesthetic gas, or (by medical personnel) to shield a patient during aseptic procedures from pathogenic organisms normally exhaled from the respiratory tract.

**masked residue,** the amino acid part of a peptide that is not accessible for activity after a condensation reaction.

**mask image,** a radiographic image made either before or immediately after contrast material has been injected but before it reaches the anatomic site being examined. The image thus produced is stored in a computer and displayed on a video monitor. It is then subtracted electronically from a series of additional images. The technique enhances the image of the tissues being studied. See also **remasking.**

**masking,** **1.** the covering or concealing of a disorder by a second condition. An example is a person's beginning a weight-loss diet while an undiagnosed wasting disease such as cancer has developed; the loss of body weight is attributed to the diet, masking the disease and delaying diagnosis and treatment. **2.** the unconscious display of a personality trait that conceals a behavioral aberration.

**masking agent,** a cosmetic preparation for covering nevi, surgical scars, and other blemishes. Masking agents are generally composed of a flesh-colored pigment in a lotion or cream base.

**masklike facies** [Fr, *masque* + L, *facies,* face], an immobile expressionless face with staring eyes and slightly open mouth. It is sometimes associated with parkinsonism.

**mask of pregnancy.** See **melasma.**

**Maslow's hierarchy of needs** /mas′lōz/ [Abraham H. Maslow, American psychiatrist, 1908–1970; Gk, *hierarches,* position of authority; AS, *nied,* obligation], (in psychology) a hierarchic categorization of the basic needs of humans. The most basic needs on the scale are the physiologic or biologic, such as the need for air, food, or water. Of second priority are the safety needs, including protection and freedom from fear and anxiety. The subsequent order of needs in the hierarchic progression are the need to belong, to love, and to be loved; the need for self-esteem; and ultimately the need for self-actualization. To progress from one need to another, the more basic need must first be satisfied.

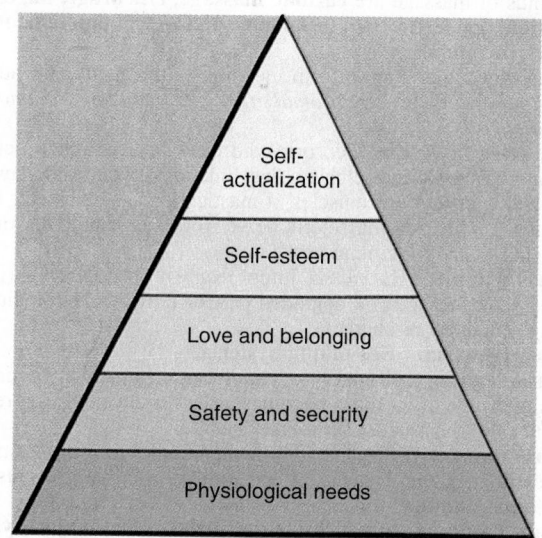

**Maslow's hierarchy of needs** *(Potter and Perry, 1997)*

**masochism** /mas′ōkiz′əm/ [Leopold von Sacher-Masoch, Austrian author, 1836–1895], pleasure or gratification derived from receiving physical, mental, or emotional abuse. The maltreatment may be inflicted by another person or by oneself. It may involve a need to experience emotional or physical pain, in reality or fantasy, to become sexually aroused. Also called **passive algolagnia.** Compare **sadism.** See also **algolagnia, sadomasochism.** —**masochistic,** *adj.*

**masochist** /mas'ōkist/ [Leopold von Sacher-Masoch], a person who derives pleasure or gratification from masochistic acts or abuse. Compare **sadist.** See also **masochism.**

**masochistic personality.** See **self-defeating personality disorder.**

**mass** [L, *massa*], **1.** the physical property of matter that gives it weight and inertia. **2.** (in pharmacology) a mixture from which pills are formed. **3.** an aggregate of cells clumped together, such as a tumor. Compare **weight.** See also **inertia.**

**mass action law, 1.** the mathematical description of reversible reactions that attain equilibrium, generally regarded as applicable to competitive assay. **2.** the rate of a chemical reaction that is proportional to the active masses of the resulting substances.

**massage** /məsäzh, məsäj'/ [Fr, *masser*, to stroke], the manipulation of the soft tissue of the body through stroking, rubbing, kneading, or tapping, to increase circulation, to improve muscle tone, and to relax the patient. The procedure is performed either with the bare hands or through some mechanical means, such as a vibrator. The most common sites for massage are the back, knees, elbows, and heels. Care is taken not to massage inflamed areas, particularly of the extremities, because of the danger of loosening blood clots; open wounds and areas of rash, tumor, or excessive sensitivity are avoided. Even if the extremities (legs) are not inflamed they should not be massaged if the client has been immobilized for an extended period of time. The procedure is performed with the patient prone or on the side, comfortably positioned, with an emollient lotion or cream applied to the area to be massaged. The caregiver's hands are warm, and excessive pressure is avoided to prevent pain or injury. Kinds of massage are **cardiac massage, effleurage, flagellation,** def. 2, **friction, frôlement, pétrissage, tapotement,** and **vibration.**

**-massage,** combining form meaning a 'therapeutic kneading of the body': *electromassage, hydromassage, phonomassage.*

**masseter** /masē'tər/ [Gk, one who chews], the thick rectangular muscle in the cheek that functions to close the jaw. It is one of the four muscles of mastication. The masseter is innervated by the masseteric nerve from the mandibular division of the trigeminal nerve.

**mass fragment** [L, *massa*, lump, *frangere*, to shatter], (in mass spectrometry) a degraded part of a molecule containing one or more charges.

**mass hysteria.** See **major hysteria.**

**massive lung collapse,** a condition in which an entire lung or one of its lobes becomes airless, frequently as a result of an obstruction in a bronchus.

**mass number (A),** the sum of the number of protons and neutrons in the nucleus of an atom or isotope. See also **atomic number.**

**mass panic, mass psychogenic illness.** See **major hysteria.**

**mass reflex,** an abnormal condition, seen in patients with transection of the spinal cord, characterized by a widespread nerve discharge. Stimulation below the level of the lesion results in flexor muscle spasms, incontinence of urine and feces, priapism, hypertension, and profuse sweating.
■ OBSERVATIONS: A mass reflex may be triggered by scratching or other painful stimulus to the skin, overdistension of the bladder or intestines, cold weather, prolonged sitting, or emotional stress. Muscle spasms may be so violent as to propel the patient off a bed or stretcher.

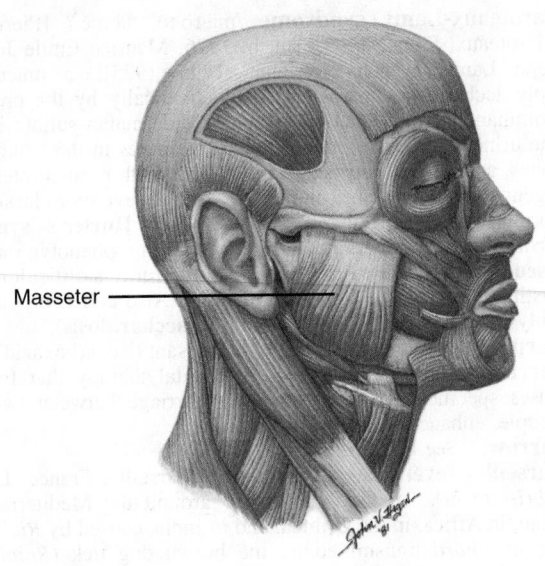

Masseter ——

**Masseter** *(Thibodeau and Patton, 1999/John V. Hagen)*

■ INTERVENTIONS: Medications to reduce mass reflexes include diazepam, dantrolene, chlordiazepoxide, and meprobamate. Hubbard baths and exercises in warm water also help. Occasionally chordotomy, rhizotomy, peripheral nerve transection, or tenotomy may be necessary.
■ NURSING CONSIDERATIONS: Nurses should avoid stimulating areas that trigger mass reflexes and should be prepared to accept them when they occur and to explain the cause to the patient. It is important to prevent decubitus ulcers and bladder infections in paraplegic and quadriplegic patients because they may also serve as triggers to initiate mass reflexes.

**mass spectrometer,** an analytic instrument for identifying a substance by sorting a stream of charged particles (ions) according to their mass. The sorting is usually accomplished by deflecting a stream of charged particles into a semicircular path as it enters a magnetic field and ultimately strikes a photographic plate or a photomultiplier tube sensor.

**mass spectrometry,** (in chemistry) a technique for the analysis of a substance in which the constituents are identified by mass and fragmentation pattern and quantified using a mass spectrometer. See also **spectrometry, spectrophotometry.**

**mass spectrum,** a characteristic pattern obtained from a mass spectrometer.

**mass transfer,** the movement of mass from one phase to another.

**MAST.** See **military antishock trousers.**

**mast-.** See **masto-.**

**mastalgia** /mastal'jə/ [Gk, *mastos*, breast, *algos*, pain], pain in the breast caused by congestion or "caking" during lactation, an infection, or fibrocystic disease, especially during or before menstruation, or in advanced cancer. The early stages of breast cancer are rarely accompanied by pain. —**mastalgic,** *adj.*

**mast cell** [Ger, *Mast*, fattening; L, *cella*, storeroom], a constituent of connective tissue containing large basophilic granules that contain heparin, serotonin, bradykinin, and histamine. These substances are released from the mast cell in response to injury and infection.

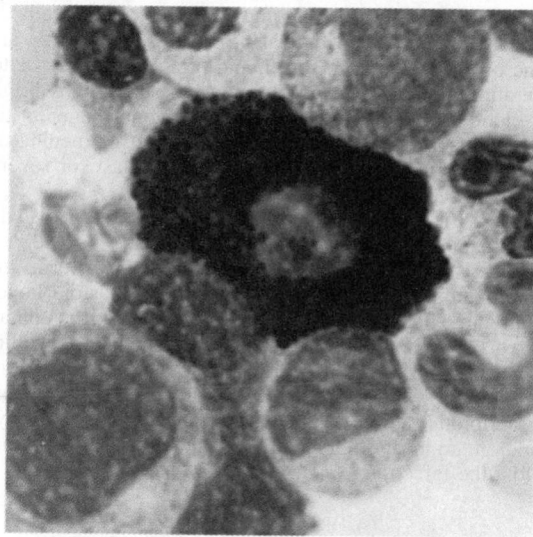

**Mast cell in bone marrow** *(Carr and Rodak, 1999)*

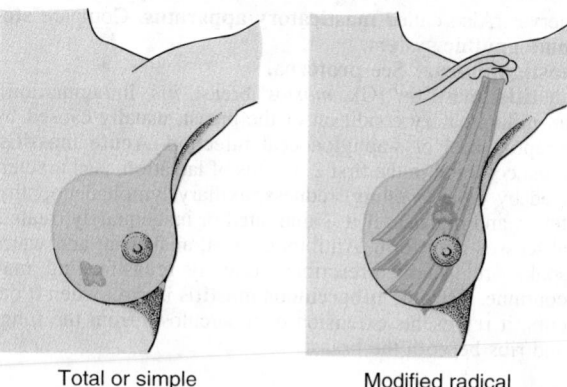

| Total or simple mastectomy | Modified radical mastectomy |

**Mastectomy** *(Beare and Myers, 1998)*

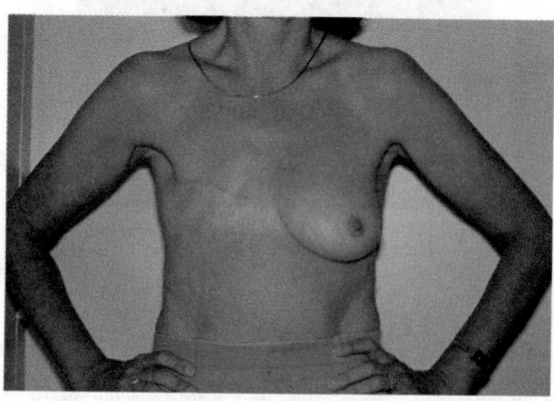

**Modified radical mastectomy**
*(Chabner, 2001/courtesy Dr. Elizabeth Chabner Thompson)*

**mast cell leukemia,** a malignant neoplasm of leukocytes characterized by connective tissue mast cells in circulating blood.

**mast cell tumor** [Ger, *Mast,* fattening; L, *cella,* storeroom; L, *tumor*], a connective tissue tumor composed of mast cells. Granules of the cells stain metachromatically with toluidine blue.

**mastectomy** /mastek′təmē/ [Gk, *mastos,* breast, *ektomē,* excision], the surgical removal of one or both breasts, most commonly performed to remove a malignant tumor. In a simple mastectomy only breast tissue is removed. In a radical mastectomy some of the muscles of the chest are removed with the breast, together with all lymph nodes in the axilla. In a modified radical mastectomy the large muscles of the chest that move the arm are preserved. The tumor is biopsied before the mastectomy. If the specimen shows a malignancy, the tumor and adjacent tissues are removed in one piece. At the end of the surgical procedure a drainage catheter is placed in the wound. The nurse inspects the wound for swelling or excessive bleeding and encourages the patient to take deep breaths hourly and, if secretions are present, to cough. The affected arm is positioned with the hand pointed upward or on pillows so that the hand is higher than the lower arm, with the lower arm above heart level. Hand and wrist movements and elbow flexion and extension are begun within 24 hours and performed regularly. The patient may be fitted with a prosthesis when the wound is completely healed or at the time of the mastectomy. Emotional support and counseling are essential. See also **breast cancer, modified radical mastectomy, radical mastectomy, simple mastectomy. —mastectomize,** *v.*

**master problem list,** a list of a patient's problems that serves as an index to his or her record. Each problem, the date when it was first noted, the treatment, and the desired outcome are added to the list as each becomes known. Thus the list provides an ongoing guide for reviewing the health status and planning the care of the patient. See also **SOAP.**

**master's degree program in nursing,** a postgraduate program in a school of nursing, based in a university setting, that grants the degree Master of Science in Nursing to successful candidates. Most programs include theory of nursing and techniques in nursing research as integral parts of the curriculum. The degree may be awarded for work in maternal-newborn nursing, medical-surgical nursing, pediatric nursing, psychiatric nursing, or other fields. Nurses with this degree function in leadership roles in clinical nursing, as consultants in various settings, in faculty positions in schools of nursing, and as nurse practitioners in various specialties.

**mastery** /mas′tərē/ [L, *magister,* chief], command or control of a situation.

**-mastia.** See **-mazia.**

**mastication** /mas′tikā′shən/ [L, *masticare,* to chew], chewing, tearing, or grinding food with the teeth while it becomes mixed with saliva. See also **bolus, digestion, ptyalin.**

**masticatory apparatus.** See **masticatory system.**

**masticatory movement** /mas′tikətôr′ē/, motion of the lower jaw in chewing.

**masticatory surface.** See **occlusal surface.**

**masticatory system** [L, *masticare,* to chew; Gk, *systema*], the combination of structures involved in chewing, including the jaws, teeth and supporting structures, mandibular and maxillary musculature, temporomandibular joints, tongue, lips, cheeks, oral mucosa, blood supply, and cranial nerves. Also called **masticatory apparatus.** Compare **stomatognathic system.**

**mastigophora.** See **protozoa.**

**mastitis** /mastī′tis/ [Gk, *mastos,* breast, *itis,* inflammation], an inflammatory condition of the breast, usually caused by streptococcal or staphylococcal infection. **Acute mastitis,** most common in the first 2 months of lactation, is characterized by pain, swelling, redness, axillary lymphadenopathy, fever, and malaise. If it is untreated or inadequately treated, abscesses may form. Antibiotics, rest, analgesia, and warm soaks are usually prescribed. Usually breastfeeding may continue. **Chronic tuberculous mastitis** is rare; when it occurs, it represents extension of tuberculosis from the lungs and ribs beneath the breast.

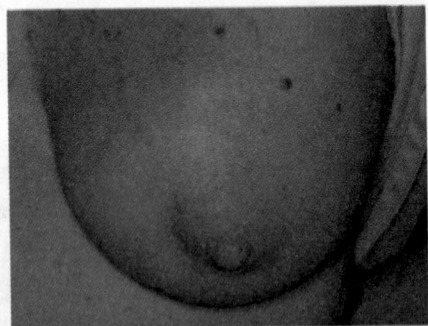

**Mastitis** *(Lemmi and Lemmi, 2000)*

**masto-, mast-,** prefix meaning 'breast': *mastochondroma, mastologist, mastoplasia.*

**mastocarcinoma** /mas′təkär′sinō′mə/, carcinoma of the mammary gland.

**mastocyte.** See **mast cell.**

**mastocytoma** /mas′təsītō′mə/, a tumor that contains mast cells.

**mastocytosis** /mas′təsītō′sis/ [Ger, *Mast,* fattening; Gk, *kytos,* cell, *osis,* condition], local or systemic overproduction of mast cells, which in rare instances may infiltrate liver, spleen, bones, the GI system, and skin. Systemic mastocytosis may precede mast cell leukemia.

**mastoid** /mas′toid/ [Gk, *mastos,* breast, *eidos,* form], **1.** pertaining to the mastoid process of the temporal bone. **2.** breast-shaped.

**mastoid-,** prefix meaning 'mastoid process': *mastoidectomy.*

**mastoid cells** [Gk, *mastos,* breast, *eidos,* form; L, *cella,* storeroom], air cells in the mastoid process of the temporal bone. Also called **mastoid air cells.**

**mastoidectomy** /mas′toidek′təmē/ [Gk, *mastos + eidos,* form, *ektomē,* excision], surgical excision of a part of the mastoid part of the temporal bone. It is performed to treat chronic suppurative otitis media or mastoiditis when systemic antibiotics are ineffective. Entry is made through the ear canal or from behind the ear. In a simple mastoidectomy with the patient under general anesthesia, diseased bone of mastoid are removed while ossicles, eardrum, and canal wall are left intact, and the eardrum is incised to drain the middle ear. Topical antibiotics are then instilled in the ear. In a radical procedure the eardrum and most middle ear structures are removed. The stapes is left intact so that a hearing

aid may be used. The opening to the eustachian tube is plugged. In a modified radical procedure the eardrum and some of the ossicles are saved, and the patient hears better than after a radical mastoidectomy. After surgery any bright red blood on the dressing may indicate hemorrhage. A stiff neck or disorientation may signal the onset of meningitis. Dizziness is usual and may be expected to last for several days. The procedure is rarely done today.

**mastoid fontanel,** a posterolateral fontanel that is usually not palpable. See also **fontanel.**

**mastoiditis** /mas′toidī′tis/ [Gk, *mastos + eidos,* form, *itis,* inflammation], an infection of one of the mastoid bones, usually an extension of a middle ear infection. It is characterized by earache, fever, headache, and malaise. Swelling of the mastoid process often displaces the pinna anteriorly and inferiorly. The infection is difficult to treat, often requiring antibiotic administered intravenously for several days. Children are most often affected. Residual hearing loss may follow the infection.

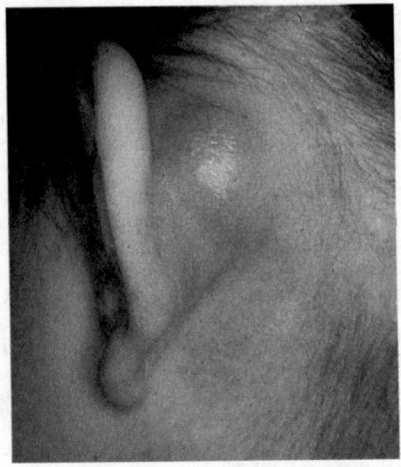

**Mastoiditis**
*(Stone and Gorbach, 2000/courtesy Dr. N. Blevins, New England Medical Center, Boston)*

**mastoid process,** the irregular conic projection of the caudal, posterior part of the temporal bone, serving as the attachment for various muscles, including the sternocleidomastoideus, splenius capitis, and longissimus capitis. A hollow section of the process contains air cells that are distinguished from a large, irregular tympanic antrum in the superior anterior part of the process. See also **temporal bone.**

**mastopathy** /mastop′əthē/, any disease of the breast.

**mastopexy,** a reconstructive procedure in cosmetic surgery to lift the breasts.

**masturbation** /mas′tərbā′shən/ [L, *masturbari,* to masturbate], sexual activity in which the penis or clitoris is stimulated, usually to orgasm, by means other than coitus. It is performed at least occasionally by most people and is considered to be normal and harmless. —**masturbate,** *v.,* **masturbatic, masturbatory,** *adj.*

**-masty.** See **-mazia.**

**mat.,** **1.** abbreviation for **maternity. 2.** abbreviation for **maturity.**

**matched group.** See **group.**

**materia** /mətir′ē·ə/, matter or material, such as materia medica.

**materia alba** /mə·tir′ē·ə al′bə/ [L, white matter], a whitish or cream-colored cheesy mass deposited around the necks of the teeth, composed of food debris, mucin, and dead epithelial cells.

**material fact** /mətir′ē·əl/ [L, *materia*, matter, *factum*], (in law) a fact that establishes or refutes an element essential to the complaint, charge, or defense. The presence of a material fact in a case being tried precludes granting of a summary judgment.

**materia medica,** 1. the study of drugs and other substances used in medicine: their origins, preparation, uses, and effects. 2. a substance or a drug used in medical treatment.

**matern.,** 1. abbreviation for **maternal.** 2. abbreviation for **maternity.**

**Materna,** trademark for a prenatal multivitamin supplement with calcium and iron.

**maternal (matern.)** /mətur′nəl/ [L, *maternus,* motherhood], 1. inherited, derived, or received from a mother. 2. motherly in behavior. 3. related through the mother's side of the family, such as a maternal grandfather.

**maternal and child health (MCH) services,** various facilities and programs organized for the purpose of providing medical and social services for mothers and children. Medical services include prenatal and postnatal services, family planning care, and pediatric care in infancy.

**maternal antibody,** an antibody transmitted from mother to fetus via the placenta. Such antibodies can provide immunity for the fetus and the newborn for up to 6 months after birth. They may also cause hemolytic anemia in newborns in cases of Rh or ABO blood group incompatibility between mother and child.

**maternal-child attachment.** See **maternal-infant bonding.**

**maternal-child separation syndrome.** See **separation anxiety.**

**maternal death,** the death of a woman during the childbearing cycle.

**maternal deprivation syndrome** [L, *maternus,* motherhood, *deprivare,* to deprive; Gk, *syn,* together, *dromos,* course], a condition characterized by developmental retardation that occurs as a result of physical or emotional deprivation. It is seen primarily in infants. Typical symptoms include lack of physical growth, with weight below the third percentile for age and size; malnutrition; pronounced withdrawal; silence; apathy; irritability; and a characteristic posture and body language, featuring unnatural stiffness and rigidity with a slow response reaction to others. Causes of the syndrome are usually multiple and complex, involving such factors as parental indifference; emotional instability or insecurity of the mother; lack of or delayed development of the mother-child attachment process; unrealistic expectations or disappointment concerning the sex, appearance, or adaptability of the child; or unfavorable socioeconomic conditions within the family. Treatment often requires hospitalization, especially in cases of severe malnutrition. Care includes assessment of the family situation, and treatment often involves psychotherapy, counseling, or special nursing instruction to help the parents learn to deal with and provide for the child. The nature and extent of the effects of the condition on later physical, emotional, intellectual, and social development vary considerably and depend on the age at which deprivation occurs, the degree and duration of the situation, the child's constitutional makeup, and the substituted care that is provided. Emotionally deprived children often remain below normal in intellectual development, fail to learn acceptable social behavior, and are unable to form trusting, meaningful relationships with others. In severe cases of early and prolonged deprivation, the damage to an infant may be irreversible. See also **failure to thrive.**

**maternal effect.** See **maternal inheritance.**

**maternal immunity,** protection against disease acquired by a fetus through the passage of maternal antibodies via the placenta. See also **maternal antibody.**

**maternal-infant bonding,** the complex process of attachment of a mother to her newborn. Disastrous effects of the disruption or absence of this attachment have long been known. The specific steps in its development and the factors that disturb or encourage it have been identified and described by anthropologists, pediatricians, psychologists, nurses, midwives, and sociologists. The process begins before birth as the parents plan for the pregnancy or discover that the mother is pregnant. The mother feels fetal movement, begins to accept the fetus as an individual, and makes plans for the baby after birth. In the first minutes and hours after birth, a sensitive period occurs during which the baby and the mother become intimately involved with each other through behaviors and stimuli that are complementary and that provoke further interactions. The mother touches the baby and holds it en face to achieve eye-to-eye contact. The infant looks back eye to eye. The mother speaks in a quiet high-pitched voice. The mother and the baby move in turn to the voice and sounds of the other, a process known as entrainment, which can be likened to a dance. The infant's movements constitute a response to the mother's voice, and she is encouraged to continue the process. The secretion of oxytocin and prolactin by the maternal pituitary gland is stimulated by the baby's sucking or licking of the mother's breasts; T and B lymphocytes and macrophages are given to the baby in the mother's milk, promoting resistance to infection. The child is also colonized by the normal flora of the mother's skin and nasal passages, improving the baby's ability to fend off infection. Physically the mother provides her body heat for the baby's warmth and comfort. Thus the extended contact in the newborn period satisfies physical and emotional needs of the mother and baby. Experts have made the following recommendations to increase the development of maternal-infant bonding: The special needs of the mother are assessed before delivery; the parents attend classes to prepare them for labor, delivery, and the puerperium; and discussions are held regarding the stresses of pregnancy and the postpartum period. In labor and delivery a companion is encouraged to stay with the mother. After the baby is born, silver nitrate drops or other medications are not placed in the baby's eyes until the mother and the baby have had time to be together en face, with eye contact for an extended period, because the drops cause a film to form over the eyes, dimming vision. During the first hour after birth the parents and the infant are not separated and are given as much privacy as possible. Skin-to-skin contact is encouraged; various methods may be used to maintain an ambient temperature adequate to maintain the baby's temperature. On the postpartum unit the mother and the baby are kept together for at least 5 hours a day, but optimally for 24 hours a day in a 24-hour rooming-in care unit. The entire family is allowed to visit. The mother has responsibility for the care of her baby, with consultation available from a midwife or a nurse. The staff does not criticize the mother's performance, because it is to the baby's inestimable benefit that the mother believes her baby is the best, most beautiful, and most perfect baby in the world and that she feels able to care for her baby.

**maternal inheritance,** the transmission of traits or conditions controlled by cytoplasmic factors within the ovum that are not self-replicating and are determined by genes within the nucleus. An example of such a characteristic is the direction of coiling in the shells of snails. Also called **maternal effect.**

**maternal inheritance mendelism.** See **inheritance.**

**maternal mortality,** **1.** the death of a woman as a result of childbearing. **2.** the number of maternal deaths per 100,000 live births. The statistic excludes women who die from ruptured ectopic pregnancy or any other condition in which there was no birth (stillbirth, septic abortion).

**maternal placenta** [L, *maternus,* motherhood, *placenta,* flat cake], the part of the placenta that develops from the decidua basalis of the uterus and is usually shed along with the fetal elements.

**maternal serum alpha-fetoprotein (MSAFP) test,** a test of a pregnant woman's blood designed to indicate an increased risk for fetal open neural tube defects, such as spina bifida. It may also indicate an increased risk for Down syndrome. See also **alpha-fetoprotein.**

**maternal status: antepartum,** a nursing outcome from the Nursing Outcomes Classification (NOC) defined as the conditions and behaviors indicative of maternal well-being from conception to the onset of labor. See also **Nursing Outcomes Classification.**

**maternal status: intrapartum,** a nursing outcome from the Nursing Outcomes Classification (NOC) defined as the conditions and behaviors indicative of maternal well-being from onset of labor to delivery. See also **Nursing Outcomes Classification.**

**maternal status: postpartum,** a nursing outcome from the Nursing Outcomes Classification (NOC) defined as the conditions and behaviors indicative of maternal well-being from delivery of placenta to completion of involution. See also **Nursing Outcomes Classification.**

**maternity (mat., matern.)** /mətur′nitē/ [L, *maternus,* motherhood], motherhood, the character and quality of a mother.

**maternity cycle** [L, *maternus,* motherhood; Gk, *kyklos,* circle], the antepartal, intrapartal, and postpartal periods of pregnancy and the puerperium, from conception to 6 weeks after birth.

**maternity nursing,** nursing care of women and their families during pregnancy and parturition and through the first days of the puerperium. Increasingly postpartum maternity nursing includes the supervision of the mothers' care of their newborns in rooming-in units and may include care of normal newborns in the nursery when they are not with their mother. Maternity nursing requires extensive instruction of the mothers in the usual behavior and needs of a newborn, in expected patterns of growth and development of the infant during the first week, and in details of care needed by the mother during the first weeks after birth. Breastfeeding, bottle feeding, baby baths, perineal care, umbilical care, nutrition, and danger signs of the puerperium are usually taught by the maternity nurse. Observation for abnormal conditions, such as thrombophlebitis, mastitis, and other infections, is a daily ongoing concern of the maternity nurse on the postpartum unit. Intrapartum maternity nursing involves the care of mothers in labor and delivery, as well as high-risk technical nursing, emotional support in labor and delivery, and ongoing observation for abnormal signs or symptoms. Often pregnant women with medical problems associated with pregnancy are cared for on a special high-risk antepartum unit by specially educated maternity nurses.

**mat gold** [Fr, *mat,* dull; AS, *geolu,* yellow], a noncohesive form of pure gold. Also called **crystal gold, sponge gold.**

**mating** /mā′ting/ [D, *mate,* companion], the pairing of individuals of the opposite sex, primarily for purposes of reproduction.

**mat. med.,** abbreviation for **materia medica.**

**matrifocal family** /mat′rifō′kəl/ [L, *mater,* mother, *focus,* hearth, *familia,* household], a family unit composed of a mother and her children. Biologic fathers may have a temporary place in the family during the first years of the children's lives, but they maintain a more permanent position in their own original families.

**matrix** /mā′triks, mat′riks/ [L, *womb*], **1.** an intercellular substance. **2.** also called **ground substance.** a basic substance from which a specific organ or kind of tissue develops. **3.** a form used in shaping a tooth surface in dental procedures. **4.** (in analytical chemistry) material of no interest in an analysis that may have an effect on the analysis. **5.** A rectangular arrangement of elements into rows and columns, often used to display a digital image.

**matrix band,** a cylindrical copper band or short tube that is seated over a tooth. The band may be filled with impression compound, which flows into a prepared cavity in order to obtain an impression, or may be used to aid in the placement and contouring of restorative materials.

**matrix holder.** See **matrix retainer.**

**matrix retainer,** a mechanical device used to secure the ends of a matrix band around a tooth. The band provides a substitute wall where a part of the tooth is missing and helps to compact a restoration into a prepared tooth cavity after the carious lesion has been removed. Also called **matrix holder.** See also **retainer.**

**matrix unguis.** See **nailbed.**

**matroclinous inheritance** /mātrō′klinəs/ [L, *mater,* mother; Gk, *klinein,* to incline], a form of heredity in which the traits of the offspring have been transmitted from the mother.

**matter** [L, *materia*], **1.** anything that has mass and occupies space. **2.** any substance not otherwise identified as to its constituents, such as gray matter, pus, or serum exuding from a wound.

**Matulane,** trademark for an antineoplastic (procarbazine hydrochloride).

**maturation** /mach′ərā′shən/ [L, *maturare,* to ripen], **1.** the process or condition of attaining complete development. In humans it is the unfolding of full physical, emotional, and intellectual capacities that enable a person to function at a higher level of competency and adaptability within the environment. **2.** the final stages in the meiotic formation of germ cells in which the number of chromosomes in each cell is reduced to the haploid number characteristic of the species. See also **meiosis, oogenesis, spermatogenesis. 3.** suppuration. —**maturate,** *v.*

**maturational crisis** /mach′ərā′shənəl/, a transitional or developmental period within a person's life, such as puberty, when psychologic equilibrium is upset.

**mature** /məchŏŏr′/ [L, *maturus,* ripe], **1.** to become fully developed; to ripen. **2.** fully developed or ripened.

**mature cataract.** See **ripe cataract.**

**mature cell leukemia.** See **polymorphocytic leukemia.**

**maturity (mat.)** /məchŏŏ′ritē/ [L, *maturus,* ripe], **1.** a state of complete growth or development, usually designated as the period of life between adolescence and old age. **2.** the stage at which an organism is capable of reproduction.

**maturity-onset diabetes.** See **type 2 diabetes mellitus.**

**max,** 1. abbreviation for *maxima.* 2. abbreviation for *maximum.*

**maxilla** /maksil′ə/, *pl.* **maxillae** [L, *mala,* jaw], one of a pair of large bones (often referred to as one bone) that form the upper jaw and teeth, consisting of a pyramidal body and four processes: the zygomatic, frontal, alveolar, and palatine.

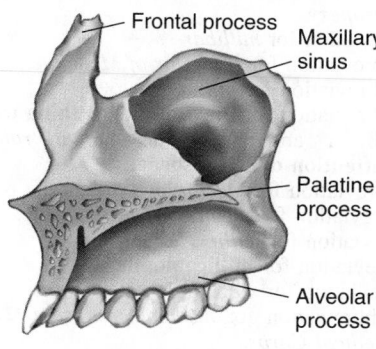

**Maxilla**

-maxilla, combining form meaning 'upper jaw or the bones composing it': *intermaxilla, submaxilla, supermaxilla.*

**maxillary** /mak′səler′ē/ [L, *maxilla,* upper jaw], pertaining to the upper jawbone.

**maxillary arch** [L, *maxilla,* upper jaw, *arcus,* bow], the curved bony ridge of the upper jawbone, in the shape of a horseshoe, including the dentition and supporting structures.

**maxillary artery** [L, *maxilla,* upper jaw; Gk, *arteria,* airpipe], either of two larger terminal branches of the external carotid arteries that rise from the neck of the mandible near the parotid gland and divide into three branches, supplying the deep structures of the face.

**maxillary fossa.** See **canine fossa.**

**maxillary process** [L, *maxilla,* upper jaw, *processus*], 1. the alveolar process of the upper jaw that contains the tooth sockets. 2. the frontal process that extends upward to articulate with the frontal and nasal bones. 3. the palatine process that helps form the hard palate. 4. the zygomatic process or anterior surface that articulates with the zygomatic bone.

**maxillary retroposition, maxillary retrusion.** See **retrognathia.**

**maxillary sinus,** one of a pair of large air cells forming a pyramidal cavity in the body of the maxilla. The apex of each sinus extends into the zygomatic arch, and its floor, formed by the alveolar process, is usually 1 to 10 mm below the floor of the nose. In the adult the volume of the sinus averages 14.75 cc. The mucous membrane of the sinus is continuous with that of the nasal cavity. In the fourth month of gestation the embryonic sinus appears as a shallow groove on the medial surface of the bone but does not reach full size until after the second teething. Also called **antrum of Highmore.** Compare **ethmoidal air cell, frontal sinus, sphenoidal sinus.**

**maxillary tuberosity,** a rounded eminence on the posterior surface of the body of the maxilla, behind the root of the third molar. It becomes prominent after the eruption and growth of the third molars.

**maxillary vein,** one of a pair of deep veins of the face, accompanying the maxillary artery and passing between the condyle of the mandible and the sphenomandibular ligament. Each maxillary vein is a tributary of the internal jugular and external jugular veins.

**maxillodental** /mak′silōden′təl/, pertaining to or affecting the upper jaw and teeth.

**maxillofacial** /mak′silōfā′shəl/ [L, *maxilla,* upper jaw, *facies,* face], pertaining to the maxilla and face.

**maxillofacial dysostosis.** See **maxillofacial syndrome.**

**maxillofacial prosthesis** [L, *maxilla,* upper jaw, *facies* face], a prosthetic replacement for part, or all, of the upper jaw, nose, or cheek. It is applied when surgical repair alone is inadequate.

**maxillofacial surgery.** See **oral and maxillofacial surgery.**

**maxillofacial syndrome,** a congenital defect of fetal ossification characterized by anteroposterior shortening of the maxilla and various other anomalies, including mandibular prognathism, slanting of the eyes, and malformation of the auricles. Also called **maxillofacial dysostosis.**

**maxillofacial trauma,** injury to the jaw and face. Fractures requiring reconstructive surgery tend to occur most frequently in motor vehicle collisions and short falls.

**maxillolacrimal suture** /-lak′riməl/, a line of union between the anterior border of the lacrimal bone and the frontal process of the maxilla. Also called **lacrimomaxillary suture.**

**maxillomandibular** /maksil′ōmandib′yŏŏlər/, pertaining to the upper and lower jaws.

**maxillomandibular fixation** [L, *maxilla,* upper jaw, *mandere,* to chew, *figere,* to fasten], stabilization of fractures of the face or jaw by temporarily connecting the maxilla and mandible by wires, elastic bands, or metal splints. See also **elastic-band fixation, nasomandibular fixation.**

**maxillomandibular relation.** See **jaw relation.**

**maxillotomy** /mak′si·lot′ə·mē/ [L, *maxilla,* upper jaw; Gk, *tomē* a cutting], surgical sectioning of the maxilla which allows movement of all or a part of the maxilla into the desired position.

**maximal breathing capacity.** See **maximum breathing capacity.**

**maximal diastolic membrane potential,** the most-negative transmembrane potential achieved by a cardiac cell during repolarization. Also called **maximum diastolic potential.**

**maximal expiratory flow.** See **maximal expiratory flow rate.**

**maximal expiratory flow rate (MEFR),** the rate of the most rapid flow of gas from the lungs during a forced expiration after a full inspiration.

**maximal expiratory pressure (MEP),** the greatest pressure of expired air achieved by a person after a full inspiration.

**maximal midexpiratory flow rate (MMFR),** the rate of the most rapid flow of gas during the middle half (in terms of volume) of a forced expiration after a full inspiration. It is measured in pulmonary function tests to detect and evaluate chronic obstructive pulmonary diseases, such as bronchitis, emphysema, and asthma.

**maximal treadmill test (MTT),** an exercise stress test in which subjects increase their heart rate during exercise to 80% to 90% of the maximal rate, which is estimated from each subject's age and sex. Newer methods of stress testing produce the same physiologic effect of exercise on the heart without using exercise. These tests use drugs such as dipyridamole to "stress" the heart.

**maximum breathing capacity (MBC)** /mak′siməl/ [L, *maximus,* greatest; AS, *braeth* + L, *capacitas*], the maximum volume of gas that a person can inhale and exhale per minute by breathing as quickly and deeply as possible. Also called **maximal breathing capacity.**

**maximum diastolic potential.** See **maximal diastolic membrane potential.**

**maximum expiratory flow, maximum expiratory flow rate.** See **maximal expiratory flow rate.**

**maximum inspiratory pressure (MIP)** /mak′səməm/ [L, *maximus,* greatest, *inspirare,* to breathe in, *premere,* to press], the maximum pressure within the alveoli of the lungs that occurs during a full inspiration.

**maximum oxygen uptake,** the greatest volume of oxygen that can be absorbed from the lungs by the blood. Also called **aerobic capacity.**

**maximum permissible dose (MPD),** the largest amount of ionizing radiation a person may receive according to radiation protection guidelines for persons working with radioactive materials or x-rays. It is 5 rem per year or a lifetime accumulation of 1 rem times the age of the person. Also called **effective dose equivalent limit.** See also **accumulated dose equivalent.**

**maximum voluntary isometric contraction (MVIC),** the peak force produced by a muscle as it contracts while pulling against an immovable object.

**maximum voluntary ventilation (MVV),** the maximum volume of gas that a person can inhale and exhale by voluntary effort per minute by breathing as quickly and deeply as possible. It is measured in pulmonary function tests.

**maxofacial surgery.** See **dentistry.**

**Mayer's reflex** /mā′ərz/ [Karl Mayer, Austrian neurologist, 1862–1932], a normal reflex elicited by grasping the ring finger and flexing it at the metacarpophalangeal joint of a person whose hand is relaxed with thumb abducted. The normal responses are adduction and apposition of the thumb. The reflex is absent in disease of the pyramidal system.

**May-Hegglin anomaly,** a rare autosomal dominant inherited blood cell disorder characterized by thrombocytopenia and granulocytes with blue-colored ribonucleic acid containing cytopathic inclusions, similar to Döhle's bodies.

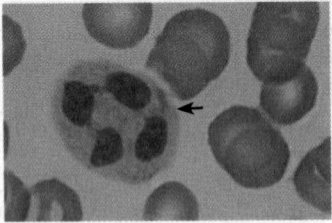

**May-Hegglin anomaly** *(Carr and Rodak, 1999)*

**Mayo scissors.** See **scissors.**

**-mazia, -mastia, -masty,** combining form meaning '(condition of the) breasts': *macromazia, pleomazia, polymazia.*

**mazindol** /mā′zindōl/, an anorexiant.

■ INDICATION: It is prescribed to decrease appetite in the treatment of exogenous obesity.

■ CONTRAINDICATIONS: Glaucoma, history of drug abuse, concomitant use of a monoamine oxidase inhibitor, or known hypersensitivity to this drug prohibits its use.

■ ADVERSE EFFECTS: Among the more serious adverse reactions are insomnia, palpitation, dizziness, dry mouth, tachycardia, and hypersensitivity reactions.

**mazo-,** combining form meaning 'breast': *mazodynia, mazology, mazopexy.*

**mb,** abbreviation for *millibar.*

**M.B.,** abbreviation for *Bachelor of Medicine.*

**mbar,** abbreviation for *millibar.*

**MBC,** abbreviation for **maximum breathing capacity.**

**MBD, M.B.D.,** abbreviation for *minimal brain dysfunction.* See **attention deficit disorder.**

**mbp,** abbreviation for *mean blood pressure.*

**mbt,** abbreviation for *mean body temperature.*

**mc,** abbreviation for *millicycle.*

**mC,** abbreviation for **millicoulomb.**

**Mc,** abbreviation for *megacycle.*

**MC,** 1. abbreviation for *medical certificate.* 2. abbreviation for *Medical Corps.*

**MCAD,** abbreviation for *medium-chain acyl-CoA dehydrogenase,* an enzyme involved in degradation of medium–chain length fatty acids. Deficiency of the enzyme **(MCAD deficiency)** is characterized by recurring episodes of hypoglycemia, vomiting, and lethargy, with urinary excretion of medium-chain dicarboxylic acids, minimal ketogenesis, and low plasma and tissue levels of carnitine.

**McArdle's disease** /məkär′dəlz/ [Brian McArdle, English neurologist, b. 1911], an inherited glycolic storage disease marked by an absence of myophosphorylase B and abnormally large amounts of glycogen in skeletal muscle. It is milder than other glycogen storage diseases, characterized by muscle fatigability and stiffness after exercise. There is no known treatment. Also called **glycogen storage disease, type V.** See also **glycogen storage disease.**

**MCAT,** abbreviation for **Medical College Aptitude Test.**

**McBurney's incision** /makbur′nēz/ [Charles McBurney, American surgeon, 1845–1913], a surgical wound that begins 2 to 5 cm above the anterior superior iliac spine and runs parallel to the external oblique muscle of the abdomen. This incision is used for an appendectomy.

**McBurney's point** [Charles McBurney; L, *pungere,* to puncture], a site of extreme sensitivity in acute appendicitis, situated in the normal area of the appendix midway between the umbilicus and the anterior iliac crest in the right lower quadrant of the abdomen. See also **appendicitis.**

**McBurney's sign** [Charles McBurney], a reaction of the patient indicating severe pain and extreme tenderness when McBurney's point is palpated. Such a reaction indicates appendicitis.

**McCall's festoon** /məkôlz′/, (in dentistry) a ring-shaped enlargement of the gingival margin on the vestibular surface (buccal or labial) of canines and premolars. It may be associated with occlusal trauma.

**McCune-Albright syndrome.** See **Albright's syndrome.**

**mcg,** abbreviation for **microgram.**

**MCH,** 1. abbreviation for **maternal and child health services.** 2. abbreviation for **mean corpuscular hemoglobin.**

**M.Ch.,** abbreviation for *Master of Surgery.*

**MCHC,** abbreviation for **mean corpuscular hemoglobin concentration.**

**mCi,** abbreviation for **millicurie.**

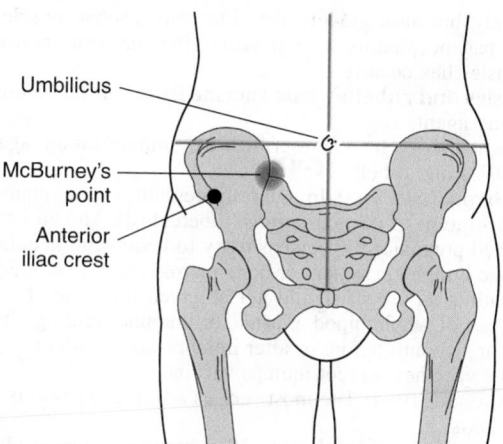

**McBurney's point** *(Phipps, Sands, and Marek, 1999)*

**mCi-hr,** abbreviation for *millicurie hour.*

**McManus, R. Louise** (1896–1993), who established the first national testing service for the nursing profession, currently the second largest educational testing program in the nation. She was also instrumental in developing a means of evaluating the nursing programs in community and junior colleges, and she established a center for education in nursing research at Teachers College, Columbia University.

**McMurray's sign** /makmur′ēz/ [Thomas P. McMurray, English surgeon, 1887–1949], an audible click heard when rotating the tibia on the femur, indicating injury to meniscal structures.

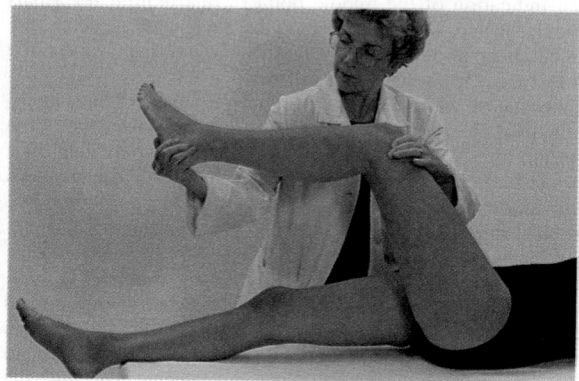

**Testing for McMurray's sign** *(Wilson and Giddens, 2001)*

**MCO,** abbreviation for **managed care organization.**

**M component,** an abnormal immunoglobulin that appears in large numbers in patients with macroglobulinemia, heavy chain disease, and multiple myeloma.

**M.C.P.,** abbreviation for **metacarpophalangeal joint dislocation.**

**M-CSF,** abbreviation for **macrophage colony-stimulating factor.**

**MCTD,** abbreviation for **mixed connective tissue disease.**

**MCV,** abbreviation for **mean corpuscular volume.**

**Md,** symbol for the element **mendelevium.**

**MD,** abbreviation for **muscular dystrophy.**

**M.D.,** abbreviation for *Doctor of Medicine.* See **physician.**

**MDA,** abbreviation for *Muscular Dystrophy Association.*

**MDI,** abbreviation for **metered dose inhaler.**

**MDR,** abbreviation for **minimum daily requirement.**

**M.D.V.,** abbreviation for *Doctor of Veterinary Medicine.*

**Me,** abbreviation for the methyl radical $CH_3$-.

**MEA,** abbreviation for **multiple endocrine adenomatosis.**

**Meals on Wheels,** a program designed to deliver hot meals to elderly, physically disabled, or other people who lack the resources to provide nutritionally adequate meals for themselves on a daily basis.

**mean** [ME, *mene,* in the middle], occupying a position midway between two extremes of a set of values or data. The **arithmetic mean** is a value that is derived by dividing the total of a set of values by the number of items in the set. The **geometric mean** is a value between the first and last of a set of values organized in a geometric progression.

**mean arterial pressure (MAP),** the arithmetic mean of the blood pressure in the arterial part of the circulation. It is calculated by adding the systolic pressure reading to two times the diastolic reading and dividing the sum by 3.

**mean corpuscular hemoglobin (MCH),** an estimate of the amount of hemoglobin in an average erythrocyte, derived from the ratio between the amount of hemoglobin and the number of erythrocytes present. The normal value of MCH is between 28 and 32 picograms of hemoglobin per red blood cell. See also **hypochromic anemia, iron deficiency anemia.**

**mean corpuscular hemoglobin concentration (MCHC),** an estimation of the concentration of hemoglobin in grams per 100 ml of packed red blood cells, derived from the ratio of the hemoglobin to the hematocrit. The normal MCHC is between 32% and 36% for adults and children and 32% and 34% in newborns.

**mean corpuscular volume (MCV),** an evaluation of the average volume of each red cell, derived from the ratio of the volume of packed red cells (the hematocrit) to the total number of red blood cells. The normal MCV is between 82 and 92 $\mu m^3$ for children and adults and 96 to 108 in newborns.

**mean marrow dose (MMD),** the estimated average annual somatic radiation received by each person in the United States. The figure is 77 mrad and represents a weighted average for people exposed to radiation and those not exposed during the period. It is expressed in terms of bone marrow because irradiation of that tissue is assumed to be a cause of leukemia.

**mean platelet volume test (MPV),** a blood test that measures the volume of a large number of platelets as determined by an automated analyzer. The MPV is very useful in the differential diagnosis of thrombocytopenic disorders.

**measles** /mē′zəlz/ [ME, *meseles,* skin spots], an acute, highly contagious viral disease involving the respiratory tract and characterized by a spreading maculopapular cutaneous rash. It occurs primarily in young children who have not been immunized and in teenagers or young adults who are inadequately immunized. Measles is caused by a paramyxovirus and is transmitted by direct contact with droplets spread from the nose, throat, and mouth of infected people, usually in the prodromal stage of the disease. Indirect transmission by uninfected people or by contaminated articles is unusual. Diagnosis is confirmed by the identification of Koplik's spots on the buccal mucosa and by sero-

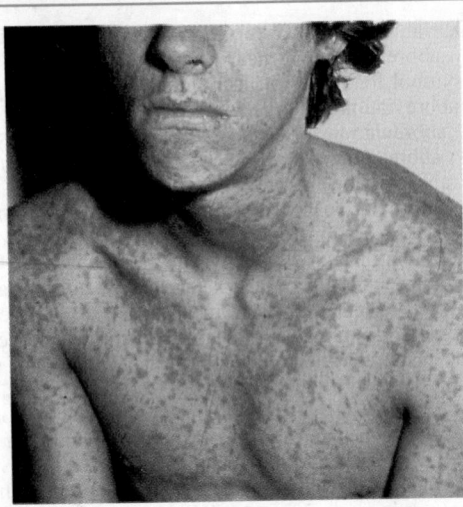

**Measles** *(Zitelli and Davis, 1997/courtesy Dr. M. Sherlock)*

logic examination. Also called **morbilli, rubeola.** See also **roseola infantum, rubella.**

■ OBSERVATIONS: An incubation period of 7 to 14 days is followed by the prodromal stage, characterized by fever, malaise, coryza, cough, conjunctivitis, photophobia, anorexia, and the pathognomonic Koplik's spots, which appear 1 to 2 days before onset of the rash. Pharyngitis and inflammation of the laryngeal and tracheobronchial mucosa develop, the temperature may rise to 103° or 104° F (39.4° to 40° C), and there is marked granulocytic leukopenia. The papules of the rash first appear as irregular brownish pink spots around the hairline, the ears, and the neck, then spread rapidly, within 24 to 48 hours, to the trunk and extremities, becoming red, maculopapular, and dense and giving a blotchy appearance. Within 3 to 5 days the fever subsides and the lesions flatten, turn a brownish color, and begin to fade, causing a fine desquamation, especially over heavily affected areas.

■ INTERVENTIONS: Routine treatment consists of bed rest, antipyretics, appropriate antimicrobials to control secondary bacterial infection, and, when necessary, application of calamine lotion, corn starch solution, oatmeal, baking soda, or cool water to relieve itching. Preventive measures include active immunization with measles virus vaccine after the infant is 1 year of age. A booster is recommended at 4 to 6 years of age or 12 years of age. Passive immunization with immune serum globulin is recommended for unvaccinated individuals exposed to the disease. One attack of the disease confers lifelong immunity.

■ NURSING CONSIDERATIONS: Bed rest, isolation, and quiet activity are recommended as long as fever and rash persist. Acetaminophen, fluids, cool sponge baths, nose drops, and cough medication may be necessary to counteract fever and respiratory symptoms. Bright sunlight may be irritating to the eyes. Special attention is given to the care and cleansing of the eyes and skin, especially in cases of severe papular eruption. An important nursing function is instruction of the parents in the proper home care of the child, because most cases are not serious enough to require hospitalization. The disease is usually benign, and mortality is rare. Complications sometimes occur; the most common are otitis media, pneumonia, bronchiolitis, obstructive laryngitis, laryngotracheitis, and occasionally encephalitis and appendicitis.

Rarely, but most gravely, the virus causes subacute sclerosing panencephalitis several years after the acute attack of measles has occurred.

**measles and rubella virus vaccine live,** an active immunizing agent.

■ INDICATIONS: It is prescribed for immunization against measles and rubella.

■ CONTRAINDICATIONS: Immunosuppression, concomitant administration of corticosteroids, tuberculosis, known or suspected pregnancy, hypersensitivity to neomycin, neoplasms of the lymphatic system or bone marrow, or active infection prohibits its use. It should not be given for 3 months after the use of whole blood, plasma, or immune serum globulin, or for 1 month before or after immunization with other live virus vaccines, except mumps vaccine.

■ ADVERSE EFFECT: The most serious adverse reaction is anaphylaxis.

**measles immune globulin.** See **immune gamma globulin.**

**measles, mumps, and rubella virus vaccine live (MMR),** an active immunizing agent.

■ INDICATION: It is prescribed for simultaneous immunization against measles, mumps, and rubella.

■ CONTRAINDICATIONS: Immunosuppression, concomitant administration of corticosteroids, tuberculosis, hypersensitivity to neomycin, neoplasms of the lymphatic system or bone marrow, known or suspected pregnancy, or acute infection prohibits its use. It is not given for 3 months after the use of whole blood, plasma, or immune serum globulin, and it is not given for 1 month before or after immunization with other live virus vaccines.

■ ADVERSE EFFECTS: The most serious adverse reaction is anaphylaxis.

**measurement** /mezh′ərment/ [L, *mensura*], the determination, expressed numerically, of the extent or quantity of a substance, energy, or time. See also **international unit, metric system.**

**measure of central tendency,** (in descriptive statistics) an indication of the middle point of distribution for a particular group. Measures include the mean average score, the median or middle score of distribution, and the mode, the most frequently occurring measure.

**measure of variability,** (in descriptive statistics) a mathematical determination of how much the performance of the group as a whole deviates from the mean or median. The most frequently used measure of variability is the standard deviation.

**meatal** /mē·ā′təl/ [L, *meatus*, channel], pertaining to a meatus.

**meatorrhaphy** /mē′ətôr′əfē/ [L, *meatus*, channel; Gk, *rhaphe*, suture], the suturing of the cut end of the urethra to the glans penis after surgery to enlarge the urethral meatus.

**meatoscopy** /mē′ətos′kəpē/ [L, *meatus* + Gk, *skopein*, to look], the visual examination of any meatus, especially the urethra, usually performed with the aid of a speculum or endoscope.

**meatus** /mē·ā′təs/, *pl.* **meatuses** [L, channel], an opening or tunnel through any part of the body, such as the external acoustic meatus that leads from the external ear to the tympanic membrane.

**meatus acusticus externus.** See **external acoustic meatus.**

**meatus acusticus internus.** See **internal acoustic meatus.**

**meatuses.** See **meatus.**

**Mebaral,** trademark for an anticonvulsant and sedative (mephobarbital).

**mebendazole** /məben'dəzōl/, an anthelmintic.
■ INDICATIONS: It is prescribed in treatment of pinworm, whipworm, roundworm, and hookworm infestations.
■ CONTRAINDICATIONS: Pregnancy or known hypersensitivity to this drug prohibits its use.
■ ADVERSE EFFECTS: Among the most serious adverse reactions are abdominal pain and diarrhea.

**MEC,** abbreviation for *minimum effective concentration,* or the minimum inhibitory concentration that allows a drug to be active. The drug is effective at any level above this threshold value.

**mecamylamine hydrochloride** /mek'əmil'əmēn/, a ganglionic blocking agent (antihypertensive).
■ INDICATION: It is prescribed in the management of severe essential hypertension and uncomplicated malignant hypertension.
■ CONTRAINDICATIONS: Coronary or cerebrovascular insufficiency, recent myocardial infarction, uremia, pyelonephritis, glaucoma, or known hypersensitivity to this drug prohibits its use.
■ ADVERSE EFFECTS: Among the most serious adverse reactions are orthostatic hypotension, paralytic ileus, urinary retention, and cycloplegia. The incidence of side effects is very high because the drug reduces all autonomic activity.

**mechanical advantage** [Gk, *mechane,* machine; L, *abante,* superior position], the ratio of the output force developed by a muscle to the input force applied to the body structure that the muscle moves. Variations in the sizes of muscles and the lengths of bones in different individuals partially account for the differences in mechanical advantage and in physical capabilities, such as speed and strength, among body types.

**mechanical condenser,** a device that delivers automatically controlled impacts for condensing restorative material in the filling of tooth cavities. It may be spring activated, pneumatic, or electrically controlled. Also called **automatic mallet condenser.**

**mechanical dead airspace** [Gk, *mechane* + AS, *dead* + Gk, *aer* + L, *spatium*], the volume of air that fills the breathing circuits of a mechanical ventilator. The mechanical dead space may be increased if necessary to control hypocapnia and respiratory alkalosis.

**mechanical heart-lung,** a device connected to the circulatory system to maintain oxygenated blood flow during surgery that requires interruption of normal heart-lung functions, such as open heart surgery. See also **blood pump.**

**mechanical restraint** [Gk, *mechane* + L, *restringere,* to confine], a device made of fabric that hinders a patient's movement, such as a safety vest, hand and wrist straps, mittens, and a stretcher equipped with belts. See also **restraint.**

**mechanical vector.** See **vector.**

**mechanical ventilation,** a nursing intervention from the Nursing Interventions Classification (NIC) defined as use of an artificial device to assist a patient to breathe. See also **Nursing Interventions Classification.**

**mechanical ventilatory weaning,** a nursing intervention from the Nursing Interventions Classification (NIC) defined as assisting the patient to breathe without the aid of a mechanical ventilator. See also **Nursing Interventions Classification.**

**mechanism** /mek'əniz'əm/, **1.** an instrument or process by which something is done, results, or comes into being. **2.** a machine or machinelike system. **3.** a stimulus-response system. **4.** a habit or drive.

**mechanism of injury,** the circumstance in which an injury occurs: for example, caused by sudden deceleration, wounded by a projectile, crushed by a heavy object.

**mechanism of labor.** See **cardinal movements of labor.**

**mechano-,** combining form meaning 'mechanical': *mechanocyte, mechanotherapy, mechanothermy.*

**mechanoreceptor** /mek'ənō'risep'tər/ [Gk, *mechane,* machine; L, *recipere,* to receive], any sensory nerve ending that responds to mechanical stimuli, such as touch, pressure, sound, and muscular contractions. See also **proprioceptor.**

**mechlorethamine hydrochloride** /mek'lôreth'əmēn/, an antineoplastic alkylating agent. Also called **nitrogen mustard.**
■ INDICATIONS: It is prescribed in the treatment of a variety of neoplasms.
■ CONTRAINDICATIONS: Bone marrow depression, pregnancy, infection, or known hypersensitivity to this drug prohibits its use.
■ ADVERSE EFFECTS: Among the most serious adverse reactions are bone marrow depression and inflammation caused by extravasation at the site of injection. Nausea, vomiting, and alopecia also may occur.

**Meckel's cartilage** /mek'elz/ [Johann Friedrich Meckel, German anatomist, 1781–1833], a cartilaginous bar (in the embryo); from it or its sheath, the sphenomandibular ligament, the malleus, and the incus develop. Also called **Meckel's rod.**

**Meckel's diverticulum** [Johann F. Meckel, German anatomist, 1781–1833], an anomalous sac protruding from the wall of the ileum between 30 and 90 cm from the ileocecal sphincter. It is congenital, resulting from the incomplete closure of the yolk stalk, and occurs in 1% to 2% of the population. The diverticulum is usually asymptomatic, but the condition is suggested by signs of appendicitis in infancy; by sudden and painless bleeding in the sac, usually in childhood; or by symptoms of intestinal obstruction. Symptomatic diverticula are most commonly resected. Surgical resection of asymptomatic diverticula is also recommended to prevent potential diverticulitis, obstruction, and blood loss. Many Meckel's diverticula are discovered incidentally during surgery for other causes and on postmortem examination.

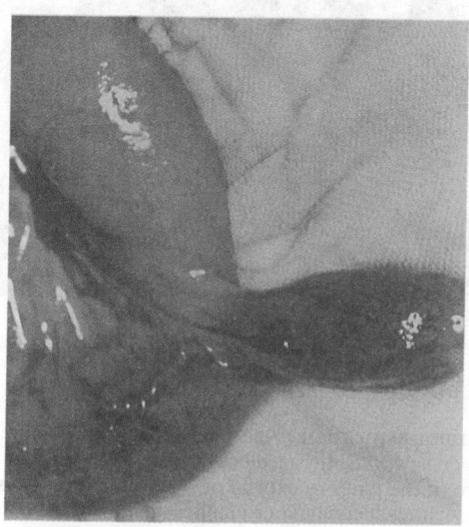

**Meckel's diverticulum** *(Zitelli and Davis, 1997)*

**Meclan,** trademark for a topical antibacterial (meclocycline sulfosalicylate).

**meclizine hydrochloride** /mek′lizēn/, an antihistamine.

- INDICATION: It is prescribed in the prevention and treatment of motion sickness.
- CONTRAINDICATIONS: Newborns and lactating mothers are not given this drug. Asthma or known hypersensitivity to it prohibits its use.
- ADVERSE EFFECTS: Among the more serious adverse effects are drowsiness, skin rash, hypersensitivity reactions, dry mouth, tachycardia, and nervousness.

**meclofenamate sodium** /mek′lōfen′əmāt/, a nonsteroidal antiinflammatory agent.

- INDICATIONS: It is prescribed in the treatment of rheumatoid arthritis and osteoarthritis.
- CONTRAINDICATIONS: Known hypersensitivity to aspirin or to nonsteroidal antiinflammatory drugs prohibits its use. It is used with caution in patients who have upper GI disease or impaired renal function.
- ADVERSE EFFECTS: Among the more serious adverse reactions are GI distress, peptic ulcers, dizziness, rashes, and tinnitus. This drug interacts with many other drugs.

**Meclomen,** trademark for an antiinflammatory agent (meclofenamate sodium).

**mecocephaly.** See **scaphocephaly.**

**meconium** /mikō′nē·əm/ [Gk, *mekon,* poppy], a material that collects in the intestines of a fetus and forms the first stools of a newborn. It is thick and sticky, usually greenish to black, and composed of secretions of the intestinal glands, some amniotic fluid, and intrauterine debris, such as bile pigments, fatty acids, epithelial cells, mucus, lanugo, and blood. With ingestion of breast milk or formula and proper functioning of the GI tract, the color, consistency, and frequency of the stools change by the third or fourth day after the initiation of feedings. The presence of meconium in the amniotic fluid during labor may indicate fetal distress.

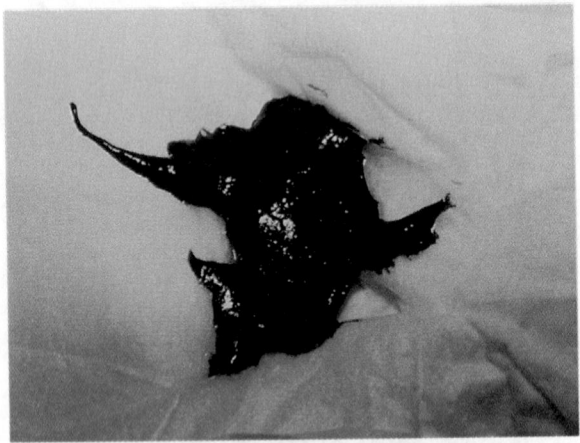

**Meconium** *(Zitelli and Davis, 1997)*

**meconium aspiration,** the inhalation of meconium by a fetus or newborn. It can block the air passages and cause failure of the lungs to expand or other pulmonary dysfunction, such as pneumonia or emphysema.

**meconium ileus,** obstruction of the small intestine in the newborn caused by impaction of thick, dry, tenacious meconium, usually at or near the ileocecal valve. Symptoms include abdominal distension, vomiting, failure to pass meconium within the first 24 to 48 hours after birth, and rapid dehydration with associated electrolyte imbalance. The condition results from a deficiency in pancreatic enzymes and is the earliest manifestation of cystic fibrosis. In uncomplicated cases in which perforation, volvulus, or atresia does not occur, the obstruction may be relieved by giving enemas with a contrast medium, such as a hypertonic solution of meglumine diatrizoate and sodium diatrizoate, under fluoroscopy. Fluid is replaced intravenously to prevent dehydration. If two or three enemas do not dislodge the obstruction, surgery is necessary. See also **meconium plug syndrome.**

**meconium plug syndrome,** obstruction of the large intestine in the newborn caused by thick, rubbery meconium that may fill the entire colon and part of the terminal ileum. Symptoms include failure to pass meconium within the first 24 to 48 hours after birth, abdominal distension, and vomiting if complete intestinal blockage occurs. A barium enema indicates the presence of a plug and in most cases dislodges it from the bowel wall. Subsequent gentle saline solution enemas may be needed to expel it. The condition may be an indication of Hirschsprung's disease or cystic fibrosis. See also **meconium ileus.**

**med,** 1. abbreviation for *medical.* 2. abbreviation for *medicine.* 3. abbreviation for *minimum effective dose.*

**MED,** 1. abbreviation for *minimal effective dose.* 2. abbreviation for *minimal erythema dose.* See also **threshold dose.**

**medcard** /med′kärd/, (in nursing) a small card listing the name, dose, and schedule of administration of each patient's medications, used in dispensing drugs to each patient.

**medevac,** abbreviation for *medical evacuation.*

**MEDEX** /med′eks/, 1. an educational program accredited by the American Medical Association for training military personnel with medical experience to become physician's assistants. 2. a physician's assistant who has gained medical experience during military service and further training in a physician's assistant program.

**medi-, medio-,** prefix meaning 'middle': *medialecithal, medicinerea, mediotarsal.*

**media.** See **medium.**

**medial** /mē′dē·əl/ [L, *medius,* middle], 1. pertaining to, situated in, or oriented toward the midline of the body. 2. pertaining to the tunica media, the middle layer of a blood vessel wall. Also **mesial.**

**medial antebrachial cutaneous nerve,** a nerve of the arm that arises from the medial cord of the brachial plexus, medial to the axillary artery. Near the axilla a cutaneous branch emerges to supply the skin over the biceps almost as far as the elbow. It descends on the ulnar side of the arm and divides into the anterior branch and the ulnar branch. The anterior branch is the larger of the two branches, innervating the skin as far as the wrist. The ulnar branch descends as far as the wrist, innervates the skin, and communicates with branches of the ulnar nerve. Compare **medial brachial cutaneous nerve.**

**medial arteriosclerosis.** See **Mönckeberg's arteriosclerosis.**

**medial brachial cutaneous nerve,** a nerve of the arm arising from the medial cord of the brachial plexus and distributed to the medial side of the arm. It passes through the axilla, pierces the deep fascia in the middle of the arm, and supplies the skin of the arm as far as the olecranon. Compare **medial antebrachial cutaneous nerve.**

**medial cerebellar nucleus.** See **fastigial nucleus.** This term is more commonly used to refer to animals other than primates.

**medial cuneiform bone,** the largest of three cuneiform bones of the foot, situated on the medial side of the tarsus, between the scaphoid bone and the first metatarsal. It serves as the attachment for various ligaments, the tendons of the tibialis anterior, and the peroneus longus. It articulates with the scaphoid, the intermediate cuneiform, and the first and second metatarsals. Also called **internal cuneiform bone.**

**medial geniculate body,** one of a pair of areas on the posterior dorsal thalamus, relaying auditory impulses from the lateral lemniscus to the auditory cortex.

**medialis** /mē′dē·ā′lis/ [L, *medius,* middle], pertaining to the middle or to the median plane.

**medial malleolus,** the rounded process of the tibia forming the internal surface of the ankle joint. Also called **internal malleolus.**

**medial pectoral nerve,** a branch of the brachial plexus that, with the lateral pectoral nerve, supplies the pectoral muscles. It joins the lateral pectoral nerve to form a loop around the artery before ending deep in the pectoralis minor. The loop branches to supply the pectoralis minor and the pectoralis major. Compare **lateral pectoral nerve.**

**medial rotation,** a turning toward the midline of the body. Compare **lateral rotation.** See also **rotation.**

**median** /mē′dē·ən/ [L, *medius,* middle], (in statistics) the number representing the middle value of the scores in a sample. In an odd number of scores arrayed in ascending order it is the middle score; in an even number of scores so arrayed it is the average of the two central scores.

**median antebrachial vein** /an′tēbrā′kē·əl/, one of the superficial veins of the upper limb, which drains the venous plexus on the palmar surface of the hand. It ascends on the ulnar side of the anterior forearm and at its terminus joins the median cubital vein. One of the veins of the median cubital complex commonly anastomoses with the deep veins of the forearm. The anastomosis holds the superficial vein in place and makes it a practical choice for venipuncture. Compare **basilic vein, cephalic vein, dorsal digital vein.**

**median aperture of fourth ventricle,** an opening between the roof of the fourth ventricle and the subarachnoid space.

**median atlantoaxial joint,** one of three points of articulation of the atlas and the axis. The median atlantoaxial joint is a pivot articulation among the dens, the axis, and the ring of the atlas and involves five ligaments. It allows rotation of the axis and the skull, the extent of rotation limited by the alar ligaments.

**median basilic vein,** one of the superficial veins of the upper limb, often formed as one of two branches from the median cubital vein. The median basilic vein courses across the palmar surface of the forearm near the elbow and is commonly used for venipuncture, phlebotomy, or IV infusion. Compare **basilic vein.**

**median cleft facial syndrome.** See **frontonasal dysplasia.**

**median effective dose (ED₅₀),** the dose of a drug that may be expected to cause a specific intensity of effect in half of the patients to whom it is given.

**median glossitis.** See **median rhomboid glossitis.**

**median jaw relation,** any jaw relation that exists when the mandible is in the median sagittal plane.

**median lethal dose (MLD, LD₅₀),** the amount of a substance or of radiation sufficient to kill one half of a population of organisms within a specified period.

**median nerve,** one of the terminal branches of the brachial plexus, which extends along the radial parts of the forearm and the hand and supplies various muscles and the skin of these parts. It arises from the brachial plexus by two large roots, one from the lateral and one from the medial cord. The roots unite to form the trunk of the nerve that courses down the arm with the brachial artery. The median nerve usually has no branches above the elbow. It has a few articular branches to the elbow joint and muscular branches to the forearm; the anterior interosseous nerve; the palmar branch; the muscular branch in the hand; the first, second, and third palmar digital nerves; and the proper digital nerves. Compare **musculocutaneous nerve, radial nerve, ulnar nerve.**

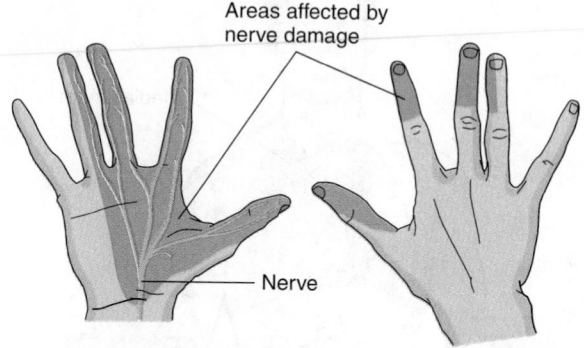

Areas affected by nerve damage

Nerve

**Median nerve distribution** *(Beare and Myers, 1998)*

**median palatine suture,** the line of junction between the horizontal parts of the palatine bones that extends from both sides of the skull to form the posterior part of the hard palate.

**median plane,** a vertical plane that divides the body into right and left halves and passes approximately through the sagittal suture of the skull. Also called **cardinal sagittal plane, midsagittal plane.** Compare **frontal plane, sagittal plane, transverse plane.**

**median rhomboid glossitis,** a red depressed, diamond-shaped area on the dorsum of the tongue, frequently irritated by alcohol, hot drinks, or spicy foods. The condition most often occurs in adult men and may be caused by candidiasis. Also called **rhomboid glossitis.**

**median sternotomy,** a chest surgery technique in which an incision is made from the suprasternal notch to below the xiphoid process. The sternum is then opened with a saw and a sternal retractor is inserted. Closure requires reunion of the sternum with stainless steel sutures. The procedure is used in coronary artery bypass and valve replacement operations. Compare **anterolateral thoracotomy, posterolateral thoracotomy.**

**median toxic dose (TD₅₀),** the dosage that may be expected to cause a toxic effect in half of the patients to whom it is given.

**mediastina.** See **mediastinum.**

**mediastinal** /mē′dē·əstī′nəl/ [L, *mediastinus,* midway], pertaining to a median septum or space between two parts of the body, such as the interval between the pleural sacs.

**mediastinitis,** an inflammation of the mediastinum.

**mediastinoscopy** /mē′dē·as′tinos′kəpē/ [L, *mediastinus,* midway; Gk, *skopein,* to view], an examination of the mediastinum through an incision in the suprasternum, using an endoscope with light and lenses.

**mediastinum** /mē′dē·əstī′nəm/, *pl.* **mediastina** [L, *mediastinus,* midway], a part of the thoracic cavity in the middle of the thorax, between the pleural sacs containing the two lungs. It extends from the sternum to the vertebral column and contains all the thoracic viscera except the lungs. It is enclosed in a thick extension of the thoracic subserous fascia and is divided into the cranial part and the caudal part. —**mediastinal,** *adj.*

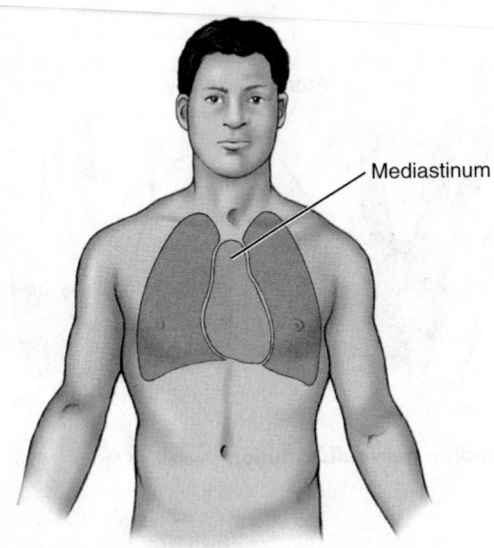

**Mediastinum** *(Herlihy and Maebius, 2000)*

**mediate** /mē′dē·āt/ [L, *medio,* in the middle],   **1.** to cause a change, as in stimulation by a hormone. **2.** to settle a dispute, as in collective bargaining. **3.** situated between two places, things, parts, or terms. **4.** (in psychology) an event that follows one process or event and precedes another; for example, in the process of cognition, perception follows stimulation and precedes thinking. —**mediating,** *adj.,* **mediator,** *n.*

**mediated transport,** the movement of a solute across a membrane with the assistance of a transport agent, such as a protein, that is specific for certain solutes.

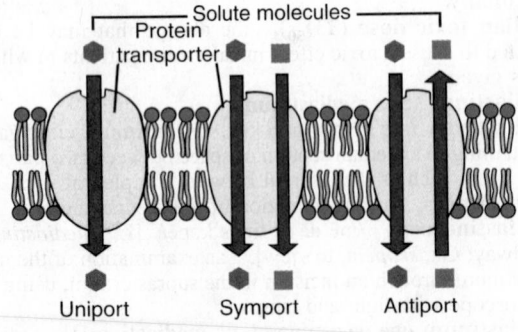

**Mediated transport** *(McCance and Huether, 1998)*

**mediate percussion.** See **percussion.**

**Mediatric,** trademark for a nutritional supplement containing multivitamins, minerals, hormones, and a central nervous system stimulant (methamphetamine hydrochloride).

**medic,** abbreviation for **paramedic.** See also **medical corpsman.**

**Medicaid** /med′ikād/, a U.S. federally funded state operated program of medical assistance to people with low incomes, authorized by Title XIX of the Social Security Act. Under broad federal guidelines the individual states determine benefits, eligibility, rates of payment, and methods of administration.

**Medicaid mill,** *informal.* a health program or facility that solely or primarily serves people eligible for Medicaid. Such facilities are found mainly in depressed areas where few other health services are available.

**medical.** See **medicine.**

**medical abortion.** See **abortion.**

**medical antishock trousers.** See **military antishock trousers.**

**medical assistant** [L, *medicare,* to heal, *assistere,* to stand by], a person who, under the direction of a physician, performs various routine administrative and nontechnical clinical tasks in a hospital, clinic, or similar facility.

**medical care,** the provision by a physician of services related to the maintenance of health, prevention of illness, and treatment of illness or injury.

**medical care plan** [L, *medicare,* to heal; OE, *caru,* sorrow, *planus,* floor], a long-range program of professional medical guidance designed to meet specific health objectives.

**medical center,** **1.** a health care facility. **2.** a hospital, especially one staffed and equipped to care for many patients and for a large number of kinds of diseases and dysfunctions, using sophisticated technology.

**Medical College Aptitude Test (MCAT),** an examination taken by persons applying to medical school; the score attained is an important criterion for acceptance. Basic science, intellectual ability, and mathematical and verbal aptitude and knowledge are tested.

**medical consultation,** a procedure whereby, on request by one physician, another physician reviews a patient's medical history, examines the patient, and makes recommendations as to care and treatment. The medical consultant often is a specialist with expertise in a particular field of medicine.

**medical corpsman** /kôr′man/ [L, *medicare,* to heal, *corpus,* body], **1.** a member of a military medical unit. **2.** a paramedic. Also called **medic.**

**medical decision level,** the concentration of analyte, or body fluid sample being analyzed, at which some medical action is indicated for proper patient care. There may be several medical decision levels for a given analyte.

**medical diagnosis** [L, *medicare* + Gk, *dia,* through, *gnosis,* knowledge], the determination of the cause of a patient's illness or suffering by the combined use of physical examination, patient interview, laboratory tests, review of the patient's medical records, knowledge of the cause of observed signs and symptoms, and differential elimination of similar possible causes.

**medical diathermy** [L, *medicare* + *dia,* through, *therme,* heat], the application of high-frequency electrical currents to generate therapeutic heat in diseased tissues.

**medical directive,** a general term for documents that provide direction on the type of care a person desires. See also **advance directive, living will.**

**medical director,** a physician who is usually employed by a hospital to serve in a medical and administrative capacity as head of the organized medical staff. He or she also may serve as liaison for the medical staff with the hospital's administration and governing board.

**medical emergency kit,** a package of drugs and devices that may be used to deal with life-threatening medical situations. The kit may include positive pressure ventilation equipment, an oxygen tank, cardiac and other medications, airway management supplies, dressings, IV fluids, suction, and splints.

**medical engineering,** a field of study of biomedical engineering and technologic concepts applied to develop equipment and instruments required in health care delivery.

**Medic Alert,** a nonprofit U.S. organization that maintains a huge data base of information about individuals who are taking one or more medications for a chronic disorder. The database also includes emergency telephone numbers for physicians treating the patients and provides bracelets or pendants to alert paramedics, interns, or other emergency medical personnel of the medical condition and prescription drugs taken by the patient, who may be unconscious or confused after an accident or episode of illness. Medic Alert maintains access to the database for emergency medical personnel through a 24-hour telephone service.

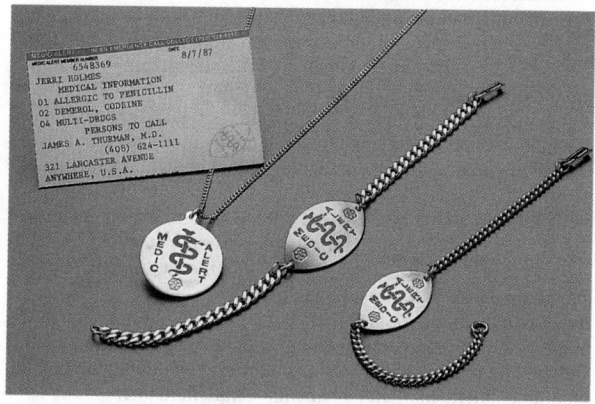

**Medic Alert** *(Judd and Ponsell, 1988)*

**medical ethics** [L, *medicare* + Gk, *ethikos*], the moral conduct and principles that govern members of the medical profession.

**medical examiner.** See **coroner.**

**medical futility,** **1.** a judgment that further medical treatment of a patient would have no useful result. **2.** a medical treatment whose success is possible but reasoning and experience suggest is highly improbable.

**medical genetics.** See **clinical genetics.**

**medical history.** See **health history.**

**medical illustrator,** an artist who creates visual material designed to record and communicate medical, biological, and related knowledge. A medical illustrator requires a strong foundation in biology, anatomy, physiology, pathology, general medicine, and the visual arts. Today most medical illustrators use a computer to create their work.

**medical indigency** /in'dijen'sē/, the lack of financial reserves adequate to pay for medical care, especially that of a person or family able to manage other basic living expenses.

**medical induction of labor.** See **induction of labor.**

**medical ionization.** See **iontophoresis.**

**medical jurisprudence** [L, *medicare* + *jus,* law, *prudentia,* knowledge], the interaction of medicine with civil and criminal law.

**medical laboratory technician,** a person who, under the supervision of a medical technologist or physician, performs microscopic and bacteriologic tests of human blood, tissue, and fluids for diagnostic and research purposes. Medical laboratory technicians are educated in either a 12-month certificate program or a 2-year associate degree program. Associate degree graduates are able to perform and interpret tests requiring discrimination between similar items.

**medical model,** the traditional approach to the diagnosis and treatment of illness as practiced by physicians in the Western world since the time of Koch and Pasteur. The physician focuses on the defect, or dysfunction, within the patient, using a problem-solving approach. The medical history, physical examination, and diagnostic tests provide the basis for the identification and treatment of a specific illness. The medical model is thus focused on the physical and biologic aspects of specific diseases and conditions. Nursing differs from the medical model in that the patient is perceived primarily as a social person relating to the environment; nursing care is formulated on the basis of a nursing assessment that assumes multiple causes for the problems experienced by the patient.

**medical outcomes study,** an evaluation of comparable medical care approaches and their relative prognoses.

**medical pathology** [L, *medicare* + Gk, *pathos,* disease, *logos,* science], the study of diseases not readily treated by surgical procedures.

**medical physics.** See **health physics.**

**medical record** [L, *medicare* + ME, *recorden,* to report], that part of a client's health record that is made by physicians and is a written or transcribed history of various illnesses or injuries requiring medical care, inoculations, allergies, treatments, prognosis, and frequently health information about parents, siblings, occupation, and military service. The record may be reviewed by a physician in diagnosing the condition. See also **chart.**

**medical record administrator,** a person who oversees maintenance of records of patients' medical histories, diagnoses, treatment, and outcome for a condition that meets medical, administrative, legal, ethical, regulatory, and institutional requirements.

**medical record technician,** a health professional responsible for maintaining components of health information systems consistent with the medical, administrative, ethical, legal, accreditation, and regulatory requirements of the health care delivery system.

**medical secretary,** a person who prepares and maintains medical records and performs related secretarial duties.

**medical snatch bag,** *informal.* a light, compact, waterproof, and shockproof container of emergency medical equipment for advanced prehospital care. It should provide all that is required to relieve an obstructed airway, provide artificial ventilation, arrest hemorrhage from a peripheral site, and establish an IV access for infusion.

**medical social worker.** See **social worker.**

**medical sonographer.** See **sonographer.**

**medical staff,** physicians and dentists who are approved and given privileges to provide health care to patients in a hospital or other health care facility. Medical staff personnel may work full time or part time and may be employed by the facility or granted admitting privileges to practice.

**medical staff, courtesy,** physicians and dentists who meet certain qualifications of the medical staff of a hospital but who admit patients only occasionally or act as consultants. They are ineligible to participate in medical staff activities.

**medical staff, honorary,** physicians and dentists, usually retired, who are recognized by the hospital medical staff for their noteworthy contributions but who may not admit patients to the hospital or participate in medical staff activities.

**medical-surgical nursing,** the nursing care of adult patients whose conditions or disorders are treated pharmacologically or surgically.

**medical technologist.** See **clinical laboratory scientist/ medical technologist.**

**medical transcriptionist,** a health professional who prepares a written record of patient data dictated by a physician. A **certified medical transcriptionist** is one who has met the qualifying standards of the American Association of Medical Transcription.

**medical vagotomy.** See **pharmacologic vagotomy.**

**medical waste,** any discarded biologic product such as blood or tissue removed from operating rooms, morgues, laboratories, or other medical facilities. The term may also be applied to bedding, bandages, syringes, and similar materials that have been used in treating patients and to animal carcasses or body parts used in research.

**Medical Women's International Association (M.W.I.A.),** an international professional organization of women physicians.

**medicamentosus** /med′ikəmen′tōsəs/ [L, *medicamentum,* drug], pertaining to a drug, particularly to an adverse reaction attributed to a medication.

**Medicare** /med′iker/, **1.** a federally funded national health insurance program in the United States for people over 65 years of age. The program is administered in two parts. Part A provides basic protection against costs of medical, surgical, and psychiatric hospital care. Part B is a voluntary medical insurance program financed in part from federal funds and in part from premiums contributed by enrollees. Medicare enrollment is offered to people 65 years of age or older who are entitled to receive Social Security or railroad retirement benefits. Other people above 65 years of age, such as federal employees and aliens, may not be eligible. Medicare was authorized by Title XVIII of the Social Security Act of 1965. **2.** (in Canada) Medicare is the name of the national health insurance program.

**medicate** /med′ikāt/ [L, *medicare,* to heal], to treat an illness by administering drugs.

**medicated bougie** /med′ikātid/ [L, *medicare,* to heal; Fr, candle], a bougie containing a medicated agent. See also **bougie.**

**medicated enema,** a medication administered via an enema. It is usually used preoperatively with patients scheduled for bowel surgery or may be used to treat infections locally.

**medicated tub bath,** a therapeutic bath in which medication is dispersed in water, usually in the treatment of dermatologic disorders.

■ METHOD: The amount of medication and the amount and temperature of the water are specified in the order for the bath. The water is run, the medication is added, and the solution is stirred with a bath thermometer to disperse the medication while testing the water temperature, usually between 96° F (35.6° C) and 100° F (37.8° C) but possibly as high as 103° F (39.4° C), as in the treatment of psoriasis vulgaris. Most medicated baths are prescribed as half-hour treatments. A folded towel or waterproof pillow is placed behind the head, and a towel is draped over the shoulders to enhance the patient's comfort. In certain conditions the patient may be asked to scrub affected areas with a brush and washcloth; in others the patient is instructed not to scrub at

all. After the bath the skin is patted dry and any ointment, cream, or other topical prescription is applied.

■ INTERVENTIONS: The reason for the treatment is explained to the patient, and instructions are given not to get out of the tub without assistance and not to add water without calling the nurse. If the patient is to scrub the affected areas, the necessary equipment is taken to the bath. The tub is thoroughly scrubbed and rinsed before and after the treatment.

■ OUTCOME CRITERIA: The medicated bath is usually soothing, relaxing, and comforting for the patient. Close attention to instructing the patient fully and to ensuring comfort during the procedure improves compliance with the treatment.

**medication** /med′ikā′shən/ [L, *medicare,* to heal], **1.** a drug or other substance that is used as a medicine. **2.** the administration of a medicine.

**medication administration,** a nursing intervention from the Nursing Interventions Classification (NIC) defined as preparing, giving, and evaluating the effectiveness of prescription and nonprescription drugs. See also **Nursing Interventions Classification.**

**medication administration: ear,** a nursing intervention from the Nursing Interventions Classification (NIC) defined as preparing and instilling otic medications. See also **Nursing Interventions Classification.**

**medication administration: enteral,** a nursing intervention from the Nursing Interventions Classification (NIC) defined as delivering medications through an intestinal tube. See also **Nursing Interventions Classification.**

**medication administration: epidural,** a nursing intervention from the Nursing Interventions Classification (NIC) defined as preparing and administering medications via the epidural route. See also **Nursing Interventions Classification.**

**medication administration: eye,** a nursing intervention from the Nursing Interventions Classification (NIC) defined as preparing and instilling ophthalmic medications. See also **Nursing Interventions Classification.**

**medication administration: inhalation,** a nursing intervention from the Nursing Interventions Classification (NIC) defined as preparing and administering inhaled medications. See also **Nursing Interventions Classification.**

**medication administration: interpleural,** a nursing intervention from the Nursing Interventions Classification (NIC) defined as administration of medication through an interpleural catheter for reduction of pain. See also **Nursing Interventions Classification.**

**medication administration: intradermal,** a nursing intervention from the Nursing Interventions Classification (NIC) defined as preparing and giving medications via the intradermal route. See also **Nursing Interventions Classification.**

**medication administration: intramuscular (IM),** a nursing intervention from the Nursing Interventions Classification (NIC) defined as preparing and giving medications via the intramuscular route. See also **Nursing Interventions Classification.**

**medication administration: intraosseous,** a nursing intervention from the Nursing Interventions Classification (NIC) defined as insertion of a needle through the bone cortex into the medullary cavity for the purpose of short-term, emergency administration of fluid, blood, or medication. See also **Nursing Interventions Classification.**

**medication administration: intravenous (IV),** a nursing intervention from the Nursing Interventions Classification (NIC) defined as preparing and giving medications via the intravenous route. See also **Nursing Interventions Classification.**

**medication administration: oral,** a nursing intervention from the Nursing Interventions Classification (NIC) defined as preparing and giving medications by mouth and monitoring patient responsiveness. See also **Nursing Interventions Classification.**

**medication administration: parenteral,** a Nursing Interventions Classification defined as preparing and giving medications via the intravenous, intramuscular, intradermal, and/or subcutaneous route. See also **Nursing Interventions Classification.**

**medication administration: rectal,** a nursing intervention from the Nursing Interventions Classification (NIC) defined as preparing and inserting rectal suppositories. See also **Nursing Interventions Classification.**

**medication administration: skin,** a nursing intervention from the Nursing Interventions Classification (NIC) defined as preparing and applying medications to the skin. See also **Nursing Interventions Classification.**

**medication administration: subcutaneous,** a nursing intervention from the Nursing Interventions Classification (NIC) defined as preparing and giving medications via the subcutaneous route. See also **Nursing Interventions Classification.**

**medication administration: topical,** a Nursing Interventions Classification defined as preparing and applying medications to the skin and mucous membranes. See also **Nursing Interventions Classification.**

**medication administration: vaginal,** a nursing intervention from the Nursing Interventions Classification (NIC) defined as preparing and inserting vaginal medications. See also **Nursing Interventions Classification.**

**medication administration: ventricular reservoir,** a nursing intervention from the Nursing Interventions Classification (NIC) defined as administration and monitoring of medication through an indwelling catheter into the lateral ventricle. See also **Nursing Interventions Classification.**

**medication error,** any incorrect or wrongful administration of a medication, such as a mistake in dosage or route of administration, failure to prescribe or administer the correct drug or formulation for a particular disease or condition, use of outdated drugs, failure to observe the correct time for administration of the drug, or lack of awareness of adverse effects of certain drug combinations. Causes of medication error may include difficulty in reading handwritten orders, confusion about different drugs with similar names, and lack of information about a patient's drug allergies or sensitivities. When the nurse is in doubt, administration of a drug should be delayed until specifically authorized by a physician.

**medication management,** a nursing intervention from the Nursing Interventions Classification (NIC) defined as facilitation of safe and effective use of prescription and over-the-counter drugs. See also **Nursing Interventions Classification.**

**medication order,** a written order by a physician, dentist, or other designated health professional for a medication to be dispensed by a pharmacy for administration to a patient.

**medication prescribing,** a nursing intervention from the Nursing Interventions Classification (NIC) defined as prescribing medication for a health problem. See also **Nursing Interventions Classification.**

**medication response,** a nursing outcome from the Nursing Outcomes Classification (NOC) defined as the therapeutic and adverse effects of prescribed medication. See also **Nursing Outcomes Classification.**

**medicinal restraint.** See **chemical restraint.**

**medicinal treatment,** therapy of disorders based chiefly on the use of appropriate pharmacologic agents.

**medicine** [L, *medicina,* art of healing], **1.** a drug or a remedy for illness. **2.** the art and science of the diagnosis, treatment, and prevention of disease and the maintenance of good health. **3.** the art or technique of treating disease without surgery. Two major divisions of medicine are academic medicine and clinical medicine. Some of the many branches of medicine are **environmental medicine, family medicine, forensic medicine, internal medicine,** and **physical medicine. —medical,** *adj.*

**medicolegal** /med′ikōlē′gəl/ [L, *medicina,* art of healing, *lex,* law], pertaining to both medicine and law. Medicolegal considerations are a significant part of the process of making many patient care decisions and determining definitions and policies for the treatment of mentally incompetent people and minors, the performance of sterilization or therapeutic abortion, and the care of terminally ill patients. Medicolegal considerations, decisions, definitions, and policies provide the framework for informed consent, professional liability, and many other aspects of current practice in the health care field.

**Medihaler-Epi,** trademark for an adrenergic (epinephrine bitartrate).

**Medihaler-Ergotamine Aerosol,** trademark for an analgesic (ergotamine tartrate).

**Medimmune,** trademark for a recombinant form of **bacille Calmette-Guérin (BCG),** a live bovine bacterium used to immunize against tuberculosis. It is inexpensive to produce and can be given orally.

**mediocarpal** /mē′dē·ō·kär′pəl/ [L, *medius,* middle; Gk, *karpos,* wrist], between the two rows of bones of the carpus. Also called **midcarpal.**

**mediolateral** /mē′dē·ō·lat′ər·əl/ [L. *medius,* middle + *latus,* side], pertaining to the middle and to one side.

**meditation** /med′itā′shən/ [L, *meditari,* to consider], a state of consciousness in which the individual eliminates environmental stimuli from awareness so that the mind has a single focus, producing a state of relaxation and relief from stress. A wide variety of techniques are used to clear the mind of stressful outside interference.

**meditation facilitation,** a nursing intervention from the Nursing Interventions Classification (NIC) defined as facilitating a person to alter his/her level of awareness by focusing specifically on an image or thought. See also **Nursing Interventions Classification.**

**meditation therapy,** a method of achieving relaxation and consciousness expansion by focusing on a mantra or a key word, sound, or image while eliminating outside stimuli from one's awareness.

**Mediterranean anemia.** See **thalassemia.**

**Mediterranean fever.** See **brucellosis.**

**Mediterranean lymphoma.** See **immunoproliferative small intestine disease.**

**medium** /mē′dē·əm/, *pl.* **media** [L, *medius,* middle], a substance through which something moves or through which it acts. A **contrast medium** is a substance that has a density different from that of body tissues, permitting visual comparison of structures when used with imaging techniques such as x-ray film. A **culture medium** is a substance that provides a nutritional environment for the growth of microorganisms or cells. A **dispersion medium** is the substance in which a colloid is dispersed. A **refractory medium** is the transparent tissues and fluid of the eye that refract light.

**medium-chain triglyceride (MCT),** a glycerine ester combined with medium-chain triglycerides distinguished from other triglycerides by having 8 to 10 carbon atoms.

Once hydrolyzed, these fatty acids can be absorbed directly into the portal system. MCTs in foods are usually high in calories and easily digested.

**medius** /mē′dē·əs/ [L], in the middle; a term used in reference to a structure lying between two other structures that are anterior and posterior, superior and inferior, or internal and external in position.

**MEDLARS** /med′lärs/, abbreviation for *Medical Literature Analysis and Retrieval System,* a computerized literature retrieval service of the National Library of Medicine in Bethesda, Maryland. MEDLARS contains more than 4,500,000 references to medical articles in professional journals and books published since 1966. The references are made available on request to more than 1000 hospitals, universities, government agencies, and other interested parties throughout the world by means of a network of computer terminals. The references are filed in 15 data bases, including MEDLINE, TOXLINE, CHEMLINE, RTECS, CANCERLIT, and EPILEPSYLINE. See also **MEDLINE.**

**MEDLINE** /med′līn/, a U.S. National Library of Medicine computer data base that covers approximately 600,000 references to biomedical journal articles published currently and in the 2 preceding years. The files duplicate the contents of the monthly and annual volumes of the *Unabridged Index Medicus,* also published by the National Library of Medicine, which indexes medical reports from 3000 professional journals in more than 70 countries. See also **MEDLARS.**

**MedRC,** abbreviation for *medical reserve corps.*

**Medrol,** trademark for a glucocorticoid (methylprednisolone disodium phosphate).

**Medrol Acetate,** trademark for a glucocorticoid (methylprednisolone acetate).

**medroxyprogesterone acetate** /medrok′sēprōjes′tərōn/, a progestin.

■ INDICATION: It is prescribed in the treatment of menstrual disorders caused by hormone imbalance.

■ CONTRAINDICATIONS: Known or suspected pregnancy, thrombophlebitis, embolism, stroke, liver dysfunction, cancer of the breast or genitals, abnormal vaginal bleeding, missed abortion, or known hypersensitivity to this drug prohibits its use.

■ ADVERSE EFFECTS: Among the more serious adverse reactions are thrombophlebitis, pulmonary embolism, stroke, hepatitis, and cerebral thrombosis.

**medrysone** /med′risōn/, a glucocorticoid that decreases the infiltration of leukocytes at the site of inflammation. It is used topically in the eye, as an antiinflammatory agent.

**Med.Sc.D.,** abbreviation for *Doctor of Medical Science.*

**Med Tech,** abbreviation for *medical technician.*

**medulla** /mədul′ə/, *pl.* **medullas, medullae** [L, marrow], **1.** the most internal part of a structure or organ, such as the renal medulla. **2.** *informal.* medulla oblongata.

**medulla oblongata,** a bulbous continuation of the spinal cord just above the foramen magnum and separated from the pons by a horizontal groove. It is one of three parts of the brainstem and mainly contains white substance with some mixture of gray substance. The medulla contains the cardiac, vasomotor, and respiratory centers of the brain; medullary injury or disease often proves fatal. Compare **mesencephalon, pons.**

**medulla of the kidney** [L, *medulla,* marrow; ME, *kidenei*], a part of the parenchyma of the kidney, beneath the cortex, including the renal pyramids and columns. It contains few, if any, glomeruli. An inner layer contains the papillae, and the outer part, which extends as far as the arcuate vessels, contains the thick ascending limbs of the loop of Henle.

**medullary** /med′əler′ē, mədul′erē, med′yəler′ē/ [L, *medulla,* marrow], **1.** pertaining to the medulla of the brain. **2.** pertaining to the bone marrow. **3.** pertaining to the spinal cord. Also **medullar.**

**medullary carcinoma,** a soft malignant neoplasm of the epithelium containing little or no fibrous tissue. Also called **carcinoma medullare, carcinoma molle, encephaloid carcinoma.**

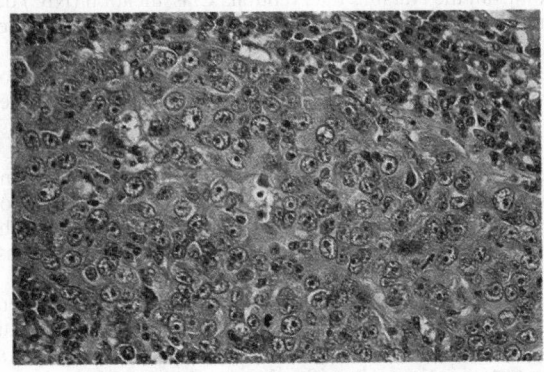

**Medullary carcinoma** *(Fletcher, 2000)*

**medullary chemoreceptor.** See **central chemoreceptor.**

**medullary cystic disease,** a chronic familial disease of the kidney, characterized by the slow onset of uremia. The disease appears in young children or adolescents, who pass large volumes of dilute urine with greater than normal amounts of sodium. Hemodialysis is the usual treatment for the disease as the uremia progresses and becomes severe. See also **uremia.**

**medullary fold.** See **neural fold.**

**medullary groove.** See **neural groove.**

**medullary nerve sheath.** See **nerve sheath.**

**medullary plate.** See **neural plate.**

**medullary sponge kidney,** a congenital defect of the kidney, leading to cystic dilation of the collecting tubules. People with this defect often develop a kidney stone or an infection of the kidney caused by urinary stasis. The condition is diagnosed by urographic techniques. Treatment includes drugs to acidify the urine and a diet low in calcium and high in fluids to discourage formation of stones.

**medullary tube.** See **neural tube.**

**medullas.** See **medulla.**

**medulla spinalis.** See **spinal cord.**

**medullated** /med′yəlā′tid/ [L, *medulla,* marrow], enclosed by a marrowlike substance, such as the myelin sheath of a nerve fiber.

**medullated neuroma.** See **fascicular neuroma.**

**medulloblastoma** /mədul′ōblastō′mə/ [L, *medulla* + Gk, *blastos,* germ, *oma,* tumor], a poorly differentiated malignant neoplasm composed of tightly packed cells of spongioblastic and neuroblastic lineage. The tumor usually arises in the cerebellum, occurs most frequently at 5 to 9 years of age, and affects more boys than girls. Medulloblastomas are extremely radiosensitive and grow rapidly; the prognosis is poor.

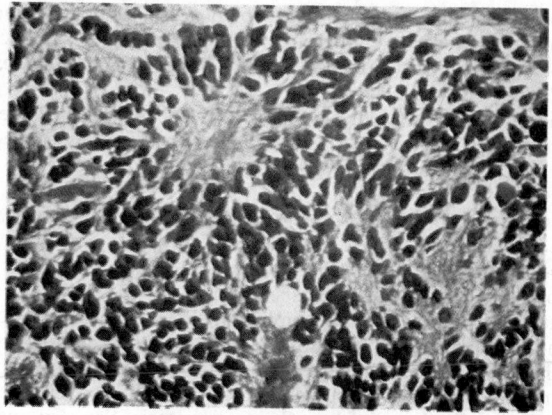

**Medulloblastoma**
*(Kumar, Cotran, and Robbins, 1997/courtesy Elisabeth Rushing, MD,
Department of Pathology, University of Texas
Southwestern Medical Center, Dallas)*

**medulloepithelioma.** See **neurocytoma**.

**mefenamic acid** /mef'ənam'ik/, a nonsteroidal antiinflammatory agent and analgesic.

■ INDICATION: It is prescribed in the treatment of mild to moderate pain.

■ CONTRAINDICATIONS: GI ulceration or inflammation, impaired renal function, or known hypersensitivity to this drug prohibits its use. It is prescribed with caution for patients with asthma.

■ ADVERSE EFFECTS: Dyspepsia and diarrhea are the most common adverse effects. Other GI symptoms, dizziness, drowsiness, or skin rash occasionally occurs. Severe blood dyscrasias develop rarely.

**mefloquine** /mef'ləkēn/, an antimalarial for the prophylaxis and treatment of chloroquine-resistant falciparum and vivax malaria.

**Mefoxin,** trademark for a cephalosporin antibiotic (cefoxitin sodium).

**MEFR,** abbreviation for **maximal expiratory flow rate.**

**mega-, megalo-, mego-,** **1.** prefix meaning 'great or huge': *megacardia, megacoccus, megadyne.* **2.** a quantity one million times a given unit: *megahertz.*

**megabladder.** See **megalocystis.**

**megacaryocyte.** See **megakaryocyte.**

**Megace,** trademark for an antineoplastic progestational agent (megestrol acetate).

**megacolon** /meg'əkōlən/ [Gk, *megas + kolon*, colon], abnormal massive dilation of the colon that may be congenital, toxic, or acquired. **Congenital megacolon** (Hirschsprung's disease) is caused by the absence of autonomic ganglia in the smooth muscle wall of the colon. **Toxic megacolon** is a grave complication of ulcerative colitis and may cause perforation of the colon, septicemia, and death. Colonoscopy and surgery are the usual treatments for toxic and congenital megacolon. **Acquired megacolon** is the result of a chronic refusal to defecate, which usually occurs in children who are psychotic or mentally retarded. The colon becomes dilated by an accumulation of impacted feces. Laxatives, enemas, and psychiatric treatment are often necessary. See also **Hirschsprung's disease.**

**megacycle.** See **megahertz.**

**megadose** /meg'ədōs/, a dose that greatly exceeds the amount usually prescribed or recommended.

**megadyne** /meg'ədīn/, a unit of force equal to one million dynes.

**megaesophagus** /meg'ə·isof'əgəs/ [Gk, *megas + oisophagos*, gullet], abnormal dilation of the lower segments of the esophagus caused by distension resulting from the failure of the cardiac sphincter to relax and allow the passage of food into the stomach. See also **achalasia.**

**megahertz (MHz)** /meg'əhurts/ [Gk, *megas*, large, *hertz*, a number of cycles per second], a unit of frequency equal to a million cycles per second. Also called **megacycle.** See also **hertz.**

**megakaryocyte** /meg'əker'ē·əsīt'/ [Gk, *megas*, large, *karyon*, nut, *kytos*, cell], an extremely large bone marrow cell measuring between 35 and 160 μm in diameter and having a nucleus with many lobes. Megakaryocytes are essential for the production and proliferation of platelets in the marrow and are normally not present in the circulating blood. Also spelled **megacaryocyte.** See also **platelet.** —**megakaryocytic,** *adj.*

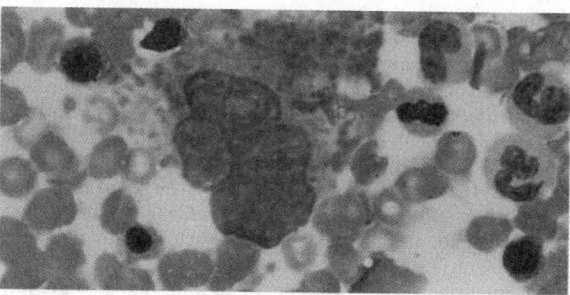

**Megakaryocyte** *(Carr and Rodak, 1999)*

**megakaryocytic leukemia** /meg'əker'ē·əsit'ik/ [Gk, *megas + karyon*, nut, *kytos*, cell], a rare malignancy of blood-forming tissue in which megakaryocytes proliferate in the bone marrow and circulate in the blood in large numbers.

**megalencephaly** /meg'əlensef'əlē/ [Gk, *megas + enkephalos*, brain], a condition characterized by pathologic parenchymal overgrowth of the brain. In some cases generalized cerebral hyperplasia is associated with mental retardation or a brain disorder, such as epilepsy. Also called **macrencephaly.** —**megalencephalic, megalencephalous,** *adj.*

**-megalia.** See **-megaly.**

**megalo-.** See **mega-.**

**megaloblast** /meg'əlōblast'/ [Gk, *megas + blastos*, germ], an abnormally large nucleated immature erythrocyte that develops in large numbers in the bone marrow and is plentiful in the circulation in anemias associated with deficiency of vitamin $B_{12}$, folic acid, or intrinsic factor. Effective treatment is the intramuscular injection of vitamin $B_{12}$. —**megaloblastic,** *adj.*

**megaloblastic anemia** /-blas'tik/, a hematologic disorder characterized by the production and peripheral proliferation of immature large dysfunctional erythrocytes. Megaloblasts are usually associated with severe pernicious anemia or folic acid deficiency anemia. See also **nutritional anemia, pernicious anemia.**

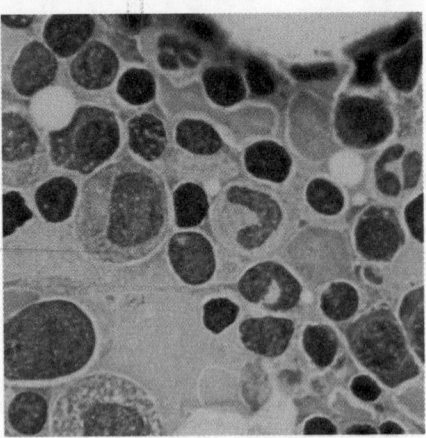

**Megaloblastic anemia** *(Carr and Rodak, 1999)*

oromandibular muscles with blepharospasm, grimacing mouth movements, and protrusion of the tongue, usually occurring in older women. Also called **Brueghel's syndrome.**, **2.** see **Milroy's disease.**

**Meigs' syndrome** /megz/ [Joe V. Meigs, American gynecologist, 1892–1963], ascites and hydrothorax associated with a fibroma of the ovaries or other pelvic tumor.

**meio-.** See **mio-.**

**meiocyte** /mī′əsīt/ [Gk, *meiosis*, becoming smaller, *kytos*, cell], any cell undergoing meiosis.

**meiogenic** /mī′əjen′ik/ [Gk, *meiosis* + *genein*, to produce], producing or causing meiosis.

**meiosis** /mī·ō′sis/ [Gk, becoming smaller], the division of a sex cell as it matures into two and then four haploid cells; the nucleus of each receives one half of the number of chromosomes present in the somatic cells of the species. Also called **reduction division.** Compare **mitosis.** See also **anaphase, metaphase, oogenesis, prophase, spermatogenesis, telophase.** —**meiotic** /mī·ot′ik/, *adj.*

**megalocephaly.** See **macrocephaly.**

**megalocornea,** an inherited disorder in which the corneal diameter is enlarged.

**megalocystis** /meg′əlōsis′tis/ [Gk, *megas* + *kystis*, bag], an abnormal condition primarily affecting girls, characterized by an enlarged and thin-walled bladder. Surgical reduction of the size of the bladder or diversion of urine through the ileum may correct the condition. Also called **megabladder.**

**megalocyte** /meg′əlōsīt/, an extremely large erythrocyte.

**megalomania** /meg′əlōmā′nē·ə/ [Gk, *megas* + *mania*, madness], an abnormal mental state characterized by delusions of grandeur in which one believes oneself to be a person of great importance, power, fame, or wealth. See also **grandiosity, mania.**

**megaloureter** /meg′əlōyŏŏrē′tər/ [Gk, *megas* + *oureter*, ureter], an abnormal condition characterized by marked dilation of one or both ureters, resulting from dysfunctional peristaltic action of the smooth muscle in the ureters. Treatment may include surgical resection.

**-megaly, -megalia,** suffix meaning an 'enlargement of a (specified) body part': *cardiomegaly, dactylomegaly, gastromegaly.*

**megavitamin therapy** /-vī′təmin/, a type of treatment that involves the administration of large doses of certain vitamins and minerals.

**megestrol acetate** /məjes′trōl/, an antineoplastic progestational agent.

■ INDICATIONS: It is prescribed to treat endometrial cancer and more commonly to palliate advanced endometrial and breast cancer.

■ CONTRAINDICATION: Hypersensitivity to the drug prohibits its use.

■ ADVERSE EFFECTS: There are no known serious adverse reactions.

**mego-.** See **mega-.**

**meibomian cyst.** See **chalazion.**

**meibomian gland** /mēbō′mē·ən/ [Heinrich Meibom, German physician, 1638–1700], one of several sebaceous glands that secrete sebum from their ducts on the posterior margin of each eyelid. The glands are embedded in the tarsal plate of each eyelid. Also called **tarsal gland, palpebral gland.**

**Meige's disease, syndrome** /mezh′əz/ [Henri Meige, French physician, 1866–1940], **1.** dystonia of facial and

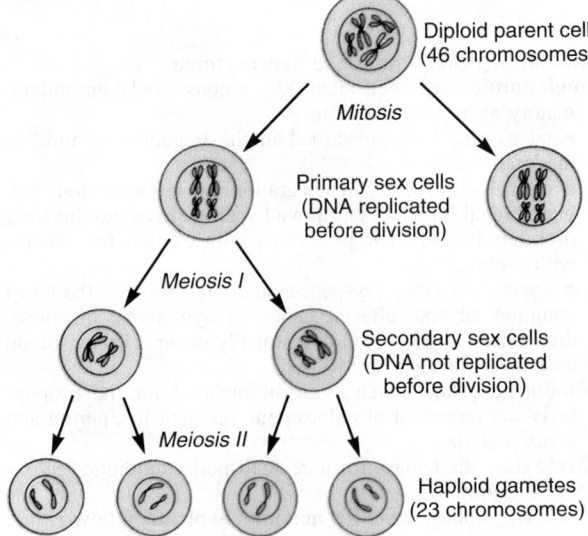

**Meiosis** *(Thibodeau and Patton, 1999/Rolin Graphics)*

**Meissner's corpuscle** /mīs′nərz/ [Georg Meissner, German anatomist, 1829–1905; L, *corpusculum*, little body], any one of a number of small, special pressure-sensitive sensory end organs with a connective tissue capsule and tiny stacked plates in the dermis of the hand and foot, the front of the forearm, the skin of the lips, the mucous membrane of the tongue, the palpebral conjunctiva, and the skin of the mammary papilla. A single nerve fiber penetrates each oval capsule, spirals through the interior, and ends as a globular mass. Also called **tactile corpuscle.** Compare **Golgi-Mazzoni corpuscles, Krause's corpuscles.**

**Meissner's plexus** [Georg Meissner; L, *plaited*], small aggregations of ganglion cells located in the submucosa of the intestine.

**mel** [L, honey], a mixture of invert sugars and polysaccharides produced from the nectar of flowers by enzymes secreted by the honeybee, *Apis mellifica.*

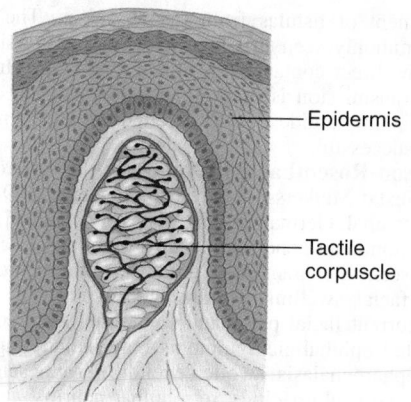

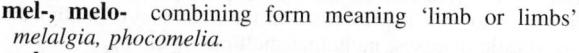

**Meissner's corpuscle** *(Thibodeau and Patton, 1999)*

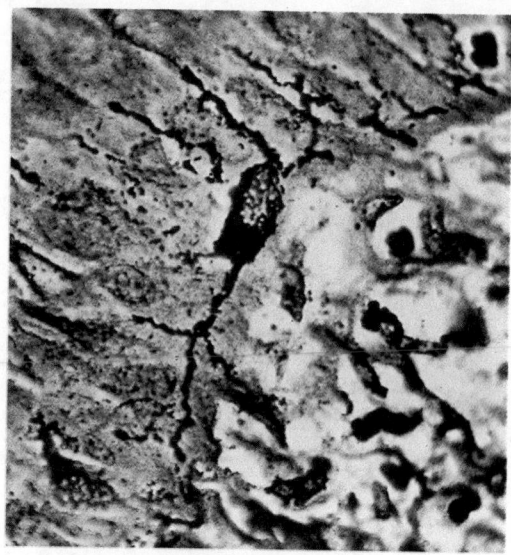

**Melanocyte** *(du Vivier, 1993)*

**mel-, melo-** combining form meaning 'limb or limbs': *melalgia, phocomelia.*

**melan-.** See **melano-.**

**melancholia** /mel′angkō′lē·ə/ [Gk, *melas*, black, *chole*, bile], a severe form of depression. See also **depression, major depressive disorder.**

**melaniferous** /mel′ənif′ərəs/ [Gk, *melas*, black; L, *ferre*, to bear], pertaining to a black pigment.

**melanin** /mel′ənin/ [Gk, *melas*, black], a black or dark brown pigment that occurs naturally in the hair, skin, and iris and choroid of the eye. See also **melanocyte.**

**melanism** /mel′əniz′əm/ [Gk, *melas*, black], an abnormal deposit of dark brown to black melanin pigment in the skin, hair, and other tissues. Also called **melanosis.**

**melano-, melan-, mel-,** combining form meaning 'black': *melanoderm, melanoleukoderma, melanophore.*

**melanoameloblastoma** /mel′ənō·am′əlōblastō′mə/, a benign neoplasm appearing as a blue-black lesion on the anterior maxilla of infants. The growth is of neuroectodermal origin and consists of small round undifferentiated tumor cells and larger melanin-producing cells. Also called **melanotic neuroectodermal tumor of infancy.**

**melanoblast** /mel′ənōblast′/ [Gk, *melas*, black, *blastos*, germ], an epithelial tissue cell containing black granules. It develops into a melanocyte from the neural crest that migrates to various parts of the body during the early stages of embryonic life and then becomes a mature melanocyte capable of forming melanin.

**melanoblastoma** /mel′ənō·blastō′mə/, a tumor of poorly differentiated melanin-producing cells.

**melanocarcinoma** /-kär′sinō′mə/, a malignant melanoma.

**melanocyte** /mel′ənōsīt′, mələn′ōsīt/ [Gk, *melas* + *kytos*, cell], a body cell capable of producing melanin. Melanocytes are distributed throughout the basal cell layer of the epidermis and form melanin pigment from tyrosine, an amino acid. Melanin granules are then transferred to adjacent basal cells and to hair. Melanocyte stimulating hormone from the pituitary controls the amount of melanin produced.

**melanocyte-stimulating hormone (MSH),** a polypeptide hormone, secreted by the anterior pituitary gland, that controls the intensity of pigmentation in pigmented cells. It is synthesized on the same large precursor polypeptide as adrenocorticotropic hormone and the enkephalins.

**melanocytic nevus** /-sit′ik/, a congenital pigmented lesion of the skin caused by a disorder involving melanocytes.

**melanoderma** /mel′ənōdur′mə/ [Gk, *melas* + *derma*, skin], any abnormal darkening of the skin caused by increased deposits of melanin or the salts of iron or silver.

**melanoma** /mel′ənō′mə/ *pl.*, **melanomas, melanomata** [Gk, *melas* + *oma*, tumor], any of a group of malignant neoplasms that originate in the skin and that are composed of melanocytes. A melanocytic nevus may be acquired or congenital. The congenital melanocytic nevus is regarded as more likely to develop into a malignant melanoma, primarily because of its larger size. Smaller melanomas tend to develop from a pigmented nevus over several months or years. They may be sporadic and occur most commonly in fair-skinned people having light-colored eyes. A previous sunburn increases a person's risk. Any black or brown spot having an irregular border; pigment appearing to radiate beyond that border; a red, black, and blue coloration observable on close examination; or a nodular surface is suggestive of melanoma and is usually excised for biopsy. Melanomas may metastasize and are among the most malignant of all skin cancers. Prognosis depends on the kind of melanoma; its size, depth of invasion, and location; and the age and condition of the patient. Because of the occurrence of melanomas and melanocytic nevi in certain families a familial atypical mole and melanoma syndrome (FAM-M) has been designated. It is defined by the occurrence of melanoma in one or more first- or second-degree relatives, a large number of moles, and moles that demonstrate certain cellular features. Patients with the syndrome have a high lifetime risk of development of melanoma. Kinds of melanoma are **amelanic melanoma, benign juvenile melanoma, lentigo maligna melanoma, nodular melanoma, primary cutaneous melanoma,** and **superficial spreading melanoma.** Compare **blue nevus.** See also **Hutchinson's freckle.**

**melanomatosis** /-mətō′sis/, **1.** a condition characterized by many widespread melanoma lesions. **2.** the development of melanomas throughout the body.

**melanosis.** See **melanism.**

**melanosis coli** /mel′ənō′sis/, an abnormal condition in which the mucous membrane of the colon is pigmented with melanin.

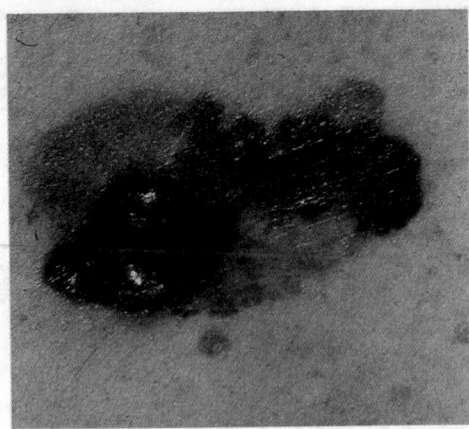

**Melanoma** *(Zitelli and Davis, 1997)*

**melanosome** /mel′ənōsōm′/, the oval pigment granules within melanocytes that synthesize melanin.

**melanotic carcinoma** /mel′ənot′ik/, a malignant pigmented skin cancer.

**melanotic neuroectodermal tumor of infancy.** See **melanoameloblastoma.**

**melanuria** /mel′ənŏŏr′ē·ə/, urine that has a dark color caused by the presence of melanin or other pigments.

**melasma.** See **chloasma.**

**melasma gravidarum** /məlaz′mə/ [Gk, *melas,* black; L, *gravida,* pregnant], a dark pigment or discoloration that may appear on the skin of pregnant women.

**MELAS syndrome,** abbreviation for *mitochondrial encephalopathy, lactic acidosis, and stroke-like episodes,* constituting a familial syndrome of maternal (mitochondrial) inheritance.

**melatonin,** a dietary supplement, also known as N-acetyl-5-methoxytryptamine.

■ USES: This supplement is used for jet lag and insomnia, for cancer protection, and as an oral contraceptive.

■ CONTRAINDICATIONS: Melatonin is not recommended during pregnancy and lactation, in children, or in those with known hypersensitivity to this product.

**Meleda disease.** See **mal de Meleda.**

**melena** /məlē′nə, məl′ənə/ [Gk, *melas,* black], abnormal black tarry stool that has a distinctive odor and contains digested blood. It usually results from bleeding in the upper GI tract and is often a sign of peptic ulcer or small bowel disease. See also **gastrointestinal bleeding.**

**melena neonatorum** [Gk, *melas,* black, *neos,* new; L, *natus,* born], the passage of dark tarry stools by a newborn. The cause is usually the alteration of blood pigment associated with hemorrhage. Normal meconium stools are greenish to black.

**meli-,** prefix meaning 'sweet, or related to honey': *melicera, melitagra, melitoptyalism.*

**-melia,** suffix meaning 'limbs': *acromelia, dolichomelia, phocomelia.*

**melioidosis** /mel′ē·oidō′sis/ [Gk, *melis,* distemper, *eidos,* form, *osis,* condition], an infection caused by the gram-negative bacillus *Burkholderia pseudomallei.* **Acute melioidosis** is fulminant and usually characterized by pneumonia, empyema, lung abscess, septicemia, and liver or spleen involvement. **Chronic melioidosis** is associated with osteomyelitis, multiple abscesses of the internal organs, and

development of fistulas from the abscesses. The disease, most commonly seen in China and Southeast Asia, is acquired by direct contact with infected animals. Human-to-human transmission is unlikely. Treatment using chloramphenicol, sulfonamides, or tetracycline for several months is usually successful.

**Melkersson-Rosenthal syndrome** /mel′kər·son·rō′zen·täl/ [Ernst Gustaf Melkersson, Swedish physician, 1898–1932; Curt Rosenthal, German psychiatrist, 20th century], an autosomal dominant condition usually beginning in childhood or adolescence, characterized chiefly by chronic noninflammatory facial swelling, localized particularly to the lips, with recurrent facial palsy and sometimes fissured tongue. Associated ophthalmic symptoms may include lagophthalmos, blepharochalasis, swollen eyelids, burning sensation of the eyes, corneal opacities, retrobulbar neuritis, and exophthalmos. Also called **Melkersson's syndrome.**

**Mellaril,** trademark for an antipsychotic agent (thioridazine).

**melon-seed body** /mel′ən/, a small, fibrous, loose body in a joint or tendon sheath.

**melphalan** /mel′fəlan/, an antineoplastic alkylating agent.

■ INDICATIONS: It is prescribed in the treatment of malignant neoplastic diseases, including multiple myeloma.

■ CONTRAINDICATIONS: Pregnancy, recent exposure to antineoplastic medication or to radiation, or known hypersensitivity to this drug prohibits its use.

■ ADVERSE EFFECTS: Among the more serious adverse reactions are bone marrow depression, nausea, and vomiting.

**melting,** **1.** the liquefaction effect of heat. **2.** the thermal denaturation of double-stranded deoxyribonucleic acid into two component strands. **3.** Conversion of the solid to the liquid phase.

**melting point (mp)** [AS, *meltan* + L, *punctus,* pricked], a characteristic temperature at which the solid and liquid forms of a substance are in equilibrium. The mp of ice is 32° F, or 0° C, at one atmosphere pressure.

**membrana tectoria** /membrā′nə/ [L, *membrana,* thin skin, *tectorium,* a covering], **1.** also called **occipitoaxial ligament.** the broad, strong ligament covering the dens and helping to connect the axis to the occipital bone of the skull. **2.** a spiral membrane projecting from the vestibular lip of the cochlea over the organ of Corti.

**membrana tympani.** See **tympanic membrane.**

**membrane** /mem′brān/ [L, *membrana,* thin skin], a thin layer of tissue composed of epithelial cells and connective tissue that covers a surface, lines a cavity, or divides a space in the body. The principal kinds of membranes are **mucous membrane, serous membrane, synovial membrane,** and **skin (cutaneous) membrane.**

**membrane attack complex (MAC),** a cluster of complement components that creates a pore in the plasma membrane of a cell, leading to the lysis of a cell.

**membrane conductance,** the degree of permeability of a cellular membrane to certain ions; the reciprocal of the membrane resistance.

**membrane diffusion coefficient,** a factor that relates the quantitative characteristics of alveolar-capillary membranes to total pulmonary diffusing capacity.

**membrane potential** [L, *membrana* + *potentia*], the difference in electrical polarization or charge between two sides of a membrane or cell wall. Also called **electric potential gradient.**

**membrane responsiveness,** the relationship between the membrane potential of a myocardial cell at the time of stimulation and the maximal rate of rise of the action potential.

**membranoproliferative glomerulonephritis (MPGN)** /mem'brənō'prōlif'ərətiv'/, a chronic form of glomerulonephritis, characterized by mesangial cell proliferation, irregular thickening of glomerular capillary walls, thickening of the mesangial matrix, and low serum levels of complement. Also called **mesangiocapillary glomerulonephritis.**

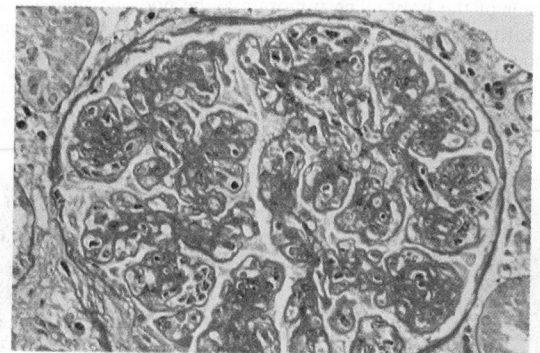

**Membranoproliferative glomerulonephritis**
*(Cotran, Kumar, and Collins, 1999/courtesy Dr. H. Rennke, Brigham and Women's Hospital, Boston)*

**membranous** /mem'brənəs/ [L, *membrana*], resembling or consisting of a membrane.

**membranous dysmenorrhea** [L, *membrana* + Gk, *dys*, bad, *men*, month, *rhein*, to flow], a form of spasmodic pain associated with menstruation, in which a cast of the uterine cavity is passed.

**membranous labyrinth** [L, *membrana* + *labyrinthos*, a maze], a network of three fluid-filled membranous semicircular ducts suspended within the bony semicircular canals of the inner ear, associated with the sense of balance. The ducts, which contain endolymph, follow the contours of the bony canals and are about one fourth of the diameter of the canals.

**membranous pharyngitis** [L, *membrana* + Gk, *pharynx*, throat], a diphtheric inflammation of the pharynx with the formation of a false membrane in the throat.

**membranous stomatitis.** See **pseudomembranous stomatitis.**

**memory**[1] /mem'ərē/ [L, *memoria*], 1. the mental faculty or power that enables one to retain and to recall, through unconscious associative processes, previously experienced sensations, impressions, ideas, concepts, and all information that has been consciously learned. 2. the reservoir of all past experiences and knowledge that may be recollected or recalled at will. 3. the recollection of a past event, idea, sensation, or previously learned knowledge. Kinds of memory include **affect memory, anterograde memory, kinesthetic memory, long-term memory, screen memory, short-term memory,** and **visual memory.** See also **amnesia, déjà vu.**

**memory**[2], a nursing outcome from the Nursing Outcomes Classification (NOC) defined as the ability to cognitively retrieve and report previously stored information. See also **Nursing Outcomes Classification.**

**memory cell.** See **lymphocyte.**

**memory image,** a sensation, impression, or sense perception as it is recalled in the memory.

**memory, impaired,** a nursing diagnosis accepted by the Eleventh National Conference on the Classification of Nursing Diagnoses. It is defined as the state in which an individual experiences the inability to remember or recall bits of information or behavioral skills. Impaired memory may be attributed to pathophysiologic or situational causes that may be either temporary or permanent.

■ DEFINING CHARACTERISTICS: Major defining characteristics are observed or reported experiences of forgetting; inability to determine whether a behavior was performed; inability to learn or retain new skills or information; inability to perform a previously learned skill; inability to recall factual information; and inability to recall recent or past events. A minor defining characteristic is forgetting to perform a behavior at a scheduled time.

■ RELATED FACTORS: Related factors are acute or chronic hypoxia, anemia, decreased cardiac output, fluid and electrolyte imbalance, neurologic disturbances, and excessive environmental disturbances. See also **nursing diagnosis.**

**memory training,** a nursing intervention from the Nursing Interventions Classification (NIC) defined as facilitation of memory. See also **Nursing Interventions Classification.**

**MEN,** abbreviation for **multiple endocrine neoplasia.**

**menadiol sodium diphosphate** /men'ədī'ol/, a water-soluble analog of vitamin K. See **menadione.**

**menadione, menaphthone** /men'ədī'ōn/, a synthetic form of vitamin $K_3$. A water-soluble injectable form of the product is menadiol sodium diphosphate.

**menarche** /menär'kē/ [Gk, *men*, month, *archaios*, from the beginning], the first menstruation and the commencement of cyclic menstrual function. It usually occurs between 9 and 17 years of age. See also **pubarche.**

**menarcheal age** /menär'kē-əl/ [Gk, *men*, month, *archaios*, beginning; L, *aetas*, age], the age at which menstruation begins. The normal range is from 9 to 17 years of age. See also **puberty.**

**Mendel-Bekhterev reflex.** See **Mendel's reflex.**

**mendelevium (Md)** /men'dəlē'vē·əm/ [Dimitrii Mendeleev, Russian chemist, 1834–1907], a synthetic element in the actinide group. Its atomic number is 101. The atomic mass of its most stable isotope is 256. It is the ninth transuranic element.

**mendelian.** See **mendelism.**

**mendelian genetics, mendelian laws.** See **Mendel's laws.**

**mendelism** /men'dəliz'əm/ [Gregor J. Mendel, Austrian geneticist, 1822–1884], the concept of inheritance derived from the application of Mendel's laws. Also called **mendelianism. —mendelian,** *adj.*

**Mendel's dorsal reflex of foot.** See **Mendel's reflex.**

**Mendel's laws** [Gregor J. Mendel], the basic principles of inheritance based on breeding experiments on garden peas by the nineteenth-century Austrian monk Gregor Mendel. These principles are usually stated as the law of segregation and the law of independent assortment. According to the law of segregation, each trait of a species is represented in the somatic cells by a pair of units, now known as genes, which are segregated during meiosis so that each gamete receives only one gene for each trait. In any monohybrid crossing, the possible ratio for the phenotypic expression of a particular dominant trait is 3:1, whereas the genotypic ratio of pure dominants to hybrids to pure recessives is 1:2:1. According to the law of independent assortment, the members of a gene pair on different chromosomes segregate independently from other pairs during meiosis so that the gametes show all possible combinations of genes. Genes on the same chromosome are affected by linkage and segregate in blocks according to the amount of crossing over that occurs, a discovery made after Mendel's work. Also called **mendelian genetics, mendelian laws.** See also **chromosome, crossing over, dominant allele, linkage, meiosis, recessive allele.**

**Mendelson's syndrome** [Curtis L. Mendelson, American obstetrician, b. 1913], a respiratory condition caused by the aspiration of acidic gastric contents into the lungs. It usually occurs when a person vomits while inebriated, stuporous from anesthesia, or unconscious, as during a seizure. It is marked by bronchoconstriction and destruction of the tracheal mucosa, progressing to a syndrome resembling acute respiratory distress syndrome. Also called **pulmonary acid aspiration syndrome.**

**Mendel's reflex** /men′dəlz/ [Kurt Mendel, German neurologist, 1874−1946], percussion of the top of the foot normally causes dorsal flexion of the second to fifth toes; in certain organic nervous conditions it causes plantar flexion of the toes. Also called **Bekhterev-Mendel reflex, cuboidodigital reflex, dorsocuboidal reflex, Mendel-Bekhterev reflex, Mendel's dorsal reflex of foot, tarsophalangeal reflex.**

**Ménétrier's disease.** See **giant hypertrophic gastritis.**

**-menia,** suffix meaning '(condition of) menstrual activity': *catamenia, ischomenia, pausimenia.*

**Ménière's disease** /mānē·erz′/ [Prosper Ménière, French physician, 1799–1862], a chronic disease of the inner ear characterized by recurrent episodes of vertigo; progressive sensorineural hearing loss, which may be bilateral; and tinnitus.

**meningeal** /mənin′jē·əl/ [Gk, *meninx,* membrane], pertaining to the meninges, the three layers of membranes covering the brain and spinal cord.

**meningeal hydrops.** See **pseudotumor cerebri.**

**meninges** /minin′jēz/, *sing.* **meninx** /mē′ningks, men′-/ [Gk, *meninx,* membrane], the three membranes enclosing the brain and the spinal cord, comprising the dura mater, the pia mater, and the arachnoid membrane. The pia mater and the arachnoid can become inflamed by bacterial meningitis, causing serious complications that may be life-threatening. —**meningeal,** *adj.*

**meningioma** /minin′jē·ō′mə/, *pl.* **meningiomas, meningiomata** [Gk, *meninx,* membrane, *oma,* tumor], a mesenchymal fibroblastic tumor of the membranes enveloping the brain and spinal cord. Meningiomas grow slowly, are usually vascular, and occur most commonly near the superior longitudinal transverse and cavernous sinuses of the dura mater of the brain. The tumors may be nodular, plaquelike, or diffuse lesions that invade the skull, causing bone erosion and compression of brain tissue. Meningiomas usually occur in adults.

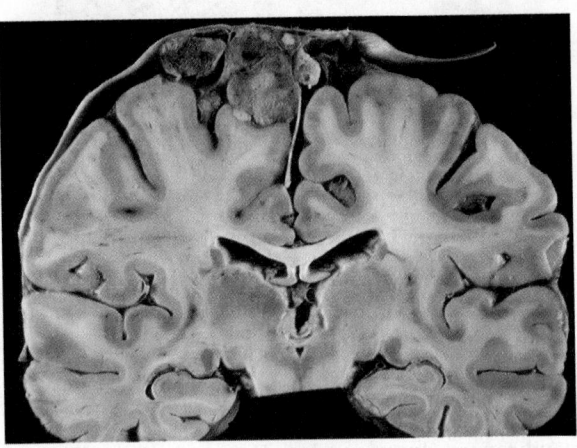

**Meningioma** *(Cotran, Kumar, and Collins, 1999)*

**meningism** /minin′jizəm/ [Gk, *meninx + ismos,* process], an abnormal condition characterized by irritation of the brain and spinal cord and by symptoms that mimic those of meningitis. In meningism, however, there is no actual inflammation of the meninges.

**meningismus** /men′injis′məs/ [Gk, *meninx,* membrane], a condition in which the patient shows signs of meningitis but examination reveals no pathologic changes in the meninges. The condition is associated with cases of pneumonia in small children. See also **meningism.**

**meningitis** /min′injī′tis/, *pl.* **meningitides** [Gk, *meninx + itis,* inflammation], any infection or inflammation of the membranes covering the brain and spinal cord. It is usually purulent and involves the fluid in the subarachnoid space. The most common causes in adults are bacterial infection with *Streptococcus pneumoniae, Neisseria meningitidis,* or *Haemophilus influenzae.* Aseptic meningitis may be caused by nonbacterial agents such as a high dose of intravenous immunoglobulin, chemicals, neoplasms, or viruses. Many of these diseases are benign and self-limited, such as meningitis caused by strains of coxsackievirus or echovirus. Others are more severe, such as those involving arboviruses, herpesviruses, or poliomyelitis viruses. Yeasts such as *Candida* and *Cryptococcus* may cause a severe, often fatal meningitis. See also **aseptic meningitis.** A kind of meningitis is **tuberculous meningitis.** Compare **encephalitis.**

■ OBSERVATIONS: The onset of meningitis is usually sudden and characterized by severe headache, stiffness of the neck, irritability, malaise, and restlessness. Nausea, vomiting, de-

Dura mater
(two layers)

Arachnoid

Pia
mater

Subarachnoid
space

Skull

Skin

Muscle

**Meningeal layers of the brain**
*(Chipps, Clanin, and Campbell, 1992)*

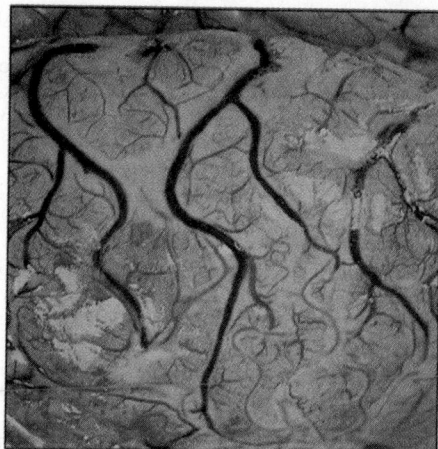

**Bacterial meningitis: purulent exudate
on surface of cerebral hemisphere**
*(Perkin, 1998)*

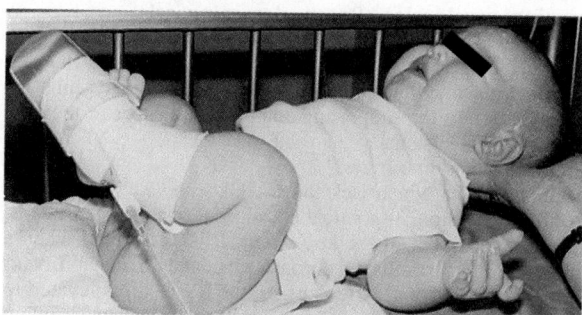

**Stiffness of the neck commonly seen in meningitis**
*(Zitelli and Davis, 1997)*

lirium, and complete disorientation may develop quickly. Temperature, pulse rate, and respirations are increased. Residual damage may include deafness, blindness, paralysis, and mental retardation. Hydrocephalus also may develop.

■ INTERVENTIONS: Bacterial meningitis is treated promptly with antibiotics specific for the causative organism; they are administered intravenously or intrathecally. Antifungal medications, such as amphotericin B, given intravenously or intrathecally for several weeks, may prevent death from fungal meningitis, but serious neurologic sequelae may occur.

■ NURSING CONSIDERATIONS: Constant skilled nursing attention is necessary to ensure early recognition of rising intracranial pressure, to prevent aspiration in the event of convulsive seizures, and to prevent airway obstruction. Except for the first day or two of meningococcal disease, strict isolation procedures are unnecessary. IV fluids and nasogastric tube feeding may be necessary for a prolonged period. Sedatives and narcotic analgesics should not be used because they may obscure important neurologic signs in addition to depressing vital functions.

**meningo-,** combining form meaning 'membranes covering the brain or spinal cord or other membranes': *meningocele, meningococcus, meningopathy.*

**meningocele** /mining'gōsēl'/ [Gk, *meninx* + *kele,* hernia], a saclike protrusion of either the cerebral or spinal meninges through a congenital defect in the skull or the vertebral column. It forms a hernial cyst that is filled with cerebrospinal fluid but does not contain neural tissue. The anomaly is designated a cranial meningocele or spinal meningocele, depending on the site of the defect; it can be easily repaired by surgery. See also **myelomeningocele, neural tube defect.**

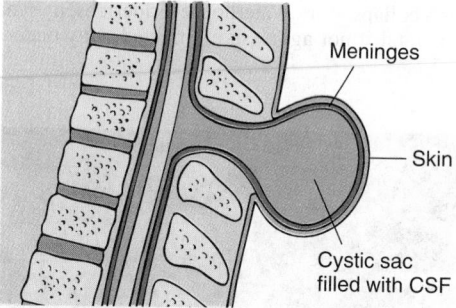

Meninges

Skin

Cystic sac
filled with CSF

**Meningocele: protrusion of meninges
through the skin**
*(Huether and McCance, 2000)*

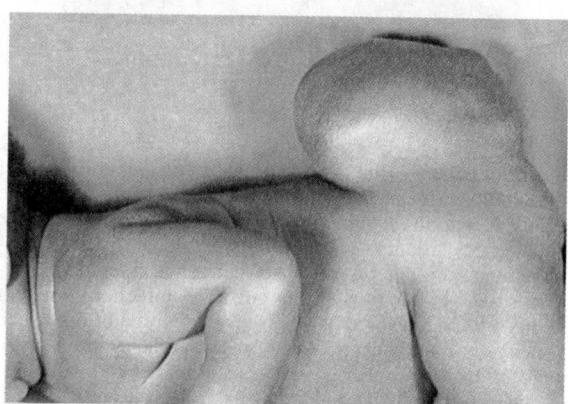

**Meningocele: clinical presentation** *(Zitelli and Davis, 1992)*

**meningococcal.** See **meningococcus.**

**meningococcal meningitis** /mi·ning'gō·kok'əl/, bacterial meningitis caused by infection with *Neisseria meningitidis,* an acute infectious disease with seropurulent meningeal inflammation. It usually appears in epidemics, and symptoms are those of acute cerebral and spinal meningitis, usually with an eruption of cutaneous erythematous, herpetic, or hemorrhagic spots. The fulminating or malignant form is known as **Waterhouse-Friderichsen syndrome.** Also called **cerebrospinal fever, epidemic cerebrospinal meningitis.**

**meningococcal polysaccharide vaccine** /-kok'əl/, either of two active immunizing agents against group A and group C meningococcal organisms.

■ INDICATION: It is prescribed for immunization against meningococcal meningitis.

■ CONTRAINDICATIONS: Immunosuppression or acute infection prohibits its use.

■ ADVERSE EFFECTS: The most serious adverse reaction is anaphylaxis.

**meningococcemia** /mining'gōkoksē'mē·ə/ [Gk, *meninx* + *kokkos,* berry, *haima,* blood], a disease caused by *Neisseria meningitidis* in the bloodstream. Onset is sudden, with chills, pain in the muscles and joints, headache, petechiae, sore throat, and severe prostration. Tachycardia is present, respirations and pulse rate are increased, and fever is intermittent. Treatment of choice is penicillin G; peripheral circulatory collapse or Waterhouse-Friderichsen syndrome, which is fatal if not aggressively treated, may occur.

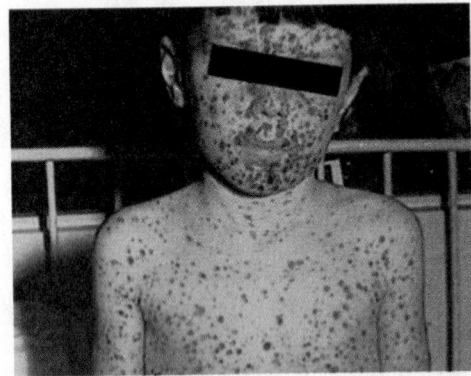

**Meningococcemia** *(Zitelli and Davis, 1997)*

**meningococcus** /mining'gōkok'əs/, *pl.* **meningococci** /-kok'sī/ [Gk, *meninx* + *kokkos,* berry], a bacterium of the genus *Neisseria meningitidis,* a nonmotile gram-negative diplococcus, frequently found in the nasopharynx of asymptomatic carriers, that may cause septicemia or epidemic cerebrospinal meningitis. Meningococcal infections are not highly communicable; however, crowded conditions, such as may be found in army camps and college dormitories, concentrate the number of carriers and reduce individual resistance to the organism. Hemorrhagic skin lesions are significant clues to the diagnosis. Stained smears of these le-

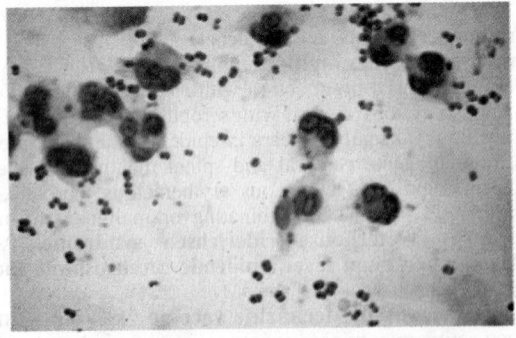

**Meningococci in cerebrospinal fluid**
*(Stone and Gorbach, 2000/courtesy Dr. Mark Drapkin, Newton Wellesley Hospital, Newton, Massachusetts)*

sions or of cerebrospinal fluid must be examined quickly because meningococci are fragile and lyse readily. Early treatment with an appropriate antibiotic such as penicillin G is essential for cure. Contacts may receive prophylaxis with rifampin. Several meningococcal vaccines are available. See also **meningitis. —meningococcal,** *adj.*

**meningoencephalitis** /-ensef'əlī'tis/ [Gk, *meninx,* membrane, *enkephalos,* brain, *itis,* inflammation], an inflammation of both the brain and the meninges, usually caused by a bacterial infection.

**meningoencephalocele** /mining'gō·ensef'əlōsēl'/ [Gk, *meninx* + *enkephalos,* brain, *kele,* hernia], a saclike cyst containing brain tissue, cerebrospinal fluid, and meninges that protrudes through a congenital defect in the skull. It may or may not contain parts of the ventricular system and is commonly associated with brain defects. Also called **encephalomeningocele.** See also **neural tube defect.**

**meningoencephalomyelitis** /mining'gō·ensef'əlōmī'əlī'tis/, a combined inflammation of the brain, spinal cord, and meninges.

**meningoencephalopathy** /mining'gō·ensef'əlop'əthē/, a noninflammatory disease of the brain and its membranes.

**meningomyelitis** /-mī'əlī'tis/ [Gk, *meninx,* membrane, *myelos,* marrow, *itis,* inflammation], an inflammation of the spinal cord and its surrounding membranes.

**meningomyelocele.** See **myelomeningocele.**

**meningovascular neurosyphilis** /-vas'kyələr/ [Gk, *meninx,* membrane; L, *vasculum,* little vessel; Gk, *neuron,* nerve, *syn,* together, *philein,* to love], a neurosyphilis inflammation of the supporting and nutrient tissues of the central nervous system.

**meninx.** See **meninges.**

**meniscectomy** /men'isek'təmē/ [Gk, *meniskos,* crescent, *ektomē,* excision], surgical excision of one of the crescent-shaped cartilages of the knee joint. It is performed when a torn cartilage results in chronic pain and in instability or locking of the joint. After surgery the leg is kept elevated to reduce swelling and exercises are performed to maintain muscle strength. See also **arthroscopy.**

**menisci.** See **meniscus.**

**meniscocyte.** See **erythrocyte.**

**meniscocytosis.** See **sickle cell anemia.**

**meniscus** /minis'kəs/, *pl.* **menisci** [Gk, *meniskos,* crescent], **1.** the interface between a liquid and air. **2.** a lens with both convex and concave aspects. **3.** a curved, fibrous cartilage in the knees and other joints. See also **meniscectomy.**

**Menkes' kinky hair syndrome** /men'kēz/ [John H. Menkes, American neurologist, b. 1928; D, *kinke,* tight twist; AS, *haer*], a familial disorder affecting the normal absorption of copper from the intestine, characterized by the growth of sparse, kinky hair. Infants with the syndrome suffer cerebral degeneration, retarded growth, and early death. Early diagnosis and IV administration of copper may prevent irreversible damage.

**meno-,** combining form meaning 'the menses': *menolipsis, menopause, menorrhea.*

**menometrorrhagia** /men'ōmet'rōrā'jē·ə/ [L, *men,* month; Gk, *metra,* womb, *rhegnyai,* to burst forth], excessive menstrual and uterine bleeding other than that caused by menstruation. It is a combination of metrorrhagia and menorrhagia and may be a sign of a urogenital malignancy.

**menopause** /men'əpôz/ [L, *men,* month; Gk, *pausis,* to cease], strictly, the cessation of menses, but commonly referring to the period of the female climacteric. Menses stop naturally with the decline of cyclic hormonal production and function usually between 45 and 55 years of age but may stop earlier in life as a result of illness or surgical removal of

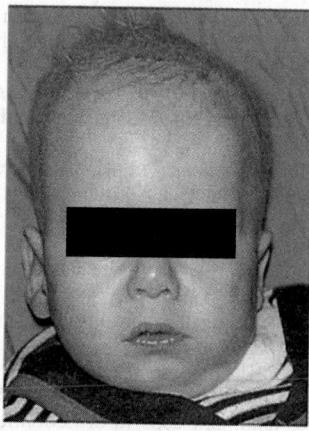

**Menkes' kinky hair syndrome:
characteristic facial appearance**
*(Newton, 1995)*

the uterus or both ovaries. As the production of ovarian estrogen and pituitary gonadotropins decreases, ovulation and menstruation become less frequent and eventually stop. Fluctuations in the circulating levels of these hormones occur as the levels decline. Hot flashes are a common symptom of menopause. They often can be controlled with estrogen but may not be so severe as to require therapy and cease in time without hormonal treatment. See also **artificial menopause.**

**menorrhagia** /men′ərā′jē·ə/ [L, *men* + *rhegnyai,* to burst forth], abnormally heavy or long menstrual periods. Menorrhagia occurs occasionally during the reproductive years of most women's lives. If the condition becomes chronic, anemia from recurrent excessive blood loss may result. Abnormal bleeding after menopause always warrants investigation to rule out malignancy. Menorrhagia is a relatively common complication of benign uterine fibromyomata; it may be so severe or intractable as to require hysterectomy. Also called **hypermenorrhea.** Compare **metrorrhagia, oligomenorrhea. —menorrhagic,** *adj.*

**menorrhalgia.** See **dysmenorrhea.**

**menorrhea** /men′ôrē′ə/ [L, *men* + Gk, *rhoia,* flow], the normal discharge of blood and tissue from the uterus. See also **menorrhagia, menstruation.**

**menostasis** /minos′təsis/ [L, *men* + Gk, *stasis,* stand still], an abnormal condition in which the products of menstruation cannot escape the uterus or vagina because of stenosis, an occlusion of the cervix or the introitus of the vagina. An imperforate hymen is a rare cause of menostasis. —**menostatic,** *adj.*

**menotropins** /men′ōtrop′inz/ [L, *men* + Gk, *trepein,* to turn], a preparation of gonadotropic hormones from the urine of postmenopausal women.

■ INDICATION: It is prescribed with chorionic gonadotropin to induce ovulation.

■ CONTRAINDICATIONS: Elevated gonadotropin levels in the urine, thyroid or adrenal dysfunction, pituitary tumor, abnormal bleeding, ovarian cyst, pregnancy, or known hypersensitivity to this drug prohibits its use.

■ ADVERSE EFFECTS: Among the more serious adverse reactions are ovarian hyperstimulation syndrome, hemoperitoneum, arterial thromboembolism, multiple gestation, and possible birth defects.

**menoxenia** /men′oksē′nē·ə/ [L, *men* + Gk, *xenos,* strange], any abnormality relating to menstruation.

**Menrium,** trademark for a fixed-combination drug for menopausal symptoms, containing esterified estrogens and a sedative (chlordiazepoxide).

**menses** /men′sēz/ [L, *men,* month], the normal flow of blood and decidua that occurs during menstruation. The first day of the flow of the menses is the first day of the menstrual cycle. Also called **catamenia,** *(nontechnical)* **period.**

**menstrual** /men′strōō·əl/ [L, *menstrualis,* monthly], pertaining to menstruation.

**menstrual age** [L, *menstrualis,* monthly, *aetas,* lifetime], the age of an embryo or fetus as calculated from the first day of the last menstrual period.

**menstrual colic** [L, *menstrualis,* monthly; Gk, *kolikos,* colon pain], a form of dysmenorrhea characterized by abdominal pain during or immediately before menstruation.

**menstrual cramps,** low abdominal pain that may range from a colicky feeling to a constant dull ache. The pain may radiate to the lower back and legs. Menstrual cramps are often associated with the beginning of menses, reaching a peak in 24 hours and subsiding after 2 days. Treatment may include administration of ibuprofen or other drugs immediately before and after the start of menses. See also **dysmenorrhea.**

**menstrual cycle,** the recurring cycle of change in the endometrium during which the decidual layer of the endometrium is shed, then regrows, proliferates, is maintained for several days, and sheds again at menstruation. The average length of the cycle, from the first day of bleeding of one cycle to the first of another, is 28 days. The duration and character vary greatly among women. Menstrual cycles begin at menarche and end with menopause. The uterine phases of the cycle are the **proliferative phase, secretory phase,** and **menstrual phase.** See also **oogenesis.**

**menstrual period** [L, *menstrualis,* monthly; Gk, *peri* + *hodos,* way], the periodic discharge of blood and cellular debris from the uterus.

**menstrual phase,** the final of the three phases of the menstrual cycle, the one in which menstruation occurs. The necrotic mucosa of the endometrium is shed, leaving the stratum basale; bleeding, primarily from the spiral arteries, occurs. The average blood loss is 30 to 80 mL. For convenience, the days of the menstrual cycle are counted from the first day of the menstrual phase. Compare **proliferative phase, secretory phase.**

**menstrual sponge,** a small natural sponge or a piece of a synthetic sponge to which a loop of string is attached. It is inserted into the vagina to absorb the menstrual flow and is removed by pulling the string. It may be washed, squeezed dry, and reused as necessary through menstruation. Menstrual sponges are not commonly used.

**menstruation** /men′strōō·ā′shən/ [L, *menstruare,* to menstruate], the periodic discharge through the vagina of a bloody secretion containing tissue debris from the shedding of the endometrium from the nonpregnant uterus. The average duration of menstruation is 4 to 5 days, and it recurs at approximately 28-day intervals throughout the reproductive life of nonpregnant women. Kinds of menstruation are **anovular menstruation, retrograde menstruation,** and **vicarious menstruation.** See also **menstrual cycle. —menstruate,** *v.*

**ment-,** prefix meaning 'mind': *mental, menticide, mentimeter.*

**mental**[1] /men′təl/ [L, *mens,* mind], **1.** of, relating to, or characteristic of the mind or psyche. **2.** existing in the mind; performed or accomplished by the mind. **3.** of, relating to, or characterized by a disorder of the mind. **4.** slang term used for clients believed to have a mental health disorder.

**mental**[2] [L, *mentum,* chin], pertaining to the chin.

**mental age (MA),** the age level at which one functions intellectually, as determined by standardized psychologic and intelligence tests and expressed as the age at which that level is average. Compare **achievement age.** See also **developmental age.**

**mental deficiency.** See **mental retardation.**

**mental disorder,** any disturbance of emotional equilibrium, as manifested in maladaptive behavior and impaired functioning, caused by genetic, physical, chemical, biologic, psychologic, or social and cultural factors. Also called **emotional illness, mental illness, psychiatric disorder.**

**mental foramen** [L, *mentum,* chin], an opening on the lateral part of the body of the mandible, inferior to the second premolar, through which the mental nerve and blood vessels pass.

**mental handicap,** any mental defect or characteristic resulting from a congenital abnormality, traumatic injury, or disease that impairs normal intellectual functioning and prevents a person from participating normally in activities appropriate for a particular age group. See also **mental retardation.**

**mental health,** a relative state of mind in which a person is able to cope with and adjust to the recurrent stresses of everyday living in an acceptable way.

**Mental Health Association (MHA),** a voluntary nonprofessional agency dedicated to the improvement of mental health facilities and services in community clinics and hospitals, the recruitment and training of volunteers, and the promotion of mental health legislation. Formerly called the **National Association for Mental Health.**

**mental health consultation,** any interaction between two or more health care professionals related to a specific issue.

**mental health nursing.** See **psychiatric nursing.**

**mental health service,** any one of a group of government, professional, or lay organizations operating at a community, state, national, or international level to aid in the prevention and treatment of mental disorders. See also **community mental health center.**

**mental hygiene,** the study concerned with the development of healthy mental and emotional habits, attitudes, and behavior and with the prevention of mental illness. Also called **psychophylaxis.**

**mental illness.** See **mental disorder.**

**mental image,** any concept or sensation produced in the mind through memory or imagination.

**mentality** /mental'itē/ [L, *mens,* mind], **1.** the functional power and capacity of the mind. **2.** intellectual character.

**mental retardation,** a disorder characterized by subaverage general intellectual function with deficits or impairments in the ability to learn and to adapt socially. The cause may be genetic, biologic, psychosocial, or sociocultural.

**mental ridge** [L, *mentum,* chin; AS, *hyrcg*], a dense elevation that extends from the symphysis menti (the center front of the mandible) to the premolar area on the anterolateral aspect of the body of the mandible.

**mental status,** the degree of competence shown by a person in intellectual, emotional, psychologic, and personality functioning as measured by psychologic testing with reference to a statistical norm. See also **mental status examination.**

**mental status examination,** a diagnostic procedure for determining the mental status of a person. The trained interviewer poses certain questions in a carefully standardized manner and evaluates the verbal responses and behavioral reactions.

**mental tubercle** [L, *mentum,* chin], one of a bilateral pair of prominences on the lower border of the body of the mandible.

**mentation** /mentā'shən/ [L, *mens,* mind, *atus,* process], any mental activity, including conscious and unconscious processes.

**menthol** /men'thol/ [L, *menta,* mint], a topical antipruritic with a cooling effect that relieves itching. It is an ingredient in many topical creams and ointments.

**mentholated camphor** /men'thəlā'tid/, a mixture of equal parts of camphor and menthol, used as a local counterirritant.

**-mentia,** suffix meaning '(condition of the) mind': *dementia, moramentia, pseudodementia.*

**menton** /men'ton/ [L, *mentum,* chin], the most inferior point on the chin in the lateral view of a cephalogram. It is a cephalometric landmark used in orthodontic treatment.

**mentor** /men'tər/ [Gk, *Mentor,* mythic educator], an older, trusted adviser or counselor who offers helpful guidance to younger colleagues.

**mentum** /men'təm/ [L, chin], **1.** the chin, especially of the fetus. **2.** a fetal reference point in designating the position of the fetus with respect to the maternal pelvis; for example, left mentum anterior (LMA) indicates that the fetal chin is presenting in the left anterior quadrant of the pelvis.

**menu** /men'yo͞o/ [Fr, small], a list of choices displayed on a computer screen from which a user selects the next action to be taken by signaling through the keyboard or another device, such as a mouse.

**MEP, 1.** abbreviation for **maximal expiratory pressure. 2.** abbreviation for *mean effective pressure.*

**mepenzolate bromide** /mepen'zəlāt/, an anticholinergic/antispasmodic agent.

■ INDICATIONS: It is prescribed as an adjunct in treating peptic ulcer.

■ CONTRAINDICATIONS: Narrow-angle glaucoma, asthma, obstruction of the genitourinary or GI tract, severe ulcerative colitis, or known hypersensitivity to this drug prohibits its use.

■ ADVERSE EFFECTS: Blurred vision, central nervous system effects, tachycardia, dry mouth, decreased sweating, or hypersensitivity reactions may occur.

**Mepergan,** trademark for a fixed-combination central nervous system drug containing an opioid analgesic (meperidine hydrochloride) and an antihistamine (promethazine hydrochloride).

**meperidine hydrochloride** /meper'idēn/, an opioid analgesic.

■ INDICATIONS: It is used to treat moderate to severe pain and to relieve pain and anxiety before surgery.

■ CONTRAINDICATIONS: It is used with caution in many conditions, including head injuries, asthma, impaired renal or hepatic function, or unstable cardiovascular status. Concomitant use of a monoamine oxidase inhibitor or known hypersensitivity to this drug prohibits its use. It is not used if the patient has convulsive disorders.

■ ADVERSE EFFECTS: Among the most serious adverse reactions are drowsiness, dizziness, nausea, constipation, sweating, respiratory and circulatory depression, and drug addiction.

**mephenytoin** /mifen'ətō'in/, an anticonvulsant.

■ INDICATION: It is prescribed for the control of seizures in epilepsy when less toxic medications have not been effective.

■ CONTRAINDICATIONS: It is not usually recommended in pregnancy. Known hypersensitivity to this drug or to any hydantoin prohibits its use.

■ ADVERSE EFFECTS: Among the most serious adverse reactions are morbilliform rash, fever, hepatotoxicity, and various blood dyscrasias. The frequent occurrence of adverse reactions limits the use of this drug.

**mephobarbital** /mef′ōbär′bitol/, an anticonvulsant and sedative.

■ INDICATIONS: It is prescribed in the treatment of anxiety, nervous tension, insomnia, and epilepsy.

■ CONTRAINDICATIONS: Porphyria or known hypersensitivity to this drug or to barbiturates prohibits its use.

■ ADVERSE EFFECTS: Among the more serious adverse reactions are drug dependence, deficiency in vitamin D, paradoxic excitement, skin rash, and GI disturbance.

**Mephyton,** trademark for a vitamin K product (phytonadione).

**mepivacaine.** See **amide local anesthetic.**

**meprobamate** /miprō′bəmāt/, an antianxiety agent.

■ INDICATIONS: It is prescribed in treatment of anxiety and tension.

■ CONTRAINDICATIONS: Intermittent porphyria or known hypersensitivity to this drug or to the chemically related drugs tybamate, mebutamate, and carisoprodol prohibits its use.

■ ADVERSE EFFECTS: Among the most serious adverse reactions are exacerbation of intermittent porphyria, augmentation of effects of other central nervous system depressants, and various allergic reactions. Drowsiness and ataxia commonly occur.

**mEq,** abbreviation for **milliequivalent.**

**mEq/L,** abbreviation for **milliequivalent per liter.**

**-mer, -mere, mero-,** 1. combining form meaning 'part, portion': *isomer, monomer, merocyte, meropia.* 2. combining form meaning 'polymer.'

**meralgia** /miral′jə/ [Gk, *meros,* thigh, *algos,* pain], the presence of pain in the thigh.

**meralgia paresthetica** /per′esthet′ikə/, a condition characterized by pain, paresthesia, and numbness on the lateral surface of the thigh in the region supplied by the lateral femoral cutaneous nerve. The cause of the condition is ischemia of the nerve caused by its entrapped position in the inguinal ligament.

**mercaptopurine** /mərkap′təpyoo′rēn/, an antineoplastic and immunosuppressive; a purine antimetabolite. Also known as **6-mercaptopurine, 6-MP.**

■ INDICATIONS: It is prescribed in the treatment of malignant neoplastic diseases, including acute lymphocytic leukemia.

■ CONTRAINDICATIONS: Known hypersensitivity to this drug prohibits its use.

■ ADVERSE EFFECTS: Among the more severe adverse reactions are bone marrow depression and acute GI disturbances, including nausea, vomiting, diarrhea, and stomatitis.

**6-mercaptopurine.** See **mercaptopurine.**

**Mercer, Ramona T.,** a nursing theorist who developed the Maternal Role Attainment model presented in her book *First-Time Motherhood: Experiences from Teens to Forties* (1986). Maternal role attainment is an interactional and developmental process. It occurs over a period during which the mother becomes attached to her infant, acquires competence in the care-giving tasks, and expresses pleasure and gratification in her role. The focus of Mercer's work went beyond the concept of the "traditional" mother to encompass a variety of mothering roles: maternal age, health status, family functioning, mother-father relationship, and infant characteristics. Mercer considers a mate's love, support, and nurturance to be important factors in enabling a woman to mother her child.

**mercurial** /mərkyoor′ē·əl/, 1. pertaining to mercury, particularly a medicine containing the element mercury. 2. an adverse effect associated with the administration of a mercurial medication, such as a mercurial tremor caused by mercury poisoning.

**mercurial diuretic,** any one of several diuretic agents that contain mercury in an organic chemical form. The principal use for the drugs is in treating edema of cardiac origin, ascites associated with cirrhosis, or oliguria in the nephrotic stage of glomerulonephritis. Immediate fatal reactions have occurred, usually as a result of ventricular failure after intravascular injection and transient high concentration of mercury in the blood. Flushing, urticaria, fever, and nausea and vomiting are common side effects. Thrombocytopenia, neutropenia, agranulocytosis, systemic mercury poisoning, and severe hypersensitivity reactions are among the more serious adverse effects of the mercurial diuretics. The drugs are contraindicated for use in the presence of renal insufficiency or acute nephritis. Because of the toxicity of these drugs, current practice usually recommends their replacement with more convenient and less toxic diuretics.

**mercurialism.** See **mercury poisoning.**

**-mercuric,** combining form meaning 'molecules of bivalent mercury or its compounds': *phenylmercuric, potassiomercuric, trimercuric.*

**mercury (Hg)** /mur′kyərē/ [L, *Mercurius,* mythic messenger of the gods], a metallic element. Its atomic number is 80; its atomic mass is 200.59. It is the only common metal that is liquid at room temperature, and it occurs in nature almost entirely in the form of its sulfide, cinnabar. Mercury is produced commercially and is used in dental amalgams, thermometers, barometers, and other measuring instruments. It forms many poisonous compounds. The air, soil, and water in many areas of the world have become contaminated by mercury because of the burning of fossil fuels that contain the element and because of the greater use of mercury in industry and agriculture. The major toxic forms of this metal are mercury vapor, mercuric salts, and organic mercurials. Elemental mercury is only mildly toxic when ingested, because it is poorly absorbed. The vapor of elemental mercury, however, is readily absorbed through the lungs and enters the brain before it is oxidized. The kidneys retain mercury longer than any of the other body tissues.

**mercury poisoning,** a toxic condition caused by the ingestion or inhalation of mercury or a mercury compound. The chronic form, resulting from inhalation of the vapors or dust of mercurial compounds or from repeated ingestion of very small amounts, is characterized by irritability, excessive saliva, loosened teeth, gum disorders, slurred speech, tremors, and staggering. Symptoms of acute mercury poisoning appear in a few minutes to a half hour and include a metallic taste in the mouth, thirst, nausea, vomiting, severe abdominal pain, bloody diarrhea, and renal failure that may result in death. The presence of mercury in the body is determined by a urine test. Free mercury, such as in thermometers, is not absorbed in the GI tract, but because it is very volatile, hazardous vapors may penetrate ordinary toxic dust respirators, causing poisoning by inhalation. Mercury compounds are found in agricultural fungicides and in certain antiseptics and pigments; they are used extensively in industry. Industrial wastes containing mercury have been identified in some areas, and seafood from contaminated waters has caused serious public health problems. Also called **hydrargyrism, mercurialism.** See also **Minamata disease.**

**mercury thermometer** [L, *Mercurius,* mythic messenger of the gods; Gk, *thermē,* heat, *metron,* measure], a thermometer in which the expandable indicator is mercury.

**mercy killing.** See **euthanasia.**

**merergasia** /mer′ərgā′zhə/ [Gk, *meros,* part, *ergein,* to work], a mild mental incapacity characterized by some emotional instability and some anxiety. —**merergastic,** *adj.*

**-meria,** suffix meaning 'related to parts': *platymeria, polymeria.*

**merisis.** See **hyperplasia.**

**Merkel cell carcinoma** /mer′kəl, mur′kəl/ [Friedrich S. Merkel, German anatomist and physiologist, 1845–1919], a rapidly growing malignant skin tumor that tends to occur on sun-exposed surfaces of older Caucasian individuals. It is composed of small cells in a trabecular pattern that contain dense core granules.

**meroanencephaly** /mer′ō·an′ən·sef′ə·lē/ [Gk, *meros,* part + *a, enkephalos,* not brain], congenital absence of part of the brain, usually the forebrain and midbrain. Compare **anencephaly.**

**meroblastic** /mer′əblas′tik/ [Gk, *meros* + *blastos,* germ], pertaining to or characterizing an ovum that contains a large amount of yolk and in which cleavage is restricted to the yolk-free part of the cytoplasm. Compare **holoblastic.**

**merocrine secretion** /mer′əkrin/ [Gk, *meros,* part, *krinein,* to separate; L, *secernere,* to separate], a secretion in which the secreting cell remains intact while producing and releasing the secretory product. Compare **apocrine secretion, holocrine secretion.**

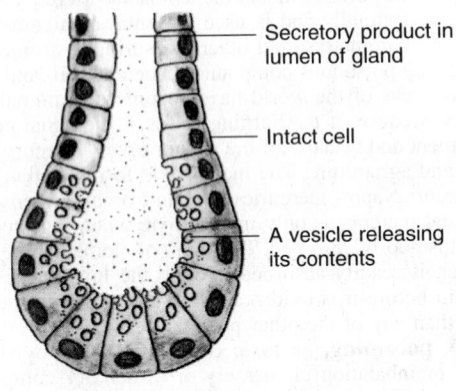

Secretory product in lumen of gland

Intact cell

A vesicle releasing its contents

Merocrine gland

**Merocrine gland** (Applegate, 2000)

**meromelia** /mer′əmē′lyə/ [Gk, *meros* + *melos,* limb], a general designation for the congenital absence of any part of a limb. It is used in reference to such conditions as adactyly, hemimelia, or phocomelia. Compare **amelia.**

**meropenem,** a miscellaneous antiinfective.

■ INDICATIONS: This drug is used to treat serious infections caused by *Streptococcus pneumoniae,* group A β-hemolytic streptococci, enterococci, *Klebsiella, Proteus, Escherichia coli, Pseudomonas aeruginosa, Bacteroides fragilis,* and *B. thetaiotaomicron.* It is also used to treat appendicitis and peritonitis caused by the *viridans* group of streptococci, as well as bacterial meningitis.

■ CONTRAINDICATIONS: Known hypersensitivity to meropenem or imipenem prohibits the use of this drug.

■ ADVERSE EFFECTS: Life-threatening effects of this drug are seizures, pseudomembranous colitis, hepatitis, eosinophilia, neutropenia, and anaphylaxis. Other adverse effects include fever, somnolence, dizziness, weakness, myoclonia, diarrhea, nausea, vomiting, glossitis, hypotension, palpitations, decreased hemoglobin and hematocrit, urticaria, pain at the injection site, phlebitis, erythema at the injection site, chest discomfort, dyspnea, and hyperventilation. Common side effects are headache, rash, and pruritus.

**merozoite** /mer′əzō′īt/ [Gk, *meros* + *zoon,* animal], an organism produced from segmentation of a schizont during the asexual reproductive phase of the life cycle of a sporozoon, specifically the malarial parasite *Plasmodium.* Merozoites can either continue the asexual phase of the life cycle by developing into trophozoites and repeating the process of schizogony or differentiate into male and female gametes and enter the sexual stage. See also *Plasmodium.*

**merozygote** /mer′əzī′gōt/, an incomplete zygote that contains only part of the genetic material of one of the parents. It occurs during conjugation in bacteria, as part of the donor chromosome is excluded by the transfer mechanism.

**MERRF syndrome,** abbreviation for *myoclonus with epilepsy and with ragged red fibers,* constituting a familial syndrome of maternal (mitochondrial) inheritance. Also called **Fukuhara syndrome.**

**Merrifield's knife,** a surgical knife with a long, narrow, triangular blade set into a shank, used for gingivectomy incisions.

**Meruvax II,** trademark for an active immunizing agent (live rubella virus vaccine).

**Merzbacher-Pelizaeus disease.** See **Pelizaeus-Merzbacher disease.**

**mes-, mesio-, meso-,** prefix meaning 'middle or median': *mesoderm, mesencephalon, mesiodens.*

**mesangial** /mesan′jē·əl/, pertaining to the mesangium.

**mesangial IgA nephropathy.** See **Berger's disease.**

**mesangiocapillary glomerulonephritis.** See **membranoproliferative glomerulonephritis.**

**mesangium** /mesan′jē·əm/, a cellular network in the renal glomerulus that helps support the capillary loops. The mesangial cells are phagocytic and frequently contain macromolecules or inflammatory agents that may aid in diagnosis of a kidney disorder when examined in a laboratory.

**Mesantoin,** trademark for an anticonvulsant (mephenytoin).

**mescaline** /mes′kəlēn, -lin/ [Mex, *mezcal*], a psychoactive poisonous alkaloid derived from a colorless alkaline oil in the flowering heads of the cactus *Lophophora williamsii.* Closely related chemically to epinephrine, mescaline causes heart palpitations, diaphoresis, pupillary dilation, and anxiety. It is a Schedule I substance. The drug, taken in capsules or dissolved in a drink, produces visual hallucinations, such as color patterns and spatial distortions, but it does not ordinarily induce disorientation. Mescaline is used in some religious ceremonies to produce euphoria and a feeling of ecstasy. Also called **peyote.**

**mescalism** /mes′kəliz′əm/ [Mex, *mezcal*], a type of chemical dependence on the effects of mescal, an intoxicant spirit obtained from a species of cactus.

**mesencephalon** /mes′ensef′əlon/ [Gk, *mesos,* middle, *enkephalos,* brain], one of the three parts of the brainstem, lying just below the cerebrum and just above the pons. It consists primarily of white substance with some gray substance around the cerebral aqueduct. Deep within the mesencephalon are nuclei of the third and the fourth cranial nerves and the anterior part of the fifth cranial nerve. The mesencephalon also contains nuclei for certain auditory and certain visual reflexes. Also called **midbrain.** —**mesencephalic** /mes′ensifal′ik/, *adj.*

**mesenchymal chondrosarcoma** /meseng′kəməl/ [Gk, *mesos,* middle, *enchyma,* infusion, *chondros,* cartilage, *sarx,* flesh, *oma*, tumor], a rare malignant tumor of soft tissue that develops in many sites. The tumors are highly vascular.

**mesenchyme** /mes'engkīm/ [Gk, *mesos* + *enchyma*, infusion], a diffuse network of tissue derived from the embryonic mesoderm. It consists of stellate cells embedded in gelatinous ground substance with reticular fibers.

**mesenchymoma** /mes'engkimō'mə/ [Gk, *mesos* + *enchyma*, infusion, *oma*, tumor], a mixed mesenchymal neoplasm composed of two or more cellular elements that are not usually associated and fibrous tissue. See also **benign mesenchymoma, malignant mesenchymoma.**

**mesenteric** /mes'enter'ik/ [Gk, *mesos*, middle, *enteron*, intestine], pertaining to the mesentery, the double layer of peritoneum suspending the intestine from the posterior abdominal wall.

**mesenteric adenitis.** See **adenitis.**

**mesenteric node** [Gk, *mesos* + *enteron*, intestine; L, *nodus*, knot], a node in one of three groups of superior mesenteric lymph glands serving parts of the intestine. An average of 125 mesenteric nodes in three different groups lie between the layers of the mesentery. The mesenteric nodes receive afferent vessels from the jejunum, ileum, cecum, vermiform appendix, ascending colon, and transverse colon. Compare **ileocolic node, mesocolic node.**

**mesentery proper** /mez'ənter'ē/ [Gk, *mesos* + *enteron*, intestine; L, *propius*, more suitable], a broad fan-shaped fold of peritoneum suspending the jejunum and the ileum from the dorsal wall of the abdomen. The root of the mesentery proper is about 15 cm long and is connected to certain structures ventral to the vertebral column. The intestinal border of the mesentery proper is about 6 m long and separates to enclose the intestine. The cranial part of the mesentery is narrow but widens to about 20 cm and suspends the small intestine and various nerves and arteries. Compare **sigmoid mesocolon, transverse mesocolon.**

**MESH** /mesh/, an abbreviation derived from *Medical Subject Headings,* the list of medical terms used by the U.S. National Library of Medicine (NLM) for its computerized system of storage and retrieval of published medical reports. The system is also used for indexing medical references published in the monthly and annual volumes of *Index Medicus,* published by the NLM. Also spelled **MeSH.** See also **MEDLARS.**

**mesh graft,** a partial or split-thickness skin graft that has had multiple slits cut into it. The slits allow the graft to be stretched to several times its original size for coverage of a

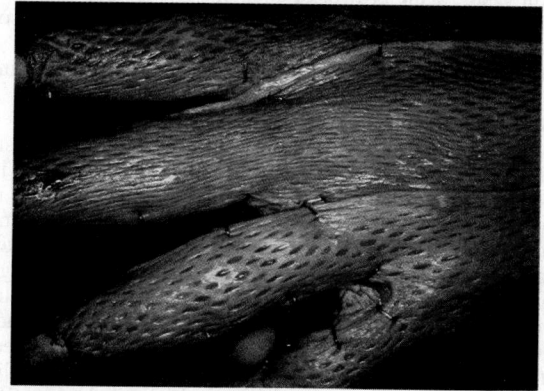

**Mesh graft covering burn to the hand** *(Wong, 1995)*

larger area on the recipient. They also facilitate acceptance of the graft by permitting fluids to escape from beneath the graft.

**mesial.** See **medial.**

**mesibucco-occlusal** /mē'zē·ōbuk'ō·okloo'zəl/ [Gk, *mesos,* middle; L, *bucca,* cheek; L, *occludere,* to close up], pertaining to the angle formed by the mesial, buccal, and occlusal surfaces of a tooth. Compare **mesiolinguo-occlusal.**

**mesiocclusion** /mē'zē·okloo'zhən/ [Gk, *mesos* + L, *occludere,* to close up], an occlusal relationship in which the lower teeth are positioned mesially to the upper teeth.

**mesiodens** /mē'zē·ədenz/ [Gk, *mesos* + L, *dens,* tooth], a supernumerary erupted or unerupted tooth that develops between two maxillary central incisors.

**mesiolinguo-occlusal,** pertaining to the angle formed by the mesial, lingual, and occlusal surfaces of a tooth. Compare **mesibucco-occlusal.**

**mesioversion** /mē'zē·ōvur'zhən/ [Gk, *mesos* + L, *vertere,* to turn], **1.** a condition in which one or more teeth are closer than normal to the midline. **2.** a condition in which the maxilla or mandible is positioned more anteriorly than normal.

**mesmerism** /mez'məriz'əm/ [Franz A. Mesmer, Austrian physician, 1734–1815], a practice of hypnotism introduced by Mesmer, who believed human health was affected by "celestial magnetic forces." Some patients were reported cured or experienced diminished symptoms by undergoing a "grand crisis," or seizure, while under hypnosis. Mesmer was regarded as a fraud by the medical profession, but his work led to serious studies of the health effects of the power of suggestion.

**meso-** /mez'ō-, mes'ō-/. See **mes-.**

**mesocolic node** /mes'ōkol'ik/ [Gk, *mesos* + *kolon,* colon; L, *nodus,* knot], a node in one of three groups of superior mesenteric lymph glands, proliferating between the layers of the transverse mesocolon, close to the transverse colon. They are best developed near the right and left colic flexures and receive afferents from the jejunum, ileum, cecum, vermiform appendix, ascending colon, and transverse colon. Their efferent vessels pass to the preaortic nodes. Compare **mesenteric node.**

**mesocolopexy** /mes'ōkō'ləpek'sē/ [Gk, *mesos* + *kolon,* colon, *pexis,* fixation], suspension or fixation of the mesocolon.

**mesoderm** /mes'ōdurm/ [Gk, *mesos* + *derma,* skin], (in embryology) the middle of the three cell layers of the developing embryo. It lies between the ectoderm and the endoderm. Bone, connective tissue, muscle, blood, vascular and lymphatic tissue, and the pleurae of the pericardium and peritoneum are all derived from the mesoderm.

**mesoduodenum** /-doo'ədē'nəm/ [Gk, *mesos,* middle; L, *duodeni,* 12 fingers long], a fold of tissue that joins the duodenum to the wall of the abdomen of the fetus. The membrane sometimes persists in later life as the **duodenal mesentery.**

**mesoepididymis** /mez'ō·ep'i·did'i·mis/ [Gk, *mesos,* middle + *epi,* above + *didymos,* pair], a fold of tunica vaginalis that sometimes connects the epididymis with the testicle.

**mesogastric** /-gas'trik/ [Gk, *mesos,* middle, *gaster,* belly], pertaining to the **mesogastrium,** a mesentery of the embryonic stomach.

**mesoglia.** See **microglia.**

**mesogluteus** /mez'ō·gloo'tē·əs/ [Gk, *mesos,* middle + *gloutos,* buttocks], the middle gluteal muscle, which abducts and rotates thigh medially.

**mesojejunum** /mez'ō·jə·joo'nəm/ [Gk, *mesos,* middle; L, *jejunus,* empty], the mesentery of the jejunum.

**mesomere** /mez'əmir/ [Gk, *mesos*, middle, *meros*, part], a row of bastomere between the macromere and micromere of the embryo. It develops into the renal tubules.

**mesometritis.** See **myometritis.**

**mesomorph** /mes'əmôrf'/ [Gk, *mesos* + *morphe*, form], a person whose physique is characterized by a predominance of muscle, bone, and connective tissue, structures that develop from the mesodermal layer of the embryo. Compare **ectomorph, endomorph.** See also **athletic habitus.**

**mesonephra, mesonephric.** See **mesonephros.**

**mesonephric duct** /-nef'rik/ [Gk, *mesos* + *nephros*, kidney; L, *ducere*, to lead], (in embryology) a duct that in the male gives rise to the ducts of the reproductive system (ductus epididymidis, ductus deferens, seminal vesicle, ejaculatory duct). In the female it persists vestigially as **Gartner's duct.** Also called **wolffian duct.**

**mesonephric tubule,** any of the embryonic renal tubules composing the mesonephros. They function as excretory structures during the early embryonic development of humans and other mammals but are later incorporated into the reproductive system. In males the tubules give rise to the efferent and aberrant ductules of the testes, the appendix epididymis, and the paradidymis; in females to the epoophoron, paroöphoron, and vesicular appendices. All of the structures are vestigial except the efferent ductules of the testes.

**mesonephros** /-nef'rəs/, *pl.* **mesonephroi, mesonephra** [Gk, *mesos* + *nephros*, kidney], the second type of excretory organ to develop in the vertebrate embryo. It consists of a series of twisting tubules that arise from the nephrogenic cord caudal to the pronephros and that at one end form the glomerulus and at the other connect with the excretory mesonephric duct. The organ is the permanent kidney in lower animals, but in humans and various other mammals it is functional only during early embryonic development and is later replaced by the metanephros, although the duct system is retained and incorporated into the male reproductive system. Also called **mesonephron, middle kidney, wolffian body.** See also **metanephros, pronephros.** —**mesonephric, mesonephroid,** *adj.*

**mesoridazine** /mez'ərid'əzēn/, a phenothiazine tranquilizer.

■ INDICATIONS: It is prescribed in the treatment of schizophrenia, behavioral problems in mental retardation, and alcoholism.

■ CONTRAINDICATIONS: Parkinson's disease, concurrent administration of central nervous system depressants, liver or renal dysfunction, severe hypotension, or known hypersensitivity to this drug or to other phenothiazine medications prohibits its use.

■ ADVERSE EFFECTS: Among the more serious adverse effects are hypotension, liver toxicity, a variety of extrapyramidal reactions, persistent tardive dyskinesia, blood dyscrasias, and hypersensitivity reactions.

**mesosalpinx** /mes'ōsal'pingks/ [Gk, *mesos* + *salpinx*, tube], the superior, free border of the broad ligament in which the uterine tubes lie.

**mesotaurodontism** /mez'ō·tô'rō·don'tiz·əm/ [Gk, *mesos*, middle; L, *taurus*, bull; Gk, *odous*, tooth], taurodontism in which the tooth roots branch only in the middle. See also **hypertaurodontism, taurodontism.**

**mesothelial** /mez'ōthē'lē·əl/, pertaining to the mesothelium cell layer.

**mesothelioma** /mes'ōthē'lē·ō'mə/, *pl.* **mesotheliomas, mesotheliomata** [Gk, *mesos* + *epi*, above, *thele*, nipple, *oma*, tumor], a rare malignant tumor of the mesothelium of the pleura or peritoneum, associated with exposure to asbestos. The lesion, composed of spindle cells or fibrous tissue, may

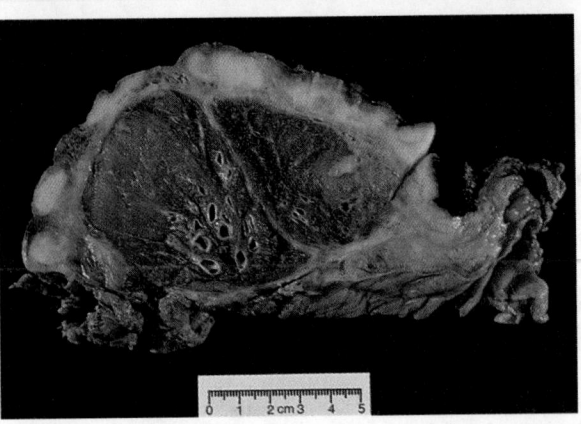

**Malignant mesothelioma** *(Kumar, Cotran, and Robbins, 1997)*

form thick sheets covering the viscera. The prognosis is poor. Also called **celothelioma.**

**mesothelium** /mes'ōthē'lē·əm/ [Gk, *mesos* + *epi*, above, *thele*, nipple], a layer of cells that line the body cavities of the embryo and continue as a layer of squamous epithelial cells covering the serous membranes of the adult.

**messenger RNA (mRNA)** /mes'ənjər/ [ME, *messangere*, message bearer; *RNA*, ribonucleic acid], (in molecular genetics) an RNA fraction that carries information from deoxyribonucleic acid to the protein-synthesizing ribosomes of cells. mRNA contains codons that are eventually encoded into amino acids via the translation process.

**Mestinon,** trademark for a neuromuscular blocking agent (pyridostigmine bromine).

**mestranol** /mes'trənōl/, an estrogen prescribed in fixed-combination drugs with a progestin as an oral contraceptive.

**Met,** abbreviation for the amino acid **methionine.**

**MET,** abbreviation for **metabolic equivalent of task.**

**meta-** /met'ə-/, 1. prefix meaning 'change or exchange': *metabasis, metallaxis, metamorphosis.* 2. prefix meaning 'after or next': *metachemical, metapneumonic, metapsychics.* 3. prefix meaning 'the 1, 3 position in derivative of benzine': *metacetone, metachloridine, metacresol.*

**meta-analysis,** a systematic method of evaluating statistical data based on results of several independent studies of the same problem.

**metabiosis** /met'əbī·ō'sis/, 1. a condition in which the growth and metabolism of one organism alter the environment to allow the growth of another organism. 2. the parasitic dependence of the existence of one organism on that of another.

**metabolic** /met'əbol'ik/ [Gk, *metabole*, change], pertaining to **metabolism.**

**metabolic acidosis,** acidosis in which excess acid is added to the body fluids or bicarbonate is lost from them. Acidosis is indicated by a pH of blood below 7.4. In starvation and in uncontrolled diabetes mellitus, glucose is not present or is not available for oxidation for cellular nutrition. The plasma bicarbonate of the body is used up in neutralizing the ketones that result from the breakdown of body fat for energy that occurs to compensate for the lack of glucose. Metabolic acidosis also occurs when oxidation takes place without adequate oxygen, as in heart failure or shock. Severe diarrhea, renal failure, and lactic acidosis also may result in metabolic acidosis. Hyperkalemia may accompany the condition. See also **diabetic ketoacidosis.**

**metabolic alkalosis,** an abnormal condition characterized by the significant loss of acid in the body or by increased levels of base bicarbonate. Loss of acid may be caused by excessive vomiting, insufficient replacement of electrolytes, hyperadrenocorticism, or Cushing's disease. Increased levels of base bicarbonate may have various causes, such as the ingestion of excessive amounts of bicarbonate of soda or other antacids during the treatment of peptic ulcers, or the administration of excessive volumes of IV fluids containing high concentrations of bicarbonate. Severe, untreated metabolic alkalosis can lead to coma and death. Compare **respiratory alkalosis.** See also **metabolic acidosis, respiratory acidosis.**

■ OBSERVATIONS: Signs and symptoms of metabolic alkalosis may include apnea, headache, lethargy, muscle cramps, hyperactive reflexes, tetany, shallow and slow respirations, irritability, nausea, vomiting, and atrial tachycardia. Confirmation of the diagnosis is commonly based on laboratory findings that show a blood pH greater than 7.45, a carbonic acid concentration greater than 29 mEq/L, and alkaline urine. The electrocardiogram of a patient with this condition may show atrial tachycardia with a low T wave merging with a P wave.

■ INTERVENTIONS: Treatment seeks to eliminate the underlying cause of alkalosis. Ammonium chloride may be given intravenously to release hydrogen chloride and restore chloride levels, except in patients with liver or kidney disease. Potassium chloride and normal saline solutions usually replace fluid losses from gastric drainage but are contraindicated in patients with associated congestive heart failure.

■ NURSING CONSIDERATIONS: Nurses closely monitor the status of the patient and cautiously administer any prescribed IV solutions. Too-rapid infusion of ammonium chloride may hemolyze red blood cells, and an excessive dosage may overcorrect alkalosis and cause acidosis. The fluid intake and output of the patient are carefully noted, and the respiration rate is regularly checked. Decreased respiratory rate indicates an effort to compensate for alkalosis and may cause respiratory acidosis.

**metabolic balance** [Gk, *metabole,* change; L, *bilanx,* having two scale trays], an equilibrium between the intake of nutrients and their eventual loss through absorption or excretion. In a positive balance the intake of a nutrient exceeds its loss; in a negative balance a nutrient is used or excreted faster than it is consumed in the diet.

**metabolic body size,** an estimate of the active tissue mass of a person, calculated by the body weight in kilograms to the 0.75 power.

**metabolic cirrhosis,** cirrhosis of the liver associated with a metabolic disorder such as Wilson's disease.

**metabolic component,** the bicarbonate component of plasma.

**metabolic disorder,** any pathophysiologic dysfunction that results in a loss of metabolic control of homeostasis in the body.

**metabolic equivalent of task (MET),** a unit of measurement of heat production by the body. One MET is equal to 50 kilogram calories (kcal) per hour per square meter of body surface of a resting individual.

**metabolic failure,** the severe and usually rapid failure of mental and physical functions, resulting in death.

**metabolic pathway,** a series of consecutive biochemical reactions or steps through which digested food is transformed into basic nutrients such as amino acids, free fatty acids, and simple carbohydrates.

**metabolic rate,** the amount of energy liberated or expended in a given unit of time. Energy is stored in the body

in energy-rich phosphate compounds (adenosine triphosphate, adenosine monophosphate, and adenosine diphosphate) and in proteins, fats, and complex carbohydrates. See also **basal metabolic rate.**

**metabolic respiratory quotient.** See **respiratory quotient.**

**metabolic waste products** [Gk, *metabole,* change; L, *vastare,* to destroy, *producere,* to produce], the products of metabolic activity after oxygen and nutrients have been supplied to a cell. These mainly include water and carbon dioxide, along with sodium chloride and soluble nitrogenous salts, which are excreted in urine, feces, and exhaled air.

**metabolism** /mətab′əliz′əm/ [Gk, *metabole,* change, *ismos,* process], the aggregate of all chemical processes that take place in living organisms, resulting in growth, generation of energy, elimination of wastes, and other body functions as they relate to the distribution of nutrients in the blood after digestion. Metabolism takes place in two steps: anabolism, the constructive phase, in which smaller molecules (such as amino acids) are converted to larger molecules (such as proteins); and catabolism, the destructive phase, in which larger molecules (such as glycogen) are converted to smaller molecules (such as glucose). Exercise, elevated body temperature, hormonal activity, and digestion can increase the metabolic rate, which is the rate determined when a person is at complete rest, physically and mentally. The metabolic rate is customarily expressed (in calories) as the heat liberated in the course of metabolism. See also **acid-base metabolism, anabolism, basal metabolism, catabolism.**

**metabolite** /mitab′əlīt/ [Gk, *metabole,* change], a substance produced by metabolic action or necessary for a metabolic process. An essential metabolite is one required for a vital metabolic process.

**metabolize** /mətab′əlīz/ [Gk, *metabole,* change], to undergo metabolism, the breaking down of carbohydrates, proteins, and fats into smaller units; reorganizing those units as tissue building blocks or as energy sources; and eliminating waste products of the processes.

**metacarpal.** See **metacarpus.**

**metacarpal phalanx** /-kär′pəl/ [Gk, *meta* + *karpos,* wrist, *phalanx,* line of soldiers], the hands and fingers, particularly phalanges that articulate with carpal bones.

**metacarpophalangeal** /-kar′pōfəlan′jē·əl/ [Gk, *meta,* beyond, *karpos,* wrist, *phalanx,* line of soldiers], pertaining to the metacarpal bones of the hand and the phalanges of fingers, as in metacarpophalangeal joints.

**metacarpophalangeal (MCP) joint dislocation** [Gk, *meta* + *karpos* + *phalanx* + L, *jungere,* to join, *dis* + *locare,* to place], the dislocation of a finger at the junction with the metacarpal bone, usually with damage to tendons and other structures.

**metacarpus** /met′əkär′pəs/ [Gk, *meta,* beyond, *karpos,* wrist], the middle part of the hand, consisting of five slender bones numbered from the thumb side, metacarpals I through V. Each metacarpal consists of a body and two extremities. —**metacarpal,** *adj., n.*

**metacentric** /met′əsen′trik/ [Gk, *meta* + *kentron,* center], pertaining to a chromosome in which the centromere is located near the center so that the arms of the chromosome are of approximately equal length. Compare **acrocentric, submetacentric, telocentric.**

**metachromasia** /-krōmā′zhē·ə/ [Gk, *meta,* beyond, *chroma,* color], a tissue staining phenomenon in which cells being examined acquire a color other than that of the dye used. Cartilage cells, for example, may appear red after being stained with a blue dye. The cause is an interaction between

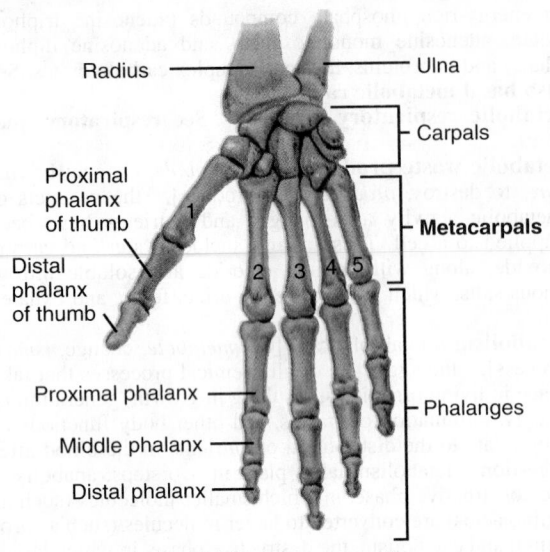

Radius — Ulna

— Carpals

Proximal
phalanx
of thumb

**Metacarpals**

Distal
phalanx
of thumb

Proximal phalanx

— Phalanges

Middle phalanx —

Distal phalanx —

Hand (right, palmar aspect)

**Metacarpal bones** *(Applegate, 2000)*

the dye molecules and the acidic radicals of the tissue cells. Also called **metachromism.**

**metachromatic leukodystrophy.**   See **sulfatide lipidosis.**

**metachromatic lipids** /-krōmat′ik/ [Gk, *meta,* beyond, *chroma,* color, *lipos,* fat], lipid molecules that accumulate in the central nervous system, peripheral nerves, and internal organs of infants who inherit a lipidosis disorder. See also **cerebroside sulfatase.**

**metachromatic stain** [Gk, *meta* + *chroma,* color; OFr, *desteindre,* to dye], a basic dye, such as toluidine, that can stain substances a different color than that of the stain.

**metachromism.**   See **metachromasia.**

**-metacin,** combining form for indomethacin-type antiinflammatory substances.

**metacommunication** /-kəmyoo̅′nikā′shən/ [Gk, *meta* + L, *communicare,* to inform], communication that indicates how verbal information should be interpreted. It is stimuli surrounding the verbal communication that also have meaning, which may or may not be congruent with that of or support the verbal talk. It may support or contradict verbal communication.

**metagenesis** /met′əjen′əsis/ [Gk, *meta* + *genein,* to produce], the regular alternation of sexual with asexual methods of reproduction within the same species. —**metagenetic, metagenic,** *adj.*

**Metahydrin,** trademark for a diuretic and antihypertensive (trichlormethiazide).

**metal** [Gk, *metallon,* a mine], any element that conducts heat and electricity, is malleable and ductile, and forms positively charged ions (cations).

**metal fume fever,** an occupational disorder caused by the inhalation of fumes of metallic oxides and characterized by symptoms similar to those of influenza. The condition occurs among workers engaged in welding, metal fabrication, casting, and other occupations dealing with the manipulation of metals. Access to fresh air and treatment of the symptoms usually alleviate the condition. Also called **brass founder's ague, zinc chill.** Compare **siderosis.**

**metallesthesia** /met′əlesthē′zhə/ [Gk, *metallon,* a mine, *aisthesia,* perception], an ability to identify a metal through the sense of touch.

**metalloprotein** /mətal′ōprō′tēn/, a protein that contains one or more metal ions.

**metallurgy** /met′əlur′jē/ [Gk, *metallon,* a mine, *ergein,* to work], the theoretic and applied sciences of the nature and uses of metals.

**metamorphopsia** /met′əmôrfop′sē·ə/ [Gk, *meta* + *morphe,* form, *opsis,* sight], a defect in vision in which objects are seen as distorted in shape, which results from disease of the retina or imperfection of the media.

**metamorphosis** /met′əmôr′fəsis/ [Gk, *meta* + *morphe,* form], a change in shape or structure, especially a change from one stage of development to another, such as the transition from the larval to the adult stage.

**metamyelocyte** /met′əmī′əlōsīt′/ [Gk, *meta* + *myelos,* marrow, *kytos,* cell], a stage in the development of the granulocyte series of leukocytes, between the myelocyte stage and the mature granulocyte. See also **leukocyte, myeloblast, myelocyte.**

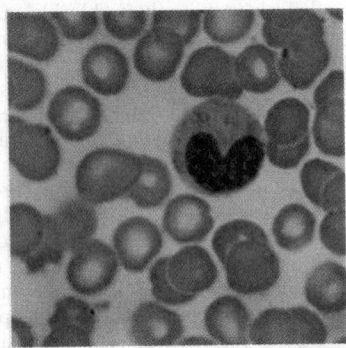

**Metamyelocyte** *(Carr and Rodak, 1999)*

**metanephra.**   See **metanephros.**

**metanephrine** /met′ənef′rin/, one of the two principal urinary metabolites of epinephrine and norepinephrine in the urine; the other is vanillylmandelic acid. The 24-hour normal adult value for total metanephrine is 1.3 mg; normally less than 1.3 mg is excreted in 24 hours.

**metanephrogenic** /met′ənef′rəjen′ik/ [Gk, *meta* + *nephros,* kidney, *genein,* to produce], capable of forming the metanephros, or fetal kidney.

**metanephros** /-nef′rəs/, *pl.* **metanephroi** [Gk, *meta* + *nephros,* kidney], the third, and permanent, excretory organ to develop in the vertebrate embryo. It consists of a complex structure of secretory and collecting tubules that develop into the kidney. In most mammals there is limited functional use of the metanephric kidney during fetal life, because waste materials are transferred across the placenta to the mother for elimination. —**metanephron,** *adj.* Also called **hind kidney.** See also **kidney, mesonephros, pronephros.**

**metaphase** /met′əfāz/ [Gk, *meta* + *phasis,* appearance], the second of the four stages of nuclear division in mitosis and in each of the two divisions of meiosis, during which the chromosomes become arranged in the equatorial plane of the spindle to form the equatorial plate, with the centromeres attached to the spindle fibers in preparation for sepa-

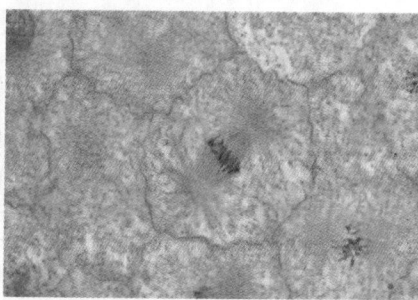

**Metaphase** (© Ed Reschke; used with permission)

ration. See also **anaphase, interphase, meiosis, mitosis, prophase, telophase.**

**metaphyseal dysostosis** /mətaf′izē′əl disostō′sis, met′əfiz′ē·əl disostō′sis/ [Gk, *meta + phyein,* to grow, *dys,* bad, *osteon,* bone], a condition characterized by abnormal mineralization of the metaphyseal area of the bones, resulting in dwarfism. Metaphyseal dysostosis is classified as the Gansen, Schmidt, or Spahar-Hartmann type or as cartilage-hair hypoplasia. The Gansen type is characterized by metaphyseal alterations similar to those of achondroplasia but not involving the skull or the epiphyses of the long bones. The Schmidt type is characterized by developmental changes from the weight-bearing age to approximately 5 years of age. The metaphyseal alterations associated with this type are similar to those of achondroplasia, resulting in moderate dwarfism. The Spahar-Hartmann type is characterized by skeletal changes and severe bowleg. Cartilage-hair hypoplasia is characterized by severe dwarfism and hair that is sparse, short, and brittle. Mental retardation is not usually associated with metaphyseal dysostosis. Radiographic examination of all types of the disease reveals characteristic widening of the metaphyses of the tubular bones, with normal diaphyseal and epiphyseal ossification centers. Treatment is supportive and symptomatic; no specific modality is used.

**metaphyseal dysplasia,** a condition characterized by disordered modeling of the long bones, in which the metaphyseal circumference is enlarged and the medullary area is reduced. Metaphyseal dysplasia most often affects the distal femur or the proximal tibia.

**metaphysis** /mətaf′əsis/ [Gk, *meta + phyein,* to grow], a region of a growing long bone in which diaphysis and epiphysis converge.

**metaplasia** /met′əplā′zhə/, the reversible conversion of normal tissue cells into another, less differentiated cell type in response to chronic stress or injury. With prolonged exposure to the inducing stimulus, cancerous transformation can occur.

**metaproterenol sulfate** /met′əprōter′inôl/, a beta₂ receptor agonist bronchodilator.

■ INDICATION: It is prescribed in the treatment of bronchial asthma.

■ CONTRAINDICATIONS: Arrhythmias associated with tachycardia or known hypersensitivity to this drug prohibits its use.

■ ADVERSE EFFECTS: Among the more serious adverse reactions are tachycardia, hypertension, and cardiac arrest.

**metaraminol bitartrate** /met′äram′inol/, an adrenergic vasopressor.

■ INDICATION: It is prescribed in the treatment of hypotension and shock.

■ CONTRAINDICATIONS: Known hypersensitivity to this drug prohibits its use. It is not used with cyclopropane or halothane anesthesia or as the sole drug for hypovolemic hypotension.

■ ADVERSE EFFECTS: Among the more serious adverse reactions are cardiac arrhythmia, tissue necrosis at the site of injection, hypertension, tremors, and nausea.

**metarubricyte** /-rōō′brisīt/ [Gk, *meta +* L, *ruber,* red, *kytos,* cell], a red blood cell possessing a nucleus. Such cells, also known as normoblasts, are not normally found in circulating blood.

**metastable solution.** See **supersaturate.**

**metastasis** /mətas′təsis/, *pl.* **metastases** [Gk, *meta + stasis,* standing], **1.** the process by which tumor cells spread to distant parts of the body. Because malignant tumors have no enclosing capsule, cells may escape, become emboli, and be transported by the lymphatic circulation or the bloodstream to implant in lymph nodes and other organs far from the primary tumor. **2.** a tumor that develops away from the site of origin. Compare **anaplasia. —metastatic,** *adj.,* **metastasize,** *v.*

**metastasizing mole.** See **chorioadenoma destruens.**

**metastatic.** See **metastasis.**

**metastatic abscess** /-stat′ik/ [Gk, *meta,* beyond, *stasis,* standing; L, *abscedere,* to go away], any secondary abscess that develops at a point distant from an original infection; the infectious particles are transported to other locations in the bloodstream.

**metastatic calcification** [Gk, *meta + stasis,* standing; L, *calx,* lime, *facere,* to make], the pathologic process whereby calcium salts accumulate in previously healthy tissues. It is caused by excessive levels of blood calcium, such as in hyperparathyroidism.

**metastatic endometriosis** [Gk, *meta,* beyond, *stasis,* standing, *endon,* within, *metra,* womb, *osis,* condition], extraperitoneal lesions that resemble metastases from a carcinoma.

**metastatic ophthalmia.** See **sympathetic ophthalmia.**

**metastatic survey** [Gk, *meta,* beyond, *stasis,* standing; OFr, *surveoir,* to examine], a method of monitoring the spread of a cancer by taking a series of periodic x-ray films.

**metatarsal** /met′ətär′səl/ [Gk, *meta + tarsos,* flat surface], **1.** pertaining to the metatarsus of the foot. **2.** any one of the five bones making up the metatarsus.

**metatarsalgia** /met′ətärsal′jə/ [Gk, *meta + tarsos + algos,* pain], a painful condition around the metatarsal bones caused by an abnormality of the foot or by recalcification of degenerated heads of metatarsal bones.

**metatarsal phalanx** /-tär′səl/ [Gk, *meta + tarsos,* flat surface, *phalanx,* line of soldiers], the bones of the foot and toes.

**metatarsal stress fracture,** a break or rupture of a metatarsal bone caused by prolonged running or walking. The condition is often difficult to diagnose with x-ray films. Also called **march fracture.**

**metatarsus** /-tär′səs/ [Gk, *meta + tarsos,* flat surface], a part of the foot, consisting of five bones numbered I to V, from the medial side. Each bone has a long, slender body; a wedge-shaped proximal end; a convex distal end; and flattened, grooved sides for the attachment of ligaments. The metatarsal bones articulate with the tarsus proximally and the first row of phalanges distally. Deformities of the metatarsus include **metatarsus valgus** and **metatarsus varus.** **—metatarsal,** *adj.*

**metatarsus adductus.** See **metatarsus varus.**

**metatarsus valgus,** a congenital deformity of the foot in which the forepart rotates outward away from the midline of

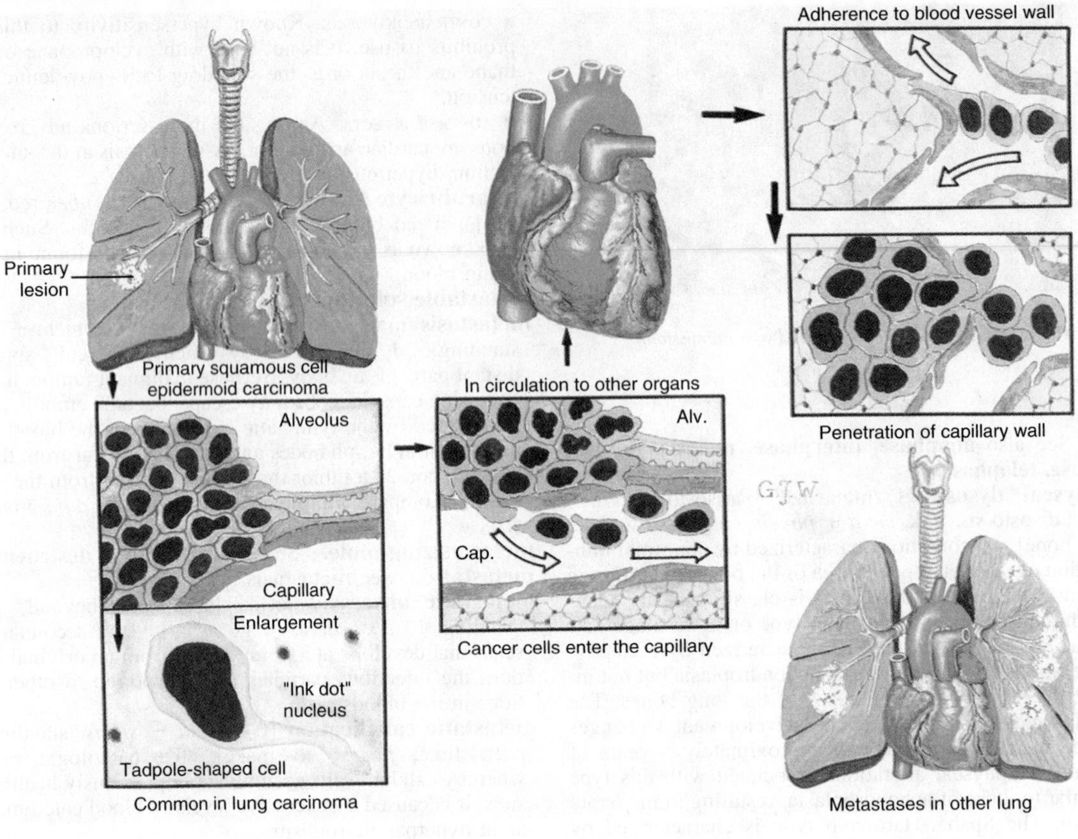

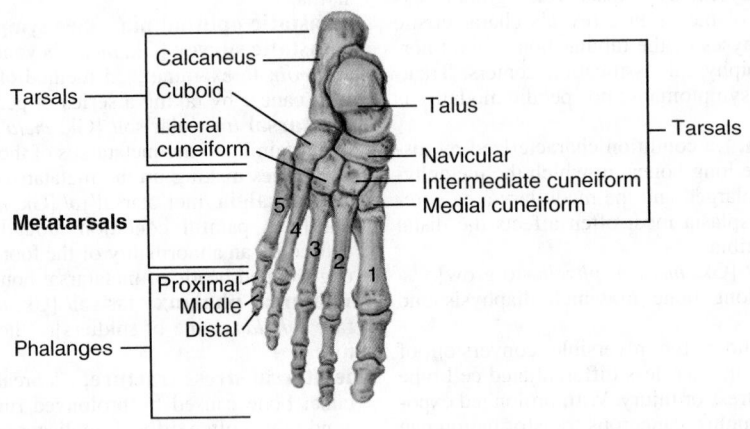

**Metastasis of cancer** *(Belcher, 1992)*

Adherence to blood vessel wall

Primary lesion

Primary squamous cell epidermoid carcinoma

Alveolus

In circulation to other organs

Penetration of capillary wall

Capillary

Enlargement

Alv.

Cap.

"Ink dot" nucleus

Tadpole-shaped cell

Cancer cells enter the capillary

Common in lung carcinoma

Metastases in other lung

Tarsals

Calcaneus

Cuboid

Lateral cuneiform

Talus

Navicular

Intermediate cuneiform

Medial cuneiform

Tarsals

**Metatarsals**

5
4
3 2 1

Proximal
Middle
Distal

Phalanges

**Metatarsal bones** *(Applegate, 2000)*

the body and the heel remains straight. Also called **duck walk, toeing out.**

**metatarsus varus,** a congenital deformity of the foot in which the forepart rotates inward toward the midline of the body and the heel remains straight. Also called **intoe, metatarsus adductus, pigeon-toed, toeing in.**

**Metatensin,** trademark for a fixed-combination cardiovascular drug containing a diuretic (trichlormethiazide) and an antihypertensive (reserpine).

**metathalamus** /met′əthal′əməs/ [Gk, *meta* + *thalamos*, chamber], one of five parts of the diencephalon. It is composed of a medial geniculate body and a lateral geniculate body on each side. The medial geniculate body acts as a relay station for nerve impulses between the inferior brachium and the auditory cortex. The lateral geniculate body is a superficial oval bulge at the posterior end of the thalamus, which accommodates the terminal ends of the fibers of the optic tract. Relay cells project to the visual cortex. Compare

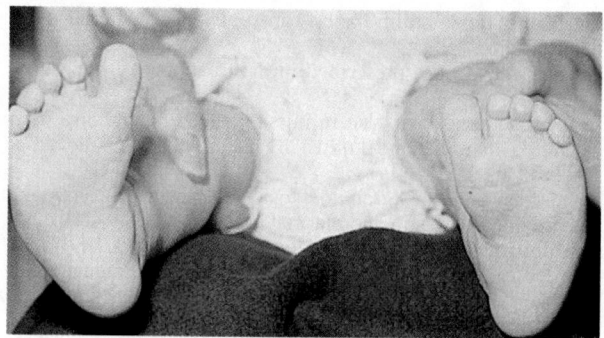

**Metatarsus varus** *(Zitelli and Davis, 1997)*

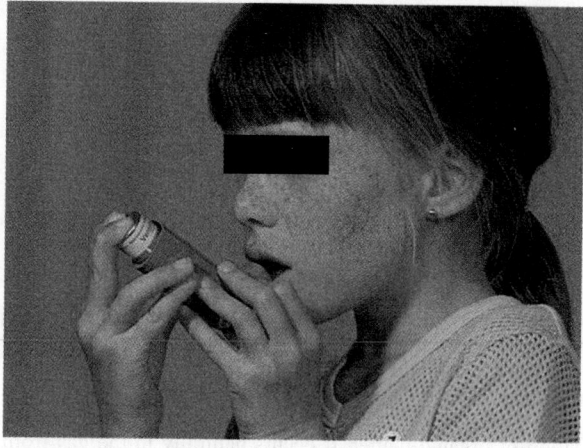

**Metered dose inhaler** *(Warner and Jackson, 1994)*

epithalamus, hypothalamus, subthalamus. **—metathalamic,** *adj.*

**metaxalone** /metak′sələn/,  a skeletal muscle relaxant.
- INDICATION: It is prescribed as an adjunct in the treatment of acute skeletal muscle spasm.
- CONTRAINDICATIONS: Significantly impaired renal or hepatic function, susceptibility to drug-induced hemolytic anemia, or known hypersensitivity to this drug prohibits its use.
- ADVERSE EFFECTS: Among the more serious adverse reactions are hemolytic anemia, leukopenia, and liver dysfunction. GI disturbances, dizziness, and nervousness may occur.

**metazoa** /-zō′ə/ [Gk, *meta* + *zoon,* animal],  a classification that includes animals that have tissues and organs. All animals except sponges are metazoa.

**Metchnikoff's theory** /mech′nikofs/ [Elie Metchnikoff, Russian-French biologist, 1845–1916; Gk, *theoria,* speculation],  the theory that living cells ingest microorganisms. The theory proved correct, as seen in the process of phagocytosis and the ingestion of injurious microbes by leukocytes.

**meteorism** [Gk, *meteorizein,* to hold up],  accumulation of gas in the abdomen or the intestine, usually with distension.

**meteorotropism** /mē′tē·ərətrō′pizəm/ [Gk, *meteoros,* high in the air, *trope,* turning],  a reaction to meteorologic influences shown by various biologic occurrences, such as sudden death, attacks of arthritis, and angina. **—meteorotropic,** *adj.*

**meter (m)** /mē′tər/ [Gk, *metron,* measure],  a metric unit of length equal to 39.37 inches.

**-meter, -metre,** **1.** /-m′ətər/ suffix meaning a 'measuring instrument': *anesthesimeter, ionometer, scopometer.* **2.** /-mē′tər/ suffix meaning 'length or measure': *centimeter, kilometer, millimeter.*

**metered dose inhaler (MDI)** /mē′tərd/,  a device designed to deliver a measured dose of an inhaled drug. It usually consists of a canister of aerosol spray, mist, or fine powder that releases a specific dose each time it is pushed against a dispensing valve. It is intended to reduce the risk of overmedication by the patient.

**metformin hydrochloride,**  an oral antidiabetic agent.
- INDICATIONS: It is prescribed in the treatment of type 2 diabetes mellitus.
- CONTRAINDICATIONS: The drug should not be given to patients with allergy to metformin, diabetes associated with high ketone levels, metabolic acidosis, or kidney disease or in radiology studies using radiopaque materials.
- ADVERSE EFFECTS: The side effects most often reported include general body discomfort, muscle pain, breathing difficulty, drowsiness, and an unpleasant metallic taste.

**methacholine challenge** /meth′əkō′lēn/,  a method of measuring airway activity by an inhalation challenge test. The patient inhales a saline aerosol as a control, followed by increasing concentrations of methacholine chloride, a cholinergic drug. The test is used to confirm the diagnosis of asthma when symptoms are present.

**methacrylic acid** /meth′əkril′ik/,  an organic acid obtained from Roman chamomile oil. It polymerizes into a ceramic-like mass. The methyl ester of methacrylic acid is used in medical and dental products such as enamel sealants. A copolymer is used in tablet coatings.

**methacycline hydrochloride** /meth′əsī′klēn/,  a tetracycline antibiotic.
- INDICATIONS: It is prescribed in the treatment of infections caused by susceptible strains of bacteria.
- CONTRAINDICATIONS: Renal or liver dysfunction, pregnancy, young age, or known hypersensitivity to this drug or to other tetracycline medications prohibits its use.
- ADVERSE EFFECTS: Among the more serious adverse reactions are GI disturbances, phototoxicity, potentially serious superinfections, and hypersensitivity reactions. Discoloration of teeth may occur in children exposed to the drug in utero or before 8 years of age.

**methadone** /meth′ədōn/,  a synthetic opioid analgesic.
- INDICATIONS: It is prescribed for relief of severe pain, for treatment in detoxification, and in treatment programs for opiate-addicted patients.
- CONTRAINDICATIONS: It is used with caution in many conditions, including head injuries, asthma, impaired renal or hepatic function, or unstable cardiovascular status. Known hypersensitivity to this drug prohibits its use.
- ADVERSE EFFECTS: Among the more serious adverse reactions are drowsiness, dizziness, nausea, constipation, respiratory and circulatory depression, and drug addiction.

**methadone hydrochloride,**  an opioid analgesic used for anesthesia or as a substitute for heroin, permitting withdrawal without development of acute abstinence syndrome. Methadone does not produce marked euphoria, sedation, or narcosis. It is not given to pregnant women or to patients with liver disease.

**methaemoglobin.**  See **methemoglobin.**

**methaemoglobinuria.**  See **methemoglobinuria.**

**methamphetamine hydrochloride** /meth′amfet′əmēn/, a central nervous system stimulant.

■ INDICATIONS: It is prescribed in the treatment of narcolepsy and hyperkinesis and the reduction of the appetite in exogenous obesity.

■ CONTRAINDICATIONS: Glaucoma, arteriosclerosis, cardiovascular disease, hypertension, hyperthyroidism, history of drug abuse, concomitant use of a monoamine oxidase inhibitor, or known hypersensitivity to this drug or to other sympathomimetic drugs prohibits its use.

■ ADVERSE EFFECTS: Among the more serious adverse reactions are various manifestations of central nervous system excitation, increase in blood pressure, arrhythmia and other cardiovascular effects, nausea, and drug dependence.

**methandriol** /methan'drē·ol/,   an anabolic hormone used as adjunctive therapy in senile and postmenopausal osteoporosis.

**methane (CH₄)** /meth'ān/,   a simple hydrocarbon in the form of colorless gas, produced by the anaerobic decomposition of organic matter. It occurs naturally in the gas from oil wells and coal mines.

**methanol (CH₃OH)** /meth'ənol/,   a clear, colorless, toxic liquid distillate of wood miscible with water, other alcohols, and ether. It is widely used as a solvent and in the production of formaldehyde. Also called **methyl alcohol, wood alcohol.**

**methanol poisoning,**   a toxic effect of ingestion, inhalation, or absorption through the skin of methanol (methyl alcohol, wood alcohol) that may impair the central nervous system; cause severe acidosis, blindness, and shock; and result in death. Also called **methyl alcohol poisoning.**

**methazolamide** /meth'əzō'ləmīd/,   a carbonic anhydrase inhibitor.

■ INDICATION: It is prescribed in the treatment of glaucoma.

■ CONTRAINDICATIONS: Hyponatremia, hypokalemia, Addison's disease, severe pulmonary obstruction, adrenocortical insufficiency, or known hypersensitivity to this drug prohibits its use.

■ ADVERSE EFFECTS: Among the more serious adverse effects are aplastic anemia, drowsiness, paresthesia, hypersensitivity reactions, and acidosis.

**methemoglobin** /met'hēməglō'bin, met·he'məglō'bin/,   a form of hemoglobin in which the iron component has been oxidized from the ferrous to the ferric state. Methemoglobin cannot carry oxygen. It is a product of various oxidative reactions that constitute normal metabolic activity and is normally present in only trace amounts (about 1%) in the blood. Maintenance of levels occurs by an active enzymatic reducing capability, the nicotinamide-adenine dinucleotide-methemoglobin reductase system present in normal red cells. Also spelled **methaemoglobin.** See also **hemoglobin.**

**methemoglobinemia** /-ē'mē·ə/,   the presence of methemoglobin in the blood.

**methemoglobinuria** /-ŏŏr'ē·ə/ [Gk, *meta,* beyond, *haima,* blood; L, *globus,* ball; Gk, *ouron,* urine],   the presence of methemoglobin in the urine. Also spelled **methaemoglobinuria.**

**methenamine hippurate and mandelete** /methē'nəmēn/,   a urinary antibacterial.

■ INDICATION: It is prescribed in the treatment of urinary tract infections.

■ CONTRAINDICATIONS: Liver or kidney dysfunction or known hypersensitivity to this drug or to mandelic acid prohibits its use.

■ ADVERSE EFFECTS: Among the most serious adverse reactions are severe GI disturbances and rashes.

**Methergine,**   trademark for an oxytocic (methylergonovine maleate).

**methimazole** /məthim'əzōl/,   an orally administered antithyroid drug.

■ INDICATIONS: It is prescribed in the treatment of hyperthyroidism.

■ CONTRAINDICATIONS: Use in nursing mothers, because it is excreted in milk, and known hypersensitivity to the drug prohibit its use.

■ ADVERSE EFFECTS: Agranulocytosis, leukopenia, thrombocytopenia, and aplastic anemia may occur.

**methionine (Met)** /methī'ənēn/,   an essential amino acid needed for proper growth in infants and for maintenance of nitrogen balance in adults. It is a source for methyl groups and sulfur in the body. It is also administered as adjunctive treatment in liver diseases. See also **amino acid, protein.**

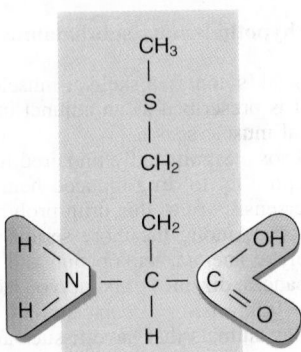

**Chemical structure of methionine**

**methisoprinol.**   See **inosiplex.**

**methocarbamol** /meth'əkär'bəmol/,   a skeletal muscle relaxant.

■ INDICATION: It is prescribed in the relief of skeletal muscle spasm.

■ CONTRAINDICATIONS: Renal dysfunction, central nervous system depression, or known hypersensitivity to this drug prohibits its use.

■ ADVERSE EFFECTS: Among the more serious adverse reactions are hypotension and tachycardia. Drowsiness, dizziness, vertigo, and nausea may occur.

**method** /meth'əd/ [Gk, *meta,* beyond, *hodos,* way],   a technique or procedure for producing a desired effect, such as a surgical procedure, a laboratory test, or a diagnostic technique.

**methodology** /meth'ədol'əjē/ [Gk, *meta + hodos + logos,* science],   **1.** a system of principles or methods of procedure in any discipline, such as education, research, diagnosis, or treatment. **2.** the section of a research proposal in which the methods to be used are described. The research design, the population to be studied, and the research instruments, or tools, to be used are discussed in the methodology. —**methodologic,** *adj.*

**methohexital sodium** /meth'ōhek'sitōl/,   an IV barbiturate of short duration.

■ INDICATION: It is used for the induction of anesthesia in short surgical procedures like cardioversion or ECT.

■ CONTRAINDICATIONS: Porphyria, status asthmaticus, or known hypersensitivity to this drug or to any barbiturate prohibits its use.

■ ADVERSE EFFECTS: Among the more serious adverse reactions are respiratory depression, skin rash, muscle tremors, hiccoughs, and cardiovascular dysfunction.

**methotrexate** /meth′ōtrek′sāt/, an antineoplastic antimetabolite.

■ INDICATIONS: It is prescribed in the treatment of severe psoriasis and a variety of malignant neoplastic diseases.

■ CONTRAINDICATIONS: Blood dyscrasias, severe renal or hepatic impairment, or known hypersensitivity to this drug prohibits its use.

■ ADVERSE EFFECTS: Among the more serious adverse reactions are diarrhea, ulcerative stomatitis, bone marrow depression, hepatotoxicity, and skin rash.

**methoxamine hydrochloride** /methok′səmēn/, an adrenergic that acts as a vasoconstrictor.

■ INDICATION: It is prescribed for use during anesthesia to maintain blood pressure and in the treatment of paroxysmal supraventricular tachycardia.

■ CONTRAINDICATIONS: It is not recommended for use as a vasoconstrictor with local anesthetics. Known hypersensitivity to this drug prohibits its use.

■ ADVERSE EFFECTS: Among the most serious adverse reactions are hypertension, bradycardia, cardiac depression, severe headache, and vomiting.

**methoxsalen** /methok′sələn/, a pigmentation agent. Also known as **8-MOP.**

■ INDICATIONS: It is used topically for enhancement of pigmentation or for repigmentation in vitiligo.

■ CONTRAINDICATIONS: Liver impairment, concomitant use of a drug that may cause photosensitization, or known hypersensitivity to this drug prohibits its use.

■ ADVERSE EFFECTS: Among the most serious adverse reactions are central nervous system effects and burns. Gastrointestinal discomfort and allergic reactions also may occur.

**methoxyflurane.** See **halogenated hydrocarbon.**

**3-methoxy-4-hydroxymandelic acid.** See **vanillylmandelic acid.**

**methscopolamine bromide** /meth′skōpō′ləmēn/, an anticholinergic/antispasmodic.

■ INDICATIONS: It is prescribed in the treatment of hypermotility of the GI tract and as an adjunct in treatment of peptic ulcer.

■ CONTRAINDICATIONS: Narrow-angle glaucoma, asthma, obstruction of the genitourinary or GI tract, severe ulcerative colitis, or known hypersensitivity to this drug prohibits its use.

■ ADVERSE EFFECTS: Blurred vision, central nervous system effects, tachycardia, dry mouth, decreased sweating, or hypersensitivity reactions may occur.

**methsuximide** /methsuk′simīd/, an anticonvulsant.

■ INDICATION: It is prescribed in the treatment of refractory petit mal epilepsy.

■ CONTRAINDICATIONS: Known hypersensitivity to this drug or to any succinimide prohibits its use.

■ ADVERSE EFFECTS: Among the more serious adverse reactions are blood dyscrasias, liver and kidney damage, and systemic lupus erythematosus.

**methyclothiazide** /məthī′klōthī′əzīd, meth′əklōthī′əzīd/, a diuretic and antihypertensive.

■ INDICATIONS: It is prescribed in the treatment of hypertension and edema.

■ CONTRAINDICATIONS: Anemia, renal or urinary disorders, or known hypersensitivity to this drug, to other thiazide medications, or to sulfonamide derivatives prohibits its use.

■ ADVERSE EFFECTS: Among the more serious adverse reactions are hypokalemia, hyperglycemia, hyperuricemia, hypotension, and hypersensitivity reactions.

**methyl (Me)** /meth′il/, the chemical radical $CH_3$.

**methyl alcohol.** See **methanol.**

**methyl alcohol poisoning.** See **methanol poisoning.**

**methylate** /meth′ilāt/ [Gk, *methy,* wine, *hyle,* matter], **1.** a compound of methyl and a base. **2.** to add a methyl group, $CH_3$, to a chemical compound.

**methylation** /-lā′shən/ [Gk, *methy,* wine, *hyle,* matter], **1.** the introduction of a methyl group, $CH_3$, to a chemical compound. **2.** the addition of methyl alcohol and naphtha to ethanol to produce denatured alcohol.

**methylbenzethonium hydrochloride** /-ben′zəthō′nē·əm/, a topical antiinfective.

■ INDICATIONS: It is prescribed for the prevention and treatment of diaper rash and other dermatoses.

■ CONTRAINDICATION: Known hypersensitivity to this drug is the only contraindication.

■ ADVERSE EFFECTS: There are no known adverse reactions. Local skin irritation may occur.

**methyldopa** /-dō′pə/, an antihypertensive; an alpha$_2$ receptor agonist agent.

■ INDICATION: It is prescribed for the reduction of high blood pressure.

■ CONTRAINDICATIONS: Use of monoamine oxidase inhibitors, liver dysfunction, or known hypersensitivity to this drug prohibits its use.

■ ADVERSE EFFECTS: Among the more serious adverse reactions are liver toxicity and blood dyscrasias. Sedation, dry mouth, nasal stuffiness, and postural hypotension may occur.

**methylene blue** /meth′əlēn/, a bluish-green crystalline substance used as a histologic stain and as a laboratory indicator. It is also used in the treatment of cyanide poisoning and methemoglobinemia.

**methylergonovine maleate** /-ərgon′əvēn/, a synthetic ergot alkaloid.

■ INDICATIONS: It is prescribed as an oxytocic to prevent or to treat postpartum uterine atony, hemorrhage, or subinvolution.

■ CONTRAINDICATIONS: It is not prescribed during pregnancy or given intravenously, except in life-threatening situations. Hypertension, toxemia, or known hypersensitivity to ergot alkaloids prohibits its use.

■ ADVERSE EFFECTS: Among the most serious adverse reactions are convulsions and death. Hypertension, nausea, blurred vision, and headaches also may occur. Adverse effects are more common after IV administration.

**3-methylfentanyl,** a potent heroin substitute and so-called designer drug. It is an analog of fentanyl and reportedly 3000 times as potent as morphine; 1 ounce represents 25 million doses of a drug with effects equivalent to that of high-grade heroin. A related designer drug is *p*-fluoro fentanyl. See also **designer drugs.**

**methylmalonicacidemia** /meth′əl·mə·lon′ik·as′i·dē′mē·ə/, **1.** an autosomal recessive aminoacidopathy characterized by an excess of the carboxylic acid methylmalonic acid in the blood and urine, with metabolic ketoacidosis, hyperammonemia, and excess glycine in the blood and urine, and presenting in infancy as failure to thrive, persistent vomiting and dehydration, respiratory distress, and hypotonia. It results from any of several defects that cause deficiency of an enzyme involved in the use of isoleucine, threonine, valine, propionate, and other odd number chain length fatty acids for fuel. Also called **methylmalonicaciduria. 2.** excess of methylmalonic acid in the blood.

**methylphenidate hydrochloride** /-fen′idāt/, a central nervous system stimulant.

■ INDICATIONS: It is prescribed in the treatment of attention deficit disorder in children and narcolepsy in adults.

■ CONTRAINDICATIONS: Glaucoma, severe anxiety, tension, mental depression, or known hypersensitivity to this drug prohibits its use. It is not given to children less than 6 years of age.

■ ADVERSE EFFECTS: Among the more serious adverse reactions are nervousness, insomnia, and anorexia. Hypersensitivity reactions and tachycardia may occur.

**methylprednisolone** /-prednis′əlōn/, a glucocorticoid.

■ INDICATIONS: It is prescribed in the treatment of inflammatory conditions, including rheumatic fever and rheumatoid arthritis.

■ CONTRAINDICATIONS: Fungal infections or known hypersensitivity to this drug prohibits its systemic use. Viral or fungal infections of the skin, impaired circulation, or known hypersensitivity to this drug prohibits its topical use.

■ ADVERSE EFFECTS: Among the more serious adverse reactions to the systemic administration of the drug are GI, endocrine, neurologic, fluid, and electrolyte disturbances. Skin reactions may result from topical administration of this drug.

**methylrosaniline chloride.** See **gentian violet.**

**methyl salicylate.** See **wintergreen oil.**

**methyltestosterone** /meth′iltəstos′tərōn/, an androgen.

■ INDICATIONS: It is prescribed in the treatment of testosterone deficiency, osteoporosis, and female breast cancer and in stimulation of growth, weight gain, and red blood cell production.

■ CONTRAINDICATIONS: Cancer of the male breast or prostate; cardiac, renal, or hepatic disease; hypercalcemia; known or suspected pregnancy; lactation; or known hypersensitivity to this drug prohibits its use.

■ ADVERSE EFFECTS: Among the more serious adverse reactions are hypercalcemia, edema, irreversible masculinization of female patients, and jaundice.

**methyprylon** /meth′əprī′lon/, a sedative and hypnotic.

■ INDICATION: It is prescribed in the treatment of insomnia.

■ CONTRAINDICATIONS: It is not given to children under 3 months of age. Intermittent porphyria or known hypersensitivity to this drug prohibits its use.

■ ADVERSE EFFECTS: Among the most serious adverse reactions are physical dependence and paradoxic excitement. Dizziness, headache, rash, and GI upset also may occur.

**methysergide maleate** /meth′isur′jīd/, a vasoconstrictor.

■ INDICATION: It is prescribed for relief of migraine headache.

■ CONTRAINDICATIONS: Pregnancy, severe infection, liver or kidney dysfunction, cardiovascular or lung disease, or known hypersensitivity to this drug prohibits its use. It is not recommended for use in children.

■ ADVERSE EFFECTS: Among the more serious adverse reactions are retroperitoneal fibrosis, hallucinations, abnormally low white cell count, pulmonary and cardiac complications, hemolytic anemia, leg cramps, and pain in the chest, abdomen, back, hands, or feet.

**Meticorten,** trademark for a glucocorticoid (prednisone).

**metoclopramide hydrochloride** /met′əklō′prəmīd/, a GI stimulant.

■ INDICATIONS: It is prescribed to stimulate motility of and increase the tone of gastric contractions of the upper GI tract and to prevent emesis.

■ CONTRAINDICATIONS: Epilepsy; concomitant use of drugs that cause extrapyramidal reactions, pheochromocytoma, GI hemorrhage, obstruction, or perforation, or known hypersensitivity to this drug prohibits its use.

■ ADVERSE EFFECTS: Among the more serious adverse reactions are extrapyramidal reactions, usually in children, and GI disturbances. Drowsiness and allergic reactions and rash also may occur.

**metocurine iodide** /met′əkyōō′rēn/, a potent neuromuscular blocking agent. Also called **dimethyl tubocurarine iodide.**

■ INDICATIONS: It is given to produce flaccid paralysis as an adjunct to anesthesia, to reduce muscle spasm in tetanus, and to assist controlled ventilation.

■ CONTRAINDICATIONS: Asthma or known hypersensitivity to this drug or to iodides prohibits its use. It is given only by medical personnel trained and equipped to maintain assisted mechanic ventilation.

■ ADVERSE EFFECTS: Among the more serious adverse reactions are hypotension, respiratory or circulatory depression, and bronchospasm.

**metolazone** /mətō′ləzōn/, a diuretic and antihypertensive.

■ INDICATIONS: It is prescribed for the treatment of edema and high blood pressure.

■ CONTRAINDICATIONS: Anuria or known hypersensitivity to this drug, to thiazides, or to sulfonamide prohibits its use.

■ ADVERSE EFFECTS: Among the more serious adverse reactions are hypokalemia, hyperglycemia, hyperuricemia, and allergic reactions.

**"me-too" drug,** informal. a drug product that is similar, identical, or closely related to a drug for which a manufacturer has obtained a new drug application. The drug is placed on the market by a company or companies other than the holder of the new drug application. On the assumption that the new drug has been recognized as safe and effective, clinical trials required of the original manufacturer are not required of the new supplier, but information regarding the manufacture, bioavailability, and labeling of the product is required to complete the abbreviated procedure for approval by the Food and Drug Administration.

**metopic** /mətō′pik/, pertaining to the forehead.

**metopo-,** combining form meaning 'forehead': *metopodynia, metopopagus, metopoplasty.*

**metoprolol tartrate** /metop′rəlol/, an antiadrenergic; a beta₁ receptor antagonist agent.

■ INDICATION: It is prescribed in the treatment of hypertension.

■ CONTRAINDICATIONS: Bradycardia, cardiogenic shock, overt cardiac failure, bronchospastic disease, or known hypersensitivity to this drug prohibits its use.

■ ADVERSE EFFECTS: Among the more serious adverse reactions are fatigue, bradycardia, bronchospasms, and GI upset.

**metr-,** combining form meaning 'measure': *metrechoscopy, metric, metrology.*

**metra-.** See **metro-.**

**metralgia** /mətral′jə/ [Gk, *metra,* womb, *algos,* pain], tenderness or pain in the uterus. Also called **hysteralgia, hysterodynia, metrodynia, uteralgia.**

**metre.** See **meter.**

**-metria, 1.** suffix meaning '(condition of the) ability to measure muscular acts': *dysmetria, hypermetria, hypometria.* **2.** suffix meaning '(condition of the) uterus': *ametria, atretometria, dimetria.*

**metric** /met′rik/, pertaining to a system of measurement that uses the meter as a basis. See also **metric system.**

**metric equivalent** [Gk, *metron,* measure; L, *aequus,* equal, *valare,* to be strong], any value in metric units of measurement that equals the same value in English units, for example, 2.54 cm equals 1 inch, and 1 L equals 1.0567 quarts.

**metric system,** a decimal system of measurement based on the meter (39.37 inches) as the unit of length, on the gram (15.432 grains) as the unit of weight or mass, and, as a derived unit, on the liter (0.908 U.S. dry quart or 1.0567 U.S. liquid quart) as the unit of volume.

**metritis** /mətrī′tis/ [Gk, *metra,* womb, *itis,* inflammation],

inflammation of the walls of the uterus. Kinds of metritis are **endometritis** and **parametritis.** Also called **uteritis.** See also **puerperal fever.**

**metro-, metra-,** prefix meaning 'uterus': *metrocele, metrofibroma, metromalacoma.*

**metrocarcinoma** /met'rōkär'sinō'mə/ [Gk, *metra,* womb, *karkinos,* crab, *oma,* tumor], a cancer of the uterus.

**metrodynia.** See **metralgia.**

**metronidazole** /met'rənī'dəzōl/, an antimicrobial.
- INDICATIONS: It is prescribed in the treatment of amebiasis, trichomoniasis, and certain bacterial infections such as trichomoniasis and bacterial vaginosis.
- CONTRAINDICATIONS: First trimester of pregnancy, blood dyscrasias, organic disease, central nervous system disorders, or known hypersensitivity to this drug prohibits its use. It is contraindicated in nursing mothers.
- ADVERSE EFFECTS: Among the more serious adverse reactions are severe GI distress, dizziness, neutropenia, and neurologic disturbances. A metallic taste in the mouth is commonly noted.

**metronoscope** /mətron'əskōp/, **1.** a tachistoscope, or device that exposes a small amount of reading matter to the eyes for brief preset periods. It is used in testing and in aiding individuals to increase reading speed. **2.** an apparatus that exercises the eyes rhythmically to improve binocular coordination.

**-metropia, -metropy,** suffix meaning '(condition of the) refraction of the eye': *allometropia, antimetropia, isometropia.*

**metroplasty** /mē'trəplas'tē/ [Gk, *metra,* womb], reconstructive surgery on the uterus. Also called **uteroplasty.**

**metrorrhagia** /met'rōrā'jē·ə/ [Gk, *metra,* womb, *rhegnynai,* to burst forth], uterine bleeding other than that caused by menstruation. It may be caused by uterine lesions and may be a sign of a urogenital malignancy, especially cervical cancer.

**-metry, -metria,** suffix meaning the 'process of measuring something' specified: *oncometry, pelvimetry, symmetry.*

**Metubine,** trademark for a neuromuscular blocking agent (metocurine iodide).

**metyrapone** /metir'əpōn/, a diagnostic test drug.
- INDICATION: It is used to test hypothalamic and pituitary function.
- CONTRAINDICATIONS: Adrenocortical insufficiency or hypersensitivity prohibits its use.
- ADVERSE EFFECTS: Among the most serious adverse reactions are nausea, dizziness, and allergic rash.

**metyrosine** /mətir'əsēn/, an antihypertensive.
- INDICATION: It is prescribed in the treatment of pheochromocytoma.
- CONTRAINDICATION: Known hypersensitivity to this drug prohibits its use.
- ADVERSE EFFECTS: Among the more serious adverse reactions are extrapyramidal reactions, including tremor, drooling, and crystalluria. Sedation is common, and diarrhea and anxiety may occur.

**Metzenbaum scissors.** See **scissors.**

**Meuse fever.** See **trench fever.**

**mev, MeV,** abbreviation for *million electron volts,* the equivalent of $3.82 \times 10^{-14}$ small calories, or $1.6 \times 10^{-6}$ ergs.

**mevalonate kinase** /məval'ənāt/, an enzyme in the liver and in yeast. It catalyzes the transfer of a phosphate group from adenosine triphosphate to produce adenosine diphosphate and 5-phosphomevalonate.

**Mexate,** trademark for an antineoplastic (methotrexate).

**Mexican bindweed.** See *Rivea corymbosa.*

**Mexican typhus** [Gk, *typhos,* fever], a form of epidemic typhus carried by lice in Mexico. Also called **tabardillo.**

**mexiletine hydrochloride** /mek'silē'tin/, an oral antiarrhythmic drug.
- INDICATIONS: It is prescribed for the treatment of symptomatic ventricular arrhythmias.
- CONTRAINDICATIONS: It is contraindicated in patients with cardiogenic shock or preexisting second- or third-degree atrioventricular block in the absence of a pacemaker.
- ADVERSE EFFECTS: Among adverse reactions reported are upper GI distress, lightheadedness, tremor, loss of coordination, diarrhea, sleep disorders, headache, visual disturbances, and palpitations.

**Mexitil,** trademark for an oral antiarrhythmic drug (mexiletine hydrochloride).

**Meynet's node** /mānāz'/, any of the numerous nodules that may develop within the capsules surrounding joints and in tendons affected by rheumatic diseases, especially in children.

**Mezlin,** trademark for a semisynthetic penicillin antibiotic (mezlocillin sodium).

**mezlocillin sodium** /mezlos'ilin/, a semisynthetic penicillin antibiotic.
- INDICATIONS: It is prescribed for the treatment of lower respiratory tract, intraabdominal, urinary tract, gynecologic, and skin infections and bacterial septicemia caused by susceptible strains of multiple microorganisms.
- CONTRAINDICATION: Hypersensitivity to any of the penicillins prohibits its use.
- ADVERSE EFFECTS: The most serious adverse reactions are anaphylaxis, convulsive seizures, epigastric pain, reduction in blood elements, and elevation in hepatic and renal parameters.

**mF,** abbreviation for *millifarad.* See **farad.**

**MFCC,** abbreviation for *Marriage, Family, and Child Counselor.*

**MFD,** abreviation for *minimum fatal dose.* See **minimum lethal dose.**

**mg,** abbreviation for **milligram.**

**Mg,** symbol for the element **magnesium.**

**MH,** **1.** abbreviation for **malignant hyperthermia. 2.** abbreviation for **mental health.**

**MHA,** abbreviation for **Mental Health Association.**

**MHC,** abbreviation for **major histocompatibility complex.**

**MHD,** abbreviation for **minimum hemolytic dose.**

**mho,** an archaic name for **siemens.**

**MHz,** abbreviation for **megahertz.**

**MI,** abbreviation for **myocardial infarction.**

**miasma** /mī·az'mə/ [Gk, *miainein,* defilement], an unwholesome, polluted atmosphere or environment, such as a marsh or swamp containing rotting organic matter. Also called **miasm** /mī'əzəm/.

**MIC,** abbreviation for **minimal inhibitory concentration.** This term is commonly used for antibiotics to describe the minimal concentration of antibiotic needed to inhibit bacterial growth.

**mica** /mī'kə/, an aluminum silicate mineral that occurs in thin laminated scales. Mica is used in paints, plastics, fire protection boards, pigments, and other industrial materials. It is used also as an electric insulator and lubricant.

**micatosis** /mī'kətō'sis/, a form of pneumoconiosis caused by inhalation of mica particles.

**micellar chromatography** /mīsel'ər/, a method of monitoring minute quantities of drugs in whole body fluids by using micellar or colloidal compounds to keep proteins in solution. The technique eliminates the need to remove proteins that usually interfere with chromatographic analysis of blood serum, urine, or saliva. Micellar chromatography is used to monitor levels of prescribed drugs, as well as illicit drugs such as lysergic acid diethylamide and tetrahydrocannabinol.

**Michaelis-Menten kinetics** [Leonor Michaelis, American biochemist, 1875–1949; Maud L. Menten, Canadian physician in U.S. practice, 1879–1960], a method of transforming drug plasma levels into a linear relationship using the parameters of drug concentration and a constant, $K_m$, which is a measure of enzyme-substrate affinity.

**-micin,** combining form for antibiotics produced by *Micromonospora* strains.

**miconazole nitrate** /mīkon'əzōl/, an antifungal.
- INDICATIONS: It is used topically to treat certain fungal infections of the skin and vagina and parenterally to treat systemic fungal infections.
- CONTRAINDICATION: Known hypersensitivity to this drug prohibits its use.
- ADVERSE EFFECTS: Among the more serious adverse reactions to topical or vaginal application are irritation, burning, and maceration of the skin. When it is used systemically, nausea, pruritus, phlebitis, and anemia may occur.

**micr-.** See **micro-.**

**micrencephalia.** See **microcephaly.**

**micrencephalon** /mī'krənsef'əlon/, an abnormally small brain. See also **microcephaly.** —**micrencephalic,** *adj., n.*

**micrencephaly.** See **microcephaly.**

**micro-, micr-, mikro-,** 1. prefix meaning 'small': microanalysis, microglossia. 2. prefix meaning one "millionth": *micrometer.*

**microabscess** /mīkrō·ab'ses/ [Gk, *mikros,* small; L, *abscedere,* to go away], a very small abscess.

**microadenoma** /mī'krō·ad'ənō'mə/, a pituitary adenoma less than 10 mM in diameter.

**microaerophile** /mī'krō·er'əfil/ [Gk, *mikros,* small, *aer,* air, *philein,* to love], a microorganism that requires free oxygen for growth but at a lower concentration than that contained in the atmosphere. Compare **aerobe, anaerobe.** —**microaerophilic,** *adj.*

**microaerotonometer** /mī'krō·er'ətonom'ətər/ [Gk, *mikros* + *aer,* air, *tonos,* tension, *metron,* measure], instrument for measuring the volume of gases in blood or other fluids.

**microaggregate recipient set** /mi'krō·ag'rəgāt/ [Gk, *mikros* + L, *ad,* to, *gregare,* to collect, *recipere,* to receive; AS, *settan*], a device composed of plastic components for the IV delivery of large volumes of stored whole blood or of packed blood cells. The components of the set include the plastic tubing, the roller clamp, and the special filter that prevents the microaggregates or deteriorated red blood cells from entering the circulatory system of the patient. The plastic tubing of this device has a larger lumen than tubing of most other IV sets, which allows the blood to be delivered more rapidly. Compare **component drip set, component syringe set, straight line blood set, Y set.**

**microalbuminuria** /mī'krō·al'binōōr'ē·ə/, the urinary excretion of small amounts of albumin, below the detection level of routine dipstick analysis. The condition is an early indicator of altered glomerular permeability in diabetes.

**microampere** /mī'krō·am'pir/, one millionth of an ampere.

**microanalysis** /mī'krō·anal'isis/, 1. analysis of minute quantities of material. 2. identification of substances by examination under a microscope.

**microaneurysm** /mi'krō·an'yəriz'əm/ [Gk, *mikros* + *aneurysma,* a widening], a microscopic aneurysm characteristic of thrombotic purpura.

**microangiopathic hemolytic anemia (MAHA)** /mī'krō·anjē·əpath'ik/, a disorder in which narrowing or obstruction of small blood vessels results in distortion and fragmentation of erythrocytes, hemolysis, and anemia.

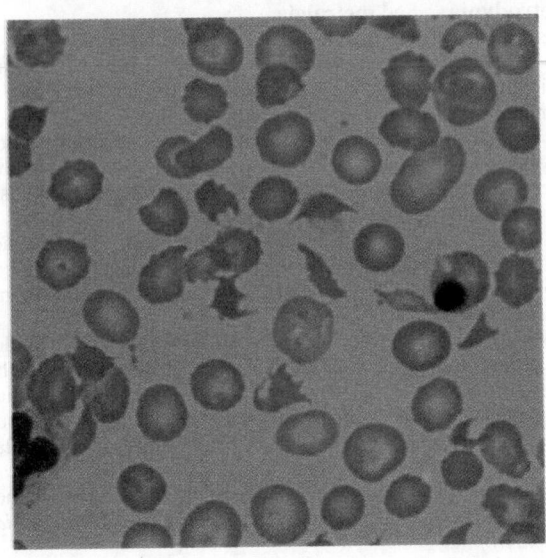

**Microangiopathic hemolytic anemia**
*(Carr and Rodak, 1999)*

**microangiopathy** /mī'krō·an'jē·op'əthē/ [Gk, *mikros* + *angeion,* vessel, *pathos,* disease], a disease of the small blood vessels. Examples are diabetic microangiopathy, in which the basement membrane of capillaries thickens, and thrombotic microangiopathy, in which thrombi form in the arterioles and capillaries.

**microbe** /mī'krōb/, a microorganism. —**microbial,** *adj.*

**-microbe,** suffix meaning a 'small living organism': *aeromicrobe, inframicrobe, ultramicrobe.*

**microbial ecology** /mīkrō'bē·əl/, the branch of biology that deals with the interaction of microorganisms with their environment.

**microbial pesticides,** pathogenic microorganisms that are toxic to a particular bacterium, insect, or other pest.

**-microbic,** suffix meaning 'referring to or consisting of microbes': *amicrobic, monomicrobic, polymicrobic.*

**microbicide** /mīkrō'bisīd/ [Gk, *mikros,* small, *bios,* life; L, *cadere,* to kill], any drug, chemical, or other agent that can kill microorganisms.

**microbiologic assay** /-bī·əloj'ik/, 1. the use of microorganisms for measuring the activity of organic compounds. 2. the calculation of the purity of nutritional factors such as vitamins by measuring the growth of certain bacteria.

**microbiology** /mī'krōbī·ol'əjē/ [Gk, *mikros* + *bios,* life, *logos,* science], the branch of biology that is concerned with the study of microorganisms, including bacteria, algae, protozoa, and fungi.

**microbiology technologist,** a medical technologist who specializes in the identification of bacteria and other microorganisms found in patient tissues and other specimens.

**microblast** /mī'krōblast'/ [Gk, *mikros,* small, *blastos,* germ], a very small immature red blood cell.

**microbody** /mī′krō·bod′ē/, any of the round membrane-bound granular cytoplasmic particles containing enzymes and other substances, which originate in the endoplasmic reticulum of vertebrate liver and kidney cells and other cells, and in protozoa, yeast, and many cell types of higher plants. An important type in vertebrates is the peroxisome.

**microbrachia** /mī′krōbrā′kē·ə/ [Gk, *mikros* + *brachion*, arm], a developmental defect characterized by abnormal smallness of the arms. —**microbrachius,** *n.*

**microcarrier** /-ker′ē·ər/, microscopic bead or sphere that increases the surface area in a tissue culture for the attachment and yield of anchorage-dependent cells.

**microcentrum.** See **centrosome.**

**microcephaly** /mī′krōsef′əlē/ [Gk, *mikros* + *kephale,* head], a congenital anomaly characterized by abnormal smallness of the head in relation to the rest of the body and by underdevelopment of the brain, resulting in some degree of mental retardation. The head is more than two standard deviations below the average circumference size for age, sex, race, and period of gestation. It has a narrow, receding forehead; a flattened occiput; and a pointed vertex. The facial features are generally normal. The condition may be caused by an autosomal-recessive disorder; a chromosomal abnormality; a toxic stimulus such as irradiation, chemical agents; maternal infection during prenatal development; or any trauma, especially during the third trimester of pregnancy or early infancy. There is no treatment, and nursing care is primarily supportive and educational, helping parents learn to care for a brain-damaged child. Also called **microcephalia, microcephalism.** Compare **macrocephaly.** —**microcephalic, microcephalous,** *adj.,* **microcephalic, microcephalus,** *n.*

**microcheiria** /mī′krōkī′rē·ə/ [Gk, *mikros* + *cheir,* hand], a developmental defect characterized by abnormal smallness of the hands. The condition is usually associated with other congenital malformations or with bone and muscle disorders. Also spelled **microchiria.**

**microcide** /mī′krəsīd/, an antimicrobial flavoprotein enzyme. It has antibacterial activity only in the presence of glucose and oxygen as it reduces the oxygen to hydrogen peroxide. The enzyme is derived from *Penicillium notatum* and other fungi.

**microcirculation** /-sur′kyələ′shən/, the flow of blood throughout the system of smaller vessels of the body, particularly the capillaries.

**microcomputer** /-kəmpyōō′tər/, a complete multiuse electronic digital computer system consisting of a central processing unit, storage facilities, input/output ports, and a chip or chips containing megabytes of high-speed internal storage. It is commonly designed for use by one person at a time. Compare **mainframe computer, minicomputer.** Also called **personal computer.**

**microcurie (μCi, μc)** /mī′krōkyŏŏr′ē/ [Gk, *mikros* + *curie,* Marie Curie], a unit of radioactivity equal to one millionth of a curie, or $3.70 \times 10^4$ disintegrations per second. See also **curie.**

**microcystic adnexal carcinoma (MAC),** a form of adnexal tumor that often appears on the face as a yellow, indurated plaque with ill-defined margins. The patient experiences fullness, pain, burning, anesthesia, or paresthesia in the area of the lesion.

**microcyte** /mī′krəsīt/ [Gk, *mikros* + *kytos,* cell], an abnormally small erythrocyte with a mean corpuscular volume of less than 80 μm³, often occurring in iron deficiency anemias.

**microcythemia** /-thē′mē·ə/ [Gk, *mikros,* small, *kytos,* cell, *haima,* blood], an excessive amount of microcytes in the blood.

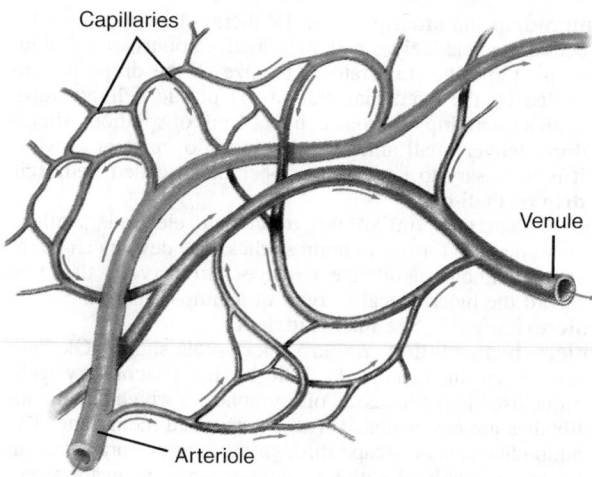

**Microcirculation** *(Thibodeau and Patton, 1999/William Ober)*

**microcytic** /mī′krōsit′ik/ [Gk, *mikros* + *kytos,* cell], (of a cell) pertaining to a smaller-than-normal cell.

**microcytic anemia,** a hematologic disorder characterized by abnormally small erythrocytes, usually associated with chronic blood loss or a nutritional anemia, such as iron deficiency anemia. Compare **macrocytic anemia.**

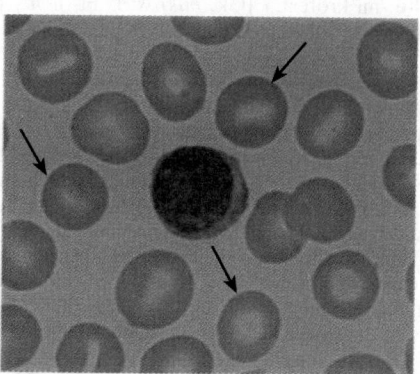

**Microcytes seen in microcytic anemia**
*(Carr and Rodak, 1999)*

**microcytosis** /mī′krōsītō′sis/ [Gk, *mikros* + *kytos* + *osis,* condition], a hematologic condition characterized by erythrocytes that are smaller than normal. Microcytosis is found in iron deficiency anemia. Compare **poikilocytosis.** See also **anisocytosis.** —**microcytic,** *adj.*

**microdactyly** /mī′krōdak′təlē/ [Gk, *mikros* + *dactylos,* finger], a developmental defect characterized by abnormal smallness of the fingers and toes. The condition is usually associated with bone and muscle disorders, such as progressive myositis ossificans.

**microdrepanocytic** /mī′krōdrep′ənōsit′ik/ [Gk, *mikros* + *drepane,* sickle, *kytos,* cell], pertaining to a blood disorder marked by the presence of both microcytes and drepanocytes, such as occurs in sickle cell-thalassemia.

**microdrip** /mī′krōdrip′/, (in IV therapy) an apparatus for delivering relatively small measured amounts of IV solutions at specific flow rates. The size of the drops is controlled by the fixed diameter of the plastic delivery tube. With a microdrip 60 drops delivers 1 mL of solution. Microdrips deliver small amounts of solution over time, as when it is necessary to keep a vein open. Also called **pediatric drip** or **Pedi-drip.**

**microelectrode** /mī′krō·ilek′trōd/, an electrode with a very small tip for use in brain studies. The device can be inserted without membrane damage into nervous tissue to record the bioelectrical activity of a simple neuron.

**microelement.** See **micronutrient.**

**microencapsulation** /mī′krō·enkap′syəlā′shən/ [Gk, *mikros + en,* in; L, *capsula,* little box], a laboratory technique used in the bioassay of hormones in which certain antibodies are encapsulated with a perforated membrane. The antibodies cannot escape through the tiny perforations, but hormones that bind with the antibodies may enter the structure to bind with them. Technicians then can measure the amount of hormone present in the specimen. The technique is used for the encapsulation of unstable enzymes and in the preparation of some drugs in slow- or time-release forms.

**microencephaly** /mī′krō·ensef′əlē/ [Gk, *mikros,* small, *egkephalos,* brain], the condition of being born with an abnormally small brain.

**microequivalent** /mī′krō·ikwiv′ələnt/, one millionth of an equivalent, the amount of a substance that corresponds to its equivalent mass in micrograms.

**microfarad** (μF) /mī′krōfer′əd/ [Gk, *mikros + farad,* Michael Faraday], a unit of capacitance that equals one millionth of a farad. See also **farad.**

**microfiche** /mī′krōfēsh′/ [Gk, *mikros* + Fr, *fiche,* peg], a sheet of microfilm that contains several separate photographic reproductions. The sheet is a convenient size for filing and enables large amounts of data to be stored in a relatively small space. See also **microfilm.**

**microfilament** /-fil′əmənt/, any of the finest of the fibrous cellular filaments, such as the tonofibrils, found in the cytoplasm of most cells, that function primarily as a supportive system. Compare **microtubule.**

**microfilaria** /mī′krōfiler′ē·ə/, *pl.* **microfilariae** [Gk, *mikros* + L, *filum,* thread], the prelarval form of any filarial worm. Certain blood-sucking insects ingest these forms from an infected host, and the microfilariae then develop in the body of the insect and become infective larvae. See also **filariasis, loiasis, onchocerciasis,** *Wuchereria.*

**microfilm** /mī′krəfilm/, a strip of 16 mM or 35 mM film that contains photographic reproductions of pages of books, documents, or other library or medical records in greatly reduced size. The film is viewed through a machine that enlarges the photographic images to normal reading size.

**microfluorometry.** See **cytophotometry.**

**microgamete** /-gam′ēt/, the small motile male gamete of certain thallophytes and sporozoa, specifically the malarial parasite *Plasmodium.* It corresponds to the sperm of the higher animals and unites in conjugation with the larger, nonmotile female gamete. See also **macrogamete.**

**microgametocyte** /-gamē′təsīt/ [Gk, *mikros + gamete,* spouse, *kytos,* cell], an enlarged merozoite that undergoes meiosis to form the mature male gamete during the sexual phase of the life cycle of certain thallophytes and sporozoa, specifically the malarial parasite *Plasmodium.* Microgametocytes are found in the red blood cells of a person infected with the malarial parasite, but they must be ingested by a female *Anopheles* mosquito to complete the maturation process and develop into microgametes.

**microgenitalia** /-jen′itā′lē·ə/, a condition characterized by abnormally small external genitalia.

**microglia** /mīkrog′lē·ə/ [Gk, *mikros + glia,* glue], small migratory interstitial cells that form part of the central nervous system. They have various forms and slender, branched processes. Microglia serve as phagocytes that collect waste products of the nerve tissue of the body. Also called **Hortega cells, mesoglia.**

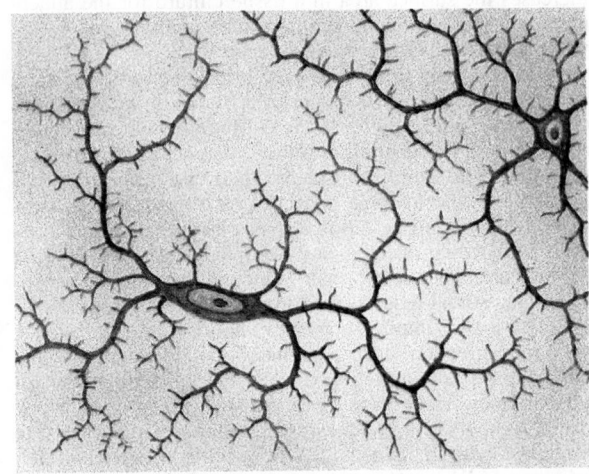

**Microglia** *(Chipps, Clanin, and Campbell, 1992)*

**microglossia** /mī′krō·glos′ē·ə/ [Gk, *mikros,* small + *glōssa,* tongue], undersized tongue.

**micrognathia** /mī′krōnā′thē·ə/ [Gk, *mikros + gnathos,* jaw], underdevelopment of the jaw, especially the mandible. Compare **macrognathia.** —**micrognathic,** *adj.*

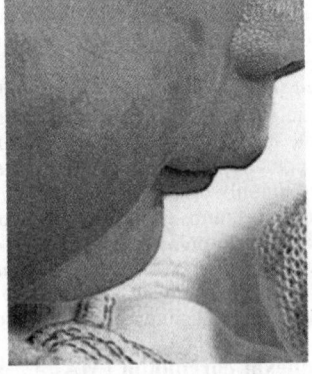

**Micrognathia**
*(Zitelli and Davis, 1997/courtesy Dr. Christine Williams, Scarsdale, New York)*

**microgram** (μg) /mī′krəgram/, a unit of measurement of mass equal to one millionth ($10^{-6}$) of a gram. See also **gram.**

**microgyri.** See **microgyrus.**

**microgyria** /mī′krōjī′rē·ə/ [Gk, *mikros* + *gyros,* turn], a developmental defect of the brain in which the convolutions are abnormally small, resulting in structural malformation of the cortex. The condition is usually associated with mental retardation and physical defects. Also called **polymicrogyria.**

**microgyrus** /mī′krōjī′rəs/, *pl.* **microgyri,** an underdeveloped, malformed convolution of the brain.

**microhm** /mī′krōm/ [Gk, *mikros* + *ohm,* George Ohm], a unit of electrical resistance equal to one millionth of an ohm. See also **ohm.**

**microinjection** /mī′krō·injek′shən/, the injection of tiny amounts of a substance into a cell, using micromanipulation instruments.

**microinjector** /mī′krō·injek′tər/, an instrument that delivers tiny amounts of a substance into a cell.

**microinvasive carcinoma** /mī′krō·invā′siv/ [Gk, *mikros* + L, *in,* within, *vadere,* to go], a squamous epithelial neoplasm that has penetrated the basement membrane, the first stage in invasive cancer. See also **carcinoma in situ.**

**microkeratome** /mī′krō·kər′ə·tōm/ [Gk, *mikros* + *keratome*], an instrument for removing a thin slice, or creating a thin hinged flap, on the surface of the cornea.

**microleakage** /mī′krō·lē′kij/ [Gk, *mikros* + ONorse *leka,* to drip], leakage of minute amounts of fluids, debris, and microorganisms through the microscopic space between a dental restoration or its cement and the adjacent surface of the cavity preparation; it may progress through the dentin into the pulp.

**microlevel interventions** /-lev′əl/, health-generating changes performed at the individual level, such as in conditioning or stimulus control therapies.

**microliter** (μL) /mī′krəlē′tər/, a unit of liquid volume equal to one millionth of a liter, or 1 mm³.

**microlith** /mī′krəlith/ [Gk, *mikros* + *lithos,* stone], a small rounded mass of mineral matter or calcified stone.

**micromanipulation** /-mənip′yəlā′shən/, surgical displacement or dissection of very small tissues, using either miniature instruments or mechanical devices that translate large motions into smaller movements.

**micromanipulator** /-mənip′yəlā′tər/, a guidance accessory to a microscope that performs displacement or dissection of very small tissues.

**micromelic dwarf** /-mē′lik/ [Gk, *mikros* + *melos,* limb], a dwarf whose limbs are abnormally short.

**micrometer** (μm) /mīkrom′ətər/, 1. an instrument used for measuring small angles or distances on objects being observed through a microscope or telescope. 2. /mī′krōmē′tər/, a unit of measurement, commonly referred to as a *micron,* that equals one thousandth ($10^{-3}$) of a millimeter.

**micromicro-,** combining form meaning '$10^{-12}$' (μμ): *micromicron.*

**micromillimeter.** See **nanometer.**

**micromyeloblastic leukemia** /mī′krōmī′əlōblas′tik/ [Gk, *mikros* + *myelos,* marrow, *blastos,* germ], a malignant neoplasm of blood-forming tissues, characterized by the proliferation of small myeloblasts distinguishable from lymphocytes only by special staining techniques and microscopic examination.

**micron** (μm) /mī′kron/ [Gk, *mikros,* small], 1. a metric unit of length equal to one millionth of a meter; micrometer (def. 2). 2. (in physical chemistry) a colloidal particle with a diameter between 0.2 and 10 μm.

**Micronase,** trademark for an oral antidiabetic drug (glyburide).

**microneurography** /-nyŏŏrog′rəfē/, the recording of impulse conduction in individual nerve fibers by means of a microelectrode. The technique is used in studies of the relationship between body mass and the sympathetic nervous system.

**micronodular** /-nod′yələr/, characterized by the presence of very small nodules.

**micronodular adrenal disease,** a rare form of Cushing's syndrome caused by multiple bilateral small, pigmented autonomous adrenocorticotropic hormone–independent cortisol-secreting adenomas. Also called **primary bilateral micronodular hyperplasia.**

**Micronor,** trademark for an oral contraceptive containing a progestin (norethindrone).

**micronucleus** /-nōō′klē·əs/, 1. a small nucleus. 2. the smaller of two nuclei in some protozoa; it functions in sexual reproduction. Compare **macronucleus.**

**micronutrient** /-nōō′trē·ənt/, any dietary element essential only in minute amounts for the normal physiologic processes of the body, including vitamins and minerals or chemical elements such as zinc or iodine. Also called **microelement, trace element.**

**microorganism** /-ôr′gəniz′əm/ [Gk, *mikros* + *organon,* instrument], any tiny, usually microscopic entity capable of carrying on living processes. It may be pathogenic. Kinds of microorganisms include **bacteria, fungi, protozoa,** and **viruses.**

**micropenis.** See **microphallus.**

**microphage** /mī′krəfāj/ [Gk, *mikros* + *phagein,* to eat], a neutrophil capable of ingesting small things, such as bacteria. Compare **macrophage.** —**microphagic,** *adj.*

**microphallus** /-fal′əs/ [Gk, *mikros* + *phallos,* penis], an abnormally small penis. When it is observed in the newborn, the nurse examines the child for other signs of ambiguous genitalia. Also called **micropenis.** See also **ambiguous genitalia.**

**microphthalmos** /mī′krəfthal′məs/ [Gk, *mikros* + *ophthalmos,* eye], a developmental anomaly characterized by abnormal smallness of one or both eyes. When the condition occurs in the absence of other ocular defects, it is called pure microphthalmos or nanophthalmos. Also spelled **microphthalmus.** Also called **microphthalmia.** —**microphthalmic,** *adj.*

**microplasia.** See **dwarfism.**

**micropodia** /-pō′dē·ə/ [Gk, *mikros* + *pous,* foot], a developmental anomaly characterized by abnormal smallness of the feet. The condition is often associated with other congenital malformations or with bone and skeletal disorders.

**microprolactinoma** /-prōlak′tinō′mə/, a prolactin-secreting pituitary tumor less than 10 mm in diameter. Microprolactinomas seldom enlarge, and some resolve spontaneously. Most patients experience a return to ovulatory menstrual cycles and fertility with treatment.

**microprosopus** /mī′krōprō′səpəs, -prəsō′pəs/ [Gk, *mikros* + *prosopon,* face], a fetus having an abnormally small or underdeveloped face.

**micropsia** /mīkrop′sē·ə/ [Gk, *mikros* + *opsis,* sight], a condition of vision in which a person perceives objects as smaller than they really are. —**microptic,** *adj.*

**microreentry** /-rē·en′trē/ [Gk, *mikros* + L, *re,* again; Fr, *entree,* entry], the reactivation of myocardial tissue by an impulse transmitted along a very small circuit within the conductive tissue of the heart.

**microscope** /mī′krəskōp′/ [Gk, *mikros,* small, *skopein,* to view], an instrument with lenses for viewing very small objects. An electron microscope uses a beam of electrons instead of visible light.

**microscopic** /mī′krəskop′ik/ [Gk, *mikros* + *skopein,* to look], 1. pertaining to a microscope. 2. very small; visible only when magnified and illuminated by a microscope. Compare **gross.**

**microscopic anatomy,** the study of the microscopic structure of the tissues and cells. Kinds of microscopic anatomy are **cytology** and **histology.**

**microscopy** /mīkros'kəpē/ [Gk, *mikros* + *skopein,* to look], a technique for observing minute materials using a microscope. Kinds of microscopy include **dark-field microscopy, electron microscopy,** and **immunofluorescent microscopy.**

**microshock** /mī'krəshok/, **1.** shock from an electric current of less than 1 milliampere. It may not be felt. **2.** the passage of current directly into the cardiac tissue.

**microsomal enzymes** /-sō'məl/, a group of enzymes associated with a certain particulate fraction of liver homogenate that plays a role in the metabolism of many drugs.

**microsome** /mī'krəsōm/, a fragment of endoplasmic reticulum associated with ribosomes, found in cells that have been homogenized and ultracentrifuged.

**microsomia** /-sō'mē·ə/ [Gk, *mikros* + *soma,* body], the condition of having an abnormally small and underdeveloped yet otherwise perfectly formed body with normal proportionate relationships of the various parts. See also **primordial dwarf.**

**microspheres** /mī'krəsfirs/, **1.** centrosomes. **2.** microscopic globules of radiolabeled material.

**microspherocytosis** /-sfir'əsītō'sis/, a hemolytic disorder characterized by the presence in the blood of an excess number of tiny spherocytes, erythrocytes whose diameter is less than normal but whose thickness is increased. See also **spherocyte.**

**Microsporida** /mī'krō·spor'i·də/ [Gk, *mikros* + *sporos,* seed], an order of parasitic protozoa found in invertebrates, especially arthropods, in lower vertebrates, and rarely in higher vertebrates.

**microsporidiosis** /mī'krō·spô·rid'ē·ō'sis/, infection with protozoa of the order Microsporida, usually seen in immunocompromised patients; the usual symptoms are diarrhea and wasting.

*Microsporum* /-spôr'əm/ [Gk, *mikros* + *sporos,* seed], a genus of dermatophytes of the family Moniliaceae. The spores are multiseptate and variable in shape and have thin or thick walls. One species is *M. audouinii,* which causes epidemic tinea capitis in children; others are *M. canis* and *M. gypseum.* Formerly called *Microsporon.*

**microstomia** /-stō'mē·ə/ [Gk, *mikros,* small, *stoma,* mouth], the condition of having an abnormally small mouth.

**microsurgery** /-sur'jərē/ [Gk, *mikros,* small, *cheirourgos,* surgery], surgery that involves dissection and manipulation of minute tissue structures under a microscope.

**microtear** /mī'krəter'/, minor damage to soft tissue.

**microthermy** /-thur'mē/ [Gk, *mikros* + *therme,* heat], the use of heat generated by radio wave conversion in physical therapy.

**microthrombus** /mī'krō·throm'bəs/ *pl.* **microthrombi** [Gk, *mikros,* small + *thrombos,* lump], a small thrombus located in a capillary or other small blood vessel.

**microtome** /mī'krətōm/ [Gk, *mikros* + *temnein,* to cut], a device that cuts specimens of tissue prepared in paraffin blocks into extremely thin slices for microscopic study.

**microtrauma** /-trô'mə/, a very slight injury or lesion.

**microtubule,** a hollow cylindrical structure (200 to 300 angstroms in diameter and of variable length) that occurs widely within plant and animal cells. Microtubules increase in number during cell division and are associated with the movement of deoxyribonucleic acid material. Compare **microfilament.**

**microvascular** /-vas'kyələr/, pertaining to the portion of the circulatory system that is composed of the capillary network.

**microvilli** /-vil'ī/ [Gk, *mikros,* small; L, *villus,* shaggy hair], tiny hairlike folds in the plasma membrane that extend from the surface of many absorptive or secretory cells. The are most clearly visible with an electron microscope but may be seen as a "brush border" with a light microscope.

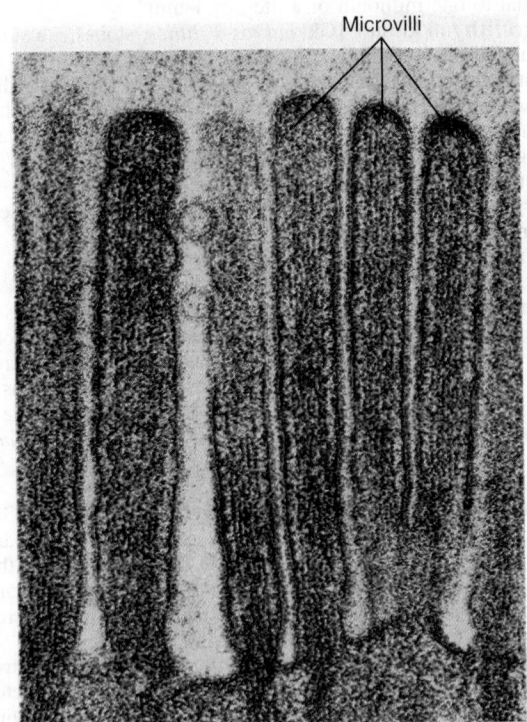

**Microvilli**
*(Thibodeau and Patton, 1999/courtesy Susumu Ito, Harvard Medical School)*

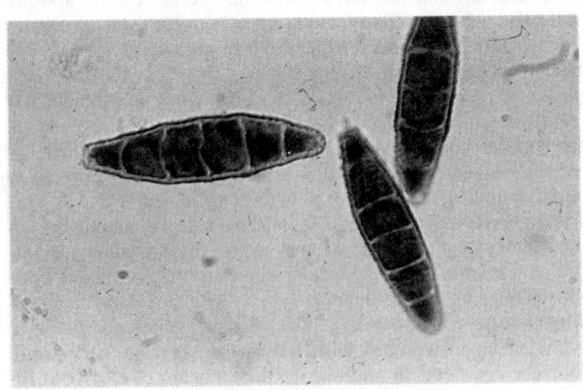

***Microsporum gypseum*** *(Murray et al, 1998)*

**microwave,** [Gk, *mikros* + AS, *wafian,* wave], electromagnetic radiation with a wavelength of 1 mm to 30 cm.

**microwave interstitial system** /mī′krəwāv/ a microwave-generated hyperthermia system that uses up to eight 50-watt applicators to create a heat field in certain accessible tumors no more than 2 inches (5.08 cm) beneath the skin. The microwaves produce a temperature of about 109° F (42.7° C) to destroy the tumor cells. The treatment can be monitored on a video terminal that shows location of the tumor and heat applicators.

**microwave thermography,** measurement of temperature through the detection of microwave radiation emitted from heated tissue.

**micturate, micturition.** See **urination.**

**micturition reflex** /mik′chərish′ən/ [L, *micturire,* to urinate, *reflectere,* to bend back], a normal reaction to a rise in pressure within the bladder, resulting in contraction of the bladder wall and relaxation of the urethral sphincter. Voluntary inhibition normally prevents incontinence; urination follows withdrawal of the inhibition.

**micturition syncope** [L, *micturire,* to urinate; Gk, *syn,* together, *koptein,* to cut], a temporary loss of consciousness that tends to affect some adult males after arising from a reclining posture to urinate in an upright posture. The effect is caused by a brief interruption of blood flow to the brain and is often associated with the use of alcohol, which contributes to vasodilation. See also **hypotension, orthostatic hypotension.**

**MICU,** abbreviation for *medical intensive care unit.*

**MID,** abbreviation for **minimal infecting dose.**

**mid-,** prefix meaning 'the middle': *midsagittal.*

**Midamor,** trademark for a diuretic (amiloride hydrochloride).

**midarm muscle circumference,** a calculation made by subtracting the triceps skin fold from the midupper arm circumference measurement. A less than expected circumference may indicate muscle wasting in the upper arm.

**midaxillary line** /midak′siler′ē/, an imaginary vertical line that passes midway between the anterior and posterior axillary folds.

**midazolam hydrochloride** /midaz′əlam/, a short-acting benzodiazepine central nervous system depressant; a benzodiazepine anxiolytic.

■ INDICATIONS: It is prescribed for preoperative sedation and impairment of memory of preoperative events, and for conscious sedation before short diagnostic or endoscopic procedures.

■ CONTRAINDICATIONS: This product is contraindicated for patients with acute narrow-angle glaucoma. It should be used with caution in those with open-angle glaucoma.

■ ADVERSE EFFECTS: Possible adverse reactions include decreased tidal volume, decreased respiratory rate, apnea, hypotension, hiccups, nausea, vomiting, oversedation, and tenderness at the site of injection.

**midbody,** 1. the middle of the body, or the midregion of the trunk. 2. a mass of granules that appears in the middle of the spindle during mitotic anaphase in a dividing cell.

**midbrain.** See **mesencephalon.**

**midcarpal.** See **mediocarpal.**

**midclavicular line** /mid′kləvik′yŏŏlər/ [AS, *midd* + L, *clavicula,* little key, *linea,* line], (in anatomy) an imaginary line that extends downward over the trunk from the midpoint of the clavicle, dividing each side of the anterior chest into two parts. The left midclavicular line is an important marker in describing the location of various cardiac phenomena, including the point of maximum impulse.

**middle adult** [AS, *middel* + L, *adultus,* grown up], an individual in the transitional age span between young adult and elderly, approximately 45 to 65 years of age, whose psychologic task, according to Erikson, is generativity versus stagnation.

**middle cardiac vein,** one of the five tributaries of the coronary sinus that drain blood from the capillary bed of the myocardium. It starts at the apex of the heart, rises in the posterior interventricular sulcus, receives tributaries from both ventricles, and ends in the right extremity of the coronary sinus. Compare **great cardiac vein, small cardiac vein.**

**middle costotransverse ligament.** See **ligament of the neck of the rib.**

**middle cuneiform bone.** See **intermediate cuneiform bone.**

**middle ear,** the tympanic cavity with the auditory ossicles contained in an irregular space in the temporal bone. It is separated from the external ear by the tympanic membrane and from the inner ear by the oval window. The auditory (pharyngotympanic or eustachian) tube carries air from the posterior nasopharynx into the middle ear. Compare **external ear, internal ear.**

**middle kidney.** See **mesonephros.**

**middle lobe syndrome,** localized atelectasis of the middle lobe of the right lung, characterized by chronic infection, cough, dyspnea, wheezing, and obstructive pneumonitis. Asymptomatic obstruction of the bronchus may occur. The condition arises when the cuff of lymphatic glands that surrounds the middle lobe bronchus becomes enlarged as a result of nonspecific or tuberculous inflammation during childhood. The bronchus is thus compressed, and bronchiectasis develops in the obstructed part of the lung. Treatment includes antituberculosis chemotherapy, administration of corticosteroids, and surgical excision. See also **atelectasis.**

**middle mediastinum,** the widest part of the mediastinum, containing the heart, ascending aorta, lower half of the superior vena cava, pulmonary trunk, and phrenic nerves. It is one of three caudal portions of the mediastinum. Compare **anterior mediastinum, posterior mediastinum, superior mediastinum.**

**middle plate.** See **nephrotome.**

**middle sacral artery,** a small visceral branch of the abdominal aorta, descending to the fourth and fifth lumbar vertebrae, the sacrum, and the coccyx. Minute branches are said to supply the posterior surface of the rectum.

**middle suprarenal artery,** one of a pair of small visceral branches of the abdominal aorta, arising opposite the superior mesenteric artery and supplying the suprarenal gland.

**middle temporal artery,** one of the branches of the superficial temporal artery on each side of the head. It arises just above the zygomatic arch, pierces the temporal fascia, branches to the temporalis, and anastomoses with the deep temporal branches of the maxillary artery. Compare **deep temporal artery, superficial temporal artery.**

**middle temporal gyrus** [AS, *middel* + L, *tempus,* time; Gk, *gyros,* turn], the middle of three gyri of the temporal area of the surface of the brain. It runs horizontally between the inferior and superior temporal sulci of the temporal lobe.

**middle umbilical fold,** the fold of peritoneum over the urachal remnant within the abdomen. Approximately 3 cm lateral to the middle umbilical fold is the lateral umbilical fold. Between the lateral and the middle folds is the medial umbilical fold. Also called **plica umbilicalis mediana.**

**midface** /mid′fās/, the middle of the face, including the nose, nasion, and glabella.

**mid forceps** [AS, *midd* + L, *forceps,* pair of tongs], an obstetric operation in which forceps are applied to the baby's head when it has reached the midplane of the mother's pelvis. An episiotomy is usually performed, and local, regional, or inhalation anesthesia is provided. In some cases, such as severe fetal distress, mid forceps may be the most rapid and the safest means of delivery, but astute selection of cases, skill, and experience are essential. Difficult mid forceps delivery is likely to be more traumatic to the baby and the mother than cesarean section. Compare **high forceps, low forceps.** See also **failed forceps, forceps delivery, obstetric forceps, trial forceps.**

**midgut** [AS, *midd* + *guttas*], the central portion of the embryonic alimentary canal, between the foregut and the hindgut. It consists of endodermal tissue, is connected to the yolk sac during early prenatal development, and eventually gives rise to some of the small intestine and part of the large intestine. Compare **foregut, hindgut.**

**midlife transition,** a period between early adulthood and middle adulthood that occurs between 40 and 45 years of age.

**midline** /mid′līn/ [AS, *midd* + L, *linea,* line], an imaginary line that divides the body into right and left halves.

**midline episiotomy.** See **episiotomy.**

**midoccipital** /mid′oksip′itəl/, pertaining to the center of the occiput.

**midodrine,** a vasopressor.

■ INDICATIONS: This drug is used to treat orthostatic hypotension.

■ CONTRAINDICATIONS: Factors that prohibit the use of this drug include known hypersensitivity to midodrine, severe organic heart disease, acute renal disease, urinary retention, pheochromocytoma, thyrotoxicosis, and persistent/excessive supine hypertension.

■ ADVERSE EFFECTS: Adverse effects of this drug include drowsiness, restlessness, headache, chills, nausea, anorexia, dry mouth, blurred vision, pruritus, piloerection, rash, urinary urgency, and supine hypertension. Common side effects are paresthesia and pain.

**midparental height** /-pəren′təl/, the average height of both parents at 25 to 45 years of age.

**midpelvic contraction.** See **contraction.**

**midposition** /mid′pəzish′ən/, the end-expiratory or end-tidal level or position of the lung-chest system under any given condition. It determines the functional residual capacity.

**Midrin,** trademark for a fixed-combination central nervous system drug containing an adrenergic (isometheptene mucate), a hypnotic (dichloralphenazone), and an analgesic (acetaminophen), used in the treatment of tension and vascular headaches.

**midsagittal plane.** See **median plane.**

**midstance** /mid′stanz/ [AS, *midd* + L, *stare,* to stand], one of the five stages in the stance phase of walking, or gait, directly associated with the period of single-leg support of body weight or the period during which the body advances over the stationary foot. During midstance the tibialis posterior and the flexor hallucis longus display their greatest activity. The midstance phase is considered in the diagnosis of many abnormal orthopedic conditions and in the analysis of the associated weaknesses of certain muscles and muscle groups. Compare **initial contact stance stage, loading response stance stage, preswing stance stage, terminal stance.** See also **swing phase of gait.**

**midsternum** /midstur′nəm/ [AS, *midd* + Gk, *sternon,* chest], the body of the breast bone (sternum).

**midstream catch urine specimen** [AS, *midd* + *stream* + L, *captere,* to capture], a urine specimen collected during the middle of a flow of urine, after the urinary opening has been carefully cleaned. Also called **clean catch urine specimen.**

**midupper arm circumference (MAC),** a measurement of the circumference of the arm at a midpoint between the tip of the acromial process of the scapula and the olecranon process of the ulna. It is an indication of upper arm muscle wasting.

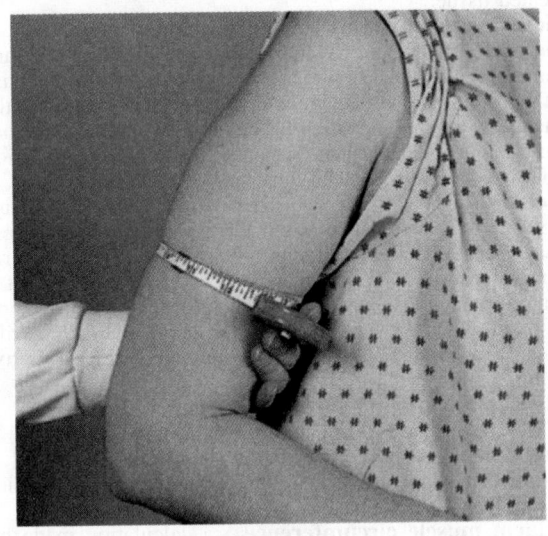

**Measurement of midupper arm circumference**
*(Seidel, 1995)*

**midwife** [AS, *midd* + *wif*], **1.** also called **obstetrix.** (in traditional use) a (female) person who assists women in childbirth. **2.** (according to the International Confederation of Midwives, World Health Organization, and Federation of International Gynecologists and Obstetricians) "a person who, having been regularly admitted to a midwifery educational program fully recognized in the country in which it is located, has successfully completed the prescribed course of studies in midwifery and has acquired the requisite qualifications to be registered and/or legally licensed to practice midwifery." Among the responsibilities of the midwife are supervision of pregnancy, labor, delivery, and puerperium. The midwife conducts the delivery independently, cares for the newborn, procures medical assistance when necessary, executes emergency measures as required, and may practice in a hospital, clinic, maternity home, or private home. The midwife, whose practice may include well-child care, family planning, and some aspects of gynecology, is often an important source of health counseling in the community. **3.** a nurse midwife or Certified Nurse Midwife.

**midwifery** /mid′wīf(ə)rē/ [AS, *midd* + *wif*], the employment of a person who is qualified by special training and experience to assist a woman in childbirth. See also **midwife.**

**MIF,** abbreviation for **macrophage inhibition factor.** See **macrophage migration inhibiting factor.**

**mifepristone** /mif′əpris′tōn/, an investigational drug that induces abortion if taken within the first 7 weeks of pregnancy. Two days after taking the drug to end the pregnancy, the woman must take a second drug to cause strong uterine contractions that expel the fetus. Mifepristone is reportedly effective 95.5% of the time, and serious complications are rare. However, the procedure may be somewhat painful, and a small percentage of patients have required blood transfusions. If the drug regimen fails to terminate the pregnancy, the woman must arrange for a surgical abortion to complete the process. Also called **RU-486.**

**miglitol,** an oral hypoglycemic.

- INDICATIONS: This drug is used to treat type 2 diabetes mellitus.
- CONTRAINDICATIONS: Factors that prohibit the use of this drug include known hypersensitivity to miglitol, diabetic ketoacidosis, cirrhosis, inflammatory bowel disease, colonic ulceration, partial intestinal obstruction, and chronic intestinal disease.
- ADVERSE EFFECTS: Hepatotoxicity is a life-threatening side effect of this drug. Other adverse effects are low iron and rash. Common side effects are abdominal pain, diarrhea, and flatulence.

**migraine** /mī′grān/ [Gk, *hemi,* half, *kranion,* skull], a recurring vascular headache characterized by unilateral onset, severe pain, photophobia, and autonomic disturbances during the acute phase, which may last for hours or days. The disorder occurs more frequently in women than in men, and a predisposition to migraine may be inherited. The exact mechanism responsible for the disorder is not known, but the head pain is related to dilation of extracranial blood vessels, which may be the result of chemical changes that cause spasms of intracranial vessels. A greatly increased amount of a vasodilating polypeptide related to bradykinin is found in tissue fluid of patients during migraine attacks. Allergic reactions, excess carbohydrates, iodine-rich foods, alcohol, bright lights, or loud noises may trigger attacks, which often occur during a period of relaxation after physical or psychic stress.

- OBSERVATIONS: An impending attack may be heralded by visual disturbances, such as aura, flashing lights or wavy lines, or by a strange taste or odor, numbness, tingling, vertigo, tinnitus, or a feeling that part of the body is distorted in size or shape. The acute phase may be accompanied by nausea, vomiting, chills, polyuria, sweating, facial edema, irritability, and extreme fatigue. After an attack the individual often has dull head and neck pains and a great need for sleep.
- INTERVENTIONS: Aspirin seldom provides relief during an attack, but ergotamine tartrate preparations that constrict cranial arteries can usually prevent the headache from developing if administered early in the onset via injection, suppository, or tablet. Ergotamine tartrate is also available in combination with other drugs, such as caffeine, phenobarbital, and belladonna; migraine patients unable to tolerate ergot preparations may use other analgesics, including acetaminophen, phenacetin, and propoxyphene.

**migraine headache.** See **headache.**

**migrainous cranial neuralgia** /mī′grānəs, mīgrā′nəs/ [Gk, *hemi,* half, *kranion,* skull; L, *osus,* having], a variant of migraine, characterized by closely spaced episodes of excruciating throbbing unilateral headaches often accompanied by dilation of temporal blood vessels, flushing, sweating, lacrimation, nasal congestion or rhinorrhea, ptosis, and facial edema. Repeated episodes usually occur in clusters within a few days or weeks and may be followed by a relatively long remission period. A typical attack begins abruptly without prodromal signs, as a burning sensation in an orbit or temple, and the resulting radiating intense pain

may last 1 or 2 hours. Histamine diphosphate injected subcutaneously in people subject to these headaches produces symptoms identical to those occurring in a spontaneous attack. The pain may be relieved by antihistamines, and ergotamine tartrate preparations may be helpful if administered at the onset of an attack. Also called **cluster headache, histamine headache, Horton's headache.** See also **migraine.**

**migrating phlebitis** /mī′grāting/ [L, *migrare,* to wander; Gk, *phleps,* vein, *itis,* inflammation], a form of phlebitis characterized by inflammation in one part of a vein and, after remission, in another part of the vein.

**migration** /mīgrā′shən/ [L, *migrare,* to wander], the passage of the ovum from the ovary into a fallopian tube and then into the uterus.

**migratory gonorrheal polyarthritis.** See **migratory polyarthritis.**

**migratory ophthalmia.** See **sympathetic ophthalmia.**

**migratory polyarthritis** /mī′grətôr′ē/, arthritis that progressively affects a number of joints and finally settles in one or more. It occurs in persons with gonorrhea and develops a few days to a few weeks after the onset of gonorrheal urethritis. The patient usually has a moderate fever and 1 to 5 days of migratory polyarthralgia with variable signs of inflammation. In more prolonged episodes initial arthritic sites may clear as new areas are affected, but persistently involved joints are usually severely inflamed and swollen. After the swelling subsides, the overlying skin may peel. Large joints are most affected. Treatment with penicillin or tetracycline generally provides some relief in 24 to 72 hours. Also called **migratory gonorrheal polyarthritis.**

**migratory thrombophlebitis,** an abnormal condition in which multiple thromboses appear in both superficial and deep veins. It may be associated with malignancy, especially carcinoma of the pancreas, often preceding other evidence of cancer by several months. Pulmonary embolism is uncommon with this condition. Also called **thrombophlebitis migrans.** See also **thrombophlebitis.**

**mikro-.** See **micro-.**

**Mikulicz's aphthae.** See **Sutton's disease.**

**Mikulicz's syndrome** /mik′yōōlich′ēz/ [Johann von Miculicz-Radecki, Polish surgeon, 1850–1905], an abnormal bilateral enlargement of the salivary and lacrimal glands. It is found in a variety of diseases, including leukemia, tuberculosis, and sarcoidosis. Also called **Mikulicz's disease.** Compare **Sjögren's syndrome.**

**mild** [AS, *milde,* soft], gentle, subtle, or of low intensity, such as a mild infection.

**mildew** /mil′dyōō/, a visible growth of any of numerous species of saprophytic fungi. Mildew causes discoloration and weakening of fabrics and fibers.

**milia.** See **milium.**

**milia neonatorum** [L, *milium,* millet; Gk, *neo,* new; L, *natus,* born], a nonpathologic dermatologic condition characterized by minute epidermal cysts consisting of keratinous debris that occur on the face and occasionally on the trunk of the newborn. They are eliminated by normal desquamation of the skin within a few weeks after birth and leave no scars.

**miliaria** /mil′ē·er′ē·ə/ [L, *milium,* millet], minute vesicles and papules, often with surrounding erythema, caused by occlusion of sweat ducts during times of exposure to heat and high humidity. Backup pressure may cause sweat to escape into adjacent tissue producing itching and prickling. Prevention and treatment include cool environment, ventilation, colloidal baths, and dusting powders. Also called **prickly heat.**

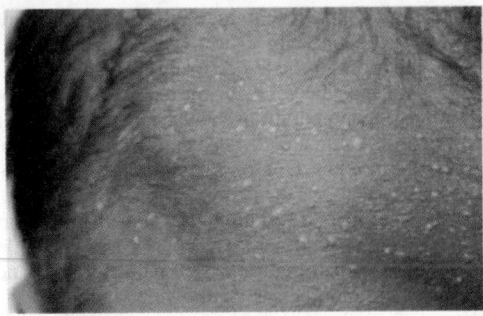

**Milia neonatorum** *(Weston and Lane, 1996)*

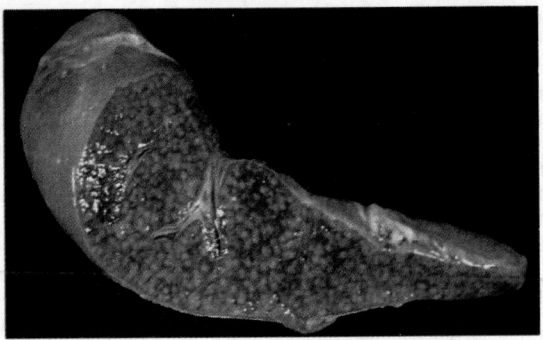

**Miliary tuberculosis of the spleen**
*(Kumar, Cotran, and Robbins, 1997)*

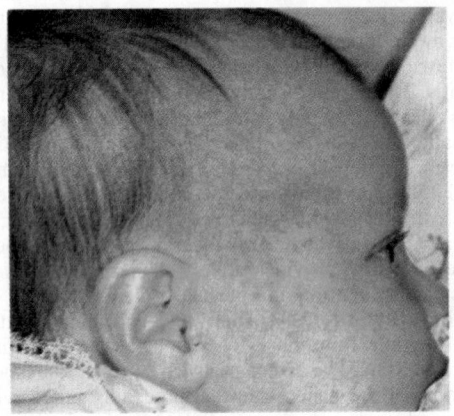

**Miliaria in infant** *(Habif, 1996)*

**miliary** /mil'ē·er'ē/ [L, *milium,* millet],  describing a condition marked by the appearance of very small lesions the size of millet seeds, such as miliary tuberculosis, which is characterized by tiny tubercles throughout the body.

**miliary carcinosis,**  a condition characterized by numerous cancerous nodules resembling miliary tubercles.

**miliary fever** [L, *milium,* millet; L, *febris*],  an inflammatory skin eruption caused by sweat retention. Sweat trapped in the dermis or epidermis causes irritation. Also called **prickly heat.**

**miliary tuberculosis,**  extensive dissemination by the bloodstream of tubercle bacilli. In children it is associated with high fever, night sweats, and often meningitis, pleural effusions, or peritonitis. A similar illness may occur in adults but with a less abrupt onset and occasionally with weeks or months of nonspecific symptoms, such as weight loss, weakness, and low-grade fever. Multiple small opacities resembling millet seeds may be evident on chest x-ray films. The liver, spleen, bone marrow, and meninges are often affected. The tuberculin test result may be negative, and diagnosis is made by biopsy of the infected tissue or organ. Combined drug therapy with isoniazid, rifampin, and pyrazinamide is usually successful if the diagnosis is not delayed. Concurrent tuberculous meningitis makes the prognosis less favorable. See also *Mycobacterium,* **tuberculosis.**

**milieu** /milyœ', milyo͞o'/, *pl.* **milieus, milieux** [Fr, middle],  the environment, surroundings, or setting. Kinds of milieus are **milieu extérieur** and **milieu intérieur.**

**milieu extérieur** /eksterē·œr'/,  the external or physical surroundings of an organism, including the social environment, especially the home, school, and recreational facilities, which play a dominant role in personality development.

**milieu intérieur** /aNterē·œr'/,  the basic concept in physiology, originated by Claude Bernard, that multicellular organisms exist in an aqueous internal environment composed of the blood, lymph, and interstitial fluid that bathes all cells and provides a medium for the elementary exchange of nutrients and waste material. All fundamental processes necessary for the maintenance and life of the tissue elements depend on the stability and balance of this environment.

**milieus.**  See **milieu.**

**milieu therapy[1],**  a type of psychotherapy in which the total environment is used in treating mental and behavioral disorders. It is primarily conducted in a hospital or other institutional setting, where the entire facility acts as a therapeutic community. The emphasis is on providing pleasant physical surroundings, structured activities, and a stable social environment where behavior modification and personal growth are promoted through patient-group interaction, staff support and understanding, and a total, humanistic approach. Individual daily routines and treatment modalities, such as drug therapy, occupational therapy, and sensitivity training, are determined by the patient's emotional and interpersonal needs. See also **situational therapy.**

**milieu therapy[2],**  a nursing intervention from the Nursing Interventions Classification (NIC) defined as use of people, resources, and events in the patient's immediate environment to promote optimal psychosocial functioning. See also **Nursing Interventions Classification.**

**milieux.**  See **milieu.**

**military antishock trousers (MAST)** [L, *ante,* opposed; Fr, *choc* + Gael, *triubhas,* trews],  a garment designed to produce pressure on the lower part of the body, thereby preventing the pooling of blood in the legs and abdomen. The trousers are used to combat shock and stabilize fractures, promote hemostasis, increase peripheral vascular resistance, and permit autotransfusion of small amounts of blood. They also are used in emergencies in the treatment of hemorrhagic shock. Also called **medical antishock trousers, pneumatic antishock garment.** See **shock trousers.**

**military attitude,**  (in obstetrics) a fetal position in which the fetal head is not flexed and the cervical spine is in extension.

**military time.** See **24-hour clock system.**

**milium** /mil′ē·əm/, *pl.* **milia** [L, millet], a minute white cyst of the epidermis caused by obstruction of hair follicles and eccrine sweat glands. One variety is seen in newborns and disappears within a few weeks. Another type is found primarily on the faces of middle-aged women. Milia may be treated with an abrasive cleanser or by incision and drainage. Compare **comedo, miliaria.**

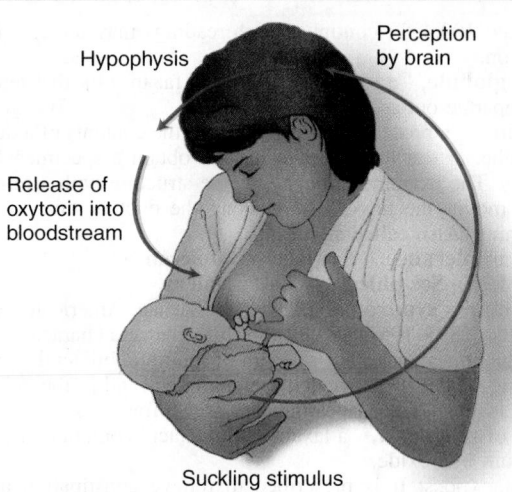

**Milk ejection reflex** *(Leonard, 2001)*

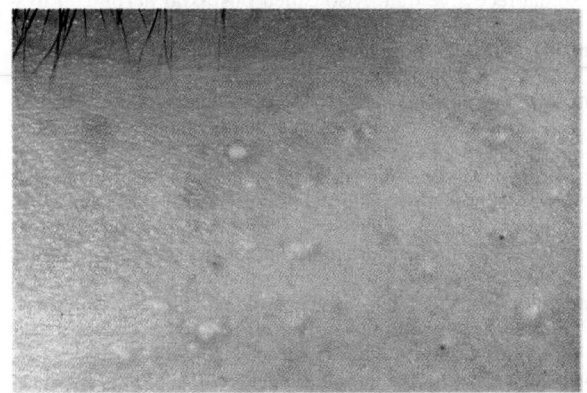

**Milia** *(du Vivier, 1993)*

**milk** [AS, *meoluc*], a liquid secreted by the mammary glands or udders of mammalian animals that suckle their young. After weaning, people consume the milk of the cow, as well as that of many other animals, including the goat, camel, mare, reindeer, llama, and yak. Milk is a basic food containing carbohydrate (in the form of lactose); protein (mainly casein, with small amounts of lactalbumin and lactoglobulin); suspended fat; the minerals calcium and phosphorus; and the vitamins A, riboflavin, niacin, thiamine, and, when the milk is fortified, vitamin D. Some individuals show a sensitivity reaction to milk caused by a deficiency of the enzyme lactase. See also **breast milk.**

**milk-alkali syndrome,** a condition of alkalosis caused by the excessive ingestion of milk, antacid medications containing calcium, or other sources of absorbable alkaline substances. The condition results in hypercalcemia, hypocalciuria, and calcium deposits in the kidneys and other tissues. The patient may experience symptoms of nausea, headache, weakness, and kidney damage. This condition occurs most frequently in older adults with peptic ulcers. Also called **Burnett's syndrome.**

**milk baby,** an infant with iron deficiency anemia caused by ingestion of excessive amounts of milk and delayed or inadequate addition of iron-rich foods to the diet. Milk babies are overweight, have pale skin and poor muscle development, and are highly susceptible to infection. See also **anemia.**

**milk bath,** a bath taken in milk for cosmetic or emollient reasons.

**milk ejection reflex,** a normal reflex in a lactating woman elicited by tactile stimulation of the nipple, resulting in release of milk from the glands of the breast. This reflex requires intact nerve connections from nipple to hypothalamus and release of the hormone oxytocin from the posterior pitu-

itary into the bloodstream. Also called **let-down reflex.** See also **oxytocin.**

**milker's nodule,** a smooth brownish-red papilloma of the fingers or palm that begins as a macule and progresses through a vesicular stage to become a nodule. The disease is acquired from pustular lesions on the udder of a cow infected with poxvirus. No treatment is necessary because immunity is produced after primary infection.

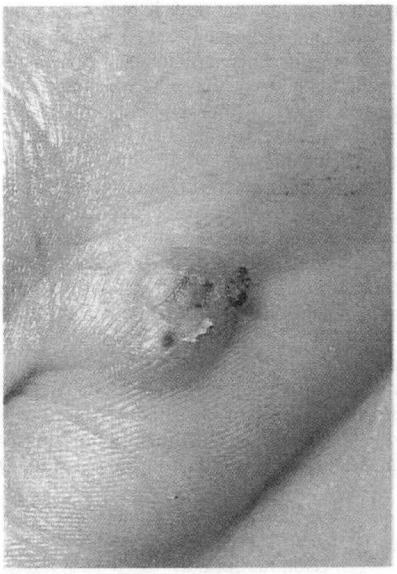

**Milker's nodule** *(Emond, Rowland, and Welsby, 1995)*

**milk fever,** *nontechnical.* postpartum fever that begins with the onset of lactation and lasts only a few hours. It was formerly considered a normal reaction to lactation. Maternal oral temperature during the puerperium does not normally exceed 100.4° F; continued high readings may indicate infection.

**milk globule,** a spherical droplet of fat in milk that tends to separate out as cream.

**milking,** a procedure used to express the contents of a duct or tube, to test for tenderness, or to obtain a specimen for study. The examiner compresses the structure with a finger and moves the finger firmly along the duct or tube to its opening. Also called **stripping.**

**milk intolerance.** See **lactose intolerance.**

**milk leg.** See **phlegmasia alba dolens.**

**Milkman's syndrome** [Louis A. Milkman, American radiologist, 1895–1951], a form of osteomalacia characterized by the appearance on x-ray film of multiple, bilateral, symmetric stripes in hypocalcified long bones and in the pelvis and scapula. The stripes indicate pseudofractures.

**milk of magnesia,** a laxative and antacid containing magnesium hydroxide.

■ INDICATIONS: It is prescribed to relieve constipation and less commonly, for acid indigestion.

■ CONTRAINDICATIONS: Renal impairment, symptoms of appendicitis, or known hypersensitivity to the drug prohibits its use.

■ ADVERSE EFFECTS: Among the most serious adverse reactions are diarrhea and hypermagnesemia, which usually occur in patients who have impaired renal function.

**milk patch.** See **macula albida.**

**milkpox.** See **alastrim.**

**milk sugar.** See **lactose.**

**milk therapy,** a nutritional treatment formerly used in the therapy of Curling's ulcer in patients who had been severely burned. Cool homogenized milk is administered in doses of 1 to 2 oz (28.3 to 56.7 g) every hour through a nasogastric tube. After instillation the tube is clamped for 5 minutes and then unclamped. Milk remaining in the stomach is allowed to flow into a basin. As the milk is better absorbed and tolerated, feedings are increased to 150 mL of milk per kilogram of body weight daily. The interval between feedings is gradually lengthened to 4 hours. As the condition improves, the nasogastric tube is withdrawn, and milk may be continued by mouth.

**milk thistle,** an herb that is native to Kashmir but is also found in North America from Canada to Mexico.

■ USES: This herb is used to protect against alcoholic cirrhosis and hepatitis, and as an antiinflammatory.

■ CONTRAINDICATIONS: Milk thistle should not be used during pregnancy and lactation, in children, or in people with hypersensitivity to this herb or other plants in the Asteraceae family.

**milky ascites.** See **chylous ascites.**

**Miller-Abbott tube** [Thomas G. Miller, American physician, 1886–1981; William O. Abbott, American physician, 1902–1943], a long small-caliber double-lumen catheter used in intestinal intubation for decompression. One lumen

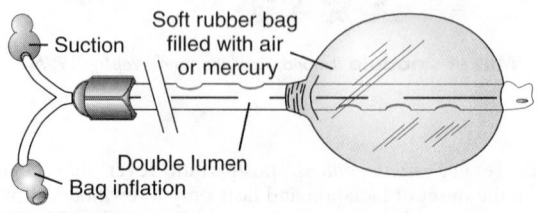

**Miller-Abbott tube** *(Lewis, Heitkemper, and Dirksen, 2000)*

ends in a perforated metal tip and the other in a collapsible balloon. These tubes are radiopaque and can therefore be seen on a radiogram. Compare **Harris tube.** See also **gastric intubation.**

**Miller syndrome** /mil′ər/ [Marvin Miller, American pediatrician, 20th century], a syndrome of extensive facial and limb defects, characterized by malar hypoplasia, downslanting palpebral fissures, micrognathia, cleft lip and palate, cup-shaped ears, lower lid ectropion, postaxial limb deficiencies, and syndactyly. Less frequently present are heart defects and hearing loss. The syndrome is probably an autosomal recessive trait. Also called **postaxial acrofacial dysostosis.**

**milli-** /mil′ē-/, prefix meaning '1/1000 part': *milliampere, millibar, milliliter.*

**milliampere (mA)** /-am′pir/ [L, *mille,* thousand; Andre Ampere], a unit of electric current that is one thousandth of an ampere. See also **ampere.**

**milliampere-second (mAs),** a measured of electric charge obtained by multiplying the electric current in milliamperes by the time in seconds. It is used to describe the exposure setting of a radiography machine and determines the density of the radiographic image.

**millicoulomb (mC)** /-kyoo′lōm/ [L, *mille,* thousand; Charles A. de Coulomb], a unit of electric charge that is one thousandth of a coulomb. See also **coulomb.**

**millicurie (mCi, mc)** /-koor′ē/ [L, *mille,* thousand; Marie Curie], a unit of radioactivity equal to one thousandth of a curie, or $3.70 \times 10^7$ disintegrations per second. See also **curie.**

**milliequivalent (mEq)** /-ikwiv′ələnt/ [L, *mille* + *aequus,* equal, *valere,* to be strong], **1.** the number of grams of solute dissolved in 1 mL of a normal solution. **2.** one thousandth of a gram equivalent.

**milliequivalent per liter (mEq/L),** one thousandth of 1 equivalent of a specific substance dissolved in 1 L of plasma.

**milligram (mg)** /-gram/ [L, *mille* + Fr, *gramme,* small weight], a metric unit of weight equal to one thousandth $(10^{-3})$ of a gram.

**milliliter (mL)** /-lē′tər/ [L, *mille* + Fr, *litre,* a measure], a metric unit of volume that is one thousandth $(10^{-3})$ of a liter, or 1 cm³.

**millimeter (mm)** /-mē′tər/, a metric unit of length equal to one thousandth $(10^{-3})$ of a meter.

**millimole (mmol, mM)** /-mōl/ [L, *mille* + *moles,* mass], a unit of metric measurement that is equal to one thousandth $(10^{-3})$ of a mole. It is equal to the formula weight of a substance in milligrams.

**milliosmol** /mil′ē·oz′mōl/, one thousandth of an osmole. See also **osmole, osmolality, osmolarity. —milliosmolar,** *adj.*

**millipede** /mil′ipēd′/ [L, *mille* + *pes,* foot], a many-legged wormlike arthropod. Certain species squirt irritating fluids that may cause dermatitis.

**millirad (mrad)** /-rad/, a unit of absorbed dose of ionizing radiation equal to one thousandth of a rad. See also **rad.**

**millirem (mrem),** a unit of ionizing radiation dose equal to one thousandth of a rem. See also **rem.**

**milliroentgen (mR, mr)** /mil′irent′gən, -jən/ [L, *mille,* thousand; Wilhelm K. Roentgen], a unit of radiation equal to one thousandth of a roentgen. See also **roentgen.**

**millisecond (msec)** /-sek′ənd/ [L, *mille,* thousand; ME, *seconde,* small part], one thousandth of a second.

**millivolt (mV, mv)** /-vōlt/ [L, *mille,* thousand; Alessandro Volta], a unit of electromotive force equal to one thousandth of a volt. See also **volt.**

**Milontin,** trademark for an anticonvulsant (phensuximide).

**Milroy's disease** /mil′roiz/ [William Forsyth Milroy, American physician, 1855−1942], congenital hereditary lymphedema of the legs caused by chronic lymphatic obstruction; other areas, including the arms, trunk, and face may be involved. Also called **congenital lymphedema, Meige's disease, Milroy's edema, Nonne-Milroy-Meige syndrome.**

**Miltown,** trademark for a sedative (meprobamate).

**Milwaukee brace** /milwô′kē/ [Milwaukee, Wisconsin; OFr, *bracier* to embrace], an orthotic device that helps immobilize the torso and neck of a patient in the treatment of scoliosis, lordosis, or kyphosis. It is usually constructed of strong but light metal and fiberglass bars lined with rubber to protect against abrasion. The bars, which commonly connect cervical supports, rib supports, and hip supports, hold the trunk and neck erect while controlling cervical flexion and hip movements. Milwaukee braces may be used in the treatment of orthopedic bed or ambulatory patients.

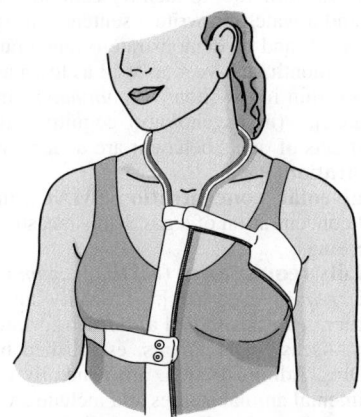

**Milwaukee brace** *(Phipps, Sands, and Marek, 1999)*

**-mimesis,** suffix meaning 'simulation, imitation': *necromimesis, neuromimesis, pathomimesis.*

**-mimetic,** suffix meaning 'simulation of (specified) effects': *andromimetic, neuromimetic, vagomimetic.*

**-mimia,** suffix meaning '(condition of) ability to express thought through gestures': *macromimia, paramimia.*

**mimicry** /mim′ikrē/ [Gk, *mimetikos,* imitation], **1.** the effort of one species or organism to resemble another to obtain an offensive or defensive advantage. **2.** an autonomic nervous system phenomenon in which facial expressions may be the unwilled and largely unconscious expression of feelings and ideas. See also **molecular mimicry.**

**mimic spasm** /mim′ik/ [Gk, *mimetikos,* imitative, *spasmos,* spasm], involuntary stereotyped movements of a small group of muscles such as of the face. The spasm is usually psychogenic and may be aggravated by stress or anxiety but is generally controllable momentarily. Multiple grimacing and blinking mimic spasms occur in Gilles de la Tourette's syndrome. Also called **tic.**

**min,** **1.** abbreviation for **minim.** **2.** abbreviation for *minute.*

**Minamata disease** /min′əmä′tə/, a severe degenerative neurologic disorder caused by the ingestion of seed grain heated with alkyl compounds of mercury or of seafood taken from waters polluted with industrial wastes contaminated by soluble mercuric salts. The term is derived from a tragedy involving Japanese who ate seafood from Minamata Bay. Mercury passes the placental barrier, causing the congenital form of the disease. Symptoms may not appear for several weeks or months; they include paresthesia of the mouth and extremities; tunnel vision; difficulties in speech, hearing, muscular coordination, and concentration; weakness; emotional instability; and stupor. Continued ingestion causes serious damage to the renal tubules and corrosion of the GI tract. Acute cases may result in coma and death. See also **mercury poisoning.**

**mind** [AS, *gemynd*], **1.** the part of the brain that is the seat of mental activity and that enables one to know, reason, understand, remember, think, feel, react to, and adapt to external and internal stimuli. **2.** the totality of all conscious and unconscious processes of the individual that influence and direct mental and physical behavior. **3.** the faculty of the intellect or understanding, in contrast to emotion and will. See also **brain, intellect, psyche.**

**mine damp.** See **damp.**

**mineral** /min′ərəl/ [L, *minera,* mine], **1.** an inorganic substance occurring naturally in the earth's crust, having a characteristic chemical composition and (usually) crystalline structure. **2.** (in nutrition) a compound containing a metal, nonmetal, radical, or phosphate that is needed for proper body function and maintenance of health. The needed substance is ingested as a part of such a compound, such as table salt (sodium chloride), instead of as a free element, and the compound is usually referred to by the name of the needed substance.

**mineral deficiency.** See specific minerals.

**mineralization** /-īzā′shən/ [L, *minera* + Gk, *izein,* to cause], the addition of any mineral to the body.

**mineral jelly.** See **petroleum jelly.**

**mineralocorticoid** /min′əral′ōkôr′tikoid/ [L, *minera* + *cortex,* bark; Gk, *eidos,* form], a hormone, secreted by the adrenal cortex, that maintains normal blood volume, promotes sodium and water retention, and increases urinary excretion of potassium and hydrogen ions. Aldosterone, the most potent mineralocorticoid with regard to electrolyte balance, and corticosterone, a glucocorticoid and a mineralocorticoid, act on the distal tubules of the kidneys to enhance the reabsorption of sodium into the plasma. Trauma and stress increase mineralocorticoid secretion. The synthetic mineralocorticoids desoxycorticosterone, which does not influence carbohydrate metabolism, and fludrocortisone, which also has glucocorticoid activity, are used in treating the salt-losing adrenogenital syndrome and the severe corticoid deficiency characteristic of Addison's disease. See also **glucocorticoid.**

**mineral oil,** a laxative, stool softener, emollient, and pharmaceutic aid used as a solvent.

■ INDICATIONS: It is prescribed to prevent constipation, to treat mild constipation, to prepare the bowel for surgery or examination, and to act as a solvent for various preparations.

■ CONTRAINDICATIONS: Appendicitis, fecal impaction, obstruction or perforation of the intestinal tract, pregnancy, or known hypersensitivity to this drug prohibits its use.

■ ADVERSE EFFECTS: Among the more serious adverse reactions are laxative dependence, lipid pneumonitis, fat-soluble vitamin deficiency, and abdominal cramps.

**mineral soap.** See **bentonite.**

**miner's cramp.** See **heat cramp.**

**miner's elbow** [L, *minera* + AS, *elboga*], an inflammation of the olecranon bursa, caused by resting the weight of the body on the elbow, as in some coal mining activities. The condition is sometimes seen in schoolchildren who lean on their elbows. Compare **lateral humeral epicondylitis.** See also **bursitis.**

**miner's pneumoconiosis.** See **anthracosis.**

**Minerva cast** /minur'və/ [L, *Minerva,* Roman goddess of wisdom; ONorse, *kasta*], an orthopedic cast applied to the trunk and head, with spaces cut out for the face and ears. The section encasing the trunk extends to the sternum and the distal rib border anteriorly and across the distal rib border posteriorly. The cast is used to immobilize the head and part of the trunk in the treatment of torticollis, cervical and thoracic injuries, and cervical spinal infections. It is not used as frequently as it once was because of advances in the field of orthotics. Also called **Minerva jacket.**

**Minerva jacket.** See **Minerva cast.**

**minicomputer** /min'ikəmpyŏŏ'tər/ [L, *minimum,* smallest, *computare,* to calculate], a medium-sized computer, intermediate in size and processing capacity between a microcomputer and a mainframe computer. Compare **mainframe computer, microcomputer.**

**minim (min)** /min'im/ [L, *minimus,* smallest], a measurement of volume in the apothecaries' system, originally one drop (of water). Sixty minims equals 1 fluid dram. One minim equals 0.06 mL.

**minimal access surgery.** See **minimally invasive surgery.**

**minimal bactericidal concentration,** the lowest concentration of drug that results in a 99.9% reduction in the initial bacterial density. Compare **minimal inhibitory concentration (MIC).**

**minimal brain dysfunction.** See **attention deficit disorder.**

**minimal care unit** /min'iməl/ [L, *minimus,* smallest], a unit for the treatment of inpatients who are ambulatory and able to meet many of their own daily living needs but require minimal nursing care.

**minimal change disease,** a kidney disorder characterized by subtle changes in renal function, including albuminuria and presence of lipid droplets in the proximal tubules. It mainly affects small children but also occurs in adults with idiopathic nephrotic syndrome. It may or may not progress to glomerulonephritis. Also called **lipoid nephrosis, nil disease.** See also **idiopathic nephrotic syndrome.**

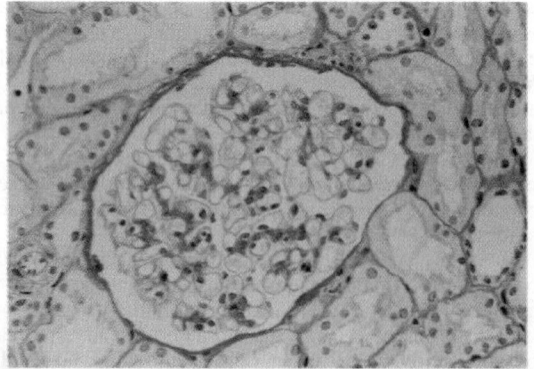

**Minimal change disease** *(Cotran, Kumar, and Collins, 1999)*

**minimal dose.** See **minimum dose.**

**minimal erythema dose.** See **threshold dose.**

**minimal infecting dose,** the smallest amount of infective material that usually produces infection.

**minimal inhibitory concentration (MIC),** the lowest concentration of an antibiotic medication in the blood that is effective against an infection, determined by injecting infected venous blood into a culture medium containing various concentrations of a proposed antibiotic. The lowest antibiotic concentration that stops microbial growth may be used in further treatment of the patient. Also called **minimum inhibitory concentration.** Compare **minimal bactericidal concentration.**

**minimally invasive surgery,** surgery done with only a small incision or no incision at all, such as through a cannula with a laparoscope or endoscope.

**minimal occlusive volume (MOV),** the volume to which an endotracheal or tracheostomy tube cuff must be inflated to obliterate an air leak during the inspiratory phase of ventilation. Also called **minimal occlusive pressure.**

**Mini-Mental State Examination (MMS),** a brief psychologic test designed to differentiate among dementia, psychosis, and affective disorders. It may include ability to count backward by 7s from 100, to identify common objects such as a pencil and a watch, to write a sentence, to spell simple words backward, and to demonstrate orientation by identifying the day, month, and year, as well as town and country.

**minimization** /min'imizā'shən/ [L, *minimum,* smallest; Gk, *izein,* to cause], (in psychology) cognitive distortion in which the effects of one's behavior are underestimated. See also **magnification.**

**minimum alveolar concentration (MAC)** /min'iməm/, the smallest concentration of a gas that is measured in the alveoli of the lungs.

**minimum daily requirement (MDR)** [L, *minimum* + OE, *daeglie* + L, *requirere,* to seek], the daily human requirement of nutrients for health and as needed for prevention of a deficiency disease. The figures, established by the U.S. Food and Drug Administration, are generally extrapolated from experimental animal studies and include an added margin for safety. See also **Estimated Safe and Adequate Daily Dietary Intake.**

**minimum dose** [L, *minimum,* smallest; Gk, *dosis,* giving], the smallest amount of a drug or other substance needed to produce a desired or specified effect. Because of individual variations in drug response, the minimal dose for one person may be either excessive or insufficient for another patient. Also called **minimal dose.**

**minimum hemagglutinating dose,** the smallest amount of hemagglutinating agent that causes a complete hemagglutinating reaction in a standard volume of red blood cells.

**minimum hemolytic dose (MHD),** the smallest amount of a reagent that produces complete lysis of a specified amount of red blood cells.

**minimum inhibitory concentration.** See **minimal inhibitory concentration.**

**minimum lethal dose (MLD)** [L, *minimum,* smallest, *lethum,* death; Gk, *dosis,* giving], the smallest dose of a drug, relative to body weight, that will kill an experimental animal. The MLD may vary with the species of animal tested. Also called *minimum fatal dose (MFD).* See also **median lethal dose.**

**Minipress,** trademark for an antihypertensive (prazosin hydrochloride); an alpha₁ receptor blocking agent.

**miniprotein** /min'iprō'tēn/, a protein that has been reduced to half its natural size without loss of its ability to function.

**Ministry of Indian Affairs.** See **Indian Health Service.**

**Minnesota Multiphasic Personality Inventory (MMPI),** a commonly used psychologic test that includes 550 statements for interpretation by the subject, used clinically for evaluating personality and for detecting various disorders.

**Minocin,** trademark for an antibacterial (minocycline hydrochloride).

**minocycline hydrochloride** /min′əsī′klēn/, a tetracycline antibiotic active against bacteria, rickettsia, and other organisms.

■ INDICATIONS: It is prescribed in the treatment of infections.

■ CONTRAINDICATIONS: It must be used with caution in cases of renal or hepatic dysfunction. Known hypersensitivity to this or other tetracyclines prohibits its use.

■ ADVERSE EFFECTS: Among the more serious adverse reactions are GI disturbances, phototoxicity, vestibular toxicity, potentially serious superinfections, and various allergic reactions. Use during pregnancy or in children less than 8 years of age may result in discoloration of teeth.

**minor** /mī′nər/ [L, smaller], (in law) a person not of legal age; a person beneath the age of majority. Minors usually cannot consent to their own medical treatment unless they are substantially independent of their parents, are married, support themselves, or satisfy other requirements specified by statute. See also **emancipated minor.**

**minor connector,** a device that links the major connector or base of a removable partial denture to other denture units, such as rests and direct and indirect retainers.

**minor epilepsy.** See **absence seizure.**

**minor hysteria** [Gk, *hystera,* womb], a mild disorder that may be expressed in emotional outbursts, repressed anxieties, or conversion of unconscious conflicts into physical symptoms.

**minor renal calyx.** See **renal calyx.**

**minor surgery,** surgical procedure for minor problems or injuries that are not considered life-threatening or hazardous. Compare **major surgery.**

**Minot-Murphy diet** [George R. Minot, American physician, 1885–1950; William P. Murphy, American physician, b. 1892], a dietary regimen developed in the 1930s for the treatment of pernicious anemia with large amounts of raw or slightly cooked liver or crude extracts of fresh calf liver. See also **pernicious anemia.**

**minoxidil** /mīnok′sidil/, a vasodilator.

■ INDICATION: It is prescribed in the treatment of severe refractory hypertension and as a topical solution for the treatment of androgenic alopecia.

■ CONTRAINDICATIONS: Pheochromocytoma or known hypersensitivity to this drug prohibits its use.

■ ADVERSE EFFECTS: Among the most serious adverse reactions are tachycardia, pericardial effusion, cardiac tamponade, salt and water retention, and excessive hair growth. GI disturbances also may occur.

**mint,** an herb that is native to Europe and is now grown widely throughout the United States and Canada.

■ USES: This herb is used for GI disorders.

■ CONTRAINDICATIONS: Mint should not be used during pregnancy and lactation, in children, or in those with known hypersensitivity or gastroesophageal reflux disease.

**Mintezol,** trademark for an anthelmintic (thiabendazole).

**minute ventilation** /min′it/ [L, *minus,* very small], the total lung ventilation per minute, the product of tidal volume and respiration rate. It is measured by expired gas collection for a period of 1 to 3 minutes. The normal rate is 5 to 10 liters per minute.

**mio-, meio-,** combining form meaning 'less': *miolecithal, mioplasmia, miosphygmia.*

**miosis** /mī·ō′sis/ [Gk, *meiosis,* becoming less], **1.** contraction of the sphincter muscle of the iris, causing the pupil to become smaller. Certain drugs and stimulation of the pupillary light reflex by an increase in light result in miosis. **2.** an abnormal condition characterized by excessive constriction of the sphincter muscle of the iris, resulting in very small, pinpoint pupils. Compare **mydriasis.**

**miotic** /mē·ot′ik/, **1.** pertaining to miosis. **2.** causing constriction of the pupil of the eye. **3.** any substance or pharmaceutic, such as pilocarpine, that causes constriction of the pupil of the eye. Such agents are used in the treatment of glaucoma.

**MIP,** abbreviation for **maximum inspiratory pressure.**

**miracidium** /mir′əsid′ē·əm/, *pl.* **miracidia** [Gk, *meirakidion,* youthfulness], the ciliated larva of a parasitic trematode that hatches from an egg and can survive only by penetrating and further developing within a host snail, whereupon the larva further develops into a maternal sporocyte that produces more larvae.

**mirage** /miräzh′/ [L, *mirari,* to look at], an optical illusion caused by the refraction of light through air layers of different temperatures, such as the illusionary sheets of water that appear to shimmer over stretches of hot sand and pavement. This phenomenon is caused by bending of horizontal light waves upward from the layer of heated air directly over the hot surface. Wind rippling the air layers may produce surprising changes in the shapes and sizes of such mirages. Individuals under severe stress are especially susceptible to interpreting these optic phenomena in bizarre, unrealistic ways.

**mirror image** /mir′ər/ [L, *mirare,* to look at, *imago*], **1.** an image formed by a reflection in a plane mirror. **2.** a kind of reversed asymmetry of characteristics often found in sets of monozygotic twins. **3.** chemical molecules with the same composition but with asymmetric arrangement of the atoms.

**mirror speech** [L, *mirari,* to look at; AS, *spaec,* speech], an abnormal manner of speaking characterized by the reversal of the order of syllables in a word.

**mirtazapine,** an antidepressant.

■ INDICATIONS: This drug is used to treat depression, dysthymic disorder, and bipolar disorder with either depression or agitation.

■ CONTRAINDICATIONS: Factors that prohibit the use of this drug include known hypersensitivity to tricyclic antidepressants, convulsive disorders, and prostatic hypertrophy. Its use is also contraindicated in patients who are in the recovery phase of a myocardial infarction.

■ ADVERSE EFFECTS: Life-threatening effects of this drug are agranulocytosis, thrombocytopenia, eosinophilia, leukopenia, seizures, paralytic ileus, jaundice, hepatitis, acute renal failure, and hypertension. Other adverse effects include confusion, headache, anxiety, tremors, stimulation, nightmares, extrapyramidal symptoms (in the elderly), increased psychiatric symptoms, nausea, vomiting, cramps, epigastric distress, stomatitis, rash, photosensitivity, palpitations, tinnitus, and mydriasis. Common side effects are dizziness, drowsiness, diarrhea, dry mouth, urinary retention, orthostatic hypotension, electrocardiogram changes, tachycardia, and blurred vision.

**mis-,** prefix meaning 'wrong or badly': *misdiagnosis.*

**miscarriage.** See **spontaneous abortion.**

**miscible** /mis′ibəl/ [L, *miscere,* to mix], able to be mixed or blended with another substance. Compare **immiscible.**

**misdemeanor** /mis′dəmē′nər/ [AS, *missan,* to miss; ME, *demenen,* conduct], (in criminal law) an offense that is considered less serious than a felony and carries a lesser penalty, usually a fine or imprisonment for less than 1 year. Conviction for a misdemeanor does not prohibit the person from holding public office or from practicing a licensed occupation.

**misfeasance** /misfē'zəns/ [AS, *missan,* to miss; L, *facere,* to make], an improper performance of a lawful act, especially in a way that may cause damage or injury. Compare **malfeasance, nonfeasance.**

**miso-,** combining form meaning 'hatred of': *misocainia, misogyny, misopedia.*

**misogamy** /misog'əmē/ [Gk, *misein,* to hate, *gamos,* marriage], an aversion to marriage. —**misogamic, misogamous,** *adj.,* **misogamist,** *n.*

**misogyny** /misoj'inē/ [Gk, *misein,* to hate, *gyne,* women], an aversion to women. —**misogynist,** *n.,* **misogynistic,** *adj.*

**misopedia** /mis'ōpē'dē·ə/ [Gk, *misein* + *pais,* children], an aversion to children. —**misopedic,** *adj.,* **misopedist,** *n.*

**misophobia, misophobic.** See **mysophobia.**

**missed abortion** [OE, *missan,* to be lacking; L, *ab,* away from, *oriri,* to be born], a condition in which a dead immature embryo or fetus is not expelled from the uterus for 2 months or more. The uterus diminishes in size, and symptoms of pregnancy abate; maternal infection and blood clotting disorders may follow. The fetus and placenta may become necrotic; less commonly the fetus becomes calcified, and the rest of the products of conception are resorbed.

**missed period** [OE, *missan,* to be lacking; Gk, *peri* + *hodos,* way], an unexplained interruption in the menstrual cycle.

**missile fracture** [L, *mittere,* to throw], a penetration fracture caused by a projectile, such as a bullet or a piece of shrapnel.

**mistura** /mistyoo'rə/ [L, mixture], any of a number of mixtures of drugs, usually containing suspensions of insoluble substances intended for internal use. Examples include **mistura kaolini et morphinae,** a mixture of kaolin and morphine, and **mistura cretae pro infantibus,** a mixture of chalk, tragacanth, chloroform water, and other ingredients formulated for the treatment of GI disorders in infants.

**mite** /mīt/ [AS], a minute arachnid with a flat, almost transparent body and four pairs of legs. Many species of these relatives of ticks and spiders are parasitic, including the chigger and *Sarcoptes scabiei,* which cause localized pruritus and inflammation. Some female mites burrow into the skin and lay eggs that hatch into larvae; the movements of the larvae cause intense itching. See also **chigger, scabies.**

**mite typhus.** See **scrub typhus.**

**Mithracin,** trademark for an antineoplastic (plicamycin).

**mithramycin.** See **plicamycin.**

**mithridatism.** See **tachyphylaxis.**

**mitleiden** /mit'līdən/ [Ger, *mit,* with, *leiden,* to suffer], psychosomatic symptoms sometimes experienced by expectant fathers.

**mito-,** combining form meaning 'threadlike': *mitochondria, mitokinetic, mitoplasm.*

**mitochondrion** /mī'tōkon'drē·on/, *pl.* **mitochondria** [Gk, *mitos,* thread, *chondros,* cartilage], a rodlike, threadlike, or granular organelle that functions in aerobic respiration and occurs in varying numbers in all eukaryotic cells except mature erythrocytes. It is bounded by two sets of membranes, a smooth outer one and an inner one that is arranged in folds, or cristae, that extend into the interior of the mitochondrion, called the matrix. Mitochondria provide the principal source of cellular energy through oxidative phosphorylation and adenosine triphosphate synthesis. They also contain the enzymes involved with electron transport and the citric acid and fatty acid cycles. Mitochondria are self-replicating and contain their own DNA, RNA polymerase, transfer RNA, and ribosomes. Also called **chondriosome.** —**mitochondrial,** *adj.*

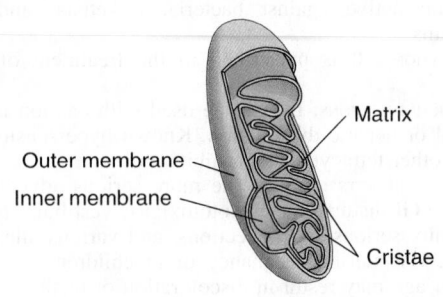

Outer membrane — Inner membrane — Matrix — Cristae

**Mitochondrion** *(Thibodeau and Patton, 1999)*

**mitogen** /mī'təjən, mit'-/ [Gk, *mitos* + *genein,* to produce], an agent that triggers mitosis. **mitogenic,** *adj.*

**mitogenesia** /mī'tōjənē'zhə/ [Gk, *mitos* + *genein,* to produce], production resulting from mitosis.

**mitogenesis** /mī'tōjen'əsis/, the induction of mitosis in a cell. —**mitogenetic,** *adj.*

**mitogenetic radiation** /-jənet'ik/, the force or specific energy that is supposedly given off by cells undergoing division. It may in turn stimulate the process of mitosis in other cells. Also called **Gurvich radiation, mitogenic radiation.**

**mitogenic factor** /-jen'ik/, a lymphokine that is released from activated T lymphocytes and stimulates the production of normal unsensitized lymphocytes.

**mitogenic radiation.** See **mitogenetic radiation.**

**mitome** /mī'tōm/, the reticular network sometimes observed within the cytoplasm and nucleoplasm of fixed cells. See also **cytomitome, karyomitome.**

**mitomycin** /mītəmī'sin/, an antineoplastic antibiotic.
- INDICATIONS: It is prescribed in the treatment of malignant neoplastic diseases.
- CONTRAINDICATIONS: Clotting deficiency, thrombocytopenia, or known hypersensitivity to this drug prohibits its use.
- ADVERSE EFFECTS: The most serious adverse reaction is bone marrow depression. GI disturbances, alopecia, and skin reactions commonly occur.

**mitosis** /mītō'sis, mit-/ [Gk, *mitos,* thread], a type of cell division that occurs in somatic cells and results in the formation of two genetically identical daughter cells containing the diploid number of chromosomes characteristic of the species. It consists of the division of the nucleus followed by the division of the cytoplasm. The former has four stages (prophase, metaphase, anaphase, and telophase), during which the two chromatids of each chromosome separate and migrate to opposite ends of the cell. Mitosis is the process by which the body produces new cells for both growth and repair of injured tissue. Kinds of mitosis are **heterotypic mitosis, homeotypic mitosis, multipolar mitosis,** and **pathologic mitosis.** Also called **indirect division.** Compare **meiosis.** See also **anaphase, interphase, metaphase, prophase, telophase.** —**mitotic,** *adj.*

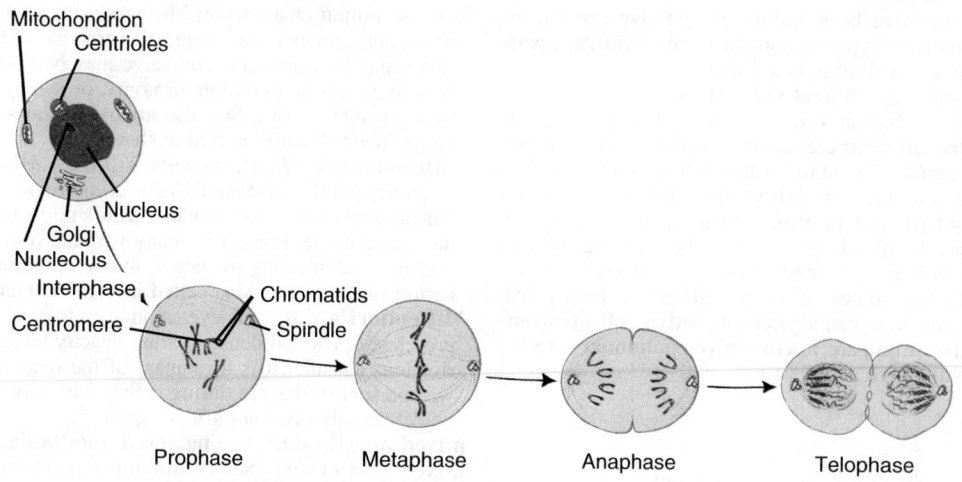

**Mitosis** *(Thibodeau and Patton, 1996/Network Graphics)*

**mitotane** /mī′tətān/,   an antineoplastic that destroys normal and neoplastic adrenal cortical cells.

■ INDICATION: It is prescribed in the treatment of carcinoma of the adrenal cortex.

■ CONTRAINDICATION: Known hypersensitivity to this drug is the only contraindication.

■ ADVERSE EFFECTS: Among the more serious adverse reactions are GI symptoms, lethargy, and adrenal insufficiency.

**mitotic** /mītot′ik/ [Gk, *mitos*, thread],   pertaining to or characterized by mitosis, the process of cell division in the formation of identical daughter cells.

**mitotic figure** [Gk, *mitos* + L, *figura*, form],   any chromosome or chromosome aggregation during any of the stages of mitosis.

**mitotic index,**   the number of cells per unit (usually 1000 cells) undergoing mitosis during a given time. The ratio is used primarily as an estimation of the rate of tissue growth.

**mitoxantrone,**   a synthetic antineoplastic anthracenedione for IV use.

■ INDICATIONS: It is prescribed in combination with other approved drugs in the initial treatment of acute lymphocytic leukemia in adults.

■ CONTRAINDICATIONS: The drug should not be given to patients with evidence of demonstrated prior hypersensitivity to it. Its use should be accompanied by close and frequent monitoring of hematologic and chemical laboratory parameters, as well as frequent patient observation.

■ ADVERSE EFFECTS: The side effects most often reported include hypotension, urticaria, dyspnea, rashes, phlebitis, myelosuppression, nausea, and vomiting.

**mitral** /mī′trəl/ [L, *mitra*, turban],   **1.** pertaining to the mitral valve of the heart. **2.** shaped like a miter.

**mitral atresia,**   a congenital absence of the mitral valve associated with transposition of the great vessels or hypoplastic left heart syndrome. See also **valvular heart disease.**

**mitral (bicuspid) valve.**   See **semilunar valve.**

**mitral commissurotomy** [L, *mitra*, turban, *commissura*, joining together; Gk, *temnein*, to cut],   a closed-heart surgical procedure in which the mitral valve is divided at the junction of its cusps for the treatment of mitral valve stenosis.

**mitral gradient,**   the difference in pressure in the left atrium and left ventricle during diastole.

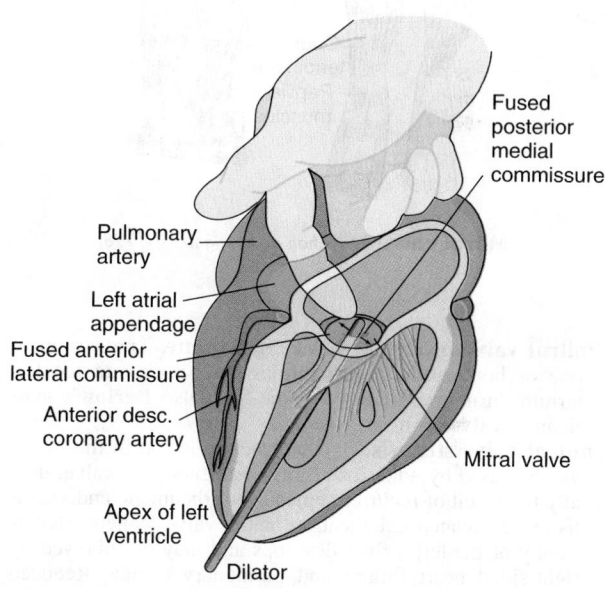

**Mitral commissurotomy** *(Beare and Myers, 1998)*

**mitral insufficiency.**   See **mitral regurgitation.**

**mitral murmur** [L, *mitra*, turban, *murmur,* humming],   a heart murmur caused by a defective mitral valve.

**mitral regurgitation,**   a backflow of blood from the left ventricle into the left atrium in systole across a diseased mitral valve. The condition may result from congenital valve abnormalities, rheumatic fever, mitral valve prolapse, endocardial fibroelastosis, myocarditis, myocardiopathy, or dilation of the left ventricle as a result of severe anemia. Symptoms include dyspnea, fatigue, intolerance of exercise, systolic murmur, and heart palpitations. Congestive heart failure may ultimately occur. Treatment depends on the severity of the condition. Surgery may be necessary in cases of refractory congestive heart failure, progressive cardiomegaly, and pulmonary hypertension. Also called **mitral insufficiency.** See also **valvular heart disease.**

**mitral stenosis.**    See **mitral valve stenosis.**

**mitral valve,** a bicuspid valve situated between the left atrium and the left ventricle; the only valve with two, rather than three, cusps. The mitral valve allows blood to flow from the left atrium into the left ventricle but prevents blood from flowing back into the atrium. Ventricular contraction in systole forces the blood against the valve, closing the two cusps and assuring the flow of blood from the ventricle into the aorta. The ventral cusp of the mitral valve is longer than the dorsal cusp. Also called **bicuspid valve, left atrioventricular valve.** Compare **aortic valve, pulmonary valve, semilunar valve, tricuspid valve.**

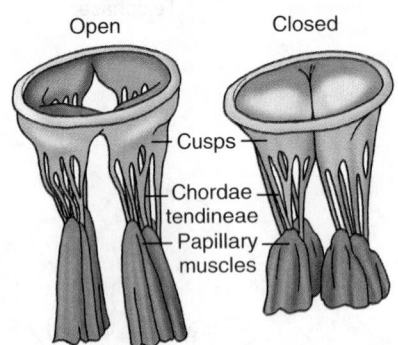

Open        Closed

Cusps
Chordae tendineae
Papillary muscles

**Mitral valve** *(Monahan and Neighbors, 1998)*

**mitral valve prolapse (MVP) syndrome,** protrusion of one or both cusps of the mitral valve back into the left atrium during ventricular systole. See also **Barlow's syndrome, valvular heart disease.**

**mitral valve stenosis,** an obstructive lesion in the mitral valve caused by adhesions on the leaflets of the valve, usually the result of recurrent episodes of rheumatic endocarditis or age-related calcification of the valve leaflets. Hypertrophy of the left atrium develops and may be followed by right-sided heart failure and pulmonary edema. Reduced

cardiac output characteristically produces fatigue, dyspnea, orthopnea, and cyanosis. Surgical correction of the defective valve may be necessary. The valve may be freed of the adhesions in a mitral commissurotomy, or it may be replaced by a prosthetic valve. See also **atrioventricular valve, valvular heart disease, valvular stenosis.**

**mittelschmerz** /mit′əlshmerts/ [Ger, *Mitte*, middle, *Schmerz*, pain], abdominal pain in the region of an ovary during ovulation, which usually occurs midway through the menstrual cycle. Present in many women, mittelschmerz is useful for identifying ovulation, thus pinpointing the fertile period of the cycle. Also called **intermenstrual pain.**

**Mittendorf's dot,** an eye anomaly characterized by the presence of a small dense floating opacity behind the posterior lens capsule. It is a remnant of the hyaloid artery that was present in the eye during embryonic development. The object usually does not affect vision.

**mixed anesthesia.**    See **balanced anesthesia.**

**mixed aneurysm.**    See **compound aneurysm.**

**mixed anxiety-depressive disorder,** a mental disorder characterized by symptoms of depression and of anxiety, but not meeting the full criteria for either a depressive disorder or an anxiety disorder.

**mixed aphasia.**    See **global aphasia.**

**mixed cell malignant lymphoma** [L, *miscere*, to mix], a lymphoid neoplasm containing lymphocytes and histiocytes (macrophages).

**mixed cell sarcoma,** a tumor consisting of two or more cellular elements, excluding fibrous tissue. Also called **malignant mesenchymoma.**

**mixed connective tissue disease (MCTD),** a systemic disease characterized by the combined symptoms of various collagen diseases, such as synovitis, polymyositis, scleroderma, and systemic lupus erythematosus. There is a high concentration of antibodies of ribonucleoprotein. Other symptoms may include arthralgia, muscle inflammation, nondeforming arthritis, swollen hands, esophageal hypomotility, and reduced diffusing capacity of the lungs. Treatment often includes the administration of corticosteroids. Recurrence is common when the steroid medication is discontinued.

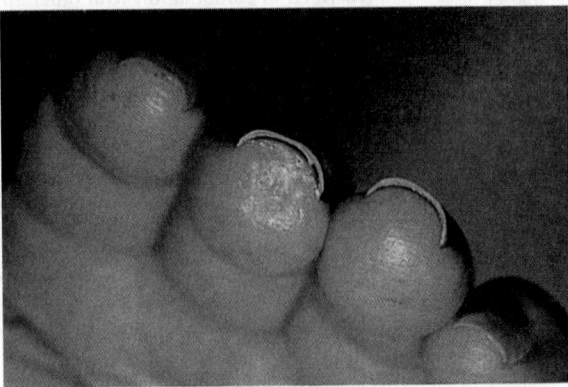

**Mixed connective tissue disease** *(White, 1994)*

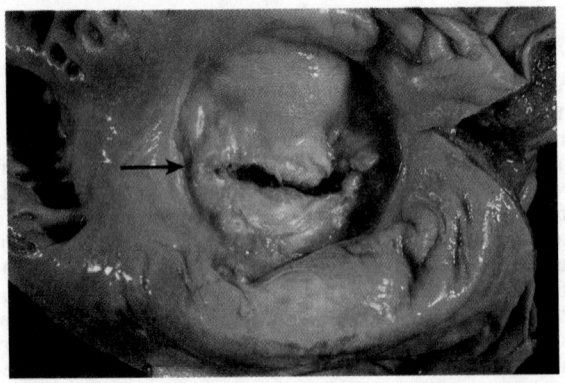

**Mitral valve stenosis** *(Cotran, Kumar, and Collins, 1999)*

**mixed culture** [L, *miscere*, to mix, *colere*, to cultivate], a laboratory culture that contains two or more different strains of organisms.

**mixed dentition,** dentition containing both deciduous and secondary teeth. It usually occurs between 6 and 13 years of age.

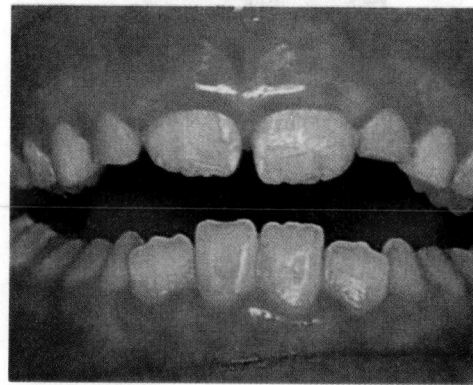

**Mixed dentition** *(Zitelli and Davis, 1997)*

**mixed dust pneumoconiosis,** pneumoconiosis that is caused by more than one type of dust.

**mixed glioma,** a tumor, composed of glial cells, that contains more than one kind of cell; the most common being nonneural cells of ectodermal origin.

**mixed hearing loss,** deafness that is both conductive and sensorineural in nature.

**mixed hyperlipemia.** See **hyperlipidemia type V.**

**mixed hypertriglyceridemia.** See **hyperlipidemia type V.**

**mixed infection,** an infection by several microorganisms, as in some abscesses, pneumonia, and infections of wounds. Numerous combinations of bacteria, viruses, and fungi may be involved. Compare **endogenous infection, germinal infection, retrograde infection, secondary infection.**

**mixed leukemia,** a malignancy of blood-forming tissues characterized by the proliferation of more than one predominant cell line.

**mixed lymphocyte culture (MLC) reaction,** an assay of the function of T cells. It is used primarily for histocompatibility testing before grafting.

**mixed neoplasm** [L, *miscere,* to mix; Gk, *neos,* new + *plasma,* something formed], a tumor or growth involving two germinal layers of tissue.

**mixed nerve** [L, *miscere,* to mix, *nervus*], a nerve that contains both sensory and motor fibers.

**mixed porphyria.** See **variegate porphyria.**

**mixed receptive-expressive language disorder,** a communication disorder involving both the expression and the comprehension of language, either spoken or signed. Patients have difficulties with language production, such as in selection of words and creation of appropriate sentences, and also have trouble understanding words, sentences, or specific types of words.

**mixed sleep apnea,** a condition marked by signs and symptoms of both central sleep apnea and obstructive sleep apnea. It often begins as central sleep apnea and develops into the obstructive form. Mixed sleep apnea may also result from obstructive sleep apnea as hypoxia and hypercapnia induce signs and symptoms of the central form. See also **central sleep apnea, obstructive sleep apnea.**

**mixed tumor,** a growth composed of more than one kind of neoplastic tissue.

**mixed vaccine,** an immunizing preparation that protects against more than one kind of pathogen, such as the diphtheria, tetanus, and pertussis vaccine or the measles, mumps, and rubella vaccine.

**mixed venous blood,** blood that is composed of the venous blood from the heart and all systemic tissues in proportion to their venous returns. In the absence of abnormalities, mixed venous blood is present in the main pulmonary artery.

**-mixis, -mixia, -mixie, -mixy, mixo-,** combining form meaning 'related to intercourse': *amphimixis, mixoscopia.*

**mixture** /miks′chər/ [L, *miscere,* to mix], **1.** a substance composed of ingredients that are not chemically combined and do not necessarily occur in a fixed proportion. **2.** (in pharmacology) a liquid containing one or more medications in suspension. The proportions of the ingredients are specific to each mixture. Compare **compound, solution.** See also **mistura.**

**-mixy.** See **-mixis.**

**mL,** abbreviation for **milliliter.**

**MLC,** abbreviation for **mixed lymphocyte culture.** See **mixed lymphocyte culture (MLC) reaction.**

**MLD,** abbreviation for **minimum lethal dose.**

**mm,** abbreviation for **millimeter.**

**mM,** abbreviation for **millimolar.**

**mm³,** abbreviation for **cubic millimeter.**

**MMFR,** abbreviation for **maximal midexpiratory flow rate.**

**M-mode,** motion modulation in diagnostic ultrasonography. It is a variation of B-mode ultrasound used in echocardiography. See also **B-mode, M-mode.**

**mmol,** abbreviation for **millimole.**

**MMPI,** abbreviation for **Minnesota Multiphasic Personality Inventory.**

**MMR,** abbreviation for **measles, mumps, and rubella virus vaccine live.**

**MMWR,** abbreviation for *Morbidity and Mortality Weekly Report.*

**Mn,** symbol for the element **manganese.**

**mne-,** combining form meaning 'memory': *mnemic, mnemism, mnemonic.*

**mnemonics** [Gk, *mnemonikos*], a system of memory training that links a new concept or image with one already established in the memory, such as associating the numbers of a combination lock with a birthday or telephone number.

**-mnesia,** suffix meaning '(condition or type of) memory': *amnesia, ecmnesia, logamnesia.*

**-mnestic, -mnesic,** suffix meaning 'memory': *amnestic, anamnestic, catamnestic.*

**MNL,** abbreviation for **mononuclear leukocyte.**

**Mo,** symbol for the element **molybdenum.**

**Moban,** trademark for an antipsychotic agent (molindone hydrochloride).

**mobile arm support (MAS)** /mō′bəl, mōbēl′/, a forearm support device that enables people with upper extremity disabilities to fulfill some activities of daily living, by helping to move the hand into position for self-feeding. It may also be used as a training device and may be mounted on a wheelchair. Sometimes called **balanced forearm orthosis (BFO), ball-bearing arm support, ball-bearing feeder,** and **arm positioner.**

**mobile unit,** an easily transportable radiography unit designed for use outside a radiology department.

**mobility** /mōbil′itē/ [L, *mobilis,* movable], the velocity a particle or ion attains for a given applied voltage and a relative measure of how quickly an ion may move in an electric field.

**-mobility.** See **-motility.**

**mobility, impaired physical,** a nursing diagnosis accepted by the Fourth National Conference on the Classification of Nursing Diagnoses. It is defined as a state in which an individual experiences a limitation of ability for independent physical movement.

■ DEFINING CHARACTERISTICS: The defining characteristics include an inability to achieve a functional level of mobility in the environment (including bed mobility, transfer, ambulation), a reluctance to move, a limited range of motion of the limbs or extremities, a decrease in the strength or control of the musculoskeletal system, an abnormal or impaired ability to coordinate movements, or any of a large number of imposed restrictions on movement such as medically required bed rest or traction. It is suggested that the limitation of injury be ranked from 0, "completely independent," to 4, "dependent, does not participate in any activity."

■ RELATED FACTORS: Related factors include a decrease in the person's strength or endurance, presence of pain or discomfort, impaired cognition or perception, depression or severe anxiety, or impaired neuromuscular or musculoskeletal function. See also **nursing diagnosis.**

**mobility level,** a nursing outcome from the Nursing Outcomes Classification (NOC) defined as the ability to move purposefully. See also **Nursing Outcomes Classification.**

**Mobitz I heart block** /mō′bits/ [Woldemar Mobitz, German physician, b. 1889; AS, *hoerte,* heart; Fr, *bloc,* block], second-degree or partial atrioventricular (AV) block in which the P-R interval increases progressively until the propagation of an atrial impulse to the ventricles does not occur. Mobitz I heart block is caused by abnormal conduction of the cardiac impulse in the AV node and may be precipitated by increased vagal tone, AV nodal ischemia, or digitalis therapy. It may be a complication of inferior myocardial infarction. Also called **type I AV block, Wenckebach heart block, Wenckebach phenomenon.**

**Mobitz II heart block,** second-degree or partial atrioventricular block, characterized by the sudden nonconduction of an atrial impulse and a periodic dropped beat without prior or subsequent lengthening of the P-R interval. This kind of block usually results from bilateral impaired conduction in the bundle branches. It may be caused by anterior myocardial infarction, myocarditis, drug toxicity, electrolyte disturbances, rheumatoid nodules, and various degenerative diseases. Syncopal attacks, which occur without warning when the patient is upright or recumbent, are common in Mobitz II heart block, which may be transient or suddenly progress to complete block. Long-term therapy may require implantation of a *pacemaker.* Also called **type II AV block.**

**Möbius' syndrome** /mē′bē·əs/ [Paul J. Möbius, German neurologist, 1853–1902], a rare developmental disorder characterized by congenital bilateral facial palsy usually associated with oculomotor or other neurologic dysfunctions, speech disorders, and various anomalies of the extremities. It is caused by a developmental defect involving the motor nuclei of the cranial nerves. Also called **congenital facial diplegia, congenital oculofacial paralysis, nuclear agenesis.**

**Moctanin,** trademark for a gallstone dissolving agent (monoctanoin).

**modafinil,** a cerebral stimulant.

■ INDICATIONS: Modafinil is used to treat narcolepsy.

■ CONTRAINDICATIONS: Factors that prohibit the use of this drug include hyperthyroidism, hypertension, glaucoma, se-

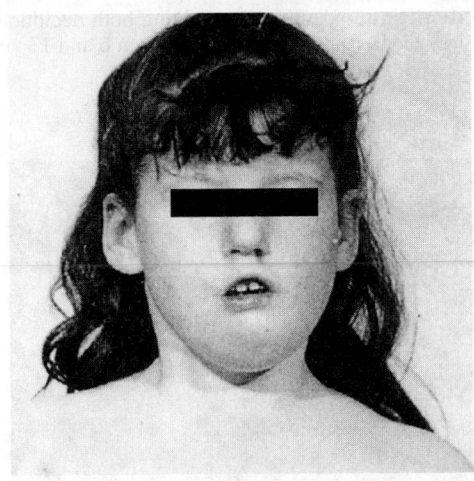

**Möbius' syndrome** *(Wright, 1995)*

vere arteriosclerosis, drug abuse, cardiovascular disease, anxiety, and known hypersensitivity to this drug.

■ ADVERSE EFFECTS: Dysrhythmias are a life-threatening effect of this drug. Other adverse effects are hyperglycemia, albuminuria, rhinitis, pharyngitis, lung disorder, dyspnea, asthma, epistaxis, abnormal vision, amblyopia, dizziness, headache, chills, stimulation, anorexia, dry mouth, diarrhea, nausea, vomiting, mouth ulcer, gingivitis, thirst, urinary retention, abnormal ejaculation, hypertension, herpes simplex, and dry skin. Common side effects include hyperactivity, insomnia, restlessness, palpitations, and tachycardia.

**modality** /mōdal′itē/, 1. the method of application of a therapeutic agent or regimen. 2. a sensory entity, such as the sense of vision or taste.

**mode** /mōd/ [L, *modus,* measure], a value or term in a set of data that occurs more frequently than other values or terms.

**model** /mod′əl/ [L, *modulus,* small measure], (in nursing research) a symbolic representation of the interrelations exhibited by a phenomenon within a system or a process. The model is presented as a conceptual framework or a theory that explains a phenomenon and allows predictions to be made about a patient or a process. A model is analogous to an equation in mathematics. Nursing models usually describe person, environment, health, and nursing.

**Model HMO Act,** a comprehensive health maintenance organization (HMO) statute adopted by several states. It requires that enrollees be entitled to receive copies of individual and group contracts and documented evidence of coverage describing the essential services and features of the HMO. It also requires filing of a premium rate schedule or method used to determine rates and establishment of a grievance procedure to resolve enrollee complaints.

**modeling** /mod′əling/, a technique used in behavior therapy in which a person learns a desired response by observing and imitating the behavior.

**Modeling and Role Modeling,** a theory developed by the nursing theorists Helen C. Erickson, Evelyn M. Tomlin, and Mary Ann P. Swain. Their book, *Modeling and Role Modeling: A Theory and Paradigm for Nursing,* was published in 1983. From a synthesis of multiple concepts related to basic needs, developmental tasks, object attachment, and adaptive coping potential, they developed their highly abstract role-modeling theory. The term *modeling* refers to the development of an understanding of the client's world. Role modeling is the nursing intervention, or nurturance, that requires unconditional acceptance. Erickson, Tomlin, and Swain believe that, although people are alike because of their holism (multiple interacting subsystems), lifetime growth, and development, they are also different because of inherent endowment, adaptation, and self-care knowledge. Role modeling provides a framework for understanding the way clients structure their world. Erickson, Tomlin, and Swain view nursing as a self-care model based on the client's perception of the world and adaptations to stressors.

**modem** /mō′dəm/, abbreviation for *modulate/demodulate*. It is a device for transforming serial binary numbers into an audible tone, and vice versa, for transmission over a telephone line to another computer. Also spelled **MODEM.**

**moderate vaginal bleeding.** See **vaginal bleeding.**

**moderator band** /mod′ərā′tər/ [L, *moderari,* to restrain; AS, *bindan,* to bind], a thick bundle of muscle in the central part of the right ventricle of the heart. Missing in some individuals and varying in size in others, it usually contains part of the atrioventricular conduction bundle. Also called **trabecula septomarginalis.**

**modesty,** propriety of dress, speech, and conduct in relations between patients and health care personnel, including draping and covering of the patient to the greatest extent possible, depending on the type of care or examination.

**Modicon,** trademark for an oral contraceptive containing an estrogen (ethinyl estradiol) and a progestin (norethindrone).

**modification** /mod′ifikā′shən/, **1.** a process whereby a substance is changed from one form to another. **2.** a change in an organism that is acquired or learned but does not involve inheritance.

**modification allele.** See **modifying gene.**

**modified jaw thrust** /mod′ifīd/, an upper airway control maneuver to maintain an open airway of an unconscious person in cases of potential spinal injury. In such persons inline stabilization of the head and neck can be obtained primarily by forward jaw thrust with minimum head extension.

**modified milk** [L, *modus,* measure, *facere,* to make], cow's milk in which the protein content has been reduced and the fat content increased to correspond to the composition of breast milk. See also **formula, infant.**

**modified radical mastectomy,** a surgical procedure in which a breast is completely removed with the underlying pectoralis minor and some of the adjacent lymph nodes. The pectoralis major is not excised. The operation is performed in treating early and well-localized malignant neoplasms of the breast. It appears to be as curative as the more extensive radical mastectomy when the tumor meets these criteria. Care of the woman before and after a modified radical mastectomy is similar to that for a radical mastectomy. Compare **radical mastectomy, simple mastectomy.** See also **lumpectomy, mastectomy, Reach to Recovery.**

**modifying gene** /mod′ifī′ing/ [L, *modus,* measure; Gk, *genein,* to produce], a gene that alters or influences the expression function of another gene, including the suppression or reduction of the usual function of the modified gene. Also called **modification allele.**

**modulation** /mod′yəlā′shən/, an alteration in the magnitude or any variation in the duration of an electrical current. Modulation, which affects physiologic responses to various waveforms, may be continuous, interrupted, pulsed, or surging.

**modulation transfer function (MTF)** [L, *modulus,* small measure; L, *transferre,* to carry, *functio,* performance], a quantitative measure of the ability of an imaging system to reproduce patterns that vary in spatial frequency. The MTF is useful in predicting image degradation in a series of radiographic components.

**Moeller's glossitis** /mel′ərz/ [Julius O.L. Moeller, German surgeon, 1819–1887], a form of chronic glossitis, characterized by burning or pain in the tongue and increased sensitivity to hot or spicy foods. Also called **glossodynia exfoliativa.** See also **glossitis.**

**moexipril,** an angiotensin-converting enzyme inhibitor.
■ INDICATIONS: It is prescribed in the treatment of high blood pressure.
■ CONTRAINDICATIONS: The drug should not be given to patients with an allergy to angiotensin-converting enzyme inhibitors. It should be used with caution in diabetes mellitus, brain-blood disease, heart or kidney disease, liver disease, scleroderma, systemic lupus erythematosus, or pregnancy.
■ ADVERSE EFFECTS: The side effects most often reported include digestive tract disorders, depression, headache, dizziness, vertigo, sleeping difficulties, chest pains, and palpitations.

**mogi-,** combining form meaning 'difficult, or with difficulty': *mogiarthria, mogigraphia, mogilalia.*

**mohel** /mō′əl, môhāl′/, in Judaism, ordained to circumcise.

**Mohr syndrome** /mor/ [Otto Lous Mohr, Norwegian geneticist, 1886–1967], an autosomal recessive disorder characterized by brachydactyly, clinodactyly, polydactyly, syndactyly, and bilateral polysyndactyly of the big toe; by cranial, facial, lingual, palatal, and mandibular anomalies; and by episodic neuromuscular disturbances. Also called **orodigitofacial dysostosis, oral-facial-digital syndrome, type II, orofaciodigital syndrome, type II.**

**moiety** /moi′itē/ [L, *medietas,* middle], a part of a molecule that exhibits a particular set of chemical and pharmacologic characteristics.

**moist cough.** See **productive cough.**

**moist crackle** [OFr, *moiste,* fresh; ME, *krakelen*], an abnormal breathing sound heard on auscultation when air bubbles through fluid or secretions in the bronchi or trachea.

**moist gangrene.** See **gangrene.**

**moist heat** [OFr, *moiste* + AS, *haetu*], the use of hot water, towels soaked in hot water, aquathermia pads, hot water bottles, or hot water vapors to reduce inflammation and pain, stimulate circulation, and/or relieve symptoms as directed by a physician. Hot towels should be wrung out to remove surplus moisture and should not be too hot to be held in the hands of the person applying moist heat.

**mol.** See **mole²**.

**molality** /mōlal′itē/ [L, *moles,* mass], the number of moles of solute per kilogram of water or other solvent; it refers to the weight of the solvent.

**molal volume.** See **mole volume.**

**molar** /mō′lər/ [L, *moles,* mass], **1.** any of the 12 teeth, 6 in each dental arch, located posterior to the premolars. The crown of each molar is nearly cubical, convex on its buccal and lingual surfaces, and flattened on its surfaces of contact. Each of the upper molars has three roots; the roots of each third upper molar are often fused. The lower molars are larger than the upper, and each has two roots; the roots of each third lower molar tend to fuse. **2.** **(M)** pertaining to the concentration of a solution, expressed as the number of moles of solute per liter of solution. See also **mole²**.

**molarity** /mōler′itē/ [L, *moles,* mass], the number of moles of solute per liter of solution; it refers to the concentration of the solution.

**molar pregnancy,** pregnancy in which a hydatid mole develops from the trophoblastic tissue of the early embryonic stage of development. The signs of pregnancy are all exaggerated: the uterus grows more rapidly than is normal, morning sickness is often severe and constant, blood pressure is likely to be elevated, and blood levels of chorionic gonadotropins are extremely high. The uterus must be evacuated, because the mole may develop into a malignant trophoblastic disease, choriocarcinoma. See also **hydatid mole.**

**molar solution,** a solution that contains one mole of solute per liter of solution.

**molar volume.** See **mole volume.**

**mold**[1], **1.** a fungus. **2.** a fungal growth.

**mold**[2], a hollow form for casting or shaping an object, as a prosthesis.

**molding** /mōl'ding/ [ME, *moulde*, shaping], the natural process by which a baby's head is shaped during labor as it is squeezed into and through the birth passage by the forces of labor. The head often becomes quite elongated, and the bones of the skull may be caused to overlap slightly at the suture lines. The biparietal diameter of the head may be compressed as much as 0.5 cm without intracranial damage. Most of the changes caused by molding resolve themselves during the first few days of life. Compare **caput succedaneum.** See also **cephalhematoma.**

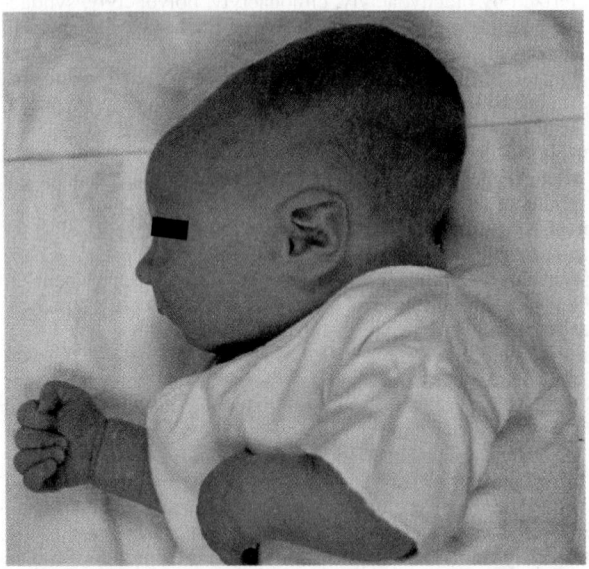

**Molding** (Lowdermilk, 1999/courtesy Kim Molloy, Knoxville, Iowa)

**mole**[1] [L, mass], *informal.* **1.** a pigmented nevus. **2.** (in obstetrics) a hydatidiform mole.

**mole**[2] [L, *molecula*, small mass], the standard unit used to measure the amount of a substance. A mole of a substance is the amount containing the same number of elementary particles as there are atoms in 12 g of carbon 12, typically $6.02 \times 10^{23}$ particles. This is called Avogadro's number. Also spelled **mol.** —**molar,** *adj.*

**molecular biology** /məlek'yələr/ [L, *molecula*, small mass; Gk, *bios*, life, *logos*, science], the branch of biology that deals with the physical and chemical interactions of molecules involved in life functions.

**molecular genetics** [L, *molecula*, small mass; Gk, *genesis*, origin], the branch of genetics that focuses on the chemical structure and the functions, replication, and mutations of the molecules involved in the transmission of genetic information, namely DNA and RNA. Molecular genetics is concerned with the arrangement of genes on DNA, the replication of DNA, the transcription of DNA into RNA, and the translation of RNA into proteins. Also called **biochemical genetics.** See also **recombinant DNA.**

**molecular lesion.** See **point lesion.**

**molecular mass,** the mass of a molecule in daltons, derived by addition of the sum of the component atomic masses. Its dimensionless equivalent is molecular weight. The term **relative molecular mass ($M_r$)** is preferable to **molecular weight.** Compare **molecular weight.**

**molecular mimicry,** an antigenic similarity between unrelated macromolecules, believed to play a role in the pathogenesis of rheumatic fever and other diseases. See also **mimicry.**

**molecular pathology** [L, *molecula*, small mass; Gk, *pathos*, disease, *logos*, science], the branch of the science of disease that is concerned with the health effects of specific molecules.

**molecular sieve,** **1.** a crystalline chemical separation device with molecular size pores that adsorbs small but not large molecules. **2.** a crosslinked polymer that forms a porous sieve used as a supporting medium for chromatographic separation of mixtures of solutes.

**molecular stutter,** a gene defect in which the three-nucleotide code for an amino acid is repeated, missing, or jumbled, causing the gene either to fail to make a specific protein or to make a protein that does not function properly. In Huntington's disease, for example, the code for glutamine may be repeated 40 or 50 times in a row in the defective gene. The symptoms of Huntington's disease develop in patients with more than 30 glutamine repeats, and the longer the string of repeats, the earlier the symptoms develop.

**molecular taxonomy,** the classification of organisms on the basis of the distribution and composition of chemical substances in them.

**molecular weight (mol wt),** the weight of a molecule of a substance as compared with the weight of an atom of carbon-12. It is equal to the sum of the weights of its constituent atoms and is dimensionless. The term **relative molecular mass ($M_r$)** is preferable. See also **atom, atomic weight, molecule.** Compare **molecular mass.**

**molecule** /mol'əkyo̅o̅l/ [L, *molecula*, small mass], the smallest unit that exhibits the properties of an element or compound. A molecule is composed of two or more atoms that are covalently bonded. See also **atom, compound.**

**mole percent,** a percentage calculation expressed in terms of moles of a substance in a mixture or solution rather than in terms of molecular mass.

**mole volume,** the volume occupied by one mole of a substance, which may be a solid, liquid, or gas. It is numerically equal to the molecular mass divided by the density. For a gas it is 22.4 liters at standard temperature and pressure. Also called **molal volume, molar volume.**

**molindone hydrochloride** /mol'indōn/, an antipsychotic agent.

■ INDICATION: It is prescribed in the treatment of schizophrenia.

■ CONTRAINDICATIONS: Severe central nervous system depression or known hypersensitivity to this drug prohibits its use.

■ ADVERSE EFFECTS: Among the most serious adverse reactions are extrapyramidal reactions, hypotension, sedation, and other reactions characteristic of the phenothiazine antipsychotics.

**molluscum** /məlus′kəm/ [L, *molluscus*, soft], any skin disease having soft, rounded masses or nodules. See also **molluscum contagiosum.**

**molluscum contagiosum,** a disease of the skin and mucous membranes caused by a poxvirus, which occurs all over the world. It is characterized by scattered flesh-toned or white papules. Palms of the hands and soles of the feet are not affected. The disease most frequently occurs in children and in adults with an impaired immune response. It is transmitted from person to person by direct or indirect contact and lasts up to 3 years, although individual lesions persist for only 6 to 8 weeks. Diagnosis is easily made by electron microscopy. Curettage or electrical or chemical desiccation helps to clear the lesions, but untreated lesions eventually resolve spontaneously without scarring.

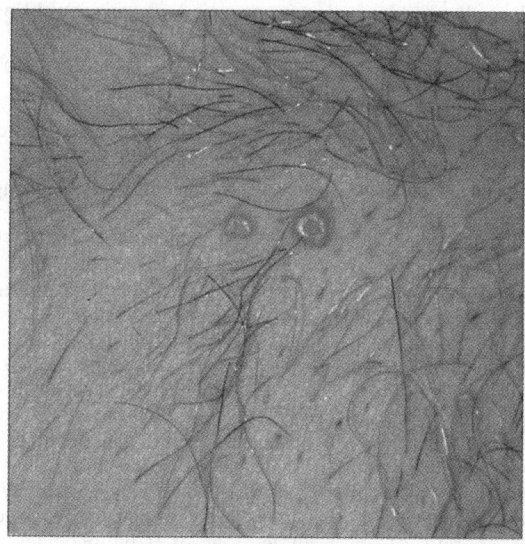

**Molluscum contagiosum**
*(Morse, Moreland, and Holmes, 1996)*

**Moloney test** [Paul J. Moloney, Canadian physician, 1870–1939], a skin test for sensitivity to diphtheria toxoid.

**mol wt,** abbreviation for **molecular weight.**

**molybdenum (Mo)** /məlib′dənəm/ [Gk, *molybdos*, lead], a grayish metallic element. Its atomic number is 42; its atomic mass is 95.94. Molybdenum is poisonous if ingested in large quantities.

**molybdenum 99,** the radionuclide that is the parent of technetium 99 and as such is present as a generator in most nuclear medicine departments.

**-monab,** combining form for monoclonal antibodies.

**monad** /mon′ad, mō′nad/, **1.** a unicellular, free-living organism. **2.** a monovalent element or radical. **3.** a haploid set of chromosomes in a spermatid or ootid.

**-monam,** combining form for monobactam (monocyclic beta-lactam) antibiotics.

**monamine.** See **monoamine.**

**monarthritis** /mon′ärthrī′tis/ [Gk, *monos*, single, *arthron*, joint, *itis*, inflammation], arthritis affecting only one joint.

**monarticular** /mon′ärtik′yələr/ [Gk, *monos*, single; L, *articulus*, joint], pertaining to only one joint.

**monascus,** a natural product derived from red yeast grown on rice, traditionally used in Chinese medicine and now in more common use as both a medicine and a foodstuff.

■ USES: This herb is used to help maintain acceptable cholesterol levels.

■ CONTRAINDICATIONS: Monascus should not be used during pregnancy and lactation, in children, or in those with known hypersensitivity to monascus or with hepatic disease such as cirrhosis or fatty liver.

**monaural** /monôr′əl/ [Gk, *monos*, single; L, *auris*, ear], pertaining to one ear.

**Mönckeberg's arteriosclerosis** /meng′kəbərgz/ [Johann G. Mönckeberg, German pathologist, 1877–1925], a form of arteriosclerosis in which extensive calcium deposits are found in the tunica media of the artery with little obstruction of the lumen. Also called **medial arteriosclerosis.**

**Monday morning fever.** See **byssinosis.**

**Monera.** See **Procaryotae.**

**Monge's disease.** See **altitude sickness.**

**Mongolian spot** /mong·gō′lē·ən/ [*Mongol,* Asian ethnic group; ME, *spotte,* stain], a benign bluish-black macule, between 2 and 8 cm, occurring over the sacrum and on the buttocks of some newborns. It is especially common in African-Americans, Native Americans, southern Europeans, and Asian-Americans and usually disappears during early childhood.

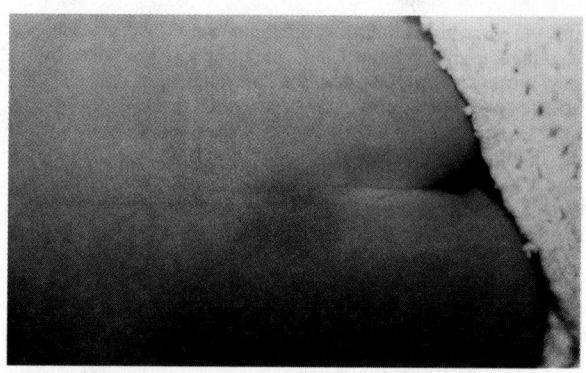

**Mongolian spot** *(Zitelli and Davis, 1997)*

**mongolism.** See **Down syndrome.**

**monilethrix** /mō·nil′ə·thriks/ [L. *monile* necklace; Gk, *thrix,* hair], an autosomal dominant condition in which the hairs exhibit multiple constrictions, with a beading effect, and are brittle, rarely reaching an inch in length before breaking.

*Monilia.* See *Candida albicans.*

**monilial vulvovaginitis, moniliasis.** See **candidiasis.**

**moniliform** /mōnil′ifôrm/, resembling a string of beads.

**Monistat,** trademark for an antifungal (miconazole nitrate).

**monitor** /mon′ətər/ [L, *monere,* to warn], **1.** to observe and evaluate a function of the body closely and constantly. **2.** a mechanical device that provides a visual or audible signal or a graphic record of a particular function, such as a cardiac monitor or a fetal monitor.

**monitrice** /mon′itris/ [Fr, female instructor], a labor coach, usually a registered nurse, who is specially trained in the Lamaze method of childbirth. The coach provides emotional support and leads the mother through labor and delivery, us-

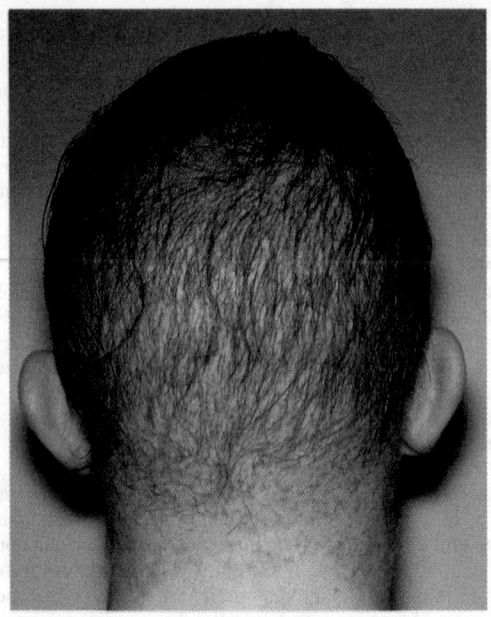

**Monilethrix** *(Hordinsky, Sawaya, and Scher, 2000)*

ing the specific techniques for breathing, concentration, and massage taught by the Lamaze method in classes for the psychophysical preparation for childbirth.

**monkeypox,** an epidemic human disease caused by exposure to a monkeypox virus with symptoms resembling those of smallpox. The virus is related antigenically to smallpox and vaccinia organisms.

**mono,** informal term for **mononucleosis.**

**mono-** /mon'ō-/, prefix meaning 'one': *monobacillary, monodal, mononeuritis.*

**monoamine** /mon'ō·am'in/, an amine containing one amine group.

**monoamine oxidase (MAO),** an enzyme that catalyzes the oxidation of amines. See also **monoamine oxidase inhibitor.**

**monoamine oxidase (MAO) inhibitor,** any of a chemically heterogeneous group of drugs used primarily in the treatment of depression. These drugs also exert an antianxiety effect, especially anxiety associated with phobia. The effects of the drugs vary greatly from patient to patient, and their specific actions leading to clinical benefits are poorly understood. Among the most common adverse effects are drowsiness, dry mouth, orthostatic hypotension, and constipation. Overdosage may cause tremor, euphoria, or manic behavior. MAO inhibitors interact with many drugs and with foods containing large amounts of the amino acid tyramine. Ingestion of these foods by a person taking a MAO inhibitor is likely to cause a severe hypertensive episode associated with headache, palpitations, and nausea. Among these foods are cheeses, red wine, smoked or pickled herring, beer, and yogurt. Among the drugs that interact with MAO inhibitors are dopamine, meperidine, and the indirect acting sympathomimetics, one of which, ephedrine, is an ingredient in many common cold remedies. MAO inhibitors are also sometimes used in the treatment of migraine headache and hypertension. See also **amine pump.**

**monobasic acid** /mon'ōbā'sik/, an acid with only one replaceable hydrogen atom, such as hydrochloric acid (HCl).

**monobenzone** /-ben'zōn/, a depigmenting agent.
- INDICATIONS: It is prescribed in final depigmentation in extensive vitiligo.
- CONTRAINDICATION: Known hypersensitivity to this drug prohibits its use.
- ADVERSE EFFECTS: The most serious adverse reaction is excessive and irreversible hypopigmentation. Common effects are irritation and allergic reactions of the skin.

**monoblast** /mon'əblast/ [Gk, *monos,* single, *blastos,* germ], an immature monocyte. Increased production of monoblasts in the marrow and the presence of these forms in the peripheral circulation occur in certain leukemias and tuberculosis. Compare **megaloblast, myeloblast.** See also **bone marrow, leukocyte.** —**monoblastic,** *adj.*

**monoblastic leukemia** /-blas'tik/, a malignancy of bloodforming organs, characterized by the proliferation of monoblasts and monocytes. The disease develops late in the course of a small but significant number of cases of plasma cell myeloma. Also called **monocytic leukemia, Schilling's leukemia.**

**monocarboxylic acid** /mon'ō·kär'bok·sil'ik/, a carboxylic acid with a single carboxyl group.

**monocephalus.** See **syncephalus.**

**monochorial twins, monochorionic twins.** See **monozygotic twins.**

**monochromatic** /-krōmat'ik/, **1.** pertaining to a single color or a single wavelength of light. **2.** describing a person who is totally color blind. **3.** pertaining to a substance that has only one color or stains with only one color.

**monochromaticity** /-krō'mətis'itē/, the specificity of light in a single defined wavelength. If the specificity is in the visible light spectrum, it is only one color.

**Monocid,** trademark for a cephalosporin-type antibiotic (cefonicid sodium).

**monoclonal** /mon'əklō'nəl/ [Gk, *monos* + *klon,* twig], pertaining to or designating a group of identical cells or organisms derived from a single cell or organism.

**monoclonal antibody (MAB)** [Gk, *monos,* single, *klon,* twig; Gk, *anti* + AS, *bodig,* body], an antibody produced in a laboratory from a single clone of B lymphocytes. All MOABs produced from the same clone are identical and have the same antigenic specificity.

**monoclonal gammopathy.** See **gammopathy.**

**monocomponent insulin** /-kəmpō'nənt/ [Gk, *monos,* single; L, *componere,* to bring together, *insula,* island]. See **single component insulin.**

**monocrotic pulse** /-krot'ik/ [Gk, *monos,* single, *krotein,* to strike; L, *pulsare,* to beat], a pulse characterized by a single wave.

**monocular diplopia** /monok'yələr/ [Gk, *monos,* single, *oculus,* eye; Gk, *diploos,* double, *opsis,* vision], a condition in which a double image is perceived with one eye. The cause is a disorder in the refracting medium of the eye, such as a cataract, or partial dislocation of the lens. In rare cases more than two images may be seen with one eye. Also called **uniocular diplopia.**

**monocular strabismus** [Gk, *monos,* single; L, *oculus,* eye; Gk, *strabismos*], a squint that is confined to one particular eye. Also called **uniocular squint.**

**monocular vision** [Gk, *monos,* single; L, *oculus,* eye, *visio,* seeing], a condition of seeing with or using only one eye at a time. Also called **uniocular vision.**

**monocutaneous candidiasis,** a cellular immunodeficiency disorder associated with fungal *(Candida)* infections of the skin, mucous membranes, nails, and hair. Patients show a lack of immune reaction after intradermal injection of *Candida,* but immunity to other infectious agents is not impaired. About half the patients also exhibit endocrine abnormalities.

**monocyte** /mon′əsīt/ [Gk, *monos* + *kytos,* cell], a large mononuclear leukocyte, 13 to 25 μm in diameter with an ovoid or kidney-shaped nucleus, containing chromatin material with a lacy pattern and abundant gray-blue cytoplasm filled with fine, reddish, and azurophilic granules. See also **monocytosis.**

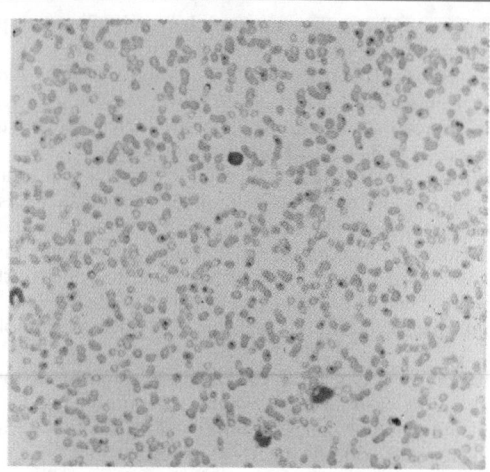

**Monocytosis** *(Zitelli and Davis, 1997)*

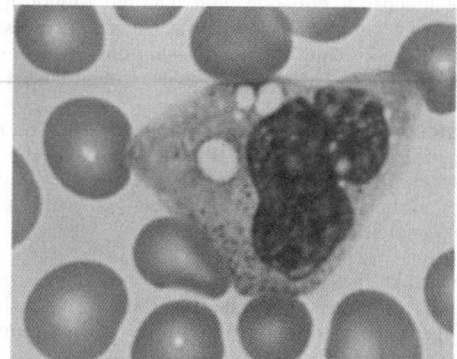

**Monocyte** *(Carr and Rodak, 1999)*

**monocytic leukemia** /mon′əsit′ik/, a malignancy of blood-forming tissues in which the predominant cells are monocytes. The disease has an erratic course characterized by malaise, fatigue, fever, anorexia, weight loss, splenomegaly, bleeding gums, dermal petechiae, anemia, and lack of responsiveness to therapy. There are two forms: **Schilling's leukemia,** in which most of the cells are monocytes that probably arise from the reticuloendothelial system, and the more common **Naegeli's leukemia,** in which a large number of the cells resemble myeloblasts. Also called **histiocytic leukemia.**

**monocytic leukopenia.** See **monocytopenia.**

**monocytopenia** /-sī′təpē′nē·ə/, an abnormally low level of monocytes in the peripheral blood, that is less than 200/mm$^3$. Also called **monocytic leukopenia.**

**monocytosis** /mon′ōsītō′sis/, an increased proportion of monocytes in the circulation.

**monodactylism** /-dak′tiliz′əm/ [Gk, *monos,* single, *daktylos,* finger or toe], a congenital defect in which the person is born with only one finger on the hand or one toe on the foot.

**monoethanolamine** /mon′ō·eth′ənol′əmēn/, an amino alcohol formed by the decarboxylation of serine. It is a component of certain cephalins and phospholipids and is used as a surfactant in pharmaceutical products. Also called **ethanolamine.**

**monofactorial inheritance** /-faktôr′ē·əl/ [Gk, *monos* + L, *factare,* to make], the acquisition or expression of a trait or condition that depends on the transmission of a single specific gene. Compare **multifactorial inheritance.**

**monogamy** /mənog′əmē/, **1.** the practice of being married to no more than one person at a time. **2.** (in biology) the habit of pairing with only one mate.

**monohybrid** /-hī′brid/ [Gk, *monos* + L, *hybrida,* mixed offspring], pertaining to or describing an individual, organism, or strain that is heterozygous for only one specific trait or that is heterozygous for the single trait or gene locus under consideration.

**monohybrid cross,** the mating of two individuals, organisms, or strains that have different alleles for only one specific trait or in which only one particular characteristic or gene locus is being followed.

**monohydric alcohol** /-hī′drik/, an alcohol containing one hydroxyl group.

**monoiodotyrosine** /mon′ō·ī·ō′dōtī′rəsin/, an iodinated amino acid involved in the synthesis of thyroxine (T$_4$) and triiodothyronine (T$_3$).

**monokaryotic** /-ker′ē·ot′ik/, having a single nucleus.

**monolayer** /-lā′ər/, a sheet of cells one cell thick, such as may be formed on the surface of a culture vessel.

**monomer** /mon′əmər/ [Gk, *monos* + *meros,* part], a molecule that repeats itself to form a polymer, such as a molecule of fibrin monomer that polymerizes to form fibrin in the blood-clotting process. **—monomeric,** *adj.*

**monomolecular elimination reaction (E1)** /-məlek′yələr/, a first-order chemical kinetic reaction in which only one molecule is involved in the slow step reaction. Also called **unimolecular reaction.**

**monomphalus** /mənom′fələs/ [Gk, *monos* + *omphalos,* navel], conjoined twins that are united at the umbilicus. Also called **omphalopagus.**

**mononeuritis multiplex.** See **multiple mononeuropathy.**

**mononeuropathy** /-nŏŏrop′əthē/ [Gk, *monos* + *neuron,* nerve, *pathos,* disease], any disease or disorder that affects a single nerve trunk. Some common causes of disorders involving single nerve trunks are electric shock, radiation, and fractured bones that may compress or lacerate nerve fibers. Casts and tourniquets that are too tight may also damage a nerve by compression or by ischemia. The peripheral nerve trunks are especially vulnerable to compression and entrapment.

**mononeuropathy multiplex,** a peripheral nerve disorder characterized by numbness, pain, and weakness in several areas of the body. The symptoms may develop suddenly in the region supplied by one peripheral nerve and days later in the region of another nerve.

**mononuclear** /-nyŏŏ′klē·ər/ [Gk, *monos,* single; L, *nucleus,* nut kernel], pertaining to one nucleus, such as a monocyte.

**mononuclear leukocyte (MNL),** a white blood cell, including lymphocytes and monocytes, with a single round or oval nucleus. Also called **mononuclear cell.** Compare **polymorphonuclear leukocyte.** See also **monocyte.**

**mononucleosis (mono)** /mon′ōnōō′klē·ō′sis/ [Gk, *monos,* single; L, *nucleus,* nut kernel; Gk, *osis,* condition], an abnormal increase in the number of mononuclear leukocytes in the blood. See also **infectious mononucleosis.**

**mononucleosis spot test,** a blood test performed to aid in the diagnosis of infectious mononucleosis (IM), a disease caused by the Epstein-Barr virus (EBV). Abnormal findings may also indicate chronic EBV infection, chronic fatigue syndrome, some forms of chronic hepatitis, and Burkitt's lymphoma, which is strongly associated with EBV.

**monooctanoin** /mon′ō·ok′tanō′in/, a gallstone-dissolving agent.
■ INDICATIONS: It is used to dissolve cholesterol gallstones.
■ CONTRAINDICATIONS: The product is contraindicated in patients with jaundice, a severe biliary tract infection, or a history of recent duodenal ulcer or jejunitis.
■ ADVERSE EFFECTS: Adverse reactions may include nausea, vomiting, diarrhea, and GI pain.

**monophagia** /-fā′jə/, the practice of eating only one kind of food.

**monophasic** /-fā′sik/, having one phase, part, aspect, or stage.

**monoploid, monoploidic.** See **haploid.**

**monopodial symmelia.** See **sympus monopus.**

**Monopril,** trademark for an angiotensin-converting enzyme inhibitor (fosinopril); an antihypertensive.

**monopus** /mon′əpəs/ [Gk, *monos* + *pous,* foot], a fetus or individual with the congenital absence of a foot or leg.

**monorchid** /monôr′kid/, a male who has monorchism.

**monorchism** /mon′ôrkiz′əm/ [Gk, *monos* + *orchis,* testicle, *ismos,* state], a condition in which only one testicle has descended into the scrotum. Also called **monorchidism.** See also **cryptorchidism.** —**monorchidic,** *adj.*

**monosaccharide** /-sak′ərīd/ [Gk, *monos* + *sakcharon,* sugar], a simple carbohydrate consisting of a single basic sugar unit with the general formula $C_n(H_2O)_n$, with $n$ ranging from 3 to 8.

**monosodium glutamate (MSG)** /-sō′dē·əm/, a food flavor enhancer derived from naturally occurring salt of glutamic acid and a cause of **Chinese restaurant syndrome.** It is also used in the treatment of encephalopathies associated with liver disorders. Also called **sodium glutamate.**

**monosodium urate monohydrate,** a uric acid salt deposited as crystals in and around joints in gout patients.

**monosome** /mon′əsōm/ [Gk, *monos* + *soma,* body], **1.** also called **accessory chromosome.** an unpaired X or Y chromosome. **2.** the single, unpaired chromosome in monosomy.

**monosomy** /mon′əsō′mē/ [Gk, *monos* + *soma,* body], a chromosomal aberration characterized by the absence of one chromosome from the normal diploid complement. In humans the monosomic cell contains 45 chromosomes and is designated $2n - 1$, such as occurs in the XO condition in Turner's syndrome. Compare **trisomy.** See also **aneuploidy.** —**monosomic,** *adj.*

**monosomy X.** See **Turner's syndrome.**

**monospecific** /-spəsif′ik/ [Gk, *monos* + L, *species,* form, *facere,* to make], pertaining to an antibody that binds to only one type of antigen.

**monosynaptic reflex** /-sinap′tik/ [Gk, *monos,* single, *synaptein,* to join; L, *reflectere,* to bend back], a reflex requiring only one afferent and one efferent neuron.

**monotherapy** /mon′ō·ther′ə·pē/ [Gk, *monos,* single + *therapeia,* treatment], treatment of a condition by means of a single drug.

**monotropy** /mənot′rəpē/ [Gk, *monos* + *trepein,* to turn], a concept named by J. Bowlby, describing the phenomenon in which a mother appears to be able to bond with only one infant at a time. The concept is used by Marshall Klaus and John Kennell in their studies of maternal-infant bonding in mothers of twins. When one twin is taken home from the hospital earlier than the other, the mother often reports that she does not feel that the baby discharged later is hers. The second baby to reach the home is much more likely to fail to thrive or to be neglected or abused. Nurses working in intensive care nurseries and adoption homes are also known to become attached to only one child at a time. Monotropy also may explain a mother's common tendency to dress twins alike, in effect making them one. —**monotropic,** *adj.*

**monounsaturated fatty acid.** See **unsaturated fatty acid.**

**monovalent** /-vā′lənt/, **1.** describing an atom or radical having the valence or combining power of one hydrogen atom. Also called **univalent.** See also **valence. 2.** describing a serum antibody capable of combining with only one antigen or complement.

**monovular.** See **uniovular.**

**monovulatory** /mənō′vyələtôr′ē/ [Gk, *monos* + L, *ovulum,* small egg, *orius,* characterized by], routinely releasing one ovum during each ovarian cycle. Compare **diovulatory.**

**monozygotic (MZ)** /-zīgō′tik/ [Gk, *monos* + *zygon,* yoke], pertaining to or developed from a single fertilized ovum, or zygote, such as occurs in identical twins. Compare **dizygotic.** —**monozygosity,** *n.,* **monozygous,** *adj.*

**monozygotic twins,** two offspring born of the same pregnancy and developed from a single fertilized ovum that splits into equal halves during an early cleavage phase in embryonic development, giving rise to separate fetuses. Such twins are always of the same sex, have the same ge-

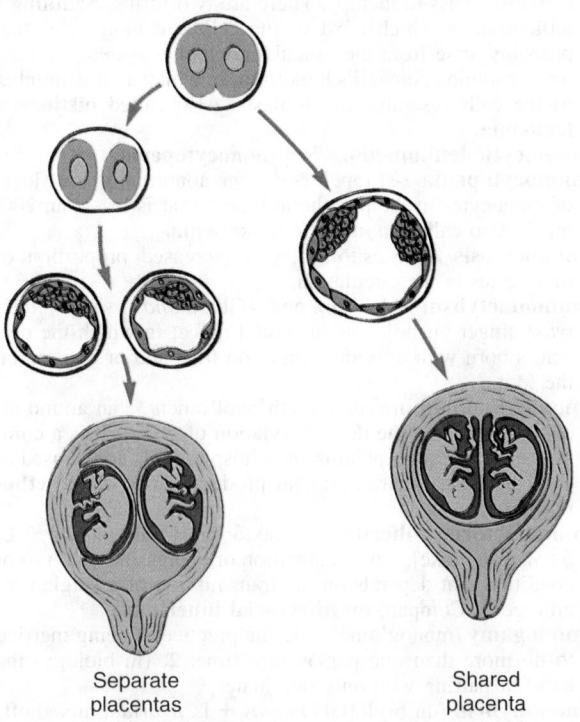

Separate placentas        Shared placenta

**Monozygotic twins** *(Carlson, 1999)*

netic constitution, possess identical blood groups, and closely resemble each other in physical, psychologic, and mental characteristics. Monozygotic twins may have single or separate placentas and membranes, depending on the time during development when division occurs. Monozygotic twinning occurs with relatively uniform frequency in all races, is unaffected by heredity, and represents approximately one third of all twin births. Also called **enzygotic twins, identical twins, true twins, uniovular twins.** Compare **dizygotic twins.** See also **Siamese twins.**

**Monro-Kellie doctrine** /mən·rō′ kel′ē/ [Alexander Monro, Scottish anatomist and surgeon, 1733−1817; George Kellie, Scottish anatomist, late 18th century],   the central nervous system and its accompanying fluids are enclosed in a rigid container whose total volume tends to remain constant; an increase in volume of one component (e.g. brain, blood, or cerebrospinal fluid) will elevate pressure and decrease the volume of one of the other elements.

**mons** /mons/ [L, mountain],   a mound or slight elevation.

**Monson curve** [George S. Monson, American dentist, 1869–1933; L, *curvus*, a bend],   the curve of occlusion in which each tooth cusp and incisal edge lie on the surface of a sphere 8 inches (20 cm) in diameter, with its center in the region of the glabella.

**mons pubis.**   See **mons veneris.**

**monstrosity** /monstros′itē/,   **1.** derogatory term for the state or condition of having severe congenital defects. **2.** anything that deviates greatly from the normal; derogatory term for a teras.

**mons veneris** /ven′əris/ [L, *mons*, mountain; *venus*, love], a pad of fatty tissue and thick skin that overlies the symphysis pubis in the woman. After puberty it is covered with pubic hair. Also called **mons pubis, mount of Venus.**

**Monteggia's fracture** /montej′əz/ [Giovanni B. Monteggia, Italian physician, 1762–1815],   a break in the ulna, associated with radial dislocation or rupture of the annular ligament and resulting in the angulation or overriding of ulnar fragments.

**montelukast,**   a leukotriene receptor.

■ INDICATIONS: Montelukast is used to treat chronic asthma.

■ CONTRAINDICATIONS: Known hypersensitivity to this drug prohibits its use.

■ ADVERSE EFFECTS: Adverse reactions to this drug include dizziness, fatigue, headache, abdominal pain, dyspepsia, abnormal liver function tests, rash, asthenia, influenza, cough, and nasal congestion.

**Montenegro test** /mon′tənā′grō/,   a test used in the diagnosis of cutaneous leishmaniasis, in which killed *Leishmania* antigens are injected intradermally. A positive reaction is indicated by the appearance of a palpable nodule in 48 to 72 hours. Also called **leishmanin test.**

**Montercaux fracture** /monterkō′/,   a break in the neck of the fibula associated with the dislocation of the ankle mortise joint.

**Montezuma's revenge.**   See **traveler's diarrhea.**

**Montgomery's gland.**   See **areolar gland.**

**Montgomery straps** /mont·gom′ərē/,   bands of adhesive tape featuring a lace-up design, which is used to secure dressings that must be changed frequently. Also called **Montgomery tapes.**

**Montgomery tapes.**   See **Montgomery straps.**

**mood,**   a prolonged subjective emotional state that influences one's whole personality and perception of the world. Examples include sadness, elation, and anger. See also **affect.**

**mood-congruent psychotic features** /-kon′grōō·ənt/ [AS, *mod*, mind; L, *congruere*, to come together],   the character-

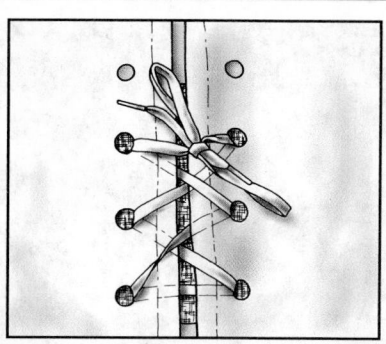

**Montgomery straps** *(Ignatavicius, Workman, and Mishler, 1999)*

istics of a psychosis in which the content of hallucinations or delusions is consistent with an elevated, expansive mood or with a depression. Mood congruence is most often noted in mood disorders, whereas schizophrenia is often a mood-incongruent disorder.

**mood disorder** [AS, *mod*, mind; L, *dis + ordo*, rank],   a variety of conditions characterized by a disturbance in mood as the main feature. If mild and occasional, the feelings may be normal. If more severe, they may be a sign of a major depressive disorder or dysthymic reaction or be symptomatic of a bipolar disorder. Other mood disorders may be caused by a general medical condition. *Mood disorder* is a *DSM-IV* term. See also *DSM.*

**mood equilibrium,**   a nursing outcome from the Nursing Outcomes Classification (NOC) defined as the appropriate adjustment of prevailing emotional tone in response to circumstances. See also **Nursing Outcomes Classification.**

**mood management,**   a nursing intervention from the Nursing Interventions Classification (NIC) defined as providing for safety, stabilization, recovery, and maintenance of a patient who is experiencing dysfunctionally depressed or elevated mood. See also **Nursing Interventions Classification.**

**mood swing,**   an oscillation between periods of feelings of well-being and depression. Occasional "blue" periods are not regarded as abnormal. The swings are longer and more intense in persons with manic-depression. See also **bipolar disorder.**

**mood theme.**   See **communication.**

**moon face** [AS, *mona*, moon; L, *facies*, face],   a condition characterized by a rounded, puffy face. It occurs in people treated with large doses of corticosteroids, such as those with chronic asthma, rheumatoid arthritis, or acute childhood leukemia. The features return to normal when the medication is stopped. Moon face is symptomatic of Cushing's disease and Cushing's syndrome. (See Figure, p. 1120)

**Moore's fracture** [Edward M. Moore, American surgeon, 1814–1902],   a break in the distal radius with associated dislocation of the ulnar head, which causes the styloid process to be secured under the annular ligaments of the wrist.

**8-MOP.**   See **methoxsalen.**

**MOPP** /mop/,   abbreviation for a combination drug regimen used in the treatment of cancer, containing three antineoplastics, Mustargen (mechlorethamine), Oncovin (vincristine sulfate), and Matulane (procarbazine hydrochloride), and prednisone (a glucocorticoid). MOPP is prescribed in the treatment of Hodgkin's disease.

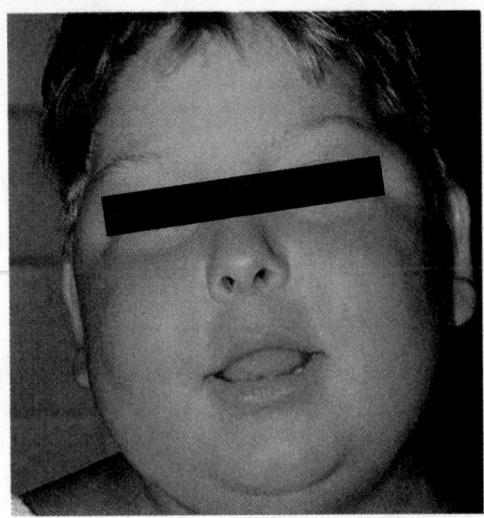

**Moon face** *(Zitelli and Davis, 1997)*

**morbilliform** /môrbil′ifôrm/ [L, *morbilli,* little disease, *forma,* form], describing a skin condition that resembles the erythematous maculopapular rash of measles, for example, a drug rash.

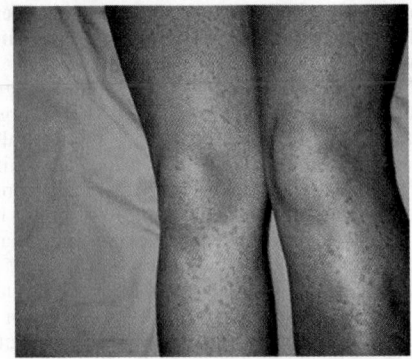

**Morbilliform eruption on legs**
*(Weston, Lane, and Morrelli, 1996)*

*Moraxella,* a genus of the Neisseriaceae family of gram-negative nonmotile cocci. They are found as pathogens and parasites on the mucous membranes of warm-blooded animals.

*Moraxella catarrhalis,* a species of aerobic nonmotile bacteria found in both the normal and the diseased nasopharynx. It is a cause of otitis media and respiratory diseases. It is a significant pathogen in children and uncompromised patients. Formerly called *Neisseria catarrhalis.*

*Moraxella lacunata,* a species of nonmotile cocci that causes corneal infections and subacute conjunctivitis or angular conjunctivitis in humans.

**morbid** [L, *morbidus,* diseased], **1.** pertaining to a pathologic or diseased condition, either physical or mental. **2.** preoccupied with unwholesome ideas.

**morbid anatomy.** See **pathologic anatomy.**

**morbidity** /môrbid′itē/ [L, *morbidus,* diseased], **1.** an illness or an abnormal condition or quality. **2.** (in statistics) the rate at which an illness or abnormality occurs, calculated by dividing the number of people who are affected within a group by the entire number of people in that group. **3.** the rate at which an illness occurs in a particular area or population.

*Morbidity and Mortality Weekly Report (MMWR),* a weekly epidemiologic report on the incidence of communicable diseases and deaths in 120 urban areas of the United States. It is published by the Centers for Disease Control and Prevention in Atlanta, Georgia. The publication also includes information on accident rates and important international health data.

**morbidity rate** [L, *morbidus,* diseased, *ratum,* calculation], the number of cases of a particular disease occurring in a single year per a specified population unit, as *x* cases per 1000. It also may be calculated on the basis of age groups, sex, occupation, or other population unit.

**morbidity statistics** [L, *morbidus,* diseased, *status,* condition], a branch of statistics that is concerned with the disease rate of a population or geographic region.

**morbid obesity** [L, *morbidus,* diseased, *obesitas,* fatness], an excess of body fat that threatens necessary body functions such as respiration.

**morbid physiology.** See **pathologic physiology.**

**morbilli.** See **measles.**

**mordant** /môr′dənt/, a substance capable of deepening the reaction of a biologic specimen to a stain. The chief mordants are alum, aniline, oil, and phenol.

**Morel's syndrome.** See **hyperostosis frontalis interna.**

**Morgagni's globule** /môrgan′yēz/ [Giovanni B. Morgagni, Italian anatomist, 1682–1771], a minute opaque sphere that may form from fluid coagulation between the eye lens and its capsule, especially in cataract. See also **globule.**

**Morgagni's tubercle** [Giovanni B. Morgagni], one of several small soft nodules on the surface of each of the areolas in women. The tubercles are produced by large sebaceous glands just below the surface of the areolae. They secrete a bacteriostatic lubricating substance during pregnancy and lactation.

**morgan** /môr′gən/ [Thomas H. Morgan, American biologist, 1866–1945], a unit of measure used in mapping the relative distances between genes on a chromosome. The measurement uses the total cross-over value as the basic unit so that 1 morgan equals 100% crossing-over or one centimorgan equals 1% recombination. One centimorgan is also equal to one map unit.

**morgue** /môrg/ [Fr, mortuary], a unit of a hospital with facilities for the storage and autopsy of the dead.

**moribund** /môr′ibund/ [L, *moribundus,* dying], near death or in the act of dying.

**morinda,** an evergreen shrub that is native to Asia, Australia, and Polynesia.

■ USES: This herb is used for headache, arthritis, and digestive, heart, and liver conditions.

■ CONTRAINDICATIONS: Morinda should not be used during pregnancy and lactation, in children, or in those with known hypersensitivity or hyperkalemia.

**Morita therapy** /môrē′tä/ [Shomei Morita, twentieth-century Japanese physician], an alternative therapy founded between 1910 and 1920. It has as its focus the symptoms of the patient. Its goal is character building, which enables the patient to live responsibly and constructively, even if the symptoms persist.

**morning after pill** [AS, *morgen* + *aefter* + *pilian,* to peel], *informal.* a large dose of an estrogen given orally, over a short period, to a woman within 24 to 72 hours after sexual intercourse to prevent conception, most commonly in an emergency such as rape or incest. The woman is warned that the medication may cause the formation of clots, severe nausea and vomiting, and teratogenic and carcinogenic effects on the fetus if pregnancy already exists or if contraception fails.

**morning dip,** a significant decline in maximal expiratory flow rate (MEFR) observed in some asthmatic patients during the early morning. The MEFR in an asthmatic person tends to follow a circadian rhythm with a morning dip and a high point in midafternoon.

**morning glory.** See *Rivea corymbosa.*

**morning ptosis,** a temporary paralysis of the upper eyelid on awakening from sleep. Also called **waking ptosis.**

**morning sickness.** See **nausea and vomiting of pregnancy.**

**morning stiffness** [OE, *morgen + stif*], a period of muscular stiffness after awakening in the morning, a common complaint of patients with arthritis or similar musculoskeletal disorders.

**Moro reflex** /môr′ō/ [Ernst Moro, German pediatrician, 1874–1951], a normal mass reflex in a young infant (up to 3 to 4 months of age) elicited by a sudden loud noise, such as by striking the table next to the child or raising the head slightly and allowing it to drop. A normal response consists of flexion of the legs, an embracing posture of the arms, and usually a brief cry. Also called **startle reflex.**

**morph-, morpho-, -morph,** combining form meaning 'form or shape': *morphallaxis, morphea, morphogenesis, endomorph.*

**morphea** /môr′fē·ə/ [Gk, *morphe*, form], a skin disease consisting of patches of yellowish or ivory-colored hard, dry, smooth skin. It is more common in females. Also spelled **morphoea.** Also called **Addison's keloid, circumscribed scleroderma, localized scleroderma.**

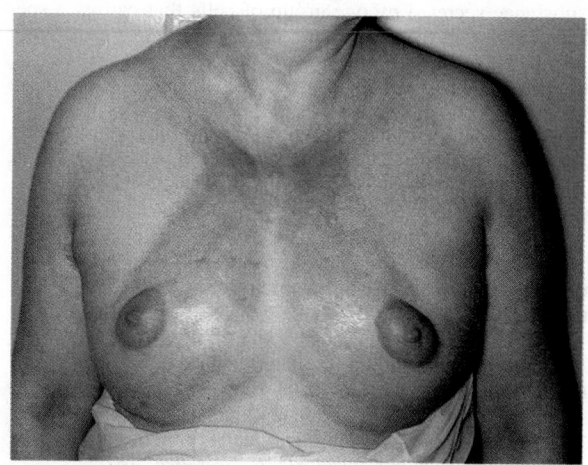

**Morphea** *(Callen et al, 1993)*

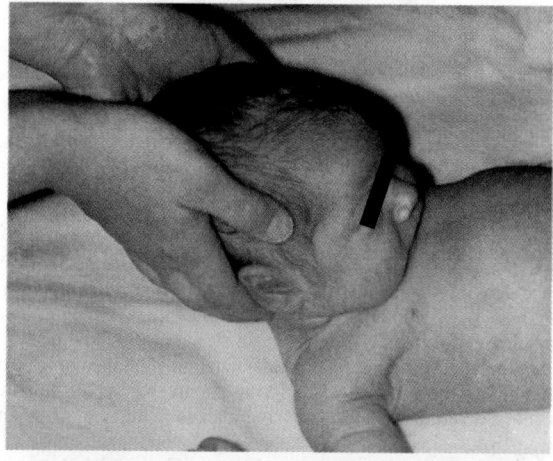

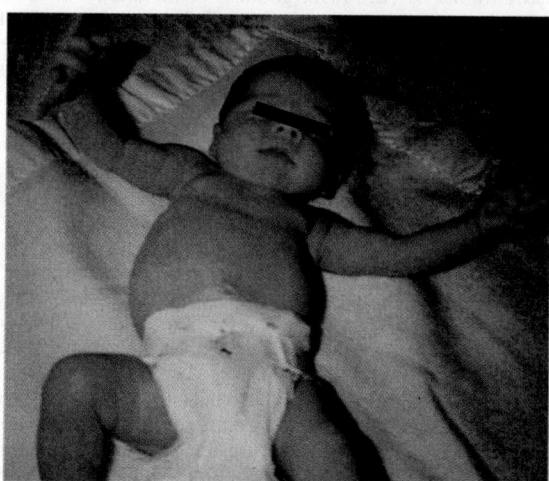

**Moro reflex** *(Zitelli and Davis, 1997)*

**-morphia, -morphy,** suffix meaning a 'condition of form': *pantamorphia, prosopodysmorphia, theromorphia.*

**morphine** /môr′fēn/ [Gk, *Morpheus*, god of sleep], a white crystalline alkaloid derived from the opium poppy, *Papaver somniferum,* the source of its principal pharmacologic activity. Morphine acts on the central nervous system to produce both depression and euphoric stimulation. It depresses the motor cortex but stimulates the spinal cord. Even in small amounts morphine depresses the respiratory system. It has a marked analgesic effect and its principal therapeutic value is pain relief. Morphine rarely provides total relief of pain, but in most cases it reduces the level of suffering. Patients with severe pain may become drowsy and relaxed but seldom achieve the sensation of euphoria associated with use of the drug. It stimulates the third cranial nerve, resulting in pupillary constriction. It is readily absorbed by mouth and is stored in skeletal muscle. Repeated use leads to physical dependence. See also **morphine sulfate, morphine tartrate.**

**morphine poisoning,** adverse effect of injection or ingestion of opioids, marked by symptoms of pinpoint pupils, drowsiness, and shallow respiration. Emergency treatment includes gastric lavage, charcoal, and respiratory support. Naloxone is administered intravenously as needed to arouse the patient and IV fluid is given to support circulation.

**morphine sulfate,** an opioid analgesic.

■ INDICATION: It is prescribed to relieve pain.

■ CONTRAINDICATIONS: Drug dependence or known hypersensitivity to this drug prohibits its use.

■ ADVERSE EFFECTS: Among the more serious adverse reactions are increased intracranial pressure, cardiovascular disturbances, respiratory depression, and drug dependence.

**morphine tartrate,** a white crystalline powder used in injections of morphine. It is more soluble in water than morphine itself and is used in various parenteral preparations.

**morphinism** /môr′finiz′əm/, a pathologic state caused by morphine addiction.

**-morphism,** suffix meaning the 'condition of having a (specified) shape': *amorphism, isomorphism, pedomorphism.*

**morpho-.** See **morph-.**

**morphoea.** See **morphea.**

**morphogen** /môr′fəjens/, **1.** a soluble substance that controls the embryonic differentiation of a cell or tissue. **2.** a substance secreted by one group of cells that causes a specific change in the growth and differentiation of a different group.

**morphogenesis** /môr′fəjen′əsis/ [Gk, *morphe* + *genein,* to produce], the development and differentiation of the structures and the form of an organism, specifically the changes that occur in the cells and tissue during embryonic development. Also called **morphogeny** /môrfoj′ənē/.

**morphogenetic** /-jənet′ik/, (in embryology) pertaining to a substance or hormone that acts as an evocator in differentiation. Also **morphogenic.**

**morphogeny.** See **morphogenesis.**

**morphology** /môrfol′əjē/ [Gk, *morphe* + *logos,* science], the study of the physical shape and size of a specimen, plant, or animal. —**morphologic** /môr′fəloj′ik/, *adj.*

**morphometry** /môrfom′ətrē/, the measurement of the structures and parts of organisms.

**-morphosis,** suffix meaning a 'development or change': *chemomorphosis, epimorphosis, heteromorphosis.*

**Morquio's disease** /môrkē′ōz/ [Luis Morquio, Uruguayan physician, 1867–1935], a familial form of mucopolysaccharidosis that results in abnormal musculoskeletal development in childhood. Dwarfism, hunchback, enlarged sternum, and knock-knees may occur. The disease may first be evident as the child, learning to walk, displays an abnormal, waddling gait. Also called **MPS IV.** See also **mucopolysaccharidosis.**

**mortal** [L, *mortalis,* perishable], **1.** subject to death. **2.** causing death.

**mortality** [L, *mortalis,* perishable], **1.** the condition of being subject to death. **2.** the death rate, which reflects the number of deaths per unit of population in any specific region, age group, disease, or other classification, usually expressed as deaths per 1000, 10,000, or 100,000.

**mortar** /môr′tər/ [L, *mortarium*], a cup-shaped vessel in which materials are ground or crushed by a pestle in the preparation of drugs.

**mortinatality** /môr′tinātal′itē/ [L, *mors,* death, *natus,* birth], the stillbirth rate. It is calculated by multiplying the number of stillbirths by 1000 and dividing by the total number of births per year. Also called **natimortality.**

**mortise joint** /môr′tis/ [ME, *mortays,* fixed in, *jungere,* to join], the articulatio talocruralis joint of the ankle.

**Morton's disease** [Thomas G. Morton, American surgeon, 1835–1903; L, *dis* + Fr, *aise,* ease], a form of foot neuralgia caused by a falling metatarsal arch, which puts pressure on the digital branches of the lateral plantar nerve. Also called **Morton's foot, Morton's neuralgia, Morton's neuroma, Morton's toe.**

**Morton's foot.** See **Morton's disease.**

**Morton's neuralgia.** See **Morton's disease.**

**Morton's neuroma.** See **Morton's disease.**

**Morton's plantar neuralgia** [Thomas G. Morton; L, *planta,* foot sole; Gk, *neuron,* nerve, *algos,* pain], a severe throbbing pain that affects the anastomotic nerve branch between the medial and the lateral plantar nerves.

**Morton's syndrome** [Dudley J. Morton, American orthopedist, 1884–1960; Gk, *syn,* together, *dromos,* course], a congenital foreshortening of the first metatarsal segment, causing pain and deformity of the front part of the foot.

**Morton's toe.** See **Morton's disease.**

**mortuary** /môr′chəwer′ē/ [L, *mortuarium,* tomb], a building where the bodies of deceased persons are held for identification, postmortem examination, and preparation for burial or cremation.

**morula** /môr′ələ/, *pl.* **morulas, morulae** [L, *morulus,* blackberry], a solid, spherical mass of cells resulting from the cleavage of the fertilized ovum in the early stages of embryonic development. It represents an intermediate stage between the zygote and the blastocyst and consists of blastomeres that are uniform in size, shape, and physiologic capabilities. —**morular,** *adj.*

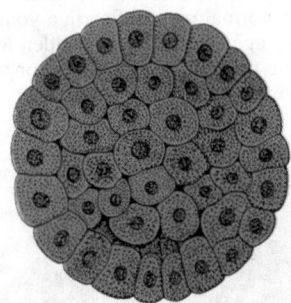

**Morula** *(Thibodeau and Patton, 1999)*

**-morula,** suffix meaning a 'clump of blastomeres formed by cleavage of a fertilized ovum': *amphimorula, archimorula, pseudomorula.*

**morulae, morulas.** See **morula.**

**Morvan's disease,** a form of syringomyelia with tissue changes in the extremities, such as a paresthesia of the forearms and hands and progressive painless ulceration of the fingertips.

**mosaic** /mōzā′ik/ [L, *Musa,* goddess of the arts], **1.** an individual or organism that developed from a single zygote but that has two or more kinds of genetically different cell populations. Mosaicism may result from a mutation, crossing over, or more commonly in humans, nondisjunction of chromosomes during early embryogenesis, which causes a variation in the number of chromosomes in the cells. The type of chromosomal aberration and the fraction of cells that are affected depend on the cleavage stage at which the causative event occurred. Because monosomic cells are nonviable, except in X monosomic conditions, most mosaic conditions caused by nondisjunction in humans represent a mixture of normal and trisomic cells, regardless of whether an autosome or the sex chromosomes are involved. The degree of clinical involvement depends on the type of tissue containing the abnormality and may vary from near normal to full manifestation of a syndrome, such as Down syndrome or Turner's syndrome. Compare **chimera.** See also **monosomy, sex chromosome mosaic, trisomy. 2.** a fertilized ovum that undergoes determinate cleavage. See also **mosaic development. —mosaicism,** *n.*

**mosaic bone,** bone tissue appearing to be made up of many tiny pieces cemented together, as seen on microscopic examination of an x-ray film of the affected bone. It is characteristic of Paget's disease.

**mosaic cleavage.** See **determinate cleavage.**

**mosaic development,** a kind of embryonic development occurring in the blastocyst. The fertilized ovum undergoes determinate cleavage, developing according to a precise, unalterable plan in which each blastomere has a characteristic position and limited developmental potency and is a precursor of a specific part of the embryo. Damage to or destruction of these cells results in a defective organism. Compare **regulative development.**

**mosaicism** /mōzā'isiz'əm/ [L, *Musa,* goddess of the arts], (in genetics) a condition in which an individual or an organism that develops from a single zygote has two or more cell populations that differ in genetic constitution. Most commonly seen in humans is a variation in the number of chromosomes in the cells, which may involve either a particular autosome, such as in Down syndrome, or the sex chromosomes, such as in Turner's syndrome and Kleinfelter's syndrome. See also **mosaic, sex chromosome mosaic.**

**mosaic wart,** a group of contiguous plantar warts.

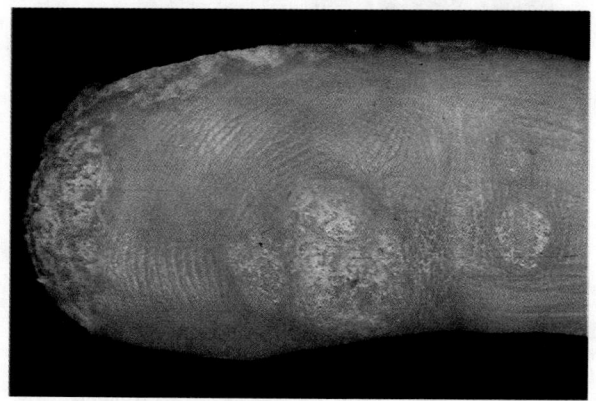

**Mosaic wart** *(du Vivier, 1993)*

**mosquito bite** /məskē'tō/ [L, *musca,* a fly; AS, *bitan,* to bite], a bite of a blood-sucking arthropod of the subfamily Culicidae that may result in a systemic allergic reaction in a hypersensitive person, an infection, or, most often, a pruritic wheal. Mosquitoes, which are attracted to hosts by moisture, carbon dioxide, estrogens, sweat, or warmth, are vectors of many infectious diseases.

**mosquito forceps,** a small hemostatic forceps. See also **Halsted's forceps,** def. 1.

**Mössbauer spectrometer** /mes'bou·ər, mœs'bou·ər/ [Rudolf L. Mössbauer, German physicist, b. 1929], an instrument that can detect small changes between an atomic nucleus and its environment, such as caused by alterations in temperature, pressure, or chemical state. The device is used in chemical and physical research with applications in medicine.

**most probable number,** a statistical value representing the viable bacterial population in a sample through the use of dilution and multiple tube inoculations.

**mot-,** prefix meaning 'movement': *motoneuron, motorgraphic, motoricity.*

**mother fixation** [AS, *modor,* mother; L, *figere,* to fasten], an arrest in psychosexual development characterized by an abnormally persistent, close, and often paralyzing emotional attachment to one's mother. Compare **father fixation.** See also **freudian fixation.**

**mother yaw.** See **yaw.**

**motile** /mō'til/ [L, *motare,* to move often], capable of spontaneous but unconscious or involuntary movement. —**motility,** *n.*

**motilin** /mōtil'in/, a peptide hormone secreted by enterochromaffin cells of the intestinal tract. It stimulates GI motility and pepsin secretion.

**-motility, -mobility,** suffix meaning the 'condition of being capable of movement': *cardiomotility, hypermotility, supermotility.*

**-motine,** combining form for antiviral quinoline derivatives.

**motion sickness.** See **kinesia.**

**motivation** /mō'tivā'shən/ [L, *movere,* to move], conscious or unconscious needs, interests, rewards, or other incentives that arouse, channel, or maintain a particular behavior.

**motivational conflict** /mō'tivā'shənəl/ [L, *movere,* to move, *alis,* relating to, *confluere,* to come together], a conflict resulting from the arousal of two or more motives that direct behavior toward incompatible goals. Kinds of motivational conflict include **approach-approach conflict, approach-avoidance conflict,** and **avoidance-avoidance conflict.**

**motoneuron** /mō'tōnŏŏr'on/ [L, *movere,* to move; Gk, *neuron,* nerve], a motor neuron. Its function is to produce muscle contractions.

**motor** [L, *movere,* to move], **1.** pertaining to motion, the body apparatus involved in movement, or the brain functions that direct purposeful activities. **2.** pertaining to a muscle, nerve, or brain center that produces or subserves motion.

**-motor,** suffix meaning 'effects of activity in a body part': *nervimotor, psychomotor, viscerimotor.*

**motor aphasia,** the inability to say remembered words, caused by a cerebral lesion in the inferior frontal gyrus (Broca's motor speech area) of the left hemisphere. The condition most commonly is the result of a stroke. The patient knows what to say but cannot articulate the words. Also called **ataxic aphasia, expressive aphasia, frontocortical aphasia, verbal aphasia.**

**motor apraxia,** the inability to carry out planned movements or to handle small objects, although cognizant of the proper use of the object. The condition results from a lesion in the premotor frontal cortex on the opposite side of the affected limb. Also called **innervation apraxia.** See also **apraxia.**

**motor area,** a portion of the cerebral cortex that includes the precentral gyrus and the posterior part of the frontal gyri and that causes the contraction of the voluntary muscles on stimulation with electrodes. Normal voluntary activity requires associations between the motor area and other parts of the cortex; removal of the motor area from one cerebral hemisphere causes paralysis of voluntary muscles, especially of the opposite side of the body. Various parts of the motor area are associated with different body structures, such as the lower limb, the face, the mouth, and the hand. The parts associated with more delicate, complicated movements, such as those of the hand, are larger than those associated with more general movements.

**motor ataxia,** an inability to perform coordinated movements. Also called **kinetic ataxia.**

**motor coordination,** the harmonious functioning of body parts that involve movement, including gross motor movement, fine motor movement, and motor planning.

**motor depressant** [L, *movere,* to move, *deprimere,* to press down], a drug or agent that reduces the normal functioning level of motor neurons, mainly in voluntary muscles.

**motor end plate,** a large special synaptic contact between motor axons and each skeletal muscle fiber. Each muscle fiber forms one end plate. See also **end plate.**

**motor fiber,** one of the fibers (axons) in the cranial and spinal nerves that transmit impulses to and cause contraction of muscle fibers.

**motor hallucination** [L, *movere,* to move, *alucinari,* wandering mind], the subjective experience of movement when there is no movement.

**motor image,** a visual concept of one's bodily movements, real or imagined.

**motor nerve,** an efferent nerve that conveys impulses to motor end plates or another terminal and is mainly responsible for stimulating muscles and glands.

**motor neuron,** one of various efferent nerve cells that transmit nerve impulses from the brain or from the spinal cord to muscular or glandular tissue. According to location, some kinds of motor neurons are the peripheral motor neurons and the upper motor neurons. Also called **motoneuron.** Compare **sensory nerve.** See also **nervous system.**

**motor neuron disease** [L, *movere,* to move, *neuron,* nerve; L, *dis* + Fr, *aise,* ease], any disease of a motor neuron, with degeneration of anterior horn cells, motor cranial nerve nuclei, and pyramidal tracts. An example is **amyotrophic lateral sclerosis (ALS).**

**motor neuron paralysis,** an injury to the spinal cord that causes damage to the motor neurons and results in various degrees of functional impairment depending on the site of the lesion. See also **lower motor neuron paralysis, upper motor neuron paralysis.**

**motor nucleus** [L, *movere,* to move, *nucleus,* nut kernel], the nucleus of a motor nerve or a collection of motor neurons.

**motor pathway** [L, *movere,* to move; AS, *paeth*], the route of motor nerve impulses, from the central neuron to a muscle or gland.

**motor planning,** the ability to plan and execute skilled nonhabitual tasks. Also called **motor praxis.**

**motor point,** **1.** a point at which a motor nerve enters a muscle. **2.** any point on the skin over a muscle at which electrical stimulation (via electrode) causes contraction of the muscle. See also **motor nerve, nervous system.**

**motor praxis.** See **motor planning.**

**motor protein,** protein that moves along a surface, propelled by the energy of adenosine triphosphate (ATP) hydrolysis.

**motor root** [L, *movere,* to move; AS, *rot*], the proximal end of a motor nerve at its attachment to the spinal cord.

**motor seizure,** a transitory disturbance in brain function caused by abnormal neuronal discharges that arise initially in a localized motor area of the cerebral cortex. The manifestations depend on the site of the abnormal electrical activity, such as tonic contractures of the thumb caused by excessive discharges in the motor area of the cortex controlling the first digit or chewing movements resulting from discharges in the lower part of the motor strip controlling mastication. The disturbance may spread, or it may end in a shower of clonic movements or a generalized convulsion. See also **epilepsy, focal seizure.**

**motor sense,** the feeling or perception enabling a person to accomplish a purposeful movement, presumably achieved by evoking a sensory engram or memory of the pattern for that specific movement. Proprioceptive signals transmitted by feedback pathways through the cerebellum and sensory areas of the motor cortex are compared with the engram and modify the movement. Experiments with animals show that a movement cannot be performed if the corresponding sensory area of the brain is removed; if the motor area is removed, the movement is accomplished by using a different group of muscles.

**motor speech areas** [L, *movere,* to move; AS, *spaec* + L, *area,* vacant place], the regions of the cerebral hemispheres that are associated with motor control of speech. For right-handed people the sites are generally located in the left hemisphere. See also **Broca's area.**

**motor tract** [L, *movere,* to move, *tractus*], an efferent nerve pathway that conveys impulses controlling movement.

**motor unit,** a functional structure consisting of a motor neuron and the muscle fibers it innervates.

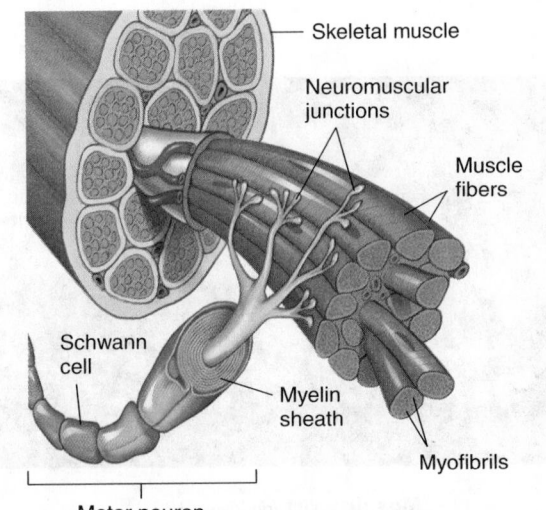

**Motor unit**

**motor unit recruitment,** the bringing into activity of additional motor neurons, which causes additional muscle fibers to contract. As more units are recruited and as the frequency of discharge increases, muscle tension increases. The pattern of motor unit recruitment varies, depending on the inherent properties of specific motor neurons.

**Motrin,** trademark for a nonsteroidal antiinflammatory (ibuprofen).

**mottle** [ME, *motley,* mixed colors], an effect observed in radiographic imaging when the dose of radiation used is reduced to a level where individual quantum effects can be seen. At very low doses, the number of photons being produced is so small that the statistical variations in x-ray production can be visualized. Also called **noise, quantum mottle.**

**mountain fever, mountain tick fever.** See **Colorado tick fever, Rocky Mountain spotted fever.**

**mountain sickness.** See **altitude sickness.**

**mounting** /mount'ing/, the preparation of specimens and slides for study.

**mount of Venus.** See **mons veneris.**

**mourning** /mōr'ning/ [AS, *murnan*, to mourn], a response to the loss of a loved object. It is through mourning that grief is resolved. See also **bereavement, grief.**

**mouse** [L, *mus*], a hand-controlled computer input device. Moving the device on a flat surface and pushing buttons on its back cause the cursor or pointer to move to target areas or select items on a computer screen. See also **joystick.**

**mouse-tooth forceps,** a kind of dressing forceps that has one or more fine sharp points on the tip of each blade. The tips turn in, and the delicate teeth interlock.

**mouth** [AS, *muth*], **1.** the nearly oval oral cavity at the superior, anterior end of the digestive tube, bounded anteriorly by the lips and containing the tongue and the teeth. It consists of the vestibule and the **oral cavity proper.** The vestibule, situated in front of the teeth, is bounded externally by the lips and the cheeks, internally by the gums and the teeth. The vestibule receives the secretion from the parotid salivary glands. The oral cavity proper is bounded by the alveolar arches and the teeth, communicates with the pharynx, and is roofed by the hard and the soft palates. The tongue forms the greater part of the floor of the cavity. The rest of the floor is formed by the reflection of the mucous membrane from the sides and the bottom of the tongue to the gum lining the inner part of the mandible. The oral cavity proper receives the secretion from the submandibular and sublingual salivary glands. **2.** an orifice.

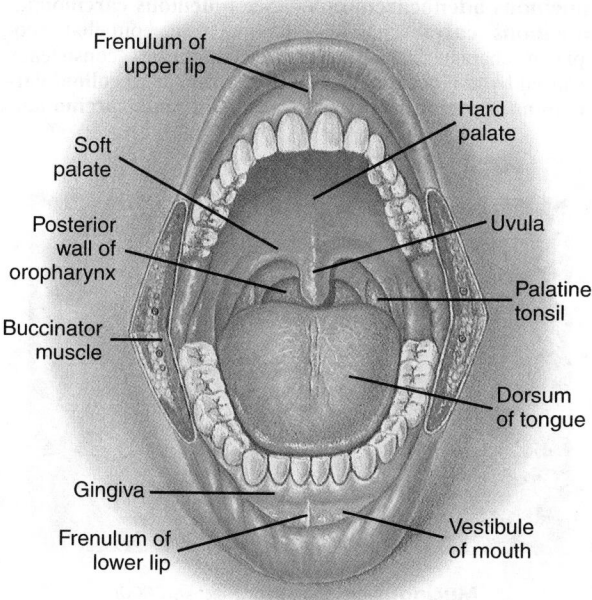

**Mouth structures** *(Seidel et al, 1999)*

Frenulum of upper lip
Hard palate
Soft palate
Posterior wall of oropharynx
Uvula
Buccinator muscle
Palatine tonsil
Dorsum of tongue
Gingiva
Frenulum of lower lip
Vestibule of mouth

**mouth breathing,** breathing through the mouth instead of the nose, usually because of some obstruction of the nasal passages.

**mouth guard,** a soft, plastic, intraoral appliance that covers the palate and all the occlusal surfaces of the teeth. It is worn in contact sports to limit damage to tissues of the mouth, lips, and other oral surfaces. Compare **biteguard.**

**mouth prop.** See **gag.**

**mouth rinse** /mouth'rins/, a solution for cleaning or treating the oral mucosa and controlling dental caries. A typical therapeutic mouth rinse may contain sodium fluoride, glycerine, alcohol, detergents, and other ingredients. Some mouth rinses only remove loose debris and add a fragrance to mask mouth odors.

**mouthstick** /mouth'stik/, a device that is gripped with the teeth and can be used to type, push buttons, turn pages, operate power wheelchairs, or modify environmental control units and other equipment using head movements. It is commonly used by individuals who have a high-level (C4 and up) quadriplegia. Also called **chinstick.**

**mouth-to-mouth resuscitation,** a procedure in artificial resuscitation, performed most often with cardiac massage. The victim's nose is sealed by pinching the nostrils closed, the head is extended, and air is breathed by the rescuer through the mouth into the lungs. See also **cardiopulmonary resuscitation.**

**mouth-to-nose resuscitation,** a procedure in artificial resuscitation in which the mouth of the victim is covered and held closed and air is breathed through the victim's nose. See also **mouth-to-mouth resuscitation.**

**mouthwash** /mouth'wôsh/, a medicated liquid used for cleaning the oral cavity and treating mucous membranes of the mouth. Many over-the-counter mouthwashes contain alcohol, which may contribute to surface softening and increased wear of dental resins and composite materials. See also **mouth rinse.**

**MOV,** abbreviation for **minimal occlusive volume.**

**movement decomposition** [L, *movere*, to move, *de*, away, *componere*, to assemble], a distortion in voluntary movement in which motion occurs in a distinct sequence of isolated steps rather than in a normal smooth, flowing pattern.

**moving grid,** an x-ray grid that is continuously moved or oscillated throughout the exposure of a radiographic film.

**moxibustion** /mok'səbus'chən/ [Jpn, *moe kusa*, burning herb; L, *comburere*, to burn up], a method of producing analgesia or altering the function of a body system by igniting moxa, wormwood, or another combustible, slow-burning substance and holding it as near the point on the skin as possible without causing pain or burning. It is also sometimes used in conjunction with acupuncture.

**moxifloxacin,** an antiinfective.

■ INDICATIONS: Moxifloxacin is used to treat acute bacterial sinusitis caused by *Streptococcus pneumoniae, Haemophilus influenzae,* and *Moraxella catarrhalis;* acute bacterial exacerbation of chronic bronchitis from *S. pneumoniae, H. influenzae, H. parainfluenzae, Klebsiella pneumoniae, Staphylococcus aureus,* and *M. catarrhalis;* and community-acquired pneumonia from *S. pneumoniae, H. influenzae, Mycoplasma pneumoniae, Chlamydia pneumoniae,* and *M. catarrhalis.*

■ CONTRAINDICATIONS: Known hypersensitivity to quinolones prohibits use of this drug.

■ ADVERSE EFFECTS: Seizures are a life-threatening effect of this drug. Other adverse effects include prolonged QT interval, dizziness, fatigue, insomnia, depression, confusion, increased ALT and AST, flatulence, heartburn, oral candidiasis, dysphagia, pruritus, urticaria, photosensitivity, flushing, fever, chills, tremor, arthralgia, and tendon rupture. Common side effects include headache, restlessness, nausea, diarrhea, and rash.

**moyamoya disease** /moi'əmoi'ə/, a cerebrovascular disorder in which the main cerebral arteries at the base of the brain are replaced by a fine network of vessels. It tends mainly to affect Japanese children and young adults and is characterized by convulsions, hemiplegia, mental retardation, and subarachnoid hemorrhage. Patients who survive into adulthood are susceptible to massive intracerebral hemorrhage caused by rupture of the fragile network of new vessels. Few patients live beyond 30 years of age.

**6-MP,** abbreviation for **6-mercaptopurine.** See **mercaptopurine.**

**MPD, M.P.D.,** abbreviation for **maximum permissible dose.**

**MPGN,** abbreviation for **membranoproliferative glomerulonephritis.**

**M.P.H.,** abbreviation for *Master of Public Health.*

**MPL + PRED,** an anticancer drug combination of melphalan and prednisone.

**MPO,** abbreviation for **myeloperoxidase.**

**MPS,** abbreviation for **mucopolysaccharidosis.**

**MPS I,** abbreviation for *mucopolysaccharidosis I.* See **Hurler's syndrome.**

**MPS II,** abbreviation for *mucopolysaccharidosis II.* See **Hunter's syndrome.**

**MPS IV,** abbreviation for *mucopolysaccharidosis IV.* See **Morquio's disease.**

**MQF,** abbreviation for *mobile quarantine facility.*

**mr, mR,** abbreviation for **milliroentgen.**

**mrad,** abbreviation for **millirad.**

**mrem,** abbreviation for **millirem.**

**MRI,** abbreviation for **magnetic resonance imaging.**

**mRNA,** abbreviation for **messenger RNA.**

**MRSA,** methicillin-resistant *Staphylococcus aureus.*

**MS,** abbreviation for **multiple sclerosis.**

**M.S.,** **1.** abbreviation for *Master of Science.* **2.** abbreviation for *Master of Surgery.*

**MSAFP test,** abbreviation for **maternal serum alphafetoprotein (MSAFP) test.**

**msec,** abbreviation for **millisecond.**

**MSG,** abbreviation for **monosodium glutamate.**

**MSH,** abbreviation for **melanocyte stimulating hormone.**

**MSLT,** abbreviation for **multiple sleep latency test.**

**MSN,** abbreviation for *Master of Science in Nursing.* See **master's degree program in nursing.**

**MSO,** abbreviation for **management service organization.**

**M.T.,** abbreviation for **medical technologist.**

**MTT,** abbreviation for **maximal treadmill test.**

**MTX + MP + CTX,** an anticancer drug combination of methotrexate, mercaptopurine, and cyclophosphamide.

**mu,** /myoo, moo/, **1.** μ, M, the twelfth letter of the Greek alphabet. **2.** μ, symbol for **micrometer, micron.**

**muc-, muco-,** combining form meaning 'mucus': *mucolytic, mucosal.*

**Mucha-Habermann disease** /moo'kä·hä'ber·män/ [Viktor Mucha; Austrian dermatologist, 1877–1919; Rudolf Habermann, German dermatologist, 1884–1941], an acute or subacute, sometimes relapsing, widespread macular, papular, or vesicular eruption that tends to crusting, necrosis, and hemorrhage, which heals, leaving pigmented depressed scars, followed by the development of a new crop of lesions. Occasionally, progression to a chronic form may occur. Also called **acute lichenoid pityriasis, acute parapsoriasis, Habermann's disease, Mucha's disease, parapsoriasis varioliformis acuta, pityriasis lichenoides et varioliformis acuta.**

**Much's granules** /mooks, mookhs/ [Hans C. Much, German physician, 1880–1932], granules and rods, found in tuberculosis sputum, that stain with Gram's stain but not by the usual methods for acid-fast bacilli.

**mucilage** /m(y)oo'səlij/, **1.** a sticky mixture of carbohydrates produced by plant cell activity. **2.** a thick aqueous solution of a gum used for suspending insoluble substances and for increasing viscosity.

**mucin** /myoo'sin/ [L, *mucus,* slime], a mucopolysaccharide, the chief ingredient in mucus. Mucin is present in most glands that secrete mucus and is the lubricant protecting body surfaces from friction or erosion.

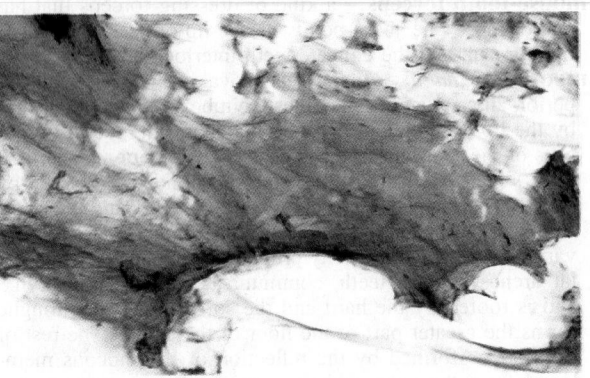

**Mucin** *(McKee, 1997)*

**mucinase.** See **mucopolysaccharidase.**

**mucinoid** /myoo'sinoid/ [L, *mucus* + Gk, *eidos,* form], resembling mucin. See also **mucoid,** def. 2.

**mucinous adenocarcinoma.** See **mucinous carcinoma.**

**mucinous carcinoma** /myoo'sinəs/, an epithelial neoplasm characterized by a sticky gelatinous consistency caused by copious mucin secretion. Also called **colloid carcinoma, gelatiniform carcinoma, gelatinous carcinoma.**

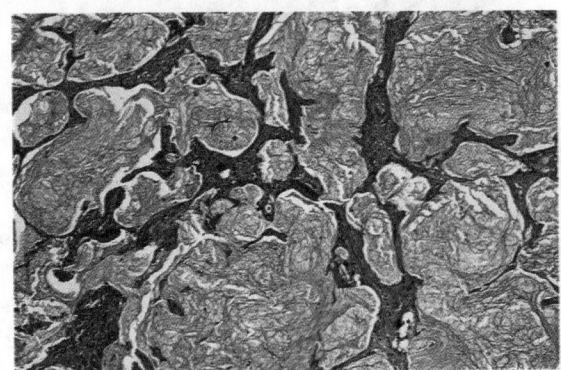

**Mucinous carcinoma** *(Fletcher, 2000)*

**mucocele** /myoo'kō·sēl/ [L, *mucus,* slime; Gk, *koilia,* cavity], **1.** dilation of a cavity with accumulated mucous secretion. **2.** see **mucus extravasation phenomenon, mucus retention cyst.**

**mucocutaneous** /myoo'kōkyootā'nē·əs/ [L, *mucus* + *cutis,* skin, *osus,* having], pertaining to the mucous membrane and the skin.

**mucocutaneous leishmaniasis.** See **American leishmaniasis.**

**mucocutaneous lymph node syndrome (MLNS),** an acute febrile illness, primarily of young children, characterized by inflamed mucous membranes of the mouth, "strawberry tongue," cervical lymphadenopathy, polymorphous rash on the trunk, and edema, erythema, and desquamation of the skin on the extremities. Other commonly associated findings include arthralgia, diarrhea, otitis, pneumonia, photophobia, meningitis, and electrocardiographic changes. The cause is unknown; no clear-cut environmental, seasonal, or geographic factors have been discovered, and person-to-person transmission is unproved. A genetic predisposition has been indicated. Treatment includes IV gammaglobulin; aspirin in large doses, which may be prescribed over a long period; and supportive care. Also called **Kawasaki disease.**

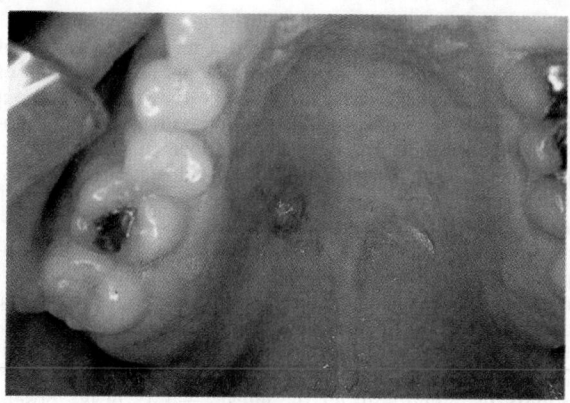

**Mucoepidermoid carcinoma**
*(Regezi, Sciubba, and Rogrel, 2000)*

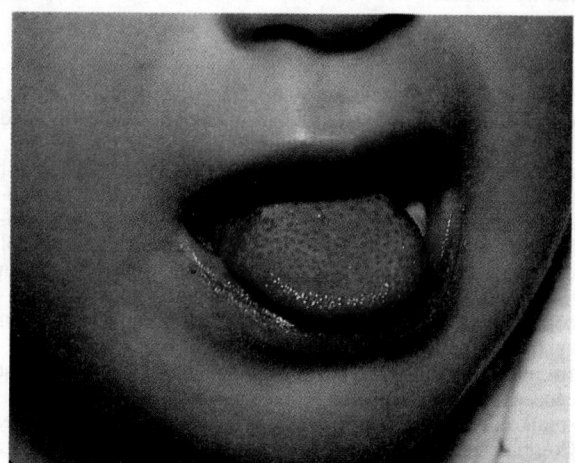

**mucogingival junction** /myo͞o′kōjinjī′vəl/ [L, *mucus* + *gingiva,* gum, *jungere,* to join], the scalloped linear area of the gums that separates the gingiva from the alveolar mucosa. It can be seen easily by pulling the mandibular lip outward and looking at the labial mucosa of the mandible.

**mucoid** /myo͞o′koid/ [L, *mucus* + Gk, *eidos,* form], **1.** resembling mucus. **2.** also **mucinoid.** a group of glycoproteins, including colloid and ovomucoid, similar to the mucins, primarily differing in solubility.

**mucoid cyst** [L, *mucus* + Gk, *eidos,* form, *kytis,* bag], a cyst formed by an overgrowth of a mucus gland or by the spread of mucus into the interstitial tissues. Also called **mucous cyst.**

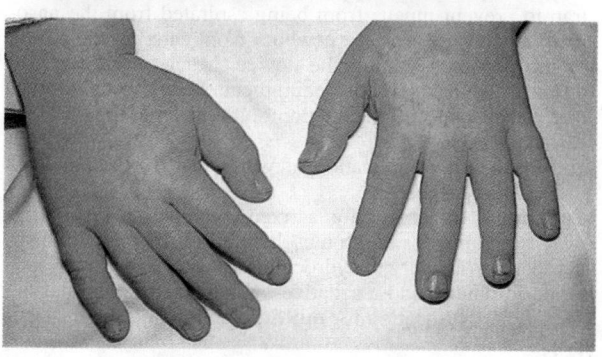

**Mucocutaneous lymph node syndrome (Kawasaki disease)**
*(Zitelli and Davis, 1997)*

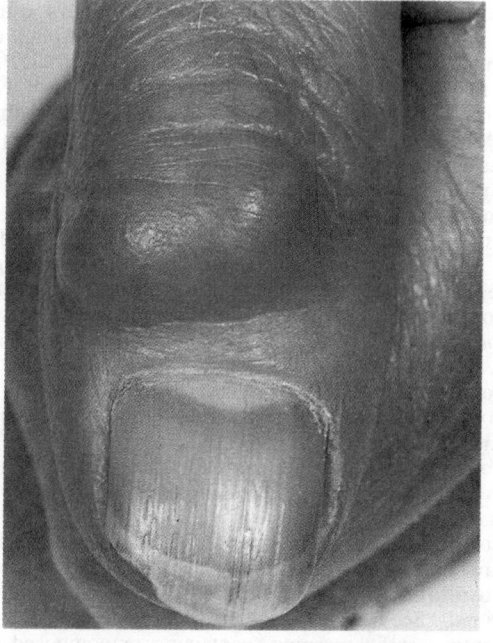

**Mucoid cyst** *(du Vivier, 1993)*

**mucoepidermoid carcinoma** /myo͞o′kō·ep′idur′moid/ [L, *mucus* + Gk, *epi,* above, *derma,* skin, *eidos,* form], a malignant neoplasm of glandular tissues, especially the ducts of the salivary glands. The tumor contains mucinous and epidermoid squamous cells.

**mucoid tissue.** See **embryonic tissue.**

**mucolipidosis** /myoo′kōlip′idō′sis/, any of a group of metabolic disorders characterized by an accumulation of mucopolysaccharides and lipids in the tissues, but without an excess of mucopolysaccharides in the urine. Mucolipidosis includes I cell disease (mucolipidosis II [ML II]) and pseudo-Hurler polydystrophy (mucolipidosis III [ML III]).

**mucolipidosis II.** See **I cell disease.**

**mucolipidosis IV,** an autosomal recessive disorder characterized by psychomotor retardation and severe visual impairment, initially manifest in infancy or childhood as corneal clouding. Sialic acid–containing gangliosides are accumulated as a result of deficient ganglioside sialidase activity; however the deficiency is not believed to be the primary defect.

**mucolytic** /myoo′kəlit′ik/ [L, *mucus* + Gk, *lysis*, loosening], **1.** exerting a destructive effect on mucus. **2.** any agent that dissolves or destroys mucus.

**mucomembranous** /myoo′kəmem′brənəs/ [L, *mucus + membrana*, thin skin, *osus*, having], pertaining to a mucous membrane, such as that of the small intestine or the bladder.

**Mucomyst,** trademark for a mucolytic (acetylcysteine).

**mucopolysaccharidase** /myoo′kōpol′ēsak′əridās′/, an enzyme that breaks down molecules of polysaccharides. Also called **mucinase.**

**mucopolysaccharide** /myoo′kōpol′ēsak′ərīd/ [L, *mucus* + Gk, *polys*, many, *sakcharon*, sugar], a polysaccharide containing hexosamine and sometimes occurring with protein, such as mucins.

**mucopolysaccharidosis (MPS)** /myoo′kōpol′ēsak′əridō′-sis/, *pl.* **mucopolysaccharidoses** [L, *mucus* + Gk, *polys*, many, *sakcharon*, sugar, *osis*, condition], one of a group of genetic disorders characterized by greater than normal accumulations of mucopolysaccharides in the tissues, with other symptoms specific to each type. The disorders are numbered MPS I through MPS VII, and each type has a specific eponym. All types are characterized by pronounced skeletal deformity (especially of the face), mental and physical retardation, and decreased life expectancy. The disorders may be detected before birth by testing fetal cells present in amniotic fluid. After birth diagnosis is established through urine testing, skeletal changes observed on radiographic films, and family history. There is no successful treatment. Kinds of mucopolysaccharidosis include **Hunter's syndrome (MPS II), Hurler's syndrome (MPS I),** and **Morquio's disease (MPS IV), Sly syndrome (MPS VII), and Sanfilippo's syndrome (MPS III)** to the list of types.

**mucoprotein** /myoo′kōprō′tēn, -tē·in/ [L, *mucus* + Gk, *proteios*, first rank], a compound, present in all connective and supporting tissue, that contains polysaccharides combined with protein. It is relatively resistant to denaturation.

**mucopurulent** /myoo′kōpyoor′yələnt/ [L, *mucus + purulentus*, pus], characteristic of a combination of mucus and pus.

**mucormycosis.** See **zygomycosis.**

**mucosa** /myoo͞okō′sə/, *pl.* **mucosae**, mucous membrane. —**mucosal**, *adj.*

**mucosal immune system** /myoo͞okō′səl/, the lymphoid tissues of the mucosal surfaces lining the GI, respiratory, and urogenital tracts.

**mucositis** /myoo′kōsī′tis/, any inflammation of a mucous membrane, such as the lining of the mouth and throat.

**mucosulfatidosis.** See **multiple sulfatase deficiency.**

**mucous.** See **mucus.**

**-mucous,** suffix meaning 'containing or composed of or secreting mucus': *fibromucous, puromucous, seromucous.*

**mucous colitis.** See **irritable bowel syndrome.**

**mucous cyst.** See **mucoid cyst.**

**mucous membrane** /myoo′kəs/ [L, *mucus + membrana*, thin skin], any one of four major kinds of thin sheets of tissue that cover or line various parts of the body. Mucous membrane lines cavities or canals of the body that open to the outside, such as the linings of the mouth, the digestive tube, the respiratory passages, and the genitourinary tract. It consists of a surface layer of epithelial tissue covering a deeper layer of connective tissue and protects the underlying structure, secretes mucus, and absorbs water, salts, and other solutes. Compare **serous membrane, skin, synovial membrane.**

**mucous plug,** (in obstetrics) a collection of thick mucus in the uterine cervix that is often expelled at the onset of dilation of the cervix, just before labor begins or in its early hours. The plug may be dry and firm, following the shape of the endocervical canal, but more often it is semifluid and mucoid, streaked with blood.

**mucous shreds.** See **shreds.**

**mucous tissue.** See **embryonic tissue.**

**mucous tumor.** See **myxoma.**

**mucoviscidosis.** See **cystic fibrosis.**

**mucus** /myoo′kəs/ [L, slime], the viscous, slippery secretions of mucous membranes and glands, containing mucin, white blood cells, water, inorganic salts, and exfoliated cells. —**mucoid,** *adj.*, **mucous** /myoo′kəs/, *adj.*

**mucus extravasation phenomenon,** extravasation of mucus into the surrounding connective tissue from a damaged minor salivary gland excretory duct, followed by an inflammatory reaction leading to the formation of a pool of macrophages and mucin surrounded by a wall of granulation tissue; visible as a small nodule or vesicle on the oral mucosa. Also called **mucocele.** Compare **mucus retention cyst.**

**mucus retention cyst,** a mucus-containing retention cyst caused by blockage of a salivary gland duct, visible as a small nodule on the oral mucosa; also called **mucocele.** Compare **mucus extravasation phenomenon.**

**mucus trap suction apparatus,** a catheter containing a trap to prevent mucus from being aspirated from the nasopharynx and trachea of a newborn from entering the mouth of the person operating the device. Mucus traps are also found in adult respiratory equipment. Mucus goes into the trap rather than into the suction bottle and can then be sent for analysis.

**mud bath,** the application of warm mud to the body for therapeutic purposes.

**Mudrane,** trademark for a fixed-combination respiratory drug containing a smooth muscle relaxant (theophylline), an adrenergic (ephedrine hydrochloride), an expectorant (potassium iodide), and a sedative-hypnotic (phenobarbital).

**MUGA,** abbreviation for **multinucleated gated angiography.**

**mulberry molar,** a malformed first molar characterized by dwarfing of the cusps and hypertrophy of the enamel surrounding the cusp with agglomeration of masses of globules, giving it the appearance of a mulberry; seen in congenital syphilis and certain other diseases. Also called **mulberry tooth.**

**mulibrey nanism** /mul′ibrī/, a rare genetic disorder, transmitted as an autosomal-recessive trait, characterized by dwarfism, constrictive pericarditis, muscular hypotonia, anomalies of the skull and face, and characteristic yellow dots in the ocular fundus. The name of the condition is an abbreviation composed of the first two letters of the anatomic sites of the principal defects: *mus*cle, *li*ver, *br*ain, and *ey*es.

**müllerian duct** /miler′ē·ən, mYl-/ [Johannes P. Müller, German physiologist, 1801–1858], one of a pair of embryonic ducts that become the fallopian tubes, uterus, and vagina in females and that atrophy in males.

**Müller's law** /mil′ərz, mYl-/ [Johannes P. Müller], the principle that each type of sensory nerve cell normally responds to only one specific stimulus and gives rise to one sensation. A cell may be excited artificially by other forms of stimuli, but the sensation evoked will be the same. Also called **law of specific nerve energies.**

**Müller's maneuver** [Johannes P. Müller], an inspiratory effort against a closed airway or glottis. The effort decreases intrapulmonary and intrathoracic pressures and expands pulmonary gas. It is used during fluoroscopic examination to help visualize esophageal varices because it also causes engorgement of intrathoracic vascular stuctures.

**multi-** /mul′ti-/, prefix meaning 'many': *multicapsular, multifamilial, multipara.*

**multiaxial joint.** See **ball-and-socket joint.**

**multicellular** /-sel′yələr/, **1.** consisting of more than one cell. **2.** containing many cavities.

**multicentric mitosis.** See **multipolar mitosis.**

**multicomponent virus** /-kəmpō′nənt/, a virus that occurs in two or more different particles; each particle contains only one part of the viral genome.

**multidisciplinary care conference,** a nursing intervention from the Nursing Interventions Classification (NIC) defined as planning and evaluating patient care with health professionals from other disciplines. See also **Nursing Interventions Classification.**

**multidisciplinary health care team** /-dis′ipliner′ē/, a group of health care workers who are members of different disciplines, each providing specific services to the patient.

**multidrug resistance,** the resistance of tumor cells to more than one chemotherapeutic agent. Resistance may be aided by a P-glycoprotein transmembrane pump that lowers the concentration of drugs in the cell.

**multifactorial** /-faktôr′ē·əl/ [L, *multus,* many, *facere,* to make], pertaining to or characteristic of any condition or disease resulting from the interaction of many factors, specifically the interaction of several genes, usually polygenes, with or without the involvement of environmental factors. Many disorders, such as spina bifida, neural tube defects, and Hirschsprung's disease, are considered to be multifactorial.

**multifactorial inheritance,** the tendency to develop a physical appearance, disease, or condition that is a condition of many genetic and environmental factors, such as stature and blood pressure. See also **polygene.**

**multifocal** /-fō′kəl/ [L, *multus* + *focus,* hearth], characterized by more than two ectopic foci that pace the heart. The foci may be atrial or ventricular.

**multiform** /mul′tifôrm/ [L, *multus,* many, *forma*], an organ, tissue, or other object that may appear in more than one shape.

**multigenerational model** /-jen′ərā′shənəl/, a model of family therapy that focuses on reciprocal role relationships over a period and thus takes a longitudinal approach. The family is viewed as an emotional system in which patterns of interacting and coping, as well as unresolved issues, can be passed down from one generation to the next and can cause stress to the family members onto whom they are projected.

**multigenerational transmission process,** the repetition of relationship patterns, including divorce, suicide, and alcoholism, associated with emotional dysfunction that can be traced through several generations of the same family.

**multigravida** /mul′tigrav′idə/ [L, *multus* + *gravidus,* pregnancy], a woman who has been pregnant more than once. Compare **multipara, primigravida.**

**multihospital system** /-hos′pitəl/, a group of two or more hospitals owned, sponsored, or managed by a central organization.

**multiinfarct dementia** /-infärkt′/ [L, *multus* + *infarcire,* to stuff, *de,* away, *mens,* mind], a form of organic brain disease characterized by the rapid deterioration of intellectual functioning, caused by vascular disease. Symptoms include emotional lability; disturbances in memory, abstract thinking, judgment, and impulse control; and focal neurologic impairment, such as gait abnormalities, pseudobulbar palsy, and paresthesia.

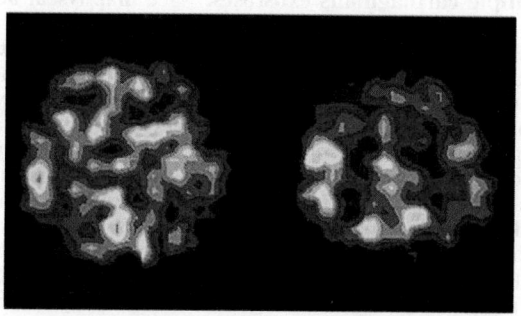

**Multiinfarct dementia** *(Perkin, 1998)*

**multilocular cyst** /-lok′yələr/ [L, *multus* + *locilus,* little place; Gk, *kystis,* bag], one of three kinds of follicular cyst, containing many spaces and not associated with a tooth. Compare **dentigerous cyst, primordial cyst.**

**multipara** /multip′ərə/, *pl.* **multiparae** [L *multus* + *parere,* to bear], a woman who has delivered more than one viable infant. Also called **pluripara.** Compare **multigravida, nullipara, primipara.**

**multiparity** /-per′itē/ [L, *multus,* many, *parere,* to give birth], the status of a mother of more than one child.

**multiparous** /multip′ərous/ [L, *multus,* many, *parere,* to give birth], having given birth to more than one child.

**multipenniform** /-pen′ifôrm/ [L, *multus* + *penna,* feather, *forma*], (of a body structure) having a shape resembling a pattern of many feathers, especially the pattern formed by the muscular fasciculi that converge to several tendons. Compare **bipenniform, penniform.**

**multiphase generator** /-fāz′/, a generator of x-rays that operates on more than single-phase power. It usually has three phases, which greatly increases the rate at which it produces x-rays.

**multiphasic screening** /-fā′sik/ [L, *multus* + *phasis,* appearance; ME, *scren*], a technique of screening populations for diseases that combines a battery of screening tests. The technique serves to identify any of several diseases being screened for in a population that is apparently healthy.

**multiple acyl CoA dehydrogenation deficiency,** glutaricaciduria, type II; see **glutaricaciduria.**

**multiple autoimmune disorder (MAD)** /mul′tipəl/, a condition in which a patient exhibits symptoms of at least two of a group of diseases, including Addison's disease, autoimmune thyroid disease, mucocutaneous candidiasis, hypoparathyroiditis, and insulin-dependent diabetes.

**multiple benign cystic epithelioma.** See **trichoepithelioma.**

**multiple carboxylase deficiency,** an inherited aminoacidopathy correctable by biotin therapy and caused by deficiency of either of two enzymes necessary for activity of several biotin-containing carboxylases; it is characterized by metabolic ketoacidosis, excretion of organic acids in the urine, hyperammonemia, and variable manifestation of breathing difficulties, hypotonia, seizures, ataxia, alopecia, skin rash, and developmental delay. The *neonatal* form, caused by deficiency of one of the enzymes, is apparently an autosomal recessive trait, often of earlier onset, and may progress rapidly to coma; the *juvenile* form, caused by deficiency of the other enzyme, is an autosomal recessive trait and is characterized additionally by sensorineural deafness and optic atrophy.

**multiple cartilaginous exostoses.** See **diaphyseal aclasis.**

**multiple endocrine adenomatosis (MEA),** a condition characterized by functioning tumors in more than one endocrine gland. The disorder is commonly associated with Zollinger-Ellison syndrome and may involve the pituitary, pancreas, and parathyroid glands. It is also seen in multiple endocrine neoplasia (MEN) type I. Also called **familial multiple endocrine adenomatosis.** See also **adenomatosis.**

**multiple endocrine neoplasia (MEN),** a hereditary hormonal disorder that occurs in an autosomal dominant pattern. The endocrine neoplasms may be expressed as hyperplasia, adenoma, or carcinoma and may develop synchronously or metachronously. Some kinds are multiple mucosal neuroma syndrome, Sipple's syndrome, and Werner's syndrome.

**multiple exostoses.** See **diaphyseal aclasis.**

**multiple factor.** See **polygene.**

**multiple family therapy** [L, *multus* + *plica*, fold], psychotherapy in which several families meet weekly to confront and deal with problems or issues that they have in common.

**multiple fission,** cell division in which the nucleus first divides into several equal parts and then the cytoplasm divides into as many cells as there are nuclei. It is the common form of asexual reproduction in certain acellular organisms. Compare **binary fission.**

**multiple fracture,** 1. a fracture break that extends several fracture lines in one bone. 2. the fracture of several bones at one time or from the same injury.

**multiple gene.** See **polygene.**

**multiple idiopathic hemorrhagic sarcoma.** See **Kaposi's sarcoma.**

**multiple lentigines syndrome.** See **LEOPARD syndrome.**

**multiple lipomatosis,** a rare inherited disorder characterized by discrete localized subcutaneous deposits of fat in the tissues of the body. This fat is not available for metabolic use, even in starvation.

**multiple mononeuropathy,** an abnormal condition characterized by dysfunction of several individual nerve trunks. It may be caused by various diseases, such as necrotizing angiopathy, uremia, diabetes mellitus, and some inflammatory immunologic disorders.

**multiple mucosal neuroma syndrome,** a condition of multiple submucosal neuromas or neurofibromas of the lips, tongue, and eyelids. The disease affects young persons and may be associated with tumors of the thyroid or adrenal medulla or with subcutaneous neurofibromatosis. See also **multiple endocrine neoplasia.**

**multiple myeloma,** a malignant neoplasm of the bone marrow. The tumor, composed of plasma cells, disrupts normal bone marrow functions, destroys osseous tissue, especially in flat bones; and causes pain, fractures, hypercalcemia, and skeletal deformities. The onset is insidious, and most people are asymptomatic until the disease is advanced. In addition, the ability of the plasma cells to make functional antibodies decreases, leaving the person immunocompromised. Characteristically abnormal proteins in the plasma and urine, anemia, weight loss, pulmonary complications secondary to rib fractures, and kidney failure are present. The cause is unknown. It occurs in middle-aged and elderly people and more frequently in males. Also called **multiple plasmacytoma of bone, myelomatosis, plasma cell myeloma.**

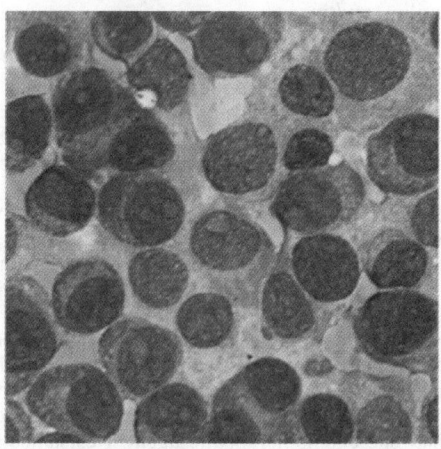

**Multiple myeloma** *(Carr and Rodak, 1999)*

**multiple myositis.** See **polymyositis.**

**multiple neuroma.** See **neuromatosis.**

**multiple peripheral neuritis,** acute or subacute disseminated inflammation or degeneration of symmetrically distributed peripheral nerves, characterized initially by numbness, tingling in the extremities, hot and cold sensations, and slight fever, progressing to pain, weakness, diminished reflexes, and in some cases flaccid paralysis. The disorder may be caused by toxic substances such as antimony, arsenic, carbon monoxide, copper, lead, mercury, nitrobenzol, organophosphates, and thallium; or by various drugs, including diphenylhydantoin, isoniazid, nitrofurantoin, thalidomide, and vincristine. Multiple peripheral neuritis may occur in alcoholism, arteriosclerosis, beriberi, chronic GI disease, diabetes, leprosy, pellagra, porphyria, rheumatoid arthritis, systemic lupus erythematosus, and many infectious diseases. Therapy consists of removal of the toxic agent or treatment of the causative disease, rest, and medication for pain. See also **Guillain-Barré syndrome.**

**multiple personality,** an abnormal condition in which the organization of the personality is fragmented. It is characterized by the presence of two or more distinct subpersonalities. Also called **split personality.**

**multiple personality disorder.** See **dissociative identity disorder.**

**multiple plasmacytoma of bone.** See **multiple myeloma.**

**multiple pregnancy,** a pregnancy in which there is more than one fetus in the uterus at the same time.

**multiple pterygium syndrome,** an autosomal recessive syndrome characterized by pterygia of the neck, axillae, and popliteal, antecubital, and intercrural areas, accompanied by hypertelorism, cleft palate, micrognathia, ptosis of eyelids, and short stature. Skeletal abnormalities include camptodactyly, syndactyly, clubfoot, and flatfoot in which the bottom of the foot resembles a rocker, as well as vertebral fusion and rib anomalies. Cryptorchidism is present in males and labia majora are absent in females. Also called **Escobar syndrome, pterygium syndrome.**

**multiple sclerosis (MS)** [L, *multus* + *plica,* fold; Gk, *sklerosis,* hardening], a progressive disease characterized by disseminated demyelination of nerve fibers of the brain and spinal cord. It begins slowly, usually in young adulthood, and continues throughout life with periods of exacerbation and remission. The first signs are paresthesias, or abnormal sensations in the extremities or on one side of the face. Other early signs are muscle weakness, vertigo, and visual disturbances, such as nystagmus, diplopia (double vision), and partial blindness. Later in the course of disease there may be extreme emotional lability, ataxia, abnormal reflexes, and difficulty in urinating. Because many other conditions affect the nervous system and produce similar symptoms, the diagnosis of MS is difficult to make. A history of exacerbation and remission of symptoms and the presence of greater than normal amounts of protein in cerebrospinal fluid are characteristic. As the disease progresses, the intervals between exacerbations grow shorter and disability becomes greater. There is no specific treatment for the disease; corticosteroids and other drugs are used to treat the symptoms accompanying acute episodes. Physical therapy may help postpone or prevent specific disabilities. The patient is encouraged to live as normal and active a life as possible. Also called **disseminated multiple sclerosis.**

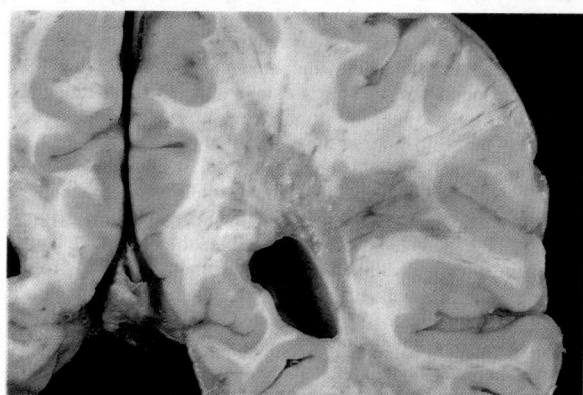

**Multiple sclerosis** *(Kumar, Cotran, and Robbins, 1997)*

**multiple self-healing squamous epithelioma.** See **keratoacanthoma.**

**multiple sleep latency test (MSLT),** a test of the propensity to fall asleep. The subject is given five 20-minute nap opportunities at 2-hour intervals. The mean latency to sleep onset and the stages of sleep that occur are determined from polygraph records. Well-rested adults have a mean MSLT of 15 minutes. A mean MSLT of less than 5 minutes indicates severe hypersomnia.

**multiple sulfatase deficiency,** an autosomal recessive lysosomal storage disease in which a deficiency of at least nine lysosomal and microsomal sulfatases leads to accumulation of sulfate-containing glycolipids, mucopolysaccharides, and steroids. The disorder generally presents as **sulfatide lipidosis** and later also shows features of **mucopolysaccharidoses,** variably combining phenotypic features of the specific enzymatic defects. Neurologic deterioration is rapid. Also called **mucosulfatidosis.**

**multiple transfusion syndrome** [L, *multus,* many, *plica,* fold, *transfundere,* to pour through; Gk, *syn,* together, *dromos,* course], a hemorrhagic reaction to massive transfusions of platelet-poor stored blood. Other clotting factors seldom contribute to the condition. Platelet concentrates may be given to correct the deficiency.

**multiplicative growth.** See **hyperplasia.**

**multipolar mitosis** /-pō′lər/ [L, *multus* + *polus,* pole], cell division in which the spindle has three or more poles and results in the formation of a corresponding number of daughter cells. Also called **multicentric mitosis, pluripolar mitosis.** See also **trisomy.**

**multiskilled worker,** a health team member with at least the education of a nurse assistant who has been trained to perform selected nursing skills and selected skills from the allied health professions under the supervision of a registered nurse. Duties may include, but are not limited to, bedmaking, bathing, assisting with elimination needs, performing phlebotomy, and recording electrocardiograms.

**multisource drug** /mul′tisôrs/ [L, *multus* + OFr, *sourse,* origin], a pharmaceutical that can be purchased under any of several trademarks from different manufacturers or distributors. See also **generic equivalent, generic name.**

**Multispecialty Medical Group.** See **Integrated Multispecialty Group.**

**multispecific** /-spes′ifik/, pertaining to an antibody that binds to more than one type of antigen.

**multisynaptic** /-sinap′tik/ [L, *multus* + Gk, *synaptein,* to join], pertaining to a nervous process or system of nerve cells requiring a series of synapses.

**multitasking,** performing two or more tasks with a computer at the same time. The computer actually processes a small part of one task at a time, switching from one to another in a commutative manner, but it can handle so many data in brief time segments that the operator or operators are not aware of the computer switching

**multivalent** /mul′tivā′lənt/ [L, *multus* + *valere,* to be strong], **1.** See **polyvalent. 2.** (in immunology) able to act against more than one strain of organism. Compare **valence.**

**multivalent vaccine** [L, *multus,* many, *valere,* value, *vaccinus,* cow], a vaccine prepared from several antigenic types within a species. Also called **polyvalent vaccine.**

**mummification** /mum′ifikā′shən/ [Per, *mum,* wax; L, *facere,* to make], a dried-up state, such as occurs in dry gangrene or a dead fetus in utero.

**mummified fetus** /mum′ifīd/, a fetus that has died in utero and has shriveled and dried.

**mumps** [D, *mompen,* to sulk], an acute viral disease, characterized by a swelling of the parotid glands, caused by a paramyxovirus. It is most likely to affect children between 5 and 15 years of age, but it may occur at any age. In adulthood the infection may be severe. Passive immunity from maternal antibodies usually prevents this disease in children younger than 1 year of age. The incidence of mumps is highest during the late winter and early spring. The mumps paramyxovirus is present in the saliva of the affected individual and is transmitted in droplets or by direct contact. The virus is present in the saliva from 6 days before to 9 days after the onset of the swelling of the parotid gland. The time of maximum communicability is believed to be the 48-hour period immediately before the start of parotid swelling. The prognosis in mumps is good, but the disease sometimes involves complications, such as arthritis, pancreatitis, myocarditis, oophoritis, and nephritis. About half of the men with mumps-induced orchitis suffer some atrophy of the testicles, but because the condition is usually unilateral, sterility rarely results. Also called **epidemic parotitis, infectious parotitis.**

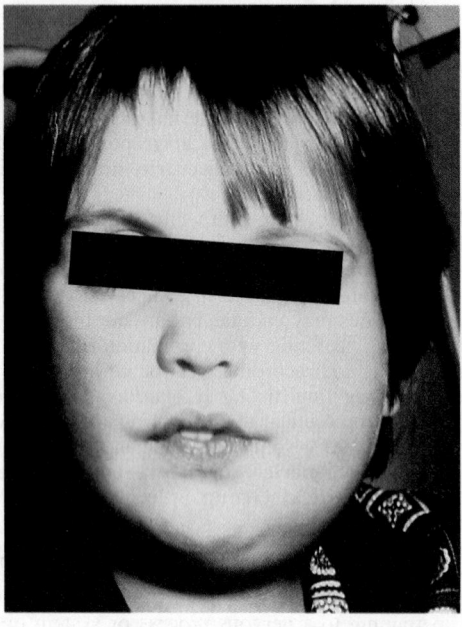

**Mumps** *(Zitelli and Davis, 1997/courtesy Dr. G.D.W. McKendrik)*

■ OBSERVATIONS: The common symptoms of mumps usually last for about 24 hours; they include anorexia, headache, malaise, and low-grade fever. These signs are commonly followed by earache, parotid gland swelling, and a temperature of 101° to 104° F (38.3° to 40° C). The patient also experiences pain when drinking acidic liquids or when chewing. The salivary glands also may become swollen. Complications, such as epididymo-orchitis and mumps meningitis, may develop. In about 25% of the postpubertal men who contract mumps, epididymoorchitis with associated testicular swelling and tenderness that may persist for several weeks develops. Mumps meningitis develops in 10% of patients with mumps and occurs in three to five times as many male as female patients. Diagnosis of mumps is usually based on typical symptoms, especially parotid gland swelling. If the parotid gland is not swollen, confirming diagnosis may be based on serologic antibody tests.
■ INTERVENTIONS: The treatment of mumps commonly includes the respiratory isolation of the patient and the administration of analgesics, antipyretics, and fluids adequate to prevent dehydration associated with fever and anorexia. IV fluids may be administered to the patient who cannot swallow as the result of severe parotitis.

■ NURSING CONSIDERATIONS: The patient is confined to bed and may be given antipyretics and tepid sponge baths to reduce fever. Patients with mumps are also encouraged to drink fluids and to avoid spicy or tart foods and those that require considerable chewing. During the acute phase of the disease, the nurse is especially alert to any signs of central nervous system involvement, such as nuchal rigidity and altered consciousness. All cases of mumps are routinely reported to local health authorities. Nurses aid public health education by stressing the importance of immunization with live attenuated mumps virus for children at 15 months of age and for susceptible people, especially males who are approaching puberty or who are past puberty. Immunization within 24 hours of exposure may prevent the disease or may minimize its effects.

**mumps orchitis,** an inflammatory disorder of the testis characterized by swelling with fever, malaise, and acute parotitis. It usually occurs in postpubertal men with a recent history of mumps and may result in testicular atrophy. Also called **orchitis parotidea.**

**Mumpsvax,** trademark for an active immunizing agent (live mumps virus vaccine).

**mumps virus vaccine live,** an active immunizing agent.
■ INDICATION: It is prescribed for immunization against mumps.
■ CONTRAINDICATIONS: Immunosuppression, concomitant use of corticosteroids, acute infection, pregnancy, or known hypersensitivity to chicken proteins, neomycin, or this drug prohibits its use.
■ ADVERSE EFFECTS: Among the most serious adverse effects are fevers, parotitis, and allergic reactions.

**Münchausen's syndrome** /mun′chousənz/ [Baron von Münchhausen, German adventurer and confabulator, 1720-1797], an unusual condition characterized by habitual pleas for treatment and hospitalization for a symptomatic but imaginary acute illness. The affected person may logically and convincingly present the symptoms and history of a real disease. Symptoms resolve with treatment, but the person may seek further treatment for another imaginary disease. Also called **pathomimicry.**

**Münchausen's syndrome by proxy** [Baron von Münchausen], a variation of Münchausen's syndrome in which the parent persistently fabricates or induces illness in a child with the intent of keeping in contact with hospitals and physicians. The child may endure dozens of surgeries and hospitalizations for illness induced by the parent; nearly 9% of the children die as a result. The mother poses as being a good parent by "saving" the child from medical catastrophe, and the child serves as a manipulative object.

**mural** /myŏŏ′rəl/ [L, *murus,* wall], something that is found on or against the wall of a cavity, such as a mural thrombus on an interior wall of the heart.

**mural thrombus** [L, *murus,* wall], a thrombus that originates in the wall of a cavity, particularly on a diseased patch of endocardium.

**Murchison fever.** See **Pel-Ebstein fever.**

**muriatic acid** /mŏŏ′rē·at′ik/ [L, *muria,* brine, *acidus,* sour], hydrochloric acid.

**murine typhus** /myŏŏ′rēn/ [L, *mus,* mouse; Gk, *typhos,* stupor], an acute arbovirus infection caused by *Rickettsia typhi* and transmitted by the bite of an infected flea. The disease is similar to epidemic typhus but less severe. It is characterized by headache, chills, fever, myalgia, and rash. After an 8- to 16-day incubation period, fever develops and lasts about 12 days. A dull-red maculopapular rash, mainly on the trunk, appears about the fifth day and lasts for 4 to 8 days. Recovery is usually rapid and complete, but death has occurred in elderly or debilitated people. Weil-Felix and complement fixation tests aid in the diagnosis. Chloramphenicol or tetracycline is usually prescribed in treatment. Prevention involves the elimination of the rodents that are the natural host of the organism and the use of appropriate insecticides to control fleas. Also called **endemic typhus, flea-borne typhus, New World typhus, rat typhus, urban typhus.** Compare **epidemic typhus, Rocky Mountain spotted fever.** See also **Brill-Zinsser disease.**

**murmur** /mur′mər/ [L, a humming], a gentle blowing, fluttering, or humming sound, such as a heart murmur, susceptible to auscultation. Types of murmurs include systolic, diastolic, and continuous murmurs.

**muromonab-Cd3** /myoo′rəmon′ab/, a parenteral immunosuppressant drug for kidney transplant rejection.
■ INDICATIONS: It is used in the control of acute renal transplant rejection.
■ CONTRAINDICATIONS: The product is not currently recommended for preventing transplant rejections of organs other than kidneys.
■ ADVERSE EFFECTS: Adverse reactions reported include pulmonary edema, fever, chills, breathing difficulty, chest pain, vomiting, nausea, diarrhea, and tremors.

**Murphy's sign,** a test for gallbladder disease in which the patient is asked to inhale while the examiner's fingers are hooked under the liver border at the bottom of the rib cage. The inspiration causes the gallbladder to descend onto the fingers, producing pain if the gallbladder is inflamed. Deep inspiration can be very much limited. The test is used in the diagnosis of carcinoma of the gallbladder, as well as cholecystitis.

**muscarine** /mus′kərēn/ [L, *musca,* fly], a choline-related alkaloid present in the poisonous mushroom *Amanita muscaria.* It is similar pharmacologically to acetylcholine, although it is not used in therapeutics.

**muscarinic** /mus′kərin′ik/ [L, *musca,* fly], **1.** stimulating the postganglionic parasympathetic receptor. **2.** pertaining to the poisonous activity of muscarine.

**musca volitans.** See **floater.**

**muscle** /mus′əl/ [L, *musculus*], a kind of tissue composed of fibers or cells that are able to contract, causing movement of body parts and organs. Muscle fibers are richly vascular, excitable, conductive, and elastic. There are two basic kinds, striated muscle and smooth muscle. Striated muscle, which composes all skeletal muscles except the myocardium, is long and voluntary; it responds very quickly to stimulation and is paralyzed by interruption of its innervation. Smooth muscle, which composes all visceral muscles, is short and involuntary; it reacts slowly to all stimuli and does not entirely lose its tone if innervation is interrupted. The myocardium is sometimes classified as a third (cardiac) kind of muscle, but it is basically a striated muscle that does not contract as quickly as the striated muscle of the rest of the body. See also **cardiac muscle, smooth muscle, striated muscle.**

**muscle albumin,** albumin present in muscle.

**muscle biopsy** [L, *musculus* + Gk, *bios,* life, *opsis,* view], an examination of surgically removed muscle tissue for diagnosis.

**muscle bridge,** a band of myocardial tissue over one or more of the large epicardial coronary vessels. It may cause constriction of the artery during systole.

**muscle cramp,** a sudden intermittent pain in almost any part of the body. It may involve involuntary contractions of variable duration and be accompanied by spasms. Cramps may develop in striated muscle as a result of exertion; high temperature; and excessive loss of sodium, potassium, and

magnesium through perspiration. Cramps can also be associated with arthritic conditions and exposure to cold. See also **heat cramp.**

**muscle excitability** /eksī′təbil′itē/, the ability of a muscle fiber to respond rapidly to a stimulating agent.

**muscle fiber,** any of the cells of skeletal or cardiac muscle tissue. Skeletal muscle fibers are cylindrical polynuclear cells containing contracting myofibrils, across which run transverse striations, enclosed in a sarcolemma. Cardiac muscle fibers contain one or sometimes two nuclei and myofibrils and are separated from one another by an intercalated disk; although striated, cardiac muscle fibers branch to form an interlacing network.

**muscle function,** a nursing outcome from the Nursing Outcomes Classification (NOC) defined as the adequacy of muscle contraction needed for movement. See also **Nursing Outcomes Classification.**

**muscle guarding,** a protective response in muscle that results from pain or fear of movement. The condition may be treated through induced relaxation of the muscle by using biofeedback to reduce electromyographic activity.

**muscle of expression.** See **facial muscle.**

**muscle overuse syndrome.** See **delayed-onset muscle soreness.**

**muscle receptor,** a sensory organ that responds to muscle stretch or tension, including muscle spindles and tendon organs. Also called **myoreceptor.**

**muscle reeducation,** the use of physical therapeutic exercises to restore muscle tone and strength after an injury or disease.

**muscle relaxant,** an agent that reduces the contractility of muscle fibers. Curare derivatives and succinylcholine compete with acetylcholine and block neural transmission at the myoneural junction. These drugs are used during anesthesia, in the management of patients undergoing mechanical ventilation, and in shock therapy, to reduce muscle contractions in pharmacologically or electrically induced seizures. Several drugs that relieve muscle spasms act at various levels in the central nervous system: baclofen inhibits reflexes at the spinal level; cyclobenzaprine acts primarily in the brainstem; and the benzodiazepines reduce muscle tension, chiefly by acting on mechanisms that control muscle tone. Dantrolene acts directly on muscles in reducing contraction and apparently achieves its effect by interfering with the release of calcium from the sarcoplasmic reticulum.

**muscle-setting exercise,** a method of maintaining muscle strength and tone by alternately contracting and relaxing a skeletal muscle or group of skeletal muscles without moving the associated body part. Such activity is useful in preventing atrophy of the muscles, especially in patients with conditions involving the joints. See also **isometric exercise.**

**muscles of mastication,** a group of muscles—the masseter, pterygoideus lateralis, pterygoideus medialis, and temporalis—responsible for movement of the jaws during the process of chewing. All four muscles are innervated by the mandibular division of the trigeminal nerve.

**muscles of ventilation** [L, *musculus* + *respirare,* to breathe], muscles that provide inspiration, partly by increasing the volume of the chest cavity so that air is drawn into the lungs, including the diaphragm and external intercostal muscles. They are aided during forced breathing by the scalenus muscles, levatores costarum, sternocleidomastoid, pectoralis major, platysma myoides, and serratus superior posterior. Muscles of forced expiration include the external and internal oblique, rectus abdominis, and transverse abdominis.

**muscle spindle** [L, *musculus* + AS, *spinel*], a specialized proprioceptive sensory organ composed of a bundle of fine striated intrafusal muscle fibers innervated by gamma nerve fibers. Their nuclei are gathered together near the center of each fiber to form a nuclear sac, which is surrounded in turn by sensory, annulospiral nerve endings, all enclosed in a fibrous sheath.

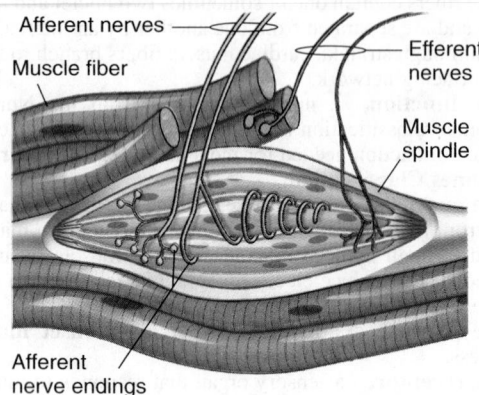

**Muscle spindle**

**muscle testing,** a method of evaluating the contractile unit, including the muscle, tendons, and associated tissues, of a moving part of the body by neurologic or resistance testing. The tests may include shortened, middle, and lengthened range-of-motion ability; isokinetic measurement of muscle strength, power, and endurance; and functional tests, such as jogging or specific agility drills, as well as radiography, arthroscopy, electromyography, and other medical tests.

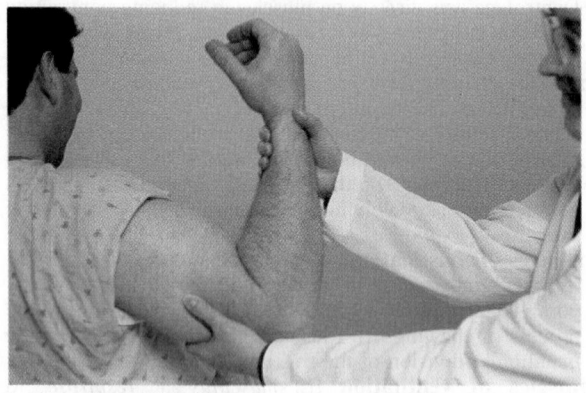

**Evaluation of muscle strength** *(Seidel et al, 1999)*

**muscle tone.** See **tonus.**
**muscular** /mus′kyələr/ [L, *musculus*], **1.** pertaining to a muscle. **2.** characteristic of well-developed musculature.
**muscular artery.** See **distributing artery.**

**muscular atrophy,** a condition of motor unit dysfunction, usually the result of a loss of efferent innervation.
**muscular branch of the deep brachial artery,** one of several similar branches of the deep brachial artery, supplying certain arm muscles, such as the coracobrachialis, biceps brachii, and brachialis.
**muscular dystrophy (MD)** [L, *musculus* + Gk, *dys,* bad, *trophe,* nourishment], a group of genetically transmitted diseases characterized by progressive atrophy of symmetric groups of skeletal muscles without evidence of involvement or degeneration of neural tissue. In all forms of muscular dystrophy an insidious loss of strength with increasing disability and deformity occurs, although each type differs in the groups of muscles affected, the age of onset, the rate of progression, and the mode of genetic inheritance. The basic cause is unknown but appears to be an inborn error of metabolism. Serum creatine phosphokinase level is increased in affected individuals and acts as a diagnostic aid, especially in asymptomatic children in families at risk. Diagnostic confirmation is made by muscle biopsy, electromyography, and genetic pedigree. Treatment of the muscular dystrophies consists primarily of supportive measures, such as physical therapy and orthopedic procedures to minimize deformity. The main types of the disease are pseudohypertrophic (**Duchenne** type) muscular dystrophy, **limb-girdle muscular dystrophy,** and facioscapulohumeral (**Landouzy-Déjérine**) muscular dystrophy. Rarer forms include **Becker's muscular dystrophy,** distal muscular dystrophy, ocular myopathy, and myotonic muscular dystrophy. Also called **myodystrophy.** See also **myotonic myopathy.**
**muscular fatigue,** a condition in which a muscle loses its ability to contract as a result of overactivity. It is usually a period after stimulation during which the muscle is unresponsive to a second stimulus.
**muscular incompetence** [L, *musculus* + *incompetens*], a failure of a cardiac valve to close properly because of a dysfunction of the papillary muscles of the heart.
**muscular sarcoidosis,** the formation of epithelioid tubercles in the skeletal muscles. The condition is characterized by interstitial inflammation, fibrosis, atrophy, and damage to the muscle fibers as the tubercles form within and replace normal muscle cells. See also **sarcoidosis.**
**muscular system,** all of the muscles of the body, including the smooth, cardiac, and striated muscles, considered as an interrelated structural group. See also the Color Atlas of Human Anatomy.
**muscular tension** [L, *musculus* + *tendere,* to stretch], the force that results from muscular contractions. Internal tension is produced when cross-bridges form between the actin and myosin filaments within each muscle fiber. The force generated by these contractile elements is transmitted to the bones via tendons and connective tissue. The bones move and produce external tension.
**muscular tone** [L, *musculus* + Gk, *tonos,* stretching], a normal degree of tension in muscles at rest.
**muscular tremor** [L, *musculus* + *tremor,* shaking], minute regular involuntary contraction of individual muscle fasciculi. If the tremors are mild and occasional, the cause may be physiologic. Profuse, persistent, or recurrent widespread muscular twitching often indicates a motor neuron disorder.
**muscular triangle.** See **inferior carotid triangle.**
**muscular tumor.** See **myoma.**
**musculature** /mus′kyələ′chər/, the arrangement and condition of the muscles.
**musculo-** /mus′kyəlō-/, combining form meaning 'muscle.'

**musculocutaneous nerve** /mus′kyəlōkyo͞otā′nē·əs/ [L, *musculus* + *cutis,* skin, *osus,* having], one of the terminal branches of the brachial plexus. It is formed on each side by division of the lateral cord of the plexus into two branches. Various branches and filaments supply different structures, such as the biceps, the brachialis, the humerus, and the skin of the forearm. Compare **median nerve, radial nerve, ulnar nerve.**

**musculoskeletal** /mus′kyo͞olōskel′ətəl/ [L, *musculus* + Gk, *skeletos,* dried up], pertaining to the muscles and the skeleton.

**musculoskeletal system,** all of the muscles, bones, joints, and related structures, such as the tendons and connective tissue, that function in the movement of body parts and organs. See also the Color Atlas of Human Anatomy.

**musculoskeletal system assessment,** an evaluation of the condition and functioning of the patient's muscles, joints, and bones and of factors that may contribute to abnormalities in these body structures.

■ METHOD: The patient is questioned about any pain and edema in muscles, joints, and bones; weakness in extremities; limitations in movements and activities; unsteadiness on the feet; fatigability; insomnia; anorexia; and weight loss. The individual's general appearance, age, blood pressure, pulse, respirations, body alignment, ability or inability to move in bed, gait, need for assistance in walking, handgrip, range of motion, and internal and external rotation of extremities are observed. The presence of contractures, deformities, paralysis, contusions, lacerations, wounds, footdrop, wristdrop, paralysis, crutches, brace, cast, prosthesis, cane, walker, pressure ulcers, allergies, skin rash, or tenseness is noted. It is ascertained whether the patient can perform activities of daily living and is able to sit up and turn; whether constipation is a complaint; and whether the individual is independent or dependent. Concurrent diseases or conditions investigated include injury to the spinal cord, nerve impairment, cerebrovascular accident, rheumatoid arthritis, osteoarthritis, bursitis, polyneuritis, multiple sclerosis, muscular dystrophy, myasthenia gravis, fracture, ruptured disk, Ménière's disease, and labyrinthitis. It is determined whether the patient previously had orthopedic or spinal surgery, poliomyelitis, hemiplegia, cerebral palsy, parkinsonism, a cerebrovascular accident, ataxia, syphilis, hyperparathyroidism, osteoporosis, rickets, osteomalacia, tuberculosis, alcoholism, and impaired vision or hearing. A family history of carcinoma, diabetes, or tuberculosis and the patient's involvement in a hazardous job or recreation, history of previous accidents, and use of tobacco or medications such as steroids, sedatives, tranquilizers, analgesics, antimalarials, acetylsalicylic acid, or indomethacin are determined. Laboratory studies important for the assessment are assays of serum and urine calcium and phosphorus and of alkaline phosphatase serum level. Diagnostic procedures that may be required include x-ray films of bones, arthrograms, myelograms, arteriograms, arthroscopy, biopsies of bone or muscle, incision and drainage of joints, and electromyograms of muscles.

■ INTERVENTIONS: Health care providers conduct the interview to obtain subjective data, make the necessary observations of the patient, and assemble the information on concurrent and previous disorders, the family history, the patient's social and medication background, and the results of laboratory studies and diagnostic procedures.

■ OUTCOME CRITERIA: A meticulous assessment of the patient's musculoskeletal system is a valuable aid in making the diagnosis, planning the course of therapy, predicting the prognosis, and ensuring the patient's safety.

**musculospiral nerve.** See **radial nerve.**

**mush bite,** a procedure for making simultaneous tooth impressions used in the construction of study models or full or partial dentures. The patient draws his or her upper and lower jaws together into a block of softened wax, thus indicating the spatial relationship between the maxilla and mandible.

**mushroom** [ME, *mucheron*], the fruiting body of the fungus of the class Basidiomycetes, especially edible members of the order Agaricales, commonly known as field mushrooms or meadow mushrooms. Mushrooms contain some protein and minerals, but they are composed largely of water.

**mushroom poisoning,** a toxic condition caused by the ingestion of certain mushrooms, particularly species of the genus *Amanita.* Muscarine in *Amanita muscaria* produces intoxication in a few minutes to 2 hours. Symptoms include lacrimation, salivation, sweating, vomiting, labored breathing, abdominal cramps, diarrhea, and in severe cases convulsions, coma, and circulatory failure. More deadly but slower-acting phalloidine in *A. phalloides* and *A. verna* causes similar symptoms, as well as liver damage, renal failure, and death in 30% to 50% of the cases. See also **phalloidine.**

**mushroom worker's lung,** a type of farmer's lung seen in those working on mushroom farms, caused by inhalation of mold spores from mushroom beds.

**music therapist,** a health professional trained to use music within a therapeutic relationship to address a client's needs, such as facilitating movement and physical rehabilitation, motivating the client to cope with treatment, providing emotional support, and providing an outlet for expressing feelings. A baccalaureate or master's degree and clinical internship are required, after which an individual may take an examination to earn the credential Music Therapist-Board Certified (MT-BC).

**music therapy**[1] [Gk, *mousike,* music, *therapeia,* treatment], a form of adjunctive psychotherapy in which music is used as a means of recreation and communication, especially with autistic children, and as a means to elevate the mood of depressed and psychotic patients.

**music therapy**[2] a nursing intervention from the Nursing Interventions Classification (NIC) defined as using music to help achieve a specific change in behavior, feeling, or physiology. See also **Nursing Interventions Classification.**

**Musset's sign** /mo͞osāz′, sīn/ [Alfred de Musset, French poet, 1810–1857], a rhythmic movement of the head and neck synchronous with each ventricular systole. The disorder is named for the patient in whom the condition was first recorded.

**mustard gas** /mus′tərd/, a poisonous gas used in chemical warfare during World War I. It causes corrosive destruction of the skin and mucous membranes, often resulting in permanent respiratory damage and death.

**mustard plaster** [L, *mustum* + Gk, *emplastron*], a mustard medication in a fabric base that can be placed close to the skin for a time as a counterirritant in the form of a poultice.

**mustard poultice.** See **poultice.**

**Mustargen,** trademark for an antineoplastic (mechlorethamine hydrochloride).

**-mustine,** combining form for antineoplastic agents, particularly [B-chlorethyl] amine derivatives.

**mutacism** /myo͞o′təsiz′əm/, mimmation, or the incorrect use of /m/ sound.

**mutagen** /myo͞o′təjən/ [L, *mutare,* to change, *genein,* to produce], any chemical or physical environmental agent that induces a genetic mutation or increases the mutation rate. —**mutagenic,** *adj.,* **mutagenicity,** *n.*

**mutagenesis** /my$\overline{oo}$′təjen′əsis/, the induction or occurrence of a genetic mutation. See also **teratogenesis.**

**mutagenic, mutagenicity.** See **mutagen.**

**Mutamycin,** trademark for an antineoplastic (mitomycin).

**mutant** /my$\overline{oo}$′tənt/ [L, *mutare,* to change], **1.** any individual or organism with genetic material that has undergone mutation. **2.** relating to or produced by mutation.

**mutant gene,** any gene that has undergone a change, such as the loss, gain, or exchange of genetic material, that affects the normal transmission and expression of a trait. Such genes can become inactive or show reduced, increased, or antagonistic activity. Kinds of mutant genes are **amorph, antimorph, hypermorph, hypomorph.**

**mutase** /my$\overline{oo}$′tās/, any enzyme that catalyzes the shifting of a chemical group or radical from one position to another within the same molecule or occasionally from one molecule to another.

**mutation** /my$\overline{oo}$otā′shən/ [L, *mutare,* to change], an unusual change in a gene occurring spontaneously or by induction. The change affects the original expression of the gene. If a mutation occurs in the genome of a gamete, the mutation may be transmitted to later generations. —**mutate,** *v.,* **mutational,** *adj.*

**mutein** /my$\overline{oo}$′tē·in, m(y)$\overline{oo}$′tēn/, a protein molecule that results from a mutation.

**mutism** /my$\overline{oo}$′tizəm/ [L, *mutus,* mute], the inability to speak because of a physical defect or emotional problem.

**muton** /my$\overline{oo}$′ton/, the smallest DNA segment whose alteration can result in a mutation.

**mutual goal setting,** a nursing intervention from the Nursing Interventions Classification (NIC) defined as collaborating with patient to identify and prioritize care goals, then developing a plan for achieving those goals. See also **Nursing Interventions Classification.**

**mutually exclusive categories** /my$\overline{oo}$′ch$\overline{oo}$·əlē/, categories on a research instrument that are sufficiently precise to allow each subject, factor, or variable to be classified uniquely, such as male/female.

**mutual support group,** a type of group in which members organize to solve their own problems. It is led by the group members themselves who share a common goal and use their own strengths to gain control over their lives.

**mv, mV,** abbreviation for **millivolt.**

**MVIC,** abbreviation for **maximum voluntary isometric contraction.**

**mVO₂,** symbol for *myocardial oxygen consumption.*

**MVP,** abbreviation for **mitral valve prolapse.**

**MVP syndrome.** See **Barlow's syndrome.**

**MVV,** abbreviation for **maximal voluntary ventilation.**

**M.W.I.A.,** abbreviation for **Medical Women's International Association.**

**MX gene,** a human gene that helps the body resist viral infections. When exposed to interferon, the MX gene inhibits the production of viral protein and nucleic acid necessary for the proliferation of new viral particles. The presence of the MX gene helps explain why some individuals are better able to resist certain viral infections, such as influenza, than other people.

**my-.** See **myo-.**

**myalgia** /mī·al′jə/ [Gk, *mys,* muscle, *algos,* pain], diffuse muscle pain, usually accompanied by malaise. Also called **myoneuralgia.**

**myalgic asthenia** /mī·al′jik/ [Gk, *mys* + *algos,* pain, *a* + *sthenos,* without strength], a condition characterized by a

general feeling of fatigue and muscular pain, often resulting from or associated with psychologic stress.

**Myambutol,** trademark for an antitubercular (ethambutol hydrochloride).

**myasthenia** /mī′əsthē′nē·ə/ [Gk, *mys* + *a* + *sthenos,* without strength], a condition characterized by an abnormal weakness of a muscle or a group of muscles that may be the result of a systemic myoneural disturbance, such as in myasthenia laryngis, which involves the vocal cord tensor muscles. See also **myasthenia gravis.** —**myasthenic,** *adj.*

**myasthenia gravis,** an abnormal condition characterized by chronic fatigability and muscle weakness, especially in the face and throat, as a result of a defect in the conduction of nerve impulses at the neuromuscular junction.

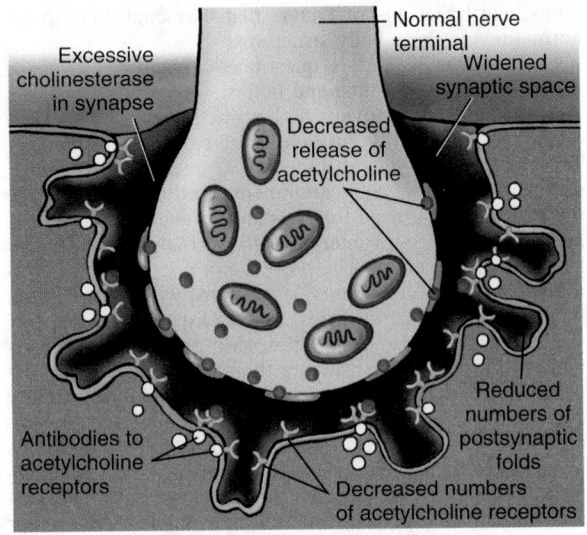

**Myasthenia gravis: changes in the neuromuscular junction**
*(Monahan and Neighbors, 1998)*

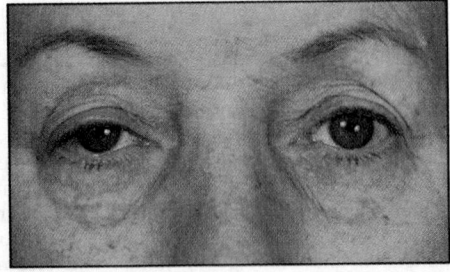

**Myasthenia gravis: typical facial expression**
*(Perkin, 1998)*

■ OBSERVATIONS: Muscular fatigability in myasthenia gravis is caused by the inability of receptors at the myoneural junction to depolarize because of a deficiency of acetylcholine; hence the diagnosis may be made by administering an anticholinesterase drug and observing improved muscle strength and stamina result. The onset of symptoms is usually gradual, with ptosis of the upper eyelids, diplopia, and weakness of the facial muscles. The weakness may then extend to other muscles innervated by the cranial nerves, particularly the respiratory muscles. Muscular exertion aggravates the symptoms, which typically vary over the course of the day. The disease occurs in younger women more often than in older women and in men over 60 years of age more often than in younger men.

■ INTERVENTIONS: Anticholinesterase drugs are given. The edrophonium test is used to determine the optimal maintenance dose. Neostigmine or pyridostigmine is the drug most often used.

■ NURSING CONSIDERATIONS: Physical activity is restricted, and bed rest encouraged. Anticholinesterase drugs are usually administered before meals, and the patient is monitored for toxic side effects. Myasthenic crisis may require emergency respiratory assistance. The patient's diet may have to be adjusted if the ability to chew and swallow is affected.

**myasthenia gravis crisis,** acute exacerbation of the muscular weakness characterizing the disease, triggered by infection, surgery, emotional stress, or an overdose or insufficiency of anticholinesterase medication.

■ OBSERVATIONS: Typical signs and symptoms include respiratory distress progressing to periods of apnea, extreme fatigue, increased muscular weakness, dysphagia, dysarthria, and fever. The patient may be anxious, restless, irritable, and unable to move the jaws or to raise one or both eyelids. If the condition is caused by anticholinesterase toxicity, anorexia, nausea, vomiting, abdominal cramps, diarrhea, excessive salivation, sweating, lacrimation, blurred vision, vertigo, and muscle cramps and spasms, as well as general weakness, dysarthria, and respiratory distress may occur.

■ INTERVENTIONS: Initial treatment is directed to maintaining airway patency. Oxygen with assisted or controlled ventilation is administered, procedures such as a tracheostomy may be performed, and bronchoscopy may be indicated. The patient is placed in a bed in which the head is elevated 30 degrees. The withdrawal or reduction of anticholinergic drugs may be ordered, or they may be given to differentiate the kind of crisis. If the eyelids are affected, the eyes may be covered with a patch and soothing eyedrops may be administered. To enable the patient to communicate, the call bell and a pad and pencil are placed within reach. Nourishment is offered between meals, and a daily intake of up to 2000 mL of fluids is encouraged. Walking as tolerated and other activities are planned at the time of the maximum effect of medication. Active or passive range-of-motion exercises of all extremities are performed several times a day, but rest periods are maintained to prevent fatigue and relapse.

■ NURSING CONSIDERATIONS: Before discharge the patient is instructed on the importance of taking the prescribed medication with milk, crackers, or bread at the scheduled time and of reporting toxic side effects and symptoms of recurrent or progressive disease. The nurse points out the need to maintain a regular diet, to exercise to tolerance, to rest, and to avoid infections and exposure to hot or cold weather and the use of alcohol and tobacco. The nurse's help in planning a schedule that conserves energy for essential activities can enable the patient to be relatively independent and self-sufficient.

**myasthenic.** See **myasthenia.**

**myasthenic crisis** /mī′asthen′ik/, an acute episode of muscular weakness. See also **myasthenia gravis crisis.**

**myc-.** See **myco-.**

**mycelium** /mīsē′lē·əm/, *pl.* **mycelia** [Gk, *mykes,* fungus, he-

*los,* nail], a mass of interwoven, branched, threadlike filaments that makes up most fungi. Also called **hypha.**

**mycetismus** /mī′sitiz′məs/, mushroom poisoning.

**myceto-.** See **myco-.**

**mycetoma** /mī′sətō′mə/ [Gk, *mykes* + *oma,* tumor], a severe fungal infection involving skin, subcutaneous tissue, fascia, and bone. One kind of mycetoma is **Madura foot.**

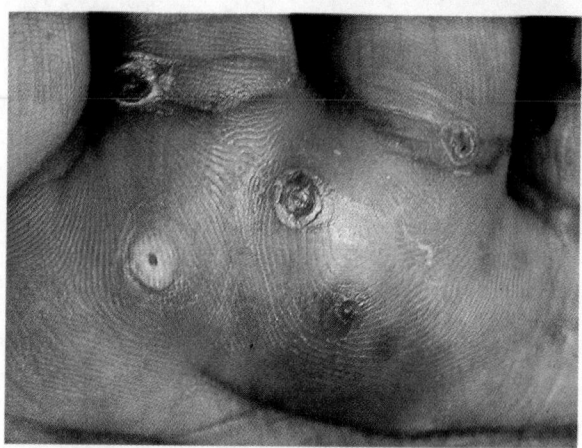

**Mycetoma** (du Vivier, 1993/courtesy Dr. Rod Hay)

**-mycin,** suffix for antibiotics produced by *Streptomyces* strains.

**Mycitracin,** trademark for a fixed-combination topical drug containing antibacterials (polymyxin B sulfate, bacitracin, and neomycin sulfate).

**myco-, myc-, myceto-, myko-,** combining form meaning 'fungus': *mycobacteriosis, mycohemia, mycophage.*

**mycobacteria** /mī′kōbaktir′ē·ə/ [Gk, *mykes* + *bakterion,* small rod], acid-fast microorganisms belonging to the genus *Mycobacterium.* —**mycobacterial,** *adj.*

**mycobacteriosis** /mī′kōbak′tirē·ō′sis/ [Gk, *mykes* + *bakterion* + *osis,* condition], a tuberculosis-like disease caused by mycobacteria other than *Mycobacterium tuberculosis.*

***Mycobacterium*** /mī′kōbaktir′ē·əm/ [Gk, *mykes* + *bakterion,* small rod], a genus of rod-shaped acid-fast bacteria having two significant pathogenic species: *Mycobacterium leprae,* which causes leprosy; *M. tuberculosis,* which causes tuberculosis. *M. avium* complex (MAC) or *M. avium-intracellulare* (MAI) disseminated infection may occur in AIDS. Children may develop cervical adenitis, and immunodeficient patients may develop pulmonary disease.

***Mycobacterium avium-intracellulare,*** a complex of slow-growing organisms that cause tuberculosis in birds and swine and are associated with human pulmonary disease, lymphadenitis in children, and serious systemic disease in immunocompromised patients. See also **mycobacteriosis, Mycobacterium avium** complex disease.

***Mycobacterium avium* complex disease,** systemic disease caused by infection with organisms of the *Mycobacterium avium-intracellulare* complex in patients with human immunodeficiency virus infection. Manifestations include bacteremia, fever, chills, fatigue, night sweats, weight loss, abdominal pain, anemia, and elevated alkaline phosphatase. Also called **MAC disease.** Compare **mycobacteriosis.**

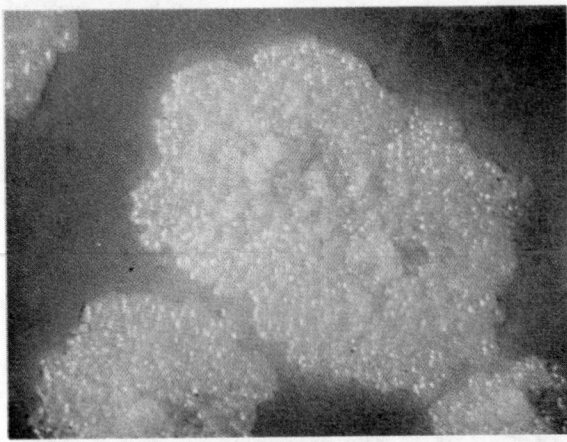

**Mycobacterium tuberculosis colonies**
*(Baron, Peterson, and Finegold, 1994)*

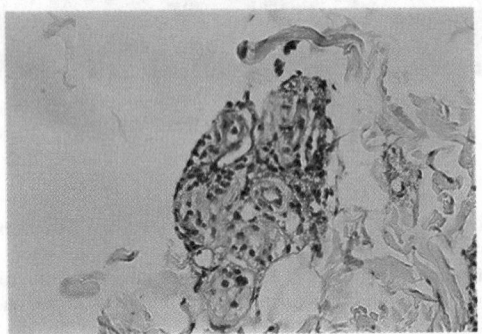

**Mycobacterium leprae from a skin biopsy from
a patient with lepromatous leprosy**
*(Mahon and Manuselis, 2000)*

**Mycobacterium bovis**, a species of bacteria that causes tuberculosis in cattle and other animals. It is transmitted to humans by drinking of raw milk contaminated by the microorganism.

**Mycobacterium kansasii**, a species of slow-growing photochromogenic bacteria that causes tuberculosis-like pulmonary infection in humans. It affects the joints, gonads, spinal fluid, lymph nodes, and viscera.

**Mycobacterium marinum**, a species of bacteria that causes a form of tuberculosis in cold-blooded animals including saltwater fish. The bacterium is also found in swimming pools and aquariums and is associated with skin lesions in humans.

**Mycolog,** trademark for a topical fixed-combination drug containing a glucocorticoid (triamcinolone acetonide), two antibacterials (neomycin sulfate and gramicidin), and an antifungal (nystatin).

**mycology** /mīkol'əjē/ [Gk, *mykes* + *logos*, science], the study of fungi and fungoid diseases. —**mycologic, mycological,** *adj.,* **mycologist,** *n.*

**mycomyringitis.** See **myringomycosis.**

**mycophenolate mofetil,** an immunosuppressant.
■ INDICATIONS: This drug is used to prevent rejection of organ transplants and for prophylaxis of organ rejection in allogenic cardiac transplants.
■ CONTRAINDICATIONS: Known hypersensitivity to this drug or to mycophenolic acid prohibits the use of mycophenolate mofetil.
■ ADVERSE EFFECTS: Life-threatening effects of this drug are leukopenia, thrombocytopenia, anemia, pancytopenia, renal tubular necrosis, and lymphoma. Other adverse effects are arthralgia, muscle wasting, and stomatitis. Common side effects are diarrhea, constipation, nausea, vomiting, rash, dyspnea, respiratory infection, increased cough, pharyngitis, bronchitis, pneumonia, tremor, dizziness, insomnia, headache, fever, peripheral edema, hypercholesterolemia, hypophosphatemia, edema, hyperkalemia, hypokalemia, hyperglycemia, urinary tract infection, hematuria, hypertension, chest pain, and nonmelanoma skin carcinoma.

**mycophenolic acid** /mī'kōfinō'lik/, a bacteriostatic and fungistatic crystalline antibiotic obtained from *Penicillium brevi compactum* and related species.

**Mycoplasma** /mī'kōplaz'mə/ [Gk, *mykes* + *plassein*, to mold], a genus of ultramicroscopic organisms lacking rigid cell walls and considered to be the smallest free-living organisms. Some are saprophytes, some are parasites, and many are pathogens. One species is a cause of mycoplasma pneumonia, tracheobronchitis, pharyngitis, and bullous myringitis. See also **pleuropneumonia-like organism.**

**mycoplasma pneumonia,** a contagious disease of children and young adults caused by *Mycoplasma pneumoniae*. It is characterized by a 9- to 12-day incubation period and followed by symptoms of an upper respiratory infection, dry cough, and fever. Also called **Eaton agent pneumonia, primary atypical pneumonia, walking pneumonia.** See also **cold agglutinin.**

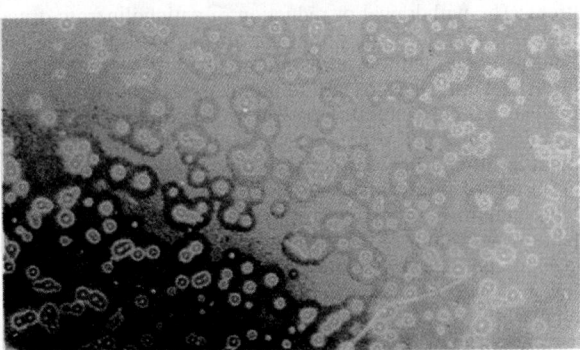

**Mycoplasma pneumoniae**
*(Baron, Peterson, and Finegold, 1994)*

■ OBSERVATIONS: Harsh or diminished breath sounds and fine inspiratory rales are frequently heard. Pulmonary infiltrates visible on chest x-ray films may resemble those of bacterial or viral pneumonia and may persist for 3 weeks in untreated cases. Rarely complications such as sinusitis, pleurisy, polyneuritis, myocarditis, or Stevens-Johnson syndrome, may follow the pneumonia. In untreated adults prolonged cough, weakness, and malaise are common. Diagnosis is suggested by physical examination and by observation of the clinical course and elevated cold agglutinin level and is confirmed by a complement fixation test. Prognosis is favorable.

■ INTERVENTIONS: Erythromycin or tetracycline, bed rest, a high-protein diet, and an adequate fluid intake are recommended. It is important that infants and people for whom a respiratory illness is particularly hazardous avoid contact with infected individuals.

**mycosis** /mīkō′sis/ [Gk, *mykes + osis,* condition], any disease caused by a fungus. Some kinds of mycoses are **athlete's foot, candidiasis,** and **coccidioidomycosis. —mycotic,** *adj.*

**mycosis fungoides** /fung·goi′dēz/, a rare chronic lymphomatous skin malignancy resembling eczema or a cutaneous tumor that is followed by microabscesses in the epidermis and lesions simulating those of Hodgkin's disease in lymph nodes and viscera. The condition is considered a distinctive entity by some specialists and a cutaneous manifestation of a malignant lymphoma by others.

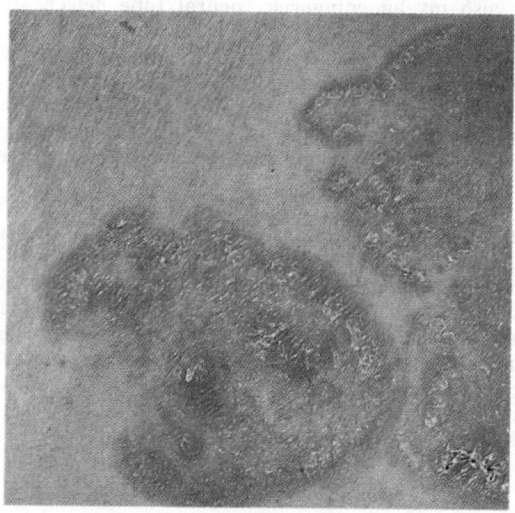

**Mycosis fungoides** *(du Vivier, 1986)*

**Mycostatin,** trademark for an antifungal (nystatin).

**mycotic** /mīkot′ik/ [Gk, *mykes,* fungus], pertaining to a disease caused by a fungus.

**mycotic aneurysm,** a localized dilation in the wall of a blood vessel caused by the growth of a fungus. It usually occurs as a complication of bacterial endocarditis. See also **bacterial aneurysm.**

**mycotic endocarditis** /mīkot′ik en′do·kär·dī′tis/ [Gk, *mykes,* fungus; Gk, *endon,* within + *kardia,* heart + *-itis,* inflammatory disease suffix], infectious endocarditis caused by a fungal infection; the most common fungi are *Candida albicans* and species of *Aspergillus* and *Histoplasma.* Symptoms are usually subacute.

**mycotic granuloma of the larynx,** a chronic throat condition characterized by white patches on an otherwise bright red mucous membrane. In the southwestern United States it is associated with histoplasmosis of the larynx. It may also be caused by candidiasis as a complication of chemotherapy or an altered immune state.

**mycotoxicosis** /mī′kōtok′sikō′sis/ [Gk, *mykes + toxikon,*

poison, *osis,* condition], a systemic poisoning caused by toxins produced by fungal organisms.

**mycotoxins** /mī′kōtok′sins/, poisons produced by fungi that are harmful to other organisms.

**mydriasis** /midrī′əsis/ [Gk, *mydros,* hot mass], **1.** dilation of the pupil of the eye caused by contraction of the dilator muscle of the iris, a muscular sheath that radiates outward like the spokes of a wheel from the center of the iris around the pupil. With a decrease in light or the pharmacologic action of certain drugs the dilator acts to pull the iris outward, enlarging the pupil. **2.** an abnormal condition characterized by contraction of the dilator muscle, resulting in widely dilated pupils. Compare **miosis. —mydriatic,** *adj.*

**mydriatic and cycloplegic agent** /mid′rē·at′ik/ [Gk, *mydros + kyklos,* circle, *plege,* stroke], any one of several ophthalmic pharmaceutic preparations that dilate the pupil and paralyze the ocular muscles of accommodation. Mydriatics stimulate the sympathetic nerve fibers or block parasympathetic nerve fibers of the eye, temporarily paralyzing the iris sphincter muscle. Cycloplegics temporarily paralyze accommodation while relaxing the ciliary muscle. These drugs are used in diagnostic and refractive examination of the eye, before and after various procedures in eye surgery, in some tests for glaucoma, and in the treatment of anterior uveitis and certain kinds of glaucoma. Blurred vision, thirst, flushing, fever, and rash may occur. In children and elderly people ataxia, somnolence, delirium, and hallucination may occur but are rare. Among these drugs are atropine, cyclopentolate, homatropine, scopolamine, and tropicamide; they are prepared in solution for topical ophthalmic application.

**myel-.** See **myelo-.**

**myelacephalus** /mī′əlāsef′ələs/ [Gk, *myelos,* marrow, *a + kephale,* without head], a fetus, usually a separate monozygotic twin, whose form and parts are barely recognizable; a slightly differentiated amorphous mass. —**myelacephalous,** *adj.*

**myelatelia** /mī′ələtē′lē·ə/ [Gk, *myelos + atelia,* unfinished], any developmental defect involving the spinal cord.

**myelauxe** /mī′əlôk′sē/ [Gk, *myelos + auxe,* increasing], a developmental anomaly characterized by hypertrophy of the spinal cord.

**myelencephalon** /mī′əlensef′əlon/, the lower part of the embryonic hindbrain, from which the medulla oblongata develops.

**-myelia,** suffix meaning '(condition of the) spinal cord': *atelomyelia, hydromyelia, syringomyelia.*

**myelin** /mī′əlin/ [Gk, *myelos,* marrow], a lipoproteinaceous substance constituting the sheaths of various nerve fibers throughout the body and enveloping the axis of myelinated nerves. It is largely composed of phospholipids and protein, which gives the fibers a white, creamy color. —**myelinic,** *adj.*

**myelinated** /mī′əlinā′tid/, (of a nerve) having a myelin sheath.

**myelination** /mī′əlinā′shən/ [Gk, *myelos + L, atio,* process], the process of furnishing or taking on myelin.

**myelin globule,** a fatlike droplet found in some sputum.

**myelinic** /mī′əlin′ik/ [Gk, *myelos + L, icus,* form of], pertaining to myelin.

**myelinic neuroma,** a neuroma neoplasm composed of myelinated nerve fibers.

**myelinization** /mī′əlin′izā′shən/ [Gk, *myelos + izein,* to cause], development of the myelin sheath around a nerve fiber. Also called **myelinogenesis.**

**myelinolysis** /mī′əlinol′isis/ [Gk, *myelos + lysein,* to loosen], a pathologic process that dissolves the myelin sheaths around certain nerve fibers, such as those of the pons in alcoholic and undernourished people who are afflicted with central pontine myelinolysis.

**myelin sheath,** a segmented fatty lamination composed of myelin that wraps the axons of many nerves in the body. The usual thickness of the myelin sheath is between 200 and 800 μm. Various diseases such as multiple sclerosis can destroy myelin wrappings.

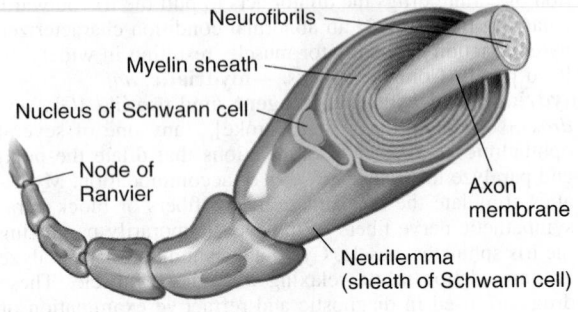

Neurofibrils
Myelin sheath
Nucleus of Schwann cell
Node of Ranvier
Axon membrane
Neurilemma (sheath of Schwann cell)

**Myelin sheath**

**myelitis** /mī′əlī′tis/, an abnormal condition characterized by inflammation of the spinal cord with associated motor or sensory dysfunction. Some kinds of myelitis are **acute transverse myelitis, leukomyelitis,** and **poliomyelitis.** —**myelitic,** *adj.*

**myelo-** /mī′əlō-/, **myel-,** prefix meaning 'spinal cord or bone marrow': *myeloblast, myelocyte, myelomenia.*

**myeloablation** /mī′ə·lō·ab·lā′shən/ [Gk, *myelos,* marrow; L, *ab, latus* carried away], severe myelosuppression; see **myelosuppression.**

**myeloblast** /mī′əlōblast′/ [Gk, *myelos + blastos,* germ], one of the earliest precursors of the granulocytic leukocytes. The cytoplasm appears light blue, scanty, and nongranular when seen in a stained blood smear through a microscope. The nucleus contains distinct chromatin material in strands, together with several nucleoli. In certain leukemias a marked increase in myeloblasts is observed in the marrow and in the peripheral blood. Compare **megaloblast, myelocyte, normoblast.** See also **myelocytic leukemia.** —**myeloblastic,** *adj.*

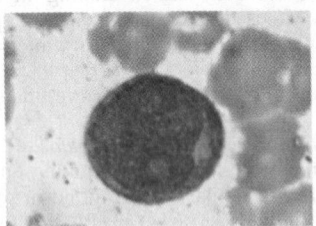

**Myeloblast** *(Carr and Rodak, 1999)*

**myeloblastemia.** See **myeloblastosis.**
**myeloblastic.** See **myeloblast.**
**myeloblastic leukemia** /-blas′tik/, a malignant neoplasm of blood-forming tissues, characterized by many myelo-

blasts in the circulating blood and tissues. The disease may be a terminal event in the course of chronic granulocytic leukemia, sometimes referred to as "blast crisis."

**myeloblastomatosis** /mī′əlōblas′tōmətō′sis/ [Gk, *myelos + blastos + oma,* tumor, *osis,* condition], abnormal localized clusters of myeloblasts in the peripheral circulation.

**myeloblastosis** /mī′əloblastō′sis/ [Gk, *myelos + blastos + osis,* condition], an excess of myeloblasts in the blood.

**myelocele** /mī′əlōsēl′/ [Gk, *myelos + kele,* hernia], a saclike protrusion of the spinal cord through a congenital defect in the vertebral column. See also **myelomeningocele, neural tube defect.**

**myeloclast** /mī′əlōklast′/ [Gk, *myelos + klastos,* broken], a cell that breaks down the myelin sheaths of nerves.

**myelocyst** /mī′əlōsist′/ [Gk, *myelos + kystis,* cyst], any benign cyst formed from the rudimentary medullary canals that give rise to the vertebral canal during embryonic development.

**myelocystocele** /mī′əlōsis′təsēl′/ [Gk, *myelos + kystis + kele,* hernia], a protrusion of a cystic tumor containing spinal cord substance through a defect in the vertebral column. See also **myelomeningocele, neural tube defect, spina bifida.**

**myelocystomeningocele** /mī′əlōsis′tōməning′gōsēl/ [Gk, *myelos + kystis + menix,* membrane, *kele,* hernia], a protrusion of a cystic tumor containing both spinal cord substance and meninges through a defect in the vertebral column. See also **myelomeningocele, neural tube defect, spina bifida.**

**myelocyte** /mī′əlōsīt′/ [Gk, *myelos + kytos,* cell], the first of the maturation stages of the granulocytic leukocytes normally found in the bone marrow. Granules are seen in the cytoplasm. The nuclear material of the myelocyte is denser than that of the myeloblast but lacks a definable membrane. The cell is flat and contains increasing numbers of granules as maturation progresses. These cells appear in the circulating blood only in certain forms of leukemia or in overwhelming infection. Compare **myeloblast.** See also **myelocytic leukemia.** —**myelocytic,** *adj.*

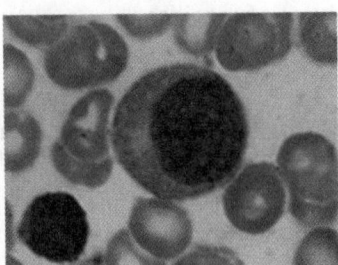

**Myelocyte** *(Carr and Rodak, 1999)*

**myelocythemia** /mī′əlōsīthē′mē·ə/ [Gk, *myelos + kytos + haima,* blood], an excessive presence of myelocytes in the circulating blood, such as in myelocytic leukemia.

**myelocytic.** See **myelocyte.**

**myelocytic leukemia** /mī′əlōsit′ik/, a disorder characterized by the unregulated and excessive production of leukocytes. Also called **granulocytic leukemia, myelogenous leukemia.** Compare **leukemoid reaction, acute lympho-**

cytic leukemia, chronic lymphocytic leukemia. See also leukocytosis.

**myelocytoma** /mī′əlō′sītō′mə/ [Gk, *myelos* + *kytos*, cell, *oma*, tumor], a localized cluster of myelocytes in the peripheral vasculature that may occur in myelocytic leukemia.

**myelocytosis.** See **myelocythemia.**

**myelodiastasis** /mī′əlōdī·as′təsis/ [Gk, *myelos* + *diastasis*, separation], disintegration and necrosis of the spinal cord.

**myelodysplasia** /mī′əlōdisplā′zhə/ [Gk, *myelos* + *dys*, bad, *plassis*, formation], a general designation for the defective development of any part of the spinal cord. The term is used primarily to describe abnormalities without gross superficial defects, especially of the lower segment, specifically spina bifida occulta.

**myelofibrosis** /mī′əlōfībrō′sis/, the replacement of bone marrow with fibrous tissue. The condition may be associated with anemia, thrombocytopenia, myeloid metaplasia, new bone formation, polycythemia vera, and other abnormalities. Also called **myelosclerosis.** See also **myeloid metaplasia.**

**myelogenesis** /-jen′əsis/ [Gk, *myelos* + *genein*, to produce], **1.** the formation and differentiation of the nervous system, in particular of the brain and spinal cord, during prenatal development. See also **neural tube formation. 2.** the development of the myelin sheath around the nerve fiber. See also **myelinization.**

**myelogenous** /mī′əloj′ənəs/, pertaining to the cells produced in bone marrow or to the tissue from which such cells originate. Also **myelogenetic, myelogenic.**

**myelogenous leukemia.** See **acute myelocytic leukemia, chronic myelocytic leukemia.**

**myelogeny** /mī′əloj′ənē/ [Gk, *myelos* + *genein*, to produce], the formation and differentiation of the myelin sheaths of nerve fibers during the prenatal and postnatal development of the central nervous system.

**myelogram** /mī′əlōgram′/, **1.** an x-ray film taken after the injection of a radiopaque medium into the subarachnoid space to demonstrate any distortions of the spinal cord, spinal nerve roots, and subarachnoid space. **2.** a graphic representation of a count of the different kinds of cells in a stained preparation of bone marrow.

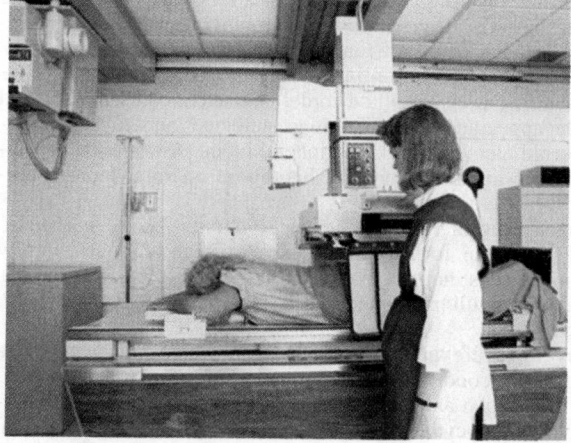

**Positioning of patient for a myelogram**
*(Chipps, Clanin, and Campbell, 1992/courtesy
Doctors Hospital, Columbus, Ohio)*

**myelography** /mī′əlog′rəfē/ [Gk, *myelos* + *graphein*, to record], a radiographic process by which the spinal cord and the spinal subarachnoid space are viewed and photographed after the introduction of a contrast medium. It is used to identify and study spinal lesions caused by trauma or disease. —**myelographic,** *adj.*

**myeloid** /mī′əloid/ [Gk, *myelos* + *eidos*, form], **1.** pertaining to the bone marrow. **2.** pertaining to the spinal cord. **3.** pertaining to myelocytic forms that do not necessarily originate in the bone marrow.

**myeloid leukemia.** See **acute myelocytic leukemia, chronic myelocytic leukemia.**

**myeloid metaplasia,** a disorder in which bone marrow tissue develops in abnormal sites. Characteristics of the condition are anemia, splenomegaly, immature blood cells in the circulation, and hematopoiesis in the liver and spleen. Myeloid metaplasia may be secondary to carcinoma, leukemia, polycythemia vera, or tuberculosis. The primary form is also called **agnogenic myeloid metaplasia.**

**myeloidosis** /mī′əloidō′sis/ [Gk, *myelos* + *eidos*, form, *osis*, condition], an abnormal condition characterized by general hyperplasia of the myeloid tissue. See also **Hodgkin's disease, multiple myeloma.**

**myeloma** /mī′əlō′mə/ [Gk, *myelos* + *oma*, tumor], an osteolytic neoplasm consisting of a profusion of cells typical of the bone marrow that may develop in many sites and cause extensive destruction of the bone. The tumor occurs most frequently in the ribs, vertebrae, pelvic bones, and flat bones of the skull. Intense pain and spontaneous fractures are common. The tumor is radiosensitive, and local lesions are curable. Kinds of myeloma are **endothelial myeloma, extramedullary myeloma, giant cell myeloma, multiple myeloma,** and **osteogenic myeloma.**

**-myeloma,** suffix meaning a 'tumor composed of cells normally found in bone marrow': *globomyeloma, lymphomyeloma, orchiomyeloma.*

**myeloma kidney disease,** a kidney disorder often characterized by irreversible renal failure. It may involve intratubular coalescence of light chain molecules and obstruction of nephronal flow.

**myelomalacia** /mī′əlōməlā′shə/ [Gk, *myelos* + *malakia*, softening], an abnormal softening of the spinal cord, caused primarily by inadequate blood supply.

**myelomatosis.** See **multiple myeloma.**

**myelomeningocele** /mī′əlō′məning′gōsēl/ [Gk, *myelos* + *menix*, membrane, *kele*, hernia], a developmental defect of the central nervous system in which a hernial sac containing a portion of the spinal cord, its meninges, and cerebrospinal fluid protrudes through a congenital cleft in the vertebral column. The condition is caused primarily by failure of the neural tube to close during embryonic development, although in some instances it may result from the reopening of the tube as a result of an abnormal increase in cerebrospinal fluid pressure. Also called **meningomyelocele.** Compare **meningocele.** See also **neural tube defect, spina bifida cystica.**

■ OBSERVATIONS: The defect, which occurs in approximately 2 in every 1000 live births, is readily apparent and easily diagnosed at birth. Although the opening may be located at any point along the spinal column, the anomaly characteristically occurs in the lumbar, low thoracic, or sacral region and extends for three to six vertebral segments. The saclike structure may be covered with a thin layer of skin or with a fine membrane that can be easily ruptured, increasing the risk of meningeal infection. The severity of neurologic dysfunction is directly related to the amount of neural tissue involved, which can be roughly estimated by the degree of the

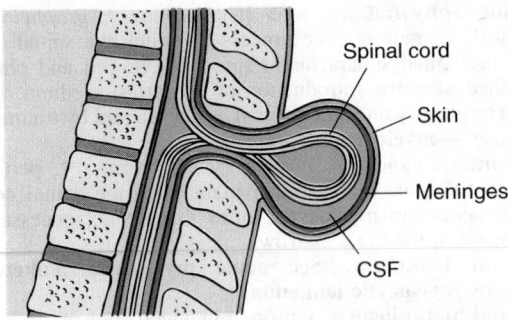

**Myelomeningocele: protrusion of meninges
and spinal cord through the skin**
*(Huether and McCance, 2000)*

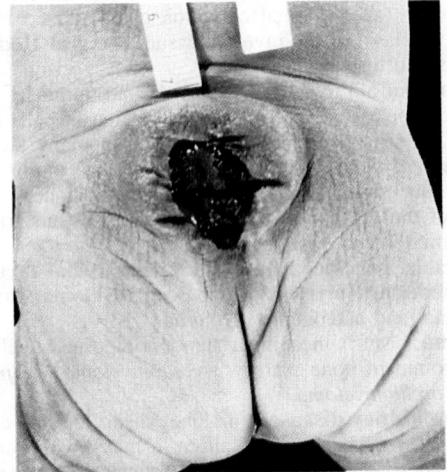

**Myelomeningocele: clinical presentation**
*(Kumar, Cotran, and Robbins, 1997)*

transillumination of the mass. Usually the condition is accompanied by varying degrees of paralysis of the lower extremities; by musculoskeletal defects such as clubfoot, flexion and joint deformities, or hip dysplasia; and by anal and bladder sphincter dysfunction, which can lead to serious genitourinary disorders. Hydrocephalus, frequently related to the Arnold-Chiari malformation, is the most common anomaly associated with myelomeningocele and occurs in approximately 90% of the cases in which the spinal lesion is located in the lumbosacral region. In most cases hydrocephalus is apparent at birth, although it may appear shortly afterward. Supplementary diagnostic procedures include x-ray examination of the spine, skull, and chest to determine the extent of the vertebral defect and the presence of other malformations in other organ systems; a computed tomographic scan of the brain to establish the ventricular size and the presence of any structural congenital anomalies; and laboratory examinations, especially urine analysis, culture, blood urea nitrogen evaluation, and creatinine clearance determination. Amniocentesis is recommended for all pregnant women who have had a child with a neural tube defect.

■ INTERVENTIONS: Immediate surgical repair is essential if the defect is leaking cerebrospinal fluid. However, surgical intervention may not be appropriate if neurologic involvement is extreme, if the lesion is infected, or if associated problems, such as hydrocephalus, are severe. When surgical repair of the spinal defect is recommended, associated problems are managed by appropriate measures, including shunt procedures for correction of hydrocephalus; antibiotic therapy to reduce the incidence of meningitis, urinary tract infections, and pneumonia; casting, bracing, traction, and surgical techniques for correction of hip, knee, and foot deformities; and prevention and treatment of renal complications. Prognosis is determined by the severity of neurologic involvement and the number of associated anomalies. With proper care and long-term maintenance most children can survive and do well. Early death is usually caused by central nervous system infection or by hydrocephalus, whereas mortality in later childhood is caused by urinary tract infection, renal failure, complications from shunt therapy, or pulmonary disease.

■ NURSING CONSIDERATIONS: Immediate care centers on the prevention of local infection and trauma by carefully handling and positioning the infant, applying sterile moist dressings to the membranous sac, avoiding fecal contamination and breakdown of sensitive skin areas, and maintaining warmth, proper nutrition, and adequate hydration and electrolyte balance. Gentle range-of-motion exercises are carried out to prevent or minimize hip and lower extremity deformity. An important function of the nurse is to involve the parents in the care of the infant as soon as possible and to teach them the essential procedures for adequate home care, including how to observe for signs of complications. The nurse also helps the parents in long-term management by planning activities appropriate to the developmental age and physical limitations of the child and by providing information for teaching all family members about the condition.

**myelomere** /mī′əlōmir′/ [Gk, *myelos* + *meros,* part], any of the embryonic segments of the brain or spinal cord during prenatal development.

**myelomonocytic leukemia.** See **monocytic leukemia.**

**myelopathic anemia.** See **myelophthisic anemia.**

**myelopathy** /mī′əlop′əthē/, **1.** any disease of the spinal cord. **2.** any disease of the myelopoietic tissues.

**myeloperoxidase (MPO)** /mī′əlōpərok′sidās/, a peroxidase enzyme occurring in phagocytic cells that can oxidize halide ions, producing a bactericidal effect.

**myeloperoxidase deficiency,** an autosomal recessive inherited disorder in which there is a lack of myeloperoxidase in the primary granules of neutrophils, causing delayed intracellular killing of fungi and bacteria by neutrophils.

**myelophthisic anemia** /mī′əlofthiz′ik/ [Gk, *myelos* + *phthisis,* wasting], a disorder characterized by anemia and the appearance of immature granulocytes and nucleated erythroid elements in the peripheral blood. Also called **myelopathic anemia.** Compare **hemolytic anemia, leukoerythroblastic anemia.**

**myelopoiesis** /mī′əlō′pō·ē′sis/ [Gk, *myelos* + *poiein,* to form], the formation and development of bone marrow or the cells that originate from it. A kind of myelopoiesis is **extramedullary myelopoiesis.** —**myelopoietic** /-pō·et′ik/, *adj.*

**myeloproliferative disorders** /mī′əlōprolif′ərətiv′/, a group of conditions characterized by proliferation of myeloid tissue, such as agnogenic myelofibrosis and myeloid metaplasia, polycythemia vera, or chronic myelogenous leukemia.

**myeloradiculodysplasia** /mī′əlō′rədik′yəlō′dis′plā′zhə/ [Gk, *myelos* + L, *radiculus,* small root; Gk, *dys,* bad, *plassein,* to form], any developmental abnormality of the spinal cord and spinal nerve roots. See also **myelomeningocele, neural tube defect.**

**myeloschisis** /mī′ǝlos′kǝsis/ [Gk, *myelos* + *schisis,* cleft], a developmental defect characterized by a cleft spinal cord that results from the failure of the neural plate to fuse and form a complete neural tube. See also **neural tube defect, neural tube formation, myelomeningocele, rachischisis, spina bifida.**

**myelosclerosis.**   See **myelofibrosis.**

**myelosuppression** /-sǝpresh′ǝn/,   See **bone marrow suppression.**

**myenteric plexus** /mī′enter′ik/ [Gk, *mys,* muscle, *enteron,* bowel; L, *plexus,* plaited], a group of autonomic nerve fibers and ganglion cells in the muscular coat of the intestine.

**myesthesia** /mī′esthē′zhǝ/,   perception of any sensation in a muscle, such as touch, direction, proprioception, contraction, relaxation, or extension.

**myiasis** /mī′yǝsis/ [Gk, *myia,* fly, *osis,* condition], infection or infestation of the body by the larvae of flies, usually through a wound or an ulcer, but rarely through intact skin.

**myitis.**   See **myositis.**

**myko-.**   See **myco-.**

**Myleran,**   trademark for an antineoplastic (busulfan).

**Mylicon,**   trademark for an antiflatulent (simethicone).

**mylohyoideus** /mī′lōhī·oi′dē·ǝs/ [Gk, *myle,* mill, *hyoeides,* upsilon, U-shaped], one of a pair of flat triangular muscles that form the floor of the cavity of the mouth. It is innervated by the mylohyoid nerve and acts to raise the hyoid bone and the tongue. Also called **mylohyoid muscle.** Compare **digastricus, geniohyoideus, stylohyoideus.**

**myo-** /mī′ō-/, **my-,** prefix meaning 'muscle': *myocardia, myocele, myolipoma.*

**myocardial.**   See **myocardium.**

**myocardial infarction (MI)** /mī′ōkär′dē·ǝl/ [Gk, *mys,* muscle, *kardia,* heart; L, *infarcire,* to stuff], necrosis of a portion of cardiac muscle caused by an obstruction in a coronary artery through either atherosclerosis, a thrombus or a spasm. Also called **heart attack.**

■ OBSERVATIONS: The onset of MI is characterized by a crushing, viselike chest pain that may radiate to the left arm, neck, jaw, or epigastrium and sometimes stimulates the sensation of acute indigestion or a gallbladder attack. The patient usually becomes ashen, clammy, short of breath, nauseated, faint, and anxious and often feels that death is imminent. Typical signs are tachycardia, a barely palpable pulse, low blood pressure, mildly elevated temperature, cardiac arrhythmia, and elevation of the S-T segment and Q wave on the electrocardiogram. Laboratory studies usually show an increased sedimentation rate, leukocytosis, and elevated serum levels of creatine kinase and its isoenzyme MB, lactic dehydrogenase and its isoenzymes, and glutamic-oxaloacetic transaminase. Potential complications in MI are pulmonary or systemic embolism, pulmonary edema, acute congestive heart failure, shock, ventricular tachycardia, ventricular fibrillation, and cardiac arrest.

■ INTERVENTIONS: Emergency treatment of MI may require cardiopulmonary resuscitation before the patient reaches the hospital emergency department. Early IV administration of

**Locations of pain from myocardial infarction**

Left of sternum or entire upper chest

Mid-chest, neck, and jaw

Mid-chest and inside arms (left more than right)

Upper abdomen

Chest, neck, jaw, and inside arms

Center of lower neck to both sides of upper neck and all of jaw

Inside right arm to below elbow, shoulder and inside left arm to waist (left side more often than right)

Between shoulder blades

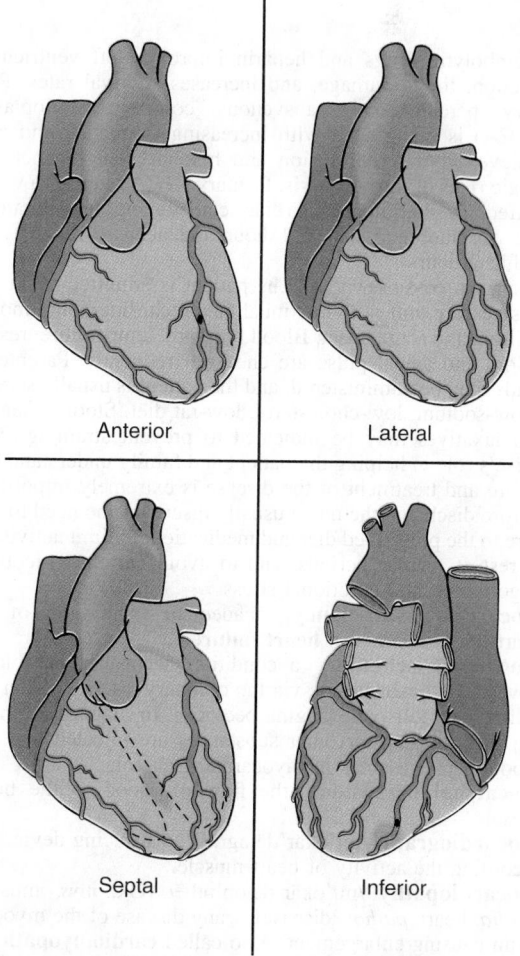

Anterior

Lateral

Septal

Inferior

**Common locations of myocardial infarction**
*(Lewis, Heitkemper, and Dirksen, 2000)*

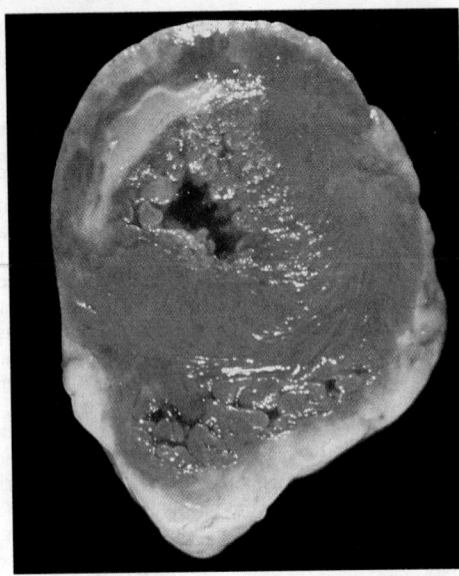

**Acute myocardial infarction, 5 to 7 days old**
*(Kumar, Cotran, and Robbins, 1997)*

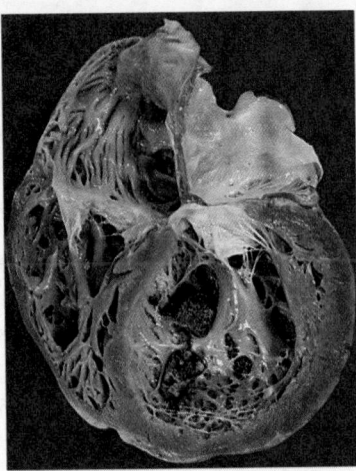

**Dilated myocardiopathy** *(Damjanov and Linder, 2000)*

thrombolytic drugs and heparin improves left ventricular function, limits damage, and increases survival rates. Primary percutaneous transvenous coronary angioplasty (PTCA) is being used with increasing frequency and can achieve prompt reperfusion and help prevent the hemorrhagic risks of thrombolysis. Primary PTCA requires a well-staffed, well-equipped cardiac catheterization laboratory that can mobilize within 1 hour and achieve reperfusion within 2 hours.

■ NURSING CONSIDERATIONS: The patient is admitted to an intensive care unit with continual electrocardiographic monitoring at the acute onset. Blood pressure, temperature, respiration, and apical pulse are checked frequently. Parenteral fluids may be administered, and the patient is usually served a low-sodium, low-cholesterol, low-fat diet. Stool softeners and laxatives may be indicated to prevent straining. The nurse's role in helping the patient and family understand the nature and treatment of the disease is extremely important. Before discharge the nurse usually discusses the need to adhere to the prescribed diet and medication, to limit activities, to rest at regular periods, and to avoid caffeine, nicotine, large meals, and emotional stress.

**myocardial insufficiency,** inadequate functioning of the heart muscle. See also **heart failure.**

**myocardial ischemia,** a condition of insufficient blood flow to the heart muscle via the coronary arteries, often resulting in chest pain (angina pectoris). In diagnostic imaging, thallium-201 or other substances are injected into the blood to reveal areas of myocardial ischemia.

**myocardial perfusion,** the flow of blood to the heart muscle.

**myocardiograph** /mī′ōkär′dē·əgraf′/, a tracing device for recording the activity of heart muscle.

**myocardiopathy** /mī′ōkär′dē·op′əthē/ [Gk, *mys,* muscle, *kardia,* heart, *pathos,* disease], any disease of the myocardium causing enlargement. Also called **cardiomyopathy.**

**myocarditis** /mī′ōkärdī′tis/ [Gk, *mys* + *kardia* + *itis,* inflammation], inflammation of the myocardium. It may be caused by viral, bacterial, or fungal infection, serum sickness, rheumatic fever, or a chemical agent, or it may be a complication of a collagen disease. Myocarditis most frequently occurs in an acute viral form and is self-limited, but it may lead to acute heart failure. Management includes treatment of the cause, analgesia, oxygen, antiinflammatory agents, constant monitoring, and rest to prevent shock or heart failure.

**myocardium** /mī′ōkär′dē·əm/ [Gk, *mys,* muscle, *kardia,* heart], a thick contractile middle layer of uniquely constructed and arranged muscle cells that forms the bulk of the heart wall. The myocardium contains a minimum of other tissue, except blood vessels, and is covered interiorly by the endocardium. The contractile tissue of the myocardium is composed of fibers with the characteristic cross-striations of muscular tissue. The fibers are about one third as large in diameter as those of skeletal muscle and contain more sarcoplasm. They branch frequently and are interconnected to form a network that is continuous except where the bundles and the laminae are attached at their origins and insertions into the fibrous trigone of the heart. Myocardial muscle contains less connective tissue than does skeletal muscle. Specially modified fibers of myocardial muscle constitute the conduction system of the heart, including the sinoatrial node, the atrioventricular (AV) node, the AV bundle, and the Purkinje fibers. Most of the myocardial fibers function to contract the heart. The metabolic processes of the myocardium are almost exclusively aerobic. Many key enzymatic reactions of the heart, such as the citric acid cycle and oxidative phosphorylation, take place in the highly concentrated myocardial sarcosomes. The process of oxidative phosphorylation produces adenosine triphosphate (ATP), the immediate energy source for myocardial contraction. Oxygen, which significantly affects ATP production and contractibility, is a critical metabolic component of the myocardium, which consumes from 6.5 to 10 mL/100 g of tissue per minute. Without this oxygen supply myocardial contractions decrease in a few minutes. The myocardium maintains a relatively constant level of glycogen in the form of sarcoplasmic granules. Compare **epicardium.** See also **cardiac muscle. —myocardial,** *adj.*

**Myochrysine,** trademark for an antirheumatic (gold sodium thiomalate).

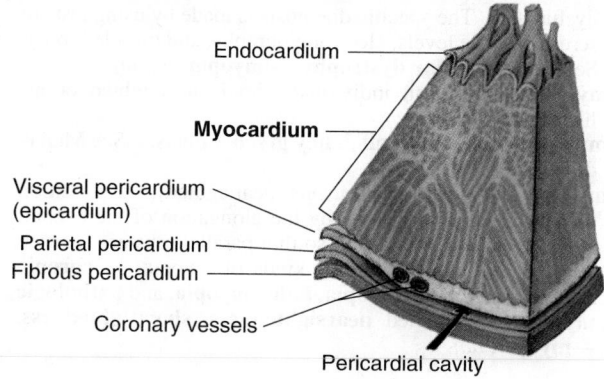

**Myocardium** *(Applegate, 2000)*

**myoclonic encephalopathy of childhood.** See **Kinsbourne syndrome.**

**myoclonus** /mī′ōklō′nəs/ [Gk, *mys* muscle; + *klonos*, contraction], a spasm of a muscle or a group of muscles. —**myoclonic,** *adj.*

**myocutaneous flap** /mī′ō·kyōō·tā′nē·əs/ [Gk, *mys,* muscle; L, *cutis,* skin], a compound flap of skin and muscle with adequate vascularity to permit sufficient tissue to be transferred to the recipient site.

**myocyte** /mī′əsīt/, a muscle cell.

**myodiastasis** /mī′ōdī·as′təsis/ [Gk, *mys* + *diastasis,* separation], an abnormal condition in which there is separation of muscle bundles.

**myodystrophy.** See **muscular dystrophy.**

**myoedema** /mī′ō·idē′mə/, *pl.* **myoedemas, myoedemata,** muscle edema. Compare **myxedema.**

**myoelectric,** pertaining to the electric property of muscle.

**myofascial** /mī·ōfā′shəl/, pertaining to a muscle and its sheath of connective tissue, or fascia.

**myofascial pain,** jaw muscle distress associated with chewing or exercise of the masticatory muscles.

**myofascial release,** a set of massage techniques used to relieve muscle pain resulting from abnormally tight fascia.

**myofibril** /-fī′bril/ [Gk, *mys* + *fibrilla,* small fiber], a slender striated strand within skeletal and cardiac muscle fibers and composed of bundles of myofilaments. Myofibrils occur in groups of branching threads running parallel to the cellular long axis of the fiber.

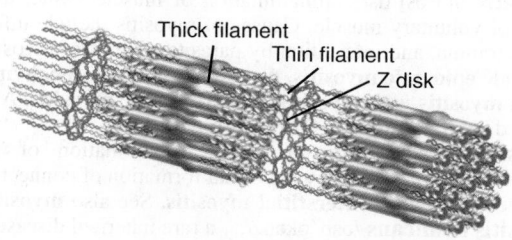

**Molecular structure of a myofibril**
*(Thibodeau and Patton, 1999/Joanna Wild)*

**myofilament** /mī′ō·fil′ə·mənt/ [Gk, *mys,* L, *filare,* to spin], any of the numerous ultramicroscopic threadlike structures occurring in bundles in the myofibrils of striated muscle fibers. The thick filaments of **myosin** and the thin filaments of **actin** are together responsible for the contractile properties of muscle. Also present are **intermediate filaments,** of uncertain function. See also **myofibril.**

**myogelosis** /mī′ōjəlō′sis/ [Gk, *mys* + L, *gelare,* to freeze; Gk, *osis*], a condition in which there are hardened areas or nodules within muscles, especially the gluteal muscles. There are no serious consequences of this condition, and no treatment is necessary.

**myogenic** /mī′ōjen′ik/ [Gk, *mys* + *genesis,* origin], generated by muscles. The term usually refers to rhythmic activity in cardiac and smooth muscles, which do not require neural input to initiate and maintain contractions.

**myoglobin** /mī′ōglō′bin/ [Gk, *mys* + L, *globus,* ball], a ferrous globin complex consisting of one heme molecule containing one iron molecule attached to a single globin chain. Myoglobin is responsible for the red color of muscle and for its ability to store oxygen. Normal blood levels of myoglobin are 0 to 85 ng/mL. Excessive myoglobin levels may result from massive burns or trauma.

**myoglobin test,** a blood test that detects levels of myoglobin, an oxygen-binding protein found in cardiac and skeletal muscle. Measurement of myoglobin is an index of damage to the myocardium in myocardial infarction or reinfarction, and also an indicator of disease or trauma of the skeletal muscle.

**myoglobinuria** /-glō′binŏŏr′ē·ə/ [Gk, *mys* + L, *globus* + Gk, *ouron,* urine], the presence of myoglobin, an oxygen-storing pigment of muscle tissue, in the urine. The condition usually occurs after massive muscle injury, physical trauma, or electrical injury.

**myoglobinuric renal failure** /-glō′binŏŏr′ik/, a kidney disease in which large amounts of filtered myoglobin coalesce in the tubules, obstructing nephronal flow and producing epithelial cell injury.

**myokinase.** See **adenylate kinase.**

**myoma** /mī·ō′mə/, *pl.* **myomas, myomata** [Gk, *mys* + *oma,* tumor], a common benign fibroid tumor of the uterine muscle. The tumor develops most frequently after 30 years of age in women, especially African-American women, who have never been pregnant. Menorrhagia, backache, constipation, dysmenorrhea, dyspareunia, and other symptoms develop in proportion to the size, location, and rate of growth of the tumor.

**myoma previum.** See **leiomyoma uteri.**

**myoma striocellulare.** See **rhabdomyoma.**

**myomata.** See **myoma.**

**myomectomy** /mī′ōmek′təmē/, the surgical removal of muscle tissue.

**myomere.** See **myotome.**

**myometria.** See **myometrium.**

**myometritis** /mī′ōmətrī′tis/, an inflammation or infection of the myometrium of the uterus.

**myometrium** /mī′ōmē′trē·əm/, *pl.* **myometria** [Gk, *mys* + *metra,* womb], the muscular layer of the wall of the uterus. The smooth muscle fibers of the myometrium course around the uterus horizontally, vertically, and diagonally.

**myonecrosis** /mī′ōnekrō′sis/ [Gk, *mys* + *necrosis,* death], the death of muscle fibers. **Progressive** or **clostridial myonecrosis** is caused by the anaerobic bacteria of the genus *Clostridium.* Seen in deep wound infections, progressive myonecrosis is accompanied by pain, tenderness, a brown serous exudate, and a rapid accumulation of gas within the muscle tissue. The affected muscle turns a blackish green.

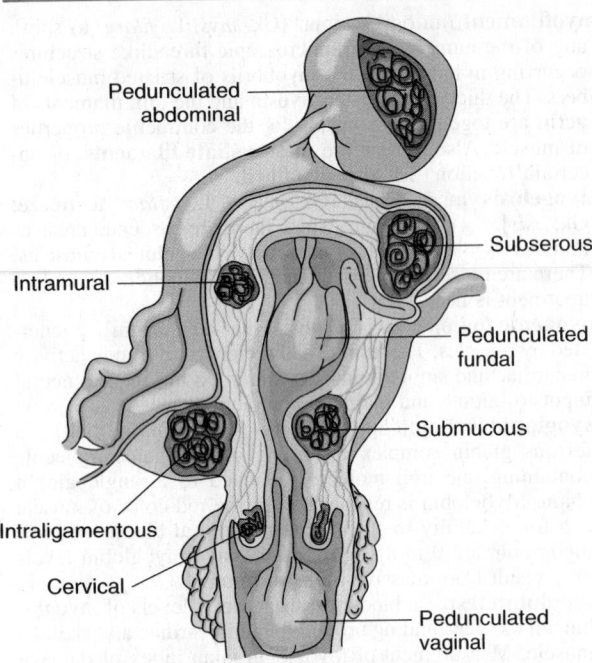

**Common locations for myomas of the uterus**
*(Phipps, Sands, and Marek, 1999)*

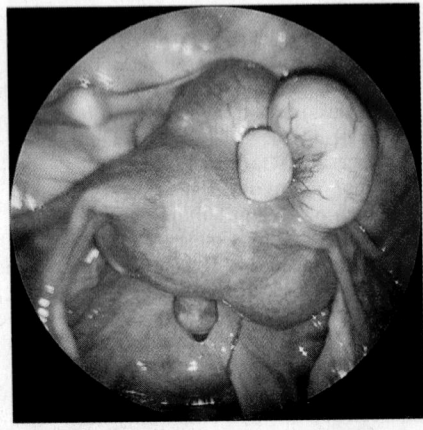

**Multiple myomas viewed laparoscopically** *(Hunt, 1999)*

Treatment includes thorough wound debridement, IV administration of penicillin, hyperbaric oxygen therapy to destroy the anaerobe and to promote healing.

**myoneural** /mī′ōnŏŏr′əl/ [Gk, *mys + neuron,* nerve], pertaining to a muscle fiber and the synapse of the motor neuron, especially to nerve endings in muscles.

**myoneuralgia.** See **myalgia.**

**myoneural junction.** See **end plate.**

**myopathy** /mī·op′əthē/ [Gk, *mys + pathos,* disease], an abnormal condition of skeletal muscle characterized by muscle weakness, wasting, and histologic changes within muscle tissue, as seen in any of the muscular dystrophies. A myopathy is distinct from a muscle disorder caused by nerve

dysfunction. The specific diagnosis is made by using tests of serum enzyme levels, electromyography, and muscle biopsy. See also **muscular dystrophy.** —**myopathic,** *adj.*

**myope** /mī′ōp/, an individual who is nearsighted or afflicted with myopia.

**myophosphorylase deficiency glycogenosis.** See **McArdle's disease.**

**myopia** /mī·ō′pē·ə/ [Gk, *myops,* nearsighted], a condition of nearsightedness caused by the elongation of the eyeball or by an error in refraction so that parallel rays are focused in front of the retina. Some kinds of myopia are **chronic myopia, curvature myopia, index myopia,** and **pathologic myopia.** Also called **nearsightedness, shortsightedness.** —**myopic,** *adj.*

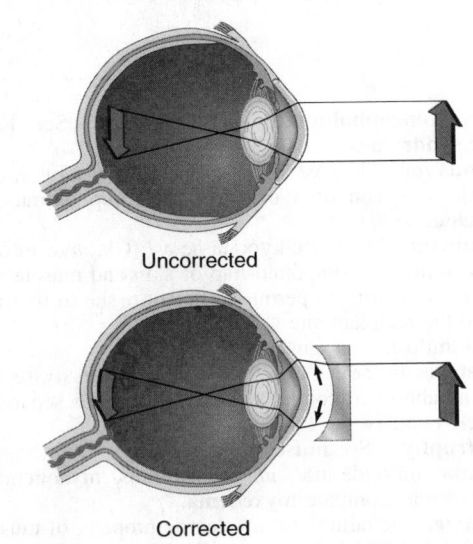

Uncorrected

Corrected

**Myopia** *(Thibodeau and Patton, 1999/Network Graphics)*

**myoreceptor.** See **muscle receptor.**

**myorrhaphy** /mī·ôr′əfē/ [Gk, *mys + rhaphe,* suture], suturing of a wound in a muscle.

**myorrhexis** /mī′ərek′sis/ [Gk, *mys + rhexis,* rupture], the tearing of any muscle. —**myorrhectic,** *adj.*

**myosarcoma** /mī′ōsärkō′mə/ [Gk, *mys + sarx,* flesh, *oma,* tumor], a malignant tumor of muscular tissue.

**myosin** /mī′əsin/ [Gk, *mys + in,* within], a protein that makes up close to one half of the total protein in muscle tissue. The interaction between myosin and another protein, actin, is essential for muscle contraction.

**myositis** /mī′əsī′tis/, inflammation of muscle tissue, usually of voluntary muscle. Causes of myositis include infection, trauma, and infestation by parasites. Kinds of myositis include **epidemic myositis, myositis fibrosa, parenchymatous myositis, polymyositis,** and **traumatic myositis.** Also called **myitis** /mī-ī′tis/. Compare **fibrositis.**

**myositis fibrosa,** an uncommon inflammation of the muscles, characterized by abnormal formation of connective tissue. Also called **interstitial myositis.** See also **myositis.**

**myositis ossificans** /əsif′əkanz/, a rare inherited disease in which muscle tissue is replaced by bone. It begins in childhood, with stiffness in the neck and back, and progresses to rigidity of the spine, trunk, and limbs. The administration of diphosphonates may prevent the abnormal deposition of bone, but there is no cure after it has occurred. Metabolism of calcium and phosphate remains normal throughout the course of the disease. Compare **myositis.**

**myositis ossificans progressiva,** a progressive disease beginning in early life, in which the muscles are gradually converted into bony tissue. Also called **fibrodysplasia ossificans progressiva, progressive ossifying myositis.**

**myositis purulenta,** any bacterial infection of muscle tissue. This condition may result in the formation of an abscess or multiple abscesses.

**myositis trichinosa** /trik′əno′sə/, inflammation of the muscles resulting from infection by the parasite *Trichinella spiralis.* See also **trichinosis.**

**myostasis** /mī′ōstā′sis/ [Gk, *mys* + *stasis,* standing], a condition of muscle weakness in which the resting length of the muscle is shorter than normal, which reduces the maximul tension the muscle can develop when it contracts. In a normal muscle, the force of contraction is greatest at the resting length. —**myostatic,** *adj.*

**myostatic reflex.** See **deep tendon reflex.**

**myostroma** /mī′əstrō′mə/ [Gk, *mys* + *stroma,* covering], the framework of muscle tissue.

**myotenotomy** /-tenot′əmē/ [Gk, *mys* + *tenon,* tendon, *temnein,* to cut], surgical division of the whole or part of a muscle by cutting through its main tendon.

**myotherapy** /-ther′əpē/, a technique of corrective muscle exercises involving pressure on fingers and joints to relieve pain or spasms.

**myotome** /mī′ətōm/ [Gk, *mys* + *temnein,* to cut], **1.** also called **myomere.** The muscle plate of an embryonic somite that develops into a voluntary muscle. **2.** a group of muscles innervated by a single spinal segment. **3.** an instrument for cutting or dissecting a muscle.

**myotomic muscle** /-tom′ik/, any of the numerous muscles of the trunk of the body, derived from the myotomes and divided into the deep muscles of the back and the thoracoabdominal muscles.

**myotomy** /mī·ot′əmē/ [Gk, *mys* + *temnein,* to cut], the dissection or cutting of a muscle, performed to gain access to underlying tissues or to relieve constriction in a sphincter, such as in severe esophagitis or pyloric stenosis. With the patient under general anesthesia, a longitudinal cut is made through the sphincter muscle but not through the mucosa lining the stomach. See also **abdominal surgery.**

**Myotonachol,** trademark for a cholinergic (bethanechol chloride).

**myotonia** /mī′ətō′nē·ə/ [Gk, *mys* + *tonos,* tone], any condition in which a muscle or a group of muscles does not readily relax after contracting. —**myotonic,** *adj.*

**myotonia atrophica.** See **myotonic muscular dystrophy.**

**myotonia congenita** /konjen′itə/, a rare mild and nonprogressive form of myotonic myopathy evident early in life. The only effects of the disorder are hypertrophy and stiffness of the muscles. Also called **Thomsen's disease.**

**myotonic.** See **myotonia.**

**myotonic muscular dystrophy** /-ton′ik/, a severe form of muscular dystrophy marked by ptosis, facial weakness, and dysarthria. Weakness of the hands and feet precedes that in the shoulders and hips. Myotonia of the hands is usually present. Electromyography is helpful in establishing the diagnosis. Although there is no specific treatment, active and passive exercises are used to alleviate symptoms. Also called **myotonia atrophica, Steinert's disease.**

**myotonic myopathy,** any of a group of disorders characterized by increased skeletal muscle tone and decreased relaxation of muscle after contraction. Kinds of myotonic my-

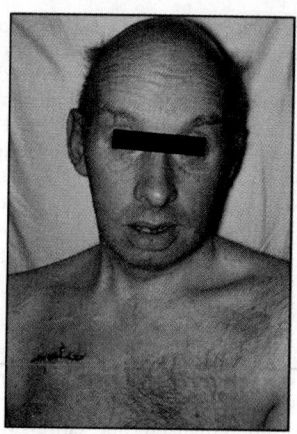

**Myotonic muscular dystrophy: characteristic facial expression**
*(Perkin, 1998)*

opathy include **myotonia congenita, myotonic muscular dystrophy.**

**myria-,** combining form meaning 'a great number': *myriapod.*

**myringa.** See **tympanic membrane.**

**myringectomy** /mir′injek′təmē/ [L, *myringa,* eardrum; Gk, *ektomē,* excision], excision of the tympanic membrane.

**myringitis** /mir′injī′tis/ [L, *myringa* + Gk, *itis*], inflammation or infection of the tympanic membrane.

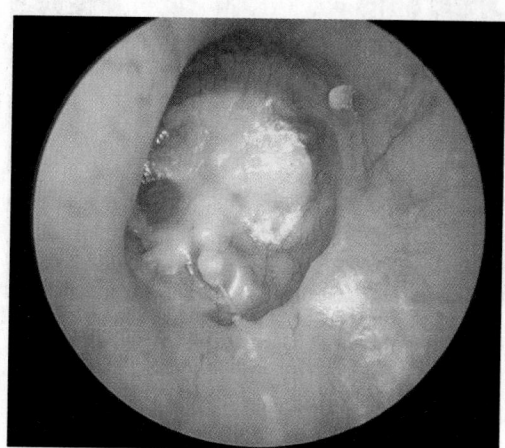

**Myringitis**
*(Stone and Gorbach, 2000/courtesy Dr. N. Blevins, New England Medical Center, Boston)*

**myringo-,** combining form meaning 'related to the tympanic membrane': *myringodectomy, myringoplasty, myringoscope.*

**myringomycosis** /miring′gōmīkō′sis/ [L, *myringa* + Gk, *mykes,* fungus, *osis,* condition], a fungal infection of the tympanic membrane. Also called **mycomyringitis.**

**myringoplasty** /miring′gōplas′tē/ [L, *myringa* + Gk, *plassein*, to mold],   surgical repair of perforations of the eardrum with a tissue graft, performed to correct hearing loss. With the patient under local or general anesthesia, the openings in the eardrum are enlarged, and the grafting material is sutured over them. Topical antibiotics are applied, then a packing of absorbable gelatin sponge to hold the graft in position. After surgery an antihistamine with an ephedrine derivative is given. The nurse keeps the outer ear clean and dry. Debris is removed by gentle suctioning about 12 days after surgery. See also **myringotomy, tympanoplasty.**

**myringotomy** /mir′ing·got′əmē/ [L, *myringa* + Gk, *temnein*, to cut],   surgical incision of the eardrum, performed to relieve pressure and release pus or fluid from the middle ear. Antibiotics are given before surgery and continued afterward. The drum is incised, and cultures may be taken; fluid is gently suctioned from the middle ear. Eardrops may be instilled, or tubes may be inserted to improve drainage. The nurse cautions against putting cotton in the canal, because the ear must drain freely. The outer ear is kept clean and dry. Careful handwashing is essential to prevent infection. If pain increases, the procedure may have to be repeated. Severe headache or disorientation must be reported. Earplugs are required for swimming and showers if tubes are used. Also called **tympanotomy.** See also **myringoplasty.**

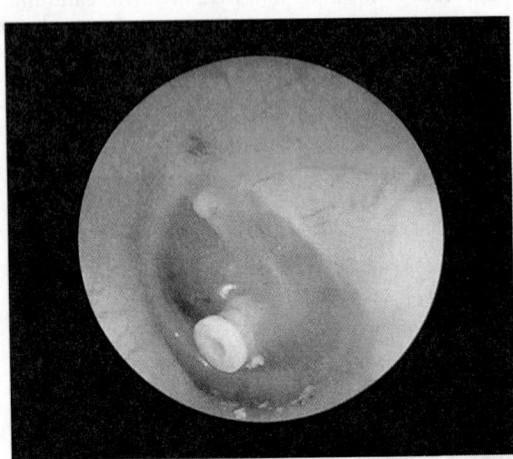

**Myringotomy (tympanostomy tube)**
*(Fireman and Slavin, 1996)*

**Mysoline,**   trademark for an anticonvulsant (primidone).

**mysophobia** /mē′sə-/ [Gk, *mysos*, anything disgusting, *phobos*, fear],   an anxiety disorder characterized by an overreaction to the slightest uncleanliness, or an irrational fear of dirt, contamination, or defilement. Also spelled **misophobia.** —**mysophobic, misophobic,** *adj.*

**myx-, myxo-,**   combining form meaning 'relating to mucus': *myxoblastoma, myxocyte, myxoma.*

**myxedema** /mik′sədē′mə/ [Gk, *myxa*, mucus, *oidema*, swelling],   the most severe form of hypothyroidism. It is characterized by swelling of the hands, face, feet, and peri-

orbital tissues. At this stage the disease may lead to coma and death. Also spelled **myxoedema.** See also **hypothyroidism.**

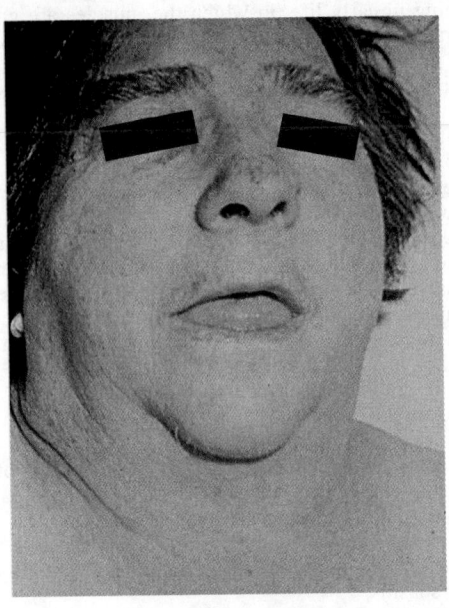

**Myxedema facies**
*(Seidel et al, 1999/courtesy Paul Ladenson MD, Johns Hopkins University and Hospital, Baltimore)*

**myxofibroma** /mik′sōfībrō′mə/ [Gk, *myxa* + L, *fibra*, fiber; Gk, *oma*, tumor],   a fibrous tumor that contains myxomatous tissue. Also called **myxoma fibrosum.**

**myxoid.**   See **mucoid,** def. 1.

**myxoma** /miksō′mə/ [Gk, *myxa* + *oma*, tumor],   a neoplasm of the connective tissue, characteristically composed of stellate cells in a loose mucoid matrix crossed by delicate reticulum fibers. These tumors may grow to enormous size and may occur under the skin but are also found in bones, the genitourinary tract, and the retroperitoneal area. —**myxomatous,** *adj.*

**-myxoma,**   suffix meaning a 'soft tumor made up of primitive connective tissues': *adenomyxoma, gliomyxoma, lipomyxoma.*

**myxoma fibrosum.**   See **myxofibroma.**

**myxoma sarcomatosum.**   See **myxosarcoma.**

**myxomatous.**   See **myxoma.**

**myxopoiesis** /mik′sōpō·ē′sis/ [Gk, *myxa* + *poiein*, to make],   the production of mucus.

**myxosarcoma** /mik′sōsärkō′mə/ [Gk, *myxa* + *sarx*, flesh, *oma*, tumor],   a sarcoma that contains some myxomatous tissue. Also called **myxoma sarcomatosum.**

**myxovirus** /mik′sōvī′rəs/ [Gk, *myxa* + L, *virus*, poison],   any of a group of medium-size ribonucleic acid viruses that are further divided into orthomyxoviruses and paramyxoviruses. Infection with these viruses is usually caused by transmission of the respiratory secretions of an infected host. Some kinds of myxoviruses are the viruses that cause influenza, mumps, and parainfluenza.

**MZ,**   abbreviation for **monozygotic.**

**N,**  1. symbol for the element **nitrogen. 2.** abbreviation for **normal. 3.** abbreviation for *node* in the TNM system for staging malignant neoplastic disease. See also **cancer staging. 4.** symbol for **Avogadro's number. 5.** symbol for *magnetic flux.*

**N/1,**  symbol for **normal solution.**

**n, 2n, 3n, 4n,**  symbols for the haploid, diploid, triploid, and tetraploid number of chromosomes in a cell, organism, strain, or individual.

**nA,**  abbreviation for *nanoampere,* one billionth of an ampere.

**Na,**  chemical symbol for the element **sodium.**

**-nab,**  combining form for cannabinol derivatives.

**nabothian cyst** /nabō'thē-ən/ [Martin Naboth, German physician, 1675–1721; Gk, *kystis,* bag],  a cyst formed in a nabothian gland of the uterine cervix. It is a common finding on routine pelvic examination of women of reproductive age, especially in women who have borne children. The cyst, which is pearly white and firm, seldom results in adverse or pathologic effects. Also called **cervical cyst.**

**nabothian gland** /nəbō'thē-ən/ [Martin Naboth; L, *glans,* acorn],  one of many small, mucus-secreting glands of the uterine cervix.

**NAD,**  abbreviation for *no appreciable disease.*

**NADH,**  abbreviation for *nicotine adenine dinucleotide, reduced.*

**nadir** /nā'dər/,  the lowest point, such as the blood count after it has been depressed by chemotherapy.

**nadolol** /nad'ənol/,  a beta-adrenergic blocking agent.

■ INDICATIONS: It is prescribed for long-term management of angina pectoris, for hypertension, and after myocardial infarction.

■ CONTRAINDICATIONS: Bronchial asthma, sinus bradycardia, greater than first-degree conduction block, cardiogenic shock, overt cardiac failure, or known hypersensitivity to this drug prohibits its use.

■ ADVERSE EFFECTS: Among the more serious adverse reactions are bronchospasm, bradycardia, precipitation of heart failure, cardiac arrhythmia, masking of signs of hypoglycemia in diabetics, fatigue, and lethargy. GI disturbances, rashes, and other allergic reactions also may occur.

**NADPH,**  abbreviation for *nicotine adenine disphosphonucleotide, reduced.*

**NADPH oxidase defect,**  a disorder in patients with chronic granulomatosis disease. It is caused by an abnormality in the enzyme (nicotinamide adenine dinucleotide phosphate oxidase) that catalyzes the conversion of oxygen to superoxide anions and hydrogen peroxide in phagocytes. Phagocytes with the abnormal enzyme are unable to destroy invading microorganisms.

**Naegeli's leukemia.**  See **monocytic leukemia.**

*Naegleria* /nā·glēr'ē-ə/ [F.P.O. Nägler, Austrian bacteriologist, 20th century],  a genus of free-living protozoa found in fresh water, soil, and sewage, which have both an ameboid and a flagellate stage in their life cycle. Certain species, especially *N. fowleri,* are capable of facultative parasitism, and some strains are highly pathogenic and may cause a highly fatal primary amebic meningoencephalitis. Infection is usually acquired by swimming in water contaminated with the organisms. See also **primary amebic meningoencephalitis.**

**naegleriasis** /nā'glə·rī'ə·sis/,  infection with *Naegleria.*

**naevus.**  See **nevus.**

**nafcillin sodium** /nafsil'in/,  an antibiotic.

■ INDICATIONS: It is prescribed in the treatment of infections caused by penicillinase-producing staphylococci.

■ CONTRAINDICATIONS: Known hypersensitivity to this drug or to other penicillins prohibits its use.

■ ADVERSE EFFECTS: Among the more serious adverse reactions are hypersensitivity reactions, nausea, and vomiting.

**Naffziger sign** /naf'zigər/ [Howard C. Naffziger, American surgeon, 1884–1961],  a diagnostic sign for sciatica or a herniated intervertebral disk. Nerve root irritation is produced by the examiner through external jugular venous compression.

**Naffziger's syndrome** [Howard C. Naffziger],  a condition of cervical vertebral muscle spasms secondary to intervertebral disk disease, cervical rib disease, or other disorders. The spasms compress the major nerve plexus of the arm, causing the patient to experience pain in the neck, shoulder, arm, and hand. Also called **scalenus anticus syndrome.** Compare **thoracic outlet syndrome.**

**Naffziger's test** /naf'zig·ərz/,  (for nerve root compression) increase or aggravation of pain or sensory disturbance over the distribution of the involved nerve root on manual compression of the jugular veins bilaterally confirms the presence of an extruded intervertebral disk or other mass.

**Nägele obliquity.**  See **asynclitism.**

**Nägele's rule** /nā'gələz/ [Franz K. Nägele, German obstetrician, 1778–1851; L, *regula,* model],  a method for calculating the estimated date of delivery based on a mean length of gestation. Three months are subtracted from the first day of the last normal menstrual period, and 1 year plus 7 days are added to that date.

**Nager's acrofacial dysostosis** /nā'gərz/ [Felix R. Nager, Swiss physician, 1877–1959; Gk, *akron,* extremity; L, *facies,* face; Gk, *dys,* bad, *osteon,* bone, *osis,* condition],  an abnormal congenital condition characterized by limb deformities such as radioulnar synostosis, hypoplasia, and the absence of the radius or of the thumbs. Also called **dysostosis mandibularis.** Compare **cleidocranial dysostosis, craniofacial dysostosis, mandibulofacial dysostosis.**

**Nahrungs-Einheit-Milch (nem)** /nä'rŏŏngz īn'hīt milsh, milkh/ [Ger, *Nahrung,* food, *Einheit,* unit, *Milch,* milk],  a nutritional unit in Pirquet's system of feeding that is equivalent to 1 g of breast milk.

**nail** [AS, *naegel*],  **1.** also called **unguis.** a flattened elastic structure with a horny texture at the end of a finger or a toe. Each nail is composed of a root, body, and free edge at the distal extremity. The root fastens the nail to the finger or the toe by fitting into a groove in the skin and is closely molded to the surface of the dermis. The nail matrix beneath the body and the root projects longitudinal vascular ridges, which are easily visible through the translucent tissue of the body. The matrix firmly attaches the body of the nail to the underlying connective tissue. The whitish lunula near the root contains irregularly arranged papillae that are less firmly attached to the connective tissue than the rest of the matrix. The cuticle is attached to the surface of the nail just ahead of the root. **2.** any of various metallic nails used in orthopedics to fasten together bones or pieces of bone.

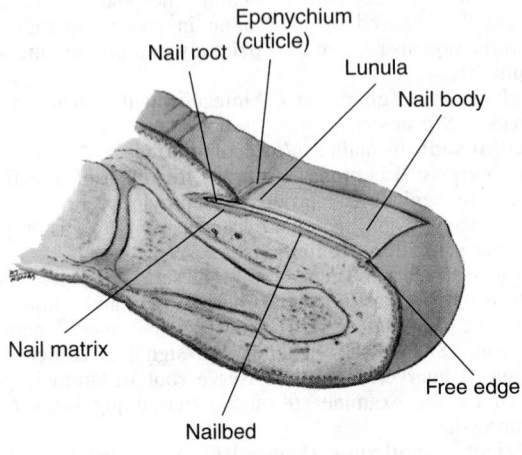

**Nail** *(Jarvis, 2000)*

**nailbed** [AS, *naegle*, nail, *bedd*, bed], the dermis beneath the nail. It appears through the clear nail as a series of longitudinal ridges. Also called **matrix unguis.**

**nail biting,** the habit of excessive biting and chewing one's fingernails and periungual skin, sometimes leading to cutaneous injury. The condition is commonly associated with body manipulations of anxious children. It is also considered a form of motor discharges of inner tension. The recommended treatment includes daily bandaging of injured fingers and frequent applications of a distasteful topical preparation. Also called **onychophagia.**

**nail care,** a nursing intervention from the Nursing Interventions Classification (NIC) defined as promotion of clean, neat, attractive nails and prevention of skin lesions related to improper care of nails. See also **Nursing Interventions Classification.**

**nail fold,** a fold of skin supporting a nail at its base.

**nail groove** [AS, *naegle* + D, *groeve*, groove], a shallow depression between the nailbed and the nail wall.

**nail matrix.** See **nailbed.**

**nail-patella syndrome,** a hereditary syndrome consisting of dystrophy of the nails, absence or hypoplasia of the patella, hypoplasia of the lateral side of the elbow joint, and bilateral iliac horns. Also called **hereditary osteo-onychodysplasia, onycho-osteodysplasia, osteo-onychodysplasia.**

**nail plate,** the rigid outer part of a nail. It extends about 8 mm under the nail fold and arises from the nailbed.

**nail plate avulsion,** a partial or complete removal of the nail plate without disruption of the underlying matrix cells.

**nal-,** prefix meaning 'narcotic agonists or antagonists related to normorphine.'

**Naldecon,** trademark for a fixed-combination drug containing two adrenergics (phenylpropanolamine hydrochlo-

ride and phenylephrine hydrochloride) and two antihistamines (chlorpheniramine maleate and phenyltoloxamine citrate).

**Nalebuff arthrodesis,** surgical fixation of the wrist accomplished with the use of a Steinmann pin.

**Nalfon,** trademark for an antiinflammatory agent (fenoprofen calcium).

**nalidixic acid** /nal'idik'sik/, an antibacterial.
- ■ INDICATIONS: It is prescribed in the treatment of certain urinary tract infections.
- ■ CONTRAINDICATIONS: Renal or hepatic insufficiency, a history of convulsive disorders, or known hypersensitivity to this drug prohibits its use.
- ■ ADVERSE EFFECTS: Among the more serious adverse reactions are mild neurologic disturbances, GI disturbances, and hemolytic anemia in glucose-6-phosphate dehydrogenase deficiency. Convulsions and increased cranial pressure may occur. Among the more serious reactions are increased intracranial pressure, seizures, hemolytic anemia in people affected with glucose-6-phosphate dehydrogenase deficiency, and GI and neurologic disturbances.

**naloxone hydrochloride** /nal'əksōn/, an opioid antagonist.
- ■ INDICATIONS: It is prescribed for reversal of narcotic depression or acute narcotic intoxication.
- ■ CONTRAINDICATION: Known hypersensitivity to this drug prohibits its use.
- ■ ADVERSE EFFECTS: Among the most serious adverse reactions when given to opioid-dependent patients are side effects associated with narcotic withdrawal.

**naltrexone hydrochloride** /naltrek'sōn/, an oral opioid antagonist.
- ■ INDICATIONS: It is prescribed to block the effects of opioid analgesics, including heroin, morphine, and methadone in patients recovering from addiction.
- ■ CONTRAINDICATIONS: Acute hepatitis or liver failure prohibits the use of the drug. Periodic liver function tests are recommended for all patients. Patients must be completely free of opioids before taking naltrexone to prevent severe withdrawal symptoms. Respiratory depression may be deep and prolonged in a patient taking a large dose of an opioid analgesic after taking naltrexone. The patient must be informed that taking an opioid while on this agent may be fatal and that an ID must be worn when taking the drug in case of the need for emergency treatment.
- ■ ADVERSE EFFECTS: The most serious adverse reactions are abdominal pain, cramps, nausea, vomiting, headache, sleep disorders, and joint and muscle pain. Some adverse effects may actually be withdrawal symptoms rather than reactions to naltrexone.

**Namaqualand hip dysplasia,** an autosomal-dominant genetic defect found in children of African heritage. It is characterized by a growth failure in the femoral epiphysis, resulting in pain and early degenerative arthritis of the hip.

**NAMI,** abbreviation for **National Alliance for the Mentally Ill.**

**NANB,** abbreviation for **non-A, non-B hepatitis.**

**Nance's leeway space.** See **leeway space.**

**NANDA,** abbreviation for **North American Nursing Diagnosis Association.**

**nandrolone decanoate** /nan'drəlōn/, an anabolic steroid.
- ■ INDICATIONS: It is prescribed in the management of the anemia of renal insufficiency. It increases hemoglobin and red cell mass.
- ■ CONTRAINDICATIONS: Cancer of the male breast or prostate, liver disease, pregnancy, suspected pregnancy, or known hypersensitivity to this drug prohibits its use.

■ ADVERSE EFFECTS: Among the most serious adverse effects are various endocrine disturbances, depending on the patient's age. Hirsutism, acne, liver toxicity, and electrolyte imbalances also occur.

**nandrolone phenpropionate,** an anabolic steroid with androgenic properties.

■ INDICATIONS: It is prescribed in the treatment of metastatic breast cancers in women.

■ CONTRAINDICATIONS: Carcinoma of the breast in males and some females, pregnancy, nephrosis, or known hypersensitivity to this drug prohibits its use.

■ ADVERSE EFFECTS: Among the more serious adverse reactions are hirsutism, acne, various endocrine effects depending on the patient's age and sex, masculinization, liver dysfunction, hypercalcemia in women taking the drug for breast cancer, and fluid and salt retention.

**nanism** /nā′nizəm, nan′-/ [Gk, nanos, dwarf], an abnormal smallness or underdevelopment of the body; dwarfism. Kinds of nanism are **mulibrey nanism, Paltauf's nanism, pituitary nanism, renal nanism, senile nanism,** and **symptomatic nanism.** Also called **nanosomia.**

**nano-,** **1.** /nā′nō-/ prefix meaning 'small, or related to smallness or dwarfism': *nanocephalia, nanomelia.* **2.** /nan′-ə-/ combining form used in measurement to mean 'billionth $(10^{-9})$': *nanocurie, nanogram, nanometer.*

**nanocephalia.** See **nanocephaly.**

**nanocephalic dwarf.** See **Seckel's syndrome.**

**nanocephaly** /nā′nōsef′əlē, nan′-/ [Gk, nanos + kephale, head], a developmental defect characterized by abnormal smallness of the head. Also called **nanocephalia, nanocephalism.** —**nanocephalous,** *adj.,* **nanocephalus,** *n.*

**nanocormia** /nā′nōkôr′mē·ə/ [Gk, nanos + kormos, trunk], abnormal disproportionate smallness of the trunk of the body in comparison with the head and limbs. —**nanocormus,** *n.*

**nanocurie (nc, nCi)** /nan′əkyŏŏr′ē/ [Gk, nanos, dwarf; Marie and Pierre Curie], a unit of radiation equal to one billionth of a curie. See also **curie.**

**nanogram (ng)** /nan′əgram/ [Gk, nanos + Fr, gramme, small weight], one billionth $(10^{-9})$ of a gram.

**-nanoid.** See **nanus.**

**nanomelia** /nā′nōmē′lyə, nan′-/ [Gk, nanos + melos, limb], a developmental defect characterized by abnormally small limbs in comparison with the size of the head and trunk. —**nanomelous,** *adj.,* **nanomelus,** *n.*

**nanometer (nm)** /nan′əmē′tər/ [Gk, nanos + metron, measure], a unit of length equal to one billionth of a meter.

**nanophthalmos** /nā′nofthal′məs, nan′-/ [Gk, nanos + ophthalmos, eye], the condition in which one or both eyes are abnormally small, although other ocular defects are not present. Also called **nanophthalmia.** See also **microphthalmos.**

**nanosecond (ns)** /nan′əsek′ənd/ [Gk, nanos, dwarf; L, secundus, second], one billionth $(10^{-9})$ of a second.

**nanosomia.** See **nanism.**

**nanosomus** /nā′nōsō′məs/ [Gk, nanos + soma, body], a person of very short stature; a dwarf.

**nanukayami** /nä′nōōkäyä′mē/ [Jpn], an acute, infectious disease caused by one of the serotypes of the spirochete *Leptospira* that is indigenous to Japan. See also **leptospirosis.**

**nanus** /nā′nəs/, **1.** a dwarf. **2.** a pygmy. —**nanoid** /nā′noid/, *adj.*

**napalm** /nā′päm/, abbreviation for *napthenate palmitate,* a form of jellied gasoline used in warfare.

**napalm burn** [AS, *baernan,* burn], a thermal burn caused by contact with flaming **napalm.**

**nape** [ME], the back of the neck.

**naphazoline hydrochloride** /nəfaz′əlēn/, an adrenergic vasoconstrictor.

■ INDICATIONS: It is prescribed in the treatment of nasal congestion and as an ophthalmic vasoconstrictor.

■ CONTRAINDICATIONS: Glaucoma or known hypersensitivity to this drug or abnormal sensitivity to sympathomimetic drugs prohibits its use.

■ ADVERSE EFFECTS: Among the most serious adverse reactions are those associated with systemic absorption, including sedation and cardiovascular effects. Irritation to mucosa and rebound congestion also may occur.

**naphthalene poisoning** /naf′thəlēn/ [Gk, naptha, flammable liquid; L, potio, drink], a toxic condition caused by the ingestion of naphthalene or paradichlorobenzene that may cause nausea, vomiting, headache, abdominal pain, spasm, and convulsions. Naphthalene and paradichlorobenzene are common ingredients in mothballs and moth crystals; paradichlorobenzene is also used as an insecticide in agriculture.

**naphthol camphor** /naf′thol/, a syrupy mixture of two parts of camphor and one part betanaphthol, used externally as an antiseptic.

**naphthol poisoning.** See **phenol poisoning.**

**napkin ring tumor** [ME, *nappekin,* tablecloth, *hring,* band; L, *tumor,* swelling], a tumor that encircles a tubular structure of the body, usually impairing its function and constricting its lumen to some degree.

**NAP-NAP,** abbreviation for **National Association of Pediatric Nurse Associates/Practitioners.**

**NAPNES,** abbreviation for **National Association for Practical Nurse Education and Services.**

**napping** [ME, *nappen,* to doze], periods of sleep, usually during the day, which may last from 15 to 60 minutes without attaining the level of deep sleep.

**Naprosyn,** trademark for a nonsteroidal antiinflammatory, antipyretic, and analgesic (naproxen).

**naproxen** /naprok′sən/, a nonsteroidal antiinflammatory agent.

■ INDICATION: It is prescribed for the relief of inflammatory symptoms of rheumatoid arthritis and osteoarthritis, relief of mild to moderate pain, treatment of primary dysmenorrhea, ankylosing spondylitis, tendinitis, bursitis, and acute gout.

■ CONTRAINDICATIONS: Impaired renal function, GI disease, or known hypersensitivity to this drug, to aspirin, or to nonsteroidal antiinflammatory drugs prohibits its use.

■ ADVERSE EFFECTS: Among the more serious adverse reactions are GI disorders and peptic ulcers. Dizziness, rashes, and tinnitus commonly occur. This drug interacts with many other drugs.

**NAPT,** abbreviation for *National Association of Physical Therapists.*

**Naqua,** trademark for a diuretic and antihypertensive (trichlormethiazide).

**naratriptan,** a migraine agent.

■ INDICATIONS: Naratriptan is used in the acute treatment of migraine with or without aura.

■ CONTRAINDICATIONS: The following factors prohibit the use of naratriptan: angina pectoris, a history of myocardial infarction, documented silent ischemia, ischemic heart disease, concurrent use of ergotamine-containing preparations, uncontrolled hypertension, hypersensitivity, severe renal disease (creatinine clearance rate 15 ml/min), and severe hepatic disease in children (Pugh grade C).

■ ADVERSE EFFECTS: Adverse reactions to this drug include nausea, myalgia, dizziness, sedation, and fatigue. Common side effects include weakness and neck stiffness.

**narc,** abbreviation for **narcotic.**

**Narcan,** trademark for an opioid antagonist (naloxone hydrochloride).

**narcissism** /när'sisiz'əm/ [Gk, *Narcissus,* mythic youth in love with himself], **1.** an abnormal interest in oneself, especially in one's own body and sexual characteristics; self-love. **2.** (in psychoanalysis) sexual self-interest that is a normal characteristic of the phallic stage of psychosexual development, occurring as the infantile ego acquires a libido. Narcissism in the adult is abnormal, representing fixation at this stage of development or regression to it. Compare **egotism.** See also **narcissistic personality, narcissistic personality disorder.**

**narcissistic personality** /när'sisis'tik/, a disposition characterized by behavior and attitudes that indicate an abnormal love of the self. Such a person is self-centered and self-absorbed, is extremely unrealistic concerning attributes and goals, vacillates between overidealizing and devaluing others, and, in general, assumes that he or she is entitled to more than is reasonable in relationships with others. Compare **narcissism.**

**narcissistic personality disorder,** a psychiatric diagnosis characterized by an exaggerated sense of self-importance and uniqueness, an abnormal need for attention and admiration, preoccupation with grandiose fantasies concerning the self, and disturbances in interpersonal relationships, usually involving the exploitation of others and a lack of empathy.

**narco-** /när'kō-/, prefix meaning 'related to stupor or a stuporous state': *narcolepsy, narcomania, narcotic.*

**narcoanalysis** /-ənal'isis/, an interview conducted while the patient is deeply sedated with medication so that inhibitions are reduced and responses will be more truthful.

**narcohypnosis** /-hipnō'sis/ [Gk, *narke,* stupor, *hypnos,* sleep], hypnosis induced with the aid of a narcotic drug such as sodium amobarbital or sodium pentothal.

**narcolepsy** /när'kəlep'sē/ [Gk, *narke,* stupor, *lambanein,* to seize], a syndrome characterized by sudden sleep attacks, cataplexy, sleep paralysis, and visual or auditory hallucinations at the onset of sleep. The syndrome begins in adolescence or young adulthood and persists throughout life. Its cause is unknown, and no pathologic lesions are found in the brain. Persons with narcolepsy experience an uncontrollable desire to sleep, sometimes many times in one day. Episodes may last from a few minutes to several hours. Momentary loss of muscle tone occurs during waking hours (cataplexy) or while the person is asleep. Narcolepsy may be difficult to diagnose because all people with the disorder do not experience all four symptoms. An electroencephalogram or other brain studies may be used to distinguish narcolepsy from an intracranial mass or encephalitis. Amphetamines and other stimulant drugs are prescribed effectively to prevent the attacks. Also called **sleep epilepsy.**

**narcoleptic** /när'kəlep'tik/, **1.** pertaining to a condition or substance that causes an uncontrollable desire for sleep. **2.** a narcoleptic drug. **3.** a person suffering from narcolepsy.

**Narcon,** abbreviation for *Narcotics Anonymous.*

**narcosis** /närkō'sis/ [Gk, *narkosis,* numbness], a state of insensibility or stupor caused by opioid drugs. See also **narcotic.**

**narcotic (narc)** /narkot'ik/ [Gk, *narkotikos,* benumbing], **1.** pertaining to a substance that produces insensibility or stupor. **2.** a narcotic drug. Narcotic analgesics, derived from opium or produced synthetically, alter perception of pain; induce euphoria, mood changes, mental clouding, and deep sleep; depress respiration and the cough reflex; constrict the pupils; and cause smooth muscle spasm, decreased peristalsis, emesis, and nausea. Repeated use of narcotics may re-

sult in physical and psychologic dependence. Among the narcotic drugs administered clinically for relief of pain are butorphanol tartrate, hydromorphone hydrochloride, morphine sulfate, pentazocine lactate, and meperidine hydrochloride. These drugs act by binding to opiate receptors in the central nervous system; narcotic antagonists such as naloxone hydrochloride, which is used in treating narcotic overdosage, apparently displace opiates from receptor sites.

**-narcotic, -narcotical,** suffix meaning 'analgesic or soporific drugs': *antinarcotic, prenarcotic, pseudonarcotic.*

**narcotic addict,** a person who is psychologically and physically dependent on narcotic drugs, a condition in which the drug is present in the body in amounts great enough to be toxic or sufficient to alter behavior.

**narcotic analgesic.** See **analgesic.**

**narcotic antagonist.** See **opioid antagonist.**

**narcotic antitussive.** See **antitussive.**

**narcotic poisoning** [Gk, *narkotikos,* stupor; L, *potio,* drink], the toxic effects of a narcotic drug that depresses the brain centers, causing unconsciousness or coma. Narcotic drugs are generally derived from opium, but other drugs, including alcohol, can produce similar effects.

**narcotize** /när'kətiz/, to subject to the influence of narcotics.

**Nardil,** trademark for an antidepressant (phenelzine sulfate).

**nares** /ner'ēz/, *sing.* **naris,** the pairs of anterior and posterior openings to the nasal cavity that allow the passage of air to the pharynx and ultimately the lungs during respiration. See also **anterior nares, posterior nares.**

**narrow-angle glaucoma.** See **glaucoma.**

**nas,** abbreviation for **nasal.**

**nas-.** See **naso-.**

**nasal (nas)** /nā'zəl/ [L, *nasus,* nose], **1.** pertaining to the nose and the nasal cavity. **2.** a speech sound produced by having air flow through the nose, such as *n, ng,* or *m.* —**nasally,** *adv.*

**nasal airway,** a flexible, curved piece of rubber or plastic, with one wide, trumpetlike end and one narrow end that can be inserted through the nose into the pharynx. Also called **nasal trumpet.**

**nasal balloon tamponade,** a procedure for the control of posterior epistaxis in which a nasal balloon is inserted into the nasal cavity and filled with saline solution. Alternatively, a Foley catheter can be placed through the nostril and used in the same manner.

**nasal cannula,** a device for delivering oxygen by way of two small tubes that are inserted into the nares.

**nasal cartilage** [L, *nasus,* nose, *cartilago*], a flat plate of cartilage in the lower anterior part of the nasal septum. Also called **septal cartilage.**

**nasal cavity,** one of a pair of cavities that open on the face through the pear-shaped anterior nares and communicate posteriorly with the pharynx. Each cavity is narrower at the top than at the bottom.

**nasal decongestant,** a drug that provides temporary relief of nasal symptoms in acute and chronic rhinitis and sinusitis. Most are over-the-counter products compounded with a small amount of vasoconstrictor such as ephedrine or phenylephrine. An antihistamine may enhance the value of a nasal decongestant in allergic rhinitis, and a corticosteroid may reduce inflammation. Prolonged use or dosage greater than recommended on the package may cause rebound vasodilation and severe congestion (rhitis medicamentosa).

**nasal drip,** a method of slowly infusing liquid into a dehydrated infant by means of a catheter inserted through the nose down the esophagus.

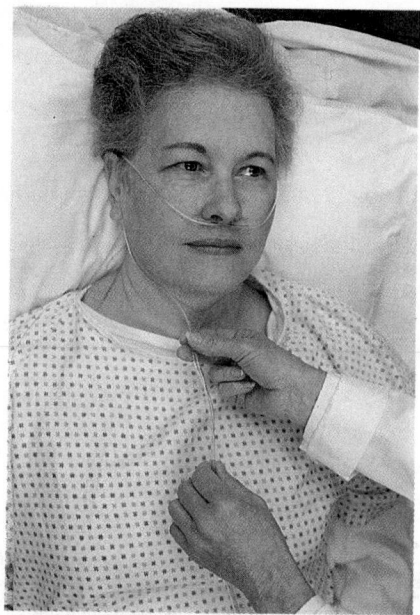

**Nasal cannula** *(Potter and Perry, 2001)*

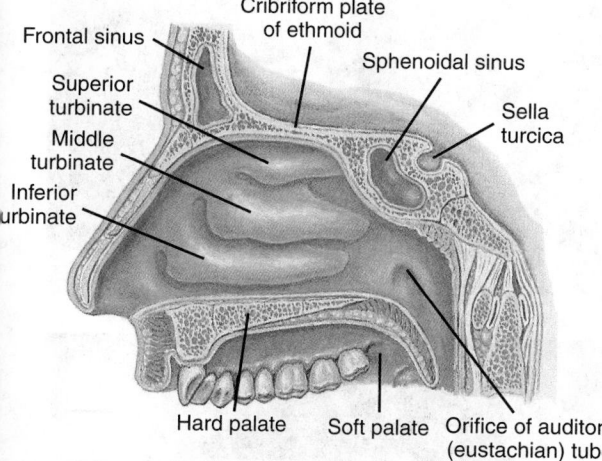

**Nasal cavity** *(Seidel et al, 1999)*

and lateral to the inferior nasal concha and contains the opening of the nasolacrimal duct. The olfactory region is located in the most superior part of the fossa and contains olfactory cells, olfactory nerves, and olfactory hairs. The respiratory region is lined with mucous membrane, numerous glands, nerves, a plexus of dilated veins, and blood spaces. The plexus is easily irritated, causing the membrane to swell, blocking the meatuses and the openings of sinuses.

**nasal glioma,**   a neoplasm characterized by the ectopic growth of neural tissue in the nasal cavity.

**nasal instillation of medication,**   the instillation of a medicated solution into the nostrils by an atomized spray from a squeeze bottle or a nasal inhaler. The patient holds one nostril closed while spraying the medication into the opposite nostril. Nasal spray is administered to the patient in a sitting position. The patient is asked to expectorate any solution that runs down the posterior nares into the throat.

**nasalis** /nāzal'is/ [L, *nasus,* nose],   one of the three muscles of the nose, divided into a transverse part and an alar part. The transverse part arises from the maxilla and covers the bridge of the nose; the alar part attaches at one end to the greater alar cartilage and at the other end to skin at the end of the nose. The transverse part serves to depress the cartilaginous part of the nose and to draw the alar toward the septum. The alar part serves to dilate the nostril. Compare **depressor septi, procerus.**

**nasally.**   See **nasal.**

**nasal obstruction** [L, *nasus,* nose, *obstruere*],   a narrowing of the nasal cavity, thereby reducing the breathing capacity, caused by an irregular or deviated septum, nasal polyps, foreign bodies, or enlarged turbinates. Sinusitis is a common complication of the condition.

**nasal polyp,**   a rounded, elongated piece of pulpy, dependent mucosa that projects into the nasal cavity.

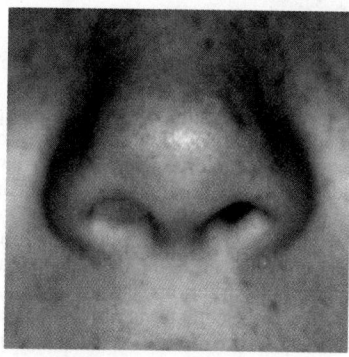

**Nasal polyp** *(Lemmi and Lemmi, 2000)*

**nasal fossa,**   one of the pair of approximately equal chambers of the nasal cavity that are separated by the nasal septum and open externally through the nares and internally into the nasopharynx through the internal nares. Each fossa is divided into an olfactory region, consisting of the superior nasal concha and part of the septum, and a respiratory region, constituting the rest of the chamber. Overhanging the three meatuses of each fossa on the lateral wall are the corresponding superior, middle, and inferior nasal conchae. The superior meatus extends obliquely about halfway along the superior border of the middle concha. The middle meatus continues into the atrium and bulges on the lateral wall at the bulla ethmoidalis. The inferior meatus courses below

**nasal septum,**   the partition dividing the nostrils. It is composed of bone and cartilage covered by mucous membrane.

**nasal sinus,**   any one of the numerous cavities in various bones of the skull, lined with ciliated mucous membrane continuous with that of the nasal cavity. The membrane is very sensitive; easily irritated, it may cause swelling that blocks the sinuses. The nasal sinuses are divided into frontal sinuses, ethmoidal air cells, sphenoidal sinuses, and maxillary sinus.

**Nasarel,**   trademark for an intranasal steroid antiinflammatory agent (flunisolide).

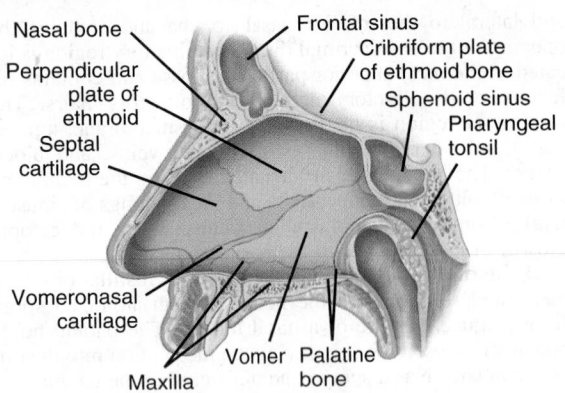

**Nasal septum** (Thibodeau and Patton, 1999)

Nasal bone
Frontal sinus
Cribriform plate of ethmoid bone
Perpendicular plate of ethmoid
Sphenoid sinus
Septal cartilage
Pharyngeal tonsil
Vomeronasal cartilage
Maxilla
Vomer
Palatine bone

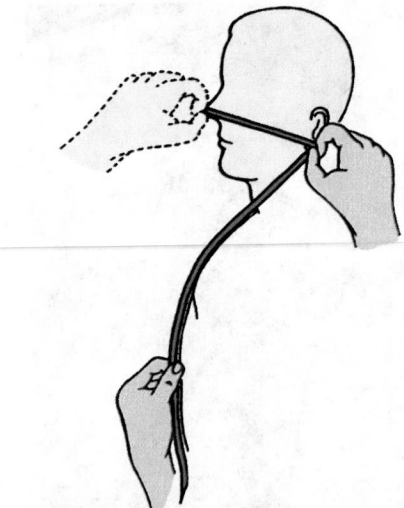

**nascent** /nas′ənt, nā′sənt/ [L, *nasci,* to be born], **1.** just born; beginning to exist; incipient. **2.** (in chemistry) pertaining to any substance liberated during a chemical reaction, which, because of its uncombined state, is more reactive.

**nascent oxygen,** oxygen that has just been liberated from a chemical compound.

**nasion** /nā′zē·on/ [L, *nasus,* nose], **1.** the anthropometric reference point at the front of the skull where the midsagittal plane intersects a horizontal line tangential to the highest points in the superior palpebral sulci. **2.** the depression at the root of the nose that indicates the junction of the intranasal and the frontonasal sutures.

**naso-** /nā′zō-/, **nas-,** combining form meaning 'nose': *nasociliary, nasolabial, nasonnement.*

**nasogastric** /nā′zō·gas′trik/ [L, *nasus,* nose; Gk, *gaster,* stomach], pertaining to the nose and stomach, as in (nasogastric) aspiration of the stomach's contents.

**nasogastric feeding.** See **gavage.**

**nasogastric intubation,** the placement of a nasogastric tube through the nose into the stomach to relieve gastric distension by removing gas, gastric secretions, or food; to instill medication, food, or fluids; or to obtain a specimen for laboratory analysis. After surgery and in any condition in which the person is able to digest food but not eat it, the tube may be introduced and left in place for tube feeding until the ability to eat normally is restored.

■ METHOD: A French size 12 to 18 plastic or rubber catheter is selected. The procedure is explained to the patient. Nares are assessed for any obstructions, deformations, deformities, or tissue irritation. If the catheter is rubber, it is soaked in ice water to stiffen and lubricate it. The patient is placed in an upright sitting position, and a towel or bib is placed over the chest. The necessary length of tube is marked off; it is the same as the distance from the tip of the nose to the ear lobe plus the distance to the xiphoid process. The tip of the tube may be lubricated with a water-soluble lubricating jelly, but, if a specimen is to be obtained for cytologic study, water or saline solution is preferred. The tube is grasped and held 7.5 cm from the tip and is placed in the nostril, where it is advanced forward and downward. When it has been passed 7.5 cm, it is in the pharynx. The patient is then asked to bend the neck forward, to take shallow rapid breaths, and to help advance the tube by swallowing. If the patient is able to drink water, he or she should sip some to facilitate swallowing; this also provides some lubrication. After the tube has been inserted the predetermined distance, it is checked to be sure it is in the stomach and not in the lungs. This may be done

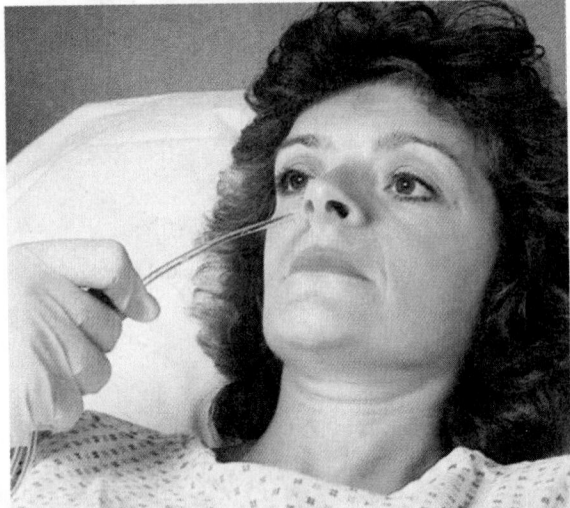

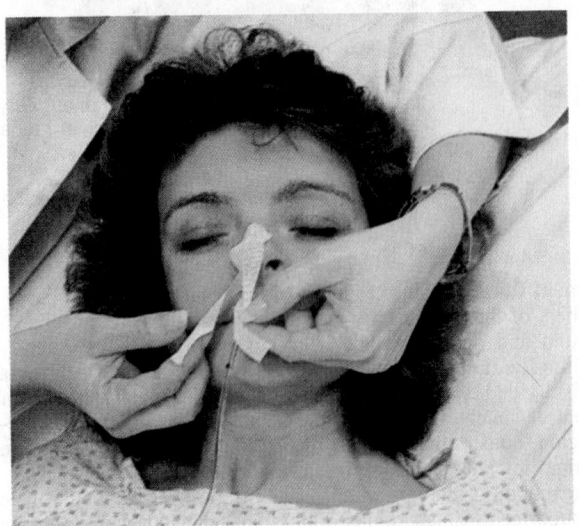

**Nasogastric intubation** (Potter and Perry, 1997)

in several ways: fluoroscopy allows visualization of the placement and is the most reliable; gastric contents may be aspirated; or air may be injected with a syringe through the tube and heard through a stethoscope as the air enters the stomach.

■ INTERVENTIONS: In many hospitals a physician inserts the tube the first time; in most hospitals, the nurse inserts it thereafter. Oral hygiene is performed regularly; and the tube, if left in place, is carefully secured with adhesive tape to the bridge of the nose. The tube is then connected to the appropriate equipment (suction, feeding tube bag, etc.) depending on the purpose for the tube and patient condition. Orders for tube feeding usually include the amount and timing of feeding, as well as the concentration and, sometimes, the ingredients of the formula. The formula is refrigerated and then warmed to room temperature. If the person is unconscious or unresponsive, suction equipment is kept at hand. An exact record of the feedings is kept.

■ OUTCOME CRITERIA: For the patient's comfort, the tube is selected to fit well and be suitable for the purpose of the procedure: a tight fit is irritating to the tissues, and a small tube might not allow the prescribed formula to pass through. Resistance, gagging, and wincing during tube insertion may be minimized by explaining the procedure, by a slow steady progress, and by proper lubrication of the tube and positioning of the patient.

**nasogastric suction,** the removal by suction of solids, fluids, or gases from the GI tract through a tube inserted into the stomach or intestines via the nasal cavity. See also **nasogastric intubation.**

**nasogastric tube,** any tube passed into the stomach through the nose. See **nasogastric intubation.**

**nasojejunal tube** /nā′zōjijōō′nəl/, a mercury-weighted tube inserted through the nose to allow natural peristaltic movement from the pylorus into the jejunum.

**nasolabial** /nā′zōlā′bē·əl/ [L, *nasus,* nose, *labium,* lip], pertaining to the nose and lip.

**nasolabial reflex** [L, *nasus,* nose, *labium,* lip], a sudden backward movement of the head, arching of the back, and extension and stretching of the limbs that occur in infants in response to a light touch to the tip of the nose with an upward sweeping motion. The reflex disappears by about 5 months of age.

**nasolacrimal** /nā′zōlak′riməl/ [L, *nasus* + *lacrima,* tear], pertaining to the nasal cavity and associated lacrimal ducts.

**nasolacrimal duct,** a channel that carries tears from the lacrimal sac to the nasal cavity.

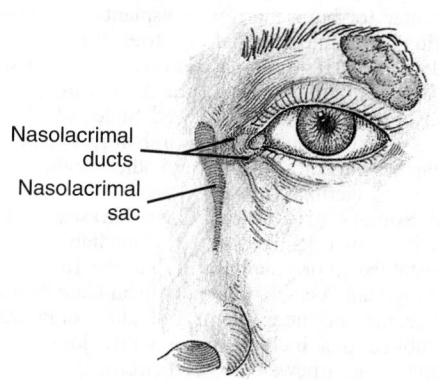

Nasolacrimal ducts

Nasolacrimal sac

**Nasolacrimal ducts** *(Potter and Perry, 2001)*

**nasolacrimal groove** [L, *nasus,* nose, *lacrima,* tear; D, *groeve,* a shallow depression], a groove on the nasal surface of the upper jaw.

**nasomandibular fixation** /nā′zōmandib′yōōlər/ [L, *nasus* + *mandere,* to chew, *figere,* to fasten], a type of maxillomandibular fixation to stabilize fractures of the jaw by using maxillomandibular splints connected to a wire through a hole drilled in the anterior nasal spine of the maxillary bone. It has been used particularly in edentulous patients. See also **maxillomandibular fixation.**

**nasomental reflex** /-men′təl/ [L, *nasus,* nose, *mentum,* chin, *reflectere,* to bend back], a reflex elicited by tapping the side of the nose, thereby causing contraction of the mentalis muscle with elevation of the lower lip and wrinkling of the skin of the chin.

**nasopharyngeal** /nā′zōferin′jē·əl/, pertaining to the cavity of the nose and the nasal parts of the pharynx. Also **rhinopharyngeal.**

**nasopharyngeal angiofibroma** [L, *nasus* + Gk, *pharynx,* throat], a benign tumor of the nasopharynx, consisting of fibrous connective tissue with many vascular spaces. The tumor usually arises in puberty and is more common in boys than in girls. Typical signs are nasal and eustachian tube obstruction, adenoidal speech, and dysphagia. Also called **juvenile angiofibroma, nasopharyngeal fibroangioma.**

**nasopharyngeal cancer,** a malignant neoplastic disease of the nasopharynx. Depending on the site of a nasopharyngeal tumor, there may be nasal obstruction, otitis media, hearing loss, sensory or motor nerve damage, bony destruction of the skull, or deep cervical lymphadenopathy. Diagnostic measures include nasopharyngoscopy, biopsy, and radiologic examination of the skull with tomographic studies. Squamous cell and undifferentiated carcinomas are the most common lesions. Nasopharyngeal cancer occurs rarely in the United States and frequently in southern China. Exposure to dusts of nickel, chromium, wood, and leather and to isopropyl oil increases the risk of developing nasopharyngeal cancer. High titers of antibodies to the Epstein-Barr virus are found in Chinese patients with the cancer, and there is evidence of genetic susceptibility, because a certain histocompatibility antigen is associated with the disease and multiple cases occur in some families. Radiation is the most effective therapy, and chemotherapy is also used.

**nasopharyngeal fibroangioma.** See **nasopharyngeal angiofibroma.**

**nasopharyngography** /-fer′ingog′rəfē/ [L, *nasus* + Gk, *pharynx,* throat, *graphein,* to record], radiographic imaging and examination of the nasopharynx.

**nasopharyngoscopy** /nā′zōfer′ing·gos′kəpē/ [L, *nasus* + Gk, *pharynx,* throat, *skopein,* to look], a technique in physical examination in which the nose and throat are visually examined using a laryngoscope, a fiberoptic device, a flashlight, and a dilator for the nares. —**nasopharyngoscopic,** *adj.*

**nasopharynx** /nā′zōfer′ingks/ [L, *nasus* + Gk, *pharynx,* throat], the uppermost of the three regions of the throat (pharynx), situated behind the nasal cavity and extending from the posterior nares to the level above the soft palate. On the posterior wall of the nasopharynx, opposite the posterior nares, are the pharyngeal tonsils. Swollen or enlarged pharyngeal tonsils can fill the space behind the posterior nares and may completely block the passage of air from the nose into the throat. Compare **laryngopharynx, oropharynx.** See also **adenoids, tonsil.** —**nasopharyngeal,** *adj.*

**nasotracheal tube** /-trā′kē·əl/ [L, *nasus* + Gk, *tracheia,* rough artery; L, *tubus*], a catheter inserted through the nasal cavity into the trachea. It is commonly attached to a mechanical ventilator or a resuscitator bag to administer oxygen.

**nat-,** prefix meaning 'birth': *natal, natality.*

**natal** /nā′təl/, **1.** [L, *natus*] pertaining to birth. **2.** [L, *nates*] pertaining to the nates, or buttocks.

**nates** /nā′tēz/, *sing.* **natis** [L, buttocks], the fleshy hillocks at the lower posterior part of the torso comprising fat and the gluteal muscles. Also called **buttocks.**

**natimortality.** See **mortinatality.**

**National Alliance for the Mentally Ill (NAMI),** a national organization for family members of psychotic patients.

**National Association for Mental Health.** See **Mental Health Association.**

**National Association for Practical Nurse Education and Services (NAPNES),** an organization concerned with the education of practical nurses and with the services provided by licensed practical nurses in the United States.

**National Association of Pediatric Nurse Associates/ Practitioners (NAP-NAP),** an organization of nurses who are prepared by education or experience to give primary care to pediatric patients in the United States. NAP-NAP works in conjunction with the American Academy of Pediatrics.

**National Bureau of Standards (NBS),** a federal agency in the Department of Commerce that sets accurate measurement standards for commerce, industry, and science in the United States. The NBS compares and coordinates its standards with those of other countries and provides research and technical service to improve computer science, materials technology, building construction, and consumer product safety. The Bureau also provides measurement services and standards for other federal agencies and state and local governments.

**National Committee for Quality Assurance (NCQA),** a U.S. independent nonprofit accrediting body for managed health care organizations. Its focus is on improving quality of care in the managed care industry by assessing compliance of health plans to NCQA-developed standards for quality improvement, utilization management, credentialing processes, member rights and responsibilities, preventive services, and record management.

**National Council Licensure Examination (NCLEX),** a comprehensive integrated examination, developed and administered by the National Council of State Boards of Nursing, designed to test basic competency for nursing practice. The NCLEX-RN test plan has three components, including nursing behaviors grouped under nursing process categories, the process of decision making that defines nursing's role, and levels of cognitive ability.

**National Eye Institute (NEI),** one of several institutes of the National Institutes of Health. NEI was established in 1968 to support research in the normal functioning of the human eye and visual system, the pathology of visual disorders, and the rehabilitation of the visually handicapped. See also **eye, vision.**

*National Formulary (NF),* a publication containing the official standards for the preparation of various pharmaceutics not listed in the *United States Pharmacopoeia.* It is revised every 5 years.

**national health insurance,** a health insurance program that is financed by taxes and administered by the government to provide comprehensive health care that is accessible to all citizens of that nation.

**National Health Planning and Resources Development Act of 1974,** U.S congressional legislation (PL 93-641) that established a nationwide network of health systems agencies. The act provides for the coordination and direction of national health policy through state and regional regulatory agencies.

**National Health Service Corps (NHSC),** a program of the U.S. Public Health Service (USPHS) in which health care personnel are placed in areas that are underserved. The Corps was established by the Emergency Health Personnel Act of 1970. Nurses, physicians, and dentists serve in rural and urban areas, usually as employees of local health care agencies. The USPHS pays most of the salary of each corps member.

**National Institute of Child Health and Human Development (NICHHD),** a branch of the National Institutes of Health that is concerned with all aspects of the growth, development, and health of the children of the United States.

**National Institute of Mental Health (NIMH),** a branch of the (U.S.) National Institutes of Health within the Alcohol, Drug Abuse, and Mental Health Administration. It is responsible for federal research and education programs dealing with mental health.

**National Institute on Aging (NIA),** a branch of the (U.S.) National Institutes of Health established in 1974. The NIA supports biomedical, social, and behavioral research and education related to aging.

**National Institutes of Health (NIH),** an agency within the U.S. Public Health Service made up of several institutions and constituent divisions, including the Bureau of Health Manpower Education, the National Library of Medicine, the National Cancer Institute, and several research institutes and divisions.

**National League for Nursing (NLN),** an organization concerned with the improvement of nursing education and nursing service and the provision of health care in the United States. Among its many activities are preadmission and achievement tests for nursing students and compilation of statistical data on nursing personnel and trends in health care delivery. The National League for Nursing Accrediting Commission (NLNAC), an entity of the NLN that is administratively and financially independent of the NLN, has the sole authority and responsibility for accreditation of nursing education schools and programs. It acts as the testing service for the State Board Test Pool Examinations for registered and practical nurse licensure. The Research Division and the Public Affairs Office are among the other sections of NLN. A monthly refereed journal, *Nursing and Health Care,* is the official publication of the organization.

**National Male Nurses Association (NMNA),** an organization that promotes the interests and practice of male nurses in the United States.

**National Marrow Donor Program (NMDP),** a coordinating center for bone marrow transplants, providing links with national and international registries of prospective volunteer donors of HLA-compatible bone marrow tissue.

**National Organization of Victims Assistance,** a private nonprofit organization in the United States of victims and witness assistance practitioners, criminal justice professionals, researchers, former victims, and others committed to the recognition of victims' rights.

**National Society of Critical Care Nurses of Canada (NSCCN),** an organization of Canadian critical care nurses, established originally in 1975 as the Toronto Chapter of the American Association of Critical-Care Nurses. The group became an independent Canadian organization in 1983. Publications include a bimonthly journal, *Critical Care Nurse,* and a newsletter, *CriticaList.*

**National Student Nurses Association (NSNA),** an organization of students in the field of nursing in the United

States. Among its purposes are the improvement of nursing education to improve health care, aid in the development of the nursing student, and encourage optimal achievement in the professional role of the nurse and the health care of people. It publishes a journal, *Imprint,* five times a year, participates in legislative activities at all levels, and gives scholarships, awards, and career workshops.

**natis.** See **nates.**

**natremia** /nātrē′mē·ə/ [L, *natrium,* sodium; Gk, *haima,* blood], the presence of sodium in the blood.

**natriuresis** /nā′trēyŏŏrē′sis/ [L, *natrium,* sodium; Gk, *ouresis,* urination], the excretion of greater than normal amounts of sodium in the urine. The condition may result from the administration of natriuretic diuretic drugs or from various metabolic or endocrine disorders.

**natriuretic** /nā′trēyŏŏret′ik/, **1.** pertaining to the process of natriuresis. **2.** a substance that inhibits the resorption of sodium ions from the glomerular filtrate in the kidneys, thus allowing more sodium to be excreted with the urine.

**natural antibody** /nach′(ə)rəl/ [L, *natura,* nature; Gk, *anti* + AS, *bodig,* body], an antibody that is present in serum in the absence of an apparent specific antigen contact.

**natural childbirth** [L, *natura,* nature; AS, *cild,* child; ME, *bwith,* birth], labor and parturition accomplished by a mother with little or no medical intervention. It is generally considered the optimal way of giving birth and being born, safest for the baby and most satisfying for the mother. Prerequisites include normal gestation, an adequate birth canal, strong maternal motivation, physical and emotional preparation, and constant and intensive support of the mother during labor and birth. See also **Lamaze method.**

**natural dentition,** the entire array of natural teeth in the dental arches at any given time, consisting of deciduous or secondary dentitions or a mixture of the two. See also **tooth.**

**natural family planning method,** any of several methods of conception control that do not rely on a medication or a physical device for effectiveness in avoiding pregnancy. Some of the methods are also used to pinpoint the time of ovulation to increase the chance of fertilization when artificial insemination or extraction of an oocyte for in vitro fertilization is to be performed. Kinds of natural family planning include **basal body temperature method of family planning, calendar method of family planning, ovulation method of family planning,** and **symptothermal method of family planning.**

**natural foods,** foods that have been grown, processed, packaged, and stored without the use of chemical additives.

**natural immunity,** a usually inherent, nonspecific form of immunity to a specific disease. Kinds of natural immunity include **individual immunity, racial immunity,** and **species immunity.** Also called **genetic immunity, innate immunity.** Compare **acquired immunity.**

**naturalistic illness** /nach′ərəlis′tik/, an illness thought to be caused by impersonal factors such as a disturbance in the Asian yin and yang equilibrium or the Hispanic model of hot and cold forces.

**natural killer (NK) cell** [L, *natura* + ME, *kullen,* to kill, *cella,* storeroom], a lymphocyte that is capable of binding to and killing virus-infected cells and some tumor cells by releasing cytotoxins. It is found in the bone marrow and spleen. Its cytotoxic activity is not antibody-dependent but is augmented by interferon. Compare **killer cell, killer T cell.** See also **null cell.**

**natural law,** a doctrine that holds there is a natural moral order or natural moral law inherent in the structure of the universe.

**naturally acquired immunity.** See **acquired immunity.**

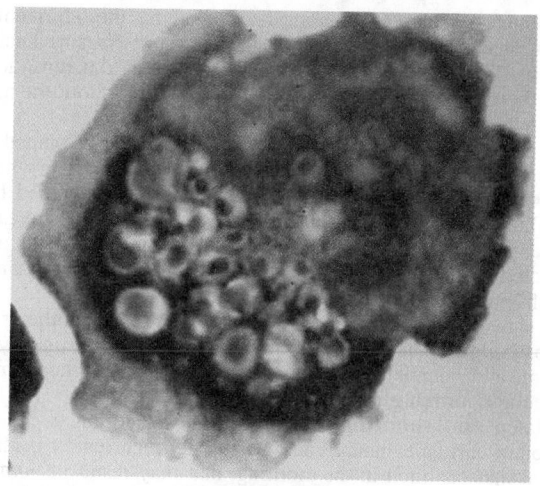

**Natural killer cell**
*(Cotran, Kumar, and Collins, 1999/courtesy Dr. Noelle Williams, Department of Pathology, University of Texas Southwestern Medical School, Dallas)*

**natural network,** (in psychiatric nursing) a patient's natural contacts in the community, including church and social groups, friends, family, and occupation that support the person's function outside the institutional environment.

**natural pacemaker,** any cardiac pacing site in the heart tissues, as opposed to an artificial pacemaker.

**natural radiation,** radioactivity that emanates from the soil, from groundwater, or from cosmic sources. Cosmic radiation includes actinic radiation from the sun and neutrinos from beyond the solar system.

**natural selection,** the natural evolutionary processes by which the organisms that are best adapted to an environment tend to survive and propagate, whereas those that are unfit are less likely to do so. Compare **artificial selection.**

**Naturetin,** trademark for a diuretic and antihypertensive (bendroflumethiazide).

**nature versus nurture** /nur′chər/, a name given to a long-standing controversy as to the relative influences of genetics versus the environment in the development of personality. Nature is represented by instincts, and genetic factors and nurture by social influences.

**naturopath** /nach′ərōpath′/ a person who practices naturopathy.

**naturopathy** /nach′ərop′əthē/ [L, *natura* + Gk, *pathos,* disease], a system of therapeutics based on natural foods, light, warmth, massage, fresh air, regular exercise, and the avoidance of medications. Advocates believe that illness can be healed by the natural processes of the body.

**Nauheim bath** /nou′hīm/ [Nauheim, Germany; AS, *baeth,* bath], a bath taken in water through which carbon dioxide is bubbled, followed by systematic exercises, used in the treatment of cardiac conditions. The procedure is named after the natural waters of Bad Nauheim, Germany. Also called **Nauheim treatment.**

**nausea**[1] /nô′zē·ə, nô′zhə/ [Gk, *nausia,* seasickness], a sensation accompanying the urge but not always leading to vomiting. Common causes are seasickness and other motion sicknesses, early pregnancy, intense pain, emotional stress, gallbladder disease, food poisoning, and various enteroviruses. —**nauseate,** *v.,* **nauseous,** *adj.*

**nausea²,** a nursing diagnosis accepted by the Thirteenth National Conference on the Classification of Nursing Diagnoses. The condition is an unpleasant, wave-like sensation in the back of the throat, epigastrium, or throughout the abdomen that may or may not lead to vomiting.

■ DEFINING CHARACTERISTICS: The sensation usually precedes vomiting, but may be experienced after vomiting or when vomiting does not occur. It is sometimes accompanied by pallor, cold and clammy skin, increased salivation, tachycardia, gastric stasis, diarrhea, and swallowing movements affected by the skeletal muscles. "Nausea" and "sick to stomach" may be reported.

■ RELATED FACTORS: Related factors include chemotherapy, post-surgical anesthesia, irritation to the gastrointestinal system, and stimulation of neuropharmacologic mechanisims. See also **nursing diagnosis.**

**nausea and vomiting of pregnancy,** a common condition of early pregnancy, characterized by recurrent or persistent nausea, often in the morning, that may result in vomiting, weight loss, anorexia, general weakness, and malaise. The causes of the condition are poorly understood. It usually does not begin before the sixth week after the last menstrual period and ends by the twelfth to the fourteenth week of pregnancy. Symptomatic relief is often obtained by eating small, easily digested meals frequently and by not allowing the stomach to be empty. In the past, antiemetic drugs were routinely prescribed for this complaint, but this practice is currently reserved for severe cases. Nausea and vomiting after the sixteenth week is an unusual complication of pregnancy, called persistent nausea and vomiting of pregnancy. If it is severe and intractable, hyperemesis gravidarum may ensue. Also called (nontechnical) **morning sickness.**

**nausea management,** a nursing intervention from the Nursing Interventions Classification (NIC) defined as prevention and alleviation of nausea. See also **Nursing Interventions Classification.**

**nauseate.** See **nausea.**

**nauseous** /nô'shəs, nô'zē·əs/ [Gk, *nausia,* seasickness], pertaining to feelings of nausea or reaction to things that may stimulate nausea.

**Navane,** trademark for a tranquilizer (thiothixene).

**navel.** See **umbilicus.**

**Navelbine,** trademark for a chemotherapeutic mitotic inhibitor (vinorelbine).

**navicular** /navik'yələr/, boat-shaped; sunken.

**navicular bone.** See **scaphoid bone.**

**navicular pads,** tarsal supports for flat feet. They are inserted directly under the arch of the foot. Also called **shoe cookies.**

**Nb,** symbol for the element **niobium.**

**n.b.,** abbreviation for the Latin *nota bene,* 'note well.'

**NBCOT,** abbreviation for *National Board for Certification in Occupational Therapy.*

**NBNA,** abbreviation for *National Black Nurses Association.*

**NBRC,** abbreviation for *National Board for Respiratory Care.*

**NBS standard,** a radioactive source standardized or certified or both by the National Bureau of Standards.

**nc, nCi,** abbreviation for **nanocurie.**

**NCI,** abbreviation for the *National Cancer Institute.* See **National Institutes of Health.**

**NCLEX-RN,** abbreviation for **National Council Licensure Examination.**

**NCQA,** abbreviation for **National Committee for Quality Assurance.**

**Nd,** symbol for the element **neodymium.**

**N.D.,** abbreviation for *Doctor of Naturopathy.*

**NDA,** abbreviation for *National Dental Association.*

**Ne,** symbol for the element **neon.**

**ne-.** See **neo-.**

**NE,** abbreviation for **niacin equivalent.**

**Neal-Robertson litter,** a modified spine board for transporting trauma patients with spinal injuries.

**near-death experience** [ME, *nere + deth* + L, *experientia,* trial], the subjective observations of people either who have been close to clinical death or who may have recovered after having been declared dead. Many claim to have witnessed similar episodes of passing through a tunnel toward a bright light and encountering people who had preceded them in death. See also **out-of-body experience.**

**near drowning** [ME, *nere,* almost, *drounen,* to drown], a pathologic state in which the victim has survived exposure to circumstances that usually cause drowning. Cardiopulmonary resuscitation is performed immediately if the patient is without pulse and/or respiration; hospitalization is always indicated. The return of consciousness does not necessarily ensure recovery. Intensive supportive therapy may be required for up to several days. Compare **drowning.** See also **hypothermia.**

**nearest neighbor analysis,** a biochemical method used to estimate the frequency with which specific pairs of bases are located next to one another.

**near field.** See **Fresnel zone.**

**nearsightedness.** See **myopia.**

**nebula** /neb'yələ/, *pl.* **nebulae** [L, cloud], **1.** a slight corneal opacity or scar that seldom obstructs vision and that can be seen only by oblique illumination. **2.** a murkiness in the urine. **3.** an oily concoction that is applied with an atomizer.

**nebulization** /neb'yəlīzā'shən/ [L, *nebula,* cloud; Gk, *izein,* to cause], a method of administering a drug by spraying it into the respiratory passages of the patient. The medication may be given with or without oxygen to help carry it into the lungs.

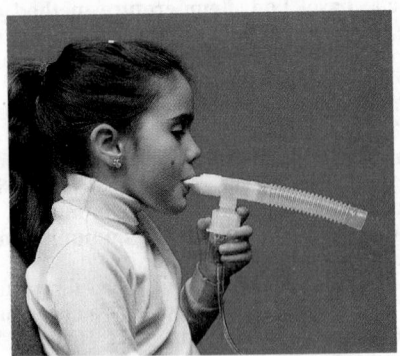

**Nebulization** *(Sanders et al, 2000)*

**nebulize** /neb'yəlīz/, to vaporize or disperse a liquid in a fine spray.

**nebulizer** /neb'yəlī'zər/, a device for producing a fine spray. Intranasal medications are often administered by a nebulizer. Also called **atomizer.**

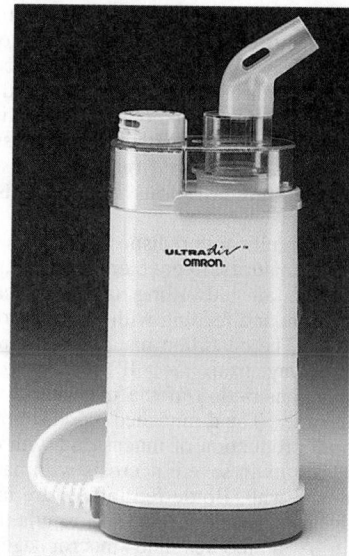

**Nebulizer**
*(Monahan and Neighbors, 1998/courtesy Omron Healthcare, Inc,
Vernon Hills, Ill)*

**NEC,** abbreviation for **necrotizing enterocolitis.**

*Necator* /nekā'tər/ [L, *necare*, to kill], a genus of nematode that is an intestinal parasite and causes hookworm disease. See also *Ancylostoma.*

**necatoriasis** /nek'ətərī'əsis/ [L, *necare*, to kill; Gk, *osis*, condition], hookworm disease, specifically that caused by *Necator americanus*, the most common North American hookworm. An estimated one third of the world's population is infected with *N. americanus*. The larvae live in the soil and reach the human digestive tract through contaminated food and water or through the skin of the feet and legs, attach to mucosa in the small bowel, and suck blood from the human host. Most infections are asymptomatic. Symptoms include diarrhea, nausea, abdominal pain, and hypochrome microcyte iron deficiency anemia in the more severe cases. Treatment consists of first correcting the anemia if present and then anthelmintic therapy, usually with pyrantel pamoate or mebendazole. Prevention includes improved sanitation for disposal of human waste to eliminate soil contamination and the avoidance of skin contact with the soil. See also **ancylostomiasis, ground itch, hookworm.**

**neck** [AS, *hnecca*], a constricted section, such as the part of the body that connects the head with the trunk. Other such constrictions are the neck of the humerus and the neck of the uterus.

**neck dissection,** surgical removal of the cervical lymph nodes, performed to prevent the spread of malignant tumors of the head and neck. With the patient under general anesthesia, the cervical chain of lymph nodes with their lymphatic channels is removed in one mass to prevent the spread of cancer cells. After surgery the patient is observed closely for signs of hemorrhage and difficulty in breathing. Compare **radical neck dissection.**

**neck of femur** [AS, *hnecca* + L, *femur*, thigh], the part of the long bone of the thigh between the head and the greater and lesser trochanters.

**neck of uterus.** See **cervix.**

**neck righting reflex,** 1. an involuntary response in newborns in which turning the head to one side while the infant is supine causes rotation of the shoulders and trunk in the same direction. The reflex enables the child to roll over from the supine to prone position. Absence of the reflex or persistence beyond about 10 months of age may indicate central nervous system damage. 2. any tonic reflex associated with the neck that maintains body orientation in relation to the head.

**neck ring,** a metal ring at the neck of a cervicothoracolumbosacral orthosis. It opens posteriorly for ease in putting on or removing the orthosis and is an attachment for a throat mold and occiput pads.

**neck shaft angle,** an angle created by the intersection of a line through the femoral shaft and a line through the femoral head and neck. Also called **femoral angle.**

**neck sign.** See **Brudzinski's sign.**

**necro-,** combining form meaning 'death or corpse': *necronectomy, necrophilia, necrosis, necrotic.*

**necrobiosis** /nek'rōbī·ō'sis/, 1. the death of a small area of cells in a large area of living tissue. 2. the normal death of tissue cells as a result of changes associated with development, aging, atrophy, or degeneration. —**necrobiotic,** *adj.*

**necrobiosis lipoidica** /lipoi'dikə/ [Gk, *nekros*, dead, *bios*, life, *lipos*, fat, *eidos*, form], a skin disease characterized by thin, shiny, yellow-to-red plaques on the shins or forearms. Telangiectases, crusting, and ulceration of these plaques may occur. Necrobiosis lipoidica is usually associated with diabetes mellitus and occurs most often in women. Treatment includes precise control of the diabetes and, possibly, intralesional application of corticosteroids.

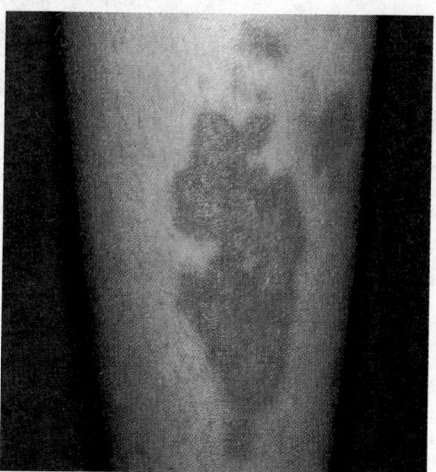

**Necrobiosis lipoidica** *(Weston, Lane, and Morrelli, 1996)*

**necrobiotic** /-bī·ot'ik/, pertaining to necrobiosis.

**necrobiotic granulomas,** granulomas that share some of the characteristics of both immunologic and nonimmunologic collections of mononuclear phagocytes. Relatively acellular areas of the skin become necrobiotic, and the collagen assumes a homogenous, amorphous appearance. See also **granuloma annulare, necrobiosis lipoidica.**

**necrogenic** /nek'rōjen'ik/ [Gk, *nekros,* dead, *genein,* to produce], **1.** capable of causing death, as of cells or tissue. **2.** originating or caused by infected dead matter. Also **necrogenous** /nekroj'ənəs/

**necrology (necrol)** /nekrol'əjē/ [Gk, *nekros,* dead, *logos,* science], the study of the causes of death, including the compilation and interpretation of mortality statistics.

**necrolysis** /nekrol'isis/ [Gk, *nekros* + *lysis,* loosening], disintegration or exfoliation of dead tissue. Compare **necrosis.** —**necrolytic,** *adj.*

**necrophilia** /nek'rōfil'yə/ [Gk, *nekros* + *philein,* to love], **1.** a morbid liking for being with dead bodies. **2.** a morbid desire to have sexual contact with a dead body, usually of men to perform a sexual act with a dead woman. —**necrophile, necrophiliac,** *n.*

**necrophobia** [Gk, *nekros,* death, *phobos,* fear], a morbid fear of death and dead bodies.

**necropsy, necroscopy.** See **autopsy.**

**necrosis** /nekrō'sis/ [Gk, *nekros* + *osis,* condition], localized tissue death that occurs in groups of cells in response to disease or injury. In **coagulation necrosis,** blood clots block the flow of blood, causing tissue ischemia distal to the clot; in **gangrenous necrosis,** ischemia combined with bacterial action causes putrefaction to set in. See also **gangrene.**

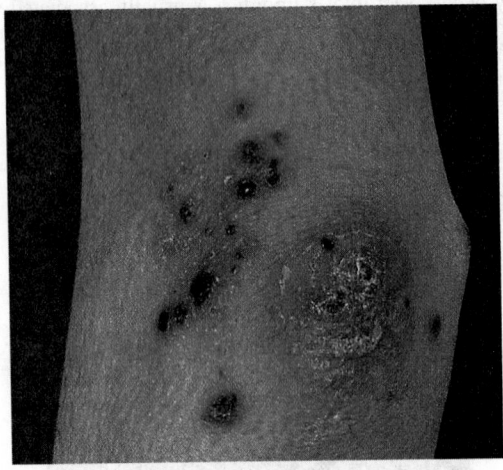

**Tissue necrosis** *(du Vivier, 1993)*

**necrotaxis** /nek'rōtak'sis/, the attraction of leukocytes to dead or dying cells.

**necrotic** /nekrot'ik/, pertaining to the death of tissue in response to disease or injury.

**necrotic arachnidism,** tissue destruction caused by spider venom. See also **spider bite.**

**necrotizing** /nek'rōtī'zing/ [Gk, *nekros,* death], causing the death of tissues or organisms.

**necrotizing angiitis.** See **periarteritis nodosa.**

**necrotizing enteritis** [Gk, *nekros* + *izein,* to cause, *enteron,* intestine, *itis*], acute inflammation of the small and large intestine by the bacterium *Clostridium perfringens,* characterized by severe abdominal pain, bloody diarrhea, and vomiting. Some people recover completely; some survive with chronic bowel obstruction; and some die of perforation of the intestine, dehydration, peritonitis, or septicemia.

**necrotizing enterocolitis (NEC),** an acute inflammatory bowel disorder that occurs primarily in preterm or low–birth weight neonates. It is characterized by ischemic necrosis of the GI mucosa that may lead to perforation and peritonitis. The cause of the disorder is unknown, although it appears to be a defect in host defenses with infection resulting from normal GI flora rather than from invading organisms. Also called **pseudomembranous enterocolitis.** See also **enteritis.**

■ OBSERVATIONS: Significant predisposing factors for the condition include prematurity, hypovolemia, respiratory distress syndrome, sepsis, an indwelling umbilical catheter, exchange transfusion, and feeding with hyperosmolar or high-caloric formulas. The condition results from a reflex shunting of blood away from the GI tract, which leads to convulsive vasoconstriction of the mesenteric vessels supplying the intestines. The diminished blood supply interferes with the normal production of mucus and with other bowel functions and results in severe necrosis with bacterial invasion of the bowel wall. Bottle-fed infants are more susceptible to the disorder, possibly because formula lacks the immunoglobulin A antibodies and macrophages found in breast milk that may protect the GI mucosa from damage and bacterial invasion. Initial symptoms, which usually develop after several days of life, include temperature instability (usually hypothermia), lethargy, poor feeding, vomiting of bile, abdominal distension, blood in the stools, and decreased or absent bowel sounds. Signs of deterioration are apnea, pallor, hyperbilirubinemia, oliguria, abdominal tenderness, and erythema and edema of the anterior abdominal wall or palpable masses, with eventual respiratory failure leading to death. Diagnosis is confirmed by x-ray visualization of the intestine or by the presence of increased peritoneal fluid or pneumoperitoneum.

■ INTERVENTIONS: Treatment includes discontinuing oral feeding, beginning IV infusion, abdominal decompression by nasogastric suction, hydration, plasma or whole blood transfusion, and administration of broad-spectrum antibiotics (usually ampicillin, gentamicin, or kanamycin). With routine supportive management, improvement usually occurs within 48 to 72 hours. Oral feedings usually are not resumed for 10 days to 2 weeks. Total parenteral nutrition is necessary during that period. Surgical resection of the affected bowel segment may be necessary, especially if signs of intestinal perforation or peritonitis develop. If a large part of bowel is affected, an ileostomy or colostomy may be necessary. Stenosis of the involved bowel segment may present later complications.

■ NURSING CONSIDERATIONS: The primary concern of the nurse is to observe high-risk, formula-fed infants for early symptoms of necrotizing enterocolitis, especially for difficulty in feeding, bile-stained regurgitation, bloody stools, temperature fluctuations, or a distended shiny abdomen. After the diagnosis is confirmed, the nurse initiates nasogastric intubation for abdominal decompression and continues to monitor the baby constantly for dehydration and electrolyte balance. Daily weight is taken. Infants who are unable to take fluids by mouth require special oral care. A pacifier helps to meet the infant's need to suck. Parents are encouraged to visit and are helped to meet the emotional needs of the infant and to provide tactile, auditory, and visual stimulation. The nurse explains the usual course of the disease and the medical and nursing procedures and keeps the parents informed of the infant's progress. Frequent visits to the care unit facilitate family-infant relationships and provide the nurse with an opportunity to teach proper care techniques before discharge.

**necrotizing vasculitis,** an inflammatory condition of blood vessels, characterized by necrosis, fibrosis, and proliferation of the inner layer of the vascular wall. Some cases result in occlusion and infarction. Necrotizing vasculitis may occur in rheumatoid arthritis and is common in systemic lupus erythematosus, periarteritis nodosa, and progressive systemic sclerosis. The condition is usually treated with corticosteroids.

**needle bath** [AS, *naedl,* needle], a shower in which fine jets of water are sprayed over the body.

**needle biopsy,** the removal of a segment of living tissue for microscopic examination by inserting a hollow needle through the skin or the external surface of an organ or tumor and rotating it within the underlying cellular layers. See also **aspiration biopsy.**

**needle filter,** a device, usually made of plastic, used for filtering medications that are drawn into a syringe before administration. Some syringe needles have built-in filters; other filters are separate units that are attached to the needle before use. Needle filters are commonly disposable items designed for one-time use.

**needle holder,** a surgical forceps used to hold and pass a suturing needle through tissue. Also called **suture forceps.**

**needlestick injuries,** accidental skin punctures resulting from contact with hypodermic syringe needles, IV cannula stylets, needles used to "piggyback" IV infusions, and needles used for drawing blood or administering parenteral injections. The contact may occur accidentally during efforts to inject a patient or as a result of carelessly touching discarded medical waste. Such injuries can be dangerous, particularly if the needle has been used in treatment of a patient with a severe blood-borne infection, such as human immunodeficiency virus. To prevent injuries, used needles are not capped or broken and are disposed of in a rigid puncture-resistant container located near the site of use.

**NEEP,** abbreviation for **negative end-expiratory pressure.**

**Neer and Horowitz classification system,** a method of classifying proximal humeral fractures in children based on the degree of separation of the epiphysis from the shaft.

**Neer classification system,** a method of classifying femoral supracondylar and intercondylar fractures. The system ranges from *type I* for minimal displacement to *type III* for conjoined supracondylar and shaft fractures. The Neer system is also applied to humeral head and neck fractures.

**nefazodone hydrochloride,** an antidepressant drug.

■ INDICATIONS: It is prescribed in the treatment of mental depression in adults.

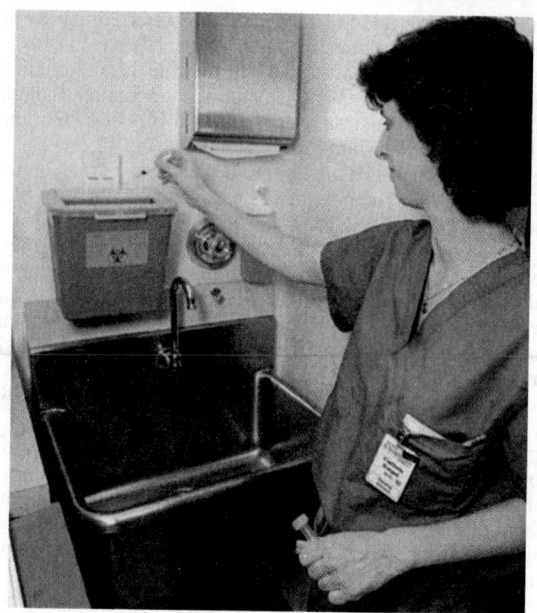

**Prevention of needlestick injuries** *(Wong, 2001)*

■ CONTRAINDICATIONS: The drug should not be given to patients with an allergy to nefazodone hydrochloride or to similar antidepressants or to patients also using monoamine oxidase inhibitors, terfenadine, or astemizole. Caution is advised in prescribing the drug for patients with a history of drug abuse, blood vessel disease, low blood pressure, or seizures.

■ ADVERSE EFFECTS: The side effects most often reported include dry mouth, impaired vision, eye pain, flulike symptoms, ringing in the ears, swollen limbs, and muscle pain.

**negative (neg)** /neg'ətiv/ [L, *negare,* to deny], **1.** (of a laboratory test) indicating that a substance or a reaction is not present. **2.** (of a sign) indicating on physical examination that a finding is not present, often meaning that there is no pathologic change. **3.** (of a substance) tending to carry or carrying a negative chemical charge.

**negative adaptation.** See **habituation.**

**negative anxiety,** (in psychology) an emotional and psychologic condition in which anxiety prevents a person's nor-

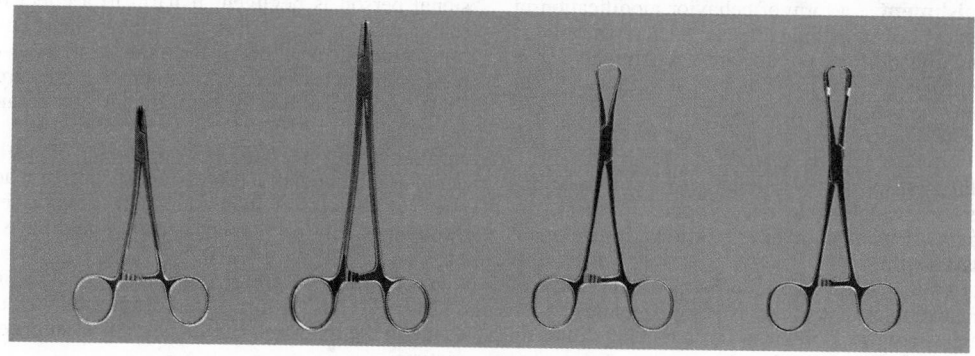

**Needle holders** *(Tighe, 1999)*

mal functioning and interrupts the person's ability to perform the usual activities of daily living.

**negative catalysis,** a decrease in the rate of any chemical reaction caused by a substance that is not consumed and not affected by the reaction. Also called **inhibition.** Compare **catalysis.** See also **catalyst.**

**negative electrode** [L, *negare,* to deny; Gk, *elektron,* amber, *hodos,* way], a cathode, or the negative pole of an electric current or of a battery or dry cell.

**negative end-expiratory pressure (NEEP),** the application of subatmospheric pressure to a patient's airway on exhalation during mechanical ventilation. The technique counterbalances the increase in mean intrathoracic pressure caused by intermittent positive-pressure breathing and is intended to reduce intrathoracic pressure for venous return to the right atrium. Generally the negative pressure is applied by using a jet or Venturi system.

**negative feedback,** **1.** (in physiology) a decrease in function in response to a stimulus; for example, the secretion of follicle-stimulating hormone decreases even as the amount of circulating estrogen increases. **2.** *informal.* a critical, derogatory, or otherwise negative response from one person to what another person has communicated.

**negative identity,** the assumption of a persona that is at odds with the accepted values and expectations of society.

**negative pathognomonic symptom** /pəthog′nəmon′ik/ [L, *negare,* to deny; Gk, *pathos,* disease, *gnomen,* index, *symptoma,* that which happens], any symptom that is not usually found in a specific condition and that, if present, would not be compatible with the diagnosis.

**negative pi meson (pion),** a form of electromagnetic radiation emitted from a proton linear accelerator.

**negative pi meson (pion) radiotherapy,** a form of radiotherapy using a beam of subatomic particles known as negative pi mesons, or pions, emitted by a proton linear accelerator. When the particles are beamed at a tumor, they cause the atomic nuclei of malignant cells to explode and scatter intensely radioactive subatomic particles through the tumor. Pion radiotherapy requires fewer rad and has a 60% greater biologic effect than conventional x-radiation techniques. It also may have less effect on normal tissue near the tumor. Some locally advanced neoplasms, especially those of the prostate, are destroyed. Gliomas and advanced cancers of the head and neck also may be well controlled with pion radiotherapy. Moderate acute toxicity occurs with treatment, but chronic toxicity is minimal.

**negative pressure,** a pressure less than ambient atmospheric pressure, as in a vacuum, at an altitude above sea level, or in a hypobaric chamber. Negative pressure may be used to help stimulate or cycle exhalation in intermittent positive-pressure breathing.

**negative punishment,** a form of behavior modification in which the removal of something after an operant (behavior) decreases the probability of the operant's recurrence.

**negative reinforcer,** (in psychology) a stimulus that, when presented immediately after occurrence of a particular behavior, will decrease the rate of occurrence of the behavior.

**negative relationship,** (in research) an inverse relationship between two variables; as one variable increases, the other decreases. Also called **inverse relationship.** Compare **positive relationship.**

**negative sequence,** the sequence of bases on the strand of a double-stranded nucleic acid that is complementary to the positive-sense strand; in DNA it is the template strand on which the mRNA is synthesized.

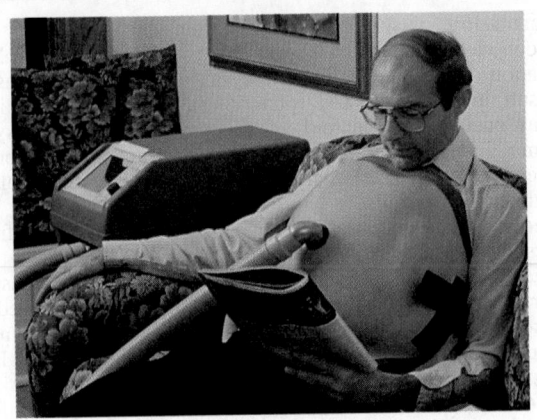

**Negative-pressure ventilator**
*(Beare and Myers, 1998/courtesy Respironics, Murrayville, Pennsylvania)*

**negative staining,** a technique in which an electron-dense substance is mixed with a specimen, resulting in an electron microscopic image in which the specimen appears translucent against an opaque or dark background.

**negativism** /neg′ətiviz′əm/ [L, *negare,* to deny], a behavioral attitude characterized by opposition, resistance, the refusal to cooperate with even the most reasonable request, and the tendency to act in a contrary manner. The resulting response may be passive such as the immobile, rigid postures observed in catatonic schizophrenia or active such as in a belligerent, impulsive, or capricious act, such as lowering the arms when asked to raise them or sitting down when asked to stand.

**negatron** /neg′ətron/, an electron or beta particle with a single negative charge.

**NegGram,** trademark for an antibacterial (nalidixic acid).

**neglect** /nəglekt′/, a condition that occurs when a parent or guardian fails to provide minimal physical and emotional care for a child or other dependent person.

**neglect recovery,** a nursing outcome from the Nursing Outcomes Classification (NOC) defined as the healing following the cessation of substandard care. See also **Nursing Outcomes Classification.**

**negligence** /neg′lijens/ [L, *negligentia,* carelessness], (in law) the commission of an act that a prudent person would not have done or the omission of a duty that a prudent person would have fulfilled, resulting in injury or harm to another person. In particular, in a malpractice suit, a professional person is negligent if harm to a client results from such an act or such failure to act, but it must be proved that other prudent members of the same profession would ordinarily have acted differently under the same circumstances. Thus negligence may be misfeasance, malfeasance, or nonfeasance.

**negligence per se,** (in law) a finding of negligence rendered in judgment of a professional action or inaction in violation of a statute or so at odds with common sense that beyond any doubt no prudent person would have been guilty of it.

**Negri bodies** /nā′grē/ [Adelchi Negri, Italian physician, 1876–1912; AS, *bodig*], intracytoplasmic inclusion bodies found in the brain and central nervous system cells of rabies victims.

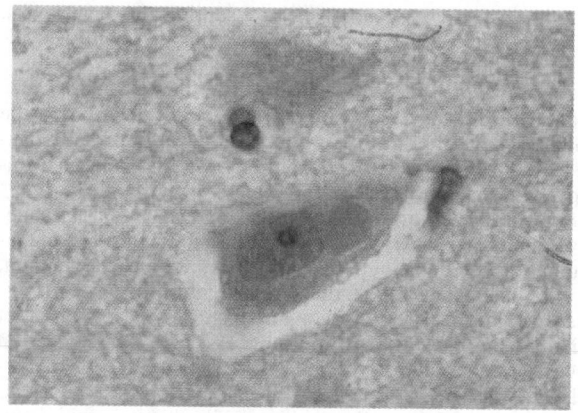

**Negri bodies** *(Murray et al, 1998)*

**NEI,** abbreviation for **National Eye Institute.**

*Neisseria* /nīser′ē·ə/ [Albert L. S. Neisser, Polish dermatologist, 1855–1916], a genus of aerobic to facultatively anaerobic bacteria of the family Neisseriaceae. The gramnegative cocci, which appear in pairs with adjacent sides flattened, are among the normal flora of genitourinary and upper respiratory tracts. Pathogenic species include gonococcus and meningococcus forms.

*Neisseria catarrhalis.* See *Moraxella catarrhalis.*

*Neisseriaceae* /nī′serē·ā′si·ē/ [Albert L. S. Neisser], a family of four genera of gram-negative aerobic cocci and rodshaped bacteria occurring singly or in pairs, chains, or clusters. They are saprophytic or parasitic. The genera are *Actinobacter, Kingella, Moraxella,* and *Neisseria.*

*Neisseria gonorrhoeae* [Albert L. S. Neisser; Gk, *gone,* seed, *rhoia,* flow], a gram-negative, nonmotile diplococcal bacterium usually seen microscopically as flattened pairs within the cytoplasm of neutrophils. It is the causative organism of gonorrhea. Also called **gonococcus.**

*Neisseria meningitidis.* See **meningococcus.**

*Neisseria sicca* [Albert L. S. Neisser], a species of dry or slimy white-to-yellow bacteria normally found in the human nasopharynx and in saliva and sputum.

*NEJM,* abbreviation for *New England Journal of Medicine.*

**Nélaton's dislocation** /nālätôNz′/ [Auguste Nélaton, French surgeon, 1807–1873], a dislocation of the ankle in which the distal ends of the tibia and fibula are separated and the talus is forced upward between the tibia and fibula.

**nelfinavir,** an antiviral.
- INDICATIONS: Nelfinavir is used to treat HIV, alone or in combination with other drugs.
- CONTRAINDICATIONS: Known hypersensitivity to protease inhibitors prohibits the use of this drug.
- ADVERSE EFFECTS: Life-threatening effects of nelfinavir include anemia, leukopenia, thrombocytopenia, and hemoglobin abnormalities. Other adverse effects include anorexia, dyspepsia, headache, asthenia, poor concentration, dermatitis, pain, bleeding, hypoglycemia, and hyperlipidemia. Common side effects include diarrhea, flatulence, and rash.

**Nelson's syndrome** [Donald H. Nelson, American physician, b. 1925], a pituitary adenoma that may follow bilateral adrenalectomy for Cushing's syndrome. It is characterized by a marked increase in the secretion of adrenocorticotropic hormone and melanocyte-stimulating hormone by the pituitary gland. Treatment includes irradiation to decrease pituitary function and in some cases hypophysectomy. See also **Cushing's disease.**

**nem,** abbreviation for **Nahrungs-Einheit-Milch.**

**nema-,** prefix meaning 'thread': *nematode, nematocide.*

**-nema,** suffix meaning a 'threadlike stage in the development of chromosomes': *chromonema, plasmonema, uronema.*

**nemaline myopathy** /nem′ə·lēn/ [Gk, *nēma,* thread], a nonprogressive myopathy of uncertain inheritance, characterized histologically by abnormal threadlike structures in muscle cells and clinically by hypotonia with diffuse weakness of the limbs and trunk, usually beginning in infancy.

**nemato-,** combining form meaning 'nematode or threadlike structure': *nematoblast, nematocide, nematodiasis.*

**nematocides** /nəmat′əsīdz/ [Gk, *nema,* thread, *eidos,* form; L, *caedere,* to kill], chemical pesticides that are used to kill nematode worms.

**nematocyst** /nem′ətōsist′/ [Gk, *nema,* thread, *eidos,* form, *kystis,* bag], a capsule containing a barbed, threadlike process found in certain cells on the external surface of cnidarians, such as the Portuguese man-of-war and jellyfish. In some cnidarians, the nematocysts can penetrate the skin and inject a poison, causing painful and potentially fatal injury.

**nematode** /nem′ətōd/ [Gk, *nema* + *eidos,* form], a multicellular, parasitic animal of the phylum Nematoda. All roundworms belong to the phylum, including *Ancylostoma duodenale, Ascaris lumbricoides, Enterobius vermicularis, Necator americanus, Strongyloides stercoralis,* and several other species.

**nematodiasis** /nem′ətōdī′əsis/ [Gk, *nema,* thread, *eidos,* form, *osis,* condition], an infestation of nematode worms.

**Nembutal,** trademark for a barbiturate (pentobarbital).

**-nemia.** suffix meaning 'blood.' See **-anemia.**

**neo-** /nē′ō-/, prefix meaning 'new': *neobiogenesis, neocyte, neonatal.*

**neoadjuvant therapy** /nē′ō·ad′jəvənt/, a preliminary cancer treatment, such as chemotherapy or radiation, that usually precedes another phase of treatment.

**neoantigen** /-an′tijən/ [Gk, *neos,* new, *anti,* against, *genein,* to produce], a new specific antigen that develops in a tumor cell.

**neobehaviorism** /-bihā′vē·əriz′əm/ [Gk, *neos* + ME, *behaven,* behavior], a school of psychology based on the general principles of behaviorism but broader and more flexible in concept. It stresses experimental research and laboratory analyses in the study of overt behavior and in various subjective phenomena that cannot be directly observed and measured, such as fantasies, love, stress, empathy, trust, and personality. See also **behaviorism.**

**neobehaviorist** /-ist/, a disciple of the school of neobehaviorism.

**neoblastic** /-blas′tik/ [Gk, *neos* + *blastos,* germ], pertaining to a new tissue or development within a new tissue.

**neocerebellum** /-ser′əbel′əm/, those parts of the cerebellum that receive input via the corticopontocerebellar pathway.

**neocortex** /-kôr′teks/ [Gk, *neos,* new; L, *cortex,* bark], the most recently evolved part of the brain. In humans the neocortex includes all of the cerebral cortex except for the hippocampal and piriform areas.

**NeoDecadron,** trademark for a topical fixed-combination drug containing a glucocorticoid (dexamethasone phosphate) and an antibacterial (neomycin sulfate).

**neodymium (Nd)** /-din′ē·əm/ [Gk, *neos* + *didymos*, twin], a rare earth element. Its atomic number is 60; its atomic mass is 144.27.

**neogenesis.** See **regeneration.**

**neoglottis** /-glot′is/, a vibrating structure that replaces the glottis in alaryngeal speech, such as after a laryngectomy. Also called **pseudoglottis.**

**neologism** /nē·ol′əjiz′əm/ [Gk, *neos* + *logos,* word], **1.** a word or term newly coined or used with a new meaning. **2.** (in psychiatry) a word coined by a psychotic or delirious patient that is meaningful only to the patient.

**neomycin sulfate** /-mī′sin/, an aminoglycoside antibiotic.

■ INDICATIONS: It is prescribed in the treatment of infections of the intestine, in hepatic coma, and topically in the treatment of skin infections.

■ CONTRAINDICATIONS: Renal dysfunction, intestinal obstruction, or known hypersensitivity to this drug or to any aminoglycoside medication prohibits its use.

■ ADVERSE EFFECTS: Among the more serious adverse reactions are nausea, vomiting, diarrhea, malabsorption, or superinfection. Prolonged treatment in patients with impaired renal function may result in the toxicities of systemic aminoglycosides. Hypersensitivity reactions may occur with topical administration of this drug.

**neon (Ne)** /nē′on/ [Gk, *neos,* new], a colorless odorless gaseous element and one of the inert gases. Its atomic number is 10; its atomic mass is 20.18. Neon has no compounds and occurs in the atmosphere in the ratio of about 18 parts per million. Some minerals and meteorites contain traces of this element. It is prepared commercially by the fractional distillation of liquefied air and is one of the first components to boil off. Neon is an excellent conductor of electricity, which ionizes the gas and causes it to emit a reddish-orange glow; this characteristic makes neon useful in devices to warn against electric current overload.

**neonatal** /-nā′təl/ [Gk, *neos* + L, *natus,* born], the period of time covering the first 28 days after birth.

**neonatal abstinence syndrome,** a behavioral pattern of irritability, tremulousness, and inconsolability exhibited in newborns exposed to heroin and methadone. Following treatment during the neonatal period, the abnormal signs usually resolve. In some infants hypertonicity has persisted for 6 months.

**Neonatal Behavioral Assessment Scale (NBAS),** a scale developed by T. Berry Brazelton for evaluating and assessing an infant's alertness, motor maturity, irritability, consolability, and interaction with people. It consists of a series of 27 reaction tests, including response to inanimate objects, pinprick, light, and to sound of a rattle or bell. It is used as a tool for the evaluation of the neurologic condition and the behavior of a newborn. Using the scale, the individuality of an infant may be demonstrated for parents, and some researchers theorize that the quality of the parent-child relationship may be predicted.

**neonatal breathing,** respiration in newborns. It begins when pulmonary fluid in the lungs is expelled by compression of the thorax during delivery and resorbed from the alveoli into the bloodstream and lymphatics. As air enters the lungs, the chest and lungs recoil to a resting position, but forceful inspirations are necessary to keep the lungs inflated. Such inspirations are triggered by changes in blood gas tension, a strong Hering-Breuer reflex, decrease in body temperature, and tactile stimuli. Irregular fetal breathing movements, which occur during rapid eye movement sleep, may be observed as early as 13 weeks of gestation. At birth the peripheral and central chemoreceptors involved in the control of respiration rate are very active, and newborns are highly sensitive to carbon dioxide during the first weeks. However, the control of rhythm breathing is not fully developed at birth.

**neonatal conjunctivitis.** See **ophthalmia neonatorum.**

**neonatal death,** the death of a live-born infant during the first 28 days after birth. Early neonatal death is usually considered to be one that occurs during the first 7 days. Compare **infant death, perinatal death.**

**neonatal developmental profile,** an evaluation of the developmental status of a newborn based on three examinations: a gestational age inventory, a neurologic examination, and a Neonatal Behavioral Assessment score.

**neonatal hepatitis,** hepatitis of unknown cause with onset in the first few weeks of life; some cases are associated with viral or bacterial infection; a few are familial. It is characterized by the transformation of hepatocytes into polynuclear giant cells and by conjugated hyperbilirubinemia with jaundice. Most patients recover completely, some develop chronic disease or fatal cirrhosis. Also called **giant cell hepatitis.**

**neonatal hyperbilirubinemia.** See **hyperbilirubinemia of the newborn.**

**neonatal intensive care unit (NICU),** a hospital unit containing a variety of sophisticated mechanic devices and special equipment for the management and care of premature and seriously ill newborns. The unit is staffed by a team of nurses and neonatologists who are highly trained in the pathophysiology of the newborn. See also **intensive care unit.**

**neonatal jaundice.** See **hyperbilirubinemia of the newborn.**

**neonatal mortality,** the statistic rate of infant death during the first 28 days after live birth, expressed as the number of such deaths per 1000 live births in a specific geographic area or institution in a given time.

**neonatal period,** the interval from birth to 28 days of age. It represents the time of the greatest risk to the infant; approximately 65% of all deaths that occur in the first year of life happen during this 4-week period.

**neonatal pustular melanosis,** a transient skin condition of the neonate characterized by vesicles present at birth that become pustular. The lesions contain neutrophils rather than eosinophils as seen in erythema toxicum neonatorum. They disappear within 72 hours, leaving dark spots that gradually fade by about 3 months of age.

**neonatal thermoregulation,** the regulation of the body temperature of a newborn, which may be affected by evaporation, conduction, radiation, and convection.

■ METHOD: To prevent the loss of body heat through evaporation, the infant is patted dry with a warm towel immediately after birth. Loss of heat by conduction is prevented by wrapping the baby in a warm blanket or placing a warm blanket over the baby as the baby lies on the mother's skin and by warming all equipment that is to be used to touch, cover, or examine the infant. Loss of heat by radiation can be minimized by placing the baby under a radiant heater, on a warmed, padded surface, or in skin-to-skin contact with the mother. Loss of body heat by convection is prevented by avoiding drafts, air conditioning vents, and low ambient temperatures. Infant bassinets have high sides to prevent cross drafts.

■ INTERVENTIONS: The infant is kept covered and protected from any means of heat loss. Because the surface area of the newborn's head is proportionately large when compared with the body, heat loss from the head may be great; therefore a cap or fold of blanket is placed around the head. Progressive family-centered maternity services, in which the

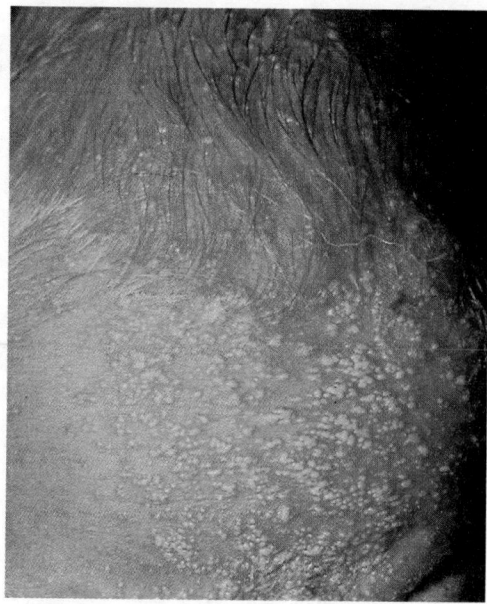

**Neonatal pustular melanosis** *(Zitelli and Davis, 1997)*

practice after delivery is to place the infant skin-to-skin with the mother, often provide caps made of stockinet. An overhead radiant heater is rolled to the delivery bed to maintain a warm ambient temperature for the infant.

■ OUTCOME CRITERIA: The axillary temperature is normally between 97.5° F (36.5° C) and 98.6° F (37° C).

**neonatal tyrosinemia.** See **tyrosinemia.**

**neonatal unit,** a unit of a hospital that provides care and treatment of newborns through the age of 28 days, and longer if necessary.

**neonatal vital signs monitor,** equipment in a specialized neonatal intensive care unit that measures mean blood pressure and mean heart rate from a plastic blood pressure cuff, with values digitally displayed on a monitor. See also **electronic fetal monitor.**

**neonate** /nē'ənāt/, an infant from birth to 28 days of age.

**neonatology** /nē'ōnātol'əjē/ [Gk, *neos* + L, *natus,* born; Gk, *logos,* science], the branch of medicine that concentrates on the care of the neonate and specializes in the diagnosis and treatment of the disorders of the newborn. —**neonatologic, neonatological,** *adj.,* **neonatologist,** *n.*

**neonatorum encephalitis** /-nātôr'əm/ [Gk, *neos,* new; L, *natus,* born; Gk, *enkephalos,* brain, *itis,* inflammation], a brain inflammation that develops in the first 4 weeks of life. Also called **encephalitis neonatorum.**

**neoplasia** /nē'ōplā'zhə/ [Gk, *neos* + *plassein,* to mold], the new and abnormal development of cells that may be benign or malignant. —**neoplastic** /-plas'tik/, *adj.*

**neoplasm** /nē'ōplaz'əm/ [Gk, *neos* + *plasma,* formation], any abnormal growth of new tissue, benign or malignant. Also called **tumor.** See **benign, cancer, malignant.** —**neoplastic,** *adj.*

**neoplastic** /nē'ōplas'tik/ [Gk, *neos,* new, *plassein,* to mold], pertaining to **neoplasty, neoplasm.**

**neoplastic fracture,** a fracture resulting from a weakness in bone tissue caused by a benign or malignant tumor. Also called **pathologic fracture.**

**neoplastic pericarditis** [Gk, *neos,* new, *plasma,* something

formed, *peri,* around, *kardia,* heart, *itis,* inflammation], inflammation of the pericardium, usually secondary to a malignant tumor within the area. Also called **carcinomatous pericarditis.**

**neoplastic transformation,** conversion of a tissue with a normal growth pattern into a malignant tumor.

**neoplasty** /nē'ōplas'tē/ [Gk, *neos,* new, *plassein,* to mold], a plastic surgery procedure to restore a part or add a new part.

**Neosporin,** trademark for a topical, fixed-combination drug containing antibacterials (polymyxin B sulfate, neomycin sulfate, and bacitracin zinc).

**neostigmine bromide** /nē'ōstig'mēn/, a cholinergic; a muscle stimulant; an anticholinesterase agent.

■ INDICATION: It is prescribed in the treatment of myasthenia gravis.

■ CONTRAINDICATIONS: Bowel obstruction, urinary tract infection, or known hypersensitivity to this drug or to other bromides prohibits its use.

■ ADVERSE EFFECTS: Among the more serious adverse reactions are severe respiratory depression, ptyalism, and intestinal cramps.

**neostriatum** /-strī·ā'təm/, the most recently evolved part of the corpus striatum, consisting of the caudate nucleus and putamen. The neostriatum receives input from the entire cerebral cortex and other brain areas and provides output to the basal nuclei.

**Neo-Synephrine,** trademark for a vasoconstrictor (phenylephrine hydrochloride).

**neoteny** /nē·ot'ənē/ [Gk, *neos,* new, *teinein,* to stretch], the attainment of sexual maturity during the larval stage of development such as in certain amphibians, especially salamanders.

**nephelometer** /nef'əlom'ətər/ [Gk, *nephele,* cloud, *metron,* measure], a photometric apparatus used to determine the concentration of solids suspended in a liquid or a gas, such as may be used to determine the number of bacteria in a specimen. See also **nephelometry.**

**nephelometry** /nef'əlom'ətrē/, a technique of determining the concentration of solids suspended in a liquid or a gas by use of a nephelometer. —**nephelometric, nephelometrical,** *adj.*

**nephr-.** See **nephro-.**

**nephrectomy** /-ek'təmē/ [Gk, *nephros,* kidney, *ektomē,* excision], the surgical removal of a kidney, performed to remove a tumor or otherwise diseased kidney. In the patient with renal failure, the kidney may be the cause of extreme hypertension and therefore one or both kidneys are removed. Before surgery the blood is typed and crossmatched for transfusion. During surgery the kidney is approached through either a flank, abdominal, or thoracoabdominal incision and removed. If the thoracic cavity is opened, a chest tube is inserted and connected to water-seal drainage. The nurse observes carefully for rapid pulse, restlessness, sweating, and a drop in blood pressure. Urinary output is measured hourly, and fluid intake and body weight are closely monitored. Deep breathing is difficult because the incision is close to the diaphragm. Pain medication is essential so the patient can deep breathe and move. The nurse reports at once any sudden shortness of breath and assesses the lungs, as this is a sign of spontaneous pneumothorax which may occur if the pleura was accidentally nicked during surgery.

**-nephric,** suffix meaning 'kidneys': *archinephric, cardionephric, splenonephric.*

**nephritic** /nəfrit'ik/ [Gk, *nephros,* kidney, *itis,* inflammation], pertaining to an inflammation of the kidney.

**nephritic calculus.** See **renal calculus.**

## Classification of neoplasms

| Parent tissue | Benign tumor | Malignant tumor |
|---|---|---|
| **Epithelium** | | |
| Skin and mucous membrane | Papilloma | Squamous cell carcinoma |
| | Polyp | Basal cell carcinoma |
| | | Transitional cell carcinoma |
| Glands | Adenoma | Adenocarcinoma |
| | Cystadenoma | |
| **Endothelium** | | |
| Blood vessels | Hemangioma | Hemangiosarcoma |
| | | Angiosarcoma |
| Lymph vessels | Lymphangioma | Lymphangiosarcoma |
| Bone marrow | | Multiple myeloma |
| | | Ewing's sarcoma |
| | | Leukemia |
| | | Lymphangioendothelioma |
| | | Reticular cell sarcoma (difficult to classify because of cell embryology) |
| | | Lymphatic leukemia |
| Lymphoid tissue | | Malignant lymphoma |
| **Connective tissue** | | |
| Embryonic fibrous tissue | Myxoma | Myxosarcoma |
| Fibrous tissue | Fibroma | Fibrosarcoma |
| Adipose tissue | Lipoma | Liposarcoma |
| Cartilage | Chondroma | Chondrosarcoma |
| Bone | Osteoma | Osteogenic sarcoma |
| Synovial membrane | Synovioma | Synovial sarcoma |
| **Muscle tissue** | | |
| Smooth muscle | Leiomyoma | Leiomyosarcoma |
| Striated muscle | Rhabdomyoma | Rhabdomyosarcoma |
| **Nerve tissue** | | |
| Nerve fibers and sheaths | Neuroma | Neurogenic sarcoma |
| | Neurinoma (neurilemoma) | |
| | Neurofibroma | Neurofibrosarcoma |
| Ganglion cells | Ganglioneuroma | Neuroblastoma |
| Glial cells | Glioma | Glioblastoma |
| | | Spongioblastoma |
| Meninges | Meningioma | |
| **Pigmented neoplasms** | | |
| Melanoblasts | Pigmented nevus | Malignant melanoma |
| | | Melanocarcinoma |
| **Miscellaneous** | | |
| Placenta | Hydatidiform mole | Chorion-epithelioma (choriocarcinoma) |
| | Dermoid cyst | Embryonal carcinoma |
| | | Embryonal sarcoma |
| | | Teratocarcinoma |

From: Phipps WJ, Sands JK, Marek JE: *Medical-surgical nursing: concepts and clinical practice,* ed 6, St Louis, 1999, Mosby.

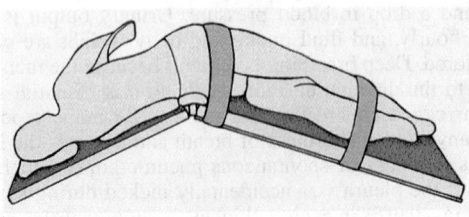

**Positioning of a patient for a nephrectomy**
*(Potter and Perry, 1997)*

**nephritic factor,** a protein found in the serum of patients with membranoproliferative glomerulonephritis. It activates alternative complement pathways.

**nephritic gingivitis** [Gk, *nephros* + L, *itis,* inflammation, *gingiva,* gum; Gk, *itis,* inflammation], inflammation of the mouth and gingiva associated with kidney failure, accompanied by pain, the odor of ammonia, and increased salivation. Also called **uremic gingivitis.**

**nephritic syndrome,** a group of signs and symptoms of a urinary tract disorder, including hematuria, hypertension, and renal failure.

**nephritis** /nəfrī′tis/ [Gk, *nephros* + *itis,* inflammation], any one of a large group of diseases of the kidney characterized by inflammation and abnormal function. Kinds of nephritis include **acute nephritis, glomerulonephritis, hereditary nephritis, interstitial nephritis, parenchymatous nephritis,** and **suppurative nephritis.**

**nephro-** /nef′rō-/, **nephr-,** prefix meaning 'kidneys': *nephroblastoma, nephrogram, nephrorrhagia.*

**nephroangiosclerosis** /nef′rō-an′jē-ō′sklerō′sis/ [Gk, *nephros + angeion,* vessel, *skleros,* hard, *osis,* condition], necrosis of the renal arterioles, associated with hypertension. This condition is present in a small number of hypertensive individuals between 30 and 50 years of age. Early signs are headaches, blurring of vision, and a diastolic blood pressure greater than 120 mm Hg. Examination of the retina reveals hemorrhages, vascular exudates, and papilledema. The heart is usually enlarged, especially the left ventricle. Proteins and red blood cells are found in the urine. Heart and kidney failure may occur if the disease remains untreated. Treatment includes measures to lower blood pressure using diet and antihypertensive medications. Hemodialysis is used when preventive measures have failed. Also called **malignant hypertension.** See also **hypertension, renal failure.**

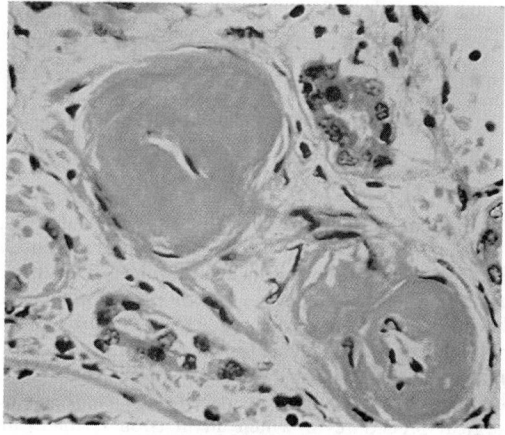

**Nephroangiosclerosis**
*(Kumar, Cotran, Robbins, 1997/courtesy Dr. M.A. Venkatachalam, Department of Pathology, University of Texas Health Sciences Center, San Antonio)*

**nephroblastoma.** See **Wilms' tumor.**

**nephrocalcinosis** /nef′rōkal′sinō′sis/ [Gk, *nephros + L, calx,* lime; Gk, *osis,* condition], an abnormal condition of the kidneys in which deposits of calcium form in the parenchyma at the site of previous inflammation or degenerative change. Infection, hematuria, anal colic, and decreased function of the kidney may occur.

**nephrocystitis** /-sistī′tis/, an inflammation involving both the kidney and the urinary bladder.

**nephrocystosis** /-sistō′sis/, the formation of cysts in the kidney.

**nephrogenic** /nef′rōjen′ik/ [Gk, *nephros + genein,* to produce], **1.** generating kidney tissue. **2.** originating in the kidney.

**nephrogenic ascites,** the abnormal presence of fluid in the peritoneal cavity of patients undergoing hemodialysis for re-

nal failure. The cause of this type of ascites is unknown. See also **ascites.**

**nephrogenic cord,** either of the paired longitudinal ridges of tissue that lie along the dorsal surface of the coelom in the early developing vertebrate embryo. It is formed from the fusion of the nephrotome tissue and gives rise to the structures making up the embryonic urogenital system. See also **mesonephros, metanephros, pronephros.**

**nephrogenic diabetes insipidus,** an abnormal condition in which the kidneys do not concentrate the urine, resulting in polyuria, polydipsia, and very dilute urine. The secretion of antidiuretic hormone (ADH) by the pituitary is normal, and all kidney function is normal, except that there is no response to ADH. See also **diabetes insipidus.**

**nephrogenous** /nəfroj′ənəs/, pertaining to the formation and development of the kidneys.

**nephrogram** /nef′rō-gram/, a radiograph of the kidney.

**nephrography** /nəfrog′rəfē/, the radiographic examination of the kidney.

**nephrohypertrophy** /-hīpur′trəfē/ [Gk, *nephros,* kidney, *hyper,* excessive, *trophe,* nourishment], enlargement of the kidney.

**nephrolith** /nef′rəlith/ [Gk, *nephros + lithos,* stone], a calculus formed in a kidney. Also called **renal calculus** or **renal stone.** —**nephrolithic,** *adj.*

**nephrolithiasis** /nef′rōlithī′əsis/, a disorder characterized by the presence of calculi in the kidney. See also **renal calculus.**

**nephrolithic.** See **nephrolith.**

**nephrolithotomy** /-lithot′əmē/, the surgical removal of renal calculi.

**nephrology** /nəfrol′əjē/ [Gk, *nephros + logos,* science], the study of the anatomy, physiology, and pathology of the kidney. —**nephrologic, nephrological,** *adj.*

**nephrolytic** /-lit′ik/ [Gk, *nephros + lysis,* loosening], pertaining to the destruction of a kidney.

**-nephroma,** combining form meaning a 'tumor of the kidney or area of the kidney': *epinephroma, paranephroma.*

**nephromere.** See **nephrotome.**

**nephron** /nef′ron/ [Gk, *nephros,* kidney], a structural and functional unit of the kidney, resembling a microscopic funnel with a long stem and two convoluted tubular sections. Each kidney contains about 1.25 million nephrons. All nephrons have a renal corpuscle and renal tubules. Juxtamedullary nephrons also have loops of Henle. Each renal corpuscle consists of a glomerulus of renal capillaries enclosed within Bowman's capsule. The renal corpuscles and the convoluted parts of the renal tubules are located in the cortex of the kidney. The loops of Henle and collecting tubules are located in the medulla. Urine is formed in the renal corpuscles and renal tubules by filtration, reabsorption, and secretion. See also **kidney, malpighian corpuscle.**

**nephronia** /nəfrō′nē-ə/, an inflammation of intrarenal connective tissue that occurs in a small percentage of patients with urinary tract infections.

**nephronophthisis.** See **medullary cystic disease.**

**nephroparalysis** /-pəral′isis/ [Gk, *nephros,* kidney, *paralyein,* to be palsied], a paralysis of the kidney resulting in a cessation of its functions.

**nephropathy** /nefrop′əthē/ [Gk, *nephros + pathos,* disease], any disorder of the kidney, including inflammatory, degenerative, and sclerotic conditions. See also **kidney disease.**

**nephropexy** /nef′rəpek′sē/ [Gk, *nephros + pexis,* fixation], a surgical operation to fixate a floating or ptotic kidney.

**nephroptosis** /nef′rəptō′sis/ [Gk, *nephros + ptosis,* falling], a downward displacement or dropping of a kidney.

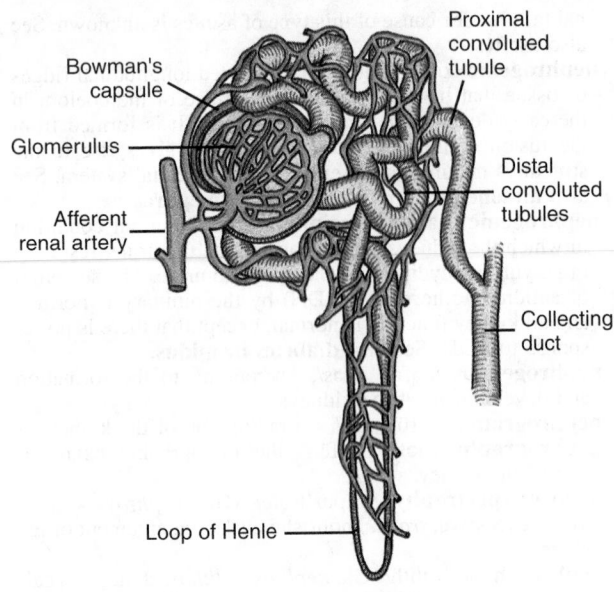

**Nephron** *(Potter and Perry, 2001)*

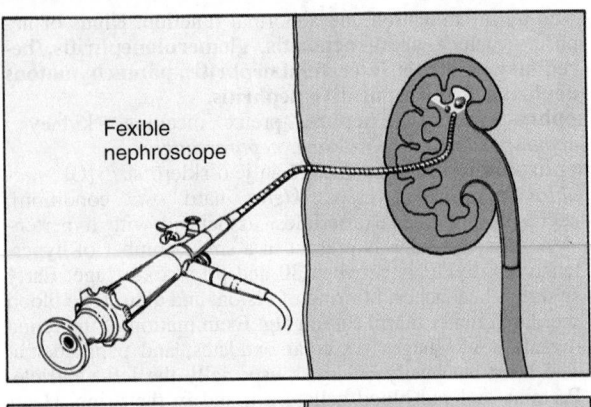

Fexible nephroscope

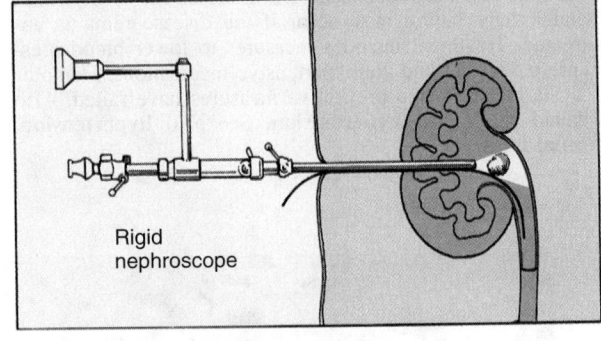

Rigid nephroscope

**Nephroscopes** *(Brundage, 1992)*

**nephrorrhaphy** /nəfrôr′əfē/ [Gk, *nephros* + *rhaphe,* suture], an operation that sutures a floating kidney in place.

**nephrosclerosis.** See **nephroangiosclerosis.**

**nephroscope** /nef′rəskōp′/ [Gk, *nephros* + *skopein,* to look], a fiberoptic instrument that is used specifically for visualization of the kidney and the disintegration and removal of renal calculi. The nephroscope is inserted percutaneously, and the calculi are located through use of x-ray films of the renal pelvis. An ultrasonic probe emitting high-frequency sound waves breaks up the calculi, which are removed by suction through the instrument.

**nephrosis.** See **nephrotic syndrome.**

**nephrostoma** /-stō′mə/, *pl.* **nephrostomas, nephrostomata** [Gk, *nephros* + *stoma,* mouth], the funnel-shaped ciliated opening of the excretory tubules into the coelom of the early developing vertebrate embryo. Also called **nephrostome.** —**nephrostomic,** *adj.*

**nephrostomy** /nəfros′təmē/, a surgical procedure in which a flank incision is made so that a catheter can be inserted into the kidney pelvis for the purpose of drainage.

**nephrotic syndrome** /nəfrot′ik/ [Gk, *nephros* + L, *icus,* like], an abnormal condition of the kidney characterized by marked proteinuria, hypoalbuminemia, and edema. It occurs in glomerular disease and thrombosis of a renal vein and as a complication of many systemic diseases, diabetes mellitus, amyloidosis, systemic lupus erythematosus, and multiple myeloma. The nephrotic syndrome occurs in a severe, primary form. The presenting symptoms include anorexia, weakness, proteinuria, hypoalbuminuria, and edema. Treatment and prognosis depend on the underlying cause of disease. Patients with primary nephrotic syndrome usually respond favorably to corticosteroids. Loop diuretics are used to control symptomatic edema, and dialysis may be necessary. Also called **nephrosis.** —**nephrotic,** *adj.*

**nephrotome** /nef′rətom/ [Gk, *nephros* + *tome,* section], a zone of segmented mesodermal tissue in the developing vertebrate embryo lying along each side of the body dorsal to the abdominal cavity between the somite-forming dorsal mesoderm and the unsegmented lateral plate mesoderm. It is the primordial tissue for the urogenital system and gives rise to the nephrogenic cord. Also called **intermediate cell mass, intermediate mesoderm, middle plate, nephromere.** See also **mesonephros, metanephros, pronephros.**

**nephrotomography** /-təmog′rəfē/ [Gk, *nephros* + *tome,* section, *graphein,* to record], sectional radiographic examination of the kidneys.

**nephrotomy** /nəfrot′əmē/ [Gk, *nephros* + *temnein,* to cut], a surgical procedure in which an incision is made in the kidney.

**nephrotoxic** /-tok′sik/ [Gk, *nephros* + *toxikon,* poison], toxic or destructive to a kidney.

**nephrotoxin** /-tok′sin/, a toxin with specific destructive properties for the kidneys.

**nephroureterolithiasis** /nef′rōyŏŏrē′tərō′lithī′əsis/, the presence of calculi in the kidneys and ureters.

**Neptazane,** trademark for a carbonic anhydrase inhibitor (methazolamide).

**neptunium (Np)** /nept(y)ŏŏ′nē·əm/ [planet Neptune], a transuranic, metallic element. Its atomic number is 93; its atomic mass is 237. Although neptunium is considered a synthetic element, traces of natural neptunium have been found in uranium ores.

**Neri's sign** /nā′rēz/ [Vincenzo Neri, Italian neurologist, 20th century], a sign of organic hemiplegia, consisting in the spontaneous bending of the knee of the affected side as the leg is passively lifted, the patient being in the dorsal position. with the patient standing, forward bending of the trunk will cause flexion of the knee on the affected side in lumbosacral and iliosacral lesions.

**Nernst equation** [Hermann W. Nernst, German physicist, 1864–1941; L, *aequare,* to make equal], an expression of the relationship between the electrical potential across a membrane and the ratio between the concentrations of a given species of permeant ion on either side of the membrane.

**nerve** /nurv/ [L, *nervus*], one or more bundles of impulse-carrying fibers, myelinated or unmyelinated or both, that connect the brain and the spinal cord with other parts of the body. Nerves transmit afferent impulses from receptor organs toward the brain, spinal cord, and efferent impulses peripherally to the effector organs. Each nerve consists of an epineurium enclosing fasciculi of nerve fibers, each fasciculus surrounded by its own sheath of connective tissue, or epineurium. Individual nerve fibers, which are microscopic, consist of formed elements within a matrix of protoplasm enclosed in endoneurium and enclosed in a neurilemmal sheath. Inside the neurilemma are nerve fibers, also enclosed in a myelin sheath. See also **axon, dendrite, neuroglia, neuron, Schwann cell.**

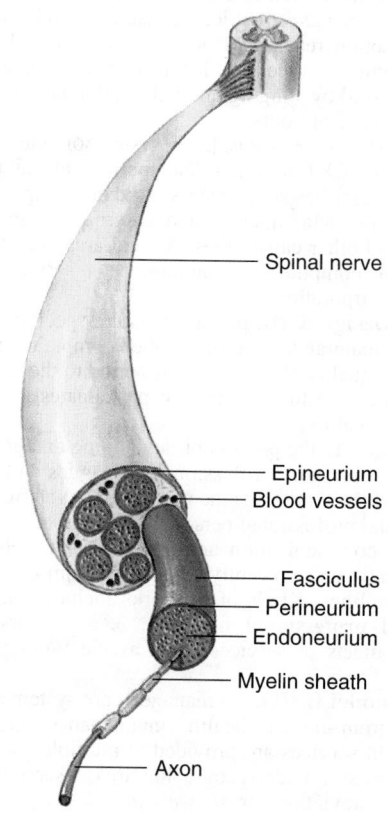

Spinal nerve

Epineurium
Blood vessels

Fasciculus
Perineurium
Endoneurium

Myelin sheath

Axon

**Cross section of a nerve** *(Applegate, 2000)*

**nerve accommodation,** the ability of nerve tissue to adjust to a constant source and intensity of stimulation so that some change in either intensity or duration of the stimulus is necessary to elicit a response beyond the initial reaction. Accommodation is probably caused by reduced sodium ion permeability, which results in an increased threshold intensity and subsequent stabilization of the resting membrane potential.

**nerve block anesthesia.** See **conduction anesthesia.**

**nerve cable graft,** a multistrand free nerve graft, taken from elsewhere in the body, to bridge a large gap in one of the main nerves in the forearm.

**nerve cell.** See **neuron.**

**nerve compression,** a pathologic event that causes harmful pressure on one or more nerve trunks, resulting in nerve damage and muscle weakness or atrophy. Any nerve that passes over a rigid prominence is vulnerable, and the degree of damage depends on the magnitude and duration of the compressive force. Various factors may contribute to susceptibility, such as inherited predisposition, malnutrition, trauma, and disease. Various activities associated with routine occupations may unduly compress especially vulnerable nerves such as the median nerve, radial nerve, femoral nerve, and plantar nerves. Rest and the cessation or modification of causative activities often heal nerve damage caused by compression. Surgery may be required to correct more severe cases. Compare **nerve entrapment.**

**nerve conduction test,** an electrodiagnostic test of the integrity of the peripheral nerves. It involves placing an electrical stimulator over a nerve and measuring the time required for an impulse to travel over a measured segment of the nerve. The test is used in the diagnosis of nerve entrapment syndrome and polyneuropathies.

**nerve deafness.** See **sensorineural hearing loss.**

**nerve endings,** the fine branchlike terminations of peripheral neurons; sensory endings are effectively dendrites lying far from the neuronal cell body and motor nerve endings are the endings of axons and are called **motor end plates.** See also **neuron.**

**nerve entrapment,** an abnormal condition and type of mononeuropathy, characterized by nerve damage and muscle weakness or atrophy. The peripheral nerve trunks of the body are especially vulnerable to entrapment in which repeated compression results in significant impairment. Nerves that pass over rigid prominences or through narrow bony and fascial canals are particularly prone to entrapment. The common signs of this disorder are pain and muscular weakness. Nerve damage by entrapment occurs more often when adjacent joints are affected by swelling and inflammation, such as in rheumatoid arthritis, pregnancy, and acromegaly. Signs of nerve entrapment also may develop after repeated bruising of certain nerves by various activities involving repeated motions, such as those associated with knitting and prolonged walking. One of the most common types of entrapment is **carpal tunnel syndrome.** Compare **nerve compression.**

**nerve excitability** [L, *nervus*, nerve, *excitare*, to rouse], the readiness of a nerve cell to respond to a stimulus. See also **all-or-none law.**

**nerve fiber,** a slender process, the axon of a neuron. Each fiber is classified as myelinated or unmyelinated. Myelinated fibers are further designated as A or B fibers; C fibers are unmyelinated. The A fibers are somatic. A alpha fibers are large fibers and transport impulses at a velocity of 60 to 100 meters per second; A beta fibers are smaller and transmit pressure and temperature impulses at a velocity of 30 to 70 meters per second; A gamma fibers transmit touch and pressure impulses. A delta fibers are the smallest and transmit impulses associated with sharp pain sensation. B fibers are more finely myelinated than A fibers. They are both afferent and efferent and are mainly associated with visceral innervation. The unmyelinated C fibers are efferent postganglionic autonomic fibers and afferent fibers that conduct impulses of prolonged, burning pain sensation from the viscera and periphery.

**nerve graft,** the transplantation of all or part of a nerve. The procedure may be performed in cases in which the gap in a severed nerve is too large to be repaired by suture alone. The graft provides a pathway that encourages the regrowth of severed axons from the central stump of the damaged nerve. Donor material may consist of heterografts, homografts, or autografts.

**nerve growth factor (NGF),** a protein whose hormone-like action affects differentiation, growth, and maintenance of neurons.

**nerve impulse.** See **impulse.**

**nerve plexus** [L, *nervus,* nerve, *plexus,* plaited], an interwoven network of nerves, such as the lumbar plexus formed by the anterior primary branch of the upper four lumbar nerves.

**nerve root impingement,** the abnormal protrusion of body tissue into the space occupied by a spinal nerve root. Causes may include disk herniation, tissue prolapse, and inflammation.

**nerve sheath** [L, *nervus,* nerve; AS, *scaeth*], any of several types of coatings or coverings for nerve fibers and nerve tracts. Kinds of nerve sheaths include **endoneurial, medullary, myelin, neurilemma,** and **notochordal.**

**nervimotor** /ner′vi·mō′tər/ [L, *nervus,* nerve + *motare,* to move], pertaining to a motor nerve.

**nervous emesis** [L, *nervus* + Gk, *emesis,* vomiting], vomiting that is functional and psychogenic. The condition is most common among young women and is regarded as a psychologic representation of a desire to reject something.

**nervous prostration** [L, *nervus* + *prosternere,* to throw down], a condition of irritable weakness and depression, which may be psychogenic or the result of a severe prolonged illness or exhausting experience.

**nervous system** [L, *nervus,* nerve; Gk, *system*], the extensive, intricate network of structures that activates, coordinates, and controls all the functions of the body. It is divided into the central nervous system, composed of the brain and the spinal cord, and the peripheral nervous system, which includes the cranial nerves and the spinal nerves. These morphologic subdivisions combine and communicate to innervate the somatic and visceral parts of the body with the afferent and efferent nerve fibers. Afferent fibers carry sensory impulses to the central nervous system; efferent fibers carry motor impulses from the central nervous system to the muscles and other organs. The somatic fibers are associated with the bones, muscles, and skin. The visceral fibers are associated with the internal organs, blood vessels, and mucous membranes. Compare **parasympathetic nervous system, sympathetic nervous system.** See also the Color Atlas of Human Anatomy.

**nervous tachypnea** [L, *nervus* + Gk, *tachys,* rapid, *pnoia,* breath], a neurotic symptom characterized by quick, shallow breathing.

**nervus abducens.** See **abducens nerve.**

**nervus accessorius.** See **accessory nerve.**

**nervus facialis.** See **facial nerve.**

**nervus glossopharyngeus.** See **glossopharyngeal nerve.**

**nervus hypoglossus.** See **hypoglossal nerve.**

**nervus oculomotorius.** See **oculomotor nerve.**

**nervus olfactorius.** See **olfactory nerve.**

**nervus opticus.** See **optic nerve.**

**nervus terminalis.** See **terminal nerve.**

**nervus trigeminus.** See **trigeminal nerve.**

**nervus trochlearis.** See **trochlear nerve.**

**nervus vagus.** See **vagus nerve.**

**Nesacaine,** trademark for a long-acting local anesthetic (chloroprocaine).

**-ness,** suffix meaning 'a quality or state of being': *illness, painless.*

**nested nails,** a pair of nails placed side by side in the medullary canal of long bones during orthopedic surgery.

**net charge,** the arithmetic sum of positive and negative charges.

**net protein utilization (NPU),** a measure of protein quality that is based on the percentage of ingested nitrogen that is retained by the body. Because NPU does not take into account differences in the digestibility of proteins, it gives a poorly digested but good-quality protein a false low value.

**net radiation,** the arithmetic difference between solar radiation received and outgoing terrestrial radiation.

**Netromycin,** trademark for an antibiotic (netilmicin).

**nettle,** a perennial herb that is native to Europe and is now found throughout the United States and parts of Canada.

■ USES: This herb is used as a diuretic and as a treatment for hay fever.

■ CONTRAINDICATIONS: Nettle should not be used during pregnancy and lactation, in children less than 2 years of age, or in people with hypersensitivity to this plant. It should be used only with caution in children and the elderly.

**nettle rash** [AS, *netele,* nettle; Fr, *rasche,* scurf], a fine, urticarial eruption resulting from skin contact with stinging nettle, a common weed with leaves containing histamine. It is characterized by stinging and itching that lasts from a few minutes to several hours.

**network** [AS, *net* + *wearc*], a system of interconnected computers or CRT terminals and peripheral equipment in which each user has some access to others using the system while sharing data, internal and external storage devices (server), and other capabilities. A local-area network is one in which the computers are interconnected serving the same facility or corporation.

**Network Design Group,** a Medicare-specific oversight group that maintains a log of enrollee complaints related to service and quality of care issues reported to the U.S. Health Care Financing Administration. It participates in investigation of complaints.

**networking,** **1.** the process of developing and using an interaction format with professional colleagues and agencies. **2.** (in psychiatric nursing) the process of developing a set of agencies and professional personnel who are able to create a system of communication and support for psychiatric patients, usually those recently discharged from inpatient psychiatric facilities. Kinds of networks include **natural network** and **professional network.** **3.** a network of supportive contacts or services, such as the Women's Health Network.

**network-model HMO,** a managed care system analogous to the group-model health maintenance organization (HMO), but services are provided at multiple sites by multiple groups so a wider geographic area is served.

**net wt,** abbreviation for *net weight.*

**Neufeld nail** /nyo͞o′fəld/ [Alonzo J. Neufeld, American surgeon, b. 1906], an orthopedic nail with a V-shaped tip and shank used for fixating an intertrochanteric fracture. The nail is driven into the neck of the femur until it reaches a round metal plate screwed onto the side of the femur. It is secured to a receptacle on the plate. Also called **Neufeld angled nail.**

**Neufeld roller traction,** a traction device for a fractured femur, consisting of a cast for the calf and thigh hinged at the knee. The cast is suspended by a line that passes from the anterior midthigh, around a pulley, to a spring attached to the anterior midleg.

**Neuman, Betty,** a nursing theorist who developed the Neuman Systems Model, first published in 1972. Her model is influenced by Gestalt theory, which states that the homeostatic process is the process by which an organism maintains its equilibrium. Major concepts include total persons approach, holism, open system, lines of resistance and defense, degree of reaction, interventions, levels of prevention, and reconstitution. A spiritual variable was added to her model later and created-environment was added to the typology. In the Neuman Systems Model, the client is presented as a whole person, an open system in constant change and in reciprocal interaction with the environment. Neuman believes the nurse should use purposeful interventions and a total-person approach to client care to help individuals, families, and groups reach and maintain a maximum level of total wellness. Nursing intervention is aimed at the reduction of stress and adverse conditions that can impact on optimal client functions.

**neur-.**   See **neuro-.**

**neural** /nŏŏr′əl/ [Gk, *neuron*, nerve],   pertaining to nerve cells and their processes.

**-neural, -neuric,**   suffix meaning 'nerve or nerves': *epineural, epithelioneural, myoneural.*

**neural canal.**   See **neurocoele.**

**neural cell-adhesion molecule,**   an immunoglobulin that functions as a molecular recognition molecule. See also **recognition site.**

**neural crest,**   the ectodermally derived cells along the outer surface of each side of the neural tube in the early stages of embryonic development. The cells migrate laterally throughout the embryo and give rise to spinal, cranial, enteric, and sympathetic ganglia, pigment cells, Schwann cells, and the adrenal medulla. Also called **ganglionic crest, ganglionic ridge.** See also **neural tube formation.**

groove and form the neural tube. Also called **medullary fold.** See also **neural tube formation.**

**neuralgia** /nŏŏral′jə/ [Gk, *neuron* + *algos,* pain],   an abnormal condition characterized by severe stabbing pain, caused by a variety of disorders affecting the nervous system. —**neuralgic,** *adj.*

**neuralgic amyotrophy** /nŏŏral′jik ā′mīot′rəfē/,   a brachial plexus disorder characterized by sudden pain and muscle weakness in the upper limbs and sometimes by muscular wasting or atrophy. The cause is unknown. Also called **Parsonage-Turner syndrome.**

**neural groove,**   the longitudinal depression that occurs between the neural folds during the invagination of the neural plate to form the neural tube in the early stages of embryonic development. Also called **medullary groove.** See also **neural tube formation.**

**neural impulse.**   See **impulse.**

**neural plate,**   a thick layer of ectodermal tissue that lies along the central longitudinal axis of the early developing embryo and gives rise to the neural tube and subsequently to the brain, spinal cord, and other tissues of the central nervous system. Also called **medullary plate.** See also **neural tube formation.**

**neural tube,**   the longitudinal tube, lying along the central axis of the early developing embryo, that gives rise to the brain, spinal cord, and other neural tissue of the central nervous system. It consists of thick ectodermal tissue and is formed by the fusion of the neural folds, resulting from the invagination of the neural plate. Failure of the tube to close results in a number of congenital defects. Also called **cerebromedullary tube, medullary tube.** See also **neural tube defect, neural tube formation.**

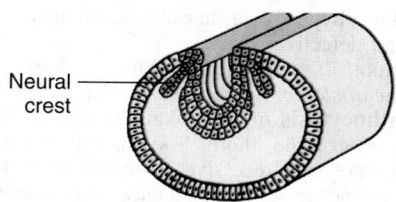

Neural crest

**Neural crest** *(Crossman and Neary, 1995)*

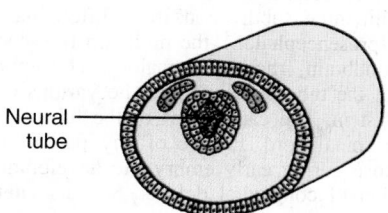

Neural tube

**Neural tube** *(Crossman and Neary, 1995)*

**neural ectoderm,**   the part of the embryonic ectoderm that develops into the neural tube. See also **neural tube formation.**

**neural fold,**   either of the paired longitudinal elevations resulting from the invagination of the neural plate in the early developing embryo. The folds unite to enclose the neural

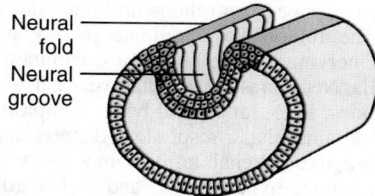

Neural fold
Neural groove

**Neural fold and neural groove** *(Crossman and Neary, 1995)*

**neural tube defect (NTD),**   any of a group of congenital malformations involving defects in the skull and spinal column that are caused primarily by the failure of the neural tube to close during embryonic development. In some instances the cleft results from an abnormal increase in cerebrospinal fluid pressure on the closed neural tube during the first trimester of development. The defect may occur at any point along the neural axis or extends the entire length of the spinal column, as in holorachischisis. The amount of deformity and disability depends on the degree of neural involvement, the most severe defect being complete cranioschisis, or the total absence of the skull and defective brain development. Other cerebral dysplasias resulting from the failure of the cranial end of the neural tube to fuse are meningoencephalocele and cranial meningocele. These defects, usually accompanied by severe mental and physical disorders, occur most often in the occipital region of the skull but may also occur in the frontal or basal regions. Most neural tube malformations are caused by incomplete fusion of one or more laminae of the vertebral column, with varying degrees of tissue protrusion and neural involvement. Such anomalies include rachischisis, spina bifida, myelocele, myelomeningocele, and meningocele. In all of these conditions there is constant risk of rupture of the saclike protrusion and danger of meningeal infection. Often immediate surgical repair is necessary. Adequate folate levels during the first month after conception are important in preventing neural tube defects; the U.S. Public Health Service recommends all women of childbearing age increase their folate intake to 400 μg per day. Many of the major neural tube defects can be determined prenatally by ultrasonic scanning of the uterus and by the presence of elevated concentrations of alpha-fetoprotein levels in the amniotic fluid. Such diagnostic tests are preferably performed during the 14th to 16th week of gestation so that termination of the pregnancy is possible. See also **anencephaly, Arnold-Chiari malformation, spina bifida cystica.**

**neural tube formation,** the various processes and stages involved in the embryonic development of the neural tube, which subsequently differentiates into the brain, the spinal cord, and other neural tissue of the central nervous system. The primitive tube originates from a flat, single layer of ectodermal tissue that extends longitudinally along the middorsal line of the embryonic disk from the area of the primitive streak forward to the cephalic extremity. This tissue, the neural plate, grows rapidly and becomes thickened, resulting in the invagination and formation of a hollow groove, the neural groove. With continued cell division the groove becomes deeper, and the folds thicken so that they eventually meet and fuse, converting the neural groove into the neural tube. The closing of the neural tube progresses toward both the caudal and the cephalic regions. At the cephalic end the tube expands into a large vesicle with three subdivisions that differentiate into the forebrain (prosencephalon), the midbrain (mesencephalon), and the hindbrain (rhombencephalon). The epithelium of the wall of the tube develops into the various cells of the nervous system. The caudal part of the tube subsequently forms the spinal cord. Failure of any part of the neural tube to close during early embryonic development results in a number of congenital defects. See also **neural tube defect.**

**neuraminidase** /nŏŏr′əmē′nədās/, an enzyme that catalyzes the cleavage of *N*-acetyl neuraminic acid from mucopolysaccharides. A hereditary deficiency of the enzyme causes sialidosis and is associated with galactogialidosis. Also called **sialidase.** See also **sialidosis.**

**neuraminidase spikes,** projections from surfaces of influenza viruses containing neuraminidase that are involved in the release of viruses from infected cells.

**neurapraxia** /nŏŏr′əprak′sē·ə/, the interruption of nerve conduction without loss of continuity of the axon.

**neurasthenia** /nŏŏr′əsthē′nē·ə/ [Gk, *neuron* + *a* + *sthenos*, without strength], **1.** an abnormal condition characterized by nervous exhaustion and a vague functional fatigue that often follows depression. **2.** (in psychiatry) a stage in the recovery from a schizophrenic experience, during which the patient is listless and apparently unable to cope with routine activities and relationships. —**neurasthenic,** *adj.*

**neurasthenic** /-əsthē′nik/ [Gk, *neuron,* nerve, *asthenia,* disability], pertaining to a disorder characterized by excessive fatigue, insomnia, weakness, anxiety, and mental and physical irritability.

**-neure,** combining form meaning a 'nerve cell': *ganglioneure, myoneure, sporadoneure.*

**neurectomy** /nŏŏrek′təmē/ [Gk, *neuron,* nerve, *ektomē,* excision], the surgical excision of a nerve segment.

**neurenteric canal** /nŏŏr′anter′ik/ [Gk, *neuron* + *enteron,* intestine; L, *canalis,* channel], a tubular passage between the posterior part of the neural tube and the archenteron in the early embryonic development of lower animals. It corresponds to the notochordal canal of humans and the higher animals. Also called **archenteric canal, blastoporic canal, Braun's canal.**

**neuresthenia.** See **fatigue state.**

**-neuria,** combining form meaning a '(specified) condition involving nerves': *acystineuria, ovariodysneuria.*

**-neuric.** See **-neural.**

**neurilemma** /nŏŏr′əlem′ə/ [Gk, *neuron* + *lemma,* sheath], a layer of cells composed of one or more Schwann cells that forms the segmented myelin sheaths of peripheral nerve fibers. It is necessary for regeneration of peripheral nerves when they have been severed. Also spelled **neurolemma.** Also called **sheath of Schwann.** —**neurilemmal, neurilemmatic, neurilemmatous,** *adj.*

**neurilemmoma.** See **schwannoma.**

**neurimotor.** See **nervimotor.**

**neurinoma** /nŏŏr′inō′mə/, *pl.* **neurinomas, neurinomata** [Gk, *neuron* + *oma,* tumor], **1.** a tumor of the nerve sheath. It is usually benign but may undergo malignant change. A kind of neurinoma is **acoustic neurinoma.** See also **schwannoma. 2.** a neuroma.

**neuritic plaque** /nŏŏrit′ik/, an extracellular deposit consisting of beta-amyloid protein mixed with branches of dying nerve cells in the brain of a patient with Alzheimer's disease.

**neuritis** /nŏŏrī′tis/, *pl.* **neuritides** [Gk, *neuron* + *itis,* inflammation], an abnormal condition characterized by inflammation of a nerve. Some of the signs of this condition are neuralgia, hypesthesia, anesthesia, paralysis, muscular atrophy, and defective reflexes.

**neuro-** /nŏŏr′ō-/, **neur-,** combining form meaning 'nerves': *neuroclonic, neurohormone, neuromast.*

**neuroacanthocytosis** /nŏŏr′ō·ə·kan′thō·sī·tō′sis/ [Gk, *neuron,* nerve + *akantha,* thorn + *kytos,* cell + *-osis,* condition], an autosomal recessive syndrome characterized by tics, chorea, and personality changes, with acanthocytes in the blood. Also called **choreoacanthocytosis.**

**neuroanatomy** /nŏŏr′ō·anat′əmē/, the branch of biology that is concerned with the structure of the nervous system.

**neuroarthropathy** /-ärthrop′əthē/ [Gk, *neuron* + *arthron,* joint, *pathos,* disease], a condition in which a disease of a joint is secondary to a disease of the nervous system.

**neurobiology** /-bī′ol′əjē/, a branch of biology that is concerned with the anatomy and physiology of the nervous system.

**neuroblast** /nŏŏr′əblast/ [Gk, *neuron* + *blastos,* germ], any embryonic cell that develops into a functional neuron; an immature nerve cell. —**neuroblastic,** *adj.*

**neuroblastoma** /nŏŏr′ōblastō′mə/, *pl.* **neuroblastomas, neuroblastomata** [Gk, *neuron* + *blastos,* germ, *oma,* tumor], a highly malignant tumor composed of primitive ectodermal cells derived from the neural plate during embryonic life. The tumor may originate in any part of the sympathetic nervous system but is most common in the adrenal medulla. Neuroblastomas metastasize early and widely to lymph nodes, liver, lungs, and bone. Symptoms may include an abdominal mass, respiratory distress, and anemia. Hormonally active adrenal lesions may cause irritability, flushing, sweating, hypertension, and tachycardia. Before metastasis, treatment with radical surgery, irradiation, and chemotherapy are often successful. Spontaneous remissions

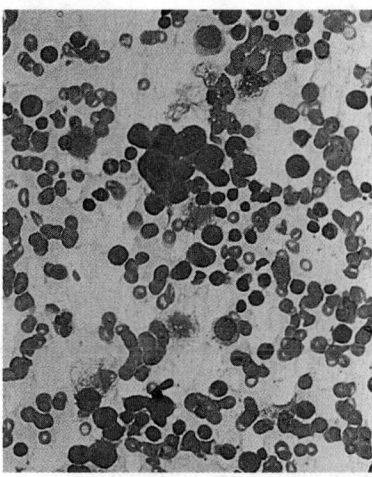

**Neuroblastoma metastasized to the bone marrow**
(Zitelli and Davis, 1997)

may occur, with the tumor undergoing maturation and forming a benign ganglioneuroma. A kind of neuroblastoma is **Pepper's syndrome.**

**neurobrucellosis** /-broo′səlo′sis/, a serious complication of a brucellosis infection that affects the nervous system and may cause meningitis, stroke, cranial nerve lesions, or mycotic aneurysms. The condition may require treatment with drugs that cross the blood-brain barrier.

**neurocanal.** See **vertebral canal.**

**neurocele.** See **neurocoele.**

**neurocentral** /-sen′trəl/ [Gk, *neuron* + *kentron,* center], pertaining to the centrum and the developing vertebrae in the early stages of embryology.

**neurocentrum** /-sen′trəm/ [Gk, *neuron* + L, *centrum,* center], the embryonic mesodermal tissue that subsequently gives rise to the vertebrae. See also **sclerotome.**

**neuro check** [Gk, *neuron* + ME, *chek,* stop], *nontechnical.* a brief neurologic assessment. The level of consciousness is evaluated as alert and oriented, lethargic, stuporous, or comatose. The movements of the extremities are determined to be voluntary or involuntary. The pupils of the eyes are observed for equality of dilation, reactivity to light, and ability to accommodate.

**neurochemistry** /-kem′istrē/, a branch of neurology that is concerned with the biochemistry of the nervous system.

**neurocirculatory asthenia** /-sur′kyələtôr′ē/ [Gk, *neuron* + L, *circulare,* to go around; Gk, *a* + *sthenos,* without strength], a psychosomatic disorder characterized by nervous and circulatory irregularities, including dyspnea, palpitation, giddiness, vertigo, tremor, precordial pain, and increased susceptibility to fatigue. The symptoms often result from or are associated with psychologic stress.

**neurocoele** /-noor′əsēl/ [Gk, *neuron* + *koilos,* hollow], a system of cavities in the central nervous system of humans and other vertebrate animals. It consists of the ventricles of the brain and the central canal of the spinal cord, which originate from the neural tube during early embryonic development. Also spelled **neurocele, neurocoel.** Also called **neural canal.**

**neurocytolysin** /-sītol′isin/, a toxic substance in snake venom that destroys nerve cell membranes.

**neurocytolysis** /-sītol′isis/, the destruction of nerve cells.

**neurocytoma** /noor′ōsītō′mə/ [Gk, *neuron* + *kytos,* cell, *oma,* tumor], a tumor composed of undifferentiated nerve cells that are usually ganglionic. Also called **neuroma.**

**neuroderm.** See **neuroectoderm.**

**neurodermatitis** /-dur′mətī′tis/ [Gk, *neuron* + *derma,* skin, *itis,* inflammation], a nonspecific, pruritic skin disorder seen in anxious, nervous individuals. Excoriations and lichenification are found on easily accessible, exposed areas of the body such as the forearms and forehead. Sometimes loosely (and incorrectly) applied to **atopic dermatitis.** See also *lichen simplex chronicus.*

**neurodevelopmental adaptation** /-dəvel′əpmen′təl/, a type of therapy that emphasizes the inhibition/integration of primitive postural patterns and promotes the development of normal postural reactions and achievement of normal tone. The therapy is used in the treatment of children with cerebral palsy.

**neuroectoderm** /noor′ō·ek′tədurm/ [Gk, *neuron* + *ektos,* outside, *derma,* skin], the part of the embryonic ectoderm that gives rise to the central and peripheral nervous systems, including some glial cells. **—neuroectodermal,** *adj.*

**neuroendocrine** /noor′ō·en′dəkrin/ [Gk, *neuron,* nerve, *endon,* within, *krinein,* to secrete], pertaining to or resembling the effects produced by endocrine glands strongly linked with the nervous system.

**neuroepithelioma** /noor′ō·ep′ithē′lē·ō′mə/ [Gk, *neuron* + *epi,* upon, *thele,* nipple, *oma,* tumor], an uncommon neoplasm of neuroepithelium in a sensory nerve. Also called **neuroepithelial tumor.**

**neurofibril** /-fī′bril/, a threadlike structure found in the cytoplasm of a neuron.

**neurofibrillary tangles** /-fī′briler′ē/, an intracellular clump of neurofibrils made of insoluble protein in the brain of a patient with Alzheimer's disease.

**neurofibroma** /noor′ōfībrō′mə/, *pl.* **neurofibromas, neurofibromata** [Gk, *neuron* + L, *fibra,* fiber; Gk, *oma,* tumor], a fibrous tumor of nerve tissue resulting from the abnormal proliferation of Schwann cells. Multiple growths in the peripheral nervous system are often associated with abnormalities in other tissues. See also **neurofibromatosis.**

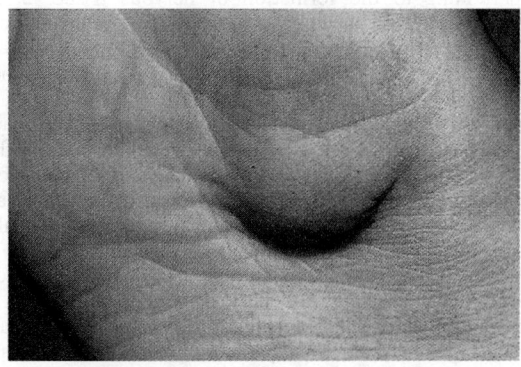

**Neurofibroma** (Weston, Lane, and Morrelli, 1996)

**neurofibromatosis** /noor′ōfī′brōmətō′sis/ [Gk, *neuron* + *fibra,* fiber; Gk, *oma,* tumor, *osis,* condition], a congenital condition transmitted as an autosomal-dominant trait, characterized by numerous neurofibromas of the nerves and skin; café-au-lait spots on the skin; and developmental anomalies of the muscles, bones, and viscera. Many large, pedunculated soft-tissue tumors may develop. Bone changes may result in skeletal deformities, especially curvature of the spine. Neurofibromas may develop in the alimentary tract, bladder, endocrine glands, and cranial nerves. Also called **multiple neuroma, neuromatosis, von Recklinghausen's disease.**

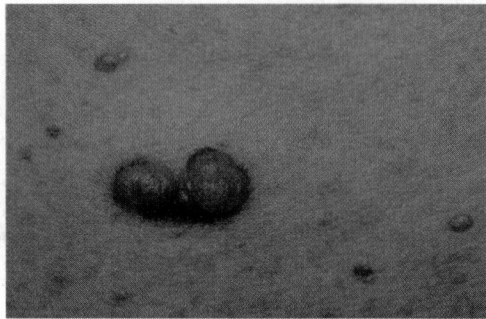

**Neurofibromatosis** *(Lemmi and Lemmi, 2000)*

**neurofilament** /nŏŏr′ō·fil′ə·ment/ [Gk, *neuron,* nerve + L, *filare,* to spin], a cytoplasmic filament approximately 10 nm in diameter occurring in the neurons; it has a cytoskeletal function and may be involved in the intracellular transport of metabolites.

**neurogen** /nŏŏr′əjən/ [Gk, *neuron* + *genein,* to produce], a substance within the early developing embryo that stimulates the primary organizer to initiate the formation of the neural plate, which gives rise to the primary axis of the body. See also **neurotransmitter.**

**neurogenesis** /-jen′əsis/ [Gk, *neuron* + *genesis,* origin], the formation of the tissue of the nervous system. —**neurogenetic,** *adj.*

**neurogenic** /-jen′ik/ [Gk, *neuron* + *genesis,* origin], **1.** pertaining to the formation of nervous tissue. **2.** the stimulation of nervous energy. **3.** originating in the nervous system.

**neurogenic arthropathy,** an abnormal condition associated with neural damage, characterized by the gradual and usually painless degeneration of a joint. One of the major causes of this condition is believed to be a minor injury that is disregarded by the affected individual because of a lack of sensation in the injured tissue. Inadequate rest and care aggravate such injuries and prevent proper healing. See also **neuropathic joint disease.**

**neurogenic bladder,** dysfunction of the urinary bladder caused by a lesion of the nervous system. Treatment is aimed at preventing infection, controlling incontinence, and preserving kidney function by enabling the bladder to empty completely and regularly. Kinds of neurogenic bladder are, **flaccid bladder, reflex bladder,** and **spastic bladder.** Also called **neuropathic bladder.**

**neurogenic claudication,** claudication accompanied by pain and paresthesias in the back, buttocks, and lower limbs that is relieved by stooping, caused by mechanical disturbances resulting from posture or by ischemia of the cauda equina.

**neurogenic fracture,** a fracture associated with the destruction of the nerve supply to a specific bone.

**neurogenic hoarseness,** a sign of unilateral vocal cord paralysis. It is asymptomatic, but there may be excessive air escape during speech as a result of incomplete closure of the glottis. Extra effort is required to generate enough air flow to make speech sounds. Untreated, there is a danger of aspiration pneumonia.

**neurogenic impotence,** penile erectile dysfunction caused by neurologic disorders. The disorders may involve the parasympathetic sacral spinal cord or the peripheral efferent autonomic fibers to the penis. See also **impotence, sexual dysfunction.**

**neurogenic shock,** a form of shock that results from peripheral vascular dilation.

**neuroglia** /nŏŏrog′lē·ə/ [Gk, *neuron* + *glia,* glue], the supporting or nonneuronal tissue cells of the central and peripheral nervous system. They perform the less specialized functions of the nerve network. Kinds of neuroglia include **astrocytes, oligodendroglia, microglia,** and **ependymal cells.** Compare **neuron.** —**neuroglial,** *adj.*

**neurography** /nŏŏrog′rəfē/, **1.** the study of the action potentials of the nerves. **2.** a technique for visualization of peripheral nerve activity by graphic representation of data obtained by media contrast radiographics or by electric recording.

**neurohormone** /nŏŏr′əhôr′mōn/, a hormone produced in neurosecretory cells such as those of the hypothalamus and released into the bloodstream, the cerebrospinal fluid, or intercellular spaces of the nervous system. The product may or may not be a true systemic hormone, such as epinephrine. When the hormone is not a true hormone, it may be a cell product that induces the release of a tropic hormone, which in turn stimulates an endocrine gland to release a systemic hormone. See also **neuromodulator, neurotransmitter.**

**neurohypophyseal hormone** /-hī′pōfiz′ē·əl/ [Gk, *neuron* + *hypo,* under, *phyein,* to grow], a hormone secreted by the posterior pituitary gland. Kinds of neurohypophyseal hormones are **oxytocin** and **vasopressin.** See also **pituitary gland.**

**neurohypophysis** /-hīpof′isis/ [Gk, *neuron* + *hypo,* under, *phyein,* to grow], the posterior lobe of the pituitary gland that is the release point of antidiuretic hormone (ADH), vasopressin, and oxytocin. Nervous stimulation from the hypothalamus controls the release of the substances into the blood. The neurohypophysis releases ADH when stimulated by the hypothalamus by an increase in the osmotic pressure of extracellular fluid in the body. The hormone acts on the cells in the distal and collecting tubules of the kidneys, making them more permeable to water and thus reducing the volume of urine. The neurohypophysis releases oxytocin under appropriate stimulation from the hypothalamus. Oxytocin produces powerful contractions of the pregnant uterus and causes milk to flow from lactating breasts. Stimulation of the nipples of the breast by a nursing infant triggers the release of this hormone. Also called **posterior pituitary gland.** Compare **adenohypophysis.**

**neuroimmunology** /nŏŏr′ō·im′yōōnol′əjē/ [Gk, *neuron* + L, *immunis,* freedom; Gk, *logos,* science], the study of relationships between the immune and nervous systems, such as autoimmune activity in neurologic diseases.

**neurol,** abbreviation for **neurology.**

**neurolemma.** See **neurilemma.**

**neurolepsis** /-lep′sis/ [Gk, *neuron* + *lepsis,* seizure], an altered state of consciousness, as induced by a neuroleptic agent, characterized by quiescence, reduced motor activity, decreased anxiety, and indifference to the surroundings. Sleep may occur, but usually the person can be aroused and can respond to commands.

**neurolepsy** /nŏŏr'əlep'sē/, a mental state characterized by the blocking of autonomic reflexes, as in hypnosis or antipsychotic drug-induced disorders.

**neurolept.** See **neuroleptic drug.**

**neuroleptanalgesia** /-lept'anəljē'zē·ə/ [Gk, *neuron + lepsis*, seizure, *a + algos*, without pain], a form of analgesia achieved by the concurrent administration of a neuroleptic such as droperidol and an analgesic such as fentanyl. Anxiety, motor activity, and sensitivity to painful stimuli are reduced; the person is quiet and indifferent to surroundings and is able to respond to commands. If nitrous oxide with oxygen is also administered, neuroleptanalgesia can be converted to neuroleptanesthesia.

**neuroleptanesthesia** /-lept'anəsthē'zhə/ [Gk, *neuron + lepsis*, seizure, *anaisthesia*, lack of feeling], a form of anesthesia achieved by the administration of a neuroleptic agent, a narcotic analgesic, and nitrous oxide with oxygen. Induction of anesthesia is slow, but consciousness returns quickly after the inhalation of nitrous oxide is stopped.

**neuroleptic** /-lep'tik/ [Gk, *neuron + lepsis*, seizure], **1.** pertaining to neurolepsis. **2.** See **neuroleptic drug.**

**neuroleptic anesthesia** [Gk, *neuron*, nerve, *lepsis*, seizure, *anaisthesia*, lack of feeling], a form of anesthesia induced by an injection of a butyrophenone derivative with a narcotic analgesic.

**neuroleptic drug,** a substance that produces a sedating or tranquilizing effect. Also called **neurolept, neuroleptic.** See also **antipsychotic, tranquilizer.**

**neuroleptic malignant syndrome** [Gk, *neuron*, nerve, *lepsis*, seizure; L, *malignus*, bad disposition; Gk, *syn*, together, *dromos*, course], a complication of psychotherapy with neuroleptic drugs given in therapeutic doses. It is characterized by hypertonicity, pallor, dyskinesia, hyperthermia, incontinence, unstable blood pressure, and pulmonary congestion.

**neurolinguistic programing** /-ling·gwis'tik/, a communication approach based on a conceptualization of levels of experience within the person and levels of the self. It involves both verbal and nonverbal messages, sensory experience, and awareness or perception through behavior patterns that can be observed and perceived.

**neurolinguistics** /noor'ō·ling·gwis'tiks/ [Gk, *neuron* + L, *lingua*, tongue], the study of language acquisition, processing, and production at the neurological level.

**neurologic, neurological.** See **neurology.**

**neurological status,** a nursing outcome from the Nursing Outcomes Classification (NOC) defined as the extent to which the peripheral and central nervous systems receive, process, and respond to internal and external stimuli. See also **Nursing Outcomes Classification.**

**neurological status: autonomic,** a nursing outcome from the Nursing Outcomes Classification (NOC) defined as the extent to which the nervous system coordinate visceral function. See also **Nursing Outcomes Classification.**

**neurological status: central motor control,** a nursing outcome from the Nursing Outcomes Classification (NOC) defined as the extent to which skeletal muscle activity (body movement) is coordinated by the central nervous system. See also **Nursing Outcomes Classification.**

**neurological status: consciousness,** a nursing outcome from the Nursing Outcomes Classification (NOC) defined as the extent to which an individual arouses, orients, and attends to the environment. See also **Nursing Outcomes Classification.**

**neurological status: cranial sensory/motor function,** a nursing outcome from the Nursing Outcomes Classification (NOC) defined as the extent to which cranial nerves convey sensory and motor function. See also **Nursing Outcomes Classification.**

**neurological status: spinal sensory/motor function,** a nursing outcome from the Nursing Outcomes Classification (NOC) defined as the extent to which spinal nerves convey sensory and motor information. See also **Nursing Outcomes Classification.**

**neurologic assessment** /-loj'ik/ [Gk, *neuron + logos*, science; L, *icus*, like, *adsidere*, to approximate], an evaluation of the patient's neurologic status and symptoms.

■ METHOD: If alert and oriented, the patient is asked about instances of weakness, numbness, headaches, pain, tremors, nervousness, irritability, or drowsiness. Information is elicited regarding loss of memory, periods of confusion, hallucinations, and episodes of loss of consciousness. The patient's general appearance, facial expression, attention span, responses to verbal and painful stimuli, emotional status, coordination, balance, cognition, and ability to follow commands are noted. Assessment of cranial nerves and deep tendon reflexes is included. If the patient is disoriented, stuporous, or comatose, demonstrated signs of these states are recorded. Observations are made of skin color and temperature; pupillary size, equality, dilation, and reactions to light; respiratory rate, rhythm, and quality; and chest movements and breath sounds. The pulse is checked; ears and nose are examined for possible drainage; strength of the handgrip is tested; and the extremities' sensations and voluntary and involuntary motions are assessed. Urinary output is determined for evidence of polyuria, and the patient's speech is evaluated for signs of slurring and aphasia. Included in the record are concurrent diseases such as hypertension, cancer, and coarctation of the aorta; past illnesses associated with head trauma; seizures, motor, sensory, or emotional disturbances; loss of consciousness; and neurologic, medical, or surgical procedures. Pertinent to the assessment are the patient's sleep pattern; medication; personality changes; relationships with family and friends; and a family history of seizures, stroke, mental illness, tumors, or sudden death. Diagnostic aids that may be required for a complete evaluation include a lumbar puncture, complete blood count, myelogram, magnetic resonance imaging, echo-

**Equipment for neurologic examination**

| Item | Purpose |
|---|---|
| Cottonball, disposable safety pin | Light touch, pain sensation, and localization |
| Tongue blade | Tongue strength, gag reflex |
| Tuning fork (512 cps) | Vibration sense |
| Ophthalmoscope | Optic nerve, pupil constriction |
| Reflex hammer | Deep tendon reflexes |
| Pencil and paper | Fine coordinated movements |
| Printed material | Reading and comprehension |
| Optional | |
|    Test tubes for cold and warm water | Temperature sensation |
|    Aromatic substances | Olfaction |
|    Sweet, sour substances | Taste |
|    Calipers | Two-point discrimination |

Modified from Barkauskas VH et al: *Health & physical assessment,* ed 2, St Louis, 1998, Mosby.

encephalogram, brain scan, computerized tomogram, and determinations of glucose, fluid, and electrolyte levels.

■ INTERVENTIONS: The nurse may conduct the interview to obtain subjective data, examines the patient, and assembles the pertinent background information and results of the diagnostic tests.

■ OUTCOME CRITERIA: A careful neurologic assessment is an important aid to the neurologist in establishing a diagnosis and the course of treatment.

**neurologic examination,** a systematic examination of the nervous system, including an assessment of mental status, of the function of each of the cranial nerves, of sensory and neuromuscular function, of the reflexes, and of proprioception and other cerebellar functions.

**neurologic monitoring,** a nursing intervention from the Nursing Interventions Classification (NIC) defined as collection and analysis of patient data to prevent or minimize neurologic complications. See also **Nursing Interventions Classification.**

**neurologist** /nŏŏrol′əjist/, a physician who specializes in the nervous system and its disorders.

**neurology (neurol)** /nŏŏrol′əjē/ [Gk, *neuron* + *logos,* science], the field of medicine that deals with the nervous system and its disorders. —**neurologic, neurological,** *adj.* **neurologist,** *n.*

**neuroma** /nŏŏrō′mə/, *pl.* **neuromas, neuromata** [Gk, *neuron* + *oma,* tumor], a benign neoplasm composed chiefly of neurons and nerve fibers, usually arising from a nerve tissue. Pain radiating from the lesion to the periphery of the affected nerve is usually intermittent but may become continuous and severe.

**-neuroma,** combining form meaning a 'tumor made up of nerve cells and fibers': *angiomyoneuroma, inoneuroma, myoneuroma.*

**neuroma cutis,** a neoplasm in the skin that contains nerve tissue and may be extremely sensitive to painful stimuli.

**neuromas, neuromata.** See **neuroma.**

**neuroma telangiectodes.** See **nevoid neuroma.**

**neuromatosis** /nŏŏr′ōmətō′sis/ [Gk, *neuron* + *oma,* tumor, *osis,* condition], a neoplastic disease characterized by numerous neuromas. Also called **multiple neuroma.** See also **neurofibromatosis.**

**neuromechanism** /-mek′əniz′əm/, a neurologic system whose components work together to produce a central nervous system function.

**neuromodulator,** a substance that alters nerve impulse transmission.

**neuromotor** /nŏŏr′ōmō′tər/ [Gk, *neuron,* nerve; L, *mover,* to move], pertaining to both the nerves and muscles or to nerve impulses transmitted to muscles.

**neuromuscular** /nŏŏr′ōmus′kyŏŏlər/ [Gk, *neuron* + L, *musculus,* muscle], pertaining to the nerves and the muscles.

**neuromuscular blockade,** the inhibition of a muscular contraction activated by the nervous system, possibly resulting in muscle weakness or paralysis.

**neuromuscular blocking agent,** a chemical substance that interferes locally with the transmission or reception of impulses from motor nerves to skeletal muscles. Nondepolarizing agents such as metocurine, pancuronium, and tubocurarine competitively block the transmitter action of acetylcholine at the postjunctional membrane. Depolarizing blocking agents such as succinylcholine chloride compete with acetylcholine for cholinergic receptors of the motor end plate. Neuromuscular blocking agents are used to induce muscle relaxation in anesthesia, endotracheal intubation, and electroshock therapy and as adjuncts in the treatment of

tetanus, encephalitis, and poliomyelitis. Neuromuscular blocking drugs can cause bronchospasm, hyperthermia, hypotension, or respiratory paralysis and are used with caution, especially in patients with myasthenia gravis or with renal, hepatic, or pulmonary impairment, and in elderly and debilitated individuals. See also **muscle relaxant.**

**neuromuscular electric stimulator (NMES),** device for improving or modulating muscular activation. It may be a portable unit for home treatment of a patient over a long period of time or a large clinical model capable of producing a wider variety of waveforms and modulations of the stimulus. The NMES generates electrical pulses that produce controlled muscle contractions similar to those that occur physiologically. Unless nerve degeneration has occurred, muscles that are weak or paralyzed because of central nervous system involvement should contract when NMES is applied. The procedure may be tested first on an uninvolved muscle on the same or another extremity to establish a normal response.

**neuromuscular junction,** the area of contact between the ends of a large myelinated nerve fiber and a fiber of skeletal muscle. Also called **myoneural junction.** See also **motor end plate, myelin, nerve.**

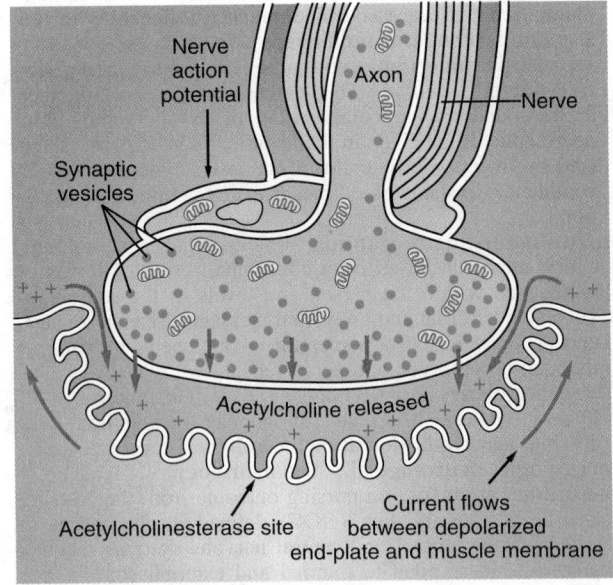

**Neuromuscular junction** *(Thompson et al, 1997)*

**neuromuscular spindle,** any one of a number of small bundles of delicate muscular fibers, enclosed by a capsule, in which sensory nerve fibers terminate. The spindles vary in length from 0.8 to 5 mm, accommodating as many as four large myelinated nerve fibers that pierce the capsule and lose their myelin sheaths. The nerve fibers end as naked axons encircling the intrafusal fibers with flattened expansions or ovoid disks.

**neuromyal transmission** /-mī′əl/ [Gk, *neuron* + *mys,* muscle; L, *transmittere,* to transmit], the passage of excitation from a motor neuron to a muscle fiber at the myoneural junction.

**neuromyelitis** /nŏŏr′ōmī′əlī′tis/ [Gk, *neuron* + *myelos,* marrow, *itis,* inflammation], an abnormal condition characterized by inflammation of the spinal cord and peripheral nerves.

**neuron** /noŏr′on/ [Gk, nerve], the basic nerve cell of the nervous system, containing a nucleus within a cell body and extending one or more processes. Neurons can be classified according to the direction in which they conduct impulses or according to the number of processes they extend. Sensory neurons transmit nerve impulses toward the spinal cord and the brain. Motor neurons transmit nerve impulses from the brain and the spinal cord to the muscles and the glandular tissue. Multipolar neurons, bipolar neurons, and unipolar neurons are classified according to the number of processes they extend to the different kinds of neurons. Multipolar neurons have one axon and several dendrites, as do most of the neurons in the brain and the spinal cord. Bipolar neurons, which are less numerous than the other types, have one axon and only one dendrite. Unipolar neurons have one axon and no dendrites. All primary sensory afferents and some autonomic neurons are unipolar. All neurons have one axon and most have one or more dendrites and have a slightly gray color when clustered, as in the nuclei of the brain and the spinal cord. As the generators and carriers of nerve impulses, neurons function according to electrochemical processes involving positively charged sodium and potassium ions and the changing electrical potential of the extracellular and the intracellular fluid of the neuron. Also spelled **neurone.**

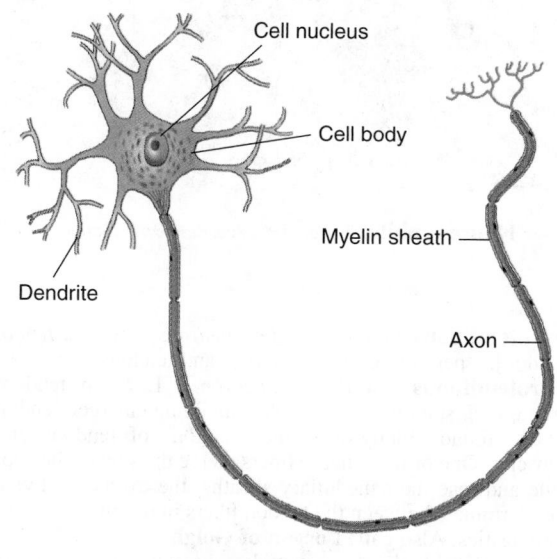

**Neuron** *(Leonard, 2001)*

**neuronal** /noŏr′ənəl, noŏrō′nəl/ [Gk, *neuron,* nerve], pertaining to or resembling a neuron.

**neuronal antibody,** an antibody found in the cerebrospinal fluid of most systemic lupus erythematosus (SLE) patients with neuropsychiatric manifestations, and in some SLE patients without such manifestations.

**neuronal sprouting,** the growth of axons or dendrites from a damaged neuron or from an intact neuron that projects to an area denervated by damage to other neurons.

**neurone.** See **neuron.**

**neuronitis** /noŏr′ənī′tis/ [Gk, *neuron* + *itis,* inflammation], inflammation of a nerve or a nerve cell, especially the cells and the roots of the spinal nerves.

**neuroparalysis** /-pəral′isis/, loss of muscle power as a result of a disorder involving the part of the nervous system affecting the muscle.

**neuropathic.** See **neuropathy.**

**neuropathic bladder.** See **neurogenic bladder.**

**neuropathic joint disease** /-path′ik/ [Gk, *neuron* + *pathos,* disease], a chronic progressive degenerative disease of one or more joints, characterized by swelling, joint instability, hemorrhage, heat, and atrophic and hypertrophic changes in the bone. Pain is usually less severe than would be expected by the appearance of the joint on an x-ray film. The disease is the result of an underlying neurologic disorder, such as tabes dorsalis from syphilis, diabetic neuropathy, leprosy, or congenital absence or depression of pain sensation. Early recognition of the disease and prophylactic protection of the joint may prevent further damage in some cases. Surgical reconstruction is not usually effective because healing is slow. Amputation may be necessary. Also called **Charcot's joint.**

**neuropathic pain syndrome,** a condition of autonomic hyperactivity that results in sharp, stinging, or stabbing pain. The disorder is usually noninflammatory but may result in the destruction of peripheral nerve tissue. It may also be accompanied by changes in skin color, temperature, and edema.

**neuropathy** /noŏrop′əthē/ [Gk, *neuron* + *pathos,* disease], inflammation or degeneration of the peripheral nerves, such as that associated with lead poisoning. **—neuropathic,** *adj.*

**neuropeptide** /noor′ō·pep′tīd/, any of several types of molecules found in brain tissue, composed of short chains of amino acids; they include endorphins, enkephalins, vasopressin, and others. They are often localized in axon terminals at synapses and are classified as putative neurotransmitters, although some are also hormones.

**neuropeptide Y (NPY),** a natural substance that acts on the brain to stimulate eating. Laboratory animals injected with NPY greatly overeat; substances that block the NPY receptor reduce the appetite. Leptin, a hormone that stimulates weight loss, reduces the output of NPY from the hypothalamus, a major production center. Another natural substance that stimulates the urge to eat is peptide YY. In animal experiments it has appeared to be at least as potent as NPY.

**neurophysin** /-fiz′in/, one of a group of proteins released from the posterior pituitary gland at the same time as the hormone vasopressin or oxytocin. It is cleared from a larger protein of which vasopressin or oxytocin is a part.

**neuroplasty** /noŏr′əplas′tē/ [Gk, *neuron,* nerve, *plassein,* to mold], plastic surgery to repair a nerve.

**neuroplegia** /noŏr′ōplē′jē·ə/ [Gk, *neuron* + *plege,* stroke], nerve paralysis caused by disease, injury, or the effect of neuroleptic drugs.

**neuropore** /noŏr′ōpôr/ [Gk, *neuron* + *poros,* pore], the opening at each end of the neural tube during early embryonic development, leading from the central canal of the neural tube to the exterior. The closure of these apertures as the tube grows and differentiates occurs with such precision that they are used to indicate horizons XI and XII in the systematic anatomic charting of human embryonic development. Kinds of neuropores are **anterior neuropore** and **posterior neuropore.** See also **horizon, neural tube formation.**

**neuropraxia** /-prak′sē·ə/ [Gk, *neuron,* nerve, *prassein,* to do], a condition in which a nerve remains in place after a severe injury, although it no longer transmits impulses.

Cell nucleus

Cell body

Myelin sheath

Dendrite

Axon

**neuroprotection** /nŏŏr′ō·prō·tek′shən/, protection against **neurotoxicity.**

**neuropsychiatrist** /-sīkī′ətrist/, a physician who deals with the relationship between neural processes and psychiatric disorders.

**neuropsychiatry** /-sīkī′ətrē/, a branch of medicine that deals with problems of psychiatry as it relates to the neurophysiology of brain functions.

**neuroradiography** /-rā′dē·og′rəfē/, the radiographic examination of the tissues of the nervous system.

**neuroradiology** /-rā′dē·ol′əjē/, the branch of radiology concerned with diagnosing diseases of the nervous system.

**neurorrhaphy** /nŏŏrôr′əfē/ [Gk, *neuron*, nerve, *rhaphe*, suture], a surgical procedure to suture a severed nerve.

**neurosarcoidosis** /-sär′koidō′sis/, a granulomatous disease that may involve any part of the nervous system but most commonly affects the cranial and spinal nerves. Cranial nerve involvement may result in facial paralysis, whereas spinal nerve involvement may manifest as mononeuritis multiplex. If the central nervous system is affected, the vasculature of the brain may be damaged, resulting in stroke.

**neurosarcoma** /-särkō′mə/ [Gk, *neuron* + *sarx*, flesh, *oma*, tumor], a malignant neoplasm composed of nerve, connective, and vascular tissues. Also called **malignant neuroma.**

**neuroscience** /nŏŏr′ōsī′əns/ [Gk, *neuron*, nerve; L, *scientia*], the study of neurology and related subjects, including neuroanatomy, neurophysiology, neuropharmacology, and neurosurgery.

**neurosis** /nŏŏrō′sis/, *pl.* **neuroses,** former name for a category of mental disorders in which the symptoms are distressing to the person, reality testing is intact, behavior does not violate gross social norms, and there is no apparent organic cause. Classified in *DSM-IV* under **anxiety disorders, dissociative disorders, mood disorders, sexual disorders,** and **somatoform disorders.**

**-neurosis,** combining form meaning a 'disease of the nerves' or a 'mental disorder': *angioneurosis, psychoneurosis, synneurosis.*

**neuroskeleton** /-skel′ətən/ [Gk, *neuron*, nerve, *skeletos*, dried up], the parts of the skeleton that surround or otherwise protect the nervous system, particularly the skull and vertebrae.

**neurosome** /nŏŏr′ō·sōm/ [Gk, *neuron*, nerve + *soma*, body], **1.** the body of a neuron. **2.** any of the minute particles found in the protoplasm of a neuron.

**neurosurgery** /-sur′jərē/ [Gk, *neuron* + *cheirourgia*, surgery], any surgery involving the brain, spinal cord, or peripheral nerves. Brain surgery is performed to treat a wound, remove a tumor or foreign body, relieve pressure in intracranial hemorrhage, excise an abscess, treat parkinsonism, or relieve pain. Before surgery skull x-ray films and a ventriculogram or an arteriogram may be taken; a diagnostic electroencephalogram, lumbar tap, or brain scan are done. A blood type and crossmatch are done. Parenteral corticosteroids are given if cerebral edema is present, and urea may be given to reduce intracranial pressure. Narcotics and hypnotics are avoided, and the nurse must confirm any that are ordered. No enemas are given. Light general or local anesthesia is used, occasionally with hypothermia. After surgery, vital signs and changes in the level of consciousness, speech, and muscle strength are monitored cosely. Any yellowish drainage from the wound may be cerebrospinal fluid and is reported immediately. Sterile dressing technique is essential. Kinds of brain surgery include craniotomy, lobotomy, and hypophysectomy. Surgery of the spine is performed to correct a defect, remove a tumor, repair a ruptured interverte-bral disk, or relieve pain. Before surgery computed tomography or magnetic resonance imaging scans are made, and a blood type and crossmatch are done. General anesthesia or a spinal block is used. After surgery the nurse keeps the patient's spine in good alignment. Return of sensation and motor function are monitored carefully. Kinds of spinal surgery include fusion and laminectomy. Surgery on the peripheral nerves is performed to remove a tumor, relieve pain, or reconnect a severed nerve. After surgery the nurse observes closely the return of sensation to the area. One kind of nerve surgery is **sympathectomy.**

**neurosyphilis** /-sif′ilis/ [Gk, *neuron* + *sys,* hog, *philein,* to love], infection of the central nervous system by *Treponema pallidum,* the causative agent of syphilis, which may invade the meninges and cerebrovascular system. If the brain tissue is affected, general paresis may result; if the spinal cord is infected, tabes dorsalis may result. See also **syphilis,** *Treponema pallidum.* —**neurosyphilitic,** *adj.*

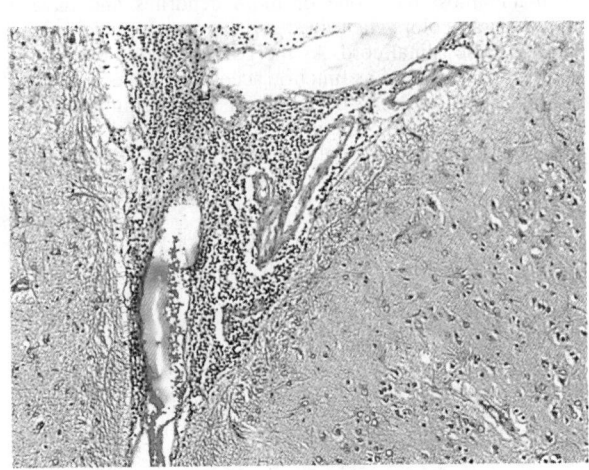

**Neurosyphilis** *(Farrar, 1993/courtesy Dr. P. Garen)*

**neurotendinous** /-ten′dinəs/ [Gk, *neuron,* nerve; L, *tendo,* tendon], pertaining to both nerves and tendons.

**neurotendinous spindle** [Gk, *neuron* + L, *tendo,* tendon; AS, *spinel,* spindle], a capsule containing enlarged tendon fibers, found chiefly near the junctions of tendons and muscles. One or more nerve fibers pierce the side of the capsule and lose their medullary sheaths; the axons subdivide and terminate between the tendon fibers in irregular disks or varicosities. Also called **organ of Golgi.**

**neurotensin** /-ten′sin/, a peptide neurotransmitter found in various parts of the brain. It is involved in vasodilation, hypotension, and pain perception.

**neurotensinoma** /-ten′sinō′mə/, a neuroendocrine tumor of the GI tract. Its major secreted product is neurotensin. The tumor originates in nonbeta islet cells but, unlike other neuroendocrine tumors, it has no distinguishing clinical features.

**neurotic** /n(y)ŏŏrot′ik/ [Gk, *neuron* + *osis,* condition; L, *icus,* like], **1.** pertaining to neurosis. **2.** pertaining to the nerves. **3.** one who is afflicted with a neurosis. **4.** *informal.* an emotionally unstable person.

**-neurotic, 1.** combining form meaning 'a (specified) abnormal condition of the nerves': *angioneurotic, aponeurotic,* *vasoneurotic.* **2.** combining form meaning 'an emotional disorder': *hyperneurotic, psychoneurotic.*

**neurotic depression.** See **dysthymic disorder.**

**neurotic personality** [Gk, *neuron*, nerve, *osis*, condition; L, *personalis*, of a person], a disposition characterized by traits and tendencies that increase the likelihood of a specific neurotic behavior. For example, the orderly, cautious, meticulous person may be prone to development of an obsessive-compulsive disorder.

**neurotmesis** /noŏr'ŏtmē'sis/ [Gk, *neuron* + *tmesis*, cutting apart], a peripheral nerve injury in which the nerve is completely disrupted by laceration or traction. It requires surgical approximation, with unpredictable recovery.

**neurotologic** /noŏr'ŏtōloj'ik/, pertaining to the study of the elements of the ear as they relate to the brain and nervous system. Also **neurotological.**

**neurotology** /noŏr'ŏtol'əjē/, a branch of otology concerned with those parts of the nervous system related to the ear, especially the inner ear and associated brainstem structures. Also called **otoneurology.**

**neurotomy** /noŏrot'əmē/, the surgical severing of a nerve or nerves.

**neurotoxic** /noŏr'ŏtok'sik/, having a poisonous effect on nerves and nerve cells, such as when ingested lead degenerates peripheral nerves.

**neurotoxicity** /-toksis'itē/ [Gk, *neuron*, nerve, *toxikon*, poison], the ability of a drug or other agent to destroy or damage nervous tissue.

**neurotoxin** /noŏr'ŏtok'sin/ [Gk, *neuron* + *toxikon*, poison], a toxin that acts directly on the tissues of the central nervous system, traveling along the axis cylinders of the motor nerves to the brain. The toxin may be secreted in the venom of certain snakes, or it may be present on the spines of a shell or in the flesh of fish or shellfish; it may be produced by certain bacteria or by the cellular disintegration of certain bacteria.

**neurotransmitter** /-transmit'ər/ [Gk, *neuron* + L, *transmittere*, to transmit], any one of numerous chemicals that modify or result in the transmission of nerve impulses between synapses. Neurotransmitters are released from synaptic knobs into synaptic clefts and bridge the gap between presynaptic and postsynaptic neurons. Each vesicle within a synaptic knob stores as many as 10,000 neurotransmitter molecules. When a nerve impulse reaches a synaptic knob, thousands of neurotransmitter molecules squirt into the synaptic cleft and bind to specific receptors. This flow allows an associated diffusion of potassium and sodium ions that causes an action potential. Excitatory neurotransmitters decrease the negativity of postsynaptic membrane potentials; inhibitory neurotransmitters increase such potentials. Kinds of neurotransmitters include **acetylcholine, gamma-aminobutyric acid,** and **norepinephrine.**

**neurotripsy** /-trip'sē/, the surgical crushing of a nerve.

**neurotrophic** /-trof'ik/, nourishing nerve cells.

**neurotropic viruses** /-trop'ik/ [Gk, *neuron*, nerve, *tropein*, to turn, *virus*, poison], viruses with an unexplained attraction to nerve tissue. The predilection also applies to certain toxic chemicals.

**neurotropism** /noŏrot'rəpiz'əm/ [Gk, *neuron*, nerve, *trepein*, to turn], **1.** the tendency for certain microorganisms, poisons, and nutrients to be attracted to nervous tissue. **2.** the tendency of basic dyes to be attracted to nervous tissue.

**neurula** /noŏr'ələ/, *pl.* **neurulas, neurulae** [Gk, *neuron*, nerve], an early embryo during the period of neurulation when the nervous system tissue begins to differentiate. The embryo at this level of growth represents a third stage in embryonic development, after the morula and blastocyst stages in humans and higher animals and the blastula and gastrula stages in lower animals. In humans the neurula stage occurs from about 19 to 26 days after fertilization.

**neurulation** /-ā'shən/ [Gk, *neuron* + L, *atus*, process], the development of the neural plate and the processes involved with its subsequent closure to form the neural tube during the early stages of embryonic development. See also **neural tube formation.**

**neutral** /n(y)oo'trəl/ [L, *neutralis*, neuter], the state exactly between two opposing values, qualities, or properties; for example, in electricity a neutral state is one in which there is neither a positive nor a negative charge; in chemistry a neutral state is one in which a substance is neither acid nor alkaline. See also **acid, base, pH.**

**neutralization** /-īzā'shən/ [L, *neutralis* + Gk, *izein*, to cause], the interaction between an acid and a base that produces a solution that is neither acidic nor basic. The usual products of neutralization are a salt and water.

**neutral rotation,** the position of a limb that is turned neither toward nor away from the body's midline. When a person is supine and the leg is neutrally rotated, the toes should point straight up.

**neutral thermal environment,** an environment created by any method or apparatus to maintain the normal body temperature to minimize oxygen consumption and caloric expenditure, such as in an incubator or Isolette for a premature, sick, or low–birth weight infant. See also **incubator, Isolette.**

**neutron** /n(y)oo'tron/ [L, *neuter*, neither; Gk, *elektron*, amber], (in physics) an elementary particle that is a constituent of the nuclei of all elements except the $^1$H form of hydrogen. It has no electric charge and is approximately the same size as a proton. Compare **electron, proton.** See also **atom.**

**neutron activation analysis,** the analysis of elements in a specimen performed by exposing it to neutron irradiation. The irradiation converts many elements in the specimen to radioactive forms which can be identified by their emissions of radiation. The method has limited application to human and animal studies.

**neutropenia** /noo'trōpē'nē·ə/ [L, *neuter*, neither; Gk, *penia*, poverty], an abnormal decrease in the number of neutrophils in the blood. The decrease may be relative or absolute. Neutropenia is associated with acute leukemia, infection, rheumatoid arthritis, vitamin B$_{12}$ deficiency, and chronic splenomegaly. Compare **leukopenia.** See also **neutrophil.**

**neutrophil** /noo'trəfil/ [L, *neuter* + Gk, *philein*, to love], a polymorphonuclear, granular leukocyte that stains easily with neutral dyes. The nucleus stains dark blue and contains three to five lobes connected by slender threads of chromatin. The cytoplasm contains fine, inconspicuous granules. Neutrophils are the circulating white blood cells essential for phagocytosis and proteolysis by which bacteria, cellular debris, and solid particles are removed and destroyed. A neutrophil count ≤ 500 may be life-threatening. See also **basophil, eosinophil, granulocyte, polymorphonuclear leukocyte.**

**neutrophil alkaline phosphatase.** See **leukocyte alkaline phosphatase.**

**neutrophilia** /-fil'yə/, an elevated number of neutrophils in the blood, a common cause of leukocytosis.

**neutrophilic leukemia.** See **polymorphocytic leukemia.**

**Neviaser procedure,** the surgical transfer of a coracoacromial ligament to the clavicle for the repair of an acromioclavicular separation.

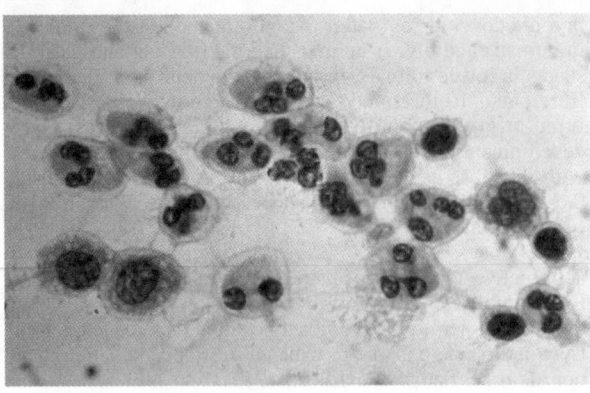

**Neutrophil** (McKee, 1997)

**nevirapine,** an antiretroviral nonnucleoside reverse transcriptase inhibitor.

■ INDICATIONS: It is prescribed in the treatment of human immunodeficiency virus infection.

■ CONTRAINDICATIONS: The drug should not be given to patients with an allergy or sensitivity to the medication. When used alone, there is a potential for viral resistance development.

■ ADVERSE EFFECTS: The side effects most often reported include rash, drug fever, and diarrhea.

**nevoid amentia.** See **Sturge-Weber syndrome.**

**nevoid basal cell carcinoma syndrome** /nē'void/, an inherited form of premalignant skin lesion. It is an autosomal-dominant trait, but the cause is unknown. It is associated with other abnormalities of the skin or bone, the nervous system, the eyes, and the reproductive system. It affects persons under the age of 20 and is accompanied by palmar pits, mandibular cysts, bifid ribs, and other birth defects.

**nevoid neuroma** [L, *naevus,* birthmark; Gk, *eidos,* form], a tumor of nerve tissue that contains numerous small blood vessels. Also called **neuroma telangiectodes.**

**nevus** /nē'vəs/ [L, *naevus,* birthmark], a pigmented congenital skin blemish that is usually benign but may become cancerous. Any change in color, size, or texture or any bleeding or itching of a nevus merits investigation. Also spelled **naevus.** Also called **birthmark, mole.** See also **blue nevus, junction nevus, nevus flammeus.**

**nevus avaneus,** See **spider telangiectasia.**

**nevus flammeus** /flam'ē·əs/, a flat capillary hemangioma that is present at birth and that varies from pale red to deep reddish purple. It most commonly occurs on the occiput and

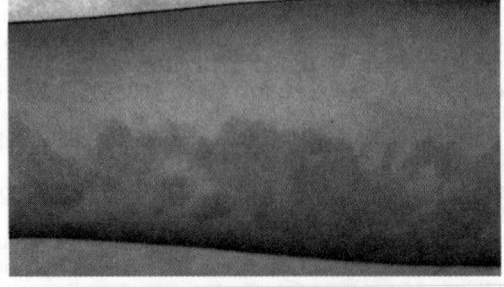

**Nevus flammeus** (Lemmi and Lemmi, 2000)

rarely causes any problems. If the lesion is on any other part of the body, it tends to be darker colored and, unlike the scalp lesions, does not regress spontaneously. These lesions most often occur on the face. The depth of the color depends on whether the superficial, middle, or deep dermal vessels are involved. On the face the lesion persists and develops a thick verrucous nodular surface. Nevus flammeus is usually unilateral, following the distribution of a cutaneous nerve. If the lesion is on the middle of the face, Sturge-Weber syndrome is suspected. Treatment is often not satisfactory. Camouflage cosmetics are used to cover the lesion, and the treatment of choice. Also called **port-wine stain.**

**nevus sebaceus of Jadassohn,** a congenital skin neoplasm with several cutaneous tissue elements. The most common location is the scalp, face, or neck. It may appear as a yellow or tan waxy patch of alopecia at birth. During puberty the lesion becomes raised, thick, and verrucous. It is usually treated with local excision. Untreated, the lesion may remain benign or become a malignant growth in later life.

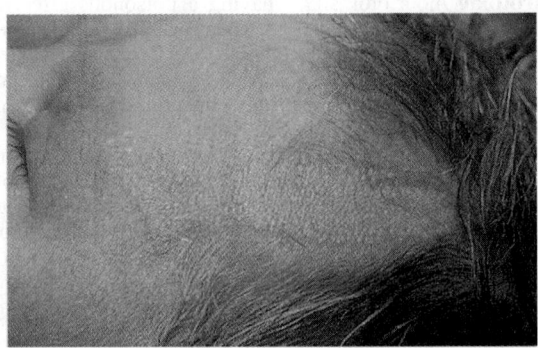

**Nevus sebaceus of Jadassohn**
(Weston, Lane, and Morrelli, 1996)

**nevus vascularis.** See **capillary hemangioma.**

**New Ballard Score,** a system of newborn assessment of gestational maturation. It provides a valid estimation of postnatal maturation for preterm infants with gestational ages greater than 20 weeks and covers a dozen categories, including posture, arm recoil, popliteal angle, skin, plantar surface, and genitals.

**newborn** [AS, *niwe,* new, *boren,* to bear], **1.** recently born. **2.** a recently born infant; a neonate.

**newborn adaptation,** a nursing outcome from the Nursing Outcomes Classification (NOC) defined as the adaptation to the extrauterine environment by a physiologically mature newborn during the first 28 days. See also **Nursing Outcomes Classification.**

**newborn care,** a nursing intervention from the Nursing Interventions Classification (NIC) defined as management of neonate during the transition to extrauterine life and subsequent period of stabilization. See also **Nursing Interventions Classification.**

**newborn intrapartal care,** care of the newborn in the delivery area during the time after birth before the mother and infant are transferred to the postpartum unit. See also **intrapartal care, postpartal care.**

■ METHOD: The nasopharynx and mouth may be suctioned to remove excess mucus as the head is born. Depending on the preference and condition of the mother and the policies of the maternity service, the baby may then be placed on the mother's abdomen and covered with a warm, dry blanket or taken by the nurse to an infant warmer. Apgar scores are assigned at 1 and at 5 minutes of age; less commonly another is assigned at 10 minutes of age. The baby is handled gently and quietly and may be put to breast if the mother wishes; bright lights are often avoided, and maternal contact is encouraged.

■ INTERVENTIONS: The nurse is usually the first person to observe and examine the baby. Most newborns are healthy and normal; if abnormal function is observed, expert assistance may be summoned and emergency measures, including tracheal suction with suction equipment and administration of oxygen by ventilator or mask, are initiated. If there are no problems, the nurse may instill erythromycin drops in the conjunctival sacs of the eyes, trim and clamp the umbilical cord, administer an injection of vitamin K, obtain footprints for identification, and diaper and wrap the baby. If the baby needs to be transferred to a nursery or special care facility, the nurse accompanies the infant and acts as the initial liaison for the mother with the nursery.

■ OUTCOME CRITERIA: Most infants born at term are healthy and do not need any medical intervention. Hemorrhage from the umbilical cord, difficult respiration, imperforate anus, endocrine dysfunction, and various other abnormal conditions may occur; but, if a baby has good color, is alert, and can cry, suck, urinate, defecate, and respond to sound and light, the nurse may reassure the mother that the baby is almost invariably healthy and normal. The individuality of each infant is remarkable and may be pointed out to the mother.

**newborn monitoring,** a nursing intervention from the Nursing Interventions Classification (NIC) defined as measurement and interpretation of physiologic status of the neonate the first 24 hours after delivery. See also **Nursing Interventions Classification.**

**new drug,** a drug for which the Food and Drug Administration requires premarketing approval.

***New England Journal of Medicine (NEJM),*** a weekly professional medical journal that publishes findings of medical research and articles about controversial political and ethical issues in the practice of medicine.

**new growth,** a neoplasm or tumor.

**Newman, Margaret A.,** a nursing theorist who contributed to the study of nursing theories and models by defining three approaches to the discovery of nursing theory: "borrowing" of theories from related disciplines, analyzing nursing practice situations in search of conceptual relationships, and creating new conceptual systems from which theories can be derived.

**newspaper sign.** See **thumb sign.**

**newton** /n(y)ōō′tən/ [Isaac Newton, English scientist, 1642–1727], a unit of force in the SI system that would impart an acceleration to 1 kilogram of mass of 1 meter per second per second.

**new tuberculin** [ME, *newe* + L, *tuber,* swelling], an extract of the tubercle bacillus from which all soluble material has been removed and glycerin added.

**New World leishmaniasis.** See **American leishmaniasis.**

**New World typhus.** See **murine typhus.**

**nexus** /nek′səs/ *pl.* nexus [L, bond], **1.** a bond, especially one between members of a series or group. 2 see **gap junction.**

**Nezelof's syndrome** /nez′əlofs/ [Christian Nezelof, French physician, b. 1922], an abnormal condition characterized by absent T cell function, deficient B cell function, fairly normal immunoglobulin levels, and little or no specific antibody production. It affects both male and female siblings, indicating that it may be transmitted as an autosomal-recessive genetic disorder. The cause is unknown. Another is that the disorder is caused by underdevelopment of the thymus gland and the consequent inhibition of T cell development. Still another holds that the disease results from a failure to produce or to secrete thymic humoral factors, especially thymosin.

■ OBSERVATIONS: Patients with Nezelof's syndrome have progressively severe, recurrent, and eventually fatal infections. Signs that often appear in infants or in children up to 4 years of age include recurrent pneumonia, otitis media, chronic fungal infections, upper respiratory tract infections, diarrhea, and hepatosplenomegaly. The lymph nodes and tonsils may be enlarged, or they may be totally absent in infants with the disease. Involved patients may develop a tendency toward malignancy. Infection may cause sepsis, which is the usual cause of death. Symptoms that often suggest Nezelof's syndrome also include weight loss and poor eating habits. Definite diagnostic evidence of the disease includes defective B cell and T cell immunity despite a normal number of circulating B cells, a moderate-to-high rise in the number of T cells, a deficiency or an increase in one or more classes of immunoglobulins, a nonreactive Schick test after DPT immunization, a reduced or an absent antibody reaction after specific antigen immunization, no thymus shadow on a chest x-ray film, thymus-dependent regions with abnormal lymphoid structure, and a decrease in the number of lymphocytes in the blood.

■ INTERVENTIONS: Initial supportive treatment of Nezelof's syndrome may include monthly injections of gamma globulin or monthly infusions of fresh frozen plasma and heavy use of antibiotics to fight infection. The plasma infusions are especially beneficial if the patient cannot produce specific immunoglobulins. Cell-mediated immune function associated with T cells can usually be temporarily restored within weeks by a fetal thymus transplant. Repeated transplants are required to maintain the immunity. Cell-mediated immunity can be only partially restored with either transfer factor therapy or repeated injection of thymosin. Histocompatible bone marrow transplants have been used, but the effectiveness of this treatment method is unclear.

■ NURSING CONSIDERATIONS: The nursing role in treating this condition is essentially supportive. Sites of gamma globulin injection in a large muscle mass are massaged after each injection, and the sites are rotated and recorded to prevent tissue damage. Gamma globulin doses greater than 1.5 mL are divided and injected into more than one site. The nurse also offers support to the parents of children affected by Nezelof's syndrome, instructs them how to recognize the signs of infection, and explains the dangers of allowing affected children to become exposed to infection.

**nF,** abbreviation for *nanofarad,* one billionth of a farad.

***N.F.,*** abbreviation for ***National Formulary.***

**NF1,** a gene associated with neurofibromatosis. The gene is normally part of a family that helps regulate the timing of cell divisions. It may become defective, leading to neurofibromatosis expression, when an itinerant sequence of a deoxyribonucleic acid molecule becomes wedged in the NF1 gene.

**ng,** abbreviation for **nanogram.**

**NGF,** abbreviation for **nerve growth factor.**

**NG tube,** abbreviation for **nasogastric tube.**

**NGU,** abbreviation for **nongonococcal urethritis.**

**NHSC,** abbreviation for **National Health Service Corps.**

**Ni,** symbol for the element **nickel.**

**NIA,** abbreviation for **National Institute on Aging.**

**niacin** /nī′əsin/, a white, crystalline water-soluble vitamin of the B complex, usually occurring in various plant and animal tissues as nicotinamide. It functions as a coenzyme necessary for the breakdown and use of all major nutrients and is essential for a healthy skin, normal functioning of the GI tract, maintenance of the nervous system, and synthesis of the sex hormones. It may be used therapeutically to help reduce high blood cholesterol levels. Rich dietary sources of both niacin and its precursor tryptophan are meats, poultry, fish, liver, kidney, eggs, nuts, peanut butter, brewer's yeast, and wheat germ. Symptoms of deficiency include muscular weakness, general fatigue, loss of appetite, various skin eruptions, halitosis, stomatitis, insomnia, irritability, nausea, vomiting, recurring headaches, tender gums, tension, and depression. Severe deficiency results in pellagra. The vitamin is not stored in the body, and daily sources are needed. Niacin toxicity is associated with large doses of nicotinic acid (may occur with as low as 50 to 100 mg). Symptoms include flushing, nausea, dizziness, diarrhea, abdominal pain, and alteration of glucose tolerance. Overdose can also exacerbate preexisting conditions such as cardiac arrhythmias and abnormal liver function. Also called **nicotinic acid.** See also **pellagra.**

**niacinamide** /nī′əsin′əmīd/, a B complex vitamin. It is closely related to niacin but has no vasodilating action. Also called **nicotinamide.**

**niacin equivalent (NE),** units used to express niacin content of food. It represents preformed niacin plus tryptophan equivalents (60 mg tryptophan = 1 mg niacin).

**NIB,** abbreviation for *National Institute for the Blind.*

**NIC,** abbreviation for **Nursing Interventions Classification.**

**nicardipine** /nikär′dipin/, a calcium channel blocker and vasodilator. It is prescribed as an antihypertensive and antianginal agent.

**niche** /nich/ [Fr, recess], a defect in an otherwise even surface, especially a depression or recess in the wall of an organ as seen on a radiograph or by the unaided eye.

**NICHHD,** abbreviation for **National Institute of Child Health and Human Development.**

**Nicholas procedure,** a surgical method for repairing severe injuries to the ligaments of the knee. It involves five procedures: medial meniscectomy, medial collateral ligament repair, vastus medialis advancement, semitendinosus advancement, and pes anserinus transfer. Also called **five-in-one repair.**

**nick** [ME, *nyke,* notch], a split in a single strand of DNA that can be made with the enzyme deoxyribonuclease or with ethidium bromide.

**nickel (Ni)** [Ger, *Kupfernickel,* copper demon], a silver-white metallic element. Its atomic number is 28; its atomic mass is 58.71. Many people are allergic to nickel. Nickel causes more cases of allergic contact dermatitis than all other metals combined. Many cases occur from exposure to jewelry, coins, buckles, and snaps and from continued use of "carbonless" business forms. Nickel carbonyl, an exremely toxic volatile liquid, may produce serious lung damage if inhaled. Nickel is now a suspected carcinogen.

**nickel dermatitis,** an allergic contact dermatitis caused by the metal nickel. Exposure comes usually from jewelry, wristwatches, metal clasps, and coins. Sweating increases the degree of rash. Treatment includes avoidance of exposure to nickel and reduction of perspiration. See also **contact dermatitis.**

**nick translation,** a method of labeling DNA in the laboratory by using the enzyme DNA polymerase.

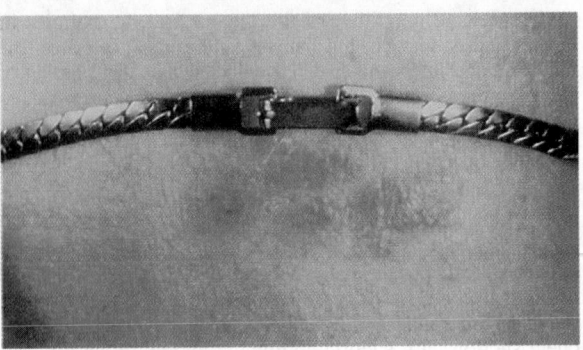

**Nickel dermatitis** *(Cohen, 1993)*

**Niclocide,** trademark for an anthelmintic (niclosamide).

**niclosamide** /niklō′səmīd/, an anthelmintic.

■ INDICATIONS: It is prescribed in the treatment of beef and fish tapeworm infestations.

■ CONTRAINDICATIONS: Known sensitivity to this drug prohibits its use. Its safety in pregnant or nursing mothers or small children has not been established.

■ ADVERSE EFFECTS: Among the most serious adverse reactions are rectal bleeding, palpitations, alopecia, edema, nausea, and vomiting.

**Nicobid,** trademark for two coenzymes, a water-soluble vitamin (B₃) (niacin and niacinamide).

**Nicola procedure,** the surgical transfer of the long head of the biceps tendon through the humeral head for chronic anterior shoulder dislocation.

**Nicorette,** trademark for a nicotine resin complex (nicotine polacrilex).

**nicotinamide.** See **niacinamide.**

**nicotine** /nik′ətēn/ [Jean Nicot Villemain, French ambassador to Portugal, 1530–1600], a colorless, rapidly acting toxic substance in tobacco that is one of the major contributors to the ill effects of smoking. It is used as an insecticide in agriculture and as a parasiticide in veterinary medicine. Ingestion of large amounts causes salivation, nausea, vomiting, diarrhea, headache, vertigo, slowing of the heartbeat, and in acute cases paralysis of respiratory muscles.

**nicotine nasal spray,** a product approved by the U.S. Food and Drug Administration for aiding tobacco smoking cessation in adults. One dose of the nasal spray administers 1 mg of nicotine directly into the nasal membranes. Because of the risk of becoming dependent on the nasal spray, it is recommended that patients not use it for more than 6 months. See also **nicotine replacement therapy.**

**nicotine poisoning,** poisoning from intake of nicotine. Nicotine poisoning is characterized by stimulation of the central and autonomic nervous systems followed by depression of these systems. In fatal cases death occurs from respiratory failure.

**nicotine polacrilex** /pōlak′rileks/, a chewing gum (nicotine resin complex) source of nicotine as an adjunct for smoking cessation.

■ INDICATIONS: It may be prescribed as an aid for patients who are trying to quit cigarette smoking.

■ CONTRAINDICATIONS: Use by postmyocardial infarction patients or those with severe or worsening angina pectoris or life-threatening arrhythmias is prohibited. It should be used cautiously in patients with hyperthyroidism, hypertension, type 1 diabetes mellitus, or peptic ulcers. Drug dosages may

have to be adjusted in patients taking other drugs with effects that may be increased or decreased when cigarette smoking ceases. Patients should be monitored to ensure that they do not become dependent on the nicotine in the gum.
■ ADVERSE REACTIONS: The most serious adverse reactions include burning and soreness of the mouth, light-headedness, headache, hiccups, nausea, vomiting, and excessive salivation.

**nicotine replacement therapy,** the use of chewing gum and skin patches as a substitute for tobacco smoke sources to satisfy nicotine cravings.

**nicotine withdrawal syndrome,** physiologic and psychologic effects of tobacco dependence that make it difficult for addicted smokers to cease use of the alkaloid. Withdrawal symptoms may be diminished by substituting nicotine chewing gum and transdermal nicotine skin patches for cigarettes.

**nicotinic acid.** See **niacin.**

**nicotinyl alcohol** /nik'ətē'nil/, an alcohol used as a vasodilator in the form of its tartrate salt in the treatment of peripheral vascular disease, vascular spasm, varicose ulcers, decubital ulcers, chilblains, Ménière's disease, and vertigo.

**NICU,** abbreviation for **neonatal intensive care unit.**

**NID,** abbreviation for *National Institute for the Deaf.*

**nid-,** prefix meaning 'to nest' or 'a place where an organism can breed': *nidal, nidus.*

**NIDA,** abbreviation for *National Institute on Drug Abuse.*

**nidation** /nīdā'shən/ [L, *nidus,* nest], the process by which an embryo burrows into the endometrium of the uterus. Also called **implantation.** See also **placenta, uterus.**

**-nidazole,** combining form for metronidazole-type antiprotozoal substances.

**NIDCR,** abbreviation for *National Institute of Dental and Craniofacial Research.*

**NIDDM,** abbreviation for **non-insulin-dependent diabetes mellitus.** See **type 2 diabetes mellitus.**

**nidus** /nī'dəs/ [L, nest], a point or origin, focus, or nucleus of a disease process.

**Niebauer prosthesis** /nē'bou·ər/, a Silastic prosthesis for interphalangeal and thumb joint replacement.

**Niemann-Pick disease** /nē'monpik'/ [Albert Niemann, German pediatrician, 1880–1921; Ludwig Pick, German pediatrician, 1868–1935], an inherited disorder of lipid metabolism in which there are accumulations of sphingomyelin in the bone marrow, spleen, and lymph nodes. The disease,

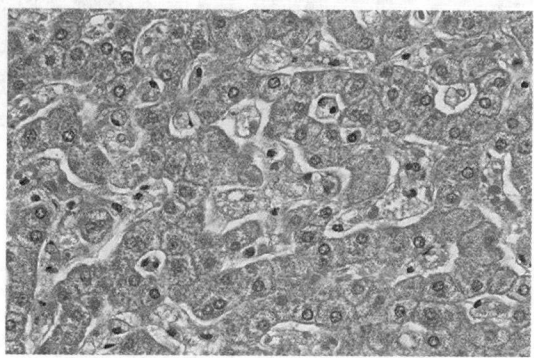

**Niemann-Pick disease in the liver**
*(Cotran, Kumar, and Collins, 1999/courtesy Dr. Arthur Weinberg, Department of Pathology, University of Texas Southwestern Medical Center, Dallas)*

which in the United States and Canada, is most common among Jewish people, begins in infancy or childhood, and is characterized by enlargement of liver and spleen, anemia, lymphadenopathy, and progressive mental and physical deterioration. There is no effective treatment, and children with the disease usually die within a few years of the onset of symptoms. See also **sphingomyelin lipidosis.**

**nifedipine** /nifed'ipēn/, a calcium channel blocker.
■ INDICATIONS: It is prescribed for the treatment of vasospastic and effort-associated angina and hypertension.
■ CONTRAINDICATION: Known hypersensitivity to this drug prohibits its use.
■ ADVERSE EFFECTS: Among the more serious adverse reactions are hypotension, peripheral edema, palpitations, dyspnea, nausea, dizziness, flushing, and headache.

**nifur-,** combining form for 5-nitrofuran derivatives.

**night blindness.** See **nyctalopia.**

**night guard.** See **biteguard.**

**Nightingale, Florence** (1820–1910), considered the founder of modern nursing. After limited formal training in nursing in Germany and Paris, she became superintendent in 1853 of a small hospital in London. Her outstanding success in reorganizing the hospital led the British government to request that she head a mission to the Crimea, where Britain was fighting a war with Russia. After her return to England in 1856, she wrote *Notes on Hospitals* and *Notes on Nursing* and founded a training school for nurses at St. Thomas' Hospital, where she attracted well-educated, dedicated women. The graduates became matrons of the most important hospitals in Great Britain, thus raising the standards of nursing across the nation and eventually around the world. Although she was, by then, bedridden much of the time, she carried on her work on the sanitary reform of India, conducted a study of midwifery, helped establish visiting nurse services, and worked for the reform of the poor laws in which she proposed separate institutions for the sick, the insane, the incurable, and children. One of Florence Nightingale's outstanding contributions was significantly decreasing the infection-related death rate through cleanliness. After Longfellow wrote *Santa Filomena,* she became known as "The Lady with The Lamp"; the Nightingale Pledge, named after her, embodies her ideals and has inspired thousands of young graduating nurses.

**Nightingale pledge,** a statement of principles for the nursing profession, formulated by a committee in 1893. It is as follows: I solemnly pledge myself before God and in the presence of this assembly: To pass my life in purity and to practice my profession faithfully. I will abstain from whatever is deleterious and mischievous, and will not take or knowingly administer any harmful drug. I will do all in my power to elevate the standard of my profession, and will hold in confidence all personal matters committed to my keeping and all family affairs coming to my knowledge in the practice of my profession. With loyalty will I endeavor to aid the physician in his work, and devote myself to the welfare of those committed to my care.

**Nightingale ward,** a kind of hospital ward designed by Florence Nightingale that revolutionized hospital design. The number of beds allowed in a ward of given size was limited to permit the circulation of air and for general cleanliness and the comfort of patients. Three sides of the ward were windowed to admit light and fresh air. Although multiple-bed wards are now obsolete in hospital design, the concerns and benefits that impelled Miss Nightingale to create them remain central to hospital planning.

**nightingalism** /nī'ting·gā'lizəm/, an ideology emphasizing self-sacrifice on the part of a nurse whose primary concern is the welfare of the patient, with minimum personal attention to the needs of the nurse. See also **Nightingale.**

**nightmare** /nīt′mer/ [AS, *niht,* night, *mara,* incubus], a dream occurring during rapid eye movement sleep that arouses feelings of intense inescapable fear, terror, distress, or extreme anxiety and that usually awakens the sleeper. Compare **pavor nocturnus, sleep terror disorder.**

**night sight.** See **hemeralopia.**

**night splint,** any splint or similar device used only at night.

**nightstick fracture,** an undisplaced fracture of the ulnar shaft caused by a direct blow.

**night sweat** [AS, *niht* + *swaetan*], sweating that occurs with a nocturnal fever, as in a wasting disease like pulmonary tuberculosis.

**night terrors** [AS, *niht* + L, *terrour*], a form of dissociated sleep, usually in children, in which there may be repeated episodes of abrupt awakening from sleep with signs of panic and anxiety. The subject may have only fragmentary dream images of a threatening nature. See also **pavor nocturnus, sleep terror disorder.**

**night vision** [AS, *niht,* night; L, *visio,* seeing], a capacity to see dimly lit objects. It stems from a chemophysical phenomenon associated with the retinal rods. The rods contain the highly light-sensitive chemical rhodopsin, or visual purple, which is essential for the conduction of optic impulses in subdued light. Night vision is sharpest at the periphery of the retina because of the concentration of rods. Night vision may be diminished by a deficiency of vitamin A, an important component of rhodopsin.

**nightwalking** [AS, *niht* + ME, *walken*], a disorder occurring during nonrapid eye movement sleep in which the subject usually sits up in bed briefly, then gets up and walks around, opening doors, eating, and so on, and eventually returns to bed. The person has no memory of the event the next day. Also called **noctambulation, sleepwalking, somnambulism.**

**nigr-,** prefix meaning 'black or a variation of the black color': *substantia nigra, nigrosin.*

**NIH,** abbreviation for **National Institutes of Health.**

**nihilistic delusion** /nī′hilis′tik/ [L, *nihil,* nothing, *icus,* form of, *deludere,* to deceive], a persistent denial of the existence of particular things or of everything, including oneself, as seen in various forms of schizophrenia. A person who has such a delusion may believe that he lives in a shadow or limbo world or that he died several years ago and that only the spirit, in a vaporous form, really exists. See also **delusion.**

**Nikolsky's sign** /nikol′skēz/ [Petr V. Nikolsky, Russian dermatologist, 1858–1940], easy separation of the stratum corneum layer of the epidermis from the basal cell layer by rubbing apparently normal skin areas; found in pemphigus and a few other bullous diseases.

**nil disease.** See **minimal change disease.**

**Nilstat,** trademark for an antifungal (nystatin).

**nilutamide,** an antineoplastic hormone.

■ INDICATIONS: This drug is used to treat stage D2 metastatic prostatic carcinoma in combination with surgical castration.

■ CONTRAINDICATIONS: Factors that prohibit the use of this drug include known hypersensitivity to nilutamide, severe hepatic impairment, and severe respiratory disease.

■ ADVERSE EFFECTS: Hepatotoxicity and interstitial pneumonitis are life-threatening effects of this drug. Other adverse effects include hot flashes, drowsiness, insomnia, dizziness, hyperthesia, depression, decreased libido, impotence, testicular atrophy, urinary tract infection, hematuria, nocturia, gynecomastia, diarrhea, nausea, vomiting, increased liver function studies, constipation, dyspepsia, rash, sweating, alopecia, dry skin, dyspnea, upper respiratory infection, pneumonia, anemia, delayed adaption to the dark, and edema.

**NIMH,** abbreviation for **National Institute of Mental Health.**

**90-90 traction.** See **traction, 90-90.**

**ninth cranial nerve.** See **glossopharyngeal nerve.**

**niobium (Nb)** /nī·ō′bē·əm/ [Gk, *Niobe,* mythic daughter of Tantalus and Amphion], a silver-gray metallic element. Its atomic number is 41; its atomic mass (weight) is 92.906. Formerly called **columbium.**

**NIOSH,** abbreviation for *National Institute for Occupational Safety and Health.*

**nipple** [ME, *neb,* beak], a small cylindric, pigmented structure that projects just below the center of each breast. The tip of the nipple has about 20 tiny openings to the lactiferous ducts. The skin of the nipple is surrounded by the lighter pigmented skin of the areola. The depth of pigmentation of the nipple and areola in nulliparas varies from rosy pink to brown, depending on the complexion of the individual. In pregnancy the skin of the nipple darkens but loses some of its pigmentation when lactation is completed. Stimulation of the nipple in men and women causes the structure to become erect through the contraction of radiating smooth muscle bundles in the surrounding areola. In women the nipple enlarges somewhat and becomes more sensitive after puberty. Also called **mammary papilla, papilla mammae, papilla mammaria.**

**nipple cancer,** an inflammatory malignant neoplasm of the nipple and areola that is usually associated with carcinoma in deeper breast structures. It represents only a small percentage of breast cancers and usually begins in the nipple and spreads to the areola. Also called **Paget's disease of the nipple.**

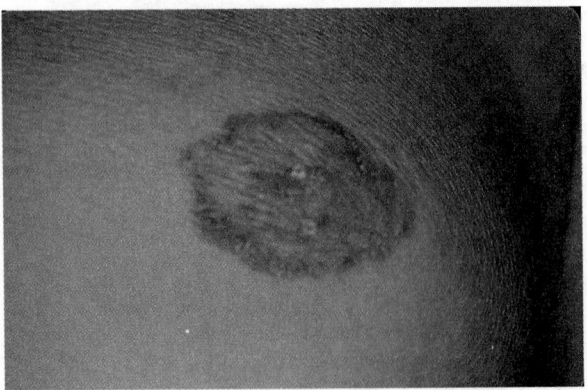

**Nipple cancer**
*(Goldstein and Goldstein, 1997/courtesy Department of Dermatology, University of North Carolina at Chapel Hill)*

**nipple discharge,** spontaneous exudation of material from the nipple. It may be normal, such as colostrum in pregnancy, or it may be a sign of endocrinologic, neoplastic, or infectious disease.

**nipple shield,** a device to protect the nipples of a lactating woman. The shield is usually made of soft latex, is 4 or 5 cm wide, and has a tab on one side with which the mother may hold it. The baby nurses from an opening at the center of the shield. It is most often used to allow sore or cracked nipples to heal while maintaining lactation. Also called **nipple protector.**

**Nipride,** trademark for a direct-acting vasodilator (sodium nitroprusside) used for marked lowering of blood pressure.

**niridazole** /nirid'əzōl/, an antischistosomal. In the United States it is available from the Centers for Disease Control and Prevention.

**Nirschl procedure** /nur'shəl/, a surgical procedure for treating chronic inflammation of the elbow. It involves excision of a segment from the hypercapsular tendon of the extensor carpi radialis brevis and removal of the head of the anterolateral condyle.

**nirvanic state** /nirvä'nik, nirvan'ik/, (in Buddhist meditation) a state in which mental processes cease, often leading to a radical alteration of the personality.

**NIS,** abbreviation for *Nursing Information System.*

**nisoldipine,** a calcium channel blocker.
- INDICATIONS: It is prescribed in the treatment of hypertension by dilating the arterioles and decreasing peripheral vascular resistance.
- CONTRAINDICATIONS: The drug should not be given with high-fat meals, which can increase peak plasma concentration, or with grapefruit juice, which can also increase blood levels.
- ADVERSE EFFECTS: The side effects of calcium channel blockers most often reported include nausea, constipation, flatulence, dizziness, lightheadedness, headache, fluid retention, and palpitations.

**Nissl body** /nis'əl/ [Franz Nissl, German neurologist, 1860–1919], any one of the large granular structures in the cytoplasm of nerve cells that stains with basic dyes and contains ribonucleoprotein.

**nit,** the egg of a parasitic insect, particularly a louse. It may be found attached to human or animal hair or to clothing fiber. See also **pediculosis.**

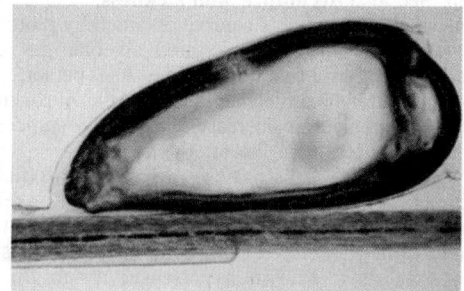

**Microscopic view of a nit** *(Zitelli and Davis, 1997)*

**nitr,** 1. abbreviation for **nitrocellulose.** 2. abbreviation for **nitroglycerin.**

**nitr-,** prefix meaning 'related to nitrogen, nitrite, and nitrate.'

**nitrate** /nī'trāt/ [Gk, *nitron* soda], 1. the ion $NO_3^-$. 2. a salt of nitric acid.

**nitric acid (HNO₃)** /nī'trik/ [Gk, *nitron,* soda; L, *acidus,* sour], a colorless, highly corrosive liquid that may give off suffocating brown fumes of nitrogen dioxide on exposure to air. Traces of nitric acid may be found in rain water during a thunderstorm. Commercially prepared nitric acid is a powerful oxidizing agent used in photoengraving and metallurgy; in the manufacture of explosives, fertilizers, dyes, and drugs; and occasionally as a cauterizing agent for the removal of warts. Organic nitrates or polyol esters of nitric acid such as nitroglycerin and amyl nitrite are effective vasodilators often used in relieving angina, but exactly how they function in dilating arterial and venous smooth muscle is not yet understood.

**nitric oxide (NO)[1],** a colorless free-radical gas commonly found in tissues of humans and other mammals. It is also prepared commercially by passing air through an electric arc. Biologically the effector molecule is commonly synthesized from the amino acid arginine. Nitric oxide participates in many biologic functions such as neurotransmission, vasodilation, cytotoxicity of macrophages, lipid lowering therapy, and inhibition of platelet aggregation. NO is involved in smooth muscle action and penile erection. It may improve oxygenation in patients with high-altitude pulmonary edema. NO deprivation may lead to high blood pressure and the formation of atherosclerotic plaque. On contact with air, NO is quickly converted to the very poisonous nitrogen dioxide ($NO_2$).

**nitric oxide (NO)[2],** a respiratory inhalant.
- INDICATIONS: Nitric oxide is used in the treatment of full-term and near-term (34 weeks) neonates with hypoxic respiratory failure associated with pulmonary hypertension. It is used with other agents and ventilatory support.
- CONTRAINDICATIONS: Two factors that prohibit this drug's use are dependence on right to left shunting of blood and known hypersensitivity.
- ADVERSE EFFECTS: Life-threatening effects of this drug are pulmonary hemorrhage, intracranial hemorrhage, sepsis, stridor, methemoglobinemia, seizures, cerebral infarction, and posttreatment infection. Other adverse effects include atelectasis, hematuria, hyperglycemia, cellulitis, withdrawal syndrome, and hypotension.

**nitrite** /nī'trīt/ [Gk, *nitron,* soda], an ester or salt of nitrous acid used as a vasodilator and antispasmodic. Among the most widely used nitrites in medicine are amyl, ethyl, potassium, and sodium nitrite.

**nitritoid reaction** /nī'tritoid/, a group of adverse effects, including hypotension, flushing, lightheadedness, and fainting, produced by administration of arsenicals or gold. The reaction is similar to that caused by administration of nitrites.

**nitro-** /nī'trō-/, combining form indicating presence of the group-$NO_2$: *nitrobenzol, nitrofuran, nitromethane.*

**nitrobenzene poisoning** /-ben'zēn/, a toxic condition caused by the absorption into the body of nitrobenzene, a pale yellow, oily liquid used in the manufacture of aniline, shoe dyes, soap, perfume, and artificial flavors. Nitrobenzene, especially its vapors, is extremely toxic. Exposure in industry is usually by inhalation of the fumes or by absorption through the skin. Symptoms of acute poisoning include headache, drowsiness, nausea, ataxia, cyanosis, and, in extreme cases, respiratory failure. Chronic exposure to nitrobenzene may cause headache, fatigue, loss of appetite, and anemia.

**Nitro-Bid,** trademark for a coronary vasodilator (nitroglycerin).

**nitrocellulose (nitr)** /-sel'yəlōs/, a mixture of nitrate esters of cellulose made by treating cotton with nitric and sulfuric acids. Solutions in a mixture of ether and alcohol are used as "plastic skin" under the name of **collodion.** See also **pyroxylin.**

**nitrofuran** /-fyōō′ran/, one of a group of synthetic antimicrobials used to treat infections caused by protozoa or by certain gram-positive or gram-negative bacteria. The precise mechanism by which nitrofurans exert their antimicrobial effects is not known. Three agents commonly prescribed are nitrofurazone, furazolidone, and nitrofurantoin. Nitrofurazone is used topically to treat superficial wounds and infections, particularly burns. Systemic toxicity is not seen when the drug is used in this way, although allergic skin reactions may occur. Furazolidone is used to treat bacterial and protozoal diarrhea and enteritis. Nitrofurantoin is used to treat urinary tract infections caused by *Escherichia coli* and other enteric pathogens of the urinary tract. Systemic administration of nitrofurans is associated with many side effects, the most common being nausea and diarrhea. Serious side effects include polyneuropathies and several hypersensitivity reactions, including pneumonitis and blood dyscrasias. Nitrofurans can cause hemolytic anemia in patients with glucose-6-phosphate dehydrogenase deficiency.

**nitrofurantoin** /nī′trōfyōōran′tō·in, -fyōō′rəntō′in/, a urinary antibacterial.
■ INDICATIONS: It is prescribed in the treatment of certain urinary tract infections.
■ CONTRAINDICATIONS: Kidney dysfunction or known hypersensitivity to this drug prohibits its use. It is not given to children under 1 month of age or to pregnant or lactating women.
■ ADVERSE EFFECTS: Among the most serious adverse reactions is hypersensitivity pneumonitis, which can lead to fibrosis, neurotoxicity, and hemolytic anemia in patients with glucose-6-phosphate dehydrogenase deficiency. GI disturbances and fever are common.

**nitrofurazone** /-fyōō′rəzōn/, a topical antibacterial.
■ INDICATIONS: It is prescribed in the prophylaxis and treatment of infections in second- and third-degree burns and of the skin and mucous membranes.
■ CONTRAINDICATION: Known hypersensitivity to this drug prohibits its use.
■ ADVERSE EFFECTS: Among the most serious adverse reactions are severe allergic reactions and superinfections.

**nitrogen (N)** /nī′trəjən/ [Gk, *nitron,* soda, *genein,* to produce], a gaseous nonmetallic element. Its atomic number is 7; its atomic mass is 14.008. Nitrogen constitutes approximately 78% of the atmosphere and is a component of all proteins and a major component of most organic substances. Nitrogen is essential to the synthesis of necessary proteins, particularly nitrogen-containing compounds or amino acids derived directly or indirectly from plant food. Nitrogen follows a cycle from atmospheric gas into nitrogen-fixing bacteria, into green vascular plants, into humans and animals, and, by decay or in excreted nitrogenous wastes, as urea, back into the soil. Denitrifying bacteria in the soil break down nitrogenous compounds and release gaseous nitrogen. During a 24-hour period in a healthy individual the nitrogen excreted in the urine, feces, and perspiration, together with the nitrogen retained in dermal structures, such as the skin and hair, equals the nitrogen consumed in food and drink. The process of protein metabolism accounts for this nitrogen balance. When protein catabolism exceeds protein anabolism, the amount of nitrogen in the urine exceeds the amount of nitrogen consumed in foods, producing a negative nitrogen balance or a state of tissue wasting. A positive nitrogen balance exists in the body when the nitrogen intake in foods is greater than that excreted in urine. Conditions usually associated with positive nitrogen balance include those related to growth, pregnancy, and convalescence from a tissue-wasting illness.

**nitrogen balance,** the relationship between the amount of nitrogen taken into the body, usually as food, and that excreted from the body in urine and feces. Most of the body's nitrogen is incorporated into protein. Positive nitrogen balance, which occurs when the intake of nitrogen is greater than its excretion, implies tissue formation and growth. Negative nitrogen balance, which occurs when more nitrogen is excreted than is taken in, indicates wasting or destruction of tissue.

**nitrogen cycle** [Gk, *nitron,* soda, *genein,* to produce, *kyklos,* circle], the circulation of nitrogen through natural processes in either of two ways: from the soil to organisms that excrete nitrogen products back into the soil or by bacterial fixation of atmospheric nitrogen through other organisms that decay and release the element back into the atmosphere.

**nitrogen dioxide ($NO_2$),** a brownish irritating gas that can be released from silage and the reaction of nitric acid with metals. It may produce symptoms of pulmonary damage in workers who perform ensilage tasks. Some studies indicate that measurable changes in pulmonary function occur when healthy individuals are exposed to nitrogen dioxide concentrations of two to three parts per million. Organic nitrates or polyol esters of nitric acid such as nitroglycerin, as well as organic nitrites or esters of nitric acid such as amyl nitrite, are effective vasodilators often used in relieving angina, but exactly how they function in dilating arterial and venous smooth muscle is not yet understood.

**nitrogen fixation,** the process by which free nitrogen in the atmosphere is converted by biologic or chemical means to ammonia and to other forms usable by plants and animals. Biologic nitrogen fixation is the more important process and is accomplished by microorganisms in the soil, either free living or in close association with root nodules of certain plants. In contrast, chemical nitrogen fixation, as is used in industry, requires extremely high temperatures and pressures.

**nitrogen mustard.** See **mechlorethamine hydrochloride.**

**nitrogen narcosis,** a condition of depressed central nervous system functions as a result of high partial pressure of nitrogen. See also **decompression sickness.**

**nitrogen washout curve,** a curve obtained by plotting the concentration of nitrogen in expired alveolar gas during oxygen breathing as a function of time. As a person inhales pure oxygen after breathing ambient air, the nitrogen concentration in exhaled air decreases. In healthy subjects, the concentration is less than 2% after 4 minutes.

**nitroglycerin (nitr)** /-glis′ərin/, a coronary vasodilator.
■ INDICATION: It is prescribed for the prevention or relief of angina pectoris. There are recommended limits to the amount of drug use before calling for emergency assistance.
■ CONTRAINDICATION: Known hypersensitivity to this drug prohibits its use.
■ ADVERSE EFFECTS: Among the most serious adverse reactions are hypotension, flushing, headache, and syncope.

**nitroglycerin tablets,** tablets of glyceryl trinitrate, a volatile ester prepared by the action of nitric and sulfuric acids on glycerol. It is prescribed for the relief of chest pain or angina. A potent smooth muscle relaxant and vasodilator, nitroglycerin is used in transdermal patches and in a paste as well as in oral and sublingual tablets.

**nitromersol** /-mur′sol/, an organic mercurial antiseptic that is not a highly effective germicide, sometimes used for the disinfecting of surgical instruments and as an antiseptic on the skin and mucous membranes.

**nitroprusside sodium.** See **sodium nitroprusside.**

**nitrosamines** /nīt′rəsam′ēnz/, potentially carcinogenic

compounds produced by reactions of nitrites with amines or amides normally present in the body. Nitrites are produced by bacteria in saliva and in the intestine from nitrates normally present in vegetables and in nitrate-treated fish, poultry, and meats. More than 70% of ingested nitrates are from vegetables.

**nitroso-,** combining form indicating presence of the group -N:O: *nitrosobacteria, nitrososubstitution.*

**nitrosourea** /nītrō′sōyŏŏrē′ə/, one of a group of alkylating drugs used as antineoplastic drugs in the chemotherapy of brain tumors, multiple myeloma, Hodgkin's disease, adenocarcinomas, hepatomas, chronic leukemias, lymphomas, myelomas, and cancers of the breast and ovaries. They have been less successful in therapy for cancers of the lungs, head, neck, and GI tract. Like other alkylating agents, they have severe toxic effects, including bone marrow depression. Nausea and vomiting are almost always present. Safe use during pregnancy has not been established, and animal studies have generally shown teratogenicity and embryotoxicity. Carmustine and lomustine are typical examples of this group. See also **alkylating agent.**

**Nitrospan,** trademark for a coronary vasodilator (nitroglycerin).

**Nitrostat,** trademark for a coronary vasodilator (nitroglycerin).

**nitrous acid (HNO₂),** a weak acid and clinical laboratory reagent formed by the action of strong acids on inorganic nitrites. In water it changes into nitric oxide and nitric acid.

**nitrous oxide (N₂O, NOx)** /nī′trəs/, a colorless, odorless, sweet-tasting, weakly anesthetic gas used in dentistry, surgery, and childbirth. It must be delivered in various concentrations with oxygen to prevent anoxia. Nitrous oxide alone does not provide enough anesthesia for surgery, for which it is supplemented with other anesthetic agents. It is often given during induction of anesthesia, preceded by the administration of a barbiturate or narcotic. Nitrous oxide is neither explosive nor flammable, and recovery is rapid. Nitrous oxide not considered suitable for prolonged surgery or for surgery requiring deep muscle relaxation and is not administered to patients with hypoxemia, respiratory disease, or intestinal occlusion. Also called **laughing gas.**

**Nix,** trademark for a topical pediculicide (permethrin).

**Nizoral,** trademark for an antifungal agent (ketoconazole).

**NK cell.** See **natural killer cell.**

**NLN,** abbreviation for **National League for Nursing.**

**nm,** abbreviation for **nanometer.**

**N-m,** abbreviation for *newton meter.*

**N/m²,** abbreviation for *newton per square meter.*

**NMDP,** abbreviation for **National Marrow Donor Program.**

**NMDS,** abbreviation for **Nursing Minimum Data Set.**

**NMES,** 1. abbreviation for **neuromuscular electrical stimulator.** 2. abbreviation for **neuromuscular electrical stimulation.** See **neuromuscular electric stimulator.**

**NMNA,** abbreviation for **National Male Nurses Association.**

**NMR,** abbreviation for **nuclear magnetic resonance.** See **magnetic resonance.**

**NMR imaging.** See **magnetic resonance imaging.**

**NNRTI,** abbreviation for **non-nucleoside reverse transcriptase inhibitors.**

**No,** symbol for the element **nobelium.**

**NO,** abbreviation for **nitric oxide.**

**N₂O,** symbol for **nitrous oxide.**

**Noack's syndrome** /no′äks/ [Margot Noack, German physician, b. 1909], an autosomal dominant type of acrocephalopolysyndactyly. See also **acrocephalopolysyndactyly.**

**nobelium (No)** /nōbel′ē·əm/ [Alfred Nobel Institute, Stockholm, Sweden], a synthetic, transuranic metallic element. Its atomic number is 102. The atomic mass of its most stable isotope is 259.

**noble gas.** See **inert gas.**

**NOC,** abbreviation for **Nursing Outcomes Classification.**

*Nocardia* /nōkär′dē·ə/ [Edmund I. E. Nocard, French veterinarian, 1850–1903], a genus of gram-positive aerobic bacteria, some species of which are pathogenic, such as *Nocardia asteroides.* See also **nocardiosis.**

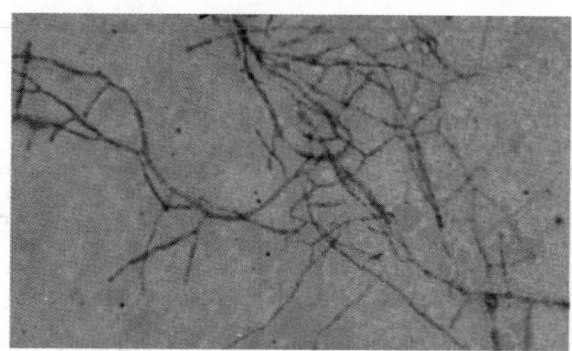

***Nocardia*** *(Baron, Peterson, and Finegold, 1994)*

**nocardiosis** /nōkär′dē·ō′sis/ [Edmund I. E. Nocard; Gk, *osis,* condition], infection with *Nocardia* species, most often *N. asteroides,* an aerobic gram-positive species of actinomycetes. It can cause pneumonia, often with cavitation, and chronic abscesses in the brain and subcutaneous tissues, and it can cause cutaneous disease through wounds contaminated with soil. The organism enters via the respiratory tract and spreads by the bloodstream, especially in immunocompromised persons such as in HIV infection, organ transplantation, and Cushing's syndrome. Surgical drainage of abscesses and sulfonamide therapy for 12 to 18 months cures between 50% and 60% of the cases treated. Combination antibiotic therapy may be required.

**noci-,** prefix meaning 'to cause harm, injury, or pain': *nociassociation, nociceptive, nociceptor.*

**nociceptive** /nō′sēsep′tiv/ [L, *nocere,* to injure, *capere,* to receive], pertaining to a neural receptor for painful stimuli.

**nociceptive reflex** [L, *nocere,* to injure, *capere,* to receive, *reflectere,* to bend back], a reflex caused by a painful stimulus.

**nociceptive stimulus** [L, *nocere,* to injure, *capere,* to receive, *stimulus,* goad], a painful, sometimes detrimental or injurious, stimulus.

**nociceptor** /nō′sēsep′tər/, a somatic and visceral free nerve ending of thinly myelinated and unmyelinated fibers. It usually reacts to tissue injury but also may be excited by endogenous chemical substances.

**no code** [AS, *na,* not; L, *caudex,* book], a note written in the patient record and signed by a qualified, usually senior or attending physician, instructing the staff of the institution not to attempt to resuscitate a particular patient in the event of cardiac or respiratory failure. This instruction is usually given only when a patient is so gravely ill that death is imminent and inevitable. Also used is **DNR** ("do not resuscitate"). See also **code,** def. 5.

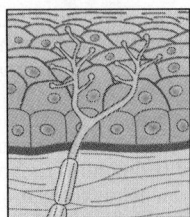

**Nociceptors** *(Thibodeau and Patton, 1999/ Network Graphics)*

**noct-,** prefix meaning 'night': *nocturia, nocturnal.*

**noct.,** abbreviation for the Latin word *nocte,* meaning 'at night.'

**noctambulation.** See **somnambulism.**

**nocturia** /noktŏŏr′ē·ə/ [L, *nocturnus,* by night; Gk, *ouron,* urine], excessive urination at night. It may be a symptom of renal or prostatic disease or bladder outlet obstruction. The condition may also occur in people who drink excessive amounts of fluids, particularly alcohol or coffee, before bedtime or in older patients who have excess body fluids that are mobilized by lying down. Also called **nycturia.** Compare **enuresis.**

**nocturnal** /noktur′nəl/ [L, *nocturnus,* by night], **1.** pertaining to or occurring during the night. **2.** describing an individual or animal that is active at night and sleeps during the day.

**nocturnal emission,** involuntary emission of semen during sleep, usually in association with an erotic dream. Also called **wet dream.**

**nocturnal enuresis** [L, *nocturnus,* by night; Gk, *enourein*], involuntary urination while asleep at night.

**nocturnal hemoglobinuria.** See **hemoglobinuria.**

**nocturnal myoclonus,** a sleep disorder that usually affects older adults and is marked by thrashing or kicking movements. The condition may be exacerbated by the use of tricyclic depressants used to induce sleep.

**nocturnal paroxysmal dyspnea.** See **paroxysmal nocturnal dyspnea.**

**nocturnal penile tumescence (NPT)** [L, *nocturnus,* by night, *penile,* pertaining to the penis, *tumescere,* to begin to swell], a normal condition of penile erection that occurs during sleep throughout most of the lifetime of a male. The occurrence of NPT is important in the diagnosis of impotence, because it indicates that impotence may be psychogenic.

**nod-,** combining form meaning 'knot': *nodal, nodose, nodulus.*

**nodal** /nō′dəl/ [L, *nodus,* knot], pertaining to a node, particularly the **atrioventricular node.**

**nodal event** /nō′dəl/, an occurrence that may cause anxiety, such as birth, death, divorce, marriage, or a child leaving home.

**node** /nōd/ [L, *nodus,* knot], **1.** a small rounded mass. **2.** a lymph node. **3.** a single computer terminal in a network of terminals and computers.

**nodular** /nod′yələr/ [L, *nodus,* knot], (of a structure or mass) small, firm, and knotty. See also **node, nodule.**

**nodular circumscribed lipomatosis,** a condition in which circumscribed, encapsulated lipomas are distributed around the neck symmetrically, randomly, or like a collar. The adipose deposits may be painful and tender.

**nodular cutaneous angiitis,** inflammation of small arteries accompanied by skin lesions.

**nodular fasciitis,** an inflammation of the fascia that causes the formation of nodules.

**nodular goiter** [L, *nodus,* knot; Gk, *guttur,* throat], an enlarged goiter that contains nodules.

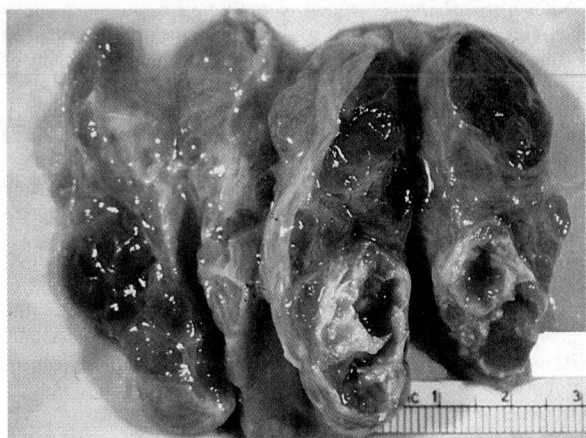

**Nodular goiter** *(Kumar, Cotran, and Robbins, 1997)*

**nodular melanoma,** a melanoma that is uniformly pigmented, usually bluish-black and nodular and sometimes surrounded by an irregular halo of pale, unpigmented skin. The lesion is always raised and may be dome-shaped or polypoid. Most often the tumor is found in middle-aged adults and occurs in 10% to 15% of patients with melanoma. See also **lentigo maligna melanoma, superficial spreading melanoma.**

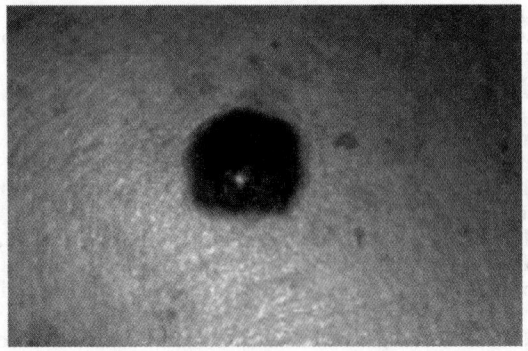

**Nodular malignant melanoma** *(Lemmi and Lemmi, 2000)*

**nodule** /nod′yōōl/ [L, *nodulus,* small knot], **1.** a small node. **2.** a small nodelike structure.

**-noia,** suffix meaning '(condition of the) mind or will': *aponoia, hypernoia, hyponoia.*

**noise,** random signals or disturbances that interfere with the normal flow of data through pathways of computers and other electronic devices.

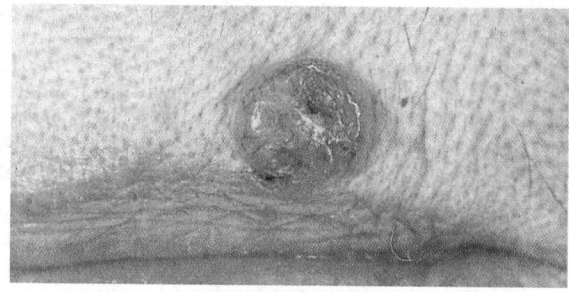

**Nodule** *(du Vivier, 1993)*

**noise-induced hearing loss,** a gradual loss of hearing caused by exposure to loud noise over an extended period of time, such as with an individual who works in a noisy environment. The hearing loss is sensorineural in nature and greatest in the higher frequencies. Although an early hearing loss may be temporary, it becomes permanent with increased exposure to noise. Compare **acoustic trauma.**

**noise pollution,** an unwanted noise level in the environment, causing discomfort and possibly threatening health.

**nok,** abbreviation for *next of kin.*

**Noludar,** trademark for a sedative (methyprylon).

**Nolvadex,** trademark for an antiestrogen (tamoxifen).

**noma** /nō′mə/ [Gk, *nome,* distribution], an acute, necrotizing ulcerative process involving mucous membranes of the mouth or genitalia. The condition is most commonly seen in severely malnourished, debilitated persons, especially children with poor nutrition and hygiene. There is rapid spreading and painless destruction of bone and soft tissue accompanied by a putrid odor caused by oral anaerobic bacteria, especially *Fusobacterium nucleatum.* Treatment involves high-dose penicillin, debridement, and improved nutrition. Healing eventually occurs but often with disfiguring defects. Also called **acute necrotizing ulcerative mucositis, gangrenous stomatitis.**

**-noma,** suffix meaning a 'spreading, invasive gangrene': *mullerianoma, pelidnoma.*

**nomen-,** combining form meaning 'a name or pertaining to names': *nomenclature.*

**nomenclature** /nō′mənklā′chər, nōmen′-/ [L, *nomen,* name, *clamare,* to call], a consistent, systematic method of naming used in a scientific discipline to denote classifications and to avoid ambiguities in names, such as binomial nomenclature in biology and chemical nomenclature in chemistry.

**-nomia,** suffix meaning 'aphasia involving names or naming ability': *anomia, paranomia, dysnomia.*

*Nomina Anatomica,* the book of official international nomenclature for anatomy as designated by the International Congress of Anatomists.

**nominal aphasia** /nom′inəl/ [L, *nomen* + Gk, *a* + *phasis,* without speech], a type of speech defect in which the person uses incorrect names in identifying objects. Minor episodes may result from anxiety, fatigue, or senility; severe cases can indicate a focal lesion on the left side of the brain. Also called **amnestic aphasia.**

**nominal damages.** See **damages.**

**nomo-,** prefix meaning 'usage or law': *nomogenesis, nomogram, nomotopic.*

**nomogram** /nom′əgram, nō′mə-/ [Gk, *nomos,* law, *gramma,* a record], **1.** a graphic representation, by any of various systems, of a numeric relationship. **2.** a graph on which a number of variables is plotted so that the value of a dependent variable can be read on the appropriate line when the values of the other variables are given.

**-nomy,** combining form meaning 'received knowledge in a field': *pathonomy, physionomy, psychonomy.*

**non-** /non-/, prefix meaning 'not': *noninvasive, noncompliant.*

**nona-, noni-,** prefix meaning 'nine': *nonan, nonigravida, nonipara.*

**nonabsorbable surgical sutures** /-əbsôr′bəbəl/ [L, *non,* not, *absorbere* + Gk, *cheirourgos,* surgeon; L, *sutura*], sutures of silk, nylon, steel, or other materials that resist absorption. They are used mainly in deep tissues where it is important for them to remain in place.

**nonadaptive immunity** /-adap′tiv/, an immune response that persists after repeated exposures to the same antigen.

**nonadherent cell** /-ədhir′ənt/, a cell such as a lymphocyte that will not adhere to a smooth surface of laboratory equipment.

**nonadherent dressing** [L, *non* + *adhesio,* sticking to; OFr, *dresser,* to arrange], a dressing designed specifically not to stick to the dried secretions of a wound.

**nonadhesive skin traction** /-ədhē′siv/ [L, *non,* not, *adhesio,* sticking to], one of two kinds of skin traction in which the therapeutic pull of traction weights is applied over the body structure involved with foam-backed traction straps that do not stick to the skin. Nonadhesive skin traction straps may be easily removed to facilitate skin care and are usually used when continuous traction is not required. The straps decrease the patient's vulnerability to skin breakdown by spreading the traction pull over a wide area of skin surface. Compare **adhesive skin traction.**

**non-A, non-B (NANB) hepatitis.** See **hepatitis C.**

**nonbacterial thrombotic endocarditis** /-baktir′ē·əl/ [L, *non* + *bakerion,* small rod], one of the three main types of endocarditis, characterized by various kinds of lesions affecting the heart valves, most often on the left side of the heart. The disease may be the first step in the development of bacterial endocarditis, and the lesions may cause peripheral arterial embolisms, resulting in death. The disease equally affects men and women between 18 and 90 years of age and causes heart murmurs in about 30% of cases. There is no successful treatment for nonbacterial thrombotic endocarditis, but anticoagulation therapy may be used to reduce

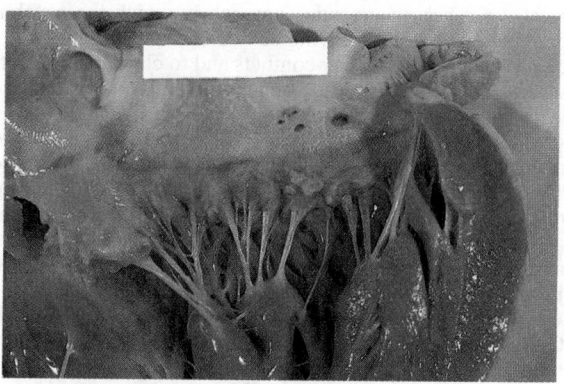

**Nonbacterial thrombotic endocarditis**
*(Kumar, Cotran, Robbins, 1997/from the teaching collection of the Department of Pathology, University of Texas Southwestern Medical School, Dallas)*

the incidence of peripheral arterial embolism. See also **Libman-Sacks endocarditis.**

**noncardiogenic pulmonary edema.** See **adult respiratory distress syndrome.**

**noncellulose polysaccharides** /-sel′yəlōs/, food substances such as hemicellulose, pectins, gums, mucilages, and algal products that absorb water and swell to a larger bulk. They slow emptying of food from the stomach, bind bile acids, provide fermentation material for the colon, and prevent spastic colon pressure.

**noncommunicating hydrocephalus.** See **hydrocephalus.**

**noncompetitive inhibition** /-kəmpet′itiv/, (in pharmacology) a form of inhibition in which a substance occupies a receptor and cannot be displaced from the receptor by increasing the number of other molecules through the principle of mass action.

**noncompliance** /-kəmplī′əns/ [L, *non* + *complere*, to complete], a nursing diagnosis accepted by the Fourth National Conference on the Classification of Nursing Diagnoses. It is defined as an informed decision on the part of the client not to adhere to a therapeutic suggestion. The nature of the noncompliance is to be specified, such as 'noncompliance: medications.'

■ DEFINING CHARACTERISTICS: The critical defining characteristic, which must be present for the diagnosis to be made, is an observation of the client's failure to adhere to a recommendation or a statement by the client or knowledgeable other person that the recommendations are not being followed. Other defining characteristics include objective tests that show noncompliance, evidence of development of complications, evidence of exacerbation of symptoms, failure to keep appointments, failure to progress, and inability to set or attain mutual goals.

■ RELATED FACTORS: The related factors include the patient's value system (health beliefs, cultural influences, spiritual values), and patient and provider relationships. See also **nursing diagnosis.**

**non compos mentis** /non′ kom′pos men′tis/ [L, not of sound mind], a legal term applied to a person declared to be mentally incompetent.

**nondepolarizing blocking agent,** a compound that causes paralysis of skeletal muscle by blocking neural transmission at the myoneural junction; it acts by competitive binding to the cholinergic receptors of the motor endplate without depolarizing the postsynaptic membrane.

**nondirective therapy** /-direk′tiv/ [L, *non* + *digere*, to direct], a psychotherapeutic approach in which the psychotherapist refrains from giving advice or interpretation as the client is helped to identify conflicts and to clarify and understand feelings and values. Compare **directive therapy.** See also **client-centered therapy.**

**nondisjunction** /-disjungk′chən/ [L, *non* + *disjungere*, to disjoint], failure of homologous pairs of chromosomes to separate during the first meiotic division or of the two chromatids of a chromosome to split during anaphase of mitosis or the second meiotic division. The result is an abnormal number of chromosomes in the daughter cells. Compare **disjunction.** See also **monosomy, trisomy.**

**nonessential amino acid** /-esen′shəl/, any amino acids that are not essential to the diet because the body can synthesize their molecules from other amino acids. See also **amino acid, essential amino acid.**

**nonfat milk.** See **skimmed milk.**

**nonfeasance** /nonfē′zəns/ [L, *non* + *facere*, to do], a failure to perform a task, duty, or undertaking that one has agreed to perform or that one had a legal duty to per-

form. Compare **malfeasance, misfeasance.** See also **negligence.**

**nongonococcal urethritis (NGU)** /-gon′əkok′əl/ [L, *non* + Gk, *gone,* seed, *kokkos,* berry], an infectious condition of the urethra in males that is characterized by mild dysuria and a small to moderate amount of penile discharge. The discharge may be white or clear, thin or mucoid, or, less often, purulent. The infection is often caused by the obligate intracellular parasite *Chlamydia trachomatis.* Untreated NGU may result in urethral stricture, epididymitis, proctitis, and chronic inflammation of the urethra. Women exposed to the exudate during coitus may develop a hypertrophic erosion of the cervix and purulent cervical mucus. An infant passing through the cervix and vagina of a mother infected with *C. trachomatis* may develop conjunctivitis and nasopharyngeal infection in the first few days after birth and pneumonia at 3 to 4 months. Diagnosis of NGU is made by excluding gonococcal urethritis through microscopic examination and by bacteriologic culture of the exudate. Nearly 50% of all cases of urethritis are nongonococcal. Most cases of NGU are successfully treated with tetracycline or erythromycin. Sexual contacts are treated whether or not they are symptomatic.

**nonheme iron** /non′hēm/, one of two forms of dietary iron. It is less efficiently absorbed than heme iron. All plant food sources and 60% of animal food sources contain nonheme iron.

**nonhemolytic jaundice** /-hē′məlit′ik/ [L, *non* + Gk, *haima,* blood, *lysein,* to loosen; Fr, *jaune,* yellow], a form of jaundice that is caused by a liver disease rather than the destruction of red blood cells.

**non-Hodgkin's lymphoma (NHL)** /- hoj′kənz/, any of a heterogenous group of malignant tumors involving lymphoid tissue. NHLs differ in their histologic, immunologic, and clinical characteristics, and as to their prognosis with therapy. An accurate diagnosis requires excision of at least one affected lymph node for biopsy evaluation by an experienced pathologist. In more than 10% of NHL patients, examination of different nodes may reveal different histologic findings. NHLs are classified into a dozen histologic grades and subtypes on the basis of nodal architecture, cell type, and clinical behavior. NHL is a disease of the middle years, usually in persons over 50 years of age. The rate of incidence is about 8.1 per 100,000 men and 5.7 per 100,000

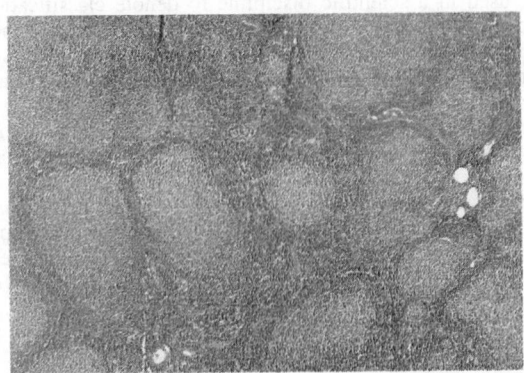

**Non-Hodgkin's lymphoma**
*(Kumar, Cotran, Robbins, 1997/courtesy Dr. Robert W. McKenna, Department of Pathology, University of Texas Southwestern Medical School, Dallas)*

women. The cause is unknown. Immunosuppressed persons have a greater incidence of NHL, suggesting the presence of an immune mechanism. The probability of acquired immunodeficiency patients developing NHL has been estimated at more than 30%. Also called **lymphosarcoma.**

**nonigravida** /nō′nigrav′idə/ [L, *nonus,* nine, *gravidus,* pregnancy], indicating a woman pregnant for the ninth time.

**nonimpact printer** /-im′pakt/, a computer printer that produces an image on a medium such as paper or by ink jet or by thermal, electromagnetic, or xerographic means. Compare **impact printer, dot-matrix printer.**

**noninfective valvular mass** /-infek′tiv/, a growth or swelling on one of the heart valves associated with autoimmune diseases or with cardiac or extracardiac malignancies. Such masses are frequently asymptomatic and are discovered only at autopsy.

**noninflammatory diarrhea** /-inflam′ətôr′ē/, a profuse watery diarrhea without fever or vomiting that begins 6 to 24 hours after ingesting food contaminated by bacterial toxins produced by either *Clostridium perfringens* or *Bacillus cereus.* The food poisoning usually involves raw meat or other proteinaceous foods exposed to warm temperatures for several hours.

**non-insulin-dependent diabetes mellitus (NIDDM).** See **type 2 diabetes mellitus.**

**noninvasive** /-invā′siv/ [L, *non + in,* into, *vadere,* to go], pertaining to a diagnostic or therapeutic technique that does not require the skin to be broken or a cavity or organ of the body to be entered. Examples include obtaining a blood pressure reading by auscultation with a stethoscope and sphygmomanometer.

**nonionic** /-ī-on′ik/, pertaining to compounds without a net negative or positive charge.

**nonionizing radiation** /-ī′ənī′zing/ [L, *non + Gk, ion,* going, *izein,* to cause], radiation for which the mechanism of action in tissue does not directly ionize atomic or molecular systems through a single interaction.

**nonipara** /nōnip′ərə/ [L, *nonus,* nine, *parere,* to bear], a woman who has given birth to nine offspring.

**nonketotic hyperglycinemia** /non-kē-tot′ik/, a usually fatal autosomal recessive aminoacidopathy with accumulation of glycine in body fluids, particularly the blood, urine, and cerebrospinal fluid; it is characterized by neonatal onset, lethargy, absence of cerebral development, seizures, myoclonic jerks, and frequently coma and respiratory failure. It is caused by a defect in one or more of the enzymes involved in the cleavage of glycine.

**nonmedullated nerve fiber.** See **nonmyelinated nerve fiber.**

**nonmyelinated nerve fiber** /-mī′əlinā′tid/ [L, *non + Gk, myelos,* marrow; L, *nervus,* nerve, *fibra,* fiber], a nerve fiber that lacks the fatty myelin insulating sheath. Such fibers form the gray matter of the nervous system, as distinguished from the white matter of myelinated fibers. Also called **nonmedullated nerve fiber.**

**Nonne-Milroy-Meige syndrome.** See **Milroy's disease.**

**nonnucleoside reverse transcriptase inhibitors (NNRTI),** a class of antiviral drugs that inhibit human immunodeficiency virus replication by interfering with the reverse transcriptase enzyme essential for viral replication. These drugs have a different mechanism of action and a distinct side effect profile from other agents. See also **nucleoside reverse transcriptase inhibitors.**

**nonnutritive sucking,** a nursing intervention from the Nursing Interventions Classification (NIC) defined as provision of sucking opportunities for the infant. See also **Nursing Interventions Classification.**

**nonnutritive sweetener** /-n͞oo′tritiv/, a chemical additive such as saccharin, acesulfame, or sucralose that gives a sweet taste to foods without contributing significant calories. The sugar substitute is either not metabolized or so intensely sweet that the calorie count is negligible.

**nonorganic hearing loss.** See **functional hearing loss.**

**nonossifying fibroma** /-os′ifī′ing/, a sharply circumscribed, eccentrically located lesion in the metaphyses of long bones in children. Microscopic examination reveals whorl patterns of spindle cells, fibrous tissue, numerous xanthoma cells, and occasional giant cells.

**nonosteogenic fibroma** /non′ostē-əjen′ik/, a common bone lesion characterized by degeneration and proliferation of the medullary and cortical tissue near the ends of the diaphyses of the large long bones of the lower extremities. Frequently the lesion causes no symptoms and is only discovered during radiographic examination of the skeleton for other reasons.

**nonpalpable testis** /pal′pəbəl/, a testis that cannot be felt and may be intraabdominal or absent.

**nonparametric test of significance** /-per′əmet′rik/ [L, *non + Gk, para,* beside, *metron,* measure], (in statistics) one of several tests that use a qualitative approach to analyze rank order data and incidence data that cannot be assumed to have a normal distribution. Kinds of nonparametric tests of significance include **chi-square, Spearman's rho.**

**nonparous** /-per′əs/ [L, *non, parere,* to bear], indicating a woman who has never given birth to a child. Also called **nulliparous.**

**nonpenetrating wound** /-pen′ətrā′ting/ [L, *non,* not, *penetrare,* to penetrate; AS, *wund*], a wound that does not break the surface of the skin.

**nonpermissive host** /-pərmis′iv/, an animal or cell that resists the replication of an infectious agent.

**nonpolar** /-pō′lər/ [L, *non + polus,* pole], pertaining to molecules that have a hydrophobic affinity, are "water hating." Nonpolar substances tend to dissolve in nonpolar solvents.

**nonpolar solvent** /-pō′lər/, a liquid solvent without significant concentration of charged groups. Liquid hydrocarbons are common examples. Also called **fat solvent.**

**nonproductive cough** /-prəduk′tiv/ [L, *non + producere,* to produce], a sudden, noisy expulsion of air from the lungs that may be caused by irritation or inflammation and does not remove sputum from the respiratory tract. In patients with respiratory tract infections, the condition may be treated by administering expectorants such as ammonium chloride, ammonium carbonate, sodium iodide, potassium iodide, ipecac, or terpin hydrate, which increase respiratory tract secretions and may result in productive coughing. If suppression of coughing is required, antitussives that depress the cough reflex may be prescribed, including codeine or dextromethorphan. Intratracheal suctioning may be necessary when secretions cause severe respiratory difficulty and coughing is unproductive. Compare **productive cough.**

**nonproprietary name** /-prəprī′əter′ē/ [L, *non + proprietas,* owner, *nomen,* name], the chemical or generic name of a drug or device, as distinguished from a brand name or trademark. A nonproprietary name may be indicated by the letters, USAN, for United States Adopted Names. See also **USAN.**

**nonprotein nitrogen (NPN)** /-prō′tēn/ [L, *non + Gk, proteios,* first rank, *nitron,* soda, *genein,* to produce], the nitrogen in the blood that is not a constituent of protein, such as the nitrogen associated with urea, uric acid, creatine, and polypeptides. Approximately one half of the nonprotein nitrogen in the blood is associated with urea.

**nonrapid eye movement.** See **sleep.**

**nonreflex bladder.** See **flaccid bladder.**

**nonresponse bias,** (in epidemiology) errors that may develop when a part of those selected and identified as study subjects cannot or will not participate in the study. The bias may occur when the group of nonrespondents differs systematically from respondents with respect to exposure or disease status. To minimize this bias, a high participation rate is necessary, or a survey is made of nonresponders to determine whether or how they might differ with regard to the risk of disease or exposure.

**nonreversible inhibitor** /-rivur′səbəl/ [L, *non* + *revertere,* to turn back, *inhibere,* to restrain], an effector substance that binds permanently to an active site of an enzyme, inhibiting the normal catalytic activity of the enzyme.

**nonsecretor** /-səkrē′tər/ [L, *non* + *secernere,* to separate], a person who does not secrete ABO blood group substances in mucous secretions of the saliva or gastric juice. The condition is genetically determined.

**nonseg.,** abbreviation for *nonsegmented.*

**nonseminomatous testicular tumors** /-sem′inom′ətəs/, any of a variety of histologic types of testicular carcinoma, including embryonal cell carcinoma, teratocarcinoma, and tumors with mixed elements. Treatment for most cases depends on the stage of the cancer at the time of diagnosis.

**nonsense mutation.** See **amber mutation.**

**nonsexual generation.** See **asexual reproduction.**

**nonshivering thermogenesis** /-shiv′əring/, a natural method by which newborns can produce body heat by increasing their metabolic rate.

**non-small-cell carcinoma of lung,** a major category of histologic types of lung carcinomas, including adenocarcinoma of the lung, large-cell carcinoma, and squamous cell carcinoma. Treatment depends on the stage of development of the cancer at the time of initial presentation. The treatment of choice for otherwise physically fit patients with early stages of disease is resection.

**nonspecific binding (NSB)** /-spəsif′ik/, in ligand binding assay, the part of a tracer used in a competitive-binding assay that is found in the bound fraction, independent of the binding reaction.

**nonspecific immunosuppression,** a therapy, including the use of immunosuppressive drugs and high doses of radiation, that blunts or abolishes the response of the immune system to all antigens.

**nonspecific urethritis (NSU)** [L, *non,* not, *species,* form], inflammation of the urethra of unknown origin. Onset of symptoms is often related to sexual intercourse. The acute phase of NSU is seldom seen in women, but the chronic phase is a common urologic difficulty among women. The condition is noted by urethral discharge in men and by reddening of the urethral mucosa in women. Treatment with antibiotics is not always successful. See also **nongonococcal urethritis.**

**nonspecific vaginitis** [L, *non,* not, *species,* form, *facere,* to make, *vagina,* sheath; Gk, *itis,* inflammation], a term formerly used for any vaginal inflammation for which no specific pathogen could be identified. Most cases of vaginitis today are found to be caused by infections of *Gardnerella vaginalis* in combination with anaerobic bacteria, although nearly one third of all cases are caused by a protozoa, *Trichomonas vaginalis.*

**nonspherocytic hemolytic anemia.** See **congenital nonspherocytic hemolytic anemia.**

**nonsteroidal antiinflammatory drug (NSAID)** /-stir′-oidəl/, any of a group of drugs having antipyretic, analgesic, and antiinflammatory effects. They counteract or reduce inflammation by inhibiting prostaglandin synthesis. NSAIDs may be indicated in the treatment of mild-to-moderate pain, rheumatoid arthritis, osteoarthritis, ankylosing spondylosis, gouty arthritis, fever, nonrheumatic inflammation, and dysmenorrhea. Examples include aspirin, ibuprofen, and ketoprofen.

**nonstress test (NST)** /non′stres/, an evaluation of the fetal heart rate response to natural contractile activity or to an increase in fetal activity. Also called **fetal activity determination (FAD).**

**nonsuppurative osteomyelitis** /-sup′yərā′tiv/, tuberculosis of the bone.

**nonthrombocytopenic purpura** /-throm′bōsī′təpē′ik/, a disorder characterized by purplish or reddish skin areas. The condition does not involve a decrease in the number of platelets.

**nontoxic** /-tok′sik/, not poisonous. Also **atoxic.**

**nontropical sprue** /-trop′ikəl/ [L, *non,* not; Gk, *tropikos,* of the solstice; D, *sprouw*], a malabsorption syndrome resulting from an inborn inability to digest foods that contain gluten. See also **celiac disease.**

**nontropic sprue.** See **tropical sprue.**

**nonulcerative blepharitis** /-ul′sərətiv′/ [L, *non* + *ilcus,* ulcer; Gk, *blepharon,* eyelid, *itis,* inflammation], a form of blepharitis characterized by greasy scales on the margins of the eyelids around the lashes and hyperemia and thickening of the skin. Nonulcerative blepharitis is often associated with seborrhea of the scalp, eyebrows, and the skin behind the ears.

**nonunion** /-yo͞o′nyən/, pertaining to a fractured bone that fails to heal properly.

**nonvenereal syphilis.** See **endemic syphilis.**

**nonverbal communication** /-vur′bəl/, the transmission of a message without the use of words. It may involve any or all of the five senses. See also **body language.**

**nonviable** /-vī′əbəl/ [L, *non* + *vita,* life], unable to exist independently after birth.

**nonvital pulp** [L, *non,* not, *vita,* life, *pulpa,* flesh], dead dental pulp caused by a disease or trauma that interferes with the blood supply. Also called **dead pulp.**

**nonvital tooth.** See **pulpless tooth.**

**Noonan's syndrome** the phenotype of Turner's syndrome (webbed neck, ptosis, hypogonadism, congenital heart disease, and short stature) without gonadal dysgenesis; formerly called *male Turner's syndrome* until the female counterpart was identified.

**nootropic** /nō·ətrop′ik/, a chemical designed to increase brain metabolism. Also called **piracetam.**

**Norcuron,** trademark for an IV neuromuscular blocking drug (vecuronium bromide).

**norepinephrine (NE)** /nôr′epinef′rin/, an adrenergic hormone (catecol amine) that acts to increase blood pressure by vasoconstriction but does not affect cardiac output. It is synthesized naturally by the adrenal medulla as well as the peripheral sympathetic nerves and the central nervous system. It is available also as a drug, levarterenol, which is used to maintain the blood pressure in acute hypotension secondary to trauma, heart disease, or vascular collapse.

**norepinephrine bitartrate,** an adrenergic vasoconstrictor.

■ INDICATIONS: It is prescribed in the treatment of cardiac arrest and in certain acute hypotensive states.

■ CONTRAINDICATIONS: Hypovolemia, vascular thrombosis, or known hypersensitivity to this drug prohibits its use. It is not used in conjunction with cyclopropane or halothane anesthesia.

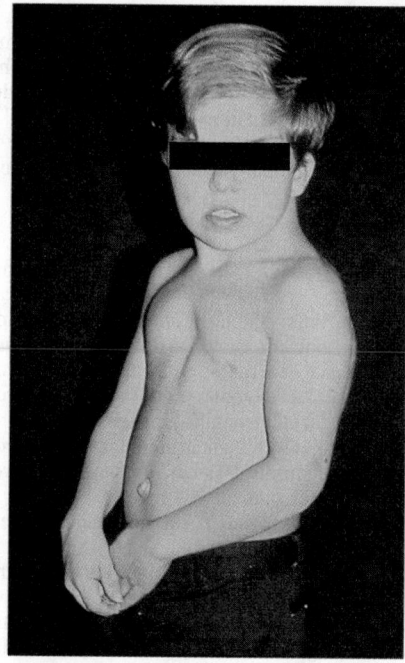

**Noonan's syndrome** *(Zitelli and Davis, 1997)*

■ ADVERSE EFFECTS: Among the more serious adverse reactions are local tissue necrosis at the site of injection, bradycardia, headache, and hypertension.

**no response (NR),** the condition for which the maximum decrease in treated tumor volume is less than 50%.

**norethindrone** /nôreth′indrōn/, a progestin.
■ INDICATIONS: It is prescribed in the treatment of abnormal uterine bleeding and endometriosis and is a component in oral contraceptive medications.
■ CONTRAINDICATIONS: Thrombophlebitis, liver dysfunction, unusual vaginal bleeding, breast cancer, missed abortion, or known hypersensitivity to this drug prohibits its use. It is not recommended for use during pregnancy.
■ ADVERSE EFFECTS: Among the more serious adverse reactions are breakthrough bleeding, amenorrhea, GI disturbances, breast changes, and masculinization of the female fetus.

**norethindrone acetate and ethinyl estradiol,** a monophasic oral contraceptive.
■ INDICATIONS: It is prescribed for contraception, endometriosis, and hypermenorrhea.
■ CONTRAINDICATIONS: Thrombophlebitis, cardiovascular disease, breast or reproductive organ cancer, unusual vaginal bleeding, gallbladder disease, liver tumor, or known hypersensitivity to this drug prohibits its use. It is not given to women over 40 years of age or during lactation, pregnancy, or suspected pregnancy. It is given with caution to women who smoke.
■ ADVERSE EFFECTS: Among the more serious adverse reactions are thrombophlebitis, uterine fibroma, porphyria, embolism, jaundice, and cerebrovascular accident.

**Norflex,** trademark for a skeletal muscle relaxant with anticholinergic properties (orphenadrine citrate).

**norfloxacin** /nôrflok′səsin/, an oral antibacterial drug.
■ INDICATIONS: It is prescribed for the treatment of bacterial urinary tract infections.
■ CONTRAINDICATIONS: This product is not recommended for children or pregnant women. Concomitant use of nitrofurantoin drugs is not recommended.
■ ADVERSE EFFECTS: Reported side effects include nausea, dizziness, and headache.

**Norgesic Forte,** trademark for a fixed-combination drug containing a muscle relaxant with anticholinergic activity (orphenadrine citrate) and APC (aspirin, phenacetin, and caffeine), used for the relief of mild-to-moderate pain of acute musculoskeletal disorders.

**norgestrel** /nôrjes′trəl/, a progestin.
■ INDICATIONS: It is prescribed alone or in combination with estrogen as a contraceptive.
■ CONTRAINDICATIONS: Thrombophlebitis, liver dysfunction, unusual vaginal bleeding, breast cancer, missed abortion, or known hypersensitivity to this drug prohibits its use.
■ ADVERSE EFFECTS: Among the more serious adverse reactions are amenorrhea, dysfunctional uterine bleeding, breast changes, and masculinization of a female fetus.

**Norinyl,** trademark for an oral contraceptive containing a progestin (norethindrone) and an estrogen (mestranol).

**Norisodrine,** trademark for an expectorant combination (isoproterenol sulfate and anydrous calcium iodide).

**Norlestrin,** trademark for an oral contraceptive containing an estrogen (ethinyl estradiol) and a progestin (norethindrone acetate).

**Norlutin,** trademark for a progestin (norethindrone).

**norm** [L, *norma,* rule], **1.** a measure of a phenomenon generally accepted as the ideal standard performance against which other measures of the phenomenon may be measured. **2.** abbreviation for **normal.**

**norma basalis** /nôr′mə basā′lis/ [L, rule; Gk, *basis,* foundation], the inferior surface of the base of the skull with the mandible removed, formed by the palatine bones, the vomer, the pterygoid processes, and parts of the sphenoid and temporal bones.

**normal (N)** /nôr′məl/ [L, *norma,* rule], **1.** describing a standard, average, or typical example of a set of objects or values. **2.** describing a chemical solution in which 1 L contains 1 g of a substance or the equivalent in replaceable hydrogen ions. **3.** people in a nondiseased population. **4.** a gaussian distribution.

**-normal,** combining form meaning 'relating to a norm': *centinormal, decanormal, prenormal.*

**normal curve.** See **bell-shaped curve.**

**normal dental function,** the correct and healthy action of opposing teeth during chewing.

**normal diet.** See **regular diet.**

**normal distribution,** (in statistics) a theoretic distribution frequency of variable data usually represented graphically by a bell-shaped curve that reaches a peak about the mean.

**normal dwarf.** See **primordial dwarf.**

**normal human plasma** [L, *norma,* rule, *humanus* + Gk, *plassein,* to mold], sterile, disease-free human blood prepared from a pooled donor supply.

**normal human serum albumin,** an isotonic preparation of pooled human serum albumin for treating hypoproteinemia, hypovolemia, and threatened or existing shock.

**normal hydrogen electrode.** See **standard hydrogen electrode.**

**normalization promotion,** a nursing intervention from the Nursing Interventions Classification (NIC) defined as assisting parents and other family members of children with chronic illnesses or disabilities in providing normal life experiences for their children and families. See also **Nursing Interventions Classification.**

**normal last shoes,** orthopedic shoes for infants and children constructed with a normal sole.

**normal phase,** a chromatographic mode in which the mobile phase is less polar than the stationary phase.

**normal pressure hydrocephalus** [L, *norma,* rule, *premere,* to press; Gk, *hydor,* water, *kephale,* head], a condition in which there is dilation of the ventricles without an increase in intracranial pressure. Classic signs and symptoms are gait disturbance, memory/cognitive problems, and urinary incontinence.

**normal saline solution** [L, *norma,* rule, *sal + solutus,* dissolved], a 0.9% w/v (grams of solute per mL of solution) sterile solution of sodium chloride in water that is isotonic with blood and injectable intravenously.

**normal sinus rhythm (NSR)** [L, *norma,* rule, *sinus,* hollow; Gk, *rhythmos*], the normal heartbeat initiated by the pacemaker in the sinus node, with a heart rate of 60 to 100/min.

**normal solution** [L, *norma,* rule, *solutus,* dissolved], a solution that contains the gram-equivalent weight of a reagent per liter. It is denoted by the symbols N/l or N.

**normal strain,** a quantity described by the quotient of the change of length of a line and its original length.

**normal stress,** (in physics) a quantity described by the quotient of distributed force and area when the force is perpendicular to the area.

**normal temperature** [L, *norma,* rule, *temperatura*], for a normal person at rest, the normal oral clinical temperature is given as 98.6° F or 37° C, but actual "normal" temperatures may range a fraction of a degree or increments of a whole degree higher or lower because of effects of sleep, exercise, eating, sleeping, metabolism, and the ambient temperature. Rectal temperature also averages a fraction of a degree higher than oral temperatures, and axillary readings are usually lower than oral temperatures.

**normo-** /nôr′mə-/, prefix meaning 'normal': *normocytic, normotensive.*

**normoblast** /nôr′məblast/ [L, *norma* + Gk, *blastos,* germ], a nucleated precursor cell in the bone marrow of the adult circulating erythrocyte. Developmental stages include the pronormoblast, the basophilic normoblast, the polychromatic normoblast, and the orthochromatic normoblast. After the extrusion of the nucleus of the normoblast, the young erythrocyte becomes known as a reticulocyte and enters the circulating blood. Compare **erythrocyte.** See also **reticulocyte. —normoblastic,** *adj.*

**normochromic** /nôr′məkrō′mik/ [L, *norma* + Gk, *chroma,* color], pertaining to a blood cell having normal color caused by the presence of an adequate amount of hemoglobin. Compare **hypochromic.** See also **red cell indexes.**

**normocyte** /nôr′məsīt/ [L, *norma* + Gk, *kytos,* cell], an ordinary, normal, adult red blood cell of average size having a diameter of 7 μ. Compare **macrocyte, microcyte. —normocytic,** *adj.*

**Normodyne,** trademark for an antihypertensive drug (labetalol hydrochloride).

**normoglycemic** /-glīsē′mik/, pertaining to a normal blood glucose level.

**normotensive** /-ten′siv/, pertaining to the condition of having normal blood pressure. **—normotension,** *n.*

**normoventilation** /-ven′tilā′shən/, the alveolar ventilation rate that produces an alveolar carbon dioxide pressure of about 40 mm Hg at any metabolic rate.

**normoxia** /nôrmok′sē-ə/, an ambient oxygen pressure of about 150 (plus or minus 10) torr, or the partial pressure of oxygen in atmospheric air at sea level.

**Noroxin,** trademark for an oral antibacterial drug (norfloxacin).

**Norpace,** trademark for an antidysrhythmic cardiac depressant (disopyramide phosphate).

**Norplant system,** trademark for subdermal contraceptive capsules containing, levonorgestrel, which are implanted beneath the skin of the upper arm of a woman. With the woman under local anesthesia, a set of six capsules, each 2.4 mm in diameter and 34 mm long, is inserted in a fan-shaped pattern through an incision about 10 cm above the elbow crease. The highly progestational drug diffuses through the walls of the capsules, maintaining a blood level of the progestin that can prevent pregnancy for up to 5 years, depending on individual differences in metabolism and body weight. The contraceptive effect can be discontinued by removing the capsules. The capsules are removed at the end of the fifth year, at which time a new set of capsules can be inserted if the woman wants to continue the protection.

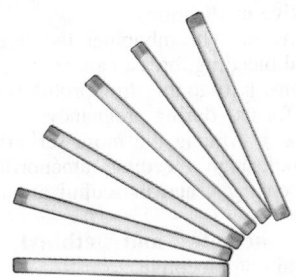

**Norplant system**
*(Thibodeau and Patton, 1999/Wyath Ayerst Laboratory)*

**Norpramin,** trademark for an antidepressant (desipramine hydrochloride).

**Nor-QD,** trademark for an oral contraceptive containing a progestin (norethindrone), but no estrogen.

**North American blastomycosis,** an infection caused by inhaling the fungus *Blastomyces dermatitidis.* It may resemble bacterial pneumonia, and x-ray films of the chest may show cavities. Painless, well-demarcated, verrucous or ulcerated skin lesions occur on the face and hands. Occa-

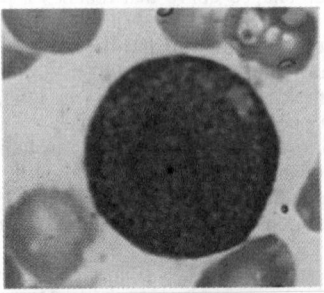

**Normoblast** *(Carr and Rodak, 1999)*

sionally lesions of the oral mucous membrane may be mistaken for squamous cell carcinoma. The disease may progress to involve bones and the brain; many viscera are infected in fatal cases. Diagnosis is made by microscopic examination of body secretions. Treatment is ketoconazole/itraconazole or amphotericin B given intravenously, depending on the severity, or in severe cases a combination of amphotericin B and sulfonamides. Also called **Gilchrist's disease.** Compare **paracoccidioidomycosis.**

**North American Nursing Diagnosis Association (NANDA),** a professional organization of registered nurses created in 1982. The purpose of the organization is 'to develop, refine, and promote a taxonomy of nursing diagnostic terminology of general use to the professional.'

**North Asian tick-borne rickettsiosis,** an infection, acquired in the Eastern Hemisphere, caused by *Rickettsia sibirica,* transmitted by ticks. It resembles Rocky Mountain spotted fever. Usual findings include a generalized maculopapular rash involving palms and soles, fever, and lymph node enlargement. It is rarely fatal and responds quickly to treatment with chloramphenicol. No vaccine is available. See also **boutonneuse fever, relapsing fever.**

**North Asian tick typhus.** See **Siberian tick typhus.**

**Northern blot test,** an electrophoretic test for identifying the presence or absence of particular mRNA molecules and nucleic acid hybridization. See also **Southern blot test.**

**nortriptyline hydrochloride** /nôrtrip'tilēn/, a tricyclic antidepressant.

■ INDICATION: It is prescribed in the treatment of mental depression.

■ CONTRAINDICATIONS: Concomitant administration of monoamine oxidase inhibitors, recent myocardial infarction, or known hypersensitivity to this drug or to other tricyclic medications prohibits its use. It is used with caution in patients having a seizure disorder or a cardiovascular disease.

■ ADVERSE EFFECTS: Among the more serious adverse effects are sedation and GI, cardiovascular, and neurologic reactions. This drug interacts with many other drugs.

**Norvir,** trademark for a protease inhibitor (ritonavir).

**Norwalk agent** [Norwalk, Ohio, site where first identified], a virus that produces gastroenteritis symptoms. The infection is transmitted from one person to another and is involved in 40% of the nonbacterial diarrhea cases in children and adults.

**Norwegian scabies** [Norway; L, *scabere,* to scratch], a severe infestation of human skin by an itch mite *(Sarcoptes scabiei).* The condition is associated with intense itching, crusting and scaling of the skin, and insect egg burrows that appear as discolored lines in the affected skin areas.

**nose** [AS, *nosu*], the structure that protrudes from the anterior part of the face and serves as a passageway for air to and from the lungs. The nose filters the air, warming, moistening, and chemically examining it for impurities that might irritate the mucous lining of the respiratory tract. The nose also contains receptor cells for smell, and it aids the faculty of speech. It consists of an internal and an external part. The external part, which protrudes from the face, is considerably smaller than the internal part, which lies over the roof of the mouth. The hollow interior part is separated into a right and a left cavity by a septum. Each cavity is divided into the superior, middle, and inferior meati by the projection of nasal conchae. The external part of the nose is perforated by two nostrils (anterior nares), and the internal part by two posterior nares. The pairs of sinuses that drain into the nose are the frontal, maxillary, ethmoidal, and sphenoidal sinuses. Ciliated mucous membrane lines the nose, closely adhering to the periosteum. The mucous membrane is continuous

with the skin through the nares and with the mucous membrane of the nasal part of the pharynx through the choanae. The mucous membrane contains the olfactory cells that form the olfactory nerve that enters the cranium.

**nosebleed** [AS, *nosu* + ME, *blod,* blood], abnormal hemorrhage from the nose. Emergency responses to nosebleed include seating the patient upright with the head thrust forward to prevent swallowing of blood. Pressure with both thumbs directly under the nostril and above the lips may block the main artery supplying blood to the nose. Alternatively, pressure with both forefingers on each side of the nostril often slows bleeding by blocking the main arteries and their branches. Continued bleeding may require the insertion of cotton or other absorbent material within the nostril and reapplication of pressure. Cold compresses on the nose, lips, and back of the head may help control hemorrhage. Continued bleeding may require cautery. Also called **epistaxis.**

**nose drops,** a medicated solution to be dropped into the nose.

**NOSIE,** abbreviation for **nurses' observation scale for inpatient evaluation.**

**noso-,** combining form meaning 'disease': *nosochthonography, nosogeny, nosophobe.*

**nosocomial** /nos'əkō'mē·əl/ [Gk, *nosokomeian,* hospital], pertaining to a hospital.

**nosocomial infection,** an infection acquired at least 72 hours after hospitalization, often caused by *Candida albicans, Escherichia coli,* hepatitis viruses, herpes zoster virus, *Pseudomonas,* or *Staphylococcus.* Also called **hospital-acquired infection.**

**nosology** /nōsol'əjē/ [Gk, *nosos,* disease, *logos,* science], the science of classifying diseases. See also **nomenclature.**

**nostrils.** See **anterior nares.**

**notch** [Fr, *noche*], an indentation or a depression in a bone or other organ, such as the auricular notch or the cardiac notch.

**nothing by mouth (NPO)** [L, *nil per os,* nothing by mouth], a patient care instruction advising that the patient is prohibited from ingesting food, beverage, or medicine. It is usually posted above the bed of a patient who is about to undergo surgery or special diagnostic procedures requiring that the digestive tract be empty or who is unable to tolerate food and fluids by mouth for some reason.

**no-threshold curve,** a linear dose-response curve that assumes there is no detectable threshold below which there is no harm. As applied in nuclear medicine, there is no identifiable concentration of radiation below which no response curve occurs.

**notifiable** [L, *nota,* mark, *facere,* to make], pertaining to certain conditions, diseases, and events that must, by law, be reported to a governmental agency, such as birth, death, smallpox, certain other communicable diseases, and certain violations of public health regulations.

**noto-,** combining form meaning 'the back': *notochord, notogenesis, notomyelitis.*

**notochord** /nō'tōkôrd/ [Gk, *noton,* back, *chorde,* cord], an elongated strip of mesodermal tissue that originates from the primitive node and extends along the dorsal surface of the developing embryo beneath the neural tube, forming the primary longitudinal skeletal axis of the body of all chordates. In humans and other vertebrate animals, the structure is replaced by vertebrae, although a remnant of it remains as part of the nucleus pulposus of the intervertebral disks. See also **neural tube. —notochordal,** *adj.*

**notochordal canal** /no'tōkôr'dəl/ [Gk, *noton* + *chorde,* cord; L, *canalis,* channel], a tubular passage that extends from the primitive pit into the head process during the early stages of embryonic development in mammals. It perforates the splanchnopleure layer so that the yolk sac and the amnion are connected temporarily. Also called **chordal canal.**

**notochordal plate.**   See **head process.**

**notogenesis** /nō′tōjen′əsis/ [Gk, *noton* + *genein*, to produce], the formation of the notochord. —**notogenetic,** *adj.*

**notomelus** /nətom′ələs/ [Gk, *noton* + *melos*, limb], a congenital malformation in which one or more accessory limbs are attached to the back.

**nourish** /nur′ish/ [L, *nutrire*, to suckle], to furnish or supply the essential foods or nutrients for maintaining life.

**nourishment** /nur′ishmənt/, **1.** the act or process of nourishing or being nourished. **2.** any substance that nourishes and supports the life and growth of living organisms.

**Novahistine,** trademark for a fixed-combination drug containing an antihistamine (chlorpheniramine maleate) and an adrenergic decongestant (phenylpropanolamine).

**Novantrone,** trademark for a synthetic antineoplastic anthracenedione (mitoxantrone).

**Novocain,** trademark for a local anesthetic (procaine hydrochloride).

**NOx,** abbreviation for **nitrous oxide,** or any mixture of oxides of nitrogen.

**noxious** /nok′shəs/ [L, *noxius,* harm], harmful, injurious, or detrimental to health.

**Noyes test** /noiz/, an orthopedic knee test performed with the knee extended and the thigh relaxed. The knee is partially dislocated anterolaterally. As the knee is gradually flexed, the dislocation is reduced at about 30 degrees of flexion.

**Np,** symbol for the element **neptunium.**

**NP,** abbreviation for **nurse practitioner.**

**NPH Iletin,** trademark for an insulin suspension (isophane).

**NPH Insulin,** trademark for an insulin suspension (isophane).

**NPN,** abbreviation for **nonprotein nitrogen.**

**NPO,** abbreviation for **nothing by mouth.**

*n*-**propyl alcohol (C₃H₇OH)** /en′prō′pil/, a clear, colorless liquid used as a solvent for resins. Also called **1-propanol.**

**NPT,** abbreviation for **nocturnal penile tumescence.**

**NPU,** abbreviation for **net protein utilization.**

**NPY,** abbreviation for **neuropeptide Y.**

**NR, 1.** abbreviation for **no response. 2.** abbreviation for *nodal rhythm.*

**NREM,** abbreviation for *nonrapid eye movement.* See **sleep.**

**NRTI,** abbreviation for **nucleoside reverse transcriptase inhibitors.**

**NSAID,** abbreviation for **nonsteroidal antiinflammatory drug.**

**NSB,** abbreviation for **nonspecific binding.**

**NSCCN,** abbreviation for **National Society of Critical Care Nurses of Canada.**

**n-s/m²,** abbreviation for *newton second per square meter.*

**NSNA,** abbreviation for **National Student Nurses Association.**

**NSR,** abbreviation for **normal sinus rhythm.**

**NSU,** abbreviation for **nonspecific urethritis.**

**N-telopeptide test (NTx),** a urine test that detects levels of N-telopeptide, a biochemical marker of bone metabolism and the most sensitive and specific indicator of bone resorption. It is used primarily to monitor the effect of antiresorptive therapy in women with osteoporosis.

**NTP, ntp,** abbreviation for *normal temperature and pressure.*

**n-type semiconductor.**   See **semiconductor.**

**nu** /n(y)ōō/,   N, *v,* the thirteenth letter of the Greek alphabet.

**Nubain,** trademark for a synthetic analgesic (nalbuphine hydrochloride), used as an adjunct to anesthesia.

**nuc,** abbreviation for *nuclear.*

**nucha** /nōō′kə/, *pl.* **nuchae** [Fr, *nuque,* nape], the nape, or back of the neck. —**nuchal,** *adj.*

**nucha-,** combining form meaning 'the neck': *nuchal, subnuchal.*

**nuchal cord** /nōō′kəl/ [Fr, *nuque,* nape; Gk, *chorde*], an abnormal but common condition in which the umbilical cord is wrapped around the neck of the fetus in utero or of the baby as it is being born. It is usually possible to slip the loop or loops of cord gently over the child's head. Sometimes it is a single loose loop, and the shoulders may deliver through it. If it is tight, it may be clamped in two places and cut with sterile, blunt tipped scissors. The condition occurs in more than 25% of deliveries, more often with long cords than with short ones.

**nuchal ligament,** a large, midline, posterior ligament in the neck from the base of the skull to the seventh cervical vertebra.

**nuchal rigidity,** a resistance to flexion of the neck, a condition seen in patients with meningitis.

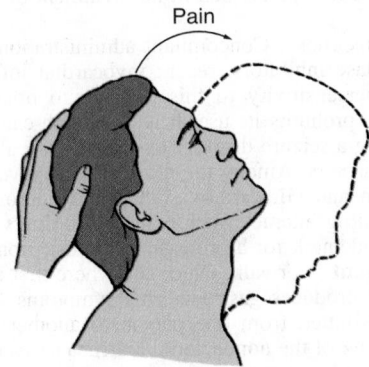

**Nuchal rigidity** *(Monahan and Neighbors, 1998)*

**nuchocephalic reflex** /nōō′kəsefal′ik/, a test for diffuse cerebral dysfunction, such as in senility. When the shoulders are turned to the left or the right, the head fails to turn in the same direction within a half-second.

**Nuck's canal, Nuck's diverticulum.**   See **processus vaginalis peritonei.**

**nucle-.**   See **nucleo-.**

**-nuclear,** combining form meaning 'nucleus': *circumnuclear, endonuclear, multinuclear.*

**nuclear agenesis.**   See **Möbius' syndrome.**

**nuclear envelope,** a double membrane that surrounds the nucleus of a eukaryotic cell. Also called **karyotheca.**

**nuclear family** /n(y)ōō′kle·ər/ [L, *nucleus,* nut kernel, *familia,* household], a family unit consisting of the biologic parents and their offspring. The nuclear family is a relatively recent product of Western society. The nuclear family unit is less efficient than an extended family unit in providing information and vital services to family members such as child rearing, child care, and care of older family members. Compare **extended family, matrifocal family.**

**nuclear fission.** See **fission.**

**nuclear hyaloplasm.** See **karyolymph.**

**nuclear isomer,** one of two or more nuclides with the same number of neutrons and protons in the nucleus (the same atomic number, or Z, and the same atomic mass, or A) but existing in different energy states.

**nuclear magnetic resonance.** See **magnetic resonance.**

**nuclear medicine,** a medical discipline that uses radiation emitted by radioactive isotopes in the diagnosis and treatment of disease. Forms of radiation important in nuclear medicine include alpha and beta particles, gamma rays, and x-rays. Radioactive elements used in nuclear medicine, called radionuclides or radiopharmaceuticals, are produced artificially. Radiopharmaceuticals are used as tracers for assessing the structure, function, secretion, excretion, and volume of a particular organ or tissue. They are also used to analyze biologic specimens and to treat specific diseases such as thyroid cancer. An important component of nuclear medicine is imaging, which involves administering radiopharmaceuticals to a patient orally, intravenously, or by inhalation to localize a specific organ or system and its structure and function. Scanning instruments convert the radioactive emissions into an image of the organ or system.

**nuclear medicine technologist,** an allied health professional who uses radioactive and stable nuclides to make diagnostic evaluations of the anatomic or physiologic conditions of the body and who provides therapy with unsealed radioactive sources. Responsibilities include application of a special knowledge of radiation physics and safety regulations to limit radiation exposure; preparation and administration of radiopharmaceuticals; use of radiation detection devices and other kinds of laboratory equipment that measure the quantity and distribution of radionuclides deposited in a patient specimen; and performance of in vivo and in vitro diagnostic procedures.

**nuclear problem,** (in psychology) an underlying reason for an individual's reaction to a precipitating event.

**nuclear radiology,** the branch of radiology that uses radioactive materials in the diagnosis and treatment of health disorders.

**nuclear sap.** See **karyolymph.**

**nuclear scanning,** a diagnostic technique that uses an injected, ingested, or inhaled radioactive material and a scanning device to determine the size, shape, location, and function of various body parts. Also called **radionuclide organ imaging.**

**nuclear spin,** an intrinsic form of angular momentum possessed by atomic nuclei containing an odd number of nucleons (protons or neutrons).

**nuclear transplantation,** the transfer of the nucleus of one cell into the cytoplasm of another.

**nucleic acid** /nōōklē'ik/ [L, *nucleus* + *acidus,* sour], a high-molecular-weight polymeric compound composed of nucleotides, each consisting of a purine or pyrimidine base, a ribose or deoxyribose sugar, and a phosphate group. Nucleic acids are involved in the determination and transmission of genetic characteristics. Kinds of nucleic acid are **deoxyribonucleic acid** and **ribonucleic acid.** See also **nucleotide.**

**nucleo-** /n(y)ōō'klē·ō-/, **nucle-,** combining form meaning 'nucleus': *nucleochylema, nucleokeratin, nucleolus.*

**nucleocapsid** /nōō'klē·ōkap'sid/ [L, *nucleus* + *capsa,* box], a viral enclosure consisting of a capsid or protein coat and a nucleic acid that it surrounds. Some viruses consist solely of bare nucleocapsids; others have more complex enclosures.

**nucleochylema** /nōō'klē·ōkīlē'mə/ [L, *nucleus* + Gk, *chylos,* juice, *haima,* blood], the ground substance of the nucleus, as distinguished from that of the cytoplasm.

**nucleochyme.** See **karyolymph.**

**nucleocytoplasmic** /nōō'klē·ōsī'tōplas'mik/ [L, *nucleus* + Gk, *kytos,* cell, *plasma,* something formed], of or relating to the nucleus and cytoplasm of a cell.

**nucleocytoplasmic ratio,** the ratio of the volume of a nucleus of a cell to the volume of the cytoplasm. The proportion is usually constant for a specific cell type, and an increase is indicative of malignant neoplasms. Also called **karyoplasmic ratio, nucleoplasmic ratio.**

**nucleohistone** /nōō'klē·ōhis'tōn/ [L, *nucleus* + Gk, *histos,* tissue], a complex that consists of DNA and a histone protein. It is the basic constituent of the chromatin in a cell nucleus.

**nucleolar organizer** /nōōklē'ələr/ [L, *nucleolus,* little nut kernel; Gk, *organon,* instrument, *izein,* to cause], a part of the nucleus of the cell, thought to consist of heterochromatin, that is responsible for the formation of the nucleolus. Also called **nucleolar zone, nucleolus organizer.**

**nucleolus** /nōōklē'ələs/, *pl.* **nucleoli** [L, little nut kernel], any one of the small, dense structures composed largely of ribonucleic acid and situated within the cytoplasm of cells. Nucleoli are essential in the formation of ribosomes that synthesize cell proteins.

**nucleolus organizer.** See **nucleolar organizer.**

**nucleon** /n(y)ōō'klē·on/, a collective term applied to protons and neutrons within the nucleus.

**nucleophilic** /-fil'ik/, pertaining to some molecules, particularly nucleic acids and proteins, having electrons that can be shared and thus form bonds with alkylating agents.

**nucleoplasm** /nōō'klē·əplaz'əm/ [L, *nucleus* + Gk, *plasma,* something formed], the protoplasm of the nucleus as contrasted with that of the cell. Also called **karyoplasm.** Compare **cytoplasm.** —**nucleoplasmic,** *adj.*

**nucleoplasmic ratio.** See **nucleocytoplasmic ratio.**

**nucleoplasmin,** an acidic protein found in the nucleus that binds to histone and participates in nucleosome assembly.

**nucleoprotein** /-prō'tēn/ [L, *nucleus* + Gk, *proteios,* first rank], a molecule in which protein is combined with nucleic acid in a cell nucleus.

**nucleoside** /nōō'klē·əsīd'/, a component of a nucleotide that consists of a nitrogenous base linked to a pentose sugar.

**nucleoside monophosphate kinase,** a liver enzyme that catalyzes the transfer of a phosphate group from adenosine triphosphate, producing adenosine diphosphate and a nucleoside diphosphate.

**nucleoside reverse transcriptase inhibitors (NRTI),** a class of antiretroviral drugs that mimic one or more of the components of human immunodeficiency deoxyribonucleic acid (DNA) or ribonucleic acid, interrupting the viral replication process. The drugs (nucleoside analogs) work by blocking the reverse transcriptase enzyme essential for viral replication. Inserting a nucleoside analog into the new viral DNA strand at a specific point terminates the viral chain, halting the replication process before it is completed. Examples of nucleoside analogs include zidovudine (AZT), didanosine (ddI), zalcitabine (ddC), stavudine (d4T), and lamivudine (3TC). See also **nonnucleoside reverse transcriptase inhibitors (NNRTI).**

**nucleosome** /nōō'klē·əsōm'/ [L, *nucleus* + Gk, *soma,* body], any one of the repeating DNA-histone complexes that appear as beadlike structures at distinct intervals along a chromosome.

**5-nucleotidase** /nōō'klē·ot'idās/, a nonlipid enzyme, elevated in some liver disorders and cancer of the pancreas. It is measured in the blood to distinguish between certain liver and bone diseases. This enzyme is widely distributed throughout the body but is found in high concentrations in the liver and pancreas. The normal accumulations in serum are 0.1 to 6 units.

**5'-nucleotidase test,**  a blood test used to help diagnose liver disease, particularly cholestasis. It provides information similar to that from the alkaline phosphatase (ALP) test. However, unlike ALP, 5'-nucleotidase is specific to the liver, so this test is used to confirm liver disease when ALP results are uncertain.

**nucleotide** /nōō′klē·ətīd′/,  a compound consisting of one or more phosphate groups, a pentose sugar, and a nitrogenous base. Chains of nucleosides form DNA and RNA; free nucleotides, such as adenosine triphosphate and guanosine triphosphate, are important energy carriers in all cells.

**nucleus** /n(y)ōō′klē·əs/ [L, nut kernel],  **1.** the central controlling body within a living cell, usually a spheric unit enclosed in a membrane and containing genetic codes for maintaining life systems of the organism and for issuing commands for growth and reproduction. **2.** a group of nerve cells of the central nervous system having a common function, such as supporting the sense of hearing or smell. **3.** the center of an atom about which electrons rotate. **4.** the central element in an organic chemical compound or class of compounds. Formerly called **cytoblast.** —**nuclear,** adj.

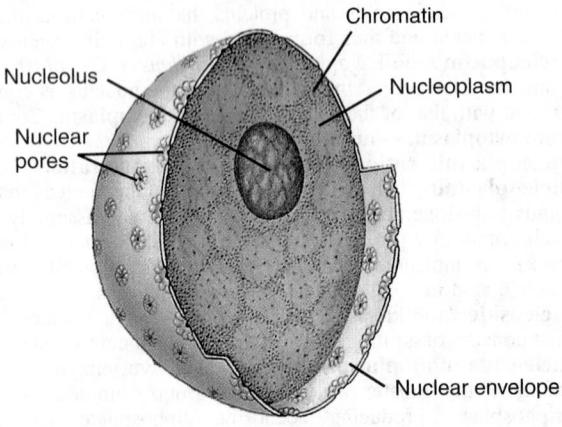

**Nucleus of a cell** *(Thibodeau and Patton, 1999/William Ober)*

Labels: Chromatin, Nucleolus, Nucleoplasm, Nuclear pores, Nuclear envelope

**nucleus pulposus,**  the central part of each intervertebral disk, consisting of a pulpy elastic substance that loses some of its resiliency with age. The nucleus pulposus may be suddenly compressed and squeeze out through the annular fibrocartilage, causing a herniated disk and extreme pain.

**nuclide** /nōō′klīd/ [L, nucleus, nut kernel],  a species of atom characterized by the constitution of its nucleus, in particular by the number of protons and neutrons. Thus, Co-59 and Co-60 are both isotopes of cobalt and are each nuclides. Co-60 is a radionuclide because it undergoes radioactive decay.

**nudge control,**  a prosthetic device with a mechanical part that can be pressed by the chin to lock or unlock one or more joints of the apparatus.

**NUG,**  abbreviation for *necrotizing ulcerative gingivitis.*

**Nuhn's gland** /noonz/ [Anton Nuhn, German anatomist, 1814–1889],  a gland on the inferior surface and near the apex and midline of the tongue.

**nuke,**  a slang term for nucleoside analog. See also **nucleoside reverse transcriptase inhibitors.**

**null cell** [L, *nullus,* not one, *cella,* storeroom],  a lymphocyte that develops in the bone marrow and lacks the characteristic surface markers of the B and T lymphocytes (surface immunoglobulin or the pan-T antigen). Null cells represent a small proportion of the lymphocyte population. Stimulated by the presence of antibody, null cells can attack certain cellular targets directly. They kill tumor or viral-infected cells, although not with the specificity of cytotoxic T cells. They are known as killer cells and natural killer (NK) cells. Compare **B cell, T cell.** See also **cytotoxin, immune gamma globulin, killer cell, natural killer cell.**

**null hypothesis (H₀),**  (in research) a hypothesis that predicts that an observed difference is caused by chance alone and not by systematic observation.

**nulli-,**  prefix meaning 'none': nullipara, nulligravida.

**nulligravida** /nul′igrav′ədə/,  a woman who has never been pregnant.

**nullipara** /nulip′ərə/, *pl.* **nulliparae** [L, *nullus,* not one, *parere,* to bear],  a woman who has not given birth to a viable infant. The designation "para 0" indicates nulliparity. Compare **multipara, primipara.**

**nulliparity** /nul′iper′itē/ [L, *nullus,* none, *parere,* to bear],  the status of a woman who has never borne a child.

**nulliparous** /nulip′ərəs/ [L, *nullus,* none, *parere,* to bear],  never having given birth.

**num,**  abbreviation for *number.*

**numbness** /num′nəs/ [ME, *nomen,* loss of feeling],  a partial or total lack of sensation in a body part, resulting from any factor that interrupts the transmission of impulses from the sensory nerve fibers. Numbness is often accompanied by tingling.

**numeric pain scale** /n(y)ōōmer′ik/,  a pain assessment system in which patients are asked to rate their pain on a scale from 1 to 10, with 10 representing the worst pain they have experienced or could imagine.

**numeric taxonomy,**  a system of classifying organisms based on the overall similarities of the measurable phenotypic characters they share. The system is used to classify strains of bacteria, as well as to separate closely related species of plants and animals.

**nummular dermatitis** /num′yələr/ [L, *nummuli,* petty cash; Gk, *derma,* skin, *itis,* inflammation],  a skin disease characterized by coin-shaped, vesicular, or scaling eczema-like lesions commonly on the forearms and front of the calves. The cause is unknown.

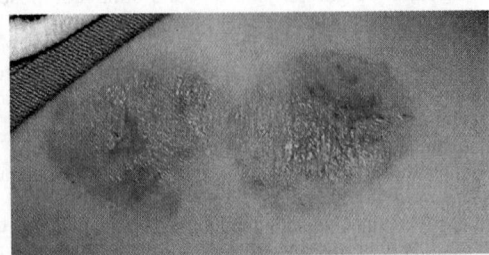

**Nummular dermatitis** *(Weston, Lane, Morrelli, 1996)*

**nummular psoriasis.** See **psoriasis.**

**Numorphan Hydrochloride,** trademark for an opioid analgesic (oxymorphone hydrochloride).

**Nupercainal,** trademark for a local anesthetic (dibucaine hydrochloride).

**Nuremberg tribunal** [Nuremberg, Germany; L, *tribunus,* platform for administration of justice], an international tribunal planned and implemented by the United Nations War Crimes Commission to detect, apprehend, try, and punish people accused of war crimes, establishing the **Nuremberg code.** In preparation for the prosecution of World War II criminals, the U.S. War Department assigned Andrew Ivy, M.D., to devise a set of principles to govern the participation of human beings in medical research. The principle and practice of informed consent was reinforced by the precedent set in the trials in which Nazi physicians were declared guilty of crimes against humanity in performing experiments on human beings who were not volunteers and did not consent. See also **Helsinki accords.**

**nurse** [L, *nutrix*], **1.** a person educated and licensed in the practice of nursing; one who is concerned with 'the diagnosis and treatment of human responses to actual or potential health problems' (American Nurses Association). The practice of the nurse includes data collection, diagnosis, planning, treatment, and evaluation within the framework of the nurse's singular concern with the patient's response to the problem, rather than to the problem itself. The concerns of the nurse are thus broader and less discrete and circumscribed than the traditional concerns of medicine. In a cooperative participatory relationship with the client or patient, the nurse acts to promote, maintain, or restore the health of the person; wellness is the goal. A collegial collaborative relationship with other health professionals who share a mission and a common data base furthers the practice of nursing. Guided by humanitarian, ethical principles, the nurse practices in a personal, nurturing, and protective manner that promotes health in all ways. The nurse may be a generalist or a specialist and, as a professional, is ethically and legally accountable for the nursing activities performed and for the actions of others to whom the nurse has delegated responsibility. **2.** to provide nursing care. See also **five-step nursing process, nursing, registered nurse.**

**nurse anesthetist,** a registered nurse qualified by advanced study in an accredited program in the specialty of nurse anesthesia to manage patient care during the administration of anesthesia in selected surgical situations. Educational requirements include a baccalaureate degree in nursing and a minimum of 1 year of acute care nursing experience, plus a 2-year or longer masters program in anesthesia. Nurse anesthetists are primarily involved in the direct administration of anesthesia to a single patient but often have other duties such as airway management in emergency situations. They practice under the supervision of an anesthesiologist.

**nurse cell,** a cell that transfers nutrients to an oocyte via a cytoplasmic bridge. Compare **Sertoli cell.**

**nurse-client interaction,** any process in which a nurse and a client exchange or share information, verbally or nonverbally. It is fundamental to communication and is an essential component of the nursing assessment.

**nurse-client relationship,** a therapeutic relationship between a nurse and a client built on a series of interactions and developing over time. All interactions do not develop into relationships but may nonetheless be therapeutic. The relationship differs from a social relationship in that it is designed to meet the needs only of the client. Its structure varies with the context, the client's needs, and the goals of the nurse and the client. Its nature varies with the context, including the setting, the kind of nursing, and the needs of the client. The relationship is dynamic and uses cognitive and affective levels of interaction. It is time-limited and goal-oriented and has three phases. During the first phase, the phase of establishment, the nurse establishes the structure, purpose, timing, and context of the relationship and expresses an interest in discussing this initial structure with the client. Data collection for the nursing care plan continues, and basic goals for the relationship are stated. During the middle, developmental, phase of the relationship, the nurse and the client get to know each other better and test the structure of the relationship to be able to trust one another. The nurse is careful to assess correctly the degree of dependency that is necessary for the particular client. Plans may be devised for improved ways of coping with problems and achieving goals. The nurse is alert to the danger of losing objectivity during this phase. The last phase, termination, ideally occurs when the goals of the relationship have been accomplished, when both the client and the nurse feel a sense of resolution and satisfaction. Often this is not possible because the nurse is transferred or the client discharged; in either case both may be left with a feeling of frustration.

**nurse clinician,** a nurse who is prepared to identify and diagnose problems of clients by using increased knowledge and skills gained through advanced study in a specific area of nursing practice. The specialist may function independently within standing orders or protocols and collaborates with associates to implement a care plan that is focused on the client.

**nurse coordinator,** a registered nurse who coordinates and manages the activities of nursing personnel engaged in specific nursing services, such as obstetrics or surgery, for two or more patient care units.

**Nurse Corps,** the branch within each of the armed services comprising the nurses within that service, such as the Army Nurse Corps. In each of the armed services, the members of the Nurse Corps have the rank, title, responsibilities, and status of commissioned officer.

**nurse educator,** a registered nurse whose primary area of interest, competence, and professional practice is the education of nurses at university level. Minimum education required is Master of Science in Nursing.

**nurse manager.** See **head nurse.**

**nurse midwife,** a registered nurse qualified by advanced education and clinical experience in obstetric and neonatal care and certified by the American College of Nurse Midwives. The nurse midwife manages the perinatal care of women having a normal pregnancy, labor, and childbirth. See also **certified nurse-midwife.**

**nurse practice act,** a statute enacted by the legislature of any of the states or by the appropriate officers of the districts or possessions. The act delineates the legal scope of the practice of nursing within the geographic boundaries of the jurisdiction.

**nurse practitioner (NP),** a registered nurse who has advanced education in nursing and clinical experience in a specialized area of nursing practice. NPs are certified by passing an examination administered by a professional organization such as the American Nurses' Credentialing Center (ANCC). They collaborate with other health care providers to deliver primary care to patients with common acute or stable chronic medical conditions in ambulatory care settings. Some NPs also function in a specialty, tertiary, or long-term care setting. NPs may offer a variety of services, such as complete physical examinations, health assessments, and patient education. Specialty certification is required for family nurse practitioner (FNP), women's health care nurse practitioner (RNC), neonatal nurse practitioner (NNP), pediatric nurse practitioner (CPNP), adult nurse practitioner (ANP), school nurse practitioner (SNP), gerontological nurse practitioner (GNP), and acute care nurse practitioner (CS). The list of NP specialties is expected to expand further in the near future to include mental health, campus health, and occupational health. The scope of all advanced nursing practice is influenced by state laws, federal laws, insurance practices, and regional acceptance. In many states NPs may obtain prescriptive authority. Some insurance organizations recognize NPs as primary health care providers and allow direct reimbursement for their services. Also called **advanced practice nurse (APN)**. See also specific kinds of nurse practitioner.

**nursery diarrhea** /nur'sərē/ [L, *nutrix*, nurse; Gk, *dia*, through, *rhein*, to flow], diarrhea of the newborn. In nurseries outbreaks of diarrhea caused by *Escherichia coli, Salmonella*, echoviruses, or adenoviruses are potentially life-threatening to the infant. The neonate may be infected at the time of birth by organisms from the mother's stool or infected later by organisms spread by the hands of hospital personnel. The most serious aspect of the disease is fluid loss, leading to dehydration and electrolyte imbalance. Care includes maintaining fluid and electrolyte balance and administering of antibiotics, if appropriate. Good handwashing technique, use of disposable nursing bottles and nipples, and early isolation of infected infants reduce the possibility of such outbreaks.

**nurse's aide,** a person who is employed to carry out basic nonspecialized tasks in the care of patients, such as bathing and feeding, making beds, and transporting patients, under the supervision and direction of a registered nurse. Many hospitals offer education and orientation programs for newly hired nurse's aides and in-service education for continued training.

**Nurses' Association of the American College of Obstetrics and Gynecology.** See **Association of Women's Health, Obstetric, and Neonatal Nurses.**

**Nurses' Coalition for Action in Politics.** See **American Nurses Association—Political Action Committee (ANA-PAC).**

**nurses' observation scale for inpatient evaluation (NOSIE),** a systematic, objective behavioral rating scale that is applied by nurses to patient behavior.

**nurses' registry,** an employment agency or listing service for nurses who wish to work in a specific area of nursing, usually for a short period of time or on a per diem basis. See also **float nurse.**

**nurses' station,** an area in a clinic, unit, or ward in a health care facility that serves as the administrative center for nursing care for a particular group of patients. It is usually centrally located and may be staffed by a unit secretary or clerk who assists with paperwork, telephone, and other communication. Before going on duty, nurses usually meet there to receive daily assignments, review the patients' charts, and update the files. In a critical care unit, the nurses' station may also contain panels of visual display terminals that allow centralized monitoring of many patients and may also have computer terminals that allow access to information in the patients' records or to a data bank of clinical information. In other parts of a hospital, the nurses' station is equipped in any of various ways appropriate to the care of the patients in that area or unit.

**nursing,** **1.** the practice in which a nurse assists "the individual, sick or well, in the performance of those activities contributing to health or its recovery (or to a peaceful death) that he would perform unaided if he had the necessary strength, will or knowledge. And to do this in such a way as to help him gain independence as rapidly as possible," (Virginia Henderson). **2.** "the diagnosis and treatment of human responses to actual or potential health problems," (American Nurses Association). There are four principal characteristics that further define nursing care: the phenomena that concern nurses; the use of theories to observe the need for nursing intervention and to plan nursing action; the nursing action taken; and an evaluation of the effects of the actions relative to the phenomena. This definition of nursing provides a framework for the nursing process, including data collection, diagnosis, planning, treatment, and evaluation. The nursing process is supported by standards of nursing practice that are congruent with the definition and that provide more specific guidelines for practice. These standards include systematic, continuous collection of data concerning the health status of the client in recorded form that is accessible and that may be communicated. A nursing diagnosis is derived from the data collected. A plan for nursing care incorporates goals derived from the nursing diagnosis and the priorities and approaches to achieve the goals as indicated by the nursing diagnosis. Nursing actions, which are selected and performed with the client's participation, provide for promotion, maintenance, or restoration of the client's health and serve to maximize the client's health care abilities. The progress or lack of progress toward the goal is mutually determined by the client and the nurse, resulting in reassessment, reordering of priorities, establishment of new goals, and revision of the plan for nursing care. Nursing touches on, intersects with, and complements other professional roles in health care, addressing itself to a wide range of health-related responses in people who are well and in those who are not. Nursing seeks to diagnose and treat the response to the problem; thus the concerns of nursing are less circumscribed and discrete than those of other health-related professions. These concerns include the following: limitations of the client's self-care ability; impaired ability to function in any fundamental area such as sleeping, breathing, eating, maintaining circulation; pain, anxiety, fear, loneliness, grief, or other physical or emotional problems related to health, illness, or treatment; impaired social or intellectual processes; impaired ability to make decisions and choices; alteration of self-image as required by the change in health; dysfunctional perception of health or health care activities; extra demands posed by such normal life-processes as birth, growth, or death; and difficulty in affiliative relationships. Various concepts, principles, processes, and actions developed and examined in nursing research guide the steps in the nursing process from initial observation and diagnosis through evaluation based on intrapersonal, interpersonal, and systems theories. The boundary for nursing practice is not static; it tends to move outward as the needs and capacities of society change. Collegial, collaborative practice with other health care professions further softens the boundaries of nursing practice. All health care professionals share a mission and a scientific data base, and to some degree their practices overlap. At its core nursing is nurturative, generative, and protective; preventive care is a part of every nurse's practice. Nurses value independence and self-respect; they are guided by an ethical and humanitarian philosophy in which every human being deserves respect, regardless of racial, social, cultural, sexual, economic, religious, or other factors. The nurse practices in the context of a relationship with the client, family, or group that is professional and yet close, in an interpersonal sense. The function of a nurse involves the physical intimacy of laying-on of hands; compassion and constant recognition of the person's dignity are essential. Nursing is practiced by specialists and generalists; generalists provide most nursing care; specialists, having added to their basic knowledge an organized and systematized body of knowledge and competencies, practice in specialized areas of nursing. Nursing care is given to people at all stages of life in the home, hospital, place of employment, school, or any environment where nursing care is needed. Nurses are ethically and legally accountable for their practice and for delegation of responsibilities to others. **3.** the professional practice of a nurse. **4.** the process of acting as a nurse, of providing care that encourages and promotes the health of the person or persons being served. See also **nursing process.**

**nursing assessment,** an identification by a nurse of the needs, preferences, and abilities of a patient. Assessment includes an interview with and observation of a patient by the nurse and considers the symptoms and signs of the condition, the patient's verbal and nonverbal communication, medical and social history, and any other information available. Among the physical aspects assessed are vital signs, skin color and condition, motor and sensory nerve function, nutrition, rest, sleep, activity, elimination, and consciousness. Among the social and emotional factors included in assessment are religion, occupation, attitude toward hospital and health care, mood, emotional tone, and family ties and responsibilities. Assessment is extremely important because it provides the scientific basis for a complete nursing care plan.

**nursing assistant,** *Canada.* a person trained in basic nursing techniques and direct patient care who practices under the supervision of a registered nurse. Also called **certified nursing assistant.** See also **licensed practical nurse.**

**nursing audit,** a thorough investigation designed to identify, examine, or verify the performance of certain specified aspects of nursing care using established criteria. A **concurrent nursing audit** is performed during ongoing nursing care. A **retrospective nursing audit** is performed after discharge from the care facility, using the patient's record. Often a nursing audit and a medical audit are performed collaboratively, resulting in a **joint audit.**

**nursing bottle caries.** See **baby bottle tooth decay.**

**nursing care plan,** a plan based on a nursing assessment and a nursing diagnosis carried out by a nurse. It has four essential components: identification of the nursing care problems or nursing diagnoses and statement of the nursing approach to solve those problems; statement of the expected benefit to the patient; statement of the specific actions by the nurse that reflect the nursing approach and achieve the goals specified; and evaluation of the patient's response to nursing care and readjustment of that care as required. The nursing care plan is begun when the patient is admitted to the health service, and, after the initial nursing assessment, a diagnosis is formulated and nursing orders are developed. The goal of the process is to ensure that nursing care is consistent with the patient's needs and progress toward self-care. A written nursing care plan should be a part of every patient's chart; an abbreviated form should be available for quick reference, such as in a Rand or Kardex file. See also **diagnosis, nursing assessment, nursing diagnosis, nursing orders, problem-solving approach to patient-centered care.**

**nursing diagnosis,** a statement of a health problem or of a potential problem in the client's health status that a nurse is licensed and competent to treat. Four steps are required in the formulation of a nursing diagnosis. A data base is established by collecting information from all available sources, including interviews with the client and the client's family, a review of any existing records of the client's health, observation of the client's response to any alterations in health status, a physical assessment, and a conference or consultation with others concerned in the client's care. The data base is continually updated. The second step includes analysis of the client's responses to the problems, healthy or unhealthy, and classification of those responses as psychologic, physiologic, spiritual, or sociologic. The third step is the organization of the data so that a tentative diagnostic statement can be made that summarizes the pattern of problems discovered. The last step is confirmation of the sufficiency and accuracy of the data base by evaluation of the appropriateness of the diagnosis to nursing intervention and by the assurance that, given the same information, most other qualified practitioners would arrive at the same nursing diagnosis. In use, each diagnostic category has three parts: the term that concisely describes the problem, the probable cause of the problem, and the defining characteristics of the problem. A number of nursing diagnoses have been identified and are listed as accepted by the North American Nursing Diagnosis Association (NANDA), and they are updated and refined at periodic meetings of the group.

**nursing differential,** an allowance added to payments to hospitals for services rendered Medicaid patients in recognition of the cost of providing nursing services to such patients that is greater than the cost to the general patient population.

**nursing director,** a nurse whose function is the administrative and clinical leadership of the nursing service of a division of a health care facility, such as a nursing supervisor of maternal and infant care nurses. Also called **nursing supervisor.**

**nursing ethics** [L, *nutrix,* nurse; Gk, *ethikos,* character], the values or moral principles governing relationships between the nurse and patient, the patient's family, other members of the health professions, and the general public. See also **Code for Nurses.**

**nursing goal,** a general goal of nursing involving activities that are desirable but difficult to measure, such as self-care, good nutrition, and relaxation. Compare **nursing objective.**

**nursing health history,** data collected about a patient's level of wellness, changes in life patterns, sociocultural role, and mental and emotional reactions to illness.

**nursing home.** See **extended care facility.**

**nursing intervention,** any act by a nurse that implements the nursing care plan or any specific objective of that plan, such as turning a comatose patient to avoid the development of decubitus ulcers or teaching insulin injection technique to a patient with diabetes before discharge from the hospital. The patient may require intervention in the form of support, limitation, medication, or treatment for the current condition or to prevent the development of further stress. As stress increases, the need to adapt and the need for nursing intervention increase. See also **adaptation, nursing process, stress.**

**nursing intervention model,** (in nursing research) a conceptual framework used to determine appropriate nursing interventions. The model is a holistic representation of the patient and the health care system. The patient's physiologic, psychologic, sociocultural, and developmental status, the patient's stressors and ability to react to them, and the levels and patterns of available health care are observed. The goal is to learn what nursing interventions would be most effective for the particular problem within the particular health care system.

**Nursing Interventions Classification (NIC),** a comprehensive, standardized system to classify treatments performed by nurses. It is a clinical tool developed by a research team at the University of Iowa that describes and defines the knowledge base for nursing curricula and practice. There are at present more than 400 nursing interventions that describe the treatments nurses perform. Each intervention has been labeled, defined, and given a list of appropriate activities. The full range of activities that nurses perform on behalf of patients are included, both independent and collaborative interventions, and both direct and indirect care. A taxonomy is provided to help the nurse find what is most relevant to her or his practice area. NIC interventions have been linked to NANDA diagnoses. It is considered part of the clinical decision making of the nurse to decide and document the nursing diagnoses, desired outcomes, interventions used, and outcomes achieved. The NIC system provides the language to document interventions.

**nursing minimum data set (NMDS),** a minimum set of items of information with uniform definitions and categories concerning the specific dimension of nursing, which meets the information needs of multiple data users in the health care system. It is the first attempt to standardize the collection of essential nursing data.

**nursing objective,** a specific aim planned by a nurse to decrease a person's stress, to improve the ability to adapt, or both. A nursing objective may be physical, emotional, social, or cultural and may involve the person's family, friends, and other patients. It is the purpose of any specific nursing order or nursing intervention. Some common nursing objectives are adequate understanding by the patient of certain details of the condition, adequate and comfortable daily elimination, a certain amount of rest, a balanced diet, and participation in specific items of self-care. Compare **nursing goal.**

**nursing observation,** an objective, holistic evaluation made by a nurse of the various aspects of a client's condition. It includes the person's general appearance, emotional affect, nutritional status, habits, and preferences, as well as body temperature, skin condition, and any obvious abnormal processes, including those of which the client complains. The client's religious preference, ethnic background, and familial relationships are also noted. Compare **nursing assessment, nursing intervention.**

**nursing orders,** specific instructions for implementing the nursing care plan, including the patient's preferences, timing of activities, details of health education necessary for the particular patient, role of the family, and plans for care after discharge. Nursing orders must be signed by the professional nurse who writes them. They should not duplicate the orders of the medical staff or of other members of the health team.

**Nursing Outcomes Classification (NOC),** a comprehensive, standardized system to classify outcomes of nursing interventions. It is a clinical tool developed by a research team at the University of Iowa that describes and defines the knowledge base for nursing curricula and practice. At present, NOC includes 190 nursing outcomes for use for individual patients or individual family caregivers in the home.

**nursing process,** the process that serves as an organizational framework for the practice of nursing. It encompasses all of the steps taken by the nurse in caring for a patient: assessment, nursing diagnosis, planning, implementation, and evaluation. The rationale for each step is founded in nursing theory. The process requires a systematic approach to a nursing assessment of the person's situation, including an evaluation and reconciliation of the perceptions by the person, the person's family, and the nurse. A plan for the nurs-

ing actions to be taken may then be made, and, with the participation of the person and the person's family, the plan may be set. The plan developed with the person and the person's family is then implemented. The outcome is evaluated with the person and the person's family. The steps follow each other at the start of the process but may need to be taken concurrently in some situations. The process does not reach completion with evaluation; the steps are begun again, allowing recurrent evaluation of the assessment, plan, goals, and actions. See also **five-step nursing process, nursing.**

**nursing process model,** a conceptual framework in which the nurse-patient relationship is the basis of the nursing process. The nursing process is represented as dynamic and interpersonal, the nurse and the patient being affected by each other's behavior and by the environment around them. Each successful two-way communication is termed a "transaction" and can be analyzed to discover the factors that promote transactions. The constraints that the various systems in the environment (personal, interpersonal, and social) place on the development of the relationship are also examined. The nurse views the patient as a person with whom to communicate to have transactions that achieve defined adaptive objectives toward the goal of health.

**nursing research,** a detailed systematic study of a problem in the field of nursing. Nursing research is practice or discipline-oriented and is essential for the continued development of the scientific base of professional nursing practice.

*Nursing Research*, a bimonthly refereed journal containing papers and other materials concerning nursing research. The goal of the journal is to stimulate research in nursing and disseminate research findings.

**nursing rounds,** chart rounds, walking rounds, teaching rounds, or grand rounds that are held specifically for nurses and that focus on nursing care. See also **rounds.**

**nursing specialty,** a nurse's selected professional field of practice, such as surgical, pediatric, obstetric, or psychiatric nursing. Compare **subspecialty.**

**nursing supervisor.** See **nursing director.**

**nursing theorist,** a person who develops integrated concepts or frameworks of nursing roles, functions, objectives, and activities and their relationships to clients and the roles of other health professionals.

**nursing theory,** an organized framework of concepts and purposes designed to guide the practice of nursing.

**nursology** /nursol′əjē/ [L, *nutrix*, nurse; Gk, *logos*, science], a conceptual framework for the study and practice of nursing. It requires the nurse to interact with the patient in an 'authentic' way, without aloofness and the distance of professionalism; the nurse must take the risk of caring. As a method, nursology requires that the nurse cut through the defenses and fears that prevent self-knowledge. The nurse tries to know the patient on an intuitive, subjective level and then, using reflection, on an objective, scientific level. The nurse recognizes that each person has an 'angular view' of the whole truth; comparison of the views of others is necessary for a perspective that allows a synthesis, often paradoxic but closer to the truth than any one person's angular view. Nursology is intended to provide a model for nursing methods and research. The nurse and the patient have the opportunity to grow, and the science of nursing may emerge from the 'angular' investigations and syntheses.

**NursoyTM,** trademark for a hypoallergenic nutritional supplement for infants.

**nurture** /nur′chər/, to feed, rear, foster, or care for, such as in the nourishment, care, and training of growing children.

**nutation** /nōotā′shən/ [L, *nutare*, to nod], the act of nodding, especially involuntary nodding as occurs in some neurologic disorders.

**nutcracker esophagus.** See **symptomatic esophageal peristalsis.**

**nutmeg poisoning,** a toxic effect of ingesting the dried kernels of the seeds of nutmeg *(Myristica fragrans)* or its volatile oils. The oils contain terpenes and myristicin, which have stimulant and carminative effects. A dose of one to three kernels may produce convulsions for up to 60 hours.

**NutramigenTM,** trademark for a milk-substitute formula that is prepared from a soy isolate base and is lactose free. It is prescribed for infants with galactosemia and as a protein supplement for people with lactose intolerance.

**nutri-,** prefix meaning 'nourishment': *nutriceptor, nutrient, nutritorium.*

**nutrient** /noo′trē·ənt/ [L, *nutriens,* food that nourishes], a chemical substance that provides nourishment and affects the nutritive and metabolic processes of the body. Nutrients are essential for growth, reproduction, and maintenance of health.

**nutrient artery of the humerus,** one of a pair of branches of the deep brachial arteries, arising near the middle of the arm and entering the nutrient canal of the humerus.

**nutrient canal.** See **interdental canal.**

**nutrient density,** the relative ratio obtained by dividing a food's contribution to the needs for a nutrient by its contribution to calorie needs.

**nutrient enema** [L, *nutriens* + Gk, *enienai,* injection], the introduction of saline or glucose into the body via the rectum. See also **enteral nutrition.**

**nutrient supplements,** vitamins and other nutrients that may not be necessary for healthy adults with an adequate intake of proper nutrients but that may be needed under certain circumstances for elderly adults or persons in a debilitated or undernourished state.

**nutriment** /noo′trimənt/ [L, *nutriens,* food that nourishes], any substance that nourishes and aids the growth and the development of the body. See also **food.**

**nutrition** /n(y)oōtrish′ən/ [L, *nutriens*], **1.** nourishment. **2.** the sum of the processes involved in the taking in of nutrients and their assimilation and use for proper body functioning and maintenance of health. The successive stages include ingestion, digestion, absorption, assimilation, and excretion. **3.** the study of food and drink as related to the growth and maintenance of living organisms.

**nutritional** /n(y)oōtrish′ənəl/ [L, *nutrire,* to nourish], pertaining to the quality of food or eating behavior that provides nourishment through assimilation of food to tissues.

**nutritional alcoholic cerebellar degeneration.** See **alcoholic-nutritional cerebellar degeneration.**

**nutritional anemia** [L, *nutrire,* to nourish; Gk, *a + haima,* without blood], a disorder characterized by the inadequate production of hemoglobin or erythrocytes caused by a nutritional deficiency of iron, folic acid, or vitamin $B_{12}$, or other nutritional disorders. See also **iron deficiency anemia, megaloblastic anemia, pernicious anemia.**

**nutritional care,** the substances, procedures, and setting involved in ensuring the proper intake and assimilation of nutriments, especially for the hospitalized patient.

■ METHOD: Depending on the patient's condition, nutritional requirements may be provided by regular meals with menus selected from the ordered diet, by tube feeding, or by parenteral hyperalimentation. Meals are served on attractive trays in an environment conducive to eating; distasteful procedures are avoided before and after mealtime. Patients who are unable to feed themselves are assisted, and abnormal intake of food is recorded and reported. Supplemental nourishment when indicated and fluids are offered between meals. The nutritional assessment includes observations of the patient's appetite, food preferences, allergies, height, intake and output, weight, measurements of the head, arms, abdomen, and skinfold thickness, skin color and turgor, and condition of the mouth, eyes, nails, and hair. Any cutaneous lesions, thyroid enlargement, dental caries, loose teeth, ill-fitting dentures, gum problems, nausea, vomiting, dehydration, diarrhea, or constipation are noted.

■ INTERVENTIONS: The nurse sees that food is presented attractively, offers a washcloth and oral hygiene before and after meals, and, when necessary, feeds the patient to maintain an adequate intake. If indicated, such as in obese patients or those with disorders requiring a highly restricted diet, the nurse restricts food intake as ordered. Tube feedings are administered as ordered.

■ OUTCOME CRITERIA: Obvious good health, maintenance of a normal weight, and the absence of GI symptoms usually indicate that the individual's nutritional requirements are being fulfilled.

**nutritional counseling,** a nursing intervention from the Nursing Interventions Classification (NIC) defined as use of an interactive helping process focusing on the need for diet modification. See also **Nursing Interventions Classification.**

**nutritional monitoring,** a nursing intervention from the Nursing Interventions Classification (NIC) defined as collection and analysis of patient data to prevent or minimize malnourishment. See also **Nursing Interventions Classification.**

**nutritional science,** a body of science that relates to the processes involved in nutrition.

**nutritional status,** a nursing outcome from the Nursing Outcomes Classification (NOC) defined as the extent to which nutrients are available to meet metabolic needs. See also **Nursing Outcomes Classification.**

**nutritional status: biochemical measures,** a nursing outcome from the Nursing Outcomes Classification (NOC) defined as the body fluid components and chemical indices of nutritional status. See also **Nursing Outcomes Classification.**

**nutritional status: body mass,** a nursing outcome from the Nursing Outcomes Classification (NOC) defined as the congruence of body weight, muscle, and fat to height, frame, and gender. See also **Nursing Outcomes Classification.**

**nutritional status: energy,** a nursing outcome from the Nursing Outcomes Classification (NOC) defined as the extent to which nutrients provide cellular energy. See also **Nursing Outcomes Classification.**

**nutritional status: food and fluid intake,** a nursing outcome from the Nursing Outcomes Classification (NOC) defined as the amount of food and fluid taken into the body over a 24-hour period. See also **Nursing Outcomes Classification.**

**nutritional status: nutrient intake,** a nursing outcome from the Nursing Outcomes Classification (NOC) defined as the adequacy of nutrients taken into the body. See also **Nursing Outcomes Classification.**

**nutrition base,** a person's normal nutritional requirements before modification to accommodate a specific condition.

**nutrition, imbalanced: less than body requirements,** a nursing diagnosis accepted by the Fourth National Conference on Nursing Diagnoses. It is defined as a state in which an individual experiences an intake of nutrients insufficient to meet metabolic needs.

■ DEFINING CHARACTERISTICS: The defining characteristics may include loss of weight with adequate food intake, body weight 20% or more under ideal for height and frame, reported intake of less food than is recommended, evidence or report of a lack of food, lack of interest in food, aversion to eating, alteration in the taste of food, feelings of fullness immediately after eating small quantities, abdominal pain with no other explanation, sores in the mouth, diarrhea or steatorrhea, pallor, weakness, and loss of hair.

■ RELATED FACTORS: A related factor is an inability, based on psychologic, biologic, or economic factors, to ingest or to digest food or to absorb nutrients in sufficient quantity for the maintenance of normal health. See also **nursing diagnosis.**

**nutrition, imbalanced: more than body requirements,** a nursing diagnosis accepted by the Fourth National Conference on Nursing Diagnoses. It is defined as a state in which an individual is experiencing an intake of nutrients that exceeds metabolic needs.

■ DEFINING CHARACTERISTICS: The critical defining characteristics, one of which must be present for the diagnosis to be made, include weight of 20% greater than the ideal for the height and body build of the client and triceps skin fold measurement greater than 15 mm in men and 25 mm in women. Other defining characteristics include a sedentary activity level and dysfunctional eating habits (including eating in response to internal cues other than hunger, pairing food with other activities, concentrating food intake at the end of the day, eating in response to external cues such as time of day and social situation).

■ RELATED FACTORS: A related factor is an excessive intake of food in relation to the body's metabolic needs. See also **nursing diagnosis.**

**nutritionist** /n(y)o͞otrish′ənist/ [L, *nutrire*, to nourish], a professional who has completed academic degrees of BS, MS, EdD, or PhD in foods and nutrition.

**nutrition management,** a nursing intervention from the Nursing Interventions Classification (NIC) defined as assisting with or providing a balanced dietary intake of foods and fluids. See also **Nursing Interventions Classification.**

**nutrition, risk for imbalanced: more than body requirements,** a nursing diagnosis accepted by the Fourth National Conference on Nursing Diagnoses. It is defined as a state in which an individual is at risk of experiencing an intake of nutrients that exceeds metabolic needs.

■ RISK FACTORS: Risk factors include hereditary predisposition; excessive energy intake during late gestational life, early infancy, and adolescence; frequent, closely spaced pregnancies; dysfunctional psychologic conditioning in relationship to food; membership in a lower socioeconomic group; reported or observed obesity in one or both parents; rapid transition across growth percentiles in infants or children; reported use of solid food as a major food source before 5 months of age; observed use of food as reward or comfort measure; reported or observed higher baseline weight at the beginning of each pregnancy; and dysfunctional eating patterns, including pairing food with other activities, concentrating food intake at the end of the day, eating in response to external cues (e.g., time of day or social situation), and eating in response to internal cues other than hunger (e.g., anxiety). See also **nursing diagnosis.**

**nutrition therapy,** a nursing intervention from the Nursing Interventions Classification (NIC) defined as administration of food and fluids to support metabolic processes of a patient who is malnourished or at high risk for becoming malnourished. See also **Nursing Interventions Classification.**

**Nutting, Mary Adelaide** (1858–1947), a Canadian-born American nursing educator and reformer. As head of Johns Hopkins School of Nursing in Baltimore beginning in 1894, she improved course content and teaching facilities, instituted the 6-month preparatory course, reduced the 12-hour day to 8 hours, and abolished the monthly payment system to students. At Teachers College, Columbia University, she created and developed the Department of Nursing and Health and became the first professor of nursing in the world. With Lavinia Dock she wrote *History of Nursing,* (published 1907–1912), a classic in nursing literature.

**nux vomica** /nuks′ vom′ikə/ [L, *nux*, nut, *vomere,* to vomit], the dried ripe seeds of a small Asian tree, *Strychnos nux vomica,* a source of the alkaloids strychnine and brucine. The seeds are powdered, and the strychnine content reduced to a little more than 1% by the addition of lactose for use as a bitter tonic and nerve stimulant.

**nvm,** abbreviation for *nonvolatile matter.*

**NVMA,** abbreviation for *National Veterinary Medical Association.*

**nyctalopia** /nik′təlō′pē·ə/ [Gk, *nyx*, night, *alaos,* obscure, *ops,* eye], poor vision at night or in dim light resulting from decreased synthesis of rhodopsin, vitamin A deficiency, retinal degeneration, or a congenital defect. Also called **day sight, night blindness. —nyctalopic,** *adj.*

**nycto-,** combining form meaning 'night or darkness': *nyctohemeral, nyctophilia, nyctophobia.*

**nyctophobia** /nik′tō-/ [Gk, *nyx* + *phobos,* fear], an anxiety reaction characterized by an obsessive, irrational fear of darkness.

**nycturia.** See **nocturia.**

**nympho-,** **1.** combining form meaning 'the labia minora': *nymphocaruncular, nymphohymeneal.* **2.** indicating a relationship to the female gender: *nymphomaniac.*

**nymphomania** /nim′fəmā′nē·ə/ [Gk, *nymphe*, maiden, *mania,* madness], a psychosexual disorder of women characterized by an insatiable desire for sexual satisfaction, often resulting from an unconscious conflict concerning personal adequacy. Compare **satyriasis.** See also **psychosexual disorder.**

**nymphomaniac** /-mā′nē·ak/, **1.** a person with or displaying characteristics of an individual possessing an insatiable desire for sexual satisfaction. **2.** pertaining to or exhibiting nymphomania. **—nymphomaniacal** /nim′fəmənī′əkəl/, *adj.*

**nystagmus** /nīstag′məs/ [Gk, *nystagmos,* nodding], involuntary, rhythmic movements of the eyes; the oscillations may be horizontal, vertical, rotary, or mixed. Jerking nystagmus, characterized by faster movements in one direction than in the opposite direction, is more common than pendular nystagmus, in which the oscillations are approximately equal in rate in both directions. Jerking nystagmus occurs normally when an individual watches a moving object, but on other occasions it may be a sign of barbiturate intoxication or of labyrinthine vestibular, vascular, or neurologic disease. Labyrinthine vestibular nystagmus, most frequently rotary, is usually accompanied by vertigo and nausea. Vertical nystagmus is considered pathognomonic of disease of the tegmentum of the brainstem; nystagmus occurring only in the abducting eye is said to be a sign of multiple sclerosis. Seesaw nystagmus, in which one eye moves up and the other down, may be observed in bilateral hemianopia. Pendular nystagmus occurs in albinism, in various diseases of the retina and refractive media, and in miners after many years of working in darkness; in miners the eye movements are very rapid, increase on upward gaze, and are often associated with vertigo, head tremor, and photophobia. **Electro-**

**nystagmography,** used in testing for vestibular disease and evaluating patients with vertigo, hearing loss, or tinnitus, records changes in the electrical field around the eyes. Nystagmus is measured as the person gazes at various objects and is placed in various positions and when cold or warm water or air is introduced into the external auditory canal. This final test causes nystagmus of equal intensity in normal individuals. In patients with an inner ear or neural disorder, nystagmus may be more intense, diminished, or absent. Also called **nystaxis. —nystagmic,** *adj.*

**nystatin** /nis′tətin/, an antifungal antibiotic; oral topical, vaginal, and mouthwash formulations.

■ INDICATIONS: It is prescribed in the treatment of fungal infections of the GI tract, vagina, and skin.

■ CONTRAINDICATION: Known hypersensitivity to this drug is the only contraindication.

■ ADVERSE EFFECTS: There are no known serious adverse reactions. Mild GI distress and mild skin reactions may occur.

**nystaxis.** See **nystagmus.**

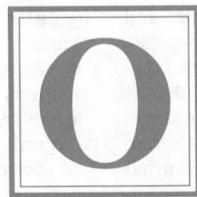

**o,** symbol for *ohm.*

**O,** symbol for the element **oxygen.**

**O₂,** symbol for *oxygen molecule.*

**oario-.** See **ovario-.**

**OASDHI,** abbreviation for **Old Age, Survivors, Disability and Health Insurance Program.**

**oat cell carcinoma** [AS, *ate,* oat; L, *cella,* storeroom; Gk, *karkinos,* crab, *oma,* tumor], a malignant, usually bronchogenic epithelial neoplasm consisting of small tightly packed round, oval, or spindle-shaped epithelial cells that stain darkly and contain neurosecretory granules and little or no cytoplasm. Tumors produced by these cells do not form bulky masses but usually spread along submucosal lymphatics. Many malignant tumors of the lung are of this type. Usually surgical resection is not possible, and chemotherapy and radiation therapy are not effective in treatment; thus the long-term prognosis is poor. Also called **small cell carcinoma.**

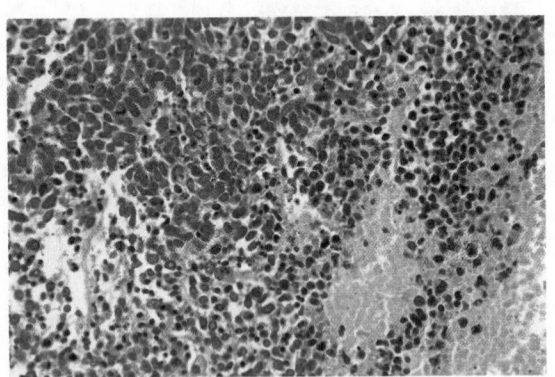

**Oat cell carcinoma** *(Fletcher, 2000)*

**oatmeal bath,** a colloid treatment for pruritus and other skin disorders. The procedure may consist of covering the patient with a layer of muslin containing oatmeal and pouring warm water over the fabric. The bath has a soothing effect. In a variation of the therapy, starch is substituted for oatmeal.

**OAV syndrome.** See **Goldenhar's syndrome.**

**OAWO,** abbreviation for **opening abductory wedge osteotomy.**

**ob.,** abbreviation for the Latin word *obit,* 'died.'

**ob-,** prefix meaning 'against, in the way, oppose': *obdormition, obduction, obtuse.*

**OB,** *informal.* **1.** abbreviation for **obstetrician. 2.** abbreviation for **obstetrics.**

**obduction** /əbduk′shən/ [L, *obductio,* a covering], a forensic medical autopsy.

**Ober and Barr procedure,** a surgical method for treating weak biceps muscles by transfer of the brachioradialis muscle.

**Ober procedure,** a surgical method for treating paralytic clubfoot by transfer of the posterior tibial tendon to the third cuneiform or metatarsal.

**Obersteiner-Redlich zone** /ō′bərshtī′nər-rād′lish, ō′bər-stē′nər-red′lik/ [H. Obersteiner, Austrian neurologist, 1847–1942; Emil Redlich, Austrian neurologist, 1866–1930], a thin line of demarcation between fibers of the peripheral nervous system and the spinal cord or brainstem. It is produced by a basal lamina separating the Schwann cells and collagen of the peripheral nervous system from the neuroglia of the central nervous system.

**Ober test** [Frank R. Ober, American surgeon, 1861–1925], an examination for tightness in the tensor fasciae latae, a muscle that flexes and rotates the thigh. The patient lies on one side with the lower hip and knee flexed on the table and the upper hip extended while the knee is flexed. Inability to place the upper knee on the table indicates tightness in the muscle.

**obese** /ōbēs′/ [L, *obesus,* swollen], pertaining to a corpulent or excessively heavy individual. Generally a person is regarded as medically obese if he or she is 20% above desirable body weight for the person's age, sex, height, and body build. Because the 'average' human body is approximately 25% fat, the proportion may be doubled for a medically defined obese person. See also **body mass index.**

**obesity** /ōbē′sitē/ [L, *obesitas,* fatness], an abnormal increase in the proportion of fat cells, mainly in the viscera and subcutaneous tissues of the body. Obesity may be exogenous or endogenous. **Hyperplastic obesity** is caused by an increase in the number of fat cells in the increased adipose tissue mass. **Hypertrophic obesity** results from an increase in the size of the fat cells in the increased adipose tissue mass.

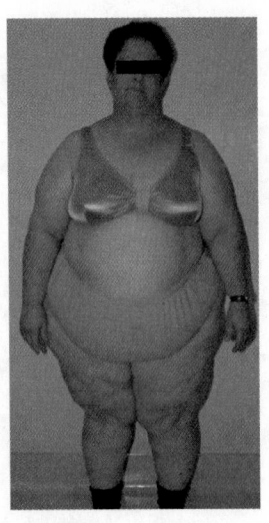

**Obesity** *(Lemmi and Lemmi, 2000)*

**Obetrol,** trademark for a fixed-combination drug containing central nervous system stimulants (dextroamphetamine and amphetamine).

**obex** /ō'beks/, a small triangular membrane formed at the caudal angle of the rhomboid fossa or fourth ventricle.

**obfuscation** /ob'fəskā'shən/ [L, *obfuscare*, to darken], the act of making something confused, clouded, or obscure.

**OBG,** abbreviation for *obstetrics and gynecology.*

**OB-Gyn,** *informal.* abbreviation for *obstetrics and gynecology.*

**object** /ob'jəkt/, (in psychology) something through which an instinct can achieve its goal. In psychoanalytic terms, a person other than self. See also **object relations.**

**object blindness,** an inability to recognize objects or analyze spatial relationships. The condition is associated with lesions of the right cerebral hemisphere in right-handed patients. Also called **visual agnosia.** See also **psychic blindness.**

**object constancy,** the ability to perceive an object as unchanging even under different conditions of observation. See **object permanence.**

**objective** /əbjek'tiv/ [L, *objectare*, to set against], **1.** a goal. **2.** pertaining to a phenomenon or clinical finding that is observed; not subjective. An objective finding is often described in health care as a sign that can be seen, heard, felt, or measured.

**objective data collection,** the process in which data relating to the client's problem are obtained by an observer through direct physical examination, including observation, palpation, percussion, and auscultation, and by laboratory analyses and radiologic and other studies. Compare **subjective data collection.**

**objective lens,** a lens that accepts light from the output phosphor of a radiographic image-intensifier tube and converts the light into a parallel beam for recording the image on film.

**objective sign** [L, *objectum*, something cast before, *signum*, sign], a clinical observation that can be seen, heard, measured, or otherwise recorded by an examining physician, nurse, or other health care provider.

**objective symptom** [L, *objectum*, something cast before; Gk, *symptoma*, that which happens], a symptom accompanied by signs that tend to confirm the patient's physical complaint and enable the examining physician, nurse, or other health care provider to deduce the cause.

**objective tinnitus,** a noise produced in the ear that can be heard by another person, particularly someone using a stethoscope. See also **tinnitus.**

**object permanence,** a capacity to perceive that something exists even when it is not seen.

**object relations,** emotional bond between one person and another, as contrasted with interest in and love for the self. It is usually described in terms of capacity for loving and reacting appropriately to others. An object relation is delayed or not achieved in borderline personality disorders.

**obligate** /ob'ligit, -gāt/ [L, *obligare*, to bind], characterized by the ability to survive only in a particular set of environmental conditions, such as an obligate parasite, which can survive only within the host organism. Compare **facultative.**

**obligate aerobe,** an organism that cannot grow in the absence of oxygen. Compare **facultative aerobe.** See also **aerobe.**

**obligate anaerobe,** an organism that cannot grow in the presence of oxygen, such as *Clostridium tetani, C. botulinum,* and *C. perfringens.* Compare **facultative anaerobe.** See also **anaerobe, anaerobic infection.**

**obligate parasite.** See **parasite.**

**obligatory water loss** /əblig'ətôr'ē/, the volume of water required for daily urinary excretion of metabolic waste products. This amount of water loss is necessary to maintain normal health. See also **optional water loss.**

**oblique** /əblēk'/ [L, *obliquus,* slanted], a slanting direction or any variation from the perpendicular or the horizontal.

**oblique bandage,** a circular bandage applied spirally in slanting turns, usually to a limb.

**oblique fiber,** any of the collagenous filaments that are bundled together obliquely in the periodontal ligament, inserted into the cementum of the teeth, and extended more occlusally in the alveolus. Oblique fibers constitute approximately two thirds of the periodontal fibers.

**oblique fissure of the lung, 1.** the groove marking the division of the lower and the middle lobes in the right lung. **2.** the groove marking the division of the upper and the lower lobes in the left lung.

**oblique fracture,** a slanted fracture of the shaft along the bone's long axis.

**oblique illumination.** See **illumination.**

**oblique presentation** [L, *obliquus,* slanted, *praesentare,* to show], a presentation in which the long axis of the fetus is oblique to the long axis of the mother.

**obliquity of pelvis** /əblik'witē/ [L, *obliquus,* aslant], an abnormal tilt of the pelvis with respect to the spinal column.

**obliquus externus abdominis.** See **external abdominal oblique muscle.**

**obliquus internus abdominis.** See **internal abdominal oblique muscle.**

**obliteration** /əblit'ərā'shən/ [L, *obliterare,* to efface], the removal or loss of function of a body part by surgery, disease, or degeneration.

**obliterative phlebitis** /əblit'ərətiv'/ [L, *obliterare,* to efface; Gk, *phleps,* vein, *itis,* inflammation], a form of phlebitis in which the inflammation results in permanent closure of the vessel. Also called **adhesive phlebitis.**

**OBS,** abbreviation for *organic brain syndrome.* See **organic mental disorder.**

**observation** [L, *observare,* to watch], **1.** the act of watching carefully and attentively. **2.** a report of what is seen or noticed, such as a nursing observation.

**observation hip,** a condition in which a patient experiences a limp, pain in the hip, and limited hip motion. Causes include toxic synovitis, infection, and avascular necrosis.

**obsession** [L, *obsidere,* to haunt], a persistent and recurrent thought or idea with which the mind is continually and involuntarily preoccupied and which cannot be expunged by logic or reasoning.

**obsessive-compulsive** /əbses'iv/ [L, *obsidere,* to haunt, *compellere,* to impel], **1.** characterized by or relating to the tendency to perform repetitive acts or rituals or think repetitive thoughts, usually as a means of releasing tension or relieving anxiety. **2.** describing a person who has an obsessive-compulsive disorder.

**obsessive-compulsive disorder,** an anxiety disorder characterized by recurrent and persistent thoughts, ideas, and feelings of obsessions or compulsions sufficiently severe to cause marked distress, consume considerable time, or significantly interfere with the patient's occupational, social, or interpersonal functioning. See also **compulsive ritual.**

**obsolescence** /ob'sələs'əns/ [L, *obsolescere,* to decay], **1.** to fall into disuse because of age or loss of function. **2.** a state of being useless.

**obstetric** /əbstet'rik/ [L, *obstetrix,* midwife], pertaining to pregnancy, childbirth.

**obstetrical.** See **obstetrics.**

**obstetric anesthesia** [L, *obstetrix,* midwife; Gk, *anaisthesia,* lack of feeling], any of various procedures used to provide anesthesia for childbirth. It includes local anesthesia for episiotomy or episiotomy repair; regional anesthesia for labor or delivery, such as by paracervical block or pudendal block; or, for a wider block, epidural, spinal, caudal, or saddle block. Anesthesia for cesarean section may be achieved with an epidural or spinal block or by general anesthesia.

**obstetric forceps,** forceps used to assist delivery of the fetal head. They vary in weight, length, shape, and mechanism of action, but all consist of a pair of instruments comprising a handle, a shank, and a blade. The blade is curved and sometimes has openings. The shank is long enough to allow the blade to reach the fetal head. The several styles of forceps are designed to assist in various clinical situations. The station of the fetus in the pelvis, the position of the head in relation to the pelvis, the size of the fetus, and the preference of the operator all affect the choice of forceps. Kinds of obstetric forceps include **Barton forceps, Elliot forceps, Kielland forceps,** and **Simpson forceps.** See also **forceps delivery.**

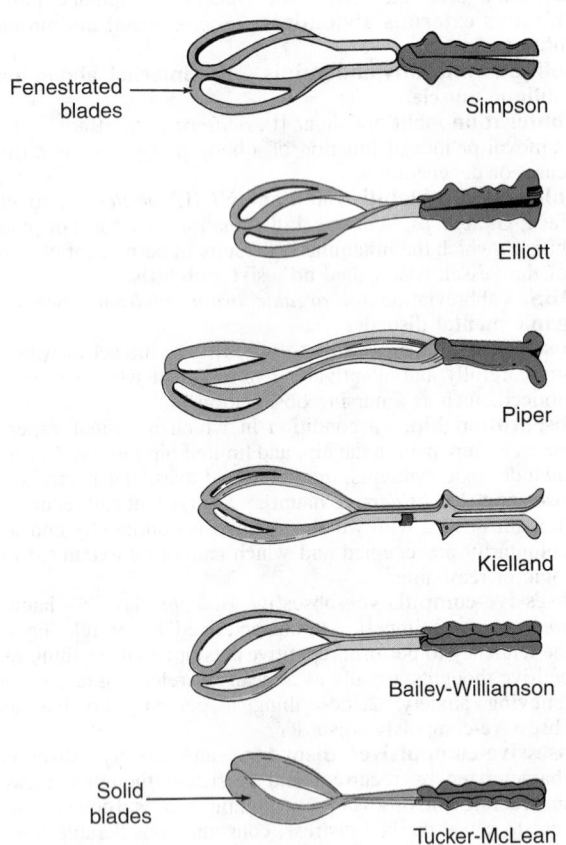

Fenestrated blades — Simpson

Elliott

Piper

Kielland

Bailey-Williamson

Solid blades — Tucker-McLean

**Obstetric forceps** (Lowdermilk, Perry, and Bobak, 2000)

**obstetrician** /ob′stətrish′ən/, a physician who specializes in the branch of medicine concerned with pregnancy and childbirth.

**obstetric position.** See **lateral recumbent position.**

**obstetrics** /əbstet′riks/ [L, *obstetrix,* midwife], the branch of medicine concerned with pregnancy and childbirth, including the study of the physiologic and pathologic function of the female reproductive tract and the care of the mother and fetus throughout pregnancy, childbirth, and the immediate postpartum period. —**obstetric, obstetrical,** *adj.*

**obstetrix.** See **midwife.**

**obstipation** /ob′stipā′shən/ [L, *obstipare,* to press], **1.** a condition of extreme and persistent constipation caused by obstruction in the intestinal system. See also **constipation. 2.** a process of blocking. —**obstipant,** *n.,* **obstipate,** *v.*

**obstruction** /əbstruk′shən/ [L, *obstruere,* to build against], **1.** something that blocks or clogs. **2.** the act of blocking or preventing passage. **3.** the condition of being obstructed or clogged. —**obstruct,** *v.,* **obstructive,** *adj.*

**obstruction series,** a test consisting of a series of x-ray films performed on the abdomen of patients with suspected bowel obstruction, paralytic ileus, perforated viscus, abdominal abscess, kidney stones, appendicitis, or foreign body ingestion.

**obstructive airways disease** /əbstruk′tiv/, any respiratory disease characterized by decreased airway size and increased airway secretions. It includes chronic bronchitis, abnormalities of the bronchi, and emphysema. See also **chronic obstructive pulmonary disease, cystic fibrosis.**

**obstructive anuria** [L, *obstruere,* to build against; Gk, *a* + *ouron,* without urine], an almost complete absence of urination caused by blockage of the urinary tract. See also **obstructive uropathy.**

**obstructive biliary cirrhosis** [L, *obstruere,* to build against, *bilis,* bile; Gk, *kirrhos,* yellow-orange, *osis,* condition], a form of secondary cirrhosis in which a stricture develops in the bile ducts. The condition may develop after cholecystectomy, gallstones, or a tumor.

**obstructive constipation** [L, *obstruere,* to build against, *constipare,* to crowd together], a condition in which feces are retained in the intestine because of a blockage in the lumen. Also called **alvine obstruction.**

**obstructive jaundice.** See **cholestasis.**

**obstructive sleep apnea,** a form of sleep apnea involving a physical obstruction in the upper airways. The condition tends to affect mainly obese people, particularly those with secondary pulmonary insufficiency or a constitutional defect. A nonobese person with a congenital abnormality of the upper airways also may experience obstructive sleep apnea. The condition is usually marked by recurrent sleep interruptions, choking and gasping spells on awakening, and drowsiness caused by loss of normal sleep. Uncorrected, the disorder often leads to central sleep apnea, pulmonary failure, and cardiac abnormalities. See also **pickwickian syndrome.**

**obstructive uropathy,** any pathologic condition that blocks the flow of urine. Causes of the condition include prostate enlargement, renal calculi, and congenital stenosis. The condition may lead to impairment of kidney function and an increased risk of urinary infection.

**obtund** /obtund′/ [L, *obtundere,* to blunt], **1.** to deaden pain. **2.** to render insensitive to unpleasant or painful stimuli by reducing the level of consciousness, such as by anesthesia or a strong opioid analgesic. —**obtundation, obtundity,** *n.,* **obtunded, obtundent,** *adj.*

**obtundation** /ob′tundā′shən/ [L, *obtundere,* to blunt, *atus,* process], the use of an agent that soothes and reduces irritation or pain by blocking sensibility at some level of the central nervous system, such as in the use of narcotics to control pain and the use of a tranquilizer as a calming agent.

**obtunded, obtundent, obtundity.** See **obtund.**

**obturation** /ob′t(y)ərā′ahən/ [L, *obturare,* to stop up], an obstruction of an opening, such as an intestinal blockage.

**obturator** /ob′tərā′tər, ob′tyərā′tər/ [L, *obturare,* to close], **1.** a device used to block a passage or a canal or to fill in a space, such as a prosthesis implanted to bridge the gap in the roof of the mouth in a cleft palate. **2.** *nontechnical.* an obturator muscle or membrane. **3.** a device that is placed into a large-bore cannula during insertion to prevent potential blockage by residual tissues.

**obturator dislocation.** See **dislocation of hip.**

**obturator externus,** the flat, triangular muscle covering the outer surface of the anterior wall of the pelvis. It arises in several pelvic structures, including the rami of the pubis and the ramus of each ischium, and inserts into the trochanteric fossa of the femur. It functions to rotate the thigh laterally. Compare **obturator internus.**

**obturator foramen,** a large opening on each side of the lower part of the hip bone, formed posteriorly by the ischium, superiorly by the ilium, and anteriorly by the pubis.

**obturator internus,** a muscle that covers a large area of the inferior aspect of the lesser pelvis, where it surrounds the obturator foramen. It functions to rotate the thigh laterally and to extend and abduct the thigh when it is flexed. Compare **obturator externus, piriformis.**

**obturator membrane,** a tough fibrous membrane that covers the obturator foramen of each side of the pelvis.

**obturator muscles** [L, *obturare,* to close, *musculus*], a pair of thigh muscles, the external and internal obturators. The external obturator flexes and rotates the thigh laterally, and the internal obturator abducts and rotates the thigh laterally.

**obturator sign** [L, *obturare,* to close, *signus,* sign], a sign of appendicitis. The internal rotation of the right leg with the leg flexed to 90 degrees at the hip and knee and a resultant tightening of the internal obturator muscle may cause abdominal discomfort, for example, in appendicitis.

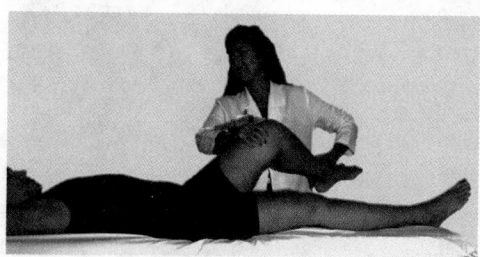

**Obturator sign** *(Lemmi and Lemmi, 2000)*

**obv,** abbreviation for *obverse.*

**oc-.** See **ob-.**

**O.C.,** abbreviation for **oral contraceptive.**

**OCA,** abbreviation for **oculocutaneous albinism.**

**occ,** abbreviation for **occipital.**

**occipit-, occipito-,** prefix meaning 'back of the head': *occipital, occipitofrontal.*

**occipita.** See **occiput.**

**occipital** /oksip′itəl/, **1.** pertaining to the back of the head. **2.** situated near the occipital bone, such as the occipital lobe of the brain.

**occipital anchorage,** an orthodontic anchorage in which the resistance is borne by the top and back of the head, and the force transmitted to the teeth by means of the headgear and heavy elastics connected with attachment on the teeth.

**occipital artery,** one of a pair of tortuous branches from the external carotid arteries that divides into six branches and supplies parts of the head and scalp. Each terminal part at the vertex of the skull is accompanied by the greater occipital nerve.

**occipital bone,** the cuplike bone at the back of the skull, marked by a large opening, the foramen magnum, that communicates with the vertebral canal. The occipital bone articulates with the two parietal bones, the two temporal bones, the sphenoid, and the atlas

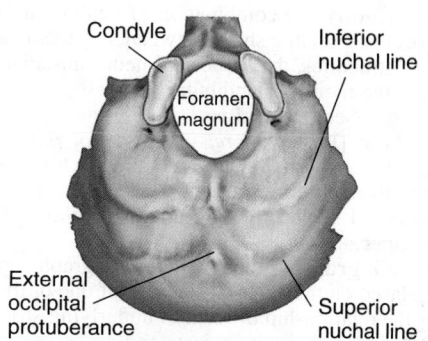

**Occipital bone**

**occipital condyle syndrome,** a condition characterized by a stiff neck and severe localized occipital pain that intensifies with neck flexion. It is associated with unilateral involvement of the twelfth nerve, dysarthria, and dysphagia.

**occipitalization** /oksip′ital′īzā′shən/, a process of bony ankylosis of the atlas with the occipital bone.

**occipital lobe,** one of the five lobes of each cerebral hemisphere, occupying a relatively small pyramidal part of the occipital pole. The occipital lobe lies beneath the occipital bone and presents medial, lateral, and inferior surfaces. Compare **central lobe, frontal lobe, parietal lobe, temporal lobe.**

**occipital sinus,** the smallest of the cranial sinuses and one of six posterior superior venous channels associated with the dura mater. Compare **inferior sagittal sinus, straight sinus, superior sagittal sinus.**

**occipito-.** See **occipit-.**

**occipitoaxial ligament.** See **membrana tectoria.**

**occipitobregmatic** /oksip′itōbregmat′ik/ [L, *occiput,* back of the head; Gk, *bregma,* front of the head], pertaining to the occiput and the bregma.

**occipitofrontal** /oksip′itōfrun′təl/ [L, *occiput* + *frons,* forehead], pertaining to the occiput and the frontal bone of the skull.

**occipitofrontalis** /oksip′itōfrəntal′is/, one of a pair of thin, broad muscles covering the top of the skull, consisting of an occipital belly and a frontal belly connected by an extensive aponeurosis. It is the muscle that draws the scalp and raises the eyebrows. Compare **temporoparietalis.**

**occipitoparietal fissure.** See **parietooccipital sulcus.**

**occiput** /ok′sipət/, *pl.* **occiputs, occipita** /oksip′itə′/, the back part of the head. Also called **occiput cranii.**

**occlude.** See **occlusion.**

**occluded** /əklōō′did/ [L, *occludere,* to close up], closed, plugged, or obstructed.

**occlusal** /əklōō′səl/ [L, *occludere,* to close up], pertaining to a closure, such as the contact between the teeth of the upper and lower jaws.

**occlusal adjustment,** the intentional mechanical grinding of the biting surfaces of teeth to improve the contact of or relationship between opposing tooth surfaces, their supporting structures, the muscles of mastication, and the temporomandibular joints. See also **bite.**

**occlusal contouring,** the modification by grinding of occlusal tooth irregularities, such as uneven marginal ridges and extruded or malpositioned teeth. See also **bite.**

**occlusal form,** the shape of the occluding surfaces of a tooth, a row of teeth, or any dentition.

**occlusal harmony,** a combination of healthy and nondisruptive occlusal relationships between the teeth and their supporting structures, the associated neuromuscular mechanisms, and the temporomandibular joints.

**occlusal lug.** See **occlusal rest.**

**occlusal plane** [L, *occludere,* to close up, *planum,* level ground], a plane passing through the occlusal or biting surfaces of the teeth. It represents the mean of the curvature of the occlusal surface. Also called **biteplane.** See also **curve of Spee.**

**occlusal radiograph,** an intraoral radiograph made with the film placed on the occlusal surfaces of one of the arches. It shows the relationship of teeth to underlying structures in the alveolar process, such as cysts and abscesses.

**occlusal recontouring,** the reshaping of an occlusal surface of a natural or artificial tooth.

**occlusal relationship,** the relationship of the mandibular teeth to the maxillary teeth when they are in a defined contact position. See also **Angle's Classification of Malocclusion.**

**occlusal rest,** a support that is part of a removable partial denture and that is placed on the occlusal surface of a posterior tooth. Also called **occlusal lug.**

**occlusal rest angle,** the angle formed by an occlusal rest with its upright minor connector. Also called **rest angle.**

**occlusal spillway,** a natural groove that crosses a cusp ridge or a marginal ridge of a tooth.

**occlusal surface** [L, *occludere,* to close up, *superficies,* surface], the surfaces of a tooth in one arch that makes contact or near contact with the corresponding surface of a tooth. Also called **biting surface, masticatory surface.**

**occlusal trauma,** injury to a tooth and surrounding structures caused by malocclusive stresses, including trauma, temporomandibular joint dysfunction, and bruxism.

**occlusion** /əklōō′zhən/ [L, *occludere,* to close up], **1.** (in anatomy) a blockage in a canal, vessel, or passage of the body; the state of being closed. **2.** (in dentistry) any contact between the incising or masticating surfaces of the maxillary and mandibular teeth. —**occlude,** *v.,* **occlusive,** *adj.*

**occlusion rim,** an artificial dental structure with occluding surfaces attached to temporary or permanent denture bases, used for recording the relation of the maxilla to the mandible and for positioning the teeth. Also called **bite block.**

**occlusive** /əklōō′siv/, pertaining to something that effects an occlusion or closure, such as an occlusive dressing.

**occlusive dressing,** a dressing that prevents air from reaching a wound or lesion and that retains moisture, heat, body fluids, and medication. It may consist of a sheet of thin plastic affixed with transparent tape.

**occlusometer.** See **gnathodynamometer.**

**occult** /əkult′/ [L, *occultare,* to hide], hidden or difficult to observe directly, such as occult prolapse of the umbilical cord or occult blood.

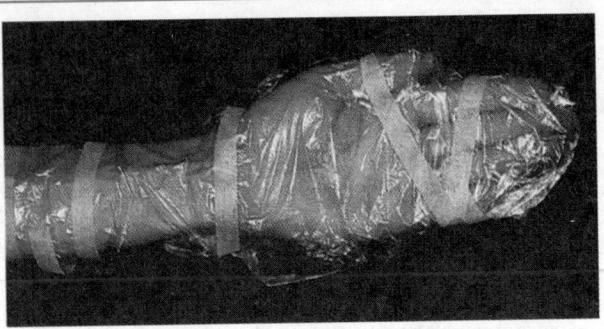

**Occlusive dressing of the hand** *(Habif, 1996)*

**occult blood,** blood that is not obvious on examination, from a nonspecific source, with obscure signs and symptoms. It may be detected by means of a chemical test or by microscopic or spectroscopic examination. Occult blood is often present in the stools of patients with GI lesions.

**occult blood test** [L, *occultare,* to hide; AS, *blod* + L, *testum,* crucible], a test for the presence of microscopic amounts of blood in the feces secondary to bleeding in the digestive tract. Normally only minimal amounts of occult blood are passed into the GI tract. Ordinarily this bleeding is not significant enough to cause a positive result for occult blood testing. Benign and malignant GI tumors, ulcers, inflammatory bowel disease, arteriovenous malformations, diverticulosis, and hematobilia can cause the appearance of occult blood in the stool, as can swallowed blood from oral or nasal pharyngeal bleeding.

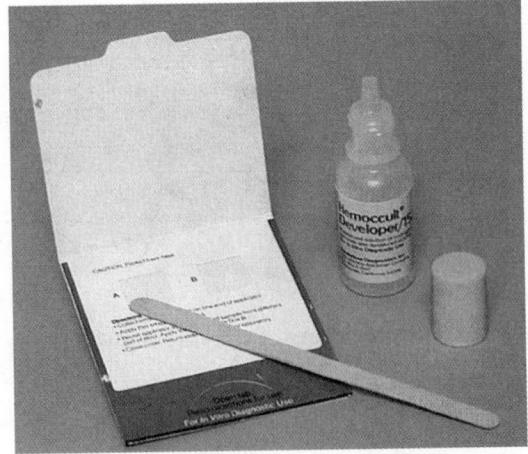

**Supplies used in testing for occult blood in stool: cardboard Hemoccult slide, wooden applicator, and Hemoccult developing solution** *(Potter and Perry, 1997)*

**occult carcinoma,** a small carcinoma that does not cause overt symptoms. The carcinoma may remain localized, be discovered only incidentally at autopsy after death resulting from another cause, or metastasize and be discovered as a result of metastatic disease. Also called **latent carcinoma.**

**occult ectopic ACTH syndrome,** a medical condition that mimics the clinical and biochemical picture of Cushing's disease. The cause is usually a tumor that secretes adrenocorticotropic hormone in the lungs, thymus, pancreas, adrenal medulla, or thyroid gland.

**occult fracture,** a fracture that cannot be detected by radiographic examination until several weeks after injury. The break is most likely to occur in the ribs, tibia, metatarsals, or navicular. It is accompanied by the usual signs of pain and trauma and may produce soft tissue edema.

**occupancy** /ok′yəpənsē′/ [L, *occupare,* to take possession of], the ratio of average daily hospital census to the total number of beds maintained during the reporting period.

**occupancy factor (T),** the level of human occupancy of an area adjacent to a source of radiation. It is used to determine the amount of shielding required in the walls. T is rated as full, for an office or laboratory next to an x-ray facility; partial, for corridors and restrooms; or occasional, for stairways, elevators, closets, and outside areas.

**occupational accident** /ok′yəpā′shənəl/ [L, *occupare,* to take possession of, *accidere,* to happen], an injury to an employee that occurs in the workplace. Occupational accidents account for over 95% of occupational disabilities. In most cases the injured worker is eligible for compensation.

**occupational asthma,** an abnormal condition of the respiratory system resulting from exposure in the workplace to allergenic or other irritating substances. The condition is most common among people working with detergents, Western red cedar, cotton, flax, hemp, grain, flour, and stone. See also **asthma, byssinosis, occupational lung disease.**

**occupational deafness,** a loss of hearing resulting from noise levels in the workplace. See also **noise-induced hearing loss.**

**occupational dermatoses,** skin disorders associated with exposure to toxic chemicals or other agents in the workplace. An estimated 80% of cases of contact dermatitis are the result of exposure to chemical irritants. Common agents of contact dermatitis in the workplace are glass fibers, cutting fluids, chemical stains, and polyhalogenated aromatic compounds such as phenol, naphthalene, and aniline herbicides intermediates. Factors influencing development of dermatoses include skin thickness, skim permeability, anatomic site, concentration of chemical, surface area of exposure, and type of substance in which the toxic chemical may be dissolved or mixed.

**occupational disability,** a condition in which a worker is unable to perform the functions required to complete a job satisfactorily because of an occupational disease or an occupational accident.

**occupational disease,** a disease that results from a particular employment, usually from the effects of long-term exposure to specific substances or continuous or repetitive physical acts.

**occupational health,** the ability of a worker to function at an optimum level of well-being at a worksite as reflected in terms of productivity, work attendance, disability compensation claims, and employment longevity.

**occupational history,** a part of the health history in which questions are asked about the person's occupation, source of income, effects of the work on worker's health or the worker's health on the job, the duration of the job, and to what degree the occupation satisfies the person. Any adverse effects known to be associated with the work or the place of work are investigated by further questions by the interviewer; for example, a tennis player might be asked about musculoskeletal problems; or a taxi driver about function of the urinary tract.

**occupational lung disease,** any of a group of abnormal conditions of the lungs caused by the inhalation of dusts, fumes, gases, or vapors in an environment where a person works. See also **chronic obstructive pulmonary disease, metal fume fever, occupational asthma, silo filler's disease.**

**occupational medicine,** a field of preventive medicine concerned with the medical problems and practices relating to occupations and especially to the health of workers in various industries.

**occupational neurosis.** See **occupational stress.**

**occupational performance tasks,** activities that can be used to measure the potential ability or actual proficiency in the handling of certain objects and use of skills related to a given occupation.

**occupational socialization,** the adaptation of an individual to a given set of job-related behaviors, particularly the expected behavior that accompanies a specific job.

**occupational stress,** a disorder associated with a job or work. The anxiety may be expressed in the form of extreme tension and anxiety and the development of physical symptoms such as headache or cramps. See also **burnout.**

**occupational therapist (OT),** an allied health professional who is nationally certified to practice occupational therapy. The OT uses purposeful activity and interventions to maximize the independence and health of any client who is limited by physical injury or illness, cognitive impairment, psychosocial dysfunction, mental illness, or a developmental or learning disability. Services include the assessment, treatment, and education of the client or family; interventions directed toward developing daily living skills, work readiness, or sensory-motor, perceptual or neuromuscular functioning, or range of motion.

**occupational therapy (OT),** a health rehabilitation profession designed to help people of all ages with physical, developmental, social, or emotional deficits regain and build skills that are important for functional independence, health and well-being. See also **occupational therapist.**

**occupational therapy aide,** a person who, under the supervision of an occupational therapist or OT assistant, performs clerical and other treatment-related tasks necessary for the implementation of occupational therapy programs.

**occupational therapy assistant.** See **certified occupational therapy assistant.**

**occurrence policy** /əkur′əns/ [L, *occurere,* to run, *politica,* pertaining to the state], a professional liability insurance policy that covers the holder during the period an alleged act of malpractice occurred. Occurrence policies are said to have a "long tail," because the statute of limitations on malpractice allegations is unlimited. Thus an individual could be sued years after an event took place. If the individual held an occurrence type of malpractice policy, there would be protection under that policy; under a claims-made policy there would not be protection unless the policy were current.

**OCD,** abbreviation for **obsessive-compulsive disorder.**

**ochre mutation.** See **amber mutation.**

**ochronosis** /ō′krənō′sis/ [Gk, *ochros,* yellow, *osis*], an inherited error of protein metabolism characterized by an accumulation of homogentisic acid, resulting in degenerative arthritis and brown-black pigment deposited in connective tissue and cartilage, often caused by alkaptonuria or poisoning with phenol. Bluish macules may be noted on the sclera, fingers, ears, nose, genitalia, buccal mucosa, and axillae. Urine color may be dark. See also **alkaptonuria.**

**OCN,** abbreviation for *Oncology Certified Nurse.*

**ocontic pressure.** See **colloid osmotic pressure.**

**OCT,** abbreviation for **oxytocin challenge test.**

**octa-, octi-, octo-,** prefix meaning 'the number eight or series of eight': *octigravida, octapeptide, octagenarian.*

**octacosanol,** a dietary supplement, also known as 1-octacosanol.

■ USES: This herb is used for herpes, inflammation of the skin, and physical endurance.

■ CONTRAINDICATIONS: Octacosanol should not be used during pregnancy and lactation or in children.

**octan** /ok'tan/, occurring at 7-day intervals, or every eighth day.

**octaploid, octaploidic.** See **polyploid.**

**octigravida** /ok'tigrav'ədə/ [L, *octo,* eight, *gravidus,* pregnancy], a woman who is pregnant for the eighth time.

**octo-,** See **octa-.**

**octopus** /ok'tə·pəs /, any of numerous carnivorous marine mollusks having eight tentacles.

**octreotide,** an antidiarrheal and hormone.

■ INDICATIONS: The two brand names of this drug are used for different purposes. Sandostatin is used to treat acromegaly, carcinoid tumors, and vasoactive intestinal peptide tumors (VIPomas). Sandostatin LAR Depot is used for long-term maintenance of acromegaly, carcinoid tumors, and VIPomas.

■ CONTRAINDICATIONS: Known hypersensitivity to this drug prohibits its use.

■ ADVERSE EFFECTS: Life-threatening effects of octreotide include seizure, dysrhythmias, congestive heart failure, hepatitis, GI bleeding, and pancreatitis. Other adverse effects are depression, anxiety, tremors, paranoia, chest pain, shortness of breath, thrombophlebitis, ischemia, hypertension, palpitations, galactorrhea, diabetes insipidus, increased liver function tests, urinary tract infection, pollakiuria, hematoma and inflammation of the injection site, bruising, rash, urticaria, and pain. Common side effects include headache, dizziness, fatigue, weakness, sinus bradycardia, conduction abnormalities, hyperglycemia, ketosis, hypothyroidism, hypoglycemia, diarrhea, nausea, abdominal pain, vomiting, flatulence, distension, constipation, and joint and muscle pain.

**ocul.,** abbreviation for the Latin word *oculis,* 'pertaining to the eyes.'

**ocular** /ok'yələr/ [L, *oculus,* eye], **1.** pertaining to the eye. **2.** an eyepiece of an optic instrument.

**ocular dysmetria,** a visual disorder in which the eyes are unable to fix the gaze on an object or follow a moving object with accuracy.

**ocular herpes** [L, *oculus,* eye; Gk, *herpein,* to creep], a herpesvirus infection of the eye. See also **herpes simplex keratitis, ophthalmic herpes zoster.**

**ocular hypertelorism,** a developmental defect involving the frontal region of the cranium, characterized by an abnormally widened bridge of the nose and increased distance between the eyes. The condition is often associated with other cranial and facial deformities and some degree of mental retardation. Also called **orbital hypertelorism.**

**ocular hypertension,** a condition of intraocular pressure that is higher than normal but that has not resulted in a constricted visual field or increased cupping of the optic nerve head. See **glaucoma.**

**ocular hypotelorism,** a developmental defect involving the frontal region of the cranium, characterized by an abnormal narrowing of the bridge of the nose and decreased distance between the eyes, with resulting convergent strabismus. The condition is often associated with other cranial and facial deformities, primarily microcephaly, trigonocephaly, and some degree of mental retardation. Also called **orbital hypotelorism.**

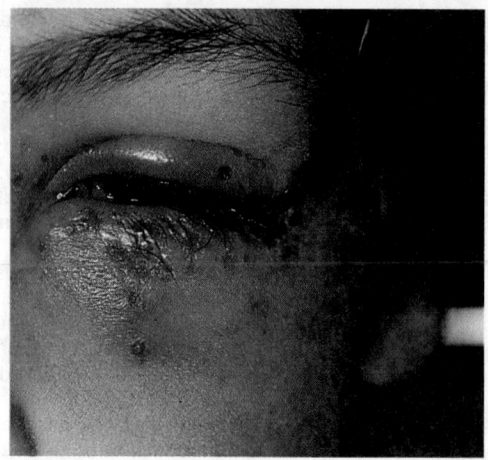

**Ocular herpes** *(Zitelli and Davis, 1997)*

**ocular melanoma,** malignant melanoma arising from the structures of the eye, usually the choroid, ciliary body, or iris, and occurring most often in the fifth and sixth decades of life; the most common site of metastasis is the liver, and such metastasis is followed rapidly by death.

**ocular myopathy,** slowly progressive weakness of ocular muscles, characterized by decreased mobility of the eye and drooping of the upper lid. The disorder may be unilateral or bilateral and may be caused by damage to the oculomotor nerve, an intracranial tumor, or a neuromuscular disease.

**ocular refraction** [L, *oculus,* eye, *refringere,* to break apart], the refraction of the eye.

**oculo-,** combining form meaning 'eye': *oculofacial, oculomycosis, oculopathy.*

**oculoauriculovertebral dysplasia.** See **Goldenhar's syndrome.**

**oculocephalic reflex** /ok'yəlō'səfal'ik/ [L, *oculus* + Gk, *kephale,* head; L, *reflectere,* to bend backward], a test of the integrity of brainstem function. When the patient's head is quickly moved to one side and then to the other, the eyes will normally lag behind the head movement and then slowly assume the midline position. Failure of the eyes to either lag properly or revert back to the midline indicates a lesion on the ipsilateral side at the brainstem level. Also called **doll's eye maneuver.**

**oculocerebral-hypopigmentation syndrome** /ok'yə·lō'sə·rē'brəl/ [L, *oculus,* eye + *cerebrum,* brain], an autosomal recessive syndrome marked by cutaneous hypopigmentation, microphthalmos, small opaque corneas, gingival hypertrophy, and cerebral defect manifested by spasticity, mental and physical retardation, and athetoid movements. Also called **Cross syndrome.**

**oculocerebrorenal syndrome.** See **Lowe's syndrome.**

**oculocutaneous albinism (OCA)** /ok'yoo·lōkyoo·tā'nē·əs/, a human albinism occurring in ten types all distinguished in their incidence and genetic, biochemical, and clinical characteristics but having in common varying degrees of decreased melanotic pigment of the skin, hair, and eyes, hypoplastic foveas, photophobia, nystagmus, and decreased visual acuity.

**oculoglandular syndrome** /ok'yəlōglan'kdyələr/, a unilateral granulomatous form of conjunctivitis. It is associated with a visibly enlarged and tender ipsilateral lymph node and a history of cat-scratch disease.

**oculogyric crisis** /ok′yəlōjī′rik/ [L, *oculus* + *gyrare*, to turn around], a paroxysm in which the eyes are held in a fixed position, usually up and sideways, for minutes or several hours, often occurring in postencephalitic patients with signs of parkinsonism. In some cases the eyes are held down or sideways, and there may be spasm or closing of the lids. Oculogyric crises may be precipitated by emotional stress, and patients with the disorder frequently show psychiatric symptoms.

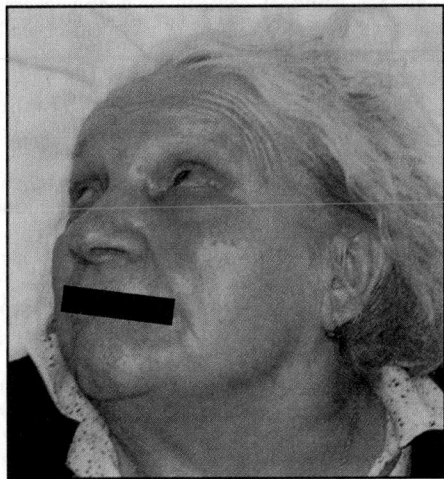

**Oculogyric crisis** *(Perkin, 1998)*

**oculomotor** /-mō′tər/ [L, *oculus*, eye, *motor*, mover], pertaining to movements of the eyeballs.

**oculomotor nerve** [L, *oculus* + *motor*, mover], one of a pair of cranial nerves essential for eye movements, supplying certain extrinsic and intrinsic eye muscles. They pass through the superior orbital fissure, connecting to the brain in nucleus III. Also called **nervus oculomotorius, third cranial nerve.**

**oculomotor nucleus** [L, *oculus*, eye, *motor*, mover, *nucleus*, nut kernel], a nucleus of a third cranial nerve arising in the midbrain.

**oculus.** See **eye.**

**Ocusert Pilo,** trademark for a cholinergic (pilocarpine).

**OD,** *informal.* abbreviation for overdose.

**O.D., 1.** abbreviation for *oculus dexter,* a Latin phrase meaning 'right eye.' **2.** abbreviation for *Doctor of Optometry.*

**odaxetic** /ō′dakset′ik/ [Gk, *odaxein,* a biting pain], causing a tactile sensation such as itching or biting.

**OD'd** /ōdēd′/, *slang.* overdosed, usually referring to a person who has suffered adverse effects from an excessively large dose of a drug of abuse.

**Oddi's sphincter** [Ruggero Oddi, Italian surgeon, 1864–1913; Gk, *sphigein,* to bind], a band of circular muscle fibers around the lower part of the common bile duct and pancreatic duct, near the common duct junction with the duodenum.

**-ode,** combining form meaning a 'type of pathway': *anode, cathode, electrode.*

**odont-.** See **odonto-.**

**odontalgia** See **toothache.**

**odontectomy** /ō′dontek′təmē/ [Gk, *odous,* tooth, *ektomē,* cut out], the extraction of a tooth by removal of the bone from around the roots before force is applied.

**-odontia, -odontic,** suffix meaning 'teeth': *periodontia, mesodontic.*

**odontiasis** /ō′dontī′əsis/, the process of teething.

**odontitis** /ō′dontī′tis/ [Gk, *odous* + *itis,* inflammation], abnormal enlargement of a tooth pulp, usually resulting from inflammation of the odontoblasts (cells responsible for dentin formation) rather than of the mature, or erupted, tooth. It may be caused by infection, tumor, or trauma.

**odonto-, odont-,** prefix meaning 'teeth': *odontoblast, odontopathy.*

**odontoblast** /ōdon′təblast′/ [Gk, *odous,* tooth, *blastos,* germ], one of the connective tissue cells in the periphery of the dental pulp that develops into the deciduous and secondary dentin of a tooth.

**odontodynia.** See **toothache.**

**odontodysplasia** /-displā′zhə/ [Gk, *odous* + *dys,* bad, *plasis,* forming], an abnormality in the development of the teeth, characterized by deficient formation of enamel and dentin. The teeth have a ghostlike appearance in radiographs. It most often affects the maxillary central and lateral incisors, usually on one side of the midline. Also called **ghost teeth.** See also **shell teeth.**

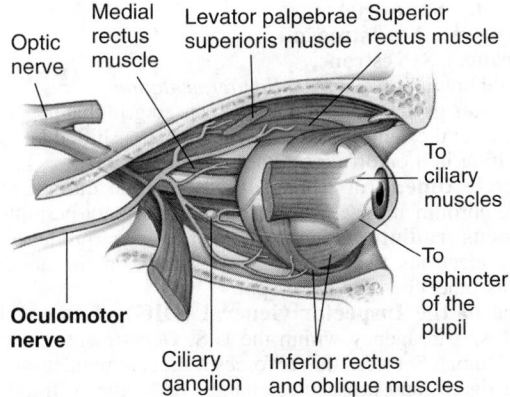

Optic nerve
Medial rectus muscle
Levator palpebrae superioris muscle
Superior rectus muscle
To ciliary muscles
To sphincter of the pupil
**Oculomotor nerve**
Ciliary ganglion
Inferior rectus and oblique muscles

**Oculomotor nerve**

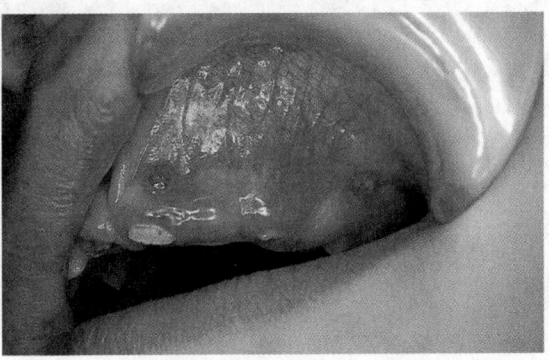

**Odontodysplasia** *(Regezi, Sciubba, and Pogrel, 2000)*

**odontogenesis** /-jen′əsis/ [Gk, *odous,* tooth, *genein,* to produce], the origin and formation of developing teeth. Also called **odontogeny** /ōdontoj′ənē/.

**odontogenesis imperfecta.** See **dentinogenesis imperfecta.**

**odontogenic** /ōdon′tōjen′ik/ [Gk, *odous* + *genein,* to produce], **1.** pertaining to the generation of teeth. **2.** developing in tissues that produce teeth.

**odontogenic cyst,** any of a variety of lesions of mouth tissues, including the relatively common dentigerous cyst, which is associated with the crown of an unerupted third molar or maxillary cuspid. Other types are ameloblastic fibroma, odontogenic myxoma, and odontoma.

**odontogenic fibroma,** a benign neoplasm of the jaw derived from the embryonic part of the tooth germ, dental follicle, or dental papilla or from the periodontal membrane.

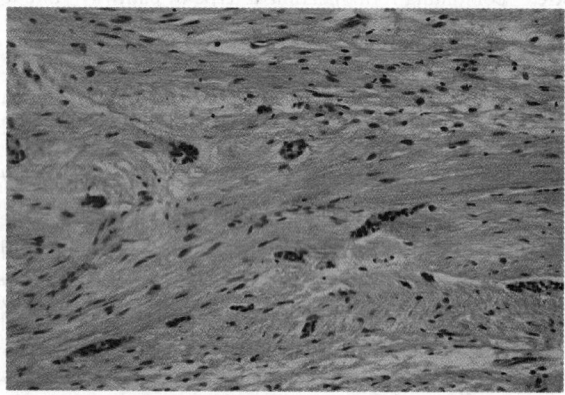

**Odontogenic fibroma** *(Regezi, Sciubba, and Pogrel, 2000)*

**odontogenic fibrosarcoma,** a malignant neoplasm of the jaw that develops in a mesenchymal component of a tooth or tooth germ.

**odontogenic myxoma,** a rare tumor of the jaw that may develop from the mesenchyme of the tooth germ.

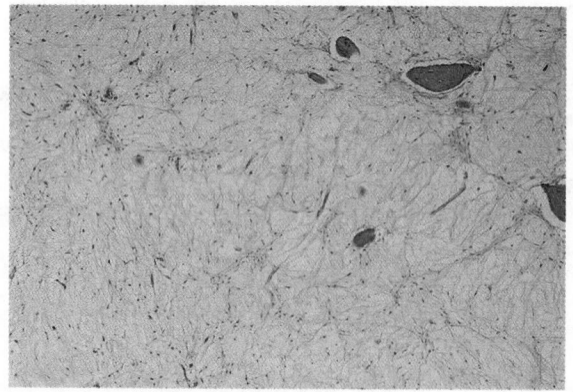

**Odontogenic myxoma** *(Regezi, Sciubba, and Pogrel, 2000)*

**odontoid ligament.** See **alar ligament.**

**odontoid process** [Gk, *odous* + *eidos,* form; L, *processus*], the toothlike projection that rises perpendicularly from the upper surface of the body of the second cervical vertebra (axis), which serves as a pivot point for the rotation of the atlas (first cervical vertebra), enabling the head to turn. Also called the **dens.**

**odontoid vertebra.** See **axis.**

**odontology** /ō′dontol′əjē/ [Gk, *odous* + *logos,* science], the scientific study of the anatomy and physiology of the teeth and of the surrounding structures of the oral cavity.

**odontoma** /ō′dontō′mə/ [Gk, *odous* + *oma,* tumor], a benign tumor consisting of cementum, dentin, enamel, and pulp tissue that may be arranged in the form of teeth. Also called **gestant anomaly.**

**odontoperiosteum.** See **periodontium** (def. 1).

**odor** /ō′dər/ [L, a smell], a scent or smell. The sense of smell is activated when airborne molecules stimulate receptors of the first cranial nerve.

**odoriferous** /ō′dərif′ərəs/ [L, *odor,* smell, *ferre,* to bear], pertaining to something that produces a smell, particularly one that is strong or offensive.

**odorous** /ō′dərəs/ [L, *odor,* smell], pertaining to something that has an odor, smell, or fragrance.

**ODTS,** abbreviation for **organic dust toxic syndrome.**

**odynacusis** [Gk, *odyne,* pain, *akouein,* to hear], a painful sensitivity to noise.

**-odyne, -odynia, odyno-,** combining form meaning 'pain': *anodyne, coccyodynia, odynolysis.*

**odynophagia** /od′inōfā′jə/ [Gk, *odyne,* pain, *phagein,* to swallow], a severe sensation of burning squeezing pain while swallowing. It is caused by irritation of the mucosa or a muscular disorder of the esophagus such as gastroesophageal reflux, bacterial or fungal infection, tumor, achalasia, or chemical irritation.

**oedema.** See **edema.**

**Oedipus complex** /ed′ipəs, ē′dəpəs/ [Gk, *Oedipus,* mythic king who slew his father and married his mother], **1.** (in psychoanalysis) a child's desire for a sexual relationship with the parent of the opposite sex, usually with strong negative feelings for the parent of the same sex. **2.** a son's desire for a sexual relationship with his mother.

**OEM,** abbreviation for *optical electron microscope.*

**OER,** abbreviation for **oxygen enhancement ratio.**

**oesophageal.** See **esophageal.**

**oesophagectomy.** See **esophagectomy.**

**oesophagitis.** See **esophagitis.**

**oesophagoscopy.** See **esophagoscopy.**

**oesophagus.** See **esophagus.**

**oestriol.** See **estriol.**

**oestrogen.** See **estrogen.**

**oestrone.** See **estrone.**

**o/f,** abbreviation for *oxidation/fermentation.*

**off-center grid,** in radiology, a focused grid that is perpendicular to the central-axis x-ray beam but is shifted laterally, resulting in a cutoff across the entire grid.

**off-cycle time,** (in managed care) a time during which open enrollment in a health plan is usually not permitted.

**off-focus radiation,** in radiology, x-rays produced by stray electrons that interact at positions on the anode at points other than the focal spot.

**Office of the Inspector General (OIG) of the United States,** an agency within the U.S. Department of Health and Human Services that enforces Medicare regulations and investigates and prosecutes charges of Medicare fraud and abuse.

**off-level grid,** in radiology, a grid that is not perpendicular to the central-axis x-ray beam. The cause is often a malpositioned x-ray tube rather than an improperly positioned grid.

**off-line,** pertaining to access to computer information not directly connected to a computer. Compare **on-line.**

**ofloxacin** /oflak'səsin/, a fluoroquinolone antibiotic.

**Ogden classification system,** a system for categorizing 17 different kinds of epiphyseal fractures.

**Ogden plate,** a long metal plate used for fixing long bone fractures. It is designed to accommodate preexisting intramedullary devices, such as rods or the stem of a prosthesis, and has slots that can accept encircling bands.

**Ogen,** trademark for an estrogen (estropipate).

**Ogsten line,** a line drawn through the knee from the adduction tubercle to the intercondylar notch, used as a guide for transection of the condyle in the surgical repair of knock-knee.

**OH,** formula for **hydroxyl.**

**o.h.,** abbreviation for the Latin term *omni hora,* 'hourly.'

**OHD,** abbreviation for *organic heart disease.*

**OHF,** abbreviation for **Omsk hemorrhagic fever.**

**ohm** [Georg S. Ohm, German physicist, 1787–1854], a unit of measurement of electrical resistance. One ohm is the resistance of a conductor in which an electrical potential of 1 volt produces a current of 1 ampere. See also **ampere, Ohm's law, volt, watt.**

**Ohm's law** [Georg S. Ohm], the principle that the strength or intensity of an unvarying electric current is directly proportional to the electromotive force and inversely proportional to the resistance of the circuit.

**-oi,** a plural-forming suffix in borrowings from Greek: *auloi, catanephroi, mesonephroi.*

**-oid,** **1.** suffix meaning 'resembling or having the appearance of' something specified: *alkaloid, spheroid, trochoid.*

**OIG,** abbreviation for **Office of the Inspector General of the United States.**

**oiko-, eco-,** prefix meaning 'house': *oikofugic, oikology, oikophobia.*

**oil** [L, *oleum*], any of a large number of greasy liquid substances not miscible in water. Oil may be fixed or volatile and is derived from animal, vegetable, or mineral matter.

**oil retention enema,** an enema containing about 200 to 250 mL of an oil-based solution given to soften a fecal mass. The patient is asked to retain the solution for 30 minutes to several hours. See also **lubricating enema.**

**ointment** [L, *unguentum,* a salve], a semisolid, externally applied preparation, usually containing a drug. Various ointments are used as local analgesic, anesthetic, antiinfective, astringent, depigmenting, irritant, and keratolytic agents. Also called **salve, unction, unguent.**

**O.L.,** abbreviation for the Latin term *oculus laevus,* 'left eye.'

**-ol** suffix designating a member of the alcohol group: *ethanol, methanol, naphthol.*

**-ol, -ole,** suffix meaning an 'oil': *benzol, furol, petrol, cholesterol.*

**olanzapine,** an antipsychotic and neuroleptic.
- ■ INDICATIONS: This drug is used to treat psychotic disorders.
- ■ CONTRAINDICATIONS: Known hypersensitivity to this drug prohibits its use.
- ■ ADVERSE EFFECTS: Neuroleptic malignant syndrome is a rare but life-threatening effect of this drug. Other adverse effects are orthostatic hypotension, tachycardia, chest pain, blurred vision, dry mouth, nausea, vomiting, anorexia, constipation, abdominal pain, weight gain, urinary retention, urinary frequency, enuresis, impotence, amenorrhea, gynecomastia, breast engorgement, premenstrual syndrome, rash, dyspnea, rhinitis, cough, pharyngitis, extrapyramidal symptoms, seizures, headache, fever, insomnia, somnolence, agitation, nervousness, hostility, dizziness, hypertonia, tremor, euphoria, joint pain, and twitching.

**Old Age, Survivors, Disability and Health Insurance Program (OASDHI),** a benefit program, administered by the U.S. Social Security Administration, that provides cash benefits to workers who are retired or disabled, their dependents, and survivors, commonly referred to as Social Security. The program also provides health insurance benefits for people over 65 and disabled people under 65, commonly referred to as Medicare. See also **Medicare.**

**old dislocation,** a dislocation in which inflammatory changes have occurred.

**Older Americans Act Amendment of 1987,** U.S. federal legislation authorizing support of Title III nutrition services for state and county programs on aging. The services include both congregate and home-delivered meals, with related nutrition education.

**old tuberculin** [ME, *ald* + L, *tubercle*], the original formula for an extract of the tubercle bacillus used in the treatment of tuberculosis by Koch, using a glycerin-broth culture of *Mycobacterium tuberculosis* after filtration and concentration of the liquid.

**Old World leishmaniasis.** See **oriental sore.**

**-ole,** suffix meaning a 'small or little example of the noun named': *arteriole.*

**oleandomycin.** See **troleandomycin.**

**oleandrism** /ō'lē·an'drizəm/, a toxic effect of ingesting or inhaling the cardiac glycoside contained in the roots, bark, flowers, and seeds of oleander *(Nerium oleander),* an evergreen ornamental shrub. Symptoms range from nausea and vomiting to bradycardia and cardiac arrest.

**olecranon** /ōlek'rənon/ [Gk, *olekranon,* tip of the elbow], a proximal projection of the ulna that forms the tip of the elbow and fits into the olecranon fossa of the humerus when

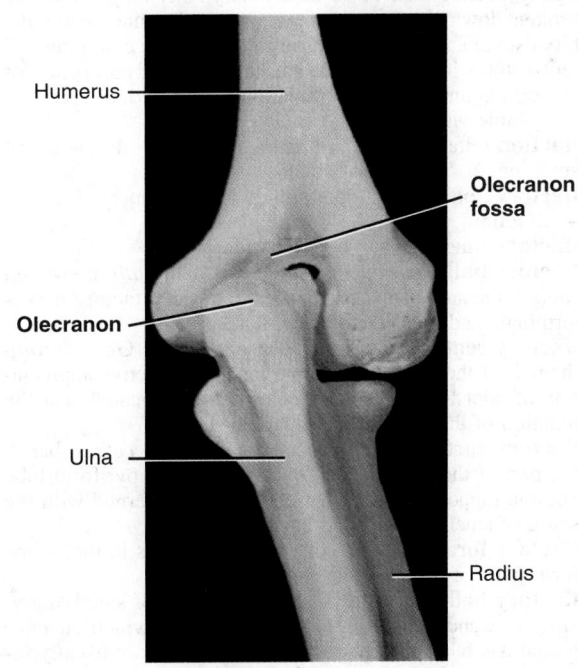

**Olecranon and olecranon fossa** *(Vidic and Suarez, 1984)*

the forearm is extended at the proximal extremity of the ulna. The anterior surface of the olecranon forms part of the trochlear notch that articulates with the humerus. Also called **olecranon process.**

**olecranon bursa,** the bursa of the elbow.

**olecranon fossa,** the depression in the posterior surface of the humerus that receives the olecranon of the ulna when the forearm is extended. Compare **coronoid fossa.**

**olecranon process.** See **olecranon.**

**olefiant gas.** See **ethylene.**

**olefin** /ō′ləfin/ [L, *oleum,* oil, *facere,* to make], any of a group of unsaturated aliphatic hydrocarbons containing one or more double bonds in the carbon chain.

**oleic acid** /ōlē′ik/ [L, *oleum,* oil, *acidus,* sour], a colorless, monounsaturated fatty acid occurring in almost all natural fats. It is a liquid at room temperature. Commercial oleic acid is used in soaps, cosmetics, ointments, lubricants, and food additives.

**oleo-, eleo-,** prefix meaning 'oil': *oleocreosote, oleodistearin, oleoresin.*

**oleoresin** /ō′lē·ō·rez′in/ [L, *oleum,* oil + *resin*], **1.** any natural combination of a resin and a volatile oil such as exudes from pines and other plants. **2.** a compound prepared by exhausting a drug by percolation with a volatile solvent, such as acetone, alcohol, or ether, and evaporating the solvent.

**oleovitamin** /ō′lē·ōvī′təmin/, a preparation of fish-liver oil or edible vegetable oil that contains one or more of the fat-soluble vitamins or their derivatives.

**oleovitamin A,** an oily preparation, usually fish-liver oil or fish-liver oil diluted with an edible vegetable oil, containing the natural or synthetic form of vitamin A. See also **vitamin A.**

**oleovitamin D$_2$.** See **calciferol.**

**OlestraTM,** a trade name for a synthetic fat substitute derived from sucrose and eight acids of vegetable oils. Olestra adds no calories or fats to the food into which it is incorporated. Because the molecules of Olestra are larger and more tightly packed than those of ordinary fats, they cannot be broken down by digestive enzymes and cannot enter the bloodstream. Adverse effects reported include cramping and loose stools in some people and inhibition of absorption of some vitamins. Newer formulation is fortified with certain fat-soluble vitamins.

**olfaction** /olfak′shən/ [L, *olfacere,* to smell], **1.** the act of smelling. **2.** the sense of smell.

**olfactory** /olfak′tərē/, pertaining to the sense of smell. —**olfaction,** *n.*

**olfactory anesthesia.** See **anosmia.**

**olfactory bulb** [L, *olfactus,* sense of smell, *bulbus,* swollen root], the area of the forebrain where the olfactory nerves terminate and the olfactory tracts arise.

**olfactory center** [L, *olfactus,* sense of smell; Gk, *kentron*], the part of the brain responsible for the subjective appreciation of odors, a complex group of neurons located near the junction of the temporal and parietal lobes.

**olfactory cortex** [L, *olfactus,* sense of smell, *cortex,* bark], the part of the cerebral cortex, including the pyriform lobe and the hippocampus formation, that is concerned with the sense of smell. Also called **archeocortex.**

**olfactory foramen,** one of several openings in the cribriform plate of the ethmoid bone.

**olfactory hallucination** [L, *olfactus,* sense of smell, *alucinari,* to wander mentally], a condition in which an individual has false perceptions of odors, which are usually repugnant or offensive. The hallucinations are sometimes associated with guilt feelings.

**olfactory lobe** [L, *olfactus,* sense of smell; Gk, *lobos,* lobe], a structure involved in the sense of smell in lower animals. Vestiges of the tissue are found in the cerebral hemispheres of humans.

**olfactory nerve,** one of a pair of nerves associated with the sense of smell. They are composed of numerous fine filaments that ramify in the mucous membrane of the olfactory area. The fibers of the olfactory nerve are nonmedullated and unite into fasciculi that form a plexus under the mucous membrane and rise in grooves or canals in the ethmoid bone. The fibers pass into the skull and form synapses with the dendrites of the mitral cells. The area in which the olfactory nerves arise is situated in the most superior part of the mucous membrane that covers the superior nasal concha. The olfactory sensory endings are modified epithelial cells and the least specialized of the special senses. The olfactory nerves connect with the olfactory bulb and the olfactory tract, which are components of the part of the brain associated with the sense of smell. Also called **first cranial nerve, nervus olfactorius.**

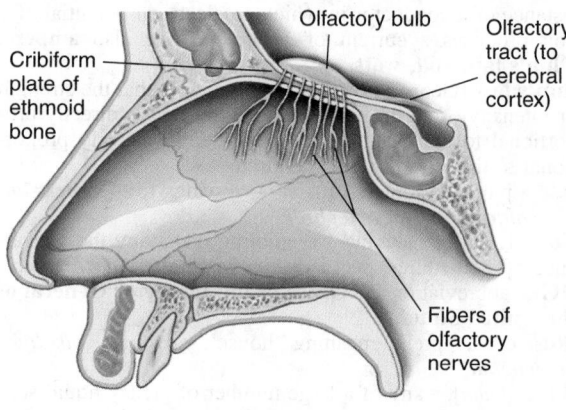

Cribiform plate of ethmoid bone

Olfactory bulb

Olfactory tract (to cerebral cortex)

Fibers of olfactory nerves

**Olfactory nerve**

**olfactory organ** [L, *olfactus,* sense of smell], the apparatus in the mucous membrane of the nose responsible for the sense of smell. It includes the sensory nerve endings and the olfactory bulb of the brain.

**olfactory receptors** [L, *olfactus,* sense of smell, *recipere,* to receive], bipolar nerve cells located in the nasal epithelium. Axons of the cells become receptors of the olfactory nerve.

**olig-.** See **oligo-.**

**oligemia** /ol′ijē′mē·ə/ [Gk, *oligos,* little, *haima,* blood], a condition of hypovolemia or reduced circulating intravascular volume. Also spelled **oligaemia.**

**oligo-** /ol′igō-/, **olig-,** combining form meaning 'few, little': *oligocholia, oligodontia, oligosialia.*

**oligoclonal banding** /ol′igōklō′nəl/, a process by which cerebrospinal fluid IgG is distributed, after electrophoresis, in discrete bands. Approximately 90% of multiple sclerosis patients show oligoclonal banding.

**oligodactyly** /ol′igōdak′tilē/ [Gk, *oligos* + *dactylos,* finger], a congenital anomaly characterized by the absence of one or more of the fingers or toes. Also called **oligodactylia, oligodactylism.** —**oligodactylic,** *adj.*

**oligodendroblastoma.** See **oligodendroglioma.**

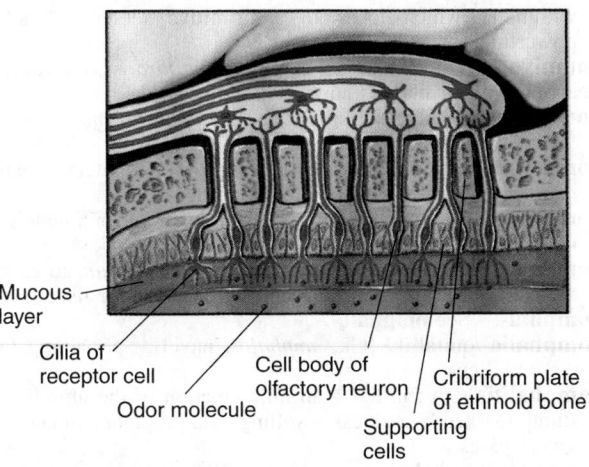

Mucous layer

Cilia of receptor cell

Odor molecule

Cell body of olfactory neuron

Supporting cells

Cribriform plate of ethmoid bone

**Olfactory receptors** (Applegate, 2000)

**oligodendrocyte** /ol'igōden'drəsīt/ [Gk, *oligos* + *dendron,* tree, *kytos,* cell], a type of neuroglial cell with dendritic projections that coil around axons of neural cells. The projections continue as myelin sheaths over the axons.

**oligodendroglia** /ol'igōdendrog'lē·ə/, one of three types of glia cells that, with the nerve cells, compose the central nervous system and are characterized by sheetlike processes that wrap around individual axons to form a myelin sheath of nerve fibers.

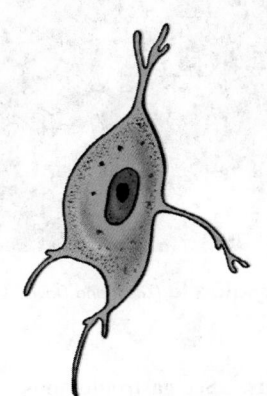

**Oligodendroglia** (Monahan and Neighbors, 1998)

**oligodendroglioma** /ol'igōden'drōglī·ō'mə/, *pl.* **oligodendrogliomas, oligodendrogliomata** [Gk, *oligos* + *dendron,* tree, *glia,* glue, *oma,* tumor], an uncommon brain tumor composed of nonneural ectodermal cells that form part of the supporting connective tissue around nerve cells. The lesion, a firm reddish-gray mass with calcified spots and a distinct margin, may be large. The tumor develops most often in frontal, parietal, and paraventricular sites but also may occur in the cerebellum. Also called **oligodendroblastoma.**

**oligodontia** /ol'igōdon'shə/ [Gk, *oligos* + *odous,* tooth], a genetically determined dental defect characterized by the development of fewer than the normal number of teeth.

**oligogenic** /ol'igōjen'ik/ [Gk, *oligos* + *genein,* to produce], pertaining to hereditary characteristics produced by one or only a few genes.

**oligohydramnios** /-hidram'nē·əs/ [Gk, *oligos* + *hydor,* water, *amnion,* fetal membrane], an abnormally small amount or absence of amniotic fluid.

**oligomeganephronia** /ol'igōmeg'ənefrō'nē·ə/ [Gk, *oligos* + *megas,* large, *nephros,* kidney], a type of congenital renal hypoplasia associated with chronic renal failure in children. The condition is characterized by a decreased number of functioning nephrons and hypertrophy of other renal elements without the presence of aberrant tissue. Also called **oligomeganephronic renal hypoplasia.** —**oligomeganephronic,** *adj.*

**oligomenorrhea** /-men'ôrē'ə/ [Gk, *oligos* + L, *men,* month, *rhoia,* flow], abnormally light or a reduction in menstruation. Also spelled **oligomenorrhoea.** —**oligomenorrheic,** *adj.*

**oligonucleotide** /-noo'klē·ətīd'/, a compound formed by linking a small number of nucleotides.

**oligopeptide** /-pep'tīd/, a peptide composed of fewer than 20 amino acids.

**oligopnea, oligopnoea.** See **bradypnea.**

**oligosaccharide** /-sak'ərīd/, a compound formed by a small number of monosaccharide units.

**oligospermia** /ol'igōspur'mē·ə/ [Gk, *oligos* + *sperma,* seed], an insufficient number of spermatozoa in the semen. Also called **oligozoospermatism.** Compare **azoospermia.**

**oligotroph** /ol'igətrof'/, an organism that can survive in a nutrient-poor environment.

**oligozoospermatism.** See **oligospermia.**

**oliguria** /ol'igyoŏr'ē·ə/ [Gk, *oligos* + *ouron,* urine], a diminished capacity to form and pass urine—less than 500 mL in every 24 hours—so that the end products of metabolism cannot be excreted efficiently. It is usually caused by imbalances in body fluids and electrolytes, renal lesions, or urinary tract obstruction. Also called **oliguresis.** Compare **anuria.** —**oliguric,** *adj.*

**olisthetic** /ōlisthet'ik/, pertaining to olisthy, or bone slippage.

**olisthy** /ōlis'thē/ [Gk, *olisthanein,* to slip], the slippage of a bone from its normal anatomic site, as in a slipped disk. —**olisthetic,** *adj.*

**olivary body** /ol'iver'ē/ [L, *oliva* + AS, *bodig*], an olivary nucleus, part of an aggregate of small densely packed nerve cells, on the medulla oblongata.

**olivopontocerebellar** /ol'ivōpon'tōser'ibel'ər/ [L, *oliva,* olive, *pons,* bridge, *cerebellum,* small brain], pertaining to the olivae, the middle peduncles, and the cerebellum.

**olivopontocerebellar atrophy (OPCA),** a group of hereditary ataxias characterized by mixed clinical features of pure cerebellar ataxia, dementia, Parkinson-like symptoms, spasticity, choreoathetosis, retinal degeneration, myelopathy, and peripheral neuropathy. Various forms of OPCA are transmitted by autosomal-dominant or autosomal-recessive inheritance.

**Ollier's disease.** See **enchondromatosis.**

**Ollier's dyschondroplasia** /ol'ē·āz'/ [Louis X.E.L. Ollier, French surgeon, 1830–1900; Gk, *dys,* bad, *chondros,* cartilage, *plasis,* formation], a rare disorder of bone development in which the epiphyseal tissue responsible for growth spreads through the bones, causing abnormal irregular growth and deformity. The long bones and the ilia are most often affected. Orthopedic procedures to correct deformities may be necessary and helpful, but invalidism is the usual prognosis. See also **hereditary multiple exostoses.**

**-ology,** suffix meaning 'the study or science of': *biology, pathology, physiology.*

**-olol,** combining form meaning 'beta blocker.'

**o.m.,** abbreviation for the Latin term *omni mane,* 'every morning.'

**oma-.** See **omo-.**

**-oma,** suffix meaning a 'tumor': *capsuloma, lymphadenoma, neurinoma.*

**Omaha System,** a method of community health nursing practice, documentation, and data management based on a nursing process model. It incorporates three standardized schemes: the *problem classification scheme,* the *intervention scheme,* and the *problem rating scale for outcomes.*

**omalgia** /ōmal'jə/ [Gk, *omos,* shoulder, *algos,* pain], pain in the shoulder.

**omarthritis** /ō'märthrī'tis/, inflammation of the shoulder joint.

**ombudsman** /om'bədzmən/ [ONorse, *umbothsmathr,* commission man], a person who investigates and mediates patients' problems and complaints in relation to a hospital's services. Also called **patient representative.**

**omega** /ōmē'gə, ōmā'gə, om'əgə/, Ω, ω, the 24th letter of the Greek alphabet.

**omega-3 fatty acid,** a fatty acid with a double bond located at the third carbon atom away from the omega (methyl) end of the molecule. Major sources are cold-water fish and vegetable oils. Omega-3 fatty acids such as eicosapentaenoic acid and docosahexanoic acid appear to have protective functions in preventing the formation of blood clots and reducing the risk of coronary heart disease. See also **essential fatty acid.**

**omega-6 fatty acid,** an unsaturated fatty acid in which the double bond closest to the omega (methyl) end of the molecule occurs at the sixth carbon from that end. Major sources are vegetable and seed oils. Diets in which the ratio of omega-6 to omega-3 fatty acids is high have been linked to promotion of some cancers.

**omega-9 fatty acid,** a polyunsaturated fatty acid found in animal and vegetable fats.

**omega-oxidation,** a metabolic pathway of fatty acid oxidation involving the carbon atom farthest removed from the original carboxyl group.

**omenta.** See **omentum.**

**omental** /ōmen'təl/ [L, *omentum,* membrane of the bowels], relating to the omentum.

**omental bursa,** a cavity in the peritoneum behind the stomach, the lesser omentum, and the lower border of the liver and in front of the pancreas and duodenum.

**omentectomy** /ō'mentek'təmē/, the surgical excision of a part of the omentum.

**omentum** /ōmen'təm/, *pl.* **omenta, omentums** [L, membrane of the bowels], an extension of the peritoneum that enfolds one or more organs adjacent to the stomach. See also **greater omentum, lesser omentum.** —**omental,** *adj.*

**omicron** /ōm'ikron/, O, o, the 15th letter of the Greek alphabet.

**omission** /ōmish'ən/ [L, *omittere,* to neglect], (in law) intentional or unintentional neglect to fulfill a duty required by law.

**omni-,** combining form meaning 'all': *omnicide, omniform.*

**omnifocal lens** /om'nēfō'kəl/ [L, *omnis,* all, *focus,* hearth, *lentil*], an eyeglass lens designed for both near and far vision with the reading part in a variable curve.

**Omnipen,** trademark for an antibacterial (ampicillin).

**omnipotence** /omnip'ətəns/, (in psychology) an infantile perception that the outside world is part of the organism and within it, which leads to a primitive feeling of all-powerfulness.

**omnivorous** /omniv'ərəs/ [L, *omnis,* all, *vorare,* to devour], eating both plants and animals.

**omn. noct,** abbreviation for the Latin term *omni nocte,* 'every night.'

**omn. quad. hor.,** abbreviation for the Latin term *omni quadrante hora,* 'every quarter of an hour.'

**omo-, oma-,** combining form meaning 'shoulder': *omoclavicular, omodynia, omohyoid.*

**omophagia** /om'ōfā'jē·ə/ [Gk, *ōmos,* raw, *phagein,* to eat], the eating of raw foods, particularly raw meat or fish.

**omphal-.** See **omphalo-.**

**omphalic** /omfal'ik/ [Gk, *omphalos,* navel], pertaining to the umbilicus.

**omphalitis** /om'falī'tis/, an inflammation of the umbilical stump marked by redness, swelling, and purulent exudate in severe cases.

**omphalo-, omphal-,** combining form meaning 'the navel': *omphalocele, omphaloma, omphalosite.*

**omphaloangiopagus.** See **allantoidoangiopagus.**

**omphalocele** /om'fəlōsēl'/ [Gk, *omphalos* + *kele,* hernia], congenital herniation of intraabdominal viscera through a defect in the abdominal wall around the umbilicus. The defect is usually closed surgically soon after birth. Compare **gastroschisis.**

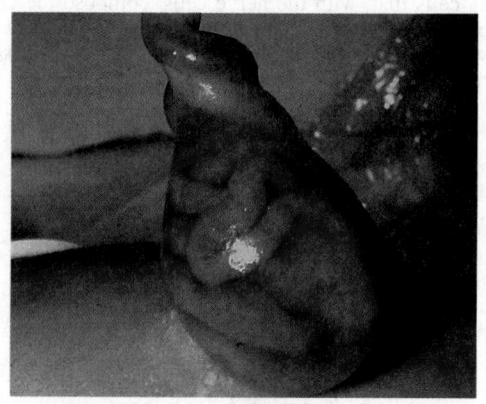

**Omphalocele** *(Zitelli and Davis, 1997)*

**omphalodidymus.** See **gastrodidymus.**

**omphalogenesis** /-jen'əsis/ [Gk, *omphalos* + *genesis,* origin], the formation of the umbilicus or yolk sac during embryonic development. —**omphalogenetic,** *adj.*

**omphalomesenteric artery.** See **vitelline artery.**

**omphalomesenteric circulation.** See **vitelline circulation.**

**omphalomesenteric duct.** See **yolk stalk.**

**omphalomesenteric vein.** See **vitelline vein.**

**omphalopagus.** See **monomphalus.**

**omphalosite** /om'falōsīt'/ [Gk, *omphalos* + *sitos,* food], the underdeveloped parasitic member of unequal conjoined twins united by the vessels of the umbilical cord. The omphalosite has no heart, derives its blood supply from the placenta of the autosite, and is incapable of independent existence after birth. See also **allantoidoangiopagus.**

**OMS,** abbreviation for **Organisation Mondiale de la Santé.** See **World Health Organization.**

**Omsk hemorrhagic fever (OHF)** /ômsk/, an acute infection seen in regions of the former U.S.S.R., caused by a flavovirus transmitted by the bite of an infected tick or by handling infected muskrats. It is characterized by fever, headache, epistaxis, GI and uterine bleeding, and other hemorrhagic manifestations. Treatment is supportive; recovery usually occurs.

**-on,** **1.** combining form meaning an 'elementary atomic particle': *electron, nucleon, proton.* **2.** combining form meaning a 'unit': *magneton, photon.* **3.** combining form meaning a '(nonmetallic) chemical element': *carbon, krypton, silicon.*

**o.n.,** abbreviation for the Latin term *omni nocte,* 'every night.'

**onanism,** /ō'nəiz'əm/ coitus interruptus; withdrawal of the penis just before ejaculation during sexual intercourse. See also **masturbation.**

**Oncaspar,** trademark for an oncolytic agent (pegaspargase).

**Onchocerca** /ong'kō·sər'kə/ [Gk, *onkos,* tumor + *kerkos,* tail], a genus of nematode parasites of the superfamily Filarioidea that infect humans and ruminants. The adults live and breed in subcutaneous fibroid nodules; the young (the microfilariae) are carried by the lymph and are found chiefly in the skin, subcutaneous connective tissues, and eyes. *O. volvulus* is a common parasite of humans that breeds in fastflowing rivers and streams in tropical regions of the Americas and Africa, particularly West Africa. It is the cause of human onchocerciasis and is transmitted by the bites of buffalo gnats.

**onchocerciasis** /ong'kōsərkī'əsis, sī'əsis/ [Gk, *onkos,* swelling, *kerkos,* tail, *osis,* condition], a form of filariasis common in Central and South America and Africa, characterized by subcutaneous nodules, pruritic rash, and eye lesions. It is transmitted by the bites of black flies that deposit *Onchocerca volvulus* microfilariae under the skin. The microfilariae migrate to the subcutaneous tissue and eyes, and fibrous nodules form around the developing adult worms. Hypersensitive reactions to the dying microfilariae include extreme pruritus, a cellulitis-like rash, lichenification, depigmentation, and rarely, elephantiasis. Involvement of the eye may include keratitis, iridocyclitis, and rarely blindness from choroidoretinitis. Diagnosis is made by demonstrating microfilariae by skin biopsy or in the eye by slit lamp. Treatment is diethylcarbamazine for the microfilariae and surgical excision of nodules to remove adult worms. Protective clothing and control of black flies with DDT are the best preventives. Also called **river blindness.**

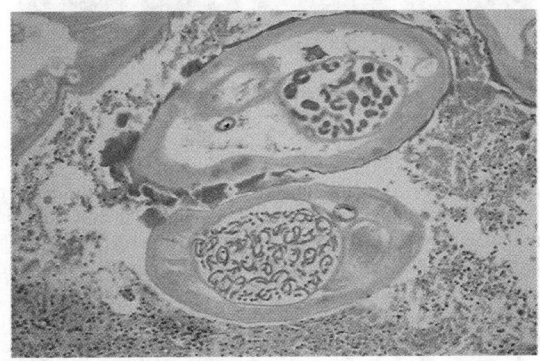

***Onchocerca volvulus*** (Cotran, Kumar, and Collins, 1999)

**onco-** /ong'kō-/, combining form meaning 'swelling, mass, or tumor': *oncology.*

**oncofetal protein** /-fē'təl/ [Gk, *onkos* + L, *fetus,* pregnant; Gk, *proteios,* first rank], a protein normally produced by fetal tissue and also by cancerous tissues in adult life.

**oncogene** /ong'kōjēn/ [Gk, *onkos* + *genein,* to produce], a potentially cancer-inducing gene. Under normal conditions such genes play a role in the growth and proliferation of cells, but, when altered in some way by a cancer-causing agent such as radiation, a carcinogenic chemical, or an oncogenic virus, they may cause the cell to be transformed to a malignant state.

**oncogenesis** /ong'kōjen'əsis/ [Gk, *onkos* + *genesis,* origin], the process initiating and promoting the development of a neoplasm through the action of biologic, chemical, or physical agents. Compare **carcinogenesis, sarcomagenesis, tumorigenesis.**

**oncogenic** /ong'kōjen'ik/ [Gk, *onkos,* swelling, *genein,* to produce], pertaining to the origin and development of tumors or cancer.

**oncogenic virus,** any one of over 100 viruses able to cause the development of a malignant neoplastic disease.

**oncogenous osteomalacia** /ongkoj'ənəs/, a bone disorder caused by mesenchymal tumors. Patients may have normal-to-low serum calcium levels, a low serum phosphorus level, and an elevated serum alkaline phosphatase level.

**oncologic emergencies** /ong'kōloj'ik/, cancer-related disorders that require emergency medical or surgical care. An example is superior vena cava syndrome, in which an expanding tumor mass compresses the thin-walled vena cava, causing obstruction in the venous blood flow from the upper part of the body. Other examples include hypercalcemia, cerebral herniation syndrome, pericardial tamponade, and spinal cord compression.

**oncologist** /ongkol'əjist/, a physician who specializes in the study and treatment of neoplastic diseases, particularly cancer.

**oncology** /ongkol'əjē/ [Gk, *onkos,* swelling, *logos,* science], **1.** the branch of medicine concerned with the study of malignancy. **2.** the study of cancerous growths.

**Oncology Nursing Society (ONS),** an organization of nurses interested or specializing in cancer patient nursing. The national publication of the ONS is *Oncology Nursing Forum.*

**oncolysis** /ongkol'isis/, **1.** the destruction or disposal of neoplastic cells. **2.** the reduction of a swelling or mass.

**oncolytic** /ong'kōlit'ik/, pertaining to the destruction of tumor cells.

**oncornavirus.** See **Oncovirinae.**

**oncotic** /ongkot'ik/ [Gk, *onkos,* a swelling], pertaining to or resulting from the presence of a swelling.

**oncotic pressure** [Gk, *onkos,* a swelling; L, *premere,* to press], the osmotic pressure of a colloid in solution, such as when there is a higher concentration of protein in the plasma on one side of a cell membrane than in the neighboring interstitial fluid. Also called **colloid osmotic pressure.**

**oncotic pressure gradient,** the difference between the osmotic pressure of blood and that of tissue fluid or lymph. It is an important force in maintaining fluid balance between the vascular space and the interstitium.

**Oncovin,** trademark for an antineoplastic (vincristine sulfate).

**Oncovirinae** /ong'kōvir'inē/, a subfamily of ribonucleic acid viruses, including types A, B, C, and D genera of oncoviruses. They are classified on the basis of morphology and type of host. Also called **oncornaviruses.** See also **onco-virus.**

**oncovirus** /ong'kōvī'rəs/ [Gk, *onkos* + L, *virus,* poison], a member of a family of viruses associated with leukemia and sarcoma in animals and, possibly, in humans.

**Ondine's curse** /ondēnz'/ [L, *Undine,* mythic water nymph; ME, *curs,* invocation], apnea caused by loss of automatic control of respiration. The term refers to a syndrome in patients with a defect in central chemoreceptor responsiveness to carbon dioxide. The condition leaves the patient with hypercapnia and hypoxemia, although fully able to breathe voluntarily. Ondine's curse may result in pickwickian syndrome or sleep apnea and may be one cause of sudden infant death syndrome. The syndrome may occur as a result of opiod or other drug overdose, after bulbar poliomyelitis or encephalitis, or after surgery involving the brainstem or the higher segments of the cervical spinal cord, as in cervical cordotomy for intractable pain.

**-one,** combining form designating organic compounds: *acetone, ketone, quinone.*

**one-and-a-half spica cast,** an orthopedic cast that covers the trunk cranially to the nipple line, one leg caudally as far as the toes, and the other leg caudally as far as the knee. For stability, a diagonal crossbar connects the parts of the cast encasing the legs. This type of cast is used for immobilization during healing of a fractured femur or after surgical hip repair or for correction and maintenance of the correction of a hip deformity. Compare **bilateral long-leg spica cast, unilateral long-leg spica cast.**

**one-child sterility.** See **acquired sterility.**

**one gene/one enzyme hypothesis,** a general rule, proposed in 1941 by G. Beadle and E. Tatum, that each gene in a chromosome controls the synthesis of one enzyme. A modification of this idea, the one gene/one polypeptide hypothesis, accommodates the fact that all gene products are polypeptides but not all polypeptides are enzymes. A further modification, the one cistron/one polypeptide concept, accommodates alternate splicing and alternative promoter sequences.

**one gene/one polypeptide,** a principle that each gene in a chromosome determines a particular polypeptide. An exception allows many genes to specify only functional ribonucleic acid.

**oneiro-,** combining form meaning 'dream': *oneirodynia, oneirology, oneiroscopy.*

**one-to-one care,** a method of organizing nursing services in an inpatient care unit by which one registered nurse assumes responsibility for all nursing care provided one patient for the duration of one shift.

**one-to-one relationship,** a mutually defined, collaborative goal-directed client-therapist relationship for the purpose of psychotherapy.

**one-way speaking valve,** a valve, placed on the end of a tracheostomy tube, that opens during inhalation and closes during exhalation, so that the exhaled air is directed over the vocal cords and out the mouth and nose, allowing a person who has had a tracheostomy to speak.

**-onide,** combining form for acetal-derived topical steroids.

**-onium,** combining form for quaternary ammonium derivatives.

**onlay** [AS, *ana,* up, *licagan,* to lie], **1.** a cast type of metal restoration retained by friction and mechanical forces in a prepared tooth, used for restoring one or more of the tooth's cusps and adjoining occlusal surfaces. **2.** an occlusal rest part of a removable partial denture, extended to cover the entire occlusal surface of a tooth.

**onlay graft,** a bone graft in which the transplanted tissue is laid directly onto the surface of the recipient bone.

**on-line,** access to information directly connected with and accessible to a computer. Compare **off-line.**

**on/off phenomenon,** a periodic loss of the efficacy of levodopa in the treatment of Parkinson's disease, without obvious relationship to the timing of levodopa administration. Also called **random off.**

**ONS,** abbreviation for **Oncology Nursing Society.**

**onset of action,** the time required after administration of a drug for a response to be observed.

**ontogenesis.** See **ontogeny.**

**ontogenetic** /on'tōjənet'ik/, **1.** of, relating to, or acquired during ontogeny. **2.** describing an association based on visible morphologic characteristics and not necessarily indicative of a natural evolutionary relationship. Also called **ontogenic.**

**ontogeny** /ontoj'ənē/ [Gk, *ontos,* being, *genein,* to produce], the development of one organism from a single-celled ovum to the time of birth, including all phases of differentiation and growth. Compare **phylogeny.** See also **comparative anatomy.**

**onych-.** See **onycho-.**

**onychia** /ōnik'ē·ə/ [Gk, *onyx,* nail], inflammation of the nailbed. Compare **paronychia.**

**-onychia,** combining form meaning a 'condition of the fingernails or toenails': *celonychia, melanonychia, pachyonychia.*

**onycho-, onych-,** combining form meaning 'the nails': *onychogenic, onychohelcosis, onychopathology.*

**onychodystrophy** [Gk, *onyx,* nail, *dys,* bad, *trophe,* nourishment], a condition of malformed or discolored fingernails or toenails.

**onychogryphosis** /on'ikōgrifō'sis/ [Gk, *onyx* + *gryphein,* to curve, *osis,* condition], thickened, curved, clawlike overgrowth of fingernails or toenails.

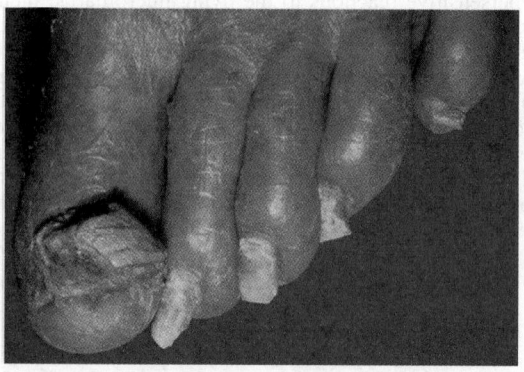

**Onychogryphosis** *(Hordinsky, Sawaya, and Scher, 2000)*

**onycholysis** /ōn'ikol'isis/ [Gk, *onyx* + *lysein,* to loosen], separation of a nail from its bed, beginning at the free margin, associated with psoriasis, dermatitis of the hand, fungal infection, *Pseudomonas* infection, and many other conditions.

**onychomycosis** /on'ikō'mīkō'sis/ [Gk, *onyx* + *mykes,* fungus, *osis,* condition], any fungus infection of the nails.

**onycho-osteodysplasia.** See **nail-patella syndrome, osteo-onychodysplasia.**

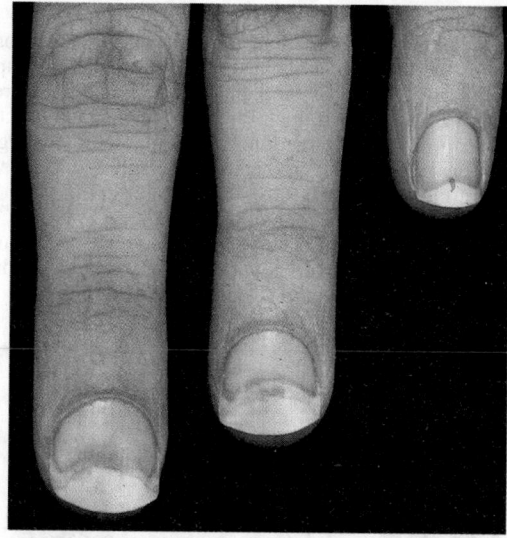

**Onycholysis** *(du Vivier, 1993/courtesy Institute of Dermatology)*

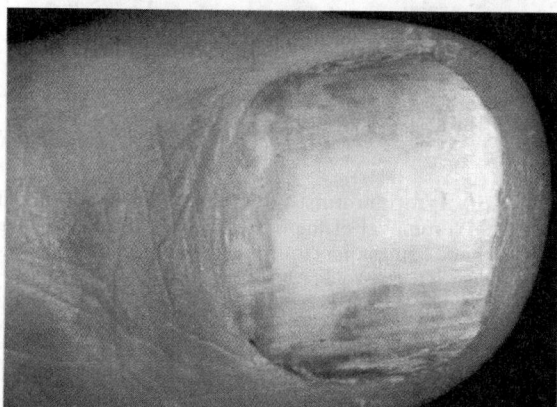

**White superficial onychomycosis** *(Habif, 1996)*

**onychophagia.** See **nail biting.**

**onychosis** [Gk, *onyx,* nail, *osis,* condition], a condition of atrophy or dystrophy of the nails, usually caused by a dermatosis such as a fungal infection.

**onychotillomania** /on′ikōtil′əmā′nē·ə/ [Gk, *onyx,* nail, *tillein,* to pluck, *mania,* madness], a nervous habit of picking at the nails to the point ot tissue damage (i.e., bleeding).

**onychotomy** /on′ikot′əmē/, a surgical incision into a nailbed.

**oo-** /ō′ə-/, prefix meaning 'egg or ovum': *ooblast, oocytase, ootid.*

**oob,** abbreviation for *out of bed.*

**oobe,** abbreviation for **out-of-body experience.**

**ooblast** /ō′əblast/ [Gk, *oon,* egg, *blastos,* germ], a female germ cell from which a mature ovum is developed.

**oocenter.** See **ovocenter.**

**oocyesis** /ō′əsī·ē′sis/ [Gk, *oon* + *kyesis,* pregnancy], an ectopic ovarian pregnancy.

**oocyst** /ō′əsist/ [Gk, *oon* + *kystis,* bag], a stage in the development of sporozoa consisting of a zygote enclosed by cyst wall. Oocysts of malarial parasites are found in the stomachs of infected mosquitoes. Oocysts of toxoplasma organisms are contained in the feces of infected cats. Compare **oocyte.**

**oocyte** /ō′əsīt/ [Gk, *oon* + *kytos,* cell], a primordial or incompletely developed ovum.

**oocytin** /ō′əsī′tin/, the substance in a spermatozoon that stimulates the formation of the fertilization membrane after penetration of an ovum.

**oogamy** /ō·og′əmē/ [Gk, *oon* + *gamos,* marriage], **1.** sexual reproduction by the fertilization of a large nonmotile female gamete by a smaller, actively motile male gamete, such as occurs in certain algae and the malarial parasite *Plasmodium.* **2.** heterogamy. Compare **isogamy.** —**oogamous,** *adj.*

**oogenesis** /ō′əjen′əsis/ [Gk, *oon* + *genesis,* origin], the formation of the female gametes, or ova. The female infant is born with the entire number of primary oocytes that will function throughout reproductive life. Only a fraction of these survive until puberty, and only a small percentage will be ovulated. Follicles containing the primary oocytes are found in varying stages of development in the ovary of the sexually mature woman. Egg and sperm formation differ considerably in the number and size of gametes resulting from gametogenesis, the total number of gametes produced in a lifetime, and the time sequence for the initiation of the meiotic divisions and the completion of the cycle. Also called **ovogenesis.** Compare **spermatogenesis.** See also **gametogenesis, meiosis, menstrual cycle, ovulation.** —**oogenetic,** *adj.*

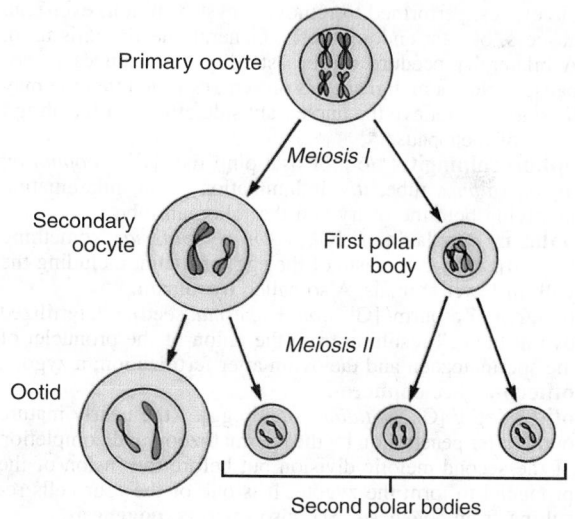

**Oogenesis** *(Thibodeau and Patton, 1999/Rolin Graphics)*

**oogonium** /ō′əgō′nē·əm/, *pl.* **oogonia** [Gk, *oon* + *gonos,* offspring], the precursor cell from which an oocyte develops in the fetus during intrauterine life. Also called **ovogonium.** See also **oogenesis.**

**ookinesis** /ō′əkinē′sis/ [Gk, *oon* + *kinesis,* movement], the chromosal movement occurring in the nucleus of the egg cell during maturation and fertilization. Also called **ookinesia.** See also **oogenesis.** —**ookinetic,** *adj.*

**ookinete** /ō'əkinēt'/ [Gk, *oon + kinein,* to move], the motile elongated zygote that is formed by the fertilization of the macrogamete during the sexual reproductive phase of the life cycle of a sporozoan, specifically the malarial parasite *Plasmodium.* It penetrates the lining of the stomach of the female *Anopheles* mosquito and attaches to the outer wall, where it forms an oocyst and gives rise to sporozoites.

**ookinetic.** See **ookinesis.**

**oolemma.** See **zona pellucida.**

**oophor-.** See **oophoro-.**

**oophoralgia** /ō'əfôral'jə/ [Gk, *oophoron,* ovary, *algos,* pain], a pain in an ovary.

**oophorectomy** /ō'əfərek'təmē/ [Gk, *oophoron,* ovary, *ektomē,* excision], the surgical removal of one or both ovaries. It is performed to remove a cyst or tumor, excise an abscess, treat endometriosis, or in breast cancer to remove the source of estrogen, which stimulates some kinds of cancer. If both ovaries are removed, sterility results, and menopause is abruptly induced; in premenopausal women one ovary or a part of one ovary may be left intact unless a malignancy is present. The operation routinely accompanies a hysterectomy in menopausal or postmenopausal women. Regional or general anesthesia is used. Unless a malignancy is present, estrogen may be given to treat the unpleasant side effects of the abrupt onset of menopause. Also called **ovariectomy.**

**oophoritis** /ō'əferī'tis/, an inflammatory condition of one or both ovaries, usually occurring with salpingitis or another infection.

**oophoro-, oophor-, ootheco-,** combining form meaning 'ovary': *oophorocytosis, oophorogenous, oophoroma.*

**oophorosalpingectomy** /ō'əfôr'əsal'pinjek'təmē/ [Gk, *oophoron + salpinx,* tube, *ektomē,* excision], the surgical removal of one or both ovaries and the corresponding fallopian tubes, performed to remove a cyst or tumor, excise an abscess, or treat endometriosis. General anesthesia is used. A bilateral procedure causees sterility and induces menopause, unless a malignancy is present, estrogen therapy may be started to relieve the unpleasant side effects of the abrupt onset of menopause.

**oophorosalpingitis** /ō'əfôr'əsal'pinjī'tis/ [Gk, *oophoron,* ovary, *salpinx,* tube, *itis,* inflammation], an inflammation involving both the ovary and the fallopian tube.

**ooplasm** /ō'əplaz'əm/ [Gk, *oon + plasma,* something formed], the cytoplasm of the egg, or ovum, including the yolk in lower animals. Also called **ovoplasm.**

**oosperm** /ō'əspurm/ [Gk, *oon + sperma,* seed], a fertilized ovum; the cell resulting from the union of the pronuclei of the spermatozoon and the ovum after fertilization; a zygote.

**ootheco-.** See **oophoro-.**

**ootid** /ō'ətid/ [Gk, *ootidion,* small egg], the nearly mature ovum after penetration by the spermatozoon and completion of the second meiotic division but before the fusion of the pronuclei to form the zygote. It is one of the four cells resulting from oogenesis. See also **meiosis, oogenesis.**

**OP,** **1.** abbreviation for *operative procedure.* **2.** abbreviation for **outpatient.**

**opacity** /ōpas'itē/ [L, *opacitus,* shadiness], pertaining to an opaque quality of a substance or object, such as cataract opacity.

**opalescent** /ō'pəl·es'ənt /, showing a milky iridescence, like an opal.

**opaque** /ōpāk'/ [L, *opacus,* obscure], **1.** pertaining to a substance or surface that neither transmits nor allows the passage of light. **2.** neither transparent nor translucent.

**OPD,** abbreviation for *Outpatient Department.*

**-ope,** combining form meaning a 'person having an eye defect': *asthenope, hyperope, protanope.*

**open amputation** [AS, *offan,* open; L, *amputare,* to cut away], a kind of amputation in which a straight, guillotine cut is made without skin flaps. Open amputation is performed if an infection is probable, developing, or recurrent. The cross section is left open for drainage, and skin traction is applied to prevent retraction. Antibiotic therapy is begun, and surgical closure is completed when the infection clears. Compare **closed amputation.** See also **gangrene.**

**open-angle glaucoma.** See **glaucoma.**

**open bite,** an abnormal dental condition in which the anterior teeth in the maxilla do not occlude those in the mandible in any mandibular position. Compare **closed bite.**

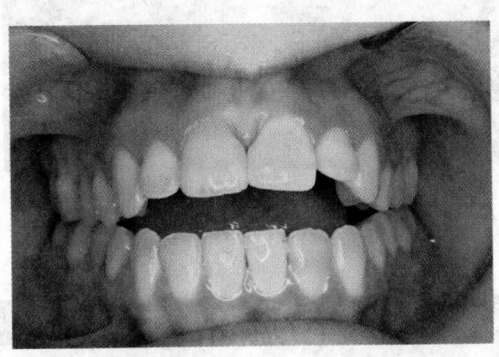

**Open bite** *(Proffit, 2000)*

**open-cavity tympanomastoidectomy,** tympanomastoidectomy with removal of the posterior wall of the ear canal, such as radical mastoidectomy and modified radical mastoidectomy. See **mastoidectomy.**

**open-chain exercise,** exercise in which the distal aspect of the extremity is free in space and not in contact with the ground.

**open charting,** a system of medical record keeping in which the patient has access to his or her chart. Open charting in varying degrees is authorized in some mental health institutions.

**open circuit,** an electric circuit in which current flow ceases.

**open-circuit breathing system,** a breathing apparatus used in cardiopulmonary therapy in which rebreathing does not occur. Gas is inspired through a breathing branch or limb that is connected to a gas source or open to the ambient atmosphere. Expired gas flows through a directional valve into a collecting reservoir or into the ambient atmosphere.

**open dislocation,** a joint displacement accompanied by a break in the skin. Formerly called **compound dislocation.**

**open drainage.** See **drainage.**

**open-drop anesthesia,** the oldest and simplest anesthetic technique. It is no longer used in the United States. A volatile liquid anesthetic agent such as halothane is dripped, one drop at a time, onto a porous cloth or mask held over the patient's face. It is difficult to control the anesthetic depth and pollution of the OR. Chloroform and ether are the major general anesthetics adaptable to open-drop administration.

**open-enrollment period,** a time during which individuals can enroll in a health care plan.

**open fracture.** See **compound fracture.**

**open fracture grading system,** a system for dividing open fractures into five categories, ranging from a clean wound that communicates to the fracture site and measures less than 1 cm to a fracture requiring repair of arteries.

**opening abductory wedge osteotomy (OAWO),** a procedure for treating a bunion deformity, in which a bone graft is used to open the wedge cut into the bone and bring the first metatarsal closer to the second.

**opening pressure,** the amount of pressure measured in a manometer after insertion of a spinal needle into the subarachnoid space.

**opening wedge osteotomy,** a procedure for treating bunion deformity in which a proximal cut is made in the metatarsal to reduce the deformity. It is performed with or without tendon transfers.

**open medical staff,** (in managed care) the opening of hospital medical staff membership to all physicians in the community who meet membership and clinical privilege requirements.

**open operation,** a surgical procedure that provides a full view of the structures or organs involved through membranous or cutaneous incisions.

**open-panel HMO,** a health maintenance organization (HMO) in which physicians treat both HMO and private patients.

**open PHO,** a physician-hospital organization in which all physicians on the hospital medical staff can participate.

**open pneumothorax** [AS, *open* + Gk, *pneuma*, air, *thorax*, chest], the presence of air or gas in the chest as a result of an open wound in the chest wall.

**open reduction** [AS, *open* + L, *reducere*, to lead back], a surgical procedure for reducing a fracture or dislocation by exposing the skeletal parts involved.

**open rhinolalia.** See **hypernasality.**

**open system,** a system that interacts with its environment.

**open-wedge osteotomy,** a straight cut made across a bone, leaving a wedge-shaped gap in the bone.

**open wound** [AS, *open* + *wund*], a wound that disrupts the integrity of the skin.

**operable** /op′ərəbəl/ [L, *operare*, to work], amenable to surgical intervention, as a disease or injury may be.

**operant** /op′ərənt/ [L, *operare*, to work], any act or response occurring without an identifiable stimulus. The result of the act or response determines whether or not it is repeated.

**operant conditioning,** a form of learning used in behavior therapy in which the person undergoing therapy is rewarded for the correct response and punished for the incorrect response. Also called **instrumental conditioning, shaping.**

**operant level,** the frequency or form of a performance under baseline conditions before any systematic conditioning procedures are introduced.

**operating microscope** /op′ərā′ting/ [L, *operare* + Gk, *mikros*, small, *skopein*, to look], a binocular microscope used in delicate surgery, especially surgery of the eye or ear. The standing type of operating microscope has a motorized zoom system operated by a foot pedal that quickly changes the magnification. The operating microscope that attaches to a surgeon's head has interchangeable lenses for different magnifications. Also called **surgical microscope.**

**operating room (OR, O.R.),** **1.** a room in a health care facility in which surgical procedures requiring anesthesia are performed. **2.** *informal.* a suite of rooms or an area in a health care facility in which patients are prepared for surgery and undergo surgical procedures.

**operating room technician,** the job title formerly used for **surgical technologist.**

**operating system (OS),** the main system programs of a computer that manage the hardware and application re-

sources of a system, including data input-output. Applications require an operating system to support and enable their function.

**operating telescope,** a magnifying lens that gives low magnification and a wide field of vision.

**operation** /op′ərā′shən/, any surgical procedure, such as an appendectomy or a hysterectomy.

**operationalization of behavior** /op′ərā′shənal′īzā′shən/, (in psychology) the stating of a patient's complaints or problems in specific, observable behavioral terms.

**operative cholangiography** /op′ərativ′/ [L, *operare* + Gk, *chole*, bile, *angeion*, vessel, *graphein*, to record], a procedure for radiographically outlining the major bile ducts during surgery. It involves the injection of a radiopaque contrast medium directly into the ducts. The procedure is usually performed to detect residual calculi in the biliary tract. See also **cholangiography.**

**operative dental surgeon.** See **dental surgeon.**

**operative dentistry,** that phase of dentistry concerned with restoration of parts of the teeth that are defective through disease, trauma, or abnormal development to a state of normal function, health, and esthetics, including preventive, diagnostic, biological, mechanical, and therapeutic techniques, as well as material and instrument science and application.

**operator gene** /op′ərā′tər/ [L, *operare* + Gk, *genein*, to produce], a section of bacterial DNA that regulates the transcription of structural genes in an operon by interacting with a repressor protein. The operator gene serves as the starting point in the coding sequence.

**operatory** /op′ər·ə·tor′ē/ [L, *operare*, to work], the working area of a dental office, in which treatment is provided to patients.

**operculum** /ōpur′kyŏŏləm/, *pl.* **opercula, operculums** [L, *lid*], a lid or covering, such as the mucous plug that blocks the cervix of the gravid uterus or the temporal operculum of the cerebral temporal hemisphere that overlaps the insula as an extension of the superior surface of the temporal lobe. —**opercular,** *adj.*

**operon** /op′əron/ [L, *operare*, to work], a section of bacterial DNA consisting of an operator gene and one or more structural genes with related functions. Transcription of the structural genes is controlled by the operator gene in conjunction with a regulator gene. See also **operator gene, regulator gene.**

**ophid-,** combining form meaning 'snake or snakelike': *ophidiophobia, ophidism, ophiasis.*

**-ophidia,** combining form meaning 'venomous snakes': *thanatophidia, toxicophidia.*

**ophth,** abbreviation for **ophthalmology.**

**ophthalm-.** See **ophthalmo-.**

**ophthalmia** /ofthal′mē·ə/ [Gk, *ophthalmos*, eye], severe inflammation of the conjunctiva or the deeper parts of the eye. Some kinds of ophthalmia are **ophthalmia neonatorum, sympathetic ophthalmia,** and **trachoma.**

**-ophthalmia,** combining form meaning a 'pathologic or anatomic condition of the eye': *allophthalmia, echinophthalmia, polemophthalmia.*

**ophthalmia neonatorum** /nē′ōnətôr′əm/, a purulent conjunctivitis and keratitis of the newborn resulting from exposure of the eyes to chemical, chlamydial, bacterial, or viral agents. Chemical conjunctivitis usually occurs as a result of the instillation of silver nitrate in the eyes of a newborn to prevent a gonococcal infection. Also called **neonatal conjunctivitis.** See also **conjunctivitis.**

**ophthalmic** /ofthal′mik/, [Gk, *ophthalmos*, eye], pertaining to the eye.

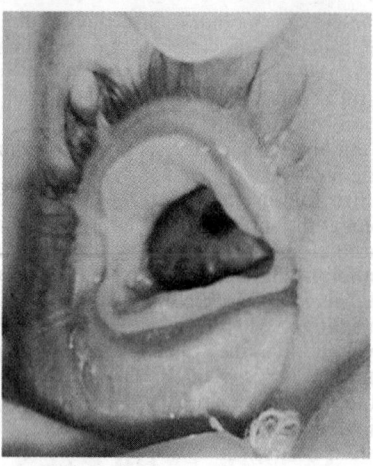

**Ophthalmia neonatorum** *(Zitelli and Davis, 1997)*

**ophthalmic administration of medication,** the administration of a drug by instillation of a cream, an ointment, or a liquid drop preparation in the conjunctival sac. The correct strength and amount of the drug are selected, and the medication is instilled into the eye or eyes as directed. The order usually specifies O.D. for right eye, O.S. for left eye, or O.U. for both eyes. Ophthalmic preparations are often refrigerated for storage but are given at room temperature. For administration the patient is positioned comfortably, lying back on a bed or examining table or sitting up with the neck hyperextended. The cul-de-sac of the conjunctival sac is exposed by gentle traction on the tissue just below the lower eyelid. The medication is placed into the sac as the patient is instructed to look away from the point of instillation. The dispenser is not allowed to touch the eye, and the medication is not placed directly on the cornea. The eyelid is slowly released, and the patient is asked to roll the eye around a few times to spread the medication over the entire surface of the eye. Applying pressure with the finger at the inner canthus may decrease systemic absorption.

**ophthalmic dispensing optician,** an allied health professional who adapts and fits corrective eyewear, including eyeglasses and contact lenses, as prescribed by an ophthalmologist or optometrist. Degree programs are usually 2 years.

**ophthalmic herpes zoster.** See **herpes zoster ophthalmicus.**

**ophthalmic laboratory technician,** a person who, working from a prescription written by an ophthalmologist or optometrist, cuts, grinds, edges, and finishes lenses and fabricates eyewear

**ophthalmic medical technician/technologist,** an allied health professional who assists ophthalmologists by collecting data and administering treatment ordered by the ophthalmologist. These specialists are qualified to take medical histories; administer diagnostic tests; make anatomic and functional ocular measurements; test ocular functions, including visual acuity, visual fields, and sensorimotor functions; administer topical ophthalmic medications; and instruct the patient in home care and the use of contact lenses. Ophthalmic medical technologists perform all duties performed by technicians but are expected to do so at a higher level of expertise.

**ophthalmic nerve** [Gk, *ophthalmos*, eye; L, *nervus*, nerve],

the first division of the trigeminal nerve (CN V), supplying the eyeball through the nasociliary branch. Branches also innervate the forehead, scalp, lacrimal gland, and dura mater.

**ophthalmic solution,** a specially prepared sterile preparation free of foreign particles for installation of a medication into the eye.

**ophthalmic vesicle.** See **optic vesicle.**

**ophthalmitis** /of'thalmī'tis/ [Gk, *ophthalmos*, eye, *itis*, inflammation], an inflammation of the eye.

**ophthalmo-** /ofthal'mō-/, **ophthalm-,** combining form meaning 'eye': *ophthalmodynia, ophthalmolith, ophthalmostat.*

**ophthalmodynamometer** /-din'əmom'ətər/ [Gk, *ophthalmos*, eye, *dynamis*, force, *metron*, measure], an instrument for measuring pressure on the sclera while the fundus is studied with an ophthalmoscope. It may be used to measure blood pressures in the ophthalmic artery.

**ophthalmodynia** /-din'ē·ə/ [Gk, *ophthalmos*, eye, *odyne*, pain], a pain in the eye.

**ophthalmologic, opthalmological.** See **ophthalmology.**

**ophthalmologist** /of'thalmol'əjist/, a physician who specializes in ophthalmology.

**ophthalmology (ophth)** /of'thalmol'əjē/ [Gk, *ophthalmos* + *logos*, science], the branch of medicine concerned with the study of the physiology, anatomy, and pathology of the eye and the diagnosis and treatment of disorders of the eye. **—ophthalmologic, ophthalmological,** *adj.*

**ophthalmopathy** /of'thəl·mop'ə·thē/ [Gk, *ophthalmos*, eye + *pathos*, disease], any disease of the eye.

**ophthalmoplasty** /ofthal'mōplas'tē/ [Gk, *ophthalmos*, eye, *plassein*, to mold], plastic surgery of the eye or the area around the eye.

**ophthalmoplegia** /ofthal'məplē'jē·ə/ [Gk, *ophthalmos* + *plege*, stroke], an abnormal condition characterized by paralysis of the motor nerves of the eye. Bilateral ophthalmoplegia of rapid onset is associated with acute myasthenia gravis, acute thiamine deficiency, botulism, and acute inflammatory cranial polyneuropathy. These diseases are potentially very destructive and require prompt attention. In some patients with myopathic ophthalmoplegia, structural abnormalities and biochemical disorders may be evident in limb muscles. Ophthalmoplegia is also associated with ocular dystrophy.

**ophthalmoplegia plus.** See **Kearns-Sayre syndrome.**

**ophthalmoscope** /ofthal'məskōp/ [Gk, *ophthalmos* + *skopein*, to look], a device for examining the interior of the eye. It includes a light, a mirror with a single aperture through which the examiner views, and a dial holding several lenses of varying strengths. The lenses are selected to allow clear visualization of the structures of the eye at any depth. If the patient or the examiner ordinarily requires extensive correction of a refractive error, the examination may require that the corrective lenses should be worn for the examination. Also called **funduscope.**

**ophthalmoscopy** /of'thalmos'kəpē/, the technique of using an ophthalmoscope to examine the eye. Also called **funduscopy.** See also **fundus microscopy.**

**ophthalmospasm** /ofthal'mōspaz'əm/ [Gk, *ophthalmos*, eye, *spasmos*], a sudden involuntary contraction of the eyeball.

**Ophthochlor,** trademark for an ophthalmic preparation of an antibacterial and antirickettsial (chloramphenicol).

**Ophthocort,** trademark for an ophthalmic, fixed-combination drug containing a glucocorticoid (hydrocortisone acetate) and antibacterials (chloramphenicol and polymyxin B sulfate).

**-opia, -opic, -opical, -ops, -opsia, -opsy, -opy,** suffix

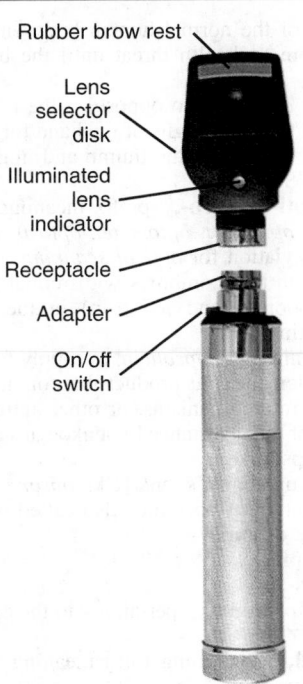

Rubber brow rest

Lens selector disk

Illuminated lens indicator

Receptacle

Adapter

On/off switch

**Ophthalmoscope** *(Seidel et al, 1999)*

meaning a '(specified) visual condition': *boopia, myopia, nonopia, senopia.*

**opiate** /ō′pē·it/ [Gk, *opion,* poppy juice], **1.** an opioid drug that contains opium, derivatives of opium, or any of several semisynthetic or synthetic drugs with opium-like activity. **2.** *informal.* any soporific or opioid drug. **3.** pertaining to a substance that causes sleep or relief of pain. Morphine and related opiates may produce unwanted side effects such as nausea, vomiting, dizziness, and constipation. Patients with reduced blood volume are more susceptible to the hypotensive effect of morphine and related drugs. Opiates are used with extreme caution in obese patients and in those with head injuries, emphysema, or other problems associated with decreased respiratory function. In patients with prostatic hypertrophy, morphine may cause acute urinary retention, requiring repeated catheterization. Also called **opioid.**

**opiate poisoning** [Gk, *opion,* poppy juice; L, *potio,* drink], toxic effects of a potent opioid, including depression of the brain centers, causing unconsciousness. Acute intoxication is characterized by euphoria, flushing, itching, and constriction of pupils, followed by reduced rate of respiration, hypotension, lowered body temperature, and abnormally slow heartbeat. Withdrawal is marked by effects generally the opposite of opiate poisoning, depending on the size of the dose and the duration of dependence.

**opiate receptor** [Gk, *opion,* poppy juice; L, *recipere,* to receive], any of a group of cells in the brain that bind to opiate drugs such as morphine. Some along the aqueduct of Sylvius and the center median have been identified as receptors associated with response to pain; others have been found in the striatum.

**-opic, -opical.** See **-opia.**

**opinion** /əpin′yən/ [L, *opinari,* to suppose], **1.** (in law) a statement by the court, usually in writing, of the reasoning behind its decision or judgment in a particular case. **2.** a statement prepared for a client by an attorney that represents the attorney's understanding of the law as it pertains to a legal question posed by the client.

**opioid** /ō′pē·oid/ [Gk, *opionm,* poppy juice, *eidos,* form], pertaining to natural and synthetic chemicals that have opium-like effects although they are not derived from opium. Examples include endorphins or enkephalins produced by body tissues or synthetic methadone.

**opioid antagonist,** a drug that is used primarily in the treatment of opioid-induced respiratory depression. The opioid antagonists nalorphine, levallorphan, and naloxone are usually administered parenterally.

**opioid receptor,** any of a number of types of receptors for opiates and opioids; at least seven different types are postulated at different locations in the body, grouped into three major classes (δ, κ, and μ) according to the specific substances they bind and to the specific physiological effect or effects that binding causes or inhibits.

**opisthion** /ō·pis′thē·on/ [Gk, *opisthion,* rear, posterior], a landmark located at the midpoint of the posterior border of the foramen magnum.

**opistho-,** combining form meaning 'backward or relating to the back': *opisthognathism, opisthoporeia, opisthotonos.*

**opisthorchiasis** /ō′pisthôrkī′əsis/ [Gk, *opisthen,* behind, *orchis,* testicle, *osis,* condition], infection with one of the species of *Opisthorchis* liver flukes commonly found in the Philippines, India, Thailand, and Laos. Carcinoma of the intrahepatic bile ducts may be a late complication. Adequate cooking of freshwater fish prevents the disease.

***Opisthorchis sinensis.*** See ***Clonorchis sinensis.***

**opisthotonos** /ō′pisthot′ənəs/ [Gk, *opisthios,* posterior, *tonos,* straining], a prolonged severe spasm of the muscles causing the back to arch acutely, the head to bend back on the neck, the heels to bend back on the legs, and the arms and hands to flex rigidly at the joints. It is related to meningitis.

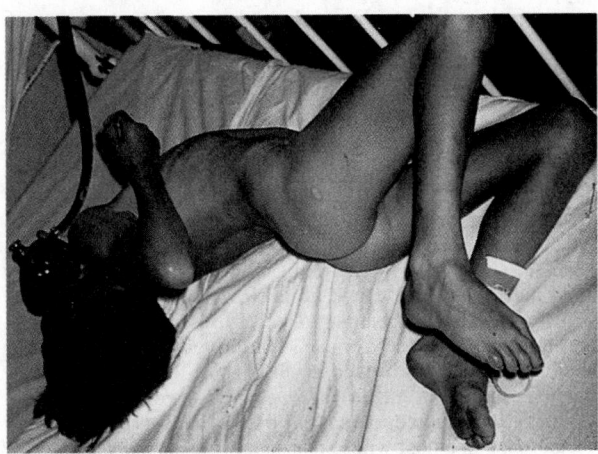

**Opisthotonos** *(Farrar, 1993)*

**Opitz syndrome** /ō′pitz/ [John Marius Opitz, German-born pediatrician in United States, b. 1935], an autosomal dominant syndrome consisting of hypertelorism and hernias, and in males hypospadias, cryptorchidism, and bifid scrotum. Cardiac anomalies, laryngotracheal malformations, imperforate anus, renal defects, lung hypoplasia, and downslanted palpebral fissures may also be present. Also called **G syndrome, hypertelorism-hypospadias syndrome.**

**opium** /ō′pē·əm/ [Gk, *opion,* poppy juice], a milky exudate from the unripe capsules of *Papaver somniferum* and *Papaver album* yielding 9.5% or more of anhydrous morphine. It is an opioid analgesic, a hypnotic, and an astringent. Opium contains several alkaloids, including codeine, morphine, and papaverine. See also **codeine, morphine sulfate, opium tincture, papaverine hydrochloride, paregoric.**

**opium alkaloid,** one of several alkaloids isolated from the milky exudate of the unripe seed pods of *Papaver somniferum,* a species of poppy indigenous to the Near East. Three of the alkaloids, codeine, papaverine, and morphine, are used clinically for the relief of pain, but their use entails the risk of physical or psychologic dependence. Morphine is the standard against which the analgesic effect of newer drugs for relief of pain is measured. The opium alkaloids and their semisynthetic derivatives, including heroin, act on the central nervous system, producing analgesia, change in mood, drowsiness, and mental slowness. The effects in a person who has pain are usually pleasant; euphoria and pain-free sleep are not uncommon, but nausea and vomiting sometimes occur. In usual doses the analgesic effects are achieved without loss of consciousness. The opium alkaloids have several other effects on the various systems of the body: Coughing is suppressed; the electrical activity pattern of the brain resembles that of sleep; the pupils constrict; respiration is depressed in rate, minute volume, and tidal exchange; the secretory activity and motility of the GI tract are diminished; and biliary and pancreatic secretions are reduced. The use of morphine as an antidiarrheal preceded its use as an analgesic by hundreds of years. Prepared in a tincture, it remains the most effective constipating agent available.

**opium tincture,** an analgesic and antidiarrheal.
■ INDICATIONS: It is prescribed in the treatment of intestinal hyperactivity, cramping, and diarrhea.
■ CONTRAINDICATIONS: Drug dependence, the presence of toxic matter in the bowel, or known hypersensitivity to this drug prohibits its use.
■ ADVERSE EFFECTS: Among the more serious adverse reactions are drug dependence, toxic megacolon, and central nervous system depression.

**opo-,** combining form meaning 'juices or certain fluids, including hormones': *opsinuria.*

**Oppenheim reflex** /op′ənhīm/ [Herman Oppenheim, German neurologist, 1858–1919], a variation of Babinski's reflex, elicited by firmly stroking downward on the anterior and medial surfaces of the tibia, characterized by extension of the great toe and fanning of other toes. It is a sign of pyramidal tract disease. Compare **Chaddock reflex, Gordon's reflex.** See also **Babinski's reflex.**

**opportunistic infection** [L, *opportunus,* convenient, *icus,* form], **1.** an infection caused by normally nonpathogenic organisms in a host whose resistance has been decreased by disorders such as diabetes mellitus, human immunodeficiency virus (HIV) infection, or cancer; a surgical procedure such as a cerebrospinal fluid shunt or a cardiac or urinary tract catheterization; or immunosuppressive drugs. Long-term use of antibiotics or other drugs also may affect the immune system, creating opportunity for microorganisms not usually pathogenic to become pathogens. People with HIV are particularly susceptible to such infections. **2.** an unusual infection with a common pathogen such as cellulitis, meningitis, or otitis media.

**opportunistic pathogen,** an organism that exists harm-

lessly as part of the normal human body environment and does not become a health threat until the body's immune system fails.

**opposition** [L, *opponere,* to oppose], the relation between the thumb and the other digits of the hand for the purpose of grasping objects between the thumb and fingers.

**-ops, -opsia.** See **-opia.**

**ops-, opto-, opti-, optico-,** prefix meaning 'visible or vision or sight': *optoblast, optometer, optostriate.*

**opscan,** abbreviation for *optical scanning.*

**opsin,** a protein that combines with retinal to form visual pigments (rhodopsin and iodopsin) in the photoreceptor cells of the retina.

**opsonin** /op′sənin/ [Gk, *opsonein,* to supply food], an antibody or complement split product that, on attaching to foreign material, microorganisms, or other antigens, enhances phagocytosis of that substance by leukocytes and other macrophages. —**opsonize,** *v.*

**opsonization** /op′sənizā′shən/ [Gk, *opsonein* + *izein,* to cause], the action of opsonin. Also called **opsonification.**

**opsonize.** See **opsonin.**

**-opsy.** See **-opia.**

**opti-.** See **ops-.**

**optic** [Gk, *optikos,* sight], pertaining to the eyes or to sight. Also **optical.**

**-optic, -optical,** combining form meaning 'vision': *bioptic, panoptic, preoptic.*

**optical.** See **optic.**

**optical activity** /op′tik/, the rotation of the plane of polarized light clockwise or counterclockwise. Substances that rotate the plane of polarized light to the right are dextrorotatory; those that rotate the plane to the left are levorotatory.

**optic angle.** See **visual angle.**

**optic atrophy,** wasting of the optic disc resulting from degeneration of fibers of the optic nerve and optic tract. In primary optic atrophy the disc is white and sharply margined, the central depression (physiologic cup) is enlarged, and the optic foramen of the sclera is clearly visible. In secondary atrophy the disc is gray, its margins are blurred, the depression is filled in, and the foramen is difficult to detect. Optic atrophy may be caused by a congenital defect, inflammation, occlusion of the central retinal artery or internal carotid artery, alcohol, arsenic, lead, tobacco, or other toxic substances. Degeneration of the disc may accompany arteriosclerosis, diabetes, glaucoma, hydrocephalus, pernicious anemia, and various neurologic disorders.

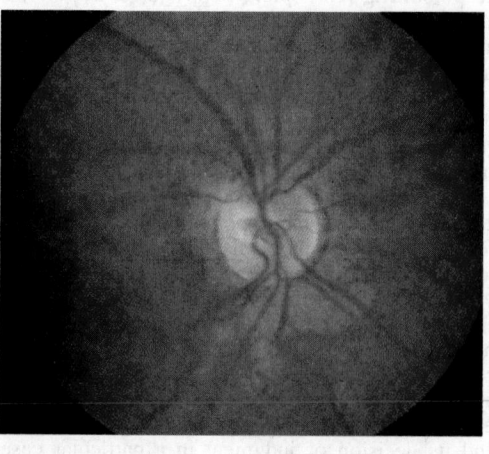

**Optic atrophy** *(Zitelli and Davis, 1997)*

**optic brightener,** a compound that absorbs ultraviolet light and emits visible light.

**optic chiasm** [Gk, *optikos,* sight, *chiasma,* crossed lines], a point near the thalamus and hypothalamus where parts of each optic nerve cross over.

**optic coupling,** the attachment of the crystal window of a scintillator to the window of a photomultiplier tube. It maximizes the transmission of light from the scintillator to the interior of the photomultiplier tube.

**optic cup,** a two-layered embryonic cavity that develops in early pregnancy. The optic cup is completed by the seventh week with the closing of the choroidal fissure. The cup initially develops from the infolding of the optic vesicle after the vesicle separates from the embryonic ectoderm. The cells of the optic cup differentiate to form the retina that first develops its layers of rods and cones in the central part of the cup, growing as the layer gradually spreads toward the cup margin. The outer layer of the cup persists as the pigmented layer of the retina; the inner layer develops the nervous elements and the supporting fibers of the retina. Compare **optic stalk.**

**optic density,** a number describing the blackening of an x-ray film in any specified location. In general, the optic density is the logarithm of the ratio of incident light intensity to the intensity of light transmitted through that area and is measured with a densitometer.

**optic disc,** the small blind spot on the surface of the retina, located about 3 mm to the nasal side of the macula. It is the point where the fibers of the retina leave the eye and become part of the optic nerve. It is the only part of the retina that is insensitive to light. At its center the porus opticus marks the point of entrance of the central artery of the retina. Also called *(informal)* **blind spot, discus nervi optici.**

**optic foramen** [Gk, *optikos,* sight, *foramen,* hole], an aperture in the root of the lesser wing of the sphenoid bone transmitting the optic nerve.

**optic glioma,** a slow-growing tumor on the optic nerve or in the chiasm. The tumor is composed of glial cells. Symptoms may include loss of vision, secondary strabismus, exophthalmos, and ocular paralysis.

**optician** /optish′ən/ [Gk, *optikos,* sight], a person who grinds and fits eyeglasses and contact lenses by prescription. To become an optician, a person must graduate from high school and complete a 4- or 5-year apprenticeship. In some states licensure is required.

**optic illusion** [Gk, *optikos,* sight; L, *illudere,* to mock], a false visual image derived from a misinterpretation of sensory stimuli caused by physical or psychologic factors or both. A common optic illusion is the appearance of railroad tracks merging in the distance.

**optic laser, optic maser.** See **laser.**

**optic nerve,** one of a pair of cranial nerves that transmit visual impulses. It consists mainly of coarse myelinated fibers that arise in the retinal ganglionic layer, traverse the thalamus, and connect with the visual cortex. At the optic chiasm the fibers from the inner or nasal half of the retina cross to the optic tract of the opposite side. The remaining fibers from the temporal or outer half of each retina are uncrossed and pass to the visual cortex on the same side. The visual cortex functions in the perception of light, shade, and objects. The optic nerve fibers correspond to a tract of fibers within the brain. Also called **nervus opticus, second cranial nerve.**

**optic neuritis** [Gk, *optikos,* sight, *neuron,* nerve, *itis,* inflammation], inflammation, degeneration, or demyelinization of an optic nerve caused by a wide variety of diseases. Loss of vision is the cardinal symptom.

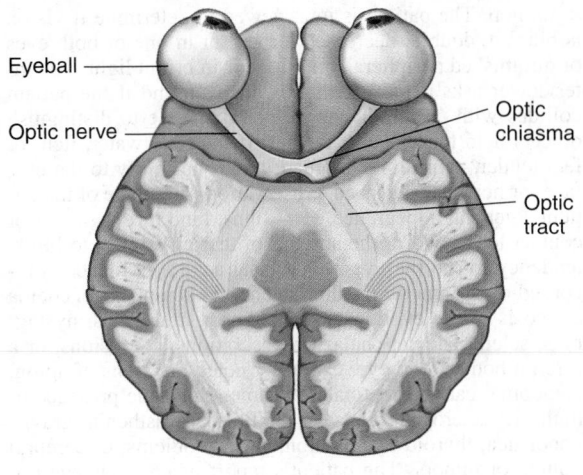

**Optic nerve**

**optic neuropathy** [Gk, *optikos,* sight, *neuron,* nerve, *pathos,* disease], a disease, generally noninflammatory, of the eye, characterized by dysfunction or destruction of the optic nerve tissues. Causes may include an interruption in the blood supply, compression by a tumor or aneurysm, a nutritional deficiency, and toxic effects of a chemical. The disorder, which can lead to blindness, usually affects only one eye.

**optico-.** See **ops-.**

**opticokinetic.** See **optokinetic.**

**optic papilla.** See **papilla.**

**optic radiation** [Gk, *optikos,* sight; L, *radiare,* to shine], a system of fibers from the lateral geniculate body of the thalamus that pass through the sublenticular part of the internal capsule to the striate area.

**optic righting,** one of the five basic neuromuscular reactions that enable a person to change body positions. It involves a reflex that automatically orients the head to a new optical or visual fixation point, depending on the body position change.

**optic righting reflex** [Gk, *optikos,* sight; AS, *riht* + L, *reflectere,* to bend back], a reflex that restores normal posture and head position with the help of visual clues.

**optics** /op′tiks/ [Gk, *optikos,* sight], **1.** (in physics) a field of study that deals with the electromagnetic radiation of wavelengths shorter than radio waves but longer than x-rays. **2.** (in physiology) a field of study that deals with vision and the process by which the functions of the eye and the brain are integrated in the perception of shapes, patterns, movements, spatial relationships, and color.

**optic stalk,** one of a pair of slender embryonic structures that become the optic nerve. In the embryo the optic stalk develops during the second week and attaches the optic vesicle to the wall of the brain. The stalk becomes complete during the seventh week of pregnancy when the choroidal fissure closes and is later converted into the optic nerve when retinal nerve fibers fill the cavity of the stalk. A few fibers grow into the stalk from the brain. About the tenth week after birth, the fibers of the optic nerve receive their myelin sheaths. Compare **optic cup.**

**optic system assessment,** an evaluation of the patient's eyes, vision, and current and past disorders or injuries that may be responsible for abnormalities in the individual's optic system.

■ METHOD: The patient is interviewed to determine if vision is blurred, double, decreased, or absent in one or both eyes or diminished peripherally at night or in bright light. The interviewer asks if halos or lights are seen and if the patient collides with unfamiliar objects or is unable to distinguish objects held too close or too far; if the eyes water, itch, or feel tender, painful, or fatigued; and if an injury to the eye, face, or head has occurred. Observations are made of the patient's general appearance, vital signs, kind of eyeglasses or contact lenses worn, the amount of tearing, ability to blink, tendency to rub the eyes, and visual acuity. Evidence is recorded of conjunctivitis, drainage, optic hemorrhage, edema or ptosis of the eyelids, exophthalmos, strabismus, nystagmus, scleral edema, chalazion, lacerations, contusions, or a foreign body in the eye. Carefully noted are signs of aging; glaucoma; cataract; retinal detachment; and the presence of multiple sclerosis, diabetes mellitus, myasthenia gravis, gonorrhea, thyroid dysfunction, sinus problems, or cerebral trauma or tumors. The patient's report of previous eye operations or treatments, head or face trauma, arteriosclerosis, glomerulonephritis, retinal degeneration, episodes of coma, therapy with oxygen, and drug misuse are investigated, as well as a family history of glaucoma or diabetes. Also explored are the possibility that the patient has a hazardous job or recreation (and note is made of any safety precautions taken); the individual's misuse of alcohol; and use of medication, especially antibiotics, antiemetics, miotics, mydriatics, and acetazolamide. Diagnostic aids available for the evaluation include a test of visual fields, x-ray film of the orbit and skull, an ophthalmoscopic examination, tonometry, brain scan, and microscopic studies of conjunctival scrapings.

■ INTERVENTIONS: A health care provider conducts the interview, observes the patient, and assembles pertinent background data and the results of the diagnostic procedures.

■ OUTCOME CRITERIA: A careful assessment of the patient's eyes and vision and of certain aspects of the medical, family, and social history is a significant aid in establishing the diagnosis of an optic system disorder.

**optic thermometer,** a temperature-measuring device in which the properties of transmission and reflection of visible light are temperature dependent, the detection of which can be related to tissue temperature.

**optic tract** [Gk, *optikos,* sight; L, *tractus*], a flat band of nerve fibers running backward and laterally around each cerebral peduncle from the optic chiasma to the lateral geniculate body.

**optic vesicle,** an early embryonic outgrowth from the ventrolateral wall of the forebrain. Its cells develop into the retina and optic nerve of the eye. Also called **ophthalmic vesicle.**

**Optimine,** trademark for an antihistamine (azatadine maleate).

**optional water loss** /op'shənəl/, a volume of average daily water loss, in addition to obligatory water loss, depending on physical activities, climate, and other factors. See also **obligatory water loss.**

**opto-.** See **ops-.**

**optokinetic** /op'tōkinet'ik/ [Gk, *optikos,* sight, *kinesis,* motion], pertaining to movement of the eyeballs in response to the movement of objects across the visual field, such as in optokinetic nystagmus. Also **opticokinetic.**

**optometrist** /optom'ətrist/ [Gk, *optikos,* sight, *metron,* measure], a person who practices optometry. An optometrist is awarded the degree of Doctor of Optometry (O.D.) after completion of at least 3 years of college followed by 4 years in an approved college of optometry. A state exami-

nation and license are also required. See also **optician, optometry.**

**optometry** /optom'ətrē/ [Gk, *optikos,* sight, *metron,* measure], the practice of primary eye care, including testing the eyes for visual acuity, diagnosing and managing eye health, prescribing corrective spectacle or contact lenses, and recommending eye exercises. See also **optician.**

**OPV,** abbreviation for **oral poliovirus vaccine.**

**-opy.** See **-opia.**

**OR, O.R.,** abbreviation for **operating room.**

**ora** /ō'rə/ *pl.* **orae** [L], an edge or margin.

**oral** /ôr'əl/ [L, *oralis,* pertaining to the mouth], pertaining to the mouth. Compare **buccal, parenteral.**

**oral administration of medication,** the administration of a tablet, a capsule, an elixir, or a solution or other liquid form of medication by mouth. An adequate amount of water should be given to lubricate or dissolve the solid medications or to dilute the liquid forms for swallowing. Preparations with a disagreeable taste may be given with something of sufficient flavor to disguise the bad taste. Substances that are harmful to the teeth are given through a straw. People who have difficulty swallowing pills or capsules may find it easier to swallow the medication if they look up as they swallow. Looking up while swallowing opens the esophagus. With patients who have difficulty swallowing, the oral cavity is always checked for pocketing the medication. Research shows that sitting up for 15 to 30 minutes after medications orally promotes dissolution of the medication and decreases gastric irritation effect. Oral administration of medication includes **buccal administration of medication** and **sublingual administration of medication.**

**oral airway,** a curved tubular device of rubber, plastic, or metal placed in the oropharynx during general anesthesia and other situations in which the level of consciousness is impaired. Its purpose is to maintain free passage of air and keep the tongue from obstructing the trachea. The artificial airway is not removed until the patient begins to awaken and regains pharyngeal, cough, and swallowing reflexes.

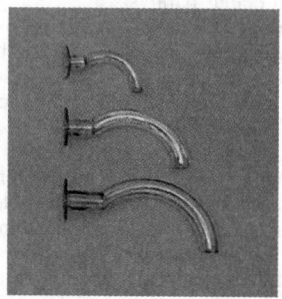

**Oral airways** *(Sanders et al, 2000)*

**oral and maxillofacial surgeon.** See **dental surgeon.**

**oral and maxillofacial surgery** [L, *oralis,* pertaining to the mouth; Gk, *cheirourgos,* surgeon], the branch of dentistry that is concerned primarily with surgery on the teeth, jaws, and surrounding soft tissues. Also called **oral surgery, maxillofacial surgery.** See also **dental surgeon.**

**oral cancer,** a malignant neoplasm on the lip or in the mouth that occurs at an average age of 60 with a frequency eight times higher in men than in women. Predisposing factors are alcoholism, heavy use of tobacco, poor oral hygiene, ill-fitting dentures, syphilis, Plummer-Vinson syndrome, betel nut chewing, and in lip cancer pipe smoking and overexposure to sun and wind. Premalignant leukoplakia or erythroplasia or a painless nonhealing ulcer may be the first sign of oral cancer; localized pain usually occurs later, but lymph nodes may be involved early in the course. Diagnostic measures include digital examination, biopsy, exfoliative cytology, x-ray film of the mandible, and chest films to detect metastatic lung lesions. Almost all oral tumors are epidermoid carcinomas; adenocarcinomas occur occasionally, whereas sarcomas and metastatic lesions from other sites are rare. Small primary lesions may be treated by excision or irradiation and more extensive oral tumors by surgery, with removal of involved lymph nodes and preoperative or postoperative radiotherapy. Among chemotherapeutic agents administered are cisplatin, methotrexate, 5-fluorouracil, bleomycin, and adriamycin.

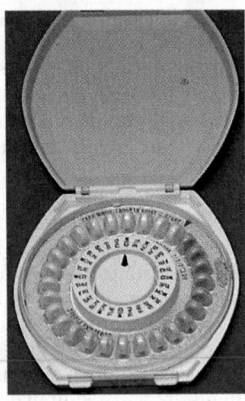

**Oral contraceptives** *(Edge and Miller, 1994)*

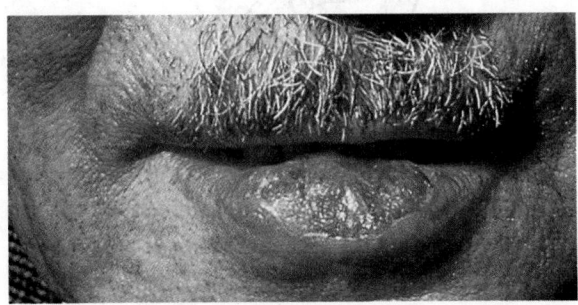

**Oral cancer** *(Hill, 1994)*

**oral cavity** [L, *oralis,* pertaining to the mouth, *cavum,* cavity], the space within the mouth, containing the tongue and teeth. See also **mouth.**

**oral character,** (in psychoanalysis) a kind of personality that exhibits patterns of behavior originating in the oral and first phase of infancy. This personality is characterized by optimism, self-confidence, and carefree generosity reflecting the pleasurable aspects of the stage; or pessimism, futility, anxiety, and sadism as manifestations of frustrations or conflicts occurring during the period. See also **oral eroticism, oral stage, psychosexual development.**

**oral contraceptive,** oral hormone medication for contraception. The two major hormones used are progestin and estrogen. The hormones act by inhibiting the production of gonadotropin-releasing hormone by the hypothalamus, and therefore the pituitary does not secrete gonadotropins to stimulate ovulation. This results in the endometrium of the uterus being thin and the cervical mucus being thick, thus preventing the penetration of sperm. Contraindications to the medication include pregnancy, diabetes mellitus, liver disease, hyperlipidemia, thrombolic complications, coronary artery disease, and sickle cell disease. Patients with depression and migraine headaches and those who are heavy cigarette smokers need to be followed up more often. The pregnancy rate when oral contraceptives are used correctly is less than 0.2% a year. See also **contraception.**

**oral decongestant,** a drug such as pseudoephedrine prescribed for the relief of nasal congestion. Oral decongestants do not appear to cause nasal swelling after long periods of use. They are commonly combined with antihistamines for

the treatment of allergic rhinitis. Abuse may cause constipation.

**oral dosage,** the administration of a medicine by mouth.

**oral eroticism,** (in psychoanalysis) libidinal fixation at or regression to the oral stage of psychosexual development, often reflected in such personality traits as passivity, insecurity, and oversensitivity. Also called **oral erotism.** Compare **anal eroticism.** See also **oral character.**

**oral examination** [L, *oralis,* pertaining to the mouth, *examinatio,* weighing], a clinical, visual, and tactile inspection and investigation of the hard and soft structures of the oral cavity for purposes of assessment, diagnosis, planning, treatment, and evaluation. Before the examination, the client's health history is obtained and studied for information concerning predisposition to bacteremia and the resulting need for premedication. If available, radiographs are used in conjunction with an oral examination.

**oral-facial-digital (OFD) syndrome, type I,** a male-lethal X-linked dominant disorder characterized by camptodactyly, polydactyly, and syndactyly; by cranial, facial, lingual, and dental anomalies; and by mental retardation, familial trembling, alopecia, and seborrhea of the face and milia. Also called **orodigitofacial dysostosis, orofaciodigital syndrome, type I.**

**oral-facial-digital (OFD) syndrome, type II.** See **Mohr syndrome.**

**oral-facial-digital (OFD) syndrome, type III,** an autosomal recessive disorder characterized by postaxial hexadactyly of the hands and feet, by ocular, lingual, and dental anomalies, and by profound mental retardation. Also called **orodigitofacial dysostosis, orofaciodigital syndrome, type III.**

**oral hairy leukoplakia.** See **hairy leukoplakia.**

**oral health,** a nursing outcome from the Nursing Outcomes Classification (NOC) defined as the condition of the mouth, teeth, gums, and tongue. See also **Nursing Outcomes Classification.**

**oral health maintenance,** a nursing intervention from the Nursing Interventions Classification (NIC) defined as maintenance and promotion of oral hygiene and dental health for the patient at risk for developing oral or dental lesions. See also **Nursing Interventions Classification.**

**oral health promotion,** a nursing intervention from the Nursing Interventions Classification (NIC) defined as promotion of oral hygiene and dental care for a patient with normal oral and dental health. See also **Nursing Interventions Classification.**

**oral health restoration,** a nursing intervention from the Nursing Interventions Classification (NIC) defined as promotion of healing for a patient who has an oral mucosa or dental lesion. See also **Nursing Interventions Classification.**

**oral herpes.** See **herpes simplex.**

**oral hygiene,** the condition or practice of maintaining the tissues and structures of the mouth. Oral hygiene includes brushing the tongue and teeth to remove food particles and residue, bacteria, and plaque; massaging the gums with a toothbrush, dental floss, or water irrigator to stimulate circulation and remove foreign matter; and cleansing dentures and ensuring their proper fit to prevent irritation. Dependent or unconscious patients are assisted in maintaining a healthy oral condition. Such care includes lubricating the lips and cleaning the inside of the cheeks, the roof of the mouth, and the tongue. In addition, the nurse checks for loose teeth that might be swallowed or aspirated.

**oral hypoglycemic agent,** an oral antidiabetic agent commonly used in the treatment of type 2 diabetes mellitus. Oral hypoglycemic agents are not prescribed as a substitute for diet and exercise but rather as adjunctive therapy.

**oral mucosa,** the mucous membrane of the cavity of the mouth, including the gums.

**oral pathology,** the branch of pathology that deals with the structural and functional changes in cells, tissues, and organs of the oral cavity that cause, or are caused by, disease.

**oral poliovirus vaccine (OPV),** an attenuated preparation of live poliovirus that confers immunity to poliomyelitis. Also called **Sabin vaccine.**

■ INDICATION: It is routinely prescribed for immunization against poliomyelitis.

■ CONTRAINDICATIONS: Immunosuppression, concomitant use of corticosteroids, cancer, immunoglobulin abnormalities, or acute infection prohibits its use.

■ ADVERSE EFFECTS: Adverse effects are uncommon. Cases of vaccine-induced paralytic disease have occurred but are very rare.

**oral prophylaxis** [L, *oralis,* pertaining to the mouth; Gk, *prophylax,* advance guard], the science and practice of preventing the onset of diseases of the teeth and adjoining mouth tissues. It involves removing bacterial plaque, food debris, stains, and calculus from the crowns and roots with hand scaling or ultrasonic scaling instruments and hand or electric polishers.

**oral rehydration solutions (ORS)** [L, *oralis,* pertaining to the mouth, *re* + *hydor,* water, *solutus,* dissolved], solutions of electrolytes and glucose used in oral rehydration therapy. The recommended electrolytes include NaCl, KCl, and trisodium citrate.

**oral rehydration therapy (ORT),** the adjustment of water, glucose, and electrolyte balance in a dehydrated patient by giving fluids with measured amounts of essential ingredients by mouth.

**oral sadism,** (in psychoanalysis) a sadistic form of oral eroticism manifested by such behavior as biting, chewing, and other aggressive impulses associated with eating habits. Compare **anal sadism.**

**oral stage,** (in psychoanalysis) according to Freud, the initial stage of psychosexual development occurring in the first 12 to 18 months of life when the feeding experience and other oral activities are the predominant source of pleasurable stimulation. See also **psychosexual development.**

**oral surgeon.** See **dental surgeon.**

**oral surgery.** See **oral and maxillofacial surgery.**

**oral temperature** [L, *oralis,* pertaining to the mouth, *temperatura*], the body temperature as recorded by a clinical thermometer placed in the mouth. It is normally around 98.6° F (37° C), but it may vary within a fraction of a degree, depending on the individual and such factors as time of day, sleep, and exercise and whether measured before or after a meal. See also **normal temperature.**

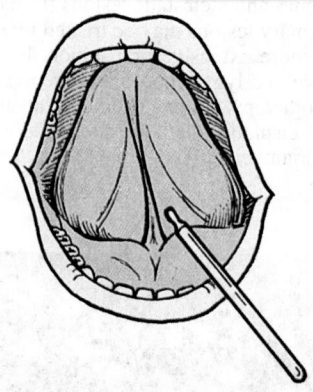

**Placement of thermometer for oral temperature measurement**
*(Potter and Perry, 1997)*

**oral tolerance therapy,** a treatment in which a patient ingests a foreign protein in an attempt to develop tolerance to that protein when it is encountered as an antigen. In addition to inhibiting allergic reactions, the therapy may suppress immune responses in general.

**Orap,** trademark for an oral neuroleptic drug (pimozide).

**ora serrata retinae,** the irregular, serrated anterior margin of the optic part of the retina, lying internal to the junction of the choroid and the ciliary body.

**orb** /ôrb/ [L, *orbis,* circle], describing something spheric or globelike.

**orbicular** /ôrbik′yələr/ [L, *orbiculus,* little circle], pertaining to something round.

**orbicular bone** [L, *orbiculus,* little circle; AS, *ban*], a knob on the end of the long process of the incus that articulates with the stapes.

**orbicularis ciliaris** /ôrbik′yo͞olär′is/ [L, *orbiculus,* little circle; *cilium,* eyelash], one of the two zones of the ciliary body of the eye, extending from the ora serrata of the retina to the ciliary processes at the margin of the iris. The orbicularis ciliaris is about 4 mm wide and increases in thickness as it approaches the ciliary processes.

**orbicularis oculi,** the muscular body of the eyelid encircling the eye and comprising the palpebral, orbital, and lacrimal muscles. It arises from the nasal part of the frontal bone, the frontal process of the maxilla in front of the lacrimal groove, and the anterior surface of the medial palpebral ligament. The palpebral muscle functions to close the eyelid gently; the orbital muscle functions to close it more energetically, such as in winking. Also called **orbicularis palpebrarum.** Compare **corrugator supercilii, levator palpebrae superioris.**

**orbicularis oris,** the muscle surrounding the mouth. It consists partly of fibers derived from other facial muscles such as the buccinator that are inserted into the lips and

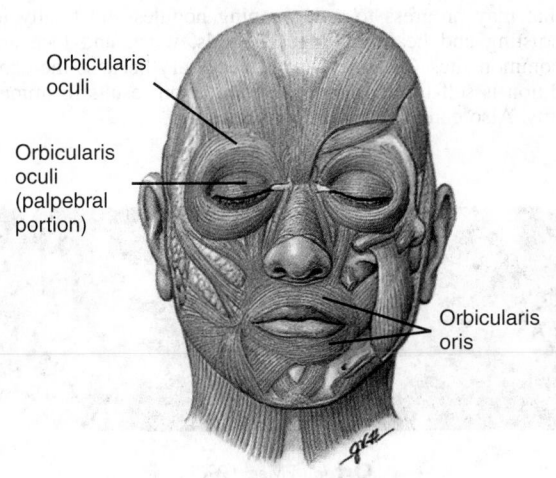

Orbicularis oculi

Orbicularis oculi (palpebral portion)

Orbicularis oris

**Muscles of the face: orbicularis oculi and orbicularis oris**
*(Thibodeau and Patton, 1999/John V. Hagen)*

partly of fibers proper to the lips. It serves to close and purse the lips.

**orbicularis palpebrarum.** See **orbicularis oculi.**

**orbicularis pupillary reflex,** a normal phenomenon elicited by forceful closure of the eyelids or attempting to close them while they are held apart, resulting first in constriction and then dilation of the pupil.

**orbit** /ôr′bit/ [L, *orbita,* wheel track], one of a pair of bony, conical cavities in the skull that accommodate the eyeballs and associated structures, such as the eye muscles, nerves, and blood vessels. The medial walls of the orbits are approximately parallel with each other and with the middle line, but the lateral walls diverge widely. The roof of each orbit is formed by the orbital plate of the frontal bone and the small wing of the sphenoid bones. The openings that communicate with each orbit are the optic foramen, the superior and the inferior orbital fissures, the supraorbital foramen, the infraorbital canal, the anterior and posterior ethmoidal foramina, the zygomatic foramen, and the canal for the nasolacrimal duct. —**orbital,** *adj.*

**orbital aperture** /ôr′bitəl/, an opening in the cranium to the orbit of the eye.

**orbitale** /ôrbitä′lē/ [L, *orbitalis,* pertaining to the orbit], an anthropometric landmark, the lowest point on the inferior margin of the orbit.

**orbital fat,** a semifluid adipose cushion that lines the bony orbit supporting the eye. Selective loss of fatty tissue caused by hormonal imbalances may produce "bulging" of the eye. Traumatic loss of the fat causes a sunken appearance of the eye. Replacement of the fat by tumor or abnormal tissue may be discovered on ophthalmologic examination. The examiner gently presses on the front of the eyes through the eyelids. Normally each eye may be displaced 0.5 cm into the socket.

**orbital fissure** [L, *orbita,* wheel track, *fissura,* cleft], the space between the floor and lateral wall of the orbit, serving as a conduit for nerves and blood vessels.

**orbital hypertelorism.** See **ocular hypertelorism.**

**orbital hypotelorism.** See **ocular hypotelorism.**

**orbital myositis,** an inflammation of the external ocular muscles. The process, which is generally autoimmune, may be associated with pain, forward displacement of the eyeball, and paralysis of the ocular muscles.

**orbital optic neuritis.** See **optic neuritis.**

**orbital pseudotumor,** a specific inflammatory reaction of the orbital tissues of the eye, characterized by exophthalmos and edematous congestion of the eyelids.

**orbitography** /ôr′bitog′rəfē/, the radiographic examination of the bony cavity containing the eye.

**orbitomeatal line** /ôr′bitō′mē·ā′təl/ [L, *orbita,* wheel track, *meatus,* passage], a positioning line used in radiography of the skull that passes through the outer canthus of the eye and the center of the external auditory meatus.

**orbitopathy** /or·bi·top′ə·thē/ [L, *orbita,* wheel track + Gk, *pathos,* disease], disease affecting the orbit and its contents.

*Orbivirus* /ôr′bivī′rəs/ [L, *orbis,* ring], a genus of the Reoviridae family of viruses that contain double-stranded ribonucleic acid. They are characterized by an outer layer of rings of capsomeres. Insects are hosts for orbiviruses. Colorado tick fever and African horse sickness are among infections caused by species of these viruses.

**orcheoplasty.** See **orchioplasty.**

**orchi-.** See **orchio-.**

**orchidectomy** /ôr′kidek′təmē/ [Gk, *orchis,* testis, *ektomē,* excision], surgical removal of one or both testes. It may be indicated for serious disease or injury to the testis or to control cancer of the prostate by removing a source of androgenic hormones. Also called **orchiectomy.**

**orchiditis.** See **orchitis.**

**orchido-.** See **orchio-.**

**orchidoplasty.** See **orchioplasty.**

**orchiectomy.** See **orchidectomy.**

**orchio-, orchi-, orchido-,** combining form meaning 'testes': *orchiocatabasis, orchiopathy, orchioscirrhus.*

**orchiopexy** /ôr′kē·ōpek′sē/ [Gk, *orchis* + *pexis,* fixation], an operation to mobilize an undescended testis, bring it into the scrotum, and attach it so that it will not retract.

**orchioplasty** /ôr′kē·ōplas′tē/ [Gk, *orchis,* testis, *plassein,* to mold], a surgical procedure involving a testis. Also called **orcheoplasty, orchidoplasty.**

**orchis.** See **testis.**

**orchitis** /ôrkī′tis/ [Gk, *orchis* + *itis,* inflammation], inflammation of one or both of the testes, characterized by swelling and pain. The condition is often caused by mumps, syphilis, or tuberculosis. Symptomatic treatment includes support and elevation of the scrotum, cold packs, and analgesics. Also called **orchiditis.** —**orchitic,** *adj.*

**orchitis parotidea.** See **mumps orchitis.**

**orciprenaline sulfate.** See **metaproterenol sulfate.**

**ordered pairs** [L, *ordo,* series, *par,* equal], pertaining to graph coordinates in which the first number of the pair represents a distance along the $x$ (horizontal) axis and the second number is plotted along the $y$ (vertical) axis.

**orderly** /ôr′dərlē/, **1.** an attendant who assists in the care of hospital patients. **2.** in order; with regular arrangements, method, or system.

**order of procedure,** the sequence in which the required steps are taken to complete an operation, such as preparation of the patient and preparation of the cavity and restoration of a tooth.

**order transcription,** a nursing intervention from the Nursing Interventions Classification (NIC) defined as transferring information from order sheets to the nursing patient care planning and documentation system. See also **Nursing Interventions Classification.**

**Orem, Dorthea E.,** author of the Self-Care Nursing Model, a nursing theory introduced in 1959. The Orem

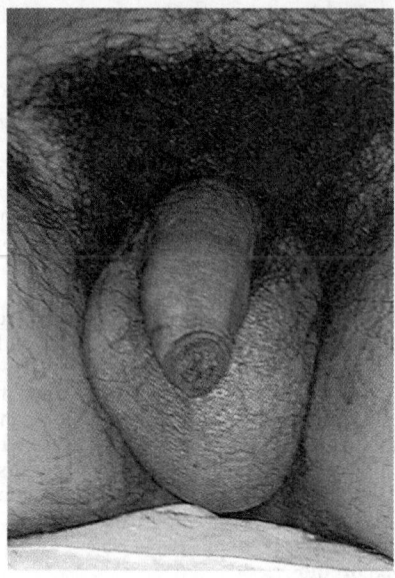

**Orchitis** *(Emond, Rowland, and Welsby, 1995)*

that may progress to red, weeping nodules and finally to crusting and healing. Fingers, hands, wrist, and face are common sites. Treatment is not necessary because the condition is self-limited, and active infection results in immunity. Also called **ecthyma contagiosum.**

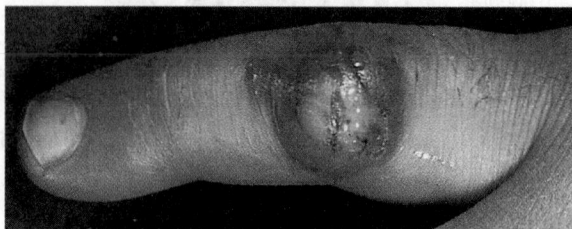

**Orf** *(du Vivier, 1993)*

theory describes the role of the nurse in helping a person experiencing inabilities in self-care. The goal of the Orem system is to meet the patient's self-care demands until the family and/or patient is capable of providing care. The process is divided into three categories: universal, which consists of self-care to meet physiologic and psychosocial needs; developmental, the self-care required when one goes through developmental stages; and health deviation, the self-care required when one has a deviation from a healthy status. Assessment is made of therapeutic self-care demand, the self-care agency, and self-care deficits in the areas of knowledge, skills, motivation, and orientation. There are three systems for meeting the patient's self-care deficits. They are wholly compensatory, in which the patient has no active role; partly compensatory, in which the patient and nurse have active roles, and educative development, in which patients can meet their need for self-care with some assistance from the nurse.

**Oretic,**   trademark for a diuretic (hydrochlorothiazide).

**Oreticyl,**   trademark for an antihypertensive, fixed-combination drug containing a diuretic (hydrochlorothiazide) and an antihypertensive (deserpidine).

**Oreton Methyl,**   trademark for an androgen (methyltestosterone).

**-orexia,**   combining form meaning '(condition of the) appetite': *cynorexia, dysorexia, anorexia.*

**orexigenic** /ôrek′sijen′ik/ [Gk, *orexis,* longing, *genein,* to produce],   a substance that increases or stimulates the appetite.

**oreximania** /ôrek′simā′nē·ə/ [Gk, *orexis* + *mania,* madness],   a condition characterized by a greatly increased appetite and excessive eating resulting from an unrealistic or exaggerated fear of becoming thin. Compare **anorexia nervosa.**

**orexis** /ôrek′sis/ [Gk, longing],   1. desire, appetite. 2. the aspect of the mind involving feeling and striving as contrasted with the intellectual aspect.

**orf** [AS],   a contagious viral skin disease acquired from infected sheep and goats, characterized by painless vesicles

**organ** [Gk, *organon,* instrument],   a structural part of a system of the body that is composed of tissues and cells that enable it to perform a particular function, such as the liver, spleen, digestive organs, reproductive organs, or organs of special sense. Each one of the paired organs can function independently of the other. The liver, pancreas, spleen, and brain may maintain normal or near normal function with over 30% of the organ damaged, destroyed, or excised. Also called **organon, organum.**

**organ albumin,**   albumin characteristic of a particular organ.

**organelle** /ôrgənel′/ [Gk, *organon,* instrument],   1. any one of various specialized macromolecular structures bound within most cells, such as the mitochondria, the Golgi apparatus, the endoplastic reticulum, the lysosomes, and the centrioles. 2. any one of the tiny structures of protozoa associated with locomotion, metabolism, and other processes. Also called **organella.**

**organic** /ôrgan′ik/ [Gk, *organikos*],   1. any chemical compound containing carbon other than simple metal carbonate, hydrogen carbonate, or cyanides. Compare **inorganic.** 2. pertaining to an organ.

**-organic,**   combining form meaning 'related to the internal organs of the body': *enorganic, homorganic, psychorganic.*

**organic brain syndrome.**   See **organic mental disorder.**

**organic chemistry,**   the branch of chemistry concerned with the composition, properties, and reactions of chemical compounds containing carbon.

**organic disease** [Gk, *organikos* + L, *dis* + Fr, *aise,* ease],   any disease associated with detectable or observable changes in one or more body organs.

**organic dust,**   dried particles of plants, animals, fungi, or bacteria that are fine enough to be windborne. Many kinds of organic dust cause various respiratory disorders if inhaled. See also **asthma, bagassosis, byssinosis, hay fever.**

**organic dust toxic syndrome (ODTS),**   any nonallergic, noninfectious respiratory illness caused by inhalation of organic dust, as from moldy silage, hay, or other agricultural products. Symptoms include shaking chills or sweats, cough or shortness of breath, headache, anorexia, and myalgia. See also **farmer's lung, hypersensitivity pneumonitis.**

**organic evolution,**   the theory that all existing forms of animal and plant life have descended with modification from previous simpler forms or from a single cell; the origin and perpetuation of species.

**organic foods,** foods that have been produced and processed without the use of commercial chemicals such as fertilizers or pesticides or synthetic substances that enhance color or flavor.

**organic headache,** a headache caused by any of a wide variety of intracranial disorders, including sinus or ear infections, brain tumors, and subdural hematomas. See also **headache.**

**organic mental disorders (OMD),** a DSM-IV class of psychiatric disorders characterized by progressive deterioration of the mental processes and caused by permanent brain damage or temporary brain dysfunction.

**organic mental syndrome,** former term for a constellation of psychological or behavioral signs and symptoms associated with brain dysfunction of unknown or unspecified cause and grouped according to symptoms. Designating certain conditions as having an organic basis, possibly implying that others do not, is currently discouraged. Compare **organic mental disorders.**

**organic mood syndrome,** a term used in a former system of classification, denoting an organic mental syndrome characterized by the presence of manic or depressive mood disturbance caused by a specific organic factor and not associated with delirium. Such disorders are now mainly classified as *substance-induced mood disorders* and *mood disorders due to a general medical condition.* See also **organic mental syndrome.**

**organic motivation.** See **physiologic motivation.**

**organic murmur,** an abnormal cardiac sound caused by a congenital or acquired heart disease.

**organic personality syndrome,** a term used in a former system of classification, denoting an organic mental syndrome characterized by a marked change in behavior or personality, caused by a specific organic factor and not associated with delirium or dementia. The most common causes are space-occupying lesions of the brain, head trauma, and cerebrovascular disease. See also **organic mental syndrome.**

**organic psychosis** [Gk, *organikos + psyche,* mind, *osis,* condition], a condition characterized by a loss of contact with reality caused by an alteration in brain tissue function.

**organic vertigo** [Gk, *organikos* + L, *vertigo,* dizziness], vertigo that is associated with a central nervous system disorder such as cerebellar lesions or tabes dorsalis.

**organification** /ôrˈganˈifikāˈshən/, a process in the thyroid gland whereby iodide is oxidized and incorporated into tyrosyl residues (tyrosine) of thyroglobulin. Organification is catalyzed by the enzyme thyroid peroxidase.

**Organisation Mondiale de la Santé.** See **World Health Organization.**

**organism** /ôrˈgənizˈəm/ [Gk, *organon,* instrument], an entity capable of carrying on life functions. All organisms are composed of cells.

**organization center** /ôrˈgənizāˈshən/ [Gk, *organon + izein,* to cause], a focal point within the developing embryo from which the organism grows and differentiates. In vertebrates this point is the chorda-mesoderm of the dorsal lip of the blastopore.

**organizer** /ôrˈgənīˈzər/ [Gk, *organon + izein,* to cause], (in embryology) any part of the embryo that induces morphologic differentiation in some other part. Those parts that are formed and in turn give rise to other parts are classified as organizers of the second degree, third degree, and so on as the embryo develops in complexity. Kinds of organizers include **nucleolar organizer, primary organizer.**

**organo-** /ôrˈgənō-/, combining form meaning 'organ or organs': *organofaction, organogenesis, organoleptic.*

**organocarbamate insecticide poisoning** /-kärˈbəmāt/, an adverse reaction to pesticides derived from esters of carbonic acid. Some of those insecticides are formulated in methyl alcohol, acquiring its added toxicity. The effects are similar to those of organophosphate insecticides, but the toxicity is less, and the duration of effects is shorter. The organocarbamate insecticides rarely produce overt central nervous system effects. See also **organophosphate insecticide poisoning.**

**organochlorine insecticide poisoning** /-klôrˈēn/, an adverse reaction to DDT-like pesticides such as chlordane and methoxychlor. Symptoms include central nervous system disorders, convulsions, increased myocardial irritability, and depressed respiration.

**organ of Corti** [Gk, *organon;* Alfonso Corti, Italian anatomist, 1822–1888], the true organ of hearing, a spiral structure within the cochlea containing hair cells that are stimulated by sound vibrations. The hair cells convert the vibrations into nerve impulses that are transmitted by the cochlear part of the vestibulocochlear nerve to the brain. Also called **spiral organ of Corti.** See also **basilar membrane.**

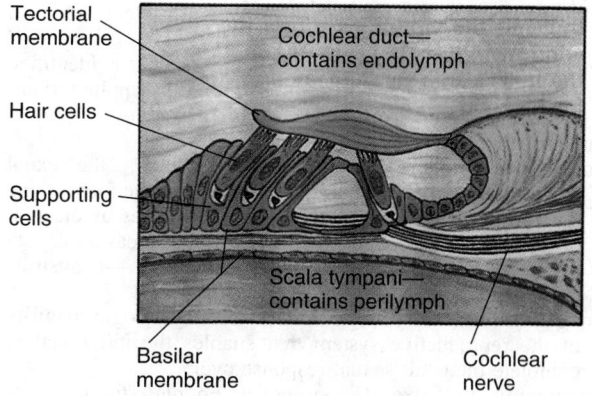

**Organ of Corti** *(Applegate, 2000)*

**organ of Giraldès.** See **paradidymis.**

**organ of Golgi.** See **neurotendinous spindle.**

**organogenesis** /-jenˈəsis/ [Gk, *organon + genesis,* origin], (in embryology) the formation and differentiation of organs and organ systems during embryonic development. In humans the period extends from approximately the end of the second week through the eighth week of gestation. During this time the embryo undergoes rapid growth and differentiation and is extremely vulnerable to environmental hazards and toxic substances. Any interference with the sequential processes involved with organogenesis causes an arrest in development and results in one or more congenital anomalies. Also called **organogeny.** See also **embryologic development, prenatal development. —organogenetic,** *adj.*

**organoid** /ôrˈgənoid/ [Gk, *organon + eidos,* form], **1.** resembling an organ. **2.** any structure that resembles an organ in appearance or function, specifically an abnormal tumor mass. See also **organelle.**

**organoid neoplasm,** a growth that resembles a body organ. Compare **heterologous tumor.**

**organoid tumor.** See **teratoma.**

**organomegaly** /-meg′əlē/ [Gk, *organon*, instrument, *megas*, large],   abnormal enlargement of an organ, particularly an organ of the abdominal cavity.

**organon.**   See **organ.**

**organophosphate insecticide poisoning** /-fos′fāt/,   an adverse reaction to organophosphate pesticides such as malathion, chlorothion, and nerve gas agents. Symptoms include nausea, vomiting, abdominal cramping, headache, blurred vision, and excessive salivation.

**organophosphates,**   a class of anticholinesterase chemicals used in certain pesticides and medications. They act by causing irreversible inhibition of cholinesterase.

**organotherapy** /-ther′əpē/ [Gk, *organon* + *therapeia*, treatment],   the treatment of disease by administering animal endocrine glands or their extracts. Whole glands are no longer implanted, but substances derived from animal organs are widely used. Also called **Brown-Séquard's treatment.** —**organotherapeutic,** *adj.*

**organotypic growth** /ôr′gənōtip′ik/ [Gk, *organon* + *typos*, mark],   the controlled reproduction of cells, such as occurs in the normal growth of tissues and organs. Compare **histiotypic growth.**

**organ procurement,**   a nursing intervention from the Nursing Interventions Classification (NIC) defined as guiding families through the donation process to ensure timely retrieval of vital organs and tissue for transplant. See also **Nursing Interventions Classification.**

**organ specificity,**   a substance or activity that is identified with a specific organ. The term is commonly applied to enzymes that function in particular organ systems.

**organum.**   See **organ.**

**orgasm** /ôr′gasəm/ [Gk, *orgein*, to be lustful],   the sexual climax, a series of strong involuntary contractions of the muscles of the genitalia, accompanied in males by ejaculation of semen, experienced as exceedingly pleasurable, set off by sexual excitation of critical intensity. —**orgasmic,** *adj.*

**orgasmic maturity** /ôrgas′mik/,   the physiologic maturity of the reproductive system that enables the individual to complete the adult sexual response cycle.

**orgasmic platform** [Gk, *orgein* + Fr, *plate-forme*, a flat form],   congestion of the lower vagina during sexual intercourse.

**orient** /ôr′ē·ənt/ [L, *oriens*, rising sun],   **1.** to make someone aware of new surroundings, including people and their roles; the layout of a facility; and its routines, rules, and services. New patients are oriented to a hospital as are new staff to a hospital unit. **2.** to help a person become aware of a situation or simply of reality, such as when a patient recovers from anesthesia. —**orientation,** *n.,* **oriented,** *adj.*

**oriental sore** /ôr′ē·en′təl/ [L, *oriens* + AS, *sar,* painful],   a dermatologic disease caused by the parasite *Leishmania tropica,* transmitted to humans by the bite of the sand fly. This form of leishmaniasis, characterized by ulcerative lesions, occurs primarily in Africa, Asia, and some Mediterranean countries. Oriental sore causes no systemic symptoms, but the sores are susceptible to secondary infections. Treatment options include infrared therapy and injection of ulcers with sodium antimony gluconate. Also called **Aleppo boil, cutaneous leishmaniasis, Delhi boil, Old World leishmaniasis, tropical sore.** See also **leishmaniasis.**

**orientation** /ôr′ē·əntā′shən/ [L, *oriens* + *itio,* process],   **1.** the direction of a fragment of nucleic acid inserted into a vector. The orientation of the fragment may be the same as that of the genetic map of the vector (the n orientation) or opposite (the u orientation). **2.** the awareness of one's physical environment with regard to time, place, and the identity of other people; the ability to adapt to such an exist-

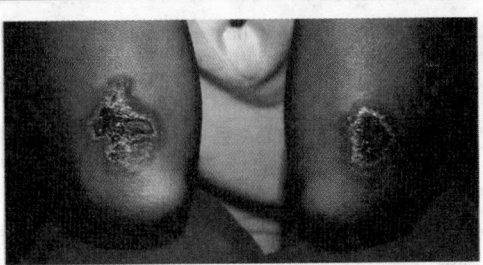

**Oriental sore** *(Auerbach, 1995/courtesy Richard Kaplan, MD)*

ing or new environment. Disorientation is usually a symptom of organic brain disease and most psychoses.

**oriented.**   See **orient.**

***Orientia tsutsugamushi*** /ôr′e·enshe′ə tso͞ots o͞og əmo͞o′she/ [L, *oriens,* east; Jpn, *tsutsuga,* illness + *mushi,* tick],   a species of organisms, formerly known as *Rickettsia tsutsugamushi,* that causes scrub typhus. It is widespread throughout southern and eastern Asia, northern Australia, Indonesia, and the Pacific islands and is transmitted from infected rodents to humans by mites of the family Trombiculidae.

**orifice** /ôr′ifis/ [L, *orificium,* opening],   the entrance or outlet of any body cavity. Also called **ostium.** —**orificial,** *adj.*

**ori gene** /ôr′ē/,   (in molecular genetics) the site or region in which deoxyribonucleic acid replication starts.

**origin** /ôr′ijin/ [L, *origo,* source],   the more fixed or most proximal attachment of two points of a muscle. Compare **insertion.**

**Orimune,**   trademark for an active immunizing agent (live oral poliovirus vaccine).

**Orinase,**   trademark for an oral sulfonylurea antidiabetic (tolbutamide).

**Orlando (Pelletier), Ida Jean,**   a nursing theorist who first described her nursing process theory in *The Dynamic Nurse-Patient Relationship* (1972). Her theory stresses the reciprocal relationship between the nurse and patient. She used the nursing process to meet the patient's need and thus alleviate distress. Three elements—patient behavior, nurse reaction, and nursing actions—comprise a nursing situation. Orlando divided actions into those that are either automatic or deliberate. Perceptions, thoughts, and feelings are not explored in automatic actions. Deliberate actions are those that may yield solutions to problems and also prevent problems. She focuses on the patient's verbal and nonverbal expressions of needs. The nurse reacts to the patient's behavior by discerning both the meaning of the distress and what would alleviate the distress. Her contribution as a theorist has advanced nursing from personal and automatic responses to disciplined and professional practice responses.

**orlistat,**   a lipase inhibitor.

■ INDICATIONS: Orlistat is used to manage obesity.

■ CONTRAINDICATIONS: Malabsorption syndrome, cholestasis, and known hypersensitivity to this drug prohibit its use.

■ ADVERSE EFFECTS: This drug's adverse effects include back pain, arthritis, myalgia, tendinitis, depression, anxiety, dizziness, headache, fatigue, nausea, vomiting, abdominal pain, infectious diarrhea, rectal pain, tooth disorder, urinary tract infection, vaginitis, menstrual irregularity, influenza, upper respiratory infection, eye-ear-nose-throat symptoms, dry skin, and rash. Common side effects include insomnia, oily spotting, flatus with discharge, fecal urgency, fatty/oily stool, oily evacuation, and fecal incontinence.

**Ornade,** trademark for a fixed-combination drug containing an adrenergic decongestant (phenylpropanolamine hydrochloride), antihistamine (chlorpheniramine maleate), and anticholinergic (isopropamide iodide).

**ornithine** /ôr′nithēn/, an amino acid, not a constituent of proteins, that is produced as an important intermediate substance in the urea cycle. It is formed by the hydrolization of arginine by arginase and is subsequently converted into citrulline. It decomposes by losing carbon dioxide, producing putrescine and a strong foul odor characteristic of decaying animal tissue. Also called **diaminovaleric acid.**

**ornithine carbamoyltransferase,** an enzyme in the blood that increases in patients with liver and other diseases. Its normal concentrations in serum are 8 to 20 mIU/ml. Also called ornithine transcarbomoylase.

**ornithine carbamoyltransferase (OCT) deficiency,** an X-linked aminoacidopathy involving the biosynthesis of urea; most hemizygous males show complete deficiency and do not survive the neonatal period; heterozygous females show varying degrees of deficiency and age of onset. Characteristic signs include hyperammonemia, neurologic abnormalities, and orotic aciduria.

**ornithine cycle.** See **urea cycle.**

**ornithine transcarbamylase.** See **ornithine carbamoyltransferase.**

***Ornithodoros*** /ôr′nithod′ərəs/ [Gk, *ornis,* bird, *doros,* leather bag], a genus of ticks, some species of which are vectors for the spirochetes of relapsing fevers.

**ornithosis.** See **psittacosis.**

**oro-,** combining form meaning 'mouth': *orolingual, oromaxillary, oropharynx.*

**orodigitofacial dysostosis.** See **oral-facial-digital syndrome, types I, II, III.**

**orofacial** /ôr′ōfā′shəl/ [L, *os, oris,* mouth, *facies,* face], pertaining to the mouth and face.

**orofaciodigital syndrome.** See **oral-facial-digital syndrome, types I, II, III.**

**oropharyngeal dysphasia** /ôr′ōfərin′jē·əl/, a difficulty in initiating a swallow, caused by a neuromuscular disorder of the hypopharynx.

**oropharynx** /ôr′ōfer′ingks/ [L, *oris,* mouth; Gk, *pharynx,* throat], one of the three anatomic divisions of the pharynx that lies posterior to the mouth and is continuous above with the nasopharynx and below with the laryngopharynx. It extends behind the mouth from the soft palate above to the level of the hyoid bone below and contains the palatine and lingual tonsils. Compare **laryngopharynx, nasopharynx. —oropharyngeal,** *adj.*

**orotic acid** /ôrot′ik/, a pyrimidine synthesized in the cell from carboxyl phosphate and aspartic acid via condensation, dehydration, and oxidation.

**orotic aciduria,** a rare autosomal recessive inherited disorder of pyrimidine metabolism. It includes signs and symptoms of macrocytic hypochromic anemia with megaloblastic changes in bone marrow, leukopenia, retarded growth, and urinary excretion of large amounts of orotic acid.

**Oroya fever.** See **bartonellosis.**

**-orphan,** combining form for morphinan-derived opioid agonists or antagonists.

**orphan disease** /ôr′fən/, any rare health disorder for which no treatment has been developed. See also **orphan drug.**

**orphan drug** /ôr′fən/ [Gk, *orphanos,* without parents; ME, *drogge*], any pharmaceutical product that may be available to physicians and patients in countries other than the United States but that has not been 'adopted' by a domestic pharmaceutical manufacturer or distributor. An orphan drug may not be available in the United States because total sales would not justify the expense of research and development, the product may not have been approved by the Bureau of Drugs of the Food and Drug Administration, or the medication may be a natural substance that cannot be effectively protected by patent laws against competition from a similar form of the product. Many orphan drugs are pharmaceutical products developed in Europe or Asia but not available in the United States until several years later. The U.S. Orphan Drug Act of 1983 offers federal financial incentives to commercial and nonprofit organizations to develop and market drugs previously unavailable in the United States.

**orphan virus** [Gk, *orphanos,* without parents; L, *virus,* poison], a virus that has been isolated and identified although it has not been associated with any particular disease.

**orphenadrine citrate** /ôrfen′ədrēn/, a skeletal muscle relaxant with anticholinergic and antihistaminic activity.

■ INDICATION: It is prescribed in the treatment of severe muscle strain.

■ CONTRAINDICATIONS: Myasthenia gravis, contraindications of anticholinergic agents, or known hypersensitivity to this drug prohibits its use.

■ ADVERSE EFFECTS: Among the most serious adverse reactions are those associated with anticholinergic activity, such as dry mouth and tachycardia, and allergic reactions.

**-orrhagia, -rrhagia, -rrhage,** suffix meaning 'excessive flow': *metrorrhagia, hemorrhage.*

**-orrhea, -rrhea,** suffix meaning 'flow or discharge': *rhinorrhea, galactorrhea.*

**-orrhexis, -rrhexis,** suffix meaning 'to rupture': *angiorrhexis, enterorrexis.*

**orrho-, oro-,** combining form meaning 'blood serum': *orrhomeningitis, orrhoreaction, orrhorrhea.*

**ORS,** abbreviation for **oral rehydration solutions.**

**ORT,** abbreviation for **oral rehydration therapy.**

**orthetist.** See **orthotist.**

**ortho,** abbreviation for *orthopedic.*

**ortho-** /ôr′thə-/, combining form meaning 'straight, normal, correct': *orthobiosis, orthodontist, orthotopic.*

**orthoboric acid.** See **boric acid.**

**orthochromatic** /or′thō-krō-mat′ik/, denoting a photographic emulsion sensitive to all colors except red.

**orthoclase ceramic feldspar** /ôr′thəklās/ [Gk, *orthos,* straight, *klassis,* breaking, *keramikos,* pottery], a plentiful clay in the solid crust of the earth, used as to fill space and give body to fused dental porcelain. Compare **feldspar.**

**Orthoclone OKT3,** trademark for an immunosuppressant drug (muromonab-CD3).

**orthodontic appliance** /-don′tik/ [Gk, *orthos* + *odous,* tooth], any device used to modify tooth position. Kinds of such appliances are **extraoral, fixed, intraoral,** and **retaining.**

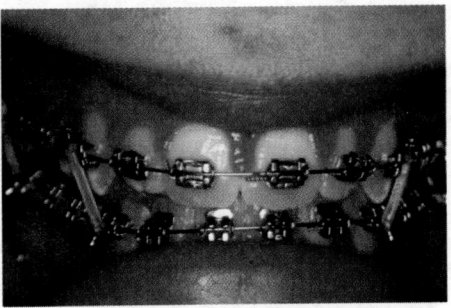

**Fixed orthodontic appliance** *(Proffit, 2000)*

**orthodontic attachment, orthodontic bracket.** See **bracket.**

**orthodontic band,** a thin metal ring, usually made of stainless steel, that is fitted over a tooth and bonded or cemented to it, for securing orthodontic attachments to the tooth.

**orthodontics and dentofacial orthopedics** /ôr′thədon′-tiks/ [Gk, *orthos* + *odous,* tooth], the specialty of dentistry concerned with the diagnosis and treatment of malocclusion and irregularities of the teeth.

**orthodontic wire.** See **arch wire.**

**orthodontist** /-don′tist/, a dentist who is concerned with the diagnosis, prevention, and correction of malocclusion of the teeth.

**orthodromic conduction** /ôr′thədrom′ik/ [Gk, *orthos* + *dromos,* course; L, *conducere,* to connect], the conduction of a neural impulse in the normal direction, from a synaptic junction or a receptor forward along an axon to its termination with depolarization. Compare **antidromic conduction.**

**orthogenesis** /ôr′thəjen′əsis/ [Gk, *orthos* + *genesis,* origin], the theory that evolution is controlled by intrinsic factors within the organism and progresses according to a predetermined course rather than in several directions as a result of natural selection and other environmental factors. —**orthogenetic,** *adj.*

**orthogenic** /-jen′ik/ [Gk, *orthos* + *genein,* to produce], **1.** pertaining to orthogenesis; orthogenetic. **2.** pertaining to the treatment and rehabilitation of children who are mentally or emotionally disturbed. See also **orthopsychiatry.**

**orthogenic evolution,** change within an animal or plant induced solely by an intrinsic factor, independent of any environmental elements. Also called **bathmic evolution.**

**orthokinetic cuff** /-kinet′ik/ [Gk, *orthos,* straight, *kinesis,* movement; ME, *cuffe*], an elastic covering for a muscle that provides tactile stimulation sufficient to induce contraction and that restricts contraction of an opposing muscle.

**orthokinetics** /-kinet′iks/ [Gk, *orthos,* straight, *kinesis,* movement], **1.** therapy for hypertrophic osteoarthritis in which an effort is made to change muscular action from one group to another to protect a joint. **2.** a therapy for spasticity that uses an orthotic device to enable contraction of one muscle while inhibiting its antagonist. **3.** the movement of microscopic particles in the same direction during sedimentation as a result of the effect of gravity on brownian motion.

**orthologous genes** /ôrthol′əgəs/, genes in different species that are similar in their nucleotide sequences, suggesting they originated from a common ancestral gene.

**orthomyxovirus** /ôr′thəmik′sōvī′rəs/ [Gk, *orthos* + *mykes,* fungus; L, *virus,* poison], a member of a family of viruses that includes several organisms responsible for human influenza infection.

**Ortho-Novum,** trademark for an oral contraceptive containing an estrogen (ethinyl estradiol) and a progestin (norethindrone).

**orthopaedics.** See **orthopedics.**

**orthopantogram** /ôr′thəpan′təgram/ [Gk, *orthos* + *pan,* all, *gramma,* record], a radiograph that is taken extraorally and shows a panoramic view of the entire dentition, alveolar bone, and other adjacent structures on a single film.

**orthopedic nurse** /-pē′dik/ [Gk, *orthos* + *pais,* child], a nurse whose primary area of interest, competence, and professional practice is the branch of nursing concerned with the prevention and correction of disorders of the locomotor system, including the skeleton, muscles, joints, and related tissues.

**orthopedic oxford,** a hard leather shoe with a leather or rubber sole, sometimes with a steel shank between the floor of the shoe and the sole, and with firmly constructed sides that support the foot in an upright position. The shoe is constructed so that assistive devices can be added. It is used to relieve pain and improve function in foot disabilities.

**orthopedics** /-pē′diks/ [Gk, *orthos,* straight, *pais,* child], a branch of health care that is concerned with the prevention and correction of disorders of the musculoskeletal system of the body. Also spelled **orthopaedics.**

**orthopedic surgery** [Gk, *orthos,* straight, *pais,* child, *cheirourgia,* surgery], the branch of medicine that is concerned with the treatment of the musculoskeletal system mainly by manipulative and operative methods.

**orthopedic traction,** a procedure in which a patient is maintained in a device attached by ropes and pulleys to weights that pull on an extremity or body part while countertraction is maintained. Traction is applied most often to reduce and immobilize fractures, but it also is used to overcome muscle spasm, stretch adhesions, correct certain deformities, and help release arthritic contractures. Traction may be applied directly to the skin if the rope-pulley-weight system is attached to bands of adhesive, moleskin, or foam rubber or to a splint affixed to the affected limb. For example, side arm traction is a kind of skin traction used to align a fractured humerus after open reduction. Skeletal traction is exerted directly on a bone by means of a wire or pin inserted under anesthesia during the open reduction of a fracture; the ends of the pin protruding through the skin on both sides of the bone are covered with corks and attached to a metal U-shaped spreader or bow, which in turn is attached to the traction rope. Skin or skeletal traction applied to a lower extremity by a balanced suspension apparatus, such as the Thomas splint and Pearson's attachment, permits the patient to move more freely in bed; the leg is balanced with countertraction, and any slack in traction caused by the patient's movements is taken up by the suspension apparatus. Bryant's traction, for treating fractures of the femur shaft in young children, uses a suspension apparatus to hold the legs at right angles to the body. A girdle that fits over the iliac crests and pelvis is used to apply traction for the relief of low back pain, and a cervical halter is used in applying traction to reduce neck pain. Cervical traction also may be used when a fracture of the cervical spine is suspected. See other specific devices and kinds of traction.

■ METHOD: To maintain the required constant pull, the traction ropes are kept taut, free to ride over the pulleys, and securely tied to the weights, which must hang free—away from the bed and off the floor. Countertraction is maintained by elevating the patient's bed under the body part to which traction is applied; a chest restraint sheet may be applied to the patient in side arm traction for countertraction if necessary. During the initial stages of traction, the involved extremity is checked every 2 hours for quality of the distal pulse, color, warmth, motion, sensation, pain, and swelling. Blood pressure, temperature, pulse, and respirations are recorded every 4 hours until stable. Pain is controlled, and the patient is positioned as ordered. If the patient is in balanced suspension, abduction of the leg and a 20-degree angle between the thigh and bed are maintained; the heel is kept free of the sling under the calf. A harness restraint is used to prevent a child in Bryant's traction from turning over, and the child's buttocks are raised slightly from the mattress. Bed linen is changed only as necessary, and an air mattress is used when required. Every 2 hours the patient is helped with deep breathing and coughing exercises; bony prominences are massaged, but vigorous rubbing is avoided. Lotion is applied to the skin, which is periodically inspected for signs of redness, abrasions, blisters, dryness, itching, excoriation, and pressure areas; for patients in skeletal traction, the pin insertion sites are inspected for signs of infection. The patient is observed every 4 hours for neurologic signs, such as tingling, numbness, and loss of sensation or motion; for thrombophlebitis in the involved extremity; and for evidence of a pulmonary blood clot or fat embolus, as indicated by decreased breath sounds, fever, tachypnea, diaphoresis, anxiety, pallor, bloody or purulent sputum, tachycardia, or acute, severe chest pain. Oral hygiene is administered every 4 hours, and, unless contraindicated, a daily intake of 2 to 3 L of fluids is encouraged. As the patient's condition improves, his or her position is changed every 4 hours; if the kind of traction permits and if the upper extremities are not involved, a trapeze is added to the bed. The patient is taught to perform range-of-motion exercises with the uninvolved extremities, dorsiflexion and plantar flexion of the ankles, and isometric exercises, such as gluteal and abdominal contraction. A high-protein, low-carbohydrate diet is served, and vitamin and iron therapy may be ordered. The immobilized patient uses a flat, fracture bedpan and usually requires stool softeners or a mild laxative.

■ INTERVENTIONS: The patient in traction often needs extensive physical care and emotional support. The patient is encouraged to verbalize feelings and concerns about prolonged hospitalization and absence from work or school. To the greatest degree possible, the nurse encourages the patient to participate in self-care and to engage in diversions, such as handicrafts, reading, watching television, and listening to the radio.

■ OUTCOME CRITERIA: The healthy young adult or adolescent in traction for the treatment of a fracture usually has an uneventful recovery, but diligent attention and nursing care are necessary to prevent pressure ulcers, infection, constipation, kidney stones, and other sequelae of immobility.

**orthopedist** /-pē′dist/, a physician who specializes in orthopedics. Also called **orthopod** *(informal).*

**orthophosphate** /-fos′fāt/, a salt of orthophosphoric acid, used in the treatment of kidney disease patients with the complication of hypophosphatemia resulting from a renal phosphate leak.

**orthopnea** /ôrthop′nē·ə/ [Gk, *orthos* + *pnoia*, breath], an abnormal condition in which a person must sit or stand to breathe deeply or comfortably. It occurs in many disorders of the cardiac and respiratory systems, such as asthma, pulmonary edema, emphysema, pneumonia, and angina pectoris. See also **dyspnea. —orthopneic,** *adj.* Also spelled **orthopnoea.**

**orthopneic position** /ôr′thopnē′ik/ [Gk, *orthos*, straight; *pnoia*, breath; L, *positio*], a body position that enables a patient to breathe comfortably. Usually it is one in which the patient is sitting up and bent forward with the arms supported on a table or chair arms. Also called **orthopnea posture.**

**orthopod.** See **orthopedist.**

**orthopsychiatry** /-sīkī′ətrē/ [Gk, *orthos* + *psyche*, mind, *iatreia*, treatment], the branch of psychiatry that specializes in correcting incipient and borderline mental and behavioral disorders, especially in children, and in developing preventive techniques to promote mental health and emotional growth and development. It involves a collaborative approach from psychology, psychiatry, and psychiatric social work. See also **mental hygiene.**

**orthoptic** /ôrthop′tik/ [Gk, *orthos* + *ops*, eye], **1.** pertaining to normal binocular vision. **2.** pertaining to a procedure or technique for correcting the visual axes of eyes improperly coordinated for binocular vision.

**orthoptic examination,** an ophthalmoscopic examination of the binocular function of the eyes. A stereoscopic instrument presents a slightly different picture to each eye. The examiner notes the degree to which the pictures are combined by the normal process of fusion. If the person has diplopia, separate pictures are seen. If the person has suppression amblyopia, only one picture is seen. Stereoscopic training may improve binocular vision in some conditions.

**orthoptic training** [Gk, *orthos,* straight; *ops,* eye; ME, *trainen*], a type of therapy for correction of squint or other ocular muscle disorders by the use of eye exercises.

**orthoptist** /ôrthop′tist/ [Gk, *orthos* + *ops,* eye], a person qualified by postsecondary training and successful completion of an examination by the American Orthoptist Council who, under the supervision of an ophthalmologist, tests eye muscles and teaches exercise programs designed to correct eye coordination defects.

**orthoroentgenography** /ôr′thō·rent′gənog′rəfē/ a radiographic method for measuring disparity of limb length. Three separate radiographs are made of the hip, knee, and ankle (for the leg) or the shoulder, elbow, and wrist (for the arm) to produce an image of the whole limb.

**orthoscopy** /ôrthos′kəpē/ [Gk, *orthos,* straight, *skopein,* to view], the use of an **orthoscope** /ôr′thəskōp′/ for examining the fundus of the eye.

**orthosis** /ôrthō′sis/ [Gk, *orthos,* straight], a force system designed to control, correct, or compensate for a bone deformity, deforming forces, or forces absent from the body. Orthosis often involves the use of special braces. **—orthotic,** *adj., n.*

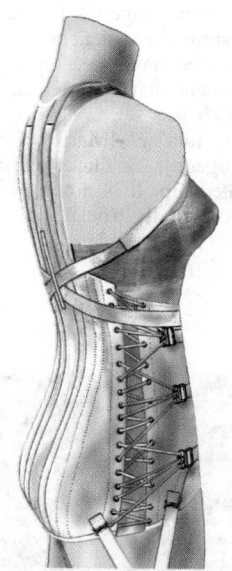

**Dorsolumbar orthosis**
*(Ignatavicius, Workman, and Mishler, 1999/courtesy Truform Orthotics and Prosthetics, Cincinnati, Ohio)*

**orthostasis** /-stā′sis/, maintenance of an upright standing posture. In some medical tests a patient may need to maintain orthostasis for a long period to stimulate a rise in aldosterone concentration.

**orthostatic** /-stat'ik/ [Gk, *orthos* + *statikos,* standing], pertaining to an erect or standing position.

**orthostatic albuminuria.** See **orthostatic proteinuria.**

**orthostatic hypotension,** abnormally low blood pressure that occurs when an individual suddenly assumes the standing posture. It can produce dizziness and fainting. Also called **postural hypotension.**

**orthostatic proteinuria,** presence of protein in the urine, especially in teenagers who have been standing for a long period. It disappears when they recline and is of no pathologic significance. Also called **orthostatic albuminuria, postural albuminuria, postural proteinuria.**

**orthotic** /ôrthot'ik/ [Gk, *orthos,* straight], pertaining to **orthosis.**

**orthotics** /ôrthot'iks/ [Gk, *orthos,* straight], the design and use of external appliances to support a paralyzed muscle, promote a specific motion, or correct a musculoskeletal deformity.

**orthotist** /ôr'thətist/ [Gk, *orthos,* straight], a person who designs, fabricates, and fits braces or other orthopedic appliances prescribed by physicians. A certified orthotist is one who passed the examination of the American Orthotist and Prosthetic Association. Also spelled **orthetist.**

**orthotonos** /ôrthot'ənəs/ [Gk, *orthos* + *tonos,* tension], a straight, rigid posture of the body caused by a tetanic spasm, resulting from strychnine poisoning or tetanus infection. The neck and all other parts of the body are in a position of extension but not as severely as in opisthotonos. Compare **emprosthotonos.**

**orthotopic liver transplantation** [Gk, *ortho,* straight, *topos,* place], a graft of liver tissue occurring at its natural place or on the proper part of the body.

**orthovoltage** /-vōl'tij/ [Gk, *orthos,* straight; Count Alessandro Volta], the energy range of 100 to 350 kiloelectron volts supplied by some x-ray generators used for radiation therapy. Such generators have been replaced in many health facilities by equipment that operates in the megaelectron volt range. See also **volt.**

**Ortolani's sign** /ôr'tərlä'nē/ [Marius Ortolani, twentieth-century Italian surgeon], a click heard in a test for a congenital dislocated hip. It is noted in infancy when the hip slips into or out of the socket. Also called **Ortolani click.**

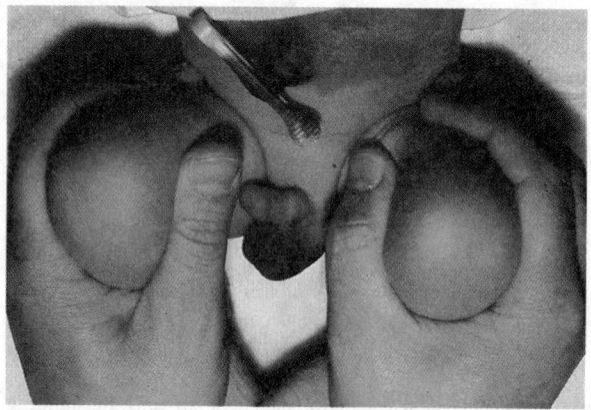

**Ortolani's test** *(Zitelli and Davis, 1997)*

**Ortolani's test** [Marius Ortolani; L, *testum,* crucible], a procedure used to evaluate the stability of the hip joints in newborns and infants. The baby is placed on his back, and the hips and knees are flexed at right angles and abducted until the lateral aspects of the knees are touching the table. The examiner's fingers are extended along the outside of the thighs, with the thumbs grasping the insides of the knees. Internal and external rotation are attempted, and symmetry of mobility is evaluated. A click or a popping sensation (Ortolani's sign) may be felt if the joint is unstable, because the head of the femur moves out of the acetabulum under pressure from the examiner's hands during rotation and abduction. See also **congenital dislocation of the hip.**

**Orudis,** trademark for a nonsteroidal antiinflammatory agent (ketoprofen).

**-ory,** suffix meaning 'pertaining to, function of, process of': *sensory.*

**os.** See **bone.**

**Os,** symbol for the element **osmium.**

**OS,** 1. abbreviation for *oculus sinister,* a Latin phrase meaning 'left eye.' 2. abbreviation for a computer **operating system.**

**-os,** suffix signaling singular nouns: *biologos, hepatomphalos, megophthalmos.*

**Osborne and Cotterill procedure,** the surgical correction of a chronic dislocated elbow by means of capsular reefing, the folding in or overlapping of soft tissue followed by surgical suture to make the joint tighter.

**Osborn wave,** an abnormal, upward deflection in the electrocardiogram (ECG) occurring at the junction of the QRS complex and the S-T segment. It is often found in ECGs of patients with moderate hypothermia and becomes more pronounced as body temperature declines. Also called **J wave.**

**osc,** 1. abbreviation for **oscillator.** 2. abbreviation for **oscilloscope.**

**os calcis.** See **calcaneus.**

**os capitatum.** See **capitate bone.**

**oscheitis** /os'kē·ī'tis/, an inflammation of the scrotum.

**oscheo-,** combining form meaning 'scrotum': *oscheocele, oscheolith, oscheoma.*

**oscillation** /os'ilā'shən/ [L, *oscillare,* to swing], 1. a back and forth motion. 2. vibration or the effects of a mechanical or electric vibrator.

**oscillator (osc)** /os'ilā'tər/ [L, *oscillare,* to swing], an electric or other device that produces oscillations, vibrations, or fluctuations, such as an alternating electric current generator.

**oscillopsia** /os'silop'sē·ə/, abnormal jerky eye movements associated with multiple sclerosis. They create a subjective sensation that the environment is oscillating.

**oscilloscope (osc)** /osil'əskōp/ [L, *oscillare,* to swing; Gk, *skopein,* to look], an instrument that displays a visual representation of electric variations on the fluorescent screen of a cathode ray tube. The graphic representation is produced by a beam of electrons on the screen. The beam is focused or directed by a magnetic field that is influenced in turn by a source such as an amplified current produced by heart contractions. As used in cardiology, the oscilloscope can function as a continuous electrocardiogram.

**os coxae.** See **innominate bone.**

**os cuboideum.** See **cuboid bone.**

**-ose,** 1. suffix meaning a 'carbohydrate': *cellulose, lactose, sucrose.* 2. suffix meaning a 'primary product of hydrolysis': *albumose, nucleose, myoproteose.*

**oseltamivir,** an antiviral.

■ INDICATIONS: This drug is used to treat type A influenza.

■ CONTRAINDICATIONS: Known hypersensitivity to this drug prohibits its use.

■ ADVERSE EFFECTS: Adverse effects of oseltamivir include fatigue, diarrhea, abdominal pain, and cough. Common side effects include headache, dizziness, insomnia, nausea, and vomiting.

**Osgood osteotomy** /oz′gŏŏd/, a surgical procedure for correcting the malrotation of a femur.

**Osgood-Schlatter disease** /-shlat′ər/ [Robert B. Osgood, American surgeon, 1873–1956; Carl Schlatter, Swiss surgeon, 1864–1934], inflammation or partial separation of the tibial tubercle caused by chronic irritation, usually as a result of overuse of the quadriceps muscle. The condition is seen primarily in muscular, athletic adolescent boys and is characterized by swelling and tenderness over the tibial tubercle that increase with exercise or any activity that extends the leg. Treatment consists primarily of preventing further irritation during the healing process, which may necessitate complete immobilization of the knee in a cast. Any residual nonunion of a proximal fragment after healing may require surgical excision. Also called **Osgood's disease, Schlatter-Osgood disease, Schlatter's disease.**

**OSHA** /ō′shä/, abbreviation for *Occupational Safety and Health Administration,* the federal agency that regulates worker safety.

**os hamatum.** See **hamate bone.**

**os hyoideum.** See **hyoid bone.**

**-osis,** 1. suffix meaning a '(specified) action, process, or result': *homeosis, narcosis, zygosis.* 2. suffix meaning 'increase in a pathologic condition': *calcicosis, psittacosis, varicosis.*

**Osler's disease.** See **Osler-Weber-Rendu syndrome, polycythemia.**

**Osler's nodes** /ōs′lərz/ [William Osler, American-British physician, 1849–1919], tender, reddish or purplish subcutaneous nodules of the soft tissue on the ends of fingers or toes, seen in subacute bacterial endocarditis and usually lasting only 1 or 2 days. The nodes represent bacterial embolisms from the infected heart valve.

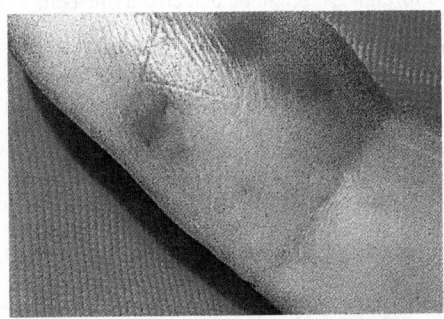

**Osler's nodes** *(Zitelli and Davis, 1997/courtesy Dr. J. F. John, Jr.)*

**Osler-Weber-Rendu syndrome** /ōs′lərweb′ərandŏŏ′/ [William Osler; Frederick P. Weber, British physician, 1863–1962; Henri J.L.M. Rendu, French physician, 1844–1902], a vascular anomaly, inherited as an autosomal-dominant trait, characterized by hemorrhagic telangiectasia of the skin and mucosa. Small, red-to-violet lesions are found on the lips, oral and nasal mucosa, tongue, and tips of fingers and toes. The thin, dilated vessels may bleed spontaneously or as a result of only minor trauma, and this condition becomes progressively more severe. Bleeding from superficial lesions is often profuse and may result in severe anemia. No specific treatment is known, but accessible bleeding lesions may be treated with pressure, styptics, and topical hemostatics. Transfusions may be indicated for acute hemorrhage, and iron deficiency anemia may require continuous treatment. Also called **hemorrhagic familial angiomatosis, hereditary hemorrhagic telangiectasia, Rendu-Osler-Weber syndrome.**

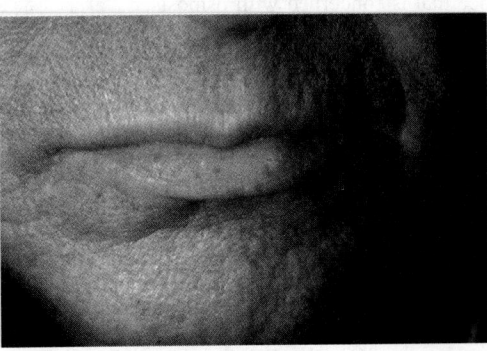

**Osler-Weber-Rendu syndrome** *(Lemmi and Lemmi, 2000)*

**os lunatum.** See **lunate bone.**

**osm,** 1. abbreviation for **osmosis.** 2. abbreviation for **osmotic.**

**os magnum.** See **capitate bone.**

**osmethesia** /os′məthē′zhə/ [Gk, *osme,* odor, *aisthesis,* feeling], the ability to perceive and distinguish odors; the sense of smell.

**-osmia,** suffix meaning '(condition of the) sense of smell': *dysosmia, hemianosmia, merosmia.*

**osmium (Os)** /oz′mē·əm/ [Gk, *osme,* odor], a hard, grayish, pungent-smelling metallic element. Its atomic number is 76; its atomic mass is 190.2. Used to produce alloys of extreme hardness, it is highly toxic.

**osmo-** /oz′mō-/, 1. prefix meaning 'odor': *osmoceptor, osmodysphoria, osmonosology.* 2. combining form meaning 'impulse or osmosis': *osmophilic, osmosology, osmotaxis.*

**osmoceptors** /-sep′tərz/ [Gk, *osme* + L, *recipere,* to receive], receptors in the anterior hypothalamus that respond to osmotic pressure, thereby regulating thirst and production of the antidiuretic hormone.

**osmol, osmolal.** See **osmole.**

**osmolal gap** /ozmōl′əl/, a difference between the observed and calculated osmolalities in serum analysis. The calculated osmolar values include sodium concentration multiplied by 2, plus glucose and blood urea nitrogen.

**osmolality** /oz′mōlal′itē/, the osmotic pressure of a solution expressed in osmols or milliosmols per kilogram of water. Normal adult blood osmolality is 285 to 295 mOsm/kg $H_2O$. Compare **osmolarity.**

**osmolal solution,** the solute concentration expressed in the number of osmoles per kilogram of solvent.

**osmolar** /osmō′lər/, pertaining to the osmotic characteristics of a solution of one or more molecular substances, ionic substances, or both, expressed in osmoles or milliosmoles.

**osmolarity** /oz'mōler'itē/,   the osmotic pressure of a solution expressed in osmoles or milliosmoles per liter of the solution. Compare **osmolality.**

**osmolar solution,**   the solute concentration expressed in the number of osmoles per liter of solution.

**osmole** /os'mōl/ [Gk, *osmos,* impulse, *osis,* condition + mole, (molecule)],   the quantity of a substance in solution in the form of molecules, ions, or both (usually expressed in grams) that has the same osmotic pressure as one mole of an ideal nonelectrolyte. Also spelled **osmol. —osmolal,** *adj.*

**osmology** /ozmol'əjē/ [Gk, *osme,* odor, *ōsmos,* impulse, *logos,* science],   **1.** the science of the sense of smell and the production and composition of odors. **2.** the branch of science that is concerned with osmosis.

**osmometer** /oz·mom'ə·tər/ [Gk, *ōsmos,* impulse + *metron,* measure],   a device for measuring osmotic concentration or pressure.

**osmometry** /ozmom'ətrē/ [Gk, *ōsmos,* impulse, *metron,* measure],   the field of study that deals with the phenomenon of osmosis and the measurement of osmotic forces. **—osmometric,** *adj.*

**Osmone-Clarke procedure,**   a surgical method for correcting splayfoot. It involves soft tissue release of the medial and lateral foot with peroneus brevis tendon transfer.

**osmoreceptor** /-risep'tər/ [Gk, *ōsmos,* impulse; L, *recipere,* to receive],   **1.** a neuron in the hypothalamus that is sensitive to the relative fluid/solute concentration in the blood plasma and regulates the secretion of antidiuretic hormone. **2.** a receptor of smell stimuli.

**osmoreceptor cell,**   a cell that recognizes changes in extracellular fluid osmolality.

**osmoregulation** /-reg'yəlā'shən/ [Gk, *ōsmos,* impulse; L, *regula,* rule],   the act of influencing or controlling the speed and extent of osmosis.

**osmosis (osm)** /ozmō'sis, os-/ [Gk, *ōsmos,* impulse, *osis,* condition],   the movement of a pure solvent such as water through a differentially permeable membrane from a solution that has a lower solute concentration to one that has a higher solute concentration. The membrane is impermeable to the solute but is permeable to the solvent. The rate of osmosis depends on the concentration of solute, the temperature of the solution, the electrical charge of the solute, and the difference between the osmotic pressures exerted by the solutions. Movement across the membrane continues until the concentrations of the solutions equalize. **—osmotic (osm),** *adj.*

Semipermeable membrane

Before osmosis      After osmosis

**Osmosis** *(Lewis, Heitkemper, and Dirksen, 2000)*

**osmotic diarrhea,**   a form of diarrhea associated with water retention in the bowel resulting from an accumulation of nonabsorbable water-soluble substances. An excessive intake of hexitols, sorbitol, and mannitol (used as sugar substitutes in candies, chewing gum, and dietetic foods) can result in slow absorption and rapid small intestine motility, leading to osmotic diarrhea. It may also occur in infants if they intake an undiluted concentrated form of formula. The severity of the condition varies directly with the amount of such sugar substitutes consumed and diminishes when intake is reduced. Also called **chewing gum diarrhea, dietetic food diarrhea.**

**osmotic diuresis,**   diuresis resulting from the presence of certain nonabsorbable substances in tubules of the kidney, such as mannitol, urea, or glucose.

**osmotic fragility,**   a sensitivity to changes in osmotic pressure characteristic of red blood cells. Exposed to a hypotonic concentration of sodium in solution, red cells take in increasing quantities of water, swell until the capacity of the cell membrane is exceeded, and burst. Exposed to a hypertonic concentration of sodium in a solution, red cells give up intracellular fluid, shrink, and break up. Laboratory findings of exceptional fragility or resistance may be diagnostic of certain conditions. Hemolysis of normal cells begins in 0.39% to 0.45% salt solution and is complete in 0.30% to 0.33% salt solution in 24 hours at 37° C (98.6° F). Also called **erythrocyte fragility.**

**osmotic pressure,**   **1.** the pressure exerted on a differentially permeable membrane separating a solution from a solvent, the membrane being impermeable to the solutes in the solution and permeable only to the solvent. **2.** the pressure exerted on a differentially permeable membrane by a solution containing one or more solutes that cannot penetrate the membrane, which is permeable only by the solvent surrounding it. See also **osmosis.**

**osmotic transfection,**   a method of inserting foreign deoxyribonucleic acid (DNA) molecules into cells by putting cells into a dilute solution that causes them to rupture. The cell membranes quickly repair themselves without irreversible injury to the cells. During the rupture period the alien DNA is added to the fluid and is absorbed into the cell nuclei. The foreign DNA can be detected in the cells as a transfection marker.

**os naviculare pedis.**   See **scaphoid bone.**

**-osphresia, -osphrasia,**   combining form meaning a 'condition of the sense of smell': *anosphresia, hyperosphresia, oxyosphresia.*

**osphresio-,**   combining form meaning 'odor': *osphresiolagnia, osphresiology, osphresiophilia.*

**osphresis** /osfrē'sis/ [Gk, smell],   olfaction; the sense of smell.

**oss-,**   combining form meaning 'bone': *osseocartilaginous, ossicle, ossific.*

**osseointegrated implant** /os'ē·ō·in'te·grā·təd/ [Gk, *osteon,* bone; L, *integrare,* to make whole],   an endosteal implant containing pores into which osteoblasts and supporting connective tissue can migrate. Metallic, ceramic, and polymeric materials have been used.

**osseous** /os'ē·əs/ [L, *os,* bone],   bony; consisting of or resembling bone.

**osseous labyrinth** [L, *os,* bone; Gk, *labyrinthos,* maze],   the bony part of the internal ear, composed of three cavities: the vestibule, the semicircular canals, and the cochlea, transmitting sound vibrations from the middle ear to the eighth cranial nerve. All three cavities contain perilymph, in which a membranous labyrinth is suspended. Also called **labyrinthus osseus.** Compare **membranous labyrinth.**

**ossicle** /os′ikəl/ [L, *ossiculum,* little bone], a small bone such as the malleus, the incus, or the stapes, which are ossicles of the middle ear. —**ossicular,** *adj.*

**ossiferous** /osif′ərəs/ [L, *os,* bone, *ferre,* to bear], pertaining to the formation of bone or bone tissue.

**ossification** /os′ifikā′shən/ [L, *os + facere,* to make], the development of bone. **Intramembranous ossification** is that preceded by membrane, such as in the process initially forming the roof and sides of the skull. **Intracartilaginous endochondral ossification** is that preceded by rods of cartilage, such as that forming the bones of the limbs.

**ossify** /os′ifī/ [L, *os,* bone, *facere,* to make], to develop into bone.

**ossifying fibroma** /os′ifī′ing/ [L, *os + facere,* to make], a slow-growing, benign neoplasm, occurring most often in the jaws, especially the mandible. The tumor is composed of bone that develops within fibrous connective tissue.

**oste-** See **osteo-.**

**ostealgia** /os′tē·al′jə/ [Gk, *osteon,* bone, *algos,* pain], any pain that is associated with an abnormal condition within a bone, such as osteomyelitis. —**ostealgic,** *adj.*

**osteanagenesis.** See **osteoanagenesis.**

**osteitis** /os′tē·ī′tis/ [Gk, *osteon + itis,* inflammation], an inflammation of bone caused by infection, degeneration, or trauma. Symptoms include swelling, tenderness, dull aching pain, and redness in the skin over the affected bone. Some kinds of osteitis are **osteitis deformans** and **osteitis fibrosa cystica.** See also **osteomyelitis, Paget's disease.**

**osteitis deformans.** See **Paget's disease.**

**osteitis fibrosa cystica,** an inflammatory degenerative condition in which normal bone is replaced by cysts and fibrous tissue. It is usually associated with hyperparathyroidism.

**osteitis fibrosa disseminata.** See **Albright's syndrome.**

**ostembryon.** See **lithopedion.**

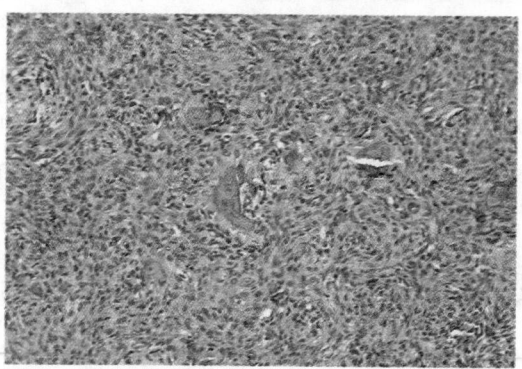

**Ossifying fibroma** *(Regezi, Sciubba, and Pogrel, 2000)*

**ostemia** /ostē′mē·ə/, an abnormal congestion of blood in a bone.

**ostempyesis** /os′təmpī·ē′sis/, an accumulation of pus within a bone.

**osteo** /os′tē·ō/, **1.** abbreviation for **osteopath. 2.** abbreviation for **osteopathy.**

**osteo-, oste-,** prefix meaning 'bone': *osteoanesthesia, osteocele, osteopathy.*

**osteoanagenesis** /os′tē·ō·an′əjen′əsis/ [Gk, *osteon + ana,* again, *genesis,* origin], the regeneration or formation of bone tissue. Also called **osteanagenesis.**

**osteoaneurysm** /-an′yəriz′əm/, a dilation of the wall of a blood vessel within a bone.

**osteoarthritis** /os′tē·ō′ärthrī′tis/ [Gk, *osteon + arthron,* joint, *itis,* inflammation], a form of arthritis in which one or many joints undergo degenerative changes, including

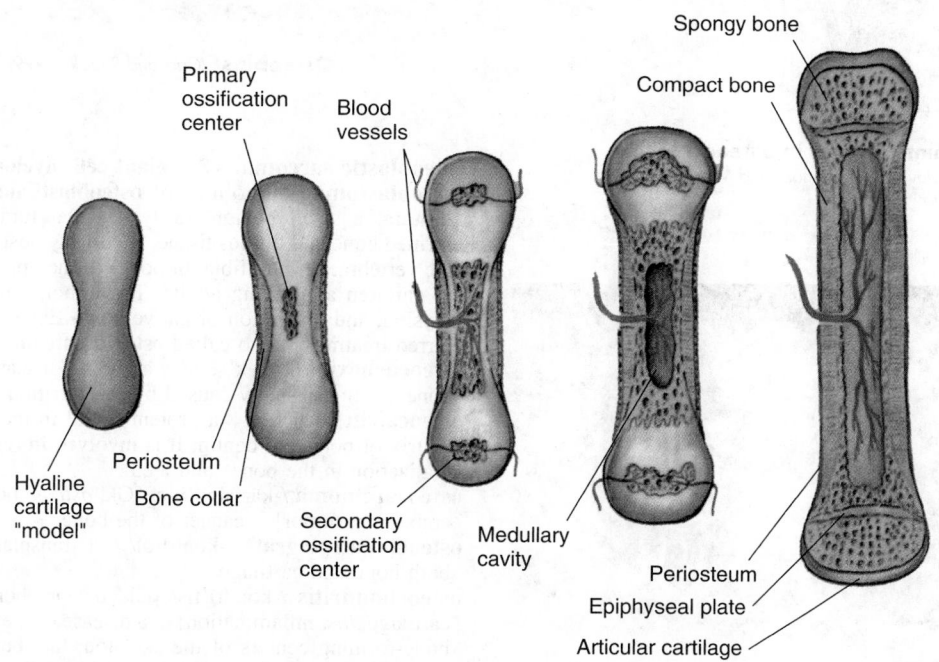

**Intracartilaginous endochondral ossification** *(Applegate, 2000)*

subchondral bony sclerosis, loss of articular cartilage, and proliferation of bone spurs (osteophytes) and cartilage in the joint. Inflammation of the synovial membrane of the joint is common late in the disease. Osteoarthritis is the most common form of arthritis, its cause is unknown but may include chemical, mechanical, genetic, metabolic, and endocrine factors. Emotional stress often aggravates the condition. The disease usually begins with pain after exercise or use of the joint. Stiffness, tenderness to the touch, crepitus, and enlargement develop; deformity, incomplete dislocation, and synovial effusion may eventually occur. Involvement of the hip, knee, or spine causes more disability than osteoarthritis of other areas. Treatment includes rest of the involved joints; use of a cane, a walker, or crutches to decrease weight-bearing; heat; and antiinflammatory drugs. Overweight patients may be advised to lose weight. Systemic corticosteroids are contraindicated, but intraarticular injections of corticosteroids may give relief. Surgical treatment is sometimes necessary and may reduce pain and greatly improve the function of a joint. Hip replacement, joint debridement, fusion, and decompression laminectomy are some of the surgical procedures used in treating advanced osteoarthritis. Compare **rheumatoid arthritis.** Also called **degenerative joint disease.**

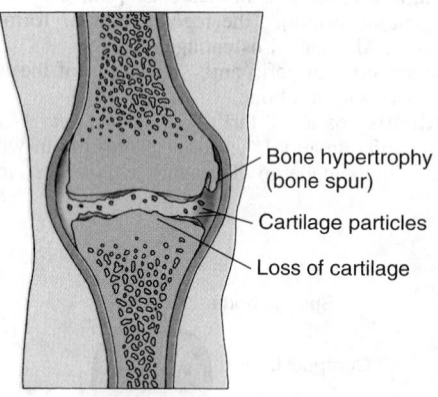

**Joint changes in osteoarthritis**
*(Ignatavicius, Workman, and Mishler, 1999)*

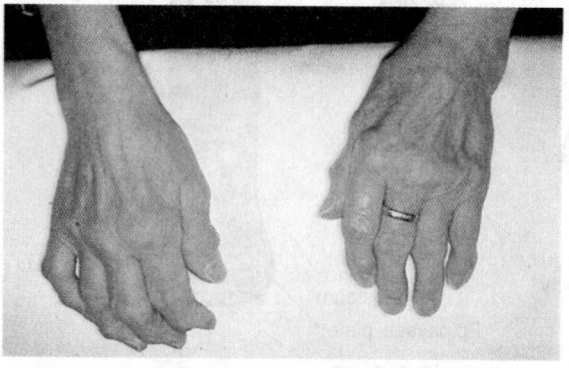

**Appearance of hands with severe osteoarthritis**
*(Kamal and Brockelhurst, 1991)*

**osteoarthritis deformans endemica.**   See **Kashin-Bek disease.**

**osteoarthropathy** /-ärthrop′əthē/ [Gk, *osteon* + *arthron,* joint, *pathos,* disease],   any disorder affecting bones and joints.

**osteoarthrosis** /-arthrō′sis/,   a condition of chronic arthritis, usually mechanical, without inflammation.

**osteoarticular** /-artik′yələr/,   pertaining to or affecting bones and joints.

**osteoarticular brucellosis,**   a form of brucellosis that affects mainly the weight-bearing joints.

**osteoarticular graft,**   a transplant of bone that contains a joint surface.

**osteoblast** /os′tē·əblast′/ [Gk, *osteon* + *blastos,* germ],   a bone-forming cell that is derived from the embryonic mesenchyme and, during the early development of the skeleton, differentiates from a fibroblast to function in the formation of bone tissue. Osteoblasts synthesize the collagen and glycoproteins to form the osteoid matrix and, with growth, develop into osteocytes. See also **ossification.** —**osteoblastic,** *adj.*

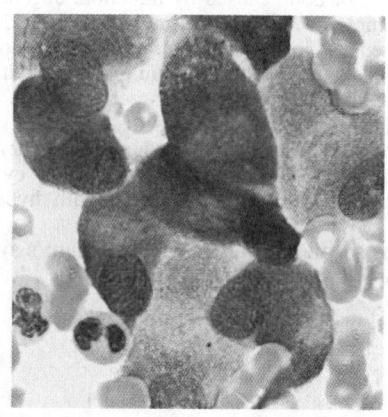

**Osteoblast** *(Carr and Rodak, 1999)*

**osteoblastic sarcoma.**   See **giant cell myeloma.**

**osteoblastoma** /-blastō′mə/, *pl.* **osteoblastomas, osteoblastomata,** a small benign, fairly vascular tumor of poorly formed bone and fibrous tissue, occurring most frequently in the vertebrae, femur, tibia, or bones of the upper extremities in children and young adults. The tumor may cause pain, erosion, and resorption of native bone. Excision is the preferred treatment. Also called **osteoid osteoma.**

**osteocachexia** /-kəkek′sē·ə/,   a chronic disease that causes bone wasting, usually caused by malnutrition.

**osteocalcin** /-kal′sin/,   a protein found in the extracellular matrix of bone and dentin. It is involved in regulating mineralization in the bones and teeth.

**osteocarcinoma** /-kär′sinō′mə/ [Gk, *osteon,* bone, *karkinos,* crab, *oma,* tumor],   cancer of the bone.

**osteochondral graft** /-kon′drəl/,   a transplant containing both bone and cartilage.

**osteochondritis** /-kəndrī′tis/ [Gk, *osteon,* bone, *chondros,* cartilage, *itis,* inflammation],   a disease of the epiphyses, or bone-forming centers of the skeleton, that begins with necrosis and tissue fragmentation and is followed by repair and regeneration. Types of the disorder include osteochondritis deformans juvenilis, osteochondritis dissecans, osteochondritis ischiopubica, osteochondritis juvenilis, and osteochondritis necroticans.

**osteochondritis dissecans** [Gk, *osteon,* bone, *chondros,* cartilage; L, *dissecare,* to cut apart], a joint disorder in which a piece of cartilage and neighboring bone tissue become detached from an articular surface.

**osteochondrodystrophy.** See **Morquio's disease.**

**osteochondrofibroma** /-kon′drōfībrō′mə/, a tumor containing tissues of osteoma, chondroma, and fibroma.

**osteochondrolysis.** See **osteochondrosis dissecans.**

**osteochondroma** /os′tē·ōkondrō′mə/ [Gk, *osteon + chondros,* cartilage, *oma,* tumor], a benign tumor composed of bone and cartilage.

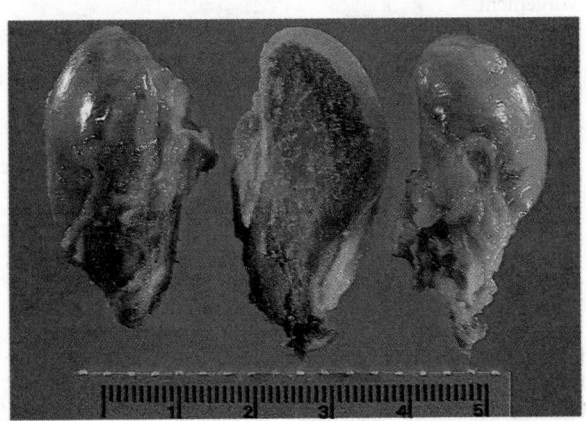

**Osteochondroma** *(Kumar, Cotran, and Robbins, 1997)*

**osteochondromatosis** /-kon′drōmətō′sis/, the transformation of synovial villi into bone and cartilage masses, causing loose bodies in the joints. It usually develops in joints affected by injury or degenerative disease.

**osteochondropathy** /kəndrop′əthē/, a condition affecting both bone and cartilage and characterized by abnormal enchondral ossification.

**osteochondrosarcoma** /-kon′drōsärkō′mə/ [Gk, *osteon,* bone, *chondros,* cartilage, *karkinos,* crab, *oma,* tumor], a cancer of the bone and cartilage.

**osteochondrosis** /-kondrō′sis/ [Gk, *osteon + chondros,* cartilage, *osis,* condition], a disease affecting the ossification centers of bone in children. It is initially characterized by degeneration and necrosis, followed by regeneration and recalcification. Kinds of osteochondrosis include **Legg-Calvé-Perthes disease, Osgood-Schlatter disease,** and **Scheuermann's disease.**

**osteochondrosis dissecans** /-dis′əkənz/, the formation of a separate center of bone and cartilage on an epiphyseal surface. The stray fragment may remain in place, be absorbed, or break off and become a loose body.

**osteoclasia** /-klā′zhə/ [Gk, *osteon + klasis,* breaking], **1.** the destruction and absorption of bony tissue by osteoclasts, such as during growth or the healing of fractures. **2.** the degeneration of bone through disease. See also **osteolysis.**

**osteoclasis** /os′tē·ōk′ləsis/, the intentional surgical fracture of a bone to correct a deformity. Also called **osteoclasty.**

**osteoclast** /os′tē·əklast′/ [Gk, *osteon + klasis,* breaking],

**1.** A large type of multinucleated bone cell with a large amount of acidophilic cytoplasm that functions to absorb and remove osseous tissue. During bone healing of fractures, or during certain disease processes, osteoclasts excavate passages through the surrounding tissue by enzymatic action. Osteoclasts become activated in the presence of parathyroid hormone and also in a lymphokine substance produced by lymphocytes in such diseases as multiple myeloma and malignant lymphomas. Also called **osteophage.** See also **ossification. 2.** a surgical instrument used in the fracturing or refracturing of bones for therapeutic purposes, such as correction of a deformity.

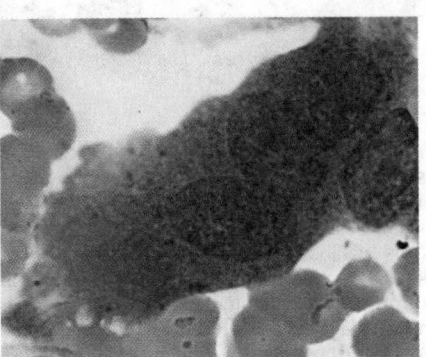

**Osteoclast in the bone marrow** *(Carr and Rodak, 1999)*

**osteoclast activating factor,** a lymphokine that promotes the resorption of bone.

**osteoclastic** /-klas′tik/, **1.** pertaining to osteoclasts. **2.** destructive to bone.

**osteoclastoma** /os′tē·ōklastō′mə/, *pl.* **osteoclastomas, osteoclastomata** [Gk, *osteon + klasis,* breaking, *oma,* tumor], a giant cell tumor of the bone that occurs most frequently at the end of a long bone and appears as a mass surrounded by a thin shell of new periosteal bone. The lesion may be malignant and may cause local pain, loss of function, weakness, and pathologic fracture. Also called **giant cell myeloma, giant cell tumor of bone.**

**osteoclasty.** See **osteoclasis.**

**osteocope** /os′tē·əkōp/, a painful, syphilitic bone disease.

**osteocystoma** /-sistō′mə/, a cystic tumor in a bone.

**osteocyte** /os′tē·əsīt/ [Gk, *osteon + kytos,* cell], a bone cell; a mature osteoblast that has become embedded in the bone matrix. It occupies a small cavity and sends out protoplasmic projections that anastomose with those of other osteocytes to form a system of minute canals within the bone matrix. **—osteocytic,** *adj.*

**osteodensitometer** /den′sitom′ətər/ [Gk, *osteon,* bone; L, *densus,* thick; Gk, *metron,* measure], an apparatus for measuring the density of bone tissue.

**osteodentin** /-den′tin/, dentin that resembles bone. It is found chiefly in the teeth of fish and certain other animals, but also occurs occasionally in humans when odontoblasts are entrapped by rapidly developing secondary dentin.

**osteodermia** /-dur′mēə/, a condition in which skeletal changes have occurred in the skin, such as a bony tumor of the skin. Also called **osteoma cutis.**

**osteodiastasis** /-dī·as′təsis/, an abnormal separation of bones.

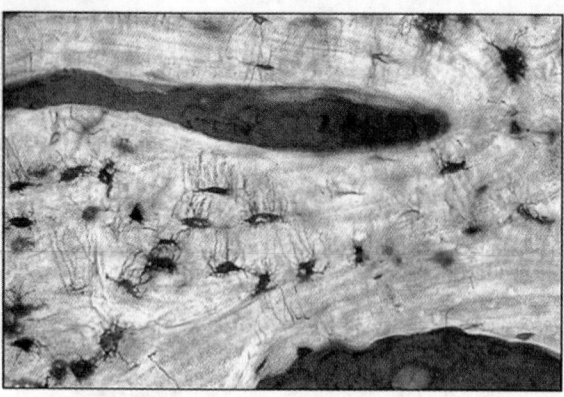

**Osteocytes** *(Aloia, 1993)*

**osteodynia** /-din′ē·ə/, bone pain.

**osteodystrophy** /-dis′trəfē/ [Gk, *osteon* + *dys,* bad, *trophe,* nourishment], any generalized defect in bone development, usually associated with disturbances in calcium and phosphorus metabolism and renal insufficiency, such as in renal osteodystrophy. Also called **osteodystrophia.**

**osteoenchondroma** /os′tē·ō·en′kəndrō′mə/, a benign bone and cartilage tumor within a bone.

**osteofibrochondrosarcoma** /-fī′brōkon′drōsärkō′mə/, a malignant tumor containing bone, cartilage, and fibrous tissues.

**osteofibroma** /-fībrō′mə/ [Gk, *osteon,* bone; L, *fibra,* fiber; Gk, *oma,* tumor], a tumor composed of both bony and fibrous tissues.

**osteogenesis** /-jen′əsis/ [Gk, *osteon* + *genesis,* origin], the origin and development of bone tissue. Also called **osteogeny.** See also **ossification.** —**osteogenetic, osteogenic, osteogenous,** *adj.*

**osteogenesis imperfecta,** a genetic disorder involving defective development of the connective tissue. It is inherited as an autosomal-dominant trait and is characterized by abnormally brittle and fragile bones that are easily fractured by the slightest trauma. Also called **brittle bones, fragilitas ossium, hypoplasia of the mesenchyme, osteopsathyrosis.**

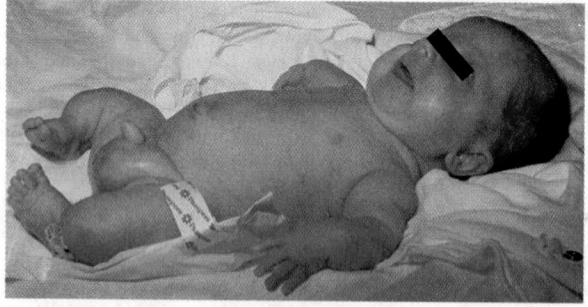

**Osteogenesis imperfecta** *(Zitelli and Davis, 1997)*

■ OBSERVATIONS: In its most severe form, the disease may be apparent at birth, when it is known as **osteogenesis imperfecta Type II.** The newborn has multiple fractures that have occurred in utero and is usually severely deformed because of imperfect formation and mineralization of bone. Most infants die shortly after birth, although a few survive as deformed dwarfs with normal mental development if no head trauma has occurred. If the disease has a later onset, it is called **osteogenesis imperfecta Type I** and usually runs a milder course. Symptoms generally appear when the child begins to walk, but they become less severe with age, and the tendency to fracture decreases and often disappears after puberty. Other manifestations of the condition include blue sclerae, translucent skin, hyperextensibility of ligaments, hypoplasia of the teeth, recurrent epistaxis, excess diaphoresis, mild hyperpyrexia, and a tendency to bruise easily and develop otosclerosis with hearing loss. There is a broad expressivity of the disease so that the number and extent of pathologic features may range from minimal to severe involvement.

■ INTERVENTIONS: Osteogenesis imperfecta has no known cure. Treatment is predominantly supportive; extreme care must be taken in handling patients, especially infants who are severely affected, to prevent fractures. In many children oral administration of magnesium oxide may decrease the fracture rate, as well as the diaphoresis, hyperpyrexia, and constipation associated with the condition.

■ NURSING CONSIDERATIONS: The primary function of the nurse is to educate the parents about the disease, especially the extent of the child's limitations, and to help them plan suitable activities that will promote optimum growth and development and at the same time protect the child from harm. Genetic counseling is also part of the goals of long-term care.

**osteogenetic.** See **osteogenesis.**

**osteogenic,** composed of or originating from any tissue involved in the development, growth, or repair of bone. Also **osteogenous.**

**osteogenic myeloma.** See **myeloma.**

**osteogenic sarcoma.** See **osteosarcoma.**

**osteogenous.** See **osteogenic.**

**osteogeny.** See **osteogenesis.**

**osteohalisteresis** /-hal′istərē′sis/, a condition of soft bones caused by a loss or deficiency of mineral elements.

**osteoid** /os′tē·oid/ [Gk, *osteon* + *eidos,* form], pertaining to or resembling bone.

**osteoid osteoma.** See **osteoblastoma.**

**osteolipochondroma** /-līp′ōkəndrō′mə/, a cartilage tumor with bone and fat elements.

**osteolipoma** /-līpō′mə/, a fatty tumor containing bone elements.

**osteology** /os′tē·ol′əgē/ [Gk, *osteon,* bone, *logos,* science], the branch of medicine concerned with the development and diseases of bone tissue.

**osteolysis** /os′tē·ol′isis/ [Gk, *osteon* + *lysis,* loosening], the degeneration and dissolution of bone caused by disease, infection, or ischemia. The condition commonly affects the terminal bones of the hands and feet, such as in acroosteolysis, and is seen in disorders involving blood vessels, such as Raynaud's disease, scleroderma, and systemic lupus erythematosus. —**osteolytic,** *adj.*

**osteolytic hypercalcemia** /-lit′ik/, a malignancy associated with excess calcium in the blood. It may be caused by either widespread skeletal metastases or extensive bone marrow involvement by a primary hematologic tumor.

**osteoma** /os′tē·ō′mə/, *pl.* **osteomas, osteomata,** a tumor of bone tissue.

**-osteoma,** combining form meaning a 'tumor composed of bone tissue, usually benign': *endosteoma, myosteoma, periosteoma.*

**osteoma cutis.** See **osteodermia.**

**osteomalacia** /-məlā'shə/ [Gk, *osteon* + *malakia*, softening], an abnormal condition of lamellar bone, characterized by a loss of calcification of the matrix and resulting in softening of the bone. It is accompanied by weakness, fracture, pain, anorexia, and weight loss. The condition is the result of an inadequate amount of phosphorus and calcium available in the blood for mineralization of the bones. This deficiency may be caused by a diet lacking these minerals or vitamin D; by a lack of exposure to sunlight and hence an inability to synthesize vitamin D; or by a metabolic disorder causing malabsorption of minerals. Osteomalacia results from and also complicates many other diseases and conditions. Treatment usually includes administration of the necessary vitamins and minerals and therapy appropriate for the underlying disorder. Also called **adult rickets.** See also **hyperparathyroidism, Paget's disease, rickets.**

**osteomas, osteomata.** See **osteoma.**

**osteomesopyknosis** /-mez'ōpiknō'sis/, a genetic disorder transmitted as an autosomal trait, characterized by osteosclerosis of the axial spine, pelvis, and proximal areas of long bones.

**osteomyelitis** /-mī·əlī'tis/ [Gk, *osteon* + *myelos*, marrow, *itis*, inflammation], local or generalized infection of bone and bone marrow. It is usually caused by bacteria introduced by trauma or surgery, by direct extension from a nearby infection, or via the bloodstream. Staphylococci are the most common causative agents.

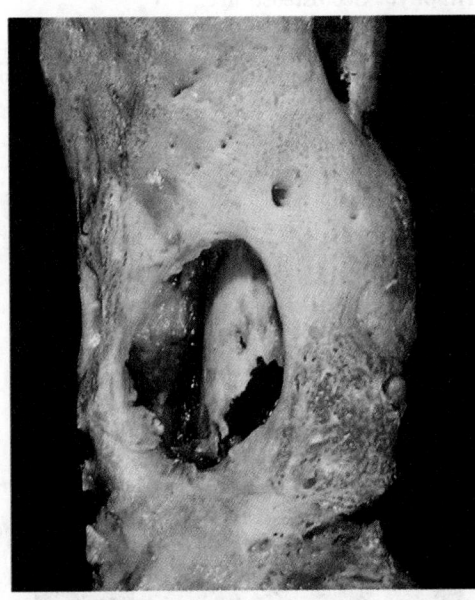

**Chronic osteomyelitis** *(Kumar, Cotran, and Robbins, 1997)*

■ OBSERVATIONS: The long bones in children and the vertebrae in adults are the most common sites of infection as a result of hematogenous spread. Persistent, severe, and increasing bone pain; tenderness; guarding on movement; regional muscle spasm; and fever suggest this diagnosis. Draining sinus tracts may accompany posttraumatic osteomyelitis or osteomyelitis from a contiguous infection. Specific diagnosis and selection of therapy depend on bacterial examination of bone, tissue, or pus.

■ INTERVENTIONS: Treatment includes bed rest and parenteral antibiotics for several weeks. Surgery may be necessary to remove necrotic bone and tissue, to obliterate cavities, to remove infected prosthetic appliances, and to apply prostheses to stabilize affected parts. Chronic osteomyelitis may persist for years with exacerbations and remissions despite treatment.

■ NURSING CONSIDERATIONS: Any drainage is disposed of using usual precautions. Absolute rest of the affected part may be necessary, with a careful positioning using pillows and sandbags for good alignment. During the early phase of infection, pain is extremely severe, and extraordinary gentleness in moving and manipulating the infected part is essential. —**osteomyelitic,** *adj.*

**osteomyelodysplasia** /os'tē·ōmī'əlō'displā'zhə/ [Gk, *osteon,* bone, *myelos,* marrow, *dys* + *plasis,* forming], a loss of bone tissue through absorption of minerals. The condition is usually associated with leukopenia and sometimes with fever. It may result from an excess of parathyroid hormone.

**osteon** /os'tē·on/ [Gk, bone], the basic central structural unit of compact bone, consisting of the haversian canal and its concentric rings of 4 to 20 lamellae. Most of the units run with the long axis of the bone. Also called **haversian system.**

**-osteon, -osteum,** combining form meaning 'bone': *melacosteon, otosteon, pleurosteon.*

**osteonal bone** /os'tē·ō'nəl/, bone tissue composed of tiny chalky tubes with an arteriole running down the middle and circular laminations of bone concentric with an artery. It is seen in mature adults.

**osteonecrosis** /os'tē·ō'nəkrō'sis/ [Gk, *osteon* + *nekros,* dead, *osis* condition], the destruction and death of bone tissue, such as from ischemia, infection, malignant neoplastic disease, or trauma. —**osteonecrotic,** *adj.*

**osteo-onychodysplasia** /os'tē·ō·on'i·kō·dis·plā'zhə/ [Gk, *osteon,* bone + *onyx,* nail + *dys,* bad + *plassein,* to form], **1.** also called **onycho-osteodysplasia.** abnormal development of nails and bones. **2.** see **nail-patella syndrome.**

**osteopath (osteo)** /os'tē·ōpath'/, a physician who specializes in osteopathy. Also called **osteopathist.**

**osteopathic.** See **osteopathy.**

**osteopathic scoliosis.** See **congenital scoliosis.**

**osteopathist.** See **osteopath.**

**osteopathology** /-pathol'əjē/ [Gk, *osteon,* bone, *pathos,* disease, *logos,* science], the study of bone diseases.

**osteopathy (osteo)** /os'tē·op'əthē/ [Gk, *osteon* + *pathos,* disease], a therapeutic approach to the practice of medicine that uses all the usual forms of medical diagnosis and therapy, including drugs, surgery, and radiation, but that places greater emphasis on the influence of the relationship between the organs and the musculoskeletal system than traditional medicine does. Osteopathic physicians recognize and correct structural problems using manipulation. See also **physician.** —**osteopathic,** *adj.*

**osteopedion.** See **lithopedion.**

**osteopenia** /-pē'nē·ə/ [Gk, *osteon* + *penes,* poverty], a condition of subnormally mineralized bone, usually the result of a rate of bone lysis that exceeds the rate of bone matrix synthesis.

**osteoperiosteal graft** /-per'ē·os'tē·əl/, a bone graft that includes the periosteal membrane covering the bone.

**osteopetrosis** /os'tē·ōpētrō'sis/ [Gk, *osteon* + *petra,* stone, *osis,* condition], an inherited disorder characterized by a generalized increase in bone density, probably caused by faulty bone resorption resulting from a deficiency of osteoclasts. In its most severe form, transmitted as an autosomal-recessive condition, there is obliteration of the bone marrow cavity, causing severe anemia, marked deformities of the skull, and compression of the cranial nerves, which may result in deafness and blindness and lead to an early death. A milder, benign form, transmitted as an autosomal-dominant trait, is characterized by short stature, fragile bones that fracture easily, and a tendency to develop osteomyelitis. Also called **ivory bones, marble bones, os-teosclerosis fragilis.** See also **Albers-Schönberg disease. —osteopetrotic,** *adj.*

**osteophage.** See **osteoclast.**

**osteophlebitis** /-fləbī′tis/, an inflammation of the veins that are a part of the vascular system of bones.

**osteophyte** /os′tē·əfīt/, a bony outgrowth, usually found around a joint.

**osteoplast.** See **osteoblast.**

**osteoplastica** /-plas′tikə/, a form of bone inflammation associated with cystic fibrosis.

**osteoplasty** /o′stē·əplas′tē/ [Gk, *osteon,* bone, *plassein,* to mold], plastic surgery performed on bone tissue.

**osteopoikilosis** /os′tē·ōpoi′kilō′sis/ [Gk, *osteon + poikilos,* mottled, *osis,* condition], an inherited condition of the bones, transmitted as an autosomal-dominant trait, characterized by multiple areas of dense calcification throughout the osseous tissue, producing a mottled appearance on x-ray examination. It is a benign condition, usually without symptoms, and of unknown cause. Also called **osteosclerosis fragilis congenita. —osteopoikilotic,** *adj.*

**osteoporosis** /os′tē·ōpərō′sis/ [Gk, *osteon + poros,* passage, *osis,* condition], a disorder characterized by abnormal loss of bone density and deterioration of bone tissue, with an increased fracture risk. It occurs most frequently in postmenopausal women, sedentary or immobilized individuals, and patients on long-term steroid therapy. The disorder may cause pain, especially in the lower back, pathologic fractures, loss of stature, and various deformities. Osteoporosis may be without a known cause or secondary to other disorders, such as thyrotoxicosis or the bone demineralization caused by hyperparathyroidism. Estrogen therapy is often used for the prevention and management of postmenopausal osteoporosis, but use of the hormone alone carries the risk of endometrial cancer. **—osteoporotic,** *adj.*

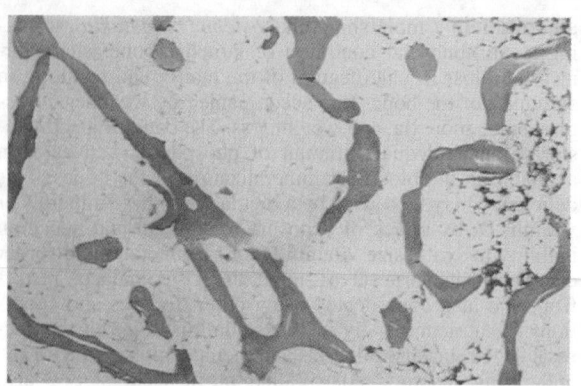

**Photomicrograph of osteoporotic bone**
*(Christiansen and Grzybowski, 1993)*

**osteoporosis of disuse** [Gk, *osteon,* bone, *poros,* passage, *osis,* condition; L, *dis,* not; ME, *usen,* to act], a decrease in bone mass that occurs in sedentary people or patients confined to bed for a long period.

**osteoporotic** /-pərot′ik/ [Gk, *osteon,* bone, *poros,* passage, *osis,* condition], pertaining to osteoporosis.

**osteopsathyrosis.** See **osteogenesis imperfecta.**

**osteorrhaphy.** See **osteosuture.**

**osteosarcoma** /os′tē·ō′särkō′mə/ [Gk, *osteon + sarx,* flesh, *oma*], a malignant tumor of the bone, composed of anaplastic cells derived from mesenchyme. Also called **osteogenic sarcoma.**

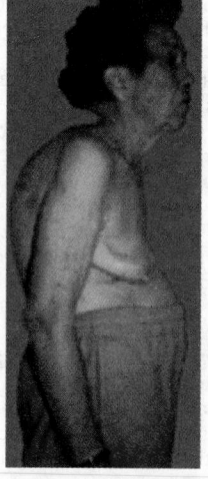

**Severe osteoporosis** *(Lemmi and Lemmi, 2000)*

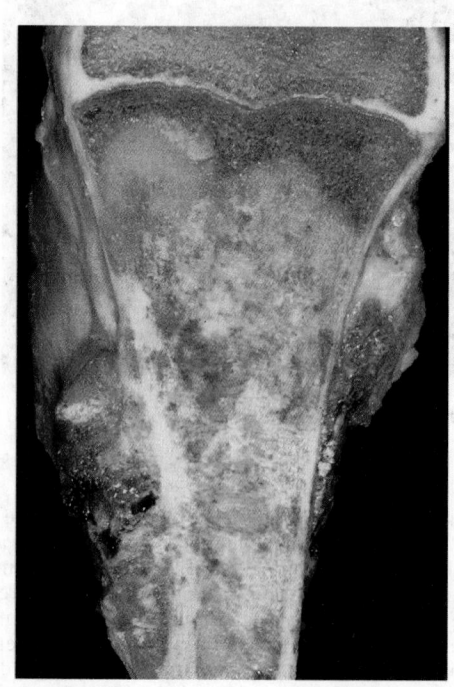

**Osteosarcoma** *(Cotran, Kumar, and Collins, 1999)*

**osteosclerosis** /os′tē·ōsklerō′sis/ [Gk, *osteon* + *skleros,* hard, *osis,* condition], an abnormal increase in the density of bone tissue. The condition occurs in a variety of disease states and is commonly associated with ischemia, chronic infection, and tumor formation. It also may be caused by faulty bone resorption as a result of some abnormality involving osteoclasts. See also **achondroplasia, osteopetrosis, osteopoikilosis. —osteosclerotic,** *adj.*

**osteosclerosis fragilis.** See **osteopetrosis.**

**osteosclerosis fragilis congenita.** See **osteopoikilosis.**

**osteosclerotic.** See **osteosclerosis.**

**osteosuture** /-sōō′chər/, the surgical repair of a fractured bone by wiring or suturing the fragments together. Also called **osteorrhaphy.**

**osteosynovitis** /-sin′ōvī′tis/ [Gk, *osteon,* bone; Gk, *syn,* together; L, *ovum,* egg; Gk, *itis,* inflammation], an inflammation of the synovial membrane of a joint and the surrounding bone tissue.

**osteosynthesis** /-sin′thəsis/, the surgical fixation of a bone using any internal mechanical means. It is usually performed in the treatment of fractures.

**osteotabes** /-tā′bēz/, a condition usually affecting infants in which bone marrow cells are destroyed and the marrow disappears.

**osteotelangiectasia** /-telan′jē·əktā′zhə/, a sarcoma of the bone characterized by dilated capillaries.

**osteothrombophlebitis** /-throm′bōfləbī′tis/, a progressive inflammation of small venules and intact bone often accompanied by clot formation.

**osteothrombosis** /-thrəmbō′sis/, a blockage of blood vessels in bone tissue.

**osteotome** /os′tē·ətōm′/ [Gk, *osteon* + *temnein,* to cut], a surgical instrument for cutting through bone.

**osteotomy** /os′tē·ot′əmē/ [Gk, *osteon* + *temnein,* to cut], the sawing or cutting of a bone. Kinds of osteotomy include block osteotomy, in which a section of bone is excised, cuneiform osteotomy to remove a bone wedge, and displacement osteotomy, in which a bone is redesigned surgically to alter the alignment or weight-bearing stress areas.

**osteotripsy** /-trip′sē/, any percutaneous reduction of a bony prominence or callus.

**-osteum.** See **-osteon.**

**ostium.** See **orifice.**

**ostium primum defect, ostium secundum defect.** See **atrial septal defect.**

**ostomate** /os′təmāt/ [L, *ostium,* mouth], a person who has undergone an ostomy.

**ostomy** /os′təmē/ [L, *ostium,* mouth], *informal.* a surgical procedure in which an opening is made to allow the passage of urine from the bladder or of intestinal contents from the bowel to an incision or stoma surgically created in the wall of the abdomen. An ostomy procedure may be performed to correct an anatomic defect, relieve an obstruction, or permit treatment of a severe infection or injury of the urinary or intestinal tract. Each procedure is named for the anatomic location of the ostomy, such as a colostomy, ureterostomy, cecostomy, or cystostomy.

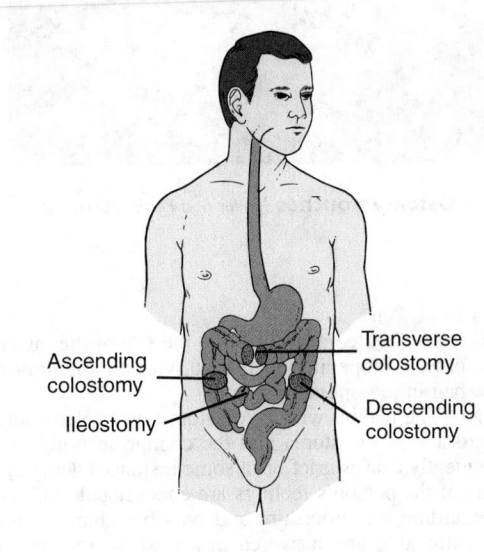

**Ostomy sites**

**-ostomy,** suffix meaning to 'form a new opening or pertaining to a mouthlike opening': *colostomy, tracheostomy.*

**ostomy care**[1], the management and support of a patient with a surgical opening created in the bladder, ileum, or colon for the temporary or permanent passage of urine or feces, necessitated by carcinoma, intestinal obstruction,

**Comparison of colostomies and ileostomy**

| | Ascending colostomy | Transverse colostomy | Sigmoid colostomy | Ileostomy |
|---|---|---|---|---|
| Stool consistency | Semiliquid | Semiliquid to semiformed | Formed | Liquid to semiliquid |
| Fluid requirement | Increased | Possibly increased | No change | Increased |
| Bowel regulation | No | Uncommon | Yes (if there is a history of a regular bowel pattern) | No |
| Pouch and skin barriers | Yes | Yes | Dependent on regulation | Yes |
| Irrigation | No | No | Possible every 24–48 hr (if patient meets criteria) | No |
| Indications for surgery | Perforating diverticulitis in lower colon; trauma; inoperable tumors of colon, rectum, or pelvis; rectovaginal fistula | Same as for ascending; birth defect | Cancer of the rectum or rectosigmoidal area; perforating diverticulum; trauma | Ulcerative colitis, Crohn's disease, diseased or injured colon, birth defect, familial polyposis, trauma, cancer |

From Lewis SM, Heitkemper MM, Dirksen SR: *Medical-surgical nursing: assessment and management of clinical problems,* ed 5, St Louis, 2000, Mosby.

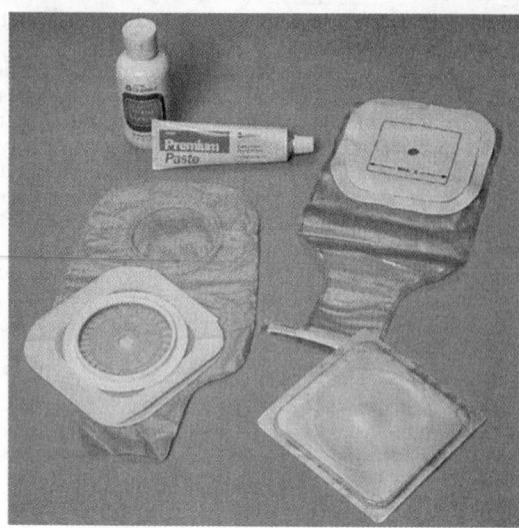

**Ostomy pouches** *(Potter and Perry, 2001)*

trauma, or severe ulceration distal to the site of the incision. In most cases the opening is covered with a temporary disposable bag in the operating room.

■ METHOD: The patient with a colostomy or an ileostomy is helped to accept the stoma and the change in body image that frequently causes grief or in some instances denial. Discussions of the person's feelings are encouraged, and questions regarding the procedure and possible changes in the person's life-style are answered in a positive manner. The disposable bag, called an appliance, is changed when necessary, and the character, color, and amount of odor and drainage are observed; mucous secretion from the stoma usually begins within 48 hours after the surgery, fecal drainage within 72 hours. The stoma is inspected periodically for color, bleeding, stricture, retraction, and infection and is measured periodically to determine the size of the appliance that is to be used. There is mild to moderate swelling of the stoma the first 2 to 3 weeks postoperatively. Size of the stoma is determined with a stoma measuring card. Each time the temporary or permanent appliance is changed, the skin around the stoma is washed with soap and water, rinsed thoroughly, and patted dry with a clean towel. If the skin is irritated or excoriated, karaya powder, alone or mixed with an ointment, is spread over the area before the appliance is reinstalled. A pouch should never be placed directly on irritated skin without the use of a skin barrier. An adhesive substance may be used to maintain a tight seal with the appliance; deodorant drops, aspirin, or various bismuth or chlorophyll preparations or mouthwash solutions are added to the ostomy bag to control odor. The diet is planned according to the kind of ostomy; ileostomates require food high in sodium and potassium, such as bananas, citrus juices, molasses, and cola, and are advised to avoid fried, highly seasoned, and rich foods, nuts, raisins, raw fruits other than bananas, and anything that produces gas or causes diarrhea. Gas-producing foods such as cabbage, beans, broccoli, cauliflower, and corn; foods causing disturbing odors such as onions, eggs, and fish; and sharp condiments are contraindicated; a low-residue diet is ordered for most ostomates. The fluid intake is carefully maintained.

■ INTERVENTIONS: Before discharge, each step in the care of the stoma and surrounding skin is rehearsed with the patient, using the equipment that will be available at home. The patient is urged to establish a regular pattern of evacuation and to report any signs of wound infection or obstruction, such as nausea, vomiting, decreased drainage from the stoma, abdominal distension, and cramps. Normal daily activity is encouraged.

■ OUTCOME CRITERIA: Visiting nurse referrals are indicated for client assessment and education. Referrals to support groups are also encouraged. Clients are encouraged to keep appointments with call providers. The ability of the patient to adjust to the ostomy procedures and equipment is greatly affected by the nursing care received in the days after surgery. A positive patient matter-of-fact approach, sensitive emotional support, and thorough teaching of self-care measures are essential aspects of ostomy nursing care.

**ostomy care**[2], a nursing intervention from the Nursing Interventions Classification (NIC) defined as maintenance of elimination through a stoma and care of surrounding tissue. See also **Nursing Interventions Classification.**

**ostomy irrigation,** a procedure for cleansing, stimulating, and regulating evacuation of an artificially created orifice. Fluids used in irrigation include tap water and saline or medicated solutions. Necessary equipment includes properly sized irrigator tips, catheters, drainage bags that allow for insertion of the catheter, water-soluble lubricants, gloves, an irrigation container, and shields to prevent leakage. Loop and double-barrel colostomies require a sequential irrigation of the proximal loop, distal loop, and rectum to prevent the accumulation of discharge.

**ostrac-, ostraco-,** combining form meaning 'like a hard shell': *astracosis, ostracod.*

**os trapezium.** See **trapezium.**

**os trapezoideum.** See **trapezoid bone.**

**os trigonum** /os′trigō′nəm/, a small foot bone just posterior to the talus. It is sometimes confused with a fracture of the posterior tubercle of the talus. Also called **Bardeleben's bone.**

**os triquetrum.** See **triangular bone.**

**OT, 1.** abbreviation for **occupational therapist. 2.** abbreviation for **occupational therapy.**

**ot-.** See **oto-.**

**otalgia** /ōtal′jə/, a pain in the ear. Also called **otodynia, otoneuralgia.**

**OTC,** abbreviation for **over the counter.**

**OTC drug.** See **patent medicine.**

**Othello syndrome** /ōthel′ō/ [Othello, jealous Shakespearean character], a psychopathologic condition characterized by suspicion of a spouse's infidelity and morbid jealousy. This condition may be accompanied by rage and violence and is frequently associated with paranoia.

**-otia,** combining form meaning '(condition of the) ear': *melotia, microtia, synotia.*

**otic** /ō′tik, ot′ik/ [Gk, *ous,* ear], pertaining to the ear. Also **auricular.**

**-otic.** See **oto-.**

**otics** /ō′tiks, ot′iks/, a group of drugs used locally to treat inflammation of the external ear canal or to remove excess cerumen.

**otic vertigo,** a sensation of rotation motion caused by an inner ear disease. Its subcategories are Meniere's disease, inner ear dysfunction, fistula or other pressure sensitivity, unilateral paresis, and benign paroxysmal positional vertigo.

**otitic** /ōtit′ik/ [Gk, *ous,* ear], pertaining to otitis.

**otitic barotrauma.** See **barotrauma.**

**otitis** /ōtī′tis/ [Gk, *ous + itis,* inflammation], inflammation or infection of the ear. Kinds of otitis are **otitis externa** and **otitis media.**

**otitis externa,** inflammation or infection of the external canal or the auricle of the external ear. Major causes are allergy, bacteria, fungi, viruses, and trauma. Allergy to nickel or chromium in earrings and to chemicals in hair sprays, cosmetics, hearing aids, and medications, particularly sulfonamides and neomycin, is common. *Staphylococcus aureus, Pseudomonas aeruginosa,* and *Streptococcus pyogenes* are common bacterial causes. Herpes simplex and herpes zoster viruses are frequently implicated. Eczema, psoriasis, and seborrheic dermatitis also may affect the external ear. Abrasions of the ear canal may become infected, and excessive swimming may wash out protective cerumen, remove skin lipids, and lead to secondary infection. Otitis externa is more prevalent during hot, humid weather. Folliculitis is particularly painful in the external auditory meatus and is a common occupational hazard in nurses, caused by irritation from the earpieces of stethoscopes. Treatment includes oral analgesics, thorough local cleansing, topical antimicrobials to treat infection, or topical corticosteroids to reduce inflammation. Prevention includes measures to reduce maceration of the skin and to avoid trauma.

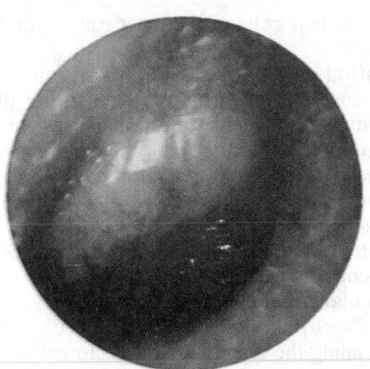

**Otitis media** *(Zitelli and Davis, 1997/courtesy Dr. Michael Hawke)*

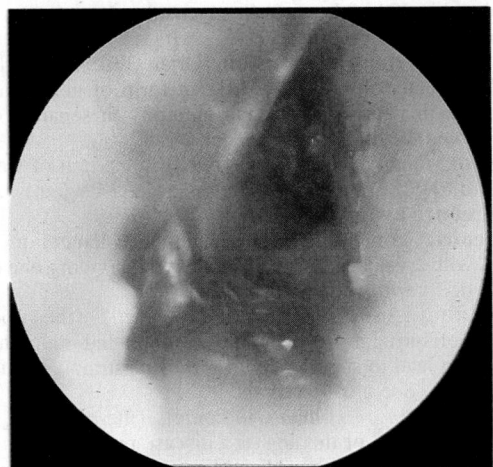

**Otitis externa** *(Zitelli and Davis, 1997)*

**otitis interna.** See **labyrinthitis.**

**otitis mastoidea** [Gk, *ous,* ear, *itis,* inflammation, *mastos,* breast, *eidos,* form], an inflammation of the middle ear associated with a mastoid infection.

**otitis media,** inflammation or infection of the middle ear. It is common in early childhood. Acute otitis media is most often caused by *Haemophilus influenzae, Moraxella catarrhalis,* or *Streptococcus pneumoniae.* Chronic otitis media is usually caused by gram-negative bacteria such as *Proteus, Klebsiella,* and *Pseudomonas.* Allergy, *Mycoplasma,* and several viruses also may be causative factors. Otitis media is often preceded by an upper respiratory infection.

■ OBSERVATIONS: Organisms gain entry to the middle ear through the eustachian tube. The small diameter and horizontal orientation of the tube in infants predisposes them to infection. Obstruction of the eustachian tube and accumulation of exudate may increase pressure within the middle ear,

forcing infection into the mastoid bone or rupturing the tympanic membrane. Symptoms of acute otitis media include a sense of fullness in the ear, diminished hearing, pain, and fever. Usually only one ear is affected. Squamous epithelium may grow in the middle ear through a rupture in the tympanic membrane; development of a cholesteatoma and hearing loss may occur if repeated infections cause an opening to persist. Pneumococcal otitis media may spread to the meninges.

■ INTERVENTIONS: Treatment includes antibiotics, analgesics, local heat, nasal decongestants, needle aspiration of secretions collected behind the membrane, and myringotomy.

■ NURSING CONSIDERATIONS: Parents are taught to recognize and watch for early warning signs of otitis media. The use of vaporizers and decongestants is often recommended during an upper respiratory tract infection as prophylaxis against otitis media. Chronic otitis media may result in hearing loss and delays in speech development.

**otitis sclerotica** [Gk, *ous,* ear, *itis,* inflammation, *sclerosis,* hardening], a sclerosing type of inflammation of the middle ear.

**oto-** /ō'tō-/, **ot-, -otic,** combining form meaning 'ear': *otoantritis, otoblennorrhea, otocyst, parotic, hematotic.*

**otoacoustic emissions,** echoes emitted by the outer hair cells of the inner ear. These echoes are used to evaluate the integrity of the inner ear and to screen hearing in newborns.

**otocephalic, otocephalous.** See **otocephaly.**

**otocephalus** /ō'tōsef'ələs/, a fetus with otocephaly.

**otocephaly** /ō'tōsef'əlē/ [Gk, *ous* + *kephale,* head], a congenital malformation characterized by the absence of the lower jaw, defective formation of the mouth, and union or close approximation of the ears on the front of the neck. See also **agnathocephaly.** —**otocephalic, otocephalous,** *adj.*

**otocranial debris,** otoliths that have been dislodged by trauma and may move about in the semicircular canals when the head changes position.

**otodynia.** See **otalgia.**

**otolaryngologist** /-ler'ing·gol'əjist/ [Gk, *ous* + *larynx* + *logos,* science], a physician who specializes in the diagnosis and treatment of diseases and injuries of the ears, nose, and throat. Also called **ENT specialist.** Compare **otologist.**

**otolaryngology** /-ler'ing·gol'əjē/ [Gk, *ous* + *larynx* + *logos,* science], a branch of medicine dealing with the diagnosis and treatment of diseases and disorders of the ears, nose, throat, and adjacent structures of the head and neck.

**otolith** /ō'təlith/ [Gk, *ous,* ear, *lithos,* stone], **1.** a calculus in the middle ear. **2.** any of the crystals of calcium carbonate attached to the hair cells of the inner ear as gravity orientation receptors.

**otolith righting reflex** [Gk, *ous* + *lithos,* stone], an involuntary response in newborns in which tilting of the body when the infant is in an erect position causes the head to return to the upright position. The reflex enables the infant to raise the head and is important for development of later gross motor skills. Absence of the reflex may indicate central nervous system damage.

**otologist** /ōtol′əjist/, a physician trained in the diagnosis and treatment of diseases and other disorders of the ear. Compare **otolaryngologist.**

**otology** /ōtol′əjē/ [Gk, *ous* + *logos,* science], the study of the ear, including the diagnosis and treatment of its diseases and disorders.

**-otomy,** suffix meaning 'to make an incision or cut into': *phlebotomy, tracheotomy.*

**otomycosis** /ō′tōmīkō′sis/, a lesion of the external ear caused by a fungus infection.

**otoneuralgia.** See **otalgia.**

**otoneurology.** See **neurotology.**

**otoplasty** /ō′təplas′tē/ [Gk, *ous* + *plassein,* to mold], a common procedure in reconstructive plastic surgery in which, for cosmetic reasons, some of the cartilage in the ears is removed to bring the auricle and pinna closer to the head.

**otopyosis** /ō′təpi·ō′sis/, a pus-producing inflammation of the ear, occurring either in the tympanic cavity or the external auditory meatus.

**otorrhea** /ō′tərē′ə/ [Gk, *ous* + *rhoia,* flow], any discharge from the external ear. Otorrhea may be serous, sanguinous, or purulent, or contain cerebrospinal fluid. **—otorrheal, otorrheic, otorrhetic,** *adj.*

**otosclerosis** /ō′tōsklərō′sis/ [Gk, *ous* + *skleros,* hard, *osis,* condition], a hereditary condition of unknown cause in which irregular ossification occurs in the ossicles of the middle ear, especially of the stapes, causing hearing loss. It is usually first noticed between 11 and 30 years of age. Women are affected twice as often as men. The condition may worsen during pregnancy. Stapedectomy or stapedotomy is usually successful in restoring hearing. Also called **otospongiosis.**

**otoscope** /ō′təskōp′/ [Gk, *ous* + *skopein,* to look], an instrument used to examine the external ear, the eardrum, and, through the eardrum, the ossicles of the middle ear. It consists of a light, a magnifying lens, a speculum, and sometimes a device for insufflation.

**otoscopy** /ōtos′kəpē/ [Gk, *ous,* ear, *skopein,* to view], an inspection of the tympanic membrane and other parts of the outer ear with an otoscope.

**otospongiosus.** See **otosclerosis.**

**ototoxic** /ō′tōtok′sik/ [Gk, *ous* + *toxikon,* poison], (of a substance) having a harmful effect on the eighth cranial nerve or the organs of hearing and balance. Common ototoxic drugs include the aminoglycoside antibiotics, aspirin, furosemide, and quinine.

**ototoxic hearing loss,** hearing loss caused by ingestion of toxic substances. Also called **toxic deafness.**

**OTR,** abbreviation for *occupational therapist, registered.* See **occupational therapist.**

**Otrivin,** trademark for an adrenergic vasoconstrictor (xylometazoline hydrochloride).

**Otto pelvis** /ot′ō/ [Adolph W. Otto, German surgeon, 1786–1845], a type of hip dislocation in which there is a gradual central displacement of the femur. The cause is unknown.

**OU,** abbreviation for *oculus uterque,* a Latin phrase meaning 'each eye.'

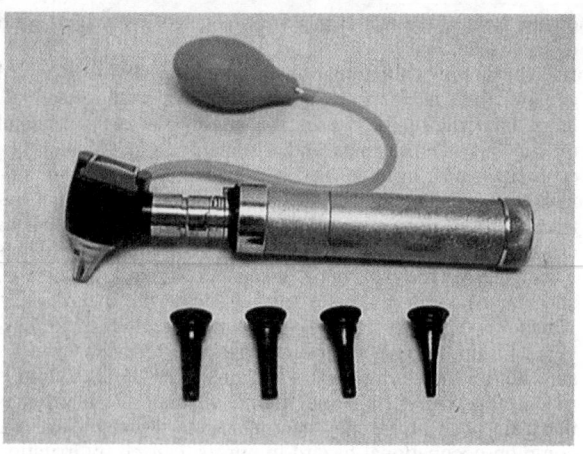

**Otoscope with pneumatic attachment** *(Seidel et al, 1999)*

**oubain** /wäbā′in/, a crystalline glycoside derived from the seeds of *Strophanthus gratus* and the wood of *Acocanthera oubaio.* It is similar in pharmaceutic action to strophanthin-K and the digitalis glycosides. It is also used as an arrow poison in Africa.

**Ouchterlony double diffusion** [Orjan T.G. Ouchterlony, Swedish bacteriologist, b. 1914], a form of gel diffusion technique in which antigen and antibody in separate cells are allowed to diffuse toward each other.

**ounce (oz)** /ouns/ [L, *uncia,* one twelfth], a unit of weight equal to 1/16 of a pound avoirdupois or 28.349 grams. Also called **ounce avoirdupois.**

**-ous, -eous,** combining form meaning an 'element or compound with a valence lower than the corresponding one ending in *-ic*': *cuprous, ferrous, hypochlorous.*

**outbreeding** [AS, *ut,* out, *bredan,* to breed], the production of offspring by the mating of unrelated individuals, which can lead to superior hybrid traits or strains. Compare **inbreeding.** See also **heterosis.**

**outcome** [AS, *ut* + *couman,* to come], the condition of a patient at the end of therapy or a disease process, including the degree of wellness and the need for continuing care, medication, support, counseling, or education.

**outcome criteria,** standards that focus on observable or measurable results of nursing and other health service activities.

**outcome data,** information collected to evaluate the capacity of a client to function at a level described in the outcome statement of a nursing care plan or in standards for patient care.

**outcome measure,** a measure of the quality of medical care, the standard against which the end result of the intervention is assessed.

**outlet** [AS, *ut* + *laetan,* to permit], an opening through which something can exit, such as the pelvic outlet.

**outlet contraction.** See **contraction.**

**outlet contracture,** an abnormally small pelvic outlet. It may be anteroposterior or transverse and is of significance in childbirth because it may impede or prevent passage of a baby through the birth canal. Anteroposterior contracture caused by fixation of the coccyx may sometimes be overcome by the force of labor, freeing the bones and allowing them to move back. Significant narrowing of the space between the ischial tuberosities is unlikely to be overcome and is most commonly associated with a heavy, android type of pelvis.

**outlet forceps.** See **low forceps.**

**outlier,** **1.** (in managed care) a case in which costs exceed the allowable amount for the specific diagnosis or treatment. The outlier amount is typically specified in advance in the contract between the provider and payer. **2.** (in research) an observation that differs from all others, suggesting that a gross error has occurred in sampling, measurement, or analysis.

**outline form** [AS, *ut* + *lin,* thread], the shape of the cavo-surface of a prepared tooth cavity, before the tooth surface or surfaces are restored.

**out-of-body experience (oobe),** a sensation that the mind has separated temporarily from the body. The feeling tends to occur when the patient is asleep, in a trance, or unconscious as during surgery. The person visualizes his or her body as an impersonal observer might. In some cases the person visualizes objects or persons who are beyond the range of normal senses. Occasionally a patient near death learns after awakening that he or she has been declared clinically dead during the moments of the experience. See also **near-death experience.**

**out of phase,** a series of events or actions that are not synchronous with a previously established periodic process or phenomenon. An oscillation or periodic process that runs in an opposite direction or pattern is sometimes described as 180 degrees out of phase.

**out-of-plan services,** services given to a patient by a provider outside the managed care system. The patient may be responsible for a larger co-payment than if the services were received within the plan.

**outpatient (OP)** [AS, *ut* + L, *patientia,* endurance], **1.** a patient, not hospitalized, who is being treated in an office, clinic, or other ambulatory care facility. **2.** pertaining to a health care facility for patients who are not hospitalized or to the treatment or care of such a patient. Compare **inpatient.**

**output** [AS, *ut* + *putian,* to put], **1.** the total of any and all measurable liquids lost from the body, including urine, vomitus, diarrhea; drainage from wounds and fistulas; and those removed by suction equipment. The output is recorded as a means of monitoring a patient's fluid and electrolyte balance. **2.** the end product of a system.

**output amplifier,** an apparatus used to increase the amplitude of the voltage output of a generator and control it at a specific level.

**output device,** any device that converts information from a computer into a form that is readable by humans or another machine, such as a printer or monitor display.

**outreach program,** a system of delivery of services to geropsychiatric clients, particularly mentally ill older adults in rural environments. They are considered most at risk because mental health and social services are usually not readily available. Outreach programs can diagnose and treat homebound clients with physical limitations or major psychiatric illnesses who are socially isolated.

**ova.** See **ovum.**

**ova and parasites test** /ō′vä/, a microscopic examination of feces for detecting parasites, such as amebas or worms and their ova, which are indicators of parasitic disorders.

**ovale malaria.** See **tertian malaria.**

**ovalocytes** /ō′vəlōsīts′/ [L, *ovalis,* egg-shaped; Gk, *kytos,* cell], oblong or oval-shaped red blood cells with pale centers that are found occasionally in patients with hemolytic anemias, thalassemias, and hereditary elliptocytosis. A genetic factor may be responsible for the presence of the abnormal blood cells. See also **elliptocytosis.**

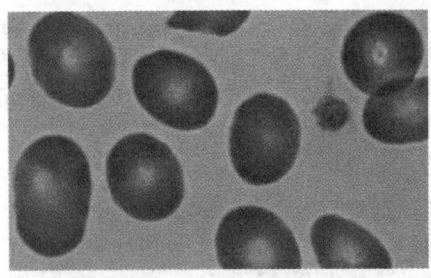

**Ovalocytes** *(Carr and Rodak, 1999)*

**ovalocytosis.** See **elliptocytosis.**

**oval window** /ō′vəl/ [L, *ovum;* ME, *windoge*], an oval-shaped aperture in the wall of the middle ear, leading to the inner ear. The footplate of the stapes vibrates in the oval window, transmitting sound waves to the cochlea.

**ovari-.** See **ovario-.**

**-ovaria,** combining form meaning '(condition of the) ovary or ovarial activity': *anovaria, hyperovaria, hypoovaria.*

**ovarian** /ōver′ē·ən/ [L, *ovum,* egg], pertaining to the ovary.

**ovarian artery,** a slender branch of the abdominal aorta, arising caudal to the renal arteries, and supplying an ovary. Compare **testicular artery.**

**ovarian cancer.** See **ovarian carcinoma.**

**ovarian carcinoma,** a malignant neoplasm of the ovaries rarely detected in the early stage and usually far advanced when diagnosed. It occurs frequently in the fifth decade of life. Ovarian cancer appears to be increasing in the United States. Risk factors of the disease are infertility, nulliparity or low parity, delayed childbearing, repeated spontaneous abortion, endometriosis, group A blood type, previous irradiation of pelvic organs, and exposure to chemical carcinogens such as asbestos and talc. After an insidious onset and asymptomatic period, the tumor may become evident as a palpable abdominal or pelvic mass accompanied by irregular or excessive menses or postmenopausal bleeding. In advanced cases the patient may have ascites, edema of the legs, and pain in the abdomen and the backs of the legs. Regular yearly pelvic examinations after 40 years of age contribute significantly to early diagnosis and the possibility of curative treatment. Characteristic of the disease as it advances are abdominal swelling and discomfort, abnormal vaginal bleeding, weight loss, dysuria or abnormal frequency of urination, constipation, and a palpable ovarian mass, especially in postmenopausal women. A Papanicolaou smear may show malignant cells if the tumor is advanced; an ultrasonic examination can demonstrate an ovarian mass but does not distinguish between a benign and malignant lesion. A computed tomographic scan may be useful in detecting ovarian cancer, but a definitive diagnosis requires surgical exploration. Most ovarian carcinomas are papillary or serous, followed in frequency by mucinous, endometrial, and undifferentiated cancers. In many cases the cancer spreads over the surface of the peritoneum, and early in the course of the lesion, tumor cells invade the lymphatic vessels under the diaphragm and the paraaortic nodes. Approximately half of the tumors diagnosed are unresectable. Treatment of resectable lesions consists of total abdominal hysterectomy, removal of both ovaries and tubes, omentectomy, and biopsies of any suspicious sites, especially in the liver and diaphragm. Chemotherapeutic agents that may be administered after surgery include chlorambucil, cisplatin, cyclophosphamide, melphalan, taxol, docetaxel, and thiotepa.

**ovarian cyst,** a globular sac filled with fluid or semisolid material that develops in or on the ovary. It may be transient and physiologic or pathologic. Kinds of ovarian cysts include **chocolate cyst,** corpus luteum cyst, and **dermoid cyst.**

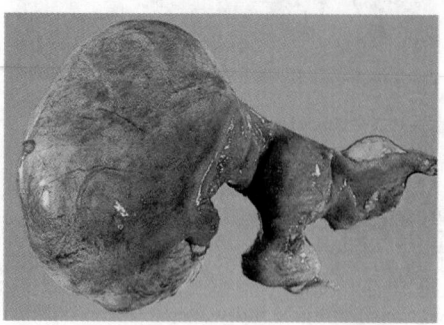

**Ovarian cyst** *(Symonds and Macpherson, 1994)*

**ovarian follicle** [L, *ovum + folliculus,* small bag], a cavity or recess in an ovary containing a liquor that divides the follicular cells into layers and surrounds an ovum.

**ovarian hormone.** See **relaxin.**

**ovarian pregnancy,** a rare type of ectopic pregnancy in which the conceptus is implanted within the ovary.

**ovarian seminoma.** See **dysgerminoma.**

**ovarian varicocele,** a varicose swelling of the veins of the uterine broad ligament. Also called **pelvic varicocele.**

**ovarian vein,** one of a pair of veins that emerge from convoluted plexuses in the broad ligament near the ovaries and the uterine tubes. The veins from each plexus ascend and unite to form single veins. The right ovarian vein opens into the inferior vena cava, and the left ovarian vein into the renal vein. In some individuals the ovarian veins contain valves and greatly enlarge during pregnancy. Compare **testicular vein.**

**ovariectomy.** See **oophorectomy.**

**ovario-, ovari-, oario-, ootheco-,** combining form meaning 'ovary': *ovariocentesis, ovariosteresis, ovariotubal.*

**ovariocele** /ōver′ē·əsēl/, a hernia of an ovary or protrusion of an ovary through the vaginal wall.

**ovariocentesis** /ōver′ē·ōsentē′sis/, surgical puncture of an ovary or of an ovarian cyst.

**ovariohysterectomy** /-his′tərek′təmē/, the surgical removal of the uterus and ovaries.

**ovary** /ō′vərē/ [L, *ovum,* egg], one of the paired female gonads found on each side of the lower abdomen, beside the uterus, in a fold of the broad ligament. At ovulation, an egg is expelled from a follicle on the surface of the ovary under the stimulation of the gonadotrophic hormones, follicle-stimulating hormone (FSH), and luteinizing hormone (LH). The remainder of the follicle (corpus luteum) secretes the hormones estrogen and progesterone, which regulate the menstrual cycle by a negative-feedback system in which an increase in estrogen decreases the secretion of FSH by the pituitary gland and an increase in progesterone decreases the secretion of LH. Each ovary is normally firm and smooth and resembles an almond in size and shape. The ovaries generally are homologous to the testes.

**Ovcon,** trademark for an oral contraceptive containing an estrogen (ethinyl estradiol) and a progestin (norethindrone acetate).

**overbite** /ō′vərbīt/ [AS, *ofer,* over, *bitan,* to bite], increased vertical overlapping of the lower teeth by the upper teeth, usually measured perpendicular to the occlusal plane. Compare **overclosure, overjet.**

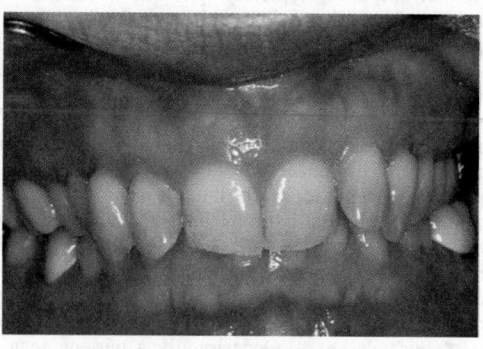

**Overbite** *(Proffit, 2000)*

**overclosure** /-klō′zhər/ [AS, *ofer* + L, *claudere,* to close], an abnormal condition in which the mandible rises beyond the point of normal occlusal contact, caused by drifting of teeth, loss of occlusal vertical dimension, change in tooth shapes through grinding, or loss of teeth.

**overcompensation** /-kom′pənsā′shən/ [AS, *ofer* + L, *compensare,* to weigh together], an exaggerated attempt to overcome a real or imagined physical or psychologic deficit. The attempt may be conscious or unconscious. See also **compensation.**

**overdenture** /-den′chər/ [AS, *ofer* + L, *dens,* tooth], a complete or partial removable denture supported by retained roots or teeth to provide improved support, stability, and tactile and proprioceptive sensation and to reduce bone resorption.

**overdose (OD)** /-dōs/, an excessive use of a drug, resulting in adverse reactions ranging from mania or hysteria to coma or death.

**overdrive suppression** /-drīv/ [AS, *ofer* + *drifan,* to drive], the inhibitory effect of a faster cardiac pacemaker on a slower one.

**overeruption** /-irup′shən/, the projection of a tooth beyond the normal occlusal plane. Also called **supereruption, supraclusion, supraocclusion.**

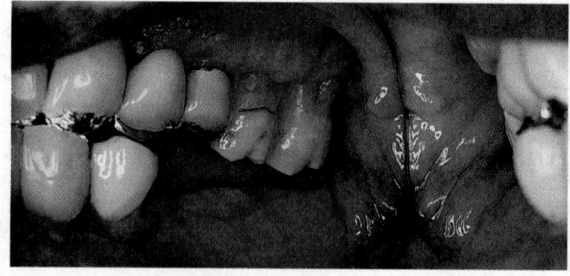

**Overeruption** *(Cranin, 1999)*

**overflow** /-flō/ [AS, *ofer* + *flowan*], the flooding or excessive discharge of a fluid, such as urine, saliva, or bile.

**overflow incontinence** [AS, *ofer* + *flowan* + L, *incontinentia,* inability to retain], an overflow of urine from a distended paralyzed bladder. See also **incontinence, urinary incontinence.**

**overgrafting** /-graf′ting/, placing an additional transplant over a previously healed tissue graft. It is sometimes performed to strengthen a split-thickness graft or to replace epithelium that may have been lost.

**overgrowth** [AS, *ofer* + ME, *growen*], an excessive growth, usually applied to organ or tissue development. Also called **hypertrophy.**

**overhang** /-hang/ [AS, *ofer* + *hangian,* to hang], an excess of dental filling material that projects beyond the margin of a tooth cavity preparation. It can trigger gingivitis or periodontitis by providing a harbor for bacteria.

**overhydration** /-hīdrā′shən/, an excess of water in the body. Also called **hyperhydration.**

**overinclusiveness** /-inkloo′sivnəs/ [AS, *ofer* + L, *includere,* to include], a type of association disorder observed in some schizophrenia patients. The individual is unable to think in a precise manner because of an inability to keep irrelevant elements outside perceptual boundaries.

**overjet** /-jet/ [AS, *ofer* + Fr, *jeter,* to throw], increased projection of the upper teeth in front of the lower teeth, usually measured parallel to the occlusal plane. Also called **horizontal overlap.** Compare **overbite, overclosure.**

**overlap** /-lap′/, to extend over and cover part of an existing surface or structure.

**overlay** /o′vərlā/, to add to an existing condition or structure.

**overlearning** /-lur′ning/, the practice of an ability that continues beyond the point where performance meets a specified standard.

**overload** /-lōd/, **1.** a burden greater than the capacity of the system designed to move or process it. **2.** (in physiology) any factor or influence that stresses the body beyond its natural limits and may impair its health.

**overnutrition** /-nootrish′ən/, a condition of excess nutrient and energy intake over time. Overnutrition may be regarded as a form of malnutrition when it leads to morbid obesity.

**overoxygenation** /-ok′sijənā′shən/ [AS, *ofer* + Gk, *oxys,* sharp, *genein,* to produce; L, *atio,* process], an abnormal condition in which the oxygen concentration in the blood and other tissues of the body is greater than normal and the carbon dioxide concentration is less than normal. The condition is characterized by a fall in blood pressure, decreased vital capacity, fatigue, errors in judgment, paresthesia of the hands and feet, anorexia, nausea, vomiting, and hyperemia.

**overresponse** /rispons′/, an abnormally strong reaction to a stimulus.

**overriding** /-rī′ding/ [AS, *ofer* + *ridan*], the overlapping or telescoping of body parts, such as when one fragment of a fractured bone rests on another.

**overripe cataract** /-rīp/ [AS, *ofer* + OE, *reap*], a cataract in which a completely opaque lens solidifies and shrinks.

**oversensing** /-sen′sing/, the sensation of stimuli, such as magnetism or static electricity, that are not normally detected by the sense organs.

**overshoot,** **1.** /ō′vərshoot′/ to go beyond or exceed a target or goal. **2.** /ō′vərshoot/ an upper part of a structure that extends beyond the lower part.

**over the counter (OTC),** (of a drug) available to the consumer without a prescription.

**overtone,** **1.** any tone produced by voice or a musical instrument that is of a higher frequency than the lowest or fundamental tone of a sound. **2.** a harmonic.

**overweight** /-wāt/ [AS, *ofer* + *gewiht,* weight], more than normal in body weight after adjustment for height, body build, and age, or 10% to 20% above the person's 'desirable' body weight. See also **body mass index.**

**overwintering** /-win′təring/, persistence of seasonal infectious agents beyond their normal period of activity, particularly warm weather pathogen vectors that remain operative into the winter months.

**ovi-, ovo-,** combining form meaning 'ovum or egg': *ovipara, oviposit, ovoplasm.*

**ovicidal** /ō′visī′dəl/, causing destruction of an ovum.

**ovicide** /ō′visīd/, an agent that destroys ova.

**oviduct.** See **fallopian tube.**

**oviferous** /ōvif′ərəs/ [L, *ovum,* egg, *ferre,* to bear], bearing or capable of producing ova (egg cells).

**oviparous** /ōvip′ərəs/ [L, *ovum* + *parere,* to bring forth], giving birth to young by laying eggs. Compare **ovoviviparous, viviparous.**

**oviposition** /ō′vipəsish′ən/ [L, *ovum* + *ponere,* to place], the act of laying or depositing eggs by a female oviparous animal.

**ovipositor** /ō′vipos′itər/ [L, *ovum* + *ponere,* to place], a specialized organ, found primarily in insects, for depositing eggs on plants or in the soil. It may be modified into a stinger as in worker bees and wasps.

**ovo-.** See **ovi-.**

**ovocenter** /ō′vəsen′tər/ [L, *ovum* + *centrum,* center], the centrosome of a fertilized ovum. Also called **oocenter** /ō′əsen′tər/.

**ovoflavin** /ō′vəflā′vin/ [L, *ovum* + *flavus,* yellow], a riboflavin derived from the yolk of eggs.

**ovogenesis.** See **oogenesis.**

**ovoglobulin** /ō′vəglob′yoŏlin/ [L, *ovum* + *globulus,* small sphere], a globulin protein derived from the white of eggs.

**ovogonium.** See **oogonium.**

**ovoid** /ō′void/, egg-shaped.

**ovoid arch** [L, *ovum* + Gk, *eidos,* form; L, *arcus,* bow], a dental arch that curves smoothly from the molars on one side to those on the opposite side to form half an oval.

**ovo-lacto-vegetarian.** See **lacto-ovo-vegetarian.**

**ovomucin** /ō′vəmyoō′sin/ [L, *ovum* + *mucus,* slime], a glycoprotein derived from the white of eggs.

**ovomucoid** /ō′vəmyoō′koid/ [L, *ovum* + *mucus,* slime; Gk, *eidos,* form], pertaining to a glycoprotein, similar to mucin, derived from the white of eggs.

**ovoplasm.** See **ooplasm.**

**ovotestis** /ō′vətes′tis/ [L, *ovum* + *testis,* testicle], a gonad that contains both ovarian and testicular tissue; a hermaphroditic gonad. —**ovotesticular,** *adj.*

**ovo-vegetarian.** See **vegetarian.**

**ovovitellin.** See **vitellin.**

**ovoviviparous** /ō′vəvivip′ərəs/ [L, *ovum* + *vivus,* living, *parere,* to bring forth], bearing young in eggs that are hatched within the body, as in some reptiles and fishes. Compare **oviparous, viviparous.**

**Ovral,** trademark for an oral contraceptive containing a progestin (norgestrel) and an estrogen (ethinyl estradiol).

**Ovrette,** trademark for an oral contraceptive containing a progestin (norgestrel).

**ovulation** /ov′yəlā′shən/ [L, *ovum* + *atio,* process], expulsion of an ovum from the ovary on spontaneous rupture of a mature follicle as a result of cyclic ovarian and pituitary endocrine function. It usually occurs on or about the eleventh to the fourteenth day before the next menstrual period and may cause brief, sharp lower abdominal pain on the side of the ovulating ovary. See also **oogenesis.** —**ovulate** /ov′yə′lāt/, *v.*

**ovulation method of family planning,** a natural method of family planning that uses observation of changes in the character and quantity of cervical mucus to determine the time of ovulation during the menstrual cycle. Because pregnancy occurs with fertilization of an ovum extruded from the ovary at ovulation, the method is used to increase or decrease the woman's chance of becoming pregnant by causing or avoiding insemination by spontaneous or artificial means during the fertile period associated with ovulation. The cyclic changes in gonadotropic hormones, especially estrogen, cause changes in the quantity and character of cervical mucus. In the first days after menstruation, scant thick mucus is secreted by the cervix. These 'dry days' are 'safe days,' with ovulation several days away. The quantity of mucus then increases; it is pearly white and sticky, becoming clearer and less sticky as ovulation approaches; these 'wet days' are 'unsafe days.' During and just after ovulation the mucus is clear, slippery, and elastic; it resembles the uncooked white of an egg. The day on which this sign is most apparent is the 'peak day,' probably the day before ovulation. The 4 days after the 'peak day' are 'unsafe'; fertilization might occur. By the end of the 4 days, the mucus becomes pearly white and sticky again and progressively decreases in quantity until menstruation supervenes to begin a new cycle. Essential to the effectiveness of this method are thorough instruction by a family planning counselor and strong self-motivation in the couple. During the first cycle, abstinence may be necessary to allow observation of the mucus without the confusing addition of semen or contraceptive foam, cream, or jelly, if being used. Daily close monitoring of the mucus is necessary even after several cycles because the length of the 'safe' and 'unsafe' periods and the time of ovulation vary from cycle to cycle, as they do from woman to woman. After delivery and during lactation the method is not effective until the menses have become regular. Effectiveness of the method in identifying the most fertile days of the cycle is augmented by using the basal body temperature method. This combined method is called the symptothermal method of planning. Proponents of the ovulation method claim the benefits of low cost, naturalness, and effectiveness. Detractors emphasize a limited public health application of the method, stating that it requires extensive teaching and self-motivation and that its effectiveness is limited by the ability of the user to observe correctly and diligently the changes in the cervical mucus. Abstinence may be necessary for up to 10 days by a woman whose menstrual cycles are long or are of irregular length. Also called **Billings method, cervical mucus method of family planning.**

**ovulatory** /ov′yələtôr′ē/ [L, *ovum*], pertaining to ovulation.

**ovulatory phase.** See **menstrual cycle, secretory phase.**

**Ovulen,** trademark for an oral contraceptive containing an estrogen (mestranol) and a progestin (ethynodiol diacetate).

**ovulocyclic** /ov′yəlōsī′klik/, pertaining to recurrent events associated with the ovulatory cycle.

**ovulocyclic porphyria,** episodes of acute abnormalities of porphyrin metabolism that tend to recur in the premenstrual period.

**ovum** /ō′vəm/, *pl.* **ova** [L, egg], **1.** an egg. **2.** the secondary oocyte (female germ cell) extruded from the ovary at ovulation.

**owl-eye cell,** an enlarged cell infected by cytomegalovirus and containing large inclusion bodies. Owl-eye cells are found mainly in the renal epithelium.

**Owren's disease** [Paul A. Owren, Norwegian hematologist, b. 1905], a rare congenital bleeding disorder caused by a deficiency of coagulation factor V. Also called **parahemophilia.**

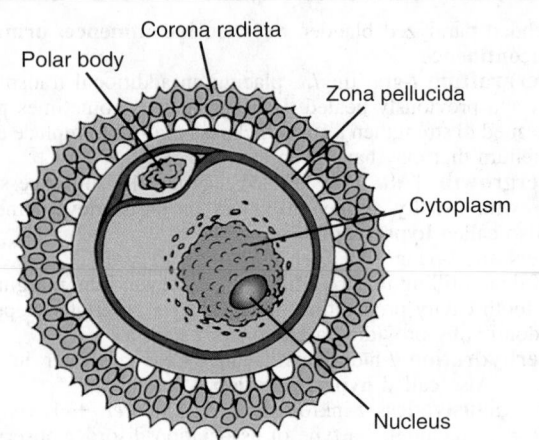

**Ovum** *(Lowdermilk, Perry, and Bobak, 2000)*

**ox-, oxi-,** combining form meaning 'presence of oxygen': *oxidize.*

**oxacillin sodium** /ok′səsil′in/, a penicillinase-resistant penicillin antibiotic.

■ INDICATION: It is prescribed in the treatment of severe bacterial infections caused by penicillinase-producing staphylococci.

■ CONTRAINDICATIONS: Known hypersensitivity to this drug or to any other penicillin prohibits its use.

■ ADVERSE EFFECTS: Among the most serious effects are anaphylaxis and other less severe allergic reactions, GI disturbances, and pruritus ani and vulvae.

**-oxacin,** combining form for nalidixic acid-type antibacterial agents.

**oxal-, oxalo-,** combining forms indicating molecules derived from oxalic acid: *oxaloacetate, oxalic.*

**oxalate** $(C_2O_4^{2-})$ /ok′səlāt/, an anion of oxalic acid.

**oxalated blood** /ok′səlā′tid/, blood to which a soluble ester of oxalic acid has been added to prevent coagulation.

**oxalemia** /ok′səlē′mē·ə/, elevated levels of oxalates in the blood.

**oxalic acid** $(H_2C_2O_4)$ /oksal′ik/, a member of a family of dibasic acids found in many common plants, such as buckwheat, wood sorrel, and rhubarb. It is an important reagent and is used in bleaching and drying. Poisonous if ingested, oxalic acid is used in veterinary medicine as a hemostatic. In dietary intake of foods containing oxalic acid, the substance binds with calcium and is sometimes found in renal calculi and urine of patients with hyperoxaluria. Also called **ethanedioic acid.**

**oxalosis** /ok′səlō′sis/, a condition in which calcium oxalate crystals accumulate in the kidneys, heart, and other organs and urinary excretion of oxalate increases. Oxalosis-inducing agents include oxalic acid, methoxyflurane, ethylene glycol, and ascorbic acid.

**oxaluric acid** /ok′səloor′ik/, a compound derived from uric acid or from parabanic acid, which occurs in normal urine.

**oxamniquine** /oksam′nəkwēn/, an antischistosomal.

■ INDICATION: It is prescribed in the treatment of infection caused by *Schistosoma mansoni.*

■ CONTRAINDICATIONS: Renal failure, congestive heart failure, or known hypersensitivity to this drug prohibits its use.

■ ADVERSE EFFECTS: Among the more serious adverse reactions are dizziness, drowsiness, and convulsions, particularly in patients with a history of epilepsy.

**-oxan,** combining form for benzodioxan-derived alpha-adrenoceptor antagonists.

**oxandrolone** /oksan'drəlōn/, an androgen.

■ INDICATIONS: It is prescribed in the treatment of bone pain accompanying osteoporosis and for the stimulation of weight gain after extensive surgery or trauma or when a pathophysiologic reason exists for failure to maintain normal weight.

■ CONTRAINDICATIONS: Cancer of the male breast or prostate, liver disease, pregnancy or suspected pregnancy, or known hypersensitivity to this drug prohibits its use.

■ ADVERSE EFFECTS: Among the more serious adverse reactions are hirsutism, acne, liver toxicity, electrolyte imbalances, and various endocrine effects in some patients.

**oxazepam** /oksā'zəpam/, a benzodiazepine tranquilizer.

■ INDICATIONS: It is prescribed to relieve anxiety and nervous tension.

■ CONTRAINDICATIONS: Acute narrow-angle glaucoma, psychotic disorders, or known hypersensitivity to this drug prohibits its use.

■ ADVERSE EFFECTS: Among the more serious adverse reactions are withdrawal symptoms resulting from discontinuation of treatment. Dizziness and fatigue commonly occur.

**-oxef,** combining form for oxacefalosporanic acid-derived antibiotics.

**-oxemia,** combining form meaning a '(specified) state of oxygen in the blood': *anoxemia, hyperoxemia, hypoxemia.*

**-oxia,** combining form meaning '(condition of) oxygenation': *anoxia, asthenoxia, hypoxia.*

**oxidant** /ok'sidənt/ [Gk, *oxys,* sharp], an oxidizing agent.

**oxidase** /ok'sidās/ [Gk, *oxys,* sharp], an enzyme that induces biologic oxidation by activating the oxygen in molecules containing the element, such as hydrogen peroxide.

**oxidation** /ok'sidā'shən/ [Gk, *oxys,* sharp, *genein,* to produce, L, *atio,* process], **1.** any process in which the oxygen content of a compound is increased. **2.** any reaction in which the positive valence of a compound or a radical is increased because of a loss of electrons. —**oxidize,** *v.,* **oxidative,** *n.*

**oxidation-reduction reaction,** a chemical change in which electrons are removed (oxidation) from an atom, ion, or molecule, accompanied by a simultaneous transfer of electrons (reduction) to another. Also called **redox.**

**oxidative phosphorylation** /ok'sidā'tiv/, an ATP-generating process in which oxygen serves as the final electron acceptor. The process occurs in mitochondria and is the major source of adenosine triphosphate generation in aerobic organisms.

**oxidative water** [Gk, *oxys,* sharp, *genein,* to produce, L, *ativus,* related to], water produced by the oxidation of molecules of food substances, such as the conversion of glucose to water and carbon dioxide.

**oxide** /ok'sīd/, **1.** a compound of oxygen and another element or radical. **2.** a dianion of oxygen, $O^{2-}$.

**oxidize** /ok'sidīz/ [Gk, *oxys,* sharp, *genein,* to produce, *izein,* to cause], (of an element or compound) to combine or cause to combine with oxygen, to remove hydrogen, or to increase the valence of an element through the loss of electrons. —**oxidation,** *n.,* **oxidizing,** *adj.*

**oxidizing agent,** a compound that readily gives up oxygen or attracts hydrogen or electrons from another compound. In chemical reactions an oxidizing agent acts as an acceptor of electrons, thereby increasing the valence of an element.

**oxidoreductase** /ok'sidō'riduk'tās/, an enzyme that catalyzes a reaction in which one substance is oxidized while another is reduced. An example is alcohol dehydrogenase.

**oximeter** /oksim'ətər/, a device used to measure oxyhemoglobin in arterial blood. See **pulse oximeter.**

**Pulse oximeter** *(Wilson and Giddens, 2001)*

**oximetry,** a photodiagnostic method of monitoring arterial blood oxygen saturation ($SaO_2$). Oximetry is commonly used to titrate levels of oxygen on hospitalized patients. It is used for monitoring the patient's oxygenation status during the perioperative period or any other time of heavy sedation, for patients receiving mechanical ventilation, and in many clinical situations such as pulmonary rehabilitation programs and stress testing.

**Oxsoralen,** trademark for a pigmentation agent (methoxsalen).

**oxtriphylline** /oks'trəfil'ēn/, a bronchodilator.

■ INDICATIONS: It is prescribed in the treatment of bronchial asthma, bronchitis, and emphysema.

■ CONTRAINDICATIONS: Known hypersensitivity to this drug or other xanthine derivatives prohibits its use. It is used with caution in patients with ulcer or with coronary disease for whom cardiac stimulation might be harmful.

■ ADVERSE EFFECTS: Among the more common adverse reactions are GI distress, palpitations, nervousness, and insomnia.

**oxy-,** **1.** combining form meaning 'sharp, quick, or sour': *oxyblepsia, oxycephalia, oxyecoia.* **2.** combining form indicating the presence of oxygen in a compound: *oxyacanthine, oxycamphor, oxyquinoline.*

**Oxy-5,** trademark for a keratolytic (benzoyl peroxide).

**oxyacoia,** an abnormal hearing acuity. Increased sensitivity to sound is sometimes associated with paralysis of the stapedius muscle.

**oxybenzene.** See **carbolic acid.**

**oxybutynin chloride** /ok'sibōō'tinin/, an anticholinergic.

■ INDICATION: It is prescribed in the treatment of neurogenic bladder.

■ CONTRAINDICATIONS: Glaucoma, obstruction of the GI or urinary tract, ulcerative colitis, paralytic ileus, toxic megacolon, or known hypersensitivity to this drug or to other anticholinergics prohibits its use.

■ ADVERSE EFFECTS: Among the more serious adverse effects are decreased sweating, urinary retention, blurred vision, tachycardia, and severe allergic reactions.

**oxycalorimeter** /ok′sēkal′ôrim′ətər/, an apparatus that measures the heat of combustion of organic materials in terms of oxygen consumed. Each liter of oxygen is roughly equivalent to 5 kilocalories,

**oxycellulose** /ok′sēsel′yəlōs/, **1.** cellulose that has been oxidized so that all or most of the glucose residues have been converted to glucuronic acid residues for use as an absorbent in chromatography. **2.** cellulose that has been partially oxidized for use as a local hemostatic.

**oxycephaly** /ok′sisef′əlē/ [Gk, *oxys* + *kephale*, head], a congenital malformation of the skull in which premature closure of the coronal and sagittal sutures results in accelerated upward growth of the head, giving it a long, narrow appearance with the top pointed or conic. Also called **acrocephaly, hypsicephaly, oxycephalia, steeple head, tower head, tower skull, turricephaly.** See also **craniostenosis.** —**oxycephalus**, *n.*, **oxycephalous**, *adj.*

**oxycodone hydrochloride** /ok′sikōdōn/, an opioid analgesic.

■ INDICATION: It is used to treat moderate to severe pain.

■ CONTRAINDICATIONS: It is used with caution in many conditions, including head injuries, asthma, impaired renal or hepatic function, or unstable cardiovascular status. Known hypersensitivity to this drug prohibits its use.

■ ADVERSE EFFECTS: Among the most serious adverse reactions are drowsiness, dizziness, nausea, constipation, respiratory and circulatory depression, and drug addiction.

**oxygen (O)** /ok′səjən/ [Gk, *oxys*, sharp, *genein*, to produce], a tasteless, odorless, colorless gas essential for human respiration. Its atomic weight (mass) is 15.9994; its atomic number is 8. In anesthesia, oxygen functions as a carrier gas for the delivery of anesthetic agents to tissues. In respiratory therapy oxygen is administered to increase the amount circulating in the blood. Overdose of oxygen can cause irreversible toxicity in people with pulmonary abnormalities, especially when complicated by chronic carbon dioxide retention. Prolonged administration of high concentrations of oxygen may cause irreversible damage to infants' eyes. An oxygen-rich environment is favorable to fire and explosion; thus smoking, open flame, or electric spark must be avoided when oxygen is being administered. See also **oxygen toxicity.**

**oxygenation** /ok′səjənā′shən/, the process of combining or treating with oxygen. —**oxygenate,** *v.*

**oxygen capacity of blood,** the maximum amount of oxygen that can combine chemically with a given amount of hemoglobin in blood. It does not include oxygen dissolved in plasma. Although 1 g of hemoglobin theoretically can bind a maximum of 1.34 mL of oxygen at standard temperature and pressure, this value is never actually achieved in vivo because of factors such as the formation of carboxyhemoglobin and the presence of methemoglobin or other inactive hemoglobins.

**oxygen concentration in blood,** the concentration of oxygen in a blood sample, including both oxygen combined with hemoglobin and oxygen dissolved in the plasma.

**oxygen consumption,** the amount of oxygen used by the body per minute. For normal aerobic metabolism, it is about 250 mL/min. Also called **oxygen uptake.**

**oxygen cost of breathing,** the rate at which the respiratory muscles consume oxygen as they ventilate the lungs.

**oxygen debt,** the quantity of oxygen that the lungs take up during recovery from exercise or apnea that is in excess of the quantity needed for resting metabolism before the exercise or apnea. Oxygen debt represents replenishment of the oxygen store that was depleted during the time that oxygen

uptake from the air was inadequate for aerobic metabolism. See also **oxygen uptake.**

**oxygen enhancement ratio (OER),** a measure of tumor sensitivity to the presence or absence of oxygen, expressed as the ratio of radiation dose required to produce a given effect with no oxygen present to the dose required to produce the same effect in 1 atmosphere of air.

**oxygen half-saturation pressure of hemoglobin,** the oxygen pressure necessary for 50% saturation of hemoglobin at body temperature and at pH 7.4 or 40 mm Hg of carbon dioxide pressure. The value is commonly used as a measure of the affinity between oxygen and hemoglobin.

**oxygen hood,** a device placed over the head of patients to deliver high concentrations of oxygen.

**oxygen mask,** a device used to administer oxygen. It is shaped to fit snugly over the mouth and nose and may be secured in place with a strap or held with the hand. The mask has inspiratory and expiratory valves allowing oxygen to be inhaled or pumped into the respiratory tract and carbon dioxide to be exhaled into the environment. Oxygen flows at a prescribed rate through a catheter to the mask. See also **Ambu-bag.**

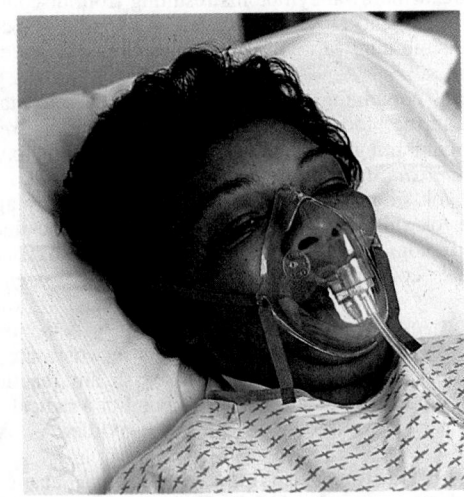

**Oxygen mask** *(Potter and Perry, 2001)*

**oxygen radicals** [Gk, *oxys*, sharp; L, *radix*, root], a substituent group of chemical elements rich in oxygen but incapable of prolonged existence in a free state. Oxygen radicals are used in some types of therapy.

**oxygen saturation,** the fraction of the hemoglobin molecules in a blood sample that are saturated with oxygen at a given partial pressure of oxygen.

**oxygen store,** the total quantity of oxygen stored in various body compartments, including the lungs, arterial and venous blood, and tissues. In a 70-kg human, blood contains about 800 mL of oxygen as oxyhemoglobin, muscles contain about 150 mL as oxymyoglobin, alveolar gas contains a few hundred milliliters, and about 50 mL is dissolved in the tissues.

**oxygen tension,** the partial pressure of oxygen molecules dissolved in a liquid, such as blood plasma.

**oxygen tent** [Gk, *oxys*, sharp; ME, *tente*], a canopy that encloses the head and neck of a patient and provides humidified oxygen. See **Croupette.**

**oxygen therapy**[1], any procedure in which oxygen is administered to a patient to relieve hypoxia.

■ METHOD: Of the many methods for providing oxygen therapy, the one selected depends on the condition of the patient and the cause of hypoxia. Low or moderate amounts of oxygen may be supplied to postoperative patients by a nasal catheter or cannula. A precise amount of oxygen may be delivered by a Venturi mask. Patients with chronic obstructive lung disease must receive low-flow oxygen to prevent eliminating their stimulus to breathe (low $O_2$ levels). If hypoxia is the result of impaired cardiac function, a high concentration of oxygen may be delivered by a nonrebreathing or partial rebreathing mask. Humidity and drugs in aerosol form may be given with oxygen using a variety of devices, such as an aerosol face mask, Croupette, or T-piece.

■ INTERVENTIONS: Thorough and careful observation of the patient's need for oxygen and response to therapy are important. The concentration of oxygen received by the patient must not be assumed by the rate and concentration at which it is delivered; a person whose respirations are rapid and shallow receives more oxygen than does a person breathing deeply and slowly. Many clinical situations require frequent laboratory evaluations of the levels of arterial blood gases or oxygen saturation levels via pulse oximetry. Thorough knowledge of the equipment used and the condition being treated enables the nurse to care safely and effectively for the patient who requires oxygen.

■ OUTCOME CRITERIA: Oxygen therapy may be used in the treatment of any condition that results in hypoxia. Although there are several kinds of hypoxia, all result in hypoxemia. Oxygen administration may relieve hypotension, cardiac arrhythmias, tachypnea, headache, disorientation, nausea, and agitation characteristic of hypoxia, as well as restore the ability of the cells of the body to carry on normal metabolic function.

**oxygen therapy**[2], a nursing intervention from the Nursing Interventions Classification (NIC) defined as administration of oxygen and monitoring of its effectiveness. See also **Nursing Interventions Classification.**

**oxygen tolerance,** an increased capacity to withstand the toxic effects of abnormally high oxygen tension as a result of any adaptive change occurring within an organism.

**oxygen toxicity,** a condition of oxygen overdosage that can result in pathologic tissue changes, such as retinopathy of prematurity or bronchopulmonary dysplasia. It can also decrease $CO_2$ drive to breathe.

**oxygen transport,** the process by which oxygen is absorbed in the lungs by the hemoglobin in circulating deoxygenated red cells and carried to the peripheral tissues. The process is made possible because hemoglobin has the ability to combine with oxygen present at a high concentration, such as in the lungs, and to release this oxygen when the concentration is low, such as in the peripheral tissues. See also **hemoglobin.**

**oxygen uptake.** See **oxygen consumption.**

**oxygen-utilization coefficient.** See **coefficient.**

**oxyhemoglobin** /ok'sēhē'məglō'bin, -hem'-/ [Gk, *oxys* + *genein*, to produce, *haima*, blood; L, *globus*, ball], the product of combining hemoglobin with oxygen. The loosely bound complex dissociates easily when the concentration of oxygen is low. Also spelled **oxyhaemoglobin.**

**oxyhemoglobin dissociation curve,** a graphic expression of the affinity between oxygen and hemoglobin, or the amount of oxygen chemically bound at equilibrium to the

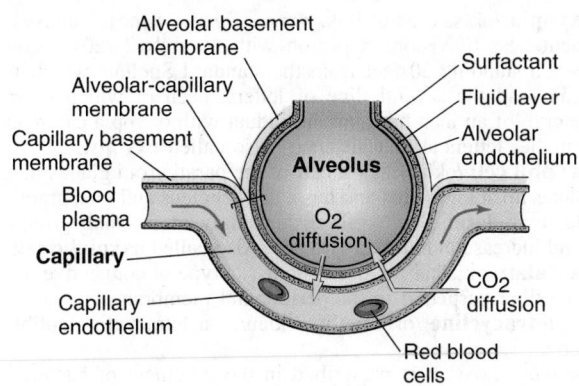

Alveolar basement membrane
Alveolar-capillary membrane
Capillary basement membrane
Blood plasma
**Capillary**
Capillary endothelium
**Alveolus**
$O_2$ diffusion
Surfactant
Fluid layer
Alveolar endothelium
$CO_2$ diffusion
Red blood cells

**Oxygen transport** (Beare and Myers, 1998)

hemoglobin in blood as a function of oxygen pressure. To define the curve completely, it should also include the pH, temperature, and carbon dioxide pressure.

**oxyhemoglobin saturation,** the amount of oxygen actually combined with hemoglobin, expressed as a percentage of the oxygen capacity of that hemoglobin.

**Oxylone,** trademark for a glucocorticoid (fluorometholone).

**oxymesterone** /ok'sēmes'tərōn/, an androgen and anabolic steroid involved in tissue building.

**oxymetazoline hydrochloride** /ok'sēmətaz'əlēn/, a decongestant.

■ INDICATION: It is prescribed in the treatment of nasal congestion and for the relief of eye redness caused by minor eye irritation.

■ CONTRAINDICATIONS: Hyperthyroidism, diabetes, use of a monoamine oxidase inhibitor within 14 days, or known hypersensitivity to this drug prohibits its use.

■ ADVERSE EFFECTS: Among the more serious adverse reactions are rebound congestion, central nervous system stimulation, and in children a severe shocklike syndrome with coma, hypotension, and bradycardia.

**oxymetholone** /ok'sēmeth'əlōn/, an anabolic steroid.

■ INDICATIONS: It is prescribed in the treatment of testosterone deficiency, osteoporosis, and female breast cancer and to stimulate growth, weight gain, and red blood cell production.

■ CONTRAINDICATIONS: Cancer of the male breast or prostate, liver disease, pregnancy or suspected pregnancy, or known hypersensitivity to this drug prohibits its use.

■ ADVERSE EFFECTS: Among the more serious adverse reactions are hirsutism, acne, liver toxicity, electrolyte imbalances, and, depending on the patient's age, various endocrine effects.

**oxymorphone hydrochloride** /ok'sēmôr'fōn/, an opioid analgesic.

■ INDICATIONS: It is prescribed for relief of moderate to severe pain, as a preoperative medication, and to support anesthesia.

■ CONTRAINDICATION: Drug dependence or known hypersensitivity to this drug prohibits its use.

■ ADVERSE EFFECTS: Among the more serious adverse reactions are drug dependence, urinary retention, and respiratory or circulatory depression.

**oxyntic cell,** a hydrochloric-acid producing cell of the stomach.

**oxyopia** /ok′sē·ō′pē·ə/ [Gk, *oxys* + *opsis* vision], unusual acuteness of vision. A person with normal (20/20) vision when standing 20 feet from the standard Snellen eye chart can read the seventh line of letters, each of which is an eighth of an inch high; an individual with oxyopia can read smaller letters at that distance. Also called **oxyopy.**

**oxyphil cell** /ok′səfil/, a cell of the parathyroid glands that takes up acidic stains and has a dark nucleus and fine, granular cytoplasm. Such cells occur singly or in small groups and increase in number with age. Also called **oxyphilic cell.**

**oxytalan** /ok′sētal′ən, oksit′ələn/, a type of connective tissue fiber particular to the periodontal membrane.

**oxytetracycline** /ok′sētet′rəsī′klēn/, a tetracycline antibiotic.

■ INDICATIONS: It is prescribed in the treatment of bacterial and rickettsial infections.

■ CONTRAINDICATIONS: Pregnancy, early childhood, or known hypersensitivity to this or other tetracyclines prohibits its use. The drug is used with caution in patients who have renal or liver dysfunction.

■ ADVERSE EFFECTS: Among the more serious adverse reactions are GI disturbances, phototoxicity, potentially serious superinfections, and various hypersensitivity reactions. Discoloration of teeth may occur in children exposed to the drug in utero or before 8 years of age.

**oxytetracycline calcium,** a tetracycline antibiotic.

**oxytocia** /ok′sētō′shə/, rapid childbirth.

**oxytocic** /ok′sitō′sik/ [Gk, *oxys* + *tokos,* birth], **1.** pertaining to a substance that is similar to the hormone oxytocin. **2.** any one of numerous drugs that stimulate the smooth muscle of the uterus to contract. The administration of an oxytocic can initiate and enhance rhythmic uterine contraction at any time, but relatively high doses are required for such responses in early pregnancy. These drugs are often used to initiate labor at term. Oxytocic agents commonly used include oxytocin, certain prostaglandins, and the ergot alkaloids. These drugs are used to induce or augment labor, control postpartum hemorrhage, correct postpartum uterine atony, produce uterine contractions after cesarean section or other uterine surgery, and induce therapeutic abortion. These drugs are used with extreme caution in parturients with severe hypotension and hypertension, partial placenta previa, cephalopelvic disproportion, or grand multiparity. The risk of using these agents is much higher in mothers who have undergone recent uterine surgery or who have suffered recent sepsis or trauma. The most serious adverse reaction is sustained tetanic contraction of the uterus, resulting in fetal hypoxia or in rupture of the uterus.

**oxytocin** /ok′sitō′sin/, an oxytocic.

■ INDICATIONS: It is prescribed to stimulate contractions in inducing or augmenting labor and to contract the uterus to control postpartum bleeding.

■ CONTRAINDICATIONS: Cephalopelvic disproportion, unfavorable fetal position, or known hypersensitivity to this drug prohibits its use.

■ ADVERSE EFFECTS: Among the more serious adverse reactions are tetanic contraction, jaundice, uterine rupture, and fetal anoxia.

**oxytocin challenge test,** a stress test for the assessment of intrauterine function of the fetus and the placenta. It is performed to evaluate the ability of the fetus to tolerate continuation of pregnancy or the anticipated stress of labor and delivery. A dilute IV infusion of oxytocin is begun, regulated by an infusion pump. The uterine activity is monitored with a tocodynamometer, and the fetal heart rate is monitored with an ultrasonic sensor as the uterus is stimulated to contract by the oxytocin. The amount of solution infused is increased as necessary to cause the uterus to contract for 30 to 40 seconds three times every 10 minutes. The fetal heart rate is observed for variability and for the timing of any marked variation from the normal in relation to uterine contractions. Decelerations of the fetal heart rate in certain repeating patterns may indicate fetal distress. One quarter of the infants diagnosed by this method as being in distress are normal; therefore other tests of fetal well-being are recommended before performing an emergency cesarean section or induction of labor.

**oxyuriasis.** See **enterobiasis.**

**oxyuricide** /ok′sē·oo′risīd/, an agent that destroys oxyur pinworms, or nematodes.

***Oxyuris vermicularis.*** Also called ***Enterobius vermicularis.***

**oz,** abbreviation for **ounce.**

**oz ap** [L, *uncia*], abbreviation for *apothecary ounce,* a unit of weight equal to 31.1035 grams.

**ozena** /ōzē′nə/ [Gk, *ozein,* to have an odor], a condition of the nose characterized by atrophy of the nasal conchae and mucous membranes. Symptoms include crusting of nasal secretions, discharge, and, especially, a very offensive odor. Ozena may follow chronic inflammation of the nasal mucosa.

**ozone (O$_3$)** [Gk, *ozein,* to have an odor], a form of oxygen consisting of three atoms. Ozone is formed when oxygen is present in an electric discharge, as might occur in a lightning storm. Ozone is used as a bleaching, cleaning, and oxidizing agent and has a faint, chlorinelike odor.

**ozone hole,** a seasonal depletion of the steady-state ozone concentration in the stratosphere, particularly over Antarctica.

**ozone shield,** the layer of ozone that hangs in the atmosphere from 20 to 40 miles above the surface of the earth and protects the earth from excessive ultraviolet radiation. Some experts claim that the manufacture of various chemicals, such as chlorofluorocarbons used as propellants in aerosol sprays, and the effects of high-flying jet aircraft are destroying this protective layer and allowing excessive amounts of ultraviolet radiation to penetrate the earth's atmosphere, thus subjecting humans to increased dangers of skin cancer and other health problems. Some chemistry experts and federal health officials also claim that an additional threat comes from nitrous oxide in nitrogenous fertilizers rising into the atmosphere and reacting unfavorably with the ozone shield. The ozone shield is implicated in certain health problems that affect some air travelers. See also **ozone sickness.**

**ozone sickness,** an abnormal condition caused by the inhalation of ozone that may seep into jet aircraft at altitudes over 40,000 feet. It is characterized by headaches, chest pains, itchy eyes, and sleepiness. Exactly why and how ozone causes this condition is not known. It is more prevalent early in the year and occurs more often over the Pacific Ocean.

**oz t** [L, *uncia*], abbreviation for *troy ounce,* a unit of weight equal to 31.103 grams.

**P, 1.** symbol for the element **phosphorus. 2.** symbol for *gas partial pressure.* See **partial pressure. 3.** symbol for *after* or **post. 4.** (in genetics) symbol for *first parental generation.* **5.** symbol for *first pulmonic sound.*

**p17,** symbol for a protein that lines the interior of the human immunodeficiency virus envelope.

**p24,** symbol for a protein that surrounds the ribonucleic acid and reverse transcriptase of the human immunodeficiency virus.

**P1E1, P2E1, P3E1, P4E1, P6E1,** trademarks for ophthalmic fixed-combination drugs containing a cholinergic (pilocarpine hydrochloride) and an adrenergic (epinephrine bitartrate). The numbers indicate the percentage of each ingredient in the solution; for example, P2E1 contains 2% pilocarpine hydrochloride and 1% epinephrine bitartrate.

**p-,** symbol for **para-.**

**P$_2$,** symbol for *second pulmonic sound.*

**P$_{50}$,** the partial pressure of oxygen at which hemoglobin is half saturated with bound oxygen.

**pA,** abbreviation for *picoampere.*

**Pa, 1.** symbol for *pascal.* **2.** symbol for the element **protactinium.**

**PA, 1.** abbreviation for **physician's assistant. 2.** abbreviation for **pulmonary artery.**

**P-A, p-a,** abbreviation for **posteroanterior.**

**P&A, 1.** abbreviation for *percussion and auscultation.* See **p and a. 2.** abbreviation for *posterior and anterior.*

**PABA,** abbreviation for **paraaminobenzoic acid,** a topical sunscreen.

**pabulin** /pab'yəlin/ [L, *pabulum,* food], products of fat and protein digestion found in the blood after a meal.

**pabulum** /pab'yələm/ [L, food], any substance that is food or nutrient.

**pac,** abbreviation for *phenacetin-aspirin-caffeine.*

**PAC,** abbreviation for **premature atrial complex.**

**PA catheter.** See **pulmonary artery catheter.**

**pacchionian foramen** /pak'ē·ō'nē·ən/ [Antonio Pacchioni, Italian anatomist, 1665–1720], a thick opening in the center of the diaphragm of sella through which the infundibulum passes. Also called **foramen diaphragmatis.**

**pacchionian granulations.** See **arachnoid villi.**

**PACE** /pās/, abbreviation for **Program of All-Inclusive Care of the Elderly.**

**PACE II,** an interdisciplinary assessment and planning system that focuses on evaluation of the physical health of nursing home residents. It includes checklists of defined (diagnosed) conditions, abnormal laboratory or other findings, risk factors, and other impairments and disabilities.

**pacemaker** [L, *passus,* step; AS, *macian,* to make], **1.** the sinoatrial node composed of specialized nervous tissue located at the junction of the superior vena cava and the right atrium. It initiates the contractions of the atria, which transmit the impulse onto the atrioventricular (AV) node, thereby initiating the contraction of the ventricles. An ectopic or idioventricular pacemaker, originating in the atria, AV node, or ventricle, may cause contractions in cases of abnormal heart functioning. **2.** also called **cardiac pacemaker.** an electric apparatus used in most cases to increase the heart rate in severe bradycardia by electrically stimulating the heart muscle. A pacemaker may be permanent or temporary, emit the stimulus at a constant and fixed rate, or fire only on demand.

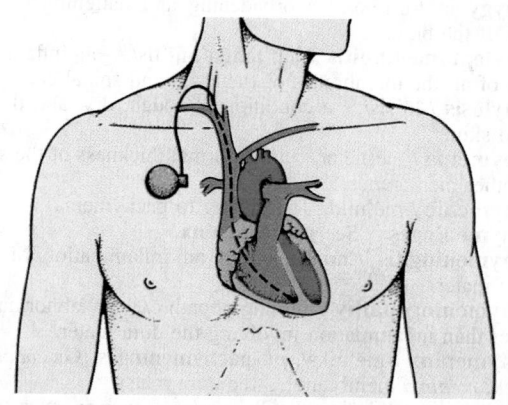

**Pacemaker** *(Thibodeau and Patton, 1999/George Wassilchenko)*

**pacemaker installation fluoroscopy,** the fluoroscopic monitoring of the insertion of an artificial pacemaker, used as an aid for correct installation of the device.

**pacer.** See **pacemaker.**

**pachometer.** See **pachymeter.**

**pachy-** /pak'i-/, combining form meaning 'thick': *pachycephaly, pachymucosa.*

**pachyblepharon** /-blef'əron/ [Gk, *pachy,* thick], a thickening of the tarsal border of the eyelid.

**pachycephalia.** See **pachycephaly.**

**pachycephalic** /-səfal'ik/, pertaining to an abnormal thickening of the skull.

**pachycephaly** /pak'ēsef'əlē/ [Gk, *pachy,* thick, *kephale,* head], an abnormal thickness of the skull, as in acromegaly. Also called **pachycephalia. —pachycephalic, pachycephalous,** *adj.*

**pachycheilia** /-kī'lē·ə/, an abnormal thickening or swelling of the lips.

**pachycholia** /-kō'lē·ə/, thickness of the bile.

**pachychromatic** /-krōmat'ik/, characterized by coarse chromatin filaments.

**pachychymia** /-kī'mē·ə/, thickness of the chyme.

**pachydactyly** /pak'ēdak'tilē/ [Gk, *pachy* + *daktylos,* finger], an abnormal thickening of the fingers or toes. **—pachydactylic, pachydactylous,** *adj.*

**pachyderma** /-dur'mə/, an overgrowth or thickening of the skin and subcutaneous tissues.

**pachyderma alba** /-dur'mə/ [Gk, *pachy* + *derma,* skin; L, *albus,* white], an abnormal state in which the buccal mucosa has an appearance suggestive of whitened elephant hide. Also called **pachyderma oralis.**

**pachyderma laryngis,** an overgrowth of epithelium over the vocal cords.

**pachyderma oralis.** See **pachyderma alba.**

**pachydermatous** /-dur'mətəs/, pertaining to a condition of pachyderma.

**pachyderma vesicae,** a potentially malignant condition of white plaques in the mucous membrane at the base of the bladder.

**pachydermoperiostosis** /-dur'moper'ē·ostō'sis/, a syndrome characterized by a thickening and folding of the facial skin, clubbing of the fingers, and new bone formation over the ends of the long bones.

**pachyglossia** /-glos'ē·ə/, an abnormal thickening of the tongue.

**pachygnathy** /-gnoth'əs/, an abnormal thickening of the jaw. See also **macrognathia. —pachygnathous,** *adj.*

**pachygyria** /-jī'rē·ə/, a broadening and flattening of the gyri of the brain.

**pachyleptomeningitis** /-lep'təmin'injī'tis/, an inflammation of all the membranes of the brain and spinal cord.

**pachylosis** /-lō'sis/, a condition of rough, dry, and thickened skin.

**pachymenia** /-mē'nē·ə/, an abnormal thickness of the skin or other membranes.

**pachymenic** /-mē'nik/, pertaining to pachymenia.

**pachymeninges.** See **pachymeninx.**

**pachymeningitis** /-min'injī'tis/, an inflammation of the dura mater.

**pachymeningopathy** /-mining'gōpath'ē/, an abnormality other than inflammation involving the dura mater.

**pachymeninx** /-mē'niks/, *pl.* **pachymeninges** [Gk, *pachys,* thick, *meninx,* membrane], the dura mater.

**pachymeter** /pakim'ətər/ [Gk, *pachy* + *metron,* measure], an instrument used to measure thickness, especially of a thin structure, such as a membrane or a tissue. Also called **pachometer.**

**pachynema** /pak'inē'mə/ [Gk, *pachy* + *nema,* thread], the postsynaptic tetradic chromosome formation that occurs in the pachytene stage of the first meiotic prophase of gametogenesis.

**pachynsis** /pakin'sis/, any thickening of tissues having a pathologic cause.

**pachyonychia** /pak'ē·ōnik'ē·ə/, an abnormal thickness of the finger or toe nails.

**pachyonychia congenita** [Gk, *pachy* + *onyx,* nail; L, *congenitus,* born with], a congenital deformity characterized by abnormal thickening and raising of the nails on the fin-

gers and the toes and hyperkeratosis of the palms of the hands and the soles of the feet. The papillae of the tongue also atrophy, causing a whitish coating over the lingual surface.

**pachyotia** /pak'ē·ō'shə/, an abnormal thickness of the auricle of the ears. Also called **boxers' ear.** See also **cauliflower ear.**

**pachypelviperitonitis** /-pel'vēper'itənī'tis/, pelvic peritonitis associated with a thickening of the tissues.

**pachyperitonitis** /-per'itənī'tis/, an inflammation and abnormal thickening of the tissues of the peritoneum.

**pachypleuritis** /-ploŏrī'tis/, an inflammation and thickening of the pleural membranes.

**pachysalpingitis.** See **parenchymatous salpingitis.**

**pachysalpingoovaritis** /-salping'gō·ō'verī'tis/, an inflammation and thickening of the tissues of the ovaries and fallopian tubes.

**pachysomia** /-sō'mē·ə/ [Gk, *pachys,* thick, *soma,* body], an abnormal thickening of the soft tissues of the body.

**pachytene** /pak'itēn/ [Gk, *pachy* + *tainia,* ribbon], the third stage in the first meiotic prophase of gametogenesis, in which the paired homologous chromosomes form tetrads. The bivalent pairs become short and thick and intertwine so that four chromatids are visible. See also **diakinesis, diplotene, leptotene, zygotene.**

**pachyvaginalitis** /-vaj'inəlī'tis/, an inflammation and thickening of the tunica vaginalis testis.

**pachyvaginitis** /-vaj'inī'tis/, an inflammation and thickening of the walls of the vagina.

**pacifier** /pas'ifī'ər/ [L, *pacificare,* to bring peace], **1.** an agent that soothes or comforts. **2.** a nipple-shaped object used by infants and children for sucking. Such devices can be dangerous if they are too small or poorly constructed, because the entire object or part of it can be aspirated or lodged in the pharynx or trachea and obstruct the passage of air. The safest pacifiers are constructed in one piece, are large enough that only the nipple fits into the mouth, and have a handle that can be easily grasped.

**pacing** [L, *passus,* step], setting of the heart's rhythm by the sinus node, by another site in the heart, or by an artificial electrical stimulator. Also called **atrial pacing, endocardial pacing, sequential pacing.** See also **programmable pacemaker.**

**pacing wire** [L, *passus,* step; AS, *wir*], the electrical connection between a pulse generator and a pacing electrode in a cardiac pacemaker.

**Pacini's corpuscles** /päsē'nēz/ [Filippo Pacini, Italian anatomist, 1812–1883; L, *corpusculum,* little body], special sensory end organs resembling tiny white bulbs. Each is attached to the end of a single nerve fiber in the subcutaneous, submucous, and subserous connective tissue of many parts of the body, especially the palm of the hand, sole of the foot, genital organs, joints, and pancreas. They average

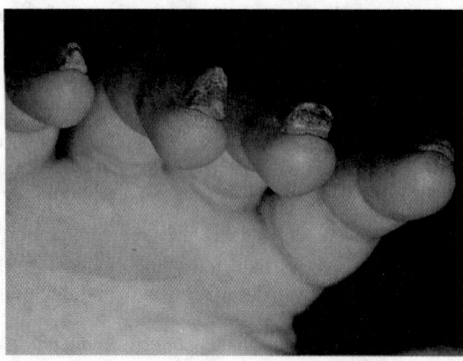

**Pachyonychia congenita**
*(Hordinsky, Sawaya, and Scher, 2000)*

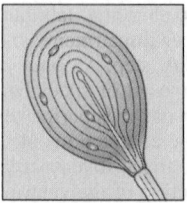

**Pacini's corpuscle**
*(Thibodeau and Patton, 1999/Network Graphics)*

about 3 mm in diameter, are pressure sensitive and vibration sensitive, contain numerous concentric layers around a central core, and in cross section resemble an onion. Also called **pacinian corpuscles.** Compare **Golgi-Mazzoni corpuscles, Krause's corpuscles.**

**pacinitis** /pas'inī'tis/, an inflammation of the pacinian corpuscles.

**pack** [ME, *pakke,* bundle], **1.** a treatment in which the entire body or a portion of it is wrapped in wet or dry towels or in ice for various therapeutic purposes, as with cold packs for reducing high temperatures and swellings or for inducing hypothermia during certain surgical procedures, especially heart surgery and organ transplantation. **2.** a tampon. **3.** the act of applying a dressing or dental cement to a surgical wound. **4.** a surgical dressing to cover a wound or to fill the cavity left from extraction of a tooth, especially a wisdom tooth.

**package insert,** a leaflet that, by order of the Food and Drug Administration (FDA), must be placed inside the package of every prescription drug. In it the manufacturer is required to describe the drug, to state its generic name, and to give the applicable indications, contraindications, warnings, precautions, adverse effects, form, dosage, and administration.

**packed cells** [ME, *pakke,* bundle; L, *cella,* storeroom], a preparation of blood cells separated from liquid plasma, often administered in severe anemia to restore adequate levels of hemoglobin and red cells without overloading the vascular system with excess fluids. Also called **packed red blood cells.** See also **bank blood, component therapy, pooled plasma.**

**packed cell volume (PCV)** [ME, *pakke* + L, *cella,* storeroom, *volumen,* paper roll], a measured quantity of blood to which an anticoagulant has been added and the cells of which have been pressed together by the force of being centrifuged at 2000 rpm. Also called **hematocrit reading.**

**packed red blood cells.** See **packed cells.**

**packer,** an instrument for tamponing or introducing a pack of gauze into a wound. See also **plugger.**

**packing** [ME, *pakke*], **1.** material used to fill a wound or cavity. **2.** the act of inserting material into a wound or cavity especially a wound with tunneling.

***P. acnes.*** See *Propionibacterium.*

**PaCO₂,** abbreviation for **partial pressure of carbon dioxide in arterial blood.**

**pad** [D, *paden,* cushion], **1.** a mass of soft material used to cushion shock, prevent wear, or absorb moisture, such as the abdominal pads used to absorb discharges from abdominal wounds or to separate viscera and improve accessibility during abdominal surgery. **2.** (in anatomy) a mass of fat that cushions various structures, such as the infrapatellar pad lying below the patella among the patellar ligament, the head of the tibia, and the femoral condyles.

**PAD,** abbreviation for **peripheral arterial disease.**

**p.ae.** [L, *partes* + *aequales*], symbol for *equal parts.*

**paed-, paedo-.** See **ped-, pedo-.**

**paediatrician.** See **pediatrician.**

**paediatrics.** See **pediatrics.**

**paedogenesis.** See **pedogenesis.**

**paedophilia.** See **pedophilia.**

**pagetoid** /paj'ətoid/, resembling Paget's disease.

**Paget-Schroetter's syndrome, Paget-von Schroetter's syndrome.** See **effort thrombosis.**

**Paget's disease** /paj'əts/ [James Paget, English surgeon, 1814–1899], a common nonmetabolic disease of bone of unknown cause, usually affecting middle-aged and elderly

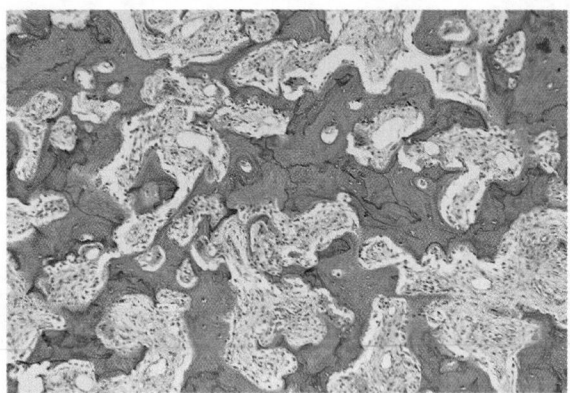

**Paget's disease** *(Regezi, Sciubba, and Pogrel, 2000)*

people, and characterized by excessive bone destruction and unorganized bone repair. Also called **osteitis deformans.**

**Paget's disease of the nipple.** See **nipple cancer.**

**pagophagia** /pā'gōfā'jē·ə/ [Gk, *pagos,* frost, *phagein,* to eat], an abnormal condition characterized by a craving to eat enormous quantities of ice. It is associated with a lack of the nutrient iron. —**pagophagic, pagophagous,** *adj.*

**-pagus,** suffix meaning 'conjoined twins': *craniopagus, pyropagus, thoracopagus.*

**PAHA,** abbreviation for **paraaminohippuric acid.**

**PAHA sodium clearance test,** a procedure formerly used for detecting kidney damage or certain muscle diseases that used the sodium salt of paraaminohippuric acid to determine the rate at which the kidneys removed this salt from the blood and urine.

**PAHO,** abbreviation for *Pan American Health Organization.*

**pain** [L, *poena,* punishment], an unpleasant sensation caused by noxious stimulation of the sensory nerve endings. It is a subjective feeling and an individual response to the cause. Pain is a cardinal symptom of inflammation and is valuable in the diagnosis of many disorders and conditions. It may be mild or severe, chronic, acute, lancinating, burning, dull or sharp, precisely or poorly localized, or referred. Experiencing pain is influenced by physical, mental, biochemical, psychological, physiological, social, cultural, and emotional factors. See also **referred pain.**

**pain, acute,** a nursing diagnosis accepted by the Fourth National Conference on the Classification of Nursing Diagnoses (revised 1996). Pain is defined as an unpleasant sensory and emotional experience arising from actual or potential tissue damage or described in terms of such damage (International Association for the Study of Pain); sudden or slow onset of any intensity from mild to severe with an anticipated or predictable end and a duration of less than 6 months.

■ DEFINING CHARACTERISTICS: Major defining characteristics are verbal or coded report, observed evidence; antalgic position; protective behavior; guarding behavior; antalgic gestures; facial mask; sleep disturbance (eyes lackluster, "hecohe look," fixed or scattered movement, grimace). Minor defining characteristics are self-focus; narrowed focus (altered time perception), impaired thought process; reduced interaction with people and environment; distraction behavior (pacing, seeking out of other people and/or activities, repetitive activities); autonomic alteration in muscle tone (may span from listless to rigid); autonomic responses (dia-

## Comparison of acute and chronic pain

| Characteristic | Acute pain | Chronic pain |
| --- | --- | --- |
| Onset | Usually sudden | May be sudden or develop insidiously |
| Duration | Transient (up to 3 months) | Prolonged (months to years) |
| Pain localization | Pain vs. nonpain areas generally well identified | Pain vs. nonpain areas less well identified; intensity becomes more difficult to evaluate (change in sensations) |
| Clinical signs | Signs of sympathetic overactivity (such as increased blood pressure) | Usually no change in vital signs (adaptation) |
| Purpose | Warning that something is wrong | Meaningless; no purpose |
| Pattern | Self-limiting or readily corrected | Continuous or intermittent; intensity may vary or remain constant |
| Prognosis | Likelihood of eventual complete relief | Complete relief usually not possible |

From Phipps WJ, Sands JK, Marek JE: *Medical-surgical nursing: concepts and clinical practice*, ed 6, St Louis, 1996, Mosby.

phoresis, blood pressure, respiration, pulse change, pupillary dilation); expressive behavior (restlessness, moaning, crying, vigilance, irritability, sighing); and changes in appetite and eating.

■ RISK FACTORS: Risk factors include injury agents (biologic, chemical, physical, psychologic). See also **nursing diagnosis.**

**pain and suffering,** (in law) an element in a claim for damages that allows recovery for the mental and physical pain, suffering, distress, and trauma that an individual has endured as a result of injury.

**pain assessment,** an evaluation of the reported pain and the factors that alleviate or exacerbate it, as well as the response to treatment of pain. Responses to pain vary widely among individuals, depending on many different physical and psychologic factors, such as specific diseases and injuries and the health, pain threshold, fear, anxiety, and cultural background of the individual involved, as well as the way the person expresses pain experiences. See also **pain intervention, pain pathway.**

■ METHOD: The patient is asked to describe the cause of the pain, if known; its intensity, location, and duration; the events preceding it; the pattern usually followed for handling pain; previous treatments and effectiveness; allergies; and ways in which the pain has affected the activities of daily living. Intensity of pain is often assessed using pain scales (numerical or face scales). Severe pain causes pallor, cold perspiration, piloerection, dilated pupils, and increases in the pulse, respiratory rate, blood pressure, and muscle tension. When brief, intense pain subsides, the pulse may be slower and the blood pressure lower than before the pain began. If pain occurs frequently or is prolonged, the pulse rate and blood pressure may not increase markedly, and, if pain persists for many days, there may be an increased production of eosinophils and 17-ketosteroids and greater susceptibility to infections. The patient's statements regarding pain; tone of voice, speed of speech, cries, groans, or other vocalizations; facial expressions; body movements; or tendency to withdraw are all noted. Pertinent background information in the assessment includes a record of the patient's chronic conditions, previous surgery, and any illnesses that caused pain; the patient's experiences with relatives and friends in pain; the role or position of the patient in the family structure; and the patient's use of alcohol and drugs, including OTC and illicit drug usage. Key aspects in evaluating pain intensity are the size of the area, the tenderness within the pain area, and the effects of movement and pressure on the pain. Duration of pain is considered in terms of hours, days, weeks, months, or years. Pain patterns are associated with various sensations such as burning, pricking, aching, rhyth-

mic throbbing, and effects on the sympathetic and the parasympathetic nervous systems. Evaluation includes the meanings the individual may attach to pain, such as a test of character, a penance, or a sign of worsening illness. Such interpretations may affect the intensity of pain and mask its significance.

■ INTERVENTIONS: The nurse establishes a relationship with the patient and uses individual or group counseling to teach the person about pain and how to modify the anxiety associated with it. Analgesics ordered for the patient are administered by the nurse before the pain becomes intense, to increase their effectiveness. In addition to helping promote rest and relaxation, the nurse decreases noxious stimuli, provides other pleasant sensory input, and helps to distract the patient by using guided imagery, walking, watching television, or reading. If the patient believes that certain acceptable measures alleviate pain, the nurse uses them.

■ OUTCOME CRITERIA: Dramatic relief of intense or chronic pain is often difficult to accomplish, but the patient can be helped to learn to handle pain effectively and to function fairly normally.

**pain, chronic,** a nursing diagnosis accepted by the Seventh National Conference on the Classification of Nursing Diagnoses (revised 1996). Chronic pain is defined as an unpleasant sensory and emotional experience arising from actual or potential tissue damage or described in terms of such damage (International Association for the Study of Pain); sudden or slow onset of any intensity from mild to severe; constant or recurring without an anticipated or predictable end; and a duration of greater than 6 months.

■ DEFINING CHARACTERISTICS: Major defining characteristics are a verbal or coded report or observed evidence of protective behavior; guarding behavior; facial mask; irritability; self-focusing; restlessness; and depression. Minor defining characteristics are atrophy of the involved muscle group; changes in sleep pattern; weight changes; fatigue; fear of reinjury; reduced interaction with people; altered ability to continue previous activities; sympathetic mediated responses (temperature, cold, changes of body position, hypersensitivity); and anorexia.

■ RELATED FACTORS: Related factors are physical and psychosocial disability. See also **nursing diagnosis.**

**pain control,** a nursing outcome from the Nursing Outcomes Classification (NOC) is defined as the personal actions to control pain. See also **Nursing Outcomes Classification.**

**pain: disruptive effects,** a nursing outcome from the Nursing Outcomes Classification (NOC) defined as the observed or reported disruptive effects of pain on emotions and behavior. See also **Nursing Outcomes Classification.**

**pain intervention,** the relief of the painful sensations experienced in suffering the physiologic and psychologic effects of disease and trauma. Effective pain intervention depends on proper evaluation of the type of pain the patient is experiencing, the physical and psychologic origins of the pain, and the behavioral patterns commonly associated with different kinds of pain. The most common method of pain intervention is the administration of narcotics, such as morphine, but many authorities believe that the exclusive use of pain-killing drugs without consideration and implementation of psychologic aids is too narrow an approach. There are few patients without a psychogenic overlay on the physical experience of pain, and comprehensive pain intervention uses methods and procedures that incorporate both psychologic and physical measures. Methods of pain intervention for acute pain are different from those for chronic pain. Acute pain, occurring in the first 24 to 48 hours after surgery, is often difficult to relieve, and narcotics seldom alleviate it completely. Some authorities believe that the individual who has undergone repeated surgical operations has a decreased tolerance for pain. The type of pain intervention usually depends on the description of the pain by the individual experiencing it. Mild pain may best be relieved by comfort measures and the distraction afforded by television, visitors, reading, and other passive activities. Moderate pain may best be relieved by a combination of comfort measures and drugs. Cognitive dissonance, often used to dampen moderate pain, encourages the patient to reflect on pleasant experiences and describe them to health care personnel. Intervention to relieve severe pain often includes the administration of narcotics, purposeful interaction between the patient and attending hospital personnel, reduction of environmental stimuli, increased comfort measures, and "waking imagined analgesia," in which the patient is encouraged to concentrate on and become distracted by former pleasant experiences, such as relaxing on a beach surrounded by cool ocean water. In the alleviation of all types of pain, dampening or decreasing stimuli that create pain is the chief goal. Pain often increases in a cold room because the muscles of the patient tend to contract, but the local application of cold, such as with an ice pack, often alleviates pain by reducing swelling. Pain intervention seeks to reduce the effects of other factors that compound pain, such as fatigue and anxiety. Coping with pain becomes increasingly difficult as the patient becomes more tired. Sensory restriction may increase pain, because it blocks otherwise effective distraction; overstimulation may cause fatigue and anxiety, thus increasing pain. Religious beliefs may be effective in helping the patient to decrease pain or increase tolerance if the pain is viewed by the patient as requiring self-discipline or as providing a catharsis for past transgressions. Religious beliefs, however, may increase pain if the patient interprets it as punishment and relates its severity to the gravity of transgressions or faults. Pain intervention by the use of drugs includes the administration of mild nonnarcotic analgesics and of much more potent and potentially addictive opioids, such as morphine. Opioid analgesics administered for the relief of pain, cough, or diarrhea provide only symptomatic treatment and are used cautiously in the care of patients with acute or chronic diseases. They may obscure the symptoms or the progress of the disease, and repeated daily administration of any opioid eventually produces some tolerance to the therapeutic effects of the drug and some physical dependence on the dosage. The risk of development of psychologic and physical dependency on any drug is always present, especially with opioids. In usual doses opioids relieve suffering by altering the emotional component of the painful experience and by effecting analgesia. Some caregivers are so concerned about the addictive dangers of opioids that they tend to prescribe initial doses that are too low or too infrequent to alleviate pain. A typical dose of 10 mg of morphine relieves postoperative pain in only two thirds of patients; some patients may require considerably more than the average dose to experience adequate relief. Some other patients with more rapid metabolisms may require such drugs at shorter intervals. Many drugs are appropriate substitutes for the potent opioids morphine and codeine. Some of the effective semisynthetic substitutes are hydrocodone, dihydrocodeine, and meperidine. The narcotic analgesics act on the central nervous system, but the salicylates and other nonnarcotic drugs act at the site of origin of the pain. Some nonnarcotic drugs, such as aspirin, indomethacin, ibuprofen, or naproxen, also have antiinflammatory and antipyretic activity. In patients who are sensitive to or are unable to take aspirin, acetaminophen is an acceptable substitute, as are the nonsteroidal antiinflammatory drugs. Pain intervention in the treatment of terminal illnesses uses numerous drugs that relieve pain and produce euphoria and tranquillity in patients who would otherwise suffer greatly. Analgesic mixtures of opioids and alcoholic solutions may be prescribed. Nerve block by the injection of alcohol, chordotomy, and other neurosurgical interventions may sometimes be used. Other techniques include acupuncture; hypnosis; behavior modification, in which treatment consists of reducing medication and gradually increasing mobility through exercise and any other appropriate modality; biofeedback; and transcutaneous electrical nerve stimulation. The latter technique is a noninvasive and nonaddictive method of modifying pain messages to the brain. See also **pain assessment.**

**pain level,** a nursing outcome from the Nursing Outcomes Classification (NOC) defined as the severity of reported or demonstrated pain. See also **Nursing Outcomes Classification.**

**pain management,** a nursing intervention from the Nursing Interventions Classification (NIC) defined as alleviation of pain or a reduction in pain to a level of comfort that is acceptable to the patient. See also **Nursing Interventions Classification.**

**pain mechanism,** the network that communicates unpleasant sensations and the perceptions of noxious stimuli throughout the body in association with physical disease and trauma involving tissue damage. The gate control theory of pain is an attempt to explain the role of the nervous system in the pain response. It states that pain signals that reach the nervous system excite a group of small neurons that form a "pain pool." When the total activity of these neurons reaches a minimum level, a theoretic gate opens up and allows the pain signals to proceed to higher brain centers. The areas in which the gates operate are considered to be in the spinal cord dorsal horn and the brainstem. The pattern theory holds that the intensity of a stimulus evokes a specific pattern, which is interpreted by the brain as pain. This perception is the result of the intensity and frequency of stimulation of a nonspecific end organ. Some authorities believe that bradykinin and histamine, two chemical substances produced by the body, cause pain. Recently discovered pain killers produced naturally by the body are the enkephalins and the endorphins. Some studies indicate that the enkephalins are 10 times as potent as morphine in reducing pain. It is known that after histamine and some other naturally occurring chemical substances are released in the body, pain sensations travel along fast-conducting and slow-conducting nerve fibers. These pain-transmitting neuropathways communicate the pain sensation to the dorsal root ganglia of the spinal cord and synapse with certain neurons in the posterior horns of the gray matter. The pain sensation is then transmitted to the reticular formation and the thalamus by neurons that form the anterolateral spinothalamic tract. It is then conveyed to various areas of the brain, such as the cortex and the hypothalamus, by synapses at the thalamus. The immediate reaction to pain is transmitted over the reflex arc by sensory fibers in the dorsal horn of the spinal cord and by synapsing motor neurons in the anterior horn. This anatomic pattern of sensory and motor neurons allows the individual to move quickly at the touch of some harmful stimulus, such as extreme heat or cold. Nerve impulses alerting the individual to move away from such stimuli are simultaneously sent along efferent nerve fibers from the brain. Also called **gate theory of pain, pain pathway.**

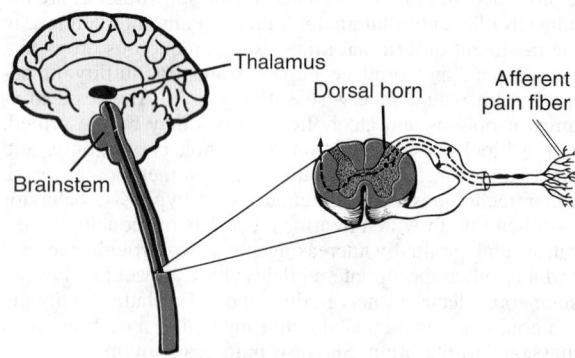

**Pain reception pathway** *(Potter and Perry, 2001)*

**pain pathway.**   See **pain mechanism.**
**pain: physiological response,**   a nursing outcome from the Nursing Outcomes Classification (NOC) defined as the cognitive and emotional response to physical pain. See also **Nursing Outcomes Classification.**
**pain receptor,**   any one of the many free nerve endings throughout the body that warn of potentially harmful changes in the environment, such as excessive pressure or temperature. The free nerve endings constituting most of the pain receptors are located chiefly in the epidermis and in the epithelial covering of certain mucous membranes. They also appear in the stratified squamous epithelium of the cornea, in the root sheaths and in the papillae of the hairs, and around the bodies of sudoriferous glands. The terminal ends of pain receptors consist of unmyelinated nerve fibers that often anastomose into small knobs between the epithelial cells. Any kind of stimulus, if it is intense enough, can stimulate the pain receptors in the skin and the mucosa, but only radical changes in pressure and certain chemicals can stimulate the pain receptors in the viscera. Referred pain results only from stimulation of pain receptors located in deep structures, such as the viscera, the joints, and the skeletal muscles, and never from pain receptors in the skin.
**paint** [Fr, *peindre*],   **1.** to apply a medicated solution to the skin, usually over a wide area. **2.** a medicated solution that is applied in this way. Kinds of paint include **antiseptics, germicides,** and **sporicides.**
**pain threshold,**   the point at which a stimulus, usually one associated with pressure or temperature, activates pain receptors and produces a sensation of pain. Individuals with

low pain thresholds experience pain much sooner and faster than those with higher thresholds; individuals' reactions to stimulation of pain receptors vary.
**pair,**   **1.** two corresponding items similar in form and function. **2.** one object composed of two joined interdependent parts. See also **base pair.**
**PAL,**   abbreviation for *posterior axillary line.*
**palatable** /pal'ətəbəl/ [L, *palatum*, palate],   pleasant to the taste, as food may be.
**palatable water.**   See **potable water.**
**palatal** /pal'ətəl/ [L, *palatum*, palate],   **1.** pertaining to the palate or palate bone. **2.** pertaining to the lingual surface of a maxillary tooth.
**palate** /pal'it/ [L, *palatum*],   a the bony muscular partition between the oral and nasal cavities that forms the roof of the mouth. It is divided into the hard palate and the soft palate. Also called *uraniscus.* —**palatal, palatine,** *adj.*
**palatine** [L, *palatum*, palate],   pertaining to or belonging to the palate.
**palatine arch** [L, *palatum* + *arcus*, bow],   the vault-shaped muscular structure forming the soft palate between the mouth and the nasopharynx. An opening in the arch connects the mouth with the oropharynx; the uvula is suspended from the middle of the posterior border of the arch.
**palatine bone,**   one of a pair of bones of the skull, forming the posterior part of the hard palate, part of the nasal cavity, and the floor of the orbit of the eye. It resembles a letter *L* and consists of horizontal and vertical parts and three processes.

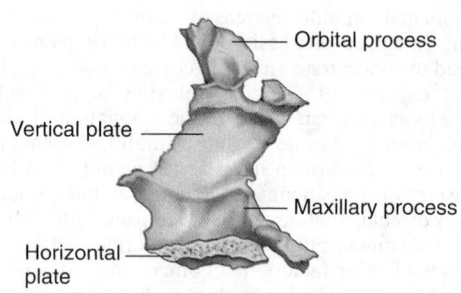

**Palatine bone**

**palatine ridge,**   any one of the four to six transverse ridges on the anterior surface of the hard palate.
**palatine suture,**   any one of a number of thin wavy lines marking the joining of the palatine processes that form the hard palate. See also **median palatine suture, transverse palatine suture.**
**palatine tonsil,**   one of a pair of almond-shaped masses of lymphoid tissue between the palatoglossal and the palatopharyngeal arches on each side of the fauces. They are covered with mucous membrane and contain numerous lymph follicles and various crypts.
**palatine uvula,**   an elongated process that hangs from the middle of the back edge of the soft palate.
**palatitis,**   an inflammation of the hard palate.
**palato-** /pal'ətō-/,   combining form meaning 'palate': *palatoglossal, palatography, palatomaxillary.*
**palatoglossal** /-glos'əl/ [L, *palatum*, palate; Gk, *glossa*, tongue],   pertaining to both the palate and the tongue.

**palatoglossus** /-glos′əs/, a muscle with an origin in the oral surface of the soft palate and an insertion at the side of the tongue. It forms the anterior pillar of the amygdaloid fossa and acts to raise the back of the tongue.

**palatognathous** /pal′ətog′nəthəs/, pertaining to a cleft palate.

**palatograph** /pal′ətōgraf′/, a device that records the movement of the palate while the person is speaking.

**palatomaxillary** /-mak′siler′ē/ [L, *palatum* + *maxilla,* jaw], pertaining to the palate and the maxilla.

**palatonasal** /-nā′zəl/ [L, *palatum* + *nasus,* nose], pertaining to the palate and the nose.

**palatopharyngeal** /-ferin′jē·əl/, pertaining to the palate and pharynx.

**palatopharyngeus** /-ferin′jē·əs/, a muscle with an origin at the back of the soft palate and an insertion on the posterior border of the thyroid cartilage and the wall of the pharynx. It acts to raise the pharynx.

**palatopharyngoplasty** /-fering′gōplas′tē/, the surgical excision of palatal and oropharyngeal tissues. The procedure may be peformed to treat cases of snoring or sleep apnea thought to be caused by obstructions in the nose or pharynx. See also **uvulopalatopharyngoplasty.**

**palatopharyngorrhaphy.** See **staphylopharyngorrhaphy.**

**palatoplasty** /pal′ətōplas′tē/, plastic surgery of the palate.

**palatoplegia** /-plē′jē·ə/, paralysis of the soft palate.

**palatorrhaphy** /pal′ətôr′əfē/, the surgical repair of a cleft palate.

**palatosalpingeus** /-salpin′jē·əs/, the tensor muscle of the soft palate. It arises from the scaphoid fossa of the sphenoid bone.

**palatoschisis** /pal′ətos′kisis/, a cleft palate.

**pale infarct** [L, *pallidus,* pallid, *infarcire,* to stuff], a wedge of dead tissue that is white because of an absence of blood. Also called **anemic infarct, white infarct.**

**paleo-,** prefix meaning 'old': *paleocerebellar, paleogenesis, paleostriatum.*

**paleocerebellum** /pal′ē-ōser′əbel′əm/, the phylogenetically oldest part of the cerebellum, including the vermis, which connects the cerebellar hemispheres, and the flocculus, or lobule on the posterior lobe. Also called *spinocerebellum.*

**paleocortex** /-kôr′teks/, the phylogenetically oldest part of the cerebral cortex, particularly the olfactory bulb.

**paleogenesis.** See **palingenesis.**

**paleogenetic** /-jənet′ik/ [Gk, *palaios,* long ago, *genesis,* origin], **1.** a trait or structure of an organism or species that originated in a previous generation. **2.** relating to the development of such a trait or structure.

**paleokinetic** /-kinet′ik/, pertaining to primitive reflexes and other automatic muscular movements.

**paleontology.** See **biology.**

**paleopathology** /-pathol′əjē/, the science of disease in ancient eras based on the condition of remains of mummies, skeletons, and other archeologic findings.

**pali-.** See **palin-.**

**palikinesia** /pal′ikīnē′zhə/, a condition in which involuntary movements are constantly repeated.

**palilalia** /pal′ilā′lyə/ [Gk, *palin,* again, *lalein,* to babble], an abnormal condition characterized by the increasingly rapid repetition of the same word or phrase, usually at the end of a sentence.

**palin′, pali-,** combining form meaning 'again': *palindromia, palinesthesia, palingenesis.*

**palindrome** /pal′indrōm′/ [Gk, *palin* + *dromos,* course], a segment of DNA in which identical or almost identical sequences of bases run in opposite directions of the complementary strands. Palindromes are often sites for attack by restriction endonucleases.

**palindromia** /pal′indrō′mē·ə/, the recurrence of a disease.

**palingenesis** /pal′injen′əsis/ [Gk, *palin* + *genesis,* origin], **1.** the regeneration of a lost part. **2.** the hereditary transmission of ancestral structural characteristics, especially abnormalities, in successive generations. Also called **paleogenesis.** Compare **cenogenesis.** —**palingenetic, palingenic,** *adj.*

**palivizumab,** a monoclonal antibody.

■ INDICATIONS: Palivizumab is used to prevent serious lower respiratory tract disease caused by respiratory syncytial virus in pediatric patients.

■ CONTRAINDICATIONS: Use of this drug is prohibited in adults, in patients with cyanotic congenital heart disease, and in patients with known hypersensitivity to this drug.

■ ADVERSE EFFECTS: Adverse reactions to this drug include nausea, vomiting, diarrhea, increased AST, upper respiratory infection, otitis media, rhinitis, pharyngitis, rash, and injection site reaction.

**palladium (Pd)** /pəlā′dē·əm/ [Gk, *Pallas Athena,* mythic goddess and protector of Troy], a hard silvery metallic element. Its atomic number is 46; its atomic mass is 106.42. Highly resistant to tarnish and corrosion, palladium is used in high-grade surgical instruments; in dental inlays, bridgework, and orthodontic appliances; and in catalytic convertors.

**pallanesthesia** /pal′anesthē′zhə/, a condition characterized by an inability to sense vibrations.

**pallesthesia** /pal′esthē′zhə/ [Gk, *pallein,* to quiver], hypersensitivity to vibration, particularly that caused by a tuning fork placed on a bony prominence.

**palliate** /pal′ē·āt/ [L, *palliare,* to cloak, to soothe or relieve. —**palliation,** *n.,* **palliative,** *adj.*

**palliative treatment** /pal′ē·ətiv′/ [L, *palliare,* to cloak, *tractare,* to handle], therapy designed to relieve or reduce intensity of uncomfortable symptoms but not to produce a cure. Some kinds of palliative treatment are the use of narcotics to relieve pain in a patient with advanced cancer, the creation of a colostomy to bypass an inoperable obstructing lesion of the bowel, and the debridement of necrotic tissue in a patient with metastatic malignancy. Compare **definitive treatment, expectant treatment.**

**pallid** /pal′id/ [L, *pallidus,* pale], lacking color.

**pallidectomy** /pal′idek′təmē/ [L, *pallidus,* pale; Gk *exome,* cutting out], the destruction of all or part of the globus pallidus by chemicals or freezing, in the treatment of Parkinson's disease.

**pallidotomy** /pal′idot′əmē/, the surgical production of lesions in the globus pallidus for the treatment of extrapyramidal disorders.

**pallidum.** See **globus pallidus.**

**pallium.** See **cerebral cortex.**

**pallor** /pal′ər/ [L, *paleness*], an unnatural paleness or absence of color in the skin.

**palm** /päm/ [L, *palma*], the flexor anterior surface of the hand, beyond the wrist to the base of the fingers, exclusive of the thumb and finger. —**palmar,** *adj.*

**palm and sole system of identification,** a method of identifying individuals by the patterns of ridges in the skin of the palms of the hands and soles of the feet. Like fingerprints, the patterns are helpful in identification of infants and others.

**palmar** /pal′mər/ [L, *palma*], pertaining to the palm.

**palmar aponeurosis** [L, *palma* + Gk, *apo,* from, *neuron,* nerve], a sheet of fascia under the skin of the palm and surrounding the muscles. Also called **palmar fascia.**

**palmar crease,** a normal groove across the palm of the hand.

**palmar erythema,** an inflammatory redness of the palms of the hands.

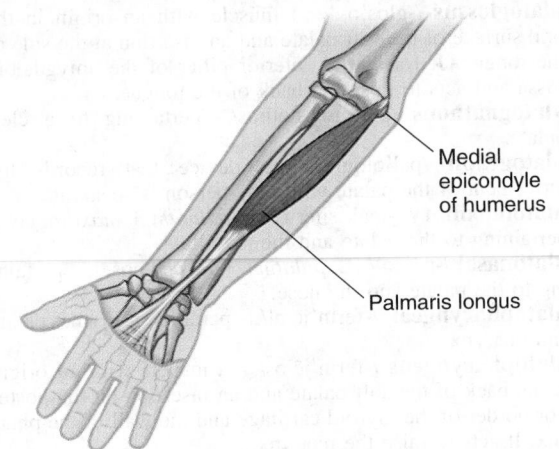

Medial epicondyle of humerus

Palmaris longus

**Palmaris longus**

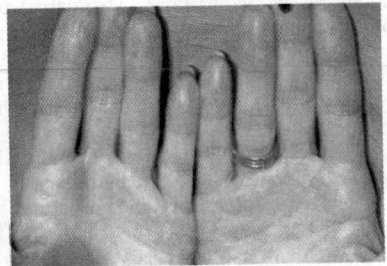

**Palmar erythema** *(Lemmi and Lemmi, 2000)*

**palmar fascia.** See **palmar aponeurosis.**

**palmar grasp reflex** [L, *palma,* palm; ONorse, *grapa,* grab], a flexion of the fingers caused by stimulation of the palm of the hand. The reflex is present at birth and usually disappears by 6 months of age.

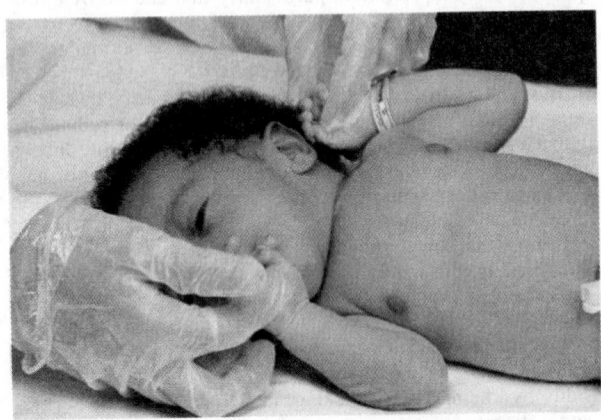

**Palmar grasp reflex in the newborn** *(Seidel et al, 1999)*

**palmaris longus** /pəlmer′is/, a long, slender, superficial fusiform muscle of the forearm, lying on the medial side of the flexor carpi radialis that functions to flex the hand. Compare **flexor carpi radialis, flexor carpi ulnaris.**

**palmar metacarpal artery,** any one of several arteries arising from the deep palmar arch, supplying the fingers.

**palmar pinch,** a thumbless grasp in which the tips of the other fingers are pressed against the palm of the hand. See also **pinch, tip pinch.**

**palmar reflex,** a reflex that curls the fingers when the palm of the hand is tickled.

**palmature** /pal′məchər/ [L, *palma*], an abnormal condition in which the fingers are webbed.

**palm-chin reflex.** See **palmomental reflex.**

**Palmer notation,** a system for designating teeth in which the mouth is divided into quadrants indicated by a right-angle symbol oriented right or left and up or down. The teeth in each quadrant are numbered from 1 to 8, starting with the central incisor and ending with the third molar. The system is no longer in general use. See also **FDI numbering system, universal tooth coding system.**

**palmitic acid (CH₃(CH₂)₁₄COOH)** /palmit′ik/ [L, *palma*], a saturated fatty acid that commonly occurs in animal and vegetable fats and oils. It is a carboxylic acid used in the production of soaps and candles. Also called **hexadecanoic acid.**

**palmitin** /pal′mitin/, a triglyceride consisting of palmitic acid present in palm oil and other vegetable and animal fats.

**palmityl alcohol.** See **cetyl alcohol.**

**palmomental reflex** /pal′məmen′təl/ [L, *palma* + *mentum,* chin, *reflectere,* to bend back], an abnormal neurologic sign, elicited by scratching the palm of the hand at the base of the thumb, characterized by contraction of the muscles of the chin and corner of the mouth on the same side of the body as the stimulus. It is occasionally seen in normal individuals, but an exaggerated reflex may occur in patients with pyramidal tract disease, latent tetany, increased intracranial pressure, and central facial paresis. Also called **palm-chin reflex.**

**palmoscopy** /palmos′kəpē/, detection of the pulse or heartbeat.

**palpable** /pal′pəbəl/ [L, *palpare,* to touch gently], perceivable by touch.

**palpate** /pal′pāt/, to use the hands or fingers to examine.

**palpation** /palpā′shən/ [L, *palpare,* to touch gently], a technique used in physical examination in which the examiner feels the texture, size, consistency, and location of certain body parts with the hands.

**palpatory percussion** /pal′pətôr′ē/ [L, *palpare,* to touch gently; *percutere,* to strike hard], a technique in physical examination in which the vibrations produced by percussion are evaluated by using light pressure of the flat of the examiner's hand.

**palpebra.** See **eyelid.**

**palpebral commissure.** See **canthus.**

**palpebral conjunctiva.** See **conjunctiva.**

**palpebral fissure** /pal′pəbrəl/ [L, *palpebra,* eyelid, *fissura,* cleft], the opening between the margins of the upper and lower eyelids.

**palpebral gland.** See **meibomian gland.**

**palpebra superior** /pal′pəbrə/, *pl.* **palpebrae superiores,** the upper eyelid, larger and more movable than the lower eyelid and furnished with an elevator muscle.

**palpebrate** /pal′pəbrāt/, **1.** to wink or blink. **2.** having eyelids.

**palpitate** /pal′pitāt/ [L, *palpitare,* to flutter], to pulsate rapidly, as in the unusually fast beating of the heart under various conditions of stress and in certain heart problems.

**palpitation** /pal′pitā′shən/ [L, *palpitare,* to flutter], a pounding or racing of the heart. It is associated with normal emotional responses and with heart disorders. Some people may complain of pounding heart and display no evidence of heart disease, whereas others with serious heart disorders may not detect associated abnormal palpitations. Some patients complain of palpitations after receiving digitalis because it increases the force of heart contractions. —**palpitate,** *v.*

**PALS,** abbreviation for **pediatric advanced life support.**

**palsy** /pôl′zē/ [Gk, *para,* beyond, *lysis,* loosening], an abnormal condition characterized by paralysis. Some kinds of palsy are **Bell's palsy, cerebral palsy,** and **Erb's palsy.**

**Paltauf's dwarf.** See **pituitary dwarf.**

**Paltauf's nanism** /päl′toufs/ [Arnold Paltauf, Czechoslovakian physician, 1860–1893; Gk, *nanos,* dwarf], dwarfism associated with excessive production or growth of lymphoid tissue.

**-pamide,** suffix for sulfamoylbenzoic acid-derived diuretics.

**-pamil,** suffix for verapamil-type coronary vasodilators.

**Pamine,** a trademark for an anticholinergic (methscopolamine bromide).

**pampiniform** /pampin′ifôrm/ [L, *pampinus,* vine tendril, *plexus,* plaited], having the shape of a tendril.

**pampiniform body.** See **epoophoron.**

**pampiniform plexus** [L, *pampinus,* vine tendril, *plexus,* plaited], a network of veins in the spermatic cord that drains the testes into the testicular vein in the lower abdomen.

**pan-** /pan-/, combining form meaning 'all': *panacea, pancarditis, pandemic.*

**panacea** /pan′əsē′ə/ [Gk, *pan,* all, *akeia,* remedy], **1.** a universal remedy. **2.** an ancient name for an herb or a liquid potion with healing properties.

**panacinar emphysema** /pan′ə·sin′ər/ [Gk, *pan,* all + L, *acinus,* grape], one of the principal types of emphysema, characterized by relatively uniform enlargement of air spaces throughout the acini. Also called **chronic hypertrophic, diffuse, ectatic, generalized, panlobular,** or **vesicular emphysema.**

**Panafil,** a trademark for a fixed-combination topical drug containing an enzyme (papain).

**panagglutinable** /pan′əglōō′tinəbəl/, pertaining to red blood cells that are agglutinable by the sera of all blood groups of the same species.

**panagglutinin** /pan′əglōō′tinin/, an antibody that causes clumping (agglutination) of red blood cells of all blood groups of a species.

**Panama fever.** See **Chagres fever.**

**panangiitis** /panan′jē·ī′tis/, an inflammation that affects all layers of a blood vessel.

**panarteritis** /-är′tərī′tis/ [Gk, *pan,* all, *arteria,* artery, *itis* inflammation], an inflammation that involves all the tissue layers of an artery.

**panarthritis** /-ärthrī′tis/ [Gk, *pan* + *arthron* joint], an abnormal condition characterized by the inflammation of many joints in the body. —**panarthritic,** *adj.*

**panatrophy** /panat′rəfē/, **1.** a general atrophy of all parts of a body or structure. **2.** a rare disorder associated with atrophy of cutaneous and subcutaneous tissue. It is characterized by prominence of underlying body structures as all levels of skin and subcutaneous tissue are reduced in thickness.

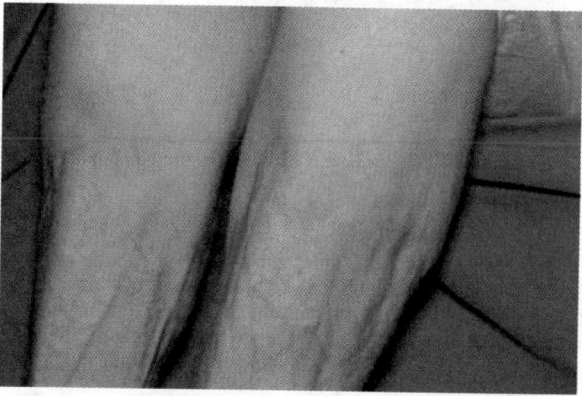

**Panatrophy** *(Lawrence and Cox, 1993)*

**panbronchiolitis** /panbrong′kē·əlī′tis/, chronic inflammation and obstruction of the bronchioles caused by the accumulation of foam cells. It usually leads to bronchiectasis.

**pancake kidney** /pan′kāk/ [ME, *panne,* pan, *kaka,* cake, *kidnere*], a congenital anomaly in which the left and right kidneys are fused into a single mass in the pelvis. The fused kidney has two collecting systems and two ureters and frequently becomes obstructed because of its abnormal position.

**pancarditis** /-kärdī′tis/ [Gk, *pan* + *kardia,* heart, *itis,* inflammation], an abnormal condition characterized by inflammation of the entire heart, including the endocardium, myocardium, and pericardium.

**Pancoast's syndrome** /pan′cōsts/ [Henry K. Pancoast, American radiologist, 1875–1939], **1.** a combination of signs associated with a tumor in the apex of the lung. The signs include neuritic pain in the arm, atrophy of the muscles of the arm and the hand, and Horner's syndrome and are caused by the damaging effects of the tumor on the brachial plexus and sympathetic ganglia. **2.** an abnormal condition caused by osteolysis in the posterior part of one or more ribs, sometimes involving associated vertebrae.

**Pancoast's tumor.** See **pulmonary sulcus tumor.**

**pancolectomy** /-kōlek′təmē/ [Gk, *pan* + *kolon,* colon, *ektomē,* excision], the excision of the entire colon, necessitating an ileostomy.

**pancreas** /pan′krē·əs/ [Gk, *pan,* all, *kreas,* flesh], an elongated grayish pink lobulated gland that stretches transversely across the posterior abdominal wall in the epigastric and hypochondriac regions of the body and secretes various substances, such as digestive enzymes, insulin, and glucagon. It is divided into a head, a flattened, elongated body, and a tail in contact with the spleen. The head of the gland, divided from the body by a small constriction, is tucked into the curve of the duodenum. The tapered left extremity of the organ forms the tail. In adults the pancreas is about 13 cm long. A compound, mixed gland composed of exocrine and endocrine tissue, it contains a main duct that runs the length

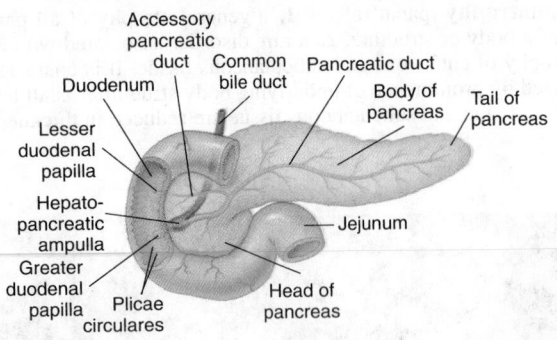

**Pancreas** *(Thibodeau and Patton, 1999/Barbara Cousins)*

of the organ, draining smaller ducts and emptying into the duodenum at the major duodenal papilla, the same site that accommodates the entrance of the common bile duct.

**pancreas scan,** a radiographic scan of the pancreas after the IV injection of a radiopaque contrast medium, used for detecting various abnormalities, such as tumors, cysts, and infections.

**-pancreat,** combining form meaning 'pancreas': *hepatico-pancreatic, lienopancreatic, splenopancreatic.*

**pancreatalgia** /pan′krē·ətal′jə/, pain in or near the pancreas.

**pancreatectomy** /pan′krē·ətek′təmē/ [Gk, *pan* + *kreas* + *ektomē*, excision], the surgical removal of all or part of the pancreas, performed to excise a cyst or tumor, treat pancreatitis, or repair trauma. The resection is done with general anesthesia. The GI tract is reconstructed, usually with an anastomosis between the common bile duct and the upper jejunum. Drains are left in the wound. After surgery the patient is given a low-sugar, low-fat diet. If the entire pancreas is removed, a brittle type of diabetes develops, requiring precise management of both diet and insulin dosage. The patient may have an insulin pump. A frequent complication is the formation of a fistula in the pancreatic bile duct, allowing digestive enzymes to contact adjacent tissues.

**pancreatemphraxis** /pan′krē·at′emfrak′sis/, hypertrophy or congestion of the pancreas caused by an obstruction in the pancreatic duct.

**pancreatic** /pan′krē·at′ik/ [Gk, *pan,* all, *kreas,* flesh], pertaining to the pancreas.

**pancreatic abscess,** an infection characterized by a collection of pus in or around the pancreas.

**pancreatic cancer** [Gk, *pan* + *kreas* + L, *cancer,* crab], a malignant neoplastic disease of the pancreas, characterized by anorexia, flatulence, weakness, dramatic weight loss, epigastric or back pain, jaundice, pruritus, a palpable abdominal mass, recent onset of diabetes, and clay-colored stools if the pancreatic and biliary ducts are obstructed. Diagnostic measures include barium radiographic studies of the stomach and duodenum, transhepatic cholangiography (endoscopic retrograde cholangiopancreatography), laboratory evaluation of liver function, celiac arteriography, computed axial tomography, and magnetic resonance imaging. Exploratory laparotomy is often required for a definitive diagnosis. About 90% of pancreatic tumors are adenocarcinomas; two thirds are in the head of the pancreas. Most tumors are not resectable at the time of diagnosis, but localized cancers in the pancreas may be treated by partial pancreatectomy with excision of the common bile duct, duodenum, and distal part of the stomach. Functioning islet cell lesions may be excised or treated with streptozocin, an antibiotic toxic to beta cells

of the pancreas. Total gastrectomy is recommended for gastrin-producing islet cell tumors that are resectable and accompanied by severe peptic ulcer disease. Radiotherapy or chemotherapy with 5-fluorouracil or mitomycin C may offer temporary palliation, but cancer of the pancreas has a poor prognosis: Few people live for more than 1 year after diagnosis. Pancreatic cancer occurs three to four times more often in men than in women. Though uncommon, it is increasing in incidence in the industrialized areas of the world. People who smoke more than 10 to 20 cigarettes a day, who have diabetes mellitus, or who have been exposed to polychlorinated biphenyl compounds are at increased risk of development of pancreatic cancer.

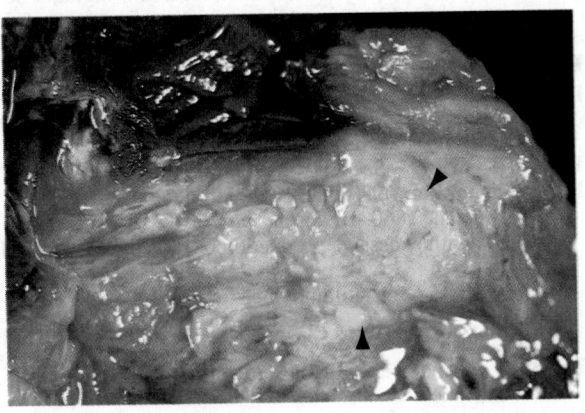

**Pancreatic cancer** *(Kumar, Cotran, and Robbins, 1997)*

**pancreatic diabetes** [Gk, *pan,* all, *kreas,* flesh, *diabainein,* to pass through], diabetes mellitus caused by a deficiency of insulin production by the islet cells of the pancreas. See also **diabetes mellitus.**

**pancreatic diverticulum,** one of a pair of membranous pouches arising from the embryonic duodenum. These two diverticula later form the pancreas and its ducts.

**pancreatic dornase,** an enzyme from beef pancreas that has been used as a mucolytic for upper respiratory infections and cystic fibrosis.

**pancreatic duct,** the primary secretory channel of the pancreas. Also called **duct of Wirsung.**

**pancreatic enzyme,** any one of the enzymes secreted by the pancreas in the process of digestion. The most important are trypsin, chymotrypsin, steapsin, and amylopsin. See also **pancreatic juice.**

**pancreatic enzyme digestion,** the action of pancreatic enzymes in the process of breaking down food into its constituents.

**pancreatic hormone,** any one of several chemical compounds secreted by the pancreas, associated with the regulation of cellular metabolism. Major hormones secreted by the pancreas are insulin, glucagon, somatostatin, and pancreatic polypeptide. Insulin and glucagon are secreted by different types of cells within the alpha and beta cells of the islands of Langerhans; somatostatin is secreted by the delta cells; and pancreatic polypeptide is secreted by a group of glandular cells arranged in a halo around each island of Langerhans.

**pancreatic insufficiency,** a condition characterized by inadequate production and secretion of pancreatic hormones or enzymes. It usually occurs secondary to a disease process destructive to pancreatic tissue. Nutritional malabsorption, anorexia, poorly localized upper abdominal or epigastric pain, malaise, and severe weight loss often occur. Alcohol-induced pancreatitis is the most common form of the condition. Supportive care, specific treatment of the cause, and replacement or augmentation of the absent or lacking substances are usually recommended as therapy for pancreatic insufficiency.

**pancreatic juice,** the fluid secretion of the pancreas, produced by the stimulation of food in the duodenum. It contains water, protein, inorganic salts, and enzymes. The juice is essential in breaking down proteins into their amino acid components, in reducing dietary fats to glycerol and fatty acids, and in converting starch to simple sugars.

**pancreaticoduodenal** /pan′krē·at′ikōdo͞o′ədē′nəl/, pertaining to the pancreas and duodenum.

**pancreaticolienal node** /pan′krē·at′ikō′lī·ē′nəl/ [Gk, *pan* + *kreas* + L, *lien,* spleen, *nodus,* knot], a node in one of three groups of lymph glands associated with branches of the abdominal and pelvic viscera that are supplied by branches of the celiac artery. The pancreaticolienal nodes accompany the splenic artery along the posterior surface and the upper border of the pancreas. Their afferent vessels, which originate from the stomach, the spleen, and the pancreas, join the celiac group of preaortic nodes. Also called **splenic gland.** Compare **gastric node, hepatic node.**

**pancreatin** /pan′krē·ətin′, -krē·ā′tin/, a concentrate of pancreatic enzymes from swine or beef cattle.

■ INDICATIONS: It is prescribed as an aid to digestion to replace endogenous pancreatic enzymes in cystic fibrosis and after pancreatectomy.

■ CONTRAINDICATIONS: Known hypersensitivity to this drug or to pork or beef protein prohibits its use.

■ ADVERSE EFFECTS: There are no known serious adverse reactions. High doses may cause nausea or diarrhea.

**pancreatitis** /pan′krē·əti′tis/ [Gk, *pan* + *kreas* + *itis,* inflammation], an inflammatory condition of the pancreas that may be acute or chronic. **Acute pancreatitis** is generally the result of damage to the biliary tract, as by alcohol, trauma, infectious disease, or certain drugs. It is characterized by severe abdominal pain (generally epigastric or upper left) radiating to the back, fever, anorexia, nausea, and vomiting. There may be jaundice if the common bile duct is obstructed. The development of pseudocysts or abscesses in pancreatic tissue is a serious complication. Treatment includes nasogastric suction to remove gastric secretions. To prevent any stimulation of the pancreas, nothing is given by mouth. The client may be given antacids to decrease the acid, which stimulates the pancreas. IV fluids and electrolytes are administered, and nonmorphine derivatives are given to relieve pain. The causes of **chronic pancreatitis** are similar to those of the acute form. When the cause is alcohol abuse, there may be calcification and scarring of the smaller pancreatic ducts. Abdominal pain, nausea, and vomiting occur, as well as steatorrhea and creatorrhea, caused by the diminished output of pancreatic enzymes. Pancreatic insulin production may be diminished, and diabetes mellitus develops in some patients. Treatment includes analgesics for pain and subtotal pancreatectomy when pain is intractable. A pancreatic extract is given orally to replace the missing enzymes; vitamin supplements are essential; calcium supplements may be needed. Both forms of pancreatitis are diagnosed by history, physical examination, radiologic studies, endoscopy, and laboratory analysis of the amount of pancreatic enzymes in the blood.

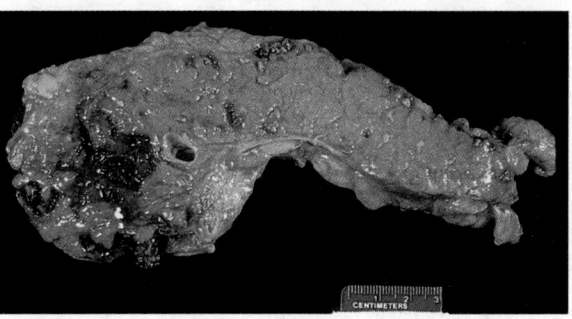

**Acute pancreatitis** *(Kumar, Cotran, and Robbins, 1997)*

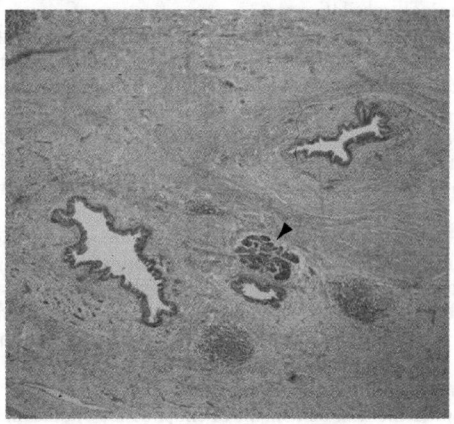

**Chronic pancreatitis** *(Kumar, Cotran, and Robbins, 1997)*

**pancreatoduodenectomy** /pan′krē·ətōdo͞o′ədənek′təmē/, [Gk, *pan* + *kreas* + L, *duodeni,* twelve fingers; Gk, *ektomē,* excision], a surgical procedure in which the head of the pancreas, the entire duodenum, a portion of the jejunum, the distal third of the stomach, and the lower third of the common bile duct are excised. Continuity is reestablished between the biliary, pancreatic, and GI systems. The operation is performed to remove the periampullary masses that occur in certain forms of biliary tract cancer. Also called **Whipple procedure.**

**pancreatoduodenostomy** /-do͞o′ədənos′təmē/, a surgical procedure to establish a fistula or duct from the pancreas into the duodenum.

**pancreatogastrostomy** /-gastros′təmē/, the surgical establishment of a fistula or duct from the pancreas to the stomach.

**pancreatogenic** /-jen′ik/, originating in the pancreas.

**pancreatography** /pan′krē·ətog′rəfē/ [Gk, *pan* + *kreas* + *graphein,* to record], visualization of the pancreas or its ducts by radiography following injection of a contrast medium into the ducts at surgery or via an endoscope, or by ultrasonography, computed tomography, or radionuclide imaging.

**pancreatojejunostomy** /-jij′o͞onos′təmē/, the surgical establishment of a fistula or duct from the pancreas to the jejunum.

**pancreatolith** /pan′krē·at′əlith/, a stone or calculus in the pancreas.

**pancreatolithiasis** /pan'kre·ətolithī'əsis/, the presence of calculi in the pancreas or pancreatic duct.

**pancreatolithotomy** /lithot'əmē/, the surgical removal of pancreatic calculi.

**pancreatolysis** /pan'krē·ətol'isis/, destruction of the pancreas by pancreatic enzymes.

**pancreatomegaly** /-meg'əlē/, an abnormal enlargement of the pancreas.

**pancreatopathy** /pan'krē·ətop'əthē/, any disease of the pancreas.

**pancreatotomy** /pan'krē·ətot'əmē/, a surgical incision in the pancreas.

**pancreatropic** /pan'krē·ətrop'ik/, exerting an influence on the pancreas. Also called **pancreatotropic.**

**pancuronium bromide** /pan'kyərō'nē·əm/, a skeletal muscle relaxant; a nondepolarizing neuromuscular blocker.
■ INDICATIONS: It is prescribed as an adjunct to anesthesia and mechanical ventilation.
■ CONTRAINDICATIONS: It is used with caution in patients with myasthenia gravis and renal and hepatic disease and in pregnancy. Known hypersensitivity to this drug or to other bromides prohibits its use.
■ ADVERSE EFFECTS: The most serious adverse reactions are prolonged muscle relaxation and respiratory depression.

**pancytopenia** /pan'sītəpē'nē·ə/ [Gk, *pan* + *kytos,* cell, *penia,* poverty], marked reduction in the number of red blood cells, white blood cells, and platelets. See also **anemia, aplasia, neutropenia. —pancytopenic,** *adj.*

**pancytopenia-dysmelia.** See **Fanconi's anemia.**

**p and a,** abbreviation for *percussion and auscultation,* as noted in the patient's chart after physical examination of the chest. See **auscultation, percussion.**

**pandemia** /-dē'mē·ə/ [Gk, *pan,* all, *demos,* people], a disease epidemic that affects all or most of a population group.

**pandemic** /-dē'mik/ [Gk, *pan* + *demos,* people], (of a disease) occurring throughout the population of a country, a people, or the world.

**pandiastolic** /-dī'əstol'ik/ [Gk, *pan* + *dia,* through, *stellein,* to set], pertaining to the complete diastole. Also called **holodiastolic.**

**panencephalitis** /pan'ənsef'əlī'tis/ [Gk, *pan* + *enkephale,* brain, *itis*], inflammation of the entire brain characterized by an insidious onset, a progressive course with deterioration of motor and mental functions, and evidence of a viral cause. **Subacute sclerosing panencephalitis** is an uncommon childhood disease thought to be caused by a "slow" latent measles virus after recovery from a previous infection. Most of the patients are younger than 11 years of age, and many more boys than girls are affected. The disease results in ataxia, myoclonus, atrophy, cortical blindness, and mental deterioration. Antiviral drugs, immunosuppressants, and interferon inducers are sometimes administered, but the disease is usually unremitting and fatal.

**panendoscope** /-en'dəskōp'/ [Gk, *pan* + *endon,* within, *skopein,* to look], a cystoscope that allows a wide view of the interior of the bladder and urethra with a special lens system.

**panesthesia** /-esthē'zhə/ [Gk, *pan* + *aisthesis,* feeling], the total of all sensations experienced by an individual at one time. Compare **cenesthesia.**

**pang,** a sudden severe but temporary pain.

**pangenesis** /-jen'əsis/ [Gk, *pan* + *genesis,* origin], an idea that each cell and particle of a parent reproduces itself in progeny.

**panhidrosis,** perspiration over the entire body.

**panhypopituitarism** /panhī'pōpitoo'itəriz'əm/ [Gk, *pan* + *hypo,* under, *pituita,* phlegm], generalized insufficiency of pituitary hormones, resulting from damage to or deficiency of the gland. **Prepubertal panhypopituitarism,** a rare disorder usually associated with a suprasellar cyst or craniopharyngioma, is characterized by dwarfism with normal body proportions, subnormal sexual development, and insufficient thyroid and adrenal function. Diabetes insipidus is frequently present; bitemporal hemianopia or complete blindness may occur; skin is often yellow and wrinkled, but mentality is usually unimpaired. X-ray films show delayed fusion of the epiphyses, suprasellar calcification, and frequently destruction of the sella turcica. The condition is treated with cortisone, thyroid and sex hormone replacement, and human growth hormone. Postpubertal panhypopituitarism may be caused by postpartum pituitary necrosis (Sheehan's syndrome), resulting from thrombosis of pituitary circulation during or after delivery. Characteristic signs of the disorder are failure to lactate, amenorrhea, weakness, cold intolerance, lethargy, and loss of libido and of axillary and pubic hair. There may be bradycardia or hypotension, and progression of the disorder leads to premature wrinkling of the skin and atrophy of the thyroid and adrenal glands. Treatment consists of the administration of adrenocorticotropic hormone, thyroid-stimulating hormone, and hormones of the target organs. Panhypopituitarism may also be caused by pituitary apoplexy, hemorrhage, or head trauma. Also called **hypophyseal cachexia, pituitary cachexia, Simmonds' disease.**

**panhysterectomy** /pan'histərek'təmē/ [Gk, *pan* + *hystera,* uterus, *ektomē,* excision], complete surgical removal of the uterus and cervix. See also **hysterectomy.**

**panic** /pan'ik/, an intense, sudden, and overwhelming fear or feeling of anxiety that produces terror and immediate physiologic changes that result in paralyzed immobility or senseless, hysteric behavior.

**panic attack** [Gk, *panikos,* of the god Pan; Fr, *attaquer*], an episode of acute anxiety that occurs unpredictably with feelings of intense apprehension or terror, accompanied by dyspnea, dizziness, sweating, trembling, and chest pain or palpitations. The attack may last several minutes and may occur again in certain situations. Compare **anxiety attack.**

**panic disorder.** See **anxiety attack.**

**panivorous** /paniv'ərəs/ [L, *panis,* bread, *vorare,* to devour], pertaining to the practice of subsisting exclusively on bread. **—panivore,** *n.*

**panlobular emphysema.** See **panacinar emphysema.**

**panmyelosis** /panmī'əlō'sis/, a pathologic condition characterized by a proliferation of bone marrow cells of all types.

**Panner's disease,** a rare form of osteochondrosis in which abnormal bony growth occurs in the capitulum of the humerus.

**panniculitis** /pənik'yəlī'tis/ [L, *panniculus,* piece of cloth; Gk, *itis,* inflammation], a chronic inflammation of subcutaneous fat in which the skin becomes hardened, particularly over the abdomen and thorax. Small subcutaneous masses of hard tissue are found in the affected areas. Some forms of the inflammation may be marked by the appearance of painless subcutaneous nodules on the lower extremities.

**panniculus** /pənik'yələs/, *pl.* **panniculi** [L, small garment], a membranous layer, the many sheets of fascia covering various structures in the body.

**pannus** /pan'əs/ [L, cloth], an abnormal condition of the cornea, which has become vascularized and infiltrated with granular tissue just beneath the surface. Pannus may develop in the inflammatory stage of trachoma or after a detached retina, glaucoma, iridocyclitis, or other degenerative eye disorder.

**panography** /pənog'rəfē/, a method of tomography that visualizes curved surfaces of the body at any depth. In dentistry it is accomplished by simultaneous radiography of the maxillary and mandibular dental arches and associated structures along two axes of rotation. Images are recorded on an intensifying screen that rotates with the radiation source around the patient's head. See also **panoramic radiograph.**

**panophobia, panophobic.** See **panphobia.**

**panophthalmitis** /pan'ofthalmī'tis/ [Gk, *pan* + *ophthalmos,* eye, *itis*], an inflammation of the entire eye, usually caused by virulent pyogenic organisms, such as strains of meningococci, pneumococci, streptococci, anthrax bacilli, and clostridia. Initial symptoms are pain, fever, headache, drowsiness, edema, and swelling. As the infection progresses, the iris appears muddy and gray, the aqueous humor becomes turbid, and precipitates form on the posterior surface of the cornea. Treatment consists of intensive systemic and local antibiotic therapy; evisceration of the globe or excision of the eye may be required, but excision is contraindicated if surrounding tissues are infected.

**panoptic** /panop'tik/ [Gk, *pan,* all, *opsis,* vision], pertaining to the enhanced visual effect produced by stains applied to microscopic specimens.

**panoramic radiograph** /pan'ôram'ik/ [Gk, *pan* + *horama,* view; L, *radiare,* to emit rays; Gk, *graphein,* to record], an x-ray image of a curved body surface, such as the upper and lower jaws, on a single film. Also called **pantomograph.**

**panotitis** /pan'ōtī'tis/, a general inflammation of the ear, including the middle ear.

**PanOxyl,** a trademark for a keratolytic (benzoyl peroxide).

**panphobia** /-fō'bē·ə/ [Gk, *pan* + *phobos,* fear], an anxiety disorder characterized by an irrational fear of everything. Also called **panophobia, pantophobia. —panphobic,** *adj.*

**panplegia** /panplē'jē·ə/, paralysis of all four extremities.

**pansclerosis** /pan'sklirō'sis/, a general hardening of a tissue or body part.

**pansystolic** /-sistol'ik/, pertaining to the entire systole. Also called **holosystolic.**

**pansystolic murmur.** See **systolic murmur.**

**pant-.** See **panto-.**

**pantalgia** /pantal'jə/, pain that affects all parts of the body.

**pantanencephaly** /pantan'ensef'əlē/, a congenital absence of all or nearly all brain tissue.

**Panteric,** a trademark for an enzyme (pancreatin).

**panthenol** /pan'thənôl/, **1.** an alcohol converted in the body to pantothenic acid, a vitamin in the B complex. **2.** a viscous liquid derived from pantothenic acid, a member of the vitamin $B_{12}$ group.

**panting** [Fr, *panteler,* to gasp], a ventilatory pattern characterized by rapid, shallow breathing. Panting usually moves gas back and forth in the anatomic dead space at a high flow rate, which evaporates water and removes heat but produces little or no alveolar ventilation and does not cause hypocapnia.

**panto-, pant-,** combining form meaning 'all, the whole': *pantophobia, pantoscopic, pantosomatous.*

**pantograph** /pan'təgraf'/, **1.** a jointed device for copying a plane figure to any desired scale. **2.** a device that incorporates a pair of face bows fixed to the jaws, used for inscribing centrically related points and arcs leading to the points on segments relatable to the three craniofacial planes.

**pantomograph** /pantom'əgraf/. See **panoramic radiograph.**

**pantomography** /-mog'rəfē/ [Gk, *pan* + *graphein,* to record], panoramic radiography for obtaining simultaneous radiographs of the maxillary and mandibular dental arches and related structures.

**pantophobia.** See **panphobia.**

**Pantopon,** a trademark for a fixed-combination opioid analgesic containing hydrochlorides of opium alkaloids.

**pantoscopic** /pan'təskop'ik/, pertaining to bifocal eyeglasses designed for both reading and distance viewing: the bottom half for close vision and the top half for far vision.

**pantothenic acid** /pan'təthen'ik/, a member of the vitamin B complex. It is widely distributed in plant and animal tissues and may be an important element in human nutrition.

**pantothenyl alcohol.** See **panthenol.**

**Panwarfin,** a trademark for an anticoagulant (warfarin sodium).

**$PaO_2$,** symbol for **partial pressure of oxygen in arterial blood.**

**$PAO_2$,** symbol for *partial pressure of alveolar oxygen.*

**pap,** any soft, soggy food.

**papain** /pəpā'ēn/, an enzyme from the fruit of *Carica papaya,* the tropical melon tree. It has been prescribed for enzymatic debridement of wounds and promotion of healing.

**Papanicolaou's test** /pap'ənik'əlou'/ [George N. Papanicolaou, Greek physician in U.S. practice, 1883–1962], a simple smear method of examining stained exfoliative cells. It is used most commonly to detect cancers of the cervix, but it may be used for tissue specimens from any organ. A smear, the **Papanicolaou's (Pap) smear,** is usually obtained during a routine pelvic examination annually beginning at 18 years of age. The technique permits early diagnosis of cancer and has contributed to a lower death rate from cervical cancer. The findings are usually reported descriptively. Also called *(informal)* **Pap test.**

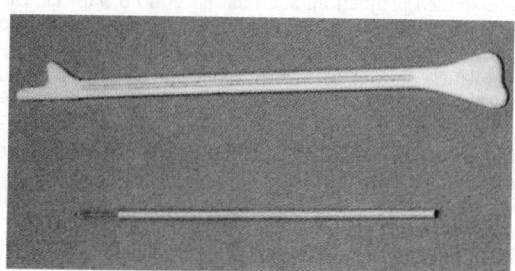

**Implements used to obtain a Pap smear**
*(Seidel et al, 1999/courtesy Cytobrush, Inc., Florida)*

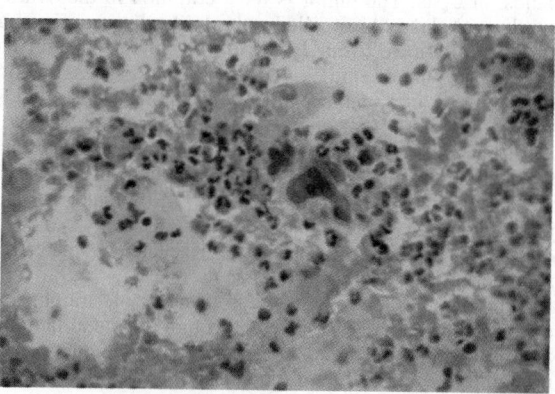

**Positive Pap smear indicative of cervical cancer**
*(Christiansen and Grzybowski, 1993)*

**papaverine hydrochloride** /papav′ərēn/, a smooth muscle relaxant.

■ INDICATIONS: It is prescribed in the treatment of cardiovascular or visceral spasms.

■ CONTRAINDICATIONS: Complete atrioventricular (AV) heart block or known hypersensitivity to this drug prohibits its use.

■ ADVERSE EFFECTS: The most serious adverse reactions include jaundice, increase in blood pressure, and arrhythmias.

**papaya** /pəpī′ə/, the fruit of the tropical *Carica papaya* (pawpaw) tree and the source of the proteolytic enzyme papain used in blood group serologic evaluation. Papain is also used to prevent adhesions and to tenderize meat.

**paper,** a material produced in sheets, usually from wood pulp or other cellulose products. It can be adapted for many purposes, such as litmus paper for testing acidity, filter paper, and articulating carbon paper used to record points of contact beween teeth of the upper and lower jaws.

**paper chromatography** [Gk, *papyros,* papyrus], the separation of a mixture into its components by filtering it through a strip of special paper.

**paper-doll fetus.** See **fetus papyraceus.**

**paper point,** in root canal therapy, a cone of variable width and taper, usually made of paper or a paper product, used to dry or maintain a liquid disinfectant in the canal. Also called **absorbent point.**

**paper radioimmunosorbent test (PRIST),** a technique for determining total immunoglobulin E levels in patients with type I hypersensitivity reactions.

**papill-,** prefix meaning 'resembling a nipple': *papilledema, papillate, papilloma.*

**papilla** /pəpil′ə/, *pl.* **papillae** [L, nipple], **1.** a small nipple-shaped projection, such as the conoid papillae of the tongue and the papillae of the dermis that extend from collagen fibers, the capillary blood vessels, and sometimes the nerves of the dermis. **2.** the optic papilla, a round white disc in the fundus oculi, which corresponds to the entrance of the optic nerve.

**papilla duodeni major.** See **hepatopancreatic ampulla.**

**papillae.** See **papilla.**

**papilla mammae.** See **nipple.**

**papilla mammaria.** See **nipple.**

**papilla of Vater.** See **hepatopancreatic ampulla.**

**papillary** /pap′əle′rē/ [L, *papilla,* nipple], pertaining to a papilla.

**papillary adenocarcinoma,** a malignant neoplasm characterized by small papillae of vascular connective tissue covered by neoplastic epithelium that projects into follicles, glands, or cysts. The tumor is most common in the ovaries and thyroid gland. Also called **polyploid adenocarcinoma.**

**papillary adenocystoma lymphomatosum,** an unusual tumor, consisting of epithelial and lymphoid tissues, that develops in the area of the parotid and submaxillary glands. Also called **adenolymphoma, Warthin's tumor.**

**papillary adenoma,** a benign epithelial tumor in which the membrane lining the glandular tissue forms papillary processes that project into the alveoli or grow out of a cavity's surface.

**papillary carcinoma,** a malignant neoplasm characterized by fingerlike projections.

**papillary duct,** any one of the thousands of straight collecting renal tubules that descend through the medulla of the kidney and join with others to form the common ducts opening into the renal papillae. Compare **loop of Henle.** See also **kidney.**

**papillary muscle,** any one of the rounded or conical muscular projections attached to the chordae tendineae in the

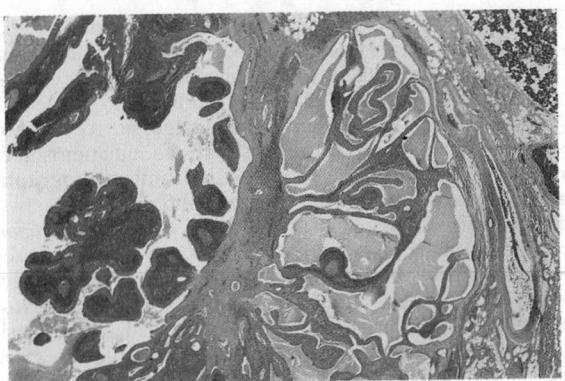

**Papillary adenocystoma lymphomatosum**
*(Fletcher, 2000)*

ventricles of the heart. The papillary muscles vary in number; the two main muscles are the anterior papillary muscle and the posterior papillary muscle. The papillary muscles are associated with the atrioventricular valves that they help open and close. Compare **chordae tendineae, trabecula carnea.**

**papillary tumor.** See **papilloma.**

**papillate** /pap′ilit/, marked by papillae or nipplelike prominences.

**papilledema** /pap′ilədē′mə/, *pl.* **papilledemas, papilledemata** [L, *papilla* + Gk, *oidema,* swelling], swelling of the optic disc, visible on ophthalmoscopic examination of the fundus of the eye, caused by increase in intracranial pressure. The meningeal sheaths that surround the optic nerves from the optic disc are continuous with the meninges of the brain; therefore increased intracranial pressure is transmitted forward from the brain to the optic disc in the eye to cause swelling. Also spelled *papilloedema.*

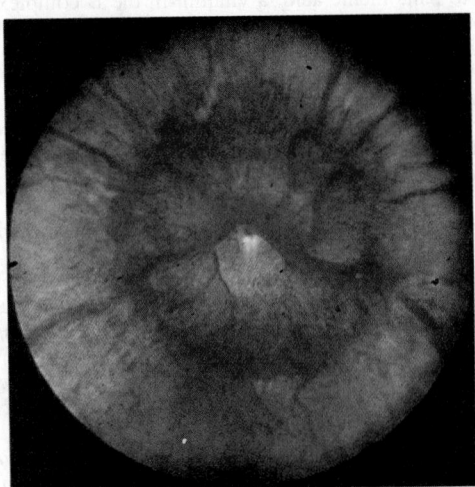

**Papilledema** *(Zitelli and Davis, 1997)*

**papilliform** /pəpil′ifôrm/, shaped like a nipple.

**papillitis** /pap′ili̅′tis/ [L, *papilla* + Gk, *itis,* inflammation],
1. inflammation of a papilla, such as the lacrimal papilla.
2. inflammation of the optic disc.

**papilloadenocystoma** /pap′ilō·ad′ənō′sistō′mə/, a benign epithelial tumor in which the lining develops in numerous small folds.

**papillocarcinoma** [L, *papilla,* nipple; Gk, *oma,* tumor, *karkinos,* crab, *oma,* tumor], a malignant tumor in which there are papillary outgrowths.

**papilloma** /pap′ilō′mə/ [L, *papilla* + Gk, *oma,* tumor], a benign epithelial neoplasm characterized by a branching or lobular tumor. Also called **papillary tumor.**

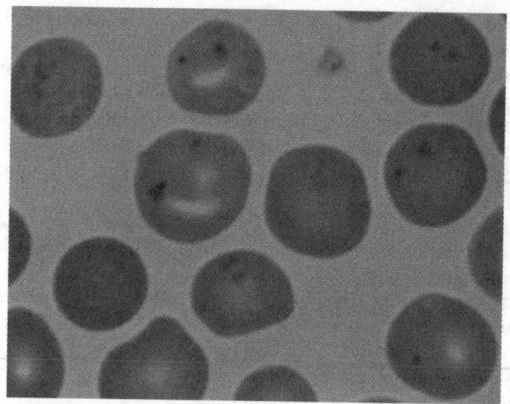
**Pappenheimer bodies** *(Carr and Rodak, 1999)*

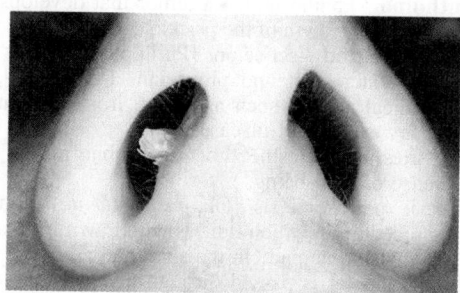
**Papilloma** *(Bingham, Hawke, and Kwok, 1992)*

**papilloma papovavirus.** See **papovavirus.**

**papillomatosis** /pap′ilōmətō′sis/ [L, *papilla* + Gk, *oma,* tumor, *osis,* condition], an abnormal condition characterized by widespread development of nipplelike growths.

**papillomatosis coronae penis.** See **hirsutoid papilloma of the penis.**

**papillomavirus** /pap′ilō′məvi̅′rəs/ [L, *papilla* + Gk, *oma,* tumor; L, *virus,* poison], the virus that causes warts in humans.

**Papillon-Lefèvre syndrome** /pä′pēyôN′ lə·fev′rə/ [M.M. Papillon, French dermatologist, 20th century; Paul Lefèvre, French dermatologist, 20th century], an autosomal recessive disorder occurring between the first and fifth years of life, characterized by palmoplantar keratoderma resembling psoriasis, which may also involve the elbows, knees, tibias, external malleoli, and other areas; ectopic calcifications of the skull; and periodontitis and premature shedding of both the deciduous and secondary teeth.

**papilloretinitis** /pap′ilōret′ini̅′tis/ [L, *papilla* + *rete,* net; Gk, *itis,* inflammation], an inflammatory occlusion of a retinal vein.

**papillotomy** /pap′ilot′əmē/, a surgical incision in the papilla of the duodenum.

**papovavirus** /pap′əvəvi̅′rəs/ [(abbreviation) *pa*pilloma, *po*lyoma, *va*cuolating, *virus*], one of a group of small deoxyribonucleic acid (DNA) viruses, some of which may be potentially cancer-producing. The human wart is caused by a kind of papovavirus, but it very rarely undergoes malignant transformation. Kinds of papovaviruses are **papilloma papovavirus, polyoma papovavirus,** and **SV-40 papovavirus.**

**pappataci fever.** See **phlebotomus fever.**

**Pappenheimer bodies** [A.M. Pappenheimer, U.S. pathologist, 1878–1955], phagosomes containing iron granules, found in red blood cells in certain disorders, including sickle cell disease and hemolytic anemia. They may contribute to spurious platelet counts by electro-optical counters.

**pappus** /pap′əs/ [Gk, *pappos,* down], the first growth of beard, characterized by downy hairs.

**Pap smear, Pap test.** See **Papanicolaou's test.**

**papula** /pap′yələ/, a small superficial elevation of the skin.

**papular** /pap′yələr/ [L, *papula,* pimple], pertaining to or resembling a papule.

**papular acrodermatitis of childhood.** See **Gianotti-Crosti syndrome.**

**papular scaling disease** [L, *papula,* pimple; AS, *scealu*], any of a group of skin disorders characterized by discrete raised dry, scaling lesions. Some kinds of papular scaling diseases are **lichen planus, pityriasis rosea,** and **psoriasis.** Also called **papulosquamous disease.**

**papular urticaria** [L, *papula,* pimple + *urtica,* nettle], a persistent cutaneous eruption representing a hypersensitivity reaction to insect bites (e.g., mites, fleas, bedbugs, gnats, mosquitoes, animal lice), seen primarily in atopic children, and characterized by crops of small urticarial papules and wheals and transitional forms of these lesions, which may become secondarily infected or lichenified owing to rubbing and scratching. Also called **lichen urticatus, strophulus.**

**papulation** /pap′yələ′shən/ [L, *papula,* pimple, *atus,* process], the development of papules.

**papule** /pap′yoo̅l/ [L, *papula,* pimple], a small solid raised skin lesion less than 1 cm in diameter, such as the lesions of lichen planus and nonpustular acne. Compare **macule.** —**papular,** *adj.*

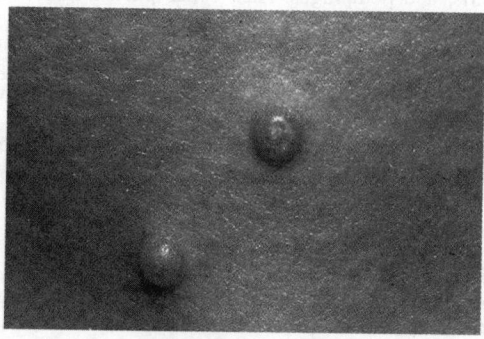
**Papules** *(du Vivier, 1993)*

**papulo-,** combining form meaning 'papules or pimples': *papular, papuliferous.*

**papuloerythematous** /pap′yəlō·er′ithem′ətəs/, pertaining to an eruption of papules on an erythematous surface.

**papulopustular** /pap′yəlōpus′tyələr/, pertaining to a skin eruption of both pustules and papules.

**papulosis** /pap′yəlō′sis/, a widespread occurrence of papules over the body.

**papulosquamous** /pap′yəlōskwā′məs/ [L, *papula,* pimple + *squama,* scale], pertaining to a skin eruption that is both papular and scaly.

**papulosquamous disease.** See **papular scaling disease.**

**papulovesicular** /pap′yəlō·vesik′yələr/, pertaining to a skin rash characterized by both papules and vesicles.

**papyraceous** /pap′irā′shəs/ [Gk, *papyros,* paper], having a paperlike quality. Also *papyraceus.*

**papyraceous fetus.** See **fetus papyraceus.**

**Paquelin's cautery** /pak′əlinz/ [Claude A. Paquelin, French physician, 1836–1905; Gk, *kauterion,* branding iron], a cauterizing device consisting of a platinum loop through which a heated hydrocarbon is passed.

**par,** a pair, specifically a pair of cranial nerves, such as the par nonum, or ninth pair.

**PAR,** abbreviation for **pulmonary arteriolar resistance.**

**par-,** combining form meaning 'aside, beyond, apart from, against': *parabacteria, parotid, parumbilical.*

**para** /par′ə/ [L, *parere,* to bear], a woman who has produced an infant regardless of whether the child was alive or stillborn. The term is used with numerals to indicate the number of pregnancies carried to more than 20 weeks' gestation, such as para 2, indicating two pregnancies, in a single pregnancy. See also **nullipara, parity.**

**para-, par-,** prefix meaning 'similar, beside, beyond, supplementary to, disordered': *paramedical, parabiosis, paranoia, paraplegia.*

**-para, -parous,** suffix meaning 'to bear or give birth': *primipara, ovovipara, pipipara.*

**paraactinomycosis** /par′ə·ak′tinō′mīkō′sis/, a chronic pulmonary infection similar to actinomycosis. The infection is caused by bacteria of the genus *Nocardia.* Also called **pseudoactinomycosis.**

**para-aminobenzenesulfonic acid.** See **sulfanilic acid.**

**paraaminobenzoic acid ($H_2NC_6H_4COOH$) (PABA)** /par′ə·amē′nōbenzō′ik/, a substance often associated with the vitamin B complex, found in cereals, eggs, milk, and meat and present in detectable amounts in blood, urine, spinal fluid, and sweat. It is widely used as a sunscreen that forms a partial chemical conjugation with constituents of the horny layer and that resists removal by water and sweat. PABA is a sulfonamide antagonist and may be an effective agent for the treatment of scleroderma, dermatomyositis, and pemphigus. Also called *para-*aminobenzoic acid.

**paraaminohippuric acid (PAHA, PHA)** /par′ə·amē′-nōhipōōr′ik/, the *p*-aminobenzamide derivative of glycerin. Its sodium salt is used for measuring effective renal plasma flow and determining kidney function.

**paraaminosalicylic acid (PAS, PASA)** /par′ə·amē′nōsal′-isil′ik/, a bacteriostatic agent.

■ INDICATIONS: It is prescribed for the treatment of pulmonary and extrapulmonary tuberculosis.

■ CONTRAINDICATIONS: Known hypersensitivity to this drug prohibits its use. It may interact with other drugs.

■ ADVERSE EFFECTS: Among the most serious reactions are nausea, vomiting, diarrhea, and abdominal pain. Fever, skin eruptions and other kinds of hypersensitivity reactions, goiter, hypokalemia, and acidosis may occur.

*para*-ammosulfonic acid. See **sulfanilic acid.**

**paraballism** /par′əbôl′izəm/ [Gk, *ballismos,* jumping about], involuntary jerking movements of the legs.

**parabiosis** /-bī·ō′sis/, the fusion of two eggs or embryos, resulting in conjoined twins.

**parabiotic syndrome** /-bī·ot′ik/ [Gk, *para,* beside, *bios,* life, *syn,* together, *dromos,* course], a blood transfer condition that can occur between identical twin fetuses as a result of placental vascular anastomoses. One twin may become anemic and the other plethoric.

**parabolic** /-bol′ik/, (in ultrasonics) pertaining to flow conditions in blood vessels. Under parabolic flow, blood cells in the middle of the vessels move the fastest, with a gradual decrease in flow velocity for points farther away from the center.

**paracanthoma** /-kanthō′mə/, a tumor that develops from the abnormal overgrowth of the prickle cell layer of the skin.

**paracelsian method** /-sel′sē·ən/ [Philippus Aureolus Paracelsus, Swiss alchemist and physician, 1493–1541], the use of chemical agents, such as sulfur, iron, lead, and arsenic, in the treatment of disease.

**paracenesthesia** /-sen′esthē′zhə/, any abnormality in the general sense of well-being.

**paracentesis** /par′əsentē′sis/ [Gk, *para* + *kentesis,* puncturing], a procedure in which fluid is withdrawn from a body cavity. An incision is made in the skin, and a hollow trocar, cannula, or catheter is passed through the incision into the cavity to allow outflow of fluid into a collecting device. Paracentesis is most commonly performed to remove excessive accumulations of ascitic fluid from the abdomen. Strict asepsis is followed. The patient needs to empty the bladder before this procedure to decrease the risk of bladder trauma. The patient is assessed for any adverse reaction.

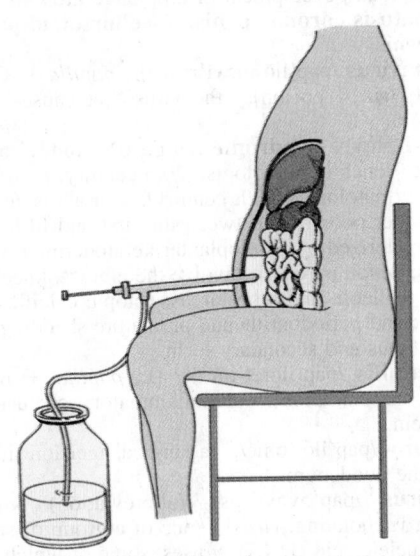

**Paracentesis** *(Elkin, Perry, and Potter, 2000)*

**paracentesis thoracis** [Gk, *para* + *kentesis,* puncturing, *thorax,* chest], the aspiration of fluid or air or both through a needle inserted into the pleural cavity.

**paracentesis tympani.** See **myringotomy.**

**paracentral** /-sen'trəl/ [Gk, *para* + *kentron*], close to a center or a central part.

**paracervical** /-sur'vikəl/ [Gk, *para* + L, *cervix*, neck], pertaining to the area adjacent to the cervix.

**paracervical block,** a form of regional anesthesia in which a local anesthetic is injected into each side of the uterine cervix to block nerve innervating the uterine cervix. Paracervical block is not the anesthesia of choice for labor and delivery, given the high incidence of fetal bradycardia and that it covers only the first stage of labor, but is an option during abortion and other gynecologic procedures.

**paracervix** /-sur'viks/, the connective tissue of the pelvic floor, extending from the uterine cervix.

**paracetamol.** See **acetaminophen.**

**paracholera** /-kol'ərə/, an infectious disease with symptoms similar to those of cholera but not caused by the true infectious agent, *Vibrio cholerae.*

**parachute reflex** /per'əshoot/, a variation of the **Moro reflex** or **startle reflex,** whereby an infant is tested for motor nerve development by suspending him or her in the prone position and then dropping him or her a short distance onto a soft surface. If the motor nerve development is normal, the infant at 4 to 6 months will extend the arms, hands, and fingers on both sides of the body in a protective movement.

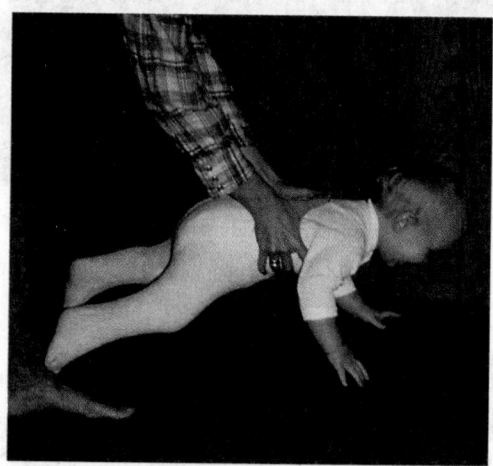

**Parachute reflex** *(Zitelli and Davis, 1997)*

**paracinesia.** See **parakinesia.**

**paracmasis.** See **paracme.**

**paracme** /perak'mē/, **1.** the phase of a fever or disease marked by a subsidence of symptoms. **2.** the point of involution, beyond the prime of life. Also called **paracmasis.**

**paracoccidioidomycosis** /per'əkoksid'ē·oi'dōmīkō'sis/ [Gk, *para* + *kokkos*, berry, *eidos*, form, *mykes*, fungus, *osis*, condition], a chronic occasionally fatal fungal infection caused by *Paracoccidioides brasiliensis.* It is characterized by ulcers of the oral cavity, larynx, and nose. Other effects include large, draining lymph nodes; cough; dyspnea; weight loss; and skin, genital, and intestinal lesions. The disease occurs in Mexico and Central and South America and is acquired by inhalation of spores of the fungus. Diagnosis is by microscopic examination of a smear prepared from a lesion. Treatment requires several years of sulfonamides or, in severe cases, IV amphotericin B followed by oral sulfon-

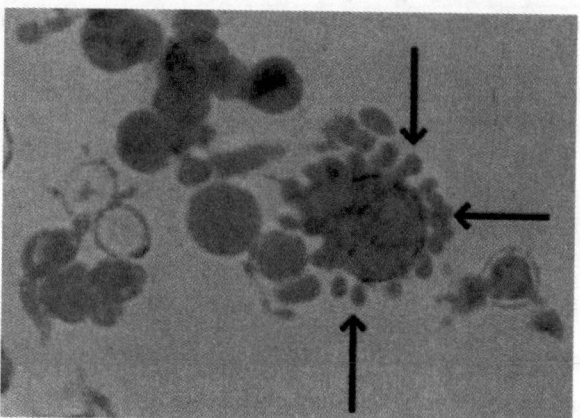

***Paracoccidioides brasiliensis***
*(Baron, Peterson, and Finegold, 1994)*

amides. Also called **paracoccidioidal granuloma, South American blastomycosis.** Compare **North American blastomycosis.**

**paracolitis** /-kōlī'tis/, an inflammation of the outer, peritoneal coat of the colon.

**paracolpium** /-kol'pē·əm/, the connective and other tissues around the vagina.

**paracortex** /-kôr'teks/, the thymus-dependent area of a lymph node between the subscapular cortex and the medullary cord.

**paracrine** /per'əkrēn/, an endocrine function in which effects of a hormone are localized to adjacent or nearby cells.

**paracusis** /per'əkoo'sis/, a disorder involving the sense of hearing, including distortions of pitch.

**paracystitis** /-sistī'tis/, an inflammation of the tissues around the urinary bladder.

**paradenitis** /-denī'tis/, an inflammation of tissues around a gland.

**paradentium.** See **periodontium** (def. 1).

**paradichlorobenzene poisoning.** See **naphthalene poisoning.**

**paradidymal** /-did'iməl/ [Gk, *para*, beside, *didymos*, twin], **1.** pertaining to the paradidymis. **2.** beside the testis.

**paradidymis** /per'ədid'imis/, *pl.* **paradidymides** /per'-ədidim'idēz/ [Gk, *para* + *epi*, above, *didymos*, twin], a rudimentary structure in the male, situated on the spermatic cord of the epididymis, that consists of vestigial remains of the caudal part of the embryonic mesonephric tubules. A similar vestigial structure, the paroophoron, is found in the female. Also called **organ of Giraldes, parepididymis.** See also **appendix epididymidis.**

**paradigm** /per'ədīm, -dim/, a pattern that may serve as a model or example.

**paradipsia** /-dip'sē·ə/, an abnormal desire for fluids unrelated to body needs.

**paradoxic** /-dok'sik/ [Gk, *paradoxos*, strange], pertaining to a person, situation, statement, or act that may appear to have inconsistent or contradictory qualities or that may be true but appears to be absurd or unbelievable. Also **paradoxical** /-dok'sikəl/.

**paradoxic aciduria,** a metabolic alkalosis condition that may involve an exchange of sodium and hydrogen ions for potassium. It may occur with prolonged nasogastric suctioning or repeated vomiting.

**paradoxic breathing** [Gk, *paradoxos* + AS, *braeth*], a condition in which a part of the lung deflates during inspiration and inflates during expiration. The condition usually is associated with a chest trauma, such as an open chest wound or rib cage damage. In such cases the condition is sometimes called internal paradoxic breathing. External paradoxic breathing may be observed during deep general anesthesia.

**paradoxic bronchospasm,** a constriction of the airways after treatment with a sympathomimetic bronchodilator.

**paradoxic incontinence.** See **retention with overflow.**

**paradoxic intention,** a logotherapeutic technique that encourages a patient to do what he or she fears and if possible to exaggerate it to the point of humor. The technique is used in the treatment of phobias.

**paradoxic pulse.** See **pulsus paradoxus.**

**paradoxic pupillary reflex,** the response of a pupil to light that is the reverse of a normal reflex, as when the pupil contracts in a darkened room.

**paradoxic thrombosis syndrome,** a condition of arterial and venous clots that may develop after a period of heparin therapy. It is thought to be caused by the production of antiplatelet antibodies that induce clotting.

**paraffin** /per'əfin/ [L, *parum*, little + *affinis*, related], any of a group of hydrocarbons or hydrocarbon mixtures of the paraffin series as indicated by the formula, $C_nH_{(2n+2)}$. Examples include methane gas, kerosene, and paraffin wax.

**paraffin bath** [L, *parum*, little, *affinis*, related], the application of heat to a specific area of the body through the use of paraffin. The part is quickly immersed in heated liquid wax and then withdrawn so that the wax solidifies to form an insulating layer. The procedure is repeated until the layer is 5 to 10 mm thick, and then the entire area is wrapped in an insulating material, such as a loose-fitting plastic bag or paper towels. The technique is effective for heating traumatized or inflamed areas, especially the hands, feet, and wrists, and is used primarily for patients with arthritis and rheumatism or any joint condition. Also called **wax bath.**

**paraffin method,** (in surgical pathology) a method used in preparing a selected portion of tissue for pathologic examination. The tissue is fixed, dehydrated, and infiltrated by and embedded in paraffin, forming a block that is cut with a microtome into slices 8 μm thick. This method, which is more commonly used than the frozen section method, is slower and therefore not used during surgery.

**paraffinoma** /per'əfinō'mə/, a tumor caused by the prosthetic or therapeutic injection of paraffin beneath the skin.

**paraffin section** [L, *parum*, little + *affinis*, related, *sectio*], a histologic section cut from tissue that has been embedded in paraffin wax.

**Paraflex,** a trademark for a skeletal muscle relaxant (chlorzoxazone).

**parafollicular C cell** /-folik'yələr/, a calcitonin-secreting cell located between follicles.

**Parafon Forte,** a trademark for a fixed-combination drug containing an analgesic-antipyretic (acetaminophen) and a skeletal muscle relaxant (chlorzoxazone), used for the relief of painful musculoskeletal conditions.

**paraganglioma** /-gang'glē·ō'mə/, a tumor derived from the chromoreceptor tissue of a paraganglion.

**paraganglion** /-gang'glē·on/, *pl.* **paraganglia** [Gk, *para* + *ganglion*, knot], any one of the small groups of chromaffin cells associated with the ganglia of the sympathetic nerve trunk and situated outside the adrenal medulla, most often near the sympathetic ganglia along the aorta and its branches. The paraganglia are also connected with the ganglia of the celiac, renal, suprarenal, aortic, and hypogastric plexuses. The paraganglia secrete the hormones epinephrine and norepinephrine. Also called **chromaffin body.** See also **chromaffin cell.**

**parageusia** /-jōō'sē·ə/, a disorder involving the sense of taste.

**paragonimiasis** /per'əgon'imī'əsis/ [Gk, *para* + *gonimos*, generative, *iasis*, condition], chronic infection by the lung fluke *Paragonimus westermani*, occurring most commonly in Asia. It is characterized by hemoptysis, bronchitis, and occasionally abdominal masses, pain and diarrhea, or cerebral involvement with paralysis, ocular pathologic conditions, or seizures. The disease is acquired by ingesting cysts in infected freshwater crabs or crayfish, the intermediate hosts. Praziquantel given orally is the usual treatment. Adequate cooking of shellfish prevents the disease.

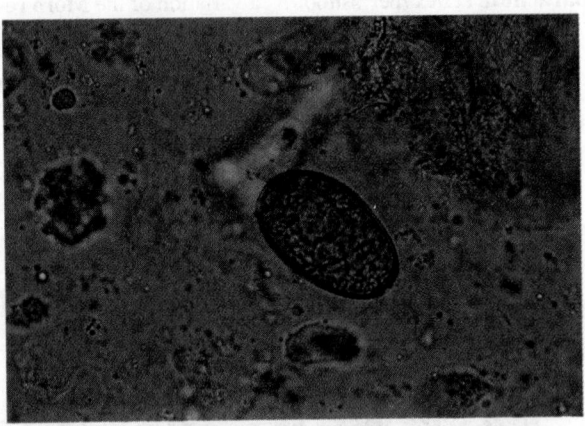

*Paragonimus westermani* **egg**
*(Mahon and Manuselis, 2000)*

**parahemophelia.** See **Owren's disease.**

**parahormone** /-hôr'mōn/, a substance that may exert a hormonal influence although it is not a true hormone.

**parahypnosis** /-hipnō'sis/ [Gk, *para* + *hypnos*, sleep], a form of disordered sleep that is observed in hypnosis and narcosis.

**parainfluenza virus** /per'ə·in'flōō·en'zə/ [Gk, *para* + It, *influenza*, influence], a myxovirus with four serotypes, causing respiratory infections in infants and young children and less commonly in adults. Type 1 and 2 parainfluenza viruses may cause laryngotracheobronchitis or croup; type 3 is a cause of croup, tracheobronchitis, bronchiolitis, and bronchopneumonia in children; types 1, 3, and 4 are associated with pharyngitis and the common cold. Compare **influenza, rhinovirus.**

**parakeratosis** /-ker'ətō'sis/, an abnormal formation of horn cells of the epidermis caused by the persistence of nuclei, incomplete formation of keratin, and moistness and swelling of the horn cells. It is observed as scaling in many conditions such as psoriasis.

**parakinesia** /-kinē'zhə/ [Gk, *para* + *kinesis*, movement], an abnormality of movement resulting from a nerve disorder in a muscle, such as an irregularity of one of the ocular muscles. Also called **paracinesia** /-sinē'zhə/.

**parakinesis.** See **telekinesis.**

**paraldehyde** /peral'dəhīd/, a clear, colorless strong-smelling liquid obtained by the polymerization of acetalde-

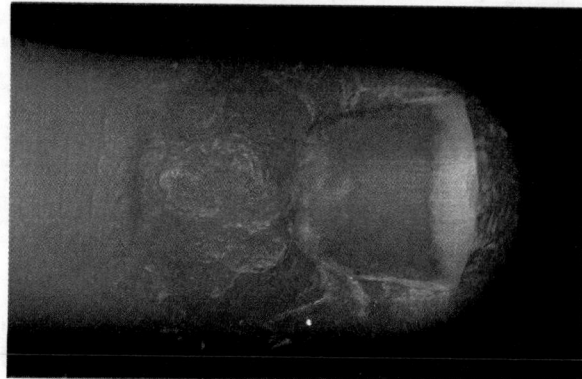

**Parakeratosis pustulosa**
*(Hordinsky, Sawaya, and Scher, 2000)*

hyde with a small amount of sulfuric acid. It is used as a solvent and may be administered orally, intravenously, intramuscularly, or rectally to induce hypnotic states or sedation.

**paralinguistic cues,** nonverbal elements (such as intonation, body posture, gestures, and facial expression) that modify the meaning of verbal communication.

**parallax** /per'əlaks/ [Gk, *parallelos,* side-by-side], the apparent displacement of an object at different distances from the eyes when viewed by both eyes together. It is the basis of stereoscopic vision and depth perception.

**parallel grid** /per'əlel/ [Gk, *parallelos,* side-by-side; ME, *gredire*], in radiography, an x-ray grid that has lead strips oriented parallel to each other.

**parallelogram condenser** /per'əlel'əgram'/ [Gk, *parallelos* + *gramma,* record; L, *condensare,* to make thick], an instrument with an end shaped like a rectangle or parallelogram, used for compacting amalgams in filling teeth.

**parallel play** [Gk, *parallelos* + AS, *plegan,* to play], a form of play among a group of children, primarily toddlers, in which each engages in an independent activity that is similar to but not influenced by or shared with the others. Compare **cooperative play.** See also **associative play, solitary play.**

**parallel talk,** a form of speech used during children's play therapy in which the clinician verbalizes activities of the child without requiring answers to questions. The parallel talk may take a form such as of "I'm making a cake. You are making a cake, too." The clinician repeats utterances of the child correctly and may parallel the child's actions.

**parallergic** /per'alur'jik/, having a nonspecific sensitivity to allergens as a result of a prior sensitization with a specific allergen.

**Paralympics** /per'əlim'piks/, [*paraplegic* + *Olympics*], an international competitive wheelchair sports event, usually held in association with the official quadrennial Olympic Games. Also called **ParaOlympics.**

**paralysis** /pəral'isis/, *pl.* **paralyses** [Gk, *paralyein,* to be palsied], the loss of muscle function, loss of sensation, or both. It may be caused by a variety of problems, such as trauma, disease, and poisoning. Paralyses may be classified according to the cause, muscle tone, distribution, or body part affected. See also **flaccid paralysis, spastic paralysis.** —**paralytic,** *adj.*

**paralysis agitans.** See **Parkinson's disease.**

**paralytic** /per'əlit'ik/ [Gk, *paralyein,* to be palsied], pertaining to the characteristics of paralysis.

**paralytic dementia.** See **paresis,** def. 2.

**paralytic ileus** [Gk, *paralyein,* to be paralyzed, *eilein,* to twist], a decrease in or absence of intestinal peristalsis. It may occur after abdominal surgery or peritoneal injury or be associated with severe pyelonephritis, ureteral stone, fractured ribs, myocardial infarction, extensive intestinal ulceration, heavy metal poisoning, porphyria, retroperitoneal hematomas, especially those associated with fractured vertebrae, or any severe metabolic disease. The most common overall cause of intestinal obstruction, paralytic ileus is mediated by a hormonal component of the sympathoadrenal system. Also called **adynamic ileus.**

■ OBSERVATIONS: Paralytic ileus is characterized by abdominal tenderness and distension, absence of bowel sounds, lack of flatus, and nausea and vomiting. There may be fever, decreased urinary output, electrolyte imbalance, dehydration, and respiratory distress. Loss of fluids and electrolytes may be extreme, and, unless they are replaced, the condition may lead to hemoconcentration, hypovolemia, renal insufficiency, shock, and death.

■ INTERVENTIONS: The patient is kept in bed in a low Fowler's position, and nothing is given by mouth. An intestinal tube may be inserted as a nasogastric tube into the duodenum and connected to intermittent suction and the patient is positioned to facilitate the advancement of the tube, which is checked at intervals, usually every 30 to 60 minutes. The character of GI drainage is monitored at intervals, usually every 2 to 4 hours, and any increase or decrease in the amount or changes in the color or consistency is reported. Bowel sounds, blood pressure, pulse, and respirations are checked every 2 to 4 hours, or as indicated in a particular circumstance, and rectal temperature usually every 4 hours. Abdominal girth is measured at least every 2 hours, and any increase is reported. Parenteral fluids with electrolytes and medication to promote peristalsis are administered as ordered; intake and output are measured, and if less than about 30 mL of urine is excreted per hour, the physician is informed. The patient is helped to turn and deep breathe every 2 to 4 hours and is given oral hygiene every 1 to 2 hours. Active or passive range-of-motion exercises are performed every 4 hours. Walking is helpful as gravity is a useful force. When intestinal output increases and bowel sounds return, the intestinal tube may be clamped and small amounts of warm tea may be given. If pain, distension, or cramps do not recur, the intestinal tube may be removed, but a rectal tube or an enema may be ordered to relieve distension.

■ NURSING CONSIDERATIONS: The concerns of the health care providers include monitoring and reporting the signs of paralytic ileus and its potential complications, ensuring that the patient is as comfortable as possible, explaining the purpose of the intestinal tube, and walking with the patient, encouraging ambulation. The patient is instructed to try to avoid mouth breathing, because swallowed air can increase distension. Before surgery, patients need reassurance that the sutures are strong and the distended abdomen will not burst.

**paralytic incontinence** [Gk, *paralyein,* to be palsied; L, *incontinentia,* inability to retain], urinary or fecal incontinence resulting from loss of or impaired motor nerve control of the sphincter muscles.

**paralytic mydriasis** [Gk, *paralyein,* to be palsied, *mydriasis,* pupil enlargement], an area of depressed vision that is on the periphery of the field.

**paralytic poliomyelitis** [Gk, *paralyein,* to be palsied, *polios,* gray, *myelos,* marrow, *itis,* inflammation], a flaccid paralysis of the limbs resulting from damaged lower motor neurons. Progressive bulbar paralysis with respiratory and vasomotor failure may result when the brainstem nuclei are involved.

**paralytic shellfish poisoning.** See **shellfish poisoning.**

**paralytic stroke** [Gk, *paralyein,* to be palsied; AS, *strac*], a sudden attack of paralysis caused by disease or injury to the brain or spinal cord.

**paralyze** /per′əlīz/ [Gk, *paralyein,* to be palsied], **1.** to produce or enter into a state of paralysis. **2.** to cause loss of muscle power.

**paramedic** /-med′ik/ [Gk, *para* + L, *medicina,* art of healing], a person who acts as an assistant to a physician or in place of a physician. —**paramedical,** *adj.*

**paramedical personnel,** health care workers other than physicians, dentists, podiatrists, and nurses who have special training in the performance of supportive health care tasks, for example, the **emergency medical technician, audiologist,** and **radiologic technologist.** Also called **allied health personnel.**

**paramesonephric duct** /per′əmēz′ōnef′rik/ [Gk, *para* + *mesos,* middle, *nephros,* kidney], one of a pair of embryonic ducts that develops into the uterus and the uterine tubes. Also called **müllerian duct.**

**parameter** /pəram′ətər/ [Gk, *para* + *metron,* measure], **1.** a value or constant used to describe or measure a set of data representing a physiologic function or system, as in the use of acid-base relationships of the blood as parameters for evaluating the function of a patient's respiratory system. **2.** a statistical value of a population group. **3.** *informal.* limit or boundary.

**parametria.** See **parametrium.**

**parametric imaging** /-met′rik/ [Gk, *para* + *metron,* measure; L, *imago,* image], **1.** a diagnostic procedure in which an image of an administered radioactive tracer is derived mathematically, such as by dividing one image by another. **2.** In positron emission tomography, a procedure in which a physiologic parameter such as blood flow is mapped according to anatomic position.

**parametric statistics,** statistics that assume a population has a symmetric, such as a gaussian or normal, distribution.

**parametritis** /per′əmetrī′tis/ [Gk, *para* + *metra,* womb, *itis*], an inflammatory condition of the tissue of the structures around the uterus. See also **pelvic inflammatory disease.**

**parametrium** /per′əmē′trē·əm/, *pl.* **parametria** [Gk, *para* + *metra,* womb], the lateral extension of the uterine subserous connective tissue into the broad ligament. Compare **endometrium, myometrium.**

**paramitome.** See **hyaloplasm.**

**paramnesia** /per′amnē′zhə/ [Gk, *para* + *amnesia,* forgetfulness], **1.** a perversion of memory in which one believes one remembers events and circumstances that never actually occurred. **2.** a condition in which words are remembered and used without comprehension of their meaning. Compare **déjà vu.**

**paramyloidosis** /peram′iloidō′sis/, **1.** an accumulation of amyloid-like protein in the tissues. **2.** any of several hereditary forms of amyloidosis characterized by sensory changes and muscle atrophy caused by amyloid deposits in somatic and visceral nerves.

**paramyxovirus** /-mik′sōvī′rəs/ [Gk, *para* + *myxa,* mucus; L, *virus,* poison], a member of a family of viruses that includes the organisms that cause parainfluenza, mumps, and some respiratory infections.

**paranasal** /-nā′zəl/ [Gk, *para* + L, *nasus,* nose], pertain-

ing to an area near or alongside the nose, such as the paranasal sinuses.

**paranasal sinus,** any one of the air cavities in various bones around the nose, such as the frontal sinus in the frontal bone lying deep to the medial part of the superciliary ridge and the maxillary sinus within the maxilla between the orbit, the nasal cavity, and the upper teeth. Compare **confluence of the sinuses, occipital sinus.**

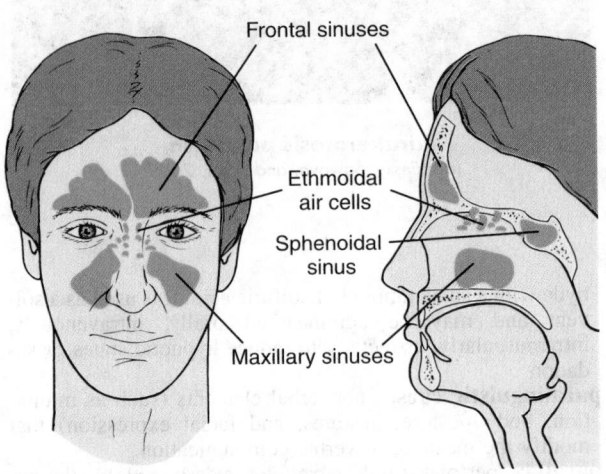

Frontal sinuses

Ethmoidal air cells

Sphenoidal sinus

Maxillary sinuses

**Paranasal sinuses** *(Lewis, Heitkemper, and Dirksen, 2000)*

**paraneoplastic cerebellar degeneration,** the most common paraneoplastic syndrome affecting the brain, occurring most commonly with ovarian and breast carcinoma and Hodgkin's disease, characterized pathologically by severe loss of Purkinje's cells and clinically by insidious and progressive truncal and appendicular ataxia, dysarthria, nystagmus, and occasionally dementia. In some women with gynecologic or breast carcinoma, it is associated with an autoantibody (anti-Yo).

**paraneoplastic syndromes** /-nē′əplas′tik/ [Gk, *para* + *neos,* new, *plassein,* to mold, *syn,* together, *dromos,* course], indirect effects of a tumor that occur distant to the tumor or metastatic site. They may result from the production of active proteins, polypeptides, or inactive hormones by the tumor.

**paranesthesia** /peran′esthē′zhə/, anesthesia affecting the lower half of the body.

**parangi.** See **yaws.**

**paranoeac.** See **paranoiac.**

**paranoia** /per′ənoi′ə/ [Gk, *para* + *nous,* mind], (in psychiatry) a condition characterized by an elaborate, overly suspicious system of thinking. It often includes delusions of persecution and grandeur usually centered on one major theme, such as a financial matter, a job situation, an unfaithful spouse, or another problem, such as being followed or monitored by the CIA, FBI, or outer space aliens; or computer tampering; or being poisoned. Also called **paranoea** /per′ənē′ə/. Compare **paranoid schizophrenia.**

**paranoiac** /per′ənoi′ak/, **1.** a person afflicted with or exhibiting characteristics of paranoia. **2.** pertaining to paranoia. Also **paranoeac.**

**paranoia querulans.** See **querulous paranoia.**

**paranoid** /per'ənoid/ [Gk, *para* + *nous*, mind, *eidos*, form], **1.** pertaining to or resembling paranoia. **2.** a person afflicted with a paranoid disorder. **3.** *informal.* a person, or pertaining to a person, who is overly suspicious or exhibits persecutory trends or attitudes.

**paranoid disorder,** any of a large group of mental disorders characterized by an impaired sense of reality and persistent delusions. Kinds of paranoid disorders include **acute paranoid disorder, paranoia,** and **shared paranoid disorder.**

**paranoid ideation,** an exaggerated, sometimes grandiose, belief or suspicion, usually not of a delusional nature, that one is being harassed, persecuted, or treated unfairly.

**paranoid personality,** a personality characterized by paranoia.

**paranoid personality disorder,** a psychiatric disorder characterized by extreme suspiciousness and distrust of others to the degree that one blames them for one's mistakes and failures and goes to abnormal lengths to validate prejudices, attitudes, or biases.

**paranoid reaction,** a psychopathologic condition that may be associated with aging and characterized by the gradual formation of delusions, usually of a persecutory nature and often accompanied by related hallucinations. Other manifestations of senile degeneration, such as memory loss and confusion, do not usually accompany the reaction, and the individual maintains orientation for time, place, and person.

**paranoid schizophrenia,** a form of schizophrenia characterized by persistent preoccupation with illogical, absurd, and changeable delusions, usually of a persecutory, grandiose, or jealous nature, accompanied by related hallucinations. The symptoms include extreme anxiety, exaggerated suspiciousness, aggressiveness, anger, argumentativeness, hostility, and violence. The condition occurs most frequently during middle age. Also called **heboid paranoia.** Compare **paranoia.** See also **schizophrenia.**

**paranoid state,** a transitory abnormal mental condition characterized by illogical thought processes and generalized suspicion and distrust, with a tendency toward persecutory ideas or delusions.

**paranormal** /-nôr'məl/ [Gk, *para* + L, *normalis*, rule], pertaining to phenomena that cannot be explained by normal scientific investigation.

**paranuclear body.** See **centrosome.**

**ParaOlympics.** See **Paralympics.**

**paraoperative,** pertaining to the accessories essential to operative surgery, such as sterilization and the care of instruments and gloves.

**paraparesis** /-pərē'sis/ [Gk, *para* + *paresis*, paralysis], a partial paralysis, usually affecting only the lower extremities.

**parapedesis** /-pedē'sis/, any secretion or excretion through an abnormal passageway.

**paraperitoneal** /-per'itənē'əl/, near or beside the peritoneum.

**paraperitoneal nephrectomy** [Gk, *para* + *peri* + *tenein*, to stretch, *nephros*, kidney, *ektome*, excision], the surgical removal of the kidney through an extraperitoneal incision.

**parapertussis** /per'əpərtus'is/ [Gk, *para* + L, *per*, very, *tussis*, cough], an acute bacterial respiratory infection caused by *Bordetella parapertussis*, having symptoms closely resembling those of pertussis. It is usually milder than pertussis, although it can be fatal. It is possible to be infected with both *B. parapertussis* and *B. pertussis* at the same time. A parapertussis vaccine is available and may be given in combination with pertussis vaccine.

**parapharyngeal abscess** /per'əfərin'jē·əl/ [Gk, *para* + *pharynx*, throat; L, *abscedere*, to go away], a suppurative infection of tissues adjacent to the pharynx, usually a complication of acute pharyngitis or tonsillitis. Infection may spread to the jugular vein, where it may cause thrombophlebitis and septic emboli. Systemic antibiotics and surgical drainage may be required. Also called **parapharyngeal space abscess.** Compare **peritonsillar abscess, retropharyngeal abscess.** See also **tonsillitis.**

**paraphasia** /-fā'zhə/ [Gk, *para* + *phrasein*, to utter], **1.** a condition in which a person hears and comprehends words but is unable to speak correctly. Incoherent words are substituted for intended words, thereby creating sentences that are unintelligible. **2.** speech that is incoherent, unintelligible, and apparently incomprehensible but may be meaningful when carefully interpreted by a psychotherapist. Also called **jargon aphasia, word hash, word salad.**

**paraphia** /pə·rā'fē·ə/ [Gk, *para*, apart from or against + *haphē*, touch], a disorder of the sense of touch. Also called **dysaphia.**

**paraphilia** /per'əfil'yə/ [Gk, *para* + *philein*, to love], sexual perversion or deviation; a condition in which the sexual instinct is expressed in ways that are socially prohibited or unacceptable or are biologically undesirable, such as the use of a nonhuman object for sexual arousal, sexual activity with another person that involves real or simulated suffering or humiliation, or sexual relations with a nonconsenting partner. Kinds of paraphilia include **exhibitionism, fetishism, pedophilia, transvestism, voyeurism,** and **zoophilia. —paraphiliac,** *adj., n.*

**paraphimosis** /per'əfīmō'sis/ [Gk, *para* + *phimoein*, to muzzle], a condition characterized by an inability to replace the foreskin in its normal position after it has been retracted behind the glans penis. Caused by a narrow or inflamed foreskin, the condition may lead to gangrene. Circumcision may be required. Compare **phimosis.**

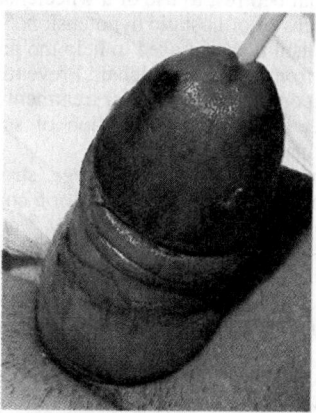

**Paraphimosis**
*(Seidel et al, 1999/courtesy Patrick C. Walsh, MD,
The Johns Hopkins University School of Medicine, Baltimore)*

**paraphrenia** /-frē'nē·ə/, a psychiatric condition that is primary to an affective illness or to an organic mental disorder. Gross disturbances of affect, volition, and function, which are characteristic of schizophrenia, are not prominent, but paranoid delusions and hallucinations are always present.

**paraplasm** /per′əplaz′əm/ [Gk, *para* + *plassein,* to mold], any abnormal growth or malformation. Compare **hyaloplasm.** —**paraplasmic,** *adj.*

**paraplastic** /-plas′tik/ [Gk, *para* + *plassein,* to mold], **1.** misshapen or malformed. **2.** showing abnormal formative power; of the nature of a paraplasm.

**paraplectic.** See **paraplegic.**

**paraplegia** /per′əplē′jē·ə/ [Gk, *para* + *plege,* stroke], paralysis characterized by motor or sensory loss in the lower limbs and trunk. Approximately 11,000 spinal cord injuries reported each year in the United States involve paraplegia. Such injuries commonly result from automobile and motorcycle accidents, sporting accidents, falls, and gunshot wounds. Paraplegia less commonly results from nontraumatic lesions, such as scoliosis, spina bifida, or neoplasms. Compare **hemiplegia, quadriplegia.** —**paraplegic,** *adj., n.*

■ OBSERVATIONS: The signs and symptoms of paraplegia may develop immediately from trauma and include the loss of sensation, motion, and reflexes below the level of the lesion. Depending on the level of the lesion and whether damage to the spinal cord is complete or incomplete, the patient may lose bladder and bowel control and sexual dysfunctions may develop. An incomplete spinal cord injury does not usually inhibit circumanal sensation, voluntary toe flexion, or sphincter control. A complete spinal cord injury destroys sensation and voluntary muscle control and usually causes the permanent loss of muscle function distal to the injury.

■ INTERVENTIONS: The treatment of paraplegia seeks to restore proper spine alignment, stabilize the injured spinal area, decompress any involved neurologic structures, and rehabilitate the patient as quickly as possible. At the accident scene when spinal cord injury is suspected the patient must not be moved until strapped and stabilized on a board. Such stabilization helps to prevent permanent damage to any injured spinal structures. Drugs such as baclofen may be administered to relieve any muscle spasms associated with dysfunction of the upper motor neurons.

■ NURSING CONSIDERATIONS: When the paraplegic patient progresses from bed rest to use of a wheelchair, the nurse is alert to any signs of orthostatic hypotension. Special binders and antiembolism hose are used to help the patient adjust to the transition from bed to wheelchair. Prevention of pressure sores is an important priority. Other treatment may include a high-bulk diet and the administration of suppositories to prevent constipation.

**paraplegic** /-plē′jik/ [Gk, *para* + *plege,* stroke], pertaining to a person affected by paraplegia or a condition resembling paraplegia. Also **paraplectic.**

**parapraxia** /-prak′sē·ə/ [Gk, *para* + *praxis,* doing], **1.** the abnormal performance of purposive actions, such as performance of one movement occurring in place of another intended movement. **2.** forgetfulness with a tendency to misplace things.

**paraproctitis** /-proktī′tis/, an inflammation affecting the tissues around the rectum and anus.

**paraprostatitis** /-pros′tətī′tis/, an inflammation of the tissues around the prostate gland.

**paraprotein** /-prō′tēn/, any of the incomplete monoclonal immunoglobulins that occur in plasma cell disorders.

**parapsoriasis** /per′əsərī′əsis/ [Gk, *para* + *psorian,* to itch], a group of chronic skin diseases resembling psoriasis, characterized by maculopapular, erythematous scaly eruptions without systemic symptoms. Parapsoriasis is resistant to all treatment.

**parapsoriasis varioliformis acuta.** See **Mucha-Habermann disease.**

**parapsychology** /-sīkol′əjē/ [Gk, *para* + *psyche,* mind,

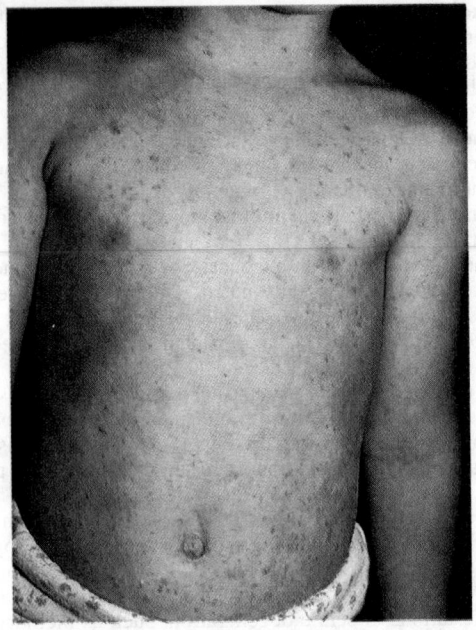

**Parapsoriasis** *(Weston, Lane, and Morrelli, 1996)*

*logos,* science], a branch of psychology concerned with the study of alleged psychic phenomena, such as clairvoyance, extrasensory perception, and telepathy.

**paraquat poisoning** /per′əkwot′/ [Gk, *para* + L, *quaterni,* four each, *potio,* drink], a toxic condition caused by the ingestion of paraquat dichloride, a highly poisonous pesticide. Characteristically progressive pulmonary fibrosis and damage to the esophagus, kidneys, and liver develop several days after ingestion. After fibrosis begins, death is inevitable, usually within 3 weeks. The mechanism of action of the poison is unknown. Most often poisoning results from accidental occupational exposure. There is considerable concern that the inhalation of the smoke of marijuana treated with the herbicide may cause intoxication, but no clinical syndrome resulting from such exposure has been documented.

**parareflexia** /-riflex′sē·ə/, any abnormal condition of the reflexes.

**pararhotacism.** See **rhotacism.**

**parasacral** /-sā′krəl/ [Gk, *para* + *sacrum*], pertaining to the area around the sacrum.

**parasalpingitis** /-sal′pinjī′tis/, an inflammation of the tissues around the fallopian tubes.

**paraseptal emphysema.** See **distal acinar emphysema.**

**parasite** /per′əsīt/ [Gk, *parasitos,* guest], **1.** an organism living in or on and obtaining nourishment from another organism. A **facultative parasite** may live on a host but is capable of living independently. An **obligate parasite** is one that depends entirely on its host for survival. **2.** see **parasitic fetus.** —**parasitic,** *adj.*

**parasitemia** /per′əsītē′mē·ə/ [Gk, *parasitos* + *haima,* blood], the presence of parasites in the blood. Compare **bacteremia, fungemia, viremia.**

**parasitic.** See **parasite.**

**parasitic fetus** /-sit′ik/ [Gk, *parasitos* + L, *icus,* like, *fetus,* pregnant], the smaller, usually malformed member of conjoined, unequal, or asymmetric twins that is attached to and dependent on the more normal fetus for growth and development. Compare **autosite.**

**parasitic fibroma,** a pedunculated uterine fibroid deriving part of its blood supply from the omentum.

**parasitic glossitis,** a mycosis of the tongue, characterized by a black or brown furry patch on the posterior dorsal surface. The patch is composed of hypertrophied filiform papillae that measure about 1 cm in length and are easily broken. The condition, caused by *Cryptococcus linguae-pilosasae* in symbiosis with *Nocardia lingualis,* produces no discomfort and may be treated with a simple mouthwash. The patch may disappear spontaneously and later reappear. Also called **black hairy tongue, glossitis parasitica, glossophytia.**

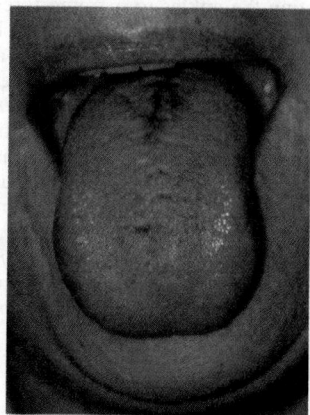

**Parasitic glossitis** *(Lemmi and Lemmi, 2000)*

**parasitic hemoptysis** [Gk, *parasitos,* guest, *haima,* blood + *ptyein,* to spit], the spitting of bright red blood caused by a parasitic infection. The condition usually involves the lung fluke *(Paragonimus)* or tapeworms *(Echinococcus).*

**parasitism** /per′əsitiz′əm/ [Gk, *parasitos,* guest], an infestation or presence of parasites.

**parasternal line.** See **costoclavicular line.**

**parasympathetic** /-sim′pəthet′ik/ [Gk, *para* + *sympathein,* to feel with], pertaining to the craniosacral division of the autonomic nervous system, consisting of the oculomotor, facial, glossopharyngeal, vagus, and pelvic nerves. The actions of the parasympathetic division are mediated by the release of acetylcholine and primarily involve the protection, conservation, and restoration of body resources. Preganglionic parasympathetic fibers, which emerge from the hypothalamus, other brain areas, and sacral segments of the spinal cord, form synapses in ganglia located near or in the walls of the organs to be innervated. Reactions to parasympathetic stimulation are highly localized and tend to counteract the adrenergic effects of sympathetic nerves. Parasympathetic fibers slow the heart; stimulate peristalsis; promote the secretion of lacrimal, salivary, and digestive glands; induce bile and insulin release; dilate peripheral and visceral blood vessels; constrict the pupils, esophagus, and bronchioles; and relax sphincters during micturition and defecation. Postganglionic parasympathetic fibers extend to the uterus, vagina, oviducts, and ovaries in females and to the prostate, seminal vesicles, and external genitalia in males, innervating blood vessels of pelvic organs in both sexes; stimulation

of these nerves causes vasodilation in the clitoris and labia minora and erection of the penis.

**parasympathetic ganglion** [Gk, *para* + *sympathein,* to feel with, *ganglion,* knot], a cluster of nerve cell bodies of the parasympathetic division of the autonomic nervous system. The nerves are functionally antagonistic to those of the sympathetic division.

**parasympathetic nervous system.** See **autonomic nervous system.**

**parasympatholytic, parasympatholytic drug.** See **anticholinergic.**

**parasympathomimetic** /per′əsim′pəthō′mimet′ik/ [Gk, *para* + *sympathein,* to feel with, *mimesis,* imitation], **1.** pertaining to a substance producing effects similar to those caused by stimulation of a parasympathetic nerve. **2.** an agent whose effects mimic those resulting from stimulation of parasympathetic nerves, especially those produced by acetylcholine. Also called **cholinergic.**

**parasympathomimetic drug.** See **cholinergic.**

**parasynovitis** /-sinəvī′tis/, an inflammation of the tissues around a joint.

**parasystole** [Gk, *para* + *systole,* contraction], an independent ectopic rhythm whose pacemaker cannot be discharged by impulses of the dominant (usually the sinus) rhythm because an area of depressed conduction surrounds the parasystolic focus. In the classic parasystole, the interectopic intervals are exact multiples of a common denominator reflecting the protected status of the parasystolic focus; however, the ectopic focus is usually influenced by the phasic events around its protection zone (modulated parasystole). Thus the sinus rhythm may modulate the parasystolic rhythm so that criteria for absolute, undisturbed regularity are not fulfilled. Fusion beats are common because of the simultaneous discharge of the ventricles by both the sinus and the parasystolic impulses.

**parataxic distortion** /per′ətak′sik/ [Gk, *para* + *taxis,* arrangement], **1.** a defense mechanism in which current interpersonal relationships are perceived and judged according to a mode of reference established by an earlier experience. **2.** Harry S. Sullivan's term for inaccuracies in judgment and perception. See also **transference.**

**parataxic mode,** a term introduced by H.S. Sullivan to identify a childhood perception of the physical and social environment as being illogical, disjointed, and inconsistent. The parataxic mode may persist into adulthood in some individuals.

**Parathar,** a trademark for a parathyroid diagnostic agent (teriparatide acetate).

**parathion poisoning** /per′əthī′on/ [Gk, *para* + *thio,* phosphate, *on* + L, *potio,* drink], a toxic condition caused by the ingestion, inhalation, or absorption through the skin of the highly toxic organophosphorus insecticide parathion. Symptoms include nausea, vomiting, abdominal cramps, confusion, headache, lack of muscular control, convulsions, and dyspnea.

**parathyroid-, parathyro-,** combining form meaning 'parathyroid glands': *parathyroidectomy.*

**parathyroidectomy** /-thī′roidek′təmē/ [Gk, *para* + *thyreos,* shield, *eidos,* form, *ektomē,* excision], the surgical removal of the parathyroid gland.

**parathyroid gland** /-thī′roid/ [Gk, *para* + *thyreos,* shield, *eidos,* form; L, *glans,* acorn], any one of several small structures, usually four, attached to the dorsal surfaces of the lateral lobes of the thyroid gland. The parathyroid glands secrete parathyroid hormone, which helps maintain the blood calcium concentration and ensures normal neuromuscular irritability, blood clotting, and cell membrane permeability.

Each parathyroid gland is an oval brownish red disk measuring about 6 by 4 mm. The parathyroids are divided, according to their location, into the superior parathyroids and the inferior parathyroids. The superior parathyroids, usually two, are commonly situated, one on each side, on the caudal border of the cricoid cartilage beside the junction of the pharynx and the esophagus. The inferior parathyroids, also usually two, may be situated on the caudal edge of the lateral lobes of the thyroid gland or adjacent to one of the inferior thyroid veins. These glands are composed of intercommunicating columns of cells bound by connective tissue with a rich supply of capillaries. Parathyroid hypofunction usually causes tetany, which can be treated by the administration of calcium salts or parathyroid extracts.

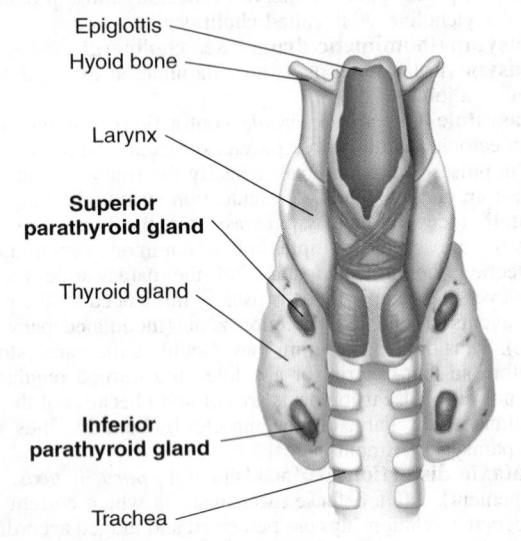

Epiglottis

Hyoid bone

Larynx

**Superior parathyroid gland**

Thyroid gland

**Inferior parathyroid gland**

Trachea

**Parathyroid glands** *(Thibodeau and Patton, 1999/Joanna Wild)*

**parathyroid hormone (PH),** a hormone secreted by the parathyroid glands that acts to maintain a constant concentration of calcium in the extracellular fluid. The hormone regulates absorption of calcium from the GI tract, mobilization of calcium from the bones, deposition of calcium in the bones, and excretion of calcium in the breast milk, feces, sweat, and urine. Surgical removal of the parathyroid glands, as may inadvertently occur in thyroidectomy, results in hypocalcemia, leading to anorexia, tetany, seizures, and death if not corrected. Normal parathyroid laboratory findings are less than 2000 pg/mL. See also **hypoparathyroidism.**

**parathyroid hormone test (PTH),** a blood test that is useful in establishing a diagnosis of hyperparathyroidism and distinguishing nonparathyroid from parathyroid causes of hypercalcemia. PTH is secreted by the parathyroid gland in response to hypocalcemia.

**parathyroid injection,** bovine parathyroid hormone.
■ INDICATION: It is prescribed to regulate blood levels of calcium, especially in the treatment of hypoparathyroidism with tetany.
■ CONTRAINDICATIONS: Hypercalcemia, tetany not caused by hypoparathyroidism, hypercalciuria, or known hypersensitivity to this drug prohibits its use.

■ ADVERSE EFFECTS: Among the most serious adverse reactions are hypercalcemia and allergic reactions.

**parathyroid tetany** [Gk, *para* + *thyreos*, shield, *tetanos,* convulsive tension], a form of tetany (hypocalcemia) that is caused by a deficiency of parathyroid secretion.

**parathyrotropic** /-thī′rōtrop′ik/, stimulating the growth or rate of activity of the parathyroid glands.

**paratonia.** See **gegenhalten.**

**paratrichosis** /-trikō′sis/, an abnormality in the distribution, growth, and quantity of scalp hair.

**paratriptic** /-trip′tik/, pertaining to an agent that causes chafing.

**paratrooper fracture** /-trOO′pər/ [Fr, *parasol* + *troupe,* company; L, *fractura,* break], a break in the distal tibia and its malleolus, commonly occurring when an individual jumps from an elevated platform and lands feet first on the ground, subjecting the ankles to extreme force.

**paratyphlitis** /-tiflī′tis/ [Gk, *para* + *typhlos* blind, *itis,* inflammation], an inflammation of the tissues around the cecum and vermiform appendix. Also called **perityphlitis.**

**paratyphoid fever** /-tī′foid/ [Gk, *para* + *typhos,* stupor, *eidos,* form; L, *febris,* fever], a bacterial infection, caused by any *Salmonella* species other than *S. typhi,* characterized by symptoms resembling typhoid fever, although somewhat milder. See also **rose spots, Salmonella, salmonellosis, typhoid fever.**

**paraurethral duct** /per′əyOOrē′thrəl/ [Gk, *para* + *ourethra,* urethra; L, *ducere,* to lead], one of a pair of ducts that drain the bulbourethral glands into the vestibule of the vagina. Also called **Skene's duct.**

**paravaccinia virus** /-vaksin′ē·ə/, a member of a subgroup of poxviruses that can infect humans through direct contact with infected livestock. It is related to the smallpox virus and is the cause of pseudocowpox, which produces milker's nodules. See also **milker's nodule.**

**paravaginitis** /-vaj′inī′tis/, an inflammation of the tissues around the vagina.

**paravertebral** /-vur′təbrəl/ [Gk, *para* + L, *vertebra,* joint], pertaining to the area alongside the spinal column or near a vertebra.

**paravertebral block** [Gk, *para* + L, *vertebra* + OFr, *bloc*], **1.** the blocking of transmission of somatic impulses by the spinal nerves by injection of a local analgesic solution near the point of their emergence. **2.** the blocking of the paravertebral sympathetic chain of nerves anterolateral to the vertebral bodies.

**paraxial** /perak′sē·əl/, pertaining to an organ or other structure located near the axis of the body.

**parchment skin** /pärch′mənt/ [Fr, *parchemin* + AS, *scinn*], thin, wrinkled, or stretched atrophic skin.

**Paredrine,** a trademark for an adrenergic (hydroxyamphetamine hydrobromide); an ophthalmic decongestant.

**paregoric** /per′əgôr′ik/, a camphorated tincture of opium.
■ INDICATIONS: It is prescribed in the treatment of diarrhea and as an analgesic.
■ CONTRAINDICATIONS: Known hypersensitivity to this drug or to any opium derivative prohibits its use. It should not be used when diarrhea is caused by a toxic substance.
■ ADVERSE EFFECTS: There are usually no adverse reactions. Occasionally GI disturbances, including constipation, occur.

**parencephalitis** /per′ensef′əlī′tis/, an inflammation of the cerebellum.

**parencephalocele** /per′ensef′əlōsēl′/, a protrusion of the cerebellum through a hole in the cranium.

**parenchyma** /pəreng′kimə/ [Gk, *para* + *enchyma,* infusion], the functional tissue or cells of an organ or gland, as distinguished from supporting or connective tissue.

**parenchymal.** See **parenchymatous.**

**parenchymal cell** /pəreng'kiməl/, any cell that is a functional element of an organ, such as a hepatocyte.

**parenchymatous** /per'əngkim'ətəs/ [Gk, *para* + *enchyma,* infusion], pertaining to or resembling the functional tissues of an organ or gland. Also **parenchymal.**

**parenchymatous myositis.** See **myositis.**

**parenchymatous nephritis.** See **nephritis.**

**parenchymatous neuritis** [Gk, *para* + *enchyma,* infusion; L, *osus,* like], any inflammation affecting the substance, axons, or myelin of the nerve. Also called **axial neuritis, central neuritis.** See also **neuritis.**

**parenchymatous salpingitis,** an inflammation and thickening of the fallopian tubes. Also called **pachysalpingitis.**

**parent** [L, *parens*], a mother or father; one who bears offspring. —**parental,** *adj.*

**parental generation (P₁)** /pəren'təl/, the initial cross between two varieties in a genetic sequence; the parents of any individual belonging to an F₁ generation.

**parental grief,** the behavioral reactions that characterize the grieving process and result in the resolution of the loss of a child from expected or unexpected death. All people who survive the loss of a loved one normally experience symptoms of both somatic and psychologic distress, such as feelings of guilt and hostility accompanied by changes in usual patterns of conduct. When the death of a child with a terminal illness is expected, there is time for anticipatory grieving, so that parents can evaluate their relationship with the child, set priorities for the duration of time involved, and prepare for the actual death of the child. In such cases parental grieving begins with the discovery of the diagnosis of a life-threatening condition. Parents' adjustment to the diagnosis involves a complete cycle of reactions that extends over an indefinite period depending on the severity and nature of the disease. The immediate reactions are shock and disbelief, followed by acute grief at the anticipation of losing the child. Periods of depression, anger, hope, fear, and anxiety alternate during induction therapy, remission, and maintenance of the disease as parents learn to accept and cope with the situation. Heightened anticipatory grieving recurs during episodes of relapse, and the parents experience increased fear, depression, and final acceptance of death during the terminal stages of the illness. Although families can prepare themselves for the expected loss, at the time of death there is a period of acute grief, during which parents need to express their deep sorrow and anger. An extended phase of mourning follows, with the eventual resolution of grief and integration into society. In sudden, unexpected death parents are denied the advantages of anticipatory grief and, because of the lack of time to prepare, usually have extreme feelings of guilt and remorse. The nurse can especially help such parents to assess their feelings so that they can work through them and progress through the resolution of grief and the mourning process, which in unexpected death take a much longer time. The function of the nurse during all phases of parental grief is primarily supportive, and the degree of intervention depends on the family's strengths and weaknesses in coping with the crisis. Nurses can act directly, or they can help find other potential sources of support for the parents, such as extended family members, other parents who have lost children, or specific community services or agencies. A large part of the nursing support involves helping families explore new ways of coping, not only to meet the present crisis but to grow and change. Always an important nursing consideration is the education of the parents about all aspects of the child's illness, especially in terminal conditions. See also **death, grief reaction.**

**parental leave.** See **family care leave.**

**parental role conflict,** a nursing diagnosis accepted by the Eighth National Conference on the Classification of Nursing Diagnoses. The condition is a state in which a parent experiences role confusion and conflict in response to a crisis.

■ DEFINING CHARACTERISTICS: Among major defining characteristics is an expression by the parent or parents of concerns or feelings of inadequacy to provide for the child's physical and emotional needs during hospitalization or in the home. A demonstrated disruption occurs in caretaking routines. The parent also expresses concerns about changes in parental role, family functioning, family communication, and family health. Minor characteristics include expressions of concern about perceived loss of control over decisions relating to the child and reluctance to participate in normal caretaking activities even with encouragement and support. Parents also verbalize or demonstrate feelings of guilt, anger, fear, anxiety, and frustration about the effect of the child's illness on the family process.

■ RELATED FACTORS: Related factors include separation from the child caused by chronic illness; intimidation by invasive or restrictive modalities (such as isolation, intubation), specialized care centers, and policies; home care of a child with special needs (such as apnea monitoring, postural drainage, and hyperalimentation); change in marital status; and interruptions of family life caused by the home care regimen (such as treatments, caregivers, and lack of respite). See also **nursing diagnosis.**

**parent-child relationship.** See **maternal-infant bonding.**

**parent education,** any experience geared to the thoughtful conveyance of information enabling the parent to provide high-quality childrearing.

**parent education: adolescent,** a nursing intervention from the Nursing Interventions Classification (NIC) defined as assisting parents to understand and help their adolescent children. See also **Nursing Interventions Classification.**

**parent education: childrearing family,** a nursing intervention from the Nursing Interventions Classification (NIC) defined as assisting parents to understand and promote the physical, psychological, and social growth and development of their toddler, preschool, or school-age child/children. See also **Nursing Interventions Classification.**

**parent education: infant,** a nursing intervention from the Nursing Interventions Classification (NIC) defined as instruction on nurturing and physical care needed during the first year of life. See also **Nursing Interventions Classification.**

**parent ego state,** (in transactional analysis) an ego state that incorporates the feelings and behavior learned from the parents or other authority figures. A part of the self that offers advice like that of one's own parents, containing messages that emphasize what one "ought to" or "should not" do.

**parenteral** /pəren'tərəl/ [Gk, *para* + *enteron,* bowel], pertaining to treatment other than through the digestive system. —**parenterally,** *adv.*

**parenteral absorption,** the taking up of substances within the body by structures other than the digestive tract.

**parenteral dosage,** pertaining to a medication administered by a route that bypasses the GI tract, such as a drug given by injection.

**parenteral fluids.** See **administration of parenteral fluids.**

**parenteral hyperalimentation.** See **total parenteral nutrition.**

**parenterally.** See **parenteral.**

**parenteral nutrition,** the administration of nutrients by a route other than the alimentary canal, such as subcutaneously, intravenously, intramuscularly, or intradermally. The parenteral fluids usually consist of physiologic saline solution with glucose, amino acids, electrolytes, vitamins, and medications. They may not be nutritionally complete but maintain fluid and electrolyte balance during the immediate postoperative period and in other conditions, such as shock, coma, malnutrition, and chronic renal and hepatic failures. See also **total parenteral nutrition.**

**parent figure** [L, *parens* + *figura,* form], **1.** a parent or a substitute parent or guardian who cares for a child, providing the physical, social, and emotional requirements necessary for normal growth and development. **2.** a person who symbolically represents an ideal parent, having those attributes that one conceptualizes as necessary for forming the perfect parent-child relationship.

**parent image,** a conscious and unconscious concept that a child forms concerning the roles and characteristics of the personality of the mother and father. See also **imago, primordial image.**

**parent-infant attachment,** a nursing outcome from the Nursing Outcomes Classification (NOC) defined as the behaviors which demonstrate an enduring affectionate bond between a parent and infant. See also **Nursing Outcomes Classification.**

**parent/infant/child attachment, impaired, risk for,** a nursing diagnosis accepted by the Eleventh National Conference on the Classification of Nursing Diagnoses. It is defined as disruption of the interactive process between parent or significant other and infant that fosters the development of a protective and nurturing reciprocal relationship.
■ RELATED FACTORS: The risk factors are inability of parents to meet the personal needs; anxiety associated with the parental role; substance abuse; prematurity of an infant; inability of an ill infant or child to initiate parental contact effectively because of altered behavioral organization; separation; physical barriers; and lack of privacy. See also **nursing diagnosis.**

**parenting,** a nursing outcome from the Nursing Outcomes Classification (NOC) defined as the provision of an environment that promotes optimum growth and development of dependent children. See also **Nursing Outcomes Classification.**

**parenting, impaired,** a nursing diagnosis accepted by the Seventh National Conference on the Classification of Nursing Diagnoses. The diagnosis describes the changes in ability of nurturing figures to create an environment that promotes the optimum growth and development of another human being.
■ DEFINING CHARACTERISTICS: The defining characteristics of the condition are multiple and may include constant complaints about the sex or the appearance of the new child, verbal self-assessment of inadequacy in the parental role, expressed disgust about the child's body functions, failure to keep health care appointments for the child, inappropriate or inconsistent disciplinary practices, slow growth and development in the child, and an observed need of the parent to receive approval from others. The critical defining characteristics, at least one of which must be present to make the diagnosis, include an observed lack of actions that demonstrate attachment to the child; inattentiveness to the child's needs; inappropriate caretaking behavior, especially in toilet training and in sleep and feeding patterns; and a history of abuse or abandonment of the child.
■ RELATED FACTORS: Related factors include lack of an available role model, ineffective role model, lack of support between/from significant others, unmet social/emotional maturation needs, interruption in the bonding process, mental and/or physical illness, presence of stress (financial, legal, recent crisis, cultural move), lack of knowledge, limited cognitive functioning, lack of role identity, lack of or inappropriate response of child to relationship, and multiple pregnancies. See also **nursing diagnosis.**

**parenting, impaired, risk for,** a nursing diagnosis accepted by the Seventh National Conference on the Classification of Nursing Diagnoses. The diagnosis is defined as the possibility of changes in ability of nurturing figures to create an environment that promotes the optimum growth and development of another human being. The cause of the problem may be complex and may involve several factors.
■ DEFINING CHARACTERISTICS: Defining characteristics include lack of parental attachment behaviors; inappropriate visual, tactile, or auditory stimulation; negative identification with or attachment of meanings to infant or child characteristics; verbalization of disappointment in or resentment toward the infant or child; noncompliance with health appointments; inappropriate caretaking behaviors; inappropriate or inconsistent discipline practices; history of child abuse or abandonment by primary caretaker; and employment of multiple caretakers without consideration for the child's needs.
■ RELATED/RISK FACTORS: Related factors include lack of an available role model; lack of support between or from significant others; interruption of the process of bonding in the newborn period; unrealistic expectations for the self, the infant, or the partner; mental or physical illness; the presence of financial, legal, or cultural stressors; a lack of knowledge; limited cognitive ability; multiple pregnancies; and a recent crisis. See also **nursing diagnosis.**

**parenting promotion,** a nursing intervention from the Nursing Interventions Classification (NIC) defined as providing parenting information, support, and coordination of comprehensive services to high-risk families. See also **Nursing Interventions Classification.**

**parenting: social safety,** a nursing outcome from the Nursing Outcomes Classification (NOC) defined as the parental actions to avoid social relationships that might cause harm or injury. See also **Nursing Outcomes Classification.**

**Parents Anonymous,** a self-help group for parents who have abused their children or who feel that they are prone to maltreat them. The organization offers support and guidance, provides a forum for discussing mutual problems, and furnishes distressed parents with a positive mechanism for coping with anger by talking to another member rather than by releasing their emotions on the child. See also **child abuse.**

**Parents Without Partners,** a self-help group for single parents, including those who are separated, divorced, or widowed.

**parepididymis.** See **paradidymis.**

**paresis** /pərē′sis, per′isis/ [Gk, *paralyein,* to be palsied], **1.** motor weakness or partial paralysis related in some cases to local neuritis. **2.** also called **dementia paralytica, general paresis, paralytic dementia.** A late manifestation of neurosyphilis, characterized by generalized paralysis, tremulous incoordination, transient seizures, Argyll Robertson pupils, and progressive dementia caused by degeneration of cortical neurons. Paresis resulting from untreated syphilis usually develops in the third to fifth decade but may occur at an early age in patients with congenital syphilis. —**paretic,** *adj.*

**-paresis,** combining form meaning 'incomplete or partial paralysis': *hemiparesis.*

**paresthesia** /per′esthē′zhə/ [Gk, *para* + *erethizein,* to excite], any subjective sensation, experienced as numbness, tingling, or a "pins and needles" feeling. Paresthesias often fluctuate according to such influences as posture, activity, rest, edema, congestion, or underlying disease. When experienced in the extremities, it is sometimes identified as acroparesthesia. Also spelled *paraesthesia*.

**paresthetic pain.** See **paresthesia.**

**paretic** /peret′ik/ [Gk, *paresis,* paralysis],   pertaining to or resembling partial paralysis.

**paretic dementia.** See **paresis.**

**pareunia.** See **coitus.**

**paricalcitol,**   a vitamin D analog.

■ INDICATIONS: This drug is used to treat hypoparathyroidism.

■ CONTRAINDICATIONS: Known hypersensitivity to this drug and hypercalcemia prohibit the use of paricalcitol.

■ ADVERSE EFFECTS: Sepsis is a life-threatening effect of this drug. Other adverse effects include nausea, vomiting, anorexia, dry mouth, lightheadedness, palpitations, pneumonia, edema, chills, fever, and flu.

**paries** /per′i·ēz/, *pl.* **parietes** /pərī′itēz/,   the wall of a hollow organ or cavity in the body.

**parietal** /pərī′ətəl/ [L, *paries,* wall],   1. pertaining to the outer wall of a cavity or organ. 2. pertaining to the parietal bone of the skull or the parietal lobe of the cerebrum.

**parietal bone,**   one of a pair of bones forming the sides of the cranium. Each parietal bone has two surfaces, four borders, and four angles and articulates with five bones: the opposite parietal, occipital, frontal, temporal, and sphenoid.

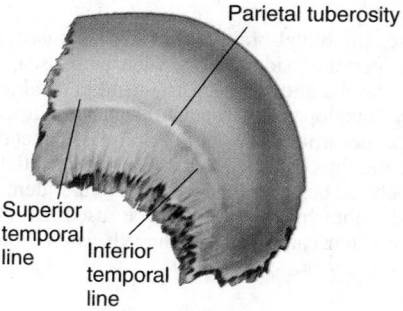

**Parietal bone**

**parietal cells** [L, *paries,* wall, *cella,* storeroom],   the cells on the periphery of the gastric glands of the stomach. They are located on the basement membrane beneath the chief cells and secrete hydrochloric acid.

**parietal hernia.** See **Richter's hernia.**

**parietal lobe,**   a portion of each cerebral hemisphere that occupies the parts of the lateral and medial surfaces that are covered by the parietal bone. On the lateral surface of the hemisphere the parietal lobe is separated from the frontal lobe by the central sulcus and from the temporal lobe by an imaginary line that extends from the posterior ramus of the lateral sulcus toward the occipital pole. It is concerned with language mechanisms and general sensory functions. Compare **central lobe, frontal lobe, occipital lobe, temporal lobe.**

**parietal lymph node,**   any one of the small oval glands that filter the lymph coursing through the lymphatic vessels in the walls of the thorax or through the lymphatic vessels

associated with the larger blood vessels of the abdomen and the pelvis. The parietal lymph nodes of the thorax include the sternal nodes, intercostal nodes, and diaphragmatic nodes. The parietal lymph nodes of the abdomen and pelvis include the common iliac nodes, epigastric nodes, external iliac nodes, iliac circumflex nodes, internal iliac nodes, lumbar nodes, and sacral nodes. See also **lymph, lymphatic system, lymph node.**

**parietal pain,**   a sharp sensation of distress in the parietal pleura, aggravated by respiration and thoracic movements and caused by pneumonia, empyema, pneumothorax, asbestosis, tuberculosis, neoplasm, or the accumulation of fluid resulting from heart, liver, or kidney disease. Pain arising from the parietal pleura lining the chest wall is perceived over the involved area, but that arising from the central part of the diaphragm is referred to the posterior shoulder area; pain from the costal portions of the diaphragm is referred to the adjacent thoracic wall.

**parietal pericardium** [L, *paries,* wall; Gk, *peri* + *kardia,* heart],   an outer layer of the serous pericardium that is not in direct contact with the heart muscle.

**parietal peritoneum,**   the portion of the largest serous membrane in the body that lines the abdominal wall. Compare **visceral peritoneum.** See also **peritoneal cavity.**

**parietes.** See **paries.**

**parietooccipital** /pərī′ətō·oksip′itəl/ [L, *paries* + *occiput,* back of the head],   pertaining to the parietal and occipital bones or cerebral lobes.

**parietooccipital sulcus,**   a groove on each cerebral hemisphere marking the division of the parietal and occipital lobes of the cerebrum. Also called **occipitoparietal fissure.**

**parietotemporal** /-tem′pərəl/ [L, *paries,* wall, *tempus,* temple],   pertaining to the temporal and parietal bones of the cranium. Also called **temporoparietal.**

**parietovisceral** /-vis′ərəl/,   pertaining to the abdominal wall and abdominal organs.

**-parin,**   combining form for heparin derivatives.

**Parinaud's oculoglandular syndrome** /per′ənōz/ [Henri Parinaud, French ophthalmologist, 1844–1905],   a term often used to refer to conjunctivitis that is usually unilateral, follicular, and followed by enlargement of the preauricular lymph nodes and tenderness. The syndrome is caused by a wide range of tularemia, cat-scratch fever, and lymphogranuloma venereum. Also called **granulomatous conjunctivitis, Parinaud's ophthalmoplegia.**

**paring board.** See **spikeboard.**

**pari passu** /per′ē pas′oo/ [L, *par,* equal, *passus,* step],   at the same time or in equal proportions.

**paritonsillar abscess.** See **parapharyngeal abscess.**

**parity** /per′itē/ [L, *parere,* to give birth],   1. (in obstetrics) the classification of a woman by the number of live-born children and stillbirths she has delivered at more than 20 weeks of gestation. Commonly parity is noted with the total number of pregnancies and represented by the letter *P* or the word *para.* A para 4 (P4) gravida 5 (G5) has had four deliveries after 20 weeks and one abortion or miscarriage before 20 weeks. Currently a more complete system is in use: the total number of pregnancies is followed by the number of deliveries at term, the number of premature infants, the number of abortions or miscarriages before 20 weeks' gestation, and the number of children living at present. This system may be abbreviated as *TPAL.* 2. (in epidemiology) the classification of a woman by the number of live-born children she has delivered. 3. (in computer processing) the condition of a set of items, either even or odd in number, used as a means for checking errors, such as in the transmission of information between various elements of the same computer.

The image shows a parietal bone with the following labels: Parietal tuberosity, Superior temporal line, Inferior temporal line.

**parkinsonian** /pär′kinsō′nē·ən/ [James Parkinson, English physician, 1755–1824],　pertaining to or resembling Parkinson's disease.

**parkinsonian facies** [James Parkinson; L, *facies,* face],　a masklike and immobile facial expression, usually occurring with Parkinson's disease. Infrequent blinking also occurs.

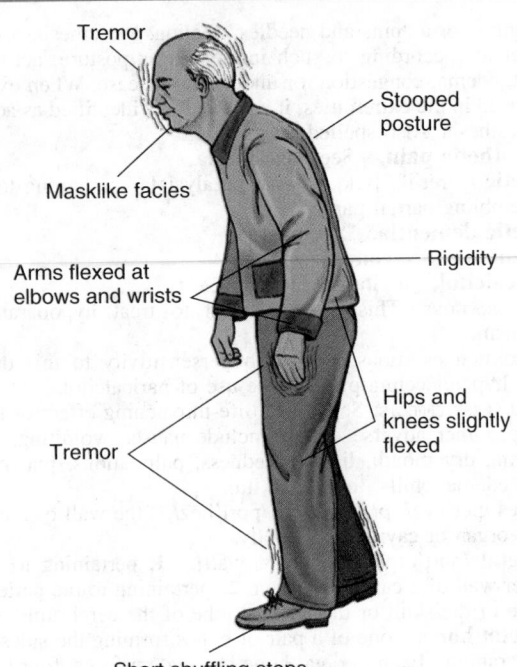

Tremor

Stooped posture

Masklike facies

Rigidity

Arms flexed at elbows and wrists

Tremor

Hips and knees slightly flexed

Short shuffling steps

**Clinical manifestations of Parkinson's disease**
*(Monahan and Neighbors, 1998)*

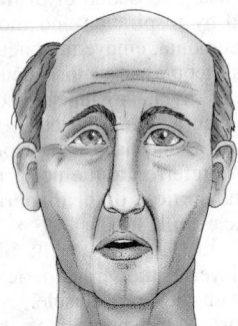

**Parkinsonian facies** *(Ignatavicius, Workman, and Mishler, 1999)*

**parkinsonian tremor** [James Parkinson; L, *tremor,* shaking],　a mild resting tremor with slow, regular oscillations of three to six per second, exacerbated by fatigue, cold, or emotion. The tremors usually, but not always, cease during voluntary movement of the affected part and during sleep.

**parkinsonism** /pär′kənsəniz′əm/ [James Parkinson],　a neurologic disorder characterized by tremor, muscle rigidity, hypokinesia, a slow shuffling gait, and difficulty in chewing, swallowing, and speaking, caused by various lesions in the extrapyramidal motor system. Signs and symptoms of parkinsonism resemble those of idiopathic Parkinson's disease and may develop during or after acute encephalitis and in syphilis, malaria, poliomyelitis, and carbon monoxide poisoning. Parkinsonism frequently occurs in patients treated with antipsychotic drugs, such as amitriptyline, chlorpromazine, fluphenazine, loxapine, thioridazine, and other phenothiazine derivatives. See also **Parkinson's disease.**

**Parkinson's disease** [James Parkinson],　a slowly progressive degenerative neurologic disorder characterized by resting tremor, pill rolling of the fingers, a masklike facies, shuffling gait, forward flexion of the trunk, loss of postural reflexes, and muscle rigidity and weakness. It is usually an idiopathic disease of people over 60 years of age; it may occur in younger people, however, especially after acute encephalitis or carbon monoxide or metallic poisoning, particularly by reserpine or phenothiazine drugs. Typical pathologic changes are destruction of neurons in basal ganglia, loss of pigmented cells in the substantia nigra, and depletion of dopamine in the caudate nucleus, putamen, and pallidum, structures in the neostriatum that normally contain high levels of the neurotransmitter dopamine. Signs and symptoms of Parkinson's disease, which include resting tremor, bradykinesias, drooling, increased appetite, intolerance to heat, oily skin, emotional instability, and defective judgment, are increased by fatigue, excitement, and frustration. Palliative and symptomatic treatment of the disease focuses on correcting the imbalance between depleted dopamine and abundant acetylcholine in the striatum, because dopamine normally appears to inhibit excitatory cholinergic activity in this brain area. Levodopa, a dopamine precursor

that crosses the blood-brain barrier, may be used, but many patients experience side effects, such as nausea, vomiting, insomnia, orthostatic hypotension, and mental confusion. Carbidopa-levodopa, which contains an inhibitor of the enzyme dopa decarboxylase, limits peripheral metabolism of levodopa and thus causes fewer side effects. Anticholinergic drugs, such as benztropine mesylate, biperiden, procyclidine, and trihexyphenidyl, may be used as therapeutic agents but often cause ataxia, blurred vision, constipation,

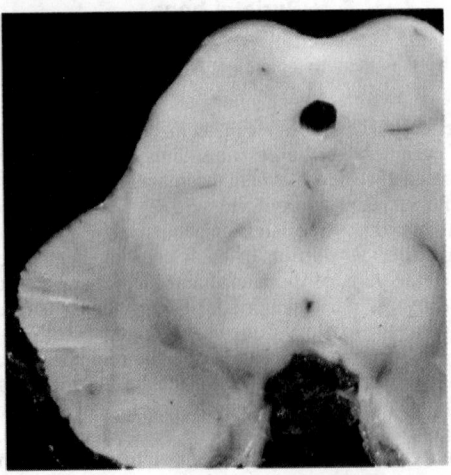

**Parkinson's disease: depigmented substantia nigra**
*(Cotran, Kumar, and Collins, 1999)*

dryness of the mouth, mental disturbances, slurred speech, and urinary urgency or retention. Amantadine hydrochloride, an antiviral drug with antiparkinsonian activity, promotes the accumulation of dopamine in extracellular or synaptic sites, but the therapeutic effectiveness may not last more than 3 months in some patients; side effects, such as mental confusion, visual disturbances, and seizures, occur infrequently. Also called **paralysis agitans.**

**Parkinson's mask** [James Parkinson; Fr, *masque*], an expressionless face with eyebrows raised, smoothing of facial muscles, but immobility of the facial muscles.

**Parlodel,** trademark for a dopamine receptor agonist (bromocriptine).

**Parnate,** trademark for an antidepressant (tranylcypromine sulfate).

**parole** /pərōl′/, (in psychiatry) a system of supervision of a patient who has been physically released from a hospital setting but is still listed as an inpatient and may be returned to the hospital without further court action.

**paromomycin sulfate** /per′əmōmī′sin/, an oral antiamebic aminoglycoside antibiotic.

■ INDICATION: It is prescribed in the treatment of intestinal amebiasis.

■ CONTRAINDICATIONS: Intestinal inflammation, intestinal obstruction, or known hypersensitivity to this drug prohibits its use.

■ ADVERSE EFFECTS: Among the most serious reactions are GI distress and diarrhea.

**paromphalocele** /perom′fəlōsēl′/, a hernia or tumor near the umbilicus.

**paronychia** /per′ənik′ē·ə/ [Gk, *para* + *onyx,* nail], an infection of the fold of skin at the margin of a nail. Treatment includes hot compresses or soaks, antibiotics, and possibly surgical incision and drainage. Compare **onychia.**

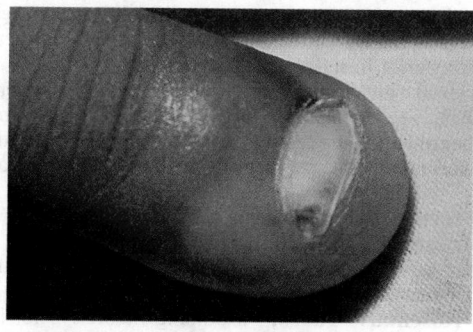

**Paronychia**
*(Zitelli and Davis, 1997/courtesy Dr. Bernard Cohen, Children's Hospital of Pittsburgh)*

**paroophoritis** /per′ō·of′ərī′tis/ [Gk, *para* + *oon,* egg, *pherein,* to bear, *itis*], **1.** inflammation of the paroophoron. **2.** inflammation of the tissues surrounding the ovary.

**paroophoron** /per′ō·of′əron/ [Gk, *para* + *oon,* egg, *pherein,* to bear], a small vestigial remnant of the mesonephros, consisting of a few rudimentary tubules lying in the broad ligament between the epoophoron and the uterus. It is most evident in very young girls. A similar vestigial structure, the aberrant ductule, is found in the male. Also called **parovarium.** Compare **epoophoron.**

**parosmia** /pəroz′mē·ə/ [Gk, *para* + *osme,* smell], any dysfunction or perversion concerning the sense of smell. See also **anosmia, cacosmia.**

**parosteitis** /per′ostē·ī′tis/, an inflammation of the tissues adjacent to or associated with a bone.

**parosteosis** /per′ostē·ō′sis/, the development of bone in an abnormal location, such as in the area of the periosteum or in the skin.

**parotid** /pərot′id/ [Gk, *para* + *ous,* ear], near the ear.

**parotid abscess,** a collection of pus in a parotid salivary gland.

**parotid duct** [Gk, *para* + *ous,* ear; L, *ducere,* to lead], a tubular canal, about 7 cm long, that extends from the anterior part of the parotid gland near the ear to the mouth. It crosses the masseter after leaving the parotid gland, pierces the buccinator, runs for a short distance obliquely forward between the buccinator and the mucous membrane of the mouth, and opens on the oral surface of the cheek through a small opening opposite the second upper molar tooth. Also called **Stensen's duct.** See also **parotid gland, salivary gland.**

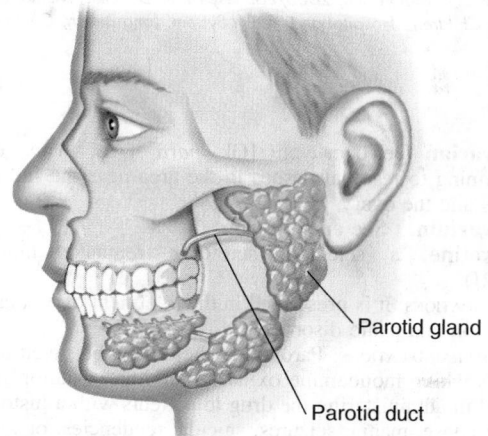

Parotid gland

Parotid duct

**Parotid duct and parotid gland**

**parotidectomy** /pərot′idek′təmē/ [Gk, *para* + *ous* + *ektomē,* excision], the surgical removal of the parotid gland.

**parotid gland** [Gk, *para* + *ous,* ear; L, *glans,* acorn], one of the largest pairs of salivary glands that lie at the side of the face just below and in front of the external ear. The main part of the gland is superficial, somewhat flattened, and quadrilateral. It is enclosed in a capsule continuous with the deep cervical fascia. The parotid duct starts at the anterior part of the gland and opens on the inside of the cheek opposite the second upper molar. Compare **sublingual gland, submandibular gland.** See also **salivary gland.**

**parotitis** /per′ətī′tis/ [Gk, *para* + *ous,* ear, *itis,* inflammation], inflammation or infection of one or both parotid salivary glands. See also **mumps.**

**parous** /per′əs/, having borne one or more viable offspring.

**-parous,** suffix meaning 'pertaining to the quantity of offspring produced simultaneously or to the method of gestation': *quadriparous, uniparous, viviparous.*

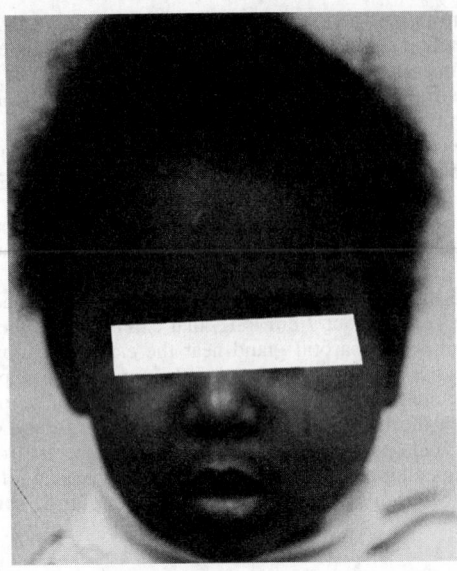

**Parotitis**
(Stone and Gorbach, 2000/courtesy Dr. A. Deveikis, Memorial Miller Children's Hospital and Health System, Long Beach, California)

**parovarian** /per′ōver′ē·ən/ [Gk, *para* + L, *ovum*, egg], pertaining to residual tissues in the area near the fallopian tubes and the ovary.

**parovarium.** See **epoophoron.**

**paroxetine,** a selective serotonin reuptake inhibitor (SSRI).

■ INDICATIONS: It is prescribed in the treatment of mental depression and panic disorder.

■ CONTRAINDICATIONS: Paroxetine should not be given to patients taking monoamine oxidase inhibitors. Caution is advised in administering the drug to patients with a history of drug abuse, mania, seizures, suicidal tendencies, or kidney or liver disease.

■ ADVERSE EFFECTS: The side effects most often reported include nausea, diarrhea, vomiting, constipation, abdominal pain, flatulence, and changes in appetite.

**paroxysm** /per′əksiz′əm/ [Gk, *paroxynein*, to stimulate], **1.** a marked, usually episodic increase in symptoms. **2.** a convulsion, fit, seizure, or spasm. —**paroxysmal,** *adj.*

**paroxysmal atrial tachycardia.** See **paroxysmal supraventricular tachycardia.**

**paroxysmal AV nodal reentry tachycardia** [Gk, *paroxysmos,* irritation; L, *nodus,* knot; Gk, *tachys,* fast, *kardia,* heart], a type of paroxysmal supraventricular tachycardia usually initiated by a premature atrial complex and sustained by an atrioventricular nodal reentry mechanism. A vagal maneuver is usually successful in restoring sinus rhythm. If it is not, adenosine or verapamil, procainamide, and cardioversion are tried, in succession.

**paroxysmal cold hemoglobinuria (PCH),** a rare autoimmune disorder characterized by hemolysis and hematuria, associated with exposure to cold.

**paroxysmal cough** [Gk, *paroxysmos,* irritation; AS, *cohhetan,* cough], a severe attack of coughing, as may accompany whooping cough, bronchiectasis, or a lung injury.

**paroxysmal hemoglobinuria,** the sudden passage of hemoglobin in urine, occurring after local or general exposure to low temperatures, as in paroxysmal cold hemoglobinuria. See also **Marchiafava-Micheli disease.**

**paroxysmal junctional tachycardia.** See **paroxysmal supraventricular tachycardia.**

**paroxysmal labyrinthine vertigo.** See **Ménière's disease.**

**paroxysmal nocturnal dyspnea (PND),** a disorder characterized by sudden attacks of respiratory distress that awaken the person, usually after several hours of sleep in a reclining position. It is most commonly caused by pulmonary edema resulting from congestive heart failure. The attacks are often accompanied by coughing, a feeling of suffocation, cold sweat, and tachycardia with a gallop rhythm. Sleeping with the head propped up on pillows may prevent PND, but treatment of the underlying cause is required to prevent fluid from accumulating in the lungs. Also called **nocturnal paroxysmal dyspnea.** See also **dyspnea.**

**paroxysmal nocturnal hemoglobinuria (PNH),** a disorder characterized by intravascular hemolysis and hemoglobinuria. It occurs in irregular episodes of several days' duration, especially at night. The basic defect in the red blood cell is an unusual sensitivity to lysis by complement or a deficiency or absence of acetylcholinesterase. The cause of the condition is unknown, but it is seen in association with abnormalities of the function of the bone marrow. Occurring predominantly in adults between 25 and 45 years of age, it is characterized by abdominal pain, back pain, dark colored urine, and headache. Its course may be complicated by thrombotic episodes and by iron deficiency caused by excessive loss of hemoglobin. Therapy includes blood transfusion and the oral or parenteral administration of iron. Corticosteroids are sometimes used and found useful; treatment of thromboses may require anticoagulant therapy.

**paroxysmal supraventricular tachycardia,** an ectopic heart rhythm with a rate of 170 to 250/min. It begins abruptly with a premature atrial or ventricular beat and is supported by an atrioventricular (AV) nodal reentry mechanism or by an AV reentry mechanism involving an accessory pathway. Formerly called **paroxysmal atrial tachycardia** or **paroxysmal junctional tachycardia.**

**paroxysmal ventricular tachycardia** [Gk, *paroxysmos,* irritation; L, *ventriculus,* little belly; Gk, *tachys* + *kardia*], a rapid heartbeat of sudden onset and termination caused by a quick succession of discharges from an ectopic site in a ventricle.

**parrot fever.** See **psittacosis.**

**parry fracture.** See **Monteggia's fracture.**

**pars** /pärs/, *pl.* **partis** [L, part], a part, such as the pars abdominalis esophagi. See also **part.**

**Parse, Rosemarie Rizzo,** a nursing theorist who, in her *Man-Living-Health: A Theory of Nursing* (1981), synthesized Martha E. Rogers' principles and concepts (Science of Unitary Human Beings) and the work of existential phenomenologists. Parse's view of nursing is based on humanism as opposed to positivism. Her theory addresses the unity of humans' lived experience, the lived experience of health. She used the term *man* to express male and female. Man chooses from options and bears responsibility for choices. Parse deduced three principles of Man-Living-Health, each interrelated with three concepts: (1) meaning (ultimate meaning and the meaning moments of life) with the concepts of imaging, valuing, and languaging; (2) rhythmicity (rhythmic patterns of living) with the concepts of revealing-concealing, enabling-limiting, and connecting-separating; and (3) cotranscendence (reaching out beyond self) with the concepts of powering, originating, and transforming. Parse proposes that nursing is a human science and rejects the traditional view of nursing as an emerging natural science. See also **Rogers.**

**pars fetalis.** See **fetal placenta.**

**Parsidol,** trademark for an antiparkinsonian (ethopropazine hydrochloride).

**Parsonage-Turner syndrome.** See **neuralgic amyotrophy.**

**pars planitis** /pärz plä·nī′tis/, a granulomatous uveitis of the ciliary disk (pars plana of the ciliary body).

**part** [L, *pars*], a part of a larger area, such as the condylar part of the occipital bone. See also **pars.**

**part-,** combining form meaning 'related to childbirth': *parturient, parturifacient, parturiometer.*

**part. aeq.** abbreviation for the Latin phrase *partes aequales,* meaning 'in equal parts.'

**parthenogenesis** /pär′thənōjen′əsis/ [Gk, *parthenos,* virgin, *genesis,* origin], a type of nonsexual reproduction in which an organism develops from an unfertilized ovum, as in many simpler animals. The development of the unfertilized ovum may be artificially induced through mechanical or chemical stimulation. **—parthenogenetic, parthenogenic,** *adj.*

**partial anodontia.** See **hypodontia.**

**partial breech extraction.** See **assisted breech.**

**partial cleavage** /pär′shəl/, mitotic division of only part of a fertilized ovum, usually the activated cytoplasmic part surrounding the nucleus. Compare **total cleavage.** See also **meroblastic.**

**partial crown,** a restoration that replaces some but not all surfaces of a tooth.

**partial denture** [L, *pars,* part, *dens,* tooth], a dental prosthesis, either fixed or removable, used to replace one or more missing teeth. Kinds of partial dentures include **articulated, bridgework, extension, fixed, fixed cantilever, removable, sectional,** and **unilateral.**

**partial dislocation** [L, *pars* + *dis* + *locare,* to place], the partial, abnormal separation of the articular surfaces of a joint. Also called **incomplete dislocation, subluxation.**

**partial hospitalization program,** an organizational entity that provides therapeutic services to patients who use only day or night hospital services or adult day health services, rather than regular inpatient hospitalization services.

**partial involution.** See **uterine subinvolution.**

**partially acid-fast** /pär′shəlē/, capable of retaining the stain carbolfuchsin during mild acid decolorization. This ability is restricted to bacteria of the genus *Nocardia,* because of the presence of unusual long-chain fatty acids in their cell walls.

**partially edentulous arch,** a dental arch in which one or more but not all natural teeth are missing.

**partial placenta previa,** placenta previa in which the placenta is implanted in the lower uterine segment and partially covers the internal os of the uterine cervix. As the cervix dilates in labor, the part of the placenta that lies over the cervix is separated, causing bleeding from the villous spaces of the uterine wall. Depending on the degree of separation, the bleeding may be scant or severe, resulting in hemorrhage that is life-threatening to the mother and the baby. Treatment may require cesarean section if the pressure of the presenting part of the baby is not sufficient to tamponade the bleeding site, stopping the hemorrhage. Diagnosis of partial placenta previa may be made before bleeding occurs by ultrasonic visualization or digital palpation in the course of prenatal examination. See also **marginal placenta previa, placenta previa.**

**partial pressure,** the pressure exerted by any one gas in a mixture of gases or in a liquid, with the pressure directly re-

lated to the concentration of that gas to the total pressure of the mixture. The concentration of oxygen in the atmosphere represents approximately 21% of the total atmospheric pressure, calculated at 760 mm Hg under standard conditions. Therefore, the partial pressure of atmospheric oxygen is about 160 mm Hg (760 × 0.21).

**partial pressure of carbon dioxide in arterial blood ($PaCO_2$),** the part of total blood gas pressure exerted by carbon dioxide. It decreases during heavy exercise, during rapid breathing, or in association with severe diarrhea, uncontrolled diabetes, or diseases of the liver or kidneys. It increases with chest injuries or respiratory disorders. The normal pressures of carbon dioxide in arterial blood are 35 to 45 mm Hg, and in venous blood, 40 to 45 mm Hg.

**partial pressure of oxygen in arterial blood ($PaO_2$),** the part of total blood gas pressure exerted by oxygen gas. It is lower than normal in patients with asthma, obstructive lung disease, or certain blood diseases and in healthy individuals during vigorous exercise. The normal partial pressure of oxygen in arterial blood is 95 to 100 mm Hg.

**partial response,** the condition in which the maximum decrease in treated tumor volume is at least 50% but less than 100%.

**partial shadowing,** (in ultrasonics) a manifestation of decreased echo signal amplitudes returning from regions lying beyond an object in which the attenuation is higher than the average attenuation in adjacent overlying regions.

**partial thromboplastin time (PTT),** a test for detecting coagulation defects of the intrinsic system by adding activated partial thromboplastin to a sample of test plasma and to a control sample of normal plasma. The time required for the formation of a clot in test plasma is compared with that in the normal plasma. A delayed clotting time suggests an abnormality in one or more factors of the intrinsic system. If indicated, specific factor abnormalities can be identified by exposing the test plasma to a series of plasma samples with known factor deficiencies and observing for coagulation, which occurs only if the test plasma provides the missing clotting factors. Partial thromboplastin time is one of the basic tests used to measure specific factor activity and to detect hemophilias. It is often performed as one test to monitor liver function and can also be used to monitor the activity of the anticoagulant heparin. The normal activated PTT in plasma is 25 to 45 seconds after the addition to the plasma sample of partial thromboplastin reagent and ionized calcium. Also called **activated partial thromboplastin time (APPT).** Compare **prothrombin time.** See also **hemostasis.**

**participant.** See **enrollee.**

**participation: health care decisions,** a nursing outcome from the Nursing Outcomes Classification (NOC) defined as the personal involvement in selecting and evaluating health care options. See also **Nursing Outcomes Classification.**

**particle** /pär′tikəl/ [L, *particula,* small part], **1.** any fundamental unit of matter. **2.** a minute fragment or speck.

**particulate** /pärtik′yəlit/, pertaining to a minute discrete particle or fragment of a substance or material.

**-partite,** combining form meaning 'having the (specified) number of parts': *bipartite, tripartite, quadripartite.*

**parts per million (PPM, ppm),** the ratio of the amount of one substance to the amount of another, expressed as a unit of solute dissolved in one million units of solution. It denotes the number of units of one substance relative to one million units of another substance. It may be further expressed in terms of mass-to-mass, volume-to-volume, or another relationship of units of measure.

**parturient** /pärt(y)oo′rē·ənt/ [L, *parturire,* to desire to bring forth], pertaining to the act of childbirth.

**parturition** /pär′t(y)o͞orish′ən/ [L, *parturire,* to desire to bring forth], the process of giving birth.

**part. vic.,** abbreviation for the Latin term *partes vicibus,* meaning 'divided doses.'

**parulis.** See **gumboil.**

**paruresis,** the inhibition of urination as a result of psychologic or other reasons.

**paruria** /pəro͝or′ē·ə/, any defect of the urination process.

**parvovirus B19** /pär′vōvī′rəs/, a small single-stranded deoxyribonucleic acid virus of the Parvoviridae family that infects humans, causing erythema infectiosum, aplastic crisis in hemolytic anemia, and other disorders. Another strain of the Parvoviridae, canine P2, causes acute enteritis and myocarditis in dogs.

**parvovirus B19 antibody test,** a blood test used to detect the presence of antibodies to the B19 parvovirus, a known human pathogen. The B19 virus is associated most commonly with erythema infectiosum (also called "fifth disease"), but also with joint inflammation, purpura, hydrops fetalis, and aplastic anemia.

**parvule** /pär′vyo͞ol/, a very small pill. Also called **pilule.**

**PAS, PASA,** abbreviation for **paraaminosalicylic acid.**

**PASCAL** /poskul′, paskal′/ [Blaise Pascal, French scientist, 1623–1662], a higher level computer compiler language, used to teach programming.

**Pascal's principle** /poskuls′, paskals′/ [Blaise Pascal], (in physics) a law stating that a confined liquid transmits pressure applied to it from an external source equally in all directions. Pascal's principle provides the basis for all hydraulic devices.

**PASG,** abbreviation for pneumatic antishock garment.

**pass.** See **conditional discharge.**

**passage** /pas′ij/, **1.** an opening, channel, route, or gap. **2.** the movement of something from one place to another, as in evacuation of the bowels.

**pass facilitation,** a nursing intervention from the Nursing Interventions Classification (NIC) defined as arranging a leave for a patient from a health care facility. See also **Nursing Interventions Classification.**

**passiflora** /pas′iflôr′ə/, the passion flower, *Passiflora incarnata,* a climbing herb. It has flowers and fruiting tops that are the source of medications used as antispasmodics and sedatives and for the treatment of burns, dysmenorrhea, hemorrhoids, and insomnia.

**passion flower,** an herbal product derived from a perennial climbing vine that is native to tropical and subtropical areas of the Americas, also found in the southeastern United States.
- ■ USES: This herb is used as an antifungal and sedative, and as a treatment for hypertension and group A hemolytic streptococcus.
- ■ CONTRAINDICATIONS: Passion flower should not be used during pregnancy and lactation, in children, or in those with known hypersensitivity.

**passive** [L *passivus*], pertaining to behavior that subordinates the individual's own interests to the demands of others.

**passive-aggressive personality** [L, *passivus + aggressus,* combative, *persona,* character], a personality characterized by a chronically negativistic disposition with passive resistance and aggression with forceful actions or attitudes expressed in an indirect, nonviolent manner, such as pouting, obstructionism, procrastination, inefficiency, stubbornness, and forgetfulness. Compare **aggressive personality, passive-dependent personality.** See also **passive-aggressive personality disorder.**

**passive-aggressive personality disorder,** a *DSM-IV* psychiatric disorder characterized by the indirect expression of resistance to occupational or social demands. It results in persistent pervasive ineffectiveness, lack of self-confidence, poor interpersonal relationships, and pessimism that can lead in severe cases to major depression, alcoholism, or drug dependence. The behavior often reflects an unexpressed hostility or resentment stemming from a frustrating interpersonal or institutional relationship on which an individual is overdependent. Treatment may consist of behavior therapy or any of the various psychotherapeutic procedures, depending on the individual and the severity of the condition.

**passive algolagnia.** See **masochism.**

**passive anaphylaxis.** See **antiserum anaphylaxis.**

**passive carrier** [L, *passivus + OFr, carier*], **1.** a healthy person whose body carries the causal organisms of an infectious disease although the person has not contracted the disease and remains symptomless. **2.** a person who carries a gene associated with a hereditary trait although the trait is not expressed in the person. Also called **symptomless carrier.**

**passive clot,** a clot that forms in an aneurysm when circulation is interrupted.

**passive congestion** [L, *passivus + congerere,* to heap together], an excessive amount of blood accumulation in an organ resulting from increased venous pressure.

**passive-dependent personality** [L, *passivus + Fr, dependre,* to depend; L, *persona,* character], a personality characterized by helplessness, indecisiveness, and a tendency to cling to and seek support from others. Compare **passive-aggressive personality.**

**passive euthanasia.** See **euthanasia.**

**passive exercise,** repetitive movement of a part of the body as a result of an externally applied force or of a voluntary effort to move another part of the body. Passive exercise can be used to prevent contractures and maintain joint mobility but does not promote muscle maintenance. Compare **active exercise.** See also **aerobic exercise, anaerobic exercise.**

**passive expiration** [L, *passivus + expirare,* to breathe out], normal exhalation that occurs without direct muscular effort, as during normal tidal breathing. Air is expelled from the lungs as a result of the recoil effect of elastic tissues in the chest, lungs, and diaphragm.

**passive immunity,** a form of acquired immunity resulting from antibodies that are transmitted naturally through the placenta to a fetus or through the colostrum to an infant or artificially by injection of antiserum for treatment or prophylaxis. Passive immunity is not permanent and does not last as long as active immunity. See also **immune response.**

**passive incontinence** [L, *passivus + incontinentia*], urine overflow that may occur when the bladder (musculus detrusor vesicae) is paralyzed and greatly distended. See also **incontinence.**

**passive lingual arch,** an orthodontic appliance that may help maintain tooth space and dental arch length when bilateral deciduous molars are prematurely lost.

**passive lung collapse** [L, *passivus + AS, lungen + L, collabi*], a condition of dyspnea, cough, and hemoptysis with pigmented cells, caused by an obstructed blood flow from the lungs to the heart.

**passive motion** [L, *passivus + motio*], involuntary motion caused by an external force rather than by voluntary muscular effort.

**passive movement,** the moving of parts of the body by an outside force without voluntary action or resistance by the individual. Also called **passive exercise.** Compare **active movement.**

**passive play,** play in which a person does not participate actively. For younger children such activity may include watching and listening to others, observing other children or animals, listening to stories, or looking at pictures. Older children are passively entertained by games and toys that require concentration and intellectual skill, such as chess, reading, listening to music, or watching television. Compare **active play.**

**passive recoil,** the return of elastic tissue to its normal length and position when applied tension on the tissue is released.

**passive sensitization** [L, *passivus* + *sentire,* to feel], a temporary form of sensitization induced by injecting serum from a sensitized individual. See also **passive immunity.**

**passive smoking,** the inhalation by nonsmokers of the smoke from other people's cigarettes, pipes, or cigars. The amount of such smoke inhaled by a nonsmoker is small compared with that inhaled by tobacco users. However, passive smoking can aggravate respiratory illnesses and contribute to serious diseases, including cancer. Infants, fetuses, and individuals with chronic heart and lung diseases or allergies to tobacco can be adversely affected by passive smoking. See also **secondhand smoke.**

**passive stretching,** stretching that involves only noncontractile elements, such as ligaments, fascia, bursae, dura mater, and nerve roots. Examples include manipulation of a muscle, such as during therapeutic massage or during isometric exercises in which there is no range of motion of the body part involved.

**passive symptom** [L, *passivus* + Gk, *symptoma,* that which happens], a symptom that attracts little or no attention. Also called **static symptom.**

**passive transfer test.** See **Prausnitz-Küstner (PK) test.**

**passive transport,** the movement of small molecules across the membrane of a cell by diffusion. Passive transport occurs when the chemicals outside a cell become concentrated and start moving into the cell, changing the intracellular equilibrium. Passive transport is essential to various processes of metabolism, such as the intake of digestive products by the cells lining the intestines. Compare **active transport, osmosis.**

**passive tremor.** See **resting tremor.**

**passivity** /pəsif′itē/ [L, *passivus*], a mental state of being submissive, dependent, or inactive, as a form of maladaptation.

**Passy-Muir valve,** a one-way speaking valve whose normal position at rest is closed, so that it is open only during inhalation and closes without exhalational pressure by the patient.

**paste** /pāst/, a topical semisolid formulation containing a pharmacologically active ingredient in a fatty base, a viscous or mucilaginous base, or a mixture of starch and petrolatum. Typically it is used externally only.

**Pasteur effect** /pastŏŏr′, pästœr′/ [Louis Pasteur, French chemist, 1822–1895], the inhibiting effect of oxygen on carbohydrate fermentation by living cells.

***Pasteurella*** /pas′tərel′ə/ [Louis Pasteur], a genus of gramnegative bacilli or coccobacilli, including species pathogenic to humans and domestic animals. *Pasteurella* infections may be transmitted to human by animal bites or scratches. The plague bacillus, *Pasteurella pestis,* is now called *Yersinia pestis; P. tularensis,* which causes tularemia, has been reclassified as *Francisella tularensis.*

***Pasteurella pestis.*** See ***Yersinia pestis.***

**pasteurellosis** /pas′tərelō′sis/ [Louis Pasteur], a local wound infection caused by the gram-negative bacillus *Pas-*

*teurella multicide,* which may be acquired through the bite or scratch of an infected animal, usually a cat.

**pasteurization** /pas′tərīzā′shən/ [Louis Pasteur; Gk, *izein,* to cause], the process of applying heat, usually to milk or cheese, for a specified period for the purpose of killing or retarding the development of pathogenic bacteria. **—pasteurize,** *v.*

**pasteurized milk** /pas′tərīzd/ [Louis Pasteur; Gk, *izein,* to cause; AS, *moluc,* milk], milk that has been treated by heat to destroy pathogenic bacteria. By law, pasteurization requires a temperature of 145° to 150° F for not less than 30 minutes, followed by a temperature of 161° F for 15 seconds, followed by immediate cooling. Pasteurized milk is sometimes produced using the high-temperature short-time method in which the milk is heated to 270° F for 1 second.

**Pasteur, Louis** [French chemist, 1822–1895], promoter of the "germ theory" of infection and developer of the "pasteurization" process to kill pathogenic organisms in milk. Pasteur also developed several vaccines and pioneered in the development of stereochemistry by separating mirror image isomers.

**Pasteur treatment** [Louis Pasteur], a method of preventing rabies by daily injections of attenuated cultures of rabies virus cultured in the central nervous system tissues of rabbits. The treatment, developed by Pasteur, is no longer used. See **human diploid cell rabies vaccine.**

**past health** [ME, *passen,* to pass; AS, *hoelth,* sound body], (in a health history) an overall summary of the person's general health to date, including past injuries, allergies, surgical procedures, immunizations, hospitalizations, and obstetric and psychiatric history. The past health information is obtained from the person or the person's family at the initial interview and becomes part of the permanent record. See also **health history.**

**Pastia's lines** /pas′te·əz/ [Chessec Pastia, 20th century Romanian physician], lines of hyperpigmentation seen in the body folds in scarlet fever.

**pastille** /pastēl′, pas′til/, **1.** a gelatin-based sweetened and molded medication impregnated with a therapeutic substance intended to be sucked. **2.** a chemically treated paper disk that undergoes color changes when exposed to radiation. Also spelled **pastil.**

**pastoral counseling department** /pas′tərəl/ [L, *pastor,* shepherd], the hospital chaplaincy service.

**past pointing** [OFr, *passer* + L, *punctus,* pricked], the inability to place a finger on another part of the body accurately, indicating a lack of coordination in voluntary movements.

**Patau's syndrome.** See **trisomy 13.**

**patch** [ME, *pacche*], a small spot of surface tissue that differs from the surrounding area in color or texture or both and is not elevated above it.

**patch test,** a skin test for identifying allergens, especially those causing contact dermatitis. The suspected substance (food, pollen, animal fur) is applied to an adhesive patch that is placed on the patient's skin. Another patch, with nothing on it, serves as a control. After a certain period (usually 24 to 48 hours) both patches are removed. If the skin under the suspect patch is red and swollen and the control area is not, the test result is said to be positive, and the person is probably allergic to that substance. Compare **radioallergosorbent test.**

**patek.** See **yaws.**

**patella** /pətel′ə/ [L, small dish], a flat, large, sesamoid bone at the front of the knee joint, having a pointed apex that attaches to the ligamentum patellae. The convex anterior surface of the bone is perforated for the passage of nu-

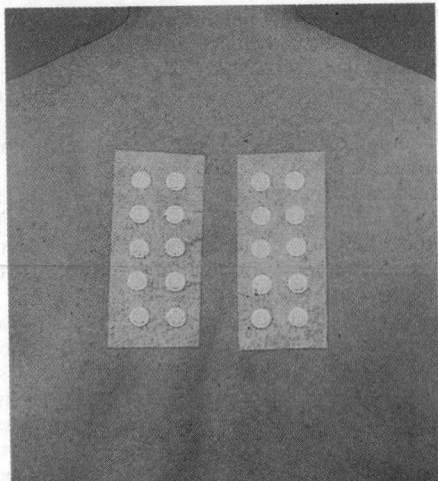

**Patch test applied to a patient's back**
*(Monahan and Neighbors, 1998/courtesy Hermal Pharmaceutical Laboratories, Delmar, New York)*

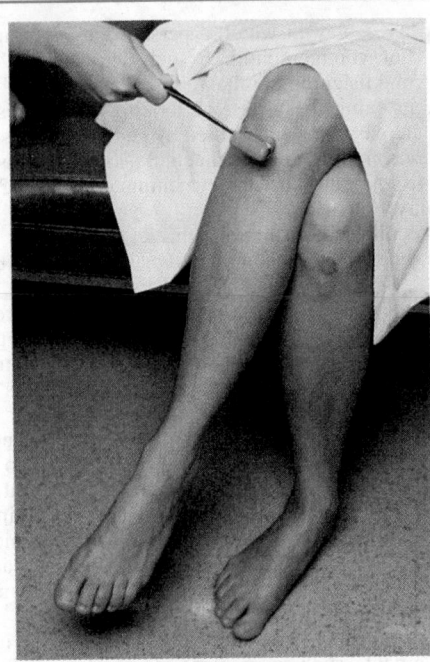

**Elicitation of the patellar reflex** *(Belcher, 1992)*

trient vessels and covered by an expansion from the tendon of the quadriceps femoris. Also called **kneecap.**

**patellar** /pətel′ər/ [L, *patella,* small dish], pertaining to the patella.

**patellar-bearing supracondylar/suprapatellar socket (PTBSC/SP),** a type of patellar-tendon below-the-knee bearing prosthesis with a socket that extends in front, medially, and laterally to accommodate both the patella and the femoral condyles. The higher socket increases knee stability, and a suspension strap is not required.

**patellar bursa** [L, *patella,* small dish; Gk, *byrsa,* wineskin], any of the fluid-filled connective tissue sacs around the knee cap. Kinds of patellar bursae include **infrapatellar, prepatellar,** and **suprapatellar.**

**patellar ligament** [L, *patella* + *ligare,* to bind], the central part of the common tendon of the quadriceps femoris. The ligament is a strong flat ligamentous band, about 8 cm long, attached proximally to the apex and the adjoining margins of the patella and distally to the tuberosity of the tibia. Its superficial fibers are continuous over the front of the patella with those of the tendon of the quadriceps femoris.

**patellar reflex,** a deep tendon reflex, elicited by a sharp tap on the tendon just distal to the patella, normally characterized by contraction of the quadriceps muscle and extension of the leg at the knee. The reflex is hyperactive in disease of the pyramidal tract above the level of the second lumbar vertebra. Also called **knee jerk reflex, quadriceps reflex.** See also **deep tendon reflex.**

**patellar-tendon bearing prosthesis (PTB),** an ankle-foot orthosis that provides prolonged stretch to the posterior leg musculature and may create extension force at the knee joint.

**patellar-tendon bearing supracondylar socket (PTB/SC),** a lower-leg prosthesis with supracondylar (above a condyle) and suprapatellar (above the patella) suspension.

**patellectomy** /pat′əlek′təmē/ [L, *patella,* small dish; Gk, *ektomē,* excision], the surgical removal of the patella.

**patency** /pā′tənsē/ [L, *patens,* open], a state of being open or exposed.

**patent** /pā′tənt/ [L, *patens,* open], open and unblocked, such as a patent airway or a patent anus.

**patent ductus arteriosus (PDA),** an abnormal opening between the pulmonary artery and the aorta caused by failure of the fetal ductus arteriosus to close after birth. It is seen primarily in premature infants. The defect allows blood from the aorta to flow into the pulmonary artery and to recirculate through the lungs, where it is reoxygenated and returned to the left atrium and left ventricle, placing an increased workload on the left side of the heart and causing increased pulmonary vascular congestion and resistance. Clinical manifestations include cardiomegaly, especially of the left atrium and left ventricle; dilated ascending aorta; bounding pulses resulting from increased systolic pressure;

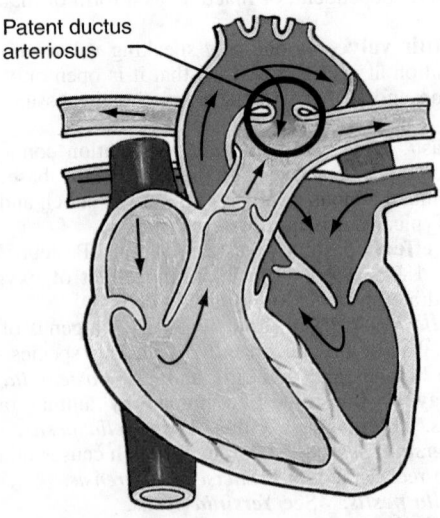

Patent ductus arteriosus

**Patent ductus arteriosus** *(Wong, 1999)*

tachycardia; and a typical machinery-like murmur that is heard during all of systole and most of diastole. Characteristic auscultatory and radiologic findings are sufficient to confirm diagnosis so that cardiac catheterization is not necessary. Correction is delayed until the child is old enough to tolerate surgery and until spontaneous closure can occur. Untreated complications include congestive heart failure, pulmonary vascular disease, calcification of the ductal site, and infective endocarditis. See also **congenital cardiac anomaly.**

**patent medicine** [L, *patens,* open, *medicina*],   a nonprescription drug available to the general public without a prescription. The ingredients and contraindications are usually listed on the label or wrapper. Also called **OTC drug, proprietary drug.**

**paternal** /pətur′nəl/ [L, *pater,* father],   pertaining to fatherhood, characteristic of a father, or related through a father.

**paternal engrossment.**   See **bonding.**

**paternity test** /pətur′nitē/ [L, *pater* + *testum,* crucible],   a test based on genetic blood groups and used mainly to exclude the possibility that a particular man could be the father of a specific child. For example, a man with group AB blood could not be the father of a child with group O blood.

**Paterson-Kelly syndrome.**   See **Plummer-Vinson syndrome.**

**Paterson-Parker dosage system** [James R.K. Paterson, English radiologist; H.M. Parker, twentieth-century American-English physicist],   a radiotherapy system that uses sources of specific relative loadings arranged according to defined rules, which lead to a homogenous dose in the implanted region.

**path** [AS, *paeth*],   a route or course along which something moves, such as a circuit of the nervous system that is followed by sensory or motor nerve impulses. See also **pathway.**

**path.,**   **1.** abbreviation for **pathologic. 2.** abbreviation for **pathology.**

**path-.**   See **patho-.**

**-path, -pathic, -pathy,**   suffix meaning 'disease or suffering': *cardiopath, naturopathic, osteopathy.*

**pathetic** /pəthet′ik/,   pertaining to something that affects emotions of sympathy, pity, and sadness.

**-pathetic, -pathetical** /pəthet′ik/,   combining form meaning 'emotions': *antipathetic, apopathetic, sympathetic.*

**pathfinder,**   a thin, flexible cylindric instrument containing a series of filiform guides, used to locate strictures.

**-pathic.**   See **-path.**

**Pathilon,**   trademark for an anticholinergic (tridihexethyl chloride).

**patho-, path-,**   prefix meaning 'disease': *pathocrinia, pathoformic, pathography.*

**pathodontia.**   See **dental pathology.**

**pathogen** /path′əjən/ [Gk, *pathos,* disease, *genein,* to produce],   any microorganism capable of producing disease. —**pathogenic,** *adj.*

**pathogenesis** /-jen′əsis/ [Gk, *pathos* + *genesis,* origin],   the source or cause of an illness or abnormal condition.

**pathogenic** /-jen′ik/ [Gk, *pathos,* disease, *genein,* to produce],   capable of causing or producing a disease. Also called **pathogenetic.**

**pathogenicity** /-jənis′itē/,   the ability of a pathogenic agent to produce a disease.

**pathogenic occlusion,**   an abnormal closure of the teeth, capable of producing pathologic changes in the teeth, supporting tissues, and related structures.

**pathognomonic** /pəthog′nəmon′ik/ [Gk, *pathos* + *gnomon,* index],   (of a sign or symptom) specific to a disease or condition, such as Koplik's spots on the buccal and lingual mucosa, which are indicative of measles.

**pathognomonic symptom.**   See **symptom.**

**pathologic (path.)** /-loj′ik/ [Gk, *pathos* + *logos,* science],   pertaining to a condition that is caused by or involves a disease process.

**pathologic absorption,**   the taking up by the blood of an excretory or morbid substance.

**pathologic amenorrhea** [Gk, *pathos,* disease, *logos,* science, *a* + *men,* month, *rhoia,* to flow],   a stoppage or absence of menstrual discharge from the uterus resulting from a disease.

**pathologic anatomy,**   (in applied anatomy) the study of the structure and morphologic characteristics of the tissues and cells of the body as related to disease.

**pathologic diagnosis,**   a diagnosis arrived at by an examination of the substance and function of the tissues of the body, especially of the abnormal developmental changes in the tissues by histologic techniques of tissue examination.

**pathologic fracture.**   See **neoplastic fracture.**

**pathologic histology** [Gk, *pathos,* disease, *logos,* science, *histos,* tissue, *logos,* science],   the study of the effects of disease on the structure, composition, and function of tissues.

**pathologic microorganisms** [Gk, *pathos,* disease, *logos,* science, *mikros,* small, *organon,* instrument, *ismos,* condi-

## Modes of transmission of some common pathogens

| Pathogen | Common reservoir |
|---|---|
| **Gram-positive cocci** | |
| *Staphylococcus aureus* | Contaminated objects, hands, and nasal tracts of health care workers, air, self |
| Group A streptococci | Direct contact, air, hands, rarely objects |
| *Enterococcus* group | Self, hands of health care workers, environmental surfaces |
| **Gram-negative rods** | |
| *Escherichia, Klebsiella, Enterobacter* | Self, hands of health care workers, contaminated solutions |
| *Proteus, Salmonella, Providencia, Serratia, Citrobacter* | Contaminated food and water, hands of health care workers, self |
| *Pseudomonas* | Contaminated environment, hands, self |
| **Anaerobic bacteria** | |
| *Clostridium, Bacteroides* | Self, contaminated environment, hands |
| **Fungal organisms** | |
| Yeasts | Self, hands of health care workers |
| Fungi | Air, contaminated environment |
| **Viruses** | |
| Varicella | Air, direct contact |
| Herpes | Self, direct contact, air |
| Rubella | Direct contact, air |
| Hepatitis B and C | Contaminated instruments or injectables, direct contact |

From Phipps WJ, Sands JK, Marek JE: *Medical-surgical nursing: concepts and clinical practice,* ed 6, St Louis, 1999, Mosby.

tion], any microscopic life form, from a virus to a nematode, that has the potential to cause disease.

**pathologic mitosis,** any cell division that is atypical, asymmetric, or multipolar and results in an unequal number of chromosomes in the nuclei of the daughter cells. It is indicative of malignancy, as occurs in cancer and the genetic anomalies.

**pathologic myopia,** a type of progressive nearsightedness characterized by changes in the fundus of the eye, posterior staphyloma, and deficient corrected acuity.

**pathologic physiology,** **1.** the study of the physical and chemical processes involved in the functioning of diseased tissues. **2.** the study of the modification of the normal functioning processes of an organism caused by disease. Also called **morbid physiology.** See also **pathophysiology.**

**pathologic reflex** [Gk, *pathos,* disease, *logos,* science; L, *reflectere,* to bend back], any abnormal reflex that is caused by a lesion in or an organic disease of the nervous system.

**pathologic retraction ring,** a ridge that may form around the uterus at the junction of the upper and lower uterine segments during the prolonged second stage of an obstructed labor. The lower segment is abnormally distended and thin, and the upper segment is abnormally thick. The ring, which may be seen and felt abdominally, is a warning of impending uterine rupture. Also called **Bandl's ring.** Compare **physiologic retraction ring, constriction ring.**

**pathologic sleep** [Gk, *pathos,* disease, *logos,* science; AS, *slaep*], excessive sleep associated with a neurologic disorder such as encephalitis lethargica, or sleeping sickness.

**pathologic triad,** the combination of three respiratory disease conditions: bronchospasm, retained secretions, and mucosal edema. It is treated with bronchodilators, hydration, mucolytics, and decongestants.

**pathologist** /pəthol′əjist/, a physician specializing in the study of disease. A pathologist usually specializes in autopsy or in clinical or surgical pathology.

**pathologists' assistant,** an allied health professional who, under the direct supervision of a licensed pathologist, participates in autopsies and in the examination, dissection, and processing of tissue specimens. Baccalaureate and masters' degree programs are available.

**pathology (path.)** /pəthol′əjē/ [Gk, *pathos,* disease, *logos,* science], the study of the characteristics, causes, and effects of disease, as observed in the structure and function of the body. **Cellular pathology** is the study of cellular changes in disease. **Clinical pathology** is the study of disease by the use of laboratory tests and methods. —**pathologic,** *adj.*

**pathomimicry.** See **Munchausen's syndrome.**

**pathophysiology** /-fiz′ē·ol′əjē/ [Gk, *pathos,* disease, *physis,* nature, *logos,* science], the study of the biologic and physical manifestations of disease as they correlate with the underlying abnormalities and physiologic disturbances. Pathophysiology does not deal directly with the treatment of disease; rather, it explains the processes within the body that result in the signs and symptoms of a disease. —**pathophysiologic,** *adj.*

**pathosis,** a disease condition.

**pathway** [AS, *paeth* + *weg*], **1.** a network of neurons that provides a transmission route for nerve impulses from any part of the body to the spinal cord and the cerebral cortex or from the central nervous system to the muscles and organs. **2.** a chain of chemical reactions that produces various compounds in critical sequence, such as the Embden-Meyerhof pathway.

**-pathy.** See **-path.**

**patient (pt.)** /pā′shənt/ [L, *pati,* to suffer], **1.** a recipient of

a health care service. **2.** a health care recipient who is ill or hospitalized. **3.** a client in a health care service.

**patient advocate.** See **ombudsman.**

**patient assignment,** a specialty capitation method in which patients choose a provider in each specialty represented. Capitation payments are then distributed accordingly to the providers selected.

**patient care committee,** a hospital staff organization, composed of medical, nursing, and other health professionals, with responsibility for monitoring all patient care practices to ensure that predetermined standards are met.

**patient care technician,** a health technician working under the supervision of a registered nurse, physician, or other health professional to provide basic patient care. Duties may include taking vital signs, obtaining blood and urine samples, performing basic diagnostic tests, and assisting the physician as needed.

**patient compensation fund,** a fund usually established by state law and commonly financed by a surcharge on malpractice premiums and used to pay malpractice claims.

**patient contracting,** a nursing intervention from the Nursing Interventions Classification (NIC) defined as negotiating an agreement with a patient that reinforces a specific behavior change. See also **Nursing Interventions Classification.**

**patient-controlled analgesia (PCA)[1],** a drug-delivery system that dispenses a preset intravascular dose of a narcotic analgesic when the patient pushes a switch on an electric cord. The device consists of a computerized pump with a chamber containing a syringe of drug. The patient administers a dose of narcotic when the need for pain relief arises. A lockout interval automatically inactivates the system if a patient tries to increase the amount of narcotic within a preset period.

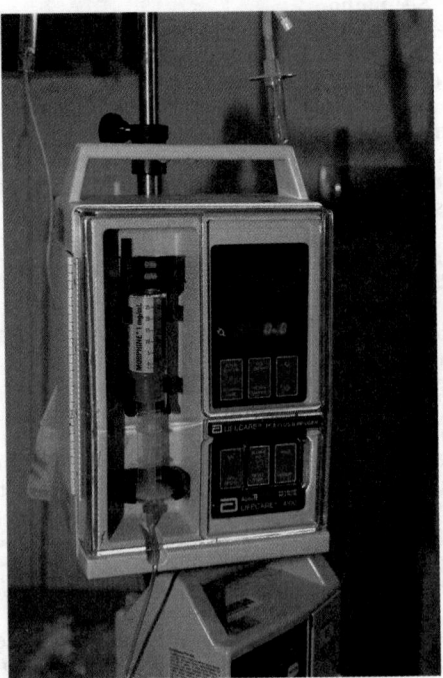

**Patient-controlled analgesia infusion pump**
*(Potter and Perry, 2001)*

**patient-controlled analgesia (PCA)**[2], a nursing intervention from the Nursing Interventions Classification (NIC) defined as facilitating patient control of analgesic administration and regulation. See also **Nursing Interventions Classification.**

**patient day (P.D.),** a unit in a system of accounting used by health care facilities and health care planners. Each day represents a unit of time during which the services of the institution or facility were used by a patient; thus 50 patients in a hospital for 1 day would represent 50 patient days.

**patient dumping,** the premature discharge of Medicare or indigent patients from hospitals for economic reasons. A 1986 U.S. federal rule requires hospitals to advise Medicare patients on admission for treatment of their right to challenge what they consider as premature discharge after treatment. The regulation was adopted after initiation of a Medicare policy of paying hospitals according to a particular illness, regardless of the length of hospitalization, as an incentive for hospitals to reduce the period of inpatient care.

**patient interview,** a systematic interview of a patient, the purpose of which is to obtain information that can be used to develop an individualized plan for care. Also called **client interview.**

**patient mix,** 1. the distribution of demographic variables in a patient population, often represented by the percentage of a given race, age, sex, or ethnic derivation. 2. the distribution of indications for admission in a patient population, such as surgical, maternity, or trauma.

**patient plan of care,** a method, formulated beforehand, to provide for a patient's needs. It is a plan of care coordinated to include appropriate participation by each member of the health care team.

**patient record,** a collection of documents that provides an account of each episode in which a patient visited or sought treatment and received care or a referral for care from a health care facility. The record is confidential and is usually held by the facility, and the information in it is released only to the patient or with the patient's written permission. It contains the initial assessment of the patient's health status, the health history, laboratory and radiologic reports of tests performed, notes by nurses and physicians regarding the daily condition of the patient and notes by consultants, as well as order sheets, medication sheets, admission records, discharge summaries, and other pertinent data. A problem-oriented medical record also contains a master problem list. The patient record is often a collection of papers held in a folder, but it may be computerized. Also called **chart.** See also **medical record.**

**patient representative.** See **ombudsman.**

**patient representative services,** hospital services provided by designated staff members relating to the investigation and mediation of patients' complaints and the promotion and protection of patients' rights. See also **ombudsman.**

**patient rights protection,** a nursing intervention from the Nursing Interventions Classification (NIC) defined as protection of health care rights of a patient, especially a minor, incapacitated, or incompetent patient unable to make decisions. See also **Nursing Interventions Classification.**

**Patient's Bill of Rights,** a list of the patient's rights promulgated by the American Hospital Association. It offers some guidance and protection to patients by stating the responsibilities that a hospital and its staff have toward them and their families during hospitalization, but it is not a legally binding document.

**Patient Self-Determination Act,** an act mandating that individuals enrolled in health care facilities are informed of their rights to formulate advance directives and to consent to or refuse treatment.

**Patient Zero,** an individual identified by the Centers for Disease Control and Prevention (CDC) as the person who introduced the human immunodeficiency virus in the United States. According to CDC records, Patient Zero, an airline steward, infected nearly 50 other persons before he died of acquired immunodeficiency syndrome in 1984.

**Patrick test,** a test for pain or dysfunction in the hip and sacroiliac joints in which overpressure is applied at the knee during flexion, abduction, and external rotation of the hip. While applying pressure on the knee, the examiner also applies counterpressure at the opposite anterior superior iliac spine. Also called **fabere sign, figure-four test.**

**patrilineal** /pat′rilin′ē-əl/ [L, *pater*, father, *linea*, line], pertaining to a line of descent through the male members of the family.

**patten** /pat′ən/, a metal support worn on a shoe to prevent weight-bearing on the opposite leg.

**patterning** /pat′ərning/ [ME, *patron*], the method of treatment or act of establishing a system or pattern of stimuli that will evoke a new set of responses. The process is commonly used to retrain people who have suffered a brain injury that disrupts normal sensory-motor activities.

**patulous** /pat′yələs/ [L, *patulus*, open], pertaining to something that is open or spread apart.

**pau d'arco,** an herbal product harvested from an evergreen flowering tree native to Florida, the West Indies, Mexico, and Central/South America.

■ USES: This herb is used for cancer, inflammation, and infection.

■ CONTRAINDICATIONS: Pau d'arco should not be used during pregnancy and lactation, in children less than 18 years of age, or in those with hemophilia, von Willebrand's disease, thrombocytopenia, or known hypersensitivity to this herb.

**Paul-Bunnell test** [John R. Paul, American physician, 1893–1971; Walls W. Bunnell, American physician, 1902–1966], a blood test for heterophil antibodies, used for confirming a diagnosis of infectious mononucleosis. See also **heterophil antibody test.**

**pauresis** /pôrē′sis/, the inhibition of urination for psychologic or other reasons.

**Pautrier microabscess** /pôtrēyā′/ [Lucien M.A. Pautrier, French dermatologist, 1876–1959; Gk, *mikros*, small; L, *abscedere*, to go away], an accumulation of intensely staining mononuclear cells in the epidermis, characterizing malignant lymphoma of the skin, especially mycosis fungoides. See also **mycosis fungoides.**

**Pauwels' fracture** /pou′əlz/ [Friedrich Pauwels, twentieth-century German surgeon; L, *fractura*, break], a break in the proximal femoral neck with varying degrees of angulation.

**Pavabid,** trademark for a smooth muscle relaxant (papaverine hydrochloride).

**pavement epithelium.** See **squamous epithelium.**

**Pavlov, Ivan Petrovich** /pav′lôv, pä′vlôf/(1849–1936), a Russian physiologist who discovered a pattern of conditioned stimulus-reflex learning, the manner in which the physiologic mechanism of digestion is controlled by the nervous system, and a theory of the causes and treatment of human neuroses.

**pavor** /pā′vôr/ [L, quaking], a reaction to a frightening stimulus characterized by excessive terror.

**pavor diurnus** /dī·ur′nəs/, a sleep disorder occurring in children during daytime sleep in which they cry out in alarm and awaken in fear and panic. See also **sleep terror disorder.**

## A patient's bill of rights

### Introduction

Effective health care requires collaboration between patients and physicians and other health care professionals. Open and honest communication, respect for personal and professional values, and sensitivity to differences are integral to optimal patient care. As the setting for the provision of health services, hospitals must provide a foundation for understanding and respecting the rights and responsibilities of patients, their families, physicians, and other caregivers. Hospitals must ensure a health care ethic that respects the role of patients in decision making about treatment choices and other aspects of their care. Hospitals must be sensitive to cultural, racial, linguistic, religious, age, gender, and other differences, as well as the needs of persons with disabilities.

The American Hospital Association presents *A Patient's Bill of Rights* with the expectation that it will contribute to more effective patient care and be supported by the hospital on behalf of the institution, its medical staff, employees, and patients. The American Hospital Association encourages health care institutions to tailor this bill of rights to their patient community by translating and/or simplifying the language of this bill of rights as may be necessary to ensure that patients and their families understand their rights and responsibilities.

### Bill of Rights*

1. The patient has the right to considerate and respectful care.

2. The patient has the right to and is encouraged to obtain from physicians and other direct caregivers relevant, current, and understandable information concerning diagnosis, treatment and prognosis. Except in emergencies when the patient lacks decision-making capacity and the need for treatment is urgent, the patient is entitled to the opportunity to discuss and request information related to the specific procedures and/or treatments, the risks involved, the possible length of recuperation, and the medically reasonable alternatives and their accompanying risks and benefits. Patients have the right to know the identity of physicians, nurses, and others involved in their care, as well as when those involved are students, residents, or other trainees. The patient also has the right to know the immediate and long-term financial implications of treatment choices, insofar as they are known.

3. The patient has the right to make decisions about the plan of care prior to and during the course of treatment and to refuse a recommended treatment or plan of care to the extent permitted by law and hospital policy and to be informed of the medical consequences of this action. In case of such refusal, the patient is entitled to other appropriate care and services that the hospital provides or transfer to another hospital. The hospital should notify patients of any policy that might affect patient choice within the institution.

4. The patient has the right to have an advance directive (such as living will, health care proxy, or durable power of attorney for health care) concerning treatment or designating a surrogate decision maker with the expectation that the hospital will honor the intent of that directive to the extent permitted by law and hospital policy. Health care institutions must advise patients of their rights under state law and hospital policy to make informed medical choices, ask if the patient has an advance directive, and include that information in patient records. The patient has the right to timely information about hospital policy that may limit its ability to implement fully a legally valid advance directive.

5. The patient has the right to every consideration of privacy. Case discussion, consultation, examination, and treatment should be conducted so as to protect each patient's privacy.

6. The patient has the right to expect that all communications and records pertaining to his/her care will be treated as confidential by the hospital, except in cases such as suspected abuse and public health hazards when reporting is permitted or required by law. The patient has the right to expect that the hospital will emphasize the confidentiality of this information when it releases it to any other parties entitled to review information in these records.

7. The patient has the right to review the records pertaining to his/her medical care and to have the information explained or interpreted as necessary, except when restricted by law.

8. The patient has the right to expect that, within its capacity and policies, a hospital will make reasonable response to the request of a patient for appropriate and medically indicated care and services. The hospital must provide evaluation, services, and/or referral as indicated by the urgency of the case. When medically appropriate and legally permissible, or when a patient has so requested, a patient may be transferred to another facility. The institution to which the patient is to be transferred must first have accepted the patient for transfer. The patient must also have the benefit of complete information and explanation concerning the need for, risk, benefits, and alternatives to such a transfer.

9. The patient has the right to ask and be informed of the existence of business relationships among the hospital, educational institutions, other health care providers, or payers that may influence the patient's treatment and care.

10. The patient has the right to consent to or decline to participate in proposed research studies or human experimentation affecting care and treatment or requiring direct patient involvement, and to have those studies fully explained prior to consent. A patient who declines to participate in research or experimentation is entitled to the most effective care that the hospital can otherwise provide.

11. The patient has the right to expect reasonable continuity of care when appropriate and to be informed by physicians and other caregivers of available and realistic patient care options when hospital care is no longer appropriate.

12. The patient has the right to be informed of hospital policies and practices that relate to patient care, treatment, and responsibilities. The patient has the right to be informed of available resources for resolving disputes, grievances, and conflicts, such as ethics committees, patient representatives, or other mechanisms available in the institution. The patient has the right to be informed of the hospital's charges for services and available payment methods.

The collaborative nature of health care requires that patients, or their families/surrogates, participate in their care. The effectiveness of care and patient satisfaction with the course of treatment depend, in part, on the patient fulfilling certain responsibilities. Patients are responsible for providing information about past illnesses, hospitalizations, medications, and other matters related to health status. To participate effectively in decision making, patients must be encouraged to take responsibility for requesting additional information or clarification about their health status or treatment when they do not fully understand information and instructions. Patients are also responsible for ensuring that the health care institution has a copy of their written advance directive if they have one. Patients are responsible for informing their physicians and other caregivers if they anticipate problems in following prescribed treatment.

## A patient's bill of rights—cont'd

Patients should also be aware of the hospital's obligation to be reasonably efficient and equitable in providing care to other patients and the community. The hospital's rules and regulations are designed to help the hospital meet this obligation. Patients and their families are responsible for making reasonable accommodations to the needs of the hospital, other patients, medical staff, and hospital employees. Patients are responsible for providing necessary information for insurance claims and for working with the hospital to make payment arrangements, when necessary.

A person's health depends on much more than health care services. Patients are responsible for recognizing the impact of their life-style on their personal health.

### Conclusion

Hospitals have many functions to perform, including the enhancement of health status, health promotion, and the prevention and treatment of injury and disease; the immediate and ongoing care and rehabilitation of patients; the education of health professionals, patients, and the community; and research. All these activities must be conducted with an overriding concern for the values and dignity of patients.

---

**pavor nocturnus** /noktur′nəs/, a sleep disorder occurring in children during nighttime sleep in which they cry out in alarm and awaken in fear and panic. See also **nightmare, sleep terror disorder.**

**Pavulon,** trademark for a neuromuscular blocking agent (pancuronium bromide).

**Paxil,** trademark for a selective serotonin reuptake inhibitor (paroxetine).

**Payr's clamp** /pī′ərz/ [Erwin Payr, German surgeon, 1871–1946; AS, *clam,* fastener], a heavy clamp used in GI surgery.

**Pb,** symbol for the element **lead.**

**PBI,** abbreviation for **protein-bound iodine.**

**PBL,** abbreviation for *peripheral blood lymphocytes.*

**PC,** **1.** abbreviation for *professional corporation.* **2.** abbreviation for *personal computer.* **3.** abbreviation for the Latin *post cibum,* 'after meals.'

**p.c.,** abbreviation for the Latin *post cibum,* 'after meals.'

**PCB,** abbreviation for **polychlorinated biphenyls.**

**pcc,** abbreviation for *precipitated calcium carbonate.*

**PCCM,** abbreviation for **primary care case management.**

**PCH,** abbreviation for **paroxysmal cold hemoglobinuria.**

**PCIS,** abbreviation for *Patient Care Information System,* an online computer system that contains full medical care data on all the residents or the patients in a facility.

**PCLN,** abbreviation for **psychiatric consultation liaison nurse.**

**PCP,** **1.** abbreviation for **phencyclidine hydrochloride.** **2.** abbreviation for *Pneumocystis carinii pneumonia.*

**P.C.P.** abbreviation for *primary care physician,* used by house staff or others to distinguish a patient's primary physician from university faculty, attending specialist physicians, or house staff. Also **L.M.D., P.M.D.**

**PCR,** abbreviation for **polymerase chain reaction.**

**PCT,** abbreviation for **porphyria cutanea tarda.**

**PCWP,** abbreviation for *pulmonary capillary wedge pressure;* see **pulmonary artery wedge pressure.**

**Pd,** symbol for the element **palladium.**

**p.d.,** abbreviation for the Latin *per diem,* 'by the day.'

**P.D., PD,** **1.** abbreviation for **patient day. 2.** abbreviation for *Doctor of Pharmacy.* **3.** abbreviation for *prism diopter.* **4.** abbreviation for *pupil diameter.* **5.** abbreviation for *pupillary distance.* **6.** abbreviation for *pulse duration.*

**PDA,** abbreviation for **patent ductus arteriosus.**

**PDL,** abbreviation for **periodontal ligament.**

**PDR,** abbreviation for *Physicians' Desk Reference.*

**PE,** abbreviation for **pulmonary embolism.**

**peak** [ME, *pec*], the amount of medication in the blood that represents the highest level during a drug administration cycle.

**peak and trough specimens,** serum samples collected to determine the level of an antibiotic or other pharmaceutic agent in the blood. Peak specimens, which represent the highest level, are generally collected one half-hour after the dose is given intravenously or 1 hour after it is given intramuscularly. Trough specimens, representing the lowest level, are generally collected approximately half an hour before the next dose. See also **peak method of dosing.**

**peak compressional pressure,** (in ultrasonics) the temporal maximum positive-pressure in a medium during the passage of a pulsed sound wave. It is expressed in pascals or megapascals.

**peak concentration,** the maximum amount of a substance or force, such as the highest concentration of a drug measured after it is administered.

**peak expiratory flow,** the greatest rate of airflow that can be achieved during forced expiration beginning with the lungs fully inflated. Also called **peak expiratory flow rate.**

**peak flow meter,** an instrument for measuring the flow of air in the early part of forced expiration.

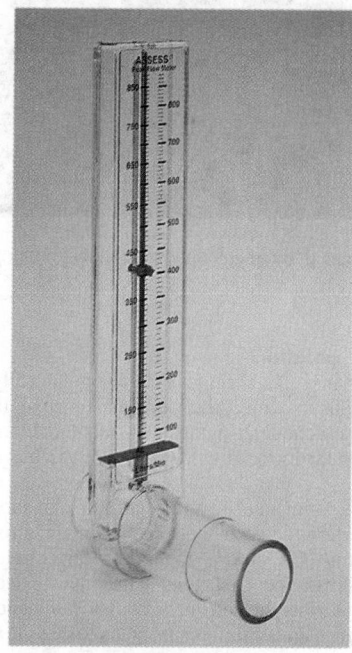

**Peak flow meter**
*(Monahan and Neighbors, 1998/courtesy HealthScan Products, Inc., Cedar Grove, New Jersey)*

**peak height velocity,** a point in pubescence in which the tempo of growth is the greatest.

**peak level,** the highest concentration, usually in the blood, that a substance reaches during the period under consideration, after which it declines, such as the highest blood glucose level attained during a glucose tolerance test.

**peak method of dosing,** the administration of a drug dosage so that a specified maximum level is reached to produce a desired effect, such as lowering the blood pressure.

**peak mucus sign,** a lubricative, cloudy to clear white cervical mucus that occurs during periods of high estrogen levels, particularly at the time of ovulation. See also **spinnbarkeit.**

**peak refractional pressure,** (in ultrasonics) the temporal maximum negative pressure in a medium occurring during the passage of a pulsed ultrasound wave. It is expressed in pascals or megapascals.

**pearly penile papules.** See **hirsutoid papilloma of the penis.**

**pearly tumor.** See **cholesteatoma.**

**Pearson's product movement correlation** [Karl Pearson, English mathematician, 1857–1936], (in statistics) a statistical test of the relationship between two variables measured in interval or ratio scales. Correlations computed fall between +1.00 and −1.00. The closer to 1 (positive or negative), the higher the correlation.

**peau d'orange** /pō′ dôräNzh′/ [Fr, skin of orange], a dimpling of the skin that gives it the appearance of the skin of an orange. It is common in advanced breast cancer.

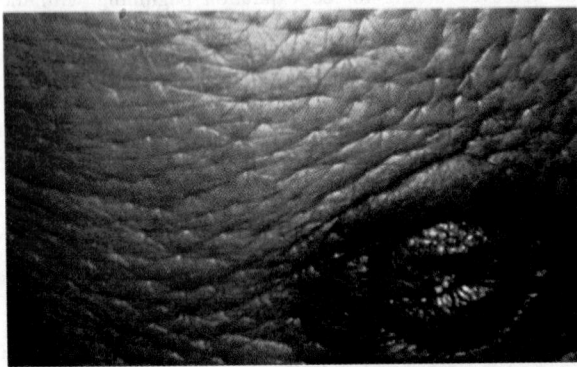

**Peau d'orange** *(Lemmi and Lemmi, 2000)*

**pecilo-.** See **poikilo-.**

**pecten** /pek′tən/, **1.** a ridge extending laterally from the pubic tubercle, to which the pectineal part of the inguinal ligament is attached. **2.** a vascular pleated membrane that extends from the optic disc to the vitreous humor in some animals.

**pectenitis** /pek′tənī′tis/, an inflammation of the anal canal, causing interference with the anal sphincter muscle.

**pectin** /pek′tin/ [Gk, *pektos,* congealed], a gelatinous carbohydrate substance found in fruits and succulent vegetables and used as the setting agent for jams and jellies and as an emulsifier and stabilizer in many foods. It also adds to the diet bulk necessary for proper GI functioning. See also **dietary fiber.**

**pectineus** /pektin′ē-əs/ [L, *pecten,* comb], the most anterior of the five medial femoral muscles. It functions to flex

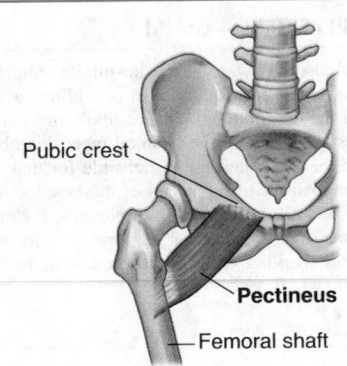

**Pectineus muscle**

and adduct the thigh and to rotate it medially. Compare **adductor brevis, adductor longus, adductor magnus, gracilis.**

**pector-,** prefix meaning 'breast': *pectoralgia, pectoriloquy, pectorophony.*

**pectoral** /pek′tərəl/ [L, *pectus,* breast], pertaining to the thorax or chest.

**pectoralgia** /pek′tôral′jə/, a pain in the thorax.

**pectoralis major** /pek′tərā′lis, pek′tərəlis′/ [L, *pectus,* breast], a large muscle of the upper chest wall that acts on the joint of the shoulder. Thick and fan-shaped, it arises from the clavicle, the sternum, the cartilages of the second to the sixth ribs, and the aponeurosis of the obliquus externus abdominis. It serves to flex, adduct, and medially rotate the arm in the shoulder joint.

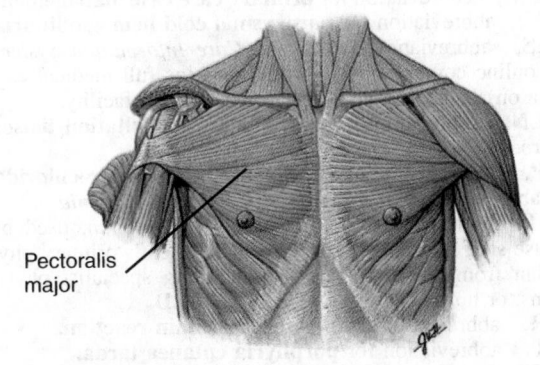

**Pectoralis major** *(Thibodeau and Patton, 1999/John V. Hagen)*

**pectoralis minor,** a thin triangular muscle of the upper chest wall beneath the pectoralis major. The base arises from the third, fourth, and fifth ribs on their upper outer surfaces. It inserts as a flat tendon into the coracoid process of the scapula. It functions to rotate the scapula, to draw it down and forward, and to raise the third, the fourth, and fifth ribs in forced inspiration. Compare **pectoralis major, subclavius.**

**pectoriloquy** /pek′təril′əkwē/, a phenomenon in which voice sounds, including whispers, are transmitted clearly through the pulmonary structures and are clearly audible

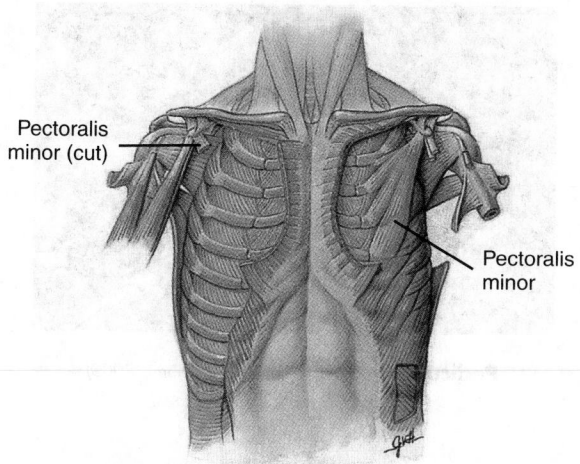

Pectoralis minor (cut)

Pectoralis minor

**Pectoralis minor** *(Thibodeau and Patton, 1999/John V. Hagen)*

through a stethoscope. It is often a sign of lung consolidation.

**pectus carinatum.** See **pigeon breast.**

**pectus excavatum.** See **funnel chest.**

**ped-.** See **pedia-.**

**pedagogy** /ped'əgōj'ē/ [Gk, *pais,* child, *agogos,* leader], the art and science of teaching children, based on a belief that the purpose of education is the transmittal of knowledge.

**pedal** /ped'əl/ [L, *pes,* foot], pertaining to the foot.

**-pedal.** See **-pedic.**

**pederosis.** See **pedophilia.**

**pedes.** See **pes.**

**pedia-, pedo-,** prefix meaning 'child': *pediatric, pediatrician, pediatrics, pedodontics, pedophilia.*

**-pedia, -paedia,** suffix meaning 'to educate or a compendium of knowledge': *pharmacopedia, logopedia.*

**Pediaflor,** trademark for a dental preparation (sodium fluoride) used in prophylaxis against dental caries in children.

**Pedialyte,** trademark for a balanced solution containing various electrolytes.

**Pediamycin,** trademark for an antibacterial (erythromycin ethylsuccinate).

**pediatric** /pē'dē·at'rik/ [Gk, *pais,* child, *iatreia,* treatment], pertaining to preventive and primary health care and treatment of children and the study of childhood diseases.

**pediatric advanced life support (PALS),** a system of critical care procedures and facilities, such as the intensive care nursery, for the basic and advanced treatment of seriously ill or injured infants and children. It includes the neonatal resuscitation program as recommended by the American Academy of Pediatrics and the American Heart Association.

**Pediatric AIDS Program,** an endeavor administered by the Federal Maternal and Child Health Bureau for children infected with human immunodeficiency virus (HIV), which produces acquired immunodeficiency syndrome (AIDS). Projects funded under the program provide comprehensive health services to the children and social support for affected families. Prevention of HIV infection among children is also a part of the Pediatric AIDS Program. Projects also stress the identification of HIV-positive pregnant women along with counseling and follow-up care.

**pediatric anesthesia** [Gk, *pais,* child, *iatreia,* treatment], a subspecialty of anesthesiology dealing with the anesthesia of neonates, infants, and children up to 12 years of age.

**pediatric dentistry,** the branch of dentistry devoted to the diagnosis and treatment of dental problems affecting children. Also called **pedodontics.**

**pediatric dosage,** the determination of the correct amount, frequency, and total number of doses of a medication to be administered to a child or infant. Such variables as the age, weight, body surface area, and ability of the child to absorb, metabolize, and excrete the medication must be considered, as well as the expected action of the drug, possible side effects, and potential toxicity. Various formulas have been devised to calculate pediatric dosage from a standard adult dose, although the most reliable method is to use the proportional amount of body surface area to body weight, based on one of the formulas. See also **Clark's rule.**

**pediatric hospitalization,** the confinement of a child or infant in a hospital for diagnostic testing or therapeutic treatment. Regardless of age or the degree of illness or injury, hospitalization constitutes a major crisis in the life of a child, and the emotional trauma elicits various behavioral reactions that the nurse must recognize and be prepared to cope with to facilitate recovery. The dominant factors influencing stress, which vary according to the child's developmental age, his or her previous experience with illness, and the seriousness of the condition, include separation from the parents and familiar environment, disruption of routine patterns of daily life, loss of independence, and worry about bodily injury or painful experiences. The nurse can minimize stress by preparing the child and family through prehospital counseling; by encouraging active parental participation in the child's care through rooming-in facilities or frequent visits; by maintaining as normal a daily routine as possible, especially with eating, sleeping, hygiene, and play activities; by explaining all hospital procedures and the immediate and long-term prognosis in terms that the child can easily understand; and by providing support and guidance for parents and siblings. The nurse also may use the hospital experience to foster an improved parent-child relationship and to teach other members of the family about proper health care. Emergency admission greatly increases the emotional trauma of hospitalization, making the nurse's role in counteracting negative reactions even more significant.

**pediatrician** /pē'dē·ətrish'ən/ [Gk, *pais,* child, *iatreia,* treatment], a physician who specializes in the development and care of infants and children and in the treatment of their diseases. Also called **pediatrist** /pē'dē·at'rist/. Also spelled **paediatrician.**

**pediatric nurse practitioner (PNP),** a nurse practitioner who, by advanced study and clinical practice, such as in a master's degree program or certificate program in pediatric nursing, has gained advanced knowledge in the nursing care of infants and children. See also **pediatric nursing.**

**pediatric nursing,** the branch of nursing concerned with the care of infants and children. Pediatric nursing requires knowledge of normal psychomotor, psychosocial, and cognitive growth and development, as well as of the health problems and needs of people in this age group. Preventive care and anticipatory guidance are integral to the practice of pediatric nursing. See also **pediatric nurse practitioner.**

**pediatric nutrition,** the maintenance of a proper well-balanced diet, consisting of the essential nutrients and the adequate caloric intake necessary to promote growth and sustain the physiologic requirements at the various stages of a child's development. Nutritional needs vary considerably with age, level of activity, and environmental conditions, and they are directly related to the rate of growth. In the prenatal period growth totally depends on adequate maternal nutrition. During infancy the need for calories, especially in the form of protein, is greater than at any postnatal period because of the rapid increase in both height and weight. From toddlerhood through the preschool and middle childhood years, growth is uneven and occurs in spurts, with a resulting fluctuation in appetite and calorie consumption. In general, the average child expends 55% of energy on metabolic maintenance, 25% on activity, 12% on growth, and 8% on excretion. The accelerated growth phase during adolescence demands greater nutritional requirements, although food habits are often influenced by emotional factors, peer pressure, and fad diets. Inadequate nutrition, especially during critical periods of growth, results in retarded development or illness, such as anemia from deficiency of iron or scurvy from deficiency of vitamin C. The role of the nurse is to educate and give nutritional guidance for good eating habits. A special problem is overfeeding in the early childhood years, which may lead to obesity or hypervitaminosis. See also **dietary allowances,** and see specific vitamins.

**pediatrics** /pē′dē·at′triks/, a branch of medicine concerned with the development and care of infants and children. Its specialties are the particular diseases of children and their treatment and prevention. Also called *(informal)* **peds.** —**pediatric,** *adj.* Also spelled **paediatrics.**

**pediatric surgery,** the special preparation and care of the child undergoing surgical procedures for injuries, deformities, or disease. In addition to the usual fears and emotional trauma of illness and hospitalization, the child is especially concerned about being anesthetized. Younger children worry more about what will happen to them and how they will feel after awakening from anesthesia, whereas older children fears the operation itself and possible death, the loss of control while under anesthesia, and any change in body image or mutilation of parts. The role of the nurse is to prepare the child psychologically and physically for the particular surgical procedure and any postoperative reactions; to offer support to the parents and involve them as much as possible in the care, both before and after surgery; and to explain immediate and long-term prognoses. See also **pediatric hospitalization.**

**pediatrist.** See **pediatrician.**

**-pedic, -pedal,** suffix meaning 'feet': *arthrosteopedic, talipedic, velocipedic, orthopedic.*

**pedicle** [L, *pediculus,* little foot], a narrow stalk, stem, or tube of tissue attached to a tumor, skin flap, bone, or organ.

**pedicle clamp** /ped′ikəl/ [L, *pediculus,* little foot; ME, *clam,* fastener], a locking surgical forceps used for compressing blood vessels or pedicles of tumors during surgery. Also called **clamp forceps.**

**pedicle flap operation,** a surgical procedure for grafting gingival tissue from a donor site to the site of an isolated defect, usually a tooth surface denuded of attached gingiva.

**pediculicide** /pədik′yōōlisīd′/ [L, *pediculus,* little foot, *caedere,* to kill], any of a group of drugs that kill lice.

**pediculosis** /pədik′yōōlō′sis/ [L, *pediculus* + *osis,* condition], an infestation with blood-sucking lice. **Pediculosis capitis** is infestation of the scalp with lice. **Pediculosis corporis** is infestation of the skin of the body with lice. **Pediculosis palpebrarum** is infestation of the eyelids and eyelashes with lice. **Pthirus pubis** (formerly called **pediculosis pubis**) is infestation of the pubic hair region with lice. An over-the-counter treatment is with pyrethrin or permethrin containing topical agents. Malathion and lindane are other treatments, although misuse can result in neurotoxicity. See also **crab louse, louse.**

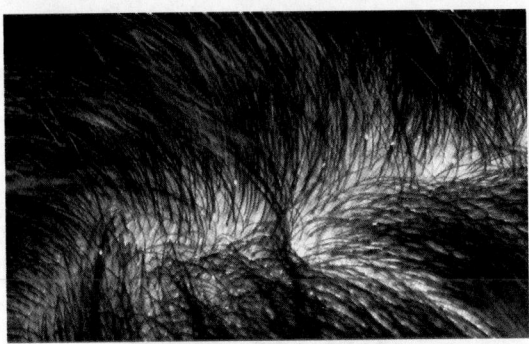

**Pediculosis capitis** *(Lemmi and Lemmi, 2000)*

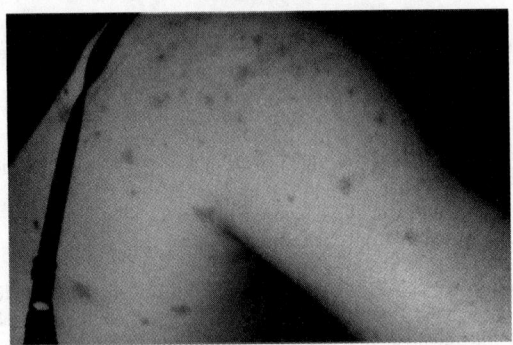

**Pediculosis corporis** *(Lemmi and Lemmi, 2000)*

**pediculous** /pədik′yələs/ [L, *pediculus*], infested with sucking lice.

***Pediculus humanus capitis,*** a species of head lice.

***Pediculus humanus corporis,*** a species of body lice.

**pedicure** /ped′ikyōōr/, care of the feet, especially trimming of the toenails.

**pedigree** /ped′əgrē/ [Fr, *pied de grue,* crane's foot pattern], **1.** line of descent; lineage; ancestry. **2.** a chart that shows the genetic makeup of a person's ancestors, used in the mendelian analysis of an inherited characteristic or disease in a particular family. It typically uses squares to represent males and circles to represent females. The figures may be unshaded, shaded, or partially shaded to designate normal individuals, those affected by the disease or trait, and those who are carriers. The generations are numbered with roman numerals at the left, with the most recent at the bottom, and members within each generation are designated by arabic numerals from left to right according to age, with the oldest at the left. The inquiry begins with the siblings of the affected person and proceeds to the parents and grandparents and any of their immediate relatives. See also **Punnett square.**

**pedo-.** See **pedia-.**

**pedodontics** See **pediatric dentistry.**

**pedogenesis** /pē′dōjen′əsis/ [Gk, *pais,* child, *genesis,* origin], the production of offspring by young or larval forms of animals, often by parthenogenesis, as in certain amphibians. Also spelled **paedogenesis.** —**pedogenetic,** *adj.*

**pedophilia** /ped′əfil′ē·ə/ [Gk, *pais,* child, *philein,* to love], **1.** an abnormal interest in children. **2.** (in psychiatry) a psychosexual disorder in which the fantasy or act of engaging in sexual activity with prepubertal children is the preferred or exclusive means of achieving sexual excitement and gratification. It may be heterosexual or homosexual. Also spelled **paedophilia.** Also called **pederosis.** See also **paraphilia. —pedophilic,** *adj.*

**-ped, -pede,**   suffix meaning 'foot or feet': *biped, taliped.*

**peds,**   abbreviation for **pediatrics.**

**peduncle** /pədung'kəl/ [L, *pes,* foot],   a stemlike connecting part, such as the pineal peduncle or a peduncle graft. **—peduncular, pedunculate,** *adj.*

**peduncular** /pədung'kyələr/,   pertaining to a pedicle or peduncle.

**pedunculate.**   See **peduncle.**

**pedunculated** /pədung'kyələ'tid/ [L, *pes,* foot],   pertaining to a structure with a stalk or peduncle.

**pedunculotomy** /pədung'kyəlot'əmē/,   a surgical incision in a cerebral peduncle.

**pedunculus** /pədung'kyələs/ [L, *pes,* foot],   a stalk, stem, or stalklike anatomic structure.

**peeling,**   the loss of epidermis, as may occur after a sunburn or exposure to a chemical.

**PEEP,**   abbreviation for **positive-end expiratory pressure.**

**Peeping Tom.**   See **voyeur.**

**peer** [L, *par,* equal],   a person deemed an equal for the purpose at hand. It is usually an "age mate," or companion or associate on roughly the same level of age or mental endowment.

**peer review**[1],   an appraisal by professional coworkers of equal status of the way an individual nurse or other health professional conducts practice, education, or research. The appraisal uses accepted standards as measures against which performance is weighed. See also **Professional Standards Review Organization.**

**peer review**[2],   a nursing intervention from the Nursing Interventions Classification (NIC) defined as systematic evaluation of a peer's performance compared with professional standards of practice. See also **Nursing Interventions Classification.**

**Peganone,**   trademark for an anticonvulsant (ethotoin).

**pegaspargase,**   an oncolytic agent and modified version of the enzyme L-asparaginase.

■ INDICATIONS: It is prescribed in the treatment of patients with acute lymphoblastic leukemia who are hypersensitive to other forms of the enzyme.

■ CONTRAINDICATIONS: The drug should not be given to patients with pancreatitis or those who have had significant hemorrhagic events associated with prior use of the enzyme or have experienced serious allergic reactions to the product.

■ ADVERSE EFFECTS: The side effects most often reported include chills, fever, edema, pain, chemical hepatotoxicities and coagulopathies.

**PEL,**   abbreviation for *permissible exposure limit.*

**Pel-Ebstein fever** /pel'eb'stēn/ [Pieter K. Pel, Dutch physician, 1852–1919; Wilhelm Ebstein, German physician, 1836–1912],   a fever recurring in cycles of several days or weeks, characteristic of Hodgkin's disease or malignant lymphoma. Also called **Murchison fever.**

**Pelger-Huët anomaly** /pel'gərhyōō'ət/ [Karel Pelger, Dutch physician, 1885–1931; G.J. Huët, Dutch physician, 1879–1970; Gk, *anomalia,* irregular],   an inherited disorder characterized by granulocytes with unusually coarse nuclear material and dumbbell-shaped or peanut-shaped nuclei. Normal nuclear segmentation does not seem to occur, but there are no associated findings. See also **band.**

**pelidnoma** /pel'idnō'mə/,   a circumscribed elevated dark patch on the skin. Also called **pelioma.**

**peliosis hepatitis** /pel'ē·ō'sis/,   the presence of blood-filled cavities in the liver. The cavities may become lined by endothelium and may be found in patients who are infected with human immunodeficiency virus or who use oral contraceptives or anabolic steroids.

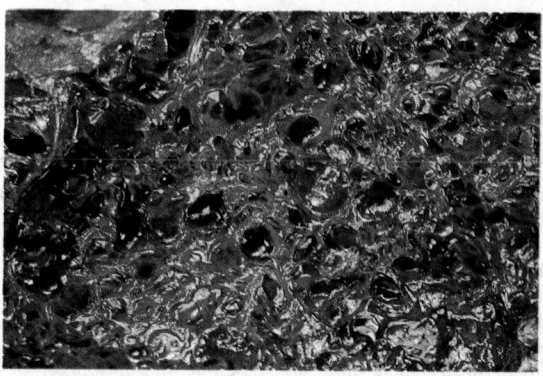

**Peliosis hepatitis** *(Fletcher, 2000)*

**Pelizaeus-Merzbacher disease** /pā'lētsā'ōos·merts'bä·kər/ [Friedrich Pelizaeus, German physician, 1850–1917; Ludwig Merzbacher, German physician, 1875–1942],   an X-linked leukoencephalopathy, occurring in early life and running a slowly progressive course into adolescence or adulthood. It is marked by nystagmus, ataxia, tremor, choreoathetoid movements, parkinsonian facies, dysarthria, and mental deterioration. Pathologically, there is diffuse demyelination in the white substance of the brain, which may involve the brainstem, cerebellum, and spinal cord. Also called **familial centrolobar sclerosis, Merzbacher-Pelizaeus disease, Pelizaeus-Merzbacher sclerosis.**

**pell-,**   prefix meaning 'skin': *pellagra, pellicle, pellicular.*

**pellagra** /pəlā'grə, pəlag'rə/ [It, *pelle,* skin, *agra,* rough],   a disease resulting from a deficiency of niacin or tryptophan or a metabolic defect that interferes with the conversion of the precursor tryptophan to niacin. It once was commonly seen in individuals whose diet consists primarily of corn, which is low in tryptophan. It is characterized by scaly dermatitis, especially of the skin exposed to the sun; glossitis;

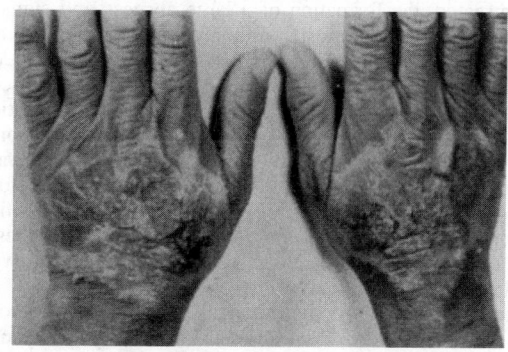

**Dermatitis caused by pellagra**
*(Cotran, Kumar, and Collins, 1999)*

inflammation of the mucous membranes; diarrhea; and mental disturbances, including depression, confusion, disorientation, hallucination, and delirium. Treatment and prophylaxis consist of administration of niacin and tryptophan, usually in conjunction with other vitamins, particularly thiamine and riboflavin, and a well-balanced diet containing foods rich in these nutrients, such as liver, eggs, milk, and meat. Kinds of pellagra are **pellagra sine pellagra** and **typhoid pellagra.** Compare **kwashiorkor.** —**pellagrous,** *adj.*

**pellagra sine pellagra** /sī′nē, sē′nə/, a form of pellagra in which the characteristic dermatitis is not present. See **pellagra.**

**pellagrous.** See **pellagra.**

**Pellegrini's disease** /pel′əgrē′nēz/ [Augusto Pellegrini, Italian surgeon, b. 1877], ossification of the upper part of the medial collateral ligament, sometimes accompanied by bony growth at the internal condyle of the femur. The condition usually follows a leg injury. Also called **Pelligrini-Stieda disease.**

**pellet** /pel′it/, a pilule or very small pill.

**pellicle** /pel′ikəl/, **1.** a thin film or skin. **2.** a scum or crust on a solution.

**pelo-,** prefix meaning 'mud': *pelohemia, pelology, pelotherapy.*

**pelotherapy** /pē′lōther′əpē/, the treatment of certain conditions with baths or packs of mud, peat, or earth on part or all of the body surface.

**pelves.** See **pelvis.**

**pelvi-,** combining form meaning 'pelvis': *pelvimetry, pelvicophalometry.*

**pelvic** /pel′vik/ [L, *pelvis,* basin], pertaining to the pelvis.

**pelvic abscess** [L, *pelvis,* basin, *abscedere,* to go away], a pus-producing lesion in the pelvic peritoneum, usually originating in the rectouterine pouch.

**pelvic axis,** an imaginary curved line that passes through the centers of the various anteroposterior diameters of the pelvis.

**pelvic bones** [L, *pelvis,* basin; AS, *ban*], a combination of the ilium, ischium, and pubis. Compare **innominate bone.**

**pelvic brim,** the curved top of the bones of the hip extending from the anterosuperior iliac crest in front on one side around and past the sacrum to the crest on the other side. Below the brim is the pelvis.

**pelvic cellulitis,** bacterial infection of the parametrium, occurring after childbirth or spontaneous or therapeutic abortion. It represents an extension of infection via the blood vessels and lymphatics from a primary wound infection in the external genitalia, perineum, vagina, cervix, or uterus. It is characterized by fever, uterine subinvolution, chills and sweats, abdominal pain that spreads laterally, and, if untreated, the formation of a large abscess and signs of peritonitis. It occurs most commonly between the third and the ninth days after delivery or abortion. Treatment includes an antibiotic, bed rest, IV fluids, and drainage of any abscess that forms. Oxytocics may be given to augment involution.

**pelvic classification,** **1.** a process in which the anatomic and spatial relationships of the bones of the pelvis are evaluated, usually to assess the adequacy of the pelvic structures for vaginal delivery. Caldwell-Moloy's system of classification is the one most commonly used. **2.** one of the types in a classification system of the pelvis. See also **Caldwell-Moloy pelvic classification.**

**pelvic congestion syndrome,** an abnormal gynecologic condition characterized by chronic low back pain, dysuria, dysmenorrhea, vague lower abdominal pain, vaginal discharge, and dyspareunia. The cause of the symptoms is not understood; formerly it was thought that the vascular bed of the area was distended with blood, but this has not been demonstrated. Women between 25 and 45 years of age are most often affected.

**pelvic diameter** [L, *pelvis,* basin; Gk, *diametros,* measuring across], **1.** at the rim of the pelvis, a line from the lumbosacral angle to the symphysis pubis. **2.** at the pelvic outlet, a line from the tip of the coccyx to the lower border of the symphysis pubis.

**pelvic diaphragm,** the inferior aspect of the body wall, stretched like a hammock across the pelvic cavity and comprising the levator ani and the coccygeus muscles. It holds the abdominal contents, supports the pelvic viscera, and is pierced by the anal canal, the urethra, and the vagina. It is reinforced by fasciae and muscles associated with these structures and with the perineum.

**pelvic examination,** a diagnostic procedure in which the external and internal genitalia are physically examined by inspection, palpation, percussion, and auscultation. It should be performed regularly throughout a woman's life. See also **female reproductive system assessment.**

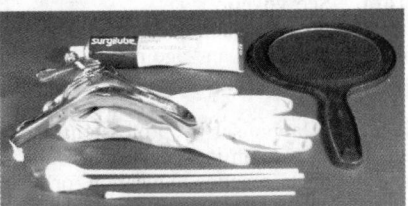

**Equipment for pelvic examination**
*(Lemmi and Lemmi, 2000)*

■ METHOD: The woman empties her bladder, disrobes, and puts on an examining gown. Breast examination is often carried out before the pelvic examination. The woman is made as comfortable as possible in the dorsal lithotomy position, her feet in stirrups and her buttocks at the very edge of the foot of the examining table, and is then draped. Particular attention is paid to the suprapubic area to detect any masses extending from the pelvis above the symphysis and to the groin to detect inguinal lymphadenopathy or hernia. If a mass is felt, percussion may be performed to delineate it. If pregnancy is suspected, palpation and percussion of the uterus and auscultation of fetal heart tones are attempted. The examiner then moves to the stool at the foot of the table between the patient's legs. The labia majora are spread apart to permit inspection of the clitoris, the urethral meatus, the labia minora, and the vaginal vestibule. Any swelling, discoloration, lesion, scar, cyst, discharge, or bleeding is noted. Skene's and Bartholin's glands and ducts are palpated and milked, and any secretions expressed are evaluated and a specimen is spread on culture medium. The tone of the perineal and paravaginal musculature is assessed. Cystocele, rectocele, or varying degrees of uterine descensus may be observed as the woman is asked to bear down. Because lubricating jelly interferes with cytologic and bacteriologic studies, the speculum examination is usually performed without using the jelly. The speculum is warmed, lubricated with warm water, and introduced gradually. The examiner is careful to direct the speculum along the axis of the vagina, which is at an angle of approximately 45 degrees to the axis of the table if the woman is lying flat. The speculum may need to be moved lightly from side to side to slip it over the vaginal rugae. The woman is advised that she may feel a stretching sensation; the speculum is gently opened and its position is adjusted to hold the vaginal folds out of the way to reveal the cervix. The color and condition of the vaginal epithelium are observed, and the position, size, and quality of the superficial epithelium are evaluated. Specimens for bacteriologic study are obtained before the Papanicolaou (Pap) test. For the Pap test scrapings of the endocervix and the cervix and a sample of the vaginal secretions are secured on a Pap stick and an applicator and lightly spread on labeled glass slides. The slides are immediately sprayed or dipped into a fixative. The speculum is then closed, rotated slightly, removed from the vagina, and, if not disposable, rinsed or placed directly into a germicidal solution. In the bimanual part of the examination two gloved fingers are well lubricated and inserted slowly and gently into the vagina. The examiner uses the opposite hand to apply pressure to the lower abdomen in several positions and directions to move the uterus, tubes, and ovaries into positions in which they may be felt. The size, shape, position, mobility, and consistency of the organs and tissues are evaluated, and any tenderness or discomfort is noted. Rectal or rectovaginal examination is then performed. Before the insertion of a finger in the anus lateral pressure is applied to the sphincter, and the woman is urged to bear down lightly to relax the muscle and minimize discomfort.

■ INTERVENTIONS: Minor thoughtlessness or inadvertent movement may cause tension and make the examination more difficult for the woman and for the examiner. Instruments, culture materials, a light, drapes, and a gown are all made ready beforehand. The table, instruments, and drapes are clean and warm. Materials from previous examinations are not in evidence. The woman is forewarned of what to expect at each step of the examination. Gentleness and quietness are exercised at all times. On completion of the examination the woman is helped to slide well back on the table before sitting up. Syncope after pelvic examination is uncommon but not rare; there is risk of injury should the patient faint and fall from the examining table. The woman is observed briefly after sitting up before being left alone. She is then given tissues, a sanitary napkin or tampon, and a private area in which to dress.

■ OUTCOME CRITERIA: Pelvic examination may demonstrate many pelvic abnormalities and diseases. Cytologic and bacteriologic specimens are conveniently obtained. A pelvic examination cannot be satisfactorily performed without the cooperation of the woman being examined; inadequate relaxation, obesity, extensive scarring, pelvic tenderness, and heavy vaginal discharge also may preclude an adequate examination.

**pelvic exenteration** /eksen′tərā′shən/, the surgical removal of all reproductive organs and their lymph nodes and en bloc removal of the rectum, distal sigmoid colon, urinary bladder, distal ureters, internal iliac vessels, entire perlvic floor, with accompanying pelvic peritoneum, levator muscles, and perineum. A partial exeneration may be done.

**pelvic floor,** the soft tissues enclosing the pelvic outlet.

**pelvic girdle** [L, *pelvis*, basin; AS, *gyrdel*], a bony ring formed by the hip bones, the sacrum, and the coccyx.

**pelvic hematoma,** an accumulation of blood in the soft tissues of the pelvis, as may occur during childbirth.

**pelvic inferior aperture.** See **pelvic outlet.**

**pelvic inflammatory disease (PID),** any inflammatory condition of the female pelvic organs, especially one caused by bacterial infection. Characteristics of the condition in-

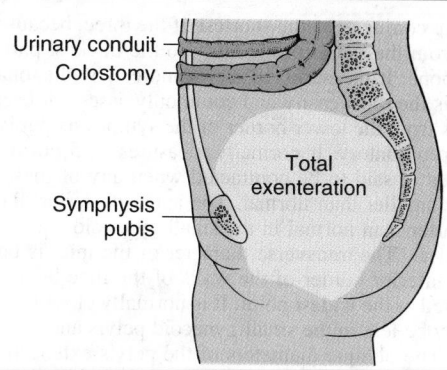

**Total pelvic exenteration** *(Beare and Myers, 1998)*

clude fever, foul-smelling vaginal discharge, pain in the lower abdomen, abnormal uterine bleeding, pain with coitus, and tenderness or pain in the uterus, affected ovary, or fallopian tube on bimanual pelvic examination. If an abscess has already developed, a soft, tender fluid-filled mass may be palpated. Bed rest and antibiotics are usually prescribed, but surgical drainage of an abscess may be required. Severe, fulminating PID may necessitate hysterectomy to prevent fatal septicemia. If the cause is infection by gonococci or chlamydiae, the woman's sexual partners are also treated with antibiotics. Severe PID is usually very painful; the woman may be prostrate and require narcotic analgesia. Recurrent or severe PID often results in scarring of the fallopian tubes, obstruction, and infertility.

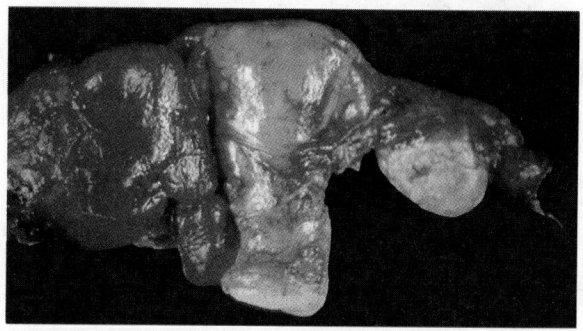

**Pelvic inflammatory disease**
*(Kumar, Cotran, and Robbins, 1997)*

**pelvic inlet,** (in obstetrics) the inlet to the true pelvis, bounded by the sacral promontory, the horizontal rami of the pubic bones, and the top of the symphysis pubis. Because the infant must pass through the inlet to enter the true pelvis and to be born vaginally, the anteroposterior, transverse, and oblique dimensions of the inlet are important measurements to be made in assessing the pelvis in pregnancy. There are three anteroposterior diameters: the true conjugate, the obstetric conjugate, and the diagonal conjugate. The true conjugate can be measured only on radiographic films, because it extends from the sacral promontory to the top of the symphysis pubis. Its normal measurement is 11 cm or more. The obstetric conjugate is the shortest of the three, because it extends from the sacral promontory to the thickest part of the pubic bone. It measures 10 cm or more. The diagonal conjugate is the most easily and commonly assessed, because it extends from the lower border of the symphysis pubis to the sacral promontory. It normally measures 11.5 cm or more. The inlet is said to be contracted when any of these diameters is smaller than normal. The anteroposterior diameters are shorter than normal in the small gynecoid and platypelloid pelvis. The transverse diameter of the inlet is bounded by the inferior border of the walls of the iliac bones and is measured at the widest point. It is normally close to 13.5 cm but may be less in the small gynecoid pelvis and anthropoid pelvis. The oblique diameters of the pelvis extend from the juncture of the sacrum and ilium to the eminence on the ilium on the opposite side of the pelvis. Each oblique diameter measures nearly 13 cm. This dimension is smaller than normal in the small gynecoid and platypelloid pelves. See also **android pelvis, anthropoid pelvis, gynecoid pelvis, platypelloid pelvis.**

**pelvic kidney.** See **ptotic kidney.**

**pelvic minilaparotomy** /min′ēlap′ərot′əmē/, a surgical operation in which the lower abdomen is entered through a small suprapubic incision. It is performed most often for tubal sterilization but also for diagnosis and treatment of ectopic pregnancy, ovarian cyst, endometriosis, and infertility. It may be performed as an alternative to laparoscopy, often on an outpatient basis. General, regional, or local anesthesia is administered. The patient is placed in the supine position, and the abdomen is prepared with antiseptic solution and covered with sterile drapes. An incision a few centimeters long is made, usually transversely, in the suprapubic fold of skin in the midline and is then carried down through the fat and fascia, between the rectus abdominis muscles, and into the peritoneal cavity. Bleeding is ligated, and a small self-retaining retractor is placed in the incision. A laparoscope may be used for visualization. The sterilization or other procedure is performed. After hemostasis is ensured, each tube is replaced in its anatomic position, and the incision is closed in layers. Because incisional pain in the postoperative period may mask the pain of intraperitoneal bleeding, vital signs are monitored frequently. Tachycardia and hypotension not alleviated by analgesia may be signs of hemorrhage or injury to the bowel. Before discharge outpatients are carefully instructed in postoperative danger signs and proper care of the incision at home. Arrangements are made for follow-up examination. Often minilaparotomy may be performed faster and less expensively than laparoscopy. Though small, the minilaparotomy incision is considerably larger than is the usual laparoscopy incision. It is therefore less pleasing cosmetically, as well as more painful in the postoperative period. Compare **laparoscopy.**

**pelvic muscle exercise,** a nursing intervention from the Nursing Interventions Classification (NIC) defined as strengthening and training the levator ani and urogenital muscles through voluntary, repetitive contraction to decrease stress, urge, or mixed types of urinary incontinence. See also **Nursing Interventions Classification.**

**pelvic outlet,** the space surrounded by the bones of the lower part of the true pelvis. In men the shape of the pelvic outlet is narrower than that in women, but this is of no clinical significance. In women the shape and size of the pelvis vary and are of importance in childbirth. The shapes are classified by the length of the diameters as compared with each other and by the thickness of the bones. The diameters of the outlet are the anteroposterior, from the symphysis pubis to the coccyx, and the intertuberous, laterally from one to the other ischial tuberosity. See also **pelvic classification.**

**pelvic pain,** pain in the pelvis, as occurs in appendicitis, oophoritis, and endometritis. The character and onset of pelvic pain and any factors that alleviate or aggravate it are significant in making a diagnosis.

**pelvic pole,** the end of the axis at which the breech of the fetus is located.

**pelvic presentation** [L, *pelvis,* basin, *praesentare,* to show], a breech presentation.

**pelvic rotation,** one of the five major kinematic determinants of gait, involving the alternate rotation of the pelvis to the right and the left of the body's central axis. The usual pelvic rotation occurring at each hip joint in most healthy individuals is approximately 4 degrees to each side of the central axis. Pelvic rotation occurs during the stance phase of gait and involves a medial to lateral circular motion. With normal locomotion or walking considered a progressive sinusoidal movement, pelvic rotation serves to minimize the vertical displacement of the body's center of gravity during walking. Analysis of pelvic rotation is often a factor in diagnosis of various orthopedic diseases, deformities, and abnormal bone conditions and in the correction of pathologic gaits. Compare **knee-ankle interaction, knee-hip flexion, lateral pelvic displacement, pelvic tilt.**

**pelvic rotunda** [L, *pelvis,* basin, *rotundus,* wheel], a part of the ear appearing as a funnel-shaped depression of the tympanum above the fenestra cochlea.

**pelvic tilt,** one of the five major kinematic determinants of gait that lowers the pelvis on the side of the swinging lower limb during the walking cycle. Through the action of the hip joint the pelvis tilts laterally downward, adducting the lower limb in the stance phase of gait and abducting the opposite extremity in the swing phase of gait. The knee joint of the non-weight-bearing limb flexes during its swing phase to allow the pelvic tilt. Pelvic tilt helps minimize the vertical displacement of the body's center of gravity, thus conserving energy during walking. It is often a factor in the diagnosis and treatment of various orthopedic diseases, deformities, and abnormal conditions and in the analysis and correction of pathologic gaits. Compare **knee-ankle interaction, knee-hip flexion, lateral pelvic displacement, pelvic rotation.**

**pelvic varicocele.** See **ovarian varicocele.**

**pelvifemoral** /pel′vēfem′ərəl/ [L, *pelvis,* basin, *femur,* thigh], pertaining to the structures of the hip joint, especially the muscles and the area around the bony pelvis and the head of the femur that make up the pelvic girdle.

**pelvifemoral muscular dystrophy.** See **Leyden-Möbius muscular dystrophy.**

**pelvimeter** /pelvim′ətər/ [L, *pelvis,* basin; Gk, *metron,* measure], a device for measuring the diameter and capacity of the pelvis.

**pelvimetry** /pelvim′ətrē/, the act or process of determining the dimensions of the bony birth canal. Kinds of pelvimetry are **clinical pelvimetry** and **x-ray pelvimetry.**

**pelviotomy.** See **pubiotomy.**

**pelvis** /pel′viz/, *pl.* **pelves** [L, basin], the lower part of the trunk of the body, composed of four bones, the two innominate bones laterally and ventrally and the sacrum and coccyx posteriorly. It is divided into the greater or false pelvis and the lesser or true pelvis by an oblique plane passing through the sacrum and the pubic symphysis. The greater pelvis is the expanded part of the cavity situated cranially and ventral to the pelvic brim. The lesser pelvis is situated distal to the pelvic brim, and its bony walls are more complete than those of the greater pelvis. The inlet and outlet of the pelvis have three important diameters: anteroposterior, oblique, and transverse. The pelvis of a woman is usually less massive but wider and more circular than that of a man. —**pelvic,** *adj.*

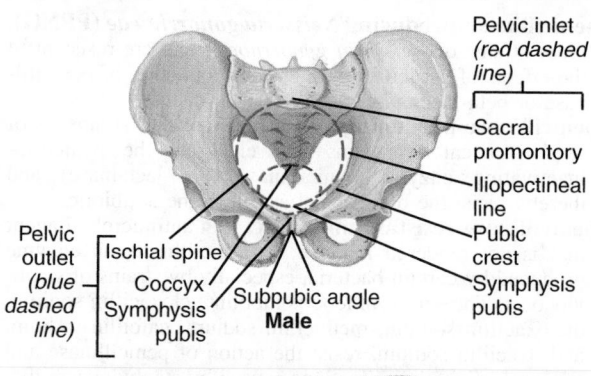

Pelvic inlet (red dashed line)

Sacral promontory

Iliopectineal line

Pubic crest

Symphysis pubis

Pelvic outlet (blue dashed line)

Ischial spine

Coccyx

Symphysis pubis

Subpubic angle

**Male**

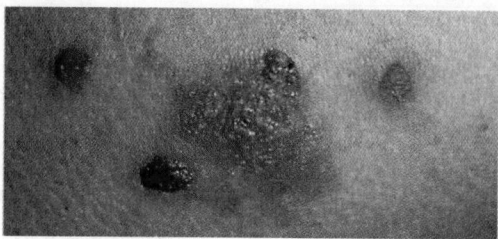

**Pemphigus vulgaris** *(du Vivier, 1993)*

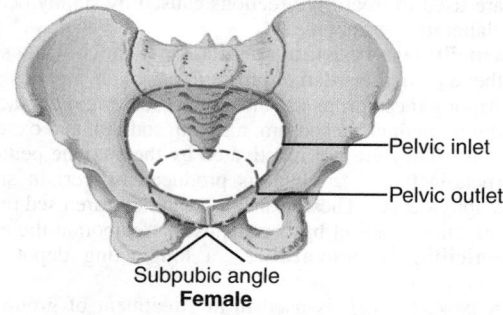

Pelvic inlet

Pelvic outlet

Subpubic angle

**Female**

**Comparison of male and female bony pelvis**
*(Thibodeau and Patton, 1999/Christine Oleksyk)*

**pelvisacral** /pel′visā′krəl/, pertaining to the pelvis and sacrum.

**pelvospondylitis ossificans** /pel′vōspon′dilī′tis/, inflammation of the pelvic part of the spine with deposits of bony material between the sacral vertebrae.

**PEM,** abbreviation for **protein-energy malnutrition.**

**pemoline** /pem′əlēn/, a central nervous system stimulant.
■ INDICATIONS: It is prescribed in the treatment of minimal brain dysfunction and attention-deficit disorder in children.
■ CONTRAINDICATION: Known hypersensitivity to this drug prohibits its use.
■ ADVERSE EFFECTS: Some of the more serious adverse reactions are insomnia, GI disturbances, rash, convulsions, and hallucinations.

**pemphigoid** /pem′figoid/ [Gk, *pemphix,* bubble, *eidos,* form], a bullous disease resembling pemphigus, distinguished by thicker walled bullae arising from erythematous macules or urticarial bases. Oral lesions are uncommon. It may rarely be associated with an internal malignancy. Spontaneous remission occasionally occurs after several years. Treatment usually uses oral corticosteroids. Compare **pemphigus.**

**pemphigus** /pem′figəs, pemfī′gəs/ [Gk, *pemphix,* bubble], an uncommon, severe disease of the skin and mucous membranes, characterized by thin-walled bullae arising from apparently normal skin or mucous membrane. The bullae rupture readily, leaving raw patches. The person loses weight, becomes weak, and is subject to major infections. Treatment with corticosteroids and other immunosuppressive medications has changed the prognosis of this disease from almost universal fatality to a controllable problem compatible with a nearly normal life. The cause is unknown. Compare **pemphigoid.**

**pemphigus chronicus.** See **pemphigus vulgaris.**

**pemphigus erythematosus.** See **erythematous pemphigus.**

**pemphigus vulgaris** [Gk, *pemphix,* bubble; L, *vulgus,* common], a chronic progressive, often fatal disease, characterized by the formation of bullae on otherwise normal skin. Also called **pemphigus chronicus.**

**Pender, Nola J.,** a nursing theorist who first presented her Health Promotion Model for nursing in her book *Health Promotion in Nursing Practice* (1982). She developed the idea that promoting optimal health supersedes preventing disease. Pender's theory identifies cognitive-perceptual factors in the individual, such as importance of health, perceived benefits of health-promoting behaviors, and perceived barriers to health-promoting behaviors. These factors are modified by demographic and biologic characteristics and interpersonal influences, as well as situational and behavioral factors. They help predict participation in health-promoting behavior. The individual's definition of health for himself or herself has more importance than a general statement about health. A major assumption in Pender's theory is that health, as a positive high-level state, is assumed to be a goal toward which an individual strives.

**pendular nystagmus** [L, *pendulus,* hanging down; Gk, *nystagmos,* nodding], an undulating involuntary movement of the eyeball.

**pendulous** /pen′dələs/, hanging loose or lacking proper support.

**pendulous abdomen** [L, *pendulus,* hanging down, *abdomen*], an abnormal condition in which the anterior abdominal wall becomes relaxed and allows the abdomen to hang down over the pubic region.

**-penem,** suffix for certain antibiotics, including analogs of penicillanic acid.

**penetrance** /pen′ətrəns/ [L, *penetrare,* to penetrate], the regularity with which an allele is expressed in a person who carries it. If an allele always produces its effect on the phenotype, it is fully penetrant. Achondroplasia is caused by a fully penetrant allele; if the allele is present, achondroplasia results. If an allele produces its effect less frequently than 100% of the time, it is not fully penetrant. Retinoblastoma develops in 90% of the children carrying the allele for the disease; in 10% of children the allele is nonpenetrant. —**penetrant,** *adj.*

**penetrate** /pen′ətrāt/ [L, *penetrare*], **1.** to enter or pierce a barrier. **2.** pertaining to the degree to which x-rays pass through matter.

**penetrating wound** /pen′ətrā′ting/ [L, *penetrare* + AS, *wund*], a wound that breaks the skin and enters into a body area, organ, or cavity.

**penetration** /pen′ətrā′shən/, **1.** a piercing or entering. **2.** intellectual discernment. **3.** a stage in establishment of a viral infection in which the viral genetic material enters the host cell through fusion, phagocytosis, or injection.

**penetrometer.** See **stepwedge.**

**-penia,** suffix meaning a '(specified) deficiency': *glycopenia, lipopenia, thyropenia.*

**penicillamine (D-penicillamine)** /pen'isil'əmēn/, a chelating agent.
- INDICATIONS: It is prescribed to bind with and remove metals from the blood in the treatment of heavy metal (especially lead) poisoning, in cystinuria, and in Wilson's disease. It is also prescribed as a palliative in the treatment of sclerosis and rheumatoid arthritis when other medications have failed.
- CONTRAINDICATIONS: Known hypersensitivity to this drug or penicillamine-related aplastic anemia prohibits its use. It is not given to patients who are pregnant or who have kidney dysfunction.
- ADVERSE EFFECTS: Among the more serious adverse reactions are fever, rashes, and blood dyscrasias. Severe bone marrow depression and immune disorders have been associated with long-term use of this drug. D-penicillamine is less toxic than the L form, and much of the reported toxicity is caused by the use of the L or DL form.

**penicillic acid** /pen'isil'ik/, an antibiotic compound isolated from various species of the fungus *Penicillium.*

**penicillin** /pen'isil'in/ [L, *penicillus,* paintbrush], any one of a group of antibiotics derived from cultures of species of the fungus *Penicillium* or produced semisynthetically. Various penicillins administered orally or parenterally for the treatment of bacterial infections exert their antimicrobial action by inhibiting the biosynthesis of cell wall mucopeptides during active multiplication of the organisms. Penicillin G (benzylpenicillin), a widely used therapeutic agent for meningococcal, pneumococcal, and streptococcal infections; syphilis; and a number of other diseases, is rapidly absorbed when injected intramuscularly or subcutaneously, but it is inactivated by gastric acid and hydrolyzed by penicillinase produced by most strains of *Staphylococcus aureus.* Penicillin V (phenethicillin) is also active against gram-positive cocci, with the exception of penicillinase-producing staphylococci, and, because it is resistant to gastric acid, it is effective when administered orally. Penicillins resistant to the action of the enzyme penicillinase (beta-lactamase) are cloxacillin, dicloxacillin, methicillin, nafcillin, and oxacillin. Ampicillin, carbenicillin, and hetacillin are broad-spectrum penicillins that are active against gram-negative organisms, including *Escherichia coli, Haemophilus influenzae, Neisseria gonorrhoeae, Proteus mirabilis,* and species of *Pseudomonas.* Hypersensitivity reactions are common in patients receiving penicillin and may appear in the absence of prior exposure to the drug, presumably because of unrecognized exposure to a food or other substance containing traces of the antibiotic. The most common hypersensitivity reactions are rash, fever, and bronchospasm, followed in frequency by vasculitis, serum sickness, and exfoliative dermatitis. In some patients severe erythema multiforme accompanied by headache, fever, arthralgia, and conjunctivitis (Stevens-Johnson syndrome) develop; the most frequent cause of anaphylactic shock is an injection of penicillin.

**penicillinase** /pen'əsil'ənās/, an enzyme elaborated by certain bacteria, including many strains of staphylococci, that inactivates penicillin and thereby promotes resistance to the antibiotic. A purified preparation of penicillinase, derived from cultures of saprophytic spore-forming *Bacillus cereus,* is used in the treatment of adverse reactions to penicillin. Also called **beta-lactamase.**

**penicillinase-producing *Neisseria gonorrhoeae* (PPNG),** those strains of *Neisseria gonorrhoeae* that are resistant to the effects of penicillin through the production of penicillinase or beta-lactamase.

**penicillinase-producing staphylococci,** strains of staphylococcal organisms that elaborate the penicillin-inactivating enzyme penicillinase (beta-lactamase) and thereby resist the bactericidal action of the antibiotic.

**penicillinase-resistant antibiotic,** an antimicrobial agent that is not rendered inactive by penicillinase, an enzyme produced by certain bacteria, especially by strains of staphylococci. The semisynthetic penicillins, cloxacillin sodium, dicloxacillin sodium, methicillin sodium, nafcillin sodium, and oxacillin sodium, resist the action of penicillinase and are used in treating infections caused by staphylococci that elaborate the enzyme.

**penicillinase-resistant penicillin,** one of the semisynthetic penicillins derived from *Penicillium,* a genus of mold. Among these drugs are cloxacillin sodium, dicloxacillin sodium, methicillin sodium, nafcillin sodium, and oxacillin sodium. They are not inactivated by the enzyme penicillinase (beta-lactamase), which is produced by certain strains of staphylococci. These resistant antibiotics are used in treating infections caused by organisms that elaborate the enzyme.

**penicillin G benzathine,** a long-acting depot form of penicillin.
- INDICATIONS: It is used in the treatment of group A beta-hemolytic streptococcal pharyngitis, group A beta-hemolytic streptococcal pyoderma, and syphilitic infection outside the central nervous system. It is given by deep intramuscular injection to achieve steady concentrations in the plasma and to slow systemic absorption from the repository in the muscle over a period of 12 hours to several days.
- CONTRAINDICATIONS: Hypersensitivity to this drug or to other penicillins prohibits its use.
- ADVERSE EFFECTS: The most serious adverse reaction is anaphylaxis. The most common side effects are diarrhea, maculopapular rash, urticarial rash, fever, bronchospasm, vasculitis, serum sickness, and exfoliative dermatitis.

**penicillin G potassium,** an antibacterial.
- INDICATIONS: It is prescribed in the treatment of many infections, including syphilis, rheumatic fever, and glomerulonephritis.
- CONTRAINDICATIONS: Known hypersensitivity to this drug or to any penicillin prohibits its use.
- ADVERSE EFFECTS: Among the more serious adverse effects are allergic reactions that vary from minor skin rashes to anaphylaxis. Nausea and diarrhea occur frequently.

**penicillin phenoxymethyl.** See **penicillin V.**

**penicillin V,** a bacterial antibiotic.
- INDICATION: It is prescribed in the treatment of susceptible infections caused by susceptible bacterial strains.
- CONTRAINDICATIONS: Known hypersensitivity to this drug or to any penicillin prohibits its use.
- ADVERSE EFFECTS: Among the more serious adverse reactions are anaphylaxis and urticaria.

**penicilliosis** /pen'isil'ē·ō'sis/ [L, *penicillus,* paintbrush; Gk, *osis,* condition], pulmonary infection caused by fungi of the genus *Penicillium.*

***Penicillium*** /pen'isil'ē·əm/ [L, *penicillus,* paintbrush], a genus of fungi, some species of which have been tentatively linked to disease in humans. Penicillin G is obtained from *Penicillium chrysogenum* and *P. notatum.*

**penile** /pē'nīl/ [L, penis], pertaining to the penis.

**penile cancer** /pē'nīl/ [L, *penis,* penis, *cancer,* crab], a rare malignancy of the penis generally occurring in uncircumcised men and associated with genital herpesvirus infection

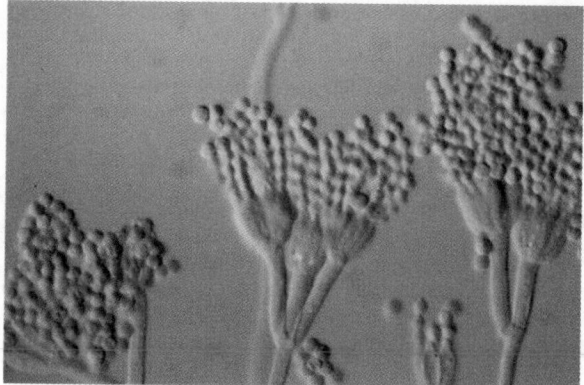

**Penicillium species** *(Mahon and Manuselis, 2000)*

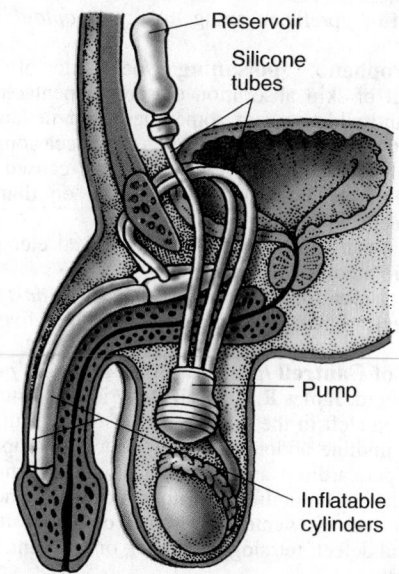

**Inflatable penile prosthesis**
*(Ignatavicius, Workman, and Mishler, 1999)*

and poor hygiene. Smegma may be a causative factor, but the specific substance and mechanism are unknown. Leukoplakia or the flat-topped papules of balanitis xerotica obliterans may be premalignant lesions, and the velvety red painful papules of Queyrat's erythroplasia are penile squamous cell carcinoma in situ. Cancer of the penis usually presents as a local mass or a bleeding ulcer and metastasizes early in its course. Surgical treatment involves partial or total amputation of the penis and excision of inguinal nodes and adjacent tissue when necessary. Radiotherapy is often used preoperatively and postoperatively. Methotrexate or bleomycin also may be administered, especially in metastatic disease.

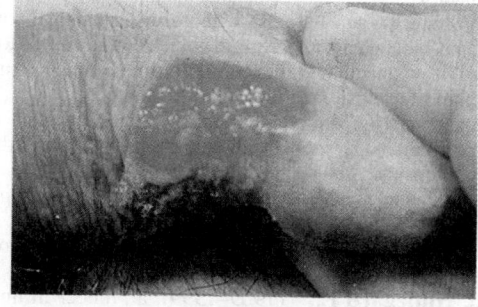

**Penile cancer**
*(Seidel et al, 1999/courtesy Patrick C. Walsh, MD, The Johns Hopkins University School of Medicine, Baltimore)*

**penile prosthesis** [L, *penis* + Gk, *prosthesis*, addition], a device that can be surgically implanted in the penis to treat erectile dysfunction. Some such devices have mechanisms that control production of an erection. Penile implants may consist of inflatable plastic cavernosal cylinders attached to a pump that forces fluid from a reservoir into the cylinders, producing an erection.

**penis** /pē′nis/ [L, male sex organ], the external reproductive organ of a man, homologous with the clitoris of a woman. It is attached with ligaments to the front and sides of the pubic arch and is composed of three cylindrical masses of cavernous tissue covered with skin. The corpora cavernosa penis surrounds a median mass called the corpus

spongiosum penis, which contains the greater part of the urethra. The subcutaneous fascia of the penis is directly continuous with that of the scrotum, which contains the testes.

**penischisis** /pēnis′kisis/ [L, *penis* + Gk, *schisis*, splitting], a penis with a fissure resulting in an abnormal opening, such as occurs in epispadias.

**penis envy,** literally, female envy of the male penis, but generally a female wish for male attributes, position, and advantages. It is believed by some psychologists to be a significant factor in female personality development.

**-pennate,** suffix meaning 'having feathers': *bipennate, pennate, unipennate.*

**penniform** /pen′ifôrm/ [L, *penna*, feather, *forma*, form], pertaining to the shape of a feather, especially the patterns of muscular fasciculi that correlate with the range of motion and the power of muscles. Penniform fasciculi converge on one side of certain tendons. Muscles with more fasciculi have greater power but less range of motion than muscles with fewer fasciculi. Compare **bipenniform, multipenniform.**

**Penrose drain** [Charles B. Penrose, American surgeon, 1862–1925; AS, *draehen*, teardrop], a thin rubber tube used as a surgical drain device.

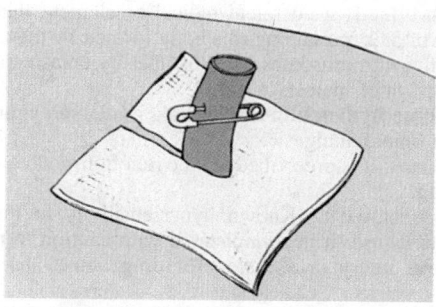

**Penrose drain** *(Potter and Perry, 2001)*

**pent-, penta-,** prefix meaning 'five': *pentaploid, pentose, pentoside.*

**pentachlorophenol poisoning** /pen′təklôr′ōfē′nol/, a toxic effect of skin absorption of sodium pentachlorophenate, an antimildew agent sometimes used in laundering. The condition has affected newborns with occasionally fatal symptoms of fever and profuse sweating, caused by skin contact with pentachlorophenate residue on diapers and nursery linens.

**pentad** /pen′tad/, **1.** a pentavalent chemical element. **2.** a relationship among five things.

**pentadactyl** /pen′tədak′til/ [Gk, *pente,* five, *daktylos,* fingers or toes], having five fingers per hand and five toes per foot.

**pentalogy of Cantrell** /pen·tal′ə·jē kan·trel/ [Gk, *pente,* five + *logos,* word; James R. Cantrell, American physician, 20th century], a cleft in the inferior part of the sternum associated with midline abdominal defects such as omphalocele, defective pericardium and diaphragm with communication between the pericardial and peritoneal cavities, and cardiac anomalies such as ventricular septal defect or less often atrial septal defect, tetralogy of Fallot, or left ventricular diverticulum.

**Pentam,** trademark for pentamidine isethionate, an antiprotozoal agent.

**Pentam 300,** trademark for a parenteral antiprotozoal drug used to treat pneumonia caused by *Pneumocystis carinii* (pentamidine isethionate).

**pentamidine** /pentam′idēn/, an antiprotozoal. It is sometimes prescribed in the treatment of trypanosomiasis and leishmaniasis, and of *Pneumocystis carinii* pneumonia in immune-compromised patients.

**pentamidine isethionate,** a parenteral antiprotozoal drug.
- INDICATIONS: It is prescribed in the treatment of pneumonia caused by *Pneumocystis carinii,* particularly in patients who have human immunodeficiency syndrome.
- CONTRAINDICATIONS: To reduce the risk of toxicity, the following tests must be carried out before, during, and after therapy: blood urea nitrogen, serum creatinine, blood glucose, complete blood and platelet counts, liver function, serum calcium, and electrocardiogram.
- ADVERSE EFFECTS: Among adverse reactions are hypotension, hypoglycemia, leukopenia, thrombocytopenia, cardiac arrhythmias, acute renal failure, hypocalcemia, Stevens-Johnson syndrome, elevated serum creatinine level, elevated liver function results, pain or induration at the injection site, nausea, anorexia, fever, and rash.

**pentaploid.** See **polyploid.**

*Pentatrichomonas hominis* /pen′tətrik′əmō′nəs/, a species of parasitic protozoan flagellate, formerly part of the genus *Trichomonas* that lives symbiotically in the colon of humans. Formerly called *Trichomonas hominis.*

**pentavalent** /pəntav′ələnt/ [Gk, *pente,* five; L, *valere,* to have worth], **1.** a chemical radical or element that has a valency of 5. **2.** pertaining to a body formed by the association of five chromosomes held together by chiasmata at the first division of meiosis.

**pentazocine hydrochloride** /pentā′zəsēn/, an agonist/antagonist opioid analgesic.
- INDICATION: It is prescribed for the relief of moderate to severe pain.
- CONTRAINDICATIONS: Known hypersensitivity to this drug prohibits its use. It is administered with caution to patients with head injury or a history of drug abuse and dependency.
- ADVERSE EFFECTS: Nausea and dizziness commonly occur. Other minor problems include constipation, hallucinations,

euphoria, and drowsiness. High doses may cause respiratory and circulatory depression. This drug can precipitate acute withdrawal symptoms in narcotic-dependent individuals.

**pentazocine lactate.** See **pentazocine hydrochloride.**

**Penthrane,** trademark for a general anesthetic (methoxyflurane).

**Pentid,** trademark for an antibacterial (penicillin G potassium).

**pentobarbital** /pen′təbär′bitol/, a sedative and hypnotic.
- INDICATIONS: It is prescribed as a preoperative sedative and in the control of acute convulsive disorders.
- CONTRAINDICATIONS: Porphyria or known hypersensitivity to this drug or to other barbiturates prohibits its use. It is used with caution in patients having impaired respiratory or liver function or a history of dependence on sedative or hypnotic drugs.
- ADVERSE EFFECTS: Among the more serious adverse reactions are respiratory or circulatory depression, paradoxic excitement, jaundice, or various hypersensitivity reactions. Nausea and hangover-like symptoms may occur.

**pentose** /pen′tōs/ [Gk, *pente,* five; L, *osus,* having], a monosaccharide made of carbohydrate molecules, each containing five carbon atoms. It is produced by the body and is elevated after the ingestion of certain fruits, such as plums and cherries, and in certain rare diseases.

**pentosuria** /pen′təsŏŏr′ē·ə/ [Gk, *pente* + L, *osus,* having; Gk, *ouron,* urine], a rare condition in which the monosaccharide pentose is found in the urine. Essential or idiopathic pentosuria is caused by an inherited error of metabolism.

**Pentothal Sodium,** trademark for a barbiturate drug (thiopental sodium).

**pentoxifylline** /pentok′sēfil′ēn/, an oral hemorrheologic drug.
- INDICATIONS: It is prescribed for the treatment of intermittent claudication associated with chronic occlusive arterial limb disease.
- CONTRAINDICATIONS: Patients with cardiovascular disorders should be closely monitored and their hypertensive dosage reduced if warranted. Patients on multiple drug regimens also should be closely monitored.
- ADVERSE EFFECTS: Among the most serious adverse reactions are nausea, dyspepsia, dizziness, angina, arrhythmia, and hypotension.

**Pen-Vee K,** trademark for an antibiotic (penicillin V potassium).

**Pepcid,** trademark for an antiulcer drug or H2 receptor antagonist (famotidine).

**Peplau, Hildegard E.,** (1909–1999), a pioneer in nursing theory development and a proponent in the 1950s of the concept that nursing is an interpersonal process. Borrowing heavily from the knowledge base of psychology, Peplau proposed hypotheses based on the premise of the interpersonal process. From the early work evolved a nursing goal to foster the assumption that humans value, strive for, and have a right to independence. In a 1952 work Peplau wrote that the nurse-patient relationship occurs in phases during which the nurse functions as a resource person, a counselor, and a surrogate. The four phases of the process are orientation, identification, exploitation, and resolution. Thus the nurse assists in orientation when a patient with a need seeks help. Identification assures the patient that the nurse can understand his or her situation. Exploitation begins when the patient uses the services available. Resolution is marked as old needs are met and newer ones emerge.

**peplos** /pep′los/, a lipoprotein coat that may surround a virion.

**peppermint,** the dried leaves and flowering tops of an

herb, *Mentha piperita.* It is a source of a volatile oil, used as a carminative and antiemetic.

**pepper spray,** an aerosolized form of oleoresins from capsicum, highly irritant to the skin and mucous membranes; used similarly to tear gas.

**Pepper syndrome** [William Pepper, American physician, 1874–1947], a neuroblastoma of the adrenal glands that usually metastasizes to the liver.

**pep pills,** *slang.* amphetamines, diet pills, or any other stimulant.

**peps-, pept-,** prefix meaning 'digestion': *pepsin, pepsiniferous, pepsitensin.*

**-pepsia, -pepsy, -peptic,** suffix meaning 'a state of the digestion': *anapepsia, colodyspepsia, oligopepsia, dyspeptic.*

**pepsin** /pep′sin/ [Gk, *pepsis,* digestion], an enzyme secreted in the stomach that catalyzes the hydrolysis of protein. Preparations of pepsin obtained from pork and beef stomachs are sometimes used as digestive aids. See also **enzyme, hydrolysis.**

**pepsinogen** /pəpsin′əjən/ [Gk, *pepsis* + *genein,* to produce], a zymogenic substance secreted by pyloric and gastric chief cells. It is converted to the enzyme pepsin in an acidic environment, as in the presence of hydrochloric acid produced in the stomach.

**pepsinuria** /pep′sinŏŏr′ē·ə/ [Gk, *pepsis,* digestion + *ouron,* urine], the presence of pepsin in urine.

**PEP syndrome.** See **POEMS syndrome.**

**pept-.** See **peps-.**

**peptic** /pep′tik/ [Gk, *peptein,* to digest], pertaining to digestion or to the enzymes and secretions essential to digestion.

**-peptic.** See **-pepsia.**

**peptic ulcer,** a sharply circumscribed loss of the mucous membrane of the stomach, duodenum, or any other part of the GI system exposed to gastric juices containing acid and pepsin. Also called **gastric ulcer.**

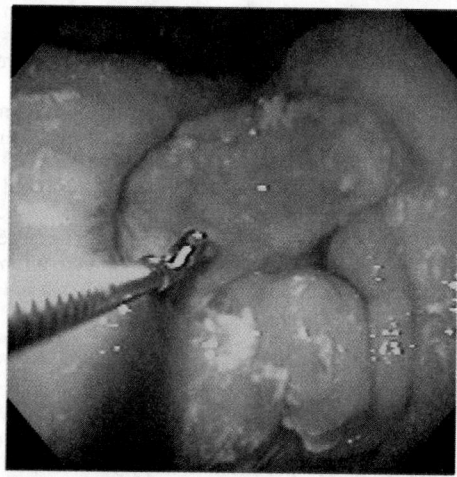

**Peptic ulcer: endoscopic view** *(Wilcox, 1995)*

■ OBSERVATIONS: Peptic ulcers may be acute or chronic. Acute lesions are almost always multiple and superficial. They may be totally asymptomatic and usually heal without scarring or other sequelae. Chronic ulcers are true ulcers.

They are deep, single, persistent, and symptomatic; the muscular coat of the wall of the organ does not regenerate; a scar forms, marking the site, and the mucosa may heal completely. Peptic ulcers are caused by a combination of poorly understood factors, including an excessive secretion of gastric acid, inadequate protection of the mucous membrane, stress, heredity, and the use of certain drugs, including the corticosteroids, certain antihypertensives, and antiinflammatory medications (especially acetylsalicylic acid and nonsteroidal antiinflammatory drugs). There is growing evidence from research that a bacterium present in the gut may be responsible for peptic ulcer disease. This bacterium is *Helicobacter pylori.* Characteristically ulcers cause a gnawing pain in the epigastrium that does not radiate to the back, is not aggravated by a change in position, and has a temporal pattern that mimics the diurnal rhythm of gastric acidity.

■ INTERVENTIONS: Symptomatic relief is provided by drugs that either neutralize or block secretion of acid, and frequent small bland meals. The underlying cause is treated if known. If *H. pylori* is present, a 2-week triple therapy regimen of tetracycline, metronidazole, and bismuth may be given. Hemorrhage caused by perforation of the muscle and blood vessels may require surgical resection of the damaged area. The diagnosis and evaluation of peptic ulcers involve serial radiographic studies using a contrast medium and endoscopy. A definitive diagnosis is important because the early signs of cancer of the stomach and duodenum resemble those of peptic ulcers.

■ NURSING CONSIDERATIONS: The patient is reassured that in most cases the ulcers heal completely and that the pain may be controlled with simple measures. The nurse emphasizes the correct use of antacids and the other medications prescribed. Usually the patient is instructed to eat frequent small meals consisting of foods known to be nonirritating. For many but not all patients, fatty, highly spiced, heavy, or fibrous foods are likely to provoke pain. The use of tobacco and alcohol is discouraged.

**peptidase** /pep′tidās/ [Gk, *peptein,* to digest, *ase,* enzyme suffix], a protein-splitting enzyme that breaks peptides into amino acids. It occurs naturally in plants, yeasts, certain microorganisms, and digestive juices.

**peptide** /pep′tīd/ [Gk, *peptein,* to digest], a molecular chain compound composed of two or more amino acids joined by peptide bonds. See also **amino acid, polypeptide, protein.**

**peptidergic** /pep′tidur′jik/, using small peptides as neurotransmitters.

**peptide YY.** See **neuropeptide Y.**

**peptogenic** /pep′təjen′ik/, pertaining to an agent that produces peptones or pepsin.

**peptone** /pep′tōn/, a derived protein, which may be produced by hydrolysis of a native protein with an acid or enzyme.

***Peptostreptococcus*** /pep′təstrep′təkok′əs/, a genus of gram-positive anaerobic chemoorganotrophic bacteria that occur in pairs or chains. The potentially pathogenic organisms are found in normal and pathologic female genital tracts and in the intestinal and respiratory tracts of normal humans. They have been associated with a variety of disorders ranging from appendicitis to putrefactive wounds.

***Peptostreptococcus anaerobius***, a potentially pathogenic species of anaerobic bacterium found throughout the body, including the mouth, the intestinal and respiratory tracts, and body cavities, particularly the vagina.

**per-,** 1. prefix meaning 'throughout, or completely': *peracephalus, perfuse, permeable.* 2. prefix meaning 'a large amount (in chemical terms)' or designating a combination of

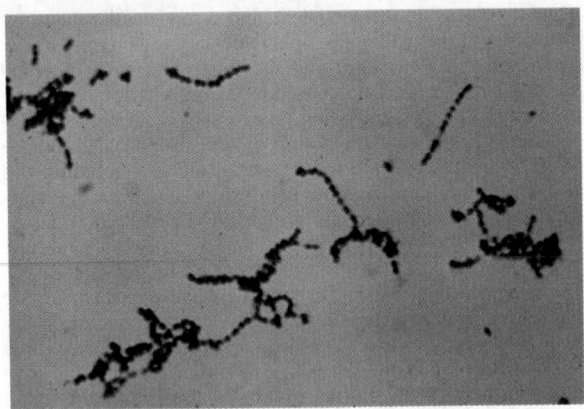

***Peptostreptococcus***
*(Mahon and Manuselis, 2000/courtesy Suzette L. Bartley,
James D. Howard, and Ray Simon, Centers for
Disease Control and Prevention, Atlanta)*

an element in its highest valence: *peracetate, peracid, per-hydride.* **3.** prefix meaning 'around, near, enclosing' *peri-apical, pericardium.*

**peracephalus** /pur'əsef'ələs/, *pl.* **peracephali** [L, *per,* completely; Gk, *a + kephale,* not head], a fetus or individual with a malformed head.

**per an.,** abbreviation for the Latin phrase *per annum,* 'yearly.'

**perceived severity** /pərsēvd'/ [L, *percipere,* to perceive, *severus,* serious], (in health belief model) a person's perception of the seriousness of the consequences of contracting a disease. Compare **perceived susceptibility.**

**perceived susceptibility,** (in health belief model) a person's perception of the likelihood of contracting a disease. Compare **perceived severity.**

**percentage depth dose** /pərsen'tij/ [L, *per,* completely, *centum,* hundred; ME, *dep,* deep; L, *dosis,* something given], the amount of therapeutic radiation delivered at a specified dose, expressed as a percentage of the skin dose.

**percentile,** the 100th part of a statistical distribution. A percentile rank of 80 indicates that 20% of the total number of cases scored above and 80% scored below in whatever characteristics were being studied.

**percent solution,** a relationship of a quantity of solute to the quantity of solution, multiplied by 100, expressed in terms of mass of solute per mass of solution. It can be expressed in terms of mass solute per mass solution, volume solute per volume solution, or mass solute (g) per volume (mL) solution. An example of a 5% by mass solution is 5 g of glucose dissolved in 95 g of water, forming 100 g of solution.

**percent systole** [L, *per + centum* + Gk, *systole,* contraction], the fraction of the duration of each heartbeat that is devoted to the contraction of the ventricles.

**percept** /pur'sept/ [L, *percipere,* to perceive], the mental impression of an object that is gained through the use of the senses.

**perception** /pərsep'shən/ [L, *percipere,* to perceive], **1.** the conscious recognition and interpretation of sensory stimuli that serve as a basis for understanding, learning, and knowing or for motivating a particular action or reaction. **2.** the result or product of the act of perceiving. Kinds of perception include **depth perception, extrasensory per-**

**ception, facial perception,** and **stereognostic perception.** —**perceptive, perceptual,** *adj.*

**perceptivity** /pur'səptiv'itē/, the ability to receive sense impressions.

**-perceptual.** See **perception.**

**perceptual constancy** /pərsep'chŏŏ·əl/ [L, *percipere,* to perceive, *cum,* together with, *stare,* to stand], (in Gestalt psychology) the phenomenon in which an object is seen in the same way under varying circumstances.

**perceptual defect,** any of a broad group of disorders or dysfunctions of the central nervous system that interfere with the conscious mental recognition of sensory stimuli. Such conditions are caused by lesions at specific sites in the cerebral cortex that may result from any illness or trauma affecting the brain at any age or stage of development. Impairment of mental activity, cognitive processes, and emotional responses may be diffuse, as occurs in organic mental disorders, such as the psychoses, delirium, and dementia, and in attention deficit disorder, or they may be manifested focally, as in aphasia, apraxia, epilepsy, disorders of memory, cerebrovascular disorders, and various intercranial neoplasms.

**perceptual deprivation,** the absence of or decrease in meaningful groupings of stimuli, which may result from a constant background noise or constant inadequate illumination.

**perceptual monotony,** a mental state characterized by a lack of variety in the normal pattern of everyday stimuli.

**perchloromethane.** See **carbon tetrachloride.**

**Percodan,** trademark for a fixed-combination central nervous system drug containing aspirin and opioid analgesics (oxycodone hydrochloride and oxycodone terephthalate).

**Percogesic,** trademark for a fixed-combination drug containing an antihistaminic (phenyltoloxamine citrate) and an analgesic (acetaminophen).

**percolation** /pur'kəlā'shən/ [L, *percolare,* to strain], **1.** the act of filtering any liquid through a porous medium. **2.** (in pharmacology) the removal of the soluble parts of a crude drug by passing a liquid solvent through it.

**per con.,** abbreviation for the Latin phrase *per contra,* 'the other side.'

**per contiguum,** spreading from one body structure to a contiguous area.

**per continuum,** describing the spread of an inflammation or other disease process from one body part to another through continuous tissue.

**Percorten,** trademark for an adrenocortical steroid (desoxycorticosterone acetate).

**percuss** /pərkus'/ [L, *percutere,* to strike hard], to perform percussion by striking, for example, the thoracic or abdominal wall, thereby producing sound vibrations that aid in diagnosis.

**percussion** /pərkush'ən/ [L, *percutere,* to strike hard], a technique in physical examination of tapping the body with the fingertips or fist to evaluate the size, borders, and consistency of some of the internal organs and to discover the presence and evaluate the amount of fluid in a body cavity. **Immediate** or **direct percussion** is percussion performed by striking the fingers directly on the body surface; **indirect, mediate,** or **finger percussion** involves striking a finger of one hand on a finger of the other hand as it is placed over the organ. See also **cupping and vibrating, percussor, pleximeter.** —**percuss,** *v.,* **percussible,** *adj.*

**percussor** /pərkus'ər/ [L, a striker], a small hammerlike diagnostic tool having a rubber head that is used to tap the body lightly in percussion. Also called **plexor.** See also **percussion.**

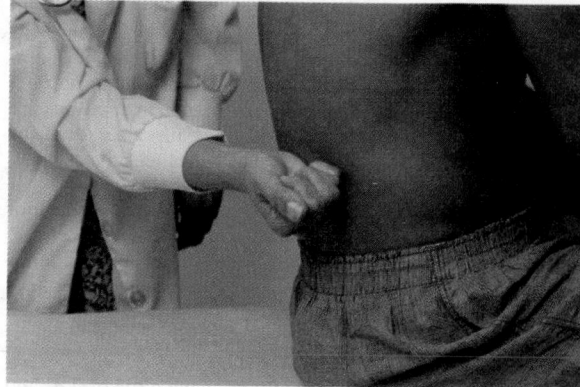

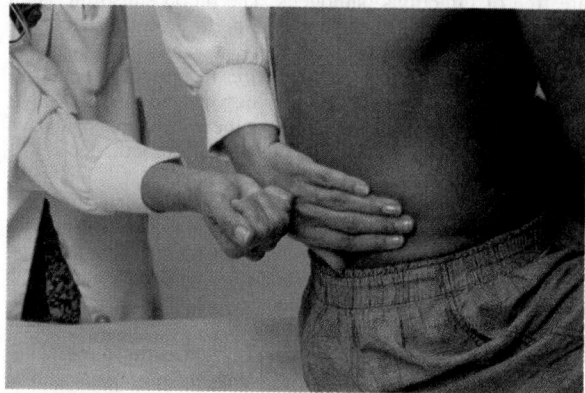

**Percussion: direct *(top)* and indirect *(bottom)***
*(Wilson and Giddens, 2001)*

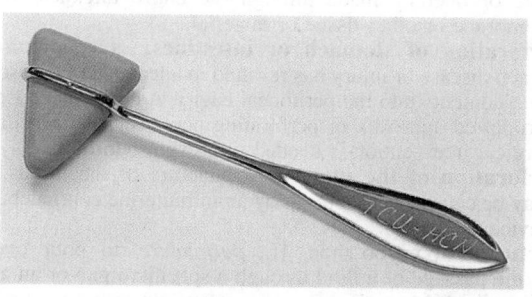

**Percussor** *(Wilson and Giddens, 2001)*

**percutaneous** /pur′kyōōtā′nē·əs/ [L, *per* + *cutis,* skin], performed through the skin, such as a biopsy; aspiration of fluid from a space below the skin using a needle, catheter, and syringe; or instillation of a fluid in a cavity or space by similar means.

**percutaneous absorption,** the process of absorption through the skin from topical application.

**percutaneous catheter placement,** a technique in which an intracatheter is introduced through the skin into an artery and placed at a site or structure to be studied by selective angiography and other diagnostic procedures. The puncture site is infiltrated with a local anesthetic before insertion of the catheter. A special needle is inserted into the artery, and

a long, flexible, spring guide is passed through the needle for approximately 15 cm. The needle is then removed, the catheter is advanced to the desired position, and the guide is withdrawn. The catheter is withdrawn at the end of the procedure.

**percutaneous endoscopic gastrostomy (PEG),** the creation of a new opening in the stomach, accomplished by puncturing the abdominal wall after the stomach has been distended by endoscopy.

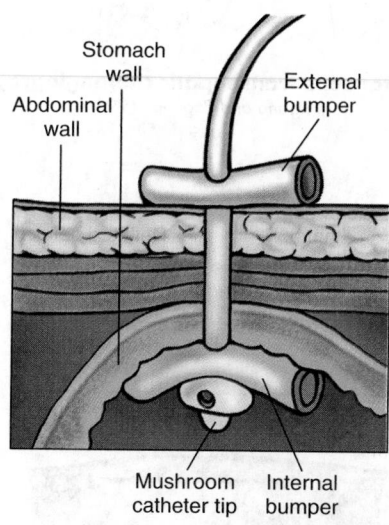

**Percutaneous endoscopic gastrostomy tube**
*(Monahan and Neighbors, 1998)*

**percutaneous nephrolithotomy,** a uroradiologic procedure performed to extract stones from within the kidney or proximal ureter by percutaneous surgery after the stones have been visualized radiologically.

**percutaneous nephroscope,** a thin fiberoptic probe that can be inserted into the kidney through an incision in the skin. Light transmitted along the fibers allows visualization of the inside of the kidney. The device is equipped with a tool that can be used to grasp and remove small kidney stones.

**percutaneous transhepatic cholangiography (PTC),** the radiographic examination of the structure of the bile ducts. A contrast medium is injected through a needle passed directly into a hepatic duct.

**percutaneous transluminal angioplasty (PTA),** a procedure for dilating blood vessels in the treatment of peripheral artery disease. Under fluoroscopic guidance a balloon-tipped catheter is inserted into a stenotic artery and the balloon is inflated. The inflated balloon may dilate the artery by stretching its elastic fibers or by flattening accumulation of plaque. See also **percutaneous transluminal coronary angioplasty (PTCA).**

**percutaneous transluminal coronary angioplasty (PTCA),** a technique in the treatment of atherosclerotic coronary heart disease and angina pectoris in which some plaques in the arteries of the heart are flattened against the arterial walls, resulting in improved circulation. The procedure involves threading a catheter through the vessel to the atherosclerotic plaque, inflating and deflating a small balloon at the tip of the catheter several times, and then remov-

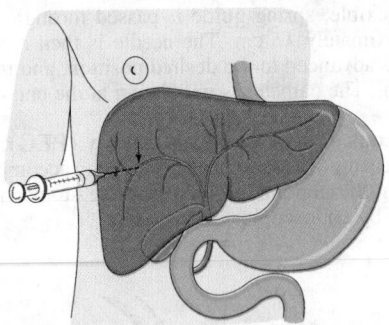

**Percutaneous transhepatic cholangiography**
*(Pagana and Pagana, 1998)*

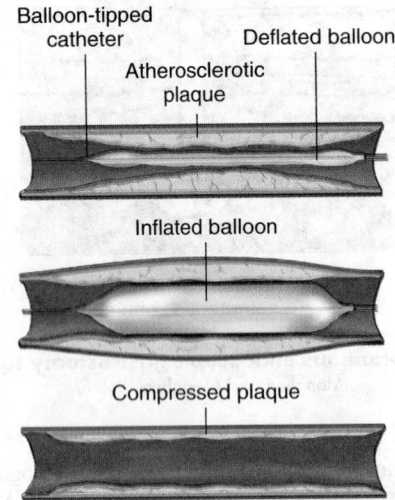

Balloon-tipped catheter

Deflated balloon

Atherosclerotic plaque

Inflated balloon

Compressed plaque

**Percutaneous transluminal coronary angioplasty**
*(Monahan and Neighbors, 1998)*

ing the catheter. The procedure is performed under radiographic or ultrasonic visualization. When it is successful, the plaques remain compressed and the symptoms of heart disease, including the pain of angina, are decreased. The alternative to this treatment is coronary bypass surgery, which is more expensive and dangerous and requires longer hospitalization and rehabilitation.

**per diem rate** /pər dē´əm, dī´əm/ [L, *per diem,* daily, *ratus,* reckoned], an established rate of payment for hospital services.

**per discharge payment,** a payment method in which costs of resources used for the entire hospital stay are the responsibility of the hospital. The hospital is then compensated according to a contractually determined amount per discharge.

**perencephaly** /per´ensef´əlē/, a condition characterized by one or more cerebral cysts.

**Perez reflex** /pərez´, per´ez/ [Bernard Perez, French physician, 1836–1903; L, *reflectere,* to bend back], the normal response of an infant to cry, flex the limbs, and elevate the head and pelvis when supported in a prone position with a finger pressed along the spine from the sacrum to the neck.

Persistence of the reflex beyond the 6 months of age may indicate brain damage.

**perfectionism** /pərfek´shəniz´əm/ [L, *perficere,* to complete], a subjective state in which a person pursues an extremely high standard of performance and, in many cases, demands the same standards of others. Failure to attain the goals may lead to feelings of defeat and other adverse psychologic consequences.

**perflation** /pərflā´shən/, a method of opening a passage or cavity entrance with air pressure.

**perfluorocarbons** /pərfloor´ōkär´bəns/, a group of chemicals with limited capacity for performing the function of hemoglobin in red blood cells by transporting oxygen through the circulatory system. They can be used for certain blood substitute purposes, regardless of the blood type of the patient; are stable at room temperatures; have a pH of 7.4; and are free of infectious pathogens. The blood substitute is an emulsion of perfluorodecalin and perfluorotripropylamine. Also called **artificial blood.**

**perforans** /pur´fôrənz/ [L, *perforare,* to pierce], penetrating. The term applies mainly to nerves, muscles, or other anatomic features that penetrate other structures, such as **perforans gasseri,** or nerves of the musculocutaneous tissues.

**perforate** [L, *perforare,* to pierce], **1.** /pur´fôrāt/ to pierce, punch, puncture, or otherwise make a hole. **2.** /purfôrit/ riddled with small holes. **3.** /pur´fôrit/ (of the anus) having a normal opening; not imperforate. —**perforation,** *n.*

**perforating fracture,** an open fracture caused by a projectile, making a small surface wound.

**perforating ulcer** /pur´fôrā´ting/ [L, *perforare,* to pierce, *ilcus*], **1.** an ulcer that penetrates the thickness of a wall or membrane, such as a peptic ulcer of the digestive tract. **2.** a deep painless ulcer, often on the sole of the foot, of a person whose skin is insensitive because of a disease such as diabetes.

**perforation** /pur´fôrā´shən/ [L, *perforare,* to pierce], a hole or opening made through the entire thickness of a membrane or other tissue or material.

**perforation of stomach or intestines,** a condition in which disease or injury has resulted in a leakage of digestive tract contents into the peritoneal cavity. A common cause is a ruptured appendix or perforating peptic ulcer. Immediate surgical intervention is needed to prevent peritonitis.

**perforation of the uterus,** a puncture of the uterus, as may be caused by a curet or by an intrauterine contraceptive device.

**perfusion** /pərfyōo´zhən/ [L, *perfundere,* to pour over], **1.** the passage of a fluid through a specific organ or an area of the body. **2.** a therapeutic measure whereby a drug intended for an isolated part of the body is introduced via the bloodstream.

**perfusionist** /pərfyōo´zhənist/ [L, *perfundere,* to pour over], an allied health professional who assists in performing procedures that involve extracorporeal circulation, such as during open-heart surgery, or hypothermia.

**perfusion lung scan,** a radiographic examination of the lungs and their function, performed after a IV injection of a radioactive material. It is performed to detect areas of lung perfusion as an aid in the diagnosis of pulmonary embolism. The procedure is usually done in conjunction with a ventilation scan, in which the patient inhales radioactive material and the lung is scanned to detect lung areas receiving ventilation. Also called **perfusion scan.**

**perfusion rate,** the rate of blood flow through the capillaries per unit mass of tissue, expressed in milliliters/minute per 100 g.

**perfusion scan.** See **perfusion lung scan.**

**perfusion technologist,** a person who, under the supervision of a physician, operates a heart-lung machine used for cardiopulmonary bypass during surgery.

**per gene,** a gene that is associated with circadian rhythms of some animal species. Mutations of the per gene locus result in alterations of their biorhythms. A similar DNA sequence occurs in the human genone, but its effect on human circadian rhythms in unknown.

**Pergonal,** trademark for human menopausal gonadotropin used to treat anovulation and infertility.

**peri-** /per′i-/, prefix meaning 'around': *periaxial, pericardial, pericolitis.*

**Periactin,** trademark for an antihistaminic and antipruritic (cyproheptadine hydrochloride).

**periadenitis** /per′i·ad′əni′tis/, an inflammation of tissues around a gland.

**periadenitis mucosa necrotica recurrens.** See **Sutton's disease.**

**perianal** /per′i·ā′nəl/ [Gk, *peri,* around; L, *anus*], pertaining to the area around the anus.

**perianal abscess** [Gk, *peri,* around; L, *anus* + *abscedere,* to go away], a focal purulent subcutaneous infection in the region of the anus. Treatment includes hot soaks, antibiotics, and possibly incision and drainage. If a rectal fistula or perianal space is found to be the cause of recurrent perianal abscesses, surgical excision is usually performed.

**periangitis.** See **periarteritis.**

**periaortic** /per′i·ā·ôr′tik/ [Gk, *peri,* around, *aerein,* to raise], pertaining to the area around the aorta.

**periaortitis** /per′i·ā′ôrtī′tis/, an inflammation of the adventitia or surrounding tissues of the aorta.

**periapical** /per′i·ap′ikəl/ [Gk, *peri* + L, *apex,* top], pertaining to the tissues around the apex of a tooth root, including the periodontal membrane and the alveolar bone.

**periapical abscess,** an infection around the root of a tooth, usually a result of spreading of dental caries. The abscess may perforate into the oral cavity or maxillary sinus; extend into nearby bone, causing osteomyelitis; or more often, spread to soft tissues, causing cellulitis and a swollen face. There may be associated fever, malaise, and nausea. Treatment includes drilling into the pulp of the tooth to establish drainage and relieve pain, followed by antibiotics and late root canal therapy or tooth extraction.

**periapical cyst.** See **radicular cyst.**

**periapical fibroma,** a mass of benign connective tissue that may form at the apex of a tooth with normal pulp. Also called **first-state cementoma.**

**periapical infection,** infection surrounding the root of a tooth, often accompanied by toothache.

**periapical radiograph,** a dental x-ray film used to detect changes in the bone surrounding the roots of the teeth.

**periappendicitis decidualis** /per′i·apen′disī′tis/, an inflammation of the vermiform appendix with the presence of decidual cells in the peritoneum of the appendix. It occurs in cases of right tubal pregnancy with adhesions between the appendix and the fallopian tubes.

**periappendicular** /per′i·ap′əndik′yələr/ [Gk, *peri,* around; L, *appendere,* to hang upon], pertaining to the area around the appendix.

**periarterial** /per′i·ärtir′ē·əl/ [Gk, *peri,* around, *arteria,* airpipe], pertaining to the area around an artery.

**periarteritis** /per′i·är′tərī′tis/ [Gk, *peri* + *arteria,* airpipe, *itis*], inflammation of the outer coat of one or more arteries and the tissue surrounding them. Kinds of periarteritis are **periarteritis nodosa** and **syphilitic periarteritis.** Also called **periangitis.**

**periarteritis gummosa.** See **syphilitic periarteritis.**

**periarteritis nodosa,** a progressive polymorphic disease of the connective tissue that is characterized by numerous large and palpable nodules or clusters of visible nodules along segments of middle-sized arteries, particularly near points of bifurcation. The disease causes occlusion of vessels, resulting in regional ischemia, hemorrhage, necrosis, and pain. Early signs of the disease include tachycardia, fever, weight loss, and pain in the viscera. Kidney, lung, and intestinal involvement is common. Other systems and organs of the body also may be affected. Periarteritis nodosa is treated with corticosteroids and cytotoxic drugs. Also called **necrotizing angiitis.**

**periarthritis** /per′i·ärthrī′tis/, inflammation of tissues around a joint.

**periarticular** /per′i·ärtik′yələr/ [Gk, *peri,* around; L, *articulus,* joint], pertaining to the area around a joint.

**peribronchial** /-brong′kē·əl/, surrounding a bronchus.

**peribronchiolar** /-brong′kē·ō′lər/ [Gk, *peri,* around, *bronchiolus*], pertaining to the area around the bronchioles.

**pericardia.** See **pericardium.**

**pericardiac** /-kär′dē·ak/ [Gk, *peri,* around, *kardia,* heart], **1.** pertaining to the pericardium. **2.** pertaining to the area around the heart. Also **pericardial.**

**pericardial.** See **pericardium.**

**pericardial adhesion** /-kär′dē·əl/ [Gk, *peri,* around, *kardia,* heart; L, *adhesio,* sticking to], an attachment of the pericardium to the heart muscle, sometimes restricting the muscle's action. In some cases a previous inflammation or surgery may result in dense fibrous adhesions that obliterate the pericardium. The condition may be general or localized and may involve adhesion between the two layers of pericardium (internal adhesive pericarditis) or between one layer and surrounding tissues (external adhesive pericarditis). Also called **adherent pericarditum.**

**pericardial artery** [Gk, *peri* + *kardia,* heart, *arteria,* airpipe], one of several small vessels branching from the thoracic aorta, supplying the dorsal surface of the pericardium.

**pericardial effusion** [Gk, *peri,* around, *kardia,* heart; L, *effundere,* to pour out], the escape of blood or other fluid into the pericardium.

**pericardial friction rub** [Gk, *peri,* around, *kardia,* heart; L, *fricare,* to rub; ME, *rubben*], the rubbing together of inflamed membranes of the pericardium, as may occur in pericarditis or after a myocardial infarction. It produces a sound audible on auscultation. Also called **pericardial murmur, pericardial rub.**

**pericardial murmur, pericardial rub.** See **pericardial friction rub.**

**pericardial tamponade.** See **cardiac tamponade.**

**pericardiectomy** /per′i·kär′dē·ek′tə·mē/ [Gk, *peri,* around + *kardia,* heart + *ektomē,* excision], excision of the pericardium.

**pericardiocentesis** /per′ikär′dē·ō′sintē′sis/ [Gk, *peri* + *kardia,* heart, *kentesis,* pricking], a procedure for drawing fluid in the pericardial space between the serous membranes by surgical puncture and aspiration of the pericardial sac. Also called **pericardicentesis.**

**pericardiotomy** /-kär′di·ot′əmē/, a surgical incision in the pericardium.

**pericarditis** /per′ikärdī′tis/ [Gk, *peri* + *kardia,* heart, *itis*], inflammation of the pericardium associated with trauma, malignant neoplastic disease, infection, uremia, myocardial infarction, collagen disease, or unknown causes.

■ OBSERVATIONS: Two stages are observed if treatment in the first stage does not halt progress of the condition to the extremely grave second stage. The first stage is characterized

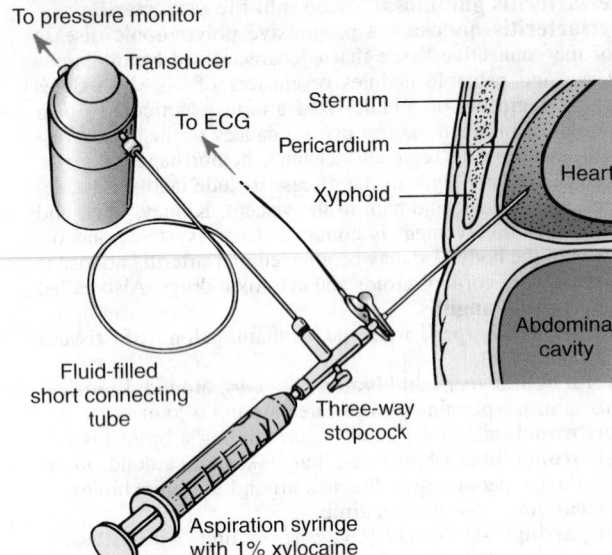

**Pericardiocentesis** *(Lewis, Heitkemper, and Dirksen, 2000)*

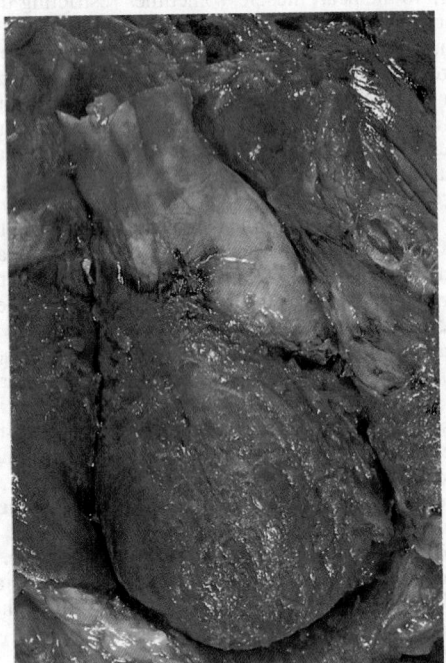

**Acute suppurative pericarditis**
*(Cotran, Kumar, and Collins, 1999)*

by fever, substernal chest pain that radiates to the shoulder or neck, dyspnea, a dry, nonproductive cough, a rapid and forcible pulse, a pericardial friction rub, and a muffled heartbeat over the apex. The patient becomes increasingly anxious, tired, and orthopneic. During the second stage a serofibrinous effusion develops within the pericardium, restricting cardiac activity; if the effusion is purulent

(caused by bacterial infection) a high fever, sweat, chills, and prostration also occur. The heart sounds become muffled, weak, and distant on auscultation, and a bulge is visible on the chest over the precordial area.

■ INTERVENTIONS: The patient is kept in bed, and the head of the bed is elevated 45 degrees to decrease dyspnea. Hypothermia treatment may be necessary to reduce the body temperature. An antibiotic or antifungal and analgesic may be ordered. Oxygen and parenteral fluids are usually given, vital signs are evaluated, and the chest is auscultated frequently. Pericardiocentesis or pericardiotomy may be performed to remove accumulated fluid or to make a diagnosis.

■ NURSING CONSIDERATIONS: Emotional support of a patient being treated for pericarditis requires remaining with the person if he or she is anxious and explaining all procedures thoroughly. During recovery rest periods are planned and the person is urged to avoid fatigue and exposure to upper respiratory infections. The patient is told to report symptoms of recurrence, including fever, chest pain, and dyspnea.

**pericardium** /per'ikär'dē·əm/, *pl.* **pericardia** [Gk, *peri* + *kardia,* heart], a fibroserous sac that surrounds the heart and the roots of the great vessels. It consists of the serous pericardium and the fibrous pericardium. The serous pericardium consists of the parietal layer, which lines the inside of the fibrous pericardium, and the visceral layer, which adheres to the surface of the heart. Between the two layers is the pericardial space containing a few drops of pericardial fluid, which lubricates opposing surfaces of the space and allows the heart to move easily during contraction. Injury or disease may cause fluid to accumulate in the space, causing a wide separation between the heart and the outer pericardium. The fibrous pericardium, which constitutes the outermost sac and is composed of tough, white fibrous tissue lined by the parietal layer of the serous pericardium, fits loosely around the heart and attaches to large blood vessels emerging from the top of the heart but not to the heart itself. It is relatively inelastic and protects the heart and the serous membranes. If pericardial fluid or pus accumulates in the pericardial space, the fibrous pericardium cannot stretch, causing a rapid increase of pressure around the heart. —**pericardial,** *adj.*

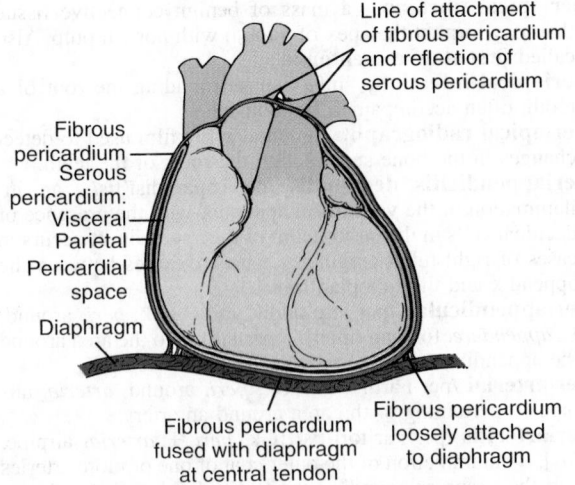

**Pericardium**
*(Thibodeau and Patton, 1999/George J. Wassilchenko)*

**pericholangitis** /per'əkō'lanjī'tis/ [Gk, *peri* + *chole*, bile, *angeion*, vessel, *itis*, inflammation], an inflammatory condition of the tissues surrounding the bile ducts in the liver. Pericholangitis is a complication of ulcerative colitis and portal hypertension. Treatment of the ulcerative colitis has little effect on the liver disease. See also **ulcerative colitis.**

**perichondrial bone** /-kon'drē·əl/ [Gk, *peri*, around, *chondros*, cartilage; AS, *ban*], bone that forms in the perichondrium of the cartilaginous template. Also called **chondrial bone, periosteal bone.**

**perichondrium** /-kon'drē·əm/, a fibrous irregular connective tissue sheath and membrane surrounding both hyaline and elastic cartilages.

**perichrome** /per'ikrōm/, a nerve cell in which the stainable chromophil substance is scattered throughout the cytoplasm.

**pericolitis** /-kōlī'tis/, an inflammation of the connective tissue around the colon.

**pericoronitis** /-kôr'ənī'tis/, inflammation of the gum tissue around the crown of a tooth, usually associated with the eruption of a third molar. Treatment depends on the severity of the condition and may include the use of antibiotics or extraction of the tooth. In most cases the inflammation subsides after the tooth has fully erupted.

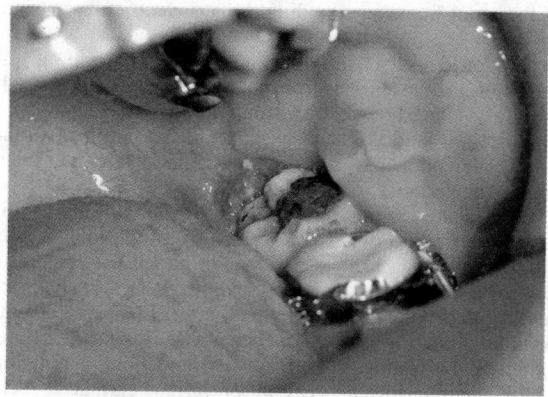

**Pericoronitis** *(Regezi, Sciubba, and Pogrel, 2000)*

**pericranium** /-krā'nē·əm/, the connective tissue membrane that surrounds the skull.

**pericystium** /-sis'tē·əm/, the tissues around a gallbladder or urinary bladder.

**periderm** /per'idurm/, the outermost layer of flattened epidermis on an embryo or fetus during the first six months of gestation.

**perididymis.** See **tunica vaginalis testis.**

**perididymitis** /-did'imī'tis/, an inflammation of the perididymis, or tunica vaginalis testis.

**peridontium.** See **periodontium** (def. 1).

**peridural anesthesia.** See **epidural anesthesia.**

**periencephalitis** /per'i·ensef'əlī'tis/, an inflammation of the membranes and surface of the brain, including the cortex.

**perifocal** /-fō'kəl/, pertaining to tissues situated around a focus of infection.

**perifollicular** /-folik'yələr/ [Gk, *peri*, around; L, *folliculus*, small bag], pertaining to the area around a follicle.

**perifolliculitis** /-folik'yəlī'tis/ [Gk, *peri* + L, *folliculus*, small bag; Gk, *itis*], inflammation of the tissue surrounding a hair follicle. Compare **folliculitis.**

**periglottic** /-glot'ik/, around the tongue, particularly the base of the tongue.

**periglottis** /-glot'is/, the mucous membrane of the tongue.

**perihepatitis** /per'i·hep'ə·ti'tis /, inflammation of the peritoneal capsule of the liver and of other nearby tissues.

**periimplantoclasia** /per'i·implan'tōklā'zhə/, a pathologic tissue reaction surrounding implanted foreign material, characterized by local inflammation.

**perikaryon** /per'iker'ē·on/ [Gk, *peri* + *karyon*, nut], the cytoplasm of a cell body exclusive of the nucleus and any processes, specifically the cell body of a neuron. Also called **cyton. —perikaryontic,** *adj.*

**perilymph** /per'ilimf/ [Gk, *peri* + L, *lympha*, water], the clear fluid separating the osseous labyrinth from the membranous labyrinth in the internal ear. Compare **endolymph.**

**perimenopause** /-men'əpôs/, a span of 4 to 6 years preceding menopause when menstrual cycles and blood flow may be irregular. As estrogen levels decline, osteoporosis begins to develop and depressive symptoms may occur.

**perimeter** /pərim'ətər/ [Gk, *peri*, around, *metron*, measure], **1.** the circumference, outer edge, or periphery of an object. **2.** an instrument for measuring visual fields. **3.** an instrument for measuring the circumference of teeth.

**perimetrium** /per'imē'trē·əm/ [Gk, *peri* + *metra*, womb], the serous membrane enveloping the uterus.

**perimetry** /pərim'ətrē/, the determination and mapping of the limits of the visual field.

**perimolysis** /-mol'isis/, decalcification of the teeth caused by exposure to gastric acid in patients with chronic vomiting, as may occur in anorexia or bulimia.

**perinatal** /per'inā'təl/ [Gk, *peri* + L, *natus*, birth], pertaining to the time and process of giving birth or being born.

**perinatal AIDS,** acquired immunodeficiency syndrome acquired by infants and children from their mothers during pregnancy, during delivery, or from ingesting infected breast milk. See **acquired immunodeficiency syndrome.**

**perinatal asphyxia.** See **asphyxia neonatorum.**

**perinatal death, 1.** the death of a fetus weighing more than 1000 g at 28 or more weeks of gestation. **2.** the death of an infant between birth and the end of the neonatal period.

**perinatal mortality,** the statistical rate of fetal and infant death, including stillbirth, from 28 weeks of gestation to the end of the neonatal period of 4 weeks after birth. Perinatal mortality is usually expressed as the number of deaths per 1000 live births in a specific geographic area or program in a given period.

**perinatal period,** an interval extending approximately from the twenty-eighth week of gestation to the twenty-eighth day after birth.

**perinatal physiology,** the physiology of the process of giving birth or being born.

**perinatologic, perinatological.** See **perinatology.**

**perinatologist** /-nātol'əjəst/, a physician who specializes in the diagnosis and treatment of disorders of pregnancy, childbirth, and the puerperium in the mother and child.

**perinatology** /-nātol'əgē/ [Gk, *peri* + L, *natus*, birth; Gk, *logos*, science], a branch of medicine concerned with the study of the anatomic and physiologic characteristics of the mother and her unborn and newborn and with the diagnosis and treatment of disorders occurring in them during pregnancy, childbirth, and the puerperium. **—perinatologic, perinatological,** *adj.*

**perindopril,** an antihypertensive.

- INDICATIONS: Perindopril is used to treat hypertension.
- CONTRAINDICATIONS: A history of angioedema and known hypersensitivity to this drug prohibit its use.
- ADVERSE EFFECTS: Life-threatening effects of this drug are agranulocytosis, neutropenia, proteinuria, and renal failure. Other adverse effects include chest pain, tachycardia, dysrhythmias, syncope, anxiety, nausea, vomiting, colitis, diarrhea, constipation, flatulence, rash, purpura, alopecia, hyperhidrosis, visual changes, double vision, dry burning eyes, increased frequency of polyuria or oliguria, rales, angioedema, and hyperkalemia. Common side effects include hypotension, insomnia, dizziness, and tinnitus.

**perineal** /per'ine-əl/ [Gk, perineos, perineum], pertaining to the perineum.

**perineal body** [Gk, perineos, perineum; AS, bodig], a mass of tissue composed of muscle and fascia between the vagina and rectum in females and between the scrotum and rectum in males.

**perineal care**[1] [Gk, perineos, perineum], a cleansing procedure prescribed for cleansing the perineum after various obstetric and gynecologic procedures. Sterile or clean perineal care may be prescribed. It is done also after elimination and as a routine part of hygiene care (bed bath) using clean technique rather than sterile.

- METHOD: In the sterile procedure the cleansing strokes always move from the vulva toward the anus and from the midline out. After each stroke, the disposable washcloth or pledget is discarded, and a new one is used for the next stroke. In sterile perineal care a sterile basin, gloves, forceps, pledgets, and pitcher or measure containing sterile solution are used. The draped patient is assisted into position on her back with a bedpan or a disposable pad beneath her buttocks, and 200 to 300 mL of solution is poured over the vulva. Then pledgets moistened with the solution are used to cleanse the area more thoroughly. The pledgets are held with sterile forceps or a sterile gloved hand. The area is dried using sterile pledgets, and the bedpan is removed. The patient then rolls to one side for cleansing and drying of the posterior area; strokes should always move away from the perineal area. In providing clean perineal care disposable washcloths and a basin or a squeeze bottle of warm water are used. A fresh disposable washcloth is used for each cleansing stroke and each drying stroke. The strokes are always from anterior to posterior. Soap may be used.
- INTERVENTIONS: Perineal care is given at prescribed intervals and after urination and defecation.
- OUTCOME CRITERIA: Sterile and clean perineal care is practiced to remove secretions or dried blood from a wound and to prevent contamination of the urethral and vaginal areas or perineal wounds with fecal matter or urine.

**perineal care**[2], a nursing intervention from the Nursing Interventions Classification (NIC) defined as maintenance of perineal skin integrity and relief of perineal discomfort. See also **Nursing Interventions Classification.**

**perineal dislocation.** See **dislocation of hip.**

**perineal pad** [Gk, perineos, perineum], a cushion of soft material used to cover the perineum to absorb the menstrual flow or to protect a wound or incision. It is abbreviated *peri pad.*

**perineo-,** combining form meaning 'related to the perineum': *perineostomy.*

**perineocele** /per'ine-əsēl'/, a hernia in the perineal area, around the rectum.

**perineorrhaphy** /per'ine-ôr'əfē/ [Gk, perineos + rhaphe, suture], a surgical procedure in which an incision, tear, or defect in the perineum is repaired by suturing.

**perineostomy** /per'ine-os'təmē/, the surgical creation of an opening between the urethra and the skin of the perineal region.

**perineotomy** /per'ine-ot'əmē/ [Gk, perineos + temnein, to cut], a surgical incision into the perineum. See also **episiotomy.**

**perinephric abscess** /-nef'rik/ [Gk, peri, around, nephros, kidney; L, abscedere, to go away], an abscess that develops in the fatty tissue around a kidney. It is usually secondary to an abscess originating earlier in the cortex of the organ. Also called **perinephritic abscess.**

**perinephrium** /-nef'rē-əm/, the connective tissue around the kidneys.

**perineum** /per'ine-əm/ [Gk, perineos], the part of the body situated dorsal to the pubic arch and the arcuate ligaments, ventral to the tip of the coccyx, and lateral to the inferior rami of the pubis and the ischium and the sacrotuberous ligaments. The perineum supports and surrounds the distal parts of the urogenital and GI tracts of the body. In the female the central fibrous perineal body is larger than in the male; the bulbospongiosus, which is a sphincter around the orifice of the vagina and a cover over the clitoris, does not exist in the male perineum. In men and women the muscles are innervated by the perineal branch of the pudendal nerve. —**perineal,** *adj.*

**perinocele,** a hernia in the perineum.

**perinodal fiber** /-nō'dəl/ [Gk, peri + L, nodus, knot], any of the atrial fibers surrounding the atrioventricular or sinus node.

**period** /pir'ē-od/, 1. an interval of time. 2. one of the stages of a disease. 3. (in physics) the duration of a single cycle of a periodic wave or event. 4. *informal.* menses.

**periodic** /pir'ē-od'ik/ [Gk, peri + hodos, way], (of an event or phenomenon) recurring at regular or irregular intervals. —**periodicity,** *n.*

**periodic apnea of the newborn,** a normal condition in the full-term newborn, characterized by an irregular pattern of rapid breathing followed by a brief period of apnea, usually associated with rapid eye movement (REM) sleep. Apnea in the newborn not associated with REM sleep or with periodic breathing is ominous because it is symptomatic of intracranial bleeding, seizure activity, infection, pneumonia, hypoglycemia, drug depression, or various cardiac defects. See also **sudden infant death syndrome.**

**periodic breathing.** See **Cheyne-Stokes respiration.**

**periodic deep inspiration,** an occasional deep breath that may be 1.5 times the normal tidal volume. Many mechanical ventilators can be set to provide a selected number of deep inspirations each hour. The process helps prevent atelectasis. Also called **sigh.**

**periodic fever** [Gk, peri, around, hodos, way; L, febris], 1. a hereditary illness with intermittent episodes of fever accompanied by abdominal or pleuritic pain. It affects mainly Sephardic Jews, Armenians, and Arabs. Onset occurs between 10 and 20 years of age. Some cases are complicated by symptoms of arthritis, splenomegaly, and renal amyloidosis that may progress to a fatal kidney disorder. 2. a common name for **familial Mediterranean fever.**

**periodic hyperinflation,** a normal phenomenon of unconscious sighing or deep breathing. It tends to occur most frequently during periods of physical inactivity. Because of the apparent need for periodic hyperinflation, an artificial sigh is often programmed into mechanical ventilators. See also **periodic deep inspiration.**

**periodicity** /pir'ē-ədis'itē/ [Gk, periodikos, periodical], events or episodes that tend to repeat at predictable intervals; for example, filarial worms may appear in cutaneous blood vessels at night but not in daylight hours and malaria may cause paroxysms at 24-, 48-, or 72-hour intervals, depending on the species of pathogen.

**periodic peritonitis, periodic polyserositis.** See **familial Mediterranean fever.**

**periodic table,** a systematic arrangement of the chemical elements. An earlier version was devised in 1869 by Dmitrii Ivanovich Mendeleev (Russian chemist, 1834–1907). By arranging the elements in order of their atomic weights, he was able to show relationships, such as valency, that occurred at regular intervals and was able to predict the properties of elements still undiscovered in the nineteenth century.

**periodontal** /per′ē·ōdon′təl/ [Gk, *peri* + *odous*, tooth], pertaining to the supporting structures of a tooth, including the cementum, alveolar bone, and gingiva.

**periodontal abscess** [Gk, *peri*, around, *odous*, tooth; L, *abscedere*, to go away], an infection in the area around a tooth. It is usually classified according to its location in the periodontal tissues, such as lateral, lateral alveolar, parietal, or peridental.

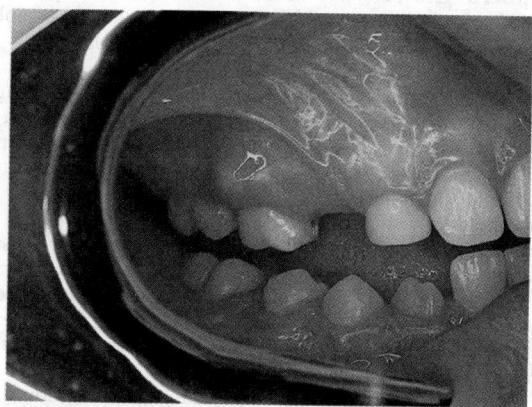
**Periodontal abscess** (Regezi, Sciubba, and Pogrel, 2000)

**periodontal cyst,** a fluid-filled, epithelium-lined sac at the apex of a tooth that has an infected pulp or, less often, lateral to a tooth root. Also called **dental root cyst, dentoalveolar cyst.**

**periodontal disease,** a pathologic condition of the tissues that support a tooth or teeth, such as an inflammation of the periodontal membrane or periodontal ligament.

**periodontal index,** a measure of an individual's periodontal condition. It is determined by adding scores based on the condition of the gingiva and dividing the sum by the number of teeth present. Individuals with clinically normal gingiva have an index of 0 to 0.2. The index reaches a maximum of 8.0 in persons with severe terminal destructive periodontitis.

**periodontal ligament (PDL),** the fibrous tissue that surrounds a tooth and attaches the tooth to the alveolus. It is composed of many bundles of collagenous tissue arranged in groups, between which lies loose connective tissue interwoven with blood vessels, lymphatic vessels, and nerves. Also called **periodontium.**

**periodontal pocket** [Gk, *peri*, around, *odous*, tooth; Fr, *pochette*], a pathologic increase in the depth of the gingival crevice or sulcus surrounding a tooth at the gingival margin. Kinds of periodontal pockets include **gingival, infrabony, intraalveolar, intrabony, relative, simple, subcrestal, suprabony,** and **supracrestal.**

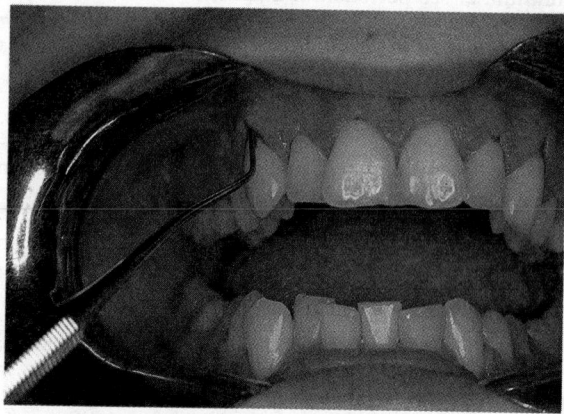
**Periodontal pocket** (Regezi, Sciubba, and Pogrel, 2000)

**periodontal probe** [Gk, *peri*, around, *odous*, tooth; L, *probare*, to test], **1.** a slender, tapered, flat or cylindric instrument with indentations spaced in millimeters, designed for introduction into the gingival sulcus for the purpose of measuring its depth. **2.** a slender tapered instrument with or without millimeter indentations for measuring furcations of the roots of premolars and molars. Also called **furcation probe.**

**periodontia.** See **periodontics.**

**periodontics** /-don′tiks/ [Gk, *peri*, around, *odous*, tooth], the branch of dentistry concerned with the diagnosis, treatment, and prevention of diseases of the periodontium. Also called **periodontia, periodontology.**

**periodontist** /-don′tist/, a dentist who specializes in treating the supporting structures of the teeth.

**periodontitis** /per′ē·ō′dontī′tis/, inflammation of the periodontium caused by a complex reaction initated when subgingival plaque bacteria are in close contact with the epithelium of the gingival sulcus. Injury arises from toxins and enzymes produced by the bacteria and from host-mediated defense responses. Apical movement of the junctional epithelium, which indicates attachment loss and alveolar bone loss, is diagnostic of periodontitis. See also **periodontal disease.**

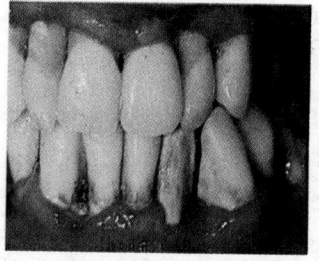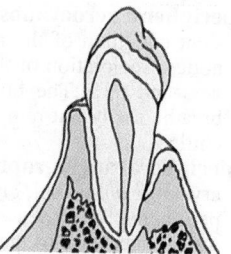
**Advanced periodontitis** (Murray et al, 1994)

**periodontium** /per'ē·ō·don'shē·əm/ *pl.* **periodontia** [Gk, *peri,* around + *odous,* tooth], **1.** the tissues that invest or help invest and support the teeth, including the periodontal ligament, gingivae, cementum, and alveolar and supporting bone. Also called **odontoperiosteum, paradentium, periodontium. 2.** see **periodontal ligament.**

**periodontoclasia** [Gk, *peri* + *odous,* tooth, *klasis,* breaking], the loosening of secondary teeth caused by breakdown and absorption of the supporting bone.

**periodontology.** See **periodontics.**

**periodontosis** /-dontō'sis/ [Gk, *peri* + *odous,* tooth, *osis,* condition], a rare disease that affects young people, especially women, and is characterized by idiopathic destruction of the periodontium without inflammation.

**perioperative** /per'i·op'ərativ/ [Gk, *peri,* around; L, *operari,* to work], pertaining to the time of the surgery. Also **paraoperative.**

**perioperative nursing** [Gk, *peri* + L, *operari,* to work, *nutrix,* nurse], nursing care provided to surgery patients during the entire inpatient period, from admission to date of discharge.

**periorbita** /per'i·ôr'bitə/ [Gk, *peri* + L, *orbita,* wheel mark], the periosteum of the orbit of the eye. It is continuous with the dura mater and the sheath of the optic nerve and extends a process at the margin of the orbit to form the orbital septum. The periorbita is loosely connected to the bones of the orbit, from which it can be easily detached.

**periorbital** /per'i·ôr'bitəl/, pertaining to the area surrounding the socket of the eye.

**periosteal** /per'i·os'tē·əl/ [Gk, *peri,* around, *osteon,* bone], pertaining to the periosteum, the membrane covering the bone.

**periosteal bone.** See **perichondrial bone.**

**periosteum** /per'i·os'tē·əm/ [Gk, *peri* + *osteon,* bone], a thick fibrous vascular membrane covering the bones, except at their extremities. It consists of an outer layer of collagenous tissue containing a few fat cells and an inner layer of fine elastic fibers. Periosteum is permeated with the nerves and blood vessels that innervate and nourish underlying bone. The membrane is thick and markedly vascular over young bones but thinner and less vascular in later life. Bones that lose periosteum through injury or disease usually scale or die.

**periostitis** /per'i·ostī'tis/ [Gk, *peri* + *osteon,* bone, *itis*], inflammation of the periosteum. The condition is caused by chronic or acute infection or trauma and is characterized by tenderness and swelling of the affected bone, pain, fever, and chills. In severe cases blood or an albuminous serous exudate forms under the membrane. In syphilitic infections periostitis may occur as an early symptom.

**peripatetic** /-pətet'ik/ [Gk, *peripatein,* to walk about], pertaining to an ambulatory typhoid patient.

**peripheral** /pərif'ərəl/ [Gk, *periphereia,* circumference], pertaining to the outside, surface, or surrounding area of an organ, other structure, or field of vision.

**peripheral acrocyanosis of the newborn,** a normal transient condition of the newborn, characterized by pale cyanotic discoloration of the hands and feet, especially the fingers and toes. The blueness fades as the baby begins to breathe easily but returns if the baby is allowed to become chilled.

**peripheral angiography** [Gk, *peri,* around, *phereia,* boundary, *angeion,* vessel, *graphein,* to record], the study of the peripheral blood vessels by radiography after radiopaque dye is injected into the circulation.

**peripheral arterial disease (PAD),** a systemic form of atherosclerosis producing symptoms in the cardiac, cerebral, and renal vascular systems. It affects up to 2% of individuals between 37 and 69 years of age and about 10% of persons over 70 years of age. The incidence is highest among males with diabetes mellitus. Other risk factors include obesity and stress. Blood flow is restricted by an intraarterial accumulation of soft deposits of lipids and fibrin that harden over time, particularly at bends or bifurcations of the arterial walls. Patients generally are not aware of the changes until the diameter of the arterial lumen has been reduced by half. Early symptoms include intermittent claudication and ischemic rest pain. See also **arterial insufficiency.**

**peripheral arteriovenography,** the radiographic examination of the blood vessels in the peripheral parts of the body, such as the arms and legs, after the injection of a contrast medium into these vessels.

**peripheral blood stem cells,** stem cells found in the peripheral blood rather than the bone marrow; their numbers can be artificially increased by exposure to hematopoietic growth factors so that they can be extracted before myeloablative chemotherapy and later infused as an autologous bone marrow transplantation. Also called **peripheral blood progenitor cells.**

**peripheral device,** any hardware device that may be attached to a computer's central processing unit via a cable, such as a printer, monitor, or external backup drive.

**peripheral glioma.** See **schwannoma.**

**peripheral lesion** [Gk, *perphereia* + L, *laesio,* hurting], an injury to any tissues distal to the main organ systems. A peripheral nerve lesion is usually traumatic and interrupts the flow of impulses between the site of the lesion and the nerve root or plexus.

**peripherally inserted central (PIC) catheter care,** a nursing intervention from the Nursing Interventions Classification (NIC) defined as insertion and maintenance of a peripherally inserted central catheter. See also **Nursing Interventions Classification.**

**peripheral motor neuron** [Gk, *periphereia* + L, *motor,* mover; Gk, *neuron,* nerve], an effector neuron located outside the central nervous system, usually in a ganglion of a sympathetic or parasympathetic nervous system.

**peripheral nervous system,** the motor and sensory nerves and ganglia outside the brain and spinal cord. The system consists of 12 pairs of cranial nerves, 31 pairs of spinal nerves, and their various branches in body organs. Sensory, or afferent, peripheral nerves transmitting information to the central nervous system and motor, or efferent, peripheral nerves carrying impulses from the brain usually travel together but separate at the cord level into a posterior sensory root and an anterior motor root. Fibers innervating the body wall are designated somatic; those supplying internal organs are termed visceral. The autonomic system includes the peripheral nerves involved in regulating cardiovascular, respiratory, endocrine, and other automatic body functions. Nerves in the sympathetic or thoracolumbar division of the autonomic system secrete norepinephrine and cause peripheral vasoconstriction, cardiac acceleration, coronary artery dilation, bronchodilation, and inhibition of peristalsis. Parasympathetic nerves, which constitute the craniosacral division of the autonomic system, secrete acetylcholine; cause peripheral vasodilation, cardiac inhibition, and bronchoconstriction; and stimulate peristalsis. Injury to a peripheral nerve results in loss of movement and sensation in the area innervated distal to the lesion.

**peripheral neuropathy,** any functional or organic disorder of the peripheral nervous system. A kind of peripheral neuropathy is **paresthesia.**

**peripheral neurovascular dysfunction, risk for,** a nursing diagnosis accepted by the Tenth National Conference on the Classification of Nursing Diagnoses. Risk for peripheral neurovascular dysfunction is defined as a state in which an individual is in danger of experiencing a disruption in circulation, sensation, or motion of an extremity.
■ RISK FACTORS: Risk factors include fractures, mechanical compression (e.g., tourniquet, cast, brace, dressing, or restraint), orthopedic surgery, trauma, immobilization, burns, and vascular obstruction. See also **nursing diagnosis.**

**peripheral odontogenic fibroma,** a fibrous connective tissue tumor associated with the gingival margin and believed to originate from the periodontium. It is a localized form of fibromatosis and commonly contains areas of calcification.

**peripheral plasma cell myeloma.** See **plasmacytoma.**

**peripheral polyneuritis.** See **multiple peripheral neuritis.**

**peripheral polyneuropathy.** See **multiple peripheral neuritis.**

**peripheral pulse** [Gk, *periphereia* + L, *pulsare,* to beat], the series of waves of arterial pressure caused by left ventricular systoles as measured in the limbs.

**peripheral resistance,** a resistance to the flow of blood determined by the tone of the vascular musculature and the diameter of the blood vessels.

**peripheral scotoma** [Gk, *periphereia* + *skotos,* darkness, *oma* tumor], a lost area of the visual field that is located peripherally and does not involve the central 30° of vision.

**peripheral sensation management,** a nursing intervention from the Nursing Interventions Classification (NIC) defined as prevention or minimization of injury or discomfort in the patient with altered sensation. See also **Nursing Interventions Classification.**

**peripheral vascular disease (PVD),** any abnormal condition that affects the blood vessels and lymphatic vessels, except those that supply the heart. Different kinds and degrees of PVD are characterized by a variety of signs and symptoms, such as numbness, pain, pallor, elevated blood pressure, and impaired arterial pulsations. Causative factors include obesity, cigarette smoking, stress, sedentary occupations, and numerous metabolic disorders. PVD in association with bacterial endocarditis may involve emboli in terminal arterioles and produce gangrenous infarctions of distal parts of the body, such as the tip of the nose, the pinna of the ear, the fingers, and the toes. Large emboli may oc-

clude peripheral vessels and cause atherosclerotic occlusive disease. Treatment of severe cases may require amputation of gangrenous body parts. Less severe peripheral vascular problems may be treated by eliminating causative factors, especially cigarette smoking, and by administering various drugs, such as salicylates and anticoagulants. Some kinds of peripheral vascular disease are **atherosclerosis** and **arteriosclerosis.**

**peripheral vision,** a capacity to see objects in the outer aspects of the field of use caused by reflected light waves that fall on areas of the retina distant from the macula.

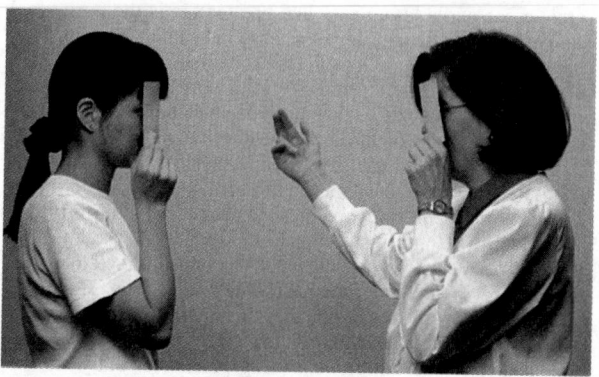

**Peripheral vision assessment** *(Wilson and Giddens, 2001)*

**periphery** /pərif′ərē/ [Gk, *peri,* around, *phereia,* boundary], **1.** parts or areas near or outside a perimeter or boundary. **2.** the outer body parts, such as the skin or limbs.

**perirectal** /-rek′təl/ [Gk, *peri,* around; L, *rectus,* straight], pertaining to the area around the rectum.

**perisinusitis** /-sī′nəsī·tis/ [Gk, *peri,* around; L, *sinus,* hollow], an inflammation of the structures around a sinus.

**peristalsis** /-stal′sis, -stôl′sis/ [Gk, *peri* + *stalsis,* contraction], the coordinated, rhythmic serial contraction of smooth muscle that forces food through the digestive tract, bile through the bile duct, and urine through the ureters.

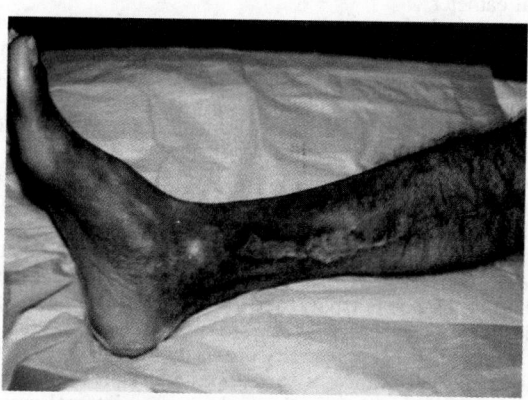

**Peripheral vascular disease of the leg**
*(Bryant, 1992/courtesy Abbott Northwestern Hospital, Minneapolis)*

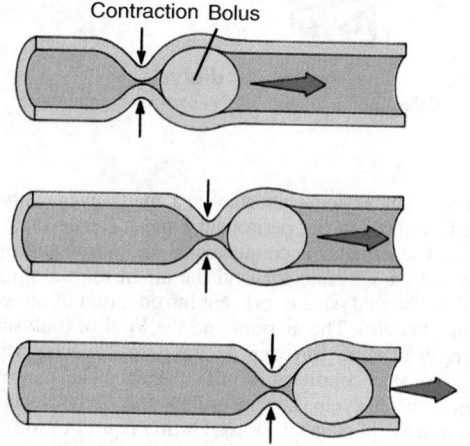

Contraction Bolus

**Peristalsis** *(Thibodeau and Patton, 1999/Rolin Graphics)*

**peristaltic** /-stal'tik, -stôl'tik/ [Gk, *peri* + *stalsis*, contraction], pertaining to peristalsis.

**peristomal** /per'istō'məl/, pertaining to the area of skin surrounding a stoma, or surgically created opening in the abdominal wall.

**peritoneal** /-tənē'əl/ [Gk, *peri* + *teinein*, to stretch], pertaining to the peritoneum.

**peritoneal abscess** [Gk, *peri* + *teinein* + L, *abscedere*, to go away], an abscess in the peritoneal cavity, the result of peritonitis and usually complicated by adhesions.

**peritoneal cavity** [Gk, *peri* + *teinein*, to stretch], the potential space between the parietal and visceral layers of the peritoneum. Normally the two layers are in contact. The peritoneal cavity is divided by a narrow constriction into a greater sac and a lesser sac. The greater sac is the peritoneal cavity, and the lesser sac is the omental bursa. The omental bursa is associated with the dorsal surface of the stomach and the surrounding structures. See also **epiploic foramen.**

**peritoneal dialysis,** a dialysis procedure performed to correct an imbalance of fluid or of electrolytes in the blood or to remove toxins, drugs, or other wastes normally excreted by the kidney. The peritoneum is used as a diffusible membrane. Peritoneal dialysis may be performed nightly for chronically ill children while they sleep and also may be carried out regularly at home. It is contraindicated in patients with extensive intraabdominal adhesions, localized peritoneal infection, and gangrenous or perforated bowels, although peritonitis may itself sometimes be treated by peritoneal lavage and antibiotics, using peritoneal dialysis.

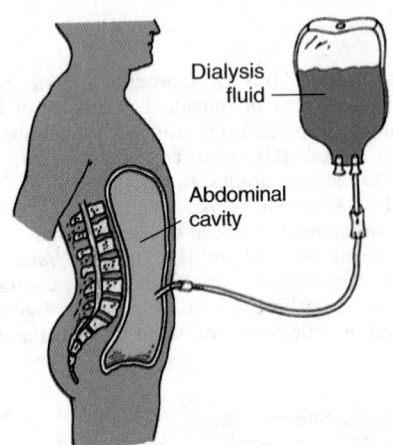

**Peritoneal dialysis**
*(Thibodeau and Patton, 1999/Barbara Stackhouse)*

■ METHOD: Under local anesthesia a many-eyed catheter is sutured in place in the peritoneum and a sterile dressing is applied. The catheter is connected to the inflow and outflow tubing with a Y connector, and the air in the tubing is displaced by the dialysate to prevent introduction of air into the peritoneal cavity. The amount and the kind of dialysate and the length of time for each exchange cycle vary with the age, size, and condition of the patient. There are three phases in each cycle. During inflow the dialysate is introduced into the peritoneal cavity. During equilibration (swell) the dialysate remains in the peritoneal cavity; by means of osmosis, diffusion, and filtration, the needed electrolytes

pass to the bloodstream via the vascular peritoneum to the blood vessels of the abdominal cavity, and the waste products pass from the blood vessels through the vascular peritoneum into the dialysate. During the third phase (drain) the dialysate is allowed to drain from the peritoneal cavity by gravity.

■ INTERVENTIONS: The fluid is warmed to body temperature before instillation, and heparin, antibiotics, or other substances may be added to the dialysate. The patient's fluid balance, respirations, pulse, blood pressure, temperature, and mental state are frequently evaluated, and blood glucose and electrolyte levels are tested regularly. The amount of fluid instilled and the amount and character of the fluid drained are noted. Bacteriologic cultures of the drainage are performed regularly. A low-sodium, high-carbohydrate, high-fat 20 to 40 g protein diet is usually offered. Medication for pain may be necessary. Much peritoneal dialysis is now done in the home, not in facility. VNA referral is done for appropriate teaching and assessment with follow-up in dialysis centers. The need for dialysis and the techniques, dangers, and advantages of peritoneal dialysis are explained to the patient and the family.

■ OUTCOME CRITERIA: Peritoneal dialysis may result in several complications, including perforation of the bowel, peritonitis, atelectasis, pneumonia, pulmonary edema, hyperglycemia, hypovolemia, hypervolemia, and adhesions. Peritonitis, the most common problem, is usually caused by failure to use aseptic technique and is characterized by fever, cloudy dialysate, leukocytosis, and abdominal discomfort. Dialysis may usually be continued while the infection is treated with antibiotics, which are given systemically or intraperitoneally. Atelectasis and pneumonia may result from compression of the thoracic cavity, with decreased respiratory excursion and blood flow to the bases of the lungs caused by an excessive volume of dialysate in the peritoneal cavity. Dyspnea, tachypnea, rales, and tachycardia require reevaluating the amount of dialysate, raising the head of the bed, and administering respiratory therapy to prevent atelectasis and pneumonia. Because patients with diabetes are at risk of development of hyperglycemia, serum and urine glucose levels are monitored, and, if necessary, sorbitol may be substituted for glucose in the dialysate. If dialysate fluid is retained in the peritoneal cavity, hypervolemia may occur, predisposing the patient to pulmonary edema and congestive failure. If the dialysate is removed too rapidly or if the dialysate used is a hypotonic glucose solution, hypovolemia may result. Adhesions often develop as a result of local irritation to the surrounding tissues caused by the intraperitoneal catheter.

**peritoneal dialysis solution,** a solution of electrolytes and other substances that is introduced into the peritoneum to remove toxic substances from the body in some patients with renal failure.

**peritoneal dialysis therapy,** a nursing intervention from the Nursing Interventions Classification (NIC) defined as administration and monitoring of dialysis solution into and out of the peritoneal cavity. See also **Nursing Interventions Classification.**

**peritoneal endometriosis** [Gk, *peri* + *teinein,* to stretch, *endon,* within, *metra,* womb], ectopic endometrial tissue found in the pelvic cavity. See also **implantation endometriosis.**

**peritoneal fluid,** a naturally produced fluid in the abdominal cavity that lubricates surfaces, thereby preventing friction between the peritoneal membrane and internal organs.

**peritoneo-,** combining form meaning 'peritoneum': *peritoneal, peritonitis.*

**peritoneoscope.** See **laparoscope.**

**peritoneoscopy** /-tō'nē·os'kəpē/ [Gk, *peri + teinein + skopein,* to view], the use of an endoscope to inspect the peritoneum through a stab incision in the abdominal wall.

**peritoneum** /per'itənē'əm/ [Gk, *peri + teinein,* to stretch], an extensive serous membrane that lines the entire abdominal wall of the body and is reflected over the contained viscera. It is divided into the parietal peritoneum and the visceral peritoneum. In men the peritoneum is a closed membranous sac. In women it is perforated by the free ends of the uterine tubes. The free surface of the peritoneum is smooth mesothelium, lubricated by serous fluid that permits the viscera to glide easily against the abdominal wall and against one another. The mesentery of the peritoneum fans out from the main membrane to suspend the small intestine. Other parts of the peritoneum are the transverse mesocolon, the greater omentum, and the lesser omentum. —**peritoneal,** *adj.*

**peritonitis** /per'itənī'tis/ [Gk, *peri + teinein,* to stretch, *itis*], an inflammation of the peritoneum. It is produced by bacteria or irritating substances introduced into the abdominal cavity by a penetrating wound or perforation of an organ in the GI tract or the reproductive tract. Peritonitis is caused most commonly by rupture of the appendix but also occurs after perforations of intestinal diverticula, peptic ulcers, gangrenous gallbladders, gangrenous obstructions of the small bowel, or incarcerated hernias, as well as ruptures of the spleen, liver, ovarian cyst, or fallopian tube, especially in ectopic pregnancy. In some cases peritonitis is secondary to the release of pancreatic enzymes, bile, or digestive juices of the upper GI tract, and there are reports of postoperative peritonitis caused by cornstarch used to powder surgical gloves. The bacteria most frequently identified as causative agents in peritonitis are *Escherichia coli, Bacteroides, Fusobacterium,* and anaerobic and aerobic streptococci. Pneumococci occasionally found in peritonitis in girls are thought to enter the abdominal cavity via the vagina and fallopian tubes. See also **appendectomy, appendicitis.**
■ OBSERVATIONS: Characteristic signs and symptoms include abdominal distension, rigidity and pain, rebound tenderness, decreased or absent bowel sounds, nausea, vomiting, and tachycardia. The patient has chills and fever; breathes rapidly and shallowly; is anxious, dehydrated, and unable to defecate; and may vomit fecal material. Leukocytosis, an electrolyte imbalance, and hypovolemia are usually present, and shock and heart failure may ensue.

**peritonitis meconium** [Gk, *peri + teinein, itis,* inflammation, *mekon,* poppy], a condition of peritonitis in a newborn resulting from rupture of the digestive tract. The inflammation is caused by leakage of meconium, or fetal contents, into the peritoneal cavity.

**peritonsillar** /-ton'silər/ [Gk, *peri + L, tonsilla*], pertaining to the area around a tonsil.

**peritonsillar abscess** [Gk, *peri + L, tonsilla,* tonsil, *abscedere,* to go away], an infection of tissue between the tonsil and pharynx, usually after acute follicular tonsillitis. The symptoms include dysphagia, pain radiating to the ear, and fever. Redness and swelling of the tonsil and adjacent soft palate are present. Treatment includes antibiotics, warm saline solution irrigation, incision and drainage with suction if there is no spontaneous rupture of the abscess, and sometimes tonsillectomy. Also called **quinsy.** Compare **parapharyngeal abscess, retropharyngeal abscess.** See also **tonsillitis.**

**Peritrate,** trademark for a vasodilator (pentaerythritol tetranitrate).

**perityphilitis.** See **paratyphlitis.**

**periumbilical** /per'i·umbil'ikəl/ [Gk, *peri,* around, *umbilicus,* navel], pertaining to the area around the umbilicus.

**periungual** /per'i·ung'gwəl/ [Gk, *peri + L, unguis,* nail], pertaining to the area around the fingernails or the toenails.

**perivascular goiter** /per'ivas'kyo͞olər/ [Gk, *peri + L, vasculum,* little vessel, *guttur,* throat], an enlargement of the thyroid gland surrounding a large blood vessel.

**perivascular spaces** [Gk, *peri,* around; L, *vasculum,* little vessel, *spatium,* space], spaces that surround blood vessels as they enter the brain. They communicate with the subarachnoid space. Also called **Virchow-Robin spaces, Virchow's spaces.**

**perivertebral** /-vur'təbrəl/ [Gk, *peri,* around, *vertebra,* joint], pertaining to the area around a vertebra.

**perivitelline** /-vitel'ēn/ [Gk, *peri + L, vitellus,* yolk], surrounding the vitellus or yolk mass.

**perivitelline space,** the space between a mammalian ovum and the zona pellucida, into which the polar bodies are released at the time of maturation. In some animals it is a fluid-filled space that separates the fertilization membrane from the vitelline membrane surrounding the ovum after the penetration of a spermatozoon.

**perle** /purl, perl/ [Fr, pearl], a soft capsule filled with medicine.

**perlèche.** See **cheilosis.**

**perlingual** /pərling'gwəl/ [L, *per + lingua,* tongue], pertaining to the administration of drugs through the tongue, which absorbs substances through its surface. See also **sublingual administration of a medication.**

**permanent dentition.** See **secondary dentition.**

**permanent pacemaker** [L, *permanere,* to remain, *passus,* step; ME, *maken*], any electric pacemaker implanted inside a patient's body for permanent use.

**permanent teeth.** See **secondary dentition.**

**permanent tooth.** See **secondary dentition.**

**permeability** /pur'mē·əbil'itē/ [L, *permeare,* to pass through], the degree to which one substance allows another substance to pass through it. See also **capillary permeability, magnetic permeability.**

**permeable** /pur'mē·əbəl/ [L, *permeare,* to pass through], a condition of allowing fluids and certain other substances to pass through, such as a permeable membrane. See also **osmosis.**

**per member per month (PMPM),** usual unit of measure for capitation payments that payers provide to providers, both hospitals and physicians. These payments also include ancillary service utilization.

**permethrin** /pərməth'rin/, a topical pediculicide/scabicide.
■ INDICATIONS: It is used for the treatment of head lice and nits.
■ CONTRAINDICATIONS: Allergies to pyrethrin, pyrethroids, or chrysanthemum flowers prohibit its use.
■ ADVERSE EFFECTS: Among reported adverse reactions are itching, mild burning or stinging, numbness, discomfort, mild erythema, or scalp rash.

**permissible dose** /pərmis'ibəl/ [L, *permittere,* to permit, *dosis,* something given], the maximum amount of radiation that may be expected to produce no significantly harmful results if given to an individual in a specified period.

**permissible exposure limit (PEL),** an occupational health standard instituted to safeguard workers against exposure to toxic material in the workplace. PELs are the result of the 1970 U.S. Occupational Safety and Health Act, which established the Occupational Safety and Health Administration (OSHA), the policing and enforcing arm of the act, and the National Institute for Occupational Safety and Health (NIOSH), which represents the research arm. OSHA publishes PELs and short-term exposure limits based on recommendations of NIOSH. Also called **permissible exposure level.**

**Permitil,** trademark for a tranquilizer (fluphenazine hydrochloride).

**pernicious** /pərnish′əs/ [L, *perniciosus,* destructive], potentially injurious, destructive, or fatal unless treated, such as pernicious anemia.

**pernicious anemia** [L, *perniciosus,* destructive; Gk, *a* + *haima,* not blood], a progressive megaloblastic macrocytic anemia that results from a lack of intrinsic factor essential for the absorption of cyanocobalamin (vitamin B$_{12}$). The maturation of red blood cells in bone marrow becomes disordered, the posterior and lateral columns of the spinal cord deteriorate, the white blood cell count is reduced, and the polymorphonuclear leukocytes become multilobed. Extreme weakness, numbness and tingling in the extremities, fever, pallor, anorexia, and loss of weight may occur. The condition is usually treated with cyanocobalamin injection and with folic acid and iron therapy. See also **atrophic gastritis, intrinsic factor, nutritional anemia.**

**pernicious vomiting** [L, *perniciosus,* destructive, *vomere,* to vomit], a severe life-threatening episode of vomiting that may occur during pregnancy. Also called **incoercible vomiting.** See also **hyperemesis gravidarum.**

**pernio.** See **chilblain.**

**pero-** /pe′rō-, pir′ō-/, combining form meaning 'maimed or deformed': *perobrachius, perodactylus, peromelus.*

**perobrachius** /pē′rōbrā′kē·əs/ [Gk, *peros,* damaged, *brachion,* arm], a fetus or individual with malformed arms.

**perochirus** /pē′rōkī′rəs/ [Gk, *peros* + *cheir,* hand], a fetus or individual with malformed hands.

**perocormus.** See **perosomus.**

**perodactylia.** See **perodactyly.**

**perodactylus** /pē′rōdak′tiləs/, a fetus or an individual with a deformity of the fingers or the toes, especially the absence of one or more digits.

**perodactyly** /pē′rōdak′tilē/ [Gk, *peros* + *daktylos,* finger], a congenital anomaly characterized by a deformity of the digits, primarily the complete or partial absence of one or more of the fingers or toes. Also called **perodactylia.**

**peromelia** /pē′rōmē′lyə/ [Gk, *peros* + *melos,* limb], a congenital anomaly characterized by the malformation of one or more of the limbs. Also called **peromely. —peromelus,** *n.*

**-perone,** suffix for certain neuroleptics or antianxiety agents.

**peroneal** /per′ənē′əl/ [Gk, *perone,* brooch], pertaining to the outer part of the leg, over the fibula and the peroneal nerve.

**peroneal muscular atrophy,** symmetric weakening or atrophy of the foot and the ankle muscles and hammertoes. This disease is a dominantly inherited condition that occurs in a hypertrophic neuropathy form or in a neuronal form. The hypertrophic neuropathy form results in demyelination of nerve fibers and characteristic onion bulb formations. Affected individuals usually have high plantar arches and an awkward gait, caused by weak ankle muscles. In the neuronal form this condition usually starts in the second decade of life and causes muscle weaknesses similar to those associated with the hypertrophic neuronal form. Both forms of the disease also may involve mild sensory loss in the lower limbs. Affected individuals may be helped by corrective surgery and leg braces that stabilize weak ankle joints.

**peroneo-,** combining form meaning 'related to the fibula or surrounding area': *peroneal.*

**peroneus brevis** /per′ənē′əs/ [Gk, *perone* + L, *brevis,* short], the smaller of the two lateral muscles of the leg, lying under the peroneus longus. It pronates and plantar flexes the foot. Compare **peroneus longus.**

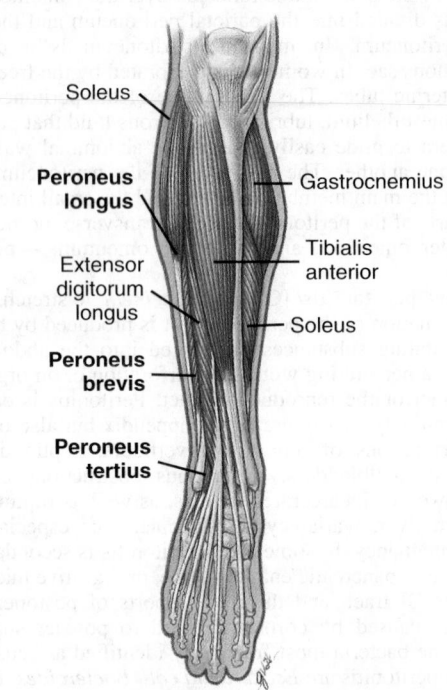

**Peroneus brevis and peroneus longus**
*(Thibodeau and Patton, 1999/John V. Hagen)*

Labels: Soleus; Peroneus longus; Extensor digitorum longus; Peroneus brevis; Peroneus tertius; Gastrocnemius; Tibialis anterior; Soleus

**peroneus longus,** the more superficial of the two lateral muscles of the leg. The muscle pronates and plantar flexes the foot. Compare **peroneus brevis.**

**peronia** /pərō′nē·ə/ [Gk, *peros,* damaged], a congenital malformation or developmental anomaly.

**peropus** /pərō′pəs/ [Gk, *peros* + *pous,* foot], a fetus or individual with malformed feet, often in association with some defect of the legs.

**per os** /pər os′/ [L], by mouth.

**perosomus** /pē′rōsō′məs/ [Gk, *peros* + *soma,* body], a fetus or individual whose body, especially the trunk, is severely malformed. Also called **perocormus.**

**perosplanchnia** /pē′rōsplangk′nē·ə/ [Gk, *peros* + *splanchnon,* viscera], a congenital anomaly characterized by the malformation of the viscera.

**peroxide.** See **hydrogen peroxide.**

**peroxisome** /pər·ok′si·sōm/, any of the microbodies present in vertebrate animal cells, especially liver and kidney cells, which are rich in the enzymes peroxidase, catalase, D-amino acid oxidase, and, to a lesser extent, urate oxidase; their functions are not fully understood, but they participate in metabolic oxidations involving hydrogen peroxide, purine metabolism, cellular lipid metabolism, and gluconeogenesis. See **microbody.**

**perphenazine** /pərfen′əzēn/, an antipsychotic; antiemetic/antivertigo agent.

■ INDICATIONS: It is prescribed in the treatment of psychotic disorders and in the control of severe nausea and vomiting in adults.

■ CONTRAINDICATIONS: Parkinson's disease, the concurrent administration of central nervous system depressants, liver or renal dysfunction, severe hypotension, or known hypersensitivity to any phenothiazine prohibits its use.

■ ADVERSE EFFECTS: Among the more serious adverse reactions are hypotension, liver toxicity, extrapyramidal reactions, blood dyscrasias, and hypersensitivity reactions.

**per primam intentionem** [L], by primary (first) intention.

**per pro.,** abbreviation for the Latin term *per procurationem,* 'on behalf of.'

**per rectum** [L], by rectum.

**PERRLA** /pur′lə/, abbreviation for *pupils equal, round, react to light, accommodation.* In the process of performing an assessment of the eyes one evaluates the size and shape of the pupils, their reaction to light, and their ability to accommodate. If all findings are normal, the abbreviation is noted in the account of the physical examination.

**Persa-Gel,** trademark for a keratolytic (benzoyl peroxide).

**Persantine,** trademark for a coronary vasodilator (dipyridamole).

**per se** [L], by itself, or of itself.

**per secundum intentionem** [L], by second intention.

**perseveration** /pur′səvərā′shən/ [L, *persevero,* to persist], the involuntary and pathologic persistence of the same verbal response or motor activity regardless of the stimulus or its duration. The condition occurs primarily in patients with brain damage or organic mental disorders, although it may also appear in schizophrenia as an association disturbance. It is caused by a neurologic deficit.

**Persian Gulf syndrome,** a diffuse collection of symptoms reported by many veterans of the 1991 Persian Gulf war. Symptoms vary widely, but include fatigue, joint pain, headache, and sleep disturbances. Musculoskeletal and connective tissue diseases are also common. The specific cause in unknown, but explanations include exposure to chemicals from burning oil wells, insecticides, and poisons linked to inoculations against biologic warfare or to chemical weapons used by the Iraqi army.

**persistent cloaca** /pərsis′tənt/ [L, *persistere,* to persist, *cloaca,* sewer], a congenital anomaly in which the intestinal, urinary, and reproductive ducts open into a common cavity resulting from the failure of the urorectal septum to form during prenatal development. Also called **congenital cloaca.**

**persistent vegetative state,** a state of wakefulness accompanied by an apparent complete lack of cognitive function, experienced by some patients in an irreversible coma. Vegetative functions and brainstem reflexes are intact, but the cortex is permanently damaged.

**persona** /pərsō′nə/, *pl.* **personae** /-nē/ [L, mask], (in analytic psychology) the personality façade or role that a person assumes and presents to the outer world to satisfy the demands of the environment or society or to express some intrapsychic conflict. The persona masks the person's inner being or unconscious self. Compare **anima.** See also **archetype.**

**personal and social history** /pur′sənəl/, (in a health history) an account of the personal and social details of a person's life that serves to identify the person. Place of birth, religion, race, marital status, number of children, military status, occupational history, and place of residence are the usual components of this part of the history, but it may often include other information, such as education, current living situation, and smoking, alcohol, and drug habits. The personal and social history is obtained at the initial interview and becomes a part of the permanent record.

**personal assistance.** See **custodial care.**

**personal care services,** the services performed by health care workers to assist patients in meeting the requirements of daily living.

**personal computer.** See **mainframe computer, microcomputer.**

**personal identity, disturbed,** a nursing diagnosis accepted by the Seventh National Conference on the Classification of Nursing Diagnoses. The diagnosis is defined as the inability to distinguish between self and nonself. The defining characteristics and related factors are to be developed at a later conference. See also **nursing diagnosis.**

**personality** /pur′sənal′itē/ [L, *personalis,* role], **1.** the composite of the behavioral traits and attitudinal characteristics by which one is recognized as an individual. **2.** the behavior pattern each person develops, both consciously and unconsciously, as a means of adapting to a particular environment and its cultural, ethnic, national, and provincial standards.

**personality disorder,** a *DSM-IV* psychiatry disorder characterized by disruption in relatedness. It is manifested in any of a large group of mental disorders characterized by rigid, inflexible, and maladaptive behavior patterns and traits that impair a person's ability to function in society by severely limiting adaptive potential. Some kinds of personality disorders are antisocial, borderline, and passive aggressive.

**personality test,** any of a variety of standardized tests used in the evaluation or assessment of various facets of personality structure, emotional status, and behavioral traits. See also **Minnesota Multiphasic Personality Inventory.** Compare **achievement test, aptitude test, intelligence test, psychologic test.**

**personal orientation, 1.** a continually evolving process in which a person determines and evaluates the relationships that appear to exist between him or her and other people. **2.** the assessment of those relationships derived by a person.

**personal protective equipment (PPE),** a part of standard precautions for all health care workers to prevent skin and mucous membrane exposure when in contact with blood and body fluid of any patient. Personal equipment includes protective laboratory clothing, disposable gloves, eye protection, and face masks. See also **Standard Precautions.**

**personal space,** the area surrounding an individual that is perceived as private by the individual, who may regard a movement into the space by another person as intrusive. Personal space boundaries vary somewhat in different cultures, but in general they are regarded as a distance of about 1 meter (3 feet) around the individual.

**personal unconscious,** (in analytic psychology) the thoughts, ideas, emotions, and other mental phenomena acquired and repressed during one's lifetime. Compare **collective unconscious.**

**personal zone,** an individual protective zone in which the boundaries may contract or expand according to contextual characteristics, usually between 18 inches and 4 feet.

**person year,** a statistical measure representing one person at risk of development of a disease during a period of 1 year.

**perspiration** /pur′spirā′shən/ [L, *per* + *spirare,* to breath], **1.** the act or process of perspiring; the excretion of fluid by the sweat glands through pores in the skin. **2.** the fluid excreted by the sweat glands. It consists of water containing sodium chloride, phosphate, urea, ammonia, and other waste products. Perspiration serves as a mechanism for excretion and for regulation of body temperature. Abnormal amounts of perspiration usually result from organic causes but may also be precipitated by severe emotional stress. Kinds of perspiration are **insensible perspiration** and **sensible perspiration**. See also **diaphoresis**.

**perspire** /pərspī′ər/ [L, *per* + *spirare,* to breathe],  to sweat or excrete sweat.

**per tertiam intentionem** [L],  by tertiary (third) intention.

**Perthes disease.**  See **Legg-Calvé-Perthes disease.**

**Pertofrane,**  trademark for an antidepressant (desipramine hydrochloride).

**perturbation** /pur′tərbā′shən/ [L, *per* + *tubare,* to disturb], a cause or a condition of disturbance, disorder, or confusion.

**pertussis** /pərtus′is/ [L, *per* + *tussis,* cough],  an acute highly contagious respiratory disease characterized by paroxysmal coughing that ends in a loud whooping inspiration. It occurs primarily in infants and in children less than 4 years of age who have not been immunized. The causative organism, *Bordetella pertussis,* is a small, nonmotile gram-negative coccobacillus. A similar organism, *B. parapertussis,* causes a less severe form of the disease called parapertussis. Also called **whooping cough.**

■ OBSERVATIONS: Transmission occurs directly by contact or by inhalation of infectious particles, usually spread by coughing and sneezing, and indirectly through freshly contaminated articles. Diagnosis consists of positive identification of the organism in nasopharyngeal secretions. The initial stages of the disease are difficult to distinguish from bronchitis or influenza. A fluorescent antibody staining technique specific for *B. pertussis* provides an accurate means of early diagnosis. The incubation period averages 7 to 14 days, followed by 6 to 8 weeks of illness divided into three distinct stages: catarrhal, paroxysmal, and convalescent. Onset of the catarrhal stage is gradual, usually beginning with coryza, sneezing, a dry cough, a slight fever, listlessness, irritability, and anorexia. The cough becomes paroxysmal after 10 to 14 days; it occurs as a series of short rapid bursts during expiration followed by the characteristic whoop, caused by a spasm of the epiglottis, a hurried, deep inhalation that has a high-pitched crowing sound. There is usually no fever, and the respiratory rate between paroxysms is normal. During the paroxysm there is marked facial redness or cyanosis and vein distension, the eyes may bulge, the tongue may protrude, and the facial expression usually indicates severe anxiety and distress. Large amounts of a viscid mucus may be expelled during or after paroxysms, which occur from 4 to 5 times a day in mild cases to as many as 40 to 50 times a day in severe cases. Vomiting frequently occurs after the paroxysms as a result of gagging or choking on the mucus. In infants, choking may be more common than the characteristic whoop. This stage lasts from 4 to 6 weeks, with the attacks being most frequent and severe during the first 1 to 2 weeks, then gradually declining and disappearing. During the convalescent stage a simple persistent cough is usual. For a period of up to 2 years after the initial attack paroxysmal coughing may accompany respiratory infections.

■ INTERVENTIONS: Routine treatment consists of bed rest, adequate nutrition, and adequate amounts of fluid. Erythromycin or another antibacterial may be prescribed to reduce transmission or to control secondary infection. Hospitalization may be necessary for infants and children with severe or prolonged paroxysms and for those with dehydration or other complications. Oxygen may be needed to relieve dyspnea and cyanosis; IV therapy may be necessary when pro-

longed vomiting interferes with adequate nutrition. Intubation is rarely necessary but may be lifesaving in infants if the thick mucus cannot be easily suctioned from the air passages. Pertussis immune globulin is available, but its efficacy has not been established and its use is not recommended. Active immunization is recommended with pertussis vaccine, usually in combination with diphtheria and tetanus toxoids in a series of injections at 2, 4, and 6 months of age and boosters at 12 to 18 months and 4 years of age. One attack of the disease usually confers immunity, although some second, usually mild episodes have occurred.

■ NURSING CONSIDERATIONS: Severe paroxysms in an infant may require oxygen, suction, and intubation. The child needs to be kept calm and protected from respiratory irritants such as dirt, smoke, or dust. Overstimulation, noise, or excitement may precipitate paroxysms. Adequate nutrition and adequate fluids are encouraged through frequent small feedings. Common complications of the disease include bronchopneumonia; atelectasis; bronchiectasis; emphysema; otitis media; convulsions; hemorrhage, including subarachnoid, and subconjunctival hemorrhage and epistaxis; weight loss; dehydration; hernia; prolapsed rectum; and asphyxia, especially in infants. Paroxysms can be fatal.

**pertussis immune globulin,**  a passive immunizing agent against whooping cough. See also **pertussis.**

■ INDICATION: It is prescribed for immunization against whooping cough.

■ CONTRAINDICATION: Known hypersensitivity to this drug prohibits its use.

■ ADVERSE EFFECTS: Among the more serious adverse reactions is anaphylaxis.

**pertussis vaccine,**  an active immunizing agent.

■ INDICATION: It is prescribed for immunization against pertussis when the administration of diphtheria, pertussis, and tetanus vaccine is contraindicated.

■ CONTRAINDICATIONS: Thrombocytopenia or known hypersensitivity to the vaccine prohibits its use.

■ ADVERSE EFFECTS: Among the most serious adverse reactions are severe allergic reactions, pain and induration at the site of injection, and fever.

**per vaginam** [L],  via the vagina.

**pervasive developmental disorder** /pərvā′siv/ [L, *pervadere,* to go through],  any of certain disorders of infancy and childhood that are characterized by severe impairment of relatedness and behavioral aberrations previously identified as childhood psychoses. The group of disorders includes infantile autism, childhood schizophrenia, and symbiotic psychosis.

**perversion** /pərvur′shən/ [L, *pervertere,* to turn about], **1.** any deviation from what is considered normal or natural. **2.** the act of causing a change from what is normal or natural. **3.** *informal.* (in psychiatry) any of a number of sexual practices that deviate from what is considered normal adult behavior. See also **paraphilia.**

**pervert** /pur′vərt/ [L, *pervertere*],  **1.** *informal.* a person whose sexual pleasure is derived from stimuli almost universally regarded as unnatural, such as a fetishist or sadomasochist; a paraphiliac. **2.** one whose sexual behavior deviates from a social or statistical norm but is not necessarily pathologic.

**pes** /pēz, pās/, *pl.* **pedes** /pē′dēz/ [L, foot],  the foot or a footlike structure.

**pes cavus.**  See **clawfoot.**

**pes equinus** [L, *pes* foot, *equinus,* pertaining to a horse],  a deformity of the foot in which the toes are extremely flexed, walking is done on the dorsal surface of the toes, and the heel does not touch the ground. Treatment is by splinting, serial casts, or surgery. Also called **talipes equinus.**

**pes planus.**   See **flatfoot.**

**pessary** /pes′ərē/ [Gk, *pessos,* oval stone],   a device inserted in the vagina to treat uterine prolapse, uterine retroversion, or cervical incompetence. It is used in the treatment of women whose advanced age or poor general condition precludes surgical repair. Pessaries are also used in younger women in evaluating symptomatic uterine retroversion and in managing cervical incompetence in pregnancy. A pessary must be removed, usually daily, for cleaning. A **Smith-Hodge pessary** is a rubber- or vinyl-covered wire rectangle that fits between the pubic bone and the posterior vaginal fornix, supporting the uterus and holding the cervix in a posterior position. A **Gellhorn pessary** is an inflexible device made of acrylic resin or plastic (Lucite) in the form of a large collar button. It has a canal through the stem that allows drainage of vaginal secretions. The large end of the pessary is placed deep in the vagina, the small end of the stem protruding at the introitus. A **doughnut pessary** is a permanently inflated flexible rubber doughnut that is inserted to support the uterus by blocking the canal of the vagina. An **inflatable pessary** is a collapsible rubber doughnut to which a flexible stem containing a rubber valve is attached. The collapsed pessary is inserted, inflated with a bulb similar to that of a sphygmomanometer, and deflated for removal. A **Bee cell pessary** is a soft rubber cube; in each face of the cube is a conical depression that acts as a suction cup when the pessary is in the vagina. A **diaphragm pessary** is a contraceptive diaphragm used for uterovaginal support. A similar device of somewhat heavier construction is sometimes used. A **stem pessary** is a slim curved rod that can be fitted into the cervical canal for uterine positioning. It is rarely used today.

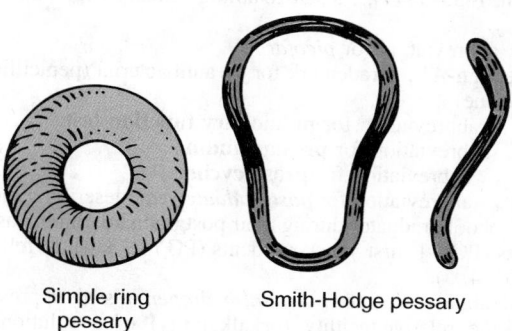

Simple ring pessary     Smith-Hodge pessary

**Pessary** *(Willson and Carrington, 1991)*

**pessary management,**   a nursing intervention from the Nursing Interventions Classification (NIC) defined as placement and monitoring of a vaginal device for treating stress urinary incontinence, uterine retroversion, genital prolapse, or incompetent cervix. See also **Nursing Interventions Classification.**

**pessimism** /pes′imiz′əm/ [L, *pessimus,* worst],   the inclination to anticipate the worst possible results from any action or situation or to emphasize unfavorable conditions, even when progress or gain might reasonably be expected. **—pessimist,** *n.*

**pesticide poisoning** /pes′tisīd/ [L, *pestis,* plague, *caedere,* to kill, *potio,* drink],   a toxic condition caused by the ingestion or inhalation of a substance used for the eradication of pests. Kinds of pesticide poisoning include **malathion poisoning** and **parathion poisoning.** See also **herbicide poisoning, rodenticide poisoning.**

**pestilence** /pes′tiləns/ [L, *pestilentia,* infectious disease],   any epidemic of a virulent infectious or contagious disease.

**pestis.**   See **bubonic plague.**

**pes valgus** [L, *pes,* foot, *valgus,* bent outward],   deviation of the foot outward at the talocalcanean joint.

**PET** /pet/,   abbreviation for **positron emission tomography.**

**peta-,**   combining form indicating a number in the range of $10^{15}$.

**petaling** /pet′əling/,   a process of smoothing the raw or ragged edges of a plaster cast to prevent skin irritation.

**petalo-,**   combining form meaning 'leaf': *petalobacteria, petalococcus.*

**petechiae** /pētē′kē·ē/, *sing.* **petechia** /-kē·ə/ [It, *petecchie,* flea-bites],   tiny purple or red spots appearing on the skin as a result of tiny hemorrhages within the dermal or submucosal layers. Petechiae range from pinpoint to pinhead size and are flush with the surface. Compare **ecchymosis. —petechial,** *adj.*

**Petechiae** *(Lemmi and Lemmi, 2000)*

**petechial** [It, *petecchie*],   pertaining to tiny red or purple spots caused by an extravasation of blood into the skin.

**petechial fever** /pitē′kē·əl/ [It, *petecchie* + L, *febris,* fever],   any febrile illness accompanied by small petechiae on the skin, such as seen with meningococcemia or in the late stage of typhoid fever.

**petechial hemorrhage** [It, *petecchie* + Gk, *haima,* blood, *rhegnynei,* to gush],   a small discrete hemorrhage under the skin.

**pethidine.**   See **meperidine hydrochloride.**

**petit mal epilepsy.**   See **minor epilepsy.**

**petit mal seizure.**   See **absence seizure.**

**petit pas gait** /pet′ē pä, ptē′pä′/   a manner of walking with short, mincing steps and shuffling with loss of associated movements. It is seen in cases of parkinsonism as well as in diffuse cerebral disease resulting from multiple small infarcts.

**Petit's sinus.**   See **aortic sinus.**

**P.E.T.N.,**   trademark for a vasodilator (pentaerythritol tetranitrate).

**petr-, petro-,** prefix meaning 'stone or the petrous region of the temporal bone': *petrifaction, petroleum, petrous.*

**Petren's gait** /pet'rənz/, a hesitant form of walking in which a patient takes a few steps, halts, and then takes a few more steps. In some cases the patient must be encouraged to begin the next brief walking period. The condition is seen in elderly people and those with paretic disease.

**Petri dish** /pē'trē, pā'trē/ [Julius R. Petri, German bacteriologist, 1852–1921], a shallow circular glass dish used to hold solid culture media.

**petrification** /pet'rifikā'shən/, the process of becoming calcified or stonelike.

**pétrissage** /pā'trisäzh'/ [Fr, *petrir,* to knead], a technique in massage in which the skin is gently lifted and squeezed. Pétrissage promotes circulation and relaxes muscles. Compare **effleurage, rolling effleurage.**

**petrolatum** /pet'rəlā'təm/ [L, *petra,* rock, *oleum,* oil], a purified mixture of semisolid hydrocarbons obtained from petroleum and commonly used as an ointment base or skin emollient. The common trade name is Vaseline.

**petrolatum gauze,** absorbent gauze permeated with white petrolatum.

**petroleum distillate poisoning** /pətrō'lē·əm/ [L, *petra* + *oleum* + *distillare,* to drop down, *potio,* drink], a toxic condition caused by the ingestion or inhalation of a petroleum distillate, such as fuel oil, lubricating oil, glue used in making model airplanes or the like, and various solvents. Nausea, vomiting, chest pain, dizziness, and severe depression of the central nervous system characterize the condition. Severe or fatal pneumonitis may occur if the substance is aspirated; therefore induced emesis is contraindicated. See also **kerosene poisoning.**

**petroleum jelly,** a nonliquid colloidal solution or gel of soft paraffin. It is an intermediate product of the distillation of petroleum and is used as a topical soothing medication for burns and abrasions. Also called **mineral jelly.** See also **petrolatum.**

**petrosphenoidal fissure** /pet'rōsfēnoi'dəl/ [L, *petra,* rock; Gk, *sphen,* wedge, *eidos,* form], a fissure on the floor of the cranial fossa between the posterior edge of the great wing of the sphenoid bone and the petrous part of the temporal bone.

**petrous** /pet'rəs/ [L, *petra,* rock], resembling a rock or stone.

**Peutz-Jeghers syndrome** /poits'jeg'ərz/ [J.L.A. Peutz, Dutch physician, 1886–1957; Harold J. Jeghers, American physician, b. 1904], an inherited disorder transmitted as an autosomal dominant trait, characterized by multiple intestinal polyps and abnormal mucocutaneous pigmentation, usually over the lips and buccal mucosa. If obstruction or bleeding occurs, surgical removal of the polyps may be indicated.

**-pexis, -pexia, -pexy,** combining form meaning 'a fixation of something specified': *glycopexis, hemopexis, splenopexis.*

**Peyer's patches,** one of a group of solitary nodules or groups of lymph nodes forming a single layer in the mucous membrane of the ileum opposite the mesenteric attachment. They are oval patches about 1 cm wide and extend for about 4 cm along the intestine. In most individuals they appear in the distal ileum, but they also appear in the jejunum of a few individuals.

**peyote** /pā·ō'tē/ [Aztec, *peyotl*], **1.** a cactus from which a hallucinogenic drug, mescaline, is derived. **2.** mescaline.

**Peyronie's disease** /pārōnēz'/ [François de la Peyronie, French physician, 1678–1747], a disease of unknown cause resulting in fibrous induration of the corpora caver-

nosa of the penis. An association with Dupuytren's contracture of the palm has been recognized. The chief symptom of Peyronie's disease is painful erection. Palliative treatment includes radiation therapy and intralesional corticosteroid injections. There is no known cure.

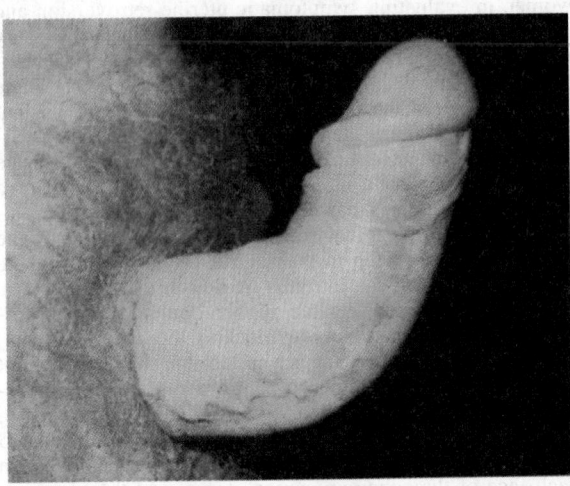

**Peyronie's disease**
*(Seidel et al, 1999/courtesy Patrick C. Walsh, MD, The Johns Hopkins University School of Medicine, Baltimore)*

**Pezzer's catheter** /pezāz/ [Oscar M. de Pezzer, French surgeon, 1853–1917], a self-retaining catheter with a bulbous tip.

**pF,** abbreviation for *picofarad.*

**Pfizerpen-AS,** trademark for an antibacterial (penicillin G procaine).

**PFT,** abbreviation for **pulmonary function test.**

**PG,** abbreviation for **prostaglandin.**

**PGI₂,** abbreviation for **prostacyclin.**

**PGY,** abbreviation for *postgraduate year,* describing medical school graduates during their postgraduate training as interns (PGY-1, first year), residents (PGY-2, 3, 4), or fellows (PGY-4, 5).

**pH,** abbreviation for *potential hydrogen,* a scale representing the relative acidity (or alkalinity) of a solution, in which a value of 7.0 is neutral, below 7.0 is acid, and above 7.0 is alkaline. The numeric pH value indicates the relative concentration of hydrogen ions in the solution compared with that of a standard (one molar) solution; it is equal to the negative log of the hydrogen ion concentration expressed in moles per liter. See also **acid, acid-base balance.**

**Ph,** symbol for **phenyl.**

**PH,** abbreviation for **parathyroid hormone.**

**Ph¹,** symbol for **Philadelphia chromosome.**

**PHA,** **1.** abbreviation for **paraaminohippuric acid. 2.** abbreviation for **phytohemagglutinin.**

**phaco-, phako-,** prefix meaning 'lens': *phacocele, phacocyst, phacoglaucoma.*

**phacomalacia** /fak'ōməlā'shə/ [Gk, *phalos,* lens, *malkia,* softness], an abnormal condition of the eye in which the lens becomes soft as a result of the presence of a soft cataract.

**phacomatosis.** See **phakomatosis.**

**phaeohyphomycosis** /fē′ōhī′fōmīkō′sis/, an opportunistic fungal infection other than mycetoma and chromoblastomycosis caused by the dematiaceous or darkly pigmented molds.

**phage.** See **bacteriophage, -phage.**

**-phage, -phag, -phagia, -phagy,** suffix meaning to 'to eat or consume': *autophage, hemophage, mycophage, osteophage.*

**phage typing** /fāj/ [Gk, *phagein,* to eat, *typos,* mark], the identification of bacteria by testing their vulnerability to bacterial viruses.

**-phagia.** See **-phage.**

**phago-,** prefix meaning 'eating or ingestion': *phagocyte, phagokaryosis, phagology.*

**phagocyte** /fag′əsīt/ [Gk, *phagein + kytos,* cell], a cell that is able to surround, engulf, and digest microorganisms and cellular debris. **Fixed noncirculating phagocytes** include the fixed macrophages and the cells of the reticuloendothelial system. **Free circulating phagocytes** include the leukocytes. —**phagocytic,** *adj.*

**phagocytic** /-sit′ik/ [Gk, *phagein,* to eat, *kytos,* cell], pertaining to phagocytes or phagocytosis.

**phagocytic vacuole.** See **phagosome.**

**phagocytize** /fag′əsitīz′/ [Gk, *phagein,* to eat, *kytos,* cell], to engulf and destroy bacteria or other foreign materials. Also **phagocytose.**

**phagocytosis** /fag′əsītō′sis/ [Gk, *phagein + kytos + osis,* condition], the process by which certain cells engulf and destroy microorganisms and cellular debris. The process includes five steps: (1) invagination, (2) engulfment, (3) internalization and formation of the phagocyte vacuole, (4) fusing of lysosomes to digest the phagocytosed material, and (5) release of digested microbial products.

**phagosome** /fag′əsōm/, a membrane-bound cytoplasmic vesicle within the phagocyte that engulfs it. The vesicle contains phagocytized materials and may fuse with a lysosome, forming a phagolysosome within which the lysosome digests the phagocytized material. Also called **phagocytic vacuole.**

**-phagy.** See **-phage.**

**-phakia,** suffix meaning a 'lens': *aphakia, microphakia, pseudophakia.*

**phako-.** See **phaco-.**

**phakomatosis** /fak′ōmətō′sis/, *pl.* **phakomatoses** [Gk, *phako,* lens, *oma,* tumor, *osis,* condition], (in ophthalmology) any of several hereditary syndromes characterized by benign tumorlike nodules of the eye, skin, and brain. The four disorders designated phakomatoses are neurofibromatosis (Recklinghausen's disease), tuberous sclerosis (Bourneville's disease), encephalotrigeminal angiomatosis (Sturge-Weber syndrome), and cerebroretinal angiomatosis (von Hippel–Lindau disease). Also spelled **phacomatosis.**

**phal,** **1.** abbreviation for **phalanges. 2.** abbreviation for **phalanx.**

**phalangeal** /fəlan′jē·al/ [Gk, *phalanx,* line of soldiers], pertaining to a phalanx.

**phalanges.** See **phalanx.**

**-phalangia,** combining form meaning a 'condition of the bones of the fingers or toes': *bradyphalangia, symphalangia, triphalangia.*

**phalanx (phal)** /fā′langks/, *pl.* **phalanges** (phal) /fəlan′jēz/ [Gk, line of soldiers], any of the 14 tapering bones composing the fingers of each hand and the toes of each foot. They are arranged in three rows at the distal end of the metacarpus and the metatarsus. The fingers each have three phalanges (proximal, middle, and distal); the thumb has two. The toes each have three phalanges; the great toe has two (proximal and distal). The phalanges of the foot are smaller and less flexible than those of the hand.

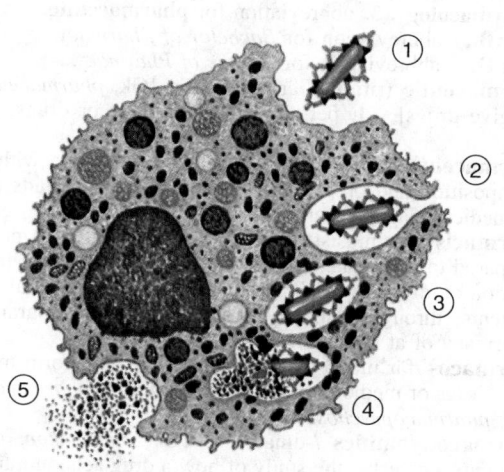

**Phagocytosis** *(Mudge-Grout, 1992)*

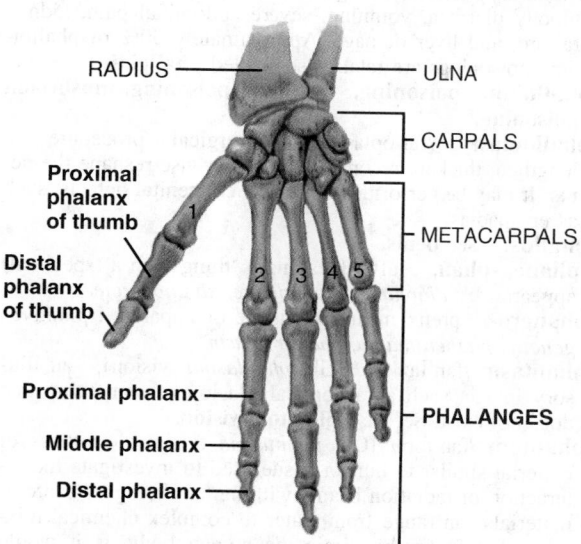

RADIUS — ULNA
CARPALS
Proximal
phalanx
of thumb
METACARPALS
Distal
phalanx
of thumb
Proximal phalanx —
Middle phalanx —
**PHALANGES**
Distal phalanx —

Hand (right, palmar aspect)

**Phalanges of the hand** *(Applegate, 2000)*

**phagolysosome,** a cytoplasmic body formed by the fusion of a phagosome or ingested particle with a lysosome containing hydrolytic enzymes. The enzymes digest most of the material within the phagosome.

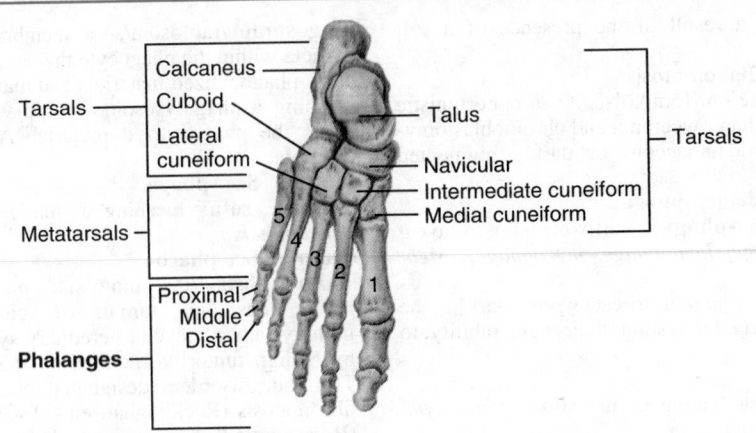

**Phalanges of the foot** *(Applegate, 2000)*

**phall-.** See **phallo-.**

**phallic** /fal′ik/ [Gk, *phallos,* penis], pertaining to the penis or penis-shaped.

**phallic stage** [L, *phallos,* penis, *stare,* to stand], (in psychoanalysis) the period in psychosexual development occurring between 3 and 6 years of age when emerging awareness and self-manipulation of the genitals are the predominant source of pleasurable experience. Fixation at this stage may lead to extreme aggressiveness in adulthood, or it may be a precipitating factor in the development of psychosexual disorders. See also **psychosexual development.**

**phallic symbol** [Gk, *phallos,* penis, *symbolon,* sign], (in psychoanalysis) any object that may be thought to resemble a penis.

**phallo-, phall-,** combining form meaning 'penis': *phallocampsis, phallodynia, phalloplasty.*

**phalloidine** /faloi′din/, a poison present in the mushroom *Amanita phalloides.* Ingestion of phalloidine results in bloody diarrhea, vomiting, severe abdominal pain, kidney failure, and liver damage. Approximately 50% of phalloidine poisonings are fatal. Also spelled **phalloidin.**

**phalloidine poisoning.** See **food poisoning, mushroom poisoning.**

**phalloplasty** /fal′ōplas′tē/, a surgical procedure to lengthen, thicken, reconstruct, or otherwise reshape the penis. It may be performed to correct congenital defects, such as epispadias.

**phallus.** See **penis.**

**-phane, -phan,** suffix meaning a 'thing with a (specified) appearance': *diaphane, rhodophane, xanthophane.*

**phanero-,** prefix meaning 'visible or apparent': *phanerogenetic, phaneromania, phaneroplasm.*

**phantasm** /fan′taz′əm/ [Gk, *phantasma,* vision], an illusory image, such as an optical illusion of something that does not exist. See also **phantom vision.**

**phantom** /fan′təm/ [Gk, *phantasma,* vision], a mass of material similar to human tissue used to investigate the interaction of radiation beams with human beings. Phantom-materials can range from water to complex chemical mixtures that faithfully mimic the human body as it would interact with radiation.

**phantom image,** an image that appears in a CT scan but is not actually in the focal plane. It is created by the incomplete blurring or fusion of the blurred margins of some structures characteristic of the type of tomographic motion used.

**phantom limb syndrome,** a phenomenon common after amputation of a limb in which sensation or discomfort is experienced in the missing limb. In some people severe pain persists. See also **pseudesthesia.**

**phantom tumor,** a swelling resembling a tumor, usually caused by muscle contraction or gaseous distension of the intestines.

**phantom vision,** a sense perception occurring in the form of a visual illusion or hallucination. It is usually regarded as a pseudohallucination in that the person sensing the perception is aware that the phenomenon is illusory. Also called **phantasm, pseudohallucination.**

**phao-.** See **pheo-.**

**phar,** 1. abbreviation for **pharmacy. 2.** abbreviation for **pharmacology. 3.** abbreviation for **pharmaceutic.**

**Phar.B.,** abbreviation for *Bachelor of Pharmacy.*

**Phar.D.,** abbreviation for *Doctor of Pharmacy.*

**pharmaceutic (phar)** /fär′məsoo̅′tik/ [Gk, *pharmakeuein,* to give drugs], 1. pertaining to pharmacy or drugs. 2. a drug.

**pharmaceutical chemistry,** the science dealing with the composition and preparation of chemical compounds used in medical diagnoses and therapies.

**pharmacist** /fär′məsist/ [Gk, *pharmakon,* drug], a person prepared to formulate, dispense, and provide clinical information on drugs or medications to health professionals and patients, through completion of a university program in pharmacy of at least 4 years' duration.

**pharmaco-** /fär′məkō-/, **pharmo-** combining form meaning 'drugs or medicine': *pharmacochemistry, pharmacomania, pharmacopsychosis.*

**pharmacodynamics** /-dīnam′iks/ [Gk, *pharmakon,* drug, *dynamis,* power], the study of how a drug acts on a living organism, including the pharmacologic response and the duration and magnitude of response observed relative to the concentration of the drug at an active site in the organism.

**pharmacogenetics** /-jənet′iks/ [Gk, *pharmakon,* drug, *genesis,* origin], the study of the effect of the genetic factors belonging to a group or to an individual has on the response of the group or the individual to certain drugs.

**pharmacokinetics** /fär′məkōkinet′iks/ [Gk, *pharmakon* + *kinesis,* motion], (in pharmacology) the study of the action of drugs within the body, including the mechanisms of absorption, distribution, metabolism, and excretion; onset of action; duration of effect; biotransformation; and effects and routes of excretion of the metabolites of the drug.

**pharmacologic agent** /-loj'ik/, any oral, parenteral, or topical substance used to alleviate symptoms and treat or control a disease process or aid recovery from an injury.

**pharmacologic treatment.** See **treatment.**

**pharmacologic vagotomy,** the use of medications to curtail functions of the vagus nerve. Also called **medical vagotomy.**

**pharmacologist** /fär'məkol'əjist/, a specialist in the preparation, properties, uses, and actions of drugs.

**pharmacology (phar)** /-kol'əjē/ [Gk, *pharmakon* + *logos*, science], the study of the preparation, properties, uses, and actions of drugs.

**pharmacopoeia** /fär'məkəpē'ə/ [Gk, *pharmakon* + *poiein*, to make], **1.** a compendium containing descriptions, recipes, strengths, standards of purity, and dosage forms for selected drugs. **2.** the available stock of drugs in a pharmacy. **3.** the total of all authorized drugs available within the jurisdiction of a given geographic or political area. Also spelled **pharmacopeia.** See also *British Pharmacopoeia, United States Pharmacopeia.*

**pharmacotherapy** /-ther'əpē/ [Gk, *pharmakon*, drug, *therapeia*], the use of drugs to treat diseases.

**pharmacy (phar)** /fär'məsē/ [Gk, *pharmakon*], **1.** the study of preparing and dispensing drugs. **2.** a place for preparing and dispensing drugs.

**Pharm Chem,** abbreviation for **pharmaceutical chemistry.**

**-pharmic,** combining form meaning 'drugs or medicinal remedies': *alexipharmic, antipharmic, polypharmic.*

**pharmo-.** See **pharmaco-.**

**pharyng-.** See **pharyngo-.**

**pharyngeal** /ferin'jē·əl/ [Gk, *pharynx*, throat], pertaining to the pharynx.

**pharyngeal aponeurosis** [Gk, *pharynx*, throat, *apo*, from, *neuron*, sinew], a sheet of connective tissue immediately beneath the mucosa of the pharynx.

**pharyngeal bursa,** a blind sac at the base of the pharyngeal tonsil.

**pharyngeal membrane,** a thin fold of ectoderm and endoderm that separates the pharyngeal pouches from the branchial clefts in a developing embryo.

**pharyngeal reflex.** See **gag reflex.**

**pharyngeal suction catheter,** a device that allows direct visualization of a pharyngeal suctioning procedure. See also **Yankauer suction catheter.**

**pharyngeal tonsil,** one of two masses of lymphatic tissue situated on the posterior wall of the nasopharynx behind the posterior nares. During childhood these masses often swell and block the passage of air from the nasal cavity into the pharynx, preventing the child from breathing through the nose. Also called **adenoid.**

**pharynges.** See **pharynx.**

**pharyngitis** /fer'inji'tis/ [Gk, *pharynx* + *itis*], inflammation or infection of the pharynx, usually causing symptoms of a sore throat. Some causes of pharyngitis are diphtheria, herpes simplex virus, infectious mononucleosis, and streptococcal infection. Specific treatment depends on the cause. The appearance of the mouth, nose, and throat and throat culture aid in differential diagnosis of a bacterial or viral cause. Symptoms may be relieved by analgesic medication, drinking of warm or cold liquids, or saline solution irrigation of the throat. See also **strep throat.**

**pharyngo-** /fəring'gō-/, **pharyng-,** combining form mean-

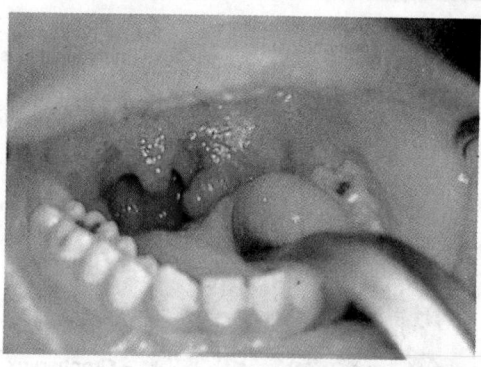

**Acute viral pharyngitis**
*(Barkauskas et al, 1998/courtesy Dr. Edward Applebaum, Head, Department of Otolaryngology, University of Illinois Medical Center, Chicago)*

ing 'pharynx': *pharyngocele, pharyngoglossus, pharyngorrhagia.*

**pharyngoconjunctival fever** /fəring'gōkon'jungktī'vəl/ [Gk, *pharnyx* + L, *conjunctivus*, connecting, *febris*, fever], an adenovirus infection characterized by fever, sore throat, and conjunctivitis. An epidemic illness, particularly prevalent in summer, spread by droplet infection and direct contact. Contaminated water in lakes and swimming pools is a common source of infection. See also **adenovirus.**

**pharyngoscope** /fəring'gəskōp/ [Gk, *pharynx* + *skopein*, to view], an endoscopic device for examining the lining of the pharynx.

**pharyngoscopy** /fer'ing·gos'kəpē/ [Gk, *pharynx*, throat, *skopein*, to view], the examination of the throat with a pharyngoscope.

**pharyngotonsillitis** /-ton'sili'tis/ [Gk, *pharynx* + L, *tonsilla* + Gk, *itis*, inflammation], an inflammation involving the pharynx and the tonsils.

**pharynx** /fer'inks/ *pl.* **pharynxes, pharynges** [Gk], the throat, a tubular structure about 13 cm long that extends from the base of the skull to the esophagus and is situated immediately in front of the cervical vertebrae. The pharynx serves as a passageway for the respiratory and digestive tracts and changes shape to allow the formation of various vowel sounds. The pharynx is composed of muscle, is lined with mucous membrane, and is divided into the nasopharynx, the oropharynx, and the laryngopharynx. It contains the openings of the right and left auditory tubes, the openings of the two posterior nares, the fauces, the opening into the larynx, and the opening into the esophagus. It also contains the pharyngeal tonsils, the palatine tonsils, and the lingual tonsils. Also called **throat.** See also **larynx.**

**phase** /fāz/ [Gk, *phasis*, appearance], in a periodic function, such as rotational or sinusoidal motion, the position relative to a particular part of the cycle.

**phase 0,** (in cardiology) the upstroke of the action potential.

**phase 1,** (in cardiology) the initial rapid repolarization phase of the action potential; seen in ventricular and His-Purkinje action potentials.

**phase 2,** (in cardiology) the plateau of the action potential; occurs during repolarization.

**phase 3,** (in cardiology) the terminal rapid repolarization phase of the action potential.

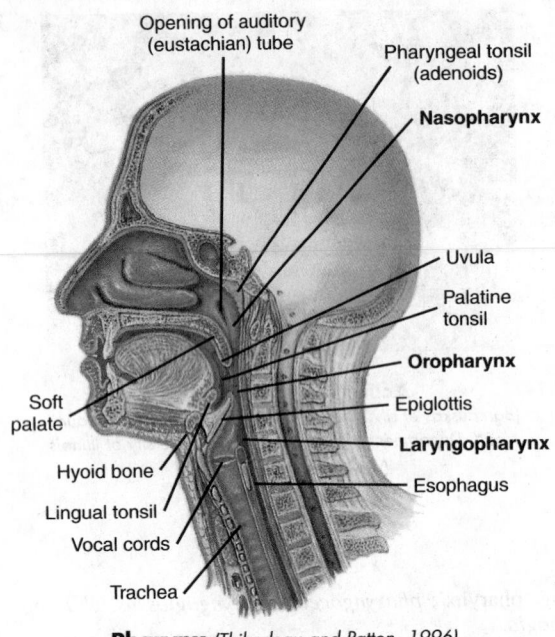

Opening of auditory (eustachian) tube

Pharyngeal tonsil (adenoids)

**Nasopharynx**

Uvula

Palatine tonsil

**Oropharynx**

Epiglottis

**Laryngopharynx**

Esophagus

Soft palate

Hyoid bone

Lingual tonsil

Vocal cords

Trachea

**Pharynx** *(Thibodeau and Patton, 1996)*

**phase 4,** (in cardiology) the period of electrical diastole. A graph of phase 4 shows a gradual upward slope in a pacemaker cell, whereas phase 4 in a nonpacemaker cell is flat.

**phase-contrast microscopy,** a type of light microscopy in which a special condenser and objective with a phase-shifting ring are used to visualize small differences in refractive index as differences in intensity or contrast. It is useful in viewing unstained specimens that appear transparent.

**phased array** /fāzd/, an array transducer assembly that has very thin rectangular elements arranged side by side. It relies on electronic beam steering to sweep sound beams over a sector-shaped scanned region. Beam steering is done using electronic time delays in the transmitting and receiving circuits.

**phase microscope,** a microscope with a special condenser and objective containing a phase-shifting ring that allows the viewer to see small differences in refraction indexes as differences in image intensity or contrast. The phase microscope is used especially for examining transparent specimens, such as living or unstained cells and tissues.

**phase of maximum slope,** the time of rapid cervical dilation and rapid fetal descent in the active phase of labor. See **Friedman curve.**

**phase one study,** a clinical trial to assess the risk that may arise from administering a new treatment modality. A **phase two study** evaluates the clinical effectiveness of the new modality, and a **phase three study** compares its effectiveness with that of the best existing treatment.

**phasic** /fā'zik/ [Gk, *phasis*], **1.** pertaining to a process proceeding in stages or phases. **2.** pertaining to a type of afferent or sensory nerve receptor of the proprioceptive system that responds to rate versus length changes in a muscle spindle. It is triggered by such stimuli as quick stretching, vibrations, and tapping.

**-phasic.** See **-phasia.**

**-phasis, -phasia, -phasic, -phasy,** suffix meaning 'speech, utterance': *allophasis, aphasia, heterophasis, aphasic.*

**Ph.D.,** abbreviation for *Doctor of Philosophy.*

**-phemia,** suffix meaning a '(specified) disorder of speech': *dysphemia, paraphemia, spasmophemia.*

**phen-,** prefix indicating derivation from benzene: *phenacitin, phenicate, phenobarbitone.*

**phenacetin** /fənas'itin/, an analgesic now little used because of its toxicity.

**Phenaphen with Codeine,** trademark for an analgesic-antipyretic (acetaminophen and codeine).

**phenazopyridine hydrochloride** /fen'əzōpī'ridēn/, a urinary tract analgesic.

■ INDICATIONS: It is prescribed to reduce the pain of cystitis or other urinary tract infections.

■ CONTRAINDICATIONS: Renal insufficiency or known hypersensitivity to this drug prohibits its use.

■ ADVERSE EFFECTS: Among the more serious adverse reactions are headache and GI disturbances.

**phencyclidine hydrochloride (PCP)** /fensī'klidēn/, a piperidine derivative administered parenterally to achieve neuroleptic anesthesia. Because of its marked hallucinogenic properties it is not used therapeutically in the United States. Its reported use as an abused substance has declined in recent years. Also called **angel dust.**

**phendimetrazine tartrate** /fen'dīmet'rəsēn/, a sympathomimetic amine used as an anorectic agent.

■ INDICATIONS: It is prescribed to reduce appetite and for short-term treatment of exogenous obesity.

■ CONTRAINDICATIONS: Cardiovascular disease, hypertension, hyperthyroidism, glaucoma, nervousness, a history of drug abuse, concomitant administration of central nervous system stimulants or monoamine oxidase inhibitors, or known hypersensitivity to this drug prohibits its use.

■ ADVERSE EFFECTS: Among the more serious adverse reactions are central nervous system stimulation, elevated blood pressure, insomnia, dry mouth, and tolerance to the drug.

**-phene, -phen,** suffix denoting members of the phenol group: *camphene, phlobaphene, phosphene.*

**phenelzine sulfate** /fē'nəlzēn/, a monoamine oxidase inhibitor.

■ INDICATIONS: It is prescribed in the treatment of endogenous and other types of depression.

■ CONTRAINDICATIONS: Liver dysfunction, congestive heart failure, pheochromocytoma, concomitant use of sympathomimetic drugs or foods high in tryptophan or tyramine, or known hypersensitivity to this drug prohibits its use.

■ ADVERSE EFFECTS: Among the most serious adverse reactions are orthostatic hypotension, vertigo, constipation, blurred vision, headache, overactivity, and dryness of the mouth. Monoamine oxidase inhibitors produce many adverse drug interactions.

**Phenergan,** trademark for a phenothiazine derivative (promethazine).

**phenic acid.** See **carbolic acid.**

**phenobarbital** /fē'nəbär'bital/, a barbiturate anticonvulsant and sedative-hypnotic.

■ INDICATIONS: It is prescribed in the treatment of seizure disorders and as a long-acting sedative.

■ CONTRAINDICATIONS: Porphyria, severe pain, respiratory problems, or known hypersensitivity to this drug or other barbiturates prohibits its use.

■ ADVERSE EFFECTS: Among the most serious adverse reactions are ataxia, porphyria, paradoxical excitement, drowsiness, occasional rashes, and rarely blood dyscrasias. It is involved in many drug interactions.

**phenobarbital-phenytoin serum levels** /-fen'itō'in/, the concentration of phenobarbital and phenytoin in the serum, monitored to maintain concentrations sufficient to control seizures but not high enough to cause toxic reactions. The control of seizures is commonly obtained in adults with plasma concentrations of phenobarbital that average 10 µg/mL per daily dose of 1 µg/kg; in children, 5 to 7 µg/mL per daily dose of 1 µg/kg. The control of seizures is commonly obtained with plasma concentrations of phenytoin that average 10 µg/mL, whereas toxic effects, such as nystagmus, typically develop with a concentration of 20 µg/mL. Ataxia may develop at a concentration of 30 µg/mL, and lethargy at a concentration of 40 µg/mL.

**phenocopy** /fē′nōkop′ē/ [Gk, *phainein*, to appear; L, *copia*, plenty], a phenotypic trait or condition that is induced by environmental factors but closely resembles a phenotype usually produced by a specific genotype. The trait is neither inherited nor transmitted to offspring. Such conditions as deafness, cretinism, mental retardation, and congenital cataracts are caused by mutant genes but also can result from a number of different agents, such as the rubella virus in the case of congenital cataracts. Because phenocopies may present problems in genetic screening and genetic counseling, all exogenous factors must be ruled out before any congenital trait or defect is labeled hereditary.

**phenol** /fē′nol/ [Gk, *phainein*, to appear; L, *oleum*, oil], **1.** a highly poisonous caustic crystalline chemical derived from coal tar or plant tar or manufactured synthetically. It has a distinctive pungent odor and in solution is a powerful disinfectant, commonly called carbolic acid. **2.** Any of a large number and variety of chemical products closely related in structure to the alcohols and containing a hydroxyl group attached to a benzene ring. The phenols are components of dyes, plastics, disinfectants, antimicrobials, and other drugs, including salicylic acid.

**phenol block,** neurolytic alcohol or block using hydroxybenzene (phenol) intended to anesthetize a particular nerve permanently. The technique is sometimes used to control spasticity in specific muscle groups or to block transmission of nerve impulses in chronic pain conditions such as cancers. Morbidity can be high and pain frequently recurs.

**phenol camphor,** an oily mixture of camphor and phenol, used as an antiseptic and toothache remedy.

**phenol coefficient,** a measure of the disinfectant activity of a given chemical in relation to carbolic acid. The activity is expressed as the ratio of a dilution of the chemical that kills in 10 minutes but not in 5 minutes to the 1:90 dilution of carbolic acid that kills in 10 minutes but not in 5 minutes.

**phenolphthalein** /fē′nolthal′ē·in, -thā′lēn/, an indicator of hydrogen ion in urine and gastric juice.

**phenol poisoning,** corrosive poisoning caused by the ingestion of compounds containing phenol, such as carbolic acid, creosote, cresol, guaiacol, and naphthol. Characteristic of phenol poisoning are burns of the mucous membranes, weakness, pallor, pulmonary edema, seizures, and respiratory, circulatory, cardiac, and renal failure. Rarely esophageal stricture may develop as a complication of extensive tissue damage.

**phenol red.** See **phenolsulfonphthalein.**

**phenolsulfonphthalein** /fē′nəlsul′fŏnfthal′ē·in/, a bright red water-soluble triphenylmethane dye used as an indicator at pH 7.7. Its sodium salt is injected intravenously and its rate of appearance in urine is used as a test for renal function. Also called **phenol red.** See also **cystochromoscopy.**

**phenomenon** /finom′ənən/, *pl.* **phenomena** [Gk, *phainomenon*, something seen], a sign that is often associated with a specific illness or condition and is therefore diagnostically important.

**phenothiazine** /fē′nōthī′əzēn/, a yellow to green crystalline compound that is a source of dyes and is used in veterinary medicine to treat infestations of threadworms and roundworms. It is too toxic for human use, but derivatives of phenothiazine are used in tranquilizers and antihistamine medications. See also **phenothiazine derivatives.**

**phenothiazine derivatives,** any of a group of drugs that have a three ring structure in which two benzene rings are linked by a nitrogen and a sulfur. They represent the largest group of antipsychotic compounds in clinical medicine. Of the many phenothiazines and their congeners that are used as adjuncts to general anesthesia, antiemetics, major tranquilizers (antipsychotic agents), and antihistamines, the most widely used are the two prototypes, chlorpromazine and prochlorperazine; closely related are trimeprazine and triflupromazine. This group of drugs has largely revolutionized the practice of psychiatric medicine. Unlike the barbiturates, which act exclusively on the central nervous system (CNS), the phenothiazines exert significant influence on many organ systems of the body at once; for example, they exert antiadrenergic, anticholinergic, and antihistaminic activity. The effects on the CNS differ according to individual drug and patient status. All phenothiazine tranquilizers are withheld from patients with severe CNS depression or epilepsy and are given with caution to those with liver disease. See also specific drugs.

**phenotype** /fē′nətīp/ [Gk, *phainein*, to appear, *typos*, mark], **1.** the complete observable characteristics of an organism or group, including anatomic, physiologic, biochemical, and behavioral traits, as determined by the interaction of both genetic makeup and environmental factors. **2.** a group of organisms that resemble each other in appearance. Compare **genotype. —phenotypic,** *adj.*

**phenoxy-,** combining form indicating the presence of a chemical group composed of phenyl and an atom of oxygen: *phenoxycaffeine.*

**phenoxybenzamine hydrochloride** /fēnok′sēben′zə mēn/, an antihypertensive.

■ INDICATIONS: It is prescribed in the control of hypertension and sweating in pheochromocytoma. If tachycardia is excessive, concomitant administration of propranolol may be necessary.

■ CONTRAINDICATIONS: Hypotension or known hypersensitivity to this drug prohibits its use.

■ ADVERSE EFFECTS: Among the more serious adverse reactions are severe hypotension, tachycardia, and GI irritation.

**phenoxymethyl penicillin.** See **penicillin V.**

**phensuximide** /fensuk′simīd/, an anticonvulsant.

■ INDICATIONS: It is prescribed to prevent and treat seizures in petit mal epilepsy.

■ CONTRAINDICATIONS: Known hypersensitivity to this drug or to any succinimide prohibits its use.

■ ADVERSE EFFECTS: Among the most serious adverse reactions are blood dyscrasias and a systemic lupuslike syndrome. Common reactions are GI disturbances and central nervous system depression with drowsiness or dizziness.

**phentermine hydrochloride** /fen′tərmēn/, a sympathomimetic amine used as an anorectic agent.

■ INDICATIONS: It is prescribed to decrease appetite and for the short-term treatment of obesity.

■ CONTRAINDICATIONS: Arteriosclerosis, cardiovascular disease, hypertension, glaucoma, hyperthyroidism, or known hypersensitivity to this drug or to other sympathomimetic drugs prohibits its use.

■ ADVERSE EFFECTS: Among the more serious adverse reactions are restlessness, insomnia, tachycardia, increased blood pressure, and dry mouth.

**phentolamine** /fentol′əmēn/, an antiadrenergic. It is administered as the hydrochloride form in tablets and as the mesylate form for injections.

■ INDICATIONS: It is prescribed in the control of symptoms of pheochromocytoma before and during surgery and for dermal necrosis and sloughing after extravasation of parenteral norepinephrine.

■ CONTRAINDICATIONS: History of myocardial infarction, angina, coronary artery disease, or known hypersensitivity to this drug prohibits its use.

■ ADVERSE EFFECTS: Among the more serious adverse reactions are tachycardia, cardiac arrhythmias, anginal pain, and hypotension.

**Phenurone,** trademark for an anticonvulsant (phenacemide).

**phenyl (Ph)** /fē′nil, fen′il/, a monovalent organic radical, $C_6H_5$, derived from benzene.

**phenylacetic acid** /fen′iləsē′tik/, a metabolite of phenylalanine excreted in urine together with glutamine in phenylketonuna.

**phenylalanine (Phe)** /fen′ilal′ənēn/, an essential amino acid necessary for the normal growth and development of infants and children and for normal protein metabolism throughout life. The normal value of this amino acid in serum is less than 3 mg/dL in adults and 1.2 to 3.5 mg/dL in newborns. It is abundant in milk, eggs, and other common foods. See also **amino acid, phenylketonuria, protein.**

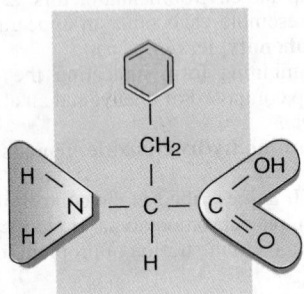

**Chemical structure of phenylalanine**

**phenylalaninemia** /fen′il′aləninē′mē·ə/, the presence of phenylalanine in the blood. See also **hyperphenylalaninemia.**

**phenyl carbinol.** See **benzyl alcohol.**

**phenylephrine hydrochloride** /-ef′rēn/, an alpha-adrenergic agent.

■ INDICATIONS: It is prescribed for maintenance of blood pressure and is used locally as a nasal or ophthalmic vasoconstrictor.

■ CONTRAINDICATIONS: Narrow-angle glaucoma, concomitant administration of monoamine oxidase inhibitors, or known hypersensitivity to this drug prohibits its use.

■ ADVERSE EFFECTS: Among the more serious adverse reactions to the systemic administration of this drug are arrhythmias and an excessive rise in blood pressure. Anxiety, congestion, and hypersensitivity reactions may result from local administration of this drug.

**phenylethyl alcohol ($C_6H_5CH_2CH_2OH$)** /-eth′il/, a colorless fragrant liquid with a burning taste, used as a bacte-

riostatic agent and preservative in medicinal solutions. Also called **benzyl carbonol, 2-phenylethanol.**

**phenylic acid, phenylic alcohol.** See **carbolic acid.**

**phenylketonuria (PKU)** /fen′əlkē′tōnyŏŏr′ē·ə, fē′nəl-/, abnormal presence of phenylketone and other metabolites of phenylalanine in the urine, characteristic of an inborn metabolic disorder caused by the absence or a deficiency of the enzyme responsible for the conversion of the amino acid phenylalanine into tyrosine. Accumulation of phenylalanine is toxic to brain tissue. Untreated individuals have very fair hair, eczema, a mousy odor of the urine and skin, and progressive mental retardation. Treatment consists of a diet low in phenylalanine. Phenylketonuria occurs approximately once in 16,000 births in the United States. Most states require a screening test for all newborns. See also **Guthrie's bacterial inhibition assay (GBIA). —phenylketonuric,** adj.

**phenylmethanol.** See **benzyl alcohol.**

**phenyl-methoxypropyl adenine (PMPA),** an investigational drug used in acquired immunodeficiency syndrome treatment. It blocks an enzyme that helps human immunodeficiency virus spread through the body. Unlike some other remedies that must be absorbed into the body's cells to be effective, PMPA can begin blocking the virus as soon as it enters the body.

**phenylpropanolamine hydrochloride** /fen′əlprō′pənol′-əmēn/, a sympathomimetic amine with vasoconstrictor action. This drug was withdrawn from the U.S. market in 2001.

■ INDICATIONS: It is prescribed to relieve nasal congestion and related cold symptoms.

■ CONTRAINDICATIONS: Hypertension, coronary artery disease, concomitant administration of monoamine oxidase inhibitors, or known hypersensitivity to this drug prohibits its use.

■ ADVERSE EFFECTS: Among the more serious adverse reactions are nervousness, insomnia, anorexia, and increased blood pressure.

**phenylpyruvic acid** /fen′ilpīrōō′vik/, a product of the metabolism of phenylalanine. The presence of phenylpyruvic acid in the urine is indicative of phenylketonuria.

**phenylpyruvic amentia.** See **phenylketonuria.**

**phenyl salicylate,** the salicylic ester of phenol. Also called **salol.** See also **salol camphor.**

**phenyltoloxamine citrate** /fen′iltəlok′səmēn/, an antihistamine usually used in a fixed-combination drug with an analgesic.

**phenytoin** /fen′ətō′in/, an anticonvulsant.

■ INDICATIONS: It is used as an anticonvulsant in grand mal and psychomotor seizure disorders and as an antiarrhythmic agent, particularly in digitalis-induced arrhythmias.

■ CONTRAINDICATIONS: Known hypersensitivity to this drug or to other hydantoins prohibits its use. It is used with caution in patients with a history of hepatic or hematologic abnormalities and in the presence of certain arrhythmias.

■ ADVERSE EFFECTS: Among the more serious adverse reactions are ataxia, nystagmus, hypersensitivity reactions, and gingival hyperplasia. Rarely a variety of severe reactions occur. This drug interacts with many other drugs.

**pheo-, phao-,** combining form meaning 'dusky': *pheochrome, pheochromoblast, pheophytin.*

**pheochromocytoma** /fē′ōkrō′mōsītō′mə/, pl. **pheochromocytomas, pheochromocytomata** [Gk, *phaios,* dark, *chroma,* color, *kytos,* cell, *oma,* tumor], a vascular tumor of chromaffin tissue of the adrenal medulla or sympathetic paraganglia, characterized by hypersecretion of epinephrine and norepinephrine, causing persistent or intermittent hypertension. Typical signs include headache, palpitation, sweating, nervousness, hyperglycemia, nausea, vomiting, and syncope. Weight loss, myocarditis, cardiac arrhythmia, and heart failure may occur. The tumor occurs most commonly at 40 to 60 years of age, and only a small percentage of the lesions are malignant. The diagnosis may be established by laboratory assays showing increased catecholamines and their metabolites in urine and by pressor tests; intravenously injected histamine causes a sharp increase in blood pressure, and the administration of phentolamine produces a marked decrease. Surgical excision is the usual treatment; patients with nonresectable tumors may be treated with adrenergic blocking agents or with methyl tyrosine, a drug that reduces norepinephrine production. Also spelled *phaeochromocytoma.*

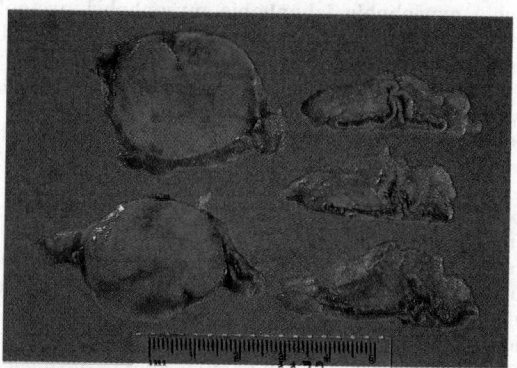

**Pheochromocytoma** *(Kumar, Cotran, and Robbins, 1997)*

**pheresis.** See **apheresis.**

**pheromone** /fer'əmōn'/ [Gk, *pherein,* to carry, *hormaein,* to stimulate], a substance secreted by an organism that elicits a particular response from another individual of the same species, usually of the opposite sex. Pheromones may be sexual stimulants or attractants or alarm or trail-making substances; in social insects they have a role in the determination of castes.

**phi** /fī/, Φ, φ, the twenty-first letter of the Greek alphabet.

**phil-,** prefix meaning 'having an affinity for or having a love for': *philanthropist, philocatalase, philoneism.*

**-phil, -philic, -philous,** combining form meaning 'of that which has an attraction to or is stained by': *chromaphil, hydrophil, lipophil.*

**Philadelphia chromosome (Ph¹)** [Philadelphia, Pennsylvania], a translocation of the long arm of chromosome 22, often seen in the abnormal myeloblasts, erythroblasts, and megakaryoblasts of patients who have chronic myelocytic leukemia.

**-phile, 1.** combining form meaning 'a lover or admirer' of something specified: *sarcophile.* **2.** combining form meaning 'having an affinity for or being strongly attracted to a specified thing': *electrophile, pedophile.*

**-philia, -phily, -philous-,** combining form meaning 'having a love, craving, affinity for': *cyanophilous, hydrophily, spasmophilia, necrophilia.*

**-philous.** See **-philia.**

**philtrum** /fil'trəm/, the vertical groove in the center of the upper lip.

**-phily.** See **-philia.**

**phimosis** /fīmō'sis/ [Gk, muzzle], tightness of the prepuce of the penis that prevents the retraction of the foreskin over the glans. The condition is usually congenital but may be the result of infection. Circumcision is the usual treatment. An analogous condition of the clitoris occurs rarely. Compare **paraphimosis.** See also **phimosis vaginalis.**

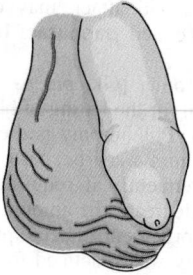

**Phimosis** *(Phipps, Sands, and Marek, 1999)*

**phimosis vaginalis** /vaj'inā'lis/, congenital narrowness or closure of the vaginal opening.

**pHisoHex,** trademark for a detergent containing a topical antiinfective (hexachlorophene).

**phleb-.** See **phlebo-.**

**phlebectomy** /fləbek'təmē/ [Gk, *phleps,* vein, *ektomē,* excision], the surgical removal of a vein or part of a vein.

**phlebitis.** See **thrombophlebitis.**

**phlebo-, phleb-** /fleb'ō-/, combining form meaning 'vein or veins': *phlebocarcinoma, phlebograph, phlebostenosis.*

**phlebogram** /fleb'əgram/ [Gk, *phleps,* vein, *gramma,* record], **1.** a radiograph obtained by phlebography. **2.** a graphic representation of the venous pulse obtained by phlebography. Also called **venogram.**

**phlebograph** /fleb'əgraf'/, a device for producing a graphic record of the venous pulse.

**phlebography** /fləbog'rəfē/ [Gk, *phleps* + *graphein,* to record], **1.** the radiographic examination of veins injected with a radiopaque contrast medium. **2.** the graphic recording of the venous pulse. Also called **venography.**

**phlebostasis** /-stā'sis/, an abnormally slow flow of blood in the veins, which are usually distended. Also called **venostasis.**

**phlebostatic axis** /-stat'ik/ [Gk, *phleps* + *stasis,* standing still], the approximate location of the right atrium, found at the intersection of the midaxillary and a line drawn from the fourth intercostal space at the right side of the sternum. The phlebostatic axis is used extensively in hemodynamics.

**phlebothrombosis** /fleb'ōthrombō'sis/ [Gk, *phleps* + *thrombos,* lump, *osis,* condition], an abnormal condition in which a clot forms within a vein. It is usually caused by hemostasis, hypercoagulability, or occlusion. In contrast to that in thrombophlebitis, the wall of the vein is not inflamed. Also called **venous thrombosis.** Compare **thrombophlebitis.**

**phlebotomist** /fləbot'əmist/ [Gk, *phleps,* vein + *ektomē*], a person with special training in the practice of drawing blood.

**phlebotomize** /fləbot'əmīz/ [Gk, *phleps,* vein, *ektomē,* excision], to open a vein to remove blood.

**phlebotomus fever** /fləbot'əməs/ [Gk, *phleps* + *tomos,* cutting; L, *febris,* fever], an acute mild infection, caused by one of five distinct arboviruses transmitted to humans by the bite of an infected sandfly, characterized by rapidly developing fever, headache, eye pain, conjunctivitis, myalgia, and occasionally a macular or urticarial rash. Aseptic meningitis also may occur. The disease is widespread in hot, dry areas where sandflies abound, and it has been seen in Panama and Brazil. Phlebotomus fever is self-limited, no fatalities have been recorded, and no specific therapy is available. Bed rest, fluids, and aspirin are recommended. A second attack may occur a few weeks after the first. Also called **pappataci fever, sandfly fever, three-day fever.**

**phlebotomy** /fləbot′əmē/ [Gk, *phleps* + *temnein*, to cut], the incision of a vein for the letting of blood, as in collecting blood from a donor. Phlebotomy is the chief treatment for polycythemia vera and may be performed every 2 to 3 months or more frequently if required. The procedure is sometimes used to decrease the amount of circulating blood and pulmonary engorgement in acute pulmonary edema. At one time phlebotomy was practiced for almost every disorder. Also called **venesection.**

**phlebotomy: arterial blood sample,** a nursing intervention from the Nursing Interventions Classification (NIC) defined as obtaining a blood sample from an uncannulated artery to assess oxygen and carbon dioxide levels and acid-base balance. See also **Nursing Interventions Classification.**

**phlebotomy: blood unit acquisition,** a nursing intervention from the Nursing Interventions Classification (NIC) defined as procuring blood and blood products from donors. See also **Nursing Interventions Classification.**

**phlebotomy: venous blood sample,** a nursing intervention from the Nursing Interventions Classification (NIC) defined as removal of a sample of venous blood from an uncannulated vein. See also **Nursing Interventions Classification.**

**phleg-.** See **phlogo-.**

**phlegm** /flem/ [Gk, *phlegma*, mucus, sluggishness], thick mucus secreted by the tissues lining the airways of the lungs.

**phlegmasia alba dolens** [Gk, *phlegmone*, inflammation; L, *albus*, white, *dolens*, painful], thrombophlebitis of the femoral vein, resulting in pain and edema of the leg. It may occur after childbirth or a severe febrile illness.

**phlegmasia cerulea dolens.** See **blue phlebitis.**

**phlegmatic** /flegmat′ik/ [Gk, *phlegma*, mucus, sluggishness], pertaining to a person who may be dull or apathetic, or calm and composed to an extent that excitation is difficult.

**phlegmon** /fleg′mon/ [Gk, *phlegmone*, inflammation], an inflammation of connective tissue.

**phlegmonous gastritis** /fleg′mənəs/ [Gk, *phlegmone* + *osis*, condition], a rare but severe form of gastritis, involving the connective tissue layer of the stomach wall. It occurs as a complication of systemic infection, peptic ulcer, cancer, surgery, or other severe stress and represents an acute abdominal emergency. Treatment includes surgery, antibiotics, and analgesics.

**phlegn-,** a combining form meaning 'mucus': *phlegmatic.*

**phlogo-, phleg-,** a rarely used combining form meaning 'inflammation': *phlogocyte, phlogogen, phlegmon.*

**phlyctenular keratoconjunctivitis** /flikten′yələr/ [Gk, *phlyktaina*, blister], an inflammatory condition of the cornea, characterized by tiny ulcerating nodules. It is seen most often in children as a response to allergens found in *Mycobacterium tuberculosis*, gonococci, *Candida albicans*, or various parasites. Vitamin deficiency may be a factor. The condition responds to topical corticosteroids, but corneal scars may remain. Also called **phlyctenulosis, scrofulous keratitis.** See also **eczematous conjunctivitis.**

**PHO,** abbreviation for **physician-hospital organization.**

**phob-,** combining form meaning 'fear, panic, or morbid dread': *phobia, phobic, phobophobia.*

**-phobe, -phobiac, -phobist,** suffix meaning 'one who fears' something specified: *dermatophobe, heliophobe, nosophobe.*

**phobia** /fō′bē·ə/ [Gk, *phobos*, fear], an obsessive, irrational, and intense fear of a specific object, such as an animal or dirt; of an activity, such as meeting strangers or leaving the familiar setting of the home; or of a physical situation, such as heights and open or closed spaces. Typical manifestations of phobia include faintness, fatigue, palpitations, perspiration, nausea, tremor, and panic. Some kinds of phobias are **agoraphobia, algophobia, claustrophobia, erythrophobia, gynephobia, laliophobia, mysophobia, nyctophobia, photophobia, xenophobia,** and **zoophobia.** Also called **phobic disorder, phobic anxiety, phobic reaction.** Compare **compulsion.** See also **simple phobia, social phobia.** —**phobic,** *adj.*

**-phobia,** suffix meaning 'abnormal fear' of the object, experience, or place specified: *agoraphobia, claustrophobia, nyctophobia.*

**phobiac** /fō′bē·ak/, a person who exhibits or is afflicted with a phobia.

**-phobiac.** See **-phobe.**

**phobic** /fō′bik/ [Gk, *phobos*, fear], pertaining to or resembling phobia.

**-phobic, -phobous, 1.** suffix meaning 'exhibiting or possessing an aversion to or fear of (something)': *Anglophobic, necrophobic, zoophobic.* **2.** combining form meaning the 'absence of a strong affinity': *chromophobic, gentianophobic, osmiophobic.*

**phobic anxiety.** See **phobia.**

**phobic desensitization** [Gk, *phobos*, fear; L, *de* + *sentire*, to feel], a method of resolving an ego dystonic or uncomfortable behavior pattern by reentry into the emotionally upsetting life situation in stages, first in fantasy and again in real life. It is similar to the psychotherapeutic techniques of **flooding** and **implosive therapy.**

**phobic disorder.** See **anxiety disorder, phobia.**

**phobic neurosis.** See **phobia.**

**phobic reaction.** See **phobia.**

**phobic state,** a condition characterized by extreme anxiety resulting from the excessive, irrational fear of a particular object, situation, or activity. See also **phobia.**

**-phobist.** See **-phobe.**

**-phobous.** See **-phobic.**

**phocomelia** /fō′kəmē′lyə/ [Gk, *phoke*, seal, *melos*, limb], a developmental anomaly characterized by absence of the upper part of one or more of the limbs so that the feet or hands or both are attached to the trunk of the body by short, irregularly shaped stumps, resembling the fins of a seal. The condition, caused by interference with the embryonic development of the long bones, is rare and is seen primarily as a side effect of the drug thalidomide taken during early pregnancy. Also called **seal limbs.** Compare **amelia.** —**phocomelic,** *adj.*

**phocomelic dwarf** /fō′kəmē′lik/, a dwarf in whom the long bones of any or all of the extremities are abnormally short.

**phocomelus** /fōkom′ələs/, an individual who has phocomelia.

**phon-.** See **phono-.**

**phonation** /fōnā′shən/ [Gk, *phone*, sound; L, *atio*, process],

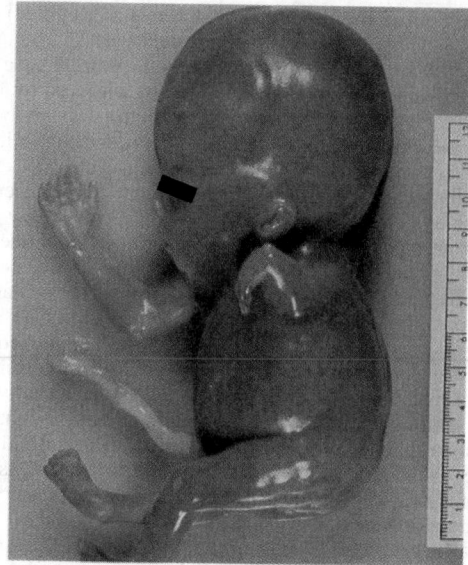

**Phocomelia of the left upper limb**
(Moore, Persaud, and Shiota, 2000/courtesy Dr. D.K. Kalousek,
Department of Pathology, University of British Columbia,
Children's Hospital, Vancouver)

the production of speech sounds through the vibration of the vocal folds of the larynx.

**-phone,** suffix meaning 'sound or voice': *osteophone.*

**phonetics** /fōnet'iks/ [Gk, *phone,* voice], the science of speech sounds used in language.

**-phonia.** See **-phony.**

**phonic,** pertaining to voice, sounds, or speech.

**-phonic.** See **-phony.**

**phono-, phon-,** /fō'no-/ prefix meaning 'sound, often specifically the sound of the voice': *phonocardiograph, phonopathy, phonopsia.*

**phonocardiogram** /-kär'dē·əgram'/, a graphic recording obtained from a phonocardiograph.

**phonocardiograph** /-kär'dē·əgraf'/ [Gk, *phone,* sound, *kardia,* heart, *graphein,* to record], an electroacoustic device that produces graphic heart sound recordings using a system of microphones and associated recording equipment. One microphone is usually placed on the chest near the base of the heart. It records the timing of the aortic and pulmonary components of the second heart sound and the loudest murmurs. Another microphone is positioned on the chest over the apex of the heart. It is connected to filters that allow the recording of low-frequency sounds, such as those associated with atrial and ventricular gallops, as well as higher-frequency sounds, such as those associated with mitral regurgitation and ventricular septal defect. To ensure an accurate recording, the examiner also uses audiophones to monitor the sounds and an oscilloscope to monitor cardiac impulses. Phonocardiographs are used in the diagnosis and monitoring of heart disorders. Also called **electrocardiophonograph. —phonocardiographic,** *adj.*

**phonocardiography** /-kär'dē·og'rəfē/ [Gk, *phone + kardia + graphein,* to record], the recording of heart sounds and murmurs by a phonocardiograph.

**phonologic disorder** /fō'nə·loj'i·k/, a communication disorder of unknown cause, characterized by failure to use age- and dialect-appropriate sounds in speaking, with errors in

the selection, production, or articulation of sounds. The most common errors are omissions, substitutions, and distortions of speech sounds.

**phonology** /fōnol'əjē/, the study of speech sounds, particularly the principles governing the way speech sounds are used in a given language.

**phonophoresis** /fō'nōfərē'sis/, a therapeutic technique in which ultrasound waves are used to force topical medicines, such as hydrocortisone, aspirin, and lidocaine, into subcutaneous tissues. Continuous phonophoresis for up to 10 minutes can drive a drug applied to the skin surface about 5 cm into muscle tissue. Because of the risk that the patient may be hypersensitive to the medication, the technique is used with caution.

**phonoreceptor** /-risep'tər/ [Gk, *phone,* sound; L, *recipere,* to receive], a device for receiving sound impulses.

**-phony, -phonia, -phonic,** suffix meaning 'sound or to a type of speech': *autophony, aphonia, organophonic.*

**phor-,** prefix meaning 'bearing, carrying': *phoresis, phoroblast, phorology.*

**-phore, -phor,** suffix meaning a 'bearer or possessor': *gluciphore, physaliphore, trochophore.*

**-phoresis,** suffix meaning a 'movement in a (specified) manner or medium': *aphoresis, cataphoresis, diaphoresis.*

**-phoria,** 1. suffix meaning '(condition of the) visual axes of the eye': *anophoria, esophoria, exophoria.* 2. combining form meaning an 'emotional state': *adiaphoria, euphoria, ideaphoria.*

**phosphatase** /fos'fətāz/, an enzyme that acts as a catalyst in chemical reactions involving phosphorus. It is present in serum, semen, the kidney, and the prostate. It is essential in the calcification of bone. See also **catalyst, enzyme.**

**phosphate** /fos'fāt/, a salt of phosphoric acid. Phosphates are extremely important in living cells, particularly in the storage and use of energy and the transmission of genetic information within a cell and from one cell to another. See also **adenosine diphosphate, adenosine triphosphate, phosphorus.**

**phosphate-bond energy,** the Gibbs energy for hydrolysis of a phosphate compound; a measure of relative phosphorylation power.

**phosphatemia** /fos'fətē'mē·ə/ [Gk, *phosphoros,* bringer of light; Gk, *haima,* blood], a condition of excessive levels of phosphates in the blood.

**phosphate test (P or PO$_4$),** a blood test used to detect hyper- and hypophosphatemia. Abnormal phosphate levels are associated with renal failure, acromegaly, hyper- or hypoparathyroidism, liver disease, advanced lymphoma or myeloma, hemolytic anemia, hypercalcemia, chronic alcoholism, vitamin D deficiency, diabetic acidosis, hyperinsulinism, and sepsis, among other conditions.

**phosphatide** /fos'fətīd/, phosphatidic acid or any of its esters. Phosphatidic acid (diacylglycerol phosphate) consists of glycerol esterified to phophoric acid and to two fatty acids. Phosphatides are major components of cell membranes. Also called **phosphatidate, phosphoglyceride.**

**phosphaturia** /fos'fətŏōr'ē·ə/ [Gk, *phosphoros,* bringer of light, *ouron,* urine], an excessive level of phosphates in the urine. Also called **phosphuria.**

**phosphoglycerate kinase** /fos'fōglis'ərāt/, an enzyme that catalyzes the reversible transfer of a phosphate group from adenosine triphosphate to D-3-phosphoglycerate, forming D-1,3-diphosphoglycerate. The reaction is one of the steps in gluconeogenesis.

**phosphoglyceride.** See **phosphatide.**

**Phospholine Iodide,** trademark for a cholinergic (echothiophate iodide).

**phospholipase** /fos′fōlī′pās/, any of a group of enzymes that catalyze the hydrolysis of phospholipids. Various phospholipases digest cell membranes, aid in the synthesis of prostaglandins, and help produce arachidonic acid, one of the essential fatty acids.

**phospholipid** /fos′fōlip′id/ [Gk, *phos,* light, *pherein,* to bear, *lipos* fat], a phosphorus-containing lipid. Two kinds of phospholipids are **phosphatides** and **sphingomyelins.**

**phospholipid as phosphorus.** See **lipid.**

**phosphomevalonate kinase** /fos′fōməval′ənāt/, an enzyme that catalyzes the transfer of a phosphate group from adenosine triphosphate to produce adenosine diphosphate and 5-pyrophosphomevalonate.

**phosphorescence** /fos′fôres′əns/ [Gk, *phos,* light, *pherein,* to bear], 1. a glow of yellow phosphorus caused by slow oxidation. 2. the emission of visible light without accompanying heat as observed in phosphorus that has been exposed to radiation, which continues after radiation has ceased.

**phosphoric acid (H₃PO₄)** /fosfôr′ik/, a clear, colorless, odorless liquid that is irritating to the skin and eyes and moderately toxic if ingested. It is used in the production of fertilizers, soaps, detergents, animal feeds, and certain drugs.

**phosphorus (P)** /fos′fərəs/ [Gk, *phos,* light, *pherein,* to bear], a nonmetallic chemical element occurring extensively in nature as a component of phosphate rock. Its atomic number is 15; its atomic mass is 30.975. Phosphorus forms a series of sulfides used commercially in the manufacture of matches. It can be prepared in yellow or white, red, and black allotropic forms. Phosphorus is essential for the metabolism of protein, calcium, and glucose. The body uses phosphorus in its combined forms, which are obtained from such nutritional sources as milk, cheese, meat, egg yolk, whole grains, legumes, and nuts. A nutritional deficiency of phosphorus can cause weight loss, anemia, and abnormal growth. Phosphorus is essential to the body for the production of adenosine triphosphate and for the process of glycolysis. Elemental white or yellow phosphorus is extremely poisonous and produces severe GI irritation. If ingested, it can produce hemorrhage, cardiovascular failure, and death. Chronic poisoning by phosphorus is characterized by anemia, cachexia, bronchitis, and necrosis of the mandible. Normal adult blood levels of phosphorus are 3 to 4.5 mg/dl or 0.97 to 1.45 mmol/L (SI units).

**phosphorus poisoning,** a toxic condition caused by the ingestion of white or yellow phosphorus, sometimes found in rat poisons, certain fertilizers, and fireworks. Intoxication is characterized initially by nausea, throat and stomach pain, vomiting, diarrhea, and an odor of garlic on the breath. After a few days of apparent recovery nausea, vomiting, and diarrhea recur with renal and hepatic dysfunction. Physical contact with the vomitus and feces of the patient is avoided.

**phosphorylase** /fosfôr′ilās/ [Gk, *phosphoros,* bringer of light + *ase,* enzyme suffix], any of a group of physiologically important enzymes that catalyze reactions between phosphates and glycogen or other starch components, yielding glucose-1-phosphate.

**phosphorylation** /fosfôr′ilā′shən/, the process of attaching a phosphate group to a protein, sugar, or other compound.

**phosphotidate.** See **phosphatide.**

**phosphuria.** See **phosphaturia.**

**phot** /fot/ [Gk, *phos,* light], the centimeter-gram-second unit of illumination, being one lumen per square centimeter.

**phot-.** See **photo-.**

**photic** /fō′tik/ [Gk, *phos,* light], pertaining to light.

**-photic,** suffix meaning 'ability to see at a (specified) light level': *euryphotic, stenophotic, sthenophotic.*

**photic epilepsy** [Gk, *phos,* light, *epilepsia,* seizure], a condition in which epileptic attacks may be triggered by flickering light. Also called **photogenic epilepsy.**

**photo-** /fō′tō-/, **phot-,** combining form meaning 'light': *photoelectric, photoreceptor, phototropism.*

**photoallergic** /-əlur′gik/ [Gk, *phos,* light, *allos,* other, *ergein,* to work], exhibiting a delayed hypersensitivity reaction after exposure to light. Compare **phototoxic.** See also **photoallergic contact dermatitis.**

**photoallergic contact dermatitis,** a papulovesicular, eczematous, or exudative skin reaction that occurs 24 to 48 hours after exposure to light in a previously sensitized person. The sensitizing substance concentrates in the skin and requires chemical alteration by light to become an active antigen. Among common photosensitizers are phenothiazines, hexachlorophene, oral hypoglycemic agents, and sulfanilamide. Prevention requires avoidance of the photosensitizer and of sunlight. Treatment is the same as that for any other inflammatory dermatitis.

**photoallergy** /-al′ərjē/ [Gk, *phos,* light, *allos,* other + *ergein,* to work], a sensitivity to light that causes allergic reactions.

**photobiology** /-bī·ol′əjē/, the study of the effects of light on organisms.

**photochemotherapy** /-kē′mōther′əpē/ [Gk, *phos* + *chemeia,* alchemy, *therapeia,* treatment], a kind of chemotherapy in which the effect of the administered drug is enhanced by exposing the patient to light. Also called **photodynamic therapy.** See also **chemotherapy.**

**photochromogen** /-krō′məjen/, 1. a pigment that develops as a result of exposure to light. 2. a type of mycobacterium that is nonpigmented in the dark but produces a yellow pigment on constant exposure to light. Also called **Runyan Group I.**

**photodisintegration** /-disin′təgrā′shən/, the emission of a nuclear fragment caused by the interaction of a high-energy x-ray with an atomic nucleus. It may occur when an x-ray photon with energy greater than 10 MeV escapes interaction with the electron cloud or nuclear force field of an atom and is absorbed directly by the nucleus.

**photodynamic therapy.** See **photochemotherapy.**

**photoelectron** /-ilek′tron/ [Gk, *phos,* light + *elektron,* amber], any electron that is discharged when light strikes a metal surface.

**photogenic epilepsy.** See **photic epilepsy.**

**photokinetic** /-kinet′ik/ [Gk, *phos,* light, *kinesis,* movement], pertaining to any movement that is stimulated by light rays.

**photometer** /fōtom′ətər/ [Gk, *phos* + *metron,* measure], an instrument that measures light intensity. It usually is composed of a source of radiant energy, a filter for wavelength selection, a cuvette holder, a detector, and a readout device.

**photomultiplier** /-mul′tiplī′ər/ [Gk, *phos,* light; L, *multiplex,* many folds], a device used in many radiation detection applications that converts low levels of light into electrical pulses. A bank of such tubes is used in gamma cameras to view a crystal.

**photon** /fō′ton/ [Gk, *phos,* light], the smallest quantity of electromagnetic energy. It has no mass and no charge but travels at the speed of light. Photons may occur in the form of x-rays, gamma rays, or quanta of light. The energy (*E*) of a photon is expressed as the product of its frequency (*v*) and Planck's constant (*h*), as in the equation $E = hv$. X-ray photons occur in frequencies of from $10^{18}$ to $10^{21}$ Hz and energies that range upward from 1 KeV.

**photophobia** /-fō′bē·ə/ [Gk, *phos + phobos,* fear],   **1.** abnormal sensitivity to light, especially by the eyes. The condition is prevalent in albinism and various diseases of the conjunctiva and cornea and may be a symptom of such disorders as measles, psittacosis, encephalitis, Rocky Mountain spotted fever, and Reiter's syndrome. **2.** (in psychiatry) a morbid fear of light with an irrational need to avoid light places. The anxiety disorder is seen more often in women than in men and is usually caused by a repressed intrapsychic conflict symbolically related to light. —**photophobic,** *adj.*

**photopic eye.**   See **light-adapted eye.**

**photopic vision** /fōtop′ik/,   daylight vision, which depends primarily on the function of the retinal cone cells.

**photoprotective** /-prətek′tiv/,   protective against the potential adverse effects of ultraviolet light.

**photoreaction** /-rē·ak′shən/ [Gk, *phos + L, re,* again, *agere,* to act],   any chemical reaction that is stimulated by the influence of light.

**photoreceptor** /-risep′tər/ [Gk, *phos,* light; L, *recipere,* to receive],   a nerve cell that is receptive to light stimuli.

**photorefractive keratectomy (PRK)** /-refrak′tiv/,   a surgical procedure in which an excimer laser is used to reshape the human cornea to improve the refractive properties of the eye and reduce or eliminate the need for eye glasses. The excimer laser does not require that incisions be made in the cornea. Rather than cutting, the laser shaves off preprogrammed outer layers of corneal tissue. The excimer laser is programmed to emit a measured and concentrated light beam to reshape a small part of the central cornea. It allows for correction of myopia of up to −10.0 diopters. See also **refractive keratotomy.** Compare **radial keratotomy.**

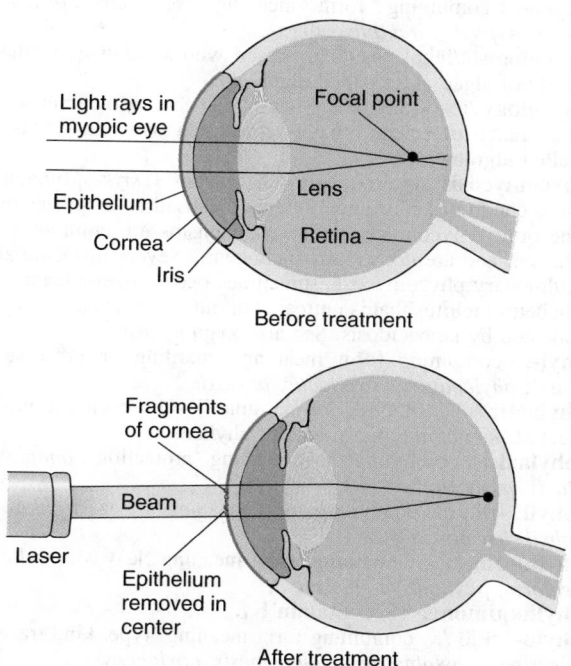

**Photorefractive keratectomy** *(Beare and Myers, 1998)*

**photoscan** /fō′tōskan′/,   a radiograph that shows the distribution of a radiopharmaceutical in the body.

**photosensitive** /-sen′sitiv/ [Gk, *phos + L, sentire,* to feel], pertaining to increased reactivity of skin to sunlight caused by a disorder, such as albinism or porphyria, or more frequently resulting from the use of certain drugs. Relatively brief exposure to sunlight or to an ultraviolet lamp may cause edema, papules, urticaria, or acute burns in individuals with endogenous or acquired photosensitivity. Drugs inducing photosensitivity include phenothiazine tranquilizers, the antibiotic tetracycline, the antimycotic griseofulvin, the antibacterial nalidixic acid, oral hypoglycemic agents, the artificial sweetener calcium cyclamate, the oral contraceptive agents mestranol and norethynodrel, and halogenated salicylamides used in antifungal soaps. Treatment involves avoidance of exposure to sunlight or the photosensitizing agent. Methoxsalen and trioxsalen are potent photosensitizers sometimes used to enhance pigmentation or increase tolerance to sunlight, but overexposure or overdosage can cause severe reactions.

**photosensitivity** /-sen′sitiv′itē/,   any abnormal response to exposure to light, specifically, a skin reaction requiring the presence of a sensitizing agent and exposure to sunlight or its equivalent. Photosensitivity includes photoallergic and phototoxic reactions and is common in systemic lupus erythematosus.

**photosensitization** /-sen′sitīzā′shən/ [Gk, *phos,* light; L, *sentire,* to feel],   the process of rendering an organism sensitive to the effects of light.

**photosynthesis** /fōtōsin′thəsis/ [Gk, *phos + synthesis,* putting together],   a process by which plants, algae, and some bacteria containing chlorophyll synthesize organic compounds, chiefly carbohydrates, from atmospheric carbon dioxide and water, using light for energy and liberating oxygen in the process.

**phototherapy** /-ther′əpē/ [Gk, *phos + therapeia* treatment], the treatment of disorders by the use of light, especially ultraviolet light. Ultraviolet light may be used in the therapy of acne, pressure ulcers and other indolent ulcers, psoriasis, and hyperbilirubinemia. Also called **lucotherapy.** See also **photochemotherapy.** —**phototherapeutic,** *adj.*

**phototherapy in the newborn,**   a treatment for hyperbilirubinemia and jaundice in the newborn that involves the exposure of an infant's bare skin to intense fluorescent light. The blue range of light accelerates the excretion of bilirubin in the skin, decomposing it by photooxidation.

■ METHOD: The infant is placed nude under the fluorescent lights with the eyes and genitalia covered. The baby is turned frequently, and the body temperature is monitored, using a skin thermistor. All vital signs are carefully noted, and details regarding position of the bulbs, time and duration of treatment, and the infant's response are charted. Adverse effects of phototherapy include dehydration: An infant may need 25% more fluid during treatment. Loose stools and "bronze baby" syndrome may occur.

■ INTERVENTIONS: The nurse performs phototherapy and may be responsible for collecting specimens for serial tests for bilirubin level in the blood. The lights may scorch the nurse's hair and irritate the eyes; as protection a cap and sunglasses may be worn. Breastfeeding may be discontinued during treatment but often is not; additional water is always given. The family is encouraged to visit and to participate in caring for the infant. They may be told that the eye shields are necessary but do not seem to bother the infant.

■ OUTCOME CRITERIA: Bilirubin levels usually decrease by 3 to 4 mg/dL in the first 8 to 12 hours of therapy; thus simple jaundice clears rapidly. Excess bilirubin and jaundice that are the result of hemolytic disease or infection may be controlled with phototherapy, but the underlying cause is treated separately. Recovery is usually complete. The long-term safety of phototherapy has not been established; short-term efficacy and practicality of use are certain.

**phototherapy: neonate,** a nursing intervention from the Nursing Interventions Classification (NIC) defined as use of light therapy to reduce bilirubin levels in newborn infants. See also **Nursing Interventions Classification.**

**phototoxic** /-tok′sik/ [Gk, *phos* + *toxikon*, poison], characterized by a rapidly developing nonimmunologic reaction of the skin when it is exposed to a photosensitizing substance and light. Compare **photoallergic.** See also **phototoxic contact dermatitis.**

**phototoxic contact dermatitis,** a rapidly appearing, sunburnlike response of areas of skin that have been exposed to the sun after contact with a photosensitizing substance. Hyperpigmentation may follow the acute reaction. Coal tar derivatives, oil of bergamot (often used in cosmetics and beverages), and many plants containing furocoumarin (cowslip, buttercup, carrot, parsnip, mustard, and yarrow) are known photosensitizing materials. Treatment includes Burow's solution, emollient creams such as Acid Mantle, and topical corticosteroids.

**-phragma, -phragm,** combining form meaning a 'septum or musculomembranous barrier between cavities': *inophragma, mesophragma, telophragma, diaphragm.*

**-phrasia,** combining form meaning an 'abnormal condition of speech': *aphrasia, echophrasia, embolophrasia.*

**phren** /fren/ [Gk, mind], **1.** the diaphragm. **2.** the mind.

**phrenetic** /frənet′ik/ [Gk, *phren*], frenzied, delirious, maniacal.

**phreni-, phrenico-, phreno-,** combining form meaning 'mind or the diaphragm': *phrenology, phrenalgia.*

**-phrenia,** combining form meaning a 'disordered condition of mental activity': *hebephrenia, ideophrenia, schizophrenia.*

**phrenic** /fren′ik/ [Gk, *phren*, mind], **1.** pertaining to the diaphragm. **2.** pertaining to the mind.

**-phrenic, 1.** combining form meaning the 'diaphragm or adjacent regions of the body': *costophrenic, postphrenic, subphrenic.* **2.** combining form meaning 'characteristic of a disorder of the mind': *hebephrenic, ideophrenic, schizophrenic.*

**phrenic nerve,** one of a pair of branches of the cervical plexus, arising from the first four cervical nerves and passing to the diaphragm. It contains about half as many sensory as motor fibers and is generally known as the motor nerve to the diaphragm, although the lower thoracic nerves also help innervate the diaphragm. The pleural branches of the phrenic nerve are very fine filaments supplying the mediastinal pleura. The pericardial branches are delicate filaments passing to the upper pericardium. The terminal branches diverge after passing separately through the diaphragm and are distributed on the abdominal surface of the diaphragm. On the right side a branch near the inferior vena cava communicates with the phrenic plexus in association with a phrenic ganglion. There is no phrenic ganglion on the left side. Also called **internal respiratory nerve of Bell.** Compare **accessory phrenic nerve.**

**phrenico-, phreno-.** See **phreni-.**

**phrenology** [Gk, *phren*, mind], the study of the conformation of the skull based on the assumption that mental faculties are localized in particular sites on the surface of the brain. According to phrenologists intelligence or other facul-

ties of a person may be mirrored through elevations in the skull overlying the particular area of the brain.

**PHSP,** abbreviation for **physician health service plan.**

***Phthirus*** /thī′rəs/ [Gk, *phtheir*, louse], a genus of bloodsucking lice that includes the species *Phthirus pubis*, the pubic louse, or crab.

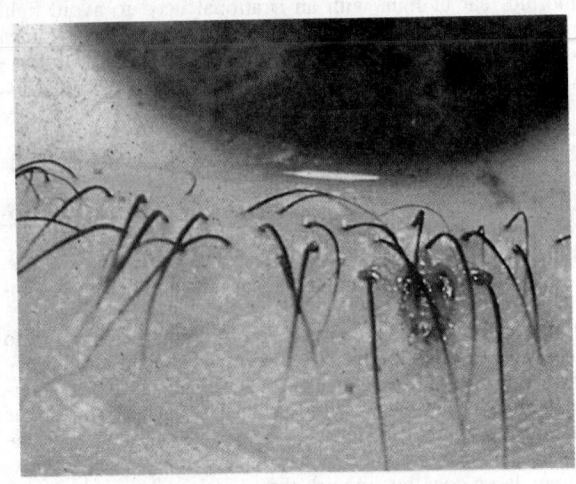

***Phthirus pubis*** (Michelson and Friedlaender, 1996)

**phthisis** /tis′is, thī′sis/ [Gk, *phthisis*, wasting away], any wasting disease involving all or part of the body, such as pulmonary tuberculosis.

**-phthongia,** combining form meaning a 'condition of speech': *aphthongia, diphthongia, heterophthongia.*

**phyco-,** combining form meaning 'seaweed': *phycochrome, phycocyan, phycology.*

**phycologist** /fēkol′əjist/, a person who specializes in the study of algae. Also called **algologist.**

**phycology** /fēkol′əjē/ [Gk, *phykos*, seaweed, *logos*, science], the branch of science that is concerned with algae. Also called **algology.**

**phycomycosis** /fī′kōmīkō′sis/ [Gk, *phykos* + *mykes*, fungus, *osis*, condition], a fungal infection caused by a species of the order Phycomycetes. These organisms are common in the soil and are not usually pathogenic. Severe nosocomial pulmonary phycomycosis sometimes occurs with advanced diabetes mellitus that is untreated or out of control and complicated by ketoacidosis. See also **zygomycosis.**

**phyl-,** combining form meaning 'guarding or preservation': *phylacagogic, phylactic, phylaxis.*

**phylactic** /filak′tik/ [Gk, *phylax*, guard], **1.** serving to protect. **2.** something that produces phylaxis.

**-phylaxis,** combining form meaning 'protection': *anaphylaxis, prophylaxis.*

**-phyll, -phyl,** combining form meaning a 'leaf': *chlorophyll, leukophyll.*

**phyllo-** /fil′ō-/, combining form meaning 'leaves': *phyllochlorin, phyllode, phyllosan.*

**phylloquinone.** See **vitamin K₁.**

**phylo-** /fī′lō-/, combining form meaning 'type, kind, race, or tribe': *phylobiology, phylogenesis, phylogeny.*

**phylogenesis.** See **phylogeny.**

**phylogenetic** /fī′lōjənet′ik/ [Gk, *phylon*, tribe, *genesis*, origin], **1.** relating to or acquired during phylogeny. **2.** based on a natural evolutionary relationship, such as a system of classification. Also called **phylogenic.**

**phylogeny** /fīloj′ənē/ [Gk, *phylon* + *genesis*], the development of the structure of a particular race or species as it evolved from earlier forms of life. Also called **phylogenesis.** Compare **ontogeny.** See also **comparative anatomy.**

**phylum** /fī′ləm/ [Gk, *phylon*, tribe], a major subdivision of a kingdom of organisms, representing one or more classes.

**-phyma,** combining form meaning a 'swelling or tumor': *adenophyma, celiophyma, onychophyma.*

**physi-.** See **physio-.**

**physiatrics.** See **physiatry.**

**physiatrist** /fiz′ē·at′rist/, a physician specializing in physical medicine and rehabilitation who has been certified by the American Board of Physical Medicine and Rehabilitation after completing residency and other requirements.

**physiatry** /fizī′ətrē/, the branch of medicine that deals with the prevention, diagnosis, and treatment of disease or injury, and the rehabilitation from resultant impairments and disabilities, using physical agents such as light, heat, cold, water, electricity, therapeutic exercise, and mechanical apparatus, and sometimes pharmaceutical agents. Also called **physiatrics, physical medicine.**

**-physical,** combining form meaning 'natural': *iatrophysical, medicophysical, psychophysical.*

**physical abuse** /fiz′ikəl/ [Gk, *physikos,* natural; L, *abuti,* to abuse], one or more episodes of aggressive behavior, usually resulting in physical injury with possible damage to internal organs, sense organs, the central nervous system, or the musculoskeletal system of another person.

**physical aging status,** a nursing outcome from the Nursing Outcomes Classification (NOC) defined as the physical changes that commonly occur with adult aging. See also **Nursing Outcomes Classification.**

**physical allergy,** a hypersensitive reaction to physical factors, such as cold, heat, light, or trauma. Common characteristics include pruritus, urticaria, and angioedema. Usually specific antibodies are found in people having physical allergies. Photosensitivity may be caused by the use of certain cosmetics or drugs. Prophylaxis typically includes an attempt to remove the stimulus, and treatment involves the use of antihistamines or steroids. Compare **contact dermatitis.** See also **atopic dermatitis.**

**physical assessment,** the part of the health assessment representing a synthesis of the information obtained in a physical examination. It involves the detailed examination of the body from head to toe using the techniques of observation/inspection, palpation, percussion, and auscultation.

**physical chemistry,** the natural science dealing with the relationship between chemical and physical properties of matter.

**physical dependence,** substance dependence in which there is evidence of tolerance, withdrawal, or both.

**physical diagnosis,** the diagnostic process accomplished by the study of the physical manifestations of health, disease, and illness revealed in the physical examination, as guided by the patient's complete history and supported by various laboratory tests. Physical diagnosis is to medicine what the health assessment is to nursing.

**physical examination,** an investigation of the body to determine its state of health, using any or all of the techniques of inspection, palpation, percussion, auscultation, and smell. The physical examination, history, and initial laboratory tests constitute the data base on which a diagnosis is made and on which a plan of treatment is developed.

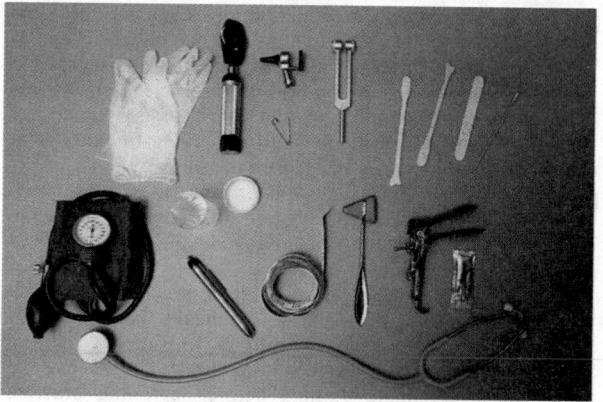

**Equipment used during a physical examination**
*(Potter and Perry, 2001)*

**physical fitness**[1], the ability to carry out daily tasks with alertness and vigor, without undue fatigue, and with enough energy reserve to meet emergencies or to enjoy leisure time pursuits.

**physical fitness**[2], a nursing outcome from the Nursing Outcomes Classification (NOC) defined as the ability to perform physical activities with vigor. See also **Nursing Outcomes Classification.**

**physical maturation: female,** a nursing outcome from the Nursing Outcomes Classification (NOC) defined as the normal physical changes in the female that occur with the transition from childhood to adulthood. See also **Nursing Outcomes Classification.**

**physical maturation: male,** a nursing outcome from the Nursing Outcomes Classification (NOC) defined as the normal physical changes in the male that occur with the transition from childhood to adulthood. See also **Nursing Outcomes Classification.**

**physical medicine.** See **physiatry.**

**physical restraint,** a nursing intervention from the Nursing Interventions Classification (NIC) defined as application, monitoring, and removal of mechanical restraining devices or manual restraints which are used to limit physical mobility of patient. See also **Nursing Interventions Classification.**

**physical science,** the study of the properties and behavior of nonliving matter. Some kinds of physical science are **chemistry,** geology, and **physics.** Compare **life science.**

**physical sign** [Gk, *physikos,* natural; L, *signum*], an objective indicator found during physical diagnosis or detected by inspection, palpation, percussion, or auscultation.

**physical therapist,** a person who is licensed in the examination, evaluation, and treatment of physical impairments through the use of special exercise, application of heat or cold, and other physical modalities. The goal is to assist persons who are physically challenged to maximize independence and improve mobility, self-care, and other functional skill necessary for daily living. A physical therapist becomes qualified by studying a 4 to 7 year college curriculum leading to a bachelor's or master's degree in physical therapy (usually B.S., M.S., or M.P.T.).

**physical therapist assistant,** a person who, under the supervision of a physical therapist, assists in carrying out patient treatment programs.

**physical therapy,** the treatment of disorders with physical agents and methods, such as massage, manipulation, therapeutic exercises, cold, heat (including paraffin, shortwave and microwave diathermy and ultrasonic heat), hydrotherapy, electrical stimulation, and light to assist in habilitating or rehabilitating patients and in restoring function after an illness or injury. Also called **physiotherapy.**

**physician** /fizish′ən/ [Gk, *physikos*, natural], a health professional who has earned a degree of Doctor of Medicine (M.D.) after completing an approved course of study at an approved medical school. Satisfactory completion of National Board Examinations, usually given during both the second and the final years of medical school and after graduation, is also required. An M.D. usually enters a hospital internship or residency program for at least 2 years of postgraduate training before beginning practice or further training in a specialty. To practice medicine, an M.D. is required to obtain a license from the state in which professional services will be performed. See also **osteopath.**

**physician assistant (PA),** a person academically and clinically prepared to practice medicine under the supervision of a licensed doctor of medicine or osteopathy. Within the physician/PA relationship, PAs exercise autonomy in medical decisions and provide a wide range of diagnostic and therapeutic services. Training programs average 25 to 27 months. National certification is available to graduates of approved training programs.

**physician extender,** a health care provider who is not a physician but who performs medical activities typically performed by a physician. It is most commonly a nurse practitioner or physician assistant.

**physician health service plan,** (in the United States) a general term relating to an arrangement for provision of professional (physician) services only.

**physician-hospital organization (PHO),** (in the United States) a management service organization in which the partners are physicians and a hospital. The PHO organization contracts for physician and hospital services.

*Physician's Desk Reference (PDR),* a compendium compiled annually, containing information about drugs, primarily prescription drugs and products used in diagnostic procedures in the United States, supplied by their manufacturers.

**physician support,** a nursing intervention from the Nursing Interventions Classification (NIC) defined as collaborating with physicians to provide quality patient care. See also **Nursing Interventions Classification.**

**physicist** /fis′isist/, a scientist who specializes in physics.

**physico-** combining form meaning 'natural or knowledge of nature': *physical, physiology.*

**physics** /fiz′iks/ [Gk, *physikos*, natural], the study of matter and energy, particularly as related to motion and force.

**-physics,** combining form meaning the 'science of the nature of': *cytophysics, medicophysics, microphysics.*

**physio-, physi-,** combining form meaning 'related to nature or to physiology': *physiochemical, physiognosis, physiotherapy.*

**physiognomy** /fiz′ē·og′nəmē/ [Gk, *physis*, nature, *gnosis*, knowledge], a method of judging the personality and other characteristics of a client by studying the face and general carriage of the body.

**physiologic** /fiz′ē·əloj′ik/ [Gk, *physis*, nature, *logos*, science], pertaining to physiology, particularly normal functions as opposed to the pathologic.

**physiologic age** [Gk, *physis*, nature, *logos*, science; L, *aetas*, age], the age of the body as determined by its stage of development in terms of functional norms for various systems.

**physiologic albuminuria** [Gk, *physis*, nature, *logos*, science; L, *albus*, white; Gk, *ouron*, urine], the presence of albumin in the urine in the absence of any disease.

**physiologic amenorrhea** [Gk, *physis*, nature, *logos*, science, *a* + *men*, month, *rhoia*, to flow], an absence of menstruation having a nonpathologic cause, such as pregnancy, lactation, menopause, or a prepubertal state of maturity.

**physiologic antidote** [Gk, *physis* + *logos* + *anti*, against, *dotos*, that which is given], a drug that has the opposite effect on the body from that caused by a poisonous or toxic substance.

**physiologic chemistry.** See **biochemistry.**

**physiologic contracture** [Gk, *physis* + *logos*, science; L, *contractio*, drawing together], a temporary condition in which muscles may contract and shorten for a considerable period. Drugs, temperature extremes, and local accumulation of lactic acid are possible causes.

**physiologic dead space.** See **dead space.**

**physiologic dwarf.** See **primordial dwarf.**

**physiologic flexion,** an excessive amount of flexor tone that is normally present at birth because of the existing level of central nervous system maturation and fetal positioning in the uterus.

**physiologic fourth heart sound.** See $S_4$.

**physiologic hypertrophy,** a temporary increase in the size of an organ or part caused by normal physiologic functions, such as occurs in the walls of the uterus and in the breasts during pregnancy.

**physiologic incompatibility,** a condition in which substances, such as drugs, may have mutually antagonistic effects on the body.

**physiologic jaundice** [Gk, *physis*, nature, *logos*, science; Fr, *jaune*, yellow], a simple jaundice of newborns that involves the breaking down of the excessive number of red blood cells that may be present at birth.

**physiologic motivation,** a body need, such as for food or water, that initiates behavior directed toward satisfying the particular need. Also called **organic motivation.** Compare **social motivation.**

**physiologic murmur.** See **functional murmur.**

**physiologic occlusion,** 1. a closure of the teeth that complements and enhances the functions of the masticatory system. 2. a closure of the teeth that produces no pathologic effects on the stomatognathic system, normally dissipating the stresses placed on the teeth and creating a balance between the stresses and the adaptive capacity of the supporting tissues. 3. an acceptable occlusion in a healthy gnathic system.

**physiologic psychology,** the study of the interrelationship of physiologic and psychologic processes, especially the effects of a change from normal to abnormal.

**physiologic retraction ring,** a ridge around the inside of the uterus that forms during the second stage of normal labor at the junction of the thinned lower uterine segment and thickened upper segment. It forms as a result of progressive lengthening of the muscle fibers of the lower segment and concomitant shortening of the muscle fibers of the upper segment. Compare **constriction ring, pathologic retraction ring.**

**physiologic saline.** See **saline solution.**

**physiologic salt solution,** a normal saline solution, usually consisting of a sterile 0.9% w/v solution of sodium chloride in distilled water. It is isotonic with normal body fluids.

**physiologic third heart sound.** See $S_3$.

**physiologic tremor** [Gk, *physis* + *logos*; L, *tremor,* shaking], any shaking or trembling caused by physiologic factors, such as fatigue, fear, or cold.

**physiologist** /fiz′ē·ol′əjist/ [Gk, *physis*, nature, *logos*, science], a person who specializes in the science of living organisms.

**physiology** /fiz′ē·ol′əjē/ [Gk, *physis* + *logos*, science], **1.** the study of the processes and function of the human body. **2.** the study of the physical and chemical processes involved in the functioning of organisms and their parts. Kinds of physiology include **comparative physiology, developmental physiology, hominal physiology,** and **pathologic physiology.** Compare **anatomy.**

**physiopathologic** /fiz′ē·əpath′əloj′ik/ [Gk, *physis*, nature, *pathos*, disease, *logos*, science], pertaining to the physiologic approach to disease.

**physiotherapy.** See **physical therapy.**

**physique** /fizēk′/, the body structure and development of a person.

**-physis,** combining form meaning a 'growth or growing': *metaphysis, onychophysis, zygapophysis.*

**physo-,** combining form meaning 'air or gas': *physocele, physocephaly, physometra.*

**physostigmine salicylate,** an anticholinergic drug antidote.

■ INDICATIONS: It is prescribed in the treatment of central nervous system effects caused by drugs in clinical or toxic dosages capable of producing anticholinergic poisoning.

■ CONTRAINDICATIONS: Asthma, gangrene, diabetes, cardiovascular disease, or mechanical obstruction of the intestines or urinary tract prohibits its use. It is also not administered to patients in any vagotonic state and to those receiving choline esters or depolarizing neuromuscular blocking agents.

■ ADVERSE EFFECTS: Among the most serious adverse reactions are hypersalivation, bradycardia, convulsions, and hypertensive reactions.

**phytanic acid storage disease** /fītan′ik/, a rare genetic disorder of lipid metabolism in which phytanic acid accumulates in the plasma and tissues. The condition is characterized by ataxia, peripheral neuropathy, retinitis pigmentosa, and abnormalities of the bone and skin. Also called **Refsum's syndrome.**

**phyte-.** See **phyto-.**

**-phyte,** combining form meaning a 'plant that grows in or on or produces': *epiphyte, paraphyte, pteridophyte.*

**phyto-, phyt-,** combining form meaning 'plant or plants': *phytobezoar, phytochemistry, phytoncide.*

**phytogenesis** /fī′tōjen′əsis/ [Gk, *phyton*, plant, *genein*, to produce], the origin and evolution of algae and plants.

**phytogenous** /fītoj′ənəs/ [Gk, *phyton*, plant, *genein*, to produce], produced by or originating in algae or plants; pertaining to phytogenesis.

**phytohemagglutinin (PHA)** /fī′tōhem′əgloo′tinin/ [Gk, *phyton*, plant, *haima*, blood; L, *agglutinare*, to glue], a hemagglutinin that is derived from a plant, specifically the lectin obtained from the red kidney bean. Also called **phytolectin.**

**phytohemagglutinin test,** a test to identify genetic carriers of cystic fibrosis, performed by exposing white blood cells to phytohemagglutinin. A normal reaction involves a noticeable increase in cell protein. Molecular genetic markers are now available for the diagnosis of cystic fibrosis.

**phytolectin.** See **phytohemagglutinin.**

**phytonadione.** See **vitamin K₁.**

**pi** /pī/, II, π, the sixteenth letter of the Greek alphabet.

**P.I., 1.** (in patient records) abbreviation for *present illness.* **2.** abbreviation for *International Pharmacopeia.*

**pia,** abbreviation for **pia mater.**

**piaarachnoid** /pī′ə·arak′noid/ [L, *pia*, tender; Gk, *arachne*, spider, *eidos*, form], pertaining to both the pia mater and arachnoid layers of the meninges covering the brain and spinal cord.

**Piaget, Jean** /zhän pē·äzhä′/, (1896–1980), a Swiss psychologist and genetic epistemologist who established the Genevan school of developmental psychology. From his original training in zoology and his early work in testing laboratory schoolchildren Piaget developed a premise that human intelligence is an extension of biologic adaptation. He assumed that human intelligence evolves in a series of stages that are related to age. At each successive stage intellectual adaptation is more general and shows a higher level of logical organization.

**piagetian** /pī′äzhe′tē·ən/, pertaining to the theories and viewpoints of **Piaget.**

**pia mater (pia)** /pē′ə mā′tər, pī′ə/ [L, *pia*, tender, *mater*, mother], the innermost of the three meninges covering the brain and the spinal cord. It is closely applied to both structures and carries a rich supply of blood vessels, which nourish the nervous tissue. The cranial pia mater covers the surface of the brain and dips into the fissures and sulci of the cerebral hemispheres. The spinal pia mater is thicker, firmer, and less vascular than the cranial pia mater and consists of two layers. The outer layer is composed of longitudinal collagenous fibers. The inner layer wraps the entire spinal cord and, at the end of the cord, is prolonged into the filum terminale. The pia mater also forms the denticulate ligament, which extends the entire length of the spinal cord on both sides. Compare **arachnoid, dura mater.** See also **meninges.**

**pian.** See **yaws.**

**pian bois.** See **forest yaws.**

**pica** /pī′kə/ [L, *magpie*], a craving to eat nonfood substances, such as dirt, clay, chalk, glue, ice, starch, or hair. The appetite disorder may occur with some nutritional deficiency states (particularly iron deficiency), with pregnancy, and in some forms of mental illness.

**Pick's disease**[1] [Arnold Pick, Czech neurologist, 1851–1924], a form of dementia occurring in middle age. This disorder mainly affects the frontal and temporal lobes of the brain and characteristically produces neurotic behavior; slow disintegration of intellect, personality, and emotions; and degeneration of cognitive abilities. See also **dementia.**

**Pick's disease**[2] [Friedel Pick, Czech physician, 1867–1926], constrictive inflammation of the mediastinum and pericardium, leading to chronic venous congestion and cirrhosis. Also called **Pick's syndrome.**

**pickwickian syndrome** /pikwik′ē·ən/ [*Pickwick Papers* by Charles Dickens], an abnormal condition characterized by obesity, decreased pulmonary function, somnolence, and polycythemia.

**pico-,** combining form meaning 'one trillionth' ($10^{-12}$) of the unit designated: *picogram, picoliter, picometer.*

**picogram (pg)** /pī′kəgram/, a unit of measure equal to one trillionth of a gram, or $10^{-12}$ gram.

**picornavirus** /pīkôr′nəvī′rəs/ [It, *pico*, small; *RNA*, ribonucleic acid; L, *virus*, poison], a member of a group of small ribonucleic acid (RNA) viruses that are ether-resistant. The two main genera are *Enterovirus* and *Rhinovirus.* These viruses cause poliomyelitis, herpangina, aseptic meningitis, encephalomyocarditis, and foot-and-mouth disease.

**picosecond (ps),** a unit of measure equal to one trillionth of a second.

**picro-,** combining form meaning 'bitter': *picroadonidin, picropyrine, picrotoxin.*

**picrotoxin** /pik′rōtok′sin/ [Gk, *pikros*, bitter, *toxikon*, poison], a central nervous system stimulant obtained from the seeds of *Anamirta cocculus,* formerly used as an antidote for acute barbiturate poisoning.

**PID,** abbreviation for **pelvic inflammatory disease.**

**PIE,** abbreviation for **pulmonary infiltrate with eosinophilia.**

**piebald** /pī′bôld/ [L, *pica*, magpie; ME, *balled*, smooth], **1.** having patches of white hair or skin caused by an absence of melanocytes in those nonpigmented areas. It is a hereditary condition. Compare **albinism, vitiligo. 2.** having two colors: black and white or brown and white; mottled. **—piebaldism,** *n.*

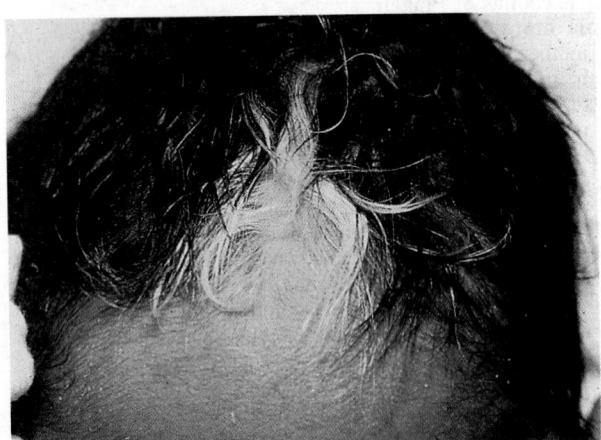

**Piebaldism** *(Zitelli and Davis, 1997)*

**Piedmont fracture** /pēd′mənt/, an oblique break in the distal radius, with fragments of bone pulled into the ulna.

**piedra** /pē·ā′drə/, fungal disease of the hair characterized by the presence of small black or white nodules. Black piedra is caused by *Piedria bortae*. White piedra (called trichosporosis) is caused by *Trichosporon biegetii*. See also **trichosporosis.**

**Pierre Robin's syndrome** /pyerob′inz, pyerōbans′/ [Pierre Robin, French histologist, 1867–1950], a complex of congenital anomalies including a small mandible, cleft lip, cleft palate, other craniofacial abnormalities, and defects of the eyes and ears, including glaucoma. Intelligence is usually normal. Plastic surgery may achieve satisfactory cosmetic repair, but speech therapy, orthodontia, and psychologic counseling and support are often necessary.

**-piesis,** suffix for certain terms relating to pressure.

**piez-,** combining form meaning 'pressure': *piezesthesia, piezallochromy, piezotherapy.*

**piezochemistry** /pī·ē′zōkem′istrē/ [Gk, *piezein*, to press, *chemeia* alchemy], a branch of chemistry concerned with reactions that occur under pressure.

**piezoelectric activity,** the changing electric of surface charges of a structure that force the structure to change shape. Also called **electropiezo activity.**

**piezoelectric effect** /pī·ē′zō·ilek′trik/ [Gk, *piezein*, to press, *elektron* amber; L *effectus*], **1.** the generation of a voltage across a solid when a mechanical stress is applied. **2.** the dimensional change resulting from the application of a voltage. **3.** (in ultrasound) the conversion of one form of energy into another, such as the conversion of electrical energy into mechanical energy.

**pigeon breast** /pij′ən/ [L, *pipio,* young bird; AS, *broest,* breast], a congenital structural defect characterized by a prominent anterior projection of the xiphoid and the lower part of the sternum and by a lengthening of the costal cartilages. It may cause cardiorespiratory complications but rarely warrants surgical correction. **—pigeon-breasted,** *adj.* Also called **pectus carinatum, pigeon chest**

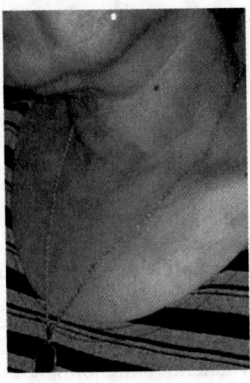

**Pigeon breast** *(Lemmi and Lemmi, 2000)*

**pigeon breeder's lung,** a respiratory disorder caused by acquired hypersensitivity to antigens in bird droppings. It is characterized by chills, fever, and difficult breathing. The symptoms subside when exposure to the allergen ceases. Also called **bird breeder's lung, bird dung lung, hen worker's lung.**

**pigeon chest.** See **pigeon breast.**

**pigeon-toed.** See **metatarsus varus.**

**piggyback port** [AS, *piken*, pick; ME, *pakke*, pack; L, *portus,* haven], a special coupling in the primary IV tubing that allows a supplementary, or piggyback, solution to run into the IV system. The piggyback port includes a back check valve that automatically prevents the primary IV solution from flowing while the piggyback solution is flowing.

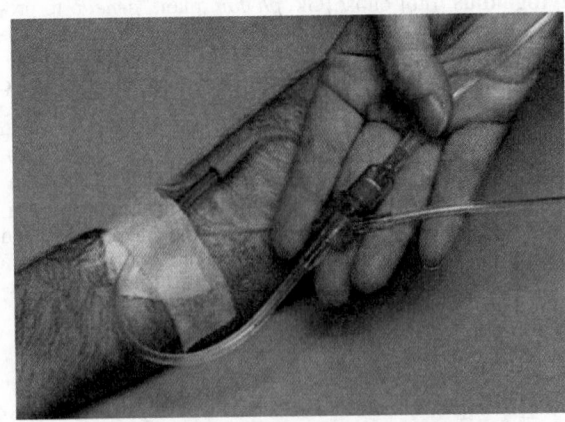

**Piggyback port** *(Potter and Perry, 1993)*

When the piggyback solution stops flowing, the back check valve allows the flow of the primary IV solution. Piggyback ports are part of piggyback IV sets, which are used solely for intermittent drug administration.

**pigment** /pig′mənt/ [L, *pigmentum,* paint], **1.** any organic coloring material produced in the body, such as melanin. **2.** any colored, paintlike medicinal preparation applied to the skin surface. —**pigmentary, pigmented,** *adj.,* **pigmentation,** *n.*

**pigmentary retinopathy** /pig′mənter′ē/, a disorder of the retina characterized by deposits of pigment and increasing loss of vision.

**pigmentation, pigmented.** See **pigment.**

**pigmented villonodular synovitis** /pig′məntid/, a disease of the joints characterized by fingerlike proliferative growths of synovial tissue, with hemosiderin deposition within the synovial tissue. The cause of the disorder is unknown.

**pigment layers,** the parts of the eye comprising the pigmented strata of the ciliary body, iris, and retina.

**pigmy.** See **pygmy.**

**pil,** abbreviation for the Latin words *pilula,* 'pill,' and *pilulae,* 'pills.'

**pilar cyst** /pī′lər/ [L, *pilus,* hair; Gk, *kystis,* bag], an epidermoid cyst of the scalp. Its keratinized contents are firmer and less cheesy than the material in epidermoid cysts found elsewhere. The cyst originates from the middle part of the epithelium of a hair follicle. Treatment is surgical excision. Also called **wen.** Compare **epidermoid cyst.**

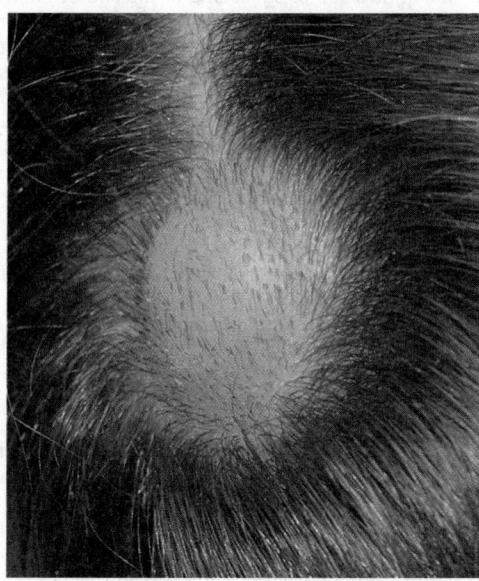

**Pilar cyst** *(Hordinsky, Sawaya, and Scher, 2000)*

**piles.** See **hemorrhoid.**

**pili.** See **pilus.**

**pili annulati** [L, *pilus,* hair + *annulus* ring], a condition in which the individual hairs appear to be marked by alternating bands of white as a result of some barrier in the hair which prevents passage of light and causes the rays to be reflected back, giving the appearance of white bands.

**piliform** /pī′lifôrm/ [L, *pilus,* hair], having the appearance of hair.

**pi lines** /pī/, radiograph artifacts that result from dirt or chemical stains on a processing roller. They occur at intervals of pi (3.14) times the diameter of the roller.

**pill.** See **tablet.**

**pillion fracture** /pil′yən/ [Gael, *pillean,* couch; L, *fractura,* break], a T-shaped break in the distal femur with displacement of the condyles posterior to the femoral shaft, caused by a severe blow to the knee.

**pilo-** /pī′lō-/, combining form meaning 'resembling or composed of hair': *pilocystic, pilomotor, pilose.*

**pilocarpine and epinephrine** /-kär′pēn/, a fixed-combination drug used in the treatment of glaucoma, containing a cholinergic (pilocarpine hydrochloride) and an adrenergic vasoconstrictor (epinephrine bitartrate).

**pilocarpine and physostigmine,** a fixed-combination drug used in the treatment of glaucoma, containing a cholinergic (pilocarpine hydrochloride) and a short-acting cholinesterase inhibitor (physostigmine salicylate). Both ingredients reduce intraocular pressure.

**pilocarpine hydrochloride,** a cholinergic derived from the leaves of the jaborandi tree and other species of *Pilocarpus.* It is used mainly as a miotic to contract the pupil in cases of glaucoma. The drug also increases the secretion of salivary, intestinal, and gastric glands when injected; reduces the heartbeat; and constricts the bronchioles.

**pilomotor reflex** /pī′lōmō′tər/ [L, *pilus,* hair, *motor,* mover, *reflectere,* to bend back], erection of the hairs of the skin caused by contraction of small involuntary arrector muscles (arrectores pilorum) in response to a chilly environment, emotional stimulus, or skin irritation. This normal reaction is abolished below the level of a transverse spinal cord lesion and may be exaggerated on the affected side in a patient with hemiplegia. Also called **gooseflesh, horripilation, piloerection.**

**pilonidal** /pī′lənī′dəl/ [L, *pilus,* hair, *nidus,* nest], a growth of hair in a cyst or other internal structure.

**pilonidal cyst** [L, *pilus + nidus,* nest], a cyst that often develops in the sacral region of the skin. Pilonidal cysts may sometimes be recognized at birth by a depression; sometimes by a hairy dimple in the midline of the back in the sacrococcygeal area. Usually these cysts do not cause any problems, but occasionally a sinus or fistula develops in early adulthood that communicates with the skin, resulting

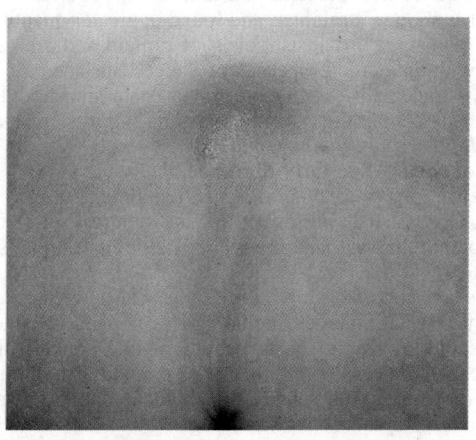

**Pilonidal cyst** *(Zitelli and Davis, 1997)*

in infection. A fistula also may develop to the spinal tract from a pilonidal cyst. If a cyst becomes infected or inflamed, it is excised, and the space is surgically closed after the infection or inflammation has been effectively treated.

**pilonidal fistula,** an abnormal channel containing a tuft of hair, situated most frequently over or close to the tip of the coccyx but also occurring in other regions of the body. Also called **pilonidal sinus.**

**pilonidal sinus** [L, *pilus* + *nidus* + *sinus,* curve], a cavity or sinus containing hair, in a dermoid cyst or the deepest layers of the skin. In most instances the hair originates in another area and becomes lodged in the sinus.

**pilosebaceous** /pī′lōsibā′shəs/ [L, *pilus* + *sebum,* fat], pertaining to a hair follicle and its oil gland.

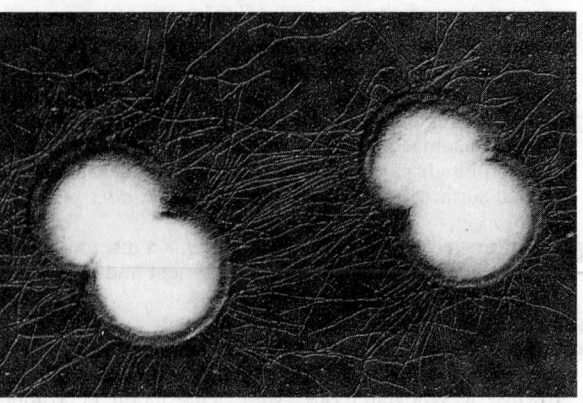

**Pili extending from the surface of *Neisseria gonorrhoeae***
*(Baron, Peterson, and Finegold, 1994/courtesy Chuen-mo To and C.C. Brinton, Jr., University of Pittsburgh)*

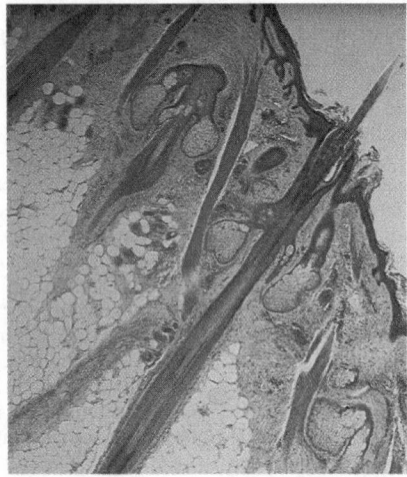

**Pilosebaceous unit in the scalp**
*(du Vivier, 1993/courtesy Dr. J.S. Dixon, University of Manchester)*

**PILOT** /pī′lət/, a computer interpreter language, similar to BASIC, used in computer-assisted instruction.

**pilule.** See **parvule.**

**pilus** /pē′ləs/, *pl.* **pili** [L, hair], **1.** a hair or hairlike structure. **2.** (in microbiology) a fine filamentous appendage found on certain bacteria and similar to flagellum except that it is shorter, straighter, and found in greater quantities in the organism. Pili consist solely of protein and are associated with antigenic properties of the cell surface.

**Pima,** trademark for an expectorant (potassium iodide).

**pimelo-,** combining form meaning 'fat': *pimeloma, pimelopterygium, pimelorrhea.*

**pimelorrhea.** See **fatty diarrhea.**

**pimozide** /pim′əzīd/, an oral neuroleptic agent.

■ INDICATIONS: It is prescribed for the suppression of motor and phonic tics associated with Gilles de la Tourette's syndrome.

■ CONTRAINDICATIONS: The drug may cause electrocardiographic (ECG) changes, including a prolonged QT interval, and should not be given to patients with a congenital prolonged QT interval or a history of cardiac arrhythmias. It also may lower the seizure threshold of patients who are also taking an anticonvulsant drug.

■ ADVERSE EFFECTS: Among the more serious adverse reactions are extrapyramidal effects, persistent tardive dyskine-

sias, sedation, drowsiness, constipation, dry mouth, visual disturbances, and electrocardiograph changes.

**pimple** [ME, *pinple*], a small papule, pustule, or furuncle.

**pin** [AS, *pinn*], **1.** (in orthopedics) to secure and immobilize fragments of bone with a nail. **2.** See **nail,** def. 2. **3.** (in dentistry) a small metal rod or peg, used as a support in rebuilding a tooth.

**pinch,** a compression or squeezing of the end of the thumb in opposition to the end of one or more of the fingers. An example is the **pulp pinch,** a type of grasp in which the pulp, or fleshy mass at the end of the fingers, is pressed against the pulp at the end of the thumb. See also **lateral pinch, palmar pinch, tip pinch.**

**pinch graft** [Fr, *pince* + Gk, *graphion,* stylus], a small circular deep graft of skin only a few millimeters in diameter. It is cut so that the center is of whole skin but the edges consist of only epidermis.

**pinch grip.** See **tip pinch.**

**pinch meter,** a type of dynamometer that measures the strength of a finger pinch.

**pindolol** /pin′dəlol/, a beta-adrenergic blocker with sympathomimetic activity.

■ INDICATIONS: It is prescribed in the treatment of hypertension, alone or concomitantly with a diuretic.

■ CONTRAINDICATIONS: Bronchial asthma, overt cardiac failure, cardiogenic shock, second- and third-degree heart block, or severe bradycardia prohibits its use. It must be used with caution in patients with diabetes.

■ ADVERSE EFFECTS: Among the most serious adverse reactions are bradycardia, hypotension, syncope, tachycardia, aggravation of bronchospasm, and GI disturbances.

**pineal** /pin′ē-əl/ [L, *pineus,* pine cone], **1.** pertaining to the pineal body. **2.** resembling a pine cone.

**pineal body** [L, *pineas,* pine cone; AS, *bodig,* body], a cone-shaped structure in the brain, situated between the superior colliculi, the pulvinar, and the splenicum of the corpus callosum. Its precise function has not been established. It may secrete the hormone melatonin, which appears to inhibit the secretion of luteinizing hormone. Also called **epiphysis cerebri, pineal gland.**

**pinealectomy** /pin′ē-əlek′təmē/ [L, *pineus* + Gk, *ektomē,* excision], the surgical removal of the pineal body.

**pineal gland.** See **pineal body.**

**pineal hyperplasia syndrome,** an abnormal condition caused by overgrowth of the pineal gland. It is characterized by severe insulin resistance, dry skin, thick nails, hirsutism, early dentition, and sexual precocity. Teeth develop prematurely and are malformed. External genitalia may reach adult size by 4 years of age. Ketoacidosis may occur despite high levels of endogenous insulin. Similar abnormalities are associated with some pineal tumors.

**pinealoma** /pin′ē·əlō′mə/, *pl.* **pinealomas, pinealomata** [L, *pineas* + Gk, *oma*, tumor], a rare neoplasm of the pineal body in the brain, characterized by hydrocephalus, pupillary changes, gait disturbances, headache, nausea, and vomiting.

**pineal peduncle** [L, *pineus*, pine cone, *peduncle*, small foot], the stalk of the pineal body.

**pineal tumor,** a neoplasm of the pineal body. See also **pinealoma.**

**pine tar** [L, *pinus*, pine; AS, *teoru*, tar], a topical antieczematic and a rubefacient. It is a common ingredient in creams, soaps, and lotions used in the treatment of chronic skin conditions, such as eczema or psoriasis.

**pinguecula** /ping·gwe′kyoo·lə/ *pl.* **pingueculae** [L, somewhat fatty], a yellowish spot of proliferation on the bulbar conjunctiva near the junction of the sclera and cornea, usually on the nasal side; seen in elderly people.

**pinhole pupil** [ME, *pyn* + *hol* + L, *pupilla*, little girl], a very small pupil, which may be a congenital condition, an effect of the use of miotics, or the result of an inflamed iris.

**pinhole retention** [ME, *pyn* + *hol* + L, *retinere*, to hold], retention developed by drilling one or more holes, 2 to 3 mm in depth, in suitable areas of a cavity preparation to supplement resistance and retention form.

**pinhole test,** **1.** a test performed on a person who has diminished visual acuity to distinguish a refractive error from organic disease. A refractive error may be corrected with glasses, whereas organic disease may signal the development of preventable blindness. Several pinholes, 0.5 to 2 mm in diameter, are punched in a card; the patient selects one and looks through it with one eye at a time, without wearing corrective lenses. If visual acuity is improved, the defect is refractive; if not, it is organic. The pinhole effect results from blocking peripheral light waves, which are most distorted by refractive error. **2.** a test to determine the size of the focal spot of an x-ray tube. **3.** a test to trace the path of x-ray tube movement.

**Pin-Index Safety System (PISS),** a system for identifying connectors for certain small cylinders of medical gases that have flush valve outlets rather than threaded outlets. The identifying code consists of a specific combination of two holes in the face of the valve into which connecting pins for a particular type of gas must fit in perfect alignment. For example, the index hole position for a cylinder of oxygen is 2-5, for nitrous oxide it is 3-5, and so on. See also **Diameter-Index Safety System.**

**pink disease.** See **acrodynia.**

**pinkeye.** See **conjunctivitis.**

**Pinkus' disease.** See **lichen nitidus.**

**pinna.** See **auricle.**

**pinocyte** /pī′nəsīt′/ [Gk, *pinein*, to drink, *kytos,* cell], a cell that can absorb liquids by pinocytosis. —**pinocytic,** *adj.*

**pinocytosis** /pī′nōsītō′sis/ [Gk, *pinein* + *kytos* + *osis*, condition], the process by which extracellular fluid is taken into a cell. The plasma membrane develops a saccular indentation filled with extracellular fluid and then pinches off the indentation, forming a vesicle or vacuole of fluid within the cell.

**pinprick test,** a test of a person's ability to detect a cutaneous pain sensation and to differentiate such sensations from

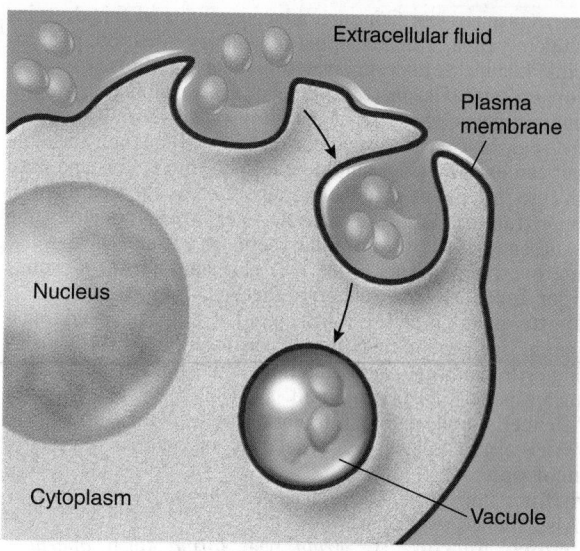

**Pinocytosis**
*(Raven and Johnson, 1992/Christy Krames; by permission of the McGraw-Hill Companies)*

pressure stimuli. The test is performed with a pin or needle gently applied to a skin area where it cannot be observed by the subject. The application of the pin or needle is alternated with the pressing of a dull object against the skin. Care is taken to prevent penetration of the dermis, and the sharp object used should be sterilized or discarded after the test.

**pinta** /pēn′tə/ [Sp, spot], an infection of the skin caused by *Treponema carateum,* a common organism in South and Central America. The bacterium gains entry into the body through a break in the skin. Prolonged exposure and close contact appear to be necessary for transmission. The primary lesion is a slowly enlarging papule with regional lymph node enlargement, followed in 1 to 12 months by a generalized red to slate-blue macular rash. Eventually these lesions become depigmented. Diagnosis is based on serologic tests and dark-field microscopic examination of scrapings from skin lesions. Treatment with penicillin G is effective. Also called **azula, carate, mal del pinto.** Compare **yaws.**

**pin track infection** [ME, *pyn* + *trak,* trace; L, *inficere,* to taint], an abnormal condition associated with skeletal traction and characterized by infection of superficial, deeper, or soft tissues or by osteomyelitis. These infections may develop at skeletal traction pin sites. Some of the signs of pin track infection are erythema at the pin sites, drainage and odor, pin slippage, elevated temperature, and pain. Superficial infection at the pin site is treated with antibiotics administered topically or orally. Deeper infection at the pin sites usually requires removal of the pins and antibiotic therapy.

**pinworm.** See *Enterobius vermicularis.*

**pio-,** combining form meaning 'fat': *pionemia, piorthopnea, pioscope.*

**$PIO_2$,** symbol for *partial pressure of inspired oxygen.*

**pioglitazone,** an oral antidiabetic.

■ INDICATIONS: Pioglitazone is used to treat stable type 2 diabetes mellitus.

■ CONTRAINDICATIONS: Lactation, diabetic ketoacidosis, and known hypersensitivity to this drug prohibit its use. Pioglitazone is also contraindicated in children.

**ADVERSE EFFECTS:** Common adverse effects of this drug include myalgia, sinusitis, upper respiratory infection, pharyngitis, headache, and aggravated diabetes mellitus.

**pion** /pī'onz/ [Gk, *pi*, 16th letter of Greek alphabet, *meson*, nuclear particle], any of a family of subatomic particles that can be created in nuclear reactions. Pions are unstable but can exist long enough to be formed into beams and used in certain types of medical therapy, such as the treatment of brain tumors. Pions of suitable energy can penetrate the skull and deliver most of their energy to a tumor while sparing overlying normal tissue. See also **negative pi meson.**

**Piper forceps.** See **obstetric forceps.**

**pipette** /pīpet', pipet'/ [Fr, little pipe], **1.** a calibrated transparent open-ended tube of glass or plastic used for measuring or transferring small quantities of a liquid or gas. **2.** use of a pipette to dispense liquid.

**Pipracel,** trademark for an antibiotic (piperacillin).

**piracetam,** orphan drug used for myoclonus. See also **nootropic.**

**piriform** /pir'ifôrm/ [L, *pirum*, pear, *forma*], pear-shaped. Also spelled **pyriform.**

**piriform aperture** [L, *pirum*, pear, *forma*, form, *apertura*, opening], the pear-shaped anterior nasal opening in the skull.

**piriformis** /pir'ifôr'mis/ [L, *pirum* + *forma*], a flat pyramidal muscle lying almost parallel with the posterior margin of the gluteus medius. It is partly within the pelvis and partly at the back of the hip joint. It is innervated by branches of the first and second sacral nerves and functions to rotate the thigh laterally and to abduct and to help extend it. Compare **obturator externus, obturator internus.**

**Pirogoff's amputation** [Nikolai I. Pirogoff, Russian surgeon, 1810–1881], an ankle joint amputation in which the posterior process of the calcaneum is retained at the skin flap and opposed to the cut end of the tibia.

**Pirquet's test** /pirkāz'/ [Clemens P. von Pirquet, Austrian physician, 1874–1929], a tuberculin skin test that consists of scratching the tuberculin material onto the skin. Also called **von Pirquet's test.** See also **tuberculin test.**

**pisiform** /pī'sifôrm, pē'-/ [L, *pisum*, pea, *forma*], pea-shaped.

**pisiform bone** [L, *pisa*, pea, *forma*, form; AS, *ban*, bone], a small pea-shaped spheroidal carpal bone in the proximal row of carpal bones. It articulates with the triangular bone and is attached to the flexor retinaculum, the flexor carpi ulnaris, and the abductor digiti minimi.

**Piskacek's sign** /pis'kə·cheks'/ [Ludwig Piskacek, Austrian obstetrician, 1854−1933], asymmetrical enlargement of the body of the pregnant uterus as a result of its enlargement in the cornual region, usually over the site of implantation.

**PISS,** abbreviation for **Pin-Index Safety System.**

**pistol-shot sound,** a sharp slapping sound heard by auscultation over the femoral pulse of a patient with aortic incompetence. It is caused by a large-volume pulse with a sharp rise in pressure.

**pit and fissure cavity** [AS, *pytt* + L, *fissura*, cleft, *cavum*, cavity], a cavity that starts in a tiny fault in tooth enamel, usually on an occlusal surface of a molar or premolar. In the classification of caries, it represents class I caries.

**pit and fissure sealant.** See **dental sealant.**

**pitch** [ME, *picchen*], the quality of a tone or sound dependent on the perception of the relative rapidity of the vibrations by which it is produced.

**pithing** /pith'ing/ [AS, *pitha*], the destruction of the central nervous system of an experimental animal in preparation for physiologic research. It is usually done by inserting a blunt probe through a foramen.

**Pitocin,** trademark for an oxytocic (oxytocin).

**Pitressin,** trademark for an antidiuretic hormone (vasopressin).

**pitting** [AS, *pytt*], **1.** small, punctate indentations in fingernails or toenails, often a result of psoriasis. **2.** an indentation that remains for a short time after pressing edematous skin with a finger. **3.** small depressed scars in the skin or other organ of the body. **4.** the removal by the spleen of material from within erythrocytes without damage to the cells.

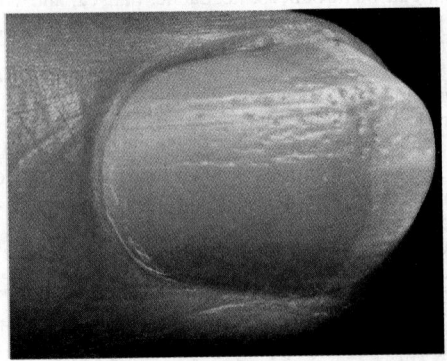

**Pitting of the fingernails** *(du Vivier, 1993)*

**pitting edema** [AS, *pytt* + Gk, *oidema*, swelling], an edema characterized by a condition in which a finger pressed into the skin over an accumulation of fluid will result in a temporary depression in the skin; normal skin and subcutaneous tissues quickly rebound when the pressure is released.

**pituicyte** /pit(y)oo'isīt/ [L, *pituita*, phlegm; Gk, *kytos*, cell], a primary cell of the posterior lobe of the pituitary gland.

**pituit-,** combining form meaning 'phlegm': *pituita, pituitary, pituitous.*

**pituitarism** /pit(y)oo'itəriz'əm/ [L, *pituita*, phlegm], any condition caused by a defect or failure of the pituitary gland.

**pituitary,** /pit(y)oo'iter'ē/ pertaining to the pituitary gland.

**pituitary adamantinoma.** See **craniopharyngioma.**

**pituitary cachexia.** See **panhypopituitarism, postpubertal panhypopituitarism.**

**pituitary dwarf** [L, *pituita*, phlegm; AS, *dweorge*], a dwarf whose retarded development is caused by a deficiency of growth hormone resulting from hypofunction of the anterior lobe of the pituitary. In most cases the cause is unknown and the defect is limited to a lack of somatotropin, although in some instances gonadotropins, adrenocorticotropic hormone, and thyroid stimulating hormone also may be deficient. The body is properly proportioned, with no facial or skeletal deformities, and mental and sexual development is normal. The condition is usually diagnosed in childhood by radiographic examination of the bones and radioimmunoassay of levels of plasma growth hormone. Also called **hypophyseal dwarf, Lévi-Lorain dwarf, Paltauf's dwarf.**

**pituitary eunuchism,** a form of impotence resulting from disease or dysfunction of the pituitary gland.

**pituitary gland** [L, *pituita*, phlegm], an endocrine gland suspended beneath the brain in the pituitary fossa of the sphenoid bone, supplying numerous hormones that govern many vital processes. It is divided into an anterior adenohypophysis and a smaller posterior neurohypophysis. The anterior lobe of the gland is composed of polygonal cells related to the production of seven hormones. The hormones, controlled by hypothalamic releasing factors, include growth hormone (somatotropin), prolactin, thyroid stimulating hormone, follicle stimulating hormone, luteinizing hormone, adrenocorticotropic hormone, and melanocyte stimulating hormone. The posterior lobe is morphologically an extension of the hypothalamus and the source of vasopressin (antidiuretic hormone) and oxytocin. Vasopressin inhibits diuresis by promoting nephron water reabsorption and raises blood pressure. Oxytocin stimulates the contraction of smooth muscle, especially in the uterus. Also called **hypophysis, hypophysis cerebri, infundibulum.** See also **adenohypophysis, neurohypophysis.**

**pituitary myxedema** [L, *pituita* + Gk, *myxa,* mucus, *oidema,* swelling], a type of hypothyroid condition secondary to an anterior pituitary disease.

**pituitary nanism,** a type of dwarfism associated with hypophyseal infantilism. See also **pituitary dwarf.**

**pituitary snuff lung,** a type of hypersensitivity pneumonitis that sometimes occurs among users of pituitary snuff. The antigens to which the hypersensitivity reaction occurs are found in serum proteins of cows and pigs and in pituitary tissue. Symptoms of the acute form of the disease include chills, cough, fever, dyspnea, anorexia, nausea, and vomiting. The chronic form of the disease is characterized by fatigue, chronic cough, weight loss, and dyspnea on exercise. Also called **pituitary snuff takers' disease.**

**pituitary stalk,** a structure that connects the pituitary gland with the hypothalamus.

**pit viper** [AS, *pytt* + L, *vipera,* snake], any one of a family of venomous snakes found in the Western Hemisphere and Asia, characterized by a heat-sensitive pit between the eye and nostril on each side of the head and hollow perforated fangs that are usually folded back in the roof of the mouth. With the exception of coral snakes, all indigenous poisonous snakes in the United States are pit vipers. See also **copperhead, cottonmouth, rattlesnake.**

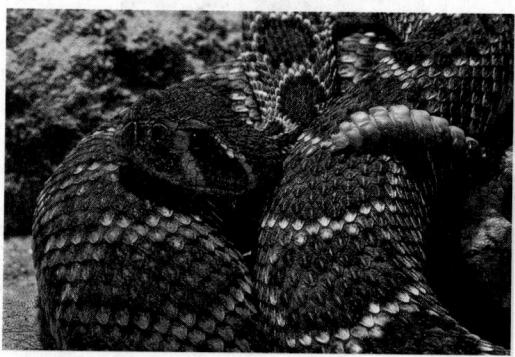

**Pit viper** *(Sanders et al, 2000/courtesy St. Louis Zoo)*

**pityriasis** /pitərī′əsis/ [Gk, *pityron,* bran], any of a number of skin diseases that have in common lesions that resemble dandrufflike scales without obvious signs of inflammation.

**pityriasis alba** [Gk, *pityron,* bran; L, *albus,* white], a common idiopathic dermatosis characterized by round or oval finely scaling patches of hypopigmentation, usually on the cheeks. The lesions are sharply demarcated and occasionally

pruritic and are found primarily in children and adolescents. The condition may recur, but spontaneous clearing is the usual prognosis. Treatment includes lubricating creams, topical corticosteroids, and less commonly coal tar creams. Compare **pityriasis rosea.**

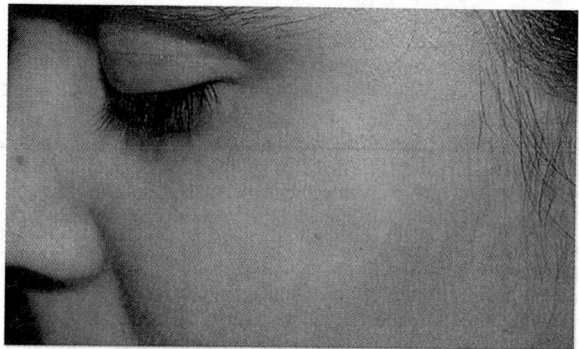

**Pityriasis alba** *(White, 1994)*

**pityriasis lichenoides et varioliformis acuta.** See **Mucha-Habermann disease.**

**pityriasis nigra.** See **tinea nigra.**

**pityriasis rosea,** a self-limited skin disease in which a slightly scaling pink macular rash spreads over the trunk and other unexposed areas of the body. A characteristic feature is the **herald patch,** a larger, more scaly lesion that precedes

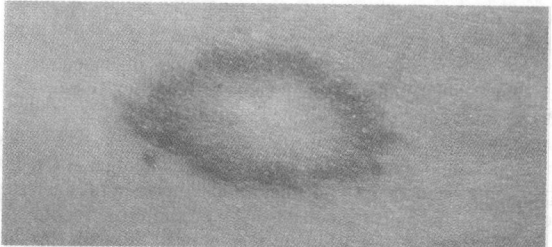

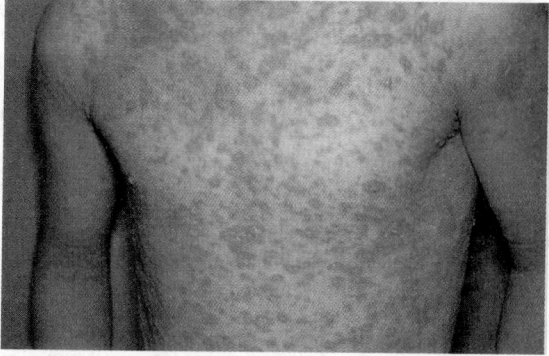

**Pityriasis rosea: herald patch *(top)* and macular rash *(bottom)*** *(Cohen, 1993)*

the diffuse rash by several days. The smaller lesions tend to line up with the long axis parallel to normal lines of cleavage of the skin. Mild itching is the only symptom. The disease lasts 4 to 8 weeks and rarely recurs. It is unusual and apparently not contagious. The cause is herpes virus hominis. Compare **pityriasis alba.**

**pityriasis rubra pilaris** [Gk, *pityron,* bran; L, *ruber* red, *pilus,* hair], a chronic inflammatory cutaneous disease characterized by tiny acuminate, reddish brown follicular papules topped by central horny plugs in which are embedded hairs; disseminated yellowish pink scaling patches; and often solid confluent hyperkeratosis of the palms and soles with a tendency to fissuring.

**Pityrosporum.** See **Malassezia.**

**pivot joint** /piv'ət/ [Fr, hinge; L, *jungere,* to join], a synovial joint in which movement is limited to rotation. The joint is formed by a pivotlike process that may turn within a ring composed partly of bone and partly of ligament. The proximal radioulnar articulation is a pivot joint in which the head of the radius rotates within the ring formed by the radial notch of the ulna and the annular ligament. Also called **trochoid joint.** Compare **ball-and-socket joint, condyloid joint, gliding joint, hinge joint, saddle joint.**

**pivot transfer,** the movement of a person from one site to another, such as from a bed to a wheelchair, when there is a loss of control of one side of the body or one side of the body is immobile. The person is helped to a position on the strong side of the body, either left or right, with both feet on the floor, heels behind the knees, and knees lower than the hips. The person stands with the weight on the strong leg, pivots on it, and carefully lowers the body into the wheelchair.

**pixels,** abbreviation for *picture elements,* small cells of information that make up the matrix of a digital image on a computer monitor screen.

**PJC,** abbreviation for *premature junctional complex.*

**PK,** abbreviation for **psychokinesis.**

**pK$_a$,** the negative logarithm of the ionization constant of an acid. A measure of the strength of an acid.

**PKA,** abbreviation for **protein kinase.**

**PKD,** abbreviation for **polycystic kidney disease.**

**PK test,** abbreviation for **Prausnitz-Küstner test.**

**PKU,** abbreviation for **phenylketonuria.**

**placebo** /pləsē'bō/ [L, shall please], an inactive substance, such as saline solution, distilled water, or sugar, or a less than effective dose of a harmless substance, such as a water-soluble vitamin, prescribed as if it were an effective dose of a needed medication. Placebos are used in experimental drug studies to compare the effects of the inactive substance with those of the experimental drug. They are also prescribed for patients who cannot be given the medication they request or who, in the judgment of the health care provider, do not need that medication.

**placebo effect,** a physical or emotional change occurring after a substance is taken or administered that is not the result of any special property of the substance. The change may be beneficial, reflecting the expectations of the patient and often those of the person giving the substance.

**placement** /plās'mənt/ [Fr, *placer,* to place], the positioning of a dental prosthesis, such as a removable denture in its planned site on the dental arch.

**placement path,** the direction of insertion and removal of a removable partial denture on its supporting oral structures. The path can be varied by altering the plane to which the guiding abutment surfaces of the denture are made parallel. The choice of a placement path is considered a compromise that best fulfills five requirements: minimal torque on abut-

ment teeth, minimal interference, maximum retention, establishment of adequate guide plane surfaces, and acceptable aesthetic qualities.

**placent-,** combining form meaning 'a cakelike mass': *placenta, placentapepton, placentogenesis.*

**placenta** /pləsen'tə/ [L, flat cake], a highly vascular fetal organ that exchanges with the maternal circulation, mainly by diffusion of oxygen, carbon dioxide, and other substances. It begins to form on approximately the eighth day of gestation when the blastocyst touches the wall of the uterus and adheres to it. Placentation begins as the trophoblast is able to digest cells of the endometrium, causing a small erosion on the uterine wall in which an embryo nidates. Human chorionic gonadotropin (HCG), which is chemically identical to luteinizing hormone, is secreted by the developing placenta and promotes survival and hormone production of the corpus luteum. The presence of HCG in the maternal blood and urine is an indicator of early pregnancy. The trophoblastic layer continues to infiltrate the maternal tissues with fingerlike projections, called chorionic villi. By the third month of pregnancy the placenta is able to secrete large amounts of progesterone, enough to relieve the corpus luteum of that function. At term the normal placenta is one seventh to one fifth of the weight of the infant. The maternal surface is lobulated and has a dark red rough, liverlike appearance. The fetal surface is smooth and shiny, covered with the fetal membranes, and marked by the large white blood vessels beneath the membranes that fan out from the centrally inserted umbilical cord. The time between the infant's birth and the expulsion of the placenta is the third and last stage of labor.

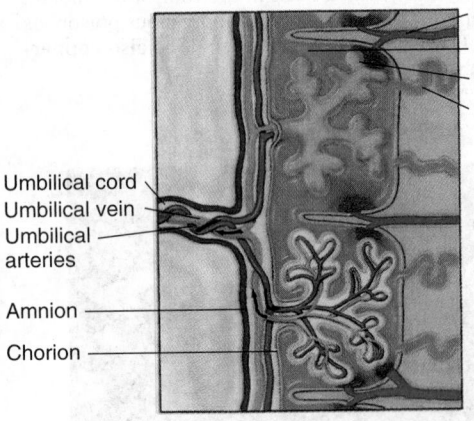

**Cross section of the placenta** *(Applegate, 2000)*

**-placenta,** combining form meaning an 'organ shaped like a flat cake': *ectoplacenta, hemiplacenta, subplacenta.*

**placenta abruptio.** See **abruptio placentae.**

**placenta accreta,** a placenta that invades the uterine muscle, making separation from the muscle difficult.

**placenta battledore.** See **battledore placenta.**

**placenta bipartitia.** See **bilobate placenta.**

**placental** /pləsen'təl/ [L, *placenta,* flat cake], pertaining to the placenta.

**placental abruption.** See **abruptio placentae.**

**placental bruit** [L, *placenta,* flat cake; Fr, *bruit,* noise], a humming noise caused by fetal circulation, heard in the pregnant uterus. It is synchronized with the mother's pulse.

**placental dysfunction.**   See **placental insufficiency.**

**placental dystocia,**   a prolonged or otherwise difficult delivery of the placenta. See also **dystocia.**

**placental hormones,**   types of hormones produced by the placenta, including human placental lactogen, chorionic gonadotropin, estrogen, progesterone, and a thyrotropin-like hormone.

**placental infarct,**   a localized ischemic hard area on the fetal or maternal side of the placenta.

**placental insufficiency,**   an abnormal condition of pregnancy, manifested clinically by a retarded rate of fetal and uterine growth. One or more placental abnormalities cause dysfunction of maternal-placental or fetal-placental circulation sufficient to compromise fetal nutrition and oxygenation. Some of the abnormalities that can result in placental insufficiency are abnormal implantation of the placenta, multiple pregnancy, abnormal attachments of the umbilical cord or anomalies of the cord itself, and abnormalities of the placental membranes. Histopathologic abnormalities that can cause placental insufficiency include intervillous thrombi, placental infarction, and breaks in the placental membrane that result in fetal bleeding into the maternal circulation. Placental insufficiency also may result from placental senescence in postmaturity; from systemic diseases, such as erythroblastosis fetalis and diabetes mellitus; or from bacterial, viral, parasitic, or fungal infections. Also called **placental dysfunction.** See also **intrauterine growth retardation, postmature infant.**

**placental membrane,**   a layer of tissue in the placenta between the fetal and maternal blood systems. The membrane regulates the diffusion of materials between the two systems.

**placental presentation** [L, *placenta,* flat cake, *praesentare,* to show],   a complication of childbirth in which the placenta is located in or near the lower uterine segment. Also called **placenta previa.**

**placental scan,**   a scan of the uterus of a pregnant woman, performed after an IV injection of a contrast medium, used for locating the fetus and placenta and for detecting intrauterine bleeding.

**placental sinus.**   See **marginal sinus.**

**placental stage of labor,**   the third stage of labor when the placenta and membranes are expelled from the uterus after birth of the child.

**placental thrombosis** [L, *placenta,* flat cake; Gk, *thrombos,* lump, *osis,* condition],   intravascular coagulation that occurs in the placenta and veins of the uterus.

**placental transmission** [L, *placenta,* flat cake; L, *transmittere,* to transmit],   the transference of a drug or other substance across the placenta.

**placenta previa** /prē′vē·ə/,   a condition of pregnancy in which the placenta is implanted abnormally in the uterus so that it impinges on or covers the internal os of the uterine cervix. It is the most common cause of painless bleeding in the third trimester of pregnancy. Its cause is unknown. The incidence of the condition increases with increased parity from approximately 1 in 1500 primiparas to approximately 1 in 20 grand multiparas. Even slight dilation of the internal os can cause enough local separation of an abnormally implanted placenta to result in bleeding. If severe hemorrhage occurs, immediate cesarean section is usually required to stop the bleeding and to save the mother's life; it is performed regardless of the stage of fetal maturity. Before hemorrhage placenta previa may be diagnosed by ultrasonography and treated with complete bed rest under close observation. Even at rest sudden massive hemorrhage can occur without warning. Vaginal examination is usually contraindicated if placenta previa is present or suspected because palpation can cause local placental separation and precipitate hemorrhage. Cautious and very gentle intracervical palpation may be performed to determine the existence and exact extent of placenta previa. Before this examination an IV infusion is begun, the woman's blood is typed and cross-matched, and preparations for immediate cesarean section are made. If the placenta is next to or near, rather than touching or covering, the cervical os, labor and vaginal delivery may be attempted. **Complete previa** refers to a placenta that has grown to cover the internal cervical os completely; **low-lying placenta** identifies a placenta that is just within the lower uterine segment; and **partial** or **marginal previa** is a condition in which the placenta partially covers the internal cervical os. See also **central placenta previa, marginal placenta previa,** and **partial placenta previa.** Also called *(informal)* **previa.** Compare **abruptio placentae.**

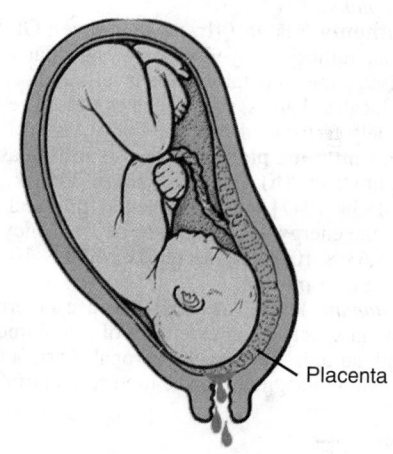

**Placenta previa** *(Thibodeau and Patton, 1999)*

**placenta previa partialis,**   a placenta that partially obstructs the internal cervical os.

**placenta souffle** [L, *placenta,* flat cake; Fr, *souffle,* puff],   a soft blowing or humming sound produced by fetal circulation at the placenta.

**placenta succenturiate,**   an accessory placenta.

**Placidyl,**   trademark for a sedative (ethchlorvynol).

**plafond fracture,**   a fracture that involves the buttress part of the malleolus of a bone.

**plagiocephaly** /plā′jē·ōsef′əlē/ [Gk, *plagios,* askew, *kephale,* head],   a congenital malformation of the skull in which premature or irregular closure of the coronal or lambdoidal sutures results in asymmetric growth of the head, giving it a twisted, lopsided appearance so that the maximum length is not along the midline but on a diagonal. Also called **plagiocephalism.** See also **craniostenosis. —plagiocephalic, plagiocephalous,** *adj.*

**plague** /plāg/ [L, *plaga,* blow],   an infectious disease transmitted by the bite of a flea from a rodent infected with the bacillus *Yersinia pestis.* Plague is primarily an infectious disease of rats: The rat fleas feed on humans only when their preferred rodent hosts, usually rats, have been killed by the plague in a rat epizootic; therefore epidemics occur after rat epizootics. Kinds of plague include **bubonic plague, pneumonic plague,** and **septicemic plague.** See also *Yersinia pestis.*

**plague vaccine,** an active immunizing agent prepared with killed plague bacilli.

■ INDICATIONS: It is prescribed for immunization against plague after probable exposure or as protection for travelers in endemic areas, such as Southeast Asia.

■ CONTRAINDICATIONS: Immunosuppression or acute infection prohibits its use.

■ ADVERSE EFFECTS: Among the most serious adverse effects are allergic reactions, inflammation at the site of injection, headache, and malaise.

**plaintiff** /plān'tif/ [ME, *plaintif,* one who complains], (in law) a person who files a lawsuit initiating a legal action. The plaintiff complains or sues for remedial relief and names a complainant in various civil actions. In criminal actions the prosecution is the plaintiff, acting in behalf of the people of the jurisdiction.

**-plakia,** combining form meaning 'a plate or flat plane, usually on a mucous membrane': *leukoplakia, malacoplakia, melanoplakia.*

**planar xanthoma** /plā'nər/ [L, *planum,* level; Gk, *xanthos,* yellow, *oma,* tumor], a yellow or orange flat macule or slightly raised papule containing foam cells and occurring in clusters in localized areas, such as the eyelids. These lesions may be widely distributed over the body. Also called **plane xanthoma, xanthoma planum.** See also **xanthelasmatosis.**

**Planck's constant (h)** /plangks/ [Max Planck, German physicist, 1858–1947], a fundamental physical constant that relates the energy of radiation to its frequency. It is expressed as $6.63 \times 10^{-27}$ erg-seconds or $6.63 \times 10^{-34}$ joule-seconds. See also **photon.**

**plane** [L, *planum,* level], **1.** a flat surface determined by three points in space. **2.** an extension of a longitudinal section through an axis, such as the coronal, horizontal, transverse, frontal, and sagittal planes, used to identify the position of various parts of the body in the study of anatomy. **3.** the act of paring or of rubbing away. **4.** a superficial incision in the wall of a cavity or between tissue layers, especially in plastic surgery. —**planar,** *adj.*

**plane xanthoma.** See **planar xanthoma.**

**-plania,** combining form meaning the 'deviation from its normal location': *choloplania, pyoplania, spiloplania.*

**planigraphic principle** /plan'igraf'ik/, a rule of tomography in which the fulcrum or axis of rotation is raised or lowered to alter the level of the focal plane but the tabletop height remains constant.

**plankton** /plangk'tən/ [Gk, *planktos,* wandering], nearly microscopic floating or weakly swimming organisms (both photosynthetic and nonphotosynthetic) found in lakes and oceans that provide the initial level in the food chain for aquatic animals.

**planned change,** an alteration of the status quo by means of a carefully formulated program that follows four steps: unfreezing the present level, establishing a change relationship, moving to a new level, and freezing at the new level. The program can be implemented by collaborative, coercive, or emulative means.

**planned parenthood,** a philosophic framework central to the development of contraceptive methods, contraceptive counseling, and family planning programs and clinics. Advocates hold that each woman has the right to decide when to conceive and bear children and that contraceptive and gynecologic care and information should be available to help her become or prevent becoming pregnant. See also **contraception.**

**planning** [L, *planum*], (in five-step nursing process) a category of nursing behavior in which a strategy is designed to achieve the goals of care for an individual patient, as established in assessing and analyzing. Planning includes developing and modifying a care plan for the patient, cooperating with other personnel, and recording relevant information. To develop the plan the nurse anticipates the patient's needs according to established priorities; involves the patient and the patient's family and significant others in designing the plan; uses all information necessary for managing the patient's care, including recorded information from other health professionals, and the age, sex, culture, ethnicity, and religion; plans for the patient's comfort, activity, and function; and chooses nursing measures that are necessary to deliver care as planned. With the cooperation of other health personnel the nurse coordinates care for the benefit of the patient and identifies resources in the health care facility or community for social or health assistance as needed by the client or the patient's family. All information relevant to the management of the patient's care plan is recorded. Planning follows analyzing and precedes implementing in the five-step nursing process. See also **analyzing, assessing, evaluating, implementing, nursing process.**

**plano-,** combining form meaning 'wandering': *planocyte, planotopokinesia.*

**plantago seed** /plantā'gō/, a bulk-forming laxative derived from *Plantago psyllium* seeds.

■ INDICATIONS: It is prescribed in the treatment of constipation and nonspecific diarrhea.

■ CONTRAINDICATIONS: Symptoms of appendicitis, intestinal obstruction, or GI ulceration prohibit its use.

■ ADVERSE EFFECTS: Among the more serious adverse effects are intestinal obstruction and allergic reactions.

**plantar** /plan'tər/ [L, *planta,* sole], pertaining to the sole of the foot. Also called **volar.**

**plantar aponeurosis,** the tough fascia surrounding the muscles of the soles of the feet. Also called **plantar fascia.**

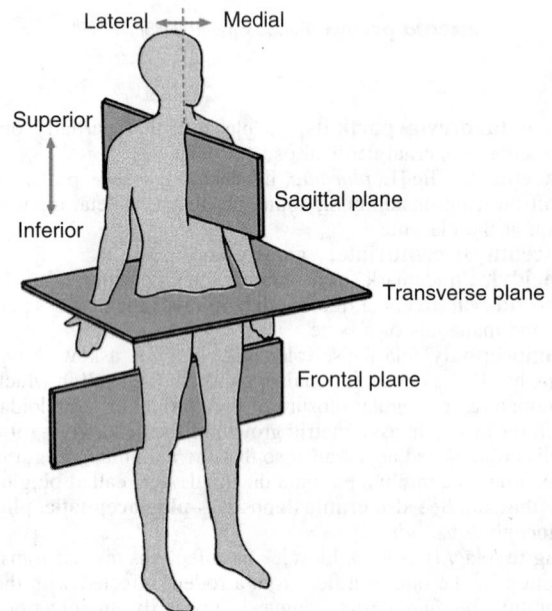

**Planes of the body** *(Potter and Perry, 2001)*

**plantar arch** [L, *planta,* sole, *arcus,* bow], the arch in the sole of the foot.

**plantar fascia.** See **plantar aponeurosis.**

**plantar flexion** [L, *planta,* sole, *flectere,* to bend], a toe-down motion of the foot at the ankle. It is measured in degrees from the 0-degree position of the foot at rest on the ground with the body in a standing position.

**plantar grasp reflex,** a reflex characterized by the flexion of the toes when the sole of the foot is stroked gently. It is present in babies at birth but should disappear after 6 weeks.

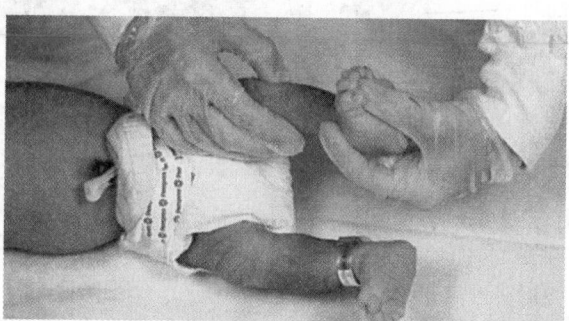

**Plantar grasp reflex in the newborn** *(Seidel et al, 1999)*

**plantaris** /planter'is, plantä'ris/ [L, *planta*], one of three superficial muscles at the back of the leg, between the soleus and the gastrocnemius. The plantaris is a small muscle that arises from the distal part of the linea aspera of the femur and from the oblique popliteal ligament of the knee joint. It has a small fusiform belly, ending in a long, slender tendon that inserts into the calcaneus. The plantaris is innervated by a branch of the tibial nerve containing fibers from the fourth and the fifth lumbar and the first sacral nerves. It plantarflexes the foot and the leg. Compare **gastrocnemius, soleus.**

**plantar neuroma,** a neuroma of the sole of the foot.

**plantar reflex,** the normal response, elicited by firmly stroking the outer surface of the sole from heel to toes, characterized by flexion of the toes. Compare **Babinski's reflex.**

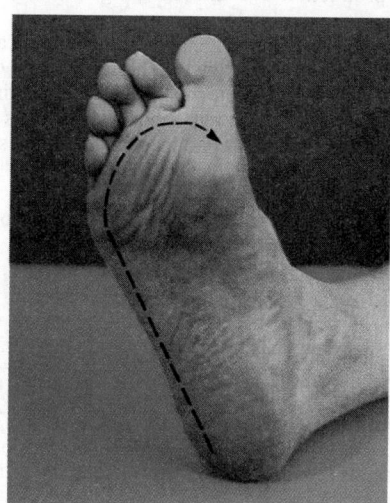

**Plantar reflex** *(Seidel et al, 1999)*

**plantar wart,** a painful verrucous lesion on the sole of the foot, primarily at points of pressure, such as over the metatarsal heads and the heel. Caused by the common wart virus, it appears as a soft central core and is surrounded by a firm hyperkeratotic ring resembling a callus. Multiple tiny black spots on the surface represent bits of coagulated blood in the wart. It is distinguished from a callus in that skin markings are interrupted by a plantar wart. Treatment methods include excision, electrodesiccation, cryotherapy, topical acids, use of cantharidin, and even mental suggestion. See also **mosaic wart.**

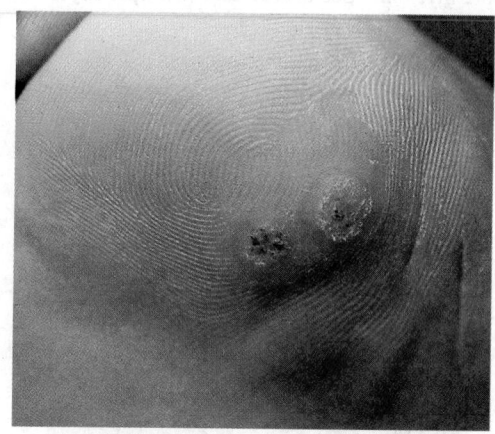

**Plantar warts** *(Zitelli and Davis, 1997)*

**plantigrade** /plan'tigrād'/ [L, *planta,* sole, *gradi,* to walk], **1.** pertaining to or characterizing the human gait; walking on the sole of the foot with the heel touching the ground. **2.** a position in which an individual is standing flexed at the hips and bearing some weight through the upper extremities.

**plant or animal classification.** See **taxonomy.**

**plant toxin** [ME, *plante* + Gk, *toxikon,* poison], any poisonous substance derived from a plant, such as ricin, which is produced by castor-oil seeds.

**plaque** /plak/ [Fr, plate], **1.** a flat, often raised patch on the skin or any other organ of the body. **2.** a patch of atherosclerosis. **3.** also called **dental plaque,** a usually thin film on the teeth. It is made up of mucin and colloidal material found in saliva and often secondarily invaded by bacteria.

**Plaquenil Sulfate,** trademark for an antimalarial, antiarthritic, and lupus erythematosus suppressant agent (hydroxychloroquine sulfate).

**-plasia, -plastia,** combining form meaning '(condition of) formation or development': *alloplasia, anosteoplasia, cacoplasia.*

**-plasm, -plasma,** combining form meaning 'cell or tissue substance': *deutoplasm, mitoplasm, phytoplasm.* See also **-plasma.**

**plasma** /plaz'mə/ [Gk, something formed], the watery straw-colored fluid part of the lymph and the blood in which the leukocytes, erythrocytes, and platelets are suspended. Plasma is made up of water, electrolytes, proteins, glucose, fats, bilirubin, and gases and is essential for carrying the cellular elements of the blood through the circulation, transporting nutrients, maintaining the acid-base balance of the body, and transporting wastes from the tissues. Plasma and interstitial fluid correspond closely in content and concentration of proteins; therefore plasma is important in maintaining the osmotic pressure and the exchange of fluids and electrolytes between the capillaries and the tissues. Compare **serum.**

**-plasma-,** combining form meaning 'the liquid part of the blood': *plasmablast, plasmacyte, plasmapheresis, ectoplasma, hydroplasma, ovoplasma.* See also **-plasm.**

**plasma cell,** a lymphoid or lymphocyte-like cell found in the bone marrow, connective tissue, and sometimes the blood. It contains an eccentric nucleus with deeply staining chromatin material arranged in a pattern like the spokes of a wheel or a clock face. Plasma cells are involved in the immunologic mechanism and are formed in large numbers in multiple myeloma. See also **B cell, multiple myeloma.**

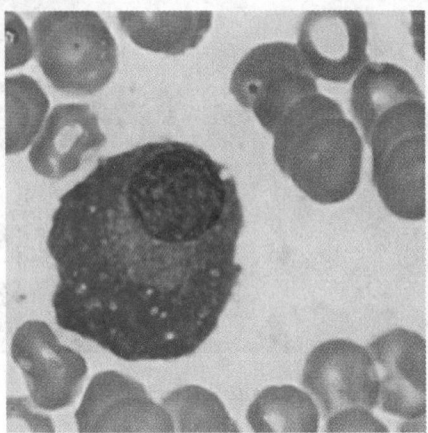

**Plasma cell** *(Carr and Rodak, 1999)*

**plasma cell leukemia,** an unusual neoplasm of blood-forming tissues in which the predominant cells are plasmacytes. The disease may develop with multiple myeloma or arise independently. Bence Jones proteinuria, abnormal serum globulins, hepatomegaly, and splenomegaly are usual in plasma cell leukemia. In most cases plasma cell leukemia is fatal, but some patients respond to treatment with alkylating agents and glucocorticoids.

**plasma cell myeloma.** See **multiple myeloma.**

**plasma cell tumor.** See **extramedullary myeloma.**

**plasmacytoma** /plaz′məsītō′mə/, *pl.* **plasmacytomas, plasmacytomata,** a focal neoplasm containing plasma cells that may develop in the bone marrow, as in multiple myeloma, or outside the bone marrow, as in tumors of the viscera and the mucosa of the nasal, oral, and pharyngeal areas. Also called **peripheral plasma cell myeloma, plasma cell tumor.**

**plasma exchange therapy** [Gk, *plassein,* to mold; L, *ex + cambire,* to change; Gk, *therapeia,* treatment], a method of treating certain diseases by removing a part of plasma from the blood supply of a patient and replacing it with plasma from a disease-free person.

**plasma expander,** a substance, usually a high-molecular-weight dextran, that is administered intravenously to increase the oncotic pressure of a patient.

**plasma membrane,** the outer covering of a cell, often having projecting microvilli and containing the cellular cytoplasm. The plasma membrane is so thin and delicate that it is barely visible with a light microscope and can be studied

in detail only with an electron microscope. The membrane controls the exchange of materials between the cell and its environment by various processes, such as osmosis, phagocytosis, pinocytosis, and secretion. Also called **cell membrane.**

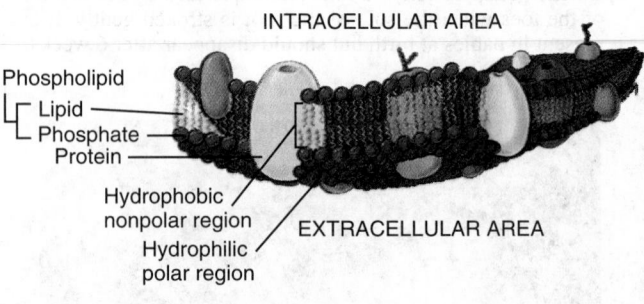

**Plasma membrane** *(Applegate, 2000)*

**plasmapheresis** /plaz′məfərē′sis/, the removal of plasma from previously withdrawn blood by centrifugation, reconstitution of the cellular elements in an isotonic solution, and reinfusion of this solution into the donor or another client who needs red cells rather than whole blood. Compare **leukapheresis, plateletpheresis.**

**plasma protein,** any of the proteins, including albumin, fibrinogen, prothrombin, and the gamma globulins, that constitute about 6% to 7% of the blood plasma in the body. These substances help maintain water balance that affects osmotic pressure, increase blood viscosity, and help maintain blood pressure. All the plasma proteins except the gamma globulins are synthesized in the liver. See also **antibody, serum.**

**plasma renin activity,** the action of the enzyme renin (produced by the kidney), measured in plasma to aid in the diagnosis of adrenal disease associated with hypertension. The normal adult value in plasma is 0.2 to 4 ng/ml/hour, depending on salt intake and the time the patient is in an upright position before a renin activity test. An upright position raises production of renin and a high salt intake lowers it.

**plasma renin assay (PRA),** a blood test that measures the rate of generation of angiotensin. The most commonly used renin assay, it is a screening procedure for detecting essential, renal, or renovascular hypertension, and it is also performed to diagnose and separate primary from secondary hyperaldosteronism.

**plasmasome.** See **plasmosome.**

**plasma thromboplastin antecedent.** See **factor XI.**

**plasma thromboplastin component deficiency.** See **hemophilia.**

**plasma volume,** the total volume of plasma in the body, elevated in diseases of the liver and spleen and in vitamin C deficiency, lowered in Addison's disease, dehydration, and shock. The normal plasma volume in males is 39 mL/kg of body weight; in females, 40 mL/kg.

**plasma volume extender** [Gk, *plassein* + L, *volumen,* paper roll, *extendere,* to stretch], an IV solution of dextran, proteins, or other substances used to treat shock caused by blood volume loss.

**plasmid** /plaz′mid/ [Gk, *plasma,* something formed], a small, circular molecule of DNA in a bacterium that is separate from the bacterial chromosome. Plasmids often carry genes that affect the ability of bacteria to respond to environmental challenges. For example, a bacterium containing the R (resistance) plasmid is able to resist many antibacterial drugs that act in different ways. Plasmids may be passed from one bacterium to another and are replicated in later generations of any bacterium carrying them. Molecular geneticists often use plasmids to insert specific genes into the chromosomes of bacteria and other organisms.

**plasmidotrophoblast.** See **syncytiotrophoblast.**

**plasmin.** See **fibrinolysin.**

**plasminogen.** See **fibrinogen.**

**plasminogen test (fibrinolysin),** a blood test used to diagnose suspected plasminogen deficiency in patients who present with multiple thromboembolic episodes. Abnormal levels of plasminogen are also characteristic of disseminated intravascular coagulation (DIC), primary fibrinolysis, cirrhosis and other severe liver diseases, pregnancy, eclampsia, and some inflammatory conditions.

**plasmo-,** combining form meaning 'of or related to plasma, or to the substance of a cell': *plasmocyte, plasmodium, plasmosome.*

***Plasmodium*** /plazmō′dē·əm/ [Gk, *plasma* + *eidos,* form], a genus of protozoa, several species of which cause malaria, transmitted to humans by the bite of an infected *Anopheles* mosquito. *Plasmodium falciparum* causes falciparum malaria, the most severe form of the disease; *P. malariae* causes quartan malaria; *P. ovale* causes mild tertian malaria with oval red blood cells; and *P. vivax* causes common tertian malaria. See also ***Anopheles,* blackwater fever, malaria.**

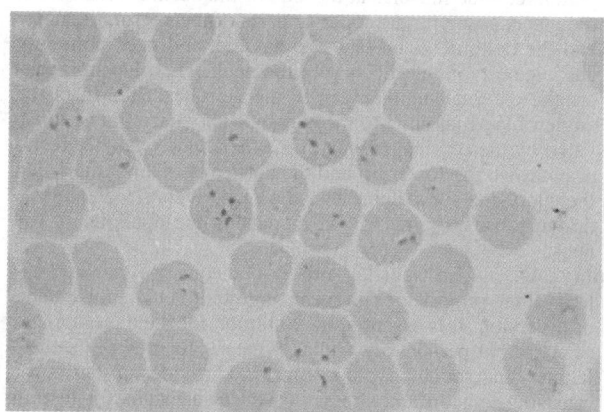

***Plasmodium falciparum*** (Murray et al, 1998)

**plasmosome** /plaz′məsōm/ [Gk, *plasma* + *soma,* body], the true nucleolus of a cell as distinguished from the karyosomes in the nucleus. Also spelled **plasmasome.**

**plast-,** combining form meaning 'to form, mold, or develop': *plastidogenetic, plastodynamia, plastogamy.*

**-plast, -plastia, -plasia, -plastic,** combining form meaning 'pertaining to the formation or development of a': *anaplastic, hemoplastic.*

**plaster** [Gk, *emplastron*], **1.** any composition of a liquid and a powder that hardens when it dries, used in shaping a cast to support a fractured bone as it heals, such as plaster of paris. **2.** a home remedy consisting of a semisolid mixture applied to a part of the body as a counterirritant or for other therapeutic reasons, such as a mustard plaster.

**plaster cast** [Gk, *emplastron,* plaster; ONorse, *kasta*], a traditional cast used to encase and immobilize a part of the body, made from a gauze roll impregnated with plaster of paris. The gauze is dipped in warm water and wrapped around the body part. Modern casts are often made of materials such as fiberglass or plastic instead of plaster of paris.

**plaster of paris** [Gk, *emplastron,* plaster; Paris, France], a white powder, calcium sulfate hemihydrate, which is mixed with water to make a paste that can be molded to encase a body part.

**-plastia.** See **-plasia, -plast, -plastic.**

**plastic** /plas′tik/ [Gk, *plastikos*], **1.** tending to build up tissues or to restore a lost part. **2.** conformable; capable of being molded. **3.** a high-molecular-weight polymeric material, usually organic, capable of being molded, extruded, drawn, or otherwise shaped and then hardened into a form. **4.** material that can be molded.

**plasticity** /plastis′itē/ [Gk, *plassein,* to mold], the quality of being plastic or formative.

**plastic surgery** [Gk, *plassein,* to mold, *cheirourgia,* surgery], the alteration, replacement, or restoration of visible parts of the body, performed to correct a structural or cosmetic defect. In performing corrective plastic surgery, the surgeon may use tissue from the patient or from another person or an inert material that is nonirritating, has a consistency appropriate to the use, and is able to hold its shape and form indefinitely. Implants are commonly used in mammoplasty for breast augmentation. Skin grafting is the most common procedure in plastic surgery. Z-plasty and Y-plasty are simpler techniques often performed instead of grafting in areas of the body covered by skin that is loose and elastic, such as the neck, axilla, throat, and inner aspect of the elbow. Dermabrasion is used to remove pockmarks, acne scars, or signs of traumatic skin damage. Chemical peeling is another technique in corrective plastic surgery; it is used primarily for removing fine wrinkles on the face. Tattooing, in which a pigment is tattooed into the skin of a graft, is performed to change the color of the graft to resemble more closely the surrounding skin. Reconstructive plastic surgery is performed to correct birth defects, to repair structures destroyed by trauma, and to replace tissue removed in other surgical procedures. Cleft lip and cleft palate repair and other maxillofacial surgical procedures, including rhinoplasty, otoplasty, and rhytidoplasty, are among these reconstructive procedures. Care of the patient before and after plastic surgery may require considerable sensitivity and tact. The patient may be exceedingly uncomfortable about the real or perceived appearance of the defect. An accepting, nonjudgmental attitude of all staff members is to the patient's benefit. Optimal nutritional status helps a graft to "take" and speeds healing. Each procedure and technique involves particular kinds of care in the preoperative and postoperative periods. Instructions and assistance in self-care activities are also specific to the various procedures. Success of most of the procedures depends greatly on the patient's cooperation and fastidious nursing care. The correction of a visible abnormality may be of inestimable benefit to the patient's assurance, self-esteem, and function in society. See also specific procedures.

**-plasty,** suffix meaning 'molding, formation, or surgical repair on a (specified) body part or by (specified) means': *bronchoplasty, cervicoplasty, uveoplasty.*

**plate** [Fr, *plat,* flat dish], **1.** a flat structure or layer, such as a thin layer of bone or the frontal plate between the sides of the ethmoid cartilage and the sphenoid bone in the fetus. **2.** a single partitioning unit of a chromatographic system.

**platelet** /plat′lit/ [Fr, small plate], the smallest cells in the blood. They are formed in the red bone marrow and some are stored in the spleen. Platelets are disk-shaped, contain no hemoglobin, and are essential for the coagulation of blood and in maintenance of hemostasis. Normally between 200,000 and 300,000 platelets are found in 1 mL$^3$ of blood. Compare **erythrocyte, leukocyte.** See also **thrombocytopenia, thrombocytosis.**

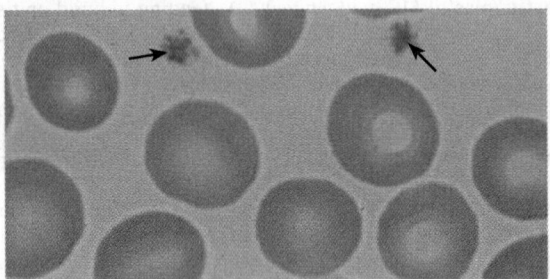

**Platelet** *(Carr and Rodak, 1999)*

**platelet aggregation,** a clumping together of platelets, part of a sequential mechanism leading to the initiation and formation of a thrombus or hemostatic plug. It can be induced in vitro, and probably in vivo, by agents such as ADP (adenosine diphosphate), thrombin, and collagen.

**platelet aggregation test,** a blood test that can detect diseases that affect either platelet number or function, thereby prolonging bleeding time. This test can provide information about prolonged platelet aggregation times, connective tissue disorders such as lupus erythematosus, recent cardiopulmonary or dialysis bypass, various myeloproliferative diseases, primary protein disease, von Willebrand's disease, uremia, and congenital disorders such as Wiskott-Aldrich syndrome, Bernard-Soulier syndrome, and glycogen storage disorders.

**platelet antibody detection test,** a blood test used to detect immune-mediated destruction of platelets. Such destruction can cause paroxysmal hemoglobinuria as well as immunologic thrombocytopenia, which includes idiopathic thrombocytopenia purpura, posttransfusion purpura, neonatal thrombocytopenia, drug-induced thrombocytopenia.

**platelet count,** a blood test that is performed on all patients who develop petechiae, spontaneous bleeding, or increasingly heavy menses. It is also used to monitor the course of the disease or therapy for thrombocytopenia or bone marrow failure. Also called **count.**

**plateletpheresis** /plat′litfer′əsis/ [Fr, *platelet* + Gk, *aphairesis,* to carry away], the removal of platelets from withdrawn blood; the remainder of the blood being reinfused into the donor. Also called **thrombapheresis, thrombotapheresis.** Compare **leukapheresis, plasmapheresis.**

**platform,** a collective term for computer hardware and software components of a particular system.

**-platin,** combining form for platinum-based antineoplastics.

**platinized gold foil** /plat′inīzd/ [Sp, *plata,* silver; AS, *geolu,* gold; L, *folium,* leaf], a thin sheet of platinum sandwiched between two sheets of gold, used for making parts of dental restorations requiring greater hardness than that obtained with other materials, such as copper amalgam.

**Platinol,** trademark for an antineoplastic (cisplatin).

**platinum (Pt)** /plat′ənəm/ [Sp, *plata,* silver], a silver-white soft metallic element. Its atomic number is 78; its atomic mass (weight) is 195.09. Platinum is used in dentistry, jewelry, and manufacture of chemical apparatus that must withstand high temperatures. Platinum is a good catalyst for a variety of chemical reactions.

**platinum foil,** a very thin sheet of pure platinum that has a high fusing point, making it an ideal matrix in various soldering procedures for fabricating orthodontic appliances and dentures. It is also commonly used as the internal form of porcelain dental restorations during fabrication.

**platy-,** combining form meaning 'broad or flat': *platybasia, platycephalous, platycnemic.*

**Platyhelminthes** /plat′ihelmin′thēz/ [Gk, *platys,* broad, *helmins,* worm], a phylum of flatworms that includes parasitic tapeworms (class Cestoda) and flukes (classes Monogenea and Trematoda) as well as mostly free-living species, such as planarians (class Turbellaria).

**platypelloid pelvis** /plat′əpel′oid/ [Gk, *platys,* broad, *pella,* bowl, *eidos,* form; L, *pelvis,* basin], a rare type of pelvis in which the inlet is round like the gynecoid type in the anterior section, but the posterior section is foreshortened by its flat and heavy border. The sacrum is hollow and inclines posteriorly, and the sidewalls are convergent. In the midplane the transverse diameter is much wider than the narrowed anteroposterior diameter. Vaginal delivery is not usually possible in the 3% of women who have platypelloid pelves.

**platysma** /plətiz′mə/ [Gk, *platys,* broad], one of a pair of platelike, wide muscles at the side of the neck. It arises from the fascia covering the superior parts of the pectoralis major and the deltoideus, crosses the clavicle, and rises obliquely and medially along the side of the neck. The platysma covers the external jugular vein as the vein descends from the angle of the mandible to the clavicle. The platysma is innervated by the cervical branch of the facial nerve and serves to draw down the lower lip and the corner of the mouth. When the platysma fully contracts, the skin over the clavicle is drawn toward the mandible, increasing the diameter of the neck.

**play** [AS, *plegan,* sport], any spontaneous or organized activity that provides enjoyment, entertainment, amusement, or diversion. It is essential in childhood for the development of a normal personality and as a means for physical, intellectual, and social development. Play provides an outlet for releasing tension and stress, as well as a means for testing and experimenting with new or fearful roles or situations. It is an indispensable part of the nursing care of children, especially in the hospital. It helps relieve the tension and anxiety of being in unfamiliar surroundings and separated from parents, and it gives the child a sense of security and a means of expressing fears and fantasies. Play also offers the nurse one of the most effective methods of communicating with and gaining the trust of the child and helping him or her to understand treatments and procedures. Kinds of play include **active play, associative play, cooperative play, dramatic play, parallel play, passive play, skill play,** and **solitary play.** See also **play therapy.**

**play participation,** a nursing outcome from the Nursing Outcomes Classification (NOC) defined as the use of activities as needed for enjoyment, entertainment, and development by children. See also **Nursing Outcomes Classification.**

**play support,** a Nursing Interventions Classification defined as purposeful use of toys or other equipment to assist a patient in communicating his/her perception of the world and mastering the environment. See also **Nursing Interventions Classification.**

**play therapy,** a form of psychotherapy in which a child plays in a protected and structured environment with games and toys provided by a therapist, who observes the behavior, affect, and conversation of the child to gain insight into thoughts, feelings, and fantasies. As conflicts are discovered, the therapist often helps the child understand and work through them.

**pleasure principle** /plezh′ər/ [Fr, *plaisir*, pleasure; L, *principium*], (in psychoanalysis) the need for immediate gratification of instinctual drives. Compare **reality principle.**

**pledget** /plej′ət/, a small flat compress made of cotton gauze, or a tuft of cotton wool, lint, or a similar synthetic material, used to wipe the skin, absorb drainage, or clean a small surface.

**-plegia, -plegic,** combining form meaning 'a (specified) paralysis': *cycloplegia, paraplegic.*

**Plegine,** trademark for an anorexiant (phendimetrazine tartrate).

**pleio-.** See **pleo-.**

**pleiotropic gene** /plī′ətrop′ik/, a gene that produces many effects in the phenotype.

**pleiotropy** /plī·ot′rəpē/ [Gk, *pleion*, more, *trepein* to turn], the production by a single gene of a complex of unrelated phenotypic effects. The effects may be a manifestation of a particular disorder, such as the cluster of symptoms in Marfan's syndrome, aortic aneurysm, dislocation of the optic lens, skeletal deformities, and arachnodactyly, any or all of which may be present. **—pleiotropic,** *adj.*

**pleocytosis** /plē′ōsītō′sis/, presence of a greater than normal number of cells in the cerebrospinal fluid.

**pleo-, pleio-,** prefix meaning 'more': *pleochromatic, pleomastia, pleomorphism.*

**plerocercoid** /plir′ōsur′koid/, the second larval stage of the cestode *Diphyllobothrium latum.* It develops in the second intermediate host, a freshwater fish, and is infective to humans if ingested.

**plessimeter.** See **pleximeter.**

**plethora** /pleth′ərə/ [Gk, *plethore*, fullness], a term applied to the beefy red coloration of a newborn. The "boiled lobster" hue of the infant's skin is caused by an unusually high proportion of erythrocytes per volume of blood. The term formerly was used to describe any red-faced person. **—plethoric,** *adj.*

**plethysmogram** /pləthiz′məgram′/ [Gk, *plethynein*, to increase, *gramma*, to record], a tracing produced by a plethysmograph.

**plethysmograph** /pləthiz′məgraf′/, an instrument for measuring and recording changes in the size and volume of extremities and organs by measuring changes in their blood volume. **—plethysmographic,** *adj.*

**plethysmography** /pleth′izmog′rəfē/ [Gk, *plethynein*, to increase, *graphein*, to record], the measurement of changes in the volume of organs or other body parts, particularly those changes resulting from blood flow.

**pleur-.** See **pleuro-.**

**pleura** /plŏŏr′ə/, *pl.* **pleurae** [Gk, rib], a delicate serous membrane enclosing the lung, composed of a single layer of flattened mesothelial cells resting on a delicate membrane of connective tissue. Beneath the membrane is a stroma of collagenous tissue containing yellow elastic fibers. The pleura divides into the visceral pleura, which covers the lung, dipping into the fissures between the lobes, and the parietal

pleura, which lines the chest wall, covers the diaphragm, and reflects over the structures in the mediastinum. The parietal and visceral pleurae are separated from each other by a small amount of fluid that acts as a lubricant as the lungs expand and contract during respiration. See also **pleural cavity, pleural space. —pleural,** *adj.*

**pleural** /plŏŏr′əl/ [Gk, *pleura*, rib], pertaining to the pleurae.

**pleural cavity** [Gk, *pleura*, rib; L, *cavum*, cavity], the space within the thorax that contains the lungs. Between the ribs and the lungs are the visceral and parietal pleurae.

**pleural effusion,** an abnormal accumulation of fluid in the intrapleural spaces of the lungs. It is characterized by fever, chest pain, dyspnea, and nonproductive cough. The fluid is an exudate or a transudate from inflamed pleural surfaces and may be aspirated or surgically drained. An exudate may result from pulmonary infarction, trauma, tumor, or infection, such as tuberculosis. The specific cause of the exudate is treated. Treatment of the effusion may include the administration of corticosteroids, diuretics, or vasodilators; oxygen therapy; or intermittent positive-pressure breathing.

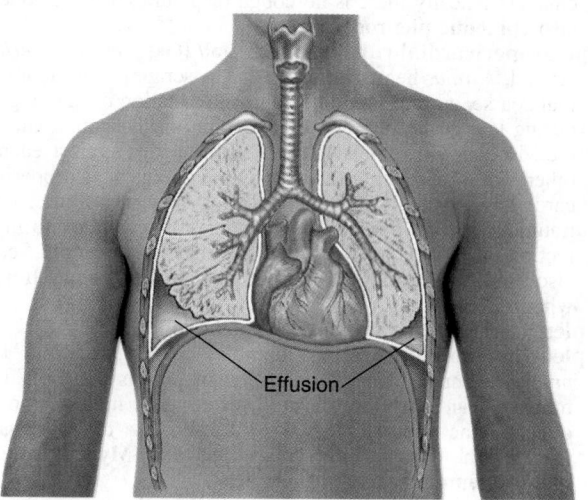

**Pleural effusion** *(Wilson and Giddens, 2001)*

**pleural friction rub.** See **pleuropericardial rub.**

**pleural space,** the potential space between the visceral and parietal layers of the pleurae. The space contains a small amount of fluid that acts as a lubricant, allowing the pleurae to slide smoothly over each other as the lungs expand and contract with respiration.

**pleura pulmonalis** [Gk, *pleura*, rib; L, *pulmo*, lung], the part of the pleural membrane that covers the lungs, as distinguished from the parietal layer of pleura that lines the inner aspect of the thoracic cavity.

**pleurisy** /plŏŏr′əsē/ [Gk, *pleura* + *itis*, inflammation], inflammation of the parietal pleura of the lungs. It is characterized by dyspnea and stabbing pain, leading to restriction of ordinary breathing with spasm of the chest on the affected side. A pleural friction rub may be heard on auscultation. Simple pleurisy with undetectable exudate is called fibrinous or dry pleurisy; pleural effusion indicates extensive inflammation with considerable amounts of exudate in the pleural spaces. Common causes of pleurisy include bronchial carcinoma, lung or chest wall abscess, pneumonia, pulmonary infarction, and tuberculosis. The condition may result in permanent adhesions between the pleura and adjacent surfaces. Treatment consists of pain relief and therapy for the primary disease. See also **pleural effusion, pleurodynia, pulmonary edema. —pleuritic,** *adj.*

**pleurisy with effusion** [Gk, *pleura* + *itis,* inflammation; L, *effundere,* to pour out], pleurisy in which there is an accumulation of fluid in the intrapleural space. The fluid has a high specific gravity as a result of a high concentration of fibrin and clots.

**pleuritic** /plŏŏrit′ik/ [Gk, *pleura,* rib], pertaining to a condition of pleurisy.

**pleuritis.** See **pleurisy.**

**pleuro-** /plŏŏr′ō-/, **pleur-,** combining form meaning 'the pleura or side': *pleurocentrum, pleurography, pleuropulmonary.*

**pleurodynia** /plŏŏr′ōdin′ē·ə/ [Gk, *pleura* + *odyne,* pain], acute inflammation of the intercostal muscles and the muscular attachment of the diaphragm to the chest wall. It is characterized by sudden, severe pain and tenderness, fever, headache, and anorexia. These symptoms are aggravated by movement and breathing. The lungs are not affected, and characteristically there is no cough or pleural effusion. See also **epidemic pleurodynia.**

**pleuropericardial rub** /-per′ikär′dē·əl/ [Gk, *pleura* + *peri,* around, *kardia,* heart; ME, *rubben,* to scrape], an abnormal coarse, grating sound heard on auscultation of the lungs during late inspiration and early expiration. It occurs when the visceral and parietal pleural surfaces rub against each other. The sound is not affected by coughing. A pleuropericardial rub indicates primary inflammatory, neoplastic, or traumatic pleural disease, or inflammation secondary to infection or neoplasm. Also called **pleural friction rub.** See also **breath sound, Kussmaul breathing, rhonchus, wheeze.**

**pleuroperitoneal cavity.** See **splanchnocoele.**

**pleuropneumonia** /plŏŏr′ōnŏŏmō′nē·ə/ [Gk, *pleura* + *pneumon,* lung], **1.** a combination of pleurisy and pneumonia. **2.** an infection of cattle resulting in inflammation of both the pleura and lungs, caused by microorganisms of the *Mycoplasma* group. See also **Mycoplasma, pleuropneumonia-like organism.**

**pleuropneumonia-like organism (PPLO),** a group of filterable organisms of the genus *Mycoplasma* similar to *M. mycoides,* the cause of pleuropneumonia in cattle.

**pleurothotonos** /plŏŏr′əthot′ənəs/ [Gk, *pleurothen,* side of the body, *tonos,* tension], an involuntary severe prolonged contraction of the muscles of one side of the body, resulting in an acute arch to that side. It is usually associated with tetanus infection or strychnine poisoning. Compare **emprosthotonos, opisthotonos, orthotonos. —pleurothotonic,** *adj.*

**plex-,** prefix meaning 'a stroke or to strike': *plexalgia, pleximeter, plexor.*

**-plex, -plexus,** suffix meaning 'a braid, nerve, network': *brachiplex, cerviplex, veniplex.*

**-plexia, -plexy,** combining form meaning 'condition resulting from a crippling or serious occurrence': *apoplexia, pagoplexia, selenoplexia.*

**plexiform neuroma** /plek′sifôrm′/ [L, *plexus,* braided, *forma,* form; Gk, *neuron,* nerve, *oma,* tumor], a neoplasm composed of twisted bundles of nerves. Also called **Verneuil's neuroma.**

**pleximeter** /pleksim′ətər/ [Gk, *plessein,* to strike, *metron,* measure], a mediating device, such as a percussor or finger, used to receive light taps in percussion. Also called **plessimeter.** See also **percussion.**

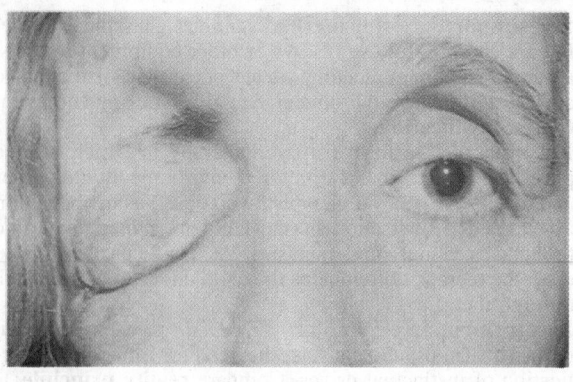

**Plexiform neuroma** *(Michelson and Friedlaender, 1996)*

**plexor.** See **percussor.**

**plexus** /plek′səs/, *pl.* **plexuses** [L, braided], a network of intersecting nerves and blood vessels or of lymphatic vessels. The body contains many plexuses, such as the brachial plexus, the cardiac plexus, the cervical plexus, and the solar plexus.

**-plexus.** See **-plex.**

**-plexy.** See **-plexia.**

**plic-,** prefix meaning a 'fold or ridge': *plicadentin, plication, plicotomy.*

**plica** /plī′kə/, *pl.* **plicae** /plī′sē/ [L, *plicare,* to fold], a fold of tissue within the body, such as the plicae transversales of the rectum and the plicae circulares of the small intestine. **—plical,** *adj.*

**plica circularis.** See **circular fold.**

**plicae transversales recti** /plī′sē/, semilunar transverse folds in the rectum that support the weight of feces. Also called **Houston's valves.** See also **rectum.**

**plicamycin** /plī′kəmī′sin/, an antineoplastic agent. Previously called **mithramycin.**

■ INDICATIONS: It is prescribed primarily in the treatment of malignant tumors of the testis. It is also prescribed in the treatment of hypercalcemia and hypercalciuria associated with cancer.

■ CONTRAINDICATIONS: Clotting disorders, thrombocytopenia, kidney or liver dysfunction, bone marrow depression, or known hypersensitivity to this drug prohibits its use.

■ ADVERSE EFFECTS: Among the more serious adverse reactions are thrombocytopenia and clotting defects. Nausea and stomatitis commonly occur.

**plica semilunaris conjunctivae.** See **semilunar fold of the conjunctiva.**

**plication** /plīkā′shən/, any operation that involves folding, shortening, or decreasing the size of a muscle or hollow organ, such as the stomach, by taking in tucks.

**plication of stomach** [L, *plicare,* to fold; Gk, *stomakhos,* gullet], a surgical treatment for obesity in which tucks are created in the wall of the stomach.

**plica umbilicalis lateralis.** See **lateral umbilical fold.**

**plica umbilicalis mediana.** See **middle umbilical fold.**

**pliers** /plī′ərz/, small tong-jawed pincers for bending metals or holding small objects; various forms are much used in dentistry.

**Plimmer's bodies** [Henry G. Plimmer, English biologist, 1857–1918], small round encapsulated bodies found in cancers and once thought to be the causative parasites. Also called **Behla's bodies.**

**-ploid, -ploidy,** combining form meaning 'having a (specified) number of chromosome sets': *heptaploid, octaploid, polyploid.*

**ploidy** /ploi'dē/ [Gk, *eidos*, form], the status of a cell nucleus in regard to the number of complete chromosome sets it contains.

**plosive.** See **stop.**

**plug** [D, *plugge*, stopper], a mass of tissue cells, mucus, or other matter that blocks a normal opening or passage of the body, such as a cervical plug.

**plugger,** an instrument for condensing or consolidating a filling material, such as a dental amalgam into a tooth restoration. See also **packer.**

**plumbism** /plum'izəm/ [L, *plumbum*, lead], a chronic form of lead poisoning caused by absorption of lead or lead salts. See also **lead poisoning.**

**Plummer's disease** [Henry S. Plummer, American physician, 1874–1937], goiter characterized by a hyperfunctioning nodule or adenoma and thyrotoxicosis. Also called **toxic nodular goiter.**

**Plummer-Vinson syndrome** /plum'ərvin'sən/ [Henry S. Plummer; Porter P. Vinson, American physician, 1890–1959], a rare disorder associated with severe and chronic iron deficiency anemia, characterized by glossitis, koilonychia, and dysphagia caused by esophageal webs at the level of the cricoid cartilage. Also called **Paterson-Kelly syndrome, sideropenic dysphagia.**

**plunging goiter.** See **diving goiter.**

**pluri-,** prefix meaning 'more': *pluriceptor, plurimenorrhea, pluritissular.*

**pluricentric blastoma.** See **blastoma.**

**pluripara** /ploorip'ərə/ [L, *plus*, more, *parere*, to bear], a woman who has borne several children.

**pluripolar mitosis.** See **multipolar mitosis.**

**pluripotential stem cell.** See **stem cell.**

**plutonium (Pu)** /plootō'nē·əm/ [planet *Pluto*], a synthetic transuranic metallic element. Its atomic number is 94; its atomic mass is 242. A highly toxic waste product of nuclear power plants, plutonium was used in the assembly of early nuclear weapons.

**plyometrics,** bounding or high-velocity exercise that entails eccentric and rapid concentric contractions, such as jumping or weighted ball throwing and catching. Also called **plyometric training.**

**pm,** abbreviation for *picometer.*

**Pm,** symbol for the element **promethium.**

***P. malariae,*** abbreviation for *Plasmodium malariae.*

**P.M.D.,** abbreviation for *private medical doctor.* Also called **L.M.D.**

**PMDD,** abbreviation for **premenstrual dysphoric disorder.**

**pmh,** abbreviation for *past medical history.*

**PMI,** abbreviation for **point of maximum impulse.**

**PMN,** abbreviation for **polymorphonuclear cell.**

**PMPA,** abbreviation for **phenyl-methoxypropyl adenine.**

**PMS, pms,** abbreviation for **premenstrual syndrome.**

**PMT,** abbreviation for *premenstrual tension.* See **premenstrual syndrome.**

**PND,** 1. abbreviation for **paroxysmal nocturnal dyspnea.** 2. abbreviation for **postnasal drip.**

**-pnea, -pnoea, pneo-,** combining form meaning 'breath or breathing': *brachypnea, dyspnea, pneoscope.*

**pneuma-.** See **pneumato-.**

**pneumatic** /noomat'ik/ [Gk, *pneuma*, air], pertaining to air or gas.

**pneumatic antishock garment (PASG).** See **military antishock trousers (MAST).**

**pneumatic condenser** [Gk, *pneuma*, air; L, *condensare*, to thicken], a pneumatic device that delivers compacting blows of variable force to restorative material used in filling tooth cavities. The frequency of the blows may be up to 360 per minute. Also called **Hollenback condenser.**

**pneumatic heart driver,** a mechanical device that regulates compressed air delivery to an artificial heart, controlling heart rate, percent systole, and delay in systole.

**pneumatic splint.** See **inflatable splint.**

**pneumatic tourniquet precautions,** a nursing intervention from the Nursing Interventions Classification (NIC) defined as applying a pneumatic tourniquet, while minimizing the potential for patient injury from use of the device. See also **Nursing Interventions Classification.**

**pneumato-, pneuma-,** combining form meaning 'air or gas, or respiration': *pneumatology, pneumatophore, pneumatothorax.*

**pneumatocele** /noomat'əsēl'/, 1. a thin-walled cavity in the lung parenchyma caused by partial airway obstruction. 2. a hernial protrusion of lung tissue. 3. a tumor or sac containing gas, especially of the scrotum. Also called **pneumonocele** /noomon'əsēl/.

**pneumatocephalus.** See **pneumocephalus.**

**pneumatogram** /noomat'əgram'/ [Gk, *pneuma*, air, *gramma*, to record], a tracing made by a pneumograph of chest movements during breathing. Also called **pneumogram.**

**pneumo-** /n(y)oo'mō-/, **pneumono-,** combining form meaning 'lungs, air, or the breath': *pneumobacillin, pneumocele, pneumolith.*

**pneumobelt** /noo'mōbelt/, a corset with an inflatable bladder that fits over the abdominal area. The bladder is connected by a hose to a ventilator that delivers positive pressure at an adjustable rate and pressure. It is used to assist in the respiratory rehabilitation of patients with high cervical injuries to alleviate strain.

**pneumocentesis** /-sentē'sis/ [Gk, *pneumon*, lung, *kentesis*, pricking], a procedure in which a lung is punctured to drain fluid contents.

**pneumocephalus** /noo'mō-sef'ə·ləs/ [Gr, *pneuma* air + *kephalē* head], the presence of air in the intracranial cavity; also called **intracranial pneumatocele, pneumatocephalus, pneumocrania, pneumoencephalocele.**

**pneumococcal** /noo'mōkok'əl/ [Gk, *pneumon*, lung, *kokkos*, berry], pertaining to bacteria of the genus *Pneumococcus.*

**pneumococcal meningitis** [Gk, *pneumon*, lung, *kokkos*, berry, *meninx*, membrane, *itis*, inflammation], meningitis caused by pneumococcal infection. Also called *Streptococcus pneumoniae.*

**pneumococcal pneumonitis,** inflammation of the lungs caused by an infection of pneumococcal bacteria.

**pneumococcal vaccine,** an active immunizing agent containing antigens of the 14 types of *Pneumococcus* associated with 80% of the cases of pneumococcal pneumonia.

■ INDICATIONS: It is prescribed for persons over 2 years of age who are at high risk of development of severe pneumococcal pneumonia, all adults over 65 years of age, and immunocompromised adults.

■ CONTRAINDICATIONS: Pregnancy, early childhood (less than 2 years of age), or known hypersensitivity to the vaccine prohibits its use.

■ ADVERSE EFFECTS: Among the more serious adverse reactions are inflammation at the site of injection, fever, and hypersensitivity.

**pneumococcus** /noo'mōkok'əs/, pl. pneumococci /-kok'sī/ [Gk, *pneumon* + *kokkos*, berry], a gram-positive diplococcal bacterium of the species *Streptococcus pneumoniae*, the most common cause of bacterial pneumonia. More than 85 subtypes of this organism are known. A vaccine protective against 35 serotypes has been developed and is recommended for those over 65 years of age, those with a chronic lung disease, or patients who have human immunodeficiency virus infection. See also **lobar pneumonia, pneumonia.**

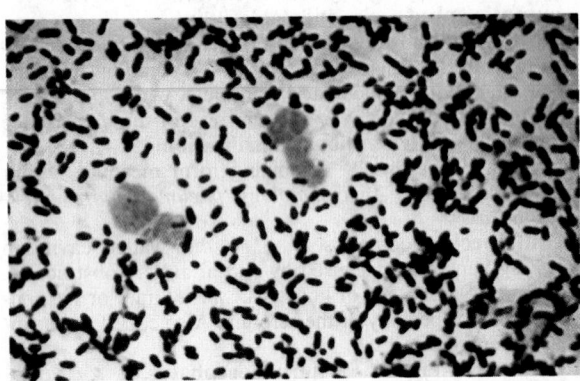

**Pneumococci in the cerebrospinal fluid**
*(Stone and Gorbach, 2000)*

**pneumoconiosis** /nōō′mōkō′nē·ō′sis/ [Gk, *pneumon + konis,* dust, *osis,* condition], any disease of the lung caused by chronic inhalation of dust, usually mineral dust of occupational or environmental origin. Some kinds of pneumoconioses are **anthracosis, asbestosis, silicosis.**

**pneumoconstriction** /nōō′mōkənstrik′shən/, an area of collapsed lung tissue that results from mechanical stimulation of an exposed part of the lung. It is produced by local reflex muscular closure of alveolar ducts and alveoli.

**pneumocrania.** See **pneumocephalus.**

***Pneumocystis carinii*** /nōō′mōsis′tis kərin′ē·ī/, a microorganism that causes pneumocystosis, a type of interstitial cell pneumonitis.

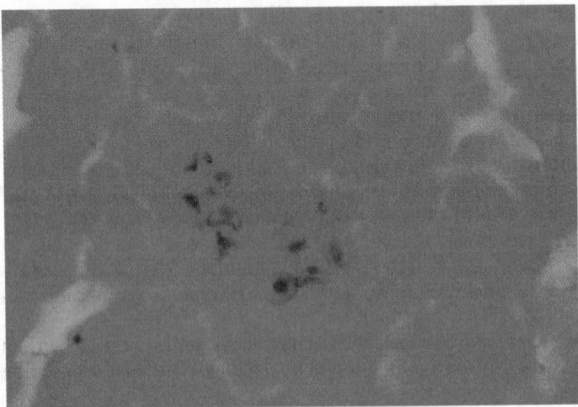

***Pneumocystis carinii* pneumonia** *(Murray et al, 1994)*

***Pneumocystis* pneumonia** [Gk, *pneuma,* air, *kystis,* bag, *pneumon,* lung], a type of interstitial plasma cell pneumonia in which the alveoli become honeycombed with an acid-

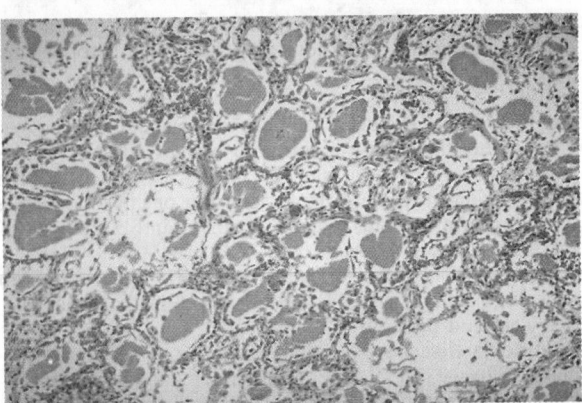

***Pneumocystis* pneumonia** *(Kumar, Cotran, and Robbins, 1997)*

ophilic material. The patient may or may not be febrile but usually is weak, dyspneic, and cyanotic.

**pneumocystosis** /nōō′mōsistō′sis/ [Gk, *pneuma,* air, *kystis,* bag, *osis,* condition], infection with the fungus *Pneumocystis carinii,* usually seen in patients with human immunodeficiency virus infection; premature, malnourished infants; or debilitated or immunosuppressed people, particularly those with hematologic malignancies. It is characterized by fever, cough, tachypnea, and frequently cyanosis. The diagnosis is difficult to make and usually requires obtaining a specimen by an induced sputum procedure or bronchoalveolar lavage and special staining techniques. Mortality rates near 100% in untreated patients. Treatment with pentamidine isethionate or a combination of trimethoprim and sulfamethoxazole, trimetrexate plus folic acid, trimethoprim plus dapsone, atovaquone, or primaquine plus clindamycin is ef-

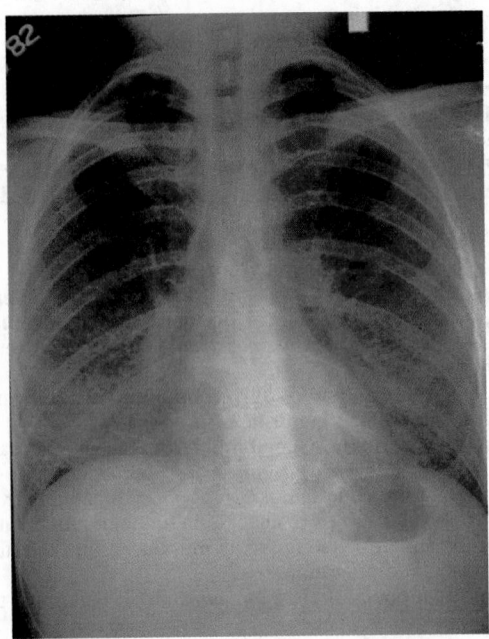

**Pulmonary pneumocystosis**
*(Monahan and Neighbors, 1998/courtesy Jonathan W.M. Gold, MD)*

fective. Patients at risk should receive prophylaxis against acute infection. Also called **interstitial plasma cell pneumonia.**

**pneumoencephalocele.** See **pneumocephalus.**

**pneumoencephalography** /nōō′mō·ensef′əlog′rəfē/ [Gk, *pneuma,* air, *enkephalos,* brain, *graphein,* to record], a procedure for the radiographic visualization of the ventricular space, basal cisterns, and subarachnoid space overlying the cerebral hemispheres of the brain. Air, helium, or oxygen is injected into the lumbar subarachnoid space after the intermittent removal of the cerebrospinal fluid by lumbar puncture. See also **encephalography, ventriculography.** —**pneumoencephalographic,** *adj.*

**pneumogastric nerve.** See **vagus nerve.**

**pneumogram.** See **pneumatogram.**

**pneumograph** /nōō′məgraf/, a device that records breathing movements by means of an inflated coil around the chest. It mainly measures the ventilatory cycle rather than the amplitude of breathing movements.

**pneumohemopericardium.** See **hemopneumopericardium.**

**pneumohemothorax** /-hem′ōthôr′aks/ [Gk, *pneuma,* air, *haima,* blood, *thorax,* chest], an accumulation of air and blood in the pleural cavity.

**pneumolysin** /nōōmol′isin/, virulence factor produced by *Streptococcus pneumoniae* associated with cytolysis.

**pneumomediastinum** /nōō′mōmē′dē·əstī′nəm/ [Gk, *pneuma,* air, *mediastinus,* midway], the presence of air or gas in the mediastinal tissues. In infants it may lead to pneumothorax or pneumopericardium, especially in those with respiratory distress syndrome or aspiration pneumonitis. In older children the condition may result from bronchitis, acute asthma, pertussis, cystic fibrosis, or bronchial rupture from cough or trauma. Also called **Hamman's disease.**

**pneumonectomy** /nōō′mənek′təmē/ [Gk, *pneumon,* lung, *ektomē,* excision], the surgical removal of all or part of a lung. See also **lobectomy.**

**pneumonia** /nōōmō′nē·ə/ [Gk, *pneumon,* lung], an acute inflammation of the lungs, often caused by inhaled pneumococci of the species *Streptococcus pneumoniae.* The alveoli and bronchioles of the lungs become plugged with a fibrous exudate. Pneumonia may be caused by other bacteria, as well as by viruses, rickettsiae, and fungi. Kinds of pneumonia are **aspiration pneumonia, bronchopneumonia, eosinophilic pneumonia, interstitial pneumonia, lobar pneumonia, mycoplasma pneumonia,** and **viral pneumonia.** See also **atypical pneumonia.**

**-pneumonia,** combining form meaning an 'inflammation of the lungs': *necropneumonia, splenopneumonia, typhopneumonia.*

**-pneumonic, 1.** combining form meaning 'related to pneumonia': *bronchopneumonic, peripneumonic, pleuropneumonic.* **2.** combining form meaning 'related to the lungs': *gastropneumonic, hepatopneumonic.*

**pneumonic plague** /nōōmon′ik/ [Gk, *pneumon,* lung; L, *plaga,* stroke], a highly virulent and rapidly fatal form of plague characterized by bronchopneumonia. There are two forms: **Primary pneumonic plague** results from involvement of the lungs in the course of bubonic plague; **secondary pneumonic plague** results from the inhalation of infected particles of sputum from a person having pneumonic plague. Compare **bubonic plague,** septicemic plague. See also **plague,** *Yersinia pestis.*

**pneumonitis** /nōō′mənī′tis/, *pl.* **pneumonitides** [Gk, *pneumon + itis*], inflammation of the lung. Pneumonitis may be caused by a virus or may be a hypersensitivity reaction to chemicals or organic dusts, such as bacteria, bird droppings, or molds. It is usually an interstitial, granulomatous, fibrosing inflammation of the lung, especially of the bronchioles and alveoli. Dry cough is a common symptom. Treatment depends on the cause but includes removal of any offending agents and administration of corticosteroids to reduce inflammation. Compare **pneumonia.**

**pneumono-.** See **pneumo-.**

**pneumonocele.** See **pneumatocele.**

**pneumonopathy** /nōō′mənop′əthē/, any disease or disorder involving the lungs.

**pneumonopleuritis** /-plŏōrī′tis/, a combined disorder of pneumonia and pleurisy.

**pneumonotherapy** /-ther′əpē/, the treatment of lung disease.

**pneumopericardium** /-per′ikär′dē·əm/, the presence of air or gas in the pericardial sac.

**pneumoperitoneum** /nōō′mōper′itənē′əm, -per′itənē′əm/ [Gk, *pneuma,* air, *peri,* around, *teinein,* to stretch], the presence of air or gas within the peritoneal cavity of the abdomen. It may be spontaneous, such as from rupture of a hollow, gas-containing organ, or induced for diagnostic or therapeutic purposes.

**pneumoperitonitis** /nōō′mōper′itənī′tis/, an acute inflammation of the peritoneal cavity accompanied by the presence of air or gas.

**pneumotachometer** /-takom′ətər/, a device that measures the flow of respiratory gases. The pressure gradient is directly related to flow, thus allowing a computer to derive a flow curve measured in liters per minute.

**pneumothorax** /nōō′mōthôr′aks/ [Gk, *pneuma,* air, *thorax,* chest], the presence of air or gas in the pleural space, causing a lung to collapse. Pneumothorax may be the result of an open chest wound that permits the entrance of air, the rup-

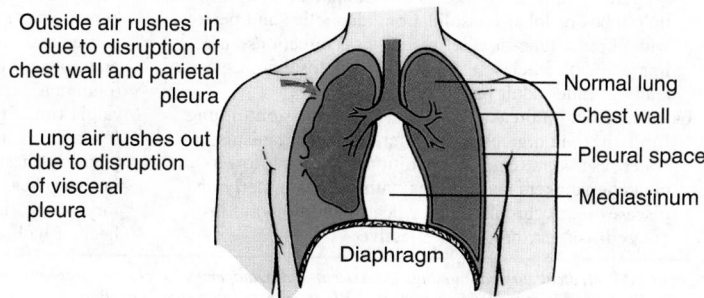

**Pneumothorax** *(Thibodeau and Patton, 1999/Rolin Graphics)*

## Comparison of types of pneumonia

| Causative agent | Characteristics | Clinical manifestations and complications |
| --- | --- | --- |
| **Gram-positive bacterial pneumonias** | | |
| Pneumococcal pneumonia (*Streptococcus pneumoniae*) | URI usually preceding, usual involvement of 1 or more lobes, incubation period of 1-3 days, peak incidence in winter and spring, damage to host by overwhelming growth of organism, necrosis of lung tissue (unusual), chest x-ray shows lobar infiltration, nasopharyngeal carriers, frequent finding of herpes labialis in association with pneumonia, risk factors of chronic heart or lung disease, diabetes mellitus, cirrhosis | Abrupt onset, elevated temperature, tachypnea, chills and rigor, productive cough (often bloody, rusty, or green), nausea, vomiting, malaise, myalgia, weakness, pleuritic chest pain, atelectasis, lung abscess (rare), pleural effusions (25%-50%), empyema, metastatic infection (meninges, joints, heart valves), bacteremia (25%) |
| Staphylococcal pneumonia (*Staphylococcus aureus*) | Acquisition via hematogenous route or via aspiration into lungs; nasopharyngeal carriers (35%-50% of population); necrotizing infection causing destruction of lung tissue; chest x-ray shows bronchopneumonia;* risk factors of chronic lung disease, leukemia, other debilitating diseases; influenza infection (10-14 days earlier) often preceding; drug abusers, diabetics, patients on long-term hemodialysis at risk as carriers; occurrence more frequent in hospitalized patients than in persons in community; prolonged antibiotic therapy usually necessary; high mortality rate in chronically debilitated patients, newborns | Abrupt onset, chills, high fever, productive cough with sputum (often bloody and purulent), tachypnea, progressive dyspnea, pleuritic chest pain, empyema, pleural effusions, lung abscess |
| Streptococcal pneumonia (*Streptococcus pyogenes*) | Occurrence in military populations after influenza epidemics and sporadically in community, often associated with strep throat, occurrence most frequent in winter, transmission to lung by inhalation or aspiration, destruction of lung tissue, chest x-ray shows bronchopneumonia | Fever (usually >102.2° F [39° C]), chills, cough, pharyngitis, hemoptysis, pleuritic chest pain, dyspnea, myalgia, empyema (common), pleural effusions, bacteremia, mediastinitis, pneumothorax, bronchiectasis |
| Anthrax pneumonia (*Bacillus anthracis*) | Association with agricultural or industrial exposure (e.g., individuals working with animal hair or contaminated animal hides or bones), transmission to lung via inhalation, formation of spores, ingestion and transport of spores to hilar lymph nodes (site of multiplication of bacteria) by alveolar macrophages, hemorrhagic pneumonitis possible | Early manifestations: insidious onset (2-4 days), mild fever, myalgia, malaise, fatigue, nonproductive cough Later manifestations: dyspnea, profuse diaphoresis, cyanosis |
| **Gram-negative bacterial pneumonias** | | |
| Friedländer's pneumonia (*Klebsiella pneumoniae*) | Most common gram-negative pneumonia acquired outside hospital; alcoholics, diabetics, persons with chronic lung disease, and postoperative patients at risk; transmission to lungs via aspiration of oropharyngeal organisms; chest x-ray shows lobar consolidation, rapid progression to lung abscess possible; high mortality and morbidity rates | Sudden onset, fever, cough, purulent sputum, hemoptysis, malaise, pleuritic chest pain, extensive lung necrosis, lung abscess, empyema, pericarditis, meningitis |
| *Pseudomonas* pneumonia (*Pseudomonas aeruginosa*) | Most common gram-negative hospital-acquired pneumonia; predisposition from endotracheal intubation, intermittent positive-pressure breathing treatments, suctioning, respiratory therapy equipment; high mortality rate in critically ill patients; chest x-ray shows nodular bronchopneumonia, persons with chronic lung disease, debilitating diseases, tracheostomies, cancer, and kidney transplants or those taking immunosuppressive drugs or broad-spectrum antibiotics at risk; high mortality rate (50%-90%) | High fever, cough, copious sputum, hypoxia, cyanosis, lung abscess |
| Influenza pneumonia (*Haemophilus influenzae*) | Increase in incidence; transmission to lung by endogenous aspiration; chest x-ray shows bronchopneumonia in multiple lobes or lobar consolidation; alcoholics and persons with chronic lung disease, recent viral infections, and immune deficiencies at risk; high mortality rate, especially in older adult patients | Usually gradual onset, sometimes abrupt; fever; chills; cough; purulent sputum; hemoptysis; sore throat; dyspnea; nausea and vomiting; pleuritic chest pain; pleural effusions; lung abscess (common); empyema (common) |
| Legionnaires' disease (*Legionella pneumophila*) | Occurrence in outbreaks or sporadic, transmission to lung from airborne organisms, proliferation of organisms in water reservoirs (e.g., air-conditioning cooling towers), cigarette smokers and persons with serious underlying diseases (e.g., chronic lung or heart conditions) at increased risk, erythromycin effective | Myalgia (initially), headache (initially), fever, chills, nonproductive cough, pleuritic chest pain, nausea and vomiting, diarrhea, mental confusion, respiratory failure (major complication), healing with fibrosis common |

From Lewis SM, Collier IC, Heitkemper MM: *Medical-surgical nursing: assessment and management of clinical problems,* ed 4, St Louis, 1996, Mosby.
*GI,* Gastrointestinal; *GU,* genitourinary; *HIV,* human immunodeficiency virus; *URI,* upper respiratory tract infection.
*Organism has characteristics of both bacteria and viruses.

## Comparison of types of pneumonia—cont'd

| Causative agent | Characteristics | Clinical manifestations and complications |
|---|---|---|
| **Anaerobic bacterial pneumonias** | | |
| Anaerobic streptococci Fusobacteria *Bacteroides* species | Transmission to lung usually by aspiration of oropharyngeal secretions but occasionally via blood from GI or GU tract or wound infections; three or four anaerobes usually causing infections; persons with poor dental hygiene, periodontal disease, and history of altered consciousness at risk; chest x-ray often shows lung abscess, empyema, necrotizing pneumonia | Similar to pneumococcal pneumonia, except for insidious onset; foul-smelling sputum; necrotizing pneumonitis (aspiration induced); lung abscess; empyema |
| ***Mycoplasma* pneumonia** | | |
| Mycoplasma pneumonia (*Mycoplasma pneumoniae*)* | Transmission from person to person by respiratory droplets; incubation period of 9-21 days; involvement of epithelial lining of respiratory system; common in children, military populations, college-age groups; increase in cold agglutinin titer in serum or complement fixation with negative bacterial culture; chest x-ray shows interstitial pneumonia, often bilaterally | Gradual onset; URI, including fever (low-grade), nasal congestion, pharyngitis; lower respiratory tract involvement (e.g., bronchitis, bronchiolitis); headache; malaise; cough (initially usually nonproductive); maculopapular rashes |
| **Viral pneumonias** | | |
| Influenza viruses Adenovirus Parainfluenza viruses Respiratory syncytial virus | Influenza A most common in civilian adults; responsible for about one half of all pneumonias; peak incidence in winter; transmission from person to person by respiratory droplets; usually self-limiting; symptomatic treatment; adverse effect on many respiratory defense mechanisms, predisposing patients to secondary bacterial pneumonia; chest x-ray shows interstitial pneumonia | Fever, chills, headache, myalgia, anorexia, sneezing, nasal congestion, cough (initially nonproductive) |
| **Protozoan pneumonia** | | |
| Interstitial plasma cell pneumonia (*Pneumocystis carinii*) | Opportunistic infection; persons with immunosuppression (e.g., recipients of organ transplants, patients with HIV infection, and those with hematologic malignancies) at highest risk; presentation similar to other atypical pneumonias | Cough (usually nonproductive), fever, night sweats, dyspnea (may be only with exertion) |

ture of an emphysematous vesicle on the surface of the lung, or a severe bout of coughing. It may also occur spontaneously without apparent cause.

■ OBSERVATIONS: The onset of pneumothorax is accompanied by a sudden sharp chest pain, followed by difficult, rapid breathing; decreased breath sounds and cessation of normal chest movements on the affected side; tachycardia; a weak pulse; hypotension; diaphoresis; an elevated temperature; pallor; dizziness; and anxiety.

■ INTERVENTIONS: The patient is assured that the condition can be treated, is urged to remain still, and is placed in bed in Fowler's position. Oxygen is administered through a nasal cannula, unless contraindicated, and the air in the pleural space is immediately aspirated. A chest tube is inserted and attached to an underwater seal; the tube is not removed until air is no longer expelled through the seal and a radiographic examination shows that the lung is completely expanded. Pain may be controlled by administering appropriate analgesics, but the use of respiratory depressants is avoided. Intermittent positive-pressure breathing may be administered.

■ NURSING CONSIDERATIONS: The patient is taught how to turn, cough, breathe deeply, and perform passive exercises and is told to avoid stretching, reaching, or making sudden movements. The patient is advised not to smoke but to drink fluids copiously, to exercise, to avoid fatigue and strenuous activity, and to report any symptoms of recurrence, such as chest pain, difficult breathing, fever, or respiratory infection.

**PNF,** abbreviation for **proprioceptive neuromuscular facilitation.**

**PNH,** abbreviation for **paroxysmal nocturnal hemoglobinuria.**

**-pnoea.** See **-pnea.**

**PNP,** abbreviation for **pediatric nurse practitioner.**

**Po,** symbol for the element **polonium.**

**p.o., P.O.,** an abbreviation for the Latin phrase *per os,* 'by mouth'; a route for administration of medications.

**PO$_2$,** symbol for *partial pressure of oxygen.* See **partial pressure.**

**pocket** /pok′ət /, a saclike space. See also **cavity, pouch, recess.**

**pockmark** [AS, *pocc + meark*], a pitted scar on the skin, usually the result of a smallpox or chickenpox pustule at the site.

**pod-.** See **podo-.**

**podagra.** See **agoraphobia.**

**podalgia.** See **tarsalgia.**

**podalic** /pōdal′ik/ [Gk, *pous,* foot], pertaining to the feet.

**podalic version,** the shifting of the position of a fetus to position the feet at the outlet during labor.

**podiatrist** /pədī′ətrist/, a health professional who diagnoses and treats disorders of the feet. Podiatrists complete a 4-year postgraduate educational program leading to a degree of Doctor of Podiatric Medicine (D.P.M.). Also called **chiropodist** in Canada.

**podiatry** /pədī′ətrē/ [Gk, *pous* + *iatros,* healer], the diagnosis and treatment of diseases and other disorders of the feet. Also called **chiropody** in Canada.

**-podium,** combining form meaning 'something footlike': *axiopodium, phyllopodium, pseudopodium.*

**podo-, pod-,** combining form meaning 'foot': *podogram, podology, podotrochilitis.*

**podophyllotoxin** /pō′dōfil′ətok′sin/ [Gk, *pous* + *phyllon,* leaf, *toxikon,* poison], any one of a group of substances derived from the roots of *Podophyllum peltatum,* a common plant species known as mayapple or American mandrake. Podophyllin, a resinous preparation of podophyllotoxin, is prescribed in the topical treatment of condyloma acuminatum and other types of warts. Several podophyllotoxin derivatives have been used as purgatives and studied for their antineoplastic effects, including the inhibition of mitosis. Podophyllotoxins are not recommended for use in early pregnancy.

**podophyllum** /pod′əfil′əm/ [Gk, *pous* + *phyllon,* leaf], the dried rhizome and roots of *Podophyllum peltatum,* from which a caustic resin is derived for use in removing certain warts.

**poecil-.** See **poikilo-.**

**POEMS syndrome,** a multisystem syndrome combining *p*olyneuropathy *o*rganomegaly, *e*ndocrinopathy, *M* component, and *s*kin changes. It may be linked to a dysproteinemia such as the presence of unusual monoclonal proteins and light chains. Also called **Crow-Fukase syndrome, PEP syndrome.**

**-poesis, -poiesis,** suffix meaning 'formation or production of': *cholanopoiesis, erythropoiesis, hemopoiesis.*

**-poetic, -poietic,** suffix meaning 'production of something specified': *cholepoetic, oenopoetic, uropoetic.*

**pogonion** /pō·gō′nē·on/ [Gk, diminutive of *pōgōn,* beard], the most anterior point in the contour of the chin in the sagittal plane.

**-poietic.** See **-poetic.**

**poikilo-, pecilo-, poecil-,** combining form meaning 'varied or irregular': *poikilocarynosis, poikiloderma, poikilothymia.*

**poikilocytosis** /poi′kilō′sītō′sis/ [Gk, *poikilos,* variation, *kytos,* cell, *osis,* condition], an abnormal degree of variation in the shape of the erythrocytes in the blood. Compare **anisocytosis, macrocytosis, microcytosis.**

**poikiloderma atrophicans vasculare** /-dur′mə/ [Gk, *poikilos,* variation, *derma,* skin, *a* + *trophe,* not nourishment; L, *vasculum,* little vessel], an abnormal skin condition characterized by hyperpigmentation or hypopigmentation, telangiectasia, and atrophy of the epidermis. It may be symmetric or patchy, localized or widespread. It tends to be permanent.

**poikiloderma congenitale.** See **Rothmund-Thomson syndrome.**

**poikiloderma of Civatte,** a common benign progressive dermatitis characterized by erythematous patches on the face and neck that become dry and scaly. As the condition progresses, pigment is deposited around the hair follicles, extending down the lateral aspects of the neck. Photosensitivity is sometimes associated with this dermatitis. Also called **reticulated pigmented poikiloderma.**

**poikilothermic.** See **cold-blooded.**

**point** [L, *punctus,* pricked], a small spot or designated area.

**point A.** See **subspinale.**

**point behavior** [L, *punctus,* pricked; AS, *bihabban,* to behave], the orientation of body parts in a certain direction within a quantum of space.

**point forceps,** a dental instrument used to hold filling

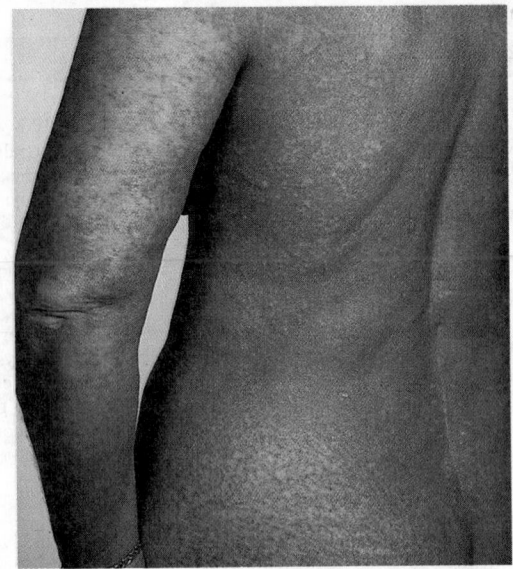

**Poikiloderma atrophicans vasculare**
*(du Vivier, 1993/courtesy St. Mary's Hospital)*

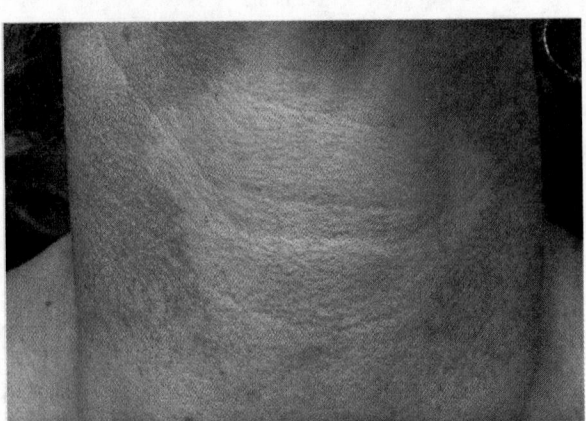

**Poikiloderma of Civatte** *(du Vivier, 1993)*

cones during their placement in root canal filling. Also called **insertion forceps, lock forceps.**

**point lesion,** a disruption of single chemical bonds caused by effects of ionizing radiation on a macromolecule. Also called **molecular lesion.**

**point mutation** [L, *punctus,* pricked, *mutare,* to change], a mutation in which only a single nucleotide of DNA is changed.

**point of maximum impulse (PMI),** the place where the apical pulse is palpated as strongest, often in the fifth intercostal space of the thorax, just medial to the left midclavicular line.

**point-of-service plan,** (in the United States) a plan in which the member may seek care outside the network, or directly from preferred providers with initial evaluation by a primary care provider, but must pay a deductible and/or co-payment.

**point Po.**   See **porion.**

**point system,**   (in the United States) a specialty capitation method in which points are assigned for each patient seen in specific diagnostic or service categories. Periodically points are totaled and income distributed proportionately.

**poise** /poiz/ [Jean L.M. Poiseuille, French physiologist, 1799–1869],   a unit of liquid or gas (fluid) viscosity expressed in terms of grams per centimeter per second $(g \times cm^{-1} \times sec^{-1})$. The centipoise, or 1/100 of a poise, is more commonly used.

**poison** /poi′zən/ [L, *potio,* drink],   any substance that impairs health or destroys life when ingested, inhaled, or absorbed by the body in relatively small amounts. Some toxicologists suggest that, depending on dosages, all substances are poisons. Many experts state that it is impossible to categorize any chemical as either safe or toxic and that the real concern is the risk or hazard associated with the use of any substance. Clinically all poisons are divided into those that respond to specific treatments or antidotes and those for which there is no specific treatment. Research continues to develop effective antitoxins for poisons, but there are relatively few effective antidotes. Maintaining respiration and circulation is the most important aspect of such treatment. See also **poisoning treatment. —poisonous,** *adj.*

**poison control center,**   one of a nearly worldwide network of facilities that provide information regarding all aspects of poisoning or intoxication, maintain records of their occurrence, and refer patients to treatment centers.

**poisoning,**   **1.** the act of administering a toxic substance. **2.** the condition or physical state produced by the ingestion of, injection of, inhalation of, or exposure to a poisonous substance. Identification of the poison ingredients and presentation of a container label are critical to expeditious diagnosis and treatment.

**poisoning, risk for,**   a nursing diagnosis accepted by the Seventh National Conference on the Classification of Nursing Diagnoses. The diagnosis describes the accentuated risk of accidental exposure to or ingestion of drugs or dangerous products in doses sufficient to cause poisoning.

■ RISK FACTORS: The risk factors may be internal (individual) or external (environmental). Internal risk factors include reduced vision, verbalization of occupational setting without adequate safeguards, lack of safety or drug education, lack of proper precautions, cognitive or emotional difficulties, and insufficient finances. External risk factors include large supplies of drugs in the house; medicines or dangerous products stored in unlocked cabinets accessible to children or confused people; availability of illicit drugs potentially contaminated by poisonous additives; flaking, peeling paint or plaster in the environment of young children; chemical contamination of food and water; unprotected contact with heavy metals or chemicals; paint or lacquer in poorly ventilated areas or without effective protection; presence of poisonous vegetation; and presence of atmospheric pollutants. See also **nursing diagnosis.**

**poisoning treatment,**   the symptomatic and supportive care given a patient who has been exposed to or who has ingested a toxic drug, commercial chemical, or other dangerous substance. In the case of oral poisoning a primary effort should be directed toward recovery of the toxic substance before it can be absorbed into the body tissues. If vomiting does not occur spontaneously, it should be induced after first identifying the poison, if possible, and calling a poison control center. If the poison is a petroleum distillate, such as kerosene, or a caustic or corrosive substance, vomiting should *not* be induced. Before any attempt to induce emesis, the victim, if conscious, should be given one or two glasses of milk or water. A carbonated beverage should never be given to an oral poisoning patient. Because of the danger of hypernatremia the patient, particularly a child, should not be given water containing salt or mustard. A family member should be instructed to call a poison control center first. Syrup of ipecac can be given, if available, to induce vomiting, and the dosage can be repeated one time. But if the ipecac fails to induce vomiting, vomiting should be encouraged by stimulating the patient's gag reflex at the back of the throat. Ipecac, which can be a GI irritant, should not be allowed to remain in the stomach. It also should not be given with milk or charcoal, both of which can interfere with its action. In certain cases an antidote may be administered to render the poison inert or to prevent its absorption, as by giving a mild solution of vinegar or citrus juice to neutralize an alkali. A physician should be summoned to take charge of the case.

**poison ivy,**   any of several species of climbing vine of the genus *Rhus,* characterized by shiny three-pointed leaves. It is common in North America and causes severe allergic contact dermatitis in many people. Localized vesicular eruption with itching and burning results and may be treated with antipruritic lotions, cool compresses, or topical corticosteroid ointment or cream. Severe cases may require corticosteroids given intramuscularly or orally. See also **rhus dermatitis, urushiol.**

---

### Interventions in accidental poisoning

1. Assess for airway patency, breathing, and circulation (ABCs) in all clients in whom accidental poisoning is suspected.
2. Remove any visible materials from areas such as the mouth and eyes to terminate exposure.
3. Identify the type and amount of substance ingested, if possible. This may help determine the antidote.
4. Call the Poison Control Center before attempting interventions.
5. If instructed to induce vomiting, give ipecac syrup, an emetic. All households with young children should have ipecac syrup on hand.
   a. Infants (up to 12 months): 5-10 mL of ipecac syrup, then 100-200 mL of water; may repeat if necessary.
   b. Children (1 to 12 years): 1 tablespoon (15 mL) of ipecac syrup, then 200-300 mL of water; may repeat once in 30 minutes.
   c. Adults: 2 tablespoons (15-30 mL) of ipecac syrup, then 200-300 mL of water; may repeat once in 30 minutes.
6. If directed, save vomitus for laboratory analysis, which may assist with further treatment.
7. Position the victim with the head to the side to prevent aspiration of vomitus and assist in keeping the airway open.
8. Never induce vomiting in an unconscious victim or in a client experiencing convulsions, since aspiration may occur.
9. Never induce vomiting if any of the following substances have been ingested: household cleaners, grease or petroleum products, or furniture polish. Vomiting may increase internal burns.
10. If instructed to take the victim to the emergency department, call an ambulance. Emergency equipment may be needed en route.

From Potter PA, Perry AG: *Fundamentals of nursing: concepts, process, and practice,* ed 5, St Louis, 2001, Mosby.

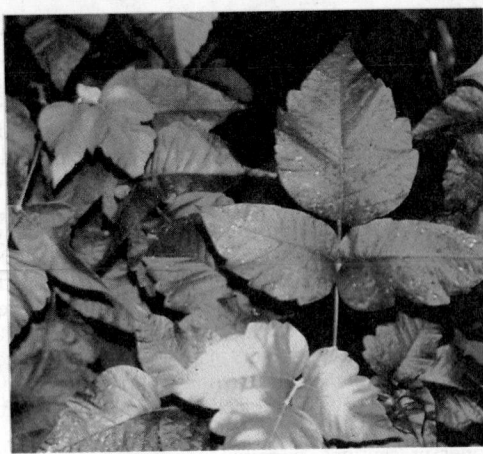

**Poison ivy** *(Zitelli and Davis, 1997)*

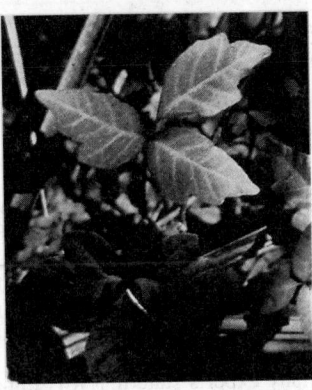

**Poison oak** *(Zitelli and Davis, 1997/courtesy Dr. Mary Jelks)*

**poison ivy dermatitis** [L, *potio,* drink; ME, *ivi* + Gk, *derma,* skin, *itis,* inflammation], an allergic contact dermatitis caused by exposure to a nonvolatile oil, toxicodendrol, present in the leaves and other plant parts of poison ivy, a member of the *Rhus toxicodendron* species. Other *Rhus* species producing the same kind of contact dermatitis are poison oak and poison sumac. Also called **rhus dermatitis.**

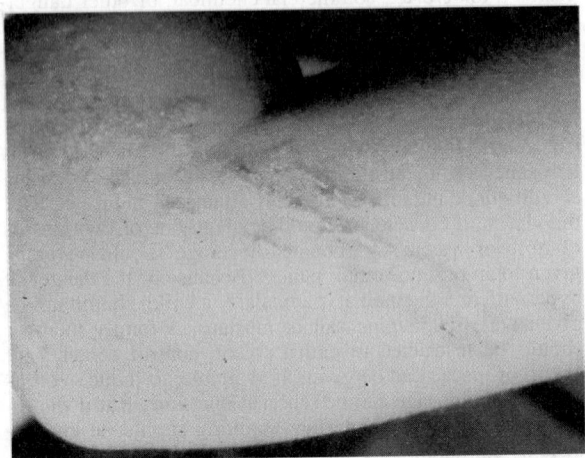

**Poison ivy dermatitis** *(Zitelli and Davis, 1997)*

**poison oak,** any of several species of shrub of the genus *Rhus,* common in North America. Skin contact results in allergic dermatitis in many people. The characteristics and treatment of the condition are similar to those of poison ivy. See also **poison ivy, rhus dermatitis, urushiol.**

**poisonous.** See **poison.**

**poison sumac** /sōō′mak/, a shrub of the genus *Rhus,* common in North America. Skin contact results in allergic dermatitis in many people. The characteristics and treatment of the condition are similar to those of poison ivy. See also **poison ivy, rhus dermatitis, urushiol.**

**poker spine.** See **bamboo spine.**

**Poland's syndrome** /pō′ləndz/ [Alfred Poland, British physician, 1820−1872], unilateral absence of the sternocostal head of the pectoralis major muscle and ipsilateral syndactyly; also called **Poland's anomaly.**

**polar** [L, *polus,* pole], pertaining to molecules that are hydrophilic, or "water-loving." Polar substances tend to dissolve in polar solvents. See also **pole, polus.**

**Polaramine,** trademark for an antihistaminic (dexchlorpheniramine maleate).

**polar body,** one of the small cells produced during the two meiotic divisions in the maturation of a female gamete, or ovum. Polar bodies are nonfunctional and incapable of being fertilized. See also **oogenesis.**

**polarity** /pōler′itē/ [L, *polus*], **1.** the existence or manifestation of opposing qualities, tendencies, or emotions, such as pleasure and pain, love and hate, strength and weakness, dependence and independence, masculinity and femininity. The concept is central to various psychotherapeutic approaches, such as client-centered therapy, in which the key to self-actualization lies in accepting polarity within oneself. **2.** (in physics) the distinction between a negative and a positive electric charge.

**polarity therapy,** a technique of massage based on the theory that the body has positive and negative energy patterns that must be balanced to establish physical harmony.

**polarization** /pō′lərīzā′shən/ [L, *polus* + Gk, *izein,* to cause], the concentration, within a population or group, of members' interests, beliefs, and allegiances around two conflicting positions.

**polarization microscope** [L, *polus,* pole; Gk, *mikros,* small, *skopein,* to view], a microscope that uses polarized light for special diagnostic purposes, such as examining crystals of chemicals found in patients with gout and related disorders.

**polarized light** /po′lərīzd/ [L, *polus* + AS, *leoht*], light that is propagated in such a way that the radiation waves occur in only one direction in the vibration plane and not at random.

**polarographic oxygen analyzer** /pō′lərōgraf′ik/, an electrochemical device used to analyze the proportion of oxygen molecules in respiratory care systems. The oxygen is measured in terms of an electron current produced after it acquires electrons from a negative electrode in a hydroxide bath. Batteries are used to polarize the electrodes in the bath.

**pole** [L, *polus*], **1.** (in biology) an end of an imaginary axis drawn through the symmetrically arranged parts of a cell, organ, ovum, or nucleus. **2.** one of a pair of opposite forces or attractants as in magnetism or electricity. **3.** (in anatomy) the point on a nerve cell at which a dendrite originates. —**polar,** *adj.*

**poles of kidney,** either end of an axis through the length of a kidney. They are designated as the **upper pole of the kidney (extremitas superior renis)** and the **inferior pole of the kidney (extremitas inferior renis).**

*pol* **gene,** a segment of a retrovirus, such as the human immunodeficiency virus, that encodes its reverse transcriptase enzyme.

**policy** /pol'isē/ [Gk, *politeia,* the state], a principle or guideline that governs an activity and that employees or members of an institution or organization are expected to follow.

**polio.** See **poliomyelitis.**

**polio-,** combining form meaning 'gray matter in the nervous system': *polioclastic, polioencephalitis, poliomyelitis.*

**polioencephalitis** /pō'lē-ō'ensef'əlī'tis/ [Gk, *polios,* gray, *enkephalos,* brain, *itis*], an inflammation of the gray matter of the brain caused by infection of the brain by a poliovirus.

**polioencephalomeningomyelitis** /pō'lē-ō'ensef'əlō'-məning'gōmī'əlī'tis/ [Gk, *polios,* gray, *enkephalos,* brain, *meninx,* membrane, *myelos,* marrow, *itis,* inflammation], an inflammation that involves the gray matter of the brain and spinal cord and also the meninges.

**polioencephalomyelitis** /pō'lē-ō'ensef'əlōmī'əlī'tis/ [Gk, *polios* + *enkephalos* + *myelos,* marrow, *itis*], inflammation of the gray matter of the brain and the spinal cord, caused by infection by a poliovirus.

**polioencephalopathy** /pō'lē-ō'ensef'əlop'əthē/ [Gk, *polios,* gray, *enkephalos,* brain, *pathos,* disease], a pathologic condition affecting the gray matter of the brain.

**poliomyelitis** /pō'lē-ōmī'əlī'tis/ [Gk, *polios* + *myelos,* marrow, *itis*], an infectious disease caused by one of the three polioviruses. Asymptomatic, mild, and paralytic forms of the disease occur. Several factors influence susceptibility to the virus and the course of the disease: More boys than girls are severely affected, stress increases susceptibility, more pregnant than nonpregnant women acquire the paralytic form of the disease, and the severity of the infection increases with age. It is transmitted from person to person through fecal contamination or oropharyngeal secretions. The disease is prevented by vaccination. Also called *(informal)* **polio.** See also **poliovirus.**

■ OBSERVATIONS: Asymptomatic infection has no clinical features, but it confers immunity. Abortive poliomyelitis lasts only a few hours and is characterized by minor illness with fever, malaise, headache, nausea, vomiting, and slight abdominal discomfort. Nonparalytic poliomyelitis is longer lasting and is marked by meningeal irritation with pain and stiffness in the back and by all the signs of abortive poliomyelitis. Paralytic poliomyelitis begins as abortive poliomyelitis. The symptoms abate, and for several days the person seems well. Malaise, headache, and fever recur; pain, weakness, and paralysis develop. The peak of paralysis is reached within the first week. In spinal poliomyelitis viral replication occurs in the anterior horn cells of the spine, causing inflammation, swelling, and, if severe, destruction of the neurons. The large proximal muscles of the limbs are most often affected. Bulbar poliomyelitis results from viral multiplication in the brainstem. Bulbar and spinal poliomyelitis often occur together.

**poliomyelitis vaccine.** See **poliovirus vaccine.**

**poliosis** /pō'lē-ō'sis/ [Gk, *polios* + *osis,* condition], depigmentation of the hair on the scalp, eyebrows, eyelashes, mustache, beard, or body. The condition may be inherited and generalized or acquired and localized in patches. Acquired localized poliosis often occurs in alopecia areata.

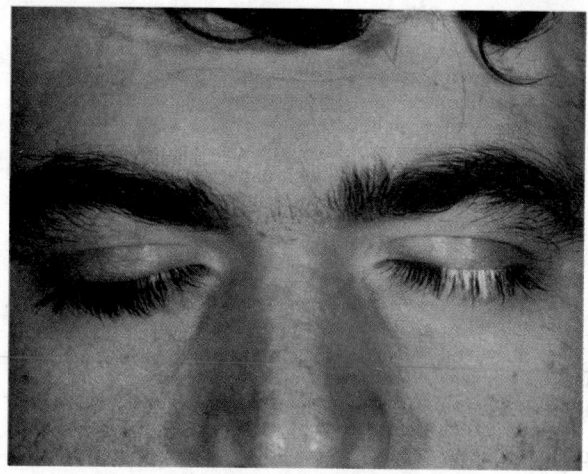

**Poliosis** *(Hordinsky, Sawaya, and Scher, 2000)*

**poliovirus** /-vī'rəs/ [Gk, *polios* + L, *virus,* poison], the causative organism of poliomyelitis. This very small ribonucleic acid virus has three serologically distinct types. Infection or immunization with one type does not protect against the others.

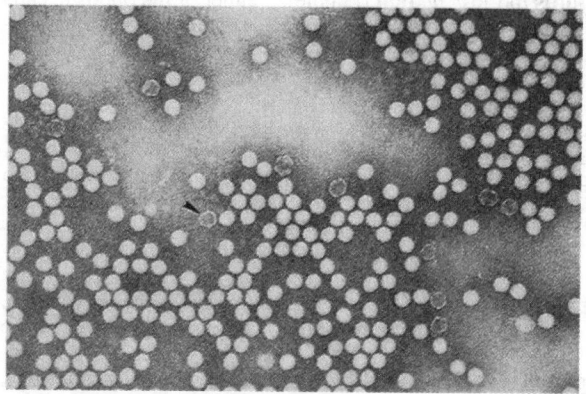

**Electron micrograph of poliovirus**
*(Murray et al, 1998/courtesy Centers for Disease Control and Prevention, Atlanta)*

**poliovirus vaccine,** a vaccine prepared from poliovirus to confer immunity to it. The trivalent live oral form of vaccine, TOPV, is recommended for all children less than 18 years of age who have no specific contraindications. The inactivated poliovirus vaccine (IPV) is a suspension of three strains of polioviruses that have been inactivated in formalin so that normal activity of the organisms has been destroyed. It is recommended for infants and children who are immunodeficient, including human immunodeficiency virus infected infants, and for unvaccinated adults. IPV is given subcutaneously. Rarely, vaccine-associated paralysis occurs after administration of TOPV; this reaction has not occurred with IPV.

**poliovirus vaccine, inactivated.**   See **poliovirus vaccine.**

**polishing** [L, *polire,* to make smooth],   a tendency of patients with right temporal lobe lesions to deny dysphoric affect and minimize socially disapproved behavior while exaggerating other qualities.

**political nursing** /pəlit′ikəl/ [Gk, *politia,* the state, *nutrix,* nurse],   the use of knowledge about power processes and strategies to influence the nature and direction of health care and professional nursing. The constituency of political nursing is patients, both diagnosed and potential, as communities, groups, or individuals.

**pollakiuria** /pol′əkēyŏŏr′ē·ə/ [Gk, *pollache,* frequent, *ouron,* urine],   abnormally frequent passage of urine. Compare **polyuria.**

**pollen coryza.**   See **hay fever.**

**pollenogenic,**   pertaining to a plant that produces pollen or something that is produced by pollen.

**pollex** /pol′eks/, *pl.* **pollices** [L],   **1.** the thumb. **2.** the big toe.

**pollinosis.**   See **hay fever.**

**pollutant** /pəlōō′tənt/ [L, *polluere,* to defoul],   an unwanted substance that occurs in the environment, usually with health-threatening effects. Pollutants may exist in the atmosphere as gases or fine particles that may be irritating to the lungs, eyes, and skin; as dissolved or suspended substances in drinking water; and as carcinogens or mutagens in foods or beverages.

**polonium (Po)** /pəlō′nē·əm/ [Polonia, Poland],   a radioactive element that is one of the disintegration products of uranium. Its atomic number is 84; its atomic mass is approximately 210.

**polus** /pō′ləs/, *pl.* **poli** [L, pole],   either of the opposite ends of any axis; the official anatomic designation for the extremity of an organ. See also **pole. —polar,** *adj.*

**poly-,**   prefix meaning 'many or much': *polyacid, polycholia, polydactylia.*

**polyacrylamide** /-akril′əmīd/,   a polymer of acrylamide and usually some crosslinking derivative.

**polyamine** /pol′ē·am′ēn/,   any compound that contains two or more amine groups, such as spermidine and spermine, which are normally found in human tissue. Many polyamines function as essential growth factors in microorganisms.

**polyanionic** /pol′ē·an′ī·on′ik/ [Gk, *polys,* many, *ana,* again, *ion,* going],   pertaining to multiple negative electric charges.

**polyarteritis** /pol′ē·är′tərī′tis/ [Gk, *polys* + *arteria,* airpipe, *itis,* inflammation],   an abnormal inflammatory condition of several arteries.

**polyarteritis nodosa,**   a severe and poorly understood collagen vascular disease in which widespread inflammation and necrosis of small and medium-sized arteries and ischemia of the tissues they serve occur. Any organ or organ system may be affected. The disease attacks men and women between 20 and 50 years of age. Its cause is unknown, although immunologic factors are suspected. Polyarteritis nodosa may be acute and rapidly fatal or chronic and wasting. It is characterized by fever, abdominal pain, weight loss, neuropathy, and, if the kidneys are affected, hypertension, edema, and uremia. Some symptoms may mimic those of GI or cardiac disorders. Diagnosis is based on the clinical signs, results of laboratory tests, and findings of biopsy of sites affected by the disease. Mortality rate in polyarteritis nodosa is high, especially if there is kidney involvement. Aggressive treatment includes massive doses of corticosteroids. Immunosuppressive drugs have been used experimentally with some success. Physical therapy helps the patient to

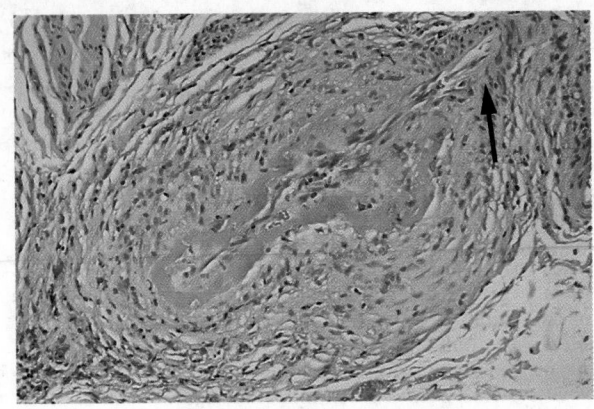

**Polyarteritis nodosa** *(Cotran, Kumar, and Collins, 1999)*

maintain muscle tone and prevents or slows the development of disability.

**polyarthralgia,** /pol′e·ärthral′jə/ [Gk, *polys* + *arthron,* joint, *algos,* pain],   pain in several joints simultaneously.

**polyarthritis** /-ärthrī′tis/,   an inflammation that involves more than one joint. The inflammation may migrate from one joint to another, or there may be simultaneous involvement of two or more joints.

**polyarticular** /-ärtik′yələr/ [Gk, *polys,* many, *articulus,* joint],   pertaining to many joints.

**polycarboxylate cement** /pol′ēkär·bok′si·lāt/,   a dental cement used as a luting agent for cementing restorations and as a cavity lining.

**polychlorinated biphenyls (PCBs)** /-klôr′inā′tid/,   a group of more than 30 isomers and compounds used in plastics, insulation, and flame retardants and varying in physical form from oily liquids to crystals and resins. All are potentially toxic and carcinogenic. The toxicity varies with the type of PCB and concurrent exposure to other substances, such as carbon tetrachloride. Mild exposure may cause chloracne; severe exposure may result in hepatic damage.

**polychondritis** /pol′ē·kon·drī′tis/ [Gk, *polys,* many + *chondros,* cartilage + *-itis,* inflammation],   inflammation involving many cartilages of the body.

**polychromasia.**   See **polychromatophilia.**

**polychromatic** /-krōmatik/ [Gk, *polys* + *chroma,* color],   a light of many colors or wavelengths. The term is usually applied to white light, although it may also refer to a defined part of the spectrum.

**polychromatophil** /pol′ēkrōmat′əfil/,   any cell that may be stained by several different dyes.

**polychromatophilia** /pol′ēkrō′matəfil′yə/ [Gk, *polys* + *chroma* + *philein,* to love],   an abnormal tendency of a cell, particularly an erythrocyte, to be dyed by a variety of laboratory stains. Also called **polychromasia.**

**Polycillin,**   trademark for an antibacterial (ampicillin).

**polyclonal** /pol′ēklō′nəl/ [Gk, *polys* + *klon,* cutting],   **1.** pertaining to or designating a group of identical cells or organisms derived from several identical cells. **2.** pertaining to or designating several groups of identical cells or organisms (clones) derived from a single cell.

**polyclonal gammopathy.**   See **gammopathy.**

**Polycose,**   trademark for a nutritional supplement containing glucose polymers derived from cornstarch.

**polycystic** /-sis′tik/ [Gk, *polys* + *kystis,* bag],   characterized by the presence of many cysts.

**polycystic kidney disease (PKD),** an abnormal condition in which the kidneys are enlarged and contain many cysts. There are three forms of the disease: **Childhood polycystic disease (CPD)** is uncommon and may be differentiated from adult or congenital polycystic disease by genetic, morphologic, and clinical facets. Death usually occurs within a few years as the result of portal hypertension and liver and kidney failure. A portacaval shunt may prolong life into the twenties. **Adult polycystic disease (APD)** may be unilateral, bilateral, acquired, or congenital. The condition is characterized by flank pain and high blood pressure. Kidney failure eventually develops and progresses to uremia and death. **Congenital polycystic disease (CPD)** is a rare congenital aplasia of the kidney involving all or only a small segment of one or both kidneys. Severe bilateral aplasia results in death shortly after birth. Minor aplasia may cause no dysfunction and may never be diagnosed.

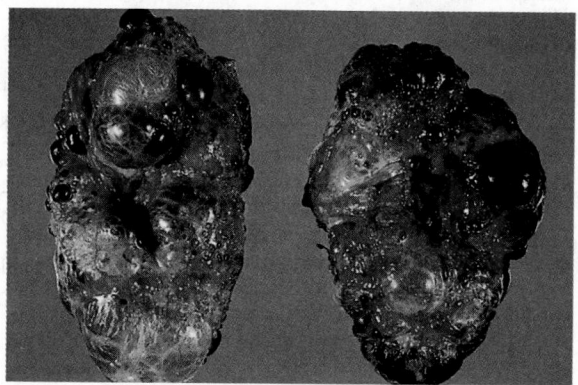

**Adult polycystic disease**
*(Silverberg, DeLellis, and Frable, 1997)*

**polycystic liver,** congenital cystic disease of the liver. Also called **polycystic liver disease.**

**polycystic ovary syndrome,** an endocrine disturbance characterized by anovulation, amenorrhea, hirsutism, and infertility. It is caused by increased levels of testosterone, estrogen, and luteinizing hormone (LH) and decreased secretion of follicle stimulating hormone (FSH). The increased level of LH associated with this disorder may be the result of an increased sensitivity of the pituitary to stimulation by releasing hormone or of excessive stimulation by the adrenal gland. It may also be associated with a variety of problems in the hypothalamic-pituitary-ovarian axis, with extragonadal sources of androgens, or with androgen-producing tumors. This condition is transmitted as an X-linked dominant or autosomal dominant trait. The depressed but continuous production of FSH associated with this disorder causes continuous partial development of ovarian follicles. Numerous follicular cysts, 2 to 6 mm in diameter, may develop. The affected ovary commonly doubles in size and is invested by a smooth pearly white capsule. The increased level of estrogen associated with this abnormality raises the risk of cancers of the breast and endometrium. Depending on the severity of symptoms and the patient's desire to become pregnant, treatment involves suppression of hormonal stimulation of the ovary, usually by use of female hormones or resection of part of one or both ovaries.

Also called *hyperandrogenic chronic anovulations, Stein-Leventhal syndrome.*

**polycythemia** /pol'ēsīthē'mē·ə/ [Gk, *polys* + *kytos,* cell, *haima,* blood], an increase in the number of erythrocytes in the blood that may be primary or secondary to pulmonary disease, heart disease, or prolonged exposure to high altitudes or may be idiopathic. Also called **Osler's disease, polycythemia vera.** Compare **hypoplastic anemia, leukemia.** See also **altitude sickness, erythrocytosis.**

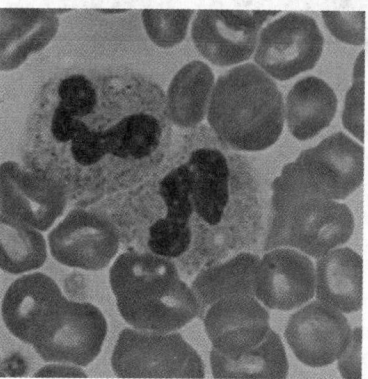

**Polycythemia** *(Carr and Rodak, 1999)*

**polycythemia rubra vera (PV)** [Gk, *polys,* many, *kytos,* cell, *haima,* blood, L, *ruber,* red, *verus,* true], a condition of unknown cause characterized by a marked increase in the red blood cell count, packed cell volume, cellular hemoglobin, leukocytes, platelets, and total blood volume. The skin and mucous membranes acquire a maroon or plum color and hepatomegaly, splenomegaly, hypertension, and neurologic symptoms develop. The condition is associated with an F chromosome defect. Also called **primary polycythemia, Vaquez's disease.**

**polycythemia vera.** See **polycythemia.**

**polydactyly** /-dak'tilē/ [Gk, *polys* + *daktylos,* finger], a congenital anomaly characterized by the presence of more than the normal number of fingers or toes. The condition is usually inherited as an autosomal dominant characteristic and can usually be corrected by surgery shortly after birth. Also called **polydactylia, polydactylism, hyperdactyly.**

**polydipsia** /pol'ēdip'sē·ə/ [Gk, *polys* + *dipsa,* thirst], **1.** excessive thirst. It is characteristic of several different conditions, including diabetes mellitus, in which an excessive concentration of glucose in the blood osmotically pulls intracellular fluid into the bloodstream and increases the excretion of fluid via increased urination, which leads to hypovolemia and thirst. In diabetes insipidus the deficiency of the pituitary antidiuretic hormone results in excretion of copious amounts of dilute urine, reduced fluid volume in the body, and polydipsia. In nephrogenic diabetes insipidus there is also copious excretion of urine with consequent polydipsia. Polyuria resulting from other forms of renal dysfunction also leads to polydipsia. The condition also may be psychogenic in origin. **2.** *(informal)* alcoholism.

**polyelectrolyte** /pol'ē·ilek'trəlīt/ [Gk, *polys* + *elektron,* amber, *lytos,* soluble], a substance with many charged or potentially charged groups.

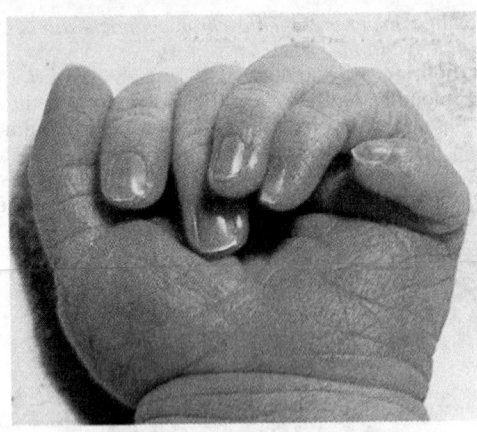

**Polydactyly**
*(Zitelli and Davis, 1997/courtesy Dr. Christine L. Williams,
New York Medical College)*

**polyendocrine deficiency syndromes.** See **polyglandular autoimmune syndromes.**

**polyesthesia** /pol'ē·esthē'zhə/ [Gk, *polys* + *aisthesis,* feeling], a sensory disorder involving the sense of touch in which a stimulus to one area of the skin is also felt at nonstimulated sites.

**polyestradiol phosphate** /-es'trədī'ôl/, an antineoplastic estrogen compound.

- INDICATIONS: It is prescribed for prostate cancer and postmenopausal breast cancer.
- CONTRAINDICATIONS: Male breast cancer, estrogen-dependent neoplasia, thrombophlebitis, or known hypersensitivity to this drug prohibits its use.
- ADVERSE EFFECTS: Among the more serious adverse reactions are loss of libido, impotence, gynecomastia, fluid retention and edema, and rarely cholestatic jaundice.

**polyethylene** /pol'ē·eth'ilēn/, a strong but flexible synthetic resin produced by the polymerization of ethylene. Polyethylene materials have been used in surgery.

**polygene** /pol'ējēn'/ [Gk, *polys* + *genein,* to produce], any of a group of nonallelic genes that individually exert a small effect but interact in a cumulative manner to produce a particular characteristic, usually of a quantitative nature, such as size, weight, skin pigmentation, or degree of intelligence. Also called **cumulative gene, multiple factor, multiple gene.** See also **multifactorial inheritance.** —**polygenic,** *adj.*

**polygenic inheritance.** See **multifactorial inheritance.**

**polyglandular autoimmune diseases.** See **polyglandular autoimmune syndromes.**

**polyglandular autoimmune syndromes,** a group of disorders manifested by subnormal functioning of more than one endocrine gland. Type I is characterized by the appearance of mucocutaneous candidiasis, often occurring in childhood, and is associated with hypoparathyroidism and adrenal insufficiency. It occurs in siblings, without involvement of other generations in the family. Type II involves primary adrenal insufficiency and primary thyroid failure occurring in the same patient for unclear reasons. Many of these patients have an autoimmune disorder, and form antibodies against cellular fractions of many endocrine glands. Type II is also called **Schmidt's syndrome.** Also called

**polyendocrine deficiency syndromes, polyglandular autoimmune diseases.**

**polyglucosan** /-glo͞o'kəsan/ [Gk, *polys* + *glykys,* sweet], a large molecule consisting of many anhydrous polysaccharides.

**polygraph** /pol'ē·graf/ [Gk, *polys* + *graphein,* to write], the most common type of **lie detector.**

**polyhybrid** /-hī'brid/ [Gk, *polys* + L, *hybrida,* offspring of mixed parents], pertaining to or describing an individual, organism, or strain that is heterozygous for more than three specific traits or gene pairs or that is the offspring of parents differing in more than three specific gene pairs.

**polyhybrid cross,** the mating of two polyhybrid individuals, organisms, or strains.

**polyhydramnios.** See **hydramnios.**

**polyleptic** /pol'ēlep'tik/ [Gk, *polys* + *lambanein,* to seize], describing any disease or condition marked by numerous remissions and exacerbations.

**polyleptic fever,** a fever occurring paroxysmally, such as smallpox and relapsing fever.

**polymenia.** See **polymenorrhea.**

**polymenorrhea,** an abnormally frequent recurrence of the menstrual cycle. Also called **polymenia.**

**polymer** /pol'imər/ [Gk, *polys* + *meros,* part], a compound formed by combining or linking a number of monomers, or small molecules. A polymer may be composed of various monomers or of many units of the same monomer.

**polymerase** /pə·lim'ər·ās /, any enzyme that catalyzes polymerization, especially of nucleotides to polynucleotides.

**polymerase chain reaction (PCR)** /pol'ēmer'ās, polim'-ərās/, a process whereby a strand of deoxyribonucleic acid can be cloned millions of times within a few hours. The process can be used to make prenatal diagnoses of genetic diseases and to identify an individual by analysis of a single tissue cell.

**polymerization** /pə·lim'ər·i·zā'shən/, the act or process of forming a compound **(polymer),** usually of high molecular weight, by the combination of simpler molecules **(monomers).**

**polymerize** /pol'əmərīz'/ [Gk, *polys,* many, *meros,* parts], to convert two or more molecules into a polymer.

**polymicrobial** /-mīkrō'bē·əl/ [Gk, *polys,* many, *mikros,* small, *bios,* life], pertaining to a number of species of microbes.

**polymicrobic infection** /-mīkrō'bik/ [Gk, *polys,* many, *mikros,* small, *bios,* life; L, *inficere,* to stain], an infection involving more than one species of pathogen. Also called **mixed infection.**

**polymicrogyria.** See **microgyria.**

**polymorphic** /-môr'fik/ [Gk, *polys,* many, *morphe,* form], pertaining to the ability to assume two or more distinct forms, such as the existence of two or more forms of chromosomes or hemoglobins in a population.

**polymorphism** /pol'ēmôr'fizəm/ [Gk, *polys* + *morphe,* form], **1.** the state or quality of existing or occurring in several different forms. **2.** the state or quality of appearing in different forms at different stages of development. Kinds of polymorphism are **balanced polymorphism** and **genetic polymorphism.** —**polymorphic,** *adj.*

**polymorphocytic leukemia** /pol'ēmôr'fəsit'ik/ [Gk, *polys* + *morphe* + *kytos,* cell, *leukos,* white, *haima,* blood], a neoplasm of blood-forming tissues in which mature segmented granulocytes are predominant. Also called **mature cell leukemia, neutrophilic leukemia.**

**polymorphonuclear** /pol'ēmôr'fōno͞o'klē·ər/ [Gk, *polys* + *morphe* + L, *nucleus,* nut kernel], having a nucleus with a number of lobules or segments connected by a fine thread.

**polymorphonuclear cell (PMN),** a leukocyte with a multilobed nucleus, such as a neutrophil.

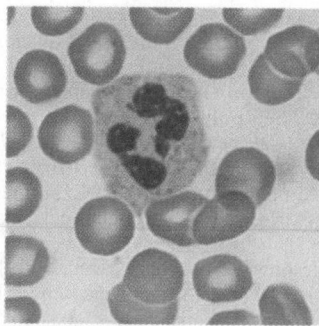

**Polymorphonuclear cell** *(Carr and Rodak, 1999)*

**polymorphonuclear leukocyte,** a white blood cell containing a segmented lobular nucleus; an eosinophil, basophil, or neutrophil. See also **granulocyte.**

**polymorphous** /pol'ēmôr'fəs/ [Gk, *polys* + *morphe,* form], occurring in many varying forms, possibly changing in structure or appearance at different stages.

**polymorphous light eruption,** a common recurrent superficial vascular reaction to sunlight or ultraviolet light in susceptible individuals. Within 1 to 4 days after exposure to the light small erythematous papules and vesicles appear on otherwise normal skin, then disappear within 2 weeks. A delayed allergic response is a possible cause. Tanning reduces the severity of the reaction.

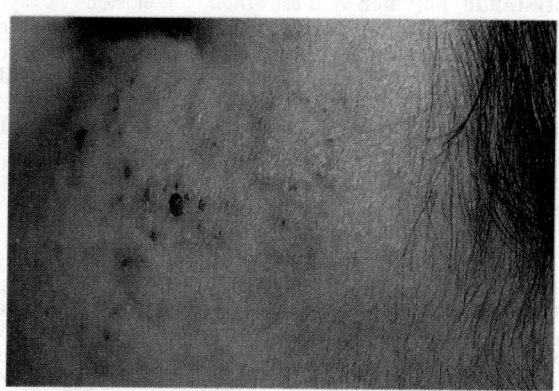

**Polymorphous light eruption**
*(Weston, Lane, and Morrelli, 1996)*

**Polymox,** trademark for an antibiotic (amoxicillin).

**polymyalgia rheumatica** /-mī·al'jə/ [Gk, *polys* + *mys,* muscle, *algos,* pain, *rheuma,* flux], a chronic, episodic, inflammatory disease of the large arteries that usually develops in people over 60 years of age. The disease primarily affects the arteries in muscles. It is characterized by pain and stiffness of the back, shoulder, or neck that is usually more severe on rising in the morning. There may also be a cranial headache, which affects the temporal and occipital arteries, causing a severe throbbing headache. Serious complications of polymyalgia rheumatica include arterial insufficiency, coronary occlusion, stroke, and blindness. Patients with the disease usually have a high erythrocyte sedimentation rate. The disease may follow a self-limited course; however, adrenocorticosteroids have proved highly effective in reducing inflammation and in speeding recovery.

**polymyositis** /pol'ēmī'ōsī'tis/ [Gk, *polys* + *mys,* muscle, *itis*], inflammation of many muscles, usually accompanied by deformity, edema, insomnia, pain, sweating, and tension. Some forms of polymyositis are associated with malignancy. See also **dermatomyositis.**

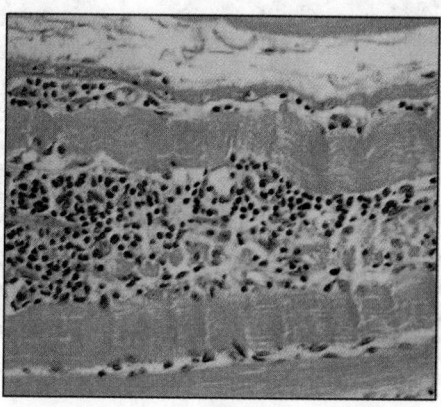

**Polymyositis: muscle biopsy** *(Perkin, 1998)*

**polymyxin** /-mik'sin/, an antibiotic.
■ INDICATIONS: It is used topically and systemically in the treatment of gram-negative bacterial infections, including meningitis, corneal ulcerations, ocular infections, and otitis media.
■ CONTRAINDICATIONS: Hypersensitivity to this drug prohibits its use. It is used with great caution in patients with impaired renal function.
■ ADVERSE EFFECTS: Among the more serious adverse reactions when this drug is used systemically are nephrotoxicity and various neurologic alterations, including blockade of the neuromuscular junction. Pain or phlebitis at the site of injection also may occur. When this drug is applied locally, irritation and allergic reactions of the skin or mucosa sometimes occur.

**polymyxin B sulfate,** an antibiotic.
■ INDICATIONS: It is prescribed for ocular infections.
■ CONTRAINDICATIONS: Known hypersensitivity to this drug prohibits its use.
■ ADVERSE EFFECTS: When it is given topically allergies are the most common problem.

**polyneuralgia** /-no͝oral'jə/ [Gk, *polys,* many, *neuron,* nerve, *algos,* pain], a type of neuralgia that affects several nerves at the same time.

**polyneuritic psychosis.** See **Korsakoff's psychosis.**

**polyneuritis** /-no͝orī'tis/ [Gk, *polys,* many, *neuron,* nerve, *itis,* inflammation], an inflammation involving many nerves.

**polyneuropathy** /-no͞orop′əthē/ [Gk, *polys,* many, *neuron,* nerve, *pathos,* disease], a condition in which many peripheral nerves are afflicted with a disorder.

**polynuclear,** having many nuclei.

**polyoma papovavirus.** See **papillocarcinoma.**

**polyopia** /pol′ē·ō′pē·ə/ [Gk, *polys* + *ops,* eye], a defect of sight in which one object is perceived as many images; multiple vision. The condition can occur in one or both eyes. See also **diplopia.**

**polyp** /pol′ip/ [Gk, *polys* + *pous,* foot], a small tumorlike growth that projects from a mucous membrane surface.

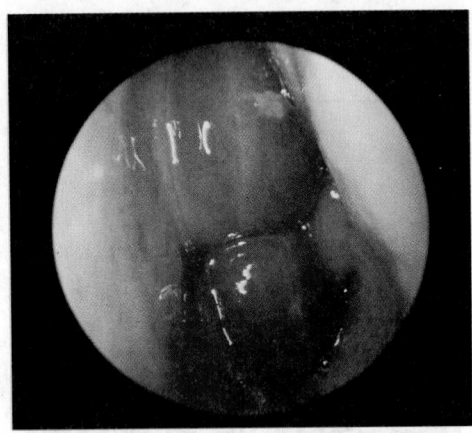

**Nasal polyp** *(Zitelli and Davis, 1997)*

**polypapilloma** /-pap′ilō′mə/ [Gk, *polys,* many; L, *papilla,* nipple; Gk, *oma*], multiple papillomas or stalked tumors.

**polypeptide** /pol′ēpep′tīd/, a long chain of amino acids joined by peptide bonds. Very long polypeptides are usually called proteins. Polypeptides may be formed by partial hydrolysis of proteins or synthesized from free amino acids.

**polyphagia** /pol′ēfā′jē·ə/ [Gk, *polys* + *phagein,* to eat], excessive uncontrolled eating. See also **bulimia.** Also called **hyperphagia.**

**polypharmacy** /-fär′məsē/, the use of a number of different drugs by a patient who may have one or several health problems.

**polyploid** /pol′əploid/ [Gk, *polys* + *plous,* times], **1.** an individual, organism, strain, or cell that has more than twice the haploid number of chromosomes characteristic of the species. The multiple of the haploid number is denoted by the appropriate prefix, as in triploid, tetraploid, pentaploid, hexaploid, heptaploid, octaploid, and so on. Polyploidy is rare in animals, producing individuals that are abnormal in appearance and usually infertile. It is common in plants, however; such plants generally are larger, have larger cells, and are hardier than diploid plants. **2.** pertaining to such an individual, organism, strain, or cell. Also called **polyploidic.** Compare **aneuploid. —polyploidy,** *n.*

**polyploid adenocarcinoma.** See **papillary adenocarcinoma.**

**polyploidic.** See **polyploid.**

**polyploidy** /pol′iploi′dē/, the state or condition of having more than two complete sets of chromosomes.

**polypoid** [Gk, *polys,* many, *pous,* foot, *eidos,* form], like a polyp or tumor on a stalk.

**polyposis** /-pōsis/ [Gk, *polys* + *pous,* foot, *osis,* condition], an abnormal condition characterized by the presence of numerous polyps on a part. See also **familial polyposis.**

**polyposis coli** [Gk, *polys,* many, *pous,* foot, *osis,* condition, *kolikos* colon], a condition of multiple polyps in the large intestine.

**polyradiculitis** /pol′ērədik′yo͞olī′tis/ [Gk, *polys* + L, *radicula,* rootlet; Gk, *itis*], inflammation of many nerve roots, such as found in Guillain-Barré syndrome.

**polyribosome.** See **polysome.**

**polysaccharide** /-sak′ərīd/ [Gk, *polys* + *sakcharon,* sugar], a carbohydrate polmer that is formed from three or more molecules of simple carbohydrates. Examples of polysaccharides are dextrin, starch, glycogen, cellulose, gums, and inulin.

**polysome** /pol′isōm/ [Gk, *polys* + *soma,* body], a group of ribosomes joined by a molecule of messenger RNA containing a portion of the genetic code that is to be translated. Polysomes are found in the cytoplasm during protein synthesis. Also called **ergosome, polyribosome.** See also **translation.**

**polysomnography** /pol′ē·som·nog′rə·fē/ [Gk, *polys,* many + L, *somnus,* sleep + Gk, *graphein,* to write or record], the polygraphic recording during sleep of multiple physiologic variables, both directly and indirectly related to the state and stages of sleep, to assess possible biological causes of sleep disorders.

**polysomy** /pol′isō′mē/, the presence of more than two copies of a chromosome in an otherwise diploid somatic cell as the result of chromosomal nondisjunction during meiosis. The chromosome may be duplicated three (trisomy), four (tetrasomy), or more times. Males with Klinefelter's syndrome may have a genotype of XXY, XXXY, or XXXXY. Polysomic females with three, four, or five X chromosomes may have a higher frequency of mental retardation.

**Polysporin,** trademark for an ophthalmic and topical fixed-combination antiinfective drug containing antibacterials (polymyxin B sulfate and bacitracin).

**polysulfide polymer** /pol′ēsul′fīd/, an elastomeric synthetic rubber used in dentistry as an impression material for fixed partial prosthodontic structures, inlays for single quadrants, and dental impressions. Also called **polysulfide rubber.**

**polysynaptic** /-sinap′tik/ [Gk, *polys,* many, *synaptein,* to join], pertaining to nerve cells that end in synapses.

**polysyndactyly** /-sindak′tilē/ [Gk, *polys,* many, *syn,* together, *daktylos,* finger or toe], multiple webbing or fusion between fingers or toes.

**polytene chromosome** /pol′itēn/ [Gk, *polys* + *tainia,* band], an excessively large type of chromosome consisting of a large number of copies of the chromosome bundled side by side. Polytene chromosomes are produced by repeated rounds of DNA synthesis without mitosis and are bundles of unseparated chromonemata filaments found primarily in the salivary glands of certain insects. See also **giant chromosome.**

**polythiazide** /-thī·az′īd/, a diuretic and antihypertensive.

■ INDICATIONS: It is prescribed in the treatment of hypertension and edema.

■ CONTRAINDICATIONS: Anuria or known hypersensitivity to this drug, other thiazides, or sulfonamide derivatives prohibits its use.

■ ADVERSE EFFECTS: Among the more serious adverse reactions are hypokalemia, hyperglycemia, hyperuricemia, and various hypersensitivity reactions.

**polyunsaturated** /-unsach′ərā′tid/ [Gk, *polys,* many; AS, *un,* not; L, *saturare,* to fill], pertaining to a chemical compound containing more than one double or triple bond that can be opened to accept more atoms in the molecule, thereby becoming saturated. A polyunsaturated fatty acid is one in which there are two or more double bonds in the chain of carbon atoms that can be opened to accept hydrogen atoms.

**polyunsaturated fatty acid.** See **unsaturated fatty acid.**

**polyuria** /pol′ēyŏŏr′ē·ə/ [Gk, *polys* + *ouron*, urine], the excretion of an abnormally large quantity of urine. Some causes of polyuria are diabetes insipidus, diabetes mellitus, use of diuretics, excessive fluid intake, and hypercalcemia.

**polyvalent,** denoting the capacity of an element to combine with two or more atoms.

**polyvalent antiserum.** See **antiserum.**

**polyvalent vaccine** /-vā′lənt/ [Gk, *polys,* many; L, *valere,* worth, *vaccinus,* cow], a vaccine prepared from several different antigenic types of a species. Also called **multivalent vaccine.**

**Poly-Vi-Flor,** trademark for an oral fixed-combination pediatric drug containing several vitamins and sodium fluoride.

**polyvinyl chloride (PVC)** /-vī′nil/, a common synthetic thermoplastic material that releases hydrochloric acid when burned and that may contain carcinogenic vinyl chloride molecules as a contaminant.

**polyvinylidene fluoride (PVF$_2$)** /-vīnil′idēn/, a commonly used piezoelectric material in a hydrophone. It is also used in imaging transducers.

**POMP** /pomp/, an abbreviation for a combination drug regimen used in the treatment of cancer, containing three antineoplastics, Purinethol (mercaptopurine), Oncovin (vincristine sulfate), and methotrexate, and prednisone (a glucocorticoid).

**Pompe's disease** [J.C. Pompe, twentieth-century Dutch physician; L, *dis,* opposite of; Fr, *aise,* ease], a form of muscle glycogen storage disease. There is a generalized accumulation of glycogen, resulting from a deficiency of acid maltase (alpha-1,4-glucosidase). It is usually fatal in infants, caused by cardiac or respiratory failure. Children with Pompe's disease appear mentally retarded and hypotonic, seldom living beyond 20 years of age. In adults muscle weakness is progressive, but the disease is not fatal. Also called **glycogen storage disease, type II.** See also **glycogen storage disease.**

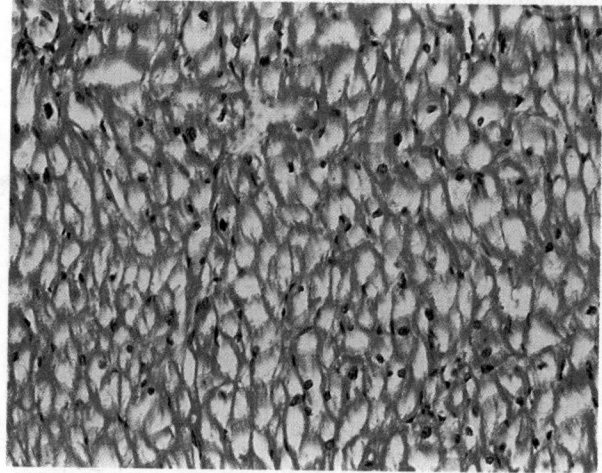

**Pompe's disease: glycogen in myocardial fibers**
*(Cotran, Kumar, and Collins, 1999/courtesy Dr. Trace Worrell, Department of Pathology, University of Texas Southwestern Medical Center, Dallas)*

**POMR,** abbreviation for **problem-oriented medical record.**

**pono-,** prefix meaning 'pain': *ponograph, ponopalmosis, ponophobia.*

**ponos.** See **kala-azar.**

**pons** /ponz/, *pl.* **pontes** /pon′tēz/ [L, bridge], **1.** a prominence on the ventral surface of the brainstem, between the medulla oblongata and the cerebral peduncles of the midbrain. The pons consists of white matter and a few nuclei and is divided into a ventral part and a dorsal part. The ventral part consists of transverse fibers separated by longitudinal bundles and small nuclei. The dorsal part comprises the tegmentum, which is a continuation of the reticular formation of the medulla. The tegmentum contains the nucleus of the abducens nerve, the nucleus of the facial nerve, the motor nucleus of the trigeminal nerve, the sensory nuclei of the trigeminal nerve, the nucleus of the cochlear division of the eighth nerve, the superior olive, and the nuclei of the vestibular division of the eighth nerve. Also called **bridge of Varolius. 2.** any slip of tissue connecting two parts of a structure or an organ of the body.

**Ponstel,** trademark for an antiinflammatory and analgesic (mefenamic acid).

**pont-,** prefix meaning 'bridge': *pontic, ponticulus, pontimeter.*

**pontes.** See **pons.**

**Pontiac fever.** See **Legionnaires' disease.**

**pontic** /pon′tik/ [L, *pons,* bridge], the suspended member of a removable partial denture or fixed bridge, such as an artificial tooth, usually occupying the space previously occupied by the natural tooth crown.

**pontine** /pon′tīn/ [L, *pons,* bridge], pertaining to the pons. Also **pontile.**

**pontine nucleus** [L, *pons,* bridge, *nucleus,* nut kernel], nerve cells in the basilar part of the pons where impulses are relayed between the cerebrum and cerebellum.

**pontine respiratory center.** See **apneustic center.**

**Pontocaine Hydrochloride,** trademark for a local anesthetic (tetracaine hydrochloride).

**pooled plasma** [AS, *pol* + Gk, *plasma,* something formed], a liquid component of whole blood, collected and pooled to prepare various plasma products or to use directly as a plasma expander when whole blood is unavailable or is contraindicated. It is useful in surgery and in the treatment of hypovolemia because of its stability and availability in freeze-dried form. It is collected from blood banks or prepared directly from donors by plasmapheresis. It is thin and colorless or slightly yellow. Of the total volume of normal blood, 55% to 65% is plasma. See also **bank blood, component therapy, packed cells.**

**poorly differentiated lymphocytic malignant lymphoma,** a lymphoid neoplasm containing cells resembling lymphoblasts that have a fine nuclear structure and one or more nucleoli. Also called **lymphoblastic lymphoma, lymphoblastic lymphosarcoma, lymphoblastoma.**

**popliteal** /poplit′ē·əl, pop′lite′əl/ [L, *poples,* ham of the knee], pertaining to the area behind the knee.

**popliteal artery** [L, *poples,* ham of the knee; Gk, *arteria,* airpipe], a continuation of the femoral artery, extending from the opening in the abductor magnus, passing through the popliteal fossa at the knee, dividing into eight branches, and supplying various muscles of the thigh, leg, and foot. Its branches are the superior muscular, sural, cutaneous, medial superior genicular, lateral superior genicular, middle genicular, medial inferior genicular, and lateral inferior genicular.

**popliteal node,** a node in one of the groups of lymph glands in the leg. Approximately seven small popliteal nodes are embedded in the fat of the popliteal fossa at the back of the knee. Compare **anterior tibial node, inguinal node.**

**popliteal pterygium syndrome,** 1. also called **popliteal web syndrome.** a congenital syndrome consisting chiefly of popliteal webs, cleft palate, lower lip pits, and dysplasia of the toenails; a wide variety of other abnormalities may be associated. 2. also called **Fèvre-Languepin syndrome.** popliteal webbing associated with cleft lip and palate, fistula of the lower lip, syndactyly, nail dysplasia, and clubfoot.

**popliteal pulse,** the pulsation of the popliteal artery, behind the knee, best palpated with the patient lying prone with the knee flexed.

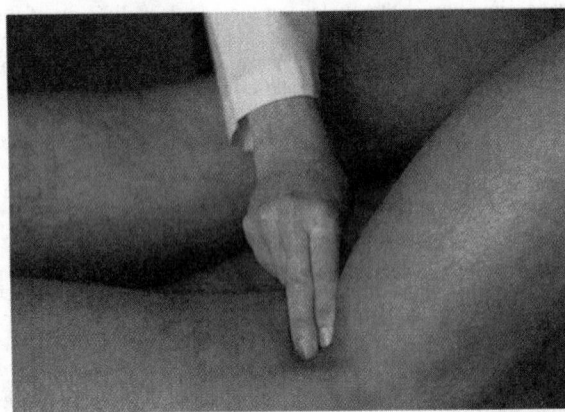

**Assessment of the popliteal pulse** (Potter and Perry, 2001)

**popliteal web syndrome.** See **popliteal pterygium syndrome.** (def. 1).

**population** /pop′yəlā′shən/ [L, *populus*, the people], 1. an interbreeding group of individuals characterized by genetic continuity through several generations. 2. a group of individuals collectively occupying a particular geographic locale. 3. any group that is distinguished by a particular trait or situation. 4. any group from which samples may be measured for some variable characteristic for statistical purposes.

**population at risk,** a group of people who share a characteristic that causes each member to be susceptible to a particular event, such as nonimmunized children who are exposed to poliovirus or immunosuppressed people who are exposed to herpesvirus. Also called **vulnerable population.**

**population genetics,** a branch of genetics that applies mendelian inheritance to groups and studies the frequency of alleles and genotypes in breeding populations. See also **Hardy-Weinberg equilibrium principle.**

**por-, poro-,** prefix meaning 'a cavity, opening, passage or pore': *porencephalia, porion, porotomy.*

**poractant alfa,** a lung surfactant extract.

■ INDICATIONS: This drug is used in the treatment (rescue) of respiratory distress syndrome in premature infants.

■ CONTRAINDICATIONS: None currently known.

■ ADVERSE EFFECTS: Concurrent illnesses that have occurred during treatment with this drug include pulmonary air leaks, pulmonary interstitial emphysema, apnea, pulmonary hemorrhage, patent ductus arteriosus, intracranial hemorrhage, severe intracranial hemorrhage, necrotizing enterocolitis, posttreatment sepsis, and posttreatment infection. Adverse effects include bradycardia, oxygen desaturation, pallor, vasoconstriction, hypotension, and hypertension.

**porcelain** /por′sə·lən/, 1. a white, translucent, dense ceramic material produced by fusing under high temperature of a mixture of feldspar, kaolin, quartz, whiting, and other substances. 2. see **dental porcelain.**

**porcine** /pôr′sīn/ [L, *porcinus,* pig-like], obtained from or related to hogs, such as porcine insulin.

**porcine graft** [L, *porcinus,* pig-like; Gk, *graphion,* plant stylus], a temporary biologic heterograft made from the skin of a pig.

**-pore,** suffix meaning an 'opening or passageway': *metapore, myelopore, neuropore.*

**porfimer,** a miscellaneous antineoplastic.

■ INDICATIONS: This drug is used to treat completely obstructing esophageal cancer and endobronchial non-small cell lung cancer.

■ CONTRAINDICATIONS: Factors that prohibit the use of this drug include porphyria, porphyrin allergy (porfimer), tracheoesophageal or bronchoesophageal fistula, and major blood vessels with eroding tumors (PDT).

■ ADVERSE EFFECTS: Life-threatening effects of this drug are cardiac failure, pleural effusion, and tracheoesophageal fistula. Other adverse effects are pneumonia, dyspnea, respiratory insufficiency, dehydration, weight decrease, anemia, photosensitivity reaction, urinary tract infection, and moniliasis. Common side effects include hypotension, hypertension, atrial fibrillation, tachycardia, abdominal pain, constipation, diarrhea, dyspepsia, dysphagia, eructation, esophageal edema/bleeding, hematemesis, melena, nausea, vomiting, anorexia, anxiety, confusion, and insomnia.

**poriomania** /pôr′ē·ōmā′nē·ə/, a tendency to leave home impulsively or to be a vagabond.

**porion** /por′ē·on/ [Gr. *poros,* passage], the most lateral point on the roof of the bony external acoustic meatus, vertically over the middle of the meatus. Also called **point Po.**

**pork tapeworm.** See *Taenia solium.*

**pork tapeworm infection** [L, *porcus,* pig, hog (male); AS, *taeppe,* tape, *wyrm,* worm; L, *inficere,* to stain], an infection of the intestine or other tissues, caused by adult and larval forms of the tapeworm *Taenia solium.* The pork tapeworm is unique in that it can use humans as both intermediate hosts for larvae and definitive hosts for the adult worm. Humans are usually infected with the adult worm after eating contaminated undercooked pork. The infection is rare in the United States but relatively common in South America, Asia, and Russia. See also **cysticercosis, tapeworm infection.**

**poro-.** See **por-.**

**porosis** /pərō′sis/ [Gk, *poros,* passage], a condition of thinning bone tissue, particularly its supporting connective tissue, as in osteoporosis.

**porous** /pôr′əs/ [Gk, *poros,* passage], pertaining to something with pores or openings.

**porphobilinogen** /pôr′fōbilin′əjən/, a chromogen substance that is an intermediate in the biosynthesis of heme and porphyrins. It appears in the urine of people with porphyria, representing an error of metabolism. See also **heme, porphyria.**

**porphyria** /pôrfir′ē·ə/ [Gk, *porphyros,* purple], a group of inherited disorders in which there is abnormally increased production of substances called porphyrins. Two major classifications of porphyria are **erythropoietic porphyria,** characterized by the production of large quantities of porphyrins in the blood-forming tissue of the bone marrow, and **hepatic porphyria,** in which large amounts of porphyrins are produced in the liver. Clinical signs common to both classifications of porphyria are photosensitivity, abdominal pain, and neuropathy. See also **uroporphyria.**

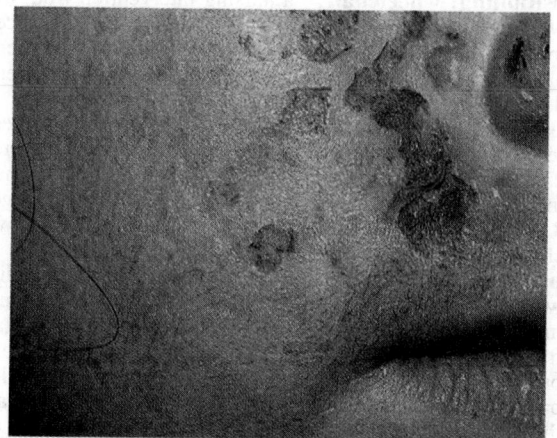

**Erythropoietic porphyria** *(Weston, Lane, and Morrelli, 1996)*

**porphyria cutanea tarda (PCT),** the most common form of porphyria, characterized by cutaneous photosensitivity that causes scarring bullae, hyperpigmentation, facial hypertrichosis, and sometimes sclerodermatous thickenings and alopecia; it is frequently associated with alcohol abuse, liver disease, or hepatic siderosis. Urinary levels of uroporphyrin and coproporphyrin are increased and activity of a specific enzyme involved in heme biosynthesis is decreased. The cause is debated, but two types are generally recognized: an autosomal dominant (or *familial* ) form in which activity of the affected enzyme is reduced to half normal in liver, erythrocytes, and fibroblasts, and a *sporadic* (but probably also familial) form in which the reduction is confined to the liver. Both types are believed to be heterozygous and clinical expression occurs in adulthood, precipitated by disease or environmental factors; a more severe homozygous form begins in childhood and is called **hepatoerythropoietic porphyria.** See also **porphyria.**

**porphyrin** /pôr′fərin/ [Gk, *porphyros*, purple], any iron- or magnesium-free pyrrole derivative occurring in many plant and animal tissues. Normal findings of porphyrins in urine are 50 to 300 mg/24 hours.

**portability** /pôr′təbil′itē/ [L, *portare*, to carry], a property of computer software that permits its use in a variety of compatible operating systems.

**portacaval shunt** /pôr′təkā′vəl/ [L, *porta*, gateway, *cavus*, cavity; ME, *shunten*], a shunt created surgically to increase blood flow from the portal circulation by carrying it into the vena cava.

**Portagen,** trademark for a nutritional supplement containing protein, carbohydrate, and fat.

**porta hepatis.** See **portal fissure.**

**portal** /pôr′təl/ [L, *porta*, gateway], **1.** an entrance. **2.** pertaining to the porta hepatis, or portal vein.

**portal circulation** [L, *porta*, gateway, *circulare*, to go around], the pathway of blood flow from the GI tract and spleen to the liver via the portal vein and its tributaries. Also called **hepatic portal circulation.**

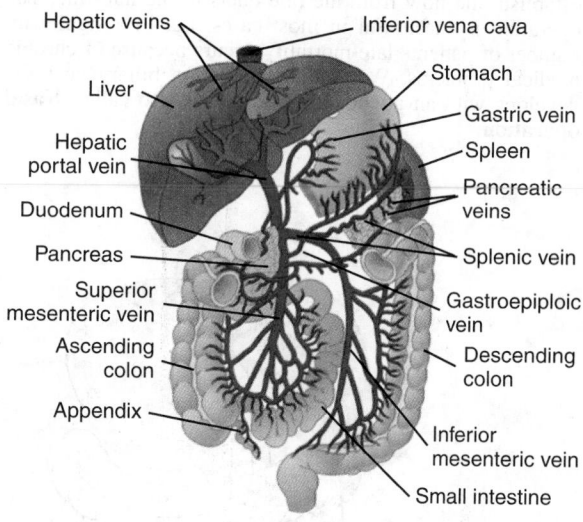

**Portal circulation**
*(Thibodeau and Patton, 1999/Network Graphics)*

**portal fissure** [L, *porta* + *fissura*, cleft], a fissure on the visceral surface of the liver along which the portal vein, the hepatic artery, and the hepatic ducts pass. Also called **porta hepatis.**

**portal hypertension,** an increased venous pressure in the portal circulation caused by compression or occlusion in the portal or hepatic vascular system. It results in splenomegaly, large collateral veins, ascites, and in severe cases systemic hypertension and esophageal varices. Portal hypertension is frequently associated with cirrhosis.

**portal of entry,** the route by which an infectious agent enters the body, such as through nonintact skin.

**portal system,** arrangement of blood vessels in which blood exiting one tissue is immediately carried to a second tissue before being returned to the heart and lungs for oxygenation and redistribution.

**portal systemic encephalopathy.** See **hepatic coma.**

**portal vein,** a vein from the small intestine that ramifies in the liver and ends in capillary-like sinusoids that convey the blood to the inferior vena cava through the hepatic veins. The portal vein passes behind the duodenum and ascends through the lesser omentum to the porta hepatis, where it divides into the right and left branches. The vein is surrounded by the hepatic plexus of nerves and is accompanied by numerous lymphatic vessels, some lymph nodes, and corresponding branches of the hepatic artery. The right branch of the portal vein enters the right lobe of the liver and the left branch enters the left lobe.

**portal venous shunt.** See **postcaval shunt.**

**Porter-Silber reaction** [Curt C. Porter, American biochemist, b. 1914; Robert H. Silber, American biochemist, b. 1915], a reaction, visible as a change in color to yellow, that indicates the amount of adrenal steroids (the 17-hydroxycorticosteroids) excreted per day in the urine. The test is used to evaluate adrenocortical function but is now largely supplanted by immunoassay techniques.

**portoenterostomy** /pôr'tō·en'təros'təmē/ [L, *porta* + Gk, *enteron,* bowel, *stoma,* mouth, *temnein,* to cut], a procedure to correct biliary atresia in which the jejunum is anastomosed by a Roux-en-Y loop to the portal fissure region to establish bile flow from the bile ducts to the intestine. The operation is successful in most cases, but in a significant number of patients late mortality occurs because of chronic medical problems. Without the operation biliary cirrhosis develops with an attendant early death. Also called **Kasai operation.**

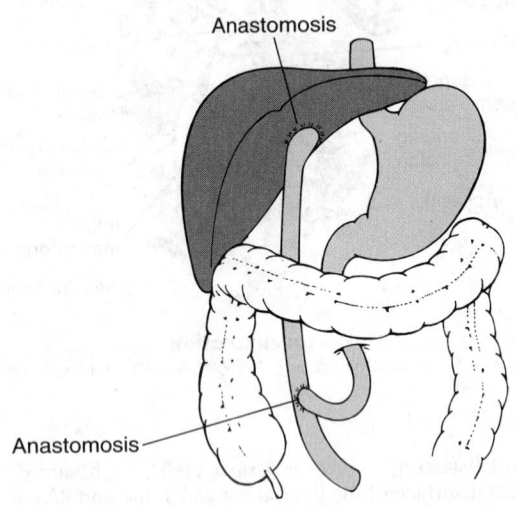

Anastomosis

Anastomosis

**Portoenterostomy** *(McCance and Huether, 1998)*

**Portuguese-Azorean disease.** See **Machado-Joseph disease.**

**port-wine stain.** See **nevus flammeus.**

**position** /pəzish'ən/ [L, *positio*], **1.** any one of many postures of the body, such as the anatomic position, lateral recumbent position, or semi-Fowler's position. See specific positions. **2.** (in obstetrics) the relationship of an arbitrarily chosen fetal reference point, such as the occiput, sacrum, chin, or scapula, on the presenting part of the fetus to its location in the maternal pelvis.

**-position,** combining form meaning the 'putting or setting in place': *electrodeposition, juxtaposition, reposition.*

**positional behavior** /pəzish'ənəl/, the orientation of the body regions to claim a quantum of space. Positional behavior involves four body regions: head and neck, upper torso, pelvis and thighs, and lower legs and feet.

**positional vertigo.** See **postural vertigo.**

**positioner** /pə·zish'ən·ər/, a resilient rubbery and plastic removable appliance fitted over the occlusal surfaces of the teeth to obtain limited tooth movement and stabilization, usually at the end of orthodontic treatment.

**positioning,** a nursing intervention from the Nursing Interventions Classification (NIC) defined as deliberative placement of the patient or a body part to promote physiological and/or psychological well-being. See also **Nursing Interventions Classification.**

**positioning: intraoperative,** a nursing intervention from

the Nursing Interventions Classification (NIC) defined as moving the patient or body part to promote surgical exposure while reducing the risk of discomfort and complications. See also **Nursing Interventions Classification.**

**positioning: neurologic,** a nursing intervention from the Nursing Interventions Classification (NIC) defined as achievement of optimal, appropriate body alignment for the patient experiencing or at risk for spinal cord injury or vertebral irritability. See also **Nursing Interventions Classification.**

**positioning: wheelchair,** a nursing intervention from the Nursing Interventions Classification (NIC) defined as placement of a patient in a properly selected wheelchair to enhance comfort, promote skin integrity, and foster independence. See also **Nursing Interventions Classification.**

**positive** /poz'itiv/ [L, *positivus,*], **1.** (of a laboratory test result) indicating that a substance or a reaction is present. **2.** (of a sign) indicating on physical examination that a finding is present, often meaning that there is pathologic change. **3.** (of a substance) tending to carry or carrying a positive chemical charge.

**positive-end expiratory pressure (PEEP),** positive airway pressure applied at the end of the exhalation phase during mechanical ventilation. Each successive breath begins from a new baseline. Air is delivered in cycles of constant pressure through the respiratory cycle. The patient is usually but not always intubated, and a ventilator cycles the air through an endotracheal tube. PEEP is used for the relief of respiratory distress secondary to prematurity, pancreatitis, shock, pulmonary edema, trauma, surgery, or other conditions in which spontaneous respiratory efforts are inadequate and arterial levels of oxygen are deficient. Close observation is necessary during PEEP therapy because PEEP may decrease venous return to the heart. Blood gases and vital signs are monitored closely. If PEEP does not significantly improve the patient's condition, its level is increased or it may be discontinued. Compare **continuous positive airway pressure.**

**positive feedback,** **1.** (in physiology) an increase in function in response to a stimulus; for example, micturition increases after the flow of urine has started, and the uterus contracts more frequently and with greater strength after it has begun to contract in labor. **2.** *informal.* an encouraging, favorable, or otherwise positive response from one person to what another person has communicated.

**positive identification,** the unconscious modeling of one's personality on that of another who is admired and esteemed. See also **identification.**

**positive mask.** See **reversal film.**

**positive pressure,** **1.** a greater-than-ambient atmospheric pressure. **2.** any technique in which compressed gas or air is delivered to the airways at greater-than-ambient pressure. Positive-pressure techniques in respiratory therapy require a flow-regulating device and a delivery system, such as a cannula, mouthpiece, endotracheal tube, or tracheostomy tube.

**positive pressure breathing unit.** See **IPPB unit.**

**positive pressure ventilation,** any of numerous types of mechanical ventilation in which gas is delivered into the airways and lungs under positive pressure, producing positive airway pressure during inspiration; it may be done via either an endotracheal tube or a nasal mask.

**positive relationship,** (in research) a direct relationship between two variables; as one increases, the other can be expected to increase. Also called **direct relationship.** Compare **negative relationship.**

**positive sequence,** the sequence of the bases on the strand of a double-stranded nucleic acid that encodes the product;

in DNA it is the strand that encodes the RNA, having thus the same base sequence except changing T for U in the RNA.

**positive signs of pregnancy,** three unmistakable signs of pregnancy: fetal heart tones, heard on auscultation; fetal skeleton, seen on x-ray film or ultrasonogram; and fetal parts, felt on palpation.

**positron** /pos′itron/, a positively charged particle emitted from neutron-deficient radioactive nuclei. The antiparticle of an electron.

**positron emission tomography (PET)** [L, *positivus* + Gk, *elektron*, amber; L, *emittere*, to send out; Gk, *tome*, section, *graphein* to record], a computerized radiographic technique that uses radioactive substances to examine the metabolic activity of various body structures. The patient either inhales or is injected with a metabolically important substance such as glucose, carrying a radioactive element that emits positively charged particles, or positrons. When the positrons combine with electrons normally found in the cells

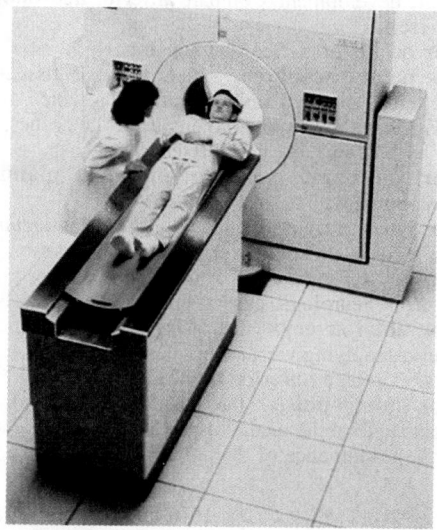

**Positioning of a patient for a PET scan**
*(Chipps, Clanin, and Campbell, 1992)*

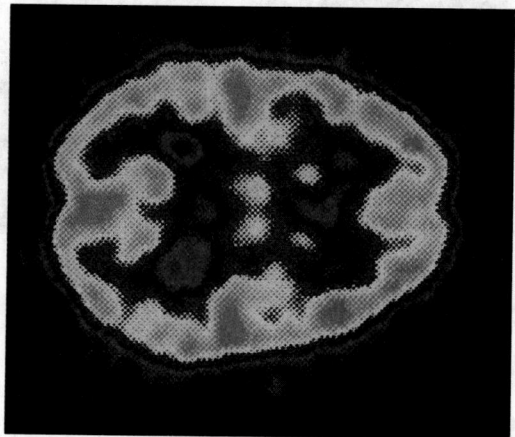

**Image produced by a PET scan after a seizure**
*(Black, Hawks, and Keene, 2001)*

of the body, gamma rays are emitted. The electronic circuitry and computers of the PET device detect the gamma rays and construct color-coded images that indicate the intensity of metabolic activity throughout the organ involved. The radioactive isotopes used in PET are very short-lived, so that patients undergoing a PET scan are exposed to very small amounts of radiation. Researchers use PET to examine blood flow and the metabolism of the heart and blood vessels; to study and diagnose cancer; and to investigate the biochemical activity of the brain.

**Posner-Schlossman syndrome.** See **glaucomatocyclitic crisis.**

**post.** See **dowel.**

**post-,** prefix meaning 'after or behind': *postabortal, postcerebellar, postdiastolic.*

**postanesthesia care,** a nursing intervention from the Nursing Interventions Classification (NIC) defined as monitoring and management of the patient who has recently undergone general or regional anesthesia. See also **Nursing Interventions Classification.**

**postanesthesia care unit (PACU),** an area adjoining the operating room to which surgical patients are taken for nursing assessment and care while recovering from anesthesia. It is also identified as the postanesthesia care unit (PACU). Vital signs, adequacy of ventilation and pain are carefully observed as the patient recovers consciousness. The PACU has nursing staff with specific skills care for patients and a nurse anesthetist or anesthesiologist is available. Also called **recovery room.** See also **postoperative care.**

**postaxial** /pōst·ak′sē·əl/ [L, *post,* after; Gk, *axon,* axis], posterior to an axis. In anatomical usage, this refers to the medial (ulnar) aspect of the upper limb, and the lateral (fibular) aspect of the lower limb.

**postaxial acrofacial dysostosis.** See **Miller syndrome.**

**postcaval shunt** /-kā′vəl/ [L, *post,* after, *vena cava* + ME, *shunten*], any of several surgical anastomoses of the portal and systemic circulations to relieve symptoms of portal hypertension. Also called **portacaval shunt; portal venous shunt.**

**postcentral gyrus** /-sen′trəl/ [L, *post,* after; Gk, *kentron,* center, *gyros,* turn], a convolution of the brain immediately posterior to the central sulcus of the cerebrum. It is the location of the sensory strip for the contralateral side of the body.

**postcoital** /-kō′itəl/ [L, *post,* after, *coire,* to come together], after sexual intercourse.

**postcommissurotomy syndrome** /-kəmis′yərot′əmē/ [L, *post,* after, *commissura,* a union; Gk, *temnein,* to cut], a condition of unknown cause occurring within the first few weeks after cardiac valvular surgery, characterized by intermittent episodes of pain and fever, which may last weeks or months and then resolve spontaneously.

**postconcussional syndrome** /-kənkush′ənəl/ [L, *post* + *concussio,* shake violently], a condition that follows head trauma, characterized by dizziness, poor concentration, headache, hypersensitivity, and anxiety. It usually resolves itself without treatment. Also called **posttraumatic syndrome.**

**postdate pregnancy** /-dāt′/ [L, *post,* after, *data* + *praegnans,* bearing child], a pregnancy that lasts more than 42 weeks. Also called **postterm pregnancy.**

**postdural puncture headache (PDPH),** headache in the erect position following procedures involving puncture of the dura mater, such as lumbar puncture and spinal anesthesia. It is thought to be caused by leakage of cerebrospinal fluid at the puncture site, with settling of the brain and stretching of the intracranial nerves.

**posterior** /postir′ē·ər/ [L, behind],   **1.** in the back part of a structure, such as of the dorsal surface of the human body. **2.** the back part of something. **3.** toward the back. Compare **anterior.**

**posterior Achilles bursitis,** a painful heel condition caused by inflammation of the bursa between the Achilles tendon and the calcaneus. It is commonly associated with Haglund's deformity.

**posterior antebrachial cutaneous nerve,** a nerve that branches off from the radial nerve, innervates the skin of the dorsal aspect of the forearm, and has a general sensory modality.

**posterior asynclitism.** See **asynclitism.**

**posterior atlantoaxial ligament,** one of five ligaments connecting the atlas to the axis. It is broad, thin, and fixed to the inferior border of the anterior arch of the atlas and to the ventral surface of the body of the axis. Compare **anterior atlantoaxial ligament.**

**posterior atlantooccipital membrane,** one of a pair of thin, broad fibrous sheets that form part of the atlantooccipital joint between the atlas and the occipital bone and contain an opening for the vertebral artery and the suboccipital nerve. Also called **posterior atlantooccipital ligament.** Compare **anterior atlantooccipital membrane.**

**posterior auricular artery,** one of a pair of small branches from the external carotid arteries, dividing into auricular and occipital branches and supplying parts of the ear, scalp, and other structures in the head.

**posterior column.** See **posterior horn.**

**posterior common ligament.** See **posterior longitudinal ligament.**

**posterior costotransverse ligament,** one of the five ligaments of each costotransverse joint, comprising a fibrous band passing from the neck of each rib to the base of the vertebra above. Compare **superior costotransverse ligament.**

**posterior drawer sign,** an orthopedic test used to determine laxity of the posterior cruciate ligament of the knee. The patient is positioned with hips at 45 degrees and knees flexed at 90 degrees while the examiner stabilizes the foot and pushes the tibia backward. Also, with both the hips and knees flexed at 90 degrees, the examiner holds the heels together and observes the knees to compare the relative posterior sag of the tibia.

**posterior fontanel,** a small triangular area between the occipital and parietal bones at the junction of the sagittal and lambdoidal sutures. See also **fontanel.**

**posterior fossa,** a depression on the posterior surface of the humerus, above the trochlea, that lodges the olecranon of the ulna when the elbow is extended.

**posterior horn** [L, behind, *cornu,* horn], the horn-shaped projection of gray matter in the posterior region of the spinal cord. Also called **dorsal column, dorsal horn,** and **posterior column.**

**posterior inferior cerebellar artery syndrome.** See **Wallenberg's syndrome.**

**posterior ligament.** See **rectovaginal ligament.**

**posterior longitudinal ligament,** a thick strong ligament attached to the dorsal surfaces of the vertebral bodies, extending from the occipital bone to the coccyx. Also called **posterior common ligament.** Compare **anterior longitudinal ligament.**

**posterior mediastinal node,** a node in one of three groups of thoracic visceral nodes, connected to the part of the lymphatic system that serves the esophagus, pericardium, diaphragm, and convex surface of the liver. Most of the efferent vessels of the posterior mediastinal nodes end in the thoracic duct, but some join the tracheobronchial nodes. Compare **anterior mediastinal node.**

**posterior mediastinum,** the irregularly shaped lower part of the mediastinum, parallel with the vertebral column. It is bounded ventrally by the pericardium, inferiorly by the diaphragm, dorsally by the vertebral column from the fourth to the twelfth thoracic vertebra, and laterally by the mediastinal pleurae. It contains the bifurcation of the trachea, two primary bronchi, the esophagus, the thoracic duct, many large lymph nodes, and various vessels, such as the thoracic part of the aortic arch. Compare **anterior mediastinum, middle mediastinum, superior mediastinum.**

**posterior nares,** a pair of posterior internal openings in the nasal cavity connecting it with the nasopharynx and allowing the inhalation and exhalation of air. Each is an oval aperture that measures about 2.5 cm vertically and is about 1.5 cm in diameter. Also called **choanae.** Compare **anterior nares.**

**posterior neuropore,** the embryonic opening at the inferior end of the neural tube from neural canal to exterior. It closes at about the 25 somite stage, which indicates the end of horizon XII in the numeric anatomic charting of human embryonic development. Compare **anterior neuropore.** See also **horizon.**

**posterior occlusion.** See **distoclusion.**

**posterior palatal seal area,** the area of soft tissues along the junction of the hard and soft palates on which displacement, within the physiologic tolerance of the tissues, can be applied by a denture to aid its retention.

**posterior pituitary, posterior pituitary gland.** See **neurohypophysis.**

**posterior rhizotomy** [L, behind; Gk, *rhiza,* root, *temnein,* to cut], a surgical procedure for cutting the posterior, or sensory, nerve root for the relief of intractable pain or to relieve spasms from neurologic causes such as cerebral palsy.

**posterior tibial artery,** one of the divisions of the popliteal artery, supplying various muscles of the lower leg, foot, and toes. Compare **anterior tibial artery.**

**posterior tibialis pulse,** the pulse of the posterior tibialis artery palpated on the medial aspect of the ankle, just posterior to the prominence of the ankle bone.

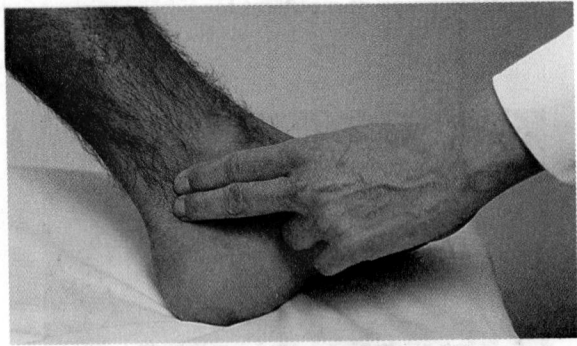

**Palpation of the posterior tibialis pulse**
*(Wilson and Giddens, 2001)*

**posterior tooth,** any of the maxillary and mandibular premolars and molars of the deciduous or secondary dentition, or of prostheses.

**posterior uveitis,** uveitis involving the posterior segment of the eye, including **choroiditis** and **chorioretinitis.**

**posterior vaginal hernia.**  See **vaginal hernia.**

**posterior vein of left ventricle,**  one of the five tributaries of the coronary sinus that drain blood from the capillary bed of the myocardium. It courses along the diaphragmatic surface of the left ventricle, accompanying the circumflex branch of the left coronary artery. In some individuals it ends in the great cardiac vein. Compare **great cardiac vein, middle cardiac vein, small cardiac vein.**

**postero-** /pos'tərō-/,  prefix meaning 'posterior part': *posteroanterior, posteromedian, posterosuperior.*

**posteroanterior** /-antīr'ē-ər/ [L, *posterus,* coming after, *anterior,* before],  the direction from back to front.

**posteroexternal** /pos'tər-ō-ek-ster'nəl/ [L, *posterus,* coming after, *externus,* outward],  situated on the outer side of a posterior aspect.

**posteroid panniculitis** /pos'təroid pənik'yəlī'tis/ [L, *panniculus,* piece of cloth],  subcutaneous nodules that may develop in children after withdrawal of corticosteroid treatment for rheumatic fever or nephrotic syndrome. The condition resolves spontaneously or with readministration of the medication.

**posteroinferior** /-infir'ē-ər/ [L, *posterus,* coming after, *inferior,* lower],  pertaining to a position that is both lower and behind.

**posterolateral** /-lat'ərəl/ [L, *posterus,* coming after, *latus,* side],  pertaining to a position behind and to the side.

**posterolateral thoracotomy,**  a chest surgery technique in which an incision is made in the submammary fold, below the tip of the scapula. The incision is continued posteriorly along the course of the ribs and upward as far as the spine of the scapula. It requires division of the trapezius, rhomboideus, latissimus dorsi, and serratus anterior muscles. Compare **anterolateral thoracotomy, median sternotomy.** See also **thoracotomy.**

**posteromedial** /pos'tər-ō-mē'dē-əl/ [L, *posterus,* coming after, *medius,* middle],  situated toward the middle of the posterior surface.

**posteromedial central arteries of posterior communicating artery,**  branches off the posterior communicating artery that supply the medial surface of the thalamus and the walls of the third ventricle.

**posteroparietal** /pos'tər-ō-pə-rī'ə-təl/ [L, *posterus,* coming after, *paries,* wall],  situated at the posterior part of the parietal bone.

**posterosuperior** /pos'tər-ō-sōō-pēr'ē-ər/ [L, *posterus,* coming after, *superior,* higher],  situated posteriorly and superiorly.

**postganglionic** /-gang'glē-on'ik/ [L, *post,* after; Gk, *ganglion,* knot],  distal to a ganglion.

**postganglionic fiber,**  the axon of a nerve cell whose cell body is situated in a ganglion.

**postganglionic neuron** [L, *post,* after; Gk, *ganglion,* knot, *neuron,* nerve],  a neuron that is distal to or beyond a ganglion.

**posthepatic cirrhosis.**  See **cirrhosis.**

**posthepatic jaundice** /pōst'hepat'ik/ [L, *post,* after; Gk, *hepar,* liver; Fr, *jaune,* yellow],  jaundice caused by obstruction of the bile ducts.

**posthumous** /pos'chəməs/ [L, *post,* after, *humare,* to bury],  after a person's death.

**posthypnotic suggestion** /-hipnot'ik/ [L, *post,* after; Gk, *hypnos,* sleep; L, *suggerere,* to suggest],  an action suggested to a hypnotized subject during a trance that the subject carries out on awakening from the trance. The action is in response to a cue and the subject usually does not know why he or she is performing it.

**postictal** /pōst'iktəl/ [L, *post* + Gk, *ikteros,* jaundice],  after a seizure. **—postictus,** *n.*

**postinfectious** /-infek'shəs/ [L, *post* + *inficere,* to stain],  after an infection.

**postinfectious encephalitis.**  See **encephalitis.**

**postinfectious glomerulonephritis,**  the acute form of glomerulonephritis, which may follow 1 to 6 weeks after a streptococcal infection, most often in childhood. Characteristics of the disease are hematuria, oliguria, edema, and proteinuria, especially in the form of granular casts. There may be slight impairment of renal function in adults, but most patients recover fully in 1 to 3 months. There is no specific treatment for this form of glomerulonephritis; the restriction of dietary protein and the prescription of diuretics may be necessary until kidney function returns to normal. See also **chronic glomerulonephritis, subacute glomerulonephritis.**

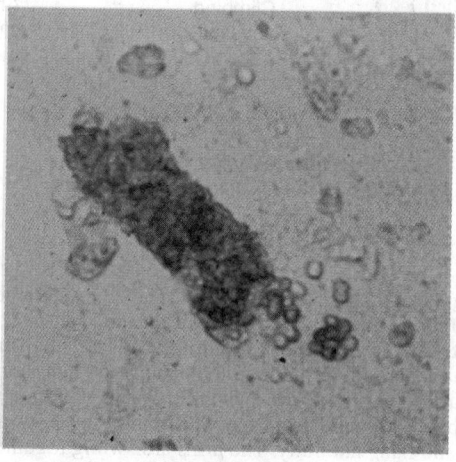

**Postinfectious glomerulonephritis: red blood cell cast**
*(Zitelli and Davis, 1997)*

**postinfectious psychosis** [L, *post,* after, *inficere,* to stain; Gk, *psyche,* mind, *osis,* condition],  psychotic behavior that follows a severe infection such as pneumonia, scarlet fever, malaria, uremia, or typhoid fever. Also called **infectious-exhaustive syndrome.**

**postlumbar puncture headache** /-lum'bar/ [L, *post,* after, *lumbus,* loin, *punctura;* AS, *heafod* + *acan*],  a headache that occurs within a few hours of a lumbar puncture and usually lasts 1 or 2 days to several weeks. It may be accompanied by nausea and vomiting and improves when the patient lies down.

**postmastectomy exercises** /-məstek'təmē/ [L, *post* + Gk, *mastos,* breast, *ektomē,* excision],  exercises essential to the prevention of shortening of the muscles, contracture of the joints, and improvement in lymph and blood circulation after mastectomy.

■ METHOD: The woman is asked to flex and extend the fingers of the affected arm in the recovery room and to pronate and supinate the forearm immediately on return to her room after recovery from anesthesia and surgery. The postoperative mastectomy exercises are begun gradually at the surgeon's discretion. Brushing her teeth and hair is encouraged as effective exercise. Other exercises are usually taught, including four specific exercises: climbing the wall, arm swinging, rope pulling, and elbow spreading. They are performed as follows: *Climbing the wall:* The patient stands

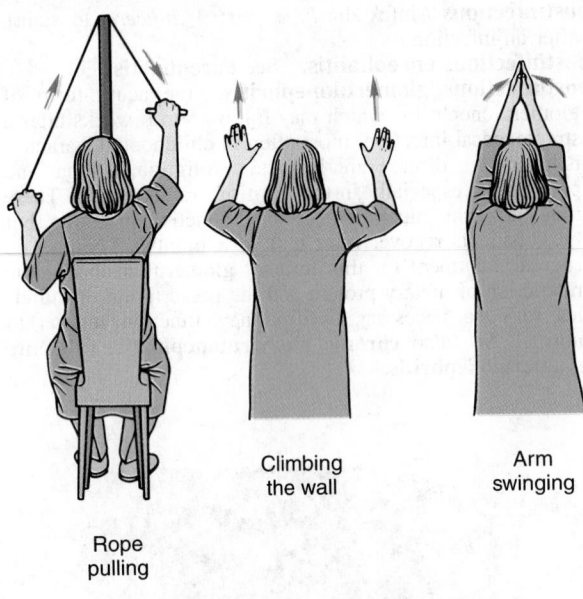

**Postmastectomy exercises**
*(Lewis, Heitkemper, and Dirksen, 2000)*

Rope
pulling

Climbing
the wall

Arm
swinging

fants often look as if they have lost weight in utero. The newborn is fed early, and the calcium and potassium levels in the blood are monitored and corrected, if necessary, to prevent seizures and neurologic damage. To prevent the syndrome labor may be induced as gestation approaches 42 weeks. To anticipate the problems associated with the syndrome, the fetus and the mother may be electronically monitored through labor.

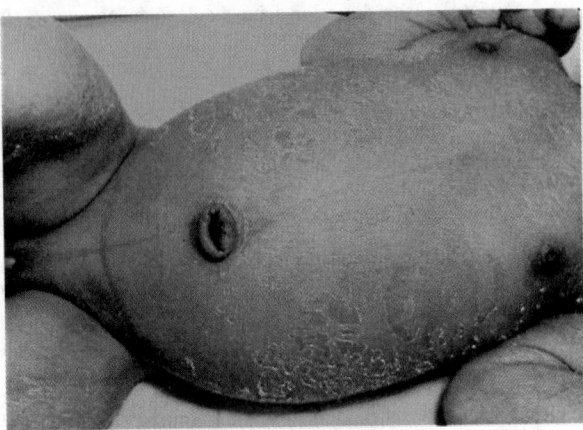

**Dry skin of postmature infant** *(Zitelli and Davis, 1997)*

facing a wall, toes close to the wall. The elbows are bent and the palms of the hands are placed on the wall at shoulder height. The hands are moved up the wall together until the woman feels pain or pulling on the incision, then returned to the starting position. *Arm swinging:* While standing, the patient bends forward from the waist, allowing both arms to relax and hang naturally. The arms are swung together from the shoulders from left to right and then in circles parallel to the floor, clockwise and counterclockwise. She straightens up slowly. *Rope pulling:* A rope is attached over a shower rod or a hook. Each end of the rope is grasped, and the patient alternately pulls each end, raising one arm after the other to the height at which incisional pain or pulling is felt. The rope is shortened until the affected arm is raised almost directly overhead. *Elbow spreading:* The hands are clasped behind the neck, and the elbows are slowly raised to chin level while the head is held erect. Gradually the elbows are spread apart to the point at which incisional pain or pulling is felt.

■ INTERVENTIONS: Specific exercises may be ordered. The patient is shown how to do them and is encouraged to continue them at home.

■ OUTCOME CRITERIA: With proper exercise full range of motion returns; both arms can be extended fully and equally high over the head. The woman benefits from having something active to do to help herself during the difficult period of adjustment after mastectomy. Many activities of daily life provide good exercise, such as reaching high shelves, hanging clothes, and gardening.

**postmature** /-məchoor´/ [L, *post* + *maturare,* to become ripe], **1.** overly developed or matured. **2.** pertaining to a postmature infant. See also **dysmaturity. —postmaturity,** *n.*

**postmature infant,** an infant born after the end of the forty-second week of gestation, bearing the physical signs of placental insufficiency. Characteristically the baby has dry, peeling skin; long fingernails and toenails; and folds of skin on the thighs and sometimes on the arms and buttocks. Hypoglycemia and hypokalemia are common. Postmature in-

**postmaturity** /-məchoo´ritē/ [L, *post,* after, *maturare,* to make ripe], beyond the normal date for maturity.

**postmenopausal** /-men´əpô´səl/ [L, *post* + *men,* month; Gk, *pauein,* to cease], pertaining to the period of life after the menopause.

**postmenopausal hemorrhage,** bleeding from the uterus after menopause.

**postmenopausal vaginitis** [L, *post,* after, *men,* month; Gk, *pauein,* to cease; L, *vagina,* sheath; Gk, *itis,* inflammation], an inflammation caused by degenerative changes in the vaginal mucosa after menopause. Also called **atrophic vaginitis.**

**postmortem** /môr´təm/ [L, *post* + *mors,* death], **1.** after death. **2.** *(informal)* **postmortem examination.**

**postmortem care,** a nursing intervention from the Nursing Interventions Classification (NIC) defined as providing physical care of the body of an expired patient and support for the family viewing the body. See also **Nursing Interventions Classification.**

**postmortem cesarean section** [L, *post,* after, *mors,* death, *secare,* to cut, *sectio*], delivery of a fetus by incision into the uterus after death of a woman.

**postmortem delivery.** See **postmortem cesarean section.**

**postmortem examination** [L, *post,* after, *mors,* death, *examinatio*], an examination of a body after death by a person trained in pathology. Also called **autopsy,** *(informal)* **postmortem.**

**postmortem graft** [L, *post,* after, *mors,* death; Gk, *graphion,* stylus], the transplanting of a cornea, artery, or other body part from a dead person to repair a defect in a living body. Also called **cadaver graft.**

**postmortem lividity,** the black and blue discoloration of the skin of a cadaver resulting from an accumulation of deoxygenated blood in subcutaneous vessels.

**postmyocardial infarction syndrome** /-mī·ə·kär′dē·əl/ [L, *post* + Gk, *mys,* muscle, *kardia,* heart; L, *infarcire,* to stuff], a condition that may occur days or weeks after an acute myocardial infarction. It is characterized by chest pain, fever, pericarditis with a friction rub, pleurisy, pleural effusion, joint pain, and elevated white blood cell count, and sedimentation rate. It tends to recur and often provokes severe anxiety, depression, and fear that another heart attack is occurring. Treatment includes aspirin, reassurance, and a short course of corticosteroids. Nursing care includes close observation and emotional support, especially when debilitating anxiety and depression are present. Also called **Dressler's syndrome.**

**postnasal** /-nā′zəl/ [L, *post,* after, *nasus,* nose], pertaining to the region posterior to the nasal cavity.

**postnasal drip (PND)** [L, *post* + *nasus,* nose; AS, *dryppan*], a drop-by-drop discharge of nasal mucus into the posterior pharynx. It is often accompanied by a feeling of obstruction, an unpleasant taste, and fetid breath, caused by rhinitis, chronic sinusitis, or hypersecretion by the nasopharyngeal mucosa. Methods of treatment include the application of drops or sprays of phenylephrine or ephedrine sulfate to constrict blood vessels and reduce hyperemia, sinus irrigation to improve drainage, and use of appropriate antibiotics. Therapy for allergies may be indicated in some cases, and surgery may be required if the nasal passages are obstructed by polyps or a deviated septum.

**postnecrotic cirrhosis** /-nekrot′ik/ [L, *post* + Gk, *nekros,* dead; *kirrhos,* yellowish, *osis,* condition], a nodular form of cirrhosis that may follow hepatitis or other inflammation of the liver. Also called **posthepatic cirrhosis.** See also **cirrhosis.**

**postoperative** /-op′ərətiv′/ [L, *post* + *operari,* to work], pertaining to the period of time after surgery. It begins with the patient's emergence from anesthesia and continues through the time required for the acute effects of the anesthetic and surgical procedures to abate.

**postoperative atelectasis,** a form of atelectasis in which collapse of lung tissue is caused by the depressant effects of anesthetic drugs. Deep breathing and coughing are encouraged at frequent postoperative intervals to prevent this condition.

**postoperative bed,** a surface prepared for a patient who is weak or unconscious, as when recovering from anesthesia. The bed is in the flat position. The bottom sheet may be covered with a cotton bath blanket that is tucked tightly beneath the mattress. The top linen is fan-folded to the far side of the bed and not tucked in. The bed is made in this way to simplify transferring a patient from a stretcher into the bed.

**postoperative care,** the management of a patient after surgery. See also **preoperative care.**
■ METHOD: Before the patient's discharge from the operating room the surgical drapes, ground plate, and restraints are removed and a sterile dressing may be applied to the incision. The patency and connections of all drainage tubes and the flow rate of parenteral infusions are checked. The patient's cleanliness and dryness are given attention, and the gown is changed, avoiding exposing the individual. The patient is transferred slowly and cautiously to a recovery room bed, maintaining body alignment and protecting the limbs. When indicated, an oral or nasal airway is inserted or a previously inserted endotracheal tube is suctioned; respiration may be supported with a pulmonator or pulse oximeter; if respiration remains impaired, the anesthetist is notified. The blood pressure, pulse, and respirations are initially reported to the anesthetist and are then checked every 15 minutes or as ordered. At similar intervals the level of consciousness, re-

flexes, and movements of extremities are observed, and the incision, drainage tubes, and IV infusion site are inspected. Nothing is given orally; medication, blood or blood components, and oxygen are administered as ordered, and fluid intake and output are measured. Pain is controlled with analgesics. The patient is kept warm and dry, and positioned for optimal ventilation and comfort. At the first sign of vomiting the head or body is turned to one side and suction is applied to prevent aspiration. Oral hygiene is administered to keep the mouth and tongue moist. The chest is auscultated for breath sounds every 30 minutes, and the patient, when reactive, is helped to turn and deep breathe. The tympanic or axillary temperature is taken every 1 to 4 hours. When completely awake, rested, able to move the extremities well, and after having exhibited stable vital signs, the patient may be transferred to the assigned room, provided the drainage tubes are functioning, the dressings show no bleeding or excessive drainage, and the anesthesiologist approves the move. The family is informed of the patient's progress and expectations for the postoperative period. The airway patency; rate, depth, and character of respirations; pulse; blood pressure; temperature; skin color; level of consciousness; and condition of dressings and drainage tubes are assessed. If respirations are noisy, the patient is assisted in coughing. A rapid, weak, thready pulse may indicate increased bleeding and is reported, especially if other signs of impending shock, such as hypotension or changes in level of consciousness, are evident. The dressing is examined at frequent intervals, and excessive drainage is reported immediately. The side rails of the bed are raised for safety and the head is slightly elevated, unless contraindicated. A cardiac monitor may be connected. Parenteral fluids and pain medication are administered as ordered. Fluid intake and output are measured; range-of-motion exercises to extremities are performed, and ambulation, when ordered, is assisted.
■ INTERVENTIONS: The postanesthesia care nurse performs the immediate postoperative procedures, and the clinical unit nurse provides ongoing care, emotional support, and instructions for the patient and family. Special attention is given to preventing trauma postoperatively, as may occur when confused or elderly patients fall getting out of bed.
■ OUTCOME CRITERIA: Meticulous postoperative care prevents falls, infections, and other complications and promotes the healing of the incision and restoration of the patient to health.

**postoperative cholangiography,** (in diagnostic radiology) a procedure for outlining the major bile ducts. A radiopaque contrast material is injected into the common bile duct via a T-tube inserted during surgery. It is usually performed after a cholecystectomy to discover any residual calculi. See also **cholangiography.**

**postoperative ileus** [L, *post* + *operari,* to work; Gk, *eilein,* to twist], an obstruction to normal intestinal function caused by a loss of peristaltic muscular action of the ileus after surgery.

**postoperative paresthesia,** prolonged paresthesia after surgery with a local anesthetic, usually around the mouth, resulting from injury of the mental nerve or mandibular nerve.

**postparalytic** /-per′əlit′ik/ [L, *post* + Gk, *paralyein,* to be palsied], pertaining to the period after paralysis.

**postpartal care**[1] /-pär′təl/ [L, *post* + *partus,* birth], care of the mother and her newborn during the first few days of the puerperium. See also **antepartal care, intrapartal care, newborn intrapartal care.**

**postpartal care**[2], a nursing intervention from the Nursing Interventions Classification (NIC) defined as monitoring and management of the patient who has recently given birth. See also **Nursing Interventions Classification.**

**postpartum** /pōstpär′təm/, after childbirth.

**postpartum blues** [L, *post,* after, *partus,* birth; ME, *bleu*], an emotional effect of childbirth experienced by mothers, consisting mainly of transient feelings of sadness for a period of about 72 hours. If the symptom persists for a longer period, the diagnosis of depression may apply. The condition may require psychotherapy, use of antidepressant medications, or both. It may occur more than once in the same person after subsequent pregnancies and may have serious consequences if untreated. See also **postpartum depression.**

**postpartum depression** [L, *post* + *partus* + *deprimere,* to press down], an abnormal psychiatric condition that occurs after childbirth, typically from 3 days to 6 weeks post partum. It is characterized by symptoms that range from mild "postpartum blues" to an intense suicidal depressive psychosis. Severe postpartum depression occurs approximately once in every 2000 to 3000 pregnancies. The cause is not proved; neurochemical and psychologic influences have been implicated. Approximately one third of patients are found to have had some degree of psychiatric abnormality predating the pregnancy. The disorder recurs in subsequent pregnancies in 25% of cases. Some women at risk for postpartum depression may be identified during the prenatal period: those who have made no preparations for the expected baby, expressed unrealistic plans for postpartum work or travel, or denied the reality of the responsibilities of parenthood. Depending on the severity of the disorder, psychoactive medication or psychiatric hospitalization may be necessary.

**postpartum hemorrhage** [L, *post,* after, *partus,* birth; Gk, *haima,* blood, *rhegnynai,* to burst forth], excessive bleeding (a loss of more than 500 mL of blood) after childbirth.

**postpartum iliofemoral thrombophlebitis** [L, *post,* after, *parturs,* birth, *ilia,* flank, *femur,* thigh; Gk, *thrombos,* lump, *phleps,* vein, *itis,* inflammation], thrombophlebitis involving the iliofemoral artery after childbirth.

**postpartum pituitary necrosis** [L, *post* + *partus* + *pituita,* phlegm; Gk, *nekros,* dead, *osis,* condition], a condition of hypopituitarism resulting from hypovolemia and shock in the immediate postpartum period. Lactation may not develop, pubic and axillary hair may be lost, and symptoms of hypoglycemia and amenorrhea are experienced. See also **Sheehan's syndrome.**

**postpartum psychosis** [L, *post,* after, *partus,* birth; Gk, *psyche,* mind], an episode of psychosis, either depressive or schizophrenic, after childbirth. Because the condition usually develops in the month after childbirth, endocrinologic factors are believed to be a cause.

**postperfusion syndrome** /-pərfyōō′zhən/ [L, *post* + *perfundere,* to pour over], a cytomegalovirus (CMV) infection, occurring between 2 and 4 weeks after the transfusion of fresh blood containing CMV. It is characterized by prolonged fever, hepatitis, rash, atypical lymphocytosis, and occasionally jaundice. No specific treatment is available.

**postpericardiotomy syndrome** /pōst′perikär′dē·ot′əmē/ [L, *post* + Gk, *peri,* around, *kardia,* heart, *temnein,* to cut], a condition that sometimes occurs days or weeks after pericardiotomy, characterized by symptoms of pericarditis, often without any fever. It appears to be an autoimmune response to damaged cells of the myocardium and pericardium. See also **pericarditis.**

**postpill amenorrhea** /-pill′/ [L, *post* + *pilla,* ball; Gk, *a,* not, *men,* month, *rhoia,* flow], failure of normal menstrual cycles to resume within 3 months after discontinuation of oral contraception. The pathophysiologic characteristics of this uncommon condition are poorly understood. Postpill amenorrhea is rarely permanent. See also **amenorrhea.**

**postpoliomyelitis muscular atrophy (PPMA)** /-pō′lē-ōmī′əlī′tis/ [L, *post,* after; Gk, *polios,* gray, *myelos,* marrow, *itis,* inflammation; L, *musculus* + Gk, *a,* not, *trophe,* nourishment], a recurrence of muscular weakness and other neuromuscular symptoms in people who had recovered from acute paralytic polio many years earlier. The condition may or may not affect the same muscles that were damaged in the earlier polio attack.

**postpolycythemic myeloid metaplasia** /-pol′isīthē′mik/ [L, *post* + Gk, *polys,* many, *kytos,* cell, *haima,* blood, *myelos,* marrow, *eidos,* form, *meta,* with, *plassein,* to mold], a late development in polycythemia vera, characterized by anemia caused by sclerosis of the bone marrow. The production of red blood cells occurs only in the liver and spleen. This condition is frequently complicated by leukemia, especially if the patient has been treated with ionizing radiation. See also **myelofibrosis, myeloid metaplasia, polycythemia.**

**postprandial,** after a meal.

**postprandial glucose test,** a blood test in which a meal acts as a glucose challenge to the body's metabolism. It is an easily performed screening test for diabetes mellitus. A 1-hour glucose screen, using a 50-gram oral glucose load, is used to detect gestational diabetes mellitus (GDM).

**postprandial pain** [L, *post,* after, *prandium,* meal, *poena,* penalty], pain that occurs after a meal.

**postprocessing** /-pros′əsing/, (in ultrasonics) manipulation and conditioning of signals and image data after they emerge from the scan converter and before they are displayed. Postprocessing is used to change the assignment of image brightness versus echo signal amplitude in memory.

**postpuberal, postpubertal.** See **postpuberty.**

**postpubertal panhypopituitarism** /-pyōō′bərtəl/ [L, *post* + *pubertas,* maturation; Gk, *pan,* all, *hypo,* below, *pituita,* phlegm], insufficiency of pituitary hormones, caused by pituitary necrosis resulting from a blood clot in the artery supplying the gland during or after birth. The disorder is characterized initially by weakness, lethargy, loss of libido, intolerance to cold, and, in females, by failure to lactate and amenorrhea. It leads eventually to loss of axillary and pubic hair, bradycardia, hypotension, premature wrinkling of the skin, and atrophy of the thyroid and adrenal glands. Treatment consists of the administration of adrenocorticotropic hormone, thyroid stimulating hormone, thyroid hormone, corticosteriods, or sex hormones. Also called **Simmonds' disease, hypophyseal cachexia, pituitary cachexia.** Compare **prepubertal panhypopituitarism.**

**postpuberty** /-pyōō′bərtē/ [L, *post* + *pubertas,* maturation], a period of approximately 1 to 2 years after puberty during which skeletal growth slows and the physiologic functions of the reproductive years are established. Also called **postpubescence.** —**postpuberal, postpubertal, postpubescent,** *adj.*

**postrenal anuria** /-rē′nəl/ [L, *post* + *renes,* kidney; Gk, *a* + *ouron,* not urine], cessation of urine production caused by obstruction of the ureters.

**postresection filling.** See **retrograde filling.**

**poststeroid lobular panniculitis** [L, *panniculus,* piece of cloth], subcutaneous nodules that may develop in a layer of fatty connective tissue in children 1 to 13 days after discontinuation of steroid therapy. The condition resolves spontaneously or without readministration of the medication.

**postsynaptic** /-sinap′tik/ [L, *post* + Gk, *synaptein,* to join],

**1.** situated after a synapse. **2.** occurring after a synapse has been crossed.

**postterm infant.** See **postmature infant.**

**postterm pregnancy.** See **postdate pregnancy.**

**posttransfusion syndrome** /-transfyo͞o′zhən/ [L, *post,* after, *transfundere,* to pour through; Gk, *syn,* together, *dromos,* course], a complex of adverse reactions that may accompany or follow IV administration of blood or blood components. Reactions may include hemolytic effects, headache and back pain, allergies to an unknown component in donor blood, circulatory overloading, effects of cold blood that chill the patient's cardiovascular system, and effects of microaggregates in stored blood.

**posttrauma response** /-trô′mə/, a nursing diagnosis accepted by the Seventh National Conference on the Classification of Nursing Diagnoses. The condition is defined as the state of an individual experiencing a sustained painful response to overwhelming traumatic events.
■ DEFINING CHARACTERISTICS: Critical defining characteristics include reexperience of the traumatic event, which may be identified in cognitive, affective, or sensory motor activities (flashbacks, intrusive thoughts, repetitive dreams or nightmares, excessive verbalization of the traumatic event, or verbalization of survival guilt or guilt about behavior required by survival). Among minor defining characteristics is psychic or emotional numbness, such as impaired interpretation of reality, confusion, dissociation or amnesia, vagueness about the traumatic event, or constricted affect. Another defining characteristic is an altered life-style characterized by self-destructiveness, including substance abuse, a suicide attempt, or other acting-out behavior; difficulty with interpersonal relationships; development of a phobia regarding the trauma; poor impulse control or irritability; and explosiveness.
■ RELATED FACTORS: Related factors include disasters, wars, epidemics, rape, assault, torture, catastrophic illness, or accident. See also **nursing diagnosis.**

**post-trauma syndrome, risk for,** a nursing diagnosis accepted by the Thirteenth National Conference on the Classification of Nursing Diagnoses. The condition is a risk for sustained maladaptive response to a traumatic, overwhelming event.
■ RISK FACTORS: Risk factors include occupation, exaggerated sense of responsibility, perception of event, a survivor's role in the event, displacement from home, inadequate social support, non-supportive environment, diminished ego-strength, and duration of the event. See also **nursing diagnosis.**

**posttraumatic** /-trômat′ik/ [L, *post,* after, Gk, *trauma,* wounded], pertaining to any emotional, mental, or physiological consequences after a major illness or injury.

**posttraumatic amnesia** [L, *post* + Gk, *trauma,* wound], a period of amnesia between a brain injury resulting in memory loss and the point at which the functions concerned with memory are restored.

**posttraumatic epilepsy.** See **traumatic epilepsy.**

**posttraumatic osteoporosis** [L, *post,* after; Gk, *trauma,* wound, *osteon,* bone, *poros,* passage, *osis,* condition], a loss of bone density that develops after an injury or other severe health episode. It may occur as a result of disease.

**posttraumatic spondylitis.** See **Kümmell's disease.**

**posttraumatic stress disorder (PTSD),** a DSM-IV psychiatric disorder characterized by an acute emotional response to a traumatic event or situation involving severe environmental stress, such as a natural disaster, airplane crash, serious automobile accident, military combat, or physical torture.

**posttraumatic syndrome.** See **postconcussional syndrome.**

**postulate** /pos′chəlāt/ [L, *postulare,* to demand], a hypothesis that is offered as true without proof or as a basis for argument or debate.

**postural albuminuria.** See **orthostatic proteinuria.**

**postural background movements** /pos′chərəl/ [L, *ponere,* to place], the spontaneous body adjustments, requiring vestibular and proprioceptive integration, that maintain the center of gravity, keep the head and body in alignment, and stabilize body parts, such as the shoulder girdle when the hand reaches for a distant object.

**postural drainage,** the use of positioning to drain secretions from specific segments of the bronchi and the lungs into the trachea. Coughing usually expels secretions from the trachea.
■ METHOD: Positions that promote drainage from the affected parts of the lungs are selected. Pillows and raised sections of the hospital bed are used to support or elevate parts of the body. The procedure is begun with the patient level, and the head is gradually lowered to a full Trendelenburg position. Inhalation through the nose and exhalation through the mouth are encouraged. Simultaneously the nurse or other health care provider may use cupping and vibration over the affected area of the lungs to dislodge and mobilize secretions. The person is then helped to a position conducive to coughing and is asked to breathe deeply at least three times and to cough at least twice. See also **cupping and vibrating.**
■ INTERVENTIONS: A patient who is dyspneic or who has hemoptysis or signs of cerebral hemorrhage, increased intracerebral pressure, or lung abscess is not placed in a head-down position without caution and a specific medical order. Suction is kept available in all cases in which the patient may not be able to expel the secretions that have drained into the trachea. The patient's tolerance for the procedure and the position is carefully observed; fatigue is prevented.
■ OUTCOME CRITERIA: Effectiveness of the procedure depends on positioning that allows drainage by gravity and on liquefaction, ciliary action, and effective breathing. As the secretions are cleared, the patient becomes better able to breathe, is more comfortable, and may move about more freely; thus the respiratory passages may remain freer of obstructing secretions and resume their expected function. Also called **bronchial drainage.**

**postural hypotension.** See **orthostatic hypotension.**

**postural proteinuria.** See **orthostatic proteinuria.**

**postural reflex** [L, *ponere,* to place, *reflectere,* to turn back], any of several reflexes associated with maintaining normal body posture.

**postural vertigo,** a severe but brief episode of vertigo associated with a change of body position, as when a patient lies down. It may be caused by an injury or disease of the utricle. Also called **positional vertigo.** See also **cupulolithiasis.**

**posture** /pos′chər/ [L, *ponere,* to place], the position of the body with respect to the surrounding space. A posture is determined and maintained by coordination of the various muscles that move the limbs, by proprioception, and by the sense of balance.

**postvaccinal encephalitis** /-vak′sinəl/ [L, *post,* after, *vaccinus,* of a cow; Gk, *enkephalos,* brain, *itis,* inflammation], acute encephalitis after vaccination, especially with vaccinia (smallpox vaccine) or the Semple rabies vaccine.

**postvaccinal encephalomyelitis** [L, *post,* after, *vaccinus,* of a cow; Gk, *enkephalos,* brain, *myelos,* marrow, *itis,* inflammation], acute encephalomyelitis after vaccination.

## Positions for postural drainage

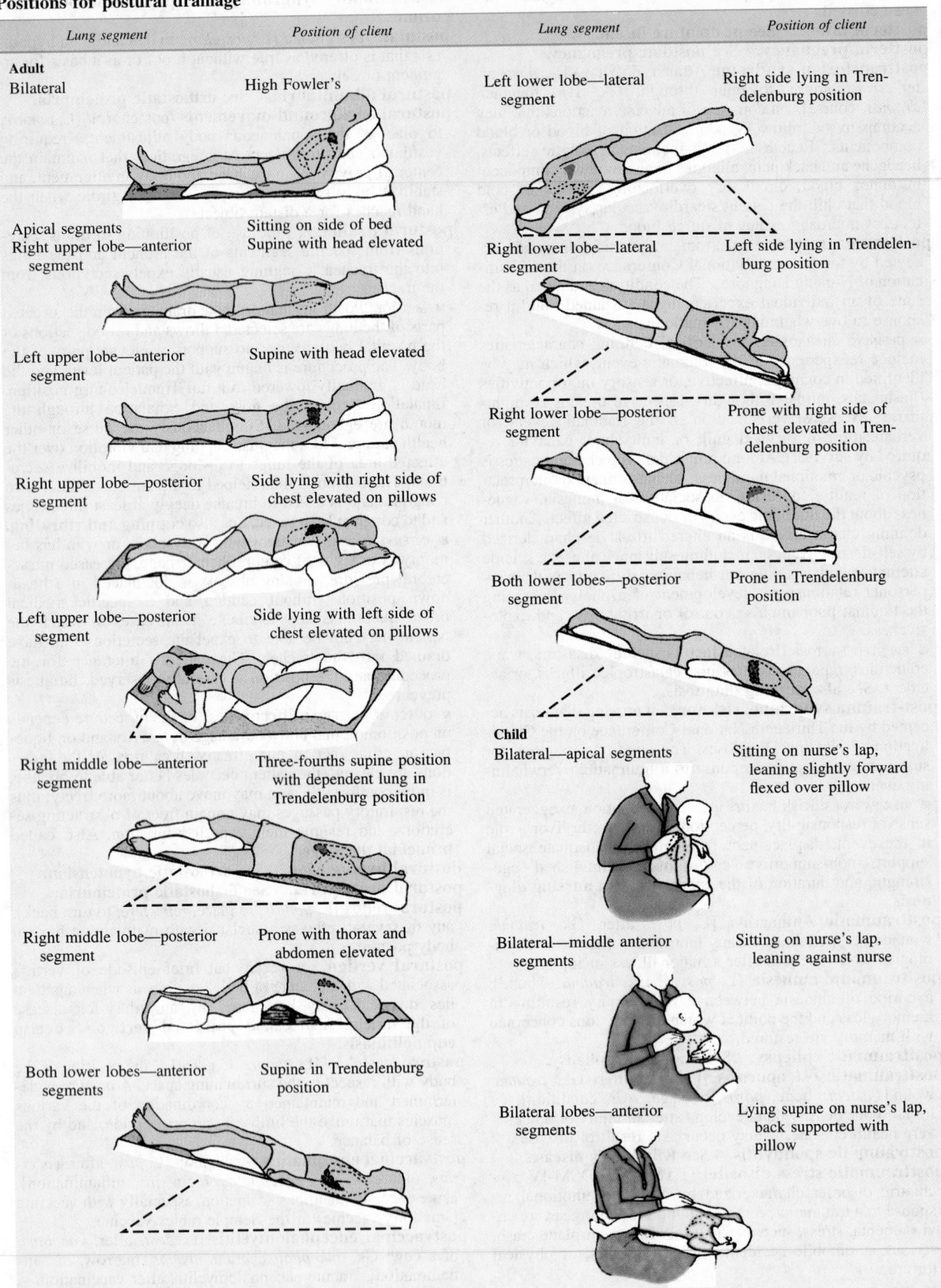

| Lung segment | Position of client | Lung segment | Position of client |
|---|---|---|---|
| **Adult** Bilateral | High Fowler's | Left lower lobe—lateral segment | Right side lying in Trendelenburg position |
| Apical segments Right upper lobe—anterior segment | Sitting on side of bed Supine with head elevated | Right lower lobe—lateral segment | Left side lying in Trendelenburg position |
| Left upper lobe—anterior segment | Supine with head elevated | Right lower lobe—posterior segment | Prone with right side of chest elevated in Trendelenburg position |
| Right upper lobe—posterior segment | Side lying with right side of chest elevated on pillows | Both lower lobes—posterior segment | Prone in Trendelenburg position |
| Left upper lobe—posterior segment | Side lying with left side of chest elevated on pillows | **Child** Bilateral—apical segments | Sitting on nurse's lap, leaning slightly forward flexed over pillow |
| Right middle lobe—anterior segment | Three-fourths supine position with dependent lung in Trendelenburg position | Bilateral—middle anterior segments | Sitting on nurse's lap, leaning against nurse |
| Right middle lobe—posterior segment | Prone with thorax and abdomen elevated | Bilateral lobes—anterior segments | Lying supine on nurse's lap, back supported with pillow |
| Both lower lobes—anterior segments | Supine in Trendelenburg position | | |

From Potter PA and Perry AG: *Fundamentals of nursing: concepts, process, and practice*, ed 5, St Louis, 2001, Mosby.

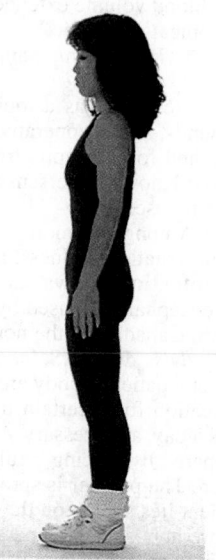

**Ideal standing posture** *(Aloia, 1993)*

**postviral fatigue syndrome** /-vīrəl/ [L, *post,* after, *virus,* poison, *fatigare,* to tire; Gk, *syn,* together, *dromos,* course], a condition of chronic muscle fatigue unrelieved by rest after a viral infection. Other symptoms may include visual and hearing difficulties, low-grade fever, stiff neck, urinary frequency, and insomnia. Also called **benign myalgic encephalomyelitis, Iceland disease, Royal Free disease.**

**pot-,** combining form meaning 'related to drinking': *potable, potocytosis, potomania.*

**potable water** /pō'təbəl/ [L, *potare,* to drink], water that can be consumed without concern for adverse health effects. Potable water does not have to taste good; on the contrary **palatable water** may taste good but is not necessarily safe to drink.

**potassemia** /pōt'əsē'meiə/ [D, *potasschen,* potash; Gk, *haima,* blood], an excess of potassium in the blood.

**potassium (K)** /pətas'ē·əm/ [D, *potasschen,* potash], an alkali metal element, the seventh most abundant element in the earth's crust. Its atomic number is 19; its atomic mass is 39.10. Potassium salts are necessary to the life of all plants and animals. Potassium in the body constitutes the predominant intracellular cation, helping to regulate neuromuscular excitability and muscle contraction. Sources of potassium in the diet are whole grains, meat, legumes, fruit, and vegetables. The average adequate daily intake for most adults is 2 to 4 g. Normal adult levels of blood potassium are 3.5 to 5 mEq/L or 3.5 to 5 mmol/L (SI units). Potassium is important in glycogen formation, protein synthesis, and correction of imbalances of acid-base metabolism, especially in association with the action of sodium and hydrogen ions. Potassium salts are very important as therapeutic agents but are extremely dangerous if used improperly. The kidneys play an important role in controlling its secretion, absorption, and secretion. Aldosterone stimulates sodium reabsorption and potassium secretion by the kidneys; the major extrarenal adaptation to this process involves the absorption of potassium by the body tissues, especially the tissues of the muscles and the liver. Potassium is most commonly depleted in the body by an increased rate of excretion by the kidneys or the GI tract. Increased renal excretion may be caused by diuretic therapy, large doses of anionic drugs, or renal disorders. Increased GI excretion of potassium may occur with the loss of GI fluid through vomiting, diarrhea, surgical drainage, or chronic use of laxatives. Potassium loss through the skin is rare but can result from perspiring during excessive exercise in a hot environment.

**potassium chloride (KCl),** a white crystalline salt used as a substitute for table salt in the diet of people with cardiovascular disorders, in administration of the potassium ion, and as a constituent of Ringer's solution.

■ INDICATIONS: It is prescribed in the treatment of hypokalemia resulting from a variety of causes and of digitalis intoxication.

■ CONTRAINDICATIONS: Hyperkalemia, concomitant use of spironolactone or triamterene, or known hypersensitivity to this drug prohibits its use.

■ ADVERSE EFFECTS: Among the most serious adverse reactions are hyperkalemia and, when given orally, ulceration of the small bowel.

**potassium hydroxide (KOH),** a white soluble highly caustic compound. Occasionally used in solution as an escharotic for bites of rabid animals, KOH has many laboratory uses as an alkalinizing agent, including the preparation of clinical specimens for examination for fungi under the microscope.

**potassium indoxyl sulfate.** See **indican.**

**potassium iodide,** an expectorant.

■ INDICATIONS: It is prescribed in the treatment of bronchitis, bronchiectasis, and asthma and in various thyroid disorders.

■ CONTRAINDICATIONS: Acute bronchitis, known or suspected pregnancy, or known hypersensitivity to this drug or to any iodide prohibits its use.

■ ADVERSE EFFECTS: Among the more serious adverse reactions are hypersensitivity, goiter, myxedema, GI disturbance, and skin lesions.

**potassium penicillin V.** See **penicillin V.**

**potassium pump,** a mechanism that involves energy-dependent pumping of potassium or the active transport of the potassium ion ($K^+$) across a biologic membrane using the energy of $K^+$-activated adenosine triphosphatase. Also called **$K^+$ pump.** See also **calcium pump, sodium-potassium pump.**

**potassium-sparing diuretic.** See **diuretic.**

**potency** /pō'tənsē/ [L, *potentia,* power], (in embryology) the range of developmental possibilities of which an embryonic cell or part is capable, regardless of whether the stimulus for growth or differentiation is natural, artificial, or experimental. See also **competence.**

**potent** /pō'tənt/ [L, *potentia,* power], powerful or strong.

**-potent,** suffix meaning 'powerful or able to do' something specified: *pluripotent, unipotent, viripotent.*

**potential** /pəten'shəl/ [L, *potentia*], an expression of the energy involved in transferring a unit of electrical charge. The gradient or slope of a potential causes the charge to move. The movement of 1 coulomb of charge from a potential of $V$ to a potential of $V - 1$ volts requires 1 joule of energy.

**potential abnormality of glucose tolerance,** a classification that includes people who have never had abnormal glucose tolerance but who have an increased risk of diabetes or impaired glucose tolerance. Factors associated with an increased risk of type 1 diabetes mellitus include having circulating islet cell antibodies, being a monozygotic twin or sibling of a type 1 diabetes patient, and being the offspring of a type 1 diabetes patient. Factors associated with an increased risk of type 2 diabetes mellitus include being a first-degree relative of a type 2 diabetes patient (particularly in a family in which there are several generations with type 2 diabetes), giving birth to a neonate weighing more than 9 pounds (4.086 kilograms), being a member of a racial or ethnic group with a high prevalence of diabetes, such as some Native American groups, and being an obese adult. See also **diabetes mellitus.**

**potential diabetes.**    See **potential abnormality of glucose tolerance.**

**potential difference,** the difference in electrical potential between two points. It represents the work involved in the energy released by the transfer of a unit quantity of electricity from one point to another.

**potential energy** [L, *potentia,* power; Gk, *energeia*], the energy contained in a body as a result of its position in space, internal structure, and stresses imposed on it. Also called **latent energy.**

**potential life,** a criterion used by the Centers for Disease Control and Prevention to gauge premature death rates. Among younger individuals, it is based on an assumption that the person would have lived to 65 years of age if life had not been interrupted by a particular disease or injury. The leading cause of loss of potential life in young people is accidents, followed by cancer and heart disease. For older people the system is based on years of potential life lost before 85 years of age, in which case cancer and heart disease rank first and second.

**potential trauma,** a change in tissue that may occur because of existing malocclusion or dental disharmony.

**potentiate** /pōten′shē-āt/, to increase the strength or degree of activity of something.

**potentiation** /pōten′shē-ā′shən/ [L, *potentia*], a synergistic action in which the effect of two drugs given simultaneously is greater than the effect of the drugs given separately.

**potentiometer** /pōten′shē-om′ətər/ [L, *potentia* + Gk, *metron,* measure], a voltage-measuring device.

**Potter-Bucky diaphragm.**    See **Potter-Bucky grid.**

**Potter-Bucky grid** [Hollis E. Potter; Gustav Bucky; twentieth-century American radiologists; ME, *gredire,* grate], an x-ray grid that oscillates during the exposure of a radiographic film, blurring the grid lines. Also called **Potter-Bucky diaphragm.** See also **grid.**

**Pott's disease.**    See **tuberculous spondylitis.**

**Pott's fracture** [Percival Pott, English physician, 1713–1788], a break in the fibula near the ankle, often accompanied by a break in the malleolus of the tibia or a rupture of the internal lateral ligament. Also called **Dupuytren's fracture.**

**potty chair** [AS, *pott* + ME, *chaire*], a small chair that has an open seat over a removable pot, used for the toilet training of young children.

**pouch** [OFr, *pouche*], any small saclike appendage or pocket, such as Rathke's pouch in the roof of the embryonic roof cavity. See also **cul-de-sac.**

**pouch of Douglas.**    See **cul-de-sac of Douglas.**

**poultice** /pōl′tis/ [L, *puls,* porridge], a soft moist pulp spread between layers of gauze or cloth and applied hot to a surface to provide heat or to counter irritation. A kind of poultice is a **mustard plaster.**

**pound** [L, *pondus,* weight] (**lb** [L, *libra*]), a unit of measure equal to 16 ounces, avoirdupois; 0.45359 kg; 7000 grains.

***P. ovale,*** abbreviation for ***Plasmodium ovale.***

**poverty** /pov′ərtē/ [L, *paupertas*], **1.** a lack of material wealth needed to maintain existence. **2.** a loss of emotional capacity to feel love or sympathy.

**povidone** /pō′vidōn/, a polymerized form of vinylpyrrolidone, a white hygroscopic powder readily soluble in water, used as a dispersing and suspending agent in drugs. It also

has been used as a blood volume extender and, in a complex with iodine, as a topical antiseptic.

**povidone-iodine** /pō′vidōnī′ədīn/, an antiseptic microbicide.

■ INDICATIONS: It is prescribed as a topical microbicide for disinfection of wounds, as a preoperative surgical scrub, for vaginal infections, and for antiseptic treatment of burns.

■ CONTRAINDICATIONS: Known hypersensitivity to this drug or to iodine prohibits its use.

■ ADVERSE EFFECTS: Among the more serious adverse reactions are local skin irritation, redness, and swelling.

**Powassan virus infection** [Powassan, Ontario], an uncommon form of encephalitis caused by a tickborne arbovirus found in eastern Canada and the northern United States.

**powder bed** [L, *pulvis,* dust; AS, *bedd*], a treatment in which large areas of a patient's body are kept in contact with a powdered medication for a certain time. It is usually repeated three times a day, as necessary. A bed that has already been made is prepared by placing a full-sized sheet lengthwise over the linen. The powder is spread on the sheet from a shaker. The patient lies supine on the powdered sheet. Areas of skin that are apposed are separated with gauze, and powder is shaken over the patient's body. The powdered sheet is then wrapped around the limbs and the trunk from the side to keep the powder in contact with the body. The patient is virtually helpless during treatment and requires close attention from the nurse.

**power centric,** the position of the mandible during a forceful bite.

**powerlessness** /pow′ərləsnes′/ [Fr, *pouvoir,* to have power; AS, *loes,* limited, *nes,* condition], a nursing diagnosis accepted by the Fifth National Conference on the Classification of Nursing Diagnoses. Powerlessness is defined as a perceived lack of control over a current situation or problem and the client's perception that any action he or she takes will not affect the outcome of the particular situation.

■ DEFINING CHARACTERISTICS: The defining characteristics may be of a severe, moderate, or low nature. Severe characteristics include the client's verbal expression of having no control or influence over self-care, the particular situation, or its outcome; apathy; or depression about physical deterioration that occurs despite compliance with regimens. Moderate characteristics include the client's nonparticipation in or lack of interest in the mode of care, in decision making regarding regimens, or in monitoring progress; the client's verbal expression of dissatisfaction and frustration regarding the inability to perform previous activities; the reluctance to express true feelings, fearing alienation of others; general irritability or passivity; and expressions of resentment, anger, guilt, or doubt regarding role performance. Low characteristics involve passivity and expressions of uncertainty about fluctuating energy levels.

■ RELATED FACTORS: Related factors include the health care environment, interpersonal interaction, a regimen related to the illness, or a generalized life-style of helplessness. See also **nursing diagnosis.**

**powerlessness, risk for,** a nursing diagnosis accepted by the Fourteenth National Conference on the classification of nursing diagnoses. The state is defined as being at risk for a perceived lack of control over a situation and/or one's ability to significantly affect the outcome.

■ RISK FACTORS: Physiological risk factors include chronic or acute illness, acute injury or progressive debilitating disease process, aging, and dying. Psychosocial factors include a lack of knowledge of illness or the health care system, a life-style of dependency with inadequate coping patterns, the absence of integrality, decreased self-esteem, and low or unstable body image. See also **nursing diagnosis.**

**power mode,** a method of color flow processing and display in which the Doppler signal amplitude or the signal intensity, averaged over a small interval, is displayed rather than the average Doppler frequency. Velocity and flow direction are not displayed and artefacts do not affect the image.

**power of attorney** [Fr, *pouvoir* + OFr, *atorne*, legal agent], a document authorizing one person to take legal actions in behalf of another, to act as an agent for the grantor. The legality of a power of attorney may be challenged if the grantor can be found to have been mentally incompetent at the time the authority was granted.

**power stroke,** a working stroke with a dental scaling instrument, used for splitting or dislodging calculus from the surface of a tooth or tooth root.

**pox** [ME, *pokkes*, pustules], **1.** any of several vesicular or pustular exanthematous diseases terminality in scars. **2.** the pitlike scars of smallpox or chicken pox. **3.** *archaic.* syphilis.

**poxvirus** /poksvī′rəs/ [ME, *pokkes* + L, *virus*, poison], a member of a family of viruses that includes the organisms that cause molluscum contagiosum, smallpox, and vaccinia.

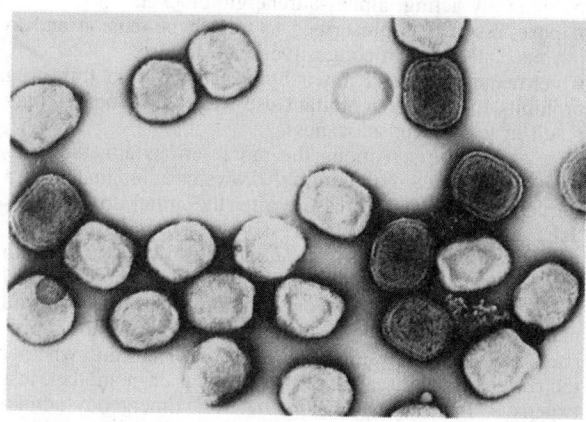

**Poxvirus**
*(Murray et al, 1994/courtesy Centers for Disease Control and Prevention, Atlanta)*

**PP,** abbreviation for (Latin) *punctum proximum*, near point of accommodation.

**PPD,** abbreviation for **purified protein derivative.**

**PPLO,** abbreviation for **pleuropneumonia-like organism.** See also *Mycoplasma.*

**PPM, ppm,** abbreviation for **parts per million.**

**PPMA,** abbreviation for **postpoliomyelitis muscular atrophy.**

**PPNG,** abbreviation for **penicillinase-producing** *Neisseria gonorrhoeae.*

**PPO,** abbreviation for **preferred provider organization.**

**PPS,** abbreviation for **prospective payment system.**

**PPV,** abbreviation for *positive pressure ventilation.* See **positive pressure,** def. 2.

**Pr,** symbol for the element **praseodymium.**

**PR,** abbreviation for **prosthion.**

**practical anatomy.** See **applied anatomy.**

**practical nurse.** See **licensed practical nurse.**

**practice guideline,** a detailed description of a process of patient care management that will facilitate improvement or maintenance of health status or slow the decline in health status in certain chronic clinical conditions. The purpose of a practice guideline is to assist health care providers to identify preferred treatment by providing linkages among diagnoses, treatments, and outcomes and by describing alternatives available for each patient. Practice guidelines provide a basis for evaluation of care and allocation of resources. See also **clinical pathway.**

**practice models** /prak′tis/ [Gk, *praktikos*, practical], the different patterns in delivery of health care services by means of which health care is made available to diverse groups of people in different settings.

**practice setting,** the context or environment within which nursing care is given.

**practice theory,** (in nursing research) a theory that describes, explains, and prescribes nursing practice in general. It serves as the basis for specific items in the curriculum of nursing education and for the development of theories in the administration of nursing and nursing education.

**practicing** /prak′tising/, the second subphase of the separation-individuation phase in Mahler's system of preoedipal development, when the child is able to move away from the mother and return to her for emotional nurturing. The child may feel elation in response to this investigation of the environment and through practicing locomotor skills.

**practicing medicine without a license,** (in law) practicing activities defined under state law in the medical practice act without physician supervision, direction, or control.

**practitioner** /praktish′ənər/ [Gk, *praktikos*], a person qualified to practice in a special professional field, such as a nurse practitioner.

**Prader-Willi syndrome** /prä′dər wil′ē/ [A. Prader, twentieth-century Swiss physician; H. Willi; Gk, *syn*, together, *dromos*, course], a metabolic condition characterized by congenital hypotonia, hyperphagia, obesity, and mental retardation. When the development of diabetes mellitus occurs with the other symptoms, the condition is called Royer's syndrome. The syndrome is associated with a below normal secretion of gonadotropic hormones by the pituitary gland.

**prae-.** See **pre-.**

**praecox** [L, premature], pertaining to something that occurred at an earlier stage of life or development.

**praevia** /prē′vē·ə/ [L], having occurred at an earlier time or in front of a place. Also **praevius.**

**-pragia,** combining form meaning 'quality of action': *bradypragia, dyspragia, tachypragia.*

**pragmatic** /pragmat′ik/, pertaining to a belief that ideas are valuable only in terms of their consequences.

**pragmatism** /prag′mətiz′əm/ [Gk, *pragma*, deed], a philosophy concerned with actual practice and practical results as opposed to theory and speculation.

**pralidoxime chloride** /pral′ədok′sēm/, a cholinesterase reactivator.

■ INDICATIONS: It is prescribed as an antidote for organophosphate poisoning and drug overdosage in the treatment of myasthenia gravis.

■ CONTRAINDICATION: Known hypersensitivity to this drug prohibits its use. It is contraindicated in poisoning by carbamate insecticides that react with pralidoxime.

■ ADVERSE EFFECTS: Among the most serious adverse reactions are dizziness, tachycardia, hyperventilation, and muscle weakness. These reactions are most common when the drug is injected too rapidly.

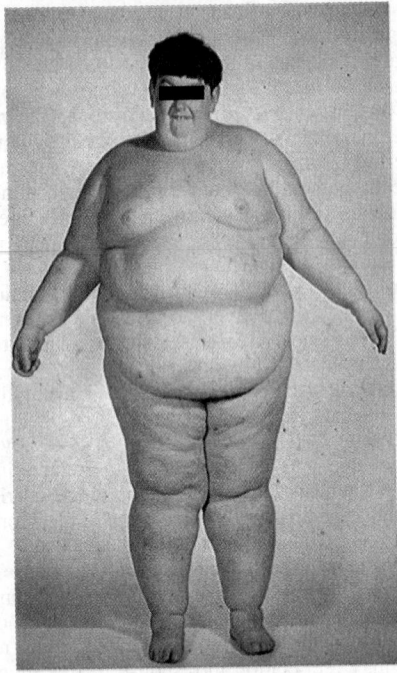

**Prader-Willi syndrome** (Bloom and Ireland, 1992)

**-pramine,** combining form for imipramine-type compounds.

**pramipexole,** an antiparkinson agent.

- INDICATIONS: Pramipexole is used to treat parkinsonism.
- CONTRAINDICATIONS: Known hypersensitivity prohibits the use of this drug.
- ADVERSE EFFECTS: Life-threatening effects of this drug are hemolytic anemia, leukopenia, and agranulocytosis. Other adverse effects include psychosis, hallucination, depression, dizziness, constipation, impotence, and blurred vision. Common side effects include agitation, insomnia, nausea, anorexia, and orthostatic hypotension.

**Pramosone,** trademark for a fixed-combination topical drug containing a glucocorticoid (hydrocortisone acetate) and a topical anesthetic (pramoxine hydrochloride).

**pramoxine hydrochloride** /prəmok′sēn/, a local anesthetic for the relief of pain and itching associated with dermatoses, anogenital pruritus, hemorrhoids, anal fissure, and minor burns.

**prandial** /pran′dē·əl/ [L, *prandium,* meal], pertaining to a meal. The term is used in relation to timing, such as postprandial or preprandial. —**prandiality,** *n.*

**praseodymium (Pr)** /prā′sē·ōdīm′ē·əm/ [Gk, *prasaios,* light-green, *didymos,* twin], a rare earth metallic element. Its atomic number is 59; its atomic mass (weight) is 140.91.

**Prausnitz-Küstner (PK) test** /prous′nitskist′nər/ [Otto C. Prausnitz, German hygienist, 1876–1963; Heinz Küstner, German gynecologist, 1897–1963], a skin test formerly used to measure the presence of immunoglobulin E. An allergic response was transferred to a nonallergic person who acts as a surrogate to permit identification of the allergen. It is no longer used because of the high risk of transfer of hepatitis or blood-borne diseases such as acquired immunodeficiency syndrome. Also, serum IgE can now be measured by in vitro assays, such as the radioallergosorbent test and radioimmunosorbent test. Also called **passive transfer test, PK test.** Compare **patch test, radioallergosorbent test.** See also **anaphylaxis.**

**-praxia,** combining form meaning 'to achieve or to do (perform)': *dyspraxia, eupraxia, hypopraxia.*

**praxis** [Gk, action], **1.** a concept that deals with actions and overt behavior, or the performance of an action, to the exclusion of metaphysical thought. **2.** the ability to plan and then execute movement.

**-praxis** /prak′sis/, combining form meaning 'to achieve, doing, an act, or treatment based on theory': *actinopraxis, echopraxis, parapraxis.*

**prazepam** /praz′əpam/, an antianxiety agent derived from benzodiazepine.

- INDICATIONS: It is prescribed for the treatment of anxiety disorders or the short-term relief of symptoms of anxiety.
- CONTRAINDICATIONS: Acute narrow-angle glaucoma or known sensitivity to this drug or other benzodiazepines prohibits its use.
- ADVERSE EFFECTS: Among the more serious, but rare, adverse reactions are confusion, tremor, palpitations, and diaphoresis.

**-prazole,** combining form for antiulcerative benzimidazole derivatives.

**prazosin hydrochloride** /prā′zəsin/, an antihypertensive, peripherally acting, alpha₁-adrenergic blocker.

- INDICATIONS: It is prescribed to treat hypertension and to decrease afterload in congestive heart disease.
- CONTRAINDICATIONS: Known hypersensitivity to this drug prohibits its use. Concomitant use with beta blockers may result in loss of consciousness.
- ADVERSE EFFECTS: Among the more serious adverse reactions are tachycardia, fainting, drowsiness, angina, and a sudden drop in blood pressure after the initial dose.

**PRE,** abbreviation for **progressive resistance exercise.**

**preadmission certification** /prē′ədmish′ən/, a system whereby physicians are required to obtain advance approval for nonemergency admission of Medicare, Medicaid, and managed care patients to hospitals, as well as most third-party payors. The system is intended to determine whether the patient can be treated as an outpatient or in another, less expensive manner than hospitalization. Emergency admissions require post hoc approval. Also called **precertification.**

**preagonal ascites** /prē·ag′ənəl/ [L, *prae,* before; Gk, *agon,* struggle, *askos,* bag], a rapid accumulation of fluid within the peritoneal cavity, representing the transudation of serum from the circulatory system. Preagonal ascites immediately precedes death in some cases. See also **ascites.**

**prealbumin test (PAB, TBPA),** a blood, 24-hour urine, or cerebrospinal fluid (CSF) analysis. It is useful as a marker of nutritional status and is a sensitive indicator of protein synthesis and catabolism. This test is done frequently on patients receiving total parenteral nutrition (TPN).

**preanal** /prē·ā′nəl/, located anterior to the anus.

**preanesthetic medication.** See **premedication.**

**preaortic node** /prē′ā·ôr′tik/ [L, *prae* + Gk, *aerein,* to raise; L, *nodus,* knot], a node in one of the three sets of lumbar lymph nodes that serve various abdominal viscera supplied by the celiac, superior mesenteric, and inferior mesenteric arteries. The preaortic nodes lie ventral to the aorta and are divided into the celiac nodes, superior mesenteric nodes, and inferior mesenteric nodes. Most of the efferent vessels from the preaortic nodes unite to form the lymphatic intestinal trunk that enters the cisterna chyli. Compare **lateral aortic node, retroaortic node.**

**preauricular** /prē′ôrik′yələr/, located anterior to the auricle of the ear.

**precancerous** /-kan′sərəs/ [L, *prae* + *cancer,* crab], pertaining to a stage of abnormal tissue growth that is likely to develop into a malignant tumor.

**precancerous dermatitis.** See **intraepidermal carcinoma.**

**precautionary labels** /prikô′shəner′ē/, information and identification that must be applied to the containers of all hazardous chemicals, including flammables, combustibles, corrosives, carcinogens, and potential carcinogens.

**precedent** /pres′ədənt/ [L, *praecedere,* to go before], a previously adjudged decision that serves as an authority in a similar case.

**Precef,** trademark for a cephalosporin-type antiinfective (ceforanide).

**precentral gyrus** /-sen′trəl/ [L, *prae* + Gk, *kentron,* center, *gyros,* turn], a convolution of the cerebral hemisphere immediately anterior to the central sulcus of the cerebrum in each hemisphere. It is the location of the motor strip that controls voluntary movements of the contralateral side of the body. Also called **anterior central gyrus.**

**preceptor: employee,** a nursing intervention from the Nursing Interventions Classification (NIC) defined as assisting and supporting a new or transferred employee through a planned orientation to a specific clinical area. See also **Nursing Interventions Classification.**

**preceptorship** /-sep′tərship′/ [L, *prae* + *capere,* to take up], the position of teacher or instructor; also a nurse who serves as a preceptor for a new graduate.

**preceptor: student,** a nursing intervention from the Nursing Interventions Classification (NIC) defined as assisting and supporting learning experiences for a student. See also **Nursing Interventions Classification.**

**precertification,** authorization for a specific medical procedure before it is done or for admission to an institution for care. It is required for payment by most U.S. managed care organizations.

**precession** /-sesh′ən/ [L, *praecedere,* to go before], a comparatively slow gyration of the axis of a spinning body, such that the axis traces out a cone, caused by the application of a torque. The magnetic moment of a nucleus with spin experiences such a torque when inclined at an angle to an applied magnetic field, resulting in precession at the Larmor frequency.

**precipitant** /-sip′ətənt/ [L, *praecipitare,* to cast down], a substance that causes another substance to settle, separate, or deposit from a solution, such as a reagent that causes certain metals to precipitate.

**precipitate** /prəsip′itāt, -it/ [L, *praecipitare,* to cast down], **1.** to cause a substance to separate or to settle out of solution. **2.** a substance that has separated from or settled out of a solution. **3.** occurring hastily or unexpectedly.

**precipitate delivery** /-sip′itit/, childbirth that occurs with such speed or in such a situation that the usual preparations cannot be made. See also **emergency childbirth.**

**precipitating factor** /-sip′itā′ting/, an element that causes or contributes to the occurrence of a disorder.

**precipitation** /-sip′itā′shən/ [L, *praecipitare,* to cast down], a process whereby solid particles are made to settle out of a solution so they can be separated from other dissolved substances.

**precipitin** /prəsip′itin/ [L, *praecipitare* + Gk, *anti,* against; AS, *bodig,* body; Gk, *genein,* to produce], an antibody that causes formation of an insoluble complex when combined with a specific soluble antigen. Compare **agglutinin.** See also **agglutination, antiglobulin.**

**precision attachment** /pri·sish′ən/ [L, *praecidere,* to cut short], a device using a precision rest to attach fixed or removable partial dentures to the crown of an abutment tooth or a restoration. Also called **precision anchorage.** See also **precision rest. 2.** see **intracoronal retainer.**

**precision rest** /prisish′ən/ [L, *praecidere,* to cut short; AS, *rest*], a rigid denture support consisting of two tightly fitting parts, the insert of which rests firmly against the gingival part of the device.

**preclinical** /-klin′ikəl/ [L, *prae* + Gk, *kline,* bed], a stage in a disease when a specific diagnosis cannot be made because adequate signs and symptoms have not yet developed.

**precocious** /-kō′shəs/ [L, *praecoquere,* to mature early], pertaining to the early, often premature, development of physical or mental qualities.

**precocious carrier.** See **amebic carrier state.**

**precocious dentition,** an abnormal acceleration of the eruption of the deciduous or secondary teeth, usually associated with an endocrine imbalance, such as excess growth hormone or hyperthyroidism. Compare **retarded dentition.**

**precocious puberty** [L, *praecoquere,* to mature early, *pubertas*], abnormally early development of sexual maturity. It is usually marked by early breast development and ovulation in girls before 8 years of age and the production of mature sperm in boys before 10 years of age.

**precognition** /-kognish′ən/, the alleged intuitive foreknowledge of events. Compare **premonition.**

**preconception counseling,** a nursing intervention from the Nursing Interventions Classification (NIC) defined as screening and providing information and support to individuals of childbearing age before pregnancy to promote health and reduce risks. See also **Nursing Interventions Classification.**

**preconscious** /-kon′shəs/ [L, *prae,* before, *conscire,* to be aware], **1.** before the development of self-consciousness and self-awareness. **2.** (in psychiatry) the mental function in which thoughts, ideas, emotions, or memories not in immediate awareness can be brought into the consciousness, usually through associations, without encountering any intrapsychic resistance or repression. **3.** the mental phenomena capable of being recalled, although not present in the conscious mind.

**precordial** /prēkôr′dē·əl/ [L, *prae* + *cor,* heart], pertaining to the precordium, which forms the region over the heart and the lower part of the thorax.

**precordial lead.** See **chest lead.**

**precordial movement,** any motion of the anterior wall of the thorax localized in the area over the heart. Variations of precordial movements include **apical impulse, left ventricular thrust,** and **right ventricular thrust.**

**precordial pain** [L, *prae,* before, *cor,* heart; *poena,* penalty], pain in the chest wall over the heart.

**precordium** /-kôr′dē·əm/ [L, *prae,* before, *cor,* heart], the part of the front of the chest wall that overlays the heart and the epigastrium.

**Precose,** trademark for an antidiabetic agent (acarbose).

**precursor** /-kur′sər/ [L, *prae* + *currere,* to run], a prognostic characteristic or feature of a patient's health data, such as a radiographic or laboratory finding, that is associated with a higher or lower risk of death than the average.

**precursor therapy,** a type of treatment involving the use of nutrients that may influence neurologic clinical conditions. An example is the use of choline, a B complex vitamin precursor of acetylcholine, in the treatment of tardive dyskinesia.

**pred-, -pred,** combining form for prednisone or prednisolone derivatives.

**predeciduous dentition** /-disid'yoo·əs/ [L, *prae* + *decidere,* to fall off], the epithelial structures in the mouth of the infant before the eruption of the deciduous teeth. See also **deciduous dentition, teething.**

**prediabetes.** See **potential abnormality of glucose tolerance, previous abnormality of glucose tolerance.**

**prediastole** /-dī·as'tələ/ [L, *prae,* before; Gk, *dia* + *stellein,* to set], the part of the cardiac cycle between late systole and the early diastole.

**prediastolic murmur** /-dī·astol'ik/ [L, *prae* + Gk, *dia* + *stellein,* to set; L, *murmur,* humming], a murmur heard during cardiac systole.

**predictive hypothesis** /-dik'tiv/ [L, *prae* + *dicere,* to say; Gk, foundation], (in research) a hypothesis that predicts the nature of a relationship among the variables to be studied.

**predictive validity,** validity of a test or a measurement tool that is established by demonstrating its ability to predict the results of an analysis of the same data using another test instrument or measurement tool. See also **validity.**

**predictor variable.** See **independent variable.**

**predisposing cause** /-dispō'sing/ [L, *prae* + *disponere,* to arrange, *causa*], any condition that enhances the specific cause of a disease, such as susceptibility caused by hereditary or life-style factors.

**predisposing factor** [L, *prae* + *disponere,* to dispose], any conditioning factor that influences both the type and the amount of resources that the individual can elicit to cope with stress. It may be biologic, psychologic, or sociocultural.

**predisposition** /-dis'pəzish'ən/ [L, *prae* + *disponere,* to dispose], a state of being particularly susceptible.

**prednisolone** /prednis'əlōn/, a glucocorticoid.
- INDICATIONS: It is prescribed as treatment for inflammation of the skin, conjunctiva, and cornea and for immunosuppression.
- CONTRAINDICATIONS: Fungal infections or known hypersensitivity to this drug prohibits its systemic use. Viral or fungal infections of the skin, impaired circulation, or known hypersensitivity to this drug prohibits its topical use.
- ADVERSE EFFECTS: Among the more serious adverse reactions to the systemic administration of this drug are GI, endocrine, neurologic, fluid, and electrolyte disturbances. Skin reactions may result from topical administration of this drug.

**prednisone** /pred'nisōn/, a glucocorticoid.
- INDICATIONS: It is prescribed in the treatment of severe inflammation and for immunosuppression.
- CONTRAINDICATIONS: Viral or fungal infections of the skin, impaired circulation, or known hypersensitivity to this drug prohibits its use.
- ADVERSE EFFECTS: Among the more serious adverse reactions to the systemic administration of the drug are GI, endocrine, neurologic, fluid, and electrolyte disturbances. Skin reactions may occur from topical administration of this drug.

**preeclampsia** /prē'iklamp'sē·ə/ [L, *prae* + Gk, *ek,* out, *lampein,* to flash], an abnormal condition of pregnancy characterized by the onset of acute hypertension after the twenty-fourth week of gestation. The classic triad of preeclampsia is hypertension, proteinuria, and edema. The cause of the disease remains unknown despite 100 years of research by thousands of investigators. It occurs in 5% to 7% of pregnancies, most often in primigravidas, and is more common in some areas of the world than others; the incidence is particularly high in the southeastern part of the United States. The incidence increases with increasing gestational age, and it is more common in cases of multiple ges-

tation, hydatidiform mole, or hydramnios. A typical lesion in the kidneys, glomeruloendotheliosis, is pathognomonic. Termination of the pregnancy results in resolution of the signs and symptoms of the disease and in healing of the renal lesion. Preeclampsia is classified as mild or severe. Mild preeclampsia is diagnosed if one or more of the following signs develop after the twenty-fourth week of gestation: systolic blood pressure of 140 mm Hg or more or a rise of 30 mm or more above the woman's usual systolic blood pressure; diastolic blood pressure of 90 mm Hg or more or a rise of 15 mm or more above the woman's usual diastolic blood pressure; proteinuria; and edema. Severe preeclampsia is diagnosed if one or more of the following is present: systolic blood pressure of 160 mm Hg or more or a diastolic blood pressure of 110 mm Hg or more on two occasions 6 hours apart with the woman at bed rest; proteinuria of 5 g or more in 24 hours; oliguria of less than 400 ml in 24 hours; ocular or cerebral vascular disorders; and cyanosis or pulmonary edema. Preeclampsia commonly causes abnormal metabolic function, including negative nitrogen balance, increased central nervous system irritability, hyperactive reflexes, compromised renal function, hemoconcentration, and alterations of fluid and electrolyte balance. Complications include premature separation of the placenta, hypofibrinogenemia, hemolysis, cerebral hemorrhage, ophthalmologic damage, pulmonary edema, hepatocellular changes, fetal malnutrition, and lowered birth weight. The most serious complication is eclampsia, which can result in maternal and fetal death. Healthy living conditions, including a diet high in protein, calories, and essential nutritional elements, and rest and exercise are associated with a decreased incidence of preeclampsia. Treatment includes rest, sedation, magnesium sulfate, and antihypertensives. Ultimately if eclampsia threatens, delivery by induction of labor or cesarean section may be necessary. See also **eclampsia.** Formerly called **toxemia of pregnancy.**

**preemie.** See **premature infant.**

**preexcitation** /prē'eksitā'shən/ [L, *prae* + *excitare,* to arouse], activation of part of the ventricular myocardium earlier than would be expected if the activating impulses traveled only down the normal routes and had experienced a normal delay within the atrioventricular (AV) node. Preexcitation may be a result of either an AV accessory pathway (Wolff-Parkinson-White syndrome), which is reflected on the electrocardiogram by a short P-R interval and a broad QRS complex, or an excessively fast intranodal pathway (Lown-Ganong-Levine syndrome), which manifests with a short P-R interval and a normal QRS complex. The degree of preexcitation is determined by the speed at which the impulse traverses the atrial tissue and the accessory pathway or the AV node. See also **accessory pathway.**

**preexisting condition** /prē'iksis'ting/ [L, *prae* + *existere,* to have reality, *conditio*], any injury, disease, or disability that may have occurred at some time in the past and may predispose an individual to limited health in the future.

**preferential anosmia** /pref'əren'shəl/ [L, *praeferens,* being preferred; Gk, *a* + *osme,* not smell], the inability to smell certain odors. The condition is often caused by psychologic factors concerning either a particular smell or the situation in which the smell occurs.

**preferred provider organization (PPO)** /-furd'/ [L, *praeferre,* to put before], an organization of physicians, hospitals, and pharmacists whose members discount their health care services to subscriber patients. A PPO may be organized by a group of physicians, an outside entrepreneur, an insurance company, or a company with a self-insurance plan. See also **health maintenance organization.**

**preformation** /-fôrmā'shən/ [L, *prae* + *formatio,* formation], an early theory in embryology in which the organism is contained in minute and complete form within the germ cell and after fertilization grows from microscopic to normal size. Compare **epigenesis.**

**preformed water** /-fôrmd'/ [L, *prae* + *forma,* form; AS, *waeter*], the water that is contained in foods.

**prefrontal lobotomy** /-frôn'təl/ [L, *prae* + *frons,* forehead; Gk, *lobos,* lobe, *temnein,* to cut], a surgical procedure in which connecting fibers between the prefrontal lobes of the brain and the thalamus are severed. An archaic technique, it is rarely used today but formerly was an accepted procedure for treating schizophrenic patients with uncontrollable, destructive behavior. After surgery patients were often apathetic, docile, and lacking social graces and decision-making abilities of even the simplest kind. If only the white fibers are severed, the procedure is called a prefrontal leukotomy.

**preg,** abbreviation for **pregnancy.**

**preganglionic neuron** /-gang'glē·on'·ik/ [L, *prae* + Gk, *gagglion,* knot, *neurom,* nerve], a neuron whose axon terminates in contact with another nerve cell located in a peripheral ganglion.

**Pregestimil,** trademark for a hypoallergenic nutritional supplement for infants.

**pregnancy (preg)** /preg'nənsē/ [L, *praegnans,* pregnant], the gestational process, comprising the growth and development within a woman of a new individual from conception through the embryonic and fetal periods to birth. Pregnancy lasts approximately 266 days (38 weeks) from the day of fertilization, but it is clinically considered to last 280 days (40 weeks; 10 lunar months; 9⅓ calendar months) from the first day of the last menstrual period. The expected date of delivery (EDD) is calculated on the latter basis even if a woman's periods are irregular. If a woman is certain that coitus occurred only once during the month of conception and if she knows the date on which coitus occurred, the EDC may be calculated as 266 days from that date. Pregnancy begins after coitus at or near the time of ovulation (usually about 14 days before a woman's next expected menstrual period). Of the millions of ejaculated sperm cells thousands reach the female ovum in the outer end of the fallopian tube, but usually only one penetrates the egg for union of the male and female pronuclei and conception. The zygote, genetically a unique entity, begins cell division as it is transported to the uterine cavity, where it implants in the uterine wall. Maternal and embryologic elements together form the beginnings of the placenta, which grows into the substance of the uterus. The placenta functions in maternal-fetal exchange of nutrients and waste products, although the maternal and fetal bloods do not normally mix. The conceptus is in some aspects like a foreign graft or transplant in the mother. Although an immune response is normally activated in the mother, all of her tissues and organs undergo change, many of them profound and some of them permanent.
■ PSYCHOLOGIC CHANGES: The emotional experiences of pregnancy, as reported by pregnant women, are normal and healthy, but extraordinary. A pregnant woman is "herself," but in a very unfamiliar way. She has a sense of heightened function and expectancy. Being keenly aware of the rapid and inevitable changes her body is undergoing, she is more intensely interested in herself. Her concern for the perfection of her baby, her anticipation of the exertion of labor, and her contemplation of the new or expanded responsibilities of motherhood all serve to intensify her emotional tone.
■ CARDIOVASCULAR CHANGES: Cardiac output increases 30% to 50% in pregnancy. The increase begins at about the sixth

week, reaches a maximum about the sixteenth week, declines slightly after the thirtieth week, and rapidly falls off after delivery. It returns to prepregnancy level about the sixth week after delivery. The stroke volume of the heart increases, and the pulse rate becomes more rapid: Normal pulse rate in pregnancy is approximately 80 to 90 beats/min. Blood pressure may drop slightly after the twelfth week of gestation and return to its usual level after the twenty-sixth week. The circulation of blood to the pregnant uterus near term is about 1 L/min, requiring about 20% of the total cardiac output. Total blood volume also increases in pregnancy; plasma volume increases more than red cell volume, and this results in a drop in the hematocrit, caused by dilution. The white blood cells increase: The normal white blood cell count in pregnancy is often above 15,000/mL.

**pregnancy epulis.** See **gingival hormonal enlargement.**

**pregnancy gingivitis,** an enlargement or hyperplasia of the gingivae caused by hormonal imbalance during pregnancy. It is usually limited to the interdental papillae.

**pregnancy luteoma.** See **luteoma.**

**pregnancy rate,** (in statistics) the ratio of pregnancies per 100 woman-years, calculated as the product of the number of pregnancies in the women observed multiplied by 12 (months), divided by the product of the number of women observed multiplied by the number of months observed. For example, if 50 women used one contraceptive method for 12 months and 5 of them became pregnant, the pregnancy rate would be 10 per 100 woman-years.

**pregnancy termination care,** a nursing intervention from the Nursing Interventions Classification (NIC) defined as management of the physical and psychological needs of the woman undergoing a spontaneous or elective abortion. See also **Nursing Interventions Classification.**

**pregnancy test.** See **HCG radioreceptor assay.**

**pregnanediol** /pregnān'dē·ol/, crystalline biologically inactive compounds in the urine of women during pregnancy or during the secretory phase of the menstrual cycle. A dihydroxy derivative of the saturated steroid pregnane, pregnanediol is the end product of metabolism of progesterone in the urine.

**pregnanediol test,** a 24-hour urine test that evaluates progesterone production by the ovaries and placenta. It is useful in documenting whether ovulation has occurred, and if so, when. The test is used primarily to monitor progesterone supplementation in patients with an inadequate luteal phase.

**pregnant** /preg'nənt/ [L, *praegnans*], gravid, with child.

**prehensile** /-hen'sil/ [L, *prehendre,* to seize], able to grasp.

**prehension** /-hen'shən/, the use of the hands and fingers to grasp or pick up objects.

**prehospital care,** any initial medical care given an ill or injured patient by a paramedic or other person before the patient reaches the hospital emergency department.

**preinfarction angina** /pre'infärc'shən/ [L, *prae* + *infarcire,* to stuff; *angina,* quinsy], angina pectoris before a myocardial infarction.

**preinvasive carcinoma.** See **carcinoma in situ.**

**preload** /prē'lōd/ [L, *prae* + AS, *lad*], the stretch of ventricular muscle fibers at end diastole. It is reflected by the ventricular pressure and volume at that part of the cardiac cycle. Cardiac output increases with preload. Also called **preload filling pressure.**

**preload filling pressure,** the load on the ventricular muscle fibers at the end of diastole or just before contraction. The preload on the heart is estimated by the left ventricular filling pressure. Cardiac performance increases with preload.

# Pregnancy table for expected date of delivery

Find the date of the last menstrual period in the top line (light-face type) of the pair of lines.
The dark number (bold-face type) in the line below will be the expected day of delivery.

|  |  |  |  |  |  |  |  |  |  |  |  |  |  |  |  |  |  |  |  |  |  |  |  |  |  |  |  |  |  |  |  | |
|---|---|---|---|---|---|---|---|---|---|---|---|---|---|---|---|---|---|---|---|---|---|---|---|---|---|---|---|---|---|---|---|---|
| **Jan.** | 1 | 2 | 3 | 4 | 5 | 6 | 7 | 8 | 9 | 10 | 11 | 12 | 13 | 14 | 15 | 16 | 17 | 18 | 19 | 20 | 21 | 22 | 23 | 24 | 25 | 26 | 27 | 28 | 29 | 30 | 31 | |
| **Oct.** | **8** | **9** | **10** | **11** | **12** | **13** | **14** | **15** | **16** | **17** | **18** | **19** | **20** | **21** | **22** | **23** | **24** | **25** | **26** | **27** | **28** | **29** | **30** | **31** | **(1** | **2** | **3** | **4** | **5** | **6** | **7** | **Nov.** |
| **Feb.** | 1 | 2 | 3 | 4 | 5 | 6 | 7 | 8 | 9 | 10 | 11 | 12 | 13 | 14 | 15 | 16 | 17 | 18 | 19 | 20 | 21 | 22 | 23 | 24 | 25 | 26 | 27 | 28 | | | | |
| **Nov.** | **8** | **9** | **10** | **11** | **12** | **13** | **14** | **15** | **16** | **17** | **18** | **19** | **20** | **21** | **22** | **23** | **24** | **25** | **26** | **27** | **28** | **29** | **30** | **(1** | **2** | **3** | **4** | **5** | | | | **Dec.** |
| **Mar.** | 1 | 2 | 3 | 4 | 5 | 6 | 7 | 8 | 9 | 10 | 11 | 12 | 13 | 14 | 15 | 16 | 17 | 18 | 19 | 20 | 21 | 22 | 23 | 24 | 25 | 26 | 27 | 28 | 29 | 30 | 31 | |
| **Dec.** | **6** | **7** | **8** | **9** | **10** | **11** | **12** | **13** | **14** | **15** | **16** | **17** | **18** | **19** | **20** | **21** | **22** | **23** | **24** | **25** | **26** | **27** | **28** | **29** | **30** | **31** | **(1** | **2** | **3** | **4** | **5** | **Jan.** |
| **April** | 1 | 2 | 3 | 4 | 5 | 6 | 7 | 8 | 9 | 10 | 11 | 12 | 13 | 14 | 15 | 16 | 17 | 18 | 19 | 20 | 21 | 22 | 23 | 24 | 25 | 26 | 27 | 28 | 29 | 30 | | |
| **Jan.** | **8** | **9** | **10** | **11** | **12** | **13** | **14** | **15** | **16** | **17** | **18** | **19** | **20** | **21** | **22** | **23** | **24** | **25** | **26** | **27** | **28** | **29** | **30** | **31** | **(1** | **2** | **3** | **4** | **5** | **6** | | **Feb.** |
| **May** | 1 | 2 | 3 | 4 | 5 | 6 | 7 | 8 | 9 | 10 | 11 | 12 | 13 | 14 | 15 | 16 | 17 | 18 | 19 | 20 | 21 | 22 | 23 | 24 | 25 | 26 | 27 | 28 | 29 | 30 | 31 | |
| **Feb.** | **5** | **6** | **7** | **8** | **9** | **10** | **11** | **12** | **13** | **14** | **15** | **16** | **17** | **18** | **19** | **20** | **21** | **22** | **23** | **24** | **25** | **26** | **27** | **28** | **(1** | **2** | **3** | **4** | **5** | **6** | **7** | **Mar.** |
| **June** | 1 | 2 | 3 | 4 | 5 | 6 | 7 | 8 | 9 | 10 | 11 | 12 | 13 | 14 | 15 | 16 | 17 | 18 | 19 | 20 | 21 | 22 | 23 | 24 | 25 | 26 | 27 | 28 | 29 | 30 | | |
| **Mar.** | **8** | **9** | **10** | **11** | **12** | **13** | **14** | **15** | **16** | **17** | **18** | **19** | **20** | **21** | **22** | **23** | **24** | **25** | **26** | **27** | **28** | **29** | **30** | **31** | **(1** | **2** | **3** | **4** | **5** | **6** | | **April** |
| **July** | 1 | 2 | 3 | 4 | 5 | 6 | 7 | 8 | 9 | 10 | 11 | 12 | 13 | 14 | 15 | 16 | 17 | 18 | 19 | 20 | 21 | 22 | 23 | 24 | 25 | 26 | 27 | 28 | 29 | 30 | 31 | |
| **April** | **7** | **8** | **9** | **10** | **11** | **12** | **13** | **14** | **15** | **16** | **17** | **18** | **19** | **20** | **21** | **22** | **23** | **24** | **25** | **26** | **27** | **28** | **29** | **30** | **(1** | **2** | **3** | **4** | **5** | **6** | **7** | **May** |
| **Aug.** | 1 | 2 | 3 | 4 | 5 | 6 | 7 | 8 | 9 | 10 | 11 | 12 | 13 | 14 | 15 | 16 | 17 | 18 | 19 | 20 | 21 | 22 | 23 | 24 | 25 | 26 | 27 | 28 | 29 | 30 | 31 | |
| **May** | **8** | **9** | **10** | **11** | **12** | **13** | **14** | **15** | **16** | **17** | **18** | **19** | **20** | **21** | **22** | **23** | **24** | **25** | **26** | **27** | **28** | **29** | **30** | **31** | **(1** | **2** | **3** | **4** | **5** | **6** | **7** | **June** |
| **Sept.** | 1 | 2 | 3 | 4 | 5 | 6 | 7 | 8 | 9 | 10 | 11 | 12 | 13 | 14 | 15 | 16 | 17 | 18 | 19 | 20 | 21 | 22 | 23 | 24 | 25 | 26 | 27 | 28 | 29 | 30 | | |
| **June** | **8** | **9** | **10** | **11** | **12** | **13** | **14** | **15** | **16** | **17** | **18** | **19** | **20** | **21** | **22** | **23** | **24** | **25** | **26** | **27** | **28** | **29** | **30** | **(1** | **2** | **3** | **4** | **5** | **6** | **7** | | **July** |
| **Oct.** | 1 | 2 | 3 | 4 | 5 | 6 | 7 | 8 | 9 | 10 | 11 | 12 | 13 | 14 | 15 | 16 | 17 | 18 | 19 | 20 | 21 | 22 | 23 | 24 | 25 | 26 | 27 | 28 | 29 | 30 | 31 | |
| **July** | **8** | **9** | **10** | **11** | **12** | **13** | **14** | **15** | **16** | **17** | **18** | **19** | **20** | **21** | **22** | **23** | **24** | **25** | **26** | **27** | **28** | **29** | **30** | **31** | **(1** | **2** | **3** | **4** | **5** | **6** | **7** | **Aug.** |
| **Nov.** | 1 | 2 | 3 | 4 | 5 | 6 | 7 | 8 | 9 | 10 | 11 | 12 | 13 | 14 | 15 | 16 | 17 | 18 | 19 | 20 | 21 | 22 | 23 | 24 | 25 | 26 | 27 | 28 | 29 | 30 | | |
| **Aug.** | **8** | **9** | **10** | **11** | **12** | **13** | **14** | **15** | **16** | **17** | **18** | **19** | **20** | **21** | **22** | **23** | **24** | **25** | **26** | **27** | **28** | **29** | **30** | **31** | **(1** | **2** | **3** | **4** | **5** | **6** | | **Sept.** |
| **Dec.** | 1 | 2 | 3 | 4 | 5 | 6 | 7 | 8 | 9 | 10 | 11 | 12 | 13 | 14 | 15 | 16 | 17 | 18 | 19 | 20 | 21 | 22 | 23 | 24 | 25 | 26 | 27 | 28 | 29 | 30 | 31 | |
| **Sept.** | **7** | **8** | **9** | **10** | **11** | **12** | **13** | **14** | **15** | **16** | **17** | **18** | **19** | **20** | **21** | **22** | **23** | **24** | **25** | **26** | **27** | **28** | **29** | **30** | **(1** | **2** | **3** | **4** | **5** | **6** | **7** | **Oct.** |

**premalignant fibroepithelioma** /-məlig′nənt/ [L, *prae* + *malignus,* bad disposition, *fibra,* fiber; Gk, *epi,* above, *thele,* nipple, *oma,* tumor], an elevated white-flesh-colored sessile neoplasm formed of interlacing ribbons of epithelial cells on a hyperplastic mesodermal stroma. The tumor occurs most often on the lower trunk of older people and may be found in association with or develop into superficial basal cell carcinoma.

**Premarin,** trademark for conjugated estrogens.

**Premarin with Methyltestosterone,** trademark for a fixed-combination hormonal drug containing Premarin and an androgen (methyltestosterone).

**premarket approval (PMA)** /-mar′kit/, permission given by the federal government to equipment manufacturers to sell their devices to the medical profession.

**premature** /-məchōōr′/ [L, *prae maturus,* too soon], **1.** not fully developed or mature. **2.** occurring before the appropriate or usual time. —**prematurity,** *n.*

**premature alopecia** [L, *praematurus,* too soon; Gk, *alopex,* fox mange], acquired baldness in a person who is not old.

**premature atrial complex (PAC),** an atrial depolarization that occurs earlier than expected. It is indicated electrocardiographically by an early P′ wave followed by a normal QRS complex. PACs may be the result of atrial enlargement or ischemia or may be caused by stress, caffeine, or nicotine. They may occur occasionally or in a regular pattern. Occasional PACs usually have no significance, but frequent PACs may lead to atrial fibrillation or to paroxysmal supraventricular tachycardia. Also called **atrial extrasystole, atrial premature beat, atrial premature complex.**

**premature beat** [L, *praematurus,* too soon; AS, *beatan*], an electrocardiogram deflection or complex that occurs earlier than expected in the ongoing rhythm pattern. Also called **premature complex, premature impulse.**

**premature complex,** any electrocardiogram deflection representing either the ventricles or atria that occurs early with respect to the dominant rhythm.

**premature ejaculation,** uncontrollable, untimely ejaculation of semen often caused by anxiety during sexual intercourse. Behavioral techniques can be learned by the man and his partner to extend the length of time between erection and ejaculation. See also **ejaculation, erection.**

**premature impulse.** See **premature beat.**

**premature infant,** any neonate, regardless of birth weight, born before 37 weeks of gestation. Because exact gestational age is often difficult to determine, low birth weight is a significant criterion for identifying the high-risk infant with incomplete organ system development. Predisposing factors associated with prematurity include multiple pregnancy, toxemia, chronic disease, acute infection, sensitization to blood incompatibility, any severe trauma that may interfere with normal fetal development, substance abuse, and teenage pregnancy. In most instances the cause is unknown. The incidence of prematurity is highest among women from low socioeconomic circumstances, for whom poor nutrition and lack of prenatal medical care are often precipitating factors. The premature infant usually appears small and scrawny, with a large head in relation to body size, and weighs less than 2500 g. The skin is thin, smooth, shiny, and translucent with the underlying vessels clearly visible. The arms and legs are extended, not flexed, as in the full-term infant. There are little subcutaneous fat, sparse hair, few creases on the soles and palms, and poorly developed ear cartilage. In boys the scrotum has few rugae and the testes may be undescended; in girls the labia gape and the clitoris is prominent. Among the common problems of the premature infant are variations in thermoregulation,

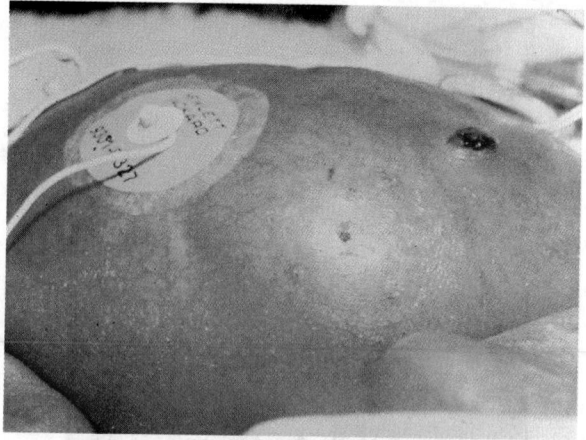

**Skin of a premature infant** *(Zitelli and Davis, 1997)*

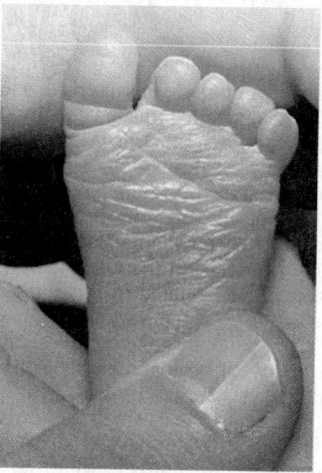

**Sole creases of a premature infant** *(Zitelli and Davis, 1997)*

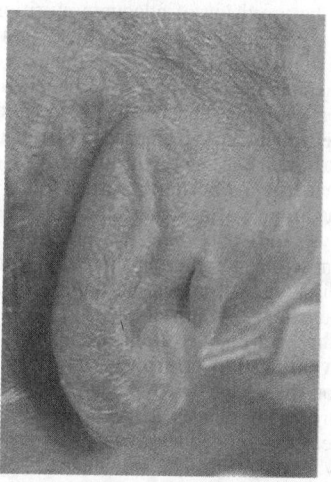

**Ear cartilage of a premature infant**
*(Zitelli and Davis, 1997)*

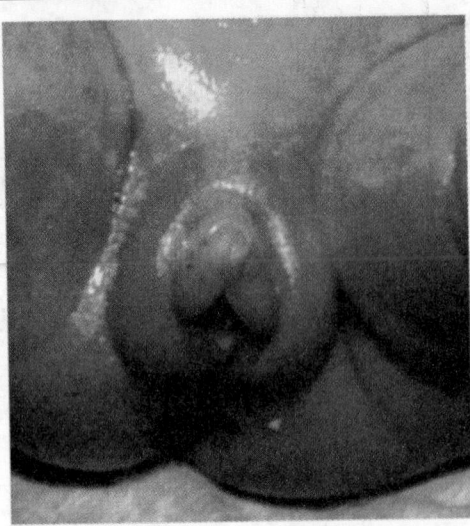

**Genitalia of premature girl** *(Zitelli and Davis, 1997)*

chilling, apnea, respiratory distress, sepsis, poor sucking and swallowing reflexes, small stomach capacity, lowered tolerance of the alimentary tract that may lead to necrotizing enterocolitis, immature renal function, hepatic dysfunction often associated with hyperbilirubinemia, incomplete enzyme systems, and susceptibility to various metabolic upsets, such as hypoglycemia, hyperglycemia, and hypocalcemia. The degree of complications and the rate of survival of premature infants are directly related to the state of physiologic and anatomic maturity of the various organ systems at the time of birth, the condition of the infant other than prematurity, and the quality of postnatal care. With treatment in a neonatal intensive care unit, survival rates improve yearly. In increasing numbers of very small babies development is normal, and those who do not have seizures or apneic spells in the first few days are unlikely to suffer neurologic or physical sequelae of their prematurity. Of primary concern for the nurse caring for the premature infant are the stabilization of body temperature by maintaining a neutral thermal environment, the maintenance of respiration, the prevention of infection, the provision of adequate nutrition and hydration, and the conservation of energy. Important functions of the nurse are to involve the parents in the care of the infant, to explain therapeutic procedures, and to facilitate attachment between the infant and family. Also called *(informal)* **preemie, preterm infant.** Compare **postmature infant.**

**premature labor.** See **preterm labor.**

**premature rupture of membranes,** the spontaneous rupture of the amniotic sac before the onset of labor.

**premature systole** [L, *praematurus* + Gk, *systole,* contraction], a ventricular contraction that occurs too early as a result of a discharge of an ectopic focus in the atria, atrioventricular junction, or ventricle.

**premature thelarche.** See **thelarche.**

**premature ventricular complex (PVC),** a ventricular depolarization that occurs earlier than expected. It appears on the electrocardiogram as an early, wide QRS complex without a preceding related P wave. PVCs may be idiopathic or caused by stress, electrolyte imbalance, ischemia, hypoxemia, hypercapnia, ventricular enlargement, or a toxic reaction to drugs. They may occur occasionally, in a regular pattern, or as several in sequence. Occasional PVCs are not

clinically significant in healthy individuals, but they may produce decreased cardiac output in people with heart disease. Frequent PVCs may be a precursor of ventricular tachycardia or fibrillation.

**prematurity** /-məchoo̅'ritē/ [L, *praematurus,* too soon], pertaining to an event that occurs before the usual or expected time, such as a premature birth.

**premed** /-med'/, abbreviation for *premedical student.*

**premedication** /-med'ikā'shən/ [L, *prae* + *medicare,* to heal], **1.** any sedative, tranquilizer, hypnotic, or anticholinergic medication administered before anesthesia to relieve anxiety and decrease pain. The choice of drug depends on such variables as the patient's age and physical condition and the specific operative procedure. **2.** the administration of such medications. —**premedicate,** *v.*

**premenarchal** /-mənär'kəl/ [L, *prae,* before, Gk, *men,* month; Gk, *archaios,* from the beginning], before the start of the first menstrual period.

**premenopausal** /-men'əpô'səl/ [L, *prae* + Gk, *men,* month; Gk, *pauein,* to cease], before the start of menopause.

**premenstrual** /-men'stroo·əl/ [L, *prae,* before, *menstrualis,* monthly], before the start of menstruation each month.

**premenstrual dysphoric disorder (PMDD),** a mental health condition in women that begins 1 or 2 weeks before menstrual flow. Symptoms include depression, tension, mood swings, irritability, decreased interest, difficulty in concentrating, fatigue, changes in appetite or sleep, physical symptoms, and a sense of being overwhelmed. The condition affects 3% of menstruating women, usually between 25 and 30 years of age. Compare **premenstrual syndrome.**

**premenstrual syndrome (PMS)** [L, *prae* + *menstrualis,* monthly, *tendere,* to stretch], a syndrome of nervous tension, irritability, weight gain, edema, headache, mastalgia, dysphoria, sleep changes, and lack of coordination occurring during the last few days of the menstrual cycle before the onset of menstruation. Several theories attempt to explain the cause of the syndrome, including nutritional deficiency, stress, hormonal imbalance, and various emotional disorders.

**premise** /prem'is/ [L, *prae* + *mittere,* to send], a proposition that is presented as the base of an argument and is usually established beforehand.

**premolar** /prēmō'lər/ [L, *prae* + *mola,* mill], one of eight teeth, four in each dental arch, located lateral and posterior to the canine teeth and in front of the molars. They are smaller and shorter than the canine teeth. The crown of each premolar is compressed anteroposteriorly and surmounted by two cusps and the neck is oval. The root is single and compressed in all premolars except the upper first, which usually have two roots. Usually an anterior and a posterior groove are also present. The upper premolars are larger than the lower premolars. Also called **bicuspid.** Compare **canine tooth, incisor, molar.**

**premonition** /-mənish'ən/, a sense of an impending event without prior knowledge of it.

**premonitory** /-mon'iter'ē/ [L, *prae* + *monere,* to warn], an early symptom or sign of a disease. The term is commonly used to describe minor symptoms that precede a major health problem.

**premorbid personality** /-môr'bid/, a personality characterized by early signs or symptoms of a mental disorder. The specific defects may indicate whether the condition will progress to schizophrenia, a bipolar disorder, or another type of condition.

**prenatal** /-nā'təl/ [L, *prae* + *natus,* birth], before birth; occurring or existing before birth, referring to both the care of the woman during pregnancy and the growth and development of the fetus. Also called **antenatal.** See also **antepartal care.**

**prenatal care¹.** See **antepartal care.**

**prenatal care²,** a nursing intervention from the Nursing Interventions Classification (NIC) defined as monitoring and management of patient during pregnancy to prevent complications of pregnancy and promote a healthy outcome for both mother and infant. See also **Nursing Interventions Classification.**

**prenatal development,** the entire process of growth, maturation, differentiation, and development that occurs between conception and birth. On approximately the fourteenth day before the next expected menstrual period ovulation usually occurs. If the egg is fertilized, it immediately begins the course to fetal maturity and birth. During the first 14 days the fertilized ovum undergoes cell division several times, becoming a morula and then a blastocyst that is able to implant in the uterine wall. From the beginning of the third to the end of the seventh week of embryonic development implantation deepens and completes. Primitive uteroplacental circulation originates between the enlarging trophoblast and the maternal endometrial tissue of the uterus. The amniotic cavity appears as an opening between the inner cell mass and the invading trophoblast. A thin lining in the cavity becomes the amnion. At this point the embryo is a two-layered embryonic disk composed of an ectoderm and an endoderm. As the disk thickens in the middle, giving rise to the third cell layer, or mesoderm, the basic structural systems of the body begin to form. The neural tube develops as a precursor of the central nervous system in the midline of the cranial part of the ectoderm. Primitive blood vessels and blood cells, a heart tube, and umbilical vessels are formed and begin to function. Arm and leg buds may appear, and rudimentary gut, lungs, and kidneys form. By the fifth week the brain has begun to grow rapidly, the heart tube is divided into chambers, the palate and the upper lip are forming, and the urogenital system is developing. By the end of the seventh week all essential systems are present. The period from the eighth week to birth is called the *fetal stage.* From the eighth to the tenth week the fetus continues to grow and development is rapid. The head is almost half of its total length, and arms, legs, and face are clearly recognizable. The fetus floats in the amniotic fluid of the amniotic sac within the uterus; the umbilical vessels in the cord extend to a rapidly growing placenta. By the twelfth week the facial features are formed and the eyelids are present but not yet closed, because they have not divided into upper and lower eyelids. The palate is fusing, a neck connects the large head and the body, and tooth buds and nailbeds have begun to form. Identification of the external genitalia is possible for the first time. From the thirteenth to the sixteenth week the arms, legs, and trunk grow rapidly, and the fetus is active. Scalp hair develops. The skeleton of the fetus is calcified and may be seen on a x-ray film. A sonogram sometimes detects respiratory movements. Between the seventeenth and the twentieth week of pregnancy the mother usually first feels the baby move. The fetus looks like a very small baby at this time. There are eyebrows and tiny nipples; during fetoscopic examination the fetus has been seen and photographed sucking its thumb and grasping its own umbilical cord. At the twenty-fourth week the external ears are smooth and soft and the skin is wrinkled and translucent. The body is covered with lanugo and vernix and weighs a little more than 1 pound. At 28 weeks subcutaneous fat begins to develop, fingernails and toenails are present, the eyelids are separate, the eyes may open, scalp hair is well developed, and in males the testes are at the internal inguinal ring or be-

low. In a modern neonatal intensive care unit most of the babies born at 28 weeks survive. By the thirty-second week the fetus weighs between 3 and 4 pounds. The hair is fine and woolly, the fingernails and toenails have grown to the tips of the fingers and toes, and there are one or two creases on the anterior part of the soles of the feet. The areolae of the breasts are visible but flat. In females the clitoris is prominent and the labia majora are small and separated. At 36 weeks the body and the limbs are fuller and more rounded, creases involve the anterior two thirds of the soles, and the skin is thicker and less translucent. As the fetus reaches term, between 38 and 42 weeks, the vernix decreases, and the ear cartilage is developed. In males the testes are in the scrotum; in females the labia majora meet in the midline and cover the labia minora and the clitoris. At 40 weeks the average fetus weighs 7¼ pounds and is between 19 and 22 inches long. Prenatal development may be adversely affected by several factors. Between 2 and 14 weeks of gestation ionizing radiation and some drugs may have profound effects on morphologic and functional development. During the first 10 days of development any damage usually kills the conceptus. Various viruses, malnutrition, trauma, or maternal disease also may affect the morphologic development of a rapidly differentiating structure or organ during the embryologic or early fetal stage. After 14 weeks, when all of the organs, systems, and body parts have formed, any adverse effects are largely functional; major morphologic damage does not occur.

**prenatal diagnosis,** any of various diagnostic techniques to determine whether a developing fetus in the uterus is affected with a genetic disorder or other abnormality. Such procedures as radiographic examination and ultrasound scanning can be used to follow fetal growth and detect structural abnormalities; amniocentesis enables fetal cells to be obtained from the amniotic fluid for culture and biochemical assay for detection of metabolic disorders and chromosomal analysis; fetoscopy enables fetal blood to be withdrawn from a blood vessel of the placenta and examined for disorders such as thalassemia, sickle cell anemia, and Duchenne's muscular dystrophy. If any of the test results are positive and the child is likely to be born with a severe defect or disease, the parents need support and advice from genetic counselors on whether to terminate the pregnancy. If the parents decide to have the baby, the nurse can help educate them about the specific disorder and prepare them for the special care required of a handicapped or genetically defective child. Also called **antenatal diagnosis.** See also **chorionic villi sampling, genetic counseling, genetic screening.**

**prenatal health behavior,** a nursing outcome from the Nursing Outcomes Classification (NOC) defined as the personal actions to promote a healthy pregnancy. See also **Nursing Outcomes Classification.**

**prenatal surgery,** any surgical procedure that is performed on a fetus. The technique has been used to correct hydrocephalus, urinary tract obstructions, and many other conditions.

**preoccupation** /prē·ok′yəpā′shən/, a state of being self-absorbed or engrossed in one's own thoughts to a degree that hinders effective contact with or relationship to external reality.

**pre-op** /prē·op′/, abbreviation for *preparation for operation* or *preoperative.*

**preoperational thought phase** /prē·op′ərā′shənəl/ [L, *prae + operari,* to work; AS, *thot +* Gk, *phainein,* to show], a piagetian phase of child development, during the period of 2 to 7 years of age, when the child focuses on the use of language as a tool to meet his or her needs.

TIMETABLE OF HUMAN PRENATAL DEVELOPMENT
1 TO 6 WEEKS

**Timetable of prenatal development**

(Moore and Persaud, 1998)

**TIMETABLE OF HUMAN PRENATAL DEVELOPMENT**
7 to 38 weeks

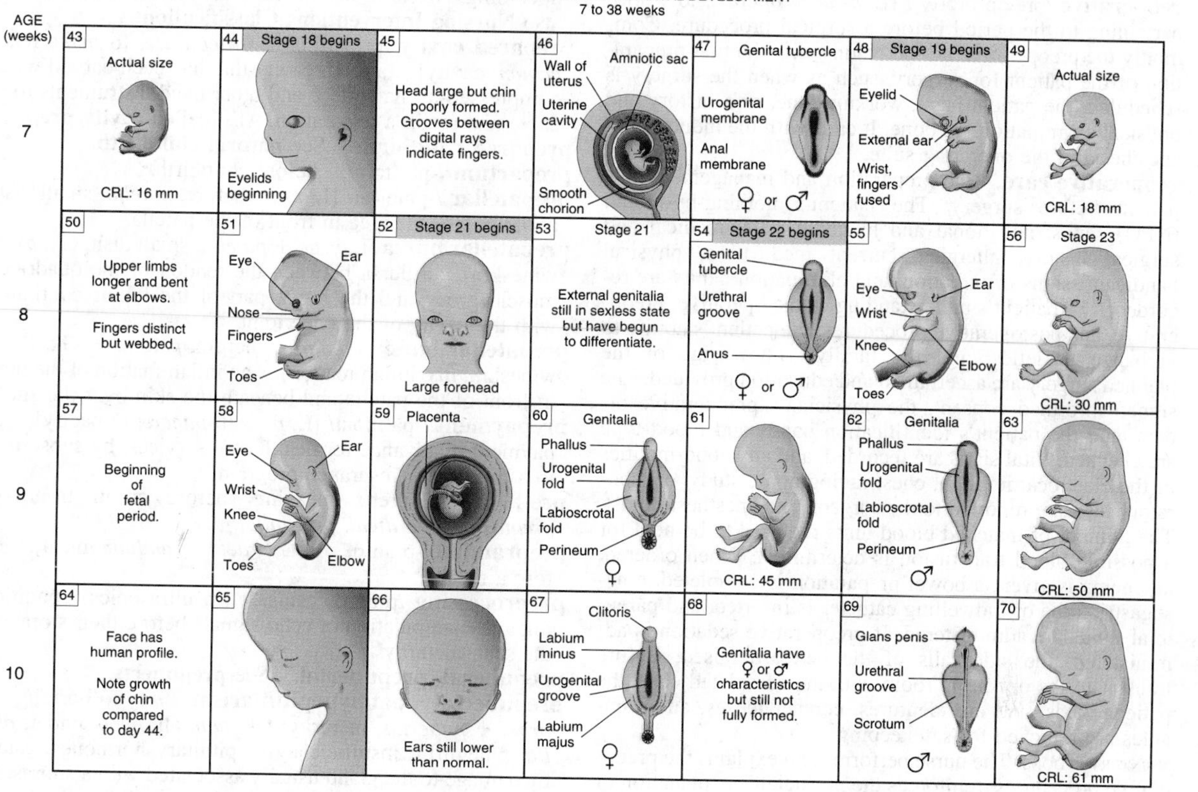

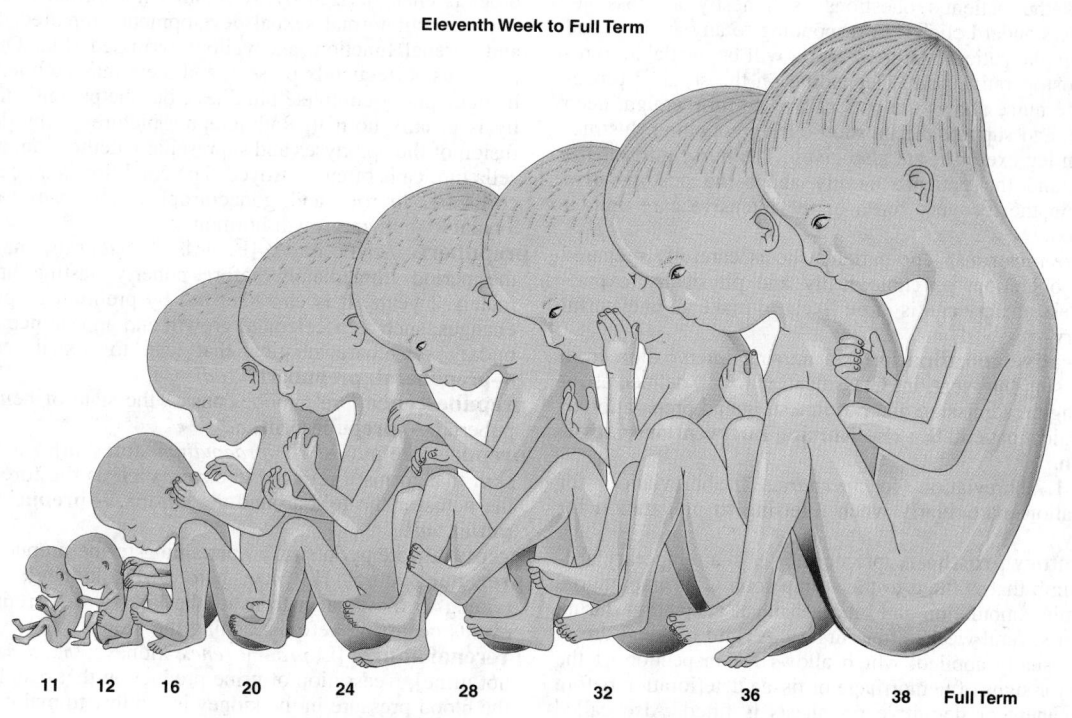

| AGE (weeks) | | | | | | | | |
|---|---|---|---|---|---|---|---|---|
| **7** | **43** Actual size — CRL: 16 mm | **44** Stage 18 begins — Eyelids beginning | **45** Head large but chin poorly formed. Grooves between digital rays indicate fingers. | **46** Wall of uterus; Amniotic sac; Uterine cavity; Urogenital membrane; Anal membrane; Smooth chorion | **47** Genital tubercle ♀ or ♂ | **48** Stage 19 begins — Eyelid; External ear; Wrist, fingers fused | **49** Actual size — CRL: 18 mm | |

Genital tubercle; Urogenital membrane; Anal membrane

| **8** | **50** Upper limbs longer and bent at elbows. Fingers distinct but webbed. | **51** Eye; Ear; Nose; Fingers; Toes | **52** Stage 21 begins — Large forehead | **53** Stage 21 — External genitalia still in sexless state but have begun to differentiate. ♀ or ♂ | **54** Stage 22 begins — Genital tubercle; Urethral groove; Anus | **55** Eye; Ear; Wrist; Knee; Elbow; Toes | **56** Stage 23 — CRL: 30 mm |

| **9** | **57** Beginning of fetal period. | **58** Eye; Ear; Wrist; Knee; Toes; Elbow | **59** Placenta | **60** Genitalia — Phallus; Urogenital fold; Labioscrotal fold; Perineum ♀ | **61** CRL: 45 mm | **62** Genitalia — Phallus; Urogenital fold; Labioscrotal fold; Perineum ♂ | **63** CRL: 50 mm |

| **10** | **64** Face has human profile. Note growth of chin compared to day 44. | **65** | **66** Ears still lower than normal. | **67** Clitoris; Labium minus; Urogenital groove; Labium majus ♀ | **68** Genitalia have ♀ or ♂ characteristics but still not fully formed. | **69** Glans penis; Urethral groove; Scrotum ♂ | **70** CRL: 61 mm |

**Eleventh Week to Full Term**

11   12   16   20   24   28   32   36   38   **Full Term**

**Timetable of prenatal development—cont'd**

**preoperative** /prē·op′ərətiv′/ [L, *prae* + *operari*, to work], pertaining to the period before a surgical procedure. Commonly the preoperative period begins with the first preparation of the patient for surgery, such as when the surgery is scheduled, the patient has a workup done, or a history and physical examination are done. It ends with the induction of anesthesia in the operating suite.

**preoperative care,** the preparation and management of a patient before surgery. The patient's nothing-by-mouth (NPO) status, nutritional and hygienic state, medical and surgical history, allergies, current medication, physical handicaps, signs of infection, and elimination habits are recorded. The patient's understanding of the operative, preoperative, and postoperative procedures; the patient's ability to verbalize anxieties; and the family's knowledge of the planned surgery are ascertained and education provided. The signed informed consent, the physician's preoperative orders, and the patient's identification bands and blood type are checked. Vital signs are recorded, and any abnormalities of the electrocardiogram, chest radiographic study, or laboratory tests are reported to the surgeon and anesthesiologist. The number of matched blood units required to be held for a possible blood transfusion is determined. When ordered, an enema is given, a bowel preparation is completed, a nasogastric tube or indwelling catheter is inserted, and parenteral fluids are administered. If preoperative sedation is administered, the side rails of the bed are raised. Before transfer to the operating room with the completed chart the patient voids, and any dentures, contact lenses, and valuables are removed for safekeeping.
■ INTERVENTIONS: The nurse performs and explains the preoperative procedures; reinforces the physician's explanation of the operation; provides instruction and emotional support; answers the patient's questions as honestly as possible, avoiding standard clichés in responding to any anxiety; and reassures the patient that medication will be available to relieve postoperative pain. Depending on the surgical procedure, the nurse shows the patient how to turn, cough, deep breathe, and support the incision during coughing. Instructions on leg exercises are also given. The nurse informs the patient and the patient's family about the postoperative period in the recovery room or the intensive care unit, if indicated.
■ OUTCOME CRITERIA: The patient who is carefully prepared for an operation, psychologically and physically, experiences less anxiety and is more likely to make an uneventful recovery.

**preoperative coordination,** a nursing intervention from the Nursing Interventions Classification (NIC) defined as facilitating preadmission diagnostic testing and preparation of the surgical patient. See also **Nursing Interventions Classification.**

**prep, 1.** abbreviation for *prepare.* **2.** abbreviation for preparation, particularly when referring to preparation for surgery.

**preparatory prosthesis** /prep′ərətôr′ē/, a temporary artificial limb that is fitted to the stump soon after amputation. It permits ambulation and biomechanical adaptation during the first several weeks after surgery. A rigid removal dressing is usually applied, which allows for inspection of the stump for signs of hemorrhage or tissue deterioration before a permanent or definitive prosthesis is fitted. Also called **temporary prosthesis.**

**preparatory sensory information,** a nursing intervention from the Nursing Interventions Classification (NIC) defined as describing in concrete and objective terms the typical sensory experiences and events associated with an upcoming stressful health care procedure/treatment. See also **Nursing Interventions Classification.**

**prepared cavity** /priperd′/ [L, *praeparare,* to make ready, *cavum,* cavity], a tooth cavity that has been carved with a compressed-air handpiece and other hand instruments to receive and retain a restoration. Also called **cavity prep.**

**prepared childbirth.** See **natural childbirth.**

**prepartum** /-pär′təm/, before childbirth.

**prepatellar** /-pətel′ər/ [L, *prae,* before, *patella,* small dish], pertaining to the area in front of the patella.

**prepatellar bursa** [L, *prae* + *patella,* small dish; Gk, *byrsa,* wineskin], a bursa between the tendon of the quadriceps muscle group and the lower part of the femur continuous with the cavity of the knee joint.

**prepatellar bursitis** [L, *prae,* before, *patella* + Gk, *byrsa,* wineskin, *itis,* inflammation], an inflammation of the bursa in front of the patella and beneath the skin over the site.

**prepayment** /-pā′mənt/ [L, *prae* + *pacere,* to pacify], the payment in advance for health care services, by subscribers to a third-party insurance program.

**pre-, prae-,** prefix meaning 'before or in front of': *preataxic, precritical, pregenital.*

**preprandial** /-pran′dē·əl/ [L, *prae* + *prandium,* meal], before a meal.

**preprocessing** /prēpros′əsing/, (in ultrasonics) conditioning and manipulation of echo signals before their storage in the scan memory.

**prepuberal, prepubertal.** See **prepuberty.**

**prepubertal panhypopituitarism** /-pyo͞o′bərtəl/ [L, *prae,* + *pubertas,* maturity; Gk, *pan,* all, *hypo,* under, *pituita,* phlegm], insufficiency of pituitary hormones, caused by damage to the gland usually associated with a suprasellar cyst or craniopharyngioma, occurring in childhood. The disorder is characterized by dwarfism with normal body proportions, subnormal sexual development, impaired thyroid and adrenal function, and yellow, wrinkled skin. Diabetes insipidus is frequently present, and there may be bitemporal hemianopia or complete blindness, but the patient's mentality is usually normal. Radiographic pictures show delayed fusion of the epiphyses and suprasellar calcification, and the sella turcica is often destroyed. The condition is treated with cortisone, thyroid and gonadotrophic hormones, and, if available, human growth hormone.

**prepuberty** /-pyo͞o′bərtē/ [L, *prae* + *pubertas,* maturity], the period immediately before puberty, lasting approximately 2 years. It is characterized by preliminary physical changes, such as accelerated growth and appearance of secondary sex characteristics, that lead to sexual maturity. —**prepuberal, prepubertal,** *adj.*

**prepubescence** /prē′pyo͞obes′əns/, the state of being prepubertal. —**prepubescent,** *adj.*

**prepuce** /prē′pyo͞os/ [L, *praeputium,* foreskin], a fold of skin that forms a retractable cover, such as the foreskin of the penis or the fold around the clitoris. —**prepucial, preputial,** *adj.*

**preputial** /prē·pyo͞o′shəl/, pertaining to the prepuce.

**prerenal** /-rē′nəl/ [L, *prae,* before, *ren,* kidney], **1.** pertaining to the area in front of the kidney. **2.** pertaining to events occurring before reaching the kidney.

**prerenal anuria** [L, *prae* + *renes,* kidneys; Gk, *a* + *ouron,* not urine], cessation of urine production that results when the blood pressure in the kidney is too low to maintain glomerular filtration pressure.

**prerenal uremia** [L, *prae,* before, *ren,* kidney; Gk, *ouron,* urine, *haima,* blood], a condition of kidney failure in which the primary cause may be outside the kidney, as in conjestive heart failure or some severe cases of alkalosis.

**presby-** /prez'bē/, combining form meaning 'aging or being elderly': *presbyopia, presbyacusia, presbyatrics.*

**presbycardia** /prez'bēkär'dē·ə/ [Gk, *presbys,* old man, *kardia,* heart], an abnormal cardiac condition that especially affects elderly individuals and may be associated with heart failure in the presence of other complications, such as heart disease, fever, anemia, mild hyperthyroidism, and excess fluid administration. Presbycardia may be associated with decreased myocardial elasticity and with mild fibrotic changes of the heart valves, but the basis for these changes and the associated pigmentation of the heart is not known.

**presbycusis** /-koo'sis/ [Gk, *presbys* + *akousis,* hearing], hearing loss associated with aging. It usually involves both a loss of hearing sensitivity and a reduction in the clarity of speech.

**presbyopia** /prez'bē·ō'pē·ə/ [Gk, *presbys* + *ops,* eye], a hyperopic shift to farsightedness resulting from a loss of elasticity of the lens of the eye. The condition commonly develops with advancing age, with the first symptoms appearing about age 40. Compare **visual accommodation.** —**presbyopic,** *adj.*

**presbyopic** /prez'bē·op'ik/ [Gk, *presbys,* old man, *ops,* eye], pertaining to a decrease in accommodation of the lens as one grows older and resulting in a shift toward hyperopia or farsightedness.

**preschizophrenic state** /prēskit'səfren'ik, prē'-/ [L, *prae* + Gk, *schizein,* to split, *phren,* mind], a period before psychosis is evident when the patient deviates from normal behavior but does not demonstrate psychotic symptoms of delusions, hallucinations, or stupor.

**prescreen** /-skrēn/ [L, *prae* + ME, *screen*], **1.** to evaluate a person or a group of people to identify those who are at greater risk of development of a specific condition in order to select those who are in particular need of special diagnostic procedures or health care. **2.** *informal.* a rapid, superficial examination of a person who does not appear to be acutely ill. It may include taking a medical history.

**prescribe** /priskrīb'/ [L, *prae* + *scribere,* to write], **1.** to write an order for a drug, treatment, or procedure. **2.** to recommend or encourage a course of action.

**prescription** /priskrip'shən/, an order for medication, therapy, or therapeutic device given by a properly authorized person, which ultimately goes to a person properly authorized to dispense or perform the order. A prescription is usually in written form; can be written, phoned, or faxed; and includes the patient's name and address, the date, the ℞ symbol (superscription), the medication prescribed (inscription), directions to the pharmacist or other dispenser (subscription), whether it is acceptable to dispense generic, directions to the patient that must appear on the label, prescriber's signature and, in some instances an identifying number.

**prescription drug** [L, prae + *scribere* + Fr, *drogue*], a drug that can be dispensed to the public only with an order given by a properly authorized person. The designation of a medication as a prescription drug is made by the U.S. Food and Drug Administration.

**prescriptive intervention mode** /priskrip'tiv/ [L, *praescriptus,* prescribed, *intervenire,* to come between, *modus,* measure], a therapeutic situation in which the health professional tells the patient explicitly how to solve a problem, so that less collaboration between the consultant and patient is needed.

**prescriptive theory,** a theory that comprises a description of a specific activity, a statement of the goal of the activity, and an analysis of the elements of the activity, which together constitute a prescription for reaching the goal.

**presence**[1] /prez'əns/, a mode of being available in a situation with the wholeness of one's individual being; a gift of self that can be given freely, invoked, or evoked.

**presence**[2], a nursing intervention from the Nursing Interventions Classification (NIC) defined as being with another, both physically and psychologically, during times of need. See also **Nursing Interventions Classification.**

**presenile** /-sē'nīl/ [L, *prae,* before, *senex,* aged], pertaining to a condition in which a person manifests signs of aging in early or middle life.

**presentation.** See **fetal presentation.**

**presentation of the cord.** See **funic presentation.**

**present health** [L, *praesentare,* to show; AS, *haelth*], (in a health history) a succinct chronologic account of any recent changes in the health of the patient and of the circumstances or symptoms that prompted the person to seek health care.

**presenting part** /prəsen'ting/ [L, *praesentare* + *pars,* part], the part of the fetus that lies closest to the internal os of the cervix.

**presenting symptom.** See **symptom.**

**preservative** /prisur'vətiv/ [L, *praeservare,* to keep], a chemical or other agent that reduces the rate of decomposition of a substance.

**presomite embryo** /prēsō'mīt/ [L, *prae* + Gk, *soma,* body, *en,* in, *bryein,* to grow], an embryo in any stage of development before the appearance of the first pair of somites (segments), which in humans usually occurs around 19 to 21 days after fertilization of the ovum.

**-pressin,** combining form for vasoconstrictors, particularly vasopressin derivatives.

**pressor** /pres'ər/ [L, *premere,* to press], describing a substance that tends to cause a rise in blood pressure.

**pressoreceptor.** See **baroreceptor.**

**pressure** /presh'ər/ [L, *premere,* to press], a force, or stress, applied to a surface by a fluid or an object, usually measured in units of mass per unit of area, such as pounds per square inch. Other units: mm Hg, bar, atm.

**pressure acupuncture,** a system of acupuncture involving the application of pressure, such as by the tip of a finger, to certain specified points of the body. See also **acupuncture.**

**pressure area,** an oral area that is subject to excessive displacement of soft tissue by a prosthesis.

**pressure control ventilation,** positive pressure ventilation in which breaths are augmented by air at a fixed rate and amount of pressure, with tidal volume not being fixed; used particularly for patients with acute respiratory distress syndrome.

**pressure dressing,** a bandage or cloth material firmly applied to exert pressure to stop bleeding, prevent edema, and provide support for varicose veins. It also is commonly used in the treatment of burns and after skin grafting.

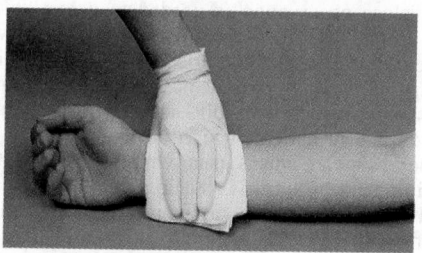

**Pressure dressing** *(Sanders et al, 2000)*

**pressure edema,** 1. edema of the lower extremities caused by pressure of a pregnant uterus against the large veins of the area. 2. edema of the fetal scalp after cephalic presentation.

**pressure management,** a nursing intervention from the Nursing Interventions Classification (NIC) defined as minimizing pressure to body parts. See also **Nursing Interventions Classification.**

**pressure necrosis.** See **pressure ulcer.**

**pressure point,** 1. a point over an artery where the pulse may be felt. Pressure on the point may be helpful in stopping the flow of blood from a wound distal to it. 2. a site that is extremely sensitive to pressure, such as the phrenic pressure point along the phrenic nerve between the sternocleidomastoid and the scalenus anticus on the right side; pressure at this site may be symptomatic of gallbladder dysfunction.

**pressure-sensitive adhesive,** a drug-delivery device that uses polymers that are permanently tacky at room temperature and adhere to the skin when slight pressure is applied.

**pressure sore.** See **pressure ulcer.**

**pressure support ventilation (PSV),** the augmentation of spontaneous breathing effort with a specific amount of positive airway pressure. The patient initiates the inspiratory flow and sets his or her own respiration rate and tidal volume.

**pressure ulcer,** an inflammation, sore, or ulcer in the skin over a bony prominence that occurs most frequently on the sacrum, elbows, heels, outer ankles, inner knees, hips, shoulder blades, and occipitae bone of high-risk patients, especially those who are obese, elderly, or suffering from chronic diseases, infections, injuries, or a poor nutritional state. It results from ischemic hypoxia of the tissues caused by prolonged pressure on them. Pressure ulcers are most often seen in aged, debilitated, immobilized, or cachectic patients. The sores are graded by stages of severity (see table). Prevention of pressure ulcers is a cardinal aspect of nursing care; treatment specific to the location and the extent of the condition is planned. Also called **bedsore, decubitus ulcer, pressure necrosis, pressure sore.**

**pressure ulcer care[1],** the management and prevention of pressure ulcers.

■ METHOD: Prevention of pressure ulcers begins with an understanding of proper body positioning, the importance of turning and repositioning, and the need for suitable support surfaces for sleeping and for sitting. Support surfaces include overlays, mattress replacements, specialty beds, and special chair cushions. "Donut" rings should not be used to relieve pressure because they reduce blood supply. Bedfast patients should be repositioned at least every two hours, and chair fast patients should be repositioned every 15 minutes. Bed linen should be kept dry and wrinkle free. To avoid shear, a sheet or mechanical lift is used to move a patient. Skin should be inspected at least once daily for redness or discoloration, and each time the patient is repositioned the bony areas should be inspected. Dark skin will not show redness; close observation is needed to detect changes in color. A prophylactic measure is daily skin care, in which all areas are washed, rinsed, and dried thoroughly, and lotion is gently applied to bony prominences. The perineal and perianal areas are washed with mild soap and warm water after defecation and urination. A high protein diet with vitamin and mineral supplements is usually required. One method of classifying pressure ulcers is staging (see table). If necrotic material exists in the ulcer, staging is not possible until it has been removed. Necrotic material can be eschar or slough. Topical wound management involves debridement, wound cleansing, the application of dressings, and possibly adjunct

therapy (electrical stimulation, hyperbaric oxygen, ultrasound). Clinical Practice Guidelines for Treatment of Pressure Ulcers may be obtained from the U.S. Department of Health and Human Services, Agency for Health Care Policy and Research (AHCPR). Normal saline is recommended for cleaning most pressure ulcers. An ideal dressing for a pressure ulcer should protect the wound and provide ideal hydration. The pressure ulcer wound bed should be moist. Devices such as heat lamps and hair dryers should not be used. Dead space within a wound should be eliminated by loosely filling all cavities with dressing materials.

■ INTERVENTIONS: The nurse plays a major role in the prevention of pressure ulcers and in their treatment if they occur, turning the patient at frequent intervals, applying the ordered medications and dressings to the lesions, avoiding rubbing in the administration of daily skin care, and encouraging good nutrition. The nurse conducts active or passive exercises with massage to the patient's extremities and, when indicated, prepares for débridement of advanced ulcers.

■ OUTCOME CRITERIA: Pressure ulcers are often resistant to treatment, and large areas of ulceration can be life-threatening and costly, especially in a debilitated patient. Prompt and continued care of early lesions can prevent invasion of underlying tissue and promote healing. The nurse may elicit the cooperation and participation of the patient in a nursing care plan that includes all preventive measures. The importance of frequent change of position, pressure, friction, moisture, shear, and good nutrition is emphasized.

**pressure ulcer care[2],** a nursing intervention from the Nursing Interventions Classification (NIC) defined as facilitation of healing in pressure ulcers. See also **Nursing Interventions Classification.**

**pressure ulcer prevention,** a nursing intervention from the Nursing Interventions Classification (NIC) defined as prevention of pressure ulcers for a patient at high risk for developing them. See also **Nursing Interventions Classification.**

**pressure ventilator,** a mechanical ventilator in which gas delivery is limited by a predetermined pressure.

**presumptive signs** /-sump′tiv/ [L, *praesumere,* to take beforehand, *signum,* mark], manifestations that indicate a pregnancy although they are not necessarily positive. Presumptive signs may include cessation of menses and morning sickness. See also **Chadwick's sign.**

**preswing stance stage** /prē′swing/ [L, *prae* + AS, *swingan,* to fling; L, *stare,* to stand; OFr, *estage,* stage], one of the five stages in the stance phase of walking or gait, a brief transitional period of double-limb support during which one leg is rapidly relieved of body-bearing weight and prepared for the swing forward. The type of preswing used by an individual is a factor in the diagnosis of many abnormal orthopedic conditions. Compare **initial contact stance stage, loading response stance stage, midstance, terminal stance.** See also **swing phase of gait.**

**presymptomatic disease** /-simp′təmat′ik/ [L, *prae* + Gk, *symptoma,* a happening], an early stage of disease when physiologic changes have begun although no signs or symptoms are observed.

**presynaptic** /-sinap′tik/ [L, *prae* + *synaptein,* to join], 1. situated near or before a synapse. 2. before a synapse is crossed.

**presystole** /-sis′təlē/ [L, *prae,* before; Gk, *systole,* contraction], the interval in the cardiac cycle immediately before systole. **—presystolic,** *adj.*

**presystolic** /-sistol′ik/ [L, *prae* + Gk, *systole,* contraction], pertaining to the period before systole.

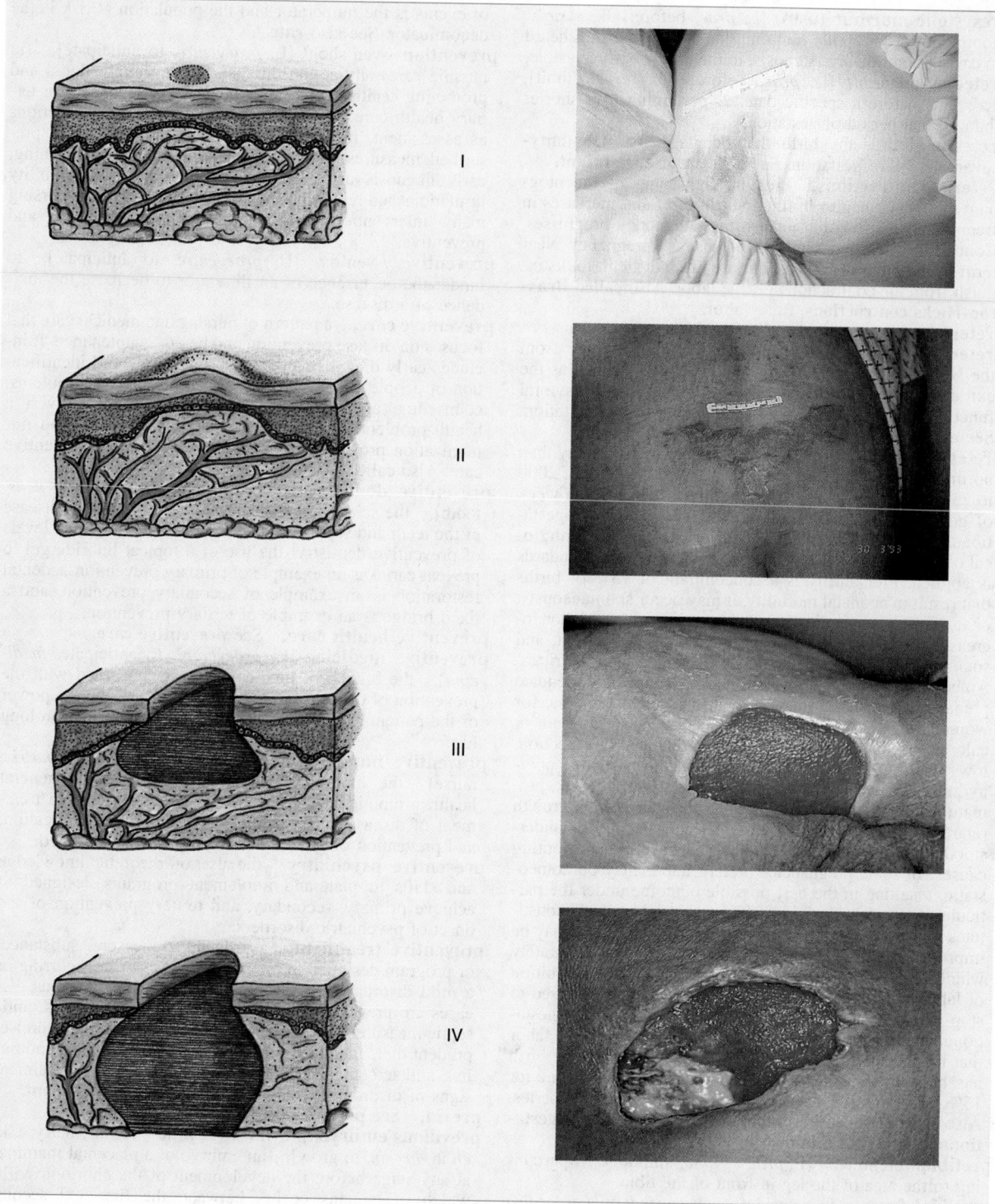

**Staging of pressure ulcers. I,** Nonblanchable erythema of intact skin—the heralding lesion of skin ulceration. **II,** Partial-thickness skin loss involving epidermis and/or dermis. **III,** Full-thickness skin loss involving damage or necrosis of subcutaneous tissue that may extend down to, but not through, underlying fascia. **IV,** Full-thickness skin loss with extensive destruction, tissue necrosis, or damage to muscle, bone, or supporting structures. Data from National Pressure Ulcer Advisory Panel: Pressure ulcers in adults: protection and prevention, US Dept of Health and Human Services, Public Health Service, Agency for Health Care Policy and Research, Rockville, Md, AHCPR Pub. No. 92-0047, May, 1992. Illustrations from Potter and Perry, 1997/courtesy Laurel Wiersma, RN, MSN, St Louis.

**presystolic murmur (psm)** [L, *prae,* before; Gk, *systole,* contraction; L, *murmur,* humming], a heart murmur heard in cases of mitral valve stenosis, immediately before systole.

**preterm** /prēturm'/ [L, *prae,* before; Gk, *terma,* limit], **1.** events before a specific date. **2.** pertaining to a shorter than normal period of gestation.

**preterm birth,** any birth that occurs before the thirty-seventh week of gestation. See also **premature infant.**

**preterm contractions,** irregular tightening of the pregnant uterus that begins in the first trimester and increases in frequency, duration, and intensity as pregnancy progresses. Contractility of uterine muscle increases in pregnancy. Near term strong preterm contractions are often difficult to distinguish from the contractions of true labor. Also called **Braxton Hicks contractions, false labor.**

**preterm infant.** See **premature infant.**

**preterm infant organization,** a nursing outcome from the Nursing Outcomes Classification (NOC) defined as the extrauterine integration of physiological and behavioral function by the infant born 24 to 37 (term) weeks gestation. See also **Nursing Outcomes Classification.**

**preterm labor,** labor that occurs earlier in pregnancy than normal, either before the fetus has reached a weight of 2000 to 2500 g or before the thirty-seventh or thirty-eighth week of gestation. No single measure of fetal weight or gestational age is used universally to designate preterm birth; local or institutional policy dictates which of several standards is applied. Prematurity is a concomitant of 75% of births that result in neonatal mortality. It may occur spontaneously, or it may be iatrogenic. The incidence of preterm labor increases in inverse proportion to maternal age, weight, and socioeconomic status. Incidence is higher for African-American women, for women who have not had adequate prenatal care or have an abnormal obstetric history, and for women who smoke or whose diet is deficient in protein or calories. Predisposing conditions include maternal infection, low weight gain, uterine bleeding, multiple gestation, polyhydramnios, uterine abnormalities, incompetent cervix, premature rupture of membranes, and intrauterine fetal growth retardation. The cause of preterm labor is poorly understood; in some cases there may be several contributing causes. In some pregnancies preterm labor may be homeostatic, resulting in the best possible outcome under the particular abnormal conditions. If preterm labor itself constitutes a threat to the fetus, the outcome of pregnancy may be improved if labor can be inhibited. Determining accurately which pregnancies are likely to benefit from the inhibition of labor and which are not is difficult. Medications used to stop labor are not always effective. Misdiagnosis of gestational age and fetal condition may lead to induction of labor that is inadvertently premature; preterm babies whose birth has been brought about inappropriately early account for 15% of admissions to newborn intensive care nurseries. Also called **premature labor.** See also **small for gestational age (SGA) infant.**

**pretibial** /prētib'ē·əl/ [L, *prae* + *tibia,* shinbone], pertaining to the area of the leg in front of the tibia.

**pretibial fever,** an acute infection caused by *Leptospira autumnalis.* It is characterized by headache, chills, fever, enlarged spleen, myalgia, low white blood cell count, and rash on the anterior surface of the legs. Also called **Fort Bragg fever.**

**pretrial discovery.** See **discovery.**

**prevalence** /prev'ələns/ [L, *praevalentia,* a powerful force], (in epidemiology) the number of all new and old cases of a disease or occurrences of an event during a particular period. Prevalence is expressed as a ratio in which the number

of events is the numerator and the population at risk is the denominator. See also **rate.**

**prevention** /-ven'shən/ [L, *praevenire,* to anticipate], (in nursing care) any action directed to preventing illness and promoting health to eliminate the need for secondary or tertiary health care. Prevention includes such nursing actions as assessment, including disease risk; application of prescribed measures, such as immunization; health teaching; early diagnosis and treatment; and recognition of disability limitations and rehabilitation potential. In acute care nursing many interventions are simultaneously therapeutic and preventive.

**preventive** /-ven'tiv/ [L, *praevenire,* to anticipate], to hinder the occurrence of an illness or to decrease the incidence of a disease.

**preventive care,** a pattern of nursing and medical care that focuses on disease prevention and health maintenance. It includes early diagnosis of disease, discovery and identification of people at risk of development of specific problems, counseling, and other necessary intervention to avert a health problem. Screening tests, health education, and immunization programs are common examples of preventive care. Also called **primary nursing.**

**preventive dentistry** [L, *praevenire,* to anticipate, *dens,* tooth], the science of the care required to prevent disease of the teeth and supporting structures. There are three levels of preventive dentistry: the use of a topical fluoride gel to prevent caries is an example of primary prevention, a dental restoration is an example of secondary prevention, and a fixed bridge is an example of tertiary prevention.

**preventive health care.** See **preventive care.**

**preventive medicine** [L, *praevenire,* to anticipate, *medicina*], the branch of medicine that is concerned with the prevention of disease and methods for increasing the power of the patient and community to resist disease and prolong life.

**preventive nursing** [L, *praevenire,* to anticipate, *nutrix,* nurse], the branch of nursing concerned with general health promotion, teaching of early recognition and treatment of disease, encouragement of life-style modification, and prevention of further deterioration of the disabled.

**preventive psychiatry,** the use of theoretic knowledge and skills to plan and implement programs designed to achieve primary, secondary, and tertiary prevention of the onset of psychiatric disorders.

**preventive treatment,** a procedure, measure, substance, or program designed to prevent a disease from occurring or a mild disorder from becoming more severe. Various diseases are prevented by immunizations with vaccines, antiseptic measures, the avoidance of smoking, regular exercise, prudent diet, adequate rest, correction of congenital anomalies, and screening programs for the detection of preclinical signs of disorders. Also called **prophylactic treatment.**

**previa.** See **placenta previa.**

**previllous embryo** /prēvil'əs/ [L, *prae* + *villus,* hairy; Gk, *en* in, *bryein,* to grow], an embryo of a placental mammal at any stage before the development of the chorionic villi, which in humans occurs between the first and second months after fertilization.

**previous abnormality of glucose tolerance** /prē'vē·əs/, an obsolete classification that includes people who previously had diabetes mellitus or impaired glucose tolerance but whose fasting and postprandial plasma glucose levels have returned to normal. Included in this category were people who had gestational diabetes but whose plasma level returned to normal after parturition and obese people whose plasma glucose level returned to normal after they lost weight. Previously called *latent diabetes, prediabetes.* See also **diabetes mellitus.**

**previtamin.** See **provitamin.**

**prevocational evaluation** /-vōkā′shənəl/, an evaluation of the abilities and limitations of a patient undergoing rehabilitation from a disabling disorder. The goal is to find eventual employment in a sheltered workshop or in the general community. The evaluation usually leads to selective placement of the patient in an appropriate business or industry.

**prevocational training,** a rehabilitation program designed to prepare a patient for the performance of useful paid work in a sheltered setting or community. It may involve training in basic work skills and counseling as required for a typical employment setting.

**PRF,** abbreviation for **pulse repetition frequency.**

**priapism** /prī′əpiz′əm/ [Gk, *priapos,* phallus], an abnormal condition of prolonged or constant penile erection, often painful and seldom associated with sexual arousal. It may result from localized infection, a lesion in the penis or the central nervous system, or the use of certain drugs. It sometimes occurs in men who have acute leukemia or sickle cell anemia.

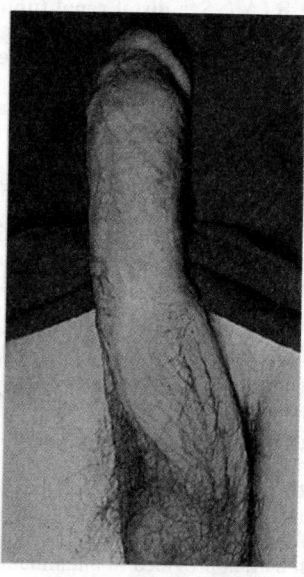

**Priapism** *(Lloyd-Davies, Gow, and Davies, 1994)*

**priapitis** /prī′əpī′tis/, inflammation of the penis.

**priapus.** See **penis.**

**prickle cell layer.** See **stratum spinosum.**

**prickly heat.** See **miliaria.**

**-pride,** combining form for sulpiride derivatives.

**-pril,** combining form for captopril-type antihypertensive agents.

**prilocaine hydrochloride** /pril′ōkān/, a local anesthetic agent of the amide family, used for nerve block, epidural, and regional anesthesia. It is not used for spinal or topical anesthesia. Prilocaine hydrochloride is about half as toxic as lidocaine but because methemoglobinemia is a possible reaction to its administration, is not used for patients with hypoxic conditions of any kind.

**prim-, primi-,** prefix meaning 'first': *primerite, primigravida, primitiae.*

**-prim,** combining form for trimethoprim-type antibacterials.

**Primacor,** trademark for a phosphodiesterase inhibitor (milrinone).

**prima facie rights** /prī′mə fā′shē·ə/, rights on the surface, or face, that may be overridden by stronger conflicting rights or by other values.

**primal scream therapy** /prī′məl/, a non-mainstream form of psychotherapy developed by Arthur Janov that focuses on repressed pain of infancy or childhood. The goal of the therapy is that the patient will surrender his or her anxiety defenses and "become real."

**primaquine phosphate** /prī′məkwin/, an antimalarial.

■ INDICATIONS: It is prescribed in the treatment of malaria and prevention of relapse during recovery from the disease.

■ CONTRAINDICATIONS: Lupus erythematosus, rheumatoid arthritis, concomitant use of bone marrow depressants or hemolytic drugs, or known hypersensitivity to this drug prohibits its use.

■ ADVERSE EFFECTS: Among the more serious adverse reactions are hemolytic anemia, agranulocytosis, and abdominal distress.

**primary** /prī′mərē/ [L, *primus,* first], **1.** first in order of time, place, development, or importance. **2.** not derived from any other source or cause, specifically the original condition or set of symptoms in disease processes, such as a primary infection or a primary tumor. **3.** (in chemistry) noting the first and most simple compound in a related series, formed by the substitution of one of two or more atoms or of a group in a molecule, such as in amine or carboxyl radicals. Compare **secondary, tertiary.**

**primary abscess** [L, *primus* + *abscedere,* to go away], an abscess that develops at the original point of infection by a pus-producing microorganism.

**primary afferent fiber.** See **gamma efferent fiber.**

**primary alveolar hypoventilation.** See **Ondine's curse.**

**primary amebic meningoencephalitis,** a rare and often fatal acute, febrile, purulent meningoencephalitis caused by usually free-living soil and water amebas of the genera *Naegleria,* or *Acanthamoeba.* Infection caused by *Naegleria* is generally seen in young persons who swim or bathe in contaminated fresh water, the pathogens gaining access to the central nervous system by penetrating the nasal mucosa and cribriform plate and then following the olfactory bulbs and nerves to the brain and meninges. By contrast, *Acanthamoeba* infections tend to be more benign, are more often seen in older or immunocompromised persons, and are sometimes associated with spontaneous recovery; the mode of transmission of these infections is not known, but hematogenous spread from amebic infection at distant sites has been reported.

**primary amenorrhea.** See **amenorrhea.**

**primary amputation,** amputation performed after severe trauma, after the patient has recovered from shock, and before infection occurs. Compare **secondary amputation.**

**primary amyloidosis.** See **amyloidosis.**

**primary anesthesia** [L, *primus,* first; Gk, *anaisthesia,* lack of feeling], any anesthetic or analgesic given a surgical patient before the administration of chemical agents that produce reversible unconsciousness.

**primary apnea,** a self-limited condition characterized by an absence of respiration. It may follow a blow to the head and is common immediately after birth in the newborn who breathes spontaneously when the carbon dioxide level in the circulation reaches a certain value. Reflexes are present and the heart is beating, but the skin may be pale or blue and muscle tone is diminished. No treatment is necessary, but careful observation, maintenance of body temperature, and oral pharyngeal aspiration are usually performed. Within seconds the newborn usually begins breathing, becomes pinker, moves the arms and legs, and cries. Compare **periodic apnea of the newborn, secondary apnea.**

**primary atelectasis,** failure of the lungs to expand fully at birth, most commonly seen in premature infants or those narcotized by maternal anesthesia. The infant is usually cared for in an incubator in which the temperature and humidity may be closely monitored. Nursing care includes changing the infant's position frequently to assist respiration, suctioning to remove bronchial secretions, and feeding very slowly to prevent abdominal distension.

**primary atypical pneumonia.** See **mycoplasma pneumonia.**

**primary bilateral micronodular hyperplasia.** See **micronodular adrenal disease.**

**primary biliary cirrhosis,** a chronic inflammatory condition of the liver. It is characterized by generalized pruritus, enlargement and hardening of the liver, weight loss, and diarrhea with pale, bulky stools. Petechiae, epistaxis, or hemorrhage resulting from hypoprothrombinemia may also be evident. Pathologic fractures and collapsed vertebrae may develop as the result of the associated malabsorption of vitamin D and calcium. Xanthomas commonly develop when the serum cholesterol level exceeds 450 mg/dL. The cause of primary biliary cirrhosis is unknown, although it is associated with autoimmune disorders. The condition most often affects women 40 to 60 years of age. The diagnosis is confirmed by liver biopsy and cholangiography. Antibody is nearly always present. Jaundice, dark urine, pale stools, and cutaneous xanthosis may occur in the later stages of this disease. Treatment commonly includes the administration of fat-soluble vitamins A, D, E, and K to prevent and correct deficiencies caused by malabsorption. Life expectancy is about 5 years for symptomatic patients after the onset of jaundice. Compare **secondary biliary cirrhosis.**

**primary bronchus,** one of the two main air passages that branch from the trachea and convey air to the lungs as part of the respiratory system. The right primary bronchus enters the right lung nearly opposite the fifth thoracic vertebra. The left primary bronchus divides into bronchi for the superior and anterior lobes of the lung. The bronchi, like the trachea, are composed of rings of hyaline cartilage, fibrous tissue, mucous membrane, and glands. The right primary bronchus has a more direct extension of the trachea than the left. Hence foreign objects entering the trachea usually drop into the right bronchus rather than the left. See also **bronchial tree.**

**primary carcinoma,** a neoplasm at the site of origin.

**primary care,** the first contact in a given episode of illness that leads to a decision regarding a course of action to resolve the health problem. Primary care often is provided by a physician, but primary care functions are also provided by nurses.

**primary care case management (PCCM),** (in the United States) a situation in which primary care receives concurrent utilization management review, and discharge planning is used to minimize resource consumption while maintaining quality of care.

**primary care physician** [L, *primus* + ME, *caru*, sorrow; Gk, *physikos*, natural], a physician who usually is the first health professional to examine a patient and who recommends secondary care physicians, medical or surgical specialists with expertise in the patient's specific health problem, if further treatment is needed.

**primary caries.** See **dental caries.**

**primary cell,** an irreversible (non-rechargeable) electromotive force cell.

**primary cell culture,** a cell line derived directly from the parent tissue. Cells in primary culture have the same karyotype and chromosome number as those in the original tissue.

**primary colors,** (in physiology and physics) a small number of fundamental colors: red, green, and blue-violet. In humans the retinal receptor cones contain pigments most sensitive to red, green, or blue light. See also **prismatic colors.**

**primary constriction.** See **centromere.**

**primary cutaneous melanoma,** the site of origin of a malignant neoplasm on the skin.

**primary dementia.** See **Alzheimer's disease.**

**primary dental caries,** dental caries developing in a tooth that was previously unaffected. Compare **secondary dental caries.**

**primary dentition.** See **deciduous dentition.**

**primary dermatitis** [L, *primus* + Gk, *derma*, skin, *itis*, inflammation], skin eruption caused by a substance that can produce cell damage on initial contact, as opposed to that which develops as a sensitivity reaction to an allergen.

**primary distal RTA.** See **distal renal tubular acidosis.**

**primary drive.** See **drive.**

**primary dysmenorrhea.** See **dysmenorrhea.**

**primary effusion lymphoma,** a B-cell lymphoma associated with human herpesvirus 8 infection, characterized by the occurrence of lymphomatous effusions in body cavities without the presence of a solid tumor.

**primary endometriosis** [L, *primus* + Gk, *endon*, within, *metra*, womb, *osis*, condition], an ingrowth of the muscle walls of the uterus by the mucous membrane lining of the organ. Also called **adenomyosis, endometriosis interna.**

**primary fissure,** a fissure that marks the division of the anterior and posterior lobes of the cerebellum.

**primary gain,** a benefit, primarily relief from emotional conflict and freedom from anxiety, attained through the use of a defense mechanism or other psychologic process. Compare **secondary gain.**

**primary gangrene** [L, *primus* + Gk, *gangraina*], a form of gangrene that occurs without preceding inflammation.

**primary health care,** a basic level of health care that includes programs directed at the promotion of health, early diagnosis of disease or disability, and prevention of disease. Primary health care is provided in an ambulatory facility to limited numbers of people, often those living in a particular geographic area. It includes continuing health care, as provided by a family nurse practitioner.

**primary hemorrhage** [L, *primus* + Gk, *haima*, blood, *rhegnynei*, to burst forth], a hemorrhage immediately after an injury.

**primary histoplasmosis.** See **histoplasmosis.**

**primary host.** See **definitive host.**

**primary hypertension.** See **essential hypertension.**

**primary intention.** See **intention.**

**primary iritis** [L, *primus* + Gk, *iris*, rainbow, *itis*, inflammation], an inflammation of the iris that results from a source within the body, such as a systemic disease. Also called **endogenous iritis.**

**primary lateral sclerosis,** a slowly progressing degenerative brain disease characterized by weakness, spasticity, hyperreflexia, and a positive Babinski sign. It involves neurons of the motor cortex but not the brainstem or spinal cord neurons. Also called **spastic primary paraplegia.**

**primary lesion** [L, *primus* + *laesio*, hurting],   a sore or wound that develops at the point of inoculation of the disease, usually applied to a syphilis chancre. Also called **initial lesion.**

**primary nurse,**   a nurse who is responsible for the planning, implementation, and evaluation of the nursing care of one or more clients 24 hours a day for the duration of the hospital stay. See also **primary nursing.**

**primary nursing,**   a system for the distribution of nursing care in which care of one patient is managed for the entire 24-hour day by one nurse who directs and coordinates nurses and other personnel; schedules all tests, procedures, and daily activities for that patient; and cares for that patient personally when on duty. In acute care the primary care nurse may be responsible for only one patient; in intermediate care, the primary care nurse may be responsible for three or more patients. Nurse midwives and other nurse practitioners practice primary nursing. Some advantages are continuity of care for the patient; accountability of the nurse for that care; patient-centered care that is comprehensive, individualized, and coordinated; and the professional satisfaction of the nurse. Compare **team nursing.**

**primary organizer,**   the part of the dorsal lip of the blastopore that is self-differentiating and induces the formation of the neural plate that gives rise to the main axis of the embryo.

**primary palate,**   a shelf formed from the medial nasal process of an embryo that separates the primitive nasal cavity from the oral cavity.

**primary physician,**   **1.** the physician who usually takes care of a patient; the physician who first sees a patient for the care of a given health problem. **2.** a family practice physician or general practitioner. See also **family medicine.**

**primary pneumonic plague.**   See **pneumonic plague.**

**primary polycythemia.**   See **polycythemia rubra vera.**

**primary prevention,**   a program of activities directed to improving general well-being while also involving specific protection for selected diseases, such as immunization against measles.

**primary processes,**   (in psychoanalytic theory) unconscious processes, originating in the id, that obey laws different from those of the ego. These processes occur in the least disguised form in infancy and in the dreams of the adult.

**primary proximal renal tubular acidosis.**   See **proximal renal tubular acidosis.**

**primary relationships,**   relationships with intimates, close friends, and family.

**primary sclerosing cholangitis,**   a progressive chronic fibrosing inflammation of the bile ducts of unknown cause, occurring most commonly in young men and frequently in association with chronic ulcerative colitis; it also occurs as a complication of HIV infection.

**primary sensation,**   a feeling or impression resulting directly from a particular stimulus. See **sensation, def. 1.**

**primary sequestrum,**   a piece of dead bone that completely separates from sound bone during the process of necrosis. Compare **secondary sequestrum.**

**primary sex character,**   an inherited trait directly concerned with the reproductive function of the primary sex organs of the individual.

**primary shock,**   a state of physical collapse comparable to fainting. It may be the result of slight pain, such as that produced by venipuncture, or may be caused by fright. Primary shock is usually mild, self-limited, and of short duration. Severe injury may prolong and merge primary shock with secondary shock. Compare **hemorrhagic shock.**

**primary sterility** [L, *primus* + *sterilis*, barren],   the inability to produce offspring caused by a functional failure of the ovaries or the testes.

**primary symptoms.**   See **symptom.**

**primary syphilis.**   See **syphilis.**

**primary tooth.**   See **deciduous dentition.**

**primary triad,**   in A.T. Beck's theory of depression the three major cognitive patterns that force the individual to view self, environment, and future in a negativistic manner.

**primary tuberculosis,**   the childhood form of tuberculosis, most commonly occurring in the lungs, the posterior pharynx, or rarely the skin. Infants lack resistance to the disease and are readily infected and especially vulnerable to rapid and extensive spread of infection through the body. In childhood the disease is usually brief and benign, characterized by regional lymphadenopathy, calcification of the tubercles, and residual immunity. The disease may reactivate later in life. The tuberculin test result will be positive for life. See also **tuberculin.**

**primate** /prī′māt, prī′mit/ [L, *primus*, first],   a member of the order of mammals that includes lemurs, monkeys, apes, and humans. Most primates a have large brain, stereoscopic vision, and hands and feet developed for grasping.

**Primaxin,**   trademark for a broad-spectrum parenteral antibiotic (imipenem/cilastatin sodium).

**prime mover** /prīm/ [L, *primus* + *movere*, to move],   a muscle that acts directly to produce a desired movement amid other muscles acting simultaneously to produce the same movement indirectly. Most movements of the body require the combined action of numerous muscles. Compare **antagonist, fixation muscle, synergist.**

**primer** /prī′mər/,   **1.** a short piece of DNA or RNA complementary to a given DNA sequence. It acts as a point at which replication can proceed, as in a polymerase chain reaction. **2.** a molecule, such as a small polymer, that induces the synthesis of a larger molecule.

**primidone** /prī′mədōn/,   an anticonvulsant.

■ INDICATIONS: It is prescribed in the treatment of seizure disorders, including grand mal, psychomotor, and focal epilepsy-like seizures.

■ CONTRAINDICATIONS: Porphyria or known hypersensitivity to this drug or to phenobarbital, a metabolite of primidone, prohibits its use.

■ ADVERSE EFFECTS: The most serious adverse reaction, seen on rare occasions, is megaloblastic anemia. Drowsiness, ataxia, and dizziness are common. Other adverse effects of phenobarbital may occur.

**primigravida** /prim′igrav′idə/ [L, *primus* + *gravidus*, pregnancy],   a woman pregnant for the first time. Also called **gravida 1.** Compare **multigravida, primipara.** —**primigravid,** *adj.*

**primipara** /primip′ərə/, *pl.* **primiparae** [L, *primus* + *parere*, to bear],   a woman who has given birth to one viable infant, indicated by the notation *para 1* on the patient's chart. Compare **multipara, nullipara, primigravida.**

**primiparity** /prim′iper′itē/ [L, *primus* + *parere*, to bear],   the condition of having borne one child.

**primiparous** /primip′ərəs/ [L, *primus* + *parere*, to bear],   pertaining to a woman who has borne one child.

**primitive** /prim′itiv/ [L, *primivus*],   **1.** undeveloped; undifferentiated; rudimentary; showing little or no evolution. **2.** embryonic; formed early in the course of development; existing in an early or simple form. Compare **definitive.**

**primitive fold.**   See **primitive ridge.**

**primitive groove,**   a furrow in the posterior region of the embryonic (primordial) disk. It indicates the cephalocaudal axis that results from the active involution of cells forming the primitive streak.

**primitive gut.**  See **archenteron.**

**primitive line.**  See **primitive streak.**

**primitive node,**  a knoblike accumulation of cells at the cephalic end of the primitive streak in the early stages of embryonic development in humans and higher animals. It consists of mesoderm cells that give rise to the notochord, and it corresponds to the dorsal lip of the blastopore in lower animals. Also called **Hensen's knot, Hensen's node.**

**primitive pit,**  a minute indentation at the anterior end of the primitive groove in the early developing embryo. It lies posterior to the primitive node and probably functions as an opening into the notochordal canal in humans and higher animals and into the neurenteric canal in lower animals.

**primitive reflex,**  any reflex normal in an infant or fetus. Its presence in an adult usually indicates serious neurologic disease. Some kinds of primitive reflexes are **grasp reflex, Moro reflex,** and **sucking reflex.**

**primitive ridge,**  a ridge that bounds the primitive groove in the early stages of embryonic development. Also called **primitive fold.** See also **primitive streak.**

**primitive streak,**  a dense area on the central posterior region of the embryonic disk. It is formed by the morphogenetic movement of a rapidly proliferating mass of cells that spreads between the ectoderm and endoderm, giving rise to the mesoderm layer. This seamlike elongation indicates the cephalocaudal axis along which the embryo develops, and it corresponds to the blastopore of lower animal groups. Also called **primitive line.**

**primordia.**  See **primordium.**

**primordial**  /prīmôr′dē·əl/  [L, *primordium,* origin], **1.** characteristic of the most undeveloped or earliest state, specifically those cells or tissues that are formed in the early stages of embryonic development. **2.** first or original; primitive.

**primordial cyst,**  one of three kinds of follicular cyst, consisting of an epithelium-lined sac that contains fluid and appears radiographically as a light area in the affected jaw. It develops from a dental enamel organ before the formation of hard tissue. Compare **dentigerous cyst, multilocular cyst.**

**primordial dwarf,**  a person of extremely short stature who is otherwise perfectly formed, with the usual proportions of body parts and normal mental and sexual development. The condition may be genetically related, involving some defect in the ability to use growth hormone, or it may occur sporadically within a particular population. Also called **hypoplastic dwarf, normal dwarf, physiologic dwarf, pure dwarf, true dwarf.** See also **pituitary dwarf, pygmy.**

**primordial germ cell,**  any of the large spheric diploid cells that are formed in the early stages of embryonic development and are precursors of the oogonia and spermatogonia. They are formed outside the gonads and migrate to the embryonic ovaries and testes for maturation. See also **oogenesis, spermatogenesis.**

**primordial image,**  (in analytic psychology) the archetype or original parent, representing the source of all life. It occurs in the memory as a stage preceding the differentiation of the actual mother and father. See also **collective unconscious.**

**primordium**  /prīmôr′dē·əm/, *pl.* **primordia**  [L, origin], the first recognizable stage in the embryonic development and differentiation of a particular organ, tissue, or structure. Also called **anlage** /un′lägə/, **rudiment.**

**principal**  /prin′sipəl/  [L, *principalis,* first in rank],  first in authority or importance.

**principal cell.**  See **chief cell.**

**Principen,**  trademark for an antibacterial (ampicillin).

**principle**  /prin′sipəl/  [L, *principium,* foundation],  **1.** a general truth or established rule of action. **2.** a prime source or element from which anything proceeds. **3.** a law on which others are founded or from which others are derived.

**principles of instrumentation,**  six rules for the use of mirrors and other hand and motor-driven devices in dentistry and dental hygiene: (1) grasp, (2) fulcrum, (3) insertion, (4) adaptation and angulation, (5) activation (lateral pressure and working stroke), and (6) rest.

**Prinivil,**  trademark for an angiotensin-converting enzyme inhibitor (lisinopril) used for hypertension.

**P-R interval,**  the interval from the beginning of the P wave to the beginning of the QRS complex on an electrocardiogram. It represents the atrioventricular conduction time, which normally is between 0.12 and 0.20 second.

**printout,**  a printed copy of information produced by a computer's printer.

**Prinzmetal's angina**  [Myron Prinzmetal, American cardiologist, 1908–1994],  chest pain caused by reversible, severe coronary artery spasm. It is associated with S-T segment elevation that reverts to normal within minutes. The S-T segment elevation indicates total occlusion of the epicardial coronary artery. Also called **variant angina.**

**prion**  /prī′on/,  one of several kinds of proteinaceous particles believed to be responsible for transmissible neurodegenerative diseases, including scrapie in sheep and kuru and Creutzfeldt-Jakob disease in humans. Because prions lack detectable nucleic acid, they are not inactivated by the usual procedures for destroying viruses. They also do not trigger an immune response.

**priority**  /prī·ôr′itē/  [L, *prius,* previously],  actions established in order of importance or urgency to the welfare or purposes of the organization, patient, or other person at a given time.

**Priscoline Hydrochloride,**  trademark for a peripheral vasodilator (tolazoline hydrochloride).

**prism**  /priz′əm/  [Gk, *prisma* that which is sawn through],  **1.** a solid figure, with a triangular or polygonal cross section, bounded by parallelograms. **2.** enamel prism, or calcified rods, surrounded by organic prism cuticle joined together to form tooth enamel. **3.** an adverse prism or verger prism used to test and train ocular muscles.

**prismatic colors**  /prizmat′ik/,  the seven rainbow hues (red, orange, yellow, green, blue, indigo, and violet) produced from white light when it is reduced to its component wavelengths by the dispersion effect of a prism.

**privacy**  /prī′vəsē/,  a culturally specific concept defining the degree of one's personal responsibility to others in regulating behavior that is regarded as intrusive. Some privacy-regulating mechanisms are physical barriers (closed doors or drawn curtains, such as around a hospital bed) and interpersonal types (lowered voices or cessation of smoking).

**private duty nurse**  /prī′vit/,  a nurse who may work in an institution, caring for a patient on a fee-for-service basis. The private duty nurse is not a member of the institution staff. Private duty care also occurs in the home.

**private practice,**  the work of a professional health care provider who is independent of economic or policy control by professional peers except for licensing and other legal restrictions.

**-privia,**  suffix meaning a '(specified) condition of loss or deprivation': *calciprivia, hormonoprivia, paraprivia.*

**privileged communication**  /priv′ilijd/,  a legal term used in court-related proceedings concerning the right to reveal information that belongs to the person who spoke. It may prevent the listener from disclosing the information without the permission of the speaker. Privileged communication may exist between a patient and a health professional only if the law specifically establishes it.

**privileges** /priv′ilij′əs/ [L, *privilegium*, private law], authority granted to a physician or dentist by a hospital governing board to provide patient care in the hospital. Clinical privileges are limited to the individual's professional license, experience, and competence. Emergency privileges may be granted by a hospital governing board or chief executive officer in an emergency and without regard to the physician's or dentist's regular service assignment or status. Temporary privileges may be granted a physician or dentist to provide health care to patients for a limited period or to a specific patient.

**Privine Hydrochloride,** trademark for an adrenergic (naphazoline hydrochloride).

**PRK,** abbreviation for **photorefractive keratectomy.**

**PRL,** abbreviation for **prolactin.**

**prn,** (in prescriptions) abbreviation for *pro re nata,* a Latin phrase meaning 'as needed.' The administration times are determined by the patient's needs. Also **p.r.n.**

**Pro,** abbreviation for **proline.**

**pro-** /prō-, prə-/, prefix meaning 'first, or in front of': *procallus, procheilon, progravid.*

**proaccelerin.** See **factor V.**

**probability** /prob′əbil′itē/ [L, *probabilitas*], **1.** a measure of the increased likelihood that something will occur. **2.** a mathematic ratio of the number of times something will occur to the total number of possible occurrences.

**probable signs** /prob′əbəl/ [L, *probabilis,* credible, *signum,* mark], clinical signs that there is a definite likelihood of pregnancy. Examples include enlargement of the abdomen, Goodell's sign, Hegar's sign, Braxton Hicks' sign, and positive hormonal test results. Compare **presumptive signs.**

**proband.** See **propositus.**

**Pro-Banthine,** trademark for an anticholinergic (propantheline bromide).

**probe,** **1.** any device used to explore an opening such as a sinus or wound. Common types of probes include a probe with a blunt leading end, a drum probe with a sounding device for the detection of metallic foreign particles, and an eyed probe with a small opening at one end for introducing a guiding thread along a fistula. **2.** any device or agent, such as a radioactively-tagged isotope or a molecular deoxyribonucleic acid fragment probe, inserted into a medium to obtain information about a structure or substance. **3.** a Doppler probe used to detect blood flow in a vessel. **4.** the act of exploring or investigating an action or unfamiliar matter.

**probenecid** /prōben′əsid/, a uricosuric and adjunct to antibiotics.

■ INDICATIONS: It is prescribed in the treatment of gout and as an adjunct to prolong the activity of penicillin or cephalosporins in some infections, such as gonorrhea.

■ CONTRAINDICATIONS: Uric acid kidney stones, blood dyscrasias, or known hypersensitivity to this drug prohibits its use. It is not initiated during an acute attack of gout but is continued if an attack intervenes during treatment. It is not given to children less than 2 years of age. Concomitant administration of salicylates decreases the effect of probenecid.

■ ADVERSE EFFECTS: Among the most serious adverse reactions are hemolytic anemia, GI disturbances, headache, urinary frequency, and minor allergic reactions. It is involved in many drug interactions, particularly salicylate drugs.

**problem** /prob′ləm/ [Gk, *proballein,* to throw forward], any health care condition that requires diagnostic, therapeutic, or educational action. Also refers, in nursing, to any unmet or partially met basic human need.

**problem-oriented medical record (POMR),** a method of recording data about the health status of a patient in a problem-solving system. The POMR preserves the data in an easily accessible way that encourages ongoing assessment and revision of the health care plan by all members of the health care team. The particular format of the system used varies from setting to setting, but the components of the method are similar. A data base is collected before beginning the process of identifying the patient's problems. The data base consists of all information available that contributes to this end, such as that collected in an interview with the patient and family or others, that from a health assessment or physical examination of the patient, and that from various laboratory and radiologic tests. It is recommended that the data base be as complete as possible, limited only by potential hazard, pain or discomfort to the patient, or excessive assumed expense of the diagnostic procedure. The interview, augmented by prior records, provides the patient's history, including the reason for contact, an identifying statement that is a descriptive profile of the person, a family illness history, a history of the current illness, a history of past illness, an account of the patient's current health practices, and a review of systems. The physical examination or health assessment makes up the second major part of the data base. The extent and depth of the examination vary from setting to setting and depend on the services offered and the condition of the patient. The next section of the POMR is the master problem list. The formulation of the problems on the list is similar to the assessment phase of the nursing process. Each problem as identified represents a conclusion or a decision resulting from examination, investigation, and analysis of the data base. A problem is defined as anything that causes concern to the patient or to the caregiver, including physical abnormalities, psychologic disturbance, and socioeconomic problems. The master problem list usually includes active, inactive, temporary, and potential problems. The list serves as an index to the rest of the record and is arranged in five columns: a chronologic list of problems, the date of onset, the action taken, the outcome of the problem (often its resolution), and its date. Problems may be added, and intervention or plans for intervention may be changed; thus the status of each problem is available for the information of all members of the various professions involved in caring for the patient. The third major section of the POMR is the initial plan, in which each separate problem is named and described, usually on the progress note in a SOAP format: *S,* subjective data from the patient's point of view; *O,* the objective data acquired by inspection, percussion, auscultation, and palpation and from laboratory and radiologic tests; *A,* assessment of the problem that is an analysis of the subjective and objective data; and *P,* the plan, including further diagnostic work, therapy, and education or counseling. After an initial plan for each problem is formulated and recorded, the problems are followed in the progress notes by narrative notes in the SOAP format or by flow sheets showing the significant data in a tabular manner. A discharge summary is formulated and written, relating the overall assessment of progress during treatment and the plans for follow-up or referral. The summary allows a review of all the problems initially identified and encourages continuity of care for the patient.

**problem-seeking interview.** See **interview.**

**problem-solving approach to patient-centered care,** (in nursing) a conceptual framework that incorporates the overt physical needs of a patient with covert psychologic, emotional, and social needs. It provides a model for caring for the whole person as an individual, not as an example of a disease or a medical diagnosis. Nursing is defined within this model as a problem-solving process. The patient is viewed as a person who is in an impaired state, less than usually able to perform self-care activities. Nursing problems are conditions experienced by the patient or the patient's family for which the nurse may provide professional service. The nurse makes a nursing diagnosis that identifies the impaired state and determines the care needed to augment the patient's ability to perform self-care. The requirements for care are classified in four levels: care given to sustain life is sustenal care; care given to assist the patient in self-care is remedial care; care that helps the patient to develop new skills and goals in self-care is restorative care; and care given to guide the patient to a level of self-help beyond the normal level is preventive care. The approach identifies 21 nursing problems and sorts them into four groups: problems relating to comfort, hygiene, and safety; physiologic balance; psychologic and social factors; and sociologic and community factors. See also **nursing care plan.**

**problem-solving interview.**   See **interview.**

**probucol** /prōbyoo′kəl/, an investigational AIDS drug.

**procainamide hydrochloride** /prōkān′əmīd/, an antiarrhythmic agent.

■ INDICATIONS: It is prescribed in the treatment of a variety of cardiac arrhythmias, including premature ventricular contractions, ventricular tachycardia, and atrial fibrillation.

■ CONTRAINDICATIONS: Myasthenia gravis, heart block, or known hypersensitivity to this drug, to procaine, or to related local anesthetics prohibits its use.

■ ADVERSE EFFECTS: Among the more serious adverse reactions are GI disturbances, hypersensitivity reactions, agranulocytosis, and a syndrome resembling lupus erythematosus.

**procaine hydrochloride** /prō′kān/, a local anesthetic of the ester family.

■ INDICATIONS: Procaine is administered for local anesthesia by infiltration and injection and for caudal, epidural, and other regional anesthetic procedures. It is not used for topical anesthesia.

■ CONTRAINDICATIONS: Known hypersensitivity to anesthetics of the ester group prohibits its use. It is not injected into inflamed or infected tissue, and large doses are not given to patients with heart block.

■ ADVERSE EFFECTS: Among the most serious adverse reactions are potentially serious neurologic and cardiovascular reactions that result from inadvertent intravascular administration. Allergic reactions also may occur.

**procarbazine hydrochloride** /prōkär′bəzēn/, an antineoplastic.

■ INDICATIONS: It is prescribed in the treatment of a variety of neoplasms, including Hodgkin's disease and lymphomas.

■ CONTRAINDICATIONS: Bone marrow depression or known hypersensitivity to this drug prohibits its use.

■ ADVERSE EFFECTS: Among the most serious adverse reactions are bone marrow depression and GI disturbances, particularly nausea and vomiting.

**Procardia,** trademark for a calcium channel blocker (nifedipine).

**procaryocyte.**   See **prokaryocyte.**

**procaryon.**   See **prokaryon.**

**procaryosis.**   See **prokaryosis.**

**Procaryotae** /prōker′ē·ō′tē/, (in bacteriology) a kingdom of bacteria, viruses, and blue-green algae that includes all microorganisms in which the nucleoplasm has no basic protein and is not surrounded by a nuclear membrane. The kingdom has two divisions: Cyanobacteria, which includes the blue-green bacteria, and bacteria. Also called **Monera.** See also **procaryocyte.**

**procaryote.**   See **prokaryote.**

**procedure** /prəsē′jər/ [L, *procedere,* to proceed], the sequence of steps to be followed in establishing some course of action.

**procercoid** /prōsur′koid/, the first stage in the life cycle of certain tapeworms that develop from the coracidium stage of *Diphyllobothrium latum.* The tapeworm develops in the body of the first intermediate host, either a crustacean or a copopod of the genus *Diaptomus.*

**procerus** /prəsir′əs/ [L, stretched], one of three muscles of the nose. It is a small pyramidal muscle that arises from the fascia of the nasal bone and the lateral nasal cartilage and inserts into the skin over the lower part of the forehead between the eyebrows. It is innervated by buccal branches of the facial nerve. The procerus functions to draw down the eyebrows and wrinkle the nose. Compare **depressor septi, nasalis.**

**process** /pros′əs/ [L, *processus*], **1.** a series of related events that follow in sequence from a particular state or condition to a conclusion or resolution. **2.** a natural growth that projects from a bone or other part. **3.** to put through a particular series of interdependent steps, as in preparing a chemical compound.

**process criteria,** standards identified by the American Nurses Association Division on Psychiatric and Mental Health Nursing Practice that focus on nursing activities.

**processor.**   See **central processing unit.**

**process recording,** (in nursing education) a system used for teaching nursing students to understand and analyze verbal and nonverbal interaction. The conversation between nurse and patient is written on special forms or in a special format. The student nurse is instructed to record observations, perceptions, thoughts, and feelings, as well as conversations. The student also is asked to analyze his or her communication, determining and naming both therapeutic and nontherapeutic techniques used within an interaction. The process recording is then studied by the nursing instructor to discover and to help the student nurse identify patterns of difficulty in communicating with the patient.

**processus vaginalis peritonei** /prəses′əs/ [L, *processus, vagina,* sheath; Gk, *peri,* around, *teinein,* to stretch], a diverticulum of the peritoneal membrane that during embryonic development extends through the inguinal canal. In males it descends into the scrotum to form the processus vaginalis testis; in females it is usually completely obliterated. Also called **Nuck's canal, Nuck's diverticulum.**

**prochlorperazine** /-klôrper′əzēn/, a phenothiazine antipsychotic and antiemetic.

■ INDICATIONS: It is prescribed in the treatment of psychotic disorders, and it may be used in the control of nausea and vomiting.

■ CONTRAINDICATIONS: Parkinson's disease, the concurrent administration of central nervous system depressants, liver or renal dysfunction, severe hypotension, or known hypersensitivity to any phenothiazine prohibits its use.

■ ADVERSE EFFECTS: Among the more serious adverse effects are hypotension, liver toxicity, extrapyramidal reactions, blood dyscrasias, and hypersensitivity reactions.

**prochlorperazine maleate.**   See **prochlorperazine.**

**prochromosome.**   See **karyosome.**

**procidentia** /-siden′shə/ [L, *procidere,* to fall forward], the prolapse of an organ. The term is usually applied to a prolapsed uterus.

**procoagulant** /-kō·ag′yələnt/, a precursor or other agent that mediates the coagulation of blood. Examples include fibrinogen and prothrombin.

**proconvertin.** See **factor VII.**

**procreate** /prō'krē·āt/ [L, *procreare,* to create], to produce offspring.

**procreation** /-krē·ā'shən/ [L, *procreare,* to create], the entire reproductive process of producing offspring. —**procreate,** *v.*

**proct-.** See **procto-.**

**proctalgia** /proktal'jə/ [Gk, *proktos,* anus, *algos,* pain], a neurologic pain in the anus or lower rectum.

**proctalgia fugax** [Gk, *proktos* + *algos,* pain; L, *fugax,* fleeting], periodic pain in the anus, possibly muscular in origin, that follows a pattern and is sometimes relieved by food and drink.

**-proctia,** combining form meaning 'anus or rectum': *ankyloproctia, cacoproctia, coloproctia.*

**proctitis** /proktī'tis/ [Gk, *proktos,* anus, *itis*], inflammation of the rectum and anus caused by infection, trauma, drugs, allergy, or radiation injury. Acute or chronic, it is accompanied by rectal discomfort and the repeated urge to pass feces and inability to do so. Pus, blood, or mucus may be present in the stools, and tenesmus may occur. Also called **rectitis.**

**procto-** /prok'tō-/, proct-, combining form meaning 'anus or rectum': *proctocele, proctorrhea, proctoscopy.*

**proctocele.** See **rectocele.**

**proctocolectomy** /prok'tōkəlek'təmē/, a surgical procedure in which the anus, rectum, and colon are removed. An ileostomy is created for the removal of digestive tract wastes. The procedure treats severe, intractable ulcerative colitis or Crohn's disease. See also **ileoanal anastomosis.**

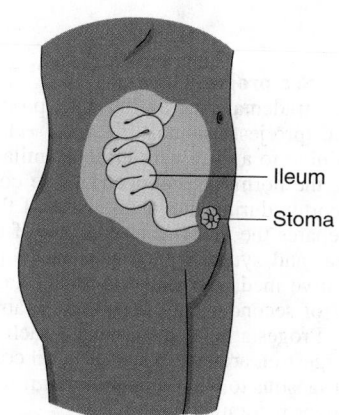

Ileum
Stoma

**Total proctocolectomy** *(Beare and Myers, 1998)*

**Proctocort,** trademark for an anorectal preparation containing a glucocorticoid (hydrocortisone).

**proctodeum** /prok'tō'dē·əm/, *pl.* **proctodea** [Gk, *proktos* + *hodiaos,* a route], a depression of the ectoderm, behind the urorectal septum of the developing embryo, that forms the anus and anal canal when the cloacal membrane ruptures. Also spelled **proctodaeum** (*pl.* **proctodaea**). Compare **stomodeum.** —**proctodeal, proctodaeal,** *adj.*

**proctodynia** /-din'ē·ə/ [Gk, *proktos* + *odyne,* pain], pain in or around the anus.

**proctologist** /proktol'əjist/, a physician who specializes in proctology.

**proctology** /proktol'əjē/ [Gk, *proktos* + *logos,* science], the branch of medicine concerned with treating disorders of the colon, rectum, and anus.

**proctoplasty** /prok'təplas'tē/ [Gk, *proktos,* anus, *plassein,* to mold], a plastic surgery procedure performed on the anus and rectum.

**proctoscope** /prok'təskōp'/ [Gk, *proktos* + *skopein,* to look], an instrument used to examine the rectum and the distal part of the colon. It consists of a light mounted on a tube or speculum. Compare **sigmoidoscope.**

**proctoscopy** /proktos'kəpē/, the examination of the rectum with an endoscope inserted through the anus.

**proctosigmoidoscopy** /prok'tōsig'moidos'kəpē/ [Gk, *proktos* + *sigmoid* + *skopein,* to view], the use of a sigmoidoscope to examine the rectum and pelvic colon.

**procumbency** /prō-kum'bensē/ [L, *procumbere,* to lean forward], excessive inclination of the incisor teeth toward the lips.

**procyclidine hydrochloride** /prōsī'klədēn/, an anticholinergic.

■ INDICATIONS: It is prescribed in the treatment of parkinsonism and drug-induced extrapyramidal dysfunction and controls sialorrhea resulting from neuroleptic medication.

■ CONTRAINDICATIONS: Narrow-angle glaucoma, asthma, obstruction of the genitourinary or GI tract, severe ulcerative colitis, or known hypersensitivity to this drug prohibits its use.

■ ADVERSE EFFECTS: Among the more serious adverse effects are confusion, disorientation, blurred vision, central nervous system effects, tachycardia, dry mouth, decreased sweating, and hypersensitivity reactions.

**prodromal** /-drō'məl/ [Gk, *pro,* before, *dromos,* course], pertaining to early symptoms that may mark the onset of a disease.

**prodromal labor** [Gk, *prodromos,* running before; L, *labor,* work], the early period in parturition before uterine contractions become forceful and frequent enough to result in progressive dilation of the uterine cervix.

**prodromal myopia,** an optical condition in which the ability to do close work without eyeglasses returns, but usually as a symptom of developing cataracts.

**prodromal phase,** a clear deterioration in function before the active phase of a mental disturbance that is not caused by a disorder in mood or a psychoactive substance. It includes some residual phase symptoms.

**prodromal rash,** a rash that precedes a potentially more serious skin eruption caused by an infectious disease.

**prodromal symptom** [Gk, *pro* + *dromos,* course, *symptoma,* that which happens], a symptom that may be the first indication of the onset of a disease.

**prodrome** /prō'drōm/ [Gk, *prodromos,* running before], **1.** an early sign of a developing condition or disease. **2.** the earliest phase of a developing condition or disease. Many infectious diseases such as chickenpox or measles are most contagious during the prodromal period. —**prodromal,** *adj.*

**prodrug** /prō'drug/, an inactive or partially active drug that is metabolically changed in the body to an active drug.

**product evaluation,** a nursing intervention from the Nursing Interventions Classification (NIC) defined as determining the effectiveness of new products or equipment. See also **Nursing Interventions Classification.**

**product evaluation committee** /prod'əkt/, a hospital committee composed of medical, nursing, purchasing, and administrative staff members whose purpose is to evaluate health care–related products and advise on their procurement. Also called **new product evaluation committee.**

**productive cough** /prəduk'tiv/ [L, *producere* + AS, *cohhetan,* to cough], a sudden, noisy expulsion of air from the lungs that effectively removes sputum from the respiratory tract and helps clear the airways, permitting air to reach the alveoli. Coughing is stimulated by irritation or inflammation of the respiratory tract, which is caused most frequently by infection. Deep breathing, with contraction of the diaphragm and intercostal muscles and forceful exhalation, promotes productive coughing in patients with respiratory infections. Mucolytic agents liquefy mucus in the respiratory tract so that it can be raised and expectorated more easily. Atropine and other anticholinergic drugs decrease pulmonary secretions. Also called **moist cough, wet cough.** See also **nonproductive cough.**

**-profen,** combining form for ibuprofen-type antiinflammatory or analgesic substances.

**Profenal,** trademark for an oral nonsteroidal antiinflammatory analgesic (suprofen).

**professional corporation (PC)** /prəfesh'ənəl/ [L, *professio,* profession], a corporation formed according to the law of a particular state for the purpose of delivering a professional service. In some states corporations may not practice law, medicine, surgery, or dentistry; in some states nurses may form or be partners in a professional corporation. According to the laws of the various states professional corporations may offer legal and tax benefits to the members of the corporation.

**professional liability,** the legal obligation of health care professionals, or their insurers, to compensate patients for injury or suffering caused by acts of omission or commission by the professionals. Professional liability is a better characterization of the responsibility of all professionals to their patients than does the concept of malpractice, but the idea of professional liability is central to malpractice.

**professional network,** (in psychiatric nursing) the network of professional resources available to support the psychiatric outpatient in the community. The network may include a therapist, hospital day treatment program, social work agency, and other agencies.

**professional organization,** an organization whose members share a professional status, created to deal with issues of concern to the professional group or groups involved.

**Professional Standards Review Organization (PSRO),** an organization formed under the U.S. Social Security Act Amendments of 1972 to review the services provided under Medicare, Medicaid, and Maternal Child Health programs. Review is conducted by physicians to ascertain the need for the program and to ensure that it is carried out in accord with certain criteria, norms, and standards, and, in institutional situations in a proper setting. The PSRO requires that regional organizations be formed to conduct these reviews throughout the nation.

**profibrinolysin.** See **fibrinogen.**

**profile** /prō'fīl/ [L, *profilare,* to outline], a short sketch, diagram, or summary relating to a person or thing.

**profunda** /prōfun'də/ [L, *profundus,* deep], pertaining to structures, mainly blood vessels, that are deeply embedded in tissues.

**profuse sweat** /prəfyōōs'/ [L, *profundere,* to pour out; AS, *swaetan*], excessive perspiration. Also called **diaphoresis.**

**progenitive** /-jen'itiv/ [Gk, *pro,* before, *genein,* to produce], capable of producing offspring; reproductive.

**progenitor** /-jen'itər/ [Gk, *pro* + *genein*], **1.** a parent or ancestor. **2.** someone or something that begets or creates.

**progeny** /proj'ənē/ [L, *progenies*], **1.** offspring; an individual or organism resulting from a particular mating. **2.** the descendants of a known or common ancestor.

**progeria** /prōjir'ē·ə/ [Gk, *pro* + *geras,* old age], an abnormal congenital condition characterized by premature aging, appearance in childhood of gray hair and wrinkled skin, small stature, absence of pubic and facial hair, and posture and habitus of an aged person. Death usually occurs before 20 years of age. Also called Hutchinson-Gelford syndrome. Compare **infantilism.**

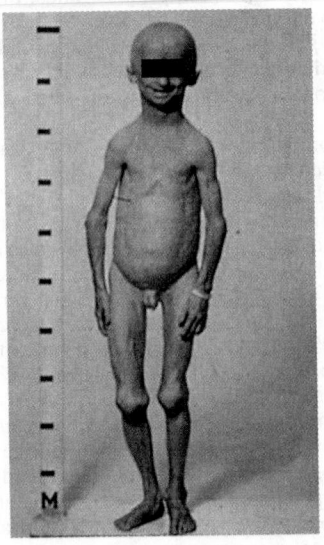

**Progeria** *(Thibodeau and Patton, 1999/Kevin Patton)*

**progestagen.** See **progestogen.**

**Progestasert,** trademark for a progestin (progesterone).

**progestational** /prō'jestā'shənəl/ [Gk, *pro* + L, *gestare,* to bear], pertaining to a drug with effects similar to those of progesterone, the hormone produced by the corpus luteum and adrenal cortex during the luteal phase of the menstrual cycle that prepares the uterus for reception of the fertilized ovum. Natural and synthetic preparations of progesterone and its derivative medroxyprogesterone acetate are used in the treatment of secondary amenorrhea and abnormal uterine bleeding. Progestational compounds, such as norethindrone and norgestrel, are constituents of oral contraceptives. The use of progestins to prevent habitual or threatened abortion is no longer recommended.

**progestational agent** [L, *pro* + *gestare,* to bear, *agere,* to do], any chemical having the same action as progesterone produced by the corpus luteum and the placenta.

**progestational phase.** See **secretory phase.**

**progesterone** /prəjes'tərōn/, a natural progestational hormone.
■ INDICATIONS: It is prescribed in the treatment of various menstrual disorders, infertility associated with luteal phase dysfunction, and repeated spontaneous abortion.
■ CONTRAINDICATIONS: Thrombophlebitis, liver dysfunction, breast cancer, missed abortion, or hypersensitivity to this drug prohibits its use.
■ ADVERSE EFFECTS: Among the more serious adverse reactions are pain at the site of injection, catabolic effects, and electrolyte disturbances.

**progesterone assay,** a blood test that is useful in documenting whether ovulation has occurred, and if so, when.

This information may be used to help women with difficulty becoming pregnant. Repeated assays may also be used to monitor the status of the placenta in high-risk pregnancy, and to monitor progesterone supplementation in patients with an inadequate luteal phase.

**progestin** /-jes′tin/, **1.** progesterone. **2.** any of a group of hormones, natural or synthetic, secreted by the corpus luteum, placenta, or adrenal cortex that have a progesterone-like effect on the uterine endometrial lining to prepare it for implantation of the blastocyst.

**progestogen** /-jes′təjən/, any natural or synthetic progestational hormone. Also spelled **progestagen.** Also called **progestin.**

**proglottid** /prōglot′id/ [Gk, *pro* + *glossa,* tongue], a sexual segment of an adult tapeworm, containing both male and female reproductive organs. Each mature segment is shed and produces additional tapeworms.

**prognathism** /prog′nəthiz′əm/ [Gk, *pro* + *gnathos,* jaw], an abnormal facial configuration in which one or both jaws project forward. It may be real or imaginary, depending on anatomic and developmental factors. Real prognathism may exist when both the mandible and the maxilla increase in length or when the maxillary length is normal and the mandibular length increases excessively. Imaginary prognathism may exist when the maxilla is underdeveloped and the mandibular length is normal. —**prognathic,** *adj.*

**prognosis** /prognō′sis/ [Gk, *pro* + *gnosis,* knowledge], a prediction of the probable outcome of a disease based on the condition of the person and the usual course of the disease as observed in similar situations.

**prognostic** /prognos′tik/ [Gk, *pro* + *gnosis,* knowledge], pertaining to signs and symptoms that may indicate the outcome of an illness or injury.

**prognosticate** /prognos′tikāt/ [Gk, *pro,* before, *gnosis,* knowledge], to forecast or predict from facts, present indications, or signs, such as the course a disease may take and the final outcome.

**Prograf,** trademark for an immunosuppressive drug (tacrolimus).

**program** /prō′grəm/ [Gk, *pro* + *gramma,* record], a sequence of instructions, written in computer programing language, that controls the functions of a computer.

**program development,** a nursing intervention from the Nursing Interventions Classification (NIC) defined as planning, implementing, and evaluating a coordinated set of activities designed to enhance wellness, or to prevent, reduce, or eliminate one or more health problems or a group or community. See also **Nursing Interventions Classification.**

**program documentation.** See **documentation.**

**programmable pacemaker** /-gram′əbəl/ [Gk, *pro* + *graphein,* to record; L, *passus,* step; ME, *maken*], an electronic pacemaker with multiple settings that can be changed after implantation.

**programmed pacing,** control of the heart rate by a programmable pacemaker. See also **pacing.**

**programmer** /prō′grəmər/, a person skilled in writing or coding computer programs.

**programming language.** See **language.**

**Program of All-inclusive Care of the Elderly (PACE /pās/),** a U.S. federally supported program of comprehensive care with a primary objective of keeping clients in the community as long as medically, socially, and financially possible. It is a team approach in which professionals assess client needs, develop a care plan, integrate primary care and other services, and arrange for implementation of services. PACE is sponsored by one or more facilities and community groups and receives funds from Medicare, Medicaid, and private donations. A forerunner of PACE is the San Francisco On Lok program, which provides comprehensive adult day care, custodial or personal care, drug treatment, dentistry, and housekeeping for older persons who have a level of impairment that usually requires admission to a nursing facility.

**progravid** /-grav′id/ [L, *pro* + *gravid,* pregnant], before pregnancy.

**progression** /-gresh′ən/, a carcinogenic process whereby cells genetically altered by initiators undergo a second (nongenetic) cell expansion that allows uncontrollable growth.

**progressive** /-gres′iv/ [L, *progredi,* to advance], describing the course of a disease or condition in which the characteristic signs and symptoms become more prominent and severe, such as progressive muscular atrophy.

**progressive assistive exercise,** an exercise designed to improve the strength of a muscle group progressively by gradually decreasing assistance required of a therapist for an active motion, thereby increasing the patient's active effort. See also **progressive resistance exercise (PRE).**

**progressive bulbar paralysis** [L, *progredi,* to advance, *bulbus,* swollen root; Gk, *paralyein,* to be palsied], a motor neuron disease characterized by weakness of the laryngeal, pharyngeal, tongue, and facial muscles. The patient experiences progressive dysarthria and dysphagia. Also called **Duchenne's paralysis.** See **association paralysis.**

**progressive histoplasmosis.** See **histoplasmosis.**

**progressive interstitial hypertrophic neuropathy.** See **Déjérine-Sottas disease.**

**progressive muscle relaxation,** a nursing intervention from the Nursing Interventions Classification (NIC) defined as facilitating the tensing and releasing of successive muscle groups while attending to the resulting differences in sensation. See also **Nursing Interventions Classification.**

**progressive myonecrosis.** See **myonecrosis.**

**progressive myopia** [L, *progredi* + Gk, *myops,* nearsighted], a condition in which myopia increases, continuing into adulthood.

**progressive ophthalmoplegia** [L, *progredi*], a form of ocular muscle paralysis that usually begins with ptosis and gradually involves all of the extraocular muscles.

**progressive ossifying myositis.** See **myositis ossificans progressiva.**

**progressive patient care,** a system of care in which patients are placed in units on the basis of their needs for care as determined by the degree of illness rather than in units based on a medical specialty. The usual levels or stages of progressive patient care are intensive care, intermediate care, and minimal care.

**progressive relaxation,** a technique for combating tension and anxiety by systematically tensing and relaxing muscle groups.

**progressive resistance exercise (PRE),** a method of increasing the strength of a weak or injured muscle by gradually increasing the resistance against which the muscle works, such as by using graduated weights over a period. Also called **graduated resistance exercise.** See also **active resistance exercise, Delorme technique, progressive assistive exercise.**

**progressive spinal muscular atrophy of infants.** See **Werdnig-Hoffmann disease.**

**progressive subcortical encephalopathy.** See **Schilder's disease.**

**progressive supranuclear palsy** [L, *supra,* above, *nucleus,* nut kernel; Gk, *paralyein*], a mild form of paralysis involving muscles innervated by the cranial nerves and primarily affecting the face, throat, and tongue.

**progressive systemic sclerosis (PSS).** See **scleroderma.**

**progress notes** [L, *progredi + nota,* mark], (in the patient record) notes made by a nurse, physician, social worker, physical therapist, and other health care professionals that describe the patient's condition and the treatment given or planned. Progress notes may follow the problem-oriented medical record format. The physician's progress notes usually focus on the medical or therapeutic aspects of the patient's condition and care; the nurse's progress notes, although recording the medical conditions of the patient, usually focus on the objectives stated in the nursing care plan. These objectives may include responses to prescribed treatments, the person's ability to perform activities of daily living, and acceptance or understanding of a particular condition or treatment. Progress notes in an in-hospital setting are recorded daily; those in a clinic or office setting are usually preceded by an episodic or interval history and are recorded as accounts of each visit.

**proinsulin** /prō·in′s(y)əlin/ [L, *pro + insula,* island], a single-chain protein molecule that is a precursor of insulin.

**projectile vomiting** /-jek′til/, expulsive vomiting that is extremely forceful.

**projection** /-jek′shən/ [L, *projectio,* thrown forward], **1.** a protuberance; anything that thrusts or juts outward. **2.** the act of perceiving an idea or thought as an objective reality. **3.** (in psychology) an unconscious defense mechanism by which an individual attributes his or her own unacceptable traits, ideas, or impulses to another. It is noted in some stages of schizophrenia.

**projection reconstruction imaging,** the techniques used in magnetic resonance (MR) imaging to obtain a cross-sectional image of an object. Such an image is computer-reconstructed from a series of MR profiles recorded all around an object by rotating the gradient field superimposed on the static magnetic field.

**projective test** /-jek′tiv/ [L, *projectio,* thrown forward], a kind of diagnostic, psychologic, or personality test that uses unstructured or ambiguous stimuli, such as inkblots, a series of pictures, abstract patterns, or incomplete sentences, to elicit responses that reflect a projection of various aspects of the individual's personality. See also **Rorschach test.**

**prokaryocyte** /prōker′ē·əsīt′/ [Gk, *protos,* first, *karyon,* nut, *kytos,* cell], a cell without a true nucleus and with nuclear material scattered throughout the cytoplasm. Prokaryocytic organisms (**Procaryotae**) include bacteria, viruses, rickettsiae, chlamydiae, mycoplasmas, actinomycetes, and blue-green algae. Also spelled **procaryocyte.** Compare **eukaryocyte.**

**prokaryon** /prōker′ē·on/ [Gk, *protos + karyon,* nut], a region within a bacterial cell that contains most of the bacterial DNA. It is not separated from the rest of the cell by a membrane. Also spelled **procaryon.** Compare **eukaryon.**

**prokaryosis** /-ker′ē·ō′sis/ [Gk, *protos + karyon + osis,* condition], the condition of having a prokaryon. Also spelled **procaryosis.** Compare **eukaryosis.**

**prokaryote** /prōker′ē·ōt/ [Gk, *protos + karyon*], a unicellular organism that does not contain a true nucleus surrounded by a double membrane; a bacterium. Division usually occurs through simple fission. Also spelled **procaryote.** Compare **eukaryote.** —**prokaryotic,** *adj.*

**prolactin (PRL)** /prōlak′tin/ [Gk, *pro,* before, *lac,* milk], a hormone produced and secreted into the bloodstream by the anterior pituitary gland. Prolactin, acting with estrogen, progesterone, thyroxine, insulin, growth hormone, glucocorticoids, and human placental lactogen, stimulates the development and growth of the mammary glands. After parturition prolactin together with glucocorticoids is essential for the initiation and maintenance of milk production. Prolactin synthesis and release from the pituitary are mediated by the central nervous system in response to suckling by the infant. When suckling or its mechanical equivalent ceases, prolactin secretion slows and milk production ceases. Prolactin is similar to growth hormone in its chemical structure. Prolactin excess is seen in the presence of prolactin-secreting pituitary tumors in both sexes. Also called **lactogenic hormone.**

**prolactin levels test (PRLs),** a blood test that is helpful for monitoring the disease activity of pituitary adenomas.

**prolapse** /prō′laps, prōlaps′/ [L, *prolapsus,* falling], the dropping, falling, sinking, or sliding of an organ from its normal position or location in the body, such as a prolapsed uterus or rectum.

**prolapsed cord** /prōlapst/, an umbilical cord that protrudes beside or ahead of the presenting part of the fetus.

**prolapsed hemorrhoid** [L, *prolapsus,* falling; Gk, *haim orrhois,* a vein that loses blood], an internal hemorrhoid that protrudes through the anal orifice.

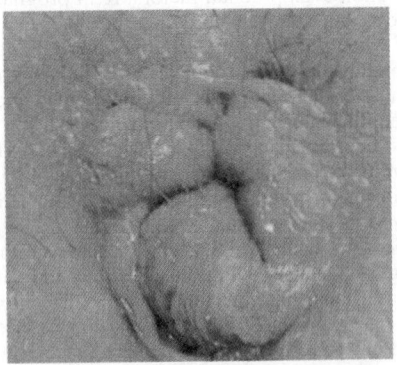

**Prolapsed hemorrhoids**
*(Seidel et al, 1999/courtesy Gershon Efron, MD, Sinai Hospital of Baltimore)*

**prolapse of anus** [L, *prolapsus,* falling, *anus*] the protrusion of the mucous membrane of the anus through the external sphincter.

**prolapse of rectum** [L, *prolapsus,* falling, *rectus,* straight], a protrusion of the mucous membrane of the lower part of the rectum through the anal orifice.

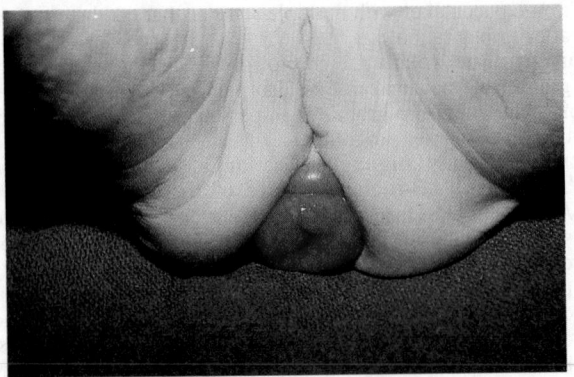

**Prolapse of the rectum** *(Zitelli and Davis, 1997)*

**prolapse of uterus** [L, *prolapsus,* falling, *uterus,* womb], the descent of the uterine cervix into the vagina, partly into the vagina, or outside the vagina.

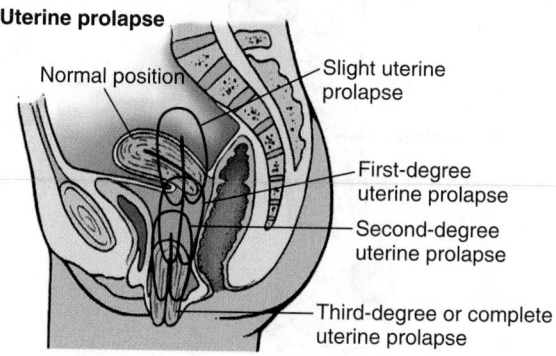

**Uterine prolapse**

Normal position

Slight uterine prolapse

First-degree uterine prolapse

Second-degree uterine prolapse

Third-degree or complete uterine prolapse

**Prolapse of the uterus** *(Monahan and Neighbors, 1998)*

**Prolastin,** trademark for alpha₁-antitrypsin (alpha₁-proteinase inhibitor, human).

**proliferate** /-lif′ərāt/ [L, *proles,* offspring, *ferre,* to bear], to grow by multiplication of cells, parts, or organisms.

**proliferation** /-lif′ərā′shən/ [L, *proles,* offspring, *ferre,* to bear], the reproduction or multiplication of similar forms. The term is usually applied to increases of cells or cysts.

**proliferation inhibiting factor,** a lymphokine that restricts cell division in tissue cultures.

**proliferative-follicular phase.** See **menstrual cycle.**

**proliferative phase** /-lif′ərətiv/, the phase of the menstrual cycle after menstruation. Under the influence of follicle stimulating hormone from the pituitary the ovary produces increasing amounts of estrogen, causing the lining of the uterus to become dense and richly vascular. The phase is terminated by rupture of a mature follicle and subsequent ovulation. Also called **proliferative-follicular phase.** Compare **menstrual phase, secretory phase.**

**prolific** /lif′ik/ [L, *proles,* offspring, *ferre,* to bear], highly productive.

**proline (Pro)** /prō′lēn/, a nonessential amino acid found in many proteins of the body, particularly collagen. See also **amino acid, protein.**

**Proloid,** trademark for a thyroid hormone preparation (thyroglobulin).

**prolonged gestation** /-longd′/ [L, *prolongare,* to lengthen, *gestare,* to bear], a pregnancy that lasts longer than the usual period of 41 weeks.

**prolonged release** [Gk, *pro,* before, *longus,* long], a term applied to a drug that is designed to deliver a dose of a medication over an extended period. The most common device for this purpose is a soft, soluble capsule containing minute pellets of the drug for release at different rates in the GI tract, depending on the thickness and nature of the oil, fat, wax, or resin coating on the pellets. Another system consists of a porous plastic carrier impregnated with the drug and a surfactant to facilitate the entry of GI fluids that slowly leach out the drug. Ion exchange resins that bind to drugs and liquids containing suspensions of slow-release drug granules are also used to provide medication over an extended period. Various mechanisms and vehicles have also been developed to prolong the release of drugs after injection.

**Proloprim,** trademark for an antibacterial (trimethoprim).

**promastigote** /prōmas′tigōt/, the flagellate stage of a trypanosome. It is found in the insect intermediate host or in culture.

**promethazine hydrochloride** /-meth′əzēn/, a phenothiazine antiemetic, antihistamine, and sedative.
■ INDICATIONS: It is prescribed in the treatment of motion sickness, nausea, rhinitis, itching, and skin rash and as an adjunct to anesthesia.
■ CONTRAINDICATIONS: Known hypersensitivity to this drug or to other phenothiazines prohibits its use.
■ ADVERSE EFFECTS: Drowsiness, hypotension, and dry mouth are the most common adverse reactions.

**promethium (Pm)** /-mē′thē·əm/ [L, *Prometheus,* mythic character who gave fire to humans], a radioactive rare earth metallic element. Its atomic number is 61; its atomic mass (weight) is 145.

**prominence** /prom′inəns/ [L, *prominentia,* sticking out], any protuberance or projection of a structural feature.

**promontory of the sacrum** /prom′əntôr′ē/ [L, *promontorium,* headland], the superior projecting part of the sacrum at its junction with the L5 vertebra.

**promoter** /-mō′tər/ [L, *promovere,* to move forward], **1.** a DNA sequence that initiates transcription of the genetic code. **2.** a cocarcinogen that encourages cells altered by initiators to reproduce more rapidly than normal, increasing the probability of malignant transformation. Examples include chlorophenothane (DDT), phenobarbital, saccharin, sunlight, and some chemicals in cigarette smoke. The effects of promoters are sometimes reversible.

**prompted voiding,** a nursing intervention from the Nursing Interventions Classification (NIC) defined as promotion of urinary continence through the use of timed verbal toileting reminders and positive social feedback for successful toileting. See also **Nursing Interventions Classification.**

**prompt insulin zinc suspension** [L, *promptus,* ready], a fast-acting noncrystalline semilente insulin prescribed in the treatment of diabetes mellitus when a prompt, intense, and short-acting response is desired. It is only slightly slower acting than insulin injection. See also **fast-acting insulin.**

**promyelocyte** /prōmī′ələsīt′/, a large mononuclear blood cell that contains a single regular, symmetric nucleus and a few undifferentiated cytoplasmic granules. As an intermediate stage in development between a myeloblast and a myelocyte promyelocyte in the circulating blood indicative of leukemia.

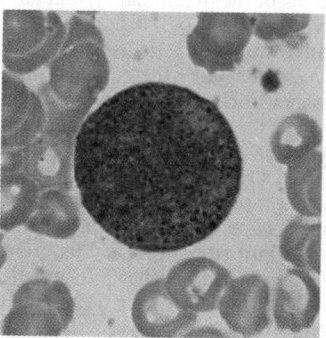

**Promyelocyte** *(Carr and Rodak, 1999)*

**pronate** /prō′nāt/ [L, *pronare*, to bend forward], to place in a prone position of lying flat with the face forward.

**pronation** /prōnā′shən/ [L, *pronare*, to bend forward], **1.** assumption of a prone position, one in which the ventral surface of the body faces downward. **2.** (of the arm) the rotation of the forearm so that the palm of the hand faces downward or backward. **3.** (of the foot) the lowering of the medial edge of the foot by turning it outward and through abduction in the tarsal and metatarsal joints. **—pronate,** *v.*

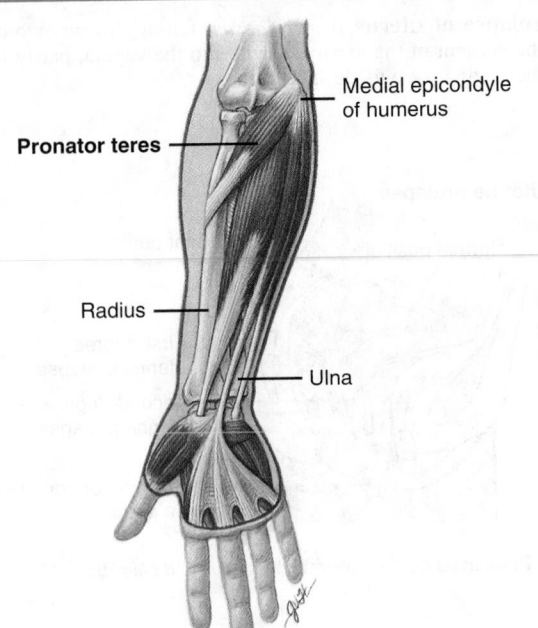

**Pronator teres** (*Thibodeau and Patton, 1999/John V. Hagen*)

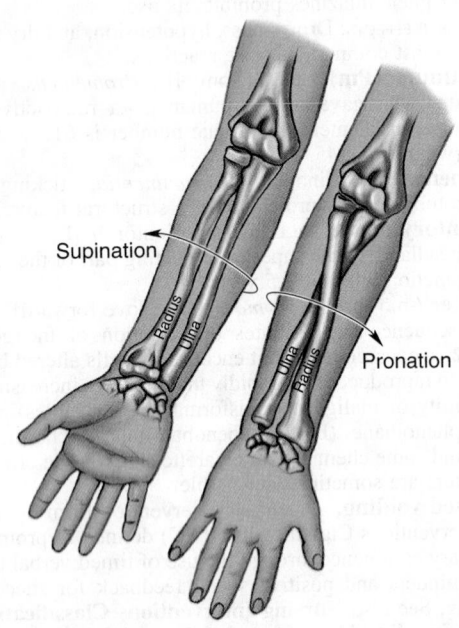

**Pronation** (*Herlihy and Meabius, 2000*)

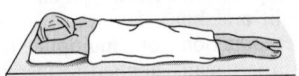

**Prone position** (*Potter and Perry, 2001*)

**pronator quadratus** /prōnā′tər/, a muscle of the forearm. It originates on the distal fourth of the anterior surface and border of the ulna and inserts onto the distal fourth of the anterior surface of the radius. It functions to pronate the forearm and hand.

**pronator reflex** [L, *pronare* + *reflectere*, to bend back], a reflex elicited by holding the patient's hand vertically and tapping the distal end of the radius or ulna, resulting in pronation of the forearm. Hyperactivity of the reflex may be seen with lesions of the pyramidal system above the level of the sixth cervical nerve root. Also called **ulnar reflex.**

**pronator syndrome** [L, *pronare*, to bend forward; Gk, *syn*, together, *dromos*, course], the compression of the median nerve in the forearm between the two heads of the pronator teres muscle.

**pronator teres** /ter′əs/, a superficial muscle of the forearm, arising from a humeral and an ulnar head and ending in a flat tendon that inserts into the radius. It functions to pronate the hand. Compare **flexor carpi radialis, flexor carpi ulnaris, flexor digitorum superficialis, palmaris longus.**

**prone** /prōn/ [L, *pronare*, to bend forward], **1.** having a tendency or inclination. **2.** (of the body) being in horizontal position when lying face downward. Compare **supine.** Also called **ventral recumbent.**

**Pronemia Hematinic Capsules,** trademark for a fixed-combination hematinic drug containing iron, vitamin $B_{12}$, intrinsic factor concentrate, vitamin C, and folic acid.

**proneness profile** /prōn′nəs/ [L, *pronare*, to bend forward, *profilare*, to outline], a screening process that evaluates the probability of developmental problems in the early years of a child's life. Screening ideally begins in the course of prenatal care and continues after birth. Several of the variables in the proneness profile that appear to be significant in selecting the infants who are at risk are the perinatal health status of the mother and infant, especially complications of pregnancy, delivery, the neonatal period, and the puerperium; characteristics of the mother, especially her temperament, educational level, perception of the life situation, and perception of the infant; characteristics of the infant, including alertness, activity pattern, and responsiveness; and behaviors of the infant and caregiver as they interact. The proneness profile is followed by a developmental profile that assesses the current status of the infant and caregiver. Three areas to be considered are characteristics of the infant, including adaptation and response to the environment, the ability to give interpretable cues, and the developmental progress as compared with established norms; characteristics of the caregiver, including adaptation to the new infant, sensitivity to cues from the infant, and techniques for relieving distress; and the healthful quality of the environment, including health, safety, comfort, and stimulation.

**prone-on-elbows,** a body position in which the person rests the upper part of the body on the elbows while lying face down. The position is used as an initial rehabilitation exercise in training a person with a cerebellar dysfunction to achieve various goals. In this position, the person can practice weight shifting through the hips to a quadruped position without the risk of falling from a standing position.

**pronephric.** See **pronephros.**

**pronephric duct** /-nef′rik/ [Gk, *pro,* before, *nephros,* kidney; L, *ducere,* to lead], one of the paired ducts that connect the tubules of each of the pronephros with the cloaca in the early developing vertebrate embryo. They later become the functional mesonephric ducts. Also called **archinephric canal, archinephric duct.**

**pronephric tubule,** any of the segmentally arranged excretory units of the pronephros in the early developing vertebrate embryo. The tubules open into the pronephric duct and communicate with the coelom through a nephrostoma. In humans and the higher vertebrates the tubules are present only in vestigial form; in lower animals they are functional.

**pronephros** /-nef′rəs/, *pl.* **pronephroi** [Gk, *pro* + *nephros,* kidney], the earliest and simplest kind of excretory organ in the developing vertebrate embryo. In humans and other mammals the structure is nonfunctional. Also called **pronephron** (*pl.* **pronephra**), **archinephron, head kidney.** See also **mesonephros, metanephros.** —**pronephric,** *adj.*

**prone posture** [L, *pronare,* to bend forward, *ponere,* to place], a posture assumed by lying flat with the face forward during certain disorders of the spine or viscera.

**pronucleus** /-nōō′klē·əs/, *pl.* **pronuclei** [Gk, *pro* + L, *nucleus,* nut kernel], the nucleus of an ovum or a spermatozoon after fertilization but before fusion of the chromosomes to form the nucleus of the zygote. Each pronucleus contains the haploid number of chromosomes, is larger than the normal nucleus, and is diffuse in appearance. The pronucleus of the ovum is formed only after it has completed its second meiotic division and the second polar body has formed, which occur after the spermatozoon has penetrated. It then loses its nuclear envelope, releasing the chromosomes so that synapsis with the chromosomes of the male pronucleus, which is contained in the head of the spermatozoon, can occur. Also called **germinal nucleus, germ nucleus.** See also **oogenesis, spermatogenesis.**

**propagation** /prop′əgā′shən/ [L, *propagare,* to generate], the process of increasing or causing to increase.

**propanoic acid.** See **propionic acid.**

**2-propanol.** See **isopropyl alcohol.**

**propantheline bromide** /-pan′thəlēn/, an anticholinergic/ antispasmodic.

■ INDICATION: It is prescribed as an adjunct in peptic ulcer therapy.

■ CONTRAINDICATIONS: Narrow-angle glaucoma, asthma, obstruction of the genitourinary or GI tract, severe ulcerative colitis, or known hypersensitivity to this drug prohibits its use.

■ ADVERSE EFFECTS: Among the more serious adverse reactions are blurred vision, central nervous system effects, tachycardia, dry mouth, decreased sweating, and hypersensitivity reactions.

**proparacaine hydrochloride** /prōper′əkān/, a rapid-acting topical anesthetic of the amide family.

■ INDICATIONS: It is used for tonometry, gonioscopy, removal of foreign objects from the eye, and other minor ophthalmologic procedures and preoperatively for major eye surgery. One drop gives 15 minutes of optic anesthesia.

■ CONTRAINDICATIONS: Proparacaine hydrochloride is not administered to individuals with cardiac disease, hyperthyroidism, or multiple allergies. People given the drug should

be warned not to touch their eyes until the anesthetic has worn off.

■ ADVERSE EFFECTS: Adverse optic reactions may occur with proparacaine, but systemic reactions are rare. Prolonged use may injure the eye. Also called **proxymetacaine.**

**properidin system.** See **alternative pathway of complement activation.**

**prophase** /prō′fāz/ [Gk, *pro* + *phasis,* appearance], the first of four stages of nuclear division in mitosis and in each of the two divisions of meiosis. In mitosis the chromosomes progressively shorten and thicken to form individually recognizable elongated double structures composed of two chromatids held together by a centromere; the nucleolus and nuclear membrane disappear, the spindle and polar bodies are formed, and the chromosomes begin to migrate toward the midplane of the developing spindle. In the first meiotic division prophase is complex and subdivided into five stages: leptotene, zygotene, pachytene, diplotene, and diakinesis. In the second meiotic division the same processes occur as in mitotic prophase. See also **anaphase, interphase, meiosis, metaphase, mitosis, telophase.**

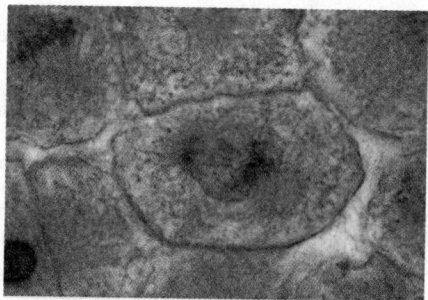

**Prophase** (© Ed Reschke; used with permission)

**prophylactic** /prō′filak′tik/ [Gk, *prophylax,* advance guard], **1.** preventing the spread of disease. **2.** an agent that prevents the spread of disease. **3.** a popular name for **condom.** —**prophylactically,** *adv.*

**prophylactic forceps.** See **low forceps.**

**prophylactic odontomy,** the surgical removal of harmful pits and fissures in the posterior primary and secondary molars to prevent the formation of caries in those areas.

**prophylactic treatment.** See **preventive treatment.**

**prophylaxis** /prō′filak′sis/ [Gk, *prophylax,* advance guard], prevention of or protection against disease, often involving the use of a biologic, chemical, or mechanical agent to destroy or prevent the entry of infectious organisms.

***Propionibacterium*** /prō′pē·on′ēbaktir′ē·əm/ [Gk, *pro* + *pion,* fat, *bakterion,* small rod], a genus of nonmotile anaerobic gram-positive bacteria found on the skin of humans, in the intestinal tract of humans and animals, and in dairy products. ***Propionibacterium acnes*** is common in acne pustules (formerly called *Corynebacterium acnes*).

**propionic acid** /prō′pē·on′ik/, an aliphatic carboxylic acid, methylacetic acid, a chemical component of sweat. It can be formed by fermentation of sugars by several species of bacteria. Also called **propanoic acid.**

**propionicacidemia** /prō′pē·on′ikas′idē′mē·ə/ [Gk, *pro* + *pion,* fat; L, *acidus,* sour; Gk, *haima,* blood], a rare inherited metabolic defect caused by the failure of the body to metabolize the amino acids threonine, isoleucine, and methionine, characterized by lethargy and mental and physical retardation. Acidosis results from the accumulation of propionic acid in the body. A diet low in these amino acids is difficult to achieve but is the only treatment. —**propionicacidemic,** *adj.*

**propionic fermentation** [Gk, *pro* + *pion* + L, *fermentare,* to cause to ferment], the production of propionic acid by the action of certain bacteria on sugars or lactic acid.

**Proplex T,** trademark for human clotting factor IX.

**proportional** /prəpôr'shənəl/, pertaining to the relationship between two quantities when a fractional variation of one is always accompanied by the same fractional change in the other.

**proportional gas detector,** a device for measuring alpha and beta forms of radioactivity.

**proportional mortality** [L, *pro* + *portio,* part, *mortalis,* subject to death], a statistical method of relating the number of deaths from a particular condition to all deaths within the same population group for the same period.

**proposition** /prop'əzish'ən/ [L, *proponere,* to place forward], **1.** a statement of a truth to be demonstrated or an operation to be performed. **2.** to bring forward or offer for consideration, acceptance, or adoption.

**propositus** /prōpoz'itəs/ [L, *proponere,* to place forward], a person from whom a genealogic lineage is traced, as is done to discover the pattern of inheritance of a familial disease or a physical trait. Also called **proband.**

**propoxyphene, propoxyphene hydrochloride** /prōpok'səfēn/, a mild centrally acting opioid analgesic.

■ INDICATION: It is prescribed to relieve mild to moderate pain.

■ CONTRAINDICATIONS: Concurrent administration of tranquilizers or antidepressant drugs, current alcohol or drug abuse, or known hypersensitivity to this drug prohibits its use. It is not recommended for use by people who are suicidal or prone to alcohol or drug addiction or by women who are pregnant, because neonatal withdrawal symptoms have been observed.

■ ADVERSE EFFECTS: Among the more serious reactions are hepatic dysfunction and severe depression of the central nervous system occurring with overdose or drug interaction. A small number of people may experience nausea, dizziness, sedation, or vomiting when correctly taking a usual prescribed dosage.

**propoxyphene hydrochloride,** an analgesic.

■ INDICATION: It is prescribed for the relief of mild to moderate pain.

■ CONTRAINDICATIONS: Known hypersensitivity to this drug or known narcotic addiction prohibits its use.

■ ADVERSE EFFECTS: Among the more serious adverse reactions are respiratory depression, paradoxical excitement, and convulsions.

**propranolol hydrochloride** /-pran'əlol/, a nonselective beta-adrenergic receptor blocking agent.

■ INDICATIONS: It is prescribed in the treatment of angina pectoris, cardiac arrhythmias, and hypertension.

■ CONTRAINDICATIONS: Asthma, COPD, certain arrhythmias, congestive heart failure, unless secondary to a tachyarrhythmia treatable with beta-blockers, or known hypersensitivity to this drug prohibits its use.

■ ADVERSE EFFECTS: Among the more serious adverse reactions are heart failure, heart block, increased airway resistance, augmentation of hypoglycemic response, GI disturbances, and hypersensitivity reactions. Withdrawal syndrome has been observed in some patients.

**proprietary** /-prī'əter'ē/ [L, *proprietas,* property], **1.** pertaining to an institution or other organization that is operated for profit. **2.** pertaining to a product, such as a drug or device, that is made for profit.

**proprietary drug.** See **patent medicine, proprietary medicine.**

**proprietary hospital,** a hospital operated as a profit-making organization. Many proprietary hospitals are owned by physicians who operate them primarily for their own patients but also accept patients from other physicians. Some proprietary hospitals are owned by investor groups or large corporations.

**proprietary medicine,** any pharmaceutic preparation or medicinal substance that is protected from commercial competition because its ingredients or method of manufacture is kept secret or is protected by trademark or copyright.

**proprioception** /prō'prē·əsep'shən/ [L, *proprius,* one's own, *capere,* to take], sensation pertaining to stimuli originating from within the body related to spatial position and muscular activity or to the sensory receptors that they activate. Compare **exteroceptive, interoceptive.** See also **autotopagnosia.**

**proprioceptive** /prō'prē·əsep'tiv/ [L, *proprius,* one's own, *capere,* to take], pertaining to the sensations of body movements and awareness of posture, enabling the body to orient itself in space without visual clues.

**proprioceptive impulse,** a nerve impulse that originates with a sensory ending in muscle, joint, or tendon. Such impulses provide information to the central nervous system about the relative position of body parts.

**proprioceptive neuromuscular facilitation (PNF),** an activity, such as a therapeutic technique, that helps initiate a proprioceptive response in a person. An example is a slow rocking movement that relaxes an anxious person by stimulating vestibular and proprioceptive nerve receptors. Techniques are used to facilitate total body responses or selective postural extensors.

**proprioceptive receptor.** See **proprioceptor.**

**proprioceptive reflex** [L, *proprius* + *capere,* to take, *reflectere,* to bend back], any reflex initiated by stimulation of proprioceptors, such as the increase in respiratory rate and volume induced by impulses arising from muscles and joints during exercise.

**proprioceptive sensation** [L, *propius* + *capere* + *sentire,* to feel], the feeling of body movement and position, including motion of the arms and legs, resulting from stimuli received by special sense organs in the muscles, tendons, joints, and inner ear. The stimuli may be produced by changes in muscle tension or stretching and reaction to the pull of gravity on the body.

**proprioceptor** /prō'prē·əsep'tər/ [L, *proprius* + *capere*], any sensory nerve ending, such as those located in muscles, tendons, joints, and the vestibular apparatus, that responds to stimuli originating from within the body related to movement and spatial position. Also called **proprioceptive receptor.** Compare **exteroceptor, interoceptor.** See also **mechanoreceptor.**

**proptosis** /proptō'sis/ [L, *pro* + *ptosis,* falling], a bulging, protrusion, or forward displacement of a body organ or area.

**propulsion** /-pul'shən/ [L, *propellere,* to drive forward], **1.** the process of pushing forward. **2.** the tendency of some patients, particularly those afflicted with nervous disorders, to push or fall forward while walking as their center of gravity is displaced.

**propylene glycol (CH₃CHOHCH₂OH)** /prop'ilēn/, a colorless viscous liquid used as a solvent in the preparation

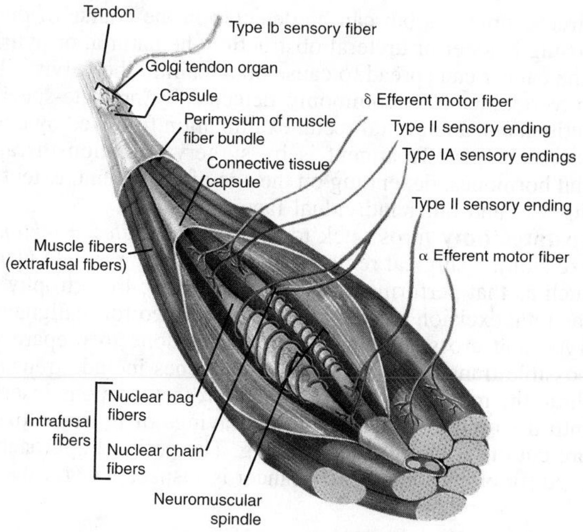


**Proprioceptors** *(Thibodeau and Patton, 1999/Christine Oleksyk)*

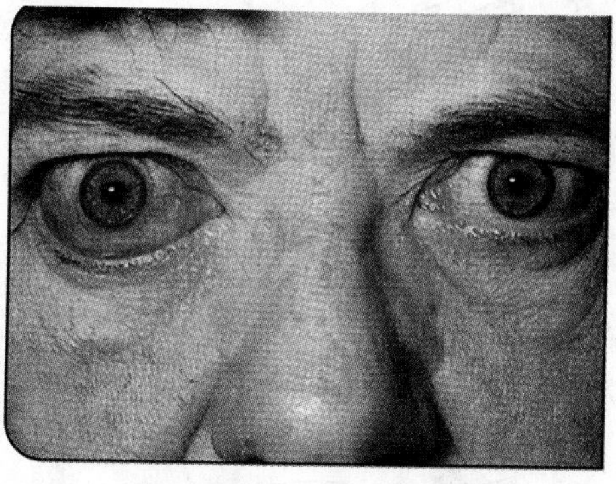

**Proptosis of the right eye** *(Kanski and Nischal, 1999)*

of certain medications. It also inhibits the growth of fungi and microorganisms and is used commercially as an antifreeze. Also called **1,2-propanediol.**

**propylformic acid.** See **butyric acid.**

**propylthiouracil** /prō′pilthī′əyo͝or′əsil/, an inhibitor of thyroid hormone biosynthesis.

■ INDICATIONS: It is prescribed in treatment of hyperthyroidism and thyrotoxic crisis and in preparation for thyroidectomy.

■ CONTRAINDICATIONS: Mental depression, cold intolerance, or known hypersensitivity to this drug prohibits its use. Caution is recommended in pregnancy.

■ ADVERSE EFFECTS: Among the more serious adverse reactions are GI distress, pruritus, and rashes. Rarely blood dyscrasia occurs.

**pro re nata.** See **prn.**

**pros-.** See **proso-.**

**proscribe** /prōskrīb′/, to forbid. **—proscriptive,** *adj.*

**prosector** /-sek′tər/ [L, *prosecare,* to cut off], a person who, under the supervision of a pathologist, performs gross dissections and prepares autopsy specimens for pathologic examination.

**prosencephalon** /pros′ensef′əlon/ [Gk, *pro* + *enkephalon,* brain], the anterior primitive cerebral vesicle which further divides into diencephalon and telencephalon. Also called **forebrain.** Compare **mesencephalon. —prosencephalic,** *adj.*

**proso-, pros-,** prefix meaning 'forward, or anterior': *prosocoele, prosodemic, prosogaster.*

**Pro Sobee,** trademark for a commercial milk-substitute formula that is prepared from a soy isolate base and is lactose free. It is prescribed for infants with galactosemia and people with lactose intolerance. It is supplemented with other nutrients, is fortified with vitamins and minerals, and is available in both powder and liquid forms. See also **Nutramigen.**

**prosopalgia.** See **trigeminal neuralgia.**

**-prosopia,** combining form meaning '(condition of the) face': *ateloprosopia, lipoprosopia, schizoprosopia.*

**prosopo-** /pros′əpō-/, combining form meaning 'face': *prosopoanoschisis, prosopodiplegia, prosoponeuralgia.*

**prosopopilary virilism** /pros′əpōpī′lərē/, a heavy growth of facial hair.

**prosopospasm** /pros′əpōspaz′əm/ [Gk, *prosopon,* face, *spasmos*], a spasm of the facial muscles, such as may occur in tetanus.

**prosoposternodidymus** /pros′əpōstur′nədid′əməs/ [Gk, *prosopon,* face, *sternon,* chest, *didymos,* twin], a fetus consisting of conjoined twins united laterally from the head through the sternum.

**prosopothoracopagus** /pros′əpōthôr′əkop′əgəs/ [Gk, *prosopon* + *thorax,* chest, *pagos,* fixed], conjoined symmetric twins who are united laterally in the frontal plane from the thorax through most of the head region.

**prospective medicine** /-spek′tiv/ [L, *proscipere,* to look forward, *medicina,* art of healing], the early identification of pathologic or potentially pathologic processes and the prescription of intervention to stop them.

**prospective payment system (PPS),** a payment mechanism for reimbursing hospitals for inpatient health care services in which a predetermined rate is set for treatment of specific illnesses. The system was originally developed by the U.S. federal government for use in treatment of Medicare recipients. See also **diagnosis-related group (DRG).**

**prospective reimbursement,** a method of payment to an agency for health care services to be delivered that is based on predictions of what the agency's costs will be for the coming year.

**prospective study,** an analytic study designed to determine the relationship between a condition and a characteristic shared by some members of a group. The population selected is healthy at the beginning of the study. Some of the members of the group share a particular characteristic, such as cigarette smoking. The researcher follows the population group over a period, noting the rate at which a condition, such as lung cancer, occurs in the smokers and in the nonsmokers. A prospective study may involve many variables or only two; it may seek to demonstrate a relationship that is an association or one that is causal. Prospective studies produce a direct measure of risk called the *relative risk.* Compare **retrospective study.**

**prost-, -prost,** combining form for prostaglandin derivatives.

**prostacyclin ($PGI_2$)** /pros′təsī′klin/, a prostaglandin. It is a biologically active product of arachidonic acid metabolism in human vascular walls and a potent inhibitor of platelet aggregation. It inhibits the vasoconstrictor effect of angiotensin and stimulates renin release.

**prostaglandin (PG)** /pros′təglan′din/ [Gk, *prostates,* standing before; L, *glans,* acorn], one of several potent unsaturated fatty acids that act in exceedingly low concentrations on local target organs. Prostaglandins are produced in small amounts and have a large array of significant effects. Those given in tablets or in solutions for oral or IV use effect changes in vasomotor tone, capillary permeability, smooth muscle tone, aggregation of platelets, endocrine and exocrine functions, and the autonomic and central nervous systems. Some of the pharmacologic uses of the prostaglandins are termination of pregnancy and treatment of asthma and gastric hyperacidity.

**prostaglandin inhibitor,** an agent that prevents the production of prostaglandins. An example is a nonsteroidal antiinflammatory drug.

**prostanoic acid** /pros′tənō′ik/, a 20-carbon aliphatic carboxylic acid that is the basic framework for prostaglandin molecules, which differ according to the location of hydroxyl and keto substitutions at various positions along the molecule.

**Prostaphlin,** trademark for an antibiotic (oxacillin sodium).

**prostate** /pros′tāt/ [Gk, *prostates,* standing before], a gland in men that surrounds the neck of the bladder and the deepest part of the urethra and produces a fluid that becomes part of semen. A firm structure about the size of a chestnut, the prostate is located in the pelvic cavity, below the inferior part of the symphysis pubis and ventral to the rectum, through which it can be felt, especially when it is enlarged. A depression on its cranial border accommodates the entry of the two ejaculatory ducts from the seminal vesicles. The prostate is composed of glandular and muscular tissue and contracts during ejaculation of seminal fluid. The prostatic secretion contains alkaline phosphatase, citric acid, prostate-specific antigen, and various proteolytic enzymes. **—prostatic,** *adj.*

**prostate,** combining form meaning 'pertaining to the prostate': *prostatectomy, prostatitis, prostalgia.*

**prostate cancer,** a slowly progressive adenocarcinoma of the prostate that affects an increasing proportion of American males after 50 years of age. It is the third leading cause of cancer deaths; more than 120,000 new cases are reported in the United States each year. The cause is unknown, but it is believed to be hormone-related. The disease may cause no direct symptoms but can be detected in the course of diagnosing bladder or ureteral obstruction, hematuria, or pyuria. The cancer can spread to cause bone pain in the pelvis, ribs, or vertebrae. It is commonly detected by prostate-specific antigen test and digital rectal examination followed by core-needle biopsy. Treatment is by surgery, radiation therapy, and hormones, depending on the age of the patient, extent of disease, and other individual factors.

**prostatectomy** /pros′tətek′təmē/ [Gk, *prostates* + *ektomē,* excision], surgical removal of a part of the prostate gland, such as that performed for benign prostatic hypertrophy, or the total excision of the gland, as performed for malignancy. Type and crossmatching of blood are done to prepare for possible transfusion. Kinds of approaches include transurethral, the most common, in which a resectoscope is inserted into the urethra, and through it shavings of prostatic tissue are cut off at the bladder opening. The perineal approach is used for biopsy when early cancer is suspected or for the re-

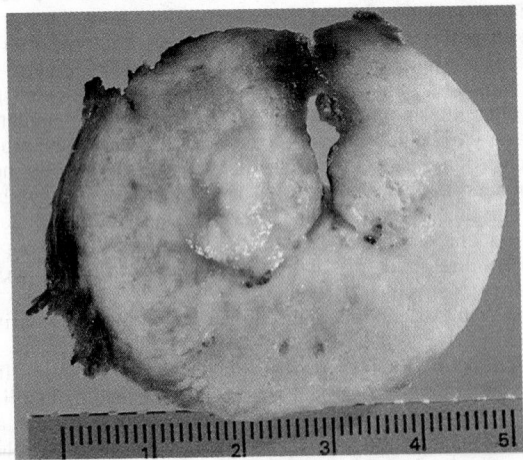

**Prostate cancer** *(Kumar, Cotran, and Robbins, 1997)*

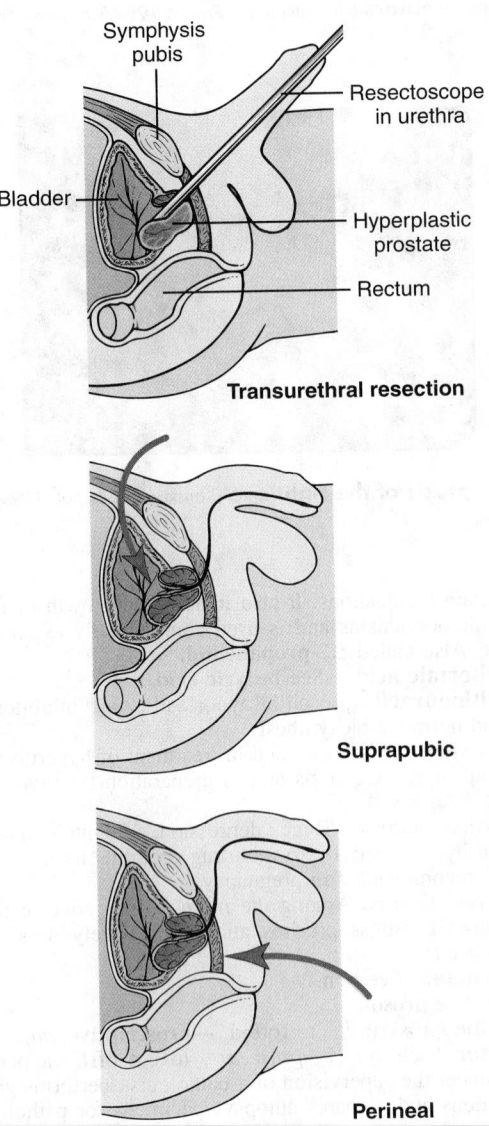

**Transurethral resection**

**Suprapubic**

**Perineal**

**Prostatectomy** *(Lewis, Heitkemper, and Dirksen, 2000)*

moval of calculi. In a suprapubic approach a large catheter is positioned into the bladder through the abdomen. Wound drains are left in place in both the perineal and the suprapubic types. After surgery hematuria is expected for several days; on the first day the bleeding is frank and usually venous. Bleeding may be controlled by increasing the pressure at the balloon end of the urethral catheter. If arterial the bleeding is bright red with clots and increased viscosity and may lead to hemorrhagic shock, requiring transfusion and surgical intervention. The bladder catheter is connected to a closed system of irrigation with drainage. Meticulous aseptic technique is required to prevent infection when tending catheters, tubings, and collection bags, as well as when changing the dressing. Catheter patency is ensured, and pain is assessed, because blockage or kinking of the drainage tubes may be the cause. Accidental removal or dislodging of catheters is prevented. Bladder spasm may occur if a catheter becomes blocked or result from the irritation of the balloon of the catheter in the bladder. Antispasmodic drugs may prevent spasm but are not given in severe cardiac disease or if glaucoma is present. The nurse also assesses the patient's ability to void in adequate amounts when the urethral catheter is removed. Complications of prostatectomy include urethral stricture, especially with the transurethral approach; urinary incontinence; and impotence, especially with the perineal approach.

**prostate-specific antigen (PSA),**    a protein produced by the prostate that may be present at elevated levels in patients with cancer or other disease of the prostate.

**prostate-specific antigen test (PSA),**    a blood test used to detect prostatic cancer and to monitor the patient's response to therapy. The PSA velocity monitors the change in PSA with time, and the percent-free PSA (%FPSA) is assessed as an independent predictor of prostate cancer risk. Currently, PSA is considered the most sensitive tumor marker for this type of cancer.

**prostatic** /prostat′ik/,    pertaining to the prostate.

**prostatic calculus** [Gk, *prostates,* standing before; L, *calculus,* pebble],    a solid calcification formed in the prostate. Typically small and multiple, prostatic calculi are often the product of chronic prostatitis and are usually composed of calcium carbonate and/or calcium phosphate. They are not clinically significant and do not require treatment.

**prostatic catheter,**    a catheter that is approximately 16 inches (41 centimeters) long and has an angled tip. It is used in male urinary bladder catheterization to pass an enlarged prostate gland obstructing the urethra. Also called **Coudé catheter.**

**prostatic ductule** /duk′tyo͞ol/ [Gk, *prostates* + L, *ductulus,* little duct],    any of 12 to 20 tiny excretory tubes that convey the alkaline secretion of the prostate and open into the floor of the prostatic part of the urethra. The ductules are joined together by areolar tissue, supported by extensions of the fibrous capsule of the prostate and its muscular stroma, and wrapped in a delicate network of capillaries.

**prostatic hypertrophy.**   See **prostatomegaly.**

**prostatic syncope** [Gk, *prostates,* standing before, *syn,* together, *koptein,* to cut],    a temporary loss of consciousness caused by restricted cerebral blood flow that may occur during a prostate examination.

**prostatic utricle,**    the part of the urethra in men that forms a cul-de-sac about 6 mm long behind the middle lobe of the prostate. It is composed of fibrous tissue, muscular fibers, and mucous membrane; numerous small glands open on its inner surface. It is homologous with the uterus in women. Also called **uterus masculinius.** See also **prostate.**

**prostatism** /pros′tətiz′əm/ [Gk, *prostates,* standing before],

an abnormal condition of the prostate, particularly an enlargement of the gland resulting in obstructed urinary flow.

**prostatitis** /pros′tətī′tis/ [Gk, *prostates* + *itis,* inflammation],    acute or chronic inflammation of the prostate gland, usually the result of infection. The patient complains of burning, urinary frequency, and urgency. Treatment consists of antibiotics, sitz baths, bed rest, and fluids. Compare **benign prostatic hypertrophy.**

**prostatomegaly** /pros′tətōmeg′əlē/ [Gk, *prostates* + *megas,* large],    hypertrophy or enlargement of the prostate.

**prosthesis** /prosthē′sis/, *pl.* **prostheses** [Gk, addition],    **1.** an artificial replacement for a missing body part, such as an artificial limb or total joint replacement. **2.** a device designed and applied to improve function, such as a hearing aid. See also **maxillofacial prosthesis, Starr-Edwards prosthesis.**

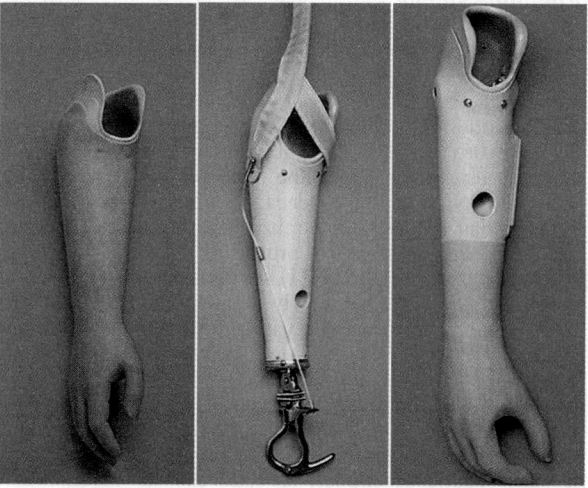

**Upper extremity prostheses *(left to right):* cosmetic, cable activated, and myoelectrically controlled**
*(Monahan and Neighbors, 1998/courtesy Otto Bock Orthopedic Industry, Inc., Minneapolis)*

**prosthesis care,**    a nursing intervention from the Nursing Interventions Classification (NIC) defined as care of a removable appliance worn by a patient and the prevention of complications associated with its use. See also **Nursing Interventions Classification.**

**prosthetic heart valve** /prosthet′ik/ [Gk, *prosthesis,* addition; AS, *hoerte* + L, *valva,* door, leaf],    an artificial heart valve.

**prosthetic restoration.**   See **restoration.**

**prosthetics** /prosthet′iks/ [Gk, *prosthesis,* addition],    the design, construction, and attachment of artificial limbs or other systems to assume the function of missing body parts. See also **orthotics.**

**prosthetist** /pros′thətist/,    a person who fabricates and fits artificial limbs and similar devices prescribed by a physician. A certified prosthetist is one who has successfully completed the examination of the American Orthotic and Prosthetic Association.

**prosthion (PR)** /pros′thē-on/ [Gk, *prosthios,* foremost],    the point of the maxillary alveolar process that projects most anteriorly in the midline of the maxilla; used for measuring upper facial height and in determining the gnathic index.

**prosthodontics** /pros'thədon'tiks/ [Gk, *prosthesis* + *odous*, tooth], a branch of dentistry devoted to the construction of artificial appliances that replace missing teeth or restore parts of the face.

**Prostigmin,** trademark for a cholinergic (neostigmine bromide).

**Prostin VR Pediatric,** trademark for a proprietary form of prostaglandin (alprostadil).

**prostration** /prostrā'shən/ [L, *prosternere*, to throw down], a condition of extreme exhaustion and inability to exert oneself further, as in heat prostration or nervous prostration. —**prostrate,** *adj.*

**prot-.** See **proto-.**

**protactinium (Pa)** /-taktin'ē·əm/ [Gk, *protos*, first, *aktis*, ray], a radioactive element. Its atomic number is 91; its atomic mass (weight) is 231.04. Its decay products are actinium and an alpha particle. See also **actinium.**

**protamine sulfate** /prō'təmēn/, a heparin antagonist derived from fish sperm.

■ INDICATION: It is prescribed to diminish or reverse the anticoagulant effect of heparin, particularly in cases of heparin overdosage.

■ CONTRAINDICATIONS: Pregnancy, allergy to fish, or known hypersensitivity to this drug prohibits its use.

■ ADVERSE EFFECTS: Among the more serious adverse reactions are hypotension, dyspnea, and bradycardia. Dosage greater than needed to neutralize heparin causes the toxic and anticoagulant effects of protamine.

**protamine zinc insulin (PZI) suspension,** a long-acting insulin that is absorbed slowly at a steady rate. Some patients can be treated with only one injection daily, but combination therapy with regular insulin may be necessary for adequate control.

**protanopia** /-tənō'pē·ə/, a form of color blindness in which the person is unable to distinguish shades of red. Also called **red blindness.**

**protaxic mode of experience** /-tak'sik/ (in psychology), a type of primitive experience characterized by sensations, feelings, and fragmented images of short duration that are not logically connected.

**protease** /prō'tē·ās/, an enzyme that is a catalyst in the breakdown of peptide bonds that join the amino acids in a protein. See also **proteolytic.**

**protease inhibitors,** 1. a group of substances that block the activity of proteases, such as in viruses. 2. See HIV protease inhibitors.

**protection, ineffective,** a nursing diagnosis accepted by the Ninth National Conference on the Classification of Nursing Diagnoses. Altered protection is defined as a state in which an individual experiences a decrease in the ability to guard the self from internal or external threats, such as illness or injury.

■ DEFINING CHARACTERISTICS: The defining characteristics are deficient immunity, impaired healing, altered clotting, maladaptive stress response, neurosensory alterations, chilling, perspiration, dyspnea, cough, itching, restlessness, insomnia, fatigue, anorexia, weakness, immobility, disorientation, and pressure sores.

■ RELATED FACTORS: Related factors are extremes of age, inadequate nutrition, alcohol abuse, abnormal blood profiles (leukopenia, thrombocytopenia, anemia, coagulation), drug therapies (antineoplastic, corticosteroid, immune, anticoagulant, thrombolytic), treatments (surgery, radiation), and diseases such as cancer and immune disorders. See also **nursing diagnosis.**

**protective** /-tek'tiv/ [L, *protegere,* to cover], guarding another person from danger or injury and providing a safe environment.

**protective apron.** See **lead apron.**

**protective isolation** [L, *protegere,* to cover in front; It, *isolare,* detached], 1. the practice of confining a patient with a virulent infectious disease in a separate area so that contact with other people can be minimized. 2. the practice of placing a highly susceptible person, such as an immunodeficient patient, in a separate area where the risk of contact with pathogenic microorganisms can be controlled.

**protein** /prō'tē·in, prō'tēn/ [Gk, *proteios,* first rank], any of a large group of naturally occurring complex organic nitrogenous compounds. Each is composed of large combinations of amino acids (usually 50 or more) containing the elements carbon, hydrogen, nitrogen, oxygen, and occasionally sulfur, phosphorus, iron, iodine, or other essential constituents of living cells. Twenty-two amino acids have been identified as vital for proper growth, development, and maintenance of health. The body can synthesize 13 of these, the nonessential amino acids, whereas the remaining 9 must be obtained from dietary sources and are termed *essential.* Protein is the major source of building material for muscles, blood, skin, hair, nails, and the internal organs. It is necessary for the formation of many hormones, enzymes, and antibodies; may act as a source of energy. Rich dietary sources are meat, poultry, fish, eggs, milk, and cheese, which are classified as complete proteins because they contain the 9 essential amino acids. Nuts and legumes, including navy beans, chick-peas, soybeans, and split peas, are also good sources but are incomplete proteins, because they do not contain all the essential amino acids in adequate amounts. Protein deficiency causes abnormal growth and tissue development in children, leading to kwashiorkor, whereas in adults it results in lack of vigor and stamina, weakness, mental depression, poor resistance to infection, impaired healing of wounds, and slow recovery from disease. Excessive intake of protein may in some conditions result in fluid imbalance.

**protein antibiotic.** See **bacteriocin.**

**proteinase** /prō'tē·inās/ [Gk, *proteios,* first rank, *ase,* enzyme suffix], a proteolytic enzyme that splits protein molecules at central linkages.

**protein calorie malnutrition.** See **energy-protein malnutrition.**

**proteinemia** /prō'tē·inē'mē·ə/ [Gk, *proteios,* first rank, *haima,* blood], an excessive level of protein in the blood. Also called **hyperproteinemia.**

**protein-energy malnutrition (PEM),** a wasting condition resulting from a diet inadequate in either protein or energy (calories) or both. These inadequacies are major problems for children in developing countries. Also called energy-protein malnutrition or protein-calorie malnutrition. See also **kwashiorkor, marasmic kwashiorkor, marasmus.**

**protein hydrolysate injection,** a fluid and nutrient replenisher.

■ INDICATIONS: It is prescribed to correct a negative nitrogen balance and to provide parenteral nutrition in other clinical situations.

■ CONTRAINDICATIONS: Renal failure, anuria, severe liver disease, hepatic coma, or known hypersensitivity to one or more of the amino acids prohibits the use of this drug.

■ ADVERSE EFFECTS: Among the more serious adverse reactions are hypotension, abdominal pain, convulsions, phlebitis, thrombosis, and edema.

**protein kinase,** a protein that catalyzes the transfer of a phosphate group from adenosine triphosphate to produce a phosphoprotein.

**protein metabolism,** the processes whereby protein foods are used by the body to make tissue proteins, together with the processes of breakdown of tissue proteins in the production of energy. Food proteins are first broken down into amino acids, then absorbed into the bloodstream, and finally used in body cells to form new proteins. Amino acids in excess of the body's needs may be converted by liver enzymes into keto acids and urea. The keto acids may be used as sources of energy via the citric acid cycle, or they may be converted into glucose or fat for storage. Urea is excreted in urine and sweat. Growth hormone, insulin, and androgens stimulate protein formation, and adrenal cortical hormones tend to cause breakdown of body proteins. Diseases affecting protein metabolism include homocystinuria, liver disease, maple sugar urine disease, and phenylketonuria.

**protein sensitization** [Gk, *proteios*, first rank; L, *sentire*, to feel], a reaction that follows parenteral introduction of a foreign protein into the body. Symptoms of varying severity, including serum sickness, occur when the same foreign protein is reintroduced into the body at a later date.

**proteinuria** /prō'tēnyŏŏr'ē·ə/ [Gk, *proteios* + *ouron*, urine], the presence in the urine of abnormally large quantities of protein, usually albumin. Healthy adults excrete less than 250 mg of protein per day. Persistent proteinuria is usually a sign of renal disease or renal complications of another disease, such as hypertension or heart failure. However, proteinuria can result from heavy exercise or fever. Also called **albuminuria.**

**proteo-,** combining form meaning 'protein': *proteocrasis, proteolysis, proteopepsis.*

**proteolipid** /prō'tē·ōlip'id/ [Gk, *proteios* + *lipos*, fat], a type of lipoprotein in which lipid material forms more than half of the molecule. It is insoluble in water and occurs primarily in the brain.

**proteolysis** /prō'tē·ol'isis/ [Gk, *proteios* + *lysis*, loosening], a process in which water added to the peptide bonds of proteins breaks down the protein molecule into simpler substances. Numerous enzymes may catalyze this process. The action of mineral acids and heat also may induce proteolysis.

**proteolytic** /prō'tē·əlit'ik/, pertaining to any substance that promotes the breakdown of protein.

*Proteus* /prō'tē·əs/ [Gk, *Proteus*, mythic god who changed shapes], a genus of motile, gram-negative bacilli often associated with nosocomial infections, normally found in feces, water, and soil. *Proteus* may cause urinary tract infections, pyelonephritis, wound infections, diarrhea, bacteremia, and endotoxic shock. Some species are sensitive to penicillin; most respond to the aminoglycoside antibiotics and cephalosporins.

*Proteus mirabilis,* a species of anaerobic, motile, rod-shaped bacteria found in putrid meat, abscesses, and fecal material. It is a leading cause of urinary tract infections.

*Proteus morgani,* a species of bacteria associated with infectious diarrhea in infants.

*Proteus syndrome* /prō'tē·us/, a rare congenital disorder with highly variable manifestations, including partial gigantism of the hands and feet with hypertrophy of the palms and soles, nevi, hemihypertrophy, subcutaneous tumors, macrocephaly and other skull abnormalities, and abdominal or pelvic lipomatosis. The cause is unknown, although a genetic origin, possibly of autosomal dominant transmission, has been conjectured.

*Proteus vulgaris*, a species of bacteria that is a frequent cause of urinary tract infections. The bacteria are found in feces, water, and soil.

**prothrombin.** See **factor II.**

**prothrombinemia** /-ē'mē·ə/ [L, *pro*, before; Gk, *thrombos*, lump, *haima*, blood], the presence of prothrombin in the blood.

**prothrombin time (PT),** a one-stage test for detecting certain plasma coagulation defects caused by a deficiency of factors V, VII, or X. Thromboplastin and calcium are added to a sample of the patient's plasma and simultaneously to a sample from a normal control. The amount of time required for clot formation in both samples is observed. Thrombin is formed from prothrombin in the presence of adequate calcium, thromboplastin, and the essential tissue coagulation factors. A prolonged PT therefore indicates deficiency in one of the factors, as in liver disease, vitamin K deficiency, or anticoagulation therapy with the drug warfarin sodium. Normal findings of prothrombin time are 11 to 12.5 seconds. Compare **partial thromboplastin time** and **International Normalized Ratio.** See also **blood clotting.**

**protist,** a member of the kingdom Protista, which includes eukaryotic, mostly unicellular organisms with animal-like (protozoa), plantlike (algae), or funguslike (slime molds) modes of nutrition.

**proto-, prot-,** prefix meaning 'first': *protoblast, protoxin, protopathic.*

**protocol** /prō'təkôl/ [Gk, *protos*, first, *kolla*, glued page], a written plan specifying the procedures to be followed in giving a particular examination, in conducting research, or in providing care for a particular condition. See also **standing orders.**

**proton** /prō'ton/ [Gk, *protos*, first], a positively charged particle that is a fundamental component of the nucleus of all atoms. The number of protons in the nucleus of an atom equals the atomic number of the element. Compare **electron, neutron.** See also **atomic weight.**

**proton density,** a measure of proton concentration, or the number of atomic nuclei per given volume. It is one of the major determinants of magnetic resonance signal strength in hydrogen imaging.

**proton pump inhibitor,** an agent that inhibits gastric acid secretion by blocking the action of $H^+, K^+$-ATPase at the secretory surface of gastric parietal cells; also called **gastric acid pump inhibitor.** See also **$H^+,K^+$-ATPase.**

**Protopam Chloride,** trademark for a cholinesterase reactivator (pralidoxime chloride).

**protopathic sensibility** /prō'təpath'ik/, pertaining to the somatic sensations of fast localized pain; slow, poorly localized pain; and temperature.

**protoplasm.** See **cytoplasm.**

**protoplasmic** /-plaz'mik/ [Gk, *protos*, first, *plasma*, something formed], pertaining to or composed of protoplasm, the substance of which animal and vegetable cells are formed.

**protoplast** /prō'təplast/ [Gk, *protos* + *plassein*, to mold], 1. (in biology) the protoplasm of a cell without its containing membrane. 2. a first entity or an original. —**protoplastic,** *adj.*

**protoporphyria** /prō'tōpôrfir'ē·ə/ [Gk, *protos* + *porphyros*, purple, *haima*, blood], increased levels of protoporphyrin in the blood and feces.

**protoporphyrin** /prō'tōpôr'firin/ [Gk, *protos* + *porphyros*], a kind of porphyrin that combines with iron and protein to form various important organic molecules, including catalase, hemoglobin, and myoglobin. See also **heme.**

**protostoma.** See **blastopore.**

**prototaxic mode** /prō'tōtak'sik/ [Gk, *protos* + *taxis*, arrangement, *modus*, measure], a stage in infancy, according to H.S. Sullivan's theory, characterized by a lack of differentiation between the self and the environment.

**prototype** /prō'tətīp/ [Gk, *protos,* first, *typos,* mark], the primary or original form of an object or organism.

**protozoon** /prō'təzō'ən/, *pl.* **protozoa** [Gk, *protos* + *zoon,* animal], a unicellular protist that ingests food. Protozoa include free-living forms, such as amebas and paramecia, as well as parasites. Approximately 30 protozoa are pathogenic to humans, including *Plasmodium,* which causes malaria, and *Trypanosoma,* which causes sleeping sickness. —**protozoal, protozoan,** *adj.*

**protozoal infection** /-zō'əl/, any disease caused by single-celled organisms of the subkingdom Protozoa. Some kinds of protozoal infections are **amebic dysentery, malaria, schistosomiasis, trichomoniasis,** and **trypanosomiasis.**

**protozoan** /-zō'ən/ [Gk, *protos,* first, *zoon,* animal], pertaining to or caused by protozoa.

**protracted dose** /prōtrak'tid/ [L, *pro,* before, *trahere,* to draw, *dosis,* something given], a low amount of therapeutic radiation delivered continuously over a relatively long period.

**protriptyline hydrochloride** /-trip'tilēn/, a tricyclic antidepressant.

■ INDICATIONS: It is prescribed in the treatment of endogenous depression marked by withdrawal and anergy.

■ CONTRAINDICATIONS: Concomitant administration of monoamine oxidase inhibitors, recent myocardial infarction, or known hypersensitivity to any tricyclic medication prohibits its use. It is used with caution when anticholinergics are contraindicated, in seizure disorders, and in cardiovascular disease.

■ ADVERSE EFFECTS: Among the more serious adverse reactions are sedation and anticholinergic side effects. A variety of GI, cardiovascular, and neurologic reactions may occur. This drug interacts with many other drugs.

**Protropin,** trademark for a synthetic human growth hormone (somatrem).

**protrusio bulbi.** See **exophthalmia.**

**protrusion** /-trōō'zhən/ [L, *protrudere,* to push forward], a state or condition of being forward or projecting.

**protrusive incisal guide angle** /-trōō'siv/, the inclination of the incisal guide of a dental articulator in the sagittal plane.

**protrypsin.** See **trypsinogen.**

**protuberance** /-t(y)ōō'bərəns/ [L, *pro* + *tuberare,* to swell], an anatomic landmark that appears as a blunt projection, eminence, or swelling, such as the chin, buttock, or bulge of the frontal bone above the eyebrow.

**proud flesh** [AS, *prud* + *flaesc*], excessive granulation tissue. See also **cicatrix, keloid, scar.**

**Proventil,** trademark for a bronchodilator (albuterol).

**Provera,** trademark for a progestin (medroxyprogesterone acetate).

**provider,** a hospital, clinic, health care professional, or group of health care professionals who provide a service to patients.

**Provincial/Territorial Nurses Association (PTNA),** an association of Canadian nurses organized at the provincial or territorial level. The Canadian Nurses' Association is a federation of the 11 PTNAs.

**provirus** /-vī'rəs/, a stage of viral replication in which the viral genetic information has been integrated into the genome of the host cell. It may be activated spontaneously or by a specific stimulus to direct the cell to produce new virions to progress to a complete virus.

**provitamin** /prōvī'təmin/, a precursor of a vitamin; a substance found in certain foods that in the body may be converted into a vitamin. Also called **previtamin.**

**provocative diagnosis** /-vok'ətiv/ [L, *provocare,* to call forth; Gk, *dia,* through, *gnosis,* knowledge], a diagnosis in which the identity and cause of an illness are discovered by inducing an episode of the condition; for example, in immunology an allergen causing an allergic response is shown to be a causative factor in the patient's allergic condition.

**prox,** abbreviation for **proximal.**

**proxemics** /proksē'miks/ [L, *proximus,* nearest], the study of spatial distances between people and their effect on interpersonal behavior, especially in relation to population density, placement of people within an area, territoriality, personal space, and the opportunity for privacy.

**proximal** /prok'siməl/ [L, *proximus*], nearer to a point of reference or attachment, usually the trunk of the body, than other parts of the body. Proximal interphalangeal joints are those closest to the hand or the surface of a tooth in relation to the abutting tooth nearer or farther from the anteroposterior median plane.

**proximal cavity,** a cavity that occurs on the mesial or distal surface of a tooth.

**proximal contact** [L, *proximus,* nearest, *contingere,* to touch], contact between the distal surface of one tooth and the mesial surface of an adjacent tooth.

**proximal contour,** the shape or form of the mesial or the distal surface of a tooth.

**proximal dental caries,** decay that may occur in the mesial or distal surface of a tooth.

**proximal radioulnar articulation,** the pivot joint between the circumference of the head of the radius and the ring formed by the radial notch of the ulna and the annular ligament. The joint allows the rotary movements of the head of the radius in pronation and supination. Also called **superior radioulnar joint.** Compare **distal radioulnar articulation.**

**proximal renal tubular acidosis (proximal RTA),** an abnormal condition characterized by excessive acid accumulation and bicarbonate excretion. It is caused by the defective reabsorption of bicarbonate in the proximal tubules of the kidney and the resulting flow of excessive bicarbonate into the distal tubules, which normally secrete hydrogen ions. This disruption impedes the formation of titratable acids and ammonium for excretion and ultimately leads to metabolic acidosis. Treatment is the same as for renal tubular acidosis. In **primary proximal RTA** the defective reabsorption of bicarbonate is the sole causative factor. In **secondary proximal RTA** the resorptive defect is one of several causative factors and may result from tubular cell damage produced by various disorders, such as Fanconi's syndrome. Compare **distal renal tubular acidosis.**

**proximate** /prok'simit/ [L, *proximus,* nearest], the nearest to a point of origin or attachment. Compare **distal.**

**proximate cause** [L, *proximus,* nearest], a legal concept of cause and effect relationships in determining, for example, whether an injury would have resulted from a particular cause.

**proximity principle** /proksim'itē/ [L, *proximus* + *principium,* origin], a rule that when two or more objects are close to each other, they may be seen as a perceptual unit.

**proximo-,** combining form meaning 'near or opposite of distal, central, or a point of attachment': *proximity, proximal, proximolabial.*

**proxymetacaine.** See **proparacaine hydrochloride.**

**Prozac,** trademark for an oral antidepressant (fluoxetine hydrochloride).

**PrP,** abbreviation for *prion protein,* a viruslike infectious agent associated with Creutzfeldt-Jakob disease.

**prune-belly syndrome,** a syndrome in which the lower part of the rectus abdominis muscle and the lower and medial parts of the oblique muscles are absent, the bladder and ureters are usually greatly dilated, the kidneys are small and dysplastic, with hydronephrosis, and the testes are undescended. The abdomen is protruding and thin-walled, with wrinkled skin, giving the syndrome its name. Also called **Eagle-Barrett syndrome.**

**prurigo** /pro͞orī′gō/ [L, an itch], any of a group of chronic inflammatory conditions of the skin characterized by severe itching and multiple dome-shaped small papules capped by tiny vesicles. Later (as a result of repeated scratching), crusting and lichenification may occur. Some causes of prurigo are allergies, drugs, endocrine abnormalities, malignancies, and parasites. Specific treatment depends on the cause. Symptomatic therapy is the same as for pruritus. A mild form of the disease is called **prurigo mitis,** a more severe form, **prurigo agria** or **prurigo ferox.** See also **pruritus.** —**pruriginous,** adj.

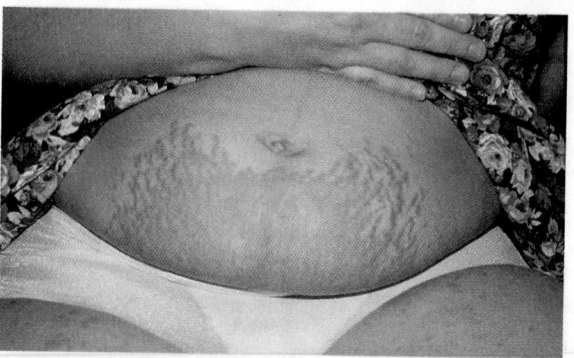

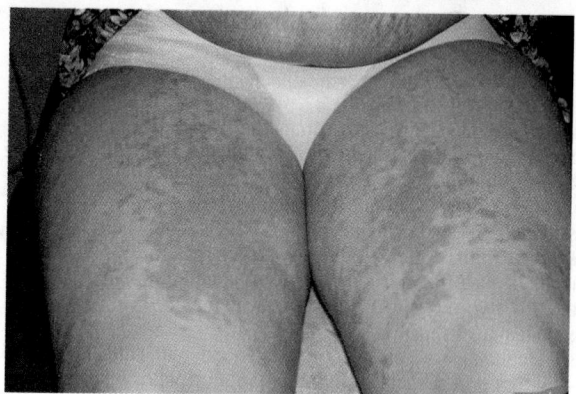

**Pruritic urticarial papules (top) and plaques (bottom) of pregnancy**
(Goldstein and Goldstein, 1997/courtesy Department of Dermatology, University of North Carolina at Chapel Hill)

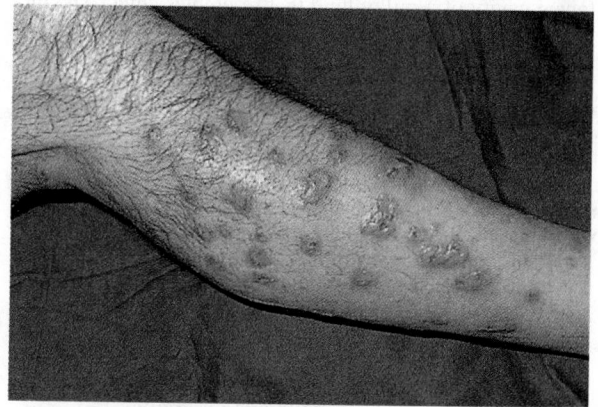

**Nodular prurigo** (Lawrence and Cox, 1993)

**pruritic urticarial papules and plaques of pregnancy (PUPPP)** /pro͞orit′ik/, small, semisolid intensely itching blisters that may appear on the abdomen of a pregnant woman and spread peripherally. They begin in the third trimester and resolve spontaneously after delivery.

**pruritus** /pro͞orī′təs/ [L, prurire, to itch], the symptom of itching, an uncomfortable sensation leading to the urge to scratch. Scratching may result in secondary infection. Some causes of pruritus are allergy, infection, jaundice, chronic renal disease, lymphoma, and skin irritation. Treatment is best directed at the cause; symptomatic relief may be obtained with antihistamines, starch baths, topical corticosteroids, cool water, or alcohol applications. —**pruritic,** adj.

**pruritus ani,** a common chronic condition of itching of the skin around the anus. Some causes are candidal infection, contact dermatitis, external hemorrhoids, pinworms, psoriasis, and psychogenic illness. Treatment is best directed at the specific cause; however, symptomatic relief may be obtained with careful cleansing, soothing creams or lotions, topical corticosteroids, antihistamines, and tranquilizers.

**pruritus management,** a nursing intervention from the Nursing Interventions Classification (NIC) defined as preventing and treating itching. See also **Nursing Interventions Classification.**

**pruritus vulvae,** itching of the external genitalia of a female. The condition may become chronic and result in lichenification, atrophy, and occasionally malignancy. Some causes of pruritus vulvae are contact dermatitis, lichen sclerosus et atrophicus, psychogenic pruritus, trichomoniasis, and vaginal candidiasis. Treatment of the condition depends on its cause.

**Prussian blue** /prush′ən/ [Prussia, Germany; ME, blew], a chemical stain used on microscopic preparations. It demonstrates the presence of copper by developing a bright blue color.

**ps,** abbreviation for **picosecond.**

**PSA, 1.** abbreviation for **pressure-sensitive adhesive. 2.** abbreviation for **prostate-specific antigen.**

**P sac,** abbreviation for pericardial cavity.

**psammo-,** combining form meaning 'sand or sandlike material': psammocarcinoma, psammoma, psammosarcoma.

**psammoma** /samō′mə/, pl. **psammomas, psammomata** [Gk, psammos, sand, oma, tumor], a neoplasm containing small calcified granules (psammoma bodies) that occurs in the meninges, choroid plexus, pineal body, and ovaries. Also called **sand tumor.**

**psammoma body,** a round layered mass of calcareous material occurring in benign and malignant epithelial and connective tissue neoplasms and in some chronically inflamed tissue.

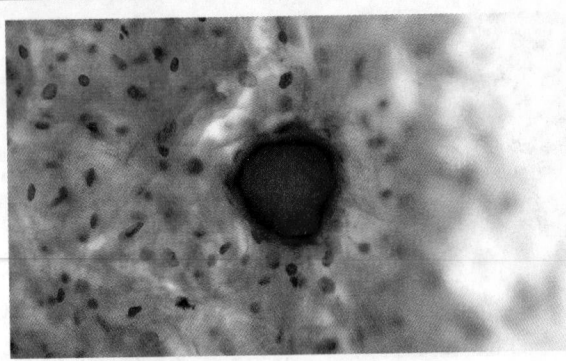

**Psammoma body** (McKee, 1997)

**psammomas, psammomata.** See **psammoma.**

**-pselaphesia, -pselaphesis,** combining form meaning '(condition of the) tactile sense': *apselaphesia, hyperpselaphesia, hypopselaphesia.*

**pseud-.** See **pseudo-.**

**pseudarthritis** /sōō′därthrī′tis/ [Gk, *pseudes,* false, *arthron,* joint, *itis,* inflammation], musculoskeletal pain that does not involve the joints.

**pseudesthesia** /sōō′desthē′zhə/ [Gk, *pseudes,* false, *aisthesis,* feeling], a sensation experienced without an external stimulus or a sensation that does not correspond to the causative stimulus, such as phantom limb pain occurring after an amputation.

**pseudo-** /sōō′dō-/, **pseud-,** prefix meaning 'false': *pseudoangina, pseudocyst, pseudorubella.*

**pseudoacanthosis nigricans** /-ak′ənthō′sis/, a condition of pigmented velvety thickening of the flexural skin, often with skin tags. It occurs most commonly in obese persons with dark complexions or in persons with endocrine disorders, and secondary to maceration of the skin from sweating.

**pseudoactinomycosis.** See **paraactinomycosis.**

**pseudoagraphia** /sōō′dō-ə·graf′ē-ə/ [Gk, *pseudes,* false + *a, graphein,* not to write], a type of dysgraphia in which the patient can copy writing, but cannot write to express ideas. Also called **echographia.**

**pseudoallele** /-əlēl′/ [Gk, *pseudes* + *allelon,* of one another], one of two or more closely linked genes on a chromosome that appear to function as a single allelic pair but occupy distinct, nearly corresponding loci on homologous chromosomes. Such gene pairs produce a mutant effect when located on homologous chromosomes but are capable of being separated by crossing over during meiosis to produce a wild-type effect when recombined on either of the homologues. —**pseudoallelic,** *adj.,* **pseudoallelism,** *n.*

**pseudoaneurysm** /-an′yəriz′əm/, **1.** a dilation of an artery caused by damage to one or more layers of the artery as a result of arterial trauma or rupture of a true aneurysm. **2.** a tortuosity of a blood vessel or cavity resulting from a herniated infarction. Also called **pulsatile hematoma.**

**pseudoankylosis** /-ang′kilō′sis/ [Gk, *pseudes,* false, *ankylosis,* joint stiffness], fixation of a joint caused by inflexibility of body structures outside the joint.

**pseudoanodontia** /-an′ōdon′shə/, an absence of teeth caused by failure of the teeth to erupt.

**pseudoanorexia** /-an′ərek′sē-ə/ [Gk, *pseudes* + *a* + *orexis,* without appetite], a condition in which an individual eats secretly while claiming a lack of appetite and inability to eat. Also called **false anorexia.**

**pseudoarthrosis.** See **false joint.**

**pseudoataxia** /-ətak′sē-ə/ [Gk, *pseudes,* false, *ataxia,* without order], a loss of control over voluntary movements that does not involve an organic lesion.

**pseudobulbar paralysis** /-bul′bər/ [Gk, *pseudes,* false; L, *bulbus,* swollen root, *paralyein,* to be palsied], a condition resembling progressive bulbar paralysis, with dysarthria and dysphagia, but in which weakness of the bulbar muscles is of the upper motor neuron type. It may result from multiple bilateral infarcts of the cerebral cortex in some cases.

**pseudocephalocele** /-sef′əlōsēl′/, a noncongenital cerebral hernia resulting from a skull injury or disease.

**pseudochancre** /-shang′kər/, an indurated genital sore resembling a chancre.

**pseudocholinesterase.** See **cholinesterase.**

**pseudochondroplasia** /-akon′drōplā′zhə/, a hereditary condition resembling achondroplasia but developing after birth.

**pseudochylous ascites** /-kī′ləs/ [Gk, *pseudes* + *chylos,* juice, *askos,* bag], the abnormal accumulation in the peritoneal cavity of a milky fluid that resembles chyle. The turbidity of the fluid is caused by cellular debris in the fluid. Pseudochylous ascites is indicative of an abdominal tumor or infection. Compare **chylous ascites.** See also **ascites.**

**pseudoclaudication** /-klô′dikā′shən/, painful cramps that are not caused by peripheral artery disease but rather by spinal, neurologic, or orthopedic disorders, such as spinal stenosis, diabetic neuropathy, or arthritis.

**pseudocoxalgia.** See **Legg-Calvé-Perthes disease.**

**pseudocyesis** /-sī-ē′sis/ [Gk, *pseudes* + *kyesis,* pregnancy], a condition in which a woman believes she is pregnant when she is not. Certain signs and symptoms suggest pregnancy, such as the absence of the menses, although conception has not occurred and therefore there is no embryonic development. The condition may be psychogenic in origin or caused by a tumor or endocrine dysfunction. Also called **false pregnancy, pseudopregnancy, spurious pregnancy.**

**pseudocyst** /sōō′dəsist/ [Gk, *pseudes* + *kystis,* bag], a space or cavity containing gas or liquid but without a lining membrane. Pseudocysts commonly occur after pancreatitis when digestive juices break through the normal ducts of the pancreas and collect in spaces lined by fibroblasts and surfaces of adjacent organs. Symptoms are caused by displacement of abdominal structures or fluid or by atelectasis at the base of the left lung. Ultrasound and computed tomography are useful in diagnosis; surgical drainage is the best therapy. See also **pancreatitis.**

**pseudodementia** /-dimen′shə/, a syndrome that mimics dementia. It needs to be differentiated from depression.

**pseudoephedrine hydrochloride** /-ef′ədrēn/, an adrenergic that acts as a vasoconstrictor and bronchodilator.

■ INDICATIONS: It is prescribed for the relief of nasal congestion and eustachian tube congestion.

■ CONTRAINDICATIONS: Known hypersensitivity to sympathomimetic drugs prohibits its use. Interaction with monoamine oxidase inhibitors may cause hypertensive crisis. It is prescribed with caution in patients who have hypertension, glaucoma, heart disease, diabetes, or urinary retention.

■ ADVERSE EFFECTS: Among the more serious adverse reactions are central nervous system stimulation, headache, and tachycardia.

**pseudoephedrine sulfate.** See **pseudoephedrine hydrochloride.**

**pseudofracture** /-frak′chər/ [Gk, *pseudes,* false; L, *fractura*], radiologic evidence of a thickened periosteum and

**pseudogene** /sōō′dōjēn′/ [Gk, *pseudes* + *genein*, to produce], a DNA sequence that resembles a gene and may be derived from one but lacks a genetic function.

**pseudoglottis.** See **neoglottis.**

**pseudogout.** See **chondrocalcinosis.**

**pseudo-Graefe's sign,** slow descent of the upper lid on looking down, and quick ascent on looking up; seen in conditions other than Graves' disease.

**pseudogynecomastia** /-gī′nəmas′tē·ə/, enlarged breasts in a male caused by fat accumulation.

**pseudohallucination.** See **phantom vision.**

**pseudohermaphrodism.** See **pseudohermaphroditism.**

**pseudohermaphrodite** /-hərmaf′rədīt/ [Gk, *pseudes,* false, *Hermaphroditos,* son of Hermes and Aphrodite], a congenital condition in which a person has either male or female gonads but external genitalia of the opposite sex, or both.

**pseudohermaphroditism** /-hərmaf′rəditiz′əm/ [Gk, *pseudes* + *Hermaphroditos,* son of Hermes and Aphrodite], a condition in which a person exhibits the somatic characteristics of both sexes though possessing the physical characteristics of either males (testes) or females (ovaries). Also spelled **pseudohermaphrodism.** See also **feminization,** def. 2, **hermaphroditism.**

**pseudo-Hurler polydystrophy,** a disorder similar to but milder than **I cell disease** (mucolipidosis II) and thought to result from the same enzyme deficiency but to a lesser extent. Also called **mucolipidosis III.**

**pseudohyperkalemia** /-hī′pərkəlē′mē·ə/, a laboratory artifact indicating an elevated blood potassium level caused by potassium released in vitro from cells in the blood sample.

**pseudohyperparathyroidism** /hī′pərper′əthī′roidiz′əm/, signs of hypercalcemia in a cancer patent in the absence of primary hyperparathyroidism or skeletal metastases.

**pseudohypertension** /-hī′pərten′shən/, a blood pressure reading that erroneously appears elevated as a result of arterial compliance. The condition occurs most often in elderly patients.

**pseudohypertrophic muscular dystrophy.** See **Duchenne's muscular dystrophy.**

**pseudohypertrophy** /-hīpur′trəfē/, abnormal enlargement of an organ or body structure caused by an overgrowth of fatty and fibrous tissues.

**pseudohypoaldosteronism** /-hī′pōaldos′tərōn′izəm/, **1.** a hereditary disorder of infancy characterized by severe salt and water depletion and other signs of aldosterone deficiency, even though normal or elevated amounts of aldosterone are secreted. Causes include aldosterone receptor defects and renal dysfunction. Some affected infants outgrow the need for dietary salt supplements in early childhood. **2.** the endocrine abnormality associated with sodium-losing nephropathy, usually resulting from chronic pyelonephritis, seen primarily in adults. See also **Gordon's syndrome.**

**pseudohyponatremia** /-hī′pōnātrē′mē·ə/, a decreased sodium concentration that does not correspond to a true hypotonic disorder. It may result instead from volume displacement by massive hyperlipidemia or hyperproteinemia.

**pseudohypoparathyroidism** /-hī′pōper′əthī′roidiz′əm/, a condition of end-organ resistance characterized by hypocalcemia, growth failure, and skeletal abnormalities such as short fingers.

**pseudoileus** /sōō′dō·il′ē·əs/, **1.** a condition resembling an intestinal obstruction caused by paralysis of a part of the bowel wall. **2.** an adynamic bowel obstruction.

**pseudoisochromatic** /sōō′dō·ī′sōkrōmat′ik/, pertaining to visual test materials in which dots that differ in color appear similar to a person with color blindness. See also **Ishihara color test.**

**pseudojaundice** /-jôn′dis/ [Gk, *pseudes* + Fr, *jaune,* yellow], a yellow discoloration of the skin that is not caused by hyperbilirubinemia. The excessive ingestion of carotene results in a form of pseudojaundice.

**pseudolymphoma** /-limfō′mə/, a benign disorder of lymphoid cells or histiocytes that produces clinical features of a malignant lymphoma.

**pseudolysogeny** /-līsoj′ənē/, a condition in which a bacteriophage is carried in a culture of a bacterial strain by infecting susceptible variants of the strain.

**pseudomamma** /-mam′ə/, a glandular structure resembling a nipple or mammary gland, sometimes found in a dermoid ovarian cyst.

**pseudomania** /-mā′nē·ə/, **1.** a condition in which a person may claim to have committed crimes of which he or she is really innocent. **2.** a deliberately pretended condition of mental illness.

**pseudomegacolon** /-meg′əkō′lon/, a dilation of the colon in an adult patient.

**pseudomembrane** /-mem′brān/ [Gk, *pseudes,* false; L, *membrana*], a membrane consisting of coagulated fibrin, bacteria, and leukocytes that forms in the throats of diphtheria patients.

**pseudomembranous** /-mem′brənəs/, describing a false membrane, as occurs in diphtheria.

**pseudomembranous colitis** /-mem′brənəs/ [Gk, *pseudes* + L, *membrana,* thin skin], a diarrheal disease frequently found in hospitalized patients who have received antibiotics that caused overgrowth of the anaerobic spore-forming toxin producing *Clostridium difficile.* Patients have profuse watery diarrhea, fever, and cramping and are found to have exudates of the colon on endoscopy. Diagnosis is made by identifying the offending toxin in the stool of the affected patient. Antidiarrheals are strictly contraindicated, as a life-threatening dilation of the bowel called toxic megacolon may result. The bacterium is passed from patient to patient by health care workers who fail to wash their hands adequately. Strict isolation of infected stools is necessary to prevent outbreaks of epidemics. Treatment with oral vancomycin or parenteral metronidazole usually will result in abatement of symptoms within 3 to 5 days.

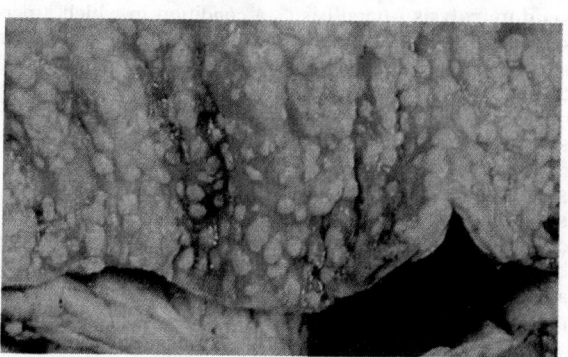

**Pseudomembranous colitis: autopsy specimen**
*(Baron, Peterson, and Finegold, 1994)*

**pseudomembranous enterocolitis.** See **necrotizing enterocolitis.**

**pseudomembranous stomatitis,** a severe inflammation of the mouth that produces a membranelike exudate. The inflammation may be caused by various bacteria or by chemical irritants. It may produce dysphagia, pain, fever, and swelling of the lymph glands, or it may remain localized and mild.

**pseudomenstruation** /-men'strōo̅-ā'shən/, bleeding from the uterus that resembles menstruation but is not associated with the usual changes in endometrial tissues.

**pseudomnesia** /sōo̅'dōmnē'zhə/, a memory aberration in which a client claims to remember events that actually have not taken place.

**pseudomonad** /sōo̅'dōmō'nad, sōo̅dom'ənad/, a bacterium of the genus *Pseudomonas.*

**Pseudomonas** /sōo̅dom'ənas/ [Gk, *pseudes* + *monas*, unit], a genus of gram-negative bacteria that includes several free-living species in soil and water and some opportunistic pathogens, such as *Pseudomonas aeruginosa*, isolated from wounds, burns, and infections of the urinary tract. Pseudomonads are notable for their fluorescent pigments and their resistance to disinfectants and antibiotics.

**Pseudomonas aeruginosa** [Gk, *pseudes*, false, *monas*, unity], a species of gram-negative nonspore-forming motile bacteria that may cause various human diseases ranging from purulent meningitis to nosocomial infected wounds. Also called *Pseudomonas pyocyanea.*

**Pseudomonas maltophilia.** See *Xanthomonas maltophilia.*

**Pseudomonas pyocyanea.** See *Pseudomonas aeruginosa.*

**pseudomutuality** /-mōo̅'tyōo̅-al'itē/ [Gk, *pseudes* + L, *mutuus*, reciprocal], (in psychotherapy) an atmosphere maintained by family members in which there are surface harmony and a high degree of agreement with one another but deep and destructive intrapsychic and interpersonal conflicts are hidden. The family acts "as if" it is close and happy, when in fact it is not.

**pseudomyopia** /-mī-ō'pē-ə/, a condition in which a person holds objects close to the eyes to see them although he or she does not have myopia.

**pseudomyxoma** /-miksō'mə/, a mucus-rich tumor.

**pseudomyxoma peritone'i,** the presence in the peritoneal cavity of mucoid matter from a ruptured ovarian cyst or a ruptured mucocele of the appendix.

**pseudonystagmus.** See **end-positional nystagmus.**

**pseudopapilledema** /-pap'ilēdē'mə/, a congenitally swollen optic disc that resembles papilledema; there are no retinal hemorrhages or exudates, nor any systemic signs of increased intraocular pressure.

**pseudoparalysis** /-pəral'isis/, a condition in which a person appears to be unable to move the arms or legs but there is no "true" paralysis. In infants, the condition may be caused by pain in joints resulting from a disease such as rickets or scurvy.

**pseudoparaplegia** /-per'əplē'jə/, a form of hysterical paralysis.

**pseudoparesis** /-pərē'sis/, a form of hysterical paralysis.

**pseudopelade** /-pelād', -pē'lād/, a scarring type of alopecia, preceded by folliculitis, in which one or more areas of baldness may appear and spread to become joined, forming an area of smooth fingerlike projections that are slightly depressed in the skin.

**pseudopericarditis** /-per'ikärdī'tis/, an auscultation sound resembling a friction rub when the diaphragm of a stethoscope is over the apex beat. It is actually caused by the movement of tissue in the intercostal space.

**pseudophakia** /-fā'kē-ə/, a failure of development of an eye in which the natural crystalline lens has been replaced by mesodermal tissue.

**pseudophakodonesis** /-fā'kōdənē'sis/, excessive movement by an intraocular lens implant.

**Pseudophyllidea** /-filid'ē-ə/, an order of tapeworms with an aquatic life cycle. The scolex usually has two opposing sucking organs.

**pseudopod** /sōo̅'dəpod/ [Gk, *pseudes*, false, *pous*, foot], a temporary cytoplasmic process of an ameba that can be extended to propel the organism or to engulf food. Also called **pseudopodium.**

**pseudopolyp** /-pol'ip/, a projecting mass of granulation tissue that may develop in ulcerative colitis and become covered by regenerating epithelium.

**pseudopregnancy.** See **pseudocyesis.**

**pseudoprognathism** /-prog'nəthiz'əm/, a condition in which the mandible is forced forward of its normal position by an occlusal disorder.

**pseudopseudohypoparathyroidism** /sōo̅'dōsōo̅'dōhī'pōpar'əthī'roidizəm/, an incomplete form of pseudohypoparathyroidism characterized by the same constitutional features but by normal levels of calcium and phosphorus in the serum. See also **pseudohypoparathyroidism.**

**pseudopsychosis** /-sīkō'sis/, a condition such as malingering that may resemble a true mental and behavioral disorder.

**pseudopterygium** /sōo̅'dopterij'ē·əm/, a fold of conjunctiva that has become attached to the cornea after an injury or disease.

**pseudoptosis** /sōo̅'doptō'sis/, an abnormally small palpebral fissure.

**pseudopuberty** /-p(y)ōo̅'pərtē/, the appearance of somatic and functional changes in an individual before the chronologic age of puberty.

**pseudorabies.** See **infectious bulbar paralysis.**

**pseudoretinitis pigmentosa** /-ret'inī'tis/, a pigmentary mottling of the retina that may follow an eye injury.

**pseudorubella.** See **roseola infantum.**

**pseudosarcoma** /-särkō'mə/, a spindle cell epithelioma on skin that has been exposed to irradiation.

**pseudosclerema.** See **adiponecrosis subcutanea neonatorum.**

**pseudostrabismus** /-strəbiz'məs/, an appearance of strabismus caused by an epicanthal fold of skin, which narrows the visible width of the sclera medial to the iris.

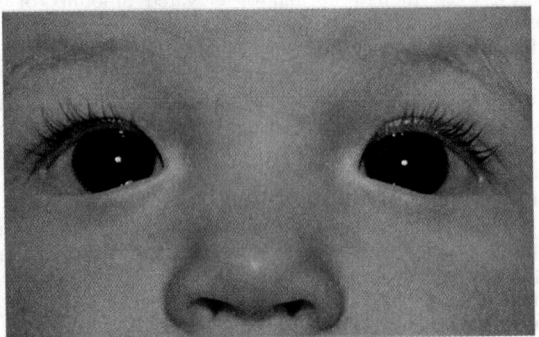

**Pseudostrabismus caused by a flat nasal bridge, wide epicanthal folds, and closely placed eyes**
*(Zitelli and Davis, 1997)*

**pseudostratified** /-stra'tifĭd/ [Gk, *pseudes*, false, *stratum*, cover],    pertaining to a type of layered epithelium in which the nuclei of adjacent cells are at different levels.

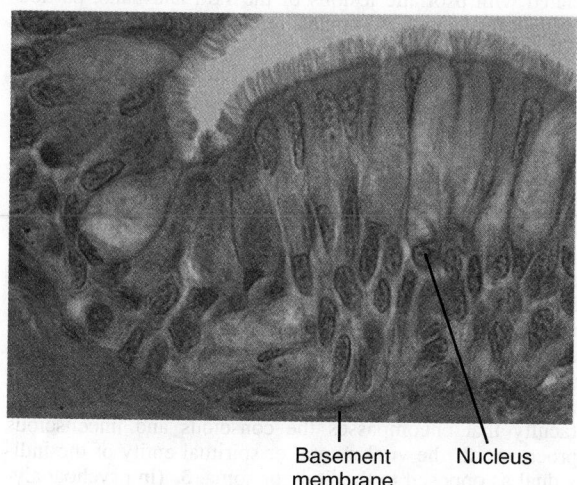

Basement    Nucleus
membrane

**Pseudostratified columnar epithelium**
*(© Ed Reschke; used with permission)*

**pseudotabes** /-tā'bēz/,    any neuropathy with symptoms like those of tabes dorsalis.

**pseudotruncus arteriosus** /-trung'kəs/,    a condition in which blood is carried to the pulmonary arteries by collateral vessels.

**pseudotubercle** /-t(y)o͞o'bərkəl/,    a nodule that resembles a tuberculosis granule but is caused by a microorganism other than *Mycobacterium tuberculosis.*

**pseudotuberculosis** /-t(y)o͞obur'kyəlo'sis/,    a pulmonary condition with symptoms resembling those of tuberculosis but not caused by *Mycobacterium tuberculosis.*

**pseudotumor** /-t(y)o͞o'mər/ [Gk, *pseudes* + L, *tumor*, swelling],    a false tumor.

**pseudotumor cerebri,**    a condition characterized by increased intracranial pressure, headache, blurring of the optic disc margins, vomiting, and papilledema without neurologic signs, except palsy of the sixth cranial nerve. Also called **benign intracranial hypertension, meningeal hydrops.**

**pseudovitamin** /-vī'təmin/,    a substance that has a chemical structure similar to that of a vitamin but lacks the physiologic effects.

**pseudoxanthoma elasticum.**    See **Grönblad-Strandberg syndrome.**

**psi** /sī/,    Ψ, ψ, the twenty-third letter of the Greek alphabet.

**p.s.i.,**    abbreviation for *pounds per square inch.*

**psia,**    abbreviation for *pounds per square inch, absolute.*

**psig,**    abbreviation for *pounds per square inch, gauge.*

**psilocin** /sī'ləsin/,    one of several indole-derived psychomimetic drugs. It is related chemically to psilocybin.

**psilocybin** /sī'lōsī'bin, -sib'in/,    a psychedelic drug and an active ingredient of various Mexican hallucinogenic mushrooms of the genus *Psilocybe mexicana.* It can produce altered states of mood and consciousness and has no acceptable medical use in the United States. Psilocybin is controlled under Schedule I of the Controlled Substances Act of 1970, which bans the prescription of psilocybin and numerous other drugs and allows their procurement and use only for special research projects authorized by the Drug Enforcement Administration of the U.S. Department of Justice.

**psittacosis** /sit'əkō'sis/ [Gk, *psittakos*, parrot],    an infectious illness caused by the bacterium *Chlamydia psittaci.* It is characterized by respiratory pneumonia-like symptoms and transmitted to humans inhaling dried secretions from by infected birds, especially pet birds and poultry. The clinical manifestations of the disease are extremely variable and resemble those of a great number of infectious diseases, but fever, cough, anorexia, and severe headache are almost always present. A history of exposure to birds is highly suggestive, because all chlamydiae are difficult to isolate and culture. A demonstrated rise in antibody titer confirms a diagnosis. Tetracycline is usually used to treat psittacosis and is continued for 10 to 14 days after the fever subsides. Isolation is advised. Also called **ornithosis, parrot fever.** See also *Chlamydia.*

**psm,**    abbreviation for **presystolic murmur.**

**psoas major** /sō'əs/ [Gk, *psoa*, loin],    a long muscle originating from the transverse processes of the lumbar vertebrae and the fibrocartilages and sides of the vertebral bodies of the lower thoracic vertebrae and the lumbar vertebrae. It joins the iliacus to form the iliopsoas deep in the pelvis as it passes under the inguinal ligament and inserts in the lesser trochanter. It acts to flex and rotate the thigh and to flex and laterally bend the spine laterally. Compare **psoas minor.**

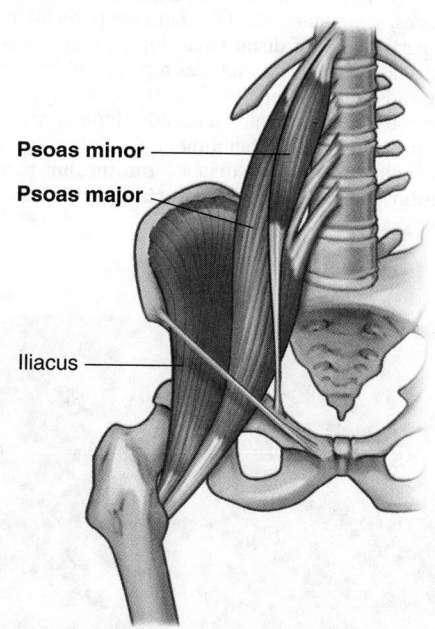

Psoas minor

Psoas major

Iliacus

**Psoas major and minor**

**psoas minor,**    a long, slender muscle of the pelvis, ventral to the psoas major. Many individuals do not have this muscle. The psoas minor functions to flex the spine. Compare **psoas major.**

**psomophagia** /sō'mōfā'jē·ə/,    the swallowing of food that has not been chewed properly.

**psor-,** combining form meaning 'itching': *psora, psorocomium, psorous.*

**psoralen-type photosensitizer** /sôr′ələn/, any one chemical compound that contains photosensitizing psoralen and that reacts on exposure to ultraviolet light to increase the melanin in the skin. Naturally occurring psoralen photosynthesizers, such as 5- and 8-methoxypsoralen, are found in buttercups, carrot greens, celery, clover, cockleburs, dill, figs, limes, parsley, and meadow grass. Some psoralen-type photosensitizers produced as pharmaceutics are methoxsalen and trioxsalen; both are used to enhance skin pigmentation or tanning in the treatment of skin diseases, such as psoriasis and vitiligo. Such drugs are carefully administered to prevent oversensitization of the skin and other complications. Psoralen-type photosensitizers are also used in the manufacture of some perfumes, colognes, and pomades. Such chemicals cause unique skin reactions, such as berlock dermatitis, in some individuals. Oil of bergamot, extracted from the peels of small oranges grown in southern France and Italy, is a photosensitizing psoralen used as a tea flavoring and in perfumes.

**psorelcosis** /sôr′əlkō′sis/, an ulceration of the skin caused by scabies.

**psorenteritis** /sôr′enterī′tis/, an inflammation of the intestines.

**psoriasis** /sərī′əsis/ [Gk, itch], a common chronic skin disorder characterized by circumscribed red patches covered by thick, dry silvery adherent scales that are the result of excessive development of epithelial cells. Exacerbations and remissions are typical. Lesions may be anywhere on the body but are more common on extensor surfaces, bony prominences, scalp, ears, genitalia, and the perianal area. An arthritis, particularly of distal small joints, may accompany the skin disease. Treatment includes topical and intralesional corticosteroids, ultraviolet light, tar solution baths, creams and shampoos, methotrexate, retinoids, topical vitamin D, cyclosporine, and photochemotherapy. Subcategories of psoriasis include **guttate psoriasis, nummular psoriasis,** and **pustular psoriasis.** See also **psoriatic arthritis.** —**psoriatic** /sôr′ē·at′ik/, *adj.*

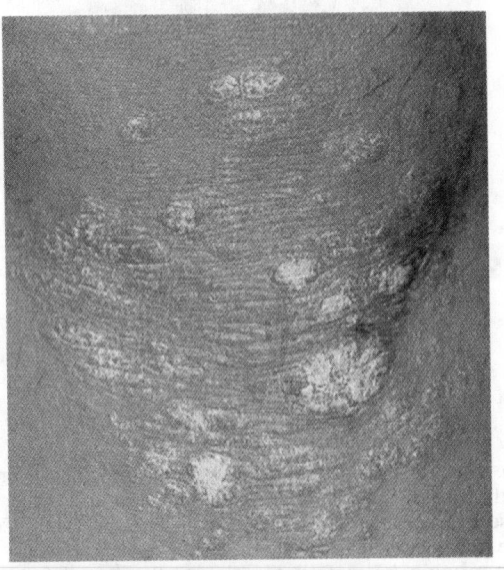

**Psoriasis** *(Habif, 1996)*

**psoriasis universalis** [Gk, *psoriasis,* itch; L, *universus,* on the whole], a severe attack of psoriasis in which most or all of the skin is involved.

**psoriatic.** See **psoriasis.**

**psoriatic arthritis** /sôr′e·at′ik/, a form of arthritis associated with psoriatic lesions of the skin and nails, particularly at the distal interphalangeal joints of the fingers and toes.

**PSRO,** abbreviation for **Professional Standards Review Organization.**

**PSS,** abbreviation for *progressive systemic sclerosis.* See **scleroderma.**

**PSSO,** abbreviation for *peer specialist second opinion, physician support services organization.*

**PSV,** abbreviation for **pressure support ventilation.**

**PSW,** abbreviation for **psychiatric social worker.**

**psych,** abbreviation for **psychology.**

**psych-.** See **psycho-.**

**psychalgia.** See **psychic pain.**

**psychataxia** /sī′kətak′sē·ə/, a condition of mental confusion and inability to concentrate or fix attention.

**psyche** /sī′kē/ [Gk, mind], **1.** the aspect of one's mental faculty that encompasses the conscious and unconscious processes. **2.** the vital mental or spiritual entity of the individual as opposed to the body or soma. **3.** (in psychoanalysis) the total components of the id, ego, and superego, including all conscious and unconscious aspects. Compare **soma.**

**psychedelic** /sī′kədel′ik/ [coined in 1956 by Humphry Osmond from Gk, *psyche* + *deloun,* to reveal], **1.** describing a mental state characterized by altered sensory perception and hallucination, accompanied by euphoria or fear, usually caused by the deliberate ingestion of drugs or other substances known to produce this effect. **2.** describing any drug or substance that causes this state, such as mescaline or psilocybin.

**psychiatric** /sī′kē·at′rik/ [Gk, *psyche,* mind, *iatreia,* treatment], pertaining to psychiatry.

**psychiatric consultation liaison nurse (PCLN),** an advanced practice nurse with a master's degree in psychiatric/mental health nursing. The practice focuses on emotional, spiritual, developmental, cognitive, and behavioral responses of patients with actual or potential physical dysfunction.

**psychiatric disorder.** See **mental disorder.**

**psychiatric emergency service** [Gk, *psyche* + *iatreia,* treatment], a hospital service that provides immediate initial evaluation and treatment to acutely disturbed mental patients on a 24-hour-a-day basis.

**psychiatric foster care,** a service for discharged psychiatric patients who receive observation and care in an approved foster home.

**psychiatric home care,** a service whereby a discharged psychiatric patient is provided observation and care in his or her place of residence. Many state laws require that the client be homebound.

**psychiatric hospital,** a health care facility providing inpatient and outpatient therapeutic services to clients with behavioral or emotional illnesses.

**psychiatric inpatient unit,** a hospital ward or similar area used for the treatment of inpatients who require psychiatric care.

**psychiatric nurse practitioner,** a nurse practitioner who, by advanced study and clinical practice, such as in a master's program in psychiatric nursing, has gained expert knowledge in the care and prevention of mental disorders. See also **psychiatric nursing.**

**psychiatric nursing,** the branch of nursing concerned with the prevention, care, and cure of mental disorders and their sequelae. It uses theories of human behavior as its scientific framework and requires the use of the self as its art or expression in nursing practice. Some of the activities of the psychiatric nurse include providing a safe therapeutic milieu; working with patients or clients on the real day-to-day problems they face; identifying and caring for the physical aspects of the patient's problems, including drug therapy reactions; assuming the role of social agent or parent for the patient in various recreational, occupational, and social situations; conducting psychotherapy; and providing leadership and clinical assistance for other nurses and health care workers. Psychiatric nurses work in many settings; their responsibilities vary with the setting and with the level of expertise, experience, and training of the individual nurse. Also called **mental health nursing.**

**psychiatric social worker (PSW),** a social worker who specializes in or works exclusively with the mentally ill.

**psychiatrist** /sīkī′ətrist/ [Gk, *psyche,* mind, *iatreia,* treatment], a physician with additional medically qualified training and experience in the diagnosis, prevention, and treatment of mental disorders.

**psychiatry** /sīkī′ətrē/ [Gk, *psyche* + *iatreia,* treatment], the branch of medical science that deals with the causes, treatment, and prevention of mental, emotional, and behavioral disorders. Some kinds of psychiatry are **community psychiatry, descriptive psychiatry, dynamic psychiatry, existential psychiatry, forensic psychiatry,** and **orthopsychiatry. —psychiatric,** *adj.*

**psychic** /sī′kik/ [Gk, *psyche,* mind], a practitioner of the systematic study of parapsychology, a category of usually alleged psychologic phenomena that cannot be explained by scientific thinking.

**-psychic,** combining form meaning 'relation between mind and body': *allopsychic, biopsychic, physiopsychic.*

**psychic blindness** [Gk, *psyche,* mind; AS, *blind*], a somatoform disorder that is manifested by the total or partial loss of vision in eyes that are organically normal. Despite the symptoms claimed, the patient usually reacts to light and avoids objects that might cause injury. The condition is frequently the result of an inner conflict or psychologic stress, such as an unconscious effort to avoid a threatening or guilt situation. See also **conversion disorder.**

**psychic contagion.** See **psychic infection.**

**psychic energy,** body energy such as thinking, perceiving, and remembering. See also **libido.**

**psychic impotence** [Gk, *psyche,* mind; L, *in* + *potentia,* power], a functional disorder of the male who is unable to perform sexual intercourse despite normal genitalia and sexual desire. The term generally applies to an inability to achieve and maintain an erection, but the disorder may be manifested in other forms such as premature ejaculation or the need for certain conditions.

**psychic infection** [Gk, *psyche* + L, *inficere,* to stain], the spread of psychic effects or influences on others on a small scale, as in folie á deux, or on a large scale, as in the dance and witch manias of the Middle Ages or the spread of hysteric or panic reactions in a crowd. Also called **psychic contagion.** See also **sympathy.**

**psychic pain** [Gk, *psyche,* mind; L, *poena,* penalty], a functional pain that, in the absence of any organic cause, is usually associated with feelings of acute anxiety. In some cases, the person may experience hallucinations or obsessions. Also called **psychalgia.**

**psychic suicide,** the termination of one's own life without the use of physical means or agents, such as by an older person, widowed after many years of marriage, who becomes sufficiently depressed to lose "the will to live."

**psychic trauma,** an emotional shock or injury or a distressful situation that produces a lasting impression, especially on the subconscious mind. Some causes of psychic trauma may include abuse or neglect in childhood, rape, and loss of a loved one. Psychotherapeutic sessions in which the injured person can ventilate feelings can help alleviate psychic trauma.

**psycho-** /sī′kō-, sī′kə-/, **psych-,** combining form meaning 'the mind': *psychoauditory, psychodynamics, psychedelic.*

**psychoacoustics** /sī′kō-əkoos′tiks/, the branch of science concerned with the physical features of sound as it relates to the psychologic and physiologic aspects of the sense of hearing in the unimpaired ear.

**psychoactive** /sī′kō-ak′tiv/ [Gk, *psyche,* mind; L, *activus*], pertaining to a drug or other agent that affects such normal mental functioning as mood, behavior, or thinking processes. Examples include stimulants, sedatives, or hallucinogens.

**psychoanalysis** /sī′kō-ənal′isis/ [Gk, *psyche* + *analyein,* to separate parts], a branch of psychiatry founded by Sigmund Freud, devoted to the study of the psychology of human development and behavior. From its systematized method for investigating the processes of the mind evolved a system of psychotherapy based on the concepts of a dynamic unconscious. Using such techniques as free association, dream interpretation, and analysis of defense mechanisms, emotions and behavior are traced to the influence of repressed instinctual drives in the unconscious. Treatment consists of helping the individual become aware of the existence of repressed emotional conflicts, analyzing their origin, and through the process of insight bringing them into the consciousness so that irrational and maladaptive behavior can be altered. See also **psychosexual development.**

**psychoanalyst** /sī′kō-an′əlist/, a psychotherapist, usually a psychiatrist, who has had special training in psychoanalysis and who applies the techniques of psychoanalytic theory.

**psychoanalytic** /sī′kō-an′əlit′ik/, **1.** pertaining to psychoanalysis. **2.** using the techniques or principles of psychoanalysis, for example, the study of the unconscious processes, in an attempt to examine causality.

**psychobiologic resilience** /-bī·əloj′ik/, a concept that proposes a recurrent human need to weather periods of stress and change successfully throughout life. The ability to weather each period of disruption and reintegration leaves the person better able to deal with the next change.

**psychobiology** /-bī′ol′əjē/ [Gk, *psyche* + *bios,* life, *logos,* science], **1.** the study of biochemical foundations of thought, mood, emotion, affect, and behavior. **2.** personality development and functioning in terms of the interaction of the body and the mind. **3.** a school of psychiatric thought introduced by Adolf Meyer that stresses total life experience, including biologic, emotional, and sociocultural factors, in assessing the psychologic makeup or mental status of an individual.

**psychocatharsis.** See **catharsis.**

**psychodiagnosis** /-dī′agnō′sis/ [Gk, *psyche,* mind, *dia* + *gnosis,* knowledge], the study of a personality through observations of behavior and mannerisms, combined with various tests.

**psychodrama** /-dram′ə/, a form of group psychotherapy, originated by J.L. Moreno, in which people act out their emotional problems through improvisational dramatizations.

**psychodynamics** /-dīnam′iks/ [Gk, *psyche* + *dynamis,* power], the study of the forces that motivate behavior. It may include the influence of past experiences on present behavior and the influence of mental and emotional forces on development and behavior.

**psychoendocrinology** /sī′kō·en′dōkrinol′əjē/,  the study of the relationship between endocrinology and psychology.

**psychoesthesia,**  a sensation of cold perceived although the body is warm.

**psychogalvanic** /-galvan′ik/,  pertaining to the effects of psychologic influences on the electrical properties of skin.

**psychogender** /-jen′dər/,  the psychologic sex as expressed in gender attitudes of a person as distinguished from biologic or somatic sex.

**psychogenesis** /sī′kōjen′əsis/ [Gk, *psyche* + *genesis,* origin],  **1.** the development of the mind or of a mental function or process. **2.** the development or production of a physical symptom or disease having a mental or psychic origin rather than an organic cause. **3.** the development of emotional states, either normal or abnormal, from the interaction of conscious and unconscious psychologic forces. Compare **somatogenesis.**

**psychogenic** /sī′kōjen′ik/ [Gk, *psyche* + *genein,* to produce],  **1.** originating within the mind. **2.** referring to any physical symptom, disease process, or emotional state that is of psychologic rather than physical origin. Also **psychogenetic.** See also **psychosomatic.**

**psychogenic pain** [Gk, *psyche,* mind; L, *poena,* penalty], a functional pain that does not have any known organic cause.

**psychogenic pain disorder,**  a *DSM-IV* psychiatric disorder characterized by persistent pain for which there is no apparent organic cause. The condition is often accompanied by other sensory or motor dysfunction, such as paresthesia or muscle spasm. The cause may be one or many unresolved needs or conflicts.

**psychogenic vomiting,**  vomiting that is stimulated by anxiety and emotional distress.

**psychogeusic** /-joo′sik/,  pertaining to the psychologic influences in taste.

**psychokinesia** /sī′kōkinē′zhə, -kīnē′zhə/ [Gk, *psyche* + *kinesis,* motion],  **1.** impulsive behavior resulting from deficient or defective inhibitions without benefit of processing between the stimulus and the response. **2.** (in parapsychology) psychokinesis.

**psychokinesis (PK)** /sī′kōkinē′sis, -kīnē′sis/ [Gk, *psyche* + *kinesis,* motion],  the alleged direct influence of the mind or will on matter to produce motion in objects without the intervention of the physical senses or a physical force.

**psychokinetics** /sī′kōkinet′iks, -kīnet′iks/,  the study of psychokinesis.

**psycholinguistics** /-ling·gwis′tiks/,  the study of language as a form of behavior, including language development, speech, and personality.

**psychologic, psychological** /sī′kəloj′ik/ [Gk, *psyche,* mind, *logos,* science],  pertaining to or involving psychology. Also **psychological.**

**psychologic miscarriage,**  an absence or deficiency of a mother's love for her infant or absence of mother-child bonding.

**psychologic test** [Gk, *psyche* + *logos,* science; L, *testum,* crucible],  any of a group of standardized tests designed to measure or ascertain such characteristics of an individual as intellectual capacity, motivation, perception, role behavior, values, level of anxiety or depression, coping mechanisms, and general personality integration. Compare **achievement test, aptitude test, intelligence test, personality test.**

**psychologist** /sīkol′əjist/,  a person who specializes in the study of the structure and function of the brain and related

mental processes of animals and humans. A clinical psychologist is one who is qualified by graduate study in psychology and training in clinical psychology and who provides testing and counseling services to patients with mental and emotional disorders.

**psychology (psych)** /sīkol′əjē/ [Gk, *psyche* + *logos,* science],  **1.** the study of behavior and of the functions and processes of the mind, especially as related to the social and physical environment. **2.** a profession that involves the practical applications of knowledge, skills, and techniques in the understanding of, prevention of, or solution to individual or social problems, especially in regard to the interaction between the individual and the physical and social environment. **3.** the mental, motivational, and behavioral characteristics and attitudes of an individual or group of individuals. Kinds of psychology include **analytic psychology, animal psychology, behaviorism, clinical psychology, cognitive psychology, educational psychology, experimental psychology, humanistic psychology, phenomenology,** and **social psychology. —psychologic, psychological,** *adj.*

**psychometrician** /-mətrish′ən/ [Gk, *psyche,* mind, *metron,* measure],  a specialist who performs quantitative estimation or measurement of personality and intelligence. The testing is not treatment oriented.

**psychometrics** /sī′kōmet′riks/ [Gk, *psyche* + *metron,* measure],  the development, administration, or interpretation of psychologic and intelligence tests. Also called **psychometry.**

**psychomotor** /-mō′tər/ [Gk, *psyche* + L, *motare,* to move about],  pertaining to or causing voluntary movements usually associated with neural activity.

**psychomotor and physical development of infants,**  a branch of pediatric psychiatry that is concerned with the development of skills requiring coordination of sensory processes and motor activities, including infant reflexes, developmental timetables, and emotional and behavioral disorders.

**psychomotor development,**  the progressive attainment by the child of skills that involve both mental and muscular activity, such as the ability of the infant to turn over, sit, or crawl at will and of the toddler to walk, talk, control bladder and bowel functions, and begin solving cognitive problems. The mean chronologic ages at which certain psychomotor skills are attained by most children follow.

| | |
|---|---|
| 12 weeks | Looks at own hand. |
| 20 weeks | Able to grasp objects voluntarily. |
| 24 weeks | Able to roll from back to front at will. |
| 11 months | Creeps with abdomen off the floor and imitates speech sounds. |
| 15 months | Able to walk without help. |
| 24 months | Has a vocabulary of 300 or more words and uses pronouns. |
| 30 months | Able to jump with both feet. |
| 3 years | Able to ride a tricycle and to feed self well. |
| 4 years | Able to hop and skip on one foot, catch and throw a ball; is independent, boasts, tattles, and shows off. |
| 5 years | Able to tie shoelaces and cut with scissors, tries to please, interested in facts about world, gets along more easily with parents. |

**psychomotor domain,**  the area of observable performance of skills that require some degree of neuromuscular coordination.

**psychomotor energy,**  a nursing outcome from the Nursing Outcomes Classification (NOC) defined as the ability to maintain activities of daily living, nutrition, and personal safety. See also **Nursing Outcomes Classification.**

**psychomotor epilepsy.** See **psychomotor seizure.**

**psychomotor learning,** the acquisition of ability to perform motor skills.

**psychomotor retardation,** a generalized slowing of motor activity related to a state of severe depression or dementia.

**psychomotor seizure,** a temporary impairment of consciousness, characterized by psychic symptoms, loss of judgment, automatic behavior, and abnormal acts. It is often associated with temporal lobe disease. No apparent convulsions occur, but there may be loss of consciousness or amnesia for the episode. During the seizure the individual may appear drowsy, intoxicated, or violent; asocial acts or crimes may be committed, but normal activities, such as driving a car, typing, or eating, may continue at an automatic level. Psychic symptoms, including visual and auditory hallucinations, a sense of unreality, and déjà vu, may be present and may be accompanied by visceral symptoms, such as chest pain, transient respiratory arrest, tachycardia, and GI discomfort, and by abnormal sensations of smell and taste. Also called **psychomotor epilepsy.**

**psychoneuroimmunology** /-nŏŏr′ō·imyŏŏnol′əjē/, a discipline that studies the relationships between psychologic states and the immune response.

**psychoneurosis.** See **neurosis.**

**psychoneurotic.** See **neurotic.**

**psychoneurotic disorder.** See **neurosis.**

**psychooncology** /sī′kō·ongkol′əjē/, the psychologic effects of cancer, particularly the psychosocial needs of the patient and the patient's family.

**psychopath** /sī′kōpath/ [Gk, *psyche + pathos,* disease], a person who has an antisocial personality disorder. Also called **sociopath.** See also **antisocial personality, antisocial personality disorder. —psychopathic,** *adj.*

**psychopathia.** See **psychopathy.**

**psychopathia sexualis** /sī′kōpā′thē·ə sek′shŏŏ·al′is/ [Gk, *psyche + pathos,* disease; L, *sexus,* male or female], a mental disease characterized by sexual perversion.

**psychopathic.** See **psychopath.**

**psychopathic personality.** See **antisocial personality.**

**psychopathologist** /-pəthol′əjist/, one who specializes in the study and treatment of mental disorders. See also **psychiatrist.**

**psychopathology** /-pəthol′əjē/, **1.** the study of the causes, processes, and manifestations of mental disorders. **2.** the behavioral manifestation of any mental disorder. See also **psychiatry.**

**psychopathy** /sīkop′əthē/, any disease of the mind, congenital or acquired, not necessarily associated with subnormal intelligence. Also called **psychopathia.**

**psychopharmaceutical** /-fär′məsŏŏ′tikəl/ a drug used in the treatment of mental health disorders.

**psychopharmacology** /-fär′məkol′əjē/, [Gk, *psyche + pharmakon,* drug, *logos,* science], the scientific study of the effects of drugs on behavior and normal and abnormal mental functions. In some age groups, psychoactive drugs are among the most commonly prescribed medications. Psychoactive drugs include antidepressants, anxiolytics, antipsychotics or neuroleptics, hypnotics, muscle relaxants, anticonvulsants, antiparkinsonian drugs, lithium for bipolar disorders, and drugs that enhance cognitive function. Each psychoactive drug category includes a choice of several agents with similar efficacy. In addition to prescribed psychoactive drugs, patients usually have access to illicit drugs such as hallucinogens, LSD, peyote, morning glory

seeds, mescaline, psilocybin, nutmeg, marijuana, inhalants, tryptamine, alcohol, and amphetamines, as well as myriad over-the-counter preparations that are ingested or inhaled to enhance the well-being of the individual and to relieve pain or digestive upset. In some cases, vitamins have found a role as psychopharmacologic drugs, as in the administration of niacin in the treatment of cerebral pathology of pellagra, thiamine for Wernicke-Korsakoff syndrome, and vitamin $B_{12}$ for certain types of dementia.

**psychophylaxis.** See **mental hygiene.**

**psychophysical** /-fiz′ikəl/, pertaining to the psychosocial and physical aspects of a client's health and illness.

**psychophysical preparation for childbirth,** a program that prepares women for giving birth by teaching them the physiologic characteristics of the process, exercises to improve muscle tone and physical stamina, and various techniques of breathing and relaxation to promote control and comfort during labor and delivery. There are several methods of psychophysical preparation for childbirth. Among the goals of all of the methods are a decrease in the mother's fear and pain, a decrease in or elimination of the use of analgesia and anesthesia in childbirth, and an increase in the mother's participation and cooperation, with a resulting reduced need for obstetric intervention. Methods of psychophysical preparation for childbirth include the **Bradley method, Lamaze method, Leboyer method,** and **Read method.**

**psychophysics** /-fiz′iks/ [Gk, *psyche + physikos,* natural], the branch of psychology concerned with the relationships between physical stimuli and sensory responses.

**psychophysiologic** /-fiz′ē·əloj′ik/ [Gk, *psyche + physikos,* natural], having physical symptoms, usually under the control of the autonomic nervous system, having emotional origins and involving a single organ system; psychosomatic.

**psychophysiologic disorder,** any of a large group of mental disorders that is characterized by the dysfunction of an organ or organ system controlled by the autonomic nervous system and that may be caused or aggravated by emotional factors. The disorders are named and classified according to the organ system involved, such as cardiovascular, respiratory, musculoskeletal, and GI. Also called **psychosomatic illness, psychosomatic reaction.**

**psychophysiology** /-fiz′ē·ol′əjē/, **1.** the study of physiology as it relates to various aspects of psychologic or behavioral function. See also **psychophysiologic disorder. 2.** the study of mental activity by physical examination and observation.

**psychoprophylactic preparation for childbirth** /-prō′filak′tik/, a system of prenatal education for giving birth using the Lamaze method of natural childbirth. See also **psychophysical preparation for childbirth.**

**psychoprophylaxis** /-prō′filak′sis/, a type of psychotherapy that is directed to prevention of emotional disorders. For example, it is used in the preparation for childbirth to reduce a woman's anxiety about pain and birth of a normal child.

**psychorelaxation** /-ri′laksā′shən/, the systematic desensitization of stress and anxiety by the practice of general body relaxation.

**psychosensory** /-sen′sərē/, pertaining to the perception and interpretation of sensory stimuli.

**psychoses.** See **psychosis.**

**psychosexual** /-sek′shŏŏ·əl/ [Gk, *psyche + L, sexus,* male or female], pertaining to the psychologic and emotional aspects of sex. See also **psychosexual development, sexual disorder. —psychosexuality,** *n.*

**psychosexual development,** (in psychoanalysis) the emergence of the personality through a series of stages from infancy to adulthood. Each stage is relatively fixed in time and characterized by a dominant mode of achieving libidinal pleasure through the interaction of the person's biologic drives and the environmental restraints.

**psychosexual disorder.** See **sexual disorder.**

**psychosexual dysfunction.** See **sexual disorder.**

**psychosexuality.** See **psychosexual.**

**psychosis** /sīkō′sis/, *pl.* **psychoses** [Gk, *psyche* + *osis,* condition], any major mental disorder of organic or emotional origin characterized by a gross impairment in reality testing; the individual incorrectly evaluates the accuracy of his or her perceptions and thoughts and makes incorrect references about external reality, even in the face of contrary evidence. It is often characterized by regressive behavior, inappropriate mood and affect, and diminished impulse control. Symptoms of psychoses include hallucinations and delusions.

**-psychosis,** combining form meaning a 'serious mental disorder': *autopsychosis, encephalopsychosis, pharmacopsychosis.*

**psychosocial** /-sō′shəl/, [Gr, *psyche* + L, *socialis,* partners], pertaining to a combination of psychologic and social factors.

**psychosocial adjustment: life change,** a nursing outcome from the Nursing Outcomes Classification (NOC) defined as the psychosocial adaptation of an individual to a life change. See also **Nursing Outcomes Classification.**

**psychosocial assessment,** an evaluation of a person's mental health, social status, and functional capacity within the community. It is generally conducted by psychiatric social workers.

**psychosocial development,** (in child development) a description devised by Erik Erikson of the normal serial development of trust, autonomy, initiative, industry, identity, intimacy, generativity, and integrity; the development begins in infancy and progresses as the infantile ego interacts with the environment. For the child to reach a new stage successfully, the tasks of the preceding one should be fully mastered. The sequence and chronology of the stages coincide with the psychosexual stages of development as described by Freud.

**psychosomatic** /sī′kōsəmat′ik/ [Gk, *psyche* + *soma,* body], **1.** pertaining to psychosomatic medicine. **2.** relating to, characterized by, or resulting from the interaction of the mind or psyche and the body. **3.** the expression of an emotional conflict through physical symptoms. See also **conversion disorder, psychogenic, psychophysiologic disorder.**

**psychosomatic approach,** the interdisciplinary or holistic study of physical and mental disease from a biologic, psychosocial, and sociocultural point of view.

**psychosomatic illness.** See **psychophysiologic disorder.**

**psychosomatic medicine,** the branch of medicine concerned with the interrelationships between mental and emotional reactions and somatic processes, in particular the manner in which intrapsychic conflicts influence physical symptoms. It maintains that the body and mind are one inseparable entity and that both physiologic and psychologic techniques should be applied in the study and treatment of illness. Also called **psychosomatics.**

**psychosomatic pain** [Gk, *psyche,* mind, *soma,* body; L, *poena,* penalty], pain that is caused in part by psychologic factors.

**psychosomatic reaction.** See **psychophysiologic disorder.**

**psychosomatics.** See **psychosomatic medicine.**

**psychosomatogenic** /-sōmat′əjen′ik/, pertaining to factors that cause or lead to the development of psychophysiologic coping measures as learned responses to stressors.

**psychostimulant** /-stim′yələnt/, an agent with mood-elevating or antidepressant effects.

**psychosurgery** /-sur′jərē/ [Gk, *psyche* + *cheirourgia*], surgical interruption of certain nerve pathways in the brain, performed to treat selected cases of chronic unremitting anxiety, agitation, or obsessional neuroses. Psychosurgery is performed when the condition is severe and when alternative treatments, such as psychotherapy, drugs, and electroshock, have proved ineffective. The procedure may be a limited prefrontal lobotomy, in which connecting fibers in the frontal region are cut, or a modified bifrontal tractotomy, in which nerve tracts of the brainstem are severed. Light general anesthesia is given. Postoperative nursing care includes observation for signs of leakage of cerebrospinal fluid. A marked alteration of personality is unavoidable. Various cognitive and affective functions also are affected, depending on the location of the induced lesion, the extent of destruction of nerve tissue, and the age, sex, and condition of the patient. Modern psychotherapeutic drugs have replaced psychosurgery in most cases.

**psychosynthesis** /-sin′thəsis/, a form of psychotherapy that focuses on three levels of the unconscious—lower, middle, and higher unconscious, or superconscious. The goal of the treatment is the re-creation or integration of the personality.

**psychotaxia,** a condition of mental confusion and inability to concentrate or fix attention.

**psychotherapeutic drugs** /-ther′əp(y)oo′tik/ [Gk, *psyche,* mind, *therapeutike,* medical practice; Fr, *drogue*], drugs that are prescribed for their effects in relieving symptoms of anxiety, depression, or other mental disorders.

**psychotherapeutics** /-tiks/ [Gk, *psyche* + *therapeia,* treatment], the treatment of personality disorders by means of psychotherapy.

**psychotherapist** /-ther′əpist/, one who practices psychotherapy, including psychiatrists, licensed psychologists, psychiatric nurses, psychiatric social workers, and individuals trained in counseling. The specific requirements for education and training differ markedly in content, breadth, and duration, depending on the form of psychotherapy practiced. Licensing procedures and definitions of practice vary from state to state. Compare **psychoanalyst.**

**psychotherapy** /-ther′əpē/ [Gk, *psyche* + *therapeia,* treatment], any of a large number of related methods of treating mental and emotional disorders by psychologic techniques rather than by physical means.

**psychotic** /sīkot′ik/ [Gk, *psyche* + *osis,* condition], **1.** pertaining to psychosis. **2.** a person exhibiting the characteristics of a psychosis. **3.** Not in contact with reality.

**psychotic disorder.** See **psychosis.**

**psychotic insight,** a stage in the development of a psychosis that follows an initial experience of confusion, bizarreness, and apprehension. At this point, an insight is reached that enables the patient to interpret the external world in terms of a delusional system of thinking. With the new insight, the factors that had previously been confusing become a part of the systematized pattern of the delusion, which, although irrational to an observer, is perceived by the patient as the attainment of exceptionally lucid thinking.

**psychotic reaction.** See **psychosis.**

**psychotogenic** /sīkot′əjen′ik/, pertaining to an agent that is capable of inducing symptoms of psychosis.

**psychotomimetic** /sīkot′ōmimet′ik/, a drug or other substance whose effects mimic the symptoms of psychosis, such as hallucinations.

**psychotropic** /-trop′ik/ [Gk, *psyche* + *trepein,* to turn], exerting an effect on the mind or modifying mental activity, as in psychotropic medications.

**psychotropic drugs,** drugs that affect the psychic functions, behavior, or experience of a person using them.

**psychro-,** combining form meaning 'cold': *psychrometer, psychrophilic, psychrophore.*

**psychroesthesia** /si′krō·esthē′zhə/, **1.** a chill. **2.** a sensation of cold although the body is warm.

**psychrometer** /sīkrom′ətər/, an instrument for calculating the degree of humidity in the atmosphere by comparing the temperatures of two thermometers, one with a wet bulb, one dry. The difference in temperature between the two thermometers indicates the relative humidity.

**psychrometry** /sīkrom′ətrē/, the calculation of relative humidity and water vapor pressure from psychrometer data and barometric pressure.

**psychrophore** /sī′krəfôr′/, a double-lumen catheter through which cold water is circulated.

**psyllium seed.** See **plantago seed.**

**Pt,** symbol for the element **platinum.**

**PT, 1.** abbreviation for **physical therapist. 2.** abbreviation for **physical therapy. 3.** abbreviation for **prothrombin time.**

**pt., 1.** abbreviation for *pint.* **2.** abbreviation for **patient.**

**PTA, 1.** abbreviation for **percutaneous transluminal angioplasty. 2.** abbreviation for **plasma thromboplastin antecedent.**

**PTB,** abbreviation for **patellar-tendon bearing prosthesis.**

**PTB/SC,** abbreviation for **patellar-tendon bearing supracondylar socket.**

**PTCA,** abbreviation for **percutaneous transluminal coronary angioplasty.**

**PTEN,** abbreviation for **pentaerythritol tetranitrate.**

**pterion** /tir′ē·on/, a point near the sphenoid fontanel of the skull, at the junction of the greater wing of the sphenoid, squamous, temporal, frontal, and parietal bones. It also intersects the course of the anterior division of the middle meningeal artery.

**pteroylglutamic acid.** See **folic acid.**

**pterygium** /tərij′ē·əm/ [Gk, *pterygion,* wing], a thick triangular patch of pale hypertrophied tissue that extends medially from the nasal border of the cornea to the inner canthus of the eye.

**-pterygium,** suffix meaning a '(specified) abnormality of the conjunctiva': *loxopterygium, pimelopterygium, symblepharopterygium.*

**pterygium colli.** See **webbed neck.**

**pterygium syndrome.** See **multiple pterygium syndrome.**

**pterygoid** /ter′igoid/ [Gk, *pteryx,* wing, *eidos,* form], pertaining to a winglike structure.

**pterygoideus lateralis.** See **external pterygoid muscle.**

**pterygoideus medialis.** See **internal pterygoid muscle.**

**pterygoid plexus,** one of a pair of extensive networks of veins between the temporalis and the pterygoideus lateralis muscles, extending between surrounding structures in the infratemporal fossa. It communicates with the facial vein through the deep facial and angular veins. Compare **maxillary vein.**

**pterygoid process** [Gk, *pteryx,* wing, *eidos,* form; L, *processus*], any one of the paired processes of the sphenoid bone.

**pterygomandibular** /ter′igōmandib′yələr/ [Gk, *pteryx,* wing, *eidos,* form; L, *mandere,* to chew], pertaining to the pterygoid process and the mandible.

**pterygomaxillary** /-mak′siler′ē/ [Gk, *pteryx,* wing, *eidos,* form; L, *maxilla,* jaw], pertaining to the sphenoid bone and the maxilla.

**pterygomaxillary notch,** a fissure at the junction of the maxilla and the pterygoid process of the sphenoid bone. Also called **hamular notch.**

**PTH,** abbreviation for **parathyroid hormone.**

*Pthirus pubis.* See **crab louse.**

**PTNA,** abbreviation for **Provincial/Territorial Nurses Association.**

**ptoma-** /tō′mə-/, combining form meaning 'corpse': *ptomaine, ptomatopsia, ptomatopsy.*

**ptomaine** /tō′mān/ [Gk, *ptoma,* corpse], an imprecise term introduced in the nineteenth century to identify a group of nitrogenous substances found in putrefied proteins. Because injection of the substances produced toxic reactions, the ptomaines were once regarded as poisonous. Later studies showed the same substances were produced by the normal digestion of proteins in the human intestine without toxic effects.

**ptomainemia** /tō′mānē′mē·ə/, a condition caused by the presence of a ptomaine, a potentially toxic amine, in the blood.

**ptosis** /tō′sis/ [Gk, falling], an abnormal condition of one or both upper eyelids in which the eyelid droops because of a congenital or acquired weakness of the levator muscle or paralysis of the third cranial nerve. The condition may be treated surgically by shortening the levator muscle. —**ptotic,** *adj.*

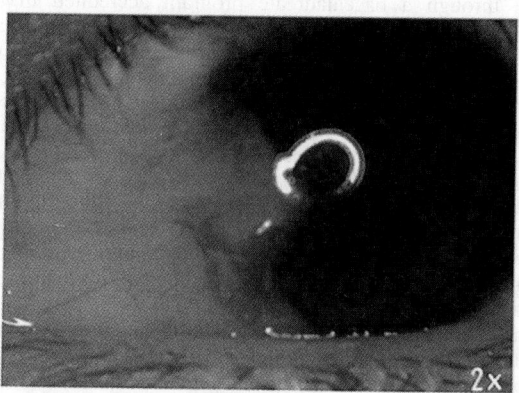

**Pterygium** *(Newell, 1996)*

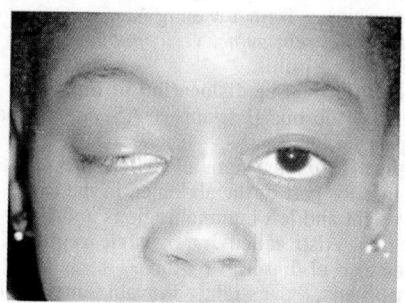

**Ptosis** *(Stein, Slatt, and Stein, 1994)*

**-ptosis,** suffix meaning a 'falling, dropping, or prolapse of an organ': *esophagoptosis, hepatoptosis, uvulaptosis.*

**ptotic kidney** /tot'ik/, a kidney that is abnormally situated in the pelvis, usually over the sacral promontory behind the peritoneum. The condition may be either congenital or secondary to trauma. It is usually asymptomatic, but during pregnancy the flow of urine from a ptotic kidney may be obstructed.

**PTSD,** abbreviation for **posttraumatic stress disorder.**

**PTT.** See **partial thromboplastin time.**

**ptyalin** /tī'əlin/ [Gk, *ptyalon,* spittle], a starch-digesting enzyme present in saliva. It hydrolyzes starch and glycogen. Its optimal pH is 6.9. Also called **amylase.**

**ptyalism** /tī'əliz'əm/ [Gk, *ptyalon,* spittle], excessive salivation, such as sometimes occurs in the early months of pregnancy. It is also a clinical sign of mercury poisoning. Also called **hyperptyalism.** See also **sialorrhea.**

**ptyalo-** /tī'əlō/, combining form meaning 'saliva': *ptyalocele, ptyalogenic, ptyalography.*

**ptyocrinous** /tī-ok'rinəs/, pertaining to the secretion of the contents of a unicellular gland in the form of extruded granules.

**p-type semiconductor.** See **semiconductor.**

**-ptysis,** combining form meaning a 'spitting of matter': *albuminoptysis, hemoptysis, plasmoptysis.*

**Pu,** symbol for the element **plutonium.**

**pub-, pubo-,** combining form meaning 'grown up or adult': *puberal, puberty, pubescence.*

**pubarche** /pyoobär'kē, pyoo'bärkē/ [L, *puber,* ripe, *arch,* beginning], onset of puberty. It is marked by the beginning of the development of secondary sexual characteristics.

**pubertal** /p(y)oo'bərtəl/ [L, *pubertas,* age of maturity], pertaining to puberty.

**puberty** /p(y)oo'bərtē/ [L, *pubertas,* age of maturity], the period of life at which the ability to reproduce begins. It is a stage of development when genitalia reach maturity and secondary sex characteristics appear. The onset normally occurs in females between 9 and 13 years of age with the development of breasts and during the phase of menarche. In males, puberty usually occurs between 12 and 14 years of age and is characterized by the ejaculation of sperm.

**puberulic acid** /pyoober'yoolik/, an antibiotic isolated from the mold *Penicillium puberulum* that prevents the replication of gram-positive bacteria.

**pubes.** See **pubis.**

**pubescent** /p(y)oobes'ənt/ [L, *pubescere,* to reach puberty], pertaining to the beginning of puberty.

**pubescent uterus** [L, *pubescere,* to reach puberty, *uterus,* womb], a uterus in which the cervix and body remain of equal length, the premenstruation state, in adult life.

**pubic** /p(y)oo'bik/ [L, *pubis*], pertaining to or involving the region of the pubic symphysis.

**-pubic,** combining form meaning 'the frontal part of the pelvis': *iliopubic, retropubic, vesicopubic.*

**pubic bone.** See **pubis.**

**pubic dislocation.** See **dislocation of hip.**

**pubic hair** /p(y)oo'bik/ [L, *pubis* + AS, *haer*], hair of the pubic region.

**pubic region** [L, *pubes,* signs of maturity, *regio,* territory], the most inferior part of the abdomen in the lower zone between the right and left inguinal regions and below the umbilical region. Also called **hypogastric region, hypogastrium.** See also **abdominal regions.**

**pubic symphysis,** the slightly movable interpubic joint of the pelvis, consisting of two pubic bones separated by a disk of fibrocartilage and connected by two ligaments. Also called **symphysis pubis.**

**pubiotomy** /p(y)oo'bi·ot'əmē/, the separation of the pubic bone, performed to increase the capacity of the pelvis to permit passage of a fetus. Also called **pelviotomy.**

**pubis** /pyoo'bis/, *pl.* **pubes** [L, *pubes*], one of a pair of pubic bones that, with the ischium and the ilium, form the hip bone and join the pubic bone from the opposite side at the pubic symphysis. The pubis forms one fifth of the acetabulum and is divisible into the body, the superior ramus, and the inferior ramus. The external surface of the pubis serves as the origin of the adductor longus, the obturator externus, the adductor brevis, and the proximal part of the gracilis. The internal surface of the pubis forms part of the anterior wall of the pelvis, giving origin to the levator ani and the obturator internus. The pubic crest affords attachment to the rectus abdominis, the pyramidalis, and the inguinal falx. The lateral part of the superior ramus of the pubis presents the superior, the inferior, and the dorsal surfaces. The superior surface presents the iliopectineal line. The inferior ramus gives origin to the gracilis, a part of the obturator externus, the adductor brevis, the adductor magnus, the obturator internus, and the constrictor urethrae. Compare **ilium, ischium.**

**public health** [L, *publicus,* of the people; AS, *haelth*], a field of medicine that deals with the physical and mental health of the community, particularly in such areas as water supply, waste disposal, air pollution, and food safety. In the United States there are more than 3000 state, county, or city public health agencies. The U.S. Public Health Service was organized in 1798 to provide hospital care for American merchant seamen. Subsequent legislation has expanded the role of the federal agency to include such services as the Food and Drug Administration; the National Library of Medicine; health care for Native Americans and Alaska Natives; protection against impure and unsafe foods, drugs, cosmetics, and medical devices; control of alcohol and drug abuse; and protection against unsafe radiation-producing projects.

**public health dentistry.** See **dental public health.**

**public health nursing,** a field of nursing that is concerned with the health needs of the community as a whole. Public health nurses may work with families in the home, in schools, at the workplace, in government agencies, and at major health facilities. A home care nursing service is provided by nurses who have special education in public health and are employed by such voluntary agencies as the Visiting Nurses Association or Visiting Nurse Service, or Victorian Order of Nurses for Canada. Public health nurses enter practice through a baccalaureate program accredited in the United States by the National League for Nursing (NLN) accrediting commission or the American Association of Colleges of Nursing (AACN), which prepares them to work as generalists. Additional recognition is offered through a certification program sponsored by the Division of Community Health Nursing of the American Nurses Association.

**public sector,** (in health care) typically, government at the federal, state, provincial, and local levels; may refer to other community organizations and lobbying groups.

**publish or perish** [L, *publicare,* to make public, *perire,* to come to naught], *informal.* a practice followed in many academic institutions in which a contract for employment is renewed at the same rank only if a candidate has demonstrated scholarship and professional status by having had work published in a book or in a reputable refereed professional or scientific journal. This work is required in addition to whatever obligations for teaching or professional practice are entailed in the position.

**pubo-.**   See **pub-.**

**pubocapsular** /p(y)o͞o′bōkap′sələr/,   pertaining to the pubis and articular capsule of the hip joint.

**pubococcygeal** /p(y)o͞o′bōkoksij′ē·əl/ [L, *pubis* + Gk, *kokkyx,* cuckoo's beak],   pertaining to the pubis and the coccyx.

**pubococcygeus exercises** /pyo͞o′bōkoksij′ē·əs/ [L, *pubes* + Gk, *kokkyx,* cuckoo's beak; L, *exercere,* to make strong],   a regimen of isometric exercises in which a woman executes a series of voluntary contractions of the muscles of her pelvic diaphragm and perineum in an effort to increase the contractility of her vaginal introitus or to improve retention of urine. Also called **Kegel exercises.**

■ METHOD: The exercise involves the familiar muscular squeezing action that is required to stop the urinary stream while voiding; that action is performed in an intensive, repetitive, and systematic way throughout each day.

■ INTERVENTIONS: The woman is instructed in how to duplicate the squeezing, pulling-up action. A woman whose muscles are particularly attenuated may have difficulty understanding or feeling the muscular action involved. It is often helpful for her to be told that the action is exactly the same as that required to stop the flow of urine. When the woman can effect the contraction required, she is asked to hold the contraction for 6 to 10 seconds, allowing the muscles to relax completely between contractions. She is then advised to perform 10 to 15 repetitions of the contraction in a series and to repeat the series three to four times each day. She is further advised that the physiologic nature of muscular exercise is such that weakened muscles may gain strength during the early phases of an exercise program, and that, with diligence, she can expect to notice significant improvement in control that will continue as she maintains the regimen of exercise.

■ OUTCOME CRITERIA: Laxity and weakness of the pubococcygeus muscles, often a result of childbirth, may predispose certain women to looseness of the vaginal introitus and to stress incontinence. These problems may be ameliorated as the strength and tone of the muscles are increased through exercise. The rapidity with which a woman can, during voiding, close off the urinary stream is taken as a measure of the strength and tone of her pubococcygeus muscles. Ideally she should be able to perform the action completely and almost instantly.

**puboprostatic** /p(y)o͞o′bōprostat′ik/,   relating to the pubis and prostate gland.

**pudenda, pudendal.**   See **pudendum.**

**pudendal block** /p(y)o͞oden′təl/ [L, *pudendus,* shameful; Fr, *bloc,* lump],   a form of regional anesthetic block administered to provide anesthesia of the perineum, which is particularly useful during the expulsive second stage of labor. The pudendal nerves are anesthetized by the injection of a local anesthetic near the trunk of each nerve as it passes over the sacrospinous ligament, just below the ischial spine. A 10 ml syringe, a long needle, and a guide are used in the procedure. The injection is most easily performed transvaginally. Pudendal block anesthetizes the perineum, vulva, clitoris, labia majora, and perirectal area without affecting the muscular contractions of the uterus. When the block is properly administered, the risk is minimal.

**pudendal canal.**   See **Alcock's canal.**

**pudendal nerve,**   one of the branches of the pudendal plexus that arises from the second, third, and fourth sacral nerves; passes between the piriformis and coccygeus; and

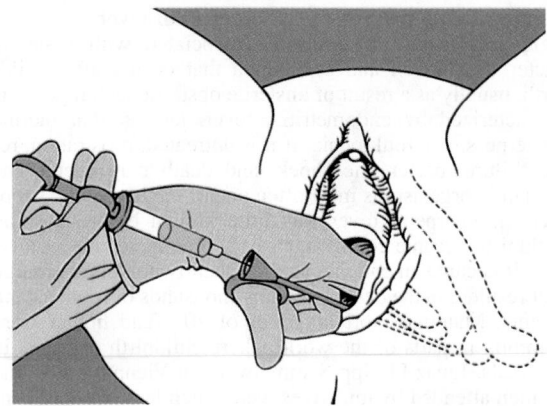

**Pudendal block** *(Lowdermilk, Perry, and Bobak, 2000)*

leaves the pelvis through the greater sciatic foramen. It divides into five branches supplying the external genital structures and the pelvic region. The branches of the pudendal nerve are the inferior rectal nerve, perineal nerve, and dorsal nerve of the penis or of the clitoris. See also **pudendal plexus.**

**pudendal plexus,**   a network of motor and sensory nerves formed by the anterior branches of the second, the third, and all of the fourth sacral nerves. It is often considered part of the sacral plexus. The pudendal plexus lies in the posterior hollow of the pelvis. The branches of the plexus are the visceral branches, the muscular branches, and the pudendal nerve. The visceral branches arise from the second, third, and fourth sacral nerves and supply the bladder, prostate, seminal vesicles, uterus, external genitalia, and some of the intestinal tract. The muscular branches arise from the fourth and sometimes the third and fifth sacral nerves and supply the levator ani, sphincter ani, and coccygeus. Compare **lumbar plexus, sacral plexus.** See also **pudendal nerve.**

**pudendum** /p(y)o͞oden′dəm/, *pl.* **pudenda** [L, *pudendus,* shameful],   the external genitalia, especially of women. In a woman it comprises the mons veneris, the labia majora, the labia minora, the vestibule of the vagina, and the vestibular glands. In a man it comprises the penis, scrotum, and testes. —**pudendal,** *adj.*

**puer-,**   combining form meaning 'child': *puericulture, puerilism, puerperium, puerperal.*

**puericulture** /pyo͝o′ərikul′chər/ [L, *pueri,* children, *colere,* to cultivate],   the rearing and training of children. —**puericulturist,** *n.*

**puerile** /pyo͞o′əril, -īl/ [L, *puerilis,* childish],   pertaining to children or childhood; juvenile. —**puerility,** *n.*

**puerilism** /pyo͞o′əriliz′əm/ [L, *puerilis,* childish],   childishness, particularly when manifested in an older adult.

**puerility.**   See **puerile.**

**puerpera** /pyo͞o·er′pərə/ [L, *puerpus,* childbirth],   a woman who has just given birth.

**puerperal** /pyo͞o·er′pərəl/ [L, *puerpus,* childbirth],   **1.** pertaining to the period immediately after childbirth. **2.** pertaining to a woman (a puerpera) who has just given birth to an infant.

**puerperal eclampsia** [L, *puerpus,* childbirth; Gk, *ek,* out, *lampein,* to flash],   a condition of coma and convulsive seizures occurring after childbirth. It is associated with hypertension, edema, and proteinuria. See also **puerperal fever.**

**puerperal endometritis.** See **puerperal fever.**

**puerperal fever,** a syndrome associated with systemic bacterial infection and septicemia that occurs after childbirth, usually as a result of unsterile obstetric technique. It is characterized by endometritis, fever, tachycardia, uterine tenderness, and foul lochia; if it is untreated, prostration, renal failure, bacteremic shock, and death may occur. The causative organism is most often one of the hemolytic streptococci. Puerperal fever was little known before hospital childbirth became common, early in the nineteenth century; then it became an endemic and frequently epidemic scourge that resulted in the deaths of many thousands of mothers and infants. Maternal mortality rates of 20% and higher were common in parts of the world where childbirth occurred in hospitals. Ignaz Philipp Semmelweis, in Vienna, noted that women attended by midwives were much less likely to contract the disease than those attended by physicians and medical students. Midwives did not perform frequent vaginal examinations during labor and did not participate in autopsies. Although the germ theory of disease had not yet been elaborated, Semmelweis deduced that the causative agent of the disease was being transmitted by doctors and students from the infected cadavers in the autopsy room to women in labor on the maternity wards. After institution of a policy requiring that the hands and instruments of obstetric attendants be disinfected, the maternal mortality rate in his clinic dropped dramatically. His work was widely ignored or discredited for almost half a century because physicians were unwilling to believe that they were the agents of transmission. Late in the nineteenth century, after Pasteur's discovery of microbes, Semmelweis was posthumously vindicated. Sterile techniques were gradually instituted, but not until the fourth decade of the twentieth century did puerperal fever cease to be the leading cause of maternal death. Postpartum uterine infection is common but is effectively treated with massive parenteral doses of antibiotics before it becomes a systemic illness. Also called **childbed fever, puerperal sepsis.**

**puerperal mania,** a rare acute mood disorder that sometimes occurs in women after childbirth, characterized by a severe manic reaction. See also **mania.** Compare **postpartum depression, postpartum psychosis.**

**puerperal mastitis** [L, *puerpus,* childbirth; Gk, *mastos,* breast, *itis,* inflammation], a form of acute mastitis in a nursing mother.

**puerperal metritis.** See **puerperal fever.**

**puerperal phlebitis** [L, *puerpus,* childbirth; Gk, *phleps,* vein, *itis,* inflammation], an inflammation that begins in a uterine vein after childbirth and spreads to other veins, particularly the iliac and femoral veins.

**puerperal psychosis.** See **postpartum psychosis.**

**puerperal sepsis,** an infection acquired during the puerperium.

**puerperium** /pyōō′ərpir′ē·əm/ [L, *puerperus*], the time after childbirth, lasting approximately 6 weeks, during which the anatomic and physiologic changes brought about by pregnancy resolve and a woman adjusts to the new or expanded responsibilities of motherhood and nonpregnant life.

**PUFA,** abbreviation for **polyunsaturated fatty acid.**

**puff** [ME *puf*] a short, soft, blowing sound heard on auscultation.

***Pulex*** /pyōō′leks/ [L, flea], a genus of fleas, some species of which transmit arthropod-borne infections, such as plague and epidemic typhus.

**pulmo-, pulmon-,** combining form meaning 'the lungs': *pulmogram, pulmolith, pulmometer.*

**pulmoaortic** /pŏŏl′mō·ā·ôr′tik/, pertaining to the lungs and aorta.

**pulmonary** /pŏŏl′məner′ē/ [L, *pulmo,* lungs], pertaining to the lungs or the respiratory system. Also called **pulmonic.**

**pulmonary acid aspiration syndrome.** See **Mendelson's syndrome.**

**pulmonary alveolar proteinosis** [L, *pulmoneus,* lungs, *alveolus,* little hollow; Gk, *proteios,* first rank, *osis,* condition], a condition in which the air sacs of the lungs become filled with protein and lipids, progressing to respiratory failure. The cause is unknown.

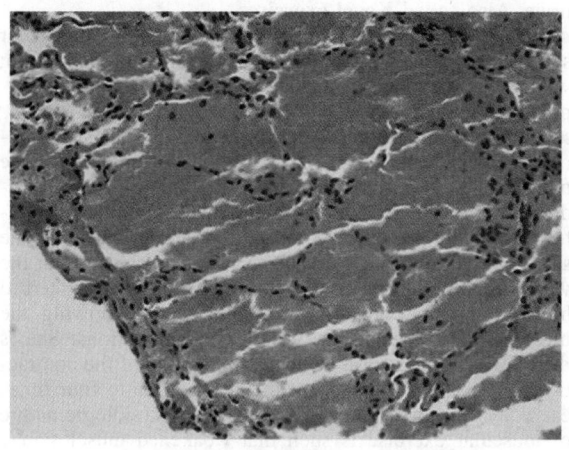

**Pulmonary alveolar proteinosis**
*(Cotran, Kumar, and Collins, 1999)*

**pulmonary alveolus,** one of the numerous terminal air sacs in the lungs where oxygen and carbon dioxide are exchanged.

**pulmonary angiography** [L, *pulmoneus,* lungs; Gk, *angeion,* vessel, *graphein,* to record], the radiographic examination of the blood vessels of the lungs after the injection of radiopaque contrast medium into the pulmonary circulation. It is used to detect pulmonary emboli.

**pulmonary anthrax.** See **woolsorter's disease.**

**pulmonary arteriolar resistance (PAR),** pressure loss per unit of blood flow from the pulmonary artery to a pulmonary vein.

**pulmonary artery** [L, *pulmoneus,* lungs; Gk, *arteria,* airpipe], either the left pulmonary artery supplying the left lung or the right pulmonary artery supplying the right lung. The lobar branches are named according to the lobe they supply, such as apical *(ramus apicalis).*

**pulmonary artery catheter** [L, *pulmoneus,* lungs; Gk, *arteria* + *katheter,* a thing lowered], a catheter inserted into a pulmonary artery to measure cardiac output, pulmonary arterial pressure, and capillary wedge pressure.

**pulmonary artery wedge pressure.** See **pulmonary wedge pressure.**

**pulmonary atresia** [L, *pulmoneus,* lungs; Gk, *a* + *tresis,* without perforation], a congenital heart defect of the right ventricular outflow tract. One form consists of an intact ventricular septum with an interatrial communication and a persistent patent ductus arteriosus. A more extreme form is the four-defect **tetralogy of Fallot.**

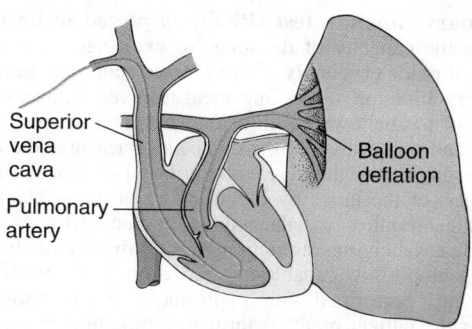

**Placement of a pulmonary artery catheter**
*(Beare and Myers, 1998)*

**pulmonary atrium,** any of the spaces at the end of an alveolar duct into which alveoli open.

**pulmonary candidiasis** [L, *pulmones,* lungs; L, *candidus,* white + Gk, *-iasis,* disease suffix], a type of fungal pneumonia caused by infection with *Candida* species, seen especially in immunocompromised patients or those with malignancies. Also called *Candida pneumonia.*

**pulmonary capillary wedge pressure.** See **pulmonary artery wedge pressure.**

**pulmonary carcinosis.** See **alveolar cell carcinoma.**

**pulmonary circulation** [L, *pulmoneus,* lungs, *circulare*], the blood flow through the network of vessels between the heart and the lungs for the oxygenation of blood and removal of carbon dioxide. Also called **lesser circulation.**

**pulmonary compliance.** See **compliance,** def. 2.

**pulmonary congestion** [L, *pulmoneus,* lungs, *congerere,* to heap together], an excessive accumulation of fluid in the lungs, usually associated with either an inflammation or congestive heart failure.

**pulmonary disease,** any abnormal condition of the respiratory system, characterized by cough, chest pain, dyspnea, hemoptysis, sputum production, stridor, and wheezing. Less common symptoms include anxiety, arm and shoulder pain, tenderness in the calf of the leg, erythema nodosum, swelling of the face, headache, hoarseness, joint pain, and somnolence. Diagnostic procedures for pulmonary diseases include bronchoscopy; cytologic, serologic, and biochemical examination of bronchial secretions; laryngoscopy; pulmonary function tests; and radiography. Obstructive respiratory disease is the result of a reduction of airway size that impedes air flow. The obstruction may result from bronchospasm, edema of the bronchial mucosa, or excessive bronchial secretions. Obstructive disease is characterized by reduced expiratory flow rates and increased total lung capacity. Acute obstructive respiratory diseases include asthma, bronchitis, and bronchiectasis; chronic obstructive diseases include emphysema, chronic bronchitis, or combined emphysema and chronic bronchitis. Patients with obstructive diseases may have acute respiratory failure from any respiratory stress, such as infections or general anesthesia. Restrictive respiratory disease is caused by conditions that limit lung expansion, such as fibrothorax, obesity, a neuromuscular disorder, kyphosis, scoliosis, spondylitis, or surgical removal of lung tissue. Pregnancy causes a self-limiting restrictive disease in the third trimester. Characteristics of restrictive respiratory disease are decreased forced expired vital capacity and total lung capacity, with increased work of breathing and inefficient exchange of gases. Acute restrictive conditions are the most common pulmonary cause of acute respiratory failure.

**pulmonary dysmaturity syndrome,** a respiratory disorder of premature infants in which the lungs contain focal emphysematous blebs and thickened alveolar walls. The infants commonly die of hypoxia.

**pulmonary edema,** the accumulation of extravascular fluid in lung tissues and alveoli, caused most commonly by congestive heart failure. Serous fluid is pushed through the pulmonary capillaries into alveoli and quickly enters bronchioles and bronchi. The condition also may occur in barbiturate and opiate poisoning, diffuse infections, hemorrhagic

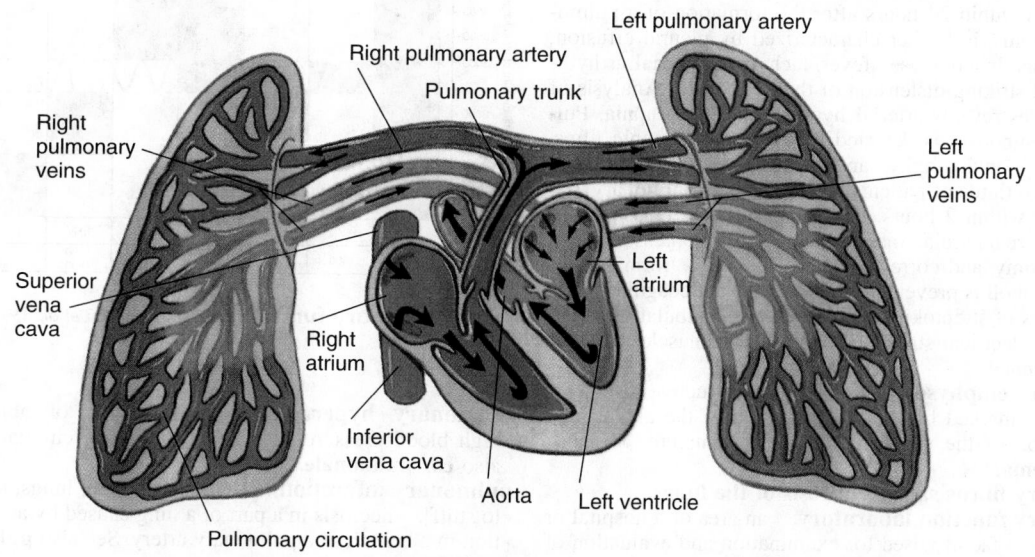

**Pulmonary circulation** *(Applegate, 2000)*

pancreatitis, and renal failure and after a stroke, skull fracture, near-drowning, inhalation of irritating gases, and rapid administration of whole blood, plasma, serum albumin, or IV fluids.

■ OBSERVATIONS: Signs and symptoms of pulmonary edema include tachypnea; labored, shallow respirations; restlessness; apprehensiveness; air hunger; cyanosis; and blood-tinged or frothy, pink sputum. The peripheral and neck veins are usually engorged; blood pressure and heart rate are increased; and the pulse may be full and pounding or weak and thready. There may be edema of the extremities, crackles in the lungs, respiratory acidosis, and profuse diaphoresis.

■ INTERVENTIONS: Acute pulmonary edema is an emergency condition requiring prompt treatment. The patient is given oxygen and placed in bed in a high Fowler's position, and IV morphine sulfate is usually administered immediately to relieve pain, to quiet breathing, and to allay apprehension. A cardiotonic, such as digitalis, and a fast-acting diuretic, such as furosemide or ethacrynic acid, may be given. Oxygen may be ordered. While the patient is acutely ill, the blood pressure, respiration, apical pulse, and breath sounds are checked frequently or continually monitored. Parenteral fluids, if indicated, are infused slowly in limited quantities; a low-sodium diet is served; and the patient's intake and output of fluids are measured. The patient is weighed daily, and any sudden weight gain is noted and reported.

■ NURSING CONSIDERATIONS: The nurse provides continued care and emotional support and directs the patient to exercise to tolerance with frequent rest periods, to report any symptoms, to avoid smoking, and to follow the regimen ordered for medication, diet, and return checkups.

**pulmonary embolism (PE),**   the blockage of a pulmonary artery by fat, air, tumor tissue, or a thrombus that usually arises from a peripheral vein (most frequently one of the deep veins of the legs). Predisposing factors include an alteration of blood constituents with increased coagulation, damage to blood vessel walls, and stagnation or immobilization, especially when associated with childbirth, congestive heart failure, polycythemia, or surgery. Pulmonary embolism is difficult to distinguish from myocardial infarction and pneumonia. It is characterized by dyspnea, sudden chest pain, shock, and cyanosis. Pulmonary infarction, which often occurs within 24 hours after the formation of a pulmonary embolus, is further characterized by pleural effusion, hemoptysis, leukocytosis, fever, tachycardia, atrial arrhythmias, and striking distension of the neck veins. Analysis of blood gases reveals arterial hypoxia and hypocapnia. Pulmonary embolism is detected by chest radiographic films, pulmonary angiography, and radioscanning of the lung fields. Two thirds of patients with a massive pulmonary embolus die within 2 hours. Initial resuscitative measures include external cardiac massage, oxygen, vasopressor drugs, embolectomy, and correction of acidosis. The formation of further emboli is prevented by the use of anticoagulants and sometimes of streptokinase or urokinase. Ambulation, exercise, and electrical stimulation of the calf muscles also are recommended.

**pulmonary emphysema,**   a chronic obstructive disease of the lungs, marked by an overdistension of the alveoli and destruction of the supporting alveolar structure. See also **emphysema.**

**pulmonary fibrosis.**   See **fibrosis of the lungs.**

**pulmonary function laboratory,**   an area of a hospital or other health facility used for examination and evaluation of patients' respiratory function.

**pulmonary function test (PFT),**   a procedure for determining the capacity of the lungs to exchange oxygen and carbon dioxide efficiently. There are two general kinds of respiratory function tests. One measures ventilation, or the ability of the bellows action of the chest and lungs to move gas in and out of alveoli; the other kind measures the diffusion of gas across the alveolar capillary membrane and the perfusion of the lungs by blood. Efficient gas exchange in the lungs requires a balanced ventilation-perfusion ratio, with areas receiving ventilation well perfused and areas receiving blood flow capable of ventilation. Basic ventilation studies are performed with a spirometer and recording device as the patient breathes through a mouthpiece and connecting tube; a nose clip prevents nasal breathing. Measurements or calculations are made of the tidal volume (TV), or gas inspired and expired in a normal breath; the inspiratory reserve volume (IRV), or the maximal volume that can be inspired after a normal respiration; the expiratory reserve volume (ERV), or the maximal volume that can be expired forcefully after a normal expiration; the residual volume (RV), or the gas remaining in the lungs after maximal expiration; and the minute volume, or the gas inspired and expired in 1 minute of normal breathing. The vital capacity of the lungs is equal to TV + IRV + ERV, and the total lung capacity to TV + IRV + ERV + RV. Bronchospirometric measurements of the ventilation and oxygen consumption of each lung separately are performed using a specially constructed double-lumen catheter with two balloons; one balloon is inflated to seal off the contralateral lung when the other lung is tested. Arterial blood gas studies, including determinations of the acidity, partial pressure of carbon dioxide and of oxygen, and oxyhemoglobin saturation, provide information on the diffusion of gas across the alveolar capillary membrane and the adequacy of oxygenation of tissues. See also **blood gas determination, forced expiratory volume, maximum breathing capacity.**

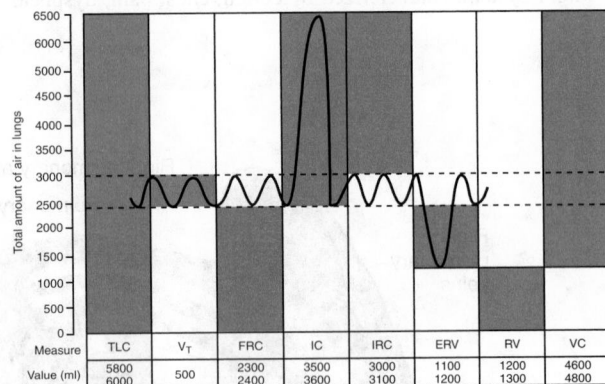

| Measure | TLC | V$_T$ | FRC | IC | IRC | ERV | RV | VC |
|---|---|---|---|---|---|---|---|---|
| Value (ml) | 5800<br>6000 | 500 | 2300<br>2400 | 3500<br>3600 | 3000<br>3100 | 1100<br>1200 | 1200<br>1300 | 4600<br>4800 |

**Pulmonary function tests** *(Thompson et al, 1993)*

**pulmonary hypertension,**   a condition of abnormally high blood pressure within the pulmonary circulation. See also **cor pulmonale.**

**pulmonary infarction (PI)** [L, *pulmoneus,* lungs, *infarcire,* to stuff],   necrosis in a part of a lung caused by an obstruction in a branch of a pulmonary artery. See also **pulmonary embolism.**

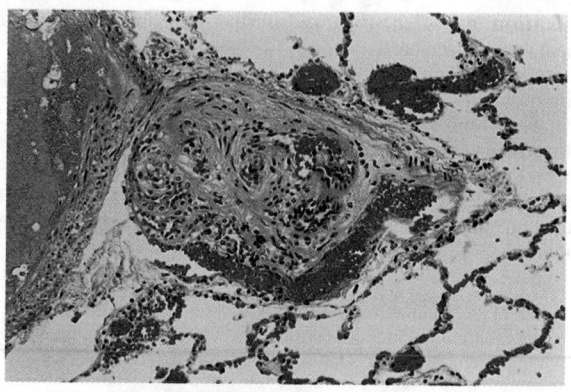

**Vascular changes in pulmonary hypertension**
*(Cotran, Kumar, and Collins, 1999)*

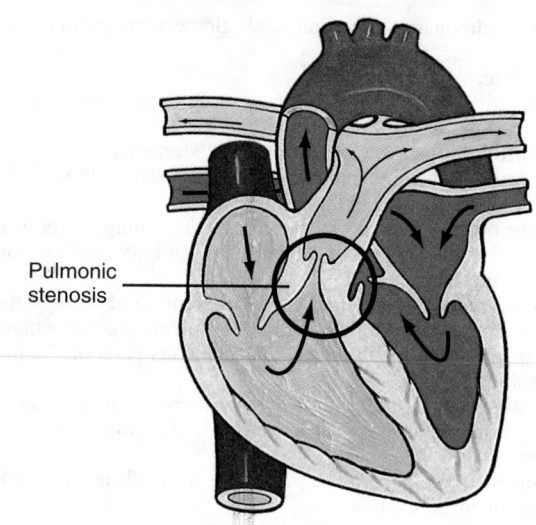

**Pulmonary stenosis** *(Wong, 1999)*

**pulmonary infiltrate with eosinophilia (PIE),** a hypersensitivity reaction characterized by infiltration of alveoli with eosinophils and large mononuclear cells, edema, and inflammation of the lungs. The simplest form of the condition, in which patchy, migratory infiltrates cause minimal symptoms, is a self-limited reaction elicited by helminthic infections and by certain drugs, such as paraaminosalicylic acid, sulfonamides, and chlorpropamide. A more prolonged illness, characterized by fever, night sweats, cough, dyspnea, weight loss, and more severe tissue reaction, occurs in certain drug allergies and in bacterial, fungal, and parasitic infections. Tropical eosinophilia with paroxysmal nocturnal asthma, dyspnea, cough, low-grade fever, and malaise is related to filarial infection, and may occur in long-standing asthma and periarteritis nodosa. See also **Löffler's syndrome.**

**pulmonary insufficiency** [L, *pulmoneus,* lungs, *in* + *sufficere,* to suffice], a failure of the pulmonary valve to close properly.

**pulmonary oxygen toxicity** [L, *pulmoneus,* lungs; Gk, *toxikon,* poison], a form of oxygen poisoning caused by breathing air having an oxygen concentration of 50% or higher for 12 to 24 hours. Pathophysiologic effects include pulmonary capillary endothelial damage and alveolar epithelial cell destruction. Clinical manifestations include cough, substernal pain, nausea, vomiting, and atelectasis.

**pulmonary stenosis,** an abnormal cardiac condition, generally characterized by concentric hypertrophy of the right ventricle with relatively little increase in diastolic volume. When the ventricular septum is intact, this condition may be caused by valvular stenosis, infundibular stenosis, or both; it produces a pressure difference during systole between the right ventricular cavity and the pulmonary artery. Pulmonary stenosis is most often congenital but also may be produced after birth by any of a number of types of lesions. Severe pulmonary stenosis may result in heart failure and death, but mild to moderate forms of this disorder are relatively well tolerated. Also called **pulmonic stenosis.** See also **congenital cardiac anomaly, valvular heart disease, valvular stenosis.**

**pulmonary sulcus tumor,** a destructive invasive neoplasm that develops at the apex of the lung and infiltrates the ribs, vertebrae, and brachial plexus. Also called **Pancoast's tumor.**

**pulmonary surfactant.** See **surfactant,** def. 2.

**pulmonary trunk,** the short, wide vessel that conveys venous blood from the right ventricle of the heart to the lungs. It is approximately 5 cm long and 3 cm in diameter, and it ascends obliquely, dividing into right and left branches.

**pulmonary tuberculosis.** See **tuberculosis.**

**pulmonary valve,** a cardiac structure composed of three semilunar cusps that close during each heartbeat to prevent blood from flowing back into the right ventricle from the pulmonary trunk. The cusps are separated by sinuses that resemble tiny buckets when they are closed and filled with blood. These flaps grow from the lining of the pulmonary trunk; when they collapse from the ejection of ventricular blood, they open the valve and allow deoxygenated blood to flow through the pulmonary artery and on to the lungs. Compare **aortic valve, mitral valve, tricuspid valve.**

**pulmonary vascular resistance (PVR),** the resistance in the pulmonary vascular bed against which the right ventricle must eject blood.

**pulmonary vein,** one of two pairs of large vessels that return oxygenated blood from each lung to the left atrium of the heart. The right pulmonary veins pass dorsal to the right atrium and the superior vena cava. The left pulmonary veins pass ventral to the descending thoracic aorta. Compare **pulmonary trunk.**

**pulmonary ventilation.** See **respiration,** def. 2.

**pulmonary wedge pressure (PWP),** the pressure produced by an inflated latex balloon against the inner wall of a pulmonary artery. A Swan-Ganz catheter or similar balloon-tipped catheter is inserted through a subclavian, jugular, or femoral vein to the vena cava and on through the right atrium and ventricle to the pulmonary artery. The balloon is inflated briefly, during which time it measures left ventricular diastolic pressure. The procedure is used in the diagnosis of congestive heart failure, myocardial infarction, and other conditions. Also called **pulmonary artery wedge pressure.**

**pulmonary Wegener's granulomatosis,** a rare fatal disease of young or middle-aged men, characterized by granulomatous lesions of the respiratory tract, focal necrotizing arteritis, and finally widespread inflammation of body organs. Pulmonary infarction and glomerulonephritis may occur.

**pulmonic.** See **pulmonary.**

**-pulmonic,** combining form meaning 'the lungs': *apulmonic, gastropulmonic, intrapulmonic.*

**pulmonic stenosis.** See **pulmonary stenosis.**

**pulmonologist** /pŏŏl'mə·nol'ə·jist/ [L, *pulmo,* lung], an individual skilled in pulmonology.

**pulmonology** /pŏŏl'mōnol'ə·jē/ [L, *pulmo,* lung], the science concerned with the anatomy, physiology, and pathology of the lungs.

**pulp** [L, *pulpa,* flesh], any soft coherent solid spongy tissue, such as that contained within the spleen, the pulp chamber of the tooth, or the distal subcutaneous pads of the fingers and the toes. —**pulpy,** *adj.*

**pulp abscess** [L, *pulpa,* flesh + *abscedere,* to go away], a pus-producing abscess that develops in the pulp cavity of a tooth.

**pulpaceous** /pulpā'shəs/, pertaining to a substance that is pulpy or macerated.

**pulpal** /pul'pəl/, pertaining to pulp.

**pulp amputation.** See **pulpotomy.**

**pulp canal,** the space occupied by the nerves, blood vessels, and lymphatic vessels in the radicular part of the tooth. Also called **root canal.**

**pulp canal therapy.** See **root canal therapy.**

**pulp cavity,** the space in a tooth bounded by the dentin and containing the dental pulp. It is divided into the pulp chamber and the pulp canal.

**pulpectomy** /pulpek'təmē/ [L, *pulpa,* flesh; Gk, *ektomē,* excision], the surgical removal of all or part of the pulp of a tooth.

**pulpifaction** /pul'pifak'shən/, the act of reducing something to a pulp.

**pulpitis** /pulpī'tis/, infection or inflammation of the dental pulp.

**pulpless tooth** /pulp'ləs/, a tooth in which the dental pulp is necrotic or has been removed. Also called **devital tooth, nonvital tooth.**

**pulpodontia.** See **endodontics.**

**pulpotomy** /pul·pot'ə·mē/, root canal therapy consisting of partial excision of the dental pulp. Also called **pulp amputation.**

**pulp pinch.** See **pinch.**

**pulp stone.** See **denticle.**

**pulp test.** See **vitality test.**

**pulpy.** See **pulp.**

**pulsate** /pul'sāt/ [L, *pulsare,* to beat], to throb or vibrate rhythmically, as does the heart during its contraction-relaxation cycle.

**pulsatile** /pul'sətil/ [L, *pulsare,* to beat], pertaining to an activity characterized by a rhythmic pulsation.

**pulsatile assist device (PAD),** a flexible, valveless balloon conduit contained within a rigid, plastic cylinder that is inserted into the arterial circulation to provide pulsatile perfusion during a cardiopulmonary bypass.

**pulsatile hematoma.** See **pseudoaneurysm.**

**pulsatility index** /pul'sətil'itē/, a measure of the variability of blood velocity in a vessel. It is equal to the difference between the peak systolic and minimum diastolic velocities, divided by the mean velocity during the cardiac cycle.

**pulsating exophthalmos** /pul'sāting/ [L, *pulsare,* to beat; Gk, *ex + ophthalmos,* eye], an eye disorder characterized by a bulging, pulsating eyeball. The cause is an arteriovenous aneurysm involving the internal carotid artery and the cavernous sinus of the orbit.

**pulsation** /pəl·sā'shən/ [L, *pulsatio*], a throb or rhythmical beat, as of the heart.

**pulse** [L, *pulsare,* to beat], **1.** a rhythmic beating or vibrating movement. **2.** a brief electromagnetic wave. **3.** the regular, recurrent expansion and contraction of an artery produced by waves of pressure caused by the ejection of blood from the left ventricle of the heart as it contracts. The pulse is easily detected on superficial arteries, such as the radial and carotid arteries, and corresponds to each beat of the heart.

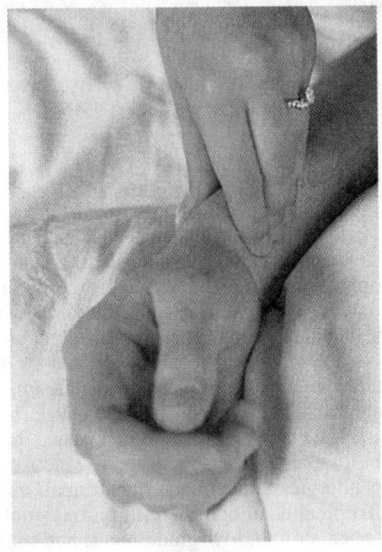

**Pulse assessment** *(Potter and Perry, 1993)*

**pulsed Doppler,** a type of Doppler device involving the transmission of a short-duration burst of sound into the region to be examined. The Doppler-shifted signals are processed from a limited depth range. The depth range is determined by a sample gate whose position and size usually can be selected by the instrument operator.

**pulse deficit,** a condition in which a peripheral pulse rate is less than the ventricular contraction rate as auscultated at the apex of the heart or seen on the electrocardiogram. The condition indicates a lack of peripheral perfusion.

**pulse duration,** (in ultrasonics) a measure of the time a transducer oscillates for each pulse. The shorter the pulse duration, the better the axial resolution.

**pulse-echo response profile,** a graph of the amplitude of an ultrasound echo from a small reflector versus the distance from the reflector beam axis. The reflector is scanned perpendicular to the axis of the ultrasound transducer beam.

**pulse-echo ultrasound,** a diagnostic technique in which short-duration ultrasound pulses are transmitted into the region to be studied, and echo signals resulting from scattering and reflection are detected and displayed. The depth of a reflective structure is inferred from the delay between pulse transmission and echo reception.

**pulse generator,** the power source for a cardiac pacemaker system, usually fueled by lithium, supplying impulses to the implanted electrodes, either at a fixed rate or in some programmed pattern.

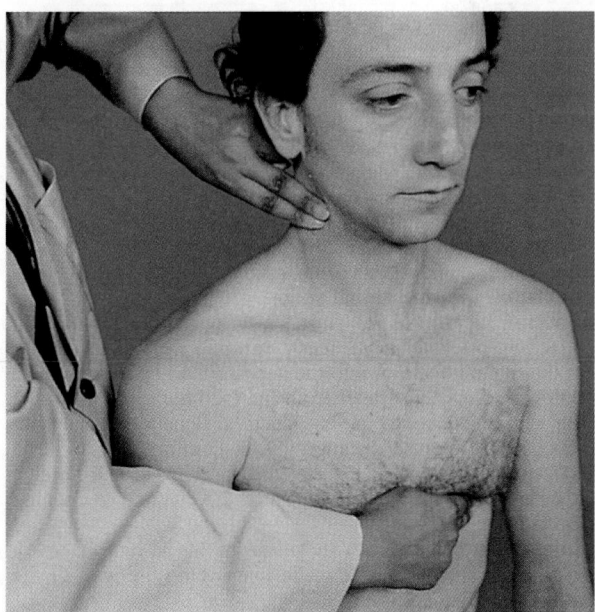

**Testing for pulse deficit** *(Barkauskas et al, 1994)*

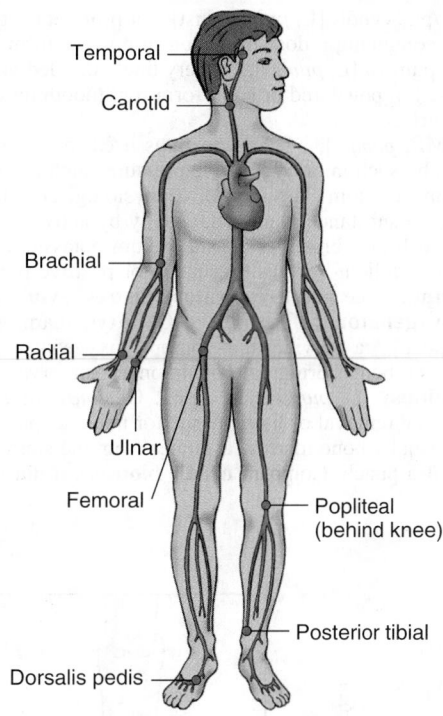

**Pulse points** *(Monahan and Neighbors, 1998)*

**pulse height analyzer,** a device that accepts or rejects electronic pulses according to their amplitude or energy. It is commonly used to select certain gamma radiation energies.

**pulseless disease.** See **Takayasu's arteritis.**

**pulse MR,** a magnetic resonance (MR) technique that uses radiofrequency pulses and Fourier transformation of the MR signal. Pulse MR has largely replaced older, continuous-wave techniques.

**pulse oximeter,** a device that measures the amount of saturated hemoglobin in the tissue capillaries. A beam of light is transmitted through the tissue to a receiver. This noninvasive method of measuring the saturated hemoglobin is a useful screening tool for determining basic respiratory function. The cliplike device may be used on either the ear lobe or the fingertip. As the amount of saturated hemoglobin alters the wavelengths of the transmitted light, analysis of the received light is translated into a percentage of oxygen saturation ($SO_2$) of the blood. Also called (informally) *pulse ox.* Compare **blood gas determination.**

**pulse point,** one of the sites on the surface of the body where arterial pulsations can be easily palpated. The most commonly used pulse point is over the radial artery at the wrist. Other pulse points include the temporal artery in front of the ear, the common carotid artery at the lower level of the thyroid cartilage, the facial artery at the lower margin of the jaw, and the femoral, popliteal, posterior tibialis, and dorsalis pedis pulse points.

**pulse pressure,** the difference between the systolic and diastolic blood pressures, normally 30 to 50 mm Hg.

**pulser** /pul'sər/, a component of an ultrasound instrument that provides signals for exciting the piezoelectric transducer in order to transmit an ultrasound beam.

**pulse rate** [L, *pulsare* + *reri,* to calculate], the number of pulse beats per minute. Normally it is the same as the heart rate. The normal pulse rate in an average adult varies from 60 to 80/min, with fluctuations occurring with exercise, injury, illness, and emotional reactions. The average pulse rate for a newborn is 120/min, which slows throughout childhood and adolescence. At about 12 years of age, females begin to have a higher pulse rate than males.

**pulse repetition frequency (PRF),** (in ultrasonics) the number of acoustic pulses transmitted per second.

**pulse wave** [L, *pulsare,* to beat; AS, *wafian*], a transient increase in blood pressure that spreads like a wave through the arterial system. It begins with the ejection of blood by the ventricles during systole.

**pulse width.** See **duration.**

**-pulsion,** combining form meaning the 'action or condition of pushing forward': *compulsion, lateropulsion, retropulsion.*

**pulsus alternans** /pul'səs ôl'tərnanz/ [L, *pulsare* + *alternare,* to alternate], a pulse characterized by a regular alternation of weak and strong beats without changes in the pulse rate. Also called **alternating pulse.**

**pulsus magnus.** See **full pulse.**

**pulsus paradoxus,** an abnormally large decrease in systolic blood pressure and pulse wave amplitude during inspiration. The normal fall in pressure is less than 10 mm Hg. An excessive decline may be a sign of tamponade, adhesive pericarditis, severe lung disease, advanced heart failure, or other conditions. Also called **paradoxic pulse.**

**pulsus parvus et tardus** [L, *pulsus,* beat, *parvus,* small, *tardus,* slow], a small pulse with low pressure that rises and falls gradually. The condition occurs in aortic stenosis.

**pulsus tardus** [L, *pulsus,* beat, *tardus,* slow], a pulse with a gradual rise and fall in amplitude.

**pultaceous,** pertaining to a substance that is pulpy or macerated.

**pulverize** /pul'vərīz/ [L, *pulvis,* dust], to reduce to a fine powder.

**pulverulent** /pulver'ələnt/, having the form of a fine powder.

**pulvule** /pul′vyo͞ol/ [L, *pulvis,* dust], a proprietary type of capsule containing a dose of a drug in powder form.

**pumice** /pum′is/ [L, *pumex*], a very finely divided volcanic rock, used in powdered or solid form for smoothing or polishing surfaces.

**pump** [ME, *pumpe*], **1.** an apparatus used to move fluids or gases by suction or by positive pressure, such as an infusion pump or stomach pump. **2.** a physiologic mechanism by which a substance is moved, usually by active transport across a cell membrane, such as a sodium-potassium pump. **3.** to move a liquid or gas by suction or positive pressure.

**pump lung.** See **adult respiratory distress syndrome.**

**pump oxygenator** [ME, *pumpe* + Gk, *oxys,* sharp, *genein,* to produce], a device that pumps oxygenated blood through the body during cardiopulmonary surgery.

**punch biopsy** [L, *pungere,* to prick; Gk, *bios,* life, *opsis,* view], the removal of living tissue for microscopic examination, usually bone marrow aspirates from the sternum, by means of a punch. Compare **needle biopsy, exfoliative cytology.**

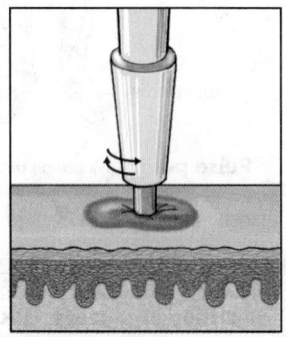
Insertion of biopsy tool

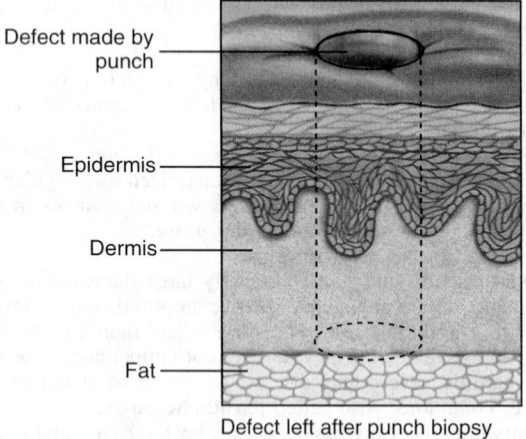

Defect made by punch

Epidermis

Dermis

Fat

Defect left after punch biopsy

**Punch biopsy** *(Monahan and Neighbors, 1998)*

**punchdrunk syndrome,** a condition in which repeated cerebral concussions result in an abnormal gait, slow movement, tremor, and slurred or halting speech.

**punch forceps,** a surgical instrument used to cut out a disk of dense or resistant tissue, such as bone and cartilage. The ends of the blades of the punch forceps are perforated to grip the involved tissue. There are several varieties of this instrument, with blades and tips specially designed for different surgical needs.

**punct-,** prefix meaning 'a point, or like a point': *punctate, punctiform, punctograph.*

**punctate** /pungk′tāt/ [L, *punctum,* point], marked with elevated or colored dots or punctures.

**punctiform** /pungk′tifôrm/, of very small size, as is a bacterial colony in a solid medium.

**punctum** /pungk′təm/, a physiologic area or point.

**punctum caecum,** blind spot.

**punctum lacrimale** /lak′rimā′lē/, *pl.* **puncta lacrimalia** [L, *punctum,* prick, *lacrima,* tear], a minute circular aperture in the medial opening into the nasolacrimal sac. The puncta drain the tears that travel from the lacrimal glands through the lacrimal ducts to the conjunctiva. Puncta clogged with mucus or dirt cause irritation and discomfort.

**puncture** /pungk′chər/ [L, *punctura*], **1.** to prick or pierce a surface, as with a needle or knife. **2.** a wound or opening made by piercing.

**puncture of the antrum** [L, *punctura* + Gk, *antron,* cave], a cavity or hollow, as is made in piercing the wall of the maxillary sinus to drain pus.

**puncture wound** [L, *punctura* + AS, *wund*], a traumatic injury caused by skin penetration by an object, such as a knife, nail, or slender fragment of metal, wood, glass, or other material. In such an injury to the eye, a lung, or a visceral organ, the object or implement is not removed until the person has been transported to a medical facility. Minor puncture wounds are treated with thorough cleansing. If a puncture wound is allowed to close at the skin before deeper healing has occurred, suppuration often results. A tetanus toxoid immunization is usually given for such wounds.

**punitive damages.** See **damages.**

**Punnett square** [Reginald C. Punnett, English geneticist, 1875–1967; OFr, *esquarre*], a matrix that shows all of the possible combinations of male and female gametes when one or more pairs of independent alleles are crossed. Letters representing the male and female gametes are placed along the left side and the top of the matrix, respectively. The genotypes of the offspring produced by each pairing of gametes occupy the cells in the matrix. See also **pedigree.**

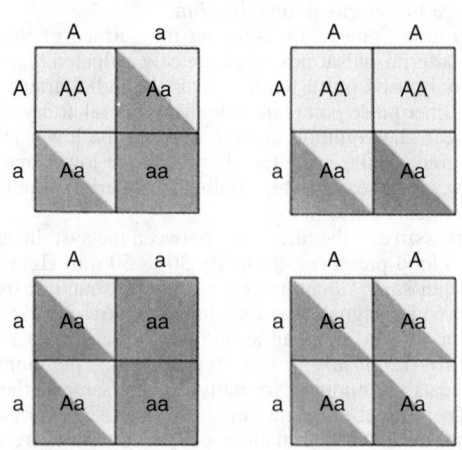

**Punnett square** *(Thibodeau and Patton, 1999/Rolin Graphics)*

**P.U.O.,** abbreviation for *pyrexia of unknown origin.*

**pupa** /pyōō'pə/ [L, doll], a stage between the larval and adult stages in the life cycle of many insects, including flies, butterflies, and beetles. It shows the basic external features of the adult form but without expanded wings.

**pupil** /pyōō'pəl/ [L, *pupa,* doll], a circular opening in the iris of the eye, located slightly to the nasal side of the center of the iris. Like the iris, the pupil lies posterior to the cornea and the anterior chamber of the eye and is anterior to the lens. Its diameter changes with contraction and relaxation of the muscular fibers of the iris as the eye responds to changes in light, emotional states, and autonomic stimulation. The pupil is the window of the eye through which light passes to the lens and the retina. See also **dilator pupillae, sphincter pupillae.** —**pupillary,** *adj.*

**pupill-.** See **pupillo-.**

**pupilla** /pyōōpil'ə/ [L], the pupil of the eye.

**pupillary** /pyōō'piler'ē/ [L, *pupilla*] pertaining to the pupil.

**pupillary reflex.** See **accommodation reflex, light reflex.**

**pupillary ruff,** a brown wrinkled rim on the edge of the pupil, derived from posterior pigment epithelium of the iris.

**pupillary skin reflex.** See **ciliospinal reflex.**

**pupillo-, pupill-,** combining form meaning 'the pupil': *pupillometer, pupilloplegia, pupillostatometer.*

**pupillometry** /pyōō'pilom'ətrē/, the measurement of the pupil.

**pupillomotor** /pyōō'pilōmō'tər/, pertaining to the autonomic nerve fibers of the smooth muscles of the iris.

**PUPPP** /pup/, abbreviation for **pruritic urticarial papules and plaques of pregnancy.**

**PUPs,** abbreviation for *previously untreated patients,* usually infants participating in clinical trials.

**pur-,** combining form meaning 'pus': *puric, puriform, purohepatitis.*

**pure** /pyōōr/, **1.** free of contamination by extraneous matter. **2.** a state in which a substance contains nothing other than itself.

**pure dwarf.** See **primordial dwarf.**

**pure science.** See **science.**

**pure tone audiometry.** See **audiometry.**

**pure vegetarian.** See **strict vegetarian, vegan.**

**purgation.** See **catharsis.**

**purgative** /pur'gətiv/ [L, *purgare,* to purge], a strong medication usually administered by mouth to promote evacuation of the bowel or to produce several bowel movements.

**purge** /purj/ [L, *purgare*], **1.** to evacuate the bowels, as with a cathartic. **2.** a cathartic. **3.** to make free of an unwanted substance. —**purgative,** *n., adj.*

**purified protein derivative (PPD)** /pyōō'rifīd/, a dried form of tuberculin used in testing for past or present infection with tubercle bacilli. This product is usually introduced into the skin during such tests and may produce a tuberculin reaction within 48 to 72 hours. Also called **PPD of Seibert, PPD-S.** See also **Mantoux test, tine test, tuberculin test, tuberculosis.**

**purine** /pyōō'rēn/ [L, *purus,* pure, *urina,* urine], any one of a large group of nitrogenous compounds. Purines are produced as end products in the digestion of certain proteins in the diet, but some are synthesized in the body. Purines are also present in many medications and other substances, including caffeine, theophylline, and various diuretics, muscle relaxants, and myocardial stimulants. Hyperuricemia may develop in some people as a result of an inability to metabolize and excrete purines. A low-purine diet or a purine-free diet may be required. Foods that are high in purines include anchovies and sardines; sweetbreads, liver, kidneys, and other organ meats; legumes; and poultry. The foods lowest in purine content include eggs, fruit, cheese, nuts, sugar, gelatin, and vegetables other than legumes.

**purine base** [L, *purus,* pure], any of the purine derivatives found in animal waste products or in nucleic acids. They include hypoxanthine, xanthine, and uric acid (waste products), and adenine and guanine (nucleic acids).

**purine-free diet,** a diet that excludes foods that are rich sources of purines. Foods high in purines particularly include organ meats, such as liver, kidney, and sweetbreads, as well as red meats, poultry, and fish. Those items can be replaced by milk, eggs, cheese, and some vegetable sources of protein. See also **purine.**

**purine-low diet,** a diet that excludes some foods rich in purines, such as certain meat products, fish, and poultry, and particularly anchovies, meat extracts, sardines, and organ meats. Also called **low-purine diet.**

**purine-restricted diet.** See **low-purine diet.**

**Purinethol,** trademark for an antineoplastic (mercaptopurine).

**Purkinje's cells** /pərkin'jēz, pur'kinjēz, -jāz/ [Johannes E. Purkinje, Czech physiologist, 1787–1869], large neurons with dendrites that extend to the molecular lay and provide the only output from the cerebellar cortex after the cortex processes sensory and motor impulses from the rest of the nervous system.

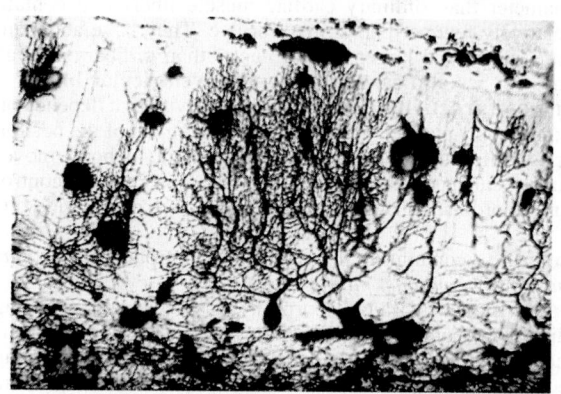

**Purkinje's cell** *(Crossman and Neary, 1995)*

**Purkinje's fiber** [Johannes E. Purkinje], one of the myocardial fibers that are the termination of the bundle branches. The fibers comprise part of the conduction system of the heart. See also **Purkinje's network.**

**Purkinje's network** [Johannes E. Purkinje], a complex fibrous network of large muscle cells that spread through the right and the left ventricles of the heart and carry the impulses that contract those chambers almost simultaneously. The fibers that connect with Purkinje's fibers start in the atrioventricular (AV) node in the right atrium of the heart, along the lower part of the interatrial septum. Impulses generated in the sinoatrial node travel through the muscle fibers of both atria of the heart, starting atrial contraction. As the impulse enters the AV node from the right atrium, it allows both atria to contract completely before the impulse spreads into the ventricles. The velocity of the impulse increases after the impulse leaves the AV node and spreads via the atrioventricular bundle (bundle of His) to the bundle branches,

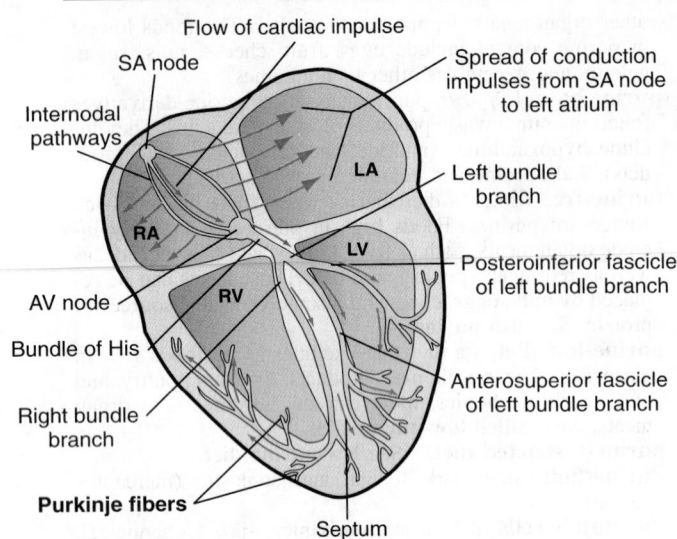

**Purkinje's network** *(Lewis, Heitkemper, and Dirksen, 2000)*

**Purpura senile** *(Lemmi and Lemmi, 2000)*

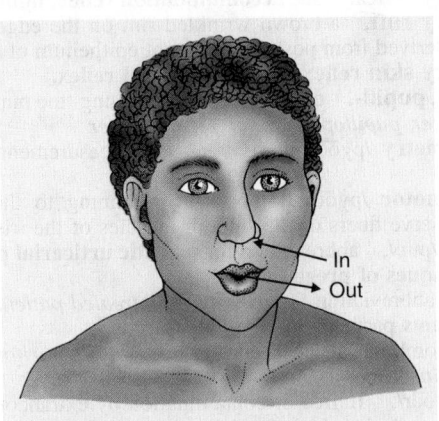

**Pursed-lip breathing**
*(Ignatavicius, Workman, and Mishler, 1999)*

and finally to Purkinje's fibers. Purkinje's fibers are larger in diameter than ordinary cardiac muscle fibers and contain relatively few peripheral myofibrillae. They have abundant sarcoplasm and larger central nuclei than ordinary cardiac muscle. See also **cardiac cycle, intraventricular block.**

**purposeful activity** /pur′pəsfo͞ol/, activity that depends on consciously planned and directed involvement of the person. It is believed that conscious involvement in body movements enhances the development of sensorimotor control and coordination during therapeutic or rehabilitative exercises.

**purpur-,** combining form meaning 'purple': *purpuriferous, purpuriparous, purpurogenous.*

**purpura** /pur′pyərə/ [L, purple], any of several bleeding disorders characterized by hemorrhage into the tissues, particularly beneath the skin or mucous membranes, producing ecchymoses or petechiae. The two major kinds of purpura are **thrombocytopenic purpura** and **nonthrombocytopenic purpura.** —**purpuric,** *adj.*

**purpura rheumatica** [L, *purpura,* purple; Gk, *rheum,* flow], a distinctive clinical sign associated with hemorrhages of the skin and other tissues. The lesions are red or purple and do not blanche on pressure. Purpura is related to either a disorder of the blood or an abnormality affecting the blood vessels.

**purpura senilis** /senē′lis/ [L, *purpura,* purple, *senilis,* aged], a skin condition affecting older people and characterized by fragile blood vessel walls that rupture on minimal trauma.

**purpuric.** See **purpura.**

**pursed-lip breathing** /purst-/, respiration characterized by deep inspirations followed by prolonged expirations through pursed lips. It is done to increase expiratory airway pressure, improve oxygenation of the blood, and help prevent early airway closure.

**purse-string suture** [L, *sutura*], a continuous suture inserted in a circle about a round wound. The opening is closed by tightly drawing the ends of the suture together.

**purulence** /pyo͞or′(y)ələns/ [L, *purulentus,* pus formation], the condition of producing or discharging pus. Also called **purulency.**

**purulent** /pyo͞or′(y)ələnt/ [L, containing pus], producing or containing pus.

**purulent conjunctivitis** [L, *purulentus,* pus formation, *conjunctivus,* connecting; Gk, *itis,* inflammation], an inflammation of the conjunctiva caused by suppurative microorganisms, including species of streptococci, gonococci, and pneumococci.

**purulent diarrhea** [L, *purulentus,* pus formation; Gk, *dia + rhein,* to flow], diarrhea in which stools contain pus, a sign of a purulent GI tract infection.

**purulent inflammation** [L, *purulentus,* pus formation, *inflammare,* to set afire], an inflammation that is accompanied by the formation of pus.

**purulent iritis** [L, *purulentus,* pus formation; Gk, *iris,* rainbow, *itis,* inflammation], an inflammation of the iris accompanied by the formation of pus.

**purulent keratitis** [L, *purulentus,* pus formation; Gk, *keras,* horn, *itis,* inflammation], a severe form of keratitis leading to disintegration of the cornea if untreated. The condition commonly begins with a bacterial infection of the lacrimal sac, occurs frequently in elderly patients who have poor nutrition, and spreads into a pus-producing ulcer.

**purulent pancreatitis** [L, *purulentus,* pus formation; Gk, *pan,* all, *kreas,* flesh, *itis,* inflammation], inflammation of the pancreas accompanied by pus formation.

**purulent rhinitis** [L, *purulentus,* pus formation; Gk, *rhis,* nose, *itis,* inflammation], an infection of the nasal mucosa that is accompanied by pus formation. The condition is often secondary to a systemic infection, such as measles.

**purulent synovitis** [L, *purulentus,* pus formation; Gk, *syn,* together; L, *ovum,* egg], an inflammation of the synovial membrane of a joint with pus formation in the cavity.

**pus** [L, corrupt matter], a creamy, viscous fluid exudate that is the result of fluid remains of liquefactive necrosis of tissues. It is usually pale yellow to yellow green, sometimes whitish, and sometimes bloody. Its main constituent is an abundance of polymorphonuclear leukocytes. Bacterial infection is its most common cause. The character of the pus, including its color, consistency, quantity, or odor, may be of diagnostic significance.

**pus cell,** a necrotic polymorphonuclear leukocyte, a major component of pus. Also called **pus corpuscle.**

**pus corpuscle.** See **pus cell.**

**push-up block.** See **handblock.**

**pus in urine** [L, *pus* + Gk, *ouron,* urine], the presence of pus in a urine sample, indicating a urinary tract infection anywhere from the kidneys to the urethra. Cloudiness in urine may be caused by either pus or chemicals, a difference determined by simple laboratory tests.

**pustular** /pus'chələr/ [L, *pustula,* blister], pertaining to or resembling pustules.

**pustular psoriasis** [L, *pustula,* blister; Gk, *psoriasis,* itch], a severe form of psoriasis consisting of bright red patches and sterile pustules all over the body. Crops of lesions lasting 4 to 7 days occur every few days in cycles over weeks or months. Recurrences are inevitable. Fever, leukocytosis, and hypoalbuminemia are associated. In rare cases, hypovolemia and kidney failure occur. Hospitalization may be necessary for fluid replacement, steroid therapy, and sedation. Compare **guttate psoriasis.** See also **psoriasis.**

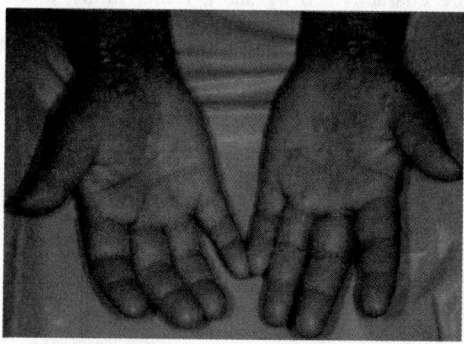

**Pustular psoriasis** *(Lemmi and Lemmi, 2000)*

**pustule** /pus'chōōl/ [L, *pustula*], a small circumscribed elevation of the skin containing fluid that is usually purulent. **—pustular,** *adj.*

**putamen** /pyōōtā'mən/ [L, *putamen,* husk], a part of the lentiform nucleus that is lateral to the globus pallidus. It is associated with the corpus striatum and receives connections from the suppressor centers of the cortex.

**putrefaction** /pyōō'trəfak'shən/ [L, *puter,* rotten, *facere,* to make], the decay of enzymes, especially proteins, that produces foul-smelling compounds, such as ammonia, hydrogen sulfide, and mercaptans. **—putrefactive,** *adj.*

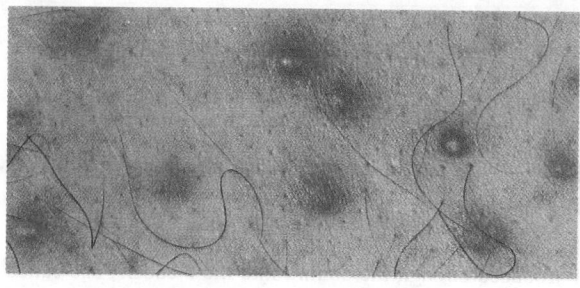

**Pustule** *(du Vivier, 1993)*

**putrefactive** /-fak'tiv/ [L, *puter,* rotten, *facere,* to make], causing, promoting, or relating to putrefaction.

**putrefy** /pyōō'trəfī/ [L, *puter,* rotten, *facere,* to make], to decay, with the production of foul-smelling substances, especially putrescine and mercaptans associated with the decomposition of animal tissues and proteins.

**putrescine** /pyōō'tresēn/, a foul-smelling toxic ptomaine produced by the decomposition of the amino acid ornithine during the decay of animal tissues, bacillus cultures, and fecal bacteria.

**putrid** /pyōō'trid/ [L, *putridus,* rotten], decomposed.

**putromaine** /pyōōtrō'mān/, any toxin produced by the decay of food within a living body.

**PUVA,** an abbreviation for a psoriasis treatment consisting of a medication called *p*soralen plus *u*ltra*v*iolet light of *A* (long) wavelength.

**P value,** (in research) the statistical probability of the occurrence of a given finding by chance alone in comparison with the known distribution of possible findings, considering the kinds of data, the technique of analysis, and the number of observations. The P value may be noted as a decimal: p .01 means that the likelihood that the phenomena tested occurred by chance alone is less than 1%. The lower the P value, the less likely the finding would occur by chance alone.

**PVB.** See **VBP.**

**PVC,** 1. abbreviation for **polyvinyl chloride.** 2. abbreviation for **premature ventricular complex.**

**PVR,** abbreviation for **pulmonary vascular resistance.**

**pW,** abbreviation for *picowatt.*

**PWA,** abbreviation for *person with AIDS.*

**P wave,** the component of the cardiac cycle shown on an electrocardiogram as an inverted U-shaped curve that follows the T wave and precedes the QRS complex. It represents atrial depolarization.

**P' wave (P prime wave),** a P wave that is generated from a site other than the sinus node; an ectopic P wave.

**PWP,** abbreviation for **pulmonary wedge pressure.**

**pyaemic embolism.** See **pyemic embolism.**

**pycno-, pykno-** [Gk, *pyknos,* thick], combining form meaning 'density or thickness': *pyknometer, pyknophrasia.*

**pyel-.** See **pyelo-.**

**pyelitis** /pī'əlī'tis/, *obsolete.* an inflammation of the pelvis of the kidney. See **pyelonephritis.**

**pyelo-, pyel-,** combining form meaning 'pelvis or kidney': *pyelocaliectasis, pyelocystitis, pyelograph.*

**pyelogram** /pī'əlōgram'/ [Gk, *pyelos,* pelvis, *gramma,* record], a radiographic picture of the kidneys and ureters taken after the IV or intraureteral injection of a radiopaque contrast medium. It shows the size and location of the kidneys, the outline of the ureters and bladder, the filling of the renal pelves, the patency of the urinary tract, and any cysts or tumors within the kidneys. Preparation for an IV pyelogram includes withholding of fluids for 8 hours and testing for sensitivity to the iodine in the contrast medium; people with known sensitivity are not tested lest anaphylaxis occur. Patients able to tolerate the contrast medium may feel warm and experience a salty taste when it is injected. Retrograde pyelograms, which demonstrate filling of the renal collecting structures, are taken after the contrast medium is injected into the ureters by means of catheters in a cystoscope introduced through the urethra into the bladder. Also called **urogram.**

**pyelography.**   See **intravenous pyelography.**

**pyelolithotomy** /pī′əlō′lithot′əmē/,   a surgical procedure in which renal calculi are removed from the pelvis of the ureter.

**pyelonephritis** /pī′əlōnəfrī′tis/ [Gk, *pyelos* + *nephros,* kidney, *itis,* inflammation],   a diffuse pyogenic infection of the pelvis and parenchyma of the kidney. **Acute pyelonephritis** is usually the result of an infection that ascends from the lower urinary tract to the kidney. *Escherichia coli* contamination of the urethral meatus is a common cause in females. Infection may spread to the kidney from other locations in the body. The onset of acute pyelonephritis is rapid, characterized by fever, chills, pain in the flank, nausea, and urinary frequency. Urinalysis reveals the presence of bacteria and white blood cells. Antimicrobial treatment is continued for 10 days to 2 weeks. Relapse or reinfection is common. **Chronic pyelonephritis** develops slowly after bacterial infection of the kidney and may progress to renal failure. Most cases are associated with some form of obstruction, such as a stone or a stricture of the ureter. Treatment includes removal of the cause of obstruction and long-term antimicrobial therapy.

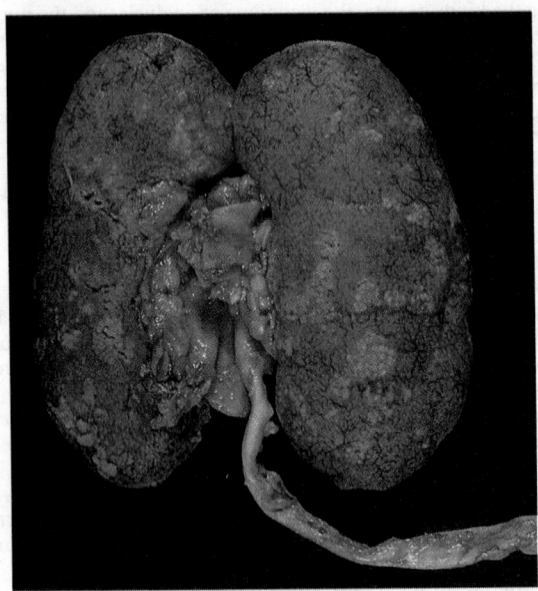

**Acute pyelonephritis** *(Cotran, Kumar, and Collins, 1999)*

**pyeloplasty** /pī′əlōplas′tē/,   the surgical reconstruction of the kidney pelvis.

**pyelorostomy,**   the surgical establishment of a fistula from the abdominal surface to the stomach at a point near the pylorus.

**pyemesis** /pī·em′əsis/,   the action of vomiting purulent material.

**pyemic embolism** /pī·ē′mik/ [Gk, *pyon,* pus, *haima,* blood, *embolos,* plug],   an infective embolus producing an abscess. Also spelled **pyaemic embolism.**

**pygeum,**   an herbal product derived from an evergreen tree native to Africa.

■ USES: This herb is used for benign prostate hypertrophy and as an antiinflammatory.

■ CONTRAINDICATIONS: Pygeum is not recommended during pregnancy and lactation, in children, or in those with known hypersensitivity to this plant.

**pygmalianism** /pigmā′lē·əniz′əm/ [Gk, *Pygmalion,* mythic sculptor who fell in love with his statue],   a psychosexual abnormality in which the individual directs erotic fantasies to an object that he or she has created.

**pygmy** /pig′mē/ [L, *pygmaeus,* dwarf],   an extremely small person whose body parts are proportioned accordingly; a primordial dwarf. Also spelled **pigmy.**

**pygo-** /pī′gō-/,   combining form meaning 'buttocks': *pygoamorphus, pygodidymus, pygopagus.*

**pygoamorphus** /pī′gō·əmôr′fəs/ [Gk, *pyge,* buttocks, *a + morphe,* not form],   asymmetric, conjoined twins in which the parasitic member is represented by an undifferentiated amorphous mass attached to the autosite in the sacral region.

**pygodidymus** /pī′gōdid′əməs/ [Gk, *pyge,* buttocks, *didymos,* twin],   **1.** a malformed fetus that has a double pelvis and hips. **2.** conjoined twins who are fused in the cephalothoracic region but separated at the pelvis.

**pygomelus** /pīgom′ələs/ [Gk, *pyge* + *melos,* limb],   a malformed fetus that has an extra limb or limbs attached to the buttock. Also called **epipygus.**

**pygopagus** /pīgop′əgəs/ [Gk, *pyge* + *pegos,* fixed],   conjoined twins consisting of two fully formed or nearly formed fetuses united in the sacral region so that they are positioned back to back.

**pyknic** /pik′nik/ [Gk, *pyknos,* thick],   describing a body structure characterized by short, round limbs; a full face with a broad head and thick shoulders; a short neck; stockiness; and a tendency to obesity. Compare **asthenic habitus, athletic habitus.** See also **endomorph.**

**pykno-.**   See **pycno-.**

**pyknodysostosis** /pik′nō·dis′os·tō′sis/ [Gk, *pyknos,* thick + *dys-,* bad + *osteon,* bone + *-osis,* condition],   an autosomal recessive symptom complex consisting of dwarfism, osteopetrosis, partial agenesis of terminal digits of hands and feet, cranial anomalies, frontal and occipital bossing, and hypoplasia of the angle of the mandible.

**pyknosis** /piknō′sis/,   the condensation of nuclear material into a solid, darkly staining mass in a dying cell.

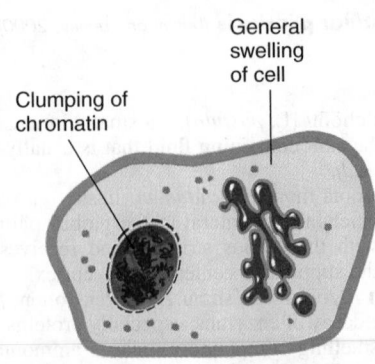

Clumping of chromatin

General swelling of cell

**Pyknosis** *(Huether and McCance, 2000)*

**pyla** /pī′lə/, the opening between the third ventricle and the cerebral aqueduct.

**pyle-,** prefix meaning 'portal vein': *pylemphraxis, pylephlebectasis, pylephlebitis.*

**pylethrombophlebitis** /pī′ləthrom′bōfləbī′tis/, inflammation of the portal vein with formation of a thrombus.

**pylon** /pī′lon/ [Gk, gate], an artificial lower limb, often a narrow vertical support consisting of a socket with wooden side supports and a rubber-clad peg end. It may be used as a temporary prosthesis.

**pylori.** See **pylorus.**

**pyloric** /pīlôr′ik/ [Gk, *pyle,* gate, *ouros,* guard], pertaining to the pylorus, the opening between the stomach and duodenum.

**pyloric canal,** the narrow, constricted region of the pyloric part of the stomach.

**pyloric obstruction and dilation** /pīlôr′ik/ [Gk, *pyle,* gate, *ouros,* guard; L, *obstruere,* to build against, *dilatare,* to widen], a reaction of the stomach to pyloric obstruction, which increases the resistance to the expulsion of partly digested food from the stomach. As a result, the stomach may become hypertrophied, then dilated. Excessive consumption of food and beverages contributes to the condition.

**pyloric orifice** [Gk, *pyle,* gate, *ouros,* guard; L, *orificium,* opening], the opening of or passage between the stomach into the duodenum lying to the right of the midline at the level of the upper border of the first lumbar vertebra. The orifice is usually indicated on the surface of the stomach by the circular duodenopyloric constriction.

**pyloric spasm.** See **pylorospasm.**

**pyloric sphincter,** a thickened muscular ring in the stomach, separating the pylorus from the duodenum. Also called **pyloric valve.**

**pyloric stenosis,** a narrowing of the pyloric sphincter at the outlet of the stomach, causing an obstruction that blocks the flow of food into the small intestine. The condition occurs as a congenital defect in 1 of 200 newborns and occasionally in older adults secondary to an ulcer or fibrosis at the outlet. Diagnosis is made in infants by the presence of forceful projectile vomiting and palpation of a hard, prominent pylorus, and in adults by x-ray examinations after a barium meal. Surgical correction is done using light general anesthesia, after the stomach is emptied. The muscle fibers of the outlet are cut, without severing the mucosa, to widen the opening. After surgery in adults, a stomach tube remains in place and observation is maintained for signs of hemorrhage or of blockage of the tube. See also **pyloromyotomy.**

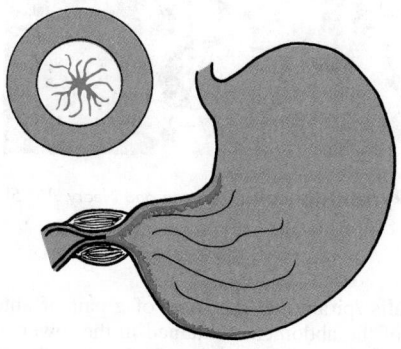

**Pyloric stenosis** *(Wong et al, 1999)*

**pyloric ulcer.** See **peptic ulcer.**

**pyloric valve.** See **pyloric sphincter.**

**pyloro-,** combining form meaning 'the pylorus': *pylorodilator, pyloroplasty, pyloroptosis.*

**pyloroduodenitis** /pilôr′ōdo͞o′ədənī′tis/, an inflammation of the pylorus and the duodenum.

**pyloromyotomy** /pīlôr′ōmī·ot′əmē/ [Gk, *pyle + ouros + mys,* muscle, *temnein,* to cut], the incision of the longitudinal and circular muscle of the pylorus, which leaves the mucosa intact but separates the incised muscle fibers. It is the treatment of choice for hypertrophic pyloric stenosis. Also called **Fredet-Ramstedt operation, Ramstedt-Fredet operation.** See also **pyloric stenosis.**

**pyloroplasty** /pīlôr′əplas′tē/ [Gk, *pyle + ouros + plassein,* to mold], a surgical procedure performed to relieve the structures of pyloric stenosis by widening the pyloric outlet. Before surgery any electrolyte imbalances or fluid deficiencies are corrected; sodium chloride and potassium chloride solutions may be given to correct ion losses from vomiting, which is characteristic of pyloric stenosis. With the patient under anesthesia the pyloric opening is dilated. Diarrhea is a common postoperative complication.

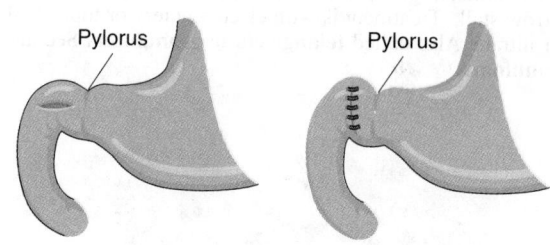

**Pyloroplasty** *(Beare and Myers, 1998)*

**pylorospasm** /pīlôr′əspaz′əm/ [Gk, *pyle, ouros + spasmos*], a spasm of the pyloric sphincter of the stomach, as occurs in pyloric stenosis.

**pylorostomy** /pī′lôros′təmē/, the surgical establishment of a fistula from the abdominal surface to the stomach at a point near the pylorus.

**pylorotomy** /pī′lôrot′əmē/ [Gk, *pyle,* gate, *ouros,* guard, *temnein,* to cut], a surgical incision of the pylorus, usually performed to remove an obstruction.

**pylorus** /pīlôr′əs/, *pl.* **pylori, pyloruses** [Gk, *pyle,* gate, *ouros,* guard], a narrow, nearly tubular part of the stomach that angles to the right from the body of the stomach toward the duodenum. The most common position of the pylorus is about 3 cm to the right of the sagittal axis. It is distinctively marked by the thickening of the pyloric sphincter, and its lining is composed of an intestinal kind of epithelium rather than the gastric kind common to the body of the stomach. —**pyloric,** *adj.*

**pyo-** /pī′ō-/, combining form meaning 'pus': *pyocalyx, pyocele, pyocyte.*

**pyocele,** an accumulation of pus in the scrotum.

**Pyocidin Otic,** trademark for a fixed-combination otic drug containing a glucocorticoid (hydrocortisone) and an antibacterial (polymyxin B sulfate).

**pyocolpos,** an accumulation of pus in the vagina.

**pyocyanic** /pī′ōsī·an′ik/, pertaining to pus that is blue or to an organism that produces blue pus, such as *Pseudomonas pyocyanea.*

**pyocyanin** /pī′ōsī′ənin/, a blue or blue-green pigment that may be extracted from *Pseudomonas aeruginosa* with chloroform.

**pyocyst** /pī′əsist/ [Gk, *pyon*, pus, *kytos*, cell], a pus-filled cyst.

**pyocystitis** /-sistī′tis/, an inflammation involving a pus-filled cyst within the urinary bladder.

**pyoderma** /pī′ōdur′mə/ [Gk, *pyon*, pus, *derma*, skin], any purulent skin disease, such as impetigo. Also called **pyodermia.**

**pyoderma gangrenosum,** a rapidly evolving, idiopathic, chronic debilitating skin disease that usually accompanies a systemic disease, especially chronic ulcerative colitis, and is characterized by irregular, boggy, blue-red ulcers with undermined borders surrounding purulent necrotic bases.

**pyogenic** /pī′əjen′ik/ [Gk, *pyon* + *genein*, to produce], pus-producing.

**pyogenic exotoxin,** extracellular toxin secreted by *Streptococcus pyogenes* that may be associated with fever and the development of renal failure, respiratory distress, and necrosis.

**pyogenic granuloma,** a small nonmalignant mass of excessive granulation tissue, usually found at the site of an injury. Most often a dull red, it contains numerous capillaries, bleeds readily, and is very tender; it may be attached by a narrow stalk. Treatment is with electrocautery or topical silver nitrate. Also called **telangiectatic granuloma.** See also **granuloma.**

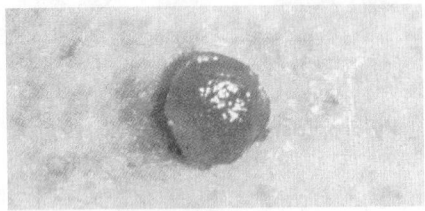

**Pyogenic granuloma**
*(Goldstein and Goldstein, 1997/courtesy Beverly Sanders, MD)*

**pyogenic infection** [Gk, *pyon*, pus, *genein*, to produce; L, *inficere*, to stain], any infection that results in pus production.

**pyogenic microorganisms** [Gk, *pyon*, pus, *genein*, to produce, *mikros*, small, *organon*, instrument], microorganisms that produce pus. They include species of bacilli, clostridia, gonococci, meningococci, pseudomonas, staphylococci, and streptococci.

**pyohemothorax** /-hem′ōthôr′aks/ [Gk, *pyon*, pus, *haima*, blood, *thorax*, chest], an accumulation of pus and blood in the pleural cavity.

**pyonephrolithiasis** /-nef′rōlithī′əsis/, an accumulation of pus and calculi in the kidney.

**pyophylactic** /-filak′tik/ [Gk, *pyon*, pus, *phylax*, protector], providing protection against purulent infections, such as administering an antibiotic before the onset of an infection.

**pyophysometra** /-fī′sōmē′trə/, an accumulation of pus and gas in the uterus.

**pyopneumopericardium** /pī′ōnōō′mōper′ikär′dē·əm/, the presence of pus and air or gas in the pericardial sac.

**pyopneumoperitonitis** /pī′ōnōō′mōper′itənī′tis/, inflammation of the peritoneal cavity caused by an accumulation of air and pus in the cavity.

**pyopyelectasis** /-pī′əlek′təsis/, a dilation of the renal pelvis of the kidney resulting from an accumulation of pus.

**pyorrhea** /pī′ərē′ə/ [Gk, *pyon* + *rhoia*, flow], **1.** a discharge of pus. **2.** a purulent inflammation of the tissues surrounding the teeth. —**pyorrheal,** *adj.* Also spelled **pyorrhoea.**

**pyorrhea-,** combining form meaning 'the flowing or discharge of pus': *ophthalmopyorrhea, otopyorrhea.*

**pyorrheal.** See **pyorrhea.**

**pyosalpinx** /pī′ōsal′pingks/ [Gk, *pyon* + *salpinx*, tube], an accumulation of pus in a fallopian tube. See also **salpingitis.**

**pyosemia.** See **pyospermia.**

**pyospermia,** a complication of chronic prostatitis marked by pus in the seminal fluid. Also called **pyosemia.**

**pyostatic** /-stat′ik/, the formation of pus.

**pyostomatitis** /-stō′mətī′tis/, an inflammation of the mouth.

**pyothorax** /-thôr′aks/, **1.** a collection of pus in the pleural cavity. **2.** purulent pleurisy.

**pyoureter** /pī′ōyŏŏr′ətər, -yōōrē′tər/, the presence of pus in the ureter.

**pyoverdin** /-vur′din/, a yellow pigment produced by some strains of *Pseudomonas aeruginosa.*

**pyramid** /pir′əmid/ [Gr, *pyramis*], a mass of tissue rising to an apex, such as the pyramids of the cerebellum and kidneys.

**pyramidal** /piram′idəl/ [Gk, *pyramis*], pertaining to the shape of a pyramid.

**pyramidal cell** [Gk, *pyramis* + L, *cella*, storeroom], a neuron with a pyramid-shaped cell body in the gray matter of the cerebral cortex.

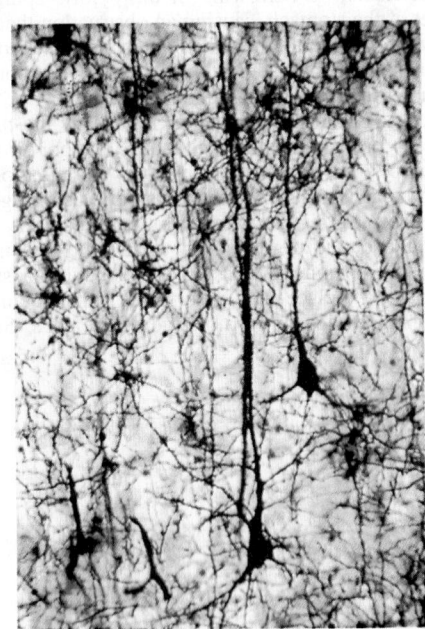

**Pyramidal cell** *(Crossman and Neary, 1995)*

**pyramidalis** /piram′idā′lis/, one of a pair of anterolateral muscles of the abdomen, contained in the lower end of the sheath of the rectus abdominis, which arises from the crest of the pubic and is inserted into the linea alba upward about halfway to the navel. It is innervated by a branch of the twelfth thoracic nerve and functions to tense the linea alba. Compare **rectus abdominis, transversus abdominis.**

**pyramidal nucleus** [Gk, *pyramis* + L, *nucleus,* nut kernel], a band of gray matter lying between the olivary nucleus and the midline that projects fibers contralaterally to the vermis of part of the cerebellum.

**pyramidal tract,** a pathway composed of groups of nerve fibers in the white matter of the spinal cord through which motor impulses are conducted to the anterior horn cells from the opposite side of the brain. These descending fibers, the nerve cell bodies of which are found in the precentral cortex, regulate the voluntary and reflex activity of the muscles through the anterior horn cells.

**pyramidotomy** /piram′idot′əmē/, the surgical severance of pyramidal tracts in the treatment of disorders associated with involuntary muscle contractions.

**pyrantel pamoate** /pīran′təl/, an anthelmintic.
■ INDICATIONS: It is prescribed in the treatment of infestation by roundworms or pinworms.
■ CONTRAINDICATION: Known hypersensitivity to this drug prohibits its use. Caution should be used in anemia or severe malnutrition.
■ ADVERSE EFFECTS: Among the more serious adverse reactions are nausea, abdominal cramps, diarrhea, dizziness, and skin rash.

**pyrazinamide** /pī′razin′əmīd/, an antimycobacterial.
■ INDICATIONS: It is prescribed in combination chemotherapy in the treatment of tuberculosis of hospitalized patients who fail to respond to other medications.
■ CONTRAINDICATIONS: Severe liver damage or known hypersensitivity to this drug prohibits its use.
■ ADVERSE EFFECTS: Among the more serious adverse reactions are hepatotoxicity and hyperuricemia.

**pyrectic** /pīrek′tik/ [Gk, *pyretos* fever], pertaining to or characterized by fever. Also called *pyretic.*

**pyrenemia** /pī′rənē′mē·ə/, a condition in which nucleated erythrocytes are present in the blood.

**pyrethrin and piperonyl butoxide** /pī′rəthrin, piper′ənil/, a fixed-combination scabicide and pediculicide.
■ INDICATIONS: It is prescribed in the treatment of infestations of head, body, and pubic lice.
■ CONTRAINDICATIONS: Known hypersensitivity to ragweed or to this drug prohibits its use.
■ ADVERSE EFFECTS: Among the more serious adverse reactions are irritation of the skin and the mucous membranes.

**pyreto-,** combining form meaning 'fever': *pyretogen, pyretography, pyretotherapy.*

**pyretogenic** /pī′rətojen′ik/ [Gk, *pyretos,* fever, *genein,* to produce], inducing, causing, or resulting from a fever.

**pyretotherapy.** See **pyrotherapy.**

**pyrexia.** See **fever.**

**-pyrexia,** combining form meaning 'febrile condition': *apyrexia, electropyrexia, physiopyrexia.*

**Pyridium,** trademark for a urinary tract analgesic (phenazopyridine hydrochloride).

**pyridostigmine bromide** /pir′idōstig′mēn/, an anticholinergic/cholinergic agent.
■ INDICATIONS: It is prescribed in the treatment of myasthenia gravis and is used as an antagonist to nondepolarizing muscle relaxants, such as curare.
■ CONTRAINDICATIONS: Intestinal or urinary obstruction, bradycardia, hypotension, or known hypersensitivity to this drug or to other anticholinesterases prohibits its use.
■ ADVERSE EFFECTS: Among the more serious adverse reactions are nausea, diarrhea, abdominal cramps, muscle cramps, and weakness.

**pyridoxal phosphate** /pir′ədok′səl/, an enzyme that acts with pyridoxamine phosphate and transaminase to catalyze the reversible transfer of an amino group from an alpha-amino acid to an alpha-keto acid, especially alpha-ketoglutaric acid. Such processes are essential to metabolism.

**pyridoxamine phosphate** /pir′ədok′səmēn/, an enzyme that participates with pyridoxal phosphate and transaminase in the reversible transfer of an amino group from an alpha-amino acid to an alpha-keto acid.

**pyridoxine** /pir′ədok′sēn/, a water-soluble white crystalline vitamin that is part of the B complex. It is derived from pyridine and converted in the body to pyridoxal and pyridoxamine for synthesis. It functions as a coenzyme essential for the synthesis and breakdown of amino acids, the conversion of tryptophan to niacin, the breakdown of glycogen to glucose 1-phosphate, the production of antibodies, the formation of heme in hemoglobin, the formation of hormones important in brain function, the proper absorption of vitamin $B_{12}$, the production of hydrochloric acid and magnesium, and the maintenance of the balance of sodium and potassium, which regulates body fluids and the functioning of the nervous and musculoskeletal systems. Rich dietary sources are meats, especially organ meats; whole-grain cereals; soybeans; peanuts; wheat germ; and brewer's yeast. Milk and green vegetables supply smaller amounts. The most common symptoms of deficiency are seborrheic dermatitis about the eyes, nose, and mouth and behind the ears; cheilosis; glossitis and stomatitis; nervousness; depression; peripheral neuropathy; and lymphopenia, leading to convulsions in infants and anemia in adults. Treatment and prophylaxis consist of administration of the vitamin and a diet rich in foods containing it. Several drugs interfere with the use of pyridoxine, notably isoniazid and penicillamine, and supplements of the vitamin are recommended with the use of these drugs. The need for increased amounts of pyridoxine is related to protein intake and occurs during pregnancy, lactation, exposure to radiation, cardiac failure, aging, and use of oral contraceptives. Also called **vitamin $B_6$.**

**pyridoxine hydrochloride.** See **pyridoxine.**

**pyriform.** See **piriform.**

**pyrimethamine** /pir′imeth′əmēn/, an antimalarial.
■ INDICATIONS: It is prescribed in the treatment of malaria and toxoplasmosis.
■ CONTRAINDICATIONS: Use in chloroguanide-resistant malaria is contraindicated. Caution is recommended in use of the drug to treat toxoplasmosis because dosages needed may be at toxic level.
■ ADVERSE EFFECTS: Among the more serious adverse reactions, primarily with large doses, are megaloblastic anemia, atrophic glossitis, leukopenia, and convulsions.

**pyrimidine** /pərim′ədēn/, an organic compound of heterocyclic nitrogen found in nucleic acids and in many drugs, including the antiviral drugs acyclovir, ribavirin, and trifluridine.

**pyro-** /pī′rō-/, prefix meaning 'fire or heat, or produced by heating': *pyrocatechin, pyrodextrin, pyromania.*

**pyrogen** /pī′rəjən/ [Gk, *pyr,* fire, *genein,* to produce], any substance or agent that tends to cause a rise in body temperature, such as some bacterial toxins. See also **fever.** —**pyrogenic,** *adj.*

**pyroglobulin** /pī′rōglob′yəlin/, an immunoglobulin that precipitates irreversibly when heated. Pyroglobulins are often present in the blood of patients with diseases such as multiple myeloma.

**pyrolagnia** /pī′rōlag′nē·ə/ [Gk, *pyr* + *lagneia,* lust], sexual stimulation or gratification from watching or setting fires.

**pyrolysis** /pīrol'isis/, the decomposition of a chemical compound by the application of heat.

**pyromania** /pī'rōmā'nē·ə/ [Gk, *pyr* + *mania,* madness], an impulse-control disorder characterized by an uncontrollable urge to set fires.

**pyromaniac** /pī'rōmā'nē·ak/, **1.** a person having or displaying characteristics of pyromania. **2.** pertaining to or exhibiting pyromania. —**pyromaniacal,** *adj.*

**pyropoikilocytosis** /pī'rōpoi'kilō'sītō'sis/, a recessive inherited disorder characterized by severe hemolysis, irregular shapes of red blood cells, and sensitivity of blood cells to fragmentation in vitro after minor temperature variations.

**pyrosis.** See **heartburn.**

**pyrotherapy** /pī'rōther'əpē/, a method of treatment in which the temperature of a patient is raised to a fever level. Also called **pyretotherapy, therapeutic fever.**

**pyroxylin.** See **nitrocellulose.**

**pyrrole (C₄H₄NH)** /pirōl', pir'ōl/ [Gk, *pyrrhos,* red], a 5-membered heterocyclic aromatic substance occurring naturally in many compounds in the body. Heme and porphyrin are pyrrole derivatives.

**Pyrroxate,** trademark for a decongestant, antihistamine, analgesic combination drug containing a decongestant (phenylpropanolamine), an antihistamine (chlorpheniramine maleate), and analgesics (acetaminophen).

**pyruvate carboxylase** /pī'rōō·vāt kär·bok'sə·lās/, an enzyme that catalyzes the irreversible carboxylation of pyruvate, a reaction necessary for gluconeogenesis from lactate or amino acids forming pyruvate and also providing four-carbon compounds for the citric acid cycle. The enzyme is a mitochondrial protein occuring in liver but not in muscle. Deficiency of the enzyme, an autosomal recessive trait, causes severe psychomotor retardation and lactic acidosis in infants; there is a particularly severe, rapidly fatal form, in which hyperammonemia, citrullinemia, and excess of lysine in the blood are also present.

**pyruvate dehydrogenase complex** /pī'rōō·vāt dē·hī'drō·jən·ās/, a multienzyme complex consisting of at least three distinct enzymes, which catalyzes the formation of acetyl coenzyme A from pyruvate and coenzyme A. The acetyl coenzyme A is used in fatty acid synthesis, for acetylations, and for oxidation via the citric acid cycle. Deficiency of any component of the complex results in excess of lactic acid in the blood, ataxia, and psychomotor retardation.

**pyruvate kinase** /pī'rəvāt/, an enzyme essential for anaerobic glycolysis in red blood cells. It catalyzes the transfer of a phosphate group from adenosine triphosphate to produce adenosine diphosphate.

**pyruvate kinase deficiency,** a congenital hemolytic disorder transmitted as an autosomal recessive trait. The homozygous condition is characterized by severe chronic hemolysis. The heterozygous form is usually asymptomatic and of no clinical significance, although mild to severe anemia may occur.

**pyruvic acid** /pīrōō'vik/, a compound formed as an end product of glycolysis, the anaerobic stage of glucose metabolism. It may enter the citric acid cycle if oxygen is present. Under anaerobic conditions it may be converted to lactic acid, which accumulates in muscle tissue.

**pyuria** /pīyōōr'ē·ə/, the presence of an excessive number of white blood cells in the urine, typically more than four leukocytes per high-power field count. It is generally a sign of an infection in the urinary tract. Bacterial pyuria usually is caused by a viral infection of the bladder and urethra. See also **bacteriuria.**

**PZI,** abbreviation for **protamine zinc insulin.** See **protamine zinc insulin (PZI) suspension.**

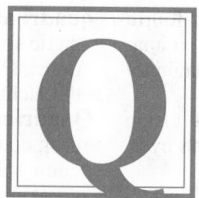

**Q, 1.** symbol for *blood volume*. **2.** symbol for *quantity*. **3.** symbol for *coulomb*.

**Q̇,** symbol for *rate of blood flow*.

**q.2h.,** (in prescriptions) abbreviation for *quaque secunda hora*, a Latin phrase meaning 'every 2 hours.'

**q.3h.,** (in prescriptions) abbreviation for *quaque tertia hora*, a Latin phrase meaning 'every 3 hours.'

**q.4h.,** (in prescriptions) abbreviation for *quaque quarta hora*, a Latin phrase meaning 'every 4 hours.'

**q.6h.,** (in prescriptions) abbreviation for *quaque sex hora*, a Latin phrase meaning 'every 6 hours.'

**q.8h.,** (in prescriptions) abbreviation for *quaque octa hora*, a Latin phrase meaning 'every 8 hours.'

**Q angle,** the angle of incidence of the quadriceps muscle relative to the patella. The Q angle determines the tracking of the patella through the trochlea of the femur. As the angle increases, the chance of patellar compression problems increases.

**QCT,** abbreviation for **quantitative computed tomography.**

**q.d., 1.** (in prescriptions) abbreviation for *quaque die* /dē′ā/, a Latin phrase meaning 'every day.' Also called **q diem, quotid. 2.** abbreviation for *quartile deviation*.

**qdrnt,** abbreviation for **quadrant.**

**Q fever** [L, *febris*], an acute febrile illness, usually respiratory, caused by the rickettsia *Coxiella burnetii (Rickettsia burnetii)*. The disease is spread through contact with infected domestic animals, by inhaling the rickettsiae from their hides, drinking their contaminated milk, or being bitten by a tick harboring the organism. Onset is abrupt, and high fever may persist for 3 weeks or more. The illness is especially common among those who work with sheep, goats, and cattle. Treatment with tetracycline is usually effective in 36 to 48 hours. People who are regularly exposed to domestic animals can be vaccinated against Q fever. Also called **Australian Q fever.** Compare **scrub typhus.**

**q.h.,** (in prescriptions) abbreviation for *quaque hora*, a Latin phrase meaning 'every hour.'

**q.i.d.,** (in prescriptions) abbreviation for *quater in die* /dē′ā/, a Latin phrase meaning 'four times a day.'

**q.l.,** abbreviation for the Latin phrase *quantum libet*, 'as much as one pleases.'

**qli,** abbreviation for *quality of life index*.

**Q-R interval,** the period from the start of the QRS complex to the peak of the R wave on an electrocardiogram.

**QRS complex,** a series of waveforms on an electrocardiogram that represent both normal and abnormal depolarization of ventricular muscle cells. It is composed of Q, R, and S waves: a Q wave is the negative deflection before the first R wave; an R wave is any positive deflection; and an S wave is the negative deflection after an R wave. If there is no R wave, the totally negative complex is designated QS. A combination of upper- and lower-case letters is used to describe the amplitude of each wave. Some variations of the QRS complex are qR, QR, qRs, rS, RS, and rSR′.

**QRST complex** [L, *complexus*], a series of waveforms on an electrocardiogram, consisting of the QRS complex, the

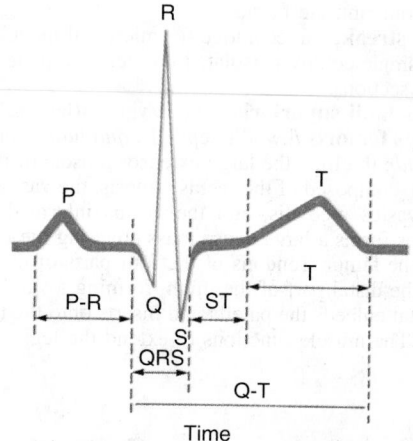

**QRS complex and Q-T interval of a normal ECG waveform**
*(Berne and Levy, 1996)*

S-T segment and the T wave. It represents depolarization and repolarization of the ventricular muscle cells.

**q.s.,** (in prescriptions) abbreviation for *quantum sufficit*, a Latin phrase meaning 'quantity required.'

**Q's test.** See **Queckenstedt's test.**

**Q-switching,** a laser technique used in glaucoma surgery to achieve high-peak power in nanosecond pulses of energy.

**qt,** abbreviation for **quart.**

**Q-T interval,** the period from the beginning of the QRS complex to the end of the T wave on an electrocardiogram. It reflects the refractory period of the heart. A long Q-T interval is associated with the life-threatening ventricular tachycardia known as torsades de pointes. Quinidine, procainamide, and disopyramide can lengthen the Q-T interval.

**Quaalude,** trademark for a sedative-hypnotic (methaqualone). It is no longer distributed in the United States.

**quack.** See **charlatan.**

**quad, 1.** abbreviation for *quadriceps*. **2.** abbreviation for *quadrilateral*. **3.** abbreviation for **quadrant. 4.** abbreviation for **quadriplegia.**

**quad coughing** /kwod/, a form of assisted coughing for patients with central nervous system disorders who are unable to generate sufficient force to clear respiratory secretions. After a maximal inspiration, the patient coughs while an assistant exerts gentle upward and inward pressure with both hands on the abdomen. The increased intraabdominal pressure produces a more forceful cough.

**quadr-, quadri-,** prefix meaning 'four': *quadrangular, quadribasic, quadrivalent.*

**quadrangular bandage** /kwodrang′gələr/, a towel or other large rectangular sheet of cloth folded over for use as a wrapping for a wound of the abdomen, chest, or head.

**quadrant (qdrnt, quad)** /kwod'rənt/ [L, *quadrans,* a fourth part], **1.** one quarter of a circle. **2.** one quarter of an anatomic area formed by the division of the area by imaginary vertical and horizontal lines bisecting each other.

**quadrantanopsia** /kwodran'tənop'sē·ə/, a loss of vision in a quarter section of the visual field of one or both eyes. The cause may vary with the quadrant affected.

**quadrantectomy** /kwod'rantek'təmē/, a partial mastectomy in which a tumor is excised in one quadrant of a breast and at least a 1-inch margin of surrounding tissue along with the pectoralis muscle fascia.

**quadrant streak,** a technique for microbial inoculation in which a single colony is isolated on a culture plate divided into four sections.

**quadratus labii superioris.** See **zygomaticus minor.**

**quadriceps femoris** /kwod'riseps/ [L, *quattuor,* four, *caput,* head, *femur,* thigh], the large extensor muscle of the anterior thigh, composed of the rectus femoris, the vastus lateralis, the vastus medialis, and the vastus intermedius. The quadriceps forms a large dense mass covering the front and sides of the femur. Tendons of the four parts of the muscle unite at the distal part of the thigh, forming a single strong tendon that embeds the patella and inserts onto the tibial tuberosity. The muscle functions to extend the leg.

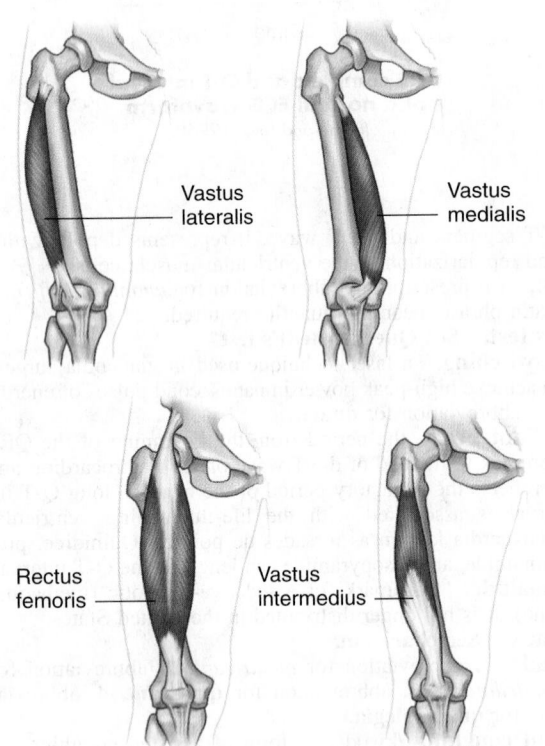

Vastus lateralis

Vastus medialis

Rectus femoris

Vastus intermedius

**Quadriceps femoris group of thigh muscles**

**quadriceps reflex.** See **patellar reflex.**

**quadridigitate,** tetradactylous; see **tetradactyly.**

**quadrigeminal** /kwod'rijem'inəl/ [L, *quadrigeminum,* fourfold], **1.** in four parts. **2.** a fourfold increase in size or frequency. **3.** having four symmetric parts.

**quadrigeminal pulse,** a pulse in which a pause occurs after every fourth beat.

**quadrilateral socket** /kwod'rilat'ərəl/, a four-sided prosthetic socket design for people with above-the-knee amputations. The posterior brim is designed to fit directly beneath the ischial tuberosity so that the person literally sits on it.

**Quadrinal,** trademark for a respiratory, fixed-combination drug containing a smooth muscle relaxant (theophylline calcium salicylate), an adrenergic (ephedrine hydrochloride), an expectorant (potassium iodide), and a sedative-hypnotic (phenobarbital).

**quadripedal extensor reflex.** See **Brain's reflex.**

**quadriplegia (quad)** /kwod'rəplē'jē·ə/ [L, *quattuor,* four; Gk, *plege,* stroke], paralysis of the arms, legs, and trunk of the body below the level of an associated injury to the spinal cord. This disorder is usually caused by spinal cord injury, especially in the area of the fifth to the seventh vertebrae. Automobile accidents and sporting mishaps are common causes. This condition affects about 150,000 Americans, the majority of whom are men between 20 and 40 years of age. Signs and symptoms commonly include flaccidity of the arms and the legs and the loss of power and sensation below the level of the injury. Cardiovascular complications also may develop from any injury that damages the spinal cord above the fifth cervical vertebra because of an associated block of the sympathetic nervous system. A major cause of death from such injury is respiratory failure. Other symptoms may include low body temperature, bradycardia, impaired peristalsis, and autonomic dysreflexia. Diagnosis is based on a complete physical and neurologic examination with radiographic pictures of the head, chest, and abdomen to rule out underlying injuries. Spinal x-ray examinations and myelography show any fractures and spinal cord blockages.
■ INTERVENTIONS: Treatment starts at the accident scene, where the patient's neck and spine are immobilized. Additional immobilization at the hospital commonly includes the use of halo traction. Diuretics and steroids are administered to decrease spinal cord edema. After an appropriate period of therapy, surgery is commonly performed to fuse unstable spinal sections and remove bone fragments.
■ NURSING CONSIDERATIONS: Nursing care includes maintaining adequate respiration and the integrity of the GI system and preventing complications such as hypothermia, bradycardia, catheter obstruction, and fecal impaction. A quadriplegic patient who suffers hypothermia is wrapped in blankets instead of being warmed with hot water bottles or electromechanic devices because such devices can burn the skin of the patient experiencing severe sensory loss. Abdominal binders and antiembolism hose are used when the patient is placed in an upright position. Patients who develop bradycardia are commonly connected to a cardiac monitor and intravenously administered an antimuscarinic drug, such as atropine. Fecal impaction may cause hypertension and is always a possible complication. Also called **tetraplegia.** Compare **hemiplegia, paraplegia.**

**quadrivalent** /kwod'rivā'lənt/, a chemical element or radical with a valence of four.

**quadruped** /kwod'roŏped'/ [L, *quattuor,* four, *pes,* foot], **1.** any four-footed animal. **2.** a human whose body weight is supported by both arms as well as both legs. See also **prone-on-elbows.**

**quadruplet** /kwod'roŏplit, kwodroŏ'plit/ [L, *quadruplex,* fourfold], any one of four offspring born of the same gestation period during a single pregnancy. See also **Hellin's law.**

**quadrupole mass filter,** a four-pole magnet system used to separate charged mass fragments in a mass spectrometer.

**qual anal,** abbreviation for **qualitative analysis.**

**quale** /kwā′lē/, *pl.* **qualia** /kwā′lē·ə/ [L, *qualis,* what kind], **1.** the quality of a particular thing. **2.** a quality considered as an independent entity. **3.** (in psychology) a feeling, sensation, or other conscious process that has its unique particular quality regardless of its external meaning or frame of reference.

**qualified** /kwol′ifīd/ [L, *qualis*], pertaining to a health professional or health facility that is formally recognized by an appropriate agency or organization as meeting certain standards of performance related to the professional competence of an individual or the eligibility of an institution to participate in an approved health care program.

**qualitative** /kwol′itā′tiv/ [L, *qualis*], pertaining to the quality, value, or nature of something.

**qualitative analysis (qual anal)** [L, *qualis,* what kind; Gk, *analysis* a loosening] **1.** (in chemistry) the study of a sample of material to determine what chemical substances are present. **2.** (in research) the analysis and interpretation of data that cannot be analyzed by statistical methods.

**qualitative melanin test,** a test for detecting melanin in the urine of patients with malignant melanomas.

**qualitative test,** a test that determines the presence or absence of a substance.

**quality** /kwol′itē/ [L, *qualis*], a descriptive specification of the penetrating nature of an x-ray beam. It is influenced by kilovoltage and filtration: a higher kilovoltage produces more penetration; filtration removes selected wavelengths and "hardens" the beam.

**quality assessment measures,** formal systematic organizational evaluation of overall patterns or programs of care, including clinical, consumer, and systems evaluation.

**quality assurance.** See **quality management.**

**quality assurance program.** See **quality management.**

**quality control,** a method of repeated assay of known standard materials and monitoring reaction parameters to ensure precision and accuracy.

**quality factor,** a term that expresses the biologic damage that radiation can produce. Doses of different types of radiation can be set equal to one another if the actual absorbed dose is multiplied by the quality factor. The product is called the dose equivalent, measured in sieverts or rem.

**quality management, 1.** (in health care) any evaluation of services provided and the results achieved as compared with accepted standards. In one form of quality assurance, various attributes of health care, such as cost, place, accessibility, treatment, and benefits, are scored in a two-part process. First, the actual results are compared with standard results; then, any deficiencies noted or identified serve to prompt recommendations for improvement. **2.** a system of review of selected hospital medical/nursing records by medical/nursing staff members, performed for the purposes of evaluating the quality and effectiveness of medical/ nursing care in relation to accepted standards.

**quality monitoring,** a nursing intervention from the Nursing Interventions Classification (NIC) defined as systematic collection and analysis of an organization's quality indicators for the purpose of improving patient care. See also **Nursing Interventions Classification.**

**quality of life**[1] [L, *qualis,* what kind; AS, *lif*], a measure of the optimum energy or force that endows a person with the power to cope successfully with the full range of challenges encountered in the real world. The term applies to all individuals, regardless of illness or handicap, on the job, at home, or in leisure activities. Quality enrichment methods can include activities that reduce boredom and allow a maximum amount of freedom in choosing and performing various tasks.

**quality of life**[2], a nursing outcome from the Nursing Outcomes Classification (NOC) defined as an individual's expressed satisfaction with current life circumstances. See also **Nursing Outcomes Classification.**

**quantitative** /kwon′titā′tiv/ [L, *quantus,* how much], capable of being measured.

**quantitative analysis** [L, *quantum,* how much; Gk, *analysis,* a loosening], **1.** (in chemistry) the determination of the amounts of constituents in a sample of material. Kinds of quantitative analysis include **gravimetric analysis, volumetric analysis,** and **spectrophotometric analysis. 2.** (in research) the use of statistical methods to analyze data.

**quantitative computed tomography (QCT),** a type of computed tomography that calculates and displays bone density in three dimensions. QCT is used mainly for lumbar spine studies but can also be applied in hip and peripheral bone mineral evaluations.

**quantitative inheritance.** See **multifactorial inheritance.**

**quantitative test** [L, *quantum,* how much, *testum,* crucible], a test that determines the amount of a substance per unit volume or unit weight.

**quantitative ultrasound,** an ultrasound technique for assessing bone mineral density. Its main advantage is the complete absence of radiation; a disadvantage is the confounding influence of soft tissue.

**quantum mechanics.** See **quantum theory.**

**quantum mottle.** See **mottle.**

**quantum theory** /kwon′təm/ [L, *quantum,* how much; Gk, *theoria,* speculation], (in physics) the theory dealing with the interaction of matter and electromagnetic radiation, particularly at the atomic and subatomic levels, according to which radiation consists of small units of energy called quanta. Radiation can be absorbed only in whole quanta, and the energy content of a quantum is inversely proportional to its wavelength. Energy and frequency are expressed as $E = h\omega$. E is the energy of the quantum; h is the Planck constant; and $\omega$ is the frequency of the radiation. Also called **quantum mechanics.**

**quarantine** /kwor′əntēn/ [It, *quarantina,* forty], **1.** isolation of people with communicable disease or those exposed to communicable disease during the contagious period in an attempt to prevent spread of the illness. **2.** the practice of detaining travelers or vessels coming from places of epidemic disease, originally for 40 days, for the purpose of inspection or disinfection.

**quart (qt)** /kwôrt/ [L, *quartus,* fourth], a unit of volume fluid measure equivalent to ¼ gallon, 2 pints, 32 ounces, or 946.24 milliliters. The British Imperial quart is equal to 1.136 liters, and the American quart for dry measure is 1.101 liters.

**quartan** /kwôr′tən/ [L, *quartanus,* relating to the fourth], recurring on the fourth day, or at about 72-hour intervals. See also **quartan malaria.**

**quartan malaria,** a form of malaria, caused by the protozoan *Plasmodium malariae,* characterized by febrile paroxysms that occur every 72 hours. Also called **quartan fever.** Compare **falciparum malaria, tertian malaria.** See also **malaria.**

**quarti-,** prefix meaning 'fourth': *quartipara, quartisect, quartisternal.*

**quartile** /kwôr′təl, kwôr′tīl/ [L, *quartus,* fourth], one-fourth of the distribution of scores. The first quartile would be the lowest 25% of scores, the second quartile would represent the 26% to 50% range of scores, and so on.

**quartz silicosis.** See **silicosis.**

**quaternary** /kwot′əner′ē, kwətur′nərē/ [L, *quattuor,* four], **1.** pertaining to a chemical compound in which four atoms or groups of elements are bonded to one atom, such as a quaternary ammonium compound in which four organic radicals are substituted for the four hydrogen molecules on an ammonium ion. **2.** fourth-level structure in proteins as in the structure of hemoglobin made up of two alpha and two beta globulins.

**quaternary ammonium derivative,** a substance whose chemical structure has four carbon groups attached to a positively charged nitrogen atom. It is usually a strong emulsifying agent, highly water soluble but relatively insoluble in lipids.

**Queckenstedt's test** /kwek′ənstets/ [Hans H. G. Queckenstedt, German physician, 1876–1918], a test for an obstruction in the spinal canal in which the jugular veins on each side of the neck are compressed alternately. The pressure of the spinal fluid is measured by a manometer connected to a lumbar puncture needle or catheter. Normally occlusion of the veins of the neck causes an immediate rise in spinal fluid pressure; if the vertebral canal is blocked, no rise occurs. If increased intracranial pressure is suspected, this test should not be performed. See also **spinal canal.**

**Queensland tick typhus,** an infection caused by *Rickettsia australis,* occurring in Australia, transmitted by ticks, and resembling mild Rocky Mountain spotted fever. Treatment includes the administration of chloramphenicol or tetracycline. Prevention depends on avoiding tick bites and on the prompt removal of attached ticks. Compare **boutonneuse fever, North Asian tick-borne rickettsiosis, Rocky Mountain spotted fever.**

**Quelidrine,** trademark for a respiratory, fixed-combination drug containing adrenergics (phenylephrine hydrochloride and ephedrine hydrochloride), an antihistaminic (chlorpheniramine maleate), an antitussive (dextromethorphan hydrobromide), and an expectorant (ammonium chloride).

**quellung reaction** /kwel′ung/ [Ger, *Quellung,* swelling; L, *re,* again, *agere,* to act], the swelling of the capsule of a bacterium, seen in the laboratory when the organism is exposed to specific antisera. This phenomenon is used to iden-

tify the genera, species, or subspecies of the bacteria causing a disease, including *Haemophilus influenzae, Neisseria meningitides,* and many kinds of streptococci.

**quenching** /kwen′ching/, **1.** a process of removing or reducing an energy source such as heat or light. **2.** stopping or diminishing a chemical or enzymatic reaction. **3.** decreasing counting efficiency in beta liquid scintillation caused by interfering materials.

**Quengle cast** /kwen′gəl/, a two-section orthopedic cast for immobilizing the lower extremity from the foot or ankle to below the knee and the upper thigh to just above the knee. The two parts of the cast are connected by hinges at knee level, medially and laterally. The Quengle cast is used for the gradual correction of knee contractures.

**quercetin** /kwur′sitin/, a yellow, crystalline, flavonoid pigment found in oak bark, the juice of lemons, asparagus, and other plants. It is used to reduce abnormal capillary fragility.

**querulous paranoia** /kwer′(y)ələs/ [L, *queri,* to complain; Gk, *para,* beside, *nous,* mind], a form of paranoia characterized by extreme discontent and habitual complaining, usually about imagined slights by others. Also called **paranoia querulans.**

**Quervain's disease** /kervānz′, kerveNz′/ [Fritz de Quervain, Swiss surgeon, 1868–1940; L, *dis;* Fr, *aise,* ease], chronic tenosynovitis of the abductor pollicis longus and extensor pollicis brevis muscles of the thumb.

**Questran,** trademark for an ion exchange resin used to lower blood cholesterol levels (cholestyramine resin).

**quetiapine,** an antipsychotic/neuroleptic.

■ INDICATIONS: Quetiapine is used in the treatment of psychotic disorders.

■ CONTRAINDICATIONS: Known hypersensitivity to this drug prohibits its use.

■ ADVERSE EFFECTS: Life-threatening effects of this drug are seizures, neuroleptic malignant syndrome, and tachycardia. Other adverse reactions include extrapyramidal symptoms, pseudoparkinsonism, akathisia, dystonia, tardive dyskinesia, drowsiness, insomnia, agitation, anxiety, orthostatic hypotension, abdominal pain, dry mouth, rhinitis, rash, asthenia, back pain, fever, and ear pain. Common side effects include headache, dizziness, nausea, anorexia, and constipation.

**Quibron,** trademark for a respiratory, fixed-combination drug containing a smooth muscle relaxant (theophylline) and an expectorant (guaifenesin).

**quick connect** [ME, *quic,* living; L, *connectere,* to bind], a plastic or similar connecting device that is attached to or implanted in a patient who will be joined to an electromechanical or other apparatus. A patient whose circulatory system is supported by an artificial heart, for example, may have a push-fit connector sewn to the natural atria, aorta, and pulmonary artery; a plastic lip on the artificial ventricle then can be securely snapped onto the quick-connect device.

**quick-cure resin.** See **self-curing resin.**

**quickening** /kwik′(ə)ning/ [ME, *quic,* living], the first feeling by a pregnant woman of movement of her baby in utero, usually occurring between 16 and 20 weeks of gestation.

**quiescent** /kwī·es′ənt/, **1.** inactive, quiet, or at rest. **2.** latent. **3.** dormant.

**quiet alert** /kwī′ət/, a period when a neonate is calm and attentive, with eyes open, ready to become acquainted with an adult person. Newborns spend about 10% of their time in this state.

**Quigley traction** /kwig′lē/, a type of traction for lateral malleolar and trimalleolar fractures in which a stockinette is placed around the leg and ankle and attached to an overhead frame, thus suspending the leg by the ankle.

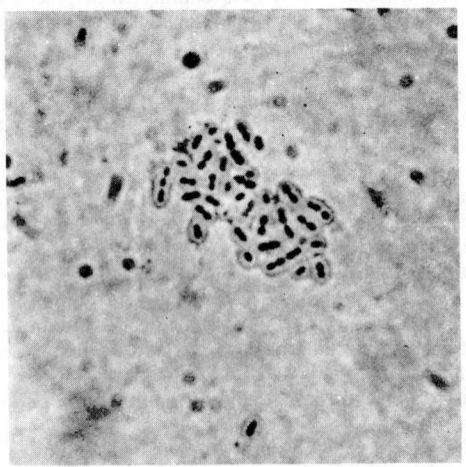

**Quellung reaction with**
*Streptococcus pneumoniae*
(Baron, Peterson, and Finegold, 1994)

**quin-,** combining form meaning 'quinine': *quiniretin, quinometry, quinotoxin.*

**-quin, -quine,** combining form naming antimalarial medicinal compounds from quinine: *aminoquin, diodoquin, Floraquin.*

**Quinaglute,** trademark for a cardiac depressant (quinidine gluconate).

**Quincke's disease** /kwing′kēz/ [Heinrich I. Quincke, German physician, 1842–1922; L, *dis* + Fr, *aise,* ease], angioneurotic edema, a potentially fatal chronic condition of subcutaneous edema, abdominal pain, urticaria, and laryngeal edema. Among its causes is anaphylactic reaction. Also called **angioedema, Quincke's edema.**

**Quincke's pulse** [Heinrich I. Quincke], an abnormal alternate blanching and reddening of the skin or nails that may be observed in several ways, such as by pressing the front edge of the fingernail and watching the blood in the nailbed recede and return. This pulsation is characteristic of aortic insufficiency and other abnormal conditions but also may occur in otherwise normal individuals. Formerly it was thought to be caused by pulsation of the capillaries; it is now known to be caused by pulsation of subpapillary arteriolar and venous plexuses. Also called **capillary pulse.**

**Quinidex,** trademark for a cardiac depressant (quinidine sulfate).

**quinidine** /kwin′ədēn, -din/, an antiarrhythmic agent used as a bisulfate, gluconate, polygalacturonate, or sulfate.
■ INDICATIONS: It is prescribed in the treatment of atrial flutter, atrial fibrillation, premature ventricular contractions, and tachycardias.
■ CONTRAINDICATIONS: Known hypersensitivity to this drug prohibits its use. It is contraindicated in some arrhythmias, particularly those associated with heart block.
■ ADVERSE EFFECTS: Among the most serious adverse reactions are cardiac arrhythmia, hypertension, and cinchonism. Rare but potentially fatal hypersensitivity reactions such as anaphylaxis and thrombocytopenia may occur. Diarrhea, nausea, and vomiting are common.

**quinidine gluconate.** See **quinidine.**

**quinine** /kwī′nīn/ [Sp, *quina,* bark], a white bitter crystalline alkaloid made from cinchona bark. Formerly used in antimalarial medications.

**quinolone** /kwin′əlōn/, any of a class of antibiotics that act by interrupting the replication of deoxyribonucleic acid (DNA) molecules in bacteria. The action involves inhibition of the bacteria's gyrase so that daughter segments of DNA cannot acquire the proper twist needed to divide. An example is ciprofloxacin.

**Quinora,** trademark for a cardiac depressant (quinidine sulfate).

**quinque-,** prefix meaning 'five': *quinquecuspid, quinquetubercular, quinquevalent.*

**quinsy.** See **peritonsillar abscess.**

**quint-,** prefix meaning 'fifth or fivefold': *quintessence, quintipara, quintuplet.*

**quintan** /kwin′tən/ [L, *quintanus,* relating to the fifth], recurring on the fifth day, or at about 96-hour intervals. See also **trench fever.**

**quintana fever.** See **trench fever.**

**quintessence** /kwintes′əns/ [L, *quinta* + *essentia,* the fifth essence], **1.** a highly concentrated extract of any substance. **2.** a tincture or extract containing the most essential components of plant materials.

**quintuplet** /kwin′tŏoplit, kwintŏo′plit/ [L, *quintuplex,* fivefold], any one of five offspring born of the same gestation period during a single pregnancy. See also **Hellin's law.**

**quotid.** See **q.d.**

**quotidian** /kwōtid′ē·ən/ [L, *quotidianus,* daily], occurring every day; for example, a malarial fever with daily attacks.

**quotient** /kwō′shənt/, the number obtained by dividing one number by another. See also **achievement quotient, intelligence quotient, respiratory quotient.**

**quot. op. sit,** abbreviation for the Latin phrase *quoties opus sit,* 'as often as necessary.'

**q.v., 1.** abbreviation for the Latin phrase *quantum vis,* 'as much as you please.' **2.** abbreviation for the Latin phrase *quod vide,* 'which see.'

**Q wave,** the first negative component of the QRS complex on an electrocardiogram. Lengthening of the wave indicates myocardial infarction. If an R wave is not present, the totally negative complex is called QS. See also **QRS complex.**

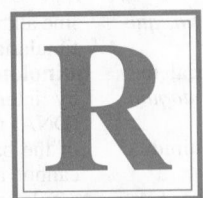

**r,** **1.** abbreviation for *right.* **2.** symbol for *resistance ohm.*
**R,** **1.** abbreviation for **resolution.** **2.** abbreviation for **respiratory exchange ratio. 3.** abbreviation for **roentgen. 4.** symbol for *gas constant.*

$R_f$, symbol for a ratio used in paper and thin-layer chromatography, representing the distance from the origin to the center of the separated zone divided by the distance from the origin to the solvent front. **2.** abbreviation for **radiofrequency.**

$R_i$, symbol for *inhibitory receptor* molecule.

$R_s$, symbol for *stimulatory receptor* molecule.

$R_x$, ℞, symbol for the Latin *recipe,* 'take.' See **prescription.**

**Ra,** symbol for the element **radium.**

**RA,** **1.** abbreviation for **rheumatoid arthritis; 2.** abbreviation for *right atrium.*

**rabbit fever.** See **tularemia.**

**rabbit test.** See **Friedman's test.**

**rabeprazole,** a proton pump inhibitor.
- INDICATIONS: Rabeprazole is used to treat gastroesophageal reflux disease (GERD), severe erosive esophagitis, poorly responsive systemic GERD, pathologic hypersecretory conditions such as Zollinger-Ellison syndrome, systemic mastocytosis, multiple endocrine adenomas, and active duodenal ulcers.
- CONTRAINDICATIONS: Known hypersensitivity to this drug prohibits its use.
- ADVERSE EFFECTS: Life-threatening effects are proteinuria, hematuria, pancytopenia, thrombocytopenia, neutropenia, and leukocytosis. Other adverse effects include abdominal swelling, anorexia, irritable colon, esophageal candidiasis, epistaxis, urticaria, alopecia, hypoglycemia, increased hepatic enzymes, weight gain, tinnitus, angina, tachycardia, bradycardia, palpitations, peripheral edema, urinary tract infection, increased creatinine, testicular pain, glycosuria, and fever. Common side effects include headache, dizziness, asthenia, diarrhea, abdominal pain, vomiting, nausea, constipation, flatulence, acid regurgitation, upper respiratory infections, cough, rash, and back pain.

**rabid** /rab'id/ [L, *rabidus,* raving], pertaining to or suffering from rabies, displaying signs of madness, agitation, delirium, hallucinations, and bizarre behavior.

**rabies** /rā'bēz/ [L, *rabere,* to rave], an acute, usually fatal viral disease of the central nervous system of mammals. It is transmitted from animals to people through infected saliva. Also called *(obsolete)* **hydrophobia. —rabid** /rab'id/, *adj.*
- OBSERVATIONS: The reservoir of the virus is chiefly wild animals, including skunks, bats, foxes, and raccoons, and unvaccinated dogs and cats. After introduction into the human body, often by a bite of an infected animal, the virus travels along nerve pathways to the brain and later to other organs. An incubation period ranges from 10 days to 1 year and is followed by a prodromal period characterized by fever, malaise, headache, paresthesia, and myalgia. After several days severe encephalitis, delirium, agonizingly painful muscular spasms, seizures, paralysis, coma, and death ensue.

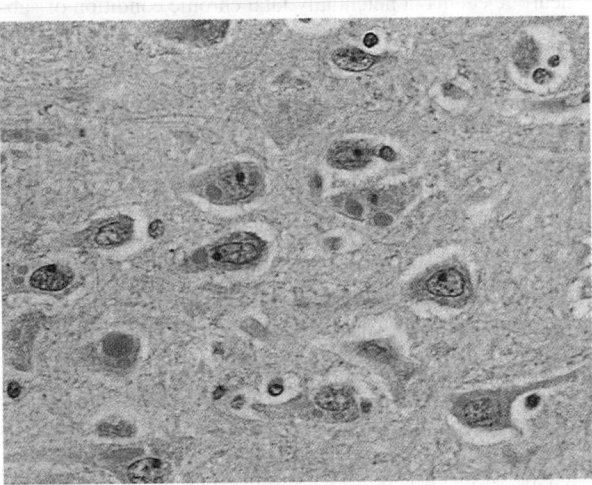

**Rabies virus in hippocampal pyramidal neurons**
*(Farrar, 1993/courtesy Dr. P. Garen)*

- INTERVENTIONS: Few nonfatal cases have been documented in humans; survival in those cases has been the result of intensive supportive nursing and medical care. There is no treatment once the virus has reached the tissue of the nervous system. Local treatment of wounds inflicted by rabid animals may prevent the disease. The wound is cleansed with soap, water, and a disinfectant. A deep wound may be cauterized, and rabies immune globulin injected directly into the base of the wound. For active immunization a series of three intramuscular injections with adsorbed vaccine (RVA), purified chick embryo cell (PCEC) vaccine, or human diploid cell rabies vaccine (HDCV) is begun. If vaccine is administered, intramuscular injection is given on days 0, 7, and 21 or 28. Great effort is made to locate and examine the animal. The animal that is suspected of being rabid is not immediately killed but put in isolation and carefully observed. If the animal is well in 10 days, there is little danger of rabies developing from the bite. Tissue from the animal's brain may be examined microscopically or by fluorescent antibody screening techniques.
- NURSING CONSIDERATIONS: Rabies virus infection can be eradicated from most communities by prophylactic immunization of domestic animals, stringent measures for the control of domestic animals, and elimination of any wild animals acting as reservoirs of infection. A preexposure vaccination is advised for those at risk, such as veterinarians, animal handlers, and some laboratory workers. The nurse and other health workers may encourage compliance with such efforts and teach the necessity of avoiding direct contact with wild animals and the importance of immediate first aid for any animal bite and reporting such contact to health care providers.

**rabies immune globulin (RIG),** a solution of antirabies immune globulin.

■ INDICATIONS: It is used in conjunction with rabies duck embryo vaccine for possible protection against rabies in persons suspected of exposure to rabies.

■ CONTRAINDICATIONS: Previous administration of this preparation or known hypersensitivity to this solution, to gamma globulin, or to thimerosal prohibits its use.

■ ADVERSE EFFECTS: Among the more serious adverse reactions are soreness at the site of injection, fever, and hypersensitivity reactions.

**rabies vaccine (DEV),** a sterile suspension of killed rabies virus prepared from duck embryo.

■ INDICATIONS: It is prescribed for immunization and postexposure prophylaxis against rabies.

■ CONTRAINDICATIONS: A history of allergic reaction to chicken or duck eggs or to protein prohibits its use.

■ ADVERSE EFFECTS: Among the most serious adverse reactions are severe hypersensitivity reactions and pain and inflammation at the site of injection.

**rabies virus group** [L, *rabere,* to rave, *virus,* poison; It, *gruppo,* knot], the genus of viruses that includes the organism that causes rabies in humans, the *lyssa* virus. See also **rhabdovirus.**

**raccoon eyes,** ecchymotic areas surrounding both eyes, suggestive of a basilar skull fracture.

**race** [It, *razza*], **1.** a vague unscientific term for a group of genetically related people who share certain physical characteristics. **2.** a distinct ethnic group characterized by traits that are transmitted through their offspring.

**racemic** /rāsē′mik/ [L, *racemus,* bunch of grapes], pertaining to a compound made up of equal amounts of dextrorotatory and levorotatory isomers, rendering it optically inactive under polarized light.

**racemic epinephrine.** See **epinephrine.**

**racemose** /ras′əmōs′/ [L, *racemus*], like a bunch of grapes. The term is used in describing a structure in which many branches terminate in nodular cystlike forms such as pulmonary alveoli.

**racemose aneurysm,** a pronounced dilation of lengthened and tortuous blood vessels, which may form a tumor. Also called **cirsoid aneurysm.**

**-racetam,** combining form for piracetam-type nootrope substances.

**rachial** /rā′kē·əl/ [Gk, *rhachis,* backbone], pertaining to the spinal column. Also **rachidial** /rākid′ē·əl/.

**rachialgia** /rā′kē·al′jə/ [Gk, *rhachis,* backbone + *algos,* pain], pain in the vertebral column; also called **rachiodynia.**

**rachio-, rachi-, rhachi-,** prefix meaning 'the spine': *rachiocampsis, rachiotome, rachiotomy.*

**rachiodynia.** See **rachialgia.**

**rachiopagus** /rā′kē·op′əgəs/ [Gk, *rachis,* backbone, *pagos,* fixed], conjoined symmetric twins united back to back along the spinal column. Also called **rachipagus.**

**rachiotomy.** See **laminotomy.**

**rachiresistance** /rā′kēresis′təns/ [Gk, *rachis,* backbone], a failure to respond adequately to spinal anesthesia.

**rachischisis** /rəkis′kəsis/ [Gk, *rachis* + *schizein,* to split], a congenital fissure of one or more vertebrae. See also **neural tube defect, spina bifida.**

**rachischisis totalis.** See **complete rachischisis.**

**rachitic** /rəkit′ik/, **1.** pertaining to rickets. **2.** resembling or suggesting the condition of one afflicted with rickets.

**rachitic dwarf,** a person whose retarded growth is caused by rickets. See also **Fanconi's syndrome.**

**rachitis** /rəkī′tis/ [Gk, *rachis* + *itis,* inflammation],

**1.** rickets. **2.** an inflammatory disease of the vertebral column.

**rachitis fetalis annularis,** congenital enlargement of the epiphyses of the long bones.

**rachitis fetalis micromelia,** congenital shortening of the long bones.

**racial immunity** /rā′shəl/ [It, *razza* + L, *immunis,* free], a form of natural immunity shared by most of the members of a genetically related population. Compare **individual immunity, species immunity.**

**racial unconscious.** See **collective unconscious.**

**rad** /rad/, abbreviation for **radiation absorbed dose.**

**radappertization** /rad′apur′tizā′shən/, the irradiation of food for the destruction of *Clostridium botulinum.*

**radarkymography** /rā′därkīmog′rəfē/ [radar + Gk, *kyma,* wave, *graphein,* to record], a technique for showing the size and outline of the heart, using a radar tracking device and a fluoroscopic screen to display images produced by electrical impulses passed over the chest surface.

**Radford nomogram** [Edward P. Radford, Jr., American physiologist, b. 1922], a mathematical chart device used in respiratory therapy to estimate combined tidal volumes and rates for mechanical ventilation. It is based on three parameters of body weight, sex, and respiratory rate.

**radi-,** combining form meaning 'root': *radiciform, radicotomy, radiectomy.*

**radial** /rā′dē·əl/ [L, *radius,* ray], pertaining to the radius.

**radial artery** [L, *radius,* ray], an artery in the forearm, starting at the bifurcation of the brachial artery and passing in 12 branches to the forearm, wrist, and hand. In the forearm it extends from the neck of the radius to the forepart of the styloid process; in the wrist, from the styloid process to the carpus; in the hand, from the carpus, across the palm, to the little finger. In the forearm the branches of the radial artery are the radial recurrent, muscular, palmar carpal, and superficial palmar; in the wrist the branches are the dorsal carpal and the first dorsal metacarpal. In the hand the branches are the princeps pollicis, radialis indicis, deep palmar arch, palmar metacarpal, perforating, and recurrent.

**radialis.** See **radial.**

**radial keratotomy (RK),** a surgical procedure in which a series of tiny shallow incisions are made in the cornea, resulting in a flattening of the cornea, thereby reducing refractive error. The operation is performed using local anesthesia

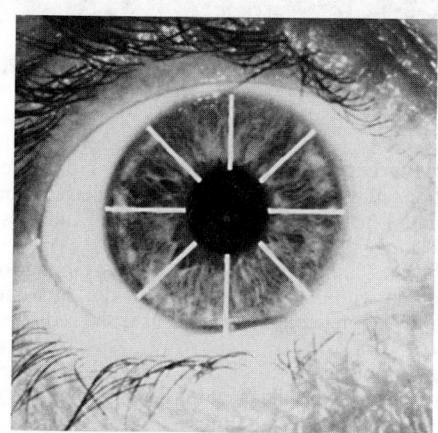

**Location of incisions in radial keratotomy**
*(Phipps, Sands, and Marek, 1999)*

and requires only 10 minutes. Hospitalization is not necessary. Radial keratotomy usually corrects mild to moderate myopia. Compare **photorefractive keratectomy.** See also **refractive keratotomy.**

**radial nerve,** the largest branch of the brachial plexus, arising on each side as a continuation of the posterior cord. It supplies the skin of the arm and forearm and their extensor muscles. The branches of the radial nerve are the medial muscular branches, the posterior brachial cutaneous nerve, the posterior muscular branches, the posterior antebrachial cutaneous nerve, the lateral muscular branches, the superficial branch, and the deep branch. Also called **musculospiral nerve.** Compare **median nerve, musculocutaneous nerve, ulnar nerve.**

**radial nerve palsy,** a type of mononeuropathy characterized by radial nerve damage with symptoms of forearm muscle weakness and sensory loss. It may be caused by excessive compression of the radial nerve against a hard surface in individuals insensitized by the intake of alcohol or sedatives. It may also be caused by the repeated compression of the nerve by various weights. Time and the withdrawal of causative compression usually ensure full recovery.

**radial notch of ulna,** the narrow lateral depression in the coronoid process of the ulna that receives the head of the radius.

**radial paralysis** [L, *radius* + Gk, *paralyein*], paralysis of muscles supplied by the radial nerve, mainly the wrist and finger extensors. See also **dropped wrist.**

**radial pulse,** the pulse of the radial artery palpated at the wrist over the radius. The radial pulse is the one most often taken, because of the ease with which it is palpated.

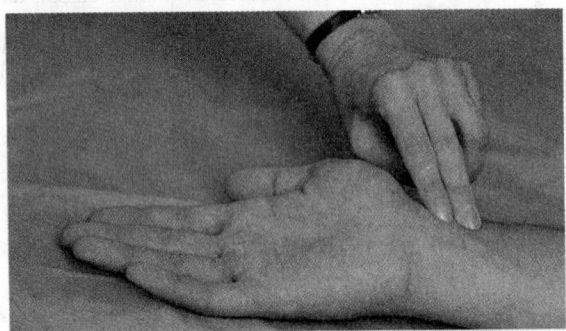

**Palpation of the radial pulse** *(Potter and Perry, 2001)*

**radial recurrent artery,** a branch of the radial artery arising just distal to the elbow, ascending between the branches of the radial nerve, and supplying several muscles of the arm and the elbow.

**radial reflex,** a normal reflex elicited by tapping over the distal radius, with the response being flexion of the forearm. Flexion of the fingers may also occur if the reflex is hyperactive.

**radial symmetry,** a form of symmetry in which body parts are arranged around a central axis, as found in animals such as jellyfish and sea urchins.

**radiant** /rā′dē·ənt/ [L, *radiare*, to emit rays], pertaining to any object that emits rays or is the center of rays that spread outward.

**radiant energy** [L, *radiare*, to emit rays; Gk *energeia*], energy emitted as electromagnetic radiation, such as radio waves, infrared radiation, visible light, ultraviolet light, x-rays, and gamma rays.

**radiant heat,** a form of infrared energy that is emitted in electromagnetic waves from a central source. It proceeds outward in wavelengths greater than those of visible light. Objects absorbing the energy experience a rise in temperature.

**radiate** /rā′dē·āt/ [L, *radiare*, to emit rays], to diverge or spread from a common point or center.

**radiate ligament,** a ligament that connects the head of a rib with a vertebra and an associated intervertebral disk.

**radiation** /rā′dē·ā′shən/ [L, *radiatio*], **1.** the emission of energy, rays, or waves. **2.** the use of a radioactive substance in the diagnosis or treatment of disease.

**radiation absorbed dose (rad),** the standard unit of absorbed dose of ionizing radiation. One rad is equal to 0.01 joule per kilogram of matter. Compare **roentgen.** See also **absorbed dose, rem.**

**radiation burn,** a burn resulting from exposure to radiant energy in the form of sunlight, x-rays, or nuclear emissions or explosion. Ionizing radiation can produce tissue damage directly by striking a vital molecule such as deoxyribonucleic acid. See also **ionizing radiation injury.**

**radiation caries,** tooth decay triggered by exposure of the head to ionizing radiation. It especially affects the cementoenamel junction and the coronal root area. Radiation makes the teeth more susceptible to caries by decreasing salivation, reducing the vitality of dental tissues, and altering oral bacteria. Radiation caries is often a side effect of radiation therapy for oral malignancies. See also **dental caries.**

**radiation cataract** [L, *radiare*, to emit rays; Gk, *katarrhaktes*, portcullis], a cataract that is caused by excessive exposure of the eye to x-rays or other types of radiation that cause a change in the protein molecules of the lens.

**radiation dermatitis** [L, *radiare*, to emit rays; Gk, *derma*, skin, *itis*, inflammation], an acute or chronic inflammation of the skin caused by exposure to ionizing radiation, as in cancer radiation therapy. Symptoms, which may not appear until 3 weeks after exposure, include redness, blistering, and sloughing of the skin. In severe cases the condition can progress to scarring, fibrosis, and atrophy. There may also be changes in skin pigmentation.

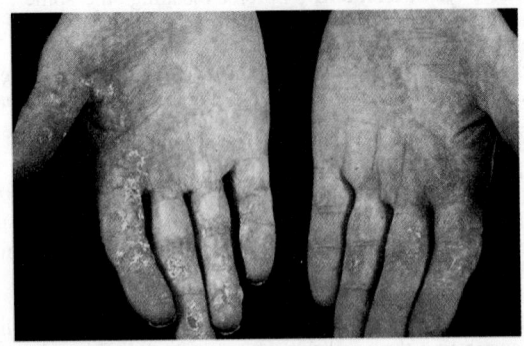

**Radiation dermatitis**
*(du Vivier, 1993/courtesy Dr. A. Warin, St. John's Hospital for Diseases of the Skin)*

**radiation detector,** a device for detecting the presence and sometimes the amount of radiation. A Geiger-Müller detector counts the number of radioactive particles reaching it and can be designed to detect cosmic radiation. An ionization chamber collects the ion pairs formed by the passage of radiation through the device.

**Radiation Effects Research Foundation (RERF),** an organization that studies the long-term effects of the atomic bombings of Hiroshima and Nagasaki during World War II on survivors. The RERF has focused on the incidence of leukemia, which reached a plateau around 1950 before beginning to decline, and has examined the varied effects related to the different types of radiation produced by the two bombs, one fueled with uranium and the other with plutonium. The RERF is the successor to the Atomic Bomb Casualty Commission.

**radiation exposure,** a measure of the ionization produced in air by x-rays or gamma rays. It is the sum of the electric charges on all ions of one sign that are produced when all electrons liberated by the radiation in a volume of air are completely stopped, divided by the mass of air in that volume. The unit of exposure is the roentgen. **Acute radiation exposure** is exposure of short duration to intense ionizing radiation, usually occurring as the result of an accidental spill of radioactive material. Exposure of the whole body to approximately 10,000 rad (100 gray) causes neurologic and cardiovascular breakdown and is fatal within 24 hours. A dose between 500 and 1200 rad (5 and 12 gray) destroys GI mucosa, produces bloody diarrhea, and may cause death in several days. A dose of 200 to 500 rad (2 to 5 gray) destroys the blood-forming organs and may cause death in a few weeks.

**radiation exposure, emergency procedures,** first aid treatment of a person who has received external body radiation through exposure to radioactive material or internal radiation contamination by inhaling or ingesting radioactive material. External radiation exposure is treated initially by cleansing and surgical isolation to protect others. One who has inhaled or ingested radioactive material should be given emergency treatment similar to a person who has been exposed to chemical poisons. Body wastes should be collected and checked for radiation levels. If the victim has also suffered a wound, care must be taken to avoid cross-contamination of exposed surfaces. In general, except for taking special precautions to control the spread of radiation effects, the patient should be given any lifesaving emergency treatment needed, and personnel handling the patient should wear surgical gowns, caps, and gloves. Also called **emergency handling of radiation accidents.**

**radiation force,** a small steady force that is produced when a sound beam strikes a reflecting or absorbing surface. It is proportional to the acoustic power.

**radiation hygiene,** the art and science of protecting human beings from injury by radiation. It reduces clinical exposure from external radiation through protective barriers of radiation-absorbing material, ensures safe distances between people and radiation sources, reduces radiation exposure times, or uses combinations of all these measures. To protect against the dangers of internal radiation, precautions seek to restrict inhalation, ingestion, and other modes of entry of radioactive substances into the body.

**radiation oncologist,** a physician with special training in the use of ionizing radiation in the treatment of cancers.

**radiation oncology,** the study of the treatment of cancer using ionizing radiation.

**radiation protection,** the use of devices, equipment, distance, and barriers to reduce the risk of exposure to ionizing radiation in a health care facility, research center, or industrial site where radiation-emitting devices are operated.

**radiation risk,** a hazard to health resulting from exposure to natural and synthetic radioactive materials. Radiation sources include cosmic rays, radon, radium, and other radionuclides in the soil, nuclear reactors, accelerators, and weapons; uranium mining and milling; and diagnostic and therapeutic x-ray devices.

**radiation safety committee,** an organization responsible for monitoring and maintaining a safe radiation environment in institutions where radiation is produced and/or used.

**radiation sensitivity,** a measure of the response of tissue to ionizing radiation.

**radiation sickness,** an abnormal condition resulting from exposure to ionizing radiation. The severity of the condition is determined by the intensity of radiation, the length of time of exposure, and the area of the body affected. Moderate exposure may cause headache, nausea, vomiting, anorexia, and diarrhea; long-term exposure may result in sterility, fetal damage in pregnant women, leukemia or other forms of cancer, alopecia, and cataracts.

**radiation symbol,** a universal symbol consisting of three red wedges arranged at positions 120 degrees apart around a central red circle on a yellow background. The symbol identifies sources or containers of radioactive materials and areas of potential radiation exposure.

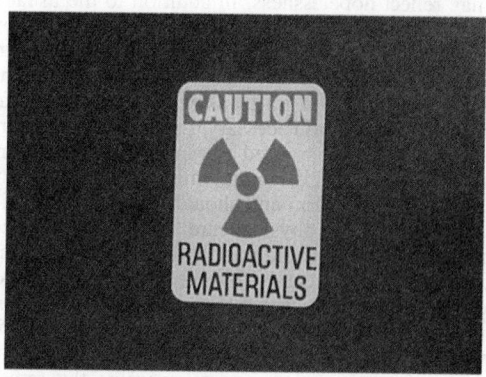

**Radiation symbol** *(Judd and Ponsell, 1988)*

**radiation syndrome.** See **radiation sickness.**

**radiation therapist,** an allied health professional who administers radiation therapy services to patients and observes patients during treatment. Duties may include tumor localization, dosimetry, patient follow-up, patient education, and record keeping.

**radiation therapy.** See **radiotherapy.**

**radiation therapy management,** a nursing intervention from the Nursing Interventions Classification (NIC) defined as assisting the patient to understand and minimize the side effects of radiation treatments. See also **Nursing Interventions Classification.**

**radiation therapy technologist.** See **radiation therapist.**

**radical** /rad′ikəl/ [L, *radix*, root], **1.** an atom or group of atoms that contains an unpaired electron. A radical does not exist freely in nature except for $O_2$, NO, and $NO_2$. **2.** pertaining to drastic therapy, such as the surgical removal of an organ, limb, or other part of the body.

**radical dissection,** the surgical removal of tissue in an extensive area surrounding the operative site. Most often it is performed to identify and excise all tissue that may possibly be malignant to decrease the chance of recurrence and often (usually) includes adjacent lymph nodes.

**radical hysterectomy.** See **hysterectomy.**

**radical mastectomy,** surgical removal of an entire breast; pectoral muscles; axillary lymph nodes; and all fat, fascia, and adjacent tissues. It is one kind of surgical treatment for breast cancer. Before surgery, in addition to giving usual preoperative care, the staff encourages verbalization of the patient's fears of the disease, the surgery, and the loss of her breast. Her self-image is usually threatened, and she characteristically grieves in anticipation of a loss of a body part. The postoperative period is physically and emotionally painful; the woman is best warned by supportive but realistic explanations before surgery. Edema of the arm on the affected side is the rule because the axillary lymphatic structures that drain the lymph from the arm are removed during surgery. Symptomatic atelectasis may develop if deep breathing is not regularly performed. The incision is expectedly painful but may be anticipated to become less so during the first few days; it should not become more inflamed or painfully swollen. A pressure dressing is usually applied and left in place until bleeding and drainage have decreased. A drain is usually left in the wound for several days. The woman may be anxious, depressed, angry, or withdrawn; or she may reflect hopelessness. In addition to the usual postoperative measures, the nurse or other health care provider elevates the affected arm above the level of the right atrium; checks the color, sensation, and motion of the fingers; checks the graft site if a graft was performed; and reinforces the pressure dressing as necessary. Later in the postoperative period, the patient is assisted in range-of-motion exercises for all extremities and is taught, with assistance, to perform gradually increasing arm and shoulder exercises. In discussion and in providing physical care, the loss of the breast is dealt with frankly; to avoid the fact is not helpful to the patient. Slowly the patient is involved in caring for herself more completely, a process that continues as she gradually resumes her normal daily activities. On discharge she is encouraged to shower daily, to apply an emollient such as cocoa butter to the incision, and to examine the remaining breast monthly. Reach to Recovery or a similar resource may be involved in counseling and support before and after a mastectomy. Chemotherapy and radiation therapy may continue after surgery. The woman is told never to allow blood to be drawn from the affected arm; IV injection is also to be avoided in that arm. Blood pressure measurement, vaccination, and other injections are best performed on the other arm. Compare **modified radical mastectomy, simple mastectomy.** See also **lumpectomy, mastectomy.**

**radical neck dissection,** dissection and removal of all lymph nodes and removable tissues under the skin of the neck, performed to prevent the spread of malignant tumors of the head and neck that have a reasonable chance of being controlled. Before surgery, thorough mouth hygiene is given, and antibiotics are begun. With the patient under general anesthesia, a tracheostomy may be done; the tumor, surrounding tissues, and the lymph nodes on the affected side are then removed in one mass from the angle of the jaw to the clavicle, forward to midline, and back to the angle of the jaw. A total laryngectomy may be done as part of the surgery. After surgery the nurse suctions the tracheostomy as necessary and observes vital signs for indications of hemor-

rhage or difficulty in breathing. A humidifier or vaporizer will ease coughing and production of mucus. IV fluids are continued in the arm not used for writing. If necessary, the patient may do extensive work with a speech pathologist to learn esophageal speech. Radiation of the tumor site may be begun, and chemotherapy may continue. Compare **neck dissection.**

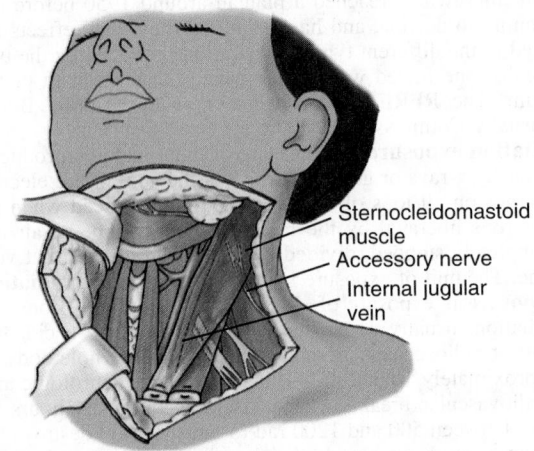

**Radical neck dissection** *(Monahan and Neighbors, 1998)*

Labels:
Sternocleidomastoid muscle
Accessory nerve
Internal jugular vein

**radical nephrectomy,** the surgical removal of a kidney, usually performed in the treatment of cancer of the kidney.

**radical surgery** [L, *radix,* root; Gk, *cheirourgia,* surgery], surgery that is usually extensive and complex and intended to correct a severe health threat such as a rapidly growing cancer. See also **radical dissection.**

**radical therapy,** 1. a treatment intended to cure, not palliate. 2. a definitive extreme treatment; not conservative, such as radical mastectomy rather than simple or partial mastectomy.

**radical vulvectomy.** See **vulvectomy.**

**radicidation** /rā′disidā′shən/, the irradiation of food to inactivate nonsporing pathogens of *Salmonella* and other microorganisms.

**radicular** /rədik′yələr/ [L, *radix,* root], pertaining to a root, such as a spinal nerve root or radical.

**radicular cyst** [L, *radix,* root; Gk, *kystis.* bag], a cyst with a wall of fibrous connective tissue and a lining of stratified squamous epithelium that is attached to the root apex of a tooth with dead pulp or a defective root canal filling. Also called **periapical cyst, root end cyst.**

**radicular retainer,** a type of retainer, such as a dowel crown, that lies within the body of a tooth, usually in the root. Resistance to displacement and shear is developed by extending an attached dowel into the root canal of the tooth. Compare **dowel.** See also **radicular retention.**

**radicular retention,** resistance to displacement of a dental prosthesis developed by placing a metal projection into the root canal of a pulpless tooth. See also **radicular retainer.**

**radiculitis** /rədik′yəlī′tis/ [L, *radix,* root; Gk, *itis,* inflammation], an inflammation involving a spinal nerve root, resulting in pain and hyperesthesia.

**radiculopathy** /rədik′yəlop′əthē/ [L, *radix,* root; Gk, *pathos,* disease], a disease involving a spinal nerve root.

**radii.** See **radius.**

**radio-** /rā′dē·ō-/, combining form meaning 'radiation,' sometimes specifically to emission of radiant energy, to radium, or to the radius: *radioactive, radiobiology, radiohumeral.*

**radioactive** /-ak′tiv/ [L, *radius,* ray, *activus,* active], giving off radiation as the result of the disintegration of atomic nuclei.

**radioactive carbon.** See **tracer.**

**radioactive contamination,** the undesirable addition of radioactive material to the body or part of the environment, such as clothing or equipment. Contamination of the body by beta radiation may occur through the ingestion, inhalation, or absorption of a beta emitter. Instruments, drapes, surgical gloves, and clothing that come in contact with serous fluids, blood, and urine of patients containing beta or gamma radiation emitters may be contaminated. The severity of the contamination is directly related to the elapsed time between the administration of the radioactive isotope and surgery. On completion of the procedure, possibly contaminated material is isolated and checked; if found to be contaminated, it is disposed of according to institutional and federal standards for the disposal of radioactive waste.

**radioactive contrast medium,** a solution or colloid containing radioactive material used for visualizing soft tissue structures. Such contrast media indicate their positions or distribution in the body by their gamma ray emissions.

**radioactive decay,** the disintegration of the nucleus of an unstable nuclide by the spontaneous emission of charged particles, photons, or both.

**radioactive element,** an element subject to spontaneous degeneration of its nucleus accompanied by the emission of alpha particles, beta particles, or gamma rays. All elements with atomic numbers greater than 83 are radioactive. Naturally occurring radioactive elements include radium, thorium, and uranium. Several radioactive elements not found in nature have been produced by the bombardment of stable elements with subatomic particles in a cyclotron. Compare **stable element.** See also **radioactivity.**

**radioactive half-life.** See **half-life.**

**radioactive implant,** a small container holding a radioactive isotope that is embedded in tissues for purposes of interstitial radiotherapy.

**radioactive iodine (RAI),** a radioactive isotope of iodine used in diagnostic radiology and radiotherapy, especially in the treatment of some thyroid conditions. A common form is $^{131}$I. Also called **radioactive iodine (RAI).**

**radioactive iodine excretion,** the elimination by the body of radioactive iodine (RAI) administered in a test of thyroid function and in the treatment of hyperthyroidism. Most RAI is excreted in urine, but small amounts may be found in sputum, perspiration, feces, and vomitus.

**radioactive iodine excretion test,** a method of evaluating thyroid function that entails measuring the amount of radioactive iodine (RAI) in urine after the patient is given an oral tracer dose of RAI in the form of the isotope $^{131}$I. Normally, 5% to 35% of the dose is absorbed by the thyroid; absorption is increased in hyperthyroidism and decreased in hypothyroidism, and the amount excreted in urine is inversely proportional to the uptake of RAI. After administration of the tracer, a scintillation detector is placed over the patient's neck at 2, 6, and 24 hours to measure the amount of RAI accumulated by the thyroid; the amount excreted is assayed in urine collected for 24 hours after the oral dose. Diarrhea can result in low levels of RAI in urine; renal failure, by de-

creasing excretion, can cause high levels. See also **radioactive iodine uptake.**

**radioactive iodine uptake (RAIU),** the absorption and incorporation by the thyroid of radioactive iodine (RAI), administered orally as a tracer dose in a test of thyroid function and as larger doses for the treatment of hyperthyroidism. The radioisotope $^{131}$I is rapidly absorbed in the stomach and concentrated in the thyroid. Normal findings: 2 hours, 4% to 12% absorbed; 6 hours, 6% to 15% absorbed; 24 hours, 8% to 30% absorbed. Patients receiving a large therapeutic dose of RAI may require hospitalization for several days. See also **radioactive iodine excretion test.**

**radioactive tracer,** a molecule containing a radioactive atom, which can be followed through a physiologic system with radiation detectors.

**radioactivity** /-activ′itē/, the emission of alpha or beta particles or gamma radiation as a consequence of nuclear disintegration. Natural radioactivity is a property exhibited by all chemical elements with an atomic number greater than 83; artificial or induced radioactivity is created through the bombardment of stable elements with subatomic particles or high levels of gamma radiation or x-radiation.

**radioallergosorbent test (RAST)** /rā′dē·ō′alur′gōsôr′-bənt/ [L, *radius* + Gk, *allos,* other, *ergein,* to work; L, *absorbere,* to swallow], a test in which a technique of radioimmunoassay is used to identify and quantify IgE in serum that has been mixed with any of 45 known allergens. If an atopic allergy to a substance exists, an antigen-antibody reaction occurs with characteristic conjugation and clumping. The test is an in vitro method of demonstrating allergic reactions. Compare **patch test, Prausnitz-Küstner (PK) test.**

**radiobiology** /-bī·ol′əjē/ [L, *radius* + *bios,* life, *logos,* science], the branch of the natural sciences dealing with the effects of radiation on biologic systems. **—radiobiologic, radiobiological,** *adj.*

**radiocarcinogenesis** /-kär′sinəjen′əsis/, the production of cancer by exposure to ionizing radiation.

**radiocarpal articulation** /-kär′pəl/ [L, *radius* + Gk, *karpos,* wrist], the condyloid joint at the wrist that connects the radius and distal surface of an articular disk with the scaphoid, lunate, and triangular bones. The joint involves four ligaments and allows all movements but rotation. Also called **wrist joint.**

**radiochemistry** /-kem′istrē/ [L, *radius* + Gk, *chemiea,* alchemy], the branch of chemistry that deals with the properties and behavior of radioactive materials and the use of radionuclides in the study of chemical and biologic problems.

**radiocurable** /-kyo͞o′rəbəl/, pertaining to the susceptibility of tumor cells to destruction by ionizing radiation.

**radiodensity.** See **radiopacity.**

**radiodermatitis** /-dur′mətī′tis/, a skin inflammation caused by exposure to ionizing radiation. The skin changes resemble those of thermal damage.

**radiofrequency (rf)** /-frē′kwənsē/ [L, *radius* + *frequens*], the part of the electromagnetic spectrum with frequencies lower than about $10^{10}$ Hz, used to produce magnetic resonance images.

**radiofrequency ablation,** unmodulated, high-frequency, alternating current flow that is applied to heart tissue to raise its temperature and injure cells for the purpose of destroying ectopic foci and accessory pathways. Radiofrequency ablation of accessory pathways is a cure for the arrhythmias associated with Wolfe-Parkinson-White syndrome and is successfully used in atrial flutter and idiopathic ventricular tachycardia. It has replaced surgical ablation.

**radiofrequency (rf) signal,**   **1.** an electrical signal whose frequency is in the rf range. **2.** a signal within an ultrasound instrument between the transducer terminals and components where rectification and filtering occur.

**radiograph** /rā′dē·əgraf′/,   an x-ray image. Also called **radiogram.**

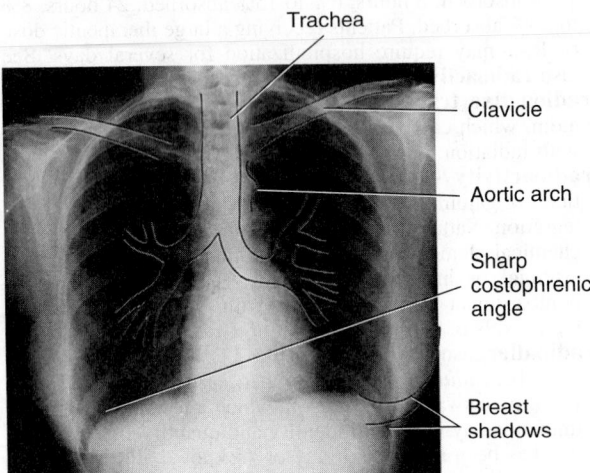

Trachea

Clavicle

Aortic arch

Sharp costophrenic angle

Breast shadows

**Normal radiograph of the chest**
*(Talbot and Meyers-Marquardt, 1997)*

**radiographer** /rā′dē·og′rəfər/. See **radiologic technologist.**

**radiographic.**   See **radiography.**

**radiographic contrast medium.**   See **radiopaque contrast medium.**

**radiographic grid** /-graf′ik/,   a device used to reduce the amount of scatter radiation reaching an x-ray film. Grids consist of parallel strips of radiopaque materials alternating with strips of radiolucent materials. See also **grid.**

**radiographic magnification,**   a procedure used to improve visualization of fine blood vessels and small bony structures during x-ray imaging. Magnification is achieved by increasing the distance of the object from the radiographic image receptor or by decreasing the distance of the x-ray source from the image receptor.

**radiographic position,**   the specific position of the body or a body part in relation to the image receptor during x-ray imaging.

**radiographic projection,**   the path taken by an x-ray beam as it passes through the body. For example, an anteroposterior projection refers to a beam that enters the anterior (front) of the body and exits the posterior (back).

**radiographic view,**   the body image as seen by the image receptor of a radiographic imaging system. It is the opposite of the radiographic projection.

**radiography** /rā′dē·og′rəfē/ [L, *radius* + Gk, *graphein*, to record],   the production of shadow images on photographic emulsion through the action of ionizing radiation. The image is the result of the differential attenuation of the radiation in its passage through the object being radiographed. **—radiographic,** *adj.*

**radiohumeral** /rā′dēō·hyōō′mər·əl/ [L, *radius,* + *humerus,* shoulder],   pertaining to the radius and humerus.

**radioimmunoassay (RIA)** /rā′dē·ō·im′yənō·as′ā/ [L, *radius* + *immunis,* free; Fr, *essayer,* to try],   a technique in radiology used to determine the concentration of an antigen, antibody, or other protein in the serum. The technique involves the injection of a known amount of a radioactively labeled substance that reacts with the protein in question.

**radioimmunofluorescence assay (RIFA)** /rā′dē·ō·im′y ənō′flōōres′əns/,   a test for the presence of antibodies sometimes used to confirm the results of ELISA or other methods.

**radioimmunosorbent test (RIST)** /rā′dē·ō·im′yənōsôr′-bənt/ [L, *radius* + *immunis* + *absorbere,* to swallow],   a test that uses serum immunoglobulin E to detect allergies to various substances such as certain cosmetics, animal fur, dust, and grasses.

**radioiodine** /rā′dē·ō·ī′ədīn/.   See **radioactive iodine (RAI).**

**radioiodine uptake,**   uptake of radioiodine from the blood by the thyroid gland; see **radioiodine uptake test.**

**radioiodine uptake test,**   one of the most common thyroid function tests; a known quantity of radioiodine is administered and 24 hours later the per cent is calculated that has been absorbed by the thyroid gland. Patients who have recently been exposed to iodine compounds, such as in dietary supplements, contrast media, medications, or antiseptics, may not be good candidates for this test.

**radioisotope** /rā′dē·ō·ī′sətōp/ [L, *radius* + Gk, *isos,* equal, *topos* place],   a radioactive form of an element, which may be used for therapeutic and diagnostic purposes.

**radioisotope scan,**   a two-dimensional representation of the gamma rays emitted by a radioisotope, showing its concentration in a body site, such as the thyroid gland, brain, or kidney. Radioisotopes used in diagnostic scanning may be administered intravenously or orally.

**radiologic.**   See **radiology.**

**radiological.**   See **radiology.**

**Radiological Society of North America (RSNA),**   a professional organization of radiologists. The group originated the certification of operators of x-ray equipment in 1920 but is no longer involved in such certification.

**radiologic anatomy** /-loj′ik/ [L, *radius* + Gk, *logos,* science],   (in applied anatomy) the study of the structure and morphology of the tissues and organs of the body based on their x-ray visualization.

**radiologic technologist,**   a person who, under the supervision of a physician radiologist, operates radiologic equipment and assists radiologists and other health professionals, and whose competence has been tested and approved by the American Registry of Radiologic Technologists. Also called **radiographer, x-ray technologist.**

**radiologist** /rā′dē·ol′əjist/,   a physician who specializes in radiology. A certified radiologist is one whose competence has been tested and approved by the American Board of Radiology. Also called **roentgenologist** /rent′gənol′əjist/.

**radiology** /-ol′əjē/ [L, *radius* + *logos,* science],   the branch of medicine concerned with radioactive substances and with the diagnosis and treatment of disease by visualizing any of the various sources of radiant energy. Three subbranches of radiology are **diagnostic radiology,** imaging using external sources of radiation; **nuclear medicine,** imaging radioactive materials that are placed into body organs; and **therapeutic radiology,** the treatment of cancer using radiation. Formerly called **roentgenology. —radiologic, radiological,** *adj.*

**radiolucency** /-lōō′sənsē/ [L, *radiare* + *lucere,* to shine],   the ability of materials of relatively low atomic number to allow most x-rays to pass through them, producing dark images on x-ray film. **—radiolucent,** *adj.*

**radiolucent** /-lōō′sənt/ [L, *radiare,* to emit rays, *lucere,* to shine],   pertaining to materials that allow x-rays to penetrate with a minimum of absorption.

**radionecrosis** /-nəkrō′sis/,   tissue death caused by radiation.

**radionuclide** /-noo′klīd/ [L, *radiare* + *nucleus,* nut kernel], an isotope that undergoes radioactive decay. Any element with an excess of either neutrons or protons in the nucleus is unstable and tends toward radioactive decay, with the emission of energy that may be measurable with a detector. The processes of radioactive decay include beta particle emission, electron capture, isomeric transition, and positron emission. Positron-emitting radionuclides are important in positron emission tomography and in medical research. Radionuclides used in scintigraphy include $^{123}$I, $^{131}$I, $^{111}$In, $^{75}$Se, $^{99m}$Tc, and $^{201}$Tl. Radionuclides of cobalt, iodine, phosphorus, strontium, and other elements are used for treatment of tumors and cancers and for nuclear imaging of internal parts of the body. See also **nuclear scanning.**

**radionuclide angiocardiography,** the radiographic examination of cardiac blood vessels after an IV injection of a radiopharmaceutical.

**radionuclide imaging,** the noninvasive examination of various parts of the body, especially the heart, using a radiopharmaceutical such as thallium-201 and a detection device such as a gamma camera, rectilinear scanner, or positron camera. See also **cardiac radionuclide imaging.**

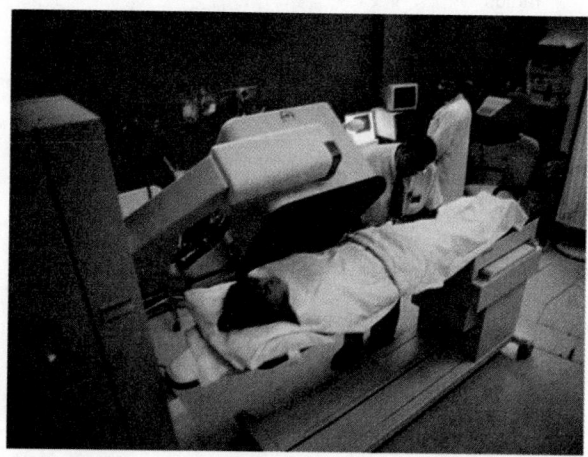

**Equipment for radionuclide imaging** *(Gray, 1992)*

**radionuclide organ imaging.** See **nuclear scanning.**

**radiopacity** /-pas′itē/ [L, *radiare,* to emit rays, *opacus,* obscure], the ability to stop or reduce the passage of x-rays. Bones have relative radiopacity and therefore show as white areas on an exposed x-ray film. Lead has marked radiopacity and therefore is widely used to shield x-ray equipment and atomic power sources. Also called **radiodensity.—radiopaque,** *adj.*

**radiopaque** /-pāk′/ [L, *radiare* + *opacus,* obscure], not permitting the passage of x-rays or other radiant energy. See also **radioactive element, radioactivity, —radiopacity,** *n.*

**radiopaque contrast medium,** a substance that stops the passage of x-rays and is used to outline the interior of hollow organs, such as heart chambers, blood vessels, respiratory passages, and the biliary tract in x-ray or fluoroscopic pictures. Also called **radiographic contrast medium.** Compare **radiolucency.**

**radiopathology** /-pəthol′əjē/, a branch of medicine involving both pathology and radiology and concerned with the effects of ionizing radiation on body tissues.

**radiopharmaceutical** /-fär′məsoo′tikəl/ [L, *radiare* + Gk, *pharmakeuein,* to give a drug], a drug that contains radioactive atoms. Kinds of radiopharmaceuticals are **diagnostic radiopharmaceutical, research radiopharmaceutical,** and **therapeutic radiopharmaceutical.**

**radiopharmacist** /-fär′məsist/, a person responsible for formulating and dispensing prescribed radioactive tracers and for the clinical aspects of radiopharmacy. Radiopharmacists are required to receive training in radioactive tracer techniques, in the safe handling of radioactive materials, in the preparation and quality control of drugs for administration to humans, and in the basic principles of nuclear medicine. Some states require that radioactive drugs be dispensed by licensed pharmacists only; others recognize radiopharmaceutic specialists who are not necessarily graduates of a school of pharmacy.

**radiopharmacy** /-fär′məsē/ [L, *radiare* + Gk, *pharmakeuein,* to give a drug], a facility for the preparation and dispensing of radioactive drugs and for the storage of radioactive materials, inventory records, and prescriptions of radioactive substances. The radiopharmacy is usually the correlation point for radioactive wastes, the unit responsible for waste disposal or storage, and a center for clinical investigations using radioactive tracers. It may also be a center for research and for the training of students and residents in radiology and nuclear medicine.

**radioprotective drugs** /-prətek′tiv/ [L, *radiare,* to emit rays, *protegere,* to cover; Fr, drogue], pharmaceuticals that protect the body against ionizing radiation. An example is Lugol's solution, an aqueous solution of iodine used to supply iodine internally, thereby blocking the uptake of radioactive iodine.

**radioresistance** /-risis′təns/ [L, *radiare* + *resistare,* to withstand], the ability of cells, tissues, organs, organisms, chemical compounds, or any other substances to remain unchanged by radiation. Compare **radiosensitivity—radioresistant,** *adj.*

**radioresistant** /-risis′tənt/, unchanged by or protected against damage by radioactive emissions such as x-rays, alpha particles, or gamma rays. Compare **radiosensitive.** See also **radioactivity.**

**radioresponsive** /-rispon′siv/, responding to radiation, whether harmful or beneficial.

**radiosensitive** /-sen′sitiv/ [L, *radiare* + *sentire,* to feel], capable of being changed by or reacting to radioactive emissions such as x-rays, alpha particles, or gamma rays. Compare **radioresistant.** See also **radioactivity.**

**radiosensitivity** /-sen′sitiv′itē/, the relative susceptibility of cells, tissues, organs, organisms, or any other substances to the effects of radiation. Cells of self-renewing tissues, such as those in the crypts of the intestine, are the most radiosensitive. Cells that divide regularly but mature between divisions, such as spermatogonia and spermatocytes, are somewhat less radiosensitive. Long-lived cells that usually do not divide unless there is a suitable stimulus, such as liver, kidney, and thyroid cells, are even less radiosensitive. Least radio sensitive are cells that have lost the ability to divide, such as neurons. Compare **radioresistance.—radiosensitive,** *adj.*

**radiosensitizers** /-sen′siti′zərs/ [L, *radiare* + *sentire* + Gk, *izein,* to cause], drugs that enhance the killing effect of radiation on cells.

**radiotherapist** /-ther′əpist/, a health professional who specializes in the use of radiation, including the application of radiopharmaceuticals, in the treatment of disease. See also **radiation oncologist.**

**radiotherapy** /-ther′əpē/ [Gk, *radiare,* to emit rays; Gk, *therapeia,* treatment], the treatment of neoplastic disease by using x-rays or gamma rays, usually from a cobalt source, to deter the proliferation of malignant cells by decreasing the rate of mitosis or impairing deoxyribonucleic acid synthesis.

**radioulnar articulation** /-ul′nər/ [L, *radius*, ray, *ulna*, elbow, arm], the articulation of the radius and the ulna, consisting of a proximal articulation, a distal articulation, and three sets of ligaments.

**radium (Ra)** /rā′dē·əm/ [L, *radius*, ray], a radioactive metallic element of the alkaline earth group. Its atomic number is 88. Four radium isotopes occur naturally and have different atomic masses: 223, 224, 226, and 228. The isotope with atomic mass 226 is the most abundant. It is formed by the disintegration of uranium 238, has a half-life of 1620 years, and decays by alpha emission to form radon 222. Radium occurs in the uranium minerals carnotite and pitchblende, which contain about $3 \times 10^{-7}$ g of radium per g of uranium. Radium salts have been used extensively as radiation sources in the treatment of cancer but are gradually being replaced in such therapy by cobalt and cesium.

**radium-226,** a radioactive isotope used for most of the twentieth century to fill the needles and tubes required for brachytherapy. It is now being replaced by cesium-137 and cobalt-60, which have similar energy characteristics but are not subject to hazardous leakage as radium sources sometimes are.

**radium insertion,** the introduction of metallic radium (Ra) into a body cavity, such as the uterus or cervix, to treat cancer.

**radium therapy** [L, *radius*, ray; Gk, *therapeia*, treatment], the use of radium and its radioactive emissions to treat disease.

**radius** /rā′dē·əs/, *pl.* **radii** [L, ray], one of the outer, shorter bones of the forearm lying parallel to the ulna and partially revolving around it. Its proximal end is small and forms a part of the elbow joint. The distal end is large and forms a part of the wrist joint. The radius receives the insertions of various muscles and articulates with the humerus, ulna, scaphoid, lunate and triangular bones.

**radix.** See **root.**

**radon (Rn)** /rā′don/ [L, *radiare*, to emit rays], a radioactive, chemically inert, gaseous element. Its atomic number is 86; its atomic mass is 222. A decay product of radium, radon is used in radiation cancer therapy. Radon is also released by rocks, soil, and groundwater and is a common source of background radiation, with an intensity that varies in different geographic areas.

**radon-222,** a radioactive decay product of radium-226 that has been used to fill permanent implants in tumors. It is being replaced by the more manageable radionuclide iodine-125.

**radon daughters,** ions that are decay products of radon. They are regarded as a potential health hazard by the U.S. Environmental Protection Agency because they tend to adhere to surfaces, such as the alveoli of the lungs, where they can cause ionizing radiation damage.

**radon seed,** a small, sealed tube of glass or gold containing radon and visible radiographically, for insertion into body tissues in the treatment of malignancies.

**ragweed** /rag′wēd/ [ME, *ragge*, rag + AS, *weod*, herb, grass, weed], any of various species of plants of the genus *Ambrosia* whose pollen can cause hay fever.

**RAI,** abbreviation for **radioactive iodine.**

**RAIU,** abbreviation for **radioactive iodine uptake.**

**RA latex test,** abbreviation for *rheumatoid arthritis latex test.* See **latex fixation test.**

**rale.** See **crackle.**

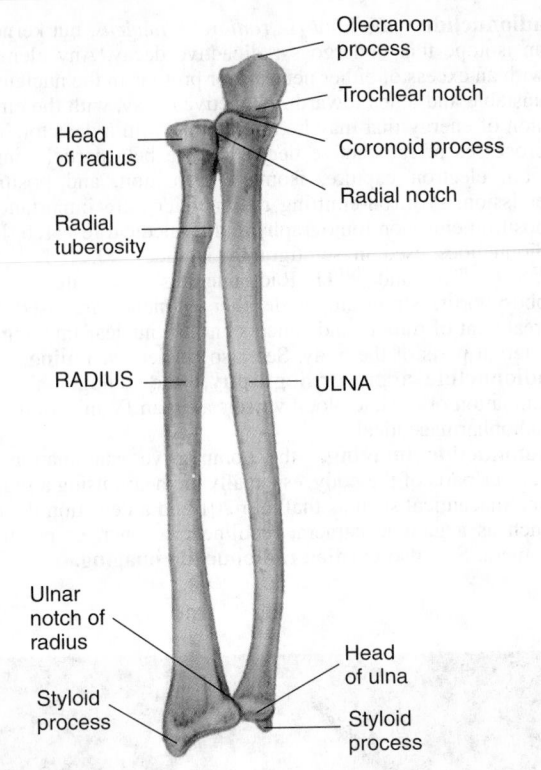

Olecranon process

Trochlear notch

Coronoid process

Radial notch

Head of radius

Radial tuberosity

RADIUS — ULNA

Ulnar notch of radius

Head of ulna

Styloid process

Styloid process

**Radius and ulna** (Applegate, 2000)

**raloxifene,** a selective estrogen receptor modulator (SERM).

■ INDICATIONS: This drug is used to prevent osteoporosis in postmenopausal women.

■ CONTRAINDICATIONS: Pregnancy, lactation, and known hypersensitivity to raloxifene prohibit the use of this drug.

■ ADVERSE EFFECTS: Adverse effects of raloxifene include insomnia, migraines, depression, hot flashes, diarrhea, anorexia, cramps, vaginitis, urinary tract infection, leukorrhea, endometrial disorder, breast pain, rash, sweating, weight gain, peripheral edema, arthralgia, myalgia, leg cramps, arthritis, sinusitis, pharyngitis, increased cough, pneumonia, and laryngitis. Nausea is a common side effect.

**RAM.** See **random-access memory.**

**rami-,** combining form meaning 'branch': *ramicotomy, ramification, ramisection.*

**ramification** /ram′ifikā′shən/ [L, *ramus*, branch, *facere*, to make], a branching, distribution.

**ramify.** See **ramus.**

**rampant dental caries,** dental caries that involve several teeth, appear suddenly, and often progress rapidly.

**Ramsay Hunt syndrome** [James Ramsay Hunt, American neurologist, 1872–1937], a neurologic condition resulting from invasion of the seventh nerve ganglia and the geniculate ganglion by varicella zoster virus, characterized by severe ear pain, facial nerve paralysis, vertigo, hearing loss, and often mild generalized encephalitis. The vertigo may last days or weeks but usually resolves itself. The facial paralysis may be permanent, and the hearing loss, which is rarely permanent, may be partial or total. Treatment usually includes the prescription of corticosteroid drugs. Also called **herpes zoster oticus.**

**Ramstedt-Fredet operation.** See **pyloromyotomy.**

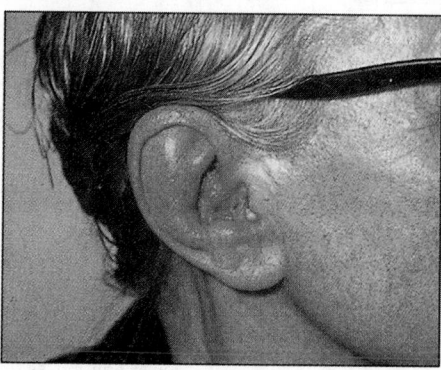

**Ramsay Hunt syndrome** *(Perkin, 1998)*

**ramus** /rā'məs/, *pl.* **rami** [L, branch], a small branchlike structure extending from a larger one or dividing into two or more parts, such as a branch of a nerve or artery or one of the rami of the blood vessel or nerve. —**ramification,** *n.* **ramify,** *v.*

**Ranchos Los Amigos Scale,** a scale of cognitive functioning, developed as a behavioral rating scale to aid in assessment and treatment of head-injured persons. Eight levels of cognitive functioning are identified, from I (no response) to VIII (purposeful and appropriate behavioral response).

**rancidity** /ransid'itē/, the unpleasant taste and smell of fatty foods that have undergone decomposition, liberating butyric acid and other volatile lipids.

**random-access memory (RAM)** /ran'dəm/, the part of a computer's memory available to execute programs and temporarily store data. It can usually be used for both reading and writing. RAM data is automatically erased when the computer is turned off unless the file has been saved. Compare **ROM.**

**random controlled trial** [ME, *randoun,* run violently; Fr, *contrôle,* check, *trier,* to grind], a study plan for a proposed new treatment in which subjects are assigned on a random basis to participate either in an experimental group receiving the new treatment or in a control group that does not.

**random genetic drift.** See **genetic drift.**

**randomization** [ME, *randoun,* run violently], the process of assigning subjects or objects to a control or experimental group on a random basis.

**random mating** [ME, *randoun,* run violently, *gemate*], a pairing of subjects when each individual has an equal chance of mating with those of other genetic backgrounds.

**random off.** See **on/off phenomenon.**

**random sampling** [ME, *randoun,* run violently; L, *exemplum*], a method of sampling for a study in which each individual has the same chance of being selected and the choice of a particular individual does not affect the chances of the others.

**random selection,** a method of choosing subjects for a research study in which all members of a particular group have an equal chance of being selected.

**random voided specimen,** a voided urine specimen obtained at any point of a 24-hour period.

**range** /rānj/ [OFr, *ranger,* to arrange in a row], the interval between the lowest and highest values in a series of data.

**range abnormalities,** uncertainties in the actual range from which Doppler signals or echo signals originate. In pulsed Doppler instruments a high pulse repetition frequency can result in range ambiguities.

**range equation,** a relationship between the distance to a reflector and the time it takes for a pulse of ultrasound to propagate to the reflector and return to the transducer.

**range of accommodation** [OFr, *ranger* + L, *accommodatio*], the distance between the farthest point that an object can be seen clearly with accommodation fully relaxed and the nearest distance that an object can be observed with full accommodation, measured in meters or centimeters.

**range of motion (ROM)** [OFr, *ranger* + L, *motio*], the extent of movement of a joint, measured in degrees of a circle.

**range-of-motion exercise** [OFr, *ranger,* to arrange in a row; L, *motio,* movement], any body action involving the muscles, joints, and natural movements, such as abduction, adduction, extension, flexion, pronation, supination, and rotation. Such exercises are usually applied actively or passively in the prevention and treatment of orthopedic deformities, in the assessment of injuries and deformities, and in athletic conditioning. See also **active range of motion.**

**ranitidine** /ranit'idēn/, a histamine $H_2$ receptor antagonist.

■ INDICATIONS: It is prescribed in the treatment of gastroesophageal reflux disease and gastric hypersecretory conditions.

■ CONTRAINDICATIONS: Known sensitivity to this drug prohibits its use. The drug should be used in pregnancy only if clearly needed.

■ ADVERSE EFFECTS: Among the most serious adverse reactions are headaches and rashes.

**Rankine scale** [William J. M. Rankine, Scottish physicist, 1820–1870], an absolute temperature scale calculated in degrees Fahrenheit. Absolute zero on the Rankine scale is $-460°$ F, equivalent to $-273°$ C. See also **Kelvin scale.**

**rank sum test,** a nonparametric statistical test for ordinal data, testing the null hypothesis that two samples are drawn from the same population against the alternative hypothesis that the two samples are drawn from two populations having probability distributions of the same shape but different locations. It is based on the value of the rank sum statistic, which is calculated as the sum of the ranks of each sample after the observations in both samples are jointly ranked in ascending order; if and only if the null hypothesis is true, the average ranks of the two samples will be similar. Also called **Mann-Whitney test** and **Mann-Whitney U** test.

**ranula** /ran'yŏŏlə/, *pl.* **ranulae** [L, *rana,* frog], a large mucocele in the floor of the mouth, usually caused by obstruction of the ducts of the sublingual salivary glands and less commonly caused by obstruction of the ducts of the submandibular salivary glands. Also called **hydroglossa.**

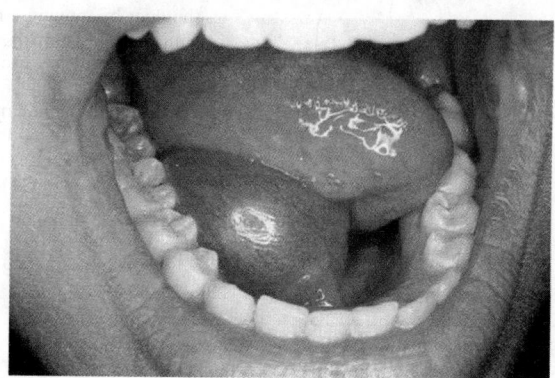

**Ranula** *(Bingham, Hawke, and Kwok, 1992)*

## Range-of-motion exercises

| Body part | Type of joint | Type of movement | Body part | Type of joint | Type of movement |
|---|---|---|---|---|---|
| Neck, cervical spine | Pivotal | Flexion: bring chin to rest on chest<br>Extension: return head to erect position | | | Circumduction: move arm in full circle (Circumduction is combination of all movements of ball-and-socket joint.) |
| | | Lateral flexion: tilt head as far as possible toward each shoulder | Elbow | Hinge | Flexion: bend elbow so that lower arm moves toward its shoulder joint and hand is level with shoulder<br>Extension: straighten elbow by lowering hand |
| | | Rotation: turn head as far as possible in circular movement | Forearm | Pivotal | Supination: turn lower arm and hand so that palm is up<br>Pronation: turn lower arm so that palm is down |
| Shoulder | Ball and socket | Flexion: raise arm from side position forward to position above head<br>Extension: move arm behind body, keeping elbow straight | | | |
| | | Abduction: raise arm to side to position above head with palm away from head<br>Adduction: lower arm sideways and across body as far as possible | Wrist | Condyloid | Flexion: move palm toward inner aspect of forearm<br>Extension: bring dorsal surface of hand back as far as possible<br>Abduction (radial flexion): bend wrist medially toward thumb<br>Adduction (ulnar flexion): bend wrist laterally toward fifth finger |
| | | Internal rotation: with elbow flexed, rotate shoulder by moving arm until thumb is turned inward and toward back<br>External rotation: with elbow flexed, move arm until thumb is upward and lateral to head | Fingers | Condyloid hinge | Flexion: make fist<br>Extension: bend fingers back as far as possible<br>Abduction: spread fingers apart<br>Adduction: bring fingers together |

Modified from Potter P, Perry AG: *Fundamentals of nursing: concepts, process, and practice*, ed 5, St Louis, 2001, Mosby.

## Range-of-motion exercises—cont'd

| Body part | Type of joint | Type of movement | Body part | Type of joint | Type of movement |
|---|---|---|---|---|---|
| Thumb | Saddle | Flexion: move thumb across palmar surface of hand<br>Extension: move thumb straight away from hand<br>Abduction: extend thumb laterally (usually done when placing fingers in abduction and adduction)<br>Adduction: move thumb back toward hand<br>Opposition: touch thumb to each finger of same hand | | | Circumduction: move leg in circle |
| Hip | Ball and socket | Flexion: move leg forward and up<br>Extension: move back beside other leg | Knee | Hinge | Flexion: bring heel back toward back of thigh<br>Extension: return leg to the floor |
| | | Hyperextension: move leg behind body | Ankle | Hinge | Dorsal flexion: move foot so that toes are pointed upward<br>Plantar flexion: move foot so that toes are pointed downward |
| | | | Foot | Gliding | Inversion: turn sole of foot medially<br>Eversion: turn sole of foot laterally |
| | | Abduction: move leg laterally away from body<br>Adduction: move leg back toward medial position and beyond if possible<br>Internal rotation: turn foot and leg toward other leg<br>External rotation: turn foot and leg away from other leg | Toes | Condyloid | Flexion: curl toes downward<br>Extension: straighten toes<br>Abduction: spread toes apart<br>Adduction: bring toes together |

**Ranvier's nodes** /ränvē-āz′, räN-/ [Louis A. Ranvier, French pathologist, 1835–1922], constrictions in the medullary substance of a nerve fiber at more or less regular intervals.

**rape** [L, *rapere,* to seize], a sexual assault, homosexual or heterosexual, the legal definitions for which vary from state to state. Rape is a crime of violence or one committed under the threat of violence, and its victims are treated for medical and psychologic trauma. See also **statutory rape.**
■ OBSERVATIONS: Characteristically the victim is frightened and feels vulnerable, humiliated, and personally violated. General physical examination may reveal cuts, bruises, and

## Rape-prevention measures

**Prevention of attack**

Set house lights to go on and off by timer

Keep light on at all entrances

Install safety locks on windows and doors

Have key ready before reaching door of house or car

Look in car before entering

Never let a stranger enter the house; insist on identification from all service personnel; check identity with agency if suspicious

Do not list first name on mailbox or in telephone directory

Make arrangements with neighbor for needed assistance

Be alert when walking; stay in lighted areas

Walk down center of street if possible

Avoid lonely or enclosed areas

**If attacked**

Run toward a lighted house; yell, "Fire"

Spit in rapist's face; act bizarre; vomit

Rip off rapist's glasses

Step hard on his foot (instep)

Aim at eyes; try to gouge eyes, scrape face

Hit throat at Adam's apple (larynx)

Use fighting and screaming with caution; this may scare some rapists, encourage others

Try talking to avoid rape

Make close observations about rapist, car, location

From Phipps WJ, Sands JK, Marek JE: *Medical-surgical nursing: concepts and clinical practice,* ed 6, St Louis, 1999, Mosby.

other injuries. Pelvic or genital examination may show traumatic injury to the internal or external genitalia or anus.

■ INTERVENTIONS: Careful physical examination should be conducted by specially trained health-care personnel, and a detailed history obtained. Evidence and medical specimens are collected as indicated. Ideally counseling is available and offered immediately to all victims of rape. In the case of a woman who has been raped by a man, a pregnancy test may be performed to document current pregnancy status. Prophylaxis against conception may be administered. Medications may be given to prevent the development of venereal disease. Arrangements for ongoing emotional support are made.

■ NURSING CONSIDERATIONS: A trained empathetic caregiver of the same gender is assigned to stay with the victim. Privacy for the history, examination, and police interview is ensured. The victim may or may not choose to report the incident to the police. The victim must sign a special form to allow specimens to be released to a law enforcement agency. In general, it is the role of the caregiver and other specially trained medical workers to examine, treat, and collect specimens as necessary but not to decide that rape has occurred. Before discharge it should be ascertained that someone can be with the victim, since depression, anger, guilt, and fear may occur after rape. See also **sexual assault.**

**rape counseling,** counseling by a trained person provided to a victim of rape. Rape counseling ideally begins at the time the crime is first reported, as in an emergency department. Initially the counselor offers sensitive support for the victim by accepting the victim in a nonprejudicial, noncritical way. The victim's response to the trauma of the assault is empathetically elicited, and three basic statements are made: the counselor is sorry that the rape happened, is glad that the injuries are not worse, and does not think that the victim was

wrong or did anything wrong. Counseling personnel may provide supportive services and advocacy and liaison between the victim and medical, legal, and law enforcement authorities. This involves staying with the victim during medical examination, during police or district attorney's questioning, and throughout the criminal justice process.

**rape-trauma syndrome,** a nursing diagnosis accepted by the Fourth National Conference on the Classification of Nursing Diagnoses. The syndrome results from the experience of being raped, which is defined as forced, violent sexual penetration against the victim's will and consent. The trauma syndrome that develops from this attack or attempted attack includes an acute phase of disorganization and a longer phase of reorganization in the victim's life.

■ DEFINING CHARACTERISTICS: The defining characteristics are divided into three subcomponents: rape trauma, compound reaction, and silent reaction. The defining characteristics of **rape trauma** in the acute phase are emotional reactions of anger, guilt, and embarrassment; fear of physical violence and death; humiliation; wish for revenge; and multiple physical complaints, including gastrointestinal distress, genitourinary discomfort, tension, and disturbance of the normal patterns of sleep, activity, and rest. The long-term phase of rape trauma is characterized by changes in the usual patterns of daily life (even a change in residence), nightmares and phobias, and a need for support from friends and family. The **compound reaction** is characterized by all of the defining characteristics of rape trauma, reliance on alcohol or drugs, or recurrence of the symptoms of previous conditions, including psychiatric illness. The **silent reaction** sometimes occurs in place of the rape trauma or compound reaction. The defining characteristics of the silent reaction are an abrupt change in the victim's usual sexual relationships, an increase in nightmares, an increasing anxiety during the interview about the rape incident, a marked change in sexual behavior, denial of the rape or refusal to discuss it, and the sudden development of phobic reactions.

■ RELATED FACTORS: Related factors include inadequate support systems; spouse-family blaming; fear of reprisal, pregnancy, and going out alone; and anxiety about potential health problems such as AIDS, venereal disease, and herpes. See also **nursing diagnosis.**

**rape-trauma treatment,** a nursing intervention from the Nursing Interventions Classification (NIC) defined as provision of emotional and physical support immediately following a reported rape. See also **Nursing Interventions Classification.**

**raphe** /rā′fē/ [Gk, *rhaphe,* seam], a crease, ridge, or seam of the halves of various symmetric parts, such as the abdominal raphe of the linea alba or the raphe penis, which appears as a narrow dark streak on the inferior surface of the penis. Also spelled **rhaphe.**

**raphe nuclei,** a subgroup of the reticular nuclei of the brain stem, found in narrow longitudinal sheets along the raphae of the medulla oblongata, pons, and mesencephalon; they include many neurons that synthesize serotonin. Their ascending fibers project to parts of the limbic system and their descending fibers project to other brainstem nuclei, the medulla oblongata, and the pons. In the group are the magnus raphe nucleus, median raphe nucleus, obscurus raphe nucleus, pallidal raphe nucleus, pontine raphe nucleus, posterior raphe nucleus, inferior linear nucleus, intermediate linear nucleus, and superior linear nucleus.

**raphe of tongue** [Gk, *rhaphe,* seam; AS, *tunge*], a fibrous wall that forms a line of union between the right and left sides of the tongue.

**rapid-acting insulin.** See **short-acting insulin.**

**rapid eye movement.** See **sleep.**

**rapid grower** /rap′id/, a saprophytic mycobacterium in group IV of the Runyon classification system that grows within 3 to 5 days.

**rapid plasma reagin (RPR) test,** an agglutination examination used in screening for syphilis. The test detects two groups of antibodies. The first is a nontreponemal antibody (reagin) directed against a lipoidal agent resulting from the *Treponema pallidum* infection. The second is an antibody directed against the *Treponema pallidum* organism itself.

**rapid pulse** [L, *rapidus,* rush, *pulsare,* to beat], a pulse faster than normal.

**rapport** /rapôr′/ [Fr, agreement], a sense of mutuality and understanding; harmony, accord, confidence, and respect underlying a relationship between two persons, which is an essential bond between a therapist and patient. It should be distinguished from transference, which is unconscious.

**rapprochement** /räprôshmäN′/ [Fr, *rapprocher,* to bring together], (in psychology) the third subphase of the separation-individuation phase of Mahler's system of preoedipal development. This subphase occurs from approximately 14 months to 2 years or more. This stage is characterized by a rediscovery of and reestablishment with mother or a significant nurturer in an attempt to have needs met after the initial separation of the practicing subphase in which the child practices autonomous behavior. The narcissistic inflation of the practicing subphase is replaced by a realization of separation and vulnerability.

**raptus** /rap′təs/ [L, *rapere,* to seize], **1.** a state of intense emotional or mental excitement, often characterized by uncontrollable activity or behavior resulting from an irresistible impulse; ecstasy; rapture. **2.** any sudden or violent seizure or attack.

**rare-earth element** [L, *rarus,* thin; AS, *earthe* + L, *elementum*], a metallic element having an atomic number between 57 to 71, inclusively. Also called **rare-earth metal.**

**rare earth screen,** an x-ray-intensifying screen made of rare-earth elements, such as yttrium and gadolinium such screens enable lower radiation doses to be used while producing acceptable film densities.

**rarefaction** /rer′əfak′shən/, reductions of density of a medium at a location in the medium accompanying the cyclic pressure reductions during the passage of a sound wave.

**RAS,** abbreviation for **reticular activating system.**

**rash** [OFr, *rasche,* scurf], a skin eruption. Kinds of rashes are **butterfly rash, diaper rash, drug rash,** and **heat rash.**

**Rashkind procedure** /rash′kind/ [William J. Rashkind, American physician, b. 1922; L, *procedere,* to go forth], the enlargement of an opening in the cardiac septum between the right and left atria. It is performed to relieve congestive heart failure in newborns with certain congenital heart defects by improving the oxygenation of the blood. The procedure allows more mixing between oxygenated blood from the lungs and systemic blood without the risk of surgery, sustaining life until the child is 2 to 3 years of age and a shunt can be created to carry systemic blood to the lungs. Before surgery a cardiac catheterization is done to pinpoint the defect. Under light general anesthesia a deflated balloon is passed pervenously through the foramen ovale into the left atrium. The balloon is inflated and pulled across the septum to enlarge the opening. After surgery the infant is observed carefully for respiratory difficulty, signs of hypoxia, or decreasing cardiac output. Humidified oxygen is administered. Fluids and electrolytes are closely monitored. Also called **balloon septostomy.**

**Rasmussen's aneurysm** /rahs′moosənz/ [Fritz Waldemar Rasmussen, Danish physician, 1834–1837], dilation of a pulmonary artery in a tuberculous cavity; rupture causes hemorrhage and hemoptysis.

**raspberry leaves,** an herbal product harvested from the raspberry plant, found worldwide.

■ USES: This herb is used to facilitate childbirth, as a uterine tonic, and as a treatment for dysmenorrhea, fever, and vomiting.

■ CONTRAINDICATIONS: Raspberry should not be used medicinally during pregnancy and lactation and is contraindicated in those with known hypersensitivity to this plant.

**raspberry tongue** /raz′berē/, a dark red tongue with a smooth surface and prominent papillae, seen after shedding of the white coating characteristic of the early stage of scarlet fever. See also **strawberry tongue.**

**RAST.** See **radioallergosorbent test.**

**rat-bite fever** [AS, *raet* + *bitan,* to bite], either of two distinct infections transmitted to humans by the bite of a rat or mouse, characterized by fever, headache, malaise, nausea, vomiting, and rash. In the United States the disease is more commonly caused by *Streptobacillus moniliformis;* its unique features are a rash on palms and soles, painful joints, prompt healing of the wound, and a duration of 2 weeks. In the Far East rat-bite fever is usually caused by *Spirillum minus* and is associated with an asymmetric rash on the extremities, no joint symptoms, a relapsing fever, swelling at the site of the wound, regional lymphadenopathy, and a duration of from 4 to 8 weeks. Relapse is common. Penicillin administered intramuscularly is effective in treating either form of the disease. Rat-bite fever resulting from infection caused by *Streptobacillus moniliformis* is also called **Haverhill fever;** infection caused by *Spirillum minus* is also called **sodoku.**

**rate** [L, *ratus,* reckoned], a numeric ratio, often used in the compilation of data concerning the prevalence and incidence of events, in which the number of actual occurrences appears as the numerator and the number of possible occurrences appears as the denominator; when 1 person in 15 fails an examination, the failure rate is said to be 1/15 (or 'one in fifteen'). Standard rates are stated in conventional units of population such as neonatal mortality per 1000 or maternal mortality per 100,000.

**rate-pressure product,** the heart rate multiplied by the systolic blood pressure. It is a clinical indicator of myocardial oxygen demand.

**rate-responsive pacer,** an electronic pacemaker whose rate can be adjusted as required to meet physiologic demands.

**Rathke's pouch** /rät′kēz/ [Martin H. Rathke, German anatomist, 1793–1860; OFr, *pouche*], a depression that forms in the roof of the mouth of an embryo, anterior to the buccopharyngeal membrane, around the fourth week of gestation. The walls of the diverticulum develop into the anterior lobe of the pituitary gland.

**Rathke's pouch tumor.** See **craniopharyngioma.**

**rating of perceived exertion (RPE),** a scale for quantifying perceived exertion, with 6 being extremely light exertion and 20 being extremely hard. The American College of Sports Medicine (ACSM) has recalibrated the scale from 1 to 10. The ACSM has also established minimal guidelines pertaining to the frequency, intensity, and duration of exercise needed to produce a training effect.

**ratio** /rā′shō/ [L, a reckoning], the relationship of one quantity to one or more other quantities expressed as a proportion of one to the others, and written either as a fraction (⅔) or linearly (8:3).

**rational** /rash′ənəl/ [L, *rationalis,* reasonable], **1.** pertaining to a measure, method, or procedure based on reason. **2.** pertaining to a therapeutic method based on an understanding of the cause and mechanisms of a specific disease and the potential effects of the drugs or procedures used in treating the disorder. **3.** sane; capable of normal reasoning or behavior.

**rationale** /rash′ənal′/ [L, *rationalis,* reasonable], a system of reasoning or a statement of the reasons used in explaining data or phenomena.

**rational emotive therapy (RET),** a form of cognitive therapy, originated by Albert Ellis, that emphasizes a reorganization and challenge of one's cognitive and emotional functions, a redefinition of one's problems, and a change in one's attitudes to develop more effective and suitable patterns of behavior. RET is conducted with individuals or with groups.

**rationalization** /rash′ənal′īzā′shən/, the most commonly used defense mechanism in which an individual justifies ideas, actions, or feelings with seemingly acceptable reasons or explanations. It is often used to preserve self-respect, reduce guilt feelings, or obtain social approval or acceptance.

**rational treatment.** See **treatment.**

**ratio solution,** the relationship of a solute to a solution expressed as a proportion, such as 1:1000, or parts per thousand.

**rattle** [ME, *ratelen*], an abnormal sound heard by auscultation of the lungs in some forms of pulmonary disease. It consists of a coarse vibration, more intense than a crackle, very much like a rhonchus, caused by the movement of moisture and the separation of the walls of small air passages during respiration.

**rattlesnake** [ME, *ratelen* + AS, *snacan,* to creep], a poisonous pit viper with a series of loosely connected, horny segments at the end of the tail that make a noise like a rattle when shaken. More than 25 species of rattlesnakes are found in the Americas, including most parts of the United States. They have a hematoxin in their venom, and they are responsible for most of the poisonous snake bites in the United States. Immediate treatment includes keeping the victim quiet and immobilizing the bite area at the level of the heart. Antivenin is available. See **snakebite.**

**rat typhus.** See **murine typhus.**

**rauwolfia** /rôwol′fē·ə, rou-, rä-/ [Leonhard Rauwolf, sixteenth century German botanist], the dried roots of *Rauwolfia serpentina* that provide the extracts for hypotensive agents and tranquilizing alkaloid drugs such as reserpine.

**rauwolfia alkaloid,** any one of more than 20 alkaloids derived from the root of a climbing shrub, *Rauwolfia serpentina,* indigenous to India and the surrounding area. Formerly used as an antipsychotic agent, it is today confined to the treatment of hypertension. Numerous trademark formulations of the principal alkaloid reserpine are available.

**rauwolfia serpentina,** the dried root from *Rauwolfia serpentina,* used as an antihypertensive in combination with bendroflumethiozide.

■ INDICATIONS: It is prescribed in the treatment of mild hypertension and hypertensive emergencies.

■ CONTRAINDICATIONS: Mental depression, peptic ulcer, ulcerative colitis, electroconvulsive therapy, or known hypersensitivity to this drug prohibits its use. It can interact adversely with monoamine oxidase inhibitors.

■ ADVERSE EFFECTS: Among the more serious adverse reactions are symptoms resembling parkinsonism, glaucoma, cardiac arrhythmias, and GI bleeding.

**Rauzide,** trademark for a cardiovascular, fixed-combination drug containing a diuretic (bendroflumethiazide) and an antihypertensive (rauwolfia serpentina).

**raw data,** the information obtained by radio reception of a magnetic resonance signal as stored by a computer. Specific computer manipulation of the data is required to construct an image.

**ray** [L, *radius*], a beam of radiation, such as heat or light, moving away from a source.

**rayl** /rāl/ [John W.S. Rayleigh, English physicist, 1842–1919], the unit for characteristic acoustic impedance. Its fundamental units are $kg/m^2/s$.

**Rayleigh scatterer** /rā′lē/ [John Rayleigh, English physicist, 1842–1919], reflecting objects whose dimensions are much smaller than the ultrasonic wavelength. The scattered intensity from a volume of Rayleigh scatterers increases rapidly with increasing frequency, being related to frequency raised to the fourth power.

**Raynaud's phenomenon** /rānōz′/ [Maurice Raynaud, French physician, 1834–1881], intermittent attacks of ischemia of the extremities of the body, especially the fingers, toes, ears, and nose, caused by exposure to cold or by emotional stimuli. The attacks are characterized by severe blanching of the extremities, followed by cyanosis, then redness; they are usually accompanied by numbness, tingling, burning, and often pain. Normal color and sensation are restored by heat. The attacks usually occur secondary to such conditions as scleroderma, rheumatoid arthritis, systemic lupus erythematosus, thoracic outlet syndrome, drug intoxications, dysproteinemia, myxedema, primary pulmonary hypertension, and trauma. The condition is called **Raynaud's disease** when there is a history of symptoms for at least 2 years with no progression of symptoms and no evidence of

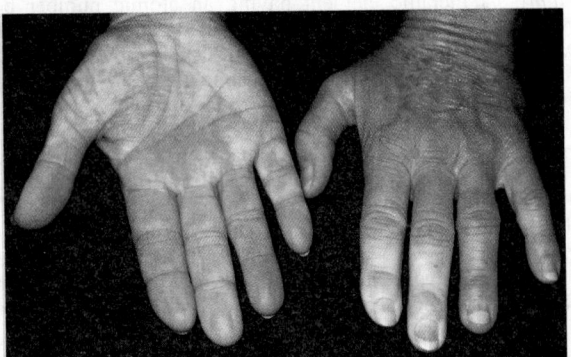

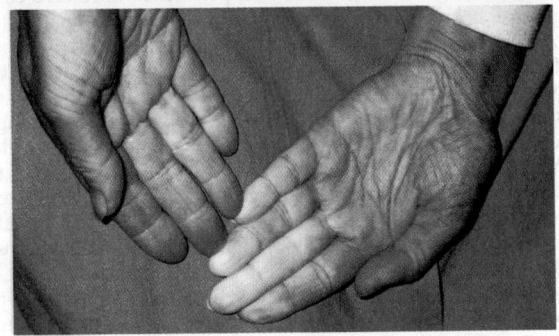

**Raynaud's phenomenon** *(Barkauskas et al, 1998)*

an underlying cause. Therapy for the secondary form depends on recognition and treatment of the underlying disease. Idiopathic forms, which occur most frequently in young women 18 to 30 years of age, may be controlled by protecting the body and extremities from the cold, by the use of mild sedatives and vasodilators, and by avoiding smoking. Biofeedback techniques have been proven useful in training the client to increase the temperature of the affected extremity, ears, or nose. Drug therapy can also provide relief of symptoms.

**Raynaud's sign.** See **acrocyanosis.**

**Rb,** symbol for the element **rubidium.**

**RBBB,** abbreviation for **right bundle branch block.**

**RBC,** abbreviation for *red blood cell.* See **erythrocyte.**

**RBE,** abbreviation for **relative biologic effectiveness.**

**RBRVS,** abbreviation for **resource-based relative value scale.**

**RCEEM,** abbreviation for **Recognized Continuing Education Evaluation Mechanism.**

**R.C.P.,** abbreviation for **Royal College of Physicians.**

**RCPSC,** abbreviation for **Royal College of Physicians and Surgeons of Canada.**

**R.C.S.,** abbreviation for **Royal College of Surgeons.**

**RD,** abbreviation for **registered dietitian.**

**RDAs,** abbreviation for **recommended dietary allowances.**

**RDH,** *Registered Dental Hygienist.*

**rdi,** abbreviation for *recommended daily intake.*

**RDS,** abbreviation for **respiratory distress syndrome of the newborn.**

**Re,** symbol for the element **rhenium.**

**re-,** prefix meaning 'back, again, contrary': *reaction, recombination, recurrent.*

**reabsorption** /rē′əbsôrp′shən/, the process of something being absorbed again, such as the removal of calcium from the bone back into the blood. Also called **resorption.**

**reacher** /rē′chər/, a pincer-type device with an extended handle that can be used to reach and grasp objects overhead or on the floor by persons with upper extremity disabilities or those who lose the ability to bend and stoop. Also called **extended arm.**

**Reach to Recovery** [AS, *reacan,* to reach; ME, *recoveren,* to get back], a national volunteer organization that offers counseling and support to women with breast cancer and to their families. Many of the members have had mastectomies themselves.

**reaction** /rē·ak′shən/ [L, *re,* again, *agere,* to act], a response to a substance, treatment, or other stimulus, such as an antigen-antibody reaction, an allergic reaction, or an adverse pharmacological reaction. —**react,** *v.,* **reactive,** *adj.*

**reaction formation,** an unconscious defense mechanism in which a person expresses toward another person or situation feelings, attitudes, or behaviors that are the opposite of what would normally be expected. It begins in early childhood and proceeds through life.

**reaction time** [L, *re,* again, *agere,* to act; AS, *tima*], the interval between the application of a stimulus and the beginning of a response.

**reactivate** /rē·ak′tivāt/ [L, *re + activus*], to make active again, as in adding fresh serum to restore the potency of an original supply of the serum.

**reactivation** /rē·ak′tivā′shən/, the restoration of impaired biologic activity caused by chemical reaction, thermal application, genetic recombination or helper elements.

**reactivation tuberculosis,** a form of secondary tuberculosis that recurs as a result of the activation of a dormant endogenous infection. Causes of the reactivation may include loss of immunity, hormonal changes, or poor nutrition.

**reactive.** See **reaction.**

**reactive arthritis** /rē·ak′tiv/ [L, *re + activus,* active], arthritis after an infection, such as urethritis caused by *Chlamydia trachomatis* or enteritis caused by *Campylobacter, Salmonella, Shigella,* or *Yersinia.* Compare **Reiter's syndrome.**

**reactive decision** /rē·ak′tiv/ [L, *re + activus*], (in psychology) a decision made by an individual in response to the influence or goals of others.

**reactive depression,** an emotional condition characterized by an acute feeling of despondency, sadness, and depressive dysphoria, which varies in intensity and duration. The condition is caused by some identifiable external situation or environmental stress and is generally relieved when the circumstance is altered or the conflict understood and resolved. The term is no longer in use. Also called **situational depression.** See also **depression.**

**reactive hypoglycemia,** low levels of glucose in the circulating blood (45 to 50 mg/dL) in an arterialized specimen after ingestion of carbohydrates. It may be related to increased insulin sensitivity or excess counterregulatory hormone secretion or action.

**reactive inflammation** [L, *re + activus + inflammare,* to set afire], an inflammation that develops as a reaction to an antigen.

**reactive schizophrenia,** a form of schizophrenia caused by environmental factors rather than by organic changes in the brain. Disease onset is usually rapid; symptoms are of brief duration, and the affected individual appears well immediately before and after the schizophrenic episode. See also brief reactive **psychosis, schizophrenia, schizophreniform disorder.**

**reactor** /rē·ak′tər/, 1. (in psychology) a family therapist who lets a family in therapy take the lead and then follows in that direction. 2. (in radiology) a cubicle in which radioisotopes are artificially produced.

**read** [AS, *raedan,* to advise], (of a computer) to retrieve or transfer data from some storage location or medium, such as a disk.

**reading** [AS, *raedan*], the linear process in which the genetic information contained in a nucleotide sequence is decoded, as in the translation of the messenger RNA into a sequence of amino acids in a polypeptide.

**reading disorder,** a language disorder in which one's reading ability is significantly below intellectual capacity. Tests show the problem does not involve mental retardation, chronologic age, or inadequate schooling but is marked by faulty oral reading, slow reading, and reduced comprehension.

**Read method** [Grantley Dick-Read, 1890–1959, English obstetrician], a method of psychophysical preparation for childbirth. It was the first 'natural childbirth' program, a term coined by Dr. Read in the 1930s. Basically Read held that childbirth is a normal, physiologic procedure and that the pain of labor and delivery is of psychologic origin—the fear-tension-pain syndrome. He countered women's fears with education about the physiologic process, encouraged a positive welcoming attitude, corrected false information, and led tours of the hospital. To decrease tension he developed a series of breathing exercises for use during the various stages of labor. To foster relaxation and optimal physical function in labor and recovery after delivery, he incorporated a series of physical exercises to be performed regularly in classes and in practice at home during pregnancy. The woman is helped to manage labor and delivery using the

Read method in the following way: During the early and mid-first stage of labor, before cervical dilation has reached 7 cm, contractions are 2 to 5 minutes apart and last for 30 to 40 seconds. The mother lies on her back with her knees bent. Abdominal breathing is used during contractions. Her hands are placed over her lower abdomen, fingers touching. She breathes deeply and slowly—in through her nose and out through her mouth. The abdominal wall rises with each inhalation, which she can feel with her hands. The rate of breathing is no more than six breaths in 30 seconds, or 12 to 18 in one contraction. During the late part of the first stage of labor, after 7 cm of cervical dilation, the contractions are 1-1/2 to 2 minutes apart and last for 40 to 60 seconds. Costal or diaphragmatic breathing is used during contractions. The mother's hands are placed on her sides, over the ribs. She breathes in more shallowly, feeling her ribs move sideways against her hands. Each breath is drawn in through her nose and exhaled through her mouth. The abdominal wall does not rise and fall with this kind of breathing. The rate of breathing is no more than six breaths in 30 seconds, or 12 to 18 in one contraction. At the end of the first stage of labor, near full dilation, contractions may be very strong, occurring every 1-1/2 to 2 minutes and lasting 60 to 90 seconds. The mother lies on her back with her knees bent. Panting respirations are used during the contractions. The mother holds one of her hands on her sternum, which rises and falls as she pants lightly and rapidly through her mouth. Panting continues through the end of the first stage to full dilation as the urge to push grows. Panting helps the woman to avoid pushing. During the second, or expulsive, stage of labor after full dilation of the cervix, the contractions occur every 1-1/2 to 2 minutes, last 60 to 90 seconds, and are accompanied with an urge to bear down and push. The woman lies back, head and shoulders supported in a semisitting position. She is helped to draw her legs up, holding them with her hands behind the lower thighs, thighs on her abdomen and spread apart. As each contraction begins, she raises her head, takes a deep breath, tucks her chin on her chest, blocks the escape of air from her lungs, and bears down. During each contraction she may need to blow the air out, refill her lungs, and push again two or three times. Throughout labor she is helped to understand what is occurring and to participate and accept the experience in anticipation of the birth of the baby. Currently many authorities who advocate use of other aspects of the Read method strongly recommend that a woman in labor not lie on her back. Supine hypotension is frequently the result of this position, because the uterus can fall back, occluding the vena cava and decreasing the volume of blood returned to the heart, thus reducing the volume of the cardiac output. Maternal hypotension follows, resulting in decreased placental perfusion and an inadequate supply of oxygen to the fetus. Today the woman using the Read method spends most of labor lying on her side or in a semisitting position with her knees, back, and head well supported. Compare **Bradley method, Lamaze method.**

**read-only memory (ROM),** the part of a computer's memory where information is permanently stored. The operator may have random access to the memory, but only for purposes of reading the contents. ROM also executes automatically when the computer is started. Special equipment is required to write or erase a read-only memory. Compare **RAM.**

**readthrough** [AS, *raedan* + *thurh*, through], transcription beyond the normal termination sequence in a DNA template, caused by the occasional failure of RNA polymerase to respond to the end-point signal.

**reagent** /rē·ā′jənt/ [L, *re*, again, *agere*, to act], a chemical substance known to react in a specific way. A reagent is used to detect or synthesize another substance in a chemical reaction. Examples include Benedict's reagent used to test for glucose and Biuret reagent used to test for protein.

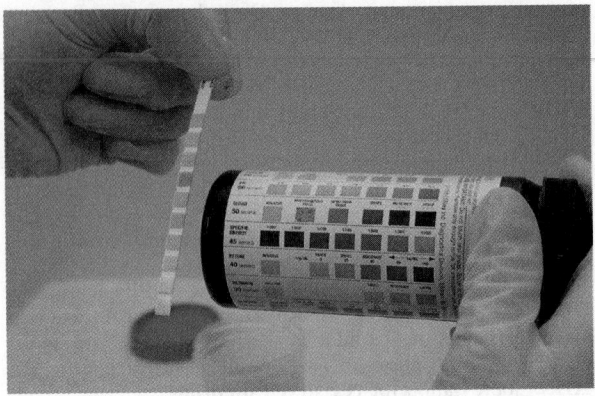

**Reagent strip** *(Zakus, 1995)*

**reagin** /rē′ājin/ [L, *re* + *agere*], **1.** an antibody associated with human atopy such as asthma and hay fever. It attaches to mast cells and basophils and sensitizes the skin and other tissues. In antigen-antibody reactions it triggers the release of histamine and other mediators that cause atopic symptoms. **2.** a nonspecific, nontreponemal antibody-like substance found in the serum of individuals with syphilis. It can combine with an antigen prepared as a lipid extract of normal tissue, a phenomenon that constitutes the basis of the serologic tests for syphilis. —**reaginic,** *adj.*

**reaginic antibody** /rē′əgin′ik/, an immunoglobulin E antibody that is more numerous in hypersensitive individuals. See also **reagin, reagin-mediated disorder.**

**reagin-mediated disorder,** a hypersensitivity reaction, such as hay fever or an allergic response to an insect sting, produced by reaginic (immunoglobulins E, or IgE) antibodies and causing degranulation and the release of histamine, bradykinin, serotonin, and other vasoactive amines. An initial sensitizing dose of the antigen induces the formation of specific IgE antibodies, and their attachment to mast cells and basophils results in hypersensitivity to a subsequent challenging dose of the antigen. Reactions range from a simple wheal and flare on the skin to life-threatening anaphylactic shock, depending on the size and route of entrance of the sensitizing dose and the challenging dose, the number and distribution of IgE antibodies, the responsiveness of the host, the timing of exposure to the allergen, and the tissues in which the antigen-antibody reaction occurs. The abundance of mast cells in the skin, nose, and lungs makes these areas susceptible to IgE-mediated reactions. Allergens that commonly cause these reactions include plant spores, pollens, animal danders, stings, serum proteins, foods, and certain drugs. See also **allergy, anaphylactic shock, hay fever.**

**reality** /rē·al′itē/ [L, *res*, factual], the culturally constructed world of perception, meaning, and behavior that members of a culture regard as an absolute.

**reality orientation**[1], a formal activity that uses specific approaches to assist confused or disoriented persons toward an awareness of reality, or the 'here and now' as by emphasizing, for example, the time, day, month, year, situation, and weather.

**reality orientation²,** a nursing intervention from the Nursing Interventions Classification (NIC) defined as promotion of patient's awareness of personal identity, time, and environment. See also **Nursing Interventions Classification.**

**reality principle,** an awareness of the demands of the environment and the need for an adjustment of behavior to meet those demands, expressed primarily by the renunciation of immediate gratification of instinctual pleasures to obtain long-term and future goals. In psychoanalysis this function is held to be performed by the ego. Compare **pleasure principle.**

**reality testing,** an ego function that enables one to differentiate between external reality and any inner imaginative world and to behave in a manner that exhibits an awareness of accepted norms and customs. Impairment of reality testing is indicative of a disturbance in ego functioning that may lead to psychosis.

**reality therapy,** a form of psychotherapy developed by William Glassner. The aims are to help define and assess basic values within the framework of a current situation and to evaluate the person's present behavior and future plans in relation to those values. The emphasis in treatment is on the present rather than the past and on behavior rather than feelings; it focuses on responsible behavior as a means of personal fulfillment.

**real time** [L, *res,* factual; AS, *tid,* tide], an application of computerized equipment that allows data to be processed with relation to ongoing external events, so that the operators can make immediate diagnostic or other decisions based on the current data output. Ultrasound scanning uses real time control systems, making results available almost simultaneously with the generation of the input data.

**real-time imaging.** See **dynamic imaging.**

**real-time scanning,** the imaging of an entire object, or a cross-sectional slice of the object, at a single moment. To produce such an image, the data must be recorded quickly over a very short time rather than by accumulation over a longer period.

**reamer** [AS, *ryman,* to make room], **1.** a tool with a straight or spiral cutting edge, used in a rotating motion to enlarge a hole or clear an opening. **2.** (in dentistry) an instrument with a tapered and loosely spiraled metal shaft, used for enlarging and cleaning root canals.

**reapproximate** /rē'əprok'simāt/ [L, *re,* again, *approximare,* to come near], to rejoin tissues separated by surgery or trauma so that their anatomic relationship is restored. —**reapproximation,** *n.*

**reasonable accommodation** /rē'zənəbəl/, an interpretation of the U.S. Americans With Disabilities Act regarding responsibility of an employer to provide an adequate work environment for a disabled but otherwise competent employee. The rule may apply in making facilities accessible, restructuring jobs, reassigning disabled employees to vacant positions, modifying work schedules, acquiring or modifying equipment, and adjusting training materials and examinations. The employer may not be required to provide reasonable accommodation if it can be shown to impose an "undue hardship" on the business operation.

**reasonable care** [L, *rationalis*], the degree of skill and knowledge used by a competent health practitioner in treating and caring for the sick and injured.

**reasonable charge, 1.** (in Medicare) the lowest customary charge by a physician for a service. **2.** the prevailing charge by a group of physicians in the area for a particular service.

**reasonable cost,** the amount a medical insurer will reimburse for a particular health service based on the cost to the provider for delivering that service.

**reasonable person,** (in law) a hypothetic person who possesses the qualities that are used as an objective standard on which to judge a defendant's action in a negligence suit. In such suits it must be decided whether or not a reasonable person, under the same circumstances, would have acted in the same way as the defendant.

**reasonably prudent person doctrine** /rē'zənəblē'/, a concept that a person of ordinary sense will use ordinary care and skill in meeting the health care needs of a patient.

**reattachment** /rē'ətach'mənt/ [L, *re,* again; OFr, *attachier*], **1.** the rejoining of accidentally severed body parts. **2.** the rejoining of periodontal membrane fibers to the cementum of a tooth and the alveolar bone to restore a loosened tooth.

**rebase** /rēbās'/ [L, *re,* again, *basis,* base], a process of refitting a denture by replacing or adding to its base material without changing the occlusal relationships of the teeth.

**rebirthing** /rēbur'thing/, a form of psychotherapy developed by Leonard Orr that focuses on the breath and breathing apparatus. Orr believes the premature severing of the umbilical cord deprives the newborn of oxygen and forces him or her to suddenly learn to breathe through fluid-filled lungs, resulting in panic and terror with every breath taken. The goal of treatment is to overcome the trauma of the birth-damaged breathing apparatus so the person is able to use the breath as a supportive and creative part of life.

**rebound** /rē'bound/ [Fr, *rebondir,* to bounce], **1.** recovery from illness. **2.** a sudden contraction of muscle after a period of relaxation, often seen in conditions in which inhibitory reflexes are lost.

**rebound congestion,** swelling and congestion of the nasal mucosa that follows the vasodilator effects of decongestant medications.

**rebound effect.** See **aftermovement.**

**rebound phenomenon** [OFr, *rebondir* + Gk, *phainomenon,* anything seen], a renewal of reflex activity after the stimulus that triggered the original action has been removed. It may be indicative of a lesion of the cerebellum.

**rebound tenderness,** a sign of inflammation of the peritoneum in which pain is elicited by the sudden release of the fingertips pressing on the abdomen. The area of pain may be diffuse or relatively sharply circumscribed. See also **appendicitis, peritonitis.**

**rebreathing** /rēbrē'thing/ [L, *re* + AS, *braeth,* breath], breathing in a closed system. Exhaled gas mixes with the gas in the system, and some of this mixture is then reinhaled. Rebreathing, which may result in progressively decreasing concentrations of oxygen and progressively increasing concentrations of carbon dioxide in the blood, can occur in poorly ventilated environments.

**rebreathing bag,** (in anesthesia) a flexible bag attached to a mask. It may function as a reservoir for anesthetic gases during surgery or for oxygen during resuscitation.

**recalcification** /rēkal'sifikā'shən/ [L, *re* + *calx,* lime, *facere,* to make], the restoration of lost calcium salts in the body needed for normal neuromuscular excitability, excitation-coupling contraction in cardiac and smooth muscle stimulus-secretion coupling, maintenance of tight junctions between cells, blood clotting, and compressional strength of bone.

**recannulate** /rēkan'yəlāt/ [L, *re* + *cannula,* small reed], to make a new opening through an organ or tissue, such as opening a passage through an occluded blood vessel.

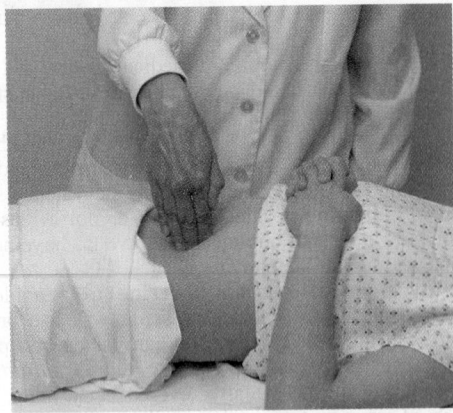

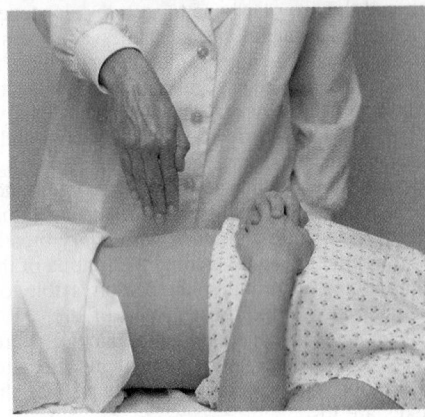

**Testing for rebound tenderness** *(Wilson and Giddens, 2001)*

**recapitulation concept** /rē'kəpit'yəlā'shən/ [L, *re + ca-pitulum,* small head], the notion, formulated by German naturalist Ernst Heinrich Haeckel (1834–1919), that an organism during the course of embryonic development passes through stages that resemble the structural form of species from which it evolved. It is summarized by the statement "ontogeny recapitulates phylogeny." The concept is now regarded as an oversimplification. Also called **biogenetic law, Haeckel's law.**

**receiver** /risē'vər/ [L, *recipere,* to receive], **1.** (in communication theory) the person or persons to whom a message is sent. **2.** the part of a hearing aid that converts electric signals to acoustic signals.

**receiving sensitivity pattern** /risē'ving/, the spatial response of an ultrasound transducer as an echo detector. For a single-element transducer it is essentially the same as the transmitted beam. For transducer arrays it can be quite different from the transmitted beam.

**receptive aphasia** /risep'tiv/, a form of sensory aphasia marked by impaired comprehension of language. It is generally precipitated by organic impairment such as stroke. Also called **Wernicke's aphasia, Wernicke's encephalopathy.**

**receptor** /risep'tər/ [L, *recipere,* to receive], **1.** a chemical structure usually of protein/carbohydrate on the surface of a cell that combines with an antigen to produce a discrete immunologic component. **2.** a sensory nerve ending that responds to various kinds of stimulation. **3.** a specific cellular protein that must first bind a hormone before cellular re-

sponse can be elicited. The protein may be in the cytoplasm or in the cell membrane and has a special affinity for toxins, amboceptors.

**receptor site** [L, *recipere,* to receive, *situs*], a location on a cell surface where certain molecules, such as enzymes, neurotransmitters, or viruses, attach to interact with cellular components.

**receptor theory of drug action,** the concept that certain drugs produce their effects by acting specifically at a receptor site on a cell or within the cell or its membrane.

**recess** /rē'ses, rises'/ [L, *recedere,* to retreat], a small hollow cavity, such as the epitympanic recess in the tympanic cavity of the inner ear or the retrocecal recess extending as a small pocket behind the cecum.

**recessive** /rises'iv/ [L, *recedere*], pertaining to or describing a gene, the effect of which is masked or hidden if there is a dominant gene at the same locus. If both genes are recessive and produce the same trait, the trait is expressed in the individual.

**recessive allele,** the member of a pair of alleles that lacks the ability to express itself in the presence of a dominant allele at the same locus; it is expressed only in the homozygous state. Compare **dominant allele.** See also **autosomal-recessive inheritance.**

**recessive trait,** an inherited characteristic that is determined by a recessive allele.

**recidivism (recid)** /risid'iviz'əm/ [L, *recidivus,* falling back], a tendency by an ill person to relapse or return to a hospital.

**recipient** /risip'ē·ənt/ [L, *recipere,* to receive], the person who receives a blood transfusion, tissue graft, or organ.

**reciprocal beat,** /risip'rəkəl/ an atrial or ventricular complex on an electrocardiogram resulting from return of an impulse to its chamber of origin. Also called **echo beat.**

**reciprocal change,** a change detected electrocardiographically in a wall of the heart opposite the site of a myocardial infarction. In acute inferior wall infarction, reciprocal changes are considered a sign of more extensive myocardial damage.

**reciprocal force,** a force applied by an orthodontic anchorage in which the resistance of one or more teeth and their adnexa is used to move one or more opposing teeth and their adnexa.

**reciprocal gene.** See **complementary gene.**

**reciprocal inhibition,** the theory in behavior therapy that, if an anxiety-producing stimulus occurs simultaneously with a response that diminishes anxiety, the stimulus may cause less anxiety, as, for example, deep chest or abdominal breathing and relaxation of the deep muscles appear to diminish anxiety and pain in childbirth. See also **systemic desensitization.**

**reciprocal roentgens,** the reciprocal of the number of roentgens needed to produce a density of 1 on x-ray film. It is used to define the speed of the film.

**reciprocal translocation,** the mutual exchange of genetic material between two nonhomologous chromosomes. Also called **interchange.** Compare **balanced translocation, robertsonian translocation.**

**reciprocation** /risip'roka'shən/, the means by which one part of a removable partial denture framework is made to counter the effect created by another part of the framework.

**reciprocity** /res'ipros'itē/ [Fr, *réciprocité*], a mutual agreement to exchange privileges, dependence, or relationships. An example is an agreement between two governing bodies to accept the medical credentials of physicians licensed in either community.

**Recklinghausen's canal** /rek'linghou'sənz/ [Friedrich D.

von Recklinghausen, German pathologist, 1833–1910], the small lymph space in the connective tissues of the body.

**Recklinghausen's disease.** See **neurofibromatosis.**

**Recklinghausen's tumor** [Friedrich D. von Recklinghausen], a benign tumor, derived from smooth muscle containing connective tissue and epithelial elements. The tumor that occurs in the wall of the oviduct or posterior uterine wall. Also called **adenomyosis of the uterus.**

**reclining** /riklī′ning/, leaning backward. —**recline,** v.

**recluse spider.** See **brown recluse spider.**

**recognition site** /rek′əgnish′ən/, a location on a nucleic acid or protein to which a specific ligand binds.

**Recognized Continuing Education Evaluation Mechanism (RCEEM),** a control process for checking that educational activities meet certain standards and establishing programs for evaluating educational opportunities and activities.

**recombinant** /rēkom′binənt/ [L, *re,* again, *combinare,* to combine], **1.** a molecule, a cell, or an organism that results from the recombination of genes, regardless of whether naturally or artificially induced. **2.** pertaining to such a molecule, a cell, or an organism. See also **recombinant DNA.**

**recombinant blood factor VIII.** See **FVIII.**

**recombinant DNA,** a DNA molecule in which rearrangement of the genes has been experimentally induced. Enzymes are used to break isolated DNA molecules into fragments that are then rearranged in the desired sequence. DNA sequences from another organism of the same or a different species may also be introduced into the molecule, which is then replicated, resulting in both genotypic and phenotypic alterations in the organism that carries the recombinant DNA. See also **genetic engineering.**

**recombinant Lyme test,** a method of identifying infection by *Borrelia burgdorferi,* the bacterium that causes Lyme disease. A protein (P-39) specific to the bacterium, produced through recombinant DNA techniques and cloning in other bacteria, is the key component in the test. It causes a strong reaction in blood cells from persons with a *B. burgdorferi* infection.

**recombinant tPA.** See **tissue plasminogen activator.**

**recombinant vaccine,** a suspension of attenuated viruses or killed microorganisms developed through recombinant DNA techniques.

**recombination** /rē′kombinā′shən/ [L, *re* + *combinare*], **1.** the formation of new arrangements of genes within the chromosomes as a result of independent assortment of unlinked genes, crossing over of linked genes, or intracistronic crossing over of nucleotides. See also **recombinant DNA. 2.** the coupling of oppositely charged ions liberated by ionizing radiation. Ionic recombination lowers the total number of charges collected by a dosimeter, thus causing the radiation dose to be underestimated. A technique for determining the magnitude of ionic recombination is routinely applied in accurate dosimetry.

**Recombivax HB,** trademark for a hepatitis B vaccine (recombinant).

**recommended dietary allowances (RDAs)** /rek′əmen′-did/ [L, *re* + *commendere,* to commend], levels of daily intake of essential nutrients judged by the Food and Nutrition Board of the National Research Council to be adequate to meet the known nutrient needs of practically all healthy people.

**recon** /rē′kon/ [L, *re* + *combinare* + Gk, *ion,* going], the smallest genetic unit that is capable of recombination, thought to be a triplet of nucleotides.

**reconstitution** /rē′konstit(y)ŌŌ′shən/ [L, *re* + *constituere,* to establish], the continuous repair of tissue damage.

**reconstruction time** /rē′kənstruk′shən/, the period between the end of a CT scan and the appearance of an image.

**record** /rek′ərd/, a written form of communication that permanently documents information relevant to the care of a patient.

**recorded detail,** /rikôr′did/, the sharpness of structural lines as recorded on a radiograph.

**Recovery** /rikuv′əry/, a self-help group that provides support for persons discharged from inpatient psychiatric hospitals.

**recovery room (RR, R.R.).** See **postanesthesia care unit.**

**recreational drug,** any substance with pharmacologic effects that is taken voluntarily for personal pleasure or satisfaction rather than for medicinal purposes. The term is generally applied to alcohol, barbiturates, amphetamines, THC, PCP, cocaine, and heroin but also includes caffeine in coffee and cola beverages.

**recreational therapy** /rē′krē·ā′shənəl/ [L, *recreare,* to renew], a form of adjunctive treatment in which games or other group activities are used as a means of modifying maladaptive behavior, awakening social interests, or improving the ability to interact and function in socially acceptable ways.

**recreation therapy,** a nursing intervention from the Nursing Interventions Classification (NIC) defined as purposeful use of recreation to promote relaxation and enhancement of social skills. See also **Nursing Interventions Classification.**

**recrudescence** /rē′krŌŌdes′əns/ [L, *re* + *crudescere,* to become hard], a return of symptoms of a disease during a period of recovery.

**recrudescent** /-ənt/ [L, *re* + *crudescere,* to become hard], the return of disease symptoms after a period of remission.

**recrudescent hepatitis,** a form of acute viral hepatitis marked by a relapse during the period of recovery. A minority of patients experience it, and the prognosis for ultimate recovery is rarely affected.

**recrudescent typhus.** See **Brill-Zinsser disease.**

**recruitment** /rikrŌŌt′mənt/, **1.** the perception of a rapid growth of loudness, commonly seen in sensorineural hearing losses that are cochlear in nature. The impaired ear cannot hear faint sounds but hears intense sounds as loudly as a normal ear. **2.** in muscle contractions, the ability to recruit additional motor units into action as the need to overcome resistance increases.

**rect-,** prefix meaning 'rectum': *rectal, rectalgia, rectorrhea.*

**recta, rectal.** See **rectum.**

**rectal abscess** /rek′təl/ [L, *rectus,* straight, *abscedere,* to go away], an abscess in the perianal area.

**rectal alimentation** [L, *rectus,* straight, *alimentum,* nourishment], the delivery of nourishment in concentrated form by injection or installation through the rectum. Also called **rectal feeding.**

**rectal anesthesia** [L, *rectus,* straight], general anesthesia achieved by the insertion, injection, or infusion of an anesthetic agent into the rectum; this procedure is sometimes used in children and other patients who may be uncooperative or unable to tolerate medications. Absorption is unpredictable.

**rectal cancer.** See **colorectal cancer.**

**rectal feeding.** See **rectal alimentation.**

**rectal instillation of medication,** the instillation of a medicated suppository, cream, or gel into the rectum. Some conditions treated by this method are constipation, pruritus ani, and hemorrhoids. The patient lies on the left side, with the lower leg extended and the upper leg flexed. The health care provider unwraps the suppository and, wearing a glove, raises the upper buttock, exposing the anus. The suppository may be self-lubricating, or it may need to be lubricated with a water-soluble lubricant. The suppository is then gently inserted past the anal sphincter. The health care provider then wipes the anus with a tissue or piece of toilet paper. Occasionally a drug may be given in a medicated enema. See also **enema.**

**rectal prolapse management,** a nursing intervention from the Nursing Interventions Classification (NIC) defined as prevention and/or manual reduction of rectal prolapse. See also **Nursing Interventions Classification.**

**rectal reflex,** the normal response (defecation) to the presence of an accumulation of feces in the rectum. Also called **defecation reflex.**

**rectal temperature** [L, *rectus*, straight, *temperatura*], body temperature as measured by a clinical thermometer placed in the rectum. Rectal temperatures average 0.5 to 0.75° F (0.3 to 0.4° C) higher than oral temperatures.

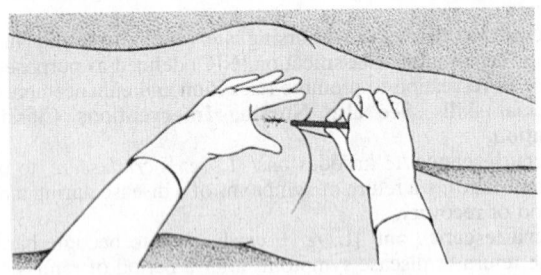

**Placement of the thermometer for rectal temperature assessment**
*(Potter and Perry, 1997)*

**rectal thermometer** [L, *rectus* + Gk, *thermē*, heat, *metron*, measure], a clinical thermometer suitable for measuring body temperature in the rectum.

**rectification** /rek′tifikā′shən/, **1.** the conversion of alternating current into pulsating direct current. **2.** a step in echo signal processing in a pulse-echo ultrasound instrument in which radiofrequency signals, which oscillate both above and below zero volts, are converted.

**rectifier** /rek′tifī′ər/, an electrical device that converts alternating current (AC) into pulsating direct current (DC). Rectifiers are used to power x-ray tubes, which require a DC electrical source.

**rectilinear scanner** /rek′tilin′ē·ər/, a device that generates an image of an anatomic structure by detecting radioactivity within the structure.

**rectitis.** See **proctitis.**

**recto-** /rek′tō-, rek′tə-/, prefix meaning 'straight or rectum': *rectoscope, rectosigmoidoscopy.*

**rectocele** /rek′təsēl′/ [L, *rectus* + Gk, *koilos*, hollow], a protrusion of the rectum and posterior wall of the vagina into the vagina. The condition, which occurs after the muscles of the vagina and pelvic floor have been weakened by childbearing, old age, or surgery, may reflect a congenital weakness in the wall and may, if severe, result in dyspareunia and difficulty in evacuating the bowel. Also called **proctocele.** Compare **cystocele.**

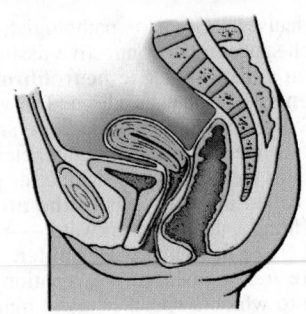

**Rectocele** *(Monahan and Neighbors, 1998)*

**rectocolitis.** See **coloproctitis.**

**rectoplasty.** See **proctoplasty.**

**rectoscope.** See **proctoscope.**

**rectosigmoid** /-sig′moid/ [L, *rectus* + Gk, *sigma*, the letter S, *eidos*, form], pertaining to the part of the large intestine that includes the lower part of the sigmoid and the upper part of the rectum.

**rectosigmoidoscopy** /-sig′moidəs′kəpē/ [L, *rectus*, straight; Gk, *sigma*, the letter S, *eidos*, form, *skopein*, to view], the examination of the rectum and pelvic colon with a sigmoidoscope.

**rectouterine excavation, rectouterine pouch.** See **cul-de-sac of Douglas.**

**rectovaginal fistula** /-vaj′ənəl/ [L, *rectus*, straight, *vagina*, sheath, *fistula*, pipe], an abnormal passage or opening between the rectum and the vagina.

**rectovaginal ligament,** one of the four main uterine support ligaments. It helps hold the uterus in position by maintaining traction on the cervix. Also called **posterior ligament.**

**rectovaginal septum,** a band of loose connective tissue between the vagina and the ampulla of the rectum.

**rectovesical** /-ves′ikəl/ [L, *rectus*, straight, *vesica*, bladder], pertaining to the rectum and bladder.

**rectum** /rek′təm/, *pl.* **rectums, recta** [L, *rectus*], the lower part of the large intestine, about 12 cm long, continuous with the descending sigmoid colon, proximal to the anal canal. It follows the sacrococcygeal curve, ends in the anal canal, and usually contains three transverse semilunar folds: one situated proximally on the right side, a second one ex-

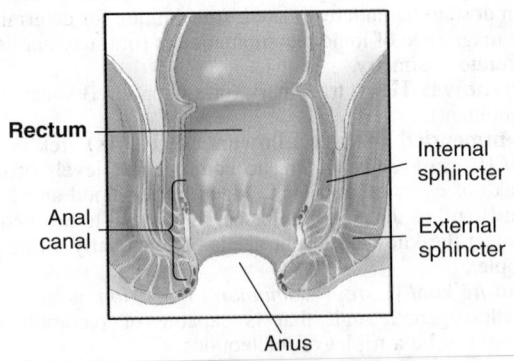

**Rectum** *(Leonard, 2001)*

tending inward from the left side, and the third and largest fold projecting caudally. Each fold is about 12 mm wide. The folds overlap when the intestine is empty or defecation occurs. —**rectal**, *adj.*

**rectus abdominis** /rek'təs/, one of a pair of anterolateral muscles of the abdomen, extending the whole length of the ventral aspect of the abdomen. The pair is separated by the linea alba. Each rectus arises in a lateral tendon from the crest of the pubis and is interlaced by a medial tendon with that of the opposite side. The rectus abdominis inserts into the fifth, sixth, and seventh ribs. It functions to flex the vertebral column, tense the anterior abdominal wall, and assist in compressing the abdominal contents. Compare **obliquus externus abdominis, obliquus internus abdominis, pyramidalis, transversus abdominis.**

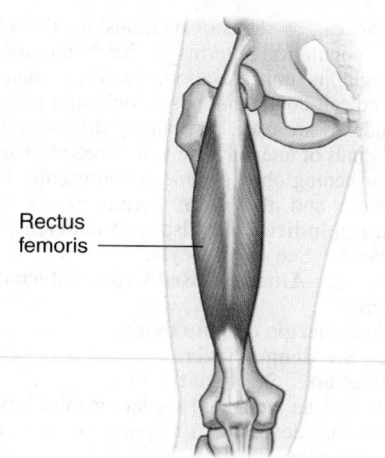

Rectus femoris

**Rectus femoris**

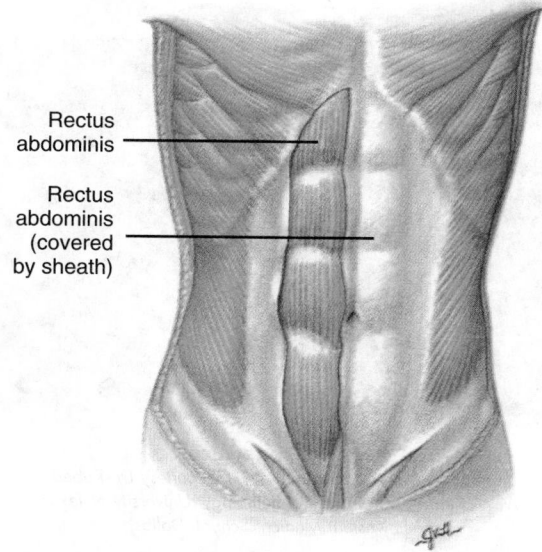

Rectus abdominis

Rectus abdominis (covered by sheath)

**Rectus abdominis muscles**
*(Thibodeau and Patton, 1999/John V. Hagen)*

**rectus capitis anterior, rectus capitis lateralis.** See **rectus muscle.**

**rectus femoris,** a fusiform muscle of the anterior thigh, one of the four parts of the quadriceps femoris. With the quadriceps group it functions to extend the lower leg. Compare **vastus intermedius, vastus lateralis, vastus medialis.** See also **quadriceps femoris.**

**rectus muscle** [L, straight, *musculus*], a muscle of the body that has a relatively straight form. Some rectus muscles are **rectus capitis anterior** and **rectus capitis lateralis.** See also **rectus abdominis.**

**recumbency** /rikum'bənsē/ [L, *recumbere*, to lie down], the state of lying down or leaning against something.

**recumbent** /rikum'bənt/ [L, *recumbere*, to lie down], lying down or leaning backward. See also **reclining.** —**recumbency,** *n.*

**recuperate** /rikōō'pərāt/ [L, *recupare*, to regain], to recover one's health and strength.

**recuperation** /rikōō'pərā'shən/ [L, *recupare*, to regain], the process of recovering health and strength.

**recurrence** /rikur'əns/ [L, *recurrere*, to run back], the reappearance of a sign or symptom of a disease after a period of remission.

**recurrence risk,** the chance that a disease found in one member of a proband will appear in other members of the same pedigree.

**recurrent** /rikur'ənt/ [L, *recurrere*, to run back], a disease sign or symptom that returns periodically.

**recurrent bandage** [L, *recurrere*, to run back], a strip of cloth that is wrapped several times around itself, usually applied to the head or amputated limb.

**recurrent fever.** See **relapsing fever.**

**recurrent inhibition.** See **Renshaw cells.**

**recurrent polyserositis.** See **familial Mediterranean fever.**

**recurrent respiratory papillomatosis,** the recurrent growth of benign squamous cell papillomas in the larynx and trachea, caused by the human papillomavirus, and leading to severe narrowing of the airway that may require frequent treatments; onset is in childhood or early adulthood.

**recurring scarring aphthae.** See **Sutton's disease.**

**recurvatum** /rē'kərvā'təm/ [L, *recurvare*, to bend back], backward thrust, or bending, for example, of the knee caused by weakness of the quadriceps or a joint disorder.

**red blindness.** See **protanopia.**

**red blood cell.** See **erythrocyte.**

**red blood cell count** [AS, *read* + *blod* + L, *cella*, storeroom; Fr, *conter*, to count], a count of the erythrocytes in a specimen of whole blood, commonly made with an electronic counting device. The normal concentrations of red blood cells in the whole blood of males are 4.6 to 6.2 million/mm$^3$; in females the concentrations are 4.2 to 5.4 million/mm$^3$.

**red blood cell (RBC) survival study,** a nuclear scan that is often performed on patients with hemolytic anemia. The test is carried out in two parts. The first determines the half-life of the RBC within the circulation, and the second images the spleen, liver, and pericardium.

***Red Book of the American Academy of Pediatrics***, a book published by the American Academy of Pediatrics, Inc., that serves as the standard reference source of immunization procedures for children and adults.

**red bug.** See **chigger.**

**red cell.** See **erythrocyte.**

**red cell indexes,** a series of relationships that characterize the red cell population in terms of size, hemoglobin content, and hemoglobin concentration. Derived mathematically from the red cell count and hemoglobin and hematocrit values, the indexes are useful in making differential diagnoses of several kinds of anemia. The values reported are the mean corpuscular hemoglobin, the mean corpuscular hemoglobin concentration, and the mean corpuscular volume. Also called **red cell indices.** See also **iron deficiency anemia.**

**red corpuscle.** See **erythrocyte.**

**Red Cross.** See **American Red Cross, International Red Cross Society.**

**redeye.** See **allergic conjunctivitis.**

**red fever.** See **dengue fever.**

**red hepatization.** See **hepatization.**

**redia** /rē'dē·ə/, an elongated second or third larval stage of a trematode that develops in a sporocyst and matures into numerous cercariae.

**red infarct** [AS, *read* + L, *infarcire,* to stuff], a pathologic change that occurs in brain tissue that has been rendered ischemic by lack of blood. With restricted blood flow, diapedesis of red blood cells occurs into the parenchyma of the brain without actually producing a well-formed hematoma but only infiltration of erythrocytes.

**red marrow** [AS, *read* + AS, *mearh,* marrow], the red vascular substance consisting of connective tissue and blood vessels containing primitive blood cells, macrophages, megakaryocytes, and fat cells. It is found in the cavities of many bones, including flat and short bones, bodies of the vertebrae, sternum, ribs, and articulating ends of long bones. Red marrow manufactures and releases leukocytes, erythrocytes, and thrombocytes into the bloodstream. Compare **yellow marrow.**

**red mite.** See **chigger.**

**red neck syndrome,** an allergic reaction to a rapid infusion of the antimicrobial agent vancomycin. It is characterized by flushing, pruritus, and erythema of the head and upper body resulting from histamine release.

**redon** /rē'don/, the smallest unit of DNA capable of recombination; it may be as small as one base pair. Compare **cistron, muton.**

**redox,** an abbreviation for *reduction-oxidation* (reaction). See **oxidation-reduction reaction.**

**red tide.** See **Gonyaulax catanella, shellfish poisoning.**

**reduce** /rid(y)ōōs'/ [L, *reducere,* to lead back], **1.** (in surgery) the restoration of a part to its original position after displacement, as in the reduction of a fractured bone by bringing ends or fragments back into alignment or of a hernia by returning the bowel to its normal position. A fracture may be reduced under local or general anesthesia. If performed by external manipulation alone, the reduction is said to be closed; if surgery is necessary, it is said to be open. See also **fracture, hernia, invagination, traction. 2.** to decrease the amount, size, extent, or number of something, as of body weight.

**reducible hernia** /rid(y)ōō'səbəl/ [L, *reducere,* to lead back, *hernia,* rupture], a hernia in which the protruding tissues can be manipulated into a normal position.

**reducing agent** /rid(y)ōō'sing/ [L, *reducere,* to lead back, *agere,* to do], a substance that donates electrons to another substance in a chemical reaction.

**reducing diet.** See **weight reduction diet.**

**reduction** /riduk'shən/ [L, *reducere*], **1.** also called **hydrogenation.** The addition of hydrogen to a substance. **2.** the removal of oxygen from a substance. **3.** the decrease in the valence of the electronegative part of a compound. **4.** the addition of one or more electrons to a molecule or atom of a substance. **5.** the correction of a fracture, hernia, or luxation. **6.** the reduction of data, as in converting interval data to an ordinal or nominal scale of measurement.

**reduction division.** See **meiosis.**

**reductionism** /riduk'shəniz'əm/, an approach that tries to explain a form of behavior or an event in terms of a specific category of phenomena, such as biologic, psychologic, or cultural, negating the possibility of an interrelation of causal phenomena.

**redux.** See **oxidation-reduction reaction.**

**Reed-Sternberg cell** [Dorothy M. Reed, American pathologist, 1874–1964; Karl Sternberg, Austrian pathologist, 1872–1935], one of a number of large, abnormal, multinucleated reticuloendothelial cells in the lymphatic system found in Hodgkin's disease. The number and proportion of Reed-Sternberg cells identified are the basis for the histopathologic classification of Hodgkin's disease.

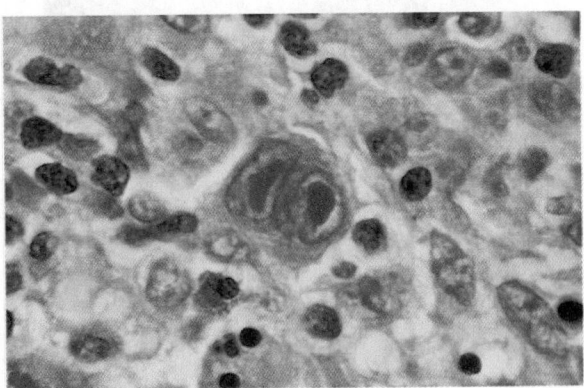

**Reed-Sternberg cell**
*(Kumar, Cotran, and Robbins, 1997/courtesy Dr. Robert W. McKenna, Department of Pathology, University of Texas Southwestern Medical School, Dallas)*

**reefer.** See **cannabis.**

**reentry** /rē·en'trē/ [L, *re,* again; Fr, *entrée*], (in cardiology) the reactivation of myocardial tissue for the second or subsequent time by the same impulse. Reentry is one of the most common arrhythmogenic mechanisms. For example, paroxysmal supraventricular tachycardia may be caused by sinus nodal reentry, atrioventricular (AV) nodal reentry, or AV reentry by way of the AV node and an accessory pathway; atrial flutter is caused by an atrial macroreentry circuit. Reentry also underlies some forms of ventricular tachycardia and extrasystoles. AV and AV nodal reentry mechanisms may be terminated by a vagal maneuver, adenosine, or procainamide.

**refereed journal** /ref'ərēd'/ [L, *referre,* to bring back, *diurnalis,* daily record], a professional or literary journal in which articles or papers are selected for publication by a panel of referees who are experts in the field. They read and evaluate each of the articles submitted for publication. The important national professional journals in medicine and nursing are refereed.

**reference electrode** /ref'ərəns/ [L, *referre,* to bring back; Gk, *elektron,* amber, *hodos,* way], an electrode that has an established potential and is used as a reference against which other potentials may be measured.

**reference group,**   a group with which a person identifies or wishes to belong.

**reference value,**   one of a battery of test results that are assumed to be typical for a population of asymptomatic persons. Each value is usually given as a range and should be interpreted according to age, sex, and race.

**referential idea.**   See **idea of reference.**

**referential index deletions** /ref′əren′shəl/,   a neurolinguistic programing term that pertains to the omission of the specific person being discussed.

**referral**[1] /rifur′əl/ [L, *referre*, to bring back],   a process whereby a patient or the patient's family is introduced to additional health resources in the community, as in helping a patient find an appropriate community health nurse after discharge from a hospital.

**referral**[2],   a nursing intervention from the Nursing Interventions Classification (NIC) defined as an arrangement for services by another care provider or agency. See also **Nursing Interventions Classification.**

**referred pain** /rifurd′/ [L, *referre* + *poena*, punishment],   pain felt at a site different from that of an injured or diseased organ or body part. Angina, the pain of coronary artery insufficiency, may be felt in the left shoulder, arm, or jaw. In gallbladder disease, pain may be felt in the right shoulder or scapular region.

Posterior

Anterior

Lungs and diaphragm
Heart
Liver
Gallbladder
Heart
Liver
Stomach
Liver
Ovaries
Appendix
Kidneys
Ureters
Kidney
Bladder

**Typical areas of referred pain**
*(Lewis, Heitkemper, and Dirksen, 2000)*

**referred sensation,**   a feeling or impression that occurs at a site other than where the stimulus is initiated. Also called **reflex sensation.** See also **sensation,** def. 1.

**refined birth rate** /rifīnd′/ [L, *re* + *finire*, to finish],   the ratio of total births to the total female population, considered during a period of 1 year. Compare **birth rate, crude birth rate, true birth rate.**

**refl,**   abbreviation for *reflexive.*

**reflecting** /riflek′ting/,   a communication technique in which the listener picks up the feeling or tone of the patient's

message and repeats it back to the patient. This often includes restatement of selected patient words. It encourages the patient to continue with clarifying comments.

**reflection** /riflek′shən/ [L, *reflectere*, to bend back],   **1.** a form of reentry in myocardial tissue in which, after encountering delay in one fiber, an impulse enters a parallel fiber and returns retrogradely to its source. **2.** the return or reentry of ultrasound waves where there is a discontinuity in the characteristic acoustic impedance along the propagation path. The intensity of the reflection is related to the difference in the characteristic acoustic impedance across the interface.

**reflective layer** /riflek′tiv/,   a thin layer of magnesium oxide or titanium oxide between the phosphor and the base of an intensifying screen used in radiography. Its function is to intercept and redirect isotropically emitted light from the phosphor to the x-ray film.

**reflex** /rē′fleks/ [L, *reflectere*, to bend back],   **1.** a backward or return flow of energy or of an image, as a reflection. **2.** a reflected action, particularly an involuntary action or movement.

**reflex action,**   the involuntary functioning or movement of any organ or body part in response to a particular stimulus. The function or action occurs immediately, without the involvement of the will or consciousness.

**reflex ankle clonus.**   See **ankle clonus.**

**reflex apnea,**   involuntary cessation of respiration caused by irritating, noxious vapors or gases.

**reflex arc** [L, *reflectere*, to bend back, *arcus*, bow],   a simple neurologic unit of a sensory neuron that carries a stimulus impulse to the spinal cord, where it connects with a motor neuron that carries the reflex impulse back to an appropriate muscle or gland.

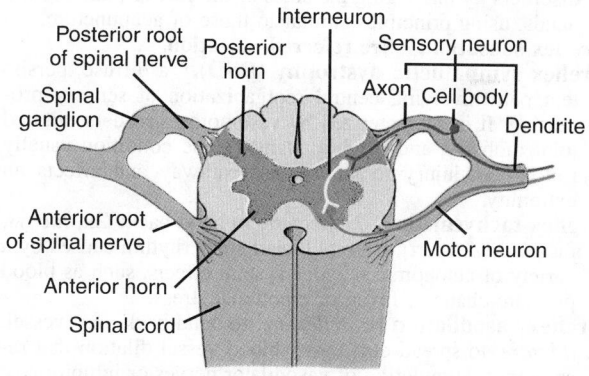

Posterior root of spinal nerve
Spinal ganglion
Anterior root of spinal nerve
Anterior horn
Spinal cord
Posterior horn
Interneuron
Sensory neuron
Axon   Cell body
Dendrite
Motor neuron

**Reflex arc** *(Chipps, Clanin, and Campbell, 1992)*

**reflex bladder.**   See **spastic bladder.**

**reflex center** [L, *reflectere*, to bend back; Gk, *kentron*],   any part of the nervous system in which reception of afferent impulses results in a discharge of efferent impulses leading to some change in a muscle or gland.

**reflex dyspepsia,**   an abnormal condition characterized by impaired digestion associated with the disease of an organ not directly involved with digestion. See also **dyspepsia.**

**reflex emesis** [L, *reflectere*, to bend back; Gk, *emesis*, vomiting],   vomiting or gagging that is induced by touching the mucous membrane of the throat or as a result of other noxious stimuli. Also called **gag reflex, vomiting reflex.**

**reflex hammer** [L, *reflectere*, to bend back; AS, *hamer*], a percussion mallet with a rubber head used to tap tendons, nerves, or muscles to elicit reflex reactions.

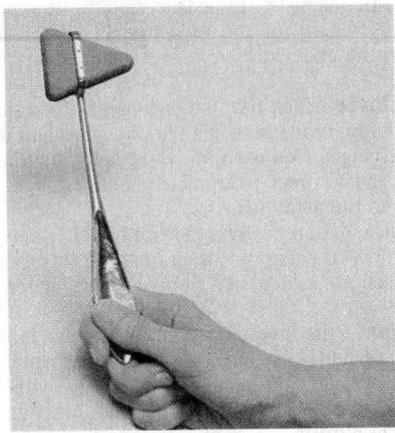

**Reflex hammer** *(Seidel et al, 1999)*

**reflex inhibiting pattern (RIP),** a conscious set of neuromuscular actions directed toward inhibition of a natural reflex. Examples include actions taken to suppress a sneeze and the learned inhibitions of toilet training.

**reflexology** /rē'fleksol'əjē/, a system of treating certain disorders by massaging the soles of the feet or palms of the hands, using principles similar to those of acupuncture.

**reflex sensation.** See **referred sensation.**

**reflex sympathetic dystrophy (RSD),** a diffuse, persistent pain involving central reorganization of sensory processing. It is characterized by vasomotor disorders, limited joint mobility, and trophic changes. The condition usually follows an injury to an afferent pathway and affects an extremity.

**reflex tachycardia** [L, *reflectere*, to bend back; Gk, *tachys*, fast, *kardia*, heart], a rapid heart sinus rhythm caused by a variety of autonomic nervous system effects, such as blood pressure changes, fever, or emotional stress.

**reflex vasodilation** [L, *reflectere*, to bend back, *vas*, vessel, *dilatare*, to spread out], any blood vessel dilation that results from stimulation of vasodilator nerves or inhibition of vasoconstrictors of the sympathetic nervous system, including epinephrine-type drugs.

**reflux** /rē'fluks/ [L, *refluere*, to flow back], an abnormal backward or return flow of a fluid. Kinds of reflux include **gastroesophageal reflux, hepatojugular reflux,** and **vesicoureteral reflux.**

**reflux esophagitis,** esophageal irritation and inflammation that result from reflux of the stomach contents into the esophagus. See also **gastroesophageal reflux.**

**reflux laryngitis,** a burning sensation in the hypopharynx and larynx caused by nocturnal gastric reflux. It occurs most commonly in older patients who sleep in the recumbent position.

**refracting angle.** See **angle of refraction.**

**refracting medium.** See **medium.**

**refraction** /rifrak'shən/ [L, *refringere*, to break apart], **1.** the change of direction of energy as it passes from one medium to another of different density. **2.** an examination to determine and correct refractive errors of the eye. **3.** (in ultrasonography) the phenomenon of bending wave fronts as the acoustic energy propagates from the medium of one acoustic velocity to a second medium of differing acoustic velocity.

**refraction of eye** [L, *refringere*, to break apart; AS, *eage*], the deflection of light from a straight path through the eye by various ocular tissues, including the cornea, lens, aqueous humor, and vitreous body.

**refractive error** /rifrak'tiv/, a defect in the ability of the lens of the eye to focus an image accurately, as occurs in nearsightedness and farsightedness.

**refractive index,** a numeric expression of the refractive power of a medium, as compared with that of air, which has a refractive index value of 1. The refractive index is related to the number, charge, and mass of vibrating particles in the material through which light is passing and may be used as a measure of the total solids in a solution.

**refractive keratotomy (RK),** a surgical procedure in which a varying number of radial or perpendicular incisions are made to flatten the cornea, resulting in the elimination or reduction of myopia or astigmatism. Incisions are made partially through the cornea sparing the central cornea. This type of refractive surgery has been largely replaced by newer methods. See also **radial keratotomy.**

**refractometer** /rē'frəktom'ətər/ [L, *refringere*, to break apart; Gk, *metron*, measure], an instrument for measuring the refractive index of a substance and used primarily for measuring the refractivity of solutions. See also **refractive index.**

**refractoriness** /rifrak'tôrines'/, the property of excitable tissue that determines how closely together two action potentials can occur.

**refractory** /rifrak'tərē/ [L, *refringere*], pertaining to a disorder that is resistant to treatment.

**refractory medium.** See **medium.**

**refractory period,** the time from phase 0 to the end of phase 3 of the action potential, divided into effective and relative. In pacing terminology, the period during which a pulse generator is unresponsive to an input signal of specified amplitude. The effective refractory period is from phase 0 to approximately −60 mV during phase 3 of the action potential, a time during which it is impossible for the myocardium to respond with a propagated action potential, or even to a strong stimulus. The **relative refractory period** is from approximately −60 mV during phase 3 to the end of phase 3 of the action potential, the time during which a depressed response is possible to a strong stimulus. Also called **refractory state, refractory phase.**

**reframing** /rē'frā'ming/, changing the conceptual and/or emotional viewpoint in relation to which a situation is experienced and placing it in a different frame that fits the "facts" of a concrete situation equally well, thereby changing its entire meaning.

**Refsum's syndrome** /ref'sŏŏmz/ [Sigvald Refsum, Norwegian physician, b. 1907], a rare hereditary disorder of lipid metabolism in which phytanic acid cannot be broken down. It is characterized by ataxia, abnormalities of the bones and skin, peripheral neuropathy, and retinitis pigmentosa. Foods containing phytanic acid must be avoided to prevent progressive deterioration. Also called **phytanic acid storage disease.**

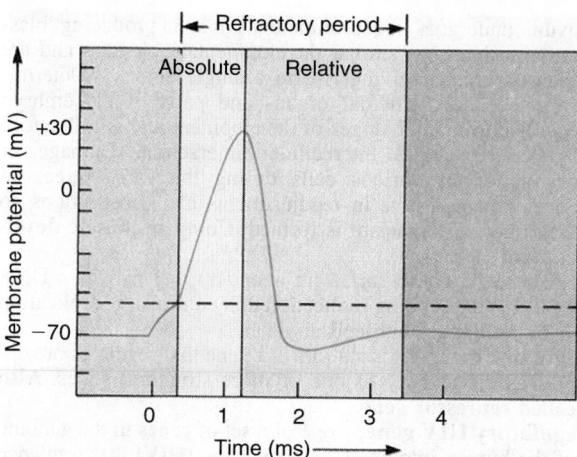

**Refractory period** *(Thibodeau and Patton, 1999/Rolin Graphics)*

**refusal of treatment,** the right of a patient to refuse treatment after the physician has informed the patient of the diagnosis, prognosis, available alternative interventions, risks and benefits of those options, and risk and probable outcome of no intervention.

**regeneration** /rijen'ərā'shən/, the process of repair, reproduction, or replacement of lost or injured cells, tissues, or organs. Also called **neogenesis.**

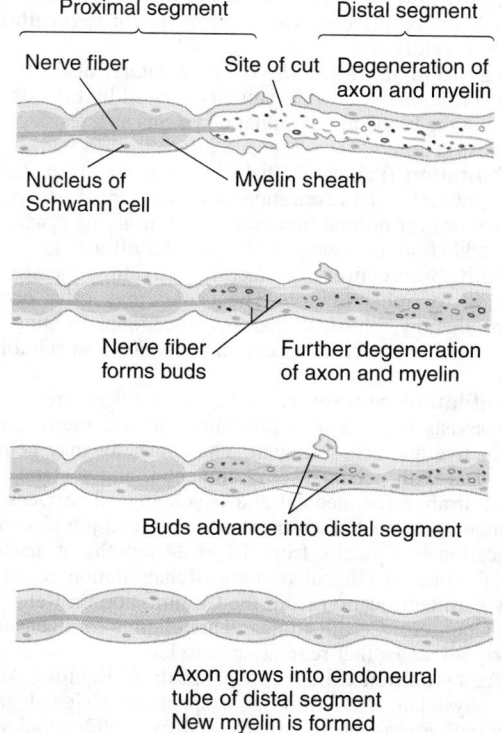

**Regeneration of a nerve** *(Beare and Myers, 1998)*

**regimen** /rej'imən/ [L, guidance], a strictly regulated therapeutic program such as a diet or exercise schedule.

**regional** /rē'jənəl/ [L, *regio,* territory], pertaining to a geographic area, such as a regional medical facility, or to a part of the body, such as regional anesthesia.

**regional anatomy,** the study of the structural relationships among the organs and the parts of the body. Kinds of regional anatomy are **surface anatomy** and **cross-sectional anatomy.**

**regional anesthesia,** anesthesia provided by injecting a local anesthetic to block a group of sensory nerve fibers. The tissues are anesthetized layer by layer, as the surgeon approaches the deeper structures of the body. Regional anesthesia has largely replaced local anesthesia for major procedures. Kinds of regional anesthesia include **brachial plexus anesthesia, caudal anesthesia, epidural anesthesia, intercostal anesthesia, paracervical block, pudendal block,** and **spinal anesthesia.** Compare **general anesthesia, local anesthesia, topical anesthesia.** See also **anesthesia.**

**regional control,** the control of cancer in sites that represent the first stages of spread from the local origin.

**regional enteritis.** See **Crohn's disease.**

**regional hyperthermia,** the elevation of temperature over an extended volume of tissue.

**regionalization** /rē'jənal'īzā'shən/, (in health care planning) the organization of a system for the delivery of health care within a region to avoid costly duplication of services and to ensure availability of essential services.

**regional medical program (RMP),** a program of community health planning that includes all the medical resources available in a region that may be mobilized to meet a specific medical objective. The RMP was authorized by the Health, Disease, Cancer and Stroke Amendments passed by the U.S. Congress in 1965. See also **regionalization.**

**region of interest (ROI),** an area on a digital image that circumscribes a desired anatomic location. Image processing systems permit drawing of ROIs on images. The average parametric value is computed for all pixels within the ROI and returned to the operator.

**region of recombination,** the first stage of amplitude of an electric signal in a gas-filled radiation detector, when the voltage is very low. No electrons are attracted to the central electrode, and ion pairs produced in the chamber will recombine.

**register** /rej'istər/ [L, *regerere,* to bring back], (in computed tomography) a device in the central processing unit that stores information for future use.

**registered dietitian (RD)** /rej'istərd/, a professional trained in foods and the management of diets (dietetics) who is credentialed by the Commission on Dietetic Registration of the American Dietetic Association. Credentialing is based on completion of a BS degree from an approved dietetic intensive or coordinated program and passing a registration examination.

**registered nurse (RN)** **1.** *(U.S.)* a nurse who has completed a course of study at a state approved school of nursing and passed the National Council Licensure Examination (NCLEX-RN). A registered nurse may use the initials RN after the signature. RNs are licensed to practice by individual states. **2.** *(Canada.)* a nurse who has completed a course of study at an approved school of nursing and who has taken and passed an examination administered by the Canadian Nurses Association Testing Service, called the Comprehensive Examination for Nurse Registration Licensure. See also **nurse, nursing.**

**registered record administrator (RRA),** a medical record administrator who has successfully completed the credentialing examination conducted by the American Medical Record Association.

**registered respiratory therapist (RRT),** an allied health professional who has successfully completed the written registry and clinical simulation examination of the National Board for Respiratory Care and who specializes in scientific knowledge and theory of clinical problems of respiratory care. Usually a 2- or 4-year college affiliation leading to an associate or bachelor's degree is required. Duties include the collection and evaluation of patient data to determine an appropriate care plan, selection and assembly of equipment, conduction of therapeutic procedures and modification of prescribed plans to achieve one or more specific objectives.

**registered technologist (RT),** a medical professional who is certified by the American Registry of Radiologic Technologists or equivalent certifying agency in one or more of the following disciplines: radiography, nuclear medicine, radiation therapy, mammography, computed tomography, magnetic resonance imaging, cardiovascular interventional technology, or quality management. See also **radiologic technologist.**

**registrar** /rej'isträr/, an administrative officer whose responsibility is to maintain the records of an institution.

**registration** /rej'istrā'shən/ [L, registratio], **1.** a learning or memory recording made in the central nervous system of an impression resulting from a stimulus. **2.** the recording of vital personal information such as health data. **3.** the recording of professional qualification information relevant to government licensing regulations.

**registry** /rej'istrē/ [L, regerere, to bring back], **1.** an office or agency in which lists of nurses and records pertaining to nurses seeking employment are maintained. **2.** (in epidemiology) a listing service for incidence data pertaining to the occurrence of specific diseases or disorders, such as a tumor registry.

**Regitine,** trademark for an alpha-adrenergic blocking agent (phentolamine hydrochloride).

**Regonol,** trademark for an anticholinesterase drug inaccurate (pyridostigmine), used as an adjunct to anesthesia.

**regression** /rigresh'ən/ [L, regredi, to go back], **1.** a retreat or backward movement in conditions, signs, or symptoms. **2.** a return to an earlier, more primitive form of behavior. **3.** a tendency in physical development to become more typical of the population than of the parents, such as a child who attains a height closer to the average than that of tall or short parents. **—regress,** v.

**Regroton,** trademark for a cardiovascular, fixed-combination drug containing a diuretic (chlorthalidone) and an antihypertensive (reserpine).

**regular diet** /reg'yələr/ [L, regula, rule], a full, well-balanced diet containing all of the essential nutrients needed for optimal growth, tissue repair, and normal functioning of the organs. Such a diet contains foods rich in proteins, carbohydrates, high-quality fats, minerals, and vitamins in proportions that meet the specific caloric requirements of the individual. Also called **full diet, normal diet.**

**regular insulin,** a fast-acting insulin prescribed in the treatment of diabetes mellitus when the desired action is prompt, intense, and short-acting. Regular insulin prepared from zinc insulin crystals is slightly longer-acting than the amorphous noncrystalline form of this type of insulin preparation.

**regulative cleavage.** See **indeterminate cleavage.**

**regulative development** /reg'yələ'tiv/ [L, regula, rule], a type of embryonic development in which the fertilized ovum undergoes indeterminate cleavage, producing blastomeres that have similar developmental potencies and are each capable of giving rise to a single embryo. Determination of the particular organs and parts of the embryo occurs during later stages of development and is influenced by inductors and intercellular interaction. Damage or destruction of various cells during the early stages of development results in readjustments and substitutions so that a normal organism is formed. Compare **mosaic development.**

**regulator** /reg'yəlā'tər/, (in genetics) that part of a DNA molecule undergoing replication that controls the replication and coordinates with cell division.

**regulator gene** /reg'yəlā'tər/, a gene that regulates or suppresses the activity of one or more structural genes. Also called **repressor gene.**

**regulatory HIV gene,** one of a set of genes in the genome of the human immunodeficiency virus (HIV) that influence the expression of other HIV genes. One regulatory gene (tat) stimulates expression, a second (nef) may inhibit expression, and a third (rev) provides feedback to the others.

**regulatory sequence** /reg'yəlatôr'ē/ [L, regula + sequi, to follow], a series of DNA nucleotides that regulate the expression of a gene.

**regurgitant menstruation.** See **retrograde menstruation.**

**regurgitant murmur** /rigur'jitənt/ [L, re + gurgitare, to flow back, murmur, humming], a heart murmur caused by the backflow of blood through the partly closed cusps of a defective valve. Kinds of regurgitant murmurs include **diastolic** and **systolic murmurs.**

**regurgitation** /rēgur'jitā'shən/ [L, re, again, gurgitare, to flow back], **1.** the backward flow from the normal direction, as the return of swallowed food into the mouth. **2.** the backward flow of blood through a defective heart valve, named for the affected valve, as in **aortic regurgitation.** See also **reflux.**

**regurgitation jaundice** [L, re + gurgitare, again to flow back; Fr, jaune, yellow], jaundice caused by bile pigment entering the blood and lymphatic systems as a result of biliary obstruction.

**rehabilitation (rehab)** /rē'habil'itā'shən/ [L, re + habitalas, aptitude], the restoration of an individual or a part to normal or near normal function after a disabling disease, injury, addiction, or incarceration. **—rehabilitate,** v.

**rehabilitation center,** a facility providing therapy and training for rehabilitation. The center may offer occupational therapy, physical therapy, vocational training, and special training such as speech therapy. See also **rehabilitation.**

**rehabilitation counselor,** a human services professional who assists persons with disabilities to become or remain productive and self-sufficient. The counselor may help clients deal with personal, environmental, and societal problems; arrange for medical and psychological services; and arrange vocational assessment, training, and job placement. Education is typically from 18 to 24 months of academic and field-based clinical training. Rehabilitation counselors may earn certification from the Commission on Rehabilitation Counselor Certification and are eligible for licensure by nearly all states that regulate counselors.

**Rehfuss stomach tube** /rā'fəs/ [Martin E. Rehfuss, American physician, 1887–1964], a specially designed gastric tube with a graduated syringe, used for withdrawing specimens of the contents of the stomach for study after a test meal.

**rehydration** /rē'hīdrā'shən/ [L, re + Gk, hydor, water],

restoration of normal water balance in a patient by giving fluids orally or intravenously.

**Reid's base line** [Robert W. Reid, Scottish anatomist, 1851–1939], the base line of the skull, a hypothetic line extending from the inferior orbital ridge to the center of the aperture of the external auditory meatus. Also called **anthropologic base line, Frankfurt line.**

**Reifenstein's syndrome** /rī′fənstīnz/ [Edward C. Reifenstein, Jr., American physician, 1908–1975], male hypogonadism of unknown origin, marked by azoospermia, undescended testes, gynecomastia, testosterone deficiency, and elevated gonadotropin titers. The condition appears to be inherited as an X-linked recessive trait, but no chromosomal abnormality has been identified.

**Reiki therapy** /rī′kē/, a complementary therapy in which a trained practitioner places his or her hands on or above a specific body area and transfers what is called "universal life energy" to the patient. That energy, it is claimed, provides "strength, harmony, and balance" necessary to treat health disturbances. The therapy, derived from an ancient Buddhist practice, involves a total of 15 hand positions covering all the body systems.

**reimbursement** /rē′imburs′mənt/ [L, *re* + *im*, in; Fr, *bourse,* purse], a method of payment, usually by a third-party payer, for medical treatment or hospital costs.

**reimplantation** /rē′im·plan·tā′shən/, the planting back of tissue or a structure, such as a tooth, in the site from which it was previously lost or removed.

**reinfection** /rē′infek′shən/, a second infection by the same microorganism, either after recovery or during the original infection.

**reinforcement** /rē′infôrs′mənt/ [L, *re* + Fr, *enforcir,* to strengthen], (in psychology) a process in which a response is strengthened by the fear of punishment or the anticipation of reward.

**reinforcement-extinction,** a process of socialization in which one learns to engage in certain behaviors (reinforcement) or to avoid certain behaviors (extinction). The anticipated result is that the reinforced behaviors become habitual and those that undergo extinction disappear.

**reinforcer** /rē′infôr′sər/, (in psychology) a consequence that increases the probability that an operant will recur.

**Reiter's syndrome** /rī′tərz/ [Hans Reiter, German physician, 1881–1969], an arthritic disorder predominantly of adult males, resulting from infection with *Shigella flexneri, Salmonella, Yersinia,* or *Chlamydia* or from enterocolitis. It most often affects the ankles, feet, and sacroiliac joints and is usually associated with conjunctivitis and urethritis. The onset may be marked by unexplained diarrhea and low-grade fever, followed in 2 to 4 weeks by conjunctivitis. Superficial ulcers may form lesions on the palms and the soles. Arthritis usually persists after the conjunctivitis and urethritis subside, but it may become episodic. Treatment includes a short course of tetracycline to treat the infection and phenylbutazone to relieve pain and inflammation in the joint. Sexual partners should also be tested. Recovery is expected, but recurrent arthritic symptoms may continue for several years. See also **dactylitis, reactive arthritis.**

**reject analysis** /rē′jekt/, the study of rejected radiographs to determine the cause for their being discarded.

**rejection** /rijek′shən/ [L, *re* + *jacere,* to throw], **1.** an immunologic attack against organisms or substances that the immune system recognizes as foreign, including grafts and transplants. **2.** the act of excluding or denying affection to another person.

**rejunctive** /rijungk′tiv/, (in contextual psychotherapy) pertaining to a relationship that is characterized by moves toward trustworthy relatedness.

**rejuvenation** /rējoo′vənā′shən/ [L, *re* + *juvenis,* youth], the restoration of youthful health and vitality.

**Rela,** trademark for a skeletal muscle relaxant (carisoprodol).

**relapse** /rilaps′/ [L, *relabi,* to slide back], **1.** to exhibit again the symptoms of a disease from which a patient appears to have recovered. **2.** the recurrence of a disease after apparent recovery.

**relapsing** [L, *relabi,* to slide back], pertaining to the return of disease after a period of apparent recovery.

**relapsing fever,** any one of several acute infectious diseases, marked by recurrent febrile episodes, caused by various strains of the spirochete *Borrelia.* The disease is transmitted by both lice and ticks and is often seen during wars and famines. It has occurred in several western states of the United States but is more commonly found in South America, Asia, and Africa. The first episode usually starts with a sudden high fever (104° to 105° F, or 40° to 40.56° C), accompanied by chills, headache, neuromuscular pains, and nausea. A rash may appear over the trunk and extremities, and jaundice is common during the later stages. Each attack lasts 2 or 3 days and culminates in a crisis of high fever, profuse sweating, and a rise in heart and respiratory rate. This is followed by an abrupt drop in temperature and a return to normal blood pressure. People typically relapse after 7 to 10 days of normal temperature and eventually recover completely. In louseborne disease there is usually only a single relapse; in tickborne disease several successively milder relapses may occur. Also called **African tick fever, famine fever, recurrent fever, spirillum fever, tick fever.**

**relapsing polychondritis,** a rare disease of unknown cause resulting in inflammation and destruction of cartilage with replacement by fibrous tissue. Autoimmunity may be involved in this condition. Most commonly the ears and noses of middle-aged people are affected with episodes of tender swelling, often accompanied by fever, arthralgias, and episcleritis. Consequences include floppy ears, collapsed nose, hearing loss, or hoarseness and airway obstruction because of laryngeal and tracheal cartilage involvement. Corticosteroids suppress the activity of the disease.

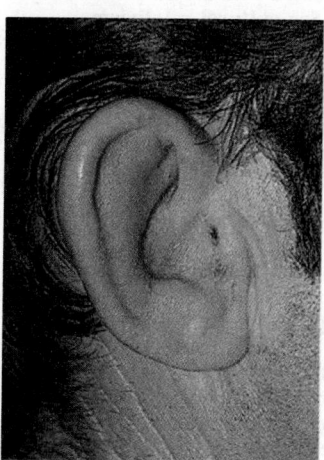

**Relapsing polychondritis** *(Lawrence and Cox, 1993)*

**relation searching** /rilā′shən/ [L, *relatio*], (in nursing research) a study design used to discover and describe relationships between and among variables. It may be used to describe various nursing situations to examine the efficacy of certain aspects of nursing care.

**relationship therapy** /rilā′shənship′/ [L, *relatio* + AS, *scieppan*, to shape], a therapy that is based on a totality of client-therapist relationship and encourages the growth of self in the client. It has been described as "an experience in living that takes place within a relationship with another person."

**relative.** See **periodontal pocket.**

**relative biologic effectiveness (RBE)** /rel′ətiv/ [L, *relatio*], a measure of the cell-killing ability of a particular radiation compared with that of 250 keV x-rays. The ratio of the number of cells killed with the test radiation over the number killed with the 250 keV radiation is the RBE.

**relative centrifugal force (RCF),** a method of comparing the force generated by various centrifuges based on the speeds of rotation and distances from the center of rotation.

**relative cephalopelvic disproportion.** See **cephalopelvic disproportion.**

**relative growth,** the comparison of the various increases in size of similar organisms, tissues, or structures at different time intervals.

**relative humidity,** the amount of moisture in the air compared with the maximum the air could contain at the same temperature.

**relative molecular mass.** See **molecular mass.**

**relative periodontal pocket.** See **periodontal pocket.**

**relative refractory period.** See **refractory period.**

**relative risk,** the ratio of the chance of a disease developing among members of a population exposed to a factor compared to a similar population not exposed to the factor. In many cases the relative risk is modified by the duration or intensity of exposure to the causative factors.

**relative sterility** [L, *relatio* + *sterilis,* barren], a condition of infertility in which one or more factors tend to reduce the chances of becoming pregnant. See also **sterility.**

**relative value unit (RVU),** a comparable service measure used by hospitals to permit comparison of the amounts of resources required to perform various services within a single department or between departments. It is determined by assigning weight to such factors as personnel time, level of skill, and sophistication of equipment required to render patient services. RVUs are a common method of physician bonus plans based partially on productivity.

**relativism.** See **cultural relativism.**

**relax** /rilaks′/ [L, *relaxare*, to ease], to reduce tension.

**relaxant** /rilak′sənt/ [L, *relaxare*, to ease], a drug or other agent that tends to reduce tension, as a muscle relaxant or bowel relaxant.

**relaxation** /rē′laksā′shən/ [L, *relaxare*, to ease], **1.** a reducing of tension, as when a muscle relaxes between contractions. **2.** (in magnetic resonance imaging) the return of excited nuclei to their normal unexcited state by the release of energy.

**relaxation oven,** a part of the xerographic plate conditioner system used to eliminate ghost images in mammograms. The plate is heated in the oven so that any residual electrostatic charge on the surface will be removed.

**relaxation response,** a protective mechanism against stress that brings about decreased heart rate, lower metabolism, and decreased respiratory rate. It is the physiologic opposite of the 'fight or flight,' or stress, response.

**relaxation therapy,** treatment in which patients are taught to perform breathing and relaxation exercises and to concentrate on a pleasant situation. An integral part of the Lamaze method of childbirth, relaxation therapy is also used to relieve various kinds of pain and physical manifestations of stress. Various yoga exercises and aspects of hypnotherapy may be included in the treatment program, and biofeedback techniques may be used to demonstrate actions that induce relaxation. Some patients learn through relaxation therapy to relax taut muscles at will, to abort migraine attacks, or to reduce their blood pressure. See also **Lamaze method.**

**relaxation time,** in magnetic resonance imaging, the characteristic time it takes for a sample of atoms, whose nuclei have first been aligned along a static magnetic field and then excited to a higher-energy state by a radiofrequency (rf) signal, to return to a lower-energy equilibrium state. Two time parameters are used to describe the return, or relaxation, to the equilibrium state once the rf signal is turned off. $T_1$ describes the relaxation of the system of spins into a condition of thermal equilibrium with its surroundings. $T_2$ describes the relaxation of the energy that is traded within the system itself. Maps of the values of $T_1$ or $T_2$ as a function of position in the cross-sectional view constitute magnetic resonance images.

**relaxin** /rilak′sin/, a hormone obtained from the corpora lutea of swine and used to relax the pelvic ligaments and dilate the cervix during labor. The medication has also been used to treat dysmenorrhea.

**release therapy** /rilēs′/ [ME, *relesen,* to release], a type of pediatric psychotherapy used to treat children with stress and anxiety related to a specific recent event.

**releasing hormone (RH),** one of several peptides produced by the hypothalamus and secreted directly into the anterior pituitary gland via a connecting vein. Each of the releasing hormones stimulates the pituitary to secrete a specific tropic hormone; thus corticotropic-releasing hormone stimulates the pituitary to secrete adrenocorticotropic hormone, whereas growth hormone–releasing hormone stimulates the secretion of growth hormone. Previously called **releasing factor.**

**releasing stimulus,** (in psychology) an action or behavior by one individual that serves as a cue to trigger a response in others. An example is yawning by one person, which results in yawning by others in the group.

**reliability** /rilī′əbil′itē/ [L, *religare,* to fasten behind], (in research) the extent to which a test measurement or device produces the same results with different investigators, observers, or administration of the test over time. If repeated use of the same measurement tool on the same sample produces the same consistent results, the measurement is considered reliable.

**relief area** [L, *relevare,* to lighten], the part of the tissue surface under a prosthesis on which pressure is reduced or eliminated.

**relieve** /rē·lēv′/ [L, *relevare,* to lighten], to mitigate or remove pain or distress.

**relieving factor** /rilē′ving/, an agent that alleviates a symptom.

**religiosity** /rilij′ē·os′itē/ [L, *religiosus*], a psychiatric symptom characterized by the demonstration of excessive or affected piety.

**religious addiction prevention,** a nursing intervention from the Nursing Interventions Classification (NIC) defined as prevention of a self-imposed controlling religious lifestyle. See also **Nursing Interventions Classification.**

**religious ritual enhancement,** a nursing intervention from the Nursing Interventions Classification (NIC) defined as facilitating participation in religious practices. See also **Nursing Interventions Classification.**

**-relin,** combining form for prehormones or hormone-release stimulating peptides.

**reline** /rēlīn'/ [L, *re* + *linea*], the resurfacing of the tissue side of a denture with new base material.

**-relix,** combining form for hormone-release inhibiting peptides.

**relocation stress syndrome,** a nursing diagnosis accepted by the Tenth National Conference on the Classification of Nursing Diagnoses (revised 2000). It is defined as the physiological and/or psychosocial disturbance following transfer from one environment to another.

■ DEFINING CHARACTERISTICS: Defining characteristics include temporary or permanent moves; voluntary or involuntary moves; aloneness, alienation, or loneliness; depression; anxiety; sleep disturbance; withdrawl; anger; loss of identity, self-worth, or self-esteem; increased verbalization of needs, unwillingness to move, or concern over relocation; increased physical symptoms or illness; dependency; insecurity; pessimism; frustration; worry; and fear.

■ RELATED FACTORS: Related factors include the unpredictability of experience; isolation from family or friends; past, concurrent, and recent losses; feelings of powerlessness; lack of adequate support system or group; lack of predeparture counseling; passive coping; impaired psychosocial health; language barrier; and decreased health status. See also **nursing diagnosis.**

**relocation stress syndrome, risk for,** a nursing diagnosis accepted by the Fourteenth National Conference on the classification of nursing diagnoses. The condition is defined as being at risk for physiological and/or psychosocial disturbance following transfer from one environment to another.

■ DEFINING CHARACTERISTICS: Defining characteristics include moderate to high degree of environmental change, temporary and/or permanent moves, voluntary or involuntary moves, the lack of an adequate support system or group, feelings of powerlessness, moderate mental competance, unpredictability of experiences, decreased psychosocial or physical health status, lack of predeparture counseling, passive coping, and past, current, or recent losses. See also **nursing diagnosis.**

**rem** /rem, är'ē'em'/, abbreviation for *roentgen equivalent man.* A dose of ionizing radiation that produces in humans the same effect as one roentgen of x-radiation or gamma radiation. See also **sievert.**

**REM** /rem, är'ē'em'/, abbreviation for **rapid eye movement.** See also **sleep.**

**remasking** /rēmas'king/, in digital fluoroscopy, the production of one or more additional mask images if the first is inadequate because of patient motion, noise, or other factors. See also **mask image.**

**remedial** /rimē'dē·əl/ [L, *remediare,* to cure], designed to improve or cure.

**remifentanil,** an opiate agonist analgesic.

■ INDICATIONS: This drug is used in combination with other drugs in general anesthesia and as a primary anesthetic in general surgery.

■ CONTRAINDICATIONS: Use of this drug is prohibited in people with hypersensitivity to remifentanil and in children less than 12 years of age.

■ ADVERSE EFFECTS: Life-threatening effects of this drug are asystole, respiratory depression, and apnea. Other adverse effects include drowsiness, confusion, sedation, euphoria, delirium, agitation, anxiety, anorexia, constipation, cramps, dry mouth, urinary retention, dysuria, rash, urticaria, bruising, flushing, diaphoresis, pruritus, tinnitus, blurred vision, miosis, diplopia, palpitations, change in blood pressure, facial flushing, syncope, and rigidity. Common side effects are dizziness, headache, nausea, vomiting, and bradycardia.

**reminiscence** /rem'inis'əns/ [L, *reminisci,* to remember], the recollection of past personal experiences and significant events.

**reminiscence therapy**[1], a psychotherapeutic technique in which self-esteem and personal satisfaction are restored, particularly in older persons, by encouraging patients to review past experiences of a pleasant nature. It is used in Alzheimer's disease when initially long-term memory stores are more intact than short-term and in other forms of dementia.

**reminiscence therapy**[2], a nursing intervention from the Nursing Interventions Classification (NIC) defined as using the recall of past events, feelings, and thoughts to facilitate pleasure, quality of life, or adaptation to present circumstances. See also **Nursing Interventions Classification.**

**remission** /rimish'ən/ [L, *remittere,* to abate], the partial or complete disappearance of the clinical and subjective characteristics of a chronic or malignant disease. Remission may be spontaneous or the result of therapy. In some cases remission is permanent, and the disease is cured. Compare **cure.**

**remittent fever** /rimit'ənt/ [L, *remittere* + *febris,* fever], diurnal variations of an elevated temperature with exacerbations and remissions but never a return to normal.

**remnant radiation** /rem'nənt/ [L, *remanere,* to remain], the radiation that passes through an object and can produce an image on an x-ray film.

**remodeling** /rēmod'əling/ [L, *re* + *modus,* to copy again], the process of changing a body part or area, as in reconstructive surgery.

**remote afterloading** /rimōt'/ [L, *removere,* to remove], a radiotherapy technique in which an applicator, such as an acrylic mold of an area to be irradiated, is placed in or on the patient and then loaded from a safe source with a high-activity radioisotope. The applicator contains grooves for the insertion of nylon tubes into which the radioactive material can be introduced. Remote afterloading is used in the treatment of head, neck, vaginal, and cervical tumors.

**remotivation** /rē'mōtivā'shən/ [L, *re* + *motus,* movement], the use of special techniques that stimulate patients to become motivated to learn and interact.

**remotivation group,** a treatment group that is organized with the purpose of stimulating the interest, awareness, and communication of withdrawn and institutionalized mental patients who experience a motivation.

**removable lingual arch** /rimoo'vəbəl/ [L, *removere,* to remove], an orthodontic arch wire designed to fit the lingual surface of the teeth and aid their orthodontic movement. Two posts soldered to each end of the wire fit snugly into the vertical tubes of molar anchor bands.

**removable orthodontic appliance,** a device placed inside the mouth to correct or alleviate malocclusion and designed to be removed or replaced by the patient.

**removable partial denture.** See **partial denture.**

**removable rigid dressing,** a dressing similar to a cast used to encase the stump of an amputated limb. It is usually applied to permit the fitting of a temporary prosthesis so that ambulation can begin soon after surgery.

**ren-,** combining form meaning 'kidney': *renicardiac, reniform, renocortical.*

**renal** /rē'nəl/ [L, *ren,* kidney], pertaining to the kidney.

**renal acidosis** [L, *ren,* kidney, *acidus,* sour; Gk, *osis,* condition], an excessive increase in the $H^+$ ions in body fluids because of impaired kidney function. The acidosis can result from excessive loss of bicarbonate or from the inability to excrete phosphoric and sulfuric acid.

**renal adenocarcinoma.** See **renal cell carcinoma.**

**renal angiography,** a radiographic examination of the renal artery and associated blood vessels after the injection of a contrast medium.

**renal anuria,** cessation of urine production caused by intrinsic renal disease.

**renal artery,** one of a pair of large, visceral branches of the abdominal aorta, arising inferior to the superior mesenteric artery at the level of the disk between the first and second lumbar vertebrae. The left renal artery is somewhat more superior than the right. Before reaching the kidney, each divides into four branches. The renal arteries supply the kidneys, suprarenal glands, and the ureters.

**renal biopsy,** the removal of kidney tissue for microscopic examination. It is conducted to establish the diagnosis of a renal disorder and to aid in determining the stage of the disease, the appropriate therapy, and the prognosis. An open biopsy involves an incision, permits better visualization of the kidney, and carries a lower risk of hemorrhage; a closed or percutaneous biopsy performed by aspirating a specimen of tissue with a needle requires a shorter period of recovery and is less likely to cause infection Contraindications to percutaneous biopsy include bleeding disorders, uncontrolled hypertension, and presence of a single kidney.

■ METHOD: Before biopsy the procedure is explained, and the patient is medically evaluated and tested for bleeding or coagulation time. Aspirin or coumadin therapy is discontinued for a period of time determined by the physician. Informed consent is obtained. The patient's blood is usually typed and crossmatched with two units of donor blood that are held for a possible transfusion until there is no threat of bleeding after the procedure. An open biopsy is generally carried out in the operating room, but the percutaneous procedure may be performed in the radiology department or the patient's room. The location of the kidney, determined by a plain x-ray film, dye contrast study, or fluoroscopic or ultrasound examination, is marked on the patient's skin in ink for a needle biopsy. The patient is then placed prone over a sandbag and soft pillow with the body bent at the level of the diaphragm, the shoulders on the bed, and the spine in straight alignment. A local anesthetic is injected, and the physician inserts the biopsy needle in the lower pole of the kidney, because this area contains the smallest number of large renal vessels. The needle is quickly withdrawn, and, after pressure is applied to the site for 30 to 60 minutes, a pressure bandage is applied; the patient is turned and kept supine and motionless for the next 4 hours. The dressing, blood pressure, and pulse are checked every 5 to 10 minutes for the first hour, then at frequency determined by institutional protocols; excessive drainage, decreased blood pressure, tachycardia, or elevated temperature is reported to the physician. Fluids are forced to the maximum allotted for the patient's condition; the amount and character of urinary output are noted, and the physician is informed if hematuria occurs. The patient is kept in bed for at least 24 hours and is cautioned not to lift any heavy objects for 10 days or to take any anticoagulants until the physician gives permission.

■ INTERVENTIONS: The nurse offers an explanation of the procedure, prepares and positions the patient for the percutaneous procedure, and, on its completion, provides care and emotional support.

■ OUTCOME CRITERIA: A biopsy is the most accurate measure for determining the nature and stage of a renal pathologic condition.

**renal calculus,** a concretion occurring in the kidney. If the stone is large enough to block the ureter and stop the flow of urine from the kidney, it must be removed by either major surgical or radiologic fluoroscopy procedures. Also called **kidney stone, nephritic calculus.** See also **nephroscope.**

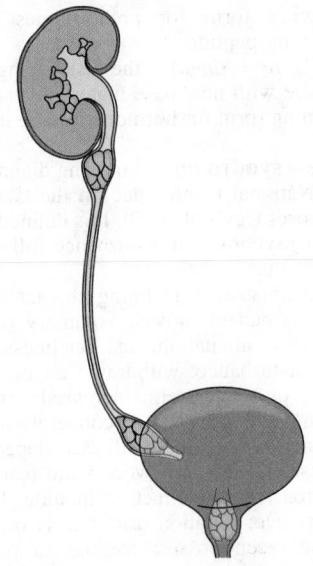

**Most common locations
for a renal calculus formation**
*(Phipps, Sands, and Marek, 1999)*

**renal calyx,** the first unit in the system of ducts in the kidney carrying urine from the renal pyramid of the medulla to the renal pelvis for excretion through the ureters. There are two divisions: the **minor renal calyx,** with several others, drains into a larger **major renal calyx,** which in turn joins other major calyces to form the renal pelvis.

**renal capsule** [L, *ren,* kidney, *capsula,* little box], a protective connective tissue capsule surrounding the kidney.

**renal cell carcinoma,** a malignant neoplasm of the kidney. Also called **adenocarcinoma of the kidney, clear cell carcinoma of the kidney.** See **kidney cancer.** See also **Wilms' tumor.**

**renal colic,** sharp, severe pain in the lower back over the kidney, radiating forward into the groin. Renal colic usually accompanies forcible dilation of a ureter, followed by spasm as a stone is lodged or passed through it. See also **urinary calculus.**

**renal corpuscle.** See **malpighian corpuscle.**

**renal cortex,** the highly vascularized granular outer layer of the kidney, containing approximately 1.25 million glomeruli and convoluted tubules, which filter body wastes from the blood, reclaim useful materials, and dispose of the remainder as urine.

**renal diabetes mellitus.** See **renal glycosuria.**

**renal dialysis** [L, *ren,* kidney; Gk, *dia,* + *lysis,* loosening], a process of diffusing blood across a semipermeable membrane to remove substances that a normal kidney would eliminate, including poisons, drugs, urea, uric acid, and creatinine. Renal dialysis may restore electrolytes and acid-base imbalances. See also **continuous ambulatory peritoneal dialysis, hemodialysis.**

**renal diet,** a diet prescribed in chronic renal failure and designed to control intake of protein, potassium, sodium, phosphorus, and fluids, depending on individual conditions. Carbohydrates and fats are the principal sources of energy. Protein is limited; the amount is determined by the patient's condition and is usually supplied from milk, eggs, and meat. Cereals, bread, rice, and pasta are the primary sources of calories. Some vegetables and fruits are included, depending on the degree of restriction of potassium and phosphorus. Special commercial flours and breads have been developed that are protein-free and low in potassium and sodium. The low potassium level of the diet also makes it useful in hyperkalemia. The diet may be nutritionally inadequate and should be supplemented with vitamins and electrolytes. See also **Giordano-Giovannetti diet.**

**renal dwarf,** a dwarf whose retarded growth is caused by renal failure.

**renal failure,** inability of the kidneys to excrete wastes, concentrate urine, and conserve electrolytes. The condition may be acute or chronic. **Acute renal failure** is characterized by oliguria and by the rapid accumulation of nitrogenous wastes in the blood (azotemia). It results from hemorrhage, trauma, burn, toxic injury to the kidney, acute pyelonephritis or glomerulonephritis, or lower urinary tract obstruction. Many forms of acute renal failure are reversible after the underlying cause has been identified. Acute renal failure may have three typical phases: prodromal, oliguric, and postoliguric. Treatment includes restricted intake of fluids and of all substances that require excretion by the kidney. Antibiotics and diuretics are also used. **Chronic renal failure** may result from many other diseases. The early signs include sluggishness, fatigue, and mental dullness. Later, anuria, convulsions, GI bleeding, malnutrition, and various neuropathies may occur. The skin may turn yellowbrown. Congestive heart failure and hypertension are frequent complications, the results of hypervolemia. Urinalysis reveals greater than normal amounts of urea and creatinine, waxy casts, and a constant volume of urine regardless of variations in water intake. Anemia frequently occurs. The prognosis depends on the underlying cause. Treatment usually includes restricted water and protein intake and the use of diuretics. When medical measures have been exhausted, long-term hemodialysis or peritoneal dialysis is often begun, and kidney transplantation is considered.

**renal fat.** See **adipose capsule.** Also called *(informal)* **kidney failure.**

**renal glycosuria** [L, *ren,* kidney; Gk, *glykys,* sweet, *ouron,* urine], a familial condition characterized by lowered renal threshold to sugar. Blood glucose levels may be normal, although sugar is excreted in the urine. Also called **renal diabetes mellitus.**

**renal hematuria** [L, *ren,* kidney; Gk, *haima,* blood, *ouron,* urine], presence of blood in the urine because of a kidney disorder.

**renal hypertension,** hypertension resulting from aortic or renal artery atherosclerosis or from kidney disease, including chronic glomerulonephritis, chronic pyelonephritis, renal carcinoma, and renal calculi. Analgesic abuse and certain drug reactions may also result in renal hypertension. Therapy depends on the cause and may include antibiotics, diuretics, or surgery. Untreated renal hypertension is likely to result in kidney damage and cardiovascular disease.

**renal insufficiency** [L, *ren,* kidney, *in + sufficere,* to suffice], partial kidney function failure characterized by less than normal urine excretion.

**renal nanism,** dwarfism associated with infantile renal osteodystrophy.

**renal osteodystrophy,** a condition resulting from chronic renal failure and characterized by uneven bone growth and demineralization. See also **renal nanism, renal rickets.**

**renal papilla.** See **papilla.**

**renal pelvis** [L, *ren + pelvis,* basin], a funnel-shaped dilation that drains urine from the kidney into the ureter.

**renal plasma flow (RPF),** the rate at which plasma flows through the renal tubules. It may be measured by *p*-aminohippurate clearance.

**renal pyramid** [L, *ren,* kidney; Gk, *pyramis*], any one of several conical masses of tissue that form the kidney medulla. The base of each pyramid adjoins the kidney's cortex; the apex terminates at a renal calyx. The pyramids consist of the loops of Henle and the collecting tubules of the nephrons.

**renal rickets,** a condition characterized by rachitic changes in the skeleton and caused by chronic nephritis. See also **renal osteodystrophy.**

**renal scan,** a radiographic scan of the kidneys performed after the IV injection of a radioactive substance. It is used to assess renal perfusion and function, particularly in renal failure and renovascular hypertension and following kidney transplantation.

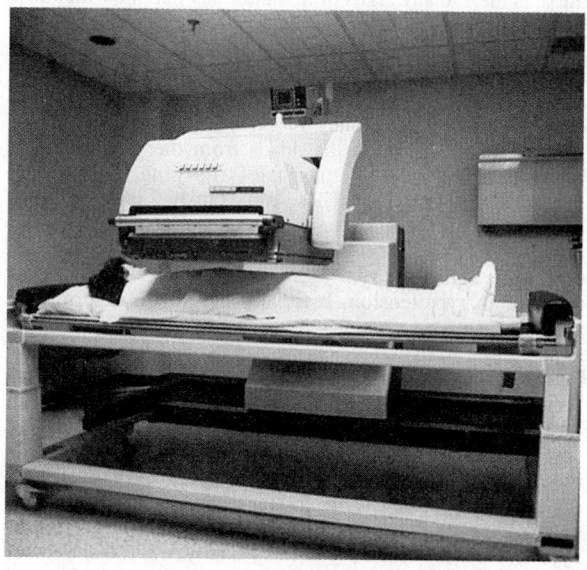

**Equipment for a renal scan** *(Brundage, 1992)*

**renal sclerosis** [L, *ren,* kidney; Gk, *skerosis,* hardening], arteriosclerosis or fibrosis of the arterioles of the kidney. See also **nephrosclerosis.**

**renal transplantation** [L, *ren,* kidney, *transplantare*], the surgical transfer of a complete kidney from a donor to a recipient.

**renal tubular acidosis (RTA),** an abnormal condition associated with persistent dehydration, metabolic acidosis, hypokalemia, hyperchloremia, and nephrocalcinosis. It is caused by the kidney's inability to conserve bicarbonate and to adequately acidify the urine. Some forms of RTA are more prevalent in women, older children, and young adults. Prolonged RTA can cause hypercalciuria and the formation of kidney stones. Prognosis depends on treatment and the extent of renal damage but is usually good. Compare **distal renal tubular acidosis, ketoacidosis, metabolic acidosis, proximal renal tubular acidosis, respiratory acidosis.**

■ OBSERVATIONS: Common signs and symptoms of RTA, especially in children, include anorexia, vomiting, constipation, retarded growth, excessive urination, nephrocalcinosis, and rickets. RTA can also cause urinary tract infections and pyelonephritis. Confirming diagnosis of distal RTA is based on laboratory tests that show impaired urine acidification in association with systemic metabolic acidosis. Confirming diagnosis of proximal RTA is based on tests that show bicarbonate wasting as a result of impaired reabsorption. Other significant laboratory findings may include decreased sodium bicarbonate, pH, potassium, and phosphorus; increased serum chloride, alkaline phosphatase, urinary bicarbonate, and potassium; and urine with low specific gravity.

■ INTERVENTIONS: Treatment includes the replacement of excessively secreted substances, especially bicarbonate, and may include the administration of sodium bicarbonate tablets, potassium, vitamin D to preserve calcium metabolism, and antibiotics to counter pyelonephritis. Surgery may be required to remove renal calculi.

■ NURSING CONSIDERATIONS: The nurse carefully monitors the results of altered laboratory tests, especially those involving potassium levels and urine pH. The patient's urine is strained to capture any kidney stones for analysis, and the nurse is alert to any signs of hematuria. A patient with a low potassium level is usually advised to eat potassium-rich foods such as bananas, oranges, and baked potatoes. The patient and family are encouraged to seek genetic counseling and RTA screening.

**renal tubule** [L, *ren,* kidney, *tubulus,* small tube], the part of the kidney's nephron that leads from the glomerulus to the collecting tubules. It consists of a looping segment and two convoluted sections. These canals resorb selected materials back into the blood and secrete, collect, and conduct urine.

**renal vein renin assay,** a blood test used to diagnose renovascular hypertension. It is very helpful in determining whether a stenosis seen on a renal angiogram is significantly contributing to hypertension.

**Rendu-Osler-Weber syndrome.** See **Osler-Weber-Rendu syndrome.**

**Renese,** trademark for a diuretic and antihypertensive (polythiazide).

**renin** /rē'nin/ [L, *ren,* kidney], a proteolytic enzyme, produced by and stored in the juxtaglomerular apparatus that surrounds each arteriole as it enters a glomerulus. The enzyme affects the blood pressure by catalyzing the change of angiotensinogen to angiotensin I, a strong pressor. Normal findings of adult plasma renin, measured in an upright position and sodium depleted, are 2.9 to 10.8 ng/mL/hr. Compare **rennin.**

**renin-angiotensin system,** the regulation of sodium balance, fluid volume, and blood pressure by renal secretions: in response to reduced perfusion, renin is secreted, which hydrolyzes a plasma globulin to release angiotensin I, which is rapidly hydrolyzed to angiotensin II; this in turn stimulates aldosterone secretion, which brings about sodium retention, increase in blood pressure, and restoration of renal perfusion, which shuts off the signal for renin release. Also called **renin-angiotensin-aldosterone system.**

**renin test.** See **plasma renin activity.**

**rennin** /ren'in/ [ME, *rennen,* to run], a milk-curdling enzyme that occurs in the gastric juices of infants and is also contained in the rennet produced in the stomach of calves and other ruminants. It is an endopeptidase that converts casein to paracasein and was formerly used extensively as a curdling agent by the cheese industry. An artificially produced microbial rennet rather than the enzyme extracted from rennet in calves is used in one half of the cheese produced in the United States today. Also called **chymosin** Compare **renin.**

**renogram** /rē'nəgram/, a radiographic image resulting from a renal scan.

**-renone,** combining form for spironolactone-type aldosterone antagonists.

**Renshaw cells** /ren'shô/ [B. Renshaw, American neurologist, b. 1911; L, *cella,* storeroom], small cells that reduce motor neuron discharge through a feedback circuit involving axon collaterals that excite interneurons. The system prevents rapid repeated firing of motor neurons.

**Reopro,** trademark for a platelet aggregation inhibitor (abcixmab).

**reovirus** /rē'ōvī'rəs/ [*respiratory* enteric *o*rphan + L, *virus*], any one of three ubiquitous, double-stranded ribonucleic acid viruses found in the respiratory and alimentary tracts in healthy and sick people. Reoviruses have been implicated in some cases of upper respiratory tract disease and infantile gastroenteritis.

**repaglinide,** an antidiabetic.

■ INDICATIONS: Repaglinide is used to treat stable type 2 diabetes mellitus.

■ CONTRAINDICATIONS: Known hypersensitivity to meglitinides, diabetic ketoacidosis, and type 1 diabetes mellitus prohibit the use of repaglinide.

■ ADVERSE EFFECTS: Hypoglycemia is a life-threatening effect of this drug. Other adverse reactions include paresthesia, nausea, vomiting, diarrhea, constipation, dyspepsia, rash, allergic reactions, back pain, arthralgia, upper respiratory infection, sinusitis, rhinitis, and bronchitis. Headache and weakness are common side effects.

**repercussion** /rē'pərkush'ən/ [L, *repercussio,* rebounding], **1.** (in obstetrics) ballottement. **2.** being driven back by a powerful resistance. **3.** the reduction of a swelling or tumor.

**reperfusion** /rē'pərfyoo'zhən/, a procedure in which blocked arteries are opened to reestablish blood flow. It may be accomplished through thrombolytic therapy or percutaneous transluminal angioplasty.

**repetition compulsion** /rep'ətish'ən/ [L, *repetere,* to repeat], an unconscious need to revert to and repeat earlier situations, behavior patterns, and acts to experience previously felt emotions or relationships. See also **compulsion.**

**repetitive stress injury** /ripet'ətiv/, tissue damage associated with tasks that require repeated movements of the hands, legs, or trunk, such as meat cutting, computer keyboarding, or playing musical instruments. Effects include chronic nerve and joint pain, spine damage, and carpal tunnel syndrome. Among recommended preventive measures are frequent rest breaks and ergonomic improvements in for the workplace.

**replacement** /riplās'mənt/ [Fr, *replacer,* to put in place again], the substitution of a missing part or substance with a similar structure or substance, such as the replacement of an amputated limb with a prosthesis or the replacement of lost blood with donor blood.

**replacement therapy, 1.** the use of a medicinal product to replace a natural hormone or enzyme that the body is no longer able to produce in sufficient amounts. **2.** a psychotherapeutic technique of replacing abnormal behavior with healthy, constructive activities.

**replacement transfusion,** the removal of all or most of a patient's diseased blood and its simultaneous replacement with an equal volume of normal blood.

**replication** /rep'likā'shən/ [L, *replicare,* to fold back], **1.** a process of duplicating, reproducing, or copying; literally, a folding back of a part to form a duplicate. **2.** (in research) the exact repetition of an experiment performed to confirm the initial findings. **3.** (in genetics) the duplication of the polynucleotide strands of deoxyribonucleic acid (DNA) or the synthesis of DNA. The process involves the unwinding of the double helix molecule to form two single strands, each of which acts as a template for the synthesis of a complementary strand. The two resulting molecules of DNA each contain one new and one parental strand, which coil to form the double helix. —**replicate,** *v.*

**replicator** /rep′likā′tər/ [L, *replicare*], a segment of DNA that initiates and controls the replication of the molecule.

**replicon** /rep′ləkon/ [L, *replicare*], a segment of DNA that is undergoing replication. It is regulated by a section of the molecule called the regulator, which controls replication and coordinates it with cell division.

**Repligen,** trademark for an human immunodeficiency virus (HIV) vaccine that contains a gp120 V3 loop. The V3 loop generates neutralizing antibodies that block the HIV virus from infecting helper T cells.

**repolarization** /rēpō′lərīzā′shən/ [L, *re* + *polus*, pole; Gk, *izein*, to cause], the process by which the membrane potential of a neuron or muscle cell is restored to the cell's resting potential. In a cardiac muscle cell, the repolarization process begins after phase 0 of the action potential and is completed by the end of phase 3; it encompasses the effective and relative refractory periods and correlates with the Q-T interval on the electrocardiogram. See also **cardiac action potential.**

**report** /ripôrt′/ [L, *re* + *portare*, to carry], (in nursing) the transfer of information from the nurses on one shift to the nurses on the following shift or before the transfer of a patient from one unit to another. Report is given systematically at the time of change of shift. The nurse manager, team leader, or primary nurse conducts the report, summarizing the progress and status of each patient, for the nurses who will next assume responsibility for the care. The provider of the information is said to 'give report,' and the oncoming staff to 'take report.' Report may be given to the assembled oncoming staff, or it may be tape recorded so that staff members can listen to it individually or in a group on their own schedule. The Kardex and medcard of each patient are updated before report, and staff members are informed of the changes during report.

**reportable diseases** /ripôr′təbəl/, diseases that must be reported by the physician to public health authorities, given their contagious nature. They include but are not limited to malaria, poliomyelitis, typhus, yellow fever, cholera, bubonic plague, and AIDS.

**repositioning** /rē′pəzish′əning/ [L, *reponere*, to put back], the restoration of an organ or body part to its natural position, as reposing an inverted uterus or changing the position of the jaws.

**representative group** /rep′rəsen′tətiv/, a group of individuals whose members represent all the various sectors of a community.

**repression** /ripresh′ən/ [L, *reprimere*, to press back], **1.** the act of restraining, inhibiting, or suppressing. **2.** (in psychoanalysis) an unconscious defense mechanism that also underlies all defense mechanisms whereby unacceptable thoughts, feelings, ideas, impulses, or memories, especially those concerning some traumatic past event, are pushed from the consciousness because of their painful guilt association or disagreeable content and are submerged in the unconscious, where they remain dormant but operant. Such repressed emotional conflicts are the source of anxiety that may lead to any of the anxiety disorders. Compare **suppression.** —**repress,** *v.* **repressive,** *adj.*

**repressive-inspirational approach** /ripres′iv/, a psychotherapeutic approach used in some groups to discourage the breaking down of defense mechanisms. Members are encouraged to focus on positive feelings and group strengths. This approach is commonly used in groups of patients with chronic mental illness.

**repressor** /ripres′ər/ [L, *reprimere*, to press back], a protein produced by a regulator gene in a bacterial genome. It binds to a sequence of nucleotides in an operator gene, blocking the transcription of one or more structural genes.

**repressor gene.** See **regulator gene.**

**reproduction** /rē′prəduk′shən/ [L, *re* + *producere*, to produce], **1.** the sum of the cellular and genetic phenomena by which organisms produce offspring similar to themselves so that the species is perpetuated. In humans the germ cells, spermatozoa in the male and ova in the female, unite during fertilization to form the new individual. Kinds of reproduction include **asexual reproduction, cytogenic reproduction,** and **sexual reproduction. 2.** the creation of a similar structure, situation, or phenomenon; duplication; replication. **3.** the recalling of a former idea or impression or of something previously learned. —**reproductive,** *adj.*

**reproductive** /rē′prəduk′tiv/ [L, *re* + *producere*, again to produce], pertaining to the process of reproduction.

**reproductive endocrinology,** the study of the maternal female hormone system, including the activities of the hypothalamus, pituitary, and ovaries from puberty through menopause.

**reproductive system,** the male and female gonads, associated ducts and glands, and external genitalia that function in the procreation of offspring. In women these include the ovaries, fallopian tubes, uterus, vagina, clitoris, and vulva. In men they include the testes, epididymis, vas deferens, seminal vesicles, ejaculatory duct, prostate, and penis. Also called **genital tract, genitourinary system, urogenital system.** See also the Color Atlas of Human Anatomy.

**reproductive technology management,** a nursing intervention from the Nursing Interventions Classification (NIC) defined as assisting a patient through the steps of complex infertility treatment. See also **Nursing Interventions Classification.**

**repulsion** /ripul′shən/ [L, *repellere*, to drive away], **1.** the act of repelling, disjoining. **2.** a force that separates two bodies or things. **3.** (in genetics) the situation in linked inheritance in which the alleles of two or more mutant genes are located on homologous chromosomes so that each chromosome of the pair carries one or more mutant and wild-type genes, which are located close enough to be inherited together. Compare **coupling.** See also **trans configuration.**

**request for proposal (RFP)** /rikwest′/ [L, *requaerere*, to require, *propronere*, to propound], a solicitation by a funding agency for proposals to accomplish a particular goal. The RFP lists the requirements a project must meet to receive funding.

**required arch length** /rikwī′ərd/ [L, *requaerere*, to require], the sum of the mesiodistal widths of all the natural teeth in a dental arch. It represents the minimum arch length that can accommodate all of the teeth in the arch.

**RES,** abbreviation for **reticuloendothelial system.**

**Rescriptor,** trademark for an antiretoviral nonucleoside reverse transcriptase inhibitor analog (delaviridine).

**research** /risurch′, rē′surch/ [Fr, *rechercher*, to investigate], the diligent inquiry or examination of data, reports, and observations in a search for facts or principles.

**research data collection,** a nursing intervention from the Nursing Interventions Classification (NIC) defined as collecting research data. See also **Nursing Interventions Classification.**

**research instrument,** a testing device for measuring a given phenomenon, such as a paper and pencil test, a questionnaire, an interview, or a set of guidelines for observation.

**research measurement,** an evaluation of the quantity or incidence of a given variable as obtained by using a research instrument.

**research radiopharmaceutical,** a drug that is labeled with a small quantity of a radioactive tracer to allow its biodistribution to be studied; it may later be used in a nonradioactive form.

**resect** /risekt′/ [L, *re* + *secare*, to cut], to remove tissue from the body by surgery.

**resection** /risek′shən/, the cutting out of a significant part of an organ or structure. Resection of an organ may be partial or complete. One type of resection is a **wedge resection.**

**reserpine** /res′ərpēn/, a peripherally acting antiadrenergic agent.
- INDICATIONS: It is prescribed in the treatment of high blood pressure and certain neuropsychiatric disorders.
- CONTRAINDICATIONS: Mental depression, peptic ulcer, ulcerative colitis, or known hypersensitivity to this drug prohibits its use.
- ADVERSE EFFECTS: Among the more serious adverse reactions are mental depression, extrapyramidal reactions, impotence, aggravation of peptic ulcer, and paradoxic excitement.

**reserve** /rizurv′/ [L, *reservare*, to save], a potential capacity to maintain vital body functions in homeostasis by adjusting to increased need, such as cardiac reserve, pulmonary reserve, and alkali reserve. See also **homeostasis.**

**reserve capacity** [L, *reservare*, to save; Gk, *aer*], the volume of air that can be exhaled with maximum effort after completion of a normal expiration. Also called **reserve air, supplemental air.**

**reserve cell carcinoma.** See **oat cell carcinoma.**

**reservoir** /rez′ərvwär/ [Fr, réservoir], a chamber or receptacle for holding or storing a fluid.

**reservoir bag,** a component of an anesthesia machine in which gas accumulates, forming a reserve supply of gas for use during manual control of ventilation. It serves as a visible monitor of respiratory rate and depth.

**reservoir host,** a nonhuman host that serves as a means of sustaining an infectious organism as a potential source of human infection. Wild monkeys are reservoir hosts for the yellow fever virus, which can spread from the jungle to infect humans.

**reservoir of infection,** a continuous source of infectious disease. People, animals, and plants may be reservoirs of infection.

**resident** /rez′idənt/ [L, *residere*, to remain], **1.** a physician in one of the postgraduate years of clinical training after the first, or internship, year. The length of residency varies according to the specialty. See also **PGY. 2.** a person who receives inpatient care in a long-term care facility.

**resident bacteria,** bacteria living in a specific area of the body.

**residential care facility** /rez′iden′shəl/, a facility that provides custodial care to persons who, because of physical, mental, or emotional disorders, are not able to live independently.

**residual** /rizij′ōo·əl/ [L, *residuum*, remainder], **1.** pertaining to the part of something that remains after an activity that removes the bulk of the substance. **2.** (in psychology), an aftereffect of an experience that influences latent behavior.

**residual air.** See **residual volume.**

**residual cyst,** an odontogenic cyst that remains in the jaw after the removal of a tooth.

**residual dental caries,** any decayed material left in a prepared tooth cavity.

**residual function** [L, *residuum*, remainder, *functio*, performance], the remaining ability to function after a serious illness or injury.

**residual ridge,** the part of the alveolar ridge that remains after the alveolar process has disappeared after extraction of the teeth.

**residual urine,** urine that remains in the bladder after urination.

**residual volume** [L, *residuum*, remainder, *volumen*, papyrus roll], the amount of air remaining in the lungs at the end of a maximum expiration.

**residue-free diet** /rez′id(y)ōo/ [L, *residuum*, remainder; AS, *freo* + Gk, *diaita*, way of life], a diet free of nondigestible cellulose or fiber, such as found in semisolid bland food.

**residue schizophrenia** [L, *residuum*], a form of schizophrenia in which the essential features include the presence of residual symptoms without evidence of delusions, hallucinations, incoherence, or gross disorganization. See also **schizophrenia.**

**resilience** /rizil′yənt/ [L, *resilere*, to spring back], the ability of a body to return to its original form after being stretched or compressed.

**resiliency promotion,** a nursing intervention from the Nursing Interventions Classification (NIC) defined as assisting individuals, families, and communities in development, use, and strengthening of protective factors to be used in coping with environmental and societal stressors. See also **Nursing Interventions Classification.**

**resin** /rez′in/ [L, *resina*], a mixture of carboxylic acids, essential oils, and terpenes (hydrocarbons of the formula $C_{10}H_{16}$), occurring as exudations on various trees and shrubs or produced synthetically. Resins are highly combustible semisolids or amorphous solids that are insoluble in water, while some are soluble in ethanol and others in carbon tetrachloride, ether, and volatile oils. Most are soft and sticky, but harden after exposure to cold.

**resins** /rez′ins/, substances used in a kind of drug therapy for lowering low-density lipoprotein C (LDL-C) levels. Bile-acid binding resins such as cholestyramine and colestipol interrupt the normal enterohepatic circulation of bile acids and indirectly increase the liver's breakdown of LDL-C.

**res ipsa loquitur** /räs′ ip′sə lok′witōor/ [L, the thing speaks for itself], a legal concept that is important in many malpractice suits, describing a situation in which an injury occurred when the defendant was solely and exclusively in control and in which the injury would not have occurred had due care been exercised. Classic examples of res ipsa loquitur are a sponge left in the abdomen after abdominal surgery or the amputation of the wrong extremity.

**resistance** /rizis′təns/ [L, *resistere*, to withstand], **1.** an opposition to a force, such as the resistance offered by the constriction of peripheral vessels to the blood flow in the circulatory system. **2.** the frictional force that opposes the flow of an electric charge, as measured in ohms. **3.** (in respiratory therapy) the process or power of acting against a force placed on it, pertaining to thoracic resistance, tissue resistance, and airway resistance.

**resistance form,** the shape given to a prepared tooth cavity to impart strength and durability to the restoration and remaining tooth structure.

**resistance-inducing factor (RIF),** an agent that interferes with multiplication of a virus or other pathogen.

**resistance-inducing factor (RIF) test.** See **Rubin's test.**

**resistance to flow,** the pressure differential required to produce a given rate of flow of a gas or liquid through a vessel.

**resistance training,** any method or form of strength training used to resist, overcome, or bear force.

**resistance transfer factor.** See **R factor.**

**resistance vessels,** the blood vessels, including small arteries, arterioles, and metarterioles that form the major part of the total peripheral resistance to blood flow.

**resistant** /rizis'tənt/, pertaining to the ability of a microorganism to remain unaffected by an antimicrobial agent.

**resistive magnet** /resis'tiv/, a simple electromagnet in which electricity passing through coils of wire produces a magnetic field.

**resocialization** /rēsō'shəlīzā'shən/ [L, *re + socialis,* partners; Gk, *izein,* to cause], the reintegration of a client into family and community life after critical or long-term hospitalization.

**resolution** [L, *re + solvere,* to solve], **1.** the state of having made a firm determination or decision on a course of action. **2.** the ability of an imaging process to distinguish adjacent structures in an object. It is an important measure of image quality. **3.** the ability of a chromatographic system to separate two adjacent peaks. The degree of separation between two peaks is represented by the symbol **R.**

**resolving power** /rizol'ving/, **1.** the ability to separate closely migrating substances, as in electrophoresis. **2.** the ability to distinguish closely positioned objects as distinct entities.

**resolving time,** the minimum time between radiation-induced ionizations that can be detected by a Geiger-Müller-type scintillation device.

**resonance** /rez'ənəns/ [L, *resonare,* to sound again], **1.** an echo or other sound produced by percussion of an organ or cavity of the body during a physical examination. **2.** the process of energy absorption by an object that is tuned to absorb energy of a specific frequency only. Other frequencies do not affect the object. An example is the effect of the vibration of a tuning fork of a particular frequency, causing only other tuning forks of the same frequency to vibrate also. —**resonant,** *adj.*

**resonance frequency,** **1.** in an ultrasound transducer, the frequency for which the response of a transducer to an ultrasound beam is a maximum. **2.** the frequency at which the transducer most efficiently converts electrical signals to mechanical vibrations. **3.** (in magnetic resonance) the frequency at which a nucleus absorbs radio energy when placed in a magnetic field.

**resonant** /rez'ənənt/ [L, *resonare,* to sound again], pertaining to a sound that vibrates on percussion or is amplified by sympathetic vibrations in another medium.

**resonating** /rez'ənā'ting/ [L, *resonare,* to sound again], pertaining to vibrations or pulsations that are synchronous with a source of sound waves or electromagnetic oscillations.

**resorb** /risôrb'/ [L, *resorbere,* to swallow again], to absorb again.

**resorbent** /risôr'bənt/ [L, *resorbere*], a material or agent that is used to absorb blood or other substances.

**resorcinated camphor** /rizôr'sinā'tid/, a mixture of camphor and resorcinol, used for the treatment of pediculosis and itching.

**resorcinol** /rizôr'sinol/, an antiseptic substance used as a keratolytic agent in the dermatoses. It is also used in dyes and pharmaceuticals and as a chemical intermediate.

**resorption** /risôrp'shən/ [L, *resorbere,* to swallow again], **1.** the loss of substance or bone by physiologic or pathologic means, such as the reduction of the volume and size of the residual ridge of the mandible or maxillae. **2.** the cementoclastic and dentinoclastic action that may occur on a tooth root.

**resource-based relative value scale (RBRVS),** a system for a Medicare fee schedule designed to address the promise of compensation to a physician for the time involved in giving physical and mental status examinations and obtaining patient history from family members.

**Respbid,** trademark for a smooth muscle relaxant (theophylline).

**Res. Phys.,** abbreviation for *resident physician.*

**respiration** /res'pirā'shən/ [L, *respirare,* to breathe], **1.** the molecular exchange of oxygen and carbon dioxide within the body's tissues. **2.** also called **breathing, pulmonary ventilation, ventilation.** The process of moving air into and out of the lungs. The rate varies with the age and condition of the person. —**respiratory,** *adj.*

**respiration of infants** [L, *respirare,* to breathe, *infans,* unable to speak], a rate of breathing that averages 40 to 50 breaths per minute at birth and declines to 15 to 20 breaths per minute at puberty.

**respiration rate** [L, *respirare,* to breathe, *ratum,* rate], the rate of breathing. It is typically from 40 to 50 breaths per minute for newborns, 20 to 25 breaths per minute for older children, and 15 to 20 breaths per minute for teenagers and adults. An adult rate of 25 breaths per minute may be regarded as accelerated, whereas a rate of less than 12 breaths per minute is abnormally low. The rate may be more rapid in fever, acute pulmonary infection, diffuse pulmonary fibrosis, gas gangrene, left ventricular failure, thyrotoxicosis, and states of tension. Slower breathing rates may result from head injury, coma, or narcotic overdose. Also called **breathing frequency, respiratory rate.** See also **bradypnea, hyperpnea, hypopnea.**

**respirator** /res'pirā'tər/ [L, *respirare*], an apparatus used to modify air for inspiration or to improve pulmonary ventilation. The term is commonly used to mean a ventilator. See also **nebulizer, IPPB unit.**

**respiratory** /res'pərətôr'ē, rispī'rətôr'ē/ [L, *respirare*], pertaining to respiration.

**respiratory acidosis,** an abnormal condition characterized by a low plasma pH resulting from reduced alveolar ventilation. The hypoventilation inhibits the excretion of carbon dioxide, which consequently combines with water in the body to produce carbonic acid, thus reducing plasma pH. Respiratory acidosis can result from disorders such as airway obstruction, medullary trauma, neuromuscular disease, chest injury, pneumonia, pulmonary edema, emphysema, and cardiopulmonary arrest. It may also be caused by the suppression of respiratory reflexes with narcotics, sedatives, hypnotics, or anesthetics. Also called **carbon dioxide acidosis.** Compare **metabolic acidosis.** See also **metabolic alkalosis, respiratory alkalosis.**

■ OBSERVATIONS: Some common signs and symptoms of respiratory acidosis are headache, dyspnea, fine tremors, tachycardia, hypertension, and vasodilation. Confirming diagnosis is usually based on a $PaCO_2$ over the normal 45 mm Hg and an arterial pH below 7.35.

■ INTERVENTIONS: Ineffective treatment of acute respiratory acidosis can lead to coma and death. Treatment seeks to remove or inhibit the underlying causes of associated hypoventilation. Any airway obstructions are immediately removed. Mechanical ventilation and oxygen therapy may be used, and IV bronchodilators and sodium bicarbonate may be administered.

■ NURSING CONSIDERATIONS: The patient with respiratory acidosis is carefully monitored for any changes in arterial blood gas pressures, electrolyte concentrations, and respiratory, cardiovascular, and central nervous system functions. In patients requiring mechanical ventilation, patent airways are maintained, and tracheal tubes are suctioned as needed. Adequate hydration is also important.

**respiratory alkalosis,** an abnormal condition characterized by a high plasma pH resulting from increased alveolar ventilation. The consequent acceleration of carbon dioxide excretion lowers the plasma level of carbonic acid, thus raising plasma pH. The hyperventilation may be caused by pulmonary and nonpulmonary problems. Some pulmonary causes are acute asthma, pulmonary vascular disease, and pneumonia. Some nonpulmonary causes are aspirin toxicity, anxiety, fever, metabolic acidosis, inflammation of the central nervous system, gram-negative septicemia, and hepatic failure. Compare **metabolic alkalosis.** See also **metabolic acidosis, respiratory acidosis.**

■ OBSERVATIONS: Deep and rapid breathing at rates as high as 40 breaths per minute is a major sign of respiratory alkalosis. Other symptoms are light-headedness, dizziness, peripheral paresthesia, tingling of the hands and feet, muscle weakness, tetany, and cardiac arrhythmia. Confirming diagnosis is often based on a $PaCO_2$ below 35 mm Hg and a pH greater than 7.45. In the acute stage blood pH rises in proportion to the fall in $PaCO_2$, but in the chronic stage it remains within the normal range of 7.35 to 7.45. The carbonic acid concentration is normal in the acute stage of this condition but below normal in the chronic stage.

■ INTERVENTIONS: Treatment of respiratory alkalosis concentrates on removing the underlying causes. Severe cases, especially those caused by extreme anxiety, may be treated by having the patient breathe into a paper bag and inhale exhaled carbon dioxide to compensate for the deficit being created by hyperventilation. Sedatives may also be administered to decrease the ventilation rate.

■ NURSING CONSIDERATIONS: The nurse monitors neurologic, neuromuscular, and cardiovascular functions, arterial blood gases, and serum electrolyte levels. The patient benefits from explanations of laboratory tests and treatment.

**respiratory arrest,** the cessation of breathing.

**respiratory assessment,** an evaluation of the condition and function of a person's respiratory system.

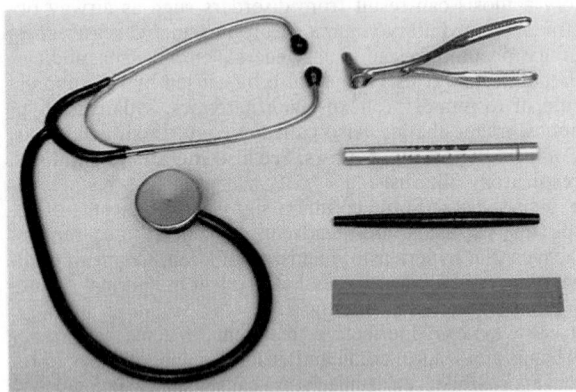

**Equipment for respiratory system assessment**
*(Wilson and Thompson, 1990)*

■ METHOD: The nurse or other health care provider asks if the person coughs, wheezes, is short of breath, tires easily, or experiences chest or abdominal pain, chills, fever, excessive sweating, dizziness, or swelling of feet and hands. Signs of confusion, anxiety, restlessness, flaring nostrils, cyanotic lips, gums, ear lobes, or nails, clubbing of extremities, fever, anorexia, and a tendency to sit upright are noted if present. The person's breathing is closely observed for evidence of slow, rapid, irregular, shallow, or Cheyne-Stokes respiration, hyperventilation, a long expiratory phase or periods of apnea, as well as for retractions in the suprasternal, supraclavicular, substernal, or intercostal areas during breathing. The presence of tachycardia, bradycardia, or sinus arrhythmia or evidence of congestive heart failure such as crackles, rhonchi, edema, hepatosplenomegaly, abdominal distension, or pain is recorded. The thorax is examined for scoliosis, kyphosis, funnel or barrel chest, or unequal shoulder height and is palpated for indications of thoracic expansion, tracheal deviation, crepitations, or fremitus. Percussion is performed to evaluate resonance, hyperresonance, tympany, and dull or flat sounds. Crackles, rhonchi, wheezing, friction rubs, the transmission of spoken words through the chest wall, and decreased or absent breath sounds are detected by auscultation. Background information pertinent to the evaluation includes allergies, recent exposure to infection, immunizations, exposure to environmental irritants, previous respiratory disorders and operations, preexisting chronic conditions, medication currently taken, the person's smoking habits, and the family history. Valuable diagnostic aids include a chest x-ray examination; complete blood count; electrocardiogram, pulmonary function tests, bronchoscopy; determination of blood gases and electrolytes; studies of sputum, throat, or nasopharyngeal cultures; gastric washings, lung scans, and biopsies.

■ INTERVENTIONS: The nurse or other health care provider collects the background information and the results of diagnostic tests and may perform the examination. In a respiratory care unit, a registered nurse, staff nurse, nurse clinician, or practitioner may interpret data from electrocardiographic tracings, set up and adjust a respirator, titrate medications, and obtain specimens for blood gas determination.

■ OUTCOME CRITERIA: An accurate and thorough assessment of respiratory function is an essential component of the physical examination and is vital to the diagnosis or ongoing care of a respiratory illness.

**respiratory bronchiole.** See **bronchiole.**

**respiratory burn,** tissue damage to the respiratory system resulting from the inhalation of a hot gas or burning particles, as may occur in a fire or explosion. Immediate hospitalization and oxygen therapy are recommended. Compare **smoke inhalation.**

**respiratory care practitioner,** a health professional with special training and experience in the treatment and rehabilitation of patients with respiratory disorders. The respiratory care practitioner typically does not diagnose but must be competent with patient assessment in a variety of clinical settings.

**respiratory center,** a group of nerve cells in the pons and medulla of the brain that control the rhythm of breathing in response to changes in levels of oxygen, carbon dioxide, and hydrogen ions in the blood and cerebrospinal fluid. Such changes activate central and peripheral chemoreceptors, which send impulses to the respiratory center, triggering an increase or a decrease in the breathing rate. In patients with retention of carbon dioxide, the respiratory center becomes insensitive to carbon dioxide, and the main stimulus to ventilation is hypoxemia. If such patients inhale air with a high oxygen content, breathing may be depressed, leading to a further rise in blood carbon dioxide levels. The respiratory center is inhibited by barbiturates, anesthetics, tranquilizing agents, and morphine. See also **hyperventilation, hypoventilation, hypoxia.**

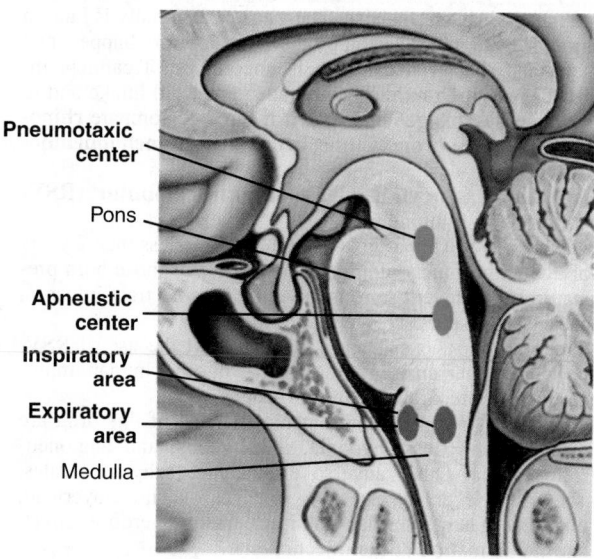

**Respiratory centers of the brainstem**
*(Thibodeau and Patton, 1999/William Ober)*

Pneumotaxic center

Pons

Apneustic center

Inspiratory area

Expiratory area

Medulla

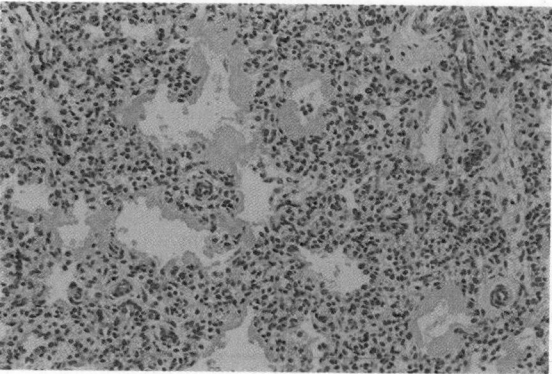

**Respiratory distress syndrome of the newborn: alternating atelectasis and dilation of the alveoli**
*(Cotran, Kumar, and Collins, 1999)*

**respiratory component ($\alpha PCO_2$),** the acid component of an acid-base control system that is modified by the respiratory status.

**respiratory cycle.** See **breathing cycle.**

**respiratory depressant** [L, *respirare,* to breathe, *depremere,* to press down], a drug or other agent that diminishes normal breathing functions. Most respiratory depressants, such as alcohol and opiates, act by depressing the central nervous system.

**respiratory depression** [L, *respirare,* to breathe, *depremere,* to press down], respiration that has a rate below 12 breaths per minute or that fails to provide full ventilation and perfusion of the lungs. Also called **respiratory insufficiency.**

**respiratory distress syndrome of the newborn (RDS),** an acute lung disease of the newborn, characterized by airless alveoli, inelastic lungs, a respiration rate greater than 60 breaths per minute, nasal flaring, intercostal and subcostal retractions, grunting on expiration, and peripheral edema. The condition occurs most often in premature babies. It is caused by a deficiency of pulmonary surfactant, resulting in overdistended alveoli and at times hyaline membrane formation, alveolar hemorrhage, severe right-to-left shunting of blood, increased pulmonary resistance, decreased cardiac output, and severe hypoxemia. The disease is self-limited; the infant dies in 3 to 5 days or completely recovers with no after effects. Treatment includes measures to correct shock, acidosis, and hypoxemia and use of continuous positive airway pressure to prevent alveolar collapse. Also called **hyaline membrane disease, idiopathic respiratory distress syndrome.** Compare **adult respiratory distress syndrome.**

**respiratory exchange ratio (R),** the ratio of the amount of carbon dioxide produced to the amount of oxygen consumed or taken up.

**respiratory failure,** the inability of the cardiovascular and pulmonary systems to maintain an adequate exchange of oxygen and carbon dioxide in the lungs. Respiratory failure may be caused by a failure in oxygenation or in ventilation. Oxygenation failure is characterized by hyperventilation and

occurs in diseases that affect the alveoli or interstitial tissues of the lungs, such as alveolar edema, emphysema, fungal infections, leukemia, lobar pneumonia, lung carcinoma, various pneumoconioses, pulmonary eosinophilia, sarcoidosis, or tuberculosis. Ventilatory failure, characterized by increased arterial tension of carbon dioxide, occurs in acute conditions in which retained pulmonary secretions cause increased airway resistance and decreased lung compliance, as in bronchitis and emphysema. Ventilation may also be reduced by depression of the respiratory center by barbiturates or opiates, hypoxia, hypercapnia, intracranial diseases, trauma, or lesions of the neuromuscular system or thoracic cage. Respiratory failure in preexisting chronic lung diseases may be precipitated by added stress, as with cardiac failure, surgery, anesthesia, or upper respiratory tract infections. Treatment of respiratory failure includes clearing the airways by suction, bronchodilators, or tracheostomy; antibiotics for infections that are usually present; anticoagulants for pulmonary thromboemboli; and electrolyte replacement in fluid imbalance. Oxygen may be administered in some cases; in others it may further decrease the respiratory reflex by removing the stimulus of a decreased level of oxygen. Chronic respiratory failure may result in cor pulmonale with congestive heart failure and respiratory acidosis. See also **airway obstruction, carbon dioxide, hypercapnia, hyperventilation, hypoxemia, hypoxia, respiratory acidosis.**

**respiratory insufficiency.** See **respiratory depression.**

**respiratory monitoring,** a nursing intervention from the Nursing Interventions Classification (NIC) defined as collection and analysis of patient data to ensure airway patency and adequate gas exchange. See also **Nursing Interventions Classification.**

**respiratory muscles,** the muscles that produce volume changes of the thorax during breathing. The inspiratory muscles include the hemidiaphragms, external intercostals, scaleni, sternomastoids, trapezius, pectoralis major, pectoralis minor, subclavius, latissimus dorsi, serratus anterior, and muscles that extend the back. The expiratory muscles are the internal intercostals, the abdominals, and the muscles that flex the back.

**respiratory quotient (RQ),** the ratio of the volume of carbon dioxide produced to the volume of oxygen consumed per unit of time by the body under steady-state conditions. Depending on the net metabolic needs of all parts of the body at a given moment, the ratio ranges from 0.7 to 1 and averages around 0.8. The RQ varies for different metabolic fuels: the RQ of fat is lower than that of protein, which is lower than that of glucose. Also called **metabolic respiratory quotient.**

**respiratory rate.** See **respiration rate.**

**respiratory rhythm,** a regular, oscillating cycle of inspiration and expiration, controlled by neuronal impulses transmitted between the respiratory centers in the brain and the muscles of inspiration in the chest and diaphragm. The normal breathing pattern may be altered by a variety of conditions. See also **apnea, apneustic breathing, Biot's respiration, Cheyne-Stokes respiration, chronic obstructive pulmonary disease, Hering-Breuer reflex, hyperventilation, hypoventilation, Kussmaul breathing, tachypnea.**

**respiratory standstill,** the cessation of respiratory movements.

**respiratory status: airway patency,** a nursing outcome from the Nursing Outcomes Classification (NOC) defined as the extent to which the tracheobronchial passages remain open. See also **Nursing Outcomes Classification.**

**respiratory status: gas exchange,** a nursing outcome from the Nursing Outcomes Classification (NOC) defined as the alveolar exchange of $CO_2$ or $O_2$ to maintain arterial blood gas concentrations. See also **Nursing Outcomes Classification.**

**respiratory status: ventilation,** a nursing outcome from the Nursing Outcomes Classification (NOC) defined as the movement of air in and out of the lungs. See also **Nursing Outcomes Classification.**

**respiratory syncytial virus (RSV, RS virus),** a member of a subgroup of myxoviruses that in tissue culture cause formation of giant cells or syncytia. It is a common cause of epidemics of acute bronchiolitis, bronchopneumonia, and the common cold in young children and sporadic acute bronchitis and mild upper respiratory tract infections in adults. Symptoms of infection with this virus include fever, cough, and severe malaise. The virus occasionally is fatal in infants. Systemic invasion by the virus does not happen, and secondary bacterial invasion is uncommon. Treatment includes rest, high humidity, and adequate fluid intake and in severe cases, oxygen and ribavirin aerosol. Compare **rhinovirus.** See also **bronchiolitis, bronchitis, bronchopneumonia, cold.**

**respiratory syncytial virus immune globulin (RSV-IGIV),** an immune serum.

■ INDICATIONS: This drug is used in children less than 2 years of age with bronchopulmonary dysplasia or those born prematurely to prevent serious lower respiratory tract infection caused by respiratory syncytial virus.

■ CONTRAINDICATIONS: Factors that prohibit the use of RSV-IGIV are hypersensitivity to this drug or other human immunoglobulin preparations and IGA deficiency.

■ ADVERSE EFFECTS: Life-threatening effects of this drug are respiratory distress, hypoxia, anaphylaxis, and angioneurotic edema. Other adverse effects are tachypnea, rales, wheezing, fever, hypertension, tachycardia, fluid overload, diarrhea, gastroenteritis, vomiting, rash, overdose effect, and inflammation at the injection site.

**respiratory system.** See **respiratory tract.**

**respiratory therapist,** a graduate of a program approved by the Commission on Accreditation of Allied Health Education Programs designed to qualify the person for the registry examination of the National Board for Respiratory Care. See also **registered respiratory therapist.**

**respiratory therapy (RT),** **1.** any treatment that maintains or improves the ventilatory function of the respiratory tract. **2.** *informal.* the department in a health care facility that provides respiratory therapy for the patients of the facility.

**respiratory therapy technician,** a graduate of a program approved by the Commission on Accreditation of Allied Health Education Programs, designed to qualify the person

**Respiratory patterns**

| Pattern | | Description |
|---|---|---|
| Eupnea | | Rhythm is smooth and even with expiration longer than inspiration. |
| Tachypnea | | Rapid superficial breathing; regular or irregular rhythm. |
| Bradypnea | | Slow respiratory rate; deeper than usual depth; regular rhythm. |
| Apnea | | Cessation of breathing. |
| Hyperpnea | | Increased depth of respiration with a normal to increased rate and regular rhythm. |
| Cheyne-Stokes respiration | | Periodic breathing associated with periods of apnea, alternating regularly with a series of respiratory cycles; the respiratory cycle gradually increases, then decreases in rate and depth. |
| Ataxic breathing | | Periods of apnea alternating irregularly with a series of shallow breaths of equal depth. |
| Kussmaul's respiration | | Deep regular sighing respirations with an increase in respiratory rate. |
| Apneusis | | Long, gasping inspiratory phase followed by a short, inadequate expiratory phase. |
| Obstructed breathing | | Long, ineffective expiratory phase with shallow, increased respirations. |

From Phipps WJ, Sands JK, Marek JE: *Medical-surgical nursing: concepts and clinical practice,* ed 6, St Louis, 1999, Mosby.

for the technician certification examination of the National Board for Respiratory Care. The program requires a special curriculum of basic sciences with supervised clinical experience.

**respiratory therapy technician, certified (CRTT),** an allied health professional who administers general respiratory care. Duties can include collection and review of clinical data; examination of the patient by inspection, palpation, percussion, and auscultation; and assembling and maintaining equipment used in respiratory care.

**respiratory tract,** the complex of organs and structures that performs the pulmonary ventilation of the body and the exchange of oxygen and carbon dioxide between ambient air and blood circulating through the lungs. It also warms the air passing into the body and assists in the speech function by providing air for the larynx and the vocal cords. Every 24 hours about 500 cubic feet of air (150 m³) passes through the respiratory tract of the average adult, who breathes in and out between 12 and 18 times a minute. The respiratory tract is divided into the upper respiratory tract and the lower respiratory tract. Also called **respiratory system.** See also the Color Atlas of Human Anatomy.

**respiratory tract infection,** any infectious disease of the upper or lower respiratory tract. **Upper respiratory tract infections** include the common cold, laryngitis, pharyngitis, rhinitis, sinusitis, and tonsillitis. **Lower respiratory tract infections** include bronchitis, bronchiolitis, pneumonia, and tracheitis.

**respiratory zone,** the air sacs where gas exchange actually occurs in the lungs, usually below the seventeenth division of bronchi.

**respirometer** /res'pirom'ətər/ [L, *respirare,* to breath; Gk, *metron,* measure], an instrument used to analyze the quality of a patient's respirations.

**respite care¹** /res'pit/ [L, *respicere,* to look back], **1.** short-term health services to the dependent older adult, either at home or in an institutional setting. **2.** the provision of temporary care for a patient who requires specialized or intensive care or supervision that is normally provided by his or her family at home. Respite care provides the family with relief from demands of the patient's care.

**respite care²,** a nursing intervention from the Nursing Interventions Classification (NIC) defined as provision of short-term care to provide relief for family caregiver. See also **Nursing Interventions Classification.**

**respite time** /res'pit/, relief time from responsibilities for the care of a patient, an individual, or a family member.

**respondeat superior** /respon'dē·at/ [L, let the master answer], the concept that an employer may be held liable for torts committed by employees acting within the scope of their employment.

**respondent conditioning.** See **classical conditioning.**

**responder** /rispon'dər/ [L, *respondere,* to promise in return], a person whose tumor shrinks in volume by at least 50% as a result of chemotherapy, radiation, or other treatment.

**response** /rispons'/ [L, *responsum,* reply], **1.** a reaction of an organism to a stimulus. **2.** (in psychology) a category of negative punishment in which the reinforcer is lost or withdrawn after an operant.

**response time, 1.** the period between the input of information into a computer and the response or output, measured in microseconds (ms) or fractions thereof. **2.** the period between the application of a stimulus and the response of a cell or cells.

**rest¹** [AS, *restan,* to rest], an extension from a prosthesis that provides vertical support for a dental restoration.

**rest²,** a nursing outcome from the Nursing Outcomes Clas-

sification (NOC) defined as the extent and pattern of diminished activity for mental and physical rejuvenation. See also **Nursing Outcomes Classification.**

**rest angle.** See **occlusal rest angle.**

**rest area,** a prepared surface on a tooth or fixed restoration into which a rest fits. Also called **rest seat.**

**resting cell,** a cell that is not undergoing division. See also **interphase.**

**resting membrane potential,** the transmembrane voltage that exists when a neuron or muscle cell is not producing an action potential.

**resting potential** [AS, *rest* + L, *potentia,* power], the electrical potential across a nerve cell membrane before it is stimulated to release the charge. The resting potential for a neuron is between 50 and 100 mV, with the excess of negatively charged ions inside the cell membrane.

**resting tremor,** an involuntary tremor occurring when the person is at rest; one of the signs of Parkinson's disease. Also called **passive tremor.** See also **tremor.**

**restitution** /res'tit(y)oo'shən/, the spontaneous turning of the fetal head to the right or left after it has extended through the vulva.

**rest jaw relation,** the postural relation of the mandible to the maxilla when the patient is resting comfortably in the upright position. The condyles are in a neutral, unstrained position in the mandibular fossae, and the mandibular musculature is in a state of minimum tonic contraction necessary to maintain the posture.

**rest joint position,** the position of a joint where the joint surfaces are relatively incongruent and the support structures are relatively lax. The position is used extensively in passive mobilization procedures.

**restless legs syndrome** [AS, *restlaes* + ONorse, *leggr*], a benign condition of unknown origin characterized by an irritating sensation of uneasiness, tiredness, and itching deep within the muscles of the leg, especially the lower part of the limb, accompanied by twitching and sometimes by pain. The only relief is walking or moving the legs. The condition may be associated with various psychiatric disorders, probably as a form of extrapyramidal hyperkinesis. Also called **anxietas tibiarum, Ekbom's syndrome, Wittmaack-Ekbom syndrome.**

**restoration** /res'tôrā'shən/ [L, *restaurare,* to restore], any tooth filling, inlay, crown, partial or complete denture, or prosthesis that restores or replaces lost tooth structure, entire teeth, or oral tissues. Also called **dental restoration, prosthetic restoration.**

**restoration contour,** the profile of the surfaces of teeth that have been restored.

**restoration of cusps,** a reduction and inclusion of tooth cusps within a tooth cavity preparation and their restoration to functional occlusion with an artificial dental material.

**restorative** /ristôr'ətiv/ [L, *restaurare*], pertaining to the power or ability to restore or renew a person to a normal state of health or consciousness.

**Restoril,** trademark for a hypnotic agent (temazepam).

**restraint** /ristrānt'/ [L, *restringere,* to confine], any one of numerous mechanical devices or chemical agents used to hinder or restrict a patient's movement. Examples of mechanical restraints are specially designed slings, jackets, or diapers. Restraints that are too tight may cause skin irritation; those that fit too loosely do not serve their purpose. When a restraining device needs to be used, it should be correctly sized for the patient and allow enough space for two fingers to fit between the patient's skin and the restraint. Restraints are usually removed every 4 hours or more frequently to assess skin integrity and provide skin care. Release of restraints at least every 2 hours is recommended to allow range-of-motion exercises and assistance with activities of daily living. Throughout the period of restraint, it is important to continue recording all physical and psychosocial assessments in accordance with hospital protocol. See also **mechanical restraint.**

**restraint in bed** [L, *restringere*, to confine; AS, *bedd*], the confinement of a person to bed rest by the use of mechanical, physical, or chemical means, if needed.

**restraint of trade,** an illegal act that interferes with free competition in a commercial or business transaction so as to restrict the production of a product or the provision of a service, affect the cost of a product or a service, or control the market in any way to the detriment of the consumers or purchasers of the service or product. The Clayton Act and the Sherman Antitrust Act are U.S. federal statutes that embody the basic concepts of the definition and the illegal nature of restraint of trade.

**restriction endonuclease** /ristrik'shən en'dōnoo'klē·ās/ [L, *restringere* + Gk, *endon*, within; L, *nucleus* nut kernel; Fr, *diastase*, enzyme], an enzyme that cleaves DNA at a specific site. Each of the many endonucleases isolated from various bacteria acts at a different site, making it possible for researchers to divide DNA molecules at selected locations. See also **restriction fragment length polymorphism.**

**restriction fragment,** a fragment of DNA produced by cleavage by a specific endonuclease.

**restriction fragment length polymorphism (RFLP),** a difference in the DNA sequences of homologous chromosomes as revealed by different lengths of the restriction fragments produced by enzymatic digestion of a selected region of chromosomes. RFLPs are believed to be inherited according to mendelian laws and have been used to locate the genes associated with several inherited disorders, including Huntington's disease.

**restrictive cardiomyopathy.** See **constrictive cardiomyopathy.**

**restrictive disease,** a respiratory disorder characterized by restriction of expansion of the lungs or chest wall, resulting in diminished lung volumes and capacities. Causes include impaired neuromuscular contraction, impaired lung expansion, thoracic deformities, and pleural-based diseases.

**rest seat.** See **rest area.**

**resume, résumé.** See **curriculum vitae.**

**resuscitation**[1] /risus'itā'shən/ [L, *resuscitare*, to revive], the process of sustaining the vital functions of a person in respiratory or cardiac failure while reviving him or her, using techniques of artificial respiration and cardiac massage, correcting acid-base imbalance, and treating the cause of failure. See also **cardiopulmonary resuscitation. —resuscitate,** *v.*

**resuscitation**[2], a nursing intervention from the Nursing Interventions Classification (NIC) defined as administering emergency measures to sustain life. See also **Nursing Interventions Classification.**

**resuscitation: fetus,** a nursing intervention from the Nursing Interventions Classification (NIC) defined as administering emergency measures to improve placental perfusion or correct fetal acid-base status. See also **Nursing Interventions Classification.**

**resuscitation: neonate,** a nursing intervention from the Nursing Interventions Classification (NIC) defined as administering emergency measures to support newborn adaptation to extrauterine life. See also **Nursing Interventions Classification.**

**resuscitator** /risus'itā'tər/, an apparatus for pumping air into the lungs. It consists of a mask snugly applied over the mouth and nose, a reservoir for air, and a manually or electrically powered pump. Often oxygen may be added to the air in the reservoir. See also **Ambu bag, bag-valve-mask resuscitator.**

**RET,** abbreviation for **rational emotive therapy.**

**retail dentistry** /rē'tāl/ [ME, *retailen,* to divide into pieces], the practice of fee-for-service dentistry in an exclusively retail environment, such as a shopping center or a department store, with the specific intention of attracting the customers of that retail environment and by using the marketing techniques of the retailers involved.

**retain.** See **retention.**

**retained placenta** /ritānd'/ [L, *retinere,* to hold, *placenta,* flat cake], the failure of the placenta to be delivered during an appropriate period, usually 30 minutes, following birth of the infant.

**retainer** [L, *retinere,* to hold], **1.** the part of a dental prosthesis that connects an abutment tooth with the suspended part of a bridge. It may be an inlay, a partial crown, or a complete crown. **2.** an appliance for maintaining teeth and jaw positions gained by orthodontic procedures. Also called **retaining orthodontic appliance. 3.** the part of a fixed prosthesis that attaches a pontic to the abutment teeth. **4.** any clasp, attachment, or device for fixing or stabilizing a dental prosthesis.

**retaining orthodontic appliance.** See **retainer.**

**retake** /rē'tāk/, the repeat of a radiograph because of inadequate technical quality, patient motion, mispositioning of the body part, or equipment malfunction.

**retard.** See **retarded.**

**retardation** /rē'tärdā'shən/ [L, *retardare,* to check], the slowing down of any mental or physical activity or failure of intellectual abilities to develop normally, as in mental retardation. Psychomotor retardation may occur in depression, and a conditioned response to an unconditioned stimulus may be retarded in appearance.

**retarded** /ritär'did/ [L, *retardare,* to check], (of physical, intellectual, social, or emotional development) abnormally slow. **—retard** /ritärd'/, *v.*

**retarded dentition,** an abnormal delay in the eruption of the deciduous or secondary teeth resulting from malnutrition, malposition of the teeth, a hereditary factor, or a metabolic imbalance, such as hypothyroidism. Compare **precocious dentition.**

**retarded depression,** the depressive phase of bipolar disorder.

**retarded ejaculation,** the inability of a male to ejaculate after having achieved an erection. This often accompanies the aging process.

**retch** [AS, *hraecan,* to spit], a strong, wrenching attempt to vomit that does not bring up anything. Compare **eructation, vomit.**

**rete** /rē'tē/ [L, net], a network, especially of arteries or veins. **—retial** /rē'tē·əl/, *adj.*

**rete arteriosum.** See **arterial network.**

**retention** /riten'shən/, **1.** a resistance to movement or displacement. **2.** the ability of the digestive system to hold food and fluid. **3.** the inability to urinate or defecate. **4.** the ability of the mind to remember information acquired from reading, observation, or other processes. **5.** the inherent property of a dental restoration to maintain its position without displacement under axial stress. **6.** a characteristic of proper tooth cavity preparation in which provision is made for preventing vertical displacement of the cavity filling. **7.** a period of treatment during which an individual wears an appliance to maintain teeth in positions to which they have been moved by orthodontic procedures. —**retain,** *v.*

**retention cyst** [L, *retinere,* to hold; Gk, *kystis,* bag], one caused by blockage of the excretory duct of a gland, so that glandular secretions are retained; also called **secretory cyst.**

**retention enema** [L, *retinere,* to hold; Gk, *enienai,* to send in], a medicinal or nutrient enema specially formulated so it will remain in the bowel without stimulating the nerve endings that would ordinarily result in evacuation. See also **oil retention enema.**

**retention form,** the provision made in a prepared tooth cavity to hold in place a restoration and to prevent its displacement.

**retention groove,** a depression formed by the opposing vertical constrictions in a prepared tooth cavity, which improves the holding ability of a restoration.

**retention of urine,** an abnormal, involuntary accumulation of urine in the bladder as a result of a loss of muscle tone in the bladder, neurologic dysfunction or damage to the bladder, obstruction of the urethra, or administration of a narcotic analgesic, especially morphine.

**retention pin,** a small metal pin that extends from a metal casting into the dentin of a tooth to improve the holding ability of a tooth restoration.

**retention procedure,** a method established by state laws or mental health codes for committing a person to a psychiatric institution. Most states recognize four types of retention: emergency, informal, involuntary, and voluntary.

**retention time ($t_a$),**   **1.** (in chromatography) the amount of time elapsed from the injection of a sample into the chromatographic system to the recording of the peak (band) maximum of the component in the chromatogram. **2.** the length of time a compound is retained on a chromatography column.

**retention with overflow** [L, *retinere,* to hold; AS, *ofer + flowan*], a complication of bladder outlet obstruction in which urine is retained after a voiding and then dribbles out. Also called **paradoxic incontinence.**

**rete peg.**   See **epithelial peg.**

**retial.**   See **rete.**

**reticul-,** combining form meaning 'netlike': *recticulation, reticulocyte, reticulopod.*

**reticular** /ritik′yələr/ [L, *reticulum,* little net], (of a tissue or surface) having a netlike pattern or structure.

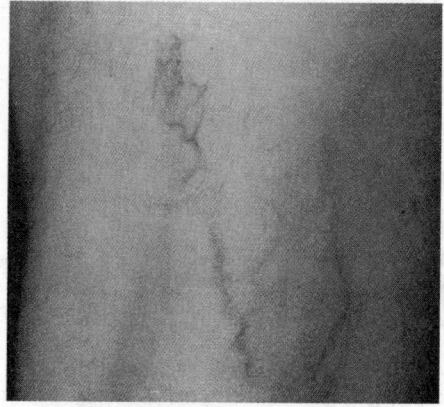

**Reticular vein** *(Goldman, 2001)*

**reticular activating system (RAS),** a functional (rather than a morphologic) system in the brain essential for wakefulness, attention, concentration, and introspection. A network of nerve fibers in the thalamus, hypothalamus, brainstem, and cerebral cortex contribute to the system.

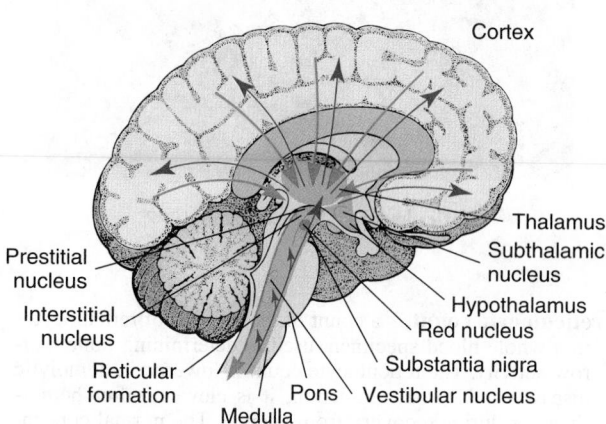

**Reticular activating system** *(Beare and Myers, 1998)*

**reticular formation,** a small, thick cluster of neurons nestled within the brainstem, including the medulla that controls the level of consciousness and other vital functions of the body. The reticular formation constantly monitors the state of the body through connections with the sensory and motor tracts. Certain nerve cells in the formation regulate the flow of hydrochloric acid in the stomach; other cells regulate swallowing, tongue movements, and movements of the face, eyes, and tongue.

**reticular membrane,** a netlike membrane over the organ of Corti; the free ends of the outer acoustic hair cells pass through its apertures. Also called **reticular lamina.**

**reticular nuclei,** nuclei found in the reticular formation of the brainstem, primarily in longitudinal columns in three groups: the median column reticular nuclei (which include the raphe nuclei), the medial column reticular nuclei, and the lateral column reticular nuclei. The term also encompasses several other nuclei that are not in any of the three columns, such as the reticular nucleus of the thalamus.

**reticulated pigmented poikiloderma.**   See **poikiloderma of Civatte.**

**reticulation film fault** /ritik′yəlā′shən/ [L, *reticulum + atio,* process], a defect in a radiograph or photograph that appears as a network of corrugations. It is usually caused during film development by an excessive temperature difference between any two of the three darkroom solutions: the developer, the fixer, and the clearing agent.

**reticulin** /ritik′yəlin/ [L, *reticulum,*], an albuminoid substance found in the connective fibers of reticular tissue.

**reticulocyte** /ritik′yələsīt′/ [L, *reticulum + Gk, kytos,* cell], an immature erythrocyte characterized by a meshlike pattern of threads and particles at the former site of the nucleus. Reticulocytes normally account for less than 2% of the circulating erythrocytes; a greater proportion reflects an increased rate of erythropoiesis in response to hypoxemia. Compare **erythrocyte.** See also **normoblast.**

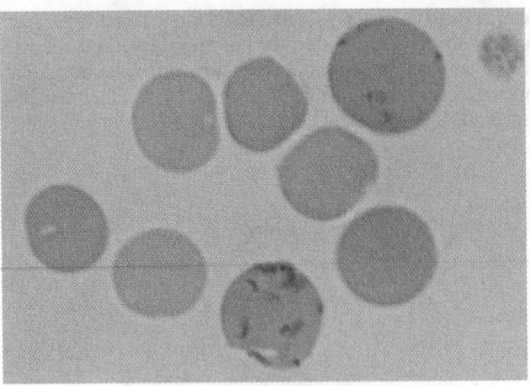

**Reticulocyte** *(Carr and Rodak, 1999)*

**reticulocyte count,** a count of the number of reticulocytes in a whole blood specimen, used in determining bone marrow activity. The reticulocyte count is lowered in hemolytic diseases and chronic infection; it is elevated after hemorrhage or during recovery from anemia. The normal concentration of reticulocytes in whole blood in adults is 0.5% to 1.5% of total RBC.

**reticulocytopenia** /ritik′yəlōsī′təpē′nē·ə/ [L, *reticulum* + Gk, *kytos,* cell, *penia,* poverty], a decrease below the normal range of 0.5% to 1.5% in the number of reticulocytes in a blood sample.

**reticulocytosis** /-sītō′sis/, an increase in the number of reticulocytes in the circulating blood that may represent a normal increase in activity of the bone marrow in response to blood loss, acclimatization to living at a higher altitude, or therapy for anemia.

**reticuloendothelial cells** /ritik′yəlō·en′dōthē′lē·əl/ [L, *reticulum* + Gk, *endon,* within, *thele,* nipple], albuminoid or scleroprotein cells lining vascular and lymph vessels and capable of phagocytosing bacteria, viruses, and colloidal particles or of forming immune bodies against foreign particles.

**reticuloendothelial system (RES),** a functional rather than anatomic system of the body involved primarily in defense against infection and in disposal of the products of the breakdown of cells. It is made up of macrophages; the Kupffer cells of the liver; and the reticulum cells of the lungs, bone marrow, spleen, and lymph nodes. Disorders of this system include **eosinophilic granuloma, Gaucher's disease, Hand-Schüller-Christian syndrome,** and **Niemann-Pick disease.**

**reticuloendotheliosis** /ritik′yəlō·en′dōthē′lē·ō′sis/, an abnormal condition characterized by increased growth and proliferation of the cells of the reticuloendothelial system. See also **reticuloendothelial system.**

**reticulogranular** /-gran′yələr/ [L, *reticulum* + *granulum,* little grain], pertaining to a cloudy appearance of the lungs on a chest radiograph of a patient with respiratory distress syndrome.

**reticulosarcoma.** See **undifferentiated malignant lymphoma.**

**reticulum cell sarcoma.** See **histiocytic malignant lymphoma.**

**-retin,** combining form for retinol derivatives.

**retin-,** combining form meaning 'retina': *retinol, retinopathy.*

**retina** /ret′inə/ [L, *rete,* net], a 10-layered, delicate nervous tissue membrane of the eye, continuous with the optic nerve, that receives images of external objects and transmits visual impulses through the optic nerve to the brain. The retina is soft and semitransparent and contains rhodopsin. It consists of the outer pigmented layer and the nine-layered retina proper. These nine layers, starting with the most internal, are the internal limiting membrane, the stratum opticum, the ganglion cell layer, the inner plexiform layer, the inner nuclear layer, the outer plexiform layer, the outer nuclear layer, the external limiting membrane, and the layer of rods and cones. The outer surface of the retina is in contact with the choroid; the inner surface with the vitreous body. The retina is thinner anteriorly, where it extends nearly as far as the ciliary body, and thicker posteriorly, except for a thin spot in the exact center of the posterior surface where focus is best. The photoreceptors end anteriorly in the jagged ora serrata at the ciliary body, but the membrane of the retina extends over the back of the ciliary processes and the iris.

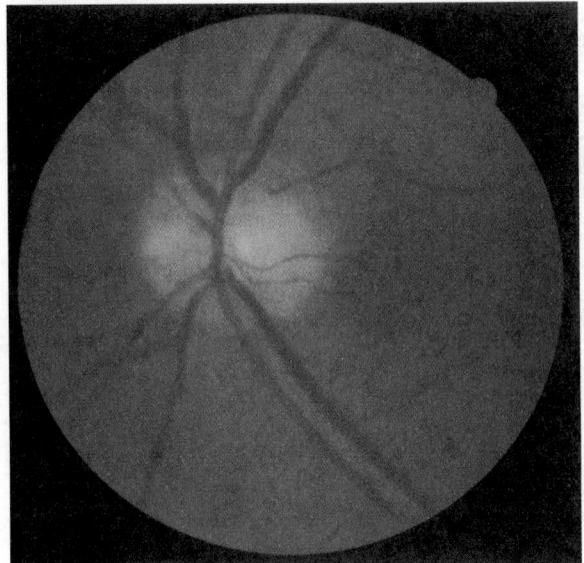

**Retina** *(Wilson and Giddens, 2001/courtesy Dr. Frances C. Gaskin)*

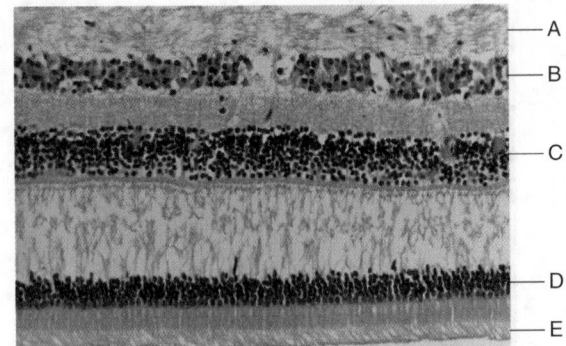

**Layers of the retina: *A,* nerve fiber layer; *B,* ganglion cell layer; *C,* inner nuclear layer; *D,* outer nuclear layer; *E,* rods and cones**

*(Cotran, Kumar, and Collins, 1999/courtesy Dr. Umberto De Girolami, Department of Pathology, Brigham and Women's Hospital, Boston)*

The retina becomes clouded and opaque if exposed to direct sunlight. See also **Jacob x membrane, macula, optic disc.**

**Retin-A,** trademark for a keratolytic (tretinoin).

**retinaculum** /ret'inak'yələm/, *pl.* **retinacula** [L, halter], **1.** a structure that retains an organ or tissue. **2.** an instrument for retracting tissues during surgery.

**retinaculum extensorum manus.** See **extensor retinaculum of hand.**

**retinaculum flexorum manus.** See **flexor retinaculum of hand.**

**retinal** /ret'inəl, ret'inal'/ [L, *rete*], **1.** an aldehyde precursor of vitamin A produced by the enzymatic dehydration of retinol. It is the active form of the vitamin necessary for night, day, and color vision. See also **retinene, vitamin A. 2.** pertaining to the retina.

**retinal detachment,** a separation of the retina from the retinal pigment epithelium in the back of the eye. It usually results from a hole or tear in the retina that allows the vitreous humor to leak between the choroid and the retina. Severe trauma to the eye, such as a contusion or penetrating wound, may be the proximate cause, but in the great majority of cases retinal detachment is the result of internal changes in the vitreous chamber associated with

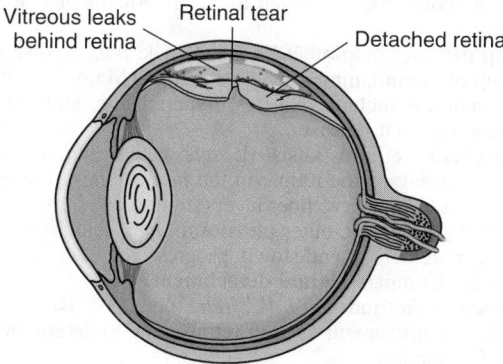

**Retinal detachment: tear in retina**
*(Phipps, Sands, and Marek, 1999)*

aging or less frequently with inflammation of the interior of the eye.

■ OBSERVATIONS: In most cases retinal detachment develops slowly. The first symptom is often the sudden appearance of a large number of floating spots loosely suspended in front of the affected eye. The person may not seek help because the number of spots tends to decrease during the days and weeks after the detachment. The person may also notice a curious sensation of flashing lights as the eye is moved. Because the retina does not contain sensory nerves that relay sensations of pain, the condition is painless. Detachment usually begins at the thin peripheral edge of the retina and extends gradually beneath the thicker, more central areas. The person perceives a shadow that begins laterally and grows in size, slowly encroaching on central vision. As long as the center of the retina is unaffected, the vision, when the person is looking straight ahead, is normal; when the center becomes affected, the eyesight is distorted, wavy, and indistinct. If the process of detachment is not halted, total blindness of the eye ultimately results. The condition does not spontaneously resolve itself.

■ INTERVENTIONS: Surgery is usually required to repair the hole and prevent leakage of vitreous humor that separates the retina from its source of nourishment, the choroid. If the condition is discovered early when the hole is small and the volume of vitreous humor lost is not large, the retinal hole may be closed by causing a scar to form on the choroid and to adhere to the retina around the hole. The scar may be produced by heat, laser energy, or cold. The scar is held against the retina by local pressure achieved by a variety of surgical techniques.

■ NURSING CONSIDERATIONS: Retinal detachment requires treatment. The degree of restoration of sight depends on the extent and duration of separation. Unless replaced, a detached retina slowly dies after several years of detachment. Blindness resulting from retinal detachment is irreversible.

**retinene** /ret'inin/ [L, *rete*], either of the two carotenoid pigments found in the rods of the retina that are precursors of vitamin A and are activated by light. See also **retinal, retinol.**

**retinitis** /ret'ini'tis/ [L, *rete*, net; Gk, *itis,* inflammation], an inflammation of the retina.

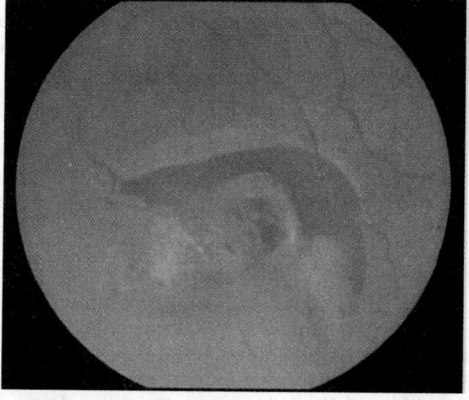

**Retinal detachment: view of fundus**
*(Black, Hawks, and Keene, 2001/courtesy Ophthalmic Photography at the University of Michigan W.K. Kellogg Eye Center, Ann Arbor)*

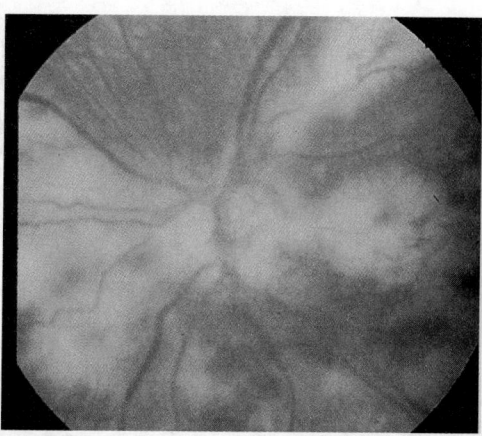

**Retinitis secondary to cytomegalovirus infection**
*(Zitelli and Davis, 1997)*

**retinitis pigmentosa** [L, *rete,* net; Gk, *itis,* inflammation; L, *pigmentum,* paint], a group of diseases, often hereditary, characterized by bilateral primary degeneration of the retina, beginning in childhood and progressing to blindness by middle age. Clinical signs include night blindness, reduced visual fields, depigmentation of the retinal pigment epithelium, and macular degeneration. Length of time to legal blindness varies widely.

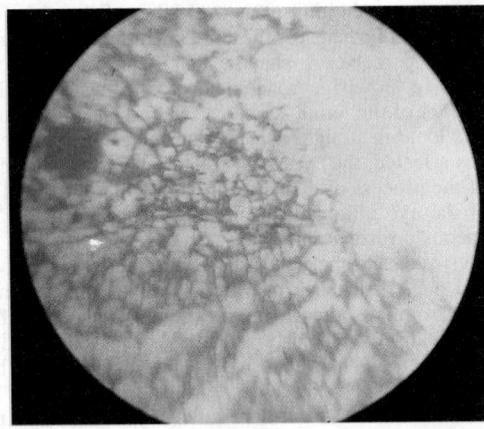

**Retinitis pigmentosa** *(Zitelli and Davis, 1997)*

**retinoblastoma** /ret′inōblastō′mə/, *pl.* **retinoblastomas, retinoblastomata** [L, *rete* + Gk, *blastos,* germ, *oma,* tumor], a congenital hereditary neoplasm developing from retinal germ cells. Characteristic signs are diminished vision, strabismus, retinal detachment, and an abnormal pupillary reflex. The rapidly growing tumor may invade the brain and metastasize to distant sites. Treatment includes removal of the eye and as much of the optic nerve as possible, followed by radiation and chemotherapy. It is bilateral in about 30% of the cases; the more affected eye is enucleated, and the other eye is treated with radiation, antibiotics, cryo-

therapy, or photocoagulation, singly or in combination. Because many of the cases are transmitted as an autosomal-dominant trait with incomplete penetration, genetic counseling is advisable.

**retinocerebral angiomatosis.** See **von Hippel–Lindau disease.**

**retinochoroiditis** /-kôr′oidī′tis/ [L, *rete,* net; Gk, *chorion,* skin, *itis,* inflammation], an inflammation of the retina and choroid coat of the eye. Compare *choroidoretinitis.*

**retinodialysis** /ret′inō′dī·al′isis/ [L, *rete* + Gk, *dia,* through, *lysis,* loosening], a separation or tear in the retina in its anterior part, in the area of the ora serrata, just behind the ciliary body.

**retinoid** /ret′inoid/ [L, *rete,* net; Gk, *eidos,* form], **1.** resembling the retina. **2.** pertaining to any of a group of compounds whose molecules contain 20 carbon atoms structurally related to retinal, retinol, and other substances, some of which exhibit vitamin A activity. Retinoid analogs have been used in the prevention and treatment of various skin cancers and the digestive and respiratory tracts. **3.** resinlike or having a resemblance to resin.

**retinol** /ret′inol/ [L, *rete*], one form of vitamin A. It is found in the retinas of mammals. Also called **vitamin A.**

**retinol equivalent (RE),** a unit used for quantifying the vitamin A value of sources of vitamin A, both including preformed retinoids in animal foods and precursor carotenoids in plant foods. RE is defined as 3.3 International Units of vitamin A.

**retinopathy** /ret′inop′əthē/ [L, *rete* + Gk, *pathos,* disease], a group of noninflammatory eye disorders. Major contributing conditions include diabetes, hypertension, and atherosclerotic vascular disease.

**retinoschisis** /ret′i·nos′ki·sis/ [L, *rete,* net + *schisis,* cleavage], splitting of the retina: in the *juvenile form* the splitting occurs in the nerve fiber layer (stratum opticum), and in the *adult form* in the outer plexiform layer. The disorder is usually more benign and slowly progressive than retinal detachment. Compare **retinal detachment.**

**retinoscope** /ret′inəskōp′/ [L, *rete,* net; Gk, *skopein,* to view], an instrument used in retinoscopy to determine errors of refraction.

**retinoscopy** /ret′inos′kəpē/ [L, *rete,* net; Gk, *skopein,* to view], a procedure for examining the eyes for possible errors of refraction. The examiner shines a light into the eye through the pupillary opening and notes the movements of reflex from the fundus, which will vary with the type of refractive error. The movements indicate the types of lenses needed to neutralize the refractive errors.

**retirement center** /ritī′ərmənt/ [Fr, *retirer,* to withdraw; Gk, *kentron,* center], a facility or organized program to provide social services and activities for senior citizens who generally do not require ongoing health care.

**retract** /ritrakt′/ [L, *retractare,* to draw back], to shrink, make shorter, or pull back.

**retracted nipple** [L, *retractare,* to draw back; ME, *neb*], a nipple drawn inward, resulting from cancer or adhesions below the skin surface or a natural condition present at birth.

**retractile mesenteritis** /rē·trak′tīl/ [L, *retractare,* to draw back; Gk, *mesos,* middle + *enteron,* intestine + *-itis,* inflammation], inflammation of the mesentery producing thickening, sclerosis, and retraction, and occasionally resulting in distortion of intestinal loops.

**retraction** /ritrak′shən/ [L, *retractare,* to draw back], **1.** the displacement of tissues to expose a part or structure of the body. **2.** a distal movement of the teeth. **3.** a distal or retrusive position of the teeth, dental arch, or jaw.

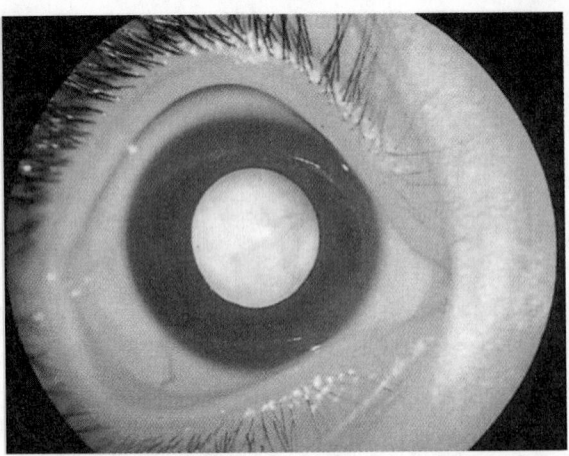

**Retinoblastoma** *(Michelson and Friedlaender, 1996)*

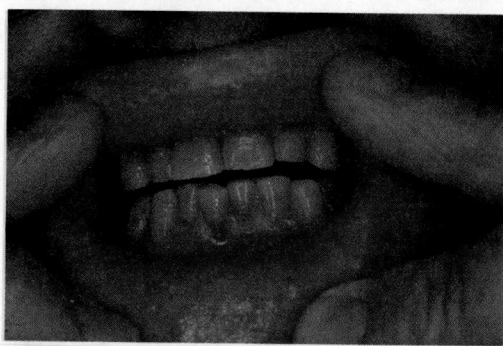

**Retraction of the gums** *(Lemmi and Lemmi, 2000)*

**retraction of the chest,** the visible sinking in of the soft tissues of the chest between and around the firmer tissue of the cartilaginous and bony ribs, as occurs with increased inspiratory effort or obstruction at some level of the respiratory tract. The extent of retraction depends on the level of an obstruction. Retraction begins in the intercostal spaces. If increased effort is needed to fill the lungs, supraclavicular and infraclavicular retraction may be seen. In infants sternal retraction occurs with only a slight increase in respiratory effort, the result of the pliability of their chests. Compare **intercostal bulging.**

**retractor** /ritrak′tər/ [L, *retractare*], an instrument for holding back the edges of tissues and organs to maintain exposure of the underlying anatomic parts, particularly during surgery.

**retro-,** prefix meaning 'backward, or located behind': *retronasal, retroperitoneal, retroversion.*

**retroanterograde amnesia** /ret′rō-anter′ōgrād/ [L, *retro,* backward, *antero,* foremost, *gradus,* step; Gk, *amnesia,* forgetfulness], a memory disorder in which current events may be assigned to the past and past events may be regarded as current.

**retroaortic node** /ret′rō-ā-ôr′tik/ [L, *retro,* backward; Gk, *aerein,* to raise], a node in one of three sets of lumbar lymph nodes that serve various structures in the abdomen and pelvis. They lie below the cisterna chyli on the bodies of the third and the fourth lumbar vertebrae and receive the lymphatic trunks from the lateral aortic nodes and preaortic nodes. The efferent vessels from the retroaortic nodes end in the cisterna chyli. Compare **lateral aortic node, preaortic node.**

**retroauricular** /ret′rō-ôrik′yələr/ [L, *retro,* backward, *auricula,* little ear], pertaining to a location behind the ear.

**retrobulbar** /-bul′bər/ [L, *retro,* backward, *bulbus,* swollen root], **1.** pertaining to the area behind the pons (posterior to the medulla oblongata). **2.** pertaining to the area behind the eyeball.

**retrobulbar neuritis** [L, *retro,* backward, *bulbus,* swollen root; Gk, *neuron + itis,* inflammation], a form of neuritis that involves the optic nerve or the optic disc. Also called **optic neuritis.**

**retrobulbar pupillary reflex,** an abnormal response of a pupil to light. After initial constriction of the pupil, dilation occurs as the stimulus continues. It is a sign of retrobulbar neuritis.

**retrocecal** /-sē′kəl/ [L, *retro,* backward, *caecus,* blind], pertaining to the region behind the cecum. Also spelled **retrocaecal.**

**retroclusion** /ret′rokloo′zhən/, a method of controlling hemorrhage from an artery by compressing it between tissues on either side. A needle is inserted through the tissues above the bleeding vessel, then turned around and down so it also passes through the tissues beneath the artery.

**retroflexion** /-flek′shən/ [L, *retro + flectere,* to bend], an abnormal position of an organ in which the organ is tilted back acutely, folded over on itself, as for example the uterus.

**retroflexion of the uterus,** a condition in which the body of the uterus is bent backward at an angle with the cervix, whose position usually remains unchanged.

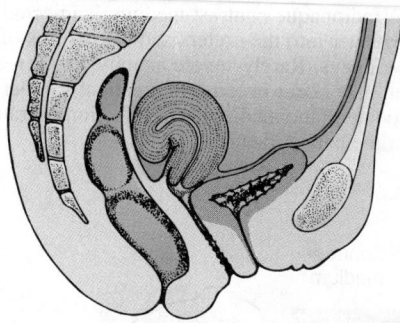

**Retroflexion of the uterus** *(Beare and Myers, 1998)*

**retrognathia** /ret′rōnā′thē·ə/ [L, *retro,* backward; Gk, *gnathos,* jaw], a condition in which either or both jaws recede with respect to the frontal plane of the forehead. According to Angle's Classification of Malocclusion, the facial profile of a person with a Class II malocclusion is retrognathic. Also called **mandibular (or maxillary) retroposition, mandibular (or maxillary) retrusion.**

**retrognathism** /ret′rōnā′thizəm/ [L, *retro + Gk, gnathos,* jaw], a facial abnormality in which a jaw, usually the mandible, or both jaws are posterior to their normal facial positions. Also called **bird-face retrognathism.**

**retrograde** /ret′rəgrād/ [L, *retro + gradus,* step], **1.** moving backward; moving in the opposite direction to that which is considered normal. **2.** degenerating; reverting to an earlier state or worse condition. **3.** catabolic.

**retrograde amnesia,** the loss of memory for events occurring before a particular time in a person's life, usually before the event that precipitated the amnesia. The condition may result from disease, brain injury or damage, or a traumatic emotional incident. Compare **anterograde amnesia.**

**retrograde cystoscopy,** a technique for radiographically examining the bladder in which a catheter is inserted through the urethra into the bladder, allowing the urine present in the bladder to pass through the catheter. A radiopaque medium is introduced, filling the bladder, and the contour of the bladder is observed, using serial x-ray films or fluoroscopy. See also **cystogram, retrograde pyelography.**

**retrograde ejaculation** [L, *retro,* backward, *gradus,* step, *ejaculari,* to throw out], an ejaculation of semen in a reverse direction into the urinary bladder. The effect is sometimes the result of prostate surgery or a congenital condition.

**retrograde filling,** a filling placed in the apical part of a tooth root to seal that part of the root canal. Also called **postresection filling.**

**retrograde flow** [L, *retro,* backward; AS, *flowan*],    the flow of fluid in a direction other than normal, as in regurgitation.

**retrograde infantilism.**    See **acromegalic eunuchoidism.**

**retrograde infection,**    an infection that spreads along a tubule or duct against the flow of secretions or excretions, as in the urinary and lymphatic systems.

**retrograde menstruation,**    a backflow of menstrual discharge through the uterine cavity and fallopian tubes into the peritoneal cavity. Fragments of endometrium may attach to the ovaries or other organs, causing endometriosis. Also called **regurgitant menstruation.**

**retrograde pyelography,**    a radiologic technique for examining the structures of the collecting system of the kidneys that is especially useful in locating a urinary tract obstruction. A radiopaque contrast medium is injected through a urinary catheter into the ureters and the calyces of the pelves of the kidneys. Rarely severe anaphylactoid reaction to the medium may occur because of a patient's hypersensitivity to the iodine in the medium, and infection or trauma may result from the catheterization.

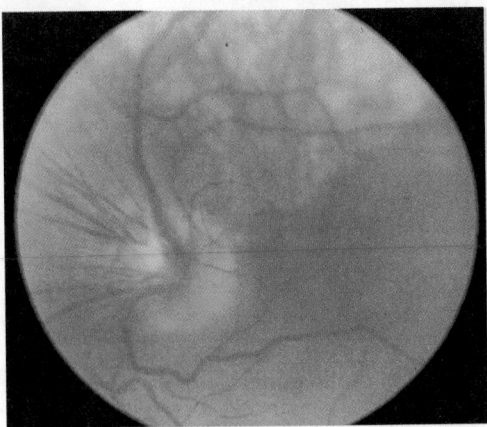

**Retrolental fibroplasia** *(Zitelli and Davis, 1997)*

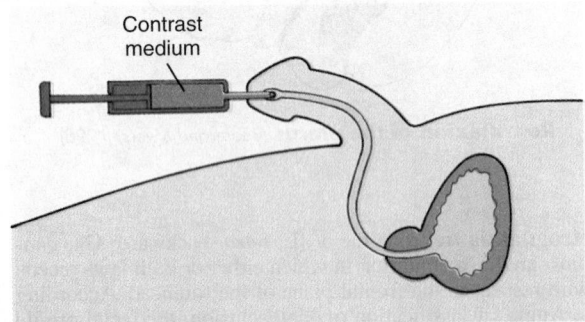

**Technique for retrograde pyelography** *(Gray, 1992)*

**retrograde urography.**    See **retrograde pyelography.**

**retrograde Wenckebach** /veng'kəbäk, -bäkh/ [Karel F. Wenckebach, Dutch-Austrian physician, 1864–1940],    a delay in the conduction of impulses from the ventricles or atrioventricular junction to the atria. The delay increases progressively until an impulse fails to reach the atria.

**retrogression** /-gresh'ən/ [L, *retro* + *gradi,* to step],    a return to a less complex state, condition, or behavioral adaptation; degeneration; deterioration. See also **regression.**

**retrolental fibroplasia** /-len'təl/ [L, *retro* + *lentil,* lens, *fibra,* fiber; Gk, *plassein,* to mold],    a formation of fibrous tissue behind the lens of the eye, resulting in blindness. The disorder is caused by administration of excessive concentrations of oxygen to premature infants.

**retromolar pad** /-mō'lər/ [L, *retro* + *mola,* mill; D, *paden,* cushion],    a mass of soft tissue, usually pear-shaped, that marks the distal termination of the mandibular residual ridge. It is composed of mucous glands and fibers of the buccinator muscle, the pterygomandibular raphe, the superior constrictor muscle, and the temporal tendon.

**retromylohyoid space** /ret'rōmī'lōhī'oid/ [L, *retro* + Gk, *myle,* mill, *hyoeides,* U-shaped; L, *spatium*],    the part of the alveolingual sulcus that is distal to the distal end of the mylohyoid ridge.

**retroperitoneal** /-per'itənē'əl/ [L, *retro* + Gk, *peri,* around, *teinein,* to stretch],    pertaining to organs closely attached to the posterior abdominal wall and partly covered by peritoneum, rather than suspended by that membrane.

**retroperitoneal abscess,**    a collection of pus between the peritoneum and the posterior abdominal wall.

**retroperitoneal fibrosis,**    a chronic inflammatory process, usually of unknown cause, in which fibrous tissue surrounds the large blood vessels in the lower lumbar area. It frequently causes constriction of the midportion of the ureters, which may lead to hydronephrosis and azotemia. Occasionally the fibrosis spreads upward to involve the duodenum, bile ducts, and superior vena cava. Symptoms include lowback and abdominal pain, weakness, weight loss, fever, and, with urinary tract involvement, frequency of urination, hematuria, polyuria, or anuria. Methysergide, taken to prevent migraine headaches, is one known cause of this condition. Treatment includes stopping methysergide and instituting surgical release of the ureters from the fibrosis with transplantation laterally or intraperitoneally.

**retroperitoneal lymph node dissection,**    surgical removal of lymph nodes bilaterally behind the peritoneum, and the lymph channels and fat around both renal pedicles, the vena cava, and the aorta. The dissection is usually performed in an attempt to eliminate sites of lymphoma or metastases from malignancies originating in pelvic organs or genitalia. Also known as **radical lymphadenectomy.**

**retroperitoneum** /-per'itənē'əm/ [L, *retro,* backward; Gk, *peri* + *teinein,* to stretch],    the space behind the peritoneum.

**retropharyngeal abscess** /-fərin'jē·əl/ [L, *retro* + Gk, *pharynx,* throat],    a collection of pus in the tissues behind the pharynx accompanied by difficulty in swallowing, fever, and pain. Occasionally the airway becomes obstructed. Treatment includes appropriate parenteral antibiotics and surgical drainage. Tracheostomy may be necessary. Compare **parapharyngeal abscess, peritonsillar abscess.**

**retroplacental** /-pləsen'təl/,    behind the placenta.

**retrospective chart audit** /-spek'tiv/ [L, *retro* + *spicere,* to look],    a format for an audit developed by the Joint Commission on Accreditation of Healthcare Organizations. The audit involves several steps that outline a procedure for evaluating the effectiveness of the care given at a particular institution and for correcting any deficiencies found by reviewing the patient's records after discharge and comparing the data with standards held to be adequate by the Commission.

**retrospective nursing audit.** See **nursing audit.**17

**retrospective study,** a study in which a search is made for a relationship between one (usually current) phenomenon or condition and another that occurred in the past. An example is a study of the family histories of young women diagnosed as having clear cell adenomas of the vagina, which yielded a relationship between the administration of diethylstilbestrol to the mothers of the women during pregnancy and the development of the condition in the daughters.

**retrosternal** /-stur′nəl/ [L, *retro,* backward; Gk, *sternon,* chest], behind the sternum.

**retrouterine** /re′trōyo͞o′tərin/, behind the uterus.

**retroversion** /-vur′zhən/ [L, *retro* + *vertere,* to turn], **1.** a common condition in which an organ is tipped backward, usually without flexion or other distortion. The uterus may be retroverted in as many as one fourth of normal women. Uterine retroversion is measured as first-, second-, or third-degree, depending on the angle of tilt with respect to the vagina. Compare **anteversion.** See also **anteflexion, retroflexion. 2.** an abnormal condition in which the teeth or other maxillary and mandibular structures are posterior to their normal positions. Also called **retrusion. —retrovert,** *v.*

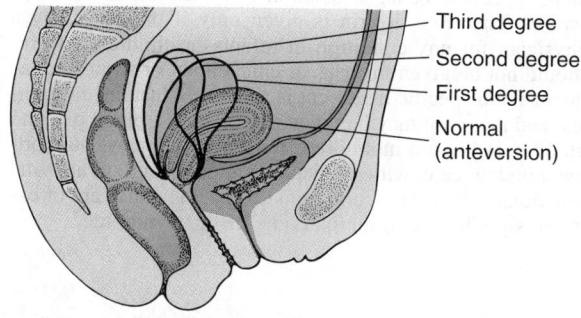

- Third degree
- Second degree
- First degree
- Normal (anteversion)

**Retroversion of the uterus** *(Beare and Myers, 1998)*

**Retrovir,** trademark for an antiretroviral drug, **zidovudine.**

**retrovirus** /-vī′rəs/ [L, *retro* + *virus*], any of a family of ribonucleic acid (RNA) viruses containing an enzyme, reverse transcriptase, in the virion. The genetic information of the virus is stored in a molecule of single-stranded ribonucleic acid. After entering the target cell, the virus uses reverse transcriptase to direct the cell to make viral deoxyribonucleic acid (DNA). The DNA becomes integrated into the DNA of the host cell. Retroviruses are enveloped and assemble their capsids in the cytoplasm of the host cell. Retroviruses are used in laboratory research to import foreign DNA into a cell. They are transmitted by sexual contact with an infected person through exposure to infected blood or blood products and perinatally from an infected mother to the child. Human immunodeficiency virus (HIV1, HIV2), which causes acquired immunodeficiency syndrome, is a retrovirus. Other retroviruses include members of the Oncornaviridae family such as human T cell lymphotropic virus type 1 (HTLV-1) and human T cell lymphotropic virus type 2 (HTLV-2), which cause adult T-cell leukemia, hairy cell leukemia, tropical spastic paresis, and HTLV-1–associated myelopathy.

**retrusion.** See **retroversion.**

**Rett syndrome** /ret/ [Andreas Rett, Austrian physician, 20th century], a pervasive developmental disorder affecting the gray matter of the brain, occurring exclusively in females and present from birth; it is progressive and is characterized by autistic behavior, ataxia, dementia, seizures, and loss of purposeful use of the hands, with cerebral atrophy, mild hyperammonemia, and decreased levels of biogenic amines. Also called **cerebroatrophic hyperammonemia.**

**revaccination** /rēvak′sinā′shən/, an immunization that is repeated although the original was successful.

**revascularization** /rēvas′kyələr′īzā′shən/ [L, *re* + *vasculum,* small vessel; Gk, *izein,* to cause], the restoration by surgical means of blood flow to an organ or a tissue, as in bypass surgery.

**reverberation** /rivur′bərā′shən/, the phenomenon of multiple reflections within a closed system.

**Reverdin's needle** /reverdaNz′/ [Jaques L. Reverdin, Swiss surgeon, 1842–1929], a surgical needle with an eye that can be opened and closed with a slide.

**reversal film** /rivur′səl/, (in radiology) a reverse-tone duplicate of an x-ray image, showing black changed to white and white to black. It is produced by exposing single-emulsion subtraction film through a standard x-ray film. Also called **diapositive, positive mask.**

**reverse anaphylaxis.** See **inverse anaphylaxis.**

**reverse Barton's fracture** /rivurs′/ [L, *revertere,* to turn back; John R. Barton, American surgeon, 1794–1871], a break in the volar articular surface of the radius with associated displacement of the carpal bones and radius.

**reverse bevel.** See **contra bevel.**

**reverse Colles' fracture.** See **Smith fracture.**

**reverse curve,** a convex curve of dental occlusion, as viewed in the frontal plane.

**reversed bandage** /rivurst′/, a roller bandage that is reversed on itself with a half twist so that it lies smoothly, conforming to the contour of the extremity. See also **roller bandage.**

**reversed coarctation.** See **Takayasu's arteritis.**

**reversed I:E ratio.** See **inverse I:E ratio.**

**reversed phase,** a chromatographic mode in which the mobile phase is more polar than the stationary phase.

**reverse isolation,** isolation procedures designed to protect a patient from infectious organisms that might be carried by the staff, other patients, or visitors or on droplets in the air or on equipment or materials. Absolute reverse isolation is rarely necessary and requires elaborate specialized equipment. Protective modified reverse isolation is less restrictive but is not prolonged needlessly, because the patient usually feels lonely and sensorially deprived. Handwashing, gowning, gloving, sterilization, or disinfection of materials brought into the area and other details of housekeeping vary with the reason for the isolation and the usual practices of the hospital.

**reverse peristalsis** [L, *revertere,* to turn back; Gk, *peristellein,* to clasp], peristalsis that propels the contents in a direction opposite to the normal outward direction.

**reverse transcriptase (RT),** an enzyme that is present in the virion of retroviruses. Also called **RNA-dependent DNA polymerase.** See also **retrovirus.**

**reverse transcriptase inhibitor,** a compound that inhibits the enzyme used by retroviruses to synthesize complementary DNA from viral RNA inside host cells.

**reverse Trendelenburg** [Friedrich Trendelenburg], a position in which the lower extremities are lower than the body and head, which are elevated on an inclined plane.

**reversible** /rivur′sibəl/, able to return to its original state or condition, as in a chemical reaction.

**reversible brain syndrome,** any of a group of acute brain disorders characterized by a disruption of cognition, as in delirium. The symptoms widely vary. The disorder is related to a variety of biologic stressors. Recovery is likely.

**reversible vascular hyperplasia,** a variation of Kaposi's sarcoma in which human immunodeficiency virus may induce cells to produce a chemical growth factor. The growth factor, in turn, makes lymphatic endothelial cells proliferate. The process may cascade as each new Kaposi's sarcoma cell produces more growth factor.

**reversion** /rivur′zhən/, **1.** the appearance in offspring of traits expressed in previous but not immediately recent generations. **2.** a return to an original phenotype, by mutation or reinstatement of the original genotype.

**review of systems (ROS)** /rivyoo′/ [Fr, *revoir,* to see again], (in a health history) a system-by-system review of the body functions. The ROS is begun during the initial interview with the patient and completed during the physical examination, as physical findings prompt further questions. Questions about family or personal history are included in each section. One outline of the systems and some of the signs and symptoms that might be noted or reported are as follows:

■ SKIN: bruising, discoloration, pruritus, birthmarks, moles, ulcers, decubiti, changes in the hair or nails, sun exposure and protection.

■ HEMATOPOIETIC: spontaneous or excessive bleeding, fatigue, enlarged or tender lymph nodes, pallor, history of anemia.

■ HEAD AND FACE: pain, traumatic injury, ptosis.

■ EARS: tinnitus, change in hearing, running or discharge from the ears, deafness, dizziness.

■ EYES: change in vision, pain, inflammation, infections, double vision, scotomata, blurring, tearing.

■ MOUTH AND THROAT: dental problems, hoarseness, dysphagia, bleeding gums, sore throat, ulcers or sores in the mouth.

■ NOSE AND SINUSES: discharge, epistaxis, sinus pain, obstruction.

■ BREASTS: pain, change in contour or skin color, lumps, discharge from the nipple.

■ RESPIRATORY TRACT: cough, sputum, change in sputum, night sweats, nocturnal dyspnea, wheezing.

■ CARDIOVASCULAR SYSTEM: chest pain, dyspnea, palpitations, weakness, intolerance of exercise, varicosities, swelling of extremities, known murmur, hypertension, asystole.

■ GASTROINTESTINAL SYSTEM: nausea, vomiting, diarrhea, constipation, quality of appetite, change in appetite, dysphagia, gas, heartburn, melena, change in bowel habits, use of laxatives or other drugs to alter the function of the gastrointestinal tract.

■ URINARY TRACT: dysuria, change in color of urine, change in frequency of urination, pain with urgency, incontinence, edema, retention, nocturia.

■ GENITAL TRACT (FEMALE): menstrual history, obstetric history, contraceptive use, discharge, pain or discomfort, pruritus, history of venereal disease, sexual history.

■ GENITAL TRACT (MALE): penile discharge, pain or discomfort, pruritus, skin lesions, hematuria, history of venereal disease, sexual history.

■ SKELETAL SYSTEM: heat, redness, swelling, limitation of function, deformity, crepitation; pain in a joint or an extremity, the neck, or the back, especially with movement.

■ NERVOUS SYSTEM: dizziness, tremor, ataxia, difficulty in speaking, change in speech, paresthesia, loss of sensation, seizures, syncope, changes in memory.

■ ENDOCRINE SYSTEM: tremor, palpitations, intolerance of heat or cold, polyuria, polydipsia, polyphagia, diaphoresis, exophthalmos, goiter.

■ PSYCHOLOGIC STATUS: nervousness, instability, depression, phobia, sexual disturbances, criminal behavior, insomnia, night terrors, mania, memory loss, perseveration, disorientation.

**Revised Trauma Score,** a system of combining cardiopulmonary assessment with the Glasgow Coma Score in estimating the degree of injury and the prognosis in a trauma patient. The cardiopulmonary factors included are respiratory rate and systolic blood pressure.

**Reye's syndrome** /rāz′/ [Ralph D. K. Reye, twentieth century Australian pathologist], a combination of acute encephalopathy and fatty infiltration of the internal organs that may follow acute viral infections. This syndrome has been associated with influenza B, chickenpox (varicella), the enteroviruses, and the Epstein-Barr virus. It usually affects people under 18 years of age, characteristically causing an exanthematous rash, vomiting, and confusion about 1 week after the onset of a viral illness. In the late stage there may be extreme disorientation followed by coma, seizures, and respiratory arrest. Laboratory tests reveal greater than normal amounts of SGOT and SGPT, bilirubin, and ammonia in the blood. A specimen obtained by liver biopsy shows fatty degeneration and confirms the diagnosis. Mortality varies between 20% and 80%, depending on the severity of symptoms. The cause of Reye's syndrome is unknown; however, there appears to be an association with the administration of aspirin. Therefore aspirin is given only if prescribed by a physician for any condition in infants or children. Aspirin should not be given in cases of chickenpox or suspected influenza. No specific treatment is available. Insulin, antibiotics, and mannitol may be given. Blood gases, blood pH, and blood pressure are monitored frequently. Intensive supportive nursing care with meticulous monitoring of all vital functions and prompt correction of any imbalance are of extreme significance in the outcome of this syndrome.

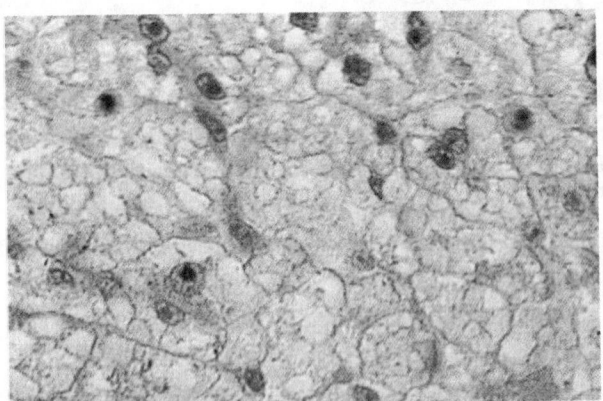

**Reye's syndrome: fatty infiltration of the liver**
*(Farrar, 1993)*

**rf,** **1.** abbreviation for **radiofrequency. 2.** abbreviation for **rheumatic fever.**

**Rf,** **1.** symbol for the element **rutherfordium. 2.** (in chromatography) abbreviation for retardation factor.

**RF,** abbreviation for **rheumatoid factor.**

**R factor,** an episome in bacteria that is responsible for drug resistance and is transmissible to progeny and to other bacterial cells by conjugation. The part of the episome involved in replication and transmission is called **resistance transfer factor.**

**RFP,** abbreviation for **request for proposal.**

**RF (rheumatoid factor) test.** See **latex fixation test.**

**RGP,** abbreviation for **rigid gas permeable.** See **rigid gas permeable (RGP) contact lens.**

**Rh, 1.** abbreviation for *rhesus.* See **Rh factor. 2.** symbol for the chemical element **rhodium.**

**-rh-.** For combining forms containing **-rh-** or **-(r)rh:** *anarrhea, arteriorrhexis.*

**r/h, 1.** abbreviation for **relative humidity. 2.** abbreviation for *roentgens per hour.*

**rhabdo-, rhabdi-,** combining form meaning 'rod-shaped' or 'pertaining to a rod': *rhabdocyte, rhabdomyoma, rhabdosarcoma.*

**rhabdomyo-,** combining form meaning 'striated or skeletal muscle': *rhabdomyolysis, rhabdomyoma.*

**rhabdomyoblast** /rab'dōmī'əblast'/ [Gk, *rhabdos,* rod, *mys,* muscle, *blastos,* germ], large round spindle-shaped cells with cross striations, found in some rhabdomyosarcomas.

**rhabdomyoblastoma.** See **rhabdomyosarcoma.**

**rhabdomyolysis** /rab'dōmī·ol'isis/, a paroxysmal, potentially fatal disease of skeletal muscle characterized by the presence of myoglobin in the urine. It is also associated with acute renal failure in heatstroke.

**rhabdomyoma** /rab'dōmī·ō'mə/, *pl.* **rhabdomyomas, rhabdomyomata** [Gk, *rhabdos,* rod, *mys,* muscle, *oma*], a tumor of striated muscle that may occur in the uterus, vagina, pharynx, tongue, or heart. Also called **myoma striocellulare.**

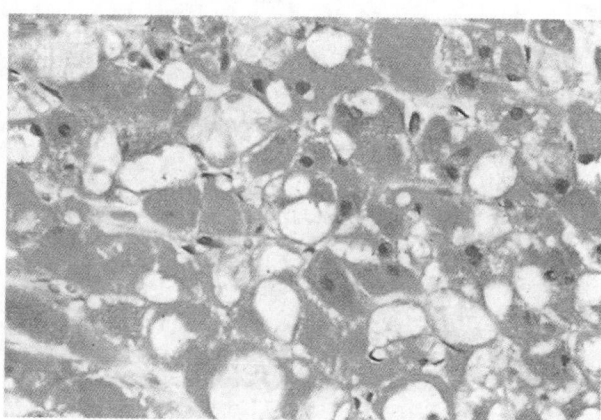

**Rhabdomyoma** *(Eveson and Scully, 1995)*

**rhabdomyosarcoma** /rab'dōmī'ō·särkō'mə/, *pl.* **rhabdomyosarcomas, rhabdomyosarcomata** [Gk, *rhabdos* + *mys,* muscle, *sarx,* flesh, *oma*], a highly malignant tumor derived from primitive striated muscle cells that occurs most frequently in the head and neck and is also found in the genitourinary tract, extremities, body wall, and retroperitoneum. In some cases the onset is associated with trauma. The initial symptoms depend on the site of tumor development and indicate local tissue or organ destruction, such as dysphagia, vaginal bleeding, hematuria, or obstructed flow of urine. Diagnostic measures may include barium x-ray studies, angiography, or tomography. Embryonal rhab-

domyosarcoma occurs in the head, neck, or trunk of young children; alveolar rhabdomyosarcoma is usually seen in the extremities of adolescents; and the pleomorphic form is most common in the legs of adults. Surgical excision is rarely possible because the tumor is poorly encapsulated and tends to spread. Amputation of an affected limb or extremity may be curative. Radiotherapy and chemotherapy with combinations of actinomycin D, adriamycin, cyclophosphamide, and vincristine may greatly increase the length of survival. Also called **rhabdomyoblastoma, rhabdosarcoma.**

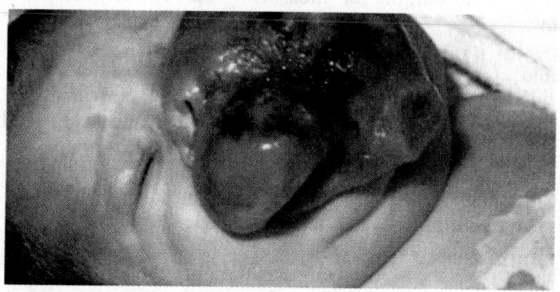

**Embryonal rhabdomyosarcoma**
*(Weston, Lane, and Morrelli, 1996)*

**rhabdosphincter** /rab'dōsfingk'tər/, a sphincter composed of striated muscle fibers.

**rhabdovirus** /rab'dōvī'rəs/ [Gk, *rhabdos* + L, *virus,* poison], a member of a family of viruses that includes the organism causing rabies.

**rhachi-.** See **rachio-.**

**rhagades** /rag'ədēz/ [Gk, chinks], cracks or fissures in skin that has lost its elasticity, especially common around the mouth. See also **cheilosis.**

**-rhage, -rrhage, -rhagia, -rrhagia,** combining, form meaning 'excessive flow': *metrorrhagia, hemorrhage.*

**Rh antiserum** [Rh, rhesus; Gk, *anti,* against; L, *serum,* whey], a serum that contains Rh antibodies.

**rhaphe.** See **raphe.**

**-rhaphy, -rrhaphy,** suffix meaning 'suturing in place': *colporrhaphy, gastrorrhaphy.*

**Rh blood group.** See **Rh factor.**

**rhd, 1.** abbreviation for *radioactive health data.* **2.** abbreviation for **rheumatic heart disease.**

**rhe** /rē/, **1.** an absolute unit of fluidity in the centimeter-gram-second (CGS) system. **2.** the reciprocal of the unit of viscosity expressed as 1/poise or 1/centipoise.

**-rhea, -rrhea,** suffix meaning 'flow or discharge': *rhinorrhea, galactorrhea.*

**rhegmatogenous** /reg'mətoj'ənəs/ [Gk, *rhegma,* breakage, *gen,* producing], arising from a tear or rupture in an organ.

**rhegmatogenous retinal detachment,** a separation of the retina associated with a hole, break, or tear in the sensory layer of the retina. The detachment occurs secondary to the formation of the opening.

**rhenium (Re)** /rē'nē·əm/ [L, *Rhenus,* Rhine], a hard, brittle metallic element. Its atomic number is 75; its atomic mass (weight) is 186.21. Rhenium has a high melting point and is used in x-ray tube anodes and in thermometers for measuring high temperatures.

**rheo-,** combining form meaning 'electric current, stream, flow': *rheobase, rheoscope, rheotaxis, rheostosis.*

**rheobase** /rē′əbās/, the least amount of electricity that will produce a stimulated response.

**rheoencephalogram** /rē′ō·ensef′əlōgram′/, a graphic representation of the changes in electrical conductivity of the head caused by blood flowing through vessels in the head.

**rheogram** /rē′əgram/, a plot of shear stress versus the shear flow of a fluid.

**rheology** /rē·ol′əjē/, the study of the flow and deformation of matter.

**Rheomacrodex,** trademark for a plasma expander (dextran 40).

**rheometry** /rē·om′ətrē/ [Gk, *rheos,* current, *metron,* measure], a technique for measuring the velocity of blood flow.

**rheostat** /rē′əstat/ [Gk, *rheos,* current, *statikos,* causing to stand], a variable resistance electrical device that can be adjusted to control the strength of a current.

**rheostosis** /rē′ostō′sis/, a condition of bone overgrowth marked by streaks in the bones.

**rhestocythemia** /res′tōsīthē′mē·ə/, the presence of damaged red blood cells in the peripheral circulation.

**Rhesus factor.** See **Rh factor.**

**rheum** /rōōm/ [Gk, *rheuma,* flow], a watery or mucous discharge from the skin or mucous membranes.

**rheumatic** /rōōmat′ik/ [Gk, *rheuma,* flux], pertaining to rheumatism.

**-rheumatic,** suffix meaning 'relating to or exhibiting traits of rheumatism': *postrheumatic, prerheumatic, pseudorheumatic.*

**rheumatic aortitis,** an inflammatory condition of the aorta, occurring in rheumatic fever. It is characterized by disseminated focal lesions that may progressively form patches of fibrosis.

**rheumatic arteritis,** a complication of rheumatic fever characterized by generalized inflammation of arteries and arterioles. Fibrin mixed with cellular debris may invade, thicken, and stiffen vessel walls and the affected vessels may be surrounded by hemorrhage and exudate.

**rheumatic carditis** [Gk, *rheuma,* flux, *kardia,* heart, *itis,* inflammation], pericarditis, myocarditis, and endocarditis that may be associated with acute rheumatic fever.

**rheumatic chorea.** See **Sydenham's chorea.**

**rheumatic endocarditis** [Gk, *rheuma,* flux, *endon,* within, *kardia,* heart, *itis,* inflammation], inflammation of the endocardium in association with acute rheumatic fever.

**rheumatic fever,** systemic inflammatory disease that may develop as a delayed reaction to an inadequately treated infection of the upper respiratory tract by group A beta-hemolytic streptococci. The disease usually occurs in young school-age children and may affect the brain, heart, joints, skin, or subcutaneous tissues. See also **rheumatic heart disease.**

■ OBSERVATIONS: The onset of rheumatic fever is usually sudden, often occurring 1 to 5 symptom-free weeks after recovery from a sore throat or scarlet fever. Early symptoms generally include fever, joint pain, nose bleeds, abdominal pain, and vomiting. The major manifestations of this disease include migratory polyarthritis affecting numerous joints and carditis, which causes palpitations, chest pain, and in severe cases symptoms of cardiac failure. Sydenham's chorea is usually the sole late sign of rheumatic fever and may initially be manifested as an increased awkwardness and tendency to drop objects. As the chorea progresses, irregular body movements may become extensive, occasionally involving the tongue and facial muscles, resulting in incapacitation. Other developments may include transient erythema marginatum with circular lesions and subcutaneous rheumatic nodules on various joints and tendons, the spine, and the back of the head. There is no specific diagnostic test for rheumatic fever. The development of serum antibodies to streptococcal antigens is a positive diagnostic sign. Affected individuals may also develop leukocytosis, moderate anemia, and proteinuria. C-reactive protein, evaluated in a specimen of blood, is abnormally high in concentration. Recurrences of rheumatic fever are common. Except for carditis, all the manifestations of the disease usually subside without any permanent effects. Mild cases may last 3 to 4 weeks. Severe cases with associated arthritis and carditis may last 2 to 3 months.

■ INTERVENTIONS: Management of rheumatic fever includes bed rest and severe restriction of normal activity. Penicillin is often administered, even if throat cultures are negative, and steroids or salicylates may be used, depending on the severity of any associated carditis and arthritis.

■ NURSING CONSIDERATIONS: Symptoms largely determine the type of nursing care. The nurse is alert to signs of toxicity associated with salicylate, steroid, and antibiotic therapies. The nurse also monitors the patient's fluid status with regard to cardiac function, helps minimize joint pains by properly positioning the patient, emotional support.

**rheumatic heart disease,** damage to heart muscle and heart valves caused by episodes of rheumatic fever. When a susceptible person acquires a group A beta-hemolytic streptococcal infection, an autoimmune reaction may occur in heart tissue, resulting in permanent deformities of heart valves or chordae tendineae. Involvement of the heart may be evident during acute rheumatic fever, or it may be discovered long after the acute disease has subsided. See also **aortic stenosis, mitral valve stenosis, rheumatic fever.**

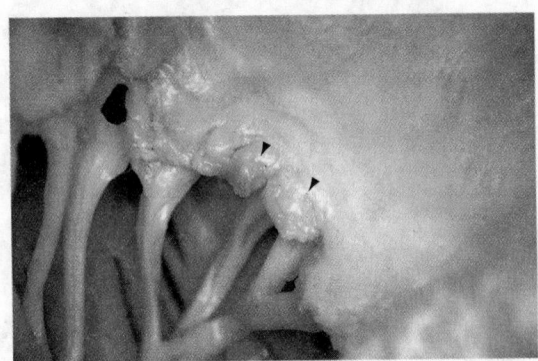

**Rheumatic heart disease** *(Kumar, Cotran, and Robbins, 1997)*

**rheumatic nodules** [Gk, *rheuma,* flux; L, *nodulus,* small knot], aggregations of fibroblasts and lymphoid cells that may accumulate in soft tissues and over bony prominences of patients afflicted with rheumatoid arthritis and rheumatic fever.

**rheumatic scoliosis** [Gk, *rheuma,* flux, *skoliosis,* curvature], a form of scoliosis associated with muscle spasms and acute inflammation. Also called **inflammatory scoliosis.**

**rheumatid** /rōō′mətid/ [Gk, *rheuma,* flux], a skin eruption that sometimes occurs with rheumatic disorders.

**rheumatism** /rōō′mətiz′əm/ [Gk, *rheuma,* flux], *nontechnical.* **1.** any of a large number of inflammatory conditions of the bursae, joints, ligaments, or muscles characterized by pain, limitation of movement, and structural degeneration of one or more parts of the musculoskeletal system. **2.** the syndrome of pain, limitation of movement, and structural degeneration of elements in the musculoskeletal system as may occur in gout, rheumatoid arthritis, systemic lupus erythematosus, ankylosing spondylitis, and many other diseases. **—rheumatic, rheumatoid,** *adj.*

**rheumatoid arteritis** /roō′mətoid/ [Gk, *rheuma,* flux, *arteria,* airpipe, *itis,* inflammation], inflammation of the arterial walls associated with a rheumatic disorder. See also **rheumatoid coronary arteritis.**

**rheumatoid arthritis** [Gk, *rheuma,* flux, *eidos,* form, *arthron,* joint, *itis,* inflammation], a chronic, inflammatory, destructive, and sometimes deforming collagen disease that has an autoimmune component. It is characterized by symmetric inflammation of synovial membranes and increased synovial exudate, leading to thickening of the membranes and swelling of the joints. Rheumatoid arthritis usually first appears when patients, most often women, are between 36 and 50 years of age. The course of the disease is variable but is most frequently marked by alternating periods of remission and exacerbation. Also called **arthritis deformans, atrophic arthritis.** See also **ankylosing spondylitis, juvenile rheumatoid arthritis.**

■ OBSERVATIONS: The medical diagnosis and prognosis of rheumatoid arthritis are based on a variety of clinical and laboratory findings. Clinical data, mainly from radiographic studies and physical examination, classify the progress of the disease into four stages. Stage I, representing early effects, is based on x-ray films showing the onset of bone changes. Stage II, moderate rheumatoid arthritis, is assigned to cases in which there is evidence of some muscle atrophy and loss of mobility, in addition to x-ray findings. Stage III, severe rheumatoid arthritis, is marked by joint deformity, extensive muscle atrophy, soft tissue lesions, and definite bone and cartilage destruction. Stage IV includes all the stage III clinical signs plus fibrous or bony ankylosis. Rheumatoid arthritis may also be classified on the basis of functional capacity: class I, no loss of function; class II, minor impairment of functional capacity with some pain and immobility; class III, capacity limited to a few tasks; and class IV, confinement to bed or a wheelchair. The disease may first be present with fatigue, weakness, poor appetite, low-grade fever, anemia, and an increased erythrocyte sedimentation rate. The diagnostic criteria listed by the American Rheumatism Association include morning stiffness, joint pain or tenderness, swelling of at least two joints, subcutaneous nodules (called arthritic nodules and usually found at pressure points such as the elbows), structural changes in joints seen on x-ray film, a positive rheumatoid factor agglutination test, decreased precipitation of mucin from synovial fluid, and characteristic histologic changes on pathologic examination of the fluid. Both blood serum and synovial fluid. Higher titers of rheumatoid factor are correlated with more severe forms of the disease, especially forms with extraar-

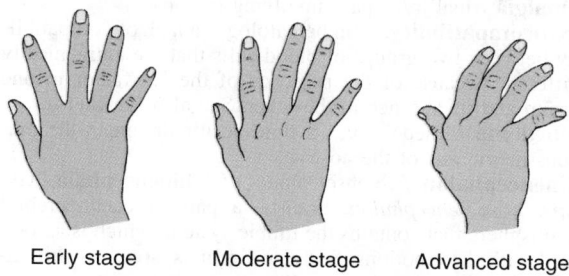

Early stage　　　Moderate stage　　　Advanced stage

**Stages in rheumatoid arthritis**
*(Monahan and Neighbors, 1998)*

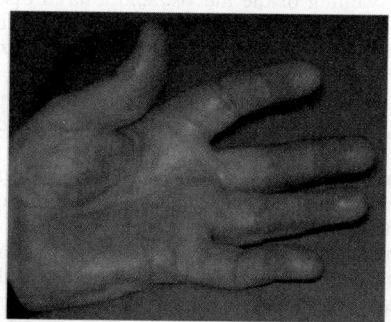

**Rheumatoid arthritis: muscle atrophy**
*(Lemmi and Lemmi, 2000)*

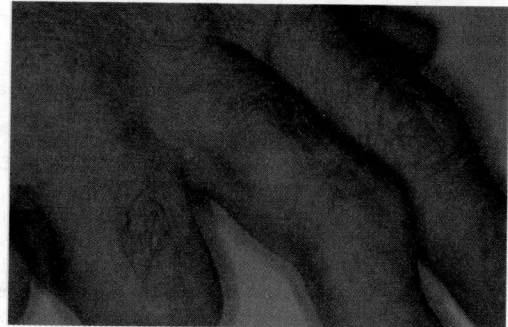

**Rheumatoid nodule** *(Lemmi and Lemmi, 2000)*

**American Rheumatism Association anatomic stages of rheumatoid arthritis**

**Stage I—early**
No destructive changes on x-ray, possible x-ray evidence of osteoporosis

**Stage II—moderate**
X-ray evidence of osteoporosis, with or without slight bone or cartilage destruction, no joint deformities (although possible limited joint mobility), adjacent muscle atrophy, possible presence of extraarticular soft tissue lesions (e.g., nodules, tenovaginitis)

**Stage III—severe**
X-ray evidence of cartilage and bone destruction in addition to osteoporosis; joint deformity, such as subluxation, ulnar deviation, or hyperextension, without fibrous or bony ankylosis; extensive muscle atrophy; possible presence of extraarticular soft tissue lesions (e.g., nodules, tenosynovitis)

**Stage IV—terminal**
Fibrous or bony ankylosis, criteria of stage III

From Lewis SL et al: *Medical-surgical nursing: assessment and management of clinical problems,* ed 5, St Louis, 2000, Mosby.

ticular manifestations, such as cardiac involvement, vasculitis, pulmonary disease, and proteinuria. There may also be a thickening of synovial membranes, called pannus formation. In long-term, severe, chronic rheumatoid arthritis, Felty's syndrome may be present. Rheumatoid arthritis is not always progressive, deforming, or debilitating; most patients may continue in their jobs.

■ INTERVENTIONS: Treatment includes sufficient rest, range-of-motion exercises to maintain joint function, medication for the relief of pain and reduction of inflammation, orthopedic intervention to prevent or correct deformities, proper nutrition, and with weight loss, if necessary. Salicylates are usually given. If improvement is not achieved, other antiinflammatory agents may be used, such as indomethacin, phenylbutazone, antimalarials, gold salts, or some antineoplastic drugs. Corticosteroids are prescribed with caution because of their side effects, including gastric ulcer, adrenal suppression, and osteoporosis. Other treatments, including diathermy, ultrasound, warm paraffin applications, exercise under water, and applications of heat, are occasionally used.

■ NURSING CONSIDERATIONS: The nurse monitors drug treatment and notes its effects; encourages the patient to get sufficient sleep and to rest both small and weight-bearing joints; suggests the most effective use of heat or cold; instructs the patient in muscle-strengthening exercises and methods for easing pain and preventing deformities, such as the proper use of pillows, splints, or molds; and offers emotional support. Because stress often precedes exacerbation of the condition, the patient is counseled to avoid situations known to cause anxiety, worry, fatigue, or infection.

**rheumatoid coronary arteritis,** an abnormal condition characterized by a thickening of the tunica intima of the coronary arteries, which may produce coronary insufficiency. Rheumatoid coronary arteritis is a collagen disease that causes inflammation and fibrinoid degeneration of connective tissue. It is commonly treated with glucocorticoids.

**rheumatoid factor (RF),** antiglobulin antibodies often found in the serum of patients with a clinical diagnosis of rheumatoid arthritis. Rheumatoid factors are present in about 70% of such cases, but they may also be found in such widely divergent diseases as tuberculosis, parasitic infections, leukemia, and connective tissue disorders. See also **latex fixation test.**

**rheumatoid factor test (RF),** a blood test whose results are positive in approximately 80% of patients with rheumatoid arthritis. Abnormal levels of RF that are lower than those characteristic of rheumatoid arthritis may indicate systemic lupus erythematosus, Sjögren syndrome, scleroderma, and other autoimmune conditions. RF is not a useful disease marker because its presence does not disappear in patients who are experiencing a remission from the disease symptoms.

**rheumatoid pneumoconiosis.** See **Caplan's syndrome.**

**rheumatoid spondylitis.** See **Strümpell-Marie disease.**

**rheumatologist** /ro̅o̅′matol′ə′jist/, a specialist in the treatment of disorders of the connective tissue.

**rheumatology** /-ol′əjē/ [Gk, *rheuma,* flux, *logos,* science], the study of disorders characterized by inflammation, degeneration, or metabolic derangement of connective tissue and related structures of the body. These disorders are sometimes referred to collectively as rheumatism.

**Rh factor,** an antigenic substance present in the erythrocytes of 85% of the people. A person having the factor is Rh$^+$ (Rh positive); a person lacking the factor is Rh$^-$ (Rh negative). If an Rh$^-$ person receives Rh$^+$ blood, hemolysis

and anemia occur. Rh+ infants may be exposed to antibodies to the factor produced in the Rh$^-$ mother's blood, resulting in red cell destruction and erythroblastosis fetalis. Transfusion, blood typing, and crossmatching depend on Rh$^+$ and ABO classification. The Rh factor was first identified in the blood of a rhesus (Rh) monkey. Also called **Rhesus factor.** See also **erythroblastosis fetalis, Rh$_O$(D) immune globulin.**

**Rh genes** [Rh, rhesus; Gk, *genein,* to produce], a series of allelic genes that account for the various Rh blood groups. The four variations of the Rh$^+$ gene are identified as R$^0$, R$^1$, R$^2$, and R$^z$, whereas the four types of Rh$^-$ gene are designated as r, r′, r″, and r$_y$.

**rhigo-,** combining form meaning 'shivering or cold': *rhigolene, rhigosis, rhigotic.*

**Rh immune globulin.** See Rh$_o$(D) **immune globulin.**

**rhin-.** See **rhino-.**

**rhinalgia** /rīnal′jə/, pain involving the nose.

**Rh incompatibility,** (in hematology) a lack of compatibility between two groups of blood cells that are antigenically different because of the presence of the Rh factor in one group and its absence in the other. See also **Rh factor.**

**rhinedema** /rī′nedē′mə/, a fluid accumulation in the mucous membrane of the nose.

**rhinencephalon** /rī′nensef′əlon/, *pl.* **rhinencephala** [Gk, *rhis,* nose, *encephalon,* brain], a part of each cerebral hemisphere that contains the limbic system, which is associated with the emotions. See also **limbic system.** —**rhinencephalic,** *adj.*

**rhinenchysis** /rī′nenkī′sis, rīnen′kisis/, douching of the nasal cavity.

**rhinitis** /rīnī′tis/ [Gk, *rhis + itis,* inflammation], inflammation of the mucous membranes of the nose, usually accompanied by swelling of the mucosa and a nasal discharge. It may be complicated by sinusitis. Rhinitis may be **acute, allergic, atrophic,** or **vasomotor.** Also called **coryza.**

**rhino-** /rī′nō-/, **rhin-,** combining form meaning 'nose or noselike structure': *rhinocephalia, rhinolalia, rhinoplasty.*

**Rhinocort,** trademark for a nasal corticosteroid (budesonide).

**rhinolaryngitis** /-ler′injī′tis/ [Gk, *rhis,* nose, *larynx,* throat, *itis,* inflammation], an inflammation of the mucous membranes of the nose and throat.

**rhinolith** /rī′nəlith/, a concretion in the nasal cavity.

**rhinolithiasis** /rī′nəlithī′əsis/, the formation of concretions in the nasal cavity.

**rhinologist** /rīnol′əjist/, a physician who specializes in the diagnosis and treatment of disorders of the nose.

**rhinology** /rīnol′əjē/, a branch of medicine specializing in the diagnosis and treatment of disorders involving the nose.

**rhinomanometer** /rī′nōmənom′ətər/, a device for measuring the air pressure in the nose. It is used in the diagnosis of nasal obstruction.

**rhinomycosis** /rī′nōmīkō′sis/, a fungal infection of the mucous membrane of the nose.

**rhinopathy** /rīnop′əthē/ [Gk, *rhis + pathos,* disease], any disease or malformation of the nose.

**rhinopharyngeal.** See **nasopharyngeal.**

**rhinophycomycosis** /rī′nōfī′kōmīkō′sis/, an infection of the nasal and paranasal sinuses caused by the phycomycete *Entomophthora coronata.* The infection often spreads to surrounding tissues, including the eye and brain.

**rhinophyma** /rī′nōfī′mə/ [Gk, *rhis + phyma,* tumor], a form of rosacea in which there is sebaceous hyperplasia, redness, prominent vascularity, swelling, and distortion of the skin of the nose. Treatment includes dermabrasion, electrosurgery, and plastic surgery. See also **rosacea.**

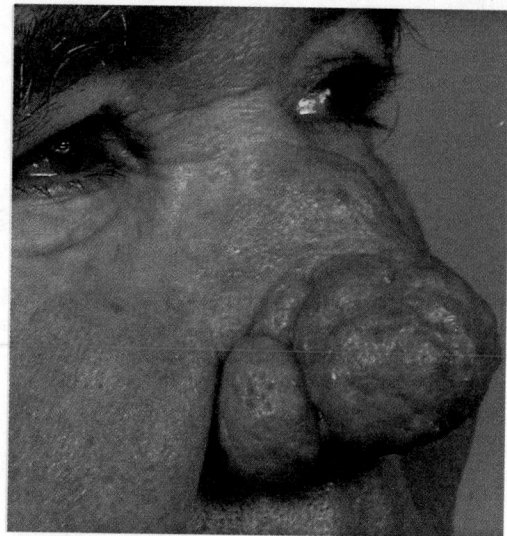

**Rhinophyma** (du Vivier, 1993)

**rhinoplasty** /rī′nəplas′tē/ [Gk, *rhis* + *plassein*, to mold], a procedure in plastic surgery in which the structure of the nose is changed. Bone or cartilage may be removed, tissue grafted from another part of the body, or synthetic material implanted to alter the shape. With the patient under local anesthesia, intranasal incisions are made, and the nose is reshaped. After surgery any respiratory difficulty is reported immediately, and the patient is kept in mid-Fowler's position. Frequent oral care is given, and ice compresses are applied to decrease the pain and edema that usually occur. Edema and discoloration around the eyes are expected to last for several days. The procedure is most frequently performed for cosmetic reasons.

**rhinorrhagia** /rī′nôrā′jə/ [Gk, *rhis*, nose, *rhegnynein*, to gush forth], a profuse nosebleed.

**rhinorrhea** /rī′nôrē′ə/ [Gk, *rhis* + *rhoia*, flow], **1.** the free discharge of a thin watery nasal fluid. **2.** the flow of cerebrospinal fluid from the nose after an injury to the head.

**rhinosalpingitis** /rī′nōsal′pinjī′tis/, an inflammation of the mucous membranes of the nose and eustachian tube.

**rhinoscleroma** /rī′nosklirō′mə/, a chronic inflammation in the nose, spreading to the larynx and pharynx. The cause is an infection of *Klebsiella rhinoscleromatis.*

**rhinoscope** /rī′nəskōp/, an instrument for examining the nasal passages through the anterior nares or through the nasopharynx.

**rhinoscopy** /rīnos′kəpē/ [Gk, *rhis* + *skopein*, to look], an examination of the nasal passages to inspect the mucosa and detect inflammation, deformities, or asymmetry, as in deviation of the septum. The nasal passages may be examined anteriorly by introducing a speculum into the anterior nares or posteriorly by introducing a rhinoscope through the nasopharynx. **—rhinoscopic,** *adj.*

**rhinosporidiosis** /rī′nōspərid′ē·ō′sis/ [Gk, *rhis* + *sporo,* seed, *osis,* condition], an infection caused by the fungus *Rhinosporidium seeberi.* It is characterized by fleshy red polyps on the mucous membranes of the nose, conjunctiva, nasopharynx, and soft palate. The disease may be acquired by swimming or bathing in infected water. The most effective treatment is electrocautery.

**rhinostenosis** /rī′nōstənō′sis/, an abnormal narrowing of a nasal passage.

**rhinotomy** /rīnot′əmē/ [Gk, *rhis* + *temnein,* to cut], a surgical procedure in which an incision is made along one side of the nose, performed to drain accumulated pus from an abscess or a sinus infection. Under local anesthesia the flap of skin and lining of the nose are turned back to provide a full view of the nasal passages for radical sinus surgery.

**rhinovirus** /rī′nōvī′rəs/ [Gk, *rhis* + L, *virus,* poison], any of about 100 serologically distinct, small ribonucleic acid viruses that cause about 40% of acute respiratory illnesses. Infection is characterized by dry scratchy throat, nasal congestion, malaise, and headache. Fever is minimal. Nasal discharge lasts 2 or 3 days. Children may also develop a cough. Type-specific antibodies may last for 2 to 4 years. The treatment is nonspecific and may include rest, analgesics, antihistamines, and nasal decongestants. Complete recovery is usual. Compare **adenovirus, parainfluenza virus, respiratory syncytial virus.** See also **cold.**

**rhitid-.** See **rhytid-.**

**rhitidoplasty.** See **rhytidoplasty.**

**rhitidosis.** See **rhytidosis.**

**rhizo-,** combining form meaning 'root': *rhizodontropy, rhizome, rhizotomist.*

**rhizoid** /rī′zoid/, resembling a root or serving to anchor.

**rhizomelia** /rī′zōmē′lyə/ [Gk, *rhizo,* root, *melos,* limb], **1.** a disorder of the hips and shoulders. **2.** an anomaly in the length of the arms and legs of an individual.

**rhizomelic** /rī′zəmel′ik/ [Gk, *rhizo,* root, *melos,* limb], pertaining to the hips and shoulder.

**rhizomeningomyelitis** /rī′zōmining′gōmī′əlī′tis/, an inflammation of the nerve roots, meninges, and spinal cord.

*Rhizopus* /rī′zōpəs/, a genus of fungi that includes some species identified as a cause of zygomycosis in humans.

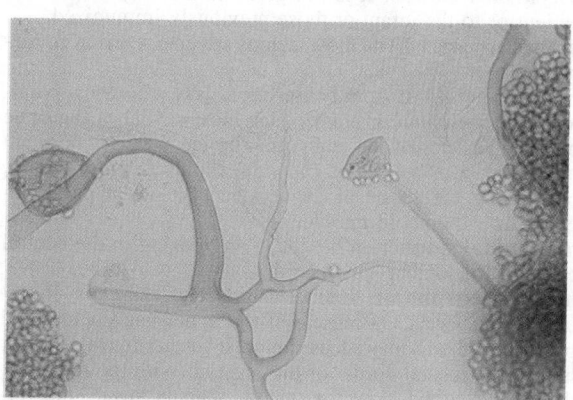

*Rhizopus* **showing rhizoids** (Mahon and Manuselis, 2000)

**rhizotomy** /rīzot′əmē/, the surgical resection of the dorsal root of a spinal nerve, performed to relieve pain and sometimes to decrease spasms.

**Rh negative.** See **Rh factor.**

**rho** /rō/, P, ρ, the seventeenth letter of the Greek alphabet.

**Rhodesian trypanosomiasis** /rōdē′zhən/, an acute form of African trypanosomiasis, caused by the parasite *Trypanosoma brucei rhodesiense.* The disease may progress rapidly, causing encephalitis, coma, and death in only a few weeks.

Also called **kaodzera.** Compare **Gambian trypanosomiasis.** See also **African trypanosomiasis.**

**rhodium (Rh)** /rō'dē·əm/ [Gk, *rhodon,* rose], a grayish-white metallic element. Its atomic number is 45; its atomic mass is 102.91. Rhodium is used for providing a hard lustrous coating on other metals and in the making of mirrors.

**rhodo-,** combining form meaning 'red': *rhodocyte, rhodopsin, rhodotoxin.*

**rhodopsin** /rōdop'sin/ [Gk, *rhodon,* rose, *opsis,* vision], the purple pigmented compound in the rods of the retina, formed by a protein, opsin, and a derivative of vitamin A, retinal. Rhodopsin gives the outer segments of the rods a purple color and adapts the eye to low-density light. The compound breaks down when struck by light, and this chemical change triggers the conduction of nerve impulses. Brief periods of darkness allow the opsin and the retinal to reconstitute the rhodopsin, which accounts for the short delay a person experiences in adapting to sudden or drastic changes in lighting, as when moving out of bright sunlight into a darkened room or from darkness into bright light. Closing the eyes is a natural reflex that allows reconstitution of rhodopsin. Compare **iodopsin.**

*Rhodotorula* /rō'dətôr'yələ/, a genus of yeasts, including species such as *R. rubra* that have been identified as causes of endocarditis and septicemia, particularly in immunocompromised patients.

**rhoencephalography,** a technique for monitoring blood flow in the brain by recording pulsatile changes in the electrical impedance of the brain.

**RhoGAM,** trademark for an immune globulin (Rh<sub>O</sub>[D] immune globulin).

**Rh<sub>O</sub>(D) immune globulin,** a passive immunizing agent. Also called **Rh immune globulin.**

■ INDICATIONS: It is prescribed to prevent Rh sensitization after abortion, miscarriage, ectopic pregnancy, or normal birth to an Rh-negative mother of an Rh-positive infant or fetus.

■ CONTRAINDICATIONS: It is not given to an Rh<sub>O</sub>(D)-positive patient or to the infant or those previously immunized.

■ ADVERSE EFFECTS: The most serious adverse reaction is anaphylaxis.

**rhombencephalon** /rom'bensef'əlon/ [Gk, *rhombos,* parallelogram, *enkephalos,* brain], the most caudal of the three primary vesicles of the embryonic brain.

**rhomboid** /rom'boid/ [Gk, *rhombos,* rhombus, *eidos,* form], resembling the shape of an oblique equilateral parallelogram, as a rhomboid muscle.

**rhomboidal sinus** /rom'boidəl/, an opening in the central canal of the lumbar spinal cord.

**rhomboideus major** /romboi'dē·əs/ [Gk, *rhombos,* rhombus, *eidos,* form], a muscle of the upper back below and parallel to the rhomboideus minor. It inserts into the lower half of the medial border of the scapula. With the rhomboideus minor, it functions to draw the scapula toward the vertebral column while supporting it and drawing it slightly upward. Compare **latissimus dorsi, levator scapulae, rhomboideus minor, trapezius.**

**rhomboideus minor,** a muscle of the upper back, above and parallel to the rhomboideus major. It arises from the ligamentum nuchae and from the spinous processes of the seventh cervical and first thoracic vertebrae. It inserts into the upper part of the medial border at the root of the spine of the scapula. With the rhomboideus major, it acts to draw the scapula toward the vertebral column while supporting the scapula and drawing it slightly upward. Compare **latissimus dorsi, levator scapulae, rhomboideus major, trapezius.**

**rhomboid glossitis.** See **median rhomboid glossitis.**

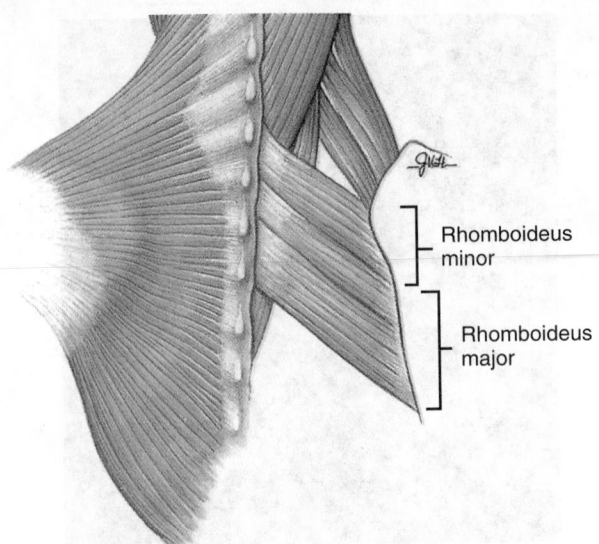

**Rhomboideus major and rhomboideus minor**
*(Thibodeau and Patton, 1999/John V. Hagen)*

**rhombomere** /rom'bəmir/, any of the nine segments of the embryonic neural tube.

**rhonchus** /rong'kəs/, *pl.* **rhonchi** /rong'kī/ [Gk, *rhonchos,* snore], an abnormal sound heard on auscultation of an airway obstructed by thick secretions, muscular spasm, neoplasm, or external pressure. The continuous rumbling sound is more pronounced during expiration and characteristically clears on coughing, whereas gurgles do not.

**rhotacism** /rō'təsizm/, a speech disorder consisting of imperfect pronouncing of the /r/ sound. Compare **lallation.** Also called **pararhotacism.**

**Rh positive.** See **Rh factor.**

**r-HuEPO,** abbreviation for *recombinant human erythropoietin.*

**rhus** /rus/, any member of the genus *Rhus.* See also **rhus dermatitis.**

*Rhus,* a genus of vines and shrubs of the family Anacardiaceae, many of them poisonous. Some species contain urushiol, a highly allergenic oleoresin mixture, and contact with them produces a severe dermatitis (**rhus dermatitis**) in sensitive persons. The most important toxic species are *R. radicans* L. (poison ivy), *R. diversiloba* L. (western poison oak), *R. quercifolia* (eastern poison oak), and *R. vernix* L. (poison sumac).

**rhus dermatitis** /rōōs/ [Gk, *rhous,* sumac], a form of contact dermatitis caused by exposure to an allergenic oil, toxicodendrol, present in any part of a plant of the genus *Rhus* such as poison ivy, poison oak, or poison sumac. Contact with a rhus plant can result in severe itching, rashes, and blistering; even the smoke of burning rhus plants may be toxic. See also **contact dermatitis.**

**rhyp-,** prefix meaning 'filth': *rhyparia, rhypophagy, rhypophobia.*

**rhythm** /rith'əm/ [Gk, *rhythmos*], the relationship of one impulse to neighboring impulses as measured in time, movement, or regularity of action.

**rhythmic nystagmus.** See **nystagmus.**

**rhythm method.** See **natural family planning method.**

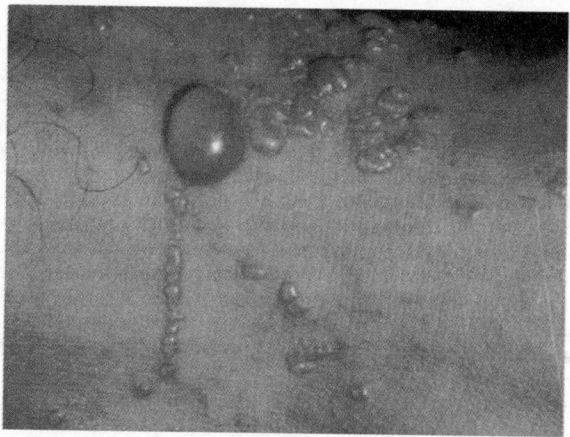

**Rhus dermatitis** *(Habif, 1996)*

**rhytid-, rhitid-,** prefix meaning 'wrinkle, or wrinkled': *rhytidectomy, rhytidosis.*

**rhytidectomy.** See **face lift.**

**rhytidoplasty** /ritid′ōplas′tē/ [Gk, *rhytis,* wrinkle, *plassein,* to mold], a procedure in reconstructive plastic surgery in which the skin of the face is tightened, wrinkles are removed, and the skin is made to appear firm and smooth. An incision is made at the hairline, and excess skin is separated from the supporting tissue and excised. The edges of the remaining skin are pulled up and back and sutured at the hairline. A pressure dressing is applied and left in place for 24 to 48 hours. Postoperative medication for pain is often necessary. The sutures are removed several days after discharge in an outpatient facility or in the surgeon's office. Also spelled **rhytidectomy, rhitidoplasty.**

**rhytidosis** /rit′idō′sis/ [Gk, *rhytis,* wrinkle, *osis,* condition], a wrinkling, especially of the cornea. Also spelled **rhitidosis.**

**RIA,** abbreviation for **radioimmunoassay.**

**rib** [AS, roof], one of the 12 pairs of arches of bone forming a large part of the thoracic skeleton. The first seven ribs on each side are called **true ribs** because they articulate directly with the sternum and vertebrae. The remaining five ribs are called **false ribs.** The first three attach ventrally to ribs above; the last two are free at their ventral extremities and are called **floating ribs.** True ribs are also known as vertebrosternal ribs; false ribs as vertebrocostal ribs; and floating ribs as vertebral ribs. See also **thorax.**

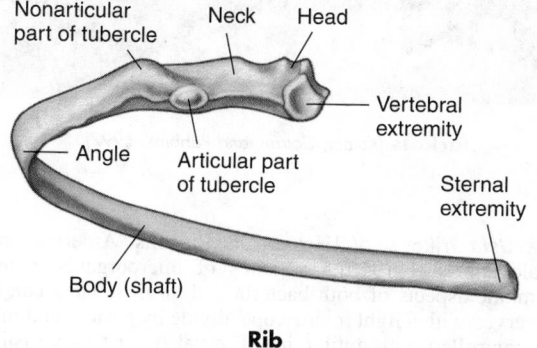

**Rib**

Nonarticular part of tubercle — Neck — Head — Vertebral extremity — Angle — Articular part of tubercle — Sternal extremity — Body (shaft)

**ribavirin** /rī′bəvir′in/, an aerosol antiviral drug.

■ INDICATIONS: It is prescribed for the treatment of respiratory syncytial virus infections for the lower respiratory tract in infants and small children.

■ CONTRAINDICATIONS: It is not recommended for infants requiring assisted ventilation.

■ ADVERSE EFFECTS: Reported side effects include bacterial pneumonia, pneumothorax, apnea, hypotension, and cardiac arrest, conditions which also may have resulted from the patient's underlying disease; deteriorated respiratory function; rash; conjunctivitis; and reticulocytosis.

**rib fracture,** a break in a bone of the thoracic skeleton caused by a blow or crushing injury or by violent coughing or sneezing. The ribs most commonly broken are the fourth to eighth; if the bone is splintered or the fracture is displaced, sharp fragments may pierce the lung, causing hemothorax or pneumothorax.

■ OBSERVATIONS: The patient with a fractured rib suffers pain, especially on inspiration, and usually breathes rapidly and shallowly. The site of the break is generally very tender to the touch, and the crackling of bone fragments rubbing together may be heard on auscultation. Breath sounds may be absent, decreased, or accompanied by rales and rhonchi. The location and nature of the fracture are determined by chest x-ray studies. The patient is observed for signs of hemoptysis, hemothorax, flail chest, atelectasis, pneumothorax, and pneumonia.

■ INTERVENTIONS: Fractured ribs may be splinted with an elastic belt or bandage or adhesive strapping; to prevent irritation the area may be shaved and painted with tincture of benzoin before the adhesive tape is applied. Increasingly, however, no splints are used, because they compromise chest expansion and predispose to pulmonary complications. If hospitalization is required, the patient is placed in a semi-Fowler's position, and the blood pressure, pulse, temperature, respirations, and breath sounds are checked every 2 to 4 hours. An analgesic may be ordered, but morphine sulfate is avoided because it depresses respiration. If strapping and analgesic medication fail to relieve pain, the physician may perform a regional nerve block by infiltrating the intercostal spaces above and below the fracture site with 1% procaine.

■ NURSING CONSIDERATIONS: The nurse assists in splinting the chest, administers the ordered medication, helps the patient to turn, and instructs the patient in how to perform deep breathing, coughing and range-of-motion exercises of the extremities.

**riboflavin** /ri′bōflā′vin/ [*ribose* + L, *flavus,* yellow], a yellow crystalline water-soluble pigment, one of the heat-stable components of the B vitamin complex. It combines with specific flavoproteins and functions as a coenzyme in the oxidative processes of carbohydrates, fats, and proteins. Small amounts of riboflavin are found in the liver and kidneys, but it is not stored to any great degree in the body and must be supplied regularly in the diet. Common sources are organ meats, milk, cheese, eggs, green leafy vegetables, meat, whole grains, and legumes. Deficiency of riboflavin is rare; it produces cheilosis; local inflammation; desquamation; encrustation; glossitis; photophobia; corneal opacities; proliferation of corneal vessels; seborrheic dermatitis about the nose, mouth, forehead, ears, and scrotum; trembling; sluggishness; dizziness; edema; inability to urinate; and vaginal itching. Also called **vitamin B₂.** See also **ariboflavinosis.**

**ribonuclear protein (RNP)** /rī′bōnoo′klē·ər/ [ribose; L, *nucleus,* nut kernel; Gk, *proteios,* first rank], a conjugated protein consisting of a protein molecule and nucleic acid.

**ribonuclease (RNase)** /-nooˈklē·ās/, a class of endonucleases that hydrolyze ribonucleic acids.

**ribonucleic acid (RNA)** /rīˈbonooklēˈik/ [*ribose* + L, *nucleus,* nut kernel, *acidus,* sour], a nucleic acid, found in both the nucleus and cytoplasm of cells, that plays several roles in the translation of the genetic code and the assembly of proteins. Kinds of RNA include **messenger RNA, ribosomal RNA,** and **transfer RNA.** See also **deoxyribonucleic acid.**

**ribonucleoside** /rīˈbonooˈklē·əsīd/, a nucleoside in which the sugar component is ribose. The ribonucleosides of RNA are adenosine, cytidine, guanosine, and uridine.

**ribonucleotide** /-nooˈklē·ətīd/, a class of nucleotides in which the pentose is D-ribose.

**ribose** /rīˈbōs/, a 5-carbon sugar that occurs as a component of RNA.

**ribosomal RNA (rRNA)** /rīˈbōsōˈməl/, the ribonucleic acid of ribosomes and polyribosomes.

**ribosome** /rīˈbəsōm/ [*ribose* + Gk, *soma,* body], an organelle composed of RNA and protein that functions in the synthesis of protein. Ribosomes interact with messenger RNA and transfer RNA to link amino acid into a polypeptide chain in a sequence determined by the sequence of nucleotides in the messenger RNA. Ribosomes may exist singly, in clusters as polysomes, or attached to the "rough" endoplasmic reticulum. See also **translation.**

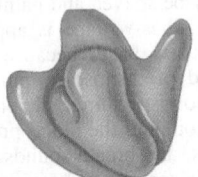

**Ribosome** *(Thibodeau and Patton, 1999/Barbara Cousins)*

**ribosome-inactivating protein (RIP),** one of a variety of enzymes that cleave the *N*-glycosidic bond of adenine in a specific ribosomal RNA sequence. Type 1 RIPs are single-chain proteins. Some type 2 RIPs, such as ricin, possess a galactose-specific lectin domain that binds to cell surfaces, making them potent toxins.

**ribosuria** /rīˈbəsŏŏrˈē·ə/, the presence of ribose in the urine, usually a sign of muscular dystrophy.

**ribovirus.** See **RNA virus.**

**rib shaking,** a procedure in physiotherapy in which constant, downward pressure is applied with an intermittent shaking motion of the hands on the rib cage over the area being drained. It is done with the flat part of the palm of the hand over the lung segment being drained during 4 to 12 prolonged exhalations by the patient through pursed lips.

**rib vibration,** a procedure in physiotherapy similar to rib shaking but done with a downward vibrating pressure with the flat part of the palm during exhalations.

**RICE,** abbreviation for *rest, ice, compression, elevation,* referring to the treatment for sprains and strains.

**rice diet** [Gk, *oryza,* rice, *diaita,* way of living], a diet consisting only of rice, fruit, fruit juices, and sugar, supplemented with vitamins and iron. Salt is forbidden. It is prescribed for the treatment of hypertension, chronic renal disease, and obesity. It should not be followed for any length of time, because the severe dietary restrictions may lead to nutritional deficiencies or imbalance. Also called **Duke diet, Kempner rice-fruit diet.**

**Richards, Linda** (1841–1930), a nurse considered to be the first American-trained nurse, being graduated in the first class of the New England Hospital for Women and Children. She then studied at the Nightingale Training School in London and in 1873 organized the Massachusetts General Hospital Training School. In 1885 she was sent to Japan to develop a training school at the Charity Hospital. In 1891 she took charge of the Philadelphia Visiting Nurse Society. She is credited with being the first to keep written records on patients, a practice she started when she worked as night superintendent at Bellevue Hospital in New York under Sister Helen.

**Richet's aneurysm.** See **fusiform aneurysm.**

**Richter's hernia** /rikˈtərz, rishˈtərs/ [August G. Richter, German surgeon, 1742–1812], a small nonpalpable visceral protrusion involving only a part of the intestinal wall. Also called **parietal hernia.**

**ricin** /rīˈsin/, a potent toxin obtained from castor beans (*Ricinus communis*) that produces agglutination of red blood cells and inflammation and hemorrhage of the respiratory and GI mucosa. Also called **ricinine.** See also **ribosome-inactivating protein.**

**rickets** /rikˈəts/ [Gk, *rachis,* backbone, *itis,* inflammation], a condition caused by the deficiency of vitamin D, seen primarily in infancy and childhood and characterized by abnormal bone formation. Symptoms include soft pliable bones causing such deformities as bowlegs and knock-knees, nodular enlargements on the ends and sides of the bones, muscle pain, enlarged skull, chest deformities, spinal curvature, enlargement of the liver and spleen, profuse sweating, and general tenderness of the body when touched. Prophylaxis and treatment include a diet rich in calcium, phosphorus, and vitamin D and adequate exposure to sunlight. Kinds of rickets include **celiac rickets, renal rickets,** and genetic forms of **vitamin D resistant rickets.** See also **osteodystrophy, osteomalacia, vitamin D.**

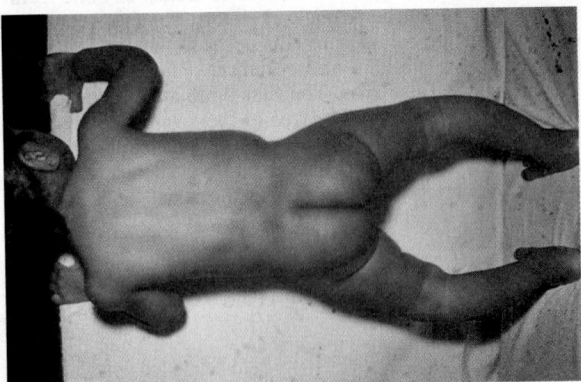

**Rickets** *(Kumar, Cotran, and Robbins, 1997)*

*Rickettsia* /riketˈsē·ə/ [Howard T. Ricketts, American pathologist, 1871–1910], a genus of microorganisms that combine aspects of both bacteria and viruses. They can be observed with a light microscope, divide by fission, and may be controlled with antibiotics. They also exist as viruslike intracellular parasites, living in the intestinal tracts of insects such as lice. Thus a human infested with lice is also likely to be infected with a form of typhus transmitted by *Rickettsia prowazeki*. Rickettsial diseases have been responsible for many of history's worst epidemics. The various species are distinguished on the basis of similarities in the diseases they cause. The spotted fever group includes Rocky Mountain spotted fever, rickettsialpox, and others; the typhus group includes epidemic typhus, murine typhus; and a miscellaneous group includes Q fever and trench fever. Rickettsial diseases are uncommon in parts of the world where insect and rodent populations are well controlled. **—rickettsial,** *adj.*

**rickettsial disease** [Howard T. Ricketts; L, *dis* + Fr, *aise,* ease], an infection caused by a species of *Rickettsia.* Examples include Rocky Mountain spotted fever and typhus.

**rickettsialpox** /riket′sē·əlpoks′/ [Howard T. Ricketts; ME, *pokkes,* pustules], a mild, acute infectious disease caused by *Rickettsia akari* and transmitted from mice to humans by mites. It is characterized by an asymptomatic crusted primary lesion, chills, fever, headache, malaise, myalgia, and a rash resembling chickenpox. About 1 week after onset of symptoms, small, discrete, maculopapular lesions appear on any part of the body, but rarely on palms or soles. These lesions become vesicular and dry and form scabs. Eventually the scabs fall off, leaving no scars. Chloramphenicol or tetracycline hastens recovery. Prevention involves the elimination of house mice. Also called **Kew Gardens spotted fever.** Compare **Rocky Mountain spotted fever.** See also *Rickettsia.*

**rickettsiosis** /riket′sē·ō′sis/, *pl.* **rickettsioses** [Howard T. Ricketts; Gk, *osis,* condition], any of a group of infectious diseases caused by microorganisms of the genus *Rickettsia.* Kinds of rickettsioses include a spotted fever group (**boutonneuse fever, rickettsialpox, Rocky Mountain spotted fever**), a typhus group (**epidemic typhus, murine typhus, scrub typhus**), and a miscellaneous group (**Q fever, trench fever**). See also **rickettsia.**

**Ridaura,** trademark for an oral antiarthritic drug (auranofin).

**rider's bone** [AS, *ridan,* to ride, *ban,* bone], a bony deposit that sometimes develops in horseback riders on the inner side of the lower end of the tendon of the adductor muscle of the thigh. Also called **cavalry bone.**

**rider's sprain** [OFr, *espreindre,* to force out], a sprain of the adductor muscles of the thigh resulting from horseback riding.

**ridge** /rij/ [AS, *hrycg*], a projection or projecting structure such as the gastrocnemial ridge or crest on the posterior surface of the femur, giving attachment to the gastrocnemius muscle.

**ridge extension,** an intraoral surgical operation for deepening the labial, buccal, or lingual sulci.

**ridge lap,** the part of an artificial tooth that is adjacent to or laps the residual ridge.

**Riedel's struma, Riedel's thyroiditis.** See **fibrous thyroiditis.**

**Rieder's cell leukemia** /rē′dərz/ [Hermann Rieder, German pathologist, 1858–1932], a malignant neoplasm of blood-forming tissues characterized by the presence in blood of large numbers of atypical myeloblasts with immature cytoplasm and relatively mature lobulated, indented nuclei.

**Riehl-Sisca, Joan,** a nursing theorist who presented her symbolic interactionism theory in Riehl and Sister Callista Roy's book, *Conceptual Models for Nursing* (1980). The Riehl Interaction Model uses the nursing process in implementing nursing care. In symbolic interactionism theory,

people interpret each other's actions based on the meaning attached to the action before reacting. It is a process of interpretation between the stimulus and response. Riehl's emphasis is on the assessment and interpretation of the patient's actions by the nurse, who then makes predictions about the patient's behavior. This is done to plan interventions with the patient and the patient's family. Riehl views the nurse and patient as actively exchanging information and collecting knowledge. The nurse then selects from multiple theories, therapies and allied health disciples in planning and implementing effective nursing interventions. See also **Roy.**

**RIF,** abbreviation for **resistance-inducing factor.**

**rifa-,** combining form for rifamycin-derived antibiotics.

**Rifadin,** trademark for an antibacterial (rifampin).

**rifampin** /rif′əmpin/, an antibacterial.
- INDICATIONS: It is prescribed in the treatment of tuberculosis, in meningococcal prophylaxis, and as an antileprotic.
- CONTRAINDICATIONS: Liver dysfunction or disease or known hypersensitivity to this drug or to rifamycin prohibits its use.
- ADVERSE EFFECTS: Among the more serious adverse reactions are liver toxicity and a syndrome resembling influenza. GI distress, aches and cramps, discoloration of urine, saliva, and sweat commonly occur. This drug interacts with many other drugs.

**rifapentine,** an antitubercular.
- INDICATIONS: Rifapentine is used to treat pulmonary tuberculosis. It must be used in combination with at least one other antitubercular.
- CONTRAINDICATIONS: Known hypersensitivity to rifamycins prohibits this drug's use.
- ADVERSE EFFECTS: Life-threatening effects of rifapentine include pancreatitis, hematuria, proteinuria, thrombocytopenia, leukopenia, neutropenia, lymphopenia, and leukocytosis. Other adverse reactions include rash, pruritus, urticaria, acne, visual disturbances, gout, arthrosis, edema, aggressive reaction, bilirubinemia, hepatitis, increased AST/ALT, pyuria, urinary casts, headache, fatigue, anxiety, dizziness, anemia, purpura, and hematoma. Common side effects include nausea, vomiting, anorexia, diarrhea, and heartburn.

**Rift Valley fever,** a bunyavirus infection of Egypt and east Africa spread by mosquitoes or by handling infected sheep, buffalo, goats, camels, and cattle. It is characterized by abrupt fever, chills, headache, and generalized aching, followed by epigastric pain, anorexia, loss of taste, and photophobia. Retinitis may cause vision loss in 1% to 10% of cases. The disease is of short duration, and recovery is usually complete. There is no specific treatment. A killed virus vaccine that provides protection for 2 years is available for those at risk such as, in the United States, laboratory workers and veterinarians.

**RIG,** abbreviation for **rabies immune globulin.**

**Riga-Fede disease** /rē′gä fā′dā/ [Antonio Riga, Italian physician, 1832–1919; Francesco Fede, Italian pediatrician, 1832–1913], an ulceration of the lingual frenum in some infants, caused by abrasion of the frenum by natal or neonatal teeth. Also called **Fede's disease.**

**right atrial catheter,** an indwelling IV catheter inserted centrally or peripherally and threaded into the superior vena cava and right atrium.

**right atrioventricular valve.** See **tricuspid valve.**

**right brachiocephalic vein** [AS, *riht* + Gk, *brachion,* arm, *kephale,* head], a vessel, about 2.5 cm long, that starts in the root of the neck at the junction of the internal jugular and the subclavian veins on the right side and descends vertically from behind the sternal end of the clavicle to join the left brachiocephalic vein and form the superior vena cava. The right brachiocephalic vein, like the left, receives various tributaries such as the vertebral vein, the internal thoracic vein, and the inferior thyroid vein. Compare **left brachioce-phalic vein.**

**right bundle branch block (RBBB),** impaired or absence of transmission of electrical impulses from the atrioventricular (AV) bundle of His to the right ventricle. The block may be complete or incomplete and may be caused by a lesion in the right bundle branch or a small, focal lesion in the AV bundle. RBBB is often associated with right ventricular hypertrophy, especially in athletes and individuals under 40 years of age. In older individuals RBBB is commonly caused by coronary artery disease. A complete RBBB commonly occurs after surgical closure of a ventricular septal defect.

**right common carotid artery,** the shorter of the two common carotid arteries, arising from the brachiocephalic trunk, passing obliquely from the level of the sternoclavicular articulation to the upper border of the thyroid cartilage, and dividing into the right internal and external carotids. Compare **left common carotid artery.**

**right coronary artery,** one of a pair of branches of the ascending aorta, arising in the right posterior aortic sinus, passing along the right side of the coronary sulcus, dividing into the right interventricular artery and a large marginal branch. It supplies both ventricles, the right atrium, and the sinoatrial node. Compare **left coronary artery.**

**right coronary vein.** See **small cardiac vein.**

**right-handedness,** a natural tendency to favor the use of the right hand. Also called **dextrality.** See also **cerebral dominance, handedness.**

**right-hand rule,** a principle of physics in which the direction of current flow in a wire is related to the position of the imaginary lines of force of the magnetic field about the wire. Thus, if the fingers of the right hand are flexed to represent the magnetic field and the thumb is extended, the thumb points in the direction of current flow.

**right-heart failure,** an abnormal cardiac condition characterized by the impairment of the right side of the heart and congestion and elevated pressure in the systemic veins and capillaries. The most common cause of right-heart failure is left-heart failure, because both sides of the heart are part of a circuit, and what affects one side will eventually affect the other. Right ventricular infarction, pulmonic stenosis, and pulmonary hypertension can also result in right-heart failure. In failure associated with either side of the heart, cardiac output is usually decreased. Also called **right-sided failure.** Compare **left-heart failure.** See also **heart failure.**

**right hepatic duct,** the duct that drains bile from the right lobe of the liver into the common bile duct.

**righting reflex** [AS, *riht* + L, *reflectere,* to bend back], any one of the neuromuscular responses to restore the body to its normal upright position when it has been displaced. The righting reflexes involve complicated mechanisms and processes associated with the structures of the internal ear, such as the utricle, the saccule, the macula, and the semicircular canals. Any change in the position of the head produces a change in the pressure on the gelatinous membrane of the macula. The fibers of the nerve (vestibular branch of the eight cranial nerve) transmit impulses to the brain, producing a sense of position. The head and trunk are thus kept in alignment. Also activating righting reflexes are proprioceptors in muscles and tendons and visual nerve impulses. Also called **body righting reflex.**

**right interventricular artery.** See **dorsal interventricular artery.**

**right lymphatic duct,** a vessel that conveys lymph from the right upper quadrant of the body into the bloodstream in the neck at the junction of the right internal jugular and the right subclavian veins. About 1.25 cm long, the duct courses over the medial border of the scalenus anterior. At its orifice are two semilunar valves that prevent venous blood from flowing backward into the duct. Lymph drains into the right lymphatic duct from numerous capillaries and vessels and from three lymphatic trunks in the right quadrant. Compare **thoracic duct.** See also **lymphatic system.**

**right pulmonary artery,** the longer and slightly larger of the two arteries conveying venous blood from the heart to the lungs. It arises from the pulmonary trunk, bends to the right behind the aorta, and divides into two branches at the root of the right lung. Compare **left pulmonary artery.**

**right-sided failure.** See **right-heart failure.**

**right subclavian artery,** a large artery that arises from the brachiocephalic artery. It has several important branches: the axillary, vertebral thoracic, and internal thoracic arteries and the cervical and costocervical trunks, perfusing the right side of the upper body.

**right-to-know laws,** laws that require employers to inform workers regarding health effects of materials they must handle, including toxic chemicals and radioactive substances. Under the authority of the U.S. Occupational Safety and Health Act of 1970, the National Institute for Occupational Safety and Health periodically revises recommendations or limits of exposure to potentially hazardous substances in the workplace. It also recommends appropriate preventive measures designed to reduce or eliminate adverse health effects of these hazards and publishes its recommendations in a variety of public documents.

**right-to-left shunt** [ME, *shunten*], a shunt in which unoxygenated venous blood bypasses the lungs and directly enters the arterial system, as in the tetralogy of Fallot and other conditions.

**right ventricle,** the relatively thin-walled chamber of the heart that pumps blood received from the right atrium into the pulmonary arteries to the lungs for oxygenation. The right ventricle is shorter and rounder than the long conical left ventricle. The chordae tendineae of the tricuspid valve of the right ventricle are finer than the coarse strands of the chordae tendineae of the left ventricle. See also **heart.**

**right ventricular thrust.** See **precordial movement.**

**rigid gas permeable (RGP) contact lens,** a rigid contact lens that allows oxygen to be transmitted through the lens material.

**rigidity** /rijid′itē/ [L, *rigere,* to be stiff], a condition of hardness, stiffness, or inflexibility. —**rigid,** *adj.*

**rigidus** /rij′idəs/ [L, stiff], a deformity characterized by limited motion, especially dorsiflexion of the great toe. This condition causes pain and may ultimately produce degenerative changes of the involved joints.

**rigor** /rig′ər/ [L, stiffness], **1.** a rigid condition of the body tissues, as in rigor mortis. **2.** a violent attack of shivering that may be associated with chills and fever.

**rigor mortis** /môr′tis/, the rigid stiffening of skeletal and cardiac muscle shortly after death.

**Riley-Day syndrome.** See **dysautonomia.**

**riluzole,** an agent used to treat amyotropic lateral sclerosis.
■ INDICATIONS: This drug is used to treat amyotropic lateral sclerosis (ALS).
■ CONTRAINDICATIONS: Known hypersensitivity to this drug prohibits its use.
■ ADVERSE EFFECTS: Neutropenia and exfoliative dermatitis are life-threatening effects of this drug. Other adverse effects are nausea, vomiting, dyspepsia, anorexia, diarrhea, flatulence, stomatitis, dry mouth, hypertonia, depression, dizziness, insomnia, somnolence, vertigo, pruritus, eczema,

alopecia, decreased lung function, rhinitis, increased cough, hypertension, tachycardia, phlebitis, palpitations, postural hypertension, urinary tract infection, and dysuria.

**rim** [OE, *rima,* edge], an outer edge, which may be curved or circular, as on an occluding surface built on a temporary or permanent denture base.

**rima** /rī′mə/, a cleft or fissure.

**Rimactane,** trademark for an antibacterial (rifampin).

**rima glottidis.** See **glottis.**

**rimose** /rī′mōs/, having many clefts or fissures.

**Rimso-50,** trademark for an antiinflammatory agent (dimethyl sulfoxide).

**rimula** /rim′yələ/ [L, small cleft], a very small fissure in the brain or spinal cord.

**ring** [AS, *hring*], **1.** a circular band surrounding a central opening. **2.** a closed chainlike linkage of atoms.

**ring chromosome** [AS, *hring*], a circular chromosome formed by the fusion of the two ends. It is the primary type of chromosome found in bacteria.

**ring-down artifact,** (in radiography) an echo pattern caused by reverberation in a bubble or other soft tissue entity.

**ring-down time,** (in ultrasonics) the time required for vibration of the transducer element at its resonance frequency to decrease to a negligible level following excitation. See also **pulse duration.**

**Ringer's lactate solution,** a fluid and electrolyte replenisher. Also called **Hartmann's solution.**

■ INDICATIONS: It is prescribed for correction of extracellular volume and electrolyte depletion.

■ CONTRAINDICATIONS: Kidney failure, congestive heart failure, or hypoproteinemia prohibits its use.

■ ADVERSE EFFECTS: Among the more serious adverse reactions are sodium excess and fluid overload, which may lead to pulmonary and peripheral edema.

**ring removal from swollen finger,** a technique for taking off a tightly fitting ring. It consists of slipping the end of a string under the ring while moving the ring toward the hand. The rest of the string is then wound around the swollen part of the finger a number of times, after which the string is unwound from the hand side, gradually easing the ring toward the finger tip. The process may need to be repeated to complete the removal.

**ringworm.** See **tinea.**

**Rinne tuning fork test** /rin′ə/ [Heinrich A. Rinne, German otologist, 1819–1868], a method of distinguishing conductive from sensorineural hearing loss. The base of a vibrating tuning fork is placed against the patient's mastoid bone. While one ear is tested, the other is masked. When the patient no longer hears the sound, the time in seconds is noted, and the fork is positioned about 1/2 inch from the ipsilateral external auditory meatus. The time sound is heard is noted. Air-conducted sound should be heard twice as long as bone-conducted sound after bone conduction stops. In sensorineural loss the sound is heard relatively longer by air conduction; in conductive hearing loss the sound is heard longer by bone conduction. The test may be performed with tuning forks of 256, 512, and 1024 cycles.

**-rinone,** combining form for amrinone-type cardiotonic agents.

**Rio Grande fever.** See **abortus fever.**

**Riopan,** trademark for an antacid (magaldrate).

**RIP,** **1.** abbreviation for **reflex inhibiting pattern. 2.** abbreviation for **ribosome-inactivating protein.**

**ripe cataract** [OE, *ripan* + Gk, *katarrhaktes,* portcullis], a mature cataract that produces swelling and opacity of the entire lens. Also called **mature cataract.**

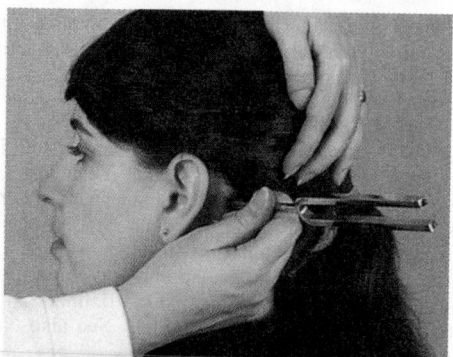

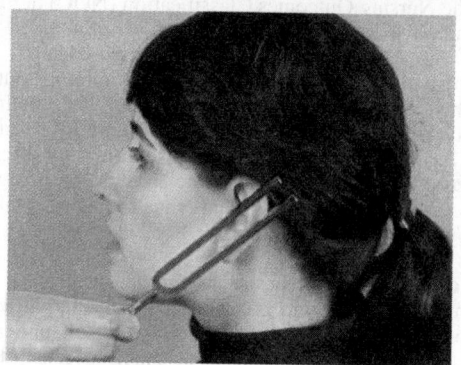

**Rinne tuning fork test** *(Seidel et al, 1999)*

**risedronate,** a bone-resorption inhibitor.

■ INDICATIONS: Risedronate is used to treat Paget's disease.

■ CONTRAINDICATIONS: Hypersensitivity to biphosphonates prohibits the use of this drug.

■ ADVERSE EFFECTS: Dizziness and headache are adverse reactions to this drug. Common side effects include abdominal pain, anorexia, diarrhea, nausea, bone pain, arthralgia, and chest pain.

**risk-benefit analysis,** the consideration as to whether a medical or surgical procedure, particularly a radical approach, is worth the risk to the patient as compared to possible benefits if the procedure is successful.

**risk control,** a nursing outcome from the Nursing Outcomes Classification (NOC) defined as the actions to eliminate or reduce actual, personal, and modifiable health threats. See also **Nursing Outcomes Classification.**

**risk control: alcohol use,** a nursing outcome from the Nursing Outcomes Classification (NOC) defined as the actions to eliminate or reduce alcohol use that poses a threat to health. See also **Nursing Outcomes Classification.**

**risk control: cancer,** a nursing outcome from the Nursing Outcomes Classification (NOC) defined as the actions to reduce or detect the possibility of cancer. See also **Nursing Outcomes Classification.**

**risk control: cardiovascular health,** a nursing outcome from the Nursing Outcomes Classification (NOC) defined as the actions to eliminate or reduce threats to cardiovascular health. See also **Nursing Outcomes Classification.**

**risk control: drug use,** a nursing outcome from the Nursing Outcomes Classification (NOC) defined as the actions to eliminate or reduce drug use that poses a threat to health. See also **Nursing Outcomes Classification.**

**risk control: hearing impairment,** a nursing outcome from the Nursing Outcomes Classification (NOC) defined as the actions to eliminate or reduce the possibility of altered hearing function. See also **Nursing Outcomes Classification.**

**risk control: sexually transmitted diseases (STD),** a nursing outcome from the Nursing Outcomes Classification (NOC) defined as the actions to eliminate or reduce the behaviors associated with sexually transmitted disease. See also **Nursing Outcomes Classification.**

**risk control: tobacco use,** a nursing outcome from the Nursing Outcomes Classification (NOC) defined as the actions to eliminate or reduce tobacco use. See also **Nursing Outcomes Classification.**

**risk control: unintended pregnancy,** a nursing outcome from the Nursing Outcomes Classification (NOC) defined as the actions to reduce the possibility of unintended pregnancy. See also **Nursing Outcomes Classification.**

**risk control: visual impairment,** a nursing outcome from the Nursing Outcomes Classification (NOC) defined as the actions to eliminate or reduce the possibility of altered visual function. See also **Nursing Outcomes Classification.**

**risk detection,** a nursing outcome from the Nursing Outcomes Classification (NOC) defined as the actions taken to identify personal health threats. See also **Nursing Outcomes Classification.**

**risk factor** [Fr, *risque,* hazard; L, *factor,* maker], a factor that causes a person or a group of people to be particularly susceptible to an unwanted, unpleasant, or unhealthful event, such as immunosuppression, which increases the incidence and severity of infection, or cigarette smoking, which increases the risk of developing a respiratory or cardiovascular disease.

**risk identification,** a nursing intervention from the Nursing Interventions Classification (NIC) defined as analysis of potential risk factors, determination of health risks, and prioritization of risk reduction strategies for an individual or group. See also **Nursing Interventions Classification.**

**risk identification: childbearing family,** a nursing intervention from the Nursing Interventions Classification (NIC) defined as identification of an individual or family likely to experience difficulties in parenting and prioritization of strategies to prevent parenting problems. See also **Nursing Interventions Classification.**

**risk identification: genetic,** a nursing intervention from the Nursing Interventions Classification (NIC) defined as identification and analysis of potential genetic risk factors in an individual, family, or group. See also **Nursing Interventions Classification.**

**risk management,** a function of administration of a hospital or other health facility directed toward identification, evaluation, and correction of potential risks that could lead to injury to patients, staff members, or visitors and result in property loss or damage.

**risorius** /risôr′ē·əs/ [L, *ridere,* to laugh], one of the 12 muscles of the mouth. A fibromusculor muscular fibrous band, it arises in the fascia over the masseter and inserts into the skin at the corner of the mouth. It acts to retract the angle of the mouth, as in a smile.

**Risser cast** /ris′ər/ [Joseph C. Risser, American surgeon, 1892–1942], an orthopedic device for encasing the entire trunk of the body, extending over the cervical area to the chin. In rare cases it extends over the hips to the knees. The Risser cast is made of plaster of paris or fiberglass and is used to immobilize the trunk in the treatment of scoliosis and in the preoperative or postoperative correction or maintenance of correction of scoliosis. Compare **body jacket, turnbuckle cast.**

**RIST,** abbreviation for **radioimmunosorbent test.**

**risus caninus** /rī′səs/ [L, *risus,* laughter, *caninus,* doglike], a grinning facial distortion caused by tension in the occipitofrontalis and other facial muscles as a result of tetanus.

**risus sardonicus** /särdon′ikəs/ [L, laughter; Gk, *sardonius,* mocking], a wry masklike grin caused by spasm of the facial muscles, as seen in tetanus.

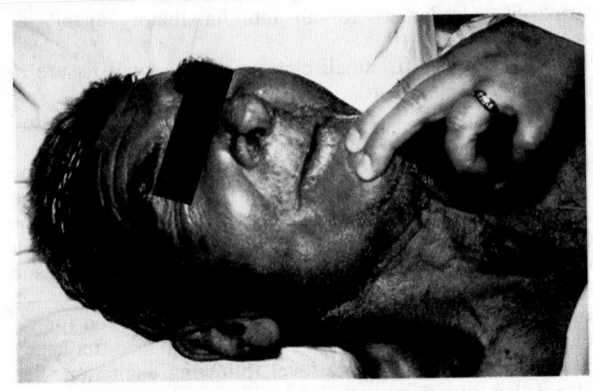

**Risus sardonicus** *(Stone and Gorbach, 2000)*

**Ritalin Hydrochloride,** trademark for a central nervous system stimulant (methylphenidate hydrochloride).

**Ritgen maneuver,** an obstetric procedure used to control delivery of the fetal head. It involves applying upward pressure from the coccygeal region to extend the head during actual delivery, thereby protecting the musculature of the perineum.

**ritodrine hydrochloride** /rit′ədrēn/, a uterine relaxant.
- INDICATION: It is prescribed in pregnancy management to stop the uterus from contracting in preterm labor.
- CONTRAINDICATIONS: It is not given before the twentieth week of gestation. Known hypersensitivity to this drug prohibits its use.
- ADVERSE EFFECTS: Among the more serious adverse reactions are tachycardia, palpitations, headache, nausea, and alterations in blood pressure. Pulmonary edema and death have occurred when it has been given concomitantly with corticosteroids to prevent the development of respiratory distress syndrome in the premature neonate.

**ritonavir,** a protease inhibitor.
- INDICATIONS: It is prescribed in the treatment of acquired immunodeficiency syndrome, either alone or in combination with nucleoside analogs.
- CONTRAINDICATIONS: The drug should not be given to patients taking clarithromycin, trimethoprim, or rifabutin, or formulations containing those drugs.
- ADVERSE EFFECTS: The side effects most often reported include nausea, vomiting, diarrhea, and numbness about the lips.

**Ritter's disease** [Gottfried Ritter von Rittershain, German physician, 1820–1883], a rare, staphylococcal infection of newborns that begins with red spots about the mouth and chin, gradually spreading over the entire body, and followed by generalized exfoliation. Vesicles and yellow crusts may also be present. Ritter's disease is usually fatal unless treated with antibiotics, which should be selected on the basis of bacterial sensitivity tests. Also called **dermatitis exfoliativa neonatorum.** Compare **toxic epidermal necrolysis.**

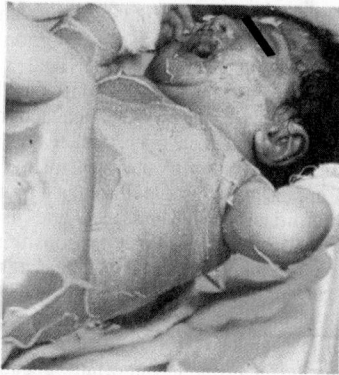

**Ritter's disease** *(Weston, Lane, and Morrelli, 1996)*

**ritual** /rich′əwəl/, **1.** a mental health disorder characterized by repetitive sequences of stereotyped daily life routines, such as repeated handwashing that interferes with an individual's level of functioning. **2.** a prescribed order of ceremonial acts or series of acts. **3.** a detailed procedure followed faithfully or regularly.

**ritual circumcision,** a surgical procedure for removing the prepuce of the male in Jewish communities or the labia minora of the female in Muslim communities as a religious rite. In Jewish families the male circumcision is usually performed on the eighth day after birth. The practice dates back to the ancient Egyptians, and in some societies it is a prerequisite for marriage. See also **circumcision, female circumcision, female genital mutilation.**

**rituximab,** a miscellaneous antineoplastic.
■ INDICATIONS: Rituximab is used to treat non-Hodgkin's lymphoma (CD20 positive, B-cell).
■ CONTRAINDICATIONS: Known hypersensitivity to this drug or to murine proteins prohibits the use of rituximab.
■ ADVERSE EFFECTS: Life-threatening effects of rituximab include leukopenia, neutropenia, thrombocytopenia, and bronchospasm. Other adverse reactions include fever, chills, asthenia, headache, angioedema, hypotension, and myalgia. Common side effects include nausea, vomiting, anorexia, irritation at the injection site, and rash.

*Rivea corymbosa,* a twining vine of the botanical family of Convulvaceae. The seeds contain indole alkaloids, a source of lysergic acid diethylamide, which have an effect of altered perception when ingested in large quantities. They have been used in religious ceremonies of indigenous Latin American cultures since the era of the Aztecs. Also called **Mexican bindweed, morning glory.**

**river blindness.** See **onchocerciasis.**

**Rivinus notch** /rēvē′nəs/ [Augustus Q. Rivinus, German anatomist, 1652–1723], a deficiency in the tympanic sulcus of the ear that forms an attachment for the flaccid part of the tympanic membrane and the mallear folds.

**rivus lacrimalis** /rī′vəs/ [L, stream of tears], a channel between the eyelids and the surface of the eye that normally allows a flow of moisture when the eyes are closed.

**rizatriptan,** a migraine agent.
■ INDICATIONS: Rizatriptan is used in the acute treatment of migraine.
■ CONTRAINDICATIONS: The following factors prohibit the use of rizatriptan: angina pectoris, a history of myocardial infarction, documented silent ischemia, Prinzmetal's angina,

ischemic heart disease, concurrent use of ergotamine-containing preparations, uncontrolled hypertension, basilar or hemiplegic migraine, and known hypersensitivity.
■ ADVERSE EFFECTS: Adverse reactions to this drug include chest tightness, chest pressure, nausea, and dry mouth. Common side effects include dizziness, headache, and fatigue.

**RK, 1.** abbreviation for **radial keratotomy. 2.** abbreviation for **refractive keratotomy.**

**R.L.E.,** abbreviation for *right lower extremity.*

**R.L.L.,** abbreviation for *right lower lobe of lung.*

**r-loop,** (in molecular genetics) a distinctive loop formation seen under an electron microscope. It is composed of a single helical strand of deoxyribonucleic acid (DNA) wound with a hybrid strand containing another single strand of DNA with a strand of ribonucleic acid.

**RLQ,** abbreviation for *right lower quadrant.*

**RMP,** abbreviation for *right mentoposterior* fetal position.

**RMSF,** abbreviation for **Rocky Mountain spotted fever.**

**RMT,** abbreviation for *right mentotransverse* fetal position.

**Rn,** symbol for the element **radon.**

**RN,** abbreviation for **registered nurse.**

**RNA,** abbreviation for **ribonucleic acid.**

**RNA-dependent DNA polymerase.** See **reverse transcriptase.**

**RNA polymerase,** an enzyme that catalyzes the assembly of ribonucleoside triphosphates into RNA, with single-stranded DNA serving as the template. Also called **RNA nucleotidyltransferase.**

**RNase,** abbreviation for **ribonuclease.**

**RNA splicing,** (in molecular genetics) the process by which base pairs that interrupt the continuity of genetic information in deoxyribonucleic acid are removed from the precursors of messenger ribonucleic acid.

**RNA virus,** any of a group of viruses whose genome is composed of RNA, including most viruses that infect animal cells. RNA viruses include arenavirus, coronavirus, orthomyxovirus, picornavirus, rhabdovirus, and togavirus. Also called **ribovirus.**

**RN, C,** abbreviation for *registered nurse, certified.*

**RN, CNA,** abbreviation for *registered nurse, certified in Nursing Administration.*

**RN, CNAA,** abbreviation for *registered nurse, certified in Nursing Administration, Advanced.*

**RN, CS,** abbreviation for *registered nurse, certified Specialist.*

**RNP,** abbreviation for **ribonuclear protein.**

**ROA,** abbreviation for *right occipitoanterior* fetal position.

**Robaxin,** trademark for a skeletal muscle relaxant (methocarbamol).

**Robb, Isabel Hampton** (1860–1910), a Canadian-born American nursing educator and writer. She was the first to institute a systematic, step-by-step course for nursing students that integrated clinical experience and classwork and the first educator to arrange for the affiliation of her students at other hospitals for specialized training. She also helped establish university affiliation for nursing education and postgraduate courses. When the Johns Hopkins School of Nursing was established in Baltimore in 1889, she became its first director, establishing the high standards for both the practical and theoretic aspects of nursing education that became the base from which she worked to establish national standards. She was one of the founders of *The American Journal of Nursing* and of the forerunner of the American Nurses Association.

**robertsonian translocation** /rob′ərtsō′nē·ən/, the exchange of entire chromosome arms, with the break occurring at the centromere, usually between two nonhomologous acrocentric chromosomes. It produces one large, metacentric chromosome and one extremely small chromosome. The latter carries little genetic material and may be lost through successive cell divisions, leading to a reduction in total chromosome number. Compare **balanced translocation, reciprocal translocation.**

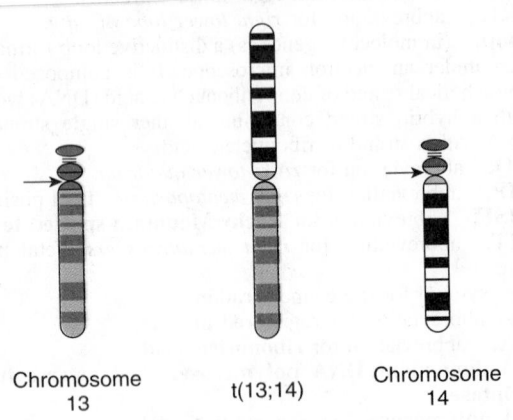

Chromosome 13    t(13;14)    Chromosome 14

**Robertsonian translocation** (Jorde et al, 2001)

**Roberts' syndrome** /rob'ərts/ [John Bingham Roberts, American surgeon, 1852–1924], a hereditary syndrome, transmitted as an autosomal recessive trait, consisting of imperfect development of the long bones of the limbs associated with cleft palate and lip and other anomalies.

**Robinow's syndrome** /rob'inouz/ [Meinhard Robinow, American physician, b. 1909], dwarfism associated with increased interorbital distance, malaligned teeth, bulging forehead, depressed nasal bridge, and short limbs. Also called **fetal face syndrome, Robinow dwarfism.**

**Robinul,** trademark for an anticholinergic (glycopyrrolate).

**Robitussin,** trademark for an expectorant (guaifenesin), also available in various fixed-combination preparations with an antihistamine, with a decongestant, or with a cough suppressant.

**robotic** /rōbot'ik/, pertaining to a robot, a mechanical or electronic device that resembles a human being, operating automatically or by remote control with the ability to perform a variety of complex tasks.

**Rocaltrol,** trademark for a regulator of calcium (calcitriol).

**Rocephin,** trademark for a cephalosporin antibiotic (ceftriaxone sodium).

**Rochalimaea** /rosh'əlimē'ə/, a genus of bacteria resembling *Rickettsia* but found extracellularly in an arthropod host. The type species, *R. quintana,* is a cause of trench fever as transmitted by the body louse. A related bacterium is a cause of bacillary angiomatosis in immunocompromised humans, including those with human immunodeficiency virus infection.

**rocker knife,** a knife with a rounded blade that cuts with a rocking motion, designed for patients who have functional use of one extremity.

**rock fever.** See **brucellosis.**

**rocking bed,** a device that rocks a patient from 30 degrees head up to 15 degrees head down several times a minute.

The rocking moves the abdominal contents, and the resulting diaphragmatic movement assists ventilation of the lungs.

**Rocky Mountain spotted fever (RMSF),** a serious tick-borne infectious disease occurring throughout the temperate zones of North and South America, caused by *Rickettsia rickettsii.* It is characterized by chills, fever, severe headache, myalgia, mental confusion, and rash. Erythematous macules first appear on wrists and ankles, spreading rapidly over the extremities, trunk, and face and usually on the palms and soles. Hemorrhagic lesions, constipation, and abdominal distension are also common. The diagnosis is based on clinical examination and confirmed by laboratory analyses, including immunofluorescent antibody screens, complement fixation test, and Weil-Felix test. Early treatment with doxycycline or tetracycline is important, because more than 20% of untreated patients die from shock and renal failure. A diet high in protein is important to avoid hypoproteinemia. Nursing care is especially important to avoid decubitus ulcers and hypostatic or aspiration pneumonia. Immunity follows recovery. Prevention includes the use of insect repellents, the wearing of protective clothing, frequent inspection of the body and careful removal of wood or dog ticks, and immunization with killed vaccine for those frequently exposed to ticks. Care must be taken not to crush ticks, because infection may be acquired through skin abrasions. Also called **mountain fever, mountain tick fever, spotted fever.** Compare **murine typhus, rickettsialpox.** See also **boutonneuse fever, scrub typhus, typhus.**

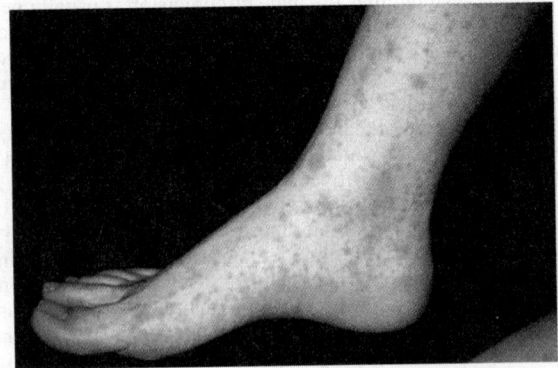

**Rocky Mountain spotted fever: typical rash**
(Goldstein and Goldstein, 1997/courtesy Medical College of Georgia, Department of Dermatology)

**rocuronium bromide,** a nondepolarizing neuromuscular blocking agent.

■ INDICATIONS: It is prescribed as an adjunct to general anesthesia in providing skeletal muscle relaxation.

■ CONTRAINDICATIONS: The drug should not be given to patients with a known hypersensitivity to the product.

■ ADVERSE EFFECTS: The side effects most often reported include nausea, vomiting, respiratory problems, arrhythmias, hiccups, injection site edema, and rash.

**rod** [AS, *rodd*], **1.** a straight cylindric structure. **2.** one of the tiny cylindric elements arranged perpendicular to the surface of the retina. Rods contain the chemical rhodopsin, which adapts the eye to detect low-intensity light and gives the rods a purple color. Each rod is 40 to 60 μm in length and about 2 μm thick and consists of a slender reactive outer segment and an inner granular segment. When bright light strikes a rod, rhodopsin rapidly breaks down; it reforms gradually in low-intensity light. Compare **cone.** See also **iodopsin, Jacob x membrane, rhodopsin.**

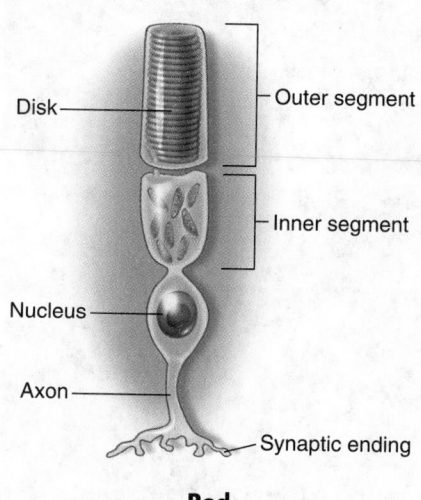

Disk — Outer segment

Inner segment

Nucleus

Axon

Synaptic ending

**Rod**

**rodenticide poisoning** /rōden′tisīd/ [L, *rodere,* to gnaw, *caedere,* to kill, *potio,* drink], a toxic condition caused by the ingestion of a substance intended for the control of rodent populations. See also **phosphorus poisoning, thallium poisoning, warfarin poisoning.**

**rodent ulcer** /rō′dənt/ [L, *rodere,* to gnaw, *ulcus,* ulcer], a slowly developing serpiginous ulceration of a basal cell carcinoma of the skin. See also **basal cell carcinoma.**

**rod-monochromat** /rod′monəkrō′mət/, a person who is totally color-blind or who lacks retinal cone function.

**rods and cones** [AS, *rodd* + Gk, *konos*], the light-sensitive cells of the retina. The rods, under the visual purple pigment epithelium, are mainly located around the periphery of the retina. The cones receive color stimuli.

**roentgen (R)** /rent′gən, ren′jən/ [Wilhelm K. Roentgen, German physicist, 1845–1923], the quantity of x- or gamma radiation that creates 1 electrostatic unit of ions in 1 mL of air at 0° and 760 mm of pressure. In radiotherapy or radiodiagnosis, the roentgen is the unit of the emitted dose. See also **rad, rem.**

**roentgen fetometry,** the use of radiographic techniques to measure the fetus in utero.

**roentgenologist.** See **radiologist.**

**roentgenology.** See **radiology.**

**roentgen ray.** See **x-ray.**

**rofecoxib,** a nonsteroidal antiinflammatory (NSAID).

■ INDICATIONS: Rofecoxib is used to treat acute, chronic osteoarthritis pain and primary dysmenorrhea.

■ CONTRAINDICATIONS: Asthma and known hypersensitivity to aspirin, iodides, and other NSAIDs prohibit the use of this drug.

■ ADVERSE EFFECTS: Life-threatening effects of rofecoxib include tachycardia, myocardial infarction, dysrhythmias, GI bleeding, nephrotoxicity (including dysuria, hematuria, oliguria, and azotemia), and blood dyscrasias. Other adverse effects include angina, purpura, pharyngitis, shortness of breath, pneumonia, and coughing. Common side effects are numerous and include fatigue, anxiety, depression, nervousness, paresthesia, palpitations, hypertension, fluid retention, tinnitus, hearing loss, blurred vision, glaucoma, cataract, conjunctivitis, eye pain, nausea, anorexia, vomiting, constipation, dry mouth, diverticulitis, gastritis, gastroenteritis, hemorrhoids, hiatal hernia, stomatitis, cystitis, urinary tract infection, epistaxis, bruising, anemia, rash, pruritus, sweating, erythema, petechiae, photosensitivity, and alopecia.

**Roferon-A,** trademark for a parenteral antineoplastic (interferon-alfa-2a).

**Rogers, Martha,** (1914–1994), a nurse theorist who developed the Science of Unitary Human Beings, a nursing theory introduced in 1970. The Rogers' theory has strong ties to the general systems theory with elements of a developmental model. It considers four "building blocks": Energy Fields, Universe of Open Systems, Pattern and Organization, and Four Dimensionality. Energy Fields refers to conceptualization of humans and their environment as matter or energy evidenced by wave patterns. Open Systems refers to views of persons as open systems who interact continuously with the environment. Pattern and Organization describes the way Energy Fields emerge, characterized by wave patterns. Four Dimensionality has been interpreted as a form of clairvoyance in which there is a "transcendence of time-space interaction," or an ability to transcend time to see into the future.

**Rohrer's constants,** the constants in an empiric equation for airway resistance. It is expressed as $R = K_1 + K_2 V$, where R is resistance, V is instantaneous volumetric flow rate, $K_1$ is a constant representing gas viscosity and airway geometry, and $K_2$ is a constant representing gas density and airway geometry.

**Rokitansky's disease.** See **Budd-Chiari syndrome.**

**Rolando's fissure** /rōlan′dōz/ [Luigi Rolando, Italian anatomist, 1773–1831; L, *fissura,* cleft], the central sulcus of the cerebrum.

**Rolando's fracture** [Luigi Rolando], a fracture of the base of the first metacarpal.

**role** [Fr, stage character], a socially expected behavior pattern associated with an individual's function in various social groups. Roles provide a means for social participation and a way to test identities for consensual validation by significant others, for example, roles within the family structure.

**role ambiguity.** See **role strain.**

**role blurring,** the tendency for professional roles to overlap and become indistinct when there is a shared body of knowledge among and between disciplines.

**role change,** a situation in which status is retained while role expectations change, as when a nurse moves from the role of a primary caregiver to that of administrator.

**role clarification,** gaining the knowledge, information, and cues needed to perform a role.

**role conflict,** the presence of contradictory and often competing role expectations.

**role enhancement,** a nursing intervention from the Nursing Interventions Classification (NIC) defined as assisting a patient, significant other, and/or family to improve relationships by clarifying and supplementing specific role behaviors. See also **Nursing Interventions Classification.**

**role incongruence.** See **role strain.**

**role model** [Fr, *role,* stage character; L, *modus,* small copy], a person who knowingly or unknowingly inspires others to imitate his or her persona. The role model may be a real person, as a parent, or a symbolic character as depicted in movies or television programs.

**role overload,** a condition in which there is insufficient time in which to carry out all of the expected role functions.

**role overqualification.** See **role strain.**

**role performance,** a nursing outcome from the Nursing Outcomes Classification (NOC) defined as the congruence of an individual's role behavior with role expectations. See also **Nursing Outcomes Classification.**

**role performance, ineffective,** a nursing diagnosis accepted by the Seventh National Conference on the Classification of Nursing Diagnoses. Altered role performance is a disruption in the way one perceives one's role performance.

■ DEFINING CHARACTERISTICS: The defining characteristics include a change in self-perception of one's role, denial of the role, a change in others' perception of one's role, conflict in roles, a change in physical capacity to resume one's role, lack of knowledge of role, and change in usual patterns of responsibility.

■ RELATED FACTORS: Related factors are to be developed. See also **nursing diagnosis.**

**role playing,** a psychotherapeutic technique in which a person acts out a real or simulated situation as a means of understanding intrapsychic conflicts.

**role-playing therapy.** See **psychodrama.**

**role reversal,** the act of assuming the role of another person to appreciate how the person feels, perceives, and behaves in relation to himself and others.

**role strain,** stress associated with expected roles or positions, experienced as frustration. **Role ambiguity** is a type of role strain that occurs when shared specifications set for an expected role are incomplete or insufficient to tell the involved individual what is desired and how to do it. **Role incongruence** is role stress that occurs when an individual undergoes role transitions requiring a significant modification in attitudes and values. **Role overqualification** is a type of role stress that occurs when a role does not require full use of a person's resources.

**Rolfing.** See **structural integration.**

**roll** [OFr, *rolle*], intrinsic joint movements on an axis parallel to the articulating surface. The axis can remain stationary or move in a plane parallel to the joint surface.

**roller bandage,** a long, tightly wound strip of material that may vary in width. It is generally applied as a circular bandage wrapped around an extremity or the trunk.

**roller clamp,** a device, usually made of plastic, equipped with a small roller that may be rolled counterclockwise to close off primary IV tubing or clockwise to open it. The roller clamp may also be manipulated to increase and decrease the flow of the IV solution and is easily moved with the thumb, thus making it a one-handed convenience in the administration of IV therapy. Compare **screw clamp, slide clamp.**

**rolling effleurage,** a circular rubbing stroke used in massage to promote circulation and muscle relaxation, especially on the shoulder and buttocks. It is performed with the hand flat, the palm and closely held fingers acting as a unit. Compare **effleurage, pétrissage.**

**ROM, 1.** abbreviation for **range of motion. 2.** abbreviation for **read-only memory. 3.** abbreviation for **rupture of membranes. 4.** abbreviation for *right otitis media.*

**Romano-Ward syndrome** /rō·mä′nō·wôrd/ [C. Romano, Italian physician, b. 1923; O.C. Ward, Irish physician, 20th century], an autosomal dominant form of the long QT syndrome, characterized by syncope and sometimes ventricular fibrillation and sudden death. See also **long QT syndrome.**

**Romberg sign** /rom′bərg/ [Moritz H. Romberg, German physician, 1795–1873; L, *signum,* mark], an indication of loss of the sense of position in which the patient loses bal-

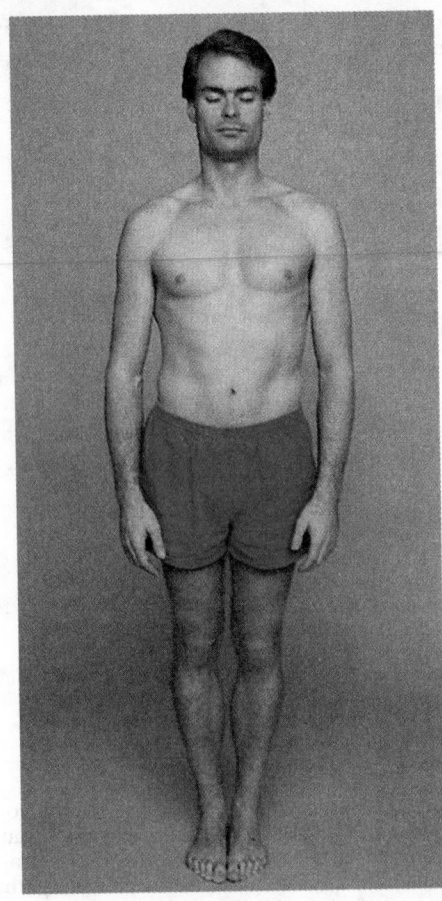

**Evaluation of the Romberg sign** *(Seidel et al, 1999)*

ance when standing erect, feet together, and eyes closed. Also called **Romberg test.**

**Rondec-DM,** trademark for a fixed-combination drug containing an antihistamine (carbinoxamine maleate), an antitussive (dextromethorphan hydrobromide), and an adrenergic decongestant and bronchodilator (pseudoephedrine hydrochloride).

**Rondomycin,** trademark for an antibiotic (methacycline hydrochloride).

**rongeur forceps** /rônzhur′, rôNzhœr′/ [Fr, *ronger,* to gnaw; L, *forceps,* pair of tongs], a kind of biting forceps that is strong and heavy, used for cutting bone. Also called **rongeur.**

**R-on-T phenomenon,** a cardiac event in which a ventricular stimulus causes premature depolarization of cells that have not completely repolarized. It is noted on the electrocardiogram as a ventricular depolarization falling somewhere within a T wave. The R-on-T phenomenon may result in ventricular tachycardia or ventricular fibrillation in patients with heart disease.

**rooming-in,** (in a hospital) a practice that allows mothers and newborn babies to share accommodations, remaining together in the hospital as they would at home rather than being separated. Also called **living-in unit.**

**room temperature** [AS, *rum* + L, *temperatura*], the air temperature as measured in a specific part of a room.

**root** /rōōt, rŏŏt/ [AS, *rot*], the lowest part of an organ or a structure by which something is firmly attached, such as the anatomic root of the tooth, which is covered by cementum. Also called *(Latin)* **radix.**

**root amputation.** See **apicectomy.**

**root canal.** See **pulp canal.**

**root canal file,** a small, metal hand instrument with tightly spiraled blades, used for cleaning and shaping a pulp canal.

**root canal filling,** a material placed in the pulp canal of a tooth to seal the space previously occupied by the dental pulp. See **canal obturation.**

**root canal therapy,** that aspect of endodontics dealing with the treatment of diseases of the dental pulp, consisting of partial (pulpotomy) or complete (pulpectomy) extirpation of the diseased pulp, cleaning and sterilization of the empty root canal, enlarging and shaping of the canal to receive sealing material, and obturation of the canal with a nonirritating hermetic sealing agent. Also called **pulp canal therapy.**

**root curettage,** the debridement and planing of the root surface of a tooth to remove accretions and induce the development of healthy gingival tissues. Also called **root planing.**

**root end cyst.** See **radicular cyst.**

**root furcation,** 1. the anatomic area at which the roots of a multirooted tooth divide. 2. abnormal intraradicular resorption of bone in multirooted teeth, resulting from periodontal disease.

**rooting reflex,** a normal response in newborns when the cheek is touched or stroked along the side of the mouth to turn the head toward the stimulated side and begin to suck. The reflex disappears by 3 to 4 months of age but in some infants may persist until 12 months of age.

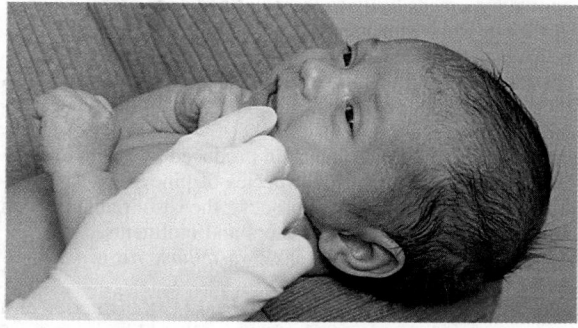

**Elicitation of the rooting reflex** *(Seidel et al, 1999)*

**root planing.** See **root curettage.**

**root resection.** See **apicectomy.**

**root resorption of teeth** [AS, *rot* + L, *resorbere*, to suck back; AS, *toth*], destruction of the cementum or dentin of tooth roots. If only the apex of the root is affected, the root may be short and blunted. If the middle of the root is affected, the pulp canal will generally be penetrated.

**root retention,** a technique that removes the crown of a root canal-treated tooth and retains enough of the root and gingival attachment to support a prosthesis.

**root submersion,** a root retention in which the tooth structure is reduced below the level of the alveolar crest and the soft tissue is allowed to heal over it. This technique is used to minimize residual ridge resorption.

**ROP,** abbreviation for *right occipitoposterior* fetal position.

**ropinirole,** an antiparkinson agent.
- INDICATIONS: Ropinirole is used to treat parkinsonism.
- CONTRAINDICATIONS: Known hypersensitivity to this drug prohibits its use.
- ADVERSE EFFECTS: Life-threatening effects of this drug are hemolytic anemia, leukopenia, and agranulocytosis. Other adverse effects include psychosis, hallucination, dystonia, depression, dizziness, constipation, dyspepsia, flatulence, rash, sweating, tachycardia, hypertension, hypotension, syncope, palpitations, blurred vision, impotence, urinary frequency, pharyngitis, rhinitis, sinusitis, bronchitis, and dyspnea. Common side effects include agitation, insomnia, nausea, vomiting, anorexia, dry mouth, and orthostatic hypotension.

**ropivacaine,** a local anesthetic.
- INDICATIONS: This drug is used to produce peripheral nerve block, caudal anesthesia, central neural block, and vaginal block.
- CONTRAINDICATIONS: Use of this drug is prohibited in children less than 12 years of age, in the elderly, in those with severe liver disease, and in those with known hypersensitivity to this drug.
- ADVERSE EFFECTS: Life-threatening effects of this drug are convulsions, loss of consciousness, myocardial depression, cardiac arrest, dysrhythmias, fetal bradycardia, status asthmaticus, respiratory arrest, and anaphylaxis. Other adverse effects are anxiety, restlessness, drowsiness, disorientation, tremors, shivering, bradycardia, hypotension, hypertension, nausea, vomiting, blurred vision, tinnitus, pupil constriction, rash, urticaria, allergic reactions, edema, burning, skin discoloration at the injection site, and tissue necrosis.

**Rorschach test** /rôr′shäk, rôr′shokh/ [Hermann Rorschach, Swiss psychiatrist, 1884–1922], a projective personality assessment test developed by Hermann Rorschach. It consists of 10 pictures of inkblots, five in black and white, three in black and red, and two multicolored, to which the subject responds by telling, in as many interpretations as is desired, what images and emotions each design evokes. Replies are evaluated according to whether the response is to the entire or only part of the image; whether color, shading, shape, or location of individual elements is significant; whether movement is seen; and the degree of complexity to which each interpretation is given. Scoring is primarily subjective and is based on both the subject's responses and the general reaction to the circumstances under which the test is administered. The test is designed to assess the degree to which intellectual and emotional factors are integrated in the subject's perception of the environment. See also **Holtzman inkblot technique.**

**ROS,** abbreviation for **review of systems.**

**rosacea** /rōzā′shē·ə/ [L, *rosaceus,* rosy], a chronic inflammatory disease seen in adults of all ages. It has two components of erythema and/or acneiform papules and pustules. It is associated with erythema, pustules, and telangiectasia, especially of the nose, forehead, and cheeks. See also **rhinophyma.**

**rose fever** [L, *rosa* + *febris,* fever], a common misnomer for seasonal allergic rhinitis caused by pollen, most frequently of grasses, that is airborne at the time roses are in bloom. Since rose pollen is not dispersed by the wind but is carried from flower to flower by insects, roses are not the cause of common spring and summer allergic reactions.

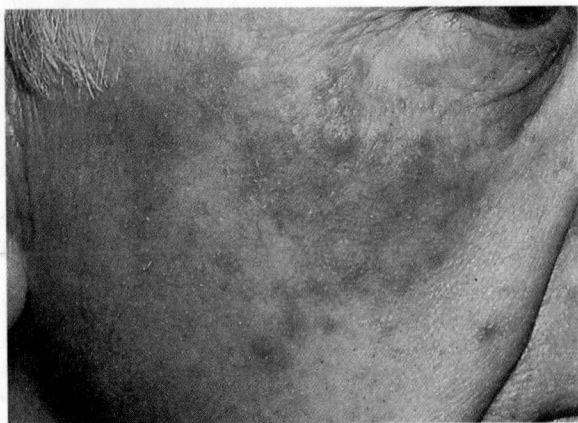

**Rosacea** (du Vivier, 1993/courtesy King's College Hospital)

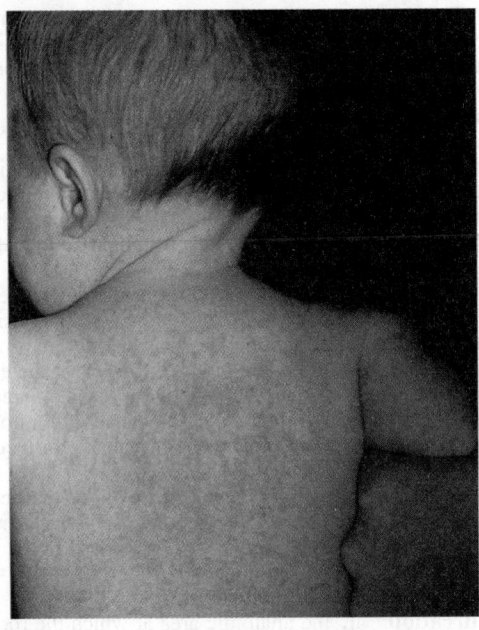

**Macular rash of roseola infantum** (Zitelli and Davis, 1997)

**rose hips,** an herbal product taken from a plant native to Europe and Asia, now grown widely in North America.
■ USES: This herb is used as a source of vitamin C and as a treatment for colds, fever, and mild infections.
■ CONTRAINDICATIONS: Rose hips should not be used during pregnancy and lactation or in people with known hypersensitivity to this plant.

**Rosenberg-Chutorian syndrome** /rō′zən·berg·chōō·tor′ē·ən/ [Roger N. Rosenberg, American physician, 20th century; Abe Milton Chutorian, American physician, b. 1929], a rare X-linked hereditary syndrome characterized by optic atrophy, progressive sensorineural hearing loss, and polyneuropathy.

**Rosenmüller's organ.** See epoophoron.

**Rosenthal's syndrome.** See hemophilia C.

**roseo-,** combining form meaning rose colored, as a roseola rash.

**roseola** /rōzē′ələ/ [L, roseus], any rose-colored rash. See also roseola infantum.

**roseola idiopathica,** a skin eruption of symmetric reddish patches in a condition not associated with any other well-defined symptoms of disease.

**roseola infantum,** a benign viral endemic illness of infants and young children, caused by human herpesvirus 6 and possibly by herpesvirus 7. It is characterized by abrupt high sustained or spiking fever, mild pharyngitis, and lymph node enlargement. Febrile seizures may occur. After 4 or 5 days the fever suddenly drops to normal, and a faint, pink, maculopapular rash appears on the neck, trunk, and thighs. The rash may last a few hours to 2 days. Diagnosis is based on high fever with rather mild illness and the rash. Sequelae may occur as a result of the seizures. There is no specific therapy or vaccine. Acetaminophen is often used to try to control fever. Also called **exanthem subitum, exanthema subitum, sixth disease, Zahorsky's disease.**

**roseola symptomatica,** a rose-colored eruption that occurs at the onset of a well-defined febrile illness.

**rose spots** [L, rosa + ME, spotte], small erythematous macules occurring on the upper abdomen and anterior thorax and lasting 2 or 3 days, characteristic of typhoid and paratyphoid fevers.

**rosette** /rōzet′/, 1. any structure resembling a rose. 2. a sporulating body of a malarial parasite.

**rosette technique,** a method of detecting antigens or antibodies on a cell surface using or antibody- or antigen-coated particles, which cause erythrocytes to form a rosette pattern.

**Rose-Waaler test.** See sheep cell agglutination test.

**rosiglitazone,** an oral antidiabetic.
■ INDICATIONS: Rosiglitazone is used to treat stable type 2 diabetes mellitus.
■ CONTRAINDICATIONS: Lactation, diabetic ketoacidosis, and known hypersensitivity to thiazolidinediones prohibit use of this drug. Rosiglitazone is also contraindicated in children.
■ ADVERSE EFFECTS: Adverse effects of this drug include upper respiratory infection, sinusitis, anemia, back pain, diarrhea, edema, fatigue, headache, and hyper- or hypoglycemia.

**rosin** /roz′in/, a solid oleo resin produced by steam distillation of balsam from various species of pine trees. After extraction of turpentine in the process, the rosin remains as an amber mass. It is used in plasters and ointments.

**rost-,** prefix meaning 'a beak': rostellum, rostrad, rostriform.

**rostellum** /rostel′əm/ [L, rostrum, beak], the anterior of a tapeworm scolex, commonly featuring hooklike jaws.

**rostral** /ros′trəl/, beak-shaped. —**rostrum,** n.

**rostrum** /ros′trəm/ [L, beak], a beaklike projection, as the rostrum of the sphenoid bone.

**rot** [AS, rotian], 1. to decay. 2. decomposition.

**ROT,** abbreviation for right occipitotransverse fetal position.

**rot-,** combining form meaning 'turned, or to turn': rotate, rotatory, rotexion.

**rotameter.** See flowmeter.

**rotary nystagmus** /rō′tərē/ [L, rotare, to rotate; Gk, nystagmos, nodding], a form of nystagmus in which the eyeball makes rotary motions around an axis.

**rotating tourniquet** /rō′tāting/ [L, rotare, to rotate; Fr, tourniquet, garrote], one of four constricting devices used in a rotating order to pool blood in the extremities. The purpose is to relieve congestion in the lungs in the treatment of acute pulmonary edema. Use of the rotating tourniquet has declined with the development of vasodilating drugs and diuretics.

**rotation** /rōtā′shən/ [L, *rotare*],   **1.** one of the four basic movements allowed by the various joints of the skeleton. It is the gyration of a bone around its central axis, which may lie in a separate bone, as in the pivot formed by the dens of the axis around which the atlas turns. Some bones, such as the humerus, rotate around their own longitudinal axis. Alternatively, the axis of rotation may not be quite parallel to the long axis of the rotating bone, as in movement of the radius on the ulna during pronation and supination of the hand. Compare **angular movement, circumduction, gliding. 2.** a turning around an axis. **3.** the turning of the fetal head to descend through the pelvis during birth.

**rotator** /rō′tātər/ [L, *rotare*, to rotate],   a muscle that rotates a structure around its axis, as the cervical, thoracic, and lumbar musculi rotatores, which function to extend and rotate the vertebral column toward the opposite side.

**rotator cuff,**   a musculotendinous structure about the capsule of the shoulder joint, formed by the inserting fibers of the supraspinatus, infraspinatus, teres minor, and subscapularis muscles, blending with the capsule, and providing mobility and strength to the shoulder joint.

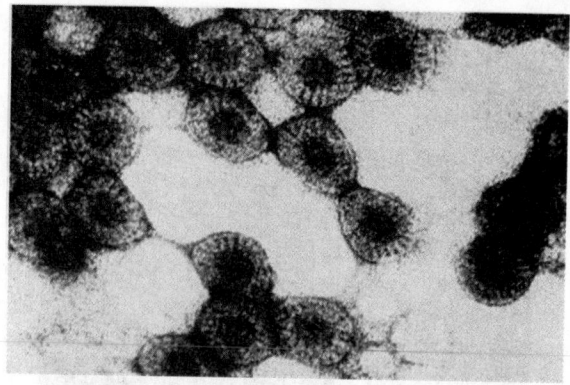

**Rotavirus** *(Baron, Peterson, and Finegold, 1994)*

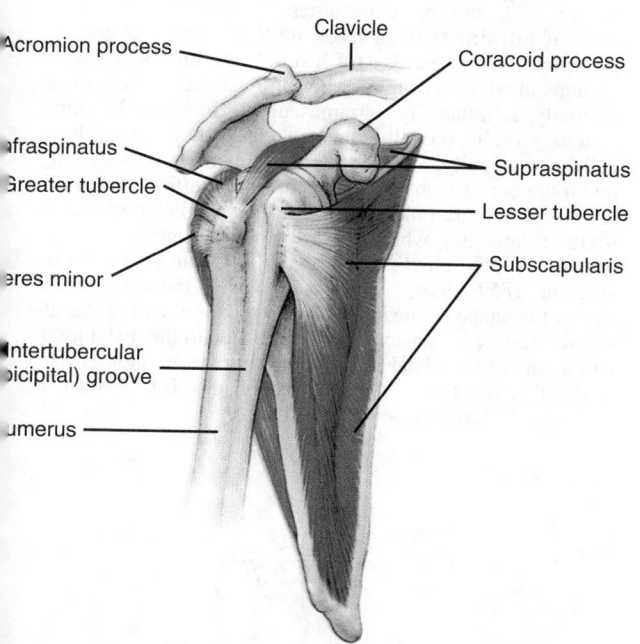

Acromion process — Clavicle — Coracoid process — Infraspinatus — Greater tubercle — Supraspinatus — Lesser tubercle — Teres minor — Subscapularis — Intertubercular (bicipital) groove — Humerus

**Rotator cuff** *(Thibodeau and Patton, 1999/John V. Hagen)*

**rotavirus** /rō′təvī′rəs/,   a double-stranded ribonucleic acid virus that appears as a tiny wheel, with a clearly defined outer layer, or rim, and an inner layer of spokes. The virus replicates in the epithelial cells of the intestine and is a cause of acute gastroenteritis with diarrhea, particularly in infants. Rotavirus is the most common cause worldwide of severe diarrheal illness in children, through fecal-oral transmission. Various strains also infect domestic and wild animals. In the United States, infections tend to peak during the winter months. A licensed live virus vaccine is no longer recom-

mended because of its association with a rare case of bowel obstruction (intussusception).

**Rothmund-Thomson syndrome** /rot′mŏŏnd·tom′son/ [August von Rothmund, Jr. German physician, 1830−1906; Mathew Sidney Thomson, English dermatologist, 1894−1969],   an autosomal recessive syndrome occurring principally in females, characterized by the presence of reticulated, atrophic, hyperpigmented, telangiectatic cutaneous plaques, often accompanied by juvenile cataracts, saddle nose, congenital bone defects, disturbances in the growth of hair, nails, and teeth, and hypogonadism. Also called **poikiloderma congenitale.**

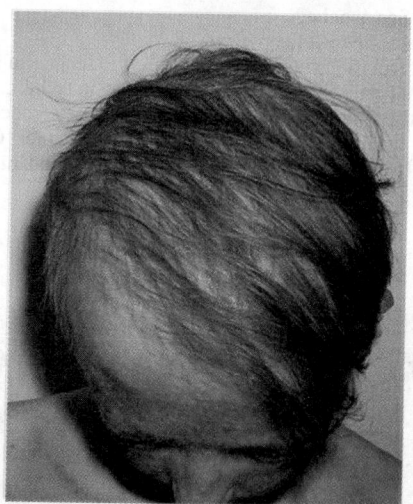

**Rothmund-Thomson syndrome**
*(Hordinsky, Sawaya, and Scher, 2000)*

**Roth spots** /roth, rōt/ [Moritz Roth, Swiss physician and pathologist, 1839–1914],   pale-centered oval hemorrhages on the retina, observed in several disorders but classically seen in bacterial endocarditis.

**Rotokinetic treatment table** /rō′tōkinet′ik/,   a special bed equipped with an automatic turning device that completely

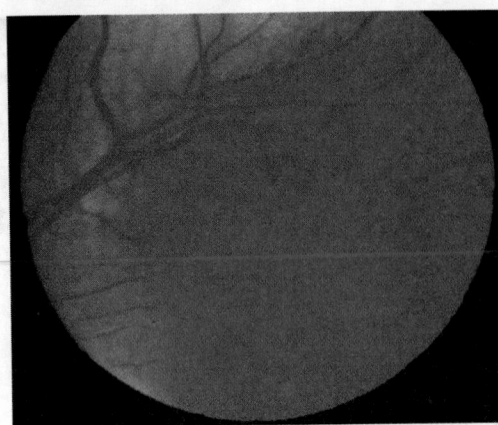

**Roth spot** (Stone and Gorbach, 2000)

immobilizes patients while rotating them from 90 to 270 degrees around a horizontal axis. As an example, the Roto-Rest, Delta Bed (Kinetic Concepts, San Antonio, Tx) rotates patients up to 124° around a horizontal axis.

**Rotor's syndrome** /rō′tər/, a rare condition of the liver inherited as an autosomal-recessive trait. It is similar to Dubin-Johnson syndrome but can be distinguished by the normal functioning of the gallbladder and lack of liver pigmentation. Jaundice occurs in childhood caused by impaired biliary excretion. See also **Dubin-Johnson syndrome, hyperbilirubinemia of the newborn.**

**rotoscoliosis** /rō′təskō′lē·ō′sis/, a condition in which there is both lateral and rotational spinal deviation.

**rotula.** See **troche.**

**roughage.** See **dietary fiber.**

**rouleaux** /rōōlō′/, *sing.* **rouleau** [Fr, cylinder], an aggregation of red cells in a roll formation that may be caused by abnormal proteins, as in multiple myeloma or macroglobulinemia, but is most often a microscopic artifact. Compare **hemagglutination.** See also **erythrocyte sedimentation rate.**

**round ligament** [L, *rotundus*, round, *ligare*, to bind], **1.** a curved fibrous band that is attached at one end to the fovea of the head of the femur and at the other to the transverse ligament of the acetabulum. **2.** a fibrous cord extending from the umbilicus to the anterior part of the liver. It is the remnant of the umbilical vein. **3.** in the female, a fibromuscular band that extends from the anterior surface of the uterus through the inguinal canal to the labium majora. The structure is homologous to the spermatic cord in the male.

**rounds,** *informal.* a teaching conference or a meeting in which the clinical problems encountered in the practice of nursing, medicine, or other service are discussed. Kinds of rounds include **grand rounds, nursing rounds, teaching rounds,** and **walking rounds.**

**round window** [L, *rotundus* + ONorse, *vindauga*], a round opening in the medial wall of the middle ear leading into the cochlea and covered by a secondary tympanic membrane. Also called **fenestra cochleae, fenestra rotunda.**

**roundworm,** any worm of the class Nematoda, including *Ancylostoma duodenale, Ascaris lumbricoides, Enterobius vermicularis,* and *Strongyloides stercoralis.*

**Roussy-Lévy disease** /rōōsē′-lāvē′/ [Gustave Roussy, French pathologist, 1874–1948; Gabrielle Lévy, French neurologist, 1886–1935], an inherited cerebellar ataxia associated with muscle wasting of the extremities, absence of tendon reflexes, and foot deformities.

**route of administration** /rōōt, rout/ [Fr, *route,* course; L, *administrare,* to serve], (of a drug) any one of the body systems in which a drug may be administered, such as intradermally, intrathecally, intramuscularly, intranasally, intravenously, orally, rectally, subcutaneously, sublingually, topically, or vaginally. Some medications can be given by only one route because absorption or maximum effectiveness occurs by that route only or because the specific substance is toxic or damaging when given by another route.

**Roux-en-Y** /rōō′enwī′, rōō′änēgrek′/ [César Roux, Swiss surgeon, 1857–1926], an anastomosis of the small intestine in the shape of the letter Y. The proximal end of the divided intestine is anastomosed end-to-side to the distal loop, and a part of the distal loop is anastomosed to another part of the digestive tract, such as the esophagus. It is performed in cases of clinically severe obesity.

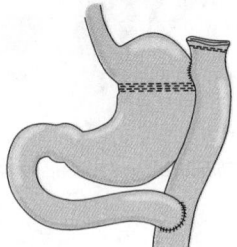

**Roux-en-Y** (Phipps, Sands, and Marek, 1999)

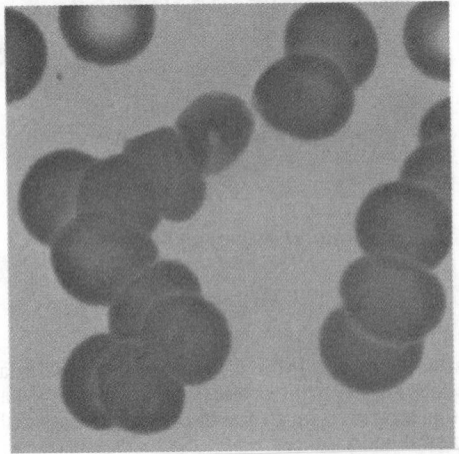

**Rouleaux** (Carr and Rodak, 1999)

**Rovsing's sign** /rov′singz/ [Nils T. Rovsing, Danish surgeon, 1862–1927], an indication of acute appendicitis in which pressure on the left lower quadrant of the abdomen causes pain in the right lower quadrant. See also **appendicitis.**

**Royal College of Physicians (R.C.P.),** a professional organization of physicians in the United Kingdom.

**Royal College of Physicians and Surgeons of Canada (RCPSC),** a national Canadian organization that recognizes and confers membership on certain qualified physicians and surgeons.

**Royal College of Surgeons (R.C.S.),** a professional organization of surgeons in the United Kingdom.

**Royal free disease.** See **postviral fatigue syndrome.**

**Royer's syndrome.** See **Prader-Willi syndrome.**

**Roy, Sister Callista,** a nursing theorist who introduced the Adaptation Model of Nursing in 1970 as a conceptual framework for nursing curricula, practice, and research. In the Roy model the human is viewed as an adaptive system. Changes occur in the system in response to stimuli. If the change promotes the integrity of the individual, it is an adaptive response. Otherwise it is a maladaptive response. The theory provides two mechanisms for coping or adapting. One, a regulator mechanism, is concerned with neural, endocrine, and perception-psychomotor processes. The other, a cognator mechanism, is concerned with perception, learning, judgment, and emotion. Four modes for effecting adaptation of a system are physiologic needs, self-concept, role function, and interdependence. The nurse achieves the goal of promoting the patient's adaptation in situations of health and sickness by manipulating stimuli. Nursing intervention is required when the coping mechanism of the patient loses effectiveness in illness.

**RPF,** abbreviation for **renal plasma flow.**

**rpm,** abbreviation for *revolutions per minute.*

**RQ,** abbreviation for **respiratory quotient.**

**R.R.A.,** abbreviation for **registered record administrator.**

**-(r)rhage,** suffix meaning a 'rupture, an excessive fluid discharge': *hemorrhage, lymphorrhage, phleborrhage.*

**-(r)rhagia,** suffix meaning a 'fluid discharge of excessive quantity': *lymphorrhagia, meningorrhagia, tracheorrhagia.*

**-(r)rhagic,** suffix meaning 'a kind or condition of excessive fluid discharge': *haemorrhagic, lymphorrhagic, serohemorrhagic.*

**-(r)rhaphy, -(r)rhaphia,** suffix meaning a 'suturing in place': *cysticorrhaphy, meningeorrhaphy, osteorrhaphy.*

**-(r)rhea, -(r)rhoea, -(r)rhoeica,** suffix meaning 'fluid discharge, flow': *anarrhea, cystirrhea, laryngorrhea.*

**-(r)rheic, -(r)rheal, -(r)rhetic, -(r)rhoeic,** suffix meaning 'fluid discharge': *cryptorrheic, diarrheic, pyorrheic.*

**-(r)rhexis,** suffix meaning a 'rupture of a (specified) body part': *arteriorrhexis, cardiorrhexis, plasmarrhexis.*

**-(r)rhine,** suffix meaning 'having a (specified sort of) nose': *leptorrhine, mesorrhine, platyrrhine.*

**-(r)rhinia,** suffix meaning '(condition of the) nose': *arrhinia, birrhinia, microrrhinia.*

**-(r)rhoeica, -(r)rhoea.** See **-(r)rhea.**

**-(r)rhythmia,** combining form meaning 'regularly occurring involuntary behavior or actions': *bradyrrhythmia, dysrrhythmia, tachyrrhythmia.*

**R-R interval,** the interval from the peak of one QRS complex to the peak of the next as shown on an electrocardiogram. It is used to assess the ventricular rate. See also **cardiac cycle.**

**rRNA,** abbreviation for **ribosomal RNA.**

**RRT,** abbreviation for **registered respiratory therapist.**

**RSD,** abbreviation for **reflex sympathetic dystrophy.**

**RSNA,** abbreviation for **Radiological Society of North America.**

**RSV, RS virus,** abbreviation for **respiratory syncytial virus.**

**RT,** abbreviation for **respiratory therapy.**

**R.T.,** abbreviation for **registered technologist.**

**RTA,** abbreviation for **renal tubular acidosis.**

**r.t.c.,** abbreviation for *return to clinic,* noted on the chart, usually followed by a date on which a subsequent appointment has been made for the patient.

**Ru,** symbol for the element **ruthenium.**

**rub** [ME, *rubben,* to scrape], the movement of one surface moving over another, thereby producing friction, as when pleural membranes produce friction rub.

**rub-, rube-,** prefix meaning 'red': *rubedo, ruber, rubor.*

**rubber.** See **condom.**

**rubber-band ligation,** a method of treating hemorrhoids by placing a rubber band around the hemorrhoidal part of the blood vessel, causing it to slough off after a period of time. The technique is used in some cases as an alternative to surgery. See also **ligation.**

**rubber dam** [ME, *rubben,* to scrape; AS, *demman,* to dam up], a thin sheet of latex rubber used to isolate one or more teeth during a dental procedure. See also **dam.**

**rubber dam clamps forceps,** a type of forceps with beaks designed to engage holes in a rubber dam clamp to facilitate its placement over teeth.

**rubbing alcohol** [ME, *rubben,* to scrape; Ar, *alkohl,* essence], a disinfectant for skin and instruments. It contains 70% isopropyl alcohol by volume, the remainder consisting of water and denaturants, with or without color or perfume. It may cause dryness of the skin. Rubbing alcohol is for external use only and is flammable.

**rubefacient** /roo′bəfā′shənt/ [L, *ruber,* red, *facere,* to make], **1.** a substance or agent that increases the reddish coloration of the skin. **2.** increasing the reddish coloration of the skin.

**rubefaction** /roo′bəfak′shən/ [L, *ruber,* red, *facer,* to make], a redness of the skin produced by a counterirritant.

**rubella** /roobel′ə/ [L, *rubellus,* somewhat red], a contagious viral disease characterized by fever, symptoms of a mild upper respiratory tract infection, lymph node enlargement, arthralgia, and a diffuse fine red maculopapular rash. The virus is spread by droplet infection, and the incubation time is from 12 to 23 days. Also called **German measles, three-day measles.** Compare **measles, scarlet fever.**

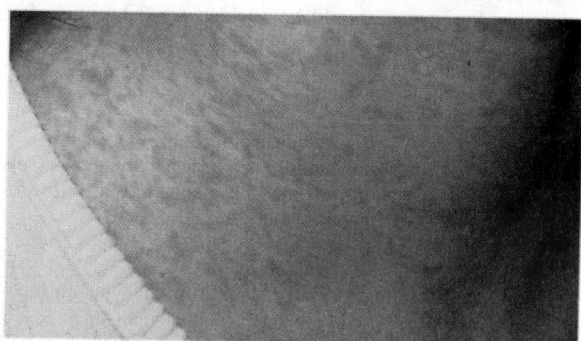

**Rubella** *(Zitelli and Davis, 1997/courtesy Dr. Michael Sherlock)*

■ OBSERVATIONS: The symptoms usually last only 2 or 3 days except for arthralgia, which may persist longer or recur. One attack confers lifelong immunity. If a woman acquires rubella in the first trimester of pregnancy, fetal anomalies may result, including heart defects, cataracts, deafness, and mental retardation. An infant exposed to the virus in utero at any time during gestation may shed the virus for up to 30 months after birth. Complications of postnatal rubella are rare.

■ INTERVENTIONS: The illness itself is mild and needs no special treatment. Live attenuated rubella vaccine is advised for all children to reduce chances of an epidemic and thus to protect pregnant women. The vaccine is not given to women already pregnant, and it is recommended that pregnancy be avoided for 3 months after the administration of rubella vaccine. Spread of the virus from a recently vaccinated individual rarely occurs. Immune serum globulin containing rubella antibodies may help prevent fetal infection in exposed susceptible pregnant women, but ordinary gamma globulin will not protect the fetus.

**rubella and mumps virus vaccine,** a suspension containing live attenuated mumps and rubella viruses.

■ INDICATIONS: It is prescribed for immunization against rubella and mumps.

■ CONTRAINDICATIONS: Acute infection or known hypersensitivity to avian proteins prohibits its use. It is not given to a patient whose immune function is compromised or to a pregnant woman. It is not given for 3 months after the use of plasma, whole blood, or an immune serum globulin. Pregnancy is avoided for 3 months after immunization.

■ ADVERSE EFFECTS: Among the more serious adverse effects are mild to severe hypersensitivity reactions.

**rubella embryopathy,** any congenital abnormality in an infant caused by maternal rubella in the early stages of pregnancy.

**rubella panencephalitis.** See **panencephalitis.**

**rubella titer** [L, *rubellus,* somewhat red; Fr, *titre,* standard], a serologic test to determine a patient's state of immunity against rubella.

**rubella virus vaccine,** a suspension containing live attenuated rubella virus.

■ INDICATION: It is prescribed for immunization against rubella.

■ CONTRAINDICATIONS: Compromised immune function, fever, acute infection, untreated tuberculosis, or hypersensitivity to proteins of the animal of the vaccine prohibits its use. It is not given to pregnant women, nor is it given for 3 months after the use of plasma, whole blood, or immune serum globulin. Pregnancy should be avoided for 3 months after immunization.

■ ADVERSE EFFECTS: Among the most serious adverse reactions are severe hypersensitivity reactions and local pain.

**rubeola.** See **measles.**

**rubeosis** /roo̅′bē·ō′sis/, a red discoloration of the skin.

**rubeosis iridis,** the formation of abnormal blood vessels on the anterior of the iris. It may be associated with thrombotic glaucoma and diabetes mellitus.

**ruber** /roo̅′bər/, *(Latin)* red.

**rubescent** /roo̅bes′ənt/, reddening.

**-rubicin,** combining form for daunorubicin-type antineoplastic antibiotics.

**rubidium (Rb)** /roo̅bid′ē·əm/ [L, *rubidus,* reddish], a soft metallic element of the alkali metals group. Its atomic number is 37; its atomic mass is 85.47. Slightly radioactive, it is used in radioisotope scanning.

**Rubinstein-Taybi syndrome** /roo̅′bin·stīn·tā′bē/ [Jack Herbert Rubinstein, American pediatrician, b. 1925; Hooshang Taybi, American radiologist, b. 1919], a congenital condition characterized by mental and motor retardation, broad thumbs and great toes, short stature, characteristic facies, including high-arched palate and straight or beaked nose, vari-

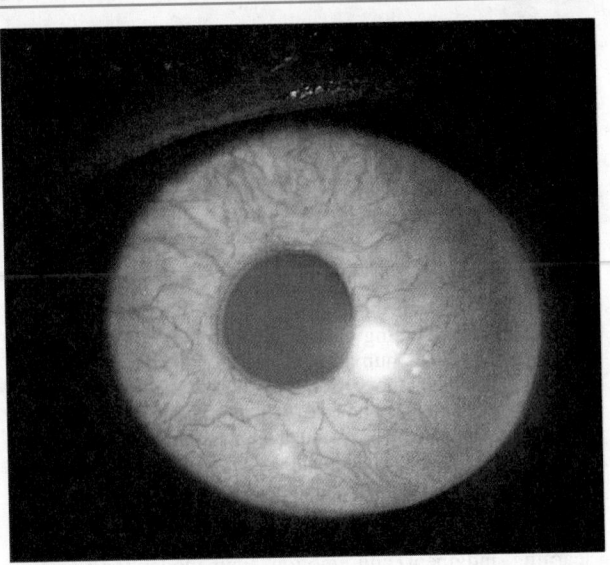

**Rubeosis iridis** *(Bloom and Ireland, 1992)*

ous eye abnormalities, pulmonary stenosis, keloid formation in surgical scars, large foramen magnum, and abnormalities of the vertebrae and sternum.

**Rubin's test** [Isador C. Rubin, American gynecologist, 1883–1958], a test performed in the process of evaluating the cause of infertility by assessing the patency of the fallopian tubes. Carbon dioxide gas ($CO_2$) is introduced into the tubes under pressure through a cannula inserted into the cervix. The $CO_2$ is passed through from a syringe connected to a manometer at pressures of up to 200 mm Hg. If the tubes are open, the gas enters the abdominal cavity, and the recorded pressure falls below 180 mm Hg. A high-pitched bubbling can be heard through the abdominal wall with the stethoscope as the gas escapes from the tubes. The patient may complain of shoulder pain from diaphragmatic irritation; an x-ray film will show free gas under the diaphragm. If the tubes are blocked, gas cannot escape from the tubes into the abdominal cavity; the pressure recorded on the manometer remains at 200 mm Hg. A tracing may be made to show tubal peristalsis, any leakage in the system, tubal spasm, or partial obstruction. After the test, the patient rests for 3 hours. Crampy pain, dizziness, nausea, and vomiting may occur; positioning with the pelvis higher than the head in genupectoral position or in Trendelenburg's position allows the gas to stay in the pelvis and gives some relief by avoiding diaphragmatic irritation. Also called **resistance-inducing factor (RIF) test.**

**rubivirus** /roo̅′bēvī′rəs/, a member of the togavirus family, which includes the rubella virus.

**rubor** /roo̅′bôr/, redness, especially when accompanying inflammation.

**rubratoxin** /roo̅′brətok′sin/, a mycotoxin produced on cereal grains by certain species of penicillin.

**rubricyte** /roo̅′brisīt/ [L, *ruber,* red; Gk, *kytos,* cell], a nucleated red blood cell; the marrow stage in the normal development of an erythrocyte.

**ructus.** See **eructation.**

**rudiment** /roo̅′dimənt/ [L, *rudimentum,* beginning], an organ or tissue that is incompletely developed or nonfunctional. —**rudimentary,** *adj.*

**rudimentary** /rōō′dimen′tərē/, [L, *rudimentum,* beginning], pertaining to something either vestigial or embryonic; undeveloped.

**Ruffini's corpuscles** /rōōfē′nēz/ [Angelo Ruffini, Italian anatomist, 1864–1929], a variety of oval-shaped, encapsulated nerve endings in the subcutaneous tissue, located principally at the junction of the dermis and the subcutaneous tissue. Ruffini's corpuscles consist of strong connective tissue sheaths enclosing nerve fibers with many branches that end in small knobs. Compare **Golgi-Mazzoni corpuscles, Krause's corpuscles, Pacini's corpuscles.**

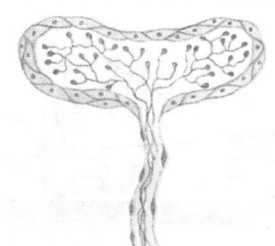

**Ruffini's corpuscles**
*(Thibodeau and Patton, 1993/Rolin Graphics)*

**RU486.** See **mifepristone.**

**ruga** /rōō′gə/, *pl.* **rugae** [L, ridge], a ridge or fold, such as the rugae of the stomach, which present large folds in the mucous membrane of that organ.

**rugae of vagina** [L, *ruga,* ridge, *vagina,* sheath], the transverse ridges on the mucous membrane lining the vagina. They allow the vagina to stretch during childbirth.

**rugitus** /rōō′jitəs/ [L, roaring], the rumbling sound of flatus in the intestines.

**rugose** /rōō′gōs/, wrinkled or corrugated. Also **rugous.**

**RUL,** abbreviation for *right upper lobe* of lung.

**rule,** a guide for conduct or action.

**rule of bigeminy** [L, *regula,* model, *bis,* double, *geminus,* twin], the tendency of a lengthened ventricular cycle to precipitate a premature ventricular complex.

**rule of confidentiality,** a principle that personal information about others, particularly patients, should not be revealed to persons not authorized to receive such information.

**rule of cooccurrence** /kō′əkur′əns/, a mandate that a person use the same level of lexic and syntactic structure when speaking as the person being spoken to.

**rule of nines,** a formula for estimating the percentage of adult body surface covered by burns by assigning 9% to the head and each arm, twice 9% (18%) to each leg and the anterior and posterior trunk, and 1% to the perineum. This is modified in infants and children because of the proportionately larger head size.

**rule of outlet,** an obstetric standard for determining whether the pelvic outlet will allow the passage of a fetus. It is calculated from the sum of the transverse and posterior sagittal diameters of the outlet, which must equal at least 15 cm.

**rule of three,** an arterial oxygen tension that is three times the value of the inspired oxygen concentration. It is regarded

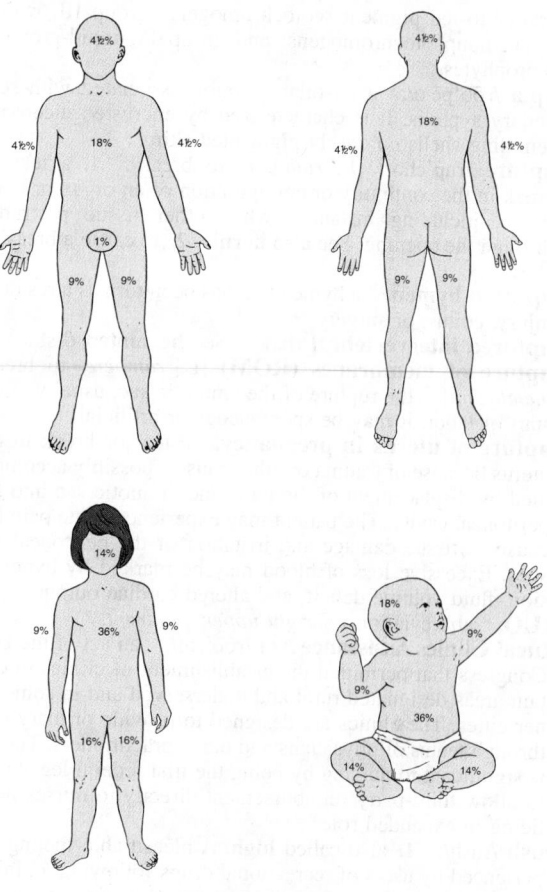

**Rule of nines**

as an empiric guide to a temporarily acceptable minimal oxygenation or expression of clinical observation and has no scientific basis.

**rum,** a spirit distilled from fermented products of sugar cane, including molasses. It may contain up to 60% of ethyl alcohol by volume.

**ruminant** /rōō′minənt/ [L, *ruminare,* to chew again], pertaining to animals that chew their cud and to human infants that may regurgitate and reswallow a meal.

**rumination** /rōō′minā′shən/ [L, *ruminare,* to chew again], habitual regurgitation of small amounts of undigested food with little force after every feeding, a condition commonly seen in infants. It may be a symptom of overfeeding, of eating too fast, or of swallowing air. It has little or no clinical significance. More copious and forceful regurgitation may indicate a more serious condition such as an allergic intestinal reaction, an infectious disease, an obstruction of the intestinal tract, or a metabolic disorder. Also called **reflux.** See also **vomit.**

**runner's high,** a feeling of euphoria experienced by some cross-country runners and joggers as they near the end of a run. The feeling of elation is believed to be associated with the body's production of endorphins during physical stress.

**Runyan classification system** /run′yən/, a system of identifying mycobacteria on the basis of pigmentation and growth condition of the organisms. It includes group I, yellow-pigment photochromogens; group II, yellow-to-orange-to-red pigment scotochromogens; group III, white-to-tan nonphotochromogens; and group IV, rapid-growing saprophytes.

**rupia** /roo′pē·ə/, a pustular eruption associated with secondary syphilis. It is characterized by encrusted ulcers resembling shells on darkly pigmented skin.

**rupture** /rup′chər/ [L, *rumpere,* to break], **1.** a tear or break in the continuity or configuration of an organ or body tissue, including instances when other tissue protrudes through the opening. See also **hernia. 2.** to cause a break or tear.

**ruptured hymen,** a hymen that has been torn as a result of injury, coitus, or surgery.

**ruptured intervertebral disk.** See **herniated disk.**

**rupture of membranes (ROM)** [L, *rumpere,* to break, *membrana*], the rupture of the amniotic sac, usually at the start of labor. It may be spontaneous or artificial.

**rupture of uterus in pregnancy,** a tear or break in the uterus because of trauma or other causes, possibly accompanied by displacement of the fetus and amniotic sac into the peritoneal cavity. The patient may experience acute pain because of tissue damage and irritation of the peritoneal tissues. Excessive loss of blood may be marked by hypotension, fluid volume deficit, and altered cardiac output.

**RUQ,** abbreviation for *right upper quadrant.*

**Rural Clinics Assistance Act** /roo′rəl/, an act of the U.S. Congress that permitted the establishment of clinics in certain areas designated rural and underserved and in some inner cities. The clinics are designed to provide primary care through teams of physicians and nurse practitioners. The act is significant to nursing by being the first federal legislation to allow third-party reimbursement directly to nurses practicing in expanded roles.

**rush** /rush/, **1.** also called **high.** A pleasurable feeling experienced by users of recreational drugs following an injection of amphetamine or heroin. An amphetamine rush is described as an abrupt awakening as distinguished from the drowsy drifting rush of heroin use. See also **flash. 2.** a strong wave of contractile activity that travels along the small intestine, usually as a result of irritation or distension.

**Russell dwarf** [Alexander Russell, twentieth century Scottish physician; AS, *dweorge*], a person affected with **Russell's syndrome,** a congenital disorder in which short stature is associated with various anomalies of the head, face, and skeleton and with varying degrees of mental retardation.

**Russell's bodies** [William Russell, Scottish physician, 1852–1940; AS, *bodig,* body], the mucoprotein inclusions found in globular plasma cells in cancer and inflammations. The bodies contain surface gamma globulins, derived from the condensation of internal cellular secretions. Also called **cancer bodies, fuchsin bodies.**

**Russell-Silver dwarfism, Russell-Silver syndrome, Silver's syndrome;** see **Silver dwarf.**

**Russell's periodontal index,** [Albert L. Russell, American dentist, b. 1905], a measure of the extent of periodontal disease in an individual that considers the amount of bone loss around the teeth and the degree of gingival inflammation.

**Russell's syndrome.** See **Russell dwarf.**

**Russell's traction** [R. Hamilton Russell, Australian surgeon, 1860–1933; L, *trahere,* to pull along], a unilateral or a bilateral orthopedic mechanism that combines suspension and traction to immobilize, position, and align the lower extremities in the treatment of fractured femurs, hip and knee contractures, and disease processes of the hip and knee. Russell's traction is applied as adhesive or nonadhesive skin traction and uses a sling to relieve the weight of the lower extremities subjected to traction pull. A jacket restraint is often incorporated to help immobilize the patient. Compare **split Russell traction.**

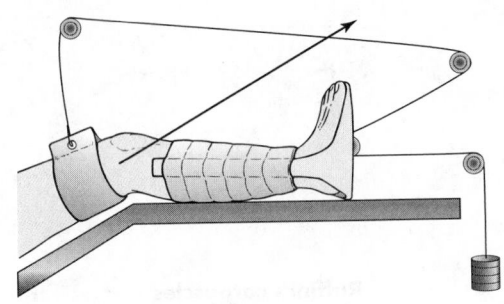

**Russell's traction** *(Lewis, Heitkemper, and Dirksen, 2000)*

**Russian bath** /rush′ən/, a hot steam bath followed by a cold plunge. Also called **Finnish bath.**

**rusts,** microbes that are pathogens of plants, particularly cereal grains. They are also important human allergens.

**rusty sputum** /rus′tē/ [AS, *rust* + L, *sputum,* spittle], sputum that is reddish, indicative of blood.

**ruthenium (Ru)** /rootHē′nē·əm/ [Ruthenia, region of western Ukraine], a hard, brittle, metallic element. Its atomic number is 44; its atomic mass is 101.07.

**rutherfordium (Rf)** [Sir Ernest Rutherford, British physicist, 1871–1937], a transuranic element, and the first transactinide element. Its atomic number is 104; its atomic mass is 261. It is produced by an induced nuclear reaction.

**rutin** /roo′tin/, a bioflavonoid obtained from buckwheat and used in the treatment of capillary fragility.

**Ruvalcaba's syndrome** /roo′väl·kā′bäz/ [R.H. Ruvalcaba, American physician, b. 1934], abnormal shortness of the metacarpal and metatarsal bones, hypogenitalism, and retardation of unknown cause but present from birth in males; it is characterized by microcephaly, skeletal abnormalities, hypoplastic genitalia, and mental and physical retardation.

**RV,** abbreviation for **residual volume.**

**RVC,** abbreviation for *responds to verbal commands.*v

**R wave.** The positive component of the QRS complex on an electrocardiogram. See also **QRS complex.**

**rxn, RXN,** symbol for drug reaction.

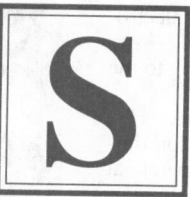

**s, 1.** abbreviation for *second* in SI units. **2.** abbreviation for **steady state. 3.** abbreviation for the Latin word *sinister,* 'left.' **4.** abbreviation for the Latin word *sine,* 'without.'

**S, 1.** symbol for **sulfur. 2.** symbol for *saturation of hemoglobin.* **3.** symbol for **siemens.**

**s̄, s,** symbol for the Latin *sine,* 'without'.

**S₁,** the first heart sound in the cardiac cycle, occurring at the outset of ventricular systole. It is associated with closure of the mitral and tricuspid valves and is synchronous with the apical pulse. Auscultated at the apex, it is longer, and lower than the second sound (S₂), which follows it. The sound of the mitral valve is loudest at the apex of the heart, and that of the tricuspid valve is loudest at the left sternal border in the fourth intercostal space.

**S1, S2, . . .,** symbols for sacral nerves.

**S₂,** the second heart sound in the cardiac cycle. It is associated with closure of the aortic and pulmonic valves at the outset of ventricular diastole. The second sound is louder and shorter than the first. The sound of the aortic valve is loudest on the right sternal border, and that of the pulmonic valve is most distinct on the left sternal border over the second intercostal space.

**S₃,** the third heart sound in the cardiac cycle. Normally, it is audible only in children and physically active young adults and usually disappears with age. In older people, it is an abnormal finding and usually indicates myocardial failure. It is heard with the bell of a stethoscope placed lightly over the apex of the heart with the patient lying down and facing left. A weak, low-pitched, dull sound, it is thought to be caused by vibrations of the ventricle walls when they are suddenly distended by blood from the atria. Also called **physiologic third heart sound, ventricular gallop.**

**S₄,** the fourth heart sound in the cardiac cycle. It occurs late in diastole on contraction of the atria. Rarely heard in normal subjects, it indicates an abnormally increased resistance to ventricular filling, as in hypertensive cardiovascular disease, coronary artery disease, cardiomyopathy, and aortic stenosis. A left-sided fourth heart sound, it may be heard with the stethoscope's bell at the apex of the heart during expiration. Also called **atrial gallop, physiologic fourth heart sound.**

**SA, 1.** abbreviation for **sinoatrial. 2.** abbreviation for **surface area. 3.** abbreviation for **surgeon's assistant.**

**saber-sheath trachea** /sā'bər/, an abnormally shaped trachea caused by chronic obstructive pulmonary disease. The diameter of the posterior part of the trachea is increased while the lateral dimension is decreased.

**saber shin,** a sharp, anterior bowing of the tibia caused by hereditary syphilis.

**Sabin-Feldman dye test** /sā'binfeld'mən/ [Albert B. Sabin, American virologist, 1906–1993; H.A. Feldman, American epidemiologist, b. 1914; AS, *deag* + L, *testum,* crucible], a serologic test for the diagnosis of toxoplasmosis that depends on the presence of specific antibodies that block the uptake of methylene blue dye by the cytoplasm of the *Toxoplasma* organisms.

**Sabin vaccine.** See **oral poliovirus vaccine.**

**sac** /sak/ [Gk, *sakkos,* sack], a pouch or a baglike organ, such as the abdominal sac of the embryo that develops into the abdominal cavity.

**saccade** /sakād', sak'ədā'/ [Fr, *saccader,* to jerk], pertaining to something jerky, broken, or abrupt, such as rapid shift of eye movement or a staccato voice.

**saccadic eye movement** /sakad'ik/, an extremely fast voluntary movement of the eyes, allowing them to accurately fix on a still object in the visual field as the person moves or the head turns.

**sacchari-.** See **saccharo-.**

**saccharide** /sak'ərīd'/, any of a large group of carbohydrates, including all sugars and starches. Almost all carbohydrates are saccharides. See also **carbohydrate, sugar.**

**saccharin** /sak'ərin/ [Gk, *sakcharon,* sugar], **1.** a white crystalline synthetic sweetening agent derived from coal tar. Although it is up to 500 times as sweet as sugar, it has no food value. **2.** having a sweet taste, especially cloyingly sweet. Also called **saccharine** /-rīn, -rin/.

**saccharo-, sacchari-,** combining form meaning 'sugar': *saccharobiose, saccharorrhea, saccharosuria.*

**saccharometabolism** /sak'ərōmətab'əliz'əm/, the functioning of sugar within a living body.

***Saccharomyces*** /sak'ərōmī'sēz/ [Gk, *sakcharon* + *mykes,* fungus], a genus of yeast fungi that cause such diseases as bronchitis, moniliasis, and pharyngitis.

**saccharomycosis** /sak'ərōmīkō'sis/ [Gk, *sakcharon* + *mykes* + *osis,* condition], infection with yeast fungi, such as the genera *Candida* or *Cryptococcus.*

**saccular** /sak'yələr/ [L, *sacculus,* small bag], pertaining to a pouch, or shaped like a sac.

**saccular aneurysm,** a localized dilation of a small area of an artery, forming a saclike swelling or protrusion. It is usually caused by trauma. Also called **ampullary aneurysm, sacculated aneurysm.** Compare **fusiform aneurysm.**

**sacculated** /sak'yəlā'tid/ [L, *sacculus,* small bag], a condition of small sacs, pouches, or saclike dilations.

**sacculated aneurysm.** See **saccular aneurysm.**

**sacculated pleurisy,** inflammation of the pleura with exudate encapsulated in several locations by adhesions.

**sacculation** /sak'yo͞o·lā'shən/ [L, *sacculus*], the quality of being sacculated, or pursed out with little pouches. See **sacculus.**

**saccule** /sak'yo͞ol/ [L, *sacculus*], a small bag or sac, such as the air saccules of the lungs. See also **sacculus. —saccular,** *adj.*

**saccule of larynx.** See **laryngocele.**

**sacculus** /sak'yo͞oləs/, *pl.* **sacculi,** a little sac or bag, especially the smaller of the two divisions of the membranous labyrinth of the vestibule, which communicates with the cochlear duct through the ductus reuniens in the inner ear. See also **saccule.**

**Sachs' disease.** See **Tay-Sachs disease.**

**SA conduction time,** the time required for an impulse to travel from the sinus node to the atrial musculature. It is measured from the sinoatrial (SA) deflection in the SA nodal electrocardiogram to the beginning of the P wave in a bipolar record, or to the beginning of the high right atrial electrogram in a unipolar record.

**sacral** /sā'krəl, sak'rəl/ [L, *sacer*, sacred],   pertaining to the sacrum.

**sacral agenesis.**   See **caudal regression syndrome.**

**sacral bone,**   a composite bone formed by the fusion during maturation of five sacral vertebrae that were separate at birth. The sacrum forms the back of the pelvis.

**sacral canal,**   an extension of the vertebral canal through the sacrum.

**sacral foramen,**   any one of several openings between the fused segments of the sacral vertebrae in the sacrum through which the sacral nerves pass.

**sacral nerves,**   the five segmental nerves from the sacral part of the spinal cord. The first four emerge through the anterior sacral foramina and the fifth from between the sacral foramen and the coccyx.

**sacral node,**   a node in one of the seven groups of parietal lymph nodes of the abdomen and the pelvis, situated within the sacrum. The sacral nodes are located in relation to the middle and the lateral sacral arteries and receive lymphatics from the rectum and the posterior wall of the pelvis. Compare **lumbar node.** See also **lymph, lymphatic system, lymph node.**

**sacral plexus,**   a network of motor and sensory nerves formed by the lumbosacral trunk from the fourth and fifth lumbar, and by the first, second, and third sacral nerves. They converge toward the lower part of the greater sciatic foramen and unite to become a large, flattened band, most of which continues into the thigh as the sciatic nerve. Compare **lumbar plexus.** See also **lumbosacral plexus.**

**sacral vertebra,**   one of the five segments of the vertebral column that fuse in the adult to form the sacrum. The ventral border of the first sacral vertebra projects into the pelvis. The bodies of the other sacral vertebrae are smaller than that of the first and are flattened and curved ventrally, forming the convex, anterior surface of the sacrum. The rudimentary spinous processes of the first several sacral vertebrae surmount the middle sacral crest, and the transverse processes of the sacral vertebrae form the lateral sacral crests. The sacral hiatus at the caudal end of the sacral canal develops from the incomplete growth of the spinous processes of the last two sacral vertebrae. The resultant widened aperture is used by anesthesiologists for the insertion of a needle to administer caudal analgesia. Compare **cervical vertebra, coccygeal vertebra, lumbar vertebra, thoracic vertebra.** See also **sacrum, vertebra.**

**sacro-** /sā'krō-/,   prefix meaning 'sacrum': *sacrococcyx, sacroiliac, sacrolumbalis.*

**sacrococcygeal** /-koksij'ē·əl/ [L, *sacer*, sacred; Gk, *kokkyx*, cuckoo's beak],   pertaining to the sacrum and the coccyx.

**sacrococcygeal teratoma,**   a common tumor of newborns, found in the primitive pit. It may represent part of the blastopore of lower vertebrates.

**sacroiliac** /sā'krō·il'ē·ak/ [L, *sacer* + *ilium*, flank],   pertaining to the part of the skeletal system that includes the sacrum and the ilium bones of the pelvis.

**sacroiliac articulation,**   an immovable joint in the pelvis formed by the articulation of each side of the sacrum with an iliac bone.

**sacroiliac joint,**   an irregular synovial joint between the sacrum and the ilium on either side.

**sacroiliitis** /sā'krō·il'ē·ī'tis/,   an inflammation of the sacroiliac joint.

**sacrolumbar.**   See **lumbosacral.**

**sacrosciatic** /sā'krōsī·at'ik/,   pertaining to the sacrum and ischium.

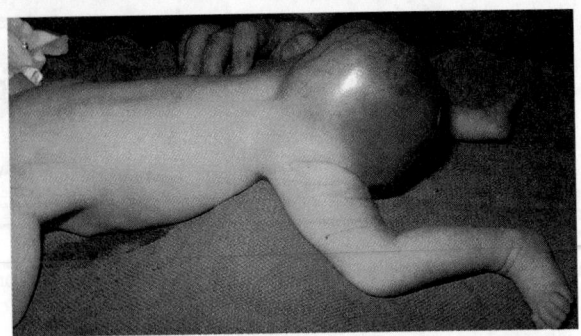

**Sacrococcygeal teratoma** *(Zitelli and Davis, 1997)*

**sacrospinalis** /sak'rōspīnal'is/ [L, *sacer* + *spina*, backbone], the superficial longitudinal muscle mass on either side of the vertebral column. It is sheathed in the fascia thoracolumbalis and arises in a broad, thick tendon from the sacrum, the ilium, and the lumbar vertebrae. It inserts into the ribs and into certain cervical vertebrae and is innervated by the branches of the dorsal primary divisions of the spinal nerves. It extends and flexes the vertebral column and the head, draws the ribs downward, and bends the trunk to the side. Also called **erector spinae, sacrospinal muscle.**

**sacrospinal muscle.**   See **sacrospinalis.**

**sacrum** /sā'krəm, sak'rəm/ [L, *sacer*, sacred],   the large, triangular bone at the dorsal part of the pelvis, inserted like a wedge between the two hip bones. The base of the sacrum articulates with the last lumbar vertebra, and its apex articulates with the coccyx; various muscles attach to its spinal crest. The sacrum is shorter and wider in women than in men. —**sacral,** *adj.*

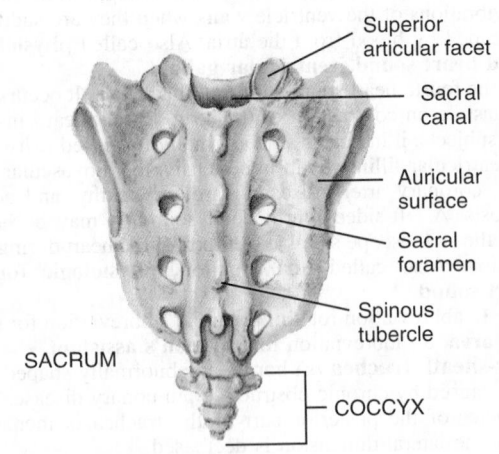

**Sacrum and coccyx** *(Applegate, 2000)*

**SAD,**   abbreviation for **seasonal affective disorder.**

**saddle** /sad'əl/ [AS, *sadol*],   **1.** a support whose shape fits the contour of the object resting on it. **2.** a saddle-shaped structure or part. **3.** see **denture base.**

**saddleback nose.**   See **saddle nose.**

**saddle block anesthesia** [AS, *sadol* + Fr, *bloc* + Gk, *anaisthesia,* lack of feeling], a form of spinal nerve block in which the area of the body that would touch a saddle, were the patient sitting astride one, is anesthetized. It is performed by injecting a local anesthetic into the subarachnoid cerebrospinal fluid space. Saddle block anesthesia is common in some centers for anesthesia during childbirth. See also **obstetric anesthesia.**

**saddle embolism,** a thrombus that straddles a dividing blood vessel. Also called **straddling embolism.**

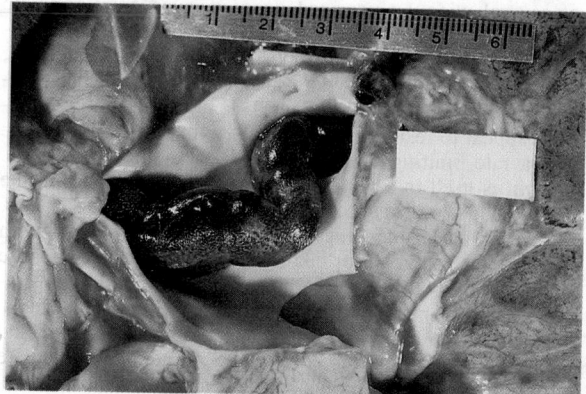

**Saddle embolism**
*(Kumar, Cotran, and Robbins, 1997/teaching collection of the Department of Pathology, University of Texas Southwestern Medical School, Dallas)*

**saddle joint,** a synovial joint in which surfaces of contiguous bones are reciprocally concavoconvex. A saddle joint permits no axial rotation but allows flexion, extension, adduction, and abduction, as in the carpometacarpal joint of the thumb. Also called **articulatio sellaris.** Compare **condyloid joint, pivot joint.**

**saddle nose** [AS, *sadol* + *nosu*], a sunken nasal bridge caused by injury or disease and resulting in damage to the nasal septum. Also called **saddleback nose.**

**sadism** /sā′dizəm, sad′izəm/ [Marquis Donatien A.F. de Sade, French writer, 1740–1814], **1.** abnormal pleasure derived from inflicting physical or psychologic pain or abuse on others; cruelty. **2.** also called **active algolagnia.** (in psychiatry) a psychosexual disorder characterized by the infliction of physical or psychologic pain or humiliation on another person, either a consenting or a nonconsenting partner, to achieve sexual excitement or gratification. The condition is usually chronic, is seen predominantly in men, may result from conscious or unconscious motivations or desires, and, in severe cases, can lead to rape, torture, and murder. Kinds of sadism are **anal sadism** and **oral sadism.** Compare **masochism.** See also **algolagnia, sadomasochism. —sadistic,** *adj.*

**sadist** /sā′dist/, a person who is afflicted with or practices sadism. Compare **masochist.**

**sadistic.** See **sadism.**

**sadomasochism** /sā′dōmas′əkiz′əm/ [Marquis de Sade; Leopold von Sacher-Masoch, Austrian author, 1836–1895], a personality disorder characterized by traits of sadism and masochism. See also **algolagnia, masochism, sadism.**

**sadomasochist** /sā′dōmas′əkist/ [Marquis de Sade; Leopold von Sacher-Masoch], a person who practices sadomasochism.

**Saethre-Chotzen syndrome** /sā′trə·kot′zən/ [Haakon Saethre, Norwegian psychiatrist, 20th century; F. Chotzen, German psychiatrist, 20th century], an autosomal dominant disorder characterized by acrocephalosyndactyly in which the syndactyly is mild and by hypertelorism, ptosis, and sometimes mental retardation. Also called **acrocephalosyndactyly, type III; Chotzen's syndrome.**

**safe period.** See **natural family planning method.**

**safe sex,** intimate sexual practices between partners who use condoms or other means to prevent the exchange of body fluids that transmit diseases. Although perfect safety is virtually impossible without abstinence, the known risks of infections by human immunodeficiency virus or other organisms transmitted through sexual contact can be reduced by safe sex practices.

**safety behavior: fall prevention,** a nursing outcome from the Nursing Outcomes Classification (NOC) defined as the individual or caregiver actions to minimize risk factors that might precipitate falls. See also **Nursing Outcomes Classification.**

**safety behavior: home physical environment,** a nursing outcome from the Nursing Outcomes Classification (NOC) defined as the individual or caregiver actions to minimize environmental factors that might cause physical harm or injury in the home. See also **Nursing Outcomes Classification.**

**safety behavior: personal,** a nursing outcome from the Nursing Outcomes Classification (NOC) defined as the individual or caregiver efforts to control behaviors that might cause physical injury. See also **Nursing Outcomes Classification.**

**safety director** /sāf′tē/ [Fr, *sauver,* to save, *directeur,* manager], a member of a hospital staff whose activities are related to safety functions, such as fire prevention, environmental safety, and disaster planning activities. Also called *safety officer.*

### Safer sexual practices to reduce the risk of HIV transmission

**Safe**
Mutual masturbation
Dry (social) kissing
Massage
Hugging
Fantasy
Nonshared sex toys

**Lower to moderate risk**
French (wet) kissing
Urine contact
Cunnilingus
Vaginal intercourse with latex condom
Fisting (manual-anal intercourse)
Fellatio with semen ingested
Anal intercourse with latex condom
Analingus or rimming (oral-anal contact)

**Highest risk**
Unprotected anal intercourse
Unprotected vaginal intercourse

From Price SA, Wilson LM: *Pathophysiology: clinical concepts of disease processes,* ed 4, St Louis, 1992, Mosby.

**safety glass,** a hard, transparent material that resists shattering on impact. It usually is made as a sandwich of two sheets of glass with an intermediate layer of plastic. Safety glass may also be produced as a tempered material that breaks into rounded granules instead of sharp shards. Also called **shatterproof glass.**

**safety glasses,** impact-resistant lenses that protect the eyes from blows or other kinds of injury. Such lenses are usually made by tempering the glass, by substituting plastic for glass, or by laminating. Also called **safety lenses.**

**safety lenses.** See **safety glasses.**

**safety status: falls occurrence,** a nursing outcome from the Nursing Outcomes Classification (NOC) defined as the number of falls in the past week. See also **Nursing Outcomes Classification.**

**safety status: physical injury,** a nursing outcome from the Nursing Outcomes Classification (NOC) defined as the severity of accidents and trauma. See also **Nursing Outcomes Classification.**

**safflower oil** /sef'lou·er/, a liquid fat containing polyunsaturated fatty acids, derived from the seeds of the safflower plant, *Carthamus tinctorius.* It is commonly mixed with other edible vegetable oils.

**sagittal** /saj'ətəl/ [L, *sagitta,* arrow], (in anatomy) pertaining to a suture or an imaginary line extending from the front to the back in the midline of the body or a part of the body, dividing into right and left parts.

**sagittal axis,** a hypothetical line through the mandibular condyle that serves as an axis for rotation of the mandible.

**sagittal fontanel,** a soft area located in the sagittal suture, halfway between the anterior and posterior fontanels. It may be found in some normal newborns and also some with Down syndrome.

**sagittal plane,** the anteroposterior plane, or the section parallel to the median plane of the body. Compare **frontal plane, median plane, transverse plane.**

**sagittal section,** an anteroposterior cross-section produced by slicing, laterally or through imaging techniques, a body or body part in a vertical plane parallel to the median plane.

**sagittal sinus** [L, *sagitta,* arrow, *sinus,* hollow], either of two venous sinuses of the dura mater. The superior venous sinus begins near the crista galli and drains backward to empty into a confluence of sinuses near the occipital area. The inferior venous sinus begins in the lower margin of the cerebral falx and follows the superior venous sinus, emptying into the straight sinus.

**sagittal suture,** the serrated connection between the two parietal bones of the skull, coursing down the midline from the coronal suture to the upper part of the lambdoidal suture.

**sago spleen** /sā'gō/, a form of amyloid spleen that mainly affects the Malpighian bodies.

**SaH, SAH,** abbreviation for **subarachnoid hemorrhage.**

**SAIN,** abbreviation for **Society for Advancement in Nursing.**

**Saint's triad** [Charles F.M. Saint, twentieth-century South African radiologist], a group of three related conditions: cholelithiasis, diverticulosis, and hiatal hernia occurring together.

**Saint Vitus' dance** /sāntvī'təs/, a motor nerve disorder characterized by irregular involuntary jerky movements of the limbs and facial muscles. Historically the condition was once confused with symptoms of a dance mania that reportedly was cured by a pilgrimage to the shrine of Saint Vitus. See also **Sydenham's chorea.**

**Sakati-Nyhan syndrome** /sä'kä·tē·nī'han/ [Nadia Sakati, American pediatrician, 20th century; William Leo Nyhan, American pediatrician, b. 1926], an autosomal dominant type of acrocephalopolysyndactyly characterized also by hypoplastic tibias and deformed, displaced fibulas. See also **acrocephalopolysyndactyly.**

**sal-, -sal,** prefix for salicylic acid derivatives.

**salaam convulsion** /säläm'/ [L, *convulsio,* cramp], a violent muscle spasm of the sternomastoid muscles marked by head bobbing or bowing. Also called **West's syndrome.**

**salbutamol.** See **albuterol.**

**salicylanilide** /sal'isilan'ilīd/, a topical antifungal prescribed in the treatment of tinea capitis caused by *Microsporum audouinii.* It is applied to the scalp in a 3% to 5% ointment; stronger concentrations cause skin irritation.

**salicylate** /səlis'əlāt/ [Gk, *salix,* willow, *hyle,* matter], any of several widely prescribed drugs derived from salicylic acid. Salicylates exert analgesic, antipyretic, and antiinflammatory actions. The most important is acetylsalicylic acid, or aspirin. Sodium salicylate also has been used systemically, and it exerts similar effects. Many of the actions of aspirin appear to result from its ability to inhibit cyclooxygenase, a rate-limiting enzyme in prostaglandin biosynthesis. Aspirin is used in a wide variety of conditions, and, in the usual analgesic dosage, it causes only mild adverse effects. Severe occult GI bleeding or gastric ulcers may occur with frequent use. Large doses taken over a long period can cause significant impairment of hemostasis. Occasionally an asthmalike reaction is produced in hypersensitive individuals. Because of the ready availability of aspirin, accidental and intentional overdosage is common. Symptoms of salicylate intoxication include tinnitus, GI disturbances, abnormal respiration, acid-base imbalance, and central nervous system disturbances. Fatalities have resulted from ingestion of as little as 10 grains of aspirin in adults or as little as 4 mL of methyl salicylate (oil of wintergreen) in children. In addition to aspirin and sodium salicylate, which are used systemically, methyl salicylate is used topically as a counterirritant in ointments and liniments. Methyl salicylate can be absorbed through the skin in amounts capable of causing systemic toxicity. Another salicylate, salicylic acid, is too irritating to be used systemically and is used topically as a keratolytic agent, for example, for removing warts. See also **salicylic acid.**

**salicylated** /səlis'ilā'tid/ [Gk, *salix,* willow, *hyle,* matter], pertaining to a chemical formed as a salt or ester of salicylic acid.

**salicylate poisoning,** a toxic condition caused by the ingestion of salicylate, most often in aspirin or oil of wintergreen. Intoxication is characterized by rapid breathing, vomiting, headache, irritability, ketosis, hypoglycemia, and, in severe cases, seizures and respiratory failure.

**salicylazosulfapyridine.** See **sulfasalazine.**

**salicylic acid** /sal'isil'ik/, a keratolytic agent.

- ■ INDICATIONS: It is prescribed in the treatment of hyperkeratotic skin conditions and as an adjunct in fungal infections.
- ■ CONTRAINDICATIONS: Diabetes, impaired circulation, or known hypersensitivity to this drug prohibits its use.
- ■ ADVERSE EFFECTS: Among the more serious adverse reactions are skin inflammation and salicylism.

**salicylism** /sal'isil'izəm/ [Gk, *salix,* willow, *hyle,* matter, *ismos,* practice], a syndrome of salicylate toxicity. See also **salicylate poisoning.**

**saline** /sā'līn/ [L, *sal,* salt], **1.** pertaining to a substance that contains a salt or salts. **2.** pertaining to something that is salty or has the characteristics of common table salt. See also **hypertonic saline, hypotonic saline.**

**saline cathartic** [L, *sal,* salt; Gk, *katharsis,* cleansing], one of a large group of cathartics administered to achieve prompt, complete evacuation of the bowel. A watery semifluid evacuation usually occurs within 3 to 4 hours. The most common indication for the administration of any of these agents is preparation of the bowel for diagnostic examination. Various preparations, including magnesium sulfate, sodium phosphate, sodium sulfate, and several naturally occurring mineral waters, may be used to achieve catharsis. The palatability, cost, and adverse systemic reactions of the saline cathartics depend on the particular agent used and the dose of the agent given.

**saline enema** [L, *sal*, salt; Gk, *enienai*, to send in], a salt-water enema. Hypertonic saline enema is used to treat worm infestations, by inducing peristalsis and evacuation. It may require 2 teaspoons of salt per 0.5 liter of warm water, sometimes with magnesium sulfate added, instilled slowly, and retained as long as possible. A normal saline enema of 1 teaspoonful of salt per 0.5 liter of water is instilled slowly and retained as long as possible to combat shock or replace lost fluids.

**saline infusion,** the therapeutic introduction of a physiologic salt solution into a vein.

**saline irrigation,** the washing out of a body cavity or wound with a stream of salt solution, usually an isotonic aqueous solution of sodium chloride.

**saline solution,** a solution containing sodium chloride. Depending on the use, it may be hypotonic, isotonic, or hypertonic with body fluids.

**saliva** /səlī′və/ [L, spittle], the clear, viscous fluid secreted by the salivary and mucous glands in the mouth. Saliva contains water, mucin, organic salts, and the digestive enzyme ptyalin. It serves to moisten the oral cavity, to initiate the digestion of starches, and to aid in the chewing and swallowing of food. Approximately 1 to 1.5 liters is produced per day.

**salivary** /sal′iver′ē/ [L, *saliva*, spittle], pertaining to saliva or to the formation of saliva.

**salivary duct,** any one of the ducts through which saliva passes. Kinds of salivary ducts are **Bartholin's duct, duct of Rivinus, parotid duct,** and **submandibular duct.**

**salivary fistula,** an abnormal communication from a salivary gland or duct to an opening in the mouth or on the skin of the face or neck.

**salivary gland,** any one of three pairs of glands secreting into the mouth, thus aiding the digestive process. The salivary glands are the parotid, the submandibular, and the sublingual. They are racemose structures consisting of numerous lobes subdivided into smaller lobules connected by dense areolar tissue, vessels, and ducts. The sublingual

gland secretes mucus; the parotid gland, serous fluid; the submandibular gland, both mucus and serous fluid. The lobules of the salivary glands are richly supplied with blood vessels and fine plexuses of nerves. The hilum of the submandibular gland contains Langley's ganglion of nerve cells.

**salivary gland cancer,** a malignant neoplastic disease of a salivary gland, occurring most frequently in a parotid gland. About 75% of tumors that develop in the salivary glands are benign, characteristically slow-growing painless mobile masses that are cystic or rubbery in consistency. In contrast, malignant tumors are rapid-growing, hard, lumpy, fixed, and frequently tender. Pain, trismus, and facial palsy may occur. Diagnostic measures include radiographic studies, with sialographic studies and mandibular and chest films to detect metastases, and cytologic studies of saliva from Stensen's duct. Direct biopsies are not recommended. The most common malignant neoplasms are mucoepidermoid, adenoid cystic, solid, and squamous cell carcinomas. Treatment usually consists of surgical removal of the lobe containing a benign tumor and total parotidectomy with a radical neck dissection if the lesion is advanced. Radiotherapy is administered for residual, recurrent, or inoperable cancers, and chemotherapy may be palliative.

**saliva substitute.** See **artificial saliva.**

**salivation** /sal′ivā′shən/, the process of saliva secretion by the salivary glands.

**salivatory** /sal′ivətôr′ē/ [L, *saliva*, spittle], stimulating the production of saliva. Also **sialogenous.**

**Salk vaccine.** See **poliovirus vaccine.**

**sallow** /sal′ō/ [ME, *salou*, dirty-gray], yellowish-gray in complexion.

**salmeterol** a sympathomimetic long-acting bronchodilator.
■ INDICATIONS: It is prescribed in the treatment of reversible bronchospasm associated with bronchial and nocturnal asthma.
■ CONTRAINDICATIONS: The drug should not be given to patients with allergy to any component of the formulation, narrow-angle glaucoma, or arrythmias.
■ ADVERSE EFFECTS: The side effects most often reported include changes in heart rhythm, muscle cramps or stiffness, parkinsonianlike symptoms, pallor, sweating, hives, tingling of the skin.

**salmon calcitonin.** See **calcitonin.**

*Salmonella* /sal′mənel′ə/ [Daniel E. Salmon, American pathologist, 1850–1914], a genus of motile gram-negative rod-shaped bacteria that includes species causing typhoid

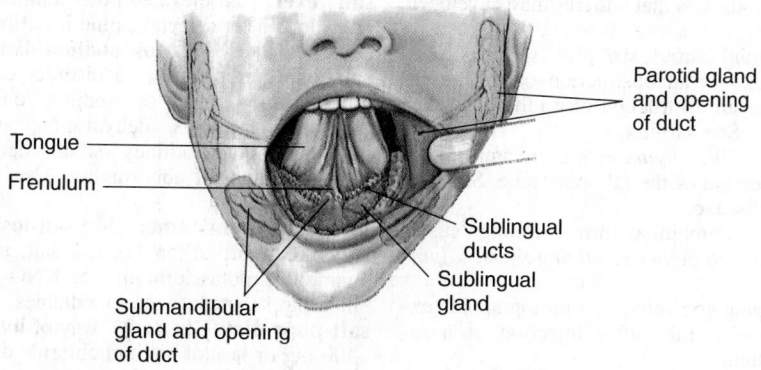

**Salivary glands** *(Jarvis, 2001)*

Tongue
Frenulum
Parotid gland and opening of duct
Sublingual ducts
Sublingual gland
Submandibular gland and opening of duct

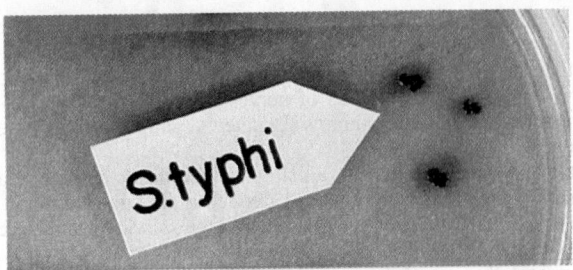

**Colonies of *Salmonella typhi* on bismuth sulfite agar**
*(Baron, Peterson, and Finegold, 1994)*

fever, paratyphoid fever, and some forms of gastroenteritis. See also **salmonellosis.**

***Salmonella enteritidis*** [Daniel E. Salmon; Gk, *enteron*, intestine], a species of *Salmonella* causing food poisoning and gastroenteritis in humans.

**salmonellosis** /sal′mənəlō′sis/ [Daniel E. Salmon; Gk, *osis*, condition], a form of gastroenteritis, caused by ingestion of food contaminated with a species of *Salmonella*. It is characterized by an incubation period of 6 to 48 hours followed by sudden colicky abdominal pain, fever, and bloody, watery diarrhea. Nausea and vomiting are common, and abdominal signs may resemble those of acute appendicitis or cholecystitis. Symptoms usually last from 2 to 5 days, but diarrhea and fever may persist for up to 2 weeks. Dehydration may occur. There is no specific treatment. Antibiotics are usually not indicated unless disease has spread beyond the intestine. Adequate cooking, good refrigeration, and careful handwashing may reduce the frequency of outbreaks. See also **food poisoning, typhoid fever.**

**salol** /sal′ol/. See **phenyl salicylate.**

**salol camphor,** a clear oily mixture of two parts of camphor and three parts of phenyl salicylate, used as a local antiseptic.

**Salonica fever.** See **trench fever.**

**salpingectomy** /sal′pinjek′təmē/ [Gk, *salpinx*, tube, *ektomē*, excision], surgical removal of one or both fallopian tubes. It is performed for removal of a cyst or tumor, excision of an abscess, or, if both tubes are removed, as a sterilization procedure or for tubal pregnancy. Often the operation is done with a hysterectomy or an oophorectomy. Either spinal block or general anesthesia may be given. Postoperatively the patient is instructed to avoid sharply flexing the thighs or the knees. Persistent low back pain or the presence of bloody or scanty urine indicates that a ureter may have been injured during surgery.

**salpingemphraxis** /salpinj′emfrak′sis/ [Gk, *salpinx*, tube, *emphraxis*, a stoppage], **1.** an obstruction of the eustachian tube of the ear. **2.** an obstruction of a fallopian tube.

**salpinges, salpingian.** See **salpinx.**

**salpingitis** /sal′pinjī′tis/ [Gk, *salpinx* + *itis*, inflammation], an inflammation or infection of the fallopian tube. See also **pelvic inflammatory disease.**

**salpingo-** /salping′gō-/, combining form meaning 'eustachian or fallopian tube': *salpingocele, salpingolysis, salpingoplasty.*

**salpingography** /sal′ping·gog′rəfē/, a radiographic examination of the fallopian tube after injection of a radiopaque contrast medium.

**salpingo-oophorectomy** /-ō′əfôrek′təmē/, the surgical removal of a fallopian tube and an ovary.

**salpingo-oophoritis** /-ō′əfôrī′tis/ [Gk, *salpinx*, tube, *oophoron*, ovary, *itis*, inflammation], an inflammation of a fallopian tube and associated ovary.

**salpingostomy** /sal′ping·gos′təmē/ [Gk, *salpinx* + *stoma*, mouth], the formation of an artificial opening in a fallopian tube. The procedure is performed to restore patency in a tube whose fimbriated opening has been closed by infection or by chronic inflammation or to drain an abscess or a fluid accumulation. Either regional or general anesthesia is used. A prosthesis may be inserted to maintain the patency of the fallopian tube and to direct the route of the ova to assist fertilization. Postoperatively the nurse cautions the patient against sharply flexing the thighs or the knees. Low back pain or scanty or bloody urine may indicate that a ureter has been injured during the procedure, requiring surgical intervention.

**salpinx** /sal′pingks/, *pl.* **salpinges** /salpin′jēz/ [Gk, tube], a tube, such as the fallopian or eustachian tube, the salpinx auditiva, or the salpinx uterina. —**salpingian,** *adj.*

**salt** /sôlt/ [L, *sal*], **1.** a compound formed by the chemical reaction of an acid and a base. Salts are usually composed of a metal cation and a nonmetal anion. **2.** sodium chloride (common table salt). **3.** a substance, such as magnesium sulfate (Epsom salt), used as a purgative.

**saltation** /saltā′shən/ [L, *saltare*, to dance], a mutation causing a significant difference in appearance between parent and offspring or an abrupt variation in the characteristics of a species. —**saltatorial, saltatoric, saltatory** /sal′tətôr′ē/, *adj.*

**saltatory conduction** /sal′tətôr′ē/ [L, *saltare* + *conducere*, to lead together], impulse transmission that skips from node to node, providing rapid transmission.

**saltatory evolution,** the appearance of a sudden change within a species, caused by mutation; the progression of a species by sudden major changes rather than by the gradual accumulation of minor changes. The phenomenon occurs predominantly in plants as a result of polyploidy. See also **emergent evolution.**

**salt cake,** sodium sulfate anhydrous; a technical grade of sodium sulfate used in detergents, dyes, soaps, and other industrial products. See also **sodium sulfate.**

**salt depletion,** the loss of salt from the body through excessive elimination of body fluids by perspiration, diarrhea, vomiting, or urination, without corresponding replacement. See also **electrolyte balance, heat exhaustion.**

**salted plasma** /sôl′tid/, a fluid part of blood that has been treated with sodium or magnesium sulfate to prevent coagulation. Also called **salted serum.**

**salted serum.** See **salted plasma.**

**Salter fracture.** See **epiphyseal fracture.**

**salt fever,** an elevated body temperature in an infant that develops after a rectal saline injection.

**salt-free diet.** See **low-sodium diet.**

**salt-losing nephritis,** a disorder characterized by abnormal kidney loss of sodium chloride, hyponatremia, azotemia, acidosis, dehydration, and vascular collapse. Causes include kidney tubule damage, endocrine dysfunction, and GI abnormality. Also called **salt-losing syndrome.**

**salt-losing syndrome.** See **salt-losing nephritis.**

**saltpeter** /sôlt′pē′tər/ [L, *sal*, salt, *petra*, rock], common name for potassium nitrate, $KNO_3$, used in gunpowder, pickling substances, and medicines.

**salt-poor diet** [Gk, *diaita*, way of living], a diet providing 500 mg or less of sodium chloride daily. To ensure that the maximum salt intake does not exceed the limit, it is necessary to record the amount of dietary sodium chloride, in-

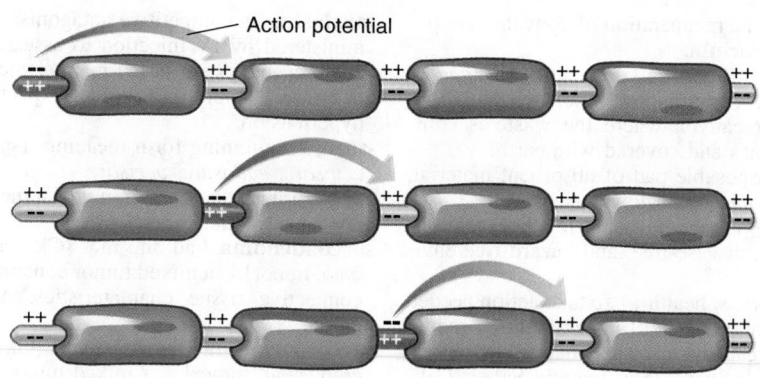

**Saltatory conduction**

cluding amounts contained in patient medications. Note: Some "salt-free" diets may contain as much as 1000 mg of sodium chloride per day.

**salt substitute,** a chemical compound for flavoring foods without adding sodium to the diet. Examples include potassium chloride, monopotassium glutamate, and glutamic acid.

**salt wasting,** inappropriate sodium excretion in the urine (natriuresis) with hyponatremia and hyperkalemia. See also **salt-losing nephritis.**

**Saluron,** trademark for an antihypertensive and diuretic (hydroflumethiazide).

**salvage therapy** /sal′vij/ [Fr, *sauver,* to save; Gk, *therapeia,* treatment], therapy administered to sites at which previous therapies have failed and the disease has recurred.

**salve.** See **ointment.**

**samarium (Sm)** /səmer′ē-əm/ [Colonel M. von Samarski, nineteenth-century Russian mine official], a metallic rare earth element. Its atomic number is 62; its atomic mass (weight) is 150.35.

**SAMHSA,** abbreviation for **Substance Abuse and Mental Health Services Administration.**

**sample** [L, *exemplum*], (in research) a group or part of the whole that can be used to demonstrate characteristics of the whole. Kinds of samples include cluster, convenience, **random,** and **stratified.**

**sanatorium.** See **sanitarium.**

**sanctuary site** /sangk′cho͞o·er′ē/ [L, *sanctus,* sacred, *situs,* location], an area of the body that is poorly penetrated by pharmacologic agents and therefore is a place in which tumor cells or infectious organisms can escape the effects of drug therapy. For example, because most drugs that are effective against the human immunodeficiency virus (HIV) do not cross the blood-brain barrier, the central nervous system provides an area in which HIV can avoid the effects of antiviral therapy and from which resistant virus can later emerge.

**sand bath,** the application of warm dry sand or of damp sand to the body.

**sand flea.** See **chigoe,** def. 1.

**sandfly fever.** See **phlebotomus fever.**

**Sandhoff's disease,** a variant of Tay-Sachs disease that includes defects in the enzymes hexosaminidase A and B. It is characterized by a progressively more rapid course and is found in the general population, not restricted as is Tay-Sachs disease. Also called **gangliosidosis type II.** See also **Tay-Sachs disease.**

**Sandoz Clinical Assessment—Geriatric,** an examination of psychologic function that is administered to elderly people to assist in the diagnostic process.

**sand tumor.** See **psammoma.**

**sandwich generation,** the middle generation who are trying to raise children and help aging parents at the same time.

**sandwich technique,** a method of identifying antibodies or antibody-synthesizing cells in a tissue preparation. A solution containing a specific antigen is applied to the preparation. If antibodies to the antigen are present in the tissue, they will bind to the antigen. Unbound antigen is washed away, and then a fluorochrome-labeled antibody specific for the antigen is added. The result is a complex of antigen sandwiched between antibodies, which can be detected by fluorescence microscopy.

**Sanfilippo's syndrome** /san·fi·lip′ōz/ [Sylvester J. Sanfilippo, American pediatrician, 20th century], four heterogeneous, biochemically distinct, but clinically indistinguishable forms of mucopolysaccharidosis characterized biochemically by excretion of the mucopolysaccharide heparan sulfate in the urine and clinically by severe, rapid mental deterioration and relatively mild somatic symptoms. Onset is from 2 to 6 years of age; the head is large, height normal; Hurler-like features are mild; hirsutism is generalized; death usually occurs before 20 years of age. The four types are **types A** through **D,** each resulting from a different enzymatic defect. Also called **mucopolysaccharidosis III.**

**sangui-,** combining form meaning 'blood': *sanguicolous, sanguiferous, sanguinolent.*

**sanguine** /sang′gwin/ [L, *sanguis,* blood], pertaining to abundant and active blood circulation, ruddy complexion, and an attitude full of vitality and confidence.

**sanguineous** /sang·gwin′ē·əs/ [L, *sanguis,* blood], pertaining to blood or containing blood, such as full-blooded. Also **sanguinous** /sang′gwinəs/.

**sanguinopurulent** /sang′gwinōpyo͞or′ələnt/, containing blood and pus.

**sanies** /sā′ni·ēz/, a thin blood-stained purulent discharge from a wound or ulcer.

**sanioserous,** containing sanies and serum.

**sanious** /sā′nē·əs/, pertaining to or resembling sanies.

**sanita-,** combining form meaning 'health': *sanitarium, sanitas, sanitation.*

**sanitarian** [L, *sanitas,* health], a health professional who is an expert in the science of public health.

**sanitarium** /san′iter′ē·əm/ [L, *sanitas,* health], a facility for the treatment of patients suffering from chronic mental or physical diseases, or the recuperation of convalescent patients. Also called **sanatorium.**

**sanitary landfill** /san′iterē/ [L, *sanitas,* health; AS, *land + fyllan,* to fill],    a solid waste disposal site. It is usually a swamp area, ravine, or canyon where the waste is compacted by heavy machines and covered with earth.

**sanitary napkin,**    a disposable pad of absorbent material, usually worn to absorb menstrual flow.

**sanitation** /san′itā′shən/ [L, *sanitas,* health],    the science of maintaining a healthful, disease-free, and hazard-free environment.

**sanitize** /san′itīz/ [L, *sanitas,* health],    to take action needed to clean the environment or a part of it, removing or reducing pathogenic microorganisms and their habitats.

**San Joaquin fever** /san′wôkēn′/ [San Joaquin Valley, California; L, *febris,* fever],    the primary stage of coccidioidomycosis.

**SA node.**    See **sinoatrial (SA) node.**

**Sanorex,**    trademark for an anorexiant (mazindol).

**Sansert,**    trademark for a vasoconstrictor (methysergide maleate).

**Santyl,**    trademark for an enzyme (collagenase).

**SaO₂,**    symbol for the percentage of oxygen *saturation of arterial blood.*

**saphenous** [Gk, *saphenes,* manifest],    pertaining to certain anatomic structures in the leg, such as arteries, veins, or nerves.

**saphenous nerve** /səfē′nəs/ [Gk, *saphenes,* manifest; L, *nervus,* nerve],    the largest and longest superficial branch of the femoral nerve, supplying the skin of the medial side of the leg and the skin over the patella. On the lateral side of the knee it joins branches of the lateral femoral cutaneous nerve to form the patellar plexus. One branch of the saphenous nerve below the knee supplies the ankle. Another branch below the knee supplies the medial side of the foot. See also **femoral nerve.**

**saphenous vein.**    See **great saphenous vein.**

**sapo-,**    combining form meaning 'soap': *sapogenin, saponaceous, sapotoxin.*

**saponaceous** /sap′ənā′shəs/ [L, *sapo,* soap],    pertaining to soap.

**saponification** /sapon′ifikā′shən/ [L, *sapo,* soap, *facere,* to make],    the production of soap.

**saponified,**    pertaining to a substance chemically hydrolyzed into soaps or acid salts and glycerol by heating with an alkali.

**saponin** /sap′ənin/ [L, *sapo,* soap],    a soapy material found in some plants, especially soapwort (Bouncing Bet) and certain lilies. It is used in demulcent medications to provide a sudsy quality. Natural saponins, which can be hemolytic toxins, have largely been replaced by synthetic preparations.

**sapro-,**    combining form meaning 'decay or putrefaction': *saprophytes, saprophagus, saprolite.*

**saprogen** /sap′rəjən/,    a microscopic saprophyte.

**saprophyte** /sap′rəfīt/ [Gk, *sapros,* rotten, *phyton,* plant],    an organism that lives on dead organic matter. —**saprophytic,** *adj.*

**saquinavir,**    an antiviral.

■ INDICATIONS: This drug is used to treat HIV in combination with zidovudine (AZT) and zalcitabine (ddC).

■ CONTRAINDICATIONS: Known hypersensitivity to this drug prohibits its use.

■ ADVERSE EFFECTS: Adverse effects of this drug include buccal mucosa ulceration, headache, musculoskeletal pain, asthenia, and hyperglycemia. Common side effects are diarrhea, abdominal pain, nausea, paresthesia, and rash.

**saralasin,**    a competitive antagonist of angiotensin. It is administered by IV injection to assess the role of the renin-angiotensin system in the maintenance of blood pressure. A decrease in blood pressure is expected in renin-dependent hypertension.

**-sarc,**    combining form meaning '(specified type of) flesh': *ectosarc, endosarc, perisarc.*

**sarco-** /sär′kō-/,    combining form meaning 'flesh': *sarcoadenoma, sarcode, sarcolyte.*

**sarcoadenoma** /-ad′ənō′mə/ [Gk, *sarx,* flesh, *aden,* gland, *oma,* tumor],    a mixed tumor containing both glandular and connective tissue characteristics. Also called **adenosarcoma.**

**sarcocarcinoma** /-kär′sinō′mə/ [Gk, *sarx,* flesh, *karkinos,* crab, *oma,* tumor],    a mixed tumor with characteristics of both sarcomas and carcinomas.

**sarcodina.**    See **protozoa.**

**sarcoidosis** /sär′koidō′sis/ [Gk, *sarx,* flesh, *eidos,* form, *osis,* condition],    a chronic disorder of unknown origin characterized by the formation of tubercles of nonnecrotizing epithelioid tissue. Common sites are the lungs, spleen, liver, skin, mucous membranes, and lacrimal and salivary glands, usually with involvement of the lymph glands. Diminished reactivity to tuberculin frequently accompanies the disorder. The lesions usually disappear over a period of months or years but may progress to widespread granulomatous inflammation and fibrosis. Also called **sarcoid of Boeck.**

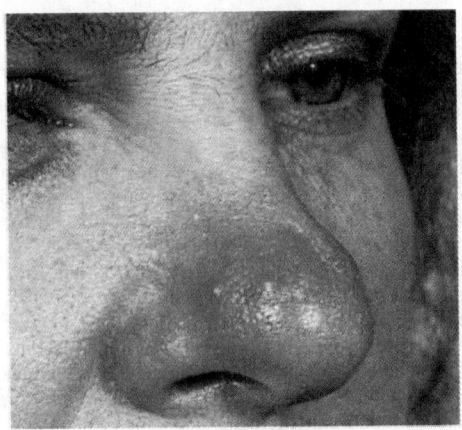

**Sarcoidosis eruption affecting the nose** *(du Vivier, 1993)*

**sarcoidosis cordis,**    a form of sarcoidosis in which granulomatous lesions develop in the myocardium. Mild cases with few infiltrates are asymptomatic. In severe cases cardiac failure may result. See also **sarcoidosis.**

**sarcolemma** /-lem′ə/ [Gk, *sarx,* flesh, *lemma,* sheath],    a membrane that covers smooth, striated, and cardiac muscle fibers.

**sarcoma** /särkō′mə/, *pl.* **sarcomas, sarcomata** [Gk, *sarx + oma,* tumor],    a malignant neoplasm of the soft tissues arising in fibrous, fatty, muscular, synovial, vascular, or neural tissue, usually first manifested as a painless swelling. About 40% of sarcomas occur in the lower extremities, 20% in the upper extremities, 20% in the trunk, and the rest in the head, neck, or retroperineum. The tumor is composed of cells in a connective tissue matrix and may be highly invasive.

Trauma probably does not play a role in the cause, but sarcomas may arise in burn or radiation scars. Small tumors may be managed by local excision and postoperative radiotherapy, but bulky sarcomas of the extremities may require amputation followed by irradiation for local control and combination chemotherapy to eliminate small foci or neoplastic cells. See specific sarcomas. —**sarcomatous,** *adj.*

**-sarcoma,** combining form meaning a 'malignant tumor from connective tissue': *angiosarcoma, hemangiosarcoma, myelosarcoma.*

**sarcoma botryoides** /bot′rē·oi′dēz/, a tumor derived from primitive striated muscle cells, occurring most frequently in young children and characterized by a painful edematous polypoid grapelike mass in the upper vagina or on the uterine cervix or the neck of the urinary bladder. See also **rhabdomyosarcoma.**

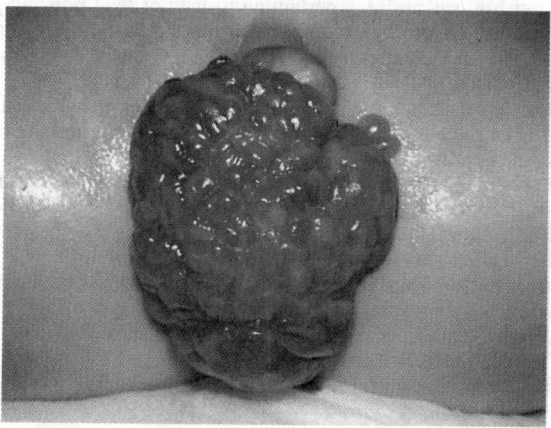

**Sarcoma botryoides** *(Zitelli and Davis, 1997)*

**sarcomagenesis** /särkō′məjen′əsis/ [Gk, *sarx* + *oma* + *genesis,* origin], the process of initiating and promoting the development of a sarcoma. Compare **carcinogenesis, oncogenesis, tumorigenesis.** —**sarcomagenetic,** *adj.*

**sarcomas.** See **sarcoma.**

**sarcomata.** See **sarcoma.**

**sarcomere** /sär′kōmir/ [Gk, *sarx* + *meros,* part], the smallest functional unit of a myofibril. Sarcomeres occur as repeating units along the length of a myofibril, occupying the region between Z lines of the myofibril.

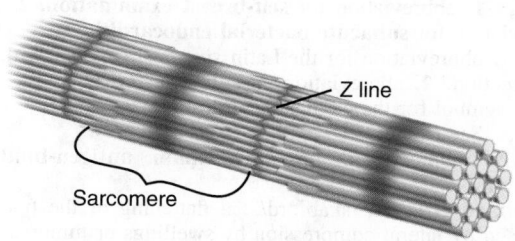

**Sarcomere** *(Thibodeau and Patton, 1999/Joanna Wild)*

**sarcopenia** /-pē′nē·ə/ [Gk, *sarx,* flesh, *penia,* poverty], a loss of skeletal muscle mass that may accompany aging. Studies indicate the loss of skeletal muscle for the average normally healthy person amounts to about 20% between about 30 and 70 years of age. The late loss may accelerate as aging progresses. Although men usually have greater muscle mass in their young adult years, the loss over a period is the same as for women. The muscle loss is replaced by fat, usually in a subtle way that is not noticed by the individual, as by padding areas of muscle loss with extra fat. Muscle strengthening and building exercises can prevent or reverse much of this problem.

**sarcoplasm** /sär′kōplaz′əm/ [Gk, *sarx,* flesh, *plassein,* to mold], the semifluid cytoplasm of muscle cells.

**sarcoplasmic reticulum** /-plas′mik/ [Gk, *sarx* + *plassein,* to mold; L, *reticulum,* little net], a network of tubules and sacs in skeletal muscle fibers that plays an important role in muscle contraction and relaxation by releasing and storing calcium ions. This network is analogous, but not identical, to the endoplasmic reticulum of other cells.

***Sarcoptes scabiei*** /särkop′tēz skā′bē·ī/ [Gk, *sarx* + *koptein,* to cut; L, *scabere,* to scratch], the genus of itch mite that causes scabies.

**sarcosine** /sär′kō·sēn /, an amino acid occurring as an intermediate in the metabolism of choline in the kidney and liver; it is normally not detectable in human blood or urine.

**SARS,** abbreviation for **severe acute respiratory syndrome.**

**sartorius** /särtôr′ē·əs/ [L, *sartor,* tailor], the longest muscle in the body, extending from the pelvis to the calf of the leg. It is a narrow ribbon-shaped muscle that arises from the anterior superior iliac spine, passes obliquely across the proximal anterior part of the thigh from the lateral to the medial

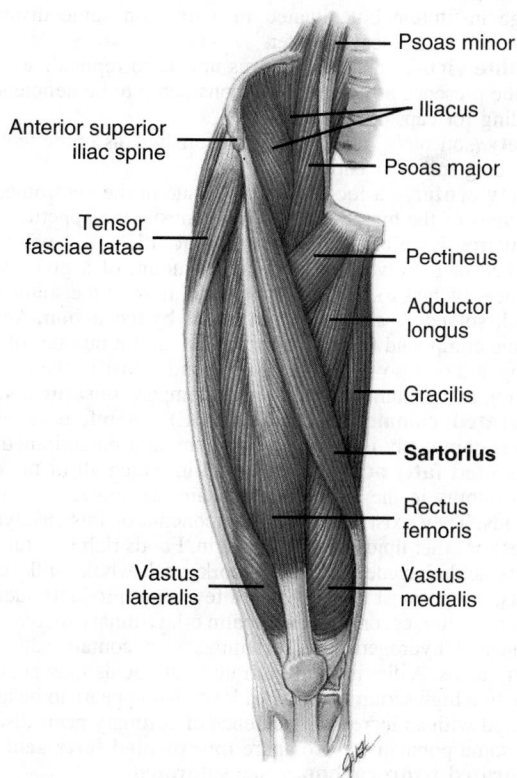

**Sartorius** *(Thibodeau and Patton, 1999/John V. Hagen)*

side, and inserts into the tibia. It acts to flex the thigh and rotate it laterally and to flex the leg and rotate it medially. Compare **quadriceps femoris.**

**satellite cells** /sat′əlīt/ [L, *satelles*, attendant, *cella*, storeroom], glial cells (astrocytes) that form around damaged nerve cells and lay close to neuron bodies in the central nervous system.

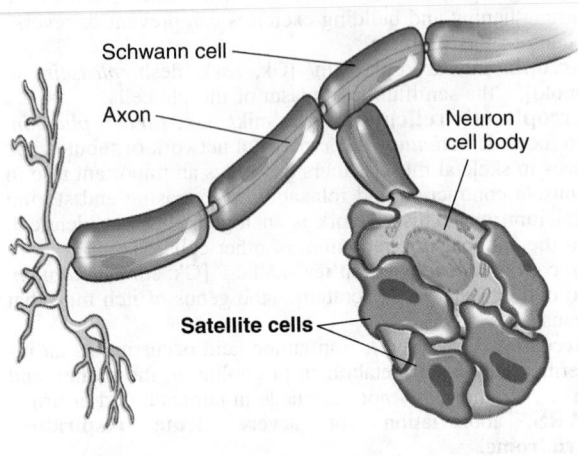

**Satellite cells**

**satellite clinic** [L, *satelles*, attendant; Gk, *kline*, bed], a health care facility usually operated under the auspices of a large institution but situated in a location some distance from the larger health center.

**satellite virus,** a strain of virus unable to replicate except in the presence of helper virus; considered to be deficient in coding for capsid formation.

**satiety** /sətī′ətē/, a state of being satisfied, as in the feeling of being full after eating.

**satiety center,** a locus of nerve tissue in the ventromedial nucleus of the hypothalamus that controls the appetite.

**saturated** /sach′ərā′tid/ [L, *saturare*, to fill], **1.** having absorbed or dissolved the maximum amount of a given substance, such as a solution in which no more of the solute can be dissolved. **2.** also called **saturated hydrocarbon.** An organic compound that contains the maximum number of hydrogen atoms so that only single bonds exist in the carbon chain, as in saturated fatty acids. Compare **unsaturated.**

**saturated calomel electrode (SCE),** a reference electrode commonly used in polarography and potentiometry.

**saturated fatty acid,** a fatty acid in which all of the carbon atoms in the hydrocarbon chain are joined by single bonds. They exist mostly as components of fats (triglycerides) or other lipids of animal origin. Foods rich in saturated fatty acids include beef, lamb, pork, veal, whole-milk products, butter, most cheeses, and a few plant products such as cocoa butter, coconut oil, and palm oil. Ordinary oleomargarine and hydrogenated shortenings also contain saturated fatty acids. A diet high in saturated fatty acids may contribute to a high serum cholesterol level and appears to be associated with an increased incidence of coronary heart disease in some populations. Compare **unsaturated fatty acid.**

**saturated hydrocarbon.** See **saturated.**

**saturated solution,** a solution in which the solvent contains the maximum amount of solute it can take up. See also **solute, solvent.**

**saturation** /sach′ərā′shən/ [L, *saturare*, to fill], **1.** a condition in which a solution contains as much solute as can remain dissolved. **2.** a measure of the degree to which oxygen is bound to hemoglobin, expressed as a percentage of the possible limit. **3.** a chemical compound in which all the valency bonds have been filled.

**saturational cuing** /sach′ərā′shənəl/, a treatment strategy for visuoconstructive disorders by presenting controlled verbal instruction on task analysis and sequence and presenting cues on spatial boundaries.

**saturation index of hemoglobin** [L, *saturare*, to fill, *index*, pointer], a measure of the amount of hemoglobin in a given amount of blood, compared with normal.

**Saturday night palsy** [Gk, *paralyein*, to be palsied], a radial nerve paralysis caused by pressure on the arm after the person has fallen asleep, usually during an alcoholic binge. See also **radial nerve palsy.**

**saturn-,** combining form meaning 'lead' /led/: *saturnine, saturnism, saturnotherapy.*

**saturnine** /sat′ərnīn/, pertaining to lead or lead poisoning.

**saturnine tremor,** a condition of involuntary muscle contractions in the extremities observed in patients with chronic lead poisoning.

**satyr ear** /sat′ər/, a congenital abnormality in which the helix of the auricle lacks the usual rolled contour and the tubercle is prominent.

**satyriasis** /sat′irī′əsis/ [Gk, *satyros*, lecherous, *osis*, condition], excessive, pathologic, or uncontrollable sexual desire in the male. The cause may be psychologic or organic. Also called **satyromania.** Compare **nymphomania.**

**sauna bath** /sô′nə/ [Finn, *sauna* + AS, *baeth*], a bath consisting of exposure to hot vapor to induce sweating, followed by rubbing or light beating of the skin. Also called **Finnish bath, Russian bath.**

**saur-,** combining form meaning 'lizard, or reptile': *sauriasis, sauriderma, sauroid.*

***S. aureus,*** abbreviation for ***Streptococcus aureus.***

**saw palmetto,** an herbal product harvested from the American dwarf palm.

■ USES: This herb is used to treat benign prostatic hypertrophy.

■ CONTRAINDICATIONS: Saw palmetto should not be used during pregnancy and lactation, in children, or in those with known hypersensitivity to this plant.

**saxitoxin** /sak′sitok′sin/, a powerful neurotoxin found in bivalve mollusks, including mussels, clams, and scallops. It is produced by certain species of dinoflagellates, which are consumed by the mollusks. Saxitoxin may cause a severe food intoxication in humans who eat the contaminated shellfish.

**Sayre's jacket** /serz/ [Lewis A. Sayre, American surgeon, 1820–1900; ME, *jaket*], a cast applied for support and immobilization in the treatment of certain abnormalities of the spinal column.

**Sb,** symbol for the element **antimony.**

**SBE, 1.** abbreviation for **self-breast examination. 2.** abbreviation for **subacute bacterial endocarditis.**

**sc, 1.** abbreviation for the Latin *sine correctione*, 'without correction.' **2.** abbreviation for *subcutaneously.*

**Sc,** symbol for the element **scandium.**

**scab.** See **eschar.**

**SCAB,** abbreviation for **single-chain antigen-binding protein.**

**scabbard trachea** /skab′ərd/, a flattening of the trachea caused by lateral compression by swellings or tumors.

**scabicide** /skab′isīd/ [L, *scabere*, to scratch, *caedere*, to kill], any one of a large group of drugs that destroy the itch mite, *Sarcoptes scabiei.* These drugs are applied topically in a lotion or cream-based preparation. All are potentially toxic and irritating to the skin. They are used with caution in treating children. Kinds of scabicides include **crotamiton** and **lindane.**

**scabies** /skā′bēz/ [L, *scabere*, to scratch], a contagious disease caused by *Sarcoptes scabiei*, the human itch mite, characterized by intense itching of the skin and excoriation from scratching. The mite, transmitted by close contact with infected humans or domestic animals, burrows into outer layers of the skin, where the female lays eggs. Two to 4 months after the first infection, sensitization to the mites and their products begins, resulting in a pruritic papular rash most common on the webs of fingers, flexor surfaces of wrists, and thighs. Secondary bacterial infection may occur. Diagnosis may be made by microscopic identification of adult mites, larvae, or eggs in scrapings of the burrows. All contacts are treated simultaneously with topical application of permethrin, crotamiton, or another scabicide. Oral antihistamines and salicylates reduce itching.

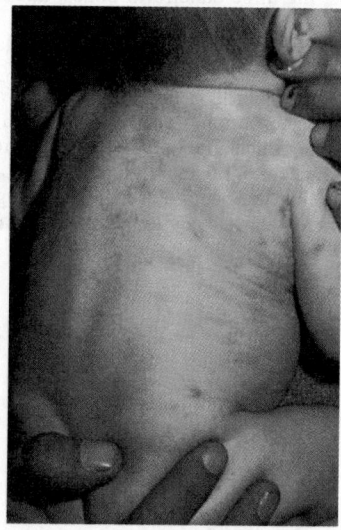

**Scabies rash on an infant** *(Weston, Lane, and Morrelli, 1996)*

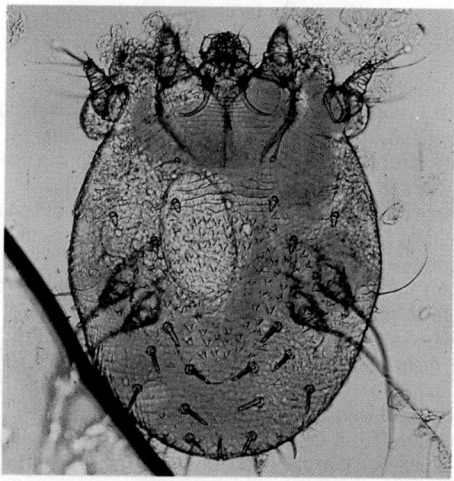

**Adult scabies mite** *(Zitelli and Davis, 1997)*

**scabietic** /skā′bē·et′ik/ [L, *scabere*, to scratch], pertaining to scabies.

**scabrities unguium** /skabrish′i·ēz/, a very pronounced thickening and distortion of the nails, separating from skin at the base.

**scag,** *slang.* heroin.

**scald** /skôld/ [L, *calidus*, hot], a burn caused by exposure of the skin to a hot liquid or vapor.

**scalded skin syndrome.** See **toxic epidermal necrolysis.**

**scale** [OFr, *escale*, husk], **1.** a small thin flake of keratinized epithelium. **2.** to remove encrusted material from the surface of a tooth.

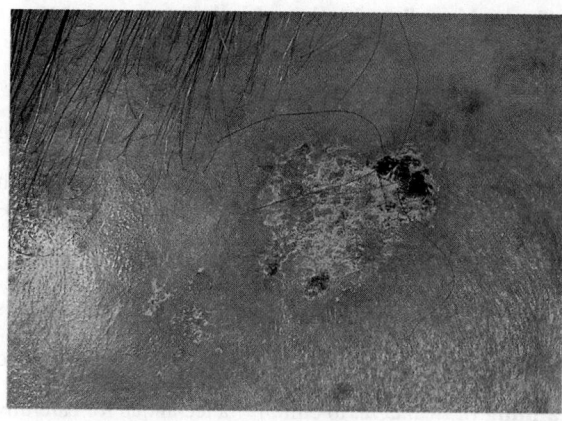

**Scale of lupus erythematosus** *(du Vivier, 1993)*

**scalene** /skā′lēn/ [Gk, *skalenos*, uneven], pertaining to one of the scalenous muscles.

**scalenus** /skālē′nəs/ [Gk, *skalenos*], one of a group of four muscles arising from the cervical vertebrae with insertions on the first or second rib.

**scalenus anticus syndrome.** See **Naffziger syndrome.**

**scaler** /skā′lər/ [OFr, *escale*, husk], a dental instrument used in removing calculus from tooth surfaces. See also **scaling.**

**scaling** /skāl′ing/ [OFr, *escale*, husk], removal of plaque and calculus from the surface of a tooth by means of a scaler.

**scalp** [ME], the skin covering the head, not including the face and ears.

**scalpel** /skal′pəl/ [L, *scalprum*, knife], a small pointed knife with a convex edge. Some scalpels use interchangeable blades for specific surgical procedures, such as operating and amputating.

**scalp medication, 1.** a cream, ointment, lotion, or shampoo used to treat dermatologic conditions of the scalp. **2.** the application of a medication to the scalp. If a cream, ointment, or lotion is to be applied, a shampoo is usually given first. The hair is dried, combed, and parted in the middle. The medication is most often spread with the fingertips. After treatment the medication may need to be washed off the scalp and hair with an alkaline shampoo. On occasion the affected area may be sharply circumscribed and may not require the scalpwide process.

**scalp tourniquet** [ME, *skalp* + OFr, *tunicle*], a bandage applied to the scalp to restrict blood flow during administration of antineoplastic drugs. The tourniquet controls the hair

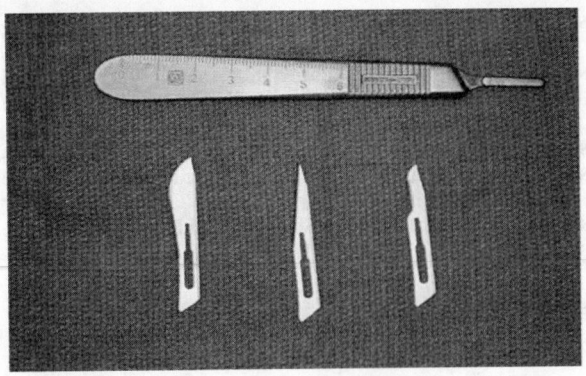

**Scalpel handle with three blades** (Grossman, 1993)

loss that commonly accompanies use of cancer-suppressing drugs.

**scalp vein needle,** a thin-gauge needle designed for use in the veins of the scalp or other small veins, especially in infants and children. Also called a **butterfly needle.**

**scan.** See **scanning.**

**scandium (Sc)** /skan′dē·əm/ [Scandinavia], a grayish metallic element. Its atomic number is 21; its atomic mass is 44.956.

**scanner** /skan′ər/ [L, *scandere*, to climb], equipment used for making scans or scanning. See **scanning.**

**scanning** [L, *scandere*, to climb], a technique for carefully studying an area, organ, or system of the body by recording and displaying an image of the area. A concentration of a radioactive substance that has an affinity for a specific tissue may be administered intravenously to enhance the image. The liver, brain, and thyroid can be examined, tumors can be located, and function can be evaluated by various scanning techniques. See specific scanning techniques. —**scan,** *n., v.*

**scanning electron microscope (SEM),** an instrument similar to an electron microscope in that a beam of electrons is used to scan the surface of a specimen. The beam is moved in a point-to-point manner over the surface of the specimen. These electrons are deflected, collected, accelerated, and directed against a scintillator. The large number of photons thus created are converted into an electrical signal that, in turn, modulates the beam scanning the surface of the specimen. The image produced appears to be three-dimensional and lifelike. Compare **electron microscope, transmission scanning electron microscope.**

**scanning electron microscopy,** the technique using a scanning electron microscope on a specimen. See also **scanning electron microscope.**

**scanning speech,** abnormal speech characterized by a staccatolike articulation in which the words are clipped and broken because the person pauses between syllables.

**scanography** /skanog′rəfē/ [L, *scandere,* to climb; Gk, *graphein,* to record], a method of producing a radiograph of an internal body organ or structure by using a series of parallel beams that eliminate size distortion. The technique is applied most in long-bone radiography. See also **orthoroentgenography.**

**scan path,** distinct eye movement patterns.

**scapegoating** /skāp′gōting/ [ME, *escapen,* to escape, *goot*], the projection of blame, hostility, or suspicion onto one member of a group by other members to avoid self-confrontation.

**scapho-,** combining form meaning 'boat-shaped': *scaphocephaly, scaphohydrocephaly, scaphoid.*

**scaphocephaly** /skaf′ōsef′əlē/ [Gk, *skaphe,* skiff, *kephale,* head], a congenital malformation of the skull in which premature closure of the sagittal suture results in restricted lateral growth of the head, giving it an abnormally long narrow appearance with a cephalic index of 75 or less. Also called **scaphocephalis, scaphocephalism, dolichocephaly, mecocephaly.** See also **craniostenosis.** —**scaphocephalic, scaphocephalous,** *adj.*

**scaphoid** /skaf′oid/ [Gk, *skaphe,* skiff, *eidos,* form], boat-shaped, such as the scaphoid bone of the wrist.

**scaphoid abdomen,** an abdomen with a sunken anterior wall.

**scaphoid bone** [Gk, *skaphe* + *eidos,* form; AS, *ban*], either of two similar proximal boat-shaped bones of the hand and the foot. The scaphoid bone of the hand is slanted at the radial side of the carpus and articulates with the radius, trapezium, trapezoideum, capitate, and lunate bones. The scaphoid bone of the foot is located at the medial side of the tarsus between the talus and cuneiform bones and articulates with the talus, the three cuneiform bones, and occasionally the cuboid bone. Also called **navicular bone.**

**scapula** /skap′yələ/, one of the pair of large flat triangular bones that form the dorsal part of the shoulder girdle. It has two surfaces, three borders, three angles, and a prominent dorsal spine. The acromion process of the scapula forms the summit of the shoulder. The coracoid process, resembling a raven's beak, accommodates the attachment of various muscles, including the pectoralis minor, and ligaments, including the trapezoid. Also called **shoulder blade.**

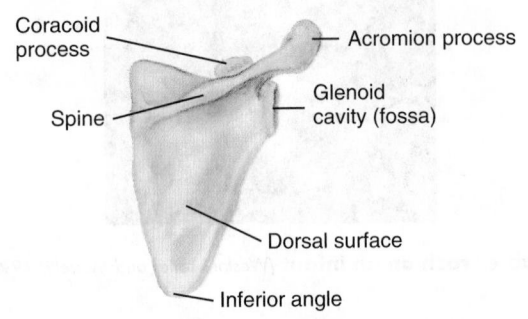

**Scapula** (Applegate, 2000)

**-scapula,** combining form meaning a 'shoulder blade or a part of it': *mesoscapula, prescapula, proscapula.*

**scapular line** /skap′yələr/, an imaginary vertical line drawn through the inferior angle of the scapula.

**scapular reflex,** a contraction of the rhomboids and approximation of the scapulae when a stimulus is applied to the midline of the back between the scapulae.

**scapulary** /skap′yəler′ē/, a suspender for holding a body bandage in place.

**scapulo-** /skap′yəlō-/ [L, *scapulae,* shoulder blades], combining form meaning 'scapula or shoulder blade': *scapulodynia, scapulopexy.*

**scapulocostal syndrome** /-kos′təl/, a condition in which pain radiates from the upper or posterior shoulder area into the neck and back of the head, down the arm, and around the chest. There may also be a tingling in the fingers. The syndrome is associated with a change in the relationship between the shoulder blade and thorax.

**scapulohumeral** /-hyoo'mərəl/ [L, *scapula* + *humerus*, shoulder], pertaining to the area around the scapula and humerus.

**scapulohumeral muscular dystrophy.** See **Erb's muscular dystrophy.**

**scapulohumeral reflex,** a normal response to tapping the vertebral border of the scapula, resulting in adduction of the arm. Absence of the reflex may indicate a lesion in the region of the fifth cervical segment of the spinal cord.

**scapus** /skā'pəs/ [Gk, *skapos*, rod], a stem or shaft, such as the scapus penis or hair (pili).

**scar.** See **cicatrix.**

**scarf skin,** the epidermis, including the cuticle.

**scarification** /sker'ifikā'shən/ [L, *scarifare*, to scratch open], multiple superficial scratches or incisions in the skin, such as those made for the introduction of a vaccine. The term is erroneously used to mean 'producing a scar.'

**scarify** /sker'əfī/ [L, *scarifare*], to make multiple superficial incisions into the skin; to scratch. Vaccination against smallpox is achieved by scarifying the skin under a drop of vaccine. See also **scarification.**

**scarlatina.** See **scarlet fever.**

**scarlatiniform** /skär'lətē'nifôrm/ [It, *scarlattina* + L, *forma*, form], resembling the rash of **scarlet fever.**

**scarlet fever** /skär'lit/ [OFr, *escarlate* + L, *febris*, fever], an acute contagious disease of childhood caused by an erythrotoxin-producing strain of group A hemolytic *Streptococcus.* The infection is characterized by sore throat, fever, enlarged lymph nodes in the neck, prostration, facial flush, strawberry tongue, accentuated petechiae on the body, lines of hyperpigmentation in the body folds (Pastia's lines), circumoral pallor, and a diffuse bright red rash. Also called **scarlatina.**

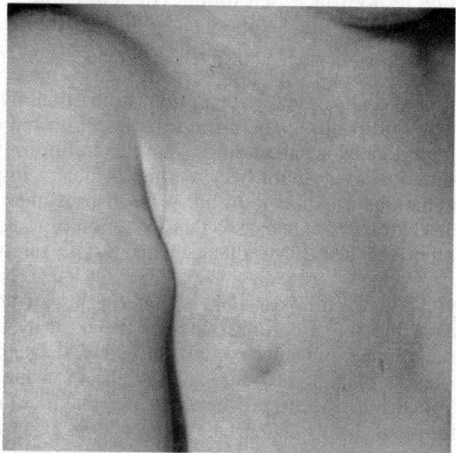

**Scarlet fever**
*(Zitelli and Davis, 1997/courtesy Dr. Michael Sherlock, American College of Rheumatology Slide Collection)*

**scarlet rash** [OFr, *escarlate* + *rasche*, scurf], any scarlatina or rosy skin eruption that accompanies an infection, such as scarlet fever or German measles.

**scarlet red,** an azo dye that has been used to impart color to pharmaceutic preparations.

**scatemia** /skətē'mē·ə/ [Gk, *skatos*, feces, *haima*, blood], a toxemic condition caused by absorption of poisonous or harmful substances from the intestinal tract.

**scato-, skato-,** combining form meaning 'dung or fecal matter': *scatophagy, scatophilia, scatoscopy.*

**scatologic** /skatəloj'ik/, pertaining to scatology.

**scatology** /skatol'əjē/ [Gk, *skatos*, dung, *logos*, science], the science of feces. Also called **coprology.**

**scattered radiation** /skat'ərd/ [ME, *scateren*, to throw away; L, *radiare*, to emit rays], photons that move in a different direction than the incident photons that produced them, after the interaction of those incident photons. Also called **backscatter radiation.**

**scattergram** /skat'ərgram'/ [ME, *scateren* + Gk, *gramma*, record], a graph representing the distribution of two variables in a sample population. One variable is plotted on the vertical axis; the second on the horizontal axis. The scores or values of each sample unit are usually represented by dots. A scattergram demonstrates the degree or tendency with which the variables occur in association with each other.

**scattering** [ME, *scateren*], a change in the direction of photons caused by the interaction between photons and matter. In **coherent scattering,** an incident photon interacts with matter and excites an atom, causing it to vibrate. The vibration causes the photon to scatter. Also called **Thompson scattering, unmodified scattering.** In **Compton scattering,** an incident photon interacts with an orbital electron, transferring some of its energy to that electron. The electron is ejected and the photon is scattered.

**scavenger cell** /skav'ənjər/ [ME, *scavager* + L, *cella*, storeroom], a phagocytic cell that removes tissue debris and some invading pathogens. It may or may not be mobile.

**scavenging system.** See **gas-scavenging system.**

**Sc.D.,** abbreviation for *Doctor of Science.*

**SCE,** abbreviation for **saturated calomel electrode.**

**scel-,** combining form meaning 'leg': *scelalgia, scelotyrbe.*

**-scelia,** combining form meaning '(condition of the) legs': *macroscelia, polyscelia, rhaeboscelia.*

**Schedule I,** a category of drugs not considered legitimate for medical use. Among the substances so classified by the Drug Enforcement Agency are mescaline, lysergic acid diethylamide, heroin, and marijuana. Special licensing procedures must be followed to use these or other Schedule I substances.

**Schedule II,** a category of drugs considered to have a strong potential for abuse or addiction but have legitimate medical use. Among the substances so classified by the Drug Enforcement Agency are morphine, cocaine, pentobarbital, oxycodone, alphaprodine, and methadone.

**Schedule III,** a category of drugs that have less potential for abuse or addiction than Schedule II or I drugs. Among the substances so classified by the Drug Enforcement Agency are glutethimide and various analgesic compounds containing codeine.

**Schedule IV,** a category of drugs that have less potential for abuse or addiction than those of Schedules I to III. Among the substances so classified by the Drug Enforcement Agency are chloral hydrate, chlordiazepoxide, meprobamate, and oxazepam.

**Schedule V,** a category of drugs that have a small potential for abuse or addiction. Among the substances so classified by the Drug Enforcement Agency are many commonly prescribed medications that contain small amounts of codeine or diphenoxylate. The specific drugs in Schedule V vary greatly from state to state.

**Schedule for Affective Disorders and Schizophrenia,** a semistructured interview administered by a professional and designed to yield diagnostic information about current and lifetime incidences of affective disorders and schizophrenia.

**Schedule of Drugs** [L, *scheda,* sheet of paper; Fr, *drogue*], a classification system that categorizes drugs by their potential for abuse. The schedule is divided into five groups: Schedules I to V. The assignment of drugs to the categories varies from state to state. Schedule I substances are not approved for medical use. All substances in Schedules II to V require a written prescription signed by a physician. Substances in Schedule V may or may not require a written prescription signed by a physician depending on state law. Specific regulations for dispensing these substances vary from state to state and from institution to institution. See also **controlled substance, Controlled Substances Act,** and specific schedules.

**Scheie's syndrome** /shāz/ [Harold Glendon Scheie, American ophthalmologist, 1909–1990], a relatively mild variant of **Hurler's syndrome,** characterized by corneal clouding, claw hand, involvement of the aortic valve, somewhat coarse facies with a broad mouth, genu valgum, and pes cavus. Stature, intelligence, and life span are normal.

**schema** /skē′mə/, an innate knowledge structure that allows a child to organize in his or her mind ways to behave in his or her environment.

**schematic** /skēmat′ik/, pertaining to a schema, model, or diagram representing, without absolute precision, a structure, strategy, or system. An anatomic chart is an example.

**schematic eye,** **1.** a simplified and enlarged illustration of the eye, featuring its anatomic details. **2.** a graphic illustration of the normal eye, with data for curvatures, indices of refraction, and distances between optical elements.

**Scheuermann's disease** /shoi′ərmonz/ [Holger W. Scheuermann, Danish surgeon, 1877–1960], an abnormal skeletal condition characterized by a fixed kyphosis that develops at puberty and is caused by wedge-shaped deformities of one or several vertebrae. The cause of the disease is unknown, but authorities have speculated that it may result from infection, inflammatory processes, aseptic necrosis, disk deterioration, mechanical influences, inadequate circulation during rapid growth, or disturbances of epiphyseal growth caused by protrusion of the intervertebral disk through deficient or defective cartilaginous plates. The most striking pathologic feature of Scheuermann's disease is the presence of wedge-shaped vertebral bodies, seen on radiographic examination, that create an excessive curvature. Scheuermann's disease occurs most frequently in children between 12 and 16 years of age, with the onset at puberty, and the incidence is greater in girls than in boys. The onset is insidious and often associated with a history of unusual physical activity or participation in sports. The most frequent symptom is poor posture with accompanying symptoms of fatigue and pain in the involved area. Tenderness and stiffness may also affect the area involved or the entire spinal column. In most affected individuals the kyphosis is within the thoracic vertebrae. If the disease is diagnosed at the onset, the associated posture may be corrected actively and passively. Otherwise, the associated posture becomes fixed within a period of 6 to 9 months. The most effective treatment of Scheuermann's disease is immobilization with a plaster cast or with a Milwaukee brace. The immobilization is continuous for 10 to 12 months, with additional immobilization at night for about the same length of time. Immobilization is usually supplemented with an exercise program that is continued after the immobilization is terminated. In adults persistent pain in the thoracic area may indicate a degenerative alteration secondary to this disease process, and spinal arthrodesis may be required to relieve the symptoms. Also called **adolescent vertebral epiphysitis, juvenile kyphosis.**

**Schick test** /shik/ [Bela Schick, Austrian-American physician, 1877–1967], a skin test formerly used to determine immunity to diphtheria in which dilute diphtheria toxin is injected intradermally. A positive reaction, indicating susceptibility, is marked by redness and swelling at the site of injection; a negative reaction, indicating immunity, is marked by absence of redness or swelling.

**Schick test control** [Bela Schick; L, *testum,* crucible; Fr, *controle,* check], a preparation used in carrying out the Schick skin test for determining diphtheria immunity.

**Schilder's disease** /shil′dərz/ [Paul F. Schilder, Austrian neurologist, 1886–1940], a group of progressive severe neurologic diseases beginning in childhood. All are characterized by demyelination of the white matter of the brain, with muscle spasticity, optic neuritis, aphasia, deafness, adrenal insufficiency, and dementia. Many of the signs resemble those of multiple sclerosis. There is no known treatment. The cause may be viral or genetic. Also called **Schilder's encephalitis, encephalitis periaxialis diffusa, Flatau-Schilder disease, progressive subcortical encephalopathy.** See also **adrenoleukodystrophy.**

**Schiller's test** /shil′ərz/ [Walter Schiller, Austrian pathologist in the United States, 1887–1960], a procedure for indicating areas of abnormal epithelium in the vagina or on the cervix of the uterus as a guide in selecting biopsy sites for cancer detection. A potassium iodide or aqueous iodine solution is painted on the vaginal walls and cervix under direct visualization. Normal epithelium contains glycogen and stains a deep brown; abnormal epithelium, containing no glycogen, will not stain, and nonstaining sites may then be included in tissue biopsy samples. The test is not specific for malignancy, because inflammation, ulceration, and keratotic lesions also may not accept the iodine stain.

**Schilling's leukemia.** See **monocytic leukemia.**

**Schilling test** /shil′ing/ [Robert F. Schilling, American hematologist, b. 1919], a diagnostic test for pernicious anemia in which vitamin $B_{12}$ tagged with radioactive cobalt is administered orally, and GI absorption is measured by determining the radioactivity of urine samples collected over a 24-hour period. Normal findings show excretion of 8% to 40% of radioactive vitamin $B_{12}$ within 24 hours. In people with pernicious anemia, the ability to absorb vitamin $B_{12}$ from the GI tract is reduced, so that excretion of radioactive material in the urine is reduced. This test is rarely used today.

**schindylesis** /skin′dilē′sis/ [Gk, splintering], an articulation (synarthrosis) of certain bones of the skull in which a thin plate of one bone enters a cleft formed by the separation of two layers of another bone, such as the insertion of the vomer bone into the fissure between the maxillae and the palatine bones.

**Schiötz' tonometer** /shē·ets′/ [Hjalmar Schiötz, Norwegian ophthalmologist, 1850–1927; Gk, *tonos,* stretching, *metron,* measure], a tonometer used to measure intraocular pressure by observing the depth of indentation of the cornea made by the weighted plunger on the device after a topical anesthetic is applied.

**Schirmer's test.** [Otto W.A. Schirmer, German ophthalmologist, 1864–1917]. See **test for lacrimation.**

**schisandra,** an herb that is native to China, Russia, and Korea.

■ USES: This herb is used for GI disorders, for liver protection, and as a tonic.

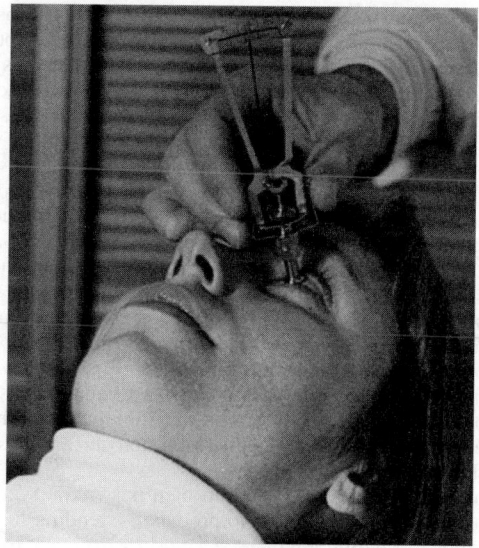

**Schiötz' tonometer** (Phipps, Sands, and Marek, 1999)

■ CONTRAINDICATIONS: Schisandra should not be used during pregnancy and lactation, in children, or in those with known hypersensitivity to this plant.

**schisto-,** combining form meaning 'split, or cleft': *schisto-celia, schistocephalus, schistomelia.*

**schistocelia** /shis'təsē'lyə/, a congenital fissure in the wall of the abdomen.

**schistocystis** /shis'təsis'tis/ [Gk, *schistos,* cleft, *kystis,* bag], a fissure in the bladder.

**schistocyte** /shis'təsīt/ [Gk, *schistos,* cleft, *kytos,* cell], an erythrocyte cell fragment characteristic of hemolysis or cell fragmentation associated with severe burns and intravascular coagulation.

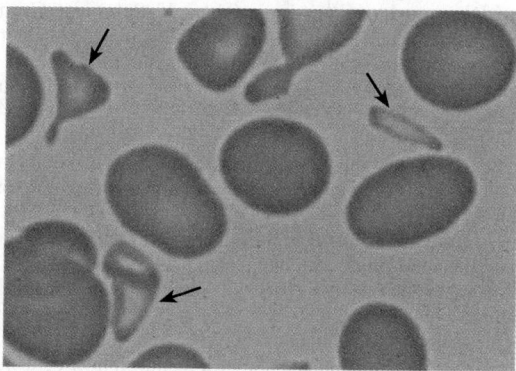

**Schistocyte** (Carr and Rodak, 1999)

*Schistosoma* /shis'təsō'mə/ [Gk, *schistos,* cleft, *soma,* body], a genus of blood flukes that may cause urinary, GI, or liver disease in humans and that requires fecal contamination of water and freshwater snails as intermediate

hosts. *Schistosoma haematobium,* found chiefly in Africa and the Middle East, affects the bladder, ureter, and pelvic organs, causing painful frequent urination and hematuria. *S. japonicum,* found in Japan, the Philippines, and Eastern Asia, causes GI ulcerations and fibrosis of the liver. *S. mansoni,* found in Africa, the Middle East, the Caribbean, and tropical America, causes symptoms similar to those caused by *S. japonicum.* Also called *Bilharzia.* See also **schistosomiasis.**

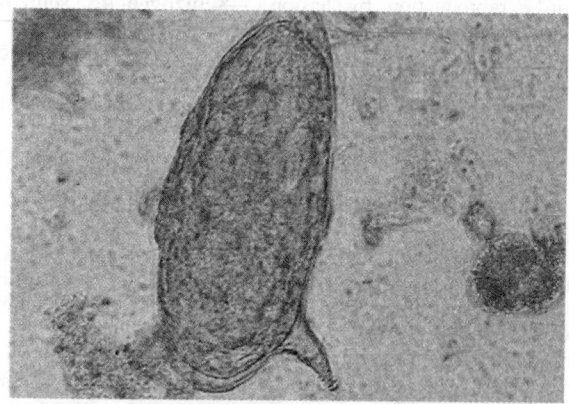

**Schistosoma mansoni egg** (Murray et al, 1998)

**schistosome dermatitis.** See **swimmer's itch.**

**schistosomiasis** /shis'təsōmī'əsis/ [Gk, *schistos* + *soma* + *osis,* condition], a parasitic infection caused by a species of fluke of the genus *Schistosoma.* It is transmitted to humans, the definitive host, by contact with water containg the infective stage of the parasite, the cercaria. A single fluke may live in one part of the body, depositing eggs frequently, for up to 20 years. The eggs are irritating to mucous membrane, causing it to thicken and become papillomatous. Symptoms depend on the part of the body infected. *Schistosoma* may be found in the bladder, rectum, liver, lungs, spleen, intestines, and portal venous system. Pain, obstruction, dysfunction of the affected organ, and anemia may result. Diagnosis requires morphologic identification of the ova or the parasite. Depending on the species, treatment may be with praziquantel, oxamniquine, or metrifonate. Prevention is more effective. Proper disposal of human urine and feces, chlorination of water, and eradication of the intermediate host, the freshwater snail *Australorbis glabratus,* are totally effective. Second only to malaria in the number of people affected, schistosomiasis is particularly prevalent in the tropics and in Asia. Also called **bilharziasis.** See also **blood fluke,** *Schistosoma.*

**schistosomicide** /shis'təsō'məsīd/ [Gk, *schistos* + *soma* + L, *caedere,* to kill], a drug destructive to schistosomes, blood flukes transmitted by snails to human hosts in many parts of Africa, Brazil, and Asia. Niridazole, metrifonate, oxamniquine hycanthone hydrochloride, and various salts of antimony, including stibophen, are potent antischistosomal agents. —**schistosomicidal,** *adj.*

**schistosternia.** See **schistothorax.**

**schistothorax** /-thôr'aks/, a congenital cleft in the wall of the thorax. Also called **schistosternia.**

**schizencephaly** /skiz′ensef′əlē/, an abnormal cleavage or other division of the brain tissues caused by maldevelopment.

**schizo-** /skit′sə-, skiz′ə-/, combining form meaning 'divided, or related to division': *schizocephalia, schizogenesis, schizophrenia.*

**schizoaffective disorder** /skit′sō·afek′tiv/ [Gk, *schizein,* to split; L, *affectus,* state of mind, *dis,* opposite of, *ordo,* rank], a psychiatric disorder in which either a major depressive or a manic episode develops concurrently, displaying the symptoms of schizophrenia.

**schizogenesis** /skit′səjen′əsis/ [Gk, *schizein* + *genesis,* origin], reproduction by fission. —**schizogenetic, schizogenic, schizogenous,** *adj.*

**schizogony,** a form of asexual reproduction characteristic of certain protozoa, including sporozoans, in which daughter cells are produced by multiple fission of the nucleus of the parasite (**schizont**) followed by segmentation of the cytoplasm to form separate masses around each smaller nucleus.

**schizogyria** /skit′səjī′rē·ə/, the presence of wedge-shaped cracks in the convolutions of the brain.

**schizoid** /skit′soid, skiz′oid/ [Gk, *schizein,* to split, *eidos,* form], **1.** characteristic of or resembling schizophrenia; schizophrenic. **2.** a person, not necessarily a schizophrenic, who exhibits the traits of a schizoid personality.

**schizoid personality,** a functioning but maladjusted person whose behavior is characterized by extreme shyness, oversensitivity, introversion, seclusiveness, and avoidance of close interpersonal relationships. See also **schizoid personality disorder, schizophrenic.**

**schizoid personality disorder,** a personality disorder (*DSM-IV*) characterized by a defect in the ability to form interpersonal relationships, as shown by emotional coldness and aloofness, withdrawn and seclusive behavior, and indifference to praise, criticism, and the feelings of others. The person is unable to express hostility and ordinary aggressive feelings and reacts to disturbing experiences with apparent detachment. Person neither desires nor enjoys personal relationships, prefers solitary activities, and has no close friends or confidants.

**schizont** /skitsənt/ [Gk, *schizein* + *genein,* to produce], **1.** reproduction by multiple fission. **2.** the multinucleated cell stage during the asexual reproductive phase in the life cycle of a sporozoon, such as the malarial parasite *Plasmodium.* Also called **agamont.** Compare **sporont.** See also **schizogony.** —**schizogonic, schizogonous,** *adj.*

**schizonticide** /skitson′təsīd/ [Gk, *schizein* + *on,* being; L, *caedere,* to kill], a substance that destroys schizonts. —**schizonticidal,** *adj.*

**schizophasia** /skit′səfā′zhə, skiz′ə-/ [Gk, *schizein* + *phasis,* speech], the disordered, incomprehensible speech characteristic of some forms of schizophrenia. See also **word salad.**

**schizophrenia** /skit′səfrē′nē·ə, skiz′ə-/ [Gk, *schizein,* to split, *phren,* mind], any one of a large group of *DSM-IV* psychotic disorders characterized by gross distortion of reality, disturbances of language and communication, withdrawal from social interaction, and disorganization and fragmentation of thought, perception, and emotional reaction. The term *schizophrenia* denotes one of the fundamental characteristics of the patients, the splitting off of a part of the psyche. The part that splits off then dominates the psychic life of the patient even though the it may express behavior that is contrary to the original personality of the patient. Apathy and confusion; delusions and hallucinations; rambling or stylized patterns of speech, such as evasiveness, incoherence, and echolalia; withdrawn, regressive, and bi-

zarre behavior; and emotional lability often occur. Most patients have both positive and negative psychotic symptoms. Positive symptoms include hallucinations; negative symptoms include anergia, flatness, and anhedonia. The condition may be mild or require prolonged hospitalization. No single cause of the disorder is known; genetic, biochemical, psychologic, interpersonal, and sociocultural factors are usually involved. Although slowly progressive deterioration of the personality may occur, dementia is not an inevitable consequence of the disorder. There may be recovery in some cases, and there may be relapse marked by intermittent episodes that begin after prolonged remission.

**schizophrenic** /skit′səfren′ik, skiz′ə-/, **1.** pertaining to schizophrenia. **2.** a person with schizophrenia.

**schizophreniform disorder** /-fren′ifôrm/ [Gk, *schizein* + *phren* + L, *forma,* form], a *DSM-IV* psychiatric disorder exhibiting the same symptoms as schizophrenia but characterized by an acute onset with resolution in 2 weeks to 6 months.

**schizophrenogenic** /skit′səfren′əjen′ik, skiz′ə-/ [Gk, *schizein* + *phren* + *genein,* to produce], tending to cause or produce schizophrenia.

*Schizotrypanum cruzi.* See **Chagas' disease.**

**schizotypal personality disorder** /skit′sōtī′pəl/ [Gk, *schizein* + *typos,* mark; L, *personalis,* of a person, *dis,* opposite of, *ordo,* rank], a *DSM-IV* psychiatric disorder characterized by oddities of thought, perception, speech, and behavior that are not severe enough to meet the clinical criteria for schizophrenia. Symptoms may include magical thinking inconsistent with cultural norms, such as superstitiousness, belief in clairvoyance and telepathy, and bizarre fantasies; ideas of reference; recurrent illusions, such as sensing the presence of a force or person not actually present; social isolation; peculiar speech patterns, including ideas expressed unclearly or words used deviantly; and exaggerated anxiety or hypersensitivity to real or imagined criticism. See also **schizoid personality disorder, schizophrenia.**

**Schlatter-Osgood disease, Schlatter's disease.** See **Osgood-Schlatter disease.**

**Schlemm's canal.** See **canal of Schlemm.**

**schlieren optics** /shlir′ən/ [Ger, *schlieren,* ulcers, streaks], a system that observes the refractive index gradient in solutions containing macromolecules.

**Schmidt's syndrome**[1] /shmits/ [Adolf Schmidt, German physician, 1865−1918], paralysis on one side, affecting the vocal cord, the soft palate, the trapezius muscle, and the sternocleidomastoid muscle; resulting from a lesion in a specific region of the brain. Also called **vagoaccessory syndrome.**

**Schmidt's syndrome**[2] [Martin Benno Schmidt, German pathologist, 1863−1949], See **polyglandular autoimmune syndrome.**

**Schneiderian carcinoma** /shnīdir′ē·ən/, an epithelial malignancy of the nasal mucosa and paranasal sinuses.

**Schönlein-Henoch purpura.** See **Henoch-Schönlein purpura.**

**school nurse practitioner (S.N.P.),** a registered nurse who is qualified through satisfactory completion of a nurse practitioner program to serve as a nurse practitioner in a school system.

**school phobia** [AS, *scol* + Gk, *phobos,* fear], an extreme separation anxiety disorder of children, usually in the elementary grades, characterized by a persistent irrational fear of going to school or being in a schoollike atmosphere. Such children are usually oversensitive, shy, timid, nervous, and emotionally immature and have pervasive feelings of inadequacy. They typically try to cope with their fears by becoming overdependent on others, especially the parents.

**Schüffner's dots** [Wilhelm A.P. Schüffner, German patholo-gist, 1867–1949], coarse pink or red granules seen in the red blood cells of patients with tertiary malaria. They are signs of *Plasmodium vivax* or *P. ovale* and are absent in blood cells of patients infected with other types of malaria.

**Schultz-Charlton phenomenon,** a reaction that occurs when scarlet fever antitoxin or scarlet fever convalescent se-rum is injected into an area of the skin showing a bright red rash. A blanching of the skin at the site of the injection oc-curs. Serum from scarlet fever patients does not produce this reaction.

**Schultze's mechanism,** the delivery of a placenta with the fetal surfaces presenting.

**Schwann cell** /shwon/ [Theodor Schwann, German anato-mist, 1810–1882], any of the cells of ectodermal origin that make up the neurilemma. They form the myelin sheath around peripheral nerve fibers.

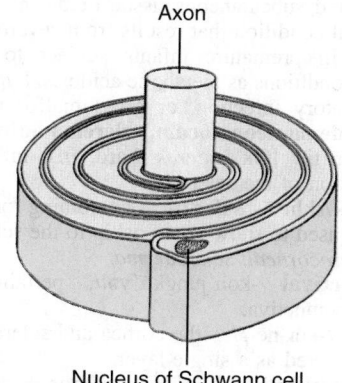

Axon

Nucleus of Schwann cell

**Schwann cell** *(Crossman and Neary, 1995)*

**schwannoma** /shwonō'mə/, *pl.* **schwannomas, schwanno-mata** [Theodor Schwann; Gk, *oma,* tumor], a benign soli-tary encapsulated tumor arising in the neurilemma (Schwann's sheath) of peripheral, cranial, or autonomic nerves. Also called **Schwann cell tumor, neurilemoma.**

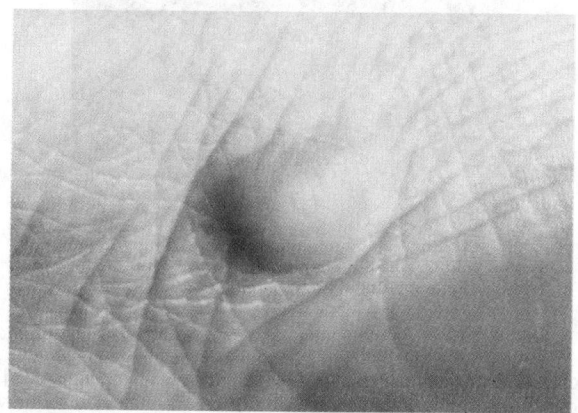

**Schwannoma on the sole of the foot** *(du Vivier, 1993)*

**schwannosis** /shwonō'sis/ [Theodor Schwann; Gk, *osis,* condition], a condition of overgrowth of the neurilemma or sheath of Schwann.

**Schwann's sheath.** See **neurilemma.**

**Schwartz bed.** See **hyperextension bed.**

**Schwartz-Jampel syndrome** /shworts·jam'pəl/ [Oscar Schwartz, American pediatrician, b. 1919; Robert Steven Jampel, American ophthalmologist, b. 1926], an autoso-mal recessive disorder characterized by myotonic myopathy, dwarfism, abnormal narrowness of the palpebral fissures in the horizontal direction, joint contractures, and flat facies. Also called **chondrodystrophic myotonia.**

**Schwartzman-Sanarelli phenomenon** /shvorts'man san'-ərel'ē/ [Gregory Schwartzman, American physician, b. 1896; Guiseppe Sanarelli, Italian bacteriologist, 1864–1940], a condition induced experimentally in the investigation of the role of coagulation in renal disease. Animals injected twice with a bacterial endotoxin experience massive dis-seminated intravascular coagulation with blood clots in the vessels of the kidneys. Also called **Schwartzman phenomenon.**

**scia-.** See **skia-.**

**sciatic** /sī·at'ik/ [Gk, *ischiadikos,* hip joint], pertaining to an area near the ischium, such as the sciatic nerve or the sci-atic vein.

**sciatica** /sī·at'ikə/, an inflammation of the sciatic nerve, usually marked by pain and tenderness along the course of the nerve through the thigh and leg. It may result in a wast-ing of the muscles of the lower leg. Also called **sciatic neuritis.**

**sciatic dislocation.** See **dislocation of hip.**

**sciatic hernia,** a protrusion of tissue through the greater sciatic notch.

**sciatic nerve,** a long nerve originating in the sacral plexus and extending through the muscles of the thigh, leg, and foot, with numerous branches.

**sciatic neuritis.** See **sciatica.**

**sciatic scoliosis,** lateral curvature of the spine caused by an asymmetric spasm of the spinal muscles, often resulting in a list to one side.

**SCID,** abbreviation for **severe combined immunodefi-ciency disease.**

**science** /sī'əns/ [L, *scientia,* knowledge], a systematic at-tempt to establish theories to explain observed phenomena and the knowledge obtained through these efforts. **Pure sci-ence** is concerned with the gathering of information solely for the sake of obtaining new knowledge. **Applied science** is the practical application of scientific theory and laws. See also **hypothesis, law, scientific method, theory.**

**Science of Unitary Human Beings,** a conceptual model and theory of nursing proposed by Martha Rogers in 1970. Its four basic concepts focus on the nature and direction of "unitary human development": (1) human and environmen-tal energy fields, (2) complete and continuous openness of the energy fields, (3) human energy fields perceived as single waves that give identity to a field, and (4) "pandimen-sionality," a nonlinear domain without spatial or temporal attributes. See also **Rogers.**

**scientific method** /sī'əntif'ik/, a systematic, ordered ap-proach to the gathering of data and the solving of problems. The basic approach is the statement of the problem followed by the statement of a hypothesis. An experimental method is established to help prove or disprove the hypothesis. The re-sults of the experiment are observed, and conclusions are drawn from observed results. The conclusions may tend to uphold or to refute the hypothesis.

**scientific rationale,** a reason, based on supporting scien-tific evidence, that a particular action is chosen.

**scimitar sign** /sim′ətər/, an arteriographic sign of encroachment on the popliteal or femoral lumen in adventitial cystic disease.

**scimitar syndrome,** a radiographic artifact caused by a congenital disorder in which the right lower pulmonary vein drains into the inferior vena cava. On a chest radiograph, the abnormal vessel configuration produces a scimitar-shaped shadow.

**scintigram** /sin′tigram/ [L, *scintillare,* to sparkle; Gk, *gramma,* record], a recording of the radioactivity emitted by a tracer in an organism or organ system.

**scintigraph** /sin′tigraf′/, a photograph showing the distribution and intensity of radioactivity in various tissues and organs after the administration of a radiopharmaceutical.

**scintillating scotoma** /sin′tilā′ting/ [L, *scintillatio,* sparkling; Gk *skotos* dark, *oma* tumor], an abnormal area of the visual field that is positive and luminous, sometimes becoming hemianopic and appearing in a migraine aura.

**scintillation detector** /sin′tilā′shən/ [L, *scintillatio,* sparkling], **1.** a device that detects the light emitted by a crystal subjected to ionizing radiation. A photomultiplier tube in the detector converts the light into an electrical signal that can be processed further. An array of scintillation detectors is used in a gamma camera. **2.** a device used to measure the amount of radioactivity in an area of the body.

**scintiscan** /sin′tiscan′/, a photographic display of the distribution of a radiopharmaceutical within the body.

**scirrho-,** combining form meaning 'hard, or related to a hard cancer or scirrhus': *scirrhoid, scirrhoma, scirrhosarca.*

**scirrhous carcinoma** /skir′əs/ [Gk, *skirrhos,* hard, *karkinos,* crab, *oma,* tumor], a hard fibrous particularly invasive tumor in which the malignant cells occur singly or in small clusters or strands in dense connective tissue. Also called **carcinoma fibrosum.** See also **breast cancer.**

**scissor gait** /siz′ər/ [L, *scindere,* to cut; ONorse, *gata,* way], a manner of walking cross-legged, as observed in spastic paraplegia.

**scissor legs** [L, *scindere,* to cut; ONorse, *leggr*], legs that are crossed because of a disorder of the adductor muscles of the thigh or a deformity of the hip.

**scissors** [L, *scindere,* to cut], a sharp instrument composed of two opposing cutting blades, held together by a central pin on which the blades pivot. The most common dissecting scissors are the straight **Mayo,** for cutting sutures; the **Snowden-Pencer,** for deep, delicate tissue; the long curved **Mayo,** for deep, heavy, or tough tissue; the short curved **Metzenbaum,** for superficial, delicate tissue; and the long, blunt curved **Metzenbaum,** for deep, delicate tissue.

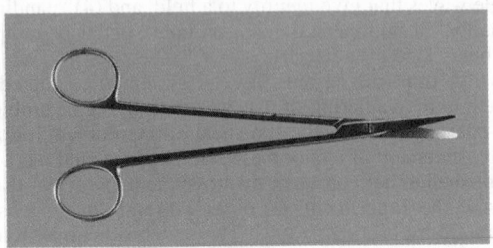

**Metzenbaum scissors** *(Tighe, 1999)*

**SCL,** abbreviation for *soft contact lens.*

**scler-.** See **sclero-.**

**sclera** /sklir′ə/ [Gk, *skleros,* hard], the tough inelastic white opaque membrane covering the posterior five sixths of the eyebulb. It maintains the size and form of the bulb and attaches to muscles that move the bulb. Posteriorly it is pierced by the optic nerve and, with the transparent cornea, makes up the outermost of three tunics covering the eyebulb.

**scleredema** /sklir′ədē′mə/ [Gk, *skleros* + *oidema,* swelling], an idiopathic skin disease characterized by nonpitting induration beginning on the face or neck and spreading downward over the body, sparing the hands and feet. There also may be tongue swelling, restriction of eye movements, and pericardial, pleural, and peritoneal effusions. Resolution occurs after several months, but recurrences are common. The condition often follows a streptococcal infection or an exanthem of childhood. There is no specific treatment. Compare **scleroderma.**

**sclerema neonatorum** /sklirē′mə/ [Gk, *skleros* + *neos,* new; L, *natus,* birth], a progressive generalized hardening of the skin and subcutaneous tissue of the newborn. It is usually a fatal condition that results from severe cold stress in severely ill premature infants subject to such life-threatening conditions as metabolic acidosis, hypoglycemia, GI or respiratory infection, or gross malformation. Also called **scleredema neonatorum, sclerema adiposum.**

**scleritis** /sklirī′tis/ [Gk, *skleros,* hard, *itis,* inflammation], an inflammation of the sclera.

**sclero-, scler-** /sklir′ō-, skler′ō-/, combining form meaning 'hard,' often used to show relationship to the sclera: *scleroadipose, sclerocorneal, scleroderma.*

**scleroconjunctival** /-kon′jungktī′vəl/, pertaining to the sclera and conjunctiva.

**sclerocornea** /-kôr′nē·ə/, the cornea and sclera of the eye surface considered as a single layer.

**sclerodactyly** /sklir′ōdak′tilē/ [Gk, *skleros* + *daktylos,* finger], a musculoskeletal deformity affecting the hands of people with scleroderma. The fingers are fixed in a semiflexed position, with subcutaneous calcification and tightened skin to the wrist. The fingertips may be ulcerated.

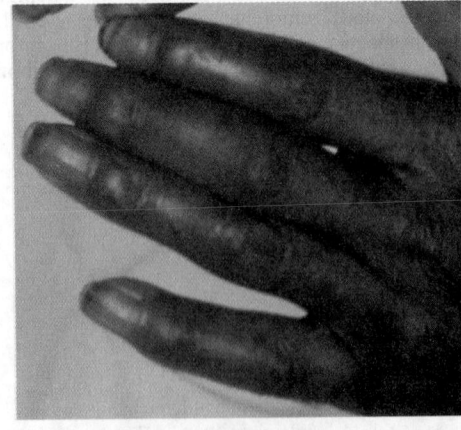

**Sclerodactyly** *(Zitelli and Davis, 1997)*

**scleroderma** /sklir′ōdur′mə/ [Gk, *skleros* + *derma,* skin], chronic hardening and thickening of the skin caused by new collagen formation, with atrophy of pilosebaceous follicles.

Scleroderma is most common in middle-aged women. It may occur in a localized form (**morphea**) or as a systemic disease (systemic sclerosis). **Progressive systemic sclerosis (PSS)** is a relatively rare autoimmune disease affecting the blood vessels and connective tissue. It is characterized by fibrous degeneration of the connective tissue of the skin, lungs, and internal organs, especially the esophagus, digestive tract, and kidneys. See also **systemic sclerosis.**

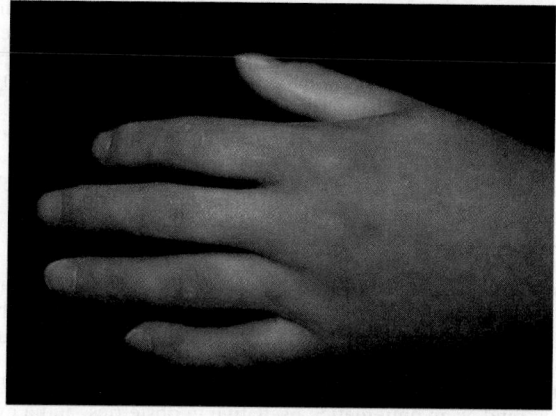

**Scleroderma**

*(Huether and McCance/courtesy Department of Dermatology, School of Medicine, University of Utah)*

■ OBSERVATIONS: The most common initial complaints are changes in the skin of the face and fingers. Raynaud's phenomenon occurs with a gradual hardening of the skin and swelling of the distal extremities. In the early stages the disease may be confused with rheumatoid arthritis or Raynaud's disease. As the disease progresses, deformity of the joints and pain on movement occur. Skin changes include edema and then pallor; then the skin becomes firm; finally it becomes slightly pigmented and fixed to the underlying tissues. At this stage the skin of the face is taut, shiny, and masklike, and the patient may have difficulty in chewing and swallowing. Patients with mild forms of scleroderma may live to 30 to 50 years of age. Those with cardiac, renal, pulmonary, or intestinal involvement may die at an earlier age. The usual indication that renal disease is present is the abrupt onset of severe arterial hypertension that does not respond to medication. Localized forms of scleroderma may occur; these cases are benign and appear only as small circumscribed patches on the skin. A biopsy of the lesion may be done to diagnose the condition. Radiographic examination of the lungs and GI tract may be diagnostic in the systemic form of the disease. Blood tests may reveal antinuclear antibodies.

■ INTERVENTIONS: There are no drugs to cure scleroderma; however, corticosteroids, immunosuppressants, antacids, and histamine receptor antagonists may be useful in treating the symptoms of the disease, and salicylates and mild analgesics are given to ease pain in the joints. Physical therapy slows the development of muscle contracture and resultant deformity and debility. Nephrectomy or renal transplantation may be performed.

■ NURSING CONSIDERATIONS: The nurse advises patients to use mild, nonalcoholic astringent soaps; to avoid extreme cold and activities that trigger pain; to wear gloves; to stop smoking; and to eat small, frequent meals. In the advanced stages of scleroderma patients often require help to eat, and mouth and skin care is particularly important. As patients become more helpless, there is a need for considerable emotional support.

**scleroderma heart,** a heart condition characterized by interstitial myocardial fibrosis and thickening of the small blood vessels in progressive systemic sclerosis.

**scleroderma neonatorum.** See **sclerema neonatorum.**

**sclerodermatitis** /-dur′mətī′tis/, an inflammation, thickening, and hardening of the skin.

**sclerokeratitis** /-ker′ətī′tis/, an inflammation of the sclera and cornea.

**-scleroma,** combining form meaning an 'induration, a hardening of the tissues': *laryngoscleroma, pharyngoscleroma, rhinoscleroma.*

**scleromalacia perforans** /sklir′ōməlā′shə/ [Gk, *skleros + malakia,* softening; L, *perforare,* to pierce], a condition of the eyes in which devitalization and sloughing of the sclera occur as a complication of rheumatoid arthritis. The pigmented uvea becomes exposed, and glaucoma, cataract formation, and detachment of the retina may result.

**sclerose** /sklərōz′/ [Gk, *skleros*], to harden or to cause hardening. —**sclerotic,** adj.

**sclerosing** /sklirō′zing/ [Gk, *skleros,* hard], pertaining to the tissue changes or other factors involved in the progress of sclerosis.

**sclerosing hemangioma** [Gk, *skleros + haima,* blood, *angeion* vessel, *oma* tumor], a solid cellular tumorlike nodule of the skin or a mass of histiocytes, thought to arise from a hemangioma by the proliferation of endothelial and connective tissue cells.

**sclerosing keratitis** [Gk, *skleros,* hard, *keras,* horn, *itis,* inflammation], 1. a form of corneal inflammation in which nodular infiltrates appear near the margin of the cornea in association with a ring of anterior scleritis. 2. a form of corneal inflammation characterized by an opaque triangle in the deep layers of the cornea, with the base of the triangle near the sclerosing area.

**sclerosing phlebitis** [Gk, *skleros,* hard, *phleps,* vein, *itis,* inflammation], inflammation of a vein that has become hardened and obstructed.

**sclerosing solution** [Gk, *skleros + L, solvere,* to dissolve], a liquid containing an irritant that causes inflammation and resulting fibrosis of tissues. It may be used in cauterizing ulcers, arresting hemorrhage, and treating hemangiomas.

**sclerosis** /sklirō′sis/ [Gk, *skleros,* hard], a condition characterized by hardening of tissue resulting from any of several causes, including inflammation, the deposit of mineral salts, and infiltration of connective tissue fibers. —**sclerotic,** adj.

**-sclerosis,** suffix meaning 'an abnormal hardening of the tissue': *atherosclerosis, arteriosclerosis, phlebosclerosis.*

**sclerotherapy** /-ther′əpē/ [Gk, *skleros,* hard, *therapeia,* treatment], the use of sclerosing chemicals to treat varicosities such as hemorrhoids or esophageal varices. The agent produces inflammation and later fibrosis and obliteration of the lumen.

**sclerotic** /sklirot′ik/ [Gk, *skleros,* hard], pertaining to induration or hardening.

**sclerotomal pain distribution** /-tō′məl/, the referral of pain from pain-sensitive tissues covering the axial skeleton along a sclerotomal segment.

**sclerotome** /sklir′ətōm/ [Gk, *skleros + temnein,* to cut], (in embryology) the part of the segmented mesoderm layer in the early developing embryo that originates from the somites and gives rise to skeletal tissue of the body, specifically the paired segmented masses of mesodermal tissue that lie on each side of the notochord and develop into the vertebrae and ribs. See also **somite.**

**sclerotylosis** /-tilō′sis/, an inherited condition of atrophic fibrosis of the skin. There is overgrowth of the nails and horny skin covering the palms of the hands and plantar surfaces of the feet. The disorder may be accompanied by cancer of the GI tract.

**scoleces.** See **scolex.**

**scoleco-,** combining form meaning 'worm': *scolecoid, scolecoidectomy, scolecology.*

**scolex** /skō′leks/, *pl.* **scoleces** /skō′ləsēz/ [Gk, worm], the headlike segment or organ of an adult tapeworm that has hooks, grooves, or suckers by which it attaches itself to the wall of the intestine.

**scolio-,** combining form meaning 'twisted or crooked': *scoliodontic, scoliokyphosis, scoliosiometry.*

**scoliokyphosis.** See **kyphoscoliosis.**

**scoliometer** /skō′lē·om′ətər/ [Gk, *skoliosis,* curvature], a device for measuring the amount of abnormal curvature in the spine.

**scoliosis** /skō′lē·ō′sis/ [Gk, *skoliosis,* curvature], lateral curvature of the spine, a common abnormality of childhood, especially in females. Causes include congenital malformations of the spine, poliomyelitis, skeletal dysplasias, spastic paralysis, and unequal leg length. Unequal heights of hips or shoulders may be a sign of this condition. Early recognition and orthopedic treatment may prevent progression of the curvature. Treatment includes braces, casts, exercises, and corrective surgery. See also **congenital scoliosis, idiopathic scoliosis, kyphoscoliosis, kyphosis, lordosis, spinal curvature.**

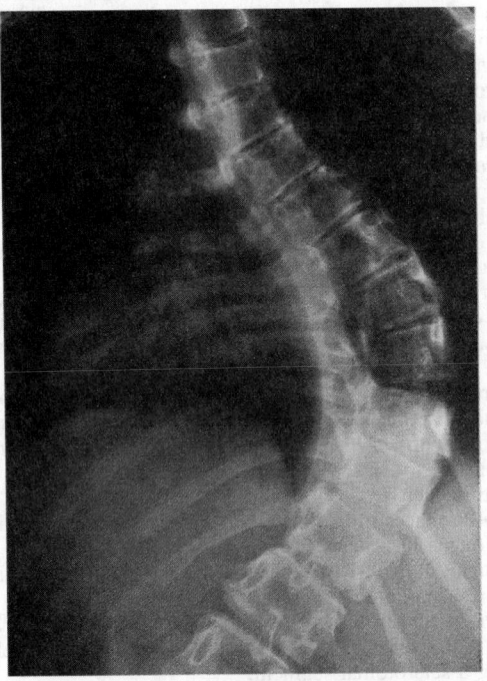

**Radiograph of the spine in scoliosis**
*(Zitelli and Davis, 1997)*

**scoliotic pelvis** /skō′lē·ot′ik/ [Gk, *skoliosis,* curvature; L, *pelvis,* basin], an effect of scoliosis in which the sacrum bends to one side, distorting the pelvis.

**scombroid** /skom′broid/ [Gk, *scombros,* mackerel, *eidos,* form], pertaining to fish of the Scombridae and Scomberescidae families, which include skipjack, mackerel, bonito, and tuna.

**scombroid poisoning,** toxic effects of eating scombroid types of fish (such as bonito or tuna) that have begun bacterial decomposition after being caught. Scombroid fish contain large amounts of free histidine in the muscle tissue, which gives rise to toxic levels of histamine under conditions of histidine decarboxylation by any of a dozen species of bacteria. Scombroid poisoning is not limited to consumption of fresh fish; the problem also may affect commercially canned tuna. Symptoms, which usually last no more than 24 hours, include nausea, vomiting, diarrhea, epigastric pain, and urticaria.

**scop-,** combining form meaning 'to examine, observe': *scopograph, scopometer, scopophilia.*

**-scope,** suffix meaning an 'instrument for observation or a visual examination': *ciliariscope, episcope, pelviscope.*

**scopolamine** /skōpol′əmēn/ [Giovanni A. Scopoli, Italian naturalist, 1723–1788], an anticholinergic alkaloid obtained from the leaves and seeds of several solanaceous plants. It is a central nervous system depressant.
■ INDICATIONS: It is prescribed for prevention of motion sickness and as an antiemetic, a sedative in obstetrics, and a cycloplegic and mydriatic.
■ CONTRAINDICATIONS: Narrow-angle glaucoma, myasthenia gravis, obstruction of the genitourinary or GI tract and known hypersensitivity prohibit its use.
■ ADVERSE EFFECTS: Among the more serious adverse reactions are blurred vision, central nervous system effects, tachycardia, dry mouth, decreased sweating, and hypersensitivity reaction. Also called **hyoscine.** See also **transdermal scopolamine.**

**scopolamine hydrobromide,** an anticholinergic.
■ INDICATIONS: It is prescribed in the treatment of nausea and vomiting, as a sedative and preanesthetic medication, and as a cycloplegic and mydriatic medication in ophthalmic procedures.
■ CONTRAINDICATIONS: Narrow-angle glaucoma, asthma, obstruction of the genitourinary or GI tract, severe ulcerative colitis, or known hypersensitivity to this drug prohibits its use.
■ ADVERSE EFFECTS: Among the more serious adverse reactions are blurred vision, central nervous system effects, tachycardia, dry mouth, decreased sweating, and hypersensitivity reaction. Also called **hyoscine hydrobromide.**

**scopophilia** /skō′pəfil′ē·ə, skop′-/ [Gk, *skopein,* to look, *philein,* to love], **1.** sexual pleasure derived from looking at sexually stimulating scenes or at another person's genitals; voyeurism. **2.** a morbid desire to be seen; exhibitionism. Also called **scoptophilia. —scopophiliac, scopophilic, scoptophiliac, scoptophilic,** *adj., n.*

**scopophobia** /skō′pə-/ [Gk, *skopein* + *phobos,* fear], an anxiety disorder characterized by a morbid fear of being seen or stared at by others. The condition is commonly seen in schizophrenia. See also **phobia.**

**scoptophilia, scoptophilic.** See **scopophilia.**

**-scopy,** suffix meaning 'observation or a visual examination': *bioscopy, stomachoscopy, thoracoscopy.*

**-scorbic,** suffix meaning 'prevention or treatment of scurvy': *antiscorbic, ascorbic, glucoascorbic.*

**-scorbutic, -scorbutical,** suffix meaning 'scurvy': *antiscorbutic, postscorbutic, scorbutic.*

**scorbutic gingivitis** /skôrby○○′tik/ [NL, *scorbutus,* scurvy; L, *gingiva,* gum; Gk, *itis,* inflammation], an abnormal condition characterized by inflamed or bleeding gums and caused by vitamin C deficiency.

**scorbutic pose,** the characteristic posture of a child with scurvy, with thighs and legs semiflexed and hips rotated outward. The child usually lies motionless in a state of pseudoparalysis, avoiding voluntary movements of the extremities because of the pain that accompanies any motion. See also **scurvy.**

**scorbutus.** See **scurvy.**

**scorpion sting** /skôr′pē·on/ [Gk, *skorpios* + AS, *stingan*], a painful wound produced by a scorpion, an arachnid with a hollow stinger in its tail. The stings of many species are only slightly toxic, but some, including *Centruroides sculpturatus* (bark scorpion) of the southwestern United States, may inflict fatal injury, especially in small children. Initial pain is followed within several hours by numbness, nausea, muscle spasm, dyspnea, and convulsion. An antivenin is available only from Arizona State University.

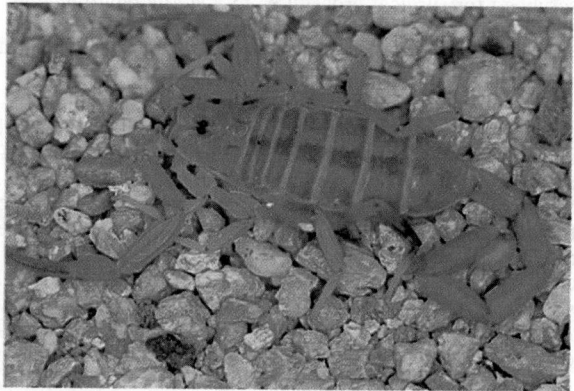

**Bark scorpion** *(Auerbach, 1995/courtesy William Banner, MD)*

**scoto-,** combining form meaning 'darkness': *scotodinia, scotogram, scotographic.*

**scotoma** /skōtō′mə/, *pl.* **scotomas, scotomata** [Gk, *skotos,* darkness, *oma,* tumor], a defect of vision in a defined area of the visual field in one or both eyes. A common prodromal symptom is a shimmering film appearing as an island in the visual field.

**scotopic vision** /skōtop′ik/ [Gk, *skotos,* darkness; L, *visio,* seeing], the ability of the eye to adjust for vision in darkness or dim light. See also **night vision.**

**scrapie** /skrā′pē/, the first of the prion diseases to be recognized, occurring in sheep and goats and characterized by severe pruritus, muscular incoordination, and increasing debility, ending in death.

**scratch test** [ME, *scratten* + L, *testum,* crucible], a skin test for identifying an allergen, performed by placing a small quantity of a solution containing a suspected allergen on a lightly scratched area of the skin. If a wheal forms within 15 minutes, allergy to the substance is indicated.

**screamer's nodule.** See **vocal cord nodule.**

**screening** [ME, *scren*], **1.** a preliminary procedure, such as a test or examination, to detect the most characteristic sign or signs of a disorder that may require further investigation. **2.** the examination of a large sample of a population to detect a specific disease or disorder, such as hypertension.

**screen memory** [ME, *scren* + L, *memoria*], a consciously tolerable memory that replaces one that is emotionally painful to recall.

**screw** /skr○○/ [MFr, *escroue*], a solid cylinder with a helical thread on its exterior surface, used to hold two objects together.

**screw artery** /skr○○/, a coiled blood vessel in either the uterine mucosa or the retinal macula. Also called **spiral artery.**

**screw clamp** [OFr, *escroe,* screw; AS, *clam,* fastener], a device, usually made of plastic, equipped with a screw that can be manipulated to close and open the primary IV tubing for regulating the flow of IV solution. Turning the screw clockwise closes the tubing; turning it counterclockwise opens it. Different positions of the screw between the open and the closed positions allow the IV fluid to flow at different rates. Compare **roller clamp, slide clamp.**

**scrib-, script-,** combining form meaning 'write': *scribble, scribomania, prescription.*

**Scribner shunt** [Belding S. Scribner, American physician, b. 1921], a type of arteriovenous bypass, used in hemodialysis, consisting of a special tube connection outside the body.

**scripting** /skrip′ting/, a technique of family therapy involving the development of new family transactional patterns.

**scrofula** /skrof′yələ/ [L, *scrofa,* brood sow], *archaic:* a form of tuberculosis cutis with abscess formation, usually of the cervical lymph nodes.

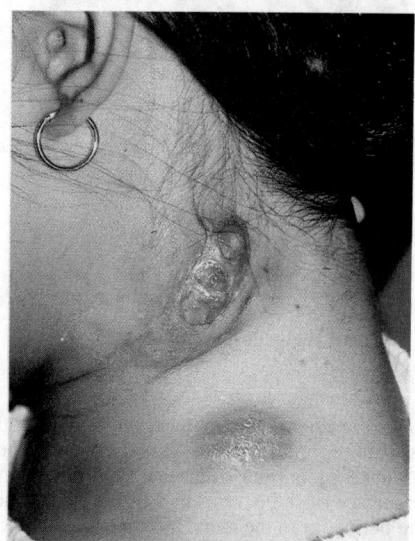

**Scrofula** *(Stone and Gorbach, 2000)*

**scroll ear** /skrōl/, a distortion of the ear in which the pinna is rolled forward.

**scrotal** /skrō′təl/, pertaining to the scrotum.

**scrotal cancer,** an epidermoid malignancy of the scrotum, characterized initially by a small sore that may ulcerate. The lesion occurs most frequently in elderly men who have been exposed to soot, pitch, crude oil, mineral oils, polycyclic hydrocarbons, or arsenic fumes from copper smelting. Treatment involves wide surgical excision of the tumor and resection of inguinal nodes. In the eighteenth century Sir Percival Pott associated scrotal cancer in chimney sweeps with exposure to soot. It is the first malignancy shown to be caused by an environmental carcinogen. Also called **chimney-sweeps' cancer, soot wart.**

**scrotal hernia,** an inguinal hernia that has descended into the scrotum.

**scrotal nuclear imaging,** a nuclear imaging scan, usually done on an emergency basis, that is helpful in diagnosing patients with a sudden onset of unilateral testicular swelling and pain. It can differentiate unilateral testicular torsion from other causes of testicular pain, such as acute epididymitis and other conditions.

**scrotal raphe,** a line of union of the two halves of the scrotum. It is generally more highly pigmented than the surrounding tissue.

**scrotal septum,** an incomplete wall of connective tissue and smooth muscle that divides the scrotum into two compartments, each containing a testis.

**scrotal swelling,** the earliest enlargement of embryonic tissue that will become half of the scrotum.

**scrotal tongue,** a nonpathologic condition in which the tongue is deeply furrowed and resembles the surface of the scrotum.

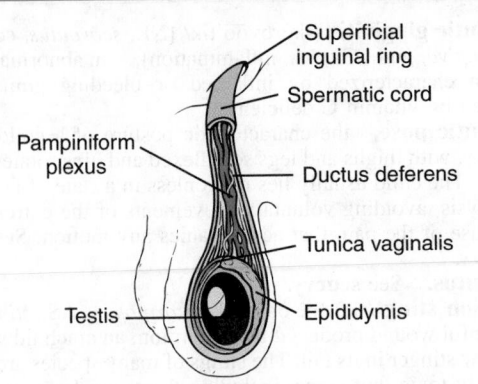

**Scrotum** *(Lewis, Collier, and Heitkemper, 2000)*

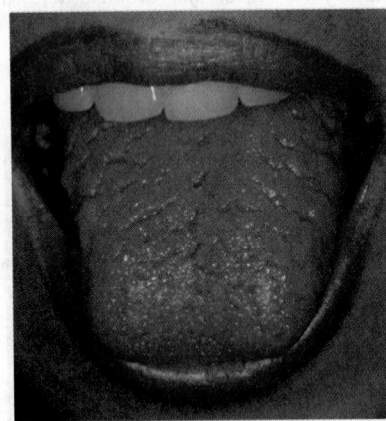

**Scrotal tongue** *(Lemmi and Lemmi, 2000)*

**scrotum** /skrō′təm/, the pouch of skin containing the testes and parts of the spermatic cords. It is divided on the surface into two lateral parts by a ridge that continues ventrally to the undersurface of the penis and dorsally along the middle line of the perineum to the anus. In young robust individuals the scrotum is short and corrugated and closely wraps the testes. In older people and debilitated individuals and in warm environments the scrotum becomes elongated and flaccid. The two layers of the scrotum are the skin and the dartos tunic. The skin is brownish and very thin is usually wrinkled, and has thinly scattered kinky hairs. The dartos tunic is composed of a thin layer of unstriated muscular fibers around the base of the scrotum. The tunic projects an internal septum that divides the pouch into two cavities for the testes, extending between the scrotal ridge and the root of the penis. The scrotum is highly vascular and contains no fat. See also **testis. —scrotal,** *adj.*

**scrub.** See **surgical scrub.**

**scrubbed team members** [ME, *scrobben,* to scrub], the surgeons, physicians, nurses, and technicians who are scrubbed for surgical procedures in a sterile environment.

**scrub itch.** See *Leeuwenhoekia australiensis.*

**scrub nurse,** a registered nurse or operating room technician who assists surgeons during operations.

**scrub room,** an operative area where surgeons and surgical teams use disposable sterile brushes and bactericidal soaps to wash and scrub their fingernails, hands, and forearms before performing or assisting in surgical operations. Scrub rooms and meticulous washing techniques improve the sterile environment of the operating room and reduce the risk of bacterial infection.

**scrub typhus,** an acute febrile disease caused by several strains of the species *Orientia tsutsugamushi* (formerly *Rickettsia tsutsugamushi*) and transmitted from infected rodents to humans by mites. It is found in Asia, India, northern Australia, and the western Pacific islands. The clinical course ranges from mild to severe and is characterized by a necrotic papule or black eschar at the site of the lesion caused by the bite of the small arachnid. Tender enlarged regional lymph nodes, fever, severe headache, eye pain, muscle aches, and a generalized rash usually occur. In severe cases the myocardium and the central nervous system may be involved. The DNA-PCR and indirect fluorescent antibody tests are useful in diagnosis. Treatment with antibiotics, such as chloramphenicol, doxycycline, or azithromycin, has reduced the mortality rate to nearly zero. Person-to-person transmission is not known to occur. No effective vaccine is available, and second attacks are common because of antigenic differences in various strains of rickettsiae. Prevention includes avoiding mite-infested terrain, reducing the rodent population, destroying scrub vegetation, and using insect repellents. Also called **Japanese flood fever, Japanese river fever, mite typhus, tsutsugamushi disease.** Compare **Q fever, Rocky Mountain spotted fever, typhus.**

**scruple** /skrōō′pəl/ [L, *scrupulus,* small stone], a measure of weight in the apothecaries' system, equal to 20 grains or 1.296 g. See also **apothecaries' weight, metric system.**

**sculpting** /skulp′ting/, a technique of family therapy involving construction of a live family portrait that depicts family alliances and conflicts.

**Scultetus bandage.** See **Scultetus binder.**

**Scultetus binder** /skəltē′təs/ [Johann Schultes, German surgeon, 1595–1645], a many-tailed binder or bandage with an attached central piece. The tails are overlapped; the last two, tied or pinned, act to secure the others. A scultetus binder may be opened or removed without moving the bandaged part of the body. Also called **Scultetus bandage.**

**scurvy** /skur'vē/ [Scand, *scurfa,* scabby], severe ascorbic acid deficiency. It is characterized by weakness; anemia; edema; spongy gums, often with ulceration and loosening of the teeth; a tendency to mucocutaneous hemorrhages, and induration of the muscles of the legs. Treatment and prophylaxis of the disease consist of administration of ascorbic acid and inclusion of fresh vegetables and fruits in the diet. Also called **scorbutus.** See also **ascorbic acid, citric acid, infantile scurvy.**

**scypho-,** combining form meaning 'a cup-shaped part': *scyphozoan, scyphus, scyphistoma.*

**SD,** 1. abbreviation for **skin dose.** 2. abbreviation for **standard deviation.**

**SDAT,** abbreviation for **senile dementia-Alzheimer type.**

**SDMS,** abbreviation for *Society of Diagnostic Medical Sonographers.*

**Se,** symbol for the element **selenium.**

**S.E.,** abbreviation for **standard error.**

**sea-blue histiocyte syndrome,** a condition of spleen enlargement and mild thrombocytopenia. Histiocytes in the bone marrow contain cytoplasmic granules that stain bright blue.

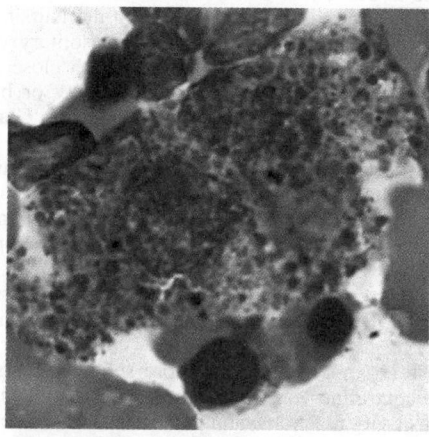

**Sea-blue histiocyte** *(Carr and Rodak, 1999)*

**seaborgium (Sg)** /sēbôr'gē·əm/ [Glenn T. Seaborg, American chemistry educator, b. 1912–1999], a synthetic radioactive element, with a half-life of 0.9 second. Its atomic number is 106; its atomic mass is 266. It was first synthesized in 1974 by scientists working independently in the United States and Russia.

**sealant** /sē'lənt/, an agent that protects against access from the outside or leakage from the inside; see also **dental sealants.**

**sealed source** [ME, *seel,* mark; Fr, *sourdre,* to spring], a source of radioactivity that is permanently encased in a container or bonding material to prevent leakage. Sealed sources, such as seeds, needles, and specially designed applicators, are used in the implantation of cesium-137, iodine-125, iridium-192, radium-226, and other radionuclides for the treatment of various malignant tumors.

**sealer cement,** a compound used in filling a pulp canal. It is applied as a plastic that fills depressions in the surface of the canal, solidifies after insertion, and helps close the apex of the root canal.

**seal limbs.** See **phocomelia.**

**seasickness.** See **motion sickness.**

**seasonal affective disorder (SAD)** /sē'zənəl/, a *DSM-IV* mood disorder associated with the shorter days and longer nights of autumn and winter. Symptoms include lethargy, depression, social withdrawal, and work difficulties. The patients also consume excess amounts of carbohydrates, gaining weight. The symptoms recede in the spring when days become longer. The condition is associated with the effect of light on melatonin secretion and is treated with light therapy for 5 to 6 hours per day.

**Seattle Foot** /sē·at'əl/, trademark for a stored-energy foot prosthesis that contains a plastic rod called a keel, which extends from the toe to the heel, where it turns upward toward the ankle. See also **keel, stored-energy foot.**

**seatworm.** See *Enterobius vermicularis.*

**sea urchin granuloma,** a type of foreign body granuloma in which nodules of granulation tissue develop in the skin several months after contact with the silicate in the spines of a sea urchin.

**sea urchin sting** /ur'chin/ [AS, *sae* + *herichon,* hedgehog], an injury inflicted by any of a variety of sea urchins, in which the skin is punctured and, in some species, venom released. A venomous sting is characterized by pain, muscular weakness, numbness around the mouth, and dyspnea. Immediate removal of the spines is necessary and may require the use of a local anesthetic. An antiseptic and a dressing are applied until the wound is healed. In all cases the broken spines cause local pain and irritation. Infection may result. See also **stingray.**

**seawater bath** [AS, *sae* + *waeter*], a bath taken in warm seawater or in saline solution.

**seb-,** combining form meaning 'sebum': *sebiferous, sebaceous, sebiparous.*

**sebaceous** /sibā'shəs/ [L, *sebum,* sweat], pertaining to sebum, the substance secreted by glands of the skin.

**sebaceous cyst,** a misnomer for an epidermoid cyst or a pilar cyst.

**sebaceous epithelioma,** a benign yellowish nodular tumor of sebaceous gland epithelium. It usually appears on the neck or face. It may resemble basal cell carcinoma but is composed mainly of baseloid and sebaceous cells.

**sebaceous follicle** [L, *sebum,* sweat, *folliculus,* small bag], a sebaceous gland that opens into a hair follicle.

**sebaceous gland,** one of the many small sacculated organs in the dermis. They are located throughout the body in close association with all types of body hair but are especially abundant in the scalp, face, anus, nose, mouth, and external ear. They are rare in the palms of the hands and the soles of the feet. Each gland consists of a single duct that emerges from a cluster of oval alveoli. The ducts from most sebaceous glands open into the hair follicles, but some open onto the skin surface, as in the labia minora and the free margin of the lips. The sebum secreted by the glands oils the hair and the surrounding skin, helps prevent evaporation of sweat, and aids in the retention of body heat. The sebaceous glands in the nose and face are large and lobulated and often swell with accumulated secretion. Compare **sudoriferous gland.**

**sebaceous horn,** a solid tissue outgrowth from a sebaceous cyst.

**seborrhea** /seb'ərē'ə/ [L, *sebum* + Gk, *rhoia,* flow], any of several common skin conditions in which an overproduction of sebum results in excessive oiliness or dry scales. Also spelled **seborrhoea.** See also **seborrheic blepharitis, seborrheic dermatitis.** —seborrheic /seb′ərē′ik/, *adj.*

**seborrhea capitis** [L, *sebum,* sweat; Gk, *rhoia,* flow; L, *caput,* the head], seborrhea of the scalp. See also **cradle cap.**

**seborrheic** /seb′ərē′ik/ [L, *sebum,* sweat], pertaining to or resembling seborrhea.

**seborrheic blepharitis,** a form of seborrheic dermatitis in which the eyelids are erythematous and the margins are covered with a granular crust.

**seborrheic dermatitis,** a common chronic inflammatory skin disease characterized by dry or moist greasy scales and yellowish crusts. Common sites are the scalp, eyelids, face, external surfaces of the ears, axillae, breasts, groin, and gluteal folds. In acute stages there may be exudate and infection resulting in secondary furunculosis. Occasionally generalized exfoliation results. In some people seborrheic dermatitis is associated with paralysis agitans, diabetes mellitus, malabsorption disorders, epilepsy, or an allergic reaction to gold or arsenic. Treatment includes selenium sulfide shampoos, topical and oral corticosteroids, topical antibiotics, proper therapy for any underlying systemic disorder, and avoidance of sweating and external irritants. Kinds of seborrheic dermatitis include **cradle cap, dandruff,** and **seborrheic blepharitis.**

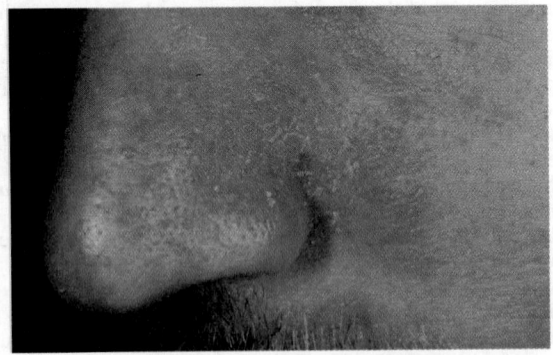

**Seborrheic dermatitis**
*(Huether and McCance, 2000/courtesy Department of Dermatology, School of Medicine, University of Utah)*

**seborrheic keratosis,** a benign, well-circumscribed, slightly raised, tan to black, warty lesion of the skin of the face, neck, chest, or upper back. The macules are loosely covered with a greasy crust that leaves a raw pulpy base when removed. Itching is common. Treatment includes curettage, electrodesiccation, or cryotherapy. Also called **seborrheic wart.**

**seborrhoea.** See **seborrhea.**

**sebum** /sē′bəm/ [L, grease], the oily secretion of the sebaceous glands of the skin, composed of keratin, fat, and cellular debris. Combined with sweat, sebum forms a moist oily acidic film that is mildly antibacterial and antifungal and protects the skin against drying.

**Seckel's syndrome,** a congenital disorder characterized by a proportionate short stature; a proportionately small head with jaw hypoplasia, large eyes, and a beaklike protrusion of the nose; mental retardation; and various other skel-

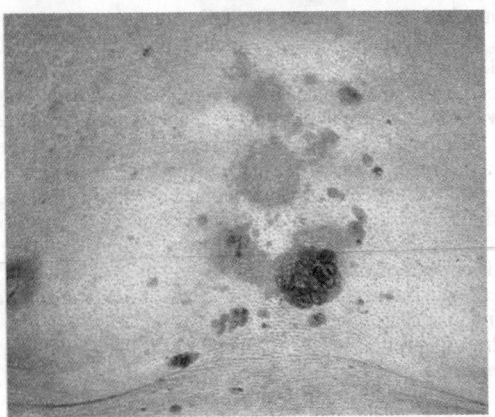

**Seborrheic keratosis** *(Habif, 1996)*

etal, cutaneous, and genital defects. People with the disorder are sometimes referred to as **nanocephalic dwarfs.**

**seclusion**[1] /siklōō′zhən/ [L, *secludere,* to isolate], (in psychiatry) the isolation of a patient in a special room to decrease stimuli that might be causing or exacerbating the patient's emotional distress, free from objects that the patient might use to cause self-harm or to harm others.

**seclusion**[2], a nursing intervention from the Nursing Interventions Classification (NIC) defined as solitary containment in a fully protective environment with close surveillance by nursing staff for purposes of safety or behavior management. See also **Nursing Interventions Classification.**

**secobarbital sodium** /sek′obär′bital/, a sedative and hypnotic. It is classified as a controlled substance.

■ INDICATIONS: It is prescribed in the treatment of insomnia and agitation, and as an anticonvulsant and preoperative sedative.

■ CONTRAINDICATIONS: Impaired liver function or known hypersensitivity to this drug or to any barbiturate prohibits its use.

■ ADVERSE EFFECTS: Among the more serious adverse reactions are central nervous system and respiratory depression, hypersensitivity reactions, and paradoxical excitement. Kidney damage may result from the polyethylene glycol that is used as a diluent in injectable preparations of the drug.

**Seconal Sodium,** trademark for a sedative-hypnotic (secobarbital sodium).

**secondary** /sek′ənder′ē/ [L, *secundus,* second], second in importance or in occurrence or belonging to the second order of sophistication or development, such as a secondary health care facility or secondary education.

**secondary allergen,** an agent that induces allergic symptoms in a person through cross-sensitivity with an agent to which the person is hypersensitive.

**secondary amenorrhea.** See **amenorrhea.**

**secondary amputation,** amputation performed after suppuration has begun after severe trauma. An area is left open for drainage, and antibiotics are given. Compare **primary amputation.**

**secondary amyloidosis.** See **amyloidosis.**

**secondary analysis,** the study of a problem using previously compiled data.

**secondary antibody response,** a rapid production of antibodies in response to an antigen in an individual who was exposed previously to the same antigen. Also called **booster response.**

**secondary apnea,** an abnormal condition in which respiration is absent and will not begin again spontaneously. Resuscitation is initiated immediately with artificial ventilation. Blood gases are analyzed, and oxygen, cardiac massage, and medication specific to the underlying cause may be administered. Secondary apnea may result from any event that severely impedes the absorption of oxygen by the bloodstream. Compare **primary apnea.**

**secondary areola,** a second ring appearing around the areola of the breast during pregnancy that is more pigmented than the areola before pregnancy.

**secondary biliary cirrhosis,** an abnormal hepatic condition characterized by obstruction of the bile duct with or without infection. It involves periportal inflammation with progressive fibrosis, destruction of parenchymal cells, and nodular degeneration. Compare **primary biliary cirrhosis.**

**secondary bronchus.** See **bronchus, primary bronchus.**

**secondary care,** the provision of a specialized medical service by a physician specialist or a hospital on referral by a primary care physician.

**secondary caries.** See **dental caries.**

**secondary dementia,** dementia resulting from another, concurrent form of psychosis. See also **dementia.**

**secondary dental caries,** dental caries developing in a tooth already affected by the condition. Often a new cavity forms adjacent to or beneath the restorative filling of an old cavity. Compare **primary dental caries.**

**secondary dentition,** the set of 32 teeth that appear during and after childhood and usually last until old age. In each jaw they include four incisors, two canines, four premolars, and six molars. The secondary teeth start to develop in the ninth week of fetal life with the thickening of the epithelium along the line of the future jaw. The permanent first molar in the lower jaw calcifies just after birth; the incisors and the canines, approximately 6 months later, the premolars during the second year, the second molar at about the end of the second year, and the third molar at about the twelfth year. The secondary teeth erupt first in the lower jaw, begining with the first molars in about the sixth year and followed by the two central incisors in about the seventh year, the two lateral incisors in about the eighth year, the first premolars in about the ninth year, the second premolars in about the tenth year, the canines between the eleventh and the twelfth years,

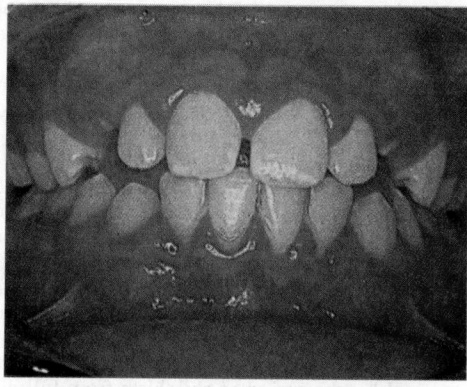

**Early secondary dentition: eruption
of 6-year molars and central incisors**
(Zitelli and Davis, 1997)

the second molars between the twelfth and the thirteenth years, and the third molars between the seventeenth and twenty-fifth years. The eruption of each secondary tooth in the upper jaw lags only slightly behind that of the corresponding tooth in the lower jaw. The third molars in many people are badly oriented or so deeply buried in bone that they must be surgically removed. In some individuals, one or all four of the third molars may not develop completely. Compare **deciduous dentition.** Also called **permanent dentition, permanent teeth, secondary teeth.** See also **tooth.**

**secondary diabetes.** See **iatrogenic diabetes mellitus.**

**secondary disease,** any disorder of bodily functions that follows or results from an earlier injury or medical episode.

**secondary distal RTA.** See **distal renal tubular acidosis.**

**secondary drive.** See **drive.**

**secondary dysmenorrhea.** See **inflammatory dysmenorrhea.**

**secondary enuresis** [L, *secundus,* second; Gk, *enourein,* to urinate], enuresis in an older child who has demonstrated bedtime control for a year or more. It is typically the result of psychologic stress but also may be an early sign of an organic disorder, such as diabetes mellitus.

**secondary fissure,** a fissure between the uvula and the pyramid of the cerebellum.

**secondary fracture.** See **neoplastic fracture.**

**secondary gain,** an indirect benefit, usually obtained through an illness or debility. Such gains may include monetary and disability benefits, personal attention, or escape from unpleasant situations and responsibilities. Compare **primary gain.**

**secondary gangrene** [L, *secundus,* second; Gk, *gaggraina*], a form of gangrene in which putrefaction follows the primary tissue necrosis, generating malodorous and toxic products.

**secondary gestation** [L, *secundus,* second, *gestare,* to bear], a pregnancy in which the ovum becomes displaced from its original site of implantation but continues development at a different location.

**secondary glandular failure,** the deficiency of a hormone secreted by a particular gland or gland atrophy caused by absence of a stimulus from another gland, as when a pituitary disorder results in hypogonadism.

**secondary health care,** an intermediate level of health care that includes diagnosis and treatment, performed in a hospital having specialized equipment and laboratory facilities.

**secondary hemorrhage** [L, *secundus,* second; Gk, *haima,* blood, *rhegnynai,* to burst forth], a hemorrhage that develops 24 hours or more after the original injury or surgery. It is often caused by an infection.

**secondary host.** See **intermediate host.**

**secondary hydrocephalus** [L, *secundus,* second; Gk, *hydor,* water, *kephale,* head], hydrocephalus that develops after an injury or infection, such as syphilis or meningitis.

**secondary hyperaldosteronism,** excessive production of aldosterone caused by an extraadrenal disorder, such as heart failure, kidney disease, cirrhosis, or hypoproteinemia.

**secondary hypertension,** elevated blood pressure associated with any of several primary diseases, such as renal, pulmonary, endocrine, and vascular diseases. Compare **essential hypertension.** See also **hypertension.**

**secondary hypertrophic osteoarthropathy.** See **clubbing.**

**secondary immunodeficiency,** a loss of immunity caused by a disease process or toxic effect of medication, rather than by a failure or defect in T or B lymphocytes.

**secondary infection,** an infection by a microorganism that follows an initial infection by another kind of organism.

**secondary infertility,** infertility occurring in patients who have previously conceived.

**secondary intention.** See **intention.**

**secondary iritis** [L, *secundus,* second; Gk, *iris,* rainbow, *itis,* inflammation], an inflammation of the iris secondary to another disorder, for example ankylosing spondylitis or unceretive colitis.

**secondary lymphoid organ,** a source of effector lymphocytes, such as the spleen, lymph nodes, or tonsils.

**secondary nutrient,** a substance that acts as a stimulant to activate the flora of the GI tract to synthesize other nutrients.

**secondary occlusal traumatism,** occlusal stress that affects previously weakened periodontal structures. The stress may not be excessive for normal tissues but can be damaging to the weakened structures.

**secondary parkinsonism,** a disease of the nervous system caused by degeneration of neurons in the corpus striatum that receive dopaminergic input from the substantia nigra. Unlike idiopathic parkinsonism, the disease does not respond to the administration of levodopa (L-dopa).

**secondary peritonitis** [L, *secundus,* second; Gk, *peri + tenein,* to stretch, *itis,* inflammation], inflammation of the peritoneum caused by the spread of infection from neighboring tissue.

**secondary pneumonia** [L, *secundus,* second; Gk, *pneumon,* lung], pneumonia that develops during the course of another disease, such as diphtheria or tularemia.

**secondary polycythemia** [L, *secundus,* second; Gk, *polys,* many, *kytos,* cell, *haima,* blood], a form of polycythemia that develops as a result of another disorder, such as a pulmonary disease.

**secondary port,** a control device for regulating the flow of a primary and a secondary IV solution. It consists of a Y-shaped plastic apparatus that attaches to the primary IV tubing and allows the primary and secondary IV solutions to flow separately or to flow simultaneously. Compare **piggyback port.**

**secondary prevention,** a level of preventive medicine that focuses on early diagnosis, use of referral services, and rapid initiation of treatment to stop the progress of disease processes or a handicapping disability.

**secondary proximal renal tubular acidosis.** See **proximal renal tubular acidosis.**

**secondary radiation,** radiation that results from the scattering of primary x-rays. Secondary radiation often accounts for fogging of radiographic film.

**secondary relationships,** relationships with those who provide or accept services, or with acquaintances and friends, as distinguished from family members and intimate friends.

**secondary sensation.** See **synesthesia.**

**secondary sequestrum,** a piece of dead bone that partially separates from sound bone during the process of necrosis but may be pushed back into position. Compare **primary sequestrum.**

**secondary sex characteristic,** any of the external physical characteristics of sexual maturity secondary to hormonal stimulation that develops in the maturing individual. These characteristics include adult distribution of hair and development of the penis or breasts and the labia.

**secondary shock,** a state of physical collapse and prostration caused by numerous traumatic and pathologic conditions. It develops over time after severe tissue damage and may merge with primary shock, accompanied by various signs, such as weakness, restlessness, low body temperature,

low blood pressure, cold sweat, and reduced urinary output. Blood pressure drops progressively in this state, and death may occur within a relatively short time after onset unless appropriate treatment intervenes. Secondary shock is often associated with heat stroke, crushing injuries, myocardial infarction, poisoning, fulminating infections, burns, and other life-threatening conditions. The pathologic characteristics of this state reflect changes in the capillaries, which become dilated and engorged with blood. Petechial hemorrhages develop in the serous membranes, edema swells the soft tissues, and the vital organs undergo degenerative changes. Compare **hemorrhagic shock, primary shock.**

**secondary symptom.** See **symptom.**

**secondary syphilis.** See **syphilis.**

**secondary teeth.** See **secondary dentition.**

**secondary thrombocytosis.** See **thrombocytosis.**

**secondary tooth.** See **secondary dentition.**

**second cranial nerve.** See **optic nerve.**

**second cuneiform bone.** See **intermediate cuneiform bone.**

**second filial generation ($F_2$),** the offspring produced by the mating of two members of the $F_1$ generation or, broadly, by the crossing of any two heterozygous strains.

**secondhand smoke,** tobacco smoke from the burning end of a cigarette, cigar, or pipe that is inhaled by nonsmokers. The American Heart Association estimated in 2001 that secondhand smoke was implicated in the deaths of 37,000 to 40,000 nonsmokers each year from heart disease and lung cancer. See also **passive smoking.**

**second-look operation,** a surgical opening of the peritoneal cavity performed within a year after removal of intraabdominal cancer to inspect for and/or resect a hidden tumor.

**second messenger,** a chemical substance inside a cell that carries information farther along the signal pathway from the internal part of a membrane-spanning receptor embedded in the cell membrane. It may be in the form of an enzyme's product or ion fluxes.

**second opinion** [L, *secundus + opinari,* to suppose], a patient privilege of requesting an examination and evaluation of a health condition by a second physician to verify or challenge the diagnosis by a first physician. The situation is most likely to arise when an examination by a first physician results in a recommendation for surgery or experimental treatment.

**second-order change,** a change that alters the system itself.

**second-order kinetics,** a chemical reaction in which the rate of the reaction is determined by the concentration of two chemical reactants involved or the square of the concentration of one chemical reactant. Also called **second-order reaction.** See also **kinetics.**

**second-set rejection,** failure of an organ or tissue graft in a host who is already immune to the histocompatibility antigens of the graft because of a previous graft with the same antigens.

**second sight,** 1. an improvement in near vision that may develop in aging as a result of increasing refractivity of the lens nucleus related to development of a nuclear sclerotic cataract. 2. an early increase in the index of refraction of the lens, resulting in a decrease in hyperopia and an increase in myopia. 3. clairvoyance, precognition. See also **senopia.**

**second stage of labor** [L, *secundus,* second; OFr, *estage +* L, *labor,* work], the period of childbirth from full dilation of the cervix to delivery of the fetus.

**secretagogue** /sikrē′əgog′/, any agent that induces exocrine, endocrine, or paracrine secretion.

**secrete** /sikrēt′/ [L, *secernere,* to separate],   to discharge a substance into a cavity, vessel, or organ or onto the surface of the skin, as by a gland. —**secretion,** *n.*

**secretin** /sikrē′tin/ [L, *secernere,* to separate],   a digestive hormone that is produced by the S cells lining the duodenum and jejunum when protein of partially digested food enters the intestine from the stomach. It stimulates the pancreas to produce a fluid high in salts but low in enzymes. Secretin has a limited stimulating effect on the production of bile. See also **pancreas.**

**secretin test,**   a test of pancreatic function after stimulation with a hormone, secretin. The test measures the volume and bicarbonate concentration of pancreatic secretions. Normal volume findings are 2 to 4 mL/kg body weight $HCO_3$ (bicarbonate): 90 to 130 mEq/L. A lower than normal volume suggests an obstructing malignancy. Reduced bicarbonate and amylase concentration is usually diagnostic of chronic pancreatitis.

**secretion** /sikrē′shən/ [L, *secernere,* to separate],   **1.** the release of chemical substances manufactured by cells of glandular organs. **2.** a substance released or eliminated.

**secretoinhibitory** /sikrē′tō·inhib′itôr′ē/ [L, *secernere,* to separate, *inhibere,* to restrain],   pertaining to a function of inhibiting secretion.

**secretor** /sikrē′tər/,   **1.** a person who releases A, B, or AB blood group antigens into saliva, gastric juice, or other exocrine secretions. **2.** the autosomal dominant allele that determines this trait.

**secretor factor,**   a substance that triggers the release of ABO blood group antigens into exocrine secretions.

**secretory** /sikrē′tərē/ [L, *secernere,* to separate],   pertaining to or contributing to the function of secretion.

**secretory component,**   a glycopeptide that is attached to immunoglobulin A (IgA). It is necessary for the secretion of IgA into mucosal spaces.

**secretory component deficiency,**   a failure of GI epithelial cells to produce secretory component, a glycopeptide occurring in secretory immunoglobulin A (IgA). It causes a lack of IgA in external secretions, such as tears, saliva, and colostrum, although serum IgA is normal.

**secretory cyst.**   See **retention cyst.**

**secretory duct** [L, *secernere*],   (of a gland) a small duct that has a secretory function and joins with an excretory duct.

**secretory IgA,**   a dimer of class A immunoglobulins, the principal agents of mucosal immunity. IgA is the only immunoglobulin isotype that can pass through mucosal membranes to reach the lumen of internal organs.

**secretory immune system,**   the part of the immune system that secretes immunoglobulins, primarily immunoglobulin A, onto mucosal surfaces.

**secretory phase,**   the phase of the menstrual cycle after the release of an ovum from a mature ovarian follicle. The corpus luteum, stimulated by luteinizing hormone (LH), develops from the ruptured follicle. It secretes progesterone, which stimulates the development of the glands and arteries of the endometrium, causing it to become thick and spongy. In a negative-feedback response to the increased level of progesterone in the blood, the secretion of LH from the pituitary decreases. In the absence of an embryo and its secretion of chorionic gonadotropin, the secretory phase ends. The corpus luteum involutes, progesterone levels fall, and menstruation occurs. Also called **luteal phase, progestational phase.** Compare **menstrual phase, proliferative phase.**

**sect-, -sect,**   combining form meaning 'to cut': *section, sector, dissect.*

**section** /sek′shən/ [L, *sectio,* a cutting],   **1.** a cut surface or slice of tissue. **2.** the act of cutting tissue.

**sectional arch wire** /sek′shənəl/ [L, *sectio,* a cutting, *arcus,* bow; AS, *wir*],   a wire attached to only a few teeth, usually on one side of a dental arch or in the anterior segment of the arch, to cause or guide orthodontic tooth movement.

**sectional denture.**   See **partial denture.**

**sectional impression** [L, *sectio,* a cutting + *imprimere,* to press into],   a dental impression that is made in sections.

**sector scan** /sek′tər/,   an ultrasound scan in which the transducer or ultrasound beam is rotated through an angle, and the center of rotation is near or behind the surface of the transducer.

**Sectral,**   trademark for a beta-adrenergic blocking agent (acebutolol).

**secund-,**   combining form meaning 'second, or following': *secundigravida, secundina, secundine.*

**secundigravida** /səkund′dəgrav′idə/ [L, *secundus,* second, *gravidus,* pregnancy],   a woman who is pregnant for the second time. Also called **gravida 2. —secundigravid,** *adj.*

**secundines** /səkun′dīnz/ [L, *secundus*],   the placenta, umbilical cord, and membranes of afterbirth.

**secundipara** /sek′əndip′ərə/ [L, *secundus* + *parere,* to bear],   a woman who has borne two viable children in separate pregnancies.

**security enhancement,**   a nursing intervention from the Nursing Interventions Classification (NIC) defined as intensifying a patient's sense of physical and psychological safety. See also **Nursing Interventions Classification.**

**SED,**   abbreviation for **skin erythema dose.** See **threshold dose.**

**sedation** /sidā′shən/ [L, *sedatio,* soothing],   an induced state of quiet, calmness, or sleep, as by means of a sedative or hypnotic medication.

**sedative** /sed′ətiv/ [L, *sedatio,* soothing],   **1.** pertaining to a substance, procedure, or measure that has a calming effect. **2.** an agent that decreases functional activity, diminishes irritability, and allays excitement. Some sedatives have a general effect on all organs; others principally affect the activities of the heart, stomach, intestines, nerve trunks, respiratory system, or vasomotor system. See also **sedative-hypnotic.**

**sedative bath,**   the immersion of the body in water for a prolonged period, used especially as a calming procedure for agitated patients.

**sedative-hypnotic,**   a drug that reversibly depresses the activity of the central nervous system, used chiefly to induce sleep and to allay anxiety. Barbiturates and many nonbarbiturate sedative-hypnotics with diverse chemical and pharmacologic properties share the ability to depress the activity of all excitable tissue, but the arousal center in the brainstem is especially sensitive to their effects. Various sedative-hypnotics and minor tranquilizers with similar effects are used in the treatment of insomnia, acute convulsive conditions, and anxiety states and in facilitation of the induction of anesthesia. Although sedative-hypnotics have a soporific effect, they may interfere with rapid eye movement sleep associated with dreaming and, when administered to patients with fever, may act paradoxically and cause excitement rather than relaxation. Sedative-hypnotics may interfere with temperature regulation, depress oxygen consumption in various tissues, and produce nausea and skin rashes; in elderly patients they may cause dizziness, confusion, and ataxia. Drugs in this group have a high potential for abuse that often results in physical and psychologic dependence; treatment of dependence involves gradual reduction of the dosage, because abrupt withdrawal frequently causes serious disorders, including convulsions. Acute reactions to an overdose of a sedative-hypnotic may be treated with an emetic, activated charcoal, gastric lavage, and measures to maintain airway patency. Among nonbarbiturate sedative-hypnotics are chloral hydrate, minor tranquilizers (chlordiazepoxide, flurazepam, diazepam), and diphenhydramine. See also **barbiturate.**

**sedentary** /sed′ənter′ē/ [L, *sedentarius,* sitting], pertaining to a condition of inaction, such as work or recreation that can be performed in the sitting posture.

**sedentary living** [L, *sedentarius* + AS, *lif*], a pattern of daily living that requires a minimum amount of physical effort.

**sediment** /sed′imənt/ [L, *sedimentum,* settling], a deposit of relatively insoluble material that settles to the bottom of a container of liquid.

**sedimentation** /sed′iməntā′shən/ [L, *sedimentum,* settling], the deposition of insoluble materials to the bottom of a liquid. The process may be accelerated by centrifugation.

**sedimentation rate (SR)** [L, *sedimentum* + *ratum,* rate], the speed of settling of red blood cells in a vertical glass column of citrated plasma. It is used to monitor inflammatory or malignant disease and to aid in the detection and diagnosis of occult diseases, such as tuberculosis. The test is nonspecific and often unreliable. See also **erythrocyte sedimentation rate.**

**sed. rate,** *informal.* erythrocyte sedimentation rate.

**Seeing Eye dog.** See **guide dog.**

**segment** /seg′mənt/ [L, *segmentum,* piece cut off], a component, part, or part of a structure, such as a lobe of the liver or part of the intestine.

**segmental bronchus** /segmen′təl/ [L, *segmentum,* piece cut off], a secondary bronchus branching from a primary bronchus to a tertiary bronchus.

**segmental fracture,** a bone break in which several large bone fragments separate from the main body of a fractured bone. The ends of the fragments may pierce the skin, as in an open fracture, or may be contained within the skin, as in a closed fracture.

**segmental reflex** [L, *segmentum* + *reflectere,* to bend back], a reflex that involves a pathway through only a single segment of the spinal cord.

**segmental resection,** a surgical procedure in which a part of an organ, gland, or other body part is excised, such as a segmental resection of a part of an ovary performed to diminish the gland's hormonal secretion by decreasing the amount of secretory tissue in the gland.

**segmentation** /seg′məntā′shən/ [L, *segmentum* + *atio,* process], **1.** the division of an animal body into repeating, similar sections, such as somites or metameres. **2.** the division of a zygote into blastomeres; cleavage.

**segmentation cavity.** See **blastocoele.**

**segmentation cell.** See **blastomere.**

**segmentation method,** a technique for filling tooth pulp canals in which a preselected gutta-percha cone is cut into segments. The tip segment is sealed into the apex of a root, and the other segments are usually warmed and condensed against the tip with a plugger. More cone segments are then added until the canal is filled.

**segmentation nucleus,** the nucleus that results from the fusion of male and female pronuclei in a fertilized ovum. Its formation is the final stage in fertilization and initiates the first cleavage of the zygote. Also called **cleavage nucleus.**

**segmented hyalinizing vasculitis** /segmen′tid/, a chronic relapsing inflammatory condition of the blood vessels of the lower legs associated with nodular or purpuric skin lesions that may become ulcerated and leave scars. Also called **livedo vasculitis.**

**segmented neutrophil,** a neutrophil with a filament between the lobes of its nucleus.

**segments of spinal cord.** See **spinal cord.**

**segregation.** See **Mendel's laws.**

**Seitelberger's disease.** See **infantile neuroaxonal dystrophy.**

**seizure** /sē′zhər/ [Fr, *saisir,* to seize], a hyperexcitation of neurons in the brain leading to a sudden, violent involuntary series of contractions of a group of muscles. It may be paroxysmal and episodic, as in a seizure disorder, or transient and acute, as after a head concussion. A seizure may be clonic or tonic; focal, unilateral, or bilateral; generalized or partial. Also called **convulsion.**

**seizure management,** a nursing intervention from the Nursing Interventions Classification (NIC) defined as care of a patient during a seizure and the postictal state. See also **Nursing Interventions Classification.**

**seizure precautions,** a nursing intervention from the Nursing Interventions Classification (NIC) defined as prevention or minimization of potential injuries sustained by a patient with a known seizure disorder. See also **Nursing Interventions Classification.**

**seizure threshold,** the amount of stimulus necessary to produce a convulsive seizure. All humans can have seizures if the provocation is sufficient. Those who have spontaneous convulsions are said to have a "low seizure threshold."

**selection** /silek′shən/ [L, *seligere,* to choose], **1.** the act or product of choosing. **2.** the process by which various factors or mechanisms determine and modify the reproductive ability of individuals with specific genotypes within a population, thus influencing evolutionary change. Kinds of selection are **artificial selection, natural selection,** and **sexual selection.**

**selective absorption.** See **differential absorption.**

**selective abstraction** /silek′tiv/ [L, *seligere,* to choose], a type of cognitive distortion in which focus on one aspect of an event negates all other aspects.

**selective angiography,** a radiographic procedure that allows selective visualization of the aorta, the major arterial systems, or a particular vessel. It is performed after a few milliliters of a radiopaque contrast medium has been injected through a percutaneous catheter. The patient is observed for signs of sensitivity to the contrast medium, including chills, tremor, and shortness of breath. After the procedure the catheter is withdrawn, and pressure is placed on the puncture site to prevent bleeding. Blood pressure is checked every 15 minutes for 2 hours.

**selective estrogen receptor modulator (SERM),** an agent that activates some estrogen receptors but not others, thereby having estrogenlike effects on target tissues without affecting other tissues that have estrogen receptors.

**selective grinding,** any modification of the occlusal forms of the teeth to improve occlusion and tooth function, produced by grinding at selected places.

**selective IgA deficiency,** a familial or acquired disorder characterized by a lack of serum and secretory immunoglobin A (IgA). The IgA-deficient patient may appear normal or asymptomatic and is diagnosed by demonstration of less than 5 mg/dL of IgA in serum. Patients have an increased risk of respiratory, GI, and urogenital infections.

**selective immunoglobulin deficiency,** a condition characterized by inadequate levels of one of the major classes of immunoglobulins.

**selective inattention,** the screening out of unwanted

stimuli, particularly the part of a message the listener does not want to hear.

**selectively permeable.**  See **semipermeable membrane.**

**selective mutism,**  a mental disorder of childhood characterized by continuous refusal to speak in social situations by a child who is able and willing to speak to selected persons.

**selective neuronal necrosis,**  a widespread destruction of neurons caused by hypoxic or ischemic events. Only a fraction of the neurons in a given region are destroyed, selected apparently at random.

**selective serotonin reuptake inhibitor (SSRI),**  an antidepressant drug. Advantages include fewer anticholinergic side effects (dry mouth, blurred vision, urinary retention), decreased drowsiness, and fewer antihistaminic side effects (sedation, weight gain).

**selectivity** /sil′ektiv′itē/ [L, *seligere*],  the capacity factor ratios of two substances measured under identical chromatographic conditions. Also called **chromatographic selectivity, separation factor.**

**selectivity coefficient,**  the degree to which an ion-selective electrode (ISE) responds to a particular ion with respect to a reference ion.

**selenium (Se)** /silē′nē·əm/ [Gk, *selene*, moon],  a metalloid element of the sulfur group. Its atomic number is 34; its atomic mass is 78.96. Selenium occurs mainly in iron, copper, lead, and nickel ores and in the form of metallic selenides. One of the chief commercial sources is the flue dust produced by the burning of pyrites to make sulfuric acid. Selenium occurs as a trace element in foods, and research continues to determine the most effective daily allowances for different age groups. Dietary experts say that the estimated safe, adequate intake of selenium for infants 6 months of age is 0.04 mg, for adults 0.05 to 0.2 mg. Although selenium deficiency can result in liver problems and degeneration of muscles in some animals, in humans its need has not yet been clearly defined. The bright orange insoluble powder selenium sulfide is used externally in the control of seborrheic dermatitis, dandruff, and other forms of dermatosis. Selenium sulfide, used as a lotion, is used in some therapeutic shampoos as 2.5% of selenium sulfide in a detergent vehicle; it is sold without prescription as a 1% detergent suspension in a scented detergent vehicle. Adverse effects may include conjunctivitis if the preparation enters the eyes, increased oiliness or dryness of the hair, and orange tinting of gray hair. The antidandruff effectiveness of selenium sulfide is thought to stem from its antimitotic activity and its residual adherence to the hair after shampooing. Normal skin absorbs very little of the drug, but inflamed or damaged skin absorbs it readily. Selenium is used in the nuclear medicine compound selenomethionine for diagnosing parathyroid tumors. The element is also used as a photoconductive layer of xeroradiographic plates. Burns and dermatitis venenata may result from prolonged skin contact.

**selenium sulfide,**  an antifungal and antiseborrheic. See also **selenium.**

■ INDICATIONS: It is prescribed for dandruff and for seborrheic dermatitis of the scalp.

■ CONTRAINDICATIONS: Acute scalp inflammation or known hypersensitivity to this drug prohibits its use.

■ ADVERSE EFFECTS: Among the more serious adverse reactions are dermatitis after prolonged skin contact and keratitis after accidental conjunctival contact.

**selenoid cells.**  See **crescent bodies.**

**self,** *pl.* **selves** /selvz/ [AS],  **1.** the total essence or being of a person; the individual. **2.** those affective, cognitive, and spiritual qualities that distinguish one person from another;

individuality. **3.** a person's awareness of his or her own being or identity; consciousness; ego. See also **personality.**

**self-acceptance** [AS, *self* + L, *accipere*, to take],  the recognition and acceptance of one's own qualities and limitations.

**self-actualization,**  (in humanistic psychology) the fundamental tendency toward the maximum realization and fulfillment of one's human potential. In Maslow's hierarchy of needs self-actualization is the highest need.

**self-alien.**  See **ego-dystonic.**

**self-alienation.**  See **depersonalization.**

**self-anesthesia,**  the self-administered inhalation anesthesia in which whiffs of anesthetic gas are inhaled from a hand-held breathing device controlled by the patient. This form of anesthesia is most common in England.

**self-antigen.**  See **autoantigen.**

**self-awareness enhancement,**  a nursing intervention from the Nursing Interventions Classification (NIC) defined as assisting a patient to explore and understand his/her thoughts, feelings, motivations, and behaviors. See also **Nursing Interventions Classification.**

**self-breast examination (SBE),**  a procedure in which a woman examines her breasts and their accessory structures for evidence of change that could indicate a malignant process. The SBE is usually performed 1 week to 10 days after the first day of the menstrual cycle, when the breasts are smallest and cyclic nodularity is least apparent. Self-examination is encouraged during all phases of a woman's adult life; a woman who regularly and carefully performs the examination is better able to detect small abnormalities than is a woman who is not familiar with her own breasts. The techniques are similar to those of the examination of the breast as performed in the health assessment or physical examination. Also called **breast self-examination (BSE).** See also **breast examination.**

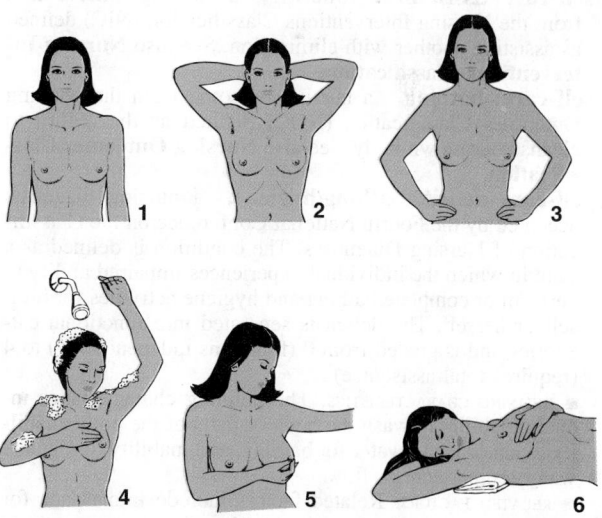

**Self-breast examination** *(Seidel et al, 1999)*

**self-care,**  **1.** the personal and medical care performed by the patient, usually in collaboration with and after instruction by a health professional. The patient's need for assistance and ability to develop a higher level of self-care must be evaluated in forming any nursing care plan. Maximal self-care appropriate to the condition and to the patient is often the ultimate goal of nursing care. Occupational therapy services also help restore, develop, or maintain the skills necessary to permit physically and mentally disabled people to perform the daily living tasks of self-care. **2.** the health care by laypeople of their families, their friends, and themselves, including identification and evaluation of symptoms, medication, and treatment. Self-care is self-limited, voluntary, and wholly outside professional health care systems but may include consultation with a physician or other health care professional as a resource. **3.** personal care accomplished without technical assistance, such as eating, washing, dressing, using the telephone, and attending to one's own elimination, appearance, and hygiene. The goal of rehabilitation medicine is maximal personal self-care.

**self-care: activities of daily living,** a nursing outcome from the Nursing Outcomes Classification (NOC) defined as the ability to perform the most basic physical tasks and personal care activities. See also **Nursing Outcomes Classification.**

**self-care assistance,** a nursing intervention from the Nursing Interventions Classification (NIC) defined as assisting another to perform activities of daily living. See also **Nursing Interventions Classification.**

**self-care assistance: bathing/hygiene,** a nursing intervention from the Nursing Interventions Classification (NIC) defined as assisting patient to perform personal hygiene. See also **Nursing Interventions Classification.**

**self-care assistance: dressing/grooming,** a nursing intervention from the Nursing Interventions Classification (NIC) defined as assisting patient with clothes and makeup. See also **Nursing Interventions Classification.**

**self-care assistance: feeding,** a nursing intervention from the Nursing Interventions Classification (NIC) defined as assisting a person to eat. See also **Nursing Interventions Classification.**

**self-care assistance: toileting,** a nursing intervention from the Nursing Interventions Classification (NIC) defined as assisting another with elimination. See also **Nursing Interventions Classification.**

**self-care: bathing,** a nursing outcome from the Nursing Outcomes Classification (NOC) defined as the ability to cleanse one's own body. See also **Nursing Outcomes Classification.**

**self-care deficit, bathing/hygiene,** a nursing diagnosis accepted by the Fourth National Conference on the Classification of Nursing Diagnoses. The condition is defined as a state in which the individual experiences impaired ability to perform or complete bathing and hygiene activities for himself or herself. The deficit is separated into functional categories and is graded from 0 (functions independently) to 4 (requires total assistance).
■ DEFINING CHARACTERISTICS: The defining characteristics include inability to wash the body or parts of the body, inability to get or get to water for bathing, and inability to regulate water temperature or flow.
■ RELATED FACTORS: Related factors include intolerance for activity caused by decreased strength and endurance, pain or discomfort, perceptual or cognitive impairment, neuromuscular impairment, musculoskeletal impairment, and depression or severe anxiety. See also **nursing diagnosis.**

**self-care deficit, dressing/grooming,** a nursing diagnosis accepted by the Fourth National Conference on the Classification of Nursing Diagnoses. It is defined as a state in which the individual experiences impaired ability to perform or complete dressing and grooming activities for himself or

herself. The deficit is separated into functional categories and is graded from 0 (functions independently) to 4 (requires total assistance).
■ DEFINING CHARACTERISTICS: The defining characteristics include impaired ability to don or to remove necessary items of clothing, to fasten clothing, to obtain or replace articles of clothing, and to maintain a satisfactory appearance.
■ RELATED FACTORS: Related factors include intolerance for activity because of decreased strength or endurance, pain or discomfort, impairment of cognitive or perceptual function, neuromuscular impairment, musculoskeletal impairment, and depression or marked anxiety. See also **nursing diagnosis.**

**self-care deficit, feeding,** a nursing diagnosis accepted by the Fourth National Conference on the Classification of Nursing Diagnoses. The condition is defined as a state in which the individual experiences impaired ability to perform or complete feeding activities for himself or herself. The deficit is separated into functional categories and is graded from 0 (functions independently) to 4 (requires total assistance).
■ DEFINING CHARACTERISTICS: The defining characteristic is an inability to carry food from a receptacle to the mouth.
■ RELATED FACTORS: Related factors include intolerance for activity because of decreased strength or endurance, pain or discomfort, impairment of cognitive or perceptual function, neuromuscular impairment, musculoskeletal impairment, and depression or marked anxiety. See also **nursing diagnosis.**

**self-care deficit, toileting,** a nursing diagnosis accepted by the Fourth National Conference on the Classification of Nursing Diagnoses. The condition is defined as a state in which the individual experiences impaired ability to perform or complete toileting activities for himself or herself. The deficit is separated into functional categories and is graded from 0 (functions independently) to 4 (requires total assistance).
■ DEFINING CHARACTERISTICS: The defining characteristics include inability to get to the toilet or to the commode, to sit down on or to arise from the toilet or commode, to get the necessary clothing on or off, and to perform the proper toilet hygiene. In addition, the person may not be able to flush the toilet or to empty the commode.
■ RELATED FACTORS: Related factors include impaired transfer ability, impaired mobility status, intolerance for activity because of decreased strength or endurance, pain or discomfort, impairment of cognitive or perceptual function, neuromuscular impairment, musculoskeletal impairment, or depression or severe anxiety. See also **nursing diagnosis.**

**self-care: dressing,** a nursing outcome from the Nursing Outcomes Classification (NOC) defined as the ability to dress self. See also **Nursing Outcomes Classification.**

**self-care: feeding,** a nursing outcome from the Nursing Outcomes Classification (NOC) defined as the ability to prepare and ingest food. See also **Nursing Outcomes Classification.**

**self-care: grooming,** a nursing outcome from the Nursing Outcomes Classification (NOC) defined as the ability to maintain kempt appearance. See also **Nursing Outcomes Classification.**

**self-care: hygiene,** a nursing outcome from the Nursing Outcomes Classification (NOC) defined as the ability to maintain one's own hygiene. See also **Nursing Outcomes Classification.**

**self-care: instrumental activities of daily living (IADL),** a nursing outcome from the Nursing Outcomes Classification (NOC) defined as the ability to perform activities needed to function in the home or community. See also **Nursing Outcomes Classification.**

**self-care: non-parenteral medication,** a nursing outcome from the Nursing Outcomes Classification (NOC) defined as the ability to administer oral and topical medications to meet therapeutic goals. See also **Nursing Outcomes Classification.**

**self-care: oral hygiene,** a nursing outcome from the Nursing Outcomes Classification (NOC) defined as the ability to care for one's own mouth and teeth. See also **Nursing Outcomes Classification.**

**self-care: parenteral medication,** a nursing outcome from the Nursing Outcomes Classification (NOC) defined as the ability to administer parenteral medications to meet therapeutic goals. See also **Nursing Outcomes Classification.**

**self-care theory,** a model, central to Dorothea Orem's concept of nursing, used to provide a conceptual framework for nursing care directed to self-care by the client to the greatest degree possible. The model requires an assessment of the client's capability for self-care and need for care. The need for care includes biophysical and psychosocial needs and the specific needs that are the result of the illness. See also **Orem, Dorothea.**

**self-care: toileting,** a nursing outcome from the Nursing Outcomes Classification (NOC) is defined as the ability to toilet self. See also **Nursing Outcomes Classification.**

**self-catheterization,** a procedure performed by a patient to empty the bladder by inserting a catheter into the urethra. The procedure is recommended for patients who cannot empty the bladder completely but can retain urine for 2 to 4 hours at a time and who have some manual dexterity and the ability to palpate the bladder.

■ METHOD: Necessary equipment consists of a pan or toilet, two 14 French catheters, a water-soluble lubricant, soap, water, and a clean washcloth and towel; women usually require a magnifying mirror initially to identify the urethral meatus, and men may prefer to perform the procedure sitting on a low stool rather than on a toilet. Women are taught to perform self-catheterization initially in a semi-Fowler's position, using a pan, but later they generally can carry out the procedure sitting on or standing over a toilet. The patient is instructed to clean the urinary meatus and labia or glans penis with soap and water, to grasp the catheter 3 or 4 inches (7.5 to 10 cm) from the tip, and to lubricate the tip before it is gently inserted into the meatus: Women insert 1-1/2 to 2 inches of the catheter, and men insert 8 inches. Urine is allowed to flow into the pan or toilet until the bladder is empty. The catheter is then removed, washed in soap and water, thoroughly rinsed, dried by rolling it in a clean towel, and placed in a clean plastic or paper bag for the next self-catheterization.

■ INTERVENTIONS: The nurse teaches the procedure and ensures that the patient understands its purpose and the need to perform it at designated times, and the importance of forcing fluids up to 3000 mL daily, unless contraindicated. The nurse makes certain that the patient is able to identify the urinary meatus.

■ OUTCOME CRITERIA: Regular self-catheterization by the patient who cannot empty the bladder allows the person to work and participate in the normal activities of daily living and to prevent kidney infection and other renal disorder.

**self-concept,** the composite of ideas, feelings, and attitudes that a person has about his or her own identity, worth, capabilities, and limitations. Such factors as the values and opinions of others, especially in the formative years of early childhood, play an important part in the development of the self-concept.

**self-confrontation,** a technique for behavior modification that depends on a patient's recognition of and dissatisfaction with inconsistencies in his or her own values, beliefs, and behaviors, or between his or her own personal system and that of a significant other.

**self-conscious, 1.** the state of being aware of oneself as an individual entity that experiences, desires, and acts. **2.** a heightened awareness of oneself and one's actions as reflected by the observations and reactions of others; socially ill at ease. —**self-consciousness,** *n.*

**self-curing resin,** any resin that can be polymerized by the addition of an activator and a catalyst without the use of external heat; used in dental restorations and repairs. Also called **activated resin, autopolymer resin, cold-curing resin, quick-cure resin.**

**self-defeating personality disorder,** a personality characterized by a type of behavior that inhibits the individual from achieving his or her own desires and goals. It is characterized by involvement in situations that continuously lead to failure, rejection, and loss even when other options for involvement are available. Also called **masochistic personality.**

**self-destructive behavior,** any behavior, direct or indirect, that if uninterrupted will ultimately lead to the death of the individual.

**self-diagnosis,** the diagnosis of one's own health problems, usually without direction or assistance from a physician.

**self-differentiation,** specialization and diversification of a tissue or body part resulting solely from intrinsic factors.

**self-direction of care,** a nursing outcome from the Nursing Outcomes Classification (NOC) defined as the directing of others to assist with or perform physical tasks, personal care, and activities needed to function in the home or the community. See also **Nursing Outcomes Classification.**

**self-disclosure,** the process by which one person lets his or her inner being, thoughts, and emotions be known to another. It is important for psychologic growth in individual and group psychotherapy.

**self-esteem[1],** the degree of worth and competence one attributes to oneself. See also **self-concept.**

**self-esteem[2],** a nursing outcome from the Nursing Outcomes Classification (NOC) defined as the personal judgment of self-worth. See also **Nursing Outcomes Classification.**

**self-esteem, chronic low,** a nursing diagnosis accepted by the Eighth National Conference on the Classification of Nursing Diagnoses (revised 1996). Chronic low self-esteem is defined as long-standing negative self-evaluation/feelings about self or capabilities.

■ DEFINING CHARACTERISTICS: The major defining characteristics are long-standing or chronic self-negating verbalization; expressions of shame/guilt; evaluation of self as unable to deal with events; rationalization/rejection of positive feedback and exaggeration of negative feedback about self; and hesitation to try new things/situations. Minor characteristics are frequent lack of success in work or other life events; overly conforming behavior and dependence on others' opinions; lack of eye contact; nonassertive/passive behavior; indecisive behavior; and excessive seeking of reassurance.

■ RELATED FACTORS: Related factors are to be developed. See also **nursing diagnosis.**

**self-esteem disturbance,** a nursing diagnosis accepted by the Eighth National Conference on the Classification of Nursing Diagnoses (revised 1996). It is defined as negative self-evaluation/feelings about the self or self capabilities, which may be directly or indirectly expressed.

■ DEFINING CHARACTERISTICS: The defining characteristics are self-negating verbalization; expressions of shame/guilt; evaluation of self as unable to deal with events; rationalization/rejection of positive feedback and exaggeration of negative feedback about self; hesitation to try new things/situations; denial of problems obvious to others; projection of blame/responsibility for problems; rationalizing about personal failures; hypersensitivity to criticism; and grandiosity.

■ RELATED FACTORS: Related factors are to be developed. See also **nursing diagnosis.**

**self-esteem enhancement,** a nursing intervention from the Nursing Interventions Classification (NIC) defined as assisting a patient to increase his/her personal judgment of self-worth. See also **Nursing Interventions Classification.**

**self-esteem, situational low,** a nursing diagnosis accepted by the Eighth National Conference on the Classification of Nursing Diagnoses (revised 2000). It is defined as the development of a negative perception of self-worth in response to a current situation.

■ DEFINING CHARACTERISTICS: Defining characteristics include verbal reports current situational challenge to self-worth, self-negating verbalizations, indecisive or nonassertive behavior, evaluation of the self as unable to deal with situations or events, and expressions of helplessness or uselessness.

■ RELATED FACTORS: Related factors include developmental changes, disturbed body image, functional impairment, loss, social role changes, lack of recognition or rewards, behavior that is inconsistent with values, and failures or rejections. See also **nursing diagnosis.**

**self-esteem, situational low, risk for,** a nursing diagnosis accepted by the Fourteenth National Conference on the classification of nursing diagnoses. The state is defined as being at risk for developing negative perception of self-worth in response to a current, specific situation.

■ RISK FACTORS: Risk factors include developmental changes; disturbed body image; functional impairment; loss, social role changes; history of learned helplessness; history of abuse, neglect or abandonment; unrealistic self-expectations; behavior that is inconsistent with values; lack of recognition or rewards; failures or rejections; decreased power or control over the environment; and physical illness. See also **nursing diagnosis.**

**self-fulfilling prophecy,** a principle that states that a belief in or the expectation of a particular resolution is a factor that contributes to its fulfillment.

**self-healing squamous epithelioma,** an inherited condition of skin tumors that appear on the head and resolve spontaneously after a few months, leaving deep-pitted scars. The tumors resemble squamous carcinoma or keratoacanthoma.

**self-help group,** a group of people who meet to improve their health through discussion and special activities. Characteristically self-help groups are not led by a professional. Compare **group therapy.**

**self-hypnosis** [AS, *self* + Gk, *hypnos,* sleep], the process of putting oneself into a trancelike state by autosuggestion, such as concentration on a single thought or object. Some subjects are more susceptible than others.

**self-ideal,** a perception of how one should behave based on certain personal standards. The standard may be either a carefully constructed image of the kind of person one would like to be or merely a number of aspirations, goals, or values one would like to achieve. See also **ego ideal.**

**self-image,** the total concept, idea, or mental image one has of oneself and of one's role in society; the person one believes oneself to be.

**self-insurance,** a system whereby hospitals or health professionals may, in lieu of commercial insurance, assume financial responsibility for their liability.

**self-insured.** See **self-insurance.**

**self-limited,** (of a disease or condition) tending to end without treatment.

**self-limited disease** [AS, *self* + L, *limes,* boundary, *dis,* not; Fr, *aise,* ease], a disease restricted in duration by its own pattern of characteristics and not by other influences.

**self-management approach,** a treatment approach in which patients assume responsibility for their behavior, changing their environment, and planning their future.

**self-modification assistance,** a nursing intervention from the Nursing Interventions Classification (NIC) defined as reinforcement of self-directed change initiated by the patient to achieve personally important goals. See also **Nursing Interventions Classification.**

**self-monitoring of blood glucose (SMBG),** the use of a glucose meter to enable a patient to recognize glycemic variations. Most self-monitoring systems use the chemical reaction between glucose oxidase and glucose as a basis for measurement. Some devices depend on hydrogen peroxide, which is a product of the same reaction.

**self-mutilation,** a nursing diagnosis accepted by the Fourteenth National Conference on the classification of nursing diagnoses. The diagnosis is defined as deliberate self-injurious behavior causing tissue damage with the intent of causing nonfatal injury to attain relief of tension.

■ DEFINING CHARACTERISTICS: Defining characteristics include cuts and scratches on the body, picking at wounds, self-inflicted burns, ingestion or inhalation of harmful substances or objects, biting, abrading, severing, insertion of objects into body orifice, hitting, and the constricting of a body part.

■ RELATED FACTORS: Related factors include a psychotic state; inability to express tension verbally; childhood sexual abuse; violence between parental figures; family divorce; family alcoholism; family history of self-destructive behaviors; adolescence; peers who self-mutilate; isolation from peers; perfectionism; substance abuse; eating disorders; sexual identity crisis; low or unstable self-esteem; low or unstable body image; labile behavior; history of inability to plan solutions or see long-term consequences; use of manipulation to obtain nurturing relationships with others; chaotic or disturbed interpersonal relationships; being emotionally disturbed or a battered child; feeling threatened with actual or potential loss of significant relationships; dissociation or depersonalization; an intolerable mounting of tension; impulsivity; inadequate coping; an irresistible urge to cut or damage oneself; need for a quick reduction of stress; childhood illness or surgery; foster, group, or institutional care; incarceration; character disorder; borderline personality disorder; developmentally delayed or autistic individual; history of self-injurious behavior; feelings of depression, rejection, self-hatred, separation anxiety, guilt, or depersonalization; poor parent-adolescent communication; and lack of family confidant. See also **nursing diagnosis.**

**self-mutilation restraint,** a nursing outcome from the Nursing Outcomes Classification (NOC) defined as the ability to refrain from intentional self-inflicted injury (nonlethal). See also **Nursing Outcomes Classification.**

**self-mutilation, risk for,** a nursing diagnosis accepted by the Tenth National Conference on the Classification of Nursing Diagnoses (revised 2000). It is defined as being at risk for deliberate self-injurious behavior causing tissue damage with the intent of causing nonfatal injury to attain relief of tension.

■ RISK FACTORS: Risk factors include a psychotic state; inability to express tension verbally; childhood sexual abuse; violence between parental figures; family divorce; family alcoholism; family history of self-destructive behaviors; adolescence; peers who self-mutilate; isolation from peers; perfectionism; substance abuse; eating disorders; sexual identity crisis; low or unstable self-esteem; low or unstable body image; history of inability to plan solutions or see long-term consequences; use of manipulation to obtain nurturing relationships with others; chaotic or disturbed interpersonal relationships; emotional disturbed and/or battered children; feeling threatened with the actual or potential loss of a significant relationship; loss of parent or parental relationships; experiences dissociation or depersonalization; experiences intolerable mounting tension; impulsivity; inadequate coping; experiences irresistible urge to cut or damage self; need of quick reduction of stress; childhood illness or surgery; foster, group, or institutional care; incarceration; character disorders; borderline personality disorders; loss of control over problem-solving situations; developmentally delayed or autistic individuals; history of self-injurious behavior; and feelings of depression, rejection, self-hatred, separation anxiety, guilt, and depersonalization. See also **nursing diagnosis.**

**self-other,** a concept that characterizes people who believe that the source of power is within the self as opposed to those who believe it is in others. See also **locus of control.**

**self-radiolysis,** a process in which a compound is damaged by radioactive decay products originating in an atom within the compound.

**self-recognition,** the ability of the body's immune system to recognize self-identifying antigens on the body's own cells.

**self-regulation,** a plan for patients to eliminate health risk behaviors. It includes self-monitoring, self-evaluation, and self-reinforcement.

**self-reinforcing adaptation,** (in occupational therapy) a therapeutic technique in which each successful stage of adjustment stimulates the next more complex step.

**self-responsibility,** a concept of holistic health by which individuals assume responsibility for their own health.

**self-responsibility facilitation,** a nursing intervention from the Nursing Interventions Classification (NIC) defined as encouraging a patient to assume more responsibility for own behavior. See also **Nursing Interventions Classification.**

**self-retaining catheter,** an indwelling urinary catheter that has a double lumen. One channel allows urine to drain from the bladder into a collecting bag; the other has a balloon at the bladder end and a diaphragm at the other end. Several centimeters of air or sterile water is injected through the diaphragm to fill the balloon in the bladder and hold the catheter in place. To remove the catheter, the water or air is withdrawn through the diaphragm. See also **Foley catheter.**

**self-stimulation,** a system in which patients control their pain by manipulating an electrical source of nerve stimulation.

**self-system,** the organization of experiences that acts as a protective mechanism against anxiety.

**self-theory,** a personality theory that uses one's self-concept in integrating the function and organization of the personality. See also **humanistic psychology.**

**self-threading pin,** a screwlike pin placed into a hole drilled in tooth dentin to improve the retention of a restoration.

**self-tolerance,** the absence of an immune response directed against a person's own tissue antigens.

**self-transcendence,** the ability to focus attention on doing something for the sake of others, as opposed to self-actualization, in which doing something for oneself is an end goal.

**sella turcica** /sel′ə tur′sikə/ [L, *sella,* seat, *turcica,* Turkish], a transverse depression crossing the midline on the superior surface of the body of the sphenoid bone and containing the pituitary gland.

**Sellick's maneuver.** See **cricoid pressure.**

**Selsun,** trademark for an antifungal and antiseborrheic (selenium sulfide).

**SEM,** abbreviation for **scanning electron microscope.**

**semantics** /siman′tiks/ [Gk, *semantikos,* significant], the study of language with special concern for the meanings of words or other symbols.

**-seme,** combining form meaning '(one) having an orbital (cephalometric) index of less than 84, more than 89, or in between' as specified by the prefix: *megaseme, mesoseme, microseme.*

**semeio-,** combining form meaning 'sign or symptom': *semeiography, semeiology, semeiotic.*

**semen** /sē′mən/ [L, seed], the thick, whitish secretion of the male reproductive organs discharged from the urethra during ejaculation. It contains spermatozoa in their nutrient plasma as well as secretions of the prostate, seminal vesicles, and other glands. Also called **seminal fluid, sperm. —seminal,** *adj.*

**semen analysis,** a fluid analysis that is one of the most important aspects of the fertility workup. This test involves measuring freshly collected semen for volume, counting the sperm, evaluating sperm motility, and studying sperm morphology.

**semi-** /sem′ē-/, prefix meaning 'one half': *semicoma, semisupination, semivalent.*

**semiautomatic external defibrillator** /sem′ē-ô′təmat′ik/, a portable apparatus used to restart a heart that has stopped. It is programmed to analyze cardiac rhythms automatically and indicate to a health professional when to deliver a defibrillating shock.

**semicanal** /-kənal′/, 1. a canal with an opening on one side. 2. a deep groove on the edge of a bone that accommodates part of an adjoining bone.

**semicircular canal** /-sur′kyələr/ [L, *semi-,* half, *circulare,* to go around, *canalis,* channel], any of three bony fluid-filled loops in the osseous labyrinth of the internal ear, associated with the sense of balance. The posterior, superior, and lateral canals, all about 0.8 mm in diameter and perpendicular to each other, open into the cochlea. The posterior canal is the longest.

**semicircular duct,** one of three ducts that make up the membranous labyrinth of the inner ear. See also **membranous labyrinth.**

**semicoma.** See **coma.**

**semicomatose** /-kō′mətōs/ [L, *semi,* half; Gk, *koma,* deep sleep], pertaining to a condition of stupor from which a patient can be aroused. See also **coma, Glasgow Coma Scale.**

**semiconductor** /-kənduk′tər/, a solid crystalline substance whose electrical conductivity is intermediate between that of a conductor and that of an insulator. An **n-type semiconductor** has loosely bound electrons that are relatively free to move about inside the material. A **p-type semiconductor** is one with holes, or positive traps, in which electrons may be bound. The holes may appear to migrate through the material.

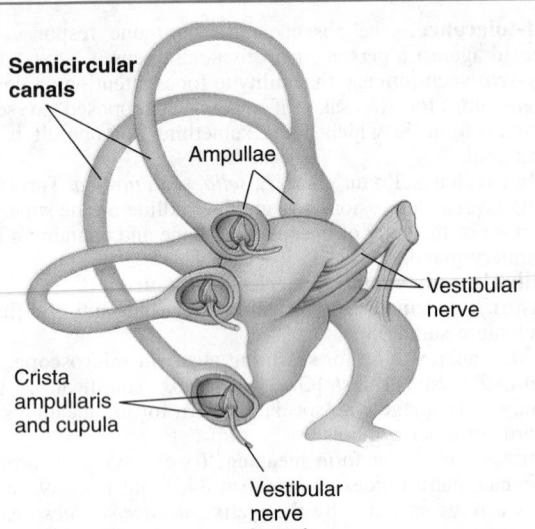

**Semicircular canals** *(Thibodeau and Patton, 1999)*

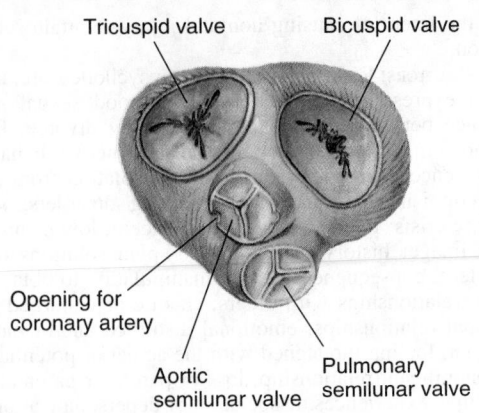

**Semilunar valves** *(Applegate, 2000)*

bers from the fifth lumbar and the first two sacral nerves. The muscle functions to flex the leg, to rotate it medially after flexion, and to extend the thigh. Compare **biceps femoris, hamstring muscle, semitendinosus.**

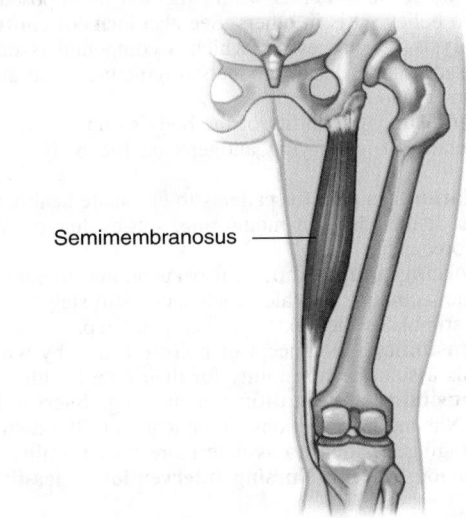

**Semimembranosus**

**semiconscious** /-kon′shəs/, an impaired state of consciousness, characterized by obtundation, stupor, or hypersomnia, from which a patient can be aroused only by energetic stimulation.

**semiflexion** /-flek′shən/, a limb position midway between full flexion and full extension.

**semi-Fowler's position** /-fou′lərz/ [L, *semi,* half; George R. Fowler, American surgeon, 1848–1906], placement of the patient in an inclined position, with the upper half of the body raised by elevating the head of the bed approximately 30 degrees.

**semihorizontal heart** /-hôr′əzon′təl/, an electrical "position" of the heart that lies between the horizontal and intermediate positions when the QRS axis is 0 degrees.

**Semilente,** trademark for a rapid-acting insulin. See **short-acting insulin.**

**semilunar bone.** See **lunate bone.**

**semilunar fold of the conjunctiva,** a fold of membrane that extends laterally from the lacrimal caruncle. It has a concave free border directed to the cornea. In some individuals it contains smooth muscular fibers. Also called **plica semilunaris conjunctivae.**

**semilunar valve** /-loo̅′nər/ [L, *semi* + *luna,* moon, *valva,* folding door], **1.** a valve with half-moon-shaped cusps, such as the aortic valve and the pulmonary valve. **2.** any one of the cusps constituting such a valve. **3.** simple cuplike valves found in the venous and lymphatic vessels. See also **heart valve, mitral valve, tricuspid valve.**

**semimembranosus** /-mem′brənō̅′səs/ [L, *semi* + *membrana,* membrane], one of three posterior femoral muscles. Situated at the back and medial side of the thigh, it originates in a thick tendon attached to the tuberosity of the ischium and inserts into the horizontal groove on the medial condyle of the tibia. The tendon of insertion passes some fibers laterally and upward to insert on the lateral condyle of the femur and form part of the oblique popliteal ligament behind the knee. The tendon of insertion forms one of the two medial hamstrings. The muscle is innervated by several branches of the tibial part of the sciatic nerve, containing fi-

**semimembranous** /-mem′brənəs/ [L, *semi,* half, *membrana*], pertaining to a muscle or other tissue that is partly membrane or fascia, such as the semimembranous hamstring muscle.

**seminal.** See **semen.**

**seminal duct** /sem′inəl/ [L, *semen,* seed, *ducere,* to lead], any duct through which semen passes, such as the vas deferens or the ejaculatory duct.

**seminal emission** [L, *semen,* seed, *emittere,* to send out], a discharge of semen.

**seminal fluid.** See **semen.**

**seminal fluid test,** any of several tests of semen to detect abnormalities in a male's reproductive system and to determine fertility. Some common factors considered are seminal fluid liquefaction time and spermatic quantity, morphologic characteristics, motility, volume, and pH. Normal values in some of these tests are as follows: sperm count, 60 million to 150 million/mL of seminal fluid; pH, more than 7 (7.7 average); ejaculation volume, 1.5 to 5.0 mL; motility, 60% of sperm.

**seminal vesicle,** either of the paired saclike glandular structures posterolateral to the urinary bladder in the male and functioning as part of the reproductive system. Each sac is pyramidal in shape and convoluted in appearance and at the anterior extremity becomes constricted into a narrow straight duct that joins the vas deferens to form the ejaculatory duct. The seminal vesicles produce a fluid that is added to the secretion of the testes and other glands to form the semen.

**seminal vesiculitis,** inflammation of a seminal vesicle.

**semination** /sem′ĭnā′shən/, the introduction of semen into the female genital tract.

**seminiferous** /sem′inif′ərəs/ [L, *semen + ferre,* to bear], transporting or producing semen, such as the tubules of the testis.

**seminiferous tubules** [L, *semen,* seed, *ferre,* to bear, *tubulus*], long, threadlike tubes packed in areolar tissue in the lobes of the testes.

**seminoma** /sem′inō′mə/, *pl.* **seminomas, seminomata** [L, *semen + oma,* tumor], a malignant tumor of the testis. It is the most common testicular tumor and is believed to arise from the seminiferous epithelium of the mature or maturing testis. The two types are classic, or typical, and spermatocytic; anaplastic seminoma is a variant of the classic type. Compare **dysgerminoma.**

**semipermeable membrane** [L, *semi + permeare,* to pass through], a membrane that prevents the passage of some substances but allows the passage of others based on differences in the size, charge, or lipid-solubility of the substances.

**semiprone** /-prōn′/ [L, *semi,* half, *pronus,* leaning forward], lying on one's side, with the thigh on the upper side flexed against the abdomen, and the arm on the lower side extended back. See also **Sims' position.**

**semiprone side position.** See Sims' position.

**semirecumbent** /-rikum′bənt/, in a reclining position.

**semisupine** /-səpīn′/, pertaining to a posture that is between a midposition and the supine position.

**semisynthetic** /-sinthet′ik/ [L, *semi,* half; Gk, *synthesis,* putting together], pertaining to a natural substance that has been partially altered by chemical manipulation.

**semitendinosus** /sem′iten′dinō′səs/ [L, *semi + tendere,* to stretch], one of three posterior femoral muscles of the thigh, remarkable for the great length of the tendon of insertion. It is a fusiform muscle located in the posterior and medial part of the thigh, arising from the tuberosity of the ischium. It ends just distal to the middle of the thigh in a long round tendon that crosses the semitendinosus and curves around the medial condyle of the tibia and inserts into the medial surface of the tibia. It functions to flex the leg, to rotate it medially after flexion, and to extend the thigh. Compare **biceps femoris, hamstring muscle, semimembranosus.**

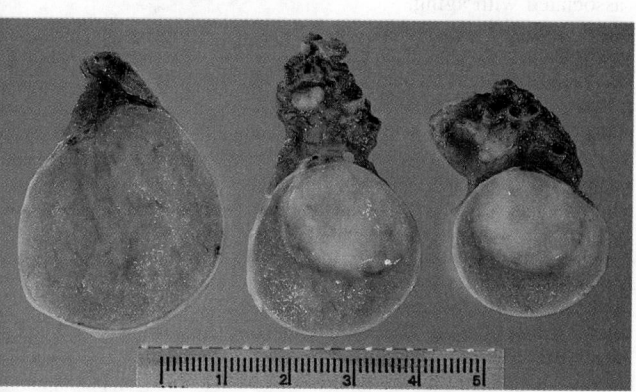

**Seminoma** *(Kumar, Cotran, and Robbins, 1997)*

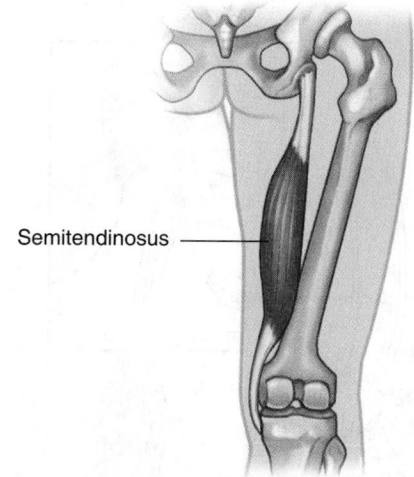

**Semitendinosus**

**semiparametric statistics** /sem′ē·par′ə·met′rik/ [L, *semi,* half + Gk, *para,* to, at, or from the side of + *metron,* measure], statistical methodology that combines both parametric and nonparametric elements; used for estimating population parameters when a function is unknown, e.g. the distribution function of a random variable that has not been observed.

**semipermeable** /-pur′mē·əbəl/ [L, *semi,* half, *permeare,* to pass through], pertaining to a membrane that allows the passage of some molecules but prevents the passage of others. Also **selectively permeable.**

**semivertical heart** /-vur′tikəl/, an electrical "position" of the heart that lies between the intermediate and vertical positions when the QRS axis is 60 degrees.

**Semprex-D,** trademark for a fixed combination drug containing an antihistamine and a decongestent (acrivastine with pseudoephedrine hydrochloride).

**semustine** /səmus′tēn/, an antineoplastic.

■ INDICATIONS: It is prescribed in the treatment of Lewis lung carcinoma, brain tumors, malignant melanoma, and Hodgkin's disease.

■ CONTRAINDICATIONS: Acute myelosuppression or known hypersensitivity to this drug prohibits its use. It is not given to pregnant or lactating women.

■ ADVERSE EFFECTS: Among the more serious adverse reactions are delayed bone marrow depression and thrombocytopenia.

**sender** [AS, *sendan,* to send], (in communication theory) the person by whom a message is encoded and sent.

**seneciosis** /senes′ē·ō′sis/, a toxic reaction to the ingestion of plants of the genus *Senecio,* which are used to make bush tea. The poison causes liver damage, particularly in malnourished patients. Common *Senecio* species include ragwort and life root, both used in herbal remedies.

**senescence** /sənes′əns/ [L, *senescere,* to grow old], the state of growing old.

**senescent** /sənes′ənt/ [L, *senescere,* to grow old], aging or growing old. See also **senile. —senescence,** *n.*

**senescent cell antigen,** an antigen that appears on old red blood cells that bind immunoglobulin G autoantibodies. It is also found on lymphocytes, platelets, and neutrophils.

**Sengstaken-Blakemore tube** [Robert W. Sengstaken, American neurosurgeon, b. 1923; Arthur H. Blakemore, American surgeon, 1897–1970], a thick catheter having a triple lumen and two balloons, used to produce pressure by balloon tamponade to arrest hemorrhaging from esophageal varices. Attached to a tube, one balloon is inflated in the stomach and exerts pressure against the upper orifice. Similarly attached, another longer and narrower balloon exerts

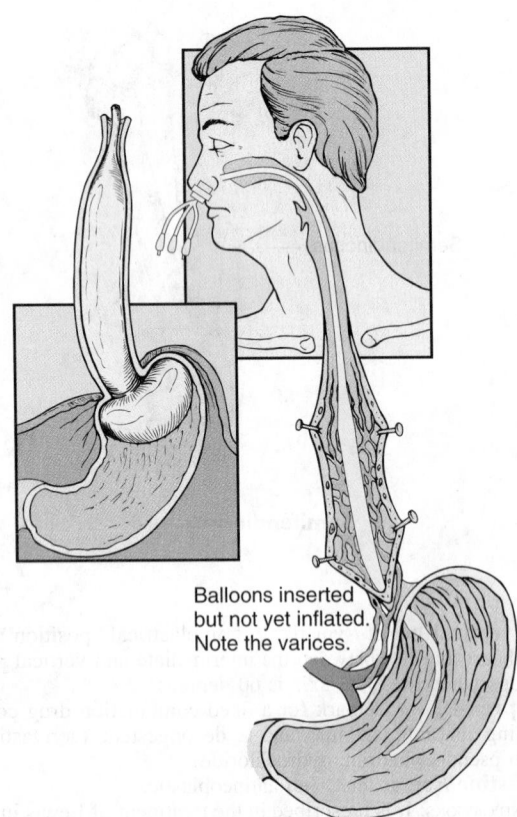

Balloons inserted but not yet inflated. Note the varices.

**Sengstaken-Blakemore tube**
*(Lewis, Collier, and Heitkemper, 2000)*

pressure on the walls of the esophagus. The third tube is used for withdrawing gastric contents.

**senile** /sē′nīl/ [L, *senilis,* aged], pertaining to or characteristic of old age or the process of aging. See also **aging. —senility,** *n.*

**senile angioma.** See **cherry angioma.**

**senile arteriosclerosis,** hardening of the arteries associated with aging.

**senile cataract,** a kind of cataract, associated with aging, in which an opacity forms in the lens of the eye. See also **cataract.**

**senile dementia.** dementia occurring in older persons, usually over the age of 65. Since most cases are due to Alzheimer's disease, the term is sometimes used as a synonym of *dementia of the Alzheimer type, late onset.*

**senile dementia–Alzheimer type. 1.** dementia occurring in older persons, usually over the age of 65, resulting from Alzheimer's disease. **2.** See **senile dementia.**

**senile dental caries,** tooth decay occurring in a person of advanced age. It is usually characterized by cavity formation in or around the cementum layer and root surfaces. See also **dental caries.**

**senile involution,** a pattern of retrograde changes occurring with advancing age and resulting in the progressive shrinking and degeneration of tissues and organs.

**senile keratosis.** See **actinic keratosis.**

**senile nanism,** dwarfism associated with progeria.

**senile psychosis,** a chronic progressive dementia associated with brain atrophy of unknown cause. Symptoms include impaired memory, impaired judgment, decreased moral and aesthetic values, inability to think abstractly, and periods of confusion, confabulation, and irritability, all of which may range from mild to severe.

**senile tremor** [L, *senilis,* aged, *tremor,* shaking], a tremor associated with aging.

**senile vaginitis** [L, *senilis,* aged, *vagina,* sheath, *itis,* inflammation], a condition of atrophy of the vagina resulting from the postmenopausal loss of estrogen secretion.

**senile wart.** See **actinic keratosis.**

**senility** /sinil′itē/ [L, *senilis,* aged], the general state of reduced mental and physical vigor associated with aging.

**senior centers** /sē′nyər/, community agencies for older adults. The centers offer nutritional, recreational, educational, health, and legal services.

**Senior Companion Program,** a service that offers personal assistance and peer support to low-income, homebound, and chronically ill older people.

**senior patient,** (in the United States) a Medicare beneficiary enrolled in a health maintenance organization.

**senna** an herbal product taken from several *Cassia* species, found across the world.

■ USES: This herb is used as a laxative.

■ CONTRAINDICATIONS: Senna should not be used during pregnancy and lactation, in children less than 12 years of age (unless prescribed by physician), or in those with known hypersensitivity to this product. Senna is also prohibited in those with intestinal obstruction, ulcerative colitis, GI bleeding, appendicitis, acute surgical abdomen, nausea, vomiting, and congestive heart failure.

**Sennetsu fever** /sə·net′sōō/, a febrile disease occurring in Japan and Malaysia and caused by the bacterium *Ehrlichia sennetsu;* symptoms include headache, nausea or vomiting, lymphocytosis, and postauricular and posterior lymphadenopathy.

**senopia** /senō′pē·ə/ [L, *senex,* old man, *opsis,* vision], an improvement in the near vision of the aged caused by the myopia associated with increasing lenticular nuclear sclerosis. This type of sclerosis commonly leads to the development of nuclear cataracts. Also called **genontopia, second sight.**

**sens-,** combining form meaning 'perception or feeling': *sensation, sensimeter, sensitinogen.*

**sensate** /sen'sāt/, capable of perceiving sensory stimuli.

**sensate focus technique,** a therapeutic program for the treatment of erectile dysfunction in males.

**sensation** /sensā'shən/ [L, *sentire*, to feel], **1.** a feeling, impression, or awareness of a body state or condition that results from the stimulation of a sensory receptor site and transmission of the nerve impulse along an afferent fiber to the brain. Kinds of sensation include **delayed sensation, epigastric sensation, primary sensation, referred sensation,** and **subjective sensation. 2.** a feeling or an awareness of a mental or emotional state, which may or may not result in response to an external stimulus.

**sense** [L, *sentire*, to feel], **1.** the faculty by which stimuli are perceived and conditions outside and within the body are distinguished and evaluated. The major senses are sight, hearing, smell, taste, touch, and pressure. Other senses include hunger, thirst, pain, temperature, proprioception, and spatial, temporal, and visceral sensations. **2.** the ability to feel; a sensation. **3.** the capacity to understand; normal mental ability. **4.** to perceive through a sense organ. **5.** pertaining to the sense strand of a nucleic acid; compare *antisense.*

**sense strand,** the strand of a double-stranded nucleic acid that encodes the product; in DNA it is the strand that encodes the RNA, having thus the same base sequence except changing T for U in the RNA. Compare **antisense strand.** Also called **coding strand.**

**sensibility** /sen'sibil'itē/, the ability to perceive sensations and impressions, both physical and psychologic.

**sensible** /sen'sibəl/, **1.** capable of sensation. **2.** possessing reason or judgment. **3.** capable of being perceived.

**sensible perspiration** [L, *sensibilis,* perceptible], loss of body fluid through the secretory activity of the sweat glands in a quantity sufficient to be observed. Compare **insensible perspiration.**

**sensitive** /sen'sitiv/ [L, *sentire,* to feel], **1.** able to perceive and transmit a sensation or stimulus. **2.** affected by low concentrations of antimicrobial drugs, said of microorganisms. **3.** abnormally susceptible to a subject, such as a drug or foreign protein.

**sensitive volume** [L, *sentire + volumen,* paper roll], the part of an object from which a magnetic resonance signal is preferentially acquired because of strong magnetic field inhomogeneity elsewhere. This preferential acquisition can be enhanced by the use of a shaped radiofrequency field that is strongest in the sensitive volume.

**sensitivity** /sen'sitiv'itē/ [L, *sentire*], **1.** capacity to feel, transmit, or react to a stimulus. **2.** susceptibility to a substance, such as a drug or an antigen. See also **allergy, hypersensitivity. 3.** the lowest level of a substance that can be detected by a laboratory test procedure. —**sensitive, diagnostic sensitivity,** *adj.*

**sensitivity test,** a laboratory method for testing the effectiveness of antibiotics. It is usually done on organisms known to be potentially resistant to antibiotic therapy in vitro. A report of a "resistant" finding means the antibiotic is not effective in inhibiting the growth of a pathogen, whereas use of an effective antibiotic results in a "sensitive" report. See also **antibiotic sensitivity test.**

**sensitivity training group,** a group that offers members a supportive atmosphere in which to experiment with and alter behavior patterns and interpersonal reactions. Sensitivity training focuses on learning what occurs during group interactions, testing and refining new behavioral responses in light of the reactions they evoke, and applying those responses to situations outside the group setting. Also called **T group.** See also **encounter group, psychotherapy.**

**sensitization** /sen'sitīzā'shən/ [L, *sentire* + Gk, *izein,* to cause], **1.** reaction in which specific antibodies develop in response to an antigen. Allergic reactions result from excess sensitization to a foreign protein. Sensitization can be induced by immunization, in which a pathogen that has been made noninfectious is introduced into the body. **2.** a photodynamic method of destroying microorganisms through the use of substances, such as fluorescent dyes, that absorb light and emit energy at wavelengths destructive to the organisms. **3.** *nontechnical.* anaphylaxis. —**sensitize,** *v.*

**sensitized** /sen'sitīzd/, pertaining to tissues that have been made reactive to antigens. See also **allergy.**

**sensitized vaccine** [L, *sentire,* to feel, *vaccinus,* of a cow], a vaccine that is prepared by suspending microorganisms in their own homologous immune serum.

**sensitometric curve.** See **characteristic curve.**

**sensor** /sen'sər/, an apparatus designed to react to physical stimuli, such as temperature, light, or movement.

**sensoriglandular** /sen'sərəglan'dyələr/, pertaining to the reflexive secretion by glands triggered by sensory stimulation of a nerve.

**sensorimotor** /sen'sərēmō'tər/ [L, *sentire,* to feel, *moveo,* to move], pertaining to both sensory and motor nerve functions.

**sensorimotor phase** [L, *sentire + moveo,* to move], the developmental phase of childhood, encompassing the period from birth to 2 years of age, according to piagetian psychology.

**sensorimotor therapy,** therapy designed to enhance the integration of reflex phenomena and the emergence of voluntary motor behaviors concerned with posture and locomotion.

**sensorimuscular** /-mus'kyələr/, pertaining to contraction of muscles triggered by sensory stimulation.

**sensorineural** /sen'sərēnoor'əl/ [L, *sentire,* to feel; Gk, *neuron,* nerve], pertaining to sensory nerves.

**sensorineural hearing loss,** a form of hearing loss in which sound is conducted normally through the external and middle ear but a defect in the inner ear or auditory nerve results in hearing loss. Sound discrimination may or may not be affected. Amplification of the sound with a hearing aid will help many people with sensorineural hearing loss; if a person demonstrates an intolerance to loud noises, the hearing aid must be adjusted properly to prevent discomfort. Compare **conductive hearing loss.**

**sensorium** /sensôr'ē·əm/, (in psychology) the part of the consciousness that includes the special sensory perceptive powers and their central correlation and integration in the brain. A clear sensorium conveys the presence of a reasonably accurate memory together with a correct orientation for time, place, and person. Sensorium may be clouded in certain stages of delirium.

**sensorivasomotor** /-vā'zōmō'tər/, pertaining to the contraction or dilation of a blood vessel in response to a sensory stimulus.

**sensory** /sen'sərē/ [L, *sentire* to feel], **1.** pertaining to sensation. **2.** pertaining to a part or all of the body's sensory nerve network.

**sensory apraxia.** See **ideational apraxia.**

**sensory area** [L, *sentire,* to feel, *area,* space], the regions of the cerebral cortex that receive impulses from sensory nerves, including thalamic, nucleic, and parietal lobes.

**sensory-based language,** the use of nonverbal behavior in neurolinguistic communication. Examples include puzzled expressions, scowling, and finger pointing.

**sensory deficit,** a defect in the function of one or more of the senses.

**sensory deprivation** [L, *sentire* + ME, *depriven,* to deprive; L, *atio,* process], an involuntary loss of physical awareness caused by detachment from external sensory stimuli. Such deprivation often results in psychologic disorders, such as panic, mental confusion, depression, and hallucinations. Sensory deprivation may be associated with various handicaps and conditions, such as blindness, heavy sedation, and prolonged isolation.

**sensory end organ** [L, *sentire,* to feel; AS, *ende* + Gk, *organon,* instrument], any of the specialized nerve endings devoted to detection of specific environmental stimuli, such as smell, sight, hearing, temperature, or touch.

**sensory function: cutaneous,** a nursing outcome from the Nursing Outcomes Classification (NOC) defined as the extent to which stimulation of the skin is sensed in an impaired area. See also **Nursing Outcomes Classification.**

**sensory function: hearing,** a nursing outcome from the Nursing Outcomes Classification (NOC) defined as the extent to which sounds are sensed, with or without assistive devices. See also **Nursing Outcomes Classification.**

**sensory function: proprioception,** a nursing outcome from the Nursing Outcomes Classification (NOC) defined as the extent to which position and movement of the head and body are sensed. See also **Nursing Outcomes Classification.**

**sensory function: taste and smell,** a nursing outcome from the Nursing Outcomes Classification (NOC) defined as the extent to which chemicals inhaled or dissolved in saliva are sensed. See also **Nursing Outcomes Classification.**

**sensory function: vision,** a nursing outcome from the Nursing Outcomes Classification (NOC) defined as the extent to which visual images are sensed, with or without assistive devices. See also **Nursing Outcomes Classification.**

**sensory integration,** the organization of sensory input for use, a perception of the body or environment, an adaptive response, a learning process, or the development of some neural function.

**sensory integrative dysfunction,** a disorder or irregularity in brain function that makes sensory integration difficult. Many, but not all, learning disorders stem from sensory integrative dysfunctions.

**sensory integrative therapy,** therapy that involves sensory stimulation and adaptive responses to it according to a child's neurologic needs. Treatment usually involves full body movements that provide vestibular, proprioceptive, and tactile stimulation. It usually does not include desk activities, speech training, reading lessons, or training in specific perceptual or motor skills. The goal is to improve the brain's ability to process and organize sensations.

**sensory nerve,** a nerve consisting of afferent fibers that conduct sensory impulses from the periphery of the body to the brain or spinal cord via the dorsal spinal roots.

**sensory neuropathy,** neuropathy or polyneuropathy of sensory nerves.

**sensory nucleus of trigeminal nerve,** a collection of nerve cells in the pons that serve as the main nucleus for reception of tactile fibers of the trigeminal area.

**sensory overload,** a condition in which the central nervous system receives much more auditory, visual, or other environmental stimuli per time frame than it can process effectively.

**sensory pathway** [L, *sentire,* to feel; AS, *paeth* + *weg*], the route followed by a sensory nerve impulse from an end organ to a reflex center in the brain or spinal cord.

**sensory perception, disturbed (visual, auditory, kinesthetic, gustatory, tactile, olfactory)** /pərsep′choo·əl/, a nursing diagnosis accepted by the Fourth National Conference on the Classification of Nursing Diagnoses. It is defined as a state in which an individual experiences a change in the amount or patterning of incoming stimuli accompanied by a diminished, exaggerated, distorted, or impaired response to such stimuli.

■ DEFINING CHARACTERISTICS: The defining characteristics include disorientation; change in the ability to abstract, conceptualize, or solve problems; change in behavior and in sensory acuity; restlessness; irritability; inappropriate response to stimuli; lack of concentration; rapid mood changes; exaggerated emotional responses; noncompliance; motor incoordination; and hallucination. Other possible defining characteristics are complaints of fatigue, changes in posture and muscular tension, inappropriate responses, and hallucinations.

■ RELATED FACTORS: Related factors include excessive or insufficient environmental stimulation, involving therapeutic restrictions, such as isolation, intensive care, or traction; those socially related, such as institutionalization, aging, mental illness, or mental retardation; changes in the reception, transmission, or integration of stimuli, because of neurologic disease or trauma, altered status of the sense organs, the inability to communicate, sleep deprivation, or pain; endogenous or exogenous chemical alteration in the perception of stimuli; or psychologic stress or disturbance. See also **nursing diagnosis.**

**sensory-perceptual overload.** See **sensory overload, sensory/perceptual alterations.**

**sensory receptor** [L, *sentire,* to feel, *recipere,* to receive], a specialized nerve ending that, when stimulated, initiates an afferent or sensory nerve impulse.

**sensory root** [L, *sentire,* to feel], the proximal end of a dorsal afferent nerve as it is attached to the spinal cord.

**sensory threshold** [L, *sentire,* to feel; AS, *therscold*], the point at which increasing stimuli trigger the start of an afferent nerve impulse. Absolute threshold is the lowest point at which response to a stimulus can be perceived.

**sensual** /sen′shoo·əl/ [L, *sensualis*], pertaining to a great interest in sex, food, or other sense satisfying topics.

**sentient** /sen′shənt/ [L, *sentire,* to feel], possessing sensitivity or powers of sensation and perception.

**sentinel gland** /sen′tinəl/ [Fr, *sentinelle* + L, *glans,* acorn], a node or growth that is associated with the presence of a nearby tumor or ulcer. An example is a supraclavicular node with cancer cells that have metastasized from an undiscovered primary cancer.

**sentinel node.** See **Virchow's node.**

**Seoul virus** /sōl/, a virus of the genus *Hantavirus* that causes mild to moderately severe epidemic hemorrhagic fever. Several species of rats are the natural hosts. See also **epidemic hemorrhagic fever.**

**SEP,** abbreviation for **somatosensory evoked potential.**

**separating spring** /sep′ə·rāt·ing/ [L, *separare,* to separate; AS, *springan,* to jump], one placed between the teeth to obtain separation.

**separating wire,** a brass wire threaded between two teeth having tight contact in an effort to wedge them slightly apart before fitting a band in the application of an orthodontic appliance.

**separation agent** /sep′ərā′shən/, a reagent used to separate bound and free tracers in radioassay.

**separation anxiety** [L, *separare,* to separate, *atio,* process], fear and apprehension caused by separation from familiar surroundings and significant people. The syndrome occurs commonly in an infant separated from its mother or mothering figure or approached by a stranger. In a separation crisis the child goes through three distinct states. The protest stage is marked by loud cries, which can last for several days and during which the child is inconsolable. In the second phase the child stops crying and becomes depressed, as a result of increasing hopelessness, grief, and mourning. The third stage is one of detachment or denial in which the child outwardly appears to have adjusted.

**separation factor.**   See **selectivity.**

**separator** /sep′ə·rā·tər/ [L, *separare*, to separate],   **1.** a device for separating one thing from another. **2.** a device or instrument for wedging teeth apart, especially proximal teeth having a tight contact, as for the examination of proximal surfaces, finishing a restoration, or before banding in orthodontic therapy. Also called **space maintainer.**

**s-EPO,**   abbreviation for *serum erythropoietin.*

**seps-,**   prefix meaning 'decay': *sepsin, sepsis, sepsometer.*

**sepsis** /sep′sis/ [Gk, *sepein*, to become putrid],   infection, contamination. Compare **asepsis.** —**septic,** *adj.*

**-sepsis,**   suffix meaning 'decay caused by a (specified) cause or of a (specified) sort': *colisepsis, endosepsis, typhosepsis.*

**sept-,**   **1.** prefix meaning 'nasal septum': *septectomy, septometer, septotomy.* **2.** prefix meaning 'seven': *septigravida, septipara, septivalent.*

**septa.**   See **septum.**

**septal** /sep′təl/ [L, *saeptum*, enclosure],   pertaining to a septum.

**septal cartilage.**   See **nasal cartilage.**

**septal defect** [L, *saeptum*, fence, *defectus*, failure],   a defect in the wall separating the left and right sides of the heart. Depending on the size and the site of the defect, various amounts of oxygenated and deoxygenated blood mix, causing a decrease in the amount of oxygen carried in the blood to the peripheral tissues. The defect is usually congenital. Kinds of septal defects are **atrial septal defect** and **ventricular septal defect.**

**septate** /sep′tāt/,   pertaining to a structure divided by a septum.

**septi-**   prefix meaning 'seven.'

**septic** /sep′tik/ [Gk, *septikos*, putrid],   pertaining to an infection with pyogenic microorganisms.

**-septic,**   suffix meaning 'decay of a sort or associated with a (specified) cause': *aseptic, colyseptic, uroseptic.*

**septic abortion** [Gk, *septikos*, putrid],   spontaneous or induced termination of a pregnancy in which the mother's life may be threatened because of the invasion of germs into the endometrium, myometrium, and beyond. The woman requires immediate and intensive care, massive antibiotic therapy, evacuation of the uterus, and often emergency hysterectomy to prevent death from overwhelming infection and septic shock. Compare **infected abortion.** See also **illegal abortion, induced abortion.**

**septicaemia.**   See **septicemia.**

**septic arthritis,**   an acute form of arthritis, characterized by bacterial inflammation of a joint caused by the spread of bacteria through the bloodstream from an infection elsewhere in the body or by contamination of a joint during trauma or surgery. The joint is stiff, painful, tender, warm, and swollen. The diagnosis is confirmed by bacteriologic identification of an organism in a specimen obtained by aspiration of the joint. Parenteral antibiotics are given to prevent destruction of the joint and are continued for several weeks after inflammation has resolved. Repeated aspiration of the joint or surgical incision and drainage may be performed to relieve pressure on it. Physical therapy as the joint heals is helpful to restore it to full range of motion. Also called **acute bacterial arthritis.**

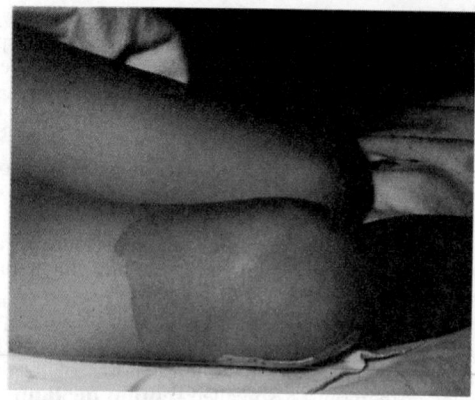

**Septic arthritis** *(Zitelli and Davis, 1997)*

**septicemia** /sep′tisē′mē·ə/ [Gk, *septikos* + *haima*, blood],   systemic infection in which pathogens are present in the circulating blood, having spread from an infection in any part of the body. It is diagnosed by culture of the blood and is vigorously treated with antibiotics. Characteristically septicemia causes fever, chill, hypotension, prostration, pain, headache, nausea, or diarrhea. Also spelled **septicaemia.** Also called **blood poisoning.** Compare **bacteremia.** See also **septic shock.** —**septicemic,** *adj.*

**-septicemia, -septicaemia,**   combining form meaning '(condition of the) blood caused by virulent microorganisms': *pyosepticemia, streptosepticemia.*

**septicemic.**   See **septicemia.**

**septicemic plague** /sep′tisē′mik/,   a rapidly fatal form of bubonic plague in which septicemia with meningitis occurs before buboes have had time to form. Compare **bubonic plague, pneumonic plague.** See also **plague,** *Yersinia pestis.*

**septic fever,**   an elevation of body temperature associated with infection by pathogenic microorganisms or in response to a toxin secreted by a microorganism.

**septic infarct** [Gk, *septikos*, putrid; L, *infarcire*, to stuff],   an infected segment of dead tissue.

**septic shock,**   a form of shock that occurs in septicemia when endotoxins or exotoxins are released from certain bacteria in the bloodstream; occasionally, septic shock may be caused by the presence of fungi or viruses in the blood. These toxins cause vasodilation, resulting in a dramatic fall in blood pressure. Fever, tachycardia, increased respiration rate, and confusion or coma also may occur. Septic shock is usually preceded by signs of severe infection, often of the genitourinary or GI system. The causative bacterium is most frequently gram negative. Antibiotics, vasopressors, and IV fluids and volume expanders are usually given. In some cases, treatment with monoclonal antibodies may be considered. Kinds of septic shock include **toxic shock syndrome** and **bacteremic shock. Compare hypovolemic shock.** See also **shock.**

**septic sore throat** [Gk, *septikos*, putrid; AS, *sar* + *throte*],   a severe throat infection, usually caused by a streptococcus strain, resulting in fever and marked exhaustion.

**septivalent.**   See **heptavalent.**

**septo-optic dysplasia** /sep′tō·op′tik dis·plā′zhə/,   a syndrome of hypoplasia of the optic disk with other ocular abnormalities, absence of the septum pellucidum, and hypopituitarism leading to growth deficiency. Also called **de Morsier's syndrome.**

**septoplasty** /sep'tō·plas'tē/ [L, *saeptum*, septum; Gk, *plassein*, to form], surgical reconstruction of the nasal septum.

**septorhinoplasty** /sep'tōrī'nəplas'tē/ [L, *saeptum*, fence], the surgical correction of defects in the nasal septum.

**septostomy** /septos'təmē/, the creation of an opening in a septum by surgery.

**Septra,** trademark for the antibacterial cotrimoxazole (a 1:5 mixture of the antibacterials trimethoprim and sulfamethoxazole).

**septum** /sep'təm/, *pl.* **septa** [L, *saeptum*, enclosure], a partition or wall, such as the interatrial septum that separates the atria of the heart.

**septum pellucidum** /sep'tum pə·lōō'si·dum/ [L, transparent septum], a triangular double membrane situated in the median plane and separating the anterior horns of the lateral ventricles of the brain. Also called **septum lucidum.**

**septuplet** /septup'lit/ [L, *septuplum*, group of seven], any one of seven children born of a single pregnancy.

**sequela** /sikwē'lə/, *pl.* **sequelae** [L, *sequi*, to follow], any abnormal condition that follows and is the result of a disease, treatment, or injury, such as paralysis after poliomyelitis, deafness after treatment with an ototoxic drug, or scar formation after a laceration.

**sequence** /sē'kwəns/ [L, *sequi*, to follow], an order of arrangement of objects or events, as the sequence of peptides in a protein molecule.

**sequential imaging,** a diagnostic procedure used to study physiologic processes by means of a series of closely timed images of the rapidly changing distribution of a radioactive tracer within the body.

**sequential line imaging,** the construction of a magnetic resonance image from successive lines through the object.

**sequential multiple analysis,** the biochemical examination of various substances in the blood, such as albumin, alkaline phosphatase, bilirubin, calcium, and cholesterol, using a computerized laboratory analyzer that produces a printout showing measured values of the substances tested.

**sequential pacing.** See **pacing.**

**sequential plane imaging,** the construction of a magnetic resonance image from successive planes through the object. The planes may be selected by oscillation of gradient magnetic fields or by selective excitation.

**sequential point imaging,** the construction of a magnetic resonance image from successive point positions in the object.

**sequester** /sikwes'tər/ [L, *sequestare*, to lay aside], to detach, separate, or isolate, such as patient sequestration to prevent the spread of an infection.

**sequestered antigens hypothesis,** a proposed explanation for autoimmunity that stresses the relationship between antigen exposure, immunogenic cells, and body cells. It maintains that immunologic tolerance depends on a certain degree of contact between immunologic cells and body cells and on a certain degree of antigen exposure. The hypothesis holds that certain sequestered antigens in the brain, the lenses of the eye, and spermatozoa are isolated from the circulation of the blood and the lymph and therefore do not contact the cells of the immune system. When body tissues are damaged, the sequestered antigens are suddenly exposed to the immune system, which treats them as foreign, triggering an autoimmune reaction. Compare **forbidden clone hypothesis.**

**sequestered edema,** edema localized in the tissues surrounding a newly created surgical wound.

**sequestra.** See **sequestrum.**

**sequestration** /sē'kwestrā'shən/ [L, *sequestare*, to lay aside], **1.** the isolation of a patient or group of patients. **2.** a method of controlling hemorrhage of the head or trunk by isolating fluid in the arms and legs from the general circulation. **3.** allowing blood from the systemic circulation to perfuse a nonfunctioning part of a lung.

**sequestrum** /sikwes'trəm/, *pl.* **sequestra** [L, a deposit], a fragment of dead bone that is partially or entirely detached from the surrounding or adjacent healthy bone.

**sequestrum forceps,** a forceps with small, powerful teeth used for extracting necrotic or sharp fragments of bone from surrounding tissue.

**sequoiasis** /sikwoi'əsis/ [sequoia (tree) + Gk, *osis*, condition], a type of hypersensitivity pneumonitis common among workers in sawmills where redwood is processed. The antigens are the fungus *Pullularia pullulans* and species of the genus *Graphium,* found in moldy redwood sawdust. Characteristics of the acute disease include chills, fever, cough, dyspnea, anorexia, nausea, and vomiting. Symptoms of the chronic disease include productive cough, dyspnea on exertion, fatigue, and weight loss.

**Ser,** abbreviation for the amino acid **serine.**

**sera.** See **serum.**

**Ser-Ap-Es,** trademark for a fixed-combination antihypertensive drug containing a diuretic (hydrochlorothiazide) and antihypertensives (reserpine and hydralazine hydrochloride).

**Serax,** trademark for a tranquilizer (oxazepam).

**serendipity** /ser'əndip'itē/ [Serendip, author Horace Walpole's mythic land of pleasant surprises], the act of accidental discovery. A number of important medications have been created through serendipity, such as the discovery of antidepressant activity in iproniazid, which was originally developed to treat tuberculosis.

**Serentil,** trademark for a phenothiazine tranquilizer (mesoridazine).

**Serevent,** trademark for a long-acting sympathomimetic bronchodilator (salmeterol).

**serial** /sir'ē·əl/ [L, *series*, row], pertaining to a succession, arrangement, or order of items.

**serial casting,** the process of using a sequence of casts to progressively correct a deformity.

**serial determination** [L, *series*, row, *determinare*, to limit], a laboratory test that is repeated at stated intervals, as in a series of repeated tests for cardiac enzymes in blood samples taken from a patient with suspected myocardial infarction.

**serial dilution,** a laboratory technique in which a substance, such as blood serum, is decreased in concentration in a series of proportional amounts. In antibody analysis, for example, a serum sample may be distributed in a series of tubes so that each has one half of the amount of the previous tube in the series, resulting in titers of 1:5, 1:10, 1:20, and so on.

**serial extraction,** a program of selective extraction of primary and sometimes secondary teeth over a period of time, with the objective of relieving crowding and of facilitating the eruption of remaining teeth into improved positions. Close supervision of ensuing eruption is essential because the closing over of spaces is common. Comprehensive orthodontic treatment should almost always be initiated during or after eruption for space management, control of tipping induced by the procedure, and correction of other problems.

**serial processing,** a specific order of information handled by various computer work centers. Information proceeds sequentially through each of the centers or processes.

**serial section** [L, *series*, in a row, *sectio*], one of a number of consecutive slices of tissue.

**serial speech,** overlearned speech involving a series of words, such as counting or reciting of days of the week.

**series** /sir′ēs/, *pl.* **series** /sir′ēs/ [L, in a row], a chain of objects or events arranged in a predictable order, such as the series of stages through which a mature blood cell develops.

**serine (Ser)** /ser′ēn/, a nonessential amino acid found in many proteins in the body (for example, cassein, vitrellin). It is a precursor of the amino acids glycine and cysteine. It can be found in urine. See also **amino acid, protein.**

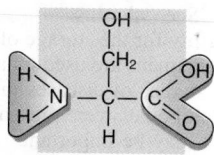

**Chemical structure of serine**

**SERM,** abbreviation for **selective estrogen receptor modulator.**

**Sernylan,** trademark for a veterinary anesthetic (phencyclidine hydrochloride), used illicitly as a euphoric called **PCP.**

**sero-** /sir′ō-/, combining form meaning 'blood serum': *seroculture, serogenesis, serolin.*

**seroconversion** /- kənvur′zhən/ [L, *serum*, whey, *conversio*, turned about], a change in serologic test results from negative to positive as antibodies develop in reaction to an infection or vaccine.

**serodiagnosis** /-dī′əgnō′sis/ [L, *serum*, whey; Gk, *dia*, through, *gnosis*, knowledge], the use of serologic tests in the diagnosis of disease.

**serofibrinous pericarditis** /-fī′brinəs/ [L, *serum*, whey, *fibra*, fibrin; Gk, *peri*, near, *kardia*, heart, *itis*, inflammation], a form of fibrinous pericarditis marked by a serous exudate.

**serofibrinous pleurisy,** an inflammation of the pleura with a watery effusion and accumulation of fibrin on the pleural membranes.

**seroimmunity** /sir′ō-imyoo͞′nitē/, immunity conferred by administration of an antiserum.

**serologic** /-loj′ik/ [L, *serum*, whey; Gk, *logos*, science], pertaining to the branch of medicine concerned with the study of blood sera. Also **serological.**

**serological.** See **serologic, serology.**

**serologic diagnosis** /siroloj′ik/ [L, *serum*, whey; Gk, *dia*, through, *gnosis*, knowledge], a diagnosis that is made through laboratory examination of antigen-antibody reactions in the serum. Also called **immunodiagnosis, serum diagnosis.**

**serologic test** [L, *serum*, whey, *testum*, crucible], any diagnostic test made with serum.

**serologist** /sirol′əjist/ [L, *serum*, + Gk, *logos*, science], a bacteriologist or medical technologist who prepares or supervises the preparation and testing of sera used to diagnose and treat diseases and to immunize people against infectious diseases.

**serology** /sirol′əjē/ [L, *serum* + Gk, *logos*, science], the branch of laboratory medicine that studies blood serum for evidence of infection by evaluating antigen-antibody reactions in vitro. —**serologic, serological,** *adj.*

**seroma** /sirō′mə/, a lump or swelling caused by an accumulation of serum within a tissue or organ.

**Seromycin,** trademark for a tuberculostatic (cycloserine).

**seronegative** /-neg′ətiv/ [L, *serum*, whey, *negare*, to deny], a serologic test with negative results.

**seropositive** /-pos′itiv/ [L, *serum*, whey, *positivus*], a serologic test with positive results.

**seroprevalence** /-prev′ələns/, the overall occurrence of a disease within a defined population at one time, as measured by blood tests. An example is human immunodeficiency virus seroprevalence.

**seroprophylaxis** /-prō′filak′sis/, the administration of a serum to prevent disease.

**seropurulent** /-pyoo͞r′ələnt/, containing serum and pus.

**serosa** /sirō′sə/ [L, *serum*], any serous membrane, such as the tunica serosa that lines the walls of body cavities and secretes a watery exudate.

**serosanguineous** /sir′ōsang·gwin′ē-əs/, (of a discharge) thin and red; composed of serum and blood. Also **serosanguinous** /sir′ōsang′gwinəs/.

**serotonin** /ser′ətō′nin, sir′-/ [L, *serum* + Gk, *tonos*, tone], a naturally occurring derivative of tryptophan found in platelets and in cells of the brain and the intestine. Serotonin is released from platelets on damage to the blood vessel walls. It acts as a potent vasoconstrictor. Serotonin in intestinal tissue stimulates the smooth muscle to contract. In the central nervous system, it acts as a neurotransmitter. Lysergic acid diethylamide interferes with the action of serotonin in the brain. The normal concentration of serotonin in the urine is 0.05 to 0.2 µg/ml. Also called **5-hydroxytryptamine.**

**serous** /sir′əs/ [L, *serum*, whey], pertaining to, resembling, or producing serum.

**serous fluid** [L, *serum* + *fluere*, to flow], a fluid that has the characteristics of serum.

**serous membrane,** one of the many thin sheets of tissue that line closed cavities of the body, such as the pleura lining the thoracic cavity, the peritoneum lining the abdominal cavity, and the pericardium lining the sac that encloses the heart. Between the visceral layer of serous membrane covering various organs and the parietal layer lining the cavity containing such organs is a potential space moistened by serous fluid. The fluid reduces the friction of the structures covered by the serous membrane, such as the lungs, which move against the thoracic walls in respiration. Compare **mucous membrane, skin, synovial membrane.**

**serovaccination** /-vak′sinā′shən/, a technique for producing mixed immunity in which a person is first injected with a serum to establish passive immunity, and then is vaccinated to produce active immunity.

**Serpasil,** trademark for an antihypertensive (reserpine).

**Serpasil-Apresoline,** trademark for a fixed-combination drug containing two antihypertensives (reserpine and hydralazine hydrochloride).

**Serpasil-Esidrix,** trademark for a fixed-combination antihypertensive drug containing a diuretic (hydrochlorothiazide) and an antihypertensive (reserpine).

**serpent ulcer** /sur′pənt/ [L, *serpens*, snake], an ulceration of the skin that heals in one area while extending to another. Also called **serpiginous ulcer.**

**-serpine,** combining form for *Rauwolfia* alkaloid derivatives.

**serrate** /ser′āt/, having an edge with notches or sawlike teeth. —**serrated,** *adj.*

**serrated suture** /ser′ātid/, a suture with sawlike edges, such as most of the sagittal suture.

**Serratia** /serā′shə/ [L, *serra,* saw teeth], a genus of motile, gram-negative bacilli capable of causing infection in humans, including bacteremia, pneumonia, and urinary tract infections. *Serratia* organisms are frequently acquired in hospitals. See also **nosocomial infection.**

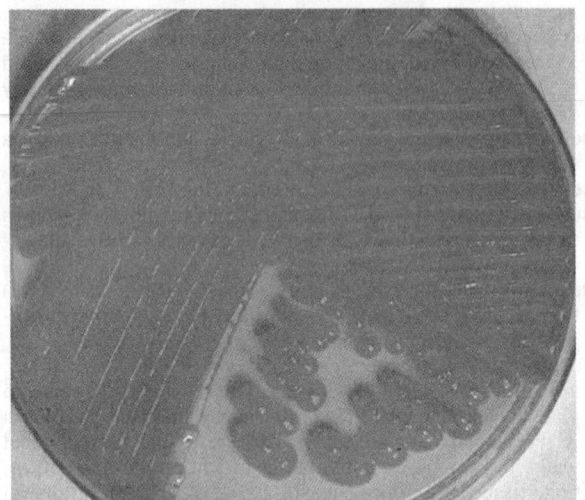

***Serratia marcescens*** *(Baron, Peterson, and Finegold, 1994)*

**serratus anterior** /serā′təs/ [L, *serra,* saw teeth], a thin muscle of the chest wall extending from the ribs under the arm to the scapula. Arising from the outer surface and upper border of the first eight or nine ribs, it inserts into the medial angle, the vertebral border, and the inferior angle of the scapula. It acts to rotate the scapula and to raise the shoulder, as in full flexion and abduction of the arm. Compare **pectoralis major, pectoralis minor, subclavius.**

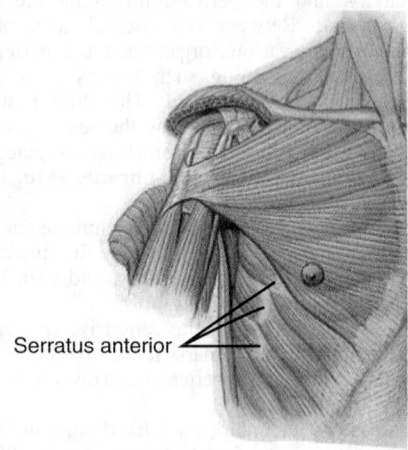

Serratus anterior

***Serratus anterior*** *(Thibodeau and Patton, 1999/John V. Hagen)*

**Sertoli cell** /sertō′lē/ [Enrico Sertoli, Italian histologist, 1842–1910; L, *cella,* storeroom], one of the supporting elongated cells of the seminiferous tubules of the testes. It functions to nourish the developing spermatocytes.

**Sertoli-cell-only syndrome** [Enrico Sertoli], a form of male sterility in which only Sertoli cells are present in the seminiferous tubules of the testes. Germinal epithelium is absent, resulting in azoospermia.

**Sertoli-Leydig cell tumor.** See **arrhenoblastoma.**

**serum** /sir′əm/, *pl.* **sera** [L, whey], **1.** also called **blood serum.** Any serous fluid that moistens the surfaces of serous membranes. **2.** any clear watery fluid that has been separated from its more solid elements, such as the exudate from a blister. **3.** the clear, thin, and sticky fluid part of the blood that remains after coagulation. Serum contains no blood cells, platelets, or fibrinogen. **4.** a vaccine or toxoid prepared from the serum of a hyperimmune donor for prophylaxis against a particular infection or poison.

**serum albumin,** a major protein in blood plasma. It is important in maintaining the osmotic pressure of the blood. Normal value is 3.5 to 5.0 g/dL.

**serumal calculus.** See **calculus.**

**serum bank,** a facility for the storage of frozen samples of blood serum. The specimens are used mainly for medical research, as in future studies of diseases in which knowledge of whether certain antibodies were present in blood samples collected in the past may be important.

**serum carnosinase deficiency,** an autosomal recessive aminoacidopathy of carnosine metabolism, characterized by urinary excretion of carnosine and accumulation of homocarnosine in the cerebrospinal fluid; this may cause myoclonic seizures, severe mental retardation, and spasticity.

**serum C-reactive protein.** See **C-reactive protein.**

**serum creatinine level,** the concentration of creatinine in the serum, used as a diagnostic sign of possible renal impairment.

**serum diagnosis.** See **serologic diagnosis.**

**serumfast** /sir′əmfast′/, **1.** resistant (as bacteria) to the destructive effects of sera. **2.** having (as a serum) little or no change in antibody titer.

**serum globulin** [L, *serum,* whey, *globulus,* small globe], one of a group of proteins in blood serum with antibody qualities. The various types of serum globulins, designated, α, β, and γ, have different specific properties.

**serum glutamic oxaloacetic transaminase (SGOT),** See **aspartate aminotransferase (AST).**

**serum glutamic pyruvic transaminase (SGPT),** See **alanine aminotransferase.**

**serum hepatitis.** See **hepatitis B.**

**serum osmolality** [L, *serum,* whey; Gk, *ōsmos,* impulse], a measure of the osmotic concentration of blood serum, expressed as the number of osmoles of solute per kilogram of plasma water.

**serum protein** [L, *serum,* whey; Gk, *proteios,* first rank], any of the proteins in blood serum. See also **serum globulin.**

**serum shock,** a life-threatening reduction in blood volume and blood pressure caused by the injection of an antitoxic or other foreign serum.

**serum sickness,** an immunologic disorder that may occur 2 to 3 weeks after the administration of an antiserum. It is caused by an antibody reaction to an antigen in the donor serum. The condition is characterized by fever, splenomegaly, swollen lymph nodes, skin rash, and joint pain. Treatment is symptomatic and supportive and may include corticosteroids. See also **angioneurotic edema, antigen-antibody reaction, Arthus reaction.**

**serum urea nitrogen.** See **urea nitrogen.**

**service dog,** a dog trained to aid disabled persons with such tasks as opening or closing doors, picking up dropped items, or pulling a wheelchair.

**service of process** /sur′vis/ [L, *servus,* a slave, *processus,* going forth], (in law) the delivery of a writ, summons, or complaint to a defendant. Once delivered or left with the party for whom it is intended, it is said to have been served. The original of the document is shown; a copy is served.

Service of process gives reasonable notice to allow the person to appear, testify, and be heard in court.

**servomechanism** /sur′vōmek′əniz′əm/,   a control system in which feedback is used to correct errors in another system. A biologic example is the mechanism that controls the size of the pupil of the eye as the intensity of light changes.

**Serzone,** trademark for an antidepressant drug (nefazodonehydrochloride).

**sesame oil** /ses′əmē/,   a liquid fat derived from the seeds of a plant, *Sesamum indicum.* The seeds are demulcent and have a laxative effect. Both seeds and oil are used as food flavorings. The oil is also used in skin lotions, as an emollient.

**sesamoid** /ses′əmoid/ [Gk, *sesamon,* sesame, *eidos,* form], nodular objects having the shape and size of sesame seeds. See **sesamoid bone.**

**sesamoid bone** [Gk, *sesamon,* sesame, *eidos,* form],   any one of numerous small round bony masses embedded in certain tendons that may be subjected to compression and tension. The largest sesamoid bone is the patella, which is embedded in the tendon of the quadriceps femoris at the knee.

**sesqui-,** combining form meaning 'one and one half': *sesquibasic, sesquibo, sesquihora.*

**sessile** /ses′əl/ [L, *sessilis,* sitting],   **1.** (in biology) attached by a base rather than by a stalk or a peduncle, such as a leaf that is attached directly to its stem. **2.** permanently connected.

**set,**   **1.** a predisposition to behave in a certain way. **2.** to reduce a fracture by moving the bones back into a normal position.

**set-,** combining form meaning 'bristle': *setaceous, setiferous, seton.*

**setaceous** /sētā′shəs/,   having or resembling bristles.

**setback,**   the surgical treatment of a bilateral cleft of the palate.

**seton** /sē′ton/,   thread, gauze, or other material passed through subcutaneous tissue or a cyst to create a sinus or fistula.

**settlement** [AS, *setlan,* to put in place],   (in law) an agreement made between parties to a suit before a judgment is rendered by a court.

**setup** [AS, *settan,* to set, *up,* on high],   **1.** an arrangement of artificial teeth on a trial denture base. **2.** a laboratory procedure in which teeth are removed from a plaster cast and repositioned in wax. It is used as a diagnostic procedure and in creation of a mold for a positioner appliance.

**seventh cranial nerve.**   See **facial nerve.**

**severe acute respiratory syndrome (SARS),**   an infectious respiratory illness first reported in Asia and characterized by a fever over 38°C, dry cough, and breathing difficulties, often accompanied by headache and body aches. It is believed to be caused by a strain of coronavirus, and severity ranges from mild illness to death. The infection appears to be spread by close contact with infected individuals by inhalation of droplet nuclei containing the organism or by contact with infected body fluids. Treatment is mainly supportive at this time, although several antivirals continue to be tested.

**severe combined immunodeficiency disease (SCID)** /sivēr′/ [L, *servus,* slave],   an abnormal condition characterized by the complete absence or marked deficiency of B cells and T cells with the consequent lack of humoral and cell-mediated immunity. The disease occurs as an X-linked recessive disorder affecting only males and as an autosomal-recessive disorder affecting both males and females. It results in a pronounced susceptibility to infection and is usually fatal. The precise cause of SCID is not known, but research indicates the disease may be caused by a cytogenic dysfunction of the embryonic stem cells that normally differentiate into B cells and T cells. The affected individual consequently has a very small thymus and little or no protection against infection.

■ OBSERVATIONS: Pronounced susceptibility to infection usually becomes obvious 3 to 6 months after birth, when maternal immunoglobulin reserves begin to diminish. Diagnosis is difficult because B cell immunity dysfunction is hard to detect in any individual until 5 months after birth, when immunoglobulin levels should reach a low point. Infants with SCID commonly fail to thrive and have a variety of complications, such as sepsis, watery diarrhea, persistent pulmonary infections, and common viral infections that are often fatal. Some infants with SCID have mild infections and low-grade fevers that last for several months while the infant uses maternal immunoglobulin stores; these conditions generally become fatal when maternal antibodies are totally depleted. Some of the more obvious symptoms after the infant has used most of the maternal immunoglobulin stores are cyanosis, rapid respirations, and normal chest sounds with an abnormal chest radiographic picture. Maternal immunoglobulin G (IgG) is persistent, and gram-negative infections usually do not appear until after the sixth month of life. Normal infants less than 5 months of age have very small amounts of IgM and IgA, and normal IgG levels only reflect maternal IgG. The combination of several symptoms may confirm the diagnosis of SCID, including the absence or severe reduction of T cell and B cell immunity; a lymph node biopsy result that shows no lymphocytes, plasma cells, or lymphoid follicles; and no skin reaction to swabbing with dinitrochlorobenzene. Most infants with SCID die from severe infection within 1 year after birth.

■ INTERVENTIONS: Treatment of SCID seeks to develop the immune system and to prevent infection. The only satisfactory treatment available to correct immunodeficiency is histocompatible bone marrow transplantation, but that may cause a graft-versus-host reaction, thus increasing the risk of infection and fatal consequences. Maintained enclosure in a completely sterile environment has prolonged the life of some infants with SCID, but this option is not successful if the infant has already had recurring infections.

■ NURSING CONSIDERATIONS: Supportive treatment is the primary approach in caring for the SCID patient. The nurse tries to promote an encouraging atmosphere of growth and development while providing the parents with emotional support in the face of the nearly inevitable early death of their child. The infant must remain in strict protective isolation and benefits from diligent nursing attention, frequent parental visits, and gifts of toys, which should be the kind that can be easily sterilized.

**Sever's disease.**   See **calcaneal epiphysitis.**

**Sevin,**   trademark for carbaryl, a widely used carbamate insecticide that causes reversible inhibition of cholinesterase. Although less toxic than parathion, carbaryl, when concentrated, may produce skin irritation and systemic poisoning characterized by nausea, vomiting, cramps, diarrhea, diaphoresis, excessive salivation, dyspnea, weakness, loss of coordination, and slurred speech; large doses may cause coma and death. Carbaryl on the skin is promptly removed by washing with water. Treatment of systemic poisoning includes the immediate IV or intramuscular injection of 1 to 4 mg of atropine sulfate, the administration of artificial respiration and oxygen, gastric lavage, and IV isotonic saline solution to correct dehydration.

**sex** [L, *sexus,* sex],   **1.** a classification of male or female based on many criteria, among them anatomic and chromosomal characteristics. **2.** coitus. Compare **gender.**

**sex-,** prefix meaning 'six': *sexdigitate, sexivalent, sextan.*

**sex chromatin,** a densely staining mass within the nucleus of all nondividing cells of normal mammalian females. It represents the heterochromatin of the inactivated X chromosome. Examination of cells obtained by amniocentesis for the presence of sex chromatin is a technique used for determining the sex of a baby before birth. Sex chromatin is also found as a drumstick-shaped mass attached to one of the nuclear lobes in polymorphonuclear leukocytes in normal females. Also called **Barr body.** See also **Lyon hypothesis.**

**sex chromosome,** a chromosome that determines the sex of individuals; it carries genes that transmit sex-linked traits and conditions. In humans and other mammals there are two distinct sex chromosomes, designated X and Y, which appear in females as XX and in males as XY. Compare **autosome.**

**sex chromosome mosaic,** an individual or organism whose cells contain variant chromosomal numbers involving the X or Y chromosomes. Such variations occur in most of the syndromes associated with sex chromosome aberrations, primarily Turner's syndrome, and may be caused by nondisjunction of the chromosomes during the second meiotic division of gametogenesis or by some error in chromosome distribution during cell division of the fertilized ovum. Sex chromosome mosaics often have sexual abnormalities, but because of the sex hormones the overall phenotype is uniform and not mosaic in external characteristics, as in certain animals and insects. Also called **sex mosaic.** See also **intersexuality.**

**sex-controlled.** See **sex-influenced.**

**sex determination** [L, *sexus,* sex, *determinare*], the process of identifying the sex of an individual, based on the presence of the XY chromosome combination in the cells of genetic males or Barr bodies in the cells of genetic females or on secondary sexual characteristics and skeletal variations.

**sex deviant,** a person whose sexual interests differ markedly from what is accepted as the norm. See also **paraphilia.**

**sex factor.** See **F factor.**

**sex hormone,** any of the androgens, estrogens, or related steroid hormones produced mainly by the testes, ovaries, and adrenal cortices.

**sex-hormone-binding globulin (SHBG),** a protein produced by the liver that binds testosterone and estradiol in the plasma. It has a greater affinity for testosterone. The plasma concentration of SHBG is influenced by liver cirrhosis, hyperthyroidism, obesity (in women), malnutrition, and estrogens.

**sexidigitate** /sek′sidij′itāt/ [L, *sex,* six], having six digits on one or both hands and feet.

**sex-influenced,** pertaining to an autosomal genetic trait, such as patterned baldness or gout, that is expressed in both homozygotes and heterozygotes in one sex but only homozygotes in the other sex. Also called **sex-controlled.**

**sexism** /sek′sizəm/, a belief that one sex is superior to the other and that the superior sex has endowments, rights, prerogatives, and status greater than those of the inferior sex. Sexism results in discrimination in all areas of life and acts as a limiting factor in educational, professional, and psychologic development. —**sexist,** *n., adj.*

**sexivalent** See **hexavalent.**

**sex-limited,** pertaining to an autosomal genetic trait that is expressed in only one sex, although the alleles for it may be carried by both sexes. Such traits are typically influenced by hormonal or environmental conditions.

**sex-linked,** pertaining to genes carried on the sex chromosomes, particularly the X chromosome, or to the traits they control. See also **sex-linked disorder, X-linked inheritance, Y-linked.** —**sex linkage,** *n.*

**sex-linked disorder,** any disease or abnormal condition that is determined by the sex chromosomes or by a defective gene on a sex chromosome. Sex-linked disorders may involve a deviation in the number of either the X or Y chromosomes, as occurs in Turner's syndrome and Klinefelter's syndrome, most occurrences of which are a result of nondisjunction during meiosis. Such aberrations in the number of sex chromosomes do not produce the severe clinical effects that are associated with autosomal aberrations, although they usually cause some degree of mental deficiency. Other sex-linked disorders are transmitted by single-gene defects carried on the X chromosome. X-linked dominant conditions, such as hypophosphatemic vitamin D–resistant rickets, are rare, and males are more seriously affected than females. In inheritance patterns, X-linked dominant conditions are transmitted by affected males to all of their daughters but none of their sons, by affected heterozygous females to one half of their children regardless of sex, and by affected homozygous females to all of their children. More common are X-linked recessive conditions, such as color blindness, ocular albinism, the Xg blood types, hemophilia, Duchenne muscular dystrophy, and inborn errors of metabolism. Such conditions are always transmitted by females. Those predominantly affected are males, because they have only one X chromosome and all of its genes, whether recessive or dominant, are expressed. Occasionally, females heterozygous for X-linked recessive disorders show varying degrees of expression, but never as severe as those of affected males. There are no known clinically significant traits or conditions associated with the genes on the Y chromosome; their only known function is to trigger the development of male characteristics.

**sex-linked ichthyosis,** a congenital skin disorder characterized by large thick dry scales with dark color; the scales cover the neck, scalp, ears, face, trunk, and flexor surfaces of the body, such as the folds of the arms and the backs of the knees. It is transmitted by females as an X-linked recessive trait and appears only in males. The condition is managed by topical applications of emollients and the use of keratolytic agents to facilitate removal of the scales. Also called **X-linked ichthyosis.** See also **ichthyosis.**

**sex mosaic.** See **sex chromosome mosaic.**

**sex ratio,** the proportion of male-to-female progeny, a relationship that varies with the stage of life. The distribution at birth is usually 106 boys to 100 girls, but the ratio shifts in adulthood, so that, because men have a lower life expectancy, the proportion of females is greater. The ratio may also vary with the effects of a particular disease or trait.

**sex role,** the expectations held by society regarding what behavior is appropriate or inappropriate for each sex.

**sex surrogate** [L, *sexus* + *surrogare,* substitute], (in sex therapy) a professional substitute trained to help the patient overcome inhibitions. Also called **surrogate partner.**

**sextuplet** /seks′tup′lit/ [L, *sex,* six], one of six children born of a single pregnancy.

**sexual** /sek′shōō·əl/, pertaining to sex.

**sexual abuse,** the sexual mistreatment of another person by fondling, rape, or forced participation in unnatural sex acts or other perverted behavior. Victims tend to experience a traumatic feeling of loss of control of themselves.

**sexual asphyxia,** accidental strangulation by ligature that occurs in an attempt to induce mild cerebral hypoxia during sexual activity for the purpose of enhancing orgasmic pleasure.

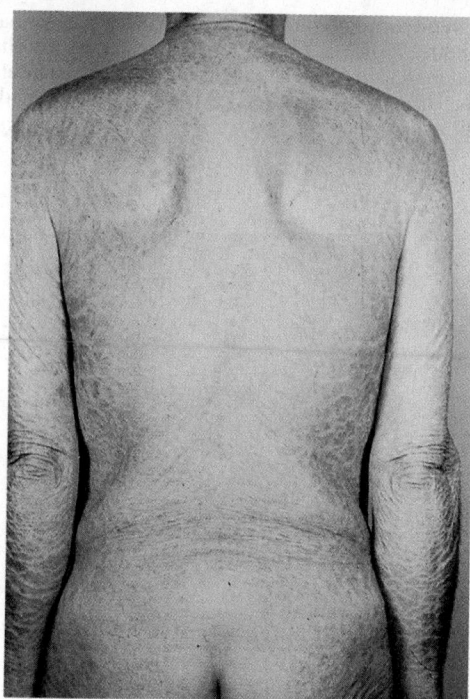

**Sex-linked ichthyosis** *(Zitelli and Davis, 1997)*

**sexual assault,** the forcible perpetration of an act of sexual contact on the body of another person, male or female, without his or her consent. Legal criteria vary among different communities.

**sexual aversion disorder,** a persistent or extreme aversion to or avoidance of all or nearly all genital sexual contact with a partner.

**sexual counseling,** a nursing intervention from the Nursing Interventions Classification (NIC) defined as use of an interactive helping process focusing on the need to make adjustments in sexual practice or to enhance coping with a sexual event/disorder. See also **Nursing Interventions Classification.**

**sexual disorder,** 1. any disorder involving sexual functioning, desire, or performance. 2. [*DSM-IV*] any such disorder that is caused at least in part by psychologic factors. Such a disorder characterized by a decrease or other disturbance of sexual desire is called a *sexual dysfunction,* and that characterized by unusual or bizarre sexual fantasies, urges, or practices is called **paraphilia.** Also called **psychosexual disorder, psychosexual dysfunction.**

**sexual dwarf,** an adult dwarf whose genital organs are normally developed.

**sexual dysfunction,** a nursing diagnosis accepted by the Fourth National Conference on the Classification of Nursing Diagnoses. It is defined as the state in which an individual experiences a change in sexual function that is viewed as unsatisfying, unrewarding, or inadequate.
■ DEFINING CHARACTERISTICS: The defining characteristics include a statement by the client of the perceived dysfunction, a physical alteration or limitation imposed by disease or treatment, a reported inability to achieve sexual satisfaction, an alteration in the sexual relationship with the partner, and a change in interest in oneself or in others.

■ RELATED FACTORS: Related factors include a biologic, psychologic, or social alteration in sexuality caused by an ineffectual or absent role model; physical abuse; psychosocial abuse, as in a harmful relationship; misinformation or lack of information; a conflict in values; a lack of privacy; or an alteration in body structure or function, as may result from pregnancy, recent childbirth, drugs, surgery, congenital anomalies, or trauma. See also **female sexual dysfunction, male sexual dysfunction, nursing diagnosis.**

**sexual fantasy,** mental images of an erotic nature that can lead to sexual arousal.

**sexual functioning,** a nursing outcome from the Nursing Outcomes Classification (NOC) defined as the integration of physical, socioemotional, and intellectual aspects of sexual expression. See also **Nursing Outcomes Classification.**

**sexual generation.** See **sexual reproduction.**

**sexual harassment,** an aggressive sexually motivated act of physical or verbal violation of a person over whom the aggressor has some power. Sexual harassment in the workplace is illegal, because it represents an abridgment of the victim's right to equal opportunity, privacy, and freedom from assault.

**sexual health** [L, *sexus* + AS, *haelth*], a condition defined by the World Health Organization as freedom from sexual diseases or disorders and a capacity to enjoy and control sexual behavior without fear, shame, or guilt.

**sexual history,** (in a patient record) the part of the patient's personal history concerned with sexual function and dysfunction. A sexual history is particularly important in gathering data from a patient who has a disease of the reproductive tract, who experiences sexual dysfunction, or who requests contraception, abortion, or sterilization. The extent of the history varies with the patient's age and condition and the reason for securing the history. A short sexual history is recommended as part of every complete physical examination. The therapist needs a detailed sexual history to understand the patient's complaint and to plan treatment. It may include the age at onset of sexual intercourse, the kind and frequency of sexual activity, and the satisfaction derived from it.

**sexual hormones,** chemical substances produced in the body that cause specific regulatory effects on the activity of reproductive organs.

**sexual identity: acceptance,** a nursing outcome from the Nursing Outcomes Classification (NOC) defined as the acknowledgement and acceptance of one's own sexual identity. See also **Nursing Outcomes Classification.**

**sexual intercourse.** See **coitus.**

**sexuality** /sek′shoo·al′ite/, 1. the sum of the physical, functional, and psychologic attributes that are expressed by one's gender identity and sexual behavior, whether or not related to the sex organs or to procreation. 2. the genital characteristics that distinguish male from female.

**sexuality patterns, ineffective,** a nursing diagnosis accepted by the Seventh National Conference on the Classification of Nursing Diagnoses. The diagnosis describes the state in which an individual expresses concern regarding his or her sexuality.
■ DEFINING CHARACTERISTICS: The defining characteristics include reported difficulties, limitations, or changes in sexual behaviors or activities.
■ RELATED FACTORS: Related factors include a knowledge or skill deficit about alternative responses to health-related transitions or altered body functions or structure (illness or medical); lack of privacy; lack of a significant other; ineffective or absent role model; conflicts with sexual orientation or variant preferences; fear of pregnancy or of sexually

transmitted disease; and an impaired relationship with a significant other. See also **nursing diagnosis.**

**sexually deviant personality** /sek'shōō·əlē'/, a sexual behavior that differs significantly from what is considered normal for a society. Either the quality or object of the sexual drives may be at variance with the accepted cultural norms for adults.

**sexually transmitted disease (STD),** a contagious disease usually acquired by sexual intercourse or genital contact. These diseases are among the most common communicable diseases, and the incidence has risen in recent years despite improved methods of diagnosis and treatment. Historically, the five venereal diseases were gonorrhea, syphilis, chancroid, granuloma inguinale, and lymphogranuloma venereum. To these have been added scabies, herpes genitalis and anorectal herpes and warts, pediculosis, trichomoniasis, genital candidiasis, molluscum contagiosum, hepatitis B, human papillomavirus infection, nonspecific urethritis, chlamydial infections, cytomegalovirus, and human immunodeficiency virus. Also called **venereal disease.** See also specific diseases.

**sexually transmitted disease cultures (STD culture),** a microscopic examination or blood test used to detect the presence of sexually transmitted diseases, such as gonorrhea, chlamydia, genital herpes, syphilis, hepatitis, AIDS, and others. Cervical cultures are usually done for women, and urethral cultures, for men; rectal and throat cultures are done for people who have engaged in anal and oral intercourse.

**sexual mores,** socially acceptable sexual behavior, usually based on fixed morally binding customs governing sexual behaviors that are harmful to others or the group, such as rape, incest, and sexual abuse of children.

**sexual orientation,** the clear persistent desire of a person for affiliation with one sex rather than the other. Also called **sexual preference.** See also **heterosexual, homosexuality.**

**sexual preference.** See **sexual orientation.**

**sexual psychopath,** an individual whose sexual behavior is openly perverted, antisocial, and criminal. See also **antisocial personality disorder.**

**sexual reassignment,** a change in the gender identity of a person by legal, surgical, hormonal, or social means.

**sexual reflex,** (in males) a reflex in which tactile or cerebral stimulation results in penile erection, priapism, or ejaculation. Also called **genital reflex.**

**sexual reproduction** [L, *sexus,* sex, *re + producere,* to produce], replication of an organism by the formation of gametes. Generally this requires the fusion of male spermatozoa and female ova; parthenogenesis is an exception. Also called **sexual generation, syngenesis.**

**sexual response cycle,** the four phases of biologic sexual response: excitement, plateau, orgasm, and resolution.

**sexual sadism.** See **sadism.**

**sexual selection,** the selection of mates based on the attraction of or preference for certain traits, such as coloration or behavior patterns, so that eventually only those particular traits appear in succeeding generations. It explains the wide variety of sexual characteristics among the various species.

**sexual tasks,** specific skills learned in various phases of development in the life cycle continuum to allow an adult to function normally in the sexual realm.

**sexual therapist,** a health care professional with specialized knowledge, skill, and competence in assisting individuals who experience sexual difficulties.

**sexual therapy,** a type of counseling that aids in the resolution of pathologic conditions so that a healthy sexuality can be maintained.

**Sézary syndrome** /sāzärēz'/ [A. Sézary, French dermatologist, 1880–1956], a condition of generalized exfoliating erythroderma, lymphadenopathy, and abnormal circulating T cells. The patient experiences pruritis, alopecia, edema, and nail and pigment changes.

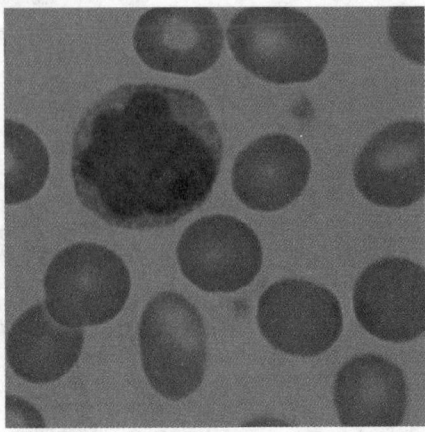

**Sézary syndrome** *(Carr and Rodak, 1999)*

**sfc,** abbreviation for *spinal fluid count.*

**SFD,** abbreviation for *small for dates.* See **small for gestational age (SGA) infant.**

**Sg,** symbol for the element **seaborgium.**

**SGA,** abbreviation for **small for gestational age.** See **small for gestational age (SGA) infant.**

**SGOT,** abbreviation for **serum glutamic oxaloacetic transaminase.**

**SGPT,** abbreviation for **serum glutamic pyruvic transaminase.**

**shadow** /shad'ō/ [AS, *sceadu*], (in psychology) an archetype that represents the unacceptable aspects and components of behavior.

**shadowcasting,** a technique for enhancing the visualization of a contoured microscopic specimen, in which a chemical film is deposited on it, making it more visible in relief.

**shadow cells.** See **ghost cells.**

**shaft,** an elongated cylindrical object, such as a long bone between the epiphyses.

**shaken baby syndrome,** a condition of whiplash-type injuries, ranging from bruises on the arms and trunk to retinal hemorrhages, coma, or convulsions, as observed in infants and children who have been violently shaken. This form of child abuse often results in intracranial bleeding from tearing of cerebral blood vessels.

**shakes** /shāks/, a popular term for the rigor, tremors, or shivering that occurs in intermittent fever or after drug withdrawal.

**shake test ("foam" test),** a qualitative test for fetal lung maturity. It is more rapid than determination of the lecithin/sphingomyelin ratio.

**shaking palsy.** See **parkinsonism.**

**shallow breathing** /shal'ō/ [ME, *schalowe,* little depth], a respiration pattern marked by slow, shallow, and generally ineffective inspirations and expirations. It is usually caused

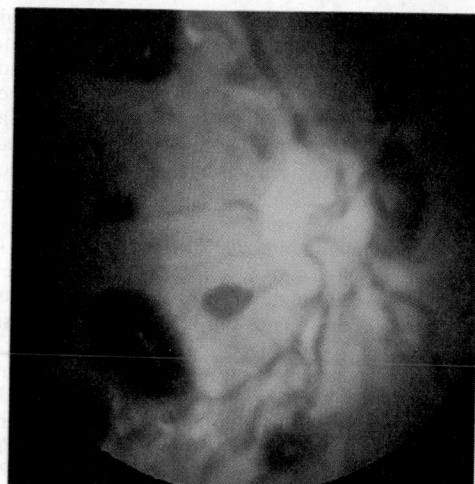

**Shaken baby syndrome: retinal hemorrhages**
*(Zitelli and Davis, 1997/courtesy Dr. Stephen Ludwig, Children's Hospital of Philadelphia)*

by drugs and indicates depression of the medullary respiratory center.

**shank,**   **1.** the tibia. **2.** the part of a device that connects the functional part to a handle.

**shaping** [AS, *scieppan,* to shape],   a procedure used for conditioning a person undergoing behavior therapy to develop new behavioral responses. Initially, any act remotely resembling the desired behavior is reinforced; gradually, the criterion is made more stringent until the desired response is attained.

**shared governance,**   an organized, systematic approach to decision making that enables all levels of nurses to participate in the resolution of clinical, professional, and administrative practice issues.

**shared paranoid disorder** [AS, *scearan,* to shear],   a psychopathologic condition characterized by identical manifestations of the same mental disorder, usually ideas, in two closely associated or related people. Also called **folie à deux.**

**shared services,**   administrative, clinical, or other service functions that are common to two or more hospitals or other health care facilities and that are used jointly or cooperatively by them.

**shark skin.**   See **dyssebacea.**

**Sharpey's fiber** [William Sharpey, Scottish anatomist, 1802–1880],   any of the many collagenous bundles of fibers of the periodontal ligament that become embedded in the cementum during its formation.

**sharps,**   any needles, scalpels, or other articles that could cause wounds or punctures to personnel handling them. See also **needlestick injuries.**

**shatterproof glass.**   See **safety glass.**

**shaving stroke** [AS, *scafan,* to shave, *strican,* to stroke],   a phase of the working stroke of a periodontal curet, used for smoothing or planing a tooth or tooth root surface.

**SHBG,**   abbreviation for **sex-hormone-binding globulin.**

**SHCC,**   abbreviation for **Statewide Health Coordinating Committee.**

**shear** /shir/ [AS, *scearan,* to cut],   an applied force or pressure exerted against the surface and layers of the skin as tissues slide in opposite but parallel planes.

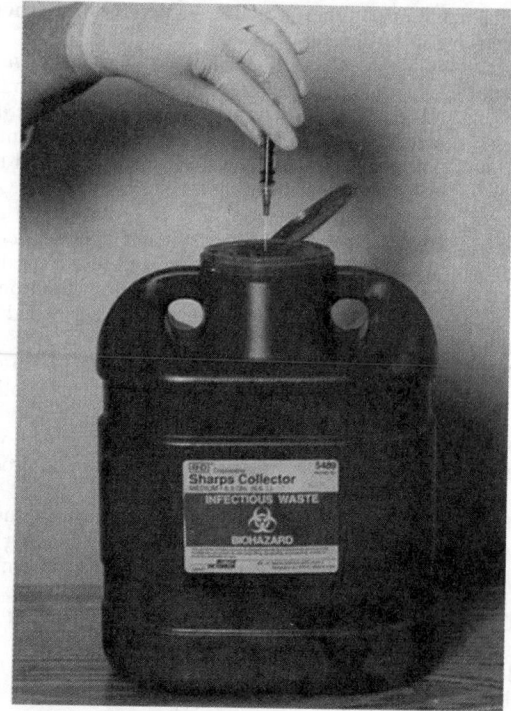

**Sharps container** *(Potter and Perry, 2001)*

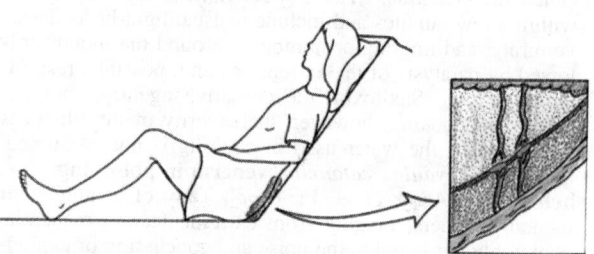

**Shearing force** *(Potter and Perry, 2001)*

**shearling** /shir′ling/,   a sheepskin placed on a bed to help prevent decubitus ulcers.

**sheath** /shēth/ [AS, *scaeth*],   a tubular structure that surrounds an organ or any other part of the body, such as the sheath of the rectus abdominis muscle or the sheath of Schwann, which covers various nerve fibers.

**sheath of Schwann** [Theodor Schwann, German anatomist, 1810–1882; AS, *scaeth*],   a neurilemma sheath of nucleated cells enclosing a nerve fiber.

**Sheehan's syndrome** [Harold L. Sheehan, English pathologist, 1900–1988],   a postpartum condition of pituitary necrosis and hypopituitarism after circulatory collapse resulting from uterine hemorrhaging. Lactation may not develop and loss of pubic and axillary hair may occur.

**sheep cell agglutination test (SCAT),**   a test for the presence of the rheumatoid factor in blood serum, using red blood cells of sheep that have been sensitized with rabbit antisheep erythrocyte immune globulin. The globulin will be agglutinated if the serum contains the rheumatoid factor.

Also called **Paul-Bunnell test, Rose-Waaler test, sheep red-cell agglutination test.**

**sheep cell test** [AS, *sceap* + L, *cella,* storeroom, *testum,* crucible], a method that mixes human blood cells with the red blood cells of sheep to determine the absence or the deficiency of human T lymphocytes. When mixed with human blood cells, the red blood cells of sheep cluster around the human T lymphocytes and form characteristic rosettes. An electron microscope is used to identify the rosettes. An absence or a decrease in the number of rosettes indicates a deficiency or absence of T cells. The sheep cell test is used to diagnose several diseases, such as DiGeorge's syndrome, that decrease or destroy the cellular immunity provided by T cells.

**sheet** /shēt/ [AS, *scēte*], **1.** a rectangular piece of cotton, linen, etc. for a bed covering. **2.** any structure resembling such a covering.

**sheet bath** [AS, *scēte* + *baeth*], the application of wet sheets to the body, used primarily as an antipyretic procedure.

**sheet wadding,** stretchable sheets of cotton padding used to cover the skin before a cast is applied. The stretching allows for some extremity edema without the cast becoming too tight.

**shelf** [AS, *scylf*], a flat, hard anatomic structure that resembles a ridge or platform.

**shell** [AS, *scell*], **1.** a hard outer protective covering that encloses material. **2.** an electron orbit surrounding the nucleus of an atom.

**shellfish poisoning** [AS, *scell* + *fisc*], a toxic neurologic condition that results from eating clams, oysters, or mussels that have ingested the toxin-producing protozoa commonly called the "red tide." The characteristic symptoms appear within a few minutes and include nausea, light-headedness, vomiting, and tingling or numbness around the mouth, followed by paralysis of the extremities and, possibly, respiratory paralysis. Saxitoxin, the causative agent, is not destroyed by cooking; however, the severity of the illness is diminished if the water used in cooking is not consumed. See also *Gonyaulax catanella,* **venerupin poisoning.**

**shell shock** [AS, *scell* + Fr, *choc*], any of a number of mental disorders, ranging from extreme fear to dementia, commonly attributed to the noise and concussion of exploding shells or bombs but actually a traumatic reaction to the stress of combat. See also **combat fatigue, posttraumatic stress disorder.**

**shell teeth,** a type of dental dysplasia in which the teeth have large pulp chambers, insufficient coronal dentin, and, usually, no roots.

**sheltered workshop** [ME, *sheltrun,* body of guards; AS, *werc* + *sceoppa,* stall], a facility or program, either for outpatients or for residents of an institution, that provides vocational experience in a controlled working environment. The workshop also offers related vocational rehabilitation services, such as job interview training, to people with physical or mental disabilities.

**shield** [AS, *scild*], a material for preventing or reducing the passage of charged particles or radiation. A shield may be designated by the radiation it is intended to absorb, such as a gamma ray shield, or by the kind of protection it is intended to give, such as a background, biologic, or thermal shield. Lucite and aluminum can be used for beta-radiation shields, but lead is required for gamma ray shields.

**shift** [AS, *sciftan,* to divide], **1.** (in nursing) the particular hours of the day during which a nurse is scheduled to work. The day shift is usually 7:00 AM to 3:00 PM or 8:00 AM to 4:00 PM. The evening shift is usually 3:00 PM to 11:00 PM or 4:00 PM to 12:00 midnight, and the night shift the remaining hours. The evening shift is also called "relief," presumably because nurses originally worked 12-hour shifts and the evening and night shift was thought to be relief for the day nurse. Many innovations in staffing practice currently allow variations on the traditional 5-day, 40-hour week, such as nurses electing to work a shorter week, preferring longer hours for fewer days. **2.** an abrupt change in an analytic system that continues at the new level.

**shift report,** a nursing intervention from the Nursing Interventions Classification (NIC) defined as exchanging essential patient care information with other nursing staff at change of shift. See also **Nursing Interventions Classification.**

**shift to the left,** (in hematology) a predominance of immature leukocytes, noted in a differential white blood cell count. It is usually indicative of an infection or inflammation. The term derives from a graph of blood components in which immature cell frequencies appear on the left side of the graph.

**shift to the right,** (in hematology) a preponderance of polymorphonuclear neutrophils having three or more lobes, indicating maturity of the cell. The phenomenon is common in severe liver disease and advanced pernicious anemia. It indicates a relative lack of blood-forming activity.

*Shigella* /shigel′ə/ [Kiyoshi Shiga, Japanese bacteriologist, 1870–1957], a genus of gram-negative pathogenic bacteria that causes gastroenteritis and bacterial dysentery, such as *Shigella dysenteriae.* It is also associated with hemolytic-uremic syndromes. See also **shigellosis.**

*Shigella dysenteriae*, a species of the bacterial family Enterobacteriaceae that causes a severe form of dysentery in humans. The *dysenteriae* species of *Shigella* is most common in Asia and is particularly virulent. Also called *Shigella shigae.*

**shigellosis** /shig′əlō′sis/ [Kiyoshi Shiga, Gk, *osis,* condition], an acute bacterial infection of the bowel, characterized by diarrhea, abdominal pain, and fever. It is transmitted by hand-to-mouth contact with the feces of individuals infected with bacteria of a pathogenic species of the genus *Shigella.* These organisms may be carried in the stools of asymptomatic people for up to several months and may be spread through contact with contaminated objects, food, or flies, especially in poor, crowded areas. The disease occurs in isolated outbreaks in the United States but is endemic in underdeveloped areas of the world. It is especially common and usually most severe in children. Diagnosis is made by isolating and identifying *Shigella* in a specimen of stool. The likelihood of encountering or engendering antibiotic-resistant organisms is very high; therefore the preferred treatment for shigellosis is supportive and the major goal is prevention of dehydration. Antimicrobials are given if the disease is severe or if the likelihood of further transmission is great. Antidiarrheal agents should be avoided. Isolation and strict handwashing precautions are instituted. Shigellosis infections must be reported to the public health department. Also called **bacillary dysentery.**

**shim,** a thin tapered piece of material used to fill a gap.

**shin bone.** See **tibia.**

**shingles.** See **herpes zoster.**

**shin splints** [AS, *scinu,* shin; ME, *splinte*], lower-leg pain caused by strain of the long flexor muscle of the toes during strenuous athletic activity, such as running. In many instances, shin splints are the result of inadequate training. Treatment usually involves rest and exercise therapy. Surgery is sometimes necessary.

**shipyard eye.** See **epidemic keratoconjunctivitis.**

**Shirodkar's operation** /shir′odkärz′/ [N. V. Shirodkar, Indian obstetrician, 1900–1971], a surgical procedure called a cerclage in which the cervical canal is closed by a purse-string suture embedded in the uterine cervix encircling the canal. It is performed to correct an incompetent cervix that has failed to retain previous pregnancies. Under spinal block or general anesthesia, a 5 mm wide band of nonabsorbable material is buried beneath the mucosa of the cervix and pulled in a purse-string manner to close the cervix. The band may be left in place permanently, in which case subsequent deliveries are by cesarean section. Occasionally, a temporary cerclage is done, sewing in the band and leaving the ends exposed in the vagina. The band is then removed before labor and vaginal delivery. Postoperatively, infection or vaginal fistula may occur. If labor begins with the suture in place, the suture is removed promptly or the infant is delivered by cesarean section, before the uterus ruptures.

**shivering** /shiv′əring/, involuntary contractions of muscles, mainly of the skin, in response to the chilling effect of low temperatures. Shivering may also occur at the onset of a fever when the body's heat balance is disturbed.

**shock** [Fr, *choc*], an abnormal condition of inadequate blood flow to the body's tissues, with life-threatening cellular dysfunction. The condition is usually associated with inadequate cardiac output, hypotension, oliguria, changes in peripheral blood flow resistance and distribution, and tissue damage. Causal factors include hemorrhage, vomiting, diarrhea, inadequate fluid intake, or excessive renal loss, resulting in hypovolemia. Kinds of shock include **anaphylactic shock, septic shock, cardiogenic shock, hypovolemic shock,** and **neurogenic shock.**
■ OBSERVATIONS: Hypovolemic shock is the most common. There is decreased blood flow with a resulting reduction in the delivery of oxygen, nutrients, hormones, and electrolytes to the body's tissues and a concomitant decreased removal of metabolic wastes. Pulse and respirations are increased. Blood pressure may decline after an initial slight increase. The patient often shows signs of restlessness and anxiety, an effect related to decreased blood flow to the brain. There also may be weakness, lethargy, pallor, and a cool, moist skin. As shock progresses, the body temperature falls, respirations become rapid and shallow, and the pulse pressure (the difference between systolic and diastolic blood pressures) narrows as compensatory vasoconstriction causes the diastolic pressure to be elevated or maintained in the face of a falling systolic blood pressure. Urinary output is reduced. Hemorrhage may be apparent or concealed, although other factors, such as vomiting or diarrhea, may account for the deficiency of body fluids.
■ INTERVENTIONS: Fluid volume must be restored quickly so there can be a rapid return of oxygenated blood to the perfusion-deprived tissues. Supplemental oxygen should be administered. Blood volume is expanded with IV fluids, such as a lactated Ringer's solution or a 5% dextrose in normal saline solution. Packed red blood cells, plasma, and plasma substitutes are also given for shock of hemorrhagic origin. Metabolic acidosis may result from anaerobic metabolism.
■ NURSING CONSIDERATIONS: After vital functions are restored and diagnosis has been made, the patient in shock must be monitored continuously until recovery is assured. The patient should remain flat in bed, but the lower extremities can be raised to improve venous return (modified Trendelenburg position). The Trendelenburg position should be avoided because it tends to push the abdominal organs against the diaphragm and increases the work of breathing. Position changes should be made slowly. Vasoactive drugs may be ordered when the blood volume is adequate. The patient's skin color, temperature, vital signs, intake and output, pulse oximetry, and level of consciousness should be monitored closely.

**shock lung.** See **adult respiratory distress syndrome.**

**shock management,** a nursing intervention from the Nursing Interventions Classification (NIC) defined as facilitation of the delivery of oxygen and nutrients to systemic tissue with removal of cellular waste products in a patient with severely altered tissue perfusion. See also **Nursing Interventions Classification.**

**shock management: cardiac,** a nursing intervention from the Nursing Interventions Classification (NIC) defined as promotion of adequate tissue perfusion for a patient with severely compromised pumping function of the heart. See also **Nursing Interventions Classification.**

**shock management: vasogenic,** a nursing intervention from the Nursing Interventions Classification (NIC) defined as promotion of adequate tissue perfusion for a patient with severe loss of vascular tone. See also **Nursing Interventions Classification.**

**shock management: volume,** a nursing intervention from the Nursing Interventions Classification (NIC) defined as promotion of adequate tissue perfusion for a patient with severely compromised intravascular volume. See also **Nursing Interventions Classification.**

**shock prevention,** a nursing intervention from the Nursing Interventions Classification (NIC) defined as detecting and treating a patient at risk for impending shock. See also **Nursing Interventions Classification.**

**shock therapy** [Fr, *choc* + GK, *therapeia*], a psychotherapeutic procedure for treating depression and other severe disorders by producing an epileptiform convulsion in the patient. The shock is induced by delivering an electric current through the brain under controlled conditions, using an anesthetic and close monitoring. See also **electroconvulsive therapy.**

**shock treatment.** See **shock therapy.**

**shock trousers,** pneumatic trousers designed to counteract hypotension associated with internal or external bleeding, and hypovolemia. They may also be used to splint or stabilize pelvic fractures. Shock trousers are contraindicated in patients with pulmonary edema, cardiogenic shock, increased intracranial pressure, or eviscerations.

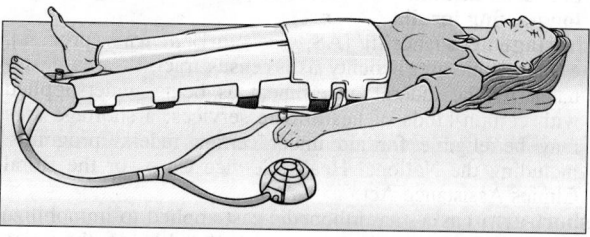

**Shock trousers** *(Lewis, Collier, and Heitkemper, 1996)*

■ METHOD: The shock trousers are used when the patient loses consciousness, has a decreased or falling blood pressure, and shows signs of respiratory distress, such as dyspnea, rapid breathing, a cough, and pink, frothy sputum. The leg pulses may be diminished or absent, and the feet may appear pale, mottled, and cold. Before the pressurized trou-

sers are applied, they are checked for tears or leaks and the proper functioning of their valves; any kinks or twists in the tubes connecting the trousers to the pneumatic pump are removed. The patient is placed in a flat, supine position over the open trousers, and the leg sections and part that encircles the abdomen just below the rib cage are firmly secured in place by closing the self-adhesive (Velcro) straps or zippers. The exact times at which the trousers' sections are inflated are recorded, and the inflated sections are checked every 15 minutes. The patient's blood pressure, respiration, and apical and peripheral pulses also are checked every 15 minutes, and chest sounds are auscultated hourly. Parenteral fluids, whole blood, plasma protein fractions, and other plasma volume expanders are administered as ordered; the flow rate of expanders is adjusted according to central venous pressure readings. An indwelling urethral catheter is connected to a closed gravity drainage system, and fluid intake and output are measured hourly; if less than 30 mL of urine per hour is excreted, renal failure may occur. Monitoring of blood gases and intermittent suctioning through a nasogastric tube may be ordered. The trousers are not deflated or removed until the blood volume replacement is stable and the patient's physician is in attendance. As each section of the trousers, starting with the abdominal section, is gradually deflated, the patient's blood pressure, respiration, and apical pulse are checked every 5 to 10 minutes; if the blood pressure drops 4 to 6 mm Hg, deflation is stopped.
■ INTERVENTIONS: The nurse checks, applies, and inflates the shock trousers and remains with the patient during the entire procedure. The vital signs are monitored at frequent intervals, parenteral fluids and plasma volume expanders are given, measures of the intake and output are taken and recorded, and emotional support is provided. Also called **military antishock trousers.**

**shoe cookies.** See **navicular pads.**

**short-acting** [AS, *sceort* + L, *agere,* to do], pertaining to or characterizing a therapeutic agent, usually a drug, with a brief period of effectiveness, generally beginning soon after the substance or measure is administered.

**short-acting insulin,** a clear preparation of regular (crystalline zinc) insulin with an immediate (15 to 30 minutes) onset of action that reaches a peak of action in 2 to 4 hours. The duration of action is 6 to 8 hours. There is considerable variation in individual patients and with different doses in the same patient; therefore these data should be considered only as rough guidelines. Also called **rapid-acting insulin.** See also **insulin.** Compare **intermediate-acting insulin, long-acting insulin.**

**shortage area** /shôr′tij/ [AS, *sceort* + L, *acticum,* process], a geographic area, county as a census tract, or area designated by the federal government as being undersupplied with certain kinds of health care services; a shortage area may be eligible for aid under certain federal programs, including the National Health Service Corps or the Rural Clinics Assistance Act.

**short-arm cast,** an orthopedic cast applied to immobilize the hand or wrist; it incorporates the hand below the wrist. The short-arm cast is used in treating fractures, for maintaining postoperative positioning, and for correcting or maintaining the correction of deformities of the hand and the wrist. Compare **long-arm cast.** See also **cast.**

**short bones,** bones that occur in clusters and usually permit movement of the extremities, such as the carpals and tarsals.

**short-bowel syndrome** [AS, *sceort* + OFr, *boel* + Gk, *syn,* together, *dromos,* course], a loss of intestinal surface for absorption of nutrients caused by the surgical removal of a section of bowel. Treatment is with parenteral nutrition in the acute phase.

**short central artery,** a branch from the precommunical part of the anterior cerebral artery.

**short course tuberculosis chemotherapy,** a 6-month treatment regimen for patients with tuberculosis who would otherwise continue to receive medications for at least 18 to 24 months after sputum has a negative finding for tubercle bacilli. The short course requires a combination of four drugs: isoniazid, rifampin, pyrazinamide, and either ethambutol, or streptomycin.

**short-gut syndrome,** **1.** any of the malabsorption conditions resulting from massive resection of the small bowel, the degree and kind of malabsorption depending on the site and extent of the resection; it is characterized by diarrhea, steatorrhea, and malnutrition. **2.** a congenital disorder in which an infant's intestine is too short or underdeveloped to allow normal food digestion. The child is maintained on parenteral nutrition until the intestine grows, develops further, or is replaced by surgical transplantation. A small child who becomes dependent on parenteral feeding may have to be taught chewing and swallowing processes when the short-gut syndrome is eventually corrected.

**shorting** [AS, *sceort*], the fraudulent practice of dispensing a quantity of drug less than that called for in the prescription and of charging for the quantity specified in the prescription. See also **kiting.**

**short-leg cast,** an orthopedic cast used for immobilizing fractures in the lower extremities from the toes to the knee. The short-leg cast is also used for treating severe sprains and torn soft tissue of the ankle, for maintaining postoperative positioning and immobilization of the foot and the ankle, and for correcting or maintaining the correction of deformities of the foot or the ankle. Compare **long-leg cast.** See also **cast.**

**short-leg cast with walker,** an orthopedic cast with rubber walkers on the bottom. It immobilizes the leg from the toes to the knee and allows the patient to walk.

**Short Portable Mental Status Questionnaire,** a 10-item questionnaire used to screen older adults for cognitive impairment. It tests orientation, remote and recent memory, practical skills, and mathematical ability.

**short-PR-normal-QRS syndrome.** See **Lown-Ganong-Levine syndrome.**

**short sight.** See **myopia.**

**shortsightedness.** See **myopia, nearsightedness.**

**short stature** [AS, *sceort,* short; L, *statura,* man's height], a body height that is less than 70% of the average for a population of the same age, culture, gender, and other peer factors.

**short-term memory,** memory of recent events, generally the first to be affected in Alzheimer's disease.

**short-wave diathermy** [AS, *sceort* + *wafian* + Gk, *dia* + *therme,* heat], a method of providing heat deep in the body by short-wave electrical currents. The high-frequency short-wave uses wavelengths of from 3 to 30 meters. It is used to treat chronic arthritis, bursitis, sinusitis, and other conditions.

**shotgun therapy** [AS, *scot* + ME, *gonne* + Gk, *therapeia,* treatment], *informal.* any treatment that has a wide range of effects and that therefore can be expected to correct an abnormal condition even though the particular cause is unknown. Shotgun therapy may cause more than an acceptable rate of side effects and is rarely desirable or necessary.

**shoulder** [AS, *sculder*], the junction of the clavicle, scapula, and humerus where the arm attaches to the trunk of the body.

**shoulder blade.** See **scapula.**

**shoulder girdle** [AS, *sculder* + *gyrdel*], a partial arch at the top of the trunk formed by the scapula and clavicle.

**shoulder-hand syndrome,** a neuromuscular condition characterized by pain and stiffness in the shoulder and arm, limited joint motion, swelling of the hand, muscle atrophy, and decalcification of the underlying bones. The condition occurs most commonly after myocardial infarction.

**shoulder joint,** the ball and socket articulation of the humerus with the scapula. The joint includes eight bursae and five ligaments, including the glenoidal labrum that deepens the articular cavity and protects the edges of articulating bones. It is the most mobile joint in the body. Also called **humeral articulation.**

**shoulder presentation** [AS, *sculder* + L, *praesentare*, to show], the part of the fetus that occupies the center of the birth canal when the presentation is associated with a transverse or oblique lie.

**shoulder spica cast,** an orthopedic cast used to immobilize the trunk of the body to the hips, the wrist, and the hand. It incorporates a diagonal shoulder support between the hip and arm parts. The shoulder spica cast is used in the treatment of shoulder dislocations and injuries and in the positioning and immobilization of the shoulder after surgery.

**shoulder subluxation,** the separation of the humeral head from the glenoid cavity, resulting in strain on the soft tissues surrounding the shoulder joint.

**show.** See **vaginal bleeding.**

**Shprintzen's syndrome.** See **velocardiofacial syndrome.**

**shreds** [AS, *screade*, piece cut off], glossy filaments of mucus in the urine, indicating inflammation in the urinary tract. Also called **mucous shreds.**

**Shulman's syndrome.** See **eosinophilic fasciitis.**

**shunt** [ME, *shunten*], **1.** to redirect the flow of a body fluid from one cavity or vessel to another. **2.** a tube or device implanted in the body to redirect a body fluid from one cavity or vessel to another. See also **left-to-right shunt, right-to-left shunt.**

**shu points** /shoo/, acupressure points.

**Shy-Drager syndrome** /shī′drā′gər/ [G. Milton Shy, American neurologist, 1919–1967; Glenn A. Drager, American physician, b. 1917], a rare progressive neurologic disorder of young and middle-aged adults. It is characterized by orthostatic hypotension, bladder and bowel incontinence, atrophy of the iris, anhidrosis, tremor, rigidity, incoordination, ataxia, and muscle wasting. Treatment includes drug therapy to control motor symptoms and to maintain adequate blood pressure. Antigravity stockings may prevent pooling of blood in the lower extremities. See also **orthostatic hypotension.**

**Shy-Magee syndrome.** See **central core disease.**

**Si,** symbol for the element **silicon.**

**SI,** abbreviation for *Système International d'Unités,* the French name for the **International System of Units.**

**SIADH,** abbreviation for **syndrome of inappropriate antidiuretic hormone secretion.**

**sial-.** See **sialo-.**

**sialadenitis** /sī′əlad′ənī′tis/, inflammation of one or more of the salivary glands. Also called **sialoadenitis.**

**sialemesis** /sī′ələmē′sis/, vomiting of saliva, or vomiting associated with excessive salivation.

**-sialia,** combining form meaning '(condition of the) saliva': *asialia, oligosialia, polsialia.*

**sialidase.** See **neuraminidase.**

**sialidosis** /sī′əlidō′sis/, a neuronal storage disease of children caused by a deficiency of the enzyme sialidase (neuraminidase). The condition is characterized by a cherry-red spot on the macula, progressive myoclonus, and seizures. There are two types. Type 1 patients have normal physical features and beta-galactosidase levels; type 2 patients also have short stature, bony abnormalities, and beta-galactosidase deficiency.

**sialo-, sial-,** combining form meaning 'saliva or the salivary glands': *sialoaerophagy, sialoangitis, sialostenosis.*

**sialoadenitis.** See **sialadenitis.**

**sialogenous.** See **salivatory.**

**sialogogue** /sī·al′əgog′/ [Gk, *sialon,* saliva, *agogos,* leading], anything that stimulates, promotes, or produces the secretion of saliva.

**sialogram** /sī·al′əgram′/ [Gk, *sialon,* saliva, *gramma,* record], a radiographic image of the salivary glands and ducts.

**sialography** /sī·əlog′rəfē/ [Gk, *sialon* + *graphein,* to record], the radiographic examination of the salivary glands after injection of a radiopaque contrast medium. —**sialographic,** *adj.*

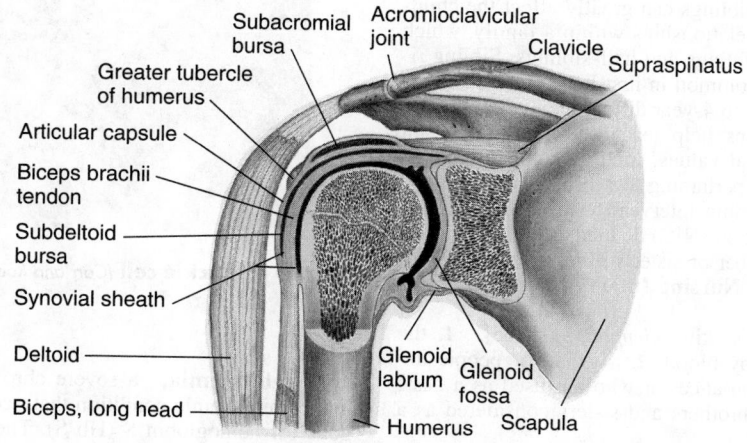

**Shoulder joint** *(Seidel, 1999)*

Labels: Subacromial bursa; Acromioclavicular joint; Clavicle; Supraspinatus; Greater tubercle of humerus; Articular capsule; Biceps brachii tendon; Subdeltoid bursa; Synovial sheath; Deltoid; Biceps, long head; Glenoid labrum; Glenoid fossa; Humerus; Scapula

**sialolith** /sī·al′əlith/ [Gk, *sialon* + *lithos,* stone], a calculus formed in a salivary gland or duct.

**sialolithiasis** /-lithī′əsis/, a pathologic condition in which one or more calculi, or stones, are formed in a salivary gland.

**sialorrhea** /sī·al′ərē′ə/ [Gk, *sialon* + *rhoia,* flow], an excessive flow of saliva that may be associated with various conditions, such as acute inflammation of the mouth, mental retardation, mercurialism, pregnancy, teething, alcoholism, or malnutrition. Also called **hypersalivation, ptyalism.**

**Siamese twins** /sī′əmēz/ [Chang and Eng, conjoined twins born in Siam (now Thailand) in 1811], conjoined equally developed twin fetuses produced from the same ovum. The severity of the condition ranges from superficial fusion, such as of the umbilical vessels, to that in which the heads or complete torsos are united and several internal organs are shared. With modern surgical techniques, most Siamese twins can be successfully separated. See also **conjoined twins.**

**sib** [AS, *sibb,* kin], pertaining to a close blood relationship. See also **sibling.**

**siberian ginseng,** an herb harvested from a shrub found throughout the world, primarily in Russia and China.
■ USES: This herb is used to improve appetite, to improve circulation, and to treat memory loss, hypertension, insomnia, rheumatism, heart ailments, diabetes, and headache.
■ CONTRAINDICATIONS: Siberian ginseng should not be used during pregnancy and lactation, in children, in those with known hypersensitivity to this product or other ginsengs, or in those with hypertension. Do not use Siberian ginseng for more than 90 days without a rest period.

**Siberian tick typhus** /sībir′ē·ən/ [Siberia], a mild acute febrile illness seen in north, central, and east Asia, caused by *Rickettsia siberica,* transmitted by ticks. It is characterized by a diffuse maculopapular rash, headache, conjunctival inflammation, and a small ulcer or eschar at the site of the tick bite. Treatment with chloramphenicol or tetracycline is associated with an excellent prognosis. Also called **North Asian tick-borne rickettsiosis.** See also **rickettsia, typhus.**

**sibilant** /sib′ilənt/ [L, *sibilare,* to hiss], a hissing sound or one in which the predominant sound is /s/.

**sibilant rhonchus.** See **wheeze** (def. 1).

**Siblin,** trademark for a bulk laxative containing psyllium seed.

**sibling** /sib′ling/ [AS, *sibb,* kin], **1.** also called *(informal)* **sib.** One of two or more children who have both parents in common; a brother or sister. The number, age differences, sex, and birth order of siblings can greatly affect the childhood environment and relationships within a family, which also may include step-siblings and half-siblings. Sibling rivalry and jealousy are common in first-born children, especially when there is a 2- to 4-year difference in age. In general, sibling relationships help teach the child important social patterns and moral values, such as competitiveness, loyalty, and sharing. **2.** pertaining to a brother or sister.

**sibling support,** a nursing intervention from the Nursing Interventions Classification (NIC) defined as assisting a sibling to cope with a brother or sister's illness/chronic condition/disability. See also **Nursing Interventions Classification.**

**sibship** /sib′ship/ [AS *sibb,* kin, *scieppan,* to shape], **1.** the state of being related by blood. **2.** a group of people descended from a common ancestor who are used as a basis for genetic studies. **3.** brothers and sisters considered as a group.

**sibutramine,** an appetite suppressant.
■ INDICATIONS: Sibutramine is used to treat obesity in conjunction with other treatments.

■ CONTRAINDICATIONS: The following factors prohibit the use of sibutramine: known hypersensitivity to this drug, hypothyroidism, anorexia nervosa, severe hepatic/renal disease, uncontrolled hypertension, cerebrovascular accident, history of coronary artery disease, congestive heart failure, dysrhythmias, pregnancy, and lactation.
■ ADVERSE EFFECTS: Tachycardia is a life-threatening effect of this drug. Other adverse reactions include headache, insomnia, seizures, stimulation, drowsiness, dizziness, nervousness, emotional lability, hypotension, palpitations, vasodilation, anorexia, constipation, dry mouth, taste aberration, nausea, increased appetite, dysmenorrhea, laryngitis, pharyngitis, rhinitis, sinusitis, rash, and sweating.

**sic** [L], thus.

**sicc-,** combining form meaning 'dry': *siccative, siccolabile, siccostabile.*

**sicca complex** /sik′ə/, abnormal dryness of the mouth, eyes, or other mucous membranes. The condition is seen in patients with Sjögren's syndrome, sarcoidosis, amyloidosis, and deficiencies of vitamins A and C.

**siccant** /sik′ənt/ [L, *siccus,* dry], **1.** drying, removing moisture. **2.** an agent that promotes drying. Also **desiccant.**

**sick,** experiencing symptoms of physical illness, such as nausea, aches and pains, dizziness, weakness, blurred vision, or malaise.

**sick building syndrome,** a condition characterized by fatigue, headache, dry eyes, and respiratory complaints affecting workers in certain buildings with limited ventilation. The symptoms seem to be caused by a combination of chemical agents in low concentrations rather than a specific irritant.

**sick cell syndrome,** a condition characterized by idiopathic hyponatremia in patients with either acute or chronic illness.

**sick euthyroid syndrome,** a nonthyroidal condition characterized by abnormalities in hormone levels and function tests findings related to the thyroid gland. The condition occurs in patients with severe systemic disease.

**sickle cell** [AS, *sicol,* crescent; L, *cella,* storeroom], an abnormal crescent-shaped red blood cell containing hemoglobin S, characteristic of sickle cell anemia.

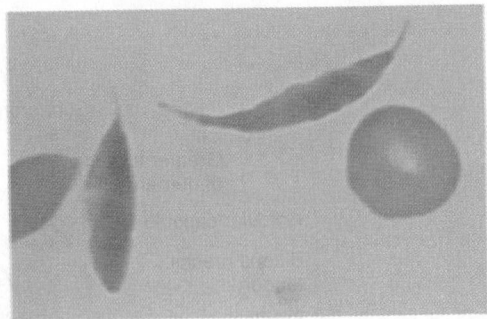

**Sickle cell** *(Carr and Rodak, 1999)*

**sickle cell anemia,** a severe chronic incurable hemoglobinopathic anemic condition that occurs in people homozygous for hemoglobin S (Hb S). The abnormal hemoglobin results in distortion and fragility of the erythrocytes. Sickle cell anemia is characterized by crises of joint pain, thrombosis, and fever and by chronic anemia, with splenomegaly,

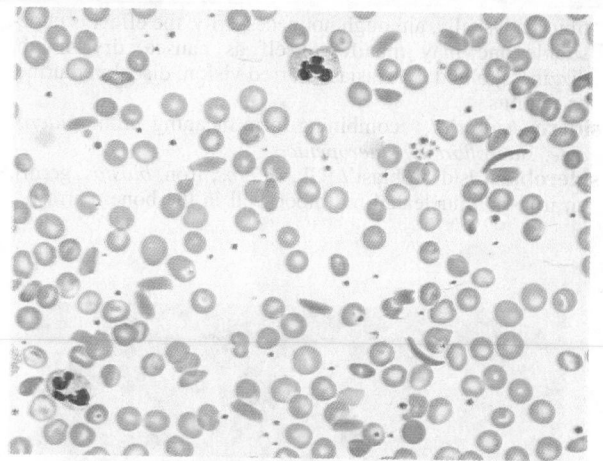

**Sickle cell anemia: peripheral blood smear**
*(Kumar, Cotran, and Robbins, 1997/courtesy
Dr. Robert W. McKenna, Department of Pathology,
University of Texas Southwestern Medical School, Dallas)*

lethargy, and weakness. See also **congenital nonspherocytic hemolytic anemia, dactylitis, elliptocytosis, hemoglobin S, sickle cell crisis.**

**sickle cell crisis,** an acute episodic condition that occurs in
children with sickle cell anemia. The crisis may be vasoocclusive, resulting from the aggregation of misshapen erythrocytes, or anemic, resulting from bone marrow aplasia,
increased hemolysis, folate deficiency, or splenic sequestration of erythrocytes. See also **hemoglobin S, sickle cell
anemia.**
■ OBSERVATIONS: Painful vasoocclusive crisis is the most
common of the sickle cell crises. It is usually preceded by an
upper respiratory or GI infection without an exacerbation of
anemia. The clumps of sickled erythrocytes obstruct blood
vessels, resulting in occlusion, ischemia, and infarction of
adjacent tissue. Characteristics of this kind of crisis are leukocytosis, acute abdominal pain from visceral hypoxia,
painful swelling of the soft tissue of the hands and feet
(hand-foot syndrome), and migratory, recurrent, or constant
joint pain, often so severe that movement of the joint is limited. Persistent headache, dizziness, convulsions, visual or
auditory disturbances, facial nerve palsies, coughing, shortness of breath, and tachypnea may occur if the central nervous system or lungs are affected. Other problems associated with vasoocclusion include priapism, hematuria, and
retinopathy. Anemic crisis is characterized by a dramatic,
rapid drop in hemoglobin levels resulting from various
causes. Aplastic crisis resulting in severe anemia occurs because red blood cell production is diminished by acute viral,
bacterial, or fungal infection. Megaloblastic anemia (another
form of anemic crisis) results from folic acid deficiency during periods of accelerated erythropoiesis. Severe anemia between crises is not common unless a generalized state of
malnutrition exists. Hyperhemolytic crisis, characterized by
anemia, jaundice, and reticulocytosis, results from glucose-
6-phosphate dehydrogenase deficiency or occurs as a reaction to multiple transfusions. Acute sequestration crisis,
which occurs in young children 6 months to 5 years of age,
results when large quantities of blood suddenly accumulate
in the spleen, causing massive splenic enlargement, severe
anemia, shock, and, ultimately, death. Susceptibility to in-

fection is a common problem of young children with sickle
cell anemia and may be greatly increased during periods of
crisis. Systemic infection and septicemia from pneumococcus or *Haemophilus influenzae* are not uncommon and may
be rapidly fatal. In older children, local infection, especially
osteomyelitis, rather than generalized septicemia is frequently a complicating factor.
■ INTERVENTIONS: Therapy consists of immediate transfusion
of packed red cells in the acute anemic crisis and alleviation
of severe abdominal and joint pain with analgesics or narcotics as needed in vasoocclusive crisis. Short-term oxygen
therapy, hydration by oral or IV means, electrolyte replacement to counteract metabolic acidosis resulting from
hypoxia, and antibiotics to treat any existing infection may
be necessary. Pneumococcal and meningococcal vaccine is
recommended for children between 2 and 5 years of age because they are highly susceptible to infection. Partial exchange transfusions are often mandatory in life-threatening
crises, such as when sickling occurs in the vessels of the
brain or lungs, and may be used as a preventive technique;
multiple transfusions, however, increase the risk of hepatitis,
hemosiderosis, and transfusion reactions. Oral anticoagulants have been used to relieve the pain of vasoocclusion,
but these increase the risk of bleeding. Priapism, a painful
condition frequently seen in vasoocclusive crisis, may be
treated by aspirating the corpora cavernosa. In children with
recurrent splenic sequestration, splenectomy may be a lifesaving procedure. The process is not routinely recommended because surgery increases the risk of acidosis and
hypoxia from anesthesia, and, in time, the spleen usually atrophies through progressive fibrotic changes. Infarction of
tissue in any organ is a potential hazard in sickle cell crisis,
and special management and treatment are warranted by the
specific site of damage. Typical complications include uremia (requiring renal transplantation or hemodialysis),
chronic functional pulmonary impairment, aseptic necrosis
of the hip, and microvascular occlusion that may lead to venous thrombosis.
■ NURSING CONSIDERATIONS: The primary concern of the nurse
during a crisis is to initiate procedures that reduce sickling.
Foremost is prevention of tissue deoxygenation and resulting hypoxia by maintaining bed rest to minimize energy expenditure and oxygen use, although some exercise is necessary to promote circulation. Hydration and electrolyte
balance are essential. A complete record of fluid intake and
output is maintained, and adequate therapy is calculated accordingly. Serum sodium level is monitored closely to prevent hyponatremia. Oxygen is given in severe anoxia, although prolonged administration depresses bone marrow
activity and thus aggravates anemia. Management of pain in
vasoocclusion is often difficult and may require experimentation with various drugs and schedules before the patient
receives adequate relief. The application of warmth is often
soothing; cold is contraindicated, because it enhances vasoconstriction and sickling. The nurse constantly monitors the
child's condition for splenomegaly, infection, evidence of
shock or cerebrovascular accident, hypervolemia, transfusion reaction, or increasing anemia. An important aspect of
nursing care is the continued emotional support of parents
whose child has a chronic illness that is potentially fatal.

**sickle cell dactylitis** [AS, *sicol* + L, *cella,* storeroom; Gk,
*daktylos,* finger, *itis,* inflammation], a painful inflammation of one or more fingers caused by an attack of sickle cell
anemia.

**sickle cell disease,** any of the diseases associated with the
presence of hemoglobin S and sickle cells, including **sickle
cell anemia, sickle cell–hemoglobin C disease, sickle
cell–hemoglobin D disease,** and **sickle cell–thalassemia.**

**sickle cell—hemoglobin C disease.**    See **hemoglobin S-C disease.**

**sickle cell—hemoglobin D disease.**    See **hemoglobin SD disease.**

**sickle cell thalassemia,** a heterozygous blood disorder in which the genes for sickle cell and for thalassemia are both inherited. A mild form and a severe form may be identified, depending on the degree of suppression of beta-chain synthesis by the thalassemia gene. In the mild form synthesis is only partially suppressed, and the red cell may contain from 25% to 35% normal hemoglobin A along with a greater concentration of hemoglobin S. The clinical course is relatively mild. In the severe form, beta-chain synthesis is completely suppressed and only hemoglobin S appears in the red cells. The clinical course is generally as severe as in homozygous sickle cell anemia. See also **hemoglobinopathy, hemoglobin S, hemoglobin SC (Hb SC) disease.**

**sickle cell trait,** the heterozygous form of sickle cell anemia, characterized by the presence of both hemoglobin S and hemoglobin A in the red blood cells. Anemia and the other signs of sickle cell anemia do not occur. People who have the trait are informed of and counseled about the possibility of having an infant with sickle cell disease if both parents have the trait. See **hemoglobin S.**

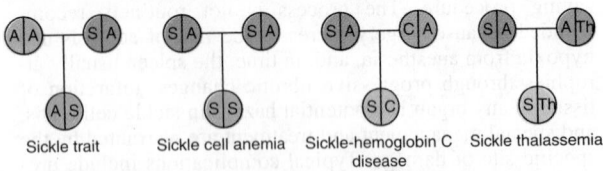

Sickle trait     Sickle cell anemia     Sickle-hemoglobin C disease     Sickle thalassemia

**Sickle cell inheritance pattern**

**sickling,** the development of sickle-shaped red blood cells, as in sickle cell anemia.

**sick role** [AS, *seoc* + Fr, stage character], a behavior pattern in which a person adopts the symptoms of a physical or mental disorder to be cared for, sympathized with, and protected from the demands and stresses of life.

**sick sinus syndrome (SSS)** [AS, *seoc* + L, *sinus,* hollow], a complex of arrhythmias associated with sinus node dysfunction. The condition may result from a variety of cardiac diseases, ranging from cardiomyopathies to inflammatory myocardial disease. It is most commonly related to either intermittent sinoatrial (SA) block or inadequate SA conduction. SSS is characterized by severe sinus bradycardia, either alone, alternating with tachycardia, or accompanied by atrioventricular block. The most common symptoms are lethargy, weakness, light-headedness, dizziness, and syncope. The severity of symptoms is related to the duration of the asystolic period. Elderly patients with episodes of near-syncope associated with a history of palpitations are most likely to be symptomatic. Accurate diagnosis requires electrocardiography. At present the only treatment is the implantation of a permanent pacemaker.

**SICU,** abbreviation for *surgical intensive care unit.*

**side effect** [AS, *side* + L, *effectus*], any reaction to or consequence of a medication or therapy. This can be an effect carried beyond the desired limit, such as hemorrhaging from an anticoagulant, or a reaction unrelated to the primary object of the therapy, such as an anaphylactic reaction to an an-

tibiotic. Usually, although not necessarily, the effect is undesirable and may manifest itself as nausea, dry mouth, dizziness, blood dyscrasias, blurred vision, discolored urine, or tinnitus.

**sidero-** /sid'ərō-/, combining form meaning 'iron': *siderocyte, siderofibrous, sideropenic.*

**sideroblast** /sid'ərōblast'/ [Gk, *sideros,* iron, *blastos,* germ], an iron-rich nucleated red blood cell in the bone marrow.

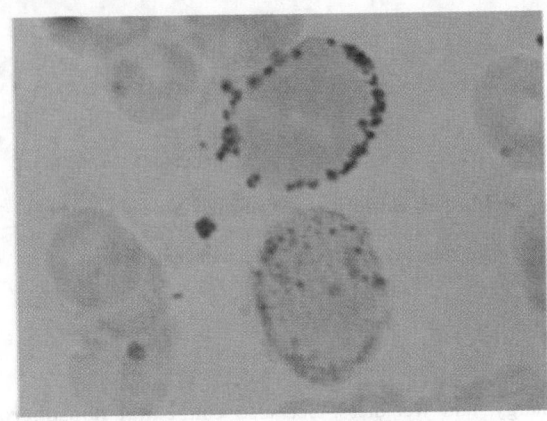

**Sideroblast** *(Carr and Rodak, 1999)*

**sideroblastic anemia** /sid'ərōblas'tik/ [Gk, *sideros,* iron, *blastos,* germ], a heterogeneous group of chronic hematologic disorders characterized by normocytic or slightly macrocytic anemia, hypochromic and normochromic red blood cells, and decreased erythropoiesis and hemoglobin synthesis. The red blood cells contain a perinuclear ring of iron-stained granules. The condition may be acquired or hereditary, and primary or secondary to another condition. The

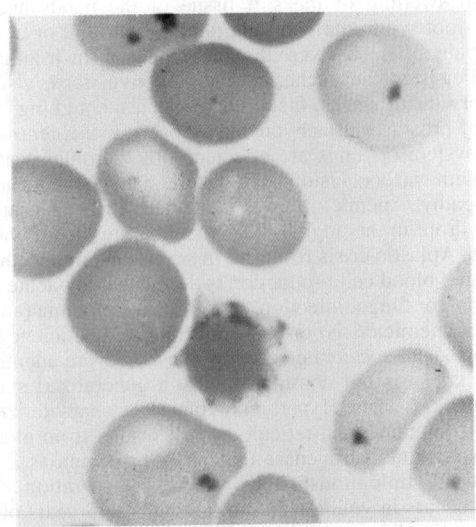

**Sideroblastic anemia** *(Zitelli and Davis, 1997)*

cause of the disease is not understood. Treatment may include extract of liver, pyridoxine, folic acid, and blood transfusion. Also spelled **sideroblastic anaemia.** Compare **iron deficiency anemia, siderosis.**

**siderocyte** /sid'ərosīt'/ [Gk, *sideros,* iron, *kytos,* cell], an abnormal erythrocyte in which particles of nonhemoglobin iron are visible.

**sideroderma** /sid'ərodur'mə/, a bronze skin coloration caused by accumulation of iron from hemoglobin degeneration.

**sideropenia** /sid'əropē'nē·ə/, an abnormally low level of serum iron.

**sideropenic dysphagia.** See **Plummer-Vinson syndrome.**

**siderosis** /sid'ərō'sis/ [Gk, *sideros + osis,* condition], **1.** a variety of pneumoconiosis caused by the inhalation of iron dust or particles. **2.** the introduction of color in any tissue caused by the presence of excess iron. **3.** an increase in the amount of iron in the blood. See also **hemochromatosis, hemosiderosis, sideroblastic anemia.**

**siderotic granules** /sid'ərot'ik/, inclusion bodies seen in the red blood cells of splenectomy patients and in cases of hemoglobin synthesis and hemolytic anemia. The granules contain iron, which takes a Prussian blue stain.

**siderotic splenomegaly,** an enlarged spleen associated with fibrosis and an excessive accumulation of iron and calcium. The condition is seen in sickle cell disease and hematochromatosis.

**side-to-side anastomosis.** See **anastomosis.**

**SIDS,** abbreviation for **sudden infant death syndrome.**

**SIECUS** /sē'kəs/, abbreviation for *Sex Information and Education Council of the United States.*

**siemens (S)** /sē'mens/ [Ernst Werner von Siemens, German electric inventor, 1816-1892], a unit of electrical conductance of a body with a resistance of 1 ohm, allowing 1 ampere of current to flow per volt applied.

**sievert (Sv)** /sē'vərt/ [R.M. Sievert, twentieth-century Swedish physicist], a measure of radiation dose. The sievert has the same units as the gray and is equal to the absorbed dose times the quality factor, which compares the health consequences of that type of radiation with those of x-rays. The rem bears the same relationship to the rad as the sievert does to the gray.

**sig.,** abbreviation for the Latin *signetur,* 'let it be labeled (according to prescription).'

**sigh.** See **periodic deep inspiration.**

**sight** /sīt/ [AS, *gesiht*], **1.** the special sense that enables the shape, size, position, and color of objects to be perceived; the faculty of vision. It is the principal function of the eye. **2.** that which is seen.

**sigma** /sig'mə/, Σ, σ and s, the eighteenth letter of the Greek alphabet.

**Sigma Theta Tau International** /sig'mə thā'tə tou'/, an international honor society for nurses. Registered nurses and student nurses are invited to join based on academic achievement or contributions to nursing.

**sigmoid** /sig'moid/ [Gk, *sigma,* the letter S, *eidos,* form], **1.** pertaining to an S shape. **2.** the sigmoid colon.

**sigmoid-,** prefix meaning 'sigmoid colon'; the section of the colon shaped like the Greek letter sigma: *sigmoidoscope, sigmoidectomy.*

**sigmoid colon,** the part of the colon that extends from the one descending colon in the pelvis to the juncture of the rectum. Also called **sigmoid flexure.**

**sigmoidectomy** /sig'moidek'təmē/ [Gk, *sigma + eidos + ektomē,* excision], excision of the sigmoid flexure of the colon, most commonly performed to remove a malignant tu-

mor. A large percentage of cancers of the lower bowel occur in the sigmoid colon.

**sigmoid flexure.** See **sigmoid colon.**

**sigmoiditis** /sig'moidī'tis/, an inflammation of the sigmoid colon.

**sigmoid mesocolon** /mez'ōkō'lən/ [Gk, *sigma + eidos + mesos,* middle, *kolon*], a fold of peritoneum that connects the sigmoid colon with the pelvic wall, forming a curved line of attachment, with the apex of the curve located at the division of the left common iliac artery. The fold is continuous with the iliac mesocolon and ends in the median plane over the rectum at the level of the third sacral vertebra. Between the two layers of the fold are the sigmoid and the superior rectal vessels. Compare **mesentery proper, transverse mesocolon.**

**sigmoid notch,** a concavity on the superior surface of the mandibular ramus between the coronoid and condyloid processes.

**sigmoidoscope** /sigmoi'dəskōp'/ [Gk, *sigma + eidos + skopein,* to look], an instrument used to examine the lumen of the sigmoid colon. It consists of a tube and a light, allowing direct visualization of the mucous membrane lining the colon. Compare **proctoscope.**

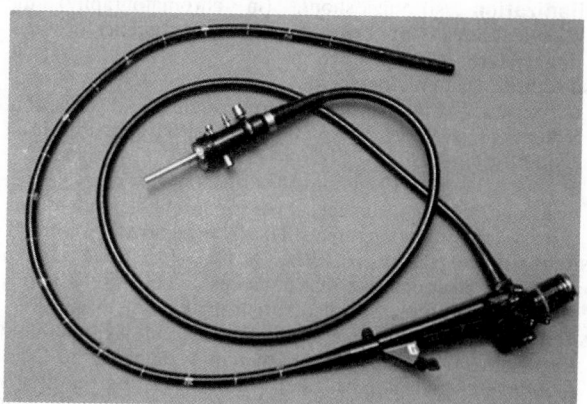

**Flexible sigmoidoscope** *(Doughty and Broadwell, 1993)*

**sigmoidoscopy** /sig'moidos'kəpē/, the inspection of the rectum and sigmoid colon by the aid of a sigmoidoscope.

**sigmoidostomy** /sig'moidos'təmē/, the surgical creation of an anus in the pelvic colon.

**sign** /sīn/ [L, *signum,* mark], an objective finding as perceived by an examiner, such as a fever, a rash, the whisper heard over the chest in pleural effusion, or the light band of hair seen in children after recovery from kwashiorkor. Many signs accompany symptoms; for example, erythema and a maculopapular rash are often seen with pruritus. Compare **symptom.**

**signal molecule** /sig'nəl/ [L, *signum,* mark], a hormone, neurotransmitter, or other agent that transfers information from one cell or organ to another. Examples include steroid hormones, insulin, and growth factors. A photon may have a similar effect on a retinal receptor.

**signal node.** See **Virchow's node.**

**signal symptom.** See **symptom.**

**signal-to-noise ratio (SNR),** the number used to describe the relative contributions to a detected signal of the true signal and random superimposed signals or "noise."

**signature** /sig'nəchər/ [L, *signare,* to mark], (in pharmacy) a part of a prescription containing instructions to the patient about dosage and manner and frequency of administration.

**signe de journal.** See **thumb sign.**

**significance** /signif'ikəns/ [L, *significare,* to signify], **1.** (in research) the statistical probability that a given finding may have occurred by chance alone. The conventional standard for attributing significance is a finding that occurs fewer than 5 times in 100 by chance alone ($p < .05$). **2.** the importance of a study in developing a practice or theory, as in nursing practice.

**significance level,** the probability of incorrectly rejecting the null hypothesis when such a hypothesis is tested. See also **Type I error.**

**significant other** /signif'ikənt/, a person who is considered by an individual as being special and as having an effect on that individual.

**sign language** [L, *signum* + *lingua,* tongue], a form of communication often used with and among deaf people consisting of hand and body movements. Many variations exist, including American Sign Language (**Ameslan**). Other forms of manual communication are Signed English and finger spelling. Compare **body language.**

**sign-off.** See **logoff.**

**sign-on.** See **login.**

**silanization** /sil'ənizā'shən/, (in chromatography) the chemical process of converting the SiOH moieties of a stationary form to the ester form.

**sildenafil,** an erectile agent.

■ INDICATIONS: Sildenafil is used to treat erectile dysfunction.

■ CONTRAINDICATIONS: Known hypersensitivity to this drug prohibits its use.

■ ADVERSE EFFECTS: Common side effects of this drug include headache, flushing, dizziness, dyspepsia, nasal congestion, urinary tract infection, abnormal vision, diarrhea, and rash.

**silent disease** /sī'lənt/ [L, *silens* + *dis* + Fr, *aise,* ease], a disease or other disorder that produces no clinically obvious signs or symptoms. See also **subclinical.**

**silent ischemia** [L, *silere,* to be silent], an asymptomatic form of myocardial ischemia that may damage the heart muscle. Ischemia is most likely to occur during the first 6 hours after a person awakens in the morning. It is triggered by mental arousal in more than 75% of patients. In contrast, cardiac ischemia accompanied by anginal pains is usually triggered by physical exertion.

**silent mutation,** an alteration in a DNA sequence that does not result in an amino acid change in a polypeptide.

**silent myocardial infarction,** an interruption in blood flow to the coronary arteries without the usual signs and symptoms of a heart attack. Such infarctions may be associated with diabetes.

**silent peritonitis** [L, *silere* + Gk, *peri* + *teinein,* to stretch, *itis,* inflammation], a case of peritonitis that develops without clinical signs or symptoms.

**silhouette sign** /sil'ōo·et'/, a radiographic artifact caused by an infiltrate that obscures the demarcating line between lung segments.

**silica (SiO₂)** /sil'i·kə/ [L, *silex,* flint], silicon dioxide, an inorganic compound occurring in nature as agate, sand, amethyst, flint, quartz, and other stones. It is one of the major constituents of dental porcelain and a common filler in resin composites; in granular form it serves as a dental abrasive and polishing agent. See also **silicosis.**

**silica gel** /sil'ikə/, a coagulated form of hydrated silica, used as an absorbent of gases and as a dehydrating agent.

**silicate cement** /sil'i·kāt/ [L, *silex,* flint + *caementum,* rough stone], a dental cement that is translucent and porcelain-like when set; formerly used for esthetic temporary and semipermanent restorations of anterior teeth.

**silicic acid** /silis'ik/, hydrated silicon dioxide. It is used in thin-layer and column chromatography.

**silico-,** combining form meaning 'silica or quartz': *silicosis, silicosiderosis, silicotuberculosis.*

**silicon (Si)** /sil'ikon/ [L, *silex,* flint], a nonmetallic element, second to oxygen as the most abundant of the elements in earth's crust. Its atomic number is 14; its atomic mass is 28.09. It occurs in nature as silicon dioxide and in silicates. The silicates are used as detergents, corrosion inhibitors, adhesives, and sealants. Elemental silicon is used in metallurgy and in transistors and other electronic components. About 60% of the rocks in the earth's crust contain silicon, and silica dusts are associated with many mining operations. Protracted inhalation of silica dusts can cause silicosis, which increases the susceptibility to other pulmonary diseases.

**silicone** /sil'ikōn/ [L, *silex,* flint], any of a large group of inert polymers. Silicones are water-repellent and stable at high temperature. They are useful in medicine as adhesives, lubricants, and sealants. They are used in glass chromatography and in coating of glassware for blood collection as they help reduce platelet loss. They are also used as a substitute for rubber, especially in prosthetic devices. Elastomeric silicone, or silicon rubber, is biologically inert. See also **silicone-gel breast implant.**

**silicone-gel breast implant,** a type of implant used in reconstructive surgery of the breast and made with synthetic polymers. The implants have been associated with adverse effects on the immune system as well as distorted and painful breasts caused by leakage of the silicone into surrounding tissues. However, a number of statistical studies have not established such a cause-and-effect relationship.

**silicone septum,** a vascular access device used in IV therapy. It consists of a silicone partition that covers the port chamber housed in the metal or plastic body of an implanted infusion port.

**silicophosphate cement** /sil'i·kō·fos'fāt/, a mixture of silicate and zinc phosphate cements, formerly used as temporary filling material and for cementation of orthodontic bands, indirect restorations, and porcelain jacket crowns.

**silicosis** /sil'ikō'sis/, a lung disorder caused by continued long-term inhalation of the dust of an inorganic compound, silicon dioxide, which is found in sands, quartzes, flints, and many other stones. Silicosis is characterized by the development of nodular fibrosis in the lungs. In advanced cases, severe dyspnea may develop. The incidence of silicosis is highest among industrial workers exposed to silica powder in manufacturing processes; in those who work with ceramics, sand, or stone; and in those who mine silica. Also called **grinder's disease, quartz silicosis.** See also **chronic obstructive pulmonary disease, inorganic dust.**

**silk suture** [AS, *seolc* + L, *sutura,* seam], a braided fine suture material, usually used to close incisions, wounds, and cuts in the skin. It is not absorbed by the body and is removed after approximately 7 days.

**silo filler's disease** /sī'lō/ [Fr, *ensilotage,* ensilage; AS, *fyllan,* to fill], a rare acute respiratory condition seen in agricultural workers who have inhaled nitrogen oxide as they work with fermented fodder in closed, poorly ventilated areas such as silos. Characteristically, symptoms of respiratory distress and pulmonary edema occur several hours after exposure. Loss of consciousness may occur. Observation in the hospital and respiratory assistance often are required. The condition is rarely fatal.

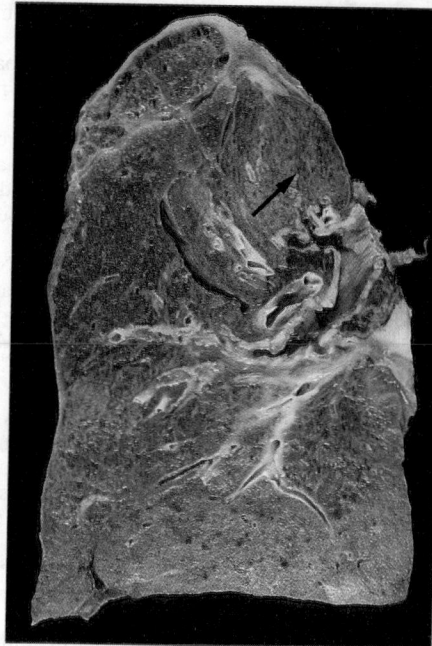

**Silicosis**
*(Kumar, Cotran, and Robbins, 1997/courtesy Dr. John Godleski, Brigham and Women's Hospital, Boston)*

**Silvadene,** trademark for an antibacterial (sulfadiazine silver).

**silver (Ag)** [AS, *seolfor*], a whitish precious metal occurring mainly as a sulfide. Its atomic number is 47; its atomic mass is 107.88. It is quite soft and is usually alloyed with small amounts of copper to increase its durability. Silver dissolves readily in nitric acid and is used extensively to produce silver halides used in photographic emulsions. It is frequently associated in small amounts with the ores of zinc, copper, and lead and is used extensively as a component of amalgams of dental fillings and in many medications, especially antiseptics and astringents. Some antiseptics containing silver are mild silver protein and strong silver protein, preparations that render silver colloidal in the presence of protein. Mild silver protein contains 19% to 23% silver. Strong silver protein contains 7.5% to 8.5% silver. Both preparations are used externally as antiseptics and do not have irritating properties. Silver nitrate is also used externally as an antiseptic and astringent, especially in the prevention of ophthalmia neonatorum. It is also used as a lubricant on the bearings of radiography tubes, and silver halides are used in x-ray films. Silver picrate, an ionizable salt of silver, is used in the treatment of trichomoniasis and of moniliasis of the vagina.

**silver amalgam** [AS, *seolfor* + Gk, *malagma*], an alloy of silver, tin, copper, mercury, and zinc used in dentistry to fill prepared tooth cavities.

**silver cone method,** a technique for filling tooth pulp canals. It is outdated because the silver corrodes over time and retreatment is necessary.

**Silver dwarf** [Henry K. Silver, twentieth-century American pediatrician], a person who has **Silver's syndrome,** a congenital disorder in which short stature is associated with lateral asymmetry; various anomalies of the head, face, and skeleton; and precocious puberty.

**silver-fork fracture.** See **Colles' fracture.**

**Silverman-Anderson score,** a system of assessing the degree of respiratory distress.

**silver nitrate,** a topical antiinfective.
- INDICATIONS: A 1% solution is prescribed for the prevention of gonococcal ophthalmia in newborns and stronger concentrations for use on wet dressings.
- CONTRAINDICATIONS: Known sensitivity to this drug prohibits its use. It should not be used with bacitracin, which inactivates it.
- ADVERSE EFFECTS: Among the more serious adverse reactions are severe local inflammation, burns, and argyria.

**silver salts poisoning,** a toxic condition caused by the ingestion of silver nitrate, characterized by discoloration of the lips, vomiting, abdominal pain, dizziness, and convulsions.

**Silver's syndrome.** See **Silver dwarf.**

**silver sulfadiazine,** a topical antibiotic.
- INDICATIONS: It is prescribed to prevent or treat infection in second- and third-degree burns.
- CONTRAINDICATIONS: Known hypersensitivity to this drug, to silver, or to sulfonamides prohibits its use. It is not given in the last weeks of pregnancy or to newborn or premature infants.
- ADVERSE EFFECTS: Among the most serious adverse reactions are rashes, fungal infections, neutropenia, and kernicterus.

**silver-wire arteries,** retinal arterioles that appear as white tubes containing a red fluid when viewed through an ophthalmoscope. The condition occurs as replacement fibrosis associated with hypertension continues and the vessel wall obscures the blood column.

**simethicone** /simeth'ikōn/, an antiflatulent.
- INDICATION: It is prescribed to decrease excess gas in the GI tract.
- CONTRAINDICATIONS: There are no significant contraindications.
- ADVERSE EFFECTS: Adverse reactions include belching and rectal flatus.

**simian crease** /sim'ē·ən / [L, *simia*, ape; ME, *creste*, crest], a single crease across the palm produced from the fusion of proximal and distal palmar creases, seen in congenital disorders, such as Down syndrome. Also called **simian line.**

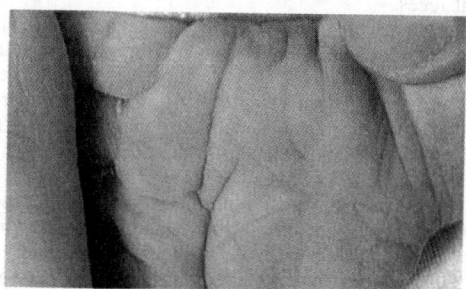

**Simian crease** *(Zitelli and Davis, 1997)*

**simian immunodeficiency virus (SIV),** a lentivirus that produces an acquired immunodeficiency syndrome-like disease in nonhuman primates. The cytopathologic changes caused by SIV are similar to those caused by the human immunodeficiency virus (HIV). SIV also shares with HIV a group of genes lacking in other retroviruses, and animals infected with either virus experience a similar decrease in the number of CD4+ lymphocytes.

**simian line.**   See **simian crease.**

**simian virus 40 (SV40),**   a vacuolating virus isolated from the kidney tissue of rhesus monkeys.

**simil-,**   combining form meaning 'like': *Similac, similimum.*

**Similac preparations,**   trademark for a group of commercial modified milk products that are prepared especially for infant feeding. They are made from a nonfat base of cow's milk supplemented with such substances as lactose, coconut and soy oils, and monosaccharides and disaccharides and fortified with vitamins and minerals. The ratio of the various nutrients, such as iron or one of the other minerals, is altered in the different preparations to accommodate infants with particular nutritional requirements or nutritional problems, such as nephrogenic diabetes insipidus. The formulas are packaged in both powder and liquid forms.

**similia similibus curantur,**   a homeopathic rule that drugs able to produce symptoms in a healthy person will also remove similar symptoms occurring as an expression of disease. See also **homeopathy.**

**Simmonds' disease.**   See **panhypopituitarism, postpubertal panhypopituitarism.**

**simplate bleeding time test,**   a blood test for determining how quickly platelets form a plug when an incision is made in the skin. Platelet plug formation is the first step in clotting and, if slower than 8 minutes, indicates platelet deficiency or the effect of a drug, such as aspirin. Also called **template bleeding time test.**

**simple, 1.** describing something composed of only one or a minimum number of parts or elements. **2.** not involved or complicated.

**simple angioma** [L, *simplex,* not mixed],   a tumor consisting of a network of small vessels or distended capillaries surrounded by connective tissue.

**simple astigmatism** [L, *simplex,* not mixed; Gk, *a + stigma,* point], **1.** simple myopic astigmatism in which one principal meridian is in focus on the retina and the other in front of it. **2.** simple hyperopic astigmatism in which one meridian is focused on the retina and the other behind it.

**simple cavity,**   a cavity that involves only one surface of a tooth.

**simple diarrhea** [L, *simplex,* not mixed; Gk, *dia + rhein,* to flow],   a form of diarrhea in which the loose stools contain normal feces.

**simple dislocation** [L, *simplex,* not mixed, *dis + locare,* to place],   displacement of a joint without a penetrating wound.

**simple figure-eight roller arm sling,**   a sling prepared by placing the patient in a supine or sitting position with the affected arm flexed and adjacent to the chest. The open sling fits under the arm and over the chest. The bandage is fixed with a single turn toward the uninjured side around the arm and chest, crossing the elbow above the external epicondyle. In the next step, the bandage is drawn forward under the tip of the elbow, after making a second turn that overlaps two thirds of the first. Then the bandage is pulled upward along the flexed arm to the base of the neck on the uninjured side. Finally, the bandage is drawn down over the scapula and across the chest and arm, overlapping and continuing in a figure-eight pattern.

**simple fission.**   See **binary fission.**

**simple fracture,**   an uncomplicated fracture in which the bone does not break the skin. It usually heals readily. Compare **compound fracture.**

**simple glaucoma** [L, *simplex,* not mixed; Gk, *glaucoma,*

cataract],   chronic open-angle glaucoma without complications but with visual field loss and optic atrophy.

**simple goiter** [L, *simplex,* not mixed, *guttur,* sore throat],   a goiter not accompanied by signs or symptoms of hyperthyroidism.

**simple guided imagery,**   a nursing intervention from the Nursing Interventions Classification (NIC) defined as purposeful use of imagination to achieve relaxation and/or direct attention away from undesirable sensations. See also **Nursing Interventions Classification.**

**simple massage,**   a nursing intervention from the Nursing Interventions Classification (NIC) defined as stimulation of the skin and underlying tissues with varying degrees of hand pressure to decrease pain, produce relaxation, and/or improve circulation. See also **Nursing Interventions Classification.**

**simple mastectomy,**   a surgical procedure in which a breast is completely removed and the underlying muscles and adjacent lymph nodes are left intact. The procedure may be performed to remove small malignant neoplasms of the breast, or it may be done as a palliative measure to remove an ulcerated carcinoma in advanced breast cancer. It also may be done prophylactically when the patient has severe fibrocystic disease and a strong family history of breast cancer. Postoperatively, the process of recovery from a simple mastectomy is less uncomfortable and faster than that from a radical or modified radical mastectomy, but nursing care is similar. Compare **modified radical mastectomy, radical mastectomy.** See also **mastectomy.**

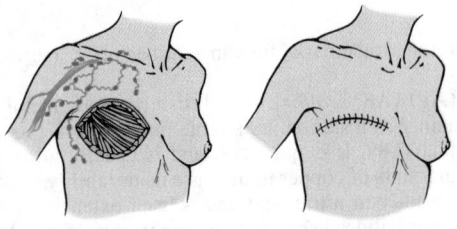

**Simple mastectomy** *(Ignatavicius, Workman, Mishler, 1999)*

**simple meningitis.**   See **sterile meningitis.**

**simple periodontal pocket.**   See **periodontal pocket.**

**simple phobia,**   an anxiety disorder characterized by a persistent, irrational fear of specific things, such as animals, dirt, light, or darkness. Compare **social phobia.** See also **phobia.**

**simple protein,**   a protein that yields amino acids as the only or chief product on hydrolysis. The class includes albumins, globulins, glutelins, alcohol-soluble proteins, albuminoids, histones, and protamines. See also **complex protein.**

**simple reflex** [L, *simplex,* not mixed, *reflectere,* to bend back],   a reflex with a motor nerve component that involves only one muscle. See also **reflex arc.**

**simple relaxation therapy,**   a nursing intervention from the Nursing Interventions Classification (NIC) defined as use of techniques to encourage and elicit relaxation for the purpose of decreasing undesirable signs and symptoms such as pain, muscle tension, or anxiety. See also **Nursing Interventions Classification.**

**simple stomatitis** [L, *simplex* + Gk, *stoma,* mouth, *itis,* inflammation],   a simple inflammation of the mucous membranes of the mouth with redness, swelling, and an excess of mucus. Also called **catarrhal stomatitis.**

**simple sugar,**   a monosaccharide, such as glucose.

**simple tubular gland,** one of the many multicellular glands with only one duct and a tube-shaped part, such as various glands within the epithelium of the intestine.

**simple vulvectomy.** See **vulvectomy.**

**Simpson forceps.** See **obstetric forceps.**

**Sims' position** [James M. Sims, American gynecologist, 1813–1883], a position in which the patient lies on the side with the knee and thigh drawn upward toward the chest. The chest and abdomen are allowed to fall forward. Left Sims' is the position of choice for administering enemas or conducting rectal examinations. Also called **semiprone side position.**

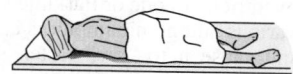

**Sims' position** *(Potter and Perry, 2001)*

**simulation** /sim'yəlā'shən/ [L, *simulare,* to imitate], a method of representing the actions of one system by those of another, as a computer program that represents the actions of something in the real world. Simulation enables a computer to explore situations that might be too expensive, dangerous, or time consuming in real life.

**simultanagnosia** /sī'multan'agnō'zhə/, a visual disorder in which a person actually perceives only one element of a picture or object at a time and is unable to absorb the whole.

**sin-, sinus-,** combining form meaning 'hollow, cavity, or to curve': *sinography, sinuses, sinusotomy.*

**sinap-,** combining form meaning 'mustard': *sinapine, sinapiscopy, sinapism.*

**sinciput** /sin'siput/ [L, half a head], the anterior or upper part of the skull. See also **bregma.**

**Sinemet,** trademark for a fixed-combination central nervous system drug containing a decarboxylase inhibitor (carbidopa) and an antiparkinsonian (levodopa).

**Sinequan,** trademark for a tricyclic antidepressant (doxepin hydrochloride).

**sinew** /sin'yoō/ [ME, *sinewe*], the tendon of a muscle, such as the thick, flattened tendon attached to the short head of the biceps brachii. See also **tendon.**

**singer's nodule.** See **vocal cord nodule.**

**single-blind study** [L, *singulus,* one by one; AS, *blind* + L, *studere,* to be busy], an experiment in which the person collecting data knows whether the subject is in the control group or the experimental group, but subjects do not. See also **double-blind study.**

**single-chain antigen-binding protein (SCAB),** a polypeptide that joins an antibody's light chain variable region to the antibody heavy chain variable region. SCABs are used as biosensors, in chemical separations, and in the treatment of cancers and heart disease.

**single component insulin** [L, *singulus* + *componere,* to bring together, *insula,* island], any highly purified insulin with less than 10 ppm of proinsulin. See also **insulin, proinsulin.**

**single footling breech.** See **footling breech.**

**single-locus probe (SLP),** a sequence of labeled DNA or RNA that can be used to identify a region of DNA tandem repeats found in the genome only once. It may be used in resolving cases of disputed parentage.

**single-parent family,** a family consisting of only the mother or the father and one or more dependent children.

**single-photon emission computed tomography (SPECT),** a variation of computed tomography in which the ray sum is defined by the collimator holes on the gamma-ray detector rotating around the patient. SPECT units usually consist of large crystal gamma cameras mounted on a gantry that permits rotation of the camera around the patient. Multiple detectors are used to reduce the imaging time.

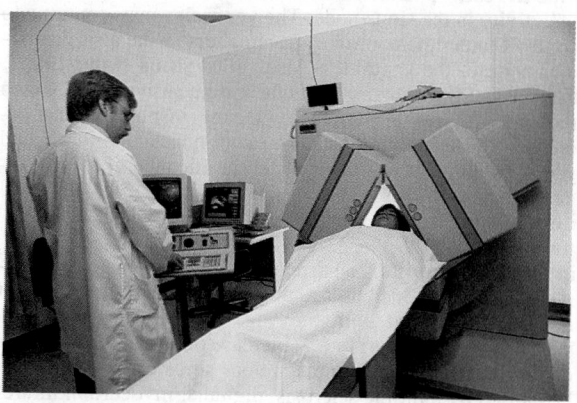

**Single-photon emission computed tomography** *(Chipps, Clanin, and Campbell, 1992)*

**single room occupant (SRO),** a single person, usually an elderly individual, who lives alone in a single room of a low-cost hotel or apartment building.

**single sweep scan,** an ultrasonic scan that is completed in a single sweep of the sensing device across the area being examined.

**singleton** /sing'gəlton/, an offspring born alone.

**singlet state** /sing'glit/, a state of an atom or molecule in which all electrons have paired spins.

**singultus.** See **hiccup.**

**sinister** /sin'istər/ [L], left, at the left side, at the left hand.

**sinistral** /sinis'trəl/ [L, *sinister,* left], relating to the left side.

**sinistrality.** See **left-handedness.**

**sinistro-,** combining form meaning 'left, or related to the left side': *sinistrocardia, sinistrophobia, sinistrotorsion.*

**sinoatrial** /sī'nō-ā'trē-əl/ [L *sinus,* hollow, *atrium,* hall], pertaining to the sinus node and atrium. Also called **sinoauricular.**

**sinoatrial (SA) block** [L, *sinus,* hollow, *atrium,* hall; Fr, *bloc*], a conduction disturbance in the heart during which an impulse formed within the sinus node is blocked or delayed from depolarizing the atria. There are two types of SA block. Type I (SA Wenckebach) is characterized on the electrocardiogram by group beating, shortening of P-P intervals, and pauses that are less than twice the shortest cycle. The P-R intervals are not affected unless there is also an atrioventricular conduction defect. In the case of a 3:2 conduction ratio, a bigeminal sinus rhythm (two sinus-conducted beats and a pause) is noted. Type II SA block is identified on the electrocardiogram by absent P waves without shortening P-P intervals. Causes include excessive vagal stimulation, acute infections, and atherosclerosis. SA block also may be an adverse reaction to quinidine or digitalis. Treatment for symptomatic SA block includes the use of atropine and isoproterenol; an electronic pacemaker is used if drug therapy is ineffective. See also **atrioventricular block, heart block, intraatrial block, intraventricular block.**

**sinoatrial (SA) node,** See **sinus node.**

**sinoauricular.** See **sinoatrial.**

**sinus** /sī'nəs/ [L, hollow], a cavity or channel, such as a cavity within a bone, a dilated channel for venous blood, or one permitting the escape of purulent material.

**sinus-.** See **sin-.**

**sinus arrest,** a heart disorder in which there is a cessation of activity in the sinus node. The ventricles may continue to contract under the control of pacemakers in the atrioventricular node or the ventricles. Also called **sinus standstill.**

**sinus arrhythmia,** an irregular cardiac rhythm in which the heart rate usually increases during inspiration and decreases during expiration. It is common in children and young adults and has no clinical significance except in elderly patients.

**sinus bradycardia,** beating of the sinus node at a rate below 60/min.

**sinus dysrhythmia,** an irregular heart rhythm characterized by alternate increases and decreases in the heart rate. It is often associated with the vagal effects of respiration, which causes the heart rate to increase on inspiration and decrease on expiration. Nonrespiratory sinus dysrhythmia can be caused by multiple sclerosis, digitalis, myocardial infarction, and increased intracranial pressure. Treatment is not necessary unless the patient is symptomatic with decreased cardiac output; then atropine is given.

**sinuses of Valsalva.** See **aortic sinus.**

**sinusitis** /sīnəsī'tis/ [L, sinus + Gk, itis, inflammation], an inflammation of one or more paranasal sinuses. It may be a complication of an upper respiratory infection; dental infection; allergy; change in atmospheric pressure, as in air travel or underwater swimming; or a structural defect of the nose. With swelling of nasal mucous membranes the openings from sinuses to the nose may be obstructed, resulting in an accumulation of sinus secretions, causing pressure, pain, headache, fever, and local tenderness. Complications include cavernous sinus thrombosis and spread of infection to bone, brain, or meninges. Treatment includes steam inhalations, nasal decongestants, analgesics, and, if infection is present, antibiotics. Surgery to improve drainage may be performed in the treatment of chronic sinusitis.

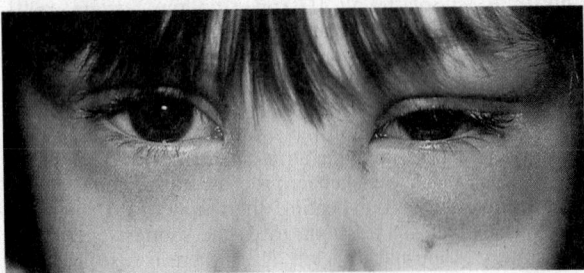

**Child with sinusitis**
(Zitelli and Davis, 1997/courtesy Dr. Ellen Wald, Children's Hospital of Pittsburgh)

**sinus node,** a cluster of hundreds of cells located in the right atrial wall of the heart, near the opening of the superior vena cava. It comprises a knot of modified heart muscle that generates impulses that travel swiftly throughout the muscle fibers of both atria, causing them to contract. Specialized pacemaker cells in the node have an intrinsic rhythm that is independent of any stimulation by nerve impulses from the brain and the spinal cord. Slender fusiform cells making up the sinoatrial node are largely filled with sarcoplasm but contain a few striated fibrillae. The cells are irregularly grouped together and, at the edge of the node, merge with the atrial musculature. The sinoatrial node will normally "fire" at a rhythmic rate of 70-75 beats/min. If the node fails to generate an impulse, pacemaker function will shift to another excitable component of the cardiac conduction system, such as the atrioventricular node or Purkinje's fibers. Certain hormones and various autonomic impulses can affect the sinoatrial node and cause it to "fire" faster, such as during strenuous physical activity. During a lifetime of 70 years the node generates about 2 billion impulses. Surgical implantation of an artificial pacemaker is a common procedure for individuals suffering from a defective sinoatrial node. Also called **Keith's bundle, Keith-Flack node, pacemaker.** Compare **atrioventricular (AV) node, Purkinje's network.** Also called **sinoatrial node, sinus pacemaker.**

**sinus node dysfunction,** any disturbance in the normal functioning of the sinus node, such as slow sinus rate or sinoatrial block, that leads to the development of arrhythmias.

**sinus of Morgagni,** sinus of Valsalva. See **aortic sinus.**

**sinusoid** /sī'nəsoid/ [L, sinus + Gk, eidos, form], an anastomosing blood vessel that is somewhat larger than a capillary and is lined with reticuloendothelial cells.

**sinus pacemaker.** See **sinus node.**

**sinus rhythm,** a cardiac rhythm stimulated by the sinus node. A rate of 60-100/min is normal.

**sinus standstill.** See **sinus arrest.**

**sinus tachycardia** [L, sinus, hollow; Gk, tachys, fast, kardia, heart], a rapid heartbeat generated by discharge of the sinus node. The rate is generally 100-180/min in the adult, although most clinicians would be suspicious of a rate of 90/min or higher. Sinus tachycardia is also indicated by a heart rate greater than 200/min in an infant and 140-200/min in a child. Sinus tachycardia is the body's normal response to exertion, congestive heart failure, cardiogenic shock, acute pulmonary embolism, acute myocardial infarction, and infarct extension.

**sinus venosus defect.** See **atrial septal defect.**

**si op. sit** (in prescriptions), abbreviation for the Latin phrase si opus sit, 'if necessary.'

**siphonage** /sī'fənij/, a process of drawing off fluid from a cavity with a tube using atmospheric pressure.

**sireniform fetus.** See **sirenomelus.**

**sirenomelia** /sī'rənəmē'lē·ə/ [Gk, seiren, mermaid, melos, limb], a congenital anomaly in which there is complete fusion of the lower extremities and no feet. Also called **apodial symmelia.**

**sirenomelus** /sī'rənom'ələs/, an infant who has sirenomelia. Also called **sireniform fetus, sympus apus.**

**siriasis** /sirī'əsis/ [Gk, sieros, scorching], sunstroke. See also **heat hyperpyrexia.**

**sirolimus,** an immunosuppressant.
- INDICATIONS: This drug is used after organ transplantation to prevent rejection. Recommended use is in combination with cyclosporine and corticosteroids.
- CONTRAINDICATIONS: Known hypersensitivity to this drug or any of its components prohibits its use.

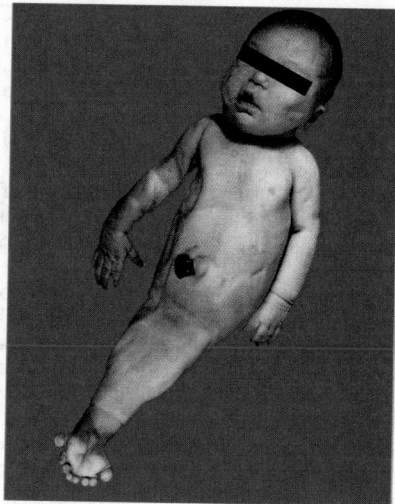

**Stillborn fetus with sirenomelia**
(Carlson, 1999/courtesy M. Barr, Ann Arbor, Michigan)

■ ADVERSE EFFECTS: Life-threatening effects of this drug are anemia, leukopenia, thrombocytopenia, purpura, albuminuria, hematuria, proteinuria, renal failure, pleural effusion, atelectasis, and lymphoma. Other adverse effects include nausea, vomiting, diarrhea, constipation, hypertension, insomnia, chills, fever, urinary tract infections, hyperglycemia, increased creatinine, edema, hypercholesterolemia, hyperlipidemia, hypophosphatemia, weight gain, hyperkalemia, hyperuricemia, hypokalemia, hypomagnesemia, blurred vision, and photophobia. Common side effects include atrial fibrillation, congestive heart failure, hypotension, palpitations, tachycardia, tremors, headache, paresthesia, dyspnea, rash, and acne.

**-sis,** suffix meaning an 'action, process, condition, state, or result of': *centesis, genesis, stasis.*

**sister,** a term used in the United Kingdom and Commonwealth for a nurse, particularly the head nurse in a hospital, a ward, or an operating room.

**Sister Joseph's nodule** [Sister Mary Joseph Dempsy, U.S. surgical assistant, 1856–1929], a malignant intraabdominal neoplasm of gastric, ovarian, colorectal, or pancreatic origin and metastatic to the umbilicus.

**Sister Kenny's treatment** [Elizabeth Kenny, Australian nurse, 1886–1952; Fr, *traitement*], poliomyelitis therapy in which the patient's limbs and back are wrapped in warm, moist woolen cloths and, after the pain subsides, the patient is taught to exercise affected muscles, especially by swimming. Equally important is passive movement of affected limbs with simultaneous stimulation at the site of muscle origins, carried out after hot packs.

**site** [L, *situs,* location], **1.** location. See also **situs. 2.** a quantum of space occupied and defined by a cluster of people.

**site visit,** a visit made by designated officials to evaluate or to gather information about a department or institution. A site visit is a step in the accreditation of an institution and in the funding of many major projects.

**-sitia,** suffix meaning '(condition of) appetite for food': *apositia, asitia, eusitia.*

**sito-, sitio-,** combining form meaning 'food': *sitomania, sitotherapy, sitiophobia.*

**sitosterol** /sītos′tərôl/ [Gk, *sitos,* food, *stereos,* solid; Ar, *alkohl,* essence], a mixture of sterols derived from plants, such as wheat germ, used for treating hyperbetalipoproteinemia and hypercholesterolemia that are unresponsive to other dietary measures. Its use is controversial, for a dispersing action in the mixture tends to cause loose bowel movements and may lead to diarrhea or interfere with the absorption of concomitantly administered medications. Use in pregnancy is not recommended.

**sitotherapy** /sī′tōther′əpē/ [Gk, *sitos,* food], a health maintenance system based on food, diet, and nutrition.

**sit-to-stand,** in the treatment of balance disorders, a movement in which the base of support is transferred from the seat to the feet. The feet begin to accept the weight first by downward pressure through the heels as the pelvis rolls anteriorly. The weight then moves to the front of the feet as the trunk moves forward and the pelvis lifts from the surface.

**situational anxiety** /sich′ōō·ā′shənəl/ [L, *situs,* location], a state of apprehension, discomfort, and anxiety precipitated by the experience of new or changed situations or events. Situational anxiety is not abnormal and requires no treatment; it usually disappears as the person adjusts to the new experience. See also **anxiety.**

**situational crisis,** (in psychiatry) an unexpected crisis that arises suddenly in response to an external event or a conflict concerning a specific circumstance. The symptoms are transient, and the episode is usually brief.

**situational depression,** (in psychiatry) an episode of emotional and psychologic depression that occurs in response to a specific set of external conditions or circumstances. See also **mood disorder.**

**situational loss,** the loss of a person, thing, or quality, resulting from alteration of a life situation, including changes related to illness, body image, environment, and death.

**situational psychosis,** (in psychiatry) a psychotic episode that results from a specific set of external circumstances.

**situational support,** a person who is available and can be depended on to help a patient solve problems.

**situational theory,** a leadership theory in which the manager chooses a leadership style to match a particular situation.

**situational therapy,** (in psychiatry) a kind of psychotherapy in which the milieu is part of the treatment program. See also **milieu therapy.**

**situation relating** /sich′ōō·ā′shən/, (in nursing research) a study design used to explain or predict phenomena in nursing practice in which a relationship is thought to exist among certain practices or characteristics of the population being studied.

**situation therapy.** See **milieu therapy.**

**situs** /sī′təs/ [L, location], the normal position or location of an organ or part of the body.

**situs inversus viscerum,** the transposition of the abdominal and thoracic organs to opposite sides of the body.

**sitz bath** /sits, zits/ [Ger, *Sitz,* seat; AS, *bæth*], a bath in which only the rectal and perineal areas are immersed in water or saline solution. The procedure is used after childbirth and after rectal or perineal surgery to decrease swelling, inflammation, and pain.

**SI units** [Fr, système international], the international units of physical amounts. Examples of these units are the mass of a kilogram, the length of a meter, and the precise amount of time in a second.

**SIV,** abbreviation for **simian immunodeficiency virus.**

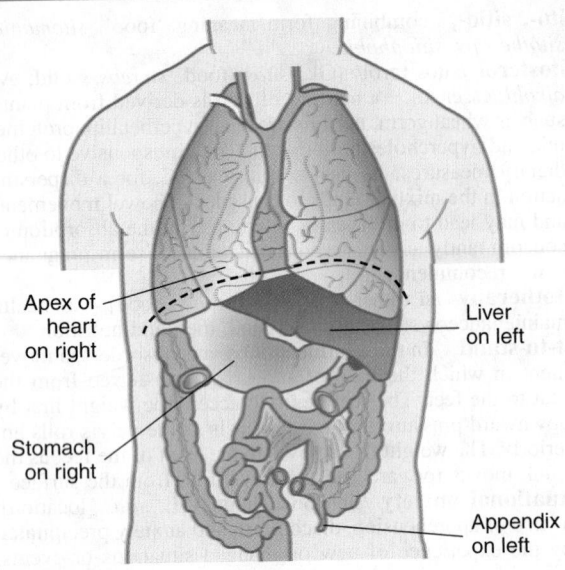

Apex of
heart
on right

Liver
on left

Stomach
on right

Appendix
on left

**Complete situs inversus in an adult** *(Carlson, 1999)*

**sixth cranial nerve.** See **abducens nerve.**

**sixth disease.** See **roseola infantum.**

**Sjögren-Larsson syndrome** /shō′grenlär′sən/ [Torsten Sjögren, Swedish pediatrician, 1859–1939; T. Larsson, twentieth-century Swedish pediatrician], a congenital condition, inherited as an autosomal recessive trait, characterized by ichthyosis, mental deficiency, and spastic paralysis.

**Sjögren's syndrome** [Henrik S.C. Sjögren, Swedish ophthalmologist, 1899–1986], an immunologic disorder characterized by deficient fluid production by the lacrimal, salivary, and other glands, resulting in abnormal dryness of the mouth, eyes, and other mucous membranes. The symptoms primarily affect women over 40 years of age. Atrophy of the lacrimal glands can lead to desiccation of the cornea and conjunctiva with damage to the tissues. Atrophy of the salivary glands results in dental disorders and loss of taste and odor sensations. When the lungs are affected, the dryness increases susceptibility to pneumonia and other respiratory infections. Sjögren's syndrome is frequently associated with Raynaud's phenomenon, rheumatoid arthritis, Waldenström's macroglobulinemia, and lymphoma. Treatment includes applying artificial tears and using soft contact lenses that can be moistened often, sipping fluids frequently to prevent mouth dryness, and avoiding medications that tend to deplete body fluids. See also **dry eye syndrome, keratoconjunctivitis sicca.**

**SK,** abbreviation for **streptokinase.**

**SK-65 Compound,** trademark for a fixed-combination drug containing analgesics (propoxyphene hydrochloride, aspirin, and phenacetin) and a stimulant (caffeine).

**SK-Ampicillin,** trademark for an antibacterial (ampicillin).

**skato-.** See **scato-.**

**SK-Bamate,** trademark for a sedative (meprobamate).

**skelalgia** [Gk, *skelos,* leg], pain in the leg.

**skeletal.** See **skeleton.**

**skeletal fixation** /skel′ətəl/ [Gk, *skeletos,* dried up; L, *figere,* to fasten], any method of holding together the fragments of a fractured bone by the attaching of wires, screws, plates, or nails. See also **external pin fixation.**

**skeletal function,** a nursing outcome from the Nursing Outcomes Classification (NOC) defined as the functional ability of the bones to support the body and facilitate movement. See also **Nursing Outcomes Classification.**

**skeletal muscle.** See **striated muscle.**

**skeletal survey,** the radiographic examination of the skeletal system for possible fractures or tumors.

**skeletal system,** all of the bones and cartilage of the body that collectively provide the supporting framework for the muscles and organs. See also the Color Atlas of Human Anatomy.

**skeletal traction,** one of the two basic kinds of traction used in orthopedics for the treatment of fractured bones and the correction of orthopedic abnormalities. Skeletal traction is applied to the affected structure by a metal pin or wire inserted into the structure and attached to traction ropes. Skeletal traction is often used when continuous traction is desired to immobilize, position, and align a fractured bone properly during the healing process. Infection of the pin tract is one of the complications that may develop with skeletal traction, and careful scrutiny of pin sites is an important precaution. Some common signs of infection of the pin tracts are erythema, drainage, noxious odor, pin slippage, temperature elevation, and pain. Superficial infection of pin tracts is often treated with antibiotic therapy. Deeper infections usually require pin removal and antibiotic therapy. Compare **skin traction.** See also **Dunlop skeletal traction.**

**skeleto-,** combining form meaning 'skeleton': *skeletogenous, skeletonic.*

**skeleton** /skel′ətən/ [Gk, *skeletos,* dried up], the supporting framework for the body, comprising 206 bones in the adult that protect delicate structures, provide attachments for muscles, allow body movement, serve as major reservoirs of blood, and produce red blood cells, platelets, and most white blood cells. The skeleton is divided into the axial skeleton, which has 74 bones; the appendicular skeleton, with 126 bones; and the 6 auditory ossicles. The four types of bones composing the skeleton are the long bones, including the humerus, the ulna, the femur, the tibia, the fibula, and the phalanges of the fingers and the toes; the short bones, including the carpals and the tarsals; the flat bones, including the frontal bone and the parietal bone of the cranium, the ribs, and the shoulder bones; and the irregular bones, including the vertebrae, the bones of the sacrum, the bones of the coccyx, and certain bones of the skull, such as the sphenoid, the ethmoid, and the mandible. The skeleton changes throughout life as bone formation and bone destruction proceed concurrently. During childhood and adolescence, bone formation proceeds faster than bone destruction. Starting at 35 to 40 years of age, bone destruction proceeds faster than bone formation. In advanced age bone destruction increases, bones become thin and brittle, vertebrae may collapse, and height decreases. See also **bone,** and see the Color Atlas of Human Anatomy. —**skeletal,** *adj.*

**Skene's duct.** See **paraurethral duct.**

**Skene's glands** /skēnz/ [Alexander J.C. Skene, American gynecologist, 1838–1900], the largest of the glands opening into the urethra of women. They contain ducts that open immediately within the urethral orifice.

**skew** /skyo͞o/ [ME, *skewen,* to escape], a deviation from a line or symmetric pattern, such as data in a research study that do not follow the expected statistical curve of distribution because of the unwitting introduction of another variable.

**skia-, scia-,** combining form meaning 'shadows, especially of internal structures as produced by roentgen rays': *skiabaryt, skiagenol, skiagraph.*

**skilled nursing facility (SNF)** [ME, *skil,* distinction], an institution or part of an institution that meets criteria for accreditation established by the sections of the Social Security Act that determine the basis for Medicaid and Medicare reimbursement for skilled nursing care. Skilled nursing care includes rehabilitation and various medical and nursing procedures. Written policies and protocols are formulated with appropriate professional consultation. Law requires that these policies designate which level of caregiver is responsible for implementation of each policy, that the care of every patient be under the supervision of a physician, that a physician be available on an emergency basis, that records of the condition and care of every patient be maintained, that nursing service be available 24 hours a day, and that at least one full-time registered nurse be employed. Other criteria stipulate that the facility have appropriate facilities for storing and dispensing drugs and biologics, that it maintain a use review plan, that all licensing requirements of the state in which it is located be met, and that an overall budget be maintained.

**Skillern's fracture** /skil′ərnz/ [Penn G. Skillern, American surgeon, b. 1882], an open fracture of the distal radius associated with a greenstick fracture of the distal ulna.

**skill play** [ME, *skil + plega,* sport], a form of play in which a child persistently repeats an action or activity until it has been mastered, such as throwing or catching a ball.

**skills training,** the teaching of specific verbal and nonverbal behaviors and the practicing of these behaviors by the patient.

**skimmed milk** [Dan, *skumme,* scum removal; AS, *meolc*], milk from which the fat has been removed. Most of the vitamin A is removed with the cream, although other nutrients remain. It is available as fluid skimmed milk, fortified skimmed milk, nonfat dry milk, and a form of buttermilk. Also called **nonfat milk, skim milk.**

**skimming** [Dan, *skumme*], a practice, sometimes used by health programs that receive their income on a prepaid or capitation basis, of seeking to enroll only relatively healthy individuals as a means of increasing profits by decreasing costs. See also **skimping.**

**skimping** [Swed, *skrympa,* to shrink], a practice, some-times used by health programs that receive their income on a prepaid or capitation basis, of delaying or denying services to enrolled members of the program as a means of increasing profits by decreasing costs. See also **skimming.**

**skin** [AS, *scinn*], the tough, supple cutaneous membrane that covers the entire surface of the body. It is composed of a thick layer of connective tissue called the dermis and an epidermis made of five layers of cells. Skin color varies according to the amount of melanin in the epidermis. Genetic differences determine the amount of melanin. The ultraviolet rays of the sun stimulate the production of melanin, which absorbs the rays and simultaneously darkens the skin. Modified skin continues into various parts of the body, such as mucous membrane, as in the lining of the vagina, the bladder, the lungs, the intestines, the nose, and the mouth. Mucous membrane lacks the heavily keratinized layer of the outside skin. The skin helps to cool the body when the temperature rises by radiating the heat of increased blood flow in expanded blood vessels and by providing a surface for the evaporation of sweat. When the temperature drops, the blood vessels constrict and the production of sweat diminishes. Also called **cutaneous membrane, integument.** See also **dermis.**

**skin barrier,** an artificial layer of skin, usually made of plastic, applied to skin before the application of tape or ostomy drainage bags. It protects the real skin from chronic irritation.

**skin button,** a plastic and fabric device that covers the drivelines of an artificial heart at their exit point from the skin. Its purpose is to prevent the transmission of pumping pressure to the surrounding tissues.

**skin cancer,** a cutaneous neoplasm caused by ionizing radiation, certain genetic defects, or chemical carcinogens, including arsenics, petroleum, tar products, and fumes from some molten metals, or by overexposure to the sun or other sources of ultraviolet light. Skin cancers, the most common and most curable malignancies, are also the most frequent secondary lesions in patients with cancer in other sites. Risk factors are a fair complexion, xeroderma pigmentosa, vitiligo, senile and seborrheic keratitis, Bowen's disease, radiation dermatitis, and hereditary basal cell nevus syndrome.

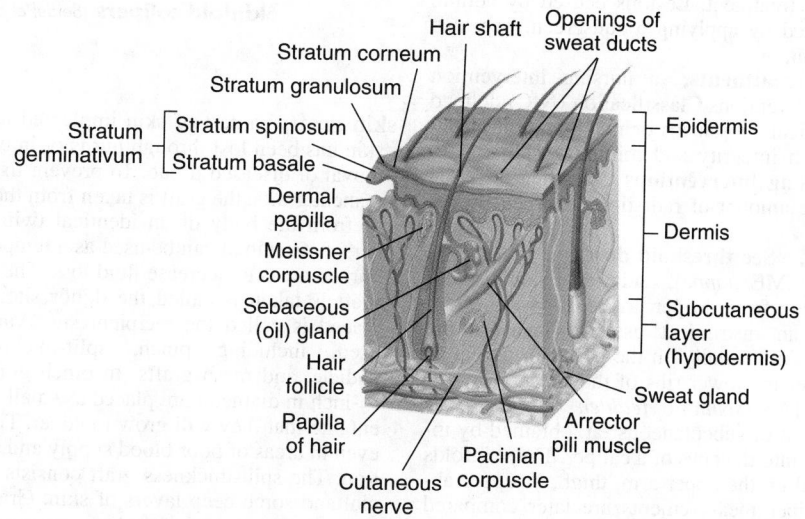

**Cross section of the skin** *(Thibodeau and Patton, 1999/Rolin Graphics)*

## Skin color variations

| Color | Condition | Causes | Assessment locations |
|---|---|---|---|
| Bluish (cyanosis) | Increased amount of deoxygenated hemoglobin (associated with hypoxia) | Heart or lung disease, cold environment | Nail beds, lips, mouth, skin (severe cases) |
| Pallor (decrease in color) | Reduced amount of oxyhemoglobin | Anemia | Face, conjunctivae, nail beds, palms of hands |
| | Reduced visibility of oxyhemoglobin resulting from decreased blood flow | Shock | Skin, nail beds, conjunctivae, lips |
| Loss of pigmentation | Vitiligo | Congenital or autoimmune condition causing lack of pigment | Patchy areas on skin over face, hands, arms |
| Yellow-orange (jaundice) | Increased deposit of bilirubin in tissues | Liver disease, destruction of red blood cells | Sclera, mucous membranes, skin |
| Red (erythema) | Increased visibility of oxyhemoglobin caused by dilation or increased blood flow | Fever, direct trauma, blushing, alcohol intake | Face, area of trauma, sacrum, shoulders, other common sites for pressure ulcers |
| Tan-brown | Increased amount of melanin | Suntan, pregnancy | Areas exposed to sun: face, arms; areolae, nipples |

From Potter PA, Perry AG: *Fundamentals of nursing: concepts, process, and practice,* ed 5, St Louis, 2001, Mosby.

The most common skin cancers are basal cell carcinomas and squamous cell carcinomas. Tumors of the sebaceous glands or sweat glands occur infrequently and are adenocarcinomas. Basal cell carcinomas, typically raised hard reddish lesions with a pearly surface, rarely metastasize. Scaly, slightly elevated squamous cell tumors may become growths with extensive ulceration and a nonhealing scab. A definitive diagnosis may be established by incisional biopsy or by excisional biopsy, which may be the only treatment required for small lesions. Surgery is usually indicated if the lesion is large, if bone or cartilage is invaded, or if lymph nodes are involved. Radiotherapy may be preferable for some smaller facial lesions and is commonly recommended for the treatment of skin tumors without distinct margins. Because of the possibility of recurrence of cancer, surgery is favored for the treatment of younger patients. Despite the curability of skin cancer, it causes many deaths because people fail to obtain treatment. Lesions caused by actinic rays may be prevented by applying a sunscreen. See also **malignant melanoma.**

**skin care: topical treatments,** a nursing intervention from the Nursing Interventions Classification (NIC) defined as application of topical substances or manipulation of devices to promote skin integrity and minimize skin breakdown. See also **Nursing Interventions Classification.**

**skin dose (SD),** the amount of radiation absorbed by the skin.

**skin erythema dose.** See **threshold dose.**

**skin flap** [AS, *scinn* + ME, *flappe*], a layer of skin, usually separated by dissection from deeper layers of tissue.

**skinfold calipers,** an instrument used to measure the breadth of a fold of skin, usually on the posterior aspect of the upper arm or over the lower ribs of the chest.

**skinfold thickness** [AS, *scinn* + *fealden* + *thicce*], a measure of the amount of subcutaneous fat, obtained by inserting a fold of skin into the jaws of a caliper. The skinfolds are usually measured on the upper arm, thigh, or upper abdomen, and the caliper measurements are later compared with precalibrated standard tables to assess an individual's body fat content indirectly.

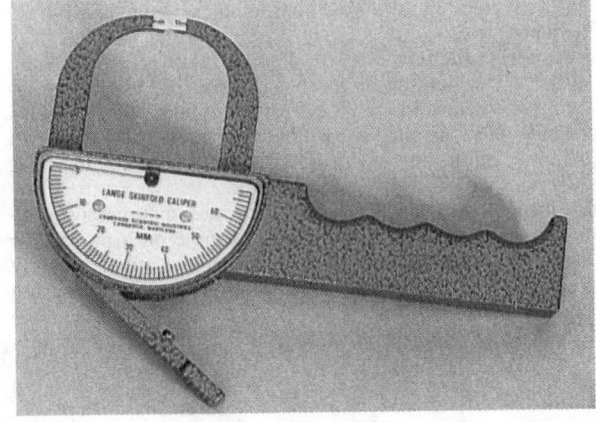

**Skinfold calipers** *(Seidel et al, 1999)*

**skin graft,** a part of skin implanted to cover areas where skin has been lost through burns or injury or by surgical removal of diseased tissue. To prevent tissue rejection of permanent grafts, the graft is taken from the patient's own body or from the body of an identical twin. Skin from another person or animal can be used as a temporary cover for large burned areas to decrease fluid loss. The area from which the graft is taken is called the donor site; that on which it is placed is called the recipient site. Various techniques are used, including pinch, split-thickness, full-thickness, pedicle, and mesh grafts. In pinch grafting, pieces of skin ¼-inch in diameter are placed as small islands on the recipient site that they will grow to cover. These grafts will grow even in areas of poor blood supply and are resistant to infection. The split-thickness graft consists of sheets of superficial and some deep layers of skin. Grafts of up to 4 inches wide and 10 to 12 inches long are removed from a flat surface—abdomen, thigh, or back—with an instrument called a dermatome. The grafts are sutured into place; compression dressings may be applied for firm contact, or the area may be left exposed to the air. A split-thickness graft cannot be used for weight-bearing parts of the body or for covering those subject to friction, such as the hand or foot. A full-thickness graft contains all skin layers and is more durable and effective for weight-bearing and friction-prone areas. A pedicle graft is one in which a part remains attached to the donor site whereas the remainder is transferred to the recipient site. Its own blood supply remains intact, and it is not detached until the new blood supply has fully developed. This type is often used on the face, neck, or hand. A successful new graft of any type is well established in about 72 hours and can be expected to survive unless a severe infection or trauma occurs. The procedure may be done with local anesthesia. Before surgery both the donor and the recipient site must be free of infection and the recipient site must have a good blood supply. After surgery stretching or movement of the recipient site is prevented. Strict sterile technique is used for handling dressings, and antibiotics may be given prophylactically to prevent infection. Good nutrition with a high-protein, high-calorie diet is essential. See also **autograft, graft, xenograft.**

**skin integrity, impaired,** a nursing diagnosis accepted by the Fourth National Conference on the Classification of Nursing Diagnoses. It is defined as a state in which an individual's skin is adversely altered.

■ DEFINING CHARACTERISTICS: The defining characteristics include disruption of the skin surface, destruction of cell layers of the skin, and invasion of body structures through the skin.

■ RISK FACTORS: Risk factors may be environmental (external) or somatic (internal). Environmental factors that may affect the development of impaired skin integrity include heat, cold, or chemical substances; mechanical factors, such as shearing force or pressure, restraint, or laceration; radiation; physical immobilization; and humidity. Somatic factors include drugs, obesity or emaciation, malnutrition, metabolic disturbance, circulatory disturbance, altered sensation or pigmentation, developmental factors, immunologic deficit, a disturbance in excretions or secretions, psychogenic factors, edema, or change in the turgor of the skin. See also **nursing diagnosis.**

**skin integrity, impaired, risk for,** a nursing diagnosis accepted by the Fourth National Conference on the Classification of Nursing Diagnoses. It is defined as a state in which an individual's skin is at risk of being adversely altered.

■ RISK FACTORS: Risk factors may be environmental (external) or somatic (internal). Environmental factors include hypothermia or hyperthermia; presence of an injurious chemical substance; shearing force or pressure, restraint, or laceration; radiation; physical immobilization; presence on the skin of excretions or secretions; and abnormally high humidity. Somatic factors include reaction to some medications; obesity or emaciation; an abnormal metabolic state; alteration in circulation, sensory function, or pigmentation; skeletal bony prominences; adverse developmental factors; decrease in normal skin turgor; and psychogenic or immunologic abnormalities. See also **nursing diagnosis.**

**Skinner box** [Burrhus F. Skinner, American psychologist, 1904–1990; L, *buxus,* boxwood], a boxlike laboratory apparatus used in operant conditioning in animals, usually containing a lever or other device that when pressed reinforces by either giving a reward, such as food or an escape outlet, or removing a punishment, such as an electric shock. Also called **standard environmental chamber.** See also **operant conditioning.**

**skin pigment** [AS, *scinn* + L, *pigmentum,* paint], any skin coloring caused by melanin deposits in skin and hair. The coloring may be modified by substances in the blood, such as the several blood pigments, bile, or malarial parasites.

**skin prep,** a procedure for cleansing the skin with an antiseptic before surgery or venipuncture. Skin preps are performed to kill bacteria and pathologic organisms and to reduce the risk of infection. Various skin prep devices are available for this procedure. Such devices are commonly constructed of plastic, filled with a specific antiseptic, and equipped with an applicator. The antiseptic is applied by rubbing the device in a circular motion over the skin. Some of the most common antiseptics contained in skin prep devices are iodine, povidone-iodine, and ethyl alcohol. Each antiseptic has associated advantages and disadvantages. The iodine skin prep kills bacteria, fungi, viruses, protozoa, and yeasts and is an inexpensive and reliable device. The disadvantages of iodine, in addition to its discoloring of the skin, are that it may burn or chap and may cause an allergic reaction. Povidone-iodine, which consists of water-soluble complexes of iodine and organic compounds, is less irritating than iodine tinctures or solutions and does not stain the skin as much as iodine. However, povidone-iodine is less effective than regular iodine solutions, may be absorbed through the skin during prolonged use, and may cause an allergic reaction. Ethyl alcohol, which is not effective against spore-forming organisms, viruses, and tubercle bacilli, is effective as a fat solvent and a germicidal when used in concentrations of 70% to 80% and may be used as a substitute skin prep antiseptic when the patient is allergic to iodine. Some disadvantages of ethyl alcohol are that it evaporates quickly, is highly flammable, and dries the skin excessively. Most skin prep devices are prepackaged and are disposable items for one-time use. To prep the skin with such a device before a venipuncture, the device is moved in a circular motion with the applicator rubbing the skin at the intended venipuncture site. The venipuncture site is swabbed with the antiseptic for about 1 minute. The antiseptic is spread over an area about 2 inches (5.08 cm) in diameter with the venipuncture site at the center.

**skin self-examination,** the practice of studying one's own skin for early signs of premalignant or malignant tumors. A 5-year study by the Sloan-Kettering Cancer Center in New York found that people who examined themselves, looking for moles that change color, shape, or size, were 44% less likely to die of melanoma than those who did not.

**skin surveillance,** a nursing intervention from the Nursing Interventions Classification (NIC) defined as collection and analysis of patient data to maintain skin and mucous membrane integrity. See also **Nursing Interventions Classification.**

**skin tag.** See **cutaneous papilloma.**

**skin test,** a test to determine the reaction of the body to a substance by observing the results of injecting the substance intradermally or of applying it topically to the skin. Skin tests are used to detect allergens, to determine immunity, and to diagnose disease. Kinds of skin tests include **patch test, Schick test,** and **tuberculin test.**

**skin traction,** one of the two basic kinds of traction used in orthopedics for the treatment of fractured bones and the correction of orthopedic abnormalities. Skin traction applies pull to an affected body structure by straps attached to the skin surrounding the structure. Kinds of skin traction are **adhesive skin traction** and **nonadhesive skin traction.** Compare **skeletal traction.** See also **Dunlop skin traction.**

**skin turgor** [AS, *scinn* + L, *turgere,* to swell], the resilience of the normal skin when subjected to physical distortion, such as by pinching or pressing. The relative speed with which the skin resumes its normal appearance after stretching or compression is an indicator of skin hydration. Turgor is slower in older people.

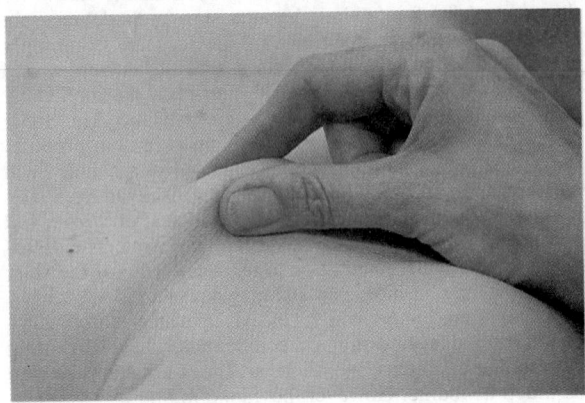

**Normal skin turgor** *(Wilson and Giddens, 2001)*

**sklero-.**   See **sclero-.**

**SK-Penicillin VK,** trademark for an antibacterial (penicillin V potassium).

**SK-Pramine,** trademark for a tricyclic antidepressant (imipramine hydrochloride).

**SK-Tetracycline,** trademark for an antibiotic (tetracycline).

**skull** [ME, *skulle,* shell], the bony structure of the head, consisting of the cranium and the skeleton of the face. The cranium, which contains and protects the brain, consists of 8 bones; the skeleton of the face is composed of 14 bones.

**skullcap,** an herb that is native to temperate regions of North America.

■ USES: This herb is used as an antibacterial and sedative.

■ CONTRAINDICATIONS: Skullcap should not be used during pregnancy and lactation, in children, or in those with known hypersensitivity to this plant.

**skull shield,** a protective plastic plate worn over a cranial defect.

**SL,** abbreviation for **soda lime.**

**slaked lime.**   See **calcium hydroxide.**

**slander** [Fr, *esclandre,* scandal], any words spoken with malice that are untrue and prejudicial to the reputation, professional practice, commercial trade, office, or business of another person. Formerly, slander included published defamation, but at present it is limited to spoken accusation. To bring legal action in slander, the slandered person must be able to demonstrate real temporal damages—except for cases in which the defamation relates to the person's business or profession or in which the malicious words question the person's chastity or accuse the him or her of being a felon or of having a loathsome disease. Compare **libel.**

**slant of occlusal plane** [ME, *slenten,* to slope], the angle between the extended occlusal plane and the axis-orbital plane.

**SLE,** abbreviation for **systemic lupus erythematosus.**

**sleep**[1] [AS, *slaepan,* to sleep], a state marked by reduced consciousness, diminished activity of the skeletal muscles, and depressed metabolism. People normally experience sleep in patterns that follow four observable, progressive stages. A device such as an encephalograph is used to record the recurrent pattern of brain waves during the stages: During stage 1 the brain waves are of the theta type, followed in stage 2 by the appearance of distinctive sleep spindles; during stages 3 and 4 the theta waves are replaced by delta waves. These four stages represent three fourths of a period of typical sleep and collectively are called **nonrapid eye movement (NREM)** sleep. The remaining time is usually occupied with **rapid eye movement (REM)** sleep, which can be detected with electrodes placed on the skin around the eyes so that tiny electric discharges from contractions of the eye muscles are transmitted to recording equipment. The REM sleep periods, lasting from a few minutes to half an hour, alternate with the NREM periods. Dreaming occurs during REM time. Individual sleep patterns normally change throughout life because daily requirements for sleep gradually diminish from as much as 20 hours a day in infancy to as little as 6 hours a day in old age. Infants tend to begin a sleep period with REM sleep, whereas REM activity usually follows the four stages of NREM sleep in adults.

**sleep**[2], a nursing outcome from the Nursing Outcomes Classification (NOC) defined as the extent and pattern of natural periodic suspension of consciousness during which the body is restored. See also **Nursing Outcomes Classification.**

**sleep apnea,** a sleep disorder characterized by periods in which respiration is absent. The person is momentarily unable to contrace respiratory muscles or to maintain airflow through the nose and mouth. See also **apnea.**

**sleep enhancement,** a nursing intervention from the Nursing Interventions Classification (NIC) defined as facilitation of regular sleep/wake cycles. See also **Nursing Interventions Classification.**

**sleep epilepsy.**   See **narcolepsy.**

**sleeping pill,** **1.** *informal.* a sedative taken for insomnia or for postoperative sedation. **2.** an over-the-counter pill, classified pharmaceutically as an aid to sleeping. Antihistamines, such as pyrilamine maleate and doxylamine succinate, depend for sedative action on side effects, which may disappear with continued use of such agents. The use of all drugs that depress the central nervous system is contraindicated for pregnant and lactating women and for asthma, glaucoma, or prostatic hypertrophy patients.

**sleeping sickness.**   See **African trypanosomiasis.**

**sleep pattern, disturbed,** a nursing diagnosis accepted by the Fourth National Conference on the Classification of Nursing Diagnoses. Sleep pattern disturbance is defined as disruption of sleep time that causes discomfort or interferes with desired life-style.

■ DEFINING CHARACTERISTICS: The critical defining characteristics, at least one of which must be present to make the diagnosis, are difficulty in falling asleep, wakening earlier than usual, interruption of sleep by periods of wakefulness, or not feeling rested after sleep. Other defining characteristics are changes in behavior and performance, including increasing irritability, restlessness, disorientation, lethargy, and listlessness; physical signs, such as mild, fleeting nystagmus, slight hand tremor, ptosis of the eyelid, and expressionless face; thick speech with mispronunciation and incorrect words; dark circles under the eyes; frequent yawning; and changes in posture.

■ RELATED FACTORS: Related factors are sensory factors, which may be either internal (illness or psychologic stress) or external (environmental changes or social cues). See also **nursing diagnosis.**

**sleep studies (polysomnography),** an electrodiagnostic test used to diagnose obstructive sleep apnea (OSA). It is performed in a sleep laboratory where the patient is monitored by electrocardiogram, pulse oximetry, electroencephalogram, and electromyography.

**sleep terror disorder** [AS, *slaepan* + L, *terrere,* to frighten], a condition occurring during stage 3 or 4 of nonrapid eye movement sleep. It is characterized by repeated episodes of abrupt awakening, usually with a panicky scream, accompanied by intense anxiety, confusion, agitation, disorientation, unresponsiveness, marked motor movements, and total amnesia concerning the event. The disorder usually occurs in children, is more common in boys than in girls, and is extremely variable in frequency but is more likely to occur if the individual is fatigued or under stress or has been given a tricyclic antidepressant or neuroleptic at bedtime. Compare **nightmare.** See also **pavor nocturnus.**

**sleep-wake schedule disorder,** a form of dyssomnia caused by a conflict between a person's circadian rhythm and the socioeconomic demands of society, such as work and travel schedules.

**sleepwalking.** See **somnambulism.**

**slice** /slīs/ [OFr, *esclice*], (in tomography) a cross-sectional plane of the body selected for imaging.

**slide clamp** [AS, *slidan* + *clam,* fastener], a device, usually constructed of plastic, used to regulate the flow of IV solution. The slide clamp has a graduated opening through which the IV tubing passes. Pushing the tube into the narrow end of the opening constricts it and reduces the flow rate of the IV solution. Sliding the wide end of the opening over the tube increases the flow rate. Compare **roller clamp, screw clamp.**

**sliding esophageal hiatal hernia,** a protrusion of the cardioesophageal junction and stomach through the esophageal hiatus.

**sliding filaments** [AS, *slidan* + L, *filamentum,* thread], interdigitated thick and thin filaments of a sarcomere. In muscle contraction they slide past each other so that the sarcomere becomes shorter although the filament lengths do not change. The action of the sliding filaments contributes to the increased thickness of a muscle in contraction.

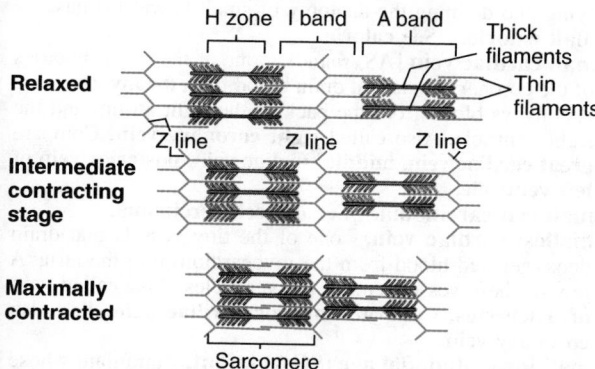

**Sliding filaments** *(Thibodeau and Patton, 1999/Rolin Graphics)*

**sliding hernia,** a protrusion of either the cecum or the sigmoid colon into the parietal peritoneum. The protrusion can be either abdominal or esophageal. Also called **slipped hernia.**

**sliding hiatal hernia,** a protrusion of the upper stomach

and cardioesophageal junction through the diaphragm into the posterior mediastinum.

**sliding transfer,** the movement of a person in a sitting position from one site to another, such as from a bed to a wheelchair, by sliding him or her along a transfer board.

**sling** [ME, *slingen,* to hurl], a bandage or device used to support an injured part of the body, especially a forearm. See also **sling restraint.**

**sling restraint,** a therapeutic device, usually constructed of felt, used to assist in the immobilization of patients, especially orthopedic patients in traction. The sling is placed over the pelvis to reduce pelvic motion with lower extremity traction or over the abdominal area as countertraction with Dunlop traction. With lower extremity traction the sling restraint is attached to both sides of the bedspring frame. Compare **diaper restraint, jacket restraint.** See also **Dunlop skeletal traction, Dunlop skin traction.**

**slip-on blood pump** [ME, *slippen,* slippery, *on*], a plastic mesh device with an attached squeeze bulb, rubber tubing, and pressure gauge, used to help administer large amounts of blood quickly. The plastic mesh slips over the blood bag and exerts pressure on it when the bulb is squeezed. The pressure gauge displays a danger zone, usually marked in red, and indicates pressure limits for safe blood administration. Excessive pressure may damage the red blood cells or may disconnect the primary IV line.

**slipped disk.** See **herniated disk.**

**slipped femoral epiphysis,** a failure of the femoral epiphyseal plate that tends to occur primarily in overweight adolescents as a result of hormonal changes. Clinical features include hip stiffness and pain, with difficulty in walking. There also may be knee pain and external rotation of the affected leg. The condition is treated by orthopedic surgery.

**slipped hernia.** See **sliding hernia.**

**slipping patella** [ME, *slippen* + L, *patella,* small dish], a patella that undergoes recurrent dislocation.

**slipping rib,** a condition in which a loose ligament allows one of the lower five ribs to slip inside or outside an adjacent rib, causing pain or discomfort. The symptoms may mimic those of a disorder of the pancreas, gallbladder, or other upper abdominal organ.

**slit lamp** [AS, *slitan* + Gk, *lampein,* to shine], an instrument used in ophthalmology for examining the external, surface, and internal segments of the eye, including the eyelid(s), lashes, conjunctiva, cornea, anterior chamber, pupil, iris, vitreous, and retina. A high-intensity beam of light is projected through a narrow slit, and a cross section of the illuminated part of the eye is examined through a magnifying lens. A second, hand-held lens is used to examine the retina.

**slit-lamp microscope,** a microscope for ophthalmic examination. It permits the viewer to examine the endothelium of the posterior surface of the cornea in a projected band of light that is shaped like a slit.

**slit scan radiography,** a technique for producing radiographs of body structures without length distortion by scanning a fan-shaped beam of x-rays through a narrow-slit collimator. The beam divergence perpendicular to the scan results in some distortion of width.

**slit tongue.** See **forked tongue.**

**slit-ventricle syndrome,** a condition of chronic headaches and cardiac disorders affecting shunt-dependent patients. Characteristics include small ventricles and slow reflux of the valve mechanism of the shunt.

**Slo-Phyllin,** trademark for a bronchodilator (theophylline).

**slough** /sluf/ [ME, *sluh,* husk], **1.** to shed or cast off dead tissue, such as cells of the endometrium, shed during menstruation. **2.** the tissue that has been shed.

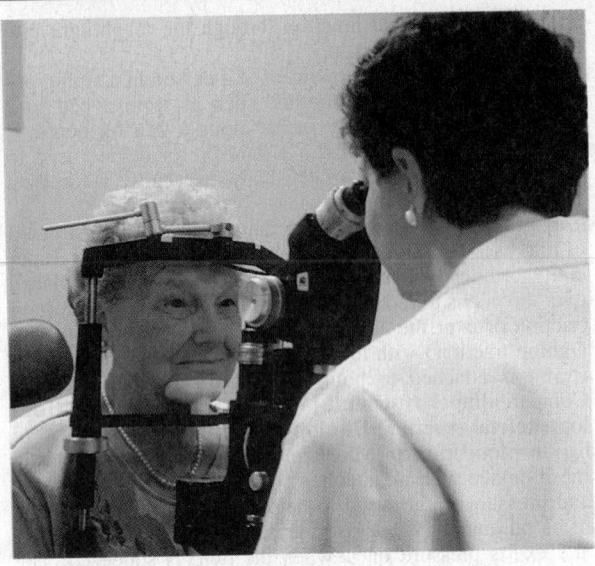

**Slit-lamp microscope**
*(Ignatavicius, Workman, and Mishler, 1999)*

**slow-acting insulin.** See **long-acting insulin.**

**slow channel,** a membrane channel that is slow to become activated. An example is the calcium channel, which allows calcium ions to diffuse across membranes. See also **calcium channel blocker.**

**slow diastolic depolarization** [AS, *slaw,* dull], the slow loss of membrane polarization that occurs between action potentials in cells of the sinus and atrioventricular nodes.

**Slow-K,** trademark for a slow-release tablet of an electrolyte replacement (potassium chloride).

**slow pain,** an unpleasant sensory experience that travels a multisynaptic route to the brain via slow-conducting, nonmyelinated nerve fibers.

**slow pulse** [AS, *slaw,* dull; L, *pulsare,* to beat], a pulse rate of less than 60/min. The rate is common among older people, conditioned athletes, and patients receiving betablockers. See also **bradycardia.**

**slow-reacting substance of anaphylaxis (SRS-A),** a group of active substances, including histamine and leukotrienes, that are released during an anaphylactic reaction. They cause the smooth muscle contraction and vascular dilation that cause the signs and symptoms of anaphylaxis.

**slow-response action potential,** a cardiac action potential produced by the influx of calcium ions without the typical and much faster influx of sodium ions. Such an action potential has a slow upstroke, low amplitude, and consequent slow conduction.

**slow stroking,** a therapeutic massage technique of slow continuous movement of the hands over the paravertebral areas along the spine from the cervical through the lumbar region. Usually a lubricant is applied to the skin, and the index and middle fingers are used to stroke both sides of the spinal column simultaneously. Also called **effleurage.**

**slow-twitch (ST) fiber,** a muscle fiber that develops less tension more slowly than a fast-twitch fiber. The ST fiber is usually fatigue resistant and has adequate oxygen and enzyme activity. Studies indicate that world-class endurance runners apparently have high percentages of ST fibers. It is called *red muscle* because of the abundance of capillaries serving the fiber muscle. The muscle also contains high amounts of the protein myoglobin which functions to store oxygen inside the muscle cell.See also **fast-twitch (FT) fiber.**

**slow vestibular stimulation,** a feeding therapy technique for disabled children, designed to promote parasympathetic loading.

**slow virus,** a virus that remains dormant in the body after initial infection. Years may elapse before symptoms occur. Several degenerative diseases of the central nervous system are believed to be caused by slow viruses, including subacute sclerosing panencephalitis and kuru.

**SLP, 1.** abbreviation for **single-locus probe. 2.** abbreviation for **speech-language pathologist.**

**slurred speech** /slurd/ [D, *sleuren,* to drag; ME, *speche*], abnormal speech in which words are not enunciated clearly or completely but are run together or partially eliminated. The condition may be caused by weakness of the muscles of articulation, damage to a motor neuron, cerebellar disease, drug use, or carelessness.

**slurry** /slur′ē/ [ME, *sloor,* mud], a thin suspension of finely divided solids in a liquid.

**Sly syndrome** /slī/ [William S. Sly, American physician, b. 1932], a mucopolysaccharidosis caused by deficiency of an enzyme important for the degradation of various mucopolysaccharides. It is characterized by excretion of mucopolysaccharides in the urine and by granular inclusions in granulocytes. Onset is between 1 and 2 years of age with mild to moderate Hurler-like features including dysostosis multiplex, pigeon breast, organomegaly, cardiac murmurs, short stature, and moderate mental retardation. Milder forms exist. Also called **mucopolysaccharidosis VII.**

**Sm,** symbol for the element **samarium.**

**SMAC,** trademark for a system that uses a small computer to perform a multiple of different blood chemical tests from a single blood sample. See **sequential multiple analysis.**

**smack,** *slang.* heroin.

**small bowel follow-through test (SBF),** a x-ray with contrast dye (usually barium) performed to identify abnormalities in the small bowel. X-ray films done at timed intervals follow the progression of the contrast medium through the small intestine. The SBF series is also helpful in identifying and defining the anatomy of small bowel fistulas.

**small calorie.** See **calorie.**

**small cardiac vein** [AS, *smael*], one of the five tributaries of the coronary sinus that drain blood from the myocardium. It conveys blood from the back of the right atrium and the right ventricle. Also called **right coronary vein.** Compare **great cardiac vein, middle cardiac vein, posterior vein of left ventricle.**

**small cell carcinoma.** See **oat cell carcinoma.**

**smallest cardiac vein,** one of the tiny vessels that drain deoxygenated blood from the myocardium into the atria. A few of these vessels end in the ventricles. Also called **vein of Thebesius.** Compare **anterior cardiac vein.** See also **coronary vein.**

**small for gestational age (SGA) infant,** an infant whose weight and size at birth fall below the tenth percentile of appropriate for gestational age infants, whether delivered at term or earlier or later than term. Factors associated with smallness or retardation of intrauterine growth other than genetic influences include any disorder causing short stature, such as dwarfism; malnutrition caused by placental insufficiency; and certain infectious agents, including cytomegalovirus, rubella virus, and *Toxoplasma gondii.* Other factors associated with the smallness of an SGA infant include cigarette smoking by the mother during pregnancy, her addiction to alcohol or heroin, and her having received methadone treatment. Asphyxia may be a significant risk for the SGA infant during labor and delivery if the condition is the result of placental insufficiency. Such an infant has a low Apgar score, becomes acidotic in labor and at birth, and is likely to experience hypoglycemia within the first hours or days of life. Given adequate nutrition and caloric intake, some SGA infants show phenomenal catch-up growth. Also called **small for dates (SFD) infant.** Compare **large for gestational age (LGA) infant.** See also **dysmaturity.**

**small intestine,** the longest part of the digestive tract, extending for about 7 m from the pylorus of the stomach to the iliocecal junction. It is divided into the duodenum, jejunum, and ileum. Decreasing in diameter from beginning to end, it is situated in the central and caudal part of the abdominal cavity, surrounded by large intestine. It functions in digestion and is the major organ of absorption of prepared food. Compare **large intestine.**

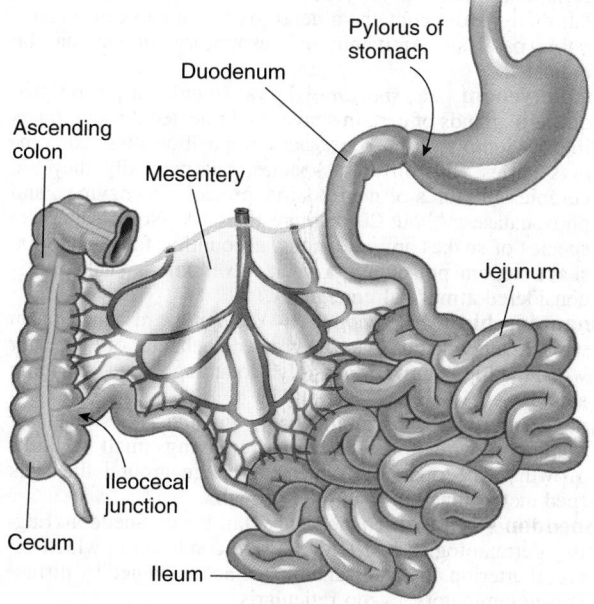

**Small intestine**

(Labels: Ascending colon; Mesentery; Duodenum; Pylorus of stomach; Jejunum; Ileocecal junction; Cecum; Ileum)

**small omentum.** See **lesser omentum.**

**smallpox** /smôl'poks/ [AS, *smael* + *pocc*], a highly contagious viral disease characterized by fever, prostration, and a vesicular, pustular rash. It is caused by one of two species of poxvirus, variola minor (alastrim) or variola major. Because human beings are the only reservoir for the virus, worldwide vaccination with vaccinia, a related poxvirus, has been effective in eradicating smallpox. The only known remaining sources of the virus are stored frozen at the U.S. Centers for Disease Control and Prevention. Smallpox is a potential agent for bioterrorism. For several years no natural case of the disease has been known to occur. Also called **variola.**

**smallpox vaccine,** a live vaccina virus vaccine prepared from calf lymph or chick embryo tissue. Some countries use it to vaccinate their military forces. In the United States, the vaccine is also indicated for health-care workers and first responders.

**small sciatic nerve** [AS, *smael* + Gk, *ischiadikos,* of the hip joint; L, *nervus*], the posterior femoral cutaneous nerve, which pierces the fascia and subdivides into fila-

ments, supplying the skin from the level of the greater trochanter to the middle of the thigh.

**SMBG,** abbreviation for **self-monitoring of blood glucose.**

**smear** [AS, *smeoru,* grease], a laboratory specimen for microscopic examination prepared by spreading a thin film of tissue on a glass slide. A dye, stain, reagent, diluent, or lysing agent may be applied to the specimen, depending on the purpose of the examination.

**smegma** /smeg'mə/ [Gk, soap], a secretion of sebaceous glands, especially the foul-smelling secretion sometimes found under the foreskin of the penis and at the base of the labia minora near the glans clitoris.

**smell** [ME, *smellen,* to detect odors], **1.** the special sense that allows perception of odors through the stimulation of the olfactory nerves; olfaction. See also **anosmia. 2.** any odor, pleasant or unpleasant.

**smelling salt** [ME, *smellen* + AS, *sealt*], aromatized ammonium carbonate to which may be added ammonia. It is used as a stimulant to arouse a person who has fainted.

**Smith fracture** [Robert W. Smith, Irish surgeon, 1807–1873], a fracture of the wrist involving volar displacement and angulation of a distal bone fragment. Also called **reverse Colles' fracture.**

**Smith-Hodge pessary.** See **pessary.**

**Smith-Lemli-Opitz syndrome** /smith·lem'lē·ō'pits/ [David W. Smith, American pediatrician, 1926−1981; Luc Lemli, American physician, 20th century; John Marius Opitz, American pediatrician, b. 1935], a hereditary syndrome, transmitted as an autosomal recessive trait, characterized by multiple congenital anomalies, including microcephaly, mental retardation, hypotonia, incomplete development of male genitalia, short nose with anteverted nostrils, and syndactyly of second and third toes.

**Smith-Petersen nail** [Marius N. Smith-Petersen, American surgeon, 1886–1953; AS, *naegel,* nail], a three-flanged, stainless steel nail used in orthopedic surgery to anchor the neck of the femur to its head in the repair of an intertrochanteric fracture. It is introduced below the prominence of the greater trochanter and passed through the fractured part into the head of the femur. See also **nail, pin.**

**smog,** a polluting combination of smoke and fog in the atmosphere.

**smoke inhalation** [AS, *smoca* + L, *in,* within, *halare,* to breathe], the inhalation of noxious fumes or irritating particulate matter that may cause severe pulmonary damage. Respiratory burns are difficult to distinguish from simple smoke inhalation. Chemical pneumonitis, asphyxiation, and physical trauma to the respiratory passages may occur.

■ OBSERVATIONS: Characteristics include irritation of the upper respiratory tract, singed nasal hairs, dyspnea, hypoxia, dusty gray sputum, rhonchi, rales, restlessness, anxiety, cough, and hoarseness. Pulmonary edema may develop up to 48 hours after exposure.

■ INTERVENTIONS: Airway maintenance and ventilatory assistance are essential. Endotracheal intubation, high-flow oxygen, and mechanical ventilation may be needed. Arterial blood gases are monitored, and corticosteroids may be given.

■ NURSING CONSIDERATIONS: The characteristics of smoke inhalation and its treatment vary with the nature of the fumes or matter inhaled and the extent of exposure; it is therefore important to know the circumstances, nature, and period of exposure and to know whether the person has a history of chronic respiratory or cardiac disease.

**smokeless tobacco** [AS, *smoca* + Sp, *tabaco*], **1.** chewing tobacco or tobacco powder that allows the stimulating components of tobacco to be absorbed through the digestive tract, or through the mucus membrane in the case of snuff. **2.** a transdermal nicotine patch that can be affixed to the upper part of the body to satisfy the person's craving for nicotine.

**smoking cessation assistance,** a nursing intervention from the Nursing Interventions Classification (NIC) defined as helping another to stop smoking. See also **Nursing Interventions Classification.**

**smooth muscle** [AS, *smoth*], one of three kinds of muscle, composed of elongated, spindle-shaped cells in muscles not under voluntary control, such as the smooth muscle of the intestines, stomach, and other viscera. The nucleated cells of smooth muscle are arranged parallel to one another and to the long axis of the muscle they form. Smooth muscle fibers are shorter than striated muscle fibers, have only one nucleus per fiber, and are smooth in appearance. Biofeedback devices may help many people gain partial control of contractions of involuntary smooth muscles. Also called **involuntary muscle, unstriated muscle.** Compare **striated muscle, cardiac muscle.**

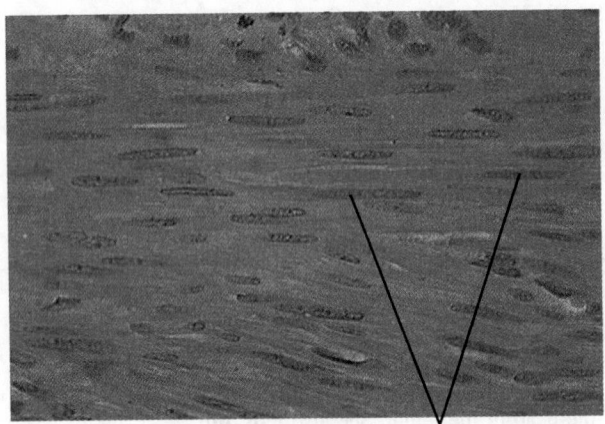

Nuclei of smooth muscle cells

**Smooth muscle** *(© Ed Reschke; used with permission)*

**smooth muscle relaxant,** an agent that reduces the tone of smooth muscle, such as a bronchodilator or vasodilator.

**smooth pursuit eye movement,** the tracking by the eyes of a slowly moving object at a steady coordinated velocity, rather than in saccades.

**smooth surface cavity,** a cavity formed by decay that starts on surfaces of teeth without pits, fissures, or enamel faults.

**SMR,** abbreviation for **submucous resection.**

**smudge cell** [ME, *sogen*, to soil], a disrupted leukocyte, sometimes seen during preparation of blood smears.

**Sn,** symbol for the element **tin.**

**S.N.,** abbreviation for *student nurse*, used in signing nursing notes (in the United States).

**SNA,** **1.** abbreviation for **State Nurses Association. 2.** abbreviation for *Student Nurses Association.*

**snail** [AS, *snagel*, slug], an invertebrate of the order Gastropoda, several of which are intermediate hosts of the blood flukes that cause schistosomiasis in humans. See also *Schistosoma,* schistosomiasis.

**snakebite** [AS, *snacan*, to creep, *bitan*], a wound resulting from penetration of the flesh by the fangs or teeth of a snake. Bites by snakes known to be nonvenomous are treated as puncture wounds; those produced by an unidentified or poisonous snake require immediate attention. The bitten area should be immobilized at heart level, the patient kept still, and prompt transportation arranged to an emergency department. Only polyvalent antivenin is available for bites of all pit vipers, including rattlesnakes, copperheads, and cottonmouths. Pit vipers are responsible for 98% of the poisonous snakebites in the United States. Bites of pit vipers are characterized by pain, redness, and edema; followed by weakness, dizziness, profuse perspiration, nausea, vomiting, or weak pulse; subcutaneous hemorrhage; and, in severe cases, shock. Treatment may include the use of antivenin, analgesics, antibiotics, and antitetanus prophylaxis to prevent infections from pathogens found in the mouths of snakes. Patients sensitive to horse serum in antivenin may require antihistamines and steroids for the control of hives, urticaria, and other allergic reactions. Coral snakes rarely bite, but their venom contains a neurotoxin that can cause respiratory paralysis. Antivenin and respiratory support may be indicated.

**snake venom** [AS, *snacan* + L, *venenum*], a poison produced in glands of certain snakes and injected through fangs into a victim's flesh. The exact composition of snake venoms varies with different species, but generally they are complex mixtures of neurotoxins, proteolytic enzymes, and phosphatases. About 20 of more than 100 North American species of snakes are venomous, accounting for about 8000 snake venom poisonings a year. A venomous snakebite is considered a medical emergency.

**snapping hip** [ME, *snappen* + AS, *hype*], a condition in which a tendon slips over the greater trochanter of the femur when the hip is moved, possibly producing a loud, snapping sound.

**snare** /sner/ [AS, *sneare*, noose], a device designed for holding a wire noose, used in removing small stalklike growths. The operator tightens the wire around the stalk (peduncle), thus removing the growth.

**Sneddon's syndrome** /sned′ənz/ [Ian Bruce Sneddon, English dermatologist, b. 1915], a rare condition in which cerebral arteriopathy and ischemia are accompanied by diffuse non-inflammatory livedo reticularis.

**sneeze** [AS, *snesen*, to sneeze], a sudden forceful involuntary expulsion of air through the nose and mouth occurring as a result of irritation to the mucous membranes of the upper respiratory tract, such as by dust, pollen, or viral inflammation. Also called **sternutation.**

**Snellen chart** [Hermann Snellen, Dutch ophthalmologist, 1834–1908], one of several charts used in testing visual acuity. Letters, numbers, or symbols are arranged on the chart in decreasing size from top to bottom.

**Snellen's reflex** [Hermann Snellen], unilateral congestion of the ear on stimulation of the distal end of the divided great auricular nerve.

**Snellen test** [Hermann Snellen], a test of visual acuity using a Snellen chart. The person being tested stands 20 feet from the chart and reads as many of the symbols as possible, reading each line and proceeding downward from the top. A score is assigned in the form of a ratio, comparing the subject's performance to that of a statistically normal subject's performance. For example, a person who can read at 20 feet what the average person can read at this distance has 20/20 vision, while a person who can read at 20 feet what the average person can read at 40 feet has 20/40 vision.

**SNF,** abbreviation for **skilled nursing facility.**

**snore** /snôr/, a harsh rough sound of breathing caused by vibration of the uvula and soft palate during sleep.

**snout reflex** [ME, *snoute*, muzzle], an abnormal sign elicited by tapping the nose, resulting in a marked facial grimace. It usually indicates bilateral corticopontine lesions.

**snowball sampling,** a method of obtaining subjects for a study by soliciting names of potential subjects from those participating in the study

**snow blindness** [AS, *snaw* + *blind*], a condition of photophobia, sometimes accompanied by keratitis or conjunctivitis, as a result of overexposure of the eyes to the glare of sun on snow.

**Snowden-Pencer scissors.** See **scissors.**

**SNP,** abbreviation for **sodium nitroprusside.**

**S.N.P.,** abbreviation for **school nurse practitioner.**

**snuff,** a powder that is inhaled through the nostrils.

**snuff dipping,** the practice of extracting juices from moist, fine-cut chewing tobacco placed in the mucobuccal fold of the mouth. The practice has been associated with an increased incidence of leukoplakia, tooth and gum diseases, and oral cancer.

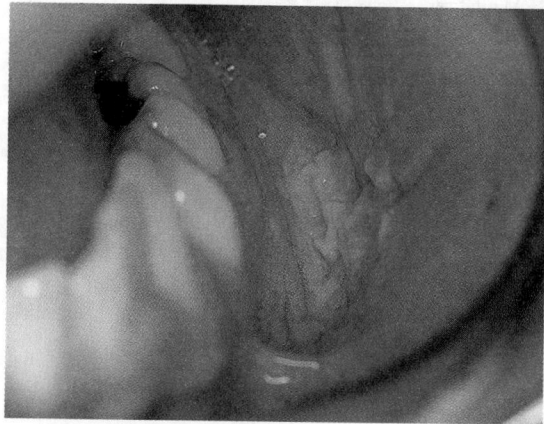

**Snuff dipper's pouch** *(Regezi, Sciubba, and Pogrel, 2000)*

**snuffles** [D, *snuffelen,* to sniff], a nasal discharge in infancy characteristic of congenital syphilis. See also **syphilis.**

**soap** [L, *sapo*], a compound of fatty acids and an alkali. Soap cleanses because molecules of fat are attracted to molecules of soap in a water solution and are pulled off the dirty surface into the water. Compare **detergent.** See also **green soap, surfactant.**

**SOAP** /sōp′, es′ō′ā′pē′/, (in a problem-oriented medical record) abbreviation for *subjective, objective, assessment,* and *plan,* the four parts of a written account of the health problem. In taking and charting the patient history and physical examination, a SOAP statement is made for each syndrome, problem, symptom, or diagnosis. Charting by this method is said to be "soaped," and charts produced using it are called "soap charts." See also **problem-oriented medical record.**

**soapsuds enema (SSE)** [L, *sapo* + D, *sudse,* marsh water; Gk, *enienai*], an evacuent enema made of 1 ounce of soft soap dissolved in 2 pints of hot water and administered at a temperature of 100° F (38° C). It acts by irritating the colon and stimulating peristalsis.

**SOB,** abbreviation for *short of breath.*

**socia** /sō′shē·ə/, an ectopic or displaced part of an organ, such as an accessory parotid gland.

**social adjustment rating scale.** See **social readjustment rating scale.**

**Social Behavior Assessment Scale** /sō′shəl/, a semistructured interview guide that elicits information from significant others regarding a patient's functioning.

**social breakdown syndrome** [L, *socius,* partner; AS, *brecan* + *dune*], the progressive deterioration of social and interpersonal skills in long-term psychiatric patients.

**social class,** a grouping of people with similar values, interests, income, education, and occupations.

**social day-care center.** See **adult day-care center.**

**social deviance,** behavior that violates social standards, engendering anger, resentment, and a desire for punishment in a significant segment of the society.

**social interaction, impaired,** a nursing diagnosis accepted by the Seventh National Conference on the Classification of Nursing Diagnoses. The condition is defined as the state in which an individual participates in an insufficient or excessive quantity or ineffective quality of social exchange. ■ DEFINING CHARACTERISTICS: Defining characteristics include verbalized or observed discomfort in social situations; verbalized or observed inability to receive or communicate a satisfying sense of belonging, caring, interest, or shared history; observed use of unsuccessful social interaction behaviors; dysfunctional interaction with peers, family, and/or others; and a family report of change of style or pattern of interaction. ■ RELATED FACTORS: Related factors include a knowledge or skill deficit about ways to enhance mutuality, communication barriers, self-concept disturbance, absence of available significant others or peers, limited physical mobility, therapeutic isolation, sociocultural dissonance, environmental barriers, and altered thought processes. See also **nursing diagnosis.**

**social interaction skills,** a nursing outcome from the Nursing Outcomes Classification (NOC) defined as an individual's use of effective interaction behaviors. See also **Nursing Outcomes Classification.**

**social involvement,** a nursing outcome from the Nursing Outcomes Classification (NOC) defined as the frequency of an individual's social interactions with persons, groups, or organizations. See also **Nursing Outcomes Classification.**

**social isolation,** a nursing diagnosis accepted by the Fifth National Conference on the Classification of Nursing Diagnoses. The diagnosis defines a condition in which a feeling of aloneness is experienced that the client acknowledges as a negative or threatening state imposed by others. ■ DEFINING CHARACTERISTICS: The defining characteristics may be objective, subjective, or both. Objective characteristics include the absence of family and friends; the absence of a supportive or significant personal relationship with another person; the client's withdrawal and preoccupation with his or her own thoughts and interests; meaningless actions or interests and activities inappropriate to the client's developmental age; a physical or mental handicap or illness; unacceptable social behavior; and a sad, dull affect. Subjective characteristics include verbal expression of feeling different from and rejected by others, acknowledgment of values unacceptable to the dominant cultural group, absence of a significant purpose in life, inability to meet the expectations of others, and the expressed feeling of insecurity in social situations. ■ RELATED FACTORS: Related factors are those that lead to unsatisfactory personal relationships, such as unaccepted social behavior or social values, the inability to engage in social situations, immature interests or attitudes inappropriate for the client's developmental age, alterations in physical appearance or mental status, or illness. See also **nursing diagnosis.**

**socialization** /sō′shəlīzā′shən/, **1.** the process by which an individual learns to live in accordance with the expectations and standards of a group or society, acquiring the beliefs, habits, values, and accepted modes of behavior primarily through imitation, family interaction, and educational systems; the procedure by which society integrates the individual. **2.** (in psychoanalysis) the process of adjustment that begins in early childhood by which the individual becomes aware of the need to accommodate inner drives to the demands of external reality. See also **internalization.**

**socialization enhancement,** a nursing intervention from the Nursing Interventions Classification (NIC) defined as facilitation of another person's ability to interact with others. See also **Nursing Interventions Classification.**

**socialized medicine** /sō′shəlīzd/, a system for the delivery of health care in which the expense of care is borne by a governmental agency supported by taxation rather than being paid directly by the client on a fee-for-service or contract basis.

**social learning theory,** a concept that the impulse to behave aggressively is subject to the influence of learning, socialization, and experience. Social learning theorists believe aggression is learned under voluntary control, by observation of aggressive behavior in others, and by direct experience.

**social margin,** the total of all resources (material, personal, and interpersonal) available to assist an individual in coping with stress.

**social medicine,** an approach to the prevention and treatment of disease that is based on the study of human heredity, environment, social structures, and cultural values.

**social mobility,** the process of moving upward or downward in the social hierarchy.

**social motivation,** an incentive or drive resulting from a sociocultural influence that initiates behavior toward a particular goal. Compare **physiologic motivation.**

**social network,** an interconnected group of cooperating significant others, who may or may not be related, with whom a person interacts.

**social network therapy,** the gathering together of patient, family, and other social contacts into group sessions for the purpose of problem solving.

**social order,** the manner in which a society is organized and the rules and standards required to maintain that organization.

**social phobia,** an anxiety disorder characterized by a compelling desire for the avoidance of and a persistent, irrational fear of situations in which the individual may be exposed to scrutiny by others. Examples of such situations are speaking, eating, or performing in public, or using public lavatories or transportation. Compare **simple phobia.** See also **phobia.**

**social psychiatry,** a field of psychiatry based on the study of social, cultural, and ecologic influences on the development and course of mental diseases. In treatment social psychiatry favors the use of milieu or other situational approaches to therapy.

**social psychology,** the study of the effects of group membership on the behavior, attitudes, and beliefs of the individual.

**social readjustment rating scale,** a scale of 43 common events associated with some degree of disruption of an indi-

vidual's life. The scale was developed by the psychologists T.J. Holmes and R. Rahe, who found that a number of serious physical disorders, such as myocardial infarction, peptic ulcer, and infections, and a variety of psychiatric disorders were associated with an accumulation of 200 or more points on the rating scale within a period of 1 year. Most disruptive on one's life, according to the psychologists, was the death of a spouse, which warranted 100 points. The lowest rated event was a minor law violation, rated at 11 points.

**social sanctions,** the measures used by a society to enforce its rules of acceptable behavior.

**Social Security Act,** a U.S. federal statute that provides for a national system of old age assistance, survivors' and old age insurance benefits, unemployment insurance and

### Social readjustment rating scale

| Life event | Mean value |
|---|---|
| 1. Death of spouse | 100 |
| 2. Divorce | 73 |
| 3. Marital separation | 65 |
| 4. Jail term | 63 |
| 5. Death of close family member | 63 |
| 6. Personal injury or illness | 53 |
| 7. Marriage | 50 |
| 8. Fired at work | 47 |
| 9. Marital reconciliation | 45 |
| 10. Retirement | 45 |
| 11. Change in health of family member | 44 |
| 12. Pregnancy | 40 |
| 13. Sex difficulties | 39 |
| 14. Gain of new family member | 39 |
| 15. Business readjustment | 39 |
| 16. Change in financial state | 38 |
| 17. Death of close friend | 37 |
| 18. Change to different line of work | 36 |
| 19. Change in number of arguments with spouse | 35 |
| 20. Mortgage or loan for major purchase (home, etc.) | 31 |
| 21. Foreclosure of mortgage or loan | 30 |
| 22. Change in responsibilities at work | 29 |
| 23. Son or daughter leaving home | 29 |
| 24. Trouble with in-laws | 29 |
| 25. Outstanding personal achievement | 28 |
| 26. Spouse begins or stops work | 26 |
| 27. Begin or end school | 26 |
| 28. Change in living conditions | 25 |
| 29. Revision of personal habits | 24 |
| 30. Trouble with boss | 23 |
| 31. Change in work hours or conditions | 20 |
| 32. Change in residence | 20 |
| 33. Change in schools | 20 |
| 34. Change in recreation | 19 |
| 35. Change in church activities | 19 |
| 36. Change in social activities | 18 |
| 37. Mortgage or loan for lesser purchase (car, TV, etc.) | 17 |
| 38. Change in sleeping habits | 16 |
| 39. Change in number of family get-togethers | 15 |
| 40. Change in eating habits | 15 |
| 41. Vacation | 13 |
| 42. Christmas | 12 |
| 43. Minor violations of the law | 11 |

Reprinted with permission from Holmes TH, Rahe RH: *J Psychosom Res* 11:213-218, 1967, Pergamon Press.

compensation, and other public welfare programs, including Medicare and Medicaid.

**social support,** a nursing outcome from the Nursing Outcomes Classification (NOC) defined as the perceived ability and actual provision of reliable assistance from other persons. See also **Nursing Outcomes Classification.**

**social support groups.** See **support groups.**

**social support programs,** services provided older persons including organizations of volunteers who visit older individuals to decrease loneliness and social isolation, volunteers who telephone older persons for similar purposes, and programs that provide a daily call with emergency procedures that go into effect if the telephone is not answered.

**social theories of aging,** concepts of social and psychologic adjustment in older persons. The theories include activity expressed in adoption of new roles and continuity, which includes retention of physical and social activities from the middle years.

**social worker,** a person with advanced education in dealing with social, emotional, and environmental problems associated with an illness or disability. A **medical social worker** usually has completed a master's degree program that includes experience in counseling patients and their families in a hospital setting. A **psychiatric social worker** may specialize in counseling individuals and families in dealing with social, emotional, or environmental problems pertaining to mental illness.

**society** /səsī'ətē/, a nation, community, or broad group of people who establish particular aims, beliefs, or standards of living and conduct.

**Society for Advancement in Nursing (SAIN),** a group established for advancement of the profession of nursing through higher education.

**sociobiology** /sō'sē·ō·bī·ol'əjē/ [L, socius, companion; Gk, bios, life, logos, science], the systematic study of biology as a basis for human behavior. Proponents contend that disease, stress, and aggression are natural pressures for maintaining an optimal level of population.

**socioeconomic status** /sō'sē·ō·ik'ənom'ik/ [L, socius, companion, oeconomicus, methodical, status, state], the position of an individual on a social-economic scale that measures such factors as education, income, type of occupation, place of residence, and in some populations heritage and religion.

**sociogenic** /-jen'ik/ [L, socius + Gk, genesis, origin], pertaining to personal or group activities that are motivated by social values and constraints.

**sociolinguistics** /-ling·gwis'tiks/, the study of the relationship between language and the social context in which it occurs.

**sociology** /sō'sē·ol'əjē/ [L, socius + Gk, logos, science], the study of group behavior within a society.

**sociopath,** popular term for antisocial personality.

**sociopathic.** See **psychopathic.**

**sociopathic personality.** See **antisocial personality.**

**sociopathy** /sō'sē·op'əthē/ [L, socius, companion; Gk, pathos, disease], a personality disorder characterized by a lack of social responsibility and failure to adapt to ethical and social standards of the community.

**sock aid,** an adaptive device that enables disabled people to pull on a pair of socks or stockings though unable to reach their feet. One type consists of a dowel with a cuphook on the end.

**socket,** the part of a prosthesis into which the stump of the remaining limb fits. Most modern prosthetic sockets are made of plastic, which is odorless and lighter and easier to clean than traditional leather sockets.

**soda** [It, sodo, solid], a compound of sodium, particularly sodium bicarbonate, or sodium carbonate.

**soda lime (SL),** a mixture of sodium and calcium hydroxides used to absorb exhaled carbon dioxide in an anesthesia rebreathing system.

**sodium (Na)** /sō'dē·əm/ [soda + L, ium (coined by Sir Humphry Davy, English chemist, 1778–1829)], a soft grayish metal of the alkaline metals group. Its atomic number is 11; its atomic mass is 22.99. Sodium is one of the most important elements in the body. Sodium ions are involved in acid-base balance, water balance, transmission of nerve impulses, and contraction of muscles. The recommended daily intake of sodium is 250 to 750 mg for infants 6 months to 1 year of age, 900 to 2700 mg for children 11 years of age or older, and 1100 to 3300 mg for adults. Sodium is an important component of more than 8 L of secretions produced by the body every day. These secretions include saliva, gastric and intestinal secretions, bile, and pancreatic fluid. The total daily secretion of sodium into these alimentary tract fluids averages between 1200 and 1400 mEq. A 154-pound adult has a total body pool of 2800 to 3000 mEq. It is also linked to chlorine, which is the most important extracellular anion in the body. Sodium is the chief electrolyte in interstitial fluid, and its interaction with potassium as the main intracellular electrolyte is critical to survival. A decrease in the sodium concentration of the interstitial fluid immediately decreases osmotic pressure, making it hypotonic to intracellular fluid osmotic pressure. The kidney is the chief regulator of sodium levels in body fluids and will excrete sodium-free urine when the body needs to conserve sodium. In high temperatures, such as those associated with fever, the body loses sodium through sweat, further diluting sodium reserves with additional water drunk by the affected individual. To prevent serious complications, depleted sodium must be replaced. Sodium salts, such as sodium bicarbonate, are widely used in medications. Sodium bicarbonate has an immediate and rapid antacid action on the stomach, but any excess rapidly enters the intestine so that the substance has a shorter action than other antacids. Sodium bicarbonate, which is very effective in rendering the urine alkaline, is an ingredient in many solutions used as douches, mouthwashes, and enemas. Sodium is also important in the transport of sodium and potassium ions through the cytoplasmic membrane.

**sodium arsenite poisoning,** a toxic condition caused by the ingestion of sodium arsenite, an insecticide and weed killer. The characteristic symptoms of arsenite poisoning are similar to those of arsenic poisoning, as is the treatment. See also **arsenic poisoning.**

**sodium barbital,** the sodium salt of 5,5-diethylbarbituric acid, a hypnotic and sedative drug.

**sodium bicarbonate,** an antacid, electrolyte, and urinary alkalinizing agent.

■ INDICATIONS: It is prescribed in the treatment of acidosis, gastric acidity, peptic ulcer, and indigestion.

■ CONTRAINDICATIONS: Pyloric obstruction, renal disease, congestive heart failure, or bleeding ulcer prohibits its use.

■ ADVERSE EFFECTS: Among the more serious adverse reactions are gastric distension, acid rebound, bicarbonate-induced alkalosis, hypernatremia, and hyperkalemia.

**sodium chloride,** common table salt (NaCl), used in various concentrations as a fluid and electrolyte replenisher, isotonic vehicle, irrigating solution, and enema.

**sodium chloride and dextrose.** See **dextrose and sodium chloride injection.**

**sodium etidronate.** See **etidronate disodium.**

**sodium fluoride poisoning,** a chronic condition of fluorine poisoning that occurs in some communities where the fluorine concentration in the water supply exceeds 1 ppm. Signs of the condition include mottling of tooth enamel and severe osteosclerosis. Also called **fluorosis.**

**sodium glutamate.** See **monosodium glutamate.**

**sodium hypochlorite solution,** a 5% aqueous solution of NaOCl used as a disinfectant for utensils not harmed by its bleaching action.

**sodium iodide,** an iodine supplement.
- INDICATIONS: It is prescribed in the treatment of thyrotoxic crisis and neonatal thyrotoxicosis, and in the management of hyperthyroidism before thyroidectomy.
- CONTRAINDICATIONS: Hyperkalemia or known hypersensitivity to this drug prohibits its use.
- ADVERSE EFFECTS: Among the more serious adverse reactions are salivary gland swelling, metallic taste, rashes, and GI disturbances. Acute poisoning may result in angioedema and pulmonary edema.

**sodium lactate injection,** an electrolyte replenisher that has been prescribed for metabolic acidosis.

**sodium nitroprusside (SNP),** a vasodilator.
- INDICATIONS: It is prescribed primarily in the emergency treatment of hypertensive crises and in heart failure.
- CONTRAINDICATIONS: Certain compensatory forms of hypertension, such as coarctation of the aorta or impaired cerebral circulation, or known hypersensitivity to the drug prohibits its use.
- ADVERSE EFFECTS: Among the most serious adverse reactions are a rapid fall in blood pressure or symptoms of cyanide poisoning (cyanide is produced by the metabolism of nitroprusside). Muscle spasms also may occur.

**sodium perborate,** an oxygen-liberating antiseptic ($NaBO_2 \cdot H_2O_2 \cdot 3H_2O$) that may be used in treating necrotizing ulcerative gingivitis and other kinds of gingival inflammation and bleaching pulpless teeth. Prolonged or indiscriminate use of the compound may cause burns of the oral mucosa and blacken the tongue.

**sodium phenobarbital,** the sodium salt of phenylethylbarbituric acid, a long-acting sedative and hypnotic. It can be administered orally or parenterally and is used in the therapeutic management of seizure disorders.

**sodium phosphate,** a saline cathartic.
- INDICATIONS: It is prescribed to achieve prompt, thorough evacuation of the bowel and, in lower dosage, for laxative effect.
- CONTRAINDICATIONS: Congestive heart failure, abdominal pain, edema, megacolon, hypovolemia, salt-restricted diet, or hypersensitivity to this drug prohibits its use. Frequent administration in any dosage is not recommended.
- ADVERSE EFFECTS: Among the more severe adverse reactions are dehydration, hypovolemia, abdominal cramping, and electrolyte imbalance.

**sodium phosphate P32,** an antineoplastic, antipolycythemic radioactive agent.
- INDICATIONS: It is prescribed for treatment of polycythemia vera, for neoplasms, including myelocytic leukemia, and for localizing tumors of the eye.
- CONTRAINDICATIONS: Polycythemia vera with leukopenia or decreased platelet count, chronic myelocytic leukemia with leukopenia or erythrocytopenia, concurrent administration of other alkalating agents, or hypersensitivity to this drug prohibits its use.
- ADVERSE EFFECT: The most serious adverse reaction is radiation sickness.

**sodium-potassium pump,** a protein that transports sodium and potassium ions across cell membranes against their concentration gradients. Sodium is normally moved from the inside of the cell, where its concentration is low, to the extracellular fluid, where its concentration is much higher. Potassium is moved in the opposite direction. Energy for the pump is obtained from the hydrolysis of adenosine triphosphate. See also **calcium pump, electrolyte balance.**

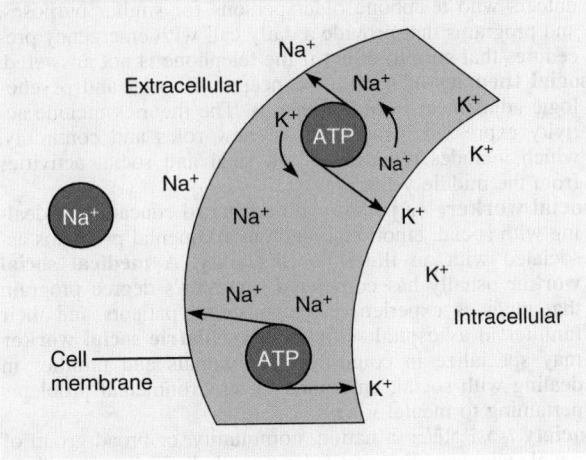

**Sodium-potassium pump** *(Lewis, Collier, and Heitkemper, 2000)*

**sodium-restricted diet.** See **low-sodium diet.**

**sodium salicylate,** an analgesic, antipyretic, and antirheumatic.
- INDICATIONS: It is prescribed to relieve pain and fever.
- CONTRAINDICATIONS: GI ulceration or bleeding or known hypersensitivity to this drug or to other salicylates prohibits its use. It is not given to newborns.
- ADVERSE EFFECTS: Among the most serious adverse reactions are GI bleeding and salicylate poisoning caused by overdose. Abdominal pain, nausea, and vomiting also may occur.

**sodium stibocaptate,** an investigational parasiticide for certain schistosomal infections. It is available from the Centers for Disease Control and Prevention. Also called **stibocaptate.**

**sodium sulfate,** a saline cathartic for chronic constipation caused by peristaltic disorders.
- INDICATIONS: It is prescribed to achieve prompt, thorough evacuation of the bowel and, in lower dosage, for laxative effect.
- CONTRAINDICATIONS: Congestive heart failure, hypovolemia, or hypersensitivity to this drug prohibits its use. Frequent administration, in any dosage, is not recommended.
- ADVERSE EFFECTS: Among the more severe adverse reactions are dehydration, hypovolemia, and electrolyte imbalance.

**sodium sulfate anhydrous.** See **salt cake.**

**Sodium Versenate,** trademark for a metal chelating agent (edetate disodium).

**sodoku.** See **rat-bite fever.**

**sodomist** /sod′əmist/ [Sodom, biblical city in ancient Palestine], a person who practices sodomy. Also called **sodomite** /sod′əmīt/.

**sodomy** /sod′əmē/ [Sodom, biblical city in ancient Palestine], **1.** anal intercourse. **2.** intercourse with an animal. **3.** a vague term for "unnatural" sexual intercourse. **sodomize,** *v.*

**soft chancre** [AS, *softe* + Fr, *canker*], a usually painless local genital ulcer that follows an infection by *Haemophilus ducreyi.* It is accompanied by suppuration of the inguinal lymphatic nodes, or inguinal buboes. Complications may include phimosis, urethral stricture or fistula, and marked tissue destruction. Also called **chancroid.**

**soft contact lens** [AS, *softe* + L, *contingere* + *lens,* lentil], a contact lens made of a flexible plastic material that can be shaped more easily to fit the eyeball than a rigid gas-permeable lens and typically provide good initial comfort. Among the disadvantages of soft lenses are that they are more easily damaged, may not provide vision as sharp as alternative methods in certain cases and must be disinfected periodically because they tend to harbor bacteria. Many people now wear disposable soft contact lenses, negating some of the disadvantages.

**soft data** [AS, *softe* + L, *datum,* something given], health information that is mainly subjective as provided by the patient and the patient's family.

**soft diet,** a diet that is soft in texture, low in residue, easily digested, and well tolerated. It provides the essential nutrients in the form of liquids and semisolid foods, such as milk, fruit juices, eggs, cheese, custards, tapioca and puddings, strained soups and vegetables, rice, ground beef and lamb, fowl, fish; mashed, boiled, or baked potatoes; wheat, corn, or rice cereals; and breads. Omitted are raw fruits and vegetables, coarse breads and cereals, rich desserts, strong spices, all fried foods, veal, pork, nuts, and raisins. It is commonly recommended for people who have GI disturbances or acute infections and those unable to tolerate a normal diet.

**softening of bones** /sô′fəning, sof′əning/ [AS, *softe* + *ban*], any disease that results in a loss of the mineral content of the bones. See also **osteomalacia.**

**soft fibroma,** a fibroma that contains many cells. Also called **fibroma molle** /mol′ē/.

**soft neurologic sign,** a mild or slight neurologic abnormality that is difficult to detect or interpret.

**soft palate,** the structure composed of mucous membrane, muscular fibers, and mucous glands, suspended from the posterior border of the hard palate forming the roof of the mouth. When the soft palate rises, as in swallowing and in sucking, it separates the nasal cavity and the nasopharynx from the posterior part of the oral cavity and the oral part of the pharynx. The posterior border of the soft palate hangs like a curtain between the mouth and the pharynx. Suspended from it is the conical, pendulous, palatine uvula. Arching laterally from the base of the uvula are the two curved musculomembranous pillars of the fauces. Compare **hard palate.**

**soft radiation,** a relatively long wavelength with less penetrating radiation than short wavelength radiation.

**soft tissue rheumatism.** See **fibrositis.**

**software,** the programs that control a computer and cause it to perform specific functions. See also **application.** Compare **hardware.**

**software bug.** See **bug.**

**soft water** [AS, *softe* + *waeter*], water that does not contain salts of calcium or magnesium, which precipitate soap solutions.

**sol,** a colloidal state in which a solid is suspended throughout a liquid, such as a soap or starch in water. The fluidity of cytoplasm depends on its sol/gel balance.

**sol.,** abbreviation for **solution.**

**-sol,** suffix meaning a 'colloidal solution': *electrosol, nitromersol, plastisol.*

**Solanaceae** /sō′lənā′si·ē/, a family of plants that includes the genus *Solanum,* or nightshades, and more than 1800 species, including deadly nightshade (belladonna), henbane, tomatoes, and potatoes.

**solanaceous** /sō′lənā′shəs/, pertaining to plants of the Solanaceae family or substances derived from them.

**solanine** /sō′lə-nēn/, a steroidal alkaloid found in several species of *Solanum,* such as the nightshades and the green spots on potatoes; it causes hemolysis, central nervous system depression, and often fatal respiratory failure.

***Solanum*** /sō-lā′nəm/ [L, nightshade], a large genus of plants of the family Solanaceae. It includes the potato, tomato, eggplant, several of the nightshades, and many poisonous and medicinal species.

**solar-,** prefix meaning 'sun': *solarium, solarization, solarize.*

**solar fever.** See **dengue fever, sunstroke.**

**solarium** /sōler′ē·əm/ [L, terrace exposed to sun], a large, sunny room or area serving as a lounge for ambulatory patients in a hospital.

**solar keratosis.** See **actinic keratosis.**

**solar plexus** /sō′lər/ [L, *sol,* sun, *plexus,* network], a dense network of nerve fibers and ganglia that surrounds the roots of the celiac and the superior mesenteric arteries at the level of the first lumbar vertebra. It is one of the great autonomic plexuses of the body in which the nerve fibers of the sympathetic system and the parasympathetic system combine. The denser part of the solar plexus lies between the suprarenal glands, on the ventral surface of the crura of the diaphragm and on the abdominal aorta. Also called **celiac plexus.**

**solar radiation,** the emission and diffusion of actinic rays from the sun. Overexposure may result in sunburn, keratosis, skin cancer, or lesions associated with photosensitivity.

**solar sneeze reflex** [L, *sol,* sun; ME, *snesen* + L, *reflectere,* to bend back], a sneeze that may be caused by exposure to bright sunlight.

**solar therapy** [L, *sol,* sun; Gk, *therapeia,* treatment], the therapeutic use of sunlight. Also called **heliotherapy.**

**solder** /sod′ər/ [L, *solidatio,* making solid], **1.** a fusible metal or alloy used to unite pieces of metals with higher fusion temperatures. **2.** to fasten together pieces of metal through the use of this material.

**sole** [L, *solea*], the plantar surface of the foot.

**soleus** /sō′lē·əs/ [L, *solea,* sole of foot], one of three superficial posterior muscles of the leg. It is a broad flat muscle lying just under the gastrocnemius. The fibers of the soleus merge near the middle of the leg with those of the gastrocnemius to form the tendo calcaneus, which inserts into the calcaneus of the foot. The soleus plantar flexes the foot. Compare **gastrocnemius, plantaris.**

**soleus pump.** See **calf muscle pump.**

**Solfoton,** trademark for an anticonvulsant and sedative-hypnotic (phenobarbital).

**Solganal,** trademark for a gold salt antirheumatic (aurothioglucose).

**solid** /sol′id/ [L, *solidus*], **1.** a dense body, figure, structure, or substance that has length, breadth, and thickness; is not a liquid or a gas; contains no significant cavity or hollowness; and has no breaks or openings on its surface. **2.** describing such a body, figure, structure, or substance.

**solitary coin lesion** /sol′iter′ē/ [L, *solitarius,* standing alone, *cuneus,* wedge, *laesus,* injury], a nodule on a chest radiographic film by clear normal lung tissue surrounding it. A coin lesion is often malignant.

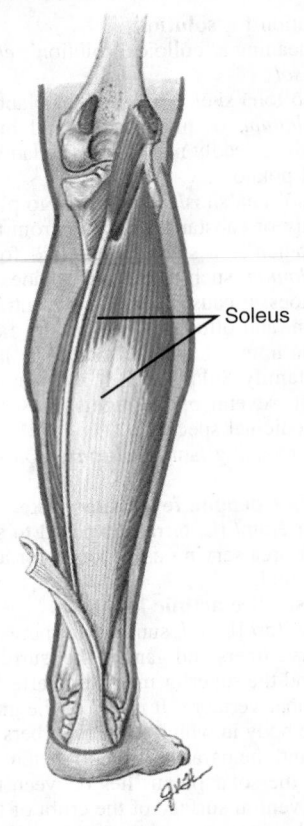

Soleus

**Soleus**
*(Seeley, Stephens, and Tate, 1995/John V. Hagen; by permission
of The McGraw-Hill Companies)*

**solitary play,** a form of play among a group of children within the same room or area in which each child engages in an independent activity using toys that are different from the others, concentrating solely on the particular activity, and showing no interest in joining in or interfering with the play of others. Compare **cooperative play.** See also **associative play, parallel play.**

**soln,** abbreviation for **solution.**

**solubility** /sol′yəbil′itē/ [L, *solubilis,* able to dissolve], **1.** the maximum amount of a solute that can dissolve in a specific solvent under a given set of conditions. **2.** the concentration of a solute in a solvent at its saturation point.

**solubility coefficient.** See **coefficient.**

**-soluble,** suffix meaning 'able to be dissolved': *acetosoluble, hydrosoluble, liposoluble.*

**Solu-Cortef,** trademark for a glucocorticoid (hydrocortisone sodium succinate).

**Solu-Medrol,** trademark for a glucocorticoid (methylprednisolone sodium succinate).

**solute** /sol′yo͞ot, sō′lo͞ot/ [L, *solutus,* dissolved], a substance dissolved in a solution.

**solution (sol., soln)** /səlo͞o′shən/ [L, *solutus*], a mixture of one or more substances dissolved in another substance. The molecules of each of the substances disperse homogenously and do not change chemically. A solution may be a gas, a liquid, or a solid. Compare **colloid, suspension.** See also **solute, solvent.**

**-solve,** combining form meaning 'to loosen': *dissolve, resolve.*

**solvent** /sol′vənt/ [L, *solvere,* to dissolve], **1.** any liquid in which another substance can be dissolved. **2.** *informal.* an organic liquid, such as benzene, carbon tetrachloride, and other volatile petroleum distillates, that when inhaled can cause intoxication as well as damage to mucous membranes of the nose and throat and the tissues of the kidney, liver, and brain. Repeated, prolonged exposure can result in addiction, brain damage, blindness, and other serious consequences, some of them fatal. See also **benzene poisoning, carbon tetrachloride, glue sniffing, petroleum distillate poisoning.**

**som-,** combining form for growth hormone derivatives.

**soma** /sō′mə/, *pl.* **somas, somata** [Gk, body], **1.** the body, as distinguished from the mind or psyche. **2.** the body, excluding germ cells. **3.** the body of a cell. —**somatic, somal,** *adj.*

**Soma,** trademark for a skeletal muscle relaxant (carisoprodol).

**soma-.** See **somato-.**

**-soma, -somus,** suffix meaning a 'body or part of a body': *hystersoma, microsoma, prosoma, pleurosomus, hemisomus.*

**somata.** See **soma.**

**-somatia, -somatic,** suffix meaning 'body': *diplosomatia, exsomatic, macrosomatia, microsomatia.*

**somatic.** See **soma, psychosomatic.**

**-somatic.** See **-somatia.**

**somatic cavity.** See **coelom.**

**somatic cell** /sōmat′ik/, any of the cells of body tissue that have the diploid number of chromosomes, as distinguished from germ cells, which contain the haploid number. Compare **germ cell.**

**somatic-cell gene therapy.** See **gene therapy.**

**somatic chromosome,** any autosome in a diploid or somatic cell.

**somatic delusion,** a false notion or belief concerning body image or body function. See also **delusion.**

**somatic mutation** [Gk, *soma,* body; L, *mutare,* to change], a sudden change in the chromosomal material in somatic cell nuclei affecting derived cells but not offspring.

**somatic therapy,** a form of treatment pertaining to the body that affects one's physiologic functioning.

**somatist** /sō′mətist/, a psychotherapist or other health professional who believes that every neurosis and psychosis has an organic cause.

**somatization** /sō′mətīzā′shən/ [Gk, *soma,* body], a process whereby a mental event is expressed in a body disorder or physical symptom. Examples include peptic ulcers and asthma. See also **conversion.**

**somatization disorder** [Gk, *soma* + *izein,* to cause], a *DSM-IV* psychiatric disorder characterized by recurrent multiple physical complaints and symptoms for which there is no organic cause. It is classified as a somatoform disorder in *DSM-IV.* The condition typically occurs in adolescence or in the early adult years and is rarely seen in men. The symptoms vary according to the individual and the underlying emotional conflict. Some common symptoms are GI dysfunction, paralysis, temporary blindness, cardiopulmonary distress, painful or irregular menstruation, sexual indifference, and pain during intercourse. Hypochondriasis may develop if the condition is untreated. Also called **Briquet's syndrome.** See also **conversion disorder.**

**somato-** /sō′mətō-, sōmat′o-/, **soma-,** combining form meaning 'body': *somatoceptor, somatogenic, somatopleural.*

**somatodyspraxia** /-disprak′sē·ə/, an impairment in the ability to plan skilled movements that are nonhabitual. Patients may be able to learn specific motor skills with practice but cannot accomplish unfamiliar tasks.

**somatoform disorder** /sōmat′əfôrm, sō′mətōfôrm′/ [Gk, *soma* + L, *forma,* form], any of a group of disorders, characterized by symptoms suggesting physical illness or disease, for which there are no demonstrable organic causes or physiologic dysfunctions. The symptoms are usually the physical manifestations of some unresolved intrapsychic factor or conflict. Kinds of somatoform disorders are **conversion disorder, hypochondriasis, psychogenic pain disorder,** and **somatization disorder.**

**somatogenesis** /sō′matəjen′əsis/ [Gk, *soma* + *genein,* to produce], **1.** (in embryology) the development of the body from the germ plasm. **2.** the development of a physical disease or of symptoms from an organic pathophysiologic cause. Compare **psychogenesis. —somatogenic, somatogenetic,** *adj.*

**somatoliberin.** See **growth hormone releasing hormone.**

**somatomedin.** See **growth hormone.**

**somatomedin C.** See **insulin-like growth factor.**

**somatomedin-C test,** a blood test most commonly used to detect levels of somatomedin-C, also called insulin-like growth factor. Screening for somatomedin-C provides an accurate reflection of the mean plasma concentration of growth hormone.

**somatomegaly** /sō′matōmeg′əlē/ [Gk, *soma* + *megas,* large], a condition in which the body is abnormally large as a result of an excessive secretion of somatotropin or an inadequate secretion of somatostatin.

**somatoplasm** /sō′mətōplaz′əm/ [Gk, *soma* + *plasma,* something formed], the nonreproductive protoplasmic material of the body cells, as distinguished from the reproductive material of the germ cells. Compare **germ plasm.**

**somatopleure** /sô′mətōploŏr′/ [Gk, *soma* + *pleura,* side], the lateral and ventral tissue layer that forms the body wall of the early developing embryo. Consisting of an outer layer of ectoderm lined with somatic mesoderm, it continues as the amnion and chorion external to the embryo. Compare **splanchnopleure. —somatopleural,** *adj.*

**somatosensory evoked potential (SEP)** /-sen′sərē/ [Gk, *soma* + L, *sentire,* to feel], evoked potential elicited by repeated stimulation of the pain and touch systems. It is the least reliable of the evoked potentials studied as monitors of neurologic function during surgery.

**somatosensory system,** the components of the central and peripheral nervous systems that receive and interpret sensory information from organs in the joints, ligaments, muscles, and skin. This system processes information about the length, degree of stretch, tension, and contraction of muscles; pain; temperature; pressure; and joint position.

**somatosplanchnic** /-splangk′nik/ [Gk, *soma* + *splanchna,* viscera], pertaining to the trunk of the body and the viscera.

**somatostatin** /sō′matōstat′in/, a hormone produced in the hypothalamus that inhibits the release of somatotropin (growth hormone) from the anterior pituitary gland. It also is produced in other parts of the body and inhibits the release of certain hormones, including thyrotropin, adrenocorticotropic hormone, glucagon, insulin, and cholecystokinin, and of some enzymes, including pepsin, renin, secretin, and gastrin. Also called **growth hormone release inhibiting hormone.**

**somatotherapy** /-ther′əpē/, the treatment of physical disorders, as distinguished from psychotherapy.

**somatotropic** /-trop′ik/ [[Gk, *soma,* body, *trope,* a turn], pertaining to an agent that influences the body or body cells.

**somatotropic hormone, somatotropin.** See **growth hormone.**

**somatotropin.** See **growth hormone.**

**somatotype** /sō′mətōtīp′/ [Gk, *soma* + *typos,* mark], **1.** body build or physique. **2.** the classification of individuals according to body build based on certain physical characteristics. The primary types are **ectomorph, endomorph,** and **mesomorph.**

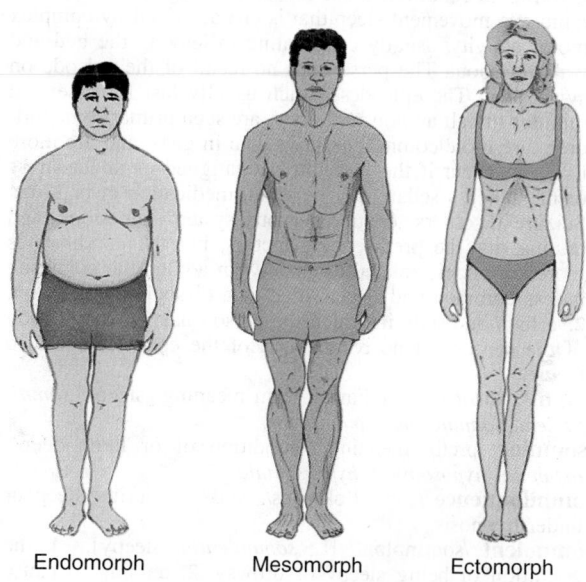

Endomorph  Mesomorph  Ectomorph

**Somatotypes** *(Thibodeau and Patton, 1999)*

**somatovisceral reflex** /-vis′ərəl/, a reflex in which visceral functions are activated or inhibited by somatic sensory stimulation.

**somatrem** /sō′mətrem/, a synthetic polypeptide growth hormone produced by recombinant deoxyribonucleic acid technology.

■ INDICATIONS: It is prescribed for growth promotion for patients not growing because of limited endogenous growth hormone secretion.

■ CONTRAINDICATIONS: This product is contraindicated for patients with closed epiphyses or evidence of underlying intracranial lesions. Concurrent use with a glucocorticoid may inhibit the effects of somatrem. The hormone may produce insulin resistance in some patients.

■ ADVERSE EFFECTS: Among reported adverse reactions are insulin resistance and hypothyroidism.

**-some,** combining form meaning 'a body' of a specified sort: *chromosome, microsome, sarcosome.*

**-somia,** combining form meaning '(condition of) possessing body': *agenosomia, diplosomia, microsomia.*

**somite** /sō′mīt/ [Gk, *soma,* body], any of the paired segmented masses of mesodermal tissue that form along the length of the neural tube during the early stage of embryonic development in vertebrates. These structures give rise to the vertebrae and differentiate into various tissues of the body, including the voluntary muscle, bones, connective tissue, and dermal layers of the skin. The first somite to appear is in the future occipital region, and the formation of new somites continues in a caudal direction until 36 to 38 have developed.

**somite embryo,**   an embryo in any stage of development between the formation of the first and the last pairs of somites, which in humans occurs in the third and fourth weeks after fertilization of the ovum.

**somn-.** See **somni-**.

**somnambulance.** See **somnambulism.**

**somnambulism** /somnam'byəliz'əm/ [L, *somnus,* sleep, *ambulare,* to walk],   **1.** also called **noctambulation, sleep-walking.** A condition occurring during stage 3 or 4 of non-rapid eye movement sleep that is characterized by complex motor activity, usually culminating in leaving the bed and walking about. The person has no recall of the episode on awakening. The episodes, which usually last from several minutes to half an hour or longer, are seen primarily in children, are more common in boys than in girls, and are more likely to occur if the individual is fatigued or under stress or has taken a sedative or hypnotic medication at bedtime. Seizure disorders, central nervous system infections, and trauma may be predisposing factors, but the condition is more commonly related to anxiety. In adults, the condition is less common and is classified as a dissociative reaction. **2.** a hypnotic state in which the person has full possession of the senses but no recollection of the episode. See also **fugue.**

**somni-, somn-,**   combining form meaning 'sleep': *somnifacient, somniferous, somnipathy.*

**-somnia,**   prefix meaning '(condition of or like) sleep': *asomnia, hyposomnia, hypersomnia.*

**somniloquence** /somnil'əkwəns/,   talking during sleep or under hypnosis.

**somnolent** /som'nələnt/ [L, *somnolentia,* sleepy],   **1.** the condition of being sleepy or drowsy. **2.** tending to cause sleepiness. —**somnolence,** *n.*

**somnolent detachment,**   (in psychology) a term introduced by H. S. Sullivan for a type of security operation in which a person falls asleep when confronted by a highly threatening, anxiety-producing experience. The mechanism originates in infancy.

**Somogyi effect (phenomenon)** [Michael Somogyi, American biochemist, 1883–1971; Gk, *phainomenon*],   a diabetes mellitus rebound effect in which an overdose of insulin induces hypoglycemia. This releases hormones that stimulate lipolysis, gluconeogenesis, and glycogenolysis, leading to hyperglycemia and ketosis. Treatment involves gradually lowering the insulin dose to achieve an optimal level.

**-somus.** See **-soma.**

**son-,**   prefix meaning 'sound': *sonitus, sonometer, sonotone.*

**sonographer** /sōnog'rəfər/,   an allied health professional with special training in the use of ultrasound equipment for diagnostic and therapeutic purposes. Also called **diagnostic medical sonographer, medical sonographer, ultrasonographer.**

**sonography.** See **ultrasonography.**

**sonorant.** See **voiced.**

**soot wart.** See **scrotal cancer.**

**sopor** /sō'pər/ [L, deep sleep],   a sleep that is as deep or sound as the state of stupor.

**soporiferous** /sop'ərif'ərəs/ [L *sopor,* deep sleep, *ferre,* to bear],   tending to cause deep sleep, such as an agent that induces deep sleep.

**soporific** /sop'ərif'ik/ [L, *sopor,* deep sleep, *facere,* to make],   **1.** pertaining to a substance, condition, or procedure that causes sleep. **2.** a soporific drug. See also **hypnotic, sedative.**

**sorbent** /sôr'bənt/ [L, *sorbere,* to swallow],   **1.** an agent that attracts and retains substances by absorption or adsorption. **2.** the property of a substance that allows it to interact with another compound, usually to make it bind.

**sorbic acid** /sôr'bik/,   a compound occurring naturally in berries of the mountain ash. Commercial sorbic acid derived from acetaldehyde is used in fungicides, food preservatives, lubricants, and plasticizers.

**Sorbitrate,**   trademark for an antianginal (isosorbide dinitrate).

**sordes** /sôr'dēz/, *pl.* **sordes** [L, *sordere,* to be dirty],   dirt or debris, especially the crusts consisting of food, microorganisms, and epithelial cells that accumulate on teeth and lips during a febrile illness or one in which the patient takes nothing by mouth. Sordes gastricae is undigested food and mucus in the stomach.

**sore** /sôr, sōr/ [AS, *sar*],   **1.** a wound, ulcer, or lesion. **2.** tender or painful.

**sore throat** [AS, *sar* + *throte*],   any inflammation of the larynx, pharynx, or tonsils.

**Sorrin's operation,**   a surgical technique for treating a periodontal abscess, used especially when the marginal gingiva appears healthy and provides no access to the abscess. A semilunar incision is made below the abscess area in the attached gingiva, leaving the gingival margin undisturbed. The tissue flap produced by the incision is raised, accessing the abscessed area for curettage, after which the wound is sutured.

**sorrow, chronic,**   a nursing diagnosis accepted by the Thirteenth National Conference on the Classification of Nursing Diagnoses. The condition is a cyclical, recurring, and potentially progressive pattern of pervasive sadness that is experienced in response to continual loss, throughout the trajectory of an illness or disability.

■ DEFINING CHARACTERISTICS: The condition is characterized by feelings that vary in intensity, are periodic, may progress and intensify over time, and may interfere with the ability to reach the highest level of personal and social well-being; expression of periodic, recurrent feelings of sadness, and expression of one or more of the following feelings: anger, being misunderstood, confusion, depression, disappointment, emptiness, fear, frustration, guilt, self-blame, helplessness, hopelessness, loneliness, low self-esteem, recurring loss, and being overwhelmed.

■ RELATED FACTORS: Related factors include the death of a loved one, chronic physical or mental illness or disability, experience of one or more trigger events, and unending caregiving as a constant reminder of loss. See also **nursing diagnosis.**

**s.o.s.,**   abbreviation for the Latin phrase *si opus sit,* 'if necessary.'

**Soto's syndrome.** See **cerebral gigantism.**

**souffle** /soō'fəl/ [Fr, breath],   a soft murmur heard through a stethoscope. When detected over the uterus in a pregnant woman, it is usually coincident with the maternal pulse and is caused by blood circulating in the large uterine arteries.

**soul food** [AS, *sawel* + *foda*],   food linked with cultural or traditional origins, especially African-American, that produces feelings of emotional significance and personal satisfaction in an individual.

**sound** [L, *sub,* under, *unde,* wave],   an emission detected by an instrument used to locate the opening of a cavity or canal, to test the patency of a canal, to ascertain the depth of a cavity, or to reveal the contents of a canal or cavity. A sound is used to determine the depth of the uterus, to detect stones in the bladder, and, less commonly, to assist in correctly inserting a urinary catheter in the urethra through the urinary meatus.

**sounds of Korotkoff.** See **blood pressure.**

**Souques's sign** /sōōks/ [Alexandre A. Souques, French neurologist, 1860–1944], in patients with a disease of the corpus striatum, the failure of a seated patient to extend the legs when the chair is pushed backward. The legs normally would be extended to prevent overbalancing. Also called **Souques's phenomenon.**

**source-to-image-receptor distance (SID),** /sôrs, sōrs/ [OFr, *sourse,* origin; L, *imago,* likeness], the distance between the focal spot on the target of an x-ray tube and the image receptor as measured along the beam.

**South African genetic porphyria.** See **variegate porphyria.**

**South American blastomycosis.** See **paracoccidioidomycosis.**

**South American trypanosomiasis.** See **Chagas' disease.**

**Southern blot test** /suth′ərn/, a gene analysis method used in identification of specific deoxyribonucleic acid (DNA) fragments and in diagnosis of cancers and hemoglobinopathies. It involves the placement of a nitrocellulose film on agarose gel surfaces with dry blotting material on the film. Liquid is then transported from a reservoir beneath the gel through the gel and nitrocellulose layer. The film adsorbs the DNA fragments. The fragments are then analyzed for rearrangements in immunoglobulin or cell receptor genes, chromosomal translocations, oncogene amplifications, and point mutations within oncogenes. Immunoglobulins and T cell receptor genes bear signatures that identify various leukemias and lymphomas. See also **Northern blot test.**

**Sp, sp., spp.,** abbreviation for **species.**

**space** [L, *spatium*], an area, region, or segment of the body, such as the complemental spaces in the pleural cavity that are not occupied by lung tissue and the lymph spaces occupied by lymph.

**space adaptation syndrome,** the ability to accommodate changes in cardiac function, bone mineral changes, and muscle atrophy while in the weightless state of a space traveler.

**space maintainer,** a fixed or removable appliance for preserving the space created by the premature loss of one or more teeth. It can be unilateral or bilateral. Types include band-loop, crown-loop, and lingual arch. See **separator.**

**space medicine,** a branch of medicine concerned with the effects of travel in space, beyond the atmosphere and pull of gravity, including weightlessness, motion sickness, and restricted physical activity.

**space obtainer,** an appliance for increasing the space between adjoining teeth.

**spacer** /spās′ər/ [L, *spatium,* space], on a metered dose inhaler, a chamber between the inhaler canister and the patient's mouth where droplets of medication can slow down and evaporate so that there is less direct impact on the oropharynx. See also **metered dose inhaler.**

**space regainer,** a fixed or removable appliance for moving a displaced secondary tooth into its normal position in a dental arch.

**space sickness.** See **air sickness; motion sickness.**

**Spanish fly.** See **cantharis.**

**spano-,** combining form meaning 'scanty or scarce': *spanogyny, spanomenorrhea, spanopnea.*

**sparfloxacin,** an antiinfective.

■ INDICATIONS: This drug is used to treat community-acquired pneumonia and chronic bronchitis caused by *Klebsiella pneumoniae, Haemophilus influenzae, H. parainfluenzae,* and *Moraxella catarrhalis.*

■ CONTRAINDICATIONS: Known hypersensitivity to quinolones and photosensitivity prohibit the use of this drug.

■ ADVERSE EFFECTS: Life-threatening effects of sparfloxacin are leukopenia and pseudomembranous colitis. Other adverse effects are eosinophilia, anemia, flatulence, diarrhea, QT interval prolongation, vasodilation, rash, pruritus, and photosensitivity. Common side effects are headache, dizziness, insomnia, nausea, vomiting, and abdominal pain.

**sparganosis** /spär′gənō′sis/ [Gk, *sparganon,* swaddling clothes, *osis,* condition], an infection with larvae of the fish tapeworm of the pseudogenus Sparganum. It is characterized by painful subcutaneous swellings or swelling and destruction of the eye. It is acquired by ingesting larvae in contaminated water or in inadequately cooked infected frog flesh. Treatment includes surgery and local injection of ethyl alcohol to kill the larvae.

**Sparine,** trademark for a phenothiazine antipsychotic and antiemetic (promazine hydrochloride).

**spasm** /spaz′əm/ [Gk, *spasmos*], **1.** an involuntary muscle contraction of sudden onset, such as habit spasms, hiccups, stuttering, or a tic. **2.** a convulsion or seizure. **3.** a sudden transient constriction of a blood vessel, bronchus, esophagus, pylorus, ureter, or other hollow organ. Compare **stricture.** See also **bronchospasm, pylorospasm.**

**-spasm,** combining form meaning 'twitching or involuntary contraction' of a specified sort: *gastrospasm, neurospasm, vasospasm.*

**spasmatic croup.** See **laryngismus.**

**spasmo-,** combining form meaning 'spasms': *spasmodermia, spasmophemia, spasmophilia.*

**-spasmodic, -spasmodical,** combining form meaning 'convulsion': *angiospasmodic, antispasmodic, postspasmodic.*

**spasmodic asthma** /spazmäd′ik/ [Gk, *spasmos + asthma,* panting], an airway obstruction caused by spasms of the bronchioles and inflammation of the bronchial mucosa and characterized by paroxysms of wheezing and coughing.

**spasmodic croup.** See **laryngismus.**

**spasmodic dysmenorrhea** /spazmod′ik/, difficult menstruation accompanied by painful contractions of the uterus.

**spasmodic dysphonia** [Gk, *spasmodes,* spasms, *dys,* bad, *phone,* voice], a speech disorder in which phonation is intermittently blocked by larynx spasms. The cause can be either organic or psychogenic. Also called **spastic dysphonia.**

**spasmodic stricture** [Gk, *spasmodes + L, strictura,* compression], a narrowing of a passage in which there is no organic change, merely muscle spasms.

**spasmodic tic** [Gk, *spasmodes + Fr, tic*], any repetitive movement in which spasmodic muscle group contractions occur at variable intervals.

**spasmodic torticollis** [Gk, *spasmodes + L, tortus,* twisted, *collum,* neck], a condition in which the head is inclined to one side as a result of episodes of spasms of the neck muscles. It is often transient, and examination seldom reveals a physical cause. In some cases, it may be brought on by severe stress.

**spasmogen** /spaz′məjən/, any substance that can produce smooth muscle contractions, as in the bronchioles; examples are histamine, bradykinin, and serotonin.

**spastic** /spas′tik/ [Gk, *spastikos,* drawing in], pertaining to spasms or other uncontrolled contractions of the skeletal muscles. See also **cerebral palsy. —spasticity,** *n.*

**spastic aphonia,** a condition in which a person is unable to speak because of spasmodic contraction of the abductor muscles of the throat.

**spastic bladder,** a form of neurogenic bladder caused by a lesion of the spinal cord above the voiding reflex center. It is marked by loss of bladder control and bladder sensation, in-

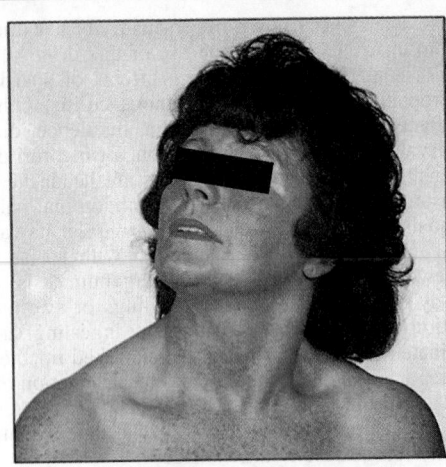

**Spasmodic torticollis: characteristic head posture**
*(Perkin, 1998)*

continence, and automatic, interrupted, incomplete voiding. It is most often caused by trauma but may result from a tumor or multiple sclerosis. Also called **reflex bladder, automatic bladder.** Compare **flaccid bladder.**

**spastic colon.**    See **irritable bowel syndrome.**

**spastic constipation** [Gk, *spasmos,* spasm; L, *constipare,* to crowd together], a form of constipation associated with neurasthenia and constrictive spasms in part of the intestine. The condition may be a sign of lead poisoning.

**spastic diplegia,** paralysis of corresponding parts on both sides of the body. See also **cerebral palsy.**

**spastic dysarthria,** a speech or language disorder caused by lesions of the corticobulbar tracts. It affects voluntary movements of the speech mechanism.

**spastic dysphonia.**    See **spasmodic dysphonia.**

**spastic dysuria,** difficulty in urination caused by bladder spasms.

**spastic entropion.**    See **entropion.**

**spastic gait** [Gk, *spasmos,* spasm; ONorse, *gata*], a pattern of walking in which the legs are stiff, the feet plantar-flexed, and movements made by circumduction. The steps also may be accompanied by toe dragging.

**spastic hemiplegia,** paralysis of one side of the body with increased tendon reflexes and uncontrolled contraction occurring in the affected muscles.

**spastic ileus** [Gk, *spasmos,* spasm, *eilein,* to twist], a form of intestinal obstruction caused by bowel spasms.

**spasticity** /spastis′ite͞/ [Gk, *spastikos,* drawing in], a form of muscular hypertonicity with increased resistance to stretch. It usually involves the flexors of the arms and the extensors of the legs. The hypertonicity is often associated with weakness, increased deep reflexes, and diminished superficial reflexes. Moderate spasticity is characterized by movements that require great effort and lack of normal coordination. Slight spasticity may be marked by gross movements that are coordinated smoothly, but combined selective movement patterns are incoordinated or impossible.

**spastic paralysis,** an abnormal condition characterized by the involuntary contraction of one or more muscles with associated loss of muscular function. Compare **flaccid paralysis.**

**spastic paraplegia** [Gk, *spasmos,* spasm, *para + plege,*

stroke], a form of partial paralysis mainly affecting older people. It is accompanied by irritability and spastic contractions of the leg muscles.

**spastic primary paraplegia.**    See **primary lateral sclerosis.**

**spastic pseudoparalysis, spastic pseudosclerosis.**    See **Creutzfeldt-Jakob disease.**

**spastic strabismus** [Gk, *spasmos + strabismos,* squint], squint caused by spasmodic contractions of ocular muscles.

**spatial dance** /spā′shəl/ [L, *spatium,* space; ME, *dauncen,* to drag along], the body shifts or movements used by individuals as they try to adjust the distance between themselves and other individuals. See also **spatial zones.**

**spatial relationships,** 1. orientation in space; the ability to locate objects in the three-dimensional external world using visual or tactile recognition and make a spatial analysis of the observed information. Spatial orientation normally is a function of the right hemisphere of the brain. 2. the relative locations of staff and equipment in an operating room with particular emphasis on what is sterile, clean, or contaminated. The operating room nurse must maintain an awareness of the arrangement of people, the height of personnel in relation to each other and to table level, and the proximity of sterile to nonsterile areas.

**spatial summation.**    See **summation,** def. 2.

**spatial zones,** the areas of personal space in which most people interact. Four basic spatial zones are the intimate zone, in which distance between individuals is less than 18 inches; the personal zone, between 18 inches and 4 feet; the social zone, extending between 4 and 12 feet; and the public zone, beyond 12 feet. See also **proxemics.**

**spatula** /spach′ə·lə/ [L], 1. a flat, blunt, usually flexible instrument, used for spreading plasters and for mixing ointments and masses. 2. a structure having a flat, blunt end.

**SPE,** abbreviation for **sucrose polyester.**

**Spearman's rho** /spir′mənz rō′/ [Charles E. Spearman, English psychologist, 1863–1945; *rho,* 17th letter in the Greek alphabet], a statistical test for correlation between two rank-ordered scales. It yields a statement of the degree of interdependence of the scores of the two scales.

**special care unit** /spesh′əl/ [L, *specialis,* individual], a hospital unit with the necessary specialized equipment and personnel for handling critically ill or injured patients, such as neonatal, burn unit, or cardiac care unit.

**special gene system,** a plasmid, transposon, or other DNA fragment that is able to transfer genetic information from one cell to another.

**specialing** /spesh′əling/, *informal.* 1. (in psychiatric nursing) the constant attendance of a professional staff member on a disturbed patient to protect the patient from harming the self or others and to observe the patient's behavior. The patient so **specialed** is accompanied in all activities by the staff member. 2. (in nursing) the giving of nursing care to only one person, such as when acting as a private duty nurse or when caring for a patient whose needs are so great that a nurse is required at all times.

**specialist** /spesh′əlist/, a health care professional who practices a specialty. A specialist usually has advanced clinical training and may have a postgraduate academic degree.

**specialist in blood bank technology.**    See **blood bank technology specialist.**

**special sense,** the sense of sight, smell, taste, touch, or hearing.

**specialty** /spesh′əlte͞/ [L, *specialis*], a branch of medicine or nursing in which the professional is specially qualified to practice by having attended an advanced program of study, by having passed an examination given by an organization of the members of the specialty, or by having gained experience through extensive practice in the specialty.

**specialty care,** specialized medical services provided by a physician specialist.

**species (Sp)** /spē′sēz, spē′shēz/, *pl.* **species (sp., spp.)** /spē′sēz, spē′shēz/ [L, *form*], the category of living things below genus in rank. A species is a genetically distinct group of demes that share a common gene pool and are reproductively isolated from all other such groups. See also **deme, genus.**

**species immunity,** a form of natural immunity shared by all members of a species. Compare **individual immunity, racial immunity.**

**species-specific** [L, *specere*, to see, *facere*, to make], **1.** characteristic of a particular species. **2.** having a characteristic effect on, or interaction with, cells, tissues, or membranes of a particular species; said of an antigen, drug, or infective agent.

**species-specific antigen,** an antigen that is restricted to a single species but occurs in all members of that species.

**species specificity.** See **specificity.**

**specific absorption rate (SAR)** /spisif′ik/ [L, *species*, form], (in hyperthermia treatment) the rate of absorption of heat energy (W) per unit mass of tissue in units of watts per kilogram (W/kg).

**specific activity,** **1.** the radioactivity of a radioisotope per unit mass of the element or compound, expressed in microcuries per millimole or disintegrations per second per milligram. **2.** the relative radioactivity per unit mass, expressed as counts per minute per milligram. For example, the specific activity of potassium in the human body is the same as that in the environment or diet; because potassium is associated chiefly with muscle tissue, a whole-body count of 40K, after administration of radioactive potassium, can be used to distinguish lean body mass from total body mass.

**specific disease,** a disorder caused by a special pathogenic organism.

**specific granule,** a secondary granule in the cytoplasm of polymorphonuclear leukocytes that contains lysozyme, vitamin $B_{12}$-binding protein, neutral proteases, and lactoferrin.

**specific granule deficiency,** an immunodeficiency state associated with pyodermas and abscesses in which neutrophils fail to make specific granules. See also **specific granule.**

**specific gravity (sp. gr.),** the ratio of the density of a substance to the density of another substance accepted as a standard. The usual standard for liquids and solids is water. Thus a liquid or solid with a specific gravity of 4 is four times as dense as water at the same temperature. Hydrogen is the usual standard for gases. See also **density, mass.**

**specific immunoglobulin,** a preparation obtained from human plasma that is preselected for its high antibody count against a specific pathogen, such as varicella zoster virus.

**specificity** /spes′əfis′itē/ [L, *species*, form, *facere*, to make], the quality of being distinctive. Kinds of specificity may include **group, species,** and **type.** See **diagnostic specificity.**

**specificity of association,** the uniqueness of a relationship between a causal factor and the occurrence of a disease.

**specific rates,** statistical rates in which the events in both the numerator and the denominator are restricted to a specific subgroup of a population.

**specific treatment.** See **treatment.**

**specific ulcer** [L, *species*, *facere*, to make, *ilcus*], ulcer associated with a specific disease, as a syphilitic ulcer.

**specific viscosity** [L, *species* + *facere*, to make, *viscosus*, sticky], the internal friction of a fluid, which may be measured by comparing the rate of flow of the fluid through a tube with the rate of a standard liquid under standard conditions.

**specimen** /spes′imən/*pl.* **specimens** [L, *specere*, to look], a small sample of something, intended to show the nature of the whole, such as a urine specimen.

**specimen management,** a nursing intervention from the Nursing Interventions Classification (NIC) defined as obtaining, preparing, and preserving a specimen for a laboratory test. See also **Nursing Interventions Classification.**

**speckled dystrophy of the cornea** /spek′əlt/, a familial condition characterized by irregular mottling of the cornea by spots that vary in shape and size, some with clear centers and sharp margins.

**speckled pattern,** an immunofluorescence pattern produced when serum from a patient with a particular connective tissue disease is placed in contact with human epithelial cells and stained with fluorochrome-labeled animal antisera. Fine, coarse, or large speckles are observed in disorders such as lupus erythematosus and rheumatoid arthritis.

**SPECT,** abbreviation for **single-photon emission computed tomography.**

**SPECTamine,** trademark for a lipid-soluble brain-imaging agent (iofetamine hydrochloride $^{123}$I).

**spectator ions** /spek′tātər/, ions that are not involved in a chemical reaction. They may be deleted when writing the equation ionically.

**Spectazole,** trademark for an antifungal (econazole nitrate).

**spectinomycin hydrochloride** /spek′tinōmī′sin/, an antibiotic.

■ INDICATIONS: It is prescribed in the treatment of gonorrhea and certain infections in penicillin-allergic patients.

■ CONTRAINDICATION: Known hypersensitivity to this drug prohibits its use.

■ ADVERSE EFFECTS: The more serious adverse reactions are oliguria, urticaria, chills, fever, dizziness, and nausea.

**spectr-,** combining form meaning 'image': *spectrograph, spectrophobia, spectrum.*

**spectra.** See **spectrum.**

**spectro-** [L, *spectrum*, image], prefix meaning relationship to a spectrum or to an image.

**Spectrobid,** trademark for a semisynthetic penicillin (bacampicillin).

**Spectrocin,** trademark for a fixed-combination topical drug containing antibacterials (neomycin sulfate and gramicidin).

**spectrometer** /spektrom′ətər/ [L, *spectrum*, image; Gk, *metron*, measure], an instrument for measuring wavelengths of rays of the spectrum, the deviation of refracted rays, and the angles between faces of a prism. See also **mass spectrometer, Mössbauer spectrometer.**

**spectrometry** /spektrom′ətrē/, the process of measuring wavelengths of light and other electromagnetic waves. See also **spectrometer. —spectrometric,** *adj.*

**spectrophotometric.** See **spectrophotometry.**

**spectrophotometric analysis.** See **quantitative analysis.**

**spectrophotometry** /spek′trōfətom′ətrē/, the measurement of color in a solution by determining the amount of light absorbed in the ultraviolet, infrared, or visible spectrum, widely used in clinical chemistry to calculate the concentration of substances in solution. **—spectrophotometric,** *adj.*

**spectroscope** /spek′trə·skōp/ [L, *spectrum*, spectrum; Gk, *skopein*, to examine], an instrument for developing and analyzing spectra.

**spectroscopy** /spek·tros′kə·pē/ [L, *spectrum*, spectrum; Gk, *skopein*, to examine], the propagation and analysis of spectra; examination by means of a spectroscope.

**spectrum** /spek′trəm/, *pl.* **spectra** [L, image], **1.** a range of phenomena or properties occurring in increasing or decreasing magnitude. Radiant or electromagnetic energy is arranged on the basis of wavelength and frequency. Electromagnetic radiation includes spectra of radio waves, infrared waves, visible light, ultraviolet waves, x-rays, and gamma rays. **2.** the range of effectiveness of an antibiotic. A broad-spectrum antibiotic is effective against a wide range of microorganisms. See also **antibiotic, electromagnetic radiation, wave.**

**speculum** /spek′yələm/ [L, mirror], a retractor used to separate the walls of a cavity to make examination possible, such as an ear speculum, an eye speculum, a nasal speculum, or a vaginal speculum.

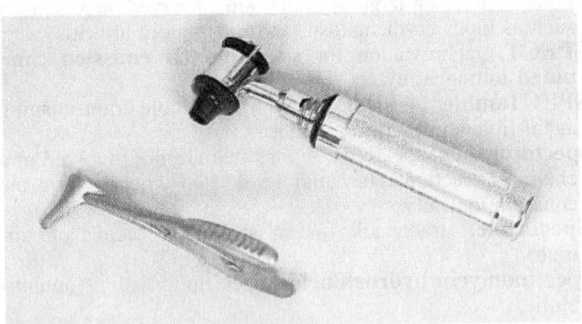

**Nasal specula** *(Seidel et al, 1999)*

**speech** [ME, *speche*], **1.** the utterance of articulate vocal sounds that form words of a language to give expression to one's thoughts or ideas. **2.** communication by means of spoken words. **3.** the faculty of language production, which involves the complex coordination of the muscles and nerves of the organs of articulation. Any neurologic or muscular injury or defect involving these organs results in various speech impediments or dysfunctions. Kinds of dysfunctions include **ataxic speech, explosive speech, mirror speech, scamping speech, scanning speech, slurred speech,** and **staccato speech.** See also **speech dysfunction.**

**speech abnormalities.** See **speech dysfunction.**

**speech audiometry.** See **audiometry.**

**speech centers** [AS, *spaec* + Gk, *kentron*], either of two motor areas involved in speech. Broca's motor speech area is a unilateral area in the posterior part of the inferior frontal gyrus and usually on the side contralateral to the dominant hand. Wernicke's second motor speech area is an area comprising the posterior part of the superior temporal gyrus next to the transverse temproal gyri and the supramarginal and temporal gyri. See also **Broca's area** and **Wernicke's center.**

**speech dysfunction,** any defect or abnormality of speech, including aphasia, alexia, stammering, stuttering, aphonia, and slurring. Speech problems may result from any of a variety of causes, among them neurologic injury to the cerebral cortex; muscular paralysis caused by trauma, disease, or cerebrovascular accident; structural abnormality of the organs of speech; emotional or psychologic tension, strain, or depression; hysteria; and severe mental retardation. See also **speech.**

**speech-language pathologist (SLP),** a health professional with graduate education in human communication, its development, and its disorders. A speech-language pathologist specializes in the measurement and evaluation of language abilities, auditory processes, speech production, and swallowing problems; clinical treatment of speech and language disorders; and research methods in the study of communication problems.

**speech-language pathology, 1.** the study of abnormalities of speech and language. **2.** the diagnosis and treatment of abnormalities of speech and language as practiced by a speech pathologist or a speech-language therapist.

**speech-language therapist.** See **speech-language pathologist.**

**speech reading** [ME, *reden,* to explain], a method of oral communication in which one uses the visual clues of the speaker's lip and facial movements, along with residual hearing. Gestures and "body language" also are observed. Formerly called **lip reading.** See also **sign language.**

**speech reception threshold,** the minimum intensity in decibels at which a patient can understand 50 per cent of spoken words; used in tests of speech audiometry. Also called **speech recognition threshold.**

**speech synthesizer** [AS, *spaec* + Gk, *synthesis,* placing together], an electronic apparatus with a keyboard that produces sounds that imitate the human voice.

**speech therapy** [AS, *spaec* + Gk, *therapeia,* treatment], the application of treatments and counseling in the prevention or correction of speech and language disorders. See also **speech-language pathologist.**

**speed** [AS, *spedan,* to hasten], **1.** the rate of change of position with time. Compare **velocity. 2.** *slang.* any stimulating drug, such as amphetamine. **3.** a reciprocal of the amount of radiation used to produce an image with various components of an x-ray imaging system, such as screens, film, and image intensifiers. There is often a tradeoff between radiation dose to the patient and the overall image quality. Thus a system using little radiation is "fast," whereas one requiring more radiation is "slow." **4.** the amount of exposure of film to light or x-rays needed to produce a desired image. X-ray film speed usually is indicated as the reciprocal of the exposure in roentgens necessary to produce a density of 1 above the base and fog levels. See also **fogged film fault.**

**speed shock,** a sudden adverse physiologic reaction to IV medications or drugs that are administered too quickly. Some signs of speed shock are a flushed face, headache, a tight feeling in the chest, irregular pulse, loss of consciousness, and cardiac arrest.

**sPEEP,** abbreviation for **spontaneous PEEP.**

**spell of illness** [ME, *spel* + *illr,* bad], a period regarded by Medicare rules as the number of days between the admission of an insured patient to a hospital and the day that marks the end of a period during which the insured has not been an inpatient in a hospital or a skilled nursing facility.

**sperm.** See **semen, spermatozoon.**

**-sperm** /spurm/, combining form meaning a 'seed': *gymnosperm, oosperm, zygosperm.*

**sperm antibody,** a glycoprotein that specifically recognizes the head or tail of a spermatozoon. The antibodies are found often in vasectomized males and infrequently in infertile males and infertile females.

**spermatic cord** /spərmat′ik/ [Gk, *sperma,* seed, *chorde,* string], a structure extending from the deep inguinal ring in the abdomen to the testis, descending nearly vertically into the scrotum. The left spermatic cord is usually longer than the right; consequently the left testis usually hangs lower than the right. Each cord comprises arteries, veins, lymphatics, nerves, and the vas deferens of the testis.

**spermatic duct.** See **vas deferens.**

**spermatic fistula,** an abnormal passage communicating with a testis or a seminal duct.

**spermatid** /spur′mətid, spərmat′id/ [Gk, *sperma*, seed], a male germ cell that arises from a spermatocyte and becomes a mature spermatozoon in the last phase of spermatogenesis.

**spermato-** /spur′mətō-, spərmat′ō-/, **spermo-,** combining form meaning 'seed, specifically the male generative element': *spermatoblast, spermatocyst, spermatogenesis.*

**spermatocele** /spərmat′əsēl′, spur′-/ [Gk, *sperma* + *kele,* tumor], a cystic swelling, either of the epididymis or of the rete testis, that contains spermatozoa. It lies above, behind, and separate from the testis. It is usually painless and requires no therapy.

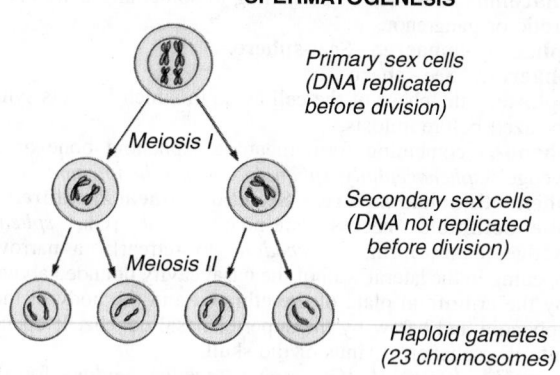

**SPERMATOGENESIS**

Primary sex cells
(DNA replicated
before division)

*Meiosis I*

Secondary sex cells
(DNA not replicated
before division)

*Meiosis II*

Haploid gametes
(23 chromosomes)

**Spermatogenesis** *(Thibodeau and Patton, 1999)*

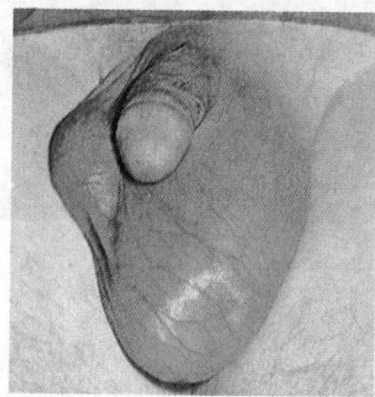

**Spermatocele** *(Lloyd-Davies et al, 1994)*

**spermatocide** /spərmat′əsīd, spur′-/ [Gk, *sperma* + L, *caedere,* to kill], a chemical substance that kills spermatozoa by reducing their surface tension, causing the cell wall to break down by a bactericidal effect or by creation of a highly acidic environment. Among many spermatocidal agents used in various contraceptive creams are lactic acid, phenylmercuric acetate, chloramine polyethylene glycol, benzethonium chloride, and certain quinine compounds. Also called **spermicide.**

**spermatocyte** /spur′mətōsīt′/ [Gk, *sperma* + *kytos,* cell], a male germ cell that arises from a spermatogonium. Each spermatocyte gives rise to two haploid secondary spermatocytes which become spermatids.

**spermatogenesis** /spərmat′əjen′əsis, spur′-/ [Gk, *sperma* + *genesis,* origin], the process of development of spermatozoa, consisting of two stages. In the first stage, spermatogonia become spermatocytes, which develop into spermatids. In the second stage, called spermiogenesis, the spermatids become spermatozoa. Also called **spermatocytogenesis, spermiogenesis.—spermatogenic, spermatogenous,** *adj.*

**spermatogonium,** /-gō′nē·əm/ *pl.* spermatogonia [Gk, *sperma* + *gone,* generation], a male germ cell that gives rise to a spermatocyte early in spermatogenesis.

**spermatopathia** /-path′ē·ə/ [Gk, *sperma,* seed, *pathos,* disease], pertaining to diseased sperm or their associated organs. Also called **spermopathy.**

**spermatozoon** /spur′mətəzō′ən, spərmat′-/, *pl.* **spermatozoa** /-zō′ə/ [Gk, *sperma* + *zoon,* animal], a mature male germ cell that develops in the seminiferous tubules of the testes. Resembling a tadpole, it is about 50 μm (1/500 inch) long and has a head with a nucleus, a neck, and a tail that provides propulsion. Developed in vast numbers after puberty, spermatozoa are the generative component of the semen. See **spermatogenesis.**

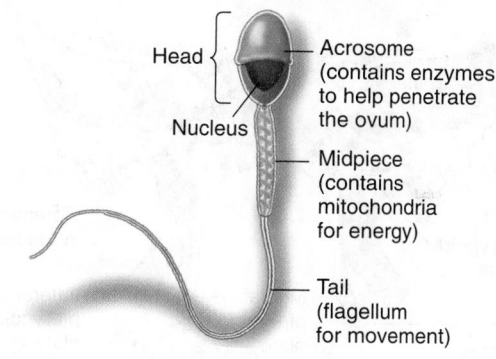

Head

Acrosome
(contains enzymes
to help penetrate
the ovum)

Nucleus

Midpiece
(contains
mitochondria
for energy)

Tail
(flagellum
for movement)

**Spermatozoon** *(Leonard, 2001)*

**sperm bank** /spurm/ [Gk, *sperma,* seed; It, *banca,* bench], a facility for storage of semen to be used for artificial insemination.

**-spermia, -spermy,** combining form meaning '(condition of) possessing or producing seed': *aspermia, asthenospermia, necrospermia.*

**spermicidal** /spur′misī′dəl/, destructive to spermatozoa.

**spermicide.** See **spermatocide.**

**spermiogenesis.** See **spermatogenesis.**

**spermo-.** See **spermato-.**

**spermopathy.** See **spermatopathia.**

**-spermy.** See **-spermia.**

**SPF,** abbreviation for **sunscreen protective factor index.**

**sp. gr.,** abbreviation for **specific gravity.**

**sphacel-,** combining form meaning 'gangrene': *sphaceloderma, sphacelotoxin, sphacelus.*

**sphacelous** /sfas′ələs/, pertaining to something that is necrotic or gangrenous.

**-sphaera, -sphaere.** See **-sphere.**

**sphaero-.** See **sphero-.**

**S-phase,** the phase of the cell cycle in which DNA is synthesized before mitosis.

**spheno-,** combining form meaning 'sphenoid bone or a wedge': *sphenocephaly, sphenoidotomy, sphenotemporal.*

**sphenoethmoidal suture.** See **ethmosphenoid suture.**

**sphenoethmoid recess** /sfē′nō·eth′moid/ [Gk, *sphen,* wedge, *eidos,* form; L, *recedere,* to retreat], a narrow opening in the lateral wall of the nasal cavity bounded above by the cribriform plate of the ethmoid and the body of the sphenoid and below by the superior nasal concha. It opens into the sphenoidal sinus of the skull.

**sphenoid** /sfē′noid/ [Gk, *sphen,* wedge, *eidos,* form], wedge-shaped. See also **sphenoid bone.**

**sphenoidal fissure** /sfēnoi′dəl/ [Gk *sphen,* wedge, *eidos* form], a cleft between the great and small wings of the sphenoid bone.

**sphenoidal sinus,** one of a pair of cavities in the sphenoid bone of the skull, lined with mucous membrane that is continuous with that of the nasal cavity. Compare **ethmoidal air cell, frontal sinus, maxillary sinus.**

**sphenoid bone,** the bone at the base of the skull, anterior to the temporal bones and the basilar part of the occipital bone. It resembles a bat with its wings extended. Also called **sphenoid.**

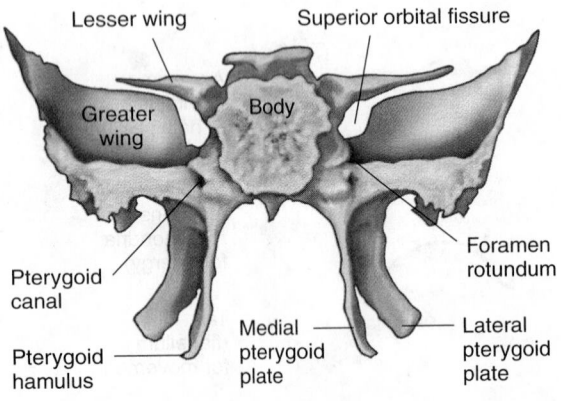

**Sphenoid bone**

**sphenoid fontanel,** an anterolateral fontanel that is usually not palpable. See also **fontanel.**

**sphenoiditis** /sfē′noidī′tis/ [Gk, *sphen,* wedge, *eidos,* form, *itis,* inflammation], an inflammation of the sphenoidal sinus.

**sphenomandibular ligament** /sfē′nōmandib′yələr/ [Gk, *sphen + eidos +* L, *mandere,* to chew], one of a pair of flat, thin ligaments comprising part of the temporomandibular joint between the mandible of the jaw and the temporal bone of the skull. It is attached to the spine of the sphenoid bone and becomes broader as it descends to the lingula of the mandibular foramen.

**sphere** /sfir/, a globe-shaped object, theoretically generated by a circle revolving on a diameter as its axis.

**-sphere** /sfir/, **-sphaera, -sphaere, 1.** suffix meaning a 'spheric body': *chondriosphere, oncosphere, somosphere.*

**2.** combining form meaning a 'realm that supports life': *biosphere, vivosphere, zoosphere.*

**sphero-, sphaero-,** combining form meaning 'round or a sphere': *spherocyte, spherolith, spherometer.*

**spherocyte** /sfir′əsīt/ [Gk, *sphaira,* sphere, *kytos,* cell], an abnormal spheric red cell that contains more than the normal amount of hemoglobin. Spherocytes can be identified under the microscope on stained blood specimens. Osmotic fragility of the red blood cells increases in the presence of increased numbers of spherocytes. —**spherocytic,** *adj.*

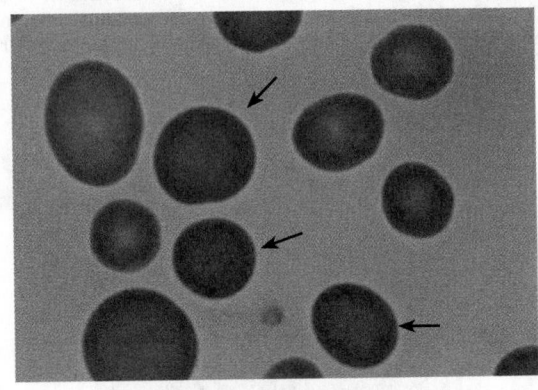

**Spherocytes** *(Carr and Rodak, 1999)*

**spherocytic anemia** /sfir′əsit′ik/, a hematologic disorder inherited as an autosomal dominant trait and characterized by hemolytic anemia caused by the presence of red blood cells that are spheric rather than round and biconcave. The cells are fragile and tend to hemolyze in the oxygen-poor peripheral circulatory system. Episodic crises of abdominal pain, fever, jaundice, and splenomegaly occur. Because repeated transfusions are often needed to treat the anemia, siderosis may develop. Splenectomy may then be necessary. Compare **congenital nonspherocytic hemolytic anemia.** See also **elliptocytosis.**

**spherocytosis** /sfir′ōsītō′sis/, the abnormal presence of spherocytes in the blood. Compare **elliptocytosis.**

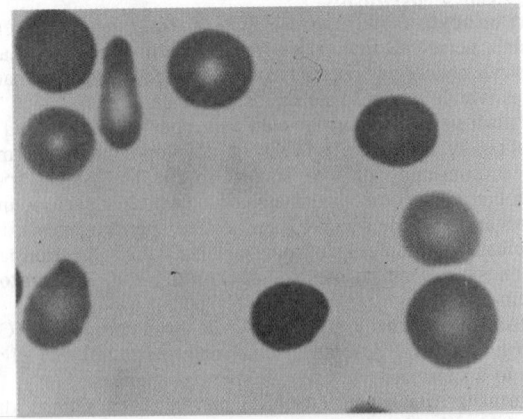

**Spherocytosis** *(Zitelli and Davis, 1997)*

**spheroidal** /sfir'oidəl/ [Gk, *sphaira*, ball, *eidos*, form], ball-shaped.

**spheroidea.** See **ball-and-socket joint.**

**spherule** /sfer'yōōl/ [Gk, *sphaira*, ball], a small ball.

**sphincter** /sfingk'tər/ [Gk, *sphingein*, to bind], a circular band of muscle fibers that constricts a passage or closes a natural opening in the body, such as the hepatic sphincter in the muscular coat of the hepatic veins near their union with the superior vena cava, and the external anal sphincter, which closes the anus.

**sphincter-,** combining form meaning 'band or sphincter': *sphincteric, sphincterectomy, sphincteral.*

**sphincter ani,** a double set of circular muscles at the opening of the anus. One, the sphincter ani internus, consists of a thickened inner circular coat of the bowel smooth muscle; the other, the sphincter ani externus, is a flat sheet of striated, voluntary muscle surrounding the anal orifice.

**sphincter choledochus** /kōled'əkəs/, a smooth muscle sphincter that encircles the lower end of the bile duct and is part of the sphincter of Oddi.

**sphincter of Oddi** [Ruggero Oddi, Italian physician, 1864–1913], a band of circular muscle fibers around the lower end of the common bile and pancreatic duct (hepatopancreatic duct).

**sphincter pupillae,** a muscle that contracts the iris, narrowing the diameter of the pupil of the eye. It is composed of circular fibers arranged in a narrow band about 1 mm wide, surrounding the margin of the pupil toward the posterior surface of the iris. The circular fibers near the free margin of the iris are closely packed; those that are near the periphery of the band are more separated and form incomplete circles. The fibers of the sphincter pupillae blend with the fibers of the dilatator pupillae near the margin of the pupil and are innervated by a motor root of the ciliary ganglion from the oculomotor nerve. Compare **dilator pupillae.**

**sphincter virginae.** See **bulbocavernosus.**

**sphingolipid** /sfing'gōlip'id/ [Gk, *sphingein*, to bind, *lipos*, fat], a compound that consists of a lipid and a sphingosine. It is found in high concentrations in the brain and other tissues of the nervous system, especially membranes.

**sphingomyelin** /sfing'gōmī'əlin/ [Gk, *sphingein* + *myelos*, marrow], any of a group of sphingolipids containing phosphorus. It occurs primarily in the tissue of the nervous system, generally in membranes, and in the lipids in the blood.

**sphingomyelin lipidosis,** any of a group of diseases characterized by an abnormality in the ability of the body to store sphingolipids. Kinds of sphingomyelin lipidosis include **Gaucher's disease, Niemann-Pick disease,** and **Tay-Sachs disease.** See also **angiokeratoma corporis diffusum.**

**sphingosine** /sfing'gōsēn/, a long-chain, unsaturated amino alcohol, a major constituent of sphingolipids, including sphingomyelins.

**sphygm-, sphygmo-,** combining form meaning 'pulse': *sphygmodynamometer, sphygmoid, sphygmomanometer.*

**-sphygmia,** combining form meaning '(condition of the) pulse': *anisosphygmia, hemisphygmia, sychnosphygmia.*

**sphygmic interval** /sfig'mik/. See **ejection period.**

**sphygmo-.** See **sphygm-.**

**sphygmogram** /sfig'məgram/ [Gk, *sphygmos*, pulse, *gramma*, record], a pulse tracing produced by a sphygmograph. A curve occurs on the tracing with each atrial pulsation. An upward, primary elevation is followed by a sudden drop to a point slightly above the baseline. The curve then gradually descends to the baseline in small decrements of amplitude. Sphygmographic abnormalities of rate, rhythm,

and form may be diagnostically useful in an assessment of cardiovascular function.

**sphygmograph** /sfig'məgraf/, an instrument that records the force of the arterial pulse on a tracing, the sphygmogram. —**sphygmographic,** *adj.*

**sphygmoid** /sfig'moid/ [Gk, *sphygmos*, pulse, *eidos*, form], pertaining to or resembling the pulse.

**sphygmomanometer** /sfig'mōmənom'ətər/ [Gk, *sphygmos* + *manos*, thin, *metron*, measure], an instrument for indirect measurement of blood pressure. It consists of an inflatable cuff that fits around a limb, a bulb for controlling air pressure within the cuff, and a mercury or aneroid manom-

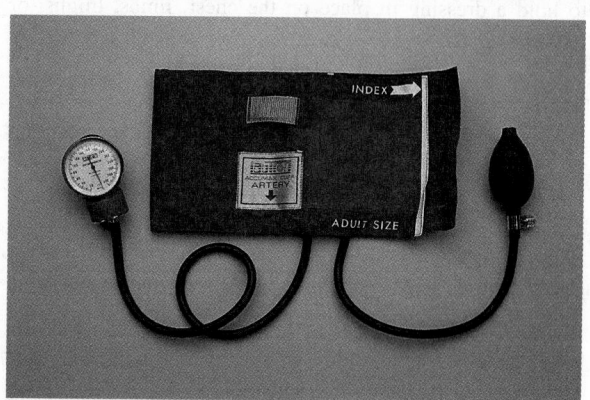

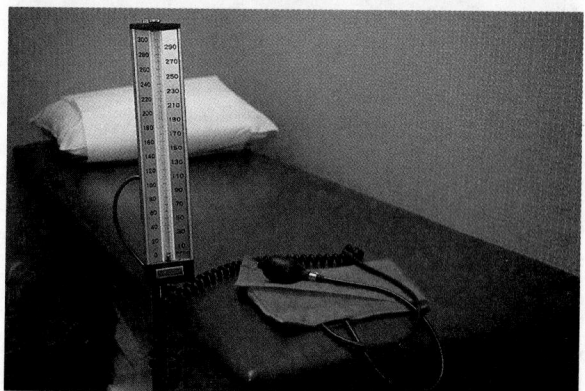

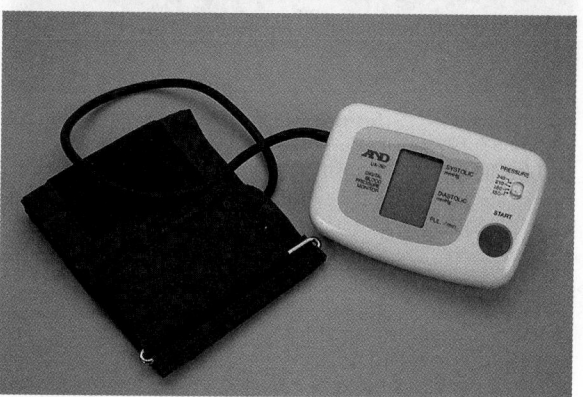

**Sphygmomanometers: aneroid *(top)*, mercury *(middle)*, and digital *(bottom)***
*(Sorrentino, 2000)*

eter. Pressure in the compressed artery is estimated by the column of mercury it balances when the cuff is inflated. See also **blood pressure, manometer.**

**sphygmoplethysmograph** /-pləthis′məgraf′/ [Gk, *sphygmos,* pulse, *plethysmos,* increase, *graphein,* to record], an instrument for measuring and recording the arterial pulse curve and blood flow in a limb.

**spica** [L, *spica,* spike, or ear of wheat], a figure-eight bandage that, when applied to a joint, resembles the head of a stalk of wheat.

**spica bandage** /spī′kə/ [L, *spica,* spike of wheat; Fr, *bande,* strip], a figure-eight bandage in which each turn generally overlaps the previous to form a succession of V-like designs. It may be used to give support, to apply pressure, or to hold a dressing in place on the chest, limbs, thighs, or pelvis.

**spica cast,** an orthopedic cast applied to immobilize part or all of the trunk of the body and part or all of one or more extremities. It is used to treat various fractures, such as of the hip and the femur, and to correct or maintain the correction of hip deformities. Kinds of spica casts are **bilateral long-leg spica cast, one-and-a-half spica cast, shoulder spica cast,** and **unilateral long-leg spica cast.** See also **cast.**

**spicule** /spik′yool/ [L, *spiculum,* point], a small sharp body with a needlelike point.

**spider angioma** [ME, *spithre* + Gk, *angeion,* vessel, *oma,* tumor], a form of telangiectasis characterized by a central elevated red dot the size of a pinhead from which small blood vessels radiate. Spider angiomas are often associated with elevated estrogen levels, such as occur in pregnancy or when the liver is diseased and unable to detoxify estrogens. Also called **spider nevus.** See also **telangiectasia.**

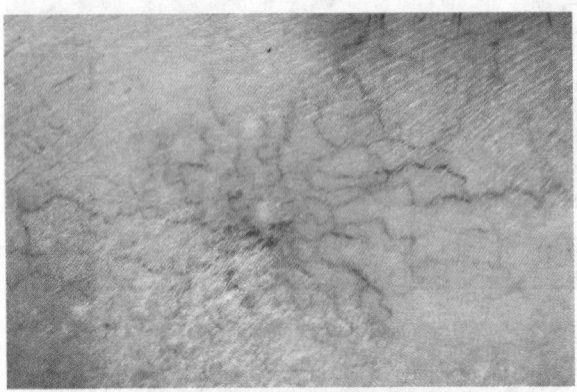

**Spider angioma**
*(Habif, 1996/courtesy American Academy of Dermatology and Institute for Dermatologic Communication, Schaumburg, Illinois)*

**spider antivenin.** See **black widow spider antivenin.**

**spider bite** [ME, *spithre* + AS, *bitan* + L, *potio,* drink], a puncture wound produced by the bite by any of nearly 60 species of venomous spiders found in North America. Most spiders have fangs that are too short or fragile to penetrate the skin, but some are dangerous to humans. These include the black widow, *Lactrodectus mactans;* the brown recluse, *Loxosceles reclusa;* and species of jumping spiders and tarantulas. Spider venom may contain enzymatic proteins, including peptides that may affect neuromuscular transmission or cardiovascular function.

**spider nevus.** See **spider angioma.**

**spider telangiectasia** [ME, *spithre* + Gk, *telos,* end, *angeion,* vessel, *ektasis,* dilation], a branched group of dilated capillary blood vessels forming a spiderlike image on the skin. Also called **nevus araneus.**

**spike,** a sharp peak in an electronic recording, such as an oscillograph.

**spikeboard** /spīk′bôrd/, a device that enables people with upper extremity disabilities to stabilize foods for meal preparation, typically used by individuals with functional use of only one hand. Sometimes called **paring board.**

**spillway** [AS, *spillan,* to destroy, *weg,* wagon track], a channel or passageway through which food normally escapes from the occlusal surfaces of the teeth during chewing.

**spin** [AS, *spinnan,* to draw threads], **1.** the intrinsic angular momentum of an elementary particle or a nucleus of an atom. **2.** intrinsic joint movements about an axis perpendicular to the articular surface.

**spina** /spī′nə/, *pl.* **spinae** [L, backbone], **1.** the spinal column. **2.** a spine or a thornlike projection, such as the bony projection on the anterior border of the ilium, forming the anterior end of the iliac crest.

**spina bifida** /bif′ədə, bī′fədə/, a congenital neural tube defect in which there is a developmental anomaly in the posterior vertebral arch. Spina bifida is relatively common, occurring approximately 10 to 20 times per 1000 births. It may occur with only a small deformed lamina separated by a midline gap, or it may be associated with the complete absence of laminae surrounding a large area. In cases where the separation is wide enough, contents of the spinal canal protrude posteriorly, and a myelomeningocele is evident. Neurologic deficits do not usually accompany the anomalies involving only bony deformity. Direct signs and symptoms are rarely noted in spina bifida, which is frequently diagnosed accidentally during radiographic examinations required for other reasons. Spina bifida that does not involve herniation of the meninges or the contents of the spinal canal (**spina bifida occulta**) rarely requires treatment. Also called **spinal dysrhaphia.**

**spina bifida anterior,** incomplete closure along the anterior surface of the vertebral column. The defect is often associated with developmental anomalies of the abdominal and thoracic viscera.

**spina bifida cystica,** a developmental defect of the central nervous system in which a hernial cyst containing meninges (meningocele), spinal cord (myelocele), or both (myelomeningocele) protrudes through a congenital cleft in the vertebral column. The protruding sac is encased in a layer of skin or a fine membrane that readily ruptures, causing the leakage of cerebrospinal fluid and an increased risk of meningeal infection. The severity of neurologic dysfunction and associated defects depends directly on the degree of nerve involvement. The most severe type is lumbosacral myelomeningocele, which is frequently associated with hydrocephalus and the Arnold-Chiari malformation. Compare **spina bifida occulta.** See also **myelomeningocele, neural tube defect.**

**spina bifida occulta,** defective closure of the laminae of the vertebral column in the lumbosacral region without hernial protrusion of the spinal cord or meninges. The defect, which is quite common, occurs in about 5% of the population. It is identified externally by a skin depression or dimple, dark tufts of hair, telangiectasis, or soft subcutaneous lipomas at the site. Because the neural tube has closed,

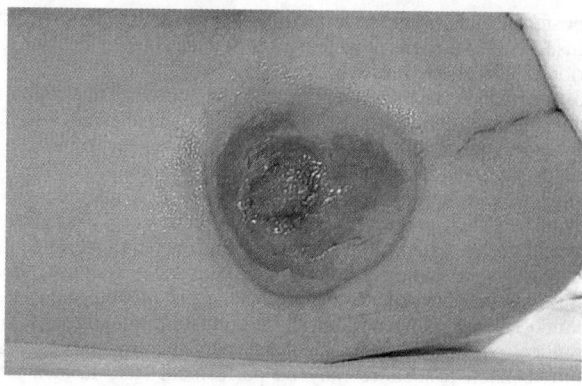

**Spina bifida cystica** *(Newton, 1995)*

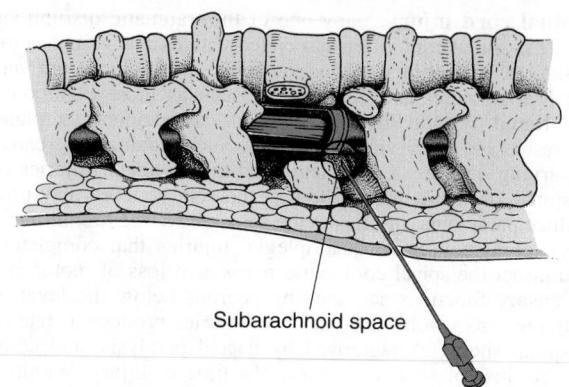

Subarachnoid space

**Spinal anesthesia** *(Ignatavicius, Workman, and Mishler, 1999)*

there are usually no neurologic impairments associated with the defect. However, any abnormal adhesion of the spinal cord to the area of the malformation may lead to neuromuscular disturbances, usually problems with gait and foot weakness and with the bowel and bladder sphincters. Compare **spina bifida cystica.**

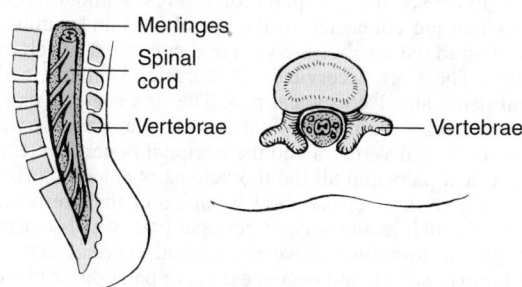

Meninges
Spinal cord
Vertebrae
Vertebrae

**Spina bifida occulta** *(Wong et al, 1999)*

**spinal** /spī'nəl/ [L, *spina*],   **1.** pertaining to a spine, especially the spinal column. **2.** *informal.* spinal anesthesia, such as saddle block or caudal anesthesia.

**spinal accessory nerve.**   See **accessory nerve.**

**spinal anesthesia** [L, *spina,* backbone; Gk, *anaisthesia,* lack of feeling],   a state of lack of sensation in the lower part of the body produced by injection of a local anesthetic drug into the subarachnoid cerebrospinal fluid space. Also called **subarachnoid block anesthesia.**

**spinal aperture,**   a large opening formed by the body of a vertebra and its arch.

**spinal block** [L, *spina,* backbone; OFr, *bloc*],   an obstruction of cerebrospinal fluid circulation. See also **subarachnoid block anesthesia.**

**spinal canal,**   the cavity within the vertebral column.

**spinal caries.**   See **tuberculous spondylitis.**

**spinal column.**   See **vertebral column.**

**spinal cord,**   a long nearly cylindric structure lodged in the vertebral canal and extending from the foramen magnum at the base of the skull to the upper part of the lumbar region. A major component of the central nervous system, the adult cord is approximately 1 cm in diameter, with an average

length of 42 to 45 cm and a weight of 30 g. The cord is an extension of the medulla oblongata of the brain that extends at the level of the first or second lumbar vertebra. The cord conducts sensory and motor impulses to and from the brain and controls many reflexes. Thirty-one pairs of spinal nerves originate from the cord: 8 cervical, 12 thoracic, 5 lumbar, 5 sacral, and 1 coccygeal. It has an inner core of gray material consisting mainly of nerve cell bodies. The cord is enclosed by three protective membranes (meninges): the dura mater, arachnoid, and pia mater. Also called **chorda spinalis, medulla spinalis.** See also **segments of spinal cord, spinal nerves.**

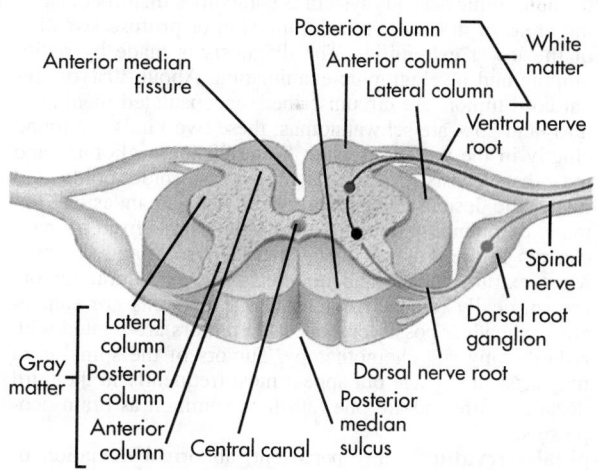

Posterior column
Anterior median fissure
Anterior column
Lateral column
White matter
Ventral nerve root
Lateral column
Gray matter
Posterior column
Anterior column
Central canal
Dorsal nerve root
Posterior median sulcus
Spinal nerve
Dorsal root ganglion

**Cross section of the spinal cord**
*(Thibodeau and Patton, 1999/Rolin Graphics)*

**spinal cord compression,**   an abnormal and often serious condition resulting from pressure on the spinal cord. The symptoms range from temporary numbness of an extremity to permanent quadriplegia, depending on the cause, severity, and location of the pressure. Causes include spinal fracture, vertebral dislocation, tumor, hemorrhage, and edema associated with contusion. See also **herniated disk, spondylolisthesis.**

**spinal cord injury,** any one of the traumatic disruptions of the spinal cord, often associated with extensive musculoskeletal involvement. Common spinal cord injuries are vertebral fractures and dislocations, such as those commonly suffered by individuals involved in car accidents, airplane crashes, or other violent impacts. Such trauma may cause varying degrees of paraplegia and quadriplegia. Injuries to spinal structures below the first thoracic vertebra may produce paraplegia. Injuries to the spine above the first thoracic vertebra may cause quadriplegia. Injuries that completely transect the spinal cord cause permanent loss of motor and sensory functions activated by neurons below the level of the lesions involved. Spinal cord injuries produce a state of spinal shock, characterized by flaccid paralysis, and complete loss of skin sensation at the time of injury. Within a few weeks the muscles affected may become spastic, and skin sensation may return to a slight degree. The motor and sensory losses that prevail a few weeks after the injury are usually permanent. Musculoskeletal complications are associated with the neurologic involvement of spinal cord injuries, and prevention of decubitus ulcers and the treatment of any loss of bladder and bowel control are continuing concerns. Treatment of spinal cord injuries varies considerably and involves numerous approaches, such as orthopedic exercises, ambulatory techniques, and special physical and psychologic therapy. See also **hemiplegia, paraplegia, quadriplegia.**

**spinal cord tumor,** a neoplasm of the spinal cord of which more than 50% are extramedullary, about 25% are intramedullary, and the rest are extradural. Symptoms usually develop slowly and may progress from unilateral paresthesia and a dull ache to lancinating pain, weakness in one or both legs, abnormal deep tendon reflexes, and, in advanced cases, monoplegia, hemiplegia, or paraplegia. Function of the autonomic nervous system is sometimes disturbed, causing areas of dry, cold, bluish pink skin or profuse sweating of the lower extremities. The diagnosis is made by radiographic and myelographic examination. About 30% of spinal cord tumors are circumscribed, encapsulated meningiomas, and 25% are schwannomas; these two kinds are found chiefly in the thoracic region. Some 20% are gliomas, and the others consist of congenital lipomas, epidermoids, and metastatic lesions. The dura is resistant to invasion, but many extradural tumors are metastatic lesions from primary cancers in the prostate, lung, breast, thyroid, and GI tract. Most extramedullary and nonmetastatic extradural tumors are surgically removed; intermedullary lesions are enucleated, whenever possible; inoperable tumors are treated with radiotherapy and chemotherapy. Tumors of the spinal cord may arise at any age but appear most frequently in the third decade of life and are one fourth as common as brain neoplasms.

**spinal curvature,** any persistent, abnormal deviation of the vertebral column from its normal position. Kinds of spinal curvature are **kyphoscoliosis, kyphosis, lordosis,** and **scoliosis.**

**spinal dysrhaphis.** See **spina bifida.**

**spinal fasciculi.** See **spinal tract.**

**spinal fluid.** See **cerebrospinal fluid.**

**spinal fusion,** the fixation of an unstable segment of the spine. It is accomplished by skeletal traction or immobilization of the patient in a body cast but most frequently by a surgical procedure. Operative ankylosis may be performed in the treatment of spinal fractures or after diskectomy or laminectomy for the correction of a herniated vertebral disk. Surgical fusion involves the stabilization of a spinal section with a bone graft or synthetic device introduced through a posterior incision in the lumbar region; in the less frequently fused cervical region the incision may be anterior or posterior. Also called **spondylosyndesis.**

**spinal headache,** a severe headache occurring after spinal anesthesia, lumbar puncture, or epidural anesthesia, caused by a leak of cerebrospinal fluid (CSF) from the subarachnoid space and the subsequent lowering of intracranial pressure. Severe spinal headache may be accompanied by diminished aural and visual acuity. Treatment usually includes keeping the patient flat in bed to relieve the meningeal irritation, promoting increased fluid intake to increase the intravascular volume and increase the production and volume of cerebrospinal fluid, and administering analgesics to reduce pain. If severe headache persists, an autologous blood patch procedure may be performed. Also known as postdural puncture headache (PDPH). See also **epidural blood patch.**

**spinal manipulation,** the forced passive flexion, extension, and rotation of vertebral segments, carrying the elements of articulation beyond the usual range of movement to the limit of anatomic range. Spinal manipulation may be used effectively in physiotherapy for the treatment of vertebral and sacroiliac dislocations, sprains, and adhesions.

**spinal meningitis,** an inflammation of the membranes of the spinal cord.

**spinal motion segment,** two adjacent vertebrae and the connecting tissues that bind them together.

**spinal muscular atrophy.** See **Duchenne's disease.**

**spinal nerves,** the 31 pairs of nerves without special names that are connected to the spinal cord and numbered according to the level of the vertebral column at which they emerge. There are 8 cervical, 12 thoracic, 5 lumbar, and 5 sacral pairs, and 1 coccygeal pair. The first cervical pair of nerves emerges from the spinal cord in the space between the first cervical vertebra and the occipital bone. The rest of the cervical pairs and all the thoracic pairs emerge horizontally through the intervertebral foramina of their respective vertebrae, such as the second cervical pair, which emerges through the foramina above the second cervical vertebra. The lumbar, sacral, and coccygeal nerve pairs descend from their points of origin at the lower end of the cord before reaching the intervertebral foramina of their respective vertebrae. Each spinal nerve attaches to the spinal cord by an anterior (or ventral) root and a posterior (or dorsal) root. The nerve impulses enter the cord by way of posterior roots. The posterior roots supply skin and muscles of much of the body with some of the nerve fibers supplying autonomic functions. The posterior roots contain sensory neurons and accompany a distended spinal ganglion within the vertebral foramina. The ventral roots contain motor neuron axons. The sacral plexus in the pelvic cavity comprises certain spinal nerve fibers from the lumbar and sacral regions and gives rise to the great sciatic nerve in the back of the thigh. See also **spinal cord.**

**spinal puncture.** See **lumbar puncture.**

**spinal reflex** [L, *spina* + *reflectere,* to bend back], any reflex with a pathway through the spinal cord but not the brain.

**spinal segment,** a division of the spinal cord containing a bilateral pair of nerve roots. From the anterior to the posterior, the segments are referred to as cervical ($C_1$-$C_8$), thoracic ($T_1$-$T_{12}$), lumbar ($L_1$-$L_5$), sacral ($S_1$-$S_5$), and coccygeal ($Co_1$-$Co_3$).

**spinal shock,** a form of shock associated with acute injury to the spinal cord. Temporary suppression of reflexes controlled by segments below the level of injury. The period of shock may last from hours to months. See also **shock.**

tary motor activity is regulated by motor nerve stimulation from the brain and brainstem to the motor neurons of the spinal cord.

**spin density,** a measure of the hydrogen concentration in magnetic resonance (MR) imaging. It is proportional to the number of hydrogen nuclei precessing at the Larmor frequency and contributing to the MR signal. See also **Larmor frequency.**

**spindle** [AS, *spinel*, to spin], **1.** the fusiform-shaped body of achromatin in the cell nucleus during the late prophase and the metaphase of mitosis. It consists of tiny fibers radiating out from the centrosomes and connecting them with one another. **2.** a type of brain wave, consisting of a short series of changes in electrical potential with a frequency of 14 per second. **3.** any one of the special receptor organs comprising the neurotendinous and neuromuscular spindles distributed throughout the body. These kinds of spindles serve as special receptor organs that detect the degree of stretch in a muscle or at the junction of a muscle with its tendon and are essential in maintaining muscle tone.

**spindle cell carcinoma,** a rapidly growing neoplasm composed of fusiform squamous cells.

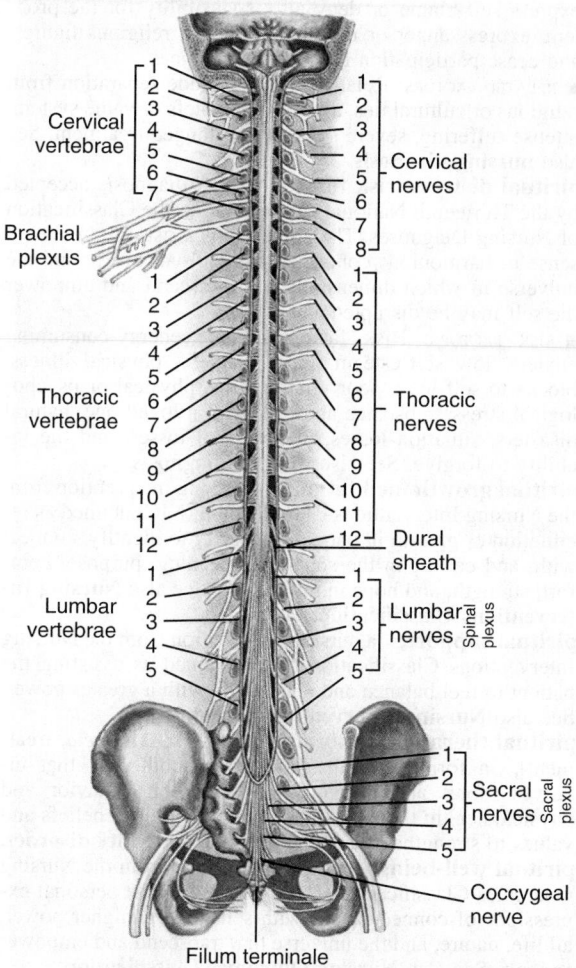

**Spinal nerves and spinal column**
*(Chipps, Clanin, and Campbell, 1992)*

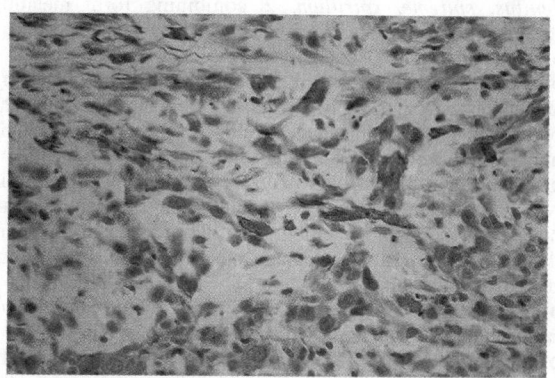

**Spindle cell carcinoma** *(Fletcher, 2000)*

**spinal stenosis,** narrowing of the vertebral canal, nerve root canals, or intervertebral foramina of the lumbar spine caused by encroachment of bone on the space; symptoms are caused by compression of the cauda equina and include pain, paresthesias, and neurogenic claudication. The condition may be either congenital or may be caused by spinal degeneration. See also **spinal cord compression.**

**spinal tract,** any one of the ascending (sensory) and descending (motor) pathways for sensory or motor nerve impulses that is found in the white matter of the spinal cord. Twenty-one different tracts lie within the dorsal, ventral, and lateral funiculi of the white substance. Ascending tracts conduct impulses up the spinal cord to the brain; descending tracts conduct impulses down the cord from the brain. The four major ascending tracts are the lateral spinothalamic, the ventral spinothalamic, the fasciculi gracilis and cuneatus, and the spinocerebellar. The four major descending tracts are the lateral corticospinal, the ventral corticospinal, the lateral reticulospinal, and the medial reticulospinal. Touch, pressure, proprioception, temperature, and pain are sensory stimuli transmitted via the spinal tracts. Reflex and volun-

**spindle cell nevus.** See **benign juvenile melanoma.**

**spine, 1.** the vertebral column, or backbone. **2.** descriptive of a spinous process.

**spinea.** See **spina.**

**spine of scapula** [L, *spina*, backbone, *scapulae*, shoulder blades], a sharp-edged plate of bone projecting posteriorly backward from the flattened scapula base.

**spin-lattice relaxation time.** See **relaxation time.**

**spinnbarkeit** /spin'bärkīt, shpin'-/ [Ger, threadability], the clear slippery elastic consistency characteristic of cervical mucus during ovulation. It has the consistency of an uncooked egg white, and it is a valuable sign of the peak fertile period in a woman's menstrual cycle. Observation of spinnbarkeit is useful in natural methods of family planning, in the clinical evaluation of infertility, and in discovering the optimal time for artificial insemination. Spinnbarkeit may be evaluated by the length to which a string of mucus can be drawn between the fingers before breaking. See also **ovulation method of family planning.**

**spino-,** combining form meaning 'spine': *spinocain, spinoglenoid, spinotransversarius.*

**spinocerebellar** /spī′nōser′əbel′ər/ [L, *spina* + *cerebellum*, small brain], pertaining to the spinal cord and the cerebellum.

**spinocerebellar disorder,** an inherited disorder characterized by a progressive degeneration of the spinal cord and cerebellum, often involving other parts of the nervous system as well. These disorders tend to occur within families and can be inherited as dominant or recessive traits. Onset is usually early, during childhood or adolescence. No effective treatment is known. Some kinds of spinocerebellar degeneration are **ataxia telangiectasia, Charcot-Marie-Tooth disease, Dejerine-Sottas disease, Friedreich's ataxia, olivopontocerebellar atrophy,** and **Refsum's syndrome.**

**spinofallopian tube shunt.** See **ventriculofallopian tube shunt.**

**spinous** /spī′nəs/ [L, *spina*, backbone], pertaining to an object that has the shape of a spine or thorn.

**spinous process** [L, *spina*, backbone, *processus*], a spine-like projection of bony tissue, such as the spinous process of a vertebra extending posteriorly from a vertebral arch. Also called **spine.**

**spin-spin relaxation time.** See **relaxation time.**

**spinth-,** combining form meaning 'spark': *spinthariscope, spintherometer, spintheropia.*

**spir-,** 1. combining form meaning 'a coil, or coiled': *spiradenitus, spireme, spirillum.* 2. combining form meaning 'breath or breathing': *spiracle, spirogram, spirophore.*

**spiral artery.** See **screw artery.**

**spiral bandage** /spī′rəl/ [Gk, *speira*, coil; Fr, *bande*, strip], any roller bandage applied around a limb that ascends the body part with each turn overlapping the previous one by half to two thirds of a bandage width.

**spiral computed tomography,** computed tomography in which the patient is moved through the scanner continuously rather than in increments, so that the path of the beam through the patient is a continuous spiral. See also **computed tomography.**

**spiral fracture** [Gk, *speira*, coil], a bone break that is spiral, oblique, or transverse to the bone's long axis.

**spiraling** /spī′rəling/, the process by which immunodeficiency allows viral replication, which further depresses the immune system, allowing further viral replication, and so on.

**spiral organ of Corti.** See **organ of Corti.**

**spiral reverse bandage,** a spiral bandage that is turned and folded back on itself as necessary to make it fit the contour of the body more securely.

**spirillary rat-bite fever, spirillum fever.** See **rat-bite fever.**

**spirit** /spir′it/ [L, *spiritus*, breath], 1. any volatile liquid, particularly one that has been distilled. 2. a volatile substance dissolved in alcohol. See also **volatile.**

**spirit of ammonia** [L, *spiritus*, breath; *Ammon*, temple in Libya], a solution of 3% ammonium carbonate in alcohol with flavorings added. It is mixed with water for use as a stimulant and carminative.

**spiritual distress** /spir′ichōo·əl/, a nursing diagnosis accepted by the Fourth National Conference on the Classification of Nursing Diagnoses. It is defined as disruption in the life principle that pervades a person's entire being and that integrates and transcends one's biologic and psychosocial nature.

■ DEFINING CHARACTERISTICS: The defining characteristics include stated anger against the deity or questions about the meaning of the suffering being experienced. The client may joke in a macabre fashion, regard the illness as punishment, have nightmares, cry, act in a hostile or apathetic manner,

express self-blame or deny all responsibility for the problem, express anger or resentment against religious figures, and cease participation in religious practices.

■ RELATED FACTORS: Related factors include separation from religious or cultural ties, a change in beliefs or value system, intense suffering, severe stress, or prolonged treatment. See also **nursing diagnosis.**

**spiritual distress, risk for,** a nursing diagnosis accepted by the Thirteenth National Conference on the Classification of Nursing Diagnoses. The condition is a risk for an altered sense of harmonious connectedness with all of life and the universe in which dimensions that transcend and empower the self may be disrupted.

■ RISK FACTORS: Risk factors include energy-consuming anxiety, low self-esteem, mental illness, physical illness, blocks to self-love, poor relationships, physical or psychological stress, substance abuse, loss of a loved one, natural disasters, situation losses, maturational losses, and the inability to forgive. See also **nursing diagnosis.**

**spiritual growth facilitation,** a nursing intervention from the Nursing Interventions Classification (NIC) defined as facilitation of growth in patient's capacity to identify, connect with, and call upon the source of meaning, purpose, comfort, strength, and hope in his/her life. See also **Nursing Interventions Classification.**

**spiritual support,** a nursing intervention from the Nursing Interventions Classification (NIC) defined as assisting the patient to feel balance and connection with a greater power. See also **Nursing Interventions Classification.**

**spiritual therapy** [L, *spiritus*, breath; Gk, *therapeia*, treatment], a form of counseling or psychotherapy that involves moral and religious influences on behavior and physical health; the use of spiritual and religious beliefs and values to strengthen the self. Also called **identity disorder.**

**spiritual well-being,** a nursing outcome from the Nursing Outcomes Classification (NOC) defined as the personal expressions of connectedness with self, others, higher power, all life, nature, and the universe that transcend and empower the self. See also **Nursing Outcomes Classification.**

**spiritual well-being, readiness for enhanced,** a nursing diagnosis accepted by the Eleventh National Conference on the Classification of Nursing Diagnoses. Spiritual well-being is the process of an individual's developing or unfolding of mystery through harmonious interconnectedness that springs from inner strengths.

■ DEFINING CHARACTERISTICS: The defining characteristics are inner strengths: a sense of awareness, self-consciousness, sacred source, unifying force, inner core, and transcendence; unfolding mystery: one's experience about life's purpose and meaning, mystery, uncertainty, and struggles; harmonious interconnectedness: relatedness, connectedness, harmony with self, others, higher power or God, and the environment. See also **nursing diagnosis.**

*Spirochaeta pallida* /spī′rəkē′tə/ [Gk, *speira*, coil, *chaite*, hair; L, *pallidus*, pale], a species of flexible spiral motile microorganisms that is the cause of human syphilis. Also called *Treponema pallidum.*

**spirochete** /spī′rəkēt′/ [Gk, *speira*, coil, *chaite*, hair], any bacterium of the genus *Spirochaeta* that is motile and spiral-shaped with flexible filaments. Kinds of spirochetes include the organisms responsible for leptospirosis, relapsing fever, syphilis, and yaws. Also spelled **spirochaete.** Compare **bacillus, coccus, vibrio.** —**spirochetal,** *adj.*

**spirochetemia** /spī′rōkātē′mē·ə/ [Gk, *speira*, coil, *chaite* + *haima*, blood], the presence of spirochetal organisms in the blood. See also **spirochete.**

**spirogram** /spī′rōgram/ [Gk, *speira* + *gramma*, record], a visual record of respiratory movements made by a spirometer, used in the assessment of pulmonary function and capacity.

**spirograph** /spī′rəgraf/ [Gk, *speira* + *graphein*, to record], a device for recording respiratory movements. See also **spirometer. —spirographic,** *adj.*

**spirometer** /spīrom′ətər/ [Gk, *speira* + *metron*, measure], an instrument that measures and records the volume of inhaled and exhaled air, used to assess pulmonary function. Volumetric information is recorded on a chart, called a spirogram. —**spirometric,** *adj.*

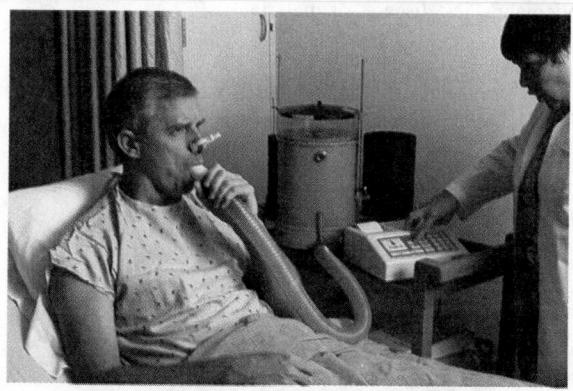

**Spirometer** *(Wilson and Thompson, 1990)*

**spirometry** /spīrom′ətrē/, laboratory evaluation of the air capacity of the lungs by means of a spirometer. Compare **blood gas determination. —spirometric,** *adj.*

**spironolactone** /spī′rənəlak′tōn/, a potassium-sparing aldosterone antagonist diuretic.

■ INDICATIONS: It is prescribed in the treatment of primary hyperaldosteronism, edema of congestive heart failure, cirrhosis of the liver accompanied by edema, nephrotic syndrome, essential hypertension, and hypokalemia.

■ CONTRAINDICATIONS: Anuria, acute renal insufficiency, significant impairment of renal function, or hyperkalemia prohibits its use.

■ ADVERSE EFFECTS: Among the most serious adverse reactions are hyperkalemia, gynecomastia, mental confusion, ataxia, impotence, amenorrhea, hirsutism, and urticaria.

**spittle** [AS, *spittan,* spew], saliva.

**Spitz nevus.** See **benign juvenile melanoma.**

**SPL.** See **Staphage Lysate.**

**splanchn-.** See **splanchno-.**

**splanchnic** /splangk′nik/, pertaining to the internal organs; visceral.

**-splanchnic,** suffix meaning 'viscera, entrails': *somaticosplanchnic, trisplanchnic, vagosplanchnic.*

**splanchnic engorgement,** the excessive filling or pooling of blood within the visceral vasculature after the removal of pressure from the abdomen, as in the excision of a large tumor, birth of a child, or drainage of a large quantity of urine from the bladder.

**splanchnic nerves** [Gk, *splanchna,* viscera, *nervus*], a network of nerves, mainly preganglionic fibers, with filaments innervating the penis and clitoris, as well as the uterus, rectum, and other structures of the abdominal cavity.

**splanchno-, splanchn-,** prefix meaning 'a viscus or splanchnic nerve': *splanchnocele, splanchnography, splanchnoptosis.*

**splanchnocele** /splangk′nōsēl′/ [Gk, *splanchna,* viscera, *kele,* hernia], hernial protrusion of any abdominal viscera. See also **splanchnocoele.**

**splanchnocoele** /splangk′nōsēl′/ [Gk, *splanchna,* viscera, *koilos,* hollow], a part of the embryonic body cavity, or coelom, that gives rise to the abdominal, pericardial, and pleural cavities. Also called **pleuroperitoneal cavity.**

**splanchnopleure** /splangk′nōploŏr′/ [Gk, *splanchna* + *pleura,* side], a layer of tissue in the early developing embryo, formed by the union of endoderm and splanchnic mesoderm. It gives rise to the embryonic gut and the visceral organs and continues external to the embryo as the yolk sac and allantois. Compare **somatopleure. —splanchnopleural,** *adj.*

**splanchnosomatic reaction.** See **viscerosomatic reaction.**

**S-plasty** /es′plas′te/, a technique of plastic surgery in which an S-shaped instead of a straight line incision is made to reduce tension and improve healing in areas where the skin is loose.

**splay** /splā/, **1.** to spread or turn out. **2.** to spread out, as said of the limbs. **3.** to open, as with the end of a tubular structure by making a longitudinal incision. **4.** to dislocate, as said of a bone.

**splayfoot** [ME, *splaien* + AS, *fot*], a foot that is flat and extremely everted, away from the midline. Also called **talipes valgus.**

**spleen** [Gk, *splen*], a soft highly vascular roughly ovoid organ situated between the stomach and the diaphragm in the left hypochondriac region of the body. It is considered part of the lymphatic system because it contains localized lymphatic nodules. It is dark purple and varies in shape in different individuals and within the same individual at different times. The precise function of the spleen has baffled physiologists for more than 100 years, but research indicates it performs various tasks, such as defense, hemopoiesis, blood storage, and destruction/recycling of red blood cells and platelets. The spleen also produces leukocytes, monocytes, lymphocytes, and plasma cells in response to an infectious agent. It produces red cells before birth and is believed to produce red cells after birth only in extreme and hemolytic anemia. If the body suffers severe hemorrhage, the spleen can contract and increase the blood volume from 350 mL to 550 mL in less than 60 seconds. In the adult the spleen is usually about 12 cm long, 7 cm wide, and 3 cm thick. Its weight increases from 17 g or less in the first year to about 170 g at 20 years of age, then slowly decreases to about 122 g at 75 to 80 years of age. The variation in the weight of

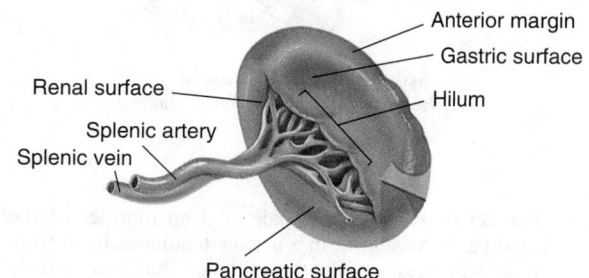

**Spleen** *(Thibodeau and Patton, 1999/Christine Oleksy)*

adult spleens is 100 to 250 g and, in extreme cases, 50 to 400 g. The size of the spleen increases during and after digestion and often increases during illness. Compare **thymus.** —**splenic** /splen'ik/, *adj.*

**spleen scan,** a radiographic scan of the spleen after the injection of radioactive red blood cells, performed to detect a tumor, damage, or other problem.

**splen-.** See **spleno-.**

**splenectomy** /splənek'təmē/ [Gk, *splen* + *ektomē,* excision], the surgical removal of the spleen. The spleen is a major phagocytic organ of the reticuloendothelial network and also serves as an important site of antibody production. Infections may follow its removal because the organ plays a vital role in the body's immune system. Splenectomized patients are particularly prone to certain bacterial infections.

**-splenia,** combining form meaning 'condition of the spleen': *asplenia, eusplenia, microsplenia.*

**splenic.** See **spleen.**

**splenic flexure** /splen'ik/ [Gk, *splen,* spleen; L, *flectere,* to bend], the left flexure of the colon, as it bends at the junction of the transverse and descending segments of the colon, near the spleen.

**splenic flexure syndrome** [Gk, *splen* + L, *flectere,* to bend], a recurrent pain and abdominal distension in the left upper quadrant of the abdomen caused by a pocket of gas trapped in the large intestine below the spleen, at the flexure of the transverse and descending colon. The symptoms are relieved by defecation or passing of flatus.

**splenic gland.** See **pancreaticolienal node.**

**splenic puncture,** a perforation of the parenchyma of the spleen to obtain pressure data or to inject radiopaque material.

**splenic vein.** See **lienal vein.**

**splenius capitis** /splē'nē·əs/ [Gk, *splenion,* bandage; L, *caput,* head], one of a pair of deep muscles of the neck and back. Arising from the ligamentum nuchae, the seventh cervical vertebra, and the first three or four thoracic vertebrae, it inserts in the occipital bone and the mastoid process of the temporal bone. It acts to rotate, extend, and bend the head.

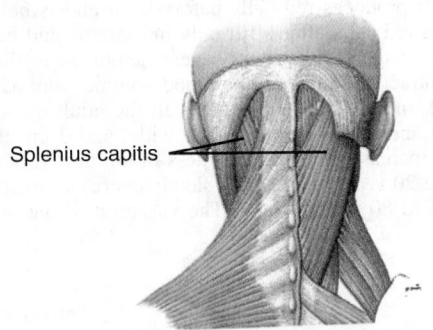

Splenius capitis

**Splenius capitis muscle**
*(Thibodeau and Patton, 1999/John V. Hagen)*

**splenius cervicis,** one of a pair of deep muscles of the neck and back. Arising from a narrow tendinous band from the spinous processes of the third through the sixth thoracic vertebrae, it inserts into the transverse processes of the upper two or three cervical vertebrae. The muscle is innervated

by the lateral branches of the dorsal primary divisions of the middle and the lower cervical nerves. The splenius cervicis acts to rotate, bend, and extend the head and neck. Also called **splenius colli.**

**spleno-, splen-,** combining form meaning 'spleen': *splenocele, splenodiagnosis, splenomalacia.*

**splenohepatomegaly** /splē'nōhep'ətōmeg'əlē/ [Gk, *splen,* spleen, *hepar,* liver, *megas,* great], an abnormal simultaneous increase in the sizes of the liver and spleen.

**splenomedullary leukemia.** See **acute myelocytic leukemia, chronic myelocytic leukemia.**

**splenomegaly** /splē'nōmeg'əlē, splen'-/ [Gk, *splen* + *megas,* large], an abnormal enlargement of the spleen, as is associated with portal hypertension, hemolytic anemia, Niemann-Pick disease, or malaria.

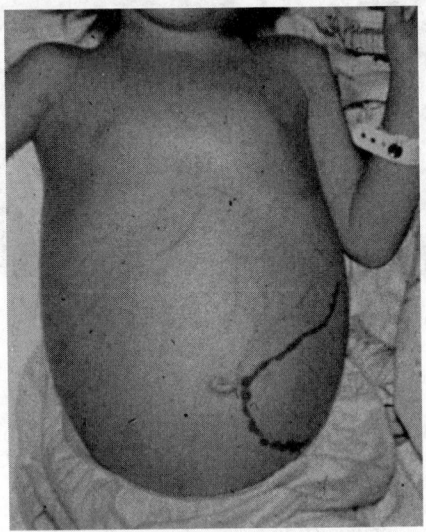

**Severe splenomegaly in a child
with beta thalassemia major**
*(Jorde et al, 1999)*

**splenomyelogenous leukemia.** See **acute myelocytic leukemia, chronic myelocytic leukemia.**

**splenosis** /splēnō'sis/, multiple splenic growths in the peritoneum resulting from splenic rupture or iatrogenic injury.

**splint** [D, *splinte,* piece of wood], **1.** an orthopedic device for immobilization, restraint, or support of any part of the body. It may be rigid (made of metal, plaster, or wood) or flexible (made of felt or leather). **2.** a device, usually made of hard acrylic and wire, for anchoring the teeth or modifying the bite. Compare **brace, cast.**

**splinter** [D, *splinte*], a sharp, pointed piece of bone or other substance.

**splinter fracture** [D, *splinte*], a comminuted fracture with thin, sharp bone fragments.

**splinter hemorrhage,** linear bleeding under a fingernail or toenail, resembling a splinter. It is seen after trauma and in bacterial endocarditis. Also spelled **splinter haemorrhage.**

**splinting**[1], the process of immobilizing, restraining, or supporting a body part.

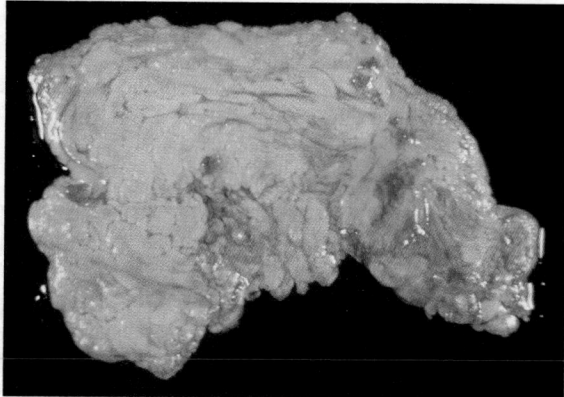

**Splenosis of the omentum** (Fletcher, 2000)

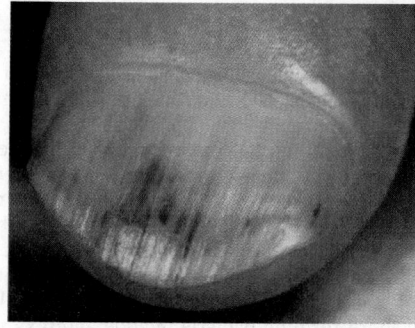

**Splinter hemorrhage** (Hordinsky, Sawaya, and Scher, 2000)

**splinting²,** a nursing intervention from the Nursing Interventions Classification (NIC) defined as stabilization, immobilization, and/or protection of an injured body part with a supportive appliance. See also **Nursing Interventions Classification.**

**split-brain state,** a condition resulting from the disconnection of the two cerebral hemispheres. It is produced when the corpus callosum is surgically divided completely or partially as a treatment for epilepsy. The cognitive effects are identified as a disconnection syndrome.

**split caliper stirrup.** See **caliper splint.**

**split gene** [D, *splitten,* to split], a gene whose continuity is interrupted.

**split-hand deformity.** See **cleft hand.**

**split personality.** See **dissociative identity disorder.**

**split Russell traction,** an orthopedic mechanism that combines suspension and traction to immobilize, position, and align the lower extremities in the correction of orthopedic deformities and in the treatment of congenital hip dislocation and hip and knee contractures. Usually applied as adhesive or nonadhesive skin traction, split Russell traction uses a sling to relieve the weight of the lower extremities. The traction weights are suspended from pulley-and-rope systems at the foot and head of the patient's bed. A jacket restraint is often incorporated to help immobilize the patient. Split Russell traction may be applied unilaterally or bilaterally. Compare **Russell traction.**

**split-skin graft.** See **split-thickness skin graft.**

**split-thickness skin graft,** a tissue transplant involving the epidermis and a part of the dermis. This type of graft is the most commonly used method of covering open burn wounds. Also called **split-skin graft.**

**splitting,** a primitive defense mechanism that when overused represents a developmental arrest. It is a failure to synthesize the positive and negative experiences and ideas one has of oneself, other people, situations, and institutions.

***S. pneumoniae,*** abbreviation for ***Staphylococcus pneumoniae.***

**spodo-,** combining form meaning 'to waste materials': *spodogenous, spodophagous, spodophorous.*

**spondyl-,** combining form meaning 'a physiologic condition or change of the vertebrae': *spondylopathy, spondylosis.*

**-spondylic** /spondil'ik/, combining form meaning 'vertebrae': *cyclospondylic, monospondylic, tectospondylic.*

**spondylitic** [Gk, *sphondylos,* vertebra], pertaining to a person afflicted with spondylitis.

**spondylitis** /spon'dəlī'tis/ [Gk, *sphondylos,* vertebra, *itis*], an inflammation of any of the vertebrae, usually characterized by stiffness and pain. The condition may be the result of traumatic injury to the spine, infection, or rheumatoid disease. See also **ankylosing spondylitis. —spondylitic,** *adj.*

**spondylitis ankylopoietica.** See **Strümpell-Marie disease.**

**spondylo-,** combining form meaning 'vertebra or the spinal column': *spondylocace, spondylodidymia, spondylolysis.*

**spondyloarthropathy** /spon'dilō'ärthrop'əthēs/, any of a set of diseases of the joints and spine. Most commonly affected are the lower extremities, sacroiliac joint, and hip. Pain and restricted motion of the hips and lower back are typical complaints. Many patients also experience eye disorders.

**spondylolisthesis** /spon'dilō'listhē'sis/ [Gk, *sphondylos + olisthanein,* to slip], the partial forward dislocation of one vertebra over the one below it, most commonly the fifth lumbar vertebra over the first sacral vertebra. See also **spinal cord compression.**

**spondylosis** /spon'dilō'sis/ [Gk, *sphondylos + osis*], a condition of the spine characterized by fixation or stiffness of a vertebral joint. See also **ankylosing spondylitis, spondylitis.**

**spondylosyndesis.** See **spinal fusion.**

**spondylothoracic dysplasia.** See **Jarcho-Levin syndrome.**

**spondylous** /spon'diləs/ [Gk, *sphondylos,* vertebra], pertaining to a vertebra.

**sponge** /spunj/ [Gk, *spongia*], **1.** a resilient absorbent mass used to absorb fluids, to apply medication, or to cleanse. The sponge may be the internal skeleton of a certain marine animal, or it may be manufactured from cellulose, rubber, or synthetic material. **2.** *informal.* a folded gauze square used in surgery.

**sponge bath,** the procedure of washing the patient with a damp washcloth or sponge, used when a full bath is not necessary or when lowering of body temperature is required.

**sponge gold.** See **mat gold.**

**spongio-,** combining form meaning 'like a sponge or related to a sponge': *spongioblast, spongiopilin, spongiosis.*

**spongioblastoma** /spun'jē-ōblastō'mə/, *pl.* **spongioblastomas, spongioblastomata** [Gk, *spongia + blastos,* germ, *oma,* tumor], a neoplasm composed of spongioblasts, embryonic epithelial cells that develop around the neural tube and transform into cells of the supporting connective tissue of nerve cells or cells of lining membranes of the ventricles and the spinal cord canal. Also called **glioblastoma, gliosarcoma, spongiocytoma.**

**spongioblastoma multiforme.** See **glioblastoma multiforme.**

**spongioblastomas, spongioblastomata.** See **spongioblastoma.**

**spongioblastoma unipolare,** a rare neoplasm composed of parallel spongioblasts. The tumor may occur near the third ventricle, in the pons and brainstem, in basal ganglia, or in the terminal filament of the spinal cord.

**spongiocytoma.** See **spongioblastoma.**

**spongy** /spun'jē/ [Gk, *spoggia*], pertaining to or resembling a sponge.

**spongy bone.** See **cancellous bone.**

**spontaneous** /spontā'nē·əs/ [L, *sponte*, willingly], occurring naturally and without apparent cause, such as spontaneous remission.

**spontaneous abortion,** a termination of pregnancy before the twentieth week of gestation as a result of abnormalities of the conceptus or maternal environment. Up to 30% of pregnancies may end as spontaneous abortions, many caused by blighted ova that have congenital defects incompatible with life. Also called **miscarriage.** Compare **induced abortion.**

**spontaneous delivery,** a vaginal birth occurring without the mechanical assistance of obstetric forceps or vacuum aspirator.

**spontaneous evolution.** See **Denman's spontaneous evolution, spontaneous version.**

**spontaneous fracture,** a fracture that occurs without trauma, as a result of bone weakness caused by osteoporosis or by a benign or malignant tumor.

**spontaneous generation.** See **abiogenesis.**

**spontaneous labor,** a labor beginning and progressing without mechanical or pharmacologic stimulation.

**spontaneous PEEP (sPEEP),** positive airway pressure applied at the end of the exhalation phase during spontaneous breathing.

**spontaneous phagocytosis** [L, *sponte*, free will; Gk, *phagein*, to eat, *kytos*, cell, *osis*, condition], ingestion of antigenic particles by phagocytes of the reticuloendothelial system.

**spontaneous pneumothorax** [L, *sponte*, free will; Gk, *pneuma*, air, *thorax*, chest], the presence of air or gas in the pleural space as a result of a rupture of the lung parenchyma and visceral pleura with no demonstrable cause.

**spontaneous remission,** 1. the reversal of progress of disease without formal treatment. 2. the disappearance of symptoms of a mentally ill patient without formal treatment.

**spontaneous ventilation,** normal, unassisted breathing in which the patient creates the pressure gradient through muscular movements that move air into and out of the lungs.

**spontaneous ventilation, impaired** a nursing diagnosis accepted by the Tenth National Conference on the Classification of Nursing Diagnoses. It is defined as a state in which the response pattern of decreased energy reserves results in an individual's inability to maintain breathing adequate to support life.

■ DEFINING CHARACTERISTICS: Major defining characteristics are dyspnea and increased metabolic rate. Minor defining characteristics are increased restlessness, apprehension, increased use of accessory muscles, decreased tidal volume, increased heart rate, decreased $pO_2$ level, increased $pCO_2$ level, decreased cooperation, and decreased $SaO_2$ level.

■ RELATED FACTORS: Related factors are metabolic factors and respiratory muscle fatigue. See also **nursing diagnosis.**

**spontaneous version** [L, *sponte*, free will, *vertere*, to turn], a change in the lie of a fetus that occurs without manipulation. Also called **spontaneous evolution.**

**spoon nail** [AS, *spon* + *naegel*], a nail of the finger or toe which has a thin and concave outer surface.

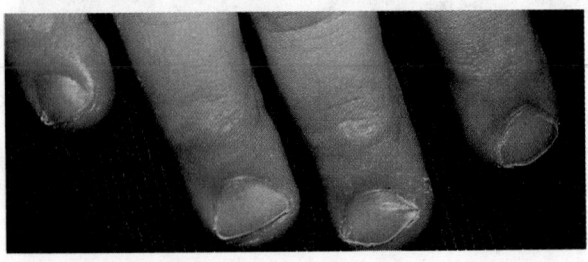

**Spoon nails** *(Zitelli and Davis, 1997)*

**spor-.** See **sporo-.**

**sporadic** /spôrat'ik/ [Gk, *sporaden*, scattered], (of a number of events) occurring at scattered, intermittent, and apparently random intervals.

**-sporangium,** combining form meaning an 'encasement of spores': *haplosporangium, oosporangium, sporangium.*

**spore** [Gk, *sporos*, seed], 1. a reproductive unit of some genera of fungi or protozoa. 2. a form assumed by some bacteria that is resistant to heat, drying, and chemicals. Under proper environmental conditions the spore may revert to the actively multiplying form of the bacterium. Diseases caused by spore-forming bacteria include anthrax, botulism, gas gangrene, and tetanus.

**-spore,** suffix meaning a 'reproductive element': *archespore, chlamydospore, hemispore.*

**sporicidal** /spôr'isī'dəl/ [Gk, *sporos*, seed; L, *caedere*, to kill], spore-killing, as are certain chemicals or other agents.

**sporicide** /spôr'isīd/ [Gk, *sporos* + L, *caedere*, to kill], any agent effective in destroying spores, such as compounds of chlorine and formaldehyde, and the glutaraldehydes.

**sporiferous** /spôrif'ərəs/, producing or bearing spores.

**spork,** a spoonlike food utensil with fork tines designed for people with upper extremity disabilities.

**sporo-, spor-,** combining form meaning 'spore': *sporocyst, sporogenesis, sporogeny.*

**sporoblast** /spôr'əblast'/ [Gk, *sporos* + *blastos*, germ], any cell that gives rise to a sporozoite or spore during the sexual reproductive phase of the life cycle of a sporozoon. It refers specifically to the cells resulting from the multiple fission of the encysted zygote of the malarial parasite *Plasmodium*, from which the sporozoites develop.

**sporocyst** /spôr'əsist/ [Gk, *sporos* + *kystis*, bag], 1. any structure containing spores or reproductive cells. 2. a saclike structure, or oocyst, secreted by the zygote of certain protists before sporozoite formation. 3. the second larval stage in the life cycle of parasitic flukes. The saclike organism develops from the miracidium, or first larval stage, in the body of a freshwater snail host and contains germinal cells that give rise either to daughter sporocysts that develop into cercariae or to rediae. See also **fluke.**

**sporogenesis** /spôr'ōjen'əsis/ [Gk, *sporos* + *genesis*, origin], 1. the formation of spores. Also called **sporogeny.** 2. reproduction by means of spores. —**sporogenic,** *adj.*

**sporogenous** /spôroj'ənəs/ [Gk, *sporos* + *genein,* to produce], describing an animal or plant that reproduces by spores.

**sporogeny.** See **sporogenesis.**

**sporogony** /spôrog'ənē/ [Gk, *sporos* + *genesis,* origin], reproduction by means of spores. It refers specifically to the formation of sporozoites during the sexual stage of the life cycle of a sporozoon, primarily the malarial parasite *Plasmodium.* Fusion of the sex cells occurs in the body of the invertebrate host, the female *Anopheles* mosquito in the case of *Plasmodium,* where the encysted zygote undergoes multiple division, giving rise to the sporozoites. Compare **schizogony.**

**sporont** /spôr'ont/ [Gk, *sporos* + *on,* being], a mature protozoan parasite in the sexual reproductive stage of its life cycle. It undergoes conjugation to form a zygote, which produces sporozoites by multiple fission. Compare **schizont.** See also **sporogony.**

**sporonticide** /spôron'tisīd/ [Gk, *sporos* + *on* + L, *caedere,* to kill], any substance that destroys sporonts, such as chloroquine and other antimalarial drugs. —**sporonticidal,** *adj.*

**sporophore** /spôr'əfôr/ [Gk, *sporos* + *pherein,* to bear], the part of an organism that produces spores.

**sporophyte** /spôr'əfīt/ [Gk, *sporos* + *phyton,* plant], the asexual, spore-bearing stage in organisms that reproduce by alternation of generations.

**sporotrichosis** /spôr'ōtrikō'sis/ [Gk, *sporos* + *thrix,* hair, *osis,* condition], a common chronic fungal infection caused by the species *Sporothrix schenckii.* It is usually characterized by skin ulcers and subcutaneous nodules along lymphatic channels. It rarely spreads to involve bones, lungs, joints, or muscles. The fungus is found in soil and decaying vegetation and usually enters the skin by accidental injury. Outbreaks have occurred in workers at plant nurseries. Treatment may include amphotericin B in severe cases or itraconazole.

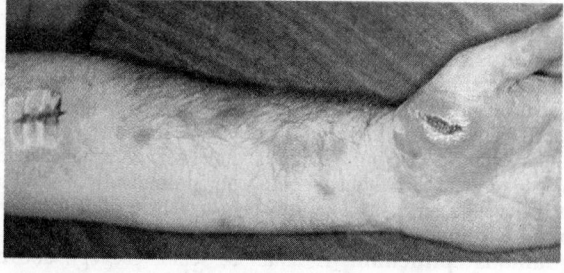

**Lymphocutaneous sporotrichosis** *(Murray et al, 1998)*

*Sporotrichum* /spôrot'rikəm/ [Gk, *sporos* + *thrix,* hair], a genus of soil-inhabiting fungi formerly thought to cause sporotrichosis.

**Sporozoa** /spôr'əzō'ə/ [Gk, *sporos* + *zoon,* animal], a class of parasite in the phylum Protozoa that is characterized by the absence of any external organs of locomotion. Included in this class are the genera *Toxoplasma* and *Plasmodium.*

**sporozoite** /spôr'əzō'īt/ [Gk, *sporos* + *zoon,* animal], any of the cells resulting from the sexual union of spores during the life cycle of a sporozoon. It refers specifically to the elongated nucleated cells produced by the multiple fission of

the zygote contained in the oocyst in the female *Anopheles* mosquito during the sexual reproductive stage of the life cycle of the malarial parasite *Plasmodium.* On release from the oocyst, the sporozoites migrate to the salivary glands of the mosquito, where they are transmitted to humans and develop within the parenchymal cells of the liver as merozoites. Also called **falciform body.** See also **malaria,** *Plasmodium.*

**sport** [ME, *disporten,* to amuse], **1.** an individual that differs drastically from its parents or others of its type because of genetic mutation; a mutant. **2.** a genetic mutation. **3.** See **lusus naturae.**

**sports-injury prevention: youth,** a nursing intervention from the Nursing Interventions Classification (NIC) defined as reducing the risk of sports-related injury in young athletes. See also **Nursing Interventions Classification.**

**sports medicine,** a branch of medicine that specializes in the prevention and treatment of injuries resulting from training for and participation in athletic events. More than 1 million people are treated for sports injuries each year in the United States. Most sports injuries involve muscle sprains, strains, and tears, which frequently result from inadequate preliminary "warm-up" exercises. Among the most common sports injuries are shin splints, runner's knee, pulled hamstring muscles, Achilles tendonitis, ankle sprain, arch sprain, charley horse, tennis elbow, baseball finger, dislocations, muscle cramps, bursitis, myofascitis, costochondritis, hernia, and "Little League elbow."

**sporulation** /spôr'yəlā'shən/ [Gk, *sporos* + L, *atus,* process], **1.** a type of reproduction that occurs in fungi, algae, and protozoa and involves the formation of spores by the spontaneous division of a cell into four or more daughter cells, each of which contains a part of the original nucleus. **2.** the formation of a refractile body, or resting spore, within certain bacteria that makes the cell resistant to unfavorable environmental conditions. The cell regains its viability when conditions become favorable. See also **spore.**

**spot** [ME, blot], (in psychotherapy) a small quantum of space that becomes the territorial object and extension of point behavior.

**spot film,** a radiograph made instantly during fluoroscopy. The technique may be used to make a permanent record of a transient effect or to record with definition and detail a small anatomic area.

**spotted fever.** See **Rocky Mountain spotted fever.**

**spotting** [ME, *spot,* blot], the appearance of a blood-stained discharge from the vagina between menstrual periods, during pregnancy, or at the beginning of labor.

**sprain,** a traumatic injury to the tendons, muscles, or ligaments around a joint, characterized by pain, swelling, and discoloration of the skin over the joint. The duration and severity of the symptoms vary with the extent of damage to the tissues. Treatment includes support, rest, and alternating cold and heat. Ultrasound therapy may speed recovery. Radiographic images are often indicated to rule out fractures.

**sprain fracture,** a fracture that results from the separation of a tendon or ligament at the point of insertion, associated with the separation of a bone at the same insertion site.

**sprain of ankle or foot** [AS, *ancleow* + *fot*], a sudden traction injury to a muscle, ligament, or capsule in the ankle or foot. The injury is not severe enough to cause a rupture of the tissue.

**sprain of back** [AS, *baec*], a sudden traction injury to muscles and related tissues of the back. The tissues may have undergone traumatic strain without being ruptured.

**spreader bar** /spred'ər/, a metal bar with curved hoop areas for attaching hooks or pins for traction.

**spreadsheet** /spred′shēt/, a computer program that simulates a business or scientific worksheet and performs the necessary calculations when data are entered or changed.

**Sprengel's deformity** /shpreng′gəlz/ [Otto Gerhard Karl Sprengel, German surgeon, 1852−1915], congenital elevation of the scapula, resulting from failure of descent of the scapula to its normal thoracic position during fetal life.

**spring** /spring/ [AS, *springan,* to jump], **1.** a piece of resilient metal, such as a hardened coiled steel wire, that will return to its original shape after bending. **2.** a resilient wire attached to a denture or other appliance.

**spring forceps** [AS, *springan,* to jump], a kind of forceps that includes a spring mechanism. They are tweezerlike and vary in thickness. With teeth, they can grasp delicate tissue. Without teeth, they can hold thick or slippery tissue. Also called **bulldog forceps.**

**spring lancet,** a very small knife with a spring-triggered blade. It may be used for collecting small specimens of blood for laboratory tests. See also **lancet.**

**sprinter's fracture** [Swe, *sprinta,* to spurt; L, *fractura,* to break], a break in the anterior superior or anterior inferior spine of the ilium, caused when the bone is forcibly pulled by a violent muscle spasm.

**sprue** /sprō̄o/ [D, *sprouw,* kind of tumor], a chronic degenerative disorder resulting from malabsorption of nutrients from the small intestine and characterized by a broad range of symptoms, including diarrhea, weakness, weight loss, poor appetite, pallor, muscle cramps, bone pain, ulceration of the mucous membrane lining the digestive tract, and a smooth, shiny tongue. It occurs in both tropical and nontropical forms and affects both children and adults. Also called **catarrhal dysentery.** See also **celiac disease, malabsorption syndrome, nontropical sprue, tropical sprue.**

**SPRX,** trademark for an anorexiant (phendimetrazine tartrate).

**SPSS (Statistical Package for the Social Sciences),** (in statistics) a computer program often used in research in clinical nursing for the analysis of complex data from large samples.

**spur** [AS, *spura*], a projection of bone from a body structure or of metal from an appliance. See also **exostosis.**

**spurious pregnancy.** See **pseudocyesis.**

**sputum** /spyō̄o′təm/ [L, spittle], material coughed up from the lungs and expectorated through the mouth. It contains mucus, cellular debris, or microorganisms, and it also may contain blood or pus. The amount, color, and constituents of the sputum are important in the diagnosis of many illnesses, including tuberculosis, pneumonia, cancer of the lung, and the pneumoconioses.

**sputum collection trap,** a plastic trap connected to a suction catheter. Sputum specimens can be contained in the trap and sent for analysis.

**sputum specimen** [L, spittle + *specere,* to look], a sample of material expelled from the respiratory passages taken for laboratory analysis to determine the presence of pathogens.

***S. pyogenes*** abbreviation for ***Staphylococcus pyogenes.***

**squam-,** combining form meaning 'scales': *squamatization, squamocellular, squamopetrosal.*

**squama** /skwā′mə/, *pl.* **squamae, 1.** a flattened scale from the epidermis. **2.** the thin, expanded part of a bone, especially in the cranial wall.

**squamocolumnar junction** /skwā′mōkəlum′nər/, a region of transition from stratified squamous epithelium to columnar epithelium in the cervical canal. It is a location where cells are obtained for Papanicolaou's (Pap) smears.

**squamous** /skwā′məs/ [L, *squama,* scale], platelike, scaly, or covered with scales.

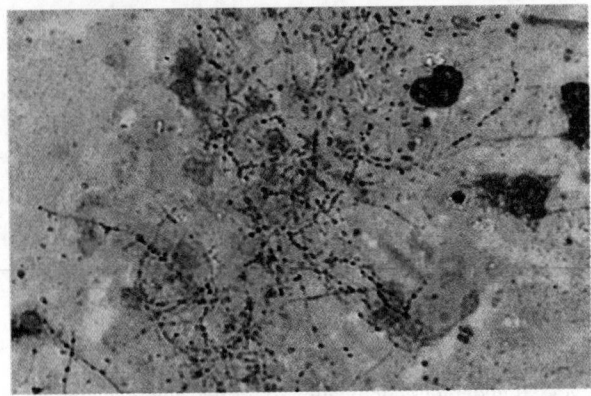

**Sputum specimen (acid-fast stain)** *(Murray et al, 1998)*

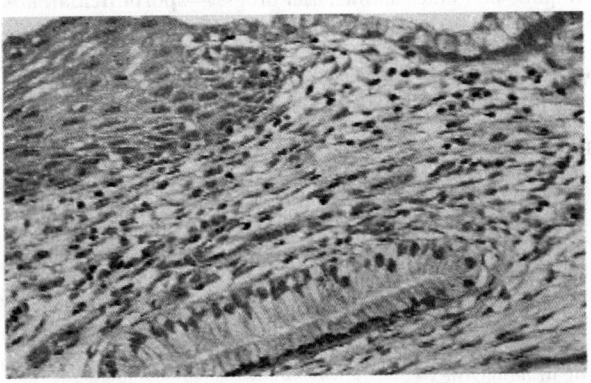

**Squamocolumnar junction** *(McKee, 1997)*

**squamous cell** [L, *squama,* scale, *cella,* storeroom], a flat, scalelike epithelial cell.

**squamous cell carcinoma,** a slow-growing malignant tumor of squamous epithelium, frequently found in the lungs and skin and occurring also in the anus, cervix, larynx, nose, and bladder. The neoplastic cells characteristically resemble prickle cells and form keratin pearls. Also called **epidermoid carcinoma.**

**squamous epithelium** [L, *squama,* scale; Gk, *epi,* above, *thele,* nipple], a sheet of flattened scalelike cells, attached together at the edges. Also called **pavement epithelium.**

**square centimeter (cm²)** /skwer/, a unit of area measurement equivalent to 1 centimeter in length multiplied by 1 centimeter in width where one centimeter equals 0.3937 inch or 0.03281 foot.

**square window** [OFr, *esquarre* + ME, *wind,* air, *owe,* eye], an angle of the wrist between the hypothenar prominence and forearm. It is used as a reference point for estimating the gestational age of a newborn.

**squatting position** /skwot′ing/ [Fr, *esquatir,* to press down], a posture in which the knees and hips are flexed and the buttocks are lowered to the level of the heels. It is adopted by children with certain heart diseases as they seek relief from exercise distress.

**squeeze dynamometer** /skwēz/ [AS, *cwesan,* to press tightly; Gk, *dynamis,* force, *metron,* measure], a device

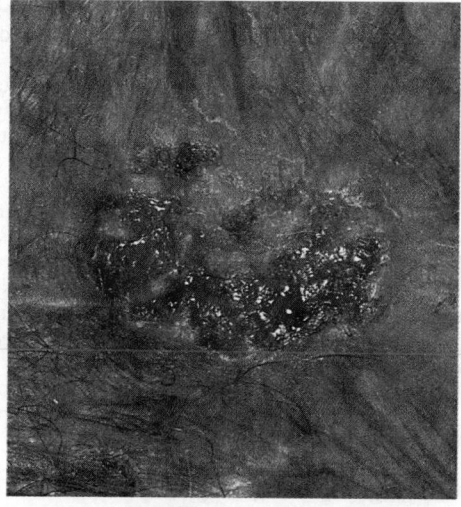

**Squamous cell carcinoma** *(du Vivier, 1993)*

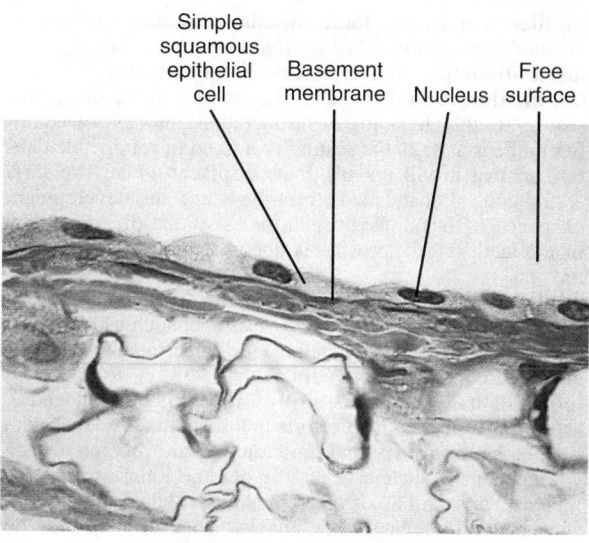

**Simple squamous epithelium**
*(© Ed Reschke; used with permission)*

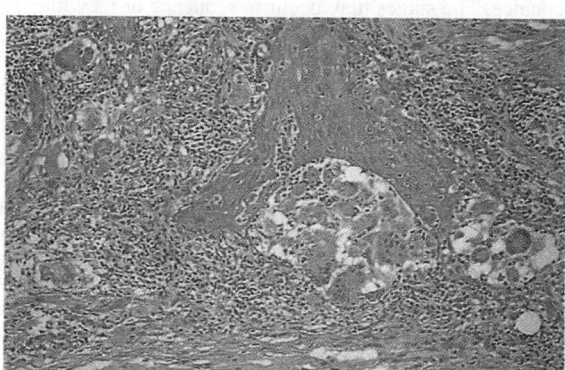

**Histopathology of squamous cell carcinoma**
*(Eveson and Scully, 1995)*

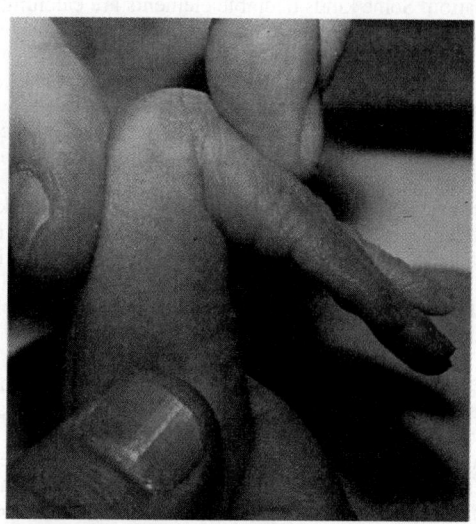

**Square window test** *(Zitelli and Davis, 1997)*

for measuring the muscular strength of the grip of the hand. See also **dynamometer.**

**squeeze-film lubrication,** the exudation of fluid from the cartilage of joints, forming a film in the transient area of impending contact.

**squint.** See **strabismus.**

**squinting eye** /skwin'ting/ [D, *schuinte,* oblique; AS, *eage*], the abnormal eye in a person with strabismus that is not aligned with the fixating eye. See also **strabismus.**

**Sr,** symbol for the element **strontium.**

**SR,** abbreviation for **sedimentation rate.**

**sRNA,** abbreviation for *soluble ribonucleic acid (RNA).*

**SRO,** abbreviation for **single room occupant.**

**SRS-A,** abbreviation for **slow-reacting substance of anaphylaxis.**

**SRY,** symbol for a "maleness" gene found on the sex-determining region of the Y chromosome. The gene is believed to function as a master control switch that can turn off or on other genes involved in sexual development.

**ss,** abbreviation for **steady state.**

**SSE, 1.** abbreviation for **skin self-examination. 2.** abbreviation for **soapsuds enema.**

**SSKI,** trademark for an expectorant (potassium iodide).

**SSRI,** abbreviation for **selective serotonin reuptake inhibitor.**

**SSS, 1.** abbreviation for *sterile saline soak.* **2.** abbreviation for **sick sinus syndrome.**

**SSSS,** abbreviation for **staphylococcal scalded skin syndrome.**

**ST,** abbreviation for slow-twitch. See **slow-twitch (ST) fiber.**

**stab** [ME, *stabbe,* piercing wound], a nonsegmented neutrophil.

**stab culture** [ME, *stabbe,* piercing wound; L, *colere,* to cultivate], a culture made by dipping a needle into an inoculum and then into a transparent gelatin or agar medium.

**stab form.** See **band.**

**-stabile,** combining form meaning 'stable, resistant to change': *coctostabile, hydrostabile, tempostabile.*

**stabile diabetes.** See **type 2 diabetes mellitus.**

**stabilization** /stab'ilīzā'shən/ [L, *stabilis,* firm, *atus,* process], **1.** the physiologic and metabolic process of attaining homeostasis. **2.** the seating of a fixed or removable denture so that it will not tilt or be displaced under pressure. **3.** the control of induced stress loads and the development of measures to counteract such forces so that the movement of the teeth or of a prosthesis does not irritate surrounding tissues.

**stabilization exercises,** exercises to develop proximal control in symptom (pain) free positions, such as sitting on a gymnastic ball and extending one knee to maintain balance and control without pain.

**stable** /stā'bəl/ [L, *stabilis,* firm], remaining unchanged.

**stable angina,** angina pectoris in which attacks occur with predictable frequency and duration and are precipitated by circumstances, such as exercise or emotional stress, that increase myocardial oxygen demands. The same circumstances tend to cause the attacks from one episode to another.

**stable condition,** a state of health or disease from which little if any immediate change is expected.

**stable element** [L, *stabilis,* firm, *elementum*], a nonradioactive element, one not subject to spontaneous nuclear degeneration. Some kinds of stable elements are calcium, iron, lead, potassium, and sodium. Compare **radioactive element.** See also **element.**

**staccato speech** /stəkä'tō/ [It, detached; ME, *speche*], abnormal speech in which the person pauses between words, breaking the rhythm of the phrase or sentence. The condition is sometimes observed in association with multiple sclerosis.

**stadium** /stā'dē·əm/, *pl.* **stadia** [Gk, *stadion,* racetrack], a significant stage in a fever or illness, such as the fastigium of a febrile illness or the prodromal stage of a viral infection.

**Stadol,** trademark for an opioid analgesic (butorphanol tartrate).

**staff** [AS, *staef*], **1.** the people who work toward a common goal and are employed or supervised by someone of higher rank, such as the nurses in a hospital. **2.** a designation by which a staff nurse is distinguished from a nurse manager or other nurse. **3.** (in nursing education) the nonprofessional employees of the institution, such as librarians, technicians, secretaries, and clerks. **4.** (in nursing service administration) the units of the organization that provide service to the line, or administratively defined hierarchy; for example, the personnel office is staff to the chief nurse executive and the nursing service administration.

**staff development[1],** a process that assists individuals in an agency or organization in attaining new skills and knowledge, gaining increasing levels of competence, and growing professionally. Various resources outside the agency employing the individuals may be used. The process may include such programs as orientation, in-service education, and continuing education.

**staff development[2],** a nursing intervention from the Nursing Interventions Classification (NIC) defined as developing, maintaining, and monitoring competence of staff. See also **Nursing Interventions Classification.**

**staffing,** the process of assigning people to fill the roles designed for an organizational structure through recruitment, selection, and placement.

**staffing pattern,** (in hospital or nursing administration) the number and types or categories of staff assigned to the particular units and departments of a hospital or other health care facility. Staffing patterns vary with the unit, department, and shift and with the patient acuity levels.

**staff of Æsculapius,** a staff carried by Æsculapius, the Greek god of medicine. It is used as the traditional symbol of the physician. A single serpent entwines the staff of Æsculapius. It is often confused with the caduceus, a staff with two serpents (which is the staff of Hermes, the Greek god of commerce and travel), symbolizing (because of this misunderstanding) the U.S. Army Medical Corps. See **Æsculapius.**

**staff supervision,** a nursing intervention from the Nursing Interventions Classification (NIC) defined as facilitating the delivery of high-quality patient care by others. See also **Nursing Interventions Classification.**

**stage** [OFr, *estage*], **1.** a platform. **2.** a period or phase.

**-stage,** combining form meaning a '(specified) phase': *aecidiostage, multistage, uredostage.*

**stages of anesthesia.** See **Guedel's signs.**

**stages of dying** [OFr, *estage,* stage; ME, *dyen,* to lose life], the five emotional and behavioral stages that may occur after a person or family first learns of approaching death. The stages, identified and described by Elisabeth Kübler-Ross, are denial and shock, anger, bargaining, depression, and acceptance. The stages may occur in sequence or they may recur, as the person moves forward and backward—especially among denial, anger, and bargaining. Caring for a dying person requires sensitivity to the signs of each stage. At first shock may be accompanied by signs of panic. The person may refuse care and deny the diagnosis and prognosis. Denial serves as a defense against the shock. Anger often follows this stage. It is characterized by abusive language, refusal to perform basic self-care responsibilities, negative criticism of anyone who wants to help, and other kinds of angry behavior. The third stage, bargaining, reflects the need of the person for time to accept the situation. A common observation of this period is the patient's attempt to make a bargain, "If I could live until Christmas, . . ." Commonly, the person goes back and forth from anger to bargaining: sometimes silent, sometimes grieving, and sometimes apathetic, depressed, insomniac, and distant. The fourth stage is a time of depression in which the person goes through a period of grieving before death, mourning over past experiences and anticipating impending losses. The final stage, acceptance, is one of inner peace and resolution that death is a certainty. The person may show his or her acceptance by being uninterested in present or future events, being preoccupied with past events, preferring to have few visitors, and wanting quiet and solitude. Nursing care includes administering adequate pain relief, ensuring privacy and dignity, and giving sensitive, honest emotional support to both patient and family. See also **emotional care of the dying patient, hospice.**

**staging** /stā'jing/, the classification of phases or periods of a disease or other pathologic process, as in the TMN clinical method of assigning numerical values to various stages of tumor development.

**stagnant anoxia** /stag'nənt/ [L, *stagnum,* standing water; Gk, *a,* without, *oxys,* sharp, *genein,* to produce], a condition in which there is inadequate blood flow in the capillaries, causing low tissue oxygen tension and reduced oxygen exchange. The condition is associated with shock, cardiac standstill, and thrombosis.

**stain** [OFr, *desteindre,* to dye], **1.** a pigment, dye, or substance used to impart color to microscopic objects or tissues to facilitate their examination and identification. Kinds of stains include **acid-fast stain, Gram's stain,** and **Wright's**

**stain. 2.** to apply pigment to a substance or tissue to examine it under a microscope. **3.** an area of discoloration.

**stained film fault,** a defect in a radiograph or photograph that appears as a streaky discoloration or abnormal opacity. It is usually caused by contaminated or exhausted development solutions, improper rinsing, inadequate washing, or damage to the film emulsion during processing.

**stalk** /stÔk/, an elongated, more or less slender anatomical structure resembling the stem of a plant; see also **peduncle, pedunculus.**

**-stalsis,** suffix meaning a 'contraction in the alimentary canal': *antistalsis, peristalsis, retrostalsis.*

**stammering** [AS, *stamerian,* to stutter], a speech dysfunction characterized by pauses, hesitations, and faltering utterances. The term is not used in the United States but is frequently used synonymously with *stuttering,* especially in Great Britain. See also **stuttering.**

**stamp cusp** [ME, *stampen* + L, *cuspis,* point], a tooth cusp that works in a fossa, such as any of the maxillary lingual cusps.

**stance phase of gait** [L, *stare,* to stand; Gk, *phainein,* to show; ME, *gate,* a way], the phase of the normal gait cycle that begins with the strike of the heel on the ground and ends with the lift of the toe at the beginning of the swing phase of gait.

**standard** [OFr, *estandart*], **1.** an evaluation that serves as a basis for comparison for evaluating similar phenomena or substances, such as a standard for the preparation of a pharmaceutic substance or a standard for the practice of a profession. **2.** a pharmaceutic preparation or a chemical substance of known quantity, ingredients, and strength that is used to determine the constituents or the strength of another preparation. **3.** of known value, strength, quality, or ingredients. **4.** predetermined criteria used to provide guidance in the operation of a health care facility to ensure high-quality performance by the personnel. **—standardize,** *v.,* **standardization,** *n.*

**standard air chamber,** a radiation-measuring device used by national and international calibration laboratories to provide exposure calibrations for ion chambers used in the diagnostic or orthovoltage energy range.

**standard bicarbonate,** the bicarbonate ion concentration of plasma separated anaerobically from whole blood that has been saturated with oxygen and equilibrated at carbon dioxide pressure of 40 torr at 100° F (38° C). It is a measure of the metabolic disturbance of acid-base balance in a sample of blood after any respiratory disturbance present has been corrected.

**standard curve,** a graphic plot of tracer binding versus the known concentration of test substances in a set of standards usually prepared by serial dilution or incremental addition.

**standard death certificate,** a form for a death certificate that is commonly used throughout the United States. It is the form preferred by the United States Census Bureau.

**standard deviation (SD),** (in statistics) a mathematic statement of the dispersion of a set of values or scores from the mean.

**standard environmental chamber.** See **Skinner box.**

**standard error (S.E.),** (in statistics) the variability in scores that can be expected if measurements are made on random samples of the same size from the same universe of populations, phenomena, or observations. The standard error provides a framework within which a determination of the difference between groups may be made. It is an element used in determining statistic significance by means of a wide variety of formulas and methods.

**standard error of the mean,** (in statistics) an indication of how well the mean of a sample estimates the mean of a population. It is measured by the standard deviation of the means of randomly drawn samples of the same size as the sample in question.

**standard hydrogen electrode,** a reference electrode that is assigned a value of 0 volt. Also called **normal hydrogen electrode.**

**standardization, standardize.** See **standard.**

**standardized death rate,** the number of deaths per 1000 people of a specified population during 1 year. This rate is adjusted to prevent distortion by the age composition of the population. A standard population is used for determining this rate. Also called **adjusted death rate.**

**standardized test,** any empirically developed examination with established reliability and validity as determined by repeated evaluation of the method and results.

**standard of care,** a written statement describing the rules, actions, or conditions that direct patient care. Standards of care guide practice and can be used to evaluate performance.

**Standard Precautions,** guidelines recommended by the Centers for Disease Control and Prevention (CDC) to reduce the risk of transmission of blood-borne and other pathogens in hospitals. The Standard Precautions synthesize the major features of Universal (Blood and Body Fluid) Precautions and Body Substance Isolation (designed to reduce the risk of pathogens from moist body substances) and applies them to all patients receiving care in hospitals regardless of their diagnosis or presumed infection status. Standard Precautions apply to (1) blood; (2) all body fluids, secretions, and excretions *excluding sweat,* regardless of whether they contain blood; (3) nonintact skin; and (4) mucous membranes. The Precautions are designed to reduce the risk of transmission of microorganisms from both recognized and unrecognized sources of infection in hospitals. See also **Transmission-based Precautions.**

**standard reference gamble,** a method of diagnostic testing in which a decision maker is faced with a choice between a certain outcome or intermediate value and a gamble involving a better or worse outcome. The outcomes are assigned arbitrary numeric values of 100 and 0, respectively. All other outcomes can be assigned values relative to the best and worst outcomes.

**standards of nursing practice,** a set of guidelines for providing high-quality nursing care and criteria for evaluating care. Such guidelines help assure patients that they are receiving high-quality care. The standards are important if a legal dispute arises over the quality of care provided a patient.

**standby guardianship,** a legal process in the United States that may name an individual to assume specified health care or financial authority for an elderly person who becomes mentally incapacitated.

**standing orders** [L, *stare,* to stand, *ordo,* rank], a written document containing rules, policies, procedures, regulations, and orders for the conduct of patient care in various stipulated clinical situations. The standing orders are usually formulated collectively by the professional members of a department in a hospital or other health care facility. Standing orders usually name the condition and prescribe the action to be taken in caring for the patient, including the dosage and route of administration for a drug or the schedule for the administration of a therapeutic procedure. Commonly used in intensive care units coronary care units, and emergency departments.

**stann-,** combining form meaning 'tin': *stanniferous, stanniform, stannoxyl.*

**stannous fluoride** /stan′əs/ [L, *stannum*, tin, *fluere*, to flow], a salt of fluorine and tin (SnF$_2$; tin (II) fluoride) used in oral hygiene products to reduce caries activity.

**stanozolol** /stənō′zəlol/, an androgenic anabolic steroid.

■ INDICATIONS: It is prescribed in the treatment of hereditary angioedema.

■ CONTRAINDICATIONS: Cancer of the breast or prostate, nephrosis, pregnancy, or known hypersensitivity to this drug prohibits its use.

■ ADVERSE EFFECTS: Among the most serious adverse reactions are various androgenic effects in males and females, hypoestrogenic effects in females, and allergic reactions. GI disturbances also may occur.

**St. Anthony's fire.** See **ergot poisoning.**

**stape-,** combining form meaning 'stapes': *stapedial, stapedectomy.*

**stapedectomy** /stā′pədek′təmē/ [L, *stapes*, stirrup; Gk, *ektomē*, excision], the removal of the stapes of the middle ear and insertion of a graft and prosthesis, performed to restore hearing in cases of otosclerosis. The stapes that has become fixed is replaced so that vibrations again transmit sound waves through the oval window to the fluid of the inner ear. Under local or general anesthesia, the stapes is removed and the opening into the inner ear is covered with a graft of body tissue. One end of a small plastic tube or piece of stainless steel wire is attached to the graft; the other end is attached to the two remaining bones of the middle ear, the malleus and the incus. Headache and dizziness are expected early in the postoperative period. The patient's hearing does not improve until the edema subsides and the packing is removed. Possible complications include infection of the outer, middle, or inner ear; displacement or rejection of the graft or the prosthesis; and leaking of perilymph around the prosthesis into the middle ear, with ringing in the ear and dizziness. Compare **incudectomy.**

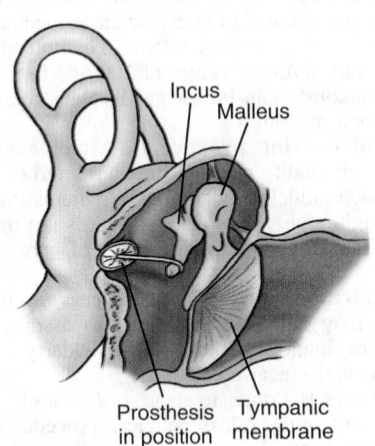

Incus
Malleus
Prosthesis in position
Tympanic membrane

**Stapedectomy** *(Monahan and Neighbors, 1998)*

**stapedius** /stəpē′dē·əs/, a small muscle on the wall of the tympanic cavity of the middle ear. With the tensor tympani, it acts reflexively in response to loud sounds to reduce excessive vibrations that could injure the internal ear by pulling the head of the stapes posteriorly out of the oval window.

**stapes** /stā′pēz/ [L, stirrup], one of the three ossicles in the middle ear, resembling a tiny stirrup, that fits into the oval window. It transmits sound vibrations from the incus to the internal ear. Compare **incus, malleus.** See also **middle ear.**

**Staphage Lysate (SPL),** trademark for an active immunizing agent (staphylococcal antigen phage lysed), used in staphylococcal infection.

**Staphcillin,** trademark for an antibacterial (methicillin sodium).

**staphyl-, staphylo-** /staf′əlo-/, combining form meaning 'grapelike clusters or conditions of the uvula': *staphyloplasty, staphyloncus;* or a micrococcal infection: *staphylolysin, staphyloderm.*

**staphylococcal** /-kok′əl/[Gk, *staphyle*, bunch of grapes *kokkos*, berry], pertaining to a genus of facultatively anaerobic gram-positive cocci.

**staphylococcal antigen phage lysed.** See **Staphage Lysate.**

**staphylococcal infection** [Gk, *staphyle*, bunch of grapes, *kokkos*, berry; L, *inficere*, to taint], an infection caused by any one of several pathogenic species of *Staphylococcus,* commonly characterized by the formation of abscesses of the skin or other organs. Staphylococcal infections of the skin include carbuncles, folliculitis, furuncles, and hidradenitis suppurativa. Bacteremia is common and may result in endocarditis, meningitis, or osteomyelitis. Staphylococcal pneumonia often follows influenza or other viral disease and may be associated with chronic or debilitating illness. Acute gastroenteritis may result from an enterotoxin produced by certain species of staphylococci in contaminated food. Treatment usually includes bed rest, analgesics, and an antimicrobial drug that is resistant to penicillinase, an enzyme secreted by many species of *Staphylococcus.* Surgical drainage, especially of deep abscesses, is often necessary.

**staphylococcal pneumonia** [Gk, *staphyle* + *kokkos* + *pneumon*, lung], pneumonia caused by a staphylococcus infection.

**staphylococcal scalded skin syndrome (SSSS),** an infection or mucous membrane colonization with toxin-producing *Staphylococcus aureus.* It is characterized by epidermal erythema, peeling, and necrosis that give the skin a scalded appearance. This disorder primarily affects infants 1 to 3 months of age and other children, but it also may affect adults. Deficient immune functions and renal insufficiency may predispose individuals to the disease. SSSS is more common in the newborn because of undeveloped immunity and renal systems.

■ OBSERVATIONS: A prodromal upper respiratory tract infection with concomitant purulent conjunctivitis is commonly associated with SSSS. Epidermal complications develop in the erythemal stage, the exfoliation stage, and the desquamation stage. Erythema often spreads around the mouth and other orifices and may extend over the entire body in wide circles as the skin becomes tender and the superficial layer of the skin sloughs from friction. The exfoliation stage follows the erythema stage by 24 to 48 hours and is commonly manifested by slight crusting and erosion, which may spread from around the orifices to wider skin areas. More severe forms of SSSS may cause large soft bullae to erupt and extend over wide skin areas. The eventual rupture of these bullae reveals areas of denuded skin. The desquamation stage of SSSS occurs after the exfoliation stage and is characterized by the drying up of affected areas and the formation of powdery scales. Normal skin replaces the scales within 5 to 7 days. Diagnosis is based on close observation of the development of SSSS through its three characteristic stages. Erythema multiforme and drug-induced toxic epidermal

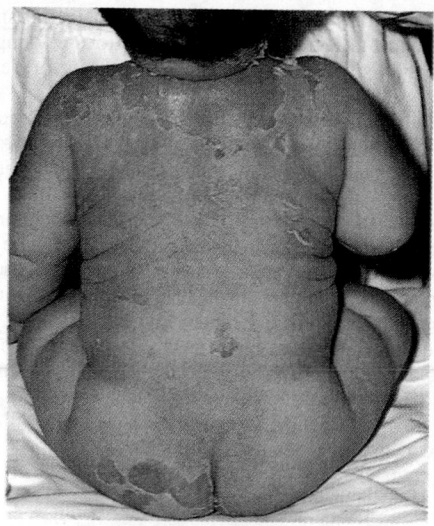

**Staphylococcal scalded skin syndrome**
*(Weston, Lane, and Morrelli, 1996)*

necrolysis are similar to SSSS but may be ruled out in differential diagnosis by exfoliative cytologic characteristics and results of biopsy. Confirming diagnosis is usually made on the basis of isolation of group II *Staphylococcus aureus* in cultures of skin lesions. The mortality rate in SSSS is 2% to 3%; death usually is caused by complications of fluid and electrolyte loss, sepsis, and involvement of other body systems.

■ INTERVENTIONS: Treatment of SSSS commonly includes the administration of systemic antibiotics to prevent secondary infections and the replacement of body fluids to maintain fluid and electrolyte balance.

■ NURSING CONSIDERATIONS: The nursing role in the treatment of this disorder focuses on special care for the neonate, such as maintenance of body temperature by placing the infant in an incubator, careful monitoring of intake and output, administration of IV fluids, maintenance of skin integrity, and careful, regular checks of vital signs. Nurses caring for SSSS patients should be especially alert for any sudden rise in temperature, which may indicate sepsis and the immediate need for aggressive treatment. A strict aseptic technique is needed to prevent any secondary infection. The aseptic technique is especially important during the exfoliation stage, during which open lesions increase the risk of infection. The patient is loosely clothed and covered to minimize friction, which sloughs off the affected skin. Cotton is inserted between the affected fingers and toes to prevent webbing. During the recovery period, warm baths and soaks aid the healing, and gentle debridement of exfoliated areas hastens the healing process. Helpful to parents is the justifiable assurance of the nurse that complications and residual scars from SSSS rarely occur.

**staphylococcemia** /-koksē'mē·ə/, **1.** the presence of staphylococci in the blood. **2.** septicemia caused by staphylococci.

***Staphylococcus*** /staf'ilōkok'əs/, *pl.* **staphylococci** [Gk, *staphyle* + *kokkos*, berry], a genus of nonmotile spheric gram-positive bacteria. Some species are normally found on the skin and in the throat; certain species cause severe purulent infections or produce an enterotoxin, which may cause nausea, vomiting, and diarrhea. Life-threatening staphylo-

coccal infections may arise within hospitals. *Staphylococcus aureus* is a species frequently responsible for abscesses, endocarditis, impetigo, osteomyelitis, pneumonia, and septicemia. *S. epidermidis,* formerly called *S. albus,* occasionally causes endocarditis in the presence of intracardiac prostheses. See also **staphylococcal infection. —staphylococcal,** *adj.*

***Staphylococcus aureus*** [Gk, *staphyle* + *kokkos* + L, *aurum,* gold], a species of *Staphylococcus* that produces a golden pigment with some color variations. It is also responsible for a number of pyogenic infections, such as boils, carbuncles, and abscesses.

**staphylokinase** /staf'ilōkī'nās/, an enzyme, produced by certain strains of staphylococci, that catalyzes the conversion of plasminogen to plasmin in various animal hosts of the microorganism.

**staphyloma** /staf'ilō'mə/, a bulging of eye contents through a thin region of the cornea or sclera.

**staphylopharyngorrhaphy.** See **palatopharyngoplasty.**

**staple** /stā'pəl/, a piece of stainless steel wire used to close certain surgical wounds.

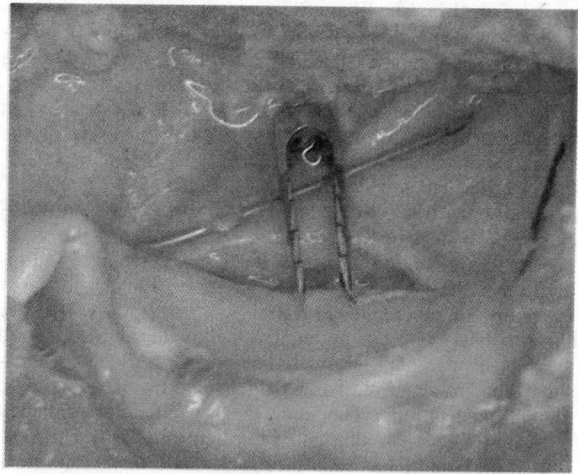

**Staple** *(Johnson, 1993)*

**stapling** [ME, *stapel,* stake], a method of fastening tissues together at the end of surgery by using a U-shaped piece of wire as a suture. The ends of the wire are bent toward the center to close the staple.

**starch** [AS, *stearc,* strong], a polysaccharide composed of long chains of glucose subunits. It is the principal molecule used for the storage of energy in plants. See also **carbohydrate, glucose, glycogen.**

**Starling's law of the heart.** See **Frank-Starling relationship.**

**Starr-Edwards prosthesis** [Albert Starr, American physician, b. 1926; M. L. Edwards, American physician, b. 1906; Gk, *prosthesis,* attachment], an artificial cardiac valve. A caged-ball form of device, it obstructs the valve opening and prevents the backward flow of blood. See also **prosthesis.**

**start codon.** See **initiation codon.**

**start hesitation,** a characteristic of parkinsonism in which the patient has difficulty initiating walking movements, as if the feet were stuck to the floor.

**startle reflex** /stär′təl/ [ME, *stertlen,* to rush; Gk, *syn,* together, *dromos,* course], a reflex response to a sudden unexpected stimulus. The reaction may be accompanied by physiologic effects including increased heartbeat and respiration, closing of the eyes, and flexion of trunk muscles. The reaction is rapid, pervasive, and uncontrollable, regardless of the unexpected stimulus, which may be as simple as a touch. It is a normal reflex in neonates. However, premature and immature infants may not show the reaction. Also called **startle reaction, startle syndrome.** See also **Moro reflex.**

**start point** [ME, *sterte* + L, *punctum,* prick], the initial nucleotide transcribed from a DNA template in the formation of messenger RNA.

**starvation** /stärvā′shən/ [ME, *sterven,* to die], **1.** a condition resulting from the lack of essential nutrients over a long period (several days) and characterized by multiple physiologic and metabolic dysfunctions. **2.** the act or state of starving or being starved. See also **malnutrition.**

**stas-,** combining form meaning 'stopped, or relation to standing or walking': *stasibasiphobia, stasidynic, stasis.*

**-stasia, -stasis, 1.** suffix meaning a '(specified) condition involving the ability to stand': *astasia, ananastasia, dysstasia.* **2.** combining form meaning '(condition of) stoppage or inhibition': *cholestasia, hemostasia, menostasia.*

**stasibasiphobia** /stas′ibas′ifō′bē·ə/, a mental health condition in which a person is convinced that walking or standing is physically impossible. The person may also express a morbid distrust of his or her ability to stand or walk.

**stasis** /stā′sis, stas′is/ [Gk, standing], **1.** a disorder in which the normal flow of a fluid through a vessel of the body is slowed or halted. **2.** stillness.

**-stasis.** See **-stasia.**

**stasis dermatitis,** a common result of venous insufficiency of the legs beginning with ankle edema and progressing to tan pigmentation, patchy erythema, petechiae, and induration. Ultimately, there may be atrophy and fibrosis of the skin and subcutaneous tissue, with ulcerations that are slow to heal. The tan pigment is hemosiderin from blood leaking through capillary walls under elevated venous pressure. The involved skin is easily irritated or sensitized to topical medications. The underlying venous insufficiency must be treated. The dermatitis is often treated by bed rest, Burow's solution for oozing lesions, antibiotics for infection, and corticosteroids for reduction of inflammation. Also called **venous stasis dermatitis.** See also **stasis ulcer.**

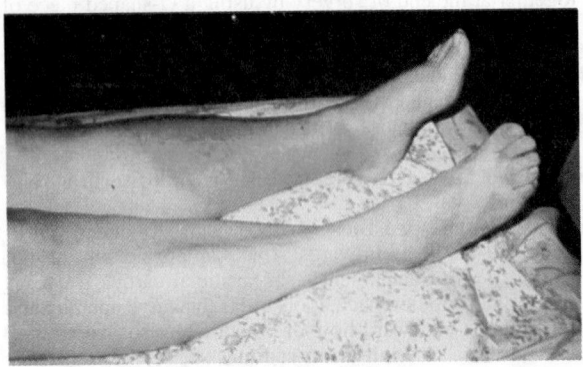

**Stasis dermatitis** *(Christiansen and Grzybowski, 1993)*

**stasis syndrome,** overgrowth of bacteria in the small intestine resulting from a variety of conditions causing stasis, particularly disturbances to intestinal motility or decreased acid secretion, but also structural abnormalities such as diverticula, fistulae between the colon and upper bowel, or chronic obstruction; it is characterized by malabsorption of vitamin $B_{12}$, steatorrhea, and anemia. Also called **bacterial overgrowth syndrome** and **blind loop syndrome.**

**stasis ulcer,** a necrotic craterlike lesion of the skin of the lower leg caused by chronic venous congestion. The ulcer is often associated with stasis dermatitis and varicose veins. Healing is slow, and care to prevent irritation and infection is essential. Potentially sensitizing agents should not be used. Bed rest, elevation, and pressure bandages are usually ordered, and appropriate antibiotics, if needed for infection. Various treatment options are available. Surgery to improve venous flow may be useful in some cases. Also called **varicose ulcer.** See also **stasis dermatitis.**

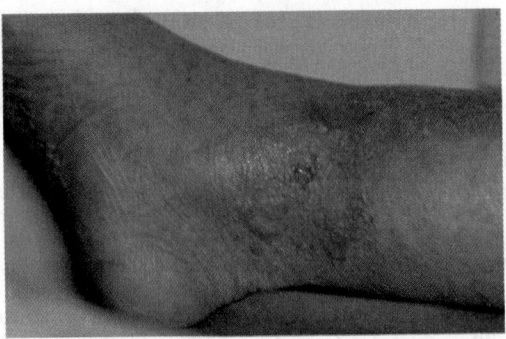

**Stasis ulcer** *(Lemmi and Lemmi, 2000)*

**stat.,** abbreviation for the Latin word *statim,* 'immediately.'

**-stat, 1.** combining form meaning a 'device for keeping something stationary': *catheterostat, hysterostat, ophthalmostat.* **2.** combining form meaning an 'instrument for the regulation of' something specified: *hemostat, rheostat, thermostat.* **3.** combining form meaning an 'apparatus for the reflection of, in one direction of' something specified: *siderostat.* **4.** combining form meaning a 'device for studying in a state of rest': *hydrostat, orbitostat, microstat.* **5.** combining form meaning an 'agent for stopping the growth of': *bacteriostat, fungistat, mycostat.*

**state** /stāt/ [L, *status,* condition], the circumstances or qualities that characterize a person, thing, or way of being at a particular time.

**-state,** combining form meaning the 'result of a (specified) process': *anastate, catastate, mesostate.*

**State Board Test Pool Examination (SBTPE),** revised and retitled in 1982 as the NCLEX-RN, an examination prepared by the National Council of State Boards of Nursing for testing the competency of a person to perform safely as a newly licensed registered nurse. Each jurisdiction within the United States and its territories regulates entry into the practice of nursing; each requires the candidate to pass the examination. The content of the examination is planned to test the candidate's knowledge of the nursing process as applied to the broad areas of nursing practice, including maternal and child health, medical and surgical nursing, and psychiatric nursing. The process includes five steps: assessing, analyzing, planning, implementing, and evaluating. Knowledge, comprehension, application, and analysis of the nursing process are tested as they apply to decision-making situations.

**state medicine.** See **socialized medicine.**

**State Nurses Association (SNA),** an association of nurses at the state level. The various State Nurses Associations are constituent units of the American Nurses Association.

**Statewide Health Coordinating Committee (SHCC),** a component of the U.S. national network of Health Systems Agencies.

**static** /stat'ik/ [Gk, *statikos,* causing to stand], without motion, at rest, in equilibrium. Compare **dynamic.**

**static cardiac work,** the energy transfer that occurs during the development and maintenance of ventricular pressure immediately before the opening of the aortic and pulmonary valves.

**static electricity film fault,** a defect in a radiograph or a developed photographic film, which appears as lightninglike streaks. It is caused by overly rapid opening of the film packet or transfer of static electricity from the user to the film.

**static equilibrium,** the ability of an individual to adjust to displacements of his or her center of gravity while maintaining a constant base of support.

**static imaging,** a diagnostic procedure for visualizing an internal organ or body compartment. A radioactive substance is administered to a patient, and an image or set of images is made of the fixed or slowly changing distribution of the radioactivity.

**static labyrinth,** the vestibule of the inner ear. It contains two communicating chambers, the saccule and the utricle, and elicits tonic reflexes on postural muscles in response to changes in head and body positions.

**static pressure** [Gk, *statikos,* causing to stand; L, *premere,* to press], a condition of equalized blood pressure throughout the body when the heartbeat is stopped. A nonmoving fluid exerts a uniform pressure in all directions.

**static reflex** [Gk, *statikos,* causing to stand; L, *reflectere,* to bend back], a reflex that helps one maintain normal posture and muscle tone when the body is at rest.

**static scoliosis** [Gk, *statikos,* causing to stand, *skoliosis,* curvature], a form of scoliosis resulting from a difference in the length of the legs.

**static symptom.** See **passive symptom.**

**static tremor,** irregular involuntary muscle contractions that occur when a patient makes an effort to hold the trunk or limbs in certain positions.

**station** /stā'shən/ [L, *stare,* to stand], the level of the biparietal plane of the fetal head relative to the level of the ischial spines of the maternal pelvis. An imaginary plane at the level of the spines is designated "zero station." Higher and lower stations are numbered at intervals of 1 cm and labeled as minus above and plus below. For example, "station minus three" is 3 cm above the spines, and "station plus two" is 2 cm below the spines. In breech presentation, the bitrochanteric diameter of the breech is used to determine station. See also **dilation, effacement, labor.**

**stationary grid** /stā'shənər'ē/ [L, *stare* + ME, *gridere,* gridiron], an x-ray grid that does not move or oscillate during the exposure of a radiographic film. The image of the lead strips that compose the grid appears on the radiograph.

**stationary lingual arch,** an orthodontic arch wire that is designed to fit the lingual surface of the teeth and is soldered to the associated anchor bands.

**statistic** /stetis'tik/ [L, *status,* condition], a number that describes a property of a set of data or other numbers.

**statistical model of patient evaluation,** a system based on gross quantitative measurements of similar cases used to determine payment for services.

**Statistical Package for the Social Sciences.** See **SPSS.**

**statistical significance** [L, *status,* condition, *significare,* to signify], an interpretation of statistical data that indicates an occurrence was probably the result of a causative factor and not simply a chance result. Statistical significance at the 1% level indicates a 1 in 100 probability that a result can be ascribed to chance.

**statistics** /stətis'tiks/, a mathematical science concerned with measuring, classifying, and analyzing objective information.

**statotonic reflex.** See **attitudinal reflex.**

**status** /stā'təs, stat'əs/ [L, *condition*], **1.** a specified state or condition, such as emotional status. **2.** an unremitting state or condition, such as status asthmaticus.

**status asthmaticus,** an acute, severe, and prolonged asthma attack. It is caused by critically diminished airway diameter resulting from ongoing bronchospasm, edema, and mucous plugging. Hypoxia, cyanosis, and unconsciousness may follow, and the attack may be fatal. Treatment includes supplemental oxygen to correct hypoxemia, bronchodilators given intravenously or by aerosol inhalation, corticosteroids, mechanical ventilation, sedation, frequent therapy, and emotional support. See also **allergic asthma, asthma.**

**status dysraphicus.** See **dysraphia.**

**status epilepticus,** a medical emergency characterized by continuous seizures occurring without interruptions lasting more than 30 minutes. Status epilepticus can be precipitated by the sudden withdrawal of anticonvulsant drugs, inadequate body levels of glucose, a brain tumor, a head injury, a high fever, or poisoning. Therapy includes IV administration of anticonvulsant drugs, nutrients, and electrolytes. An adequate airway is usually maintained with a nasopharyngeal or endotracheal tube.

**status lacunaris.** See **lacunar state.**

**status marmoratus,** the presence in full-term infants of basal nucleus lesions resulting from acute total asphyxia. The lesions have a marbled appearance caused by neuronal loss and an overgrowth of myelin in the putamen, caudate, and thalamus.

**statute of limitations** /stach' oot/ [L, *statuere,* to set up, *limes,* boundary], (in law) a statute that sets a limit of time during which a suit may be brought or criminal charges may be made. In a malpractice suit, dispute may arise as to whether the time set by the particular statute of limitations begins to run at the time of the injury or at the time of the discovery of the injury.

**statutory rape** /stach'ətôr'ē/ [L, *statuere,* to place, *rapere,* to seize], (in law) sexual intercourse with a female below the age of consent, which varies from state to state. See also **rape.**

**stavudine,** a synthetic thymidine nucleoside analog.

■ INDICATIONS: It is prescribed in the treatment of adults with advanced human immunodeficiency virus (HIV) infection who are intolerant of other approved therapies. However, patients should be advised that the product is not a cure for HIV infection, that they may continue to acquire opportunistic infections associated with acquired immunodeficiency syndrome, and that long-term effects of this therapy are unknown.

■ CONTRAINDICATIONS: Hypersensitivity to this drug or to any of its components prohibits its use.

■ ADVERSE EFFECTS: The side effects most often reported include peripheral neuropathies, elevation of hepatic transaminase levels, headache, chills, fever, asthenia, abdominal pain, diarrhea, nausea, and vomiting.

**STD,** abbreviation for **sexually transmitted disease.**

**steady state (s, ss)** /sted′ē/ [AS, *stedefast,* firm in its place; L, *status,* condition], a basic physiologic concept implying that the various forces and processes of life are in a state of homeostasis. Living organisms are in constant flux, working to balance the internal and external environments in an effort to prevent a deficiency or an excess that might cause illness. Steady state is a complete state of well-being involving total adaptation.

**steam sterilization** [ME, *steme,* vapor; L, *sterilis,* barren], the destruction of all forms of microbial life on an object by exposing the object to moist heat for 15 minutes at 121° F (49.44° C).

**steap-, stear-.** See **stearo-.**

**-stearic,** combining form meaning '(specified) fat or fat derivatives': *aleostearic, ketostearic, neurosteric.*

**Stearns' alcoholic amentia** /sturnz/ [A. Warren Stearns, American physician, 1885–1959; Ar, *alkohl,* essence; L, *ab,* from, *mens,* mind], a form of insanity brought on by alcohol, characterized by an emotional disturbance of a less severe nature than that of delirium tremens but of longer duration and with greater mental clouding and amnesia.

**stearo-, steap-, stear-, steato-,** combining form meaning 'fat': *stearoconotum, stearodermia, stearopten.*

**stearrhea** [Gk, *stear,* fat, *rhoia,* flow], excessive secretion of fat.

**stearyl alcohol,** a solid substance, prepared by the catalytic hydrogenation of stearic acid, used in various ointments.

**steato-.** See **stearo-.**

**steatorrhea** /stē′ətərē′ə/ [Gk, *stear,* fat, *rhoia,* flow], greater than normal amounts of fat in the feces, characterized by frothy foul-smelling fecal matter that floats, as in celiac disease, some malabsorption syndromes, and any condition in which fats are poorly absorbed by the small intestine.

**steatorrhea simplex.** See **seborrhea.**

**Steele-Richardson-Olszewski syndrome** [John C. Steele, Canadian neurologist, 1951–1968; J. Clifford Richardson, Canadian neurologist, b. 1909; Jerzy Olszewski, Canadian neurologist, 1913–1966], a rare progressive neurologic disorder of unknown cause, occurring in middle age, more often in men. It is characterized by paralysis of eye muscles, ataxia, neck and trunk rigidity, pseudobulbar palsy, and parkinsonian facies. Dementia and inappropriate emotional responses also are common. Treatment usually includes the antiparkinsonian drug levodopa for control of extrapyramidal symptoms. Also called **progressive supranuclear palsy.** See also **Parkinson's disease.**

**steeple head.** See **oxycephaly.**

**steering wheel injury,** a traumatic injury most commonly to the anterior chest wall caused by forward propulsion of the body of an automobile driver into the steering wheel during collision. Injuries include broken ribs and sternum, cardiac and pulmonary damage, and tearing of major blood vessels.

**Steinert's disease.** See **myotonic muscular dystrophy.**

**Stein-Leventhal syndrome.** See **polycystic ovary syndrome.**

**Steinmann pin** /stīn′mən/ [Fritz Steinmann, Swiss surgeon, 1872–1932; AS, *pinn*], a wide diameter pin used for heavy skeletal traction, as in the tibia or femur.

**Stelazine,** trademark for a phenothiazine tranquilizer (trifluoperazine).

**stell-,** combining form meaning 'star': *stellate, stellectomy, stellula.*

**stellate** /stel′it, -āt/ [L, *stella,* star], star-shaped or arranged in the pattern of a star.

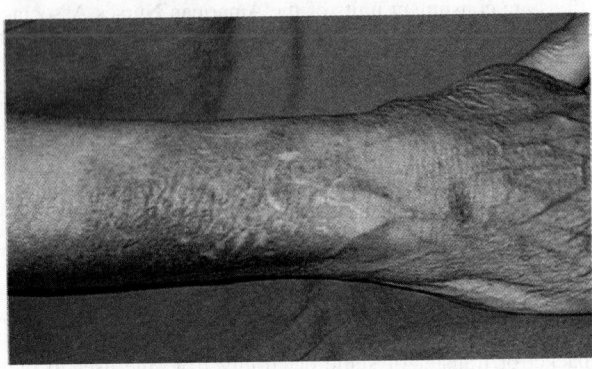

**Stellate scar** *(Lawrence and Cox, 1993)*

**stellate fracture,** a fracture in which there are numerous fissures radiating from the central point of impact or injury throughout surrounding bone tissue.

**stellate ganglion** [L, *stella,* star; Gk, *gagglion,* knot], a large irregular ganglion on the lowest part of the cervical sympathetic trunk fused with the first thoracic ganglion. Its branches communicate with the seventh and eighth cervical nerves.

**stem cell** [AS, *stemm,* tree, trunk; L, *cella,* storeroom], a formative cell; a cell whose daughter cells may give rise to other cell types. A **pluripotential stem cell** is one that has the potential to develop into several different types of mature cells, including lymphocytes, granulocytes, thrombocytes, and erythrocytes. See also **hematopoietic stem cell.**

**stem cell leukemia,** a neoplasm of blood-forming organs in which the predominant malignant cell is too immature to classify. The acute disease has a rapid, relentless course. Also called **embryonal leukemia, hemoblastic leukemia, hemocytoblastic leukemia, lymphoidocytic leukemia, undifferentiated cell leukemia.**

**stem cell lymphoma.** See **undifferentiated malignant lymphoma.**

**steno-,** prefix meaning 'short, contracted, or narrow': *stenobregmate, stenocephaly, stenothorax.*

**stenosis** /stinō′sis/ [Gk, *stenos,* narrow, *osis,* condition], an abnormal condition characterized by the constriction or narrowing of an opening or passageway in a body structure. Kinds of stenosis include **aortic stenosis** and **pyloric stenosis. —stenotic,** *adj.*

**-stenosis,** suffix meaning 'narrowed or constricted': *angiostenosis, aortostenosis.*

**stenotic** [Gk, *stenos,* narrow], pertaining to a structure that is narrowed or strictured.

**Stensen's duct.** See **parotid duct.**

**stent** [Charles R. Stent, nineteenth-century English dentist], **1.** a compound used in making dental impressions and medical molds. **2.** a mold or device made of stent, used in anchoring skin grafts. **3.** a rod or threadlike device for sup-

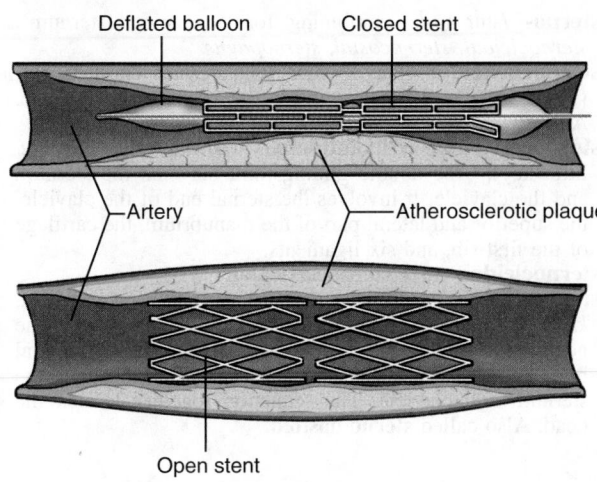

Coronary stent *(Monahan and Neighbors, 1998)*

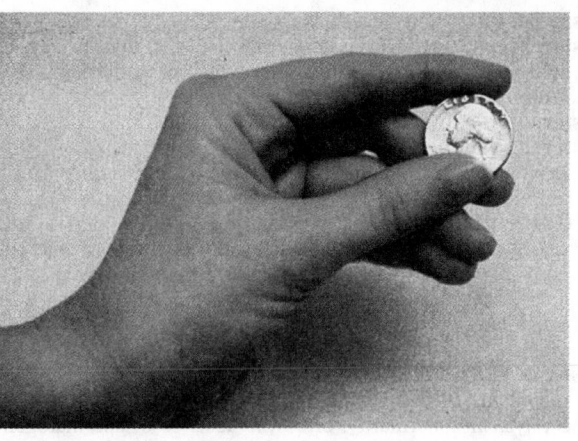

**Assessment of stereognosis** *(Seidel et al, 1999)*

porting tubular structures during surgical anastomosis or for holding arteries open during angioplasty.

**step-care therapy,** a therapeutic program that begins with a simple, conservative type of treatment but may advance to more complex stages as needed to achieve control of a disease or disorder. An example is step-care therapy of hypertension, in which the first step is limited to nonpharmacologic treatments such as weight control, low-salt diet, and exercise. If the first step fails to produce results, the next step may be the prescription of diuretics, followed by the use of beta blockers, angiotensin-converting enzyme inhibitors, or other drugs, until an effective form of treatment is found.

**steppage gait** /step'ij/ [AS, *staepe* + ONorse, *gata,* way], a gait in which the legs are raised abnormally high, as in patients with footdrop.

**stepping reflex.** See **dance reflex.**

**step reflex.** See **dance reflex.**

**stepwedge** /step'wej/, an aluminum device that, when exposed to x-rays, displays a range of exposure intensities on a radiograph. These exposure "steps" are analyzed to determine the speed characteristics of the radiographic film. Also called **penetrometer.**

**Sterane,** trademark for a glucocorticoid (prednisolone).

**Sterapred,** trademark for a glucocorticoid (prednisone).

**sterco-,** combining form meaning 'feces': *stercobilin, stercolith, stercoremia.*

**stereo-** /stir'ē'·ō-/, combining form meaning 'solid, three dimensional, or firmly established': *stereoblastula, stereograph, stereopsis.*

**stereognosis** /stir'·ē·ōgnō'sis/ [Gk, *stereos,* solid, *gnosis,* knowledge], **1.** the faculty of perceiving and understanding the form and nature of objects by the sense of touch. **2.** perception by the sense of the solidity of objects. —**stereognostic,** *adj.*

**stereognostic perception** /stir'ē·ōgnos'tik/ [Gk, *stereos,* solid, *gnosis,* knowledge], the ability to recognize objects by the sense of touch.

**stereoisomer** /stir'ē·ō·ī'səmər/ [Gk, *stereos,* solid, *isos,* equal, *meros,* part], one of two or more chemical compounds that contain the same atoms linked in the same way but are organized differently in space. For example, one may be the mirror image of the other.

**stereoisomeric specificity** /-ī'səmer'ik/ [Gk, *stereos* + *isos,* equal, *meros,* part], specificity of an enzyme for one enantiomer of a racemic mix.

**stereoophthalmoscope** /stir'·ē·ō'ofthal'məskōp/, an ophthalmoscope fitted with two eyepieces so the examiner can view the three-dimensional interior of the eye.

**stereopsis,** binocular perception of depth or three-dimensional space.

**stereoradiographs.** See **stereoscopic radiograph.**

**stereoradiography** /-ra'dē·og'rəfē/ [Gk, *stereos* + L, *radiare,* to emit rays; Gk, *graphein,* to record], a technique for producing radiographs that give a three-dimensional view of an internal body structure. The stereoradiographs are produced by combining two separate x-ray films, each made from a slightly different angle without movement of the body part being x-rayed. The developed films are then viewed through a device that allows the two images to be perceived as one.

**stereoscopic microscope** /-skop'ik/ [Gk, *stereos* + *skopein,* to look], a microscope that produces three-dimensional images through the use of double eyepieces and double objectives. The three-dimensional image is created because the double optic systems have independent light paths. Also called **Greenough microscope.**

**stereoscopic parallax.** See **binocular parallax.**

**stereoscopic radiograph,** a composite of two radiographs made through **stereoradiography.** Also called **stereoradiograph.**

**stereotaxic instrument** /-tak'sik/, an apparatus that fits on the head and helps locate structures in the brain by means of coordinates.

**stereotaxic neuroradiography** [Gk, *stereos* + *taxis,* arrangement, *neuron,* nerve; L, *radiare,* to emit rays; Gk, *graphein,* to record], a radiographic procedure commonly performed during neurosurgery to guide the insertion of a needle into a specific area of the brain.

**stereotaxic radiosurgery,** stereotaxic surgery in which lesions are produced by ionizing radiation. See also **stereotaxic surgery.**

**stereotaxic surgery,** any of several techniques for the production of sharply circumscribed lesions in specific tiny areas of pathologic tissue in deep-seated structures of the central nervous system. The site to be worked on is localized with three-dimensional coordinates, and methods of producing lesions include heat, cold, x-rays, and ultrasound. Also called **stereotaxy.**

**stereotaxy.** See **stereotaxic surgery.**

**stereotype** /stir′ē·ətīp/ [Gk, *stereos* + *typos*, mark], a generalization about a form of behavior, an individual, or a group.

**stereotypical.** See **stereotypy.**

**stereotypic behavior** /stir′ē·ōtip′ik/, a pattern of body movements that has autistic and symbolic meaning for an individual. It may occur in persons with schizophrenia.

**stereotypy** /ster′ē·ətī′pē/ [Gk, *stereos* + *typos*, mark], the persistent inappropriate mechanical repetition of actions, body postures, or speech patterns, usually occurring with a lack of variation in thought processes or ideas. It is often seen in patients with schizophrenia. —**stereotypical,** *adj.*

**sterile** /ster′il/ [L, *sterilis*, barren], **1.** free of living microorganisms. **2.** barren; unable to produce children because of a physical abnormality, often the absence of spermatogenesis in a man or blockage of the fallopian tubes in a woman. Compare **impotence.** —**sterility,** *n.* **3.** aseptic.

**sterile field,** **1.** a specified area, such as within a tray or on a sterile towel, that is considered free of microorganisms. **2.** an area immediately around a patient that has been prepared for a surgical procedure. The sterile field includes the scrubbed team members, who are properly attired, and all furniture and fixtures in the area.

**sterile meningitis** [L, *sterilis*, barren; Gk, *meninx*, membrane, *itis*, inflammation], a form of nonbacterial meningitis, usually involving a viral infection but it also may be drug-induced, in which there is a primarily lymphocytic response in the cerebrospinal fluid. Also called **benign lymphocytic meningitis, simple meningitis.** See also **aseptic meningitis.**

**sterile technique.** See **aseptic technique.**

**sterility** /stəril′itē/ [L, *sterilis*, barren], a condition of being unable to conceive or reproduce the species.

**sterilization** /ster′ilīzā′shən/ [L, *sterilis* + Gk, *izein*, to cause], **1.** a process or act that renders a person unable to produce children. See also **hysterectomy, tubal ligation, vasectomy. 2.** a technique for destroying microorganisms or inanimate objects, using heat, water, chemicals, or gases. —**sterilize,** *v.*

**sterilize** /ster′ilīz/ [L, *sterilis*, barren], **1.** to make powerless to reproduce, such as by surgery. **2.** to destroy all living organisms and viruses in a material.

**sternal** /stur′nəl/ [Gk, *sternon*, chest], pertaining to the sternum.

**-sternal,** suffix meaning 'sternum': *adsternal, presternal, suprasternal.*

**sternal node** [Gk, *sternon*, chest; L, *nodus*, knot], a node in one of the three groups of thoracic parietal lymph nodes. They are situated at the anterior ends of the intercostal spaces, adjacent to the internal thoracic artery. The afferent vessels of the sternal nodes drain the lymph from the breast, the diaphragmatic surface of the liver, and the deep ventral thoracic wall. Also called **internal mammary node.** Compare **diaphragmatic node, intercostal node.** See also **lymphatic system, lymph node.**

**sternal puncture** [Gk, *sternon*, chest; L, *punctura*], a diagnostic procedure in which a needle is inserted into the marrow of the sternum to remove bone marrow samples for diagnosis.

**Sternberg-Reed cell.** See **Reed-Sternberg cell.**

**Sternheimer-Malbin stain** /sturn′hīmərmal′bin/, a crystal violet and safranin stain used in urinalyses to provide additional contrast for certain casts and cells.

**-sternia,** combining form meaning '(condition of the) sternum': *asternia, koilosternia, schistosternia.*

**sterno-** /stur′nō-/, combining form meaning 'sternum': *sternocleidal, sternocostal, sternopagus.*

**sternoclavicular** /-klavik′yələr/ [Gk, *sternon*, chest; L, *clavicula*, little key], pertaining to the sternum and clavicle. Also **sternocleidal.**

**sternoclavicular articulation** [Gk, *sternon* + L, *clavicula*, little key], the double gliding joint between the sternum and the clavicle. It involves the sternal end of the clavicle, the superior and lateral part of the manubrium, the cartilage of the first rib, and six ligaments.

**sternocleidal.** See **sternoclavicular.**

**sternocleidomastoid** /-klī′dōmas′toid/ [Gk, *sternon*, chest, *kleis*, key, *mastos*, breast, *eidos*, form], a muscle of the neck that is attached to the mastoid process of the temporal bone and superior nuchal line and by separate heads to the sternum and clavicle. They function together to flex the head. Also called **sternomastoid.**

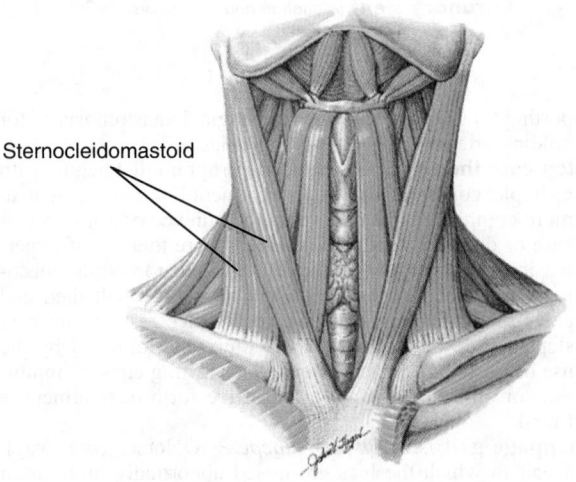

Sternocleidomastoid

**Sternocleidomastoid**
*(Seeley, Stephens, and Tate, 1995/John V. Hagen; by permission of The McGraw-Hill Companies)*

**sternocostal articulation** /-kos′təl/ [Gk, *sternon* + L, *costa*, rib], the gliding articulation of the cartilage of each true rib and the sternum, except the articulation of the first rib, in which the cartilage is directly united with the sternum to form a synchondrosis. Each sternocostal articulation also involves five ligaments.

**sternohyoideus** /stur′nōhī·oi′dē·əs/ [Gk, *sternon* + *hyoeides*, upsilon, U-shaped], one of the four infrahyoid muscles. It acts to depress the hyoid bone. Also called **sternohyoid muscle.** Compare **sternothyroideus.**

**sternomastoid.** See **sternocleidomastoid.**

**sternothyroideus** /stur′nōthīroi′de·əs/ [Gk, *sternon* + *thyreos*, shield, *eidos*, form], one of the four infrahyoid muscles. It acts to depress the thyroid cartilage. Also called **sternothyroid muscle.** Compare **sternohyoideus.**

**sternum** /stur′nəm/ [Gk, *sternon*], the elongated flattened bone forming the middle part of the thorax. It supports the clavicles, articulates directly with the first seven pairs of ribs, and comprises the manubrium, the gladiolus (body), and the xiphoid process. It is composed of highly vascular tissue covered by a thin layer of bone.

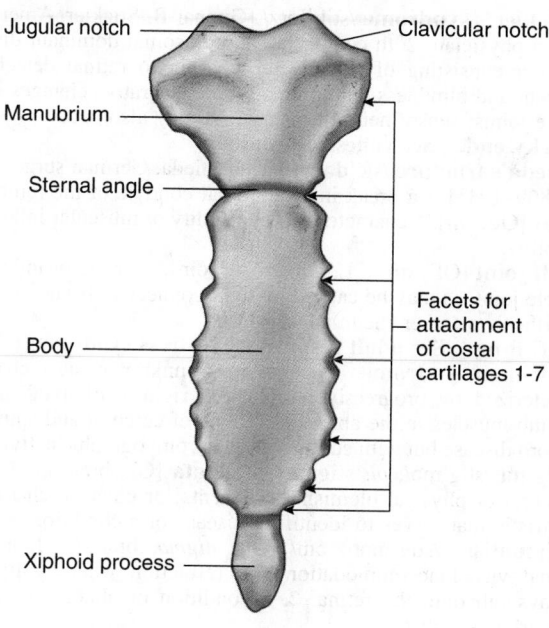

**Sternum**

**stethoscope** /steth′əskōp/ [Gk, *stethos*, chest, *skopein*, to look], an instrument consisting of two earpieces connected by means of flexible tubing to a diaphragm, which is placed against the skin of the patient's chest or back to hear heart and lung sounds. It is also used to hear bowel sounds.

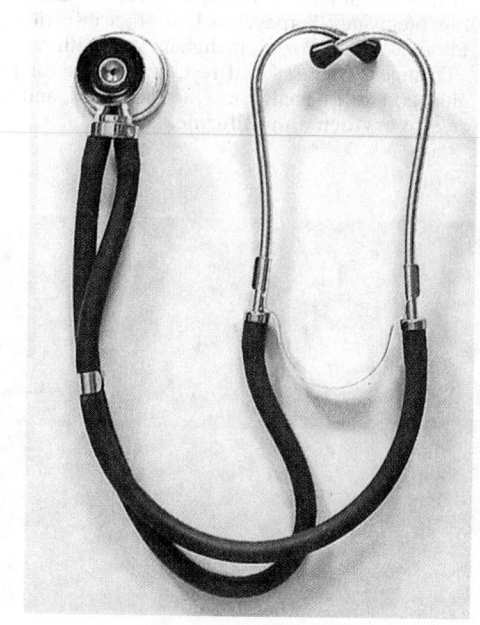

**Stethoscope** *(Seidel et al, 1999)*

**sternutation.** See **sneeze.**

**steroid** /stir′oid/ [Gk, *stereos* + *eidos*, form], any of a large number of hormonal substances with a similar basic chemical structure, produced mainly in the adrenal cortex and gonads. Steroids are chemically related to sterols.

**steroid acne** [Gk, *stereos*, solid; L, *oleum*, oil; Gk, *eidos*, form, *akme*, point], a form of acne caused by the use of corticosteroids.

**steroid cell antibody,** an immunoglobulin G glycoprotein that interacts with antigens in the cytoplasm of gonadal or adrenal cells that produce steroids.

**steroid hormones** [Gk, *stereos*, solid; L, *oleum*, oil; Gk, *eidos*, form, *hormaein*, to set in motion], any of the ductless gland secretions that contain the basic steroid nucleus in their chemical formulae. The natural steroid hormones include the androgens, estrogens, and adrenal cortex secretions.

**steroid hormone therapy** [Gk, *stereos* + L, *oleum*, oil; Gk, *eidos*, form, *hormaein*, to set in motion, *therapeia*, treatment], treatment with any of the steroid hormones, such as the use of estrogen to reduce symptoms of postmenopausal disorders.

**steroidogenesis** /stiroi′dōjen′əsis/, the biologic synthesis of steroid hormones.

**sterol** /stir′ôl/ [Gk, *stereos* + Ar, *alkohl*, essence], a large subgroup of steroids containing a hydroxyl group at position 3 and a branched aliphatic side chain of eight or more carbon atoms at position 17. Kinds of sterols include **cholesterol** and **ergosterol.**

**stertorous** /stur′tərəs/ [L, *stertere*, to snore], pertaining to a respiratory effort that is strenuous or struggling; having a snoring sound.

**stetho-, steth-,** combining form meaning 'the chest': *stethometer, stethomyitis, stethospasm.*

**stethomimetic** /steth′ōmimet′ik/, pertaining to any condition causing or associated with a reduction of chest volume below its normal value. The condition may be congenital, temporary, or permanent.

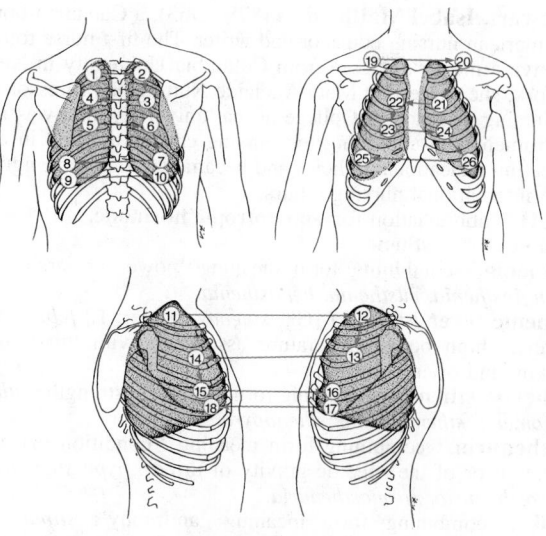

**Stethoscope placement for auscultation of lung sounds**
*(Potter and Perry, 2001)*

**Stevens-Johnson syndrome** [Albert M. Stevens, American pediatrician, 1884–1945; F.C. Johnson, American physician, 1894–1934], a serious, sometimes fatal, inflammatory disease affecting children and young adults. It is characterized by the acute onset of fever, bullae on the skin, and ulcers on the mucous membranes of the lips, eyes, mouth, nasal passage, and genitalia. Other complications are pneumonia, pain in the joints, prostration, and perforation of the cornea. It may be an allergic reaction to certain drugs, or it may follow pregnancy, herpesvirus I, or other infection. It is seen rarely in association with malignancy or with radiation therapy. Treatment includes bed rest, antibiotics for pneumonia, glucocorticoids, analgesics, mouthwashes, and sedatives. See also **erythema multiforme.**

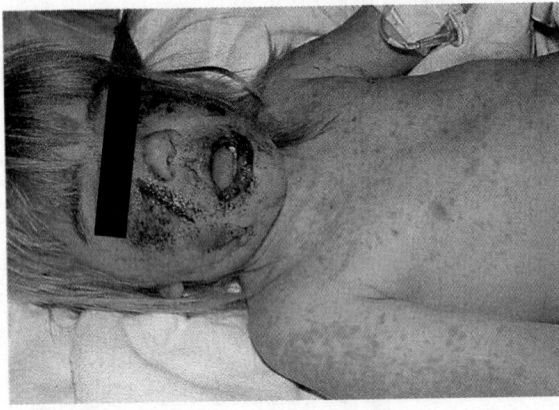

**Stevens-Johnson syndrome** *(Zitelli and Davis, 1997)*

**Stewart, Isabel Maitland** (1878–1963), a Canadian-born American nursing educator and writer. The first nurse to receive a master's degree from Columbia University in New York, she succeeded Mary Adelaide Nutting as Professor of Nursing at Teachers College at that university. She was instrumental in upgrading the nursing curriculum and in directing educational policies and became an important figure in international nursing affairs.

**STH,** abbreviation for **somatotropic hormone.**

**sthen-.** See **stheno-.**

**-sthenia,** combining form meaning 'power or strength': *angiosthenia, eusthenia, hyposthenia.*

**sthenic fever** /sthen'ik/ [Gk, *sthenos,* power; L, *febris,* fever], high body temperature associated with thirst, dry skin, and often delirium.

**stheno-, sthen-,** combining form meaning 'strength': *sthenometer, sthenoplastic, sthenopyra.*

**-sthenuria,** combining form meaning '(condition of) urination or of the specific gravity of urine': *hypersthenuria, isosthenuria, normosthenuria.*

**stib-,** combining form meaning 'antimony': *stibamine, stibophen, stiburea.*

**stibocaptate.** See **sodium stibocaptate.**

**stibogluconate sodium** /stib'ōgloo'kənāt/, an antileishmanial available from the Centers for Disease Control and Prevention. It is a drug of choice for the visceral form of leishmaniasis and has some effect on other forms.

**stich-, -stichia,** combining form meaning 'rows': *stichochrome, polystichia.*

**Stickler's syndrome** /stik'lərz/ [Gunnar B. Stickler, American physician, 20th century], an autosomal dominant disorder consisting of myopia progressing to retinal detachment and blindness, and premature degenerative changes in the joints; sensorineural hearing loss may also occur.

**sticky end.** See **cohesive terminus.**

**Stieda's fracture** /stē'dəz/ [Alfred Stieda, German surgeon, 1869–1945], a break in the internal condyle of the femur.

**stiff** [OE, *stif*], characterized by rigidity or muscular inflexibility.

**stiff joint** [OE, *stif* + L, *jungere,* to join], a rigid or inflexible joint, as may be caused by tight connective tissue or by arthritis or other rheumatic disorders.

**stiff lung.** See **adult respiratory distress syndrome.**

**stiff-man syndrome,** a condition of unknown cause characterized by progressive fluctuating rigidity of axial and limb muscles in the absence of signs of cerebral and spinal cord disease but with continuous electromyographic activity.

**stigma** /stig'mə/, *pl.* **stigmas, stigmata** [Gk, brand], **1.** a moral or physical blemish. **2.** a mental or physical characteristic that serves to identify a disease or a condition.

**stigmatism** /stig'mətiz'əm/ [Gk, *stigma,* brand], **1.** normal visual accommodation and refraction whereby light rays fall onto the retina. **2.** a condition of abnormal skin markings.

**stilbestrol.** See **diethylstilbestrol.**

**stilet, stilette.** See **stylet.**

**stillbirth** [AS, *stille* + ME, *burth*], **1.** the birth of a fetus that died before or during delivery. **2.** a fetus, born dead, that weighs more than 500 g and would usually have been expected to live.

**stillborn** [AS, *stille* + *boren*], **1.** an infant that was born dead. **2.** pertaining to an infant that was born dead.

**Still's disease.** See **juvenile rheumatoid arthritis.**

**Stilphostrol,** trademark for an estrogen (diethylstilbestrol diphosphate).

**stimulant** /stim'yələnt/ [L, *stimulare,* to incite], any agent that increases the rate of activity of a body system.

**stimulant cathartic,** a cathartic that acts by promoting the motility of the bowel, especially the longitudinal peristalsis of the colon. Kinds of stimulant cathartics are **cascara** and **senna.**

**stimulate** /stim'yəlāt/ [L, *stimulare,* to incite], to excite, as in the process of increasing a vigorous functional activity.

**stimulating bath,** a bath taken in water that contains an aromatic substance, an astringent, or a tonic.

**stimulation** /stim'yəlā'shən/ [L, *stimulare,* to incite], the condition of being stimulated.

**stimulus** /stim'yələs/, *pl.* **stimuli** [L, *stimulare,* to incite], anything that excites or incites an organism or part to function, become active, or respond. —**stimulate,** *v.*

**stimulus control,** a strategy for self-modification that depends on manipulating the causes of behavior to increase goals or behaviors desired by a patient while decreasing those that are undesired.

**stimulus duration,** the length of time a stimulus must be applied for the resulting nerve impulse to produce excitation in the receptor tissue. In general, more intense stimuli require shorter excitation times to effect cellular response. Any stimulus that acts too briefly to overcome the threshold intensity of the receptor cell will not elicit a response.

**stimulus generalization,** a type of conditioning in which the reaction to one stimulus is reinforced to allow transfer of the reaction to other occurrences.

**sting** [AS, *stingan*], an injury caused by a sharp, painful penetration of the skin, often accompanied by exposure to an irritating chemical or the venom of an insect or other animal. In cases of hypersensitivity, a highly venomous sting, or multiple stings, anaphylactic shock may occur. Kinds of stings include bee, jellyfish, scorpion, sea urchin, and shellfish stings. See also **stingray, wasp.**

**stingray** /sting′rā/ [AS, *stingan* + L, *raia,* ray-fish], a flat, long-tailed fish bearing barbed spines on its back that are connected to sacs of venom. Spasm of the skeletal muscles, severe local pain, seizures, and dyspnea may occur if the skin is broken by the spines. See also **sea urchin sting.**

**stippling** [D, *stippen,* to prick], **1.** the appearance of colored dots in some cells when stained. Red stippling in blood cells stained with eosin hematoxylin is a sign of malaria. **2.** the appearance of the retina, as if dotted with light and dark points. See also **gingival stippling.**

**stitch** [ME, *stiche*], **1.** a suture. **2.** a sudden sharp pain.

**stitch abscess** [ME, *stiche* + L, *abscedere,* to go away], an abscess that develops around a suture.

**St. John's wort,** an herb that is native to Europe and Asia, also now grown in the United States.

■ USES: This herb is used as an antidepressant and antiviral.

■ CONTRAINDICATIONS: St. John's wort is not recommended during pregnancy and lactation, in children, or in those with known hypersensitivity to this product.

**St. Louis encephalitis** /săntloo′is/ [St. Louis, Missouri; Gk, *enkephalon,* brain, *itis,* inflammation], a flavovirus infection of the brain transmitted from birds to humans by the bite of an infected mosquito. It occurs most commonly in the central and southern parts of the United States and is characterized by headache, malaise, fever, stiff neck, delirium, and convulsions. Sequelae may include visual and speech disturbances, difficulty in walking, and personality changes. Convalescence may be prolonged, and death may result. Compare **California encephalitis, equine encephalitis.** See also **encephalitis.**

**stocking aid.** See **sock aid.**

**stock vaccine,** an immunizing agent made from a stock microbial strain.

**stoker's cramp.** See **heat cramp.**

**Stokes-Adams syndrome.** See **Adams-Stokes syndrome.**

**-stole,** suffix meaning 'contraction, retraction, or dilation of various organs': *anastole, diastole, peristole.*

**stoma** /stō′mə/, *pl.* **stomas, stomata** [Gk, mouth], **1.** a pore, orifice, or opening on a surface. **2.** an artificial opening of an internal organ on the surface of the body, created surgically, such as for a colostomy, ileostomy, or tracheostomy. **3.** a new opening created surgically, between two body structures, such as for a gastroenterostomy, pancreaticogastrostomy, pancreatoduodenostomy, or pyeloureterostomy.

**-stoma, -stome,** suffix meaning a 'mouth or opening': *hypostoma, metastoma, tetrastoma.*

**stomach** /stum′ək/ [Gk, *stomakhos,* gullet], the food reservoir and first major site of digestion, located just under the diaphragm and divided into a body and a pylorus. It receives partially processed food and drink funneled from the mouth through the esophagus and gradually feeds liquefied food (chyme) into the small intestine. The stomach lies in the epigastric and left hypogastric regions bounded by the anterior abdominal wall and the diaphragm between the liver and the spleen. The shape of the stomach is modified by the amount of contents, stage of digestion, development of gastric musculature, and condition of the intestines. It is lined with a mucous coat, a submucous coat, a muscular coat, and a serous coat, all richly supplied with blood vessels and nerves, and contains fundic, cardiac, and pyloric gastric glands. Also called **gaster.**

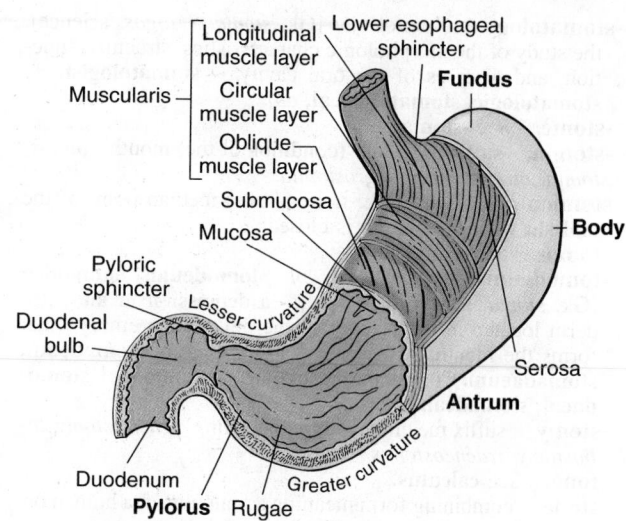

**Stomach** *(Lewis, Heitkemper, and Dirksen, 2000)*

**stomach ache** [Gk, *stomakhos,* gullet; ME, *aken,* pain], pain in the stomach area. Also called **gastralgia, gastrodynia, stomachalgia.**

**stomach cancer.** See **gastric cancer.**

**stomach drops,** a medication that promotes gastric activity.

**stomach pump,** a pump for withdrawing the contents of the stomach through a tube passed through the mouth or nose into the stomach.

**stomach tube,** a tube used to introduce nutrients into the stomach, remove fluids and ingested poisons, or decompress the stomach. Also called **gastrostomy tube, G tube.**

**stomadaeum, stomadeal, stomadeum.** See **stomodeum.**

**stomal** /stō′məl/ [Gk, mouth], pertaining to one or more stomata or mouthlike openings. Also **stomatal.**

**stomal peptic ulcer,** a marginal peptic ulcer. See also **marginal peptic ulcer, peptic ulcer.**

**stomata.** See **stoma.**

**stomatal.** See **stomal.**

**stomatitis** /stō′mətī′tis/ [Gk, *stoma* + *itis,* inflammation], any inflammatory condition of the mouth. It may result from infection by bacteria, viruses, or fungi; from exposure to certain chemicals or drugs from vitamin deficiency; or from a systemic inflammatory disease. Kinds of stomatitis include **aphthous stomatitis, pseudomembranous stomatitis, thrush,** and **Vincent's infection.** See also **candidiasis.**

**stomatitis parasitica** [Gk, *stoma,* mouth, *itis,* inflammation, *parasitos,* guest], an inflammation of the mucous membranes of the mouth by a yeast fungus, *Candida albicans,* typically expressed by a white coating on the tongue. It may affect infants or immunosuppressed people with human immunodeficiency virus, or appear as an outgrowth secondary to antibiotic therapy. Also called **thrush.**

**stomato-, stomo-,** combining form meaning 'mouth': *stomatodysodia, stomatogastric, stomatopathy.*

**stomatognathic system** /stō′mətōnath′ik/ [Gk, *stoma* + *gnathos,* jaw, *systema*], the combination of organs, structures, and nerves involved in speech and reception, mastication, and deglutition of food. This system is composed of the teeth, the jaws, the masticatory muscles, the tongue, the lips, surrounding tissues, and the nerves that control these structures.

**stomatology** /stō′mətol′əjē/ [Gk, *stoma* + *logos,* science], the study of the morphologic characteristics, structure, function, and diseases of the oral cavity. —**stomatologist,** *n.,* **stomatologic, stomatological,** *adj.*

**-stome.** See **-stoma.**

**-stomia,** suffix meaning '(condition of the) mouth': *atelostomia, atretostomia, hygrostomia.*

**stomion** /stō′mē·on/ [Gk, *stoma*], the median point of the oral slit when the mouth is closed.

**stomo-.** See **stomato-.**

**stomodeum** /stom′ədē′əm/, *pl.* **stomodeums, stomodea** [Gk, *stoma* + *odaios,* a way], a depression in the ectoderm located in the foregut of the developing embryo that forms the mouth. Also spelled **stomodaeum, stomadeum, stomadaeum.** Compare **proctodeum.** —**stomodeal, stomodaeal, stomadeal,** *adj.*

**-stomy,** suffix meaning 'surgical opening': *gastrostomy, lobostomy, tracheostomy.*

**stone.** See **calculus.**

**-stone,** combining form meaning a 'calculus in a human organ or duct': *bilestone, gallstone, wombstone.*

**stone disease,** urolithiasis that may have complications when obstructive uropathy or infection develops. See also **urinary calculus.**

**stool.** See **feces.**

**stool for occult blood test (stool for OB),** a stool test performed as part of every routine physical examination to detect the presence of occult blood in the GI tract. Presence of OB in the stool may indicate benign and malignant GI tumors, ulcers, inflammatory bowel disease, arteriovenous malformation, diverticulosis, and hematobilia.

**stool softener.** See **fecal softener.**

**stop** [AS, *stoppian,* to stop], a consonantal speech sound produced by closing off the oral cavity and then releasing with a burst of air, such as an initial /p/. Also called **plosive.**

**stopcock,** a valve or turning plug that controls the flow of fluid from a container through a tube. A three-way stopcock can be used on IV tubing to turn off one solution and turn on another.

**stop needle** [AS, *stoppian,* to stop, *naedel*], a needle with a shoulder flange that prevents it from penetrating beyond a certain distance.

**storage capacity** /stôr′ij/, the amount of data that can be held on a computer disk or tape, usually expressed in kilobytes (one thousand bytes), megabytes (one million bytes), gigabytes (one billion bytes), or terabytes (one trillion bytes).

**storage disease,** a metabolic disorder in which certain cells accumulate excessive amounts of lipids, proteins, or other substances.

**storage pool disease,** a blood coagulation disorder caused by failure of platelets to release adenosine diphosphate in response to aggregating agents.

**stored-energy foot,** a lower-limb prosthesis designed to imitate the springlike action of a natural foot and leg. A device in the prosthesis stores energy when weight is put on the prosthesis. When the weight is shifted to the other leg, the stored energy is released, returning the prosthesis to its original shape.

**stork bite.** See **telangiectatic nevus.**

**storm fermentation** [OE, *sturm,* storm; L, *fermentum,* leaven], the rapid gaseous clotting of milk caused by *Clostridium perfringens.*

**Stoxil,** trademark for an antiviral (idoxuridine).

**STP,** *slang.* a psychedelic agent, dimethoxy-4-methylamphetamine. STP is an abbreviation for *serenity, tranquillity, and peace.*

**STPD conditions of a volume of gas,** (standard temperature, standard pressure, dry) the conditions of a volume of gas at 0° C and 760 torr and containing no water vapor (dry). It should contain a calculable number of moles of a particular gas.

**Str.,** abbreviation for *Streptococcus.*

**strab-,** combining form meaning 'squinting': *strabismometer, strabometry, strabismus.*

**strabismal** /strabiz′məl/ [Gk, *strabismos,* squint], pertaining to the condition of strabismus.

**strabismus** /strabiz′məs/ [Gk, *strabismos,* squint], an abnormal ocular condition in which the visual axes of the eyes are not directed at the same point. There are two kinds of strabismus, paralytic and nonparalytic. Paralytic strabismus results from the inability of the ocular muscles to move the eye because of neurologic deficit or muscular dysfunction. The muscle that is dysfunctional may be identified by watching as the patient attempts to move the eyes to each of the cardinal positions of gaze. If the affected eye cannot be directed to a position, the examiner infers that the associated ocular muscle is the dysfunctional one. Because this kind of strabismus may be caused by tumor, infection, or injury to the brain or the eye, an ophthalmologic examination is recommended. Nonparalytic strabismus is a defect in the position of the two eyes in relation to each other. The condition is inherited. The person cannot use the two eyes together but has to fixate with one or the other. The eye that looks straight at a given time is the fixing eye. Some people have alternating strabismus, using one eye and then the other; some have monocular strabismus, which affects only one eye. Visual acuity diminishes with diminished use of an eye, and suppression amblyopia may develop. Nonparalytic strabismus and suppression amblyopia are treated most successfully in early childhood. The primary treatment consists mainly of covering the fixing eye, forcing the child to use the deviating eye. The earlier it is begun, the more rapid and effective is the treatment. By 6 years of age, a deviating eye has usually become so suppressed that treatment is not effective and permanent visual loss has occurred. The eyes might be straightened by surgery, but suppression amblyopia will not be corrected. Also called **squint.** See also **convergent squint, divergent squint.** —**strabismal, strabismic, strabismical,** *adj.*

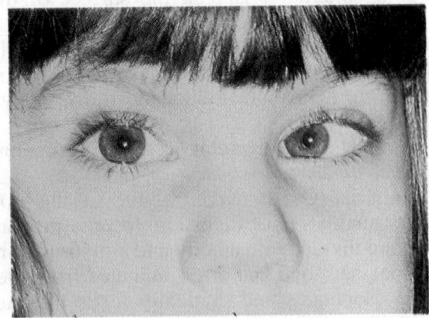

**Strabismus** *(Zitelli and Davis, 1997)*

**straddling embolism.** See **saddle embolism.**

**straight-leg-raising (SLR) test,** a physical examination technique to determine abnormality of the sciatic nerve or tightness of the hamstrings. The presence of sciatica is confirmed by sciatic nerve pain radiating down the limb when the supine person attempts to raise the straightened limb.

**straight line blood set** /strāt/ [ME, *streght*], a common device, composed of plastic components, for delivering blood infusions. It includes plastic tubing, a clamp, a drip chamber, and a filter. Some kinds of straight-line blood sets contain filters within drip chambers; others have separate filters. The latter kind can be filled by squeezing the attached drip chamber but must not be squeezed itself or it may rupture. The former kind can be filled by squeezing the section of the blood set that contains the filter and the drip chamber. Before infusion, the filter of either kind is tapped with the fingers to dislodge any trapped air bubbles. Compare **component drip set, component syringe set, microaggregate recipient set, Y-set.**

**straight sinus** [ME, *streght* + L, *sinus*, hollow], one of the six posterior-superior venous channels of the dura mater, draining blood from the brain into the internal jugular vein. It has no valves and is located at the junction of the falx cerebri with the tentorium cerebelli. Compare **inferior sagittal sinus, superior sagittal sinus, transverse sinus.**

**straight wire fixed orthodontic appliance,** a fixed orthodontic appliance used for correcting and improving malocclusion. It is a variation of the edgewise orthodontic appliance. Its design and placement of arch wire brackets and tubes are intended to limit the need for arch wire adjustments.

**strain** [ME, *streinen*], **1.** to exert physical force in a manner that may result in injury, usually muscular. **2.** to separate solids or particles from a liquid with a filter or sieve. **3.** damage, usually muscular, that results from excessive physical effort. **4.** a taxon that is a subgroup of a species. **5.** an emotional state reflecting mental pressure or fatigue.

**straitjacket** /strāt'jakit/ [OFr, *estreit*, strict, *jaquette*, short coat], a coatlike garment of canvas with long sleeves that can be tied behind the wearer's back to prevent arm movement. It is used for restraining violent or uncontrollable people. Also called **camisole restraint.**

**strangle** /strang'gəl/ [L, *strangulare*, to choke], to cause an interruption of breathing by compressing or constricting the trachea. Also called **strangulate. —strangulated,** *adj.*

**strangulated** /strang'gyəlā'tid/ [L, *strangulare*, to choke], pertaining to a constriction or compression of the trachea or other upper airway structure that interrupts the normal flow of air.

**strangulated hemorrhoid** [L, *strangulare*, to choke; Gk, *haimorrhoise*, vein that discharges blood], a prolapsed hemorrhoid that has become trapped by the anal sphincter, causing the blood supply to become occluded by the sphincter's constricting action.

**strangulated hernia** [L, *strangulare*, to choke, *hernia*, rupture], a hernia in which the blood vessels have become constricted by the neck of the hernial sac, resulting in ischemia and possible gangrene if blood circulation is not quickly restored.

**strangulation** /strang'gyəlā'shən/ [L, *strangulare*, to choke], the constriction of a tubular structure of the body, such as the trachea, a segment of bowel, or the blood vessels of a limb, that prevents function or impedes circulation. See also **intestinal strangulation.**

**strap** [AS, *stropp*], **1.** a band, such as that made of adhesive plaster, that is used to hold dressings in place or to attach one thing to another. **2.** to bind securely.

**strapping,** the application of overlapping strips of adhesive tape to an extremity or body area to exert pressure and hold a structure in place, performed in the treatment of strains, sprains, dislocations, and certain fractures. See **strata, stratum.**

**strata.** See **stratum.**

**strati-,** combining form meaning 'layer': *stratification, stratiform, stratigraphy.*

**stratified** /strat'ifīd/ [L, *stratum + facere*, to make], arranged in layers.

**stratified clot,** a semisolid mass of coagulated blood that forms in layers within an aneurysm.

**stratified epithelium** [L, *stratum + facere*; Gk, *epi*, above, *thele*, nipple], closely packed sheets of epithelial cells arranged in layers over the external surface of the body and lining most of the hollow structures. The layers may include stratified squamous, stratified columnar, or stratified columnar ciliated types of cells. There are various subtypes of stratified epithelium, named for the type of cells on the surface, e.g., stratified squamous epithelium, stratified columnar epithelium.

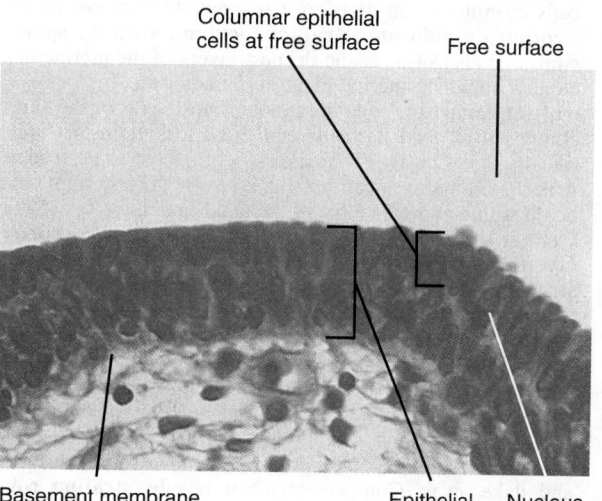

**Stratified columnar epithelium**
*(© Ed Reschke; used with permission)*

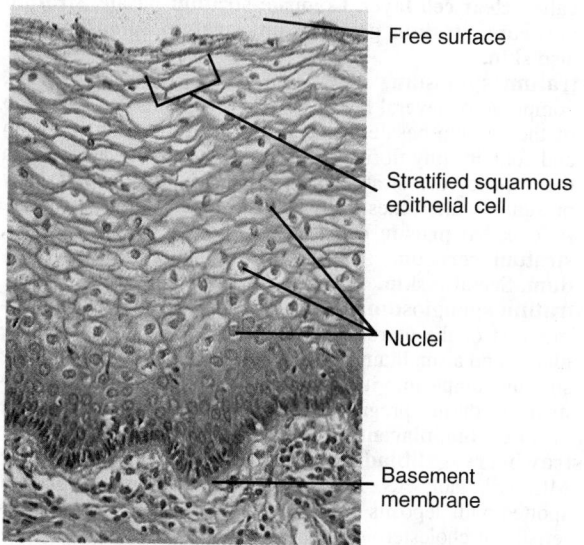

**Stratified squamous epithelium**
*(© Ed Reschke; used with permission)*

**stratified sample.**   See **sample.**

**stratiform cartilage.**   See **fibrocartilage.**

**stratiform fibrocartilage** /strat′ifôrm/ [L, *stratum,* layer, *forma,* form, *fibra,* fiber, *cartilago,* cartilage], a structure made of fibrocartilage that forms a thin coating of osseous grooves through which tendons of certain muscles glide. Small masses of stratified fibrocartilage also develop in the tendons of some muscles that glide over bones, as in the tendons of the peroneus longus and the tibialis posterior. Compare **circumferential fibrocartilage, connecting fibrocartilage, interarticular fibrocartilage.**

**stratum** /strā′təm, strat′əm/, *pl.* **strata** [L, layer], a uniformly thick sheet or layer, usually associated with other layers, such as the stratum basale of the epidermis.

**stratum basale,**   **1.** also called **basal layer, stratum germinativum.** The deepest of the five layers of the epidermis, composed of cuboidal-shaped cells. This layer provides new cells by mitotic cell division. Compare **stratum corneum, stratum granulosum, stratum lucidum, stratum spinosum.** See also **skin. 2.** the deepest layers of the uterine decidua, containing uterine gland terminals.

**stratum corneum,**   the horny, outermost layer of the skin, composed of dead flat cells converted to keratin that continually flakes away. The thickness of the layer is correlated with the normal wear of the area it covers. The stratum corneum is thick on the palms of the hands and the soles of the feet but relatively thin over most areas. Also called **horny layer.** Compare **stratum basale, stratum granulosum, stratum lucidum, stratum spinosum.** See also **skin.**

**stratum germinativum.**   See **stratum basale.**

**stratum granulosum,**   one of the layers of the epidermis, situated just below the stratum corneum except in the thick skin of the palms of the hands and the soles of the feet, where it lies just under the stratum lucidum. The stratum granulosum contains visible granules in the cytoplasm of its cells, which die, become keratinized, move to the surface, and flake away. Compare **stratum basale, stratum corneum, stratum lucidum, stratum spinosum.** See also **skin.**

**stratum lucidum,**   one of the layers of the epidermis, situated just beneath the stratum corneum and present only in the thick skin of the palms of the hands and the soles of the feet. It contains translucent eleidin that forms keratin. Also called **clear cell layer.** Compare **stratum basale, stratum corneum, stratum granulosum, stratum spinosum.** See also **skin.**

**stratum spinosum,**   one of the layers of the epidermis, composed of several layers of polygonal cells. It lies on top of the stratum basale and beneath the stratum granulosum and contains tiny fibrils within its cellular cytoplasm. When the cells of the stratum spinosum are pulled apart, they present minute spines, called desmosomes, at their surfaces. Also called **prickle cell layer.** Compare **stratum basale, stratum corneum, stratum granulosum, stratum lucidum.** See also **skin.**

**stratum spongiosum,**   one of the three layers of the endometrium of the uterus, containing tortuous, dilated uterine glands and a small amount of interglandular tissue. With the stratum compactum it forms the functional part of the endometrium during pregnancy. Compare **stratum basale.** See also **decidua, placenta.**

**strawberry gallbladder** /strô′berē/ [AS, *strawberig* + ME, *gal,* gall; AS, *blaedre*], a tiny yellow gallbladder spotted with deposits on the red mucous membrane, characteristic of cholesterolosis.

**strawberry hemangioma, strawberry mark.**   See **capillary hemangioma.**

**strawberry tongue,**   a strawberry-like coloration of the inflamed tongue papillae. It is a clinical sign of scarlet fever and is also seen in Kawasaki disease.

**stray light** [OFr, *estraier,* to wander; AS, *leoht,* illumination], radiant energy that reaches a photodetector and that consists of wavelengths other than those defined by the filter or monochromator.

**stray radiation.**   See **leakage radiation.**

**streak** [AS, *strican,* to stroke], a line or a stripe, such as the primitive streak at the caudal end of the embryonic disk.

**street virus,**   a natural infectious agent, such as rabies, that may be transmitted from a domestic animal or may be obtained in the wild, outside the laboratory.

**strength** [AS, *strengou*], the ability of a muscle or a person to produce or resist a physical force.

**strength of association,**   the degree of relationship between a causal factor and the occurrence of a disease, usually expressed in terms of a relative risk ratio.

**strength training,**   a method of improving muscular strength by gradually increasing the ability to resist force through the use of free weights, machines, or the person's own body weight. Strength training sessions are designed to impose increasingly greater resistance, which in turn stimulates development of muscle strength to meet the added demand.

**strepho-, streph-,**   combining form meaning 'twisted': *strephopodia, strephosymbolia, strephotome.*

**streptavidin** /strep′təvī′din/,   a biotin-binding protein isolated from streptomyces and used to identify antigens in surgical pathologic diagnosis.

**strep throat** [*Streptococcus* + AS, *throte*], *informal.* an infection of the oral pharynx and tonsils caused by a hemolytic species of *Streptococcus,* usually belonging to group A. The infection is characterized by sore throat, chills, fever, swollen lymph nodes in the neck, and sometimes nausea and vomiting. The symptoms usually begin abruptly a few days after exposure to the organism in airborne droplets or after direct contact with an infected person. Also called **streptococcal sore throat.**

■ OBSERVATIONS: The throat is diffusely red, and tonsils often are covered with a yellow or white exudate. Diagnosis is confirmed by bacteriologic culture and identification of the streptococcal bacteria in a specimen taken from the throat. Complications of strep throat are otitis media, scarlet fever, and sinusitis; other complications include acute glomerulonephritis and acute rheumatic fever.

■ INTERVENTIONS: Treatment usually includes intramuscular injection of penicillin G benzanthine or the administration of penicillin for 10 days. Erythromycin may be given to people allergic to penicillin. For recurrent infections, tonsillectomy may be recommended.

**strepticemia.**   See **streptococcemia.**

**strepto-** /strep′tō-/,   combining form meaning 'twisted': *streptobacilli, streptococcal, streptomicrodactyly.*

**streptobacillary rat-bite fever.**   See **Haverhill fever.**

***Streptobacillus moniliformis*** [Gk, *streptos,* curved; L, *bacillum,* small rod, *monile,* necklace, *forma,* form], a species of necklace-shaped bacteria that can cause rat-bite fever in humans.

**streptococcal** /strep′təkok′əl/ [Gk, *streptos,* curved, *kokkos,* berry], pertaining to any of the species of streptococcus.

**streptococcal angina** [Gk, *streptos* + *kokkos,* berry; L, *angina,* quinsy], a condition in which feelings of choking, suffocation, and pain result from a streptococcal infection.

**streptococcal infection,**   an infection caused by pathogenic bacteria of one of several species of the genus *Streptococcus* or their toxins. Almost any organ of the body may be involved. The infections occur in many forms, including cellulitis, endocarditis, erysipelas, impetigo, meningitis, pneumonia, scarlet fever, tonsillitis, and urinary tract infection. See also **strep throat.**

**streptococcal sore throat.** See **strep throat.**

**streptococcemia** /-koksē′mē-ə/ [Gk, *streptos,* curved, *kokkos,* berry], a condition of the presence of streptococci bacteria in the blood. Also called **streptcemia, streptosepticemia.**

**Streptococcus** /strep′təkok′əs/ [Gk, *streptos + kokkos,* berry], a genus of nonmotile gram-positive cocci classified by serologic types (Lancefield groups A through T), by hemolytic action (α, β, γ) when grown on blood agar, and by reaction to bacterial viruses (phage types 1 to 86). The various species occur in pairs, short chains, and chains. Some are facultative aerobes, and some are anaerobic. Some species also are hemolytic, and others are nonhemolytic. Many species cause disease in humans. *Streptococcus faecalis,* a penicillin-resistant group D enterococcus and normal inhabitant of the GI tract, may cause infection of the urinary tract or endocardium. *S. pneumoniae* (formerly *Diplococcus pneumoniae*) causes a majority of the cases of bacterial pneumonia in the United States. *S. pyogenes* belongs to group A and may cause tonsillitis and respiratory, urinary, or skin infections. Some β-hemolytic strains may lead to rheumatic fever or to glomerulonephritis. *S. viridans,* a member of the normal flora of the mouth, is the most common cause of bacterial endocarditis, especially when introduced into the bloodstream during dental procedures.

**streptococcus β-hemolytic, Group B,** a strain of streptococcus that causes human infections such as neonatal sepsis, endocarditis, and septic arthritis.

**streptococcus β-hemolytic, Group A,** a strain of streptococcus, group A in the Lancefield classification, that causes necrotizing fasciitis toxic shock syndrome.

**Streptococcus pneumoniae** [Gk, *streptos,* curved, *kokkos,* berry, *pneumon,* lung], any of 70 antigenic types of pneumococcal bacteria that cause pneumonia and other diseases in humans.

**Streptococcus pyogenes** [Gk, *streptos,* curved, *kokkos,* berry, *pyon,* pus, *genein,* to produce], a species of streptococcus with many strains that are pathogenic to humans, including the beta-hemolytics in Lancefield group A. It causes suppurative diseases, such as scarlet fever and strep throat.

**Streptococcus viridans** [Gk, *streptos,* curved, *kokkos,* berry], a species of streptococcus similar to *S. pyogenes* strains. It produces alpha-hemolysis in cultures and is a common cause of subacute bacterial endocarditis and other infections in humans.

**streptokinase** /strep′təkī′nās/ [Gk, *streptos + kinesis,* motion, (ase) enzyme], a fibrinolytic activator that enhances the conversion of plasminogen to the fibrinolytic enzyme plasmin. It is produced by strains of streptococci. It is used in the treatment of certain cases of pulmonary and coronary embolism.

**streptokinase-streptodornase** /-strep′tōdôr′nās/, two enzymes derived from a strain of *Streptococcus hemolyticus.*
- INDICATIONS: It is prescribed for débridement of purulent exudates, clotted blood, radiation necrosis, or fibrinous deposits resulting from trauma or infection.
- CONTRAINDICATIONS: Active hemorrhage, acute cellulitis, or danger of reopening bronchopleural fistulas prohibits its use.
- ADVERSE EFFECTS: Among the more serious adverse reactions are pyrogenic reactions and irritation.

**streptolysin** /streptol′isis/ [Gk, *streptos + lysein,* to loosen], a filterable substance, produced by streptococci, that liberates hemoglobin from red blood cells.

**streptomycin sulfate** /strep′təmī′sin/, an aminoglycoside antibiotic.
- INDICATIONS: It is prescribed in the treatment of tuberculosis, endocarditis, and certain other infections.
- CONTRAINDICATIONS: Labyrinthine disease or known hypersensitivity to this drug prohibits its use. It must be used with caution in individuals who have impaired renal function and in the elderly.
- ADVERSE EFFECTS: Among the most serious adverse reactions are ototoxicity, nephrotoxicity, muscle weakness, and allergic reactions.

**streptosepticemia.** See **streptococcemia.**

**streptozocin** /strep′təzō′sin/, an antineoplastic used in the treatment of neoplasms, including metastatic islet cell tumors of the pancreas. It is an antibiotic substance from *Streptomyces acromogenes.*

**stress** [OFr, *estrecier,* to tighten], any emotional, physical, social, economic, or other factor that requires a response or change. Examples include dehydration, which can cause an increase in body temperature, and a separation from parents, which can cause a young child to cry. Stress can be positive or negative. Ongoing chronic stress can result in physical illness. Stress has been theorized as a major contributing factor in many physical diseases, for example, asthma. Stress also may be applied therapeutically to promote change, such as implosive therapy for phobic patients, in which the patient is given support while being exposed to the situation that produces anxiety and is thereby gradually desensitized. The nature and degree of stress observed in a patient are frequently evaluated by the nurse as part of the ongoing holistic nursing assessment. See also **general adaptation syndrome.**

**stress-adaptation theory,** a concept that stress depletes the reserve capacity of individuals, thereby increasing their vulnerability to health problems.

**stress amenorrhea** [OFr, *estrecier,* Gk, *a + men,* month, *rhoia,* to flow], a cessation in menstruation caused by a physical change or mental stress.

**stress-bearing area.** See **basal seat area.**

**stress behavior,** a change from a person's normal behavior in response to a stressor.

**stress fracture,** a fracture, often in one or more of the metatarsal bones, caused by repeated, prolonged, or abnormal stress.

**stress incontinence.** See **incontinence.**

**stress inoculation,** a procedure useful in helping patients control anxiety by substituting positive coping statements for statements that bring about anxiety.

**stress kinesic,** a type of behavioral characteristic of personal conversation, such as the use of body shifts or movements, that marks the flow of speech and generally coincides with linguistic stress patterns.

**stress management,** methods of controlling factors that require a response or change within a person by identifying the stressors, eliminating negative stressors, and developing effective coping mechanisms to counteract the response constructively. Examples include progressive muscular relaxation, guided imagery, biofeedback, breathing techniques, and active problem solving.

**stressor** /stres′ər/ [OFr, *estrecier,* to tighten], anything that causes wear and tear on the body's physical or mental resources. See also **general adaptation syndrome.**

**stress radiography,** the radiographic examination of a body area for soft tissue tears or ruptures. The lesions may appear as abnormal gaps between joint surfaces.

**stress reaction,** an acute maladaptive emotional response to an actual or perceived stressor.

**stress response syndrome.** See **posttraumatic stress disorder.**

**stress test,** a test that measures the function of a system of the body when subjected to carefully controlled amounts of physiologic stress, usually exercise but sometimes specific drugs. The data produced allow the examiner to evaluate the condition of the system being tested. Cardiopulmonary function, respiratory function, and intrauterine fetal placental function are tested with stress tests. Also called **thallium stress test, treadmill stress test.** See also **exercise electrocardiogram, oxytocin challenge test.**

**stress ulcer,** a gastric or duodenal ulcer that develops in previously unaffected individuals subjected to severe stress, such as a severe burn. See also **Curling's ulcer.**

**stretching of contractures** [AS, *streccan* + L, *contractura,* drawing together], any of several procedures for release of muscle and other structures that have been shortened because of paralysis, spasm, disuse, or fibrosis. The procedures include stretching exercises, tissue grafts, scar tissue removal, tendon transfer, and incision of a joint capsule.

**stretch mark.** See **stria.**

**stretch pressure,** a rehabilitation technique in which the thumb, fingertips, or palm of the hand is used to stretch a target muscle, followed by briefly maintained pressure.

**stretch receptors** [AS, *streccan* + L, *recipere,* to receive], specialized sensory nerve endings in muscle spindles or tendons that are stimulated by stretching movements.

**stretch reflex** [AS, *streccan* + L, *reflectere,* to bend back], a reflex muscle contraction after it is stretched as a result of stimulation of proprioceptors in the muscle. Tendon reflexes function in a similar manner. Also called **myotatic reflex.**

**stretch release,** a rehabilitation technique in which the fingertips are placed over the belly of a large muscle and then spread apart in an effort to stretch the skin and underlying muscle. The stretch is done firmly enough to deform the soft tissue temporarily, stimulating cutaneous and muscle efferents and producing facilitation of the underlying muscle.

**stri-,** combining form meaning 'line, stripe, or streak': *striation, striocellular, striomuscular.*

**stria** /strī′ə/, *pl.* **striae** [L, furrow], a streak or a linear scar that often results from rapidly developing tension in the skin, such as seen on the abdomen after pregnancy. Purplish striae are among the classic findings in hyperadrenocorticism. Also called **stretch mark.**

**stria atrophica.** See **linea alba.**

**striae.** See **stria.**

**stria gravidarum,** irregular depressions with red to purple coloration that appear in the skin of the abdomen, thighs, and buttocks of pregnant women.

**striatal** /strī·ā′təl, strī′ətəl/ [L, *striatus,* striped], pertaining to the corpus striatum.

**striatal toe,** hyperextension of the great toe.

**striate** /strī′āt/ [L, *striatus,* striped], identifying something that is striped, is marked by parallel lines, or has structural lines. Also called **striated.**

**striated muscle** /strī′ātid/ [L, *striatus,* striped, *musculus,* muscle], any muscle, including all the skeletal muscles, in which the fibers are divided by bands of cross striations (stripes) as a result of overlapping of thick and thin myofilaments. Contractions in such muscles are voluntary. The heart, a striated involuntary muscle, is an exception. Cardiac muscle is often placed in its own category because it has microanatomic and contraction physiologic characteristics very different from those of most striated muscle. Also called **skeletal muscle, voluntary muscle.** Compare **cardiac muscle, smooth muscle.**

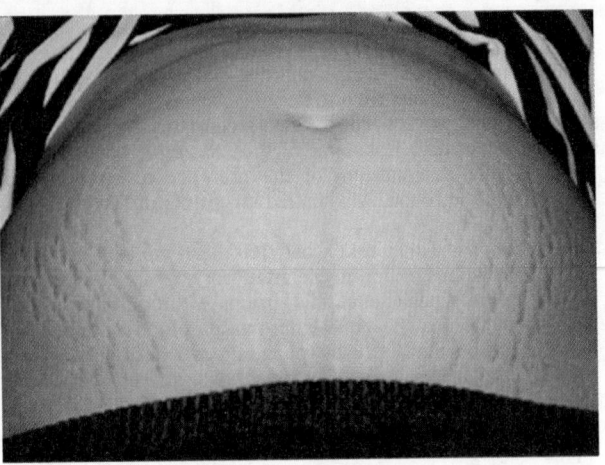

**Striae gravidarum**
(Lowdermilk, Perry, and Bobak, 2000/courtesy
Michael S. Clement, Mesa, Arizona)

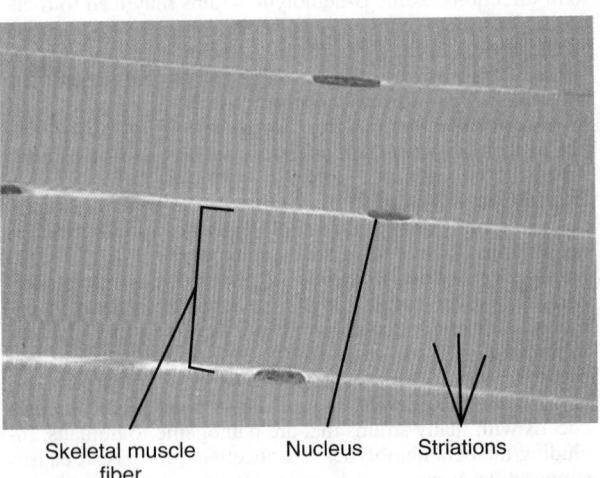

Skeletal muscle  Nucleus  Striations
fiber

**Striated muscle** (© Ed Reschke; used with permission)

**stria terminalis,** a slender, compact fiber bundle that functions as a limbic pathway running from the amygdaloid complex to the hypothalamus and septum.

**stricture** /strik′chər/ [L, *stringere,* to tighten], an abnormal temporary or permanent narrowing of the lumen of a hollow organ, such as the esophagus, pylorus of the stomach, ureter, or urethra. It is caused by inflammation, external pressure, or scarring. Treatment varies depending on the cause. Compare **spasm.**

**strict vegetarian** [L, *stringere* + *vegetare,* to grow, *arius,* believer], a vegetarian whose diet excludes the use of all foods of animal origin. Such diets, unless adequately planned, may be inadequate in many essential nutrients, particularly vitamin $B_{12}$. Also called **pure vegetarian, vegan.**

**stridor** /strī′dôr/ [L, harsh sound], an abnormal, high-pitched, musical sound caused by an obstruction in the trachea or larynx. It is usually heard during inspiration. Stridor may indicate several neoplastic or inflammatory conditions, including glottic edema, asthma, diphtheria, laryngospasm, and papilloma.

**strike** [AS, *strican*, to advance swiftly], an action taken collectively by the employees of a company or institution in which they stop reporting for work in an effort to cause the employer to accede to certain demands. A strike usually follows unsuccessful negotiations between representatives of the union and management.

**string,** a cord, usually made of fiber, configured in a long thin line.

**string carcinoma** [AS, *strenge*, cord; Gk, *karkinos*, cancer, *oma*, tumor], a malignancy of the large intestine, usually the ascending or transverse colon. On radiologic visualization, it causes the intestine to appear to be tied in segments like a string of large beads.

**stringiness** /string′inəs/, an abnormal tissue texture caused by fine or stringlike myofascial structures.

**string sign,** a narrow pyloric canal with congenital pyloric stenosis, or a narrowed bowel segment with regional ileitis. Use of a radiopaque contrast medium causes the narrowed lumen to appear as a thin string on radiographs.

**striocerebellar tremor** /strī′ōser′əbel′ər/, a combination of static, active, and intentional voluntary muscle contractions with both striatal and cerebellar components. It is associated with hereditary ataxia and diffuse degeneration of the central nervous system.

**strip membranes** [Ger, *strippe*, strap; L, *membrana*, thin skin], (in obstetrics) a procedure in which an examiner, with the fingers, frees the membranes of the amniotic sac from the wall of the lower segment of the uterus in the small area around the cervical os. It is done to stimulate labor, but, because infection or hemorrhage may result, it is not recommended.

**stripping,** 1. *nontechnical.* a surgical procedure for the removal of the long and short saphenous veins of the legs. See also **milking, varicose vein. 2.** the mechanical removal of a very small amount of enamel from the mesial or distal surfaces of teeth to alleviate crowding.

**stroke.** See **cerebrovascular accident.**

**stroke prone profile** [AS, *strac*], a predictive index using a complex of risk factors that indicate susceptibility of a person to cerebrovascular accident (CVA). The factors include advanced age, hypertension, a history of transient ischemic attacks, cigarette smoking, heart disorders, associated embolism, family history of CVA, use of oral contraceptives, diabetes mellitus, physical inactivity, obesity, hypercholesteremia, and hyperlipidemia.

**stroke volume,** the amount of blood ejected by a ventricle during contraction.

**stroke volume index,** stroke volume divided by the body surface area.

**stroking** /strō′king/, running the entire hand over large parts of the body to relax the muscles reflexively and eliminate muscle spasm, improve circulation, or produce a parasympathetic response. See also **effleurage.**

**stroma** /strō′mə/, *pl.* **stromas, stromata** [Gk, covering], the supporting tissue or the matrix of an organ, as distinguished from its parenchyma. Some kinds of stromata are the vitreous stroma, which encloses the vitreous humor of the eye, and Rollet's stroma, which contains the hemoglobin of a red blood cell. —**stromatic,** *adj.*

**stroma-,** prefix meaning 'connective tissue forming framelike support for an organ': *stromatin, stromatogenous, stromatosis.*

**-stroma,** suffix meaning 'supporting tissue of an organ': *blastostroma, mesostroma, myostroma.*

**stromata, stromatic.** See **stroma.**

---

*Strongyloides* /stron′jiloi′dēz/ [Gk, *strongylos*, round, *eidos*, form], a genus of parasitic intestinal nematode. A species of *Strongyloides, S. stercoralis,* causes strongyloidiasis.

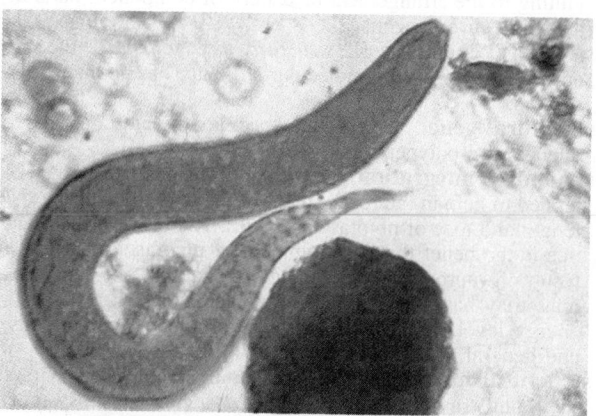

***Strongyloides stercoralis* larvae** *(Murray et al, 1998)*

**strongyloidiasis** /stron′jəloidī′əsis/, infection of the small intestine by the roundworm *Strongyloides stercoralis.* It is acquired when larvae from the soil penetrate intact skin, incidentally causing a pruritic rash. The larvae pass to the lungs via the bloodstream, sometimes causing pneumonia. They then migrate up the air passages to the pharynx, are swallowed, and develop into adult worms in the small intestine. Bloody diarrhea and intestinal malabsorption may result. Rarely, fatal disseminated strongyloidiasis occurs. Diagnosis depends on finding larvae in freshly passed feces. Treatment often includes administration of thiabendazole, ivermectin, and albendazole. Proper sanitary methods for the disposal of excrement can eliminate the disease. Wearing shoes prevents contagion from contaminated soil. Also called **threadworm infection.** See also **Löffler's syndrome.**

**strontium (Sr)** /stron′sh(ē)əm/ [Strontian, Scotland], a metallic element. Its atomic number is 38; its atomic mass is 87.62. Chemically similar to calcium, it is found in bone tissue. Isotopes of strontium are used in radioisotope scanning procedures of bone. Strontium 85 ($^{85}$Sr) and strontium 87 ($^{87}$Sr) mimic calcium metabolism and are used in studies of bone physiologic characteristics and disorders. These radionuclides can be counted with any standard detector or imaged at a very early stage in bone disease, whereas radiographic films of bone without the use of a radioactive tracer can show decreased density only after approximately 50% of bone is decalcified. Most $^{85}$Sr or $^{87}$Sr is deposited in bone within 1 hour after injection; increased deposition of these radionuclides is strongly linked to osteoblastic activity and new bone formation. In addition to 4 naturally occurring isotopes ($^{88}$Sr, $^{87}$Sr, $^{86}$Sr, and $^{84}$Sr), 12 artificial strontium isotopes are produced by nuclear reactions. Strontium 90, the longest-lived, is the most dangerous constituent of fallout from atomic bomb tests. It can replace some of the calcium in food, become concentrated in teeth and bones, and continue to emit electrons that can cause death in the host. Strontium 90 becomes concentrated in cow's milk.

**-strophe, -strophy,** suffix meaning 'turning or twisting': *cardianastrophe, enstrophe, phallanastrophe.*

**stropho-,** combining form meaning 'twisted': *strophocephalus, strophosomus.*

**strophulus.** See **papular urticaria.**

**-strophy.** See **-strophe.**

**structural** /struk'chərəl/ [L, *structura,* arrangement], pertaining to the arrangement or pattern of component parts of an object or organism.

**structural chemistry** [L, *structura,* arrangement], the science dealing with the molecular structure of chemical substances.

**structural gene,** a gene that specifies the amino acid sequence of a polypeptide.

**structural integration,** a technique of deep massage intended to help in the realignment of the body by altering the length and tone of myofascial tissues. The basis of the practice is the belief that misalignment of myofascial tissues, a result of improper posture and emotional and physical traumas, may have an overall detrimental effect on a person's energy level, self-image, muscular efficiency, perceptions, and general health. Also called **Rolfing.**

**structural model,** a model of family therapy that views the family as an open system and identifies subsystems within the family that carry out specific family functions. When faced with demands for change, individual family members, family subsystems, or the family as a whole may respond with growth behaviors or with maladaptive behaviors. The goal of family therapy is to help family members learn new scripts or transactional patterns.

**structure** /struk'chər/ [L, *structura*], a part of the body, such as the heart, a bone, a gland, a cell, or a limb.

**structure-activity relationship (SAR),** the relationship between the chemical structure of a drug and its activity.

**structured learning therapy** /struk'chərt/, a rehabilitation technique used with schizophrenic patients.

**strum-,** combining form meaning 'a goiter or scrofula': *strumectomy, strumiform, strumitis.*

**struma lymphomatosa.** See **Hashimoto's disease.**

**Strümpell-Marie disease** /strim'pəlmärē'/ [Ernst A. von Strümpell, German neurologist, 1853–1925; Pierre Marie, French neurologist, 1853–1940; L, *dis* Fr, *aise,* ease], ankylosing spondylitis. Also called **rheumatoid spondylitis, Marie-Strümpell arthritis, spondylitis ankylopoietica.**

**strychnine** /strik'nin, strik'nīn/ [Gr, *strychnos,* nightshade], a white crystalline alkaloid obtained from the leaves of the *Strychnos nux-vomica* plant. It is extremely toxic to the central nervous system, producing as a classic strychnine poisoning symptom an arched back (opisthotonus).

**strychnine poisoning** [Gk, *strychnos* + L, *potio,* a drink], toxic effects of ingesting strychnine, a central nervous system stimulant. Symptoms include restlessness and hyperacuity of hearing and vision. Minor stimuli may produce convulsions, but there may be complete muscle relaxation between convulsions. One classic sign of strychnine poisoning is an arched back(opisthotonus).

**Stryker wedge frame,** trademark for an orthopedic bed that allows the patient to be rotated as required to either the full supine or the full prone position. It is used in the immobilization of patients with unstable spines, postoperative management of multilevel spinal fusions, and management of severe burn patients. Compare **CircOlectric (COL) bed, Foster bed, hyperextension bed.**

**S-T segment,** an isoelectric line after the QRS complex on the electrocardiogram. It represents phase 2 of the cardiac action potential. Elevation or depression of the S-T segment is the hallmark of myocardial ischemia or injury and coronary artery disease.

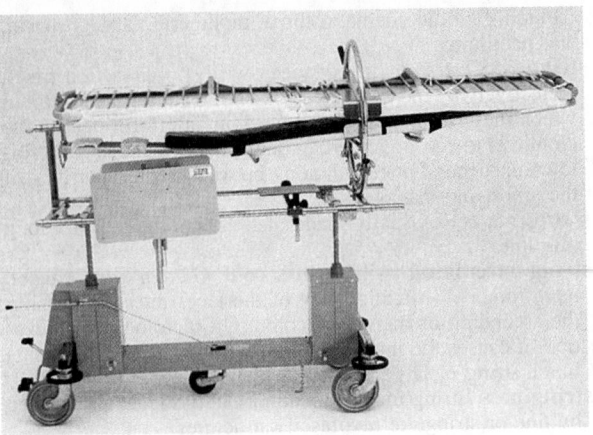

**Stryker wedge frame**
*(Sorrentino, 1992/courtesy The Stryker Corporation, Kalamazoo, Michigan)*

**Stuartnatal Plus,** trademark for a fixed-combination oral prenatal drug containing vitamins and minerals.

**Stuart-Power factor.** See **factor X.**

**stump** [ME, *stumpe*], the part of a limb that remains after amputation.

**stump hallucination,** the sensation of the continued presence of an amputated limb. See also **hallucination, phantom limb syndrome.**

**stunned myocardium,** a condition of impaired myocardial contractile function, cellular biochemical characteristics, and microvasculature function in the absence of gross myocardial necrosis. It can last for minutes to days and is caused by ischemia that is either brief or occurs in the area immediately outside an infarct zone.

**stupefacient** /st(y)oo'pəfā'shənt/ [L, *stupere,* to stun, *facere,* to make], an opioid or other agent that has the effect of making a person stuporous.

**stupor** /st(y)oo'pər/ [L, *stupere,* to stun], a state of unresponsiveness in which a person seems unaware of the surroundings. The condition occurs in neurologic and psychiatric disorders. The person may be totally or almost totally immobile and unresponsive, even to painful stimuli. Kinds of stupor are **anergic stupor, benign stupor, delusion stupor,** and **epileptic stupor.**

**stuporous** /st(y)oo'pərəs/ [L, *stupere,* to stun], in a state of reduced consciousness and diminished spontaneous movement.

**Sturge-Weber syndrome** /sturj'web'ər/ [William A. Sturge, English physician, 1850–1919; Frederick P. Weber, English physician, 1863–1962], a congenital neurocutaneous disease marked by a port-wine-colored capillary hemangioma over a sensory dermatome of a branch of the trigeminal nerve of the face. Radiographic examination of the skull reveals intracranial calcification. The cerebral cortex may atrophy, and generalized or focal seizures, angioma of the choroid, secondary glaucoma, optic atrophy, and new cutaneous hemangiomas may develop. There is no known cure. Treatment is supportive and includes anticonvulsive medication. Also called **encephalotrigeminal angiomatosis.**

**stuttering** [D, *stotteren*], a speech dysfunction usually characterized by excessive abnormal hesitations, blocks, part-word and whole-word repetitions, and audible or silent prolongation of sounds. The cause of stuttering is unknown;

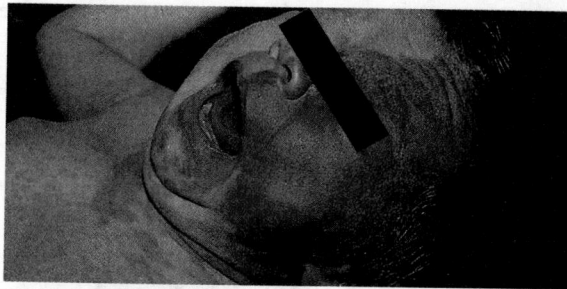

**Sturge-Weber syndrome** *(Zitelli and Davis, 1997)*

it may be hereditary or may result from developmental processes or neurologic impairment. Hesitancy and lack of fluency in speech are typical characteristics of normal speech and language development during the preschool years, when a child's physical, psychologic, and speech/ language development do not match the linguistic demands of talking. The child may become conscious of speaking difficulties associated with acquisition and a fear of speaking may develop. Early prevention and evaluation are recommended. The health care professional may educate parents by making them aware of the normal dysfluent patterns in a child's speech and by suggesting ways to encourage a child's speech development. If stuttering persists, parents should be encouraged to seek the advice of a speech-language pathologist. See also **stammering.**

**sty** [ME, *styanye,* eyelid tumor], a purulent infection of a meibomian or sebaceous gland of the eyelid, often caused by a staphylococcal organism. Also spelled **stye.** Also called **hordeolum.**

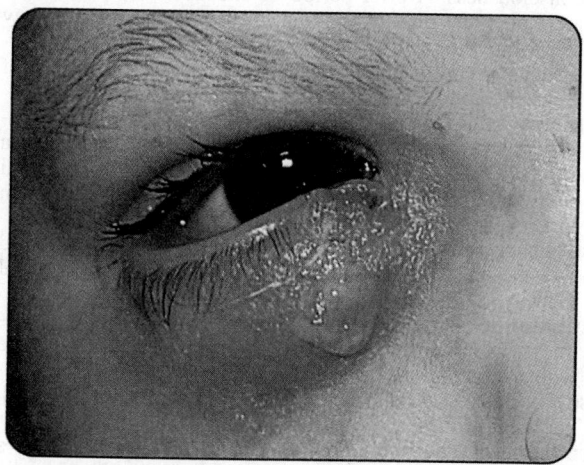

**Sty** *(Kanski and Nischal, 1999)*

**-style,** combining form meaning a 'bone attached to an internal structure': *cephalostyle, sarcostyle, zygostyle.*

**stylet** /stī'lət, stīlet'/ [It, *stiletto,* dagger], a thin metal probe for inserting into or passing through a needle, tube, or catheter to clean the hollow bore or for inserting into a soft, flexible catheter to make it stiff as the catheter is placed in a

vein or passed through an orifice of the body. Also spelled **stilet, stilette.**

**stylo-,** combining form meaning 'like a pillar, stake, or pole': *stylomastoid, stylomyloid, stylostixis, styloid.*

**stylohyoideus** /stī'lōhī·oi'dē·əs/ [Gk, *stylos,* pillar, *hyoeides,* U-shaped], one of four suprahyoid muscles, lying anterior and superior to the posterior belly of the digastricus. It is a slender muscle that arises from the styloid process and inserts into the hyoid bone. It serves to draw the hyoid bone up and back. Also called **stylohyoid bone.** Compare **digastricus, geniohyoideus, mylohyoideus.**

**stylohyoid ligament** /stī'lōhī'oid/, the ligament attached to the tip of the styloid process of the temporal bone and to the lesser cornu of the hyoid bone. It frequently contains a small cartilage in its center and is often partially ossified.

**styloid** /stī'loid/ [Gk, *stylos,* pillar, *eidos,* form], long and tapered, like a pen or stylus.

**styloid process** [Gk, *stylos* + *eidos* + L, *processus*], any of several projections of bone tissue, particularly a projection on the temporal bone.

**stylomandibular ligament** /stī'lōmandib'yələr/ [Gk, *stylos* + L, *mandere,* to chew, *ligare,* to bind], one of a pair of specialized bands of cervical fascia, forming an accessory part of the temporomandibular joint. It extends from the styloid process of the temporal bone to the ramus of the mandible between the masseter and pterygoideus muscles and separates the parotid gland from the submandibular gland. Compare **sphenomandibular ligament.**

**stylus** /stī'ləs/, 1. a fine probe. 2. a wire inserted into a catheter to stiffen it. 3. a device that imprints electrical activity and wave patterns on electrocardiographic, electroencephalographic, or similar graphic recordings.

**styptic** /stip'tik/ [Gk, *styptikos,* astringent], 1. a substance used as an astringent, often to control bleeding. A chemical styptic induces coagulation of blood. A cotton pledget used as a compress to control bleeding is a mechanical styptic. 2. acting as an astringent or agent to control bleeding.

**subacromial** /sub'əkrō'mē·əl/ [L, *sub,* beneath; Gk, *akron,* extremity, *omos.* shoulder], pertaining to the area below the acromion process.

**subacromial bursa** [L, *sub,* under; Gk, *akron,* extremity, *omos,* shoulder, *byrsa,* wineskin], the bursa separating the acromion process and deltoid muscle from the insertion of the supraspinatus muscle and the greater tubercle of the humerus.

**subacute** /-əkyōōt'/ [L, *sub* + *acutus,* sharp], 1. less than acute. 2. pertaining to a disease or other abnormal condition present in a person who appears to be clinically well. The condition may be identified or discovered by means of a laboratory test or radiologic examination.

**subacute bacterial endocarditis (SBE),** a chronic bacterial infection of the valves of the heart. It is characterized by a slow, quiet onset with fever, heart murmur, splenomegaly, and development of clumps of abnormal tissue, called vegetations, around an intracardiac prosthesis or on the cusps of a valve. Various species of *Streptococcus* or *Staphylococcus* are commonly the cause of SBE. Dental procedures are associated with infection by *Streptococcus viridans,* surgical procedures with *Streptococcus faecalis,* and self-infection (especially by drug abusers) with *Staphylococcus aureus.* See also **bacterial endocarditis, endocarditis, Janeway lesion.**

■ OBSERVATIONS: The infected vegetations may separate from the valve or prosthesis and form emboli. Osler's nodes, petechiae, Roth's spots, and splinter hemorrhages under the fingernails are common manifestations of blood-borne metastases of these emboli. Bacteriologic examination of cultures of the blood may allow specific diagnosis and treatment.

■ INTERVENTIONS: Treatment requires prolonged and regular administration of an antibiotic that is known to be effective against the causative organism. If a prosthesis has become infected, it is usually removed. Before surgery or a dental procedure prophylactic antibiotics are given. During the acute phase of illness the fever is treated with antipyretic medication and bed rest; adequate high-protein diet and fluids are encouraged.

■ NURSING CONSIDERATIONS: Bed rest and hospitalization may be necessary for several weeks. Emotional and psychologic support may help the patient adjust to the necessary inactivity and to understand that SBE is a chronic illness.

**subacute care,** **1.** a level of treatment that is between chronic and acute. **2.** treatment of a disease that is of moderate severity or duration.

**subacute combined degeneration of the spinal cord.** See **combined system disease.**

**subacute glomerulonephritis,** an uncommon noninfectious disease of the glomerulus of the kidney characterized by proteinuria, hematuria, decreased production of urine, and edema. Of unknown cause, the disease may progress rapidly, and renal failure may occur. Kidney transplantation and dialysis are the only treatments available. See also **chronic glomerulonephritis, postinfectious glomerulonephritis, uremia.**

**subacute infection** [L, *sub*, beneath, *acutus*, sharp, *inficere*, to stain], a disease condition that is not chronic and that runs a rapid and severe, but less than acute, course.

**subacute inflammation,** a reactive sign of inflammation with a gradual onset, later increasing to a chronic or severe type of reaction.

**subacute myelooptic neuropathy (SMON),** a condition of muscular pain and weakness, usually below the T12 vertebra; painful dysesthesia of the limbs; and, in some cases, optic atrophy. The patient usually experiences a significant alteration of gait.

**subacute necrotizing encephalomyelopathy, subacute necrotizing encephalopathy.** See **Leigh disease.**

**subacute necrotizing lymphadenitis.** See **Kikuchi's lymphadenitis.**

**subacute sclerosing panencephalitis,** a rare disorder occuring with primary measles infection in children 2 years of age or younger. It has a period of latency for 6 to 8 years. It is characterized by diffuse inflammation of brain tissue, personality change, seizures, ataxia myoclonus, visual disturbances, dementia, fever, and death. The condition occurs in children and in adolescents who have had measles at a very early age. Live measles virus can be cultured from brain tissue. No effective therapy is known. See also **slow virus.**

**subacute thyroiditis.** See **de Quervain's thyroiditis.**

**subaortic** /-ā-ôr′tik/ [L, *sub* + Gk, *aerein*, to raise], pertaining to the area of the body below the aorta.

**subaortic stenosis** [L, *sub*, beneath; Gk, *aerein*, to raise, *stenos*, narrow, *osis* condition], a narrowing of the left ventricle outflow tract below the aortic valve. Also called **aortic valvular stenosis.**

**subapical** /-ap′ikəl/, below the peak or apex.

**subaponeurotic** /-ap′ŏnŏŏrot′ik/ [L, *sub*, beneath; Gk, *apo*, from, *neuron*, nerve; L, *tendo*], beneath an aponeurosis.

**subarachnoid** /sub′ərak′noid/ [L, *sub* + Gk, *arachne*, spider, *eidos*, form], pertaining to the area under the arachnoid membrane and above the pia mater.

**subarachnoid block anesthesia.** See **spinal anesthesia.**

**subarachnoid hemorrhage (SaH, SAH),** an intracranial hemorrhage into the cerebrospinal fluid-filled space between the arachnoid and pial membranes on the surface of the brain. The hemorrhage may extend into the brain if the force of the bleeding from the broken vessel is sudden and severe. The cause may be trauma, rupture of an aneurysm, or an arteriovenous anomaly.

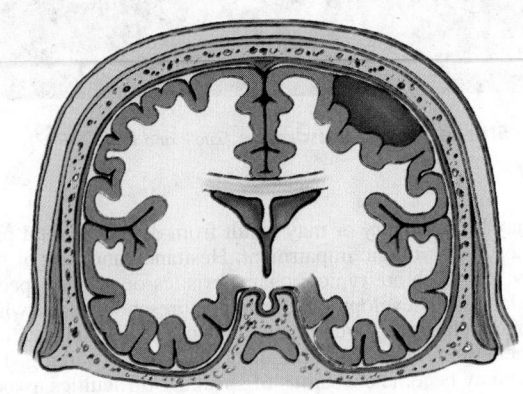

**Subarachnoid hemorrhage** *(Monahan and Neighbors, 1998)*

■ OBSERVATIONS: The first symptom of a subarachnoid hemorrhage is a sudden extremely severe headache that begins in one localized area and then spreads, becoming dull and throbbing. The localized pain results from vascular distortion and injury. The generalized ache is the result of meningeal irritation by blood in the subarachnoid space. Other characteristics of subarachnoid hemorrhage can include dizziness, rigidity of the neck, pupillary inequality, vomiting, seizures, drowsiness, sweating and chills, stupor, and loss of consciousness. A brief period of unconsciousness immediately after the rupture is common; severe hemorrhage may result in continued unconsciousness, coma, and death. Delirium and confusion often persist through the first weeks of recovery, and permanent brain damage is common.

**subarachnoid hemorrhage precautions,** a nursing intervention from the Nursing Interventions Classification (NIC) defined as reduction of internal and external stimuli or stressors to minimize risk of rebleeding prior to aneurysm surgery. See also **Nursing Interventions Classification.**

**subarachnoid space,** the space between the arachnoid and pia mater membranes and containing cerebrospinal fluid.

**subatomic** /-ətom′ik/ [L, *sub*, beneath; Gk, *atomos*, indivisible], pertaining to the particles and phenomena that are within an atom.

**subaxillary** /-ak′siler′ē/ [L, *sub*, beneath, *axilla*, wing], pertaining to the area beneath the axilla.

**subcapital fracture** /-kap′itəl/ [L, *sub* + *caput*, head], a fracture located just below the head of a bone that pivots in a ball-and-socket joint, such as the femur.

**subcapsular** /-kap′s(y)ələr/ [L, *sub*, beneath, *capsula*, little box], pertaining to the area below a capsule.

**subcapsular cataract** [L, *sub* + *capsula*, little box], a condition marked by opacity or cloudiness beneath the anterior or posterior capsule of the lens of the eye.

**subclavian** /səbklā′vē-ən/ [L, *sub* + *clavicula*, little key], situated under the clavicle, such as the subclavian vein.

**subclavian artery,** one of a pair of arteries passing under the clavicle that vary in origin, course, and the height to which they rise in the neck but have six similar main branches supplying the vertebral column, spinal cord, ear, and brain. See also **left subclavian artery, right subclavian artery.**

**subclavian steal syndrome,** a vascular syndrome caused by an occlusion in the subclavian artery proximal to the origin of the vertebral artery. It results in a reversal of the normal blood pressure gradient in the vertebral artery and decreased blood flow distal to the occlusion. It is characterized by episodes of flaccid paralysis of the arm, pain in the mastoid and occipital areas, and a diminished or absent radial pulse on the involved side. Markedly different blood pressure measurements obtained from each arm are sometimes indicative of the condition.

**subclavian vein,** the continuation of the axillary vein in the upper body, extending from the lateral border of the first rib to the sternal end of the clavicle, where it joins the internal jugular to form the brachiocephalic vein. It usually contains a pair of valves near its junction with the internal jugular vein. The subclavian vein receives deoxygenated blood from the external jugular vein and, on the left side, at the junction with the internal jugular vein, receives lymph from the thoracic duct. On the right side, at the corresponding junction, it receives lymph from the right lymphatic duct.

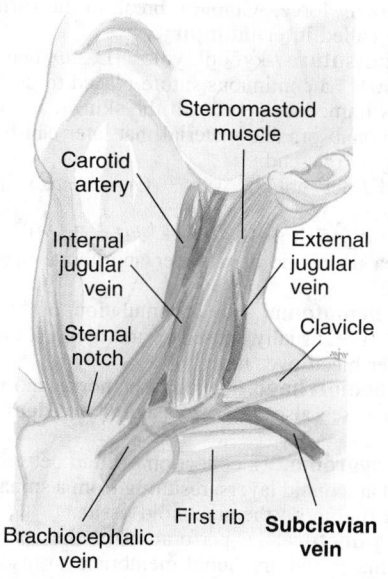

Carotid artery

Sternomastoid muscle

Internal jugular vein

External jugular vein

Sternal notch

Clavicle

Brachiocephalic vein

First rib

**Subclavian vein**

**Subclavian vein** *(Sanders et al, 2000)*

**subclavius** /səbklā′vē·əs/ [L, *sub* + *clavicula*], a short muscle of the chest wall. It is a small cylindric muscle between the clavicle and the first rib and arises in a short thick tendon from the junction of the first rib and its cartilage under the clavicle. It inserts into the groove on the inferior surface of the clavicle between the costoclavicular and conoid ligaments. The subclavius is innervated by a special nerve from the lateral trunk of the brachial plexus, which contains fibers from the fifth and sixth cervical nerves. It acts to draw the shoulder down and forward. Compare **pectoralis major, pectoralis minor, serratus anterior.**

**subclinical** /-klin′ikəl/ [L, *sub* + Gk, *kline*, bed], pertain-

ing to a disease or abnormal condition that is so mild it produces no symptoms.

**subclinical diabetes.** See **impaired glucose tolerance.**

**subcollateral gyrus** /-kəlat′ərəl/ [L, *sub* + *con* + *lateralis* + Gk, *gyros*, turn], a convolution below the collateral fissure or sulcus of the cerebrum.

**subconscious** /-kon′shəs/ [L, *sub* + *conscire*, to be aware], imperfectly or partially conscious. —**subconsciousness,** *n.*

**subconscious memory,** a thought, sensation, or feeling that is not immediately available for recall to the conscious mind.

**subconsciousness.** See **subconscious.**

**subcrestal periodontal pocket.** See **periodontal pocket.**

**subculture** /sub′kulchər/ [L, *sub* + *colere*, to cultivate], an ethnic, regional, economic, or social group with characteristic patterns of behavior and ideals that distinguish it from the rest of a culture or society.

**subcutaneous** /sub′kyoŏotā′nē·əs/ [L, *sub* + *cutis*, skin], beneath the skin.

**subcutaneous adipose tissue** [L, *sub,* beneath, *cutis,* skin, *adeps,* fat; OFr, *tissu*], fat deposits beneath the skin.

**subcutaneous emphysema,** the presence of air or gas in the subcutaneous tissues. The air or gas may originate in the rupture of an airway or alveolus and migrate through the subpleural spaces to the mediastinum and neck. The face, neck, and chest may appear swollen. Skin tissues can be painful and may produce a crackling or popping sound as air moves under them. The patient may experience dyspnea and appear cyanotic if the air leak is severe. Treatment may require an incision to release the trapped air. Also called **aerodermectasia.**

**subcutaneous fascia,** a continuous layer of connective tissue over the entire body between the skin and the deep fascial investment of the specialized structures of the body, such as the muscles. It comprises an outer normally fatty layer and an inner thin elastic layer. Between the two layers lie superficial blood vessels, nerves, lymphatics, the mammary glands, most of the facial muscles, and the platysma. Also called **subcutaneous layer.** Compare **deep fascia, subserous fascia.**

**subcutaneous fat necrosis.** See **adiponecrosis subcutanea neonatorum.**

**subcutaneous infusion.** See **hypodermoclysis.**

**subcutaneous injection,** the introduction of a hypodermic needle into the subcutaneous tissue beneath the skin, usually on the upper arm, thigh, or abdomen. A 24- or 27-gauge needle 2 cm long is used. The drug is prepared and drawn into the syringe. The cleansed area of skin is held by the thumb and forefinger to tense and steady the injection site. The needle is inserted at an angle of 45 to 90 degrees, piercing the skin quickly and advancing steadily to minimize the pain. The barrel or plunger is withdrawn slightly to ascertain whether the syringe of the needle has inadvertently entered a blood vessel. If no blood is aspirated, the drug is injected slowly, the needle is withdrawn, and the skin is massaged gently (unless contraindicated) with a sterile alcohol sponge. Certain drugs that are extremely irritating to the skin are injected into the deep subcutaneous tissues by using a variation of the technique. The skin tissue overlying the injection site is grasped with the thumb and forefinger but elevated in a roll, rather than tensed and flattened. The angle of injection may be as great as 90 degrees to the skin. Heparin, insulin, and emetine are injected in this way. If subcutaneous injections are repeated, each is performed at least 5 cm from the previous site. A diagram of a plan for the rotation of injection sites helps to prevent overuse of one area of skin.

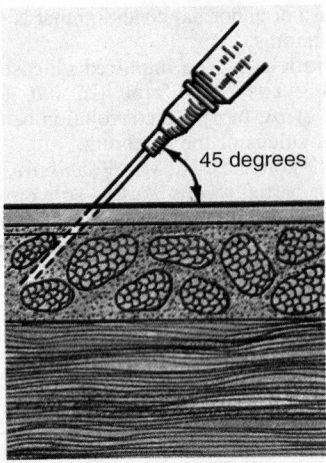

45 degrees

**Subcutaneous injection: insertion of the needle**
*(Potter and Perry, 2001)*

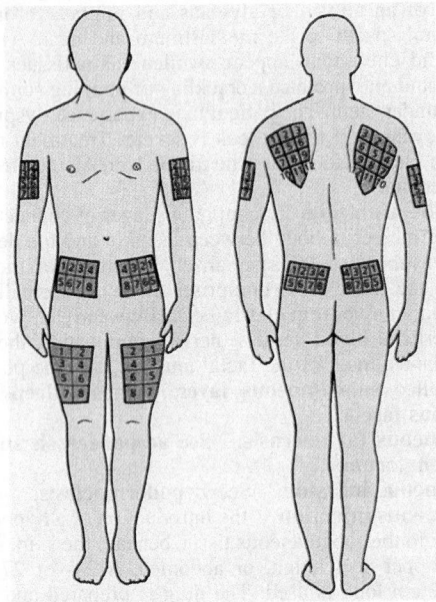

**Subcutaneous injections: rotation of sites**
*(Potter and Perry, 2001)*

**subcutaneous layer.** See **subcutaneous fascia.**

**subcutaneous mastectomy,** a surgical procedure in which all the breast tissue of one or both breasts is removed, leaving the skin, areola, and nipple intact. The adjacent lymph nodes, pectoralis major, and pectoralis minor are not removed. It may be performed on women who are at great risk of development of breast cancer. Reconstruction of the breasts is performed, with the assistance of a plastic surgeon, through the insertion of prostheses to return the normal contour to the breasts. Also called **adenomammectomy.**

**subcutaneous nodule,** a small, solid mass, or node, beneath the skin that can be detected by touch. Subcutaneous

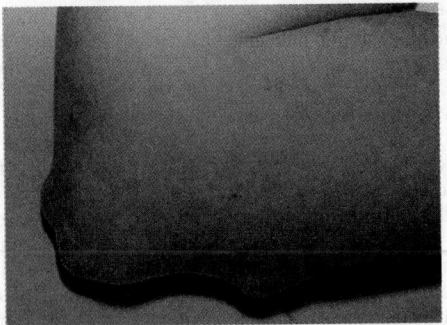

**Subcutaneous nodules** *(Zitelli and Davis, 1997)*

nodules consisting chiefly of Aschoff bodies are found in patients with rheumatic fever. Minute subcutaneous nodules formed by the perivascular infiltration of mononuclear cells occur in typhus.

**subcutaneous test.** See **intradermal test.**

**subcutaneous tunnel,** a tunnel under the skin between the exit site of an atrial catheter and the entrance into the vein.

**subcutaneous wound** [L, *sub,* beneath, *cutis,* skin; AS, *wund*], an injury to internal organs, such as by crushing or another violent force, without a break in the surface of the skin. Also called **internal injury.**

**subcuticular suture** /-kyo͞otik′yələr/ [L, *sub,* beneath, *cutis,* skin, *sutura*], a continuous suture placed to draw together the tissues immediately beneath the skin. It is frequently a suture of nonabsorbable material that later can be removed by pulling on one end.

**subdermal** /-der′məl/ [L, *sub* + Gr, *derma,* skin] beneath the dermis.

**subdural** /-d(y)o͞o′rəl/ [L, *sub* + *durus,* hard], pertaining to the area under the dura mater and above the arachnoid membrane.

**subdural hematoma,** an accumulation of blood in the subdural space, usually caused by an injury. It can be acute or a slower bleed over time.

**subdural hemorrhage,** cerebral hemorrhage into the subdural space; see also **cerebrovascular accident, subdural hematoma.**

**subdural hygroma,** a collection of fluid between the dura mater and arachnoid layers, resulting from a spinal fluid leak through a rupture in the arachnoid tissue.

**subdural puncture,** a perforation of the space between the dura mater and arachnoid membrane to insert a needle for the injection of diagnostic or therapeutic medications or for aspiration of blood or other fluid.

**subdural space** [L, *sub,* beneath, *dura, mater,* hard mother, *spatium*], the potential space between the dura mater and the arachnoid membrane.

**subendocardial infarction** /-en′dōkär′dē·əl/, a myocardial infarction that involves the innermost layer and in some cases parts of the middle layer of the myocardium but does not extend to the epicardium.

**subepidermal** /-ep′idur′məl/ [L, *sub,* beneath; Gk, *epi,* above, *derma,* skin], beneath the epidermis.

**subgerminal cavity.** See **blastocoele.**

**subgingival calculus.** See **calculus.**

**subgingival curettage,** the debridement of an ulcerated epithelial attachment and subjacent gingival corium to eliminate inflammation and to shrink and restore gingival tissue.

**subglottic** /-glot'ik/, beneath the glottis. Also **infraglottic**.

**subiculum** /səbik'yələm/, a part of the hippocampal formation consisting of the transition zone between the parahippocampal gyrus and Ammon's horn.

**subintimal** /-in'timəl/ [L, *sub* + *intimus,* innermost], pertaining to the area beneath the intima or membrane lining a blood vessel, usually a large artery.

**subinvolution.** See **uterine subinvolution.**

**subjective** /-jek'tiv/ [L, *subjectus,* subject], **1.** pertaining to the essential nature of an object as perceived in the mind rather than to a thing in itself. **2.** existing only in the mind. **3.** that which arises within or is perceived by the individual, as contrasted with something that is modified by external circumstances or something that may be evaluated by objective standards. **4.** pertaining to a person who places excessive importance on his own moods, attitudes, or opinions; egocentric.

**subjective data collection,** the process in which data relating to the his or her problem are elicited from a patient. The data are retrieved from the patient's description of an event rather than from a physical examination, which provides objective data. The interviewer encourages a full description of the onset, the course, and the character of the problem and any factors that aggravate or ameliorate it. Compare **objective data collection.**

**subjective sensation,** a feeling or impression that is not associated with or does not directly result from any external stimulus. See also **sensation,** def. 1.

**subjective symptoms** [L, *subjectus,* subject; Gk, *symptoma*], symptoms that are observed only by the patient and cannot be objectively confirmed.

**subjective vertigo,** an inappropriate sensation of bodily movement.

**subjects** /sub'jekts/, people, animals, or events selected for a study to examine a particular variable or condition, such as the effects of a new medication or therapy.

**sublethal allele** [L, *sub* + *letum,* death; Gk, *genein,* to produce], an allele whose presence causes abnormalities or impairs the functioning of an organism but does not cause its death. Compare **lethal allele.**

**sublethal dose** /-lē'thəl/ [L, *sub,* beneath, *letum,* death; Gk, *dosis,* giving], a dose of a potentially lethal substance that is not large enough to cause death.

**subleukemic leukemia.** See **aleukemic leukemia.**

**sublimate** /sub'limāt/ [L, *sublimare,* to lift up], to refine or divert instinctual impulses and energy from their immediate goal to one that can be expressed in a social, moral, or aesthetic manner acceptable to the person and the society.

**sublimation** /-limā'shən/ [L, *sublimare*], **1.** an unconscious defense mechanism by which an unacceptable instinctive drive is diverted to and expressed through a personally approved, socially accepted means. **2.** (in psychoanalysis) the process of diverting certain components of the sex drive to a socially acceptable, nonsexual goal. Compare **displacement. 3.** change in a physical state from the solid phase directly to the gas phase.

**Sublimaze,** trademark for an opioid analgesic (fentanyl).

**subliminal** /-lim'inəl/ [L, *sub* + *limen,* threshold], taking place below the threshold of sensory perception or outside the range of conscious awareness.

**subliminal self** [L, *sub,* beneath, *limen,* threshold; AS, *self*], a level of mental activity at which an individual under normal waking conditions may function without consciousness. See also **preconscious, unconscious.**

**sublingual** /səbling'gwəl/ [L, *sub* + *lingua,* tongue], pertaining to the area beneath the tongue.

**sublingual administration of a medication,** the administration of a drug, usually in tablet form, by placing it beneath the tongue until the tablet dissolves.

**sublingual caruncle** [L, *sub,* beneath, *lingua,* tongue, *caruncula,* small piece of flesh], a small fleshy growth under the tongue.

**sublingual duct.** See **Bartholin's duct, duct of Rivinus.**

**sublingual gland,** one of a pair of small salivary glands situated under the mucous membrane of the floor of the mouth, beneath the tongue. It is a narrow, almond-shaped structure and has from 8 to 20 ducts, some of which join to form the sublingual duct. The sublingual gland secretes mucus produced by its alveoli. Compare **parotid gland, submandibular gland.**

**subluxation.** See **incomplete dislocation.**

**subluxation complex** /-luksā'shən/, a theoretic chiropractic model of motion-segment dysfunction that incorporates the complex interaction of pathologic changes in nervous, muscular, ligamentous, vascular, and connective tissues.

**subluxation syndrome,** an aggregate of signs and symptoms in chiropractic that relate to pathophysiologic characteristics or dysfunction of spinal and pelvic motion segments or to peripheral joints.

**submandibular** /-məndib'yələr/ [L, *sub* + *mandible*], pertaining to the area beneath the mandible, or lower jaw. Also called **inframandibular.**

**submandibular duct** [L, *sub* + *mandere,* to chew], a duct through which a submandibular gland secretes saliva. Also called **submaxillary duct of Wharton, Wharton's duct.**

**submandibular gland,** one of a pair of round walnut-sized salivary glands in the submandibular triangle that open on a small papilla at the side of the frenulum linguae. The gland secretes both mucus and a thinner serous fluid, which aid the digestive process. Compare **sublingual gland, parotid gland.** See also **salivary gland.**

**submarginal** /sub·mär'ji·nəl/ [L, *sub,* beneath + *margo,* margin], situated inferior to or beneath a margin.

**submaxillary** /-mak'siler'ē/ [L, *sub* + *maxilla*], pertaining to the area below the maxilla, or upper jaw.

**submaxillary duct of Wharton.** See **submandibular duct.**

**submeatal** /-mē·ā'təl/ [L, *sub,* beneath, *meatus,* passage], pertaining to tissues beneath a meatus, such as the mastoid air cells under the acoustic meatus or the hard palate beneath the nasal meatus.

**submental** /-men'təl/ [L, *sub* + *mentum,* chin], pertaining to the area beneath the chin.

**submentovertex** /-men'tōvur'teks/ [L, *sub* + *mentum,* chin, *vertex,* peak], pertaining to a radiographic projection of the skull in which x-rays enter just behind the chin and exit at the top of the head.

**submetacentric** /sub'metəsen'trik/ [L, *sub* + Gk, *meta,* besides, *kentron,* center], pertaining to a chromosome in which the centromere is located approximately equidistant between the center and one end so that the arms of the chromosomes are not equal in length. Compare **acrocentric, metacentric, telocentric.**

**submucous** /-m(y)ōō'kəs/, pertaining to a location beneath a mucous membrane.

**submucous resection (SMR)** [L, *sub* + *mucous* + *re* + *secare,* to cut], a surgical procedure for correcting a deviated nasal septum, leaving the mucous membrane of the septum intact.

**subnormal temperature** /-nôr'məl/, any degree of sensible heat below the normal body level of 98.6° F (37° C).

**suboccipitobregmatic** /-aksip'itō'bregmat'ik/ [L, *sub* + *occiput,* back of the head; Gk, *bregma,* front of the head], pertaining to the smallest anteroposterior diameter of an infant's neck when it is well flexed during labor.

**subperiosteal fracture** /sub′perē·os′tē·əl/ [L, *sub* + Gk, *peri*, around, *osteon*, bone], a fracture in a bone beneath the periosteum that does not disrupt the periosteum.

**subphrenic** /-fren′ik/ [L, *sub* + Gk, *phren*, diaphragm], pertaining to the area under the diaphragm.

**subphrenic abscess** [L, *sub*, beneath; Gk, *phren*, diaphragm; L, *abscedere*, to go away], an abscess that develops on or near the undersurface of the diaphragm, usually as a result of peritonitis or from another visceral site.

**subpoena** /-pē′nə/ [L, *sub* + *poena*, penalty], (in law) a document from a court commanding that a person appear at a certain time and place to testify on a specific matter. Subpoenas are governed by federal rules for criminal and civil procedures.

**subpoena duces tecum,** (in law) a subpoena commanding a person to take books, papers, records, or other items to the court.

**subpubic dislocation.** See **dislocation of hip.**

**subscapularis** /-skap′yəler′is/ [L, *sub*, beneath, *scapulae*, shoulder blades], the muscle arising from the subscapular fossa with insertion in the humerus. It functions to rotate the arm medially.

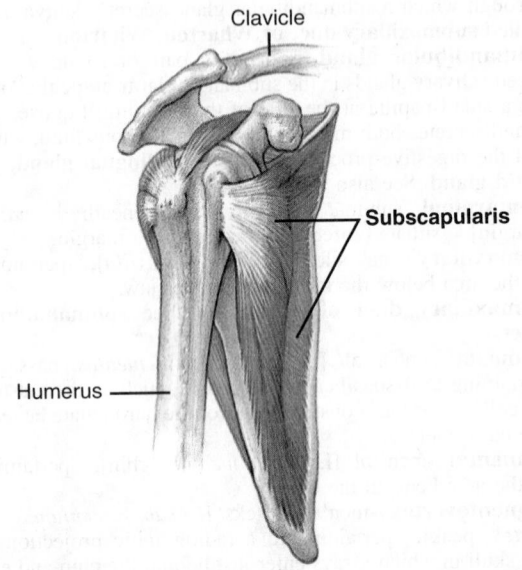

**Subscapularis** *(Thibodeau and Patton, 1999/John V. Hagen)*

**subscriber,** (in managed care) an individual, agency, or employer that has contracted for services under a health plan.

**subserous fascia** /-sir′əs/ [L, *sub* + *serum*, whey, *fascia*, band], one of three kinds of fascia, lying between the internal layer of deep fascia and the serous membranes lining the body cavities in much the same manner as the subcutaneous fascia lies between the skin and the deep fascia. It is thin in some areas, such as between the pleura and the chest wall, and thick in other areas, where it forms a pad of adipose tissue. Compare **deep fascia, subcutaneous fascia.**

**subsistence** /-sis′təns/ [L, *subsistere*, to stand still], the

state of being sustained or remaining alive with a minimum of life essentials.

**subspecialty** /-spesh′əltē/ [L, *sub* + *specialis*, individual], (in nursing) a nurse's particular highly specific professional field of practice, such as dialysis, oncology, neurology, or newborn intensive care nursing. Compare **specialty.**

**subspinale** /sub′spī·nā′lē /, the deepest midline point on the maxilla on the concavity between the anterior nasal spine and the prosthion. Also called **point A.**

**substance** /sub′stəns/ [L, *substantia*, essence], **1.** any drug, chemical, or biologic entity. **2.** any material capable of being self-administered or abused because of its physiologic or psychologic effects.

**substance abuse,** the overindulgence in and dependence on a stimulant, depressant, or other chemical substance, leading to effects that are detrimental to the individual's physical or mental health, or the welfare of others.

**Substance Abuse and Mental Health Services Administration (SAMHSA),** an agency of the United States Department of Health and Human Services with the function of disseminating accurate and up-to-date information about and providing leadership in the prevention and treatment of addictive and mental disorders.

**substance addiction consequences,** a nursing outcome from the Nursing Outcomes Classification (NOC) defined as the compromise in health status and social functioning due to substance addiction. See also **Nursing Outcomes Classification.**

**substance dependence,** a maladaptive pattern of substance abuse, leading to clinically significant impairment or distress as manifested by three or more episodes within a 12-month period of tolerance, withdrawal, use of larger amounts or over a longer period, a peristent desire or unsuccessful effort to control substance abuse, or investment of a great deal of time in activities necessary to obtain the substance.

**substance P,** a polypeptide neurotransmitter that stimulates vasodilation and contraction of intestinal and other smooth muscles. It also plays a part in salivary secretion, diuresis, natriuresis, and pain sensation. It has been isolated from certain cells of the GI and biliary tracts.

**substance use prevention,** a nursing intervention from the Nursing Interventions Classification (NIC) defined as prevention of an alcoholic or drug use life-style. See also **Nursing Interventions Classification.**

**substance use treatment,** a nursing intervention from the Nursing Interventions Classification (NIC) defined as supportive care of patient/family members with physical and psychosocial problems associated with the use of alcohol or drugs. See also **Nursing Interventions Classification.**

**substance use treatment: alcohol withdrawal,** a nursing intervention from the Nursing Interventions Classification (NIC) defined as care of the patient experiencing sudden cessation of alcohol consumption. See also **Nursing Interventions Classification.**

**substance use treatment: drug withdrawal,** a nursing intervention from the Nursing Interventions Classification (NIC) defined as care of the patient experiencing drug detoxification. See also **Nursing Interventions Classification.**

**substance use treatment: overdose,** a nursing intervention from the Nursing Interventions Classification (NIC) defined as monitoring, treatment, and emotional support of a patient who has ingested prescription or over-the-counter drugs beyond the therapeutic range. See also **Nursing Interventions Classification.**

**substandard** /-stan′dərd/ [L, *sub*, beneath; OFr, *estandart*], below the predetermined model or measure.

**substantia alba** /-stan'shə/ [L, *substantia*, essence, *albus*, white], the part of the central nervous system that is enclosed in myelin sheaths. The myelin contributes a white coloring to otherwise gray nerve tissue.

**substantia gelatinosa**, the apical part of the posterior horn of the spinal cord's gray matter. It appears gelatinous because of its lack of myelinated nerve fibers.

**substantia innominata**, a region of the forebrain that lies ventral to the anterior half of the lentiform nucleus. It contains the basal forebrain, which receives afferent input from the reticular formation, hypothalamus, and limbic cortex.

**substantia nigra** [L, *substantia*, essence, *niger*, black], a dark band of gray matter lying between the tegmentum of the midbrain and the crus cerebri.

Cerebral aqueduct

Superior colliculus

Substantia nigra, pars compacta

Substantia nigra, pars reticulata

Crus cerebri

**Substantia nigra** *(Crossman and Neary, 1995)*

**substantive epidemiology** /sub'stəntiv/ [L, *subtantia* + Gk, *epi*, upon, *demos*, people, *logos*, science], the body of knowledge derived from epidemiologic studies, including for each disease the natural history of the disorder, patterns of occurrence, and risk factors for development of the disorder.

**substantivity** /-stəntiv'itē/, the property of continuing therapeutic action despite removal of the vehicle, such as applied to certain shampoos.

**substernal** /-stur'nəl/ [L, *sub* + Gk, *sternon*, chest], pertaining to the area beneath the sternum.

**substernal goiter** [L, *sub* + Gk, *sternon*, chest; L, *guttur*, throat], a nonbacterial inflammation of the lower thyroid isthmus, often preceded by a viral infection causing fever, tenderness, and enlargement of the thyroid gland. Symptoms may last 2 to 4 months and are usually resolved by corticosteroids. See also **thyroiditis.**

**substitution** /-stit(y)o͞o'shən/, a mental defense mechanism, operating unconsciously, by which an unattainable or unacceptable goal, emotion, or object is replaced by one that is more attainable or acceptable.

**substitutive therapy** /sub'stit(y)o͞o'tiv/ [L, *substituere*, to put in place of; Gk, *therapeia*, treatment], a treatment that

effects a condition incompatible with or antagonistic to the condition being treated. Also called **allopathy.**

**substrate** /sub'strāt/ [L, *sub* + *stratum*, layer], a chemical acted on and changed by an enzyme in a chemical reaction.

**substrate depletion phase**, a period during an enzyme assay when the concentration of substrate is falling and the assay is not following zero-order kinetics.

**substratum** /-strā'təm/ [L, *sub* + *stratum*, layer], any underlying layer; a foundation.

**sub-, suf-, sup-,** prefix meaning 'under, below, down, near, almost, or moderately': *subacid, subdental.*

**subsystem** /sub'sistəm/, a smaller component of a large system composed of individuals or dyads, formed by generation, gender, interest, or function.

**subtask work**, a part of the whole task in a rehabilitation program but distinguished by changes in speed or direction.

**subthalamus** /-thal'əməs/ [L, *sub* + Gk, *thalamos*, chamber], a part of the diencephalon that serves as a correlation center for optic and vestibular impulses relayed to the globus pallidus. It is a transition zone between the thalamus and the tegmentum mesencephali. Compare **epithalamus, hypothalamus, metathalamus, thalamus. —subthalamic,** *adj.*

**subtle** /sut'əl/ [L, *subtilis*], having a low intensity; not severe and having no serious sequelae, such as a mild infection or inflammation.

**subtotal** /sub'tōtəl/ [L, *sub*, beneath, *totus*, whole], less than complete.

**subtotal hysterectomy** [L, *sub* + *totus* + Gk, *hystera*, womb, *extome*, excision], the surgical removal of the body of the uterus without removing the cervix. See also **supracervical hysterectomy, supravaginal hysterectomy.**

**subtrochanteric osteotomy** /-trō'kənter'ik/ [L, *sub* + Gk, *trochanter*, runner, *osteon*, bone, *temnein*, to cut], a surgical procedure that divides the shaft of the femur below the lesser trochanter to correct ankylosis of the hip joint.

**subungual** /səbung'gwəl/ [L, *sub* + *unguis*, nail], under a fingernail or toenail.

**subungual hematoma**, a collection of blood beneath a nail that usually results from trauma. The pain accompanying this condition may be quickly alleviated by burning or drilling a small hole through the nail to release the blood.

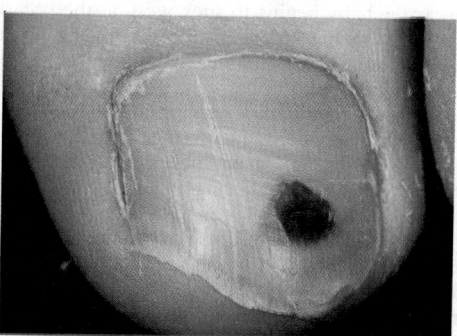

**Subungual hematoma** *(du Vivier, 1993)*

**subunit vaccine** /sub'yo͞onit/, a viral immunizing agent that has been treated to remove traces of viral nucleic acid, so that only protein subunits remain. The subunits have little likelihood of causing adverse reactions.

**subventricular zone** /-ventrik′yələr/, an area located between the ventricular and intermediate zones in the fetal forebrain, in which neurons of the cerebrum are generated.

**succ-,** combining form meaning 'juice': *succagogue, succorrhea, succus.*

**succenturiate placenta.** See **accessory placenta.**

**succi.** See **succus.**

**succinic acid (HOOC(CH₂)₂COOH)** /suksin′ik/, a dicarboxylic acid found in certain hydatid cysts and in lichens, amber, and fossils. Commercial succinic acid, produced by the fermentation of ammonium tartrate, is used in lacquer and dyes. Succinic acid was formerly used in the treatment of diabetic ketoacidosis. Also called **butanedioic acid.**

**succinylcholine chloride** /suk′sinilkō′lēn/, a depolarizing neuromuscular blocker that is a skeletal muscle relaxant.

■ INDICATIONS: It is prescribed to provide an adjunct to anesthesia, to reduce muscle contractions during surgery or mechanical ventilation, and to facilitate endotracheal intubation.

■ CONTRAINDICATIONS: Known hypersensitivity to this drug prohibits its use. Caution is used in administering it to patients with low pseudocholinesterase levels and those with myasthenia gravis or renal failure.

■ ADVERSE EFFECTS: Among the more serious adverse reactions are cardiac arrhythmia and severe respiratory depression.

**succus** /suk′əs/, *pl.* **succi** /suk′sī/ [L, *juice*], a juice or fluid, usually one secreted by an organ, such as succus prostaticus of the prostate.

**succussion splash** /səkush′ən/ [L, *succutere,* to shake up; ME, *plasche,* puddle], the sound elicited by shaking the body of a person who has free fluid and air or gas in a hollow organ or body cavity. This sound may be present over a normal stomach but also may be heard with hydropneumothorax, large hiatal hernia, or intestinal or pyloric obstruction.

**suck** [L, *sugere,* to suck], **1.** to draw a liquid or semiliquid into the mouth by creating a partial vacuum through motions of the lips and tongue. **2.** to hold on the tongue and dissolve by the movements of the mouth and action of the saliva. **3.** to draw fluid into the mouth, specifically to draw milk from the breast or nursing bottle.

**sucking blisters,** the pale soft pads on the upper and lower lips of a baby that look like blisters but are not. They form as soon as the baby begins to suck well, at the breast or on a bottle. They seem to augment the seal of the lips around the nipple or breast. Some babies, who have sucked on their own fingers, hand, or arm before birth, are born with them.

**sucking reflex,** involuntary sucking movements of the circumoral area in newborns in response to stimulation. The reflex continues throughout infancy and often occurs without stimulation, such as during sleep. Compare **rooting reflex.**

**suckle** [L, *sugere*], **1.** to provide nourishment, specifically to breastfeed. **2.** to take in nourishment, especially by feeding from the breast.

**suckling,** an infant that has not been weaned.

**Sucostrin,** trademark for a depolarizing neuromuscular-blocker agent (succinylcholine).

**sucrose** /sōō′krōs/ [Fr, *sucre,* sugar], a disaccharide sugar derived from sugar cane, sugar beets, and sorghum and made up of one molecule of glucose and one of fructose joined together in a glycosidic linkage.

**sucrose polyester (SPE),** a synthetic nonabsorbable fat that, when added to the diet, reduces plasma cholesterol levels by increasing the excretion of cholesterol in the feces. It is formulated to have the characteristic texture, taste, and consistency of regular margarine or vegetable oil and adds no calories to the diet.

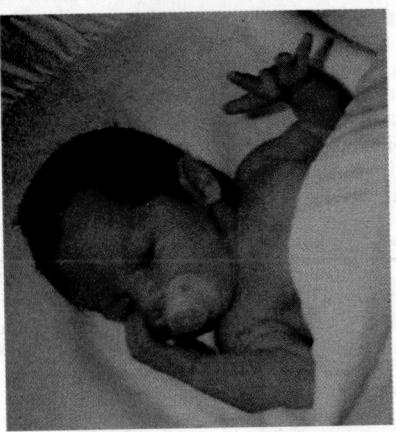

**Sucking reflex** *(Zitelli and Davis, 1997)*

**suction** /suk′shən/ [L, *sugere,* to suck], the aspiration of a gas or fluid by reducing air pressure over its surface, usually by mechanical means.

**suction biopsy** [L, *sugere,* to suck; Gk, *bios,* life, *opsis,* view], a procedure for obtaining tissue or fluid samples from lymph nodes or a deep lesion by using suction and a trochar or cannula. Also called **aspiration biopsy.**

**suction curettage.** See **vacuum aspiration.**

**suction drainage.** See **drainage.**

**suction lipectomy.** See **liposuction.**

**Sudafed,** trademark for an adrenergic vasoconstrictor and decongestant (pseudoephedrine hydrochloride).

**sudden death** [ME, *sodain,* to come up; AS, *death*], death that occurs unexpectedly and from 1 to 24 hours after the onset of symptoms, with or without known preexisting conditions.

**sudden infant death syndrome (SIDS)** [ME, *sodain,* to come up; L, *infans,* unable to speak; AS, *death* + Gk, *syn,* together, *dromos,* course], the unexpected and sudden death of an apparently normal and healthy infant that occurs during sleep and with no physical or autopsic evidence of disease. It is the most common cause of death in children between 2 weeks and 1 year of age, with an incidence rate of 1 in every 300 to 350 live births. The origin is unknown, but multiple causes have been proposed, including lack of biotin in the diet, abnormality of the endogenous-opioid system, mechanical suffocation, a defect in respiratory mucosal defense, prolonged apnea, an unknown virus, anatomic abnormality of the larynx, and immunoglobulin abnormalities. It is known that the condition occurs more often in infants 10 to 14 weeks of age, especially those born prematurely; in boys more than in girls; and more frequently during the winter months; and that it is seen more often among babies who have recently had a minor illness such as upper respiratory infection or infants born to women less than 20 years of age who have had at least one previous child, who begin prenatal care in the third trimester, or who smoke or are anemic or drug dependent. The syndrome is neither contagious nor hereditary, although there is a greater than average risk of its occurrence within the same family, which may indicate the influence of polygenic factors. Infants should be placed for sleep supine or on their side as a preventive measure. Nursing considerations consist predominantly of support and counseling, such as assessing how the parents feel about the death to help them through the resolution of grief, learning what they know about the syndrome, supplying them with whatever information and literature they need, and finding out how they are coping with any guilt feelings and how the siblings, if any, are coping with the death. The nurse also can supply information about local groups of parents who have lost a child from SIDS. Also called **cot death, crib death.** See also **parental grief.**

**sudo-,** combining form meaning 'sweat': *sudogram, sudokeratosis, sudorrhea.*

**sudor** /sōō'dôr/ [L, sweat], perspiration.

**sudoriferous duct** /sōō'dərif'ərəs/ [L, *sudor,* sweat, *facere,* to make], a duct leading from a sweat gland to the surface of the skin. Each sweat duct is the most superficial part of a coiled tube that forms the body of each sweat gland and opens onto the surface through a funnel-shaped opening. The sweat ducts in the armpits and in the groin are larger than in other parts of the body. Also called **sweat duct.**

**sudoriferous gland,** one of about two million tiny structures within the dermis that produce sweat. The average quantity of sweat secreted in 24 hours varies from 700 to 900 g. Most of these glands are eccrine glands, producing sweat that carries away sodium chloride, the waste products urea and lactic acid, and the breakdown products from garlic, spices, and other substances. Apocrine sweat glands associated with the coarse hair of the armpits and the pubic region are larger and secrete fluid that is much thicker than that secreted by the eccrine glands. Each sudoriferous gland

### Epidemiology of SIDS

| Factors | Occurrence |
|---|---|
| Incidence | 0.6:1000 live births (1998) |
| Peak age | 2 to 4 months; 95% occur by 6 months |
| Sex | Higher percentage of males affected |
| Time of death | During sleep |
| Time of year | Increased incidence in winter; peak in January |
| Racial | Greater incidence in Native Americans, blacks, and Hispanics |
| Socioeconomic | Increased occurrence in lower socioeconomic class |
| Birth | Higher incidence in: Premature infants, especially infants of low birth weight Multiple births* Neonates with low Apgar scores Infants with central nervous system disturbances and respiratory disorders such as bronchopulmonary dysplasia Increasing birth order (subsequent siblings as opposed to firstborn child) Infants with a recent history of illness |
| Sleep habits | Prone position; use of soft bedding; overheating (thermal stress), co-sleeping with adult, especially on sofa |
| Feeding habits | Lower incidence in breast-fed infants |
| Siblings | May have greater incidence |
| Maternal | Young age; cigarette smoking, especially during pregnancy; poor prenatal care, substance abuse (heroin, methadone, cocaine) |

Wong DL: *Whaley and Wong's essentials of pediatric nursing,* ed 6, St Louis, 2001, Mosby.
*Although a rare event, simultaneous death of twins from SIDS can occur.

consists of a single tube with a deeply coiled body and a superficial duct. The number of glands per square centimeter of skin varies in different parts of the body; the sudoriferous glands are very plentiful on the palms of the hands and on the soles of the feet, least numerous in the neck and the back, and completely absent in the deeper parts of the external auditory meatus, the prepuce, and the glans penis. Also called **sweat gland.** Compare **sebaceous gland.**

**sudorific** /sōō'dərif'ik/ [L, *sudor,* sweat, *facere,* to make], **1.** pertaining to a substance or condition, such as heat or emotional tension, that promotes sweating. **2.** a sudorific agent. Sweat glands are stimulated by cholinergic drugs. The alkaloid pilocarpine is a potent sudorific drug, but it is rarely used for that purpose in modern medicine. Also called **diaphoretic.**

**suf-.** See **sub-.**

**Sufenta,** trademark for an IV analgesic-anesthetic (sufentanil citrate).

**sufentanil citrate** /sufen'tənil/, an IV analgesic and anesthetic.

■ INDICATIONS: It is used as an adjunct to general anesthesia and as a primary anesthetic with 100% oxygen.

■ CONTRAINDICATIONS: Sufentanil can cause respiratory depression and musculoskeletal rigidity; ready availability of drugs and equipment is required to reduce such adverse effects. Sufentanil is a Schedule II drug under the Controlled Substance Act.

■ ADVERSE EFFECTS: Among the more serious adverse reactions are hypotension, hypertension, bradycardia, and chest wall rigidity.

**suffering level,** a nursing outcome from the Nursing Outcomes Classification (NOC) defined as the severity of anguish associated with a distressing symptom, injury, or loss with potential long-term effects. See also **Nursing Outcomes Classification.**

**suffocation** /suf'əkā'shən/ [L, *suffocare,* to choke], an interruption in breathing with oxygen deprivation, usually caused by an obstruction in the airways. The condition may be accidental, or intentional or may result from disease or inadequate levels of respirable gases in the atmosphere.

**suffocation, risk for,** a nursing diagnosis accepted by the Seventh National Conference on the Classification of Nursing Diagnoses. The diagnosis is defined as the accentuated risk of accidental suffocation (inadequate air available for inhalation).

■ RISK FACTORS: The risk factors may be internal (individual) or external (environmental). Internal risk factors include reduced olfactory sensation, reduced motor abilities, lack of safety education, lack of safety precautions, cognitive or emotional difficulties, and disease or injury processes. External risk factors include a pillow or a propped bottle placed in an infant's crib, a vehicle warming in a closed garage, children's playing with plastic bags or inserting small objects into their mouths or noses, discarded or unused refrigerators or freezers without removed doors, lack of monitoring of children in bathtubs or pools, household gas leaks, smoking in bed, consumption of overly large mouthfuls of food, use of fuel-burning heaters not vented to the outside, low-strung clotheslines, and a pacifier hung around an infant's neck. See also **nursing diagnosis.**

**suffocative goiter** /suf'əkā'tiv/ [L, *suffocare,* to choke, *guttur,* throat], an enlargement of the thyroid gland that causes a sensation of suffocation when pressed.

**sugar** /shŏŏg'ər/ [Gk, *sakcharon*], any of several water-soluble simple carbohydrates. The principal categories of sugars are monosaccharides, disaccharides, and polysaccharides. A monosaccharide is a single sugar, such as glucose, fructose, or galactose. A disaccharide is a double sugar, such as sucrose (table sugar) or lactose. A polysaccharide is a sugar made up of repeating units of glucose, such as cellulose, starch, and glycogen. See also **carbohydrate, fructose, galactose, glucose, saccharide, sucrose.**

**sugar alcohol,** an alcohol produced by the reduction of an aldehyde or ketone of a sugar.

**sugar cataract,** a visual disorder associated with diabetes in which sorbitol collects within the lens, causing an osmotic gradient of fluid in the lens. This condition leads to a disruption of the lens matrix and loss of transparency.

**suggestibility** /səjes'tibil'itē/, pertaining to a person's susceptibility to having his or her ideas or actions influenced or altered by others.

**suggestion** /səjes'chən/ [L, *suggerere,* to propose], **1.** the process by which one thought or idea leads to another, as in the association of ideas. **2.** the use of persuasion, exhortation, or another technique to implant an idea, thought, attitude, or belief in the mind of another as a means of influencing or altering behavior or states of mind. See also **hypnosis. 3.** an idea, belief, or attitude implanted in the mind of another. Compare **autosuggestion.**

**suicidal** /soo̅'isī'dəl/ [L, *sui,* of oneself, *caedere,* to kill], of, relating to, or tending toward self-destruction.

**suicide** /soo̅'isīd/ [L, *sui,* of oneself, *caedere,* to kill], **1.** the intentional taking of one's own life. **2.** *informal.* the ruin or destruction of one's own interests. **3.** a person who commits or attempts self-destruction. Early signs of suicidal intent include depression; expressions of guilt, tension, and agitation; insomnia; loss of weight and appetite; neglect of personal appearance; giving away of personal or valued possessions; and direct or indirect threats to commit suicide.

**suicide gesture,** (in psychiatric nursing) an apparent attempt by a patient to cause self-injury without lethal consequences and generally without actual intent to commit suicide. A suicide gesture serves to attract attention to the patient's disturbed emotional status but is not as serious as a suicide attempt, although it may result in suicide, intentional or not.

**suicide prevention,** a nursing intervention from the Nursing Interventions Classification (NIC) defined as reducing the risk for self-inflicted harm with intent to end life. See also **Nursing Interventions Classification.**

**suicide prevention center,** a crisis-intervention facility dealing primarily with people preoccupied with suicidal thoughts. Such facilities are usually operated by professional social workers with special training in counseling possible suicide victims in person or by telephone.

**suicide, risk for,** a nursing diagnosis accepted by the Fourteenth National Conference on the classification of nursing diagnoses. The condition is defined as being at risk for self-inflicted, life-threatening injury.

■ RISK FACTORS: Risk factors include a history of prior suicide attempts; impulsiveness; buying of a gun; stockpiling of medicines; the making or changing of a will; giving away possessions; the sudden euphoric recovery from major depression; marked changes in behavior, attitude, or school performance; threats of killing oneself; a stated desire to die or end it all; living alone; being retired; relocation; institutionalization; economic instability; loss of autonomy or independence; the presence of a gun in the home; adolescents living in nontraditional settings; a family history of suicide; alcohol and substance use or abuse; psychiatric illness or disorder; abuse in childhood; guilt; gay or lesbian youth; physical illness; terminal illness; chronic pain; loss of important relationship; disrupted family life; grief or bereavement; a poor support system; loneliness; hopelessness; helplessness; social isolation; legal or disciplinary problems; cluster suicides; being elderly, a young adult male, or adolescent; being Native American or caucasian; being male; and being divorced or widowed. See also **nursing diagnosis.**

**suicide self-restraint,** a nursing outcome from the Nursing Outcomes Classification (NOC) defined as the ability to refrain from gestures and attempts at killing self. See also **Nursing Outcomes Classification.**

**suicidology** /soo̅'isīdol'əjē/ [L, *sui* + *caedere* + Gk, *logos,* science], the study of the prevention and causes of suicide. —**suicidologist,** *n.*

**Sular,** trademark for a calcium channel blocker (nisoldipine).

**sulcate, sulci.** See **sulcus.**

**sulcoplasty.** See **vestibuloplasty.**

**sulculus** /sul'kyələs/ [L, *sulcus*], a small sulcus.

**sulcus** /sul'kəs/, *pl.* **sulci** /sul'sī/ [L, furrow], a shallow depression, or furrow on the surface of an organ, such as cerebral sulcus that separates the convolutions of the cerebral hemisphere. A sulcus is usually not as deep as a fissure, but, in the terminology of anatomy, the words *sulcus* and *fissure* are often used interchangeably. —**sulcate,** *adj.*

**sulcus centralis cerebri.** See **central sulcus.**

**sulcus pulmonalis,** a depression on each side of the vertebral bodies that accommodates the posterior part of the lung.

**sulfa-,** combining form for sulfonamide antimicrobials.

**sulfacetamide** /sul'fəset'əmīd/, a topical antibacterial.

■ INDICATIONS: It is most commonly prescribed for the prophylaxis of infection after injury to the cornea and in the treatment of bacterial conjunctivitis and urinary tract infections.

■ CONTRAINDICATIONS: Known hypersensitivity to the drug or to other sulfonamides or impaired kidney function prohibits its use.

■ ADVERSE EFFECTS: Among known adverse reactions are local pain, overgrowth of nonsusceptible pathogens, and hypersensitivity reaction.

**Sulfacet-R,** trademark for a fixed-combination topical drug containing a scabicide (sulfur), an antibacterial (sulfacetamide sodium), and an antiseptic and astringent (zinc oxide).

**sulfadiazine** /sul'fədī'əzēn/, a sulfonamide antibacterial.

■ INDICATIONS: It is prescribed in the treatment of infection, particularly of the urinary tract, and in rheumatic fever prophylaxis.

■ CONTRAINDICATIONS: Porphyria, urinary tract obstruction, or known hypersensitivity to sulfonamides prohibits its use.

■ ADVERSE EFFECTS: Among the more serious adverse effects are crystalluria, photosensitivity, severe allergic reactions, and blood dyscrasias.

**sulfa drugs** /sul'fə/, a group of bacteriostatic agents that inhibit the biosynthesis of folic acid.

**sulfamethizole** /sul'fəmeth'izōl/, a sulfonamide antibiotic.

■ INDICATIONS: It is prescribed in the treatment of infection, particularly pyelonephritis, pyelitis, and cystitis.

■ CONTRAINDICATIONS: Porphyria, urinary tract obstruction, or known hypersensitivity to sulfonamides prohibits its use.

■ ADVERSE EFFECTS: Among the more serious adverse reactions are crystalluria, photosensitivity, blood dyscrasias, and severe allergic reactions.

**sulfamethoxazole** /sul'fəmethok'səzōl/, a sulfonamide antibacterial.

■ INDICATIONS: It is prescribed in the treatment of otitis media, prostatitis, epididimytis, bronchitis, and certain urinary tract infections.

■ CONTRAINDICATIONS: It is not given during the last trimester of pregnancy, during lactation, or to children under 2 months of age. Known hypersensitivity to this drug or other sulfonamides prohibits its use.

■ ADVERSE EFFECTS: Among the more serious adverse reactions are crystalluria and rash, fever, and other allergic reactions.

**sulfamethoxazole and trimethoprim** /trīmeth'əprim/, a fixed-combination antibacterial.

■ INDICATIONS: It is prescribed in the treatment of urinary tract infections, otitis media, and shigellosis.

■ CONTRAINDICATIONS: It is used with caution in patients with impaired renal or hepatic function, possible folate deficiency, or known hypersensitivity to either drug or to sulfonamides. It is not recommended for use in infants less than 2 months of age or in the third trimester of pregnancy.

■ ADVERSE EFFECTS: Among the more serious adverse reactions are crystalluria and rashes, fever, and other allergic reactions.

**Sulfamylon,** trademark for a topical antiinfective (mafenide acetate).

**sulfanilic acid** /sul'fənil'ik/, a red-tinged white crystalline compound used in the synthesis of sulfonamides and as a reagent in tests for phenol, fecal matter in water, albumin, aldehydes, and glucose. Also called *para*-**aminobenzenesulfonic acid.**

**sulfasalazine** /sul'fəsəlaz'ēn/, a sulfonamide; a sulfonamide antibiotic; also called **salicylazosulfapyridine.**

■ INDICATIONS: It is prescribed in the treatment of mild to moderate ulcerative colitis and as adjunctive therapy in severe cases.

■ CONTRAINDICATIONS: Urinary obstruction, porphyria, or known hypersensitivity to this drug, to other sulfonamide medications, or to salicylates prohibits its use. It is not given during the last trimester of pregnancy.

■ ADVERSE EFFECTS: Among the more serious adverse reactions are crystalluria, blood dyscrasias, and severe hypersensitivity reactions. GI symptoms and anorexia commonly occur.

**sulfatase** /sul'fə·tās /, any of a group of enzymes that catalyze the cleavage of inorganic sulfate from sulfate esters to form alcohols.

**sulfate ($SO_4{}^{2-}$)** /sul'fāt/, an anion of sulfuric acid. A sulfate is usually a combination of a metal with sulfuric acid. Natural sulfate compounds, such as sodium sulfate, calcium sulfate, and potassium sulfate, are plentiful in the body.

**sulfatide lipidosis** /sul'fətīd/, an inherited lipid metabolism disorder of childhood caused by a deficiency of cerebroside sulfatase enzyme. It results in an accumulation of metachromatic lipids in tissues of the central nervous system, kidney, spleen, and other organs, leading to dementia, paralysis, and death by 10 years of age. Also called **metachromatic leukodystrophy.** See also **lipidosis.**

**sulfhemoglobin** /sulfhem'əglō'bin/, a form of hemoglobin found in the blood in trace amounts that contains an irreversibly bound sulfur molecule that prevents normal oxygen binding. Also spelled **sulphaemoglobin.**

**sulfhemoglobinemia** /-ē'mē·ə/, the presence of abnormal sulfur-containing hemoglobin circulating in the blood.

**sulfinpyrazone** /sul'finpir'əzōn/, a uricosuric.

■ INDICATIONS: It is prescribed in the treatment of chronic gout and intermittent gouty arthritis.

■ CONTRAINDICATIONS: Peptic ulcer, ulcerative colitis, renal dysfunction, or known hypersensitivity to this drug or to phenylbutazone prohibits its use. It is not usually given during an acute attack of gout.

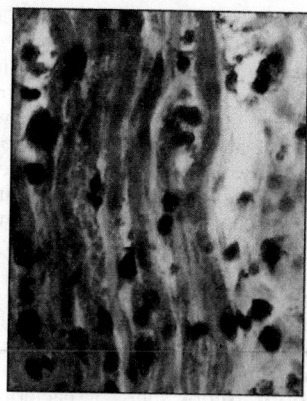

**Sulfatide lipidosis** *(Perkin, 1998)*

■ ADVERSE EFFECTS: Among the more serious adverse reactions are GI ulcers, blood dyscrasias, and dermatitis.

**sulfisoxazole** /sul'fisok'səzōl/, a sulfonamide antibiotic.

■ INDICATIONS: It is prescribed in the treatment of conjunctivitis and urinary tract infections, including vaginitis, cystitis, and pyelonephritis.

■ CONTRAINDICATIONS: Porphyria, urinary tract obstruction, or known hypersensitivity to this drug or to sulfonamide medications prohibits its use. It is not given during the last trimester of pregnancy or to children less than 2 months of age.

■ ADVERSE EFFECTS: Among the more serious adverse reactions are crystalluria, blood dyscrasias, and severe hypersensitivity reactions.

**sulfiting agents** /sul'fīting/, food preservatives composed of potassium or sodium bisulfite or potassium metabisulfite. Sulfiting agents are used in processing of beer, wine, baked goods, soup mixes, and some imported seafoods and by restaurants to impart a "fresh" appearance to salad fruits and vegetables. The chemicals can cause a severe allergic reaction in people who are hypersensitive to sulfites. The reactions are marked by flushing, faintness, hives, headache, GI distress, breathing difficulty, and, in extreme cases, loss of consciousness and death.

**sulfo-** /sul'fō-, sul'fə-/, combining form naming chemical compounds, showing presence of divalent sulfur or of the group $SO_2OH$: *sulfonamide, sulfomethane, sulfophenol.*

**sulfobromophthalein** /sul'fəbrō'məfthal'ēn, -ē·in/, a substance used in its disodium salt form for evaluating the function of the liver.

**sulfonamide** /səlfon'əmīd/, one of a large group of synthetic bacteriostatic drugs that are effective in treating infections caused by many gram-negative and gram-positive microorganisms. They are bacteriostatic rather than bactericidal. Some sulfonamides are short-acting, some are intermediate-acting, and some are long acting, depending on the speed with which they are excreted. They are used in treating many urinary tract infections. Some people are hypersensitive to the drugs. Sulfonamides are given with caution to people who have impaired liver or kidney function, and they are not given in the last trimester of pregnancy or to young infants, because mental retardation sometimes can result. Hemolytic anemia, agranulocytosis, thrombocytopenia, or aplastic anemia, drug fever, and jaundice may occur, particularly with long-acting sulfonamides given for more than 10 days. Most sulfonamides are given orally.

**sulfonates** /sul′fənāts/, a class of anticholinesterase compounds used as insecticides.

**sulfonylurea** /sul′fənilyo̅o̅r′ē·ə/, an oral antidiabetic agent that stimulates the pancreatic production of insulin. Hypersensitivity to sulfonamides is a contraindication for using such agents, and ethanol consumption is incompatible with all sulfonylureas. The safety of these drugs for use in pregnant women has not been established, making insulin the preferred drug in treating diabetes in pregnancy. Aspirin or other salicylates taken with any sulfonylurea may intensify the hypoglycemic effect.

**sulfosalicylic acid** /sul′fōsalisil′ik/, a white or faintly pink crystalline substance that is highly water-soluble and is used as a reagent in tests for albumin and as an intermediate compound in the manufacture of dyes and surfactants.

**sulfoxone sodium** /sulfok′sōn/, a bacteriostatic sulfone derivative.
- INDICATIONS: It is prescribed in the treatment of leprosy and dermatitis herpetiformis.
- CONTRAINDICATIONS: Advanced renal amyloidosis or known sensitivity to this drug prohibits its use.
- ADVERSE EFFECTS: Among the most serious adverse reactions are hemolysis, hemolytic anemia, toxic epidermal necrolysis, and several blood dyscrasias.

**Sulfoxyl,** trademark for a fixed-combination topical drug containing a disinfectant (benzoyl peroxide) and a scabicide (sulfur).

**sulfur (S)** /sul′fər/ [L], a nonmetallic polyvalent tasteless, odorless chemical element that occurs abundantly in yellow crystalline form or in masses, especially in volcanic areas. Its atomic number is 16; its atomic mass is 32.07. It is used in the production of sulfuric acid and used in metallurgy, rubber vulcanization, petroleum refining, and many other industrial processes. Sulfur has been used in the treatment of gout, rheumatism, and bronchitis and as a mild laxative. The sulfonamides, or sulfa drugs, are used in the treatment of various bacterial infections. Also spelled **sulphur.**

**-sulfuric** /sulf(y)oo̅′rik/, **-sulphuric**, combining form meaning 'compounds containing sulfur, especially in its highest valences': *hydrosulfuric, persulfuric, thiosulfuric.*

**sulfuric acid** ($H_2SO_4$), a clear, colorless, oily highly corrosive liquid that generates great heat when mixed with water. An extremely toxic substance, sulfuric acid causes severe skin burns, blindness on contact with the eyes, serious lung damage if the vapors are inhaled, and death if it is ingested. In industry, sulfuric acid is used in the manufacture of fertilizers, dyes, glue, and other acids; in the purifying of petroleum; and in the pickling of metals. Weak solutions of sulfuric acid are used in the treatment of gastric hypoacidity and serous diarrhea. It was formerly called **oil of vitriol.**

**sulfurous acid** ($H_2SO_3$) /sul′fərəs/, a weak inorganic acid used as a chemical reducing and bleaching agent. It has been used in medicine in skin lotions and nasal and throat sprays. Sulfites formed by the acid may be included in antiseptics, antifermentatives, and antizymotics.

**sulindac** /sulin′dek/, a nonsteroidal antiinflammatory agent.
- INDICATIONS: It is prescribed in the treatment of osteoarthritis, rheumatoid arthritis, and ankylosing spondylitis.
- CONTRAINDICATIONS: Pregnancy, lactation, or known hypersensitivity to this drug, to aspirin, or to nonsteroidal antiinflammatory drugs prohibits its use. It is used with caution in patients who have upper GI tract disease or impaired renal function.
- ADVERSE EFFECTS: Among the more serious adverse reactions are GI upset, peptic ulcer, dizziness, tinnitus, and skin rash.

**sulphaemoglobin.** See **sulfhemoglobin.**

**sulphur.** See **sulfur.**

**Sultrin Triple Sulfa,** trademark for a fixed-combination vaginal drug containing antibacterials (sulfathiazole, sulfacetamide, and sulfabenzamide).

**sumac** [Ar, *summaq*], any of a number of species of trees and shrubs in the Anacardiaceae family, including the Rhus species, which have poisonous properties. See **poison ivy, poison oak, poison sumac, rhus dermatitis.**

**summary judgment** [L, *summa,* total, *jus,* law, *dicere,* to state], (in law) a judgment requested by any party to a civil action to end the action when it is believed that there is no genuine issue or material fact in dispute. Summary judgment may be directed toward part or all of a claim or defense and may be based on the proceedings in court or on affidavits or other outside materials.

**summation** [L, *summa,* total], 1. an accumulative effect or action; a total aggregate; totality. 2. (in neurology) the concentration of a neurotransmitter at a synapse, either by increasing the frequency of nerve impulses in each fiber (temporal summation) or by increasing the number of fibers stimulated (spatial summation), so that the threshold of the postsynaptic neuron is overcome and an impulse is transmitted. See also **facilitation,** def. 2.

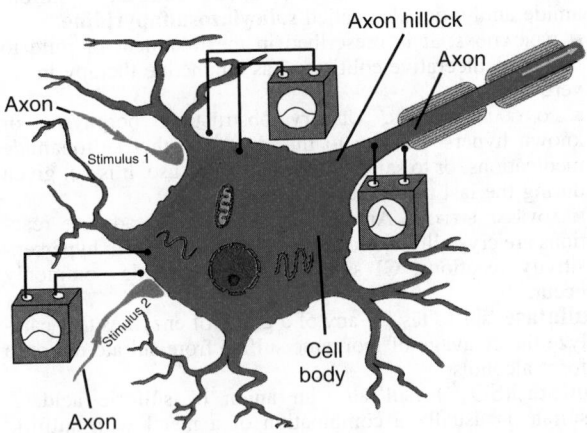

**Spatial summation** *(Thibodeau and Patton, 1999)*

**summation gallop,** a gallop rhythm in which the third and fourth heart sounds are superimposed, appearing as one loud sound; it may occur in some patients with tachycardia but is usually associated with cardiac disease. See also **gallop.**

**summons** /sum′əns/ [OFr, *somondre,* to remind secretly], (in law) a document issued by a clerk of the court on the filing of a complaint. A sheriff, marshal, or other appointed person serves the summons, notifying a person that an action has been begun against him or her. See also **service of process.**

**sump drain,** a drainage device consisting of two tubes, one to allow fluid to be drained from a cavity and the other to allow air to enter the cavity to replace the fluid. It may be attached to a suction apparatus.

**Sumycin,** trademark for an antibiotic (tetracycline hydrochloride).

**sunbath** [AS, *sunne* + *baeth*], the exposure of the naked body to the sun.

**sunburn,** a skin injury characterized by redness, tenderness, and possible blistering that results from exposure to actinic radiation from the sun.

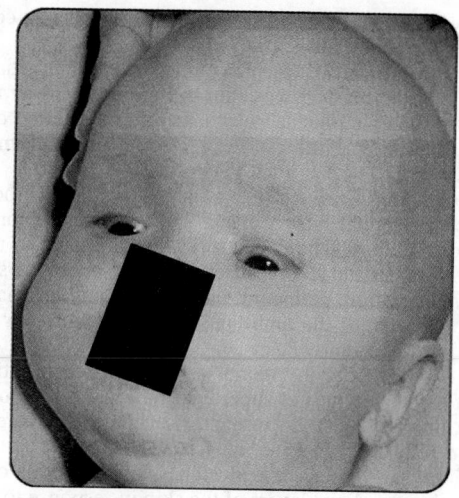

**Sun-setting sign** (Kanski and Nischal, 1999)

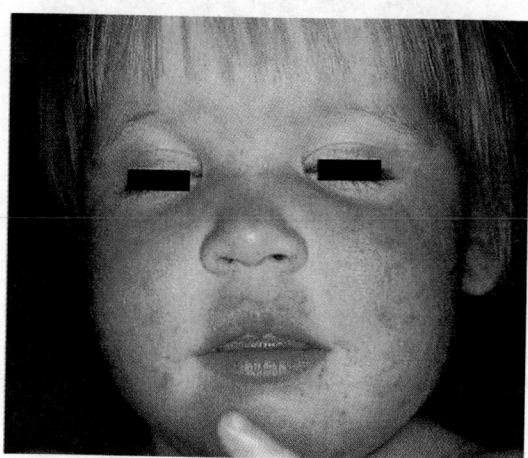

**Sunburn of an infant's face**
(Weston, Lane, and Morrelli, 1996)

**SunDare,** trademark of an ultraviolet screen (cinoxate).

**sundowning** /sun'douning/ [AS, *sunne* + *ofdune*, off the hill], a condition in which persons with cognitive impairment and elderly people tend to become confused or disoriented at the end of the day. Many of them have diminished visual acuity and varying degrees of sensorineural and conduction hearing loss. With less light, they lose visual cues that help them to compensate for their sensory impairments. It may also be a result of decreased sensory stimulation, especially in the evening, when there is less environmental activity and less structure. Sundowning is most common with dementia, Alzheimer's type, and is seen with delirium.

**sunrise syndrome,** a condition of unstable cognitive ability on arising in the morning. Compare **sundowning.**

**sunscreen protective factor index (SPF),** a system of evaluating the effectiveness of various formulations for protecting the skin from actinic rays of the sun. Protective agents are rated from 1 to 50 by the U.S. Food and Drug Administration. A sun protective factor of 15 means that the sunscreen provides 15 times the protection of unprotected skin. Among the most highly rated sunscreen lotions are nonopaque combinations of paraaminobenzoic acid ester and benzophenone.

**sun-setting sign,** a characteristic of hydrocephalus in which an infant's eyes appear to look only downward, with the sclera prominent over the iris.

**sunstroke** [AS, *sunne* + *strac*, stroke], a morbid condition caused by overexposure to the sun and characterized by a high temperature and altered level of consciousness. See also **heat hyperpyrexia.**

**sup-.** See **sub-.**

**Supen,** trademark for an antibacterial (ampicillin).

**super-** /sōo'pər-/, prefix meaning 'above, more than normal, or implying excess': *superduct, superfunction, supernumerary.*

**superantigen,** one of a family of related substances including staphylococcal and streptococcal exotoxins that can short-circuit the normal sequence of events leading to activation of helper T cells. Superantigens initiate an uncontrolled proliferation of T cells but do not require processing and presentation by macrophages. The result is either an acute and potentially life-threatening disease, such as toxic shock syndrome, or a chronic inflammatory process, such as rheumatic fever.

**supercomputers,** high-performance computing equipment capable of handling massive amounts of research and clinical data at speeds more than 1000 times that of most computer equipment. Supercomputer hardware and software may offer a potential of connecting thousands of research facilities and transmitting data at rates up to one billion bits per second. Proposed high-performance computers could quickly analyze archived medical data about worldwide populations, determining, for example, the "normal" human blood pressure on the basis of records of millions of patients.

**superego** /ē'gō/ [L, *super,* over; *ego,* I], (in psychoanalysis) that part of the psyche, functioning mostly in the unconscious, that develops when the standards of the parents and of society are incorporated into the ego. The superego has two parts, the conscience and the ego ideal. Also known as the structure of the psyche that is governed by one's moral code. See also **ego, ego ideal, id.**

**supereruption.** See **overeruption.**

**superfecundation** /-fekəndā'shən/ [L, *super* + *fecundare,* to be fruitful], the impregnation of two or more ova released during the same ovulation by spermatozoa from successive coital acts.

**superfetation** /-fētā'shən/ [L, *super* + *fetus,* pregnancy], the fertilization of a second ovum after the onset of pregnancy, resulting in the simultaneous development of two fetuses of different degrees of maturity within the uterus. Also called **superimpregnation.**

**superficial** /-fish'əl/ [L, *superficies,* surface], **1.** pertaining to the surface. **2.** not grave or dangerous.

**superficial abscess** [L, *superficialis* + *abscedere,* to go away], an abscess that develops above the fascia layer.

**superficial fading infantile hemangioma,** a superficial temporary salmon-colored patch in the center of the forehead, face, or occiput of many newborns. It fades during the first 2 years of life, but it may temporarily deepen in color if the child becomes flushed or angry.

**superficial implantation,** (in embryology) the partial embedding of the blastocyst within the uterine wall so that it and later the chorionic sac protrude into the uterine cavity. Also called **central implantation, circumferential implantation.**

**superficial inguinal node,** a node in one of the two groups of inguinal lymph glands in the upper femoral triangle of the thigh. The nodes form a chain distal to the inguinal ligament and receive afferent vessels from the skin of the penis, scrotum, perineum, buttocks, and abdominal wall below the level of the umbilicus. Compare **anterior tibial node, popliteal node.**

**superficial reflex,** any neural reflex initiated by stimulation of the skin. Kinds of superficial reflexes are **abdominal reflex, anal reflex,** and **cremasteric reflex.** Compare **deep tendon reflex.**

**superficial sensation,** the awareness or perception of feelings in the superficial layers of the skin in response to touch, pressure, temperature, and pain. Such sensations are conveyed to the brain via the spinothalamic system. Compare **deep sensation.**

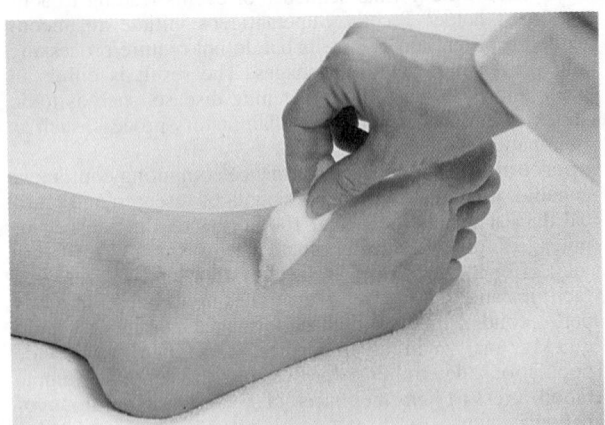

**Superficial tactile sensation** *(Seidel et al, 1999)*

**superficial spreading melanoma,** the most common melanoma that grows outward, spreading over the surface of the affected organ or tissue. It occurs most commonly on the lower legs of women and the torso of men. The lesion is raised and palpable, unevenly pigmented, and irregularly shaped and has an unclear border. See also **lentigo maligna melanoma, nodular melanoma.**

**superficial temporal artery,** an artery at each side of the head that can be easily felt in front of the ear and is often used for taking the pulse. It is the smaller of the two terminal branches of the external carotid. Compare **deep temporal artery, middle temporal artery.**

**superficial vein,** one of the many veins between the subcutaneous fascia just under the skin. Compare **deep vein.**

**superimpregnation.** See **superfetation.**

**superinfection** /-infek′shən/ [L, *super* + *inficere*, to stain], an infection occurring during antimicrobial treatment for another infection. It is usually a result of change in the normal tissue flora favoring replication of some organisms by di-

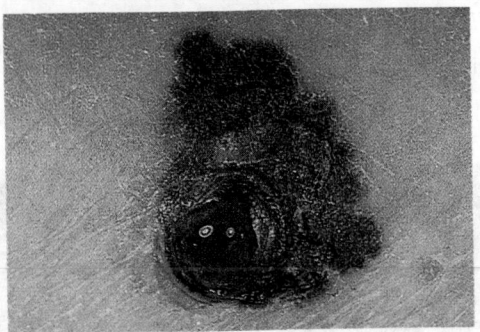

**Superficial spreading melanoma** *(du Vivier, 1993)*

minishing the vitality and then the number of competing organisms, as yeast microbes flourish during penicillin therapy prescribed to cure a bacterial infection.

**superior** /səpir′ē·ər/ [L, higher], situated above or oriented toward a higher place, as the head is superior to the torso. Compare **inferior.**

**superior aperture of minor pelvis,** an opening bounded by the crest and pecten of the pubic bones, the arch-shaped lines of the ilia, and the anterior margin of the base of the sacrum.

**superior aperture of thorax,** an elliptic opening at the summit of the thorax bounded by the first thoracic vertebra, the first ribs, and the upper margin of the sternum.

**superior carotid triangle** [L, *superior,* higher; Gk, *karos,* heavy sleep; L, *triangulus*], a triangle bounded by the sternocleidomastoid muscle, in front and below by the omohyoid muscle, and above by the stylohyoid and digastric muscles.

**superior conjunctival fornix,** the space in the fold of the conjunctiva created by the reflection of the conjunctiva covering the eyeball and the lining of the upper lid. Compare **inferior conjunctival fornix.**

**superior costotransverse ligament,** one of five ligaments associated with each costotransverse joint, except that of the first rib. It passes from the neck of each rib to the transverse process of the vertebra immediately above and is associated with the intercostal vessels and the intercostal nerves. The first rib has no superior costotransverse ligament. Compare **posterior costotransverse ligament.**

**superior gastric node,** a node in one of two sets of gastric lymph glands, accompanying the left gastric artery. The node is divided into the upper group of nodes on the stem of the artery, the lower group of nodes accompanying branches of the artery along the cardiac half of the lesser curvature of the stomach, and the paracardial group of nodes around the neck of the stomach. The superior gastric nodes receive their afferent vessels from the stomach and pass their efferent vessels to the celiac group of preaortic nodes. Compare **inferior gastric node.**

**superior hemorrhagic polioencephalitis.** See **Wernicke's encephalopathy.**

**superior mediastinum,** the upper part of the mediastinum in the middle of the thorax, containing the trachea, the esophagus, the aortic arch, and the origins of the sternohyoidei and the sternothyroidei. Compare **anterior mediastinum, middle mediastinum, posterior mediastinum.**

**superior mesenteric artery,** a visceral branch of the abdominal aorta, arising inferior to the celiac artery, dividing into five branches, and supplying most of the small intestine and parts of the colon. The branches are the inferior pancreaticoduodenal, intestinal, ileocolic, right colic, and middle colic.

**superior mesenteric node,** a node in one of the three groups of visceral lymph nodes that serve the viscera of the abdomen and the pelvis. The superior mesenteric nodes are associated with branches of the superior mesenteric artery and are divided into mesenteric nodes, iliocolic nodes, and mesocolic nodes. Compare **gastric node, inferior mesenteric node.**

**superior mesenteric vein,** a tributary of the portal vein that drains the blood from the small intestine, the cecum, and the ascending and transverse colons. See also **portal vein.**

**superior olivary nucleus** [L, *supurus + oliva + nucleus,* nut kernel], a collection of nerve cells appearing as a clump of gray matter in the pons. The nucleus receives fibers from the cochlear nerve receptors on the same and opposite sides through the trapezoid body. It assists in the localization of sound by comparing the time difference between sounds received by the left and right ears.

**superior orbital fissure,** an elongated cleft between the small and great wings of the sphenoid bone, which transmits various nerves and vessels.

**superior profunda artery.** See **deep brachial artery.**

**superior radioulnar joint.** See **proximal radioulnar articulation.**

**superior sagittal sinus,** one of the six venous channels in the posterior of the dura mater, draining blood from the brain into the internal jugular vein. It has no valves. The superior sagittal sinus receives the superior cerebral veins, veins from the diploe and near the posterior extremity of the sagittal suture, the anastomosing emissary veins from the pericranium, and the veins from the dura mater. It also anastomoses with veins of the nose, the scalp, and the diploe. Compare **inferior sagittal sinus, straight sinus, transverse sinus.**

**superior subscapular nerve** /səbskap′yələr/, one of a pair of small nerves on opposite sides of the body that arise from the posterior cord of the brachial plexus. It supplies the superior part of the subscapularis. Compare **inferior subscapular nerve.**

**superior temporal gyrus,** a rounded elevation on the lateral surface of either temporal lobe of the brain.

**superior thyroid artery,** one of a pair of arteries in the neck, usually arising from the external carotid artery, that supplies the thyroid gland and several muscles in the head.

**superior ulnar collateral artery,** a long slender division of the brachial artery, arising just distal to the middle of the arm, descending to the elbow, and anastomosing with the posterior ulnar recurrent and inferior ulnar collateral arteries.

**superior vena cava,** the second largest vein of the body, returning deoxygenated blood from the upper half of the body to the right atrium. It is about 2 cm in diameter and 7 cm long. The section of the superior vena cava closest to the heart composes about one half of the vessel's length and is within the pericardial sac, covered by the serous pericardium. It has no valves. Compare **inferior vena cava.**

**superior vena cava syndrome,** a condition of edema and engorgement of the veins of the upper body caused by obstruction of the superior vena cava by thrombi or primary pulmonary tumors. Signs and symptoms include a nonproductive cough, breathing difficulty, cyanosis, central nervous system disorders, and edema of the conjunctiva, trachea, and esophagus.

**supernatant** /-nā′tənt/ [L, *super + natare,* to swim], **1.** situated above or on top of something. **2.** the clear upper liquid part of a mixture (a liquid and a solid) after it has been centrifuged.

**supernormal excitability** /-nôr′məl/, the ability of the myocardium to respond at the end of phase 3 of the cardiac action potential to a stimulus that would be ineffective at other times.

**supernormal period,** a period of supernormal excitability of the myocardium.

**supernumerary nipples** /-nōō′mərer′ē/ [L, *super + numerus,* number; ME, *neb,* beak], an excessive number of nipples, which are usually not associated with underlying glandular tissue. They may vary in size from small pink dots to that of normal nipples.

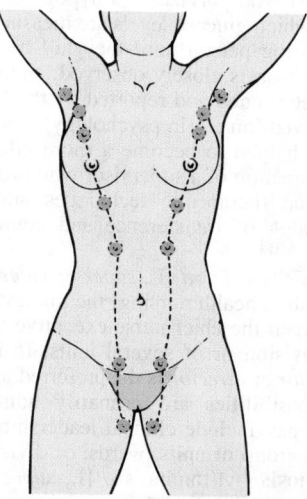

**Supernumerary nipples**

**supernumerary tooth** [L, *super,* above, *numerus,* number; AS, *toth*], any tooth in addition to the normal 32 teeth in secondary dentition or the 20 teeth in deciduous dentition.

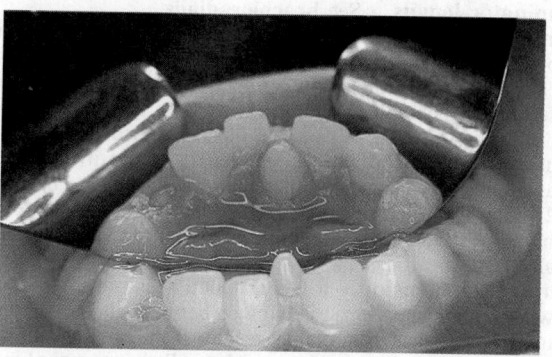

**Supernumerary tooth** *(Regezi, Sciubba, and Pogrel, 2000)*

**superoxide** /-ok′sīd/, a common reactive form of oxygen that is formed when molecular oxygen gains a single electron. Superoxide radicals can attack susceptible biologic targets, including lipids, proteins, and nucleic acids.

**superoxide dismutase (SOD),** an enzyme composed of metal-containing proteins that converts superoxide radicals into less toxic agents. It is the main enzymatic mechanism for clearing superoxide radicals from the body.

**supersaturate** /-sach′ərāt/ [L, *super*, above, *saturare*, to fill], a solution that contains solute above the saturation point at a given temperature. Also called **metastable solution.**

**supertwins,** multiple births of more than two infants. Children of multiple births are more prone to premature birth and are likely to suffer from congenital defects, according to studies. The rate of cerebral palsy in multiple births is six times that for single births.

**superversion.** See **sursumversion.**

**supervised fast** /so͞o′pərvīzd/, a hypoglycemic diagnostic procedure in which glucose levels are measured every 4 to 6 hours in a fasting person until they fall below 50 mg/dL. The fasting person is closely observed, and glucose values are rapidly determined and reported by the laboratory.

**supervision** /-vizh′ən/, (in psychology) a process whereby a therapist is helped to become a more effective clinician through the direction of a supervisor who provides theoretic knowledge and therapeutic techniques and supports the working through of transference and countertransference reactions.

**supervisor** /so͞o′pərvī′zər/ [L, *super* + *videre*, to see], (in hospital or public health nursing) the midlevel management position between the chief nurse executive and nurse managers of a division or of several units. In many hospitals *clinical director* or *director* is the preferred term. The supervisor's responsibilities are primarily administrative, although they may include clinical leadership for the nurses working in a group of units, wards, or divisions.

**supervitaminosis** /-vī′təminō′sis/ [L, *super*, above, *vita* + *amine* + Gk, *osis*, condition], a condition of ingesting an excessive amount of vitamins in the forms of supplements. Signs and symptoms vary with specific vitamin excesses. See also **hypervitaminosis.**

**supinate** /so͞o′pənāt/, pertaining to a supine position or upturning of the palm.

**supination** /so͞o′pinā′shən/ [L, *supinus*, lying on the back], **1.** one of the kinds of rotation allowed by certain skeletal joints, such as the elbow and the wrist joints, which permit the palm of the hand to turn up. **2.** assumption of a supine position, one of lying on the back, face up. Compare **pronation.** —**supinate,** *v.*

**supinator jerk reflex.** See **supinator longus reflex.**

**supinator longus.** See **brachioradialis.**

**supinator longus reflex** /so͞o′pinā′tər/ [L, *reflectere*, to bend back], a contraction of the brachioradialis muscle, causing flexion at the elbow joint, on tapping the point of insertion of the supinator longus muscle at the lower end of the radius. Also called **radial reflex, supinator jerk reflex.**

**supine** /səpīn′, so͞o′pīn/ [L, *supinus*], **1.** position of the arms or body in which the palms of the hands face upward. **2.** lying horizontally on the back. Also called **dorsal decubitus position, dorsal recumbent.** Compare **prone.** See also **body position.**

**supine hypotension,** a fall in blood pressure that occurs when a pregnant woman is lying on her back. It is caused by impaired venous return that results from pressure of the gravid uterus on the vena cava. Also called **vena caval syndrome.**

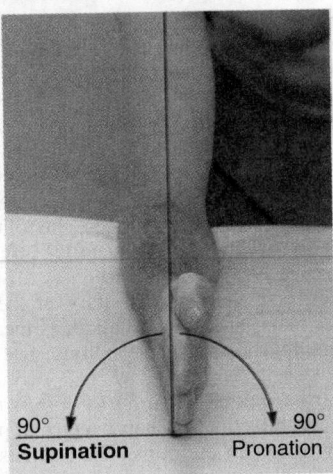

**Supination and pronation** *(Seidel et al, 1999)*

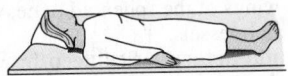

**Supine position** *(Potter and Perry, 2001)*

**supplemental air.** See **reserve capacity.**

**supplemental inheritance** /sup′ləmen′təl/ [L, *supplere*, to complete, *in*, in, *hereditare*, hereditary], the acquisition or expression of a genetic trait or condition through the presence of two independent pairs of nonallelic genes that interact in such a way that one gene supplements the action of the other.

**supplementary gene** /sup′ləmen′tərē/ [L, *supplere* + Gk, *genein*, to produce], one of two pairs of nonallelic genes that interact in such a way that one pair needs the presence of the other to be expressed, whereas the second pair can produce an effect independently of the first.

**supply management,** a nursing intervention from the Nursing Interventions Classification (NIC) defined as ensuring acquisition and maintenance of appropriate items for providing patient care. See also **Nursing Interventions Classification.**

**support** /səpôrt′/ [L, *supportare*, to bring up], **1.** to sustain, hold up, or maintain in a desired position or condition, as in physically supporting the abdominal muscles with a scultetus binder or emotionally supporting a client under stress. **2.** the assistance given to this end, such as physical support, emotional support, or life support.

**support group,** a nursing intervention from the Nursing Interventions Classification (NIC) defined as use of a group environment to provide emotional support and health-related information for members. See also **Nursing Interventions Classification.**

**support groups, 1.** organizations that serve as a link in the network for family caregivers and patients, such as those who are homebound, mentally ill, elderly, or suicidal or who have a specific disorder, such as multiple sclerosis. The groups help families and patients find a balance of responsibility. The groups are supported by various national and local organizations. **2.** organizations for people who share a common problem. See also **social support groups.**

**supporting area** [L, *supportare* + *area*, space],  any of the areas of maxillary or mandibular edentulous ridges that are considered best suited to bear the forces of chewing with functioning dentures.

**supporting cells,**  cells that serve to provide support and protection and perhaps contribute to the nutrition of principal or other cells of certain organs; such cells are found in the labyrinth of the inner ear, organ of Corti, olfactory epithelium, taste buds, and seminiferous tubules. Also called **sustentacular cells.**

**supportive psychotherapy** /səpôr'tiv/,  a form of psychotherapy that concentrates on creating an effective means of communication with an emotionally disturbed person rather than on trying to produce psychologic insight into the underlying conflicts. Through such supportive measures as reassurance, reinforcement of the person's defenses, direction, suggestion, and persuasion, the therapist participates directly in the solution of specific problems. Compare **nondirective therapy.**

**supportive treatment.**  See **treatment.**

**support system enhancement,**  a nursing intervention from the Nursing Interventions Classification (NIC) defined as facilitation of support to patient by family, friends, and community. See also **Nursing Interventions Classification.**

**suppository** /səpoz'ətôr'ē/ [L, *sub*, under, *ponere*, to place],  an easily melted medicated mass for insertion into the rectum, urethra, or vagina. Theobroma oil, glycerinated gelatin, and high-molecular-weight polyethylene glycols are common vehicles for drugs in suppositories that are cone- or spindle-shaped for insertion into the rectum, globular or egg-shaped for use in the vagina, and pencil-shaped for insertion into the urethra. Drugs administered by rectal suppository are absorbed systemically, and this route is especially useful in babies, in uncooperative patients, and in cases of vomiting or certain digestive disorders.

**suppressant** /səpres'ənt/ [L, *supprimere*, to press down],  an agent that suppresses or diminishes a physical or mental activity.

**suppressed menstruation** /səprest'/ [L, *supprimere*, to press down, *menstruare*],  a failure of menstruation to occur when expected, as in amenorrhea, or menstration that is suppressed, as with Gn Rit agonists.

**suppression** /səpresh'ən/ [L, *supprimere*],  (in psychoanalysis) the conscious inhibition of or effort to conceal unacceptable or painful thoughts, desires, impulses, feelings, or acts. Compare **repression.**

**suppression amblyopia,**  a partial loss of vision, usually in one eye, caused by cortical suppression of central vision to prevent diplopia. It occurs commonly in strabismus in the eye that deviates and does not fixate. Early recognition of strabismus and amblyopia is essential because occlusive therapy that forces use of the bad eye may dramatically improve the child's vision if begun early. It becomes progressively less effective with increasing age but may improve vision even up to 9 years of age. Near-blindness in the affected eye may result.

**suppression of menses.**  See **suppressed menstruation.**

**suppressor gene** /səpres'ər/,  a gene that is able to reverse the effect of a specific kind of mutation in other genes.

**suppressor mutation,**  a mutation that partially or completely restores a function lost by a primary mutation occurring at a different locus.

**suppressor T cell.**  See **T cell.**

**suppurate** /sup'yərāt/ [L, *suppurare*, to form pus],  to produce purulent matter. —**suppuration,** *n.,* suppurative, *adj.*

**suppuration** /sup'yərā'shən/ [L, *suppurare*, to form pus],  the production and exudation of pus.

**suppurative** /sup'yərā'tiv/ [L, *suppurare*, to form pus],  pus-forming.

**suppurative arthritis,**  inflammation of a joint with exudation of pus into the joint fluid.

**suppurative fever** [L, *suppurare*, to form pus, *febris*, fever],  a fever accompanied by pus formation.

**suppurative pancreatitis** [L, *suppurare*, to form pus; Gk, *pan*, all, *kreas*, flesh, *itis*, inflammation],  a form of pancreatic inflammation accompanied by the appearance of small abscesses.

**suppurative phlebitis** [L, *suppurare*, to form pus; Gk, *phleps*, vein, *itis*, inflammation],  a vein inflammation that results from septicemia or a nearby pyogenic infection.

**supra-** /sŏŏ'prə-/,  prefix meaning 'above or over': *suprabuccal, supradural, suprarenalism.*

**suprabony periodontal pocket.**  See **periodontal pocket.**

**supracallosus gyrus** /-kəlō'ses/ [L, *supra*, above, *callosus*, hard; Gk, *gyros*, turn],  the gray matter covering the corpus callosum of the brain.

**supracervical hysterectomy** /-sur'vikəl/ [L, *supra*, above, *cervix*, neck; Gk, *hystera*, womb, *ektomē*, excision],  a subtotal hysterectomy in which the body of the uterus is removed, leaving the cervix.

**supraclavicular** /-kləvik'yələr/ [L, *supra*, above, *clavicula*, little key],  pertaining to the area above the clavicle, or collar bone.

**supraclavicular nerve,**  one of a pair of cutaneous branches of the cervical plexus, arising from the third and the fourth cervical nerves, mostly from the fourth nerve. The anterior group supplies the skin of the infraclavicular region, the middle group supplies the skin over the pectoralis major and the deltoideus, and the posterior group supplies the skin of the cranial and dorsal parts of the shoulder.

**supraclavicular triangle** [L, *supra*, above, *clavicula*, little key, *triangulus*],  the lower and anterior areas of the neck, bounded by the omohyoid muscle above, the sternocleidomastoid muscle in front, and the clavicle below. The first rib is in the base of the triangle.

**supraclusion.**  See **overeruption.**

**supracondylar** /-kon'dilər/ [L, *supra*, above; Gk, *kondylos*, knuckle],  pertaining to an area above a condyle.

**supracondylar fracture** [L, *supra* + *kondylos*, knuckle],  a fracture involving the area between the condyles of the humerus or the femur.

**supracrestal periodontal pocket.**  See **periodontal pocket.**

**supragingival calculus.**  See **calculus.**

**suprahyoid muscles,**  a group of four muscles that attach the hyoid bone to the skull. See also **digastricus, geniohyoideus, mylohyoideus, stylohyoideus.**

**suprainfection** /-infek'shən/ [L, *supra* + *inficere*, to stain],  a secondary infection usually caused by an opportunistic pathogen, such as a fungal infection after the antibiotic treatment of another infection or pneumonia in a patient debilitated by another illness.

**supramentale** /sŏŏ'prə·men·tā'lē/ [L, *supra*, above + *mentum*, chin],  in radiographic cephalometry, the most posterior midline point in the concavity between the infradentale and pogonion, determined on the lateral head film.

**supranasal** /sŏŏ'prə·nā'zəl/ [L, *supra*, above + *nasus*, nose],  superior to the nose.

**supranuclear gaze disturbance** /-nŏŏ'klē·ər/,  an inability to direct the eyes to the side contralateral to a lesion in the frontal lobe. If the frontal lobe lesions are bilateral, the patient can maintain fixation and follow visual targets but cannot shift the gaze in any direction in the absence of a target. See also **gaze palsy.**

**supraocclusion.** See **overeruption.**

**supraoptic nucleus** /-op'tik/ [L, *supra*, above; Gk, *optikos* + L, *nucleus*, nut kernel], a hypothalamic nucleus that lies above the optic chiasma with fibers extending to the posterior lobe of the pituitary.

**supraorbital** /sŏŏ'prə·or'bi·təl/ [L, *supra*, above + *orbita*, wheel track], superior to the orbit.

**suprapatellar** /-pətel'ər/ [L, *supra*, above, *patella*, small dish], pertaining to a location above the patella.

**suprapelvic** /sŏŏ'prə·pel'vik/ [L, *supra*, above + *pelvis*, basin], above the pelvis.

**suprapubic** /-p(y)ŏŏ'bik/ [L, *supra* + *pubes*, signs of maturity], pertaining to a location above the symphysis pubis.

**suprapubic aspiration of urine,** a procedure for draining the bladder by inserting a sterile needle through the skin above the pubic arch and into the bladder. The bladder may also be emptied by inserting a catheter through a suprapubic incision when conditions prohibit use of the conventional insertion. Also called **suprapubic puncture.**

**suprapubic catheter** [L, *supra* + *pubis* + Gk, *katheter*, a thing lowered into], a urinary bladder catheter inserted through the skin about 1 inch above the symphysis pubis. It is inserted under a general or local anesthetic. It is used for closed drainage and may be left in place for a time, sutured to the abdominal skin. Benefits include a lower incidence of urinary tract infection, ease of voiding naturally when the catheter is clamped, and ease of ambulation. Disadvantages are that they must be inserted through the abdominal wall by a physician and the insertion site must be cleaned daily using sterile technique.

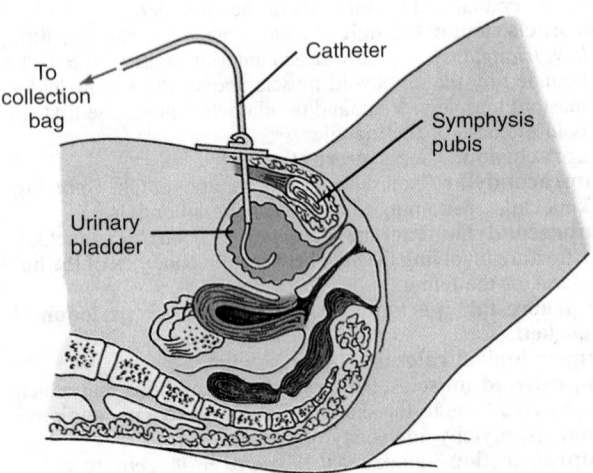

**Suprapubic catheter** *(Elkin, Perry, and Potter, 2000)*

**suprapubic lithotomy.** See **high lithotomy.**

**suprapubic puncture.** See **suprapubic aspiration of urine.**

**suprarenal** /-rē'nəl/ [L, *supra* + *ren*, kidney], pertaining to a location above the kidney, such as the suprarenal gland.

**suprarenal gland.** See **adrenal gland.**

**suprascapular ligament** /-skap'yələr/ [L, *supra*, above, *scapula*, shoulder blade, *ligare*, to bind], a ligament that extends from the base of the coracoid process to the medial end of the suprascapular notch.

**suprascapular nerve** [L, *supra* + *scapulae*, shoulder

blades], one of a pair of branches from the cords of the brachial plexus. It supplies the shoulder joint, scapula, and associated muscles.

**suprasellar** /-sel'ər/, above the sella turcica.

**suprasellar cyst.** See **craniopharyngioma.**

**supraspinal** /-spī'nəl/ [L, *supra*, above, *spina*, backbone], pertaining to an area above the spine.

**supraspinal ligament** [L, *supra* + *spina*, backbone], the ligament that connects the apices of the spinous processes from the seventh cervical vertebra to the sacrum.

**supraspinatus** /sŏŏ'prə·spī·nā'tus/ [L, *supra*, above + *spina*, spine], a muscle originating in the supraspinous fossa and inserting in the greater tubercle of the humerus. It functions to abduct the humerus.

**supraspinatus syndrome** /-spīnā'təs/, pain and tenderness involving the supraspinatus tendon of the arm, restricting abduction of the shoulder.

**supraspinous fossa** /-spī'nəs/ [L, *supra*, above, *spina*, backbone, *fossa*, ditch], a depressed area on the dorsal surface of the scapula, above the spine.

**suprasternal** /-stur'nəl/, pertaining to a location above the sternum, adjacent to the neck.

**supratentorial** /-tentôr'ē·əl/ [L, *supra*, above, *tentorium*, tent], pertaining to a location above a tentorium.

**supravaginal hysterectomy** /-vaj'inəl/ [L, *supra*, above, *vagina*, sheath; Gk, *hystera*, womb, *ektomē*, excision], a subtotal hysterectomy in which the body of the uterus is removed but the cervix remains.

**supraventricular tachycardia (SVT)** /-ventrik'yələr/ [L, *supra* + *ventriculus*, little belly], any cardiac rhythm with a rate exceeding 100/min that originates above the branching part of the atrioventricular bundle, that is, in the sinus node, atria, or AV junction.

**supraversion** /sŏŏ'prə·ver'zhən/ [L, *supra*, above + *vertere*, to turn], **1.** malocclusion in which a tooth or other maxillary or mandibular structure extends farther away from the alveolus than normal, the occluding surfaces of the teeth extending beyond the normal occlusal line. **2.** see **sursumversion.**

**suprofen** /səprō'fən/, an oral nonsteroidal antiinflammatory analgesic.

■ INDICATIONS: It is used in the treatment of mild to moderate pain and primary dysmenorrhea.

■ CONTRAINDICATIONS: This drug is contraindicated for patients who experience asthma, rhinitis, urticaria, or other allergic reactions from the use of aspirin or other nonsteroidal antiinflammatory drugs. It is not recommended for patients with a history of peptic ulcers or risk of other types of GI bleeding.

■ ADVERSE EFFECTS: Reported side effects include severe flank pain, nausea, vomiting, dyspepsia, abdominal pain, diarrhea, constipation, flatulence, headache, dizziness, sedation, and sleep disturbances.

**sural region** /sŏŏ'rəl/ [L, *sura*, calf of the leg], the calf of the leg. It is formed by the bellies of the gastrocnemius and soleus muscles.

**suramin sodium** /sŏŏ'rəmin/, an antitrypanosomal and an antifilarial available from the Centers for Disease Control and Prevention. It is used primarily for treatment and prophylaxis of African trypanosomiasis and onchocerciasis.

**surcharge,** (in the United States) an additional fee charged to health plan enrollees for benefits not provided in the health plan contract.

**surface anatomy** /sur'fəs/ [L, *superficies*, surface], the study of the structural relationships of the external features of the body to the internal organs and parts. Compare **cross-sectional anatomy.**

**surface anesthesia.** See **topical anesthesia.**

**surface area (SA),** the total area exposed to the outside environment. The surface area of an object increases with the square of the its linear dimensions; volume increases as the cube of the object's linear dimensions. Thus the larger of two objects of the same shape will have less surface area per unit volume than the smaller object. Most loss of body heat is from the body surface.

**surface biopsy,** the removal of living tissue for microscopic examination by scraping the surface of a lesion. It is done primarily to diagnose cancer of the uterine cervix. See also **exfoliative cytology, Papanicolaou's test.**

**surface tension,** the tendency of a liquid to minimize the area of its surface by contracting. This property causes liquids to rise in a capillary tube, affects the exchange of gases in the pulmonary alveoli, and alters the ability of various liquids to wet another surface.

**surface therapy,** a form of radiotherapy administered by placing one or more radioactive sources on or near an area of body surface. The resulting array of sources is called a surface mold, surface applicator, or plaque.

**surface thermometer,** a device that detects and indicates the surface temperature of any part of the body.

**surfactant** /sərfak′tənt/ [L, *superficies*], **1.** an agent, such as soap or detergent, dissolved in water to reduce its surface tension or the tension at the interface between the water and another liquid. **2.** certain lipoproteins that reduce the surface tension of pulmonary fluids, allowing the exchange of gases in the alveoli of the lungs and contributing to the elasticity of pulmonary tissue. Also called **pulmonary surfactant.** See also **alveolus, atelectasis, surface tension.**

**Surfadil,** trademark for a topical fixed-combination drug containing an antihistaminic (methapyrilene hydrochloride) and a topical anesthetic (cyclomethycaine sulfate).

**Surfak,** trademark for a stool softener (docusate calcium).

**surfer's nodules** [ME, *suffe*, rush; L, *nodus*, knot], nodules on the skin of the knees, ankles, feet, or toes of a surfer caused by repeated contact of the skin with an abrasive, sandy surfboard. The nodules slowly diminish in size and disappear if surfing is discontinued. When treatment is necessary, injection of corticosteroids is usually effective.

**surgeon** /sur′jən/, a physician who treats injuries, deformities, and diseases by operative methods.

**surgeon general,** (in the United States) the chief medical officer of the Army, Navy, Air Force, and Public Health Service. In other countries, the title may indicate any physician with the rank of general.

**surgeon's assistant (SA)** /sur′jənz/ [Gk, *cheirourgos*, surgeon; L, *assistere*, to cause to stand], a medical professional trained to assist during surgery and in the preoperative and postoperative periods under the supervision of a licensed physician qualified to practice surgery.

**surgery** /sur′jərē/ [Gk, *cheirourgia*], the branch of medicine concerned with diseases and trauma requiring operative procedures. —**surgical,** *adj.*

**-surgery,** combining form meaning the 'treatment of illness or deformity': *cardiosurgery, chemosurgery, radiosurgery.*

**surgical** /sur′jikəl/ [Gk, *cheirourgia*], pertaining to the treatment of disease by manipulative and operative methods.

**surgical abdomen.** See **acute abdomen.**

**surgical anatomy,** (in applied anatomy) the study of the structure and morphologic characteristics of the tissues and organs of the body as they relate to surgery.

**surgical asepsis.** See **asepsis.**

**surgical assistance,** a nursing intervention from the Nursing Interventions Classification (NIC) defined as assisting the surgeon/dentist with operative procedures and care of the surgical patient. See also **Nursing Interventions Classification.**

**surgical diathermy.** See **electrocoagulation.**

**surgical fever** [Gk, *cheirourgia* + L, *febris*], a fever that develops after surgery. As a result of modern aseptic techniques fever is unlikely to accompany an operation.

**surgical gut.** See **catgut.**

**surgical induction of labor.** See **induction of labor.**

**surgical ligature,** the exposure of an unerupted tooth by placing a metal ligature around its cervix. The free ends of the ligature are fixed to a fine, precious-metal chain attached to an orthodontic appliance. These components act together to produce traction on the unerupted tooth and force it through the gingival tissues.

**surgical menopause** [Gk, *cheirourgia* + L, *men*, month; Gk, *pauein*, to cease], the creation of a menopausal state by surgical removal of the ovaries.

**surgical microscope.** See **operating microscope.**

**surgical neck of humerus** [Gk, *cheirourgia* + AS, *hnecca* + L, *humerus*, shoulder], the shaft of the humerus distal to the tuberosities. It is a region particularly vulnerable to fracture and surgical correction.

**surgical pathology,** the study of disease by the analysis of tissue specimens obtained during surgery. The surgical pathologist often examines specimens during surgery to determine how the operation should be modified or completed. Various techniques are used. The appearance of the specimen is first noted; then slices of the tissue are prepared by the paraffin or frozen section method and microscopically examined by a physician trained in pathology.

**surgical precautions,** a nursing intervention from the Nursing Interventions Classification (NIC) defined as minimizing the potential for iatrogenic injury to the patient related to a surgical procedure. See also **Nursing Interventions Classification.**

**surgical preparation,** a nursing intervention from the Nursing Interventions Classification (NIC) defined as providing care to a patient immediately prior to surgery and verification of required procedures/tests and documentation in the clinical record. See also **Nursing Interventions Classification.**

**surgical scrub, 1.** a bactericidal soap or solution used by surgeons and surgical nurses before performing or assisting in surgery. **2.** the act of washing the fingernails, hands, and forearms in a prescribed manner for a specific period, with a bactericidal soap or solution before a surgical procedure.

**surgical sectioning,** an oral surgery procedure for dividing a tooth to facilitate its removal. A variety of instruments are used for surgical sectioning, including osteotomes and power-driven burs.

**surgical shock** [Gk, *cheirourgia* + Fr, *choc*], a condition of shock that may occur intraoperatively or follow surgery, with signs of low blood volume, decreased urine, increased heart rate, restlessness, and cyanosis of the extremities.

**surgical suite,** a group of one or more operating rooms and adjunct facilities, such as a sterile storage area, scrub room, and recovery room.

**surgical technologist,** an allied health professional who prepares the operating room by selecting and opening sterile supplies; assembles, adjusts, and checks nonsterile equipment to ensure it is in good working order; and operates sterilizers, lights, suction machines, electrosurgical units, and diagnostic equipment. Surgical technologists have primary responsibility for maintaining the sterile field and being constantly vigilant that all members of the surgical team adhere to aseptic technique.

**surgical treatment.**   See **treatment.**

**Surmontil,**   trademark for an antidepressant (trimipramine maleate).

**surrogate** /sur'əgāt/ [L, *surrogare*, to substitute],   **1.** a substitute; a person or thing that replaces another. **2.** a person who represents and acts as a parent, taking the place of the father or mother. **3.** (in psychoanalysis) a substitute parental figure, a symbolic image or representation of another, as may occur in a dream. The identity of the person represented often remains in the unconscious.

**surrogate parenting,**   a form of artificial insemination in which a fertile woman who is not the wife of the sperm donor agrees to be impregnated by him and to carry the child to term, at which time the offspring is surrendered to the care of the infertile wife. The surrogate mother usually receives a fee for bearing the child.

**surrogate partner.**   See **sex surrogate.**

**sursum-,**   combining form meaning 'upward': *sursumduction, sursumvergence, sursumversion.*

**sursumversion** /sur'sum·ver'zhən/ [L. *sursum* upward + *vertere,* to turn],   binocular conjugate upward rotation of both eyes; also called **superversion, supraversion.**

**surveillance**[1] /sərvā'ləns/ [Fr, *surveiller,* to watch over],   **1.** supervising or observing a patient or a health condition. It may include the use of closed circuit television cameras and monitors to cover unattended locations from a central office. **2.** a detailed examination or investigation for the accurate collection of data to record changes in the character of a population as at a particular time or, in a prospective or longitudinal surveillance, over a period. Retrospective surveillance might study the characteristics of a population in which a previous event occurred. The collection of data may include hospital records, morbidity and mortality statistics, death certificates, records of immunization, age groups, and various ecologic and weather factors for the period of investigation, particularly if insect vectors are possible influences.

**surveillance**[2],   a nursing intervention from the Nursing Interventions Classification (NIC) defined as purposeful and ongoing acquisition, interpretation, and synthesis of patient data for clinical decision making. See also **Nursing Interventions Classification.**

**surveillance: community,**   a nursing intervention from the Nursing Interventions Classification (NIC) defined as purposeful and on-going acquisition, interpretation, and synthesis of data for decision making in the community. See also **Nursing Interventions Classification.**

**surveillance: late pregnancy,**   a nursing intervention from the Nursing Interventions Classification (NIC) defined as purposeful and ongoing acquisition, interpretation, and synthesis of maternal-fetal data for treatment, observation, or admission. See also **Nursing Interventions Classification.**

**surveillance: remote electronic,**   a nursing intervention from the Nursing Interventions Classification (NIC) defined as purposeful and ongoing acquisition of patient data via electronic modalities (telephone, video conference, e-mail) from distant locations, as well as interpretation and synthesis of patient data for clinical decision making with individuals or populations. See also **Nursing Interventions Classification.**

**surveillance: safety,**   a nursing intervention from the Nursing Interventions Classification (NIC) defined as purposeful and ongoing collection and analysis of information about the patient and the environment for use in promoting and maintaining patient safety. See also **Nursing Interventions Classification.**

**surveyed height of contour** /sərvād'/ [OFr, *surveir,* to survey; AS, *heah,* high; It, *contornare,* to surround],   a line, scribed or marked on a cast, that designates the greatest convexity relative to a selected path of denture placement and removal.

**survival curve** /sərvī'vəl/ [Fr, *survivre,* to survive; L, *curvus,* bent],   a plot of the number or percentage of organisms surviving for a given period as a function of radiation dose.

**survivor guilt** /sərvī'vər/ [OFr, *survivre* + ME, *gilt,* sin],   feelings of guilt for surviving a tragedy in which others died. In some cases, the person may believe the tragedy occurred because he or she did something bad; in others, the person may feel guilty for not taking proper steps to avert the tragedy. Also called **survival guilt.**

**susceptibility** /səsep'tibil'itē/ [L, *suscipere,* to undertake],   the condition of being vulnerable to a disease or disorder.

**susceptible** /səsep'tibəl/ [L, *suscipere,* to undertake],   being predisposed, liable, or sensitive to the effects of an infectious disease, allergen, or other pathogenic agent; lacking immunity or resistance.

**suspension** /səspen'shən/ [L, *suspendere,* to hang],   **1.** a liquid in which small particles of a solid are dispersed, but not dissolved, and in which the dispersal is maintained by stirring or shaking the mixture. If left standing, the solid particles settle at the bottom of the container. See also **colloid, solution. 2.** a treatment, used primarily in spinal disorders, consisting of suspending the patient by the chin and shoulders. **3.** a temporary cessation of pain or of a vital process.

**suspension sling,**   a sling usually made of muslin or lightweight canvas and used primarily to provide support, such as against the gravitational pull on an injured arm. An example is a common triangular sling.

**suspensory ligament** /səspen'sərē/ [L, *suspendere,* to hang, *ligare,* to bind],   any of a number of ligaments that help support an organ or body structure, such as the suspensory ligaments inside the eye that hold the lens in tension.

**suspensory ligament of the lens.**   See **zonula ciliaris.**

**sustained release.**   See **prolonged release.**

**sustenance** /sus'tənəns/ [L, *sustenare,* to sustain],   **1.** the act or process of supporting or maintaining life or health. **2.** the food or nutrients essential for maintaining life.

**sustenance support,**   a nursing intervention from the Nursing Interventions Classification (NIC) defined as helping a needy individual/family to locate food, clothing, or shelter. See also **Nursing Interventions Classification.**

**sustentacular** /sus'ten·tak'yōō·lər/ [L, *sustentare,* to support],   pertaining to a support or serving to support.

**sustentacular cells.**   See **supporting cells.**

**susto** /sōōs'tō/,   a culture-bound syndrome found in Central American populations. It is related to stress engendered by a self-perceived failure to fulfill sex-role expectations.

**Sutton's disease** /sut'ənz/ [Richard Lightburn Sutton, American dermatologist, 1878–1952],   a recurrent disease of the mucous membranes of unknown cause, generally considered to be a severe form of aphthous stomatitis, characterized by deep crater-like ulcers with inflamed borders that leave scars after healing. It usually involves the mucosa of the lips, cheeks, tongue, palate, and anterior tonsillar pillars, but the pharynx, larynx, and genitalia may also be affected. Also called **Mikulicz's aphthae, periadenitis mucosa necrotica recurrens, recurring scarring aphthae.** See also **aphthous stomatitis.**

**sutura** /sōōchōō'rə/, *pl.* **suturae** [L, suture],   an immovable fibrous joint in which certain bones of the skull are connected by a thin layer of fibrous tissue. Compare **gomphosis, syndesmosis.**

**sutura dentata,**   an immovable fibrous joint that is one kind of true suture in which toothlike processes interlock along the margins of connecting bones of the skull. Compare **sutura limbosa, sutura serrata.**

**suturae cranii.** See **cranial sutures.**

**sutura limbosa,** an immovable fibrous joint that is one kind of true suture in which beveled and serrated edges of certain connecting bones of the skull, such as the parietal and temporal bones, overlap and interlock. Compare **sutura dentata, sutura serrata.**

**sutura plana,** a fibrous joint that is one kind of false suture in which rough contiguous edges of certain bones of the skull, such as the maxillae, form a connection. Compare **sutura squamosa.**

**sutura serrata,** an immovable fibrous joint that is one kind of true suture in which connecting bones interlock along serrated edges that resemble fine-toothed saws. Compare **sutura dentata, sutura limbosa.**

**sutura squamosa,** an immovable fibrous joint that is one kind of false suture in which overlapping beveled edges unite certain bones of the skull, such as the temporal and the parietal bone. Compare **sutura plana.**

**suture** /soo′chər/ [L, *sutura*], **1.** a border or a joint, such as between the bones of the cranium. **2.** to stitch together cut or torn edges of tissue with suture material. **3.** a surgical stitch taken to repair an incision, tear, or wound. **4.** material used for surgical stitches, such as absorbable or nonabsorbable silk, catgut, wire, or synthetic material.

**suture forceps.** See **needle holder.**

**suturing,** a nursing intervention from the Nursing Interventions Classification (NIC) defined as approximating edges of a wound using sterile suture material and a needle. See also **Nursing Interventions Classification.**

**Sv,** abbreviation for **sievert.**

**SV40,** abbreviation for **simian virus 40.**

**SV40 papovavirus.** See **papovavirus.**

**S. viridans** abbreviation for *Staphylococcus viridans.*

**SvO₂,** symbol for the percentage of oxygen saturation of mixed venous blood.

**SVR,** abbreviation for **systemic vascular resistance.**

**SVT,** abbreviation for **supraventricular tachycardia.**

**swab** /swob/ [D, *swabber,* ship's drudge], a stick or clamp holding absorbent gauze or cotton, used for washing, cleansing, or drying a body surface; for collecting a specimen for laboratory examination; or for applying a topical medication.

**swaddling** /swod′ling/ [OE, *swethel,* swaddling band], **1.** long narrow bands of cloth once used to wrap a newborn. **2.** a method of wrapping a newborn, especially a premature or at risk newborn, that provides maximal comfort and containment.

**swage** /swāj/ [OFr, *souage*], **1.** to shape metal by hammering or by adapting it to a die. **2.** to fuse suture material to a needle, especially an eyeless needle. **3.** a tool or form, often one of a pair, for shaping metal by pressure.

**Swain, Mary Ann P.** See **Modeling and Role Modeling.**

**swallowing** /swol′ō·ing/ [AS, *swelgan*], the process that usually involves movement of food from the mouth to the stomach via the esophagus. Coordination of muscles is needed from the tongue to the esophageal sphincter. See **swallowing reflex.**

**swallowing examination,** an X-ray with contrast dye (usually barium) that is performed to pinpoint problems that exist in a patient who is unable to swallow. The examination is used to detect tumors, upper esophageal diverticula, inflammation, extrinsic compression of the upper GI tract, problems resulting from surgery to the oropharyngeal tract, motility disorders of the upper GI tract, and neurologic disorders such as stroke, Parkinson's disease, and neuropathies.

**swallowing, impaired,** a nursing diagnosis accepted by the Seventh National Conference on the Classification of Nursing Diagnoses. It is defined as the state in which an individual has decreased ability to pass fluids and/or solids from the mouth to the stomach voluntarily.

■ DEFINING CHARACTERISTICS: The defining characteristics are observed evidence of difficulty in swallowing, such as stasis of food in the oral cavity, coughing, or choking, and evidence of aspiration.

■ RELATED FACTORS: Among related factors are neuromuscular impairment, such as decreased or absent gag reflex, and decreased strength or excursion of muscles involved in mastication. Other factors are perceptual impairment, facial paralysis, mechanical obstruction (such as edema, tracheostomy tube, or tumor), tumor, fatigue, limited awareness, and an irritated oropharyngeal cavity. See also **nursing diagnosis.**

**swallowing reflex** [AS, *swelgan* + L, *reflectere,* to bend back], a sequence of reflexes that begins when a bolus of food is manipulated by the tongue and other oral cavity muscles to the palate or the pharynx.

**swallowing status,** a nursing outcome from the Nursing Outcomes Classification (NOC) defined as the extent of safe passage of fluids and/or solids from the mouth to the stomach. See also **Nursing Outcomes Classification.**

**swallowing status: esophageal phase,** a nursing outcome from the Nursing Outcomes Classification (NOC) defined as the adequacy of the passage of fluids and/or solids from the pharynx to the stomach. See also **Nursing Outcomes Classification.**

**swallowing status: oral phase,** a nursing outcome from the Nursing Outcomes Classification (NOC) defined as the adequacy of preparation, containment, and posterior movement of fluids and/or solids in the mouth for swallowing. See also **Nursing Outcomes Classification.**

**swallowing status: pharyngeal phase,** a nursing outcome from the Nursing Outcomes Classification (NOC) defined as the adequacy of passage of fluids and/or solids from the mouth to the esophagus. See also **Nursing Outcomes Classification.**

**swallowing therapy,** a nursing intervention from the Nursing Interventions Classification (NIC) defined as facilitating swallowing and preventing complications of impaired swallowing. See also **Nursing Interventions Classification.**

**swamp fever.** See **leptospirosis, malaria.**

**Swan-Ganz catheter** /swän′ganz′/ [Harold J.C. Swan, American physician, b. 1922; William Ganz, American cardiologist, b. 1919; Gk, *katheter,* something lowered], a long thin cardiac catheter with a tiny balloon at the tip. It is used to determine left ventricular function by measuring pulmonary capillary wedge pressure.

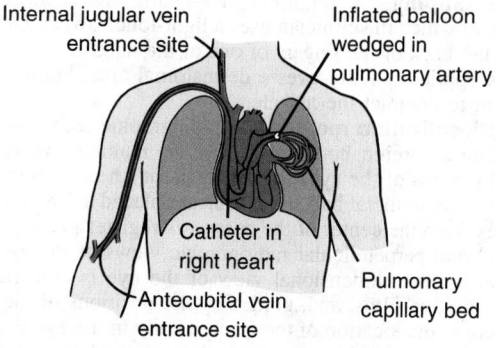

**Swan-Ganz catheter**

**swan neck deformity** /swän/ [D, *zwaan* + AS, *hnecca,* neck; L, *deformis,* misshapen],　**1.** an abnormal condition of the finger characterized by flexion of the distal interphalangeal joint and hyperextension of the proximal interphalangeal joint. It is caused by a taut profundus tendon in the presence of a weakened distal interphalangeal joint and may be combined with a volar plate rupture. The condition is seen most often in rheumatoid arthritis. Also called **zig-zag.** **2.** a structural abnormality of the kidney tubules associated with rickets. The kidney tubule connecting the glomerulus with the convoluted part of the tubule is narrowed into a configuration referred to as "swan neck." There are also a thinning and atrophy of the distal tubule and a shortening of the convoluted part.

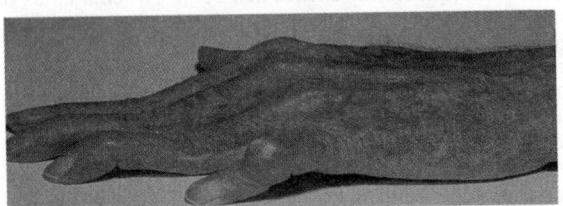

**Swan neck deformity** *(Phipps, Sands, and Marek, 1999)*

**S wave,** the negative component after the R wave in each QRS complex on an electrocardiogram.

**sway,** to rock, teeter, wobble, or swing back and forth.

**sweat.** See **perspiration.**

**sweat bath,** a bath given to induce sweating.

**sweat duct.** See **sudoriferous duct.**

**sweat gland.** See **sudoriferous gland.**

**sweating.** See **diaphoresis.**

**sweat test,** a method for evaluating sodium and chloride excretion from the sweat glands, often the first test performed in the diagnosis of cystic fibrosis. The sweat glands are stimulated with a drug, such as pilocarpine, and the perspiration produced is analyzed. The eccrine glands of patients with cystic fibrosis produce sodium and chloride concentrations that are three to six times normal. Chloride levels above 60 mEq/L and sodium levels above 90 mEq/L are considered diagnostic for the disease. The test is very reliable, and although it may be useful at any age, it is usually performed on infants from 2 weeks to 1 year of age. See also **cystic fibrosis.**

**Swedish massage** /swē′dish/ [Fr, *masser*], a regimen of massage combined with physical exercises.

**sweep tapping,** a proprioceptive-tactile treatment technique in which the clinician uses a light-touch sweep pattern over the back of the fingers of one of the hands. The stimulus is applied quickly over a dermatomal area, helping the patient to contract the muscle.

**Sweet localization method,** a radiographic technique for locating a foreign body in the eye by making two radiographic films of the eye while the patient's head is immobilized. A small metal ball and a cone are placed at precise distances from the center of the cornea as register marks while lateral and perpendicular radiographic views of the eye are made. A three-dimensional view of the eye is constructed from the two films, and, guided by the positions of the ball and cone, the location of the foreign body in the eye is plotted from the intersection of lines through the ball and cone.

**Sweet's syndrome** /swēts/ [Robert Douglas Sweet, English dermatologist, 20th century], a condition usually seen on the upper body of middle-aged women, characterized by one or more large, rapidly extending, erythematous, tender or painful plaques, accompanied by fever and dense infiltration of neutrophils in the upper and middle dermis. Also called **acute febrile neutrophilic dermatosis.**

**Swift's disease.** See **acrodynia.**

**swimmer's ear** [AS, *swimman,* to swim, *eare*], *informal.* otitis externa resulting from infection transmitted in the water of a swimming pool. See also **otitis externa.**

**swimmer's itch,** an allergic dermatitis caused by sensitivity to schistosome cercarias that die under the skin, leading to erythema, urticaria, and a papular rash lasting 1 or 2 days. Treatment usually includes oral antihistamines and antipruritic lotions. See also **schistosomiasis.**

**swimming reflex,** a primitive fetal activity, marked by well-coordinated movements, that is exhibited when the infant's face is placed in water. It normally disappears at 6 months of age.

**swing phase of gait** [AS, *swingan* + Gk, *phasis,* appearance; ME, *gata,* a way], the phase of the normal gait cycle during which the foot is off the ground. The swing phase follows the stance phase and is divided into the initial swing, the midswing, and the terminal swing stages.

**switch site,** a point on a chromosome where gene segments unite during segment rearrangement, as in the production of immunoglobulins.

**swoon** [OE, *geswogen,* unconscious], a fainting spell.

**sy-.** See **syn-.**

**sycosis barbae** /sikō′sis/ [Gk, *sycon,* fig, *osis,* condition; L, *barba,* beard], an inflammation of hair follicles of skin that has been shaved. Treatment includes light and infrequent shaving, topical and systemic antibiotics, and daily plucking of infected hairs. Also called **barber's itch, sycosis vulgaris.**

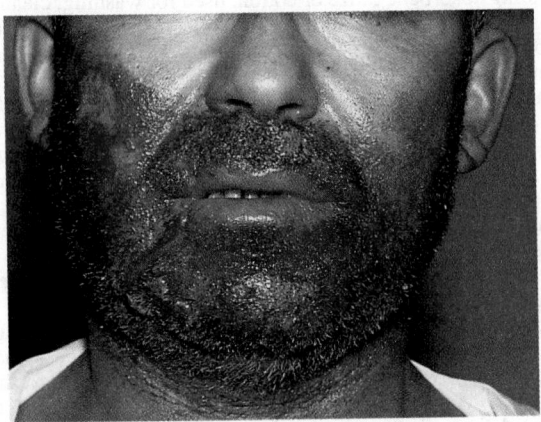

**Sycosis barbae** *(du Vivier, 1993)*

**Sydenham's chorea** /sīd′ənhamz/ [Thomas Sydenham, English physician, 1624–1689; Gk, *choreia,* dance], a form of chorea associated with rheumatic fever, usually occurring during childhood. The cause is a streptococcal infection of the vascular and perivascular tissues of the brain. The choreic movements increase over the first 2 weeks, reach a plateau, and then diminish. The child usually recovers within 10 weeks. With undue exertion or emotional strain, the condition may recur. Also called **chorea minor, rheumatic chorea.**

**syl-.** See **syn-.**

**sylvatic plague** /silvat′ik/ [L, *sylva*, forest, *plaga*, stroke], an endemic disease of wild rodents caused by *Yersinia pestis* and transmitted to humans by the bite of an infected flea. It is found on every continent except Australia. See also **bubonic plague.**

**sylvian aqueduct** /sil′vē·ən/ [Franciscus Sylvius, Dutch anatomist, 1614–1672], L, *aquaductus,* canal], a narrow canal from the third to the fourth ventricle of the midbrain. Also called **Sylvius′ aqueduct.**

**sylvian fissure** [Franciscus Sylvius; L, *fissura*, cleft], the lateral sulcus of the cerebral hemisphere. Also called **sylvian sulcus.**

**Sylvius′ aqueduct.** See **sylvian aqueduct.**

**sym-.** See **syn-.**

**symbiosis** /sim′bē·ō′sis/ [Gk, *syn*, together, *bios*, life], **1.** a mode of living characterized by a close association between organisms of different species. **2.** a state in which two people are emotionally dependent on each other. **3.** a pathologic inability of a child to separate from its mother emotionally and sometimes physically. —**symbiotic,** *adj.*

**symbiotic** /sim′bē·ot′ik/ [Gk, *syn,* together, *bios,* life], characterized by or concerned with symbiosis or living together.

**symbiotic phase,** in Mahler's system of preoedipal development, the stage between 1 and 5 months when the infant participates in a "symbiotic orbit" with the mother. All parts of the mother, including voice, gestures, clothing, and space in which she moves, are joined with the infant.

**symbol** /sim′bəl/ [Gk, *symbolon,* sign], **1.** an image, object, action, or other stimulus that represents something else by reason of conscious association, convention, or another relationship, such as a flag or a statue. **2.** an object, mode of behavior, or feeling that disguises a repressed emotional conflict through an unconscious association rather than through an objective relationship, as in dreams and anxiety.

**-symbolia,** suffix meaning '(condition involving) the ability to interpret symbols': *asymbolia, dyssymbolia, strephosymbolia.*

**symbolism** /sim′bəlizəm/, **1.** the representation or evocation of one idea, action, or object by the use of another, as in systems of writing, poetic language, or dream metaphor. **2.** (in psychiatry) an unconscious mental mechanism characteristic of all human thinking in which a mental image stands for but disguises some other object, person, or thought, especially one associated with emotional conflict. The mechanism is a principal factor in the formation of dreams and in various symptoms resulting from such anxious and psychotic conditions as conversion reactions, obsessions, and compulsions. Also called **symbolization.**

**symelus.** See **symmelus.**

**symmelia** /simē′lyə/ [Gk, *syn,* together, *melos,* limb], a fetal anomaly characterized by the fusion of the lower limbs with or without feet. Kinds of symmelia are **apodial symmelia, dipodial symmelia, monopodial symmelia,** and **tripodial symmelia.**

**symmelus** /sim′ələs/, a malformed fetus characterized by symmelia. Also spelled **symelus.**

**Symmers′ disease.** See **giant follicular lymphoma.**

**Symmetrel,** trademark for an antiviral and antiparkinsonian (amantadine hydrochloride).

**symmetric** /simet′rik/ [Gk, *syn + metron,* measure], (of the body or parts of the body) pertaining to equality in size or shape; very similar in relative placement or arrangement

about an axis. Also **symmetrical.** Compare **asymmetric.** —**symmetry,** *n.*

**symmetric lipomatosis.** See **nodular circumscribed lipomatosis.**

**symmetric orientation,** (in neonatal care) midline positioning of the head with similar alignment of the trunk and extremities. The orientation helps promote even development of tone and function in both sides of the body.

**symmetric tonic neck reflex,** a normal response in infants to assume the crawl position by extending the arms and bending the knees when the head and neck are extended. The reflex disappears when neurologic and muscular development allows independent limb movement for actual crawling. Also called **crawling reflex.** See also **tonic neck reflex.**

**symmetry** /sim′ətrē/ [Gk, *syn,* together, *metron,* measure], (in anatomy) the correspondence of parts on opposite sides of the body, or equality of parts on both sides of a dividing line.

**sympathectomize** /sim′pəthek′təmiz/ [Gk, *sympathein,* to feel with, *ektomē,* excision], to interrupt the conduction of nerve impulses along part of the sympathetic trunk by surgery or drugs.

**sympathectomy** /sim′pəthek′təmē/ [Gk, *sympathein,* to feel with, *ektomē,* excision], a surgical interruption of part of the sympathetic nerve pathways. It is performed for the relief of chronic pain or the promotion of vasodilation in vascular diseases, such as arteriosclerosis, claudication, Buerger's disease, and Raynaud's phenomenon. The sheath around an artery carries the sympathetic nerve fibers that control constriction of the vessel. Removal of the sheath causes the vessel to relax and expand and allows more blood to pass through it. The operation also may be done with a vascular graft, to increase the blood flow through the graft area. Preoperatively the physician may assess the effect of surgery by injecting sympathetic ganglia with a local anesthesia to interrupt temporarily the sympathetic nerve impulses. The nerves lie along the spinal column and are approached through the back or the neck, using local anesthesia. Postoperatively, the adequacy of circulation and peripheral nervous supply in the affected extremity is monitored. An arteriogram shows a widened pathway.

**sympathetic** /sim′pəthet′ik/ [Gk, *sympathein,* to feel with], **1.** displaying of compassion for another's grief. **2.** pertaining to a division of the autonomic nervous system.

**sympathetic eye.** See **sympathizing eye.**

**sympathetic ganglion** [Gk, *sympathein,* to feel with, *ganglion,* knot], a collection of multipolar nerve cells along the course of the sympathetic trunk. Nearly two dozen of the ganglia serve as "cell stations" on efferent pathways between the cervical and sacral parts of the sympathetic trunk.

**sympathetic imbalance** [Gk, *sympathein,* to feel with; L, *in + balance*], pertaining to vagotony, or vagus nerve tension and hyperexcitability of the parasympathetic nervous system, as opposed to the sympathetic nervous system. Also called **vagotonia.**

**sympathetic irritation** [Gk, *sympathein,* to feel with; L, *irritare,* to tease], inflammation of one organ after inflammation of a related organ, such as when trauma to an eye is followed by similar symptoms in the uninjured eye.

**sympathetic nerve** [Gk, *sympathein,* to feel with; L, *nervus*], any nerve of the sympathetic branch of the autonomic nervous system.

**sympathetic nervous system.** See **autonomic nervous system.**

**sympathetic ophthalmia,** a granulomatous inflammation of the uveal tract of both eyes occurring after an injury to the uveal tract of one eye. Corticosteroids may be helpful in treatment, but surgical enucleation of the originally injured eye may be necessary to preserve vision in the uninjured eye. Also called **metastatic ophthalmia, migratory ophthalmia.**

**sympathetic pain,** distress that occurs in the hemiplegic shoulder as a result of muscle imbalance, with a loss of joint range. It results from loss of active and passive motion, loss of ability to bear weight, and long-standing subluxation without support.

**sympathetic symptom** [Gk, *sympathein*, to feel with, *symptoma*, that which occurs], a symptom occurring in one body area when the causative lesion is actually in another area. See also **referred pain.**

**sympathetic trunk,** one of a pair of chains of ganglia extending along the side of the vertebral column from the base of the skull to the coccyx. Each trunk is part of the sympathetic nervous system and consists of a series of ganglia connected by various types of fibers. Each sympathetic trunk distributes branches with postganglionic fibers to the autonomic plexuses, the cranial nerves, the individual organs, the nerves accompanying arteries, and the spinal nerves.

**sympathize.** See **sympathy.**

**sympathizing eye** /sim′pəthī′zing/, (in sympathetic ophthalmia) the fellow eye that becomes inflamed by lymphatic or blood-borne metastasis of the causative antigen or microorganism. Also called **sympathetic eye.**

**sympatholytic, sympatholytic agent.** See **antiadrenergic.**

**sympathomimetic** /sim′pəthō′mimet′ik/ [Gk, *sympathein* + *mimesis*, imitation], denoting a pharmacologic agent that mimics the effects of stimulation of organs and structures by the sympathetic nervous system. It functions by occupying adrenergic receptor sites and acting as an agonist or by increasing the release of the neurotransmitter norepinephrine at postganglionic nerve endings. Various sympathomimetic agents are used as decongestants of nasal and ocular mucosa, such as bronchodilators in the treatment of asthma, bronchitis, bronchiectasis, and emphysema; and vasopressors and cardiac stimulants in the treatment of acute hypotension and shock; they are also used for maintaining normal blood pressure during operations using spinal anesthesia. Drugs in this group include cyclopentamine, dobutamine, dopamine, ephedrine, isoproterenol, metaproterenol, metaraminol, mephentermine, methoxamine, methoxyphenamine, naphazoline, norepinephrine, phenylephrine, phenylpropanolamine, propylhexedrine, protokylol, pseudoephedrine, terbutaline sulfate, tetrahydrozoline, tuaminoheptane, xylometazoline, and epinephrine, a synthetic isomer of the hormone secreted by the adrenal medulla. Adverse effects of sympathomimetic drugs may be nervousness, severe headache, anxiety, vertigo, nausea, vomiting, dilated pupils, glycosuria, and dysuria. Also called **adrenergic drug.**

**sympathomimetic amine.** See **adrenergic.**

**sympathomimetic bronchodilator,** a medication that reduces bronchial muscle spasm through action that mimics the sympathetic nervous system in producing smooth muscle relaxation. It is commonly a beta₂ receptor agonist agent.

**sympathy** /sim′pəthē/ [Gk, *sympathein*], **1.** an expressed interest or concern regarding the problems, emotions, or states of mind of another. Compare **empathy. 2.** the relation that exists between the mind and body, causing the one to be affected by the other. **3.** mental contagion or the influence exerted by one individual or group on another and the ef-

fects produced, such as the spread of panic, uncontrollable laughter, or yawning. **4.** the physiologic or pathologic relationship between two organs, systems, or parts of the body. —**sympathetic,** *adj.,* **sympathize,** *v.*

**symphalangia** /sim′fəlan′jē·ə/ [Gk, *syn,* together, *phalanx,* finger], **1.** a condition, usually inherited, characterized by ankylosis of the fingers or toes. **2.** a congenital anomaly in which webbing of the fingers or toes occurs in varying degrees, often in conjunction with other defects of the hands or feet. Also called **symphalangism.** See also **syndactyly.**

**symphocephalus** /sim′fōsef′ələs/ [Gk, *symphes,* growing together, *kephale,* head], twin fetuses joined at the head. The term is often used as a general designation for fetuses with varying degrees of the anomaly. See also **craniopagus, syncephalus.**

**symphyseal angle** /simfiz′ē·əl/ [Gk, *symphysis,* growing together; L, *angulus,* corner], the angle of the chin, which may be classified as protruding, straight, or receding.

**symphyses, symphysic.** See **symphysis.**

**symphysic teratism** /simfiz′ik/, a congenital anomaly in which there is a fusion of normally separated parts or organs, such as a horseshoe kidney, or in which parts close prematurely, such as the skull bones in craniostenosis.

**symphysis** /sim′fəsis/, *pl.* **symphyses** [Gk, growing together], **1.** also called **fibrocartilaginous joint.** A line of union, especially a cartilaginous joint in which adjacent bony surfaces are firmly united by fibrocartilage. **2.** *informal.* symphysis pubis. —**symphysic,** *adj.*

**symphysis menti,** **1.** the junction between the two halves of the mandible. **2.** the prominence of the chin.

**symphysis pubis.** See **pubic symphysis.**

**sympodia** /simpō′dē·ə/ [Gk, *syn,* together, *pous,* foot], a congenital developmental anomaly characterized by fusion of the lower extremities. See also **sirenomelus, sympus.**

**symptom** /simp′təm/ [Gk, *symptoma,* that which happens], a subjective indication of a disease or a change in condition as perceived by the patient. For example, the halo symptom of glaucoma is seen by the patient as colored rings around a single light source. Many symptoms are accompanied by objective signs, such as pruritus, which is often reported with erythema and a maculopapular eruption on the skin. Some symptoms may be objectively confirmed, such as numbness of a body part, which may be confirmed by absence of response to a pin prick. **Primary symptoms** are symptoms that are intrinsically associated with a disease. **Secondary symptoms** are a consequence of illness and disease. Compare **sign.**

**symptomatic** /simp′təmat′ik/ [Gk, *symptoma,* that which happens], having characteristics of a symptom or indications of a specific disease.

**symptomatic esophageal peristalsis,** a condition in which peristaltic progression in the body of the esophagus is normal but contractions in the distal esophagus are increased in amplitude and duration. Also called **esophageal spasm, nutcracker esophagus.**

**symptomatic impotence** [Gk, *symptoma,* that which happens; L, *in* + *potentia,* power], impotence that is the result of poor health or the use of medications.

**symptomatic nanism,** dwarfism associated with defects in bone growth, tooth formation, and sexual development.

**symptomatic neuralgia** [Gk, *symptoma,* that which happens, *neuron,* nerve, *algos,* pain], nerve pain that is secondary to a disease condition.

**symptomatic torticollis** [Gk, *symptoma* + L, *tortus,* twisted, *collum,* neck], stiff neck caused by a disease in the neck, such as rheumatoid torticollis or myogenic torticollis.

**symptomatic treatment.** See **treatment.**

**symptomatology** /simp'təmətol'əjē/ [Gk, *symptoma* + *logos*, science], the science of symptoms of disease in general or of the symptoms of a specific disease.

**symptom-bearer,** (in psychology) a family member frequently seen as the patient who is functioning poorly because family dynamics interferes with functioning at a higher level. Also known as the *identified patient.*

**symptom complex.** See **syndrome.**

**symptom control,** a nursing outcome from the Nursing Outcomes Classification (NOC) defined as the personal actions to minimize perceived adverse changes in physical and emotional functioning. See also **Nursing Outcomes Classification.**

**symptomless carrier.** See **passive carrier.**

**symptom severity,** a nursing outcome from the Nursing Outcomes Classification (NOC) defined as the extent of perceived adverse changes in physical, emotional, and social functioning. See also **Nursing Outcomes Classification.**

**symptom severity: perimenopause,** a nursing outcome from the Nursing Outcomes Classification (NOC) defined as the extent of symptoms caused by declining hormonal levels. See also **Nursing Outcomes Classification.**

**symptom severity: premenstrual syndrome (PMS),** a nursing outcome from the Nursing Outcomes Classification (NOC) defined as the extent of symptoms caused by cyclic hormonal fluctuations. See also **Nursing Outcomes Classification.**

**symptothermal method of family planning** /simp'-təthur'məl/ [Gk, *symptoma* + *therme*, heat], a natural method of family planning that incorporates the ovulation and basal body temperature methods of family planning. It is more effective than either method used alone and requires fewer days of abstinence from sexual intercourse because it allows the fertile period of the menstrual cycle to be more precisely identified.

**sympus** /sim'pəs/ [Gk, *syn*, together, *pous*, foot], a malformed fetus in which the lower extremities are completely fused or rotated and the pelvis and genitalia are defective. Kinds of sympuses are **sirenomelus, sympus dipus,** and **sympus monopus.** See also **symmelus.**

**sympus apus.** See **sirenomelus.**

**sympus dipus** /dē'pəs/, a malformed fetus in which the lower extremities are fused and both feet are formed.

**sympus monopus** /mon'əpəs/, a malformed fetus in which the lower extremities are fused and one foot is formed. Also called **monopodial symmelia, uromelus.**

**syn-, sy-, syl-, sym-,** prefix meaning 'union, or association': *synalgia, syncephalus, synchronous.*

**synactive model of infant behavior** /sinak'tiv/, a major theoretic framework for establishing physiologic stability as the foundation for the organization of motor, behavioral state, and attentive/interactive behaviors in neonates.

**synadelphus** /sin'ədel'fəs/, pl. **synadelphi** [Gk, *syn* + *adelphos*, brother], a conjoined twin with a single head and trunk and eight limbs. Also called **syndelphus, cephalothoracoiliopagus.**

**Synalar,** trademark for a glucocorticoid (fluocinolone acetonide).

**Synanon,** a residential center that provides a therapeutic community approach to rehabilitation of drug abusers.

**synapse** /sin'aps, sinaps'/ [Gk, *synaptein*, to join], **1.** the region surrounding the point of contact between two neurons or between a neuron and an effector organ, across which nerve impulses are transmitted through the action of a neurotransmitter, such as acetylcholine or norepinephrine. When an impulse reaches the terminal point of one neuron, it causes the release of the neurotransmitter. The neurotransmitter diffuses across the gap between the two cells to bind with receptors in the other neuron, muscle, or gland, triggering electrical changes that either inhibit or continue the transmission of the impulse. Synapses are polarized so that nerve impulses normally travel in only one direction; they are also subject to fatigue, oxygen deficiency, anesthetics, and other chemical agents. Kinds of synapses include **axoaxonic synapse, axodendritic synapse, axodendrosomatic synapse, axosomatic synapse,** and **dendrodendritic synapse.** Compare **ephapse. 2.** to form a synapse or connection between neurons. **3.** (in genetics) to form a synaptic fusion between homologous chromosomes during meiosis. —**synaptic,** *adj.*

**synapsis** /sinap'sis/, *pl.* **synapses,** the pairing of homologous chromosomes during early meiotic prophase in gametogenesis to form double or bivalent chromosomes.

**synaptic** /sinap'tik/ [Gk, *synaptein*, to join], pertaining to or resembling a synapse.

**synaptic cleft,** the microscopic extracellular space at the synapse that separates the membrane of the terminal nerve endings of a presynaptic neuron and the membrane of a postsynaptic cell. Nerve impulses are transmitted across this cleft by means of a neurotransmitter. See also **neuromuscular junction.** Also called **synaptic gap.**

**synaptic junction,** the membranes of both the presynaptic neuron and the postsynaptic receptor cell together with the synaptic cleft. See also **synapse.**

**synaptic transmission,** the passage of a neural impulse across a synapse from one nerve fiber to another by means of a neurotransmitter. Compare **ephaptic transmission.**

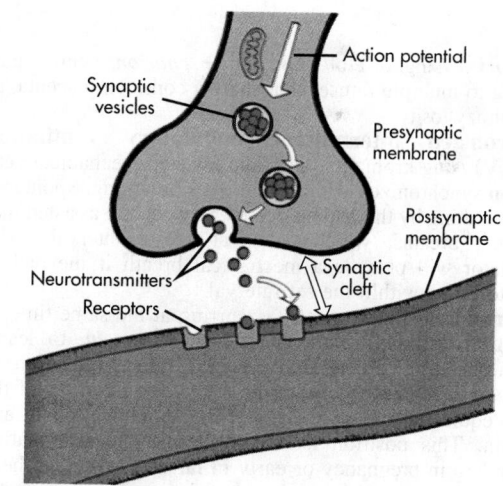

**Synaptic transmission** *(Chipps, Clanin, and Campbell, 1992)*

**synaptogenesis** /sinap'tōjen'əsis/, the formation of synapses between neurons. In humans it begins early in gestation but occurs most rapidly from 2 months before birth to 2 years after birth.

**synaptosome** /sinap'təsōm'/, a presynaptic nerve terminal that has been separated from the rest of the neuron and isolated from homogenates of brain tissue. It appears as a membrane-bound structure containing synaptic vesicles.

**synarthrosis,** any of several immovable articulations. See also **fibrous joint.**

**syncephalus** /sinsef′ələs/ [Gk, *syn* + *kephale,* head], a conjoined twin having a single head and two bodies. Also called **monocephalus.**

**synchilia** /singkē′lyə/ /singkē′lē·ə/ [Gk, *syn* + *cheilos,* lip], a congenital anomaly in which there is complete or partial fusion of the lips; atresia of the mouth. Also spelled **syncheilia.**

**synchondrosis** /sing′kondrō′sis/, *pl.* **synchondroses** [Gk, *syn* + *chondros,* cartilage], a cartilaginous joint creating a union between two immovable bones, such as the synchondroses of the cranium, the pubic symphysis, the sternum, and the manubrium.

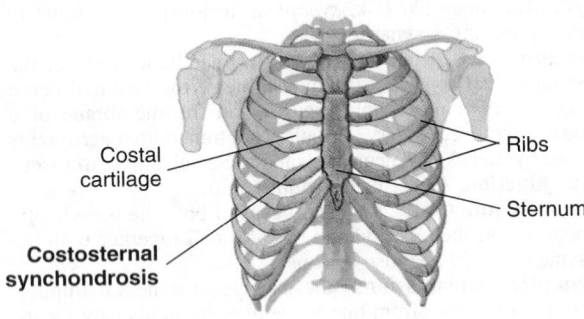

Costal cartilage
Ribs
Sternum
**Costosternal synchondrosis**

**Synchondroses of the ribs and sternum**
*(Thibodeau and Patton, 1999/David J. Mascaro and Associates)*

**synchorial** /singkôr′ē·əl/ [Gk, *syn* + *chorion,* skin], pertaining to multiple fetuses that share a common placenta, as in monozygosity.

**synchronized intermittent mandatory ventilation (SIMV)** /sing′krənīzd/, periodic assisted mechanical ventilation synchronized with the patient's breathing. Spontaneous breathing by the patient occurs between the assisted mechanical breaths, which occur at preset intervals. The ventilator will provide a mechanical breath if the patient fails to do so within the set interval.

**synchronous** /sing′krənəs/, occurring at the same time.

**synclitism** /sing′klitiz′əm/ [Gk, *syn* + *klinein,* to lean], **1.** (in obstetrics) a condition in which the sagittal suture of the fetal head is in line with the transverse diameter of the inlet, equidistant from the maternal symphysis pubis and sacrum. This position is usually found on examination either late in pregnancy or early in labor, as the fetal head descends into the pelvic inlet. As labor progresses, posterior asynclitism develops, and, as the head descends farther, anterior asynclitism is evident because of the shape of the true pelvis below the inlet. **2.** (in hematology) the normal condition in which the nucleus and the cytoplasm of the blood cells mature simultaneously and at the same rate.

**syncope** /sing′kəpē/ [Gk, *synkoptein,* to cut short], a brief lapse in consciousness caused by transient cerebral hypoxia. It is usually preceded by a sensation of light-headedness and often may be prevented by lying down or by sitting with the head between the knees. It may be caused by many different factors, including emotional stress, vagal stimulation, vascular pooling in the legs, diaphoresis, and a sudden change in environmental temperature or body position. Also called **fainting.**

**syncretic thinking** /singkret′ik/ [Gk, *synkretismos,* combined beliefs; AS, *thencan,* to think], a stage in the development of the cognitive thought processes of the child. During this phase thought is based purely on what is perceived and experienced. The child is incapable of reasoning beyond the observable or of making deductions or generalizations. Through imaginative play, questioning, interaction with others, and the increasing use of language and symbols to represent objects, the child begins to learn to make associations between ideas and to elaborate concepts. In Piaget's classification, this stage occurs between 2 and 7 years of age and is preceded by the sensorimotor stage of development, when the child progresses from reflex activity to repetitive and imitative behavior. Compare **abstract thinking, concrete thinking.** —**syncresis,** *n.*

**syncytia.** See **syncytium.**

**syncytial** /sinsish′əl/, pertaining to a syncytium.

**syncytial virus,** a virus that induces the formation of syncytia, particularly in cell cultures.

**syncytiotrophoblast** /sinsish′ē·ōtrof′əblast′/ [Gk, *syn* + *kytos,* cell, *trophe,* nutrition, *blastos,* germ], the outer syncytial layer of the trophoblast of an early mammalian embryo. It erodes the uterine wall during implantation and gives rise to the villi of the placenta. Also called **plasmidotrophoblast, syncytial trophoblast, syntrophoblast.** Compare **cytotrophoblast.** —**syncytiotrophoblastic,** *adj.*

**syncytium** /sinsit′ē·əm/, *pl.* **syncytia** [Gk, *syn* + *kytos,* cell], a group of cells in which the cytoplasm of one cell is continuous with that of adjoining cells, resulting in a multinucleate unit. —**syncytial,** *adj.*

**syndactyl, syndactylia, syndactylism, syndactylous.** See **syndactyly.**

**syndactylus** /sindak′tiləs/, a person with webbed fingers or toes.

**syndactyly** /sindak′təlē/ [Gk, *syn* + *daktylos,* finger], a congenital anomaly characterized by the fusion of the fingers or toes. It varies in degree of severity from incomplete webbing of the skin of two digits to complete union of digits and fusion of the bones and nails. Also called **syndactylia, syndactylism.** —**syndactyl, syndactylous,** *adj.*

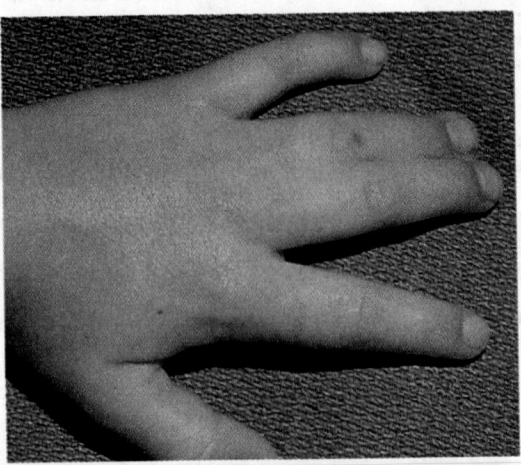

**Mild syndactyly of the fingers** *(Zitelli and Davis, 1997)*

**syndelphus.** See **synadelphus.**

**syndesis** /sin′dəsis/ [Gk, *syn*, together, *dein*, to bind], surgical fixation of a joint. Also called **arthrodesis.**

**syndesmo-,** combining form meaning 'connective tissue or particularly the ligaments': *syndesmochorial, syndesmography, syndesmoma.*

**syndesmophyte** /sindez′məfīt/, a bony growth attached to a ligament. It is found between adjacent vertebrae in ankylosing spondylitis.

**syndesmosis** /sin′desmō′sis/, *pl.* **syndesmoses** [Gk, *syndesmos*, ligament], a fibrous union in which two bones are connected by interosseous ligaments, such as the anterior and the posterior ligaments in the radioulnar and tibiofibular articulations. Compare **gomphosis, sutura.**

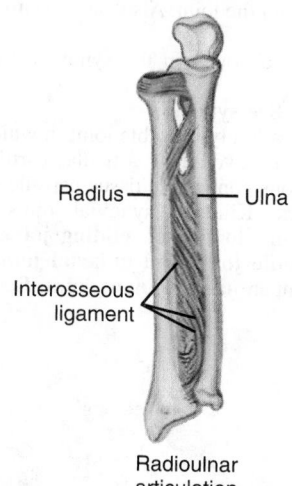

Radius — — Ulna

Interosseous ligament

Radioulnar articulation

**Syndesmosis** *(Thibodeau and Patton, 1999)*

**syndrome** /sin′drəm/ [Gk, *syn*, together, *dromos*, course], a complex of signs and symptoms resulting from a common cause or appearing, in combination, to present a clinical picture of a disease or inherited abnormality. See also specific syndromes. Also called **symptom complex.**

**syndrome of inappropriate antidiuretic hormone secretion (SIADH),** an abnormal condition characterized by the excessive release of antidiuretic hormone (ADH) that alters the body's fluid and electrolytic balances. It results in various malfunctions, such as the inability to produce and secrete dilute urine, water retention, increased extracellular fluid volume, and hyponatremia. SIADH develops in association with diseases that affect the osmoreceptors of the hypothalamus. Oat cell carcinoma of the lung is the most common cause, affecting about 80% of involved patients. Less common causes are disorders that affect the central nervous system, such as brain tumors and lupus erythematosus; pulmonary diseases, such as pneumonia; cancers of the pancreas and the prostate; and pathologic reactions to various drugs, such as chlorpropamide, vincristine sulfate, carbamazepine, and clofibrate. Prognosis depends on the underlying disease, promptness of diagnosis and treatment, and the response to treatment.

■ OBSERVATIONS: Common signs and symptoms of SIADH are weight gain despite anorexia, vomiting, nausea, muscle weakness, and irritability. In some patients SIADH may produce coma and convulsions. Most of the free water associated with this syndrome is intracellular, and associated edema is rare unless excess water volume exceeds 4 mOsm. Confirming diagnosis is based on urine osmolality that exceeds 150 mOsm/kg of water and serum osmolality of less than 280 mOsm/kg of water. Normal urine osmolality is 1.5 times serum osmolality. Other significant results include less than normal concentrations of blood urea nitrogen, serum creatinine, and albumin and a concentration of sodium in the urine higher than normal.

■ INTERVENTIONS: Treatment of SIADH commonly includes restriction of water intake and may require administration of normal saline solution to raise the serum sodium level if water intoxication is severe. Furosemide may be administered to block circulatory overload, and drugs, such as demeclocycline hydrochloride and lithium, may be administered to block renal response to ADH. Surgery and chemotherapy are other alternatives to remove or destroy neoplasms that may be the underlying causes of this syndrome.

■ NURSING CONSIDERATIONS: The SIADH patient is monitored for any signs of hyponatremia, weight change, and fluid imbalance. The patient is carefully advised on the importance of restricted water intake to prevent water intoxication and is closely observed for any indications of restlessness, congestive heart failure, and convulsions.

**syndrome X,** a condition characterized by hypertension with obesity, type 2 diabetes mellitus, hypertriglyceridemia, increased peripheral insulin resistance, hyperinsulinemia, and elevated catecholamine levels.

**synechia** /sinek′ē·ə/, *pl.* **synechiae** [Gk, continuity], an adhesion, especially of the iris to the cornea or lens of the eye. It may develop from glaucoma, cataracts, uveitis, or keratitis or as a complication of surgery or trauma to the eye. Synechiae may prevent or impede flow of aqueous fluid between the anterior and posterior chambers of the eye, resulting in angle closure glaucoma. Treatment consists of dilation of the pupils with a mydriatic agent and/or intraocular injection of tissue plasminogen activator enzyme (TPA) to melt the synechialytic tissue.

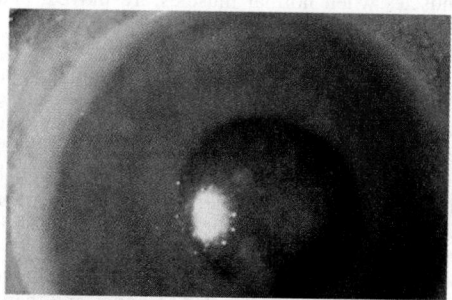

**Synechia** *(Michelson and Friedlaender, 1996)*

**synechiotomy** /sinek′ē·ot′əmē/ [Gk, *synechia*, continuity, *temnein*, to cut], the surgical division of an adhesion.

**Synemol,** trademark for a glucocorticoid (fluocinolone acetonide).

**syneresis** /siner′əsis/ [Gk, *syn* + *hairein*, to draw], the drawing together or coagulation of particles of a gel with separation from the medium in which the particles were suspended, such as occurs in blood clot retraction.

**synergic.**   See **synergistic.**

**synergism.**   See **synergy.**

**synergist** /sin′ərjist/ [Gk, *syn* + *ergein*, to work],   an organ, agent, or substance that augments the activity of another organ, agent, or substance.

**synergistic** /sin′ərjis′tik/ [Gk, *syn*, together, *ergein*, to work],   pertaining to the acting or working together of a number of components, as when groups of muscles function in a coordinated manner. Also **synergic** /sinūr′jik/.

**synergistic agent,**   a substance that augments or adds to the activity of another substance or agent. See also **synergy,** def. 4.

**synergistic muscles,**   groups of muscles that contract together to accomplish the same body movement.

**synergy** /sin′ərjē/ [Gk, *syn* + *ergein*, to work],   **1.** the process in which two organs, substances, or agents work simultaneously to enhance the function and effect of one another. **2.** the coordinated action of a set of muscles that work together to produce a specific movement, as in a reflex action. **3.** a combined action of different parts of the autonomic nervous system, as in the sympathetic and parasympathetic innervation of secreting cells of the salivary glands, with both systems having a secretory effect. **4.** the interaction of two or more drugs to produce a certain effect, as in the exaggerated response to tyramine in a person who is treated with a monoamine oxidase inhibitor. Also called **synergism.**

**synesthesia** /sin′esthē′zhə/,   a phenomenon in which sensations of two or more modalities accompany one another, as when a visual sensation is experienced when a particular sound is heard. Also called **secondary sensation.**

**syngeneic** /sin′jənē′ik/ [Gk, *syn* + *genesis*, origin],   **1.** denoting an individual or cell that has the same genotype as another individual or cell. **2.** denoting tissues that are antigenically similar. Also called **isogeneic.** Compare **allogenic, xenogeneic.**

**syngenesis.**   See **sexual reproduction.**

**Synkayvite,**   trademark for a brand of menadione, synthetic vitamin K₃.

**synkinesis** /sin′kinē′sis/ [Gk, *syn*, together, *kinesis*, movement],   an involuntary movement by one part of the body when an intentional movement is made by another part. In imitative synkinesis, movement may be detected in paralyzed muscles when normal muscles are moved, and vice versa.

**synophthalmia.**   See **cyclopia.**

**Synophylate GG,**   trademark for a bronchodilator (theophylline sodium glycinate).

**synopsis** /sinop′sis/ [Gk, *syn*, together, *opsis*, vision],   a brief review, condensation, summary, or abridgment.

**synostosis** /sin′ostō′sis/ [Gk, *syn*, together, *osteon*, bone],   the joining of two bones by the ossification of connecting tissues. It occurs normally in the fusion of cranial bones to form the skull.

**synostotic joint** /sin′ostot′ik/ [Gk, *syn* + *osteon*, bone],   a joint in which bones are connected to bones and there is no movement between them, as in the bones of the adult sacrum or skull.

**synotia** /sīnō′shə/ [Gk, *syn* + *ous*, ear],   a congenital malformation characterized by the union or approximation of the ears in front of the neck, often accompanied by the absence or defective development of the lower jaw. Compare **agnathia.** See also **otocephaly.**

**synotus** /sīnō′təs/,   a fetus with synotia.

**synovectomy** /sin′ōvek′təmē/ [Gk, *syn* + L, *ovum*, egg; Gk, *ektomē*, excision],   the removal of a synovial membrane of a joint.

**synovia** /sinō′vē·ə/,   a clear, viscous fluid, resembling the white of an egg, secreted by synovial membranes and acting as a lubricant for many joints, bursae, and tendons. It contains mucin, albumin, fat, and mineral salts. Also called **synovial fluid.**

**synovial** /sinō′vē·əl/,   pertaining to, consisting of, or secreting synovia, the lubricating fluid of the joints, bursae, and tendon sheaths.

**synovial bursa,**   one of the many closed sacs filled with synovial fluid in the connective tissue between the muscles, the tendons, the ligaments, and the bones. The synovial bursae facilitate the gliding of muscles and tendons over bony and ligamentous prominences. Compare **synovial membrane, synovial tendon sheath.**

**synovial chondroma,**   a rare cartilaginous growth developing in the connective tissue below the synovial membrane of the joints, tendon sheaths, or bursa. Foci on the surface may develop stalks and then detach, resulting in numerous loose bodies within the joint. Also called **synovial chondromatosis.**

**synovial crypt,**   a pouch in the synovial membrane of a joint.

**synovial fluid.**   See **synovia.**

**synovial joint,**   a freely movable joint in which contiguous bony surfaces are covered by articular cartilage and connected by a fibrous connective tissue capsule lined with synovial membrane. Kinds of synovial joints are **ball and socket joint, condyloid joint, gliding joint, hinge joint, pivot joint, saddle joint,** and **uniaxial joint.** Also called **diarthrosis.** Compare **cartilaginous joint, fibrous joint.**

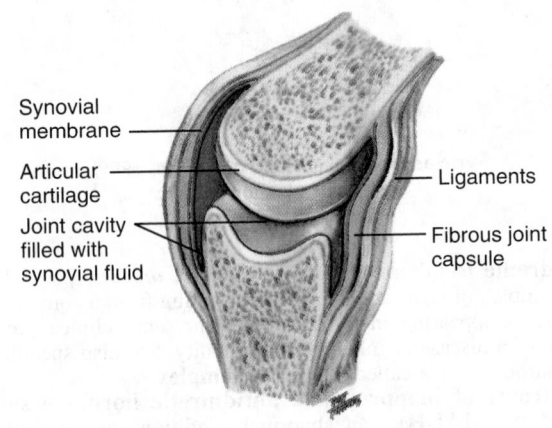

Synovial membrane —
Articular cartilage —
Joint cavity filled with synovial fluid —
— Ligaments
— Fibrous joint capsule

**Synovial joint** *(Applegate, 2000)*

**synovial membrane,**   the thin layer of tissue lining the articular capsule surrounding a freely movable joint. The synovial membrane is loosely attached to the external fibrous capsule. It secretes into the joint a thick fluid that normally lubricates the joint but that may accumulate in painful amounts when the joint is injured. Compare **synovial bursa, synovial tendon sheath.**

**synovial sac,**   a herniation of a synovial membrane beyond the confines of a joint.

**synovial sarcoma,**   a malignant tumor, composed of synovioblasts, that begins as a soft swelling and often metastasizes through the bloodstream to the lung before it is discovered.

**synovial sheath,** any one of the membranous sacs enclosing a tendon of a muscle and facilitating the gliding of a tendon through a fibrous or a bony tunnel, such as that under the flexor retinaculum of the wrist.

**synovial tendon sheath,** one of the many membranous channels or tubes enclosing various tendons that glide through fibrous and bony tunnels in the body, such as those under the flexor retinaculum of the wrist. One layer of the synovial sheath lines the tunnel; the other covers the tendon. The sheath secretes synovial fluid, which lubricates the tendon. Compare **synovial bursa, synovial membrane.**

**synovitis** /sin′əvī′tis/, an inflammatory condition of the synovial membrane of a joint as the result of an aseptic wound or a traumatic injury, such as a sprain or severe strain. The knee is most commonly affected. Fluid accumulates around the capsule; the joint is swollen, tender, and painful; and motion is restricted. In most cases, the inflammation subsides, and the fluid is resorbed without medical or surgical intervention.

**synovium** /sinō′vē-əm/, a synovial membrane.

**syntactic aphasia** /sintak′tik/ [Gk, *syn,* together, *taxis,* arrangement, *a, phasis,* not speech], an inability to arrange words in a logical sequence, with the result that what is spoken is not understood.

**syntax** /sin′taks/ [Gk, *syn + taxis,* arrangement], word order; sentence order; a property of language involving structural cues for the arrangement of words as elements in a phrase, clause, or sentence.

**syntaxic mode** /sintaks′ik/, the ability to perceive whole, logical, coherent pictures as they occur in reality, according to the H.S. Sullivan theory of psychology.

**synteny** /sin′tənē/ [Gk, *syn + taina,* ribbon], (in genetics) the presence on the same chromosome of two or more genes that may or may not be transmitted as a linkage group but that appear to be able to undergo independent assortment during meiosis. The term is used primarily in human genetics, where linked inheritance patterns are more difficult to determine. See also **linkage.**

**synthermal** /sinthur′məl/, possessing the same temperature.

**synthesis** /sin′thəsis/ [Gk, *synthenai,* to put together], a level of cognitive learning in which the individual puts together the elements of previous learning levels to create a unified whole.

**-synthesis,** combining form meaning 'putting together or formation of': *narcosynthesis, psychosynthesis, velosynthesis.*

**synthesize** /sin′thəsīz/ [Gk, *synthesis,* putting together], to form by building, as in forming complex chemical compounds such as proteins from simpler units of amino acids.

**synthetic** /sinthet′ik/, pertaining to a substance that is produced by an artificial rather than a natural process or material.

**synthetic chemistry,** the science dealing with the formation of more complex chemical compounds from simpler substances.

**synthetic human growth hormone,** a synthetic form of somatotropin produced by recombinant deoxyribonucleic acid techniques from a strain of *Escherichia coli* bacteria. The polypeptide hormone consists of 191 amino acid residues in a sequence identical to that of natural human growth hormone.

**synthetic insulin** [Gk, *synthesis,* putting together; L, *insula,* island], a form of insulin synthesized in a non-disease-producing strain of *Escherichia coli* bacteria or in yeast cells that has been genetically altered by the addition of the human gene for insulin production.

**synthetic oleovitamin D.** See **viosterol.** See **artificial saliva.**

**synthetic saliva.** See **artificial saliva.**

**synthetic vaccines,** prophylactic immunization substances prepared by artificial techniques, such as through peptide synthesis or cloning of deoxyribonucleic acid.

**Synthroid,** trademark for a thyroid hormone (levothyroxine sodium).

**Syntocinon,** trademark for an oxytocic (oxytocin).

**syntrophism** /sin′trəfiz′əm/, **1.** mutual dependence for food or other resources. **2.** a condition in which two strains of bacteria can grow together in a mixed culture in a medium that would not support either alone; each strain produces a nutrient required by the other.

**syntrophoblast.** See **syncytiotrophoblast.**

**syntropy** /sin′trəpē/ [Gk, *syn,* together, *trepein,* to turn] a tendency for two diseases to merge into one.

**syphilis** /sif′ilis/ [from the name of a literary figure (1530) who was thus infected (literally, L, lover of swine)], a sexually transmitted disease caused by the spirochete *Treponema pallidum,* characterized by distinct stages of effects over a period of years. Any organ system may become involved. The spirochete is able to pass through the human placenta, producing congenital syphilis. Also called **lues.**

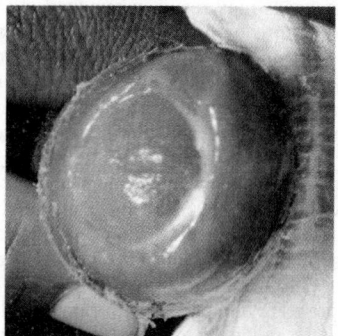

**Primary syphilis**
*(Greenberger and Hinthorn, 1992/courtesy Dr. W.S. Royster, U.S. Public Health Service, Kansas City, Missouri)*

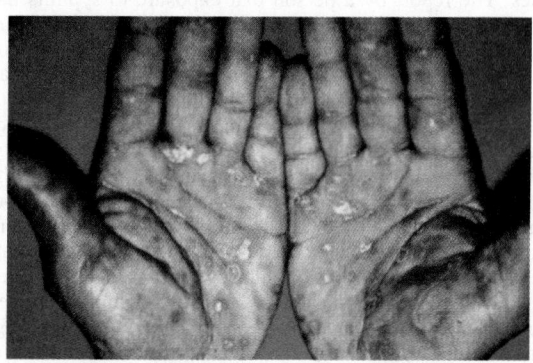

**Secondary syphilis** *(Goldstein and Goldstein, 1997)*

■ OBSERVATIONS: The first stage (**primary syphilis**) is marked by the appearance of a small painless red pustule on the skin or mucous membrane between 10 and 90 days after exposure. The lesion may appear anywhere on the body where contact with a lesion on an infected person has occurred, but it is seen most often in the anogenital region. It quickly erodes, forming a painless, bloodless ulcer, called a *chancre,* exuding a fluid that swarms with spirochetes. The chancre may not be noticed by the patient, and many people may become infected. It heals spontaneously within 10 to 40 days, often creating the mistaken impression that it was not a serious symptom. The second stage (**secondary syphilis**) occurs about 2 months later, after the spirochetes have increased in number and spread throughout the body. This stage is characterized by general malaise, anorexia, nausea, fever, headache, alopecia, bone and joint pain, or the appearance of a morbilliform rash that does not itch, flat white sores in the mouth and throat, or condylomata lata papules on the moist areas of the skin. The disease remains highly contagious at this stage and can be spread by kissing. The symptoms usually continue for from 3 weeks to 3 months but may recur over a period of 2 years. The third stage (**tertiary syphilis**) may not develop for 3 to 15 or more years. It is characterized by the appearance of soft rubbery tumors, called *gummas,* that ulcerate and heal by scarring. Gummas may develop anywhere on the surface of the body and in the eye, liver, lungs, stomach, or reproductive organs. Tertiary syphilis may be painless, unnoticed except for gummas, or it may be accompanied by deep, burrowing pain. The ulceration of the gummas may result in punched-out areas of the palate, nasal septum, or larynx. Various tissues and structures of the body, including the central nervous system, myocardium, and valves of the heart, may be damaged or destroyed, leading to mental or physical disability and premature death. **Congenital syphilis** resulting from prenatal infection may result in the birth of a deformed or blind infant. In some cases, the infant appears to be well until, at several weeks of age, snuffles, sometimes with a blood-stained or mucopurulent discharge, and skin lesions, particularly on the palms and soles or in the genital region, are observed. Such children also may have visual or hearing defects, and progeria and poor health may develop. Diagnosis of syphilis is made by dark field microscopy of fluid from primary or secondary stage lesions, by bacteriologic study of blood samples, and by an examination of cerebrospinal fluid. Because of the slow development of the disease during the early stages, the various serologic tests, including the obsolete Wassermann, may not produce accurate findings until months after exposure. Repeated tests and cross-checking with more than one test may be required in some cases. The report by a person that exposure to syphilis has occurred is often the only evidence available to the clinician. ■ INTERVENTIONS: Patients with primary or secondary syphilis are usually given benzathine, penicillin G benzathine, or an equivalent in a single dose of 2.4 million units intramuscularly. The objective is to maintain penicillin in the bloodstream for a number of days, because *Treponema pallidum* divides at an average rate of once every 33 hours, and the antibiotic is most effective during the stage of cell division. Larger doses of penicillin, 7.2 million units total, are administered in 3 doses 1 week apart for tertiary syphilis. Infants and small children with congenital syphilis are usually given 50,000 units/kg intramuscularly. Treatment of an infected mother with penicillin during the first 4 months of pregnancy usually prevents the development of congenital syphilis in the fetus. Treating the mother with antibiotics later in the pregnancy eliminates the infection but may not protect the fetus. Patients should be reexamined clinically and serologically 3 months and 6 months after treatment. Human immunodeficiency virus-infected patients (also infected with syphilis) should be seen at 1, 2, 3, 6, 9, and 12 months for follow-up observation. ■ NURSING CONSIDERATIONS: Special care and aseptic precautions are taken while handling the highly contagious fluid from syphilitic lesions used in diagnostic testing, because the infection may be acquired through a cut or break in the skin. The nurse discusses with the patient the disease course, its treatment, and ways of preventing future infections. The extremely contagious nature of the infection is explained, and the importance of treatment for all who may have been exposed is emphasized. Tact, patience, and understanding are required to reassure the patient and to secure the patient's cooperation in accepting treatment and in assisting in the identification and location of others needing treatment. Active, serologically documented cases of syphilis must, by law, be reported to local departments of health throughout the United States. See also **chancre, Hutchinson's teeth, Hutchinson's triad, snuffles.**

**syphilitic,** pertaining to, resembling, or infected with syphilis. Also **luetic** /loo·et′ik/.

**syphilitic aortitis,** inflammation of the aorta occurring in tertiary syphilis. It is characterized by diffuse dilation with gray, wheal-like plaques containing calcium on the inside and scars and wrinkles on the outside of the aorta. The middle layer of the aortic wall is usually infiltrated with plasma cells and contains fragments of damaged elastic tissue and many newly formed blood vessels. There may be damage to the cardiac valves, narrowing of the mouths of the coronary arteries, and formation of thrombi. Cerebral embolism may result. Signs of syphilitic aortitis are substernal pain, dyspnea, bounding pulse, and high systolic blood pressure. Penicillin may slow the course of the disease, but it cannot reverse the structural damage to the vessels and the heart. Also called **Döhle-Heller disease, luetic aortitis.**

**syphilitic dementia** [L, *de* + *mens,* mind], a form of dementia resulting from a syphilis infection. Specific symptoms may vary from memory impairment to personality changes and are severe enough to interfere with social and occupational activities. If untreated, the disease may progress to dementia paralytica, paralysis, and death.

**syphilitic endocarditis** [L, *endon,* within, *kardia,* heart, *itis,* inflammation], a thickening and stretching of the cusps of the aortic valve, with aortic valve incompetence, caused by a syphilis infection of the aorta.

**syphilitic fever** [L, *febris*], pyrexia that is caused by a syphilis infection.

**syphilitic heart disease.** See **cardiovascular disease.**

**syphilitic meningoencephalitis.** See **general paresis.**

**syphilitic periarteritis,** an inflammatory condition of the outer coat of one or more arteries occurring in tertiary syphilis and characterized by soft gummatous perivascular lesions infiltrated with lymphocytes and plasma cells. Also called **periarteritis gummosa.** See also **syphilitic aortitis.**

**syphilitic retinopathy** [L, *rete,* net; Gk, *pathos,* disease], an invasion of the retina and optic nerve by a spreading syphilis infection. Primary retinal lesions are associated with the blood vessels, and the choroid layer is often affected first. There may be occlusion of the retinal vessels.

**syr.,** abbreviation for the Latin *syrupus,* 'syrup.'

**syring-.** See **syringo-.**

**syringe** /sərinj′, sir′inj/ [Gk, *syrinx,* tube], a device for withdrawing, injecting, or instilling fluids. A syringe for the injection of medication usually consists of a calibrated glass or plastic cylindric barrel having a close-fitting plunger at one end and a small opening at the other to which the head of a hollow-bore needle is fitted. Medication of the desired amount may be pulled up into the barrel by suction as the plunger is withdrawn and injected by pushing the plunger back into the barrel, forcing the liquid out through the needle. A syringe for irrigating a wound or body cavity or for extracting mucus or another body fluid from an orifice or body cavity is usually larger than the kind used for injection. It often has a rubber bulb at one end and a blunt soft-tipped flexible tube with an opening at the other end. The bulb is squeezed to eject a fluid and is released to withdraw one. Kinds of syringes include **Asepto syringe, bulb syringe, hypodermic syringe, Luer-Lok syringe,** and **tuberculin syringe.**

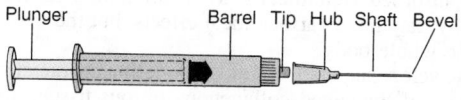

Plunger      Barrel   Tip   Hub   Shaft   Bevel

**Syringe** (Potter and Perry, 2001)

**syringectomy** /sir′injek′təmē/ [Gk, *syrinx*, tube, *ektomē*, excision],   a surgical procedure for excising the walls of a fistula.

**syringo-, syring-** /siring′gō-/,   combining form meaning 'tube or a fistula': *syringobulbia, syringocystoma, syringomyelitis.*

**syringobulbia** /si·ring′gō·bul′bē·ə/ [Gk, *syrinx*, tube; L, *bulbus*, swollen root],   syringomyelia in which the cavity extends to involve the medulla oblongata. See also **syringomyelia.**

**syringoencephalomyelia** /siring′gō·ensef′əlō′mī·ē′lyə/,   a progressive disorder characterized by cavitation of the spinal cord. It may occur anywhere from the medulla oblongata to the thoracic segments but usually appears in cervical segments.

**syringoma,** *pl.* **syringomata** /sir′ing·gō′mə/,   a benign tumor derived from an eccrine sweat gland. It appears as a small smooth papule the color of the underlying skin, often on the upper body of a postpubertal woman. Some are typically multiple, often appearing on the lower eyelids.

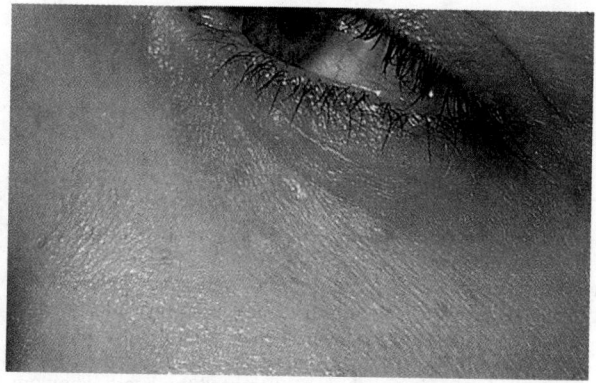

**Syringoma** (Lawrence and Cox, 1993)

**syringomeningocele** /-məning′gōsēl′/ [Gk, *syrinx*, tube, *meninx*, membrane, *kele*, hernia],   a meningocele that is connected to the central canal of the spinal cord. See also **spina bifida.**

**syringomyelia** /-mī·ē′lyə/ [Gk, *syrinx*, tube, *myelos*, marrow],   a chronic progressive disease of the spinal cord, marked by elongated central fluid-containing cavities, surrounded by gliosis or a proliferation of neurologic tissue. Symptoms begin early in adulthood, usually involving the cervical region with muscular wasting in the upper limbs. The disease is more common in males.

**syringomyelocele** /siring′gōmī′əlōsēl′/ [Gk, *syrinx* + *myelos*, marrow, *kele*, hernia],   a hernial protrusion of the spinal cord through a congenital defect in the vertebral column. The cerebrospinal fluid within the central cavities of the cord is greatly increased so that the cord tissue forms a thin-walled sac that lies close to the membrane of the cavity. See also **myelomeningocele, neural tube defect, spina bifida.**

**syrup of ipecac** /sir′əp/,   an emetic preparation of ipecac fluid extract, glycerin, and syrup used to treat certain types of poisonings and drug overdoses. See also **ipecac.**

**system** /sis′təm/ [Gk, *systema*],   **1.** a collection or assemblage of parts that, unified, make a whole. Physiologic systems, such as the cardiovascular or reproductive system, are made up of structures specifically able to engage in processes that are essential for a vital function in the body. **2.** a set of computer programs and hardware that work together for some specific purpose.

**systematic** /sis′təmat′ik/ [Gk, *systema*],   pertaining to a system.

**systematic error** [Gk, *systema* + L, *errare*, to wander],   a nonrandom statistical error that affects the mean of a population of data and defines the bias between the means of two populations.

**systematic heating,**   the elevation of the temperature of the whole body.

**systematic tabulation,**   (in research) mechanical or manual techniques for recording and classifying data for statistical analysis.

**system documentation.**   See **documentation.**

**systemic** /sistem′ik/ [Gk, *systema*],   pertaining to the whole body rather than to a localized area or regional part of the body.

**systemic circulation** [Gk, *systema* + L, *circulare,* to go around],   the general blood circulation of the body, not including the lungs. Also called **greater circulation.**

**systemic desensitization,**   a technique used in behavior therapy for eliminating maladaptive anxiety associated with phobias. The procedure involves the construction by the person of a hierarchy of anxiety-producing stimuli and the general presentation of these stimuli until they no longer elicit the initial response of fear. Also called **desensitization.** Compare **flooding.** See also **reciprocal inhibition.**

**systemic heart,**   side of the heart, which moves oxygenated blood through the systemic circulation.

**systemic hypertension.**   See **cardiovascular disease.**

**systemic immunoblastic proliferation,**   a condition of immature lymphocyte production resulting in rash, breathing difficulty, enlarged spleen, lymphadenopathy, and increased incidence of immunoblastic lymphoma.

**systemic infection** [Gk, *systema* + L, *inficere*, to stain],   an infection in which the pathogen is distributed throughout the body rather than concentrated in one area.

**systemic lesion** [Gk, *systema* + L, *laesio,* attack],   a pathologic disturbance that involves a system of tissues with a common function.

**systemic lupus erythematosus (SLE),** a chronic inflammatory disease affecting many systems of the body. It is an example of a collagen disease. The pathophysiologic characteristics of the disease includes severe vasculitis, renal involvement, and lesions of the skin and nervous system. The primary cause of the disease has not been determined; viral infection or dysfunction of the immune system has been suggested. Adverse reaction to certain drugs also may cause a lupuslike syndrome. Four times more women than men have SLE. Also called **disseminated lupus erythematosus, lupus erythematosus.**

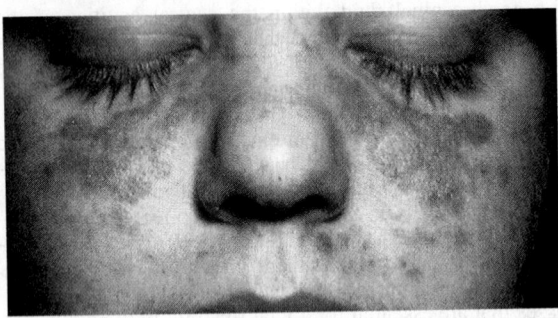

**Classic butterfly rash of systemic lupus erythematosus**
*(Goldstein and Goldstein, 1997/courtesy Department of Dermatology, University of North Carolina at Chapel Hill)*

■ OBSERVATIONS: The initial manifestation is often arthritis. An erythematous rash ("butterfly rash") over the nose and malar eminences, weakness, fatigue, and weight loss also are frequently seen early in the disease. Photosensitivity, fever, skin lesions on the neck, and alopecia where the skin lesions extend beyond the hairline may occur. The skin lesions may spread to the mucous membranes and other tissues of the body. They do not ulcerate but cause degeneration of the affected tissues. Depending on the organs involved, the patient also may have glomerulonephritis, pleuritis, pericarditis, peritonitis, neuritis, or anemia. Renal failure and severe neurologic abnormalities are among the most serious manifestations of the disease. Diagnosis of SLE is made by subjective and objective findings based on physical examination and laboratory findings, including antinuclear antibody in the cerebrospinal fluid and a positive lupus erythematosus (LE) cell reaction in a lupus erythematosus preparation (LE prep). Other laboratory examinations may be useful, depending on the organs, tissues, and systems affected by the disease.
■ INTERVENTIONS: In many cases SLE may be controlled with corticosteroid medication administered systemically. Care and treatment vary with the severity and nature of the disease and the body systems that are affected. Topical steroids may be applied to the rash; salicylates may be given to alleviate pain and swelling in the joints. Fatigue and stress are prevented, and all body surfaces are protected from direct sunlight. Antimalarial drugs are sometimes given to treat cutaneous lesions, but retinal damage may occur with prolonged use.
■ NURSING CONSIDERATIONS: The timing, dosage, side effects, and toxic reactions to the medications are explained before

discharge. The steroids must be taken exactly as prescribed, and, in the event that the patient cannot take them, the doctor is to be consulted promptly. An identification card is carried bearing the patient's diagnosis, a list of all medications and their dosage, and the doctor's name and telephone number. As in any disease marked by chronic remission and exacerbation of many distressing symptoms, the patient may require extensive emotional and psychologic support.

**systemic mycosis** [Gks, *systema* + *mykes,* fungus, *osis,* condition], a fungal infection that involves more than one body system or area.

**systemic oxygen consumption,** the amount of oxygen consumed by the body per minute.

**systemic remedy,** a medicinal substance that is given orally, parenterally, or rectally to be absorbed into the circulation for treatment of a health problem. Many remedies or medications administered locally or regionally are to some degree absorbed systemically. Medication administered systemically may have various local effects, but the intent is to treat the whole body.

**systemic sclerosis,** a form of scleroderma characterized by formation of thickened collagenous fibrous tissue, thickening of the skin, and adhesion to underlying tissues. The disease, which may be preceded by Raynaud's phenomenon, progresses to involve the tissues of the heart, lungs, muscles, genitourinary tract, and kidneys. See also **scleroderma.**

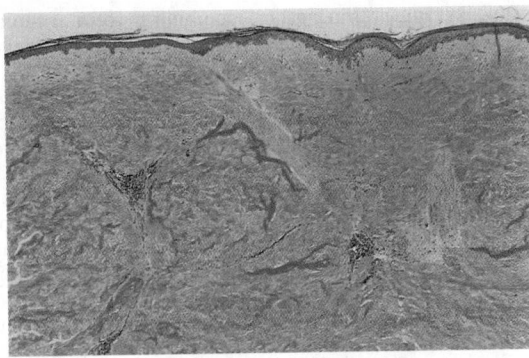

**Systemic sclerosis**
*(Kumar, Cotran, and Robbins, 1997/courtesy Dr. Trace Worrell, Department of Pathology, University of Texas Southwestern Medical School, Dallas)*

**systemic toxin clearance: dialysis,** a nursing outcome from the Nursing Outcomes Classification (NOC) defined as the extent to which toxins are cleared from the body with peritoneal or hemodialysis. See also **Nursing Outcomes Classification.**

**systemic vascular resistance (SVR),** the resistance the left ventricle must overcome to pump blood through the systemic circulation. As peripheral blood vessels constrict, the SVR increases.

**systemic vein,** one of a number of veins that drain deoxygenated blood from most of the body, as opposed to the pulmonary circulation. Systemic veins arise in tiny plexuses that receive blood from capillaries and converge into trunks that increase in size as they pass toward the heart. They are larger and more numerous than the arteries, have thinner walls, and collapse when they are empty. Groups of systemic veins include the coronary veins, the superior vena cava and its tributaries in the upper body, and the inferior vena cava and its tributaries in the lower body.

**systemic venous hypertension,** elevation of the venous pressure, usually detected by inspection of the jugular veins and most often caused by disease of the right heart or pericardium.

**system of care** /sis'təm/, a framework within which health care is provided, comprising health care professionals; recipients, consumers, or patients; energy resources or dynamics; organizational and political contexts or frameworks; and processes or procedures. Current theory recognizes that an analysis of the provision of health care requires knowledge of the systems of care.

**system overload,** an inability to cope with messages and expectations from a number of sources within a given time limit.

**systems integration,** the unification of disparate computer hardware and software to achieve usability and transferability of data, such as throughout a managed care or provider network.

**systems software,** a group of computer utilities programs that control the execution of applications programs.

**systems theory,** a holistic medical concept in which the human patient is viewed as an integrated complex of open systems rather than as semiindependent parts. The health care approach in this theory requires the incorporation of family, community, and cultural factors as influences to be considered in the diagnosis and treatment of the patient.

**systole** /sis'təlē/ [Gk, *systole,* contraction], the contraction of the heart, driving blood into the aorta and pulmonary arteries. The occurrence of systole is indicated by the first heart sound heard on auscultation, by the palpable apex beat, and by the peripheral pulse.—**systolic,** *adj.*

**-systole,** suffix meaning 'types and locations of the higher blood pressure measurement': *dyssystole, hysterosystole, tachysystole.*

**systolic** /sistol'ik/ [Gk, *systole,* contraction], pertaining to or resulting from a heart contraction.

**systolic click** [Gk, *systole,* contraction; Fr, *cliqueter,* to click], a sharp, clicking sound heard in mid- or late systole, and believed to originate from the abnormal motion of the mitral valve. The most frequent cause of systolic clicks is prolapse of a mitral valve leaflet, in which case there may be an associated late systolic regurgitant murmur, sometimes called the *click-murmur syndrome.* Compare **ejection click.**

**systolic click-murmur syndrome.** See **Barlow's syndrome.**

**systolic dysfunction,** a loss of cardiac muscle with volume overload and decreased contractility.

**systolic ejection period,** the amount of time the ventricles spend in systole per minute.

**systolic gradient,** the difference between the pressure in the left atrium and that in the left ventricle during systole.

**systolic murmur,** a cardiac murmur occurring during systole. Systolic murmurs include **ejection murmurs,** often heard in pregnant women or in people with anemia, thyrotoxicosis, or aortic or pulmonary stenosis; **pansystolic murmurs,** heard in people with incompetence of the mitral or tricuspid valve; and late systolic murmurs, also caused by mitral valve incompetence.

**systolic pressure,** the blood pressure measured during the period of ventricular contraction (systole). In blood pressure readings, it is the higher of the two measurements.

**t,** symbol for **time.**

**T,** 1. symbol for **temperature.** 2. abbreviation for **tumor.** See **cancer staging.**

**T₁/₂,** symbol for the half-life of a radioactive isotope.

**T₁, T₂.** See **relaxation time.**

**T₃,** symbol for **triiodothyronine.**

**T₄,** symbol for **thyroxine.**

**T1, T2, . . .,** symbols for thoracic nerves.

**T-4 cell,** a thymus-derived lymphocyte of the body's immune system that destroys or neutralizes cells or substances identified as "nonself." T-4 cells secrete a substance, interleukin-2, which stimulates the activity of natural killer cells, gamma interferon, and suppressor T-8 cells. The human immunodeficiency virus commonly targets T-4 cells, with the result that the body's immune defenses are severely damaged and opportunistic infections are allowed to flourish.

**Ta,** symbol for the element **tantalum.**

**TA,** abbreviation for **transactional analysis.**

**ta-.** See **tono-.**

**tabardillo.** See **Mexican typhus.**

**tabe-,** combining form meaning 'wasting (away)': *tabefaction, tabescent, tabetiform.*

**tabes** /tā´bēz/ [L, *tabes,* wasting], a gradual, progressive wasting of the body in any chronic disease.

**tabes dorsalis** [L, *tabes,* wasting, *dorsum,* the back], an abnormal condition characterized by the slow degeneration of all or part of the body and the progressive loss of deep tendon reflexes. This disease involves the posterior columns and posterior roots of the spinal cord and destroys the large joints of affected limbs in some individuals. A wide-base ataxic gait is usually present. It is often accompanied by incontinence and impotence and severe flashing pains in the abdomen and extremities. The cause of tabes dorsalis is syphilitic.

**tabetic crisis** /tābet´ik/ [L, *tabes,* wasting; Gk, *krisis,* turning point], an exacerbation of pain in tabes dorsalis because of syphilis.

**tabetic gait** [L, *tabes,* wasting; ONorse, *gata,* a way], a high-stepping gait associated with tabes dorsalis, a disease in which the posterior or dorsal columns of the spinal cord and the sensory nerve trunks degenerate.

**tabetic neuritis** [L, *tabes,* wasting; Gk, *neuron,* nerve, *itis,* inflammation], a form of neuritis that accompanies a syphilitic infection or tabes dorsalis, involving the dorsal posterior column spinal pathways.

**table** [L, *tabula*], 1. any structure with a flat surface. 2. a chart showing columns of data.

**tablespoon (Tbs, tbsp),** a household spoon that may be used to measure a dose of liquid medicine, equivalent to about 4 fluid drams or 1/2 fluid ounce or 15 mL.

**tablet** /tab´lit/ [Fr, *tablette,* lozenge], a small, solid dosage form of a medication. It may be compressed or molded in its manufacture; and it may be of almost any size, shape, weight, and color. Most tablets are intended to be swallowed whole; but some may be dissolved in the mouth, chewed, or dissolved in liquid before swallowing; and some may be placed in a body cavity.

**taboo** /tab̄oo´/, something that is forbidden by a society as unacceptable or improper. Incest is a taboo common to many societies.

**taboparesis** /tā´bōpərē´sis/ [L, *tabes,* wasting; Gk, *paralyein,* to be palsied], a form of paralysis associated with cerebral syphilis. Also called **taboparalysis.**

**tabula rasa** /tä´bōōlä rä´sä, tab´yəle rä´sə/, a term used to describe a child's mind at birth as a receptive 'blank slate.'

**tache** /täsh/ [Fr], a spot, stain, blot, or mark.

**tache laiteuse.** See **macula albida.**

**tache noire** /täshnô·är´/ [Fr, black spot], a local ulcerous lesion marking the point of infection in certain rickettsial diseases such as African tick typhus and scrub typhus.

**tachistoscope** /təkis´təskōp´/ [Gk, tachistos, rapid, *skopein,* to view], a device used to increase the speed of visual perception by displaying visual stimuli only extremely briefly.

**tacho-,** combining form meaning 'swift or rapid': *tachogram, tachography, tachometer.*

**tachometer** /təkom´ətər/, a device for measuring speed, such as the rate of blood flow in a vessel.

**tachy-** /tak´ē-/, combining form meaning 'swift or rapid': *tachycardia, tachyphrenia, tachysystole.*

**tachyarrythmia** /tak´ē·ərith´mē·ə/ [Gk, *tachys,* fast, *a + rhythmos,* rhythm], an abnormally rapid heartbeat accompanied by an irregular rhythm.

**tachycardia** /tak´ēkär´dē·ə/ [Gk, *tachys,* fast, *kardia,* heart], a condition in which the heart contracts at a rate greater than 100/min. It may occur normally in response to fever, exercise, or nervous excitement. Pathologic tachycardia accompanies anoxia, such as that caused by anemia, congestive heart failure, hemorrhage, or shock. Tachycardia acts to increase the amount of oxygen delivered to the cells of the body by increasing the rate at which blood circulates through the vessels. —**tachycardiac,** *adj.*

**tachycardia-bradycardia syndrome.** See **bradycardia-tachycardia syndrome.**

**tachycardiac** /-kär´dē·ak/ [Gk, *tachys,* fast, *kardia,* heart], pertaining to or affected by tachycardia.

**tachykinin.** See **substance P.**

**tachyphagia** /-fā´jē·ə/, rapid or hasty eating.

**tachyphylaxis** /tak´ēfəlak´sis/ [Gk, *tachys + phylax,* guard], 1. (in pharmacology) a phenomenon in which the repeated administration of some drugs results in a marked decrease in effectiveness. 2. also called **mithridatism.** (in immunology) a rapidly developing immunity to a toxin because of previous exposure, such as from previous injection of small amounts of the toxin.

**tachypnea** /tak´ēpnē´ə/ [Gk, *tachys + pnoia,* breathing], an abnormally rapid rate of breathing (more than 20 breaths per minute in adults), such as seen with hyperpyrexia. Also spelled **tachypnoea.**

**tack,** the degree of stickiness of an adhesive required to affix a therapeutic foreign substance such as a transdermal delivery device to the skin.

1676

**tacrolimus,** an immunosuppressive drug.

■ INDICATIONS: The drug is prescribed to suppress the immune system after transplantation of the liver or other organs.

■ CONTRAINDICATIONS: The drug should not be given to patients with allergy to tacrolimus or those receiving potassium-sparing diuretics, cyclosporine, or other immunosuppressive agents, with the exception of adrenal corticosteroids.

■ ADVERSE EFFECTS: The side effects most often reported include tremor, headache, diarrhea, hypertension, nausea, and renal dysfunction.

**tact-,** prefix meaning 'touch': *tactile, tactilogical, taction.*

**-tactic, -tactical, -taxic, 1.** suffix meaning 'exhibiting agent-controlled orientation or movement': *chemotactic, eosinotactic, thermotactic.* **2.** suffix combining form meaning 'having an arrangement of something': *cytotactic, leukotactic, phyllotactic.*

**tactile** /tak′təl/, tak′tīl/ [L, *tactus,* touch], pertaining to the sense of touch.

**tactile amnesia** [L, *tactus* + Gk, *amnesia,* forgetfulness], a loss of the ability to determine the shape of objects through the sense of touch. See also **astereognosis.**

**tactile anesthesia,** the absence or lack of the sense of touch in the fingers, possibly resulting from injury or disease. This condition can be congenital or psychosomatic and may cause the patient to incur severe burns, serious cuts, contusions, or abrasions. See also **traumatic anesthesia.**

**tactile corpuscle.** See **Meissner's corpuscle.**

**tactile defensiveness,** a sensory integrative dysfunction characterized by tactile sensations that cause excessive emotional reactions, hyperactivity, or other behavior problems.

**tactile discrimination** [L, *tactus* + *discrimen,* division], the ability to discriminate among objects by the sense of touch.

**tactile fremitus,** a tremulous vibration of the chest wall during speaking that is palpable on physical examination. Fremitus may be decreased or absent when vibrations from the larynx to the chest surface are impeded by obstruction, pleural effusion, or pneumothorax. Tactile fremitus is increased in pneumonia.

**tactile hair** [L, *tactus* + AS, *haer*], a hair shaft that is sensitive to the sensation of touch.

**tactile hallucination** [L, *tactus* + *alucinare,* to wander in mind], a subjective experience of touch in the absence of tactile stimulation. It is most common in delirium tremens or alcoholic hallucinosis.

**tactile hyperesthesia** [L, *tactus* + Gk, *hyper,* excessive, *aesthesis,* sensitivity], an abnormal increase in the sense of touch.

**tactile image,** a mental concept of an object as perceived through the sense of touch. See also **image.**

**tactile localization** [L, *tactus* + *locus,* place], the ability to identify, without looking, the exact point on the body where a tactile stimulus is applied. The localization test is applied in sensory evaluation tests.

**tactile sensation** [L, *tactus* + *sentire,* to feel], the sensation of touch.

**tactile system** [L, *tactus* + Gk, *systema*], the part of the nervous system that is concerned with the sense of touch.

*Taenia* /tē′nē·ə/ [Gk, *tainia,* ribbon], a genus of large parasitic intestinal flatworm of the family Taeniidae, class Cestoda, having an armed scolex and a series of segments in a chain. Taeniae are among the most common parasites infecting humans and include *T. saginata,* the beef tapeworm, and *T. solium,* the pork tapeworm.

**taenia-.** See **tenia-.**

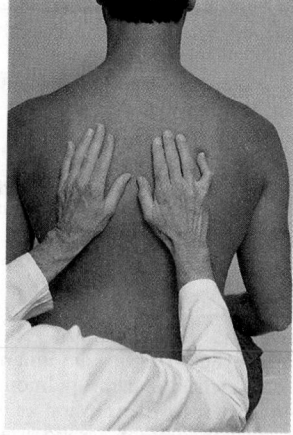

With palmer surface of hands

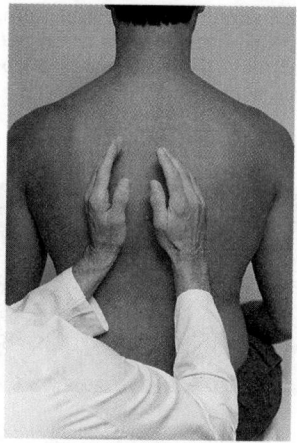

With ulnar aspect of hands

**Evaluation of tactile fremitus** *(Seidel et al, 1999)*

*Taenia saginata,* a species of tapeworm that inhabits the tissues of cattle during its larval stage and infects the intestine of humans in its adult form. *T. saginata* may grow to a length of between 12 and 25 feet and is the tapeworm species that most often infects humans. Also called **beef tapeworm.** See also **tapeworm, tapeworm infection.**

**taeniasis** /tēnī′əsis/ [Gk, *tainia* + *osis,* condition], an infection with a tapeworm of the genus *Taenia.* Transmission is through ingestion of undercooked pork containing cysticercus or food contaminated with pig feces containing eggs. See also **tapeworm infection.**

*Taenia solium,* a species of tapeworm that most commonly inhabits the tissues of pigs during its larval stage and infects the intestine of humans in its adult form. Infrequently humans serve as the intermediate hosts for this tapeworm, and larval infestation of the muscle and brain tissue may occur. Also called **pork tapeworm.** See also **cysticercosis, tapeworm, tapeworm infection.**

**TAF,** abbreviation for **tumor angiogenesis factor.**

**tag,** a small piece of epidermal and dermal fibrovascular tissue attached by one margin or a pedicle to a main structure.

**TAG,** abbreviation for *3,4,6-tri-o-acetyl-D-glucal.*

**Tagamet,** trademark for a histamine $H_2$ receptor antagonist (cimetidine).

**tail,** the caudal extremity of an organ or body, such as an axillary tail of a mammary gland.

**tail bud.** See **end bud.**

**tail fold** [AS, *taegel + fealdan,* to fold], a curved ridge formed at the caudal end of the early developing embryo. It consists of the tail bud, which in lower animals gives rise to the caudal appendage and in humans forms the hindgut.

**tail of Spence,** the upper outer tail of breast tissue that extends into the axilla.

**tailor's bunion.** See **bunionette.**

**Takayasu's arteritis** /tä′kəyä′sōōz/ [Mikito Takayasu, Japanese surgeon, 1860–1938], an inflammation of the aorta, its major branches, and the pulmonary artery. It is characterized by progressive occlusion of the innominate, left subclavian and left common carotid arteries above their origin in the aortic arch. Signs of the disorder are absence of a pulse in both arms and in the carotid arteries, transient paraplegia, transient blindness, and atrophy of facial muscles. Also called **brachiocephalic arteritis, Martorell's syndrome, pulseless disease, reversed coarctation.** See also **aortic arch syndrome.**

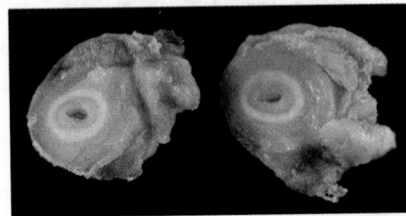

**Takayasu's arteritis** *(Cotran, Kumar, and Collins, 1999)*

**take,** a popular term for a satisfactory response, as of a vaccination or tissue graft.

**talc** /talk/ [Ar, *talq*], a native, hydrous magnesium silicate, sometimes containing a small proportion of aluminum silicate, used as a dusting powder and adsorbent in clarifying liquids. Also called **talcum.**

**talcosis** /talkō′sis/, a silicosis-like respiratory disorder caused by inhalation of magnesium silicate dust.

**talcum.** See **talc.**

**talip-,** combining form meaning 'a nontraumatic (usually congenital) twisting defect or clubfooted': *taliped, talipes, talipomanus.*

**talipes** /tal′ipēz/ [L, *talus,* ankle, *pes,* foot], a deformity of the foot and ankle, usually congenital, in which the foot is twisted and relatively fixed in an abnormal position. Talipes refers to deformities that involve the foot and ankle, whereas pes refers only to deformities of the foot. Kinds of talipes include **talipes calcaneovalgus, talipes calcaneovarus,** and **talipes equinovarus.** See also **clawfoot, flatfoot.**

**talipes calcaneovalgus.** See **clubfoot.**

**talipes cavus.** See **pes cavus.**

**talipes equinovarus.** See **clubfoot.**

**talipes equinus.** See **pes equinus.**

**talipes valgus.** See **splayfoot.**

**talipes varus.** See **pigeon-toed.**

**tallow** /tal′ō/, **1.** a hard fat obtained from the bodies of ruminant animals such as cattle and sheep and used in soaps and lubricants. **2.** a vegetable fat obtained from plants, such as the wax myrtle.

**talo-,** prefix meaning 'ankle': *talocalcaneal, talocrural, talofibular.*

**talofibular** /tā′lōfib′yələr/, pertaining to the talus and the fibula.

**talonavicular** /tā′lōnəvik′yələr/ [L, *talon,* bird claw, *naviculus,* scaphoid], pertaining to the talus and the navicular bones.

**talus** /tā′ləs/, *pl.* **tali** [L, ankle], the second largest tarsal bone. It supports the tibia, rests on the calcaneus, and articulates with the malleoli and navicular bones. It consists of a body, neck, and head. Also called **ankle bone, astragalus.**

**Talwin,** trademark for an antagonist/agonist analgesic (pentazocine).

**Tambocor,** trademark for an oral antiarrhythmic drug (flecainide acetate).

**tambour** /tam′bōōr/, a cylindric drumlike device connected to an air tube and stylus, used to record sphygmograph or other physiologic data.

**Tamm-Horsfall protein (THP)** [Igor Tamm, American virologist, b. 1922; Frank L. Horsfall, American virologist, 1906–1971], a mucoprotein found in the matrix of renal tubular casts. THP is secreted in the loop of Henle.

**tamoxifen** /təmok′səfin/, a nonsteroidal antiestrogen used in the palliative treatment of advanced breast cancer in premenopausal and postmenopausal women whose tumors are estrogen-dependent.

**tampon** /tam′pon/ [Fr, plug], a packed cotton, a sponge or other material for checking bleeding or absorbing secretions in cavities or canals or for holding displaced organs in position.

**tamponade** /tam′pənād′/ [Fr, *tamponner,* to plug up], stoppage of the blood flow to an organ or a part of the body by pressure, such as by a tampon or a pressure dressing applied to stop a hemorrhage or by the compression of a part by an accumulation of fluid, such as in cardiac tamponade.

**tamsulosin,** a selective $\alpha_1$-adrenergic blocker.

■ INDICATIONS: This drug is used to treat benign prostatic hyperplasia.

■ CONTRAINDICATIONS: Known hypersensitivity to this drug prohibits its use.

■ ADVERSE EFFECTS: Adverse reactions to this drug include chest pain, dizziness, headache, asthenia, nausea, diarrhea, decreased libido, abnormal ejaculation, amblyopia, back pain, rhinitis, pharyngitis, and cough.

**tangentiality** /tanjen′chē·al′itē/ [L, *tangere,* to touch], expressions or responses characterized by a tendency to digress from an original topic of conversation, in which a common word connects two unrelated thoughts. For example, the boy caught a ball; balls of fire exploded from the house. Tangentiality can destroy or seriously hamper the ability of people to communicate effectively. It is frequently seen in schizophrenia.

**tangible elements** /tan′jibəl/ [L, *tangere + elementum,* first principle], objects that can be seen or touched as distinguished from emotions, knowledge, or abstractions.

**Tangier disease** /tanjir′/ [Tangier Island, Virginia], a rare familial deficiency of high-density lipoproteins, characterized by low blood cholesterol and an abnormal orange or yellow discoloration of the tonsils and pharynx. There also may be enlarged lymph nodes, liver, and spleen; muscle atrophy; and peripheral neuropathy. No specific treatment is known.

**tangle** /tang′gəl/, a dense mass of interlacing of fibers, sometimes appearing as a loose knot, such as intraneural fibrillary tangle.

**tannic acid** /tan′ik/ [Celt, *tann*, oak; L, *acidus*, sour], a substance obtained from the bark and fruit of various trees and shrubs, particularly the nutgalls of oak trees. The acid is used as an astringent and protein precipitant. Also called **tannin.**

**tanning** [Fr, *tanner*, to tan], a process in which the pigmentation of the skin deepens as a result of exposure to ultraviolet light. Skin cells containing melanin darken immediately. New melanin is formed within 2 to 3 days and moves upward rapidly, allowing the darkening process to continue.

**tantalum (Ta)** /tan′tələm/ [Gk, *Tantalus*, mythic king of Phrygia], a silvery metallic element. Its atomic number is 73; its atomic mass (weight) is 180.95. Relatively inert chemically, tantalum is used in prosthetic devices such as skull plates and wire sutures.

**tantrum** /tan′trəm/, a sudden outburst or violent display of rage, frustration, and bad temper, usually occurring in a maladjusted child and certain emotionally disturbed people. The activity is usually not directed at anyone or anything specific but toward the environment in general and is used primarily as a device for attempting to control others and the surroundings. It most commonly occurs at age 2 to 2-1/2 years. Also called **temper tantrum.**

**TAO,** trademark for an antibacterial (troleandomycin).

**tap** [ME, *tappen*], **1.** to strike lightly, as in percussion or testing of reflexes. **2.** to draw off fluid through a small opening.

**tape** [AS, *taeppe*], strips of material, usually with adhesive, used to secure bandages.

**tape-compression folliculitis,** inflammation of the hair follicles caused by tape dressings placed over foam or cotton-ball pads under a graduated compression stocking. The condition is more likely to occur on patients with hairy legs who may perspire during the summer months.

**tapering arch** /tā′pəring/ [AS, *tapor*, slender, *arcus*, bow], a dental arch that converges from the molars to the central incisors to such a degree that lines passing through the central grooves of the molars and premolars intersect within 1 inch (2.5 cm) anterior to the central incisors.

**tapetoretinopathy** /tapē′tōret′inop′əthē/, a hereditary visual disorder characterized by degeneration of the sensory retina and pigmentary epithelium. It occurs in pigmentary retinopathy and other eye diseases.

**tapetum,** **1.** a carpetlike layer or covering of tissue. **2.** a thin sheet of fibers covering parts of the brain and continuous with the corpus callosum. **3.** the reflective part of the choroid coat of the eye in many mammals.

**tapeworm** /tāp′wurm/ [AS, *taeppe* + *wyrm*], a parasitic intestinal worm belonging to the class Cestoda and having a scolex and a ribbon-shaped body composed of segments in a chain. Humans usually acquire tapeworms by eating the undercooked meat of intermediate hosts contaminated by the cysticercus or larval form of the tapeworm. In the human alimentary canal the worm develops into an adult with an attaching head, or scolex, and numerous hermaphroditic segments, or proglottids, each of which is capable of producing eggs. Kinds of tapeworm include *Diphyllobothrium latum, Taenia saginata,* and *Taenia solium.* Also called **cestode.**

**tapeworm infection,** an intestinal infection by one of several species of parasitic worms, caused by eating raw or undercooked meat infested with tapeworm or its larvae or food contaminated with feces containing tapeworm eggs. Tapeworms live as larvae in one or more vertebrate intermediate hosts and grow to adulthood in the intestine of humans. Symptoms of intestinal infection with adult worms are usually mild or absent; but diarrhea, epigastric pain, and weight loss may occur. Diagnosis is made when eggs or parts of the adult worm are passed in the stool. Treatment is with praza-

quantel and albendazole. Sanitary disposal of fecal material from affected patients is necessary to prevent the passage of larvae or eggs to humans or other hosts. Certain species of tapeworm can infect humans during the larval stage, causing a serious, often cystic, condition of larval infestation. Also called **cestodiasis.** See also **cysticercosis, tapeworm.**

**tapho-,** combining form meaning 'the grave': *taphophilia, taphophobia.*

**tapioca** /tap′ē·ō′kə/, tiny starchy balls (pearls) or flakes made from the dried paste of grated cassava root, *Janipha manihot.* It is used as a thickener in a variety of easily digested food items, particularly cereals, soups, and puddings.

**tapotement** /täpôtmäN′/ [Fr, *tapoter*, to pat], a type of massage in which the body is tapped in a rhythmic manner with the tips of the fingers or the sides of the hands, using short, rapid, repetitive movements. The procedure is often used on the chest wall of patients with bronchitis to help loosen the mucus in the air passages. See also **massage.**

**tar** /tär/ [AS, *teoru*], a dark, viscid organic mixture produced by the distillation of coal, wood, or vegetable matter. Some forms of tar are used to treat eczema and other skin disorders.

**Taractan,** trademark for a tranquilizer (chlorprothixene).

**tarantula** /təran′chələ/, popular name for any of a number of species of large, hairy spiders. Although potentially poisonous, most are relatively harmless to humans. A bite by some species may produce an area of superficial skin destruction.

**tardive** /tär′div/ [L, *tardus*, late], describing a disease in which a period of time passes between exposure and the first symptoms.

**tardive dyskinesia** [L, *tardus*, late; Gk, *dys*, difficult, *kinesis*, movement], an abnormal condition characterized by involuntary repetitious movements of the muscles of the face, limbs, and trunk. This disorder most commonly affects older people who have been treated for extended periods with phenothiazine. The involuntary movements associated with the condition may slacken or disappear after weeks or months and have been significantly reduced in some individuals by the administration of cholinergic drugs. See also **antiparkinsonian.**

**tardy peroneal nerve palsy** [L, *tardus* + Gk, *perone*, brooch; L, *nervus* + *paralyein*, to be palsied], an abnormal condition and a type of mononeuropathy in which the peroneal nerve is excessively compressed where it crosses the head of the fibula. Such compression may occur when an individual falls asleep with the legs crossed.

**tardy ulnar nerve palsy,** an abnormal condition characterized by atrophy of the first dorsal interosseous muscle and difficulty in performing fine manipulations. It may be caused by injury of the ulnar nerve at the elbow and commonly affects individuals with a shallow ulnar groove or those who persistently rest their weight on their elbows. Signs and symptoms of this disorder may include numbness of the small finger, of the contiguous half of the proximal and middle phalanges of the ring finger, and of the ulnar border of the hand. Treatment concentrates on the prevention of further injury to the ulnar nerve. Therapy may include the use of a doughnut cushion for the elbow to relieve the pressure on the ulnar nerve. Severe cases of this disorder may be corrected by surgical procedures that mobilize and transplant the nerve to a site in front of the medial epicondyle.

**target** /tär′git/ [OFr, *targuete*, small shield], **1.** any object area subjected to bombardment by radioactive particles or another form of diagnostic or therapeutic radiation. **2.** a device used to contain stable materials and subsequent radioactive materials during bombardment by high-energy nuclei from a cyclotron or other particle accelerator. **3.** the part of the anode struck by electrons in an x-ray tube.

**target cell,**    **1.** also called **leptocyte.** an abnormal red blood cell characterized by a densely stained center surrounded by a pale unstained ring circled by a dark, irregular band. Target cells occur in the blood after splenectomy, in anemia, in hemoglobin C disease, and in thalassemia. Compare **discocyte, spherocyte. 2.** any cell having a specific receptor that reacts with a specific hormone, antigen, antibody, antibiotic, sensitized T cell, or other substance.

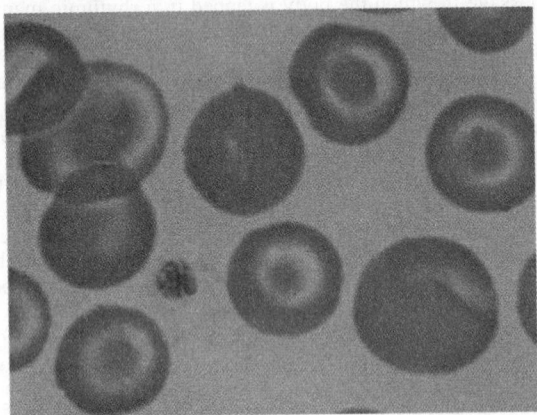

**Target cell, definition 1** *(Carr and Rodak, 1999)*

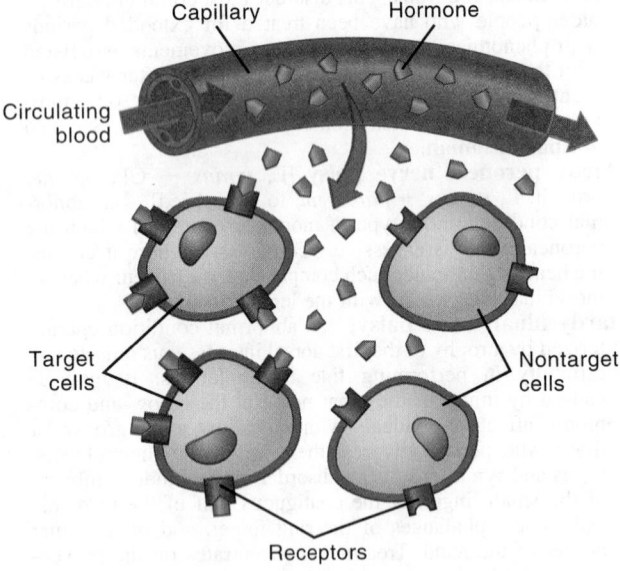

**Target cell, definition 2**
*(Thibodeau and Patton, 1999/Network Graphics)*

**target organ,**    **1.** an organ intended to receive a therapeutic dose of irradiation, such as the kidney when high-energy x-rays or gamma rays are beamed to the renal area for the treatment of a tumor. **2.** an organ intended to receive the

greatest concentration of a diagnostic radioactive tracer, such as the liver, which accumulates 99Tc sulfur colloid when it is injected intravenously to detect hepatic lesions. **3.** an organ most affected by a specific hormone, such as the thyroid gland, which is the target organ of thyroid stimulating hormone secreted by the anterior pituitary gland.

**target symptoms,**   symptoms of an illness that are most likely to respond to a specific treatment such as a particular psychopharmacologic drug.

**tarsal** /tär′səl/ [Gk, *tarsos,* flat surface],   pertaining to the tarsus, or ankle bone.

**tarsal arches** [Gk, *tarsos,* flat surface; L, *arcus,* rainbow], the superior and inferior branches of the palpebral artery supplying the eyelid.

**tarsal bone,**   any one of seven bones making up the tarsus of the foot, consisting of the talus, calcaneus, cuboid, navicular, and the three cuneiforms.

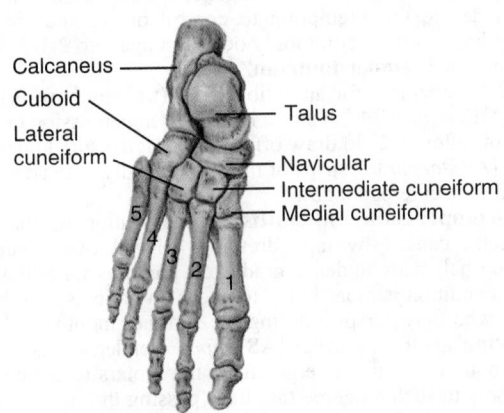

**Tarsal bones** *(Applegate, 2000)*

**tarsal cartilage.**   See **tarsus.**

**tarsalgia** /tärsal′jə/,   foot pain, usually involving fallen arches. Also called **podalgia.**

**tarsal gland,**   any one of numerous modified sebaceous glands on the inner surfaces of the eyelids. Acute localized bacterial infection of a tarsal gland may cause a sty or a chalazion. Also called **meibomian gland.** Compare **ciliary gland.**

**tarsal plate.**   See **tarsus.**

**tarsal tunnel syndrome,**   an abnormal condition and a kind of mononeuropathy characterized by pain and numbness in the sole of the foot. This disorder may be caused by fractures of the ankle that compress the posterior tibial nerve. It may be corrected by appropriate orthopedic therapy or surgery.

**tarso-,**   prefix meaning 'instep of the foot or the edge of the eyelid': *tarsoclasis, tarsomalacia, tarsometatarsal.*

**tarsometatarsal** /tär′sōmet′ətär′səl/ [Gk, *tarsos,* flat surface, *meta,* beyond, *tarsos*],   pertaining to the metatarsal bones and the tarsus of the foot, especially the articulations of the metatarsal bones with the cuneiform and cuboid bones at the instep of the foot.

**tarsophalangeal reflex.**   See **Mendel's reflex.**

**tarsorrhaphy** /tärsôr′əfē/,   a surgical procedure for uniting the upper and lower eyelids. It usually is performed in pro-

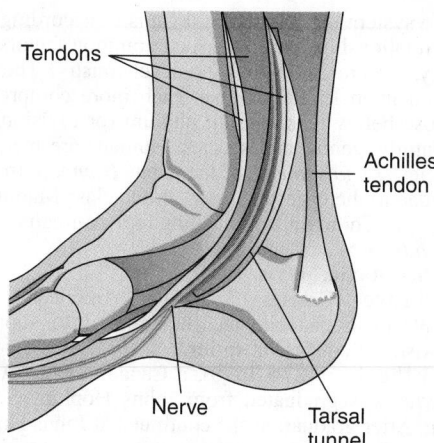

**Locations of tarsal tunnel syndrome**
*(Beare and Myers, 1998)*

sweet, salty, sour, and bitter. The front of the tongue is most sensitive to salty and sweet substances; the sides of the tongue are most sensitive to sour substances; and the back of the tongue is most sensitive to bitter substances. The middle of the tongue produces virtually no taste sensation. Chemoreceptor cells in the taste buds of the tongue detect different substances. Adults have about 9000 taste buds, most of them situated on the upper surface of the tongue. The sense of taste is intricately linked with the sense of smell, and taste discrimination is very complex. Many experts believe the capacity to perceive different tastes involves a synthesis of chemoreactive nerve impulses and coordinating brain processes, still not completely understood.

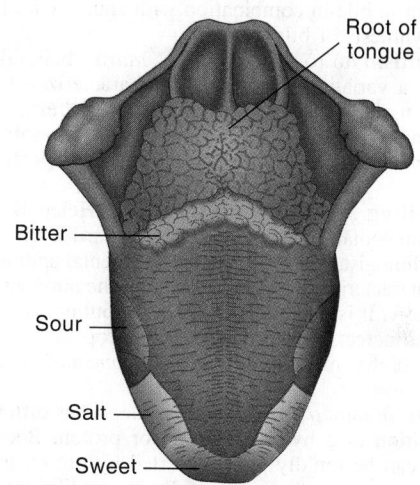

**Taste regions of the tongue**
*(Thibodeau and Patton, 1999/Network Graphics)*

cedures to protect the cornea and may involve only the lateral parts of the eyelids.

**tarsus** /tär′səs/, *pl.* **tarsi** [Gk, *tarsos,* flat surface], **1.** the flat area of articulation between the foot and the leg or the edge of the eyelid. **2.** also called **tarsal plate.** Any one of the fibrous plates of cartilage about 2.5 cm long that form the eyelids. One tarsal plate shapes and gives solidarity to the edge of each eyelid.

**TAR syndrome.** See **thrombocytopenia−absent radius syndrome.**

**tart,** abbreviation for the *tartrate carboxylate anion.*

**tartar** /tär′tär/ [Fr, *tartre*], **1.** See **calculus. 2.** any of several compounds containing tartrate, the salt of tartaric acid.

**tartaric acid** [**HOOC(CH₂O)₂COOH**] /tärter′ik/, a colorless or white powder found in various plants and prepared commercially from maleic anhydride and hydrogen peroxide. It is used in baking powder, certain beverages, and tartar emetic.

**tartrate** /tä′trāt/, **1.** a dianion of tartaric acid. **2.** any salt or ester of tartaric acid.

**Tarui's disease** /tah′roo·ē/, a form of glycogen storage disease in which abnormally large amounts of glycogen are deposited in the skeletal muscle. The disorder is characterized by cramping on exercise but no rise in blood lactate, as well as hemolysis. Biopsy of the affected organ reveals the absence of the enzyme phosphofructokinase. Also called **glycogen storage disease type VII.** See also **glycogen storage disease.**

**-tas,** a noun-forming combining form: *fragilitas, graviditas, infertilitas.*

**task functions,** behaviors that focus or direct activities toward movements with work or labor overtones.

**task group,** a group in which structured verbal or nonverbal exercises are used to help a person gain emotional, physical, and other personal awareness.

**task-oriented behavior,** actions involving a person's cognitive abilities in an attempt to solve problems, resolve conflicts, and gratify the person's needs to reduce or avoid distress.

**taste** [ME, *tasten*], the sense of perceiving different flavors in soluble substances that contact the tongue and trigger nerve impulses to special taste centers in the cortex and thalamus of the brain. The four basic traditional tastes are

**taste bud,** any one of many peripheral taste organs distributed over the tongue and the roof of the mouth. The four basic taste sensations registered by chemical stimulation of the taste buds are sweet, sour, bitter, and salty. All other tastes perceived are combinations of these four basic flavors plus the input from olfactory receptors. Each taste bud rests in a spheric pocket, which extends through the epithelium. Gustatory cells and supporting cells form each bud, which has a surface opening and an opening in the basement membrane. Also called **gustatory organ.**

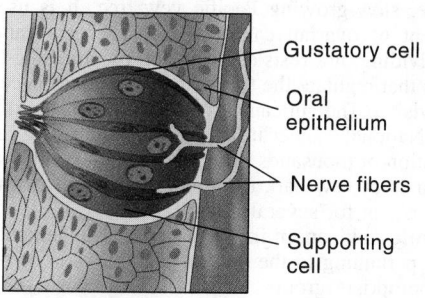

**Taste bud** *(Thibodeau and Patton, 1999/Network Graphics)*

**taste papilla** [OFr, *taster* + L, *papilla*, nipple], small nipplelike elevations on the tongue. They contain sense organs that are sensitive to the chemicals identified with tastes, which vary with their location on the tongue.

**TAT,** abbreviation for **tetanus antitoxin.**

**tattoo** /tatoō′/ [Tahitian, *tatau*, marks], a permanent coloration of the skin by the introduction of foreign pigment. A tattoo may be created deliberately or may accidentally occur when a bit of graphite from a broken pencil point is embedded in the skin. Small tattoos can be removed by surgical excision. Dermabrasion or laser is preferred for removal of extensive areas of pigment. **—tattoo,** *v.*

**tau** /tou, tō/, T, τ, the nineteenth letter of the Greek alphabet.

**taurine** /tôr′in/, a derivative of the amino acid cysteine. It is present in bile in combination with cholic acid. It is used in the synthesis of bile salts.

**taurodontism** /tô′rō·don′tiz·əm/ [L, *taurus*, bull; Gk, *odous*, tooth], a variation in tooth form characterized by prism-shaped molars with large pulp spaces, resulting from branching of the root only in the middle **(mesotaurodontism),** or in the apical third or not at all **(hypertaurodontism).**

**Taussig-Bing syndrome** /tô′sig-bing′/ [Helen B. Taussig, American pediatrician, 1898–1986; Richard J. Bing, American cardiologist, b. 1909], a developmental anomaly of the heart, characterized by transposition of the aorta and pulmonary artery. It is accompanied by a subpulmonary ventricular septal defect and ventricular hypertrophy.

**tauto-,** prefix meaning 'same': *tautomenial, tautomeral, tautomerism.*

**tautomer** /tôtəmər/, structural isomers that differ only in the position of a hydrogen atom, or proton. Because tautomers can be rapidly interconverted by proton transfer in aqueous solutions, they are usually in equilibrium with one another. Keto and enol isomers are common examples of tautomers.

**Tavist,** trademark for an antihistaminic agent (clemastine).

**tax-,** combining form meaning 'order or arrangement': *taxis, taxology, taxonomy.*

**-taxia, -taxis, -taxy,** combining form meaning '(condition of) internal ordering or arrangement': *acrotaxia, diataxia, cataxia, heterotaxia, prostaxia.* See also **-taxis.**

**-taxic.** See **-tactic.**

**taxis** /tak′sis/, **1.** movement away from or toward a stimulus. **2.** the reduction of a hernia. **3.** a dislocation of a hernia by means of manipulation.

**-taxis, -taxia, -taxy, 1.** combining form meaning a '(specified) arrangement': *biotaxis, heterotaxis, homotaxis.* **2.** combining form meaning a 'movement of an organism in response to a stimulus': *aerotaxis, electrotaxis, geotaxis.* See also **-taxia.**

**Taxol** /tak′sol/, an anticancer drug derived from the bark of the rare, slow-growing Pacific yew tree. It is used in the treatment of ovarian cancer. Taxol prevents cancer cells from dividing; it arrests cell division by attaching to microtubules that regulate the formation of spindles necessary for cell division. The anticancer effect of Taxol was discovered by the National Cancer Institute in 1963 during a routine investigation of thousands of plant compounds. It takes about 60 pounds of yew bark to produce enough Taxol to treat a single patient for several weeks.

**taxonomic** /tak′sənom′ik/ [Gk, *taxis*, arrangement, *nomos*, law], pertaining to the orderly classification of organisms into appropriate groups, or taxa, on the basis of interrelationships, with the use of suitable names.

**taxonomy** /takson′əmē/ [Gk, *taxis*, arrangement, *nomos*, rule], a system for classifying organisms according to their natural relationships based on such common factors as embryology, structure, or physiologic chemistry. The system has seven main levels, or taxa, each more comprehensive than those below it: kingdom, phylum (or division), class, order, family, genus, and species. Humans are members of the species *Homo sapiens,* of the genus *Homo,* in the family Hominidae in the order Primates, in the class Mammalia, in the phylum Chordata, in the kingdom Animalia. **—taxonomic,** *adj.*

**-taxy.** See **-taxia, -taxis.**

**Taylor brace** [Charles F. Taylor, American surgeon, 1827–1899], a padded steel brace used to support the spine. Also called **Taylor splint.**

**Taylor, Effie J.** (1874–1970), a Canadian-born American nurse who was graduated from Johns Hopkins School of Nursing. After graduation she continued at Johns Hopkins at the Phipps Psychiatric Institute, served as a nurse in World War I, and went to Yale University School of Nursing in 1923, succeeding Annie Goodrich as dean in 1934. She served as president of the International Council of Nurses during World War II.

**Tay-Sachs disease** /tā′saks′/ [Warren Tay, English ophthalmologist, 1843–1927; Bernard Sachs, American neurologist, 1858–1944], an inherited, neurodegenerative disorder of lipid metabolism caused by a deficiency of the enzyme hexosaminidase A, which results in the accumulation of sphingolipids in the brain. The condition, which is transmitted as an autosomal-recessive trait, occurs predominantly in families of Eastern European Jewish origin, specifically the Ashkenazic Jews. It is characterized by progressive mental and physical retardation and early death. Symptoms first appear by 6 months of age, after which no new skills are learned and there is progressive loss of those skills already acquired. Convulsions and atrophy of the optic nerve head occur after 1 year, followed by blindness, with a cherry-red spot on each retina, spasticity, dementia, and paralysis. Most children die between 2 and 4 years of age. There is no specific therapy for the condition, and intervention is purely symptomatic and supportive. The disease can be diagnosed in utero through amniocentesis. Also called **amaurotic familial idiocy, gangliosidosis type I, infantile cerebral sphingolipidosis, Sachs' disease.** See also **Sandhoff's disease.**

**Tay's spot.** See **cherry red spot.**

**Tazicef,** trademark for a cephalosporin antibiotic (ceftazidime).

**Tb,** symbol for the element **terbium.**

**TB, 1.** abbreviation for **tuberculosis. 2.** abbreviation for *tubercle bacillus.*

**T bandage,** a bandage in the shape of the letter T. It is used for the perineum and sometimes for the head. Also called **crucial bandage.**

**TBI, 1.** abbreviation for **total body irradiation. 2.** abbreviation for **traumatic brain injury.**

**TBP, 1.** abbreviation for **bithionol. 2.** abbreviation for *total bypass.*

**Tbs,** abbreviation for **tablespoon.**

**TBSA,** abbreviation for *total body surface area.* See **surface area (SA).**

**tbsp,** abbreviation for **tablespoon.**

**TBT,** abbreviation for **tracheobronchial tree.**

**TBW,** abbreviation for **total body water.**

**TBZ,** abbreviation for *tetrabenazine,* an anesthetic adjuvant.

**Tc,** symbol for the element **technetium.**

**TC,** abbreviation for **therapeutic community.**

**t.c.,** abbreviation for *telephone call.*

**TCDD,** abbreviation for **(2,3,7,8-tetrachlorodibenzoparadioxin).** See **dioxin.**

**T cell,** a small circulating lymphocyte produced in the bone marrow that matures in the thymus. T cells primarily mediate cellular immune responses such as graft rejection and delayed hypersensitivity. One kind of T cell, the **helper cell,** affects the production of antibodies by B cells; a **suppressor T cell** suppresses B cell activity. Compare **B cell.** See also **antibody, immune response.**

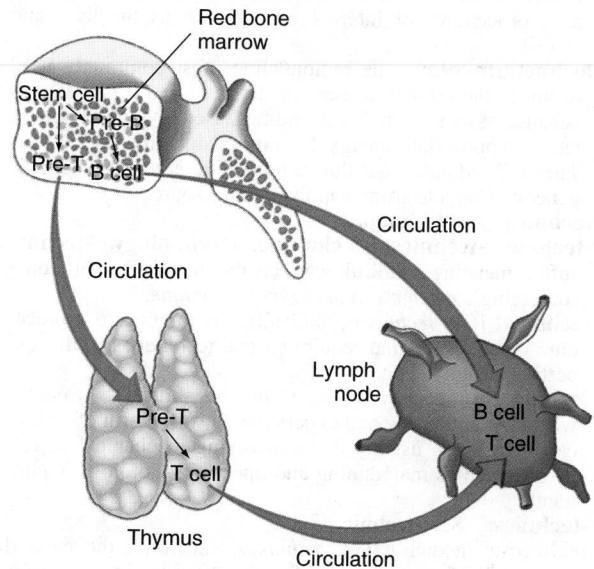

**Development of T cells**
*(Thibodeau and Patton, 1999/Network Graphics)*

**T cell antigen receptor,** a protein present on T cells that combines with antigens to produce discrete immunologic components.

**T-cell lymphomas,** a heterogenous group of lymphoid tumors representing malignant transformation of the T lymphocytes. Some types of tumors formerly included in this group have been found to be mixtures of T cells and B cell precursors.

**T cell−mediated hypersensitivity reaction,** type IV hypersensitivity reaction; see **hypersensitivity reaction.**

**T cell–mediated immunity.** See **cellular immunity, immune response, T cell.**

**Td,** abbreviation for **tetanus and diphtheria toxoids.**

**TD,** abbreviation for **toxic dose.**

**TD50.** See **median toxic dose.**

**TDD,** abbreviation for **transdermal drug delivery.**

**tDNA,** abbreviation for **transfer DNA.**

**t.d.s.,** abbreviation for Latin phrase '*ter die sumendum,*' (to be taken) three times a day.

**Te,** symbol for the element **tellurium.**

**tea** [Chin, *ch'a*], **1.** a beverage prepared from the leaves and leaf buds of an evergreen shrub, *Thea sinensis.* A member of the camellia family, the plant is grown mainly in Asia. Its pharmacologically active components include caffeine, theobromine, theophylline, and tannin. **2.** maté tea, a caffeine beverage prepared from the leaves of *Ilex paraguayensis,* a shrub grown in South America.

**teacher's nodule.** See **vocal cord nodule.**

**teaching: disease process,** a nursing intervention from the Nursing Interventions Classification (NIC) defined as assisting the patient to understand information related to a specific disease process. See also **Nursing Interventions Classification.**

**teaching: group,** a nursing intervention from the Nursing Interventions Classification (NIC) defined as development, implementation, and evaluation of a patient teaching program for a group of individuals experiencing the same health condition. See also **Nursing Interventions Classification.**

**teaching hospital** [AS, *taecan,* to show how], a hospital associated with a university that has accredited programs in various specialties of medical practice.

**teaching: individual,** a nursing intervention from the Nursing Interventions Classification (NIC) defined as a planning, implementation, and evaluation of a teaching program designed to address a patient's particular needs. See also **Nursing Interventions Classification.**

**teaching: infant care,** a Nursing Interventions Classification defined as instruction on nurturing and physical care needed during the first year of life. See also **Nursing Interventions Classification.**

**teaching: infant nutrition,** a nursing intervention from the Nursing Interventions Classification (NIC) defined as instruction on nutrition and feeding practices during the first year of life. See also **Nursing Interventions Classification.**

**teaching: infant safety,** a nursing intervention from the Nursing Interventions Classification (NIC) defined as instruction on safety during first year of life. See also **Nursing Interventions Classification.**

**teaching: preoperative,** a nursing intervention from the Nursing Interventions Classification (NIC) defined as assisting a patient to understand and mentally prepare for surgery and the postoperative recovery period. See also **Nursing Interventions Classification.**

**teaching: prescribed activity/exercise,** a nursing intervention from the Nursing Interventions Classification (NIC) defined as preparing a patient to achieve and/or maintain a prescribed level of activity. See also **Nursing Interventions Classification.**

**teaching: prescribed diet,** a nursing intervention from the Nursing Interventions Classification (NIC) defined as preparing a patient to correctly follow a prescribed diet. See also **Nursing Interventions Classification.**

**teaching: prescribed medication,** a nursing intervention from the Nursing Interventions Classification (NIC) defined preparing a patient to safely take prescribed medications and monitor for their effects. See also **Nursing Interventions Classification.**

**teaching: procedure/treatment,** a nursing intervention from the Nursing Interventions Classification (NIC) defined as preparing a patient to understand and mentally prepare for a prescribed procedure or treatment. See also **Nursing Interventions Classification.**

**teaching: psychomotor skill,** a nursing intervention from the Nursing Interventions Classification (NIC) defined as preparing a patient to perform a psychomotor skill. See also **Nursing Interventions Classification.**

**teaching rounds,** informal conferences held regularly, often at the beginning of the day. Various members of the department and staff may attend, including nurses, residents, interns, students, attending physicians, and faculty. Specific problems in the care of current patients, as well as case presentation of patients with specific diseases, are discussed. See also **nursing rounds.**

**teaching: safe sex,** a nursing intervention from the Nursing Interventions Classification (NIC) defined as providing instruction concerning sexual protection during sexual activity. See also **Nursing Interventions Classification.**

**teaching: sexuality,** a nursing intervention from the Nursing Interventions Classification (NIC) defined as assisting individuals to understand physical and psychosocial dimensions of sexual growth and development. See also **Nursing Interventions Classification.**

**teaching: toddler nutrition,** a nursing intervention from the Nursing Interventions Classification (NIC) defined as instruction on nutrition and feeding practices during the second and third years of life. See also **Nursing Interventions Classification.**

**teaching: toddler safety,** a nursing intervention from the Nursing Interventions Classification (NIC) defined as instruction on safety during the second and third years of life. See also **Nursing Interventions Classification.**

**team nursing** [AS, *team,* family; L, *nutrix,* nurse], a decentralized system in which the care of a patient is distributed among the members of a group working in coordinated effort. The charge nurse delegates authority to a team leader who must be a professional nurse. This nurse leads the team—usually of 4 to 6 members—in the care of between 15 and 25 patients. The team leader assigns tasks, schedules care, and instructs team members in details of care. A conference is held at the beginning and end of each shift to allow team members to exchange information and the team leader to make changes in the nursing care plan for any patient. Compare **primary nursing.**

**team practice,** professional practice by a group of professionals that may include physicians, nurses, and others, such as a social worker, nutritionist, or physical therapist, who manage the care of a specified number of patients as a coordinated group, usually in an outpatient setting.

**tear** /ter/ [ME, *teren,* to rend], to rip, rend, or pull apart by force.

**teardrop fracture** /tir′drop/ [AS, *tear* + *dropa* + L, *fractura,* break], an avulsion fracture of one of the short bones, such as a vertebra, causing a tear-shaped disruption of bone tissue.

**tear duct** /tir/ [AS, *tear* + L, *ducere,* to lead], any duct that carries tears, including the lacrimal ducts, nasolacrimal ducts, and excretory ducts of the lacrimal glands.

**tear gas** /tēr/, a gas that produces severe lacrimation by irritating the conjunctivae.

**tearing** /tir′ing/, watering of the eye usually caused by excessive tear production, such as by strong emotion, infection, or mechanic irritation by a foreign body. If the normal amount of fluid tears is produced but not drained into the lacrimal punctum at the nasal border of the eye, tear overflow will occur. If the lacrimal punctum, sac, canaliculi, or nasolacrimal duct becomes blocked, tears also will overflow. Also called **epiphora.**

**tears** /tirz/ [ME, *tere*], a watery saline or alkaline fluid secreted by the lacrimal glands to moisten the conjunctiva and cornea. Also called **dacryon.**

**tears of the perineum** /ters/ [ME, *teren* + Gk, *perineos*], a rending of the tissues between the vulva and anus caused by overstretching of the vagina during child delivery. The degree of damage ranges from a tear of the superficial tissues without injury to the surrounding muscle to a rupture of the perineal skin, vaginal and rectal mucosa, and anal sphincter. The damage is usually repaired by surgery.

**teaspoon (tsp),** a small spoon that may be used to measure a dose of a liquid medication, equivalent to about 1 fluid dram or 5 mL.

**tea tree oil,** an herbal product taken from a species of myrtle tree native to coastal Australia.

■ USES: This herb is used topically for infections and as an inhalant for respiratory disorders.

■ CONTRAINDICATIONS: Tea tree oil should not be used during pregnancy and lactation or in those with known hypersensitivity to this plant.

**tebutate,** a contraction for tertiary butyl acetate.

**technetium (Tc)** [Gk, *technectos,* artificial], a radioactive, metallic element. Its atomic number is 43; its atomic mass is 99. The first synthetic element, technetium also occurs in nature. Isotopes of technetium are used in radioisotope scanning procedures of internal organs such as the liver and spleen.

**technetium-99m,** the radionuclide most commonly used to image the body in nuclear medicine scans. It is preferred because of its short half-life and because the emitted photon has an appropriate energy for normal imaging techniques. The "m" indicates that this radionuclide is metastable. It is generated on site from a molybdenum source.

**technic.** See **technique.**

**-technic, -technics, -technique, -technology, -techny,** suffix meaning 'skillful way or the mechanics of doing something': *mnemotechnics, zymo-technique.*

**technical** [Gk, *technikos,* skillfull], pertaining to a procedure or its results that require special techniques, skills, expertise, or knowledge.

**technician** /teknish′ən/ [Gk, *technikos,* skillful], a person with special training and experience in some form of technical procedures, usually those involving mechanical adjustments, such as maintaining and operating radiologic equipment.

**-technics.** See **-technic.**

**technique** /teknēk′/ [Gk, *technikos,* skillful], the method and details followed in performing a procedure, such as those used in conducting a laboratory test, a physical examination, a psychiatric interview, a surgical operation, or any process requiring certain skills or an ordered sequence of actions. Also spelled **technic.**

**-technique.** See **-technic.**

**techno-,** combining form meaning 'art': *technopsychology, technocausis, technology.*

**technologist** /teknol′əjist/ [Gk, *techne,* art, *logos,* science], a person who studies the application of processes for making natural resources beneficial for humans. A medical technologist may work under the supervision of a physician in general clinical laboratory procedures.

**technology** /teknol′əjē/ [Gk, *techne,* art, *logos,* study], **1.** the application of science or the scientific method to commercial or industrial objectives. **2.** the knowledge and use of science applied to the conversion of natural resources for the benefit of humans.

**technology management,** a nursing intervention from the Nursing Interventions Classification (NIC) defined as use of technical equipment and devices to monitor patient condition or sustain life. See also **Nursing Interventions Classification.**

**-technology, -techny.** See **-technic.**

**tecto-,** prefix meaning 'rooflike': *tectocephalic, tectorial, tectum.*

**tectonic** /tekton′ik/, **1.** pertaining to variations in structure in the cornea or other parts of the eye. **2.** pertaining to plastic surgery or tissue transplants.

**tectorial** /tektôr′ē·əl/, pertaining to a rooflike structure or cover.

**tectorium** /tektôr′ē·əm/, a body structure that serves as an overlying structure or roof.

**Tedral,** trademark for a respiratory fixed-combination drug containing a bronchodilator (theophylline), an adrenergic (ephedrine hydrochloride), and a sedative-hypnotic (phenobarbital).

**teenager.** See **adolescent.**

**teeth.** See **tooth.**

**teether** /tē'ther/, an object such as a plastic or rubber teething ring on which an infant can bite or chew during the teething process.

**teething** /tē'thing/ [AS, *toth*], the physiologic process of the eruption of the deciduous teeth through the gums. It normally begins around the sixth month of life and occurs periodically until the complete set of 20 teeth has appeared at about 30 to 36 months. Discomfort and inflammation result from the pressure exerted against the periodontal tissue as the crown of the tooth breaks through the membranes. General signs of teething include excessive drooling, biting on hard objects, irritability, difficulty in sleeping, and refusal of food. Fever or diarrhea often occurs during teething but may be indicative of illness rather than of teething. The pain and inflammation usually may be soothed by cold, such as with a frozen teething ring, cold metal spoon, or ice wrapped in a wash cloth. Use of teething powders and procedures such as rubbing or cutting the gums are discouraged because of the possibility of infection or complications from ingestion of the medication. —**teethe,** *v.*

**teething ring.** See **teether.**

**Teflon,** trademark for a substance (polytetrafluorethylene) used for the construction of surgical implants in restorative surgery.

**teg-,** combining form meaning 'a cover': *tegmen, tegmental, tegument.*

**Tegison,** trademark for an antipsoriatic vitamin A derivative (etretinate).

**tegmen** /teg'mən/, a covering, such as the bone that covers the tympanic cavity.

**tegmental** /tegmen'təl/ [L, *tegmentum*, cover], of or relating to an integument.

**Tegopen,** trademark for an antibacterial (cloxacillin sodium).

**Tegretol,** trademark for an analgesic and anticonvulsant (carbamazepine).

**TEIB,** abbreviation for *triethylene-immunobenzoquinone.*

**tela-,** combining form meaning 'a web or weblike structure': *telalgia, telangiectasia, telangitis.*

**-tela,** combining form meaning a 'weblike membrane': *aulatela, epitela, metatela.*

**telangiectasia** /təlan'jē·ektā'zhə/ [Gk, *telos,* end, *angeion,* vessel, *ektasis,* swelling], permanent dilation of groups of superficial capillaries and venules. Common causes are actinic damage, atrophy-producing dermatoses, rosacea, elevated estrogen levels, and collagen vascular diseases. See also **Osler-Weber-Rendu syndrome, spider angioma.**

**telangiectasia lymphatica** [Gk, *telos,* end, *angeion,* vessel, *ektasis,* swelling; L, *lympha,* water], a congenital or acquired condition of obstructed dilated lymphatic vessels, resulting in lymphangiomas.

**telangiectatic angioma** /təlan'jē·ektat'ik/, a tumor composed of dilated blood vessels.

**telangiectatic epulis,** a benign red tumor of the gingiva, containing prominent blood vessels. Low-grade or chronic irritation is a risk factor.

**telangiectatic fibroma.** See **angiofibroma.**

**telangiectatic glioma,** a tumor composed of glial cells and a network of blood vessels, which give the mass a vivid pink appearance.

**telangiectatic granuloma.** See **pyogenic granuloma.**

**Telangiectasia** *(Lemmi and Lemmi, 2000)*

**telangiectatic lipoma.** See **angiolipoma.**

**telangiectatic nevus,** a common skin condition of neonates, characterized by flat, deep-pink localized areas of capillary dilation that occur predominantly on the back of the neck, lower occiput, upper eyelids, upper lip, and bridge of the nose. The areas disappear permanently by about 2 years of age. Also called **capillary flames, stork bite.**

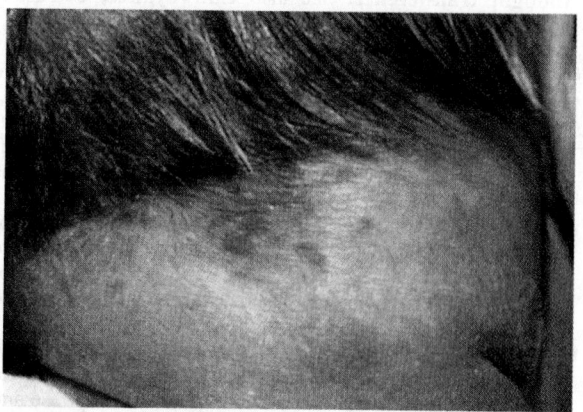

**Telangiectatic nevus** *(Weston, Lane, and Morelli, 1996)*

**telangiectatic sarcoma,** a malignant tumor of mesodermal cells with an unusually rich vascular network.

**tele-, teleo-,** combining form meaning 'end or occurring at a distance': *telekinesis, telosynapsis.*

**telediagnosis** /tel'ədī'əgnō'sis/ [Gk, *tele,* far off, *dia,* through, *gnosis,* knowledge], a process whereby a disease diagnosis, or prognosis, is made by the electronic transmission of data between distant medical facilities.

**telehealth,** the use of telecommunication technologies to provide health care services and access to medical and surgical information for training and educating health care professionals and consumers, to increase awareness and educate the public about health-related issues, and to facilitate medical research across distances.

**telekinesis** /tel'əkinē'sis/ [Gk, *tele,* far off, *kinesis,* movement], a concept of parapsychology that one can control external events such as the movement of a solid object by the powers of the mind. For example, practitioners of telekinesis may believe it possible, by thought processes alone, to influence the roll of dice. Also called **parakinesis, psychokinesis.**

**telemedicine,** the use of telecommunication equipment and information technology to provide clinical care to individuals at distant sites and the transmission of medical and surgical information and images needed to provide that care.

**telemetry** /telem′ətrē/ [Gk, *tele,* far off, *metron,* measure], the electronic transmission of data between distant points, such as the transmission of cardiac monitoring data.

**telencephalization** /tel′ensef′əlīzā′shən/, a stage in fetal development in which the forebrain begins to assume control over nervous system functions previously directed by more primitive neural centers. Also called **corticalization.**

**telencephalon** /tel′ensef′əlon/ [Gk, *telos,* end, *egekephalos,* brain], the paired brain vesicles or endbrain from which the cerebral hemispheres are derived.

**teleo-.** See **tele-.**

**teleology** /tel′ē·ol′əjē/ [Gk, *telos,* end, *logos,* science], **1.** the study of ultimate purpose or design in natural phenomena. **2.** a theory that everything is directed toward some final purpose.

**telepathist** /təlep′əthist/, **1.** a person who believes in telepathy. **2.** a person who claims to have telepathic powers.

**telepathy** /təlep′əthē/ [Gk, *tele,* far off, *pathos,* feeling], the alleged communication of thought from one person to another by means other than the physical senses. Also called **thought transference.** See also **clairvoyance, extrasensory perception, parapsychology. —telepathic,** *adj.,* **telepathize,** *v.*

**telephone consultation,** a nursing intervention from the Nursing Interventions Classification (NIC) defined as eliciting patient's concerns, listening, and providing support, information, or teaching in response to patient's stated concerns, over the telephone. See also **Nursing Interventions Classification.**

**telephone counseling,** a strategy system to provide support by telephone for patients or family caregivers who are homebound. The system may offer safety provisions and social contacts for frail older persons or the visually impaired as well as suicide-prevention counseling.

**telephone follow-up,** a nursing intervention from the Nursing Interventions Classification (NIC) defined as providing results of testing or evaluating patient's response and determining potential for problems as a result of previous treatment, examination, or testing, over the telephone. See also **Nursing Interventions Classification.**

**telereceptive** /tel′ərisep′tiv/, pertaining to the exteroceptors of hearing, sight, and smell that detect stimuli distant from the body.

**teletherapy** /tel′əther′əpē/ [Gk, *tele + therapeia,* treatment], radiation therapy administered by a machine that is positioned at some distance from the patient. Typically a teletherapy unit can rotate around a patient, thus allowing the use of multiple beams that intersect at the tumor and lowering the dose to surrounding normal tissue.

**telluric** /teloo′rik/ [L, *tellus,* earth], pertaining to the soil and its possible pathogenic influence.

**tellurium (Te)** /teloo′rē·əm/ [L, *tellus,* earth], an element exhibiting metallic and nonmetallic chemical properties. Its atomic number is 52; its atomic mass (weight) is 127.60. Inhaling vapors of tellurium results in a garlicky breath.

**telmisartan,** an antihypertensive.

■ INDICATIONS: Telmisartan is used to treat hypertension, either alone or in combination with other drugs.

■ CONTRAINDICATIONS: Known hypersensitivity to this drug prohibits its use.

■ ADVERSE EFFECTS: Adverse reactions to telmisartan include dizziness, insomnia, dyspepsia, and cough. Common side effects include anxiety, diarrhea, anorexia, vomiting, myalgia, pain, and upper respiratory infection.

**telo-,** combining form meaning 'end': *telobiosis, telodendron, telosynapsis.*

**telocentric** /tel′əsen′trik/ [Gk, *telos,* end, *kentron,* center], pertaining to a chromosome in which the centromere is located at the end so that the chromosome appears as a straight filament. Compare **acrocentric, metacentric, submetacentric.**

**telogen.** See **hair.**

**telomerase** /tə·lō′mər·ās/, a DNA polymerase involved in the formation of telomeres and the maintenance of telomere sequences during replication.

**telomere** /tel′ō·mēr /, either of the ends of a chromosome, which possess special properties, among them a polarity that prevents their reunion with any fragment after a chromosome has been broken.

**telophase** /tel′əfāz/ [Gk, *telos + phasis,* appearance], the final of the four stages of nuclear division in mitosis and in each of the two divisions in meiosis. The newly produced daughter chromosomes from the preceding stage (anaphase) assemble at the poles of the spindle and become long and slender, the nuclear membrane forms around them, the nucleolus reappears, and the cytoplasm begins to divide. See also **anaphase, interphase, meiosis, metaphase, mitosis, prophase.**

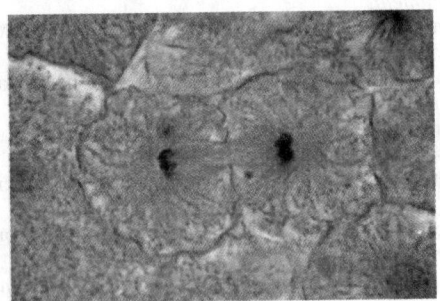

**Telophase** (© Ed Reschke; used with permission)

**Temaril,** trademark for an antihistamine (trimeprazine tartrate).

**temazepam** /temaz′əpam/, a benzodiazepine hypnotic agent.

■ INDICATIONS: It is prescribed for the relief of transient and intermittent insomnia.

■ CONTRAINDICATIONS: Pregnancy or lactation prohibits its use. It is not recommended for patients under 18 years of age. Patients should avoid use of alcohol while also using temazepam.

■ ADVERSE EFFECTS: The most serious adverse reactions are confusion, euphoria, anorexia, ataxia, palpitations, hallucinations, horizontal nystagmus, and paradoxic reactions.

**Temovate,** trademark for a topical corticosteroid (clobetasol propionate).

**temozolomide,** a miscellaneous antineoplastic agent.

■ INDICATIONS: Temozolomide is used to treat anaplastic astrocytoma with relapse.

■ CONTRAINDICATIONS: Pregnancy, lactation, and known hypersensitivity to this drug or to carbazine prohibit the use of temozolomide.

■ ADVERSE EFFECTS: Life-threatening effects of this drug are thrombocytopenia, leukopenia, and seizures. Other adverse effects include anemia, urinary incontinence, urinary tract infection, urinary frequency, upper respiratory infection, pharyngitis, sinusitis, cough, headache, fatigue, asthenia, fever, edema, back pain, weight increase, and diplopia. Common side effects include nausea, anorexia, vomiting, hemiparesis, dizziness, poor coordination, amnesia, insomnia, paresthesia, somnolence, paresis, ataxia, anxiety, dysphagia, depression, confusion, rash, and pruritus.

**temper** [L, *temperare,* to moderate],  **1.** to moderate or soften the effects. **2.** a state of mind regarding calmness or anger.

**temperament** /temp′(ə)rəmənt/ [L, *temperamentum,* mixture in proper proportions],  the features of a persona that reflect an individual's emotional disposition, or the way he or she behaves, feels, and thinks.

**temperance** /tem′pərəns/,  behavior that emphasizes moderation and self-restraint, particularly in the use of alcohol.

**temperate phage** /tem′pərit/ [L, *temperare,* to moderate; Gk, *phagein,* to eat],  a bacteriophage whose genome is incorporated into the host bacterium. It persists through many cell divisions of the bacterium without destroying the host, in contrast to a virulent phage, which lyses and kills its host.

**temperature** /tem′pə(r)chər/ [L, *temperatura*],  **1.** a relative measure of sensible heat or cold. **2.** (in physiology) a measure of sensible heat associated with the metabolism of the human body, normally maintained at a constant level of 98.6° F (37° C) by the thermotaxic nerve mechanism that balances heat gains and heat losses. **3.** *informal.* a fever.

**temperature of infant** [L, *temperatura + infans,* infant],  the neonatal temperature, which normally ranges from 96° to 99.5° F (35.5° to 37.5° C). It is unstable because of immature physiologic mechanisms.

**temperature regulation,**  a nursing intervention from the Nursing Interventions Classification (NIC) defined as attaining and/or maintaining body temperature within a normal range. See also **Nursing Interventions Classification.**

**temperature regulation: intraoperative,**  a nursing intervention from the Nursing Interventions Classification (NIC) defined as attaining and/or maintaining desired intraoperative body temperature. See also **Nursing Interventions Classification.**

**temperature sense.**  See **thermic sense.**

**temper tantrum.**  See **tantrum.**

**template** /tem′plit/ [L, *templum,* section],  the strand of DNA that acts as a model for the synthesis of messenger RNA. The messenger RNA contains a complementary sequence of nucleotides and travels to the ribosomes, which are located in the cytoplasm, for the synthesis of proteins.

**template bleeding time test.**  See **simplate bleeding time test.**

**tempo-,**  **1.** prefix meaning 'time': *tempolabile, temporal, tempostabile.* **2.** prefix meaning 'the temples, in the lateral regions of the head': *temporal, temporalis, temporomandibular.*

**temporal** /tem′pərəl/ [L, *tempus,* time; *tempora,* the temples],  **1.** pertaining to a limited time. **2.** relating to the temple of the skull. **3.** pertaining to the temporal bone of the skull.

**temporal arteritis** [L, *temporalis,* temporary, *arteria,* airpipe, *itis,* inflammation],  a progressive inflammatory disorder of cranial blood vessels, principally the temporal artery. It occurs most frequently in women over 70 years of age. Characteristic changes in the involved vessels include granulomatous disruption of the elastic layer and engulfment of fiber fragments by giant cells in the intimal and medial layers. The temporal artery is typically tender, swollen, and pulseless but may be clinically normal. Symptoms are intractable headache, difficulty in chewing, weakness, rheumatic pains, and loss of vision if the central retinal artery becomes occluded. Also called **cranial arteritis, giant cell arteritis, Horton's arteritis.**

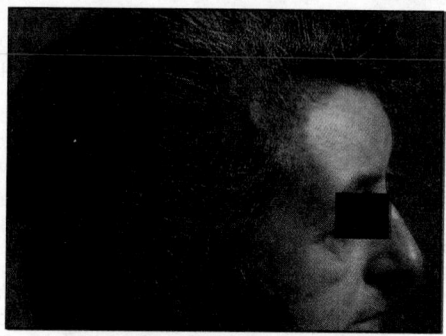

**Temporal arteritis** *(Perkin, 1998)*

**temporal artery,**  any one of three arteries on each side of the head: the superficial temporal artery, the middle temporal artery, and the deep temporal artery.

**temporal bone,**  one of a pair of large bones forming part of the lower cranium and containing various cavities and recesses associated with the ear, such as the tympanic cavity and the auditory tube. Each temporal bone consists of four parts: the mastoid, the squama, the petrous, and the tympanic.

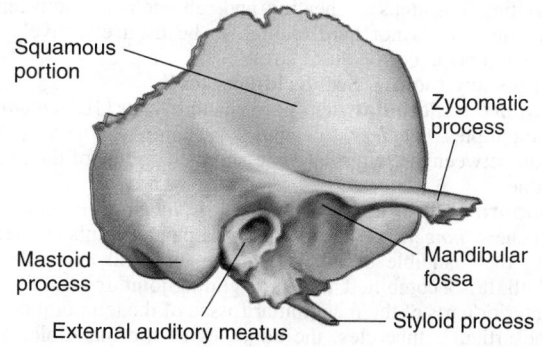

Squamous portion · Zygomatic process · Mastoid process · Mandibular fossa · External auditory meatus · Styloid process

**Temporal bone**

**temporal bone fracture,**  a break in the temporal bone of the skull, sometimes characterized by bleeding from the ear. Diminished hearing, facial paralysis, or infection of the tympanic cavity leading to meningitis may occur.

**temporal gyrus,**  any of three convolutions, inferior, middle, or superior, on the lateral surface of the temporal lobe of the brain.

**temporalis** /tem′pəral′is/, one of the four muscles of mastication. It is a broad radiating muscle that acts to close the jaws and retract the mandible. Also called **temporal muscle.** Compare **masseter, pterygoideus lateralis, pterygoideus medialis.**

**temporal lobe,** the lateral region of the cerebrum, below the lateral fissure. Within the temporal lobe of the brain is the center for smell, some association areas for memory and learning, and a region where choice is made of thoughts to express. Compare **frontal lobe, occipital lobe, parietal lobe.**

**temporal lobe epilepsy.** See **psychomotor seizure.**

**temporal muscle.** See **temporalis.**

**temporal subtraction,** the subtraction of two or more digitized x-ray images that were acquired at different times. The subtraction process eliminates information in the image that was static. If contrast material is introduced into the organ during the period between two image acquisitions, the subtracted image will show only the space filled with the contrast material.

**temporal summation.** See **summation,** def. 2.

**temporary absence.** See **conditional discharge.**

**temporary base.** See **baseplate.**

**temporary pacemaker** /tem′pərer′ē/ [L, *temporalis,* temporary, *passus,* step; ME, *maken*], an electronic pacemaker used as an interim treatment when the heart rate is excessively low. It consists of either a pulse generator and battery attached outside the patient's body and connected to a transvenous electrode in the right ventricle, or conductive pads placed on the chest and connected to an external pulse generator by cables.

**temporary prosthesis.** See **preparatory prosthesis.**

**temporary removable splint** [L, *temporalis,* temporary, *remover* + D, *splint*], any of a variety of dental appliances, including occlusal splints, used when limited stability of the teeth is required. It may be placed on or removed from teeth at will. Examples include Haley's orthodontic appliance and Elbrecht's cast metal splint.

**temporary stopping** [L, *temporalis* + AS, *stoppian,* to stop up], a mixture of gutta-percha, zinc oxide, white wax, and coloring, used for temporarily sealing dressings in tooth cavities. It softens on heating and rehardens at room temperature but is not hard enough to be used effectively in tooth areas under occlusal stress.

**temporary tooth.** See **deciduous tooth.**

**temporomandibular** /tem′pərō′mandib′yələr/ [L, *tempora,* the temples, *mandere,* to chew], pertaining to the articulation between the temporal bone and the condyle of the mandible.

**temporomandibular joint (TMJ)** [L, *tempora* + *mandere,* to chew, *jungere,* to join], one of a pair of joints connecting the mandible of the jaw to the temporal bone of the skull. It is a combined hinge and gliding joint, formed by the anterior parts of the mandibular fossae of the temporal bone, the articular tubercles, the condyles of the mandible, and five ligaments.

**temporomandibular joint capsule,** a fibrous protective sheath enclosing the temporomandibular joint of the lower jaw.

**temporomandibular joint (TMJ) pain dysfunction syndrome,** an abnormal condition characterized by facial pain and by mandibular dysfunction, apparently caused by a defective or dislocated temporomandibular joint. Some common indications of this syndrome are clicking of the joint when the jaws move, limitation of jaw movement, subluxation, and temporomandibular dislocation.

**temporomandibular ligament** [L, *temporalis* + *mandere,*

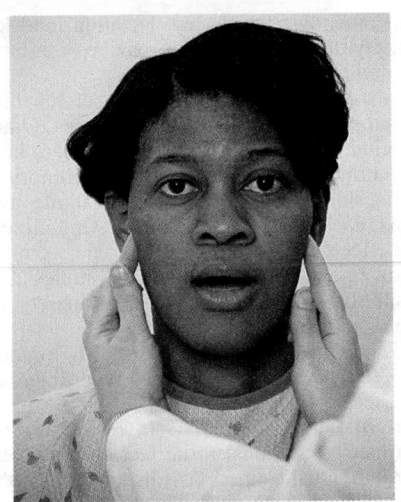

**Assessment of the temporomandibular joint**
*(Seidel et al, 1999)*

to chew, *ligare,* to bind], an oblique band of connective tissue that extends downward and backward from the zygomatic process to the neck of the mandible.

**temporomaxillary** /-mak′siler′ē/, pertaining to the area of the temporal and maxillary bones.

**temporooccipital** /tem′pərō·oksip′itəl/, pertaining to the area of the temporal and occipital bones.

**temporoparietal.** See **parietotemporal.**

**temporoparietalis** /tem′pərōpərī′ətal′is/ [L, *temporalis* + *paries,* wall], one of a pair of broad, thin muscles of the scalp, divided into three parts, which fan out over the temporal fascia and insert into the galea aponeurotica. The three parts include an anterior temporal part, a superior parietal part, and a triangular part in between. On both sides it acts in combination with the occipitofrontalis to wrinkle the forehead, widen the eyes, and raise the ears. It is innervated by branches of the facial nerve. Compare **occipitofrontalis.**

**TEN,** abbreviation for **toxic epidermal necrolysis.**

**tenacious** /tenā′shəs/ [L, *tenax,* holding fast], pertaining to secretions that are sticky or adhesive or otherwise tend to hold together, such as mucus and sputum.

**tenacity** /tenas′itē/ [L, *tenax,* holding fast], the ability to be persistent or remain attached.

**tenaculum** /tənak′yələm/, *pl.* **tenacula** [L, holder], a clip or clamp with long handles used to grasp, immobilize, and hold an organ or a piece of tissue. Kinds of tenacula include the **abdominal tenaculum,** which has long arms and small hooks, the **forceps tenaculum,** which has long hooks and is used in gynecologic surgery, and the **uterine** or **cervical tenaculum,** which has short hooks or open, eye-shaped clamps used to hold the cervix.

**tenalgia** /tenal′jə/, pain referred to a tendon. Also called **tenodynia.**

**tender,** responding with a sensation of pain to pressure or touch that would not normally cause discomfort.

**tendinitis** /ten′dənī′tis/ [L, *tendere,* to stretch; Gk, *itis,* inflammation], inflammation of a tendon, usually resulting from strain. Treatment may include rest, corticosteroid injections, application of ice or heat, and support. Also spelled **tendonitis.**

**tendino-.** See **teno-.**

**tendinous** /ten'dinəs/ [L, *tendere*, to stretch],   pertaining to or resembling a tendon.

**tendinous cords.**   See **chordae tendineae.**

**tendo** /ten'dō/,   a tendon, such as the tendo calcaneus, the Achilles tendon.

**tendo-.**   See **teno-.**

**tendo calcaneus.**   See **Achilles tendon.**

**tendon** /ten'dən/ [Gk, *tenon*],   any one of many white, glistening bands of dense fibrous connective tissue that attach muscle to bone. Except at points of attachment, tendons are parallel bundles of collagenous fibers sheathed in delicate fibroelastic connective tissue. Larger tendons contain a thin internal septum, a few blood vessels, and specialized stereognostic nerves. Tendons are extremely strong, flexible, and inelastic and occur in various lengths and thicknesses. Compare **ligament.** —**tendinous,** *adj.*

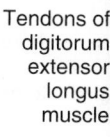

Tendons of digitorum extensor longus muscle

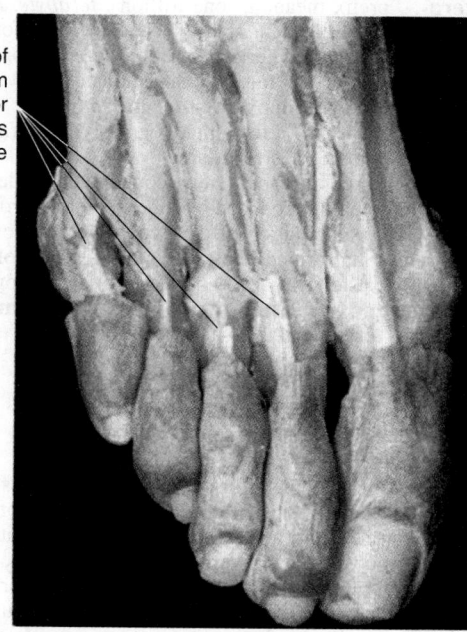

**Tendons** *(Vidic and Suarez, 1984)*

**tendonitis.**   See **tendinitis.**

**tendon of Achilles.**   See **Achilles tendon.**

**tendon reflex.**   See **deep tendon reflex.**

**tendosynovitis.**   See **tenosynovitis.**

**tenesmic** /tənez'mik/ [Gk, *tenedere*, to stretch],   pertaining to or resembling tenesmus.

**tenesmus** /tənez'məs/ [Gk, *tenedere*, to stretch],   persistent, ineffectual spasms of the rectum or bladder, accompanied by the desire to empty the bowel or bladder. Intestinal tenesmus is a common complaint in inflammatory bowel disease and irritable bowel syndrome. —**tenesmic,** *adj.*

**tenia** /tē'nē·ə/,   **1.** any anatomic bandlike structure, such as a band of muscle fibers. **2.** a bandage or tape.

**tenia-, taenia-,**   combining form meaning 'ribbon, band': *taeniasis, teniafuge, taenidium.*

**teniasis** /tēnī'əsis/,   an infection of intestinal tapeworms of the genus *Taenia.*

**tennis elbow.**   See **lateral humeral epicondylitis.**

**teno-, tenonto-, tendo-, tendino-,**   prefix meaning 'tendon': *tenodesis, tenodynia, tenomyotomy.*

**tenodesis splint** /tənod'əsis, ten'ōdē'sis/,   the fixation of a tendon, sometimes performed by suturing one of its ends to a different point.

**tenodynia.**   See **tenalgia.**

**tenofibril.**   See **tonofibril.**

**Tenon's capsule.**   See **fascia bulbi.**

**tenonto-.**   See **teno-.**

**tenophony** /tenof'ənē/,   a heart murmur associated with a defect in the chordae tendineae.

**Tenormin,**   trademark for a beta-blocker (atenolol).

**tenosynovitis** /ten'ōsin'əvī'tis/ [Gk, *tenon*, tendon, *syn*, together; L, *ovum*, egg; Gk, *itis*],   inflammation of a tendon sheath caused by calcium deposits, repeated strain or trauma, high levels of blood cholesterol, rheumatoid arthritis, gout, or gonorrhea. In some instances, movement causes a crackling noise over the tendon. Most cases not associated with systemic disease respond to rest. Local injections of corticosteroids may provide relief; surgery is indicated if the condition persists. Also called **tendosynovitis.**

**tenotomy** /tenot'əmē/ [Gk, *tenon*, tendon, *temnein*, to cut],   the total or partial severing of a tendon, performed to correct a muscle imbalance, such as in the correction of strabismus of the eye or in clubfoot.

**TENS,**   abbreviation for **transcutaneous electrical nerve stimulation.**

**Tensilon,**   trademark for an anticholinesterase drug (edrophonium).

**Tensilon test,**   a diagnostic technique for verifying the signs of myasthenia gravis by testing the power of skeletal muscles before and after injection of edrophonium hydrochloride.

**tensiometer** /ten'sē·om'ətər/ [L, *tendere*, to stretch; Gk, *metron*, measure],   a device for measuring the surface tension of a liquid.

**tension** /ten'shən/ [L, *tendere*, to stretch],   **1.** the act of pulling or straining until taut. **2.** the condition of being taut, tense, or under pressure. **3.** a state or condition resulting from the psychologic and physiologic reaction to a stressful situation. It is characterized physically by a general increase in muscle tonus, heart rate, respiration rate, and alertness and psychologically by feelings of strain, uneasiness, irritability, and anxiety. See also **stress.**

**-tension.**   See **-tention.**

**tension headache,**   a pain that affects the head as the result of overwork or emotional strain and involving tension in the muscles of the neck, face, and shoulder.

**tension pneumothorax** [L, *tendere*, to stretch; Gk, *pneuma*, air, *thorax*],   the presence of air in the pleural space caused by a rupture through the chest wall or lung parenchyma associated with the valvular opening. Air passes through the valve during coughing but cannot escape on exhalation. Unrelieved pneumothorax can lead to respiratory arrest.

**tensor** /ten'sər/ [L, *tendere*, to stretch],   any one of the muscles of the body that tenses a structure, such as the tensor fasciae latae of the thigh. Compare **abductor, adductor, depressor, sphincter.**

**tensor fasciae latae,**   one of the 10 muscles of the gluteal region, arising from the outer lip of the iliac crest, the iliac spine, and the deep fascia lata. It inserts between the two layers of fascia lata in the proximal third of the thigh. The tensor fasciae latae functions to flex the thigh and rotate it slightly medially. Also called **tensor fasciae femoris.**

**tensor tympani** /ten'sər tim'pə·nē/,   a muscle originating in the cartilaginous portion of the auditory tube and insert-

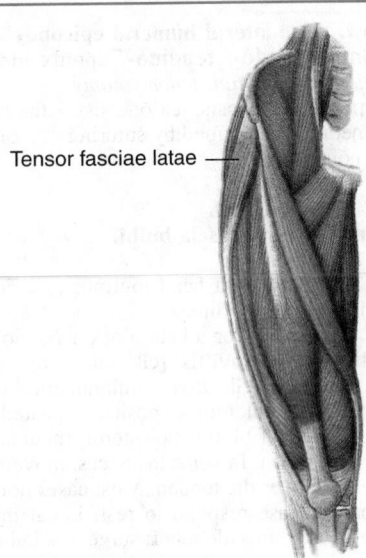

Tensor fasciae latae

**Tensor fasciae latae**
*(Thibodeau and Patton, 1999/John V. Hagen)*

ing in the manubrium of the malleus; it functions to tense the tympanic membrane.

**tent** [ME, *tente*],    **1.** a transparent cover, usually of plastic, supported over the upper part of a patient by a frame. Used in the treatment of respiratory conditions, it provides a controlled environment into which steam, oxygen, vaporized medication, or droplets of cool water may be sprayed, such as an oxygen tent. **2.** a cone made of various materials inserted into a cavity or orifice of the body to dilate its opening, such as a laminaria tent. **3.** a pack placed in a wound to hold it open to ensure that healing progresses from the base of the wound upward to the skin.

**tentative** /ten′tətiv/ [L, *tentare*, to touch],    not final or definite, such as an experimental finding that has not been validated.

**tenth cranial nerve.**    See **vagus nerve.**

**tenth-value layer (TVL)** [ME, *tenpe* + L, *valere*, to be worth; AS, *lecgan*, to lie],    the thickness of material required to attenuate a beam of radiation to one tenth of its original intensity. See also **half-value layer.**

**tenting of skin** /ten′ting/,    a slow return of the skin to its normal position after being pinched, a sign of either dehydration or aging, or both.

**-tention,**    suffix meaning the 'condition of being held': *histroretention, retention.*

**-tention, -tension,**    suffix meaning 'condition of being stretched or strained, or in which pressure is exerted': *attention, distension, intention.*

**tentorial herniation** /tentôr′ē·əl/ [L, *tentorium*, tent, *hernia*, rupture],    the protrusion of brain tissue into the tentorial notch, caused by increased intracranial pressure resulting from edema, hemorrhage, or a tumor. Characteristic signs are severe headache, fever, flushing, sweating, abnormal pupillary reflex, drowsiness, hypotension, and loss of consciousness. Also called **transtentorial herniation.**

**tentorial notch** [L, *tentorium*, tent; OFr, *enochier*],    an area occupied by the midbrain and enclosed by the free border of the tentorium cerebelli and the sphenoid bone.

**tentorium** /tentôr′ē·əm/, *pl.* **tentoria** [L, tent],    any part of the body that resembles a tent, such as the tentorium of the hypophysis that covers the hypophyseal fossa.

**tentorium cerebelli,**    one of the membranous covers of the dura mater that separates the cerebellum from the occipital lobe of the cerebrum. Compare **falx cerebelli, falx cerebri.**

**Tenuate,**    trademark for an anorexiant (diethylpropion hydrochloride).

**tenure** /ten′yər/ [L, *tenere*, to hold],    (in a university) a faculty appointment with few limits on the number of years it may be held; a permanent appointment usually awarded to a person who has advanced to the rank of associate professor and who demonstrates scholarship, community service, and teaching excellence in a specific field of study.

**-tepa,**    combining form for antineoplastic thiotepa derivatives.

**tephr-,**    prefix meaning 'gray or ash-colored': *tephromalacia, tephromyelitis, tephrosis.*

**tepid,**    moderately warm to the touch.

**teprotide** /tep′rōtīd/,    a bradykinin-potentiating peptide.

**tera-,**    prefix meaning 'one trillion': *terabyte, terahertz.*

**teramorphous** [Gk, *teras*, monster, *morphe*, form],    of the nature of or characteristic of a teratic embryo.

**teras** /ter′əs/, *pl.* **terata** [Gk, monster],    a severely deformed fetus; a **monster. —teratic,** *adj.*

**teratic embryo**    a fetus that is grossly malformed and usually nonviable. See **teratism.**

**teratism** /ter′ətiz′əm/,    any congenital or developmental anomaly that is produced by inherited or environmental factors or a combination of the two; any condition in which a severely malformed fetus is produced. Kinds of teratism include **atresic teratism, ceasmic teratism, ectopic teratism, ectrogenic teratism, hypergenetic teratism,** and **symphysic teratism.** Also called **teratosis.**

**terato-,**    combining form meaning 'monster': *teratoblastoma, teratogenesis, teratoma.*

**teratoblastoma** /ter′ətō′blastō′mə/,    a teratoma in which not all germ layers are present.

**teratogen** /ter′ətəjen′/ [Gk, *teras* + *genein,* to produce],    any substance, agent, or process that interferes with normal prenatal development, causing the formation of one or more developmental abnormalities in the fetus. Teratogens act directly on the developing organism or indirectly, affecting such supplemental structures as the placenta or some maternal system. The type and extent of the defect are determined by the specific kind of teratogen, its mode of action, the embryonic process affected, genetic predisposition, and the stage of development at the time the exposure occurred. The period of highest vulnerability in the developing embryo is from about the third through the twelfth week of gestation, when differentiation of the major organs and systems occurs. Susceptibility to teratogenic influence decreases rapidly in the later periods of development, which are characterized by growth and elaboration. Among the known teratogens are chemical agents, including such drugs as thalidomide, alkylating agents, and alcohol; infectious agents, especially the rubella virus and cytomegalovirus; ionizing radiation, particularly x-rays; and environmental factors, such as the age and general health of the mother or any intrauterine trauma that may affect the fetus, especially during the later stages of pregnancy. Compare **mutagen. —teratogenic,** *adj.*

**teratogenesis** /ter′ətōjen′əsis/,    the development of physical defects in the embryo. Also called **teratogeny** /ter′ətoj′ənē/. **—teratogenetic,** *adj.*

**teratogenic agent.**    See **teratogen.**

**teratogenous** /ter′ətoj′ənəs/ [Gk, *teras,* monster, *genein,* to produce],    developed from fetal membranes.

## Well-established human teratogens

Drugs and chemicals
   Thalidomide
   Diethylstilbestrol
   Warfarin
   Hydantoin
   Trimethadione
   Excessive alcohol
   Valproic acid
   Aminopterin/methotrexate
   Tetracycline
   Isotretinoin
   Angiotensin-converting enzyme inhibitors
   Penicillamine
   Antithyroid drugs
   Androgen/masculinizing progestogen
   Methylmercury
   Polychlorobiphenyls
Maternal infections
   Rubella
   Cytomegalovirus
   Toxoplasmosis
   Varicella
   Venezuela equine encephalitis
   Syphilis
   Parvovirus
Maternal states
   Diabetes mellitus
   Phenylketonuria
   Systemic lupus erythematosus
   Graves disease
Ionizing radiation

From Jorde LB, Carey JC, White RL: *Medical genetics, revised for 1997*, St Louis, 1995, Mosby.

**teratogeny.** See **teratogenesis.**

**teratoid** /ter′ətoid/ [Gk, *teras* + *eidos,* form], pertaining to malformed physical development; grossly misplaced. misshapen parts.

**teratoid tumor.** See **dermoid cyst.**

**teratologist** /ter′ətol′əjist/, one who specializes in the causes and effects of congenital anomalies and developmental abnormalities.

**teratology** /-tol′əgē/ [Gk, *teras* + *logos,* science], the study of the causes and effects of congenital malformations and developmental abnormalities. **—teratologic, teratological,** *adj.*

**teratoma** /ter′ətō′mə/, *pl.* **teratomas, teratomata,** a tumor composed of different kinds of tissue, none of which normally occur together or at the site of the tumor. Teratomas are most common in the ovaries or testes.

**teratosis.** See **teratism.**

**terazosin** /ter′əzō′sin/, a drug approved for the treatment of benign prostatic hypertrophy. It acts by relaxing the smooth muscle fibers of the prostate through its alpha receptor blockage mechanisms. It is also used alone or in combination for the treatment of hypertension.

**terbium (Tb)** /tur′bē·əm/ [Yterby, Sweden], a rare earth metallic element. Its atomic number is 65; its atomic mass (weight) is 158.294.

**terbutaline sulfate** /terbyoo′təlēn/, a beta₂-adrenergic stimulant.

■ INDICATIONS: It is prescribed as a bronchodilator in the treatment of asthma, bronchitis, and emphysema and as a uterine relaxant to treat premature labor.

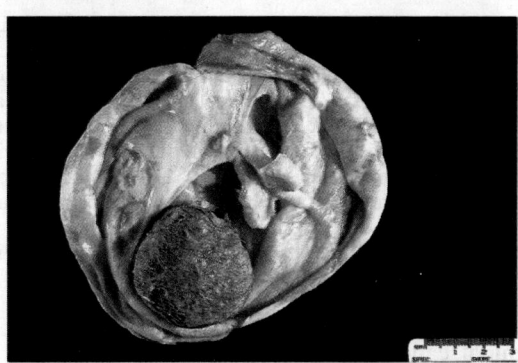

**Cystic teratoma of the ovary**
*(Kumar, Cotran, and Robbins, 1997/courtesy Dr. Christopher Crum, Brigham and Women's Hospital, Boston)*

■ CONTRAINDICATIONS: Cardiac arrhythmias or known hypersensitivity to this drug prohibits its use. It may interact with monoamine oxidase inhibitors and other beta-adrenergic blockers.

■ ADVERSE EFFECTS: Among the most serious reactions are dizziness and palpitations. Nervousness and tremor are common reactions.

**teres** /tir′ēz, ter′ēz/, *pl.* **teretes** /ter′ətēz/ [L, rounded], a long cylindric muscle such as the teres minor or the teres major. **—teres,** *adj.*

**teres major,** a thick flat muscle of the shoulder. It functions to adduct, extend, and rotate the arm medially. Compare **teres minor.**

**teres minor,** a cylindric, elongated muscle of the shoulder. It functions to rotate the arm laterally, weakly adduct the arm, and draw the humerus toward the glenoid fossa of the scapula, strengthening the shoulder joint. Compare **teres major.**

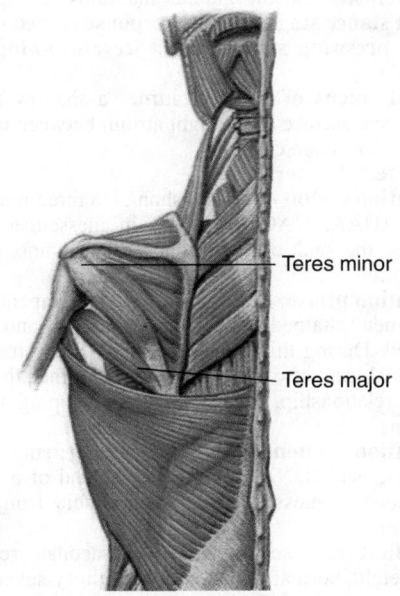

**Teres major and teres minor**
*(Thibodeau and Patton, 1999/John V. Hagen)*

**term** [L, *terminus,* limit], **1.** a specified period of time. **2.** the normal gestation period.

**terminal** /tur´minəl/ [L, *terminus,* boundary], **1.** (of a structure or process) near or approaching its end, such as a terminal bronchiole or a terminal disease. **2.** an input/output (I/O) device that has two-way communication capability with a computer. A terminal usually has a keyboard and a cathode-ray or video display screen, or a text printing facility. —**terminate,** *v.,* **terminus,** *n.*

**terminal arteriole** [L, *terminus,* boundary, *arteriola,* little artery], an arteriole that divides into capillaries.

**terminal artery.** See **end artery.**

**terminal bronchiole.** See **bronchiole.**

**terminal cancer** [L, *terminalis* + *cancer,* crab], an advanced stage of a malignant neoplastic disease with death as the inevitable prognosis.

**terminal drop,** a rapid decline in cognitive function and coping ability that occurs 1 to 5 years before death.

**terminal illness** [L, *terminalis* + ON, *illr,* bad], an advanced stage of a disease with an unfavorable prognosis and no known cure.

**terminal insomnia,** a chronic sleep disturbance occurring at the end of a sleep period. It may be indicative of an underlying depressive disorder and treated with an antidepressant.

**terminal nerve,** a small nerve originating in the cerebral hemisphere in the region of the olfactory trigone, classified by most anatomists as part of the olfactory, or first cranial, nerve. It courses anteriorly along the olfactory tract and passes through the ethmoid bone. It communicates in the nasal cavity with the ophthalmic division of the trigeminal nerve.

**terminal stance,** one of the five stages in the stance phase of a walking gait, directly associated with the continuation of single limb support or the period during which the body moves forward on the supporting foot. Double limb support is initiated during the latter part of terminal stance, which is often a factor in the analysis of many abnormal orthopedic conditions and the diagnosis of weaknesses that may develop in certain muscles used in walking, such as the quadriceps femoris and the gluteus maximus. Compare **initial contact stance stage, loading response stance stage, midstance, preswing stance stage.** See also **swing phase of gait.**

**terminal sulcus of right atrium,** a shallow channel on the external surface of the right atrium between the superior and inferior venae cavae.

**terminate.** See **terminal.**

**termination codon** /tur´minā´shən/, a three-nucleotide sequence (UAA, UAG, or UGA) in messenger RNA that specifies the end of the sequence of amino acids in a polypeptide.

**termination phase,** the last stage of a therapeutic relationship when attained goals are evaluated and outcomes achieved. During this stage practitioners also may help patients establish networks of support, other than the therapist-patient relationship, that may help in coping with future problems.

**termination sequence,** (in molecular genetics) a deoxyribonucleic acid (DNA) segment at the end of a unit that is transcribed to messenger ribonucleic acid from the DNA template.

**term infant** [L, *terminus,* limit], any neonate, regardless of birth weight, born after the end of the thirty-seventh and before the beginning of the forty-third week of gestation. Infants delivered at term usually measure from 48 to 53 cm from head to heel and weigh between 2700 and 4000 g.

**terminus** /tur´minəs/ [L, the end], a boundary or limit.

**terpin** /tur´pin/, **1.** a diterpene alcohol derived from turpentine oil. **2.** an expectorant ingredient produced through the action of nitric and sulfuric acids on pine oil.

**terpin hydrate and codeine elixir** /tur´pin/, a preparation of the expectorant terpin hydrate, with sweet orange peel tincture, benzaldehyde, glycerin, alcohol, syrup, water, and the antitussive opiate codeine. Terpin hydrate diminishes secretions and promotes healing of the mucous membrane, and codeine depresses the cough center in the medulla oblongata; prolonged use may lead to addiction.

**Terra-Cortril,** trademark for a topical fixed-combination drug containing a glucocorticoid (hydrocortisone) and an antibiotic (oxytetracycline).

**Terramycin,** trademark for an antibiotic (oxytetracycline).

**territorial** /ter´ətôr´ē·əl/ [L, *territorium,* district], a type of body movement that aids in communication. A territorial will frame an interaction and define an individual's "territory." See also **territoriality.**

**territoriality** /ter´itôr´ē·al´itē/, an emotional attachment to and defense of certain areas related to one's existence. Humans and animals generally establish a claim to or occupy a defined or undefined area over which they can maintain some degree of control.

**terti-,** combining form meaning 'third': *tertiary, tertigravida, tertipara.*

**tertian** /tur´shən/ [L, *tertius,* third], occurring every 48 hours, including the first day of occurrence, such as vivax or tertian malaria, in which fever occurs every third day. Compare **quartan.** See also **malaria.**

**tertian malaria,** a form of malaria caused by the protozoan *Plasmodium vivax* or *P. ovale,* characterized by febrile paroxysms that occur every 48 hours. **Vivax malaria,** caused by *P. vivax,* is the most common form of malaria; although it is rarely fatal, it is the most difficult form to cure. Relapses are common. **Ovale malaria,** caused by *P. ovale,* is usually milder and causes only a few short attacks. Both types of tertian malaria are treated with chloroquine. Compare **falciparum malaria, quartan malaria.** See also **malaria.**

**tertiary** /tur´shē·er´ē, tursh´ərē/ [L, *tertius,* third], third in frequency or order of use; belonging to the third level of sophistication of development, such as a tertiary health care facility.

**tertiary health care,** a specialized, highly technical level of health care that includes diagnosis and treatment of disease and disability. Specialized intensive care units, advanced diagnostic support services, and highly specialized personnel are usually characteristic of tertiary health care. It offers highly centralized care to the population of a large region and in some cases to the world.

**tertiary intention.** See **intention.**

**tertiary prevention,** a level of preventive medicine that deals with the rehabilitation and return of a patient to a status of maximum usefulness with a minimum risk of recurrence of a physical or mental disorder.

**tertiary syphilis** [L, *tertius,* third], the most advanced stage of syphilis, resulting in infections of the cardiovascular and neurologic systems and marked by destructive lesions involving many tissues and organs. Late-stage syphilis is symptomatic but not contagious.

**tervalent.** See **trivalent.**

**tesla** /tes´lə/ [Nikola Tesla, American engineer, 1856–1943], a unit of magnetic flux density, defined by the International System of Units as 1 weber per square meter, the equivalent of 1 volt/second per square meter, or 10,000 gauss.

**Teslac,** trademark for an antineoplastic (testolactone).

**Tessalon,** trademark for a local anesthetic agent (benzonatate).

**test** [L, *testum,* crucible], **1.** an examination or trial intended to establish a principle or determine a value. **2.** a chemical reaction or reagent that has clinical significance. **3.** to detect, identify, or conduct a trial. See also **laboratory test.**

**test-,** combining form meaning 'testicles': *testicond, testitoxicosis, testosterone.*

**testa** /tes'tə/ [L, a shell], **1.** an eggshell. **2.** powdered oyster shells used in antacids. **3.** the outer coat of a seed.

**Testacealobosia** /tes'təse'lōbō'zhə/, a subclass of ameboid protozoa in which the cells are enclosed in a chitinous or membranous envelope, vest, or shell. It includes both marine and freshwater forms.

**testamentary capacity** /tes'təmen'tərē/, a person's competency to make a will, including that he or she be aware that a will is being made, of the nature and extent of property covered by the will, and of the identities of beneficiaries.

**testcross** [L, *testum + crux,* cross], **1.** a cross between a dominant and a recessive phenotype to determine either the degree of genetic linkage or whether the dominant phenotype is a result of a homozygous or a heterozygous genotype. **2.** a subject undergoing such a test. See also **backcross.**

**testes.** See **testis.**

**testes determining factor (TDF)** /tes'tēz/, a gene on the Y chromosome that is believed to determine male sexual development. Individuals with the normal female sex chromosome combination (XX) may develop as males if the TDF gene has migrated to one of the X chromosomes. Also, individuals with the normal male sex chromosome pair (XY) may develop as females if the TDF gene is missing from the Y chromosome.

**test for acetone in urine,** a part of routine urinalysis. Normal findings are negative, since acetone and other ketones are not normally present in urine. Exceptions include such cases as poorly controlled diabetic patients, alcoholics, and people who may be fasting or on special high-protein diets.

**test for lacrimation,** a test for possible dry eye and/or keratoconjunctivitis sicca conducted by placing a 35-mm long piece of filter paper in the lower fornix of the conjunctiva for 5 minutes. Failure of tears to wet as much as 10 mm of the strip indicates inadequate tear production. Also called **Schirmer's test.**

**testicle.** See **testis.**

**testicular** /testik'yələr/ [L, *testiculus,* testicle], pertaining to the testicle.

**testicular artery,** one of a pair of long, slender branches of the abdominal aorta, arising inferior to the renal arteries and supplying the testis.

**testicular cancer,** a malignant neoplastic disease of the testis occurring most frequently in men between 20 and 35 years of age. An undescended testicle is often involved. In many cases the tumor is detected after an injury, but trauma is not considered a causative factor. Patients with early testicular cancer are often asymptomatic, and metastases may be present in lymph nodes, the lungs, and the liver before the primary lesion is palpable. In the later stages there may be pulmonary symptoms, ureteral obstruction, gynecomastia, and an abdominal mass. Diagnostic measures include transillumination of the scrotum, excretory urography, lymphangiography, and a urine or serum test to evaluate circulating levels of tumor markers. Tumors develop more often in the right than in the left testis. Testis cancers are often curable. Chemotherapeutic agents, used in various combinations, are increasing the survival of patients with testicular cancer. Some of these drugs are actinomycin D, bleomycin, *cis*-platinum, cyclophosphamide, methotrexate, and vincristine.

**testicular duct.** See **vas deferens.**

**testicular feminization.** See **feminization.**

**testicular hormone,** any androgenic steroid hormone secreted by the Leydig cells in the interstitial tissues of the male gonads. Testosterone is the principal hormone secreted by the cells, which also secrete estrogen, the female sex hormone. Testosterone may be converted into estrogen and other steroid hormones, such as dihydrotestosterone, in certain tissues. The secretion of testicular hormones is controlled by luteinizing hormone and follicle-stimulating hormone, both secreted by the anterior pituitary gland.

**testicular self-examination (TSE),** a procedure recommended by the National Institutes of Health for detecting tumors or other abnormalities in the male testes. The TSE is conducted in four simple steps, starting by standing in front of a mirror and looking for any swelling on the skin of the scrotum. One testicle may appear larger than the other, and one may hang lower, which is usually normal. Next, each testicle is examined with both hands, placing the fingers under the testicle while the thumbs are placed on top. The testicle is then rolled gently between the thumbs and fingers. In the next step the epididymis, a normal cordlike structure on the top and back of each testicle, should be found. A small pea-sized lump is felt for on the front or side of a testicle. The lump is usually painless. TSE should be performed once a month, usually after a warm bath or shower because the heat causes scrotal skin to relax, thereby increasing the chances of detecting any tissue abnormality. Testicular cancer almost always occurs in only one testicle. It is highly curable when detected at an early stage.

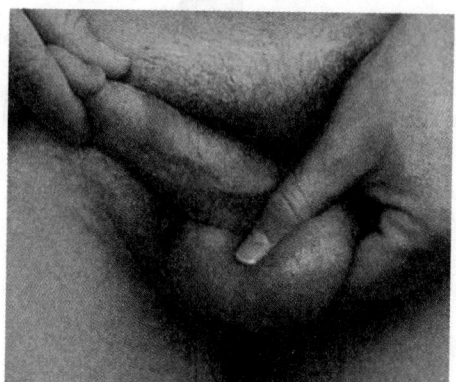

**Testicular self-examination** (Seidel et al, 1999)

**testicular vein,** one of a pair of veins emerging from convoluted venous plexuses, forming the greater mass of the spermatic cords. The right testicular vein opens into the inferior vena cava; the left testicular vein into the left renal vein. Both testicular veins contain valves. Compare **ovarian vein.**

**testimony** /tes'timō'nē/ [L, *testimonium,* evidence], the statement of a witness, usually made orally and given under oath, such as at a court trial.

**testis** /tes′tis/, *pl.* **testes** /tes′tēz′/, one of the pair of male gonads that produce sperm and testosterone. The adult testes are suspended in the scrotum by the spermatic cords; in early fetal life they are contained in the abdominal cavity behind the peritoneum. Before birth they normally descend into the scrotum. The coverings of the testes are the skin and the dartos tunic of the scrotum, the external spermatic fascia, the cremasteric layer, the internal spermatic fascia, and the tunica vaginalis. Each testis is a laterally compressed oval body about 4 cm long and 2.5 cm wide, and weighs about 12 g. It is positioned obliquely in the scrotum, with the cranial extremity directed ventrally and slightly laterally and the caudal end directed dorsally and slightly medially. The anterior border, lateral surfaces, and extremities of the organ are convex, free, smooth, and covered by the tunica vaginalis. The convoluted epididymis lying on the posterior border of the testis contains a tightly coiled tube that is about 20 feet long and connects with the vas deferens through which spermatozoa pass during ejaculation. Each testis consists of several hundred conical lobules containing the tiny coiled seminiferous tubules, each about 75 mm long, in which spermatozoa develop. In early life the tubules are pale in color, but in old age become invested with yellow fatty matter. The tubules converge to form the rete testis, which is drained by the efferent ducts into the head of the epididymis. The testes are supplied with blood by the two internal spermatic arteries that arise from the aorta, are served by the testicular veins that form the pampiniform plexuses constituting the greater part of the spermatic cords, and are innervated by the spermatic plexuses of nerves from the celiac plexuses of the autonomic nervous system. Also called **testicle.** Compare **ovary.** See also **scrotum.** —**testicular,** *adj.*

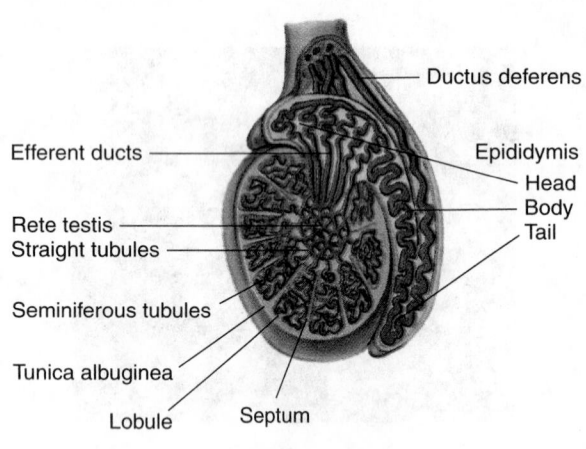

Labels (clockwise):
Ductus deferens
Epididymis
Head
Body
Tail
Septum
Lobule
Tunica albuginea
Seminiferous tubules
Straight tubules
Rete testis
Efferent ducts

**Testis** *(Applegate, 2000)*

**test method,** a method chosen for experimental testing or study by means of method evaluation.

**test of patency of tear duct,** a procedure in which drops of a weak sugar solution are placed in the eye. If the patient then detects a sweet taste, the tear duct is assumed open.

**testolactone** /tes′təlak′tōn/, an antineoplastic androgen analog.

■ INDICATIONS: It is prescribed in the treatment of postmenopausal breast cancer and in premenopausal women whose ovarian function has been terminated.

■ CONTRAINDICATIONS: Pregnancy, lactation, or known hypersensitivity to this drug prohibits its use. It is not given to men.

■ ADVERSE EFFECTS: Among the more serious adverse reactions are hypercalcemia and peripheral neuropathies with numbness or tingling.

**testosterone** /testos′tərōn/, a naturally occurring androgenic hormone.

■ INDICATIONS: It is prescribed for androgen deficiency, for female breast cancer, and for stimulation of growth, weight gain, and red blood cell production.

■ CONTRAINDICATIONS: Cancer of the male breast or prostate, liver disease, pregnancy or suspected pregnancy, or known hypersensitivity to this drug prohibits its use.

■ ADVERSE EFFECTS: Among the more serious adverse reactions are fluid retention, masculinization, acne, and erythrocythemia.

**testosterone cyclopentylpropionate.** See **testosterone cypionate.**

**testosterone cypionate,** a long-acting form of testosterone.

**testosterone derivative.** See **anabolic steroid.**

**testosterone enanthate,** a long-acting form of testosterone.

**testosterone propionate,** an androgen given intramuscularly. See also **testosterone.**

**testosterone test,** a blood test that detects levels of circulating testosterone in men and women. It may be used to evaluate ambiguous sex characteristics, precocious puberty, virilizing syndromes in the female, and infertility in the male. It can also be used as a tumor marker for rare tumors of the ovary and testicle.

**test tube,** a thin glass container with one open end and one closed end. It is used in many common laboratory procedures. Compare **Veillon tube.** See also **tube.**

**test tube baby,** a popular term for an infant conceived through in vitro fertilization, using an ovum removed from the mother. After fertilization the zygote is transplanted to the mother's uterus to develop normally. See also **in vitro fertilization.**

**-tetanic** /tetan′ik/, combining form meaning 'tetanus or tetany': *antitetanic, posttetanic, subtetanic.*

**tetanic contraction** [Gk, *tetanos,* extreme tension; L, *contractio,* drawing together], a condition of continuous contraction in a voluntary muscle caused by a steady stream of efferent nerve impulses.

**tetanic convulsion** [Gk, *tetanos,* extreme tension; L, *convulsio,* cramp], **1.** a generalized tonic muscular contraction. **2.** a prolonged violent involuntary muscular contraction. See also **tonic convulsion.**

**tetano-,** combining form meaning 'tetanus': *tetanolysin, tetanometer, tetanophilic.*

**tetanus** /tet′ənəs/ [Gk, *tetanos,* extreme tension], an acute, potentially fatal infection of the central nervous system caused by an exotoxin, tetanospasmin, elaborated by an anaerobic bacillus, *Clostridium tetani.* More than 50,000 people a year die of tetanus infection worldwide. The toxin is a neurotoxin and one of the most lethal poisons known. *C. tetani* infects only wounds that contain dead tissue. The bacillus is a common resident of the superficial layers of the soil and a normal inhabitant of the intestinal tracts of cows and horses; therefore barnyards and fields fertilized with manure are heavily contaminated.

■ OBSERVATIONS: The bacillus may enter the body through a puncture wound, abrasion, laceration, or burn; via the uterus into the bloodstream in septic abortion or postpartum sepsis; or through the stump of the umbilical cord of the newborn. The dead tissue of the area is low in oxygen; this is the en-

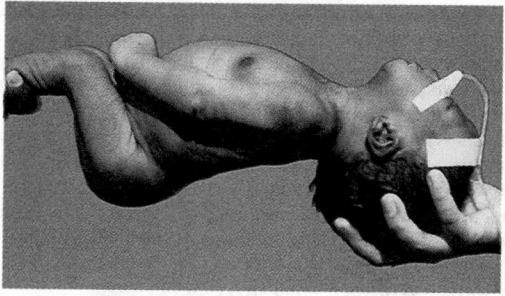

**Tetanus: characteristic muscle spasms**
*(Farrar, 1993/courtesy Dr. T.F. Sellers Jr.)*

vironment essential for the replication of *C. tetani*. The infection occurs in two clinical forms: one with an abrupt onset, high mortality, and a short incubation period (3 to 21 days); the other with less severe symptoms, a lower mortality, and a longer incubation period (4 to 5 weeks). Wounds of the face, head, and neck are the ones most likely to result in fatal infection. The disease is characterized by irritability, headache, fever, and painful spasms of the muscles resulting in lockjaw, risus sardonicus, opisthotonos, and laryngeal spasm; eventually every muscle of the body is in tonic spasm. The motor nerves transmit the impulses from the infected central nervous system to the muscles. There is no lesion; even at autopsy no organic lesion is seen and the cerebrospinal fluid is clear and normal.

■ INTERVENTIONS: Prompt and thorough cleansing and debridement of the wound are essential for prophylaxis. A booster shot of tetanus toxoid is given to previously immunized people; tetanus immune globulin and a series of three injections of tetanus toxoid are given to those not immunized. People who are known to have been adequately immunized within 5 years do not usually require immunization. Treatment of people who have the infection includes maintenance of an airway, administration of an antitoxin as soon as possible, sedation, control of the muscle spasms, and assurance of a normal fluid balance. The room is kept quiet, and benzodiazepines may be given to reduce hypertonicity; penicillin G is administered for infection; and a tracheostomy is performed and oxygen given for ventilation.

■ NURSING CONSIDERATIONS: The nurse may encourage everyone to be actively immunized against the infection. The vaccine is safe and effective.

**tetanus and diphtheria toxoids (Td),** an active immunizing agent containing detoxified tetanus and diphtheria toxoids that slowly produce an antigenic response to the diseases.

■ INDICATIONS: It is prescribed for immunization against tetanus and diphtheria in children under 7 years of age when pertussis vaccine present in the usual diphtheria, pertussis, and tetanus trivalent vaccine is contraindicated.

■ CONTRAINDICATIONS: Immunosuppression, concomitant use of corticosteroids, or acute infection prohibits its use.

■ ADVERSE EFFECTS: Among the most serious adverse reactions are allergic reactions and stinging at the site of injection.

**tetanus antitoxin (TAT),** a tetanus immune serum that neutralizes exotoxins in tetanus infection.

■ INDICATIONS: It is prescribed for short-term immunization against tetanus after possible exposure to the organism and in tetanus treatment.

■ CONTRAINDICATIONS: It is not given if the more effective tetanus immune globulin is available or if there is a known sensitivity to equine serum.

■ ADVERSE EFFECTS: Among the most serious adverse reactions are allergic reactions and pain and inflammation at the site of injection.

**tetanus immune globulin (TIG),** an injectable solution prepared from the globulin of an immune human. It is effective and much safer than tetanus antitoxin.

■ INDICATIONS: It is prescribed for short-term immunization against tetanus after possible exposure to the organism and tetanus treatment.

■ CONTRAINDICATIONS: Known hypersensitivity to this drug prohibits its use. It should not be substituted for tetanus toxoid.

■ ADVERSE EFFECTS: The most serious adverse reaction is anaphylaxis. Fever, pain, and inflammation at the site of injection may occur.

**tetanus toxoid,** an active immunizing agent prepared from detoxified tetanus toxin that produces an antigenic response in the body, conferring permanent immunity to tetanus infection.

■ INDICATION: It is prescribed for primary active immunization against tetanus.

■ CONTRAINDICATIONS: Immunosuppression or immunoglobulin abnormalities, acute infection, or illness prohibits its use.

■ ADVERSE EFFECTS: The most serious adverse reaction is hypersensitivity. Pain and inflammation at the site of injection may occur.

**tetany** /tet′ənē/ [Gk, *tetanos,* extreme tension], a condition characterized by cramps, convulsions, twitching of the muscles, and sharp flexion of the wrist and ankle joints. These symptoms are sometimes accompanied by attacks of stridor. Tetany is a manifestation of an abnormality in calcium metabolism, which can occur in association with vitamin D deficiency, hypoparathyroidism, alkalosis, or the ingestion of alkaline salts. Kinds of tetany are **duration tetany, gastric tetany, hyperventilation tetany,** and **hypocalcemic tetany.**

**tetart-,** combining form meaning 'fourth': *tetartanopia, tetartocone, tetartoconoid.*

**tetra-** /tet′rə/, **tetro-,** combining form meaning 'four': *tetracycline, tetrahydric, tetranopsia.*

**tetrabasic** /tet′rəbā′sik/, **1.** describing a compound that has four acidic hydrogen atoms replaced by metal ions. **2.** an alcohol containing four hydroxyl groups.

**tetracaine hydrochloride,** a local anesthetic used for spinal nerve blockage and topical anesthesia.

**2,3,7,8-tetrachlorodibenzoparadioxin.** See **dioxin.**

**tetrachloroethane** /-klôr′ō·eth′ān/, a potentially toxic solvent with a sweet, chloroform-like odor. It is used to dissolve fats, waxes, oils, and resins and in the manufacture of paints, varnishes, and rust removers. Symptoms of overexposure include nausea, vomiting, abdominal pain, finger tremors, skin disorders, and liver damage.

**tetrachloromethane.** See **carbon tetrachloride.**

**tetracycline** /tet′rəsī′klēn/, a broad-spectrum antibiotic.

■ INDICATIONS: It is prescribed for the treatment of many bacterial and rickettsial infections.

■ CONTRAINDICATIONS: Significantly impaired liver or renal function or known hypersensitivity to this drug prohibits its use. Because it may cause permanent discoloration of the teeth, its use is contraindicated in the last half of pregnancy and during a child's first 8 years.

■ ADVERSE EFFECTS: Among the more serious adverse reactions are renal toxicity, hepatotoxicity, severe GI disturbances, photosensitivity, enterocolitis, inflammatory lesions

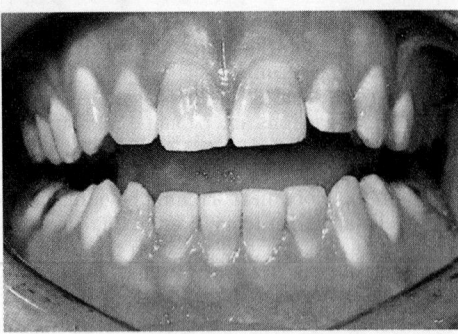

**Discoloration of the teeth caused by tetracycline**
*(Christensen, 1994)*

with monilial overgrowth in the anogenital area, hemolytic anemia, thrombocytopenia, eosinophilia, and rashes.

**tetracycline hydrochloride,** an antibiotic.

■ INDICATIONS: It is prescribed in the treatment of bacterial infections.

■ CONTRAINDICATIONS: Known hypersensitivity to this drug or to other tetracyclines prohibits its use. Use during pregnancy or in children under 8 years of age may result in discoloration of the child's teeth. It is to be administered with caution with renal or liver impairment.

■ ADVERSE EFFECTS: Among the most serious reactions are potentially serious superinfections, allergic reactions, phototoxicity, and GI disturbances.

**tetrad** /tet′rad/ [Gk, *tetra,* four], a group of four chromatids of a synapsed pair of homologous chromosomes during the first meiotic prophase of gametogenesis. The group is formed in preparation for the two meiotic divisions in the maturation of gametes. —**tetradic,** *adj.*

**tetradactyly** /-dak′tilē/ [Gk, *tetra* + *dactylos*], the presence of only four fingers on each hand or four toes on each foot (quadridigitate).

**tetraethyl lead** /tet′rə·eth′il led/, a potentially toxic, antiknock gasoline additive. Effects of overexposure include insomnia, lassitude, anxiety, nausea, tremor, pallor, hypothermia, anorexia, and psychosis.

**tetrahydrobiopterin** /tet′rə·hī′drō·bī·op′tər·in/, a compound related to folic acid, which functions as a coenzyme in the reactions hydroxylating phenylalanine, tryptophan, and tyrosine by carrying electrons to oxygen. Defects in its biosynthesis or regeneration affect all three hydroxylation reactions, interfere with production of the corresponding neurotransmitter precursors, and result in malignant hyperphenylalaninemia.

**tetrahydrocannabinol (THC)** /-hi′drōkənab′inol/, the active principle, occurring as two psychomimetic isomers, in the hemp plant *Cannabis sativa,* used in the preparation of marijuana, hashish, bhang, and ganja. THC, a rapidly metabolized beta-adrenergic agonist, increases pulse rate; causes conjunctival reddening and a feeling of euphoria; and has variable effects on blood pressure, respiratory rate, and pupil size. The drug affects memory, cognition, and the sensorium; decreases motor coordination; and increases appetite. Nonintoxicating doses of THC are used experimentally in the treatment of glaucoma and to relieve nausea and increase the appetite in patients receiving cancer chemotherapy. See also **cannabis.**

**tetrahydrozoline hydrochloride** /-hīdroz′əlēn/, an adrenergic vasoconstrictor.

■ INDICATIONS: It is prescribed for the treatment of nasal and nasopharangeal congestion and as an ophthalmic vasoconstrictor.

■ CONTRAINDICATIONS: Glaucoma or known hypersensitivity to this drug or to other vasoconstrictors prohibits its use. It is used with caution in patients who have cardiovascular disease.

■ ADVERSE EFFECTS: Among the more serious adverse reactions are irritation to mucosa, rebound nasal congestion, and effects associated with systemic absorption, including sedation and alterations in cardiovascular function.

**tetraiodothyronine.** See **thyroxine.**

**tetralogy** /tetrol′əjē/ [Gk, *tetra,* four, *logos,* word], any group of four writings, symptoms, or other related factors. See **tetralogy of Fallot.**

**tetralogy of Fallot** /falō′/ [Gk, *tetra,* four, *logos,* word; Etienne-Louis A. Fallot, French physician, 1850–1911], a congenital cardiac anomaly that consists of four defects: pulmonary stenosis, ventricular septal defect, malposition of the aorta so that it arises from the septal defect or the right ventricle, and right ventricular hypertrophy. The primary symptoms in the infant are cyanosis, hypoxia, difficulty in feeding, failure to gain weight, and poor development. In older children a squatting position and clubbing of the fingers and toes are evident. A pansystolic murmur is usually heard, and the second heart sound is faint or absent. Diagnosis of the condition is primarily based on the patient's history and physical symptoms, although cardiac catheterization is performed to evaluate the severity of the defects. Treatment consists mainly of supportive measures and palliative surgical procedures, primarily systemic to pulmonary anastomoses to decrease tissue hypoxia and prevent complications until the child is old enough to tolerate total corrective surgery. The optimal age for surgical repair is approximately 1 year. Also called **Fallot's syndrome.** See also **blue baby, trilogy of Fallot.**

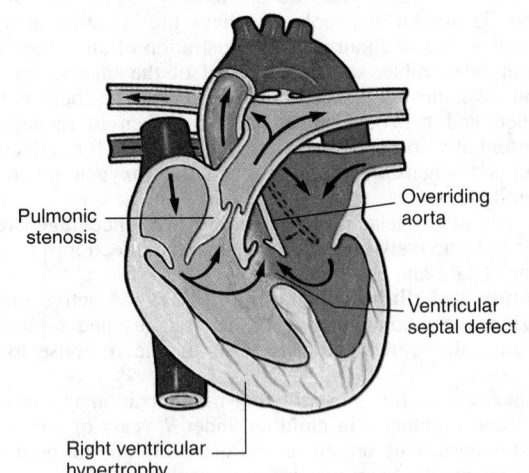

**Tetralogy of Fallot** *(Wong, 1999)*

**tetramer** /tet′rəmer/ [Gk, *tetra* + *meros,* part], something that is composed of four parts, such as a protein composed of four polypeptide subunits.

**tetraodon poisoning,** a reaction caused by a toxin in

puffer fish and marine sunfish. It may result in myalgia, paresthesia, and other neuromuscular disorders. Death may result from respiratory paralysis. See also **ciguatera poisoning, fish poisoning, scombroid poisoning.**

**tetraparesis** /tet′rə·pərē′sis/ [Gk, *tetra*, four + *paresis*, relaxation], muscular weakness affecting all four extremities.

**tetrapeptide** /-pep′tīd/, a compound formed by four amino acids united by peptide links.

**tetraplegia.** See **quadriplegia.**

**tetraploid (4n)** /tet′rəploid/ [Gk, *tetraploos*, fourfold, *eidos*, form], **1.** an individual, organism, strain, or cell that has four complete sets of chromosomes, quadruple the haploid number characteristic of the species. In humans the tetraploid number is 92; it occurs extremely rarely, in aborted or stillborn fetuses. **2.** also **tetraploidic.** Pertaining to such an individual, organism, strain, or cell. Compare **diploid, haploid, triploid.** See also **polyploid. —tetraploidy,** *n.*

**tetraploidy** /tet′rəploi′dē/, the state or condition of having four complete sets of chromosomes.

**tetrasaccharide** /-sak′ərīd/, a sugar containing four molecules of monosaccharide.

**tetrascelus** /tetras′ēləs/, a fetal anomaly with four legs.

**tetravalent** /-vā′lənt/, pertaining to a chemical with a valency of four.

**tetro-.** See **tetra-.**

**TFIIE,** a general transcription factor involved in complementary DNA encoding. TFIIE consists of two subunits, TFIIE-alpha and TFIIE-beta.

**T fracture** /tē′frakchər/, an intercondylar fracture in which the fracture lines are T-shaped.

**TGF,** abbreviation for **transforming growth factor.**

**T group.** See **sensitivity training group.**

**Th,** symbol for the element **thorium.**

**thalamic** /thalam′ik/ [Gk, *thalamos,* chamber], pertaining to the thalamus.

**thalamic peduncle** [Gk, *thalamos,* chamber; L, *pes,* foot], a group of fibers linking the thalamus with the hypothalamus.

**thalamic syndrome** [Gk, *thalamos* + *syn,* together, *dromos,* course], a vascular disorder involving the ventral and posterolateral nuclei of the thalamus and related nerve fibers. It causes disturbances of sensation and partial or complete paralysis of one side of the body. A major effect is an increased threshold to all stimuli on the opposite side of the body so that any stimuli may cause an exaggerated response. Also called **Dejerine-Roussy syndrome.**

**thalamo-,** combining form meaning 'relating to the thalamus': *thalamocortical, thalamotomy.*

**thalamotomy** /thal′əmot′əmē/, the surgical production of lesions within the nuclei of the thalamus, generally performed to treat diseases of the basal ganglia.

**thalamus** /thal′əməs/, *pl.* **thalami** [Gk, *thalamos,* chamber], one of a pair of large oval nervous structures made of gray matter and forming most of the lateral walls of the third ventricle of the brain and part of the diencephalon. It relays sensory information, excluding smell, to the cerebral cortex. It is composed mainly of gray substance and translates impulses from appropriate receptors into crude sensations of pain, temperature, and touch. It also participates in associating sensory impulses with pleasant and unpleasant feelings, in the arousal mechanisms of the body, and in the mechanisms that produce complex reflex movements. Compare **epithalamus, hypothalamus, subthalamus. —thalamic,** *adj.*

**thalassemia** /thal′əsē′mē·ə/ [Gk, *thalassa*, sea, *a* + *haima*, without blood], a hemolytic hemoglobinopathy anemia characterized by microcytic, hypochromic, and short-lived red blood cells caused by deficient synthesis of hemoglobin polypeptide chains and are classified according to the chain involved, with alpha-thalassemia and beta-thalassemia being the two major categories. All types are transmitted by autosomal recessive genes, and people of Mediterranean origin are more often affected than others. Beta-thalassemia occurs in two forms, called thalassemia major and thalassemia minor. **Thalassemia major (Cooley's anemia),** the homozygous form, evident in infancy, is recognized by anemia, fever, failure to thrive, and splenomegaly and is confirmed by characteristic changes in the red blood cells on microscopic examination. Frequent transfusions are necessary to maintain oxygen-carrying capacity of the blood. Red cells are rapidly destroyed, freeing large amounts of iron to be deposited in the skin, which becomes bronzed and freckled. The iron is also deposited in the heart, liver, and pancreas, which become fibrotic and dysfunctional. The spleen may become so enlarged that respiratory excursion is impeded and the abdominal organs are crowded. Headache, abdominal pain, fatigue, and anorexia often occur. No cure exists. The nurse is aware that the child is uncomfortable and that growth and sexual development are usually retarded. Rarely a child with thalassemia major is able to function without transfusions, thereby avoiding the massive ill effects of accumulated iron deposits. **Thalassemia minor,** the heterozygous form, is characterized only by a mild anemia

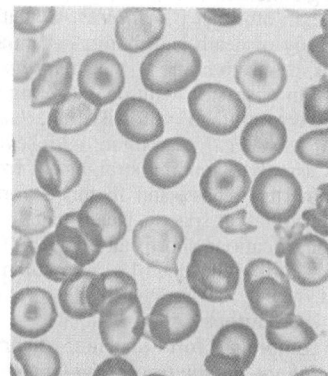

Thalassemia major

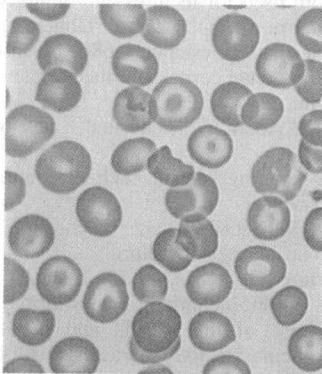

Thalassemia minor

**Thalassemia** *(Damjanov and Linder, 2000)*

and minimal red blood cell changes. Thalassemia minima is a form that lacks clinical symptoms, although patients show hematologic evidence of the disease. Ill effects of transfusion, should be monitored and the patient should be educated and counseled about the disease and referred for genetic counseling. See also **hemochromatosis, hemosiderosis.**

**thalasso-,** combining form meaning 'the sea': *thalassophobia, thalassotherapy.*

**thalassotherapy** /thalas'ōther'əpē/ [Gk, *tahassa*, seal], a treatment system based on sea bathing and exposure to sea air.

**thalidomide** /thalid'əmīd/, a sedative-hypnotic sometimes prescribed for the treatment of leprosy. It is never given to women who are or who might become pregnant.

**thallium (Tl)** /thal'ē·əm/ [Gk, *thallos*, green line], a soft, bluish-white metallic element that exhibits some nonmetallic chemical properties. Its atomic number is 81; its atomic mass is 204.38. Many of its compounds are highly toxic. Thallium sulfate is widely used as a rat poison.

**thallium poisoning,** a toxic condition caused by the ingestion or absorption through the skin of thallium salts, especially thallium sulfate. Characteristic of the condition are abdominal pain, vomiting, bloody diarrhea, tremor, delirium, and alopecia. Thallium has been used in insect and rodent poisons, fireworks, and some cosmetic hair removers; but this extremely toxic and cumulative poison was banned for use in household products in 1965.

**thallium stress test.** See **stress test.**

**thanato-,** combining form meaning 'death': *thanatobiologic, thanatognomonic, thanatology.*

**thanatology** /than'ətol'əjē/ [Gk, *thanatos*, death, *logos*, science], the study of death and dying. —**thanatologist,** *n.*

**thanatomania** /than'ətōmā'nē·ə/ [Gk, *thanatos*, death, *mania*, frenzy], an obsession with death, dying, or suicide.

**thanatophoric dwarf** /than'ətōfôr'ik/ [Gk, *thanatos* + *phoros*, bearer; AS, *dweorge*], an infant with severe micromelia, the limbs usually extending straight out from the trunk, an extremely narrow chest, and flattened vertebral bodies with wide intervertebral spaces. Death usually occurs from respiratory complications shortly after birth.

**Thanatos** /than'ətəs/ [Gk, death], a freudian term for the death instinct.

**thanotopsy.** See **autopsy.**

**thaumato-,** combining form meaning 'marvel or miracles': *thaumatology, thaumaturgic, thaumaturgy.*

**THC,** abbreviation for **tetrahydrocannabinol.**

**theater** /thē'ətər/, **1.** an operating room or suite of rooms. **2.** a large room used for lectures and demonstrations.

**thebesian foramen** /thəbē'zē·ən, tābā'zē·ən/ [Adam C. Thebesius, German physician, 1686–1732], any of the openings of the venae cordis minimae, or small veins, into the right atrium.

**thebesian vein** [Adam C. Thebesius], any of the smallest cardiac veins.

**thec-,** prefix meaning 'sheath, such as of a tendon': *thecal, thecitis, thecodont.*

**theca** /thē'kə/, *pl.* **thecae** /thē'sē/, a sheath or capsule, such as the theca cordis or pericardium.

**theca cell tumor** [Gk, *theke*, sheath; L, *cella*, storeroom; *tumor*, swelling], an uncommon benign fibroid tumor of the ovary, composed of theca cells and usually containing granulosa (follicular) cells. Characteristically solid masses with yellow fatty streaks, these tumors are frequently associated with excessive estrogen production and tend to develop cystic degeneration. Also called **fibroma thecocellulare xanthomatodes, thecoma** /thēkō'mə/.

**thecal** /thē'kəl/ [Gk, *theke*, sheath], pertaining to a theca or sheath.

**-thecium,** combining form meaning a 'sack or container': *bdellepithecium, epithecium, perithecium.*

**thecoma,** a tumor derived from ovarian mesenchyme, consisting of spindle-shaped cells that may contain fat droplets. It is sometimes associated with excessive estrogen production and precocious sexual development in prepubertal girls.

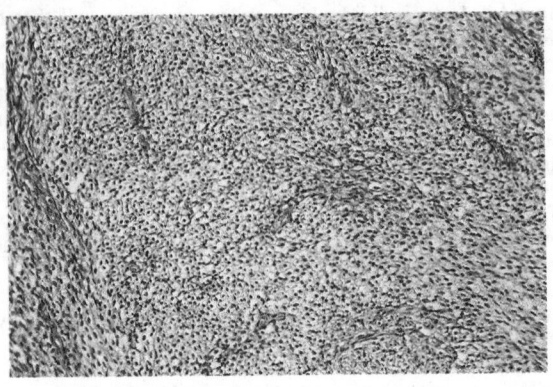

**Thecoma** *(Fletcher, 2000)*

**Theden's bandage** /tā'dənz/ [Johann C.A. Theden, German surgeon, 1714–1797], a roller bandage applied below the injury and continued upward over a compress, used to stop bleeding. Also called **Genga's bandage.**

**thel-,** combining form meaning 'nipple': *thelalgia, theleplasty, thelitis.*

**thelarche** /thilär'kē/ [Gk, *thele*, nipple, *archaios*, beginning], the beginning of female pubertal breast development normally occurring between 9 and 13 years of age. Thelarche is before puberty at the beginning of the phase of rapid growth. **Premature thelarche** is precocious breast development in a female without other evidence of sexual maturation. Compare **menarche.**

**-thelia,** suffix meaning '(condition of the) nipples': *epithelia, hyperthelia, microthelia.*

**-thelioma,** suffix meaning a 'tumor in a cellular tissue': *celiothelioma, hemendothelioma, perithelioma.*

**-thelium,** suffix meaning a 'layer of (specified kind of) cellular tissue': *desmepithelium, mesothelium.*

**thely-,** combining form meaning 'female': *thelyblast, thelygenic, thelyplasty.*

**thenar** /thē'när/ [Gk, palm of the hand], pertaining to any structure in relation to the palm of the hand.

**thenar eminence** [Gk, *thenar*, palm of the hand; L, *eminentia*, projection], a raised fleshy area on the palm of the hand near the base of the thumb.

**theo-,** combining form meaning 'a god': *theomania, theophobia, theotherapy.*

**Theobid,** trademark for a bronchodilator (theophylline).

**theobroma oil** /thē'ōbrō'mə/, a liquid fat derived from seeds of *Theobroma cacao*, the cocoa plant. It contains a number of fatty acids used in suppositories, ointments, and lubricants.

**theobromine** /thē'əbrō'min/, a substance (methylxanthine) that is related chemically to caffeine and theophylline and differs from them by the number and distribution of

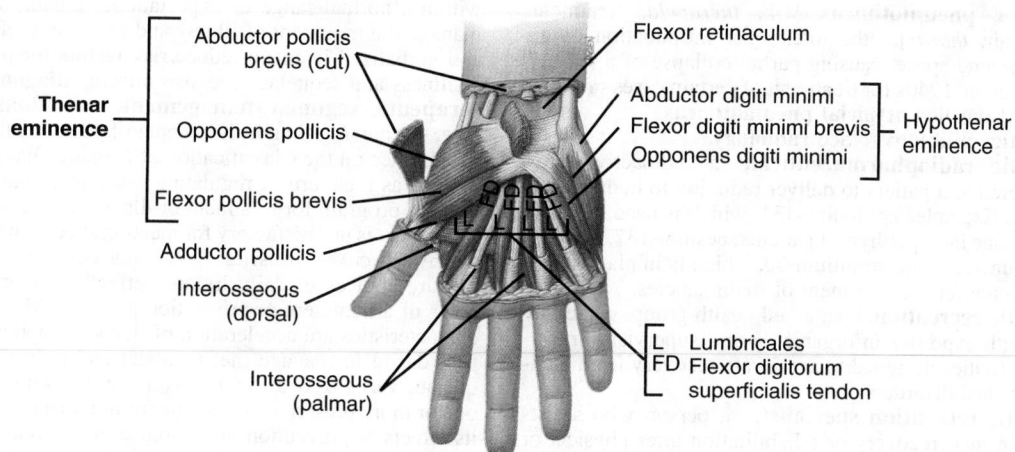

**Thenar eminence** *(Thibodeau and Patton, 1999/John V. Hagen)*

methyl groups. Theobromine occurs naturally in cocoa, cola nuts, and tea. It acts as a diuretic, vasodilator, cardiac stimulant, and smooth muscle relaxant.

**Theo-Dur,** trademark for a bronchodilator (theophylline).

**Theolair,** trademark for a bronchodilator (theophylline).

**theophylline** /thē-əfil′ēn/ [L, *thea,* tea; Gk, *phyllon,* leaf], a bronchodilator.

■ INDICATIONS: It is prescribed to relax the smooth muscle of the bronchial passages in the treatment of bronchospasm in bronchial asthma, bronchitis, and emphysema.

■ CONTRAINDICATIONS: Hypertension, cardiac disease, liver disease, renal disease, or concurrent treatment with other xanthines may prohibit its use.

■ ADVERSE EFFECT: Among the most serious adverse reactions are hypersensitivity, GI bleeding, palpitations, and seizures.

**theorem** /thē′ərəm/ [Gk, *theorein,* to look at], **1.** a proposition to be proved by a chain of reasoning and analysis. **2.** a rule expressed by symbols or formulae.

**theoretic effectiveness** /thē-əret′ik/ [Gk, *theorein* + L, *efficere,* to do], (of a contraceptive method) the effectiveness of a medication, device, or method in preventing pregnancy if used consistently and exactly as intended, without error. Compare **use effectiveness.**

**theoretic plate number (N),** a number defining the efficiency of a chromatographic column.

**theory** /thē′ərē/ [Gk, *theorein,* to look at], an abstract statement formulated to predict, explain, or describe the relationships among concepts, constructs, or events. Theory is developed and tested by observation and research, using factual data.

**theotherapy** /thē′ōther′əpē/ [Gk, *theos,* god, *therapeia,* treatment], a therapeutic approach to the prevention, diagnosis, and treatment of disease and dysfunction based on religious or spiritual beliefs.

**Theovent,** trademark for a bronchodilator (theophylline).

**therapeutic** /ther′əpyōō′tik/ [Gk, *therapeuein,* to treat], **1.** beneficial. **2.** pertaining to a treatment.

**-therapeutic, -therapeutics,** suffix meaning 'medical treatment by (specified) techniques': *kinetotherapeutic, orthotherapeutic, radiotherapeutics.*

**therapeutic abortion, 1.** a termination of early pregnancy deemed necessary by a physician. **2.** *informal.* any legal induced abortion. Compare **elective abortion.** See also **induced abortion.**

**therapeutic communication,** a process in which the nurse consciously influences a client or helps the client to a better understanding through verbal or nonverbal communication.

**therapeutic community (TC),** (in mental health) a treatment facility in which the entire milieu is part of the treatment. The physical environment, the other clients, the staff, and the policies of the facility influence the function of the individual in the activities of daily living in the community. The concept of a therapeutic community is integral to milieu therapy.

**therapeutic dose** [Gk, *therapeia,* treatment, *dosis,* giving], the dose that may be required to produce a desired effect.

**therapeutic drug monitoring test (TDM),** a blood test that entails taking measurements of blood drug levels to determine effective drug dosages and to prevent toxicity. It is also used to identify noncompliant patients.

**therapeutic equivalent,** a drug that has essentially the same effect in the treatment of a disease or condition as one or more other drugs. A drug that is a therapeutic equivalent may or may not be chemically equivalent, bioequivalent, or generically equivalent. See also **bioequivalent, chemical equivalent, generic equivalent.**

**therapeutic exercise,** any exercise planned and performed to attain a specific physical benefit, such as maintenance of the range of motion, strengthening of weakened muscles, increased joint flexibility, or improved cardiovascular and respiratory function.

**therapeutic fever.** See **pyrotherapy.**

**therapeutic gain,** the ratio of the biologic effect of a therapy on a tumor compared with the effect on surrounding normal tissue. Higher therapeutic gains mean lower complications of therapy.

**therapeutic index,** the difference between the minimum therapeutic and minimum toxic concentrations of a drug.

**therapeutic play,** a nursing intervention from the Nursing Interventions Classification (NIC) defined as purposeful and directive use of toys or other materials to assist children in communicating their perception and knowledge of their world and to help in gaining mastery of their environment. See also **Nursing Interventions Classification.**

**therapeutic pneumothorax** [Gk, *therapeia,* treatment, *pneuma,* air, *thorax*], the intentional introduction of air into the pleural space, causing partial collapse of a lung. It was used in the 1940s for treatment of certain cases of tuberculosis. Also called **artificial pneumothorax.**

**therapeutic radiology.** See **radiology.**

**therapeutic radiopharmaceutical,** a radioactive drug administered to a patient to deliver radiation to body tissues internally. Examples are iodine-131, which is used to ablate thyroid tissue in hyperthyroid patients; cesium-137; iridium-192; radium-226; and strontium-90, which is implanted in a sealed source for the treatment of malignancies.

**therapeutic recreation,** an allied health group, staffed by people with expertise in organizing and supervising recreational activities designed to accelerate recovery from mental or physical disorders.

**therapeutic recreation specialist,** a person who assists patients in their recovery or rehabilitation after physical or emotional illness or disability by planning and supervising recreation programs.

**therapeutic regimen management, community, ineffective,** a nursing diagnosis accepted by the Eleventh National Conference on the Classification of Nursing Diagnoses. It is defined as a pattern of regulating and integrating into community processes programs for treatment of illness and sequelae of illness that are unsatisfactory for meeting health-related goals.
■ DEFINING CHARACTERISTICS: The defining characteristics are deficits in persons and programs to be accountable for illness care of aggregates; deficits in advocates for aggregates; deficits in community activities for secondary and tertiary prevention; illness symptoms above the norm expected for the number and type of population; number of health care resources insufficient for the incidence or prevalence of illness(es); and unexpected acceleration of illness. See also **nursing diagnosis.**

**therapeutic regimen management, family, ineffective,** a nursing diagnosis accepted by the Eleventh Conference on the Classification of Nursing Diagnoses. It is defined as a pattern of regulating and integrating into family processes a program for treatment of illness and the sequelae of illness that are unsatisfactory for meeting specific health goals.
■ DEFINING CHARACTERISTICS: A major defining characteristic is inappropriate family activities for meeting the goals of a treatment or prevention program. Minor defining characteristics are acceleration (expected or unexpected) of illness symptoms of a family member; lack of attention to illness and its sequelae; verbalized desire to manage the treatment of illness and prevention of the sequelae; verbalized difficulty with regulation/integration of one or more effects or prevention of complications; and verbalizing that the family did not take action to reduce risk factors for progression of illness and sequelae.
■ RELATED FACTORS: The related factors are complexity of the health care system, complexity of the therapeutic regimen, decisional conflicts, economic difficulties, excessive demands on the individual or family, and family conflicts. See also **nursing diagnosis.**

**therapeutic regimen management, individual, effective,** a nursing diagnosis accepted by the Eleventh National Conference on the Classification of Nursing Diagnoses. It is defined as a pattern of regulating and integrating into daily living a program for treatment of illness and its sequelae that is satisfactory for meeting specific health goals.
■ DEFINING CHARACTERISTICS: The defining characteristics are appropriate choices of daily activities for meeting the goals of a treatment or prevention program; illness symptoms

within a normal range of expectation; verbalized desire to manage the treatment of illness and prevention of sequelae; and verbalized intent to reduce risk factors for progression of illness and sequelae. See also **nursing diagnosis.**

**therapeutic regimen management, individual, ineffective,** a nursing diagnosis accepted by the Tenth National Conference on the Classification of Nursing Diagnoses. It is defined as a pattern of regulating and integrating into daily living a program for treatment of illness and the sequelae of illness that is unsatisfactory for meeting specific health goals.
■ DEFINING CHARACTERISTICS: The major defining characteristics are choices of daily living ineffective for meeting the goals of a treatment or prevention program. Minor defining characteristics are acceleration of illness symptoms, verbalized desire to manage the treatment and prevention of sequelae, verbalized difficulty with regulation/integration of one or more prescribed regimens for treatment of illness and its effects or prevention of complications, verbalization that intimates that the patient would not attempt to include treatment regimens in daily routines, and verbalization that intimates that the patient would not attempt to reduce risk factors for progression of illness and sequelae.
■ RELATED FACTORS: Related factors include complexity of the health care system, complexity of the therapeutic regimen, decisional conflicts, economic difficulties, excessive demands made on the individual or family, family conflict, family patterns of health care, inadequate number and types of cues to action, knowledge deficits, mistrust of regimen and/or health care personnel, perceived seriousness, perceived susceptibility, perceived barriers, perceived benefits, powerlessness, and social support deficits. See also **nursing diagnosis.**

**therapeutics** /ther′əpyōō′tiks/ [Gk, *therapeia,* treatment], a branch of health care that is concerned with the treatment of disease, seeking to relieve symptoms or produce a cure.

**therapeutic temperature,** (in hyperthermia treatment) temperatures between 107° to 113° F (42° to 45° C).

**therapeutic touch,** a nursing intervention from the Nursing Interventions Classification (NIC) defined as attuning to the universal healing field, seeking to act as an instrument for healing influence, and using the natural sensitivity of the hands to gently focus and direct the intervention process. See also **Nursing Interventions Classification.**

**-therapia, -therapy,** suffix meaning 'a specific type of medical care': *balneotherapia, odontotherapia, hypnotherapy.*

**therapist** /ther′əpist/, a person with special skills, obtained through education and experience, in one or more areas of health care.

**therapy** /ther′əpē/ [Gk, *therapeia*], the treatment of any disease or a pathologic condition, such as inhalation therapy, which administers various medicines for patients suffering from diseases of the respiratory tract.

**-therapy.** See **-therapia.**

**therapy group,** a nursing intervention from the Nursing Interventions Classification (NIC) defined as application of psychotherapeutic techniques to a group, including the utilization of interactions between members of the group. See also **Nursing Interventions Classification.**

**therio-,** combining form meaning 'beasts': *theriomimicry, theriotherapy, theriotomy.*

**therm-.** See **thermo-.**

**-therm, -thermia, -thermy,** suffix meaning 'a state of heat': *allotherm, azothermia, hypothermia, poikilotherm.*

**thermal** /thur′məl/ [Gk, *thermē,* heat], pertaining to the production, application, or maintenance of heat. Also **thermic.**

**thermal burn,** tissue injury, usually of the skin, caused by exposure to extreme heat. See also **burn.**

**thermal dilution.** See **thermodilution.**

**thermal field size,** the area over which therapeutic heating is likely to be produced.

**thermalgesia** /thur′məljē′zhə/ [Gk, *thermē,* heat, *algos,* pain], pain caused by exposure to high temperatures.

**thermalgia** /thurmal′jə/, a sensation of intense burning pain sometimes experienced following nerve injuries.

**thermal radiation** [Gk, *thermē,* heat; L, *radiare,* to shine], the emission of energy in the form of heat.

**-thermia.** See **-therm.**

**thermic fever.** See **heat hyperpyrexia.**

**thermic sense** /thur′mik/ [Gk, *thermē,* heat; L, *sentire,* to feel], the network of sense organs and connecting pathways that allow an appreciation of temperature changes. Also called **temperature sense.**

**thermionic emission** /ther′mī·on′ik/, the emission of electrons and ions by incandescent bodies.

**thermistor** /thərmis′tər/ [Gk, *thermē* + L, *resistere,* to withstand], a kind of thermometer for measuring minute changes in temperature. The resistance of a thermistor varies with the ambient temperature, thereby enabling accurate measurements of small temperature changes. See also **temperature, thermometer.**

**thermo-, therm-,** combining form meaning 'heat': *thermochemistry, thermogenesis, thermopalpation.*

**thermocautery** /thur′mōkô′tərē/ [Gk, *thermē* + *kauterion,* branding iron], the use of a needle or snare heated by direct flame, a heated hydrocarbon vapor, or an electrical current in the destruction of tissue. See also **Paquelin's cautery.**

**thermochemistry** /-kem′istrē/ [Gk, *thermē,* heat, *chemia,* alchemy], a branch of chemistry that is concerned with the heat changes involved in chemical reactions.

**thermocoagulation** /-kō·ag′yəlā′shən/ [Gk, *thermē,* heat; L, *coagulare*], the use of high-frequency electrical currents to destroy tissue through heat coagulation.

**thermocouple** /thur′məkup′əl/ [Gk, *thermē* + Fr, *couple,* pair], a temperature-measuring device that relies on the production of a temperature-dependent voltage at the junction of two dissimilar metals.

**thermodilution** /-dilyōō′zhən/, a method of cardiac output determination. A bolus of solution of known volume and temperature is injected into the right atrium, and the resultant change in blood temperature is detected by a thermistor previously placed in the pulmonary artery with a catheter. Also called **thermal dilution.**

**thermodynamics** /-dīnam′iks/ [Gk, *thermē,* heat, *dynamis,* power], the science of the interconversion of heat and work.

**thermogenesis** /thur′mōjen′əsis/ [Gk, *thermē* + *genesis,* origin], production of heat, especially by the cells of the body. —**thermogenetic,** *adj.*

**thermogenic center.** See **thermoregulatory center.**

**thermograph** /thur′məgraf′/ [Gk, *thermē* + *graphein,* to record], **1.** a photographic record of the amount of heat radiated from the surface of the body, revealing 'hot spots' of potential tumors or other disorders. **2.** a device consisting of a thermometer, inked stylus, and chart for continuous recording of the ambient temperature.

**thermography** /thərmog′rəfē/, a technique for sensing and recording on film hot and cold areas of the body by means of an infrared detector that reacts to blood flow. Disease states that manifest increased or decreased blood flow present thermographic patterns that can be distinguished from those of normal areas. —**thermographic,** *adj.*

**thermoinhibitory center.** See **thermoregulatory center.**

**thermointegrator** /thur′mō·in′təgrā′tər/, an instrument used to create a thermal model of an environment, measuring the warmth and coldness as it might be experienced by a living organism in that environment.

**thermokeratoplasty** /-ker′ətōplas′tē/, a procedure to correct myopia by applying heat to flatten the cornea. The heat shrinks the collagen in the substantia propria layer of the cornea.

**thermolabile** /thur′məlā′bəl/ [Gk, *thermē* + L, *labilis,* slipping], easily destroyed or altered by heat. Also called **heat labile.** Compare **thermostable.**

**thermoluminescent dosimetry** /-lōō′mines′ənt/ [Gk, *thermē* + L, *lumen,* light; Gk, *dosis,* something given, *metron,* measure], a method of measuring the ionizing radiation to which a person is exposed by means of a device that contains a radiation-sensitive crystalline material. The material stores the radiations energy by changing structure. When the material is heated at some later time, it releases the energy as ultraviolet or visible light. The light emitted is detected by a photomultiplier tube that generates an electric signal whose magnitude reflects the amount of ionizing radiation originally received.

**thermomassage** /-məsäzh′/, a physical therapy technique that combines heat and massage.

**thermometer** /thermom′ətər/ [Gk, *thermē* + *metron,* measure], an instrument for measuring temperature. Originally, it consisted of a sealed glass tube, marked in degrees Celsius or Fahrenheit, and contained liquid such as mercury or alcohol. The liquid rises or falls as it expands or contracts according to changes in temperature. See also **clinical thermometer, electronic thermometer, mercury thermometer, rectal thermometer, surface thermometer, tympanic membrane thermometer, wet-and-dry-bulb thermometer.**

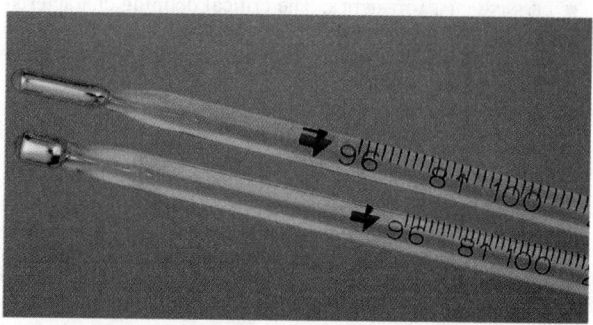

**Thermometers: oral (*top*) and rectal (*bottom*)**
*(Zakus, 1995)*

**thermoneutral environment** /-nōō′trəl/ [Gk, *thermē* + L, *neutralis,* neutral; ME, *environ,* around], **1.** an environment that keeps body temperature at an optimum point at which the least amount of oxygen is consumed for metabolism. **2.** an environment that enables a neonate to maintain a body temperature of 97.7° F (36.5° C) with a minimal requirement of energy and oxygen.

**thermonuclear** /-nōō′klē·ər/ [Gk, *thermē,* heat; L, *nucleus,* nut kernel], pertaining to a reaction in which isotopes of hydrogen (protium, deuterium, or tritium) can be fused at temperatures of nearly 100,000,000° C into heavier nuclei of helium atoms. The process is the source of energy of the sun and is used in the explosion of thermonuclear weapons.

**thermopenetration** /-pen′ətrā′shən/ [Gk, *thermē* + L, *penetrale*, passing through], the use of diathermic techniques to produce warmth within the body tissues for therapeutic purposes. Also called **transthermia.**

**thermophilic** /-fil′ik/ [Gk, *thermē*, heat, *philein*, to love], pertaining to organisms that thrive in very hot environments (for example, up to 80° C for some bacteria that live in hot springs).

**thermophore** /thur′məfôr/, a procedure in which heat is applied locally to a body part.

**thermoplastic** /ther′mō·plas′tik/ [Gk, *thermē*, heat + *plassein*, to mold], softening under heat and capable of being molded into shape with pressure, then hardening on cooling without undergoing chemical change.

**thermoradiotherapy** /-rā′dē·ō·ther′əpē/, a therapeutic process that applies ionizing radiation to any part of the body in which the temperature has been raised by artificial means. Thermoradiography seeks to increase the radiosensitivity of the body part being treated.

**thermoreceptor** /-risep′tər/ [Gk, *thermē*, heat; L, *recipere*, to receive], nerve endings that are sensitive to heat or a rise in body temperature.

**thermoregulation**[1] /-reg′yəlā′shən/ [Gk, *thermē* + L, *regula*, rule], the control of heat production and heat loss, specifically the maintenance of body temperature through physiologic mechanisms activated by the hypothalamus.

**thermoregulation**[2], a nursing outcome from the Nursing Outcomes Classification (NOC) defined as the balance among heat production, heat gain, and heat loss. See also **Nursing Outcomes Classification.**

**thermoregulation, ineffective,** a nursing diagnosis accepted by the Seventh National Conference on the Classification of Nursing Diagnoses. Ineffective thermoregulation is defined as the state in which an individual's temperature fluctuates between hypothermia and hyperthermia.
■ DEFINING CHARACTERISTICS: The critical defining characteristic is the fluctuation in body temperature above or below the normal range. See also defining characteristics of **hypothermia** and **hyperthermia.**
■ RELATED FACTORS: Related factors include trauma or illness, immaturity, aging, and fluctuating environmental temperature. See also **nursing diagnosis.**

**thermoregulation: neonate,** a nursing outcome from the Nursing Outcomes Classification (NOC) defined as the balance among heat production, heat gain, and heat loss during the neonatal period. See also **Nursing Outcomes Classification.**

**thermoregulatory center** /-reg′yələtôr′ē/ [Gk, *thermē*, heat; L, *regula*, rule; Gk, *kentron*, center], center located in the hypothalamus concerned mainly with the regulation of heat production, heat inhibition, and heat conservation to maintain a normal body temperature. Kinds of thermoregulatory centers include **thermogenic center, thermoinhibitory center,** and **thermotaxic center.**

**thermoresistance** /-risis′təns/, an ability to tolerate heat, as in certain thermophilic bacteria.

**thermosetting** /ther′mō·set·ing/ [Gk, *thermē*, heat; AS, *settan*, to set], (of resins) becoming hard or solid when heat is applied and remaining that way on being recooled; the change is not reversible.

**thermostable** /-stā′bəl/, unaffected by or resistant to change by an increase in temperature. Compare **thermolabile.**

**thermostasis** /-stā′sis/, maintenance of a stable body temperature, as in mammals and birds.

**thermostat** /thur′məstat/ [Gk, *thermē* + *statos*, standing], a device for the automatic control of a heating or cooling system. —**thermostatic,** *adj.*

**thermotaxic center.** See **thermoregulatory center.**

**thermotaxis** /-tak′sis/ [Gk, *thermē* + *taxis*, arrangement], **1.** the normal adjustment and regulation of body temperature. **2.** the movement of an organism in response to heat, either toward the stimulus (positive thermotaxis) or away from the stimulus (negative thermotaxis). Also called **thermotropism.**

**thermotherapeutic penetration** /-ther′əpyōō′tik/, the depth to which heating to therapeutic temperatures is likely to extend.

**thermotherapy** /-ther′əpē/ [Gk, *thermē* + *therapeia*, treatment], the treatment of disease by the application of heat. Thermotherapy may be administered as dry heat with heat lamps, diathermy machines, electrical pads, or hot water bottles or as moist heat with warm compresses or immersion in warm water. Warm soaks or compresses may be used to treat local infections, relax muscles and relieve pain in patients with motor problems, and promote circulation in peripheral vascular disorders such as thrombophlebitis. —**thermotherapeutic,** *adj.*

**thermotropism.** See **thermotaxis.**

**-thermy.** See **-therm.**

**theta** /thē′tə, thā′tə/, Θ, θ, the eighth letter of the Greek alphabet.

**theta wave** [Gk, *theta*, eighth letter of Greek alphabet; AS, *wafian*], one of the several types of brain waves, characterized by a relatively low frequency of 4 to 7 Hz and a low amplitude of 10 μV. Theta waves are the 'drowsy waves' of the temporal lobes of the brain and appear in electroencephalograms when the individual is awake but relaxed and sleepy. Also called **theta rhythm.** Compare **alpha wave, beta wave, delta wave.**

**-thetic, -thetical,** suffix meaning 'to put, place, set': *metathetic, prosthetic, synthetic.*

**thiabendazole** /thī′əben′dəzōl/, an anthelmintic.
■ INDICATIONS: It is prescribed in the treatment of worm infestations, including hookworms, roundworms, and pinworms.
■ CONTRAINDICATIONS: Erythema multiforme, Stevens-Johnson syndrome, or known hypersensitivity to this drug prohibits its use.
■ ADVERSE EFFECTS: Among the more serious adverse reactions are anorexia, central nervous system effects, severe GI disturbances, dizziness, and hypotension.

**thiaminase** /thī·am′inās/, an enzyme present in raw fish that destroys thiamine. A diet containing a substantial amount of raw fish could result in a thiamine deficiency because of the enzyme. A heat-stable form also exists.

**thiamine** /thī′əmin/ [Gk, *theion*, containing sulfur, *amine*, ammonia], a water-soluble, crystalline compound of the B vitamin complex, essential for normal metabolism and health of the cardiovascular and nervous systems. Thiamine plays a key role in the metabolic breakdown of glucose to yield energy in body tissues. Rich sources are pork; organ meats; green leafy vegetables; legumes; sweet corn; egg yolk; corn meal; brown rice; yeast; and the germ and husks of grains, berries, and nuts. It is not stored in the body and must be supplied daily. A deficiency of thiamine affects chiefly the nervous system, the circulation, and the GI tract. Symptoms include irritability, emotional disturbances, loss of appetite, multiple neuritis, increased pulse rate, dyspnea, reduced intestinal motility, and heart irregularities. Severe deficiency causes beriberi. Also spelled **thiamin.**

Also called **antiberiberi factor, antineuritic vitamin, vitamin B₁**.

**thiazide diuretic.** See **diuretic.**

**thiemia** /thī·ē′mē·ə/ [Gk, *theion,* sulfur, *haima,* blood], an excess of sulfur in the blood.

**thiethylperazine** /thī·eth′ilper′əzēn/, a phenothiazine antiemetic.

■ INDICATIONS: It is prescribed to control nausea and vomiting.

■ CONTRAINDICATIONS: Parkinson's disease, central nervous system disorders, liver or renal dysfunction, severe hypotension, or known hypersensitivity to phenothiazine medications prohibits its use.

■ ADVERSE EFFECTS: Among the more serious adverse effects are hypotension, liver toxicity, extrapyramidal reactions, blood dyscrasias, and hypersensitivity reactions.

**thigh** [AS, *theoh*], the section of the lower limb between the hip and the knee.

**thigh bone.** See **femur.**

**thigm-,** suffix meaning 'touch': *thigmesthesia, thigmocyte, thigmotropic.*

**thinking** [AS, *thencan,* to think], **1.** the cognitive process of forming mental images or concepts. **2.** the process of cognitive problem solving through the sorting, organizing, and classification of facts. Kinds of thinking include **abstract thinking, concrete thinking,** and **syncretic thinking.** See also **imagination.**

**thin-layer chromatography (TLC),** a method of separating two or more chemical compounds in a solution through their differential migrations across a thin layer of adsorbent spread over a glass or plastic plate.

**thio-** /thī′ō-/, prefix designating the presence of sulfur: *thioarsenite, thiocyanate.*

**thioamide derivative** /thī′ō·am′īd/, one of a group of antithyroid drugs prescribed in the treatment of hyperthyroidism. Thioamide drugs act by inhibiting the synthesis of thyroid hormone. The principal thioamides are propylthiouracil, methimazole, methylthiouracil, and carbimazole. Adverse reactions include agranulocytosis, hypersensitivity, and a mild transient pruritus. Because agranulocytosis may occur very rapidly, serial white blood cell counts are not useful in diagnosing that complication of treatment. Instead, the patient is requested to report immediately instances of sore throat and fever, which often herald the onset of agranulocytosis. Prompt discontinuation of the drug before serious depletion of granulocytic white cells develops usually results in complete recovery. Use of antithyroid medications in pregnancy may result in fetal hypothyroidism, goiter, and cretinism.

**thioctic acid** /thī·ok′tik/, a pyruvate oxidation factor found in liver and yeast, used in bacterial culture media.

**thioester** /thī′ō·es′tər/, an important group of biologic chemicals formed by the hydrosulfides and carboxylic acids and identified by an ester bond involving the —SH radical. Examples include the coenzyme A thioesters.

**thioethanolamine acetyltransferase** /thī′ō·eth′ənol′əmin/, an enzyme that catalyzes the transfer of acetyl groups from acetyl CoA to the sulfur atom of thioethanolamine, producing CoA and *S*-acetylthioethanolamine.

**thioflavine T** /thī′oflā′vin/, a yellow dye used as a fluorochrome in histopathology.

**thioguanine** /thī′ōgwä′nēn/, a purine analog.

■ INDICATIONS: It is prescribed in the treatment of a variety of malignant neoplastic diseases, including the acute leukemias.

■ CONTRAINDICATIONS: Known hypersensitivity or resistance to this drug prohibits its use. It is not given during pregnancy.

■ ADVERSE EFFECTS: Among the most serious adverse reactions are bone marrow depression, GI distress, and stomatitis.

**thiopental sodium** /-pen′təl/, a widely used, potent, and ultrashort-acting barbiturate used as a general anesthetic induction agent. It is administered intravenously in adults; in children it is occasionally given rectally. By depressing the central nervous system, thiopental sodium induces hypnotic sleep in less than 1 minute. It has no analgesic properties and therefore must be supplemented by analgesics. It is a powerful respiratory and myocardial depressant. See also **barbiturate.**

**thioridazine hydrochloride** /-rid′əzēn/, a phenothiazine antipsychotic.

■ INDICATIONS: It is prescribed in the treatment of childhood behavioral disorders, geriatric mental disorders, depression, and alcohol withdrawal.

■ CONTRAINDICATIONS: Parkinson's disease, concurrent administration of central nervous system depressants, hepatic or renal dysfunction, severe hypotension, or known hypersensitivity to this drug or to other phenothiazine medications prohibits its use.

■ ADVERSE EFFECTS: Among the more serious adverse reactions are hypotension, hepatotoxicity, extrapyramidal reactions, blood dyscrasias, and hypersensitivity reactions.

**Thiosulfil Forte,** trademark for a sulfonamide antibiotic (sulfamethizole).

**thiotepa** /thī′ōtep′ə/, an antineoplastic alkylating agent.

■ INDICATIONS: It is prescribed in the treatment of malignant neoplastic diseases, including adenocarcinoma of the breast and ovary, and urinary bladder carcinomas.

■ CONTRAINDICATIONS: Bone marrow depression, pregnancy, liver or kidney dysfunction, or known hypersensitivity to this drug prohibits its use.

■ ADVERSE EFFECTS: Among the most serious adverse reactions are bone marrow depression, anorexia, nausea, and headache.

**thiothixene** /-thī′ksēn/, a thioxanthene antipsychotic.

■ INDICATIONS: It is prescribed in the treatment of acute agitation and mild-to-severe psychotic disorders.

■ CONTRAINDICATIONS: Parkinson's disease, concurrent administration of central nervous system depressants, hepatic or renal dysfunction, severe hypotension, or known hypersensitivity to this drug or to phenothiazine medications prohibits its use. It is not recommended for children under 12 years of age.

■ ADVERSE EFFECTS: Among the more serious adverse reactions are hypotension, hepatotoxicity, extrapyramidal reactions, blood dyscrasias, and hypersensitivity reactions.

**thiouracil** /thī′ōyŏŏr′əsil/ [Gk, *theion,* sulfur, *ouron,* urine], a chemical compound derived from thiourea that inhibits the formation of thyroxine in the thyroid gland and is used to treat hyperthyroidism.

**thioxanthene derivative** /thī·oksan′thēn/, any one of a group of antipsychotic drugs, each of which is similar to the phenothiazenes in indication, action, and adverse effects.

**third cranial nerve.** See **oculomotor nerve.**

**third cuneiform bone.** See **lateral cuneiform bone.**

**third-degree AV heart block.** See **complete heart block.**

**third-party reimbursement,** reimbursement for services rendered to a person in which an entity other than the receiver of the service is responsible for the payment. Third-party reimbursement for the cost of a subscriber's health care is commonly paid in full or in part by a health insurance plan, such as Blue Shield or Blue Cross, Medicare, or Medicaid.

**third stage of labor,** the expulsion of the placenta, membranes, and a small amount of blood and amniotic fluid, occurring within 5 to 30 minutes after delivery of the fetus.

**third ventricle** [Gk, *triotus*, below second rank; L, *ventriculus*, little belly], a cavity of the brain bounded on each side by a thalamus and the hypothalamus. It communicates anteriorly with the lateral ventricles and posteriorly with the aqueduct of the midbrain.

**third ventriculostomy** /ventrik′yələs′təmē/ [L, *tertius*, three, *ventriculus*, little belly; Gk, *stoma*, mouth], a surgical procedure for draining cerebrospinal fluid into the cisterna chiasmatis of the subarachnoid space in hydrocephalus, usually in the newborn. The procedure is not commonly performed and is used chiefly when the cisterna magna is not available for ventriculocisternostomy. The third ventriculostomy makes an opening on the anterior wall of the floor of the third ventricle into the interpeduncular cistern and is performed to correct an obstructive type of hydrocephalus.

**thirst** /thurst/ [AS, *Thurst*], a perceived desire for water or other fluid. The sensation of thirst is usually referred to the mouth and throat.

**Thiry-Vella fistula** /thī′rēvel′ə/ [Ludwig Thiry, Austrian physiologist, 1817–1897; Luis Vella, Italian physiologist, 1825–1886], an artificial passage from the abdominal surface of an experimental animal to an isolated intestinal loop, created surgically for the study of intestinal secretions. The continuity of the animal's gut is restored by anastomosis of the severed sections, and the vascular connections and mesenteric attachment of the isolated loop are preserved. The ends of the isolated segment are attached to two openings in the skin of the abdomen to form a closed internal loop.

**thixo-,** combining form meaning 'touch': *thixolabile, thixotropic, thixotropy.*

**thixotropy** /thiksot′rəpē/ [Gk, *this*, touch, *terpin*, to turn], a property of certain gels or colloids that become less viscous when shaken or agitated but revert to their original viscosity after standing.

**Thomas' splint** [Hugh O. Thomas, English surgeon, 1834–1891], **1.** a rigid splint constructed of steel bars that are curved to fit the involved limb and are held in place by a cast or a rigid bandage. It is used in the treatment of chronic joint diseases. **2.** a rigid metal splint that extends from a ring at the hip to beyond the foot. It is used to treat a fractured leg and, in conjunction with various traction and suspension devices, to immobilize and position a fractured femur in a preoperative or postoperative patient. Also called **Thomas' knee splint, Thomas' ring splint.**

**Thompson scattering.** See **scattering.**

**Thomsen's disease.** See **myotonia congenita.**

**thoracentesis** /thôr′əsentē′sis/ [Gk, *thorax* + *centesis*, puncture], the surgical perforation of the chest wall and pleural space with a needle to aspirate fluid for diagnostic or therapeutic purposes or to remove a specimen for biopsy. The procedure is usually performed using local anesthesia, with the patient in an upright position. Thoracentesis may be used in the treatment of pleural effusion, as may occur in bronchogenic carcinoma. Fluid samples may be examined for erythrocyte, leukocyte, and differential white cell counts, as well as protein, glucose, and amylase concentrations, and may be cultured for studies of microorganisms that may be present. Also called **thoracocentesis.**

**thoracic** /thôras′ik/, pertaining to the thorax.

**-thoracic,** combining form meaning 'the chest': *abdominothoracic, extrathoracic, intrathoracic.*

**thoracic actinomycotics.** See **actinomycosis.**

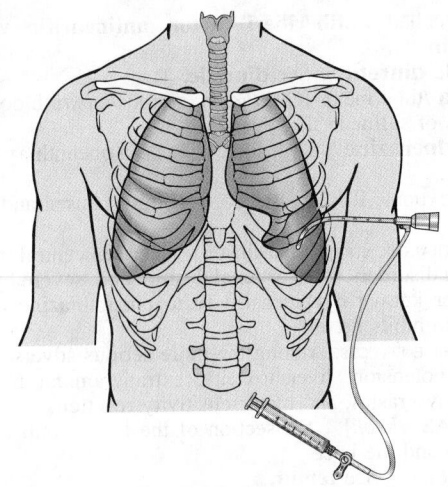

**Thoracentesis**
*(Lewis, Heitkemper, and Dirksen, 2000/courtesy Sherwood Medical, St Louis)*

**thoracic aorta** [Gk, *thorax*, chest, *aerein*, to raise], the large upper part of the descending aorta, starting at the lower border of the fourth thoracic vertebra, dividing into seven branches, and supplying many parts of the body such as the heart, ribs, chest muscles, and stomach. Its seven branches are the pericardial, bronchial, esophageal, mediastinal, posterior intercostal, subcostal, and superior phrenic. See also **descending aorta.** Compare **abdominal aorta.**

**thoracic cage** [Gk, *thorax*, chest; L, *cavus*, hollow], the bony framework that surrounds the organs and soft tissues of the chest. It consists of 12 thoracic vertebrae, 12 pairs of ribs, and the sternum.

**thoracic cavity** [Gk, *thorax*, chest; L, *cavum*], the cavity enclosed by the ribs, the thoracic part of the vertebral column, the sternum, the diaphragm, and associated muscles.

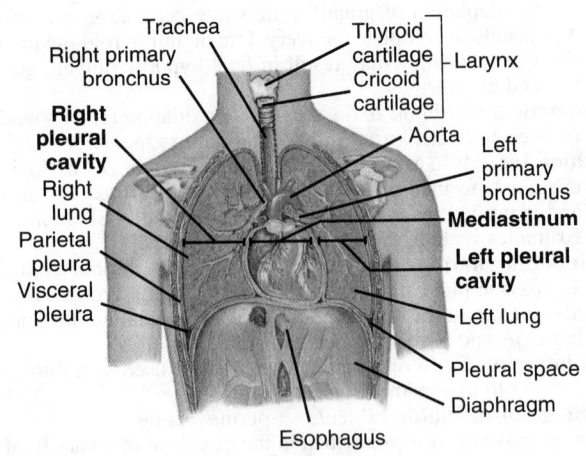

**Thoracic cavity**
*(Thibodeau and Patton, 1999/George J. Wassilchenko)*

**thoracic duct,** the common trunk of all the lymphatic vessels in the body, except those on the right side of the head, the neck, and the thorax, the right upper limb, the right lung, the right side of the heart, and the diaphragmatic surface of the liver. In the adult it is 38 to 45 cm long and 3 to 5 mm in diameter. Compare **right lymphatic duct.** See also **lymphatic system.**

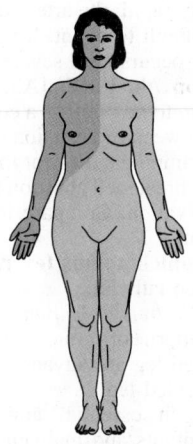

**Thoracic duct drainage (blue)**
*(Thibodeau and Patton, 1999/Barbara Cousins)*

**thoracic fistula,** an abnormal opening in the chest wall that ends blindly or communicates with the thoracic cavity.

**thoracic medicine,** the branch of medicine concerned with the diagnosis and treatment of disorders of the structures and organs of the chest, especially the lungs.

**thoracic nerves,** the 12 pairs of spinal nerves emerging from the spinal cord at the level of the thorax, including 11 intercostal nerves and one subcostal nerve. They are distributed mainly to the walls of the thorax and the abdomen. The thoracic nerves do not enter a plexus but follow independent courses, making them different from other spinal nerves. The first two intercostal nerves innervate the upper limb and the thorax; the next four supply only the thorax; and the lower five supply the walls of the thorax and the abdomen. Each subcostal thoracic nerve innervates the abdominal wall and the skin of a buttock. See also **autonomic nervous system.**

**thoracic outlet syndrome,** an abnormal condition and a type of mononeuropathy characterized by paresthesia. It may be caused by a nerve root compression by a cervical disk.

**thoracic parietal node,** one of the lymph glands in the thorax, associated with various lymphatic vessels and divided into sternal nodes, intercostal nodes, and diaphragmatic nodes. See also **lymphatic system, lymph node.**

**thoracic surgery** [Gk, *thorax,* chest, *cheirourgia,* surgery], the branch of medicine that deals with disease and injuries of the thoracic area by manipulative and operative methods.

**thoracic vertebra,** one of the 12 bony segments of the spinal column of the upper back designated T1 to T12 or D1 to D12. T1 is just below the seventh cervical vertebra (C7), and T12 is just above the first lumbar vertebra (L1). The tho-

racic part of the spine is flexible and has a concave ventral curvature. Each vertebra has a broad thick lamina; long, obliquely directed spinous processes; and thick strong articular facets. The thoracic vertebrae are unique in having small lateral facets for articulation with the ribs. The vertebrae are separated from each other by intervertebral disks. The vertebrae become thicker and heavier in descending order from T1 to T12. Compare **cervical vertebra, lumbar vertebra, sacral vertebra.**

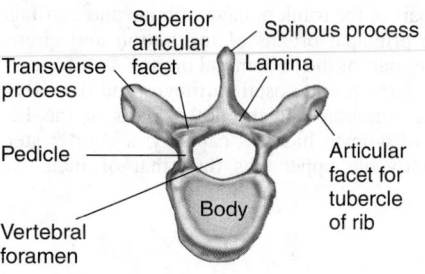

**Thoracic vertebra** *(Applegate, 2000)*

**thoracic visceral node,** a node in the three groups of lymph nodes connected to the part of the lymphatic system that serves certain structures within the thorax such as the thymus, pericardium, esophagus, trachea, lungs, and bronchi. The thoracic visceral nodes include the anterior mediastinal nodes, posterior mediastinal nodes, and tracheobronchial nodes. Compare **thoracic parietal node.** See also **lymph, lymphatic system, lymph node.**

**thoraco-** /thôr′əkō-/, combining form meaning 'the chest': *thoracobronchotomy, thoracocentesis, thoracomyodynia.*

**thoracocentesis.** See **thoracentesis.**

**thoracodorsal nerve** /thôr′əkōdôr′səl/ [Gk, *thorax* + L, *dorsum,* back], a branch of the brachial plexus, usually arising between the two subscapular nerves. It courses along the posterior wall of the axilla and terminates in branches that supply the latissimus dorsi.

**thoracodynia** /-din′ē·ə/ [Gk, *thorax,* chest, *odyne,* pain], chest pain.

**thoracolumbar fascia** /thôr′əkōlum′bər/, a noncontractile structure that functions in a manner similar to a ligament in the lumbar area. It extends from the iliac crest and sacrum to the thoracic cage and envelops the paravertebral musculature.

**thoracolumbosacral orthosis (TLSO)** /thôr′ə·kōlum′bō·sā′krəl/ [Gk, *thorax,* chest; L, *lumbus,* loin; + *sacrum,* sacred], a spinal orthosis that goes over the lumbar, sacral, and thoracic regions and thus limits movement of the thorax; different types vary in rigidity and in the kind of support given to the thorax. See also **body jacket.**

**thoracopathy** /thôr′əkop′əthē/, any disorder involving the thorax or the organs it contains.

**thoracoplasty** /thôr′əkoplas′tē/, the surgical reduction in the size of abnormal spaces in the thoracic cavity, such as may result from a collapsed lung.

**thoracoscopy,** an endoscopic procedure used to directly visualize the pleura, lungs, and mediastinum and to obtain tissue for testing. It is also helpful in staging and dissection of lung cancers.

**thoracostomy** /thôr′əkos′təmē/ [Gk, *thorax* + *stoma*, mouth], an incision made into the chest wall to provide an opening for the purpose of drainage.

**thoracostomy tube,** a catheter inserted through the chest wall to drain fluid from the pleural space.

**thoracotomy** /thôr′əkot′əmē/ [Gk, *thorax* + *temnein*, to cut], a surgical opening into the thoracic cavity.

**Thoraeus filters** /thôrē′əs/, a combination of metals, usually tin, copper, and aluminum, used to modify the quality of orthovoltage x-ray beams and thus improve their penetrating ability.

**thorax** /thôr′aks/, *pl.* **thoraxes, thoraces** [Gk, chest], the upper part of the trunk or cage of bone and cartilage containing the principal organs of respiration and circulation and covering part of the abdominal organs. It is formed ventrally by the sternum and costal cartilages and dorsally by the 12 thoracic vertebrae and the dorsal parts of the 12 ribs. The thorax of women has less capacity, a shorter sternum, and more movable upper ribs than that of men. Also called **chest.**

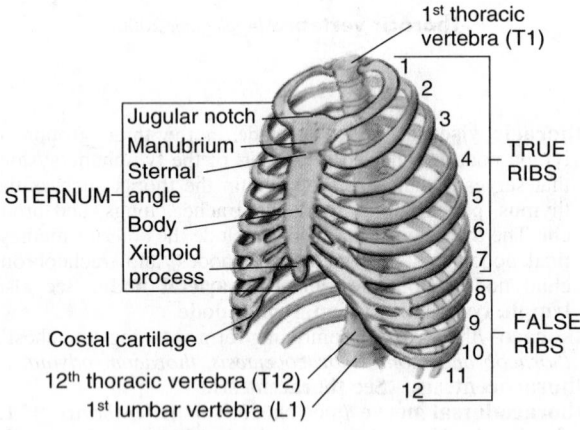

1st thoracic vertebra (T1)

Jugular notch
Manubrium
Sternal angle
STERNUM
Body
Xiphoid process

Costal cartilage

12th thoracic vertebra (T12)
1st lumbar vertebra (L1)

TRUE RIBS

FALSE RIBS

**Thorax** (Applegate, 2000)

**Thorazine,** trademark for a phenothiazine antiemetic and tranquilizer (chlorpromazine).

**thorium (Th)** /thôr′ē·əm/ [ONorse, *Thor*, god of thunder], a heavy grayish radioactive metallic element. Its atomic number is 90; its atomic mass is 232.04. Thorium is used in nuclear medicine and in radiation therapy.

**thought broadcasting** /thôt/ [AS, *thot*], a symptom of psychosis in which the patient believes that his or her thoughts are "broadcast" beyond the head so that other people can hear them.

**thought insertion,** a belief by some mentally ill patients that thoughts of other people can be inserted into their own minds.

**thought processes, disturbed,** a nursing diagnosis accepted by the Fourth National Conference on the Classification of Nursing Diagnoses (revised). Altered thought processes is defined as a state in which an individual experiences a disruption in cognitive operations and activities.

■ DEFINING CHARACTERISTICS: The defining characteristics are inaccurate interpretation of environment, cognitive dissonance, distractibility, memory deficit/problems, egocentric-

ity, and hypervigilance or hypovigilance. Another possible characteristic is inappropriate nonreality-based thinking.

■ RELATED FACTORS: Related factors are to be developed. See also **nursing diagnosis.**

**thought transference.** See **telepathy.**

**Thr,** abbreviation for **threonine.**

**threadworm.** See *Enterobius vermicularis.*

**threadworm infection.** See **strongyloidiasis.**

**thready pulse** /thred′ē/ [AS, *thraed* + L, *pulsare*, to beat], an abnormal pulse that is weak, somewhat difficult to palpate, and often fairly rapid; the artery does not feel full, and the rate may be difficult to count. It is characteristic of hypovolemia, such as occurs with severe hemorrhage.

**threatened abortion** /thret′ənd/ [AS, *threat*, coercion; L, *ab*, away from, *oriri*, to be born], a condition in pregnancy before the twentieth week of gestation characterized by uterine bleeding and cramping sufficient to suggest that miscarriage may result. A threatened abortion is generally managed with rest and observation. Compare **incomplete abortion, inevitable abortion.**

**3-day fever.** See **phlebotomus fever.**

**3-day measles.** See **rubella.**

**three-point gait** [Gk, *treis* + L, *pungere*, to prick; ONorse, *gata*, way], a pattern of crutch-walking in which the crutches and affected leg are advanced together, in alternation with the unaffected leg.

**threonine (Thr),** an essential amino acid needed for proper growth in infants and maintenance of nitrogen balance in adults. See also **amino acid, protein.**

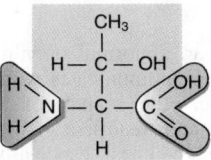

**Chemical structure of threonine**

**threp-,** combining form meaning 'nutrition': *threpsis, threpology, threptic.*

**threshold** /thresh′ōld/ [AS, *therscold*], the point at which a stimulus is great enough to produce an effect; for example, a pain threshold is the point at which a person becomes aware of pain.

**threshold dose** [AS, *therscold* + Gk, *dosis*, giving], a measure of a dose of radiation exposure defined in terms of conditions needed to produce a visible erythema in a given proportion of people exposed. Also called **minimal erythema dose (MED), skin erythema dose (SED), threshold erythema dose (TED).**

**threshold limit values,** the maximum concentration of a chemical to which workers can be exposed for a fixed period, such as 8 hours per day, without developing a physical impairment.

**threshold of consciousness** [AS, *therscold* + L, *conscire*, to be aware], the lowest limit of perception of a stimulus.

**threshold stimulus** [AS, *therscold* + L, *stimulare*, to incite], a stimulus that is just sufficient to produce a response. Below that level, no action or response is likely without additional intensity of the stimulus. Also called **limen, liminal stimulus.**

**thrill** [AS, *thyrlian,* to pierce], a fine vibration, felt by an examiner's hand on a patient's body over the site of an aneurysm or on the precordium, the result of turmoil in the flow of blood, indicating the presence of an organic murmur of grade 4 or greater intensity. A thrill can also be felt over the carotids if a bruit is present and over an arteriovenous fistula in the patient undergoing hemodialysis. Compare **bruit, murmur.**

**thrix** /thriks/ [Gk], hair.

**throat.** See **pharynx.**

**throat and nose cultures,** a microscopic examination used to isolate and identify pathogens such as streptococci, meningococci, gonococci, *Bordetella pertussis,* and *Corynebacterium diphtheriae.* Identification of streptococci is particularly important in a throat culture, since rheumatic heart disease or glomerulonephritis may follow a streptococcal pharyngitis. Nasopharyngeal cultures are often done to screen for infections and carrier states caused by various other organisms such as *Staphylococcus aureus, Haemophilus influenzae, Neisseria meningitidis,* respiratory syncytial virus (RSV), and viruses causing rhinitis.

**throb** [ME, *throbben,* to beat intensely], a deep, pulsating kind of discomfort or pain. —**throbbing,** *adj., n.*

**thrombapheresis.** See **plateletpheresis.**

**thrombasthenia** /throm′basthē′nē·ə/ [Gk, *thrombos,* lump, *a + sthenos,* not strength], a rare hemorrhagic disease characterized by a defect in platelet-mediated hemostasis caused by an abnormality in the membrane surface of the platelet. It is inherited as an autosomal-recessive trait. The platelets do not aggregate, a clot does not form, and hemorrhage ensues. Transfusion with platelets is effective in controlling the hemorrhage. The condition is an inherited autosomal-recessive trait.

**thrombectomy** /thrombek′təmē/ [Gk, *thrombos + ektomē,* excision], the removal of a thrombus from a blood vessel, performed as emergency surgery to restore circulation to the affected part. Anticoagulant therapy may begin before surgery. An arteriogram is done to locate the thrombus. During surgery a longitudinal incision is made into the blood vessel, and the clot is removed. After surgery the blood pressure is maintained close to its preoperative level because a decrease would predispose to further clotting. Compare **embolectomy.**

**thrombi.** See **thrombus.**

**thrombin** /throm′bin/, an enzyme formed from prothrombin, calcium, and thromboplastin in plasma during the clotting process. Thrombin causes fibrinogen to change to fibrin, which is essential in the formation of a clot. See also **blood clot.**

**thrombo-** /throm′bō-/, combining form meaning 'clot': *thromboarteritis, thrombocystis, thrombolysis.*

**thromboangiitis** /throm′bō·an′jē·ī′tis/, an inflammation of the blood vessels associated with thrombosis and accompanied by destruction of the intima.

**thromboangiitis obliterans** [Gk, *thrombos + angeion,* vessel, *itis,* inflammation; L, *obliterare,* to cancel], an occlusive vascular condition, usually of a leg or a foot, in which the small and medium-sized arteries become inflamed and thrombotic. Early signs of the condition are burning, numbness, and tingling of the foot or leg distal to the lesion. Phlebitis and gangrene may develop as the disease progresses. Pulsation in the limb below the damaged blood vessels is often absent. The goal of therapy is to avoid all factors that decrease the blood supply to the extremity, such as cigarette smoking, and to use all means possible to increase the supply. Amputation may be necessary if the condition progresses to gangrene with chronic infection and extensive

tissue destruction. Men are affected more often than women; most affected men smoke and are between 20 and 40 years of age. Also called **Buerger's disease.**

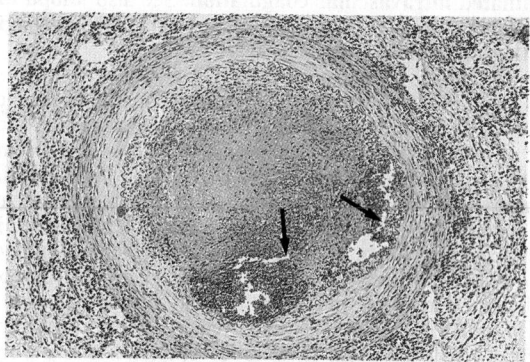

**Thromboangiitis obliterans**
*(Kumar, Cotran, and Robbins, 1997)*

**thromboarteritis** /throm′bō·är′tərī′tis/, arterial inflammation with thrombus formation.

**thrombocyst** /throm′bəsist/, a membranous sac enclosing a thrombus.

**thrombocyt-,** combining form meaning 'platelet': *thrombocytopenia, thrombocytosis.*

**thrombocytapheresis.** See **plateletpheresis.**

**thrombocyte.** See **platelet.**

**thrombocythaemia, thrombocythemia.** See **thrombocytosis.**

**thrombocytopathy** /throm′bōsītop′əthē/ [Gk, *thrombos + kytos,* cell, *pathos,* disease], any disorder of the blood coagulation mechanism caused by an abnormality or dysfunction of platelets. Kinds of thrombocytopathies include **thrombocytopenia** and **thrombocytosis.** —**thrombocytopathic,** *adj.*

**thrombocytopenia** /throm′bōsī′təpē′nē·ə/ [Gk, *thrombos + kytos + penia,* poverty], reduction in the number of platelets. There may be decreased production of platelets, decreased survival of platelets, and increased consumption of platelets or splenomegaly. Thrombocytopenia is the most common cause of bleeding disorders. Bleeding is usually from small capillaries. Treatment requires a specific diagnosis of the cause. All drugs are stopped because nearly any drug may cause the condition. Adrenal corticosteroids and transfusion may be necessary.

**thrombocytopenia—absent radius syndrome,** an autosomal recessive syndrome consisting of thrombocytopenia associated with absence or hypoplasia of the radius and sometimes congenital heart disease and renal anomalies. Also called **TAR syndrome.**

**thrombocytopenic purpura** /-sī′təpē′nik/ [Gk, *thrombos + kytos,* cell, *penia,* poverty; L, *purpura,* purple], a bleeding disorder characterized by a marked decrease in the number of platelets, resulting in multiple bruises, petechiae, and hemorrhage into the tissues. Causes include infection and drug sensitivity and toxicity. A diagnosis is reached only by the exclusion of other causes. Considered to be a manifestation of an autoimmune response, two distinct entities, acute and chronic thrombocytopenia, can be differentiated on clinical manifestations alone. The acute form usually occurs in children between 2 and 6 years of age and is benign, with complete recovery usually apparent within 6 weeks. The chronic form usually occurs in adults between 20 and 50 years of age. Recovery is rarely spontaneous and often requires adrenocortical steroids or splenectomy. Compare **disseminated intravascular coagulation.** See also **idiopathic thrombocytopenic purpura, hemophilia, hemorrhagic diathesis, thrombasthenia.**

**thrombocytosis** /throm′bōsītō′sis/ [Gk, *thrombos* + *kytos* + *osis*, condition],   an abnormal increase in the number of platelets in the blood. **Benign thrombocytosis,** or **secondary thrombocytosis,** is asymptomatic and usually occurs after splenectomy, inflammatory disease, hemolytic anemia, hemorrhage, or iron deficiency; as a response to exercise; after chemotherapy; in chronic myelogeneous leukemia; or in advanced carcinoma, Hodgkin's disease, or other lymphomas. **Essential thrombocythemia** is characterized by episodes of spontaneous bleeding alternating with thrombotic episodes. The platelets may reach levels exceeding 1,000,000/μL. Compare **thrombocytopenia.** See also **polycythemia.**

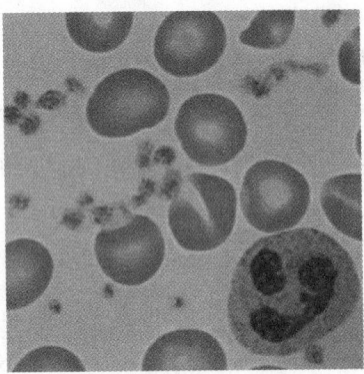

**Thrombocytosis** *(Carr and Rodak, 1999)*

**thromboembolism** /-em′bəliz′əm/ [Gk, *thrombos* + *embolos*, plug],   a condition in which a blood vessel is obstructed by a clot (thrombus) carried in the bloodstream from its site of formation. The area supplied by an obstructed artery may tingle and become cold, numb, and cyanotic. Treatment includes quiet bed rest, warm wet packs, and anticoagulants to prevent the formation of additional thrombi. Embolectomy may be indicated, especially if the aorta or common iliac artery is obstructed. A thromboembolus in the lungs causes a sudden, sharp thoracic or upper abdominal pain, dyspnea, cough, fever, anxiety, and hemoptysis. Obstruction of the pulmonary artery or one of its main branches may be fatal. Thromboemboli are diagnosed by x-ray films and other radiologic techniques, including lung scans and angiography.

**thrombogenesis** /-jen′əsis/,   formation of a thrombus or blood clot.

**thrombogenic** /-jen′ik/ [Gk, *thrombos* + *genein*, to produce],   pertaining to a thrombus or a factor that causes a thrombus.

**thromboid** /throm′boid/,   **1.** clotlike.   **2.** resembling a thrombus.

**thrombokinase.**   See **factor X.**

**thrombolysis** /thrombol′isis/,   the dissolution of a thrombus.

**thrombolytic** /-lit′ik/ [Gk, *thrombos* + *lysis,* a loosening],   pertaining to a drug or other agent that dissolves thrombi.

**thrombolytic therapy (TT),**   administration of a thrombolytic agent such as tissue plasminogen activator, urokinase, or streptokinase to dissolve an arterial clot, such as a clot in a coronary artery in a patient with an acute myocardial infarction. TT is also used to dissolve clots (thrombus) in venous access devices.

**thrombopathy** /thrombop′əthē/,   a condition in which is a clotting ability is deficient for reasons other than thrombocytopenia.

**thrombopenia** /-pē′nē·ə/ [Gk, *thrombos,* lump, *penia,* poverty]. See **thrombocytopenia.**

**thrombopenic purpura.**   See **hemorrhagic purpura.**

**thrombophlebitis** /-fləbī′tis/ [Gk, *thrombos* + *phleps,* vein, *itis*],   inflammation of a vein accompanied by the formation of a clot. It occurs most commonly as the result of trauma to the vessel wall; hypercoagulability of the blood; infection; chemical irritation; postoperative venous stasis; prolonged sitting, standing, or immobilization; or a long period of IV catheterization. Also called **phlebitis.**

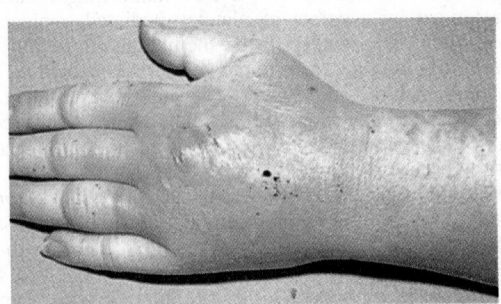

**Thrombophlebitis** *(Greig and Garden, 1996)*

■ OBSERVATIONS: Thrombophlebitis of a superficial vein is generally evident; the vessel feels hard and thready or cord-like and is extremely sensitive to pressure; the surrounding area may be erythematous and warm to the touch, and the entire limb may be pale, cold, and swollen. Deep vein thrombophlebitis is characterized by aching or cramping pain, especially in the calf when the patient walks or dorsiflexes the foot (Homans' sign).

**thrombophlebitis migrans.**   See **migratory thrombophlebitis.**

**thrombophlebitis purulenta,**   inflammation of a vein associated with the formation of a soft, purulent thrombus that infiltrates the wall of the vessel.

**thromboplastic** /-plas′tik/,   **1.** causing clot formation.   **2.** pertaining to the role of thromboplastin in forming a clot.

**thromboplastin.**   See **factor III.**

**thrombosed** /throm′bōst/,   **1.** clotted.   **2.** pertaining to a blood vessel in which a thrombus has formed.

**thrombosis** /thrombō′sis/,   *pl.* **thromboses,** an abnormal condition in which a clot (thrombus) develops within a blood vessel. See also **blood clotting.**

**thrombotapheresis.**   See **plateletpheresis.**

**thrombotic** /thrombot′ik/ [Gk, *thrombos,* lump],   caused or characterized by thrombosis.

**thrombotic microangiopathy,** the formation of thrombi in the arterioles and capillaries, as occurs in **thrombotic thrombocytopenic purpura** and **hemolytic uremia syndrome.**

**thrombotic phlegmasia.** See **phlegmasia alba dolens.**

**thrombotic thrombocytopenic purpura (TTP)** [Gk, *thrombos*, lump, *thrombos* +*kytos*, cell, *penia*, poverty; L, *purpura*, purple], a disorder characterized by thrombocytopenia, hemolytic anemia, and neurologic abnormalities. It is accompanied by a generalized purpura with the deposition of microthrombi within the capillaries and smaller arterioles. It includes a chronic form and an acute fulminating form that may be fatal in weeks. Therapy includes corticosteroids, splenectomy, and therapeutic plasma exchange. Compare **disseminated intravascular coagulation.** See also **thrombocytopenic purpura.**

**thromboxane,** any of several compounds synthesized by platelets and other cells that cause platelet aggregation and vasoconstriction.

**thromboxane A$_2$ (TXA$_2$)** /thrombok'sān/, a highly unstable, biologically active compound derived from prostaglandin G$_2$. It increases in concentration after injury to blood vessels and stimulates the primary hemostatic response and irreversible platelet aggregation.

**thromboxane-A synthase,** an enzyme that catalyzes the conversion in platelets of prostaglandin G$_2$ to thromboxane A$_2$. A deficiency of the enzyme causes a defect in the release of platelets. See also **thromboxane A$_2$.**

**thromboxane B$_2$ (TXB$_2$),** a stable metabolite of thromboxane A$_2$ that has an effect on polymorphonuclear cells and may possess chemotactic activity. It is released during anaphylaxis in laboratory animals. See also **thromboxane A$_2$.**

**thrombus** /throm'bəs/, *pl.* **thrombi** [Gk, *thrombos*, lump], an aggregation of platelets, fibrin, clotting factors, and the cellular elements of the blood attached to the interior wall of a vein or artery, sometimes occluding the lumen of the vessel. Kinds of thrombi include **agonal thrombus, hyaline thrombus, laminated thrombus,** and **white thrombus.** Also called **blood clot.** Compare **embolus.**

**through-and-through drainage** /thrōō/ [ME, *thurgh* +S, *drachen*, tear drop], a method of irrigating a body organ by inserting two tubes, one to introduce the fluid and another to drain the fluid that accumulates within the organ.

**through transmission,** a type of ultrasound imaging in which the sound field is transmitted through a specimen and the transmitted energy is picked up on a far surface by a receiving transducer.

**thrush** [Dan, *troeske*, dryness], candidiasis of the tissues of the mouth. The condition is characterized by the appearance of creamy white patches of exudate on an inflamed tongue or buccal mucosa. It is usually a benign condition in normal children but may be a sign of human immunodeficiency virus infection. See also **candidiasis, stomatitis parasitica.**

**thulium (Tm)** /thōō'lē·əm/ [L, *Thule*, northern island], a rare earth metallic element. Its atomic number is 69; its atomic mass is 168.93. Thulium that has been irradiated in a nuclear reactor gives off gamma radiation.

**thumb** /thum/ [AS, *thuma*], the first and shortest digit on the radial side of the of the hand, classified by some anatomists as one of the fingers because its metacarpal bone ossifies in the same manner as those of the phalanges. Other anatomists classify the thumb separately, noting that it has a much different articulation with the metacarpal bone (a saddle joint) and is composed of one metacarpal bone and only two phalanges. The nerves that innervate the various muscles controlling the thumb include branches of the radial

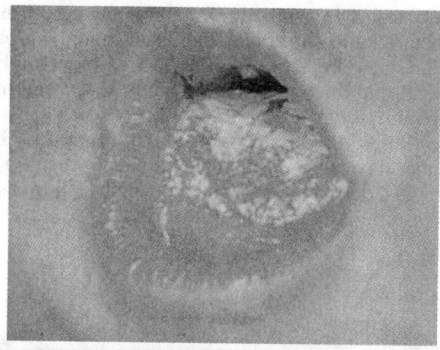

**Thrush**
*(Seidel et al, 1999/courtesy Mead Johnson and Co., Evansville, Indiana)*

nerve, the deep palmar branch of the ulnar nerve, and a branch of the median nerve.

**thumb forceps,** a surgical instrument used to grasp soft tissue, especially while suturing. Also called **tissue forceps.**

**thumb sign** [AS, *thuma* + L, *signum*], the flexing of the terminal phalanx of the thumb against the flexed index finger, as in holding a piece of paper. It is observed in patients who are unable to adduct the thumb because of an ulnar lesion. Also called **Froment sign, newspaper sign, signe de journal.**

**thumbsucking,** the habit of sucking the thumb for oral gratification. It is normal in infants and young children as a pleasure-seeking or comforting device, especially when the child is hungry or tired. The habit reaches its peak when the child is between 18 and 20 months of age, and it normally disappears as the child develops and matures. Thumbsucking beyond 4 to 6 years of age may lead to malocclusion of the teeth and deformation of the bony tissue of the thumb. Excessive thumbsucking, especially in older children, may be indicative of some emotional problem.

**thumps, 1.** hiccups. **2.** spasmodic contractions of the diaphragm.

**thyme** /tīm, thim/ [Gk, *thymon*], the dried leaves and flowering tops of an herb, *Thymus vulgaris*, which produces a pungent mintlike aroma. It is the source of a volatile oil, tannin, and gum but is used mainly as a flavoring agent.

**thymectomy** /thīmek'təmē/ [Gk, *thymus*], the surgical removal of the thymus.

**thymi.** See **thymus.**

**-thymia,** combining form meaning '(condition of the) mind or will': *amphithymia, barythymia, poikilothymia.*

**thymic** /thī'mik/, pertaining to the thymus gland.

**thymic hypoplasia, thymic parathyroid aplasia.** See **DiGeorge's syndrome.**

**thymidine (dThd)** /thī'mədēn/, one of the four major nucleosides in DNA. It is formed by the condensation of thymine with deoxyribose.

**thymine,** a pyrimidine base, in animal cells usually occurring condensed with deoxyribose to form the nucleoside deoxythymidine, a component of deoxyribonucleic acid. See also **cytosine, guanine, uracil.**

**thymo-, 1.** combining form meaning 'thymus gland': *thymocyte, thymolysis, thymoma.* **2.** combining form meaning 'the spirit or mind': *thymogenic, thymopathy, thymopsyche.*

**thymol** /thī′mol/,   a synthetic or natural thyme oil, used as an antibacterial and antifungal, that is an ingredient in some over-the-counter preparations for the treatment of hemorrhoids, acne, and tinea pedis. It is also used as a stabilizer in various pharmaceutic preparations.

**thymoma** /thīmō′mə/, *pl.* **thymomas, thymomata** [Gk, *thymos,* thyme, flowers, *oma* tumor],   a usually benign tumor of the thymus gland that may be associated with myasthenia gravis or an immune deficiency disorder.

puberty, when it weighs about 35 g. After puberty the organ undergoes involution. With aging the gland may change from pinkish-gray to yellow and in the elderly individual may appear as small islands of thymic tissue covered with fat and surrounded by the yellowish capsule. The normal involution of the thymus may be superseded by rapid accidental involution caused by starvation or by acute disease. Compare **spleen.**

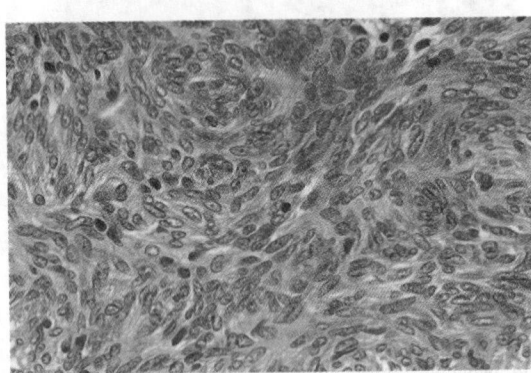

**Benign thymoma**
*(Cotran, Kumar, and Collins, 1999/courtesy Dr. David Dorfman, Department of Pathology, Brigham and Women's Hospital, Boston)*

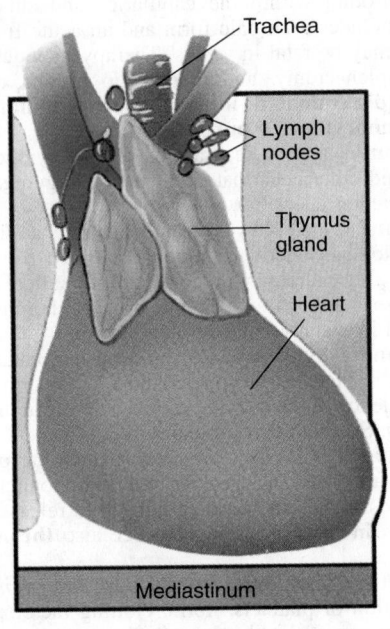

**Thymus** *(Thibodeau and Patton, 1999/Nadine Sokol)*

**thymosin** /thī′məsin/,   **1.** a naturally occurring immunologic hormone secreted by the thymus gland. It is present in greatest amounts in young children and decreases in amount throughout life. **2.** an investigational drug derived from bovine thymus extracts and prescribed as an immunomodulator in experimental treatments for certain diseases such as systemic lupus erythematosus or rheumatoid arthritis.

**thymus** /thī′məs/, *pl.* **thymuses, thymi** [Gk, *thymos,* thyme, flowers],   a single unpaired lymphoid organ that is located in the mediastinum, extending superiorly into the neck to the lower edge of the thyroid gland and inferiorly as far as the fourth costal cartilage. The thymus is the primary central gland of the lymphatic system. The endocrine activity of the thymus is believed to depend on the hormone thymosin, which is composed of biologically active peptides critical to the maturation and the development of the immune system. The T cells of the cell-mediated immune response develop in this gland before migrating to the lymph nodes and spleen. The gland consists of two lateral lobes closely bound by connective tissue, which also encloses the entire organ in a capsule. Superficial to the gland is the sternum. Lying deep to the thymus are the great vessels and the cranial part of the pericardium. The two lobes of the gland differ in size, and, in many individuals the right lobe overlaps the left lobe. The thymus is about 5 cm long, 4 cm wide, and 6 mm thick. The lobes are composed of numerous lobules, which are separated by delicate connective tissue. Each lobule is composed of a dense cellular cortex and an inner, less dense medulla. The thymus develops in the embryo from the third branchial pouch and increases in size until attaining a weight of 12 to 14 g before birth. The size of the organ relative to the rest of the body is largest when the individual is about 2 years of age. The thymus usually attains its greatest absolute size at

**thymus-dependent antigen,**   an antigen that requires the interaction between T and B cells to initiate antibody production.

**thymus-independent antigen,**   an antigen that induces antibody (immunoglobulin M) production without direct cooperation from T cells.

**Thypinone,**   trademark for the synthetic thyrotropin-releasing hormone (protirelin), used as an adjunctive agent in the diagnostic assessment of thyroid function.

**Thyrar,**   trademark for thyroid hormone.

**-thyrea, -thyreosis, -thyroidism,**   combining form meaning a 'condition of the thyroid gland': *athyrea, hypothyrea, hyperthyrea.*

**thyro-** /thī′rō-/,   **thyroido-, threo-,** combining form meaning 'a shield or pertaining to the thyroid gland': *thyroactive, thyroidectomy, thyroiditis.*

**thyroaplasia** /thī′rō-aplā′zhə/,   variations in any of several defects in the thyroid gland and deficiencies of its secretions.

**thyrocalcitonin.**   See **calcitonin.**

**thyrocervical trunk** /-sur′vikəl/ [Gk, *thyreos,* shield, *eidos,* form; L, *cervix,* neck, *truncus*],   one of a pair of short thick arterial branches arising from the first part of the subclavian arteries close to the medial border of the scalenus anterior and supplying numerous muscles and bones in the head, neck, and back. Each is divided into three branches: the inferior thyroid, suprascapular, and transverse cervical.

**thyrocricotomy** /-krīkot′əmē/ [Gk, *thyreos,* shield, *eidos,* form, *krikos,* ring, *temnein,* to cut], a tracheotomy procedure in which the cricovocal membrane is divided.

**thyrogenic** /-jen′ik/ [Gk, *thyreos,* shield, *eidos,* form, *genein,* to produce], pertaining to an origin in the thyroid gland. Also **thyrogenous** /thīroj′ənəs/.

**thyroglobulin** /-glōb′yəlin/, a purified extract of porcine thyroid. See also **thyroid hormone.**

■ INDICATIONS: It is prescribed in the treatment of cretinism, myxedema, goiter, and other hypothyroid states.

■ CONTRAINDICATIONS: Cardiovascular disease, hypopituitarism, or known hypersensitivity to this drug may prohibit its use.

■ ADVERSE EFFECTS: Among the more serious adverse reactions are tremors, nervousness, palpitation and tachycardia, and arrhythmias when given in excessive doses.

**thyroglossal** /-glos′əl/, pertaining to an embryonic duct connecting the thyroid gland and the tongue. Also **thyrolingual.**

**thyroid.** See **thyroid gland, thyroid hormone.**

**thyroid acropathy** /thī′roid/ [Gk, *thyreos,* shield, *eidos,* form, *akron,* extremity, *pathos,* disease], swelling of subcutaneous tissue of the extremities and clubbing of the digits, occurring rarely in patients with thyroid disease and usually associated with pretibial myxedema or exophthalmos.

**thyroid cancer,** a neoplasm of the thyroid gland, usually characterized by slow growth and a slower and more prolonged clinical course than that of other malignancies. A significant carcinogenic effect of exposure to ionizing radiation is demonstrated by the high rate of thyroid cancer in survivors of exposure to atomic bomb explosions and in individuals who have been treated with radiotherapy for an enlarged thymus in infancy or for acne or other skin disorders in adolescence. Nontoxic colloid goiters and follicular adenomas may be precursors of malignant thyroid tumors. The first sign of cancer may be an increased size of the thyroid gland, a palpable nodule, hoarseness, dysphagia, dyspnea, or pain on pressure. Diagnostic measures include x-ray examination, transillumination of the gland, radioisotope scanning, needle biopsy, and ultrasonic examination. More than half of thyroid malignancies are papillary carcinomas, about one third are follicular carcinomas, and the rest consist of rapidly growing invasive anaplastic carcinomas; medullary carcinomas that secrete calcitonin; and metastatic lesions from primary tumors in the breast, kidneys, or lungs. Total or subtotal thyroidectomy with excision of involved lymph nodes is usually recommended. Radioactive iodine may be administered after surgery, and high doses of exogenous thyroid are often used to suppress thyroid-stimulating hormone (TSH) in an effort to cause the regression of residual tumor dependent on TSH. Various chemotherapeutic agents, especially adriamycin, may be effective in patients with metastatic thyroid cancer that is unresponsive to conventional treatment. Thyroid cancer is twice as common in women as in men. Although it is diagnosed most frequently in people between 30 and 50 years of age, it may also occur in children and older individuals.

**thyroid cartilage,** the largest cartilage of the larynx, consisting of two laminae fused together at an acute angle in the midline of the anterior neck to form the Adam's apple. Compare **cricoid.**

**thyroid crisis** [Gk, *thyreos,* shield, *eidos,* form, *krisis,* turning point], a sudden exacerbation of symptoms of thyrotoxicosis characterized by fever, sweating, tachycardia, extreme nervous excitability, and pulmonary edema. It usually occurs in a patient whose thyrotoxicosis treatment is inadequate, and the paroxysm is triggered by a stressful infection or injury. If untreated, the crisis is often fatal. Also called **thyroid storm, thyrotoxic crisis.** See also **Graves' disease.**

**thyroid dermoid cyst,** a tumor derived from embryonal tissues that is believed to have developed in the thyroid gland or in the thyrolingual duct.

**thyroidectomized** /thī′roidek′təmīzd/ [Gk, *thyreos,* shield, *eidos,* form, *ektomē,* excision], pertaining to a patient or condition in which the thyroid gland has been removed.

**thyroidectomy** /thī′roidek′təmē/ [Gk, *thyreos* + *eidos,* form, *ektomē,* excision], the surgical removal of the thyroid gland. It is performed for colloid goiter, tumors, or hyperthyroidism that does not respond to iodine therapy and antithyroid drugs. All but 5% to 10% of the gland is removed; regrowth usually begins shortly after surgery, and thyroid function may return to normal. For cancer of the thyroid, the entire gland is removed, along with surrounding structures from neck to collarbone, in a radical neck dissection. Before surgery the basal metabolism rate is lowered to normal by giving iodine and antithyroid drugs. If a tumor is present, a frozen section of the affected tissue is examined by a pathologist. If malignant cells are found, all the gland is removed. After surgery the patient is most comfortable in semi-Fowler's position with continuous mist inhalation administered to liquefy oral secretions. Oral suctioning may be necessary. A tracheotomy set and oxygen are kept in the room. Calcium gluconate is on hand for use if the patient develops tetany. After surgery the patient is observed for signs of hemorrhage, respiratory difficulty caused by edema of the glottis, and the muscular twitching of tetany from inadvertent removal of a parathyroid gland.

**thyroid function test,** any of several laboratory tests performed to evaluate the function of the thyroid gland. Thyroid function tests include protein-bound iodine, butanol-extractable iodine, $T_3$, $T_4$, free thyroxine index, thyroxin-binding globulin, thyroid stimulating hormone, long-acting thyroid stimulator, radioactive iodine uptake, and radioactive iodine excretion. Often several of the tests are performed simultaneously.

**thyroid gland** [Gk, *thyreos,* shield, *eidos,* form], a highly vascular organ at the front of the neck, usually weighing about 30 g, consisting of bilateral lobes connected in the middle by a narrow isthmus. It is slightly heavier in women than in men and enlarges during pregnancy. The majority of the thyroid gland secretes the hormone thyroxin, and other clusters of cells produce the hormone calcitonin. These hormones are secreted directly into the blood; thus the thyroid is part of the endocrine system of ductless glands. It is essential to normal body growth in infancy and childhood, and its removal greatly reduces the oxidative processes of the body, producing a lower metabolic rate characteristic of hypothyroidism. The thyroid is activated by the pituitary thyrotrophic hormone and requires iodine to elaborate thyroxine. Compare **parathyroid gland.**

**thyroid hormone,** an iodine-containing compound secreted by the thyroid gland, predominantly as thyroxine ($T_4$) and in smaller amounts, but four times more potent, triiodothyronine ($T_3$). These hormones increase the rate of metabolism; affect body temperature; regulate protein, fat, and carbohydrate catabolism in all cells; maintain growth hormone secretion, skeletal maturation, and the cardiac rate, force, and output; promote central nervous system development; stimulate the synthesis of many enzymes; and are necessary for muscle tone and vigor. Derivatives of thyronine, $T_4$ and $T_3$, are synthesized in the thyroid gland by a complex process involving the uptake, oxidation, and incorporation of iodide and the production of thyroglobulin, the form in which the hormones apparently are stored in thyroid follicu-

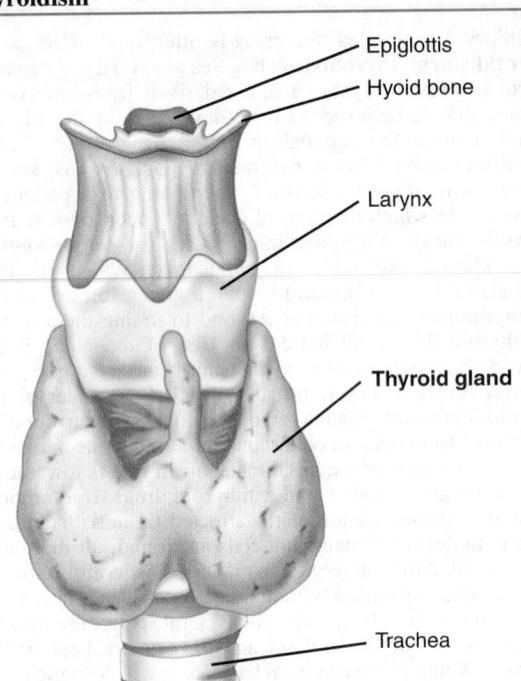

Epiglottis
Hyoid bone
Larynx
Thyroid gland
Trachea

**Thyroid gland** *(Thibodeau and Patton, 1999/Joanna Wild)*

lar colloid. After the proteolysis of thyroglobulin, $T_4$ and $T_3$ are released and transported in the blood in strong, but noncovalent, association with certain plasma proteins; $T_4$ accounts for approximately 90% of iodine in circulation, and $T_3$ for 5%. All phases of the production and release of $T_4$ and $T_3$ are regulated by the thyroid-stimulating hormone secreted by the anterior pituitary gland. Production of thyroid hormones is excessive in Graves' disease and toxic nodular goiter (Plummer's disease), diminished in myxedema, and absent in cretinism. The normal 6-to-7-day half-life of $T_4$ in blood is reduced to 3 or 4 days in hyperthyroidism and extended to 9 or 10 days in myxedema. $T_3$ has a normal half-life of 2 days or less and, like $T_4$, is metabolized most actively in the liver. Pharmaceutic preparations of thyroid hormones extracted from animal glands and the synthetic compounds levothyroxine sodium and liothyronine sodium are used as replacement therapy in patients with hypothyroidism. The dosage is initially low and is gradually increased to the optimal level based on the patient's clinical response and tests of the findings on thyroid function studies. Overdosage or a rapid increase in the dosage may result in signs of hyperthyroidism such as nervousness, tremor, tachycardia, cardiac arrhythmia, and menstrual irregularity.

**-thyroidism.** See **-thyrea.**

**thyroiditis** /thī'roidī'tis/, inflammation of the thyroid gland. Acute thyroiditis caused by staphylococcal, streptococcal, or other infections is characterized by suppuration and abscess formation and may progress to subacute diffuse disease of the gland. Subacute thyroiditis is marked by fever, weakness, sore throat, and a painfully enlarged gland containing granulomas composed of colloid masses surrounded by giant cells and mononuclear cells. Chronic lymphocytic thyroiditis (Hashimoto's disease), characterized by

lymphocyte and plasma cell infiltration of the gland and diffuse enlargement, seems to be transmitted as a dominant trait, may be associated with various autoimmune disorders, and is more common in women. Another chronic form of thyroiditis is Riedel's struma, a rare progressive fibrosis, usually of one lobe of the gland but sometimes involving both lobes, the trachea, and surrounding muscles, nerves, and blood vessels. Radiation thyroiditis occasionally occurs 7 to 10 days after the treatment of hyperthyroidism with radioactive iodine 131.

**thyroid notch,** **1.** (superior) a separation above the anterior border of the thyroid cartilage. **2.** (inferior) a depression in the middle of the lower border of the thyroid cartilage.

**thyroido-.** See **thyro-.**

**thyroid-releasing hormone.** See **thyrotropin-releasing hormone.**

**thyroid scanning,** a radionuclear scan that determines the size, shape, position, and physiologic function of the thyroid gland. It is useful in patients with neck or substernal masses, thyroid nodules, hyperthyroidism, metastatic tumors without a known primary site, and well-differentiated forms of thyroid cancer. The scan may focus either on the neck area only, or the whole body (done in patients previously treated for thyroid cancer).

**thyroid-stimulating hormone (TSH),** a substance secreted by the anterior lobe of the pituitary gland that controls the release of thyroid hormone and is necessary for the growth and function of the thyroid gland. The secretion of TSH is regulated by thyrotropin-releasing hormone, elaborated in the median eminence of the hypothalamus. Normal adult blood levels are 2 to 10 mU/L (SI units). Also called **thyrotropin.** See also **thyroid hormone.**

**thyroid stimulating hormone test (TSH),** a blood test that measures TSH concentration, helping to differentiate primary from secondary hypothyroidism. It is also used to monitor exogenous thyroid replacement.

**thyroid storm,** a crisis of uncontrolled hyperthyroidism caused by the release into the bloodstream of increased amounts of thyroid hormone. Thyroid storm may occur spontaneously or be precipitated by infection, stress, or a thyroidectomy performed on a patient who is inadequately prepared with antithyroid drugs. Characteristic signs are fever that may reach 106° F, a rapid pulse, acute respiratory distress, apprehension, restlessness, irritability, and prostration. The patient may become delirious, lapse into a coma, and die of heart failure. Also called **thyroid crisis.**

**Thyrolar,** trademark for a thyroid hormone (liotrix).

**thyroliberin** /thī'rōlib'ərin/, a tripeptide hormone produced by the hypothalamus that stimulates the anterior pituitary gland to release thyrotropin. Also called **thyrotropin-releasing hormone.**

**thyrolingual.** See **thyroglossal.**

**thyromegaly** /-meg'əlē/ [Gk, *thyreos,* shield, *eidos,* form, *megas,* large], enlargement of the thyroid gland.

**thyrotonine (T₃) triiodothyronine.** See **thyroid hormone.**

**thyrotoxic crisis.** See **thyroid crisis.**

**thyrotoxic myopathy** /-tok'sik/, a condition in thyrotoxicosis consisting of severe weakness in the limb and trunk muscles, including those used in speech and swallowing.

**thyrotoxicosis.** See **Graves' disease.**

**thyrotoxin** /-tok'sin/, a theoretic cytotoxin of the thyroid gland, assumed to be a cause of the signs and symptoms of thyrotoxicosis.

**thyrotrophic** /-trof'ik/ [Gk, *thyreos,* shield, *eidos,* form, *trophe,* nutrition], influencing the thyroid gland, such as the thyroid-stimulating hormone. Also **thyrotropic.**

**thyrotropic hormone.** See **thyroid-stimulating hormone.**

**thyrotropin.** See **thyroid-stimulating hormone.**

**thyrotropin (systemic)** /-trō′pin/, a preparation of bovine thyroid-stimulating hormone that increases the uptake of radioactive iodine in the thyroid and the secretion of thyroxine by the thyroid.

■ INDICATIONS: It is prescribed in diagnostic tests and to enhance uptake of [131]I in the treatment of thyroid cancer.

■ CONTRAINDICATIONS: Coronary thrombosis or known hypersensitivity to this drug prohibits its use. It should not be given in untreated Addison's disease or after myocardial infarction.

■ ADVERSE EFFECTS: Among the most serious adverse reactions are symptoms of hyperthyroidism, allergic reactions, hypotension, and arrhythmias.

**thyrotropin-releasing hormone,** a substance produced in the hypothalamus that stimulates the release of thyrotropin (thyroid-stimulating hormone) from the anterior lobe of the pituitary gland. Previously called **thyrotropin-releasing factor (TRF), TSH-releasing factor.**

**thyroxine ($T_4$)** /thīrok′sēn/, a hormone of the thyroid gland, derived from tyrosine, that influences metabolic rate. Also called **tetraiodothyronine.**

**thyroxine-binding globulin,** a plasma protein that binds with and transports thyroxine in the blood.

**thyroxine-binding globulin test (TBG),** a blood test used to detect levels of TBG, the major thyroid hormone protein carrier. Elevated TBGs may indicate porphyria or infectious hepatitis, among other conditions, while decreased TBGs may signify various causes of hypoproteinemia (nephrotic syndrome, GI malabsorption, malnutrition).

**Thytropar,** trademark for bovine thyrotropin.

**Ti,** symbol for the element **titanium.**

**TI,** abbreviation for *therapeutic index.*

**TIA,** abbreviation for **transient ischemic attack.**

**tiagabine,** an anticonvulsant.

■ INDICATIONS: This drug is used as an adjunct treatment for partial seizures.

■ CONTRAINDICATIONS: Known hypersensitivity to this drug prohibits its use.

■ ADVERSE EFFECTS: Adverse reactions to this drug include dizziness, anxiety, somnolence, ataxia, amnesia, unsteady gait, depression, vasodilation, nausea, vomiting, diarrhea, pruritis, rash, pharyngitis, and coughing.

**tibia** /tib′ē·ə/ [L, shin bone], the second longest bone of the skeleton, located at the medial side of the leg. It articulates with the fibula laterally, the talus distally, and the femur proximally, forming part of the knee joint. It attaches to the quadriceps femoris group of muscles via the patellar tendon and attaches to the ligament of the patella and to various muscles, including the popliteus and the flexor digitorum longus. Also called **shin bone.**

**tibia-,** combining form meaning 'the tibia': *tibial, tibialis, tibiafemoral.*

**tibial** /tib′ē·əl/ [L, *tibia,* shin bone], pertaining to the largest long bone of the lower leg.

**tibialis anterior** /tib′ē·ā′lis/ [L, *tibia + anticus,* in front], one of the anterior crural muscles of the leg, situated on the lateral side of the tibia. It is a thick fleshy muscle proximally and tendinous distally. The muscle dorsiflexes and supinates the foot. Also called **tibialis anticus.** Compare **extensor digitorum longus.**

**tibial torsion** [L, *tibia + torquere,* to twist], a lateral or a medial twisting rotation of the tibia on its longitudinal axis. It is similar to pronation of the hand because of the contraction of the pronator teres and the pronator quadratus, or su-

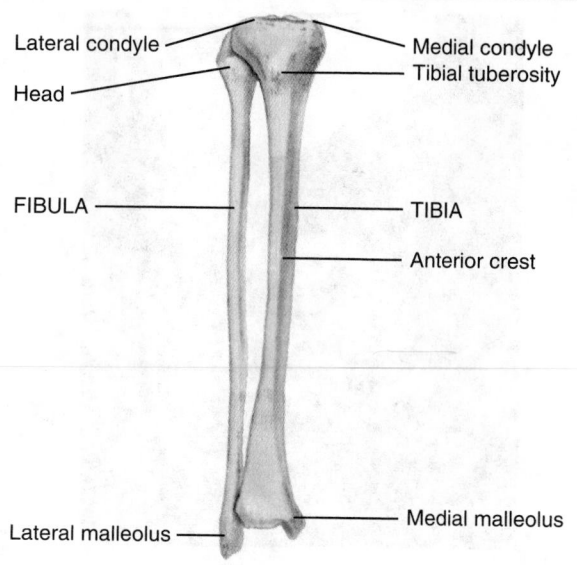

Lateral condyle — Medial condyle
— Tibial tuberosity
Head — 

FIBULA — TIBIA

— Anterior crest

Lateral malleolus — Medial malleolus

Anterior view (right)

**Tibia** *(Applegate, 2000)*

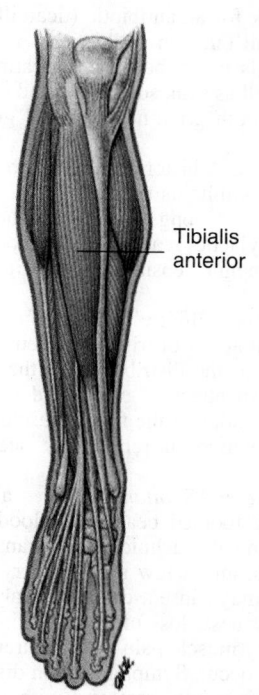

Tibialis anterior

**Tibialis anterior** *(Thibodeau and Patton, 1999/John V. Hagen)*

pination of the hand, caused by the contraction of the supinator muscle. Compare **femoral torsion.**

**tibia valga** [L, *tibia,* shin bone, *valgus,* bowlegged], a bowed tibia with the convex surface toward the outside of the leg.

**tic.** See **mimic spasm.**

**-tic,** suffix meaning 'pertaining to': *paralytic, therapeutic.*

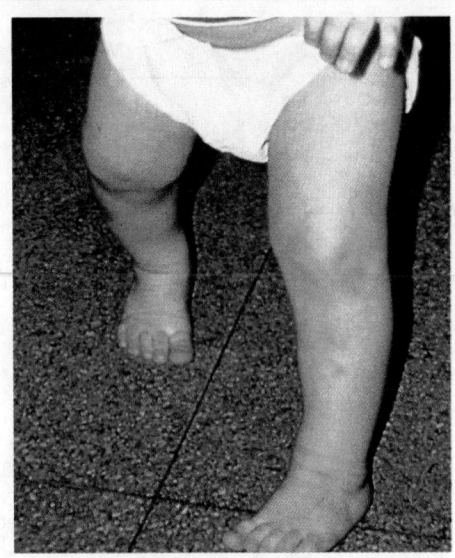

**Tibial torsion** *(Zitelli and Davis, 1997)*

**Ticar,** trademark for an antibiotic (ticarcillin).

**ticarcillin** /tik′ärsil′in/, an antibiotic.

■ INDICATIONS: It is prescribed in the treatment of bacterial septicemia, as well as skin, soft tissue, and respiratory infections caused by both gram-negative and gram-positive organisms.

■ CONTRAINDICATION: A history of allergic reaction to any of the penicillins prohibits its use.

■ ADVERSE EFFECTS: Among the most serious adverse reactions are anaphylactic reactions, thrombocytopenia, leukopenia, neutropenia, eosinophilia, vein irritation, and phlebitis.

**tic douloureux** /tikdo͞olo͞oro͞e′/ [Fr, painful spasm], a brief extremely painful attack of trigeminal neuralgia. It is unilateral and limited to the distribution of the trigeminal (fifth cranial) nerve. An attack is easily and unexpectedly provoked by any stimulus of the facial muscles, from touching to speaking, and may occur repetitively. See also **trigeminal neuralgia.**

**tick bite** [ME, *tike* + AS, *bitan,* to bite], a puncture wound produced by the toothed beak of a blood-sucking tick, a small, tough-skinned arachnid. Ticks transmit several diseases to humans, and a few species carry a neurotoxin in their saliva that may cause ascending paralysis beginning in the legs. Nervousness, loss of appetite, tingling, and headache, followed by muscle pain and in extreme cases respiratory failure may occur. Symptoms often disappear when the attached tick is carefully removed with forceps. See also **Lyme disease, Q fever, relapsing fever, Rocky Mountain spotted fever, tularemia.**

**tick-borne relapsing fever.** See **Dutton's relapsing fever.**

**tick-borne rickettsiosis** [ME, *tike* + *beren* + *Rickettsia* + Gk, *osis,* condition], any disease transmitted by Ixodid ticks carrying the *Rickettsia* pathogens, microorganisms smaller than bacteria but larger than viruses. A common infectious species in North America is *Rickettsia rickettsii,* the cause of Rocky Mountain spotted fever.

**tick fever.** See **relapsing fever.**

**tickling,** a gentle stimulation of the skin surface that produces pleasurable reflexes.

**tick paralysis,** a rare progressive reversible disorder caused by several species of ticks that release a neurotoxin that causes weakness, incoordination, and paralysis. The tick must feed on the host for several days before the symptoms appear, and removal of the tick leads to rapid recovery. Because respiratory or bulbar paralysis can cause death, it is important to search for ticks, frequently hidden in scalp hair, on a patient with these symptoms.

**t.i.d.,** (in prescriptions) abbreviation for the Latin phrase *ter in die* /dē′ā/, 'three times a day.'

**tidal** /tī′dəl/ [AS, *tid,* time], pertaining to an alternating process, such as a rise-and-fall, ebb-and-flow, or periodic lapse of time.

**tidal drainage.** See **drainage.**

**tidal volume (TV, V$_t$)** [AS, *tid,* time; L, *volumen,* paper roll], the amount of air inhaled and exhaled during normal ventilation. Inspiratory reserve volume, expiratory reserve volume, and tidal volume make up vital capacity. See also **pulmonary function test.**

**tide** [AS, *tid*], a variation, increase or decrease, in the concentration of a particular component of body fluids, such as acid tide, fat tide. —**tidal,** *adj.*

**tidemark,** a transitional zone, appearing as a wavy line, that marks the junction between calcified and uncalcified cartilage.

**Tietze's syndrome** /tēt′sēz/ [Alexander Tietze, German surgeon, 1864–1927], **1.** a disorder characterized by nonsuppurative swellings of one or more costal cartilages that may accompany chronic respiratory infections. It causes pain that may radiate to the neck, shoulder, or arm, mimicking the pain of coronary artery disease. If the pain is severe, infiltration with procaine and hydrocortisone may provide relief. **2.** albinism, except for normal eye pigment, accompanied by deaf mutism and hypoplasia of the eyebrows.

**TIG,** abbreviation for **tetanus immune globulin.**

**Tigan,** trademark for an antiemetic (trimethobenzamide hydrochloride).

**tight junction** /tīt/ [ME, *thight,* strong; L, *jungere,* to join], the zonula occludens of the junctional complex between cells in which the plasma membranes of adjacent cells are in direct contact and where there is no intercellular space.

Cell membranes
of adjacent cells

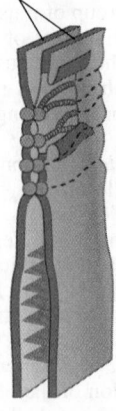

**Tight junction** *(Thibodeau and Patton, 1999/Network Graphics)*

**tilt table** [AS, *tealt,* unsteady; L, *tabula,* board], an examining table that allows a patient to be raised to an approximate 60-degree angle during study of the response of the patient's circulatory system to gravitational forces. A tilt table is also used to assist recovery from orthostatic hypotension after prolonged immobility.

**tiludronate,** a parathyroid agent (calcium regulator).

■ INDICATIONS: This drug is used to treat Paget's disease.

■ CONTRAINDICATIONS: Factors that prohibit the use of this drug include known hypersensitivity to biphosphonates, pathologic fractures, colitis, and severe renal disease with creatinine 5 mg/dL. Use of this drug is also contraindicated in children.

■ ADVERSE EFFECTS: Adverse effects of this drug include dry mouth, gastritis, vomiting, flatulence, gastric ulcers, rhinitis, rales, sinusitis, upper respiratory infection, headache, somnolence, dizziness, anxiety, vertigo, nervousness, involuntary movements, hyperparathyroidism, rash, epidermal necrosis, pruritus, sweating, nephrotoxicity, decreased mineralization of nonaffected bones, and pathologic fractures. Common side effects include nausea, diarrhea, and bone pain.

**timbre** /tim′bər/ [Fr], **1.** a characteristic sound quality of a voice or musical instrument, as determined by the harmonics of the sound. **2.** a second metallic sound heard in aortic dilation.

**time (t)** [AS, *tima*], **1.** a measure of duration. **2.** an interval separating two points in a continuum between the past and future.

**time agnosia.** See **dischronation.**

**time constant,** a mathematic term of fixed value used in expressing the rate of change of some variable, such as air flow in the airways, as a function of time.

**timed collection,** the collection of a specimen such as a urine or stool sample for a specific period of time.

**time delay,** a period between the application of an input and the beginning of the response.

**timed release.** See **prolonged release.**

**timed vital capacity.** See **forced expired vital capacity.**

**time-sharing.** See **multitasking.**

**timolol maleate** /tim′əlōl/, a beta-adrenergic receptor blocking agent.

■ INDICATIONS: It is prescribed for reducing intraocular pressure in chronic open-angle, aphakic, and secondary glaucoma.

■ CONTRAINDICATIONS: Bronchial asthma, chronic obstructive pulmonary disease, sinus bradycardia, or known hypersensitivity to this drug prohibits its use. It is used with caution in patients with contraindications to systemic use of beta-adrenergic receptor blocking agents.

■ ADVERSE EFFECTS: The most serious adverse reaction is blurring of vision. Mild eye irritation also may occur.

**Timoptic,** trademark for a beta-adrenergic receptor blocking agent (timolol maleate).

**tin (Sn)** [AS], a whitish metallic element. Its atomic number is 50; its atomic mass is 118.69. Tin (IV) oxide is used in dentistry as a polishing agent for teeth and in some restorative procedures. See **stannous fluoride.**

**Tinactin,** trademark for an antifungal (tolnaftate).

**tincture (tinct.)** /tingk′chər/, a substance in a solution that is diluted with alcohol.

**tincture of iodine** [L, *tinctura* + Gk, *ioeides,* violet], a mixture of sodium iodide in an alcohol-water solution used as a skin disinfectant. The term is no longer in official use.

**tine,** a sharp projecting point, as a prong of a fork.

**tinea** /tin′ē-ə/ [L, worm], a group of fungal skin diseases caused by dermatophytes of several kinds. The condition is characterized by itching, scaling, and sometimes painful lesions. Tinea is a spread by direct contact between humans and even domestic dogs or cats. Diagnosis is made by demonstrating fungus on smear or by culture. Also called **ringworm.** See also **tinea corporis, tinea cruris, tinea pedis, tinea unguium.**

**tinea capitis,** a superficial fungal infection of the scalp, most common in children. Most infections are caused by species of *Trichophyton.* The infection may lead to hair loss and become secondarily infected with bacteria, causing a severe inflammation. Symptoms include severe itching and scaling of the scalp. Treatment with oral antifungal agents such as griseo fulvin, as well as appropriate antibiotics, is necessary. Oral steroids may be necessary to prevent scarring hair loss. Also called **ringworm.**

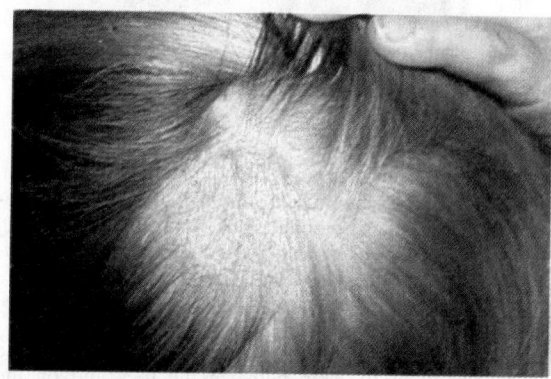

**Tinea capitis**
*(Goldstein and Goldstein, 1997/courtesy Department of Dermatology, University of North Carolina at Chapel Hill)*

**tinea corporis,** a superficial fungal infection of the nonhairy skin of the body, most prevalent in hot, humid climates and usually caused by species of *Trichophyton* or *Microsporum.* Topical fungicides such as miconazole are used for moderate cases; severe infection calls for griseofulvin.

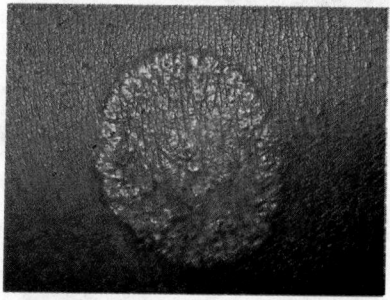

**Tinea corporis** *(Zitelli and Davis, 1997)*

**tinea cruris** /krōō′ris/, a superficial fungal infection of the groin caused by species of *Trichophyton* or *Epidermophyton floccosum.* It is most common in the tropics and among males. Topical antifungals such as miconazole and clotrima-

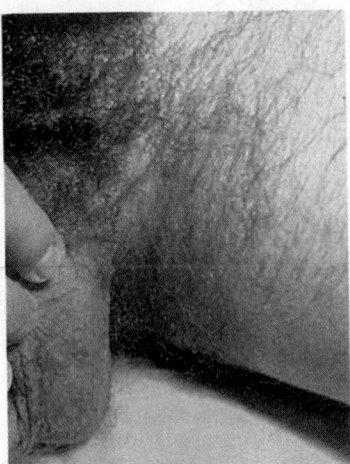

**Tinea cruris** *(Lookingbill and Marks, 1993)*

**tinea unguium** /un'gwē·əm/, a superficial fungal infection of the nails caused by various species of *Trichophyton* and occasionally by *Candida albicans*. It is more common on the toes than the fingers and can cause complete crumbling and destruction of the nails. Itraconazole and terbinafine are the drugs of choice, but they must be continued until the nail has regrown completely. See also **onychomycosis.**

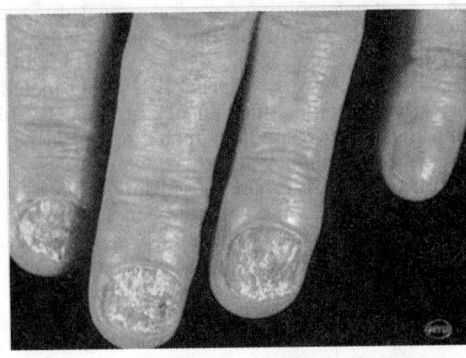

**Tinea unguium**
*(Seidel et al, 1999/courtesy American Academy of Dermatology)*

zole are often prescribed. Griseofulvin is used only for severe resistant cases. Also called **jock itch.**

**tinea nigra,** a minor fungal infection, caused by *Malassezia furfur* or *Exophiala werneckii*, characterized by dark lesions on the skin of the hands or occasionally other areas. Also called **pityriasis nigra.**

**tinea pedis,** a chronic superficial fungal infection of the foot, especially of the skin between the toes and on the soles. It is common worldwide and is usually caused by *Trichophyton mentagrophytes, T. rubrum,* and *Epidermophyton floccosum.* Adults are most susceptible, and the wearing of constricting footwear such as sneakers seems to induce the infection. Drying the feet well after bathing and applying powder between the toes help prevent it. Griseofulvin is the most effective treatment, but miconazole and tolnaftate are also used. Recurrence is common. Also called **athlete's foot.**

**tinea versicolor,** a fungal infection of the skin caused by *Malassezia furfur* and characterized by finely desquamating, pale tan patches on the upper trunk and upper arms that may itch and do not tan. In dark-skinned people the lesions may be depigmented. The fungus fluoresces under Wood's light and may be easily identified in scrapings viewed under a microscope. Treatment usually includes an application of selenium sulfide left on overnight and rinsed off by thorough showering in the morning for 10 consecutive days. Topical and oral antifungal agents may be used. The pale patches

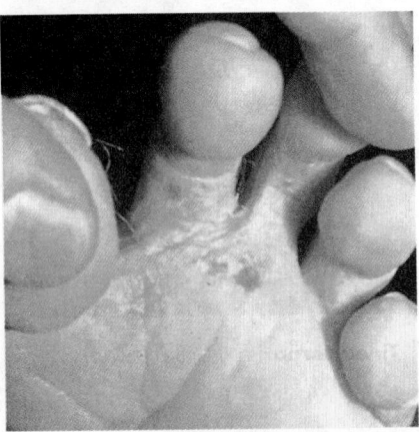

**Tinea pedis**
*(Greenberger and Hinthorn, 1993/courtesy Loren H. Amundson, University of South Dakota, Sioux Falls)*

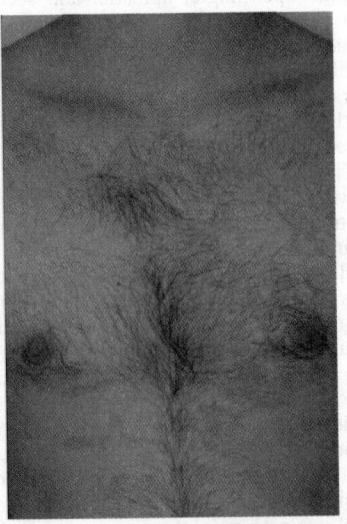

**Tinea versicolor: pigmented phase**
*(Lemmi and Lemmi, 2000)*

may persist for up to 1 year after successful treatment and recurrence is common.

**Tinel's sign** /tinelz'/ [Jules Tinel, French neurosurgeon, 1879–1952], an indication of irritability of a nerve, resulting in a distal tingling sensation on percussion of a damaged nerve. The sign is often present in carpal tunnel syndrome and is produced by tapping over the median nerve on the volar aspect of the wrist.

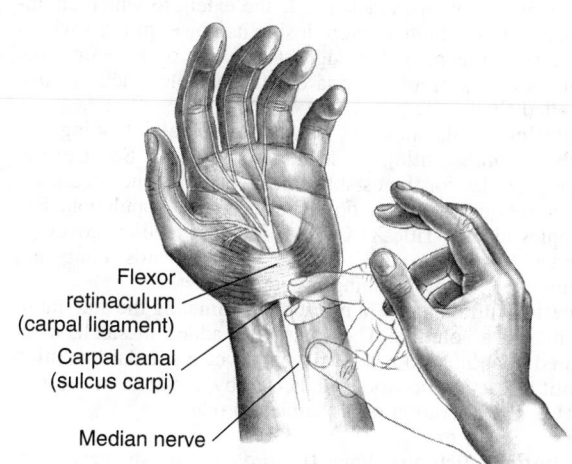

Flexor retinaculum (carpal ligament)

Carpal canal (sulcus carpi)

Median nerve

**Evaluation of Tinel's sign** *(Seidel et al, 1999)*

**tine test** /tīn/ [ME, *tind*, rake tooth; L, *testum*, crucible], a tuberculin skin test in which a small disposable disk with multiple tines bearing tuberculin antigen is used to puncture the skin. The method is widely used to test for sensitivity to the tuberculin antigen. Induration around the puncture site indicates previous exposure or active disease, requiring further testing. See also **tuberculin test.**

**tingling** [ME, *tinklen*, to tinkle], a prickly sensation in the skin or a body part, accompanied by diminished sensitivity to stimulation of the sensory nerves.

**tinnitus** /tinī'təs/ [L, *tinnire*, to tinkle], a subjective noise sensation, often described as ringing, heard in one or both ears. It may be a sign of acoustic trauma, Ménière's disease, otosclerosis, presbycusis, or an accumulation of cerumen impinging on the eardrum or occluding the external auditory canal. It occasionally occurs for no apparent reason.

**tint,** a shade or gradation of a color, usually a pale or less saturated version of the basic shade.

**tinted denture base,** a denture base that has a color close to that of natural oral tissue.

**-tion,** suffix meaning 'act of, process of, result of': *elongation, irritation.*

**tip,** 1. the end of a pointed object. 2. an attachment fitted to the end of something else. 3. a point.

**tipped uterus** /tipt/ [ME, *tipen*, upset; L, *uterus*, womb], a uterus that is displaced from its normal position. See **uterine anteflexion, uterine anteversion, uterine retroflexion, uterine retroversion.**

**tip pinch,** a grasp in which the tip of the thumb is pressed against any or each of the tips of the other fingers. Also called **pinch grip.** See also **palmar pinch, pinch.**

**tipping,** a tooth movement in which the angle of the tooth's long axis is changed.

**TIPS,** abbreviation for **transjugular intrahepatic portosystemic shunt.**

**tip seal,** the closure of an ampule accomplished by melting a bead of glass at the neck of the ampule.

**tirofiban,** an antiplatelet agent.

■ INDICATIONS: Tirofiban is used to treat acute coronary syndrome.

■ CONTRAINDICATIONS: The following factors prohibit the use of tirofiban: known hypersensitivity to this drug, active internal bleeding, stroke, major surgery, severe trauma, intracranial neoplasm, aneurysm, and hemorrhage.

■ ADVERSE EFFECTS: Bleeding is a life-threatening effect of tirofiban. Other adverse reactions include bradycardia, dizziness, dissection, coronary artery edema, pain in the legs and/or pelvis, and sweating. Rash is a common side effect.

**tisane** /tizān', tizän'/, a tealike infusion or light drink of a vegetable herb consumed for a claimed medicinal effect.

**tissue** /tish'ōō/ [Fr, *tissu*, fabric], a collection of similar cells acting together to perform a particular function.

**tissue activator.** See **fibrinokinase.**

**tissue bank,** a facility for storing and maintaining a collection of tissues for future use in transplants.

**tissue-base relationship,** the relationship of the bottom of a removable dental prosthesis to underlying structures.

**tissue committee,** a group that evaluates all surgery performed in a hospital or other health care facility. The evaluation is usually made on the basis of the extent of agreement of the preoperative, postoperative, and pathologic diagnoses and on the relevance and acceptability of the diagnostic procedures. See also **tissue review.**

**tissue culture** [OFr, *tissu* + L, *colere*, to cultivate], the maintenance of growth in vitro, under artificial conditions, of tissue or organ specimens.

**tissue dextrin.** See **glycogen.**

**tissue dose,** the amount of radiation absorbed by tissue in the region of interest, expressed in rad.

**tissue fixation,** a process in which a tissue specimen is placed in a fluid that preserves the cells as nearly as is possible in their natural state.

**tissue fixative,** a fluid that preserves cells in their natural state so they may be identified and examined.

**tissue forceps.** See **thumb forceps.**

**tissue integrity, impaired,** a nursing diagnosis accepted by the Seventh National Conference on the Classification of Nursing Diagnoses. Impaired tissue integrity is defined as a state in which an individual experiences damage to mucous membrane or corneal, integumentary, or subcutaneous tissue.

■ DEFINING CHARACTERISTICS: The principal characteristic is damaged or destroyed tissue.

■ RELATED FACTORS: Related factors are altered circulation, nutritional deficit or excess, fluid deficit or excess, knowledge deficit, and impaired physical mobility. Other factors are irritants, such as chemical (including body excretions, secretions, and medications), thermal (temperature extremes), mechanical (pressure, shear, friction), and radiation (including therapeutic radiation). See also **nursing diagnosis.**

**tissue integrity: skin and mucous membranes,** a nursing outcome from the Nursing Outcomes Classification (NOC) defined as the structural intactness and normal physiological function of skin and mucous membranes. See also **Nursing Outcomes Classification.**

**tissue kinase.** See **fibrinokinase.**

**tissue macrophage** [OFr, *tissu* + Gk, *makros*, large, *phagein*, to eat], a large, mobile, highly phagocytic cell derived from monocytes. These cells become mobile when stimulated by inflammation and migrate to the affected area.

**tissue perfusion: abdominal organs,** a nursing outcome from the Nursing Outcomes Classification (NOC) defined as the extent to which blood flows through the small vessels of the abdominal viscera and maintains organ function. See also **Nursing Outcomes Classification.**

**tissue perfusion: cardiac,** a nursing outcome from the Nursing Outcomes Classification (NOC) defined as the extent to which blood flows through the coronary vasculature and maintains heart function. See also **Nursing Outcomes Classification.**

**tissue perfusion: cerebral,** a nursing outcome from the Nursing Outcomes Classification (NOC) defined as the extent to which blood flows through the cerebral vasculature and maintains brain function. See also **Nursing Outcomes Classification.**

**tissue perfusion, ineffective (renal, cerebral, cardiopulmonary, gastrointestinal, peripheral),** a nursing diagnosis accepted by the Fourth National Conference on the Classification of Nursing Diagnoses. It is defined as a state in which an individual experiences a decrease in nutrition and oxygenation at the cellular level caused by a deficit in capillary blood supply.
■ DEFINING CHARACTERISTICS: The defining characteristics include coldness of the affected extremity, paleness on elevation of the extremity, diminished arterial pulses, and changes in the arterial blood pressure when measured in the affected extremity. Claudication, gangrene, brittle nails, slowly healing ulcers or wounds, shiny skin, and lack of hair are also common.
■ RELATED FACTORS: Related factors include interruption of the venous or arterial circulation to the affected part of the body, hypovolemia or hypervolemia, or a condition that causes abnormal exchange of fluids and nutrients to or from the cells to or from the circulation. See also **nursing diagnosis.**

**tissue perfusion: peripheral,** a nursing outcome from the Nursing Outcomes Classification (NOC) defined as the extent to which blood flows through the small vessels of the extremities and maintains tissue function. See also **Nursing Outcomes Classification.**

**tissue perfusion: pulmonary,** a nursing outcome from the Nursing Outcomes Classification (NOC) defined as the extent to which blood flows through intact pulmonary vasculature with appropriate pressure and volume, perfusing alveoli/capillary units. See also **Nursing Outcomes Classification.**

**tissue plasminogen activator (TPA),** a clot-dissolving substance produced naturally by cells in the walls of blood vessels. It is also manufactured synthetically by genetic engineering techniques. TPA activates plasminogen to dissolve clots and has been used therapeutically to open occluded coronary arteries.

**tissue response,** any reaction or change in living cellular tissue when it is acted on by disease, toxin, or other external stimulus. Some kinds of tissue responses are **immune response, inflammation,** and **necrosis.**

**tissue review,** a review of the surgery performed in a hospital or other health care facility. The evaluation is usually made on the basis of the extent of agreement of the preoperative, postoperative, and pathologic diagnoses and on the relevance and acceptability of the diagnostic procedures. See also **tissue committee.**

**tissue typing,** a systematized series of tests to evaluate the intraspecies compatibility of tissues from a donor and a recipient before transplantation. Typing is accomplished by identifying and comparing a large series of human leukocyte antigens in the cells of the body. See also **HLA, immune system, transplant.**

**titanium (Ti)** /tītā′nē·əm/ [Gk, *Titan,* mythic giant], a grayish brittle metallic element. Its atomic number is 22; its atomic mass is 47.88. An alloy of titanium is used in the manufacture of orthopedic prostheses. Titanium dioxide is the active ingredient in a number of topical ointments and lotions.

**titer** /tī′tər/ [Fr, *titre,* to make a standard] **1.** the normality of a solution or substance, determined by titration to find the equivalence of two reactants. **2.** the extent to which an antibody can be diluted before losing its power to react with a specific antigen. **3.** the highest dilution of a serum that causes clumping of bacteria or other visible reaction. Also spelled **titre.**

**titillation** /tit′ilā′shən/ [L, *titillare,* to tickle], tickling.

**Title** [L, *titulus,* title], a section of the Social Security Act that provides for the establishment, funding, and regulation of a service to a specific segment of the population. Examples include Title XIX, which includes medical coverage under Medicaid, and Title X, which awards lump-sum grants for family planning programs.

**titration** /tītrā′shən/, a method of estimating the amount of solute in a solution. The solution is added in small, measured quantities to a known volume of a standard solution until a reaction occurs, as indicated by a change in color or pH or the liberation of a chemical product.

**titre.** See **titer.**

**titubation** /tich′əbā′shən/ [L, *titubare,* to stagger], unsteady posture characterized by a staggering or stumbling gait and a swaying head or trunk while sitting. It may be a manifestation of cerebellar disease. Compare **ataxia.**

**tizanidine,** a skeletal muscle relaxant and a$_2$-adrenergic agonist.
■ INDICATIONS: This drug is used in the acute/intermittent management of increased muscle tone associated with spasticity.
■ CONTRAINDICATIONS: Known hypersensitivity to this drug prohibits its use.
■ ADVERSE EFFECTS: Adverse reactions to this drug include dry mouth, vomiting, increased ALT, abnormal liver function studies, constipation, somnolence, dizziness, speech disorder, dyskinesia, nervousness, hallucination, psychosis, urinary tract infection, blurred vision, urinary frequency, flulike syndrome, pharyngitis, and rhinitis.

**Tl,** symbol for the element **thallium.**

**TLC, 1.** abbreviation for **total lung capacity. 2.** abbreviation for **thin-layer chromatography.** *informal.* **3.** abbreviation for *tender loving care.*

**TLI,** abbreviation for **total lymphoid irradiation.**

**TLR,** abbreviation for **tonic labyrinthine reflex.**

**TLSO,** abbreviation for **thoracolumbosacral orthosis.**

**T lymphocyte.** See **lymphocyte, T cell.**

**Tm,** symbol for the element **thulium.**

**TM,** abbreviation for **transcendental meditation.**

**TMJ,** abbreviation for **temporomandibular joint.**

**TMP/SMX,** abbreviation for *trimethoprim sulfamethoxazole.* See **sulfamethoxazole, trimethoprim.**

**TNF,** abbreviation for **tumor necrosis factor.**

**TNM,** a system for staging malignant neoplastic disease. See also **cancer staging.**

**t.n.t.c.,** abbreviation for *too numerous to count,* usually applied to organisms or cells viewed on a slide under a microscope.

**t.o.,** abbreviation for *telephone order.*

**toadstool poisoning** /tōd′stool/ [AS, *tadige + stol + L, potio,* drink], a toxic condition caused by ingestion of certain varieties of poisonous mushrooms. See also **mushroom poisoning.**

**tobacco** /təbak′ō/ [Sp, *tabaco*], a plant whose leaves are dried and used for smoking and chewing, and in snuff. See also **nicotine.**

**tobacco withdrawal syndrome,** a change in mood or performance associated with the cessation of or reduction in exposure to nicotine. Symptoms may range from lack of concentration to anxiety and temper outbursts. A multitude of physical symptoms can also emerge.

**TOBEC,** abbreviation for **total body electric conductivity.**

**tobramycin sulfate** /tō′brəmī′sin/, an aminoglycoside antibiotic.

■ INDICATIONS: It is prescribed in the treatment of external ocular infection, septicemia, and lower respiratory tract and central nervous system infections.

■ CONTRAINDICATIONS: Kidney dysfunction, use of potent diuretics, or known hypersensitivity to this or other aminoglycosides prohibits its use.

■ ADVERSE EFFECTS: Among the more serious adverse reactions are ototoxicity and nephrotoxicity.

**Tobruk plaster** /tō′brook/, a plaster cast splint with tapes for skin traction coming through openings in the plaster and connected with a Thomas' splint. It covers and immobilizes the leg from foot to groin. Also called **Tobruk splint.**

**tocainide hydrochloride** /tōkā′nīd/, an oral lidocaine-type antiarrhythmic.

■ INDICATIONS: It is prescribed for the suppression of symptomatic ventricular arrhythmias.

■ CONTRAINDICATIONS: Tocainide may cause adverse cardiovascular effects such as worsened arrhythmias and hypotension. It should not be given to patients with second- or third-degree atrioventricular block who do not also have an artificial ventricular pacemaker. It should not be administered to a patient with an uncorrected potassium deficit, and it may interact with beta-blockers, particularly in patients with known heart failure.

■ ADVERSE EFFECTS: Among the most serious adverse reactions are hypotension, arrhythmias, dizziness, paresthesias, numbness, tremor, nausea, vomiting, rash, and headache.

**-tocia,** **1.** combining form meaning 'conditions of labor': *mogitocia, omotocia, tomotocia.* **2.** combining form meaning the 'product of parturition': *deuterotocia, dystrophiadystocia, odontocia.*

**-tocin,** combining form for oxytocin derivatives.

**toco-, toko-** /tō′kō-/, prefix meaning 'childbirth or labor': *tocodynamometer, tocography, tocomania.*

**tocodynamometer** /tō′kōdī′nəmom′ətər/ [Gk, *tokos*, birth, *dynamis*, force, *metron*, measure], an electronic device for monitoring and recording uterine contractions in labor. It consists of a pressure transducer that is applied to the fundus of the uterus by means of a belt, which is connected to a machine that records the duration of the contractions and the interval between them on graph paper. The relative intensity of the contractions is also indicated but cannot be quantified. The tocodynamometer is a component of external monitoring in childbirth. Also spelled **tokodynamometer.** See also **electronic fetal monitor.**

**tocolytic drug** /-lit′ik/, any drug used to suppress premature labor.

**tocopherol.** See **vitamin E.**

**tocopherolquinone (TQ)** /tōkof′ərōlkwī′nōn/, an oxidized form of tocopherol, or vitamin E.

**tocotransducer** /-transd(y)ōo′sər/ [Gk, *tokos* + L, *trans*, through, *ducer*, to lead], an electronic device used to measure uterine contractions. See also **tocodynamometer.**

**toddler** [ME, *toteren*, to walk unsteadily], a child between 12 and 36 months of age. During this period of development the child acquires a sense of autonomy and independence through the mastery of various specialized tasks such as control of body functions, refinement of motor and language skills, and acquisition of socially acceptable behavior, especially toleration of delayed gratification and acceptance of separation from the mother or parents. The period is characterized by exploration of the environment and rapid cognitive development as the child strives for self-assertion and personal interaction with others while struggling with parental discipline and sibling rivalry. Of primary importance for the nurse is an understanding of the dynamics of the growth and development of the toddler to help parents deal effectively with appropriate nutrition, toilet training, temper tantrums, prevention of accidental injury (primarily from falls, poisoning, and burns), and childhood fears, especially anxiety as a result of separation from the parents.

**toddlerhood** /tod′lərhood′/, the state or condition of being a toddler.

**Todd's paralysis** [Robert Bentley Todd, English physician, 1809–1860; Gk, *paralyein,* to be palsied], postepileptic hemiplegia or monoplegia lasting a few minutes, hours, or occasionally, several days after a seizure.

**toe,** any one of the digits of the feet.

**toe clonus** [AS, *tá* + Gk, *klonos*], an increased reflex activity in the large toe caused by a sudden extension of the first phalanx.

**toe drop** [AS, *tá* + *dropa*], a condition in which the toes droop and cannot be lifted because of paralysis of the tibial muscles.

**toeing in.** See **metatarsus varus.**

**toeing out.** See **metatarsus valgus.**

**toenail** [AS, *ta* + *naegel*], one of the heavy ungual structures covering the terminal phalanges of the toes. Also called **unguis** /ung′gwis/.

**Tofranil,** trademark for a tricyclic antidepressant (imipramine hydrochloride).

**togaviruses** /tō′gəvī′rəsəs/ [L, *toga,* cloak, *virus,* poison], a family of arboviruses that includes the organisms causing encephalitis, dengue, yellow fever, and rubella.

**toilet training,** the process of teaching a child to control the functions of the bladder and bowel. Training programs vary, but all emphasize a positive, consistent, nonpunitive, nonpressured approach; each program is individualized, depending on the mental and physical age and state of the child, the parent-child relationship, and readiness of the child to learn. Training often begins around 24 months of age, when voluntary control of the anal and urethral sphincters is achieved by most children. When the child has mastered some motor skills, is aware of his or her ability to control the body, and can communicate adequately, training is likely to be easy. Resistance occurs if the parents try to train the child before the child is physiologically and psychologically ready. Bowel training is usually accomplished before bladder training because the urge to evacuate the bowel is stronger than the urge to empty the bladder, and the need is less frequent and more regular. Nighttime bladder control may not be achieved until the child is 4 or 5 years of age or older. Behavior modification, using a system of rewards for each of the various phases of the training, has been successful with both normal and mentally retarded children. A major nursing function is to identify the readiness of the child to learn and to work with the parents, advising them in a nonauthoritarian way of the various techniques.

**-toin,** combining form for hydantoin derivative antiepileptics.

**token economy** [AS, *tacen,* to show; Gk, *oikonomia,* household management], a technique of reinforcement used in behavior therapy in the management of a group of people, such as in hospitals, institutions, or classrooms. Individuals are rewarded for specific activities or behavior with tokens they can exchange for desired objects or privileges.

**toko-.** See **toco-.**

**tokodynamometer.** See **tocodynamometer.**

**tolazamide** /tolaz'əmīd/, an oral sulfonylurea antidiabetic.
- INDICATIONS: It is prescribed in the treatment of stable or non-insulin-dependent diabetes mellitus and for some patients sensitive to other types of sulfonylureas or who have failed to respond to other similar drugs.
- CONTRAINDICATIONS: Unstable diabetes, serious impairment of renal, hepatic, or thyroid function, pregnancy, or known hypersensitivity to this drug or other sulfonylurea medications prohibits its use.
- ADVERSE EFFECTS: Among the more serious adverse effects are hypoglycemia and skin reactions. Blood dyscrasias may occur.

**tolazoline hydrochloride** /tolaz'əlēn/, an antiadrenergic/sympatholytic.
- INDICATIONS: It is prescribed in the treatment of persistent pulmonary hypertension of the newborn.
- CONTRAINDICATIONS: Hypersensitivity to this drug prohibits its use.
- ADVERSE EFFECTS: Among the more serious adverse reactions are cardiac arrhythmia, hypotension or hypertension, exacerbation of stress ulcer, hemorrhage, and mitral stenosis.

**tolbutamide** /tolboo'təmīd/, an oral sulfonylurea antidiabetic.
- INDICATIONS: It is prescribed in the treatment of stable non-insulin-dependent diabetes mellitus uncontrolled by diet alone and for some patients changing from insulin to oral therapy.
- CONTRAINDICATIONS: Unstable diabetes, serious impairment of renal, hepatic, or thyroid function, pregnancy, or known hypersensitivity to this drug or to other sulfonylurea medications prohibits its use.
- ADVERSE EFFECTS: Among the more serious adverse reactions are hypoglycemia and skin reactions. Blood dyscrasias may occur.

**tolcapone,** an antiparkinson agent.
- INDICATIONS: Tolcapone is used in the treatment of parkinsonism.
- CONTRAINDICATIONS: Known hypersensitivity to this drug prohibits its use.
- ADVERSE EFFECTS: Life-threatening effects of tolcapone include hemolytic anemia, leukopenia, and agranulocytosis. Other adverse reactions include dystonia, dyskinesia, dreaming, psychosis, hallucinations, dizziness, chest pain, hypotension, cataract, eye inflammation, diarrhea, constipation, urinary tract infection, urine discoloration, uterine tumor, micturition disorder, sweating, and alopecia. Common side effects include fatigue, headache, confusion, orthostatic hypotension, nausea, vomiting, anorexia, and abdominal distress.

**Tolectin,** trademark for a nonsteroidal antiinflammatory agent (tolmetin sodium).

**tolerance** /tol'ərəns/ [L, *tolerare,* to endure], a phenomenon by which the body becomes increasingly resistant to a drug or other substance through continued exposure to the substance. A kind of tolerance is **work tolerance.**

**tolerance dose.** See **maximum permissible dose.**

**tolerance test,** 1. an investigation of the ability of the body to metabolize a drug or nutrient, as in a glucose tolerance test. 2. a physical activity drill administered to evaluate the efficiency of blood circulation or of another body system.

**Tolinase,** trademark for an antidiabetic (tolazamide).

**tolmetin sodium** /tol'mətin/, a nonsteroidal antiinflammatory agent.
- INDICATIONS: It is prescribed primarily in the treatment of rheumatoid arthritis, juvenile rheumatoid arthritis, and osteoarthritis.
- CONTRAINDICATIONS: Impaired renal function, GI disease, or known hypersensitivity to this drug, to aspirin, or to nonsteroidal antiinflammatory medications prohibits its use.
- ADVERSE EFFECTS: Among the more serious adverse reactions are peptic ulcer and GI distress. Dizziness, skin rash, and tinnitus commonly occur. This drug interacts with many other drugs.

**tolnaftate** /tolnaf'tāt/, an antifungal.
- INDICATIONS: It is prescribed in the treatment of superficial fungus infections of the skin, including tinea pedis, tinea cruris, and tinea versicolor.
- CONTRAINDICATION: Known hypersensitivity to this drug prohibits its use.
- ADVERSE EFFECTS: Among the more common adverse reactions are hypersensitivity reactions and mild irritation of the skin.

**Tolosa-Hunt syndrome** /tō·lō'sä·hunt/ [Eduardo S. Tolosa, Spanish neurosurgeon, 20th century; William Edward Hunt, American neurosurgeon, b. 1921], unilateral ophthalmoplegia associated with pain behind the orbit and in the area supplied by the first division of the trigeminal nerve; it is thought to result from nonspecific inflammation and granulation tissue in the superior orbital fissure or cavernous sinus. Compare **cavernous sinus syndrome.**

**tolterodine,** a muscarinic receptor antagonist.
- INDICATIONS: Tolterodine is used to treat overactive bladder (frequency and urgency).
- CONTRAINDICATIONS: Factors that prohibit the use of this drug include known hypersensitivity, uncontrolled narrow-angle glaucoma, urinary retention, and gastric retention.
- ADVERSE EFFECTS: Adverse reactions to tolterodine include paresthesia, fatigue, headache, chest pain, hypertension, vision abnormalities, xerophthalmia, abdominal pain, constipation, dry mouth, dyspepsia, dysuria, urinary retention, urinary frequency, urinary tract infection, rash, pruritus, bronchitis, cough, pharyngitis, and upper respiratory infection. Common side effects include anxiety, dizziness, nausea, vomiting, and anorexia.

**toluene** ($C_6H_5CH_3$) /tol'yoo·ēn/, an aromatic colorless flammable liquid produced from coal tar, petroleum, or Peruvian tolu balsam. It is used in dyes, explosives, gums, and lacquers and in the manufacture of drugs and the extraction of organic chemicals from plants.

**-tome,** 1. combining form meaning a 'cutting instrument': *labiotome, neurotome, thyrotome.* 2. combining form meaning a '(specified) segment or region': *dermomyotome, pleurotome, viscerotome.*

**-tomic, -tomical,** suffix meaning 'incisions or sections of tissue': *dermatomic, phlebotomic, somatomic.*

**Tomlin, Evelyn M.** See **Modeling and Role Modeling.**

**tomo-,** combining form meaning 'preparation of a section or layer': *tomograph.*

**tomogram** /tō'məgram'/ [Gk, *tome,* section, *gramma,* record], a radiograph produced by tomography.

**tomograph** /tō'məgraf'/ [Gk, *tome,* section, *graphein,* to record], a radiographic apparatus that makes an image of layers of body tissues at various depths.

**tomographic DSA** /-graf'ik/, the visualization of blood vessels in the body in three dimensions. See also **digital subtraction angiography.**

**tomography** /təmog'rəfē/ [Gk, *tome* + *graphein,* to record], 1. sectional imaging. 2. a radiographic technique in which the tube and film are moved synchronously during exposure, producing a blurred radiograph in which objects within the focal plane are seen more clearly than objects outside the focal plane. **3.** a radiographic technique that produces a film representing a detailed cross section of tissue at a predetermined depth. It is a valuable diagnostic tool for the discovery and identification of space-occupying lesions such as might be found in the brain, liver, pancreas, and gallbladder. See also **computed tomography, positron emission tomography (PET).**

**-tomy,** suffix meaning a 'surgical incision': *cystotomy, oncotomy, phlebotomy.*

**tonaphasia.** See **amusia.**

**tone.** See **tonus.**

**tone deafness** [Gk, *tonos,* stretching; AS, *deaf*], an inability to detect the pitch or changing pitch of a musical note or a voice change.

**tongue** /tung/ [AS, *tunge*], the principal organ of the sense of taste that also assists in the mastication and deglutition of food. It is located in the floor of the mouth within the curve of the mandible. Its root is connected to the hyoid bone posteriorly. It is also connected to the epiglottis, soft palate, and pharynx. The apex of the tongue rests anteriorly against the lingual surfaces of the lower incisors. The mucous membrane connecting the tongue to the mandible reflects over the floor of the mouth to the lingual surface of the gingiva and in the midline of the floor is raised into a vertical fold. The dorsum of the tongue is divided into symmetric halves by a median sulcus, which ends posteriorly in the foramen cecum. A shallow sulcus terminalis runs from this foramen laterally and forward on either side to the margin of the organ. From the sulcus the anterior two thirds of the tongue are covered with papillae. The posterior third is smoother and contains numerous mucous glands and lymph follicles. The use of the tongue as an organ of speech is not anatomic but a secondary acquired characteristic. Also called **glossa, lingua.**

during the act of swallowing. It may result in forward displacement of the maxilla with consequent malocclusion of the teeth.

**tongue-tie.** See **ankyloglossia.**

**-tonia, -tony,** suffix meaning '(condition or degree of) muscle tension': *angiotonia, hemotonia, neurotony, vagotony, vasotonia.*

**tonic** /ton'ik/, pertaining to a type of afferent or sensory nerve receptor that responds to length changes placed on the noncontractile part of a muscle spindle. It may be triggered by a mechanical external force such as positioning or by an internal stretch caused by intrafusal muscle contraction.

**-tonic, 1.** combining form meaning the 'quality of muscle contraction or tonus': *hypertonic, myatonic, normotonic.* **2.** combining form meaning a 'solution with a comparative concentration': *hypertonic, hypotonic, isotonic.*

**tonic-clonic seizure,** an epileptic seizure characterized by a generalized involuntary muscular contraction and cessation of respiration followed by tonic and clonic spasms of the muscles. Breathing resumes with noisy respirations. The teeth may be clenched, the tongue bitten, and control of the bladder or bowel lost. As this phase of the seizure passes, the person may fall asleep or experience confusion. Usually the person has no recall of the seizure on awakening. A sensory warning, or aura, can precede each tonic-clonic seizure. These seizures may occur singly, at intervals, or in close succession. Anticonvulsant medications are usually prescribed as prophylaxis against tonic-clonic seizures. Also called **grand mal seizure.** Compare **absence seizure, focal seizure, psychomotor seizure.**

**tonic convulsion** [Gk, *tonos,* stretching; L, *convulsio,* cramp], a prolonged generalized contraction of the skeletal muscles.

**tonicity** /tōnis'itē/ [Gk, *tonikos,* stretching], the quality of possessing tone, or tonus.

**tonic labyrinthine reflex** [Gk, *tonikos + labyrinthos,* maze; L, *reflectere,* to bend back], a normal postural reflex in animals, abnormally accentuated in decerebrate humans, characterized by extension of all four limbs when the head is positioned in space at an angle above the horizontal in quadrupeds or in the neutral erect position in humans. Also called **decerebrate rigidity.**

**tonic neck reflex,** a normal response in newborns to extend the arm and the leg on the side of the body to which the head is quickly turned while the infant is supine and to flex

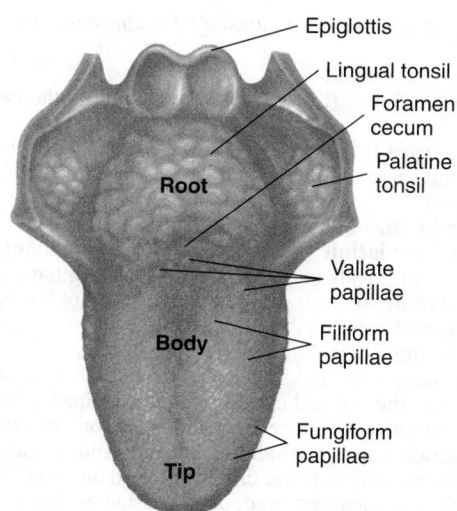

**Tongue** *(Thibodeau and Patton, 1999/Rolin Graphics)*

- Epiglottis
- Lingual tonsil
- Foramen cecum
- Palatine tonsil
- Vallate papillae
- Filiform papillae
- Fungiform papillae

**Root**
**Body**
**Tip**

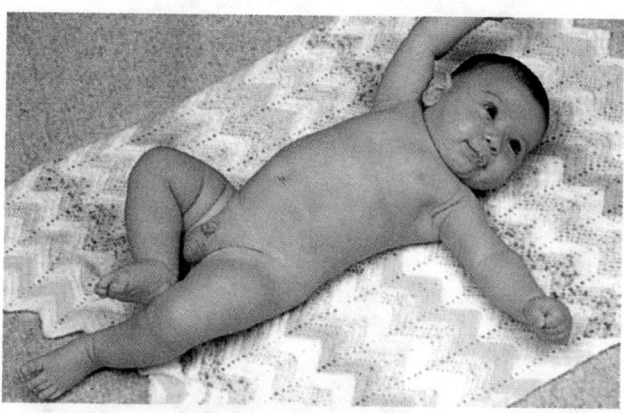

**Tonic neck reflex**
*(Lowdermilk, Perry, and Bobak, 2000/courtesy Marjorie Pyle, Lifecircle, Costa Mesa, California)*

**tongue deviation.** See **deviation of tongue.**

**tongue-thrust swallow,** an immature form of swallowing in which the tongue is projected forward instead of retracted

the limbs of the opposite side. The reflex, which prevents the infant from rolling over until adequate neurologic and motor development occurs, disappears by 3 to 4 months of age to be replaced by symmetric positioning of both sides of the body. Absence or persistence of the reflex may indicate central nervous system damage. Also called **asymmetric tonic neck reflex.** See also **symmetric tonic neck reflex.**

**tonic pupil.** See **Adie's pupil.**

**tonic spasm** [Gk, *tonos,* stretching, *spasmos*], a sustained contraction of a muscle as distinguished from a transient clonic contraction.

**tonitrophobia** /tonit′rōfō′bē·ə/, an abnormal fear of thunder.

**tono-,** combining form meaning 'tone or tension': *tonoclonic, tonoscillograph, tonoplast.*

**Tonocard,** trademark for a lidocaine-type oral antiarrhythmic drug (tocainide hydrochloride).

**tonoclonic** /ton′əklon′ik/ [Gk, *tonos,* stretching, *klonos,* tumult], pertaining to muscular spasms that are tonic and then clonic.

**tonofibril** /ton′əfī′bril/ [Gk, *tonos,* stretching, *fibrilla,* small fiber], a bundle of fine filaments found in the cytoplasm of epithelial cells. The individual strands, or **tonofilaments,** spread throughout the cytoplasm and extend into the intercellular bridge to converge at the desmosome. The system of fibers functions as a supportive element within the cytoskeleton. In keratinizing epithelium the strands are the main precursor of keratin. Also called **epitheliofibril, tenofibril.** See also **keratohyalin.**

**tonofilament** /ton′ōfil′əmənt/ [Gk, *tonos,* stretching], a proteinaceous fiber found in epithelial cells. Bundles of tonofilaments form a tonofibril, which has a supporting function.

**tonograph** /ton′əgraf/, an apparatus that makes a record of tension measurements.

**tonography** /tōnog′rəfē/, **1.** the measurement over time of intraocular pressure with graphic documentation. **2.** the measurement of tension.

**tonometer** /tōnom′ətər/ [Gk, *tonos* + *metron,* measure], an instrument used in measuring tension or pressure, especially intraocular pressure.

**tonometry** /tōnom′ətrē/, the measuring of intraocular pressure by determining the resistance of the eyeball to indentation by an applied force. Several kinds of tonometers are used. The air-puff tonometer, which does not touch the eye, records deflections of the cornea from a puff of pressurized

air. The Schiötz impression and the applanation tonometers record the pressure needed to indent or flatten the corneal surface. Applanation tonometry is considered most accurate. Schiötz tonometry is rarely done today.

**tonoscillograph** /ton′əsil′əgraf′/, an apparatus that records arterial and capillary pressures with a corresponding pulse tracing.

**tonsil** /ton′səl/ [L, *tonsilla*], a small rounded mass of tissue, especially lymphoid tissue, such as that composing the palatine tonsils in the oropharynx. Compare **intestinal tonsil, lingual tonsil, palatine tonsil, pharyngeal tonsil.** Also called **tonsilla.**

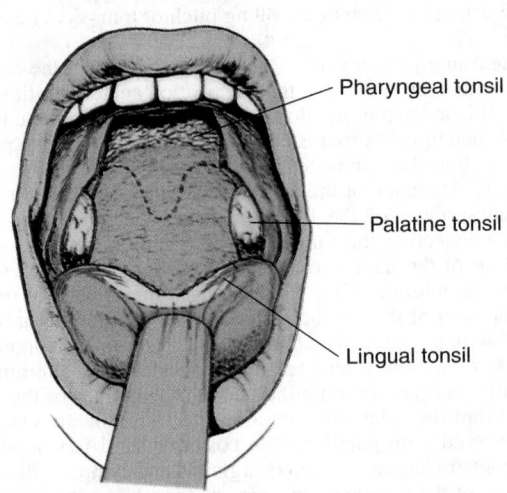

**Tonsils** *(Thibodeau and Patton, 1999/Rolin Graphics)*

**tonsill-,** prefix meaning 'tonsils': *tonsillectomy, tonsillith, tonsillitis.*

**tonsilla.** See **tonsil.**

**tonsillar** /ton′silər/ [L, *tonsilla*], pertaining to the palatine tonsil.

**tonsillar crypt** [L, *tonsilla* + Gk, *kryptos,* hidden], a small tubular invagination on the surface of a palatine or pharyngeal tonsil.

**tonsillar fossa.** See **amygdaloid fossa.**

**tonsillar herniation** [L, *tonsilla* + *hernia,* rupture], the herniation of tonsils of the cerebellum through the foramen magnum of the skull. It may occur as a result of intracranial pressure from an injury or tumor.

**tonsillar ring.** See **Waldeyer's throat ring.**

**tonsillectomy** /ton′silek′təmē/ [L, *tonsilla* + Gk, *ektomē,* excision], the surgical excision of the palatine tonsils, performed to prevent recurrent tonsillitis. Before surgery several laboratory tests, including a bleeding and clotting time, complete blood count, and urinalysis are done. Tonsillar tissue is dissected and removed, usually using general anesthesia, and bleeding areas are sutured or cauterized. An airway remains in place until swallowing returns. An increase in pulse rate, falling blood pressure, restlessness, or frequent swallowing warns of possible hemorrhage. When the patient has recovered from anesthesia, ice chips or clear liquids without a drinking straw may be offered. Tonsillectomy is often combined with adenoidectomy.

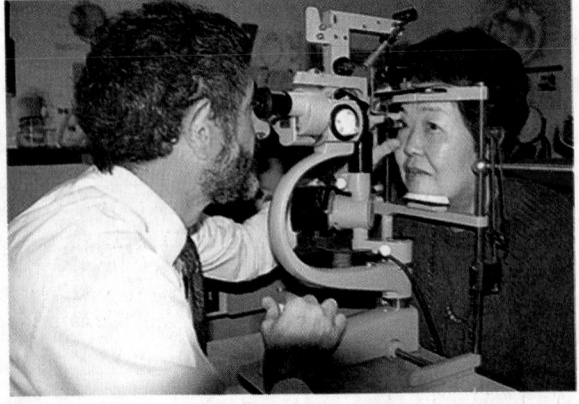

**Applanation tonometry** *(Lewis, Heitkemper, and Dirksen, 2000)*

**tonsillitis** /-ī′tis/,　an infection or inflammation of a tonsil. Acute tonsillitis, frequently caused by *Streptococcus* infection, is characterized by severe sore throat, fever, headache, malaise, difficulty in swallowing, earache, and enlarged tender lymph nodes in the neck. Acute tonsillitis may accompany scarlet fever. Treatment includes systemic antibiotics, analgesics, and warm irrigations of the throat. Soft foods and ample fluids are given. Tonsillectomy is sometimes performed for recurrent tonsillitis or tonsillar abscess. See also **acute tonsillitis, peritonsillar abscess, scarlet fever, strep throat.**

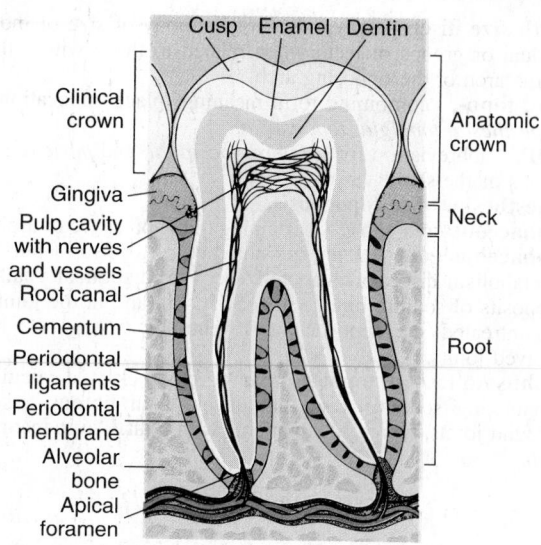

**Tooth** *(Beare and Myers, 1998)*

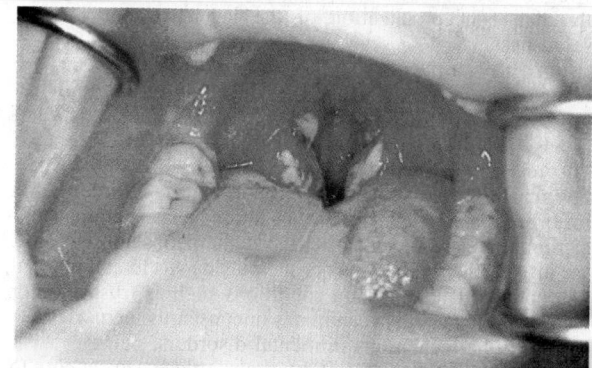

**Tonsillitis**
*(Wong, 1999/courtesy Dr. Edward L. Applebaum, University of Illinois Medical Center)*

**tonsilloadenoidectomy** /ton′silō·ad′ənoidek′təmē/ [L, *tonsilla* + Gk, *aden*, gland, *eidos*, form, *ektomē*, excision], the surgical removal of tonsil and adenoid tissues.

**tonus** /tō′nəs/ [Gk, *tonos*, stretching],　**1.** the normal state of balanced tension in the body tissues, especially the muscles. Partial contraction or alternate contraction and relaxation of neighboring fibers of a group of muscles hold the organ or the part of the body in a neutral functional position without fatigue. Tonus is essential for many normal body functions, such as holding the spine erect, the eyes open, and the jaw closed. Also called **muscle tone. 2.** the state of the body tissues being strong and fit. Also called **tone.**

**-tony.** See **-tonia.**

**tooth,** *pl.* **teeth** [AS, *toth*],　any one of numerous dental structures that develop in the jaws. Although derived from modified bone, they are typically classified as part of the digestive system and are used to cut and grind food in the mouth for ingestion. Each tooth consists of a crown, which projects above the gum; two to four roots embedded in the alveolus; and a neck, which stretches between the crown and the root. Each tooth also contains a cavity filled with pulp, richly supplied with blood vessels and nerves that enter the cavity through a small aperture at the base of each root. The solid part of the tooth consists of dentin, enamel, and a thin layer of bone on the surface of the root. The dentin composes the bulk of the tooth. The enamel covers the exposed part of the crown. Two sets of teeth appear at different periods of life: the 20 deciduous teeth appear during infancy, the 32 secondary teeth during childhood and early adulthood. See also **deciduous dentition, secondary dentition.**

**tooth abscess** [AS, *toth* + L, *abscedere*, to go away],　a collection of pus on a tooth, usually close to the root and often the result of an untreated cavity. If untreated, the pressure of the abscess may destroy the alveolar bone and adjoining soft tissues. Also called **dental abscess.** See also **periapical abscess.**

**toothache** /too͞′thāk/ [AS, *toth* + *aeca*],　pain in a tooth, usually caused by caries that have extended into the dentin or pulp or by traumatic occlusion. Also called **dentalgia, odontalgia, odontodynia.** See also **pulpitis.**

**tooth alignment,**　the arrangement of the teeth in relation to their supporting bone or alveolar process, adjacent teeth, and opposing dentition.

**tooth bleaching,**　the process of removing stains or color from teeth by applying chemicals, such as hydrogen peroxide.

**tooth-borne,**　describing a dental prosthesis or part of a prosthesis that depends entirely on abutment teeth for support.

**tooth-borne base,**　a denture base restoring an edentulous area that has abutment teeth at each end for support. The tissue that it covers is not used to support the base.

**toothbrush,**　an implement of various design, with bristles fixed to a head at the end of a handle, used for cleaning the teeth and cleaning and massaging the gingival tissues.

**tooth eruption,**　the final stage of odontogenesis, in which a tooth breaks out from its crypt through surrounding tissue.

**tooth form,**　the identifying curves, lines, angles, and contours of a tooth that differentiate it from other teeth.

**tooth fulcrum,**　the axis of movement of a tooth subjected to lateral forces. It is considered to be at the middle third of the part of the tooth root embedded in the alveolus.

**tooth germ,**　a primitive cell in the embryo that is the precursor of a tooth.

**tooth inclination,**　the angle of slope of a tooth or teeth from the vertical plane. Inclinations may be mesial, distal, lingual, buccal, or labial.

**toothpaste.** See **dentifrice.**

**tooth rotation** [AS, *toth* + L, *rotare*, to rotate],　**1.** the turning of a tooth around its longitudinal axis. **2.** the process by which a tooth is turned.

**tooth size discrepancy,** lack of harmony of size of individual or groups of teeth when related to those within the same arch or the opposing arch.

**top-, topo-,** combining form meaning 'place or location': *topesthesia, topalgia, topognosia.*

**TOP,** abbreviation for *temporal, occipital,* and *parietal* regions of the skull.

**topesthesia.** See **topognosis.**

**tophaceous** /tōfā′shəs/, pertaining to the presence of tophi.

**tophaceous gout** [L, *tufa,* porous rock], a form of purine metabolism disorder characterized by formation of chalky deposits of sodium biurate under the skin and in the joints. If untreated, the deposits may eventually destroy the involved joints.

**tophus** /tō′fəs/, *pl.* **tophi** [L, *tufa,* porous rock], a calculus containing sodium urate that develops in fibrous tissue around joints, typically in patients with gout. –**tophaceous,** *adj.*

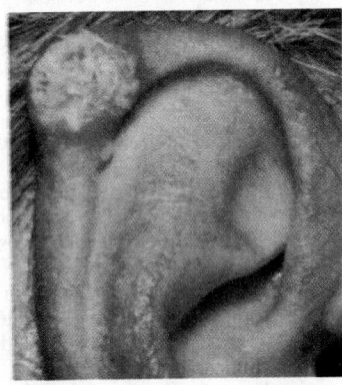

**Tophus** *(Sigler and Schuring, 1993)*

**-topia, -topy,** combining form meaning '(condition of) placement of organs in the body': *heterotopia, normotopia, skeletopia.*

**topical** /top′ikəl/ [Gk, *topos,* place], **1.** pertaining to the surface of a part of the body. **2.** pertaining to a drug or treatment applied topically.

**topical anesthesia,** surface analgesia produced by application of a topical anesthetic in the form of a solution, gel, or ointment to the skin, mucous membrane, or cornea. The most common ingredients include benzocaine, dibucaine, lidocaine, hexylcaine, and tetracaine. Cocaine may be applied in solution to the mucous membranes of the nasal passages in certain otolaryngeal or maxillofacial procedures. Also called **surface anesthesia.** Compare **general anesthesia, local anesthesia, regional anesthesia.**

**Topicort,** trademark for a topical glucocorticoid (desoximetasone).

**topiramate,** a miscellaneous anticonvulsant.
- ■ INDICATIONS: This drug is used to treat partial seizures, with or without generalization in adults.
- ■ CONTRAINDICATIONS: Known hypersensitivity to this drug prohibits its use.
- ■ ADVERSE EFFECTS: Adverse effects of topiramate include upper respiratory infection, pharyngitis, sinusitis, diplopia, vision abnormality, rash, weight loss, leukopenia, dizziness, fatigue, cognitive disorder, insomnia, anxiety, depression,

paresthesia, weight loss, diarrhea, anorexia, nausea, dyspepsia, abdominal pain, constipation, dry mouth, breast pain, dysmenorrhea, and menstrual disorder.

**topo-.** See **top-.**

**topoanesthesia.** See **atopognosia.**

**topognosis** /top′ognō′sis/ [Gk, *topos* + *gnosis,* recognition], the ability to recognize tactile stimuli. Also called **topesthesia.**

**topogometer** /top′ōgom′ətər/ [Gk, *topos,* place, *gonia,* angle, *metron,* measure], a movable fixation target attached to an instrument for measuring the radius of curvature of the cornea. It is used in fitting contact lenses of correct curvature.

**topographic** /top′əgraf′ik/, (in psychiatry) pertaining to a freudian conceptualization of the layers of human consciousness.

**topographic anatomy** [Gk, *topos,* place, *graphein,* to record, *ana* + *temnein,* to cut], the study of a specific region of a body structure such as a lower leg, including all of the systems in the part and their relationship to each other. Also called **regional anatomy.**

**topographic disorientation,** a psychiatric disorder based on Freud's topographic model of the mental apparatus, consisting of conscious, preconscious, and unconscious systems for interpreting perceptions of the outside world and internal perceptions. Under certain conditions such as frustration or sleep, psychic energy reanimates unconscious memories, resulting in hallucinations in mental disorders.

**topography** /təpog′refē/ [Gk, *topos,* place, *graphein,* to record], the anatomic description of a body part in terms of the region in which it is located.

**topology** /təpol′əjē/, **1.** orientation of the presenting part of a fetus. **2.** the study of special regions of anatomy. **3.** the science of properties of geometric configuration.

**topotecan,** an antineoplastic hormone.
- ■ INDICATIONS: This drug is used to treat metastatic carcinoma of the ovary after failure of traditional chemotherapy.
- ■ CONTRAINDICATIONS: Factors that prohibit the use of this drug are known hypersensitivity to topotecan, lactation, and severe bone marrow depression.
- ■ ADVERSE EFFECTS: Life-threatening effects of this drug are neutropenia, leukopenia, thrombocytopenia, anemia, and sepsis. Other adverse effects are abdominal pain, constipation, diarrhea, obstruction, nausea, stomatitis, vomiting, increased ALT and AST, anorexia, arthralgia, asthenia, headache, myalgia, pain, dyspnea, and total alopecia.

**TOPV,** abbreviation for *trivalent oral polio vaccine.*

**TORCH** /tôrch/, abbreviation for *to*xoplasmosis, *o*ther, *ru*bella virus, *c*ytomegalovirus, and *h*erpes simplex viruses, a group of agents that can infect the fetus or the newborn, causing a constellation of morbid effects called the TORCH syndrome.

**TORCH syndrome,** infection of the fetus or newborn by one of the TORCH agents. The Outcomes of a pregnancy complicated by a TORCH agent may be abortion, stillbirth, intrauterine growth retardation, or premature delivery.
- ■ OBSERVATIONS: At delivery and during the first days after birth an infant infected with any one of the organisms may demonstrate various clinical manifestations such as fever, lethargy, poor feeding, petechiae on the skin, purpura, pneumonia, hepatosplenomegaly, jaundice, hemolytic and other anemias, encephalitis, microcephaly, hydrocephalus, intracranial calcifications, hearing deficits, chorioretinitis, and microphthalmia. In addition, each of the agents is associated with several other abnormal clinical findings involving abnormal immune response, cataracts, glaucoma, vesicles, ulcers, and congenital cardiac defects.

■ INTERVENTIONS: Before pregnancy women may be tested for susceptibility to the rubella virus and inoculated against it if not immune. There are currently no vaccines that confer immunity to the other TORCH agents, but the mother may be serologically tested for antibody levels to them. During pregnancy toxoplasmosis is asymptomatic in about 90% of cases, making diagnosis unlikely. If infection is suspected, serial paired serologic tests are performed; a high, rising titer indicates recent infection. Transplacental infection occurs in 35% of mothers infected during pregnancy. If the mother contracts infection in the first trimester, before the placenta is fully developed, the infant may not become infected; if the fetus contracts the infection, severe congenital manifestations of the syndrome usually occur. If the fetus is infected after the first trimester, the baby is usually born with asymptomatic or mild disease; the infection may be spread from the baby during the newborn period. Sulfadiazine, pyrimethamine, and folic acid are sometimes given to treat the infection. Primary cytomegalovirus infection during pregnancy is usually asymptomatic. If the infection is suspected, serologic testing may be performed to demonstrate primary infection, because infants born to mothers infected for the first time during pregnancy are much more likely to develop severe congenital anomalies than if the infection is a reactivation of previous cytomegalovirus infection. There is no specific treatment. The child is considered to be infectious, but contagion among newborns from a congenitally infected infant has not been proven. Transplacental rubella virus infection in pregnancy during the first 8 weeks is likely to cause infection in 50% of fetuses and to result in demonstrable defects in 85% of those infected. The risk becomes less as gestation increases to 24 weeks, after which time infection has not been known to result in defects. Rubella is the only TORCH virus that is usually symptomatic, and therefore it is often recognized. Many mothers infected during the first trimester choose to abort the pregnancy. There is no treatment for the infection, but screening and immunization before pregnancy could prevent virtually all cases of congenital rubella. Herpesvirus infection in pregnancy is rarely transplacentally transmitted to the fetus. Primary infection during pregnancy sometimes results in spontaneous abortion or premature delivery. In the newborn the infection is usually systemic and life-threatening. The fetus is most apt to become infected by the virus shed from an active genital lesion during vaginal delivery or as the result of vaginal examination or the placement of an intrauterine catheter or a fetal scalp electrode during labor. If the mother has active genital herpesvirus lesions, intrapartal internal monitoring is contraindicated, vaginal examinations are often omitted, regional anesthetic techniques are avoided, and the infant is delivered by cesarean section. The TORCH infections caused by other agents are asymptomatic in pregnancy, revealing themselves by the syndrome after birth. The congenital effects are not amenable to change or to amelioration by any known treatment.

**TORCH test,** a series of tests for diseases that exert recognized detrimental effects on the fetus (tests include *Toxo*plasmosis, *O*ther [including syphilis], *R*ubella, *C*ytomegalovirus, and *H*erpes), such as precipitating abortion or premature labor.

**Torecan,** trademark for a phenothiazine antiemetic (thiethylperazine maleate).

**toremifene,** an antineoplastic.

■ INDICATIONS: Toremifene is used to treat advanced breast carcinoma that is not responsive to other therapy in estrogen-receptor-positive patients (usually postmenopausal).

■ CONTRAINDICATIONS: Known hypersensitivity to this drug and pregnancy prohibit its use.

■ ADVERSE EFFECTS: Life-threatening effects of this drug are thrombocytopenia and leukopenia. Other adverse effects include altered taste (anorexia), vaginal bleeding, pruritus vulvae, rash, alopecia, chest pain, depression, hypercalcemia, ocular lesions, retinopathy, corneal opacity, and blurred vision (high doses). Common side effects include nausea, vomiting, hot flashes, headache, and light-headedness.

**Torkildsen's procedure.** See **ventriculocisternostomy.**

**Tornalate,** trademark for an orally inhaled bronchodilator (bitolterol mesylate).

**torose** /tôr′ōs/ [L, *torosus,* bulging], knoblike, knobby, or bulging.

**torpor** /tôr′pər/, **1.** a state of mental or physical inactivity. **2.** an absence or slowness of response to a stimulus.

**torque** /tôrk/ [L, *torquere,* to twist], **1.** a twisting force produced by contraction of the medial femoral muscles that tend to rotate the thigh medially. **2.** (in dentistry) a force applied to a tooth to rotate it on a mesiodistal or buccolingual axis. **3.** a rotary force applied to a denture base. Compare **torsion.**

**torr** /tôr/ [Evangelista Torricelli, Italian physicist, 1608–1647], a unit of pressure equal to 1333.22 dynes/$cm^2$, or 1.33322 millibars. One torr is the pressure required to support a column of mercury 1 mm high when the mercury is of standard density and subjected to standard acceleration. These standard conditions are 0° C and 45° latitude, where the acceleration of gravity is 980.6 $cm/sec^2$. In reading a mercury barometer at other temperatures and latitudes, corrections commonly exceeding 2 torr may be required to compensate for the thermal expansion of the measuring scale used.

**tors-,** combining form meaning 'twisted': *torsiometer, torsive, torsiversion.*

**torsades de pointes** /tôrsäd′ de pô·aNt′, tôr′säd də point′/ [Fr, *torsader,* to twist together, *pointes,* tips], a type of ventricular tachycardia with a spiral-like appearance ("twisting of the points") and complexes that at first look positive and then negative on an electrocardiogram. It is precipitated by a long Q-T interval, which often is induced by drugs (quinidine, procainamide, or disopyramide), but which may be the result of hypokalemia or profound bradycardia. The first line of treatment is IV magnesium sulfate. See also **long QT syndrome.**

**torsiometer** /tôr′sē·om′ətər/, a device for measuring the amount of torsion of an eye around its anteroposterior axis.

**torsion** /tôr′shən/ [L, *torquere,* to twist], **1.** the process of twisting in a positive (clockwise) or negative (counterclockwise) direction. **2.** the state of being turned. **3.** (in dentistry) the twisting of a tooth on its long axis.

**torsion dystonia.** See **dystonia musculorum deformans.**

**torsion fracture,** a spiral fracture, usually caused by a torsion injury.

**torsion of the testis,** the axial rotation of the spermatic cord that cuts off the blood supply to the testicle, epididymis, and other structures. Complete ischemia for 6 hours may result in gangrene of the testis. Partial loss of circulation may result in atrophy. Certain testes are anatomically predisposed to torsion because of inadequate connective tissue, but the condition may be caused by trauma with severe swelling. Torsion of the testis occurs more often on the left than on the right side and is most frequent in the first year of life and during puberty. Surgical correction is required in most cases; if performed within 5 hours of the onset of symptoms, the testis can usually be saved.

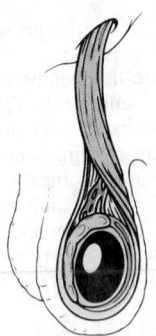

**Torsion of the testis** (Lewis, Heitkemper, and Dirksen, 2000)

**torsion spasm.** See **dystonia musculorum deformans.**

**torso** /tôr′sō/ [L, *thyrsus,* stem], the body excluding the head and limbs. Also called **trunk.**

**tort** [L, *tortus,* twisted], (in law) a civil wrong, other than a breach of contract. Torts include negligence, false imprisonment, assault, and battery. The elements of a tort are: a legal duty owed by the defendant to the plaintiff, a breach of duty, and damage from the breach of duty. A tort may be constitutional, in which one person deprives another of a right or immunity guaranteed by the Constitution; personal, in which a person or a person's reputation or feelings are injured; or intentional, in which the wrong is a deliberate act that is unlawful. Many other kinds of torts exist. —**tortious,** *adj.*

**torticollis** /tôr′tikol′is/ [L, *tortus,* twisted, *collum,* neck], an abnormal condition in which the head is inclined to one side as a result of the contraction of muscles on that side of the neck. It may be congenital or acquired. Treatment may include surgery, heat, support, or immobilization, depending on the cause and severity of the condition. Also called **wryneck.** See also **spasmodic torticollis.**

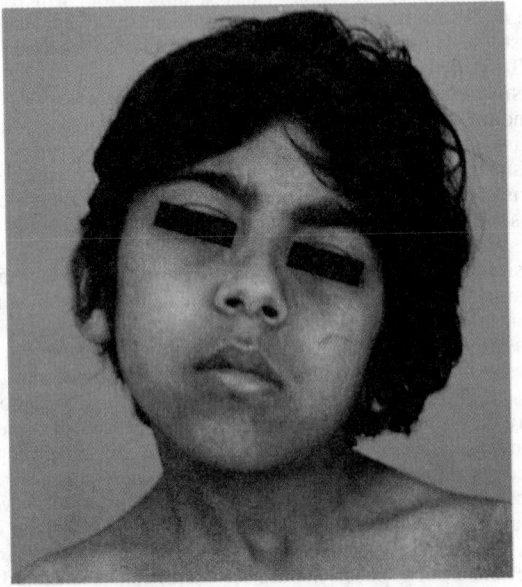

**Torticollis** (Bingham, Hawke, and Kwok, 1992)

**tortious.** See **tort.**

**tortipelvis** /-pel′vis/ [L, *tortus,* twisted, *pelvis,* basin], a form of muscular dystonia resulting in a distortion of the pelvis or the spine and hips.

**tortuous** /tôr′chōō·əs/ [L, *tortus,* twisted], having or making twists and turns.

*Torula histolytica.* See *Cryptococcus neoformans.*

*Torulopsis,* a genus of Fungi Imperfecti of the family Cryptococcaceae; it is closely related to *Candida* and some authorities have considered it the same genus. Some species are normal inhabitants of the skin, respiratory tract, GI tract, and urogenital region but may also cause opportunistic infections.

*Torulopsis glabrata,* a species of fungus that is part of the normal flora of the human mouth, gut, and urinary tract but that in weak or immunocompromised patients may cause opportunistic infections such as meningitis, pneumonia, cystitis, and fungemia. Also called *Candida glabrata.*

**torulopsosis** /tôr′yəlopsō′sis, tôr′yōōlop′səsis/ [L, *torulus,* small swelling; Gk, *opsis,* appearance, *osis,* condition], an infection with the yeast *Torulopsis glabrata,* a normal inhabitant of the oropharynx, GI tract, and skin. *T. glabrata* causes disease in severely debilitated patients, in those with impaired immune function, or sometimes in patients having prolonged urinary catheterization. Systemic infection is usually treated with amphotericin B.

**torulosis.** See **cryptococcosis.**

**torus fracture.** See **lead pipe fracture.**

**torus palatinus** [L, *torus,* swelling, *palatum,* palate], a bony ridge along the hard palate at the line of fusion of the left and right jawbone segments. It is a hereditary feature.

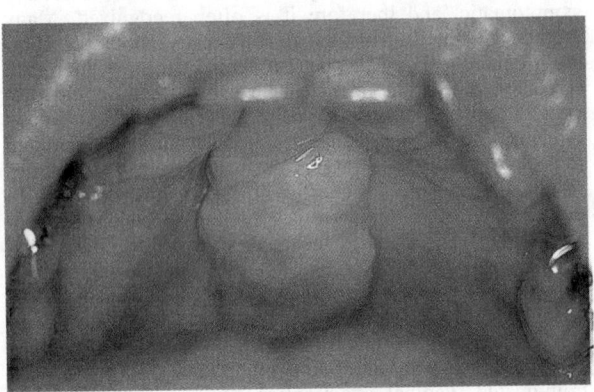

**Torus palatinus** (Bull, 1995)

**total allergy syndrome,** a condition of hypersensitivity to a wide range of substances, including pesticides, insecticides, pharmaceuticals, certain metals, and chemicals used in the manufacture of plastics and epoxy resins. Also called **twentieth-century syndrome.**

**total anomalous venous return** [L, *totus,* whole; Gk, *anomalos,* uneven; L, *vena,* vein; ME, *retournen,* to turn back], a rare congenital cardiac anomaly in which the pulmonary veins attach to the right atrium or to various veins draining into the right atrium rather than to the left atrium. Clinical manifestations include cyanosis, pulmonary congestion, and heart failure. Other cardiac defects also may be present, such as atrial septal defect, which shunts blood from the right atrium to the left atrium and helps decompress the right atrium. Corrective surgery is indicated, usually after 1 year of age, but may be necessary at an earlier age if pulmonary venous obstruction or severe congestive heart failure is present. See also **congenital cardiac anomaly.**

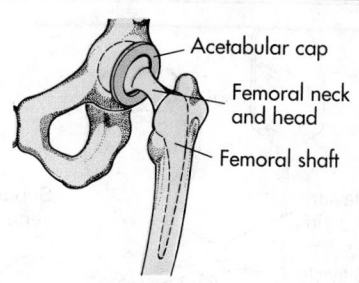

**Total hip replacement** *(Beare and Myers, 1998)*

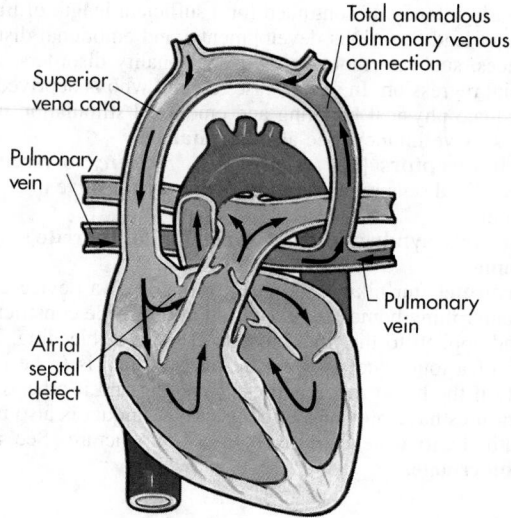

**Total anomalous venous return** *(Wong, 1999)*

**total body electric conductivity (TOBEC),** a method of measuring body composition by the differences in electrical conductivity of fat, bone, and muscle. It is used for monitoring fitness of athletes; in clinical studies of weight control in which physicians want to determine if weight loss is caused by fat, water, or other tissues; and in measurement of fat content of dietary meats. See also **bioelectric impedance analysis.**

**total body radiation,** radiation that exposes the entire body and, theoretically, all cells in the body.

**total body water (TBW),** all the water within the body, including intracellular and extracellular water plus the water in the GI and urinary tracts.

**total cleavage,** mitotic division of a fertilized ovum into blastomeres. Compare **partial cleavage.**

**total color blindness.** See **color blindness.**

**total communication,** the combined use of oral language and manual communication by a person with hearing loss.

**total hip arthroplasty.** See **total hip replacement.**

**total hip replacement,** a surgical procedure to correct a hip joint damaged by degenerative disease, often arthritis. The head of the femur and the acetabulum are replaced with metal components. The acetabulum is plastic coated to avoid metal-to-metal articulating surfaces. Also called **total hip arthroplasty.** See also **total joint replacement.**

**total hysterectomy.** See **hysterectomy.**

**total intravenous anesthesia (TIVA),** anesthesia using only IV agents without the use of inhalational agents. Drugs used are generally of short duration of action and half-life in order to reduce the risks associated with accumulation. TIVA avoids unwanted effects of inhalational agents and the need for complex apparatus.

**total iron,** the total iron concentration in the blood. The normal concentrations in serum are 50 to 150 μg/dL.

**total joint arthroplasty.** See **total joint replacement.**

**total joint replacement,** a surgical procedure for the treatment of severe arthritis and other disorders in which the normal articulating surfaces of a joint are replaced by metal and plastic prostheses. The operation most commonly involves replacement of the hip joint, although the knee and other joints may also be replaced. Also called **total joint arthroplasty.**

**total lung capacity (TLC),** the volume of gas in the lungs at the end of a maximum inspiration. It equals the vital capacity plus the residual capacity.

**total lymphoid irradiation (TLI),** a method of inducing a strong immunosuppressive effect in patients undergoing bone marrow transplants, treatment of certain lymphomas, or other therapies requiring immunosuppression. TLI involves exposing all lymph nodes, the thymus, and spleen to a total of 2000 rad in 100-rad doses from a linear accelerator before graft implantation.

**total macroglobulins,** the heavy serum macroglobulins that are elevated in various diseases, such as cancer, and infections. The normal concentrations in serum are 70 to 430 mg/dL.

**total parenteral nutrition (TPN),** the administration of a nutritionally adequate hypertonic solution consisting of glucose, protein hydrolysates, minerals, and vitamins through an indwelling catheter into the superior vena cava or other main vein. Fat is also provided in a three-in-one solution or "piggy-backed." The high rate of blood flow results in rapid dilution of the solution, and full nutritional requirements can be met indefinitely. The procedure is used in prolonged coma, severe uncontrolled malabsorption, extensive burns, GI fistulas, and other conditions in which feeding by mouth cannot provide adequate amounts of the essential nutrients. In infants and children it is used when feeding via the GI tract is impossible, inadequate, or hazardous, such as in chronic intestinal obstruction from peritoneal sepsis or adhesions, inadequate intestinal length, or chronic nonremitting severe diarrhea. The hyperalimentation solution is infused through conventional tubing with an IV filter attached to remove any contaminates. In adults the catheter is placed directly into the subclavian vein and threaded through the right innominate vein into the superior vena cava. In infants and small children the catheter is usually threaded to the central venous location by way of the jugular vein, which is entered through a subcutaneous tunnel beneath the scalp. Strict asepsis must be maintained because infection is a grave and present danger of this therapy. Also called **hyperalimentation, intravenous alimentation, parenteral hyperalimentation, total parenteral alimentation.**

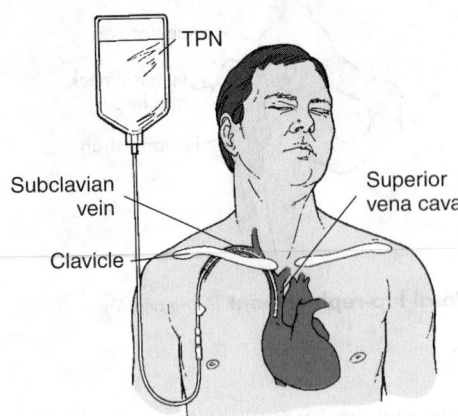

**Total parenteral nutrition: adult**

**total parenteral nutrition (TPN) administration,** a nursing intervention from the Nursing Interventions Classification (NIC) defined as preparation and delivery of nutrients intravenously and monitoring of patient responsiveness. See also **Nursing Interventions Classification.**

**total peripheral resistance,** the overall resistance to blood flow through the systemic blood vessels.

**total quality management (TQM),** an approach to the improvement of the provision of services based on the premise that the overwhelming majority of quality failures are the result of flaws in processes and that quality can be improved by controlling these processes. TQM replaces traditional methods of quality management based on the identification and correction of problems as they occur and requires the participation of all members of an organization in improving processes, products, services, and the culture in which they work. TQM involves creation of an organizational structure for identifying and improving processes, the use of data-based statistical analysis to study processes, and the empowerment of employees to take responsibility for their own tasks in a way that encourages both continuous learning and personal responsibility. In a health care setting, this means a shift from an emphasis on tasks to emphasis on Outcomess of care, which provide the data. See also **continuous quality improvement (CQI).**

**total renal blood flow (TRBF),** the total volume of blood that flows into the renal arteries. The average TRBF in a normal adult is 1200 mL per minute. Compare **glomerular filtration rate.**

**total thyroxine test ($T_4$),** a blood test that directly measures the total amount of $T_4$ present in the patient's blood, with abnormal values indicating either hyper- or hypothyroid states. This test is also used to monitor replacement suppressive therapy.

**totem** /tō′təm/, an animal, plant, force of nature, or inanimate object that represents the tribal ancestor of a clan. It also serves as a tutelary spirit and protector and may communicate through oracles.

**totipotency** /tō′tipō′tənsē/, the ability of a cell, particularly a zygote, to differentiate into any of a number of specialized cells and thus form a new organism or regenerate a body part. Also called **totipotence.**

**touch¹** /tuch/ [Fr, *toucher,* to touch], **1.** the ability to feel objects and to distinguish their various characteristics; the

tactile sense. **2.** the ability to perceive pressure when it is exerted on the skin or mucosa of the body. **3.** to palpate or examine with the hand, such as the digital examination of the abdomen, rectum, or vagina.

**touch²,** a nursing intervention from the Nursing Interventions Classification (NIC) defined as providing comfort and communication through purposeful tactile contact. See also **Nursing Interventions Classification.**

**touch deprivation,** a lack of tactile stimulation, especially in early infancy. If continued for a sufficient length of time, it may lead to serious developmental and emotional disturbances, such as stunted growth, personality disorders, and social regression. In severe cases a child who is deprived of adequate physical handling and emotional stimulation may not survive infancy. See also **hospitalism.**

**touch receptors** [Fr, *toucher* + L, *recipere,* to receive], specialized sensory nerve endings that are sensitive to tactile stimuli.

**Tourette's syndrome.** See **Gilles de la Tourette's syndrome.**

**tourniquet** /tur′nikit, tŏŏr′-/ [Fr, turnstile], a device used in controlling hemorrhage, consisting of a wide constricting band applied to the limb close to the site of bleeding. The use of a tourniquet is a drastic measure and is to be used only if the hemorrhage is life-threatening and if other safer measures have proved ineffective. A tourniquet is also used routinely to distend veins before venipuncture. See also **hemorrhage.**

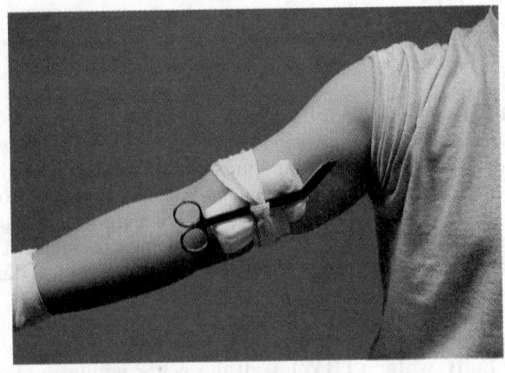

**Tourniquet** *(Sanders et al, 2000)*

**tourniquet infusion method,** a technique of intraarterial regional chemotherapy used in the treatment of osteogenic sarcoma. The technique uses one or two external tourniquets, depending on the location of the tumor, that slow or interrupt the blood flow to a limb temporarily while an anticancer drug, such as adriamycin, is infused into the area. The method increases the concentration of an antineoplastic drug by as much as 100 times compared with an alternative technique of injecting the drug into the circulation without application of a tourniquet, which results in rapid dilution of the drug by the normal blood volume.

**tourniquet test,** a test of capillary fragility caused by an abnormality in the capillary wall or thrombocytopenia, in which a blood pressure cuff is applied for 5 minutes to a person's arm and inflated to a pressure halfway between the diastolic and systolic blood pressure. The number of petechiae within a circumscribed area of the skin may be counted, or the results may be reported in a range from negative (no petechiae) to +4 positive (confluent petechiae).

**tower head, tower skull.** See **oxycephaly.**

**tox-, toxi-, toxico-, toxo-** combining form meaning 'toxins or poisons': *toxin, toxicology.*

**toxaemia.** See **toxemia.**

**-toxaemia.** See **-toxemia.**

*Toxascaris leonina* /toksas′kəris/, a species of nematode found mainly in domestic animals. It differs from related species in that it spends its entire developmental cycle in the digestive tract, rather than migrating through the lungs.

**toxemia** /toksē′mē·ə/ [Gk, *toxikon,* poison, *haima,* blood], the presence of bacterial toxins in the bloodstream. Also spelled **toxaemia.** Also called **blood poisoning.** See also **preeclampsia.** —**toxemic,** *adj.*

**-toxemia, -toxaemia,** suffix meaning a '(specified) toxic substance in the blood': *ectotoxemia, gonotoxemia, ophiotoxemia.*

**toxemia of pregnancy.** See **preeclampsia.**

**toxi-.** See **tox-.**

**-toxia,** combining form meaning 'condition resulting from a poison in a (specified) region of the body': *neurotoxia, thyrotoxia, urotoxia.*

**toxic** /tok′sik/ [Gk, *toxikon*], **1.** pertaining to a poison. **2.** (of a disease or condition) severe and progressive.

**-toxic, -toxical,** combining form meaning 'poison': *cardiotoxic, hematoxic, spermatoxic.*

**toxic albuminuria** [Gk, *toxikon,* poison; L, *albus,* white; Gk, *ouron,* urine], a condition of serum albumin in the urine caused by the presence of toxic substances in the body.

**toxic allergic syndrome.** See **Löffler's syndrome, PIE.**

**toxic amblyopia,** partial loss of vision because of retrooptic bulbar neuritis, resulting from poisoning with quinine, lead, wood alcohol, nicotine, arsenic, or certain other poisons.

**toxicant** /tok′sikənt/, any poisonous agent.

**toxic deafness.** See **ototoxic hearing loss.**

**toxic delirium** [Gk, *toxikon,* poison; L, *delirare,* to rave], a symptom of disordered mental status as a result of poisoning.

**toxic dementia,** dementia resulting from excessive use of or exposure to a poisonous substance. See also **dementia.**

**toxic dilation of colon** [Gk, *toxikon* + L, *dilatare,* to widen; Gk, *kolon*], a condition of transverse colon dilation as a complication of amebic colitis, ulcerative colitis, or other bowel disease. Symptoms may include cramping, fever, rapid heartbeat, and mental confusion.

**toxic dose (TD),** (in toxicology) the amount of a substance that may be expected to produce a toxic effect. See also **median toxic dose.**

**toxic encephalitis** [Gk, *toxikon,* poison, *enkephalos,* brain, *itis,* inflammation], encephalitis caused by heavy metal poisoning. It is characterized by convulsions and cerebral edema.

**toxic epidermal necrolysis (TEN),** a rare skin disease, characterized by epidermal erythema, superficial necrosis, and skin erosions. This condition, which affects mainly adults, makes the skin appear scalded, often leaving scars. The cause of TEN is unknown, but it may result from toxic or hypersensitive reactions. It is commonly associated with drug reactions, such as those associated with butazones, sulfonamides, penicillins, barbiturates, and hydantoins. Other drugs may be involved, and the disease also has been associated with airborne toxins such as carbon monoxide. TEN also may indicate an immune response, or it may be associated with severe physiologic stress. A similar skin disorder may be the result of a staphylococcal infection.

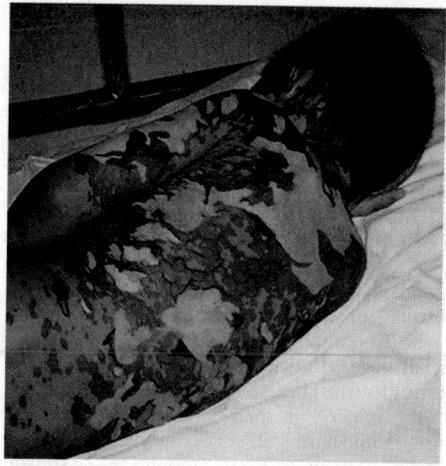

**Toxic epidermal necrolysis** *(Shah and Laude, 2000)*

■ OBSERVATIONS: Early signs of the condition include inflammation of the mucous membranes, fever, malaise, a burning sensation in the conjunctivae, and pervasive tenderness of the skin. The first phase of TEN is manifested by diffuse erythema. The second phase involves vesiculation and blistering. The third phase is marked by extensive epidermal necrolysis and desquamation. As the disease progresses, large flaccid bullae develop and rupture, exposing wide expanses of denuded skin. Tissue fluids and electrolytes are consequently lost, resulting in extensive systemic complications, such as pulmonary edema, bronchopneumonia, GI and esophageal hemorrhage, sepsis, shock, renal failure, and disseminated intravascular coagulation. These extreme conditions contribute to the high mortality associated with TEN, which is about 30%, especially among the infirm and the elderly. Confirming diagnosis is based on symptoms in the third phase of the disease, such as skin denuded by even slight friction, affecting the areas of erythema. Diagnosis is commonly supported by bacteriologic culture and Gram's stains of lesions to determine whether infection exists. The presence of leukocytosis, fluid and electrolyte imbalances, albuminuria, and elevated transaminase levels are characteristic and help confirm the diagnosis. Erythema multiforme and exfoliative dermatitis may be ruled out by exfoliative biopsy and cytology.

■ INTERVENTIONS: Treatment of TEN commonly involves the administration of IV fluids to replace body fluids and maintain electrolyte balance. Frequent laboratory analyses are necessary to monitor hematocrit and hemoglobin, serum proteins, electrolytes, and blood gases.

■ NURSING CONSIDERATIONS: Nursing care of patients with TEN requires meticulous monitoring of vital signs, central venous pressure, and urinary output. Any signs of renal failure, such as decreased urinary output, and bleeding are of immediate concern. It is important to detect and quickly treat any septic infection. Temperature elevations are reported immediately, and all laboratory work, such as blood cultures and sensitivity tests, are performed promptly. Ocular lesions are common with TEN, and frequent eye care is often needed to remove exudate. Protective isolation and prophylactic antibiotic therapy may be required to prevent secondary infection. That the TEN patient avoids tight clothing and is covered loosely to minimize the friction that causes skin sloughing. A Stryker frame or a CircOlectric bed may be helpful in caring for the patient. Analgesics are administered as needed, and cool sterile compresses may be applied to relieve discomfort. Psychologic and emotional support for the patient and family is also a key nursing concern. Also called **scalded skin syndrome.**

**toxic erythema** [Gk, *toxikon* poison, *erythema,* redness], an inexact term sometimes applied to reddish skin eruptions of undetermined origin.

**toxic erythema of the newborn.** See **erythema neonatorum.**

**toxic gastritis.** See **corrosive gastritis.**

**toxic goiter,** an enlargement of the thyroid gland associated with exophthalmia and systemic disease. See also **Graves' disease, thyroiditis.**

**toxic hemoglobinuria.** See **hemoglobinuria.**

**toxicity** /toksis'itē/ [Gk, *toxikon*], **1.** the degree to which something is poisonous. **2.** a condition that results from exposure to a toxin or to toxic amounts of a substance that does not cause adverse effects in smaller amounts.

**toxic neuritis** [Gk, *toxikon,* poison, *neuron,* nerve, *itis,* inflammation], a painful nerve inflammation caused by a metallic, bacterial, or other poison.

**toxic nodular goiter,** an enlarged thyroid gland characterized by numerous discrete nodules and hypersecretion of thyroid hormones. It occurs most frequently in elderly individuals. Typical signs of thyrotoxicosis such as nervousness, tremor, weakness, fatigue, weight loss, and irritability are usually present, but exophthalmia is rare; anorexia is more common than hyperphagia, and cardiac arrhythmia or congestive heart failure may be a predominant manifestation. When clinical findings suggest thyrotoxicosis, a therapeutic trial of antithyroid drugs such as propylthiouracil or methimazol, is indicated, but after the diagnosis is established, radioactive iodine is considered the treatment of choice, and large doses are usually required.

**toxico-.** See **tox-.**

*Toxicodendron* /tok'sikōden'dron/, a genus of plants that includes poison ivy, poison oak, and poison sumac. The toxic agent in the plants is a nonvolatile oil, toxicodendrol. See also **rhus dermatitis.**

**toxicokinetics** /tok'sikō'kinet'iks/, the passage through the body of a toxic agent or its metabolites, usually in an action similar to that of pharmacokinetics.

**toxicologist** /tok'sikol'əjist/, a specialist in poisons, their effects, and antidotes.

**toxicology** /-ol'əjē/, the scientific study of poisons, their detection, their effects, and methods of treatment for conditions they produce. —**toxicologic, toxicological,** *adj.*

**toxicology screening,** a blood or urine test that detects the most commonly abused nonprescription mood altering drugs. Testing for drug overdose and poisoning is best done on blood, while screening for use or abuse of nonprescription drugs is usually done on urine. Toxicology studies are used to incriminate drugs as a cause or factor in the death of a person.

**toxic or drug-induced hepatitis,** hepatitis resulting from a chemical, parasitic, or metabolic poison.

**toxicosis** /tok'sikō'sis/ [Gk, *toxikon,* poison, *osis,* condition], a disease condition caused by the absorption of metabolic or bacterial poisons.

**toxic psychosis,** psychosis that results from the poisonous effects of chemicals or drugs, including those produced by the body itself.

**toxic shock syndrome (TSS),** a severe acute disease caused by infection with strains of *Staphylococcus aureus,* phage group I, that produces a unique toxin, enterotoxin F. It is most common in menstruating women using high-

absorbency tampons but has been seen in newborns, children, and men.

■ OBSERVATIONS: The onset of the syndrome is characterized by sudden high fever, headache, sore throat with swelling of the mucous membranes, diarrhea, nausea, and erythroderma. Acute renal failure, abnormal liver function, confusion, and refractory hypotension usually follow, and death may occur. It is probable that mild forms of the syndrome are not reported and therefore are not diagnosed. No seasonal or geographic factor appears involved in the cause of the disease, and there is no evidence of contagion among household members or through sexual contacts of people who have TSS. Bacteremia, or discernible local infection, is absent in most cases. *S. aureus* may be cultured from many sites, including the pharynx, nares, and cervix, but the drastic effects of infection are the result of the toxin released from the organism rather than from the infection itself.

■ INTERVENTIONS: Aggressive volume expansion by the administration of large amounts of IV fluids, assisted ventilation, and administration of vasopressors may be necessary in treating severe TSS. Early recognition and active supportive treatment greatly improve the survival rates and decrease both prolonged morbidity and recurrence.

**toxic substance** [Gk, *toxikon,* poison; L, *substantia,* essence], any poison.

**toxin** /tok'sin/, a poison, usually one produced by or occurring in a plant or microorganism. See also **endotoxin, exotoxin.**

**-toxin,** combining form meaning 'poison': *cynotoxin, hypnotoxin, zootoxin.*

**toxin-antitoxin** [Gk, *toxikon,* poison, *anti,* against, *toxikon*], a mixture of toxin and antitoxin. Diphtheria toxin-antitoxin was formerly used for active immunization.

**toxinology** /tok'sinol'əjē/, the study of poisons, with particular emphasis on relatively unstable proteinaceous substances. See also **toxicology.**

**toxo-.** See **tox-.**

*Toxocara* /tok'səker'ə/, a genus of ascarid nematodes. *T. canis* affects mainly dogs. *T. mustax* affects cats but may also infect humans, particularly children, causing intestinal and respiratory symptoms and damage to the spleen and liver. See also **toxocariasis.**

**toxocariasis** /tok'sōkarī'əsis/ [Gk, *toxo,* bow, *kara,* head, *osis,* condition], infection with the larvae of *Toxocara canis,* the common roundworm of dogs, and with *T. cati,* of cats. Human ingestion of viable eggs, commonly found in

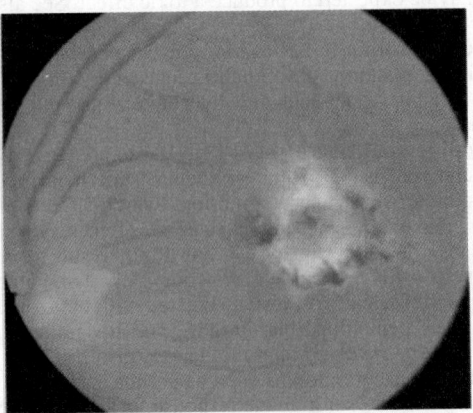

**Toxocariasis: histology of an infected eye**
*(Zitelli and Davis, 1997)*

soil, leads to the spread of tiny larvae throughout the body, resulting in respiratory symptoms, enlarged liver, skin rashes, eosinophilia, and delayed ocular lesions. Children who eat dirt are particularly subject to this disease. Specific drug therapy is not very useful; the Outcomes is usually good without therapy. Regular worming of pets helps prevent infection. Also called **visceral larva migrans.**

**toxoid** /tok'soid/ [Gk, *toxikon*, poison, *eidos*, form], a toxin that has been treated with chemicals or heat to decrease its toxic effect but that retains its antigenic power. It is given to produce immunity by stimulating the creation of antibodies. See also **toxin, vaccine.**

**toxophore** /tok'səfôr'/, the part of a toxic molecule that is responsible for the poisonous effect.

*Toxoplasma* /tok'sōplaz'mə/ [Gk, *toxikon* + *plasma*, something formed], a genus of protozoa with only one known species, *Toxoplasma gondii,* an intracellular parasite of cats and other hosts that causes toxoplasmosis in humans.

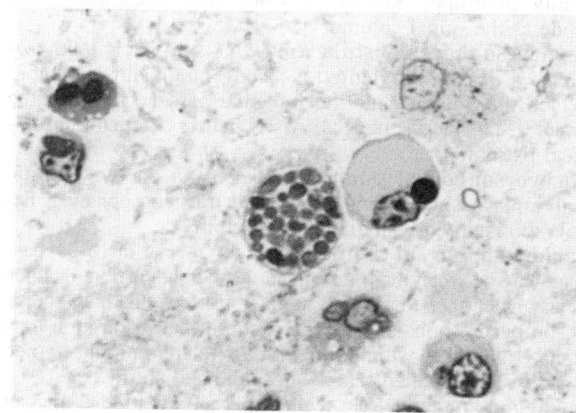

**Toxoplasma gondii cysts in brain section**
(Tilton et al, 1992)

**toxoplasmosis** /tok'sōplazmō'sis/ [Gk, *toxikon* + *plasma* + *osis,* condition], a common infection with the protozoan intracellular parasite *Toxoplasma gondii.* The congenital form is characterized by liver and brain involvement with cerebral calcification, convulsions, blindness, microcephaly or hydrocephaly, and mental retardation. The acquired form is characterized by rash, lymphadenopathy, fever, malaise, central nervous system disorders, myocarditis, and pneumonitis.

■ OBSERVATIONS: Cats acquire the organism by eating infected birds and mice. Cysts of the organism are transmitted from cat feces to humans or by human ingestion of inadequately cooked meat containing the cysts. Transplacental transmission occurs only during acute infection of the mother, but the disease is very serious in the fetus and in those with human immunodeficiency virus or other immunosuppressive conditions or impaired immune system. Diagnosis is made by demonstrating rising antibody titers or by immunofluorescent antibody tests. Infection confers immunity.

■ INTERVENTIONS: Combinations of sulfonamides with pyrimethamine are recommended as treatment, possibly reducing the severity of the illness in the fetus.

■ NURSING CONSIDERATIONS: All meat should be heated to at least 140° F (60° C) throughout to kill this parasite. Pregnant

women who are not immune are advised not to handle cats, cat feces, or litter boxes.

**Toynbee maneuver** /toin'bē/ [Joseph *Toynbee,* English otologist, 1815−1866], pinching the nostrils and swallowing; if the auditory tube is patent, the tympanic membrane will retract medially.

**Toynbee test** /toin'bē/ [Joseph *Toynbee*], performance of the Toynbee maneuver (q.v.) and monitoring of pressure changes in the middle ear. Subsequent middle ear negative pressure or negative pressure followed by ambient pressure usually indicates normal function of the auditory tube.

**TPA,** abbreviation for **tissue plasminogen activator.**

**TPAL.** See **parity.**

**TPN,** abbreviation for **total parenteral nutrition.**

**TPR,** abbreviation for *temperature, pulse, respiration.*

**TQ,** symbol for **tocopherolquinone.**

**TQM,** abbreviation for **total quality management.**

**TR,** abbreviation for **tricuspid regurgitation.**

**trabecula carnea** /trəbek'yələ/, *pl.* **trabeculae carneae** [L, little beam, *carneus,* flesh], any one of the irregular bands and bundles of muscle projecting from the inner surfaces near the apex of the ventricles of the heart. Compare **chordae tendineae.** See also **heart, left ventricle, right ventricle.**

**trabeculae,** (in ophthalmology) the part of the eye in front of the canal of Schlemm and within the angle created by the iris and the cornea.

**trabecular pattern** /trəbek'yələr/ [L, little beam], an irregular meshwork of stress and stress-related struts within a cancellous bone.

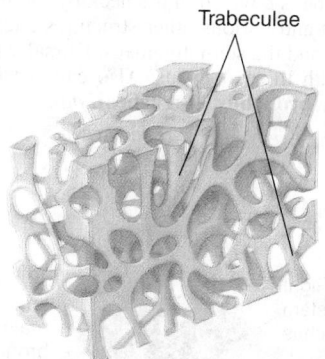

Trabeculae

**Trabecular pattern**
(Thibodeau and Patton, 1999/Christine Oleksyk)

**trabecula septomarginalis.** See **moderator band.**

**trabeculectomy,** creation of a fistula between the anterior chamber of the eye and the subconjunctival space by surgical removal of a portion of the trabecular meshwork, performed to facilitate drainage of the aqueous humor in glaucoma.

**trabeculoplasty** /trabek'yəlōplas'tē/, a plastic surgery procedure used in the treatment of glaucoma. An argon laser beam is used to blanch the trabecular network of the eye, thereby permitting drainage of the excess fluid that is causing increased pressure within the eyeball.

**trabeculotomy** /-ot'əmē/, a surgical opening in an orbital trabecula to increase the outflow of aqueous humor.

**trace element** [L, *trahere*, to draw, *elementum*, first principle], an element essential to nutrition or physiologic processes, found in such minute quantities that analysis yields a presence of only trace amounts.

**trace gas,** a gas or vapor that escapes into the atmosphere during an anesthetic procedure. Because these substances may have adverse effects on the health of personnel exposed to them, scavenging equipment is often installed in operating rooms to prevent the escape of waste gas into the atmosphere. See also **gas-scavenging system.**

**tracer** [L, *trahere*, to draw], **1.** a radioactive isotope that is used in diagnostic x-ray techniques to allow a biologic process to be seen. After introduction into the body, the tracer binds with a specific substance and is followed with a scanner or fluoroscope as it passes through various organs or systems. Kinds of tracers include **radioactive iodine (RAI)** and **radioactive carbon** ($^{14}$C). See also **radioisotope scan.** **2.** a mechanical device that graphically records the outline or movements of an object or part of the body. **3.** a dissecting instrument that is used to isolate vessels and nerves. —**trace,** *v.*

**tracer depot method,** a technique used to determine local blood flow through skin or muscle, based on the rate at which a radioactive tracer deposited in a tissue is removed by diffusion into the capillaries and washed out by the local blood supply. If blood flow is diminished or absent, as in dead skin, the deposited tracer does not wash out.

**trachea** /trā′kē·ə/ [Gk, *tracheia*, rough artery], a nearly cylindric tube in the neck, composed of C-shaped cartilage and membrane, that extends from the larynx at the level of the sixth cervical vertebra to the fifth thoracic vertebra, where it divides into two bronchi. The trachea conveys air to the lungs; it is about 11 cm long and 2 cm wide. The ventral surface of the tube is covered in the neck by the isthmus of the thyroid gland and various other structures such as the sternothyroideus and the sternohyoideus. Dorsally the trachea is in contact with the esophagus. Also called **windpipe.** See also **primary bronchus. —tracheal,** *adj.*

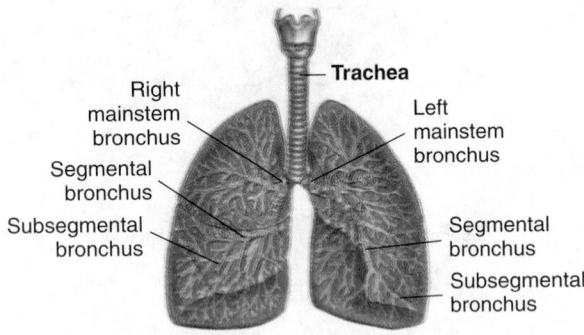

**Trachea** *(Wilson and Giddens, 2001)*

Right mainstem bronchus
Segmental bronchus
Subsegmental bronchus
Trachea
Left mainstem bronchus
Segmental bronchus
Subsegmental bronchus

**tracheal** /trā′kē·əl/ [Gk, *tracheia*, rough artery], pertaining to the trachea.

**tracheal breath sound.** See **bronchial breath sound.**

**tracheal tugging** [Gk, *tracheia*, rough artery; ME, *toggen*], an effect of an aortic aneurysm in which the trachea is pulled downward with each heart contraction.

**tracheitis** /trā′kē·ī′tis/, any inflammatory condition of the trachea. It may be acute or chronic, resulting from infection, allergy, or physical irritation. Also called **trachitis.**

**trachelagra.** See **agoraphobia.**

**trachelo-,** combining form meaning 'neck or necklike structure': *trachelobregmatic, trachelocystitis, tracheloschisis.*

**trachelodynia.** See **cervicodynia.**

**tracheo-** /trā′kē·ō-/, combining form meaning 'trachea': *tracheobronchial, tracheomalacia, tracheorrhaphy.*

**tracheobronchial** /trā′kē·ō·brong′kē·əl/, pertaining to the trachea and bronchi. Also called **bronchotracheal.**

**tracheobronchial tree (TBT)** /-brong′kē·əl/ [Gk, *tracheia* + *bronchos*, windpipe], an anatomic complex that includes the trachea, bronchi, and bronchial tubes. It conveys air to and from the lungs and is a primary structure in respiration. See also **bronchial tree.**

**tracheobronchitis** /trā′kē·ōbrongkī′tis/, inflammation of the trachea and bronchi, a common symptom of pulmonary infection.

**tracheobronchomegaly** /-brong′kōmeg′əlē/, an abnormally large upper airway, in which the trachea may be as wide as the spinal column.

**tracheoesophageal fistula** /trā′kē·ō·ē′səfā′jē·əl/ [Gk, *tracheia* + *oisophagos*, gullet], a congenital malformation in which there is an abnormal tubelike passage between the trachea and the esophagus. Also spelled **tracheooesophageal fistula.**

**tracheoesophageal puncture (TEP),** a one-way plastic valve placed in a surgically-created tracheoesophageal fistula to restore speech after laryngectomy.

**tracheoesophageal shunt,** surgical formation of a passageway between the trachea and the esophagus that enables a laryngectomee to speak. The operation results in an ability to produce esophageal speech with normal respiration as a source of air and without the need to belch to produce voice sounds. Also spelled **tracheooesophageal shunt.**

**tracheolaryngeal** /-lerin′jē·əl/, pertaining to the trachea and larynx.

**tracheomalacia** /trā′kē·ōmələā′shə/, an eroding of the trachea, usually caused by excessive pressure from a cuffed endotracheal tube.

**tracheooesophageal fistula.** See **tracheoesophageal fistula.**

**tracheooesophageal shunt.** See **tracheoesophageal shunt.**

**tracheopharyngeal** /-ferin′jē·əl/, pertaining to the trachea and pharynx.

**tracheoplasty** /trā′kē·ōplas′tē/, plastic surgery of the trachea.

**tracheostenosis** /-stəno′sis/, constriction of the lumen of the trachea.

**tracheostomy** /trā′kē·os′təmē/ [Gk, *tracheia* + *stoma*, mouth], an opening through the neck into the trachea through which an indwelling tube may be inserted. After tracheostomy the patient's chest is auscultated for breath sounds indicative of pulmonary congestion, mucous membranes and fingertips are observed for cyanosis, and humidified oxygen is given via tent or directly into the tracheostomy tube. The patient is reassured that the tube is open and that air can pass through it. The tube is suctioned frequently to keep it free from tracheobronchial secretions using a suction catheter attached to a Y-connector. The catheter is inserted 6 to 8 inches into the tube. The catheter is rotated, and intermittent suction is applied for no longer than 10 seconds. Complications of tracheostomy include pneumothorax, respiratory insufficiency, obstruction of the tracheostomy tube or its displacement from the lumen of the trachea, pulmonary infection, atelectasis, tracheoesophageal fistula, hemorrhage, and mediastinal emphysema. If the procedure was done as an emergency, the tracheostomy is closed after normal breathing is restored. If the tracheostomy is permanent, such as with a laryngectomy, the patient is taught self-care. Compare **tracheotomy.**

an incision is made through the skin and through the second, third, or fourth tracheal ring. A small hole is made in the fibrous tissue of the trachea, and the opening is then dilated to allow air intake. In an emergency any available instrument may be used as a dilator, even the barrel of a ballpoint pen with the inner part removed. If the blockage persists, a tracheostomy tube is inserted; if not, the incision is closed after normal respirations are established. After surgery the patient is observed for recurrent respiratory difficulty or cyanosis. Compare **tracheostomy.**

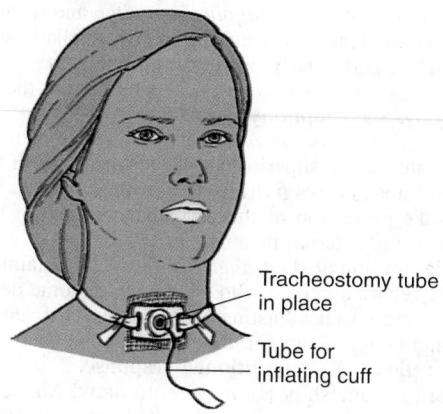

**Tracheostomy** *(Thibodeau and Patton, 1999)*

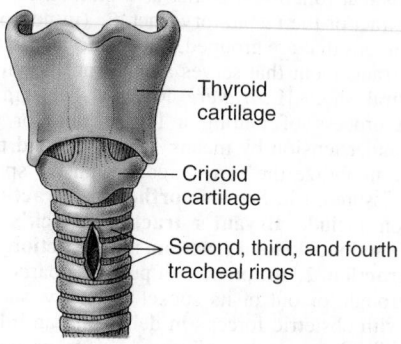

**Tracheotomy incision**
*(Ignatavicius, Workman, and Mishler, 1999)*

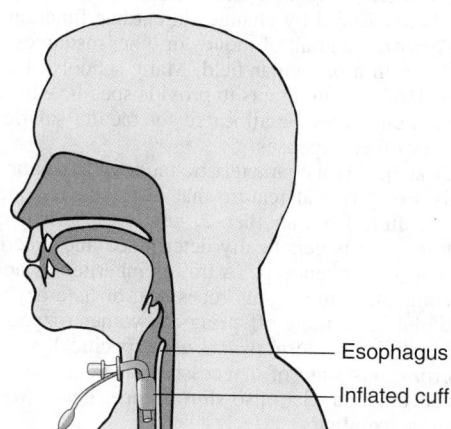

**Tracheostomy tube** *(Lewis, Heitkemper, and Dirksen, 2000)*

**tracheostomy care** [Gk, *tracheia,* rough artery, *stoma,* mouth], care of the tracheostomy patient, consisting of maintenance of a patent airway, adequate humidification, aseptic wound care, and sterile tracheal aspiration. Complications can include injury to the vocal cords, gastric distension and regurgitation, occlusion of the endotracheal tube, and an increased risk of infection.

**tracheotomy** /trā′kē·ot′əmē/ [Gk, *tracheia* + *temnein,* to cut], an incision made into the trachea through the neck below the larynx, performed to gain access to the airway below a blockage with a foreign body, tumor, or edema of the glottis. The opening may be made as an emergency measure at an accident site, at a hospitalized patient's bedside, or in the operating room. Local or general anesthesia may be used, if available. The patient's neck is hyperextended, and

**tracheotomy tube** [Gk, *tracheia,* rough artery, *temnein,* to cut; L, *tubus*], a curved hollow tube of rubber, metal, or plastic surgically inserted in the trachea to relieve a breathing obstruction.

**trachitis.** See **tracheitis.**

**trachoma** /trəkō′mə/ [Gk, roughness], a chronic infectious disease of the eye caused by the bacterium *Chlamydia trachomatis.* It is characterized initially by inflammation, pain, photophobia, and lacrimation. If untreated, follicles form on the upper eyelids and grow larger until the granulations invade the cornea, eventually causing blindness. Tetracycline, erythromycin, and topical sulfonamides usually provide effective treatment. Scarred eyelids may be surgically repaired. Trachoma is a significant cause of blindness and is

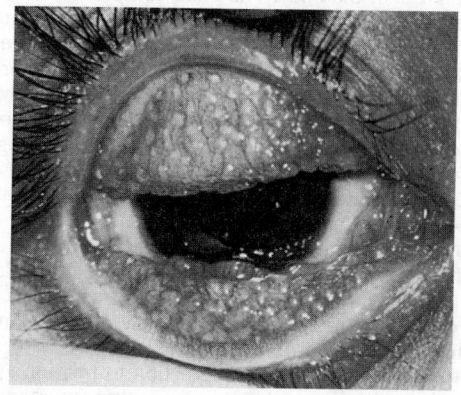

**Severe active trachoma** *(Stone and Gorbach, 2000)*

endemic to hot, dry, poverty-ridden areas. In the United States it is found in the Southwest. Teaching an affected population about the spread of trachoma and having an adequate water supply for washing hands, towels, and handkerchiefs are important factors in eliminating the disease. Also called **Egyptian ophthalmia, granular conjunctivitis.**

**tracing** [L, *trahere*, to draw], a graphic record of a physical event, such as an electrocardiograph tracing made by pens on a moving sheet of paper while recording the electrical impulses of heart muscle contractions.

**trackball.** See **joystick.**

**tract** [L, *tractus*, trail], 1. an elongated group of tissues and organs that function together as a pathway, such as the digestive tract or the respiratory tract. 2. (in neurology) the neuronal axons that are grouped together to form a pathway; a serial arrangement that serves a common function.

**traction** /trak'shən/ [L, *trahere*, to draw], 1. (in orthopedics) the process of putting a limb, bone, or group of muscles under tension by means of weights and pulleys to align or immobilize the part to reduce muscle spasm or to relieve pressure on it. See also **orthopedic traction.** Kinds of traction include **Bryant's traction, Buck's traction, Russell traction, skeletal traction, skin traction,** and **split Russell traction.** 2. the process of pulling a part of the body along, through, or out of its socket or cavity, such as axis traction with obstetric forceps in delivering an infant.

**traction, 90-90,** an orthopedic mechanism, used especially in pediatrics, that combines skeletal traction and suspension with a short-leg cast or a splint to immobilize and position the lower extremity in the treatment of a displaced fractured femur. This type of traction is usually unilateral with the opposite leg in Buck's traction or in split Russell traction for immobilization. The pin used in this kind of skeletal traction is inserted into bone in the knee area and attached to a riser running through a pulley on an overhead traction frame to a pulley and weight system fitted over the foot of the bed. The pulley and weight system at the foot of the bed also accommodates additional attachments to the short-leg cast or splint of the involved lower limb. Application of 90-90 traction also may incorporate a jacket restraint to help immobilize the patient. A variation of this type of traction is often used with adults in the treatment of low back pain.

**traction frame,** an orthopedic apparatus that supports the pulleys, ropes, and weights by which traction is applied to various parts of the body or by which various parts of the body are suspended. Traction frames are used in the treatment of bone fractures, dislocations, and disease processes of the musculoskeletal system; in the correction of various orthopedic deformities; and in the general immobilization of specific areas of the body. The main components of a traction frame are metal uprights that attach to the bed and support an overhead metal bar. In addition to traction equipment, traction frames are often rigged with trapeze bars that the patient can grasp to help in changing positions and to exercise the muscles of the arms and the trunk. The components of a traction frame are securely clamped together when in use but can be easily disassembled and reassembled. Compare **IV-type traction frame, claw-type traction frame, Balkan traction frame.**

**traction/immobilization care,** a nursing intervention from the Nursing Interventions Classification (NIC) defined as management of a patient who has traction and/or a stabilizing device to immobilize and stabilize a body part. See also **Nursing Interventions Classification.**

**traction response,** the body's reaction to traction applied to the spine. Alterations of certain signs and symptoms of a musculoskeletal disorder may be revealed by traction tests.

For example, if traction relieves a symptom, it may indicate impingement of a nerve root. Traction also may be used therapeutically to increase joint range, overcome muscle spasms, shorten soft tissues, or neutralize pressure and relieve pain in various joints.

**trademark,** a word, symbol, or device assigned to a product by its manufacturer, registered or not registered, as a part of its identity. See also **generic name.**

**tragacanth** /trag'əkanth/, a white tasteless vegetable gum derived from a shrub, *Astragalus gummifer,* and related species. It is used as a suspending agent in pharmaceutical preparations, particularly powders and tinctures.

**tragal** /trā'gəl/ [Gk, *tragos,* goat], pertaining to the tragus. **tragophony.** See **egophony.**

**tragion** /traj'ēən/ [Gk, *tragos,* goat], a cephalometric landmark located at the superior margin of the tragus of the ear.

**tragus** /trā'gəs/, *pl.* **tragi** /trā'jī/ [Gk, *tragos,* goat], a small tongue-like projection of the auricular cartilage of the ear, anterior to the external meatus.

**trainable** /trā'nəbəl/ [L, *trahere,* to draw], pertaining to a mentally retarded person who is capable of some degree of self-care and social adjustment in a supervised setting but would not benefit from formal education.

**trained reflex.** See **conditioned response.**

**traineeship** /trānē'ship/ [L, *trahere,* to draw; AS, *scieppan,* to shape], a grant of money allocated to an individual for advanced study in a given field. In nursing many graduate students have been awarded federal traineeships that provide funds for tuition and living expenses.

**training effect,** a rehabilitation effect for heart patients that can be measured by changes in cardiac function.

**training grant,** a grant of money or other resources to provide training in a particular field. Many schools of nursing receive federal or state grants to provide specific educational programs. Funds may be allocated for faculty salaries, student aid, or other expenses.

**trait** [Fr, trace], 1. a characteristic mode of behavior or any mannerism or physical feature that distinguishes one individual or culture from another. 2. any characteristic quality or condition that is genetically determined and inherited as part of a specific phenotype. A trait is inherited as homozygous dominant, homozygous recessive, or heterozygous in the ratio of 1:2:1 among offspring of two heterozygous parents. In medicine the term *trait* is used specifically to denote the heterozygous state of a recessive disorder, such as the sickle cell amemia. See also **dominance, gene, Mendel's laws, recessive allele.**

**tramadol,** a central analgesic.

■ INDICATIONS: This drug is used to manage moderate to severe pain.

■ CONTRAINDICATIONS: Factors that prohibit the use of this drug are known hypersensitivity to this drug or acute intoxication with any central nervous system depressant.

■ ADVERSE EFFECTS: Seizures and GI bleeding are life-threatening effects of this drug. Other adverse effects are dizziness, central nervous system stimulation, somnolence, headache, anxiety, confusion, euphoria, hallucination, nausea, constipation, vomiting, dry mouth, diarrhea, abdominal pain, anorexia, flatulence, vasodilation, orthostatic hypotension, tachycardia, hypertension, abnormal electrocardiograms, pruritus, rash, urticaria, vesicles, urinary retention/frequency, menopausal symptoms, dysuria, and menstrual disorders.

**TRAM flap,** an autogenous myocutaneous flap that uses transverse rectus abdominal muscle (TRAM) to carry lower abdominal skin and fat to the breast for reconstruction. See also **myocutaneous flap.**

**trance** [L, *transire*, to pass across], **1.** a sleeplike state characterized by the complete or partial suspension of consciousness and loss or diminution of motor activity, as seen in hypnosis, dissociative disorders, and various cataleptic and ecstatic states. **2.** a dazed or bewildered condition; stupor. **3.** a state of detachment from one's immediate surroundings, such as in deep concentration or daydreaming. Kinds of trances are **alcoholic trance, death trance, hypnotic trance,** and **induced trance.**

**Trandate,** trademark for an antihypertensive drug (labetalol hydrochloride).

**trandolapril,** an antihypertensive.

■ INDICATIONS: Trandolapril is used to treat hypertension, heart failure, and postmyocardial infarction/left ventricular dysfunction.

■ CONTRAINDICATIONS: Factors that prohibit the use of this drug include known hypersensitivity, a history of angioedema, and 2nd- or 3rd-trimester pregnancy.

■ ADVERSE EFFECTS: Life-threatening effects of trandolapril include myocardial infarction, stroke, agranulocytosis, neutropenia, leukopenia, anemia, proteinuria, and renal failure. Other adverse effects include palpitations, angina, transient ischemic attacks, bradycardia, dysrhythmias, paresthesias, headache, fatigue, drowsiness, depression, sleep disturbances, nausea, vomiting, cramps, diarrhea, constipation, ileus, pancreatitis, hepatitis, rash, purpura, dyspnea, hyperkalemia, hyponatremia, and impotence. Common side effects include hypotension, dizziness, dyspepsia, cough, and myalgia.

**tranquilizer** /trang′kwilī′zər/ [L, *tranquillus*, calm], a drug prescribed to calm anxious or agitated people, ideally without decreasing their consciousness. Major tranquilizers are generally used in the treatment of psychoses. Minor tranquilizers usually prescribed for the treatment of anxiety, irritability, tension, or psychoneurosis. Tranquilizers tend to induce drowsiness and have the potential for causing physical and psychologic dependence. Also spelled **tranquillizer.** See also **antipsychotic.**

**trans-** /trans-, tranz-/, prefix meaning 'across, through, over': *transabdominal, transferase, transplacental.*

**transabdominal** /-abdom′inəl/ [L, *trans*, across, *abdomen*, belly], pertaining to a procedure through the abdominal wall.

**transactional analysis (TA)** /-ak′shənəl/ [L, *transigere*, to drive through; Gk, *analyein*, to loosen], a form of psychodynamic psychotherapy developed by Eric Berne, based on a role theory that three different coherent organized egos exist throughout life simultaneously in every person, representing the child, the adult, and the parent. Interactions between people are transactions, originating from a person in one of the ego states, and received by another person who may be in a complementary or a crossed ego state. Transactions are motivated by a need for recognition and contact called 'strokes.' Transactions occur in six kinds of 'time structure': withdrawal, rituals, pastimes, games, activities, and intimacy. The way in which a person structures time reflects internal conflicts and patterns adopted to cope with those conflicts. The goal of transactional analysis is to enable clients to communicate from the ego state appropriate to the situation and the responses of the individuals, thereby decreasing conflict.

**transaminase** /-transam′inās/ [L, *trans*, across, *amine*, ammonia; Fr, *diastase*, enzyme], an enzyme that catalyzes the transfer of an amino group from an alpha-amino acid to an alpha-keto acid, with pyridoxal phosphate and pyridoxamine phosphate acting as coenzymes. Glutamic-oxaloacetic transaminase (GOT), normally present in serum and various tissues, especially in the heart and liver, is released by damaged cells. As a result, a high serum level of GOT may be diagnostic in myocardial infarction or hepatic disease. Glutamic-pyruvic transaminase, a normal constituent of serum and various tissues, especially in the liver, is released by injured tissue and may be present in high concentrations in the sera of patients with acute liver disease. Also called **aminotransferase.**

**transamination** /-am′inā′shən/, the reaction between an amino acid and an alpha-ketoacid in which the enzyme transaminase induces transfer of the amino group to the alpha-ketoacid.

**transanimation** /-an′imā′shən/, the resuscitation effort to induce a newborn to breathe.

**transaortic** /-ā-ôr′tik/ [L, *trans*, across; Gk, *aerein*, to raise], through the aorta.

**trans arrangement.** See **trans configuration.**

**transcellular water** /-sel′yələr/ [L, *trans* + *cella*, storeroom], the part of extracellular water that is enclosed by an epithelial membrane and whose volume and composition are determined by the cellular activity of that membrane.

**transcendence** /transen′dəns/ [L, *trans* + *scandere*, to climb], the rising above one's previously perceived limits or restrictions.

**transcendental meditation (TM),** a psychophysiologic exercise designed to lower levels of tension and anxiety and increase tolerance of frustration. TM has been described as a state of consciousness that does not require any physical or mental control. During meditation, the person enters a hypometabolic state in which there is reduced activity of the adrenergic component of the autonomic nervous system.

**transcervical fracture** /-transur′vikəl/ [L, *trans*, across, *cervix*, neck, *fractura*], a fracture through the neck of the femur.

**transcondylar fracture** /-transkon′dilər/ [L, *trans* + Gk, *kondylos*, condyle], a fracture that occurs transverse and distal to the epicondyles of any one of the long bones.

**trans configuration** /-kənfig′yərā′shən/ [L, *trans* + *configurare*, to form from], **1.** an arrangement in which the dominant allele of one pair of genes and the recessive allele of another pair are on the same chromosome. **2.** an arrangement in which at least one mutant gene and one wild-type gene of a pair of pseudoalleles are present on each chromosome of a homologous pair. Also called **trans arrangement, trans position.** Compare **cis configuration. 3.** (in chemistry) a form of isomerism in which two substituent groups occur on opposite sides of a structure such as a ring or a double bond. Compare **cis configuration.**

**transcortical** /-trans·kor′ti·kəl/ [L, *trans*, across + *cortex*, bark], connecting two different parts of the cerebral cortex; also, dependent on disease of the tracts connecting different parts of the cerebral cortex.

**transcortical apraxia.** See **ideomotor apraxia.**

**transcortin** /-kôr′tin/, a diglobulin protein that binds a majority of cortisol in the plasma. Also called **corticosteroid-binding globulin.**

**transcriptase** /transkrip′tās/, an enzyme that induces transcription.

**transcription** /transkrip′shən/ [L, *trans* + *scribere*, to write], the process by which messenger RNA is formed from a DNA template. See also **anticodon, genetic code.**

**transcription factor,** a specific protein required for the initiation of transcription by an RNA polymerase; each polymerase has its own set of transcription factors.

**transcultural nursing** /-kul′chərəl/ [L, *trans* + *colere*, to cultivate, *nutrix*, nurse], a field of nursing, founded by Madeleine Leininger, in which the nurse transcends ethnocentricity and practices nursing in other cultural environments. Because current nursing process and theory are not culturally bound and the needs of each person are considered individually, transcultural nursing is a part of all nursing practice.

**transcutaneous** /-k(y)o͞ota′ne-əs/ [L, *trans* + *cutis,* skin], pertaining to a procedure that is performed through the skin.

**transcutaneous electrical nerve stimulation (TENS)[1]**, a method of pain control by the application of electric impulses to the nerve endings. This is done through electrodes that are placed on the skin and attached to a stimulator by flexible wires. The electric impulses generated are similar to those of the body, but different enough to block transmission of pain signals to the brain. TENS is noninvasive and nonaddictive, with no known side effects. It is contraindicated in patients with a demand-type cardiac pacemaker. See **galvanic electric stimulation.**

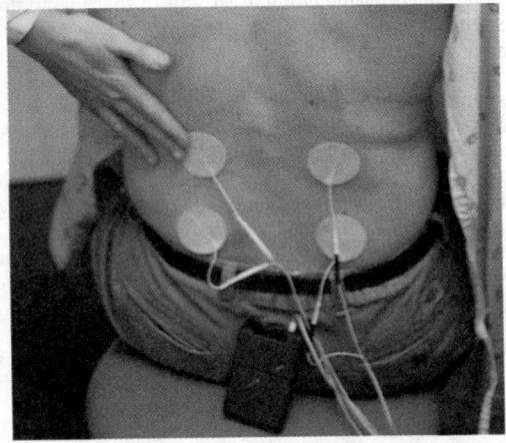

**Transcutaneous electric nerve stimulation**
*(Ignatavicius, Workman, and Mishler, 1999)*

**transcutaneous electrical nerve stimulation (TENS)[2]**, a nursing intervention from the Nursing Interventions Classification (NIC) defined as stimulation of skin and underlying tissues with controlled, low-voltage electrical vibration via electrodes. See also **Nursing Interventions Classification.**

**transcutaneous nerve stimulation.** See **transcutaneous electrical nerve stimulation.**

**transcutaneous oxygen/carbon dioxide monitoring,** a method of measuring the oxygen or carbon dioxide in the blood by attaching electrodes to the skin. Oxygen is commonly measured through an oximeter, which contains heating coils to raise the skin temperature and increase blood flow at the surface. Oxygen content is calculated in terms of light absorption at various wavelengths. Transcutaneous carbon dioxide electrodes are similar to blood gas electrodes, with a Teflon membrane tip that is permeable to gases.

**transdermal drug delivery (TDD)** /-dur′məl/ [L, *trans* + Gk, *derma,* skin], a method of applying a drug to unbroken skin. The drug is absorbed continuously through the skin and enters the systemic system. It is used particularly for the administration of nicotine, nitroglycerin, and scopolamine.

**transdermal scopolamine,** a method of administration of the motion sickness drug scopolamine by application of a skin patch containing the medication.

**transducer** /-d(y)o͞o′sər/ [L, *trans* + *ducere,* to lead], a hand-held device that sends and receives ultrasound signals. It changes electrical impulses into soundwaves, receives reflected soundwaves, and converts them back into electrical energy.

**transductant** /-duk′tənt/, a cell that has acquired a new character by the transfer of genetic material.

**transduction** /-duk′shən/, a method of genetic recombination by which DNA is transferred from one cell to another by a viral vector. Various bacteriophages transfer DNA from one species of bacteria to another.

**transect** /transekt′/ [L, *trans* + *secare,* to cut], to sever or cut across, as in preparing a cross section of tissue. See **transection, transsection.**

**transection.** See **transsection.**

**transesophageal echocardiography (TEE),** an endoscopic/ultrasound test that provides ultrasonic imaging of the heart from a retrocardiac vantage point, thus preventing the interposed subcutaneous tissue, bony thorax, and lungs from interfering with the ultrasound. It is performed to better visualize the mitral valve or atrial septum, to differentiate intracardiac from extracardiac masses and tumors, to diagnose thoracic aortic dissection, to detect valvular vegetation as seen with endocarditis, to determine cardiac sources of arterial embolism, to detect coronary artery disease, and to monitor high-risk patients for ischemia intraoperatively.

*trans*—fatty acids, stereoisomers of the naturally occurring *cis*—fatty acids, found in margarines and shortenings as artifacts after hydrogenation; pregnant women and certain other individuals should restrict intake of these.

**transfection** /-fek′shən/ [L, *trans* + *inficere,* to taint], the process by which a bacterial cell is infected with purified DNA or RNA isolated from a virus after a specific pretreatment. Acute transfection is short-term infection.

**transfer,** to move a person or object from one site to another.

**transfer ability, impaired,** a nursing diagnosis accepted by the Thirteenth National Conference on the Classification of Nursing Diagnoses. The condition is a limitation of independent movement between two nearby surfaces.

■ DEFINING CHARACTERISTICS: The condition is characterized by the impaired ability to transfer from bed to chair and chair to bed, the impaired ability to transfer on or off a toilet or commode, the impaired ability to transfer in and out of a bathtub or shower, the impaired ability to transfer between uneven levels, the impaired ability to transfer from chair to car or car to chair, the impaired ability to transfer from chair to floor or floor to chair, and the impaired ability to transfer from standing to floor or floor to standing.

■ RELATED FACTORS: Related factors are to be developed. See also **nursing diagnosis.**

**transfer agreement** /trans′fur/ [L, *transferre,* to carry over, *ad,* toward, *gratus,* pleasure], a written hospital agreement between two health care institutions for the transfer of patients from one to another and the orderly exchange of pertinent clinical information on the patients transferred.

**transferase** /trans′fərās/ [L, *transferre* + Fr, *diastase,* enzyme], any of a group of enzymes that catalyzes the transfer of a chemical group or radical, such as the phosphate, methyl, amine, or keto groups, from one molecule to another.

**transfer DNA (tDNA),** DNA transferred from its original source and present in transformed cells.

**transference** /-fur′əns/ [L, *transferre*], **1.** the shifting of symptoms from one part of the body to another, as occurs in conversion disorder. **2.** (in psychiatry) an unconscious defense mechanism whereby feelings and attitudes originally associated with important people and events in one's early life are attributed to others in current interpersonal situations. **3.** (in psychoanalysis and psychotherapy) the feelings, either positive or negative, of a patient for the analyst to whom the patient has attributed or assigned the qualities, attitudes, and feelings of a person or people significant in his or her emotional development, usually a figure from childhood. The phenomenon is used as a tool in understanding the emotional problems of the patient and their origins. See also **countertransference, parataxic distortion.**

**transference love,** (in psychoanalytic therapy) a projection of libidinal drives expressed by the patient for the psychoanalyst who has "unconsciously" come to represent a person from the patient's past.

**transfer factor,** a leukocyte extract that transfers delayed hypersensitivity from one person to another. Transfer factor has been studied for its possible use in the treatment of chronic mucocutaneous candidiasis and Wiskott-Aldrich syndrome and as a means of transferring antitumor immunity to patients with various types of cancer.

**transfer factor of lungs.** See **diffusing capacity of lungs.**

**transfer performance,** a nursing outcome from the Nursing Outcomes Classification (NOC) defined as the ability to change body locations. See also **Nursing Outcomes Classification.**

**transferrin** /transfer′in/, a trace protein present in the blood that is essential in the transport of iron from the intestine into the bloodstream, making it available to the normoblasts in the bone marrow. It also may take part in a slower exchange with ferritin, hemosiderin, and other iron forms in the tissues. See also **hemosiderin, iron transport.**

**transferring** /-fur′ing/ [L, *trans*, across, *ferre*, to bring], relocating a person in need from one location to another.

**transfer RNA (tRNA),** a kind of RNA that carries an anticodon (three nucleotide bases) and a specific amino acid. The identity of the amino acid is determined by the sequence of nucleotides in the anticodon. There are 64 possible anticodons and about two dozen amino acids that are found in proteins. This means that several anticodons may specify to the same amino acid. Each anticodon is complementary to a specific codon in the messenger RNA. The tRNAs (with their amino acids attached) translate the sequence of codons in messenger RNA into a sequence of amino acids in a polypeptide. Also called **adaptor RNA.**

**transfixation** /-fiksā′shən/, a surgical procedure in which, in an amputation, the soft tissues are cut through from one side to the other, close to the bone. The muscles are then divided from within outward.

**transformation** /-fôrmā′shən/ [L, *transformare*, to change shape], the integration of exogenous genes into chromosomes in a form that is recognized by the replicative and transcriptional apparatus of the host cell. Transformation occurs rarely in most cell populations.

**transformer** /-fôr′mər/ [L, *transformare*, to change shape], an electrical apparatus that changes alternating current of one voltage into a different voltage of the same frequency.

**transforming growth factor (TGF),** a group of proteins produced by the cells of a tumor that, when inoculated into a normal cell culture, causes a disorderly increase in the number of cells in the culture.

**transfuse** /-fyo͞oz′/, to transfer blood or blood components from one person to another.

**transfusion** /-f(y)o͞o′zhən/ [L, *trans* + *fundere*, to pour], the introduction into the bloodstream of whole blood or blood components, such as plasma, platelets, or packed red cells. Whole blood may be infused into the recipient directly from a donor matched for the ABO blood group and antigenic subgroups, but more frequently the donor's blood is collected and stored by a blood bank. See also **blood transfusion.**

**transfusion reaction,** a systemic response by the body to the administration of blood incompatible with that of the recipient. The causes include red cell incompatibility; allergic sensitivity to the leukocytes, platelets, plasma protein components of the transfused blood; or potassium or citrate preservatives in the banked blood. See also **hemolysis.**

■ OBSERVATIONS: Fever is the most common transfusion reaction; urticaria is a relatively common allergic response. Asthma, vascular collapse, and renal failure occur less commonly. A hemolytic reaction from red cell incompatibility is serious and must be diagnosed and treated promptly. Symptoms develop shortly after beginning the transfusion, before 50 mL have been given, and include a throbbing headache, sudden deep severe lumbar pain, precordial pain, dyspnea, and restlessness. Objective signs include ruddy facial flushing followed by cyanosis and distended neck veins, rapid, thready pulse, diaphoresis, and cold, clammy skin. Profound shock may occur within 1 hour.

■ INTERVENTIONS: When a hemolytic reaction is suspected, the transfusion is promptly terminated, and the infusion line kept open with a normal solution of IV fluid. The remaining bank blood is saved for a repeat type and crossmatch against a fresh sample of blood from the recipient. Direct and indirect antiglobulin tests are usually ordered to detect hemolytic antibodies, and a sample of urine is examined for free hemoglobin. Immediate treatment may include IV mannitol and a solution of 5% dextrose in water to maintain urine flow of more than 100 mL per hour. In the presence of oliguria, the possibility of acute renal failure is evaluated, and the patient is managed accordingly. Hypovolemia is corrected with saline or plasma expanders, but the administration of more whole blood is avoided, if possible.

■ NURSING CONSIDERATIONS: The need for exceptional care to ensure that typed and crossmatched blood conforms to compatibility standards is emphasized. The identifying information on the blood container is always checked against the transfusion records and the patient's identification on the band. Questioning the patient about previous transfusions may elicit warning indications of possible adverse reactions. After the transfusion is started, the patient is watched for objective signs of a transfusion reaction and is questioned for subjective symptoms. Routine temperature checks are done to detect febrile reactions that can be controlled by antipyretic drugs.

**transgender reassignment,** the surgical alteration of external sexual characteristics so that they resemble those of the opposite sex. Also called **transsexual surgery.**

**transgene** /trans′jēn/, a gene that has been transferred from one genome into another. For example, a mouse with a rat hormone gene grows much larger than normal. —**transgenic,** *adj.*

**transient** /tran′shənt, tran′zē-ənt/ [L, *transire*, to go through], pertaining to a condition that is temporary, such as transient ischemic attack.

**transient global amnesia (TGA)** [L, *transire*, to go through, *globus*, ball; Gk, *amnesia*, forgetfulness], a temporary short-term memory loss followed by full recovery. The disorder tends to affect middle-aged adults and may be

## Immunologic reactions to blood transfusion

| Clinical manifestations | Management | Prevention |
|---|---|---|
| **Acute hemolytic**<br>Chills, fever, low back pain, flushing, tachycardia, tachypnea, hypotension, vascular collapse, hemoglobinuria, hemoglobinemia, bleeding, acute renal failure, shock, cardiac arrest, death | Treat shock.<br>Draw blood samples for serologic testing. To avoid hemolysis from the procedure, use a new venipuncture (not an existing central line) and avoid small-gauge needles. Send urine specimen to the laboratory.<br>Maintain blood pressure with IV colloid solutions. Give diuretics as prescribed to maintain urine flow.<br>Insert indwelling catheter or measure voided amounts to monitor hourly urine output. Dialysis may be required if renal failure occurs.<br>Do not transfuse additional red blood cell–containing components until the transfusion service has provided newly crossmatched units. | Meticulously verify and document patient identification from sample collection to component infusion.<br>Transfuse blood slowly for first 15-20 minutes with nurse at patient's side. |
| **Febrile, nonhemolytic (most common)**<br>Sudden chills and fever (rise in temperature of greater than 1° C [2° F]), headache, flushing, anxiety, muscle pain | Give antipyretics as prescribed. Do not give aspirin to thrombocytopenic patients.<br>*Do not restart transfusion.* | Consider leukocyte-poor blood products (filtered, washed, or frozen). |
| **Mild allergic**<br>Flushing, itching, urticaria (hives) | Give antihistamines as directed.<br>If symptoms are mild and transient, restart transfusion slowly.<br>Do not restart transfusion if fever or pulmonary symptoms develop. | Treat prophylactically with glucocorticoid steroids or antihistamines (Decadron, Benadryl) given 30-60 min before transfusion. |
| **Anaphylactic**<br>Anxiety, urticaria, wheezing, tightness and pain in chest, difficulty swallowing, progressing to cyanosis, shock, and possible cardiac arrest | Initiate cardiopulmonary resuscitation if indicated.<br>Have epinephrine ready for injection (0.4 ml of a 1:1000 solution subcutaneously or 0.1 ml of 1:1000 solution diluted to 10 ml with saline for IV use).<br>*Do not restart transfusion.* | Transfuse extensively washed red blood cell products from which all plasma has been removed. Alternatively, use blood from immunoglobulin A–deficient donor. |
| **Delayed hemolytic**<br>Fever, chills, back pain, jaundice, anemia, hemoglobinuria | Monitor adequacy of urinary output and degree of anemia.<br>Treat fever with acetaminophen (Tylenol).<br>May need further blood transfusion. | Do more specific type and crossmatch when giving patient blood. |
| **Graft-versus-host disease-PT**<br>Anorexia, nausea, diarrhea, high fever, rash, stomatitis, liver dysfunction | No effective treatment.<br>Administer steroids. | Give irradiated blood products. |
| **Noncardiac pulmonary edema**<br>Fever, chills, hypotension, cough, orthopnea, cyanosis, shock | Stop transfusion.<br>Continue IV saline.<br>Give oxygen as necessary.<br>Administer steroids as directed.<br>Give furosemide (Lasix) and epinephrine as ordered. | — |

From Phipps WJ, Sands JK, Marek JE: *Medical-surgical nursing: concepts and clinical practice*, ed 6, St Louis, 1999, Mosby.

attributed to cerebral ischemia. It is usually not accompanied by other mental deficiencies.

**transient ischemic attack (TIA),** an episode of cerebrovascular insufficiency, usually associated with partial occlusion of a cerebral artery by an atherosclerotic plaque or an embolus. The symptoms vary with the site and degree of occlusion. Disturbance of normal vision in one or both eyes, dizziness, weakness, dysphasia, numbness, or unconsciousness may occur. The attack usually lasts a few minutes; in rare cases symptoms continue for several hours.

**transient myopia** [L, *transire,* to go through; Gk, *myops,* nearsighted], a temporary change in visual accommodation secondary to trauma, high blood sugar level, sulfanilamide therapy, and other conditions.

**transillumination** /-ilō̄o'minā'shən/ [L, *trans,* through, *illuminare,* to light up], **1.** the passage of light through a solid or liquid substance. **2.** the passage of light through body tissues for the purpose of examining a structure interposed between the observer and the light source. A diaphanoscope is an instrument introduced into a body cavity to transilluminate tissues.

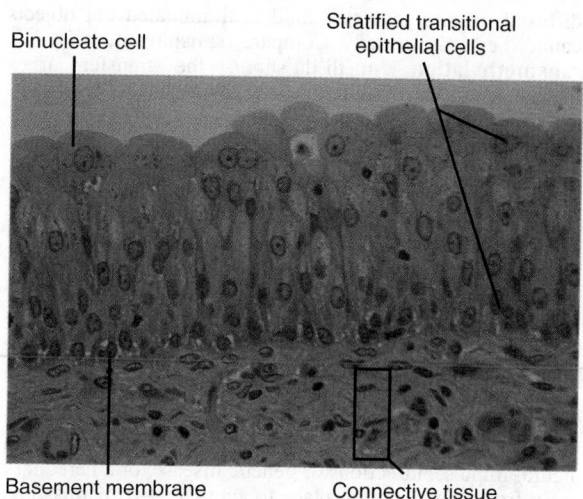

Binucleate cell

Stratified transitional epithelial cells

Basement membrane

Connective tissue

**Transitional epithelium** *(© Ed Reschke; used with permission)*

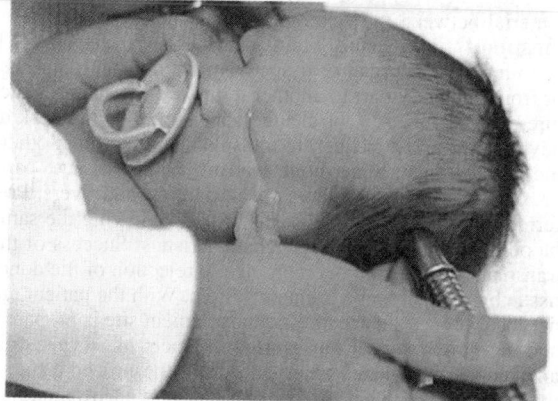

**Transillumination of an infant's scalp** *(Seidel et al, 1999)*

**transition** /tranzish'ən/ [L, *transire,* to go through], the last phase of the first stage of labor, sometimes indicated by cervical dilation of 8 to 10 cm.

**transitional** /tranzish'ənəl/ [L, *transire,* to go through], between a previous and a succeeding state, or in a state of becoming something else.

**transitional cell carcinoma,** a malignant, usually papillary tumor derived from transitional stratified epithelium, occurring most frequently in the bladder, ureter, urethra, or renal pelvis. The majority of tumors in the collecting system of the kidney are of this kind. They have a better prognosis than squamous cell carcinomas in the same site.

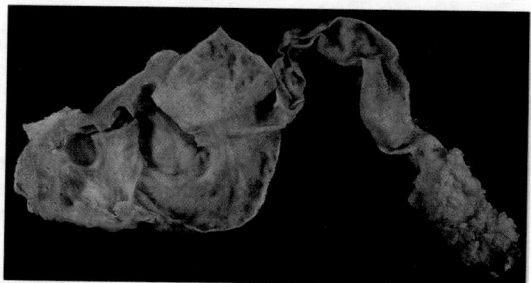

**Transitional cell carcinoma of the ureter** *(Fletcher, 2000)*

**transitional dentition.** See **mixed dentition.**

**transitional epithelium,** a form of pseudostratified epithelium found characteristically in the mucous membrane of kidney, ureter, and bladder; in the contracted condition it consists of many cell layers, whereas in the stretched condition usually only two layers can be distinguished.

**transitional object,** an object used by a child to provide comfort and security while he or she is away from a secure base, such as mother or home.

**transitional zone** [L, *transire,* to go through; Gk, *zone,* belt], a part of the crystalline lens of the eye where epithelial-capsule cells change into lens fibers.

**transitory mania** /tran'sitôr'ē/ [L, *transire,* to go through; Gk, *mania,* madness], a mood disorder characterized by the sudden onset of manic reactions that are of short duration, usually lasting from 1 hour to a few days. See also **mania.**

**transjugular intrahepatic portosystemic shunt (TIPS)** /tranz·jug'yo͞o·lər/, percutaneous creation of a shunt between the hepatic and portal veins within the liver followed by placement of an expandable stent in the tract created, performed by a transjugular route under radiologic guidance; done for the treatment of bleeding esophageal varices.

**translation** /-lā'shən/ [L, *translatio,* handing over], the process in which the genetic information carried by nucleotides in messenger RNA directs the amino acid sequence in the synthesis of a specific polypeptide. See also **anticodon, genetic code.**

**translocation** /-lōkā'shən/ [L, *trans + locus,* place], the rearrangement of DNA within a chromosome or the transfer of a segment of one chromosome to a nonhomologous one. In simple translocations, an end segment of one chromosome is transferred onto the end of another, involving a single break in only one of the chromosomes. Translocations in which material from the middle of one chromosome is shifted to the middle of another one are more complex and involve at least three breaks in the participating chromosomes. Such shifting of genetic material can result in serious disorders, such as Down syndrome, which can be caused by a 14/21 translocation, and chronic granulocytic leukemia, in which part of the long arm of chromosome 22 is translocated to the short arm of chromosome 9. Kinds of translocations are **balanced translocation, reciprocal translocation,** and **robertsonian translocation.**

**translucent** /-lō̄o'sənt/ [L, *trans,* across, *lucens,* shining], pertaining to a medium through which light can pass in a diffused manner so that a field is illuminated but objects cannot be seen distinctly. Compare **transparent.**

**transmethylation** /-meth'ilā'shən/, the transfer of a methyl group from one compound to another.

**transmigration** /-mīgrā'shən/ [L, *trans* + *migrare*, to migrate], a movement from one side to another, from inside to outside, or from outside to inside.

**transmissible** /-mis'ibəl/ [L, *transmittere*, to transmit], capable of being passed from one person or place to another, as in the transmission of a disease.

**transmissible spongiform encephalopathy,** a group of neurodegenerative diseases that are unique in having either infectious or genetic causes. Examples include **Creutzfeldt-Jakob disease (CJD)** and **Gerstmann-Straussler syndrome,** a homozygous prion protein genotype predisposes individuals to susceptibility to the diseases.

**transmission** /-mish'ən/ [L, *transmittere*, to transmit], the transfer or conveyance of a thing or condition, such as a neural impulse, infectious or genetic disease, or a hereditary trait, from one person or place to another. —**transmissible,** *adj.*

**transmission-based precautions,** safeguards designed for patients documented or suspected to be infected with highly transmissible or epidemiologically important pathogens for which additional precautions beyond standard precautions are needed to interrupt transmission in hospitals. There are three types of transmission-based precautions: airborne precautions, droplet precautions, and contact precautions. They may be combined for diseases that have multiple routes of transmission. When used either singularly or in combination, they are to be used in addition to standard precautions. See also **airborne precautions, droplet precautions, contact precautions, standard precautions.**

**transmission electron microscopy.** See **electron microscopy.**

**transmission scanning electron microscope,** an instrument that transmits a highly magnified, well-resolved, three-dimensional image on a television screen, thus combining the advantages of the electron and the scanning electron microscopes. Compare **electron microscope, scanning electron microscope.**

**transmission scanning electron microscopy (TSEM),** a technique using a transmission scanning electron microscope in which the atomic number of the part of the sample being scanned is determined and used to modulate a beam of electrons in a cathode-ray tube and in the beam scanning the sample. The image produced is clear, three-dimensional, and highly magnified. Compare **electron microscopy, scanning electron microscopy.**

**transmitted light** [L, *transmittere*, to transmit; AS, *leoht*], light that has been transmitted through a transparent medium.

**transmitter substance.** See **neurotransmitter.**

**transmural** /-m(y)ōō'rəl/ [L, *trans* + *murus*, wall], pertaining to the entire thickness of the wall of an organ, such as a transmural myocardial infarction, or through any wall such as the body or cyst of a hollow structure.

**transmural infarction,** death of myocardial tissue that extends from the endocardium to the epicardium as a result of a myocardial infarction.

**transmutation** /-m(y)ōōtā'shən/ [L, *transmutare*, to change], **1.** a mutation that causes a significant species change during evolution. **2.** the conversion of one chemical element into another by radioactive bombardment.

**transovarial transmission** /-ōver'ē·əl/ [L, *trans* + *ovum*, egg], the transfer of pathogens to succeeding generations through invasion of the ovary and infection of the eggs, such as occurs in arthropods, primarily ticks and mites.

**transparent** /-per'ənt/ [L, *trans*, across, *parere*, to appear], pertaining to a clear medium that allows for the transmission of light so that objects on the other side are distinguishable. Compare **translucent.**

**transpeptidase** /-pep'tidās/, an enzyme that catalyzes the transfer of an amino group from one peptide chain to another.

**transpeptidation** /-pep'tidā'shən/, the transfer of an amino acid from one peptide chain to another.

**transplacental** /trans'pləsen'təl/ [L, *trans* + *placenta*, flat cake], across or through the placenta, specifically in reference to the exchange of nutrients, waste products, and other material between the developing fetus and the mother.

**transplant** /trans'plant, transplant'/ [L, *transplantare*], **1.** to transfer an organ or tissue from one person to another or from one body part to another to replace a diseased structure, restore function, or change appearance. Skin and kidneys are the most frequently transplanted structures; others include cartilage, bone, bone marrow, corneal tissue, parts of blood vessels and tendons, hearts, lungs, and livers. Preferred donors are identical twins or people having the same blood type and immunologic characteristics. Success of the transplant depends on overcoming the rejection of the donor tissue by the recipient's immune system. With the patient under local or general anesthesia, the recipient site is prepared, and the donor structure is grafted in place; its oxygenation and blood supply are preserved during the procedure until the circulation can be restored at the new site. After surgery circulation in the area is observed for signs of impairment. Antirejection drugs are given, with steroids, to suppress the production of antibodies to the foreign tissue proteins. Signs of rejection reaction include fever, pain, and loss of function, usually occurring in the first 4 to 10 days after transplantation. An abscess may form if the reaction is not subdued promptly. The grafted structure may require several weeks to become established. Late rejection may occur several months or even 1 year later. **2.** any tissue or organ that is transplanted. **3.** pertaining to a tissue or organ that is transplanted, a recipient of a donated tissue or organ, or a phenomenon associated with the procedure. Also called **graft, transplantation.**

**transplantation** /-plantā'shən/ [L, *transplantare*, to transplant], the transfer of tissue from one site to another or from one person or organism to another.

**transplantation endometriosis** [L, *transplantare*, to transplant; Gk, *endon*, within, *metra*, womb, *osis*, condition], endometrial tissue that is accidentally transplanted to the incision wound during pelvic surgery.

**transport**[1] /trans'pôrt/ [L, *trans*, across, *portare*, carry], the movement or transference of biochemical substances from one site to another. Active transport involves an expenditure of energy, whereas passive transport allows movement down a gradient without an energy expenditure.

**transport**[2], a nursing intervention from the Nursing Interventions Classification (NIC) defined as moving a patient from one location to another. See also **Nursing Interventions Classification.**

**transposable element.** See **transposon.**

**transposase** /trans'pəzās/, an enzyme involved in the movement of a DNA fragment from one site in the genome to another.

**trans position** /-pəsish'ən/ [L, *transponere*], **1.** an abnormality occurring during embryonic development in which a body part normally on the left is found on the right or vice versa. **2.** the shifting of genetic material from one chromosome to another at some point in the reproductive process, often resulting in a congenital anomaly. —**transpose,** *v.*

**transposition of the great vessels,** a congenital cardiac anomaly in which the pulmonary artery arises from the left ventricle and the aorta from the right ventricle and there is no communication between the systemic and pulmonary circulations. Life is impossible with this anomaly unless there are associated cardiac defects, such as a septal defect or a patent ductus arteriosus, that enable the mixing of oxygenated and unoxygenated blood. The severity of the condition depends on the type and size of the associated defect. The primary symptoms are cyanosis and hypoxia, especially in infants with small septal defects, although cardiomegaly is usually evident a few weeks after birth. Signs of congestive heart failure develop rapidly, especially in infants with large ventricular septal defects. Definitive diagnosis is based on cardiac catheterization. Surgical correction of the defect is postponed, if possible, until after 6 months of age, when the infant can better tolerate the procedure. Immediate palliative surgical procedures such as the Rashkind procedure may be performed to decrease pulmonary vascular resistance and prevent congestive heart failure. See also **blue baby.**

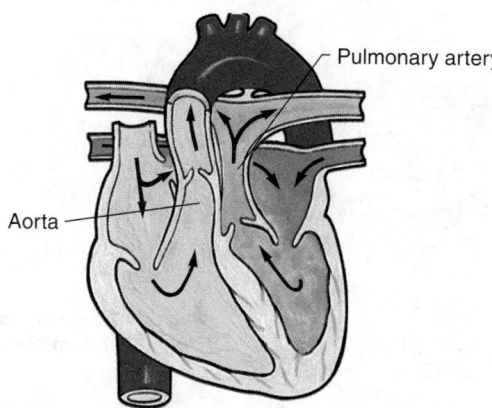

**Transposition of the great vessels** *(Wong, 1999)*

**transposon** /transpō'sən/ [L, *transponere* + on], a segment of DNA that can move from one place to another in a cell's genome or between a bacterial cell and a plasmid or virus. Viruses may even carry a transposon from one bacterium to another. Also called **jumping gene, transposable element.**

**transpulmonary pressure** /-pul'məner'ē/, the difference between intraalveolar and intrapleural pressure, or the pressure acting across the lung from the pleural space to the alveoli.

**transsect.** See **transect.**

**transsection** /transek'shən/ [L, *trans,* across, *sectio*], a cross-section of a biologic specimen or a cut across the long axis. Also spelled **transection.**

**transseptal fiber** /transep'təl/ [L, *trans* + *saeptum,* wall], any of the many filamentous tissues of the gingival system that extend mesially from the supraalveolar cementum of one tooth, through the interdental-attached gingiva above the septum of the alveolar bone, to the distal cementum of an adjacent tooth.

**transsexual** /transek'choo·əl/, a person whose gender identity is opposite his or her biologic sex.

**transsexualism** /-iz'əm/, a condition in which a person has an intense desire to discard one's biologic sex and live as a member of the opposite sex. It is considered a psychiatric disorder if the condition continues for more than 2 years. Some transsexual individuals crossdress and seek medical or surgical help to change their physical sex characteristics.

**transsexual surgery.** See **transgender reassignment.**

**transtentorial herniation** /trans'tentôr'ē·əl/ [L, *trans* + *tentorium,* tent, *hernia,* rupture], a bulge of brain tissue out of the cranium through the tentorial notch, caused by increased intracranial pressure. See also **tentorial herniation.**

**transthermia.** See **thermopenetration.**

**transthoracic** /trans'thôras'ik/, across or passing through the thorax.

**transthoracic pacemaker** /-thôras'ik/ [L, *trans,* across; Gk, *thorax,* chest; L, *passus,* step; ME, *maken*], a permanent pacemaker with the pulse generator located in the abdominal wall and the pacing wires attached directly to the epicardium.

**transtracheal oxygen** /-trā'kē·əl/ [L, *trans,* across; Gk, *tracheia,* rough artery, *oxys,* sharp, *genein,* to produce], the administration of oxygen via a low-flow catheter inserted directly into the trachea. It is sometimes preferred to the administration of oxygen through a nasal cannula.

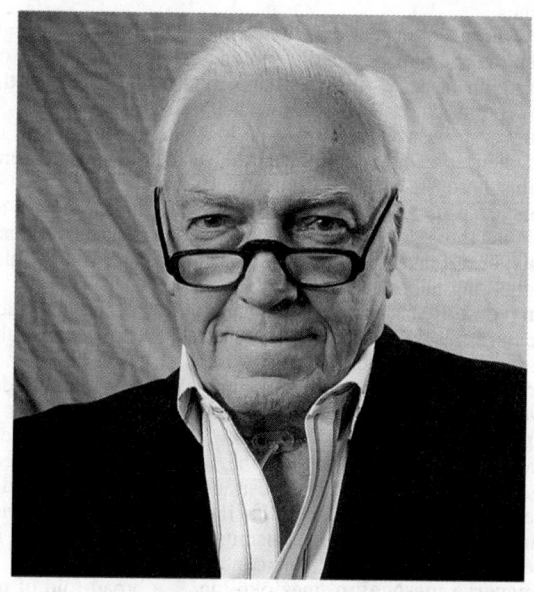

**Transtracheal oxygen catheter**
*(Beare and Myers, 1998/courtesy Transtracheal Systems, Englewood, Colorado)*

**transtrochanteric osteotomy** /-trō'kənter'ik/ [L, *trans,* across; Gk, *trochanter,* runner, *osteon* + *temnein,* to cut], a surgical division of the upper end of the femur through the area of the trochanters.

**transubstantiation** /trans'əbstan'chē·ā'shən/, the replacement or substitution of one kind of tissue for another.

**transudate** /trans′yədāt/ [L, *trans* + *sudare*, to sweat], a fluid passed through a membrane or squeezed through a tissue or into the space between the cells of a tissue. It is thin and watery and contains few blood cells or other large proteins. See also **edema.**

**transudation** /-yədā′shən/, **1.** the passage of a substance through a membrane as a result of a difference in hydrostatic pressure. **2.** the passage of a fluid through a membrane with nearly all the solutes of the fluid remaining in solution or suspension.

**transudative ascites** /transyoo̅′dətiv/, an abnormal accumulation in the peritoneal cavity of a fluid that characteristically contains scant amounts of protein and cells. Ascitic fluids with protein levels of less than 2.5 g/mL are considered to be transudates. Transudative ascites is indicative of cirrhosis or congestive heart failure rather than infection, inflammation, or a tumor.

**transurethral resection (TUR)** /trans′yoo̅re̅′thrəl/ [L, *trans* + Gk, *ourethra*, urethra; L, *re*, again, *secare*, to cut], the surgical removal of a structure performed through the urethra.

**transurethral resection of the prostate (TURP),** resection of the prostate by means of a cystoscope passed through the urethra.

**transvaginal** /trans·vaj′i·nəl/ [L, *trans*, across + *vagina*, sheath], performed through the vagina.

**transverse** /-vurs′/ [L, *transversus*, oblique], at right angles to the long axis of any common part, such as the planes that cut the long axis of the body into upper and lower parts and are at right angles to the sagittal and frontal planes.

**transverse colon,** the segment of the colon that extends from the end of the ascending colon at the hepatic flexure on the right side across the midabdomen to the beginning of the descending colon at the splenic flexure on the left side.

**transverse fissure,** a fissure dividing the dorsal surface of the diencephalon and the ventral surface of the cerebral hemisphere. Also called **fissure of Bichat.**

**transverse foramen** [L, *transversus* + *foramen*, hole], an opening through the transverse process of a cervical vertebra.

**transverse fracture,** a fracture that occurs at right angles to the longitudinal axis of the bone involved.

**transverse lie,** abnormal presentation of a fetus in which the long axis of the baby's body is across the long axis of the mother's body; unless the baby turns spontaneously or is turned by means of external or internal version, vaginal delivery is impossible.

**transverse ligament of the atlas,** a thick, strong ligament stretched across the ring of the atlas, holding the dens against the anterior arch. The transverse ligament divides the circular opening of the atlas into posterior and anterior parts. The posterior part transmits the spinal cord and its membranes; the anterior part contains the dens.

**transverse mesocolon** /mez′ōkō′lən/, a broad fold of the peritoneum connecting the transverse colon to the dorsal wall of the abdomen. It is continuous with the greater omentum along the ventral surface of the transverse colon and contains between its layers the vessels that supply the transverse colon. Its two layers diverge along the anterior border of the pancreas. Compare **mesentery proper, sigmoid mesocolon.**

**transverse myelitis** [L, *transversus* + Gk, *myelos*, marrow, *itis*, inflammation], an acute attack of spinal cord inflammation involving both sides of the cord.

**transverse palatine suture,** the line of junction between the processes of the maxilla and the horizontal parts of the palatine bones that form the hard palate.

**transverse plane,** any one of the planes cutting across the body perpendicular to the sagittal and the frontal planes, dividing the body into superior and inferior parts. Also called **cardinal horizontal plane.** Compare **frontal plane, median plane, sagittal plane.**

**transverse presentation** [L, *transversus* + *praesentare*, to show], a presentation of the fetal body in an oblique or transverse position across the birth canal.

**transverse relaxation time.** See **relaxation time.**

**transverse sinus,** one of a pair of large venous channels in the posterior superior group of sinuses serving the dura mater. Compare **confluence of the sinuses, inferior sagittal sinus, occipital sinus, straight sinus, superior sagittal sinus.**

**transversus abdominis** /-vur′səs/, one of a pair of transverse abdominal muscles that are the anterolateral muscles of the abdomen, lying immediately under the internal abdominal oblique. Arising from the inguinal ligament, the iliac crest, the thoracolumbar fascia, and the last six ribs, it inserts into the linea alba. It serves to constrict the abdomen and, by compressing the contents, to assist in micturition, defecation, emesis, parturition, and forced expiration. Compare **pyramidalis, rectus abdominis.**

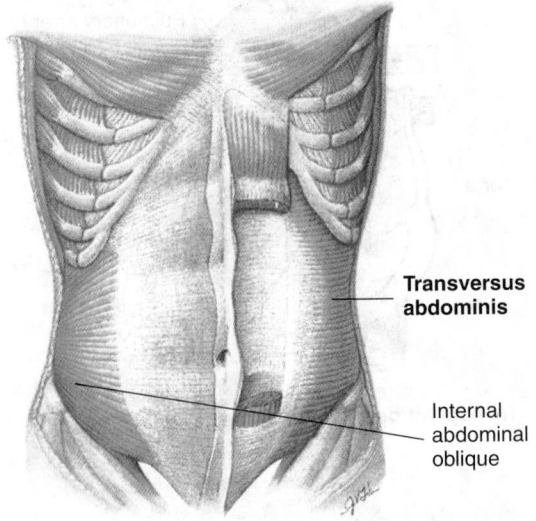

**Transversus abdominis**
*(Thibodeau and Patton, 1999/John V. Hagen)*

**transvestism** /-ves′tizəm/, a tendency to achieve psychic and sexual relief by dressing in the clothing of the opposite sex.

**Tranxene,** trademark for a benzodiazepine tranquilizer (clorazepate dipotassium).

**tranylcypromine sulfate** /tran′əlsip′rəmēn/, a monoamine oxidase inhibitor that acts as an antidepressant.

■ INDICATIONS: It is prescribed in the treatment of severe reactive or endogenous mental depression.

■ CONTRAINDICATIONS: Cerebrovascular or cardiovascular diseases, paranoid schizophrenia, liver dysfunction, alcoholism, pheochromocytoma, or known hypersensitivity to this drug prohibits its use. It is not given to children under 16 years of age.

■ ADVERSE EFFECTS: Among the most serious adverse reactions are severe hypertensive episodes that can be precipitated by ingestion of foods rich in tyramine or by concurrent administration of many sympathomimetic drugs. Common side effects include headache, vertigo, dry mouth, blurred vision, and orthostatic hypotension.

**trapeze bar** /trapēz′/, a triangular metal apparatus above a bed, used to help the patient move and support weight during transfer or position change.

**trapezium** /trəpē′zē·əm/, *pl.* **trapeziums, trapezia** [Gk, *trapezion,* small table], a carpal bone in the distal row of carpal bones. The trapezium articulates with the scaphoid proximally, the first metacarpal distally, and the trapezoideum and the second metacarpal medially. Also called **greater multangular, os trapezium.**

**trapezius** /trəpē′zē·əs/ [Gk, *trapezion,* small table], a large, flat triangular muscle of the shoulder and upper back. It arises from the occipital bone, the ligamentum nuchae, and the spinous processes of the seventh cervical and all the thoracic vertebrae. It acts to rotate the scapula, raise the shoulder, and abduct and flex the arm.

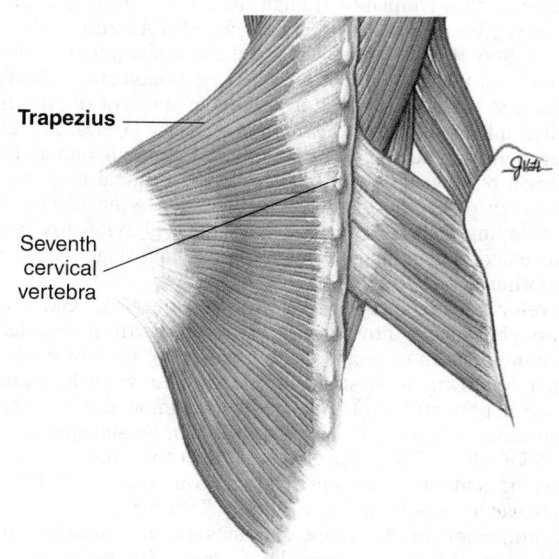

Trapezius

Seventh
cervical
vertebra

**Trapezius** *(Thibodeau and Patton, 1999/John V. Hagen)*

**trapezoid** /trap′əzoid/ [Gk, *trapezion,* small table, *eidos,* form], having the shape of a trapeze, an irregular four-sided figure with one set of parallel sides.

**trapezoidal arch** /trap′əzoidəl/ [Gk, *trapezion* + *eidos,* form; L, *arcus,* bow], a dental arch that has slightly less convergence than that of a tapering arch. The anterior teeth in the arch are somewhat square or abruptly rounded from tip to tip of the canines, which are at the corners of the arch.

**trapezoid bone** [Gk, *trapezion* + *eidos* + AS, *ban*], the smallest carpal bone, located in the distal row of carpal bones between the trapezium and the capitate. It resembles a wedge, with the broad end at the dorsal surface, the narrow end at the palmar surface. Also called **lesser multangular bone, os trapezoideum.**

**trastuzumab,** a miscellaneous antineoplastic.

■ INDICATIONS: Trastuzumab is used in the treatment of metastatic breast cancer with the overexpression of HER2.

■ CONTRAINDICATIONS: Factors that prohibit the use of trastuzumab include known hypersensitivity to this drug or to Chinese hamster ovary cell protein.

■ ADVERSE EFFECTS: Life-threatening effects of this drug are tachycardia, congestive heart failure, and leukopenia. Other adverse reactions include depression, insomnia, neuropathy, peripheral neuritis, acne, herpes simplex, nausea, vomiting, anorexia, diarrhea, anemia, arthralgia, bone pain, edema, peripheral edema, cough, dyspnea, pharyngitis, rhinitis, and sinusitis. Common side effects include dizziness, numbness, paresthesias, rash, and flulike syndrome (fever, headache, chills).

**trauma** /trou′mə, trô′mə/ [Gk, wound], **1.** physical injury caused by violent or disruptive action or by the introduction into the body of a toxic substance. **2.** psychic injury resulting from a severe emotional shock. —**traumatic,** *adj.,* **traumatize,** *v.*

**-trauma,** combining form meaning a 'wound or injury, psychic or physical': *arthrotrauma, barotrauma, neurotrauma.*

**trauma center,** a service providing emergency and specialized intensive care to critically ill and injured patients.

**trauma registry,** a repository of data on the incidence, diagnosis, and treatment of acute trauma victims treated by emergency service personnel.

**trauma, risk for,** a nursing diagnosis accepted by the Seventh National Conference on the Classification of Nursing Diagnoses. It is defined as the accentuated risk of accidental tissue injury, such as a wound, burn, or fracture.

■ RISK FACTORS: The risk factors may be internal (individual) or external (environmental). Internal risk factors include weakness; poor vision; balancing difficulties; reduced temperature or tactile sensation; reduced muscle or eye-hand coordination; lack of safety education, precautions, or equipment; cognitive or emotional difficulties; and history of previous trauma. External risk factors include slippery floors, stairs, or walkways (such as highly waxed, wet, or icy); a bathtub without hand grip or antislip equipment; unsteady chairs or ladders; defective electric wires or appliances; obstructed passageways; potential igniting gas leaks; unscreened fires or heaters; inadequately stored combustibles or corrosives; contact with intense cold or heat (such as very hot water); overexposure to sun, sunlamps, or radiotherapy; and exposure to dangerous machinery. Others include unsafe driving (drunk driving, excessive speeds, absent visual aids), nonuse or misuse of seat restraints, nonuse of headgear for motorized cyclists, and unsafe road or road-crossing conditions. Some external risk factors affecting children are a lack of safe stair rails or safety gates, unsafe window protection, highly flammable children's toys or clothing, and children playing with matches or fireworks. See also **nursing diagnosis.**

**traumatic** /trômat′ik/ [Gk, *trauma,* wound], pertaining to an injury, usually a serious and unexpected injury.

**traumatic abscess,** a pus collection that develops in tissue that has been damaged by a wound or injury.

**traumatic anesthesia** [Gk, *trauma* + *anaisthesia,* lack of feeling], a total lack of normal sensation in a part of the body, resulting from injury, destruction of nerves, or interruption of nerve pathways.

**traumatic delirium,** delirium after severe head injury, characterized by alertness and consciousness, with disorientation, confabulation, and amnesia apparent. See also **delirium.**

**traumatic dislocation** [Gk, *trauma*, wound; L, *dis* + *locare*], a dislocation caused by an injury.

**traumatic epilepsy** [Gk, *trauma*, wound, *epilepsia*, seizure], a form of motor or sensory seizures caused by a brain injury. Also called **posttraumatic epilepsy.**

**traumatic fever,** an elevation in body temperature secondary to mechanical trauma, particularly a crushing injury. Such fevers may last 1 or 2 days. The increased body temperature may help provide resistance to subsequent infection, and increased wound temperature may accelerate local healing.

**traumatic gangrene** [Gk, *trauma*, wound, *gaggraina*], gangrene that follows a severe injury resulting in damage to blood vessels.

**traumatic herpes** [Gk, *trauma*, wound, *herpein*, to creep], herpes that develops at the site of an injury.

**traumatic meningitis** [Gk, *trauma*, wound, *meninx*, membrane, *itis*, inflammation], meningitis that develops as a result of injury to the skull or spinal column.

**traumatic myelitis** [Gk, *trauma*, wound, *myelos*, marrow, *itis*, inflammation], a spinal cord inflammation resulting from an injury.

**traumatic myositis,** an inflammation of the muscles resulting from a wound or other trauma.

**traumatic neuritis** [Gk, *trauma*, wound, *neuron*, nerve, *itis*, inflammation], neuritis that is caused by injury to a nerve.

**traumatic neuroma,** a mass of nerve elements and fibrous tissue produced by the proliferation of Schwann cells and fibroblasts after severe injury to a nerve. A kind of traumatic neuroma is **amputation neuroma.**

**traumatic occlusion,** repeated excessive force in closure of the teeth that injures the teeth, the periodontal tissues, the residual ridge, or other oral structures. The closure extends beyond the reparative ability of the attachment apparatus (cementum, periodontal ligaments, and alveolar bone).

**traumatic psychosis** [Gk, *trauma*, wound, *psyche*, mind, *osis*, condition], a psychiatric disorder that results from injury to the head, with symptoms usually indicating brain trauma. It is differentiated from psychic trauma in which personality damage can be traced to an unpleasant experience such as sexual assault.

**traumatic rhabdomyolysis,** skeletal muscle destruction after a crush injury. During reperfusion of the damaged tissue after crushing pressure has been relieved, myoglobin, potassium, and phosphorus are released into the circulation, causing symptoms of renal failure, hypovolemic shock, and hyperkalemia.

**traumatic shock** [Gk, *trauma*, wound; Fr, *choc*], the emotional or psychologic state after trauma that may produce abnormal behavior. The most common types are hypovolemic shock from blood loss and neurogenic shock caused by a disruption of the integrity of the spinal cord.

**traumatic spondylopathy.** See **Kümmell's disease.**

**traumatic thrombosis** [Gk, *trauma*, wound, *thrombos*, lump, *osis*, condition], intravascular coagulation of a vein or other blood vessel after injury or irritation. The condition may develop as an adverse effect of an IV injection that damages the wall of a vein. See also **thrombophlebitis.**

**traumato-,** combining form meaning 'trauma, injury, wound': *traumatogenic, traumatopnea, traumatopyra.*

**traumatology** /trô′mətol′əjē/ [Gk, *trauma* + *logos*, science], **1.** the study of wounds and injuries. **2.** a surgical specialty dealing with the treatment of wounds, injuries, and resulting disabilities. —**traumatologic, traumatological,** *adj.*

**traumatopathy** /trô′mətop′əthē/ [Gk, *trauma* + *pathos*, disease], a pathologic condition resulting from a wound or injury. —**traumatopathic,** *adj.*

**traumatophilia** /trô′mətofil′ē·ə/ [Gk, *trauma* + *philein*, to love], a psychologic state in which the individual derives unconscious pleasure from injuries and surgical operations. —**traumatophiliac,** *n.,* **traumatophilic,** *adj.*

**traumatopnea** /trô′mətop′nē·ə/ [Gk, *trauma* + *pnein*, to breathe], partial asphyxia with collapse of the patient, caused by a penetrating thoracic wound permitting air to enter the pleural space and compress the lungs. Also called **open pneumothorax.**

**traumatopyra** /trô′mətōpī′rə/ [Gk, *trauma* + *pyr*, fire], an elevated temperature resulting from a wound or injury.

**traumatotherapy** /-ther′əpē/ [Gk, *trauma* + *therapeia*, treatment], the medical, surgical, and psychologic treatment of wounds, injuries, and disabilities resulting from trauma. —**traumatotherapeutic,** *adj.*

**traumatropism** /trômat′rəpiz′əm/ [Gk, *trauma* + *trepein*, to turn], the tendency of damaged tissue to attract microorganisms and promote their growth, frequently causing infections after injuries, especially burns.

**travail** /trəvāl′/ [OFr, *travaillier*, to work], **1.** physical or mental exertion, especially when distressful. **2.** (in obstetrics) the effort of labor and childbirth.

**Travase,** trademark for a proteolytic enzyme (sutilains).

**Travelbee, Joyce** (1926–1973), a nursing theorist who developed the Human-to-Human Relationship Model and theory, presented in her book *Interpersonal Aspects of Nursing* (1966, 1971). Travelbee based the assumptions of her theory on the concepts of logotherapy. Logotherapy theory was first proposed by Viktor Frankel, a survivor of Auschwitz, in his book *Man's Search for Meaning* (1963). Travelbee believed nursing is accomplished through human-to-human relationships that begin with the original encounter and then progresses through stages of emerging identities, developing feelings of empathy, and later of sympathy. The nurse and patient attain a rapport in the final stage. See also **logotherapy.**

**traveler's diarrhea** [OFr, *travailler*, to work; Gk, *dia*, through, *rhein*, to flow], any of several diarrheal disorders commonly seen in people visiting regions of the world other than their own. Some strains of *Escherichia coli*, which produce a powerful exotoxin, are the common cause. Other causative organisms include *Giardia lamblia* and species of *Salmonella* and *Shigella*. Symptoms last for a few days and include abdominal cramps, nausea, vomiting, slight fever, and watery stools. Relapse is rare. Treatment depends on identification of the cause and includes rehydration with beverages containing electrolytes. Preventive measures include using pure or boiled water and beverages for drinking and brushing the teeth and eating only fruits and vegetables with a skin or peel that can be removed and discarded before consumption. Also called **Montezuma's revenge, turista.**

**traverse** /travurs′/, **1.** to travel or pass across, over, or through. **2.** a single, complete movement of the x-ray tube around the object being scanned in computed tomography.

**TRBF,** abbreviation for **total renal blood flow.**

**Treacher Collins syndrome** [Edward Treacher Collins, English ophthalmologist, 1862–1919], an inherited disorder, characterized by mandibulofacial dysostosis. See also **Pierre Robin's syndrome.**

**treadmill stress test.** See **stress test.**

**treatment** [Fr, *traitement*], **1.** the care and management of a patient to combat, ameliorate, or prevent a disease, disorder, or injury. **2.** a method of combating, ameliorating, or preventing a disease, disorder, or injury. Active or curative treatment is designed to cure; palliative treatment is directed to relieve pain and distress; prophylactic treatment is for the prevention of a disease or disorder; causal treatment focuses on the cause of a disorder; conservative treatment avoids

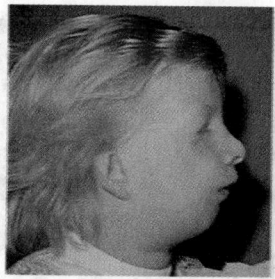

**Treacher Collins syndrome** *(Zitelli and Davis, 1997)*

radical measures and procedures; empiric treatment uses methods shown to be beneficial by experience; rational treatment is based on a knowledge of a disease process and the action of the measures used. Treatment may be pharmacologic, using drugs; surgical, involving operative procedures; or supportive, building the patient's strength. It may be specific for the disorder, or symptomatic to relieve symptoms without effecting a cure.

**treatment behavior: illness or injury,** a nursing outcome from the Nursing Outcomes Classification (NOC) defined as the personal actions to palliate or eliminate pathology. See also **Nursing Outcomes Classification.**

**treatment guardian,** a person who is appointed by the court for the purpose of consenting to or refusing medical treatment for a patient.

**treatment plan** [Fr, *traitement* + L, *planta*], (in dentistry) a schedule of procedures and appointments designed to restore, step by step, a patient's oral health. The plan contains the advantages, disadvantages, costs, alternatives, and sequelae of treatment. It must be presented to the patient for approval.

**treatment room,** a room in a patient care unit, usually in a hospital, in which various treatments or procedures requiring special equipment are performed, such as removing sutures, draining a hematoma, packing a wound, or performing an examination.

**Trecator-SC,** trademark for a tuberculostatic (ethionamide).

**Trechona** /trikōn′ə/, a genus of spiders, family Dipluridae, the bite of which is toxic and irritating to humans.

**tree** [AS, *treow*], **1.** (in anatomy) an anatomic structure with branches that spread out like those of a tree, such as the bronchial tree and the tracheobronchial tree. **2.** a pattern of searching for information in a computer data base, following a series of branching options from a general category to reach specific desired items while eliminating unwanted possibilities. MEDLINE and other computer data bases are organized in a 'logic tree' pattern.

**-trema,** **1.** combining form meaning a 'hole, orifice, opening': *gonotrema, helicotrema, peritrema.* **2.** combining form meaning 'creatures possessing an opening': *Eurytrema, Monotrema, Troglotrema.*

**Trematoda** /trem′ətō′də/, a class of flatworms, Platyhelminthes, that includes flukes. The adults are external or internal parasites of vertebrates. Intestinal infections in North America are rare except through flukes in foods imported from Asia or the tropics.

**trematode** /trem′ətōd/ [Gk, *trematodes*, pierced], any species of flatworm of the class Trematoda, some of which are parasitic to humans, infecting the liver, the lungs, and the intestines. Kinds of trematodes include the organisms causing **clonorchiasis, fascioliasis, paragonimiasis,** and **schistosomiasis.** See also **fluke.**

**trembles** /trem′bəls/, a toxic reaction experienced by cattle that have eaten white snakeroot or rayless goldenrod, pasture weeds that contain tremetone, a ketone. The toxic chemical is eliminated in the milk of the cows, causing sickness in humans who drink the milk.

**tremor** /trem′ər, trē′mər/ [L, shaking], rhythmic, purposeless, quivering movements resulting from the involuntary alternating contraction and relaxation of opposing groups of skeletal muscles occurring in some elderly individuals, certain families, and patients with various neurodegenerative disorders. Senile tremor is characterized by fine quick movements, especially of the hands, rhythmic head nodding, and increased trembling during purposeful movements. Familial tremor, which may be hereditary, and the tremor occurring in multiple sclerosis also increase during voluntary movement and may be intensified by anxiety, excitement, and self-consciousness. The tremors of Graves' disease, alcoholism, mercury poisoning, and other toxicoses are usually less rhythmic; the tremor in lead poisoning often affects the lips. The fine quick continuous tremor present in Parkinson's disease sometimes disappears during purposeful movements. Kinds of tremors are **resting tremor** and **intention tremor.**

**tremulous** /trem′yələs/ [L, *tremulare,* to tremble], pertaining to tremors, or involuntary muscular contractions.

**tremulous pulse** [L, *tremulare,* to tremble, *pulsare,* to beat], a feeble, fluttering pulse.

**trench fever** [OFr, *trenchier,* to cut; L, *febris,* fever], a self-limited infection, caused by *Bartonella,* a rickettsial organism transmitted by body lice, characterized by weakness, fever, rash, and leg pains. It was common during World War I but is now rare. Also called **quintana fever.**

**trench foot** [OFr, *trenchier,* to cut; AS, *fot*], a condition of moist gangrene of the foot caused by the freezing of wet skin.

**trench mouth.** See **acute necrotizing ulcerative gingivitis.**

**Trendelenburg gait** /trendel′ənbərg, tren′d(e)lənbŏŏrg′/ [Friedrich Trendelenburg, German surgeon, 1844–1924], an abnormal gait associated with a weakness of the gluteus medius. It is characterized by the dropping of the pelvis on the unaffected side of the body at the moment of heelstrike on the affected side. In this deviation the pelvic drop during the walking cycle lasts until heelstrike on the unaffected side and is accompanied by an apparent lateral protrusion of the affected hip. The person with a Trendelenburg gait also shortens the step on the unaffected side and displays a lateral deviation of the entire trunk and the affected side during the stance phase of the affected lower limb. This gait is one of the more common gait deviations. Also called **uncompensated gluteal gait.** Compare **compensated gluteal gait.**

**Trendelenburg position** [Friedrich Trendelenburg], a position in which the head is low and the body and legs are on an inclined plane. It is sometimes used in pelvic surgery to displace the abdominal organs upward, out of the pelvis, or

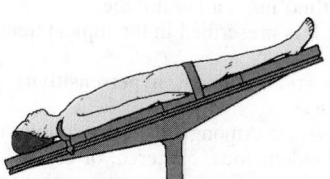

**Trendelenburg position**

to increase the blood flow to the brain in hypotension and shock.

**Trendelenburg test** [Friedrich Trendelenburg], a simple test for incompetent valves in a person who has varicose veins. The person lies down and elevates the leg to empty the vein, then stands, and the vein is observed as it fills. If the valves are incompetent, the vein fills from above; if the valves are normal, they do not allow backflow of blood, and the vein fills from below.

**Trental,** trademark for an oral hemorheologic drug (pentoxifylline).

**trepan.** See **trephine.**

**trephination** /trif′inā′shən/, the surgical excision of a circular piece of bone or other tissue accomplished with a cylindric saw.

**trephine** /trifīn′, trifēn′/ [Gk, *trypan*, to bore], a circular sawlike instrument used in removing pieces of bone or tissue, usually from the skull. Also called **trepan.**

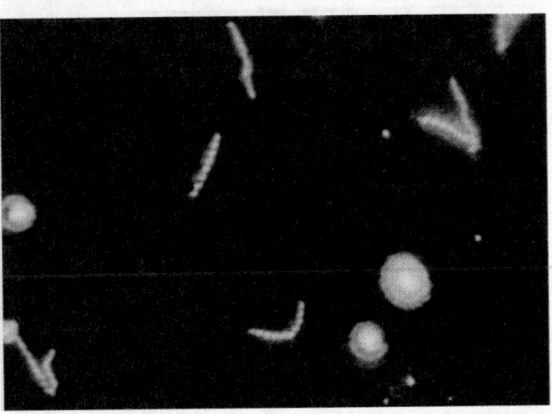
***Treponema pallidum*** *(Baron, Peterson, and Finegold, 1994)*

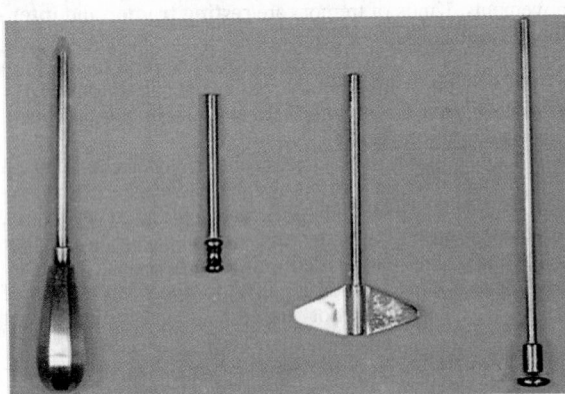
**Trephines** *(Aloia, 1993)*

**trepidation** /trep′idā·shən/ [L, *trepidare*, to tremble], a state of anxiety.

***Treponema*** /trep′ənē′mə/ [Gk, *trepein*, to turn, *nema*, thread], a genus of spirochetes, including some pathogenic to humans, such as the organisms causing bejel, pinta, syphilis, and yaws.

***Treponema pallidum***, an actively motile, slender spirochetal organism that causes syphilis.

**treponematosis** /trep′ənē′mətō′sis/, *pl.* **treponematoses** [Gk, *trepein* + *nema* + *osis*, condition], any disease caused by spirochetes of the genus *Treponema.* All these infections are effectively treated with penicillin; often one dose, given intramuscularly, results in cure. Kinds of treponematoses are **bejel, pinta, syphilis,** and **yaws.**

**-tresia,** combining form meaning 'perforation': *atresia, proctotresia, sphenotresia.*

**tretinoin** /tret′inō′in/, a keratolytic.
■ INDICATION: It is prescribed in the topical treatment of acne vulgaris.
■ CONTRAINDICATION: Known hypersensitivity to this drug prohibits its use.
■ ADVERSE EFFECTS: Among the more serious adverse reactions are red, edematous, blistered, or crusted skin.

**Trevor's disease.** See **dysplasia epiphysealis hemimelica.**

**Trexan,** trademark for an oral opioid antagonist (naltrexone hydrochloride).

**-trexate,** suffix for folic acid analogs used as antimetabolites.

**TRF,** abbreviation for **thyrotropin-releasing factor.** See **thyrotropin-releasing hormone.**

**TRH,** abbreviation for **thyrotropin-releasing hormone.**

**tri-,** prefix meaning 'three or thrice': *triage, tribrachia, tridermoma.*

**triacetin** /trī·as′itin/, an antifungal.
■ INDICATIONS: It is prescribed in the treatment of superficial fungus infections of the skin, including athlete's foot.
■ CONTRAINDICATIONS: There are no known contraindications.
■ ADVERSE EFFECTS: There are no known serious adverse effects.

**triacetyloleandomycin.** See **troleandomycin.**

**triad** /trī′əd/ [Gk, *trias*, three], a combination of three, such as two parents and a child.

**triage**[1] /trē·äzh′/ [Fr, *trier*, to sort out], **1.** (in military medicine) a classification of casualties of war and other disasters according to the gravity of injuries, urgency of treatment, and place for treatment. **2.** a process in which a group of patients is sorted according to their need for care. The kind of illness or injury, the severity of the problem, and the facilities available govern the process, as in a hospital emergency department. **3.** (in disaster medicine) a process in which a large group of patients is sorted so that care can be concentrated on those who are likely to survive.

**triage**[1], a Nursing Interventions Classification defined as establishing priorities of patient care for urgent treatment while allocating scarce resources. See also **Nursing Interventions Classification.**

**triage: disaster,** a nursing intervention from the Nursing Interventions Classification (NIC) defined as establishing priorities of patient care for urgent treatment while allocating scarce resources. See also **Nursing Interventions Classification.**

**triage: emergency center,** a nursing intervention from the Nursing Interventions Classification (NIC) defined as establishing priorities and initiating treatment for patients in an emergency center. See also **Nursing Interventions Classification.**

**triage: telephone,** a nursing intervention from the Nursing Interventions Classification (NIC) defined as determining the nature and urgency of a problem(s) and providing direc-

## Triage rating systems

**Five-tier system** (used in military triage)
Dead or will die
Life-threatening—readily correctable
Urgent—must be treated within 1 to 2 hours
Delayed—noncritical or ambulatory
No injury—no treatment necessary

**Four-tier system**
Immediate—seriously injured, reasonable chance of survival
Delayed—can wait for care after simple first aid
Expectant—extremely critical, moribund
Minimal—no impairment of function, can either treat self or be treated by a nonprofessional

**Three-tier system**
Life-threatening—readily correctable
Urgent—must be treated within 1 to 2 hours
Delayed—no injury, noncritical, or ambulatory

**Two-tier system**
Immediate versus delayed
Immediate—life-threatening injuries that are readily correctable on scene and those that are urgent
Delayed—no injury, noncritical injuries, ambulatory victims, moribund, or dead

tions for the level of care required, over the telephone. See also **Nursing Interventions Classification.**

**trial,** a process of quality testing.

**trial forceps** /trī′əl/ [Fr, *trier,* to sort out], an obstetric operation consisting of an attempt to deliver an infant with obstetric forceps. The forceps are applied to the baby's head, and moderate traction is applied. The delivery is continued only if the trial indicates that delivery can be accomplished safely. The procedure is abandoned if proper application of the forceps or rotation of the baby's head is not possible or if the trial indicates that completion of the delivery with forceps will require inordinately heavy traction likely to be more traumatic to mother or baby than cesarean section. Trial forceps is usually performed with a double setup so that cesarean section can be carried out immediately if necessary. Compare **failed forceps.** See also **double setup.**

**trial of labor** [Fr, *trier,* to sort out; L, *labor,* work], childbirth in which there is doubt as to whether the head of the fetus will pass through the pelvic brim. The situation must be monitored and assessed carefully to avoid fetal or maternal distress.

**triamcinolone** /trī′amsin′əlōn/, a corticosteroid.

■ INDICATIONS: It is prescribed as an antiinflammatory agent in the treatment of dermatoses, stomatitis, and lichen planus lesions.

■ CONTRAINDICATIONS: Fungal infections or known hypersensitivity to this drug prohibits its systemic use. Viral or fungal infections of the skin, impaired circulation, or known hypersensitivity to this drug prohibits its topical use.

■ ADVERSE EFFECTS: Among the more serious adverse reactions to the systemic administration of the drug are GI, endocrine, neurologic, fluid, and electrolyte disturbances. Skin reactions may occur from topical administration of this drug.

**triamterene** /trī·am′tərēn/, a potassium-sparing diuretic.

■ INDICATIONS: It is usually prescribed alone or with another diuretic in the treatment of edema, hypertension, and congestive heart failure.

■ CONTRAINDICATIONS: Anuria, severe liver or kidney dysfunction, hyperkalemia, or known hypersensitivity to this drug prohibits its use.

■ ADVERSE EFFECTS: Among the most serious adverse reactions are electrolyte disturbances, particularly hyperkalemia. GI disturbances also may occur.

**triangle** [L, *triangulus,* three-cornered], a predictable emotional process that takes place when there is difficulty in a relationship. Triangles represent dysfunctional efforts to reduce fusion or conflict in a relationship. The three corners of a triangle can be composed of three people or two people and an object, group, or issue.

**triangular bandage** /trī·ang′gyələr/, a square of cloth folded or cut into the shape of a triangle. It may be used as a sling, a cover, or a thick pad to control bleeding.

**triangular bone,** the pyramidal carpal bone in the proximal row on the ulnar side of the wrist. Also called **cuneiform bone, os triquetrum.**

**triangular dullness.** See **Korányi's sign.**

**triangularis** /trī·ang′gyōo·lar′is/ [L], triangular.

**Triavil,** trademark for a central nervous system fixed-combination drug containing a phenothiazine tranquilizer (perphenazine) and a tricyclic antidepressant (amitriptyline hydrochloride).

**triazolam** /tri·az′əlam/, a benzodiazepine hypnotic agent.

■ INDICATIONS: It is prescribed in the short-term treatment of insomnia.

■ CONTRAINDICATIONS: Known sensitivity to this drug or other benzodiazepines prohibits its use. It is not given to pregnant women, lactating mothers, or patients younger than 18 years.

■ ADVERSE EFFECTS: Among the most serious adverse reactions are anterograde amnesia, paradoxic reactions, tachycardia, depression, confusion or memory impairment, and visual disturbances.

**tribe** [L, *tribus*], a taxonomic division of organisms, subordinate to a family and superior to a genus, or subtribe.

**-tribe,** suffix meaning a 'surgical instrument used to crush a body part': *cephalotribe, sphenotribe, vasotribe.*

**tribology** /tribol′əjē/ [Gk, *tribo,* to rub, *logos,* science], the study of friction, wear, and lubrication of articulating surfaces.

**TRIC** /trik/, abbreviation for *trachoma inclusion conjunctivitis* agent, which refers to *Chlamydia trachomatis,* the organism that causes both inclusion conjunctivitis and trachoma. See also **Chlamydia.**

**tricarboxylic acid cycle.** See **citric acid cycle.**

**triceps brachii** /trī′seps brak′ē·ī/ [L, three-headed, *brachium,* arm], a large muscle that extends the entire length of the posterior surface of the humerus. Proximally it has a long head, a lateral head, and a medial head. The three parts of the muscle converge in a long tendon and insert in the posterior aspect of the olecranon. It functions to extend the forearm and to adduct the arm. Also called **triceps, triceps extensor cubiti.** Compare **biceps brachii.**

**triceps reflex,** a deep tendon reflex elicited by tapping sharply the triceps tendon proximal to the elbow with the forearm in a relaxed position. The response is a definite extension movement of the forearm. The reflex is accentuated by lesions of the pyramidal tract above the level of the seventh or eighth vertebra. See also **deep tendon reflex.**

**triceps skinfold,** the thickness of a fold of skin around the triceps muscle. It is measured primarily to estimate the amount of subcutaneous fat.

**triceps surae limp,** an abnormal action in the walking or gait cycle, associated with a deficiency in the elevating and propulsive factors on the affected side of the body, espe-

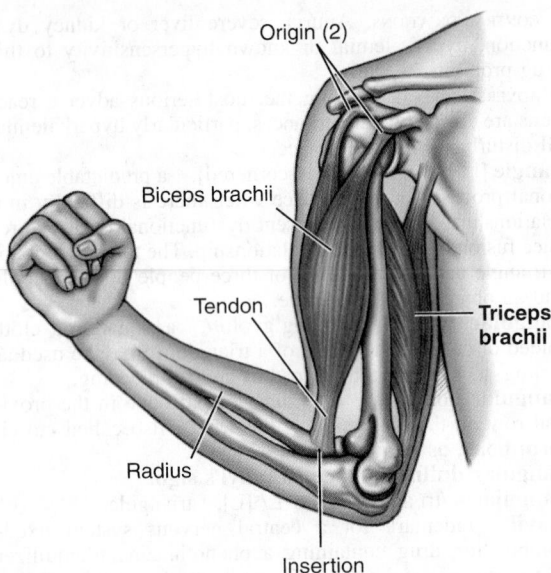

**Triceps brachii** *(Herlihy and Maebius, 2000)*

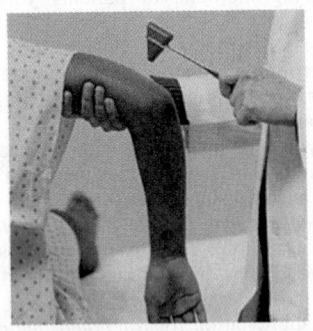

**Triceps reflex test** *(Seidel et al, 1999)*

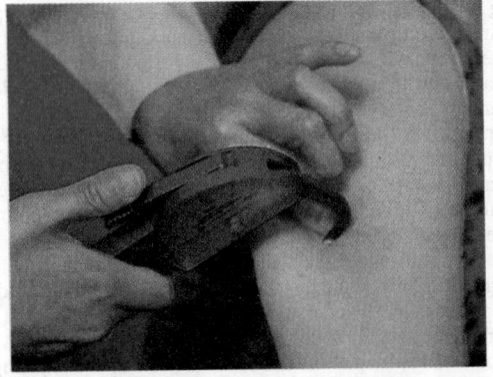

**Triceps skinfold measurement** *(Barkauskas et al, 1998)*

cially a deficiency of the triceps surae. Such a deficiency prevents the triceps surae from raising the pelvis and carrying it forward during the walking cycle. The pelvis consequently sags below its normal level and lags behind in the walking movement.

**trichi-, tricho-, -trichia, -trichosis,** combining forms meaning 'hair', *trichinosis, trichophagia, glossotrichia.*

**trichiasis** /trikī'əsis/ [Gk, *thrix,* hair, *osis,* condition], an abnormal inversion of the eyelashes that irritates the eyeball. It usually follows infection or inflammation. Compare **ectropion.**

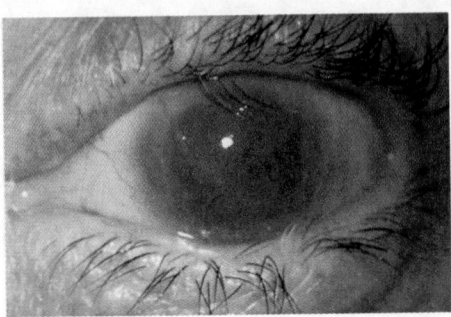

**Trichiasis in late trachoma** *(Stone and Gorbach, 2000)*

**trichinosis** /trik'inō'sis/ [Gk, *thrix + osis,* condition], infestation with the parasitic roundworm *Trichinella spiralis,* transmitted by eating raw or undercooked meat containing cysts (pork, bear, or other wild game). Early symptoms of infection include abdominal pain, nausea, fever, and diarrhea; later, muscle pain, tenderness, fatigue, and eosinophilia are observed. Light infections may be asymptomatic. Also called **trichinellosis, trichiniasis.**
■ OBSERVATIONS: Encysted larvae in improperly cooked pork mature in the intestines of the host, with mature worms depositing their larvae in the intestinal wall. The larvae penetrate the intestinal mucosa and move to other parts of the body through the blood and lymphatic systems, ultimately invading skeletal muscles, especially the diaphragm and the chest muscles, where they encyst. Larval penetration of the brain or heart may result in death. Serologic tests, skin sensitivity tests, and microscopic examination of specimens of infested muscle obtained by a biopsy often contribute to the diagnosis.
■ INTERVENTIONS: There is no specific treatment. Analgesics, thiabendazole, and corticosteroids may relieve symptoms. Bed rest is recommended to prevent relapse and possible death. After 2 or 3 months, the organisms are completely encysted and cause no further symptoms.

**trichiuriasis.** See **trichuriasis.**

**trichlormethiazide** /trī'klôrməthī'əzīd/, a thiazide diuretic and antihypertensive.
■ INDICATIONS: It is prescribed in the treatment of hypertension and edema.
■ CONTRAINDICATIONS: Anuria or known hypersensitivity to this drug, to thiazide medications, or to sulfonamide derivatives prohibits its use.
■ ADVERSE EFFECTS: Among the more serious adverse effects are hypokalemia, hyperglycemia, hyperuricemia, and various hypersensitivity reactions.

**trichloroethylene** /trīklôr′ō·eth′ilēn/, a general anesthetic, administered by mask with $N_2O$, for dentistry, minor surgery, and the first stages of labor. It is too cardiotoxic for deep anesthesia; even in light planes of anesthesia. It is not currently used in clinical anesthesia practice in developed countries.

**tricho-.** See **trichi-.**

**trichobasalioma hyalinicum.** See **cylindroma,** def. 2.

**trichoepithelioma** /trik′ō·ep′ithē′lē·ō′mə/, *pl.* **trichoepitheliomas, trichoepitheliomata** [Gk, *thrix* + *epi,* above, *thele* nipple, *oma* tumor], a cutaneous tumor derived from the basal cells of the follicles of fine body hair. One form of trichoepithelioma is an inherited condition and usually occurs as multiple growths. Also called **acanthoma adenoides cysticum, epithelioma adenoides cysticum.**

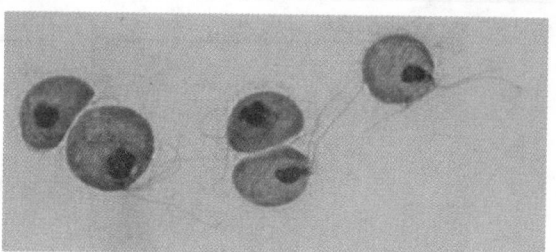
***Trichomonas vaginalis* trophozoites**
*(Cotran, Kumar, and Collins, 1999)*

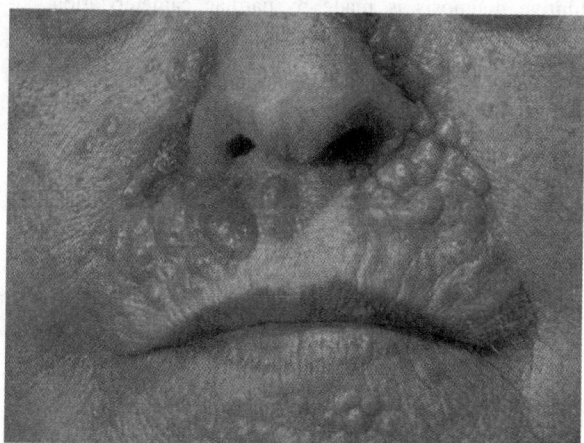
**Trichoepithelioma** *(Hordinsky, Sawaya, and Scher, 2000)*

**trichoid** /trik′oid/, resembling a hair.

**trichologia** /trik′əlō′jē·ə/ [Gk, *thrix* + *legein,* to pull], an abnormal condition in which a person pulls out his or her own hair, usually seen only in delirium.

**trichology** /trikol′əjē/, the study of the anatomy, development, and diseases of the hair.

**trichomania.** See **trichotillomania.**

**trichomatous** /trikom′ətəs/ [Gk, *trichoma,* hairy growth], **1.** pertaining to an introversion of the margin of the eyelid. **2.** pertaining to matted hair or ingrowing hair.

**trichomonacide** /trik′ōmon′əsīd/ [Gk, *thrix* + *monas,* unit; L, *caedere,* to kill], an agent destructive to *Trichomonas vaginalis,* a parasitic protozoan flagellate that causes a refractory type of vaginitis, cystitis, and urethritis. Metronidazole is used in the treatment of women with trichomoniasis and their asymptomatic partners. **—trichomonacidal,** *adj.*

*Trichomonas* /trik′əmon′əs/, a genus of flagellate protozoa, which includes many species that are parasitic. Some live in the mouth of humans and are found around carious teeth; other species are found in the vagina and urethra of women. They are a cause of trichomoniasis.

*Trichomonas tenax,* a species of protozoa that is found in the human mouth, particularly in cases of pyorrhea.

*Trichomonas vaginalis* [Gk, *thrix* + *monas* + L, *vagina,* sheath], a motile protozoan parasite that causes vaginitis with a copious malodorous discharge and pruritus. See also **trichomoniasis.**

**trichomoniasis** /trik′əmənī′əsis/ [Gk, *thrix* + *monas* + *osis,* condition], a vaginal infection caused by the protozoan *Trichomonas vaginalis.* It is characterized by itching, burning, and frothy, pale yellow to green, malodorous vaginal discharge. With chronic infection all symptoms may disappear, although the organisms are still present. In men infection is usually asymptomatic but may be evidenced by a persistent or recurrent urethritis. Infection is transmitted by sexual intercourse, rarely by moist washcloths, or, in newborns, by passage through the birth canal. Diagnosis is by microscopic examination of fresh vaginal secretions. Treatment is by oral metronidazole and tinidazole. Reinfection is common if sexual partners are not treated simultaneously.

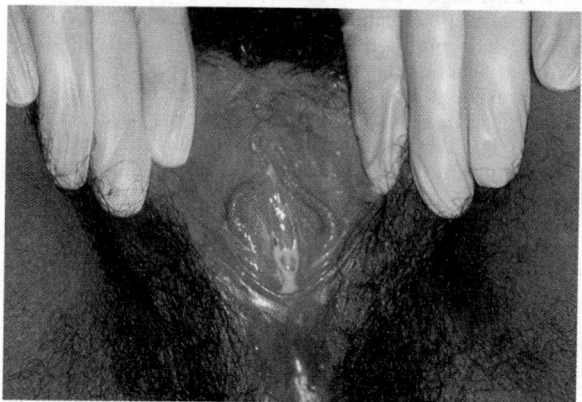
**Trichomoniasis vaginal discharge**
*(Monahan and Neighbors, 1998/courtesy Leonard Wolf, MD, New York)*

**trichopathy** /trikop′əthē/ [Gk, *thrix,* hair, *pathos,* disease], any disease condition involving the hair.

**trichophytic granuloma.** See **Majocchi's granuloma.**

*Trichophyton* /trikof′iton/ [Gk, *thrix* + *phyton,* plant], a genus of fungi that infects skin, hair, and nails. See also **dermatomycosis, dermatophyte.**

**trichosis** /trikō′sis/ [Gk, *thrix,* hair, *osis,* condition], any abnormal condition of hair growth, including alopecia, excessive female hair growth, or abnormal hair color.

**-trichosis.** See **trichi-.**

**trichosporosis** [Gk, *thrix,* hair, *spora,* seed, *osis,* condition], a fungus disease of the hair shaft, giving the hair a metallic

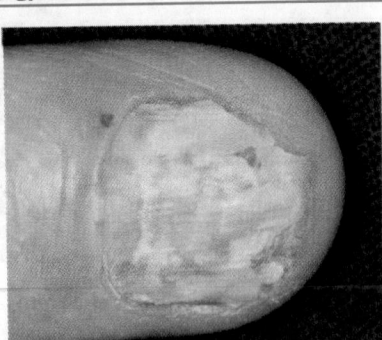

***Trichophyton rubrum*** *(Hordinsky, Sawaya, and Scher, 2000/courtesy Dr. J. Del Rosso, Las Vegas)*

appearance and caused by *Trichosporon biegetii.* Also called **white piedra.** See also **piedra.**

**trichostrongyliasis** /trik′ōstron′jəlī′əsis/ [Gk, *thrix* + *strongylos,* round, *osis,* condition], infestation with *Trichostrongylus,* a genus of nematode worm. Also called **trichostrongylosis.** See also **nematode.**

***Trichostrongylus*** /trik′ōstron′jiləs/ [Gk, *thrix* + *strongylos*], a genus of roundworm, some species of which are parasitic to humans, such as *T. orientalis.* See also **trichostrongyliasis.**

**trichotillomania** /trik′ōtil′ōmā′nē·ə/ [Gk, *thrix* + *tillein,* to pull, *mania* madness], an impulse disorder characterized by a desire to pull out one's hair, frequently seen in cases of severe mental retardation and delirium. Also called **trichomania, hair pulling.** See also **trichologia.** —**trichotillomanic, trichomanic,** *adj.*

**trichuriasis** /trik′yərī′əsis/ [Gk, *thrix* + *oura,* tail, *osis,* condition], infestation with the roundworm *Trichuris trichiura.* The condition is usually asymptomatic, but heavy infestation may cause nausea, abdominal pain, diarrhea, and occasionally anemia and rectal prolapse. It is common in tropical areas with poor sanitation. Eggs are passed in feces. Contamination of the hands, food, and water results in ingestion of the eggs, which hatch in the intestines where the adult worms embed two thirds of their length in the intestinal mucosa. The worms may live 15 to 20 years. Treatment is with mebendazole; prevention includes proper disposal of feces and good personal hygiene. Also called **trichiuriasis** /trik′ē-/.

***Trichuris*** /trikyŏŏr′is/ [Gk, *thrix* + *oura*], a genus of parasitic roundworms of which the species *T. trichiura* infects the intestinal tract. Adult worms, which are 30 to 50 mm long, resemble a whip, with a threadlike anterior and a thicker posterior. Also called **whipworm.** See also **trichuriasis.**

***Trichuris trichiura,*** a species of whipworms, commonly found in warm, moist regions of the world. Ingestion of whipworm eggs results in infection in humans; the parasites live mainly in the cecum or large intestine. Heavy infections cause symptoms of abdominal pain and diarrhea; very heavy infections may result in anemia because of intestinal blood loss.

**trick knee.** See **locked knee.**

**tricrotic pulse** /trīkrot′ik/, an abnormal pulse that has three peaks of elevation on a sphygmogram, representing the pressure wave from the heart in systole followed by two pressure waves in diastole.

**tricuspal.** See **tricuspid.**

**tricuspid** /trīkus′pid/ [Gk, *treis,* three; L, *cuspis,* point], **1.** pertaining to three points or cusps. **2.** pertaining to the tricuspid valve of the heart. **3.** a tooth with three points or cusps, rare in humans. Also called **tricuspal, trident, tridentate.**

**tricuspid area** [Gk, *treis,* three; L, *cuspis,* point], the region of the chest near the left lower sternum and opposite the fourth and fifth costal cartilages, where sounds of the tricuspid heart valve are best heard by auscultation. Also called **tricuspid-valve area.**

**tricuspid atresia,** a congenital cardiac anomaly characterized by the absence of the tricuspid valve so that there is no opening between the right atrium and right ventricle. Other cardiac defects, such as atrial and ventricular septal defects, are usually present, allowing some shunting of blood into the lungs. Clinical manifestations include severe cyanosis, dyspnea, anoxia, and signs of right-sided heart failure. Definitive diagnosis is made by cardiac catheterization, although radiographic studies usually reveal a small, underdeveloped right ventricle and large atria, giving the heart a round shape, and decreased pulmonary vascularity. Immediate palliative treatment includes pulmonary artery anastomoses to increase blood flow to the lungs and atrial septostomy if the atrial septal defect is small. Total corrective surgery has been successful in a limited number of older children.

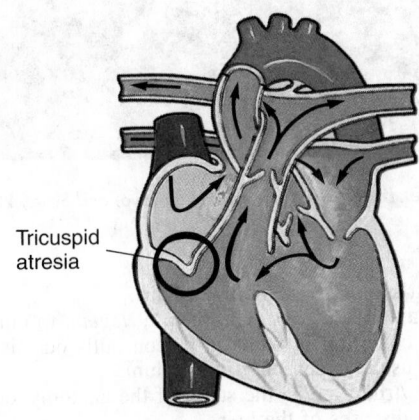

Tricuspid atresia

**Tricuspid atresia** *(Wong, 1999)*

**tricuspid murmur** [Gk, *treis,* three; L, *cuspis* point, *murmur,* humming], one of the heart murmurs caused by a defective tricuspid valve. The tricuspid diastolic and systolic murmurs resemble mitral valve diastolic and systolic murmurs.

**tricuspid regurgitation (TR)** [Gk, *treis,* three; L, *cuspis,* point plus; *re, gurgitare,* again to flow back], the backflow of blood from the right ventricle into the right atrium, resulting from imperfect functioning (insufficiency) of the tricuspid valve.

**tricuspid stenosis,** narrowing or stricture of the tricuspid valve. It is relatively uncommon and usually associated with lesions of other valves caused by rheumatic fever. Clinical characteristics include a diastolic pressure gradient between the right atrium and right ventricle, jugular vein distension, pulmonary congestion, and in severe cases hepatic congestion and splenomegaly.

**tricuspid valve,** a valve with three main cusps situated between the right atrium and right ventricle of the heart. The cusps of the tricuspid valve include the ventral, dorsal, and medial cusps. The cusps are composed of strong fibrous tissue and are anchored to the papillary muscles of the right ventricle by several tendons. As the right and left ventricles relax during the diastolic phase of the heartbeat, the tricuspid valve opens, allowing blood to flow into the ventricle. In the systolic phase of the heartbeat, both blood-filled ventricles contract, pumping out their contents, while the tricuspid and mitral valves close to prevent any backflow. Also called **right atrioventricular valve.** Compare **aortic valve, mitral valve, pulmonary valve, semilunar valve.** See also **atrioventricular valve, heart valve.**

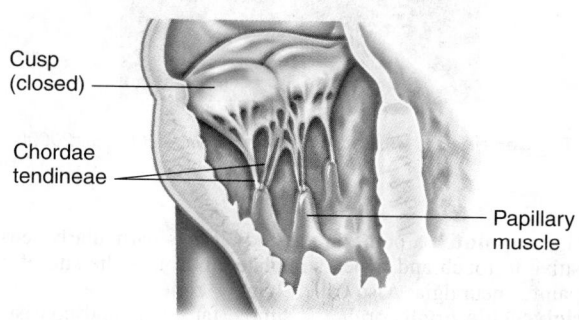

Cusp
(closed)

Chordae
tendineae

Papillary
muscle

**Tricuspid valve**

**tricuspid-valve area.** See **tricuspid area.**

**tricyclic antidepressant,** any of group of antidepressant drugs that contain three fused rings in their chemical structure and that potentiate the action of catecholamines; they block the reuptake of amine neurotransmitters, but their exact mechanism of their effect is unknown. The tricyclic antidepressants include a number of compounds, which may be grouped into four classes on the basis of chemical structure: dibenzazepines, dibenzocycloheptadienes, dibenzoxazepines, and dibenzoxepines. Besides their use to treat depression, various tricyclic antidepressants are used for other conditions, such as obsessive-compulsive disorder, panic disorder, and neurogenic pain.

**tricyclic compound** /trīsik′lik/ [Gk, *treis* + *kyklos,* circle; L, *componere,* to put together], a chemical substance containing three rings in the molecular structure, especially a tricyclic antidepressant drug used in the treatment of reactive or endogenous depression. These drugs also have anticonvulsant, antihistaminic, anticholinergic, hypotensive, and sedative effects. See also **antidepressant.**

**trident, tridentate.** See **tricuspid.**

**Tridesilon,** trademark for a glucocorticoid (desonide).

**tridihexethyl chloride** /trī′dīhek′səthil/, an anticholinergic antispasmodic.

■ INDICATIONS: It is prescribed in the treatment of GI muscle spasm and to reduce gastric secretion and GI motility.

■ CONTRAINDICATIONS: Narrow-angle glaucoma, asthma, obstruction of the genitourinary or GI tract, severe ulcerative colitis, or known hypersensitivity to this drug prohibits its use.

■ ADVERSE EFFECTS: Among the more serious adverse effects are blurred vision, tachycardia, dry mouth, decreased sweat-

ing, and hypersensitivity reactions. It may cause prostatic hypertrophy in elderly men.

**Tridione,** trademark for an anticonvulsant (trimethadione).

**trientine hydrochloride** /trī·en′tēn/, an oral medication for treatment of an inherited defect in copper metabolism (Wilson's disease).

■ INDICATIONS: It is prescribed for the relief of symptoms of Wilson's disease.

■ CONTRAINDICATIONS: Known hypersensitivity to this drug prohibits its use.

■ ADVERSE EFFECTS: The most serious side effects are possible iron deficiency and hypersensitivity reactions.

**triethanolamine polypeptide oleate-condensate** /trī-eth′-ənol′əmēn/, a ceruminolytic agent prescribed to reduce excessive earwax, used as a solution in propylene glycol. A possible serious adverse effect is severe contact dermatitis.

**trifacial nerve.** See **trigeminal nerve.**

**trifluoperazine hydrochloride** /trī′floo·ōper′əzēn/, a phenothiazine tranquilizer.

■ INDICATIONS: It is prescribed in the treatment of anxiety, schizophrenia, and other psychotic disorders and as an antiemetic.

■ CONTRAINDICATIONS: Parkinson's disease, concurrent administration of central nervous system depressants, hepatic or renal dysfunction, severe hypotension, or known hypersensitivity to this drug prohibits its use.

■ ADVERSE EFFECTS: Among the more serious adverse effects are hypotension, hepatotoxicity, extrapyramidal reactions, blood dyscrasias, and hypersensitivity reactions.

**trifluorothymidine** /trīfloor′ōthī′mədēn/, an antiviral. Also called **trifluridine.**

■ INDICATIONS: It is prescribed in the treatment of keratoconjunctivitis, herpetic keratitis, and other forms of keratitis caused by herpes simplex virus.

■ CONTRAINDICATIONS: Known hypersensitivity to this drug prohibits its use. Ocular toxicity may result from continued use beyond 21 days.

■ ADVERSE EFFECTS: Among the more serious adverse effects are hypersensitivity reactions, stromal edema, and increased ocular pressure.

**triflupromazine hydrochloride** /trī′floopprō′məzēn/, a phenothiazine tranquilizer/antiemetic.

■ INDICATIONS: It is prescribed in the treatment of severe agitation and other psychotic disorders and for the control of severe vomiting.

■ CONTRAINDICATIONS: Parkinson's disease, concurrent administration of central nervous system depressants, liver or renal dysfunction, severe hypotension, or known hypersensitivity to this drug or to other phenothiazine medications prohibits its use.

■ ADVERSE EFFECTS: Among the more serious adverse effects are hypotension, liver toxicity, extrapyramidal reactions, blood dyscrasias, and hypersensitivity reactions.

**trifluridine.** See **trifluorothymidine.**

**trifocal lens** /trīfō′kəl/ [Gk, *treis,* three; L, *focus,* hearth, *lens,* lentil], an eyeglass lens ground with three foci to allow correction of near, intermediate, and far vision.

**trifurcation** /-furkā′shən/ [Gk, *treis,* three; L, *furca,* fork], pertaining to a vessel or other structure with three branches.

**trigeminal** /trījem′inəl/ [Gk, *treis,* three; L, *geminus,* twins], pertaining to the three-branch trigeminal (fifth cranial) nerve innervating the face, eyes, nose, mouth, and jaws.

**trigeminal nerve** [Gk, *treis* + *geminus,* twin], either of the largest pair of cranial nerves, essential for the act of chewing, general sensibility of the face, and muscular sensibility of the obliquus superior. The trigeminal nerves have sensory, motor, and intermediate roots and connect to three

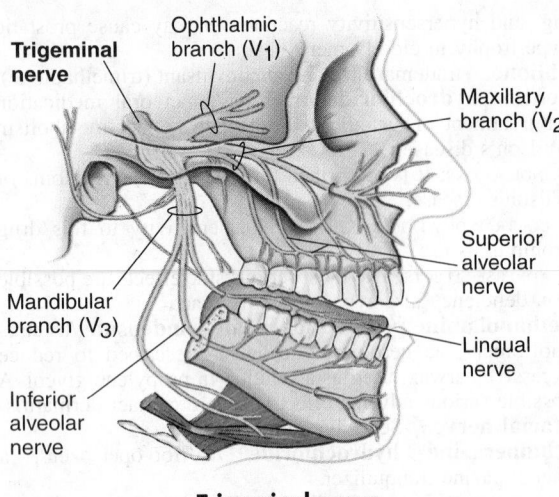

**Trigeminal nerve**

Ophthalmic branch (V₁)
Trigeminal nerve
Maxillary branch (V₂)
Superior alveolar nerve
Mandibular branch (V₃)
Lingual nerve
Inferior alveolar nerve

areas in the brain. Also called **fifth cranial nerve, nervus trigeminus, trifacial nerve, trigeminus.**

**trigeminal neuralgia,** a neurologic condition of the trigeminal facial nerve, characterized by paroxysms of flashing, stablike pain radiating along the course of a branch of the nerve from the angle of the jaw. It is caused by degeneration of the nerve or by pressure on it. Any or all of the three branches of the nerve may be affected. Neuralgia of the first branch results in pain around the eyes and over the forehead; of the second branch, in pain in the upper lip, nose, and cheek; of the third branch, in pain on the side of the tongue and the lower lip. The momentary bursts of pain recur in clusters lasting many seconds; paroxysmal episodes of the pains may last for hours. Also called **prosopalgia, tic douloureux.**

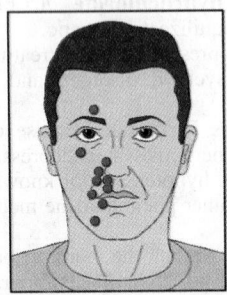

**Trigeminal neuralgia: distribution of trigger zones**
(Perkin, 1998)

**trigeminal pulse,** an abnormal pulse in which every third beat is absent. See also **bigeminal pulse, trigeminy.**

**trigeminus.** See **trigeminal nerve.**

**trigeminy** /trījem′inē/ [Gk, *treis* + L, *geminus,* twin], **1.** a grouping in threes. **2.** a cardiac arrhythmia characterized by the occurrence of three heartbeats in a repeating pattern: two normal beats coupled to an ectopic beat, or two ectopic beats coupled to a normal beat. —**trigeminal,** *adj.*

**trigger** [D, *trekker,* that which pulls], a substance, object, or agent that initiates or stimulates an action.

**triggered activity** [D, *trekker,* that which pulls; L, *activus*], rhythmic cardiac activity that results when a series of after depolarizations reach the threshold potential.

**trigger finger,** a phenomenon in which the movement of a finger is halted momentarily in flexion or extension and then continues with a jerk. Also called **jerk finger.**

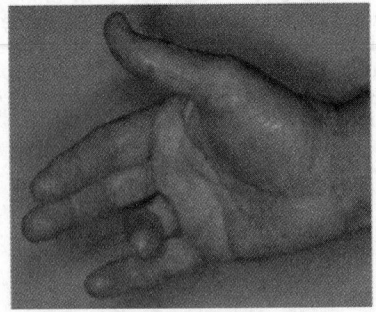

**Trigger finger, locked position** (Lemmi and Lemmi, 2000)

**trigger point,** a point on the body that is particularly sensitive to touch and, when stimulated, becomes the site of a painful neuralgia. Also called **trigger zone.**

**triglyceride** /trīglis′ərīd/, a simple fat compound consisting of three molecules of fatty acid (e.g., oleic, palmitic, or stearic) and glycerol. Triglycerides make up most animal and vegetable fats and are the principal lipids in the blood, where they circulate, within lipoproteins. The total amount of triglyceride and the amount, proportion, and kinds of lipoproteins are important in the diagnosis and treatment of many diseases and conditions, including diabetes, hypertension, and heart disease. Normally the total amount of triglyceride in the blood does not exceed 200 mg to 300 mg/dL.

**triglycerides test (TGs),** a blood test that detects levels of fats existing within the bloodstream that are transported by very low-density lipoproteins (VLDLs) and low-density lipoproteins (LDLs). It is done as part of a lipid profile, which also evaluates cholesterol and lipoproteins to assess the risk of coronary and vascular disease.

**trigone** /trī′gōn/ [Gk, *trigonos,* three-cornered], **1.** a triangular space, especially one at the base of the shoulder. **2.** the first three dominant cusps, considered collectively, of an upper molar.

**trigonelline** /trig′ōnel′ēn/, an alkaloid derived from various kinds of plant products, including coffee beans, fenugreek, and seeds of *Cannabis sativa,* as well as from sea urchins and jellyfish. Trigonelline is used in the manufacture of poultices and other medicinals.

**trigone of the bladder** /trīgō′n/, a triangular area of the bladder between the opening of the ureters and the orifice of the urethra. Also called **trigonum vesicae**

**trigonitis** /trī′gənī′tis/, inflammation of the trigone of the bladder, which often accompanies urethritis.

**trigonum vesicae.** See **trigone of the bladder.**

**trihexyphenidyl hydrochloride** /trīhex′ifen′idil/, an anticholinergic agent.

■ INDICATIONS: It is prescribed in the treatment of Parkinson's disease and to control drug-induced extrapyramidal reactions.

■ CONTRAINDICATIONS: Narrow-angle glaucoma, asthma, obstruction of the genitourinary or GI tract, severe ulcerative colitis, or known hypersensitivity to this drug prohibits its use.

■ ADVERSE EFFECTS: Among the more serious adverse effects are blurred vision, central nervous system effects, tachycardia, dry mouth, decreased sweating, and hypersensitivity reactions.

**trihybrid** /trīhī′brid/ [Gk, *treis* + *hybrida,* mixed offspring], pertaining to an individual, organism, or strain that is heterozygous for three specific traits, that is the offspring of parents differing in three specific gene pairs, or that is heterozygous for three particular traits or gene loci being followed.

**trihybrid cross,** the mating of two individuals, organisms, or strains that have different gene pairs that determine three specific traits or in which three particular characteristics or gene loci are being followed.

**trihydric alcohol** /trīhid′rik/, an alcohol containing three hydroxyl groups. An example is **glycerin.**

**triiodothyronine (T3)** /trī′ī·ō′dōthī′rənēn/, a hormone that helps regulate growth and development, helps control metabolism and body temperature, and, by a negative-feedback system, acts to inhibit the secretion of thyrotropin by the pituitary gland. Triiodothyronine is produced mainly from the metabolism of thyroxine in the peripheral tissues but is also synthesized by and stored in the thyroid gland as an amino acid residue of the protein thyroglobulin. Triiodothyronine circulates in the plasma, where it is bound mainly to thyroxine-binding globulin and thyroxine-binding prealbumin, proteins that protect the hormone from metabolism and excretion during its half-life of 2 days or less before it is degraded in the liver. The hormone is the most active thyroid hormone and affects all body processes, including gene expressions. It is a component of various drugs, such as liotrix and liothyronine sodium, used in the treatment of hypothyroidism and simple goiter. Normal adult blood levels are 110 to 230 ng/dL. See also **thyroid hormone.**

**triiodothyronine (T3) test,** a test used to accurately measure thyroid function. Since nonthyroidal diseases can convert $T_4$ to $T_3$ in the liver, and because there is considerable overlap between hypothyroid states and normal thyroid function, $T_3$ is less useful in indicating hypothyroid states. It is used primarily to determine hyperthyroidism.

**Trilafon,** trademark for a phenothiazine tranquilizer (perphenazine).

**trilaminar blastoderm** /trīlam′inər/ [Gk, *treis* + L, *lamina,* plate; Gk, *blastos,* germ, *derma,* skin], the stage of embryonic development in which all three of the primary germ layers, the ectoderm, mesoderm, and entoderm, have formed. Compare **bilaminar blastoderm.**

**trill** [It, *trillare* to make a ringing sound], a vibratory, quavering, warbling sound, as produced by human voice, birds, insects, or musical instruments.

**trilogy of Fallot** /tril′əjē, falō′/ [Gk, *treis* + *logos,* word; Etienne-Louis A. Fallot, French physician, 1850–1911], a congenital cardiac anomaly consisting of pulmonary stenosis, interatrial septal defect, and right ventricular hypertrophy. For discussion of diagnosis and treatment, see **tetralogy of Fallot.**

**trimalleolar fracture.** See **Cotton's fracture.**

**trimester** /trīmes′tər, trī′-/ [L, *trimestris,* three months], one of the three periods of approximately 3 months into which pregnancy is divided. The first trimester includes the time from the first day of the last menstrual period to the end of 12 weeks. The second trimester, closer to 4 months in length than 3, extends from the twelfth to the twenty-eighth week of gestation. The third trimester begins at the twenty-eighth week and extends to the time of delivery.

**trimethadione** /trī′methədī′ōn/, an anticonvulsant.

■ INDICATIONS: It is prescribed to prevent seizures in petit mal epilepsy, particularly seizures that are resistant to other therapies.

■ CONTRAINDICATIONS: Severe renal or hepatic impairment, blood dyscrasias, or known hypersensitivity to this drug prohibits its use.

■ ADVERSE EFFECTS: Among the more serious adverse reactions are exfoliative dermatitis, blood dyscrasias, and aplastic anemia. Sedation and hemeralopia may occur.

**trimethaphan camsylate** /trīmeth′əfan/, a ganglionic blocking agent.

■ INDICATIONS: It is prescribed to produce controlled hypotension during surgery and to lower blood pressure in hypertensive emergencies.

■ CONTRAINDICATIONS: It is not used where hypotension places a patient in undue risk or when hypersensitivity to this drug prohibits its use.

■ ADVERSE EFFECTS: The most serious adverse reaction is severe hypotension.

**trimethobenzamide hydrochloride** /trīmeth′ōben′zəmīd/, an anticholinergic and antiemetic.

■ INDICATION: It is prescribed for the relief of nausea and vomiting.

■ CONTRAINDICATIONS: Reye's syndrome or known hypersensitivity to this drug prohibits its use.

■ ADVERSE EFFECTS: Among the most serious adverse reactions with high doses are drowsiness, diarrhea, allergic reactions, and extrapyramidal reactions. Adverse reactions are rare at usual dosages.

**trimethoprim** /trīmeth′əprim/, an antibacterial.

■ INDICATIONS: It is prescribed in the treatment of infections, particularly of the urinary tract, middle ear, and bronchi.

■ CONTRAINDICATIONS: Known hypersensitivity to this drug prohibits its use. It should not be used to treat streptococcal pharyngitis.

■ ADVERSE EFFECTS: Among the more serious adverse reactions are blood dyscrasias and allergic, GI, and central nervous system disorders.

**trimethoprim and sulfamethoxazole.** See **sulfamethoxazole and trimethoprim.**

**trimipramine maleate** /trimip′rəmēn/, an antidepressant.

■ INDICATIONS: It is prescribed in the treatment of anxiety, depression, and insomnia.

■ CONTRAINDICATIONS: Concomitant use of a monoamine oxidase inhibitor within 14 days or known hypersensitivity to this drug prohibits its use. It is not given during recovery from myocardial infarction or to schizophrenic patients. It is not recommended for children.

■ ADVERSE EFFECTS: Among the more serious adverse reactions are tachycardia, seizures, parkinsonism, blurred vision, hypotension, and aggravation of glaucoma.

**Trimox,** trademark for an antibiotic (amoxicillin trihydrate).

**Trimpex,** trademark for an antibacterial (trimethoprim).

**Trinalin Repetabs,** trademark for an antihistamine (azatadine maleate).

**Trinsicon,** trademark for a hematinic fixed-combination drug containing iron, vitamin $B_{12}$, and intrinsic factor concentrate.

**trinucleotide.** See **codon.**

**trioxsalen** /trī·ok′sələn/, a melanizing agent.

■ INDICATIONS: It is prescribed to enhance pigmentation, for repigmentation of the skin in idiopathic vitiligo, and to increase tolerance to sunlight.

■ CONTRAINDICATIONS: Diseases associated with photosensitivity, such as porphyria, acute lupus erythematosus, or leukoderma of infectious origin, or the concomitant use of drugs having any photosensitizing activity prohibits its use.

■ ADVERSE EFFECTS: Among the most serious adverse reactions are severe burns from excessive exposure to ultraviolet light. Gastric irritation and nausea also may occur.

**tripelennamine hydrochloride** /trī'pelen'əmēn/, an antihistamine.

■ INDICATIONS: It is prescribed in the treatment of rhinitis and hypersensitivity reactions of the skin.

■ CONTRAINDICATIONS: Asthma, glaucoma, difficulty in emptying the bladder, concomitant administration of a monoamine oxidase inhibitor, or known hypersensitivity to this drug prohibits its use. It is not given to premature or newborns or to lactating mothers.

■ ADVERSE EFFECTS: Among the more serious adverse reactions are sedation, tachycardia, and GI upset.

**tripe palms,** a condition of thickened velvet or moss-textured palms with pronounced skin ridge pattern. Tripe palms has been associated with certain malignancies, including lung and stomach cancers and pulmonary carcinomas.

**triphasic** /trīfā'zik/ [Gk, *treis,* three, *phasis,* appearance], having three phases or stages.

**triple-dye treatment,** a therapy for burns in which three dyes, 6% gentian violet, 1% brilliant green, and 0.1% acriflavine base, are applied.

**triplegia** /trīplē'jə/ [Gk, *treis,* three, *plege,* stroke], a condition of paralysis on one side of the body plus paralysis of an arm or leg on the opposite side.

**triple lumen catheter** [L, *triplus,* triple; L, *lumen,* light; Gk, *katheter,* a thing lowered into], any catheter with three separate passages. In a triple-lumen urinary catheter, one passage is for irrigation, one for drainage, and one for inflation of the bulb.

**triple point,** the combination of temperature and pressure in which a given substance may exist in solid, liquid, and vapor forms at the same time. Every substance has a theoretic triple point.

**triple response,** a triad of phenomena that occur in sequence after the intradermal injection of histamine. First, a red spot develops, spreading outward for a few millimeters, reaching its maximal size within 1 minute and then turning bluish. Next, a brighter red flush of color spreads slowly in an irregular flare around the original red spot. Finally, a wheal filled with fluid forms over the original spot. Also called **triple response of Lewis.**

**triple sugar iron reaction,** any one of several reactions seen in certain bacterial cultures growing on triple sugar iron agar, a culture medium used to aid in the identification of *Escherichia coli, Proteus, Salmonella, Shigella,* and other pathogenic enteric bacteria.

**triple sulfonamides.** See **trisulfapyrimidines.**

**triplet** /trip'lit/ [L, *triplus*], **1.** any one of three offspring born of the same gestation period during a single pregnancy. See also **Hellin's law. 2.** (in genetics) the unit of three consecutive bases in one polynucleotide chain of deoxyribonucleic acid or RNA that codes for a specific amino acid. See also **codon, genetic code.**

**triple X syndrome.** See **XXX syndrome.**

**triploid** (3*n*) /trip'loid/ [L, *triplus* + *eidos*], **1.** an individual, organism, strain, or cell that has three complete sets of chromosomes, triple the haploid number characteristic of the species. In humans the triploid number is 69; it is found in rare cases of aborted or stillborn fetuses. Of triploid fetuses born alive, all are characterized by gross and multiple malformations; they live for only a few hours. **2.** also **triploidic.** pertaining to such an individual, organism, strain, or

cell. Compare **diploid, haploid, tetraploid.** See also **polyploid. —triploidy,** *n.*

**triploidy** /trip'loidē/, the state or condition of having three complete sets of chromosomes.

**tripod** /trī'pod/ [Gk, *treis,* three, *pous,* foot], any object with three legs or three feet.

**tripodial symmelia** /trīpō'dē·əl/ [Gk, *treis,* three, *pous,* foot, *syn,* together, *melos,* limb], a fetal anomaly characterized by the fusion of the lower extremities and the presence of three feet.

**triprolidine hydrochloride** /trī-prol'idēn/, an antihistamine.

■ INDICATIONS: It is prescribed in the treatment of hypersensitivity reactions, including rhinitis, skin rash, and pruritus.

■ CONTRAINDICATIONS: Asthma or known hypersensitivity to this drug prohibits its use. It is not given to newborns or lactating mothers. Adverse reactions may occur in elderly patients.

**tripsis** /trip'sis/ [Gk rubbing], **1.** massage. **2.** the process of reducing the particle size of a substance by grinding it with a mortar and pestle. Also called **trituration.**

**-tripsis,** combining form meaning 'to crush, break, or pulverize': *anatripsis, entripsis, syntripsis.*

**-tripsy,** combining form meaning 'to crush, break, or pulverize': *basiotripsy, lithotripsy, sarcotripsy.*

**trisaccharide** /trīsak'ərīd/ [Gk, *treis,* three, *sakcharon,* sugar], a carbohydrate composed of three monosaccharide units linked together.

**trismus** /triz'məs/ [Gk, *trismos,* gnashing], a prolonged tonic spasm of the muscles of the jaw. Also called (*informal*) **lockjaw.** See also **tetanus.**

**trisomy** /trī'səmē/ [Gk, *treis* + *soma,* body], a chromosomal aberration characterized by the presence of one more than the normal number of chromosomes in a diploid complement; in humans the trisomic cell contains 47 chromosomes and is designated $2n + 1$. The additional member can join any of the normal homologous pairs, although most human trisomies involve the small chromosomes such as those in the E or G group or the sex chromosomes. Partial trisomy occurs when only a part of a chromosome attaches to another. In genetic nomenclature trisomies are indicated by the exact chromosome or karyotypic group in which the addition is made, such as trisomy 13 or trisomy D. Also called **trisomia.** Compare **monosomy.** See also **aneuploidy, multipolar mitosis, trisomy syndrome. —trisomic,** *adj.*

**trisomy 8,** a congenital condition associated with the presence of an extra chromosome 8 within the C group. Those with the condition are slender and of normal height and have a large asymmetric head, prominent forehead, deep-set eyes, low-set prominent ears, and thick lips. There is mild to severe mental and motor retardation, often with delayed and poorly articulated speech. Skeletal anomalies and joint limitation, especially permanent flexion of one or more fingers, may occur. There are unusually deep palmar and plantar creases, which are diagnostically significant. Most trisomy 8 individuals are mosaic, with no abnormal or only slight clinical manifestations, or they are only partially trisomic, with part of the extra chromosome 8 missing, and show varying degrees of the clinical symptoms. In general, trisomy 8 is a less severe condition than other trisomies, especially trisomy 13 and trisomy 18, so that mortality is low. Also called **trisomy C syndrome.**

**trisomy 13,** a congenital condition caused by the presence of an extra chromosome in the D group, predominantly chromosome 13, although in rare instances chromosome 14 or 15. It occurs in approximately 1 in 5000 births and is characterized by multiple midline anomalies and central nervous system defects, including holoprosencephaly, microcephaly, myelomeningocele, microphthalmos, and cleft lip and palate. There is also severe mental retardation; polydactyly; deafness; convulsions; and abnormalities of the heart, viscera, and genitalia. Most infants with the condition are severely affected and do not survive beyond the first 6 months of life. The symptom combination of cleft lip/palate, polydactylism, and microcephaly is sometimes identified as the triad. Also called **Patau's syndrome, trisomy D syndrome, trisomy 13-15.**

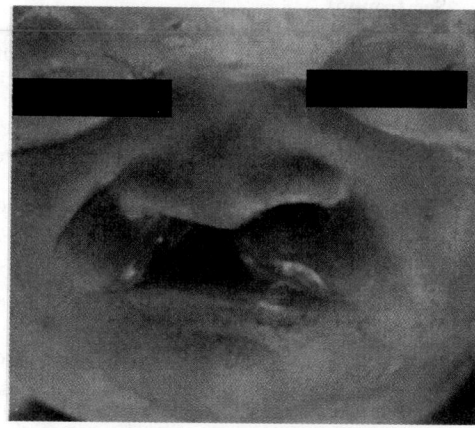

**Trisomy 13: midline defect**
*(Zitelli and Davis, 1997/courtesy Dr. T. Kelly, University of Virginia Medical Center, Charlottesville)*

**trisomy 18,**   a congenital condition caused by the presence of an extra chromosome 18, characterized by severe mental retardation and multiple deformities. Among the most common defects are scaphocephaly or other skull abnormalities; micrognathia; abnormal facies with low-set malformed ears and prominent occiput; cleft lip and palate; clenched fists with overlapping fingers, especially the index over the third finger; clubfeet; and syndactyly. Ventricular septal defect, patent ductus arteriosus, atrial septal defect, and renal anomalies are also common. The condition occurs in about 1 in 3000 births and predominantly in females, according to a 3:1 sex ratio, and survival for more than a few months is

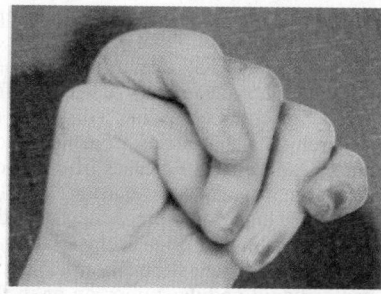

**Trisomy 18: clenched hand showing the typical pattern of overlapping fingers**
*(Zitelli and Davis, 1997)*

rare. Also called **Edwards' syndrome, trisomy E syndrome, trisomy 16-18.**

**trisomy 21.**   See **Down syndrome.**

**trisomy 22,**   a congenital condition caused by the presence of an extra chromosome 22 in the G group, characterized by psychomotor retardation and various developmental anomalies. Common defects include microcephaly, micrognathia, hypotonia, hypertelorism, abnormal ears with preauricular tags or fistulas, and congenital heart disease. In partial trisomy 22 the extra chromosome is much smaller than the normal pair and causes coloboma of the iris, anal atresia, or both, as well as various other defects. See also **cat-eye syndrome.**

**trisomy C syndrome.**   See **trisomy 8.**

**trisomy D syndrome.**   See **trisomy 13.**

**trisomy E syndrome.**   See **trisomy 18.**

**trisomy syndrome,**   any condition caused by the addition of an extra member to a normal pair of homologous autosomes or to the sex chromosomes or by the translocation of a part of one chromosome to another. Most trisomies occur as a result of complete or partial nondisjunction of the chromosomes during cell division. The more severe conditions are related to trisomies of the autosomes rather than the sex chromosomes. The most common trisomy syndromes with clearly established clinical manifestations are trisomy 8, trisomy 13, trisomy 18, trisomy 21, and trisomy 22. See also **trisomy.**

**Trisoralen,**   trademark for a pigmentation agent (trioxsalen).

**trisplanchnic** /trīsplangk′nik/,   pertaining to three visceral body cavities: skull, thorax, and abdomen.

**trisulfapyrimidines** /trīsul′fəpirim′idīnz/,   three antibacterials in combination (sulfadiazine, sulfamerazine, and sulfamethazine), rarely prescribed today.

**tritium ($^3$H)** /trit′ē·əm, trish′əm/ [Gk, *tritos,* third],   the radioactive isotope of the hydrogen atom, used as a tracer; a β emitter. See also **deuterium.**

**trituration.**   See **tripsis.**

**trivalence** /trīvā′ləns/ [Gk, *treis* + L, *valere,* to be worth],   a triple state, an ability of a group of atoms to replace three monovalent elements in a compound.

**trivalent** /trīvā′lənt/ [Gk, *treis* + L, *valere,* to be worth],   **1.** pertaining to an atom or group of atoms with the capability of bonding with or replacing three monovalent elements. **2.** designating a vaccine that can prevent diseases or conditions.

**trivial name** /triv′ē·əl/,   a chemical name that lacks a systematic notation that would indicate its molecular structure or other information about its relationship to other chemicals. The name may be accepted as an official nonproprietary designation because of common usage. Examples include caffeine, folic acid, and aspirin.

**Tri-Vi-Flor,**   trademark for an oral pediatric fixed-combination drug containing sodium fluoride and vitamins A, C, and D.

**tRNA,**   abbreviation for **transfer RNA.**

**Trobicin,**   trademark for an antibacterial (spectinomycin hydrochloride).

**trocar** /trō′kär/ [Fr, *trois,* three, *carres,* sides],   a sharp, pointed rod that fits inside a tube. It is used to pierce the skin and the wall of a cavity or canal in the body to aspirate fluids, to instill a medication or solution, or to guide the placement of a soft catheter. The trocar is usually removed; and the catheter, tube, or instrument is left in place. See also **cannula.**

**trochanter** /trōkan′tər/ [Gk, runner],   one of the two bony projections on the proximal end of the femur that serve as the point of attachment of various muscles. The two protuberances are the trochanter major and the trochanter minor.

**trochanter major** [Gk, *trochanter,* runner; L, *major,* great], a large projection from the proximal end of the shaft of the femur. It is a point of attachment for the gluteus minimus and gluteus medius muscles. Also called **greater trochanter.**

**trochanter minor.** See **lesser trochanter.**

**troche** /trō′kē/ [Gk, *trochos,* lozenge], a small oval, round, or oblong tablet containing a medicinal agent incorporated in a flavored, sweetened mucilage or fruit base that dissolves in the mouth, releasing the drug. Also called **lozenge, rotula, trochiscus.**

**trochlea** /trok′lē·ə/, a pulley-shaped part or structure. —**trochlear,** *adj.*

**trochlear** /trok′lē·ər/ [L, *trochlea,* pulley], **1.** pertaining to a trochlea or something that is pulley shaped. **2.** relating to the trochlear (fourth cranial) nerve.

**trochlear nerve** [L, *trochlea,* pulley; *nervus,* nerve], either of the smallest pair of cranial nerves, essential for eye movement and eye muscle sensibility. The trochlear nerves branch to supply the superior oblique muscle and communicate with the ophthalmic division of the trigeminal nerve, connecting with two areas in the brain. Also called **fourth cranial nerve, nervus trochlearis.**

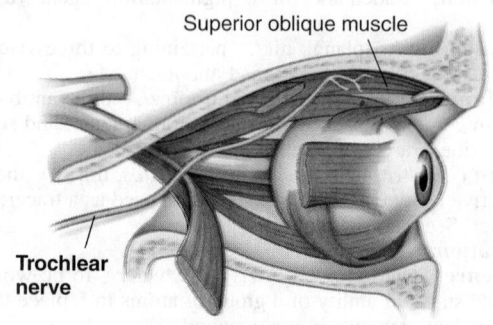

Superior oblique muscle

Trochlear nerve

**Trochlear nerve**

**trochlear notch of ulna,** a large depression in the ulna, formed by the olecranon and coronoid processes, that articulates with the trochlea of the humerus.

**trochoid joint.** See **pivot joint.**

**trolamine** /trol′əmēn/, a contraction for *triethanolamine.*

**troleandomycin** /trol′ē·an′dōmī′sin/, a macrolide antibiotic.

■ INDICATIONS: It is prescribed in the treatment of certain infections, including pneumococcal pneumonia and group A streptococcal infections of the upper respiratory tract.

■ CONTRAINDICATION: Known hypersensitivity to this drug prohibits its use.

■ ADVERSE EFFECTS: Among the more serious adverse effects are GI disturbances, mild to severe allergic reactions (including anaphylaxis), and hepatotoxicity.

**Trombiculidae** /trom′bikyoo′lidē/, a family of mites, including harvest mites, red bugs, and chiggers. The larvae are parasitic and the adults are free-living. The mites are disease vectors of typhus, rickettsiae, scrub itch, tsutsugamushi disease, and other infections.

**trombiculosis** /trombik′yəlō′sis/ [Gk, *tromein,* to tremble,

*osis,* condition], an infestation with mites of the genus *Trombicula,* some species of which carry scrub typhus.

**-tron,** combining form meaning a '(specified) type of vacuum tube': *dynatron, magnetron, thyratron.*

**Tronothane Hydrochloride,** trademark for a local anesthetic (pramoxine hydrochloride).

**trop-, -trop,** combining form for atropine derivatives.

**trop-, tropo-,** combining form meaning 'turn, turning' or 'tendency, affinity': *tropism, tropomyosin.* See also **tropho-,** with which this combining form is sometimes confused.

**-tropal.** See **-tropia.**

**-trope,** suffix meaning 'influencing or influenced by': *gonadotrope, heliotrope, rheotrope.*

**troph-.** See **tropho-.**

**-troph,** **1.** suffix meaning 'that which nourishes an embryo': *embryotroph, hemotroph, histotroph.* **2.** suffix meaning an 'organism that gets nourishment from a (specified) source': *autotroph, metatroph, prototroph.*

**trophectoderm.** See **trophoblast.**

**trophic** /trof′ik/ [Gk, *trophe,* nutrition], pertaining to a nutritive effect on or quality of cellular activity.

**-trophic,** combining form meaning 'a type of nutrition or nutritional requirement': *chondrotrophic, lipotrophic, viscerotrophic.*

**trophic action** [Gk, *trophe,* nutrition; L, *agere,* to do], the stimulation of cell reproduction and enlargement by nurturing and causing growth.

**trophic fracture,** a fracture resulting from the weakening of bone caused by nutritional disturbances.

**trophic hormones,** hormones secreted by the adenohypophysis that stimulate target organs.

**trophic ulcer,** a pressure ulcer caused by external trauma to a part of the body that is in poor condition resulting from disease, vascular insufficiency, or loss of afferent nerve fibers. Trophic ulcers may be painless or associated with severe causalgia. See also **pressure ulcer.**

**trophism** /trof′izəm/ [Gk, *trophe,* nutrition], the influence of nourishment.

**tropho-** /trof′ə-, trō′fə-/, **troph-,** combining form meaning 'food or nourishment': *trophoblast, trophoedema, trophoneurosis.* See also **trop-.**

**trophoblast** /trof′əblast′/ [Gk, *trophe* + *blastos,* germ], the outermost layer of tissue that forms the wall of the blastocyst of placental mammals in the early stages of embryonic development. It functions in the implantation of the blastocyst in the uterine wall and in supplying nutrients to the embryo. At implantation the cells differentiate into two layers: the inner cytotrophoblast, which forms the chorion, and the syncytiotrophoblast, which develops into the outer layer of the placenta. Also called **trophectoderm.** —**trophoblastic,** *adj.*

**trophoblastic cancer** /-blas′tik/, a malignant neoplastic disease of the uterus derived from chorionic epithelium, characterized by the production of high levels of human chorionic gonadotropin (HCG). The tumor may be an invasive hydatid mole (chorioadenoma destruens) formed by grossly enlarged vesicular chorionic villi or a malignant uterine choriocarcinoma that arises from nonvillous chorionic epithelium. One half of the cases of choriocarcinoma follow a molar pregnancy, 25% an abortion, 22.5% a normal pregnancy, and 2.5% an ectopic pregnancy. A hydatid mole invades the myometrium and often forms extrauterine nodules that may spread to distant sites. Choriocarcinoma forms a dark red hemorrhagic nodular tumor on or in the uterine wall and metastasizes early in its course to the lungs, brain, liver, bones, vagina, or vulva. Initial symptoms are vaginal bleeding and a profuse, foul-smelling discharge; a persistent cough or hemoptysis signals pulmonary involvement. As the disease progresses, there may be frequent hemorrhage, weakness, and emaciation. Diagnostic measures include serial assays to determine whether the HCG level in the blood is elevated and histologic examination of specimens obtained by curettage. Hysterectomy is indicated in most cases, but surgery does not eliminate the possibility of a recurrence. Chemotherapy is effective in curing a large percentage of patients with trophoblastic tumors. Also called **trophoblastic disease.** See also **choriocarcinoma, hydatid mole.**

**trophotropic** /trof'ətrop'ik/ [Gk, *trophe* + *trepein,* to turn], pertaining to a combination of parasympathetic nervous system activity, somatic muscle relaxation, and cortical beta rhythm synchronization, such as in a resting or sleep state.

**trophotropism** /trof'ətrop'izəm/, movement toward or away from nutrient sources.

**trophozoite** /trof'əzō'īt/ [Gk, *trophe* + *zoon,* animal], an immature ameboid protozoon. Diseases in which trophozoites may be isolated by bacteriologic studies include amebic dysentery, malaria, and trichomonas vaginitis. When fully developed, a trophozoite may be identified as a schizont.

**-trophy, -trophia,** combining form meaning a 'condition of nutrition or growth': *cyotrophy, embryotrophy, lipotrophy.*

**-tropia, -tropic, -tropal, -tropous, 1.** suffix meaning a 'turn or deviation from normal': *anatropic, hemitropic, stereotropic.* **2.** combining form meaning a 'tendency to have an influence on, or be influenced by: *corticotropic, pancreatropic, radiotropic.*

**tropical acne** /trop'ikəl/, a form of acne that is caused or aggravated by high temperature and humidity. It is characterized by large nodules or pustules on the neck, back, upper arms, and buttocks.

**tropical medicine** [Gk, *tropikos,* of the solstice; L, *medicina*], the branch of medicine concerned with the diagnosis and treatment of diseases commonly occurring in tropic and subtropic regions of the world, generally between 30 degrees north and south of the equator.

**tropical sore.** See **oriental sore.**

**tropical spastic paraparesis.** See **chronic progressive myelopathy.**

**tropical sprue,** a malabsorption syndrome of unknown cause that is endemic in the tropics and subtropics. It is characterized by abnormalities in the mucosa of the small intestine, resulting in protein malnutrition and multiple nutritional deficiencies, often complicated by severe infection. Symptoms include diarrhea, anorexia, and weight loss. Megaloblastic anemia may result from folic acid and vitamin $B_{12}$ deficiency. Treatment includes administration of antibiotics, particularly tetracycline, folic acid, iron, calcium, and vitamins A, D, K, and B complex, as well as a balanced diet high in protein and normal in fat content. See also **nontropic sprue.**

**tropical typhus.** See **scrub typhus.**

**-tropin,** suffix meaning 'stimulating effect of a hormone or other substance on a target organ or system': *somatotropin.*

**-tropism.** See **-tropy.**

**-tropo.** See **-trop.**

**tropocollagen** /trop'əkol'əjən/ [Gk, *trepein,* to turn, *kolla,* glue, *genein,* to produce], fundamental units of collagen fibrils obtained by prolonged extraction of insoluble collagen with dilute acid.

**tropomyosin** /trop'əmī'əsin/ [Gk, *trepein* + *mys,* muscle], a protein component of sarcomere filaments, which, together with troponin, regulates interactions of actin and myosin in muscle contractions.

**troponin** /trō'pənin/ [Gk, *trepein,* to turn], a protein in the striated cell ultrastructure that modulates the interaction between actin and myosin molecules. It is believed to be part of the calcium-binding complex of the thin myofilaments. See also **tropomyosin.**

**troponins test,** a blood test that measures levels of cardiac troponins, which are considered a promising biochemical marker for cardiac disease. This test assists in evaluating patients with suspected acute coronary ischemic syndrome. It is particularly useful in differentiating cardiac from noncardiac chest pain, evaluating patients with unstable angina, detecting reperfusion associated with coronary recanalization, estimating myocardial infarction size, and detecting perioperative myocardial infarction.

**-tropous.** See **-tropia.**

**-tropy, -tropism,** combining form meaning 'influenced by or having an affinity for' something specified: *allotropy, ergotropy, syntropy.*

**trough** /trôf/ [AS, *trog*], a groove or channel, such as the gingival trough around the neck of a tooth.

**Trousseau's sign** /trōōsōz'/ [Armand Trousseau, French physician, 1801–1867; L, *signum,* mark], **1.** a test for latent tetany in which carpal spasm is induced by inflating a sphygmomanometer cuff on the upper arm to a pressure exceeding systolic blood pressure for 3 minutes. A positive test may be seen in hypocalcemia and hypomagnesemia. **2.** a reddened streak, the result of drawing a finger across the skin. It is seen with a variety of nervous system disorders.

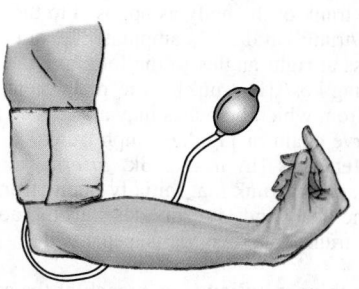

**Trousseau's sign** *(Monahan and Neighbors, 1998)*

**Trousseau's syndrome** [Armand Trousseau], superficial migratory thrombophlebitis associated with visceral cancer.

**Trp,** abbreviation for **tryptophan.**

**true ankylosis.** See **ankylosis.**

**true birth rate** [ME, *treue,* faith, *burthe* + L, *reri,* to calculate], the ratio of total births to the total female population of childbearing age, between 15 and 45 years of age. Compare **birth rate, crude birth rate, refined birth rate.**

**true chondroma.** See **enchondroma.**

**true conjugate,** a radiographic measurement of the distance from the upper margin of the symphysis pubis to the sacral promontory. It is usually 1.5 to 2 cm less than the diagonal conjugate. See also **conjugate.**

**true denticle.** See **denticle.**

**true diverticulum** [ME, *treue,* faith; L, *diverticulare,* to turn aside], diverticulum that includes all the same tissue layers as the organ from which it originates.

**true dwarf.** See **primordial dwarf.**

**true glottis.** See **glottis.**

**true hermaphroditism** [ME, *treue,* faith; Gk, *Hermaphroditos,* son of Hermes and Aphrodite], a condition in which an individual is born with both male and female gonads.

**true labor,** uterine contractions that result in a change in the cervix and birth of an infant.

**true neuroma,** any neoplasm composed of nerve tissue.

**true oxygen,** the calculated concentration as either a percentage or a fraction that, when multiplied by the expiratory minute volume at STPD, gives oxygen uptake.

**true pelvis.** See **pelvis.**

**true rib.** See **rib.**

**true shunt.** See **zero V/Q.**

**true suture,** an immovable fibrous joint of the skull in which the edges of bones interlock along a series of processes and indentations. The three kinds of true sutures are the sutura dentata, the sutura limbosa, and the sutura serrata. Compare **false suture.**

**true twins.** See **monozygotic twins.**

**true value,** (in statistics) a value that is closely approximated by the definitive value and somewhat less closely by the reference value.

**true vocal cords** [ME, *treue,* faith; L, *vocalis,* of the voice; Gk, *chorde,* string], the vocal folds of the larynx (plicae vocales), as distinguished from the vestibular folds (plicae vestibulares), called false vocal cords. They are located inferior to the false vocal cords. See also **vocal cord.**

**truncal** /trung′kəl/ [L, *truncus*], pertaining to the trunk of the body or to any arterial or nerve trunk.

**truncal ataxia,** a loss of coordinated muscle movements for maintaining normal posture of the trunk.

**truncal obesity,** obesity that preferentially affects or is located in the trunk of the body as opposed to the extremities.

**truncated** /trung′kātid/, **1.** amputated from the trunk. **2.** cut across at right angles to the long axis.

**truncus** /trung′kəs/ [L, trunk], the main stem of an anatomic part from which branches may arise, such as the sympathetic nerve chain or jugular lymph trunk.

**truncus arteriosus** [L, trunk; Gk, *arteria,* airpipe], the embryonic arterial trunk that initially opens from both ventricles of the heart and later divides into the aorta and the pulmonary trunk, the two parts separated by the bulbar septum.

**truncus brachiocephalicus,** a branch of the aorta that divides into the right common carotid and right subclavian arteries.

**trunk** [L, *truncus*], **1.** the main stalk of an anatomic structure with many branches, such as an artery or nerve. **2.** the body excluding the head and appendages. Also called **torso.**

**trunk balance,** the ability to maintain postural control of the trunk, including the shifting and bearing of weight on each side to free an extremity for a particular function such as reaching and grasping. Weight shifting can be anterior, posterior, lateral, or diagonal and involve righting, equilibrium, and protective reactions. Head and neck control allows for dissociation of the shoulder and pelvic girdles from the trunk.

**trunk incurvation reflex.** See **Galant reflex.**

**Trusopt,** trademark for a carbonic anhydrase inhibitor (dorzolamide hydrochloride).

**truss** [Fr, *trousser,* to pack up], an apparatus worn to prevent or retard the herniation of the intestines or other organ through an opening in the abdominal wall.

**trust** [ME, protection], a risk-taking process whereby an individual's situation depends on the future behavior of another person.

**truth** [AS, *treowo*], a rule or statement that conforms to fact or reality.

**truth serum,** a common name for any of several sedatives, such as the short-acting barbiturates, that have been administered intravenously in subjects to elicit information that may have been repressed. It has been used successfully in helping to identify amnesia victims.

**truth telling,** a nursing intervention from the Nursing Interventions Classification (NIC) defined as use of whole truth, partial truth, or decision delay to promote the patient's self-determination and well-being. See also **Nursing Interventions Classification.**

**Trypanosoma** /trip′ənōsō′mə/ [Gk, *trypanon,* borer, *soma,* body], a genus of parasitic organisms, several species of which can cause significant diseases in humans. Most *Trypanosoma* organisms live part of their life cycle in insects and are transmitted to humans by insect bites. See also **trypanosome, trypanosomiasis.**

**Trypanosoma brucei gambiense.** See **Gambian trypanosomiasis.**

**Trypanosoma brucei rhodesiense.** See **Rhodesian trypanosomiasis.**

**Trypanosoma cruzi.** See **Chagas' disease.**

**trypanosomal infection.** See **trypanosomiasis.**

**trypanosome** /trip′ənōsōm′, tripan′-/, any organism of the genus *Trypanosoma.* See also **trypanosomiasis. —trypanosomal,** *adj.*

**trypanosomiasis** /trip′ənō′sōmī′əsis/ [Gk, *trypanon* + *soma* + *osis,* condition], an infection by an organism of the *Trypanosoma* genus. Kinds of trypanosomiasis are **African trypanosomiasis** and **Chagas' disease.**

**trypanosomicide** /trip′ənōsō′misīd/ [Gk, *trypanon* + *soma* + L, *caedere,* to kill], a drug destructive to trypanosomes, especially the species of the protozoan parasite transmitted to humans by various insect vectors common in Africa and Central and South America. Various arsenic preparations are used to treat African sleeping sickness, caused by *Trypanosoma gambiense* and *T. rhodesiense,* and Chagas' disease, caused by *T. cruzi,* in the Americas. **—trypanosomicidal,** *adj.*

**trypsin** /trip′sin/ [Gk, *tripsis,* rubbing], a proteolytic digestive enzyme produced by the exocrine pancreas that catalyzes in the small intestine the breakdown of dietary proteins to peptones, peptides, and amino acids.

**trypsin, crystallized,** a proteolytic enzyme from the pancreas of the ox, *Bos taurus,* that has been used as a debriding agent for open wounds and ulcers.

**trypsin inhibitor,** one of a group of peptides, present in such varied sources as soybeans, egg white, and human colostrum, that mask or inhibit the active site of the trypsin molecule. Also called **kunitz inhibitor.**

**trypsinogen** /tripsin′əjən/ [Gk, *tripsis* + *genein,* to produce], the inactive precursor form of trypsin. Trypsinogen is secreted in pancreatic juice and converted to active trypsin through the action of enterokinase in the intestine. Also called **protrypsin.**

**tryptases.** See **proteinase.**

**tryptophan (Trp)** /trip′təfan/, an amino acid essential for normal growth and nitrogen balance. Tryptophan is the precursor of several important biomolecules, including serotonin and niacin. See also **amino acid, protein.**

**TSEM,** abbreviation for **transmission scanning electron microscopy.**

**tsetse fly** /tset′sē, tsē′tsē/ [Afr, *tsetse* + AS, *flyge*], a bloodsucking fly found in regions of Africa, mainly south of the Sahara desert. It is an insect of the *Glossina* genus and a secondary host of trypanosomes, which cause African sleeping sickness and other diseases in humans and domestic and wild animals. Also spelled **tzetze fly.** See also **trypanosomiasis.**

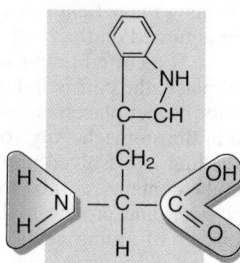

**Chemical structure of tryptophan**

**TSH,** abbreviation for **thyroid-stimulating hormone.**

**TSH releasing factor.** See **thyrotropin-releasing hormone.**

**tsp,** abbreviation for **teaspoon.**

**TSS,** abbreviation for **toxic shock syndrome.**

**TSTA,** abbreviation for *tumor-specific transplantation antigen.*

**tsutsugamushi disease.** See **scrub typhus.**

**TT,** abbreviation for **thrombolytic therapy.**

**t test,** a statistic test used to determine whether there are differences between two means or between a target value and a calculated mean.

**TTP,** abbreviation for **thrombotic thrombocytopenic purpura.**

**T tube, 1.** a tubular device in the shape of a T, inserted through the skin into a cavity or a wound, used for drainage. **2.** an apparatus used to connect a source of humidified oxygen to the endotracheal tube so that a spirometer can be attached for the evaluation of tidal volume.

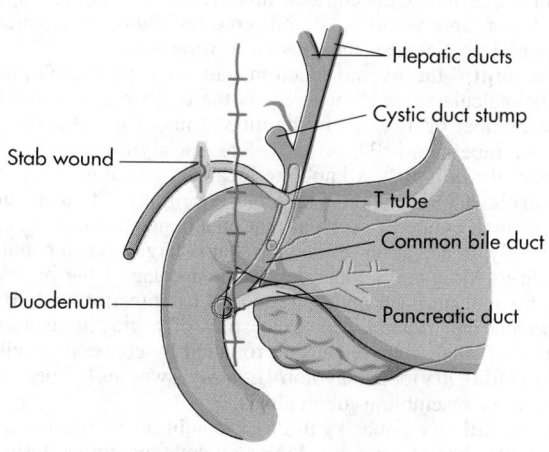

**T tube in the common bile duct for
T-tube cholangiography**
*(Beare and Myers, 1998)*

**T-tube cholangiography,** a type of biliary tract radiographic examination in which a water-soluble iodinated contrast medium is injected into the bile duct through an indwelling, T-shaped rubber tube. The tube is inserted in the common bile duct as a routine postoperative procedure to provide drainage.

**T tubule system,** a system of tubular invaginations along the surface of all striated muscle cell membranes, providing an extension of the membrane into the cells. The system is believed to be part of an extensive endomembrane system involved in storing calcium ions and in the movement of action potentials into the cells. T tubules are likely to be the link between membrane stimulation and the triggering of the release of calcium ions from the sarcoplasmic reticulum.

**T.U., 1.** abbreviation for *toxic unit.* **2.** abbreviation for *toxin unit.* **3.** abbreviation for *tuberculin unit.*

**tubal abortion** /t(y)o͞o′bəl/ [L, *tubus* + *ab*, away from, *oriri*, to be born], a condition of pregnancy in which an embryo, ectopically implanted, is expelled from the uterine tube into the peritoneal cavity. Tubal abortion is often accompanied by significant internal bleeding, causing acute abdominal and pelvic pain. It may be asymptomatic, the products of conception being resorbed. Rarely the conceptus reimplants on the peritoneum and continues growing to become an abdominal pregnancy. See also **abdominal pregnancy, ectopic pregnancy, tubal pregnancy.**

**tubal dermoid cyst,** a tumor derived from embryonal tissues that develops in an oviduct.

**tubal ligation,** one of several sterilization procedures in which both fallopian tubes are blocked to prevent conception from occurring. Through a small abdominal incision, the fallopian tubes are ligated in two places with laser; and the intervening segment is burnt, crushed, or excised. The procedure is less commonly performed vaginally. Complications of the procedure, which are rare but serious, include pulmonary embolism, hemorrhage, infection, and tubal pregnancy. The requirements for informed consent for sterilization procedures vary among states and institutions.

**tubal pregnancy,** an ectopic pregnancy in which the conceptus implants in the fallopian tube. Approximately 2% of all pregnancies are ectopic; of these, approximately 90% are tubal. Tubal pregnancy seldom occurs in primigravidas. The most important predisposing factor is prior tubal injury. Pelvic infection, scarring and adhesions from surgery, or intrauterine device complications may result in damage that diminishes the motility of the tube. Transport of the ovum through the tube after fertilization is slowed, and implantation takes place before the conceptus reaches the uterine cavity. Most often the tube, which cannot long contain the growing fetus, ruptures, precipitating an intraperitoneal hemorrhage; if not stopped, the hemorrhaging can lead rapidly to shock and often death. Some conceptuses apparently die and are resorbed in the tube. Diagnosis of tubal pregnancy is often difficult. With rupture of the fallopian tube, women commonly experience sudden sharp pain in one side of the lower abdomen, but signs and symptoms of tubal pregnancy are insidiously variable, and the classic triad of amenorrhea, pelvic pain, and a tender adnexal mass are present only 50% of the time. Recovery of blood from the cul-de-sac by means of culdocentesis is highly suggestive of a ruptured fallopian tube and tubal pregnancy; it requires immediate surgical exploration of the abdomen. Absence of blood on culdocentesis does not rule out the presence of an unruptured tubal pregnancy; laparotomy may be required, particularly if a woman's pregnancy test is positive, the pelvic findings are suggestive, and sonography of the pelvis cannot demonstrate an intrauterine pregnancy. Because of the lethal potential of an undiagnosed tubal pregnancy, women who report any of the characteristic symptoms early in their pregnancies, particularly during the time before the existence of a normal intrauterine pregnancy can be confirmed, must be considered susceptible. In women who have a history of prior pelvic disease and in those who have symptoms or signs of tubal pregnancy, emergency treatment requires an immediate IV infusion via a large-bore IV catheter, type and crossmatch of blood for blood replacement, and treatment of shock as necessary. Treatment is surgical and involves laparotomy, removal of the entire products of conception and any intraperitoneal blood present, and the removal or repair of the involved tube. Conditions that predispose to a first tubal pregnancy also predispose to a second; a woman who has had one tubal pregnancy has one chance in five of having another in a subsequent pregnancy. Depending on the location of the developing embryo, the condition is classified as an ampullary, fimbrial, or interstitial tubal pregnancy.

**tube** /t(y)o͞ob/ [L, *tubus*], a hollow, cylindric piece of equipment or structure of the body.

**tube care,** a nursing intervention from the Nursing Interventions Classification (NIC) defined as management of a patient with an external drainage device exiting the body. See also **Nursing Interventions Classification.**

**tube care: chest,** a nursing intervention from the Nursing Interventions Classification (NIC) defined as management of a patient with an external water-seal drainage device exiting the chest cavity. See also **Nursing Interventions Classification.**

**tube care: gastrointestinal,** a nursing intervention from the Nursing Interventions Classification (NIC) defined as management of a patient with a gastrointestinal tube. See also **Nursing Interventions Classification.**

**tube care: umbilical line,** a nursing intervention from the Nursing Interventions Classification (NIC) defined as management of a newborn with an umbilical catheter. See also **Nursing Interventions Classification.**

**tube care: urinary,** a nursing intervention from the Nursing Interventions Classification (NIC) defined as management of a patient with urinary drainage equipment. See also **Nursing Interventions Classification.**

**tube care: ventriculostomy/lumbar drain,** a nursing intervention from the Nursing Interventions Classification (NIC) defined as management of a patient with an external cerebrospinal fluid drainage system. See also **Nursing Interventions Classification.**

**tube feeding,** the administration of nutritionally balanced liquefied foods or nutrients through a tube inserted into the esophagus, stomach, duodenum, or jejunum. The conditions for which tube feeding is administered include after mouth or gastric surgery, in severe burns, in paralysis or obstruction of the esophagus, in severe cases of anorexia nervosa, and for unconscious patients or those unable to chew or swallow. Also called **esophageal feeding, gavage feeding, jejunostomy feeding, nasogastric feeding.** See also **drip gavage, enteral tube feeding.**

**tube feeding care,** the nursing care and management of a patient receiving nourishment through a nasogastric tube.

■ METHOD: The tip of a nasogastric tube is lubricated with a water-soluble lubricant, inserted into a nostril, and rapidly advanced into the stomach as the patient, if conscious, is asked to swallow hard repeatedly. Correct placement of the tube may be best determined by x-rays. Placement also may be checked, although not as reliably, by listening for a bubbling sound through a stethoscope placed over the stomach, as 5 mL of air is injected into the tube. The pH of secretions may also be checked. If the patient coughs forcefully when 1 or 2 mL of water is injected into the tube, it is placed in the upper respiratory tract rather than the stomach. The tube, held securely and comfortably by a tape across the nose or upper lip, may be left in place in adults and older children but usually is removed and reinserted for each feeding in in-

fants. Before each feeding the patient is helped up to a semi-Fowler's position or is turned on the right side and elevated slightly if unconscious. If a cuffed tracheostomy tube or endotracheal tube is in place, the cuff is inflated. The nasogastric tube is checked for proper placement and for the amount of residual formula in the stomach. Any solid medication to be given with the feeding is dissolved in water. The normal liquefied diet formula contains a mixture of milk, eggs, sugar, skim milk powder, and protein hydrolysates. A low-residue formula consists of amino acids, sugars, vitamins, and minerals. Blue food coloring can be added to the formula to help distinguish gastric contents from respiratory secretions to detect aspirations. Depending on the patient's preference, the formula is at or below room temperature when administered slowly by gravity at a rate of no more than 300 mL an hour. During feeding the patient is observed for respiratory distress, nausea, vomiting, abdominal cramps, and restlessness. At the completion of the procedure, the tube is flushed with water as ordered and then clamped. The patient receives oral hygiene and lubrication and cleaning of the nares and is maintained in the same position for 30 minutes after feeding; at that time the cuff on the tracheostomy or endotracheal tube is deflated.

■ INTERVENTIONS: The nurse positions the patient for feeding, checks the tube placement, notes and replaces the amount of residual formula, and reports residual volume in excess of 100 ml, or 75% of previous feeding. Bags and tubing need to be changed per institutional protocol to prevent bacterial growth. The nurse administers the feeding, ensures that the patient and family members understand the purpose of the procedure, and cautions the patient to report symptoms such as nausea, abdominal cramps, diarrhea, or constipation.

■ OUTCOME CRITERIA: A formula containing the proper proportions of protein, carbohydrate, and fat administered through a nasogastric tube can provide adequate nutrition over a short term. A high content of simple sugars may cause diarrhea. Concentrated mixtures containing too little water or large volumes administered rapidly may dehydrate the patient. See also **nasogastric intubation.**

**tube gain,** the overall electron gain of a photomultiplier tube, calculated as $g^n$, where $g$ is the dynode gain and $n$ is the number of dynodes in the tube. Thus, if $g$ is 3 and $n$ is 8, the tube gain is $3^8$, or 6561. See also **dynode.**

**tuber** /t(y)o͞o′bər/, a knoblike localized swelling.

**tubercle** /t(y)o͞o′bərkəl/ [L, *tuber*, swelling], 1. a nodule or a small eminence, such as that on a bone. 2. a nodule, especially an elevation of the skin that is larger than a papule, such as Morgagni's tubercles of the areolae of the breasts. 3. a small rounded nodule produced by infection with *Mycobacterium tuberculosis*, consisting of a gray translucent mass of small spheric cells surrounded by connective cells.

**tubercular** /t(y)o͞obur′kyələr/ [L, *tuber*, swelling], pertaining to or resembling tuberculosis.

**tuberculid** /t(y)o͞obur′kyəlid/, a condition in tuberculous patients characterized by skin or mucous membrane lesions in which the tubercle bacillus is absent. It is the result of sensitivity to mycobacterial antigens.

**tuberculin.** See **tuberculin test, tuberculosis.**

**tuberculin purified protein derivative** /to͞obur′kyo͞olin/, a solution containing a purified protein fraction derived from isolated culture filtrates of strains of *Mycobacterium tuberculosis*. It is used as an aid in the diagnosis of tuberculosis, in the Mantoux test, and, for the same purpose in a dried form, in multiple puncture devices. See also **Mantoux test, tine test.**

**tuberculin reaction,** hardening or blistering as a delayed reaction at the site of a tuberculin test, a positive result.

**tuberculin test** [L, *tuber* + *testum*, crucible], a test to determine past or present tuberculosis infection based on a positive skin reaction, using one of several methods. A purified protein derivative of tubercle bacilli, called **tuberculin**, is introduced into the skin by scratch, puncture, or intradermal injection. If a raised, red, or hard zone forms surrounding the tuberculin test site, the person is said to be sensitive to tuberculin, and the test is read as positive. However, a negative tuberculin reaction does not rule out a diagnosis of previous or active tuberculosis. Sputum and gastric cultures, acid-fast staining, and x-ray studies often are needed to establish a diagnosis of tuberculosis. Kinds of tuberculin tests include **Heaf test, Mantoux test, Pirquet's test,** and **tine test.**

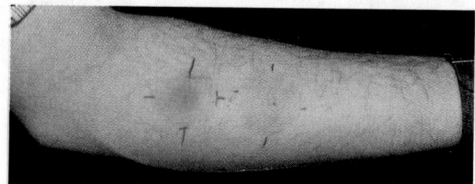

**Positive tuberculin skin test**
*(Zitelli and Davis, 1997/courtesy Dr. Kenneth Schuitt)*

**tuberculin tine test** [L, *tuber* + ME, *tind* + L, *testum*, crucible], a test for the presence of tubercle bacilli. It is performed by applying a device with multiple sharp prongs to the skin. The prongs penetrate the skin and inject tuberculin, a purified protein derivative of tubercle bacilli. A hardened raised area at the test site 48 to 72 hours later indicates the presence of the pathogens in the blood. Because of variations in sensitivity and strength of tuberculin units administered, a negative test result does not necessarily exclude a diagnosis of tuberculosis. See also **Mantoux test.**

**tuberculoid leprosy.** See **leprosy.**

**tuberculoma** /t(y)o͞obur′kyəlō′mə, to͞obur′kyo͞olō′mə/ [L, *tuber* + Gk, *oma*, tumor], a rare tumorlike growth of tuberculous tissue in the central nervous system, characterized by symptoms of an expanding cerebral, cerebellar, or spinal

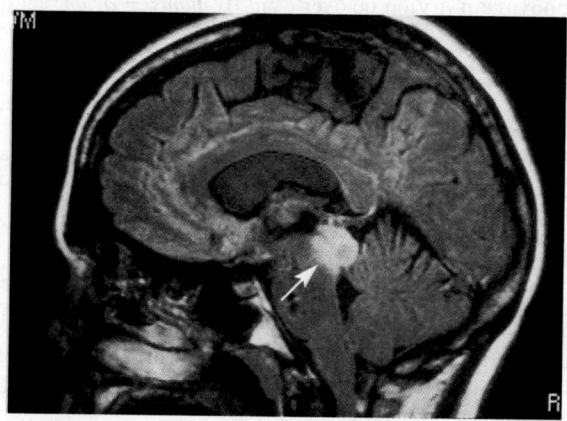

**Tuberculoma**
*(Stone and Gorbach, 2000/courtesy Dr. Carl Heilman, New England Medical Center, Boston)*

mass. Treatment consists of the administration of antimicrobial drugs to resolve the primary growth and to prevent meningitis.

**tuberculosis (TB)** /t(y)o͞obur′kyəlō′sis/ [L, *tuber* + Gk, *osis,* condition], a chronic granulomatous infection caused by an acid-fast bacillus, *Mycobacterium tuberculosis.* It is generally transmitted by the inhalation or ingestion of infected droplets and usually affects the lungs, although infection of multiple organ systems occurs. Persons who are immunodeficient, such as those infected with human immunodeficiency virus, may have extrapulmonary tuberculosis. This includes disseminated tuberculosis, which involves multiple organs such as the liver, lung, spleen, bone marrow, and lymph nodes. Diagnosis is through biopsy, stain, sputum and gastric cultures, and x-ray studies. Central nervous system tuberculosis may occur as inflammation of the meninges or a mass lesion (tuberculoma).

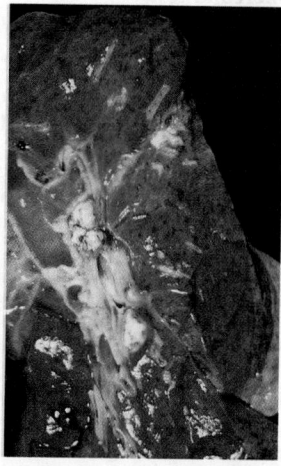

**Primary pulmonary tuberculosis**
*(Kumar, Cotran, and Robbins, 1997)*

■ OBSERVATIONS: Listlessness, vague chest pain, pleurisy, anorexia, fever, and weight loss are early symptoms of pulmonary tuberculosis. Night sweats, pulmonary hemorrhage, expectoration of purulent sputum, and dyspnea develop as the disease progresses. The lung tissues react to the bacillus by producing protective cells that engulf the disease organism, forming tubercles. Untreated, the tubercles enlarge and merge to form larger tubercles that undergo caseation, eventually sloughing off into the cavities of the lungs. Hemoptysis occurs as a result of cavitary spread.

■ INTERVENTIONS: The bacillus is generally sensitive to isoniazid, pyrazinamide, paraaminosalicylic acid, streptomycin, rifampin, ethambutol, dihydrostreptomycin, ultraviolet radiation, and heat. A combination of drugs is prescribed, with regular tests of the function of the kidneys, liver, eyes, and ears to discover early signs of drug toxicity. This is particularly important because drug therapy will usually continue for up to 1 year. The person may be hospitalized for the first weeks of treatment to limit the possible spread of infection, to encourage rest and excellent nutrition, to ensure complete compliance with the prescribed drug regimen, and to observe for adverse drug effects. Samples of sputum are regularly examined. The disease is not infectious after the bacillus is no longer present in the sputum. Care of an outpatient includes continued medication, evaluation for adverse drug effects, sputum analyses, and encouragement to complete the long course of treatment. All contacts are tested periodically with purified protein derivative. People who are at increased risk of infection may be treated empirically, without a positive diagnosis having been made. BCG vaccination has been widely used worldwide but may not be effective at preventing tuberculosis.

■ NURSING CONSIDERATIONS: Before discharge the patient is taught how to prevent the spread of the disease; the elements of good nutrition; the name, dose, action, and side effects of all medications prescribed; the need to take the drugs regularly; and how and where to get the next supply of drugs. Plans for follow-up care are discussed; they include date, time, and place of the next laboratory tests; referral to community nurses is made. The patient is reminded that a cough, weight loss, fever, night sweats, and hemoptysis are danger signals that are to be reported immediately. See also **miliary tuberculosis, tuberculin test.**

**tuberculosis vaccine.** See **BCG vaccine.**

**tuberculous** /t(y)ōōbur′kyələs/ [L, *tuber*], pertaining to tuberculosis.

**tuberculous arthritis,** a joint inflammation caused by invasion of the joint by tuberculosis bacilli that have migrated from a primary infection, usually in the chest.

**tuberculous lymphadenitis** [L, *tuber* + *lympha*, water; Gk, *aden*, gland, *itis*, inflammation], an inflammation of the lymph glands caused by the presence of *Mycobacterium tuberculosis.*

**tuberculous meningitis.** See **meningitis.**

**tuberculous peritonitis** [L, *tuber* + Gk, *peri* + *teinein*, to stretch, *itis*, inflammation], an inflammation of the peritoneum that is secondary to a tuberculous infection in the viscera.

**tuberculous pneumonia** [L, *tuber* + Gk, *pneumon*, lung], a complication of tuberculosis in which caseous material is inhaled into the bronchi, leading to bronchopneumonia or lobar pneumonia.

**tuberculous spondylitis,** a rare, grave form of tuberculosis caused by the invasion of *Mycobacterium tuberculosis* into the spinal vertebrae. The intervertebral disks may be destroyed, resulting in the collapse and wedging of affected vertebrae and the shortening and angulation of the spine. Thoracic vertebrae are more frequently involved than the vertebrae of the lumbar, cervical, or sacral segments of the spine. More than one area of the spine may be affected, and normal vertebrae may be evident between affected and unaffected sections. The infection characteristically dissects vertebrae anterolaterally and produces abscesses. The pressure of the abscess may cause ischemic paralysis in the subjacent spinal cord, and abscesses in the cervical area may displace or obstruct the trachea and the esophagus. Also called **Pott's disease, spinal caries.** See also **tuberculosis.**

**tuberculum** /t(y)ōōbur′kyələm/, a tubercle, nodule, or rounded elevation.

**tuberosity** /t(y)ōō′bəros′itē/ [L, *tuber*], an elevation or protuberance, especially of a bone.

**tuberosity of the tibia,** a large oblong elevation at the proximal end of the tibia to which the ligament of the patella attaches.

**tuberous carcinoma** /t(y)ōō′bərəs/ [L, *tuber* + Gk, *karkinos*, crab, *oma*, tumor], a scirrhous carcinoma of the skin, characterized by nodular projections. Also called **carcinoma tuberosum.**

**tuberous sclerosis,** a familial, neurocutaneous disease characterized by epilepsy, mental deterioration, adenoma se-

baceum, nodules and sclerotic patches on the cerebral cortex, retinal tumors, depigmented leaf-shaped macules on the skin, tumors of the heart or kidneys, and cerebral calcifications. There is no effective treatment. Also called **Bourneville's disease, epiloia.** See also **adenoma sebaceum.**

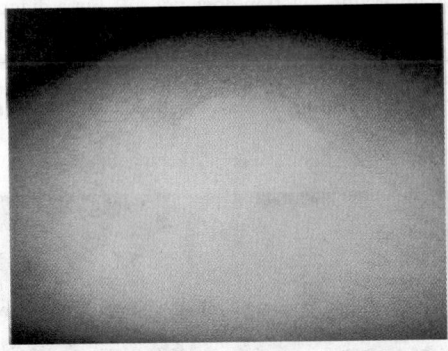

**Ash leaf spot in tuberous sclerosis**
*(Goldstein and Goldstein, 1997/courtesy Beverly Sanders, MD)*

**tuberous xanthoma.** See **xanthoma tuberosum.**

**Tubex unit,** trademark for a unit consisting of a cartridge with an attached needle that screws onto a plunger. The cartridge may be empty or prefilled with a standard dose of a medication. As the plunger is depressed, forcing the diaphragm into the cartridge, medication is forced out through the needle. The cartridge needle unit is disposable. The plunger requires no special care and is reusable.

**tubo-** /t(y)ōō′bō-, t(y)ōō′bə-/, combining form meaning 'tube or tubing': *tubular.*

**tuboabdominal gestation** /-abdom′inəl/ [L, *tubus* + *abdomen*, belly; L, *gestare,* to bear], an ectopic pregnancy in which the embryo develops while partly in the abdominal cavity and partly in the fallopian tube. The condition usually begins as a tubal pregnancy and extends into the abdomen as development continues. Also called **tuboabdominal pregnancy.**

**tubocurarine chloride.** See **curare.**

**tuboovarian** /t(y)ōō′bō·ōver′ē·ən/ [L, *tubus* + *ovum*, egg], pertaining to the ovary and fallopian tube. Also **tuboovarial.**

**tuboovarian abscess** [L, *tubus* + *ovum* + *abscedere,* to go away], an abscess involving the ovary and fallopian tube. It is commonly associated with salpingitis.

**tuboovarian cyst** [L, *tubus* + *ovum* + Gk, *kystis,* bag], a cyst that forms by adhesion of the ovary at the fimbriated end of the fallopian tube.

**tuboovarian gestation** [L, *tubus* + *ovum* + *gestare,* to bear], an ectopic pregnancy that develops partly in the fallopian tube and partly in the ovary. Also called **tuboovarian pregnancy.**

**tuboplasty** /t(y)ōō′bōplas′tē/ [L, *tubus,* tube; Gk, *plassein,* to mold], a surgical procedure in which severed or damaged fallopian tubes are repaired in hopes of restoring fertility.

**tubular.** See **tubule.**

**tubular necrosis** [L, *tubulus,* little tube; Gk, *nekros,* dead, *osis,* condition], the death of cells in the small tubules of the kidneys as a result of disease or injury.

**tubule** /t(y)o͞o′byo͞ol/ [L, *tubulus*], a small tube, such as one of the collecting tubules in the kidneys, the seminiferous tubules of the testes, or Henle's tubules between the distal and proximal convoluted tubules. —**tubular,** *adj.*

**tuft** [Fr, *touffe,* a tuft], an object resembling a tassle, such as a tuft of hair.

**tuft fracture** [Fr, *touffe,* tuft; L, *fractura,* break], a break in any one of the distal phalanges.

**tug** [ME, *toggen,* to pull], a dragging or hauling movement or sensation.

**tularemia** /to͞o′lərē′mē·ə/ [Tulare, California; Gk, *haima,* blood], an infectious disease of animals caused by the bacillus *Francisella (Pasteurella) tularensis,* which may be transmitted by insect vectors or direct contact. It is characterized in humans by fever, headache, and an ulcerated skin lesion with localized lymph node enlargement or by eye infection, GI ulcerations, or pneumonia, depending on the site of entry and the response of the host. Treatment includes streptomycin, chloramphenicol, and tetracycline. Recovery produces lifelong immunity. A vaccine is available. Also called **deerfly fever, rabbit fever.** Also spelled **tularaemia.**

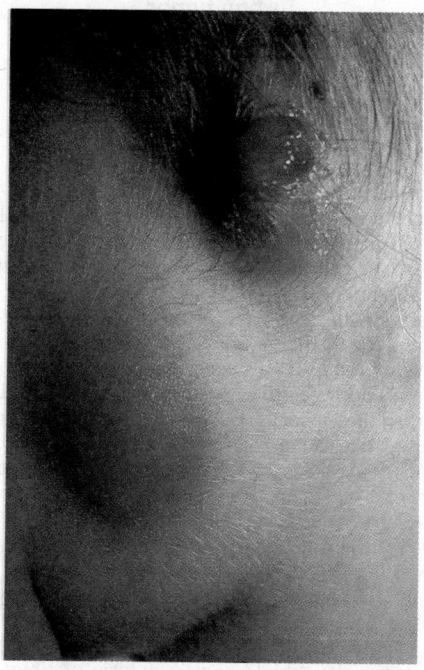

**Tularemia** *(Stone and Gorbach, 2000)*

**tumescence** /t(y)o͞omes′əns/ [L, *tumescere,* to begin to swell], a state of swelling or edema.

**-tumescence,** suffix meaning a 'swelling': *detumescence, intumescence, tumescence.*

**tumescent anesthesia,** administration of a local infiltration anesthetic (lidocaine) through the use of large volumes of fluid. The technique is applied in liposuction surgery, varicose vein treatment, scalp surgery, dermabrasion, and soft tissue reconstruction.

**tummy tuck.** See **abdominoplasty.**

**tumor** /t(y)o͞o′mər/ [L], **1.** a swelling or enlargement occurring in inflammatory conditions. **2.** also called **neo-**

**plasm.** A new growth of tissue characterized by progressive, uncontrolled proliferation of cells. The tumor may be localized or invasive, benign or malignant. A tumor may be named for its location, for its cellular makeup, or for the person who first identified it.

**tumor albus,** a white swelling occurring in a tuberculous bone or joint.

**tumor angiogenesis factor (TAF),** a protein that stimulates the formation of blood vessels in tumors. See also **angiogenin.**

**tumoricide** /t(y)o͞omôr′isīd/, a substance capable of destroying a tumor. —**tumoricidal,** *adj.*

**tumorigenesis** /t(y)o͞o′mərijen′əsis/, the process of initiating and promoting the development of a tumor. Compare **carcinogenesis, oncogenesis, sarcomagenesis. —tumorigenic,** *adj.*

**tumorigenic** /-jen′ik/ [L, *tumor,* swelling; Gk, *genein,* to produce], capable of producing tumors.

**tumor marker,** a substance in the body that may be associated with the presence of a cancer.

**tumor necrosis factor (TNF),** a natural body protein, also produced synthetically, with anticancer effects. The body produces it in response to the presence of toxic substances such as bacterial toxins. Adverse effects are toxic shock and cachexia.

**tumor registry,** a repository of data on the incidence of cancers and personal characteristics, treatment, and treatment Outcomess of patients diagnosed with cancer.

**tumor-specific antigen,** an antigen produced by a particular type of tumor that does not appear on normal cells of the tissue in which the tumor developed.

**tumor suppressor gene.** See **antioncogene.**

**tumor viruses** [L, *tumor,* swelling, *virus,* poison], viruses that are capable of directly or indirectly inducing tumor formation. Direct tumor formation may result from inoculation of living cells with tumorigenic viruses. Tumor formation may result from the influence of the virus on normal cells that are transformed into tumor cells.

**tumor volume,** a part of an organ or tissue that includes both the tumor and adjacent areas of invasion.

***Tunga penetrans*.** See **chigoe.**

**tungiasis** /tung·gī′ə·sis/, infestation of the skin with the chigoe (*Tunga penetrans*). See also **chigoe.**

**tungsten (W)** /tung′stən/ [SW, *tung,* heavy, *sten,* stone; *wolfram,* the German word for tungsten], a metallic element. Its atomic number is 74; its atomic mass is 183.85. It has the highest melting point of all metals and is used as a target material in x-ray tubes and as filaments in incandescent light bulbs.

**tunica** /t(y)o͞o′nikə/ [L, tunic], an enveloping coat or covering membrane.

**tunica adventitia,** the outer layer or coat of an artery or other tubular structure. See also **arterial wall.**

**tunica albuginea** [L, *tunica* + *albus,* white], a tissue covering of white collagenous fibers, such as the sclerotic coat of the eyeball and the testes.

**tunica dartos** /to͞o′ni·kə där′tōs/ [L, *tunica;* Gk, flayed], the thin layer of subcutaneous tissue underlying the skin of the scrotum, consisting mainly of nonstriated muscle fibers (the dartos muscle). Also called **dartos.**

**tunica intima,** the membrane lining an artery. See also **arterial wall.**

**tunica media,** a muscular middle coat of an artery. See also **arterial wall.**

**tunica vaginalis testis,** the serous membrane surrounding the testis and epididymis.

**tunica vasculosa bulbi.** See **uvea.**

**tuning fork** /t(y)o͞o′ning/ [Gk, *tonos*, stretching; L, *furca*, fork], a small metal instrument consisting of a stem and two prongs that produces a constant pitch when either prong is struck. It is used by physicians as a screening test of air and bone conduction.

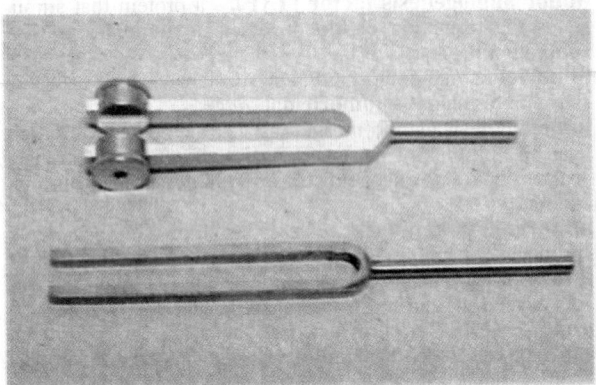

**Tuning forks** *(Seidel et al, 1999)*

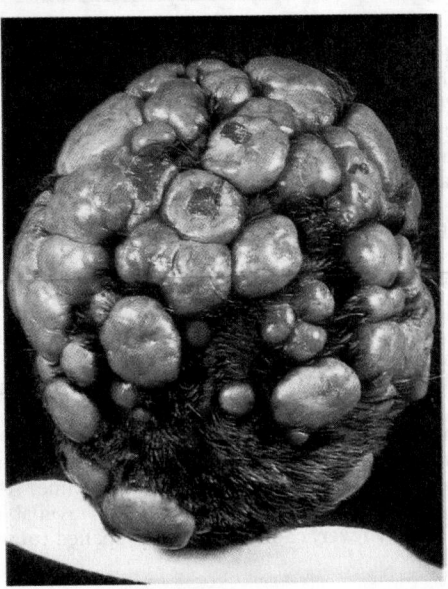

**Turban tumor**
*(Du Vivier, 1993/courtesy Queen Victoria Hospital, East Grinstead, England)*

**tunnel** [OFr, *tonnel*, fowl trap], a canal or passage, such as the carpal tunnel.

**tunnel vision** [OFr, *tonnel*, fowl trap; L, *videre*, to see], a defect in sight in which there is a great reduction in the peripheral field of vision, as if looking through a hollow tube or tunnel. The condition occurs in advanced glaucoma.

**tunnel wound** [OFr, *tonnel* + AS, *wund*], a break in the surface of the body or an organ in which the entry and exit wounds are the same size.

**TUR,** abbreviation for **transurethral resection.**

**turban tumor** /tur′bən/ [Turk, *tulbend*, headdress; L, *tumor*, swelling], a benign neoplasm consisting of pink or maroon nodules that may cover the entire scalp, trunk, and extremities. The growth is familial and often recurs after excision.

**turbid** /tur′bid/ [L, *turbidus*, confused], clouded or obscured, as in solids in suspension in a solution.

**turbidimetry** /tur′bidim′ətrē/ [L, *turbidus,* confused; Gk, *metron,* measure], measurement of the turbidity (cloudiness) of a solution or suspension in which the amount of transmitted light is quantified with a spectrophotometer or estimated by visual comparison with solutions of known turbidity.

**turbidity** /tərbid′itē/ [L, *turbidus*], a condition of light scattering in a liquid resulting from the presence of suspended particles. Turbidity increases with the concentration of particles and depends on their shapes and sizes.

**turbinate** /tur′binit/ [L, *turbinum*, top-shaped], 1. pertaining to a scroll shape. 2. pertaining to the concha nasalis.

**turgid** /tur′jid/ [L, *turgidus*], swollen, hard, and congested, usually as a result of an accumulation of fluid. —**turgor,** *n.*

**turgor** /tur′gər/ [L, *turgere*, to be swollen], the expected resiliency of the skin caused by the outward pressure of the cells and interstitial fluid. Dehydration results in decreased skin turgor, manifested by lax skin that, when grasped and raised between two fingers, slowly returns to a position level with the adjacent tissue. Marked edema or ascites results in increased turgor manifested by smooth, taut, shiny skin that cannot be grasped and raised. Elderly people normally do not have "good" skin turgor because of a lack of skin elasticity, an expected part of aging. An evaluation of the skin turgor is an essential part of physical assessment.

**turista.** See **traveler's diarrhea.**

**turnbuckle cast** [AS, *tyrnan* + ME, *bocle,* small shield; ONorse, *kasta*], an orthopedic device used to encase and immobilize the entire trunk, one upper arm to the elbow, and the opposite upper leg to the knee. It is constructed of plaster of paris or fiberglass and incorporates hinges as part of its design in the treatment of scoliosis. The hinges are placed at the level of the apex of the curvature. It is used for preoperative and postoperative positioning, although less frequently than the Risser cast. An adaptation of the turnbuckle cast is used occasionally as a hyperextension cast for the treatment of kyphosis or kyphoscoliosis. Compare **Risser cast.**

**Turner's sign.** See **Grey Turner's sign.**

**Turner's syndrome** [Henry H. Turner, American endocrinologist, 1892–1970], a chromosomal anomaly seen in about 1 in 3000 live female births, characterized by the absence of one X chromosome; congenital ovarian failure, genital hypoplasia; cardiovascular anomalies; dwarfism; short metacarpals; "shield chest"; extosis of tibia; and underdeveloped breasts, uterus, and vagina. Spatial disorientation and moderate degrees of learning disorders are common. Treatment includes genetic counseling, hormone therapy (estrogens, androgens, pituitary growth hormone), and often surgical correction of cardiovascular anomalies and the webbing of the neck skin. Also called **Bonnevie-Ullrich syndrome, monosomy X.** See also **Noonan's syndrome.**

**turnkey** /turn′kē/, a term referring to a computer system or installation that is complete on delivery and ready to operate without modification.

**TURP,** abbreviation for **transurethral resection of the prostate.**

**turricephaly.** See **oxycephaly.**

**-tuse,** 1. combining form meaning 'dull or blunt': *obtuse.* 2. combining form meaning 'to beat or bruise': *contuse.*

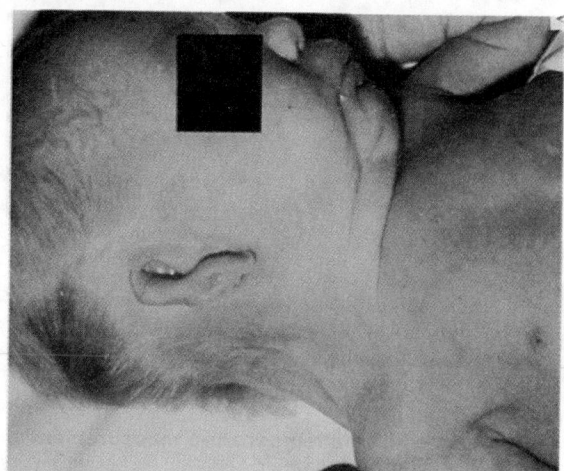

**Webbed neck, widespread nipples, abnormal ears, and micrognathia associated with Turner's syndrome** (Zitelli and Davis, 1997)

**Tussionex,** trademark for a fixed-combination drug containing an antitussive (hydrocodone bitartrate) and an antihistamine (phenyltoloxamine citrate).

**tussis** /tus′is/ [L, *tussis,* cough], a cough or pertussis.

**tussive fremitus** /tus′iv/ [L, *tussis,* cough, *fremitus,* murmuring], a vibratory cough that can be felt by a hand over the chest of the patient.

**tutorial** /t(y)o̅o̅tôr′ē·əl/ [L, *tueri,* to look with care], a form of instruction in which the student is guided step-by-step through the application of a computer program.

**TV,** abbreviation for *tidal volume,* the amount of air in milliliters per breath. Also called **V_t.** $V_t$.

**TVL,** abbreviation for **tenth-value layer.**

**T wave,** the component of the cardiac cycle shown on an electrocardiogram as a short, inverted, U-shaped curve after the S-T segment. It represents membrane repolarization phase 3 of the cardiac action potential.

**Tweed triangle** [Charles Tweed, American dentist, 1895–1970; L, *triangulus,* three-cornered], the triangle formed by the mandibular plane, the Frankfurt horizontal plane, and the long axis of the lower central incisor. It is used as a diagnostic aid.

**twelfth cranial nerve.** See **hypoglossal nerve.**

**twentieth-century syndrome.** See **total allergy syndrome.**

**24-hour clock system,** a method of designating time by using the numeric sequence from 00 to 23 for the hours and the numbers 00 to 59 for the minutes in a daily cycle beginning with 0000 (midnight) and ending with 2359 (1 minute before the next midnight). The system provides a clear distinction between prenoon and afternoon time without requiring the designations AM and PM. Also called **military time.**

**twilight state** [Ger, *Zwielicht,* twilight; L, *status*], an impaired state of consciousness in which the patient may experience visual or auditory hallucinations and responds to them with irrational behavior. The person may be unaware of the surroundings at the time of the experience and have no memory of it later, except perhaps to recall a related dream. It may be induced with certain anesthetics.

**twin** [AS, *twinn,* double], either of two offspring born of the same pregnancy and developed from either a single ovum or from two ova that were released from the ovary simultaneously and fertilized at the same time. The incidence of twin births is approximately 1 in 80 pregnancies. Kinds of twins include **conjoined twins, dizygotic twins, interlocked twins, monozygotic twins, Siamese twins,** and **unequal twins.** See also **Hellin's law.**

**twinge** /twinj/ [ME, *twengen,* to pinch], a sudden brief darting pain.

**twinning** [AS, *twinn*], **1.** the development of two or more fetuses during the same pregnancy, either spontaneously or through external intervention for experimental purposes in animals. **2.** the duplication of like structures or parts by division.

**twin-to-twin transfusion,** an intrauterine abnormality of fetal circulation in monozygotic twins, in which blood is shunted directly from one twin to the other.

**twin—twin transfusion syndrome,** a syndrome caused by twin-to-twin transfusion; the donor twin develops hypovolemia, hypotension, anemia, microcardia, and growth retardation, while the recipient develops hypervolemia, hypertension, polycythemia, cardiomegaly, and congestive heart failure; hydramnios frequently occurs.

**twin-wire orthodontic appliance,** a fixed orthodontic appliance that typically uses a pair of 0.01-inch (0.25-mm) wires to form the midsection of the arch wire. It is used to correct the crowding of anterior teeth and to expand the dental arch.

**twitch** [AS, *twiccian*], **1.** the contraction of small muscle units, manifested as a quick, simple, spasmodic contraction of a muscle. **2.** to jerk convulsively.

**twitching** [AS, *twiccian*], a series of contractions by small muscle units. Twitching that involves large groups of muscle fibers is identified as **fascicular twitching.**

**two-point discrimination test,** a test of the ability of a person to differentiate touch stimuli at two nearby points on the body at the same time. It is used in studies of possible damage to the parietal regions of the brain.

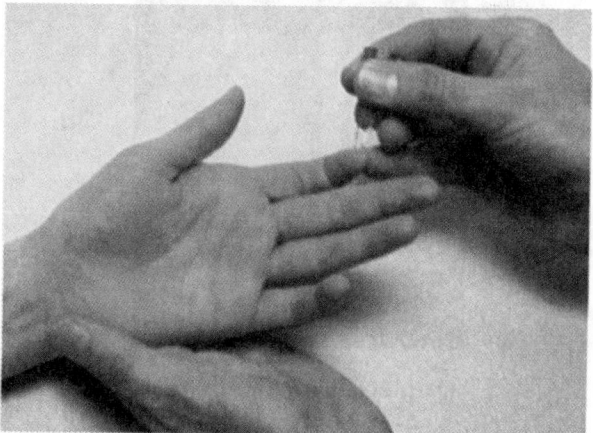

**Two-point discrimination test** (Seidel et al, 1999)

**two-point gait** [OE, *twa* + L, *punctus,* pricked; ONorse, *gata,* way], a pattern of crutch-walking in which the right foot and left crutch advance together, followed by the left foot and right crutch. See also **three-point gait.**

**two-way catheter** [AS, *twa* + *weg* + Gk, *katheter,* something lowered], a catheter that has a double lumen, one channel for injection of medication or fluids and the other for removal of fluid or specimens.

**TXA$_2$,** abbreviation for **thromboxane A$_2$.**

**TXB$_2$,** abbreviation for **thromboxane B$_2$.**

**Tylenol,** trademark for an analgesic and antipyretic (acetaminophen).

**tylosis** /tīlō′sis/, formation of a callus.

**tyloxapol** /tīlok′səpôl/, an ocular lubricant used to lubricate, clean, and wet artificial eyes to improve wearing comfort.

**tympan-,** combining form meaning 'the tympanic membrane': *tympanoplasty, tympanotomy.*

**tympanal.** See **tympanic.**

**tympanectomy** /tim′pənek′təmē/ [Gk, *tympanon,* drum, *ektomē*], the surgical removal of the tympanic membrane.

**tympanic** /timpan′ik/ [Gk, *tympanon,* drum], pertaining to a structure that resonates when struck; drumlike, such as a **tympanic abdomen** that resonates on percussion because the intestines are distended with gas. Also **tympanal.** —**tympanum** /tim′pənəm (*pl.* **tympana**), *n.*

**tympanic antrum,** a relatively large, irregular cavity in the superior anterior part of the mastoid process of the temporal bone, communicating with the mastoid air cells and lined by the extension of the mucous membrane of the tympanic cavity. The bony tegmen tympani separates the tympanic antrum from the middle fossa of the cranial cavity, and the lateral semicircular canal of the internal ear projects into the antrum. See also **mastoid process.**

**tympanic cavity.** See **middle ear.**

**tympanic membrane,** a thin semitransparent membrane in the middle ear that transmits sound vibrations to the internal ear by means of the auditory ossicles. It is nearly oval in form, with a vertical diameter of about 10 mm, and separates the tympanic cavity from the bottom of the external acoustic meatus. Also called **eardrum, membrana tympani.**

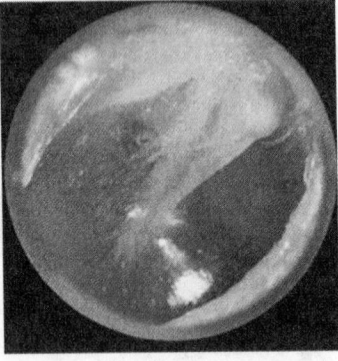

**Normal tympanic membrane**
*(Seidel et al, 1999/courtesy Dr. Richard A. Buckingham, Abraham Lincoln School of Medicine, University of Illinois, Chicago)*

**tympanic membrane thermometer,** a device that measures the temperature of the tympanic membrane by detecting infrared radiation from the tissue. Results are obtained within 2 seconds and directly reflect the body's core temperature. Tympanic thermometer is the common term. See also **ear thermometry.**

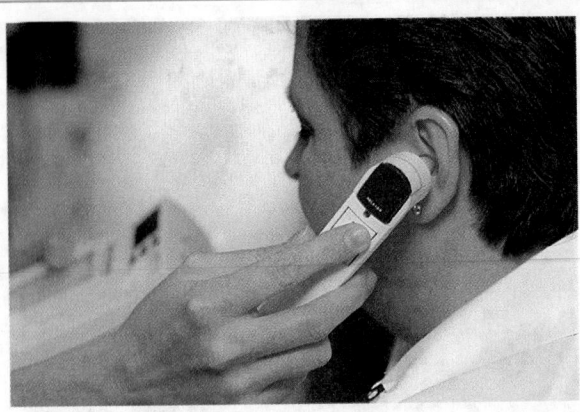

**Tympanic membrane temperature measurement**
*(Potter and Perry, 2001)*

**tympanic reflex,** the reflection of a beam of light shining on the eardrum. In a normal ear a bright, wedge-shaped reflection is seen; its apex is at the end of the malleus, and its base is at the anterior inferior margin of the eardrum. In disorders of the middle ear or eardrum, this shape may be distorted.

**tympanic resonance** [Gk, *tympanon* + L, *resonare,* to sound again], a drumlike or hollow sound heard over a large air space of the body such as the pneumothorax.

**tympanic sulcus** [Gk, *tympanon,* drum; L, *sulcus,* furrow], a narrow circular groove at the medial end of the osseous part of the external acoustic meatus that holds the tympanic membrane.

**tympanic temperature,** the body temperature as measured electronically at the tympanic membrane. See also **tympanic membrane thermometer.**

**tympano-** combining form meaning 'ear drum or tympanic membrane': *tympanoplasty, tympanotomy.*

**tympanogram** /timpan′əgram/, a graphic representation of the acoustic impedance and air pressure of the middle ear and mobility of the tympanic membrane, measured as part of the audiologic test battery. In the normal middle ear the air pressure is the same as the atmospheric pressure, as shown by a peak in the middle of the tympanogram. Various middle ear pathologies such as otitis media, otosclerosis, or tympanic membrane perforations each yield distinctive tympanograms. See also **acoustic impedance.**

**tympanomastoidectomy,** mastoidectomy with tympanectomy, done as either closed-cavity or open-cavity tympanomastoidectomy.

**tympanoplasty** /timpan′əplas′tē/ [Gk, *tympanon* + *plassein,* to mold], any of several operative procedures on the eardrum or ossicles of the middle ear designed to restore or improve hearing in patients with conductive hearing loss. These operations may be used to repair a perforated eardrum, for otosclerosis, or for dislocation or necrosis of one of the small bones of the middle ear. See also **myringoplasty, stapedectomy.**

**tympanostomy.** See **myringotomy.**

**tympanotomy.** See **myringotomy.**

**tympanum.** See **tympanic.**

**tympany** /tim′pənē/ [Gk, *tympanon,* drum], a loud, high-pitched musical sound percussed over the upper gastric area or a puffed-out cheek.

**-type,** combining form meaning a 'representative form or class': *lysotype, serotype, somatotype.*

**type 1 diabetes mellitus,** an inability to metabolize carbohydrate because of absolute insulin deficiency, occurring in children and adults. It is characterized by excessive thirst, increased urination, increased desire to eat, loss of weight, diminished strength, and marked irritability. The clinical onset is usually rapid, but approximately one third of patients have a remission within 3 months; this stage may continue for days or years, but type 1 diabetes then progresses quickly to a state of total dependence on insulin. Occasionally the disease is asymptomatic and is discovered only by postprandial elevated blood glucose level or abnormal results of glucose tolerance tests. Type 1 patients are sensitive to insulin and physical activity and diet and likely to experience ketoacidosis. Evidence suggests that type 1 diabetes may be triggered by environmental factors, such as a viral infection ingenetically susceptible individuals. Previously called **brittle diabetes, insulin-dependent diabetes mellitus, juvenile diabetes, juvenile-onset diabetes, JOD, juvenile onset–type diabetes, ketosis-prone diabetes, type I diabetes mellitus.** Compare **type 2 diabetes mellitus.** See also **diabetes mellitus.**

**type I AV block.** See **Mobitz I heart block.**

**type I error,** in a test of a statistical hypothesis, the probability of rejecting the null hypothesis when it is true and should be accepted. Also called **alpha error, error of the first kind.**

**type I hyperlipidemia.** See **hyperlipidemia type I.**

**type I hypersensitivity.** See **anaphylactic hypersensitivity.**

**type II AV block.** See **Mobitz II heart block.**

**type 2 diabetes mellitus,** a type of diabetes mellitus in which patients are not insulin-dependent or ketosis prone, although they may use insulin for correction of symptomatic or persistent hyperglycemia and they can develop ketosis under special circumstances such as infection or stress. Onset is usually after 40 years of age but can occur at any age. Two subclasses are the presence or absence of obesity. About 60% to 90% are obese; in these patients glucose tolerance is often improved by weight loss. Hyperinsulinemia and insulin resistance characterize some patients. There are probably multiple causes for the derangement of carbohydrate metabolism. Familial aggregation implies genetic factors, and this class includes diabetes presenting in childhood and adults in whom autosomal-dominant inheritance is clearly established. Environmental factors superimposed on genetic susceptibility are probably involved in the onset. Previously called **adult-onset diabetes, ketosis-resistant diabetes, maturity-onset diabetes, maturity-onset type diabetes, MOD, non–insulin-dependent diabetes mellitus, stable diabetes.** Also called **type II diabetes mellitus.** See also **diabetes mellitus.**

**type II error,** in a test of a statistical hypothesis, the probability of accepting the null hypothesis when it is false and should be rejected. Also called **beta error, error of the second kind.**

**type II hypersensitivity.** See **cytotoxic anaphylaxis.**

**type III hypersensitivity.** See **immune complex hypersensitivity.**

**type IV hypersensitivity.** See **cell-mediated immune response.**

**type A personality** [Gk, *typos,* mark], a parent ego state characterized by a behavior pattern described by Meyer Friedman and Ray Rosenman as associated with individuals who are highly competitive and work compulsively to meet deadlines. The behavior also is associated with a higher than usual incidence of coronary heart disease.

**type B personality,** a child ego state characterized by a form of behavior associated by Friedman and Rosenman with people who appear free of hostility and aggression and who lack a compulsion to meet deadlines, are not highly competitive at work and play, and have a lower risk of heart attack.

**type E personality,** a term introduced by Harriet Braiker to describe professional women who fit neither type A nor type B personality categories, but who have a marked sense of insecurity and strive to convince themselves that they are worthwhile. Type E women try to be 'all things to all people,' according to Braiker, and tend to suffer psychologic strain. Also called **adult ego state.**

**type specificity.** See **specificity.**

**typhlitis.** See **cecitis.**

**typhlo-,** 1. combining form meaning 'cecum': *typhlocolitis, typhlostenosis, typhlostomy.* 2. combining form meaning 'blindness': *typhlolexia, typhlology, typhlosis.*

**typho-,** combining form meaning 'fever' and related to typhus and typhoid fevers.

**typhoid** /tī′foid/ [Gk, *typhos,* fever, *eidos,* form], pertaining to or resembling typhus.

**-typhoid,** combining form meaning 'typhus': *bronchotyphoid, meningotyphoid, nephrotyphoid, antityphoid, paratyphoid, posttyphoid.*

**typhoid carrier,** a person without signs or symptoms of typhoid fever who carries the bacteria that cause the disease and sheds the pathogens in body excretions. The typical typhoid carrier has recovered from an attack of the disease.

**typhoid fever** [Gk, *typhos,* fever, *eidos,* form; L, *febris,* fever], a bacterial infection usually caused by *Salmonella typhi,* transmitted by contaminated milk, water, or food. It is characterized by headache, delirium, cough, watery diarrhea, rash, and a high fever. Also called **enteric fever.** Compare **cholera, paratyphoid fever, salmonellosis.**

**typhoid nodules** [Gk, *typhos,* fever; L, *nodulus,* small knot], a liver nodule consisting of a cluster of monocytes and lymphocytes surrounding the typhoid fever pathogen, *Salmonella typhi.*

**typhoid pellagra,** a form of pellagra in which the symptoms also include continued high temperatures.

**typhoid vaccine,** a bacterial vaccine prepared from an inactivated dried strain of *Salmonella typhi.*

■ INDICATIONS: It is prescribed for primary immunization against typhoid fever for adults and children.

■ CONTRAINDICATIONS: Acute infection or concomitant use of corticosteroids prohibits its use.

■ ADVERSE EFFECTS: Among the more serious adverse reactions are anaphylaxis and pain and inflammation at the site of injection.

**typhomania** /tīfōmā′nē·ə/, a condition characterized by coma and delirium associated with typhus, typhoid fever, and similar febrile infections.

**typhous** /tī′fəs/ [Gk, *typhos,* fever], pertaining to typhus fever.

**typhus** /tī′fəs/ [Gk, *typhos,* fever], any of a group of acute infectious diseases caused by various species of *Rickettsia* and usually transmitted from infected rodents to humans by the bites of lice, fleas, mites, or ticks. These diseases are all characterized by headache, chills, fever, malaise, and a maculopapular rash. Kinds of typhus are **epidemic typhus, murine typhus,** and **scrub typhus.** See also **Brill-Zinsser disease, Rocky Mountain spotted fever.**

**typhus vaccine,** any one of three vaccines, each of which is prepared for the different rickettsial organisms that cause epidemic typhus, murine typhus, or Brill-Zinsser disease.

■ INDICATIONS: Each of the vaccines is prescribed for immunization against a form of typhus.

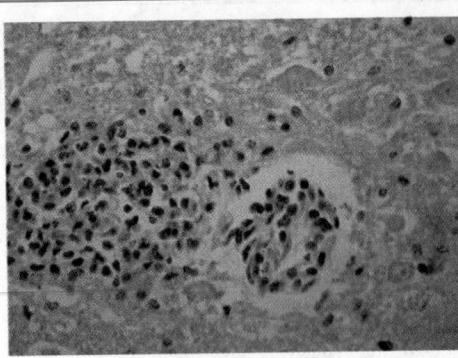

**Typhus nodule in the brain**
*(Cotran, Kumar, and Collins, 1999)*

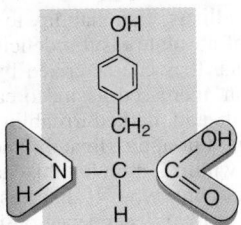

**Chemical structure of tyrosine**

■ CONTRAINDICATIONS: Acute infection, debilitating disease, concomitant use of corticosteroids, or hypersensitivity to eggs prohibits its use.

■ ADVERSE EFFECTS: Among the most serious adverse reactions are anaphylaxis and various allergic reactions. Pain at the site of injection also may occur.

**-typia,** combining form meaning '(condition of) conformity to type': *atypia, ectypia, zelotypia.*

**typical** /tip'ikəl/ [L, *typicus,* characteristic of a kind], a representative example.

**typing** [Gk, *typos,* mark], the process of classifying a specimen of blood, tissue, or other substance according to common traits or characteristics. See also **blood typing, tissue typing.**

**typo-,** combining form meaning 'a particular type': *typology, typography.*

**Tyr,** abbreviation for **tyrosine.**

**tyramine** /tī'rəmēn/ [Gk, *tyros,* cheese, *amine,* ammonia], an amino acid synthesized in the body from the essential amino acid tyrosine. Tyramine stimulates the release of the catecholamines epinephrine and norepinephrine. It is important that people taking monoamine oxidase inhibitors avoid the ingestion of foods and beverages containing tyramine, particularly aged cheeses and meats, bananas, yeast-containing products, and certain alcoholic beverages, such as red wines. See also **amine, catecholamine, epinephrine, norepinephrine, sympathomimetic, vasoconstriction.**

**tyro-,** combining form meaning 'cheese': *tyrogenous, tyroid, tyrometosis.*

**tyroma** /tūrō'mə/, *pl.* **tyromas, tyromata** [Gk, *tyros* + *oma,* tumor], a new growth or nodule with a caseous or cheesy consistency.

**tyromatosis** /tī'rōmətō'sis/ [Gk, *tyros* + *oma* + *osis,* condition], a process in which necrotic tissue is broken down and degenerates to a granular, amorphous, caseous mass.

**tyrosine (Tyr)** /tī'rəsēn/ [Gk, *tyros*], an amino acid synthesized in the body from the essential amino acid phenylalanine. Tyrosine is found in most proteins and is a precursor of melanin and several hormones, including epinephrine and thyroxin. See also **amino acid, hormone, melanocyte.**

**tyrosinemia** /tī'rōsinē'mē·ə/ [Gk, *tyros* + *haima,* blood], **1.** also called **neonatal tyrosinemia.** a benign, transient condition of the newborn, especially premature infants, in which an excessive amount of the amino acid tyrosine is found in the blood and urine. The disorder is caused by an anomaly in amino acid metabolism, usually delayed development of the enzymes necessary to metabolize tyrosine,

and is controlled by dietary measures and vitamin C therapy. The metabolic defect disappears with treatment, or it may disappear spontaneously. **2.** also called **hereditary tyrosinemia.** a hereditary disorder involving an inborn error of metabolism of the amino acid tyrosine. The condition, which is transmitted as an autosomal-recessive trait, is caused by an enzyme deficiency and results in liver failure or hepatic cirrhosis, renal tubular defects that can lead to renal rickets and renal glycosuria, generalized aminoaciduria, and mental retardation. Treatment consists of a diet low in tyrosine and phenylalanine and high in vitamin C. In severe cases prognosis is extremely poor, and a liver transplantation may be the only lifesaving measure.

**tyrosinosis** /tī'rōsinō'sis/ [Gk, *tyros* + *osis,* condition], a rare condition resulting from a defect in amino acid metabolism and transmitted as an autosomal-recessive trait. It is characterized by the excretion of an excessive amount of parahydroxyphenylpyruvic acid, an intermediate product of tyrosine, in the urine. There is no known treatment. See also **tyrosinemia.**

**tyrosinurea** /tī'rōsinŏŏr'ē·ə/ [Gk, *tyros* + *ouron,* urine], the presence of tyrosine in the urine.

**Tyzine,** trademark for an alpha-adrenergic drug (tetrahydrozoline hydrochloride).

**Tzanck test** /tsangk/ [Arnault Tzanck, Russian dermatologist in France, 1886–1954], a microscopic examination of cellular material from skin lesions to help diagnose certain vesicular diseases. The tissue is scraped from the base of a vesicle, placed on a slide, and stained with Wright's or Giemsa's stain. Multinucleated giant cells are diagnostic of herpesvirus or varicella. Typical pemphigus and other cells also can be identified.

**tzetze fly.** See **tsetse fly.**

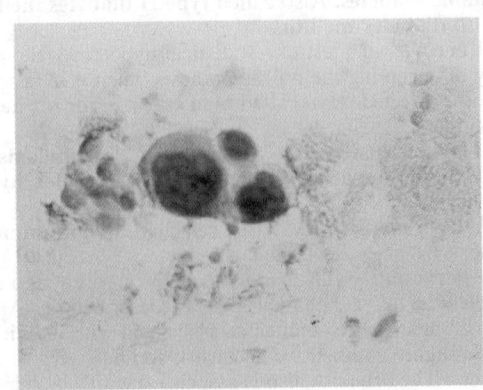

**Tzanck test** *(Zitelli and Davis, 1997)*

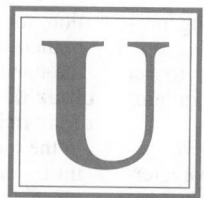

**u,** symbol sometimes used to stand for **micro-** (properly μ), as in "ul" or "um," representing μL or μm.

**U,** **1.** abbreviation for **unit. 2.** symbol for the element **uranium.**

**UAO,** abbreviation for **upper airway obstruction.**

**ubiquinone** /yo̅o̅bik′winōn/, a quinone derivative that occurs in the lipid core of mitochondrial membranes and functions in the electron transport chain as a carrier. Formerly called **coenzyme Q.**

**ubiquitin** /yo̅o̅bik′witin/, a small polypeptide that is involved in histone modification. It is found in all cells of higher organisms.

**UGI,** abbreviation for **upper GI.**

**UICC,** abbreviation for *International Union Against Cancer, Unión internacional contra el cancer, Union internationale contre le cancer, Unio internationalis contra cancrum,* or *Unione internazionale contro il cancro.*

**-ula,** suffix meaning 'small, little, minute': *macula.*

**-ular, 1.** suffix meaning 'pertaining to' something specified: *appendicular, molecular, pedicular.* **2.** combining form meaning 'resembling' something specified: *circular, globular, tubular.*

**ulcer** /ul′sər/ [L, *ulcus,* a sore], a circumscribed, craterlike lesion of the skin or mucous membrane resulting from necrosis that accompanies some inflammatory, infectious, or malignant processes. An ulcer may be shallow, involving only the epidermis, as in pemphigus, or deep, as in a rodent ulcer. Some kinds of ulcers are **pressure ulcer, peptic ulcer,** and **serpent ulcer. —ulcerate,** *v.,* **ulcerative,** *adj.*

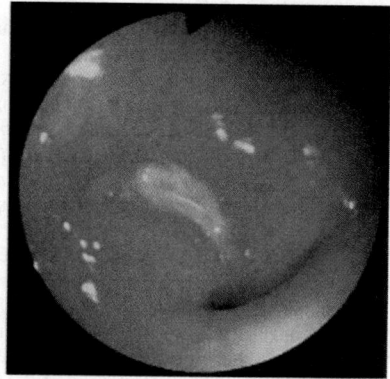

**Duodenal ulcer** *(Misiewicz et al, 1994)*

**ulcerate** /ul′sərāt/ [L, *ulcus,* a sore], to form an ulcer.

**ulceration** /ul′sərā′shən/ [L, *ulcus,* a sore], the process of ulcer formation.

**ulcerative blepharitis** /ul′sərā′tiv, ul′sərətiv′/ [L, *ulcus + atus,* relating to; Gk, *blepharon,* eyelid, *itis,* inflammation], a form of blepharitis in which a staphylococcal infection of the follicles of the eyelashes and glands of the eyelids results in sticky crusts forming on the lid margins. If the crusts are pulled off, the skin beneath bleeds. Tiny pustules develop in the follicles of the eyelashes and break down to form shallow ulcers. Other symptoms include burning, itching, swelling, and redness of the eyelids; a loss of eyelashes; irritation of the conjunctiva with tearing; photophobia; and gluing together of the eyelids during sleep by the dried secretions. Compare **nonulcerative blepharitis.**

**ulcerative colitis,** a chronic, episodic, inflammatory disease of the large intestine and rectum. It is characterized by profuse watery diarrhea containing varying amounts of blood, mucus, and pus. Some of the many systemic complications of ulcerative colitis include peripheral arthritis, ankylosing spondylitis, kidney and liver disease, and inflammation of the eyes, skin, and mouth. People with severe disease may develop toxic megacolon, a dangerous complication that may lead to perforation of the bowel, septicemia, and death. Also called **inflammatory bowel disease (IBD).** See also **Crohn's disease.**

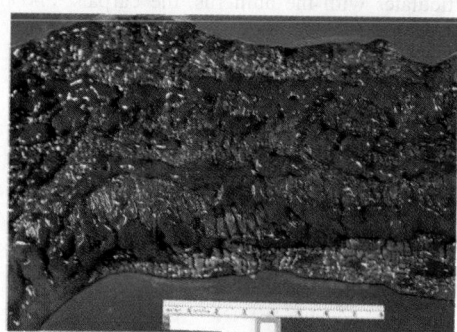

**Ulcerative colitis** *(Rosai, 1996)*

■ OBSERVATIONS: The attacks of diarrhea are accompanied by tenesmus, severe abdominal pain, fever, chills, anemia, and weight loss. Children with the disease may suffer retarded physical growth. The debilitating symptoms often prevent people with ulcerative colitis from carrying on the normal activities of daily living. Diagnosis of the disease is based on clinical signs, the results of barium x-ray films of the colon, and colonoscopy with biopsy. It is often difficult to differentiate between ulcerative colitis and Crohn's disease.

■ INTERVENTIONS: Medical treatment with corticosteroids or other antiinflammatory agents may help control the symptoms in some people. Those with severe disease or life-threatening complications may require surgery. Total proctocolectomy with ileostomy is a permanent cure. Ulcerative colitis carries an increased risk of developing cancer of the colon, and periodic colonoscopy is performed to rule out this complication. A person with ulcerative colitis is suffering from a chronic, life-threatening illness and requires frequent evidence of support and understanding during prolonged hospitalization.

**ulcerative inflammation** [L, *ulcus* + *inflammare*, to set afire], the development of an ulcer over an area of inflammation.

**ulcerative stomatitis** [L, *ulcus* + Gk *stoma*, mouth, *itis*, inflammation], an infectious disease of the mouth characterized by swollen spongy gums, ulcers, and loose teeth. Also called **trench mouth, ulceromembranous stomatitis, Vincent's angina.**

**ulcerogenic drug** /ul'sərōjen'ik/, a drug that produces or exacerbates peptic ulcers, such as aspirin and NSAID medications.

**ulceromembranous** /ul'sərōmem'brənəs/, describing an ulcer with a membranous exudation.

**ulceromembranous stomatitis.** See **ulcerative stomatitis.**

**ulcerous** /ul'sərəs/, pertaining to ulcers.

**ULD,** abbreviation for **upper level discriminator.**

**ule-.** See **ulo-.**

**-ule.** See **-ulum, -ulus.**

**ulegyria** /yōō'ləjī'rē·ə/, a cerebral cortex abnormality in which the gyri are narrow and distorted by scars.

**-ulent,** suffix meaning 'full of, characterized by': *feculent, pulverulent, succulent.*

**ulerythema** /yōō'lərithē'mə/, a skin eruption characterized by redness and scarring.

**ulna** /ul'nə/ [L, elbow], the bone on the medial or little finger side of the forearm, lying parallel with the radius. Its proximal end bulges into the olecranon and the coronoid processes and dips into the trochlear and radial notches. The ulna articulates with the humerus, the carpals, and the radius. Also called **elbow bone.** See also **radius.**

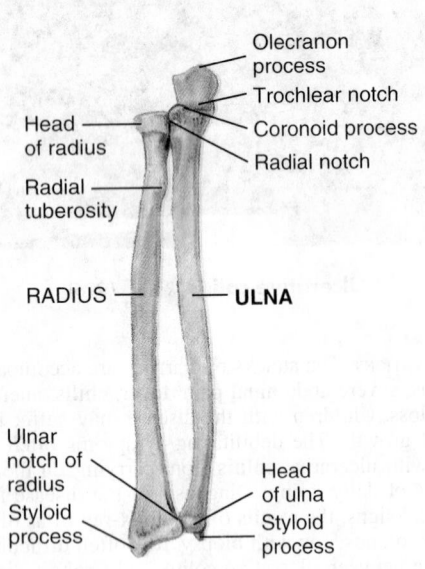

Olecranon process
Trochlear notch
Coronoid process
Radial notch
Head of radius
Radial tuberosity
RADIUS — ULNA
Ulnar notch of radius
Styloid process
Head of ulna
Styloid process

**Ulna and radius**

**ulnar** /ul'nər/ [L, *ulna*, elbow], pertaining to the long medial bone of the forearm.

**ulnar artery,** a large artery branching from the brachial artery, supplying muscles in the forearm, wrist, and hand. Arising near the elbow, it passes obliquely in a distal direction to become the superficial palmar arch. It has nine branches: four in the forearm, two in the wrist, and three in the hand.

**ulnar deviation.** See **ulnar drift.**

**ulnar drift** [L, *ulna*, elbow; AS, *drifan*, to drive], a change in the metacarpophalangeal joints because of rheumatoid arthritis and chronic synovitis. The long axis of the fingers make an angle with the long axis of the wrist so that the fingers are deviated to the ulnar side of the hand.

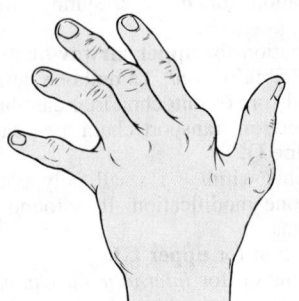

**Ulnar drift** *(Lewis, Collier, and Heitkemper, 1996)*

**ulnar nerve,** one of the terminal branches of the brachial plexus that arises on each side from the medial cord of the plexus. It receives fibers from both cervical and thoracic nerve roots and supplies the muscles and skin on the ulnar side of the forearm and the hand. It can be easily palpated as the 'funny bone' of the elbow as it courses along the groove between the olecranon process and the medial epicondyle of the humerus. Compare **median nerve, musculocutaneous nerve, radial nerve.**

**ulnar reflex.** See **pronator reflex.**

**ulnocarpal** /ul'nōkär'pəl/, pertaining to the ulna and carpus or ulnar area of the wrist.

**ulnoradial** /ul'nōrā'dē·əl/, pertaining to the ulna and radius and the ligaments associated with them.

**ulo-,** **1.** combining form meaning 'scar or cicatrix': *ulodermatitis, uloid, ulotomy.* **2.** also **ule-.** combining form meaning 'gums or gingivae': *ulocase, ulorrhagia, ulotripsis.*

**ulocarcinoma** /yōō'lōkär'sinō'mə/, *pl.* **ulocarcinomas, ulocarcinomata** [Gk, *oule*, scar, *karkinos*, crab, *oma*, tumor], any malignant neoplasm of the gums that is classified as a carcinoma.

**ulodermatitis** /yōō'lōdur'mətī'tis/, dermatitis resulting in the destruction of tissue and scar formation.

**uloid** /yōō'loid/, resembling scar tissue.

**ulterior transactions** /ultir'ē·ər/, (in transactional analysis), communication that is bilevel. The first level is overt (social), usually of relevant verbal statements. The second level is usually covert (psychologic) and nonverbal and has hidden psychologic meaning. For example, "Come up to my apartment to see my etchings."

**ultimate strain** /ul'timit/, the strain at the point of failure.

**ultimate stress,** the highest load that can be sustained by a material at the point of failure.

**ultra-** /ul'trə-/, prefix meaning 'beyond, farther, beyond a certain limit': *ultragaseous, ultrasound, ultravirus.*

**ultrabrachycephalic** /-brak'ēsəfal'ik/, describing an extremely short, broad skull.

**Ultracef,** trademark for a cephalosporin antibiotic (cefadroxil monohydrate).

**ultracentrifuge** /ul'trəsen'trifyo͞oj/ [L, *ultra,* beyond; Gk, *kentron,* center; L, *fugere,* to flee], a high-speed centrifuge with a rotation rate fast enough to produce sedimentation of protein and viruses, even in blood plasma. Use of an attached microscope may make it possible to see the sediment.

**ultradian** /rā'dē·ən/ [L, *ultra* + *dies,* day], pertaining to a biorhythm that occurs in cycles of less than 24 hours.

**ultrafilter** /-fil'tər/, a semipermeable membrane with pores of a known diameter used to separate colloids and large molecules from water and other small molecules.

**ultrafiltrate** /-fil'trāt/ [L, *ultra* + Fr, *filtre,* filter], a solution that has passed through a semipermeable membrane with very small pores. It usually contains only low-molecular weight solutes.

**ultrafiltration** /-filtrā'shən/, a type of filtration, sometimes conducted under pressure, through filters with very small pores, such as used by an artificial kidney. It can separate large molecules from smaller molecules in body fluids.

**ultra-high-speed handpiece,** a device for holding rotary instruments, such as burrs, that permits rotational speeds of 100,000 to 450,000 rpm. It is used primarily for tooth cavity preparation.

**Ultralente,** trademark for an insulin zinc suspension.

**ultralente insulin.** See **long-acting insulin.**

**ultraligation** /-līgā'shən/, tying or closing off a blood vessel beyond the point where it branches.

**ultramicroscopy.** See **darkfield microscopy.**

**ultramicrotome** /-mī'krətōm'/, a microtome that cuts very thin slices for examination by electron microscopy.

**ultrasonic** /ul'trəson'ik/ [L, *ultra,* beyond + *sonus,* sound], pertaining to ultrasound, or sound frequencies so high (greater than 20 kilohertz) that they cannot be perceived by the human ear.

**ultrasonic cardiography.** See **echocardiography.**

**ultrasonic cleaner,** a device that transmits high-energy, high-frequency sound waves into a fluid-filled container, used to remove deposits from instruments and appliances.

**ultrasonic cleaning,** the use of high-frequency vibrations to dislodge deposits from teeth or other objects.

**ultrasonic nebulizer,** a humidifier in which an electric current is used to produce high-frequency vibrations in a container of fluid. The vibrations break up the fluid into aerosol particles.

**ultrasonics** /-son'iks/, the science dealing with sound waves having frequencies above the approximately 20-kHz range of human hearing. Ultrasound evolved from the World War II sonar underwater detection apparatus and was first adapted for medical diagnostic purposes in the 1950s. It uses a transducer and generates very short pulses of high-frequency sound that are transmitted into the body. Echoes from interfaces within the body are displayed on a cathode ray tube so that images of normal and abnormal structures can be viewed.

**ultrasonic scaler,** an ultrasonic instrument with a tip for supplying high-frequency vibrations, used to remove adherent deposits from the teeth and bits of inflamed tissue from the walls of the gingival crevice. See also **scaler.**

**ultrasonic wave** [L, *ultra,* beyond, *sonus,* sound], a sound wave transmitted at a frequency greater than 20,000 per second, or beyond the normal hearing range of humans. The specific wavelength is equal to the velocity divided by the frequency.

**ultrasonographer.** See **sonographer.**

**ultrasonography** /-sənog'rəfē/ [L, *ultra* + *sonus,* sound; Gk, *graphein,* to record], the process of imaging deep structures of the body by measuring and recording the reflection of pulsed or continuous high-frequency sound waves. It is valuable in many medical situations, including the diagnosis of fetal abnormalities, gallstones, heart defects, and tumors. Also called **sonography.**

**ultrasonography: limited obstetric,** a nursing intervention from the Nursing Interventions Classification (NIC) defined as performance of ultrasound exams to determine ovarian, uterine, or fetal status. See also **Nursing Interventions Classification.**

**ultrasound** /ul'trəsound/ [L, *ultra* + *sonus*], sound waves at the very high frequency of over 20 kHz (vibrations per second). Ultrasound has many medical applications, including fetal monitoring, imaging of internal organs, and, at an extremely high frequency, the cleaning of dental and surgical instruments. —**ultrasonic,** *adj.*

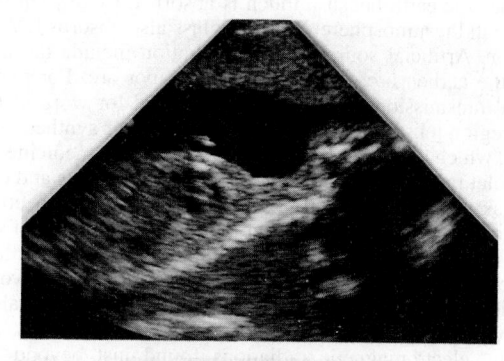
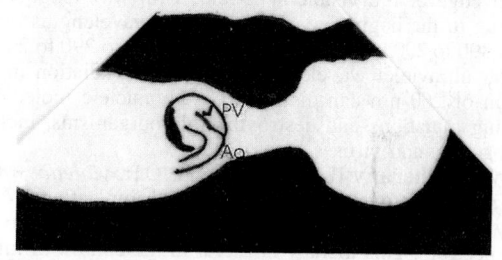

**Ultrasound: image of a fetus in the second trimester**

**ultrasound imaging,** the use of high-frequency sound (several MHz or more) to image internal structures by the differing reflection signals produced when a beam of sound waves is projected into the body and bounces back at interfaces between those structures. Ultrasound diagnosis differs from radiologic diagnosis in that there is no ionizing radiation involved. Also called **ultrasound diagnosing.**

**ultrastructure** /-struk'chər/, a structure so small it can be viewed only with an ultramicroscope or electron microscope.

**ultraviolet (UV)** /-vī'ələt/ [L, *ultra* + Fr, *violette*], light beyond the range of human vision, at the short end of the spectrum, or that part of the electromagnetic spectrum with wavelengths between about 10 and 400 nm. Equivalently, an ultraviolet photon has an energy between 5 and 500 eV. It occurs naturally in sunlight; it burns and tans the skin and converts precursors in the skin to vitamin D. Ultraviolet lamps are used in the control of infectious airborne bacteria and viruses and in the treatment of psoriasis and other skin conditions. Black light is ultraviolet light used in fluoroscopy. See also **angstrom, light, radiation, spectrum.**

**ultraviolet lamp** /-vī′ələt/, a lamp that emits electromagnetic radiation in a range between 4 and 400 nm, or beyond the violet spectrum of visible light. Equipped with a nickel oxide filter, an ultraviolet lamp radiating at wavelengths around 360 nm can be used to examine hairs infected with certain agents. The pathogens reflect the ultraviolet light with a greenish-yellow fluorescence. See also **Wood's light.**

**ultraviolet microscopy.** See **fluorescent microscopy.**

**ultraviolet radiation,** a range of electromagnetic waves extending from the violet or short-wavelength end of the visible spectrum to the beginning of the x-ray spectrum. Near-UV radiation covers a range of wavelengths from 400 to 320 nm; middle-UV from 320 to 280 nm; and far-UV from 280 to about 10 nm. About 5% of the energy from the sun consists of UV radiation, but little of this type of it reaches the earth because much is absorbed by oxygen and ozone in the atmosphere. Window glass also absorbs UV radiation. Artificial sources of UV radiation include the iron arc, the carbon arc, and the mercury vapor arc. For maximum transmission, prisms and lenses used for work in the UV region must be made of quartz, fluorite, or synthetic halides, which are transparent to UV radiation. In medicine ultraviolet radiation is used in the treatment of rickets and certain skin conditions. Milk and some other foods become activated with vitamin D when exposed to this type of energy. UV radiation also causes certain substances to fluoresce or phosphoresce, a useful characteristic in such diverse applications as lighting and the identification of minerals.

**ultraviolet rays** [L, *ultra,* beyond; OFr, *violette* + L, *radius*], electromagnetic radiations found just beyond the violet edge of the visible spectrum, with wavelengths extending to the beginning of x-rays. The wavelengths range from 390 to 290 nm for near ultraviolet rays to 290 to 20 nm for far ultraviolet wavelengths. Ultraviolet radiation in the region of 260 nm can distort deoxyribonucleic molecules, causing mutations and destroying microorganisms, including bacteria and viruses.

**ultraviolet therapy** [L, *ultra,* beyond; OFr, *violette* + Gk, *therapeia,* treatment], the therapeutic application to the body of electromagnetic radiation in the ultraviolet region of the spectrum. This therapy is useful in the control of infectious airborne bacteria and viruses and in the treatment of psoriasis and other skin conditions.

**-ulum, -ule,** suffix meaning 'small one': *ovulum, speculum, venule.*

**-ulus, -ule,** suffix meaning 'small one': *homunculus, nodulus, ramulus.*

**-um,** suffix identifying singular nouns: *cerebellum, dextrum, quantum.*

**umbilical** /umbil′ikəl/ [L, *umbilicus,* navel], **1.** pertaining to the umbilicus. **2.** pertaining to the umbilical cord.

**umbilical artery catheter** [L, *umbilicus,* navel; Gk, *arteria,* airpipe, *katheter,* a thing lowered], a catheter inserted into the umbilical artery of a newborn. See **umbilical catheterization.**

**umbilical catheterization,** a procedure in which a radiopaque catheter is passed through an umbilical artery to provide a newborn with parenteral fluid, to obtain blood samples, or both, or through the umbilical vein for an exchange transfusion or the emergency administration of drugs, fluids, or volume expanders.

■ METHOD: Within 1 hour of insertion of the catheter, the position of the tip is validated by x-ray examination. The infant

is maintained in a neutral thermal environment as parenteral fluids are delivered by an infusion pump; the rate of flow is checked hourly, and the IV bottle is never allowed to empty. All connections to the umbilical line are checked every 30 to 60 minutes, and only grounded electric equipment is used on or near the infant. At hourly intervals the young patient is repositioned, and the cardiac and respiratory rates are monitored; the axillary temperature is taken every 2 to 3 hours, and the pedal pulses are checked every 2 to 4 hours. The condition of the cord is observed every 2 to 3 hours for signs of infection such as redness, edema, or drainage at the catheter insertion site; the IV tubing is retaped when required, the cord dressing is changed, and antibiotic or antiseptic ointment is applied as ordered. If the umbilical line is displaced, pressure is quickly applied to the cord with a sterile 4 × 4-inch gauze, and an associate is delegated to notify the physician immediately. Fluid intake and output are measured. The infant is observed for oliguria or anuria; signs of vasospasm such as blanching, mottling, or darkening of the legs and absence of peripheral pulses; evidence of sepsis, hemorrhage, or oozing at the catheter insertion site; thromboembolism; and abdominal distension and vomiting, which may indicate necrotizing enterocolitis.

■ INTERVENTIONS: The nurse provides ongoing care, monitoring the catheterized infant for any signs of complications, which are promptly reported. The family is included in the care of the infant as much as possible.

■ OUTCOME CRITERIA: Umbilical catheterization can be an effective method of administering therapeutic fluids and agents or of obtaining diagnostic blood samples from a high-risk newborn, but great care is required in inserting and monitoring the tube.

**umbilical cord,** a flexible structure connecting the umbilicus with the placenta in the gravid uterus and giving passage to the umbilical arteries and vein. In the newborn it is about 2 feet long and 1/2 inch in diameter. First formed during the fifth week of pregnancy, it contains the yolk sac and the body stalk with the enclosed allantois. Also called the **chorda umbilicalis, funiculus umbilicalis.** See also **allantois.**

**umbilical duct.** See **vitelline duct.**

**umbilical fissure,** a groove on the inferior surface of the liver that holds the ligamentum teres and separates the right and left lobes of the liver.

**umbilical fistula,** an abnormal passage from the umbilicus to the intestine or more frequently to the remnant of the canal in the median umbilical ligament that connects the fetal bladder with the allantois.

**umbilical hernia,** a soft, skin-covered protrusion of intestine and omentum through a weakness in the abdominal wall around the umbilicus. It usually closes spontaneously within 1 to 2 years, although large hernias may require surgical closure.

**umbilical region,** the part of the abdomen surrounding the umbilicus, in the middle zone between the right and left lateral regions. See also **abdominal regions.**

**umbilical vasculitis,** an inflammation of the umbilical cord and its blood vessels.

**umbilical vein,** one of a pair of embryonic vessels that return the blood from the placenta and fuse to form a single trunk in the body stalk.

**umbilical vesicle,** a pear-shaped structure formed from the yolk sac at about the fourth week of prenatal development that protrudes into the cavity of the chorion and connects to the developing embryo by the yolk stalk at the region of the future midgut.

**umbilication** /um′bilikā′shən/ [L, *umbilicus,* navel], the

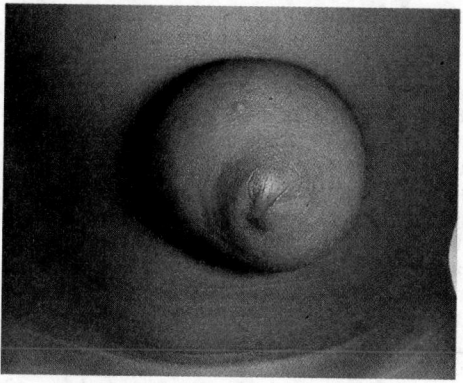

**Umbilical hernia** *(Zitelli and Davis, 1997)*

process of becoming dimpled or pitted or acquiring a depressed area.

**umbilicus** /umbilī'kəs, umbil'ikəs/ [L, navel], the point on the abdomen at which the umbilical cord joined the fetal abdomen. In most adults it is marked by a depression; in some it is marked by a small protrusion of skin. It interrupts the linea alba about halfway between the infrasternal notch and the pubic symphysis. It is located at the level of the interspace of the third and the fourth lumbar vertebrae. Also called **belly button, navel.**

**umbo** [L, knob], a projection on any rounded surface, such as the inner surface of the tympanic membrane where the malleus is attached.

**umbrella filter** /umbrəl'ə/, a small, porous, umbrella-shaped device that can be inserted into a vena cava or other blood vessel to trap blood clots.

**un-** prefix meaning 'not': *unconscious.*

**uncal** [L, *uncus,* hook], pertaining to the uncus.

**uncal herniation** /ung'kəl/ [L, *uncus,* hook, *hernia,* rupture], a condition in which the medial part of the temporal lobe protrudes over the tentorial edge as a result of increased intracranial pressure. If uncorrected, the progressive disorder causes pressure on the brainstem after first impinging on the third cranial nerve. A dilated pupil on the side of the herniation is a diagnostic sign of the disorder.

**unciform bone.** See **hamate bone.**

*Uncinaria* /un'siner'ē·ə/ [L, *uncinus,* hook], a genus of nematode that causes hookworm in dogs, cats, and other carnivores.

**uncinate** /un'sināt/, having hooks or barbs.

**uncipressure** /un'sipresh'ər/, pressure with a hook to control a hemorrhage.

**uncompensated care** /unkom'pənsā'tid/ [ME, *un,* against, not; L, *compendere,* to be equivalent], services provided by a hospital or a physician or other health care professional for which no charge is made and for which no payment is expected.

**uncompensated gluteal gait.** See **Trendelenburg gait.**

**uncompetitive inhibitor** /un'kəmpet'itiv/ [ME, *un* + L, *competere,* to compete, *inhibere,* to restrain], an enzymatic inhibitor that appears to bond only to the enzyme-substrate complex and not to free enzyme molecules.

**uncomplemented,** not united with proteins of the body's immune system and therefore inactive.

**unconditioned response** /un'kəndish'ənd/ [ME, *un* + L, *conditio,* condition, *respondere,* to reply], a normal, instinctive, unlearned reaction to a stimulus; one that occurs naturally and is not acquired by association and training. Also called **inborn reflex, instinctive reflex, unconditioned reflex.** Compare **conditioned response.**

**unconjugated bilirubin.** See **bilirubin.**

**unconjugated monoclonal antibody** /unkon'jəgā'tid/, One of a population of antibodies produced from a single clone of B lymphocytes and used for highly selective targeting of tumor cells. The antibodies can destroy malignant cells by direct lysis, by binding to cell receptors, and by mobilization of various killer cells.

**unconscious** /unkon'shəs/ [ME, *un* + L, *conscire,* to be aware], **1.** unaware of the surrounding environment; insensible; incapable of responding to sensory stimuli. **2.** (in psychiatry) the part of the mental function in which thoughts, ideas, emotions, or memories are beyond awareness and rarely subject to ready recall. It contains data that have never been conscious or that were conscious at one time, usually for a brief period, and later repressed. Compare **preconscious.** See also **collective unconscious, personal unconscious.**

**unconsciousness** /unkon'shəsnəs/, a state of complete or partial unawareness or lack of response to sensory stimuli as a result of hypoxia caused by respiratory insufficiency or shock; from metabolic or chemical brain depressants such as drugs, poisons, ketones, or electrolyte imbalance; or from a form of brain pathologic condition such as trauma, seizures,

### Possible causes of alterations in consciousness

1. Resulting from primary brain injury or disease
   a. Trauma (concussion, contusion, laceration, or traumatic intercerebral hemorrhage, subdural hematoma, epidural hematoma)
   b. Vascular disease (intracerebral hemorrhage, subarachnoid hemorrhage, infarction)
   c. Infections (meningitis, encephalitis, abscess, human immunodeficiency virus)
   d. Neoplasms (primarily intracranial, metastatic, or non-metastatic complication of malignancy)
   e. Seizures
   f. Degeneration (Alzheimer's disease)
2. Resulting from systemic conditions that secondarily affect the brain
   a. Metabolic encephalopathies (hypoglycemia, diabetic ketoacidosis, hyperglycemic nonketotic hyperosmolar states, uremia, hepatic encephalopathy, hyponatremia, hypokalemia, myxedema, acid-base imbalances, hypercalcemia)
   b. Urinary or respiratory infections
   c. Hypoxic encephalopathies (severe congestive heart failure with decompensation, severe anemia, hypertensive encephalopathies, hemorrhage)
   d. Toxicity (drugs, especially alcohol, anticholinergics, those with central nervous system effects)
   e. Physical causes (heatstroke, hypothermia)
   f. Nutritional causes (Wernicke's encephalopathy)
3. Resulting from psychologic causes that affect the brain
   a. Stress
   b. Depression
   c. Anxiety
4. Resulting from environmental conditions that affect the brain
   a. Sensory deprivation
   b. Sensory overload

From Phipps WJ, Sands JK, Marek JE: *Medical-surgical nursing: concepts and clinical practice,* ed 6, St Louis, 1999, Mosby.

cerebrovascular accident, brain tumor, or infection. Various degrees of unconsciousness can occur during stupor, fugue, catalepsy, and dream states. See also **coma.**

**unction.** See **ointment.**

**uncus** /ung′kəs/ [L, hook],   **1.** the hooklike anterior end of the hippocampal gyrus on the temporal lobe of the brain. **2.** a hook-shaped structure.

**undecylenic acid** /un′desilen′ik/,   a topical antifungal agent.

■ INDICATIONS: It is prescribed in the treatment of athlete's foot and ringworm.

■ CONTRAINDICATIONS: Known hypersensitivity to this drug prohibits its use. It is not used in the eyes or on mucous membranes. Caution is advised when the patient is diabetic.

■ ADVERSE EFFECTS: Among the more serious adverse effects are skin irritation and hypersensitivity reactions.

**undercut,**   **1.** the part of a tooth or artificial crown that lies between the height of contour and the gingivae, only if that part has a smaller diameter than the height of the contour. **2.** the contour of a cross section of a residual ridge that would prevent the placement of a denture or other prosthesis. **3.** the contour of flasking stone that interlocks so as to prevent the separation of parts. **4.** the part of a prepared cavity that creates a mechanical lock or area of retention. It may be desirable in a cavity to be filled with gold foil or amalgam but is undesirable in a cavity prepared for a restoration to be cemented.

**underdamping** /un′dərdam′ping/ [AS, *under,* beneath, *dampen,* to check],   the transmission of all frequency components in electrocardiography without a reduction in amplitude.

**underlying assumption** /un′dərlī′ing/,   a set of rules one holds about oneself, others, and the world. These rules are regarded by the individual as unquestionably true.

**undernutrition** /-nōōtrish′ən/,   malnutrition caused by an inadequate food supply or an inability to use the nutrients in food.

**underwater exercise** /un′dərwô′tər/ [AS, *under* + *woeter*],   any physical activity performed in a pool or large tub, such as a Hubbard tank, where the buoyancy of the water facilitates the movement of weak or injured muscles. Sometimes called **aquatherapy** or **aquatic exercise.** See also **exercise.**

**underwater seal,**   a seal formed by water allowed to flow over a tube that exits from the chest cavity of a patient. The water acts as a one-way valve and permits the outflow of air but prevents the ingress of air. Also called **water trap.**

**underweight** /un′dərwāt′/ [AS, *under* + *wiht*],   less than normal in body weight after adjustment for height, body build, and age. See also **body mass index.**

**undescended testis.** See **cryptorchidism, monorchism.**

**undifferentiated cell** /undif′ərən′shē·ā′tid/ [AS, *un* not; L, *differentia,* difference, *cella,* storeroom],   a cell that has not yet expressed signs of its future specific type.

**undifferentiated cell leukemia.** See **stem cell leukemia.**

**undifferentiated family ego mass,**   an emotional fusion in a family in which all members are similar in emotional expression and know each others' thoughts, feelings, and fantasies.

**undifferentiated malignant lymphoma** [ME, *un* + L, *differe,* to differ, *atus,* process, *malignus,* evil, *lympha,* water; Gk, *oma,* tumor],   a lymphoid neoplasm containing stem cells that have large nuclei, a small amount of pale cytoplasm, and ill-defined borders. Also called **reticulosarcoma, stem cell lymphoma.**

**undifferentiation** /un′difərən′shē·ā′shən/,   the lack or absence of normal cell differentiation into an identifiable cell type.

**undisplaced fracture** /un′displāst, un′displāst′/,   a bone break in which cracks in the bone may radiate in several directions but the bone fragments do not separate.

**undoing** /undōō′ing/ [ME, *un* + AS, *don*],   the performance of a specific action that is intended to negate in part a previous action or communication. According to some psychologists, undoing is related to the magical thinking of childhood. For example, a spouse brings home flowers after having a lunchtime affair with another. Also known as an unconscious defense mechanism.

**undulant** /un′dyələnt/ [L, *unda,* wave],   wavelike, such as a vibration, fluctuation, or oscillation.

**undulant fever.** See **brucellosis.**

**undulate** /un′dyəlit/,   to have wavelike fluctuations or oscillations.

**undulating pulse** /un′dyəlā′ting/,   a pulse characterized by a succession of waves without force.

**unengaged head** /un′engājd′/ [ME, *un* + Fr, *engager,* to involve; AS, *heafod*],   the head of a floating fetus. See **engagement.**

**unequal cleavage** /unē′kwəl/ [ME, *un* + L, *aequare,* to make equal; AS, *cleofan,* to split],   mitotic division of a fertilized ovum into blastomeres that are larger near the yolky part of the cell (the vegetal pole) and smaller near the nucleus (the animal pole). Compare **equal cleavage.**

**unequal pulse** [AS, *un,* not; L, *aequare,* to make equal, *pulsare,* to beat],   a pulse in which the beats vary in intensity.

**unequal twins,**   two nonjoined fetuses born of the same pregnancy in which only one of the pair is fully formed, with the other showing various degrees of developmental defects.

**unfinished business** /unfin′isht/,   the concerns of a dying patient that require resolution before death can be accepted by the patient. Unfinished business may range from financial matters to personal relationships.

**ung.,**   abbreviation for the Latin word *unguentum,* 'unguenta', 'or ointment.'

**ungual** /ung′gwəl/,   pertaining to the fingernails.

**ungual phalanx.** See **distal phalanx.**

**unguent.** See **ointment.**

**unguis.** See **nail.**

**uni-** /yōō′nē-/ prefix meaning 'one or single': *unipara, unipolar, unicellular.*

**uniaxial joint** /yōō′nē·ak′sē·əl/ [L, *unus,* one, *axis,* axle, *jungere,* to join],   a synovial joint in which movement is only in one axis, such as a pivot or hinge joint.

**UNICEF** /yōō′nisef′/,   abbreviation for **United Nations International Children's Emergency Fund.**

**unicellular reproduction.** See **parthenogenesis.**

**unicentric blastoma.** See **blastoma.**

**unicuspid.** See **cuspid.**

**unidirectional block** /-direk′shənəl/ [L, *unus* + *dirigere,* to direct; Fr, *bloc*],   a pathologic failure of cardiac impulse conduction in one direction while conduction is possible in the opposite direction.

**unidisciplinary health care team** /-dis′ipliner′ē/,   a group of health care workers who are members of the same discipline.

**unidose.** See **unit dose.**

**unification model** /-kā′shən/ [L, *unus* + *ficare,* to make whole, *atus,* process, *modulus,* small measure],   a theoretic framework based on the close relationship of nursing education and clinical nursing service at the University of Rochester (New York). The faculty of the school of nursing hold joint appointments to the school and the hospital, teaching nursing students and providing clinical leadership in nursing service in the hospital. See also **joint appointment.**

**uniform** /yōō′nifôrm/, **1.** having only one form or shape. **2.** distinctive clothing worn by members of a group.

**uniform reporting,** the reporting of service and financial data by a hospital in conformance with prescribed standard definitions to permit comparisons with other health facilities.

**unilaminar** /-lam′inər/, composed of only one layer.

**unilateral** /-lat′ərəl/ [L, *unus,* one, *latus,* side], involving only one side.

**unilateral denture.** See **partial denture.**

**unilateral hypertrophy** [L, *unus* + *latus,* side; Gk, *hyper,* above, *trophe,* nourishment], enlargement of one side or a part of one side of the body.

**unilateral long-leg spica cast,** an orthopedic cast applied to immobilize one leg and the trunk of the body cranially as far as the nipple line. It is used to treat a fractured femur or for the correction or the maintenance of the correction of a hip deformity. See also **cast.** Compare **bilateral long-leg spica cast, one-and-a-half spica cast.**

**unilateral neglect,** a nursing diagnosis accepted by the Seventh National Conference on the Classification of Nursing Diagnoses. The condition is defined as a state in which an individual is perceptually unaware of and inattentive to one side of the body.

■ DEFINING CHARACTERISTICS: The defining characteristics are consistent inattention to stimuli on the affected side, inadequate self-care (as in positioning and/or safety precautions in regard to the affected side), lack of looking toward the affected side, and leaving food on the plate on the affected side.

■ RELATED FACTORS: Related factors include effects of disturbed perceptual abilities, such as hemianopsia; one-sided blindness; and neurologic illness or trauma. See also **nursing diagnosis.**

**unilateral neglect management,** a nursing intervention from the Nursing Interventions Classification (NIC) defined as protecting and safely reintegrating the affected part of the body while helping the patient adapt to disturbed perceptual abilities. See also **Nursing Interventions Classification.**

**unilateral paralysis.** See **hemiplegia.**

**unilobular** /-lob′yəlar/, having only one lobe.

**unilocular** /-lok′yəlar/, having only one locus, chamber, or cell.

**unimolecular reaction.** See **monomolecular elimination reaction (E1).**

**uninterrupted suture** /unin′tərup′tid/ [AS, *un,* not; L, *interrumpere,* to sever, *sutura*], a continuous suture running forward and backward without interruption.

**uniocular diplopia.** See **monocular diplopia.**

**uniocular squint.** See **monocular strabismus.**

**uniocular vision.** See **monocular vision.**

**union** /ūn′yən/ [L, *unio*], the process of healing; the renewal of continuity in a broken bone or between the edges of a wound. See also **healing.**

**uniovular** /yōō′nē·ov′yələr/ [L, *unus* + *ovum,* egg], developing from a single ovum, as in monozygotic twins as contrasted with dizygotic twins. Also **monovular.** Compare **binovular.**

**uniovular twins.** See **monozygotic twins.**

**Unipen,** trademark for an antibiotic (nafcillin sodium).

**unipolar** /-pō′lər/ [L, *unus,* one, *polus*], pertaining to a nerve cell with only one pole, such as a nerve cell in which the axon and dendrite are fused into a single process a short distance from the cell body.

**unipolar depression,** a major disorder of mood that is characterized by symptoms of depression only. See **depression, major affective disorder.**

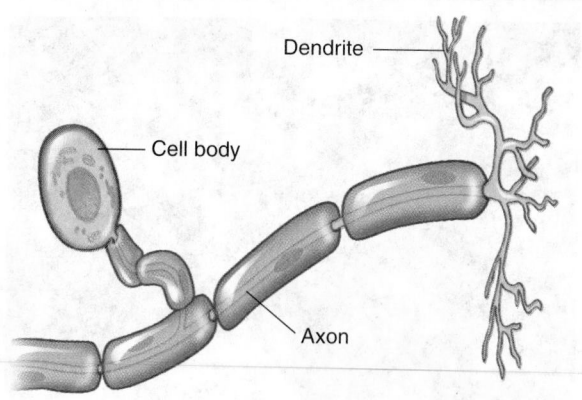

**Unipolar neuron**

**unipolar disorder.** See **major depressive disorder.**

**unipolar lead** [L, *unus* + *polus,* pole; AS, *laedan,* to lead], **1.** an electrocardiographic conductor in which the exploring electrode is placed on the precordium or a limb while the indifferent electrode is in the central terminal. **2.** *informal.* a tracing produced by such a lead on an electrocardiograph.

**unique radiolytic product** /yōōnēk′/, a product such as a food substance that has undergone chemical changes as a result of exposure to ionizing radiation.

**uniseptate** /-sep′tāt/, having only one septum.

**unisex** /yōō′niseks/ [L, *unus,* one, *sexus,* sex], **1.** concerning only one sex or having reproductive organs of only one sex. **2.** an interchange of sex roles in clothing and hair styles, work assignments, shared restrooms, and activities, such as encouraging boys to play with dolls.

**unit (U)** /yōō′nit/ [L, *unus*], **1.** a single item. **2.** a quantity designated as a standard of measurement. **3.** an area of a hospital that is staffed and equipped for treatment of patients with a specific condition or other common characteristics.

**unitary human conceptual framework** /yōō′niter′ē/, a complex theory in nursing that emphasizes the importance of holistic health care and an understanding of the human being in relation to the universal environment.

**unit clerk,** a person who performs routine clerical and reception tasks in a hospital inpatient care unit.

**unit dose,** a method of preparing medications in which individual doses of patient medications are prepared by the pharmacy and delivered in individual labeled packets to the patient's unit to be administered by the nurses on the ordered schedule. One intent of unit dose is to decrease administration error. Also called **unidose.**

**unit-dose system,** a system of drug distribution in which a portable cart containing a drawer for each patient's medications is prepared by the hospital pharmacy with a 24-hour supply of the medications.

**United Nations International Children's Emergency Fund (UNICEF)** /yōō′nisef′/, a fund established by the General Assembly of the United Nations in 1946 to aid children in devastated areas of the world. It is funded by contributions from the member nations and acts to prevent disease, including tuberculosis, whooping cough, and diphtheria, and provides food and clothing to needy children in more than 50 countries. In 1953 UNICEF was made a permanent organization of the United Nations.

**United Network for Organ Sharing (UNOS)** /yōō′nos/, a national organization for the collection and distribution of

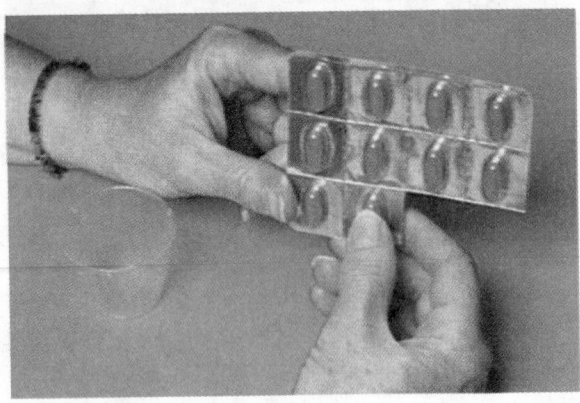

**Unit-dose medication** *(Potter and Perry, 2001)*

body organs that can be used in transplants. Hospitals advise relatives of newly deceased patients about the availability of UNOS service in arranging organ donations.

*United States Pharmacopeia* (USP), a compendium recognized officially by the Federal Food, Drug, and Cosmetic Act that contains descriptions, uses, strengths, and standards of purity for selected drugs and for all of their forms of dosage.

**United States Public Health Service (USPHS),** an agency of the federal government responsible for the control of the arrival from abroad of any people, goods, or substances that may affect the health of U.S. citizens. The agency sets standards for the domestic handling and processing of food and the manufacture of serums, vaccines, cosmetics, and drugs. It supports and performs research, aids localities in times of disaster and epidemics, and provides medical care for certain groups of Americans.

**unit of blood,** a standard measure of approximately 1 pint of whole blood.

**unit of service,** any individual, family, aggregate, organization, or community given nursing care. The level at which service is delivered varies with the particular unit entity.

**univalent** See also **monovalent.**

**univalent antiserum.** See **antiserum.**

**univalent reduction,** a phenomenon during intracellular metabolism involving oxygen-reduction reactions in which superoxide radicals are produced because oxygen accepts electrons only one at a time. In the short period between acceptance of the first and second electrons, one electron is unpaired, and oxygen is a superoxide radical. The superoxide may then be converted to a second free radical.

**Univasc,** trademark for an angiotensin-converting enzyme inhibitor (moexipril).

**universal** /yōō′nivur′səl/ [L, *universus*, whole world], occurring everywhere and in all things.

**universal antidote** [L, *universus*, whole world; Gk, *anti*, against, *dotos*, something given], a mixture of 50% activated charcoal, 25% magnesium oxide, and 25% tannic acid, formerly thought to be useful as an antidote for most types of acid, heavy metal, alkaloid, and glycoside poisons. It is now believed that the mixture is no more effective than activated charcoal given with water.

**universal choking signal.** See **Heimlich sign.**

**universal cuff,** an adaptive device worn on the hand to hold items such as utensils, shaver, or pencil, allowing a patient with a weak grasp to participate more in self-care.

**universal donor,** a person with type O, Rh factor negative red blood cells. Packed red blood cells of this type may be used for emergency transfusion with minimal risk of incompatibility. Blood plasma is not universal plasma. See also **blood donor, blood group, transfusion.**

**universalizability principle** /yōō′nivur′səlī′zəbil′itē/, a principle that an act is good if everyone should, in similar circumstances, do the same act without exception.

**universal precautions,** an approach to infection control designed to prevent transmission of bloodborne diseases such as human immunodeficiency virus, hepatitis B, and hepatitis C in health care settings. Universal precautions were initially developed in 1987 by the Centers for Disease Control and Prevention in the United States and in 1989 by the Bureau of Communicable Disease Epidemiology in Canada. The guidelines for universal precautions include specific recommendations for use of gloves and masks and protective eyewear when contact with blood or body secretions containing blood is anticipated.

**universal qualifiers,** (in neurolinguistic programming) the use of terms that give general impressions of limitations, such as all, common, every, only, and never.

**universal recipient** [L, *universus* + *recipere*, to receive], a person with blood type AB, who can receive a transfusion of any blood type without agglutination or precipitation effects.

**universal tooth coding system,** a tooth-numbering system in which the secondary teeth are numbered from 1 (the maxillary right third molar) to 32 (the mandibular left third molar). The deciduous teeth are similarly numbered from 1 to 20, with the numbers preceded by the letter D (for deciduous). The universal tooth coding system is similar to the ADA numbering system, except that the latter uses the letters A to T to identify the deciduous teeth. See also **FDI numbering system, Palmer notation.**

**unlicensed assistive personnel,** health care workers who are not licensed and who are prepared to provide certain elements of patient care under the supervision of a registered nurse. Unlicensed assistive personnel include patient care technicians, nurses' aides, and certified nursing assistants.

**unmedullated.** See **unmyelinated.**

**unmodified scattering.** See **scattering.**

**unmyelinated** /unmī′əlinā′tid/ [AS, *un*, not; Gk, *myelos*, marrow], describing a nerve fiber that is not coated with a myelin sheath. An unmyelinated fiber, lacking the whitish sheath, appears as gray matter in the brain.

**Unna's paste boot** /ōō′nəz/ [Paul G. Unna, German dermatologist, 1850–1929; L, *pasta*, paste; ME, *bote*], a dressing for varicose ulcers formed by applying a layer of a gelatin-glycerin-zinc oxide paste to the leg and then a spiral bandage covered with successive coats of paste to produce a rigid boot.

**UNOS** /yōō′nos/, abbreviation for **United Network for Organ Sharing.**

**unresolved grief** /un′rizolvd′/, a severe, chronic sorrow reaction in which a person does not complete the resolution stage of the mourning process within a reasonable time.

**unsaturated** /unsach′ərātid/ [ME, *un* + L, *saturare*, to fill], **1.** describing a solution that is capable of dissolving more of the solute; not saturated. **2.** also called **unsaturated hydrocarbon.** an organic compound in which one or more pairs of carbon atoms are united by double or triple bonds, as in unsaturated fatty acids. Compare **saturated.**

**unsaturated alcohol,** an alcohol derived from an unsaturated hydrocarbon, such as an alkene or olefin.

**unsaturated compound** [AS, *un*, not; L, *saturare*, to fill, *componere*, to put together], a chemical compound that contains double or triple bonds.

**unsaturated fatty acid,** a fatty acid in which some of the carbon atoms in the hydrocarbon chain are joined by double or triple bonds. These bonds are easily split in chemical reactions, and other substances may be joined to the carbon atoms involved. Monounsaturated fatty acids have only one double or triple bond per molecule and are found as components of fats (triglycerides) in such foods as fowl, almonds, pecans, cashew nuts, peanuts, and olive oil. Polyunsaturated fatty acids have more than one double or triple bond per molecule and are found in fish, corn, walnuts, sunflower seeds, soybeans, cottonseeds, and safflower oil. Diets high in polyunsaturated fatty acids and low in saturated fatty acids have been correlated with low serum cholesterol levels in some study populations. Compare **saturated fatty acid.**

**unsaturated hydrocarbon.** See **unsaturated.**

**unscrubbed team members** /unskrubd´/, the members of a surgical team, including the anesthetist and circulating nurse, who wear surgical attire but are not gowned or gloved and do not enter the sterile field.

**unsocialized aggressive reaction** /unsō´shəlīzd/ [ME, *un* + L, *socialis,* companion, *aggressio,* an attack, *re,* again + *agere,* to act], a behavior disorder of childhood characterized by overt and covert hostility, disobedience, physical and verbal aggression, vengefulness, quarrelsome behavior, and destructiveness, often manifested in acts such as lying, stealing, temper tantrums, vandalism, and physical violence against others.

**unstable** /unstā´bəl/, **1.** in an excited or active state, such as an atom with a nucleus possessing excess energy. **2.** easily broken down.

**unstable angina** [AS, *un,* not, *stabilis,* firm, *angina,* quinsy], thoracic pain that may mark the onset acute myocardial infarction. It typically has a sudden onset, sudden worsening, and stuttering recurrence over days and weeks. It carries a more severe short-term prognosis than stable chronic angina.

**unstriated muscle.** See **smooth muscle.**

**Unverricht's disease** /un´vərikts, ŏŏn´ferishts/ [Heinrich Unverricht, German physician, 1853–1912], an inherited condition characterized by progressive degeneration of gray matter, resulting in myoclonic epilepsy. It appears in patients 8 to 13 years of age and is marked by general neurologic and intellectual decline.

**unvoiced.** See **voiceless.**

**upper airway obstruction (UAO),** any abnormal condition of the mouth, nose, or larynx that interferes with breathing when the rest of the respiratory system is functioning normally.

**upper extremity suspension,** an orthopedic procedure used in the treatment of fractures and in the correction of orthopedic abnormalities of the upper limbs. The procedure uses traction equipment, including metal frames, ropes, and pulleys, to relieve the weight of the involved upper limb rather than to exert traction. Upper extremity suspension is usually unilateral but also may be used bilaterally in postoperative, posttraumatic, or postreduction control of edema. Compare **balanced suspension, lower extremity suspension.**

**upper GI,** pertaining to the upper gastrointestinal tract, from the esophagus to and including the duodenum. The term is commonly applied to radiographic or fluoroscopic diagnostic views after ingestion of a barium sulfate solution. Normal findings include normal size, contour, patency, filling, positioning, and transmission of barium through the lower esophagus, stomach, and duodenum. Also called **UGI, upper GI series.**

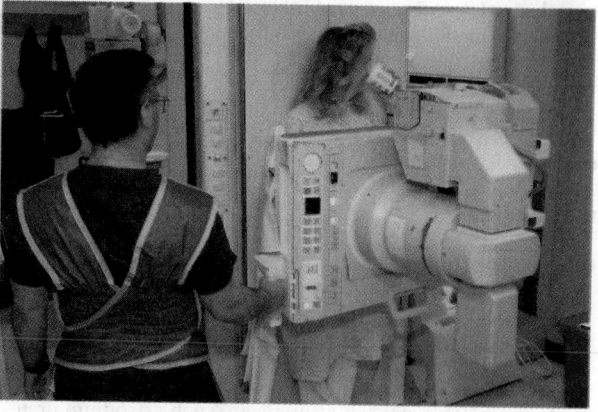

**Upper GI barium study** *(Zakus, 1995)*

**upper level discriminator (ULD),** an electronic device used in nuclear medicine to discriminate against all radionuclide pulses whose heights are above a given level.

**upper motor neuron paralysis,** an injury to or lesion in the brain or spinal cord that causes damage to the cell bodies, axons, or both of the upper motor neurons, which extend from the cerebral centers to the cells in the spinal column. Clinical manifestations include weakness or paralysis, increased muscle tone and spasticity of the muscles involved with little or no atrophy, hyperactive deep tendon reflexes, diminished or absent superficial reflexes, the presence of pathologic reflexes, such as Babinski's and Hoffmann's reflexes, and no local twitching of muscle groups. Compare **lower motor neuron paralysis.**

**upper pole of kidney,** the extremitas superior renis. See **poles of kidney.**

**upper respiratory infection.** See **respiratory tract infection.**

**upper respiratory tract (URT),** one of the two divisions of the respiratory system. The URT consists of the nose, nasal cavity, ethmoidal air cells, frontal sinuses, sphenoidal sinuses, maxillary sinus, larynx, and trachea. The URT conducts air to and from the lungs and filters, moistens, and warms the air during each inspiration. Infection and irritation of the URT are common and often spread to the lower respiratory tract, where they may cause serious complications. See also **larynx, nose, trachea.** Compare **lower respiratory tract.**

**UPPP,** abbreviation for *uvulopalatopharyngoplasty;* see **palatopharyngoplasty.**

**upsilon** /yŏŏp´silon, up´-/, Υ, υ, the twentieth letter of the Greek alphabet.

**uptake** /up´tāk/ [AS, *uptacan*], the drawing up or absorption of a substance.

**upward-and-downward squint.** See **vertical strabismus.**

**UR,** abbreviation for **utilization review.**

**ur-.** See **uro-.**

**urachus** /yŏŏr´əkəs/ [Gk, *ourachos,* urinary tract], an epithelial tube connecting the apex of the urinary bladder with the allantois. Its connective tissue forms the median umbilical ligament.

**uracil,** a pyrimidine base found in RNA.

**-uracil,** suffix for uracil derivatives used as thyroid antagonists and as antineoplastics.

**uragogue,** an agent that increases production of urine.

**uranium (U)** /yo͞orā′nē·əm/ [planet Uranus], a heavy, radioactive metallic element. Its atomic number is 92; its atomic mass is 238.03. Uranium is the heaviest of the natural elements. Isotopes of uranium are used in nuclear power plants to provide neutrons for the nuclear reactions that result in release of energy.

**urano-,** combining form meaning 'the palate': *uranoplasty, uranoplegia, uranoschism.*

**uranoschisis** /yo͞o′rənos′kisis/, [Gk, *ouranos,* palate, *schisis,* fissure], cleft palate.

**uranostaphyloplasty** /-staf′ilōplas′tē/ [Gk, *ouranos,* palate, *staphyle,* uvula, *plassein,* to mold], the surgical repair of a cleft palate.

**uranostaphyloschisis** /yo͞o′rənōstaf′ilos′kisis/, a fissure that extends from the hard palate to the soft palate.

**urarthritis,** inflammation of a joint caused by gout.

**urate** /yo͞or′āt/, any salt of uric acid, such as sodium urate. Urates are found in urine, blood, and tophi or calcareous deposits in tissues. They also may be deposited as crystals in joints. See also **gout, uric acid.**

**uraturia** /yo͞or′əto͞or′ē·ə/, the presence of uric acid salts in the urine.

**urban typhus.** See **murine typhus.**

**urceiform** /o͞orsē′ifôrm/, pitcher-shaped.

**Ur-defenses** /o͞or′dəfen′səs/, a set of three fundamental beliefs essential for psychologic integrity of the individual, as proposed by Jules Masserman. They are a delusion of invulnerability and immortality, faith in a celestial order, and a wishful fantasy that fellow human beings are potential friends available for mutual service.

**urea** /yo͞orē′ə/ [Gk, *ouron,* urine], a systemic osmotic diuretic and topical emollient.
■ INDICATIONS: It is prescribed to reduce cerebrospinal and intraocular fluid pressure and is used topically as a keratolytic agent.
■ CONTRAINDICATIONS: Severely impaired kidney function, active intracranial bleeding, marked dehydration, or liver damage prohibits its systemic use.
■ ADVERSE EFFECTS: Among the more serious adverse reactions are pain and necrosis at the site of injection, headache, GI disturbances, and dizziness. There are no known severe reactions to topical use.

**-urea,** suffix meaning a 'compound containing urea': *glycolylurea, plenylurea, solurea.*

**urea cycle,** a series of complex enzymatic reactions by which ammonia is detoxified in the liver. In the series of steps for disposing of the ammonia molecule, a waste product of protein metabolism, five enzymatic reactions occur as $NH_2$ radicals are combined with carbon and oxygen atoms from carbon dioxide to form urea, which is excreted. The amino acid arginine is synthesized during the same process. Also called **Krebs-Henseleit cycle.**

**ureagenesis** /yo͞or′ē·əjen′əsis/, the process by which urea becomes the final waste product of amino acid metabolism and the detoxification of ammonia from the blood.

**urea nitrogen.** See **blood urea nitrogen.**

**urea nitrogen blood test (BUN),** a blood test that detects levels of urea nitrogen in the blood, which serve as an index of liver and kidney function and indicate diseases of these organs, as well as other conditions that affect their function. BUN is interpreted in conjunction with the creatinine test as in a series known as renal function studies.

*Ureaplasma urealyticum* /-plaz′mə/, a sexually transmitted microorganism that is a common inhabitant of the urogenital systems of men and women in whom infection is asymptomatic. Neonatal death, prematurity, and perinatal morbidity are statistically associated with colonization of the chorionic surface of the placenta by *Ureaplasma urealyticum.* The mechanisms by which the unfavorable effects on pregnancy occur are not understood. There is no characteristic lesion in the fetus or newborn.

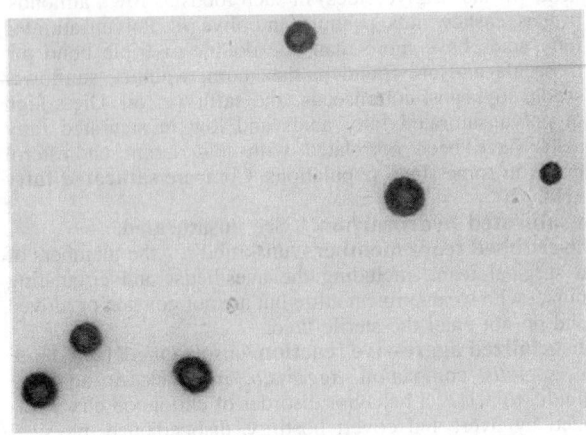

***Ureaplasma urealyticum* colonies on agar**
(Baron, Peterson, and Finegold, 1994)

**urease** /yo͞or′ē·ās/, **1.** an enzyme used in the determination of urea in the blood or urine. **2.** an enzyme that catalyzes the hydrolysis of urea to carbon dioxide and ammonia. **3.** an antitumor enzyme.

**Urecholine,** trademark for a cholinergic (bethanechol chloride).

**uremia** /yo͞orē′mē·ə/ [Gk, *ouron* + *haima,* blood], the presence of excessive amounts of urea and other nitrogenous waste products in the blood, as occurs in renal failure. Also called **azotemia.** See also **chronic glomerulonephritis, subacute glomerulonephritis. —uremic,** *adj.*

**uremic** /yo͞orē′mik/ [Gk, *ouron,* urine, *haima,* blood], pertaining to a toxic level of urea in the blood.

**uremic coma** [Gk, *ouron,* urine, *koma,* deep sleep], a stuporous condition resulting from acidosis and the toxic effects of uremia.

**uremic convulsion,** an episode of involuntary muscle contractions caused by uremia or retention in the blood of substances that would normally be excreted by the kidneys.

**uremic frost,** a pale frostlike deposit of white crystals on the skin caused by kidney failure and uremia. Urea compounds and other waste products of metabolism that cannot be excreted by the kidneys into the urine are excreted through the small superficial capillaries into the skin, where they collect on the surface.

**uremic gingivitis.** See **nephritic gingivitis.**

**-uret,** combining form designating a binary compound: *bromuret, phosphuret, sulphuret.*

**ureter** /yo͞or′ətər, yo͞orē′tər/ [Gk, *oureter*], one of a pair of tubes, about 30 cm long, that carries urine from the kidney into the bladder. Each tube is composed of a fibrous, a muscular, and a mucous coat and divides into an abdominal part and a pelvic part. The abdominal part lies behind the peritoneum on the medial side of the psoas major and enters the pelvic cavity by crossing either the termination of the common iliac artery or the commencement of the external iliac artery. In men the pelvic part of the ureter runs caudal along the lateral wall of the pelvic cavity and reaches the lateral angle of the bladder just ventral to the upper tip of the seminal vesicle. In women the pelvic part of the ureter forms the posterior boundary of the ovarian fossa and runs medially and ventrally along the upper part of the vagina. The ureter enters the bladder through a tunnel that functions as a valve to prevent backflow of urine into the ureter when the bladder contracts. Connecting with the kidneys, the ureters expand into funnel-shaped renal pelves that branch into calyces. Urine is pumped through the ureters by peristaltic waves that occur an average of three times a minute. —**ureteral,** *adj.*

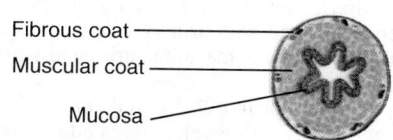

Fibrous coat
Muscular coat
Mucosa

**Cross section of a ureter** *(Applegate, 2000)*

**ureter-, uretero-,** combining form meaning 'ureter': *ureterorrhagia, ureterostenosis, ureterosigmoidoscopy.*

**ureteral dysfunction** /yŏŏrē′terəl/ [Gk, *oureter* + *dys*, bad; L, *functio*, performance], a disturbance of the normal peristaltic flow of urine through a ureter, resulting from dysfunction of ureteral motor nerves. See also **megaloureter.**

**uretercystoscope** /yŏŏr′ētər-sis′təskōp′/ [Gk, *oureter*, ureter, *kystis*, bladder, *skopein*, to view], a cystoscope equipped with ureteric catheters that can be inserted into either ureter.

**ureteritis** /yŏŏrē′tərī′tis/ [Gk, *oureter* + *itis*], an inflammatory condition of a ureter caused by infection or by the mechanic irritation of a stone.

**uretero-.** See **ureter-.**

**ureterocele** /yŏŏrē′tərōsēl′/ [Gk, *oureter* + *kele*, hernia], a prolapse of the terminal part of the ureter into the bladder. The condition may lead to obstruction of the flow of urine, hydronephrosis, and loss of renal function. Cystoscopy and pyelography reveal the prolapsed ureter. Surgical correction is performed to prevent permanent damage to the kidney. Compare **cystocele.**

**ureterodialysis** /-dī·al′isis/ [Gk, *oureter*, ureter, *dialysis*, a breaking], the rupture of a ureter. Also called **ureterolysis.**

**ureterography** /yŏŏrē′tərog′rəfē/ [Gk, *oureter* + *graphein*, to record], the radiologic imaging of a ureter, usually conducted as part of an examination of the urinary tract. The examination may involve injection of a radiopaque medium through a urinary catheter with the aid of a ureterocystoscope (the ascending method), or by IV injection of a contrast medium that permits the filtering of the substance through the kidneys (the descending method) to the ureters.

**ureterohydronephrosis.** See **hydronephrosis.**

**ureterolysis.** See **ureterodialysis.**

**ureteroplasty** /yŏŏrē′tərōplas′tē/ [Gk, *oureter* + *plassein*, to mold], a surgical procedure performed to restructure a ureter, such as when a stricture blocks the normal flow of urine.

**ureteropyelonephritis** /-pī′əlō′nəfrī′tis/ [Gk, *oureter* + *pyelos*, pelvis, *nephros*, kidney, *itis*, inflammation], an inflammation of the kidney, pelvis, and ureter.

**ureterosigmoidostomy** /-sig′moidos′təmē/ [Gk, *oureter* + *sigma*, S-shaped, *eidos*, form, *stoma*, mouth], a surgical

procedure in which a ureter is implanted in the sigmoid flexure of the intestinal tract.

**ureterostomy** /-os′təmē/ [Gk, *oureter* + *stoma*, mouth], the surgical creation of a new opening through which a ureter empties onto the surface of the body or into another outlet, such as the rectum.

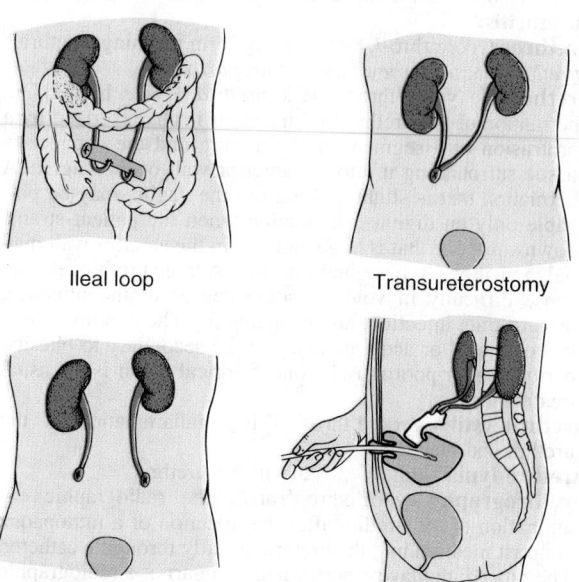

Ileal loop

Transureterostomy

Double ureterostomy

Continent urinary diversion

**Ureterostomy** *(Potter and Perry, 2001)*

**ureterotomy,** an incision into a ureter.

**ureterovaginal** /-vaj′inəl/, pertaining to the ureters and vagina.

**urethra** /yŏŏrē′thrə/ [Gk, *ourethra*], a small tubular structure that drains urine from the bladder. In women it is about 3 cm long and lies directly behind the symphysis pubis, anterior to the vagina. In men it is about 20 cm long and begins at the bladder, passes through the center of the prostate gland, goes between two sheets of tissue connecting the pubic bones, and finally passes through the urinary meatus of the penis. In men the urethra is joined by the ejaculatory duct and serves as a passageway for semen during ejaculation, as well as a canal for urine during voiding. See also **ureter.**

**urethral** /yŏŏrē′thrəl/, pertaining to the urethra.

**urethral caruncle** [Gk, *ourethra* + L, *caruncula*, small piece of flesh], a small, painful growth in the mucous membrane of the female urethral meatus. It may be a source of bleeding.

**urethral hematuria** [Gk, *ourethra* + *haima*, blood, *ouron*, urine], blood in the urine as a result of a urethral lesion.

**urethral orifice,** 1. the external opening of the urethra in the glans penis of a male or the vestibule of a female. 2. internal opening of the urethra at the anterior and inferior angle of the trigone.

**urethral papilla.** See **papilla.**

**urethral sphincter,** the voluntary muscle at the neck of the bladder that relaxes to allow urination.

**urethral swab** [Gk, *ourethra* + D, *zwabber*], an absorbent pad on a slender rod used to treat lesions or to remove secretions.

**urethritis** /yŏŏr'ithrī'tis/, inflammation of the urethra. The condition is characterized by dysuria and is usually the result of an infection in the bladder or kidneys. An antibiotic, a urinary antiseptic, and an analgesic are usually prescribed after the causative organism is identified by bacteriologic culture of a urine specimen. See also **nongonococcal urethritis.**

**urethro-** /yŏŏrē'thrō-/, combining form meaning 'urethra': *urethrocele, urethrocystitis, urethrophraxis.*

**urethrocele** /yŏŏrē'thrəsēl/ [Gk, *urethra* + *kele,* hernia], a herniation of the urethra in females. It is characterized by a protrusion of a segment of the urethra and the connective tissue surrounding it into the anterior wall of the vagina. A herniation that is slight and high in the vagina may be palpable only on digital examination when the patient strains downward; one that is large and low in the anterior wall may bulge visibly at the vaginal introitus. A large urethrocele can cause difficulty in voiding, some degree of incontinence, urinary tract infection, and dyspareunia. The condition may be congenital or acquired and may be secondary to obesity, parturition, or poor muscle tone. Surgical repair is the usual treatment.

**urethrocystitis** /yŏŏrē'thrōsistī'tis/, inflammation of the urethra and bladder.

**urethrodynia** /-din'ē·ə/, pain in the urethra.

**urethrography** /yŏŏr'ēthrog'rəfē/, the radiographic examination of the urethra after the injection of a radiopaque contrast medium into the urethra, usually through a catheter. The procedure may be performed as a part of a radiographic examination of the lower urinary tract.

**urethroplasty** /yŏŏrē'thrəplastē'/, a surgical procedure for the repair of a urethra, as in the correction of hypospadias.

**urethroscope** /-skōp/ [Gk, *ourethra,* urethra, *skopein,* to view], an instrument used to examine the internal surfaces of the urethra.

**urethrospasm** /-spaz'əm/, a spasm of the musculature of the urethra.

**urethrostenosis** /-stənō'sis/ [Gk, *ourethra,* urethra, *stenosis,* a narrowing], a stricture of the urethra.

**Urex,** trademark for an antibacterial (methenamine hippurate).

**urgency** /ur'jensē/ [L, *urgere,* to drive on], a feeling of the need to void urine immediately.

**-urgy,** suffix meaning the 'art of working with (specified) tools': *chemurgy, micrurgy, zymurgy.*

**URI,** abbreviation for **upper respiratory infection.** See **respiratory tract infection.**

**-uria, 1.** suffix meaning the 'presence of a substance in the urine': *ammoniuria, calciuria, enzymuria.* **2.** combining form meaning '(condition of) possessing urine': *paruria, polyuria, pyuria.*

**uric acid** /yŏŏr'ik/, a product of the metabolism of protein that is present in the blood and excreted in the urine. Normal adult levels of blood uric acid range from 2.0 to 8.5 mg/dL, with slightly higher values for elderly patients. See also **gout, kidney, liver, purine, urine.**

**uricaciduria** /yŏŏr'ikas'idŏŏr'ē·ə/ [Gk, *ouron* + L, *acidus,* sour; Gk, *ouron*], an elevated amount of uric acid in the urine, often associated with urinary calculi or gout.

**urico-,** combining form meaning 'uric acid': *uricocholia, uricosuria, uricotelic.*

**uricosuric drugs** /yŏŏr'ikōsŏŏr'ik/ [Gk, *ouron* + L, *acidus,* sour; Gk, *ouron* + Fr, *drogue*], drugs administered to relieve the pain of gout or to increase the elimination of uric acid.

**-uridine,** suffix for uridine derivatives used as antiviral agents and as antineoplastics.

**urinal** /yŏŏr'inəl/, an external plastic or metal receptacle for collecting urine.

**urinalysis** /yŏŏr'inal'isis/ [Gk, *ouron* + *analysein,* to loosen], a physical, microscopic, or chemical examination of urine. The specimen is physically examined for color, turbidity, and specific gravity. Then it is spun in a centrifuge to allow collection of a small amount of sediment, which is examined microscopically for blood cells, casts, crystals, pus, and bacteria. Chemical analysis may be performed to measure the pH and to identify and measure the levels of ketones, sugar, protein, blood components, and many other substances.

**urinary** /yŏŏr'iner'ē/, pertaining to urine or the formation of urine.

**urinary albumin** [Gk, *ouron,* urine; L, *albus,* white], the presence of albumin, a protein, in the urine. Normally protein is not found in the urine because the spaces in the glomerular membrane of the kidney are too small to allow escape of protein molecules. If the membrane is damaged, however, as in some kidney diseases, albumin molecules can leak through into the urine. Normal findings are: none or as high as 8 mg/dL; 50 to 80 mg/24 hours at rest; less than

## Urinalysis findings

| Test | Normal | Abnormal |
|------|--------|----------|
| Color | Amber-yellow | Red indicates hematuria (possibly urinary obstruction, renal calculi, tumor, renal failure, cystitis) |
| Clarity | Clear | Cloudy: debris, bacterial sediment (urinary infection) |
| pH | 4.6-8.0 (average 6.0) | Alkaline on standing or with urinary tract infection<br>Increased acidity with renal tubular acidosis |
| Specific gravity | 1.010-1.026 | Usually reflects fluid intake; the less the fluid intake, the higher the specific gravity<br>If specific gravity remains low (1.010-1.014), renal disease or pituitary disease (deficit of ADH) is suspected |
| Protein | 0-8 mg/dl | Proteinuria may occur with high-protein diet and exercise (particularly prolonged)<br>Seen in renal disease |
| Sugar | 0 | Glycosuria occurs after a high intake of sugar or with diabetes mellitus |
| Ketones | 0 | Ketonuria occurs with starvation and diabetic ketoacidosis |
| RBCs | 0-4 | Injury to kidney tissue (see color, above) |
| WBCs | 0-5 | Urinary tract infection |
| Casts | 0 | Urinary tract infection, renal disease |

From Phipps WJ, Sands JK, Marek JE: *Medical-surgical nursing: concepts and clinical practice,* ed 6, St Louis, 1999, Mosby.

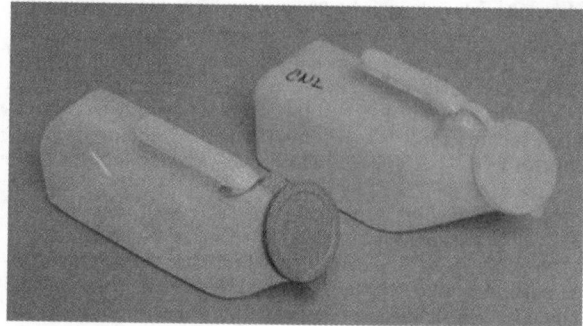

**Urinals** *(Potter and Perry, 2001)*

250 mg/24 hours after strenuous exercise. Also called **urine protein.** See also **proteinuria.**

**urinary bladder** [Gk, *ouron* + AS, *blaedre*], the muscular membranous sac in the pelvis that stores urine for discharge through the urethra. It is connected anteriorly with the two ureters and posteriorly with the urethra.

**urinary bladder training,** a nursing intervention from the Nursing Interventions Classification (NIC) defined as improving bladder function for those with urge incontinence by increasing the bladder's ability to hold urine and the patient's ability to suppress urination. See also **Nursing Interventions Classification.**

**urinary calculus,** a mineral concretion formed in any part of the urinary tract. Calculi may be large enough to obstruct the flow of urine or small enough to be passed with the urine. Kinds of urinary calculi are **renal calculus, vesicla calculus.** See also **calculus.**

**urinary casts** [Gk, *ouron*, urine; ONorse, *kasta*], cells or particles excreted in the urine having the shape of renal-collecting tubule cells.

**urinary catheterization,** a nursing intervention from the Nursing Interventions Classification (NIC) defined as insertion of a catheter into the bladder for temporary or permanent drainage of urine. See also **Nursing Interventions Classification.**

**urinary catheterization: intermittent,** a nursing intervention from the Nursing Interventions Classification (NIC) defined as regular periodic use of a catheter to empty the bladder. See also **Nursing Interventions Classification.**

**urinary continence,** a nursing outcome from the Nursing Outcomes Classification (NOC) defined as the control of the elimination of urine. See also **Nursing Outcomes Classification.**

**urinary elimination,** a nursing outcome from the Nursing Outcomes Classification (NOC) defined as the ability of the urinary system to filter wastes, conserve solutes, and collect and discharge urine in a healthy pattern. See also **Nursing Outcomes Classification.**

**urinary elimination, impaired,** a nursing diagnosis accepted by the Fourth National Conference on the Classification of Nursing Diagnoses. It is defined as the state in which an individual experiences a disturbance in urine elimination.

■ DEFINING CHARACTERISTICS: The defining characteristics are dysuria, urinary frequency, urinary hesitancy, urinary incontinence, nocturia, urinary retention, and urinary urgency.

■ RELATED FACTORS: Related factors are sensory motor impairment, neuromuscular impairment, and mechanical trauma. See also **nursing diagnosis; incontinence, functional; incontinence, reflex; incontinence, stress; incontinence, total; incontinence, urge.**

**urinary elimination management,** a nursing intervention from the Nursing Interventions Classification (NIC) defined as maintenance of an optimum urinary elimination pattern. See also **Nursing Interventions Classification.**

**urinary frequency,** frequent urination or urgency without an increase in the total daily volume of urine. The condition may result from a bladder or urethral infection, a diminished bladder capacity or other structural abnormalities. See also **cystitis, cystocele, ureterocele, urethritis, urethrocele.**

**urinary habit training,** a nursing intervention from the Nursing Interventions Classification (NIC) defined as establishing a predictable pattern of bladder emptying to prevent incontinence for persons with limited cognitive ability who have urge, stress, or functional incontinence. See also **Nursing Interventions Classification.**

**urinary hesitancy,** a decrease in the force of the stream of urine, often with difficulty in beginning the flow. Hesitancy is usually the result of an obstruction or stricture between the bladder and the external urethral orifice; in men it may indicate an enlargement of the prostate gland, in women stenosis of the orifice. Cold, stress, dehydration, and various neurogenic and psychogenic factors are common causes of this condition.

**urinary ileostomy** [Gk, *ouron,* urine; L, *ilia,* intestines; Gk, *stoma,* mouth], the surgical creation of a passage between the urinary bladder and the ileum for the diversion of urine.

**urinary incontinence,** inability to control urination. Several forms are recognized. Functional incontinence is the result of cerebral clouding and/or physical factors that make it difficult to get to bathroom facilities in time. Overflow incontinence occurs when the urinary tract is obstructed or when the detrusor muscle fails to contract as bladder capacity is reached; spinal cord injury or benign prostatic hypertrophy may be the cause. Stress incontinence is precipitated by coughing, sneezing, or straining; it occurs more often in women and is commonly related to anatomical changes, such as occur in stroke or multiple sclerosis. Treatment depends on the underlying cause and may include anticipatory toileting, bladder retraining, exercise of perineal muscles, anticholinergic medications, and surgery. See also **incontinence, retention with overflow.**

**urinary incontinence care,** a nursing intervention from the Nursing Interventions Classification (NIC) defined as assistance in promoting continence and maintaining perineal skin integrity. See also **Nursing Interventions Classification.**

**urinary incontinence care: enuresis,** a nursing intervention from the Nursing Interventions Classification (NIC) defined as promotion of urinary continence in children. See also **Nursing Interventions Classification.**

**urinary infection.** See **urinary tract infection.**

**urinary meatus,** the external opening of the urethra.

**urinary output,** the total volume of urine excreted daily, normally between 700 and 2000 mL. The smaller number represents the minimum volume needed to excrete waste products. Various metabolic and renal diseases may increase or decrease urinary output. See also **anuria, oliguria, polyuria.**

**urinary overflow,** a condition that occurs when a patient's bladder is extremely distended with urine and the patient voids or leaks only a small amount of it. See **retention with overflow.**

**urinary retention,** a nursing diagnosis accepted by the Seventh National Conference on the Classification of Nursing Diagnoses. The condition is described as the state in which an individual experiences incomplete emptying of the bladder.

■ DEFINING CHARACTERISTICS: Defining characteristics are bladder distension; small, infrequent voiding or absence of urine output; a sensation of bladder fullness; dribbling; residual urine; dysuria; and overflow incontinence.

■ RELATED FACTORS: Related factors include high urethral pressure caused by a weak detrusor, inhibition of reflex arc, strong sphincter, and blockage. See also **nursing diagnosis.**

**urinary retention care,** a nursing intervention from the Nursing Interventions Classification (NIC) defined as assistance in relieving bladder distension. See also **Nursing Interventions Classification.**

**urinary sediment** [Gk, *ouron,* urine; L, *sedimentum,* a settling], solid matter that settles to the bottom of a urine sample that has been allowed to stand for several hours.

**urinary system.** See **urinary tract.**

**urinary system assessment,** an evaluation of the condition and functioning of the kidneys, ureters, bladder, and urethra and an investigation of concurrent and previous disorders that may be factors in abnormalities in these structures. The assessment aids the urologist in diagnosing the abnormalities.

■ METHOD: In an interview the patient is asked whether painful urination, frequency or burning on urination, dribbling, a decreased urinary stream, nocturia, stress incontinence, headache, back pain, or increased thirst has occurred. The color, odor, and amount of urine voided and obtained via catheter are determined. The patient's vital signs; any bladder distension; skin condition; neurologic changes; the location, duration, and character of pain; and the presence of bladder spasms are recorded. It is determined whether the patient has hypertension, diabetes, a venereal disease, vaginal or urethral drainage or discharge, or a history that includes cystitis, pyelonephritis, kidney stones, prostatectomy, renal surgery, a kidney transplant, or a venereal infection. The patient's sexual activity; use of coffee, tea, cola beverages, alcohol, perfumed soaps, feminine hygiene sprays, and prescribed and over-the-counter medication; and habit of bathing in a tub or shower are ascertained. A family history of polycystic kidney disease, hypertension, diabetes, or cancer is noted in the assessment, together with laboratory studies of the specific gravity of the patient's urine, casts, protein, red and white cells in the urine, and serum creatinine level. Diagnostic procedures may include cystoscopy, excretory and IV urography, renal angiography, retrograde studies, and x-ray film of the kidneys, ureters, and bladder.

■ INTERVENTIONS: The nurse interviews the patient, records the objective and subjective data, and assembles the background information and the results of the diagnostic tests.

■ OUTCOME CRITERIA: A comprehensive assessment of the patient's urinary system aids the urologist in establishing the diagnosis.

**urinary tract,** all organs and ducts involved in the secretion and elimination of urine from the body.

**urinary tract infection (UTI),** an infection of one or more structures in the urinary system. Most UTIs are caused by gram-negative bacteria, most commonly *Escherichia coli* or species of *Klebsiella, Proteus, Pseudomonas,* or *Enterobacter.* The condition is more common in women than in men. UTI may be asymptomatic but is usually characterized by urinary frequency, burning pain with voiding, and, if the infection is severe, visible blood and pus in the urine. Fever and back pain often accompany kidney infections. Diagnosis of the cause and location of the infection is made by microscopic examination and bacteriologic culture of a urine specimen, physical examination of the patient, and, if necessary, various radiologic techniques such as retrograde py-

elography or cystoscopy. Treatment includes antibacterial, analgesic, urinary antiseptic drugs and increased fluid intake up to 3L/day unless contraindicated. Teaching the patient about increased fluid intake, frequent voiding, and good perineal hygiene is also helpful. Kinds of urinary tract infections include **cystitis, pyelonephritis,** and **urethritis.**

**urinate** /yōŏr′ināt/ [Gk *ouron* urine], to excrete urine from the bladder.

**urination** /yōŏr′inā′shən/ [Gk, *ouron* + L, *atus,* process], the act of passing urine. Also called **micturition.**

**urine** /yōŏr′in/ [Gk *ouron*], the fluid secreted by the kidneys, transported by the ureters, stored in the bladder, and voided through the urethra. Normal urine is clear, straw-colored, and slightly acid; has the odor of urea; and has a specific gravity between 1.003 and 1.035. Its normal constituents include water, urea, sodium chloride, potassium chloride, phosphates, uric acid, organic salts, and the pigment urobilin. Abnormal constituents indicative of disease include ketone bodies, protein, bacteria, blood, glucose, pus, and certain crystals. See also **bacteriuria, glycosuria, hematuria, ketoaciduria, proteinuria. —urinary,** *adj.*

**urine culture and sensitivity (C&S),** a microscopic study of the urine culture performed to determine the presence of pathogenic bacteria in patients with suspected urinary tract infection.

**urine flow studies,** a noninvasive, uncomplicated urodynamic test that measures the volume of urine expelled from the bladder per second. It is indicated to investigate dysfunctional voiding or suspicious outflow tract obstruction, and is done before and after any procedure designed to modify the function of the urologic outflow tract.

**urine glucose test,** a qualitative urine test that is usually done as part of a routine urinalysis to screen for the presence of glucose in the urine, which may indicate diabetes mellitus or other causes of glucose intolerance. Other tests are then used to confirm the diagnosis.

**urine osmolality,** the osmotic pressure of urine, usually greater than the osmolality of serum. The normal values are 500 to 800 mOsm/L after overnight water deprivation.

**urine osmolality test,** a urine test used in the precise evaluation of the concentrating ability of the kidney. It is also used to monitor fluid and electrolyte imbalance and is valuable in the workup of patients with renal disease, the syndrome of inappropriate antidiuretic hormone (SIADH) secretion, and diabetes insipidus.

**urine pH,** the hydrogen ion concentration of the urine, or a measure of its acidity or alkalinity. The normal pH value for urine is 4.6 to 8.0.

**urine potassium test ($K^+$),** a 24-hour urine test that detects the urine concentration of potassium, the major cation within cells. Abnormal findings are associated with chronic and acute renal failure, Cushing's syndrome, hyperaldosteronism, alkalosis, diuretic therapy, dehydration, Addison's disease, malnutrition, and malabsorption, among other conditions.

**urine protein.** See **urinary albumin.**

**urine sodium test ($Na^+$),** a 24-hour urine test that evaluates sodium balance in the body by determining the amount of sodium excreted in urine during a 24-hour period. It is useful for evaluating patients with volume depletion, acute renal failure, adrenal disturbances, and acid-base imbalances; it is especially important when the serum sodium concentration is low.

**urine specific gravity,** a measure of the degree of concentration of a sample of urine. The normal range of urine specific gravity is 1.003 to 1.035, depending on the patient's previous fluid intake, renal perfusion, and renal function.

**urinoma** /yŏŏr'inō'mə/, *pl.* **urinoma, urinomata,** a cyst filled with urine.

**urinometer** /yŏŏr'inom'ətər/ [Gk, *ouron* + *metron,* measure], any device for determining the specific gravity of urine. Also called **urometer.** See also **hydrometer.**

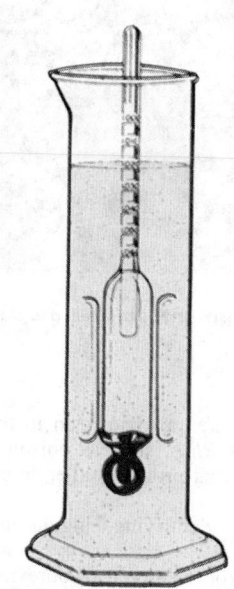

**Urinometer** *(Potter and Perry, 1993)*

**Urised,** trademark for a urinary fixed-combination drug containing an antibacterial (methenamine), an analgesic (phenyl salicylate), anticholinergics (atropine sulfate and hyoscyamine sulfate), an antifungal (benzoic acid), and an antiseptic (methylene blue).

**Urispas,** trademark for a smooth muscle relaxant (flavoxate hydrochloride).

**uro-** /yŏŏr'ō-/, **ur-, urono-,** combining form meaning 'urine, the urinary tract, or urination': *urocrisia, uromancy, uropterin.*

**urobilin** /yŏŏr'əbī'lin/, a brown pigment formed by the oxidation of urobilinogen, normally found in feces and in small amounts in urine.

**urobilinogen** /yŏŏr'əbilin'əjən/, a colorless compound formed in the intestine after the breakdown of bilirubin by bacteria. Some of this substance is excreted in feces, and some is resorbed and excreted again in bile or urine. See also **urobilin.**

**urobilinuria** /yŏŏr'ōbī'linŏŏr'ē·ə/, the presence of excess urobilin in the urine.

**Urobiotic,** trademark for a urinary fixed-combination drug containing antibacterials (oxytetracycline hydrochloride and sulfamethizole) and an analgesic (phenazopyridine hydrochloride).

**urodynamics** /-dīnam'iks/ [Gk, *ouron,* urine, *dynamis,* force], the study of the hydrology and mechanics of urinary bladder filling and emptying.

**urogenital** /yŏŏr'ōjen'itəl/ [Gk, *ouron* + L, *genitalis,* fruitful], pertaining to the urinary and the reproductive systems. Also called **genitourinary.**

**urogenital sinus,** one of the elongated cavities, formed by the division of the cloaca in early embryonic development, into which open the ureter, mesonephric and paramesonephric ducts, and bladder. It also gives rise to the vestibule, urethra, and part of the vagina in the female and part of the urethra in the male.

**urogenital system,** all of the urinary and genital organs and their associated structures, including the kidneys, ureters, bladder, and urethra; the ovaries, fallopian tubes, uterus, clitoris, and vagina (in women); and the testes, seminal vesicles, seminal ducts, prostate, and penis (in men). Also called **genitourinary system.** See also the Color Atlas of Human Anatomy.

**urogram** /yŏŏr'əgram'/, an x-ray film of the urinary tract, obtained by urography. See also **pyelogram.**

**urography** /yŏŏrog'rəfē/ [Gk, *ouron* + *graphein,* to record], the radiographic examination of the urinary system. A radiopaque substance is injected, and radiographs are taken as the substance is passed through or excreted from the part of the system being studied. Some kinds of urography are **cystoscopic urography, intravenous pyelography,** and **retrograde pyelography.**

**urokinase** /yŏŏr'əkī'nās/, an enzyme produced in the kidney and found in urine that is a potent plasminogen activator of the fibrinolytic system. A pharmaceutic preparation of urokinase is administered intravenously in the treatment of pulmonary embolism.

**urolagnia** /yŏŏr'əlag'nē·ə/, sexual stimulation gained from acts involving urine, such as watching people urinate or being urinated on.

**urolithiasis,** /yŏŏr'ōlithī'əsis/, the presence of calculi in the urinary system.

**urologic** /-loj'ik/ [Gk, *ouron,* urine, *logos,* science], pertaining to the scientific study of the urinary tract.

**urologist** /yŏŏrol'əjist/, a licensed physician who has completed an approved residency program and who specializes in the practice of urology.

**urology** /yŏŏrol'əjē/ [Gk, *ouron* + *logos,* science], the branch of medicine concerned with the study of the anatomy, physiology, disorders, and care of the urinary tract in men and women and of the male genital tract. —**urologic,** *adj.*

**uromelus.** See **sympus monopus.**

**urometer** /yŏŏrom'ətər/ [Gk, *ouron,* urine, *metron,* measure], a type of hydrometer used to measure the specific gravity of a urine sample. Also called **urinometer.**

**urono-.** See **uro-.**

**uropathy** /yŏŏrop'əthē/ [Gk, *ouron* + *pathos,* disease], any disease or abnormal condition of any structure of the urinary tract. —**uropathic,** *adj.*

**uroporphyria** /yŏŏr'ōpôrfir'ē·ə/ [Gk, *ouron* + *porphyros,* purple], a rare genetic disease characterized by excessive secretion of uroporphyrin in the urine, blistering dermatitis, photosensitivity, splenomegaly, and hemolytic anemia. Corticosteroid ointments may be helpful for the skin lesions; splenectomy may be necessary to alleviate the hemolytic anemia. Most patients die from hematologic complications before they reach middle age. See also **porphyria.**

**uroporphyrin** /yŏŏr'ōpôr'firin/, a porphyrin normally excreted in the urine in small amounts. See also **uroporphyria.**

**uroradiology** /-rā'dē·ol'əjē/, the radiologic study of the urinary tract.

**urorectal septum** /-rek'təl/ [Gk, *ouron* + L, *rectus,* straight, *saeptum,* wall], a ridge of mesoderm covered with endoderm that in the early developing embryo divides the endodermal cloaca into the urogenital sinus and the rectum. Also called **cloacal septum.**

**uroscopy** /yo͝oros′kəpē/ [Gk, *ouron,* urine, *skopein,* to view], diagnostic examination of urine samples.

**urostomy** /yo͝oros′təmē/, the diversion of urine away from a diseased or defective bladder through a surgically created opening, or stoma, in the skin.

**urotoxicity** /yo͝or′ōtoksis′itē/, toxicity of urine.

**ursodeoxycholic acid** /ur′sōdē·ok′sikol′ik/, a secondary bile salt. It is used in vivo to dissolve cholesterol gallstones. See also **chenodeoxycholic acid.**

**urticaria** /ur′tiker′ē·ə/ [L, *urtica,* nettle], a pruritic skin eruption characterized by transient wheals of varying shapes and sizes with well-defined erythematous margins and pale centers. It is caused by capillary dilation in the dermis that results from the release of vasoactive mediators, including histamine, kinin, and the slow reactive substance of anaphylaxis associated with antigen-antibody reaction. Treatment includes antihistamines and removal of the stimulus or allergen. Cholinergic urticaria appears as wheals surrounded by a large axon flare. It may be caused by drugs, food, insect bites, inhalants, emotional stress, exposure to heat or cold, and exercise. Also called **hives.** See also **angioneurotic edema. —urticarial,** *adj.*

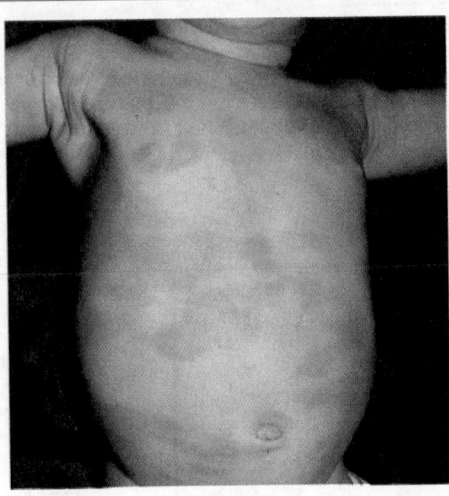

**Urticaria pigmentosa** *(Zitelli and Davis, 1997)*

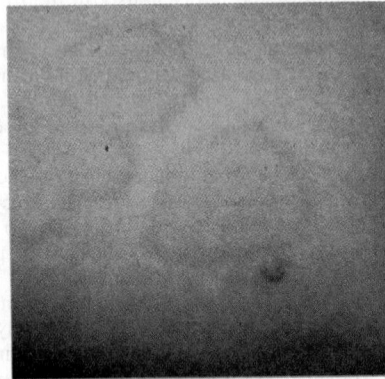

**Urticaria**
*(Zitelli and Davis, 1997/courtesy Dr. Donald W. Kress, Children's Hospital of Pittsburgh)*

**urticaria bullosa** [L, *urtica,* nettle, *bulla,* bubble], a skin eruption in which the lesions are capped by blisters.

**urticaria hemorrhagica.** See **hemorrhagic urticaria.**

**urticaria maculosa** [L, *urtica,* nettle, *macule,* spot], a chronic skin eruption in which red lesions form with little or no edema present.

**urticaria medicamentosa** [L, *urtica,* nettle, *medicina*], a form of skin eruption that follows the use of certain medications, including those containing quinine.

**urticaria papulosa** [L, *urtica,* nettle, *papula,* pimple], a form of skin eruption affecting mainly children and characterized by reddish macules on which papules develop.

**urticaria pigmentosa,** an uncommon form of mastocytosis characterized by pigmented skin lesions that usually begin in infancy and become urticarial on mechanical or chemical irritation. Although duration of the condition is unpredictable, prognosis is good. Treatment is symptomatic and usually includes antihistamines for relief of itching. See also **mastocytosis.**

**urushiol** /əro͞o′shē·ôl/, a toxic resin in the sap of certain plants of the genus *Rhus,* such as poison ivy, poison oak, and poison sumac, that produces allergic contact dermatitis in many people.

**-us,** suffix usually identifying singular nouns: *echolalus, thalamus, tonus.*

**USAN** /yo͞o′san, yo͞o′es′ā′en′/, abbreviation for *United States Adopted Names,* an organization that works with pharmaceutical manufacturers to designate names for nonproprietary drugs. A list of USAN-approved drugs is published by U.S. Pharmacopeial Convention, Inc. See also **nonproprietary name.**

**use effectiveness** [L, *usus,* make use of, *efficere,* to produce], (of a contraceptive method) the actual effectiveness of a medication, device, or method in preventing pregnancy. Inconsistent use and human error usually reduce the theoretic effectiveness of any particular method of contraception. Compare **theoretic effectiveness.**

**useful radiation,** the part of direct radiation that is permitted to pass from an x-ray tube housing through the tube head port, aperture, or collimator. Also called **useful beam.**

**user documentation.** See **documentation.**

**user friendly,** presenting operating information or instructions in a form that is familiar and easy to understand.

**user interaction.** See **interactive terminal.**

**use test,** a procedure used to identify offending allergens in foods, cosmetics, or fabrics by the systematic elimination and addition, one at a time, of specific items associated with the life-style of the patient involved. Allergic reactions to the use test may be immediate or spread over a considerable period of time. Some patients undergoing the test become frustrated and discouraged, requiring regular encouragement to continue the search for sources of their allergies by this method. See also **allergy testing.**

**U-shaped arch,** a dental arch in which there is little difference in width between the first premolars and the last molars and in which the curve from canine to canine is abrupt and U-shaped.

**Usher's syndrome,** an inherited disorder characterized by retinitis pigmentosa and a sensorineural hearing deficit.

**USP.** See *United States Pharmacopeia.*

**USPHS,** abbreviation for **United States Public Health Service.**

**USP unit,** a dose unit as recommended by the *United States Pharmacopoeia,* the primary legally recognized national drug-standard compendium.

**uta** /yōo′tə/ [Sp, facial ulcers], a mild cutaneous form of American leishmaniasis, occurring in the Andes of Peru and Argentina, caused by *Leishmania peruana.* The lesions are small and usually occur on the exposed surfaces of the skin, which ordinarily heal spontaneously within 1 year. The disease has been slowly disappearing because of the increased use of insecticides.

**ut dict.,** abbreviation for the Latin phrase *ut dictum,* 'as directed.'

**utend.,** abbreviation for the Latin phrase *utendus,* 'to be used.'

**uter-, utero-,** combining form meaning 'relating to the uterus': *uterotomy, uteroplasty.*

**uteralgia.** See **metralgia.**

**uterine** /yōo′tərēn/ [L, *uterus,* womb], pertaining to the uterus.

**uterine anteflexion** [L, *uterus,* womb, *ante,* before, *flectere,* to bend], an abnormal position of the uterus in which the uterine body is bent forward on itself at the juncture of the isthmus of the uterine cervix and the lower uterine segment.

**uterine anteversion,** a position of the uterus in which the body of the uterus is directed ventrally. Mild degrees of anteversion are of no clinical significance. On speculum examination of the vagina, acute anteversion of the uterus may be deduced from the location of the cervix in the posterior of the vaginal vault. Slight anteversion is the most common uterine position; on speculum examination the cervix is in the middle of the top of the vagina vault and protrudes directly downward toward the vaginal orifice.

**uterine bleeding** [L, *uterus* + ME, *blod*], any loss of blood from the uterus.

**uterine bruit,** a sound made by the passage of blood through the arteries of the pregnant uterus. The sounds are synchronized with the maternal heart rate. See also **uterine souffle.**

**uterine cancer,** any malignancy of the uterus, including the cervix or endometrium. See also **cervical cancer, endometrial cancer.**

**uterine colic** [L, *uterus* + Gk, *kolikos,* pain in the colon], a spasmodic pain originating in the uterus. It is usually caused by dysmenorrhea or extrusion of a fibroid polyp.

**uterine fibroid** [L, *uterus* + *fibra,* fiber; Gk, *eidos,* form], a growth of fibrous tissue in the uterus, usually a fibroma, fibromyoma, or leiomyofibroma.

**uterine fibroma,** a benign encapsulated uterine tumor. It affects about 20% of women over the age of 30. The tumor may develop in the wall of the uterus or be attached to a stalk of tissue originating in the wall. Symptoms may include menstrual disorders such as menorrhagia; symptoms are also likely to be related to the location of the tumor with respect to neighboring organs, as when a uterine fibroma causes pressure on the urinary bladder, producing symptoms of dysuria. Uterine fibromas rarely spread or become life-threatening.

**uterine hemorrhage,** bleeding from the uterus. Types of uterine hemorrhage include fetomaternal hemorrhage, in which fetal blood cells leak into the maternal circulation; postmenopausal bleeding; and dysfunctional uterine bleeding. See also **hemorrhage, intrapartum hemorrhage, postpartum hemorrhage.**

**uterine inertia,** abnormal relaxation of the uterus during labor, causing a lack of obstetric progress, or after childbirth, causing uterine hemorrhage.

**uterine ischemia,** a decreasing or ineffective blood supply to the uterus.

**uterine prolapse,** the falling, sinking, or sliding of the uterus from its normal location in the body.

**uterine retroflexion,** a position of the uterus in which its body is bent backward on itself at the isthmus of the cervix and the lower uterine segment. This condition has no clinical significance; it does not prevent conception or adversely affect pregnancy. On speculum examination of the vagina, the condition may be deduced by the location of the cervix in the anterior vaginal vault.

**uterine retroversion,** a position of the uterus in which the body of the uterus is directed away from the midline, toward the back. Mild degrees of retroversion are common and have no clinical significance. Severe retroversion may be accompanied by vague persistent pelvic discomfort and dyspareunia and may prevent the fitting and use of a contraceptive diaphragm. Compare **uterine anteversion.** See also **uterine retroflexion.**

**uterine sinus,** one of the small irregular vascular channels in the endometrium of the pregnant uterus.

**uterine souffle,** a soft, blowing sound made by the blood in the arteries of a pregnant uterus. It is synchronized with the maternal pulse.

**uterine subinvolution** [L, *uterus* + *sub,* under, *involere,* to roll up], delayed or absent involution of the uterus during the postpartum period. The causes of subinvolution include retained fragments of placenta, uterine fibromyomas, and infection. Regardless of the cause of the condition, it is characterized by longer and heavier bleeding after childbirth and, on pelvic examination, a larger and softer uterus than would be expected at that time. Treatment includes ergonovine given by mouth for 2 or 3 days, and, if an infection is present, an antibiotic. The hemoglobin or hematocrit is also evaluated, and iron is given if necessary. A follow-up examination is performed 2 weeks later. Also called **partial involution.**

**uterine swab** [L, *uterus* + D, *zwabber*], an absorbent material on a rod or flattened wire used to obtain specimens or to remove secretions from the uterus.

**uterine tenaculum.** See **tenaculum.**

**uterine tetany,** a condition characterized by uterine contractions that are extremely prolonged.

**uterine tube.** See **fallopian tube.**

**uteritis.** See **metritis.**

**utero-.** See **uter-.**

**uteroabdominal pregnancy** /yōo′tərō·abdom′inəl/ [L, *uterus* + *abdomen* + *pregnans*], a twin pregnancy in which one fetus develops in the uterus and the other develops in the abdomen.

**uteroglobulin.** See **blastokinin.**

**uteroovarian varicocele** /yōo′tərō·ōver′ē·ən/ [L, *uterus* + *ovum,* egg, *varix,* varicose vein; Gk, *kele,* tumor], a swelling of the veins of the pampiniform plexus of the female pelvis. Compare **ovarian varicocele, varicocele.**

**uteroplacental apoplexy.** See **Couvelaire uterus.**

**uteroplacental sinus** /yōo′tərōpləsen′təl/, one of the spaces in the zone of the placenta and the uterine wall where blood is exchanged between the circulations of the fetus and the mother.

**uteroplasty.** See **metroplasty.**

**uterosalpingography** /yōo′tərōsal′ping·gog′rəfē/ [L, *uterus* + Gk, *salpinx,* tube, *graphein,* to record], a radiographic examination of the uterus and fallopian tubes.

**uterotomy** /yōo′tərot′əmē/ [L, *uterus* + Gk, *temnein,* to cut], a surgical incision into the uterus, such as in a cesarean section.

**uterovaginal** /yo͞o′tərovaj′inəl/, pertaining to the uterus and vagina.

**uterovesical.** See **vesicouterine.**

**uterus** /yo͞o′tərəs/ [L, womb], the hollow pear-shaped internal female organ of reproduction in which the fertilized ovum is implanted and the fetus develops and from which the decidua of menses flows. Its anterior surface lies on the superior surface of the bladder, separated by a fold of peritoneum, the vesicouterine pouch. Its posterior surface, also covered with peritoneum, is adjacent to the sigmoid colon and some of the coils of the small intestine. The uterus is composed of three layers: the endometrium, the myometrium, and the parametrium. The endometrium lines the uterus and becomes thicker and more vascular in pregnancy and during the second half of the menstrual cycle under the influence of the hormone progesterone. The myometrium is the muscular layer of the organ. Its muscle fibers wrap around the uterus obliquely, laterally, and longitudinally. The muscle fibers contract during childbirth to expel the fetus. After childbirth the meshlike network of fibers contracts again, creating a mass of natural ligatures that stops the flow of blood from the large blood vessels supplying the placenta. The parametrium is the outermost layer of the uterus. It is composed of serous connective tissue and extends laterally into the broad ligament. In the adult the organ measures about 7.5 cm long and 5 cm wide at its fundus and weighs approximately 40 g. During pregnancy it is able to grow to many times its usual size, almost entirely by cellular hypertrophy.

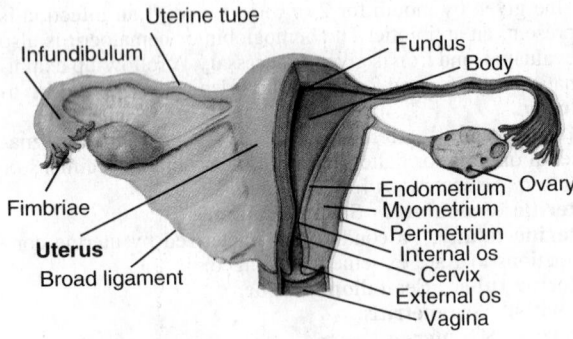

Uterine tube
Infundibulum
Fundus
Body
Fimbriae
Endometrium
Myometrium
Perimetrium
Internal os
Cervix
External os
Vagina
Ovary
**Uterus**
Broad ligament

**Uterus** (Applegate, 2000)

**uterus bicornis** [L, *uterus* + *bis* + *cornu,* horn], a uterus that is divided into two parts, usually separate at the upper end and joined at the lower end.

**uterus masculinus.** See **prostatic utricle.**

**UTI,** abbreviation for **urinary tract infection.**

**utilitarianism** /yo͞o′tiliter′ē·əniz′əm/ [L, *utilis,* useful, *isma,* practice], a doctrine of ethics that the purpose of all action should be to bring about the greatest happiness for the greatest number of people and that the value of anything is determined by its utility. The philosophy is often applied in the distribution of health care resources, as in decisions regarding the expenditure of public funds for health services.

**utilization review (UR)** /yo͞o′tilīzā′shən/ [L, *utilis* + *atus,* process], an assessment of the appropriateness and economy of an admission to a health care facility or a con-

tinued hospitalization. The length of the hospital stay also is compared with the average length of stay for similar diagnoses.

**utricle** /yo͞o′trikəl/ [L, *utriculus,* small bag], the larger of two membranous pouches in the vestibule of the membranous labyrinth of the inner ear. It is an oblong structure that communicates with the semicircular ducts by five openings and receives utricular filaments of the vestibular branch of the vestibulocochlear nerve. Compare **saccule.**

**utriculosaccular duct** /yo͞otrik′yəlosak′yələr/ [L, *utriculus* + *sacculus,* small sack, *ducere,* to lead], a duct connecting the utricle with an endolymphatic duct of the membranous labyrinth.

**UV,** abbreviation for **ultraviolet.**

**uvea** /yo͞o′vē·ə/ [L, *uva,* grape], the vascular, pigmented, middle coat of the eye. Also called **tunica vasculosa bulbi, uveal tract.** —**uveal,** *adj.*

**uveal malignant melanoma** /yo͞o′vē·əl mə·lig′nənt mel′-ə·nō′mə /, the most common type of ocular melanoma, consisting of overgrowth of uveal melanocytes and often preceded by a uveal nevus. See also **ocular melanoma.**

**uveitis** /yo͞o′vē·ī′tis/ [L, *uva* + Gk, *itis*], inflammation of the uveal tract of the eye, including the iris, ciliary body, and choroid. It may be characterized by an irregularly shaped pupil, inflammation around the cornea, pus in the anterior chamber, opaque deposits on the cornea, pain, and lacrimation. Causes include allergy, infection, trauma, diabetes, collagen disease, and skin diseases. A major complication may be glaucoma. See also **chorioretinitis, choroiditis, iritis.**

**uvula** /yo͞o′vyələ/, *pl.* **uvulae** [L, *uva,* grape], the small cone-shaped process suspended in the mouth from the middle of the posterior border of the soft palate, especially the uvula palatina. —**uvular,** *adj.*

**uvular** /yo͞o′vyələr/ [L, *uva,* grape], pertaining to the palatine uvula.

**uvulectomy** /yo͞o′vyəlek′təmē/ [L, *uva,* grape; Gk, *ektomē,* excision], the surgical removal of the uvula.

**uvulitis** /yo͞o′vyəlī′tis/, an inflammation of the uvula. Common causes are allergy and infection.

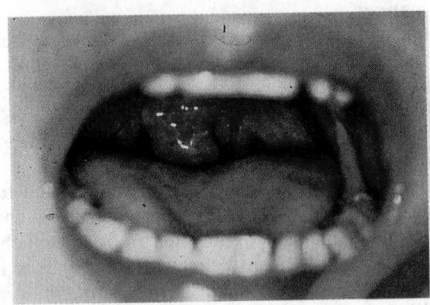

**Uvulitis** (Zitelli and Davis, 1997)

**uvulopalatopharyngoplasty.** See **palatopharyngoplasty.**

**uvulotomy** /yo͞o′vyəlot′əmē/, the surgical removal of all or part of the uvula.

**U wave,** a small, rounded wave that follows the T wave on an electrocardiogram. Normally its polarity is that of the T wave. Its mechanism is unknown. The U wave becomes taller in hypokalemia and inverted in heart disease. It may signify decreased potassium levels in the blood.

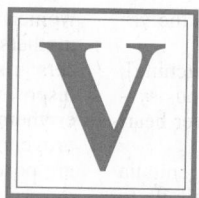

**v, 1.** abbreviation for **vein. 2.** abbreviation for **venous blood.**

**V, 1.** symbol for the element **vanadium. 2.** symbol for *ventilation capacity of the lung.*

**V̇** symbol for *rate of gas flow.*

**V̇max,** the maximum rate of catalysis.

**Vt,** abbreviation for *tidal volume,* the amount of air in milliliters per breath. Also called **TV.**

**VAC,** an anticancer drug combination of vincristine, dactinomycin, and cyclophosphamide.

**vaccinal** /vak′si·nəl/ [L, *vaccinus*], **1.** pertaining to vaccinia, to vaccine, or to vaccination. **2.** having protective qualities when used by way of inoculation.

**vaccination (vacc)** /vak′sinā′shən/ [L, *vaccinus,* relating to a cow], any injection of attenuated or killed microorganisms, such as bacteria, viruses, or rickettsiae, administered to induce immunity or to reduce the effects of associated infectious diseases. Historically the first vaccinations were administered to immunize against smallpox. Vaccinations are now available to immunize against many diseases such as typhoid, measles, and mumps. —**vaccinate,** *v.*

**vaccine** /vaksēn′, vak′sēn, -sin/ [L, *vaccinus*], a suspension of attenuated or killed microorganisms administered intradermally, intramuscularly, orally, or subcutaneously to induce active immunity to infectious disease. Viruses and rickettsiae used in some vaccines are grown in avian embryos, rabbit brain tissue, or monkey kidney tissue, and the organisms are usually inactivated by formalin, phenol, or beta-propiolactone. Bacteria for some vaccines may be inactivated by acetone, formalin, heat, or phenol. Vaccines may be used as single agents or in combinations. Compare **antiserum.**

**-vaccine,** combining form meaning a 'preparation containing microorganisms for producing immunity to disease': *autovaccine, enterovaccine, heterovaccine.*

**vaccinia** /vaksin′ē·ə/ [L, *vaccinus*], an infectious disease of cattle caused by a poxvirus that may be transmitted to humans by direct contact or deliberate inoculation as a vaccine against smallpox. A pustule develops at the site of infection, usually followed by malaise and fever that last for several days. After 2 weeks the pustule becomes a crust that eventually drops off, leaving a scar. Satellite lesions may occur, and the virus may be spread to other sites by scratching. Individuals with eczema or other preexisting skin disease may develop generalized vaccinia. Rarely, a severe encephalitis follows vaccinia. Also called **cowpox.** Compare **smallpox.** See also **vaccination.**

**vaccinia immune globulin,** a hyperimmune gamma globulin developed for the treatment of skin reactions to immunization against the viral disease vaccinia.

**vaccinotherapeutics** /vak′sinōther′əpyōō′tiks/, a form of therapy that involves injections of bacterial antigens.

**vacuole** /vak′yōō·ōl/ [L, *vacuus,* empty], **1.** a clear or fluid-filled space or cavity within a cell, such as occurs when a droplet of water is ingested by the cytoplasm. **2.** a small space in the body enclosed by a membrane, usually

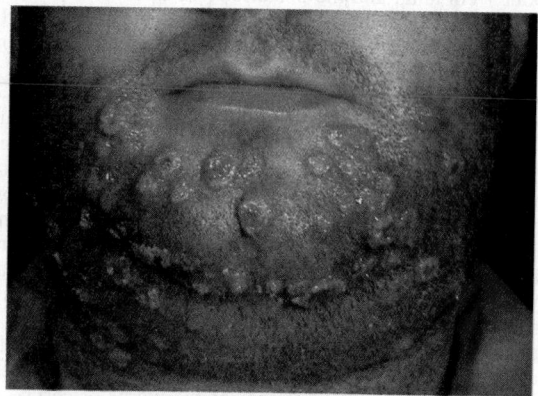

**Vaccinia** *(du Vivier, 1993)*

containing fat, secretions, or cellular debris. —**vacuolar, vacuolated,** *adj.*

**Vacutainer tube,** a glass tube with a rubber stopper in which air can be removed to create a vacuum, usually used to draw blood.

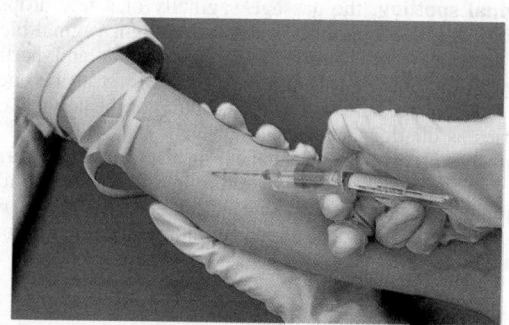

**Obtaining a blood sample with a Vacutainer**
*(Sanders et al, 2000)*

**vacuum aspiration** /vak′yōō·əm/ [L, *vacuus,* empty, *aspirare,* to breathe upon], a method of removing tissues from the uterus by suction for diagnostic purposes or to remove elements of conception. With the patient under local or light general anesthesia, the cervix is dilated, and the uterus is emptied with suction. Postoperative care includes the close observation of vital signs for symptoms of blood loss. Also called **suction curettage.** Compare **dilation and curettage.** See also **elective abortion, therapeutic abortion.**

**VAD,** abbreviation for **vascular access device.**

**vade mecum** /vā′dē mē′kəm/ [L, go with me], something carried by a person for constant use.

**vagal** /vā'gəl/ [L, *vagus,* wandering],    pertaining to the vagus nerve.

**vagal tone** [L, *vagus,* wandering; Gk, *tonos,* stretching], **1.** the level of activity in the parasympathetic nervous system. **2.** the inhibitory control of the vagus nerve over heart rate and atrioventricular conduction.

**vagina** /vəjī'nə/ [L, sheath],    the part of the female genitalia that forms a canal from the orifice through the vestibule to the uterine cervix. It is behind the bladder and in front of the rectum. In the adult woman the anterior wall of the vagina is about 7 cm long, and the posterior wall is about 9 cm long. The canal is actually a potential space; the walls usually touch. The muscles of the vagina are innervated by the pudendal nerve and perfused by the vaginal artery.

**vaginal atrophy** /vaj'ənəl/,    a postmenopausal condition of gradually declining tissue activity in the female reproductive tract. It is caused by a cessation of follicular inhibin and estrogen secretion. This leads to decreased negative feedback on the release of follicle-stimulating hormone and luteinizing hormone by the anterior pituitary gland. Tissue effects related to estrogen deficiency include atrophy and dystrophy of the vulva and vagina, pruritus vulvae, dyspareunia, cystourethritis, ectropion, and uterovaginal prolapse.

**vaginal bleeding,**    an abnormal condition in which blood is passed from the vagina, other than during the menses. It may be caused by abnormalities of the uterus or cervix, an abnormal pregnancy, endocrine abnormalities, abnormalities of one or both ovaries or one or both fallopian tubes, or an abnormality of the vagina. The following terms are commonly used in describing the approximate amount of vaginal bleeding: **heavy vaginal bleeding,** which is greater than heaviest normal menstrual flow; **moderate vaginal bleeding,** which is equal to heaviest normal menstrual flow; **light vaginal bleeding,** which is less than heaviest normal menstrual flow; **vaginal staining,** a very light flow of blood barely requiring the use of a sanitary napkin or tampon; **vaginal spotting,** the passage vaginally of a few drops of blood; and **bloody show,** an episode of light vaginal bleeding as often occurs in early labor, during labor, and, particularly, at the time of full dilation of the cervix at the end of the first stage of labor because of rupture of the cervical capillaries as dilation occurs.

**vaginal cancer,**    a malignancy of the vagina occurring rarely as a primary neoplasm and more often as a secondary lesion or extension of vulvar, cervical, endometrial, or ovarian cancer. Clear cell adenocarcinoma occurs in young women exposed in utero to diethylstilbestrol, given to their mothers to prevent abortion; but most primary vaginal cancers arise in Causasian women over 50 years of age. A predisposing factor is cervical carcinoma. Vaginal leukoplakia, erythematosus, erosion, or granulation of the mucosa may prove to be carcinoma in situ. Symptoms of invasive lesions are postmenopausal bleeding, purulent discharge, pain, and dysuria. Diagnostic measures include cervical, endocervical, and vaginal Papanicolaou smears, colposcopy, biopsy, and Schiller's iodine test in which malignant cells do not stain dark brown. Ninety percent of vaginal cancers are squamous cell carcinomas; others are clear cell or undifferentiated adenocarcinomas, malignant melanomas, and sarcomas. Depending on the patient's age and condition and the site and extent of the lesion, treatment may be by irradiation or vaginectomy and radical hysterectomy with lymph node dissection. Cryosurgery, topical 5-fluorouracil, and dinitrochlorobenzene may be used, but chemotherapy is not usually effective.

**vaginal candidiasis.**    See **vulvovaginal candidiasis.**

**vaginal cornification test,**    a test for the level of estrogen in a urine sample of a woman. Confirmation is indicated by the appearance of cornified epithelia cells in a vaginal smear of a laboratory animal.

**vaginal cyst** [L, *vagina,* sheath; Gk, *kytis,* bag],    an abnormal closed sac or pouch in the vaginal tissues.

**vaginal delivery,**    birth of a fetus through the vagina.

**vaginal discharge,**    any discharge from the vagina. A clear or pearly-white discharge occurs normally. Throughout the reproductive years the amount varies greatly from woman to woman, and the amount and character vary in each woman at different times in her menstrual cycle. Before menarche and after menopause, the quantity of discharge is usually less than during the reproductive years. The discharge is largely composed of secretions of the endocervical glands. Inflammatory conditions of the vagina and cervix often cause an increase in the discharge, which may then have a foul odor and cause pruritus of the perineum and external genitalia.

**vaginal fornix,**    a recess in the upper part of the vagina caused by the protrusion of the uterine cervix into the vagina.

**vaginal hernia,**    **1.** a hernia into the vagina. **2.** a downward protrusion of the cul-de-sac of Douglas between the posterior vaginal wall and the rectum. Also called **posterior vaginal hernia.**

**vaginal hysterectomy** [L, *vagina,* sheath; Gk, *hystera,* womb, *ektomē,* excision],    the surgical removal of the uterus through the vagina.

**vaginal instillation of medication,**    the instillation of a medicated cream, suppository, or gel into the vagina, usually to treat a local infection of the vagina or uterine cervix. The woman voids before the treatment. She then lies back, recumbent or semirecumbent. The nurse or other designated health care provider, wearing gloves, separates the labia majora, exposing the vaginal orifice. The medication is instilled gently. A cream or gel is squeezed into an applicator from a tube and is then placed in the vagina by depressing the plunger of the applicator while withdrawing the device from the vagina. A tablet or suppository is usually placed in the vagina near the cervix with another style of applicator that holds the medication in a slotted receptacle at its tip. The woman remains recumbent after the instillation to prevent escape of the medication from the vagina. Most applicators may be washed after each instillation and reused for the same woman for the next dose. They are discarded after a course of treatment.

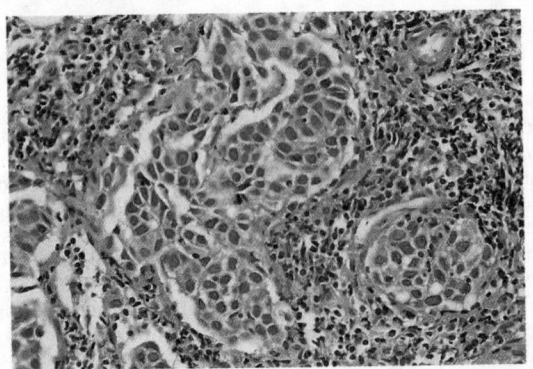

**Vaginal cell squamous cell carcinoma** *(Fletcher, 2000)*

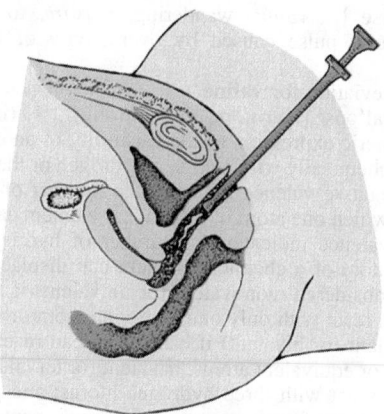

**Vaginal instillation of medicine** *(Potter and Perry, 2001)*

**vaginal jelly,** a contraceptive product containing a spermicide in a jelly medium. It is usually used in conjunction with a contraceptive diaphragm or cervical cap. Some antimicrobial medications are also supplied in the form of a vaginal jelly.

**vaginal lubricant,** an ointment or cream used to reduce friction in the vagina.

**vaginal mucification test** /myōō'sifikā'shən/, a test for the presence of progestins in a urine sample of a woman. Confirmation is indicated by the stimulation of mucus production in the vaginal epithelium of a laboratory animal.

**vaginal speculum** [L, *vagina,* sheath; L, *speculum,* mirror], a bivalved instrument, with two blades used to hold open the vaginal opening for inspection of the vaginal cavity.

**vaginal spotting, vaginal staining.** See **vaginal bleeding.**

**vaginismus** /vaj'iniz'məs/ [L, *vagina* + *spasmus,* spasm], a psychophysiologic genital reaction of women, characterized by intense contraction of the perineal and paravaginal musculature, tightly closing the vaginal introitus. It occurs in response to fear of painful intercourse before coitus or of pelvic examination. Vaginismus is considered abnormal if it occurs in the absence of genital lesions and if it conflicts with a woman's desire to participate in sexual intercourse or to permit examination, but it may be a normal or physiologic response if painful genital conditions exist or if forcible or premature intromission is anticipated. Abnormal vag-

inismus is uncommon. Sexual adjustment often can be achieved through educative and supportive measures that lead to improved sexual self-awareness and response. In some cases the condition is a manifestation of serious mental illness and requires formal psychiatric evaluation and treatment. Gender identity conflict, a history of trauma from rape or incest, or an intense suppression of sexuality in childhood and adolescence are factors that often are associated with vaginismus. See also **dyspareunia.**

**vaginitis** /vaj'inī'tis/, an inflammation of the vaginal tissues, such as trichomonas vaginitis. See also **atrophic vaginitis.**

**vagino-,** combining form meaning 'vagina': *vaginodynia, vaginolabial, vaginopexy.*

**vaginography** /vaj'inog'rəfē/, the radiographic examination of the vagina after the injection of a radiopaque contrast medium. The procedure is performed in the investigation of congenital abnormalities, vaginal fistulae, and other pathologic conditions.

**vaginolabial hernia** /vaj'inōlā'bē·əl/, an inguinal hernia that reaches the tissue of the labium majus.

**vaginoperineoplasty** /vaj'inōper'inē'əplas'tē/, plastic surgery of the vagina and perineum.

**Vagisec,** trademark for a vaginal douche containing polyoxyethylene nonyl phenol, edetate sodium, and dioctyl sodium sulfosuccinate, used to treat trichomoniasis.

**vagoaccessory syndrome.** See **Schmidt's syndrome[1].**

**vagosympathetic** /vā'gōsim'pəthet'ik/ [L, *vagus,* wandering; Gk, *sympathein,* to feel with] pertaining to the vagus nerve and the cervical part of the sympathetic nervous system.

**vagotomy** /vāgot'əmē/ [L, *vagus,* wandering, *temnein,* to cut], the cutting of certain branches of the vagus nerve, performed with gastric surgery, to reduce the amount of gastric acid secreted and lessen the chance of recurrence of a gastric ulcer. With the patient under general anesthesia, a gastrectomy is performed, and the appropriate branches of the vagus nerve are excised. Because peristalsis will be diminished, a pyloroplasty or an anastomosis of the stomach to the jejunum may be done to ensure proper emptying of the stomach. See also **anastomosis, gastrectomy, gastric ulcer, pyloroplasty, vagus nerve.**

**vagotonia.** See **sympathetic imbalance.**

**vagotonus** /vā'gətō'nəs/ [L, *vagus* + Gk, *tonos,* tension], an abnormal increase in parasympathetic activity caused by stimulation of the vagus nerve, especially bradycardia with decreased cardiac output, faintness, and syncope. Vagotonus may occur in suctioning the oropharynx of a newborn as the syringe, laryngoscope blade, or catheter is inadvertently

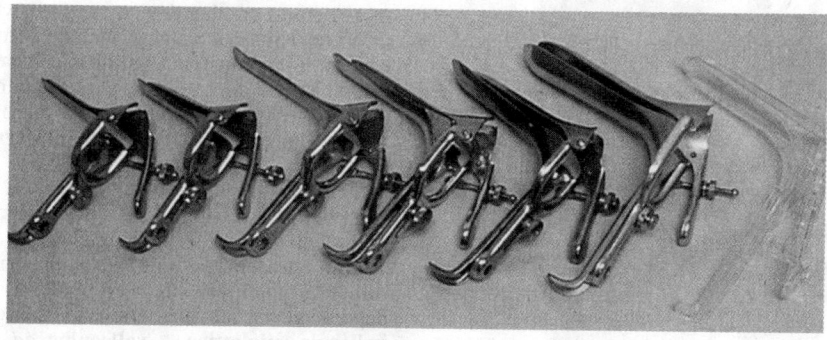

**Vaginal specula** *(Seidel et al, 1999)*

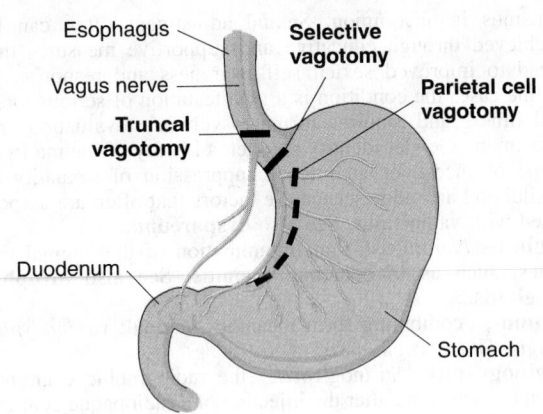

**Vagotomy procedures** *(Beare and Myers, 1998)*

pressed on the back of the throat, stimulating the nerve. It also occurs in some women after surgical treatment or simple manipulation of the uterine cervix.

**vagovagal reflex** /vā′gōvā′gəl/ [L, *vagus* + *vagus* + *reflectere*, to bend back], a stimulation of the vagus nerve by reflex in which irritation of the larynx or the trachea results in slowing of the pulse rate.

**vagueness** /vāg′nəs/, a communication pattern involving the use of global pronouns and loose associations that lead to ambiguity and confusion in communication.

**vagus nerve** /vā′gəs/ [L, *vagus*, wandering, *nervus*, nerve], either of the longest pair of cranial nerves mainly responsible for parasympathetic control over the heart and many other internal organs, including thoracic and abdominal viscera. The vagus nerves communicate through 13 main branches, connecting to four areas in the brain. Also called **nervus vagus, pneumogastric nerve, tenth cranial nerve.**

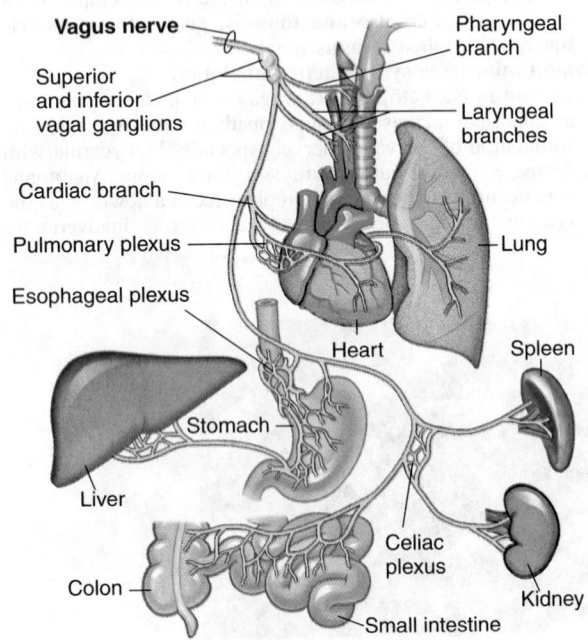

**Vagus nerve**

**vagus pulse** [L, *vagus,* wandering, *pulsare,* to beat], a slow, regular pulse caused by overactivity of the vagus nerve.

**Val,** abbreviation for **valine.**

**valence** /vāl′əns/ [L, *valere,* to be strong], **1.** (in chemistry) a numeric expression of the capability of an element to combine chemically with atoms of hydrogen or their equivalent. A negative valence indicates the number of hydrogen atoms to which one atom of a chemical element can bond. A positive valence indicates the number of hydrogen atoms that one atom of a chemical element can displace. An element is considered monovalent (or univalent) if each of its atoms can react with only one hydrogen atom or its equivalent; divalent (or bivalent) if each atom can react with two hydrogen or equivalent atoms; trivalent (or tervalent) if each atom can react with three hydrogen atoms; and polyvalent (or multivalent) if each atom can react with many hydrogen atoms. **2.** (in immunology) an expression of the number of antigen-binding sites for one molecule of any given antibody or the number of antibody-binding sites for any given antigen. Most antibody molecules, and those belonging to the IgG, IgA, and IgE immunoglobulin classes, have two antigen-binding sites. Most large antigen molecules are multivalent.

**-valence, -valency,** a combining term meaning the 'combining capacity of an atom compared with that of one hydrogen atom': *quantivalence, trivalence, univalence.*

**valence electron,** any of the electrons in the highest principal energy level of an atom or ion. They are responsible for the bonding of atoms to form crystals, molecules, and compounds.

**-valent,** combining form meaning 'having a valency of a (specified) magnitude': *octavalent, pentavalent, tetravalent.*

**valerian,** a perennial herb native to Eurasia that is now grown worldwide.

■ USES: This herb is used as a sedative.

■ CONTRAINDICATIONS: Valerian should not be used during pregnancy and lactation, in those with known hypersensitivity to this herb, or those with hepatic disease. It should be used only with caution in children, since research is lacking.

**valeric acid (CH₃(CH₂)₃COOH)** /vəler′ik/, an organic acid with a foul odor found in the roots of *Valeriana officinalis.* Commercially prepared, it is used in the production of perfumes, flavors, lubricants, and certain drugs. Also known as **pentanoic acidi.**

**valgus** /val′gəs/ [L, bent], describing an abnormal position in which a part of a limb is bent or twisted outward, away from the midline, such as the heel of the foot in **talipes valgus (splayfoot).** Compare **varus.** See also **hallux valgus.**

**validation** /val′idā′shən/, an agreement of the listener with certain elements of the patient's communication.

**validity** /valid′itē/, (in research) the extent to which a test measurement or other device measures what it is intended to measure. Kinds of validity include **content validity, current validity, construct validity,** and **predictive validity.**

**valine (Val)** /val′ēn/, an essential amino acid needed for optimal growth in infants and for nitrogen equilibrium in adults. See also **amino acid, maple syrup urine disease, protein.**

**valinemia.** See **hypervalinemia.**

**Valisone,** trademark for a glucocorticoid (betamethasone valerate).

**Valium,** trademark for a benzodiazepine (diazepam).

**vallecula** /vəlek′yələ/ [L, little valley], **1.** any crevice or depression on the surface of an organ or structure. **2.** See **vallecula epiglottica. —vallecular,** *adj.*

**vallecula epiglottica,** a furrow between the glossoepiglot-

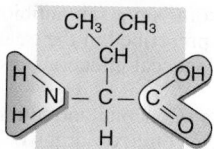

**Chemical structure of valine**

tic folds of each side of the posterior oropharynx. Also called (informal) **vallecula.**

**vallecular dysphagia** /vəlek'yələr/, difficulty or pain on swallowing caused by inflammation of the vallecula epiglottica. Compare **contractile ring dysphagia, dysphagia lusoria.**

**valley fever.** See **coccidioidomycosis.**

**valproic acid** /valprō'ik/, an anticonvulsant.
- INDICATIONS: It is prescribed to treat epilepsy, mania associated with bipolar disorder, and migraines.
- CONTRAINDICATIONS: It is not recommended for use during pregnancy or lactation. Hepatic disease or dysfunction and known hypersensitivity to this drug prohibit its use.
- ADVERSE EFFECTS: Among the more severe adverse reactions are decreased platelet function and hepatotoxicity. GI disturbances are common; alopecia, rash, headache, and insomnia also may occur.

**valrubicin,** an antibiotic antineoplastic.
- INDICATIONS: Valrubicin is used to treat bladder cancer.
- CONTRAINDICATIONS: Factors that prohibit the use of valrubicin include known hypersensitivity to anthracyclines or Cremophor E1, urinary tract infection, and small bladder size.
- ADVERSE EFFECTS: Life-threatening side effects of this drug include thrombocytopenia and leukopenia. Common side effects include anemia, nausea, vomiting, anorexia, diarrhea, urinary tract infection, urinary retention, hematuria, rash, and chest pain.

**Valsalva maneuver** /valsal'və/ [Antonio M. Valsalva, Italian surgeon, 1666–1723; OFr, maneuvre, work done by hand], any forced expiratory effort against a closed airway, such as when an individual holds the breath and tightens the muscles in a concerted, strenuous effort to move a heavy object. Most healthy individuals perform Valsalva maneuvers during normal daily activities without any injurious consequences. However, such efforts are dangerous for many patients with cardiovascular disease, especially if they become dehydrated, increasing the viscosity of their blood and the attendant risk of blood clotting. Constipation increases the risk of cardiovascular trauma in such patients, especially if they perform a Valsalva maneuver in trying to move their bowels. On relaxation after each muscular effort with held breath, the blood of such individuals rushes to the heart, often overloading the cardiac system and causing cardiac arrest. Orthopedic patients often use a Valsalva maneuver in changing their position in bed with the aid of an overhead trapeze bar. Patients who may be endangered by performing a Valsalva maneuver are commonly instructed to exhale instead of holding their breath when they move. Exhalation decreases the risk of cardiovascular trauma.

**Valsalva's test** [Antonio Valsalva; L, testum, crucible], a method for testing the patency of the eustachian tubes. With mouth and nose kept tightly closed, the patient makes a forced expiratory effort; if the eustachian tubes are open, air will enter into the middle ear cavities, and the subject will hear a popping sound. See also **Valsalva maneuver.**

**valsartan,** an antihypertensive.
- INDICATIONS: This drug is used to treat hypertension, either alone or in combination with other agents.
- CONTRAINDICATIONS: Factors that prohibit the use of this drug are known hypersensitivity to valsartan, pregnancy, severe hepatic disease, and bilateral renal artery stenosis.
- ADVERSE EFFECTS: Life-threatening effects of this drug are cerebrovascular accident, myocardial infarction, hepatotoxicity, and nephrotoxicity. Other adverse effects are depression, drowsiness, vertigo, angina pectoris, 2nd degree atrioventricular block, hypotension, conjunctivitis, abdominal pain, nausea, impotence, neutropenia, cramps, myalgia, musculoskeletal pain, and stiffness. Common side effects are dizziness, insomnia, dysrhythmias, diarrhea, anemia, and cough.

**value** /val'yōō/ [L, valere, to be strong], a personal belief about the worth of a given idea or behavior.

**values clarification**[1], a method whereby a person can discover his or her own values by assessing, exploring, and determining what those personal values are and how they affect personal decision making.

**values clarification**[2], a nursing intervention from the Nursing Interventions Classification (NIC) defined as assisting another to clarify her/his own values in order to facilitate effective decision making. See also **Nursing Interventions Classification.**

**value system,** the accepted mode of conduct and the set of norms, goals, and values binding any social group. Such guidelines for determining what is right or wrong, good or bad, and desirable or undesirable serve as a frame of reference for the individual in reaching decisions and in achieving a meaningful life.

**valve** /valv/ [L, valva, folding door], a natural structure or artificial device in a passage or vessel that prevents reflux of the fluid contents passing through it. Valves in veins are membranous folds that prevent backflow of blood. —**valvular,** adj.

**-valve,** suffix meaning 'a thing that regulates the flow of': bivalve, pseudovalve, trivalve.

**valve of Kerkring.** See **circular fold.**

**valve of lymphatics,** any one of the tiny semilunar structures in the vessels and trunks of the lymphatic system that helps regulate the flow of lymph and prevents venous blood from entering the system. There are no valves in the capillaries of the system, but there are many in the collecting vessels. The valves are attached by their convex edges to the walls of the vessels, leaving their concave edges free and directed along the course of the current of lymph. Usually two valves of equal size are found opposite each other. They are more numerous near the lymph nodes and more prevalent in the lymphatic vessels of the neck and the arms than in the vessels of the legs. The wall of the vessel just above the attachment of each valve bulges with a small sinus that gives the vessel its beaded appearance. See also **lymphatic system.**

**valvotomy** /valvot'əmē/ [L, valva + Gk, temnein, to cut], the incision into a valve, especially one in the heart, to correct a defect and allow proper opening and closure. Before surgery a cardiac catheterization is performed. With the patient under general anesthesia, the damaged valve is repaired, if possible, or removed; a prosthetic or biologic valve suture is put in its place. Complications peculiar to prosthetic valve surgery are displacement of the valve caused by broken sutures, heart block, leakage and regurgitation from chamber to chamber, infection, and embolus.

**valvular endocarditis.** See **chronic endocarditis.**

**valvular heart disease** [L, *valva* + AS, *hoert* + L, *dis,* opposite of; Fr, *aise,* ease],   an acquired or congenital disorder of a cardiac valve. It is characterized by stenosis and obstructed blood flow and by valvular degeneration and regurgitation of blood. Diseases of aortic and mitral valves are most common and may be caused by congenital defects, bacterial endocarditis, syphilis, or, most frequently, rheumatic fever. Episodes of rheumatic fever cause the cardiac valves to degenerate and remain open or cause the cusps of the valves to become stiff, calcified, constricted, and fused. Valvular dysfunction results in changes in intracardiac pressure and pulmonary and peripheral circulation. It may lead to cardiac arrhythmia, heart failure, and cardiogenic shock. Cardiotonics, diuretics, analgesics, sodium restriction, and antibiotics, if indicated, are used in the conservative treatment of valvular heart disease; surgery is usually performed when the symptoms are incapacitating. A diseased valve may be repaired by removing the calcium deposits and opening the fused commissures or by removing a cusp and reconstructing the valve, or it may be replaced with a porcine or artificial valve. Types of valvular heart disease include **aortic regurgitation, mitral regurgitation, aortic stenosis, mitral valve stenosis, pulmonary stenosis, tricuspid stenosis.**

**valvular regurgitation** [L, *valva,* folding door, *re* + *gurgitare,* to flow],   a backflow of blood that occurs when the heart contracts but a heart valve fails to close properly.

**valvular stenosis,**   a narrowing or stricture of any of the heart valves. The condition may result from a congenital defect or may be caused by disease. See also **aortic stenosis, congenital cardiac anomaly, mitral valve stenosis, pulmonary stenosis.**

**valvulitis** /val'vyəlī'tis/,   an inflammation of a valve, especially a cardiac valve. Inflammatory changes in the aortic, mitral, and tricuspid valves of the heart are caused most commonly by rheumatic fever and less frequently by bacterial endocarditis and syphilis. Infected valves degenerate, or their cusps become stiff and calcified, resulting in stenosis and obstructed blood flow.

**valvuloplasty** /val'vyəlōplas'tē/ [L, *valva,* folding door; Gk, *plassein,* to shape],   the use of a balloon-tipped catheter to dilate a cardiac valve.

**VAMP** /vamp/,   abbreviation for a combination drug regimen, used in the treatment of cancer, containing three antineoplastics (vincristine sulfate, methotrexate, and mercaptopurine) and a glucocorticoid (prednisone).

**vanadium (V)** /vənā'dē·əm/ [ONorse, *Vanadis,* (Freya) goddess of fertility],   a grayish metallic element. Its atomic number is 23; its atomic mass is 50.942. Absorption of vanadium compounds results in a condition called **vanadiumism,** characterized by anemia, conjunctivitis, pneumonitis, and irritation of the respiratory tract.

**van Bogaert's disease** /vanbō'gərts/ [Ludo van Bogaert, Belgian neurophysiologist, b. 1897],   a rare familial disorder of lipid metabolism in which the substance cholestanol is deposited in the nervous system, blood, and connective tissue. Individuals with the disease develop progressive ataxia and dementia, premature atherosclerosis, cataracts, and xanthomas of the tendons. No effective treatment has been found. Also called **cerebrotendinous xanthomatosis.**

**Van Buchem's syndrome.** See **endosteal hyperostosis.**

**Vanceril,**   trademark for a glucocorticoid (beclomethasone dipropionate).

**Vancocin Hydrochloride,**   trademark for an antibacterial (vancomycin hydrochloride).

**vancomycin** /van'kōmī'sin/,   an antibiotic.

■ INDICATIONS: It is prescribed in the treatment of infections, particularly staphylococcal infections resistant to other antibiotics.

■ CONTRAINDICATIONS: Concomitant administration of neurotoxic, nephrotoxic, or ototoxic drugs or known hypersensitivity to this drug prohibits its use.

■ ADVERSE EFFECTS: Among the more serious adverse reactions are anaphylaxis, dizziness, and tinnitus.

**Van Deemter's equation** /vandēm'tərz/,   an expression of a gas chromatography relationship between the height equivalent to the theoretic plate and the linear velocity of the carrier gas.

**Van de Graaff generator** /van'dəgräf'/ [Robert J. Van de Graaff, American physicist, 1901–1967],   a device in which electrically charged particles are sprayed on a moving belt and carried by it to an insulated terminal, where they cause a large electrostatic charge to build up. The charged particles are then accelerated along a discharge path through a vacuum tube by the potential difference between the insulated terminal and the opposite end of the device. The generator often is used to inject charged particles into a larger accelerator.

**van den Bergh's test** /van'dənburgs'/ [Albert A. H. van den Bergh, Dutch physician, 1869–1943],   a test for the presence of bilirubin in the blood serum. Blood is obtained from a patient who has fasted overnight, and the diluted serum is added to diazo reagent. A blue or violet color indicates the presence of bilirubin. The rate and magnitude of the color change are noted. See also **bilirubin.**

**van der Waals forces** /van'derwäls', fän-/ [Johannes D. van der Waals, Dutch physicist and Nobel laureate, 1837–1923],   weak attractive forces between neutral atoms and molecules. They occur because a fluctuating dipole moment in one molecule induces a dipole moment in another and the two dipole moments interact in an attractive manner. The activity accounts for some deviation from Boyle's law at very low temperatures or very high pressures. Also called **dispersion forces.**

**vanillylmandelic acid (VMA)** /vənil'ilməndel'ik/,   a urinary metabolite of epinephrine and norepinephrine. It may be measured in the urine to determine the levels of the catecholamines (adrenaline and noradrenaline). A greater than normal amount of VMA is characteristic of a pheochromocytoma and neuroblastomas. Increased concentrations of this acid may raise the blood pressure and indicate the presence of tumors of the adrenal glands or nervous system, muscular dystrophy, and myasthenia gravis; they may be caused by stress, exercise, or certain drugs or foods. Normal amounts in the urine of adults after 24-hour collection are 1.5 to 7.5 mg; in the urine of infants, 83 µg/kg of body weight. Also called **3-methoxy-4-hydroxymandelic acid.**

**vanillylmandelic acid (VMA) and catecholamines test,**   a 24-hour urine test that is performed primarily to diagnose hypertension secondary to pheochromocytoma. It is also used to detect the presence of neuroblastomas and rare adrenal tumors.

**vanishing twin** /van'ishing/,   a twin embryo or fetus that is aborted during pregnancy.

**vanity surgery** /van'itē/,   plastic surgery performed primarily to make the patient appear more youthful.

**Vanoxide,**   trademark for a topical fixed-combination drug containing an antibacterial (benzoyl peroxide) and a keratolytic drying agent (chlorhydroxyquinoline).

**Van Rensselaer, Euphenia** /vanren'səlir/,   (1840–1912), an American socialite who entered the first class of the Bellevue Hospital Training School for Nurses in New York. She designed the first nurses' uniform, a blue and white seersucker dress with collar and cuffs, apron, and cap. She succeeded Sister Helen as superintendent of Bellevue and later joined the Sisters of Charity, for whom she established a mission in Nassau, New York. She organized the Seton Hospital for Tuberculosis in New York.

**Vaponefrin,** trademark for an adrenergic agent (epinephrine hydrochloride).

**vapor** /vā'pər/ *pl.* **vapores, vapors** [L], **1.** an atmospheric dispersion of a substance that in its normal state is a liquid or solid. **2.** steam, gas, or an exhalation.

**vapor bath** /vā'pər/, the exposure of the body to vapor, such as steam.

**vaporization** /vā'pərīzā'shən/ [L, *vapor,* steam], the changing of a liquid or solid (such as dry ice) to a gaseous state.

**vaporizer,** a device for reducing medicated liquids to a vapor useful for inhalation or application to accessible mucous membranes.

**vapor pressure depression,** a phenomenon in which the addition of a solute molecule to a solvent will decrease the vapor pressure of the solvent in equilibrium with the vapor phase and the liquid phase.

**vapor therapy,** the therapeutic use of vapors or sprays. See also **vaporizer.**

**Vaquez's disease.** See **polycythemia rubra vera.**

**variability** /ver'ē·əbil'itē/ [L, *variare,* to diversify], the degree of divergence or ability of an object to vary from a given standard or average.

**variable** /ver'ē·əbəl/, a factor in an experiment or scientific test that tends to vary, or take on different values, while other elements or conditions remain constant. See also **dependent variable, independent variable.**

**variable behavior** [L, *variare,* to diversify; AS, *bihabban,* to behave], a response, activity, or action that may be modified by individual experience. Compare **invariable behavior.**

**variable interval (VI) reinforcement,** reinforcement that is offered after varying lapses of time.

**variable-performance oxygen delivery system.** See **low-flow oxygen delivery system.**

**variable ratio (VR) reinforcement,** reinforcement that requires variable numbers of responses.

**variable region,** the part of an immunoglobulin in which the amino acid sequence can differ among molecules of that class of immunoglobulin. The variable region includes the antigen-binding site. Compare **constant region.**

**variance** /ver'ē·əns/ [L, *variare*], **1.** (in statistics) a numeric representation of the dispersion of data around the mean in a given sample. It is represented by the square of the standard deviation and is used principally in performing an analysis of variance. **2.** *nontechnical.* the general range of a group of findings.

**variant** /ver'ē·ənt/ [L, *variare,* to diversify], an individual or subpopulation that differs from other individuals or subpopulations of its species.

**variant angina.** See **Prinzmetal's angina.**

**varicella.** See **chickenpox.**

**varicella gangrenosa** /ver'isel'ə/, a potentially fatal form of varicella characterized by gangrenous lesions. A fulminating subvariety of the skin disorder may become fatal within a few hours if complicated by hemolytic streptococcus.

**varicella-zoster immune globulin** /zos'tər/ [L, *varius,* diverse; Gk, *zoster,* girdle; L, *immunis,* free from, *globulus,*

small globe], an immune globulin obtained from the blood of uninfected individuals who have high levels of antibodies against varicella zoster virus. The immune globulin can be administered to people exposed to chickenpox to prevent or modify symptoms of the infection. See also **immune globulin.**

**varicella zoster virus (VZV)** [L, *varius,* diverse; Gk, *zoster,* girdle; L, *virus,* poison], a member of the herpesvirus family, which causes the diseases varicella (chickenpox) with primary infection and herpes zoster (shingles) of the virus reactivator. The virus has been isolated from vesicle fluid in chickenpox, is highly contagious, and may be spread by direct contact or droplets. Dried crusts of skin lesions do not contain active virus particles. Herpes zoster is produced by reactivation of latent varicella virus, usually several years after the initial infection. There is no simple test for measuring antibodies to this virus; however, zoster immune globulin (ZIG) obtained from convalescing zoster patients, if injected within 3 days of exposure, will prevent varicella in susceptible children. The temporary nature of this protection and the relative scarcity of ZIG warrant reservation of its use to children receiving immunosuppressive therapy or suffering from immune deficiency diseases. Herpes zoster should be treated promptly with acyclovir, desciclovir, valaciclovir, or penciclovir to speed healing. (Famciclovir is used for postherpetic neuralgia.) A licensed vaccine is available and highly effective. See also **chickenpox, herpes zoster.**

**varicelliform** /ver'isel'ifôrm/, resembling the rash of chickenpox.

**varices.** See **varix.**

**varicocele** /ver'əkōsēl'/ [L, *varix,* varicose vein; Gk, *kele,* tumor], a dilation of the pampiniform venous complex of the spermatic cord. The varicocele forms a soft, elastic swelling that can cause pain. It is usually more pronounced and painful when the patient is standing. Varioceles are most common in men between 15 and 25 years of age and affects the left spermatic cord more often than the right. Compare **ovarian varicocele, uteroovarian varicocele.**

**varicose** /ver'əkōs/ [L, *varix*], abnormally swollen or dilated.

**varicose aneurysm,** a blood-filled, saclike projection that connects an artery and one or several veins and that is formed from a localized dilation of the adjoining vessels.

**varicose ulcer.** See **stasis ulcer.**

**varicose vein,** a tortuous, dilated vein with incompetent valves. Causes include congenitally defective valves, thrombophlebitis, pregnancy, and obesity. Varicose veins are common, especially in women, and are usually painless. The saphenous veins of the legs are most often affected. Elevation of the legs and use of elastic stockings are frequently sufficient therapy for uncomplicated cases. Ligation of the vein above the varicosity and removal of the distal part of the vessel may be indicated for more severe cases if deeper vessels can maintain the return of venous blood. Injection of sclerosing solutions helps prevent or treat postphlebitic syndrome.

**varicosis** /ver'ikō'sis/ [L, *varix* + Gk, *osis,* condition], a common condition characterized by one or more tortuous, abnormally dilated usually in the legs or the lower trunk. It most often occurs in persons between 30 and 60 years of age. Varicosis may be caused by congenital defects of the valves or walls of the veins or by congestion and increased intraluminal pressure resulting from prolonged standing, poor posture, pregnancy, abdominal tumor, or chronic systemic disease. Symptoms include pain and muscle cramps

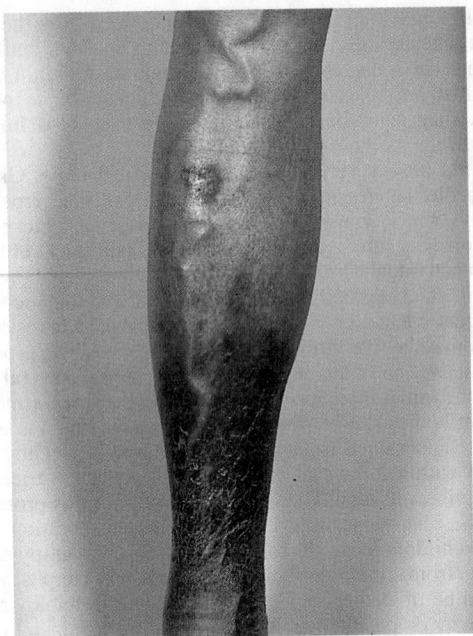

**Varicose veins** *(du Vivier, 1993)*

with a feeling of fullness and heaviness in the legs. Dilation of superficial veins is often evident before the condition produces discomfort.

**varicosity** /ver′ikos′itē/, **1.** an abnormal condition, usually of a vein, characterized by swelling and tortuosity. **2.** a vein in this condition.

**variegate** /ver′ē·əgāt′/ [L, *varius*, diverse], having characteristics that vary, especially as to color.

**variegate porphyria,** an uncommon form of hepatic porphyria, characterized by skin lesions and photosensitivity. The condition may be congenital or acquired. The congenital form is more serious, resulting in crises of acute abdominal pain and certain neurologic complications. See also **porphyria.**

**variola minor.** See **alastrim.**

**variola, variola major.** See **smallpox.**

**varioloid** /ver′ē·əloid′/ [L, *varius* + Gk, *eidos,* form], **1.** resembling smallpox. **2.** a mild form of smallpox in a vaccinated person or one who has previously had the disease.

**varix** /ver′iks/, *pl.* **varices** /ver′əsēz/ [L, varicose vein], a tortuous, dilated vein, artery, or lymphatic vessel.

**varnish** /vär′nish/, a solution of natural resins and gums used as a protective coating over the surfaces of a dental cavity preparation before restorative material is applied or over a tooth surface after sealing and root planing.

**varus** /ver′əs/ [L, bent], describing an abnormal position in which a part of a limb is turned inward toward the midline, such as the great toe in **hallux varus.** Compare **valgus.**

**vas** /vas/, *pl.* **vasa** /vā′sə/ [L, vessel], any one of the many vessels of the body, especially those that convey blood, lymph, or spermatozoa.

**vas afferens,** a small arteriole that supplies blood to a renal glomerulus. Also called **afferent glomerular arteriole.**

**vasa vasorum** [L, *vas,* vessel], small blood vessels that supply the walls of the arteries and veins.

**vascular** /vas′kyələr/ [L, *vasculum,* little vessel], pertaining to a blood vessel.

**vascular access device (VAD),** an indwelling catheter, cannula, or other instrumentation used to obtain venous or arterial access.

**vascular endothelium,** the endothelium that lines the blood vessels.

**vascular hemophilia.** See **von Willebrand's disease.**

**vascular insufficiency,** inadequate peripheral blood flow. Causes include occlusion of vessels by atherosclerotic plaques, thrombi, or emboli; damaged, diseased, or intrinsically weak vascular walls; arteriovenous fistulas; hematologic hypercoagulability; and heavy smoking. Signs of vascular insufficiency include pale, cyanotic, or mottled skin over the affected area; swelling of an extremity; absent or reduced tactile sensation; tingling; diminished sense of temperature; muscle pain, such as intermittent claudication in the calf; and, in advanced disease, ulcers and atrophy of muscles in the involved extremity. Diagnosis may be made by comparing peripheral pulses in contralateral extremities or by angiography, plethysmography, ultrasonography, and skin temperature tests. Treatment of vascular insufficiency may include a diet low in saturated fats, moderate exercise, sleeping on a firm mattress, avoidance of tobacco products, proper standing or sitting posture, elevation of the involved extremity, use of a vasodilating drug, and, if indicated, repair of an arteriovenous fistula or aneurysm or bypass surgery. See also **arterial insufficiency.**

**vascularity** /vas′kyələr′itē/ [L, *vasculum,* little vessel], the state of blood vessel development and functioning in an organ or tissue.

**vascularization** /vas′kyələr′īzā′shən/, the process by which body tissue develops proliferating capillaries. It may be natural or induced by surgical techniques. —**vascularize,** *v.*

**vascular leiomyoma,** a neoplasm that has developed from smooth muscle fibers of a blood vessel.

**vascular sclerosis** [L, *vasculum* + Gk, *skerosis,* hardening], a condition of hyaline degeneration of the blood vessels with hypertrophy of the tunica media and subintimal fibrosis. There also may be a weakening and loss of elasticity in the artery walls.

**vascular spider.** See **spider angioma.**

**vascular tumor.** See **aneurysm.**

**vasculature** /vas′kyələ′chər/ [L, *vasculum*], the blood vessels in an organ or tissue.

**vasculitis** /vas′kyəlī′tis/, inflammation of the blood vessels. It may be caused by a systemic disease or an allergic reaction. Kinds of vasculitis are **allergic vasculitis, necrotizing vasculitis,** and **segmented hyalinizing vasculitis.** See also **angiitis.**

**vasculogenic impotence** /vas′kyəlōjen′ik/ [L, *vasculum,* little vessel; Gk, *genein,* to produce; L, *in* + *potentia,* power], impotence resulting from an inadequate supply of arterial blood to the penis.

**vasculomotor.** See **vasomotor.**

**vas deferens** /def′ərənz/, *pl.* **vasa deferentia** /def′əren′shē·ə/ [L, *vas* + *deferens,* carrying away], the extension of the epididymis of the testis that ascends from the scrotum into the abdominal cavity and joins the seminal vesicle to form the ejaculatory duct. It is enclosed by fibrous connective tissue with blood vessels, nerves, and lymphatics and passes through the inguinal canal as part of the spermatic cord. Also called **deferent duct, ductus deferens, spermatic duct, testicular duct.** See also **testis.**

**vasectomy** /vasek′təmē/ [L, *vas* + Gk, *ektomē,* excision], a procedure for male sterilization involving the bilateral surgical removal of a part of the vas deferens. Vasectomy is most commonly performed at an outpatient surgery center

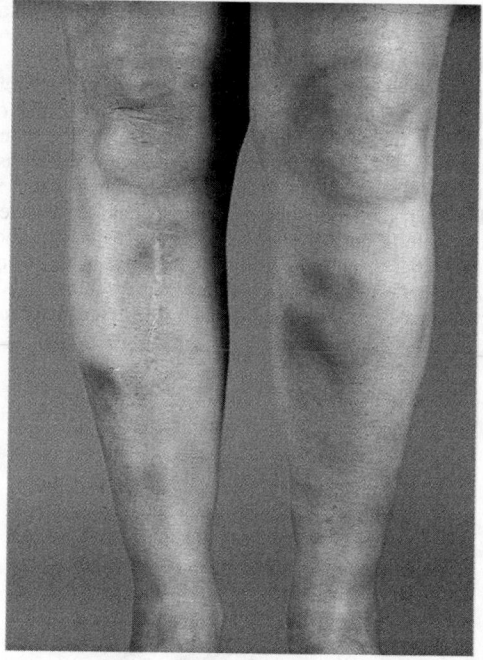

**Nodular vasculitis** (du Vivier, 1993)

using local anesthesia. The procedure is also performed routinely before removal of the prostate gland to prevent inflammation of the testes and epididymides. Potency is not affected.

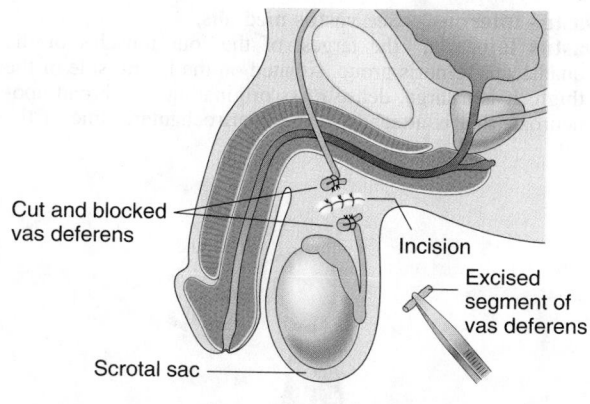

Cut and blocked
vas deferens

Incision

Excised
segment of
vas deferens

Scrotal sac

**Vasectomy** (Chabner, 2001)

**vasectomy reversal.** See **vasovasostomy.**

**vaso-** /vas′ō-, vā′sō/, combining form meaning 'vessel or duct': *vasoconstrictor, vasodilation, vasoganglion.*

**vasoactive** /vā′zō·ak′tiv/ [L, *vas* + *activus*, active], (of a drug) tending to cause vasodilation or vasoconstriction.

**vasoactive intestinal polypeptide (VIP),** a glucagon-secretin hormone found in the pancreas, intestine, and central nervous system. The hormone stimulates insulin and glucagon release. Gastric secretion, gastric motility, and pe-

ripheral vasodilation, as well as hyperglycemia by hepatic glycogenolysis, are inhibited. See also **vipoma.**

**vasoconstriction** [L, *vas* + *constrigere,* to tighten], a decrease in the diameter of a blood vessel. It plays an important role in the control of blood pressure and the distribution of blood throughout the body. Vasoconstriction is triggered by stimulation of the vasomotor constriction center in the medulla. Impulses from this center travel along sympathetic nerve fibers and cause contraction of the smooth muscle layers of arteries, arterioles, and, to a lesser extent, venules, and veins, bringing about constriction of these vessels. Vasoconstriction is also induced by vasomotor pressure reflexes, chemical reflexes, the medullary ischemic reflex, and impulses from the cerebral cortex and the hypothalamus. Compare **vasodilation**—**vasoconstrictive,** *adj.*

**vasoconstrictive** /-kənstrik′tiv/ [L, *vas,* vessel, *constringere,* to draw tight], able to cause a constriction of blood vessels.

**vasoconstrictor** /-kənstrik′tər/ [L, *vas* + *constrigere*], **1.** pertaining to a process, condition, or substance that causes the constriction of blood vessels. **2.** an agent that promotes vasoconstriction. Cold, fear, stress, and nicotine are common exogenous vasoconstrictors. Internally secreted epinephrine and norepinephrine cause blood vessels to contract by stimulating adrenergic receptors of peripheral sympathetic nerves. Other endogenous vasoconstrictors are angiotensin, which is formed in the blood through the action of renin, and antidiuretic hormone, which is secreted by the pituitary. Adrenergic sympathomimetic drugs cause some degree of vasoconstriction, and several of these agents are used for this action in maintaining blood pressure during anesthesia and in treating pronounced hypotension resulting from hemorrhage, myocardial infarction, septicemia, sympathectomy, or drug reactions. Among these therapeutic agents are methoxamine hydrochloride, metaraminol bitartrate, and norepinephrine. Also called **vasopressor.**

**vasodepressor syncope,** a sudden loss of consciousness, resulting from cerebral ischemia; secondary to decreased cardiac output, peripheral vasodilation, and bradycardia; and associated with vagal activity. The condition may be triggered by pain, fright, or trauma and accompanied by symptoms of nausea, pallor, and perspiration. Also called **vasovagal syncope.**

**vasodilatation.** See **vasodilation.**

**vasodilation** /-dīlā′shən/ [L, *vas* + *dilatare*], an increase in the diameter of a blood vessel. It is caused by a relazation of the smooth muscles in the vessel wall. Also called **vasodilatation.** Compare **vasoconstriction.**

**vasodilator** /vā′zōdī′lātər/ [L, *vas* + *dilatare*], a nerve or agent that causes dilation of blood vessels by promoting the relaxation of vascular smooth muscle. Chemical vasodilators include hydralazine, nitroglycerin, nitroprusside, and trimethaphan. They have been useful in the treatment of acute heart failure in myocardial infarction, in cases associated with severe mitral regurgitation, and in failure resulting from myocardial disease.

**vasoganglion** /-gang′glē·on/, a spherical mass of small blood vessels.

**vasogenic shock** /-jen′ik/ [L, *vas* + *genein,* to produce; Fr, *choc*], shock resulting from peripheral vascular dilation produced by factors such as toxins that directly affect the blood vessels. Examples of vasogenic shock include **anaphylactic shock** and **septic shock.**

**vasohypertonic** /-hī′pərton′ik/, causing constriction of blood vessels.

**vasoinhibitor** /vas′ō·inhib′itər/, an agent that opposes the action of vasomotor nerves, thereby causing arterial dilation and reduced blood pressure.

**vasoinhibitory** /vas′ō·inhib′itôr′ē/, inhibiting the activity of vasomotor nerves.

**vasomotor** /-mō′tər/ [L, *vas* + *movere,* to move], pertaining to the nerves and muscles that control the diameter of the blood vessels. Circularly arranged smooth muscle fibers of arteries and arterioles can contract, causing vasoconstriction, or they can relax, causing vasodilation. Also called **vasculomotor.**

**vasomotor center,** a collection of cell bodies in the medulla oblongata of the brain that regulates or modulates blood pressure and cardiac function primarily via the autonomic nervous system.

**vasomotor epilepsy,** a form of epilepsy characterized by episodes of autonomic dysfunction and extreme contractions of the arteries. Also called **autonomic epilepsy.**

**vasomotor paralysis,** hypotonia of blood vessels caused by blockage of activity in nerves that stimulate vascular constriction. Also called **vasoparalysis.** See also **vasoparesis.**

**vasomotor reflex** [L, *vas,* vessel, *movere,* to move, *reflectere,* to bend back], any reflex response of the circulatory system caused by stimulation of vasodilator or vasoconstrictive nerves.

**vasomotor rhinitis,** chronic rhinitis and nasal obstruction, without allergy or infection, characterized by sneezing, rhinorrhea, nasal obstruction, and vascular engorgement of the mucous membranes of the nose. A vaporizer or humidifier and systemic vasoconstrictive agents are used to alleviate discomfort. Nose drops and nasal sprays are avoided, because continued use may cause further vasodilation of the mucous membrane and aggravation of the condition. Topical vasoconstrictors should also be avoided because the nasal mucous membrane loses sensitivity to stimuli. Vasomotor rhinitis is common in pregnancy.

**vasomotor spasm.** See **angiospasm.**

**vasomotor system,** the part of the nervous system that controls the constriction and dilation of the blood vessels. See also **vasoconstriction, vasodilation.**

**vasoparalysis.** See **vasomotor paralysis.**

**vasoparesis,** a mild form of vasomotor paralysis.

**vasopressin.** See **antidiuretic hormone.**

**vasopressor.** See **vasoconstrictor.**

**vasospasm.** See **angiospasm.**

**vasospastic** /-spas′tik/, **1.** relating to a spasmodic constriction of a blood vessel. **2.** any agent that produces spasms of the blood vessels.

**vasospastic angina,** chest pain caused by spasms of the coronary arteries. It has features that differ from those of angina pectoris. See also **Prinzmetal's angina.**

**vasostimulation** /-stim′yəlā′shən/ [L, *vas,* vessel, *stimulare,* to incite], the promotion of vasomotor activity.

**Vasotec,** trademark for an angiotensin-converting enzyme inhibitor (enalapril maleate).

**vasovagal reflex,** a stimulation of the vagus nerve by reflex in which irritation of the larynx or the trachea results in slowing of the pulse rate.

**vasovagal syncope.** See **vasodepressor syncope.**

**vasovasostomy** /vas′ōvəsos′təmē/ [L, *vas* + *vas* + Gk, *stoma,* mouth], a surgical procedure in which the function of the vas deferens on each side of the testes is restored, having been cut and ligated in a preceding vasectomy. The procedure is performed if a man wants to regain his fertility. In most cases the patency of the canals is achieved, but in many cases, fertility does not result, probably because of circulating autoantibodies that disrupt normal sperm activity. The antibodies apparently develop after vasectomy because the developing sperm cannot be excreted through the urogenital tract.

**Vasoxyl,** trademark for an alpha-adrenergic (methoxamine hydrochloride).

**vastus intermedius** /vas′təs/ [L, *vastus,* enormous, *inter,* between, *mediare,* to divide], one of the four muscles of the quadriceps femoris group, situated in the center of the thigh under the rectus femoris. It arises from the front and lateral surfaces of the femur and the lateral intermuscular septum. Its fibers end in a superficial aponeurosis that forms the deep part of the quadriceps femoris tendon, inserted under the patella and onto the tibial tuberosity. It functions with the other three muscles of the quadriceps to extend the leg. Also called **crureus.** Compare **rectus femoris, vastus lateralis, vastus medialis.** See also **quadriceps femoris.**

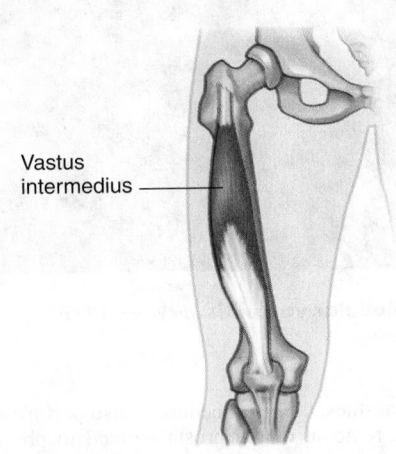

Vastus intermedius

**Vastus intermedius**

**vastus internus.** See **vastus medialis.**

**vastus lateralis,** the largest of the four muscles of the quadriceps femoris group, situated on the lateral side of the thigh. It is a large, dense mass originating in a broad aponeurosis that is attached to the intertrochanteric line of the

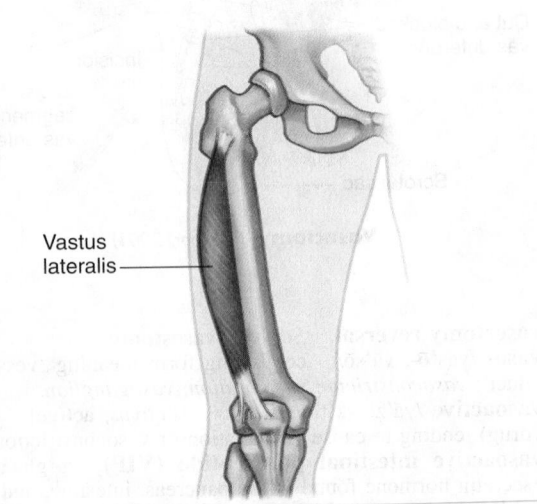

Vastus lateralis

**Vastus lateralis**

femur, the greater trochanter, the lateral lip of the gluteal tuberosity, and the lateral lip of the linea aspera. The fibers of the muscle are gathered to form a strong aponeurosis that converges to become a flat tendon before inserting under the patella and onto the lateral condyle of the tibia. The muscle functions to help extend the leg. Compare **rectus femoris, vastus intermedius, vastus medialis.** See also **quadriceps femoris.**

**vastus medialis,** one of the four muscles of the quadriceps femoris group, situated in the medial part of the thigh. It originates from the intertrochanteric line of the femur, the linea aspera, the medial supracondylar line, the tendons of the adductor longus and the adductor magnus, and the medial intermuscular septum. The vastus medialis extends to the lower anterior aspect of the thigh and inserts by an aponeurosis under the patella as part of the quadriceps femoris tendon and onto the medial condyle of the femur. An expansion of the aponeurosis passes to the capsule of the knee joint. The muscle functions in combination with other parts of the quadriceps femoris to extend the leg. Also called **vastus internus.** Compare **rectus femoris, vastus intermedius, vastus lateralis.** See also **quadriceps femoris.**

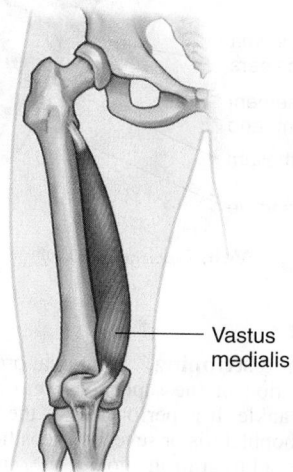

Vastus medialis

**Vastus medialis**

**VATER complex,** a nonrandom association of congenital anomalies consisting of *v*ertebral defects, imperforate *a*nus, *t*racheo*e*sophageal fistula, and *r*adial and *r*enal dysplasia.

**Vater-Pacini corpuscles** /fä′tərpäse̅′ne̅/ [Abraham Vater, German anatomist, 1684–1751; Filippo Pacini, Italian anatomist, 1812–1883], kinesioceptors located in joint capsules and ligaments. They may transmit nerve impulses at an increasing rate as a joint approaches its maximal range of motion and are believed to have a protective function of signaling the cerebral cortex when a joint has reached the end position of its range. They are the most complicated of the nerve endings.

**Vater's ampulla** /fä′tərz/ [Abraham Vater 1684–1751; L, *ampulla,* jug], a flask-shaped dilation at the end of the common bile duct where the duct joins with the duodenum. Also called **hepatopancreatic ampulla.**

**VBP,** an anticancer drug combination of vinblastine, bleomycin, and cisplatin. Also called **PVB.**

**VC,** abbreviation for **vital capacity.**

**VCO₂,** symbol for carbon dioxide output per unit of time.

**VCU,** abbreviation for **voiding cystourethrography.**

**VD,** abbreviation for **venereal disease.** See **sexually transmitted disease.**

**V deflection** /diflek′shən/, a deflection on the His bundle electrogram that represents ventricular activation.

**VDRL,** abbreviation for *Venereal Disease Research Laboratories.*

**VDRL test,** abbreviation for *Venereal Disease Research Laboratory test,* a serologic flocculation test for syphilis. It is also positive in other treponemal diseases such as yaws. False-positive and false-negative results may occur. A positive test must be confirmed by further, more definitive testing.

**VDT,** abbreviation for **video display terminal.**

**V̇e,** symbol for *expired volume.*

**V̇E,** symbol for *volume expired in 1 minute.*

**vector** /vek′tər/ [L, carrier], **1.** a quantity having direction and magnitude, usually depicted by a straight arrow; the length of the arrow represents magnitude and the head represents direction. **2.** a carrier, especially one that transmits disease. A **biologic vector** is usually an arthropod in which the infecting organism completes part of its life cycle. A **mechanical vector** transmits the infecting organism from one host to another but is not essential to the life cycle of the parasite. Kinds of vectors include dogs, which carry rabies; mosquitoes, which transmit malaria; and ticks, which carry Rocky Mountain spotted fever. **3.** a retrovirus that has been modified by alteration of its genetic component. Through recombinant deoxyribonucleic acid techniques, genes that cause harmful effects such as cancer, are removed, and genes that mediate synthesis of essential enzymes are added. The vector then can be injected into a patient who suffers from an enzyme deficiency, such as Lesch-Nyhan syndrome. —**vector,** *v.,* **vectorial,** *adj.*

**vectorcardiogram** /-kär′de̅·əgram′/ [L, *vector,* carrier; Gk, *kardia,* heart, *gramma,* record], a tracing of the direction and magnitude of the heart's electrical activity during a cardiac cycle. It is produced by the simultaneous recording of three standard leads, using an oscilloscope.

**vectorcardiography** /-kär′de̅·og′rəfe̅/ [L, *vector,* carrier; Gk, *kardia,* heart, *graphein,* to record], a method of recording the direction and magnitude of the heart's electrical activity.

**vecuronium bromide** /vek′yərō′ne̅·əm/, an IV neuromuscular blocking drug.

■ INDICATIONS: It is used as an adjunct to general anesthesia, to facilitate endotracheal intubation, and to relax skeletal muscles during surgery or mechanical ventilation.

■ CONTRAINDICATIONS: The drug should be used cautiously in patients with myasthenia gravis or other neuromuscular disorders, or who have been given drugs that produce or increase neuromuscular block. Effects of vecuronium may be prolonged in patients with liver disease.

■ ADVERSE EFFECTS: No serious adverse reactions have been reported.

**VEE,** abbreviation for **Venezuelan equine encephalitis.** See **equine encephalitis.**

**Veetids,** trademark for an antibacterial (penicillin V potassium).

**vegan.** See **strict vegetarian.**

**veganism** /vej′əniz′əm/ [L, *vegetare,* to grow, *ismus,* practice], the adherence to a strict vegetarian diet, with the exclusion of all protein of animal origin.

**vegetable albumin** /vej′(i)təbəl/, albumin protein produced in plants.

**vegetal pole** /vej′ətəl/ [L, *vegetare* + *polus,* pole], the relatively inactive part of an ovum where the yolk is situated, usually opposite the animal pole. Also called **vegetative pole, antigerminal pole.** Compare **animal pole.**

**vegetarian** /vej′əter′ē·ən/ [L, *vegetare*], a person who eats only foods of plant origin, including fruits, grains, and nuts. Many vegetarians eat eggs and milk products but avoid all animal flesh. Kinds of vegetarians are **lacto-ovo-vegetarian, lacto-vegetarian, ovo-vegetarian,** and **strict vegetarian.**

**vegetarianism** /vej′əter′ē·əniz′əm/, the theory or practice of eating only foods of plant origin, including fruits, grains, and nuts.

**vegetation** /vej′ətā′shən/, an abnormal growth of tissue around a valve, composed of fibrin, platelets, and bacteria.

**vegetative** /vej′ətā′tiv, vej′ətətiv′/ [L, *vegetare*], **1.** pertaining to nutrition and growth. **2.** pertaining to the plant kingdom. **3.** denoting involuntary function, as produced by the parasympathetic nervous system. **4.** resting, not active; denoting the stage of the cell cycle in which the cell is not replicating. **5.** leading a secluded, dull existence without social or intellectual activity; sluggish; lacking animation. **6.** (in psychiatry) emotionally withdrawn and passive, as may occur in schizophrenia and depression or in unipolar depression in severe cases. —**vegetate,** *v.*

**vegetative endocarditis** [L, *vegetare,* to grow; Gk, *endon,* within, *kardia,* heart, *itis,* inflammation], a subacute form of bacterial endocarditis characterized by vegetation on the heart valves. The vegetation may cause ulceration and perforation of the heart valve cusps.

**vegetative pole.** See **vegetal pole.**

**vegetative state,** a physical condition in which a previously comatose patient continues to be unable to communicate or respond to stimuli, despite at times giving the appearance of wakefulness. The eyes may be open, but, because of senile brain disease, cerebral arteriosclerosis, or injury to the cerebral cortex, the patient remains immobile and must be fed and toileted, and all other physical needs attended to. It is important to speak to the patient, since it is not known whether the patient can hear.

**vehicle** /vē′ikəl/ [L, *vehiculum,* conveyance], **1.** an inert substance with which a medication is mixed to facilitate measurement and administration or application. **2.** any fluid or structure in the body that passively conveys a stimulus. **3.** any substance, such as food or water, that can serve as a mode of transmission for infectious agents.

**vehicle safety promotion,** a nursing intervention from the Nursing Interventions Classification (NIC) defined as assisting individuals, families, and communities to increase awareness of measures to reduce unintentional injuries in motorized and nonmotorized vehicle. See also **Nursing Interventions Classification.**

*Veillonella* /vā′yənel′ə/ [Adrien Veillon, French bacteriologist, 1864–1931], a genus of gram-negative anaerobic bacteria. The species *Veillonella parvula* is normally present in the alimentary tract, especially in the mouth.

**Veillon tube** /vāyōn′/, a transparent tube, the ends of which are closed with removable stoppers, one cotton and one rubber. It is used for the laboratory growth of bacteriologic cultures.

**vein (v)** /vān/ [L, *vena*], any one of the many vessels that convey blood from the capillaries as part of the pulmonary venous system, the systemic venous network, or the portal venous complex. Most of the veins of the body are systemic veins that convey blood from the whole body (except the lungs) to the right atrium of the heart. Each vein is a macroscopic structure enclosed in three layers of different kinds of tissue homologous with the layers of the heart. The outer tunica adventitia of each vein is homologous with the epicardium, the tunica media with the myocardium, and the tunica intima with the endocardium. Deep veins course through the more internal parts of the body, and superficial veins lie near the surface, where many of them are visible through the skin. Veins have thinner coatings and are less elastic than arteries and collapse when cut. They also contain semilunar valves at various intervals to control the direction of the blood flow back to the heart. Compare **artery.** See also **portal vein, pulmonary vein, systemic vein.**

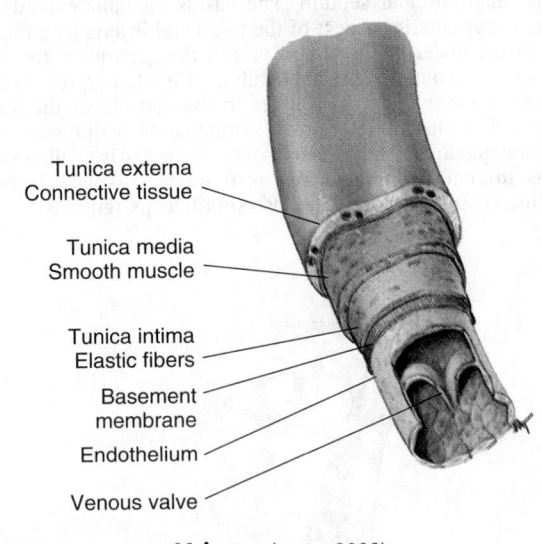

Tunica externa
Connective tissue

Tunica media
Smooth muscle

Tunica intima
Elastic fibers

Basement membrane

Endothelium

Venous valve

**Vein** *(Applegate, 2000)*

**vein ligation and stripping,** a surgical procedure consisting of the ligation of the saphenous vein and its removal from groin to ankle. It is performed for the treatment of recurrent thrombophlebitis or severe varicosities or for obtaining a blood vessel to graft in another site, such as in a coronary bypass operation.

**vein lumen,** the central opening through which blood flows in a vein.

**vein of Thebesius.** See **smallest cardiac vein.**

**veins of the vertebral column,** the veins that drain the blood from the vertebral column, adjacent muscles, and meninges of the spinal cord. Along the entire vertebral column these veins form plexuses that are divided into internal and external groups according to their locations inside or outside the vertebral canal. The plexuses and veins of the vertebral network are the external plexus, internal plexus, basivertebral veins, intervertebral veins, and spinal cord veins.

**Velban,** trademark for an antineoplastic (vinblastine sulfate).

**Velcro,** trademark for a type of fastening device with a surface of tiny hooks that adheres to the opposite side, used mainly on fabric products.

**vellus hair.** See **lanugo.**

**velocardiofacial syndrome** /vel′ō·kär′dē·ō·fā′shəl /, an autosomal dominant syndrome of cardiac defects and characteristic craniofacial abnormalities including cleft palate, jaw abnormalities, and prominent nose; it is often associated with abnormalities of chromosome 22. Learning disabilities occur often; short stature, slender hyperextensible hands and digits, scoliosis, mental retardation, inguinal hernia, auricular abnormalities, and microcephaly occur less frequently. Also called **Shprintzen's syndrome.**

**velocity** /vəlos'itē/ [L, *velox,* quick],   the rate of change in the position of a body moving in a particular direction. Velocity along a straight line is linear velocity. Angular velocity is that of a body in circular motion. Compare **speed.**

**velocity of growth,**   the rate of growth or change in growth measurements over a period of time.

**velocity of ultrasound,**   the speed of ultrasound waves in a particular medium. The velocity varies from 331 meters per second (m/sec) in air to 1450 m/sec in fat, 1570 m/sec in blood, and 4080 m/sec in the skull.

**velocity spectrum rehabilitation,**   a rehabilitation program that uses strength training at multiple speeds of movement from slow to fast.

**velopharyngeal closure,**   closure of nasal air escape by the elevation of the soft palate and contraction of the posterior pharyngeal wall.

**velopharyngeal insufficiency,**   an abnormal condition resulting from a congenital defect in the structure of the velopharyngeal sphincter: Closure of the oral cavity beneath the nasal passages is not complete, as seen in cleft palate. Food may be regurgitated through the nose, and speech is impaired. Surgical correction is usually successful.

**Velosef,**   trademark for a cephalosporin antibiotic (cephradine).

**Velpeau's bandage** /velpōz'/ [Alfred A. L. M. Velpeau, French surgeon, 1795–1867],   a roller bandage that immobilizes the elbow and shoulder by holding the brachium against the side and the flexed forearm on the chest. The palm of the hand rests on the clavicle of the opposite side.

**vena cava** /vē'nə kā'və/, *pl.* **venae cavae** [L, *vena,* vein, *cavum,* cavity],   one of two large veins returning blood from the peripheral circulation to the right atrium of the heart. See also **inferior vena cava, superior vena cava. —vena caval,** *adj.*

**vena caval foramen,**   an opening in the diaphragm through which the inferior vena cava and vagus nerve pass.

**vena caval syndrome.**   See **supine hypotension.**

**vena comes** /kō'mēz/, *pl.* **venae comites** /kom'itēz/,   one of the deep paired veins that accompany the smaller arteries on each side of the artery. The three vessels are wrapped together in one sheath. Some of the arteries accompanied by such venous pairs are the brachial, the ulnar, and the tibial.

**vena cordis magna.**   See **great cardiac vein.**

**veneer** /vənir'/ [Fr, *fournir,* to furnish],   **1.** a layer of tooth-colored material, usually porcelain or acrylic, attached to the surface of a crown or artificial tooth by direct fusion. **2.** See **serumal calculus.**

**venepuncture.**   See **venipuncture.**

**venereal** /vənir'ē·əl/ [L, *Venus,* goddess of love],   pertaining to or caused by sexual intercourse or genital contact.

**venereal bubo** [L, *Venus,* goddess of love; Gk, *boubon,* groin],   a swollen, inflamed lymph gland or node, usually in the groin and sometimes purulent. It is associated with a sexually transmitted disease.

**venereal disease.**   See **sexually transmitted disease.**

**venereal sore.**   See **chancre.**

**venereal ulcer.**   See **chancroid.**

**venereal urethritis,**   an inflammation of the male urethra caused by sexually transmitted microorganisms. See **gonorrheal urethritis.**

**venereal wart.**   See **condyloma acuminatum, genital wart.**

**venereologist** /vənir'ē·ol'əjist/ [L, *Venus,* goddess of love;

Gk, *logos,* science],   a health professional who specializes in the study of the causes and treatments of venereal diseases.

**venereology** /-ol'əjē/,   the study of the causes and treatments of venereal diseases. **—venereologic, venereological,** *adj.,* **venereologist,** *n.*

**venerupin poisoning** /ven'ərōō'pin/,   a potentially fatal form of shellfish poisoning that results from ingestion of oysters or clams contaminated with venerupin, a toxin that causes impaired liver functioning, GI distress, and leukocytosis. The shellfish toxin occurs in waters around Japan. About one third of the cases are fatal. See also **shellfish poisoning.**

**venesection.**   See **phlebotomy.**

**Venezuelan equine encephalitis.**   See **equine encephalitis.**

**Venezuelan hemorrhagic fever,**   a hemorrhagic fever caused by an arenavirus transmitted to humans by contact with or inhalation of aerosolized excreta of infected rodents. The disease occurs in west central Venezuela, primarily in settlers moving into areas of cleared forest. Initially it is characterized by the gradual onset of fever, malaise, myalgia, and anorexia, followed by prostration, dizziness, headache, back pain, and GI disturbances. Bleeding of the gums is a typical finding, and there may be petechiae on the palate and axillae. Neurologic manifestations, such as tremor of tongue and hands, diminished deep tendon reflexes, lethargy, and hyperesthesia, often occur. Most patients begin to improve after 1 or 2 weeks, but the disease takes a more serious course in about a third; some patients develop a hemorrhagic diathesis, some develop severe neurologic deterioration marked by delirium, coma, and convulsions, and still others develop a mixed hemorrhagic-neurologic syndrome with shock. Treatment is supportive, with careful attention to fluid and electrolyte balance. If untreated, the case fatality rate may reach 30% or more; with aggressive treatment, the usual prognosis is complete recovery.

**venipuncture** /ven'əpungk'chər/ [L, *vena* + *pungere,* to prick],   the transcutaneous puncture of a vein by a sharp rigid stylet or cannula carrying a flexible plastic catheter or by a steel needle attached to a syringe or catheter. It is done to withdraw a specimen of blood, perform a phlebotomy, instill a medication, start an IV infusion, or inject a radiopaque substance for radiologic examination of a part or system of the body. Also spelled **venepuncture.**

■ METHOD: The specific steps in performing a venipuncture vary with the purpose of the procedure and the equipment to be used, but in most instances it begins as follows. The nurse dons disposable gloves. A convenient vein is selected, usually on the outside of the forearm, on the back of the hand, or in the antecubital fossa. The vein is palpated, and to dilate the vein a tourniquet is wrapped around the arm proximal to the intended site of puncture. After cleansing the intended insertion site, the examiner avoids touching the site with the gloved finger(s). The vein is immobilized by applying traction on the skin around the puncture site. The stylet or needle is held at an angle of 30 degrees for direct venipuncture. In performing direct venipuncture, the tip of the needle is pointed in the direction of the flow of blood and advanced through the skin directly into the vein. The tip is usually inserted bevel side up; however, if a large-bore needle must be used in a small vein, it is preferable to insert the needle bevel side down, because it is less likely to perforate the posterior wall of the vein. After the skin is punctured, little resistance is felt as the tip passes through the subcutaneous tissue, but a sudden slight resistance may be felt as the tip hits the wall of the vein. At this point the tip

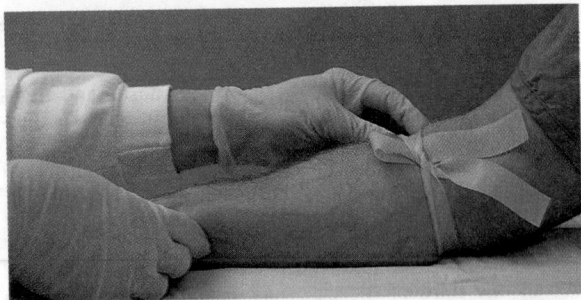

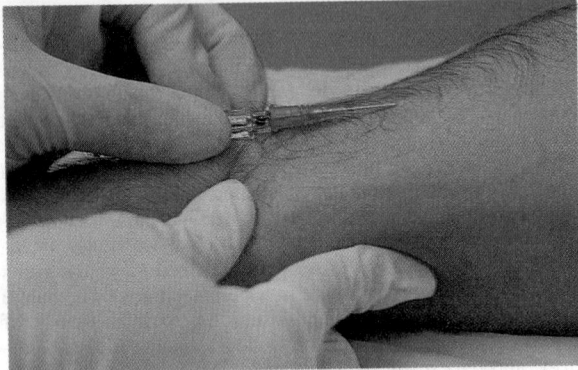

**Venipuncture** (Potter and Perry, 2001)

is cautiously advanced, with the needle or stylet held nearly flush with the skin. Slight upward pressure aids in keeping the tip in the vein as it is advanced into the lumen of the IV space. Blood flows back into the hub of the needle or into the catheter attached to the needle or covering the stylet, and the tip of the needle usually can be felt to be in the vein. If these signs are absent, the tip is not in the vein, in which case it is usually best to remove the needle or stylet, apply pressure to the puncture site, and start the procedure again, using new equipment.

■ INTERVENTIONS: Wing-tipped 'butterfly' needles, various kinds of intracatheters, and single or multiple venipuncture needles require familiarity and practice for correct insertion and stabilization. A sterile dressing and an antimicrobial ointment are applied over the insertion site. The cleansing agent used to prepare the injection site may be iodine, povidone-iodine, or ethyl alcohol. If an iodine preparation or solution is to be used, the patient is first asked about any previous allergic reaction to iodine. To aid insertion of the tip into the vein, the patient may be asked to clench the fist to further dilate the vein. The use of the gloves helps to protect the health care worker from inadvertent contact with the patient's blood.

■ OUTCOME CRITERIA: Aseptic technique is required to avoid infection. A quick, skillful insertion is nearly painless for the patient. Specific sequelae to venipuncture vary with the techniques and equipment used. See also **intravenous infusion, phlebotomy.**

**veno-,** combining form meaning 'vein': *venoclysis, venopressor, venovenostomy.*

**venoatrial** /vē′nō·ā′trē·əl/, pertaining to either vena cava and the right atrium.

**venogram.** See **phlebogram.**

**venography.** See **phlebography.**

**venom** /ven′əm/ [L, *venenum,* poison], a toxic fluid substance secreted by some snakes, arthropods, and other animals and transmitted by their stings or bites.

**venom extract therapy,** the administration of antivenin as prophylaxis against the toxic effects of the bite of a specific poisonous snake or spider or other venomous animal.

**venom immunotherapy,** the reduction of sensitivity to a specific venom by the administration of gradually increasing amounts of that venom. See also **immunotherapy.**

**venomous snake** /ven′əməs/, a snake that secretes a poison. See also **coral snake, pit viper, snakebite, snake venom.**

**venospasm** /vēn′əspaz′əm/ [L, *vena,* vein; Gk, *spasmos,* spasm], a spasmodic constriction of a vein.

**venostasis.** See **phlebostasis.**

**venothrombotic** /vē′nəthrombot′ik/, producing a venous thrombus.

**venotomy** /vēnot′əmē/, the surgical opening of a vein.

**venous** /vē′nəs/, pertaining to a vein.

**-venous,** combining form meaning 'veins': *endovenous, lymphovenous, perivenous.*

**venous access device,** a catheter designed for continuous access to the venous system. Such devices may be required for long-term parenteral feeding or the administration of IV fluids or medications for a period of several days.

**venous access devices (VAD) maintenance,** a nursing intervention from the Nursing Interventions Classification (NIC) defined as management of the patient with prolonged venous access via tunneled and nontunneled (percutaneous) catheters, and implanted ports. See also **Nursing Interventions Classification.**

**venous blood (v)** [L, *vena,* vein; AS, *blod*], dark red blood that has been deoxygenated during passage from the left ventricle through the systemic circulation, en route to the right atrium.

**venous blood gas** [L, *venosus,* full of veins; AS, *blod* + Gk, *chaos,* gas], the oxygen and carbon dioxide levels in venous blood. Venous blood gas is measured by various methods to assess the adequacy of oxygenation and ventilation and to determine the acid-base status. The oxygen tension of venous blood normally averages 40 mm Hg; the dissolved oxygen content, 0.1% by volume; the total oxygen content, 15.2%; and the oxygen saturation of venous hemoglobin, 75%. The carbon dioxide tension normally averages 46 mm Hg; the dissolved carbon dioxide content, 2.9% by volume; and the total carbon dioxide content, 50%. The normal average pH of venous plasma is 7.37. Venous blood gas in an extremity pertains chiefly to that limb. A sample from a central venous catheter is usually an incomplete mix of venous blood from various parts of the body; a sample of completely mixed venous blood may be obtained from the pulmonary artery for an accurate determination of venous blood gas.

**venous capillaries** [L, *vena,* vein, *capillaris,* hairlike], capillaries that terminate in venules.

**venous circulation** [L, *vena,* vein, *circulare,* to go around], the movement of blood from the venules, which drain deoxygenated blood from the capillaries, through the veins to the venae cavae, and from there through the right atrium and ventricle to the pulmonary circulation of the lungs.

**venous cutdown,** a small surgical incision made in a vein of a patient who has suffered vascular collapse to permit the introduction of IV fluids or drugs. A cutdown also may be performed for the insertion of a cannula for the withdrawal of blood.

**venous hemorrhage,** the escape of blood from a vein.

**venous hum,** a continuous murmur heard on auscultation over the major veins at the base of the neck and around the umbilicus. It is most audible in the neck when the patient is anemic, upright, and looking to the contralateral side. It is also heard in some healthy, young individuals.

**venous insufficiency,** an abnormal circulatory condition characterized by decreased return of venous blood from the legs to the trunk of the body. Edema is usually the first sign of the condition; pain, varicosities, and ulceration may follow. Treatment usually consists of elevation of the legs, use of elastic hose, and correction of the underlying condition.

**venous lake,** small blue-purple sessile, compressible papules or blebs seen most often on the lips, ears, and face of elderly persons, which histologically represent dilated capillaries filled with red blood cells and lined with flattened endothelial cells.

**venous ligation,** the ligation of varicose veins whose valves are ineffective, performed to remove weakened parts of tissues in which thrombi might lodge. During surgery the saphenous vein is ligated at the groin, where it joins the femoral vein. A wire device, called a stripper, is threaded through the lumen of the vein from groin to ankle. The wire and the vein are then pulled from the groin incision. Incisions may be made at several sites along the leg. Bleeding is minimal. After surgery a pressure bandage is applied from foot to thigh, and the foot of the bed is elevated 6 to 9 inches, raising the legs above heart level. The patient is encouraged to walk but discouraged from standing or sitting. Cyanosis of the toes indicates possible constriction by the dressings. Elastic bandages remain in place until the seventh day after surgery, when the sutures are usually removed. Possible complications include hemorrhage, infection, nerve damage, and thrombosis.

**venous plethysmography,** a manometric test that measures changes in the volume of an extremity. It is usually performed on a leg to exclude deep-vein thrombosis.

**venous pressure,** the blood pressure in the veins. It is elevated in congestive heart failure, acute or chronic constrictive pericarditis, and venous obstruction caused by a clot or external pressure against a vein. Indications of increased venous pressure are continued distension of veins on the back of the hand when it is raised above the sternal notch and distension of the neck veins when the individual is sitting with the head elevated 30 to 45 degrees.

**venous pulse,** the pulse of a vein usually palpated over the internal or external jugular veins in the neck. The pulse in the jugular vein is taken to evaluate the pressure of the pulse and the form of the pressure wave, especially in a person with a cardiac conduction defect or cardiac arrhythmia.

**venous return,** the return of blood to the heart via the superior and inferior venae cavae and the coronary sinus.

**venous sinus,** any one of many sinuses that collect blood from the dura mater and drain it into the internal jugular vein. Each sinus is formed by the separation of the two layers of the dura mater, the outer coat of the sinus consisting of fibrous tissue, and the inner coat consisting of endothelium continuous with that of the veins.

**venous stasis,** a disorder in which the normal flow of blood through a vein is slowed or halted.

**venous stasis dermatitis.** See **stasis dermatitis.**

**venous thrombosis.** See **phlebothrombosis.**

**ventilate** /ven′tilāt/ [L, *ventilare,* to fan], **1.** to provide with fresh air. **2.** to provide the alveoli of the lungs with air from the atmosphere and to aerate or oxygenate blood in the pulmonary capillaries. **3.** to open discussion of something, such as one's feelings. —**ventilatory,** *adj.*

**ventilation.** See **respiration,** def. 2.

**ventilation assistance,** a nursing intervention from the Nursing Interventions Classification (NIC) defined as promotion of an optimal spontaneous breathing pattern that maximizes oxygen and carbon dioxide exchange in the lungs. See also **Nursing Interventions Classification.**

**ventilation lung scan,** a radiographic examination of the lungs, performed while the patient inhales a radioactive gas as a contrast medium and the lungs are scanned to detect nonfunctional or impaired lung areas or other abnormalities.

**ventilation perfusion defect,** a disorder in which one or more areas of the lungs receive air but no blood flow or receive blood flow but no air.

**ventilation/perfusion (V/Q) ratio,** the ratio of pulmonary alveolar ventilation to pulmonary capillary perfusion, both quantities expressed in the same units.

**ventilator** /ven′tilā′tər/, any of several devices used in respiratory therapy to provide assisted respiration and intensive positive-pressure breathing. Kinds of ventilators are **pressure ventilator** and **volume ventilator.** See also **IPPB unit.**

**ventilator-associated pneumonia,** the most common type of nosocomial pneumonia, a frequently fatal type seen in patients breathing with a ventilator; it is usually caused by aspiration of contaminated secretions or stomach contents and may be bacterial, viral, or fungal.

**ventilatory compliance** /ven′tilətôr′ē/, the sum of the dynamic compliance of the lung and the compliance of the thoracic cage.

**ventilatory rate** [L, *ventilare,* to fan, *ratum,* to calculate], the volume of air passing into and out of the lungs per minute. Compare **respiration rate.**

**ventilatory standstill** [L, *ventilare,* to fan; AS, *standan + stille*], the complete cessation of breathing activity. Compare **apnea.**

**ventilatory weaning process, dysfunctional (DVWR),** a nursing diagnosis accepted by the Tenth National Conference on the Classification of Nursing Diagnoses. It is defined as a state in which an individual cannot adjust to lowered levels of mechanical ventilatory support, which interrupts and prolongs the weaning process. DVWR may be classified as mild, moderate, or severe.

■ DEFINING CHARACTERISTICS: For mild DVWR, the major defining characteristic is a response to lowered levels of mechanical ventilator support with restlessness or a respiratory rate slightly increased from baseline. The minor defining characteristic is a response to lowered levels of mechanical ventilator support with expressed feelings of increased need for oxygen, breathing discomfort, fatigue, or warmth, queries about possible machine malfunction, and increased concentration on breathing. For moderate DVWR, the major defining characteristic is a response to lowered levels of mechanical ventilator support with a slight increase from baseline blood pressure (less than 20 mm Hg), a slight increase from baseline heart rate (less than 20 beats/min), and a baseline increase in respiratory rate (less than 5 breaths per minute). Minor defining characteristics are hypervigilance to activities, inability to respond to coaching, inability to cooperate, apprehension, diaphoresis, eye widening, decreased air entry on auscultation, color changes (pale, slight cyanosis), and slight respiratory accessory muscle use. For severe DVWR, the major defining characteristic is a response to lowered levels of mechanical ventilator support with agitation, deterioration in arterial blood gas levels from current baseline, increase from baseline blood pressure of greater than 20 mm Hg, increase from baseline heart rate of greater than 20 beats/min, and significant increase in respiratory rate. Minor defining characteristics are profuse diaphoresis, full respiratory accessory muscle use, shallow gasping breaths, paradoxic abdominal breathing, discoordinated breathing with the ventilator, decreased level of consciousness, adventitious breath sounds, audible airway secretions, and cyanosis.

■ RELATED FACTORS: Related factors may be physical, psychologic, or situational. Physical factors are ineffective airway clearance, sleep pattern disturbance, inadequate nutrition, and uncontrolled pain or discomfort. Psychologic factors are knowledge deficit of the weaning process/patient role, patient-perceived inefficacy in the ability to wean, decreased motivation, decreased self-esteem, moderate or severe anxiety, fear, hopelessness, powerlessness, and insufficient trust in the nurse. Situational factors are uncontrolled episodic energy demands or problems, inappropriate pacing of diminished ventilator support, inadequate social support, an adverse environment (noisy, active, negative events in the room, low nurse-patient ratio, extended nurse absence from the bedside, unfamiliar nursing staff), a history of ventilator dependence longer than 1 week, and a history of multiple unsuccessful weaning attempts. See also **nursing diagnosis.**

**venting** [Fr, *vent*, breath], (in IV therapy) a method for allowing air to enter the vacuum of the IV bottle and displace the IV solution as it flows out. Glass IV bottles are usually equipped with a venting tube attached to the primary IV tubing or to a vent port incorporated with the bottle stopper. Venting is not required with a plastic IV bag, because the bag collapses as the fluid runs out. The air vent attached to primary IV tubing is removable to allow the injection of medication.

**Ventolin,** trademark for a bronchodilator (albuterol).

**ventral** /ven'trəl/ [L, *venter,* belly], pertaining to a position toward the anterior surface of the body; frontward. Compare **dorsal.**

**-ventral,** suffix meaning 'of the stomach or abdominal region': *biventral, dorsoventral, uteroventral.*

**ventral column.** See **anterior horn.**

**ventral corticospinal tract.** See **anterior corticospinal tract.**

**ventral hernia.** See **abdominal hernia.**

**ventral horn** [L, *venter,* belly, *cornu*], see **anterior horn.**

**ventral recumbent.** See **prone.**

**ventral root** [L, *venter,* belly; AS, *rot*], the anterior or motor division of each spinal nerve.

**ventri-.** See **ventro-.**

**ventricle** /ven'trikəl/ [L, *ventriculus,* little belly], a small cavity, such as the right and the left ventricles of the heart or one of the cavities filled with cerebrospinal fluid in the brain.

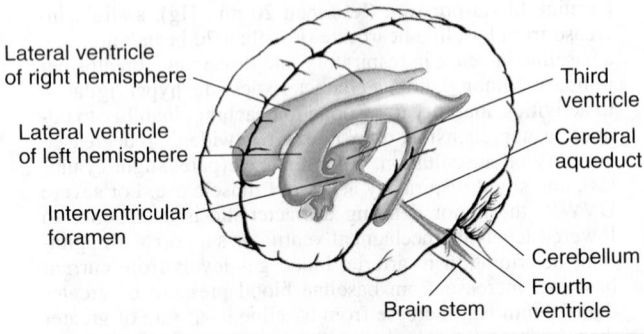

Lateral ventricle of right hemisphere

Lateral ventricle of left hemisphere

Interventricular foramen

Third ventricle

Cerebral aqueduct

Cerebellum

Brain stem

Fourth ventricle

**Ventricles of the brain** *(Applegate, 2000)*

**ventricles of the brain,** the cavities within the brain that are filled with cerebrospinal fluid, including the two lateral, the third, and (linked by the aqueduct) the fourth ventricles. They are lined by ependyma which, in certain regions, is invaginated by vascular fringes of pia mater to form the choroid plexuses.

**ventricular** /ventrik'yələr/ [L, *ventriculus,* little belly], pertaining to a ventricle.

**ventricular aberration.** See **aberrant ventricular conduction.**

**ventricular aneurysm,** a localized dilation or saccular protrusion in the wall of a ventricle, occurring most often after a myocardial infarction. Scar tissue is formed in response to the inflammatory changes of the infarction. This tissue weakens the myocardium, allowing its walls to bulge outward when the ventricle contracts. A typical sign of the lesion is a recurrent ventricular arrhythmia that does not respond to treatment with conventional antiarrhythmic drugs. Diagnostic measures are echocardiography and cardiac catheterization. Treatment may involve surgical removal of the scar tissue. Also called **cardiac aneurysm.**

**ventricular assist device (VAD),** a circulatory support device that augments function of the left ventricle, the right ventricle, or both; it consists of one or two implanted or extracorporeal pumps with afferent and efferent conduits attached so as to provide mechanically assisted pulsatile blood flow.

**ventricular bigeminy** [L, *ventriculus + bis + geminus,* twin], a cardiac arrhythmia in which every other beat consists of a premature ventricular beat.

**ventricular block** [L, *ventriculus* + OFr, *bloc*], an obstruction of the flow of cerebrospinal fluid. Causes usually are closure of the foramina of Magendie or Luschka. The condition results in a distension of the brain ventricles because of an increased accumulation of cerebrospinal fluid.

**ventricular compliance,** a property of a heart ventricle in its resting state that determines the relation between the filling of the ventricle and its diastolic pressure.

**ventricular dysfunction,** an abnormality in the contraction of the ventricles or the motion of the calls.

**ventricular ejection** [L, *ventriculus + ejicere,* to cast out], the forceful expulsion of blood from the ventricles into the aorta and the pulmonary arteries.

**ventricular escape** [L, *ventriculus* + OFr, *escaper*], the discharge of a normal ventricular pacemaker cell when the sinus or junctional rate of discharge falls below that of the ventricular pacemaker cells.

**ventricular extrasystole,** a premature beat arising from a ventricle.

**ventricular fibrillation (VF),** a cardiac arrhythmia marked by rapid depolarizations of the ventricular myocardium. The condition is characterized by a complete lack of organized electric activity, and of ventricular ejection. Blood pressure falls to zero, resulting in unconsciousness. Death may occur within 4 minutes. Cardiopulmonary resuscitation must be initiated immediately with defibrillation and resuscitative medications given according to advanced cardiac life support protocol.

**ventricular flutter,** a condition of very rapid contractions of the ventricles of the heart. Electrocardiograms show poorly defined QRS complexes occurring at a rate of 250/min or higher. Cardiac output is severely compromised or absent. The condition is fatal if untreated. Compare **ventricular fibrillation.**

**ventricular gallop.** See $S_3$.

**ventricular gradient,** the sum of the areas within the QRS complex and the T wave on the electrocardiogram.

**ventricular hypertrophy** [L, *ventriculus* + Gk, *hyper,* excessive, *trophe,* nourishment], abnormal enlargement of the heart ventricles. It is often caused by hypertension, a valvular disease, or heart failure.

**ventricular pacing.** See **pacing.**

**ventricular remodeling,** progressive myocardial ventricular dilation, eccentric ventricular hypertrophy, and distortion of left ventricular geometry that persist in the noninfarcted myocardium after a myocardial infarction has healed. It is associated with impaired functional capacity, congestive heart failure, and premature death. Angiotensin-converting enzyme inhibitors can limit the ventricular dilation.

**ventricular rhythm** [L, *ventriculus* + Gk, *rhythmos*] the recurrent beating of the ventricles, normal or abnormal.

**ventricular septal defect (VSD),** the most common congenital cardiac anomaly, charaterized by one or more abnormal openings in the septum separating the ventricles. The openings, which may range in size from 1 to 2 mm to several centimeters, permit oxygenated blood to flow from the left to the right ventricle and to recirculate through the pulmonary artery and lungs. Small defects may close spontaneously, and children with such defects are usually asymptomic. Large defects may lead to bacterial endocarditis, lower respiratory tract infections, pulmonary vascular obstructive disease, aortic regurgitation, or congestive heart failure. Children with large defects may show rapid breathing, poor weight gain, restlessness, and irritability. Diagnosis is established by electrocardiography, cardiac catheterization, and angiography. Treatment consists of surgical repair of the defect, preferably in early childhood.

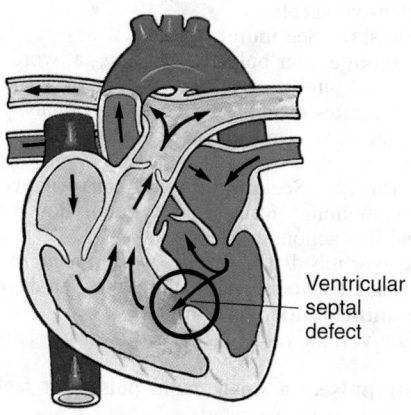

**Ventricular septal defect** *(Wong, 1999)*

**ventricular septum** See **interventricular septum.**

**ventricular standstill,** a complete cessation of electrical and mechanical activity in the ventricles of the heart.

**ventricular systole** [L, *ventriculus* + Gk, *systole,* contraction], the contraction of the heart ventricles. It begins with the first heart sound.

**ventricular tachycardia,** tachycardia of at least three consecutive ventricular complexes with a rate greater than 100/min. It usually originates in a focus distal to the branching of the atrioventricular bundle.

**ventriculo-** /ventrik′yəlō-/, combining form meaning 'ventricle of the heart or brain': *ventriculocisternostomy, ventriculopuncture, ventriculostium.*

**ventriculoatrial shunt** /ventrik′yəlō·ā′trē·əl/ [L, *ventriculus* + *atrium,* hall; ME, *shunten*], a surgically created passageway, consisting of plastic tubing and one-way valves, implanted between a cerebral ventricle and the right atrium of the heart to drain excess cerebrospinal fluid from the brain in hydrocephalus.

**ventriculoatriostomy.** See **auriculoventriculostomy.**

**ventriculocisternostomy** /-sis′tərnos′təmē/ [L, *ventriculus* + *cisterna,* vessel; Gk, *stoma,* mouth], a surgical procedure performed to treat hydrocephalus. An opening is created that allows cerebrospinal fluid to drain through a shunt from the ventricles of the brain into the cisterna magna. Also called **Torkildsen's procedure, ventriculostomy.**

**ventriculofallopian tube shunt** /-fəlō′pē·ən/, a surgical procedure with limited effectiveness for diverting cerebrospinal fluid into the peritoneal cavity. A polyethylene tube is passed from the lateral ventricle or from the spinal subarachnoid space into a ligated fallopian tube and finally into the peritoneal cavity, where the shunted cerebrospinal fluid is absorbed. This procedure is used to correct both the obstructive and the communicating types of hydrocephalus. Also called **spinofallopian tube shunt.**

**ventriculogram** /ventrik′yəlōgram′/, a radiograph of the cerebral ventricles or the ventricles of the heart.

**ventriculography** /ventrik′yəlog′rəfē/ [L, *ventriculus* + *graphein,* to record], **1.** the radiographic examination of a ventricle of the heart after injection of a radiopaque contrast medium. **2.** the radiographic examination of the head following cerebrospinal fluid removal from the cerebral ventricles and its replacement by a contrast medium, usually air.

**ventriculoperitoneal shunt** /-per′itənē′əl/ [L, *ventriculus* + Gk, *peri,* around, *teinein,* to stretch; ME, *shunten*], a surgically created passageway consisting of plastic tubing and one-way valves between a cerebral ventricle and the peritoneum for the draining of excess cerebrospinal fluid from the brain in hydrocephalus.

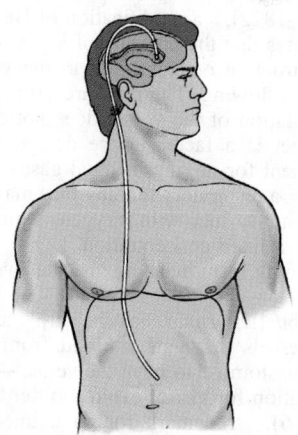

**Ventriculoperitoneal shunt** *(Monahan and Neighbors, 1998)*

**ventriculoperitoneostomy** /ventrik′yəlōper′itō′nē·os′təmē/ [L, *ventriculus* + Gk, *peri,* around, *teinein,* to stretch, *stoma,* mouth], a surgical procedure for temporarily diverting cerebrospinal fluid in hydrocephalus, usually in the newborn. In this procedure, which spares the kidney but is less efficient than a ventriculoureterostomy, a polyethylene tube is passed from the lateral ventricle subcutaneously down the dorsal spine and is reinserted into the peritoneal cavity, where the diverted fluid is absorbed. This procedure is used to correct both the communicating and the obstructive types of hydrocephalus.

**ventriculopleural shunt** /-plŏŏr′əl/ [L, *ventriculus* + Gk, *pleura*, rib; ME, *shunten*], a surgical procedure for diverting cerebrospinal fluid from engorged ventricles in hydrocephalus, usually in the newborn. In this procedure cerebrospinal fluid is diverted from the lateral ventricle into the pleural cavity. It is used to correct both the obstructive and the communicating types of hydrocephalus.

**ventriculostomy.** See **ventriculocisternostomy.**

**ventriculoureterostomy** /ventrik′yəlō′yŏŏrē′təros′təmē/ [L, *ventriculus* + Gk, *oureter*, ureter, *stoma*, mouth], a surgical procedure for directing cerebrospinal fluid into the general circulation. It is performed in the treatment of hydrocephalus, usually in the newborn. In this procedure a polyethylene tube is passed from the lateral ventricle down the dorsal spine subcutaneously to the twelfth rib; the tube is inserted through the paraspinal muscles into a ureter. Rarely used, the method is an alternative to auriculoventriculostomy, especially if the obstruction to cerebrospinal fluid includes the basilar and cerebral subarachnoid spaces, the posterior fossa, and the spinal subarachnoid spaces. The procedure is performed to correct an obstructive type of hydrocephalus.

**ventriculovenous shunt,** an artificially created communication between a cerebral ventricle and the internal jugular vein by means of a plastic tube with an in-line pressure-flow regulator, to permit drainage of cerebrospinal fluid for relief of hydrocephalus.

**ventro-, ventri-,** combining form meaning 'belly or to the front of the body': *ventrodorsal, ventrolateral, ventroptosia.*

**ventrolateral** /ven′trōlat′ərəl/, pertaining to the part of the body opposite the back and away from the midline.

**ventromedial** /ven′trōmē′dē·əl/, pertaining to the part of the body opposite the back and near the midline.

**Venturi effect** /ventŏŏ′rē/ [Giovanni B. Venturi, Italian physicist, 1746–1822], a modification of Bernoulli's principle, which states that the pressure of a gas is reduced just beyond an obstruction or restriction in the vessel through which the gas is flowing. The pressure drop can be nearly eliminated if dilation of the vessel does not exceed 15 degrees. The effect is a factor in the design of respiratory therapy equipment for mixing medical gases.

**Venturi mask,** a respiratory therapy face mask designed to allow inspired air to mix with oxygen, which is supplied through a jet at a fixed concentration.

**venul-,** combining form meaning 'venule': *venulitis, venuloma.*

**venule** /ven′yŏŏl/ [L, *venula*, small vein], any one of the small blood vessels that gather blood from the capillary plexuses and anastomose to form the veins. —**venular,** *adj.*

**VEP,** abbreviation for **visual-evoked potential.**

**VePesid (VP-16),** trademark for an antineoplastic agent (etoposide).

**verapamil** /verap′əmil/, a calcium channel blocker.
- INDICATIONS: It is prescribed for the treatment of vasospastic and exertional angina, supraventricular tachycardia, atrial fibrillation, and atrial flutter.
- CONTRAINDICATIONS: Severe left ventricular dysfunction, hypotension, cardiogenic shock, sick sinus syndrome, or second- or third-degree atrioventricular (AV) block prohibits its use.

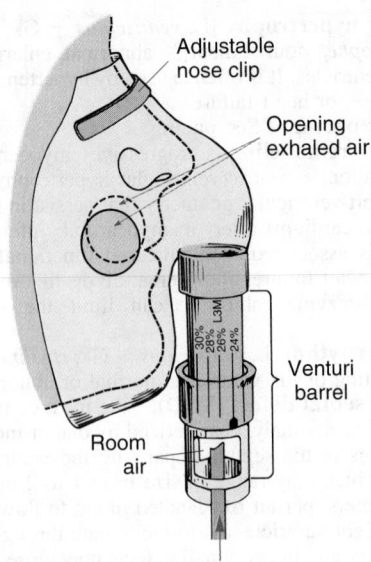

**Venturi mask** *(Potter and Perry, 2001)*

- ADVERSE EFFECTS: Among the more serious adverse reactions are hypotension, peripheral edema, AV block, bradycardia, congestive heart failure, pulmonary edema, and dizziness.

*Veratrum* /vərā′trəm/ [L, hellebore], a genus of poisonous herbs of the lily family. The dried rhizomes of the British and American hellebore provide alkaloids that are used as antihypertensive agents.

**verbal aphasia.** See **motor aphasia.**

**verbal language** /vur′bəl/ [L, *verbum*, a word, *lingua*, tongue], a culturally organized system of vocal sounds that communicates meaning between individuals.

**vergence** /vur′jəns/, movement of the two eyes in opposite directions.

**vergence ability.** See **amplitude of convergence.**

**-verine,** combining form for spasmolytics having a papaverine-like action.

**vermicide** /vur′misīd/ [L, *vermis*, worm, *caedere*, to kill], an agent that kills worms, particularly those in the intestine. Compare **anthelmintic, vermifuge.**

**vermicular** /vərmik′yələr/ [L, *vermis*, worm], resembling a worm.

**vermicular pulse,** a small, rapid pulse that feels like a writhing worm when palpated.

**vermiform** /vur′mifôrm/ [L, *vermis*, worm, *forma*, form], resembling a worm. Also **lumbrical.**

**vermiform appendix** [L, *vermis* + *forma*, form, *appendix*, appendage], a wormlike blunt process extending from the cecum. Its length varies from 7 to 15 cm, and its diameter is about 1 cm. Also called **appendix vermiformis, cecal appendix.** See also **appendicitis.**

**vermifuge** /vərmifyōōj′/ [L, *vermis* + *fugare*, to chase away], an agent that causes the evacuation of intestinal parasitic worms.

**vermilion border** /vərmil′yən/ [L, *vermillium*, bright red; OFr, *bordure*, frame], the external pinkish-to-red area of the upper and lower lips. It extends from the junction of the lips with the surrounding facial skin on the exterior to the labial mucosa within the mouth.

**vermin** /vur′min/ [L, *vermis*, worm], any parasitic insects, such as a louse or bedbug, regarded as a destructive or disease-carrying pest.

**vermis** /vur′mis/, *pl.* **vermes** [L],   **1.** a worm. **2.** a structure resembling a worm, such as the median lobe of the cerebellum. —**vermiform,** *adj.*

**vermis cerebelli** /vər′mis ser′ə·bel′ī/ [L, worm of cerebellum],   the narrow median part of the cerebellum, between the two lateral hemispheres; the cranial or superior portion extends from the lingula to the folium vermis, and the inferior or caudal portion from the tuber vermis to the nodulus. Also called **vermis of cerebellum.**

**Vermox,**   trademark for an anthelmintic (mebendazole).

**vernal conjunctivitis** /vur′nəl/ [L, *vernare,* springlike, *conjunctivus,* connecting; Gk, *itis,* inflammation],   a chronic, bilateral inflammation of the conjunctiva, thought to be allergic in origin, that occurs most frequently in men under 20 years of age during the spring and summer. The most-common symptoms include intense itching and a crusting discharge. Topical corticosteroids may be applied, and desensitization to pollen may be helpful. Compare **allergic conjunctivitis.**

**Vernet's syndrome** /vernāz′/ [Maurice Vernet, French neurologist, b. 1887],   a neurologic disorder caused by injury to the ninth, tenth, and eleventh cranial nerves as they pass through the jugular foramen when leaving the skull. Symptoms include unilateral flaccid paralysis of the palatal, pharyngeal, and intrinsic laryngeal muscles and the sternocleidomastoid and trapezius muscles. The patient also experiences dysphagia, the voice is nasal and hoarse, and there may be some loss of taste sensations. Also called **jugular foramen syndrome.**

**Verneuil's neuroma.**   See **plexiform neuroma.**

**vernix caseosa** /vur′niks kas′ē·ō′sə/ [Gk, resin; L, *caseus,* cheese],   a grayish-white cheeselike substance, consisting of sebaceous gland secretions, lanugo, and desquamated epithelial cells, that covers the skin of the fetus and newborn. It acts as a protective agent during intrauterine life and is thought to have an insulating effect against heat loss.

**verocytotoxin** /ver′ō·sī′tō·tok′sin/,   either of two toxins found in certain strains of *Shigella dysenteriae* and *Escherichia coli,* causing a type of hemolytic uremic syndrome. Humans are infected by ingesting undercooked meat, unpasteurized milk, and foods contaminated with cattle feces.

**verruca** /vərōō′kə/ [L, wart],   a benign viral warty skin lesion with a rough papillomatous surface. It is caused by a common contagious papovavirus. Methods of treatment include salicylic acid, cantharidin, electrodesiccation, currette excision, laser excision solid carbon dioxide, liquid nitrogen, and mental suggestion. Also called **verruca vulgaris, wart.** —**verrucose, verrucous,** *adj.*

**verruca acuminata.**   See **genital wart.**

**verruca plana,**   a small, slightly elevated, smooth tan or flesh-colored wart, sometimes occurring in large numbers on the face, neck, back of the hands, wrists, and knees, especially in children. Also called **flat wart.**

**verruca senilis.**   See **basal cell papilloma.**

**verruca vulgaris.**   See **verruca.**

**verrucous carcinoma** /vərōō′kəs/,   a well-differentiated squamous cell neoplasm of soft tissue of the oral cavity, larynx, or genitalia. A slow-growing tumor with displacement of surrounding tissue rather than invasion or metastasis occurs.

**verrucous dermatitis,**   any skin rash with wartlike lesions.

**verrucous endocarditis** [L, *verruca,* wart; Gk, *endon,* within, *kardia,* heart, *itis,* inflammation],   a form of heart

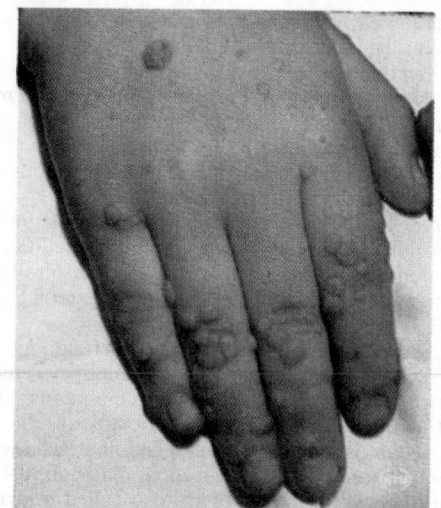

**Verruca**
*(Wilson and Giddens, 2001/courtesy American Academy of Dermatology and Institute for Dermatologic Communication and Education, Schaumburg, Illinois)*

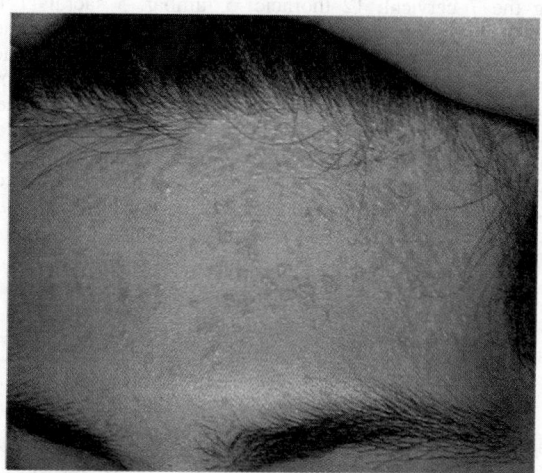

**Verruca plana** *(Habif, 1996)*

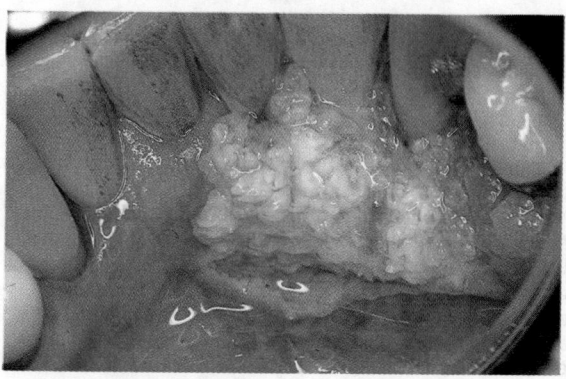

**Verrucous carcinoma** *(Regezi, Sciubba, and Pogrel, 2000)*

inflammation characterized by the development of wartlike growths on the heart valves.

**verruga peruana.**   See **bartonellosis.**

**-verse,**   **1.** suffix meaning 'to turn': *reverse, sacrotransverse, transverse.* **2.** combining form meaning 'turned, changed': *inverse, reverse.*

**Versed,**   trademark for a parenteral central nervous system depressant (midazolam hydrochloride).

**version** /vur′zhən/ [L, *vertere,* to turn],   the changing of the fetal position in the uterus, usually done to facilitate delivery. Version may occur spontaneously as a result of uterine contractions or be performed by internal or external manipulation by the physician.

**version and extraction,**   an obstetric operation in which a fetus presenting head first is turned and delivered feet first. It is performed by reaching deeply into the uterus, grasping the feet and pulling them down, and extracting the infant. The procedure is considered outmoded and hazardous and has been replaced by cesarean section, although it still may be done to deliver a second twin. Also called **internal podalic version and total breech extraction.** Compare **external version.** See also **breech birth.**

**-vert,**   combining form meaning a 'person who has turned (metaphorically)' in a specified direction: *extrovert, introvert, invert.*

**vertebra** /vur′təbrə/ *pl.* **vertebrae** [L, joint],   any one of the 33 bones (26 in the adult) of the spinal column, comprising the 7 cervical, 12 thoracic, 5 lumbar, 5 sacral (1 in adult), and 4 coccygeal vertebrae (1 in adult). The vertebrae, with the exception of the first and second cervical vertebrae, are much alike and are composed of a body, an arch, a spinous process for muscle attachment, and pairs of pedicles and processes. The first cervical vertebra is called the atlas and has no vertebral body. The second cervical vertebra is called the axis and forms the pivot on which the atlas rotates, permitting the head to turn. The body of the axis also extends into a strong, bony process (the dens).

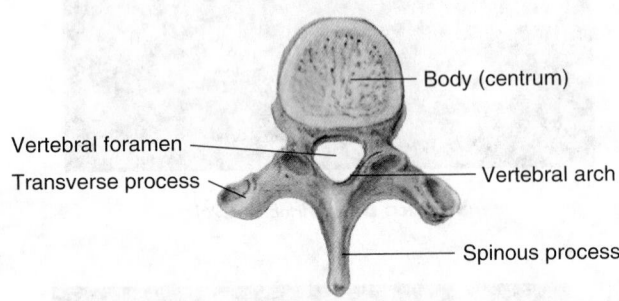

**General features of a vertebra** *(Applegate, 2000)*

**vertebral** /vur′təbrəl/ [L, *vertebra,* joint],   pertaining to one or more vertebrae.

**-vertebral,**   combining form meaning "spinal column": *paravertebral, pelvivertebral, subvertebral.*

**vertebral angiography** [L, *vertebra* + Gk, *angeion* + *graphein,* to record],   the radiographic examination of blood circulation in the spinal area after the injection of radiopaque contrast medium. See **angiography.**

**vertebral arch** [L, *vertebra,* joint, *arcus,* bow],   the arch formed on the back of the vertebral body by the pedicles and laminae.

**vertebral artery,**   one of a pair of arteries branching from the subclavian arteries, arising deep in the neck from the cranial and dorsal subclavian surfaces. Each vertebral artery divides into two cervical and five cranial branches, supplying deep neck muscles, the spinal cord and spinal membranes, and the cerebellum.

**vertebral-basilar system,**   an arterial complex in which two vertebral arteries join at the base of the skull to form the basilar artery.

**vertebral body,**   the weight-supporting, solid central part of a vertebra. The pedicles of the arch project from its dorsolateral surfaces.

**vertebral canal** [L, *vertebra,* joint, *canalis*],   the passage formed anterior to the vertebral arches and posterior to the vertebral bodies and occupied by the spinal cord. The vertebral canal courses within the vertebral column and contains the spinal cord. The canal is formed by the posterior arches of the vertebrae and is large and triangular in the cervical and lumbar sections of the column, the most flexible parts. The canal is small and rounded in the thoracic region, where motion is more restricted.

**vertebral column,**   the flexible structure that forms the longitudinal axis of the skeleton. In the adult it includes 26 vertebrae arranged in a straight line from the base of the skull to the coccyx. The vertebrae are separated by intervertebral disks. They provide attachment for various muscles such as the iliocostalis thoracis and the longissimus thoracis that give the column strength and flexibility. In the adult the five sacral and four coccygeal vertebrae fuse to form the sacrum and the coccyx. The average length of the vertebral column in men is about 71 cm. The cervical part measures about 12.5 cm, the thoracic part about 28 cm, the lumbar part about 18 cm, and the sacrum and the coccyx about 12.5 cm. The vertebral column in women measures approximately 61 cm. Several curves in the column increase its strength, such as the cervical, thoracic, lumbar, and pelvic curves. The cervical curve is convex ventrally from the apex of the dens to the middle of the second thoracic vertebra and is the least marked of all the curves. The thoracic curve, concave ventrally, starts at the middle of the second and ends at the middle of the twelfth thoracic vertebra. The lumbar curve, more pronounced in women than in men, begins at the middle of the last thoracic vertebra and ends at the sacrovertebral angle. The pelvic curve starts at the sacrovertebral articulation and ends at the point of the coccyx. The thoracic and the sacral curves constitute primary curves, present during fetal life; the cervical and lumbar curves constitute secondary curves, which develop after birth. Also called **spinal column, spine.** See also **vertebra, vertebral canal.**

**vertebral foramen** [L, *vertebra,* joint, *foramen,* a hole],   the opening between the neural arch and the body of a vertebra through which the spinal cord passes.

**vertebral groove** [L, *vertebra,* joint; D, *groeve*],   a shallow depression on each side of the spinous processes of the vertebrae, occupied by the deep back muscles.

**vertebral notch** [L, *vertebra,* joint; OFr, *enochier,* notch],   either of the concavities on the lower or upper border of a vertebral pedicle.

**vertebral rib,**   one of two lower ribs on either side that are not attached anteriorly. Also called **floating rib.** See also **rib.**

**vertebral-venous system,**   a group of four interconnected venous networks surrounding the vertebral column.

**vertebrate** [L, *vertebra,* joint],   any animal that possesses a backbone and thus is a member of the subphylum Vertebrata of the phylum Chordata. Vertebrates include fish, amphibians, birds, reptiles, and mammals.

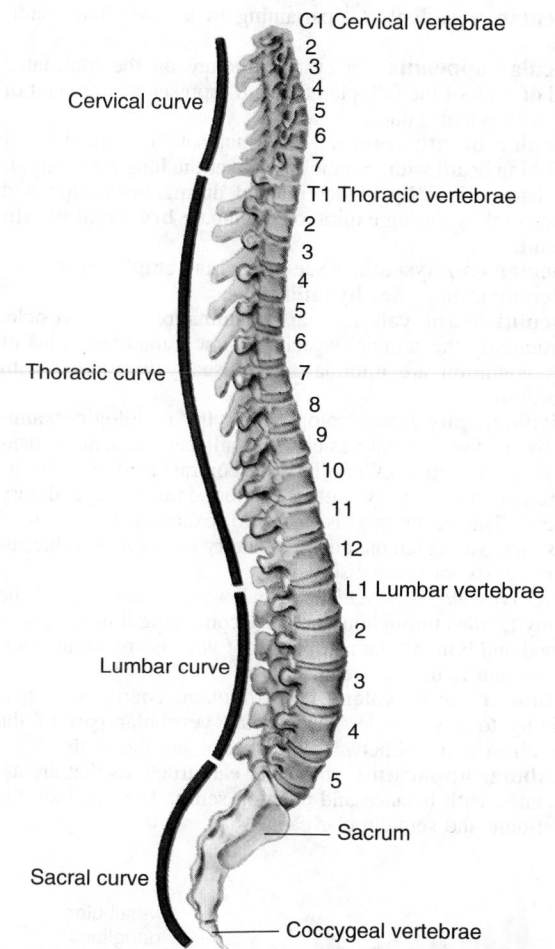

C1 Cervical vertebrae
2
3
4
5
6
7
T1 Thoracic vertebrae
2
3
4
5
6
7
8
9
10
11
12
L1 Lumbar vertebrae
2
3
4
5
Sacrum
Coccygeal vertebrae

Cervical curve

Thoracic curve

Lumbar curve

Sacral curve

**Vertebral column: right lateral view** *(Applegate, 2000)*

**vertebro-,** combining form meaning 'vertebral column or vertebra': *vertebrocostal, vertebrodymus, vertebrosternal.*

**vertebrochondral** /vur′təbrōkon′drəl/, pertaining to a vertebra and a costal cartilage.

**vertebrocostal** /-kos′təl/, pertaining to a vertebra and a rib, or a vertebra and a costal cartilage.

**vertebrocostal rib,** one of the eighth, ninth, and tenth ribs on either side that articulate posteriorly with the vertebrae and have their costal cartilages connected anteriorly by capsular ligaments. Also called **false rib.** See also **rib.**

**vertebrosternal rib** /-stur′nəl/, one of the seven upper ribs on either side that have cartilage articulating directly with the sternum. Also called **true rib.** See also **rib.**

**vertex** /vur′teks/ [L, summit], **1.** the top of the head; crown. **2.** the apex or highest point of any structure.

**vertex presentation,** (in obstetrics) a fetal presentation in which the vertex of the fetus is the part nearest to the cervical os and can be expected to be born first. Compare **breech presentation.**

**vertical** /vur′tikəl/ [L, *vertex,* summit], perpendicular or at a right angle to the plane of the horizon.

**vertical angulation** [L, *vertex + angulus,* corner], the angle within the vertical plane, relative to a reference in the horizontal or occlusal plane, at which the central x-ray beam is directed during radiography of oral structures.

**vertical coordination,** a system of community health nurses who serve as links between their level in the organization and those above and below their level. They also serve as links between the agency and the patient.

**vertical diplopia** [L, *vertex* + Gk, *diploos,* double, *opsis,* vision], a form of double vision in which one image is displaced vertically above the other.

**vertically-integrated health care,** a health delivery system in which the complete spectrum of care, including financial services, is provided within a single organization, such as a health maintenance organization.

**vertical nystagmus,** a visual abnormality in which the eyes involuntarily move up and down.

**vertical plane.** See **cardinal frontal plane.**

**vertical resorption,** a pattern of bone loss in which the alveolar bone adjacent to an affected tooth is destroyed without simultaneous crestal loss. See also **resorption.**

**vertical squint.** See **vertical strabismus.**

**vertical strabismus** [L, *vertex* + Gk, *strabismos,* squint], a deviation of one eye in a vertical direction from a point of fixation. A common cause is overaction by the inferior oblique muscles, resulting in a quick vertical movement of the eyeball on adduction. Also called **upward-and-downward squint, vertical squint.**

**vertical transmission,** the transfer of a disease, condition, or trait from one generation to the next, either genetically or congenitally, such as the spread of an infection through breast milk or through the placenta.

**vertical vertigo,** a sense of instability caused by looking up or down.

**verticosubmental** /vur′tikō′submen′təl/ [L, *vertex* + *sub,* below, *mentum,* chin], pertaining to a radiographic projection of the head in which the central ray passes from the vertex of the skull through its base.

**vertigo** /vur′tigō, vurtī′gō/, a sensation of instability, giddiness, loss of equilibrium, or rotation, caused by a disturbance in the semicircular canal of the inner ear or the vestibular nuclei of the brainstem. The sensation that one's body is rotating in space is called subjective vertigo, whereas the sensation that objects are spinning around the body is termed objective vertigo. See also **dizziness, postural vertigo, vestibular neuronitis.**

**very-low-density lipoprotein (VLDL),** a plasma lipoprotein that is composed chiefly of triglycerides with small amounts of cholesterol, phospholipid, fat-soluble vitamins, and protein. It transports triglycerides primarily from the liver to peripheral sites in the tissues for use or storage. The triglycerides are quickly converted to smaller, more soluble intermediate lipoproteins and eventually to low-density lipoproteins (LDLs). Elevations in VLDL are associated with increased risk of atherosclerosis. See also **high-density lipoprotein (HDL), low-density lipoprotein (LDL).**

**vesical** /ves′ikəl/ [L, *vesica,* bladder], pertaining to a fluid-filled sac, usually the urinary bladder.

**vesical fistula** [L, *vesica,* bladder, *fistula,* pipe], an abnormal passage communicating with the urinary bladder. Vesical fistulae may communicate with the skin, vagina, uterus, or rectum.

**vesical hematuria** [L, *vesica,* bladder; Gk, *haima,* blood + *ouron,* urine], the presence of blood in the urine caused by bleeding in the bladder. The urine is bright red.

**vesical reflex,** the sensation of a need to urinate when the bladder is moderately distended. See also **micturition reflex.**

**vesical sphincter,** a circular muscle surrounding the opening of the urinary bladder. It is normally contracted to prevent leakage from the bladder.

**vesicant** /ves′ikənt/, a drug capable of causing tissue necrosis when extravasated.

**vesicle** /ves′ikəl/ [L, *vesicula*], a small bladder or blister, such as a small, thin-walled raised skin lesion containing clear fluid. Compare **bulla. —vesicular,** *adj.*

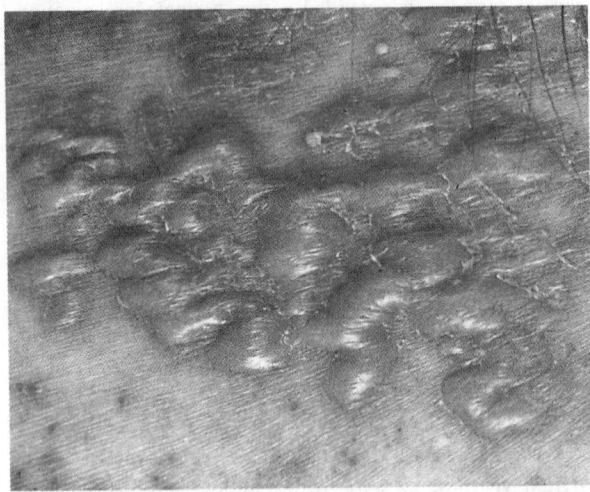

**Vesicles** (du Vivier, 1993)

**vesicle calculus,** a calculus found in the urinary bladder. Also called **bladder stone, cystolith.**

**vesicle lithotomy.** See **cystolithotomy.**

**vesico-,** combining form meaning 'bladder or blister': *vesicocavernous, vesicosigmoid, vesicourethral.*

**vesicoabdominal** /ves′ikō-abdom′inəl/, pertaining to the urinary bladder and abdominal wall.

**vesicocele.** See **cystocele.**

**vesicoureteral reflux** /ves′ikōyŏŏrē′tərəl/ [L, *vesica* + Gk, *oureter,* ureter; L, *refluxus,* backflow], an abnormal backflow of urine from the bladder to the ureter, resulting from a congenital defect, obstruction of the outlet of the bladder, or infection of the lower urinary tract. Reflux increases the hydrostatic pressure in the ureters and kidneys and may cause permanent damage. The condition is characterized by abdominal or flank pain, enuresis, pyuria, hematuria, proteinuria, and bacteriuria accompanied by persistent or recurrent urinary tract infections. Diagnosis is made by cystoscopy and voiding cystourethrography. Obstruction of the ureter or defective implantation of the ureter in the bladder may be surgically corrected. Antibacterial medication, urinary tract antiseptics, and analgesia are usually prescribed for any infection that causes or results from this condition.

**vesicouterine** /ves′ikōyŏŏ′tərin, -ēn/ [L, *vesica* + *uterus,* womb], pertaining to the bladder and uterus. Also called **uterovesical.**

**vesicovaginal** /ves′ikōvaj′inəl/, pertaining to the urinary bladder and vagina.

**vesicovaginal fistula,** a fistula between the bladder and the vagina.

**vesicula** /vəsik′yələ/ [L], a vesicle or small bladder.

**vesicular** /vesik′yələr/, pertaining to a blisterlike condition.

**vesicular appendix,** a cystic structure on the fimbriated end of each of the fallopian tubes. It represents a remnant of the mesonephric ducts.

**vesicular breath sound,** a normal sound of rustling or swishing heard with a stethoscope over the lung periphery. It is characteristically higher pitched during inspiration and fades rapidly during expiration. Compare **bronchial breath sound.**

**vesicular emphysema.** See **panacinar emphysema.**

**vesicular mole.** See **hydatid mole.**

**vesiculitis** /vəsik′yəlī′tis/, an inflammation of any vesicle, particularly the seminal vesicles. Clinical manifestations of this condition are minimal; it is usually associated with prostatitis.

**vesiculography** /vəsik′yəlog′rəfē/, the radiologic examination of the seminal vesicles and adjacent structures, usually after injection of a radiopaque contrast medium into the deferent ducts or, by catheterization, into the ejaculatory ducts. The technique is used to examine the seminal vesicles, vas deferens, and ejaculatory duct for possible tumors, cysts, or other disorders.

**vessel** /ves′əl/ [L, *vascellum,* small vase], any one of the many tubules throughout the body conveying fluids, such as blood and lymph. The main kinds of vessels are the arteries, veins, and lymphatic vessels.

**vestibular** /vestib′yələr/ [L, *vestibulum,* courtyard], pertaining to a vestibule, such as the vestibular part of the mouth, which lies between the cheeks and the teeth.

**vestibular apparatus,** the inner ear structures that are associated with balance and position sense. They include the vestibule and semicircular canals.

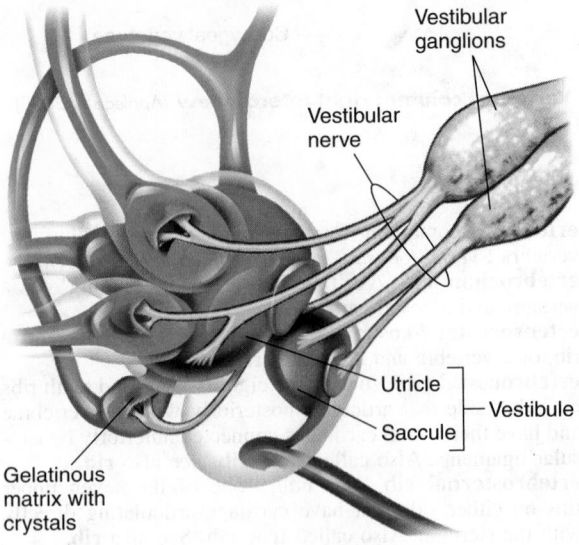

**Vestibular apparatus**

**vestibular extension.** See **vestibuloplasty.**

**vestibular function,** the sense of balance.

**vestibular gland,** any one of four small glands, two on each side of the vaginal orifice. One pair of the small structures constitutes the greater vestibular glands; the other pair constitutes the lesser vestibular glands. The vestibular glands secrete a lubricating substance. Compare **Cowper's gland.** See also **Bartholin's gland.**

**vestibular nerve** [L, *vestibulum,* courtyard, *nervus*], a branch of the eighth cranial nerve associated with the sense of equilibrium. It arises in the vestibular ganglion (Scarpa's ganglion) of the ear.

**vestibular neuronitis,** a sudden, severe attack of vertigo without symptoms of deafness or tinnitus. It usually affects young or middle-aged adults, is temporary, and follows an upper respiratory infection.

**vestibular surface,** the surface of a tooth that is directed outward toward the vestibule of the mouth, including the buccal and labial surfaces, and opposite the lingual (or oral) surface.

**vestibular toxicity,** toxic effects (commonly of drugs) on the vestibule of the ear, resulting in dizziness, vertigo, and loss of balance.

**vestibular window.** See **oval window.**

**vestibule** /ves′tibyo͞ol/ [L, *vestibulum,* courtyard], a space or a cavity that serves as the entrance to a passageway, such as the vestibule of the vagina or the vestibule of the ear.

**vestibule of the ear,** the central part of the inner ear, within the osseous labyrinth, involved with the sensation of position and movement.

**vestibule of the mouth,** the portion of the oral cavity bounded on one side by the teeth and gingivae, or the residual alveolar ridges, and on the other side by the lips (labial vestibule) and cheeks (buccal vestibule).

**vestibulocochlear nerve,** either of a pair of cranial nerves composed of fibers from the cochlear nerve and the vestibular nerve in the inner ear, conveying impulses of both the sense of hearing and the sense of balance. Also called **acoustic nerve, eighth cranial nerve.**

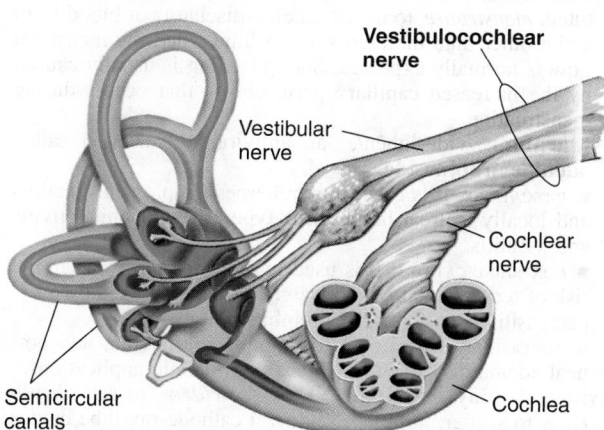

**Vestibular nerve** — labels:
**Vestibulocochlear nerve**
Vestibular nerve
Cochlear nerve
Semicircular canals
Cochlea

**Vestibulocochlear nerve**

**vestibuloocular reflex** /vestib′yəlō-ok′yələr/, a normal reflex in which eye position compensates for movement of the head. It is induced by excitation of the vestibular apparatus.

**vestibuloplasty** /vestib′yəlōplas′tē/ [L, *vestibulum,* courtyard; Gk, *plassein,* to shape], plastic surgery of the oral vestibule, particularly modification of the gingival tissues. Also called **sulcoplasty, vestibular extension.**

**vestige** /ves′tij/ [L, *vestigium,* trace], an imperfectly developed, relatively useless organ or other structure of the body

that had a vital function at an earlier stage of life or in a more primitive form of life. The vermiform appendix is a vestigial organ. **—vestigial,** *adj.*

**veterinarian** /vet′əriner′ē-ən/ [L, *veterinarius,* beast of burden], a health professional who specializes in the causes and treatment of diseases and disorders of domestic and wild animals.

**veterinary medicine** /vet′əriner′ē/, the field of medicine concerned with the health and diseases of animals other than humans.

**VF,** **1.** abbreviation for **ventricular fibrillation. 2.** abbreviation for **visual field. 3.** abbreviation for **vocal fremitus.**

**VH,** abbreviation for **viral hepatitis.**

**VI,** abbreviation for *variable interval.* See **variable interval (VI) reinforcement.**

**via** /vī′ə, vē′ä/ [L, a way], any passage or course, such as the esophagus or trachea.

**viability** /vī′əbil′itē/ [L, *vita,* life], the ability to continue living.

**viable** /vī′əbəl/ [Fr, likely to live], capable of developing, growing, and otherwise sustaining life, such as a normal human fetus at 24 weeks of gestation. **—viability,** *n.*

**viable infant,** an infant who at birth weighs at least 500 g or is 24 weeks or more of gestational age.

**vial** /vī′əl/, a glass container with a metal-enclosed rubber seal.

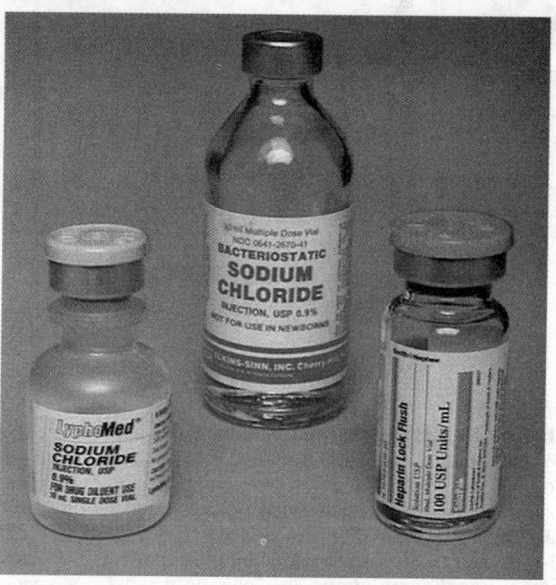

**Vials** *(Potter and Perry, 2001)*

**Vibramycin,** trademark for a tetracycline antibiotic (doxycycline hyclate).

**Vibramycin Monohydrate,** trademark for a tetracycline antibiotic (doxycycline monohydrate).

**vibrating.** See **cupping and vibrating.**

**vibration** /vībrā′shən/ [L, *vibrare,* to vibrate], a type of massage administered by quickly tapping with the fingertips or alternating the fingers in a rhythmic manner or by a mechanical device. See also **massage.**

**vibratory** /vī′brətôr′ē/ [L, *vibrare,* to vibrate], causing vibrations or a state of vibration.

**vibratory massage,** the manipulation of body surfaces with an instrument that produces a rapid tapping sensation. Also called **vibrotherapeutics.**

**vibratory sense** [L, *vibrare,* to vibrate, *sentire,* to feel], the ability to perceive vibratory sensations. Vibration receptors in the body are found in a variety of locations, from the skin surface to the membranes covering bones. Some respond only to certain vibration frequencies.

**vibrio** /vib′rē-ō/ [L, *vibrare*], any bacterium that is curved and motile, such as those belonging to the genus *Vibrio.* Cholera and several other epidemic forms of gastroenteritis are caused by members of the genus.

***Vibrio cholerae,*** the species of comma-shaped, motile bacillus that is the cause of cholera.

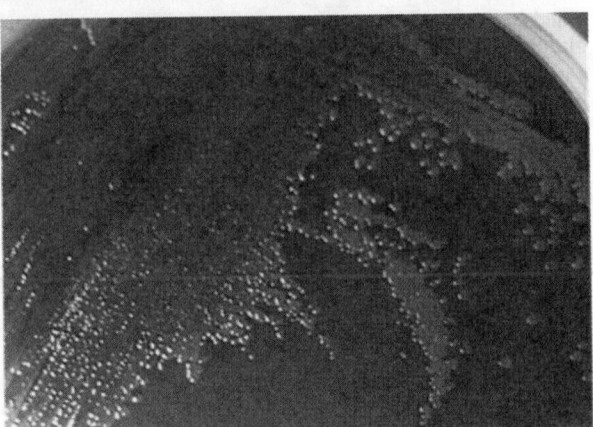

**Vibrio parahaemolyticus colonies on TCBS agar**
*(Baron, Peterson, and Finegold, 1994)*

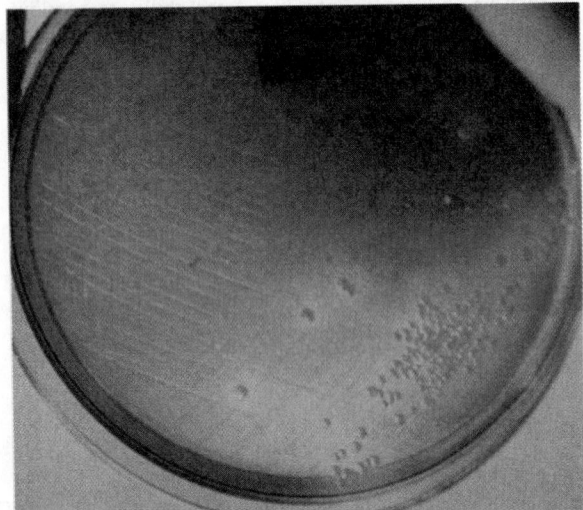

**Vibrio cholerae colonies on TCBS agar**
*(Baron, Peterson, and Finegold, 1994)*

***Vibrio fetus.*** See ***Campylobacter.***

**vibrio gastroenteritis,** an infectious disease caused by *Vibrio parahaemolyticus* acquired from contaminated seafood. It is characterized by nausea, vomiting, abdominal pain, and diarrhea. Headache, mild fever, and bloody stools also may be present. Spontaneous recovery usually occurs in 2 to 5 days. Compare **salmonellosis, shigellosis.**

***Vibrio parahaemolyticus*** /per′əhē′mōlit′ikəs/, a species of microorganisms of the genus *Vibrio,* the causative agent in food poisoning associated with the ingestion of raw or undercooked shellfish, especially crabs and shrimp. This microorganism is a common cause of gastroenteritis in Japan, aboard cruise ships, and in the eastern and southeastern coastal areas of the United States. Thorough cooking of seafood prevents the infection associated with *Vibrio parahaemolyticus,* which causes watery diarrhea, abdominal cramps, vomiting, headache, chills, and fever. This microorganism has an incubation period of 2 to 48 hours, after which the symptoms of infection appear. The food poisoning from this agent usually subsides spontaneously within 2 days but may be more severe, even fatal, in debilitated and elderly people. Confirming diagnosis must rule out other causes of food poisoning and acute GI disorders and requires bacteriologic

examination of the vomitus, stool, and blood. Treatment usually includes bed rest and the oral replacement of fluids. IV replacement of fluids is seldom required.

***Vibrio vulnificus,*** a halophilic (salt-tolerant) species whose strains are similar to *V. parahaemolyticus* but differ in that they can ferment lactose. Infection by eating raw seafood causes septicemia and cellulitis, and may be especially severe or even fatal in those with preexisting hepatic disease. Wound infection may occur following exposure to sea water or from injury when handling crabs.

**vibrotherapeutics.** See **vibratory massage.**

**vicarious menstruation** /vīker′ē·əs/ [L, *vicarius,* substituted, *menstruare,* to menstruate], discharge of blood from a site other than the uterus at the time when the menstrual flow is normally expected. Such bleeding is usually caused by the increased capillary permeability that occurs during menstruation.

**vidarabine** /vider′əbēn/, an antiviral agent. Also called **adenine arabinoside.**

■ INDICATIONS: It is used to treat herpes simplex encephalitis and locally to treat herpesvirus type 1 keratoconjunctivitis and keratitis.

■ CONTRAINDICATIONS: It is used in pregnancy only when the risk of teratogenicity is outweighed by benefits. Known hypersensitivity to this drug prohibits its use.

■ ADVERSE EFFECTS: Local irritation, photophobia, and corneal edema may occur in topical ophthalmic applications.

**video display terminal (VDT)** [L, *videre,* to see, *displicare,* to scatter, *terminus,* end], a cathode-ray tube device with a surface similar to a television screen, used in word processors, computer terminals, and similar equipment. Use of video display terminals has been associated with a variety of environmental health complaints, including burning and itching eyes, headaches, and back and arm pain. Published studies indicate the health effects are caused by inadequate or improper office environments, such as unsuitable furniture or light levels, rather than VDT radiation.

**Videx,** trademark for an antiretroviral acquired immunodeficiency syndrome drug (dideoxyinosine or ddI).

**vigilambulism** /vij′ilam′byəliz′əm/, a condition in which walking or other motor acts are performed in an unconscious but waking state.

**vigilance** /vij′iləns/ [L, *vigil,* awake], a state of being attentive or alert.

**vigil coma** /vij′əl/ [L, *vigil* + Gk, *koma,* deep sleep], a semiconscious state of delirium in which the patient may appear awake, with eyes open and staring, and may make verbal sounds.

**villi.** See **villus.**

**villoma** /vilō′mə/, *pl.* **villomas, villomata** [L, *villus,* hair; Gk, *oma,* tumor], a villous neoplasm or papilloma, occurring in the bladder or rectum. Also called **villioma.**

**villous adenoma** /vil′əs/ [L, *villus,* hair], a slow-growing, soft, spongy, potentially malignant papillary growth of the mucosa of the large intestine.

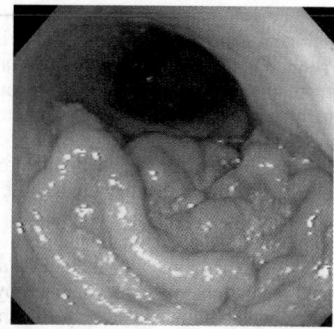

**Villous adenoma: endoscopic view** *(Wilcox, 1995)*

**villous carcinoma,** an epithelial tumor with many long velvety papillary outgrowths. Also called **carcinoma villosum.**

**villous papilloma,** a benign tumor with long, slender processes, usually occurring in the bladder, breast, or a cerebral ventricle.

**villus** /vil′əs/, *pl.* **villi** [L, shaggy, hair], one of the many tiny projections, barely visible to the naked eye, clustered over the entire mucous surface of the small intestine. The villi are covered with epithelium that diffuses and transports fluids and nutrients. They are larger in some parts of the intestine than in others and flatten out when the intestine distends. Each villus has a core of delicate areolar and reticular connective tissue supporting the epithelium, various capillaries, and often a single lymphatic lacteal that fills with

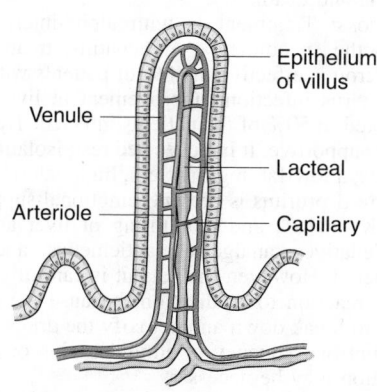

**Villus** *(Phipps, Sands, and Marek, 1999)*

milky white chyle during the digestion of a fatty meal. —**villous,** *adj.*

**vin-, -vin,** combining form for antiviral substances.

**vinblastine sulfate** /vinblas′tēn, -tin/, an antimitotic antineoplastic.

■ INDICATIONS: It is prescribed in the treatment of many neoplastic diseases such as choriocarcinoma, testicular carcinoma, Hodgkin's disease, and non-Hodgkin's lymphoma.

■ CONTRAINDICATIONS: Leukopenia, bacterial infection, or known hypersensitivity to this drug prohibits its use. It is not prescribed in pregnancy.

■ ADVERSE EFFECTS: Among the most serious adverse reactions are leukopenia and neurotoxicity. Nausea, diarrhea, stomatitis, and alopecia also may occur.

**Vincent's angina, Vincent's infection.** See **acute necrotizing ulcerative gingivitis.**

**Vincent's stomatitis** [Henri Vincent, French physician, 1862–1950; Gk, *stoma,* mouth, *itis,* inflammation], an infection of the mouth. See **acute necrotizing ulcerative gingivitis.**

**vincristine sulfate** /vinkris′tēn, -tin/, an antimitotic antineoplastic.

■ INDICATIONS: It is prescribed in the treatment of many neoplastic diseases such as leukemia, neuroblastoma, lymphomas, and sarcomas.

■ CONTRAINDICATIONS: Pregnancy, leukopenia, preexisting neuromuscular disease, or known hypersensitivity to this drug prohibits its use.

■ ADVERSE EFFECTS: Among the most serious adverse reactions are neurotoxicity and leukopenia. Constipation, abdominal pain, alopecia, and inflammation at the site of injection also may occur.

**vindesine sulfate** /vin′dəsēn/, an investigational antineoplastic.

■ INDICATIONS: It is prescribed in the treatment of acute lymphoblastic leukemia, breast cancer, malignant melanoma, lymphosarcoma, and non-small-cell lung carcinoma.

■ CONTRAINDICATIONS: Leukopenia, bacterial infections, or known sensitivity to this drug prohibits its use.

■ ADVERSE EFFECTS: Among the most serious adverse reactions are neurotoxicity, leukopenia, thrombocytopenia, phlebitis, and alopecia.

**Vineberg's operation** /vīn′bərgs/ [Arthur M. Vineberg, Canadian thoracic surgeon, 1903–1988], a technique in which the internal mammary artery is implanted into the myocardium to improve blood flow to the heart. Common in the 1950s, the procedure has been replaced by others, such as saphenous vein grafting.

**vinegar acid.** See **acetic acid.**

**vinorelbine,** a chemotherapeutic mitotic inhibitor that prevents cancer cells from dividing.

■ INDICATIONS: It is prescribed in the treatment of unresectable, advanced non–small cell lung cancer.

■ CONTRAINDICATIONS: The drug should not be given to patients with low granulocytic blood counts or persons with allergy or sensitivity to vinorelbine. Caution is advised in administering the drug to patients with compromised bone marrow; bronchospasm; infections; or kidney, liver, or lung disease.

■ ADVERSE EFFECTS: The side effects most often reported include anemia or other blood disorders, abnormal skin sensations, skin discoloration, chest pain, or phlebitis.

**vinorelbine tartrate,** an anticancer mitotic inhibitor.

■ INDICATIONS: It is prescribed in the treatment of non-small cell lung cancer.

■ CONTRAINDICATIONS: The drug should not be given to patients with low blood counts or those who may have an allergy or sensitivity to vinorelbine. It should be used with caution in patients with comprised bone marrow, bronchospasm, or kidney, liver, or lung disease.

■ ADVERSE EFFECTS: The side effects most often reported include granulocytopenia, leukopenia, or anemia.

**Vioform,**   trademark for an antiamebic and topical antiinfective (iodochlorhydroxyquin).

**Viokase,**   trademark for an enzyme (pancreatin).

**violence, other-directed, risk for,**   a nursing diagnosis accepted by the Fourth National Conference on the Classification of Nursing Diagnoses (revised 1996). It is defined as behaviors in which an individual demonstrates that he or she can be physically, emotionally, and/or sexually harmful to others.

■ RISK FACTORS: Presence of risk factors such as history of violence: (1) against others (hitting, kicking, spitting at someone, scratching, throwing objects at someone, biting, attempted rape, rape, sexual molestation, urinating/defecating on a person; (2) threats (verbal threats against property and/or against person, social threats, cursing, threatening notes/letters, threatening gestures, sexual threats); (3) against self (suicidal threats or attempts, hitting or injuring self, banging head against wall); (4) social (stealing, insistent borrowing, insistent demands for privileges, insistent interruptions of meetings, refusal to eat and/or to take medication, ignoring instructions); (5) indirect (tearing off clothes, ripping objects off walls, urinating and/or defecating on floor, stamping feet, temper tantrum, running in corridors, yelling, throwing objects, breaking a window, slamming doors, sexual advances). Many other factors may be present, including neurologic impairment (positive electroencephalogram, computed tomographic scan, or magnetic resonance imaging, head trauma, positive neurologic findings, seizure disorders); cognitive impairment (learning disabilities, attention deficit disorder, decreased intellectual functioning); history of childhood abuse; history of witnessing family violence; cruelty to animals; fire-setting; prenatal and perinatal complications/abnormalities; history of drug/alcohol abuse; and pathologic intoxication.

■ RELATED FACTORS: The related factors are antisocial character; battered women; catatonic excitement; child abuse; manic excitement; organic brain syndrome; panic states; rage reactions; suicidal behavior; temporal lobe epilepsy; and toxic reactions to medication. See also **nursing diagnosis.**

**violence, self-directed, risk for,**   a nursing diagnosis accepted by the Eleventh National Conference on the Classification of Nursing Diagnoses. It is defined as behaviors in which an individual demonstrates that he or she can be physically, emotionally, and/or sexually harmful to himself or herself.

■ RISK FACTORS: Risk factors may include age (15 to 19 or over 45); marital status (single, widowed, or divorced); employment (unemployed, recent job loss or failure); occupation (executive, administrative owner of business, professional, semiskilled worker); interpersonal relationships (conflictual); family background (chaotic or conflictual, history of suicide); sexual orientation (active bisexual, inactive homosexual); physical health (hypochondriac, chronic or terminal illness); mental health (severe depression, psychosis, severe personality disorder, alcoholism or drug abuse); emotional status (hopelessness, despair, increased anxiety, panic, anger, hostility, history of multiple attempts); suicidal ideation (frequent, intense prolonged); suicidal plan (clear and specific); lethality (methods and availability of destructive means); personal resources (poor achievement, poor insight, affect unavailable and poorly controlled); social re-

sources (poor rapport, socially isolated, unresponsive family); verbal clues (writing forlorn love notes, directing angry messages at a significant other who has rejected the person, giving away personal items, taking out a large life insurance policy); and persons who engage in autoerotic sexual acts.

**viosterol** /vī·os′tərôl/,   synthetic vitamin D$_2$ in an oil base. Also called **synthetic oleovitamin D.** See also **calciferol, ergosterol.**

**VIP,   1.** abbreviation for **vasoactive intestinal polypeptide. 2.** abbreviation for *very important person.* A VIP suite in a hospital is one reserved for such people.

**vipoma** /vipō′mə/,   a type of pancreatic tumor that causes changes in secretion of vasoactive intestinal polypeptide (VIP). VIP causes dilation of blood vessels throughout the body and secretion of fluid and salt in the intestinal tract, resulting in diarrhea. The VIP effects mimic the symptoms of cholera and can result in death from dehydration and subsequent kidney failure if treatment is not begun early. See also **vasoactive intestinal polypeptide.**

**vir-, -vir,**   combining form for antiviral substances.

**Vira-A,**   trademark for an antiviral (vidarabine).

**viraemia.**   See **viremia.**

**viral disease.**   See **viral infection.**

**viral dysentery** /vī′rəl/ [L, *virus,* poison; Gk, *dys,* bad, *enteron,* intestine],   a form of dysentery caused by a virus and usually characterized by an acute watery diarrhea.

**viral gastroenteritis,**   an inflammation of the intestine caused by a virus. The symptoms usually include abdominal cramps, diarrhea, nausea, and vomiting.

**viral hepatitis (VH),**   a viral inflammatory disease of the liver caused by one of the hepatitis viruses, A, B, C, delta, E, F, G, or H. All have chronic forms except hepatitis A. The disease is transmitted sexually and through blood transfusions and is common among people with behavior risks or human immunodeficiency virus infection. Speed of onset and probable course of the illness vary with the kind and strain of virus, but the characteristics of the disease and its treatment are the same. See also **hepatitis A, hepatitis B, hepatitis C, delta hepatitis.**

■ OBSERVATIONS: Diagnosis is made through antibody (A + C) or antigen (B + D). Characteristic of viral hepatitis are anorexia, malaise, headache, pain over the liver, fever, jaundice, clay-colored stools, dark urine, nausea and vomiting, and diarrhea. Laboratory analyses reveal increased amounts of aspartate aminotransferase (AST) and bilirubin and an abnormal coagulation of the blood. Severe infection, especially with hepatitis B virus, may be prolonged and result in tissue destruction, cirrhosis, and chronic hepatitis or in hepatic coma and death.

■ INTERVENTIONS: Treatment is with alpha-interferon. Depending on the specific type of hepatitis, treatment with alpha-interferon is effective in 40% of patients with chronic hepatitis B virus infection; improvement in liver function has been noted in 50% of the patients infected. Treatment is also largely supportive. It includes bed rest; isolation, if necessary; fluids; a low-fat, high-protein, high-calorie diet; special skin care if pruritus is present; emotional support; vitamins B$_{12}$, K, and C; and monitoring of liver and kidney function. Sedatives, analgesics, antiemetics, and steroids may be ordered. However, the patient is carefully observed for adverse reaction to medication, because the liver may not be able to break down and detoxify the drugs. Decrease in the amount or frequency of administration or change of the medication may be necessary.

■ NURSING CONSIDERATIONS: The person is taught the importance of rest and avoiding fatigue, washing the hands carefully after urinating or defecating to avoid spreading the virus, eating well, following written dietary instructions after discharge, and avoiding alcohol, usually for at least 1 year. The patient is encouraged to have certain blood tests performed periodically, including AST and serum bilirubin, to report any symptoms of recurrence immediately, and to avoid contact with people having infections. The person is told not to donate blood and not to take over-the-counter drugs without medical consultation.

**viral infection,** any of the diseases caused by one of approximately 200 viruses pathogenic to humans. Some are the most communicable and dangerous diseases known; some cause mild and transient conditions that pass virtually unnoticed. If cells are damaged by the viral attack, disease exists. The signs of the infection reflect the anatomic location of the damaged cells. Viruses are introduced into the body through nonintact skin or mucous membranes or through a transfusion into the bloodstream or transplantation, by droplet infection through the respiratory tract, or by ingestion through the digestive tract into the GI system. The pathogenicity of the particular virus depends on the rapidity of replication, the enzymes released, the part of the body infected, and the particular action of the virus. After it enters the body, the virus attaches to and enters a cell. The virus directs the cell to produce new virions using chemical building blocks and energy available in the parasitized cell. The virus has now taken over the cell. After a variable period of time, masses of fully grown viruses appear, each able to survive outside the cell until more susceptible cells are found. In poliovirus infection one parasitized cell may produce more than 100,000 poliovirus particles in a few hours. Techniques used in viral identification and immunization are based on the essential fact that viruses can multiply only inside living cells. Inoculation of susceptible animals, tissue culture media, and chick embryos allows cultivation of viruses for study and identification and for the preparation of vaccine. Diagnosis of the cause of viral infection also is possible using various other techniques, including serologic tests, fluorescent antibody microscopic examination, microscopic examination, and skin tests. In many viral diseases, including mumps, smallpox, and measles, one attack confers permanent immunity. In others immunity is short-lived. The incubation period for viral infection is usually short, the viruses do not circulate in the bloodstream, antibodies do not form, and most often immunity does not develop. Exposure to a few viruses results in immunity to that virus and to other closely related viruses. Some vectors are able to spread several viruses, but only one at a time. Other mechanisms of natural resistance to viral infection are poorly understood, but susceptibility to a particular virus is somehow species-specific; for example, chickenpox, caused by the varicella zoster virus, is seen only in humans. A protective substance, interferon, is elaborated naturally in small amounts in the body. It is cell-specific and species-specific but not virus-specific. Interferon may act as a broad spectrum antiviral agent, protecting the body from the effects of many viral infections stopping the synthesis of viral nucleic acid within the parasitized cell. See also **specific viral infections.**

**viral keratoconjunctivitis** [L, *virus*, poison; Gk, *keras*, horn; L, *conjunctivus*, connecting; Gk, *itis*, inflammation], a combination of inflammation of the cornea and conjunctiva caused by a viral infection.

**viral load,** measurement of the amount of human immunodeficiency virus in the blood expressed as copies per milliliter. Plasma viremia is used to guide treatment decisions and monitor response to treatment. See also **viremia.**

**viral meningitis,** meningitis caused by various viruses, such as the coxsackieviruses, mumps virus, and the virus of lymphocytic choriomeningitis, characterized by malaise, fever, headache, nausea, cerebrospinal fluid pleocytosis (principally lymphocytic), abdominal pain, siffness of the neck and back, and a short uncomplicated course. See also **aseptic meningitis.**

**viral myocarditis,** inflammation of the myocardium caused by coxsackie virus.

**viral pneumonia,** pulmonary infection caused by a virus.

**viral therapy,** the use of genetically altered viruses to deliver genes to specific sites.

**Viramune,** trademark for an antiretroviral nonnucleoside analog (nevirapine).

**Virazole,** trademark for an aerosol antiviral drug (ribavirin).

**Virchow-Robin space.** See **perivascular space.**

**Virchow's node** /fir′shōz/ [Rudolf L. K. Virchow, German pathologist, 1821–1902], a firm supraclavicular lymph node, particularly on the left side, that is so enlarged that it is palpable. Also called **sentinel node, signal node.**

**Virchow's space.** See **perivascular space.**

**viremia** /vīrē′mē·ə/ [L, *virus* + Gk, *haima*, blood], the presence of viruses in the blood. Compare **bacteremia, fungemia, parasitemia.**

**virgin** /vur′jən/, **1.** a person who has never had sexual intercourse. **2.** uncontaminated.

**virginity** /vurjin′itē/, the state of being a virgin.

**virile** /vir′əl/ [L, *virilis*, masculine], **1.** pertaining to or characteristic of an adult male; masculine; manly. **2.** possessing or exhibiting masculine strength, vigor, force, or energy. **3.** pertaining to the male sexual functions; capable of procreation. Compare **virilism. —virility,** *n.*

**virilism** /vir′əliz′əm/ [L, *virilis* + *ismus*, practice], **1.** See **virilization. 2.** pseudohermaphroditism in a female. **3.** premature development of masculine characteristics in the male. Kinds of virilism are **adrenal virilism** and **prosopopilary virilism.**

**virilization** /vir′əlīzā′shən/ [L, *virilis* + *atus*, process], a process in which secondary male sexual characteristics are acquired by a female, usually as the result of adrenal dysfunction or hormonal medication. Also called **masculinization.** See also **adrenal virilism.**

**virion** /vir′ē·on, vī′rē·on/ [L, *virus*, poison], a single virus particle with a central nucleoid surrounded by a protein coat or capsid. The complete nucleocapsid with a nucleic acid core may constitute a complete virus, such as the adenoviruses and the picornaviruses, or it may be surrounded by an envelope, as in the herpesviruses and the myxoviruses. Such an envelope is a membrane that contains lipids, proteins, and carbohydrates and projects spikelike structures from its surface. See also **capsid.**

**virocytes** /vī′rəsīts/ [L, *virus* + Gk, *kytos*, cell], lymphocytes altered in appearance and in staining that are seen in blood smears from patients with viral diseases.

**viroid** /vī′roid/, a small infective segment of nucleic acid, usually ribonucleic acid (RNA). It is not translated and is replicated by host cell enzymes. Viroids include segments that are complementary to introns and may bind to intron RNA. Viroids are responsible for several plant diseases. Although they have not been associated with animal diseases, viroidlike deoxyribonucleic acid has been found in cancer cells, and some authorities believe viroids can evolve into infectious animal viruses. See also **intron, plasmid, transposon.**

**virologist** /vīrol′əjist, vir-/, a specialist who studies viruses and diseases caused by viruses.

**virology** /-l'əjē/ [L, *virus* + Gk, *logos,* science], the study of viruses and viral diseases. —**virologic, virological,** *adj.*

**Viroptic,** trademark for an ophthalmic antiviral (trifluridine).

**virtual reality** /vur'cho͞o·əl/, a system of computer-generated, three-dimensional, imaginary environments with which a person can subjectively interact. Examples include medical research to monitor brain activity in the hippocampus of subjects trying to solve maze problems. It is also used for simulations and gaming.

**virucidal** /vī'rəsī'dəl/, pertaining to the destruction of viruses.

**virucide** /vī'rəsīd/ [L, *virus* + *caedere,* to kill], any agent that destroys or inactivates a virus.

**virulence** /vir'yələns/ [L, *virulentus,* poisonous], the power of a microorganism to produce disease.

**virulent** /vir'yələnt/ [L, *virulentus*], pertaining to a very pathogenic or rapidly progressive condition.

**virus** /vī'rəs/ [L, poison], a minute parasitic microorganism much smaller than a bacterium that, having no independent metabolic activity, may replicate only within a cell of a living plant or animal host. A virus consists of a core of nucleic acid (deoxyribonucleic acid or ribonucleic acid) surrounded by a coat of antigenic protein sometimes surrounded by an envelope of lipoprotein. The virus provides the genetic code for replication, and the host cell provides the necessary energy and raw materials. More than 200 viruses have been identified as capable of causing disease in humans. Some kinds of viruses are **adenovirus, arenavirus, enterovirus, herpesvirus,** and **rhinovirus.** See also **viral infection.** —**viral,** *adj.*

**virus shedding,** the movement by any route of a virus from an infected host.

**virustatic** /vī'rəstat'ik/, pertaining to the inhibition of the growth and development of viruses, as distinguished from their destruction.

**vis** /vis, vēs/ [L, force], energy or power.

**viscera** /vis'ərə/, *sing.* **viscus** /vis'kəs/ [L, *viscus,* internal organs], the internal organs enclosed within a body cavity, including the abdominal, thoracic, pelvic, and endocrine organs.

**visceral** /vis'ərəl/ [L, *viscus,* internal organs], pertaining to the viscera, or internal organs in the abdominal cavity. Also **splanchnic.**

**visceral afferent fibers,** the nerve fibers of the visceral nervous system that receive stimuli, carry impulses toward the central nervous system, and share the sensory ganglia of the cerebrospinal nerves with the somatic sensory fibers. Peripheral distribution of the visceral afferent fibers constitutes the main difference between them and the somatic afferents. The visceral afferent fibers produce sensations different from those of the somatic afferent fibers. The visceral efferent fibers connect with both the somatic and visceral afferent fibers; the number and extent of the visceral afferent fibers is not clearly established. Their peripheral processes reach the ganglia by various routes. Most of the visceral afferent fibers accompany blood vessels for part of their course, and various afferent fibers run in the cerebrospinal nerves. Some of the parts of the body with visceral afferent fibers are the face, scalp, nose, mouth, descending colon, lungs, abdomen, and rectum. See also **autonomic nervous system.**

**visceral cavity** [L, *viscus,* internal organs, *cavum*], **1.** the abdominal cavity containing the viscera. **2.** the cavity of any viscus, such as the stomach.

**visceral efferent system** [L, *viscus,* internal organs, *effere,* to bear out; Gk, *systema*], the part of the autonomic nervous system that supplies efferent nerve fibers from the central nervous system to the visceral organs.

**visceral larva migrans,** infestation with parasitic larvae, *Toxocara,* or, occasionally, *Ascaris, Strongyloides,* or other nematodes. See **toxocariasis.**

**visceral leishmaniasis.** See **kala-azar.**

**visceral lymph node,** a small oval nodular gland that filters lymph circulating in the lymphatic vessels of the thoracic, abdominal, and pelvic viscera. The visceral lymph nodes of the thorax include the anterior mediastinal nodes, posterior mediastinal nodes, and tracheobronchial nodes. The visceral lymph nodes of the abdomen and pelvis include those that follow the course of the celiac artery, superior mesenteric artery, and inferior mesenteric artery. Compare **parietal lymph node.** See also **lymph, lymphatic system, lymph node.**

**visceral nervous system,** the visceral part of the peripheral nervous system that comprises the whole complex of nerves, fibers, ganglia, and plexuses by which impulses travel from the central nervous system to the viscera and from the viscera to the central nervous system. It contains the usual afferent fibers that receive stimuli and carry impulses toward the central nervous system and efferent fibers that carry impulses from the appropriate centers to the active effector organs, such as the nonstriated muscle, cardiac muscle, and glands of the body. Also called **involuntary nervous system.** See also **autonomic nervous system, visceral afferent fibers.**

**visceral pain,** abdominal pain caused by any abnormal condition of the viscera. It is characteristically severe, diffuse, and difficult to localize.

**visceral pericardium** [L, *viscus* + Gk, *peri,* around, *kardia,* heart], the surface of the pericardial membrane that is in direct contact with the heart. Also called **epicardium.**

**visceral peritoneum,** one of two parts of the largest serous membrane in the body that invests the viscera. The free surface of the visceral peritoneum is a smooth layer of mesothelium exuding a serous fluid that lubricates the viscera and allows them to glide freely against the wall of the abdominal cavity or over each other. The attached surface of the membrane is connected to the viscera and the abdominal wall by subserous fascia. Compare **parietal peritoneum.** See also **peritoneal cavity.**

**visceral pleura,** the inner layer of pleura that is adjacent to the external lung tissue.

**visceral protein status,** the amount of protein that is contained in the internal organs.

**visceral reflex.** See **viscerosomatic reaction.**

**visceral skeleton** [L, *viscus* + Gk, *skeletos,* dried up], the part of the skeleton, including sternum, ribs, pelvis, and vertebrae, that enclose the viscera.

**visceral swallow,** an immature swallowing pattern of an infant, resembling wavelike contractions of peristalsis.

**viscero-,** combining form meaning 'organs of the body': *viscerocranium, visceropleural, visceral, viscerosomatic.*

**visceromotor** /vis'ərōmō'tər/, **1.** pertaining to nerve impulses that control visceral smooth muscle. **2.** pertaining to movement of the viscera.

**viscerosomatic reaction** /vis'ərō'sōmat'ik/ [L, *viscus* + Gk, *soma,* body; L, *re* + *agere,* to act], a muscular response to stimulation of a nerve-receptor organ in a visceral organ. Also called **splanchnosomatic reaction, visceral reflex.**

**viscid** /vis'id/ [L, *viscidus,* sticky], sticky or glutinous. Also **viscous.**

**viscoelasticity** /vis'kō·ē'lastis'itē/, the quality or condition of being both viscous and elastic.

**viscosity** /viskos'itē/ [L, *viscosus,* sticky],   the ability or inability of a fluid solution to flow easily. A solution that has high viscosity is relatively thick and flows slowly because of the adhesive effect of adjacent molecules.

**viscous** /vis'kəs/ [L, *viscosus,* sticky],   pertaining to something thick, viscid, sticky, or glutinous. Also **viscid.**

**viscous fermentation** [L, *viscosus*],   the formation of viscous material in milk, urine, or wine by the action of various bacilli.

**viscus.**  See **viscera.**

**visibility** /vis'əbil'itē/ [L, *visibilitas,* being seen],   a condition of being visible under the circumstances of light, distance, and other factors.

**visible** /viz'ibəl/ [L, *visibilis,* visible],   perceptible to the eye.

**visible light** [L, *visus,* sight; AS, *leoht*],   the radiant energy in the electromagnetic spectrum that is visible to the human eye. The wavelengths cover a range of approximately 390 to 780 nm.

**visible radiation** [L, *visibilis,* vision, *radiare,* to shine],   electromagnetic radiation in the wavelengths between infrared and ultraviolet that can be perceived by most normal humans.

**visible spectrum** [L, *visibilis,* vision, *spectrum,* image],   the colors of the spectrum that can be observed by most people, from violet at about 4000 angstrom units (400 nm) through blue, green, yellow, and orange, to red, at about 6500 angstrom units (650 nm).

**vision** /vizh'ən/ [L, *visus,* vision],   the capacity for sight.

**vision compensation behavior,**   a nursing outcome from the Nursing Outcomes Classification (NOC) defined as the actions to compensate for visual impairment. See also **Nursing Outcomes Classification.**

**visit** /viz'it/ [L, *visitare,* to see often],   **1.** a meeting between a practitioner and a client or patient. In the hospital and the home, the practitioner makes a visit to the patient; in the clinic or office the patient makes a visit to the practitioner. **2.** (of a patient) to meet a practitioner to obtain professional services or (of a practitioner) to see a patient or client to render a professional service.

**visitation facilitation,**   a nursing intervention from the Nursing Interventions Classification (NIC) defined as promoting beneficial visits by family and friends. See also **Nursing Interventions Classification.**

**visiting nurse,**   a nurse who is responsible for a group of patients in a home setting, usually in a defined geographic area. The nurse makes visits to provide skilled nursing care as prescribed by a physician, particularly for persons unable to leave home for professional care, and to educate patients in matters of self-care. See also **home health nurse.**

**Visken,**   trademark for a beta blocker (pindolol).

**Vistaril,**   trademark for an antianxiety/antihistamine (hydroxyzine hydrochloride).

**visual** /vizh'ŏŏ·əl/ [L, *visus,* vision],   pertaining to the sense of sight.

**visual accommodation,**   a process by which the eye adjusts and is able to focus, producing a sharp image at various, changing distances from the object seen. The convexity of the anterior surface of the lens may be increased or decreased by contraction or relaxation of the ciliary muscle. With increasing age the lens becomes harder and less flexible, resulting in a loss of accommodation and usually of the ability to focus on nearby objects. Compare **presbyopia.**

**visual acuity** [L, *visus,* vision, *acuitas,* sharpness],   **1.** a measure of the resolving power of the eye, particularly with its ability to distinguish letters and numbers at a given distance. **2.** the sharpness or clearness of vision.

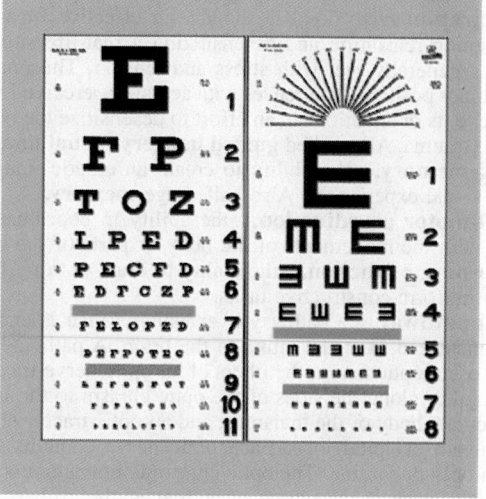

**Visual acuity test for distance vision**
*(Lemmi and Lemmi, 2000)*

**visual agnosia,**   an inability to recognize objects by sight although vision is intact. See also **object blindness.**

**visual amnesia** [L, *visus,* vision; Gk, *amnesia,* forgetfulness],   an inability to recognize objects, including written words, previously seen.

**visual angle** [L, *visus,* vision, *angulus*],   the angle between two lines passing from the extremities of an object looked at, through the nodal point of the eye. Also called **optic angle.**

**visual aphasia** [L, *visus,* vision; Gk, *a + phasis,* not speech],   the inability to understand written language caused by a lesion in the left visual cortex and the connections between the right visual cortex and the left hemisphere.

**visual center,**   the center of the brain concerned with vision.

**visual center of the cornea,**   the point of intersection of the line of sight with the cornea.

**visual-evoked potential (VEP),**   an evoked potential elicited by a repeatedly flashing light or a pattern stimulus. It may be used to confirm optic nerve or visual pathway damage.

**visual field (VF),**   the area of physical space visible to an eye in a given position. The average VF is 65 degrees upward, 75 degrees downward, 60 degrees nasally, and 90 degrees temporally.

**visual field defect,**   one or more spots or defects in the vision that remain constant in position, unlike a floater. This fixed defect is usually caused by damage to the retina or visual pathways, such as by retinal detachments, chorioretinitis, traumatic injury, macular degeneration, glaucoma, or a vascular occlusion of the eye or the brain. Sudden loss of a noticeable part of the visual field warrants ophthalmologic examination. Amsler grid detects defects only in the central 30°—not the entire visual field.

**visual hallucinations** [L, *visus,* vision, *alucinari*],   a subjective visual experience in the absence of objective evidence of a corresponding stimulus. Such hallucinations are most likely to be associated with acute organic disorders such as toxic confusional psychoses, delirium, and focal brain diseases and may occur with any stage of schizophrenia.

**visual imagery.**   See **visualization.**

**visualization** /vizh′ o͞o·əlīzā′shən/,   an effective means of deepening relaxation and desensitizing a real-life situation that is generally met with stress and tension. The imagery combines positive experiences with actual or perceived negative events or situations in an effort to desensitize the person to the trauma. Also called **guided imagery, visual imagery.**

**visual memory,**   the ability to create an eidetic image of past visual experiences. Also called **eye memory.**

**visual-motor coordination,**   the ability to coordinate vision with the movements of the body or parts of the body.

**visual-motor function,**   the ability to draw or copy forms or to perform constructive tasks.

**visual pathway,**   a pathway over which a visual sensation is transmitted from the retina to the brain. A pathway consists of an optic nerve, the fibers of an optic nerve traveling through or along the sides of the optic chiasm to the lateral geniculate body of the thalamus, and an optic tract terminating in an occipital lobe. Each optic nerve contains fibers from only one retina. The optic chiasm contains fibers from the nasal parts of the retinas of both eyes; these fibers cross to the opposite side of the brain at the optic chiasm. The fibers from the temporal part of each eye bypass the optic chiasm, pass through the lateral geniculate body on the same side of the brain, and continue back to the occipital lobe. Thus the optic tracts, occipital lobe, lateral geniculate bodies of the thalamus, and optic chiasm each contain nerve fibers from both eyes. If the right optic tract were destroyed, a person would lose partial vision in both eyes—the right nasal and the left temporal fields of vision.

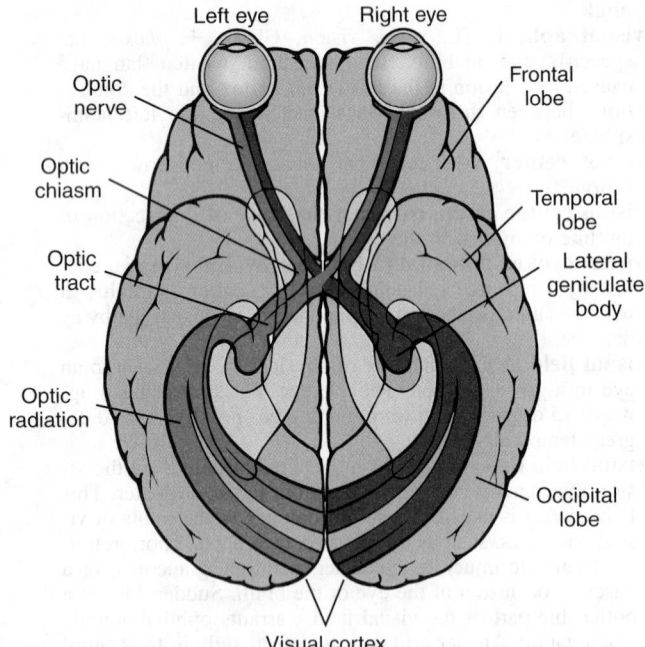

Labels: Left eye, Right eye, Optic nerve, Frontal lobe, Optic chiasm, Temporal lobe, Optic tract, Lateral geniculate body, Optic radiation, Occipital lobe, Visual cortex

**Visual pathway** *(Lewis, Heitkemper, and Dirksen, 2000)*

**visual plane,**   the plane in which the two optic axes lie.
**visual purple.**   See **rhodopsin.**
**visual response audiometry (VRA),**   a technique for

testing the hearing of older infants and children between the ages of 12 and 30 months. Sounds such as speech and tones are presented through loudspeakers. When the child looks toward the source of the sound, he or she is rewarded by seeing a toy on top of the speaker move or light up. See also **conditioned orientation response (COR).**

**visual-spatial agnosia,**   an inability to analyze spatial relationships or to perform simple constructional tasks under visual control.

**visuospatial** /vizh′ o͞o·ospā′shəl/,   pertaining to the ability to comprehend visual representations and their spatial relationships.

**vita-,**   combining form meaning 'life': *vitaglass, vital, vitascope.*

**vital** /vī′təl/ [L, *vita,* life],   pertaining to or contributing to life forces.

**vital capacity (VC)** [L, *vita,* life, *capacitas,* capacity],   the maximum volume of air that can be expelled at the normal rate of exhalation after a maximum inspiration, representing the greatest possible breathing capacity. The VC equals the inspiratory reserve volume plus the tidal volume plus the expiratory reserve volume. The average normal value of 4 to 5 L is are affected by age, the physical dimensions of the chest cage, physical fitness, posture, and gender. The VC may be reduced by a decrease in the amount of functioning lung tissue resulting from atelectasis, edema, fibrosis, pneumonia, pulmonary resection, or tumors; by limited chest expansion resulting from ascites, chest deformity, neuromuscular disease, pneumothorax, or pregnancy; or by airway obstruction. Compare **forced expiratory volume, forced expired vital capacity, residual volume.**

**vitality test** /vītal′itē/,   a group of thermal, transillumination, and electric tests used to evaluate the health of dental pulp. Also called **pulp test.**

**vital signs,**   the measurements of pulse rate, respiration rate, and body temperature. Although not strictly a vital sign, blood pressure is also customarily included. Abnormalities of vital signs are often clues to diseases, and alterations in vital signs are used to evaluate a patient's progress. See also **blood pressure, pulse, respiration, temperature.**

**vital signs monitoring,**   a nursing intervention from the Nursing Interventions Classification (NIC) defined as collection and analysis of cardiovascular, respiratory, and body temperature data to determine and prevent complications. See also **Nursing Interventions Classification.**

**vital signs status,**   a nursing outcome from the Nursing Outcomes Classification (NOC) defined as temperature, pulse, respiration, and blood pressure within expected range

**Vital signs: normal ranges**

| | Pulse (beats/min) | Respirations (breaths/min) | Blood pressure (mm Hg) |
|---|---|---|---|
| Newborn | 120 to 160 | 30 to 50 | 60 to 96/30 to 62 |
| Toddlers (1-3 years) | 90 to 140 | 20 to 30 | 78 to 112/48 to 78 |
| Preschool (4-6 years) | 80 to 110 | 18 to 26 | 78 to 112/50 to 82 |
| School age (7-11 years) | 75 to 110 | 16 to 22 | 85 to 114/52 to 85 |
| Adolescent (12-16 years) | 60 to 100 | 14 to 20 | 94 to 136/58 to 88 |
| Adult | 60 to 110 | 12 to 20 | 100 to 140/60 to 90 |

From Thompson JM: *Quick reference for clinical nursing,* ed 2, St Louis, 1997, Mosby.

for the individual. See also **Nursing Outcomes Classification.**

**vital stain** [L, *vita,* life; OFr, *desteindre,* to dye], any dye used to impart color to tissues or cells of living organisms.

**vital statistics,** data relating to births or natality, deaths or mortality, marriages, health, and disease or morbidity.

**vital ultraviolet,** the ultraviolet wavelengths between 320.0 and 290.0 nm, which are believed to be necessary or helpful for normal growth and health. Ultraviolet radiation at this wavelength converts vitamin D to its first active form.

**vitamin** /vī′təmin/ [L, *vita* + *amine,* ammonia], an organic compound essential in small quantities for normal physiologic and metabolic functioning of the body. With few exceptions, vitamins cannot be synthesized by the body and must be obtained from the diet or dietary supplements. No one food contains all the vitamins. Vitamin deficiency diseases produce specific symptoms usually alleviated by the administration of the appropriate vitamin. Vitamins are classified according to their fat or water solubility, their physiologic effects, or their chemical structures; they are designated by alphabetic letters and chemical or other specific names. The fat-soluble vitamins are A, D, E, and K; the B complex and C vitamins are water soluble. See also **avitaminosis, hypervitaminosis, oleovitamin, provitamin,** and see the specific vitamins.

**vitamin A,** a fat-soluble, solid terpene alcohol essential for skeletal growth, maintenance of normal mucosal epithelium, reproduction, and visual acuity. It is derived from various carotenoids, mainly beta-carotene and is present in leafy green vegetables and yellow fruits and vegetables as a precursor and is found preformed in fish liver oils, liver, milk, cheese, butter, and egg yolk. Deficiency leads to atrophy of epithelial tissue resulting in keratomalacia, xerophthalmia, night blindness, and lessened resistance to infection of mucous membranes. Symptoms of hypervitaminosis A are irritability, fatigue, lethargy, abdominal discomfort, painful joints, severe throbbing headache, increased intracranial pressure, insomnia and restlessness, night sweats, loss of body hair, and brittle nails. Also called **antiinfection vitamin, antixerophthalmic vitamin.**

**vitamin A₁,** one of the two forms of vitamin A that occur in nature. It is a fat-soluble unsaturated alcohol formed by hydrolysis of beta-carotene, one molecule of which yields two molecules of vitamin A₁. Natural sources include fish-liver oils, butterfat, and egg yolk. The vitamin is needed for healthy vision and skin epithelium. Also called **retinol.**

**vitamin A₂,** an alternative form of vitamin A found in the tissues of freshwater fish but not in mammals or saltwater fish. Differences in ultraviolet light absorption spectra are used to distinguish the vitamin A forms.

**vitamin B₁.** See **thiamine.**

**vitamin B₂.** See **riboflavin.**

**vitamin B₆.** See **pyridoxine.**

**vitamin B₉.** See **folic acid.**

**vitamin B₁₂.** See **cyanocobalamin.**

**vitamin B₁₂ test (cyanocobalamin),** a blood test that measures levels of vitamin B₁₂, which is necessary for conversion of the inactive form of folate to the active form, a process that is crucial in the formation and function of red blood cells. Abnormal levels may indicate leukemia, severe liver dysfunction, myeloproliferative disease, pernicious anemia, malabsorption syndromes, inflammatory bowel disease, and Zollinger-Ellison syndrome, among other conditions.

**vitamin B₁₇.** See **Laetrile.**

**vitamin B complex,** a group of water-soluble vitamins differing from each other structurally and in their biologic effect. All of the B vitamins are found in large quantities in liver and yeast, and they are present separately or in combination in many foods. Heat and prolonged cooking, especially cooking with water, can destroy B vitamins. See also **folic acid** and vitamins **B₁** through **B₁₂.**

**vitamin C.** See **ascorbic acid.**

**vitamin D,** a fat-soluble vitamin chemically related to the steroids and essential for the normal formation of bones and teeth and for the absorption of calcium and phosphorus from the GI tract. The vitamin is present in natural foods in small amounts, and requirements are usually met by artificial enrichment of various foods, especially milk and dairy products, and exposure to sunlight. Ultraviolet rays activate a form of cholesterol in an oil of the skin which is converted to a form of the vitamin in the kidney. The natural foods containing vitamin D are of animal origin and include saltwater fish, especially salmon, sardines, and herring; organ meats; fish-liver oils; and egg yolk. Deficiency of the vitamin results in rickets in children, osteomalacia, osteoporosis, and osteodystrophy. Hypervitaminosis D produces a toxicity syndrome characterized by anorexia, vomiting, headache, drowsiness, diarrhea, and calcification of the soft tissues of the heart, blood vessels, renal tubules, and lungs. Treatment consists of discontinuing the vitamin dosage and initiating a low-calcium diet until symptoms resolve. See also **calciferol, vitamin D₃.**

**vitamin D₂.** See **calciferol.**

**vitamin D₃,** an antirachitic white odorless crystalline unsaturated alcohol that is the predominant form of vitamin D of animal origin. It is found in most fish-liver oils, butter, brain, and egg yolk and is formed in the skin, fur, and feathers of animals and birds exposed to sunlight or ultraviolet rays. Also called **activated 7-dehydrocholesterol, cholecalciferol.**

**vitamin deficiency,** a state or condition resulting from the lack of or inability to use one or more vitamins. The symptoms and manifestations of each deficiency vary, depending on the specific function of the vitamin in promoting growth and development and maintaining body health.

**vitamin D resistant rickets,** a genetic disease clinically similar to rickets but resistant to treatment with large doses of vitamin D. It is caused by a congenital defect in renal tubular resorption of phosphate and usually occurs in men. See also **rickets.**

**vitamin E,** any or all of the group of fat-soluble vitamins that consist of the tocopherols and are essential for normal reproduction, muscle development, resistance of erythrocytes to hemolysis, and various other biochemical functions. It is a fat-soluble antioxidant and acts in maintaining the stability of polyunsaturated fatty acids and other fatlike substances, including vitamin A and hormones of the pituitary, adrenal, and sex glands. Deficiency is rare and may take from months to years to occur but results in muscle degeneration, vascular system abnormalities, megaloblastic anemia, hemolytic anemia, infertility, creatinuria, and liver and kidney damage and is associated with the aging process. The richest dietary sources are wheat germ; soybean, cotton seed, peanut, and corn oils; margarine; whole raw seeds and nuts; soybeans; eggs; butter; liver; sweet potatoes; and the leaves of many vegetables such as turnip greens. It is stored in the body for long periods of time so that any deficiency is rare. It is considered nontoxic except in hypertensive patients and those with chronic rheumatic heart disease. Alpha-tocopherol is the most physiologically active form of the group. Toxicity is also rare. Also called **tocopherol.**

**vitamin H.** See **biotin.**

**vitamin K,** a group of fat-soluble vitamins known as quinones that are essential for the synthesis of prothrombin in the liver and of several related proteins involved in the clotting of blood. The vitamin is widely distributed in foods, especially leafy green vegetables, pork liver, yogurt, egg yolk, kelp, alfalfa, fish-liver oils, and blackstrap molasses and is synthesized by the bacterial flora of the GI tract. It is also produced synthetically. Deficiency results in hypoprothrombinemia, characterized by poor coagulation of the blood and hemorrhage, and usually occurs from inadequate absorption of the vitamin from the GI tract or the inability to use it in the liver. It is used to reduce the clotting time in patients with obstructive jaundice and in hemorrhagic states associated with intestinal diseases and diseases of the liver; it is given prophylactically to infants to prevent hemorrhagic disease of the newborn. Natural vitamin K is stored in the body and produces no toxicity. Excessive doses of synthetic vitamin K may cause anemia in newborns and hemolysis in people with glucose-6-phosphate deficiency. See also **vitamin $K_1$, vitamin $K_2$, menadione.**

**vitamin $K_1$,** a yellow, viscous, oil-soluble vitamin, occurring naturally, especially in alfalfa, and produced synthetically. It is used as a prothrombinogenic agent. Also called **phylloquinone.**

**vitamin $K_2$,** a pale yellow fat-soluble crystalline vitamin of the vitamin K group that is more unsaturated than vitamin $K_1$ and slightly less active biologically. It is isolated from putrefied fish meal and synthesized by various bacteria in the GI tract. See also **vitamin K.**

**vitamin $K_3$.** See **menadione.**

**vitamin loss** [L, *vita,* life, *amine*], reduction in vitamin content of food resulting from the handling and preparation of fresh foods during harvesting, heating, pickling, salting, milling, canning, and other food-processing techniques. Further vitamin losses can occur because of digestive disorders that prevent nutrient absorption and the use of drugs such as isoniazid that are vitamin antagonists.

**vitaminology** /vī′təminol′əjē/ [L, *vita* + *amine* + Gk, *logos,* science], the study of vitamins, including their structures, modes of action, and function in maintaining body health.

**vitamin P.** See **bioflavonoid.**

**vitamin supplements,** any vitamins or provitamins consumed in addition to nutrients in the food eaten.

**vitellin** /vitel′in/ [L, *vitellus,* yolk], a lipoprotein containing lecithin, found in the yolk of eggs. Also called **ovovitellin. —vitelline** /-ēn/, *adj.*

**vitelline artery** /vitel′in, -ēn/ [L, *vitellus* + Gk, *arteria,* airpipe], any of the embryonic arteries that circulate blood from the primitive aorta of the early developing embryo to the yolk sac. Also called **omphalomesenteric artery.**

**vitelline circulation,** the circulation of blood and nutrients between the developing embryo and the yolk sac by way of the vitelline arteries and veins. Also called **omphalomesenteric circulation.** See also **fetal circulation.**

**vitelline duct,** (in embryology) the narrow channel connecting the yolk sac with the intestine. Also called **umbilical duct.**

**vitelline membrane,** the delicate cytoplasmic membrane surrounding the ovum. Also called **yolk membrane.** See also **zona pellucida.**

**vitelline sac.** See **yolk sac.**

**vitelline sphere.** See **morula.**

**vitelline vein,** any of the embryonic veins that return blood from the yolk sac to the primitive heart of the early developing embryo. Also called **omphalomesenteric vein.**

**vitellogenesis** /vitel′ōjen′əsis/ [L, *vitellus* + Gk, *genein,* to produce], the formation or production of yolk. **—vitellogenetic,** *adj.*

**vitellus.** See **yolk.**

**vitiligo** /vit′ilē′gō, -ī′gō/ [L, *vitium,* blemish], a benign acquired skin disease of unknown cause, consisting of irregular patches of various sizes totally lacking in pigment and often having hyperpigmented borders. Exposed areas of skin are most often affected. Treatment using 8-methoxypsoralen requires extreme care and carefully regulated sun exposure. Waterproof, sun protective cosmetics are often used to cover the patches. Compare **albinism, piebald. —vitiliginous,** *adj.*

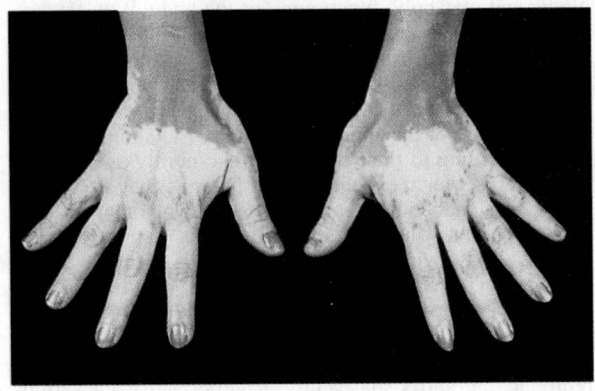

**Vitiligo** *(du Vivier, 1993)*

**vitrectomy** /vitrek′təmē/ [L, *vitreus,* glassy; Gk, *ektomē,* excision], a surgical procedure for removing the contents of the vitreous chamber of the eye, which is then replaced by oil, air, or a vitreous substitute.

**vitreous** /vit′rē·əs/ [L, *vitreus,* glassy], pertaining to the vitreous body of the eye located in the posterior chamber of the eye.

**vitreous body.** See **vitreous humor.**

**vitreous cavity** [L, *vitreus,* glassy, *cavum,* cavity], the cavity in the eye posterior to the lens that contains the vitreous body and vitreous membrane and is transected by the vestigial remnants of the hyaloid canal.

**vitreous degeneration** [L, *vitreus,* glassy, *degenerare,* to deviate from kind], a form of hyaline degeneration; the formation of glassy material in the connective tissue of blood vessels and other tissues.

**vitreous hemorrhage,** a hemorrhage into the vitreous humor of the eye.

**vitreous humor,** a transparent, semigelatinous substance contained in a thin hyoid membrane filling the cavity behind the crystalline lens of the eye. Some indications of the hyaloid canal may persist in the vitreous humor, which is not penetrated by any blood vessels and is nourished at its periphery by vessels of the retina and the ciliary processes. The vitreous humor is concave anteriorly to accommodate the crystalline lens and is closely applied to the retina around the wall of the eyeball. Also called **corpus vitreum, vitreous body.**

**vitreous membrane,** a membrane that lines the posterior cavity of the eye and surrounds the vitreous body.

**vitrification** /vit′rifikā′shən/, the conversion of a silicate material by heat and fusion to a glassy substance. Heat converts the material into a viscous liquid, which hardens on cooling.

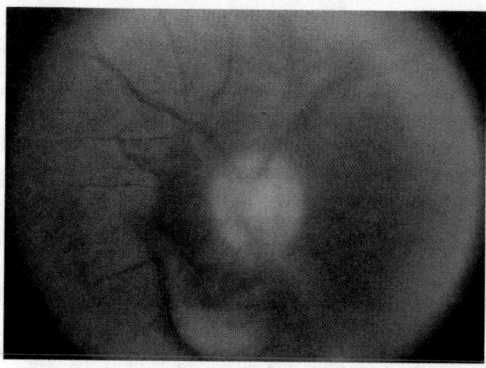

**Vitreous hemorrhage** (Zitelli and Davis, 1997)

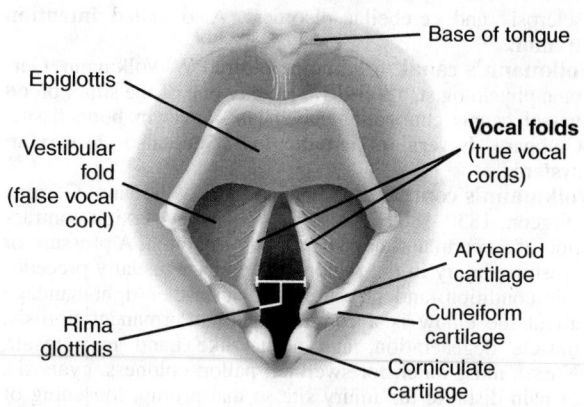

**Vocal cords** (Thibodeau and Patton, 1999/Christine Oleksky)

**vitriol, oil of.** See **sulfuric acid.**

**Vivactil,** trademark for a tricyclic antidepressant (protriptyline hydrochloride).

**vivax malaria.** See **tertian malaria.**

**vivi-,** combining form meaning 'being alive': *vivisection, viviparous.*

**viviparous** /vivip'ərəs/ [L, *vivus,* alive, *parere,* to bear], bearing living offspring rather than laying eggs, such as most mammals and some fishes and reptiles. Compare **oviparous, ovoviviparous.**

**vivisection** /viv'əsek'shən [L, *vivus,* alive, *secare,* to cut], the performance of surgical operations on living animals, particularly experimental surgery for the purpose of research.

**Vivonex,** trademark for a nutritional supplement containing protein, carbohydrate, and fat.

**VLDL,** abbreviation for **very low–density lipoprotein.**

**VMA,** abbreviation for **vanillylmandelic acid.**

**VNA,** abbreviation for *Visiting Nurses Association.*

**VO₂,** symbol for *oxygen uptake.*

**vocal apparatus** /vō'kəl/ [L, *vocalis,* voice, *ad* + *parare,* to prepare], the larynx, pharynx, and oral and nasal cavities involved in the production of sound.

**vocal cord** [L, *vocalis,* voice; Gk, *chorde,* string], one of a pair of strong bands of yellow elastic tissue in the larynx enclosed by membranes called vocal folds and attached ventrally to the angle of the thyroid cartilage and dorsally to the vocal process of the arytenoid cartilage. Also called **true vocal cord, vocal ligament.** Compare **false vocal cord.**

**vocal cord nodule,** a small inflammatory or fibrous growth that develops on the vocal cords of people who constantly strain their voices. Also called **screamer's nodule, singer's nodule, teacher's nodule.** See also **chorditis.**

**vocal cues,** a category of nonverbal communication that includes all the noises and sounds that are extra-speech sounds.

**vocal folds** [L, *vocalis* + AS, *fealdan*], the true vocal cords.

**vocal fremitus (VF),** the vibration of the chest wall as a person speaks or sings that allows the person's voice to be heard by auscultation of the chest with a stethoscope. Vocal fremitus is decreased in emphysema, pleural effusion, pulmonary edema, and bronchial obstruction.

**vocal paralysis,** paralysis of the vocal cords.

**vocal resonance** [L, *vocalis* + *resonare,* to sound again], **1.** auscultation. **2.** modification of the laryngeal tone as it passes through the pharynx and oral cavity to produce an increase in the intensity and quality of the sound.

**voice,** the acoustic component of speech that is normally produced by vibration of the vocal folds of the larynx.

**voice box.** See **larynx.**

**voiced** /voist/ [L, *vox,* voice], said of speech sounds produced with vibration of the vocal cords, such as *b, d,* or *z.* Also called **sonorant.**

**voiceless** /vois'ləs/ [L, *vox,* voice + AS, *laes,* less], said of speech sounds produced without vibration of the vocal cords, such as *p, t,* or *s.* Also called **unvoiced.**

**voiceprint** /vois'print/, a graphic representation of a person's speech pattern electronically recorded. Like a fingerprint, the speech pattern for any individual is distinctive.

**voice sounds,** auscultatory sounds heard over the lungs or airways when the patient speaks; increased resonance indicates consolidation or an airless lung underlying an effusion. Types include bronchophony, egophony, and pectoriloquy.

**void** /void/ [ME, *voide,* empty], to empty or evacuate, such as urine from the bladder.

**voiding cystourethrography (VCU)** [ME *voide,* empty; Gk, *kystis,* bag + *ourethra,* urethra + *graphein,* to record], cystourethrography in which radiographs are made before, during, and after voiding. See also **cystourethrography.**

**voiding urethrography** [ME, *voide,* empty; Gk, *ourethra* + *graphein,* to record], radiography of the urethra during micturition after the introduction of a radiopaque fluid into the bladder.

**vol.,** abbreviation for **volume.**

**vol.%,** abbreviation for *volume percent.*

**volar** /vō'lər/ [L, *vola,* palm, sole], pertaining to the palm of the hand or the sole of the foot.

**volar ligament.** See **retinaculum flexorum manus.**

**volatile** /vol'ətəl/ [L, *volatilis,* flying], (of a liquid) easily vaporized.

**volatile solvent,** an easily vaporized solvent.

**-volemia,** combining form meaning '(condition of the) volume of plasma in the body': *hypervolemia, hypovolemia, normovolemia.*

**volition** /vōlish'ən/ [L, *voluntas,* inclination], **1.** the act, power, or state of willing or choosing. **2.** the conscious impulse to perform or to abstain from an act. —**volitional,** *adj.*

**volitional** /vōlish'ənəl/ [L, *velle,* to wish], pertaining to the use of one's own will in performing or abstaining from an action.

**volitional tremor** [L, *velle,* to wish, *tremor,* shaking], a trembling that begins during voluntary effort, sometimes spreading throughout the body. It may occur in multiple sclerosis and cerebellar disorders. Also called **intention tremor.**

**Volkmann's canal** /fōlk'munz/ [Alfred W. Volkmann, German physiologist, 1800–1877], any one of the small blood vessel canals connecting haversian canals in bone tissue. Compare **haversian canaliculus.** See also **haversian system.**

**Volkmann's contracture** [Richard von Volkmann, German surgeon, 1830–1889], a serious persistent flexion contraction of forearm and hand caused by ischemia. A pressure or crushing injury in the region of the elbow usually precedes this condition, and pressure from a cast or tight bandage about the elbow is a common cause. Permanent fibrosis, muscle degeneration, and a clawlike hand may result. Nurses must watch for swelling, pallor, coldness, cyanosis, or pain distal to the injury site so that prompt loosening of constriction can restore circulation. Also called **ischemic contracture, Volkmann's paralysis.**

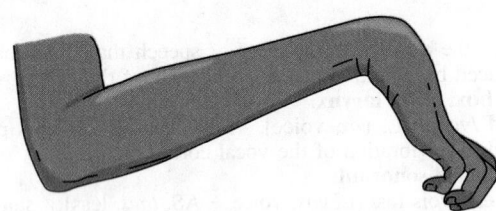

**Volkmann's ischemic contracture**
*(Phipps, Sands, and Marek, 1999)*

**Volkmann's paralysis.** See **Volkmann's contracture.**

**Volkmann's splint** [Richard von Volkmann; AS, *splinte,* thin board], a splint that supports and immobilizes the lower leg. A footpiece extends from the foot to the knee on both sides of the splint, allowing ambulation.

**volsella forceps** /volsel'ə/ [L, *vosella,* tweezers, *forceps,* tongs], a kind of forceps having a small, sharp-pointed hook at the end of each blade. Also called **volsella, volsellum forceps, vulsella forceps.**

**volt (V)** /vōlt/ [Alessandro Volta, Italian physicist, 1745–1827], the unit of electrical potential. In an electric circuit a volt is the force required to send 1 ampere of current through 1 ohm of resistance, or the difference in potential between two points on a conductor carrying a charge of 1 ampere when there is a dissipation of 1 watt between them. See also **ampere, circuit, current, ohm, watt.**

**voltage** /vō'tij/ [Alessandro Volta], an expression of electromotive force in terms of volts.

**voltammetry** /voltam'ətərē/, the measurement of an electric current as a function of potential.

**voltmeter** /vōlt'mētər/, an instrument such as a galvanometer that measures in volts the differences in potential between different points of an electric circuit.

**volume (vol.)** /vol'yəm, -yoōm/ [L, *volumen,* paper roll], the amount of space occupied by a body, expressed in cubic units.

**volume ATPS,** abbreviation for ambient temperature, ambient pressure, saturated with water vapor conditions of a volume of gas. The conditions exist in a water-sealed spirograph or gasometer when the water temperature equals ambient temperature.

**volume BTPS,** abbreviation for body temperature, ambi-

ent pressure, saturated with water vapor conditions of a volume of gas. For humans normal respiratory tract temperature is measured at 37° C, the pressure as ambient pressure, and the partial pressure of water vapor at 37° C as 47 mm Hg.

**volume control fluid chamber,** any one of several types of transparent plastic reservoirs with graduated volumetric markings, used to regulate the flow of IV solutions. These devices are components of IV volume control sets and accommodate the injection and mixing of medications by means of special built-in ports. The volume control fluid chamber contains a filter that must be primed to function.

**volume dose.** See **integral dose.**

**volume imaging,** magnetic resonance (MR) imaging techniques in which MR signals are gathered at once from the whole object volume to be imaged. Many sequential plane imaging techniques can be categorized as volume imaging, at least in principle. Advantages include potential improvement in the signal-to-noise ratio as a result of the inclusion of signals from the whole volume; disadvantages include a bigger computational task for image reconstruction and longer image acquisition times, although the entire volume can be imaged from one set of data.

**volumetric analysis.** See **quantitative analysis.**

**volumetric flow rate** /vol'yəmet'rik/, the rate at which a volume of fluid flows past a designated point, usually measured in liters per second.

**volumetric glassware,** (in chemistry) glassware designed and marked to contain or to deliver specific volumes of liquid solutions.

**volume unit (VU),** a unit of a logarithmic scale for expressing the power level of a complex audio-frequency electrical signal such as that transmitting sound.

**volume ventilator,** a ventilator that delivers a predetermined volume of gas with each cycle.

**voluntary** /vol'ənter'ē/ [L, *voluntas,* inclination], referring to an action or thought originated, undertaken, controlled, or accomplished as a result of a person's free will or choice.

**voluntary abortion.** See **elective abortion.**

**voluntary agency,** a service agency legally controlled by volunteers rather than by owners or a paid staff.

**voluntary hospital system,** a nationwide complex of autonomous, self-established, and self-supported private not-for-profit and investor-owned hospitals in the United States.

**voluntary muscle.** See **striated muscle.**

**volunteer** /vol'əntir'/ [Fr, *volontaire*], a person who serves without pay, augmenting but not replacing paid personnel and professional staff members.

**-volute,** combining form meaning 'to roll or turn around, or convoluted': *circumvolute, involute, revolute.*

**volution.** See **will.**

**volvulus** /vol'vyələs/ [L, *volvere,* to turn], a twisting of the bowel on itself, causing intestinal obstruction. The condition is frequently the result of a prolapsed segment of mesentery and occurs most often in the ileum, the cecum, or the sigmoid parts of the bowel. If it is not corrected, the obstructed bowel becomes necrotic, peritonitis and rupture of the bowel occur, and death may ensue. Severe gripping pain, nausea and vomiting, an absence of bowel sounds, and a tense distended abdomen suggest the diagnosis, which is confirmed by x-ray examination. Compare **intussusception.**

**volvulus neonatorum,** an intestinal obstruction in a newborn resulting from a twisting of the bowel caused by malrotation or nonfixation of the colon. Typical symptoms include abdominal distension; persistent regurgitation, often accompanied by fecal vomiting; and nonpassage of stools. Characteristic barium enema x-ray studies confirm the diag-

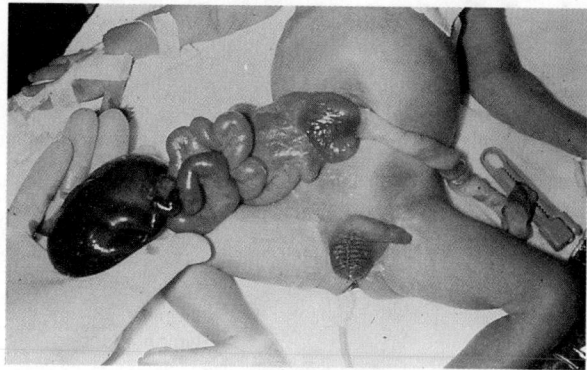

**Volvulus neonatorum** *(Zitelli and Davis, 1997)*

nosis. The condition requires immediate surgical correction to prevent necrosis and gangrene of the affected segment of bowel.

**vomer** /vō′mər/ [L, plowshare], the plow-shaped bone forming the posterior and inferior part of the nasal septum and having two surfaces and four borders.

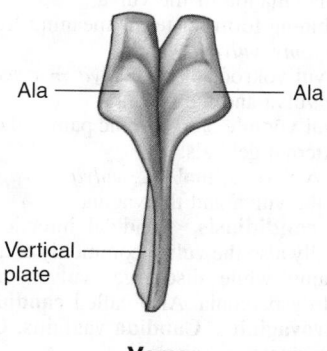

**Vomer**

**vomeronasal organ,** a structure on each side of the nasal septum believed to be a chemical sensory center for "sixth sense" detection of pheromones.

**vomit** /vom′it/ [L, *vomere*, to vomit], **1.** to expel the contents of the stomach through the esophagus and out of the mouth. **2.** also called **emesis, vomitus.** the material expelled.

**vomiting** [L, *vomere*, to vomit], the forcible voluntary or involuntary emptying of the stomach contents through the mouth.

**vomiting management,** a nursing intervention from the Nursing Interventions Classification (NIC) defined as prevention and alleviation of vomiting. See also **Nursing Interventions Classification.**

**vomiting of pregnancy,** vomiting that occurs during the early months of pregnancy. Factors contributing to the condition include delayed stomach emptying during pregnancy, relaxation of the esophageal sphincter at the opening into the stomach, and relaxation of the diaphragmatic hiatus, which increase the risk of gastric reflux. See also **vomiting reflex; morning sickness.**

**vomiting reflex.** See **reflex emesis.**

**vomitus** /vom′itəs/ [L, *vomere*, to vomit], pertaining to the material expelled from the stomach during vomiting. Vomitus is sometimes classified by color or other appearances as an indicator of the cause of illness, such as a 'coffee-ground' vomitus being a clinical sign of gastric bleeding.

**VON,** abbreviation for *Victorian Order of Nurses.*

**von Economo's encephalitis.** See **epidemic encephalitis.**

**von Gierke's disease** /fôngir′kəz/ [Edgar von Gierke, German pathologist, 1877–1945], a form of glycogen storage disease in which abnormally large amounts of glycogen are deposited in the liver and kidneys. The disorder is characterized by hypoglycemia, metabolic acidosis, dyslipidemia, and hepatomegaly. Biopsy of the affected organs reveals the absence of glucose-6-phosphatase, an enzyme necessary for glycogen metabolism. There is no effective treatment for the disorder. Medical efforts are directed at preventing hypoglycemia and acidosis. Also called **glycogen storage disease, type Ia.** See also **glycogen storage disease.**

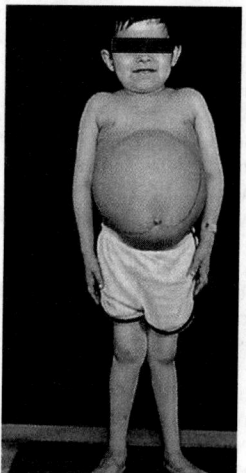

**Von Gierke's disease** *(Newton, 1995)*

**von Hippel–Lindau disease** [Eugen von Hippel, German ophthalmologist, 1867–1939; Arvid Lindau, Swedish pathologist, 1892–1958], a hereditary disease characterized by congenital, tumorlike vascular nodules in the retina and hemangioblastomas of the cerebellar hemispheres. Similar spinal cord lesions, cysts of the pancreas, kidneys, and other viscera, seizures, and mental retardation may be present. Also called **cerebroretinal angiomatosis, Lindau–von Hippel disease, retinocerebral angiomatosis.** Compare **Hippel's disease.**

**von Pirquet's test.** See **Pirquet's test.**

**von Recklinghausen's canal.** See **Recklinghausen's canal.**

**von Recklinghausen's disease.** See **neurofibromatosis.**

**von Recklinghausen's tumor.** See **Recklinghausen's tumor.**

**von Willebrand's disease** [Erick A. von Willebrand, Finnish physician, 1870–1949], an inherited disorder characterized by abnormally slow coagulation of the blood and spontaneous epistaxis and gingival bleeding caused by a deficiency of a component of factor VIII. Excessive bleeding is common after delivery, during menstruation, and after injury or surgery. Also called **angiohemophilia.** See also **hemophilia, thrombasthenia.**

**voracious** [L, *vorax*], greedy or gluttonous, with an insatiable appetite.

**-vorous,** combining form meaning 'feeding on something': *leguminivorous, panivorous.*

**vortex,** *pl.* **vortexes, vortices** [L, whirl], a whirlpool effect produced by the whirling of a more or less cylindric mass of fluid (liquid or gas). The velocity of the motion increases as the radius of the circle described by the motion decreases; the velocity decreases as the radius increases. Tornadoes and whirlpools are examples of free vortexes.

**voxel** /vok'səl/, abbreviation for *vo*lume element, the three-dimensional version of a pi*xel.*

**voyeur** /voiyur', vô·äyœr'/ [Fr, *voir,* to see], one whose sexual desire is gratified by the practice of voyeurism. Also called **Peeping Tom.** The female counterpart is a **voyeuse.**

**voyeurism** /voi'yəriz'əm, voiyur'izəm/ [Fr, *voyeur* + L, *ismus,* practice], a psychosexual disorder in which a person derives sexual excitement and gratification from looking at the naked bodies and genital organs or observing the sexual acts of others, especially from a secret vantage point. See also **compulsion.**

**VP-L-asparaginase,** an anticancer drug combination of vincristine, prednisone, and asparaginase.

**V/Q,** abbreviation for *ventilation/perfusion.* See **ventilation/perfusion ratio.**

**VR,** abbreviation for *variable ratio.* See **variable ratio (VR) reinforcement.**

**V.S.,** 1. abbreviation for **vesicular sound.** 2. abbreviation for *Veterinary Surgeon.* 3. abbreviation for **vital signs.** 4. abbreviation for *volumetric solution.*

**VSD,** abbreviation for **ventricular septal defect.**

**VU,** abbreviation for **volume unit.**

**vulgaris** /vulger'is/ [L, *vulgus,* common people], common or ordinary.

**vulnerable** /vul'nərəbəl/ [L, *vulnus,* wound], being in a dangerous position or condition and thereby susceptible to being infected or injured.

**vulnerable period,** a short period in the cardiac cycle during which activation may result in an ectopic beat. The ventricular vulnerable period corresponds to the apex of the T wave toward its ascending side.

**vulnerable population.** See **population at risk.**

**vulsella forceps.** See **volsella forceps.**

**vulva.** See **pudendum.**

**vulvar** /vul'vər/, pertaining to the vulva.

**vulvar dystrophy,** a disorder characterized by skin eruptions of white atrophic pustules, squamous cell hyperplasia, and lichen sclerosis et atrophicus.

**vulvectomy** /vulvek'təmē/ [L, *vulva,* wrapper; Gk, *ektomē,* excision], the surgical removal of part or all of the tissues of the vulva, performed most frequently in the treatment of malignant or premalignant neoplastic disease. **Simple vulvectomy** includes the removal of the skin of the labia minora, labia majora, and clitoris. **Radical vulvectomy** in-

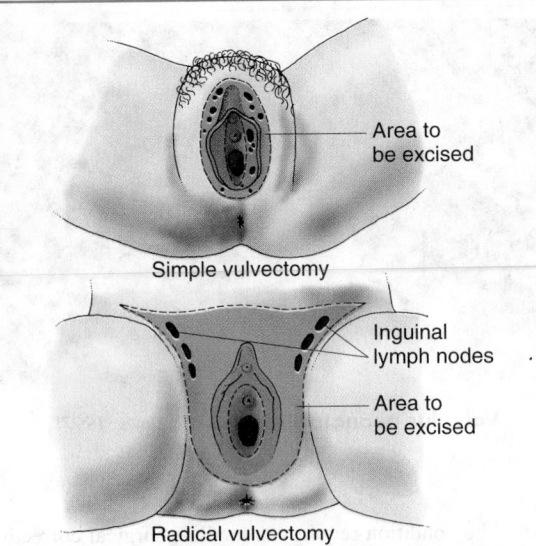

**Vulvectomy** *(Ignatavicius, Workman, Mishler, 1998)*

volves excision of the labia majora, labia minora, clitoris, surrounding tissues, and pelvic lymph nodes.

**vulvitis** /vulvī'tis/ [L, *vulva,* wrapper; Gk, *itis,* inflammation], an inflammation of the vulva.

**vulvo-,** combining form for terms meaning 'relating to the vulva': *vulvectomy, vulvovaginal.*

**vulvocrural** /vul'vōkrōō'rəl/ [L, *vulva* + *crus,* leg], pertaining to the vulva and the thigh.

**vulvodynia** /vul'vōdin'ē·ə/, chronic pain and discomfort in the female external genitals.

**vulvovaginal** /vul'vōvaj'inəl/ [L, *vulva* + *vagina,* sheath], pertaining to the vulva and the vagina.

**vulvovaginal candidiasis,** candidal infection of the vagina, and usually also the vulva, commonly characterized by pruritus, creamy white discharge, vulvar erythema and swelling, and dyspareunia. Also called **candidal vaginitis, candidal vulvovaginitis, Candida** vaginitis, **Candida** vulvovaginitis, vaginal candidiasis.

**vulvovaginitis** /vul'vōvaj'inī'tis/, an inflammation of the vulva and vagina, or of the vulvovaginal glands.

**vv,** 1. an abbreviation for *veins.* 2. an abbreviation for *vice versa.*

**v/v,** 1. symbol for *volume of dissolved substance per volume of solvent.* 2. symbol for *volume per volume.*

**v/w,** symbol for *volume of substance per unit of weight of another component.*

**V-Y plasty** /vē'wī'plas'tē/, a surgical incision made in a V shape and sutured in a Y shape to lengthen the tissue area. In a variation of the procedure, the incision is made in a Y shape and sutured in a V shape to shorten the tissue area. Also called **V-Y flap.**

**VZIG,** abbreviation for **varicella-zoster immune globulin.**

**VZV,** abbreviation for **varicella zoster virus.**

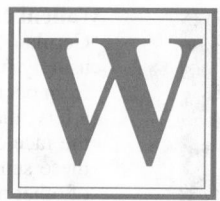

**w,** the amount of energy required to ionize a molecule of air, as expressed by w = 33.85 eV/ion pair. This is an important quantity for radiation dosimetry because it allows the extraction of dose from ionization measurements.

**W,** 1. abbreviation of **watt.** 2. symbol for the element **tungsten.**

**Waardenburg's syndrome** /vär′den·bərgz/ [Petrus Johannes Waardenburg, Dutch ophthalmologist, 1886−1979], **1.** an autosomal dominant disorder characterized by wide bridge of the nose resulting from lateral displacement of the inner canthi and puncta, pigmentary disturbances, including white forelock, heterochromia iridis, white eyelashes, leukoderma, and sometimes cochlear deafness. **2.** also called **acrocephalosyndactyly, type IV; Klein-Waardenburg syndrome.** an autosomal dominant disorder characterized by acrocephaly, orbital and facial deformities, and brachydactyly with mild soft tissue syndactyly; cleft palate, congenital glaucoma, cardiac malformation, and contractures of the elbows and knees may also be present.

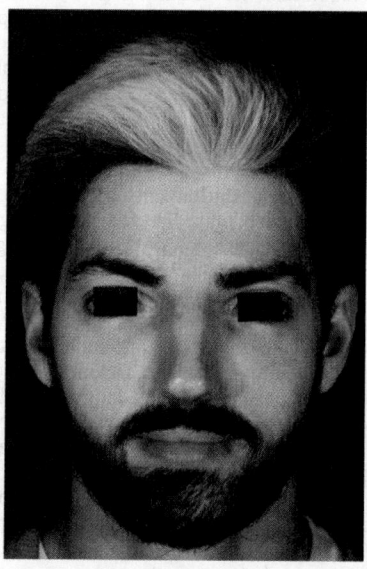

**Waardenburg's syndrome**
*(Hordinsky, Sawaya, and Scher, 2000)*

**waddling gait** /wod′ling/ [ME, *waden,* to wade; ONorse, *gata,* way], a gait characterized by exaggerated lateral trunk movements and hip elevations. It is observed in pregnancy and in patients with osteoarthritis of the hip or progressive muscular dystrophy.

**WAGR syndrome,** a syndrome of *W*ilms' tumor, *a*niridia, *g*enitourinary abnormalities or *g*onadoblastoma, and mental *r*etardation, resulting from a small interstitial deletion on chromosome 11.

**Wagstaffe's fracture** /wag′stafs/ [William Wagstaffe, English surgeon, 1834–1910; L, *fractura,* break], a fracture characterized by separation of the medial malleolus of the tibia.

**waiting list,** a roll of persons waiting to fill a vacancy, such as a list of candidates waiting for an organ transplant.

**wakefulness** /wāk′fulnəs/, **1.** an alert state of mind. **2.** sleeplessness or insomnia.

**waking imagined analgesia (WIA)** [AS, *wacian,* to awaken; L, *imaginari,* to picture oneself; Gk, *a* + *algos,* without pain], the pain relief experienced by a patient who uses the psychologic technique, usually with the help of an attending nurse or a hospital aide, of concentrating on previous pleasant personal experiences that produced tranquillity, such as lying on a summer beach beside cooling ocean water or drifting down a quiet river in a canoe. The patient using the WIA technique is encouraged to verbalize such experiences, thereby reinforcing recollection with attendant soothing biologic responses. This technique is often effective in reducing mild to moderate pain, especially when used with a mild nonnarcotic analgesic and the compassionate interaction of an attending health care professional. See also **pain assessment, pain intervention, pain pathway.**

**waking ptosis.** See **morning ptosis.**

**Wald** /wôld/, **Lillian** (1867–1940), an American public health nurse, settlement leader, and social reformer. She founded the Henry Street Settlement in New York to bring nursing care into the homes of the poor. This led to the development of the Visiting Nurse Service of New York. She was also instrumental in establishing the school nursing system, the federal government's Children's Bureau, and the Nursing Service Division of the Metropolitan Life Insurance Company. She was the first nurse to be elected into the Hall of Fame for Great Americans.

**Waldenström's macroglobulinemia.** See **macroglobulinemia.**

**Waldeyer's throat ring** /wäl′dī·ərz/ [Heinrich W.G. von Waldeyer, German anatomist, 1836–1921; AS, *hring*], the palatine, pharyngeal, and lingual tonsils that encircle the pharynx. Also called **lymphoid ring, tonsillar ring.**

**walker** /wô′kər/ [AS, *wealcan,* to roam], **1.** an extremely light, movable apparatus, about waist high, made of metal tubing, used to aid a patient in walking. It has four widely placed, sturdy legs. The patient holds onto the walker and takes a step and then moves the walker forward and takes another step. Some walkers have wheels on the rear two legs. A walker can be used by an individual with a lower extremity that is full, partial, or non-weight-bearing. It should be used only on flat, level surfaces. **2.** A small, rubber or plastic heel attached to the bottom of a walking cast to prevent the cast from slipping on hard surfaces. Also called **walking heel.** Compare **crutch.**

**Walker-Warburg syndrome** /waw′kər·vär′bŏŏrg/ [Arthur Earl Walker, American surgeon, b. 1907; Mette Warburg, Danish ophthalmologist, 20th century], a congenital syndrome, usually fatal before the age of one year, consisting of hydrocephalus, agyria, various ocular anomalies such as

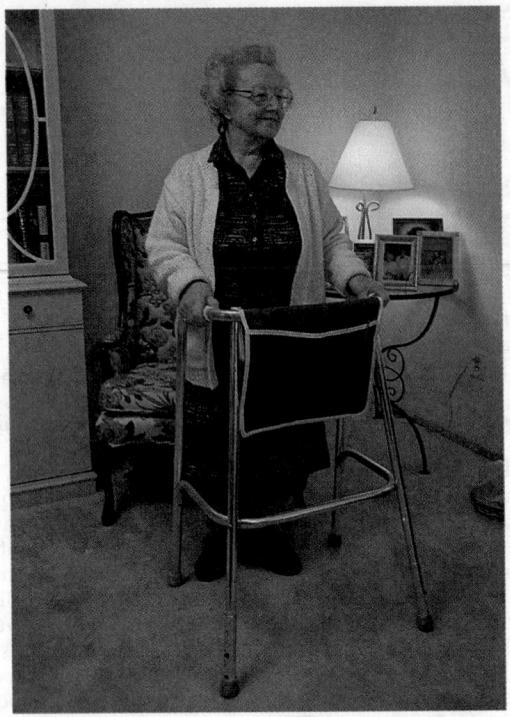

**Walker** *(Sorrentino, 2000)*

retinal dysplasia, corneal opacity, or microphthalmia, and sometimes encephalocele. Also called **HARD syndrome, Walker's lissencephaly, Warburg's syndrome.**

**walking belt,** a leather or nylon device with handles that fastens around the patient's waist and assists the health care provider with the patient's ambulation. Also called **gait belt.**

**walking cast** [AS, *wealcan,* to roam; ONorse, *kasta*], a cast that permits a patient to walk. See also **long-leg cast with walker, short-leg cast with walker.**

**walking heel.** See **walker.**

**walking pneumonia.** See **mycoplasma pneumonia.**

**walking program,** an aerobic exercise regimen of walking 30 to 45 minutes a day 5 or 6 days a week. It may be part of a program to condition the heart or lower blood pressure.

**walking reflex,** a series of steplike motions of an infant's legs when the infant is held under the arms and with the feet in contact with a surface. The reflex disappears at approximately 4 to 8 weeks of age.

**walking rounds** [AS, *wealcan* + Fr, *rond*], rounds in which the clinician responsible leads a group of junior clinicians on a tour to visit the patients for whom they are collectively responsible. In some hospitals nurses may participate in walking rounds in lieu of or in addition to report.

**walking typhoid** [AS, *wealcan,* to roam; Gk, *typhos,* fever, *eidos,* form], an ambulatory subclinical case of typhoid fever. The person may be infected with typhoid but have mild symptoms that do not interfere with the activities of daily living.

**walking wounded** [AS, *wealcan,* to roam, *wund*], a triage term for an injured person who is ambulatory and has minor injuries.

**wall** [L, *vallum,* palisade], a limiting structure within the body, such as the wall of the abdominal, thoracic, or pelvic cavities or the wall of a cell.

**Wallenberg's syndrome** /väl′en·bergz/ [Adolf Wallenberg, German physician, 1862−1949], a syndrome resulting usually from occlusion of the vertebral artery, and less often from occlusion of its branch, the posterior inferior cerebellar artery; marked by loss of temperature and pain sensations of the face on the same side as the legion, contralateral loss of these sensations in the trunk and extremities, and a variety of other neurologic and ocular symptoms including Horner's syndrome. Also called **lateral medullary syndrome, posterior inferior cerebellar artery syndrome.**

**wallerian degeneration** /waler′ē·ən/ [Augustus V. Waller, English physician, 1816–1870; L, *degenerare,* to degenerate], the fatty degeneration of a nerve fiber after it has been severed from its cell body.

**wall stress,** the tension within the wall of the left ventricle. It is determined by the pressure in the ventricle, the internal radius of the ventricle, and the thickness of the wall. Also called **wall tension.**

**wander** /won′dər/ [AS, *wandrian*], **1.** to move about purposelessly. **2.** to cause to move back and forth in an exploratory manner; for example, in inserting an intrauterine catheter, the tip of the inserter usually must be wandered around the fetal head in the cervix to find a space through which the catheter may be passed upward into the uterus.

**wandering,** a nursing diagnosis accepted by the Fourteenth National Conference on the classification of nursing diagnoses. The diagnosis is defined as meandering, aimless or repetetive locomotion that exposes the individual to harm. It is frequently incongruent with boundaries, limits, or obstacles.

■ DEFINING CHARACTERISTICS: Defining characteristics include frequent or continuous movement from place to place, often revisiting the same destinations; persistent locomotion in search of "missing" or unattainable people or places; haphazard locomotion; locomotion into unauthorized or private spaces; locomotion resulting in unintended leaving of a premise; long periods of locomotion without apparent destination; fretful locomotion or pacing; inability to locate significant landmarks in a familiar setting; locomotion that cannot be easily dissuaded or redirected; following behind or shadowing a caregiver's locomotion; trespassing; hyperactivity; scanning, seeking, or searching behaviors; periods of locomotion interspersed with periods of nonlocomotion; and getting lost.

■ RELATED FACTORS: Related factors include cognitive impairment, specifically memory and recall deficits, disorientation, poor visuoconstructive ability, and language defects; cortical atrophy; premorbid behavior; separation from familiar people and places; sedation; emotional state, especially frustration, anxiety, boredom, or depression; over or understimulating social or physical environment; physiological state or need; and time of day. See also **nursing diagnosis.**

**wandering abscess** [AS, *wandrian* + L, *abscedere,* to go away], an abscess that moves through tissue openings to a point some distance from its origin.

**wandering atrial pacemaker** [AS, *wandrian* + L, *passus* + ME, *maken*], a sinus arrhythmia with an atrial or junctional escape rhythm during the slow phase of the sinus rhythm. Frequently there are atrial fusion beats when impulse from the two pacing sources collide within the atrial. An accelerated junctional rhythm that competes with the sinus rhythm is often mislabled "wandering pacemaker."

**wandering goiter.** See **diving goiter.**

**wandering rash.** See **geographic tongue.**

**wandering spleen.** See **floating spleen.**

**Wangensteen apparatus** /wang′ənstēn/ [Owen H. Wangensteen, American surgeon, 1898–1981; L, *ad* + *parare,* to prepare], a nasogastroduodenal catheter and suction apparatus used for constant gentle drainage and decompression of the stomach or duodenum. It may be used to relieve abdominal distension that often occurs after surgery or that may complicate a GI disorder, especially an intestinal obstruction. See also **Wangensteen tube.**

**Wangensteen tube** [Owen H. Wangensteen], the catheter part of a Wangensteen apparatus.

**Warburg's syndrome.** See **Walker-Warburg syndrome.**

**ward** /wôrd/ [AS, *weard*, guard], a hospital room designed and equipped to house more than four patients.

**warfarin poisoning** /wôr′fərin/ [Wisconsin Alumni Research Foundation + coumarin], a toxic condition caused by the ingestion of warfarin, accidentally in the form of a rodenticide or by overdose with the substance in its pharmacologic anticoagulant form. The poison accumulates in the body and results in nosebleed, bruising, hematuria, melena, and internal hemorrhage. Vitamin K is the antidote to warfarin.

**warfarin sodium,** an oral anticoagulant.

■ INDICATIONS: It is prescribed for the prophylaxis and treatment of thrombosis, atrial fibrillation, and embolism.

■ CONTRAINDICATIONS: Pregnancy, severe renal or hepatic disease, hemorrhage, or known hypersensitivity to this drug prohibits its use.

■ ADVERSE EFFECTS: The most serious adverse reaction is hemorrhage. Many other drugs interact with this drug to increase or decrease its effects.

**warm-blooded** [AS, *wearm* + *blod*], having a relatively high and constant body temperature, such as the temperatures maintained by humans, other mammals, and birds, despite changes in environmental temperatures. Heat is produced in the warm-blooded human body by the catabolism of foods in proportion to the amount of work performed by the tissues in the body. Heat is lost from the body by evaporation, radiation, conduction, and convection. About 80% of the body heat that is dissipated in humans is lost through the skin; the rest is lost through the mucous membranes of the respiratory, the digestive, and the urinary systems. The average temperature of the healthy human is 98.6° F (37° C). Also called **homoiothermal, homothermal.** Compare **cold-blooded.**

**warmup,** light calisthenics and stretching exercises intended to increase flexibility, minimize risk of musculoskeletal complications, and gradually increase heart rate before the start of strenuous athletic activity.

**war neurosis.** See **combat fatigue.**

**wart.** See **verruca.**

**Warthin's tumor.** See **papillary adenocystoma lymphomatosum.**

**washout** /wosh′out/ [AS, *wascan*, to wash; ME, *oute*], the elimination or expulsion of one gas or volatile anesthetic agent by the administration of another.

**wasp** /wosp/ [L, *vespa*], a thin, narrow-waisted hymenopteran insect with two pairs of membranous wings that are folded lengthwise when at rest like parts of a fan. Many species of wasps can give painful stings that produce severe effects in hypersensitive individuals. Treatment is as for bee stings. See also **yellow jacket venom.**

**Wassermann blood test** /was′ərmən, vos′ərmun/ [August P. von Wassermann, German bacteriologist, 1866–1925], the first standard diagnostic blood test (no longer used) for syphilis based on the complement fixation reaction.

**wasted ventilation,** the volume of air that ventilates the physiologic dead space in the respiratory system.

**waste products** [L, *vastare*, to destroy, *producere*, to produce], the products of metabolic activity after oxygen and

nutrients have been supplied to a cell. These include mainly carbon dioxide and water, along with sodium chloride and soluble nitrogenous salts, which are excreted in feces, urine, and exhaled air.

**wasting** [L, *vastare*, to destroy], a process of deterioration marked by weight loss and decreased physical vigor, appetite, and mental activity. See also **wasting syndrome.**

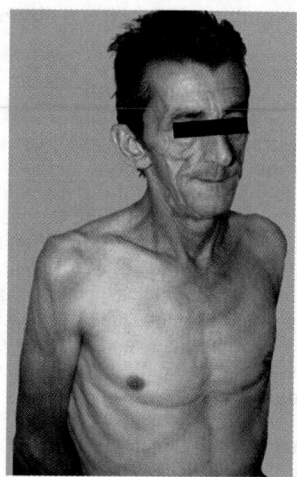

**Weight loss and muscular wasting**
*(Lemmi and Lemmi, 2000)*

**wasting palsy.** See **amyotrophic lateral sclerosis.**

**wasting syndrome,** a condition characterized by weight loss associated with chronic fever and diarrhea. Over a period of 1 month, the patient may lose 10% of baseline body weight. In cases of human immunodeficiency virus infection, the malnutrition of wasting exacerbates the condition.

**watchfulness** /woch′fəlnes/, continuous supervision, either open or unobtrusive, as the situation indicates.

**water ($H_2O$)** /wô′tər/ [AS, *waeter*], a chemical compound, one molecule of which contains one atom of oxygen and two atoms of hydrogen. Almost three quarters of the earth's surface is covered by water. Essential to life as it exists on this planet, water makes up more than 70% of living things. Pure water freezes at 32° F (0° C) and boils at 212° F (100° C) at sea level.

**waterbed,** a closed rubber bag filled with water and used as a mattress to prevent or treat pressure ulcers by equalizing the patient's weight against the support. Also called **water mattress.**

**waterborne,** carried by water, such as a waterborne epidemic of typhoid fever.

**water-hammer pulse.** See **collapsing pulse, Corrigan's pulse.**

**Waterhouse-Friderichsen syndrome** /wô′tərhous′ frid′-ərik′sən/ [Rupert Waterhouse, English physician, 1873–1958; Carl Friderichsen, Danish physician, b. 1886], overwhelming cerebrospinal meningitis, most often caused by meningoccal infection, characterized by the sudden onset of fever, cyanosis, petechiae, and collapse from massive, bilateral adrenal hemorrhage. It requires immediate emergency treatment, hospitalization, and intensive care. Emergency treatment includes vasopressor drugs, IV fluids, plasma, and oxygen. No sedatives or narcotics are given. Specific treatment is intensive antibiotic therapy, given parenterally and continued for several days after symptoms subside. Nursing care includes close observation and maintaining adequate provision of fluids and nutrients.

**water intoxication,** an increase in the volume of free water in the body, resulting in dilutional hyponatremia. Common causes are excessive ingestion of water, increased infusions of hypotonic IV solutions, or excess secretions of antidiuretic hormone. Clinical manifestations are abdominal cramps, nausea, vomiting, lethargy, and dizziness. It can potentially lead to convulsions and coma.

**water mattress.** See **waterbed.**

**water moccasin.** See **cottonmouth.**

**water pollution,** the contamination of lakes, rivers, and streams by industrial or community sources of pollutants.

**water purification, emergency,** methods of purifying unclean water for drinking purposes in emergencies. The three basic techniques include boiling the water and straining it through a cloth, adding 3 drops of tincture (alcoholic solution) of iodine per each quart of the water, and adding 10 drops of 1% chlorine bleach per each quart of water. When purifying chemicals are added, they should be thoroughly mixed with the water, and the mixture allowed to stand for 30 minutes. Also called **emergency preparation of safe drinking water.**

**waters.** See **amniotic fluid.**

**watershed infarct** /wô'tərshed/, an area of necrosis in the brain caused by an insufficiency of blood where the distributions of cerebral arteries overlap. The condition resembles that of an agricultural field irrigation system, in which the most distant sections may not be irrigated if there is a fall in water pressure.

**water-soluble contrast medium,** an iodinated contrast medium that is absorbed by the blood and excreted by the kidneys. Among the advantages of a water-soluble contrast medium are that it does not need to be removed after a procedure and it may reduce the length of the procedure.

**water trap.** See **underwater seal.**

**Watson, Jean,** a nursing theorist who proposed a philosophy and science of caring in 1979 in an effort to reduce the dichotomy between theory and practice. Her Theory of Human Caring reflects an existential phenomenologist's view of psychology and humanities. Caring is a universal social phenomenon that is only effectively practiced interpersonally. Watson identified 10 caring factors: (1) the formation of a humanistic-altruistic system of values; (2) the instillation of faith-hope; (3) the cultivation of sensitivity to self and others; (4) the development of a helping-trust relationship; (5) the promotion and acceptance of the expression of positive and negative; (6) the systematic use of the scientific problem-solving method for decision making; (7) the promotion of interpersonal teaching-learning; (8) the provision for a supportive, protective, or corrective mental, physical, sociocultural, and spiritual environment; (9) assistance with the gratification of human needs; and (10) the allowance for existential-phenomenologic forces. According to Watson, caring is a nursing term, and nursing concerns itself with health promotion, restoration, and prevention of illness as opposed to curing. Clients require holistic care that promotes humanism, health, and quality of living.

**watt (W)** /wot/ [James Watt, Scottish engineer, 1736–1819], the unit of electric power or work in the meter/kilogram/second system of notation. The watt is the product of the voltage and the amperage. One watt of power is dissipated when a current of 1 ampere flows across a difference in potential of 1 volt. See also **ampere, current, ohm, volt.**

**watt per square centimeter (W/cm²),** a unit of power density or intensity used in ultrasonography.

**wave** [AS, *wafian,* to fluctuate], a periodic disturbance in which energy moves through a medium without permanently altering the constituents of the medium. Electromagnetic waves, such as light, x-rays, and radio waves, can travel through a vacuum. Sound waves can be transmitted only through matter. See also **electromagnetic radiation, light, sound, x-ray.**

**waveform,** 1. the graphic representation of a wave, derived by plotting a characteristic wave against time. 2. the form of an arterial pressure pulse or displacement wave. 3. the representation of a neuromuscular electrical stimulation unit, which is usually a symmetric or asymmetric biphasic pulse with two phases in each pulse. The two phases continually alternate or reverse in direction between positive and negative polarity.

**wavelength,** the distance between a given point on one wave cycle and the corresponding point on the next successive wave cycle. A pure color is produced by light of a specific wavelength. Electromagnetic waves of different wavelengths account for many of the transmission characteristics of radio and television.

**wax.** a low-melting, high-molecular-weight organic mixture or compound similar to fats and oils but lacking glycerides. See **cerumen.**

**wax bath.** See **paraffin bath.**

**waxy flexibility.** See **cerea flexibilitas.**

**Wb,** abbreviation for Weber.

**WBC,** abbreviation for **white blood cell.** See **leukocyte.**

**wbt,** abbreviation for *wet bulb thermometer.*

**wc,** abbreviation for **wheelchair.**

**W chromosome and Z chromosome,** the sex chromosomes of certain insects, birds, and fish. Females of such animals are heterogametic and have one W and one Z chromosome, whereas males are homogametic and have two Z chromosomes. The ZZ-ZW nomenclature was chosen to differentiate this system from the XX-XY system, which occurs in humans and various other animals and in which the female is homogametic and the male is heterogametic.

**W/cm²,** abbreviation for **watt per square centimeter.**

**W/D,** abbreviation for *well developed,* often used in the initial identifying statement in a patient record. It is used so frequently as to have lost all meaning or use in identifying or describing the patient.

**weakness** /wēk'nəs/, a condition of being feeble, fragile, frail, or decrepit or lacking physical strength, energy, or vigor. Causes of weakness include muscle disuse and nerve injury. Partially denervated muscle shows some degree of weakness, whereas completely denervated muscle becomes flaccid. Concomitant with partial denervation is a patient's complaint of rapid fatigue and diminished capacity to perform activities of daily living. Deep tendon reflexes are diminished or absent, and electromyographic readings are abnormal.

**wean** [AS, *wenian,* to accustom], 1. to induce a child to give up breastfeeding and accept other food in place of breast milk. Many children are ready for weaning during the second half of the first year; some wean themselves. 2. to withdraw a person from something on which he is dependent. 3. to remove a patient gradually from dependency on mechanical ventilation.

**weanling,** a child who has recently been weaned.

**wear-and-tear theory** /wer/, one theory of biologic aging in which structural and functional changes occur during the aging process (e.g., osteoarthritis).

**weaver's bottom** [AS, *wefan,* to weave, *botm,* undersurface], a form of bursitis affecting the ischial bursae in people whose work requires prolonged sitting in one position. See also **bursitis.**

**web,** a network of fibers and cells forming a tissue or a membrane.

**webbed neck** /webd/, a congenital thick fold of skin and fascia that stretches from the mastoid process to the clavicle on the lateral aspect of the neck. It occurs in such genetic conditions as Noonan's syndrome and Turner's syndrome. Also called **pterygium colli.**

**webbed toes** [AS, *wefan,* to weave, *t*], an abnormality in which the toes are connected by webs of skin.

**webbing,** skinfolds connecting adjacent structures such as fingers or toes or the neck from the acromion to the mastoid, associated with genetic anomalies.

**weber (Wb)** /web′ər/ [Wilhelm Edward Weber, German physicist, 1804–1891], a unit of magnetic flux equal to $1 \text{ m}^2\text{kg/s}^2\text{A}$.

**Weber's sign** /web′ərz/ [Hermann D. Weber, English physician, 1823–1918], ipsilateral oculomotor nerve paresis and contralateral paralysis of the face, tongue, and extremities caused by a midbrain lesion. Also called **Weber's paralysis.**

**Weber's tuning fork test,** a method of screening auditory acuity. It is especially useful in determining whether a hearing loss in one ear is a conductive or a sensorineural loss. The test is performed by placing the stem of a vibrating tuning fork in the center of the person's forehead, or the midline vertex. The loudness of the sound is equal in both ears if hearing is normal or if there is a symmetrical hearing loss. If the person has a sensorineural loss in one ear, the unaffected ear perceives the sound as louder. When conductive hearing loss is present in one ear, the sound is perceived as louder in that ear because it does not hear ordinary background noise conducted through the air and receives only vibrations by bone conduction.

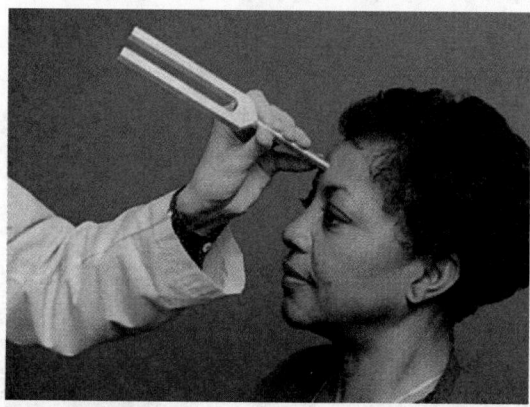

**Weber's tuning fork test** *(Sigler and Schuring, 1994)*

**web of causation,** an interrelationship of multiple factors that contribute to the occurrence of a disease.

**Webril,** trademark for a stretchable cotton material applied over the skin to protect it from plaster irritation.

**Wechsler intelligence scales** /weks′lər/ [David Wechsler, American psychologist, b. 1896], a series of standardized tests designed to measure the intelligence at several age levels, from preschool through adult, by means of questions that examine general information, arrangement of pictures and objects, vocabulary, memory, reasoning, and other abilities.

**wedge** /wej/ [AS *wecg*], **1.** a piece of material thick at one end and tapering to a thin edge at the other end. **2.** to force something into a space of limited size. See **wedge pressure.**

**wedge fracture** /wej/ [AS, *wecg*, peg; L, *fractura*, break], a fracture of the vertebral body with anterior compression.

**wedge pressure,** the blood pressure in the left atrium, determined with a cardiac catheter wedged in the most distal segment of the pulmonary artery. See also **pulmonary wedge pressure.**

**wedge resection,** the surgical excision of part of an organ, such as part of an ovary containing a cyst. The segment excised may be wedge-shaped.

**WEE,** abbreviation for **western equine encephalitis.** See **equine encephalitis.**

**weed.** See **cannabis.**

**weeping** [AS, *wepan,* to cry], **1.** crying, lacrimating. **2.** oozing or exuding fluid, such as a sore or rash.

**weeping eczema** [AS, *wepan,* to cry; Gk, *ekzein,* to boil over], an inflammatory form of skin disease marked by a fluid exudate.

**weeping lubrication,** a form of hydrostatic lubrication in which the interstitial fluid of hydrated articular cartilage flows onto its surface when a load is applied.

**Wegener's granulomatosis** /wā′gənərz/ [Friedrich Wegener, German pathologist, 1907–1990; L, *granulum*, little grain; Gk, *oma,* tumor, *osis,* condition], an uncommon disease occurring mainly in the fifth decade and characterized by granulomatosis vasculitis of the upper and lower respiratory tract, necrotizing glomerulonephritis, and varying degrees of small-vessel vasculitis. Symptoms may include sinus pain; bloody, purulent nasal discharge; saddle-nose deformity; chest discomfort and cough; weakness; anorexia; weight loss; and skin lesions. Renal involvement is seen in 80% of cases. Use of cytotoxic drugs, especially cyclophosphamide, has produced long-term remissions in many patients.

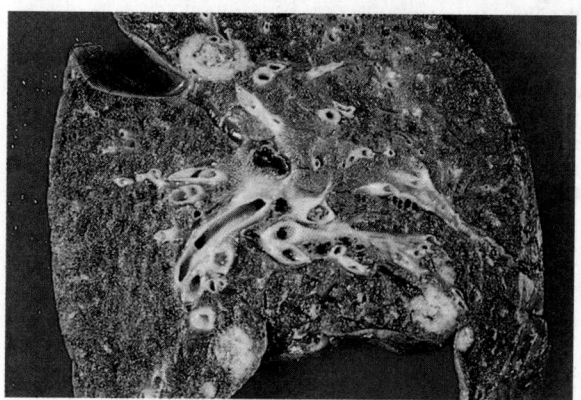

**Wegener's granulomatosis**
*(Silverberg, DeLellis, and Frable, 1997)*

**weight (wt)** /wāt/ [AS, *gewiht*], the force exerted on a body by gravitational attraction. As a body moves away from the earth, the weight of the body decreases, but the mass remains constant. In empty space a body has mass but no weight. Weight is sometimes measured in units of force such as newtons or poundals, but it is usually expressed in pounds or kilograms, as is mass. See also **mass.**

**weight control,** a nursing outcome from the Nursing Outcomes Classification (NOC) defined as the personal actions resulting in achievement and maintenance of optimum body weight for health. See also **Nursing Outcomes Classification.**

**weight gain assistance,** a nursing intervention from the Nursing Interventions Classification (NIC) defined as facilitating gain of body weight. See also **Nursing Interventions Classification.**

**weight holder,** a metal, T-shaped bar that holds weights for traction.

**weightlessness** [AS, *gewiht* + ME, *les*], a state of absence of apparent weight, as in being beyond the effects of gravitational force in space travel. See also **space medicine.**

**weightlifter's headache,** a type of headache sometimes experienced by weightlifters and others engaged in resistance forms of exercise. The headache is commonly occipital or upper cervical and comes on suddenly while straining, perhaps as a result of cervical ligament damage. The pain may be severe, steady, burning, or boring and may last for days.

**weightlifting,** a resistance form of exercise that involves the lifting of maximum heavy weights in a prescribed manner.

**weight loss,** a reduction in body weight. The loss may be the result of a change in diet or life-style or a febrile disease. To lose 1 pound a week a person must consume 500 fewer calories daily. See also **wasting.**

**weight management,** a nursing intervention from the Nursing Interventions Classification (NIC) defined as facilitating maintenance of optimal body weight and percent body fat. See also **Nursing Interventions Classification.**

**weight per volume (w/v) solution,** the relationship of a solute to a solvent expressed as grams of solute per milliliter of the total solution. An example is 50 g of glucose in 1 L of water, considered a 5% w/v solution, even though it is not a true percent solution.

**weight reduction assistance,** a nursing intervention from the Nursing Interventions Classification (NIC) defined as facilitating loss of weight and/or body fat. See also **Nursing Interventions Classification.**

**weight reduction diet,** a diet that is low in calories, used to decrease body weight. The diet must supply fewer calories than the individual expends each day while supplying all the essential nutrients for maintaining health. A diet of this type may provide 1200 calories per day from the food guide pyramid. Current reduction diets recommend that fatty meat servings be reduced and continue to advise: 55%+ calories from carbohydrate, 10% to 15% protein, and 30% or less fat. Foods to be avoided are sweetened carbonated beverages, fried foods, pastries, and most snack foods. Vitamin and mineral deficiencies may result if such a diet is not carefully planned by a registered dietition. Also called **low-caloric diet, reducing diet.**

**weights and measures,** a system of establishing units or parts of quantities of substances, including standards of mass or volume

**weight traction** [AS, *gewiht* + L, *trahere*, to draw], traction applied to a limb or part of a limb by means of a suspended weight.

**weight training,** a type of resistance-training exercise using barbells, dumbbells, or machines to increase muscle strength. See also **strength training.**

**Weill-Marchesani syndrome** /vīl mär·kə·sä′nē/ [Georges Weill, French ophthalmologist, 1866−1952; Oswald Marchesani, German ophthalmologist, 1900−1952], a congenital disorder of connective tissue, autosomal dominant or recessive, characterized by brachycephaly, shortened digits, short stature with broad chest and heavy musculature, reduced joint mobility, and a variety of ocular defects. Also called **Marchesani's syndrome.**

**Weil's disease.** See **leptospirosis.**

**Weiss' sign.** See **Chvostek's sign.**

**well baby care** [AS, *wyllan*, to wish; ME, *babe* + L, *garrire*, to chatter], periodic health supervision for infants and children to promote optimal physical, emotional, and intellectual growth and development. Such health care measures include routine immunizations to prevent disease, screening procedures for early detection and treatment of illness, and parental guidance and instruction in proper nutrition, accident prevention, and specific care and rearing of the child at various stages of development. The recommended preventive health care schedule for children who are developing normally is at months 1, 2, 4, 6, 9, 12, 15, 18, and 24 and at years 3, 4, 5, 8, 10, 12, 14, 16, and 18. Well baby care may be provided in a clinic, a convenient local meeting place, a private doctor's office, the office of a community health nursing service, or a school. Nurses or nurse practitioners frequently provide the care.

**well baby clinic,** a clinic that specializes in medical supervision and services for healthy infants.

**well-being**[1] [AS, *wyllan* + *beon*, to be], achievement of a good and satisfactory existence as defined by the individual.

**well-being**[2], a nursing outcome from the Nursing Outcomes Classification (NOC) defined as an individual's expressed satisfaction with health status. See also **Nursing Outcomes Classification.**

**well-differentiated lymphocytic malignant lymphoma** /-dif′ərⁿen′shē·ā′tid/, a lymphoid neoplasm characterized by the predominance of mature lymphocytes. Also called **lymphocytic lymphoma, lymphocytic lymphosarcoma, lymphocytoma.**

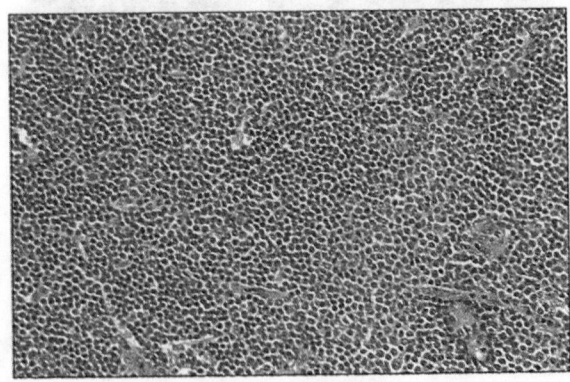

**Well-differentiated lymphocytic malignant lymphoma**
*(Eveson and Scully, 1995)*

**Wellens' syndrome,** the electrocardiographic signs of critical proximal left anterior descending coronary artery stenosis in patients with unstable angina. The signs are: normal or minimally elevated enzyme; little or no S-T segment elevation; no loss of precordial R waves; and progressive, deep, symmetric inversion of the T waves in leads V2 and V3, and sometimes other leads. The signs are seen when the patient is without pain and represent reperfusion following transient occlusion.

**wellness,** a dynamic state of health in which an individual progresses toward a higher level of functioning, achieving an optimum balance between internal and external environments.

**Wells's syndrome** /welz/ [G.C. Wells, British dermatologist, 20th century], cellulitis with erythema, edema, and often blistering of the skin accompanied by eosinophilia, flame figures, and a mild fever; a single episode lasts 2 to 6 weeks and recurrences or exacerbations are common. Also called **eosinophilic cellulitis.**

**welt** [OE, *wealtan*, to roll], a raised ridge on the skin, usually caused by a blow.

**wen.** See **pilar cyst.**

**Wenckebach heart block, Wenckebach phenomenon.** See **Mobitz I heart block.**

**Werdnig-Hoffmann disease** /verd'nighôf'mun/ [Guido Werdnig, Austrian neurologist, 1844–1919; Johann Hoffmann, German neurologist, 1857–1919], a genetic disorder beginning in infancy or young childhood, characterized by progressive atrophy of the skeletal muscle resulting from degeneration of the cells in the anterior horn of the spinal cord and the motor nuclei in the brainstem. Onset occurs within the first year of life, with the condition usually apparent at birth. Symptoms include congenital hypotonia; absence of stretch reflexes; flaccid paralysis, especially of the trunk and limbs; lack of sucking ability; fasciculations of the tongue and sometimes of other muscles; and often, dysphagia. Treatment is symptomatic, and death generally occurs in early childhood, often from respiratory complications. The condition is transmitted as an autosomal-recessive trait and occurs more frequently in siblings than in successive generations. Also called **familial spinal muscular atrophy, Hoffmann's atrophy, infantile spinal muscular atrophy, progressive spinal muscular atrophy of infants, Werdnig-Hoffmann paralysis.** See also **floppy infant syndrome.**

**Werlhof's disease.** See **thrombocytopenic purpura.**

**Werner's syndrome** /wur'nərz, wer'nərz/, an inherited condition of progeria with scleroderma, juvenile cataracts, diabetes mellitus, and hypogonadism.

**Wernicke-Korsakoff syndrome,** the coexistence of Wernicke's encephalopathy and Korsakoff's syndrome.

**Wernicke's aphasia** /ver'nikēz/ [Karl Wernicke, Polish neurologist, 1848–1905], a form of aphasia affecting comprehension of written and spoken words, possibly caused by a lesion in Wernicke's center. The client may articulate normally, but speech is incoherent, with malformed or substitute words and grammatic errors.

**Wernicke's center** [Karl Wernicke; Gk, *kentron,* center], a sensory speech center located in the posterior temporal gyrus and adjacent angular gyrus in the dominant hemisphere. Wernicke observed in 1874 that patients with brain damage in that area also suffered a loss of speech comprehension. Also called **Wernicke's area, Wernicke's zone.** See also **speech centers.**

**Wernicke's encephalopathy** [Karl Wernicke], an inflammatory, hemorrhagic, degenerative condition of the brain. It is characterized by lesions in several parts of the brain, including the hypothalamus, mammillary bodies, and tissues surrounding ventricles and aqueducts, double vision, involuntary and rapid movements of the eyes, lack of muscular

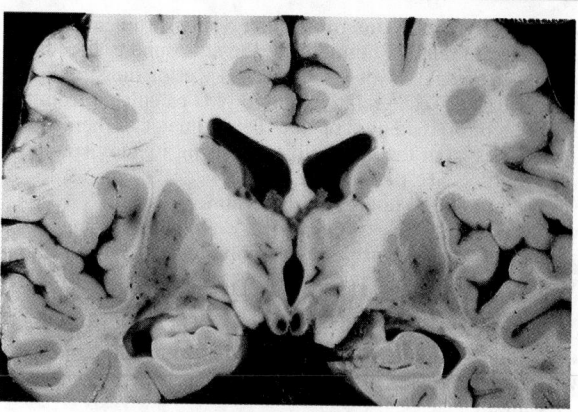

**Wernicke's encephalopathy**
*(Kumar, Cotran, and Robbins, 1997)*

coordination, and decreased mental function, which may be mild or severe. Wernicke's encephalopathy is caused by a thiamine deficiency and is seen in association with chronic alcoholism. It also occurs as a complication of GI tract disease and hyperemesis gravidarum associated with malabsorption and malnutrition. Also called **Wernicke's syndrome.**

**Wernicke's field.** See **Wernicke's center.**

**Wernicke's syndrome.** See **Wernicke's encephalopathy.**

**Wernicke's zone.** See **Wernicke's center.**

**West African sleeping sickness.** See **Gambian trypanosomiasis.**

**Westcort,** trademark for a glucocorticoid (hydrocortisone valerate).

**Westermark's sign** [Neil Westermark, German radiologist, b. 1904], on a radiograph of the lung, the absence of blood vessel markings beyond the location of a pulmonary embolism.

**Western blot test,** a laboratory blood test to detect the presence of antibodies to specific antigens. It is regarded as more precise than the enzyme-linked immunosorbent assay (ELISA) and is sometimes used to check the validity of ELISA tests.

**western equine encephalitis.** See **equine encephalitis.**

**West Nile encephalitis** /west nīl/ [West Nile River valley and region in northern Uganda, where the disease was first observed in 1937], a mild, febrile, sporadic disease caused by the West Nile virus, transmitted by *Culex* mosquitoes and occurring chiefly in the summer; infection often does not lead to encephalitis. It may be of sudden onset, and symptoms may include drowsiness, severe frontal headache, maculopapular rash, abdominal pain, loss of appetite, nausea, and generalized lymphadenopathy. Also called **West Nile fever.**

**West Nile virus** /west nīl /, a virus of the genus *Flavivirus* that causes West Nile encephalitis. It is transmitted by *Culex* mosquitoes, with wild birds serving as the reservoir, and occurs widely in Africa, Europe, the Middle East, and Asia; it has recently been reported in the United States.

**West nomogram,** a graph used in estimating the body surface area. See also **nomogram.**

**West's syndrome,** an infantile encephalopathy characterized by spasms, arrest of psychomotor development, and an electroencephalogram abnormality of random high-voltage slow waves and spikes from multiple loci.

**wet-and-dry-bulb thermometer,** an instrument used to measure the relative humidity of the atmosphere. It consists of a thermometer with a bulb that is wet or moist and one that is kept dry. The relative humidity is calculated from the difference in readings of the thermometers when water evaporates from the wet bulb, decreasing its temperature.

**wet cough.** See **productive cough.**

**wet dream.** See **nocturnal emission.**

**wet dressing** [AS, *waet* + Ofr, *dresser,* to arrange], a moist dressing used to relieve symptoms of some skin diseases. As the moisture evaporates, it cools and dries the skin, softens dried blood and sera, and stimulates drainage. Medication may be added if necessary.

**wet lung.** See **adult respiratory distress syndrome.**

**wet nurse,** a woman who cares for and breastfeeds another's infant.

**wet pack** [AS, *waet,* moist; ME, *pakke*], a therapy that involves wrapping the patient in wet sheets with a top covering of a dry blanket, usually to reduce fever.

**wet pleurisy** [AS, *waet* + Gk, *pleuritis*], pleurisy in which the inflammation has progressed to an effusive state. The escaped fluid has a high specific gravity because of the presence of blood clots and fibrin.

**wet-tap,** accidental puncture of the dura mater while performing extradural anesthesia, so called from the leakage of cerebrospinal fluid from the needle hub.

**wetting agent,** a detergent such as tyloxapol used as a mucolytic in respiratory therapy.

**wet to dry dressing,** a wet dressing that is allowed to dry and then is removed. In removal it lightly debrides the wound.

**W/F,** abbreviation for *white female,* often used in the initial identifying statement in a patient record.

**Wharton's duct.** See **submandibular duct.**

**Wharton's jelly** /wôr′tənz/ [Thomas Wharton, English anatomist, 1614–1673; L, *gelare,* to congeal], a gelatinous tissue that remains when the embryonic body stalk blends with the yolk sac within the umbilical cord.

**wheal** /wēl/ [AS, *walu,* pimple], an individual lesion of urticaria.

**wheal-and-flare reaction** [AS, *walu* + *flare* + ME, *fleare,* to blaze up; L, *re,* again, *agere,* to act], a skin eruption that may follow injury or injection of an antigen. It is characterized by swelling and redness caused by a release of histamine. The reaction usually occurs in three stages, beginning with the appearance of an erythematous area at the site of injury, followed by development of a flare surrounding the site; finally a wheal forms at the site as fluid leaks under the skin from surrounding capillaries.

**wheat weevil disease,** a hypersensitivity pneumonitis caused by allergy to weevil particles found in wheat flour.

**wheel,** **1.** a rigid circular frame designed to revolve about an axis in the center of the disk. **2.** a round cutting or polishing dental instrument.

**wheelchair (wc),** a mobile chair equipped with large wheels and brakes. If long-term use of the chair is expected, a physical therapist may prescribe certain personalized requirements, such as size, left- or right-hand propulsion, type of brakes, height of armrests, and special seat pads.

**wheelie** /wē′lē/, a wheelchair mobility skill in which the front casters are raised and balance is maintained over the large rear wheels. It is used for negotiating steep ramps, steps, curbs, and other rough terrain.

**wheeze** [AS, *hwesan,* to hiss], **1.** a form of rhonchus, characterized by a high-pitched or low-pitched musical quality. It is caused by a high-velocity flow of air through a narrowed airway and is heard during both inspiration and expi-

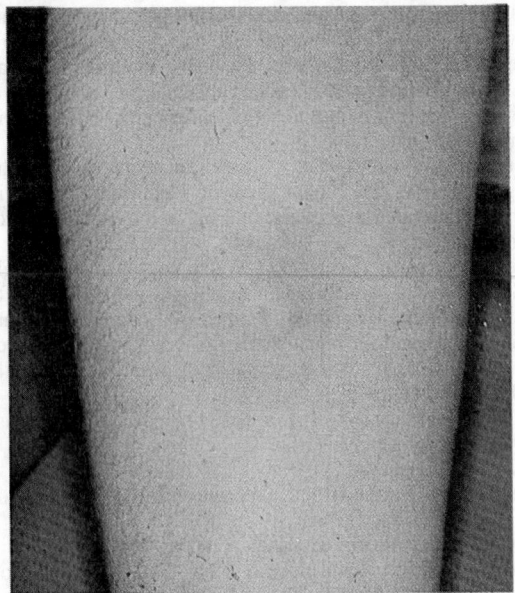

**Wheal-and-flare reaction** *(Fireman and Slavin, 1996)*

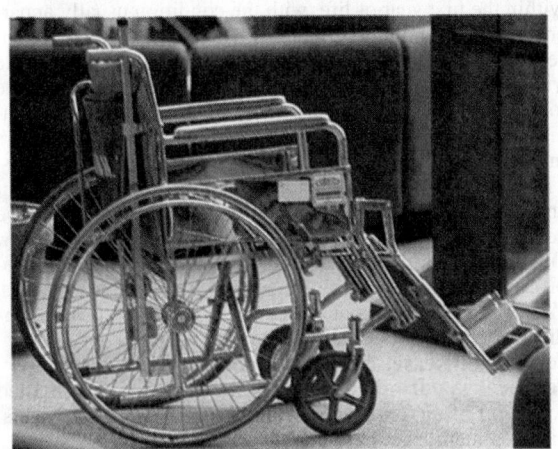

**Wheelchair** *(Potter and Perry, 2001)*

ration. It may be caused by bronchospasm, inflammation, or obstruction of the airway by a tumor or foreign body. Wheezes are associated with asthma and chronic bronchitis. Unilateral wheezes are characteristic of bronchogenic carcinoma, foreign bodies, and inflammatory lesions. In asthma expiratory wheezing is more common, although inspiratory and expiratory wheezes are heard. **2.** to breathe with a wheeze. Compare **crackle, rhonchus.**

**whiplash injury** [ME, *whippen* + *lasshe* + L, *ijuria*], *informal.* an injury to the cervical vertebrae or their supporting ligaments and muscles marked by pain and stiffness. It usually results from sudden acceleration or deceleration, such as in a rear-end car collision that causes violent back-and-forth movement of the head and neck.

**Whipple procedure** /hwip′əl/ [Allen O. Whipple, American surgeon, 1881–1963], radical pancreatoduodenectomy with removal of the distal third of the stomach, the entire duodenum, and the head of the pancreas, with gastrojejunostomy, choledochojejunostomy, and pancreaticojejunostomy. See also **pancreatoduodenectomy.**

**Whipple's disease** [George Hoyt Whipple, American pathologist, 1878–1976], a rare intestinal disease characterized by severe intestinal malabsorption, steatorrhea, anemia, weight loss, arthritis, and arthralgia. People with the disease are severely malnourished and have abdominal pain, chest pain, and a chronic nonproductive cough. The diagnosis is made by jejunal biopsy. Penicillin and tetracycline may alleviate the symptoms. See also **malabsorption syndrome.**

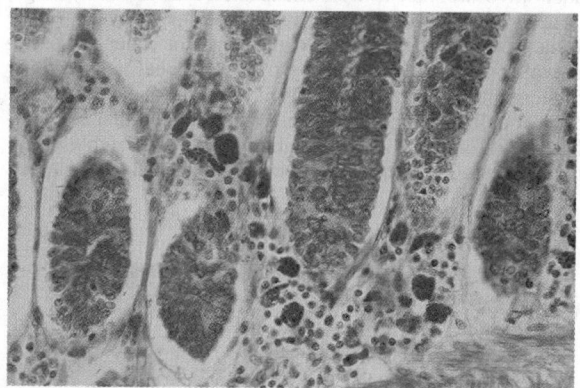

**Whipple's disease** *(Cotran, Kumar, and Collins, 1999)*

**whipworm.** See *Trichuris.*

**whirlpool bath** /(h)wurl/, the immersion of the body or a part of the body in a tank of warm water agitated by a jet of equally hot water and air, often used to clean infected wounds.

**whistling face syndrome, whistling face−windmill vane hand syndrome.** See **Freeman-Sheldon syndrome.**

**white blood cell.** See **leukocyte.**

**white blood cell (WBC) count and differential count,** a two-component blood test that first counts the total number of WBCs (leukocytes) in 1 cubic millimeter of peripheral venous blood and then measures the percentage of each type of leukocyte present in the same specimen (the differential count). The WBC and differential count are routinely measured as part of a complete blood count and, when done serially, have both diagnostic and prognostic value.

**white cell,** *informal.* white blood cell. See also **leukocyte.**

**white corpuscle.** See **leukocyte.**

**white damp.** See **damp.**

**white fibrocartilage** [AS, *hwit* + L, *fibra,* fiber, *cartilago*], a mixture of tough, white fibrous tissue and flexible cartilaginous tissue. It is divided into four types: interarticular fibrocartilage, connecting fibrocartilage, circumferential fibrocartilage, and stratiform fibrocartilage. Compare **hyaline cartilage, yellow cartilage.**

**white gold,** a gold alloy with a high content of palladium or platinum used in dental restorations, such as prepared tooth cavities and gold crowns. It has a higher fusion range, lower ductility, and greater hardness than a yellow gold alloy.

**whitehead.** See **milium.**

**white infarct.** See **pale infarct.**

**white leg.** See **phlegmasia alba dolens.**

**white line.** See **linea alba.**

**white matter.** See **white substance.**

**white noise,** a sound in which the intensity is the same at all frequencies within a designated band.

**white piedra.** See **trichosporosis.**

**white radiation,** a form of radiation that results from the rapid deceleration of high-speed electrons striking a target, as occurs when the electron beam of a tungsten cathode strikes the tungsten or molybdenum target of the anode in an x-ray tube. Most of the x-rays emitted from a diagnostic or therapeutic x-ray unit represent white radiation. Also called **braking radiation, bremsstrahlung radiation, general radiation.**

**white spots film fault,** a defect in a radiograph or photograph that appears as scattered white spots throughout the image area. It is caused by air bubbles clinging to the emulsion during development or by fixing solution splattered on the film before processing.

**white substance,** the tissue of the central nervous system and much of the part of the cerebrum, consisting mainly of myelinated nerve fibers, but with some unmyelinated nerve fibers, embedded in a spongy network of neuroglia. It is subdivided in each half of the spinal cord into three funiculi: the anterior, the posterior, and the lateral column. Each column subdivides into tracts that are closely associated in function. The anterior column divides into two ascending tracts and five descending tracts. The posterior column divides into two large ascending tracts, one small descending tract, and one intersegmental tract. The lateral column divides into six ascending tracts and four descending tracts. Also called **white matter.** Compare **gray substance.** See also **cerebrum, spinal cord, spinal tract.**

**white thrombus,** a clot composed of some combination of blood platelets, fibrin, clotting factors, and white blood cells but containing few or no erythrocytes.

**whitlow** /(h)wit′lō/ [Scand, *whick,* nail, *flaw,* crack], an inflammation of the end of a finger or toe that results in suppuration. See also **felon.**

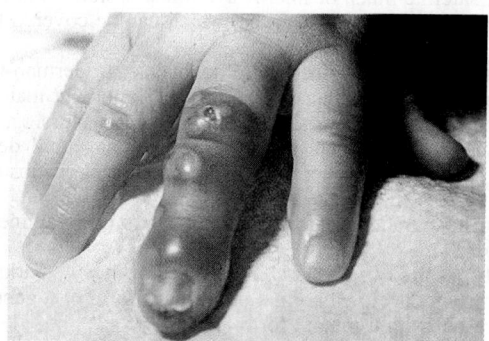

**Herpetic whitlow**
*(Stone and Gorbach, 2000/courtesy Dr. Mark Drapkin, Newton Wellesley Hospital, Newton, Massachusetts)*

**WHO,** abbreviation for **World Health Organization.**

**whole blood** /hōl/ [AS, *hal* + *blod*], blood that is unmodified except for the presence of an anticoagulant. Whole blood may be used for transfusion. Various components and factors may be separated from whole blood for infusion to replace or to augment a deficient or nonfunctional component or factor.

**whole-body irradiation,** ionizing radiation exposure that affects the entire body. Short-term whole-body irradiation can cause injury or death in humans, mainly from damage to the GI tract and the bone marrow. However, such injury occurs only with doses far beyond the diagnostic range, such as with exposure to nuclear weapons. The absorbed dose equivalent limit for whole-body occupational exposure is 5 rem per year. The nonoccupational absorbed dose equivalent limit is 0.5 rem per year. Also called **total body radiation.**

**whole bowel irrigation,** a method of treating poisoned patients by flushing large volumes of fluid through the GI tract.

**whole milk,** cow's milk from which no constituent such as fat has been removed. To be called whole milk it must contain 3.5% fat, 8.5% nonfat milk solids, and 88% water.

**whoop** /hoop, (h)woop/, a noisy spasm of inspiration that terminates a coughing paroxysm in cases of pertussis. It is caused by a sudden sharp increase in tension on the vocal cords.

**whooping cough.** See **pertussis.**

**whorl** /(h)wurl/ [ME, *hwarwy*], a spiral turn, such as one of the turns of the cochlea or of the dermal ridges that form fingerprints.

**WIA,** abbreviation for **waking imagined analgesia.**

**wick humidifier,** a respiratory care device in which a piece of paper, sponge, or similar material that absorbs water by capillary action is inserted in the path of the air flow. With the addition of heat, high levels of humidity can be achieved over a wide range of flows and temperatures.

**Widal's test** /vēdäls'/ [Georges F. I. Widal, French physician, 1862–1929], an agglutination test used to aid in the diagnosis of *Salmonella* infections such as typhoid fever. A fourfold increase in titer of agglutinins to O or H antigens is highly suggestive of active infection. A high titer may persist for years after the disease or after immunization against typhoid fever.

**wide-angle glaucoma.** See **glaucoma.**

**wide area network (WAN),** a computer network that uses long-distance communications methods, such as telephone lines, satellite links, or microwave transmission, to cover a geographic area larger than that which can be covered by a local area network (LAN).

**Wiedenbach, Ernestine,** /wē′dənbak/, a German-born American nursing educator and writer. She taught maternal and newborn health nursing at Yale School of Nursing, was a leader in family-centered maternity nursing, and developed the full range of the art and science of obstetric nursing.

**Wigraine,** trademark for a vasoconstrictor (ergotamine tartrate).

**wild-type allele** [AS, *wilde,* untamed; Gk, *typos,* mark, *genein,* to produce], a normal or standard form of a gene, as contrasted with a mutant form.

**will** [AS, *wyllan*], **1.** the mental faculty that enables one consciously to choose or decide on a course of action. **2.** the act or process of exercising the power of choice. **3.** a wish, desire, or deliberate intention. **4.** a disposition or attitude toward another or others. **5.** determination or purpose; willfulness. **6.** (in law) an expression or declaration of a person's wishes as to the disposition of property to be performed or take effect after death. Also called **volution.**

**Williams syndrome** /wil′yəmz/ [J.C.P. Williams, New Zealand cardiologist, 20th century], supravalvular aortic stenosis, mental retardation, elfin facies, and transient hypercalcemia in infancy. Also called **elfin facies syndrome.**

**Willis' circle.** See **circle of Willis.**

**willow fracture.** See **greenstick fracture.**

**will to live,** a nursing outcome from the Nursing Outcomes Classification (NOC) defined as the desire, determination, and effort to survive. See also **Nursing Outcomes Classification.**

**Wilms' tumor** /vilms/ [Max Wilms, German surgeon, 1867–1918], a malignant neoplasm of the kidney occurring in young children before the fifth year in 75% of the cases. The most frequent early signs are hypertension, a palpable mass, pain, and hematuria. Diagnosis can be established by an excretory urogram with tomography. The tumor, an embryonal adenomyosarcoma, is well encapsulated in the early stage, but it may extend into lymph nodes, the renal vein, or the vena cava and metastasize to the lungs or other sites. Removal of resectable tumors by transperitoneal nephrectomy is recommended. Radiotherapy is used before or after surgery or palliatively in inoperable cases. Chemotherapy combined with surgery and irradiation is proving highly effective. Also called **nephroblastoma.** See also **kidney cancer.**

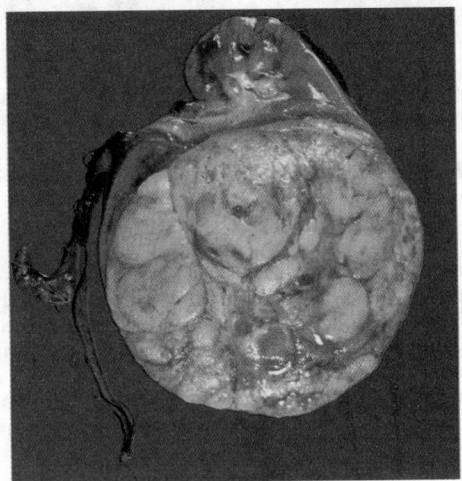

**Wilms' tumor** *(Kumar, Cotran, and Robbins, 1997)*

**Wilson's disease** [Samuel A. K. Wilson, English neurologist, 1878–1937], a rare inherited disorder whereby a decrease in ceruloplasmin causes copper to accumulate slowly in the liver, to then be released, and to be taken up in other parts of the body. Hemolysis and hemolytic anemia occur as the copper accumulates in the red blood cells. Accumulation in the brain destroys certain tissue and may cause tremors, muscle rigidity, poorly articulated speech, and dementia. Kidney function is diminished; the liver becomes cirrhotic. Treatment of Wilson's disease includes a reduction of copper in the diet and the prescription of copper-binding agents and penicillamine. Also called **hepatolenticular degeneration.**

**Winckel's disease.** See **hemoglobinuria.**

**windburn** /wind′burn/ [AS, *wind,* air, *baernan*], a skin disorder caused by exposure to winds.

**windchill** /win′chil/, the loss of heat from the body when it is exposed to wind of a given speed at a given temperature and humidity.

**windchill factor** [AS, *wind,* air, *cele,* cold], the amount of chilling of the body, beyond that resulting from a cold ambient temperature, because of exposure to cool air currents. The windchill factor is expressed in degrees Celsius or Fahrenheit as the effective temperature felt by a person exposed to the weather. Because windchill factors are based on exposure of dry skin to cool air currents, air blowing at the same speed over a wet skin surface would cause additional loss of body heat and a greater windchill.

**windchill index,** a chart that compares temperatures of the atmosphere with various wind speeds, enabling one to calculate the windchill factor. The comparison is expressed in kilocalories per hour per square meter of skin surface.

**winding sheet** /wīn'ding/, a shroud for wrapping a dead body.

**window** [AS, *wind,* air, *owe,* eye], **1.** a surgically created opening in the surface of a structure or an anatomically occurring opening in the surface or between the chambers of a structure. **2.** a specific time period during which a phenomenon can be observed, a reaction monitored, or a procedure initiated.

**windowed** /win'dōd/, referring to an orthopedic cast that has an opening designed to relieve pressure that may irritate and inflame the skin or to provide access to an incision or a wound.

**windpipe.** See **trachea.**

**winegrower's lung** /wīn'grō·ərs/, a type of hypersensitivity pneumonitis caused by contact with mold on grapes.

**winged scapula** /wingd/ [ONorse, *vaengr* + L, *scapulae,* shoulderblades], an abnormal prominence of the scapula caused either by projection of posterior angles of the ribs in a flat chest or by paralysis of the serratus anterior muscle.

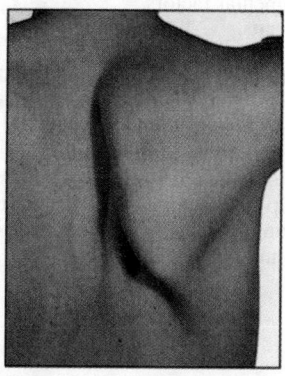

**Winged scapula** *(Perkin, 1998)*

**wink reflex,** an automatic closure of the eyelids in response to an appropriate stimulus. Also called **eye-closure reflex.**

**Winstrol,** trademark for an androgen (stanozolol) used as an anabolic agent.

**winter cough** [AS, *winter* + *cohhetan*], *nontechnical.* a chronic condition characterized by a persistent cough occasioned by cold weather. See also **cough.**

**wintergreen oil,** a volatile oil with a characteristic odor and taste; used as a counterirritant in ointments or liniments

for muscle pain and also as a flavoring agent. Also called **methyl salicylate.**

**winter itch,** pruritus occurring in cold weather in people who have dry skin, particularly in those who have atopic dermatitis. Warmer temperature, increased humidity, and topical, antipruritic emollients may offer relief.

**wire** /wīr/, **1.** *n.,* a long, slender, flexible structure of metal, used in surgery and dentistry. **2.** *v.,* to insert such metal strands into a body structure, as into a broken bone to immobilize fragments, or into an aneurysm to promote clot formation.

**wire suture** [AS, *wir* + L, *sutura*], a stainless steel or silver wire used for uniting bone fracture fragments or in dentistry.

**wiry pulse** /wī'(ə)re/ [AS, *wir* + L, *pulsare,* to beat], an abnormal pulse that is strong but small.

**wisdom tooth** [AS, *wisdom* + *toth*], a third molar; either of the last teeth on each side of the upper and lower jaw. The wisdom teeth are the last teeth to erupt, usually between 17 and 25 years of age, often causing considerable pain, dental problems, and the need for extraction. Also called **dens serotinus.** See also **molar.**

**wish fulfillment** [AS, *wiscan,* to wish, *fullfyllan,* to fill full], **1.** the gratification of a desire. **2.** (in psychology) the satisfaction of a desire or the release of emotional tension through such processes as dreams, daydreams, and neurotic symptoms. **3.** (in psychoanalysis) one of the primary motivations for dreams in which an unconscious desire or urge, unacceptable to the ego and superego because of sociocultural restrictions or feelings of personal guilt, is given expression.

**wishful thinking** [AS, *wiscan* + *thencan,* to think], the interpretation of facts or situations according to one's desires or wishes rather than as they exist in reality, usually used as an unconscious device to avoid painful or unpleasant feelings.

**Wiskott-Aldrich syndrome** /wis'kotôl'drich/ [Alfred Wiskott, German pediatrician, 1898–1978; Robert Anderson Aldrich, American pediatrician, b. 1917], an immunodeficiency disorder inherited as a recessive X-linked trait, characterized by thrombocytopenia, eczema, inadequate T and B cell function, and an increased susceptibility to viral, bacterial, and fungal infections and to cancer. Treatment includes the prescription of appropriate antibiotics for specific infectious organisms and the administration of transfer factor from activated lymphocytes to increase the resistance to infection and to clear the eczema. See also **transfer factor.**

**witch doctor,** a shamanistic healer whose primary function is to cure the sick members of the community.

**witch hazel** [AS, *wican,* to bend; Ger, *hasel*], **1.** a shrub, *Hamamelis virginiana,* indigenous to North America, from which an astringent extract is derived. **2.** also called **hamamelis water.** A solution comprising the extract, alcohol, and water, used as an astringent.

**witch's milk,** a milklike substance secreted from the breast of the newborn, caused by circulating maternal lactating hormone. Also called **hexenmilch.**

**withdrawal** /withdrô'əl/ [ME, *with* + *drawen,* to take away], a common response to physical danger or severe stress characterized by a state of apathy, lethargy, depression, retreat into oneself, and in grave cases catatonia and stupor. It is pathologic if it interferes with a person's perception of reality and ability to function in society, such as in the various forms of schizophrenia. See also **schizophrenia.**

**withdrawal behavior,** the physical or psychologic removal of oneself from a stressor.

**withdrawal bleeding,** the passage of blood from the uterus, associated with the shedding of endometrium that has been stimulated and maintained by hormonal medication. It occurs when the medication is discontinued. In the endocrine evaluation of a woman with amenorrhea, withdrawal bleeding constitutes evidence that the woman's endometrium is responsive to hormonal stimulation and that the cause of her amenorrhea is probably not uterine.

**withdrawal method,** a contraceptive technique in coitus wherein the penis is withdrawn from the vagina before ejaculation. It is not reliable because small amounts of seminal fluid carrying millions of spermatozoa may be emitted without sensation before full ejaculation. Also called **coitus interruptus.**

**withdrawal reflex.** See **flexor withdrawal reflex.**

**withdrawal symptoms,** the unpleasant, sometimes life-threatening physiologic changes that occur when some drugs are withdrawn after prolonged, regular use. The effects may occur after use of a narcotic, tranquilizer, stimulant, barbiturate, alcohol, corticosteroid, or other substance to which the person has become physiologically or psychologically dependent or addicted. Other drug therapy may be used to relieve symptoms of withdrawal, such as methadone used for heroin withdrawal or Librium for alcohol withdrawal. Withdrawal symptoms can also be managed with a planned schedule of tapering the drug dose by gradually reducing the dosage over time, as with the tapering of corticosteroids.

**withdrawal syndrome** [ME, *with* + *drawen,* to take away; Gk, *syn,* together, *dromos,* course], a physical and mental response after cessation or severe reduction in intake of a substance such as alcohol or opiates that has been used regularly to induce euphoria, intoxication, or relief from pain or distress. The body tissues become dependent on the regular reinforcing effect of the chemical so that interruption of the dosage induces an organic mental state characterized by anxiety, restlessness, insomnia, irritability, impaired attention, and often physical illness.

**withdrawn behavior,** a condition in which there is a blunting of the emotions and a lack of social responsiveness.

**witness,** a person who is present and can testify that he or she has personally observed an event, such as the signing of a will or consent form.

**Wittmaack-Ekbom syndrome.** See **restless legs syndrome.**

**W/M,** abbreviation for *white male,* often used in the initial identifying statement in a patient record.

**W/N,** abbreviation for *well nourished,* often used in the initial identifying statement in a patient record. It is used so frequently as to have lost all meaning or use in identifying or describing the patient.

**WOB,** abbreviation for **work of breathing.**

**wobble** /wob′əl/, an eccentric rotation that permits increased resolution of tomographic imaging devices composed of discrete detector systems. Typical eccentric excursions are 1 to 2 cm.

**WOCN,** an abbreviation for the Wound, Ostomy and Continence Nurses (WOCN) Society. An organization of nurses who manage conditions such as stomas, draining wounds, fistulas, vascular ulcers, pressure ulcers, neuropathic wounds, urinary incontinence, fecal incontinence, and functional disorders of the bowel and bladder. See **enterostomal therapist.**

**Wohlfart-Kugelberg-Welander disease.** See **juvenile spinal muscular atrophy.**

**Wolff-Chaikoff effect** /woolf′chī′kəf/, the decreased formation and release of thyroid hormone in the presence of an excess of iodine.

**wolffian body.** See **mesonephros.**

**wolffian cyst** /wôl′fē·ən/ [Kaspar F. Wolff, German anatomist, b. 1733–1794; Gk, *kystis,* bag], **1.** a cyst of the wolffian duct. **2.** a cyst of a broad ligament of the uterus.

**wolffian duct.** See **mesonephric duct.**

**Wolff-Parkinson-White syndrome** /woolf′pär′kinsən-(h)wīt′/ [Louis Wolff, American physician, 1898–1972; John Parkinson, English cardiologist, 1885–1976; Paul Dudley White, American cardiologist, 1886–1973], a disorder of atrioventricular (AV) conduction involving an accessory pathway. This syndrome is often identified by a characteristic delta wave seen on an electrocardiogram at the beginning of the QRS complex. See also **Lown-Ganong-Levine syndrome.**

**Wolff's law** /wôlfs/ [Julius Wolff, German anatomist, 1836–1902], the principle that changes in the form and function of a bone are followed by changes in its internal structure.

**Wolf-Herschorn syndrome,** a genetic disorder of infants characterized by psychomotor and growth retardation, hypertonicity, seizures, and microcephaly. Other features include craniofacial anomalies, ocular malformations, cleft lip or palate, heart malformations, and scoliosis.

**wolfram.** See **tungsten.**

**Wolfram syndrome** /wool′frəm/ [D.J. Wolfram, American physician, 20th century], an autosomal recessive syndrome, first evident in childhood, consisting of diabetes mellitus, diabetes insipidus, optic atrophy, and neural deafness. Also called **DIDMOAD syndrome.**

**Wolman's disease.** See **cholesteryl ester storage disease.**

**woman,** an adult female human.

**woman-year** [AS, *wifman* + *gear*], (in statistics) 1 year in the reproductive life of a sexually active woman; a unit that represents 12 months of exposure to the risk of pregnancy. Woman-years are used in calculating a pregnancy rate in the assessment of the effectiveness of the various methods of family planning and of the adverse effect on the birth rate of various environmental factors.

**womb.** See **uterus.**

**wood alcohol.** See **methanol.**

**Wood's lamp** [Robert W. Wood, American physicist, 1868–1955; AS, *glaes*], an illuminating device with a nickel oxide filter that holds back all light except for a few violet rays of the visible spectrum and ultraviolet wavelengths of about 365 nm. It is used extensively to help diagnose fungus infections of the scalp and erythrasma. The light causes hairs infected with a fungus such as *Tinea capitis* to become brilliantly fluorescent. Also called **black light.**

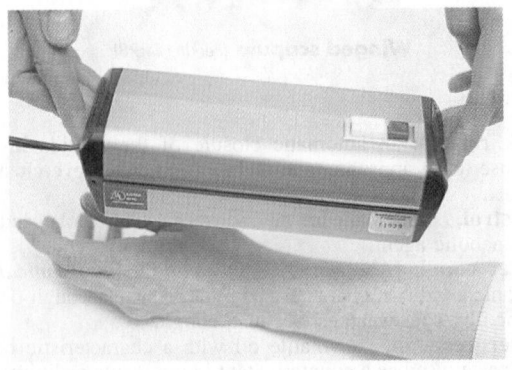

**Wood's lamp** *(Wilson and Giddens, 2001)*

**Wood's light.**   See **ultraviolet lamp.**

**wood tick** [AS, *wudu* + ME, *tike*], a hardshelled tick of the Ixodidae family and a natural reservoir of *Rickettsia rickettsii.* One species of wood tick, *Dermacentor andersoni,* is the principal vector in western North America of **Rocky Mountain spotted fever,** transmitted by *R. rickettsii.*

**wool fat,** a fatty substance obtained from sheep's wool and of which lanolin is a common chemical component. It consists primarily of lanosterol, cholesterol and its esters.

**woolsorter's disease** [AS, *wull* + Fr, *sorte* + L, *dis,* opposite of; Fr, *aise,* ease], the pulmonary form of anthrax, so named because it is an occupational hazard to those who handle sheep's wool. Early symptoms mimic those of influenza, but the patient soon develops high fever, respiratory distress, and cyanosis. If the disease is not treated at this stage, it is often fatal. Also called **pulmonary anthrax.** See also **anthrax.**

**word association.**   See **controlled association.**

**word association test.**   See **association test.**

**word blindness** [AS, *word* + *blind*], an inability to understand written language; a form of receptive aphasia caused by lesions in the parietal or parietal-occipital areas of the brain. The condition may be congenital or acquired as a result of disease or injury. Also called **alexia.**

**word deafness.**   See **auditory amnesia.**

**word processor,** a computer software application designed for the keyboarding, formating, correcting, and storing of text, including correspondence, reports, manuscripts, and books or other publications.

**word salad,** a jumble of words and phrases that lacks logical coherence and meaning, often characteristic of disoriented individuals and persons with schizophrenia. See **jargon aphasia.**

**work hardening,** a highly structured, goal-oriented, individualized treatment program designed to maximize a person's ability to return to work. Work hardening uses work (real or simulated) as a treatment modality.

**working occlusion** [AS, *weorc* + L, *occludere,* to shut], the occlusal contacts of teeth on the side of the jaw toward which the mandible is moved.

**working phase,** (in psychology) the second stage of the therapist-client relationship. During this stage clients explore their experiences. Therapists assist clients in this process by helping them to describe and clarify their experiences, to plan courses of action and try out the plans, and to begin to evaluate the effectiveness of their new behavior. Should new behavior prove ineffective, therapists can assist clients in revising their courses of action.

**working pressure,** the recommended pressure, usually about 34 Pa (50 p.s.i.), for oxygen or compressed air leaving a cylinder. It is reduced by a pressure regulator for clinical use in respiratory therapy.

**working through,** a process by which repressed feelings are released and reintegrated into the personality.

**workload,** an amount of work to be performed within a specific time period.

**work of breathing (WOB),** the effort required to inspire air into the lungs. WOB accounts for 5% of total body oxygen consumption in a normal resting state but can increase dramatically during acute illness.

**work of worrying,** a coping strategy in which inner preparation through worrying increases the level of tolerance for subsequent threats.

**workout,** **1.** a test of ability and endurance. **2.** a physical exercise session.

**work simplification,** the use of special equipment, ergonomics, functional planning, and behavior modification to reduce the physical and psychologic stresses of home maintenance for disabled people or their family members.

**workstation,** **1.** an area, as in an office equipped with a computer or computer terminal. **2.** an electronic monitor such as a computer or television screen with controls for manipulating images.

**work therapy** [AS, *weorc* + Gk, *therapeia,* treatment], a therapeutic approach in which the client performs a useful activity or learns an occupation, as in occupational therapy.

**work tolerance,** the kind and amount of work that a physically or mentally ill person can or should perform.

**work-up,** the process of performing a complete patient evaluation, including history, physical examination, laboratory tests, and x-ray or other diagnostic procedures to acquire an accurate data base on which a diagnosis and treatment plan may be established.

**World Health Organization (WHO),** an intergovernmental organization within the United Nations system whose purpose is to aid in the attainment of the highest possible level of health by all people. Programs include education for current health issues, proper food supply and nutrition, safe water and sanitation, maternal and child health, immunization against major infectious diseases, and prevention and control of diseases. WHO is coordinating global strategies to control and prevent acquired immunodeficiency syndrome. Its functions include furnishing technical assistance, stimulating and advancing epidemiologic investigation of diseases, recommending health regulations, promoting cooperation among scientific and professional health groups, and providing information and counsel relating to health matters. Its headquarters are in Geneva, Switzerland.

**worm** /wurm/ [AS, *wyrm*], any of the soft-bodied, elongated invertebrates of the phyla Annelida, Nemathelminthes, or Platyhelminthes. Some kinds of worms parasitic for humans are **hookworm, pinworm,** and **tapeworm.** See also **fluke, roundworm.**

**wormian bone** /vôr′mē-ən/ [Olaus Worm, Danish anatomist, 1588–1654; AS, *ban*], any of several tiny smooth bones, usually found at the serrated borders of the sutures between the cranial bones.

**worthlessness** /wurth′ləsnəs/, a component of low self-esteem, characterized by feelings of uselessness and inability to contribute meaningfully to the well-being of others or to one's environment.

**wound** /wo͞ond/ [AS, *wund*], **1.** any physical injury involving a break in the skin, usually caused by an act or accident rather than by a disease, such as a chest wound, gunshot wound, or puncture wound. **2.** to cause an injury, especially one that breaks the skin.

**wound care,** a nursing intervention from the Nursing Interventions Classification (NIC) defined as prevention of wound complications and promotion of wound healing. See also **Nursing Interventions Classification.**

**wound care: closed drainage,** a nursing intervention from the Nursing Interventions Classification (NIC) defined as maintenance of a pressure drainage system at the wound site. See also **Nursing Interventions Classification.**

**wound culture and sensitivity (C&S),** a microscopic examination done to determine the presence of pathogens in patients with suspected wound infections, which are most often causing by pus-forming organisms. Most organisms require approximately 24 hours to grow in the laboratory, but when antibiotic therapy needs to be instituted before lab results are available, Gram's stain of the specimen smeared on a slide can be reported in less than 10 minutes to help determine the organism's possible identity and decide an appropriate antibiotic treatment.

**wound healing,** a process to restore to a state of soundness any injury that results in an interruption in the continuity of external surfaces of the body. Also called **wound repair.** See also **healing, intention.**

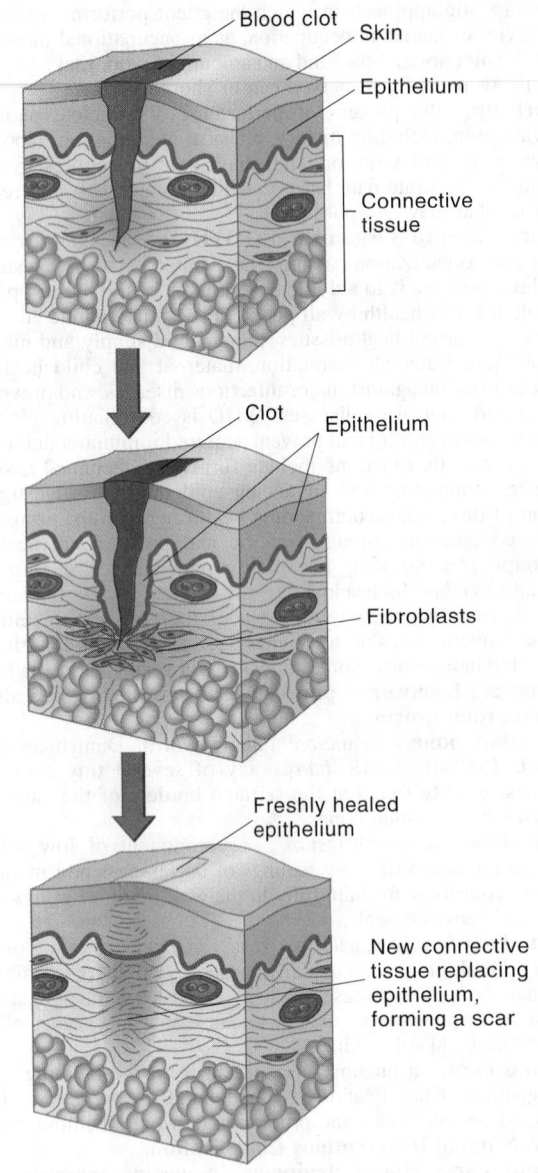

Blood clot
Skin
Epithelium
Connective tissue

Clot
Epithelium
Fibroblasts

Freshly healed epithelium
New connective tissue replacing epithelium, forming a scar

**Stages of wound healing** *(Thibodeau and Patton, 1999)*

**wound healing: primary intention,** a nursing outcome from the Nursing Outcomes Classification (NOC) is defined as the extent to which cells and tissues have regenerated following intentional closure. See also **Nursing Outcomes Classification.**

**wound healing: secondary intention,** a nursing outcome from the Nursing Outcomes Classification (NOC) defined as the extent to which cells and tissues in an open wound have regenerated. See also **Nursing Outcomes Classification.**

**wound irrigation**[1], the rinsing of a wound or the cavity formed by a wound using a medicated solution, water, or saline, or antimicrobial liquid preparation.

■ METHOD: A sterile irrigating solution is poured into a sterile bowl. It is then warmed in a basin of warm water unless the solution's action depends on antibiotic or enzyme activity, which would be inhibited by warming. An emesis or kidney-basin is then fitted snugly against the patient's body beneath the wound. It may be held in place by the patient or by an assistant. A catheter is held with sterile gloves or forceps and gently inserted into the wound to a prescribed depth and at a prescribed angle. A syringe filled with irrigating solution is then attached to the catheter, and the solution is gently instilled. The catheter is pinched before the empty syringe is removed to prevent aspiration of the return irrigation flow during disconnection. The syringe is filled and attached again, and the wound is irrigated until the returning solution runs clear. If a catheter is not used, the solution is sprayed directly on the wound from the syringe until the wound looks clean. After irrigation is completed, the body area is dried with sterile sponges working from the wound out to the area around it, and a dry sterile dressing is applied.

■ INTERVENTIONS: Frequency of irrigation, type of solution, and amount of solution to be used are specifically prescribed. The condition of the wound, amount of irrigating solution used, and appearance of the returned solution should be documented.

**wound irrigation**[2], a nursing intervention from the Nursing Interventions Classification (NIC) defined as flushing of an open wound to cleanse and remove debris and excessive drainage. See also **Nursing Interventions Classification.**

**wound repair.** See **wound healing.**

**Wright's stain** /rīts/ [James H. Wright, American pathologist, 1869–1928; Fr, *teindre,* to dye], a stain containing methylene blue and eosin that is used to color blood specimens for microscopic examination, such as for complete blood count and particularly for malarial parasites.

**wrinkle test** /ring′kəl/ [AS, *gewrinclian,* to wind; L, *testum,* crucible], a test for nerve function in the hand by observing the presence of skin wrinkles after the hand has been placed in warm water for 20 to 30 minutes. Denervated skin does not wrinkle.

**wrist.** See **carpus.**

**wrist clonus reflex** /rist/, a sustained clonic muscle spasm caused by the sudden hyperextension of the wrist joint.

**wrist drop** [AS, *wrist + dropa*], a condition caused by paralysis of the extensor muscles of the hand and fingers or by injury of the radial nerve, resulting in flexion of the wrist.

**wrist ganglion,** a cystic enlargement of a tendon sheath on the back of the wrist.

**wrist joint.** See **radiocarpal articulation.**

**writer's cramp** [AS, *writan,* to write, *crammian,* to fill], a painful, involuntary contraction of the muscles of the hand in a person attempting to write. It often occurs after long periods of writing. Also called **chirospasm** /kir′əspaz′əm/, **graphospasm.**

**wrongful birth** /rông′fəl/ [OE, *wrang,* twisted; ME, *burth*], a belief that a birth could have been avoided if the parents had been properly advised by a physician that a pregnancy could occur or that a fetus would be deformed.

**wrongful death statute** [AS, *wrang + death + L, statuere,* to place], (in law) a statute existing in all states that provides that the death of a person can give rise to a cause of legal action brought by the person's beneficiaries in a civil suit against the person whose willful or negligent acts caused the death. Before the existence of these statutes, a suit could be brought only if the injured person survived the injury.

**wrongful life** [OE, *wrang,* twisted; AS, *lif*]. See **wrongful birth.**

**wrongful life action,**    (in law) a civil suit usually brought against a physician or health facility on the basis of negligence that resulted in the wrongful birth or life of an infant. The parents of the unwanted child seek to obtain payment from the defendant for the medical expenses of pregnancy and delivery, for pain and suffering, and for the education and upbringing of the child. Wrongful life actions have been brought and won in several situations, including malpracticed tubal ligations, vasectomies, and abortions. Failure to diagnose pregnancy in time for abortion and incorrect medical advice leading to the birth of a defective child also have led to malpractice suits for a wrongful life.

**wryneck.**   See **torticollis.**

**wt,**   abbreviation for **weight.**

*Wuchereria* /vo͞oˈkərēˈrē·ə/ [Otto Wucherer, German physician, 1820–1873], a genus of filarial worms found in warm, humid climates. *Wuchereria bancrofti,* transmitted by mosquitoes, is the cause of elephantiasis. See also **filariasis.**

**W/V,**   abbreviation for *weight per volume.* See **weight per volume (W/V) solution.**

**w/w,**   abbreviation for *weight per weight.*

**Wyburn-Mason's syndrome** /wīˈbərn·māˈsənz/ [Roger Wyburn-Mason, British physician, 20th century], arteriovenous aneurysms on one or both sides of the brain, with ocular anomalies, especially in the retina, facial nevi, and sometimes mental retardation.

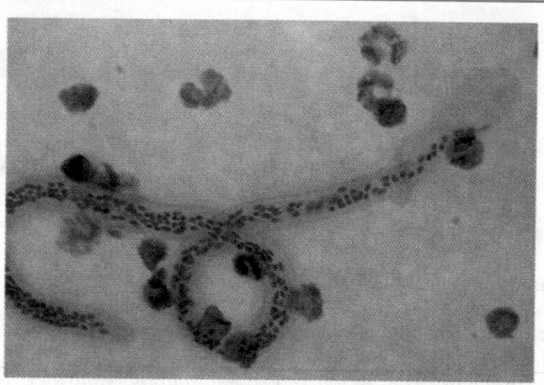

***Wuchereria bancrofti* microfilaria**
*(Mahon and Manuselis, 2000)*

**Wycillin,**   trademark for an antibacterial (penicillin G procaine).

**Wydase,**   trademark for an enzyme (hyaluronidase).

**Wymox,**   trademark for an antibiotic (amoxicillin).

**Wytensin,**   trademark for an antihypertensive agent (guanabenz).

**Wyvac,**   trademark for a rabies virus vaccine (rabies human diploid cell vaccine).

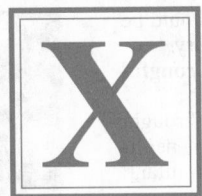

**Xanax,** trademark for a benzodiazepine antianxiety agent (alprazolam).

**-xanox,** combining form for antiallergic respiratory tract drugs of the xanoxic acid group.

**xanthelasma** /zan′thəlaz′mə/ [Gk, *xanthos*, yellow + Gk. *elasma*, plate], a planar xanthoma involving the eyelid(s). Also called **xanthoma palpebrarum.**

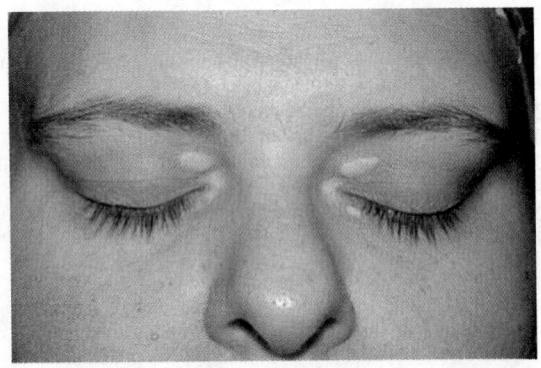

**Xanthelasma**
*(Seidel et al, 1999/courtesy John W. Payne, MD, The Wilmer Ophthalmological Institute, The Johns Hopkins University and Hospital, Baltimore)*

**xanthelasmatosis** /zan′thilaz′mətō′sis/ [Gk, *xanthos*, yellow, *elasma*, plate, *osis*, condition], a disseminated, generalized form of planar xanthoma frequently associated with reticuloendothelial disorders, especially multiple myeloma.

**xanthemia.** See **carotenemia.**

**xanthene** /zan′thēn/ [Gk, *xanthos*, yellow], a crystalline organic compound in which two benzene rings are fused to a central pyran ring. The pyran oxygen bridges the two benzene rings. It is a parent chemical structure of many medicinal elements.

**xanthine** /zan′thīn/ [Gk, *xanthos*, yellow], a nitrogenous by-product of the metabolism of nucleoproteins. It is normally found in the muscles, liver, spleen, pancreas, and urine. —**xanthic,** *adj.*

**xanthine base** [Gk, *xanthos*, yellow], a purine compound occurring in plants and animals as a metabolite of adenine and guanine. It is the parent structure of the methyl xanthine alkaloids that include caffeine in coffee, theophylline in tea, and theobromine in cocoa.

**xanthine derivative,** any one of the closely related alkaloids caffeine, theobromine, and theophylline. They are found in plants widely distributed geographically and are variously ingested as components in beverages such as coffee, tea, cocoa, and cola drinks. The xanthine derivatives ore

methylxanthines have pharmacologic properties that stimulate the central nervous system, produce diuresis, and relax smooth muscles. Theobromine has low potency and is seldom used as a pharmaceutic. Caffeine produces greater central nervous system stimulation than theophylline or theobromine. Caffeine and theophylline also affect the circulatory system, tending to dilate the systemic blood vessels but increasing cerebrovascular resistance with an associated decrease in cerebral blood flow and the oxygen tension of the brain. The ability of the xanthine derivatives to relax smooth muscle is especially important in certain treatments of asthma. Theophylline is most effective in such treatment and markedly increases vital capacity. The methylxanthines reinforce the release of certain secretions of various endocrine and exocrine tissues, except for mast cells and, possibly, certain other mediators of inflammation. Consumption of xanthine beverages may cause various problems, including restlessness and inability to sleep, GI irritation, and excessive myocardial stimulation characterized by premature systole and tachycardia.

**xanthinuria** /zan′thinyŏor′ē·ə/ [Gk, *xanthos* + *ouron*, urine], **1.** the presence of excessive quantities of xanthine in the urine. **2.** a rare disorder of purine metabolism, resulting in the excretion of large amounts of xanthine in the urine because of the absence of an enzyme, xanthine oxidase, that is necessary in xanthine metabolism. This inherited deficiency may cause the development of kidney stones made of xanthine precipitate.

**xanthism** /zan′thizəm/, a genetic pigment anomaly characterized by yellow or yellowish-red hair, copper-red skin, and reddish-brown irises.

**xantho-,** combining form meaning 'yellow': *xanthochroia, xanthogen, xanthophore.*

**xanthochromia** /zan′thəkrō′mē·ə/, a pale yellow or straw-colored discoloration of cerebrospinal fluid. It is caused by the presence of hemoglobin breakdown products.

**xanthochromic** /zan′thəkrō′mik/ [Gk, *xanthos* + *chroma*, color], having a yellowish color, such as cerebrospinal fluid that contains blood or bile. Also **xanthochromatic.**

**xanthoderma** /zan′thədur′mə/, skin that has a yellow coloration, as in jaundice.

**xanthogranuloma** /zan′thəgran′yəlō′mə/, *pl.* **xanthogranulomas, xanthogranulomata** [Gk, *xanthos* + L, *granulum*, little grain; Gk, *oma*, tumor], a tumor or nodule of granulation tissue containing lipid deposits. A kind of xanthogranuloma is **juvenile xanthogranuloma.**

**xanthoma** /zanthō′mə/, *pl.* **xanthomas, xanthomata** [Gk, *xanthos* + *oma*, tumor], a benign fatty fibrous yellowish plaque, nodule, or tumor that develops in the subcutaneous layer of skin, often around tendons. The lesion is characterized by the intracellular accumulation of cholesterol and cholesterol esters.

**xanthoma disseminatum,** a benign chronic condition in which small orange or brown papules and nodules develop on many body surfaces, especially on the mucous membrane of the oropharynx, larynx, and bronchi and in skin folds and fissures. Also called **xanthoma multiplex.**

**1838**

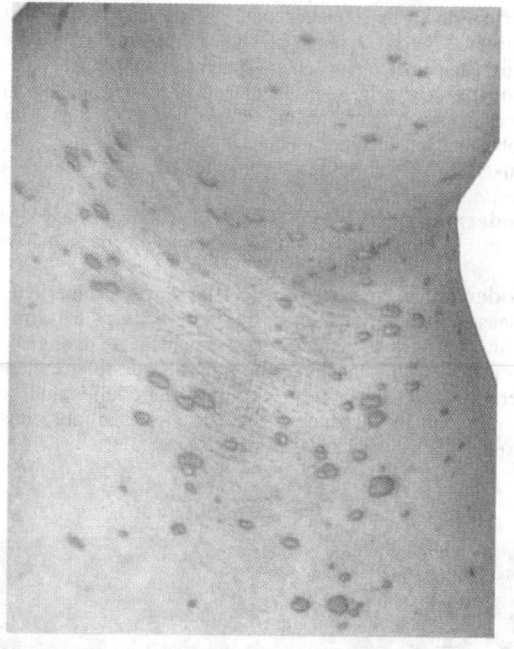

**Xanthoma disseminatum** *(du Vivier, 1993)*

**xanthoma eruptivum.**  See **eruptive xanthoma.**
**xanthoma multiplex.**  See **xanthoma disseminatum.**
**xanthoma palpebrarum.**  See **xanthelasma.**
**xanthoma planum.**  See **planar xanthoma.**
**xanthomasarcoma** /zan'thōmǝsärkō'mǝ/, *pl.* **xantho-masarcomas, xanthomasarcomata** [Gk, *xanthos* + *oma* + *sarx*, flesh, *oma*, tumor],  a giant cell sarcoma of the tendon sheaths and aponeuroses that contains xanthoma cells.
**xanthoma striatum palmare,**  a yellow or orange flat plaque or slightly raised nodule occurring in groups on the palms of the hands.

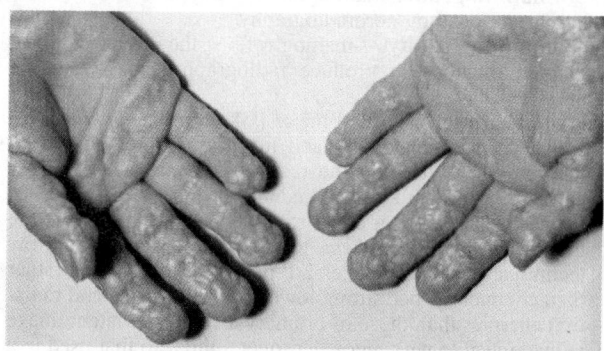

**Xanthoma striatum palmare** *(du Vivier, 1993)*

**xanthoma tendinosum,**  a yellow or orange elevated or flat round papule or nodule occurring in clusters on tendons, especially the extensor tendons of the hands and feet, of individuals with hereditary lipid storage disease.

**xanthomatosis** /zan'thōmǝtō'sis/ [Gk, *xanthos* + *oma* + *osis,* condition],  an abnormal condition in which there are deposits of yellowish fatty material in the skin, internal organs, and reticuloendothelial system. It may be associated with hyperlipoproteinemia, paraproteinemia, lipoid storage diseases, and other disorders of adipose tissue. Also called **xanthosis.** See also **lipemia, xanthoma, xanthoma palpebrarum.**
**xanthomatosis bulbi,**  a fatty degeneration of the cornea.
**xanthoma tuberosum,**  a yellow or orange flat or elevated round papule occurring in clusters on the skin of joints, especially the elbows and knees, usually in people who have a hereditary lipid storage disease such as hyperlipoproteinemia. The xanthomatous papules also may be associated with biliary cirrhosis and myxedema. Also called **tuberous xanthoma, xanthoma tuberosum multiplex.**

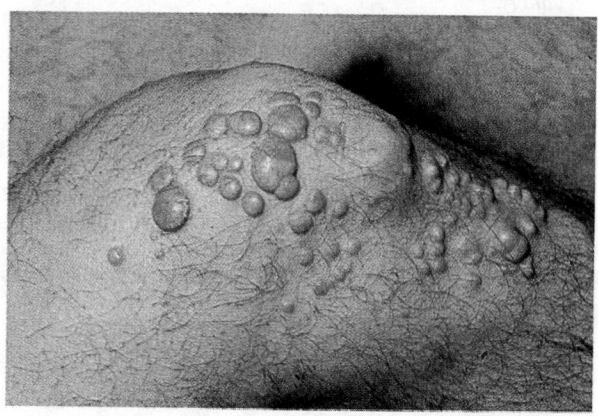

**Xanthoma tuberosum** *(Bloom and Ireland, 1992)*

*Xanthomonas* /zan'thǝmon'ǝs/,  a genus of gram-negative rod-shaped aerobic bacteria that produces a yellow pigment.
*Xanthomonas maltophilia*,  a species of *Xanthomonas* bacteria commonly found in water, milk, and frozen food and in the upper respiratory tract, blood, and urine of humans. It is an opportunistic cause of infections in hospitalized and immunocompromised patients. Also called *Pseudomonas maltophilia.*
**xanthopsia** /zanthop'sē-ǝ/ [Gk, *xanthos* + *opsis,* sight],  an abnormal visual condition in which everything appears to have a yellow hue. It is sometimes associated with jaundice or digitalis toxicity.
**xanthosis** /zanthō'sis/ [Gk, *xanthos* + *osis,* condition],  **1.** a yellowish discoloration sometimes seen in degenerating tissues of malignant diseases. **2.** See **xanthomatosis. 3.** also called **carotenosis.** A reversible yellow discoloration of the skin most commonly caused by the ingestion of large amounts of yellow or orange leafy vegetables containing carotene pigment. The antimalarial drug quinacrine, if taken over a prolonged period, may produce a similar skin color. Xanthosis may be differentiated clinically from jaundice because the sclerae are colored yellow in jaundice but are not discolored in xanthosis. See also **carotenemia.**
**xanthosis of retina,**  a generalized yellow discoloration of the posterior pole of the fundus, sometimes found in diabetic retinopathy.
**xanthotoxin.**  See **methoxsalen.**

**xanthurenic acid** /zan'thŏōrē'nik/, a metabolite of tryptophan that occurs in normal urine and in elevated levels in patients with vitamin B$_6$ deficiency.

**xanthurenic aciduria,** a genetic disorder of tryptophan metabolism characterized by a deficiency of the kynureninase liver enzyme. It is also seen in vitamin B deficiency.

**X chromosome,** a sex chromosome that in humans and many other animals is present in both sexes, appearing singly in the cells of normal males and in duplicate in the cells of normal females. The chromosome is present in all of the female gametes and one half of the male gametes, is much larger than the Y chromosome, and has many sex-linked genes associated with clinically significant disorders, such as hemophilia, Duchenne's muscular dystrophy, and Hunter's syndrome. Compare **Y chromosome.**

**Xe,** symbol for the element **xenon.**

**xeno-** /zē'ne-, zen'ō-/, combining form meaning 'strange or pertaining to foreign matter': *xenodiagnosis, xenogenous, xenology.*

**xenoantibody,** an antibody produced in one species to an antigen derived from a different species.

**xenoantigen** /zē'nō·an'təjən/, an antigen that occurs in organisms of more than one species.

**xenobiotic** /-bī·ot'ik/ [Gk, *xenos,* strange, *bios,* life], pertaining to organic substances that are foreign to the body, such as drugs or organic poisons.

**xenodiagnosis** /-dī·agnō'sis/, a method of diagnosing a vector-transmitted infection such as Chagas' disease, in which a laboratory-reared, pathogen-free insect is allowed to suck blood from a patient. The intestinal contents of the insect are then examined for the presence of the pathogen.

**xenogeneic** /-jənē'ik/ [Gk, *xenos* + *genein,* to produce], **1.** denoting individuals or cell types of different species and different genotypes. **2.** denoting tissues from different species that are therefore antigenically dissimilar. Also **heterologous.** Compare **allogenic, syngeneic.**

**xenogenesis** /zen'əjen'əsis/, **1.** alternation of traits in successive generations; heterogenesis. **2.** the theoretic production of offspring that are totally different from both of the parents. —**xenogenetic, xenogenic,** *adj.*

**xenograft** /zen'əgraft'/ [Gk, *xenos* + *graphion,* stylus], tissue from another species used as a temporary graft in certain cases, as in treating a severely burned patient when sufficient tissue from the patient or from a tissue bank is not available. It is quickly rejected but provides a cover for the burn for the first few days, reducing fluid loss from the open wound. Also called **heterograft.** Compare **allograft, autograft, isograft.** See also **graft.**

**xenology** /zēnol'əjē/ [Gk, *xenos,* stranger, *logos,* science], the study of parasites.

**xenoma** /zēnō'mə/, a tumor that develops on tissue infected with certain parasites.

**xenon (Xe)** /zen'on, zē'non/ [Gk, *xenos,* strange], a nonreactive gaseous nonmetallic element. Its atomic number is 54; its atomic mass is 131.30.

**xenon-133** [Gk, *xenos,* strange], a radioactive isotope of zenon gas, used in radiographic studies of the lung.

**xenoparasite** /-per'əsīt/, an ectoparasite that has become pathogenic as a result of weakened resistance of the host.

**xenophobia** /-fō'bē·ə/ [Gk, *xenos* + *phobos,* fear], an anxiety disorder characterized by a pervasive, irrational fear or uneasiness in the presence of strangers, especially foreigners, or in new surroundings.

*Xenopsylla* /zen'ōsil'ə/, a genus of parasitic fleas responsible for the transmission of bubonic plague and other infections. Many of more than 30 species of *Xenopsylla* are vectors of pathogens, including *X. cheopis,* a rat flea found

worldwide. It is a vector of *Yersinia pestis,* the bacterial source of murine typhus, as well as of the plague.

**xenotransplant.** See **cross-species transplant.**

**xenotype** /zen'ətīp/, molecular variation based on differences in structure and antigenic specificity, such as immunoglobulin from different species.

**xero-** /zir'ō-/, combining form meaning 'dryness': *xerocheilia, xeromenia, xerophthalmia.*

**xeroderma** /zir'ədur'mə/ [Gk, *xeros,* dry, *derma,* skin], a chronic skin condition characterized by dryness and roughness.

**xeroderma pigmentosum (XP),** a rare, inherited skin disease characterized by extreme sensitivity to ultraviolet light, exposure to which results in freckles, telangiectases, keratoses, papillomas, carcinoma, and possibly, melanoma. Keratitis and tumors developing on the eyelids and cornea may result in blindness. Exposure to sunlight must be avoided. See also **Kaposi's disease.**

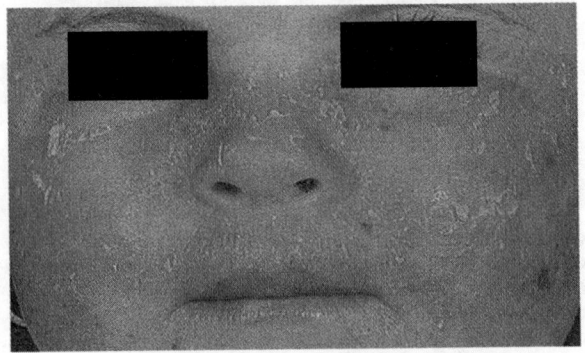

**Xeroderma pigmentosum** *(du Vivier, 1993)*

**xerogram** /zir'əgram'/ [Gk, *xeros* + *gramma,* record], an x-ray image produced by xeroradiography.

**xerography.** See **xeroradiography.**

**xeromammogram** /-mam'əgram'/, a type of breast radiograph produced by xeroradiography.

**xeromammography** /-mamog'rəfē/, the use of xerographic methods to produce radiographic images of the breasts.

**xerophthalmia** /zir'ofthal'mē·ə/ [Gk, *xeros* + *ophthalmos,* eye], a condition of dry and lusterless corneas and conjunctival areas, usually the result of vitamin A deficiency and associated with night blindness.

**xeroradiography** /-rā'dē·og'rəfē/ [Gk, *xeros* + L, *radiare,* to emit rays; Gk, *graphein,* to record], a diagnostic x-ray technique in which images are produced electrically rather than chemically, permitting lower exposure times and radiation energies than those of ordinary x-rays. The latent image is made visible with a powder toner similar to that used in a copying machine. The powder image is transferred and heat-fused to a sheet of paper. The images exhibit "edge contrast" because of the shape of the electrical fields that pull toner onto the plate. Such edge contrast is useful for identifying minute calcifications in the breast. Xeroradiography is used primarily for mammography. Also called **xerography.**

**xerosis.** See **dry skin.**

**xerostomia** /zir'əstō'mē·ə/ [Gk, *xeros* + *stoma,* mouth], dryness of the mouth caused by cessation of normal salivary

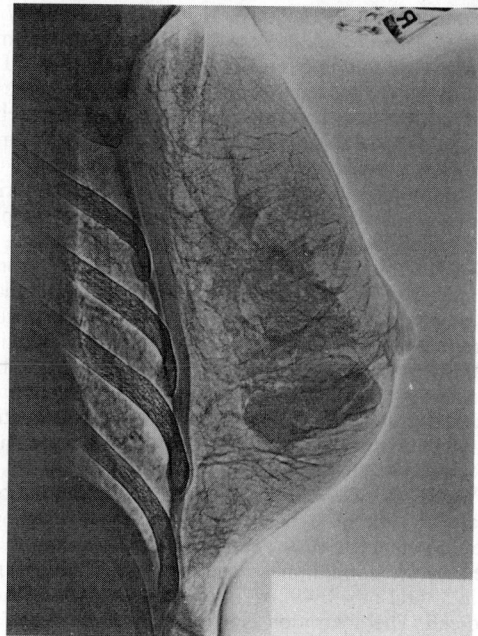

**Xerogram** *(Ballinger, 1995)*

secretion. The condition is a symptom of various diseases such as diabetes, acute infections, hysteria, and Sjögren's syndrome and can be caused by paralysis of facial nerves. It is also a common adverse reaction to drugs.

**xerotic eczema** /zi·rot′ik ek′zə·mə /,   See **asteatosis.**

**xerotic keratitis** /zirot′ik/ [Gk, *xeros,* dry, *keras,* horn, *itis,* inflammation],   an inflammation of the cornea resulting from dryness of the conjunctiva. Underlying causes may be malnutrition, a deficiency of vitamin A, or autoimmune diseases.

**xi** /zī, sī/,   Ξ, ξ, the fourteenth letter of the Greek alphabet.

**X-inactivation.**   See **Lyon hypothesis.**

**xiphi-.** See **xipho-.**

**xiphisternal articulation** /zif′istur′nəl/ [Gk, *xiphos,* sword, *sternon,* chest; L, *articulare,* to divide into joints],   the cartilaginous connection between the xiphoid process and the body of the sternum. This joint usually ossifies at puberty. Compare **manubriosternal articulation.**

**xiphisternum.**   See **xiphoid process.**

**xipho-, xiphi-,**   combining form meaning 'sword or xiphoid process': *xiphodymus, xiphoiditis, xiphopagus.*

**xiphodynia** /zī′fōdin′ē·ə/,   a pain in the xiphoid process.

**xiphoid** /zif′oid/ [Gk, *xiphos,* sword, *eidos,* form],   **1.** shaped like a sword. **2.** See **xiphoid process.**

**xiphoid process** /zif′oid/ [Gk, *xiphos* + *eidos,* form; L, *processus,* going forth],   the smallest of three parts of the sternum, articulating with the inferior end of the body of the sternum above and laterally with the seventh rib. Several muscles of the abdominal wall are attached to the xiphoid process, including the rectus abdominis. Also called **ensiform cartilage, ensiform process, xiphisternum, xiphoid, xiphoid appendix.** Compare **manubrium.**

**xiphopagus** /zīfop′əgəs/,   conjoined twins united at the xiphoid process of the sternum.

**X-linked** /eks′lingkt/,   pertaining to genes or to the characteristics or conditions they transmit that are carried on the X chromosome. Compare **Y-linked.** See also **sex-linked disorder. —X linkage,** *n.*

**X-linked bulbospinal neuropathy,**   a hereditary disorder of the spinal cord and medulla oblongata in males, with associated endocrine features, including azoospermia, gynecomastia, glucose intolerance, and feminized skin changes.

**X-linked disorders,**   diseases and disorders associated with genetic abnormalities on the X chromosomes. Examples are the muscular dystrophies and hemophilias.

**X-linked dominant inheritance,**   a pattern of inheritance in which the transmission of a dominant allele on the X chromosome causes a characteristic to be manifested. Hypophosphatemic vitamin D–resistant rickets is an example of such inheritance. X-linked dominant inheritance closely resembles autosomal-dominant inheritance. Compare **X-linked recessive inheritance.** See also **sex-linked disorder.**

**X-linked ichthyosis.**   See **sex-linked ichthyosis.**

**X-linked inheritance,**   a pattern of inheritance in which the transmission of traits varies according to the sex of the person, because the genes on the X chromosome have no counterparts on the Y chromosome. The inheritance pattern may be recessive or dominant. The trait determined by a gene on the X chromosome is always expressed in males. Transmission from father to son does not occur. Kinds of X-linked inheritance are **X-linked dominant inheritance** and **X-linked recessive inheritance.** Compare **autosomal inheritance.** See also **sex-linked.**

**X-linked lymphoproliferative syndrome,**   a rare X-linked immunodeficiency in which there is a normal response to childhood infection but infection with Epstein-Barr produces a fatal lymphoproliferative disorder. Most patients die of acute infection. Others develop hypogammaglobulinemia, B-cell lymphoma, aplastic anemia, or agranulocytosis.

**X-linked mucopolysaccharidosis.**   See **Hunter's syndrome.**

**X-linked recessive inheritance,**   a pattern of inheritance in which the transmission of a recessive allele on the X chromosome results in a carrier state in females and characteristics of an abnormal condition in males. Affected people have unaffected parents (except for the rare situation in which the father is affected and the mother is a carrier). One half of the female siblings of an affected male carry the trait. Unaffected male siblings do not carry the trait. Sons of affected males are unaffected, and daughters of affected males are carriers. Unaffected male children of a carrier female do not carry the trait. Compare **X-linked dominant inheritance.**

**XO,**   the designation of a cell in which or individual in whom only one sex chromosome is present; either the other X or the Y chromosome is missing so that each cell is monosomic and contains a total of 45 chromosomes. All XO individuals are females with **Turner's syndrome.** Individuals with only a Y chromosome do not survive.

**XP,**   abbreviation for **xeroderma pigmentosum.**

**x radiation.**   See **x-ray.**

**x-ray, 1.** Electromagnetic radiation with wavelengths between about 0.005 and 10 nm. X-rays are produced when electrons traveling at high speed strike certain materials, particularly heavy metals such as tungsten. They can penetrate most substances and are used to investigate the integrity of certain structures, to therapeutically destroy diseased tissue, and to make radiographic images for diagnostic purposes, as in radiography and fluoroscopy. Also called **roentgen ray, x radiation. Discrete x-rays** are those with precisely fixed energies that are characteristic of differences between electron binding energies of a particular element.

Tungsten, for example, has 15 different effective energies and no more, representing emissions from 5 different electron shells. **2.** also called **x-ray film.** A radiograph made by projecting x-rays through organs or structures of the body onto a photographic film. Structures that are relatively radiopaque (allow few x-rays to pass through), such as bones and cavities filled with a radiopaque contrast medium, cast a shadow on the film. Also called **x-ray film. 3.** to make a radiograph. See also **contrast medium, electron, fluoroscopy, radiopaque. —x-ray,** adj.

**x-ray dermatitis,** a skin inflammation caused by exposure to x-rays. Excessive exposure to x-rays can lead to skin cancer.

**x-ray film.** See **x-ray.**

**x-ray fluoroscopy,** real-time imaging using an x-ray source that projects through the patient onto a fluorescent screen or image intensifier. Image-intensified fluoroscopy has replaced conventional fluoroscopy in current practice.

**x-ray microscope,** a microscope that produces images using x-rays and records them on fine-grain film or projects them as enlargements. Film images produced by x-ray microscopes may be examined at large magnifications with a light microscope.

**x-ray pelvimetry,** a radiographic examination used to determine the dimensions of the bony pelvis of a pregnant woman and, if possible, the biparietal diameter of her baby's head. It is performed when doubt exists as to whether the head can pass safely through the pelvis in labor. Images of the pelvis and the baby are projected radiographically onto film. After the film is developed, the images are measured. The measurements are corrected for distortion, and the true dimensions of the birth canal and head are calculated. Often the cephalopelvic relationship cannot be accurately evaluated from the films because the baby's head may be positioned in such a way that the biparietal diameter cannot be visualized. Because minor degrees of cephalopelvic disproportion are often overcome safely in labor by molding of the fetal skull and because major disproportions may be detected by clinical pelvimetry without x-rays, the value of x-ray pelvimetry is frequently judged to be insufficient to warrant the risk of radiation exposure. Other diagnostic tools, among them ultrasonography, often provide the necessary information with less apparent risk. Compare **clinical pelvimetry.** See also **cephalopelvic disproportion, contraction, dystocia.**

**x-ray technologist.** See **radiologic technologist.**

**x-ray tube,** a large vacuum tube containing a tungsten filament cathode and an anode that often is a tungsten disk. When heated to incandescence, the cathode emits a cloud of electrons that produce x-rays when they strike the surface of the anode at high speed. The anode is designed to deflect the x-rays toward an object to be radiographed. X-ray tubes are produced in a variety of designs for different purposes. Low-kilovoltage x-ray tubes may contain anodes made of molybdenum rather than tungsten; some anodes are stationary and others rotate at high speed. Because of the intense heat generated by x-ray production, the specific design usually includes devices to help dissipate the heat.

**x-tra density** /ek'strə/, an image on an x-ray film caused by the presence of a foreign object, such as a bullet or surgical clip in the patient's body.

**XX** /ekseks'/, the designation for the normal sex chromosome complement in the human female. See also **X chromosome.**

**XXX syndrome** /trip'əleks'/, a human sex chromosomal aberration characterized by the presence of three X chromosomes and two Barr bodies instead of the normal XX

complement, so that somatic cells contain a total of 47 chromosomes; trisomy X. The condition occurs approximately once in every 1000 live female births and is confirmed diagnostically by the presence of the extra Barr body in the cells. Individuals with the anomaly show no significant clinical manifestations, although there is usually some degree of mental retardation. Because selective migration of the X chromosome occurs during meiosis, half of the offspring of a trisomy X female will be both chromosomally and phenotypically normal. Also called **triple X syndrome.**

**XXXX, XXXXX** /fôreks', fīveks'/, the designations for abnormal sex chromosome complements in the human female in which there are, respectively, four or five instead of the normal two X chromosomes so that each somatic cell contains a total of 48 or 49 chromosomes. Although there is no consistent phenotype associated with such aberrations, the risk of congenital anomalies and mental retardation in the affected individual increases significantly as the number of X chromosomes increases.

**XXXY, XXXXY, XXYY** /thrē'ekswī, fôr'ekswī, dob'əleks'dob'əlwī'/, the designations for abnormal sex chromosome complements in the human male in which there are more than the normal one X and one Y chromosome resulting, in a total of 48, 49, or more chromosomes in each somatic cell. The aberration is a variant of Klinefelter's syndrome. In general, the more X chromosomes there are, the greater is the number of congenital defects and the severity of mental retardation in the affected individual. See also **Klinefelter's syndrome.**

**XXY syndrome.** See **Klinefelter's syndrome.**

**XY** /ekswī'/, the designation for the normal sex chromosome complement in the human male. See also **X chromosome, Y chromosome.**

**xylitol** /zī'litôl/, a sweet crystalline pentahydroxy alcohol obtained by the reduction of xylose and used as a sweetener in confectionary items such as gum.

**xylo-,** combining form meaning 'wood': *xyloketosuria, xylose, xylosuria.*

**Xylocaine,** trademark for a local anesthetic (lidocaine).

**xylometazoline hydrochloride** /zī'lōmetaz'əlēn/, an adrenergic vasoconstrictor.

■ INDICATIONS: It is prescribed in the treatment of nasal congestion in colds, hay fever, sinusitis, and other upper respiratory allergies.

■ CONTRAINDICATIONS: Glaucoma or known hypersensitivity to this drug or to sympathomimetic medications prohibits its use. It is used with caution in patients having cardiovascular disease.

■ ADVERSE EFFECTS: Among the more serious adverse reactions are irritation to the mucosa, rebound nasal congestion, and effects associated with systemic absorption, including sedation and alterations in cardiovascular function.

**xylose** /zī'lōs/, an aldopentose sugar produced by hydrolyzing straw and corn cobs. It is incompletely absorbed when taken by mouth and is used in diagnostic studies of the digestive tract.

**xylose absorption test,** a laboratory test for intestinal absorption of the monosaccharide D-xylose. Absorption of D-xylose occurs readily in the normal intestine but is diminished in malabsorption patients.

**xysma** /zis'mə/, membranous shreds sometimes found in the feces of patients with diarrhea.

**XYY syndrome** /eks'dob'əlwī'/, the phenotypic manifestation of an extra Y chromosome, which tends to have a positive effect on height and may have a negative effect on mental and psychologic development. However, the anomaly also occurs in normal males. See also **trisomy.**

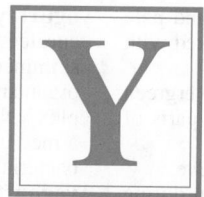

**Y,** symbol for the element **yttrium.**

**-y,** suffix meaning 'a condition or processor having the nature or quality of': *gouty, myopathy.*

**YAC,** abbreviation for **yeast artificial chromosome.**

**YAG,** abbreviation for *yttrium aluminum garnet,* a crystal used in some types of lasers.

**Yallow, Rosalyn Sussman** [U.S, medical physicist, b. 1921], co-winner with Roger Guillemin and Andrew Schally of the 1977 Nobel prize for medicine or physiology for her work in endocrinology and development of the radioimmunoassay technique.

**yang,** a polarized aspect of ch'i that is active or positive energy. See also **ch'i, yin.**

**Yankauer suction catheter,** a rigid hollow tube with a curve at the distal end to facilitate the removal of thick pharyngeal secretions during oral pharyngeal suctioning.

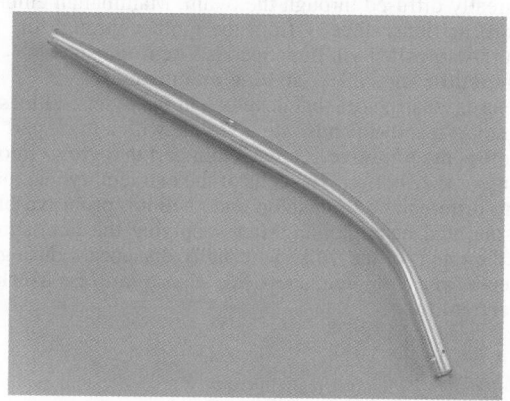

**Yankauer suction catheter** *(Sanders et al, 2000)*

**yarrow,** an herb native to Europe and Asia, now grown in North America.

■ USES: This herb is used to decrease bleeding, to improve circulation, and to treat GI disorders, hypertension, and thrombi.

■ CONTRAINDICATIONS: Yarrow should not be used during pregnancy and lactation. It is also contraindicated in those with known hypersensitivity to this plant or other members of the Compositae family, such as *Chamomilla recutita, Tanacetum parthenium,* or *T. vulgare.*

**yaw** /yô/ [Carib, *VaVa*], a lesion of the syphilis-like tropical disease of yaws. The initial lesion or primary sore is identified as the **mother yaw.**

**yawn** /yôn/ [AS, *geonian*], an involuntary act of opening the mouth wide and taking a deep breath. It tends to occur when a person is bored, drowsy, or depressed and may be accompanied by upper body movements or the act of stretching to aid chest expansion.

**yaws** /yôs/ [Afr, *yaw,* raspberry], a chronic nonvenereal infection caused by the spirochete *Treponema pallidum* subsp.

*pertenue,* transmitted by direct contact. It is characterized by chronic, ulcerating sores anywhere on the body but usually on the legs, with eventual tissue and bone destruction, leading to crippling if untreated. It is a disease of unsanitary tropical living conditions and may be effectively treated with penicillin G. All serologic tests for syphilis may be positive in yaws. The infection may afford protection against syphilis. Also called **bouba, buba, frambesia, framboesia, parangi, patek, pian.** Compare **bejel, pinta, syphilis.**

**Yb,** symbol for the element **ytterbium.**

**Y-cartilage,** a Y-shaped band of connective tissue that extends through the acetabulum to join the ilium, ischium, and pubis. Also called **hypsiloid cartilage.**

**Y chromosome,** a sex chromosome that in humans and many other animals is present only in the male, appearing singly in the normal male. It is present in one half of the male gametes and none of the female gametes, is much smaller than the X chromosome, and has genes associated with triggering the development and differentiation of male characteristics. Compare **X chromosome.**

**years of potential life lost (YPLL),** an evaluation of the economic, social, and other consequences of premature death in a population from injury or disease as compared to the potential productivity of the deceased if they had lived normal lifespans.

**yeast** /yēst/ [AS, *gist*], any unicellular, usually oval, nucleated fungus that reproduces by budding. *Candida albicans* is a kind of pathogenic yeast.

**yeast artificial chromosome (YAC),** a yeast chromosome used in recombinant DNA procedures. It can carry large segments of foreign DNA.

**yellow cartilage.** See **elastic cartilage.**

**yellow fever,** an acute arbovirus infection transmitted by mosquitoes. It is characterized by headache, fever, jaundice, vomiting, and bleeding. There is no specific treatment, and mortality is about 5%. Recovery is followed by lifelong immunity. Immunization for travelers to endemic areas is advised. Nonhuman primates are a reservoir of infection.

**yellow fever vaccine,** a vaccine produced from live, attenuated yellow fever virus grown in chick embryos.

■ INDICATION: It is prescribed for immunization against yellow fever.

■ CONTRAINDICATIONS: Immunosuppression, pregnancy, or known hypersensitivity to chicken or egg protein prohibits its use.

■ ADVERSE EFFECTS: Among the more serious adverse effects are fever, malaise, and hypersensitivity reactions.

**yellow hepatization.** See **hepatization.**

**yellow jacket venom,** a toxin injected by the stings of wasps and hornets. It can induce potentially fatal anaphylactic shock.

**yellow marrow,** bone marrow in which the fat cells predominate in the meshes of the reticular network. See also **bone marrow.**

**yellow nail syndrome,** a condition in which there is complete or almost complete cessation of nail growth and loss of cuticle. Nails become thickened, convex, opaque, and pale yellow to yellowish green. The condition is associated with pulmonary disorders and lymphedema.

**yerba maté,** an herbal product taken from an evergreen tree belonging to the holly family that is native to parts of South America.

- ■ USES: This herb is used as a diuretic and depurative.
- ■ CONTRAINDICATIONS: Yerba maté should not be used during pregnancy and lactation, in children, or in those with anxiety disorders, hypertension, or known hypersensitivity to this plant.

*Yersinia* /yersin′ē·ə/ [Alexandre E.J. Yersin, French bacteriologist, 1862–1943], a genus of nonmotile ovoid or rod-shaped gram-negative bacteria of the Enterobacteriaceae family.

*Yersinia* **arthritis** [Alexandre E. J. Yersin], a polyarticular inflammation occurring a few days to 1 month after the onset of infection caused by *Yersinia enterocolitica* or *Y. pseudotuberculosis* and usually persisting longer than 1 month. Knees, ankles, toes, fingers, and wrists are most often affected. Cultures of synovial fluid yield no infectious organism. The clinical presentation may mimic juvenile rheumatoid arthritis, rheumatic fever, or Reiter's syndrome and may be associated with erythema nodosum or erythema multiforme. Treatment is with antibiotics.

*Yersinia* **enterocolitica,** a ubiquitous species isolated from mammals, birds, and frogs, and from material contaminated by feces; it is transmitted by infected food and water and by person-to-person contact and causes yersiniosis in humans.

*Yersinia* **pestis** [Alexandre E. J. Yersin; L, *pestis,* plague], a species of small gram-negative bacteria that causes plague. The primary host is the rat, but other small rodents also harbor the organism. A person without symptoms may be a carrier, but this happens rarely. *Yersinia pestis* is hardy, living for long periods in infected carcasses, the soil of the host's habitat, or sputum. Also called *Pasteurella pestis.* See also **plague.**

*Yersinia* **pseudotuberculosis,** a species found in the intestinal tract of birds, rodents, and other animals; it causes mesenteric adenitis and pseudotuberculosis in humans who have contact with infected food or animals.

**yersiniosis** /yər·sin′·ē·ō′sis /, infection with bacteria of the genus *Yersinia,* especially *Y. enterocolitica,* which causes symptoms such as acute gastroenteritis and mesenteric adenitis in children and arthritis, septicemia, and erythema nodosum in adults.

**Y fracture,** a Y-shaped fracture of the tissue between condyles.

**yield,** **1.** an amount or quantity produced in return for an effort or investment. **2.** the energy released by a nuclear reaction.

**yin,** a polarized aspect of ch′i that is passive or negative energy. See also **ch′i, yang.**

**-yl,** suffix used in naming radicals: *benzoyl, ethyl, hydroxyl.*

**-ylene,** suffix for chemical terms relating to a bivalent hydrocarbon radical, as in the reagent aminoxylene.

**Y-linked** /wī′lingkt/, pertaining to genes or to the characteristics or conditions they transmit that are carried on the Y chromosome. Excess hair on the pinna of the ear may be Y-linked. Compare **X-linked.** See also **sex-linked. —Y linkage,** *n.*

**Yodoxin,** trademark for an antiamebic (diiodohydroxyquin).

**yoga,** a discipline that focuses on the body's musculature, posture, breathing mechanisms, and consciousness. The goal of yoga is attainment of physical and mental well-being through mastery of the body, achieved through exercise, holding of postures, proper breathing, and meditation.

**yogurt** /yō′gərt/ [Turk, *yoghurt*], a slightly acid, semisolid, curdled milk preparation made from either whole or skimmed cow's milk and milk solids by fermentation with organisms from the genus *Lactobacillus.* It is rich in B complex vitamins and a good source of protein. It also provides a medium in the GI tract that retards the growth of harmful bacteria and aids in mineral absorption. Also spelled **yoghurt.**

**yohimbe,** an herbal product taken from the bark of a tree that is native to areas of West Africa.

- ■ USES: This herb is used to treat male organic impotence.
- ■ CONTRAINDICATIONS: Yohimbe should not be used during pregnancy and lactation, in children, or in those with known hypersensitivity to this plant. Prolonged use is contraindicated, as is the use of this herb in those with renal or hepatic disease, hypertension, angina pectoris, gastric or duodenal ulcers, bipolar disorder, anxiety disorder, schizophrenia, suicidal tendencies, and prostatitis.

**yoke** /yōk/ [L, *jungere,* to join], a connector used to link small cylinders of medical gases, such as portable oxygen tanks, to respiratory equipment.

**yolk** /yōk,yelk/ [AS, *geolca*], a material rich in fats and proteins that is contained in an ovum and that supplies nourishment to the developing embryo. The amount and distribution of the yolk within the ovum depend on the species of animal and the type of reproduction and development of offspring. In humans and most other mammals, yolk is absent or greatly diffused through the ovum. Mammalian embryos absorb nutrients directly from the mother through the placenta. Also called **vitellus.** See also **deutoplasm.**

**yolk membrane.** See **vitelline membrane.**

**yolk sac,** a structure that develops in the inner cell mass of the embryo and expands into a vesicle with a thick part that becomes the primitive gut and a thin part that grows into the cavity of the chorion. The cells of the extraembryonic mesoderm differentiate to develop endothelium, primitive blood plasma, and hemoglobin. After supplying the nourishment for the embryo, the yolk sac usually disappears during the seventh week of pregnancy. See also **allantois, Meckel's diverticulum.**

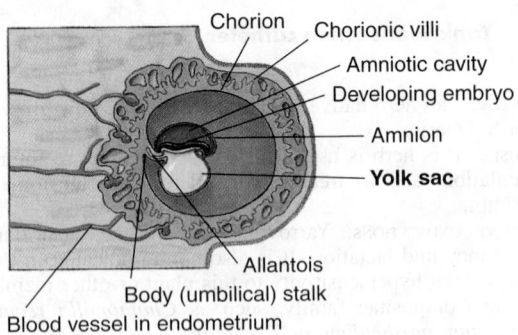

Yolk sac (Applegate, 2000)

**yolk sphere.** See **morula.**

**yolk stalk,** the narrow duct connecting the yolk sac with the midgut of the embryo during the early stages of prenatal development. It connects at the region of the future ileum and usually undergoes complete obliteration but occasionally may appear as a diverticulum. Also called **ompha-lomesenteric duct, umbilical duct, vitelline duct.** See also **Meckel's diverticulum.**

**young and middle adult,** the stages of life from 22 to 65 years of age.

**Young-Helmholtz theory of color vision** [Thomas Young, English physician, 1773–1829; Hermann L.F. von Helmholtz, German physician, physicist, and physiologist, 1821–1894], the concept that all color sensations are mediated by three types of retinal receptors, which correspond to three primary colors: red, green, and blue-violet. By their individual and combined activities, the receptors produce the perception of all visible hues.

**young offender.** See **juvenile delinquent.**

**Young prostatic tractor** [Hugh Young, American urologist, 1870–1945], a short straight surgical instrument with blades operated by a knob, for use in open perineal prostatectomy. The device can be inserted through the prostatic urethra and by direct traction used to draw down the prostate gland into the operative field.

**Young's operation** [Hugh Young, American, urologist, 1870-1945], **1.** the surgical construction of a new urethra to repair a structural defect of the penis. **2.** perineal prostatectomy.

**Y-plasty** /wī′plas′tē/, a method of surgical revision of a scar, using a Y-shaped incision to reduce scar contractures. See also **Z-plasty.**

**YPLL,** abbreviation for **years of potential life lost.**

**Y-set,** a device composed of plastic components, used for delivering IV fluids through a primary IV line connected to a combination drip chamber filter section from which two separate plastic tubes lead to fluid sources. The Y-set also includes three clamps, one for the primary IV line and one for each of the two separate tubes. It is often used to transfuse blood cells used for any type of blood administration that must be diluted with saline solution to decrease their viscosity. In such a transfusion one of the tubes is connected to the container of blood cells; the other tube is connected to the container of saline solution. Compare **component drip set, component syringe set, microaggregate recipient set, straight line blood set.**

**ytterbium (Yb)** /itur′bē·əm/ [Ytterby, Sweden], a rare earth metallic element. Its atomic number is 70; its atomic mass (weight) is 173.04.

**yttrium (Y)** /it′rē·əm/ [Ytterby, Sweden], a scaly, grayish metallic element. Its atomic number is 39; its atomic mass (weight) is 88.905. Radioactive isotopes of yttrium have been used in cancer therapy.

**Yutopar,** trademark for a beta-adrenergic drug (ritodrine hydrochloride).

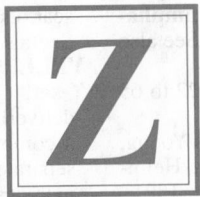

**zafirlukast,** a bronchodilator.
- INDICATIONS: This drug is used for prophylaxis and chronic treatment of asthma in adults and in children less than 12 years of age.
- CONTRAINDICATIONS: Known hypersensitivity to this drug prohibits its use.
- ADVERSE EFFECTS: Adverse reactions to this drug include headache, dizziness, nausea, diarrhea, abdominal pain, vomiting, infections, pain, asthenia, myalgia, fever, dyspepsia, and increased ALT.

**Zahorsky's disease.** See **roseola infantum.**

**Zakrzewski, Marie** /zakshef′ skē/ (1829–1902), a Polish-German-American midwife who studied medicine in Berlin before emigrating to the United States. In New York she met Elizabeth Blackwell, who encouraged her to continue her medical studies. After receiving her medical degree in Cleveland, she worked at Blackwell's New York Infirmary before going to Boston. In 1872 she organized the first successful American school of nursing at the New England Hospital for Women and Children.

**zalcitabine,** an antiretroviral nucleoside reverse transcriptase inhibitor analog. Also known as **ddC, dideoxycytidine.**
- INDICATIONS: It is prescribed in the treatment of human immunodeficiency virus infections.
- CONTRAINDICATIONS: The drug should not be given to patients with an allergy to zalcitabine or any of its components. Zalcitabine is not a cure, and acquired immunodeficiency syndrome patients may continue to acquire symptoms associated with the disease. Caution is recommended in patients with low CD4 cell counts, esophageal ulcers, numbness or tingling in the extremities, or a history of pancreatitis or alcohol abuse.
- ADVERSE EFFECTS: The side effects most often reported include nausea, appetite loss, stomach pain, headache, dizziness, fatigue, dry mouth, and night sweats.

**zaleplon,** a sedative/hypnotic.
- INDICATIONS: This drug is used to treat insomnia.
- CONTRAINDICATIONS: Known hypersensitivity to this drug prohibits its use.
- ADVERSE EFFECTS: Adverse reactions to this drug include dizziness, confusion, anxiety, amnesia, depersonalization, hallucinations, hypesthesia, paresthesia, somnolence, tremor, vertigo, nausea, abdominal pain, constipation, anorexia, colitis, dyspepsia, dry mouth, vision changes, ear/eye pain, hyperacusis, parosmia, asthenia, fever, headache, myalgia, and dysmenorrhea. Common side effects include lethargy, drowsiness, and daytime sedation.

**zanamivir,** an antiviral.
- INDICATIONS: Zanamivir is used to treat type A influenza in patients who have had symptoms for no more than 2 days.
- CONTRAINDICATIONS: Known hypersensitivity to this drug prohibits its use.
- ADVERSE EFFECTS: Adverse reactions to this drug include fatigue, ear-nose-throat infections, diarrhea, nasal symptoms, cough, sinusitis, and bronchitis. Common side effects include headache, dizziness, nausea, and vomiting.

**Zarontin,** trademark for an anticonvulsant (ethosuximide).

**Zaroxolyn,** trademark for a diuretic and antihypertensive (metolazone).

**Z band.** See **Z line.**

**Z chromosome.** See **W chromosome and Z chromosome.**

**Z disk.** See **Z line.**

**ZDV,** abbreviation for **zidovudine.**

**Zeeman effect** /sē′man, tsā′mon/ [Pieter Zeeman, Dutch physicist and Nobel Laureate, 1865–1945], a splitting of lines in an emission spectrum into three or more symmetrically placed lines when the radiation source is in a magnetic field.

**ZEEP,** abbreviation for **zero-end expiratory pressure.**

**Zeitgeist** /tsīt′gīst/ [Ger], literally, the spirit of the time, a climate of opinion, a convention of thought, or implicit assumptions.

**Zellweger syndrome** [Hans Ulrich Zellweger, American pediatrician, 1909–1990], See **cerebrohepatorenal syndrome.**

**Zemuron,** trademark for a nondepolarizing neuromuscular blocking agent (rocuronium bromide).

**Zenker's diverticulum** /tseng′kerz/ [Friedrich A. Zenker, German pathologist, 1825–1898; L, *diverticulare,* to turn aside], a circumscribed herniation of the mucous membrane of the pharynx as it joins the esophagus. It is the most common type of diverticulum of the esophagus. Food may become trapped in the diverticulum and can be aspirated. Diagnosis is confirmed by x-ray studies. In most cases the herniation is small, causes no dysfunction, is not diagnosed, and requires no treatment.

**zeolites,** hydrated silicates of aluminum used in ion exchange water softeners. Synthetic zeolites are used as porous molecular containers for reagents and drugs.

**Zephiran Chloride,** trademark for a disinfectant (benzalkonium chloride).

**zeranol** /zer′ənol/, an estrogenic substance used to fatten livestock. Consumption of beef from zeranol-treated cattle has been associated with precocious puberty in some boys and girls.

**Zerit,** trademark for a synthetic thymidine nucleoside analog (stavudine).

**zero** /zir′ō/ [Ar, *sifr,* cipher], **1.** nothing. **2.** the point on most scales from which measurements begin. **3.** absolute zero (0 K) on the Kelvin scale, the temperature at which there is no molecular movement, corresponding to $-273.15°$ C or $-459.67°$ F.

**zero dose,** the absence of added ligand. Also called **B₀.**

**zero-end expiratory pressure (ZEEP)** [Ar, *zefiro* + ME, *ende*], pressure in the airways that has returned to ambient or atmospheric pressure at the end of exhalation.

**zero fluid balance,** a state in which the amount of fluid intake is equal to the amount of fluid output.

**zero gravity,** a physical state of weightlessness in space or during flight when the centrifugal thrust on a body in a parabolic glide exactly counteracts the force of gravity.

**zero order kinetics,** a state at which the rate of an enzyme reaction is independent of the concentration of the substrate.

**zero population growth (ZPG),** a situation in which there is no population increase during a given year because the total of live births is equal to the total of deaths.

**zero-to-three infant stimulation groups,** groups that provide therapeutic services for children from birth to 3 years of age, an age group not yet eligible for public school placement.

**zero V/Q,** an intrapulmonary shunt that allows blood to pass through the lungs without entering alveolar capillaries, causing hypoxemia. Also called **true shunt.**

**Zestril,** trademark for an angiotensin-converting enzyme inhibitor and antihypertensive (lisinopril).

**zeta** /zē′tə, zā′tə/, Z, ζ, the sixth letter of the Greek alphabet.

**zeta potential** [Gk, *zeta,* sixth letter of Greek alphabet; L, *potentia,* power], the potential produced by the effective charge of a macromolecule, usually measured at the boundary between what is moving in a solution with the macromolecule and the rest of the solution.

**Zetar,** trademark for a topical antieczematic containing coal tar.

**zeugmatography** /zoōg′mətog′rəfē/ [Gk, *zeugnynai,* to join, *graphein,* to record]. See **magnetic resonance imaging.**

**zidovudine (ZDV)** /zīdov′ədēn/, a pyrimidine nucleoside analog active against human immunodeficiency virus. Formerly called **azidothymidine (AZT).**

■ INDICATIONS: Its function is to inhibit the reverse transcriptase enzyme of the human immunodeficiency virus (HIV). It is used in the management of patients with HIV infection who have some evidence of impaired immunity. It also may be used for prophylaxis after exposure to HIV.

■ CONTRAINDICATIONS: It must be used cautiously in patients with impaired renal or hepatic function; it must also be used cautiously in patients with preexisting bone marrow suppression.

■ ADVERSE EFFECTS: Headache, GI disturbances, insomnia, flulike symptoms, rash, fatigue, myalgia, and central nervous system symptoms may occur during the first weeks of therapy. The drug may cause granulocytopenia and macrocytic anemia, particularly in patients with advanced HIV disease.

**Ziehl-Neelsen test** /zēl′nēl′sən/ [Franz Ziehl, German bacteriologist, 1857–1926; Friedrich K. A. Neelsen, German pathologist, 1854–1894], one of the most widely used methods of acid-fast staining, commonly used in the microscopic examination of a smear of sputum suspected of containing *Mycobacterium tuberculosis.* See also **acid-fast stain.**

**Ziehl's stain.** See **carbol-fuchsin stain.**

**Zieve's syndrome** [Leslie Zieve, American physician, b. 1915], a mild spherocytic anemia with transient jaundice and hyperlipidemia found in patients with acute alcoholism and liver cirrhosis.

**ZIFT,** abbreviation for **zygote intrafallopian transfer.**

**ZIG,** abbreviation for **zoster immune globulin.**

**zig-zag.** See **swan neck deformity.**

**zileuton,** a bronchodilator and leukotriene pathway inhibitor.

■ INDICATIONS: This drug is used to treat allergic rhinitis and asthma.

■ CONTRAINDICATIONS: Factors that prohibit the use of this drug are hepatic disease, liver function test results three times higher than upper limits, and known hypersensitivity to zileuton.

■ ADVERSE EFFECTS: Adverse reactions to this drug include dizziness, insomnia, fatigue, paresthesias, headache, nausea, abdominal pain, dyspepsia, diarrhea, liver function test abnormalities, hives, myalgia, and asthenia.

**Zimmermann reaction** /zim′ərman, tsim′ərmon/ [Wilhelm Zimmermann, German physician, b. 1910], a chromogen reaction previously used for detecting androgens with the 17-keto configuration. It involves a reaction between an alkaline solution of meta-dinitrobenzene and an active methylene group.

**Zinacef,** trademark for a cephalosporin antibiotic (cefuroxime sodium).

**zinc (Zn)** /zingk/ [Ger, *Zink*], a bluish-white crystalline metal commonly associated with lead ores. Its atomic number is 30; its atomic mass is 65.38. It is ductile in its pure form and occurs abundantly in minerals such as sphalerite, zincite, and franklinite. It has many commercial uses, such as a protective coating for steel and in printing plates. It is an essential nutrient in the body and is used in numerous pharmaceutics, such as zinc acetate, zinc oxide, zinc permanganate, and zinc stearate. Zinc acetate is used as an emetic, a styptic, and an astringent. Zinc oxide is used internally as an antispasmodic and as a protective in ointments. Zinc permanganate is used as an astringent and in the treatment of urethritis by injection or douche in a 1:4000 solution. Zinc stearate is used as a water-repellent protective agent in the treatment of acne, eczema, and other skin diseases.

**zinc chill.** See **metal fume fever.**

**zinc deficiency,** a condition resulting from insufficient amounts of zinc in the diet. It is characterized by abnormal fatigue, decreased alertness, a decrease in taste and odor sensitivity, poor appetite, retarded growth, delayed sexual maturity, prolonged healing of wounds, and susceptibility to infection and injury. Other conditions that may precipitate the deficiency include alcoholic cirrhosis and other liver diseases, and ulcers, myocardial infarction. Prophylaxis and treatment consist of a diet of foods high in protein, which are also rich in zinc, including meats, eggs, liver, seafood, legumes, nuts, peanut butter, milk, and whole-grain cereals.

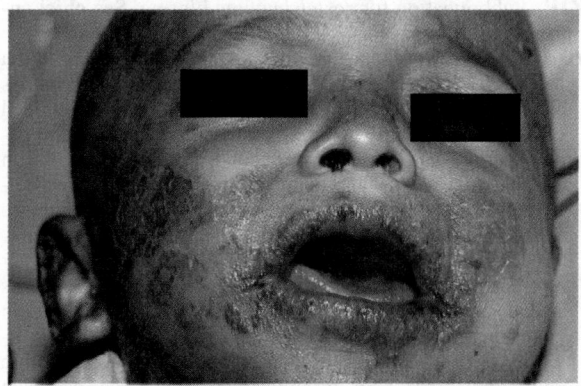

**Zinc deficiency causing hemorrhagic dermatitis**
*(Kumar, Cotran, and Robbins, 1997)*

**zinc finger,** a loop of a transcription factor that is stabilized by a zinc atom linked to four carbon atoms in the protein. It is an important step in the cloning and sequencing of human general transcription factors because individual proteins appear to be involved in the regulation of transcription and in RNA transport.

**zinc gelatin,** a topical protectant for varicosities and other lesions of the lower limbs. It is available as a smooth jelly containing zinc oxide (10%), gelatin (15%), glycerin (40%), and purified water (35%). It is also available impregnated in gauze.

**zinc ointment** [Ger, *Zink* + OFr, *oignement*], a preparation of 20% zinc oxide in mineral oil or a white petrolatum semisolid base, used as a local surface treatment for various skin disorders. Some preparations also may contain salicylic acid.

**zinc oxide,** a topical protectant used for a wide range of minor skin irritations.

**zinc oxide and eugenol (ZOE),** a dental cement composed primarily of zinc salts, eugenol, and rosin, used chiefly in temporary tooth fillings. It has low relative strength and abrasion resistance, but its nearly neutral pH causes minimal irritation to dental pulp. It is intended as a sedative dressing until pain subsides and a more permanent filling can be inserted. Also called **zinc oxide eugenol dental cement.**

**zinc phosphate dental cement,** a material for coating or attaching dental inlays, crowns, bridges, and orthodontic appliances and for some temporary restorations of teeth. It is prepared by mixing a powder composed of zinc and magnesium oxides and a liquid composed of phosphoric acid, water, and buffering agents.

**zinc salt poisoning,** a toxic condition caused by the ingestion or inhalation of a zinc salt. Symptoms of ingestion include a burning sensation of the mouth and throat, vomiting, diarrhea, abdominal and chest pain, and in severe cases shock and coma. Inhalation of zinc salts may cause metal fume fever; skin contact may produce blisters. A lethal dose of 10 g of zinc sulfate has been reported.

**zinc sulfate,** an ophthalmic astringent given in drops for nasal congestion or irritation of the eye, applied topically in deodorants, and given orally in tablets to promote healing and as a dietary supplement.

**Zinecard,** trademark for a cardioprotective agent against cardiac toxicity induced by doxorubicin (dexrazoxane).

**ZIP,** abbreviation for *zoster immune plasma.* See **chickenpox.**

**zirconium (Zr)** /zərkō′nē·əm/ [Ar, *zarqun,* zircon], a steel-gray, tetravalent metallic element. Its atomic number is 40; its atomic mass is 91.22. It occurs widely in combined form, especially in zircon and baddeleyite. It is usually extracted from sands containing zircon by heating with carbon and chlorine and passing the resulting volatile zirconium tetrachloride into hot molten magnesium or into sodium to yield a spongy form of the free metal. A component of zirconium dioxide was formerly used in some ointments for the treatment of poison ivy skin rashes, but such ointments caused skin granulomas in some individuals. Similar skin conditions developed in individuals using deodorants containing zirconium sodium lactate, and the use of zirconium compounds, except for zirconyl hydroxychloride, has been discontinued in the manufacture of skin ointments. Zirconyl hydroxychloride is still used in antiperspirants.

**zirconium granuloma,** an inflammatory lesion, usually occurring in the axilla as a reaction to zirconium salts in antiperspirants.

**Zithromax,** trademark for an antibiotic (azithromycin).

**Z line,** a narrow, darkly staining cross-striation that bisects the I band of skeletal muscles. The distance between Z lines is the length of the sarcomere. Also called **intermediate disk, Z band, Z disk.** See also **I band, sarcomere.**

**Zn,** symbol for the element **zinc.**

**zoacanthosis** /zō′akanthō′sis/, a dermatitis caused by retention in the skin of foreign bodies such as insect stingers, animal hairs, or bristles.

**zoanthropy** /zō·an′thrəpē/ [Gk, *zoon,* animal, *anthropos,* human], the delusion that one has assumed the form and characteristics of an animal. —**zoanthropic,** *adj.*

**ZOE,** abbreviation for **zinc oxide and eugenol.**

**-zoite,** combining form meaning a 'simple organism' of a specified sort: *merozoite, saprozoite, sporozoite.*

**Zollinger-Ellison syndrome** /zol′injərel′isən/ [Robert M. Zollinger, American surgeon, 1903–1992; Edwin H. Ellison, American physician, 1918–1970], a condition characterized by severe peptic ulceration, gastric hypersecretion, elevated serum gastrin, and gastrinoma of the pancreas or the duodenum. The syndrome is uncommon and occurs in a bipolar distribution such as in early childhood but is seen more frequently in people between 20 and 50 years of age. Two thirds of the tumors are malignant. Total gastrectomy may be necessary, but the administration of cimetidine in large doses may control gastric hypersecretion and allow the ulcers to heal. See also **peptic ulcer.**

**zolmitriptan,** a migraine agent.

■ INDICATIONS: This drug is used in the acute treatment of migraine with or without aura.

■ CONTRAINDICATIONS: Factors that prohibit the use of this drug include angina pectoris, a history of myocardial infarction, documented silent ischemia, ischemic heart disease, concurrent use of ergotamine-containing preparations, uncontrolled hypertension, known hypersensitivity to this drug, and basilar or hemiplegic migraine.

■ ADVERSE EFFECTS: Adverse reactions to this drug include palpitations, abdominal discomfort, myalgia, and chest tightness and pressure. Common side effects include weakness, neck stiffness, tingling, hot sensation, burning, a feeling of pressure and tightness in the head, numbness, dizziness, and sedation.

**zombie** /zom′bē/, a supernatural power that supposedly can enter into and reanimate a corpse.

**zona** /zō′nə/, *pl.* **zonae** [Gk, *zone,* belt], a zone, or girdle-like segment of a rounded or spheric structure. See also **zone.**

**zona ciliaris.** See **ciliary zone.**

**zona fasciculata,** the middle part of the adrenal cortex, which is the site of production of glucocorticoids and sex hormones.

**zona glomerulosa,** the outer part of the adrenal cortex, where mineralocorticoids are produced.

**zona pellucida** /pəloo′sidə/, the thick, transparent, noncellular membrane that encloses a mammalian ovum. It is secreted by the maturing oocyte during its development in the ovary and is retained until near the time of implantation. Also called **oolemma.** See also **vitelline membrane.**

**zona radiata,** a zona pellucida that has a striated appearance caused by radiating canals within the membrane. Also called **zona striata.**

**zona reticularis,** the innermost part of the adrenal cortex, which borders on the adrenal medulla part of the gland. It acts in consort with the zona fasciculata in producing various sex hormones and glucocorticoids.

**zona striata.** See **zona radiata.**

**zonate** /zō′nāt/, having ringed layers with differing colors or textures.

**zone** [Gk, belt], an area with specific boundaries and characteristics, such as the epigastric, mesogastric, and hypogastric zones of the abdomen, or the breasts, lips, or genitals. See also **zona.**

**zone of equivalence,** a region of an antibody-antigen reaction in which concentrations of both reactants are equal.

**zonesthesia** /zō'nesthē'zhə/ [Gk, *zone* + *aisthesis,* feeling], a painful sensation of constriction, as of a bandage bound too tightly, especially experienced around the waist or abdomen. Also called **girdle sensation.**

**zone therapy,** the treatment of a disorder by mechanical stimulation and counterirritation of a body area in the same longitudinal zone as the affected organ or region.

**zonifugal** /zōnif'yəgəl/ [Gk, *zone,* belt; L, *fugere,* to flee], moving from within a zone or area outward.

**zonography** /zōnog'rəfē/ [Gk, *zone* + *graphein,* to record], an x-ray imaging technique used to produce films of body sections similar to those made by tomography. A very narrow exposure angle of less than 10 degrees is used in zonography, producing a focal zone of less than 1 inch in thickness.

**zonula** /zōn'yələ/, *pl.* **zonulae** [Gk, *zone,* belt], a small zone or band. Also called **zonule.**

**zonula adherens** [L, *zone,* belt, *adhaerere,* to stick], a continuous zone running around the outer surface of a cell in which there is an intercellular space of about 15 to 20 nm width. A component of the junctional complex between cells, the zone contains dense filamentous material.

**zonula ciliaris,** a ligament composed of straight fibrils radiating from the ciliary body of the eye to the crystalline lens, holding the lens in place and relaxing by the contraction of the ciliary muscle. Relaxation of the ligament allows the lens to become more convex. Also called **zonule of Zinn.**

**zonulae, zonule.** See **zonula.**

**zonula occludens** [L, *zona,* belt, *occludere,* to close up], a component of the junctional complex between cells in which there is no intercellular space and the plasma membranes of adjacent cells are in direct contact.

**zonule of Zinn.** See **zonula ciliaris.**

**zoo-, zo-** /zō'ə-/, combining form meaning 'animal': *zooamylon, zoogony, zoonosis.*

**zoobiology** /-bī·ol'əjē/ [Gk, *zoon,* animal, *bios,* life, *logos,* science], the biology of animals.

**zoochemistry** /-kem'istrē/ [Gk, *zoon,* animal, *chemeia,* alchemy], the biochemistry of animals.

**zooerastia.** See **bestiality.**

**zoogenous** /zō·oj'ənəs/ [Gk, *zoon,* animal, *genein,* to produce], acquired from or originating in animals. See also **zoonosis.**

**zoograft** /zō'əgraft/ [Gk, *zoon* + *graphion,* stylus], tissue of an animal transplanted to a human, such as a heart valve from a pig to replace a damaged heart valve in a human.

**zoologist** /zō·ol'əjist/ [Gk, *zoon,* animal, *logos,* science], a person concerned with the scientific study of animals.

**zoology** /zō·ol'əjē/, the study of animal life.

**zoom** /zoom/, a system of camera lenses that allows an object to remain in focus when the camera approaches or recedes or when the object is viewed close-up or at a distance.

**zoomania** /zō·əmā'nē·ə/ [Gk, *zoon* + *mania,* madness], a psychopathologic state characterized by an excessive fondness for and preoccupation with animals. **—zoomaniac,** *n.*

**-zoon,** combining form meaning a 'living being': *dermatozoon, entozoon, hepatozoon.*

**zoonosis** /zō·on'əsis, zō'ənō'sis/ [Gk, *zoon* + *nosis,* disease], a disease of animals that is transmissible to humans from its primary animal host. Some kinds of zoonoses are **equine encephalitis, leptospirosis, rabies,** and **yellow fever.**

**zooparasite** /zō·əper'əsīt/ [Gk, *zoon* + *parasitos,* guest], any parasitic animal organism. Kinds of zooparasites are **arthropods, protozoa,** and **worms. —zooparasitic,** *adj.*

**zoopathology** /-pəthol'əjē/, the study of the diseases of animals.

**zoophilia** /zō·əfil'ē·ə/ [Gk, *zoon* + *philein,* to love], **1.** an abnormal fondness for animals. **2.** (in psychiatry) a psychosexual disorder in which sexual excitement and gratification are derived from the fondling of animals or from the fantasy or act of engaging in sexual activity with animals. Also called **zoophilism** /zō·of'iliz'əm/. See also **paraphilia. —zoophile,** *n.,* **zoophilic, zoophilous,** *adj.*

**zoophobia** /-fō'bē·ə/ [Gk, *zoon* + *phobos,* fear], an anxiety disorder characterized by a persistent, irrational fear of animals, particularly dogs, snakes, insects, and mice. The condition is seen more often in women than in men, nearly always begins in childhood, and can typically be traced to some frightening or unpleasant experience involving an animal. Treatment consists of psychotherapy to uncover the cause of the phobic reaction followed by behavior therapy, specifically the techniques of systemic desensitization and flooding.

**zoopsia** /zō·op'sē·ə/ [Gk, *zoon* + *opsis,* vision], a visual hallucination of animals or insects, often occurring in delirium tremens.

**zootoxin** /zō'ətok'sin/ [Gk, *zoon* + *toxikon,* poison], a poisonous substance from an animal, such as the venom of snakes, spiders, and scorpions. **—zootoxic,** *adj.*

**zoster.** See **herpes zoster.**

**zoster auricularis** /zos'tər/, an acute earache with herpetic blebs on the eardrum and external auditory meatus.

**zosteriform** /zoster'ifôrm/ [Gk, *zoster,* girdle; L, *forma,* form], resembling the pocks seen in herpes zoster infection.

**zoster immune globulin (ZIG)** [Gk, *zoster* + L, *immunis,* freedom, *globulus,* small sphere], a passive immunizing agent currently in limited experimental use for preventing or attenuating herpes zoster virus infection in immunosuppressed individuals who are at great risk of severe herpes zoster virus infection.

**zoster ophthalmicus** [Gk, *zoster,* girdle, *ophthalmos,* eye], a herpes infection of the eye, particularly of the optic nerve. The infection frequently involves the cornea. There may be lid edema, ciliary and conjunctival involvement, and pain. Keratitis may be severe. Scarring and glaucoma are common sequelae. Topical corticosteroids are commonly prescribed, and intraocular pressure is monitored.

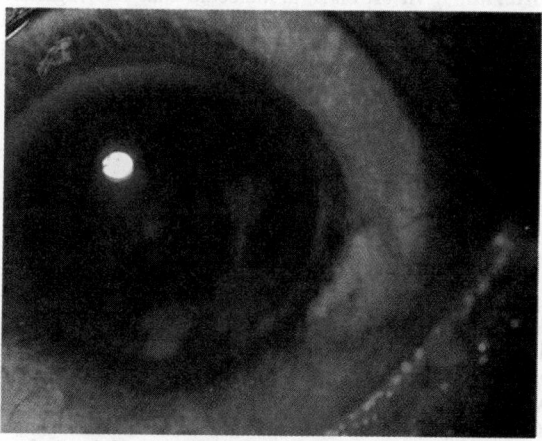

**Zoster ophthalmicus** *(Apple and Rabb, 1998)*

**Zovirax,**   trademark for an antiviral (acyclovir).

**ZPG,**   abbreviation for **zero population growth.**

**Z-plasty** /zē′plas′tē/,   a method of surgical revision of a scar or closure of a wound using a Z-shaped incision to reduce contractures of the adjacent skin. See also **Y-plasty.**

**Zr,**   symbol for the element **zirconium.**

**z score.**   See **z value.**

**z test,**   a statistical test using normalized data (z values) to compare differences in proportions between sets of data or between individual members of different sets of data.

**Z-track,**   a technique for injecting irritating preparations into muscle without tracking residual medication through sensitive tissues.

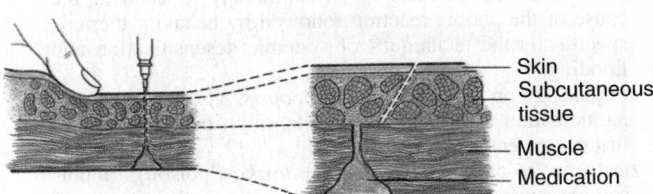

Skin
Subcutaneous tissue
Muscle
Medication

**Z-track method of intramuscular injection**
*(Potter and Perry, 1993)*

**Zung Self-Rating Depression Scale,**   a 'self-report test' of 20 descriptors of depression on which clients rate themselves on a four-point scale ranging from 'a little of the time' to 'most of the time.' The scale is useful in determining the depth or intensity of a client's depression.

**z value,**   a normalized value created from a member of a set of data by expressing it in terms of standard deviations from the mean, using the equation $z = \dfrac{x - \bar{x}}{\sigma}$ where $x$ is an item of data, $\bar{x}$ is the mean of the data, and $\sigma$ is the standard deviation. The mean and standard deviation of the set of such z values are 0 and 1, respectively. Also called **z score.**

**zwieback** /zwī′bak, zwē′-/ [Ger, *zwie,* twice, *backen,* to bake],   a sweetened bread that is enriched with eggs and baked, then sliced and toasted until dry and crisp. It is used as a snack food for children, especially teething infants, or an early food given during convalescence.

**zwitterion** /tsvit′ərī′ən/,   a molecule that has regions of both negative and positive charge. Amino acids such as glycine are almost always present as zwitterions when in neutral solutions. Also called **dipolar ion.**

**zygapophyseal joints.**   See **facet joint.**

**zygo-** /zī′gō-/,   **zyg-,** combining form meaning 'union or fusion, yoked or joined, a junction or a pair': *zygomatic, zygogenesis, zygote.*

**zygocyte.**   See **zygote.**

**zygogenesis** /zī′gōjen′əsis/ [Gk, *zygon,* yoke, *genesis,* origin],   **1.** the formation of a zygote. **2.** reproduction by the union of gametes. —**zygogenetic, zygogenic,** *adj.*

**zygoma** /zīgō′mə, zig-/ [Gk, *zygon,* yoke],   **1.** a long slender zygomatic process of the temporal bone, arising from the lower part of the squamous part of the temporal bone, passing forward to join the zygomatic bone, and forming part of the zygomatic arch. **2.** the zygomatic bone that forms the prominence of the cheek.

**zygomatic** /-mat′ik/ [Gk, *zygon,* yoke],   pertaining to the zygoma, or malar bone of the face.

**zygomatic arch** [Gk, *zygon* + L, *arcus,* bow],   an arch formed by the temporal process of the zygomatic bone with the zygomatic process of the temporal bone. The tendon of the temporal muscle passes beneath it.

**zygomatic bone** [Gk, *zygon* + *ban*],   one of the pair of bones that forms the prominence of the cheek, the lower part of the orbit of the eye, and parts of the temporal and infratemporal fossae.

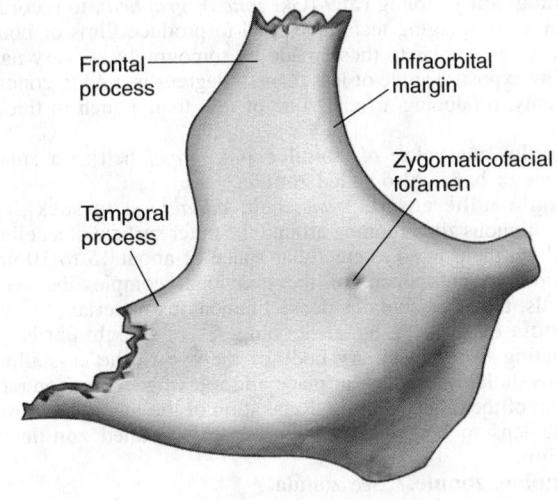

Frontal process

Infraorbital margin

Zygomaticofacial foramen

Temporal process

**Zygomatic bone**

**zygomatic head.**   See **zygomaticus minor.**

**zygomaticofacial** /zī′gōmat′ikōfā′shəl/,   pertaining to the facial surface of the zygomatic bone.

**zygomatic process** [Gk, *zygon* + L, *processus*],   **1.** a projection of the frontal bone forming the lateral boundary of the superciliary arch. **2.** a process of the maxilla. **3.** a process of the temporal bone.

**zygomatic reflex** [Gk, *zygon* + L, *reflectere,* to bend back],   movement of the lower jaw toward the percussed side when the zygoma is tapped lightly but sharply.

**zygomaticus major** /zī′gōmat′ikəs/,   one of the 12 muscles of the mouth. Arising from the zygomatic bone and inserting into the corner of the mouth, it acts to draw the angle of the mouth up and back to smile or laugh. Also called **zygomaticus.** Compare **zygomaticus minor.**

**zygomaticus minor,**   one of the 12 muscles of the mouth. Arising from the malar surface of the zygomatic bone and inserting into the upper lip, it acts to deepen the nasolabial furrow in a sad facial expression. Also called **quadratus labii superioris, zygomatic head.** Compare **zygomaticus major.**

**zygomaxillare.**   See **key ridge.**

**zygomycosis** /zī′gōmīkō′sis/ [Gk, *zygon* + *mykes,* fungus],   an acute, often fulminant, and sometimes fatal fungal infection caused by a class of phycomycetal water molds. It occurs primarily in patients with chronic debilitating diseases, especially uncontrolled diabetes mellitus. Characteristically it begins with fever, pain, and discharge in the nose and paranasal sinuses that progresses to invade the eye and lower respiratory tract. The fungus may enter blood vessels and spread to the brain and other organs. Transmission is usually by inhalation. The diagnosis is confirmed by biopsy and pathologic examination of sputum. Treatment includes improved control of diabetes mellitus, extensive debridement of craniofacial lesions, and amphotericin B administered intravenously. Also called **mucormycosis.** Compare **phycomycosis.**

**zygonema** /zī'gənē'mə/ [Gk, *zygon* + *nema*, thread], the synaptic chromosome formation that occurs in the zygotene stage of the first meiotic prophase of gametogenesis. **—zygonematic,** *adj.*

**zygopodium** /zī'gōpō'dē·əm/, the part of an embryonic limb consisting of the radius and ulna or the tibia and fibula.

**zygosis** /zīgō'sis/, a form of sexual reproduction in unicellular organisms, consisting of the union of the two cells and fusion of their nuclei. **—zygotic,** *adj.*

**zygosity** /zīgos'itē/, the characteristics or conditions of a zygote. The form occurs primarily as a suffix denoting genetic makeup, referring specifically to whether the paired alleles determining a particular trait are identical (homozygosity) or different (heterozygosity) or to the condition in twins of having developed from the fertilization of one ovum (monozygosity) or two (dizygosity).

**zygospore** /zī'gōspôr'/ [Gk, *zygon* + *sporos,* seed], the spore resulting from the conjugation of two isogametes, as in certain fungi and algae. Also called **zygosperm.**

**zygote** /zī'gōt/ [Gk, *zygon,* yoke], the combined cell produced by the union of a sperm pronucleus and an egg pronucleus at the completion of fertilization until the first cleavage. Also called **zygocyte.**

**zygote intrafallopian transfer (ZIFT),** retrieval of oocytes from the ovary, followed by their fertilization and culture in the laboratory and placement of the resulting zygotes in the fallopian tubes by laparoscopy 24 hours after oocyte retrieval; used as a means of establishing pregnancy in treatment of infertility.

**zygotene** /zī'gətēn/ [Gk, *zygon* + *tainia,* band], the second stage in the first meiotic prophase of gametogenesis, in which synapsis of homologous chromosomes occurs. See also **diakinesis, diplotene, leptotene, pachytene.**

**Zyloprim,** trademark for a xanthine oxidase inhibitor (allopurinol).

**-zyme, zymo-,** combining form meaning a 'ferment or enzyme': *lysozyme, serozyme, zymophore.*

**zymogen granules** /zi'məjən/ [Gk, *zyme,* ferment, *genein,* to produce; L, *granulum,* little grain], granules found in some secretory exocrine cells. They contain the precursors of enzymes that become active after the granules leave the cell.

**zymogenic cell.** See **chief cell.**

**zymoprotein** /-prō'tēn/ [Gk, *zyme,* ferment, *proteios,* first rank], **1.** a yeast protein. **2.** any protein that functions as an enzyme.

**zymorphic** /zīmôr'fik/ [Gk, *zyme,* ferment, *morphe,* form], pertaining to fermentation properties. Also **zymorphous** /zīmôr'fəs/.

**Z.Z.'Z.",** symbol for increasing strength or intensity of contraction.

# ILLUSTRATION CREDITS

Aloia JF: *A Color atlas of osteoporosis,* London, 1993, Mosby-Wolfe.

American College of Rheumatology: *Clinical slide collection of the rheumatic diseases,* Atlanta, 1991, 1995, 1997, American College of Rheumatology.

Apple DJ, Rabb MF: *Ocular pathology,* ed 5, St Louis, 1998, Mosby.

Applegate E: *The anatomy and physiology learning system,* ed 2, Philadelphia, 2000, WB Saunders.

Auerbach PS: *Wilderness medicine: management of wilderness and environmental emergencies,* ed 3, St Louis, 1995, Mosby.

Auerbach PS: *Wilderness medicine: management of wilderness and environmental emergencies,* ed 4, St Louis, 2001, Mosby.

Ball K: *Lasers; the perioperative challenge,* ed 2, St Louis, 1995, Mosby.

Ballinger PW: *Merrill's atlas of radiographic positions and radiologic procedures,* ed 9, St Louis, 1999, Mosby.

Baran R, Dawber RPR, Levene GM: *Color atlas of the hair, scalp, and nails,* London, 1992, Mosby-Wolfe.

Barkauskas VH et al: *Health and physical assessment,* ed 2, St Louis, 1998, Mosby.

Baron EJ, Peterson LR, Finegold SM: *Bailey and Scott's diagnostic microbiology,* ed 9, St Louis, 1994, Mosby.

Beare PG, Myers JL: *Adult health nursing,* ed 3, St Louis, 1998, Mosby.

Beeching NJ, Cheesbrough J: *Illustrated case histories in infectious disease,* London, 1993, Mosby-Wolfe.

Beeching NJ, Nye F: *Diagnostic picture tests in clinical infectious diseases,* London, 1996, Mosby-Wolfe.

Belcher AE: *Cancer nursing,* St Louis, 1992, Mosby.

Berne RM, Levy MN: *Principles of physiology,* ed 2, St Louis, 1996, Mosby.

Berne RM, Levy MN: *Principles of physiology,* ed 3, St Louis, 2000, Mosby.

Besser GM, Thorner MO: *Clinical endocrinology,* ed 2, London, 1994, Times Mirror International Publishers.

Bingham BJG, Hawke M, Kwok P: *Atlas of clinical otolaryngology,* St Louis 1992, Mosby.

Black JM, Hawks JH, Keene AM: *Medical-surgical nursing: clinical management for positive outcomes,* ed 6, Philadelphia, 2001, WB Saunders.

Black JM, Matassarin-Jacobs E: *Medical-surgical nursing: clinical management for continuity of care,* ed 5, Philadelphia, 1997, WB Saunders.

Bloom A, Ireland J: *Color atlas of diabetes,* ed 2, London, 1992, Mosby-Wolfe.

Bodansky HJ: *Pocket picture guide to diabetes,* London, 1989, Gower Medical Publishing.

Brooks Tighe SM: *Instrumentation for the operating room: a photographic manual,* ed 4, St Louis, 1994, Mosby.

Brundage DJ: *Renal disorders,* St Louis, 1992, Mosby.

Bryant RA: *Acute and chronic wounds: nursing management,* St Louis, 1992, Mosby.

Bryant RA: *Acute and chronic wounds: nursing management,* ed 2, St Louis, 2000, Mosby.

Bull TR: *Color atlas of E.N.T. diagnosis,* ed 3, London, 1995, Times Mirror International Publishers.

Callen JP, Greer KE, Paller AS et al: *Color atlas of dermatology,* Philadelphia, 1993, WB Saunders.

Cannobio MM: *Cardiovascular disorders,* St Louis, 1990, Mosby.

Carlson BM: *Human embryology and developmental biology,* ed 2, St Louis, 1999, Mosby.

Carr JH, Rodak BF: *Clinical hematology atlas,* Philadelphia, 1999, WB Saunders.

Chabner D: *The language of medicine,* ed 6, Philadelphia, 2001, WB Saunders.

Chipps EM, Clanin NJ, Campbell VG: *Neurologic disorders,* St Louis 1992, Mosby.

Christensen GJ: *A consumer's guide to dentistry,* St Louis, 1994, Mosby.

Christiansen JL, Grzybowski JM: *Biology of aging,* St Louis, 1993, Mosby.

Cohen BA: *Atlas of pediatric dermatology,* London, 1993, Wolfe.

Cotran RS, Kumar V, Collins T: *Robbins' pathologic basis of disease,* ed 6, Philadelphia, 1999, WB Saunders.

Cranin AN: *Atlas of oral implantology,* ed 2, St Louis, 1999, Mosby.

Crossman AR, Neary D: *Neuroanatomy: an illustrated color text,* Edinburgh, 1995, Churchill Livingstone.

Damjanov I, Linder J: *Anderson's pathology,* ed 10, St Louis, 1996, Mosby.

Damjanov I, Linder J: *Pathology: a color atlas,* St Louis, 2000, Mosby.

Doughty DB, Broadwell-Jackson D: *Gastrointestinal disorders,* St Louis, 1993, Mosby.

du Vivier A: *Atlas of clinical dermatology,* ed 2, London, 1993, Gower Medical Publishing.

Earis JE, Pearson MG: *Respiratory medicine,* London, 1995, Times Mirror International Publishers.

Edge V, Miller M: *Women's health care,* St Louis, 1994, Mosby.

Elkin MK, Perry AG, Potter PA: *Nursing interventions and clinical skills,* St Louis, 1996, Mosby.

Elkin MK, Perry AG, Potter PA: *Nursing interventions and clinical skills,* ed 2 St Louis, 2000, Mosby.

Emond RTD, Rowland HAK, Welsby PD: *Color atlas of infectious diseases,* ed 2, London, 1995, Times Mirror International Publishers.

Eveson JW, Skully C: *Color atlas of oral pathology,* London, 1995, Times Mirror International Publishers.

Farrar WE: *Atlas of infections of the nervous system,* London, 1993, Mosby-Wolfe.

Fewkes JL, Cheney ML, Pollack SV: *Illustrated atlas of cutaneous surgery,* London, 1992, Gower Medical Publishing.

Fireman P, Slavin RG: *Atlas of allergies,* ed 2, London, 1996, Gower Medical Publishing.

Fletcher CDM: *Diagnostic histopathology of tumors,* ed 2, London, 2000, Churchill Livingstone.

Fletcher CDM, McKee PH: *An atlas of gross pathology,* London, 1987, Gower Medical Publishing.

Gill KA: *Abdominal ultrasound: a practitioner's guide,* Philadelphia, 2001, WB Saunders.

Gitlin N, Strauss RM: *Atlas of clinical hepatology,* Philadelphia, 1995, WB Saunders.

Goldman MP: *Sclerotherapy,* ed 3, St Louis, 2001, Mosby.

Goldman MP, Fitzpatrick RE: *Cutaneous laser surgery: the art and science of selective photothermolysis,* St Louis, 1994, Mosby.

Goldman MP, Fitzpatrick RE: *Cutaneous laser surgery: the art and science of selective photothermolysis,* ed 2, St Louis, 1999, Mosby.

Goldstein BJ, Goldstein AO: *Practical dermatology,* St Louis, 1992, Mosby.

Goldstein BJ, Goldstein AO: *Practical dermatology,* ed 2, St Louis, 1997, Mosby.

Gray M: *Genitourinary disorders,* St Louis, 1992, Mosby.

Greenberger NJ, Hinthorn DR: *History taking and physical examination: essentials and clinical correlates,* St Louis, 1993, Mosby.

Greig JD, Garden OJ: *Color atlas of surgical diagnosis,* London, 1996, Times Mirror International Publishers.

Grossman FA: *Atlas of minor injuries and repairs,* London, 1993, Gower Medical Publishing.

Grundy FR, Glyn Jones J: *A color atlas of clinical operative dentistry: crowns and bridges,* ed 2, London, 1993, Mosby-Wolfe.

Habif TP: *Clinical dermatology: a color guide to diagnosis and therapy,* ed 2, St Louis, 1990, Mosby.

Habif TP: *Clinical dermatology: a color guide to diagnosis and therapy,* ed 3, St Louis, 1996, Mosby.

Hart CA, Broadhead RL: *Color atlas of pediatric infectious diseases,* London, 1992, Mosby-Wolfe.

Herlihy B, Maebius NK: *The human body in health and illness,* Philadelphia, 2000, WB Saunders.

Heuman DM, Mills AS, McGuire HH: *Gastroenterology,* Philadelphia, 1997, WB Saunders.

Hill MJ: *Skin disorders,* St Louis, 1994, Mosby.

Hordinsky MK, Sawaya ME, Scher RK: *Atlas of hair and nails,* Philadelphia, 2000, Churchill Livingstone.

Huether SE, McCance KL: *Understanding pathophysiology,* ed 2, St Louis, 2000, Mosby.

Hunt RB: *Text and atlas of female infertility surgery,* ed 3, St Louis, 1999, Mosby.

Ignatavicius DD, Workman ML, Mishler MA: *Medical-surgical nursing across the health care continuum,* ed 3, Philadelphia, 1999, WB Saunders.

Jaffe NS: *Atlas of ophthalmic surgery,* ed 2, London, 1996, Times Mirror International Publishers.

Jarvis C: *Physical examination and health assessment,* ed 3, Philadelphia, 2000, WB Saunders.

Johnson LL: *Diagnostic and surgical arthroscopy: the knee and other joints,* ed 2, St Louis, 1981, Mosby.

Jordan RE: *Esthetic composite bonding, techniques and materials,* ed 2, St Louis, 1993, Mosby.

Jorde LB et al: *Medical genetics,* ed 2, St Louis, 2000, Mosby.

Judd RL, Ponsell PP: *Mosby's first responder,* ed 2, St Louis, 1988, Mosby.

Kamal A, Brockelhurst JC: *Color atlas of geriatric medicine,* ed 2, St Louis, 1991, Mosby.

Kanski J, Nischal KK: *Ophthalmology: clinical signs and differential diagnosis,* London, 1999, Mosby International.

Kumar V, Cotran RS, Robbins SL: *Basic pathology,* ed 6, Philadelphia, 1997, WB Saunders.

Lawrence CM, Cox NH: *Physical signs in dermatology: color atlas and text,* London, 1993, Mosby Europe.

Lemmi FO, Lemmi CAE: *Physical assessment findings CD-ROM,* Philadelphia, 2000, WB Saunders.

Leonard PC: *Building a medical vocabulary,* ed 5, Philadelphia, 2001, WB Saunders.

Lewis SM, Collier IC, Heitkemper MM: *Medical-surgical nursing: assessment and management of clinical problems,* ed 4, St Louis, 1996, Mosby.

Lewis SM, Heitkemper MM, Dirksen SR: *Medical-surgical nursing: assessment and management of clinical problems,* ed 5, St Louis, 2000, Mosby.

Lloyd-Davies et al: *Color atlas of urology,* ed 2, London, 1994, Mosby.

Lookingbill DM, Marks JG: *Principles of dermatology,* ed 2, Philadelphia, 1993, WB Saunders.

Lowdermilk DL, Perry SE, Bobak IM: *Maternity and women's health care,* ed 7, St Louis, 2000, Mosby.

Mahon CR, Manuselis G: *Textbook of diagnostic microbiology,* ed 2, Philadelphia, 2000, WB Saunders.

McCance KL, Huether SE: *Pathophysiology: the biologic basis for disease in adults and children,* ed 3, St Louis, 1998, Mosby.

McKee GT: *Cytopathology,* London, 1997, Mosby-Wolfe.

McKenry LM, Salerno E: *Mosby's pharmacology in nursing,* ed 20, St Louis, 1998, Mosby.

McKinney ES et al: *Maternal-child nursing,* Philadelphia, 2000, WB Saunders.

McLaren DS: *Color atlas and text of diet-related disorders,* London, 1992, Mosby-Wolfe.

Michelson JB, Friedlaender MH: *The eye in clinical medicine,* London, 1996, Times Mirror International Publishers.

Miesiewicz JJ et al: *Atlas of clinical gastroenterology,* ed 2, London, 1994, Gower Medical Publishing.

Monahan FD, Neighbors M: *Medical-surgical nursing: foundations for clinical practice,* ed 2, Philadelphia, 1998, WB Saunders.

Moore KL, Persaud TVN, Shiota K: *Color atlas of clinical embryology,* ed 2, Philadelphia, 2000, WB Saunders.

Moore KL, Persaud TVN: *The developing human: clinical oriented embryology,* ed 6, Philadelphia, 1998, WB Saunders.

Morse SA, Moreland A, Holmes K: *Atlas of sexually transmitted diseases and AIDS,* ed 2, London, 1996, Gower Medical Publishing.

Mourad LA: *Orthopedic disorders,* St Louis, 1991, Mosby.

Mudge-Grout C: *Immunologic disorders,* St Louis, 1992, Mosby.

Murray PR et al: *Medical microbiology,* St Louis, 1990, Mosby.

Murray PR et al: *Medical microbiology,* ed 2 St Louis, 1994, Mosby.

Murray PR et al: *Medical microbiology,* ed 3 St Louis, 1998, Mosby.

Newell FW: *Ophthalmology: principles and concepts,* ed 8, St Louis, 1996, Mosby.

Newton RW: *Color atlas of pediatric neurology,* London, 1995, Times Mirror International Publishers.

Pagana KD, Pagana TJ: *Mosby's manual of diagnostic and laboratory tests,* St Louis, 1998, Mosby.

Pagana KD, Pagana TJ: *Mosby's diagnostic and laboratory test reference,* ed 4, St Louis, 1999, Mosby.

Perkin GD: *Mosby's color atlas and text of neurology,* London, 1998, Times Mirror International Publishers.

Perkin GD et al: *Atlas of clinical neurology,* London, 1986, Gower Medical Publishing.

Phipps WJ, Sands J, Marek JF: *Medical-surgical nursing: concepts and clinical practice,* ed 5, St Louis, 1999, Mosby.

Potter PA, Perry AG: *Fundamentals of nursing,* ed 3, St Louis, 1993, Mosby.

Potter PA, Perry AG: *Fundamentals of nursing,* ed 4, St Louis, 1997, Mosby.

Potter PA, Perry AG: *Fundamentals of nursing,* ed 5, St Louis, 2001, Mosby.

Potter PA, Perry AG: *Basic nursing,* ed 3, St Louis, 1995, Mosby.

Potter PA, Perry AG: *Basic nursing,* ed 4, St Louis, 1999, Mosby.

Regezi JA, Sciubba JJ, Pogrel MA: *Atlas of oral and maxillofacial pathology,* Philadelphia, 2000, WB Saunders.

Rosai J: *Ackerman's surgical pathology,* ed 8, St Louis, 1996, Mosby.

Rudy EB: *Advanced neurologic and neurosurgical surgery,* St Louis, 1984, Mosby.

Sanders M et al: *Mosby's paramedic textbook,* ed 2, St Louis, 2000, Mosby.

Schoen FJ: *Interventional and surgical cardiovascular pathology: clinical correlations and basic principles,* Philadelphia, 1989, WB Saunders.

Seeley RS, Stephens TD, Tate P: *Anatomy and physiology,* ed 3, St Louis, 1995, Mosby.

Seidel HM et al: *Mosby's guide to physical examination,* ed 3, St Louis, 1995, Mosby.

Seidel HM et al: *Mosby's guide to physical examination,* ed 4, St Louis, 1999, Mosby.

Shah BR, Laude TA: *Atlas of pediatric clinical diagnosis,* Philadelphia, 2000, WB Saunders.

Shipley M: *A colour atlas of rheumatology,* ed 3, London, 1993, Mosby Europe.

Sigler BA, Schuring LT: *Ear, nose and throat disorders,* St Louis, 1994, Mosby.

Silverberg SG, DeLellis RA, Frable WJ: *Principles and practice of surgical pathology and cytopathology,* ed 3, New York, 1997, Churchill Livingstone.

Skarin AT: *Atlas of diagnostic oncology,* ed 2, London, 1996, Times Mirror International Publishers.

Sleisenger MH, Fordtran JS: *Gastrointestinal and liver disease: pathophysiology, diagnosis, and management,* ed 5, Philadelphia, 1993, WB Saunders.

Sorrentino SA: *Mosby's textbook for nursing assistants,* ed 3, St Louis, 1992, Mosby.

Sorrentino SA: *Mosby's textbook for nursing assistants,* ed 4, St Louis, 1996, Mosby.

Sorrentino SA: *Mosby's textbook for nursing assistants,* ed 5, St Louis, 2000, Mosby.

Stanford Project: *Clinical anatomy principles,* St Louis, 1996, Mosby.

Stein HA, Slatt BJ, Stein RM: *The ophthalmic assistant: a guide for ophthalmic medical personnel,* ed 7, St Louis, 2000, Mosby.

Stein HA, Slatt BJ, Stein RM: *The ophthalmic assistant: a guide for ophthalmic medical personnel,* ed 6, St Louis, 1994, Mosby.

Stevens A, Lowe J: *Pathology,* St Louis, 1995, Mosby.

Stone DR, Gorbach SL: *Atlas of infectious diseases,* Philadelphia, 2000, WB Saunders.

Stoy WA: *Mosby's first responder textbook,* St Louis, 1997, Mosby.

Symonds EM, MacPherson MBA: *Color atlas of obstetrics and gynecology,* London, 1994, Mosby-Wolfe.

Talbot LA, Myers-Marquardt M: *Pocket guide to critical care assessment,* ed 3, St Louis, 1997, Mosby.

Thibodeau GA, Patton KT: *Anatomy and physiology,* ed 4, St Louis, 1999, Mosby.

Thompson JL et al: *Mosby's clinical nursing,* ed 2, St Louis, 1989, Mosby.

Thompson JL et al: *Mosby's clinical nursing,* ed 3, St Louis, 1993, Mosby.

Thompson JM et al: *Mosby's clinical nursing,* ed 4, St Louis, 1997, Mosby.

Tighe SMB: *Instrumentation for the operating room: a photographic manual,* ed 5, St Louis, 1999, Mosby.

Tilton RC, Ballows A, Hohnadel DC: *Clinical laboratory medicine,* St Louis, 1992, Mosby.

US Department of Agriculture: USDA Human Nutrition Information Pub No. 249, Washington, DC, 1992, US Government Printing Office.

Vidic B, Suarez FR: *Color atlas of the human body,* St Louis, 1984, Mosby.

Warner JO, Jackson WF: *Color atlas of pediatric allergy,* London, 1994, Mosby Europe.

Weston WL, Lane AT , Morrelli JG: *Color textbook of pediatric dermatology,* ed 2, St Louis, 1996, Mosby.

White GM: *Color atlas of regional dermatology,* London, 1994, Times Mirror International Publishers.

Wilcox CM: *Atlas of clinical gastrointestinal endoscopy,* Philadelphia, 1995, WB Saunders.

Willson JR, Carrington ER: *Obstetrics and gynecology,* ed 9, St Louis, 1991, Mosby.

Wilson SF, Thompson JM: *Respiratory disorders,* St Louis, 1990, Mosby.

Wilson SF, Giddens JF: *Health assessment for nursing practice,* ed 2, St Louis, 2001, Mosby.

Wong DL: *Whaley & Wong's essentials of pediatric nursing,* ed 4, St Louis, 1993, Mosby.

Wong DL: *Whaley & Wong's essentials of pediatric nursing,* ed 6, St Louis, 2001, Mosby.

Wong DL: *Whaley & Wong's nursing care of infants and children,* ed 5, St Louis, 1995, Mosby.

Wong DL: *Whaley & Wong's nursing care of infants and children,* ed 6, St Louis, 1999, Mosby.

Wright KW: *Pediatric ophthalmology and strabismus,* St Louis, 1995, Mosby.

Youmans JR: *Neurological surgery: a comprehensive reference guide to the diagnosis and management of neurosurgical problems,* Philadelphia, 1982, WB Saunders.

Zakus SM: *Clinical procedures for medical assistants,* ed 3, St Louis, 1995, Mosby.

Zitelli BJ, Davis HW: *Atlas of pediatric physical diagnosis,* ed 3, St Louis, 1997, Mosby.

# APPENDIXES

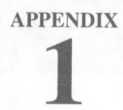

# UNITS OF MEASUREMENT

## 1-1 Conversion factors

| Units To convert from | Conventional units | |
|---|---|---|
| | To | Multiply by |
| **Energy** | | |
| Calories (c) | Joules | 0.23 |
| | Kilocalories | .001 |
| Joules (J) | Calories | 4.184 |
| Kilocalories (C or Kc) | Calories | 1000 |
| **Length** | | |
| Centimeters (cm) | Feet | 0.0328 |
| | Inches | 0.3937 |
| | Meters | 0.01 |
| | Micrometers | 10,000 |
| | Millimeters | 10 |
| | Yards | 0.0109 |
| Feet (ft) | Centimeters | 30.48 |
| | Inches | 12 |
| | Meters | 0.3048 |
| | Yards | 0.3333 |
| Inches (in) | Centimeters | 2.54 |
| | Feet | 0.0833 |
| | Meters | 0.0254 |
| Meters (m) | Centimeters | 100 |
| | Feet | 3.2808 |
| | Inches | 39.370 |
| | Millimeters | 1000 |
| | Yards | 1.0936 |
| Micrometers (μm) | Centimeters | $1 \times 10^{-4}$ |
| | Feet | $3.2808 \times 10^{-6}$ |
| | Inches | $3.9370 \times 10^{-5}$ |
| | Meters | $1 \times 10^{-6}$ |
| | Millimeters | 0.001 |
| Millimeters (mm) | Centimeters | 0.1 |
| | Decimeters | 0.01 |
| | Dekameters | $1 \times 10^{-4}$ |
| | Feet | $3.2808 \times 10^{-3}$ |
| | Inches | 0.0394 |
| | Meters | 0.001 |
| | Micrometers | 1000 |
| | Mils | 39.370 |
| Yards (yd) | Centimeters | 91.44 |
| | Feet | 3 |
| | Inches | 36 |
| | Meters | 0.9144 |
| | Quarters | 4 |
| **Mass** | | |
| Centigrams (cg) | Grains | 0.1543 |
| | Grams | 0.01 |
| Drams (apoth. or troy) (dr ap, ℨ) | Drams (avdp.) | 2.1943 |
| | Grains | 60 |
| | Grams | 3.8879 |
| | Ounces (apoth. or troy) | 0.125 |
| | Ounces (advp.) | 0.1371 |
| | Scruples (apoth.) | 3 |

*Continued*

| Units<br>*To convert from* | Conventional units | |
| --- | --- | --- |
| | *To* | *Multiply by* |
| **Mass—cont'd** | | |
| Drams (avdp.) (dr avdp) | Drams (apoth. or troy) | 0.4557 |
| | Grains | 27.344 |
| | Grams | 1.7718 |
| | Ounces (apoth. or troy) | 0.0570 |
| | Ounces (avdp.) | 0.0625 |
| | Pennyweights | 1.1393 |
| | Pounds (apoth. or troy) | $4.7472 \times 6^{-3}$ |
| | Pounds (avdp.) | $3.9063 \times 10^{-3}$ |
| | Scruples (apoth.) | 1.3672 |
| Grains (gr) | Carats (metric) | 0.3240 |
| | Drams (apoth. or troy) | 0.0167 |
| | Drams (avdp.) | 0.0366 |
| | Dynes | 63.546 |
| | Grams | 0.0648 |
| | Milligrams | 64.799 |
| | Ounces (apoth. or troy) | $2.0833 \times 10^{-3}$ |
| | Ounces (avdp.) | $2.8571 \times 10^{-3}$ |
| | Pennyweights | 0.0417 |
| | Pounds (apoth. or troy) | $1.7361 \times 10^{-4}$ |
| | Pounds (avdp.) | $1.4286 \times 10^{-4}$ |
| | Scruples (apoth.) | 0.05 |
| Grams (g) | Carats (metric) | 5 |
| | Decigrams | 10 |
| | Dekagrams | 0.1 |
| | Drams (apoth. or troy) | 0.2572 |
| | Drams (avdp.) | 0.5644 |
| | Grains | 15.432 |
| | Kilograms | 0.001 |
| | Micrograms | $1 \times 10^{6}$ |
| | Myriagrams | $1 \times 10^{-4}$ |
| | Ounces (apoth. or troy) | 0.3215 |
| | Ounces (avdp.) | 0.3527 |
| | Pennyweights | 0.6430 |
| | Poundals | 0.0709 |
| | Pounds (apoth. or troy) | $2.6792 \times 10^{-3}$ |
| | Pounds (avdp.) | $2.2046 \times 10^{-3}$ |
| | Scruples (apoth.) | 0.7716 |
| Hectograms (hg) | Grams | 100 |
| | Poundals | 7.0932 |
| | Pounds (apoth. or troy) | 0.2679 |
| | Pounds (avdp.) | 0.2205 |
| Kilograms (kg) | Drams (apoth. or troy) | 257.21 |
| | Drams (avdp.) | 564.38 |
| | Grains | 15,432 |
| | Hundredweights (long) | 0.0197 |
| | Hundredweights (short) | 0.0220 |
| | Ounces (apoth. or troy) | 32.151 |
| | Ounces (avdp.) | 35.274 |
| | Pennyweights | 643.01 |
| | Poundals | 75.932 |
| | Pounds (apoth. or troy) | 2.6792 |
| | Pounds (advp.) | 2.2046 |
| | Scruples (apoth.) | 771.62 |
| Micrograms (μg) | Grams | $1 \times 10^{-6}$ |
| | Milligrams | 0.001 |
| Milligrams (mg) | Carats (1877) | $4.871 \times 10^{-3}$ |
| | Carats (metric) | 0.005 |
| | Drams (apoth. or troy) | $2.5721 \times 10^{-4}$ |
| | Drams (advp.) | $5.6438 \times 10^{-4}$ |
| Ounces (apoth. or troy) (oz, ℥) | Dekagrams | 1.7554 |
| | Drams (apoth. or troy) | 8 |
| | Drams (advp.) | 17.554 |
| | Grains | 480 |

| Units<br>To convert from | Conventional units | |
|---|---|---|
| | To | Multiply by |
| **Mass—cont'd** | | |
| Ounces (apoth. or troy) (oz, ℥)—cont'd | Grams | 31.103 |
| | Milligrams | 31,103 |
| | Ounces (avdp.) | 1.0971 |
| | Pennyweights | 20 |
| | Pounds (apoth. or troy) | 0.0833 |
| | Pounds (avdp.) | 0.0686 |
| | Scruples (apoth.) | 24 |
| Ounces (avdp.) (oz) | Drams (apoth. or troy) | 7.2917 |
| | Drams (avdp.) | 16 |
| | Grains | 437.5 |
| | Grams | 28.350 |
| | Hundredweights (long) | $5.5804 \times 10^{-4}$ |
| | Hundredweights (short) | $6.25 \times 10^{-4}$ |
| | Ounces (apoth. or troy) | 0.91146 |
| | Pennyweights | 18.229 |
| | Pounds (apoth. or troy) | 0.0760 |
| | Pounds (avdp.) | 0.0625 |
| | Scruples (apoth.) | 21.875 |
| Pennyweights (dwt) | Drams (apoth. or troy) | 0.4 |
| | Drams (avdp.) | 0.8777 |
| | Grains | 24 |
| | Grams | 1.5552 |
| | Ounces (apoth. or troy) | 0.05 |
| | Ounces (avdp.) | 0.0549 |
| | Pounds (apoth. or troy) | $4.167 \times 10^{-3}$ |
| | Pounds (avdp.) | 0.0034 |
| Poundals | Dynes | 13,825 |
| | Grams | 14.098 |
| | Pounds (avdp.) | 0.3108 |
| Pounds (apoth. or troy) (lb ap) | Drams (apoth. or troy) | 96 |
| | Drams (avdp.) | 210.65 |
| | Grains | 5760 |
| | Grams | 373.24 |
| | Kilograms | 0.3732 |
| | Ounces (apoth. or troy) | 12 |
| | Ounces (avdp.) | 13.166 |
| | Pennyweights | 240 |
| | Pounds (avdp.) | 0.8229 |
| | Scruples (apoth.) | 288 |
| Pounds (avdp.) (lb avdp.) | Drams (apoth. or troy) | 116.67 |
| | Drams (avdp.) | 256 |
| | Grains | 7000 |
| | Grams | 453.59 |
| | Kilograms | 0.4536 |
| | Ounces (apoth. or troy) | 14.583 |
| | Ounces (avdp.) | 16 |
| | Pennyweights | 291.67 |
| | Poundals | 32.174 |
| | Pounds (apoth. or troy) | 1.2153 |
| | Scruples (apoth.) | 350 |
| | Slugs | 0.0311 |
| Quintals (metric) | Grams | 100,000 |
| | Hundredweights (long) | 1.9684 |
| | Kilograms | 100 |
| | Pounds (avdp.) | 220.46 |
| Scruples (apoth.) (s apoth) | Drams (apoth. or troy) | 0.3333 |
| | Drams (avdp.) | 0.7314 |
| | Grains | 20 |
| | Grams | 1.2960 |
| | Ounces (apoth. or troy) | 0.0417 |
| | Ounces (avdp.) | 0.0457 |
| | Pennyweights | 0.8333 |
| | Pounds (apoth. or troy) | $3.4722 \times 10^{-3}$ |
| | Pounds (avdp.) | $2.8571 \times 10^{-3}$ |

*Continued*

| Units To convert from | Conventional units | |
|---|---|---|
| | *To* | *Multiply by* |
| **Pressure** | | |
| Atmospheres, standard (atm) | Bars | 1.0133 |
| | Grams/square centimeter | 1033.2 |
| | Inches of Hg (32° F) | 29.921 |
| | Kilograms/square centimeters | 1.0332 |
| | Millimeters of Hg (0° C) | 760 |
| | Pounds/square inch | 14.696 |
| Meters of Hg (0° C) | Atmospheres | 1.3158 |
| | Feet of $H_2O$ (60° F) | 44.647 |
| | Inches of Hg (32° F) | 39.370 |
| | Kilograms/square centimeters | 1.3595 |
| | Pounds/square inch | 19.337 |
| Millimeters of Hg (0° C) (mm Hg) | Atmospheres | $1.3158 \times 10^{-3}$ |
| | Bars | $1.3322 \times 10^{-3}$ |
| | Grams/square centimeter | 1.3595 |
| | Kilograms/square meter | 13.595 |
| | Pounds/square foot | 2.7845 |
| | Pounds/square inch | 0.0193 |
| | Torrs | 1 |
| **Substance concentration** | | |
| Parts per million* (ppm) | Grains/gallon (Brit.) | 0.0702 |
| | Grains/gallon (U.S.) | 0.0584 |
| | Grams/liter | 0.001 |
| | Milligrams/liter | 1 |
| **Surface area** | | |
| Square inches ($in^2$) | Square centimeters | 6.4516 |
| | Square decimeters | 0.0645 |
| | Square feet | $6.9444 \times 10^{-3}$ |
| | Square meters | $6.4516 \times 10^{-4}$ |
| | Square millimeters | 645.16 |
| | Square mils | $1 \times 10^6$ |
| Square meters ($m^2$) | Square centimeters | 10,000 |
| | Square feet | 10.764 |
| | Square inches | 1550.0 |
| Square millimeters ($mm^2$) | Square centimeters | 0.01 |
| | Square inches | $1.550 \times 10^{-3}$ |
| | Square meters | $1 \times 10^{-6}$ |
| **Volume and capacity** | | |
| Centiliters (cL) | Cubic centimeters | 10 |
| | Cubic inches | 0.6103 |
| | Liters | 0.01 |
| | Ounces (U.S., fluid) | 0.3381 |
| Cubic centimeters ($cm^3$) | Cubic feet | $3.5315 \times 10^{-5}$ |
| | Cubic inches | 0.0610 |
| | Cubic meters | $1 \times 10^{-6}$ |
| | Cubic yards | $1.3080 \times 10^{-6}$ |
| | Drams (U.S., fluid) | 0.2705 |
| | Gallons (Brit.) | $2.1997 \times 10^{-4}$ |
| | Gallons (U.S., dry) | $2.2702 \times 10^{-4}$ |
| | Gallons (U.S., fluid) | $2.6417 \times 10^{-4}$ |
| | Gills (Brit.) | $7.0390 \times 10^{-3}$ |
| | Gills (U.S.) | $8.4535 \times 10^{-3}$ |
| | Liters | 0.001 |
| | Ounces (Brit., fluid) | 0.0352 |
| | Ounces (U.S., fluid) | 0.0338 |
| | Pints (U.S., dry) | $1.8162 \times 10^{-3}$ |
| | Pints (U.S., fluid) | $2.1134 \times 10^{-3}$ |
| | Quarts (Brit.) | $8.7990 \times 10^{-4}$ |
| | Quarts (U.S., dry) | $9.0808 \times 10^{-4}$ |
| | Quarts (U.S., fluid) | $1.0567 \times 10^{-3}$ |
| Cubic decimeters ($dm^3$) | Cubic centimeters | 1000 |
| | Cubic feet | 0.0353 |
| | Cubic inches | 61.024 |

*Based on density of 1 g/ml for the solvent.

| Units To convert from | Conventional units | |
|---|---|---|
| | To | Multiply by |
| **Volume and capacity—cont'd** | | |
| Cubic decimeters (dm$^3$)—cont'd | Cubic meters | 0.001 |
| | Cubic yards | $1.3080 \times 10^{-3}$ |
| | Liters | 1 |
| Cubic dekameters (dam$^3$) | Cubic decimeters | $1 \times 10^6$ |
| | Cubic feet | 35,315 |
| | Cubic inches | $6.1024 \times 10^7$ |
| | Cubic meters | 1000 |
| | Liters | $1 \times 10^6$ |
| Cubic feet (ft$^3$) | Cubic centimeters | 28,317 |
| | Cubic meters | 0.0283 |
| | Gallons (U.S., dry) | 6.4285 |
| | Gallons (U.S., fluid) | 7.4805 |
| | Liters | 23.317 |
| | Ounces (Brit., fluid) | 996.61 |
| | Ounces (U.S., fluid) | 957.51 |
| | Pints (U.S., fluid) | 59.844 |
| | Quarts (U.S., dry) | 25.714 |
| | Quarts (U.S., fluid) | 29.922 |
| Cubic inches (in$^3$) | Cubic centimeters | 16.387 |
| | Cubic feet | $5.7870 \times 10^{-4}$ |
| | Cubic meters | $1.6387 \times 10^{-5}$ |
| | Drams (U.S., fluid) | 4.4329 |
| | Gallons (Brit.) | $3.6047 \times 10^{-3}$ |
| | Gallons (U.S., dry) | $3.7202 \times 10^{-3}$ |
| | Gallons (U.S., fluid) | $4.3290 \times 10^{-3}$ |
| | Liters | 0.0164 |
| | Milliliters | 16.387 |
| | Ounces (Brit., fluid) | 0.5767 |
| | Ounces (U.S., fluid) | 0.5541 |
| | Pints (U.S., dry) | 0.0298 |
| | Pints (U.S., fluid) | 0.0346 |
| | Quarts (U.S., dry) | 0.0149 |
| | Quarts (U.S., fluid) | 0.0173 |
| Cubic meters (m$^3$) | Cubic centimeters | $1 \times 10^6$ |
| | Cubic feet | 35.315 |
| | Cubic inches | 61,024 |
| | Gallons (Brit.) | 219.97 |
| | Gallons (U.S., fluid) | 264.17 |
| | Liters | 1000 |
| | Pints (U.S., fluid) | 2113.3 |
| | Quarts (U.S., fluid) | 1056.7 |
| Cubic millimeters (mm$^3$) | Cubic centimeters | 0.001 |
| | Cubic inches | $6.1024 \times 10^{-5}$ |
| | Cubic meters | $1 \times 10^{-9}$ |
| | Minims (Brit.) | 0.0169 |
| | Minims (U.S.) | 0.0162 |
| Deciliters (dL) | Milliliters | 100 |
| | Cubic centimeters | 100 |
| Drams (U.S., fluid) (fl dr) | Cubic centimeters | 3.6967 |
| | Cubic inches | 0.2256 |
| | Gills (U.S.) | 0.0313 |
| | Milliliters | 3.6966 |
| | Minims (U.S.) | 60 |
| | Ounces (U.S., fluid) | 0.125 |
| | Pints (U.S., fluid) | $7.8125 \times 10^{-3}$ |
| Gallons (Brit.) (gal) | Barrels (Brit.) | 0.0278 |
| | Cubic centimeters | 4546.1 |
| | Cubic feet | 0.1605 |
| | Cubic inches | 277.42 |
| | Firkins (Brit.) | 0.1111 |
| | Gallons (U.S., fluid) | 1.2009 |
| | Gills (Brit.) | 32 |
| | Liters | 4.5460 |
| | Minims (Brit.) | 76,800 |

*Continued*

| Units<br>To convert from | Conventional units | |
|---|---|---|
| | To | Multiply by |
| **Volume and capacity—cont'd** | | |
| Gallons (Brit.) (gal)—cont'd | Ounces (Brit., fluid) | 160 |
| | Ounces (U.S., fluid) | 153.72 |
| | Pecks (Brit.) | 0.5 |
| | Pounds of $H_2O$ (62° F) | 10 |
| Gallons (U.S., dry) | Cubic centimeters | 4404.9 |
| | Cubic feet | 0.1556 |
| | Cubic inches | 268.80 |
| | Gallons (U.S., fluid) | 1.1636 |
| | Liters | 4.4048 |
| Gallons (U.S., liq.) (gal) | Cubic centimeters | 3785.4 |
| | Cubic feet | 0.1337 |
| | Cubic inches | 231 |
| | Cubic meters | $3.7854 \times 10^{-3}$ |
| | Gallons (Brit.) | 0.8327 |
| | Gallons (U.S., dry) | 0.8594 |
| | Gills (U.S.) | 32 |
| | Liters | 3.7854 |
| | Minims (U.S.) | 61,440 |
| | Ounces (U.S. fluid) | 128 |
| | Pints (U.S. fluid) | 8 |
| | Quarts (U.S. fluid) | 4 |
| Gills (Brit.) | Cubic centimeters | 142.07 |
| | Gallons (Brit.) | 0.0313 |
| | Gills (U.S.) | 1.2009 |
| | Liters | 0.1421 |
| | Ounces (Brit., fluid) | 5 |
| | Ounces (U.S., fluid) | 4.8038 |
| | Pints (Brit.) | 0.25 |
| Gills (U.S.) | Cubic centimeters | 118.29 |
| | Cubic inches | 7.2188 |
| | Drams (U.S., fluid) | 32 |
| | Gallons (U.S., fluid) | 0.0313 |
| | Gills (Brit.) | 0.8327 |
| | Liters | 0.1183 |
| | Minims (U.S.) | 1920 |
| | Ounces (U.S., fluid) | 4 |
| | Pints (U.S., fluid) | 0.25 |
| | Quarts (U.S., fluid) | 0.125 |
| Liters (L*) | Cubic centimeters | 1000 |
| | Cubic feet | 0.0353 |
| | Cubic inches | 61.025 |
| | Cubic meters | 0.001 |
| | Drams (U.S., fluid) | 270.52 |
| | Gallons (Brit.) | 0.2200 |
| | Gallons (U.S., dry) | 0.2270 |
| | Gallons (U.S., fluid) | 0.2642 |
| | Gills (Brit.) | 7.0392 |
| | Gills (U.S.) | 8.4537 |
| | Minims (U.S.) | 16,231 |
| | Ounces (Brit., fluid) | 35.196 |
| | Ounces (U.S., fluid) | 33.815 |
| | Pints (Brit.) | 1.7598 |
| | Pints (U.S., dry) | 1.8162 |
| | Pints (U.S., fluid) | 2.1134 |
| | Quarts (Brit.) | 0.8799 |
| | Quarts (U.S., dry) | 0.9081 |
| | Quarts (U.S., fluid) | 1.0567 |
| Milliliters (mL) | Cubic centimeters | 1 |
| | Cubic inches | 0.0610 |
| | Drams (U.S., fluid) | 0.2705 |
| | Gills (U.S.) | $8.4537 \times 10^{-3}$ |
| | Liters | 0.001 |
| | Minims (U.S.) | 16.231 |

*It is recommended in the United States that the capital "L" be the accepted symbol for liter since most typefaces give insufficient distinction between "l" and the numeral one "1."

| Units<br>To convert from | Conventional units | |
|---|---|---|
| | To | Multiply by |
| **Volume and capacity—cont'd** | | |
| Milliliters (mL)—cont'd | Ounces (Brit., fluid) | 0.0352 |
| | Ounces (U.S., fluid) | 0.3381 |
| | Pints (Brit.) | $1.7598 \times 10^{-3}$ |
| | Pints (U.S., fluid) | $2.1134 \times 10^{-3}$ |
| Minims (Brit.) (min, ♏) | Cubic centimeter | 0.0592 |
| | Cubic inches | $3.6122 \times 10^{-3}$ |
| | Milliliters | 0.0592 |
| | Ounces (Brit., fluid) | $2.0833 \times 10^{-3}$ |
| | Scruples (Brit., fluid) | 0.05 |
| Minims (U.S.) (min, ♏) | Cubic centimeters | 0.0616 |
| | Cubic inches | $3.7598 \times 10^{-3}$ |
| | Drams (U.S., fluid) | 0.0167 |
| | Gallons (U.S., fluid) | $1.6276 \times 10^{-5}$ |
| | Gills (U.S.) | $5.2083 \times 10^{-4}$ |
| | Liters | $6.1610 \times 10^{-5}$ |
| | Milliliters | 0.0616 |
| | Ounces (U.S., fluid) | $2.0833 \times 10^{-3}$ |
| | Pints (U.S., fluid) | $1.3021 \times 10^{-4}$ |
| Ounces (Brit., fluid) (oz) | Cubic centimeters | 28.413 |
| | Cubic inches | 1.7339 |
| | Drachms (Brit., fluid) | 8 |
| | Drams (U.S., fluid) | 7.6861 |
| | Gallons (Brit.) | $6.25 \times 10^{-3}$ |
| | Milliliters | 28.412 |
| | Minims (Brit.) | 480 |
| | Ounces (U.S., fluid) | 0.96076 |
| Ounces (U.S., fluid) (oz) | Cubic centimeters | 29.574 |
| | Cubic inches | 1.8047 |
| | Cubic meters | $2.9574 \times 10^{-5}$ |
| | Drams (U.S., fluid) | 8 |
| | Gallons (U.S., dry) | $6.7138 \times 10^{-3}$ |
| | Gallons (U.S., fluid) | $7.8125 \times 10^{-3}$ |
| | Gills (U.S.) | 0.25 |
| | Liters | 0.0296 |
| | Minims (U.S.) | 480 |
| | Ounces (Brit., fluid) | 1.0408 |
| | Pints (U.S., fluid) | 0.0625 |
| | Quarts (U.S., fluid) | 0.0313 |
| Pints (Brit.) (pt) | Cubic centimeter | 568.26 |
| | Gallons (Brit.) | 0.125 |
| | Gills (Brit.) | 4 |
| | Gills (U.S.) | 4.8038 |
| | Liters | 0.5682 |
| | Minims (Brit.) | 9600 |
| | Ounces (Brit., fluid) | 20 |
| | Pints (U.S., dry) | 1.0321 |
| | Pints (U.S., fluid) | 1.2009 |
| | Quarts (Brit.) | 0.5 |
| | Scruples (Brit., fluid) | 480 |
| Pints (U.S., dry) (pt) | Cubic centimeters | 550.61 |
| | Cubic inches | 33.600 |
| | Gallons (U.S., dry) | 0.125 |
| | Gallons (U.S., fluid) | 0.1455 |
| | Liters | 0.5506 |
| | Quarts (U.S., dry) | 0.5 |
| Pints (U.S., liq.) (pt) | Cubic centimeters | 473.18 |
| | Cubic feet | 0.0167 |
| | Cubic inches | 28.875 |
| | Drams (U.S., fluid) | 128 |
| | Gallons (U.S., fluid) | 0.125 |
| | Gills (U.S.) | 4 |
| | Liters | 0.4732 |
| | Milliliters | 473.16 |
| | Minims (U.S.) | 7680 |

*Continued*

| Units<br>To convert from | Conventional units | |
| --- | --- | --- |
| | To | Multiply by |
| **Volume and capacity—cont'd** | | |
| Pints (U.S., liq.) (pt)—cont'd | Ounces (U.S., fluid) | 16 |
| | Pints (Brit.) | 0.8327 |
| | Quarts (U.S., fluid) | 0.5 |
| Quarts (Brit.) (qt) | Cubic centimeters | 1136.5 |
| | Cubic inches | 69.355 |
| | Gallons (Brit.) | 0.25 |
| | Gallons (U.S., fluid) | 0.3002 |
| | Liters | 1.1365 |
| | Quarts (U.S., dry) | 1.0321 |
| | Quarts (U.S., fluid) | 1.2009 |
| Quarts (U.S., dry) (qt) | Bushels (U.S.) | 0.0313 |
| | Cubic centimeters | 1101.2 |
| | Cubic feet | 0.0389 |
| | Cubic inches | 67.201 |
| | Gallons (U.S., dry) | 0.25 |
| | Gallons (U.S., fluid) | 0.2909 |
| | Liters | 1.1012 |
| | Pints (U.S., dry) | 2 |
| Quarts (U.S., liq.) (qt) | Cubic Centimeters | 946.35 |
| | Cubic feet | 0.0334 |
| | Cubic inches | 57.75 |
| | Drams (U.S., fluid) | 256 |
| | Gallons (U.S., dry) | 0.2148 |
| | Gallons (U.S., fluid) | 0.25 |
| | Gills (U.S.) | 8 |
| | Liters | 0.9463 |
| | Ounces (U.S., fluid) | 32 |
| | Pints (U.S., fluid) | 2 |
| | Quarts (Brit.) | 0.83267 |
| | Quarts (U.S., dry) | 0.8594 |
| Scruples (Brit., fluid) | Minims (Brit.) | 20 |
| Square feet (ft$^2$) | Square centimeters | 929.03 |
| | Square inches | 144 |
| | Square meters | 0.0929 |

## 1-2   Conversion between conventional and SI units

| | Conventional units | x | Factor | = | SI units |
|---|---|---|---|---|---|
| Gram | g/mL | | $\dfrac{10^{15}}{mw}$ | | pmol/L |
| | g/100 mL | | $10$ | | g/L |
| | g/100 mL | | $\dfrac{10}{mw}$ | | mol/L |
| | g/100 mL | | $\dfrac{10^4}{mw}$ | | mmol/L |
| | g/d | | $\dfrac{1}{mw}$ | | mol/d |
| | g/d | | $\dfrac{10^3}{mw}$ | | mmol/d |
| | g/d | | $\dfrac{10^9}{mw}$ | | nmol/d |
| Microgram | μg/100 mL | | $\dfrac{10}{mw}$ | | μmol/L |
| | μg/d | | $\dfrac{1}{mw}$ | | μmol/d |
| | μg/d | | $\dfrac{10^3}{mw}$ | | nmol/d |
| Micromicrogram | μμg | | $\dfrac{10^3}{mw}$ | | fmol |
| | μμg/mL | | $\dfrac{10^3}{mw}$ | | pmol/L |
| Milliequivalent | mEq/L | | $\dfrac{1}{valence}$ | | mmol/L |
| | mEq/kg | | $\dfrac{1}{valence}$ | | mmol/kg |
| | mEq/d | | $\dfrac{1}{valence}$ | | mmol/d |
| Milligram | mg/100 mL | | $10^{-2}$ | | g/L |
| | mg/100 mL | | $\dfrac{10^{-2}}{mw}$ | | mol/L |
| | mg/100 mL | | $\dfrac{10}{mw}$ | | mmol/L |
| | mg/100 mL | | $\dfrac{10^4}{mw}$ | | μmol/L |
| | mg/100 g | | $10$ | | mg/kg |
| | mg/100 g | | $\dfrac{10}{mw}$ | | mmol/kg |
| | mg/d | | $\dfrac{1}{mw}$ | | mmol/d |
| | mg/d | | $\dfrac{10^3}{mw}$ | | μmol/d |
| Milliliter | ml/100 g | | $10$ | | ml/kg |
| | ml/min | | $1.667 \times 10^{-2}$ | | ml/s |
| Millimeters of mercury | mm Hg | | $1.333$ | | mbar |
| | mm Hg | | $0.133$ | | kPa |
| Minute | min | | $60$ | | s |
| | min | | $0.06$ | | ks |
| Percent | % | | $10^{-2}$ | | 1 (unity) |
| | % (g/100 gm) | | $10$ | | g/kg |
| | % (g/100 gm) | | $10^{-2}$ | | kg/kg |
| | % (g/100 mL) | | $10$ | | g/L |
| | % (g/100 mL) | | $\dfrac{10}{mw}$ | | mol/L |
| | % (g/100 mL) | | $\dfrac{10^4}{mw}$ | | mmol/L |
| | % (ml/100 mL) | | $10^{-2}$ | | L/L |

## 1-3   Pounds to kilograms conversion

Numbers in the farthest left column are 10-pound increments; numbers across the top row are 1-pound increments. The kilogram equivalent of weight in pounds is found at the intersection of the appropriate row and column. For example, to convert 34 pounds, read down the left column to 30 and then across that row to 4: 34 pounds = 15.42 kilograms.

| Pounds | 0 | 1 | 2 | 3 | 4 | 5 | 6 | 7 | 8 | 9 |
|---|---|---|---|---|---|---|---|---|---|---|
| 0 | 0.00 | 0.45 | 0.90 | 1.36 | 1.81 | 2.26 | 2.72 | 3.17 | 3.62 | 4.08 |
| 10 | 4.53 | 4.98 | 5.44 | 5.89 | 6.35 | 6.80 | 7.25 | 7.71 | 8.16 | 8.61 |
| 20 | 9.07 | 9.52 | 9.97 | 10.43 | 10.88 | 11.34 | 11.79 | 12.24 | 12.70 | 13.15 |
| 30 | 13.60 | 14.06 | 14.51 | 14.96 | 15.42 | 15.87 | 16.32 | 16.78 | 17.23 | 17.69 |
| 40 | 18.14 | 18.59 | 19.05 | 19.50 | 19.95 | 20.41 | 20.86 | 21.31 | 21.77 | 22.22 |
| 50 | 22.68 | 23.13 | 23.58 | 24.04 | 24.49 | 24.94 | 25.40 | 25.85 | 26.30 | 26.76 |
| 60 | 27.21 | 27.66 | 28.12 | 28.57 | 29.03 | 29.48 | 29.93 | 30.39 | 30.84 | 31.29 |
| 70 | 31.75 | 32.20 | 32.65 | 33.11 | 33.56 | 34.02 | 34.47 | 34.92 | 35.38 | 35.83 |
| 80 | 36.28 | 36.74 | 37.19 | 37.64 | 38.10 | 38.55 | 39.00 | 39.46 | 39.91 | 40.37 |
| 90 | 40.82 | 41.27 | 41.73 | 42.18 | 42.63 | 43.09 | 43.54 | 43.99 | 44.45 | 44.90 |
| 100 | 45.36 | 45.81 | 46.26 | 46.72 | 47.17 | 47.62 | 48.08 | 48.53 | 48.98 | 49.44 |
| 110 | 49.89 | 50.34 | 50.80 | 51.25 | 51.71 | 52.16 | 52.61 | 53.07 | 53.52 | 53.97 |
| 120 | 54.43 | 54.88 | 55.33 | 55.79 | 56.24 | 56.70 | 57.15 | 57.60 | 58.06 | 58.51 |
| 130 | 58.96 | 59.42 | 59.87 | 60.32 | 60.78 | 61.23 | 61.68 | 62.14 | 62.59 | 63.05 |
| 140 | 63.50 | 63.95 | 64.41 | 64.86 | 65.31 | 65.77 | 66.22 | 66.67 | 67.13 | 67.58 |
| 150 | 68.04 | 68.49 | 68.94 | 69.40 | 69.85 | 70.30 | 70.76 | 71.21 | 71.66 | 72.12 |
| 160 | 72.57 | 73.02 | 73.48 | 73.93 | 74.39 | 74.84 | 75.29 | 75.75 | 76.20 | 76.65 |
| 170 | 77.11 | 77.56 | 78.01 | 78.47 | 78.92 | 79.38 | 79.83 | 80.28 | 80.74 | 81.19 |
| 180 | 81.64 | 82.10 | 82.55 | 83.00 | 83.46 | 83.91 | 84.36 | 84.82 | 85.27 | 85.73 |
| 190 | 86.18 | 86.68 | 87.09 | 87.54 | 87.99 | 88.45 | 88.90 | 89.35 | 89.81 | 90.26 |
| 200 | 90.72 | 91.17 | 91.62 | 92.08 | 92.53 | 92.98 | 93.44 | 93.89 | 94.34 | 94.80 |

## 1-4   Temperature

To *convert centigrade or Celsius degrees to Fahrenheit degrees:* multiply the number of centigrade degrees by 9/5 and add 32 to the result. *To convert Fahrenheit degrees to centigrade degrees:* Subtract 32 from the number of Fahrenheit degrees and multiply the difference by 5/9.

### Fahrenheit and Celsius equivalents: body temperature range

| F° | C° | F° | C° | F° | C° | F° | C° | F° | C° |
|---|---|---|---|---|---|---|---|---|---|
| 94.0 | 34.44 | 97.0 | 36.11 | 100.0 | 37.78 | 103.0 | 39.44 | 106.0 | 41.11 |
| 94.2 | 34.56 | 97.2 | 36.22 | 100.2 | 37.89 | 103.2 | 39.56 | 106.2 | 41.22 |
| 94.4 | 34.67 | 97.4 | 36.33 | 100.4 | 38.00 | 103.4 | 39.67 | 106.4 | 41.33 |
| 94.6 | 34.78 | 97.6 | 36.44 | 100.6 | 38.11 | 103.6 | 39.78 | 106.6 | 41.44 |
| 94.8 | 34.89 | 97.8 | 36.56 | 100.8 | 38.22 | 103.8 | 39.89 | 106.8 | 41.56 |
| 95.0 | 35.00 | 98.0 | 36.67 | 101.0 | 38.33 | 104.0 | 40.00 | 107.0 | 41.67 |
| 95.2 | 35.11 | 98.2 | 36.78 | 101.2 | 38.44 | 104.2 | 40.11 | 107.2 | 41.78 |
| 95.4 | 35.22 | 98.4 | 36.89 | 101.4 | 38.56 | 104.4 | 40.22 | 107.4 | 41.89 |
| 95.6 | 35.33 | 98.6 | 37.00 | 101.6 | 38.67 | 104.6 | 40.33 | 107.6 | 42.00 |
| 95.8 | 35.44 | 98.8 | 37.11 | 101.8 | 38.78 | 104.8 | 40.44 | 107.8 | 42.11 |
| 96.0 | 35.56 | 99.0 | 37.22 | 102.0 | 38.89 | 105.0 | 40.56 | 108.0 | 42.22 |
| 96.2 | 35.67 | 99.2 | 37.33 | 102.2 | 39.00 | 105.2 | 40.67 | | |
| 96.4 | 35.78 | 99.4 | 37.44 | 102.4 | 39.11 | 105.4 | 40.78 | | |
| 96.6 | 35.89 | 99.6 | 37.56 | 102.6 | 39.22 | 105.6 | 40.89 | | |
| 96.8 | 36.00 | 99.8 | 37.67 | 102.8 | 39.33 | 105.8 | 41.00 | | |

# APPENDIX 2

# SYMBOLS AND ABBREVIATIONS

## 2-1 Symbols

| Symbol | Meaning | Symbol | Meaning |
|---|---|---|---|
| @ | At | ↓ | Decreased |
| ℥ | Dram | → | Yields; leads to |
| f℥ | Fluid dram | ← | Resulting from; secondary to |
| ℥ | Ounce | △ | Change |
| f℥ | Fluid ounce | # | Number; following a number, pounds |
| O | Pint | ÷ | Divided by |
| lb | Pound | × | Multiplied by; magnification |
| ℞ | Recipe; take | = | Equals |
| M | Misce; mix | ≅ | Approximately equals |
| A, Å | Angstrom unit | ≠ | Not equal to |
| $E_0$ | Electroaffinity | > | Greater than; from which is derived |
| $F_1$ | First filial generation | < | Less than; derived from |
| $F_2$ | Second filial generation | ≮ | Not less than |
| mμ | Millimicron, micromillimeter | ≯ | Not greater than |
| μg | Microgram | ≦, ≤ | Equal to or less than |
| mEq | Milliequivalent | ≧, ≥ | Equal to or greater than |
| mg | Milligram | / | Divided by; per |
| m% | Milligrams percent; milligrams per 100 ml | √ | Root; square root; radical |
| Q $O_2$ | Oxygen consumption | ²√ | Square root |
| m- | Meta- | ³√ | Cube root |
| o- | Ortho- | ∞ | Infinity |
| p- | Para- | : | Ratio; "is to" |
| $Po_2$ | Partial pressure of oxygen | ∴ | Therefore |
| $Pco_2$ | Partial pressure of carbon dioxide | ° | Degree |
| μm | Micrometer | % | Percent |
| μ | Micron | π | 3.1416—ratio of circumference of a circle to its diameter; pi |
| μμ | Micromicron | □, ♂ | Male |
| + | Plus; excess; acid reaction, positive | O, ♀ | Female |
| − | Minus; deficiency; alkaline reaction; negative | ⇌ | A reversible reaction |
| ± | Plus or minus; either positive or negative; indefinite | | |
| ↑ | Increased | | |

## 2-2   Abbreviations

Note: Abbreviations in common use can vary widely from place to place. Each institution's list of acceptable abbreviations is the best authority for its records.

| Abbreviation | Meaning | Abbreviation | Meaning | Abbreviation | Meaning |
|---|---|---|---|---|---|
| A | Accommodation; acetum; Angström unit; anode; anterior | alt. hor. | Alternate hours (*alternis horis*) | BCLS | Basic cardiac life support |
| | | alt. noct. | Alternate nights (*alternis noctes*) | BE | Barium enema |
| a | Accommodation; ampere; anterior; area | | | Be | Beryllium |
| | | Am | Mixed astigmatism | BFP | Biologically false positivity (in syphilis tests) |
| $\bar{a}$ | Before | AM | Morning | | |
| $A_2$ | Aortic second sound | ama | Against medical advice | Bi | Bismuth |
| abd | Abdominal/abdomen | AMI | Acute myocardial infarction | Bib | Drink |
| ABG | Arterial blood gases | | | bid; b.i.d. | Twice a day (*bis in die*) |
| ABO | Three basic blood groups | amp | Ampule; amputation | BK | Below the knee |
| AC | Alternating current; air conduction; axiocervical; adrenal cortex | amp. | Ampere | BM | Bowel movement |
| | | amt | Amount | BMR | Basal metabolic rate |
| | | ANA | Antinuclear antibody | BP | Blood pressure; buccopulpal |
| acc. | Accommodation | ana | So much of each, or $\bar{a}\bar{a}$ | | |
| ACE | Adrenocortical extract; angiotensin-converting enzyme | anat | Anatomy or anatomic | bp | Boiling point |
| | | ant. | Anterior | BPH | Benign prostatic hypertrophy |
| | | AO | Anodal opening; atrioventricular valve openings | | |
| ACh | Acetylcholine | | | bpm | Beats per minute |
| ACH | Adrenocortical hormone | AOP | Anodal opening picture | BRP | Bathroom privileges |
| ACLS | Advanced cardiac life support | AOS | Anodal opening sound | BSA | Body surface area |
| | | A-P; AP; A/P | Anterior-posterior | BSE | Breast self-examination |
| ACTH | Adrenocorticotropic hormone | | | BSP | Bromsulphalein |
| | | A.P. | Anterior pituitary gland | BUN | Blood urea nitrogen |
| AD | Right ear (*auris dextra*) | APA | Antipernicious anemia factor | BW | Birthweight |
| ADD | Attention deficit disorder | | | Bx | Biopsy |
| add | Add to (*adde*) | AQ | Achievement quotient | C | Carbon; centigrade; Celsius |
| ADDH | Attention deficit disorder, hyperactivity | AR | Alarm reaction | $\bar{c}$ | With |
| | | ARC | Anomalous retinal correspondence, AIDS-related complex | $C_{alb}$ | Albumin clearance |
| ADH | Antidiuretic hormone | | | $C_{cr}$ | Creatinine clearance |
| ADHD | Attention deficit-hyperactivity disorder | | | $C_{in}$ | Inulin clearance |
| | | ARD | Acute respiratory disease | CA | Chronologic age; cervico-axial |
| ADL | Activities of daily living | arg | Silver | | |
| ADS | Antidiuretic substance | As | Arsenic | Ca | Calcium; cancer; carcinoma |
| AF | Atrial fibrillation | As. | Astigmatism | | |
| AFB | Acid-fast bacillus | AS | Left ear (*auris sinistra*) | CABG | Coronary artery bypass graft |
| AFP | Alpha-fetoprotein | ASCVD | Arteriosclerotic cardiovascular disease | | |
| A/G; A-G ratio | Albumin/globulin ratio | | | CABS | Coronary artery bypass surgery |
| | | ASD | Atrial septal defect | $CaCO_3$ | Calcium carbonate |
| Ag | Silver, antigen | AsH | Hypermetropic astigmatism | CAD | Coronary artery disease |
| $AgNO_3$ | Silver nitrate | ASHD | Arteriosclerotic heart disease | CAH | Chronic active hepatitis |
| ah | Hypermetropic astigmatism | | | Cal | Large calorie |
| AHF | Antihemophilic factor | AsM | Myopic astigmatism | cal | Small calorie |
| AICD | Automatic implantable cardiac defibrillator | ASS | Anterior superior spine | C&S | Culture and sensitivity |
| | | AST | Aspartate aminotransferase (formerly SGOT) | CAT | Computed (axial) tomography |
| AIDS | Acquired immunodeficiency syndrome | Ast | Astigmatism | cath. | Catheter |
| | | ATS | Anxiety tension state; antitetanic serum | CBC or cbc | Complete blood count |
| aj | Ankle jerk | | | | |
| AK | Above the knee | AU | Angström unit | CC | Chief complaint |
| Al | Aluminum | Au | Gold | cc | Cubic centimeter |
| Alb | Albumin | A-V; AV; A/V | Arteriovenous; atrioventricular | $CCl_4$ | Carbon tetrachloride |
| ALH | Combined sex hormone of the anterior lobe of the hypophysis | | | CCU | Coronary care unit; critical care unit |
| | | Av | Average or avoirdupois | | |
| | | ax | Axis | CF | Cystic fibrosis |
| ALS | Advanced life support, amyotrophic lateral sclerosis | B | Boron; bacillus | cf | Compare or bring together |
| | | Ba | Barium | | |
| | | BAC | Buccoaxiocervical | CFT | Complement-fixation test |
| ALT | Alamine aminotransferase (formerly SGPT) | Bact | Bacterium | Cg; Cgm | Centigram |
| | | BBB | Blood-brain barrier | | |
| alt. dieb. | Every other day (*alternis diebus*) | BBT | Basal body temperature | | |

| Abbreviation | Meaning | Abbreviation | Meaning | Abbreviation | Meaning |
|---|---|---|---|---|---|
| CH | Crown-heel (length of fetus) | DCA | Deoxycorticosterone acetate | ER | Emergency room (hospital); external resistance |
| $CHCL_3$ | Chloroform | Dcg | Degeneration; degree | ERG | Electroretinogram |
| $CH_3COOH$ | Acetic acid | dg | Decigram | ERPF | Effective renal plasma flow |
| CHD | Congenital heart disease; coronary heart disease | DIC | Desseminated intravascular coagulation | ERV | Expiratory reserve volume |
| ChE | Cholinesterase | diff | Differential blood count | ESR | Erythrocyte sedimentation rate |
| CHF | Congestive heart failure | dil | Dilute or dissolve | | |
| $C_5H_4N_4O_3$ | Uric acid | dim | One half | ESRD | End-stage renal disease |
| CHO | Carbohydrate | DJD | Degenerative joint disease | EST | Electroshock therapy |
| $C_2H_6O$ | Ethyl alcohol | DKA | Diabetic ketoacidosis | Et | Ethyl |
| $CH_2O$ | Formaldehyde | dL | Deciliter | ext | Extract |
| $CH_4O$ | Methyl alcohol | DM | Diabetes mellitus, diastolic murmur | F | Fahrenheit; field of vision; formula |
| CI | Cardiac index; cardiac insufficiency; cerebral infarction | DNA | Deoxyribonucleic acid | FA | Fatty acid |
| | | DNR | Do not resuscitate | FANA | Fluorescent antinuclear antibody test |
| CK | Creatinine kinase | DOA | Dead on arrival | F & R | Force and rhythm (pulse) |
| Cl | Chlorine | DOB | Date of birth | FAS | Fetal alcohol syndrome |
| cm | Centimeter | DOE | Dyspnea on exertion | FBS | Fasting blood sugar |
| CMR | Cerebral metabolic rate | DPT | Diphtheria-pertussis-tetanus | FD | Fatal dose; focal distance |
| CMV | Cytomegalovirus | | | Fe | Iron |
| CNS | Central nervous system | dr | Dram | $FeCl_3$ | Ferric chloride |
| c/o | Complaints of | DRG | Diagnosis-related groups | ferv. | Boiling |
| CO | Carbon monoxide; cardiac output | DSD | Discharge summary dictated, dry sterile dressing | FEV | Forced expiratory volume |
| $CO_2$ | Carbon dioxide | | | FH, Fhx | Family history |
| Co | Cobalt | DT | Delirium tremens | FHR | Fetal heart rate |
| COLD | Chronic obstructive lung disease | DTR | Deep tendon reflex | Fl, fld | Fluid |
| | | D5W | Dextrose 5% in water | fl dr | Fluid dram |
| COPD | Chronic obstructive pulmonary disease | Dx | Diagnosis | fl oz | Fluid ounce |
| | | E | Eye | FR | Flocculation reaction |
| CP | Cerebral palsy; cleft palate | EAHF | Eczema, asthma, and hay-fever | FSH | Follicle-stimulating hormone |
| CPAP | Continuous positive airway pressure | EBV | Epstein-Barr virus | ft | Foot |
| | | EC | Electroconvulsive therapy | FTT | Failure to thrive |
| CPC | Clinicopathologic conference | ECF | Extended care facility; extracellular fluid | FUO | Fever of unknown origin |
| CPD | Cephalopelvic disproportion | ECG | Electrocardiogram, electro-cardiograph | fx | Fracture |
| | | | | Gm; g; gm | Gram |
| CPK | Creatinine phosphokinase | ECHO | Echocardiography | GA | Gingivoaxial |
| CPR | Cardiopulmonary resuscitation | ECMO | Extracorporeal membrane oxygenation | Galv | Galvanic |
| | | | | GB | Gallbladder |
| CR | Crown-rump length (length of fetus) | ECT | Electroconvulsive therapy | GBS | Gallbladder series |
| | | ED | Emergency department; erythema dose; effective dose | GC | Gonococcus or gonorrheal |
| CS | Cesarean section | | | GDM | Gestational diabetes mellitus |
| CSF | Cerebrospinal fluid | | | | |
| CSM | Cerebrospinal meningitis | $ED_{50}$ | Median effective dose | GFR | Glomerular filtration rate |
| CT | Computed tomography | EDD | Estimated date of delivery (formerly EDC, estimated date of confinement) | GH | Growth hormone |
| Cu | Copper | | | GI | Gastrointestinal |
| $CuSO_4$ | Copper sulfate | | | GL | Greatest length (small flexed embryo) |
| CV | Cardiovascular; closing volume | | | | |
| | | EEG | Electroencephalogram, electroencephalograph | GLA | Gingivolinguoaxial |
| CVA | Cerebrovascular accident; costovertebral angle | EENT | Eye, ear, nose, and throat | GP | General practitioner; general paresis |
| CVP | Central venous pressure | EKG | Electrocardiogram, electro-cardiograph | G6PD | Glucose-6-phosphate dehydrogenase |
| CVS | Chorionic villi sampling; clean voided specimen | ELISA | Enzyme-linked immunosorbent assay | gr | Grain |
| CXR | Chest x-ray | | | Grad | By degrees (gradatim) |
| cyl | Cylinder | Em | Emmetropia | GRAS | Generally recognized as safe |
| D | Dose; vitamin D; right (dexter) | EMB | Eosin-methylene blue | | |
| | | EMC | Encephalomyocarditis | Grav I, II, III, etc. | Pregnancy one, two, three, etc. (Gravida) |
| d | Day; diem | EMF | Erythrocyte maturation factor | | |
| DAH | Disordered action of the heart | | | GSW | Gunshot wound |
| | | EMG | Electromyogram | gt | Drop (gutta) |
| D & C | Dilation (dilatation) and curettage | EMS | Emergency medical service | GTT | Glucose tolerance test |
| | | | | gtt | Drops (guttae) |
| db, dB | Decibel | ENT | Ear, nose, and throat | GU | Genitourinary |
| DC | Direct current | EOM | Extraocular movement | Gyn | Gynecology |
| dc, DC, D/C | Discontinue | EPR | Electrophrenic respiration | H | Hydrogen |
| | | | | $H^+$ | Hydrogen ion |

*Continued*

| Abbreviation | Meaning | Abbreviation | Meaning | Abbreviation | Meaning |
|---|---|---|---|---|---|
| H & E | Hematoxylin and eosin stain | Ig | Immunoglobulin | LP | Lumbar puncture |
| H & P | History and physical | IH | Infectious hepatitis | LPF | Leukocytosis-promoting factor |
| HAV | Hepatitis A virus | IM | Intramuscular; infectious mononucleosis | LR | Lactated Ringer's |
| Hb; Hgb | Hemoglobin | | | LTD | Lowest tolerated dose |
| $H_3BO_3$ | Boric acid | IOP | Intraocular pressure | LTH | Luteotrophic hormone |
| HBV | Hepatitis B virus | IPPB | Intermittent positive pressure breathing | LUE | Left upper extremity |
| HC | Hospital corps | | | LUL | Left upper lobe |
| HCG | Human chorionic gonadotropin | IQ | Intelligence quotient | LUQ | Left upper quadrant |
| | | IRV | Inspiratory reserve volume | LV | Left ventricle |
| HCHO | Formaldehyde | IS | Intercostal space | LVH | Left ventricular hypertrophy |
| HCl | Hydrochloric acid | IU | Immunizing unit | L & W | Living and well |
| HCN | Hydrocyanic acid | I.U. | International Unit | M | Myopia; meter; muscle; thousand |
| $H_2CO_3$ | Carbonic acid | IUD | Intrauterine device | | |
| HCT | Hematocrit | IV | Intravenous | m | Meter |
| HD | Hearing distance | IVP | Intravenous pyelogram, intravenous push | MA | Mental age |
| HDL | High density lipoprotein | | | Mag | Large (magnus) |
| HDLW | Distance at which a watch is heard by the left ear | IVT | Intravenous transfusion | MAP | Mean arterial pressure |
| | | IVU | Intravenous urogram/urography | MBD | Minimal brain dysfunction |
| HDRW | Distance at which a watch is heard by the right ear | JRA | Juvenile rheumatoid arthritis | mc; mCi | Millicurie |
| | | | | μc | Microcurie |
| He | Helium | K | Potassium | mcg | Microgram |
| HEENT | Head, eye, ear, nose, and throat | k | Constant | MCH | Mean corpuscular hemoglobin |
| | | Ka | Cathode or kathode | | |
| Hg | Mercury | KBr | Potassium bromide | MCHC | Mean corpuscular hemoglobin concentration |
| Hgb | Hemoglobin | kc | Kilocycle | | |
| HHC | Home health care | KCl | Potassium chloride | MCV | Mean corpuscular volume |
| Hib | Haemophilus influenzae type B | kev | Kilo electron volts | MD | Muscular dystrophy |
| | | kg | Kilogram | MDI | Medium dose inhalants; metered dose inhaler |
| HIV | Human immunodeficiency (AIDS) virus | KI | Potassium iodide | | |
| | | kj | Knee jerk | Me | Methyl |
| HME | Home medical equipment | km | Kilometer | MED | Minimal erythema dose; minimal effective dose |
| $HNO_3$ | Nitric acid | KOH | Potassium hydroxide | | |
| h/o | History of | KUB | Kidney, ureter, and bladder | mEq | Milliequivalent |
| $H_2O$ | Water | kv | Kilovolt | μEq | Microequivalent |
| $H_2O_2$ | Hydrogen peroxide | KVO | Keep vein open | mEq/L | Milliequivalent per liter |
| HOP | High oxygen pressure | kw | Kilowatt | ME ratio | Myeloid/erythroid ratio |
| HPI | History of present illness | L | Left; liter; length; lumbar; lethal; pound | Mg | Magnesium |
| HR | Heart rate | | | mg | Milligram |
| $H_2SO_4$ | Sulfuric acid | lab | Laboratory | μg | Microgram |
| HSV | Herpes simplex virus | L & A | Light and accommodation | MHD | Minimal hemolytic dose |
| Ht | Total hyperopia | L & D | Labor and delivery | MI | Myocardial infarction |
| HT, HTN | Hypertension | lat. | Lateral | MID | Minimum infective dose |
| HTLV-III | Human T lymphotropic virus type III | lb | Pound (libra) | ML | Midline |
| | | LB | Large bowel (x-ray film) | mL | Milliliter |
| hx, Hx | History | LBW | Low birth weight | MLD | Median or minimum lethal dose |
| Hy | Hyperopia | LCM | Left costal margin | | |
| I | Iodine | LD | Lethal dose; perception of light difference | MM | Mucous membrane |
| $^{131}I$ | Radioactive isotope of iodine (atomic weight 131) | | | mm | Millimeter, muscles |
| | | LDL | Low density lipoprotein | mm Hg | Millimeters of mercury |
| | | LE | Lower extremity; lupus erythematosus | mmm | Millimicron |
| $^{132}I$ | Radioactive isotope of iodine (atomic weight 132) | | | MMR | Maternal mortality rate; measles-mumps-rubella |
| | | le | Left extremity | | |
| | | l.e.s. | Local excitatory state | mμ | Millimicron |
| I & O | Intake and output | LFD | Least fatal dose of a toxin | μm | Micrometer |
| IB | Inclusion body | LGA | Large for gestational age | μμ | Micromicron |
| IBW | Ideal body weight | LH | Luteinizing hormone | Mn | Manganese |
| IC | Inspiratory capacity; intracutaneous | Li | Lithium | mN | Millinormal |
| | | LIF | Left iliac fossa | MRI | Magnetic resonance imaging |
| ICP | Intracranial pressure | lig | Ligament | | |
| ICS | Intercostal space | Liq | Liquor | MS | Multiple sclerosis |
| ICSH | Interstitial cell-stimulating hormone | LLE | Left lower extremity | MSL | Midsternal line |
| | | LLL | Left lower lobe | MT | Medical technologist; membrane tympani |
| ICT | Inflammation of connective tissue | LLQ | Left lower quadrant | | |
| | | LMP | Last menstrual period | mu | Mouse unit |
| ICU | Intensive care unit | LNMP | Last normal menstrual period | MVA | Motor vehicle accident |
| Id. | The same (idem) | | | MW | Molecular weight |
| IDDM | Insulin-dependent diabetes mellitus | LOC | Level/loss of consciousness | My | Myopia |
| | | | | N | Nitrogen |

| Abbreviation | Meaning | Abbreviation | Meaning | Abbreviation | Meaning |
|---|---|---|---|---|---|
| n | Normal | P-A; P/A; PA | Posterior-anterior | PMS | Premenstrual syndrome |
| N/A | Not applicable | | | PN | Percussion note |
| Na | Sodium | PAB; PABA | Para-aminobenzoic acid | PND | Paroxysmal nocturnal dyspnea |
| NaBr | Sodium bromide | | | | |
| NaCl | Sodium chloride | PALS | Pediatric Advanced Life Support | PNH | Paroxysmal nocturnal hemoglobinuria |
| Na$_2$CO$_3$ | Sodium carbonate | | | | |
| Na$_2$C$_2$O$_4$ | Sodium oxalate | P & A | Percussion and auscultation | PO; p.o. | Orally (per os) |
| NAD | No appreciable disease | | | PPD | Purified protein derivative (TB test) |
| NaF | Sodium fluoride | Pap test | Papanicolaou smear | | |
| NaHCO$_3$ | Sodium bicarbonate | Para I, II, III, etc. | Unipara, bipara, tripara, etc. | ppm | Parts per million |
| Na$_2$HPO$_4$ | Sodium phosphate | | | Pr | Presbyopia; prism |
| NAI | Sodium iodide | PAS; PASA | Para-aminosalicylic acid | PRN, p.r.n | As required (pro re nata) |
| N & V, N/V | Nausea and vomiting | | | pro time | Prothrombin time |
| | | PAT | Paroxysmal atrial tachycardia | PSA | Prostate-specific antigen |
| NaNO$_3$ | Sodium nitrate | | | PSP | Phenolsulfonphthalein |
| Na$_2$O$_2$ | Sodium peroxide | Pb | Lead | pt | Pint |
| NaOH | Sodium hydroxide | PBI | Protein-bound iodine | Pt | Platinum; patient |
| Na$_2$SO$_4$ | Sodium sulfate | PCA | Patient-controlled analgesia | PT | Prothrombin time; physical therapy |
| n.b. | Note well | PCP | Phencyclidine, Pneumocystis carinii pneumonia, primary care physician, pulmonary capillary pressure | | |
| NCA | Neurocirculatory asthenia | | | PTA | Plasma thromboplastin antecedent |
| Ne | Neon | | | | |
| NG, ng | Nasogastric | | | PTC | Plasma thromboplastin component |
| NH$_3$ | Ammonia | | | | |
| Ni | Nickel | PCV | Packed cell volume | PTT | Partial thromboplastin time |
| NICU | Neonatal intensive care unit | PCWP | Pulmonary capillary wedge pressure | Pu | Plutonium |
| NIDDM | Noninsulin-dependent diabetes mellitus | PD | Interpupillary distance | PUO | Pyrexia of unknown origin |
| | | pd | Prism diopter; pupillary distance | | |
| NIH | National Institutes of Health | | | PVC | Premature ventricular contraction |
| | | PDA | Patent ductus arteriosus | | |
| NKA | No known allergies | PDR | Physician's Desk Reference | Px | Pneumothorax |
| nm | Nanometer | PE | Physical examination | PZI | Protamine zinc insulin |
| NMR | Nuclear magnetic resonance | PEEP | Positive end expiratory pressure | Q | Electric quantity |
| N.O. | Nursing order | | | q | Every |
| NPN | Nonprotein nitrogen | PEFR | Peak expiratory flow rate | qns | Quantity not sufficient |
| NPO; n.p.o. | Nothing by mouth (non per os) | PEG | Pneumoencephalography | q.o.d. | Every other day |
| | | PERRLA | Pupils equal, regular, react to light and accommodation | qt | Quart |
| NRC | Normal retinal correspondence | | | Quat | Four (quattuor) |
| | | PET | Positron emission tomography | R | Respiration; right; Rickettsia; roentgen |
| NS | Normal saline | | | | |
| NSAID | Nonsteroidal anti-inflammatory drug | PFF | Protein-free filtrate | ℞ | Take |
| | | PGA | Pteroylglutamic acid (folic acid) | RA | Rheumatoid arthritis |
| NSR | Normal sinus rhythm | | | Ra | Radium |
| NTP | Normal temperature and pressure | PH | Past history | rad | Unit of measurement of the absorbed dose of ionizing radiation; root |
| | | pH | Hydrogen ion concentration (alkalinity and acidity in urine and blood analysis) | | |
| NYD | Not yet diagnosed | | | | |
| O | Oxygen; oculus; pint | | | RAI | Radioactive iodine |
| O$_2$ | Oxygen; both eyes | | | RAIU | Radioactive iodine uptake |
| O$_3$ | Ozone | Pharm; Phar. | Pharmacy | RBC; rbc | Red blood cell; red blood count |
| OB | Obstetrics | | | | |
| OBS | Organic brain syndrome | PI | Previous illness; protamine insulin | RCD | Relative cardiac dullness |
| OD | Optical density; overdose; right eye (Oculus dexter) | | | RCM | Right costal margin |
| | | PICC | Percutaneously inserted central catheter | RDA | Recommended daily/dietary allowance |
| OOB | Out of bed | | | | |
| OPD | Outpatient department | PID | Pelvic inflammatory disease | RDS | Respiratory distress syndrome |
| OR | Operating room | | | | |
| ORIF | Open reduction and internal fixation | PK | Psychokinesis | RE | Right eye; reticuloendothelial tissue or cell |
| | | PKU | Phenylketonuria | | |
| OS | Left eye (oculus sinister) | PL | Light perception | Re | Rhenium |
| Os | Osmium | PM | Postmortem; evening | re | Right extremity |
| OT | Occupational therapy | PMB | Polymorphonuclear basophil leukocytes | Rect | Rectified |
| OTC | Over-the-counter | | | Reg umb | Umbilical region |
| OTD | Organ tolerance dose | PME | Polymorphonuclear eosinophil leukocytes | RES | Reticuloendothelial system |
| OU | Each eye (oculus uterque) | | | Rh | Symbol of rhesus factor; symbol for rhodium |
| oz; ℨ | Ounce | PMH | Past medical history | RhA | Rheumatoid arthritis |
| P | Phosphorus; pulse; pupil | PMI | Point of maximal impulse | RHD | Relative hepatic dullness; rheumatic heart disease |
| p | After | PMN | Polymorphonuclear neutrophil leukocytes (polys) | | |
| P$_2$ | Pulmonic second sound | | | RLE | Right lower extremity |

Continued

| Abbreviation | Meaning | Abbreviation | Meaning | Abbreviation | Meaning |
|---|---|---|---|---|---|
| RLL | Right lower lobe | sss | Layer upon layer (*stratum super stratum*) | TST | Triple sugar iron test |
| RLQ | Right lower quadrant | | | TUR; TURP | Transurethral resection |
| RM | Respiratory movement | St | Let it stand (*stet; stent*) | Tx | Treatment |
| RML | Right middle lobe of lung | Staph | Staphylococcus | U | Uranium; unit |
| Rn | Radon | stat | Immediately (*statim*) | UA | Urinalysis |
| RNA | Ribonucleic acid | STD | Sexually transmitted disease; skin test dose | UBI | Ultraviolet blood irradiation |
| R/O | Rule out | | | | |
| ROM | Range of motion | STH | Somatotrophic hormone | UE | Upper extremity |
| ROS | Review of systems | Strep | Streptococcus | UIBC | Unsaturated iron-binding capacity |
| RPF | Renal plasma flow | STS | Serologic test for syphilis | | |
| RPM; rpm | Revolutions per minute | STU | Skin test unit | Umb; umb | Umbilicus |
| RPR | Rapid plasma reagin | SV | Stroke volume; supraventricular | URI | Upper respiratory infection |
| RPS | Renal pressor substance | | | US | Ultrasonic |
| RQ | Respiratory quotient | sv | Alcoholic spirit (*spiritus vini*) | USP | *U.S. Pharmacopeia* |
| RR | Recovery room; respiratory rate | | | UTI | Urinary tract infection |
| | | Sx | Symptoms | UV | Ultraviolet |
| RT | Radiation therapy; reading test; respiratory therapy | Sym | Symmetrical | V | Vanadium; vision; visual acuity |
| | | T | Temperature; thoracic | | |
| R/T | Related to | t | Temporal | v | Volt |
| RU | Rat unit | T₃ | Triiodothyronine | VA | Visual acuity |
| RUE | Right upper extremity | T₄ | Thyroxine | V & T | Volume and tension |
| RUL | Right upper lobe | TA | Toxin-antitoxin | VC | Vital capacity |
| RUQ | Right upper quadrant | Ta | Tantalum | VD | Venereal disease |
| S | Sulfur | TAB | Vaccine against typhoid, paratyphoid A and B | VDA | Visual discriminatory acuity |
| S. | Sacral | | | VDG | Venereal disease— gonorrhea |
| s̄ | Without | Tab | Tablet | | |
| S-A; S/A; SA | Sinoatrial | TAH | Total abdominal hysterectomy | VDM | Vasodepressor material |
| | | | | VDRL | Venereal Disease Research Laboratories (sometimes used loosely to mean venereal disease report) |
| SAS | Sodium acetate solution | TAM | Toxoid-antitoxoid mixture | | |
| SB | Small bowel (x-ray film); sternal border | T & A | Tonsillectomy and adenoidectomy | | |
| Sb | Antimony | TAT | Toxin-antitoxin, tetanus antitoxin | VDS | Venereal disease—syphilis |
| SC | Closure of semilunar valves | | | VEM | Vasoexciter material |
| | | TB | Tuberculin; tuberculosis; tubercle bacillus | Vf | Field of vision |
| SD | Skin dose | | | VHD | Valvular heart disease |
| Se | Selenium | Tb | Terbium | VIA | Virus inactivating agent |
| Sed rate | Sedimentation rate | TCA | Tetrachloracetic acid | VLBW | Very low birth weight |
| SGA | Small for gestational age | Te | Tellurium; tetanus | VLDL | Very low density lipoprotein |
| SGOT | Serum glutamic oxaloacetic transaminase | TEM | Triethylene melamine | | |
| | | TENS | Transcutaneous electrical nerve stimulation | VMA | Vanillylmandelic acid |
| SGPT | Serum glutamic pyruvic transaminase | | | vol | Volume |
| | | Th | Thorium | VR | Vocal resonance |
| SH | Serum hepatitis | TIA | Transient ischemic attack | VS | Volumetric solution |
| SI | International system of units (stroke index) | TIBC | Total iron-binding capacity | VS, v.s. | Vital signs |
| | | Tl | Thallium | Vs | Venisection |
| S.I. | Soluble insulin | TM | Tympanic membrane | VsB | Bleeding in arm (*venaesectio brachii*) |
| Si | Silicon | Tm | Thulium; symbol for maximal tubular excretory capacity (kidneys) | | |
| SIDS | Sudden infant death syndrome | | | VSD | Ventricular septal defect |
| | | TMJ | Temporomandibular joint | VW | Vessel wall |
| SLE | Systemic lupus erythematosus | TNT | Trinitrotoluene | VZIG | Varicella zoster immune globulin |
| | | TNTM | Too numerous to mention | | |
| SLP | Speech-language pathology | TP | Tuberculin precipitation | W | Tungsten |
| Sn | Tin | TPI | *Treponema pallidum* immobilization test for syphilis | w | Watt |
| SNF | Skilled nursing facility | | | WBC; wbc | White blood cell; white blood count |
| SOB | Shortness of breath | | | | |
| sol | Solution, dissolved | | | WD | Well developed |
| SP | Spirit | TPN | Total parenteral nutrition | WL | Wavelength |
| sp. gr., SG, s.g. | Specific gravity | TPR | Temperature, pulse, and respiration | WN | Well nourished |
| | | | | WNL | Within normal limits |
| sph | Spherical | tr | Tincture | WR | Wassermann reaction |
| SPI | Serum precipitable iodine | Trans D | Transverse diameter | wt | Weight |
| spir | Spirit | TRU | Turbidity reducing unit | X-ray | Roentgen ray |
| SR | Sedimentation rate | TS | Test solution | y, yr | Year |
| Sr | Strontium | TSE | Testicular self-examination | yo | Years old |
| s/s | Signs and symptoms | TSH | Thyroid-stimulating hormone | Z | Symbol for atomic number |
| SSS | Specific soluble substance, sick sinus syndrome | | | Zn | Zinc |
| | | TSP | Trisodium phosphate | Zz | Ginger |

## 2-3   Common abbreviations used in writing prescriptions

| Abbreviation | Derivation | Meaning | Abbreviation | Derivation | Meaning |
|---|---|---|---|---|---|
| $\overline{aa}$ | ana | of each | o.d. | omni die | every day |
| a.c. | ante cibum | before meals | o.h. | omni hora | every hour |
| ad | ad | to, up to | o.m. | omni mane | every morning |
| ad lib. | ad libitum | freely as desired | o.n. | omni nocte | every night |
| agit. ante sum. | agitare ante | shake before taking | os | os | mouth |
| | | | oz | uncia | ounce |
| alt. dieb. | alternis diebus | every other day | p.c. | post cibum | after meals |
| alt. hor. | alternis horis | alternate hours | per | per | through or by |
| alt. noct. | alternis noctibus | alternate nights | pil. | pilula | pill |
| aq. | aqua | water | p.o. | per os | orally |
| aq. dest. | aqua destillata | distilled water | p.r.n. | pro re nata | when required |
| b.i.d. | bis in die | two times a day | q | quaque | every |
| b.i.n. | bis in nocte | two times a night | q.d. | quaque die | every day |
| c., c̄ | cum | with | q.h. | quaque hora | every hour |
| Cap. | capiat | let him take | q. 2 h. | | every two hours |
| caps. | capsula | capsule | q. 3 h. | | every three hours |
| c.m.s. | cras mane sumendus | to be taken tomorrow morning | q. 4 h. | | every four hours |
| | | | q.i.d. | quater in die | four times a day |
| c.n. | cras nocte | tomorrow night | q.l. | quantum libet | as much as desired |
| c.n.s. | cras nocte sumendus | to be taken tomorrow night | q.n. | quaque nocte | every night |
| | | | q.p. | quantum placeat | as much as desired |
| comp. | compositus | compound | q.v. | quantum vis | as much as you please |
| Det. | detur | let it be given | | | |
| Dieb. tert. | diebus tertiis | every third day | q.s. | quantum sufficit | as much as is required |
| dil. | dilutus | dilute | | | |
| elix. | elixir | elixir | ℞ | recipe | take |
| ext. | extractum | extract | Rep. | repetatur | let it be repeated |
| fld. | fluidus | fluid | s, s̄ | sine | without |
| Ft. | fiat | make | seq. luce. | sequenti luce | the following day |
| g | gramme | gram | Sig. or S. | signa | write on label |
| gr | granum | grain | s.o.s. | si opus sit | if necessary |
| gt | gutta | a drop | sp. | spiritus | spirits |
| gtt | guttae | drops | ss | semis | a half |
| h. | hora | hour | stat. | statim | immediately |
| h.d. | hora decubitus | at bedtime | syr. | syrupus | syrup |
| h.s. | hora somni | hour of sleep (bedtime) | t.d.s. | ter die sumendum | to be taken three times daily |
| M. | misce | mix | t.i.d. | ter in die | three times a day |
| m. | minimum | a minim | t.i.n. | ter in nocte | three times a night |
| mist. | mistura | mixture | tr. or tinct. | tinctura | tincture |
| non rep. | non repetatur | not to be repeated | ung. | unguentum | ointment |
| noct. | nocte | in the night | ut. dict. | ut dictum | as directed |
| O | octarius | pint | vin. | vini | of wine |
| ol. | oleum | oil | | | |

# MEDICAL TERMINOLOGY

The ability to break down medical terms into separate components or to recognize a complete word depends on the mastery of the combining forms (a stem or root with an "o" attached), roots or stems that appear in medical terms, and prefixes and suffixes that alter or modify meaning and usage of a term.

## PREFIXES

Prefixes, the most frequently used elements in the formation of Greek and Latin words, consist of one or more syllables (prepositions or adverbs) placed before words or roots to show various kinds of relationships. They are never used independently, but when added before verbs, adjectives, or nouns, they modify the meaning. Most prefixes are a part of words in ordinary speech and do not refer specifically to medical or scientific terminology, but many occur frequently in medical terminology.

## SUFFIXES

Suffixes are the one or more syllables or elements added to the root or stem of a word (the part that indicates the essential meaning) to alter the meaning or indicate the intended part of speech.

To make a word pronounceable, the last letter or letters of the root to which the suffix is attached may be changed. The last vowel may be changed to an "o" or an "o" may be inserted if it is not already present before a suffix beginning with a consonant, as in cardiology. The final vowel in the root may be dropped before a suffix beginning with a vowel, as in neuritis.

Most suffixes are in common use in English, but some are peculiar to medical science. The suffixes most commonly used to indicate disease are *itis*, meaning inflammation; *oma*, meaning tumor; and *osis*, meaning a condition, usually morbid. The suffixes listed occur often in medical terminology, but they are also in use in ordinary language. These suffixes apply to Greek and Latin words.

| Form | Meaning | Example(s) |
|---|---|---|
| a-, an- | without, lack of, not | Aphasia (without speech)<br>Anemia (lack of blood) |
| ab- | away from | Abductor (leading away from)<br>Aboral (away from mouth) |
| abdomin/o | abdomen | Abdominoplasty (plastic repair of the abdomen) |
| -ac,-al | pertaining to, relating to | Cardiac (pertaining to the heart)<br>Neural (pertaining to nerves) |
| acanth/o | thorny, spiny | Acanthocyte (abnormal red blood cell with spiny projections) |
| acetabul/o- | acetabulum | acetabulum |
| acou/o | hearing | Acoumeter (instrument used to measure hearing) |
| acr/o | extremities, height | Acrophobia (fear of heights) |
| ad- | toward, to, near | Adductor (leading toward)<br>Adrenal (near the kidney) |
| aden/o- | gland | adenofibroma |
| adenoid/o | adenoids | Adenoiditis (inflammation of the adenoids) |
| adip/o- | fat | adipokinesis |
| adren/o-, adrenal/o- | adrenal gland | adrenocortical |
| aer/o | air, gas | Aerobic (pertaining to the presence of air or oxygen) |
| -agra | excessive pain | Cardiagra (excessive chest or heart pain) |
| albumin/o | albumin | Albuminuria (excess albumin in the urine) |
| albus | white | albumin |
| algesi/o | pain | Analgesic (agent used to decrease pain) |
| -algia | pain | Neuralgia (pain in nerves) |
| alveol/o | alveolus | Alveoloplasty (surgical repair of the alveolus) |
| ambi-, ampho- | both | Ambidextrous (ability to use both hands equally)<br>Amphogenic (producing young of both sexes) |
| ambly/o | dull, dim | Amblyopia (dulled or reduced vision in an eye) |
| amni/o, amnion/o | amnion | Amnionitis (inflammation of the amnion) |
| amphi- | on both sides, double | Amphibious (living both on land and in water)<br>Amphithymia (dual mental state of depression and elation) |
| amyl/o- | starch | amylolysis |
| amyl/o | starch | Amyloid (resembling a starch) |
| ana- | up, toward, apart | Anatomy (to cut apart)<br>Anacatharsis (vomiting up) |
| andr/o | male | Androgen (hormone that increases male characteristics) |
| angi/o- | vessel, usually a blood vessel | angiography |
| ankyl/o- | bent, crooked, stiff, fixed | Ankyloglossia (tongue-tie)<br>Ankylosis (stiff or fixed joint) |
| an/o | anus | Anoplasty (surgical repair of the anus) |

| Form | Meaning | Example(s) |
|---|---|---|
| ante- | before, in front of, forward | Antecubital (before the elbow) |
| | | Anteflex (to bend forward) |
| anti- | against, opposing | Antisepsis (against infection) |
| | | Anticarious (against cavities) |
| antr/o | antrum | Antrectomy (excision of the antrum) |
| aort/o | aorta | Aortogram (x-ray of the aorta) |
| ap-, apo- | separated from, derived from | Apobiosis (death of a part) |
| | | Apocleisis (aversion to food) |
| -apheresis | removal | Leukapheresis (removal of white blood cells from blood) |
| aponeur/o | aponeurosis | Aponeurorrhaphy (suture of an aponeurosis) |
| appendic/o | appendix | Appendicitis (inflammation of the appendix) |
| aqua, hydr/o- | water | aqueous hydroadipsia |
| -ar, -ary | pertaining to | Alveolar (pertaining to alveoli) |
| arteri/o- | artery | arteriofibrosis |
| arteriol/o- | arteriole | arteriolosclerosis |
| arthr/o- | joint | arthritis |
| articul/o | joint | Articular (relating to a joint) |
| -ase | enzyme | Lipase (enzyme that breaks down lipids) |
| -asthenia | weakness | Myasthenia (muscle weakness) |
| -ate | use, subject to | Impregnate (to make pregnant) |
| atel/o | imperfect, incomplete | Atelectasis (incomplete expansion of the lung) |
| ather/o | yellowish, fatty plaque | Atherogenesis (formation of plaques in the arteries) |
| -atresia | absence of a normal body opening, occlusion, closure | Urethatresia (abnormal occlusion or closure of the urethra) |
| atri/o- | atrium or upper heart chamber | atrioventricular |
| audi/o- | hearing | Audiometer (hearing test device) |
| | | Audiology (study of hearing) |
| aur/i, aur/o | ear | Auricle (outer ear) |
| aut-, auto- | self | Autoanalysis (self-analysis) |
| | | Autoerotism (sexual self-love) |
| aut/o | self | Autoactivation (self-activation) |
| axill/o | armpit | Axillary (pertaining to the armpit) |
| azot/o | urea, nitrogen | Azoturia (excess nitrogen in the urine) |
| bacteri/o | bacteria | Bacteriolysis (breakdown of bacteria) |
| balan/o- | glans penis or glans clitoridis | balanoposthis |
| bi-, bin- | two, double, twice | Bifocal (two foci) |
| | | Biarticulate (double joint) |
| bil/i | bile | Biliuria (presence of bile in the urine) |
| bio-, bi/o- | life | Biology (study of living things) |
| | | Biogenesis (origin of life) |
| blast/o | developing cell | Blastolysis (destruction of the blastoderm) |
| blephar/o- | eyelid or eyelash | blepharitis |
| brachi/o- | arm | brachial artery |
| brachy- | short | Brachydactylia (short fingers) |
| | | Brachygnathous (receding underjaw) |
| brady- | slow | Bradycardia (slow heartbeat) |
| | | Bradypepsia (slow digestion) |
| brev/i- | short | Brevicollis (short neck) |
| | | Breviflexor (short flexor muscle) |
| bronch/i-, bronch/o- | bronchus | bronchial |
| bronchiol/o- | bronchiolus | bronchiolar |
| bucc/o- | cheek | buccal mucosa |
| burs/o | bursa (cavity) | Bursectomy (excision of abursa) |
| calc/i | calcium | Calcinosis (excessive calcium deposits) |
| cancer/o | cancer | Cancerous (resembling a cancer) |
| canth/o- | corner of eye | canthorraphy |
| capit/o- | head | capitulum |
| -capnia | carbon dioxide | Hypocapnia (low arterial carbon dioxide level) |
| carcin/o | cancer | Carcinogen (cancer-causing agent) |
| cardi/o- | heart | cardiogenic |
| carp/o- | wrist | carpal |
| cata- | down, under, lower, against | Catabolism (breaking down) |
| | | Catalepsy (reduced movement) |
| caud/o | tail, toward the lower part of the body | Caudocephalad (movement from the tail toward the head) |
| caus-, caut- | burn | Causalgia (burning pain) |
| | | Cautery (device to scar or burn) |
| cec/o | cecum | Cecostoma (surgical opening into the cecum) |

*Continued*

| Form | Meaning | Example(s) |
|------|---------|------------|
| cel-, celi/o-, coel- | hollow, cavity | Celiac (pertaining to the abdominal cavity)<br>Coelom (body cavity of embryo) |
| -cele | protrusion (hernia) | Cystocele (bladder hernia)<br>Rectocele (protrusion of the rectum into the vagina) |
| -centesis | surgical puncture to remove fluid | Paracentesis (removal of fluid from a body cavity)<br>Thoracentesis (removal of fluid from the chest cavity) |
| cephal/o- | head | cephalic |
| cerebell/o- | cerebellum of brain | cerebellopontine |
| cerebr/i-, cerebr/o- | cerebrum of brain | cerebroid |
| cerumen, cerumin/o- | earwax | ceruminolytic |
| cervic/o- | neck | cervix |
| cheil/o-, chil/o- | lip | cheilosis |
| cheir/o-, chir/o- | hand | chiropractor |
| chlor/o-, chloros | green | chlorephidrosis |
| cholangi/o- | bile duct | cholangioma |
| chol/e-, chol/o- | bile | cholesterase |
| choledoch/o- | common bile duct | choledocholithiasis |
| chondr/i, chond/io-, chondr/o- | cartilage | chondroclast |
| chord/o- | vocal cord or spermatic cord | chordiod |
| chori/o | chorion | Choriogenesis (development of the chorion) |
| chrom/o- | color (as compared with no color) | chromatopsia |
| chyle | milky fluid (product of digestion) | chylomicron |
| -cidal | killing | Bacteriocidal (pertaining to a substance that destroys bacteria) |
| cili/o- | eyelid, eyelash, or small hairlike process | ciliary body |
| circum- | around | Circumflex (winding around)<br>Circumarticular (around a joint) |
| cirrhos | orange-yellow | cirrhosis |
| clas- | break | Osteoclasis (surgical fracture)<br>Clastothrix (splitting of hair) |
| -clasia, -clasis, -clast | break | Osteoclast (cell that contributes to the breakdown of bone tissue) |
| clavic/o-, clavicul/o- | clavicle (collar bone) | clavicle |
| -cle, -cule | small | Follicle (small sac)<br>Molecule (small unit of matter) |
| cleid/o- | clavicle | cleidocostal |
| -clysis | irrigating, washing | Hydroclysis (irrigating with water) |
| -coccus (*pl.* cocci) | berry-shaped (a form of bacterium) | Staphylococcus (berry-shaped bacteria arranged in grape-like clusters) |
| co-,* com-,** con- | with, together | Commissure (coming together)<br>Conductor (leading together) |
| collagen/o- | fibrous protein of connective tissue, cartilage, bone, and skin | collagenoblast |
| col/o- | colon | colonoscopy |
| colp/o- | vagina | colpalgia |
| coni/o | dust | Otoconia (small dust particles in the ear) |
| conjunctiv/o | conjunctiva | Conjunctivitis (inflammation of the conjunctiva) |
| contra- | opposed, against | Contralateral (opposite side)<br>Contraception (prevention of conception) |
| cor/e, cor/o- | pupil of eye | cornea |
| corne/o | cornea | Corneoiritis (inflammation of the cornea and iris) |
| coron/o | heart | Coronary (pertaining to the heart) |
| cortic/o | cortex (outer layer of body organ) | Corticoid (resembling the cortex) |
| cost/o- | rib | costochondral |
| crani/o | cranium (skull) | Craniotomy (surgical opening into the cranium) |
| -crit | to separate | Hematocrit (separated blood to determine percentage of erythrocytes in whole blood) |
| cry/o- | cold | Cryotherapy (treatment using cold)<br>Cryoanesthesia (freezing of a body part) |
| crypt/o- | hidden | Cryptorchidism (undescended testis)<br>Cryptomnesia (subconscious memory) |
| culd/o | cul-de-sac | Culdoscopy (visual examination of the Douglas' cul-de-sac) |
| cutane/o- | skin | cutaneous |
| cyan/o- | blue | cyanotic |

*co- before a vowel.
**com- before b, m, and p.

| Form | Meaning | Example(s) |
|---|---|---|
| cyes/i-, cyes/o- | pregnancy | Cyesiology (the study of pregnancy) |
| cyst/i-, cyst/o- | bladder, cyst, or sac | cystocele |
| -cyte | cell | Leukocyte (white blood cell) |
| | | Erythrocyte (red blood cell) |
| cyt/o- | cell | cytogenesis |
| dacry/o-, lacrima | tears | dacryostenosis lacrimation |
| dactyl/o- | finger, sometimes toe | dactylion |
| de- | down, from | Dehydrate (remove water from) |
| | | Decay (break down) |
| denti/i-, dent/o- | tooth or teeth | dentibuccal |
| derm/a-, derm/o-, dermat/o- | skin | dermatitis |
| -desis | surgical fixation, fusion | Arthrodesis (surgical fixation of a joint) |
| dextr/o- | right, right side | Dextrocardia (heart on right side) |
| | | Dextromanual (righthanded) |
| di- | two, twice | Dicephalous (two-headed) |
| | | Dichromic (having two colors) |
| dia- | between, through, apart, across, completely | Diapedesis (ooze through) |
| | | Diaphragm (wall across) |
| | | Diagnosis (complete knowledge) |
| diaphor/o- | sweat | Diaphoresis (excessive sweating) |
| diaphragmat/o- | diaphragm | Diaphragmatocele (hernia of the diaphragm) |
| dipl/o- | double, twice | Diplocoria (double pupil in eye) |
| | | Diplopia (double vision) |
| dips/o- | thirst | Polydipsia (excessive thirst) |
| dis- | apart from, free from | Disinfection (free from infection) |
| | | Dissect (cut apart) |
| | | Disarticulation (separation at a joint) |
| disk/o- | intervertebral disk | Diskitis (inflammation of an intervertebral disk) |
| diverticul/o- | diverticulum | diverticulum |
| dolich/o- | long | Dolichocephalic (long head) |
| | | Dolichoderus (long neck) |
| dors/i-, dors/o- | posterior or back | dorsiflexion |
| -drome | run, running | Syndrome (group of symptoms that run or occur together) |
| -duct- | lead | Abduct (lead away from) |
| | | Duct (tube leading to or from) |
| duoden/o- | duodenum of intestine | duodenostomy |
| dur/o- | hard, duramater | Duritis (inflammation of the dura mater) |
| dynam/o- | power or strength | Dynamometer (a device to measure the strength of muscle contractions) |
| -dynia, -odynia | pain | Mastodynia (pain in the breast) |
| dys- | difficult, bad, painful | Dyskinesis (difficult motion) |
| | | Dyspepsia (bad digestion) |
| | | Dyspareunia (painful coitus) |
| -eal | pertaining to | Perotoneal (pertaining to the peritoneum) |
| ech/o- | sound | Echocardiogram (a record of the heart activities using sound waves) |
| -ectas- | dilate | Phlebectasia (dilation of veins) |
| | | Venectasia (dilation of veins) |
| -ectasis | stretching out, dilatation, expansion | Atelectasis (incomplete expansion of a lung) |
| ect-, ecto- | outer, outside, situated on | Ectal (on the surface) |
| | | Ectoderm (outer skin) |
| | | Ectocytic (outside of the cell) |
| -ectomy | cutting out | Lobectomy (cutting out of a lobe) |
| | | Appendectomy (cutting out of the appendix) |
| -ectopia | displacement | Tarsectopia (displacement of the tarsal bone) |
| ectop/o- | located away from usual place | Ectopic pregnancy (pregnancy outside the uterus) |
| -edem- | swelling | Cephaledema (swelling of head) |
| | | Edematous (swollen) |
| e-, ec- | out of, from, away from | Enucleate (remove whole from) |
| | | Ectopic (out of place) |
| electr/o- | electricity, electrical activity | Electroanesthesia (the use of an electric current to produce anesthesia) |
| ele/o-, ole/o- | oil | eleoma oleoresin |
| embry/o- | embryo, to be full | Embryonic (resembling an embryo) |
| em-,* en- | in | Empyema (pus in a body cavity) |
| | | Encranial (in the cranium) |

*em- before b, m, and p.

Continued

| Form | Meaning | Example(s) |
|------|---------|-----------|
| -emesis | vomit | Hematemesis (vomiting of blood)<br>Hyperemesis (excessive vomiting) |
| -emia | blood condition | Leukemia (malignant disease of the blood)<br>Anemia (lack of red blood cells) |
| emmetr/o | a normal measure | Emmetropia (normal condition of an eye) |
| encephal/o- | brain | encephalodysplasia |
| end-, endo-, ent-, ento- | within, inner | Endaural (within the ear)<br>Endocranial (within the cranium)<br>Entiris (inner eye color)<br>Entocele (internal hernia) |
| endocrin/o | endocrine | Endocrinology (study of the endocrine system) |
| -ent, -er | person or agent | Recipient (one who receives)<br>Examiner (one who examines) |
| enter/o- | intestine | enterocolitis |
| ep-, epi- | upon, on, over | Epicostal (upon a rib)<br>Epidermis (outer skin layer)<br>Eponychia (infection over the nail bed) |
| epididym/o | epididymis | Epididymitis (inflammation of the epididymis) |
| epiglott/o- | epiglottis | epiglottitis |
| episi/o- | vulva | episiotomy |
| epitheli/o | epithelium | Epithelioma (a neoplasm derived from the epithelium) |
| erythr/o- | red | erythromelalgia |
| -esis | state or condition | Paresis (partial paralysis) |
| eso- | within, inward | Esophoria (crossed eye)<br>Esodeviation (a turning inward) |
| esophag/o- | esophagus | esophagocele |
| -esthes-, esthesi/o- | sensation | Anesthesia (without sensation)<br>Esthesiogenic (producing sensation) |
| eti/o | cause (of disease) | Etiology (study of the cause of a disease) |
| eu-, | normal, good, well, healthy | Eucrasia (normal health)<br>Euplastic (healing well) |
| eury- | wide, broad | Eurysomatic (thickset body)<br>Eurycephalic (unusually broad head) |
| ex-, exo- | outside, outward | Exostosis (outgrowth of bone)<br>Exogenic (originating outside) |
| extra-, extro- | outside of, beyond, outward | Extraoral (outside of the mouth)<br>Extroversion (turning insideout) |
| faci/o | face | facial |
| femor/o | femur (upper leg bone) | Femoral (pertaining to the femur) |
| ferrum | iron | ferrous |
| fet/i, fet/o | fetus, unborn child | Fetometry (measurement of the size of the fetus) |
| fibr/o- | fiber | fibroblastoma |
| fibul/o | fibula (lower leg bone) | Fibular (pertaining to the fibula) |
| fiss- | split, cleft | Fissure (cleft or groove)<br>Fissile (capable of being split) |
| -flect-, flex- | bend | Anteflect (bend forward)<br>Flexion (bending) |
| -form | resembling, shaped like | Fusiform (spindle-shaped) |
| galact/o-, lac | milk | galactosemia lactotherapy |
| gangli/o, ganglion/o | ganglion | Ganglionectomy (excision of a ganglion) |
| gastr/o- | stomach | gastrectasia |
| -genesis | beginning process, origin | Pathogenesis (origin of disease)<br>Homogenesis (young same as parent) |
| -genic, -gen | producing, originating, causing | Pathogen (disease causing agent) |
| gen/o- | producing | Genesis (origin or beginning)<br>Genophobia (fear of sexuality) |
| ger/o, geront/o | old age, aged | Gerontology (study of the aging process) |
| gingiv/o- | gums | gingivitis |
| gli/o- | neuroglia or gluey substance | gliococcus |
| glomerul/o | glomerulus | Glomerulonephritis (inflammation of the glomerulus of the kidney) |
| gloss/o- | tongue | glossopathy |
| glyc/o-, gluc/o- | sugar, sweet | Glycemia (glucose in the blood)<br>Glycogeusia (sweet taste) |
| glyc/o-, glycos/o-,<br>sacchar/o-,<br>sacchar/i- | sugar | glycogen saccharobiose |
| gnath/o- | jaw | gnathostatics |

| Form | Meaning | Example(s) |
|------|---------|-----------|
| -gram, -graphy | recording, written record | Mammogram (x-ray of the breast) |
| | | Cardiography (heart action record) |
| -graph | instrument that records | Cardiograph (instrument for measuring heart action) |
| | | Encephalograph (instrument for measuring brain function) |
| gravid/o | pregnancy | Gravida (pregnant woman) |
| gynec/o, gyn/o | woman | Gynecopathic (pertaining to women's diseases) |
| hal/o- | a salt | halogen |
| hapl/o- | simple, single | Haploid (single or half set of chromosomes) |
| | | Haplopathy (uncomplicated disease) |
| hem/a-, hemat/o-, hem/o- | blood | hemapoiesis |
| heme | iron-based, pigmented part of hemoglobin | hemoglobin |
| hemi- | half | Hemiepilepsy (epilepsy on one side of the body) |
| | | Hemilingual (half of the tongue) |
| hepat/ico-, hepat/o- | liver | hepatobiliary |
| herni/o | hernia | Herniorrhaphy (suturing of a hernia) |
| heter/o- | other, different | Heterocellular (pertaining to different cells) |
| | | Heterohypnosis (induced by another) |
| hidr/o-, sudor | sweat | hidrosadenitis sudoriferous |
| hist/o- | tissue | histology |
| hom/eo-, hom/o- | same, alike | Homeomorphous (similar in shape) |
| | | Homozygous (having identical genes) |
| horomone | body-produced chemical substance | hormesis |
| humer/o- | humerus (upper arm bone) | humeral |
| hyal/o-, hyalin | glassy, translucent substance | hyalinuria |
| hydr/o- | wet, water | Hydremia (excess water in blood) |
| | | Hydroadipsia (absence of thirst) |
| hymen/o | hymen | Hymenotomy (incision of the hymen) |
| hyper- | excessive, above, beyond | Hyperactive (overactive) |
| | | Hypertension (above-normal blood pressure) |
| hyp-, hypo- | under, deficient, beneath | Hypalgia (reduced pain sense) |
| | | Hypothyroidism (deficiency of thyroid activity) |
| hypn/o | sleep | Hypnosis (trance like state resembling sleep) |
| hyster/o- | uterus | hysteroscopy |
| -ia, -iasis, -ism, -ity | state or condition | Anesthesia (loss of sensation) |
| | | Psoriasis (skin condition) |
| | | Priapism (persistent erection) |
| | | Acidity (excess acid) |
| -iatr/o- | treatment | Geriatrics (treatment of aging) |
| | | Pediatrics (treatment of children) |
| -iatry | physician, treatment | Psychiatry (branch of medicine that deals with treating mental disorders) |
| -ible, -ile | capable, able | Flexible (capable of bending) |
| | | Contractile (able to contract) |
| ichthy/o | fish | Ichthyoid (resembling fishlike structures) |
| -ic, -ial | pertaining to, relating to | Hemorrhagic (relating to bleeding) |
| -ictal | seizure, attack | Preictal (occurring before a seizure or attack) |
| ile/o- | ileum of intestine | ileocecal |
| ili/o- | ilium (upper part of hip bone) | iliofemoral |
| im-,† in- | in, into, within | Implant (insert into) |
| | | Injection (forcing fluid into) |
| im-,† in- | not | Immature (not mature) |
| | | Involuntary (not voluntary) |
| immun/o | immune | Immunocompromised (weakened immune system) |
| infra- | below, beneath | Infraorbital (beneath the eyes) |
| | | Infracostal (below a rib) |
| inter- | between | Intercostal (between ribs) |
| | | Internodal (between nodes) |
| intra- | within | Intracardiac (within the heart) |
| | | Intraocular (within the eye) |
| intro- | into, within | Introversion (turning inward) |
| | | Introrsus (turned in) |
| irid/o- | iris of eye | iridectomy |
| iri/o | iris | Iritis (inflammation of the iris) |
| ischi/o- | ischium | ischiodidymus |
| isch/o | deficiency, blockage | Ischemia (deficient blood supply to a body part) |
| is/o- | equal, alike | Isocellular (having similar cells) |
| | | Isocoria (equal-sized pupils) |

†im- before b, m, and p.

*Continued*

| Form | Meaning | Example(s) |
|------|---------|------------|
| -ist,-ician | person or agent | Oculist (eye physician) |
| -ites,-itis | inflammation | Tympanites (drumlike swelling of the abdomen) |
|  |  | Adenitis (inflammation of a gland) |
| -ize | use, subject to | Visualize (to use the imagination) |
| jejun/o- | jejunum of intestine | jejunostomy |
| kal/i | potassium | Kaliuresis (excretion of potassium in the urine) |
| kary/o | nucleus | Karyogenesis (formation of a nucleus) |
| kerat/o- | horny tissue or cornea of eye | keratosis |
| kin/e-, kin/o-, kinesi/o- | movement, motion | Kinetogenic (producing movement) |
|  |  | Kinomometer (device to measure motion) |
| kyph/o | hump | Kyphosis (abnormal hump or curvature of the thoracic-spine) |
| labi/o- | lip, especially lips of mouth | labiodental |
| labyrinth/o | labyrinth | Labryinthectomy (excision of the labyrinth) |
| lamin/o | lamina (thin, flat plate or layer) | Laminectomy (surgical removal of the lamina of the vertebral arch) |
| lapar/o- | loin or flank, sometimes abdomen | laparoscopy |
| lapis | stone | lapis dentalis |
| laryng/o- | larynx | laryngeal |
| later/o- | side | lateral |
| lei/o- | smooth | Leiodermia (smooth, glossy skin) |
|  |  | Leiotrichous (smooth hair) |
| -lepsy | seizure | Epilepsy (disorder characterized by recurrent seizures) |
| lept/o- | slender, small, thin | Leptodactylous (slender fingered) |
|  |  | Leptodermic (thin-skinned) |
| leuc/o-, leuk/o- | white | leukopenia |
| lev/o- | left, to the left | Levoduction (eyes turn left) |
|  |  | Levorotation (turning to the left) |
| lien/o- | spleen | lienography |
| lingu/o- | tongue | lingual |
| lip/o-, lipid | fat, fatty acids | lipolytic |
| lith/o- | stone or calculus | lithotripsy |
| lob/o | lobe | Lobotomy (incision into a lobe) |
| lord/o | bent forward | Lordosis (forward curvature of the lumbar spine) |
| lutein | saffron yellow | luteinization |
| lymph/o- | lymph | lymphedema |
| lymph/o- | lymphatic vessels or lymphocytes | lymphopoiesis |
| ly/o-, lys/o- | dissolve | Lyotropic (readily soluble) |
|  |  | Lysogen (producing dissolution) |
| -lysis | loosening, dissolution, separating | Hemodialysis (removal or separation of impurities from the blood) |
| -lytic | destroy, reduce | Leukolytic (pertaining to destruction of leukocytes) |
| macr/o- | large | Macrencephaly (large brain) |
|  |  | Macrobiosis (long life) |
| mal- | ill, bad | Malady (illness) |
|  |  | Malaise (general discomfort) |
| -malacia | softening | Osteomalacia (softening of the bones) |
| malac/o- | soft, softening | Malacia (softening) |
|  |  | Malacotomy (incision of soft parts) |
| mamm/a-, mamm/o- | breast | mammography |
| mandibul/o | mandible (lower jawbone) | Mandibular (pertaining to the mandible) |
| mast/o- | breast | mastocarcinoma |
| mastoid/o | mastoid | Mastoiditis (inflammation of the mastoid bones of the ear) |
| maxill/o | maxilla (upper jawbone) | Maxillofacial (pertaining to the maxilla and the face) |
| meat/o- | meatus (opening) | Meatoscopy (visual examination of a meatus) |
| -megaly | enlargement | Organomegaly (enlargement of an organ) |
| meg/a-, megal/o-, megaly- | large, oversized | Megalgia (severe pain) |
|  |  | Megalomania (grandiose delusions) |
|  |  | Hepatomegaly (enlarged liver) |
| melan/o- | black | melancholia |
| mel/i- | honey or sugar | melitagra |
| mel/o- | limb | melalgia |
| mening/o-, mening/i- | membranes covering brain and spinal cord | meningismus |
| menisc/o | meniscus (crescent) | Meniscectomy (surgical excision of the meniscus of the knee) |
| men/o | menstruation | Menopause (cessation of menstruation) |
| ment/o | mind | Mental (relating to the mind) |

| Form | Meaning | Example(s) |
|------|---------|------------|
| mes-, meso- | middle | Mesencephalon (midbrain) |
| | | Mesonasal (middle of the nose) |
| meta- | change, beyond | Metachrosis (color change) |
| | | Metabasis (disease changes) |
| -meter, -metry | instrument used to measure; measurement | Thermometer (instrument used to measure temperature) |
| metr/a-, metr/o-, metr/i- | uterus | metralgia |
| micr-, micro- | small | Micracoustic (faint sounds) |
| | | Microbe (minute organism) |
| mi/o- | less, decrease | Miopragia (decreased activity) |
| | | Miosis (contraction of pupil) |
| mon/o | one | Monoplegia (paralysis of one limb) |
| -morph | form, shape | Ectomorph (body shape or physique characterized by slenderness and fragility) |
| morph/o- | form, structure, shape | Amorphous (having no definite form) |
| | | Polymorphic (having many forms) |
| mucus, muc/o | secretion of mucous membranes | mucoviscidosis |
| mult-, multi- | many | Multiarticular (many joints) |
| | | Multiform (many shapes) |
| myc/o | fungus | Mycology (the study of fungi and fungal diseases) |
| myel/o-, myelon/o- | bone marrow or spinal cord | myelodiastasis |
| my/o-, myos/o- | muscle | myocele |
| myring/o | eardrum | myringomycosis |
| myx/o- | mucus | myxedema |
| narc/o | stupor | Narcosis (state of stupor caused by narcotic drugs) |
| nas/o- | nose | nasopharyngeal |
| nat/o | birth | Natal (pertaining to birth) |
| natrium | sodium | natremia |
| necr/o- | death | Necrophobia (fear of death) |
| | | Necropsy (autopsy) |
| neo- | new, recent | Neoblastic (new tissue growth) |
| | | Neonatal (newborn) |
| nephr/o- | kidney | nephroangiosclerosis |
| neur/o- | nerve, nerves, or nervous system | neurofibroma |
| noct/i | night | Nocturia (excessive urination at night) |
| nulli- | none | Nulligravida (a woman who has never been pregnant) |
| nyct/o, nyctal/o | night | Nyctophobia (fear of night or darkness) |
| occipit/o- | back of head | occipitobregmatic |
| ocul/o- | eye | oculomotor |
| odont/o- | tooth or teeth | odontogenesis |
| -oid | resembling, shaped like | Ovoid (egg-shaped) |
| -ole, -ola | small | Arteriole, arteriola (small artery) |
| olig/o- | few, little | Oligomenorrhea (scanty menses) |
| | | Oligosymptomatic (having few symptoms) |
| -ologist | one who studies and practices (specialist) | Gastroenterologist (one who studies diseases of the GI tract) |
| -ology, -logy | study of | Biology (science of life) |
| | | Histology (study of tissues) |
| -oma | tumor | Carcinoma (malignant growth) |
| | | Sarcoma (cancerous tumor) |
| om/o- | shoulder | omalgia |
| omphal/o- | navel or umbilicus | omphalocele |
| onc/o | tumor | Oncogenic (causing tumors) |
| onych/o- | nail or nails | onychomycosis |
| oo- | egg, ovum | Oocyte (incompletely developed ovum) |
| oophor/o- | ovary | oophorogenous |
| ophthalm/o- | eye or eyes | opthalmia |
| -opia | vision (condition) | Myopia (nearsightedness) |
| -op/ia | vision | Myopia (nearsightedness) |
| | | Hyperopia (farsightedness) |
| opisth/o- | backward, behind, dorsal | Opisthocheilia (recession of lips) |
| | | Opisthoporeia (walking backward) |
| -opsy | to view | Biopsy (removal of tissue to be viewed microscopically) |
| opt/ico-, opt/o- | seeing | Opticokinetic (pertaining to eye movement) |
| | | Optometer (device for refraction) |
| -or | person or agent | Donor (one who donates) |

*Continued*

| Form | Meaning | Example(s) |
|------|---------|------------|
| orchi/o-, orchi/do-, orch/o- | testis or testes | orchioscirrhus |
| organ/o | organ | Organoid (resembling an organ) |
| or/o- | mouth | oral |
| -orrhagia | rapid flow of blood | Menorrhagia (rapid or heavy menstrual flow) |
| -orrhaphy | suturing, repairing | Cystorrhaphy (suturing the bladder) |
| -orrhea | flow, excessive discharge | Seborrhea (excessive discharge of sebum) |
| -orrhexis | rupture | Hysterorrhexis (rupture of the uterus) |
| orth/o- | straight, normal, correct | Orthodontics (straightening of teeth) Orthograde (walking erect) |
| osche/o- | scrotum | oscheoma |
| -osis | state or condition | Narcosis (drugged state) |
| oss/eo-, oss/i-, ost/e-, ost/eo- | bone or bones | osteoanagenesis |
| -ostomy | creation of an artificial opening | Colostomy (opening into the colon) |
| ot/o- | ear | otopyosis |
| -ous | relating to | Delirious (relating to mental disturbance) |
| ov/i, ov/o | egg | Oviparous (giving birth by laying eggs) |
| -oxia | oxygen | Hypoxia (state of decreased oxygen) |
| ox/i, ox/o | oxygen | Oximeter (instrument used to measure oxygen levels in the blood) |
| oxy- | sharp, quick | Oxyesthesia (overly acute senses) Oxyrhine (sharp-pointed nose) |
| pachy- | thick | Pachyderma (abnormally thick skin) Pachyonychia (overly thick nails) |
| pachy-, pachy/o- | thick | Pachyderma (abnormally thick skin) Pachyonychia (overly thick nails) |
| palat/o- | palate | palatine |
| pale/o- | old, primitive | Paleogenetic (originating in past) Paleologic (primitive reasoning) |
| pan- | all, entire | Panacea (cure-all) Pantalgia (entire-body pain) |
| pancreat/o- | pancreas | pancreatolith |
| papill/o- | nipple or nipple-shaped projection | papilloretinitis |
| para- | beside, beyond, after | Paracardiac (beside the heart) Paracyesis (pregnancy outside the uterus) |
| parathyroid/o | parathyroid gland | Parathyroidoma (tumor of the parathyroid gland) |
| -paresis | slight paralysis | Hemiparesis (weakness/slight paralysis affecting one side of the body) |
| par/o, part/o | bear, give birth to, labor | Parturition (the process of giving birth) |
| patell/o | patella (kneecap) | Patellectomy (surgical excision of the patella) |
| path/o | disease | Pathogenic (producing disease) |
| -pathy | disease | Myopathy (muscle disease) |
| pector/o | chest | Pectoralgia (chest pain) |
| ped/o | child, foot | Pedodontics (dentistry devoted to children) |
| pelv/i, pelv/o | pelvis, pelvic bone | Pelvimetry (measurement of the size of the pelvis) |
| -penia | deficiency of, lack of | Glycopenia (sugar in tissues) Leukopenia (white blood cells) |
| -pepsia | digestion | Bradypepsia (slow digestion) |
| per- | through, excessive | Permeable (may pass through) Peracute (excessively sharp) |
| peri- | around | Periosteum (membrane around bone) Peribulbar (around the eye bulb) |
| perine/o | perineum | Perineorrhaphy (suturing of the perineum) |
| peritone/o | peritoneum | Peritoneal (pertaining to the peritoneum) |
| petrous; petr/o- | stony hardness, stone | petrolatum |
| -pexy, -pexis | fixation, storing | Nephropexy (of floating kidney) Glycopexis (glycogen in liver) |
| phac/o, phak/o | lens of the eye | Phacomalacia (softening of the lens of the eye) |
| -phagia, -phagy | eating, devouring | Geophagia (eating dirt or clay) Aerophagy (swallowing air) |
| phag/o- | eating | Phagomania (food craving) Phagophobia (fear of eating) |
| phalang/o | phalanx (finger or toe bone) | Phalangectomy (excision of aphalanx) |
| phall/o- | penis | phallic |
| phan/ero- | visible, manifest | Phanerosis (process of becoming visible) Phantasm (unreal mental image) |

| Form | Meaning | Example(s) |
|------|---------|-----------|
| pharyng/o- | pharynx | pharyngorrhagia |
| -phas-, phas/o- | speech | Aphasia (loss of speech functions) |
| | | Dysphasia (difficulty in speaking) |
| phil- | affinity, love for | Philanthropy (love of humankind) |
| | | Philoneism (love of change) |
| -philia, -phily | love, attraction for | Hydrophilia (attraction to water molecules) |
| phleb/o- | vein or veins | phlebostasis |
| -phobia | abnormal fear or intolerance | Acrophobia (fear of heights) |
| | | Photophobia (of light) |
| -phonia | sound or voice | Aphonia (absence of voice) |
| -phoria | feeling | Euphoria (feeling of elation) |
| phot/o | light | Photophobia (fear of light) |
| phren/i-, phren/ico-, phren/o- | diaphragm or mind | phrenology |
| -physis | growth | Symphysis (growing together) |
| pil/o- | hair | pilonidal |
| -plasia | formation, development, a growth | Hypoplasia (incomplete development) |
| -plasm | growth, substance, formation | Somatoplasm (body substance) |
| plasma, plasm/o- | fluid portion of blood | plasmapheresis |
| -plasty | surgical shaping or formation | Rhinoplasty (nose formation) |
| | | Otoplasty (external ear) |
| platy- | flat, wide | Platyglossal (wide, flat tongue) |
| | | Platycephaly (flattened skull) |
| -plegia | paralysis | Hemiplegia (one-sided paralysis) |
| | | Paraplegia (paralysis of lower trunk andlegs) |
| ple/o- | more | Pleonexia (excessive greediness) |
| | | Pleonosteosis (excessive bone growth) |
| pleur/o- | pleura or rib | pleurocentrum |
| -pnea | breathing | Apnea (absence of breathing) |
| | | Dyspnea (difficult breathing) |
| pneum/a-, pneum/o-, pneum/ato-, pneum/ono- | lungs or respiration | pneumoconstriction |
| pod/o- | foot or foot-shaped part | podalic |
| -poiesis | formation, production | Hemopoiesis (blood cell formation) |
| | | Leukopoiesis (white blood cell production) |
| poikil/o- | irregular, varied | Poikiloderma (mottled skin) |
| | | Poikilothermic (cold-blooded) |
| poli/o- | gray (pertaining to gray matter of the nervous system) | polioencephalitis |
| poly- | many, much, excessive | Polycystic (with many cysts) |
| | | Polydipsia (excessive thirst) |
| polyp/o | polyp, small growth | Polyposis (abnormal presence of numerous polyps) |
| post- | after, behind | Postoperative (after surgery) |
| | | Postocular (behind the eye) |
| poster/o | back (of body) | Posteroanterior (the direction from back to front) |
| -prandial | meal | Postprandial (after a meal) |
| pre-, pro- | before, in front of | Prenatal (before birth) |
| | | Project (throw forward) |
| prim/i | first | Primigravida (woman in her first pregnancy) |
| proct/o- | rectum or anus | proctology |
| prostat/o- | prostate gland | prostatectomy |
| pseud/o | false | Pseudocyesis (false pregnancy) |
| pseud-, pseudo- | false | Pseudarthrosis (false joint) |
| | | Pseudocyesis (false pregnancy) |
| psych/o | mind | Psychopathy (disease of the mind) |
| -ptosis | prolapse, downward displacement | Proctoptosis (prolapse of anus) |
| | | Nephroptosis (prolapse of kidney) |
| ptyal/o- | saliva | ptyalogenic |
| -ptysis | spitting | Hemoptysis (spitting up blood) |
| pub/o | pubis | Pubofemoral (pertaining to the pubis and femur) |
| puerper/o | childbirth | Puerperal (pertaining to the period immediately following childbirth) |
| pulm/o-, pulmon/o- | lungs | pulmogram |
| pupill/o | pupil | Pupillometer (instrument to measure width and diameter of a pupil) |
| pus | liquid portion of inflammation | pustule |
| pyel/o- | plevis of kidney | pyelocaliectasis |

*Continued*

| Form | Meaning | Example(s) |
|---|---|---|
| pylor/o- | pylorus (pyloric sphincter) | pyloroplasty |
| py/o- | pus | pyocyst |
| pyr/o | fever, heat | Pyrogen (a substance that causes fever) |
| quadr/i | four | Quadriplegia (paralysis of four limbs) |
| rachi/o- | spine | rachiotome |
| radic/o, radicul/o, rhiz/o | nerve root | Radicotomy (incision into a nerve root) |
| radi/o | radius (lower arm bone) | Radioulnar (pertaining to the radius and ulna) |
| re- | again, backward | Reflex (bend back) |
| | | Regurgitation (vomiting) |
| rect/o- | rectum | rectosigmoidoscopy |
| ren/i-, ren/o- | kidney | renin |
| retin/o | retina | Retinopathy (disease of the retina) |
| retro- | backward, behind | Retrograde (going backward) |
| | | Retrolingual (behind the tongue) |
| rhabd/o | rod-shaped, striated | Rhabdomyoma (tumor of striated muscle) |
| rhin/o- | nose | rhinology |
| rhod/o- | red | rhodopsin |
| rhytid/o | wrinkles | Rhytidoplasty (plastic repair of wrinkles) |
| -rrhage, -rrhagia | excessive flow | Hemorrhage (excessive blood flow) |
| | | Metrorrhagia (abnormal menses) |
| -rrhaphy | suturing in place | Herniorrhaphy (repair of hernia) |
| | | Osteorrhaphy (wiring of bone) |
| -rrhea | flow or discharge | Rhinorrhea (nasal discharge) |
| | | Galactorrhea (breast milk) |
| -rrhexis | rupture | Enterorrhexis (intestinal rupture) |
| | | Metrorrhexis (rupture of uterus) |
| ruber, rubor | red, redness | rubedo |
| sacr/o- | sacrum | sacrococcygeal |
| sal | salt | saline |
| salping/o- | fallopian tube or Eustachian tube | salpingostomy |
| -salpinx | fallopian tube | Hydrosalpinx (water in the fallopian tube) |
| sangui-, sanguin/o- | blood, bloody | sanguineous |
| sarc/o- | flesh or muscular substance | sarcoadenoma |
| -sarcoma | malignant tumor | Myosarcoma (malignant tumor of muscular tissue) |
| scapul/o- | scapula | scapulohumeral |
| -schisis | split, fissure | Cranioschisis (fissure of the skull) |
| schist/o-, schiz/o- | split, cleft, division | Schistocystis (bladder fissure) |
| | | Schizonychia (splitting of nails) |
| -scler/o- | hardness | Sclerosis (hardening) |
| | | Arteriosclerosis (hardening of artery) |
| -sclerosis | hardening | Arteriosclerosis (hardening of arteries) |
| scoli/o- | twisted, crooked | Scoliokyphosis (curvature of spine) |
| | | Scoliosis (crooked spine) |
| -scope | instrument for examining | Microscope (minute objects) |
| | | Cystoscope (urinary bladder) |
| -scopy, -scopic | act of examining | Microscopy (minute objects) |
| | | Cystoscopy (urinary bladder) |
| sebum, seb/o- | sebaceous gland secretion (sebum) | seborrhea |
| semi- | half | Semiconscious (partly aware) |
| | | Seminormal (half normal) |
| -sepsis | infection | Antisepsis (destruction of microorganisms to prevent infection) |
| sept/o | septum | Septotomy (incision into the nasal septum) |
| serum | clear portion of blood fluid | serum globulin |
| sial/o- | saliva, salivary glands | sialorrhea |
| sigmoid/o | sigmoid | Sigmoidoscopy (visual examination of the sigmoid) |
| sinistr/o- | left, to the left | Sinistrocular (left-eyed) |
| | | Sinistromanual (left-handed) |
| sinus/o | sinus | Sinusotomy (incision of a sinus) |
| -sis | state or condition | Narcosis (drugged state) |
| somat/o-, somatic/o- | body | somatotype |
| somn/i | sleep | Insomnia (in ability to sleep or remain asleep) |
| son/o | sound | Sonometer (instrument used to measure sound) |
| -spasm | sudden involuntary muscle contraction | Laryngospasm (contraction of the larynx) |
| spasm/o- | spasm | Spasmogenic (causing spasms) |
| | | Spasmolysis (relieving a spasm) |

| Form | Meaning | Example(s) |
|---|---|---|
| spermat/o, sperm/o | spermatozoan, sperm | Spermatolysis (destruction of sperm) |
| sphygm/o | pulse | Sphygmograph (instrument that records the force of the arterial pulse) |
| spir/o | breathe, breathing | Spirograph (a device for recording breathing) |
| splanchn/e-, splanchn/o- | viscera or splachnic nerve | splanchnopleure |
| splen/o- | spleen | splenomegaly |
| spondyl/o- | vertebra or spinal column | spondylosis |
| -stalsis | contraction | Peristalsis (contraction of the digestive tract muscles) |
| staped/o- | stapedes (middle earbone) | stapedius |
| staphyl/o | grapelike clusters | Staphylococcus (bacteria arranged in grapelike clusters) |
| -stasis | standing still, stoppage | Epistasis (film on standing liquid)<br>Hemostasis (stoppage of blood flow) |
| sten/o- | narrow | Stenosed (narrowed, contracted)<br>Stenostomia (narrow oral cavity) |
| -stenosis | constriction, narrowing | Tracheostenosis (construction of the trachea) |
| stere/o- | solid, three-dimensional | Stereoscopic (solid appearance)<br>Stereopsis (three-dimensional vision) |
| stern/o- | sternum | sternocleidal |
| steth/o- | chest | stethomimetic |
| stom-, stomat/o- | mouth | stomatology |
| -stomy | surgical opening | Colostomy (colon to body surface)<br>Gastrostomy (into stomach) |
| strept/o | twisted chains | Streptococcus (bacteria arranged in twisted chains) |
| sub- | under, beneath | Subcutaneous (under the skin)<br>Subungual (under the nail) |
| super-, supra- | above, superior, excess | Superactivity (overactivity)<br>Suprarenal (above the kidneys) |
| sym-,* syn- | together, with | Symmelia (fusion of limbs)<br>Synclinal (bent together) |
| synovi/o | synovia, synovial membrane | Synoviosarcoma (tumor of the synovial membrane) |
| system/o | system | Systematic (pertaining to a system) |
| tachy- | rapid, fast | Tachyphagia (bolting one's food)<br>Tachylogia (rapid speech) |
| tal/o- | ankle or ankle bone | talocalcaneal |
| tars/o- | instep of foot or eyelid edge | tarsomalacia |
| tel/e-, tel/o- | distant, end | Telalgia (pain from another area)<br>Telencephalon (end brain) |
| tend/o-, ten/o-, tenont/o-, tendin/o- | tendon | tenosynovitis |
| test/o | testis, testicle | Testitis (inflammation of the testes) |
| tetra- | four | Tetradactyly (having only 4 fingers on each hand or 4 toes on each foot) |
| thel/o- | nipple | theleplasty |
| therm/o- | heat | Thermogenic (producing heat)<br>Thermolabile (alteration or destruction by heat) |
| thorac/o- | chest or thorax | thoracentesis |
| -thorax | chest | Pneumothorax (air in the chest) |
| thromb/o | clot | Thrombosis (abnormal development of a clot within a blood vessel) |
| thym/o- | thymus gland | thymoma |
| thyr/o-, thyroid/o- | thyroid gland | thyroaplasia |
| tibi/o- | tibia | tibial |
| -tic | pertaining to | Acoustic (pertaining to sound) |
| -tion | state or condition | Inhalation (state of inhaling) |
| -tocia | birth, labor | Embryotocia (birth of an embryo) |
| -tome | instrument for | Cystotome (cutting into bladder)<br>Neurotome (dissecting nerves) |
| tom/o | cut, section | Dermatome (instrument used to cut thin slices of skin for grafting) |
| -tomy | cutting, incision | Cystotomy (of urinary bladder)<br>Phlebotomy (incision of vein) |
| ton/o | tension, pressure | Tonometry (measurement of pressure within the eye) |
| tonsill/o | tonsils | Tonsillitis (inflammation of the tonsils) |
| top/o- | place, location | Topalgia (localized pain)<br>Toponarcosis (localized anesthesia) |
| toxic/o | poison | Toxicosis (a disease condition caused by poisons) |
| trachel/o- | neck or necklike structure | tracheloschisis |

*sym- before b, m, p, and ph.

*Continued*

| Form | Meaning | Example(s) |
|------|---------|------------|
| trache/o- | trachea | tracheomalacia |
| trans- | across, through | Transection (cut across) |
| | | Transaortic (through the aorta) |
| tri- | three | Tricuspid (having 3 points or cusps) |
| trich/o- | hair or hairlike structure | trichopathy |
| -tripsy | surgical crushing | Lithotripsy (surgical crushing of a stone) |
| troph/o- | nourishment, food | Trophism (nutrition) |
| | | Dystrophy (defective nutrition) |
| -trophy | nourishment, development | Nephrohypertrophy (excessive development of the kidney) |
| tympan/o- | eardrum (middle ear) | tympanoplasty |
| -ule, -ulum, -ulus | small | Nodule (small node) |
| | | Ovulum (small egglike structure) |
| | | Homunculus (small human) |
| uln/o | ulna (lower arm bone) | Ulnar (relating to the ulna) |
| ultra- | beyond, excess | Ultravirus (very small virus) |
| | | Ultrasonic (beyond the upper limit of human hearing) |
| ungu/o- | nail or nails | ungual |
| uni- | one | Unilateral (involving only 1 side) |
| ureter/o- | ureter | ureterostenosis |
| urethr/o- | urethra (tube from bladder to outside) | urethrocystitis |
| ur/e-, ure/a-, ure/o-, urin/o-, ur/o- | urine, urea | urobilinuria |
| -uria | urine, urination | Pyuria (pus in the urine) |
| uter/o- | uterus | uterotomy |
| uvul/o | uvula | Uvulectomy (surgical removal of the uvula) |
| vagin/o | vagina | Vaginography (radiographic examination of the vagina) |
| valv/o, valvul/o | valve | Valvotomy (incision into a valve) |
| vas/o- | vessel or duct | vasodilation |
| ven/e-, ven/i-, ven/o- | vein or veins | venoatrial |
| ventricul/o | ventricle | Ventriculography (x-ray examination of a ventricle) |
| ventr/i-, ventr/o- | front of body or belly | ventrolateral |
| vertebr/o | vertebra, spinal or vertebral column | Vertebrocostal (pertaining to the vertebrae and ribs) |
| vesic/o- | bladder or blister | vesicoureteral |
| vesicul/o | seminal vesicles | Vesiculography (radiologic examination of the seminal vesicles) |
| viscer/o- | viscera | viscerosomatic |
| vulv/o | vulva | Vulvovaginitis (inflammation of the vulva and vagina) |
| xanth/o- | yellow, yellowish | xanthoma |
| xer/o- | dry | Xerochilia (drylips) |
| | | Xerostomia (dry mouth) |
| -y | state or condition | Therapy (treatment condition) |

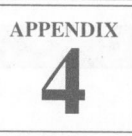

APPENDIX
4

# TABULAR ATLAS OF HUMAN ANATOMY AND PHYSIOLOGY

## 4-1 Basic structures and functions of the body

### Major cell structures and functions

| Cell structure | Functions |
|---|---|
| **MEMBRANOUS** | |
| Plasma membrane | Serves as the boundary of the cell, maintaining its integrity; protein molecules embedded in plasma membrane perform various functions; for example, they serve as markers that identify cells of each individual, as receptor molecules for certain hormones and other molecules, and as transport mechanisms |
| Endoplasmic reticulum (ER) | Ribosomes attached to rough ER synthesize proteins that leave cells via the Golgi complex; smooth ER synthesizes lipids incorporated in cell membranes, steroid hormones, and certain carbohydrates used to form glycoproteins |
| Golgi apparatus | Synthesizes carbohydrate, combines it with protein, and packages the product as globules of glyco-protein |
| Lysosomes | A cell's "digestive system" |
| Peroxisomes | Contain enzymes that detoxify harmful substances |
| Mitochondria | Catabolism; ATP synthesis; a cell's "power plants" |
| Nucleus | Houses the genetic code, which in turn dictates protein synthesis, thereby playing essential role in other cell activities, namely, cell transport, metabolism, and growth |
| **NONMEMBRANOUS** | |
| Ribosomes | Synthesize proteins; a cell's "protein factories" |
| Cytoskeleton | Acts as a framework to support the cell and its organelles; functions in cell movement; forms cell extensions (microvilli, cilia, flagella) |
| Cilia and flagella | Hairlike cell extensions that serve to move substances over the cell surface (cilia) or propel sperm cells (flagella) |
| Nucleolus | Plays an essential role in the formation of ribosomes |

From Thibodeau GA, Patton KT: *Anatomy and physiology,* ed 3, St Louis, 1996, Mosby.

### Tissues

| Tissue | Location | Function |
|---|---|---|
| **EPITHELIAL** **Membranous** | | |
| Simple squamous | Alveoli of lungs | Absorption by diffusion of respiratory gases between alveolar air and blood |
| | Lining of blood and lymphatic vessels (called endothelium; classified as connective tissue by some histologists) | Absorption by diffusion, filtration, osmosis |
| | Surface layer of pleura, pericardium, peritoneum (called mesothelium; classified as connective tissue by some histologists) | Absorption by diffusion and osmosis; also, secretion |
| Stratified squamous | Surface of mucous membrane lining mouth, esophagus, and vagina | Protection |
| | Surface of skin (epidermis) | Protection |
| Transitional | Surface of mucous membrane lining urinary bladder and ureters | Permits stretching |
| Simple columnar | Surface layer of mucous lining of stomach, intestines, and part of respiratory tract | Protection; secretion; absorption; moving of mucus (by ciliated columnar epithelium) |
| Stratified columnar | Lining of portions of the male urethra; mucous membrane near anus (rare) | Protection |
| Pseudostratified columnar | Surface of mucous membrane lining trachea, large bronchi, nasal mucosa, and parts of male reproductive tract (epididymis and vas deferens); lines large ducts of some glands (e.g., parotid) | Protection |

From Thibodeau GA, Patton KT: *Anatomy and physiology,* ed 3, St Louis, 1996, Mosby.

*Continued*

## Tissues—cont'd

| Tissue | Location | Function |
|---|---|---|
| **EPITHELIAL—cont'd** | | |
| **Membranous—cont'd** | | |
| Simple cuboidal | Ducts and tubules of many organs, including exocrine glands and kidneys | Secretion; absorption |
| Stratified cuboidal | Ducts of sweat glands; lining of pharynx; covering portion of epiglottis | Protection |
| Glandular | Glands | Secretion |
| **CONNECTIVE** | | |
| **Fibrous** | | |
| Loose, ordinary (areolar) | Between other tissues and organs | Connection |
| | Superficial fascia | Connection |
| Adipose (fat) | Under skin | Protection |
| | Padding at various points | Insulation |
| | | Support |
| | | Reserve food |
| Reticular | Inner framework of spleen, lymph nodes, bone marrow | Support |
| | | Filtration |
| Dense fibrous | | |
|   Regular | Tendons | Flexible but strong connection |
| | Ligaments | |
| | Aponeuroses | |
|   Irregular | Deep fascia | Connection |
| | Dermis | Support |
| | Scars | |
| | Capsule of kidney, etc. | |
| **Bone** | Skeleton | Support |
| | | Protection |
| | | Calcium reservoir |
| Cartilage | | |
|   Hyaline | Part of nasal septum | Firm but flexible support |
| | Covering articular surfaces of bones | |
| | Larynx | |
| | Rings in trachea and bronchi | |
|   Fibrocartilage | Disks between vertebrae | |
| | Symphysis pubis | |
|   Elastic | External ear | |
| | Eustachian tube | |
| Blood | In blood vessels | Transportation |
| | | Protection |
| **MUSCLE** | | |
| Skeletal (striated voluntary) | Muscles that attach to bones | Movement of bones |
| | Extrinsic eyeball muscles | Eye movements |
| | Upper third of esophagus | First part of swallowing |
| Smooth (nonstriated, involuntary, or visceral) | In walls of tubular viscera of digestive, respiratory, and genitourinary tracts | Movement of substances along respective tracts |
| | In walls of blood vessels and large lymphatic vessels | Change diameter of blood vessels, thereby aiding in regulation of blood pressure |
| | In ducts of glands | Movement of substances along ducts |
| | Intrinsic eye muscles (iris and ciliary body) | Change diameter of pupils and shape of lens |
| | Arrector muscles of hairs | Erection of hairs (gooseflesh) |
| Cardiac (striated involuntary) | Wall of heart | Contraction of heart |
| **NERVOUS** | Brain | Excitability |
| | Spinal cord | Conduction |
| | Nerves | |

| 4-2 | **Skeletal system** |
|---|---|

### Bones of the skeleton (206 total)*

| Part of body | Name of bone | Number | Identification |
|---|---|---|---|
| **APPENDICULAR SKELETON (126 bones)** | | | Bones that are appended to axial skeleton; upper and lower extremities, including shoulder and hip girdles |
| **Upper extremities** (including shoulder girdle) (64 bones) | Clavicle | 2 | Collar bones; shoulder girdle joined to axial skeleton by articulation of clavicles with sternum; scapula does not form joint with axial skeleton |
| | Scapula | 2 | Shoulder blades; scapulae and clavicles together comprise shoulder girdle |
| | Humerus | 2 | Long bone of upper arm |
| | Radius | 2 | Bone of thumb side of forearm |
| | Ulna | 2 | Bone of little finger side of forearm; longer than radius |
| | Carpals (scaphoid, lunate, triquetrum, pisiform, trapezium, trapezoid, capitate, and hamate) | 16 | Wrist bones; arranged in two rows at proximal end of hand |
| | Metacarpals | 10 | Long bones forming framework of palm of hand |
| | Phalanges | 28 | Miniature long bones of fingers, 3 in each finger, 2 in each thumb |
| **Lower extremities** (62 bones) | Ossa coxae or innominate bones | 2 | Large hip bones; with sacrum and coccyx, these 3 bones form basin-like pelvic cavity; lower extremities attached to axial skeleton by pelvic bones |
| | Femur | 2 | Thigh bone; largest, strongest bone of body |
| | Patella | 2 | Kneecap; largest sesamoid bone of body*; embedded in tendon of quadriceps femoris muscle |
| | Tibia | 2 | Shin bone |
| | Fibula | 2 | Long, slender bone of lateral side of lower leg |
| | Tarsals (calcaneus, talus, navicular, first, second, and third cuneiforms, cuboid) | 14 | Bones that form heel and proximal or posterior half of foot |
| | Metatarsals | 10 | Long bones of feet |
| | Phalanges | 28 | Miniature long bones of toes; 2 in each great toe, 3 in other toes |
| **AXIAL SKELETON (80 bones)** | | | Bones that form upright axis on body—skull, hyoid, vertebral column, sternum, and ribs |
| **Skull (28 bones)** | | | |
| Cranium (8 bones) | | | Cranium forms floor for brain to rest on and helmet-like covering over it |
| | Frontal | 1 | Forehead bone; also forms most of roof of orbits (eye sockets) and anterior part of cranial floor |
| | Parietal | 2 | Prominent, bulging bones behind frontal bone; form top sides of cranial cavity |
| | Temporal | 2 | Form lower sides of cranium and part of cranial floor; contain middle and inner ear structures |
| | Occipital | 1 | Forms posterior part of cranial floor and walls |
| | Sphenoid | 1 | Keystone of cranial floor; forms its midportion; resembles bat with wings outstretched and legs extended downward posteriorly; lies behind and slightly above nose and throat; forms part of floor and sidewalls of orbit |
| | Ethmoid | 1 | Complicated irregular bone that helps make up anterior portion of cranial floor, medial wall of orbits, upper parts of nasal septum, and sidewalls and part of nasal roof; lies anterior to sphenoid and posterior to nasal bones |

From Thibodeau GA, Patton KT: *Anatomy and physiology,* ed 4, St Louis, 2000, Mosby.

*An inconstant number of small, flat, round bones known as *sesamoid bones* (because of their resemblance to sesame seeds) is found in various tendons in which considerable pressure develops. Because the number of these bones varies greatly between individuals, only 2 of them, the patellae, have been counted among the 206 bones of the body. Generally, 2 of them can be found in each thumb (in flexor tendon near metacarpophalangeal and interphalangeal joints) and great toe plus several others in the upper and lower extremities. *Wormian bones,* the small islets of bone frequently found in some of the cranial sutures, have not been counted in the list of 206 bones because of their variable occurrence.

*Continued*

## Bones of the skeleton (206 total)—cont'd

| Part of body | Name of bone | Number | Identification |
|---|---|---|---|
| **AXIAL SKELETON (80 bones)—cont'd** | | | |
| **Skull (28 bones)—cont'd** | | | |
| Face (14 bones) | Nasal | 2 | Small bones forming upper part of bridge of nose |
| | Maxillary | 2 | Upper jaw bones; form part of floor of orbit, anterior part of roof of mouth, and floor and part of side-walls of nose |
| | Zygomatic (malar) | 2 | Cheekbones; form part of floor and sidewall of orbit |
| | Mandible | 1 | Lower jawbone; largest, strongest bone of face |
| | Lacrimal | 2 | Thin bones about size and shape of fingernail; posterior and lateral to nasal bones in median wall or orbit; help form sidewall of nasal cavity, often missing in dry skull |
| | Palatine | 2 | Form posterior part of hard palate floor and part of sidewalls of nasal cavity and floor of orbit |
| | Inferior conchae (turbinates) | 2 | Thin scroll of bone forming a kind of shell along inner surface of sidewall of nasal cavity; lies above roof of mouth |
| | Vomer | 1 | Forms lower and posterior part of nasal septum; shaped like ploughshare |
| Ear bones (6 bones) | Malleus (hammer) | 2 | Tiny bones referred to as auditory ossicles in middle ear cavity in temporal bones; resemble, respectively, miniature hammer, anvil, and stirrup |
| | Incus (anvil) | 2 | |
| | Stapes (stirrup) | 2 | |
| **Hyoid bone** | | 1 | U-shaped bone in neck between mandible and upper part of larynx; claims distinction as only bone not forming a joint with any other bone; suspended by ligaments from styloid processes of temporal bones |
| **Sternum and ribs** (25 bones) | | | Sternum, ribs, and thoracic vertebrae together form bony cage known as *thorax;* ribs attach posteriorly to vertebrae, slant downward anteriorly to attach to sternum (see description of false ribs below) |
| | Sternum | 1 | Breastbone; flat dagger-shaped bone |
| | True ribs | 14 | Upper seven pairs; fasten to sternum by costal carti-lages |
| | False ribs | 10 | False ribs do not attach to sternum directly; upper three pairs of false ribs attach by means of costal cartilage of seventh ribs; last two pairs do not attach to sternum at all; therefore called "floating" |
| **Vertebral column** (26 bones) | | | Not actually a column but a flexible segmented rod shaped like an elongated letter S; forms axis of body; head balanced above, ribs and viscera suspended in front, and lower extremities attached below; encloses spinal cord |
| | Cervical vertebrae | 7 | First, or upper, seven vertebrae |
| | Thoracic vertebrae | 12 | Next 12 vertebrae; 12 pairs of ribs attached to these |
| | Lumbar vertebrae | 5 | Next five vertebrae |
| | Sacrum | 1 | Five separate vertebrae until about 25 years of age; then fused to form one wedge-shaped bone |
| | Coccyx | 1 | Four or five separate vertebrae in child but fused into one in adult |

From Thibodeau GA, Patton KT: *Anatomy and physiology,* ed 4, St Louis, 2000, Mosby.

## Special features of the skull

| Feature | Description | Feature | Description |
|---------|-------------|---------|-------------|
| **SUTURES** | Immovable joints between skull bones | **AIR SINUSES** | Spaces or cavities within bones; those that communicate with nose called *paranasal sinuses* (frontal, sphenoidal, ethmoidal, and maxillary); mastoid cells communicate with middle ear rather than nose, therefore not included among paranasal sinuses |
| Squamous | Line of articulation along top curved edge of temporal bone | | |
| Coronal | Joint between parietal bones and frontal bone | | |
| Lambdoidal | Joint between parietal bones and occipital bone | | |
| Sagittal | Joint between right and left parietal bones | **ORBITS FORMED BY** | |
| | | Frontal | Roof of orbit |
| **FONTANELS** | "Soft spots" where ossification is incomplete at birth; allow some compression of skull during birth; also important in determining position of head before delivery; six such areas located at angles of parietal bones | Ethmoid | Medial wall |
| | | Lacrimal | Medial wall |
| | | Sphenoid | Lateral wall |
| | | Zygomatic | Lateral wall |
| | | Maxillary | Floor |
| | | Palatine | Floor |
| Frontal (or anterior) | At intersection of sagittal and coronal sutures (juncture of parietal bones and frontal bone); diamond shaped; largest of fontanels; usually closed by 1½ years of age | **NASAL SEPTUM FORMED BY** | Partition in midline of nasal cavity; separates cavity into right and left halves |
| | | Perpendicular plate of ethmoid bone | Forms upper part of septum |
| Occipital (or posterior) | At intersection of sagittal and lambdoidal sutures (juncture of parietal bones and occipital bone); triangular in shape; usually closed by second month | Vomer bone | Forms lower, posterior part |
| | | Cartilage | Forms anterior part |
| | | **WORMIAN BONES** | Small islets of bones with suture |
| Sphenoid (or anterolateral) | At juncture of frontal, parietal, temporal, and phenoid bones | **MALLEUS, INCUS, STAPLES** | Tiny bones, referred to as auditory ossicles, in middle ear cavity in temporal bones; resemble, respectively, miniature hammer, anvil, and stirrup |
| Mastoid (or posterolateral) | At juncture of parietal, occipital, and temporal bones; usually closed by second year | | |

From Thibodeau GA, Patton KT: *Anatomy and physiology,* ed 3, St Louis, 1996, Mosby.

## Cranial bones and their markings

| Bones and markings | Description | Bones and markings | Description |
|--------------------|-------------|--------------------|-------------|
| **FRONTAL** | Forehead bone; also forms most of roof of orbits (eye sockets) and anterior part of cranial floor | **SPHENOID** | Keystone of cranial floor; forms its midportion; resembles bat with wings outstretched and legs extended downward posteriorly; lies behind and slightly above nose and throat; forms part of floor and sidewalls of orbit |
| Supraorbital margin | Arched ridge just below eyebrow, forms upper edge of orbit | | |
| Frontal sinuses | Cavities inside bone just above supraorbital margin; lined with mucosa; contain air | Body | Hollow, cubelike central portion |
| | | Greater wings | Lateral projections from body, form part of outer wall of orbit |
| Frontal tuberosities | Bulge above each orbit; most prominent part of forehead | Lesser wings | Thin, triangular projections from upper part of sphenoid body; form posterior part of roof of orbit |
| Superciliary ridges | Ridges caused by projection of frontal sinuses; eyebrows lie superficial to these ridges | | |
| | | Sella turcica (or *Turk's saddle*) | Saddle-shaped depression on upper surface of sphenoid body; contains pituitary gland |
| Supraorbital foramen (sometimes notch) | Foramen or notch in supraorbital margin slightly medial to its midpoint; transmits supraorbital nerve and blood vessels | | |
| | | Sphenoid sinuses | Irregular air-filled mucosa-lined spaces within central part of sphenoid |
| Glabella | Smooth area between superciliary ridges and above nose | Pterygoid processes | Downward projections on either side where body and greater wing unite; comparable to extended legs of bat if entire bone is likened to this animal; form part of lateral nasal wall |
| **PARIETAL** | Prominent, bulging bones behind frontal bone; forms top sides of cranial cavity | | |

From Thibodeau GA, Patton KT: *Anatomy and physiology,* ed 3, St Louis, 1996, Mosby.

*Continued*

## Cranial bones and their markings—cont'd

| Bones and markings | Description | Bones and markings | Description |
|---|---|---|---|
| **SPHENOID—cont'd** | | **TEMPORAL—cont'd** | |
| Optic foramen | Opening into orbit at roof of lesser wing; transmits optic nerve | Stylomastoid foramen | Opening between styloid and mastoid processes where facial nerve emerges from cranial cavity |
| Superior orbital fissure | Slitlike opening into orbit; lateral to optic foramen; transmits third, fourth, and part of fifth cranial nerves | Jugular fossa | Depression on undersurface of petrous portion; dilated beginning of internal jugular vein lodged here |
| Foramen rotundum | Opening in greater wing that transmits maxillary division of fifth cranial nerve | Jugular foramen | Opening in suture between petrous portion and occipital bone; transmits lateral sinus and ninth, tenth, and eleventh cranial nerves |
| Foramen ovale | Opening in greater wing that transmits mandibular division of fifth cranial nerve | Carotid canal (or foramen) | Channel in petrous portion; best seen from undersurface of skull; transmits internal carotid artery |
| Foramen lacerum | Opening at the junction of the sphenoid, temporal, and occipital bones; transmits branch of the ascending pharyngeal artery | **OCCIPITAL** | Forms posterior part of cranial floor and walls |
| Foramen spinosum | Opening in greater wing that transmits the middle meningeal artery to supply meninges | Foramen magnum | Hole through which spinal cord enters cranial cavity |
| **TEMPORAL** | Form lower sides of cranium and part of cranial floor; contain middle and inner ear structures | Condyles | Convex, oval processes on either side of foramen magnum; articulate within depressions on first cervical vertebra |
| Squamous portion | Thin, flaring upper part of bone | External occipital protuberance | Prominent projection on posterior surface in midline short distance above foramen magnum; can be felt as definite bump |
| Mastoid portion | Rough-surfaced lower part of bone posterior to external auditory meatus | Superior nuchal line | Curved ridge extending laterally from external occipital protuberance |
| Petrous portion | Wedge-shaped process that forms part of center section of cranial floor between sphenoid and occipital bones; name derived from Greek word for stone because of extreme hardness of this process; houses middle and inner ear structures | Inferior nuchal line | Less well-defined ridge paralleling superior nuchal line a short distance below it |
| Mastoid process | Protuberance just behind ear | Internal occipital protuberance | Projection in midline on inner surface of bone; grooves for lateral sinuses extend laterally from this process and one for sagittal sinus extends upward from it |
| Mastoid air cells | Air-filled mucosa-lined spaces within mastoid process | | |
| External auditory meatus (or canal) | Tube extending into temporal bone from external ear opening to tympanic membrane | **ETHMOID** | Complicated irregular bone that helps make up anterior portion of cranial floor, medial wall of orbits, upper parts of nasal septum, and sidewalls and part of nasal roof; lies anterior to sphenoid and posterior to nasal bones |
| Zygomatic process | Projection that articulates with malar (or zygomatic) bone | Horizontal (cribriform) plate | Olfactory nerves pass through numerous holes in this plate |
| Internal auditory meatus | Fairly large opening on posterior surface of petrous portion of bone; transmits eighth cranial nerve to inner ear and seventh cranial nerve on its way to facial structures | Crista galli | Meninges (membranes around the brain) attach to this process |
| Mandibular fossa | Oval-shaped depression anterior to external auditory meatus; forms socket for condyle of mandible | Perpendicular plate | Forms upper part of nasal septum |
| | | Ethmoid sinuses | Honeycombed, mucosa-lined air spaces within lateral masses of bone |
| Styloid process | Slender spike of bone extending downward and forward from undersurface of bone anterior to mastoid process; often broken off in dry skull; several neck muscles and ligaments attach to styloid process | Superior and middle conchae (turbinates) | Help to form lateral walls of nose |
| | | Lateral masses | Compose sides of bone; contain many air spaces (ethmoid cells or sinuses); inner surface forms superior and middle conchae |

From Thibodeau GA, Patton KT: *Anatomy and physiology,* ed 3, St Louis, 1996, Mosby.

## Facial bones and their markings

| Bones and markings | Description | Bones and markings | Description |
|---|---|---|---|
| **PALATINE** | Form posterior part of hard palate, floor, and part of sidewalls of nasal cavity and floor of orbit | **MAXILLA** | Upper jaw bones; form part of floor of orbit, anterior part of roof of mouth, and floor of nose and part of sidewalls of nose |
| Horizontal plate | Joined to palatine processes of maxillae to complete part of hard palate | Alveolar process | Arch containing teeth |
| | | Maxillary sinus (antrum of Highmore) | Large air-filled mucosa-lined cavity within body of each maxilla; largest of sinuses |
| **MANDIBLE** | Lower jawbone; largest, strongest bone of face | Palatine process | Horizontal inward projection from alveolar process; forms anterior and larger part of hard palate |
| Body | Main part of bone; forms chin | | |
| Ramus | Process, one on either side, that projects upward from posterior part of body | Infraorbital foramen | Hole on external surface just below orbit; transmits vessels and nerves |
| Condyle (or head) | Part of each ramus that articulates with mandibular fossa of temporal bone | Lacrimal groove | Groove on inner surface; joined by similar groove on lacrimal bone to form canal housing nasolacrimal duct |
| Neck | Constricted part just below condyles | | |
| Alveolar process | Teeth set into this arch | | |
| Mandibular foramen | Opening on inner surface of ramus; transmits nerves and vessels to lower teeth | **NASAL** | Small bones forming upper part of bridge of nose |
| Mental foramen | Opening on outer surface below space between two bicuspids; transmits terminal branches of nerves and vessels that enter bone through mandibular foramen; dentists inject anesthetics through these foramina | **ZYGOMATIC** | Cheekbones; form part of floor and sidewall or orbit |
| | | **LACRIMAL** | Thin bones about size and shape of fingernail; posterior and lateral to nasal bones in medial wall of orbit; help form sidewall of nasal cavity, often missing in dry skull |
| Coronoid process | Projection upward from anterior part of each ramus; temporal muscle inserts here | | |
| Angle | Juncture of posterior and inferior margins of ramus | **INTERIOR NASAL CONCHAE (turbinates)** | Thin scroll of bone forming kind of shelf along inner surface of sidewall of nasal cavity; lies above roof of mouth |
| | | **VOMER** | Forms lower and posterior part of nasal septum; shaped like ploughshare |

From Thibodeau GA, Patton KT: *Anatomy and physiology,* ed 3, St Louis, 1996, Mosby.

## Hyoid, vertebrae, and thoracic bones and their markings

| Bones and markings | Description | Bones and markings | Description |
|---|---|---|---|
| **HYOID** | U-shaped bone in neck between mandible and upper part of larynx; distinctive as only bone in body not forming a joint with any other bone; suspended by ligaments from styloid processes of temporal bones | **VERTEBRAL COLUMN—cont'd** **General features—cont'd** | |
| | | Body | Main part; flat, round mass located anteriorly; supporting or weight-bearing part of vertebra |
| | | Pedicles | Short projections extending posteriorly from body |
| **VERTEBRAL COLUMN** | Not actually a column but a flexible, segmented curved rod; forms axis of body; head balanced above, ribs and viscera suspended in front, and lower extremities attached below; encloses spinal cord | Lamina | Posterior part of vertebra to which pedicles join and from which processes project |
| | | Neural arch | Formed by pedicles and laminae; protects spinal cord posteriorly; congenital absence of one or more neural arches is known as *spina bifida* (cord may protrude right through skin) |
| **General features** | Anterior part of each vertebra (except first two cervical) consists of body; posterior part of vertebrae consists of neural arch, which, in turn, consists of two pedicles, two laminae, and seven processes projecting from laminae | Spinous process | Sharp process projecting inferiorly from laminae in midline |
| | | Transverse processes | Right and left lateral projections from laminae |

From Thibodeau GA, Patton KT: *Anatomy and physiology,* ed 3, St Louis, 1996, Mosby.

*Continued*

## Hyoid, vertebrae, and thoracic bones and their markings—cont'd

| Bones and markings | Description | Bones and markings | Description |
|---|---|---|---|
| **VERTEBRAL COLUMN—cont'd** **General features—cont'd** | | **SACRUM—cont'd** | |
| Superior articulating processes | Project upward from laminae | Coccyx | Four or five separate vertebrae in child but fused into one in adult |
| Inferior articulating processes | Project downward from laminae; articulate with superior articulating processes of vertebrae below | **CURVES** | Curves have great structural importance because they increase carrying strength of vertebral column, make balance possible in upright position (if column were straight, weight of viscera would pull body forward), absorb jolts from walking (straight column would transmit jolts straight to head), and protect column from fracture |
| Spinal foramen | Hole in center of vertebra formed by union of body, pedicles, and laminae; spinal foramina, when vertebrae, superimposed one on other, form spinal cavity that houses spinal cord | | |
| Intervertebral foramina | Opening between vertebrae through which spinal nerves emerge | | |
| **CERVICAL VERTEBRAE** | First or upper seven vertebrae; foramen in each transverse process for transmission of vertebral artery, vein, and plexus of nerves; short bifurcated spinous processes except on seventh vertebra, where it is extra long and may be felt as protrusion when head bent forward; bodies of these vertebrae small, whereas spinal foramina large and triangular | Primary | Column curves at birth from head to sacrum with convexity posteriorly; after child stands, convexity persists only in *thoracic* and *sacral* regions, which therefore are called *primary curves* |
| | | Secondary | Concavities in *cervical* and *lumbar* regions; cervical concavity results from infant's attempts to hold head erect (2 to 4 months); lumbar concavity, from balancing efforts in learning to walk (10 to 18 months) |
| Atlas | First cervical vertebra; lacks body and spinous process; superior articulating processes concave ovals that act as rockerlike cradles for condyles of occipital bone; named *atlas* because it supports the head as Atlas supports the world in Greek mythology | **STERNUM** | Breastbone; flat dagger-shaped bone; sternum, ribs, and thoracic vertebrae together from body cage known as *thorax* |
| | | Body | Main central part of bone |
| | | Manubrium | Flaring, upper part |
| Axis (epistropheus) | Second cervical vertebra, so named because atlas rotates about this bone in rotating movements of head; *dens,* or odontoid process, peglike projection upward from body of axis, forming pivot for rotation of atlas | Xiphoid process | Projection of cartilage at lower border of bone |
| | | **RIBS** | |
| | | **True ribs** | Upper seven pairs; fasten to sternum by costal cartilages |
| **THORACIC VERTEBRAE** | Next 12 vertebrae; 12 pairs of ribs attached to these; stronger, with more massive bodies than cervical vertebrae; no transverse foramina; two sets of facets for articulations with corresponding rib: one on body, second on transverse process; upper thoracic vertebrae with elongated spinous process | **False ribs** | False ribs do not attach to sternum directly; upper three pairs of false ribs attach by means of costal cartilage of seventh ribs; last two pairs do not attach to sternum at all, therefore called "floating" ribs |
| | | Head | Projection at posterior end of rib; articulates with corresponding thoracic vertebra and one above, except last three pairs, which join corresponding vertebrae only |
| **LUMBAR VERTEBRAE** | Next 5 vertebrae; strong, massive; superior articulating processes directed medially instead of upward; inferior articulating processes, laterally instead of downward; short, blunt spinous process | Neck | Constricted portion just below head |
| | | Tubercle | Small knob just below neck; articulates with transverse process of corresponding thoracic vertebra; missing in lowest 3 ribs |
| | | Body or shaft | Main part of rib |
| **SACRUM** | Five separate vertebrae until about 25 years of age; then fused to form one wedge-shaped bone | Costal cartilage | Cartilage at sternal end of true ribs; attaches ribs (except floating ribs) to sternum |
| Sacral promontory | Protuberance from anterior, upper border of sacrum into pelvis; of obstetrical importance because its size limits anteroposterior diameter of pelvic inlet | | |

From Thibodeau GA, Patton KT: *Anatomy and physiology,* ed 3, St Louis, 1996, Mosby.

## Upper extremity bones and their markings

| Bones and markings | Description | Bones and markings | Description |
|---|---|---|---|
| **CLAVICLE** | Collar bones; shoulder girdle joined to axial skeleton by articulation of clavicles with sternum (scapula does not form joint with axial skeleton) | **RADIUS—cont'd** | |
| | | Styloid process | Protuberance at distal end on lateral surface (with forearm in anatomical position) |
| **SCAPULA** | Shoulder blades; scapulae and clavicles together comprise shoulder girdle | **ULNA** | Bone of little finger side of forearm; longer than radius |
| Borders | | Olecranon process | Elbow |
|   Superior | Upper margin | Coronoid process | Projection on anterior surface of proximal end of ulna; trochlea of humerus fits snugly between olecranon and coronoid processes |
|   Vertebral | Margin toward vertebral column | | |
|   Axillary | Lateral margin | | |
| Spine | Sharp ridge running diagonally across posterior surface of shoulder blade | Semilunar notch | Curved notch between olecranon and coronoid process into which trochlea fits |
| Acromion process | Slightly flaring projection at lateral end of scapular spine; may be felt as tip of shoulder; articulates with clavicle | Radial notch | Curved notch lateral and inferior to semilunar notch; head of radius fits into this concavity |
| Coracoid process | Projection on anterior surface from upper border of bone; may be felt in groove between deltoid and pectoralis major muscles, about 1 inch below clavicle | Head | Rounded process at distal end; does not articulate with wrist bones but with fibrocartilaginous disk |
| | | Styloid process | Sharp protuberance at distal end; can be seen from outside on posterior surface |
| Glenoid cavity | Arm socket | **CARPALS** | Wrist bones; arranged in two rows at proximal end of hand; proximal row (from little finger toward thumb)—*pisiform, triquetrum, lunate,* and *scaphoid;* distal row—*hamate, capitate, trapezoid,* and *trapezium* |
| **HUMERUS** | Long bone of upper arm | | |
| Head | Smooth, hemispherical enlargement at proximal end of humerus | | |
| Anatomical neck | Oblique groove just below head | | |
| Greater tubercle | Rounded projection lateral to head on anterior surface | | |
| Lesser tubercle | Prominent projection on anterior surface just below anatomical neck | **METACARPALS** | Long bones forming framework of palm of hand; numbered I through V |
| Intertubercular groove | Deep groove between greater and lesser tubercles; long tendon of biceps muscle lodges here | **PHALANGES** | Miniature long bones of fingers, three (proximal, middle, distal) in each finger, two (proximal, distal) in each thumb |
| Surgical neck | Region just below tubercles; so named because of its liability to fracture | | |
| Deltoid tuberosity | V-shaped, rough area about midway down shaft where deltoid muscle inserts | **COXAL** | Large hip bone; with sacrum and coccyx, forms basinlike pelvic cavity; lower extremities attached to axial skeleton by coxal bones |
| Radial groove | Groove running obliquely downward from deltoid tuberosity; lodges radial nerve | | |
| | | Ilium | Upper, flaring portion |
| | | Ischium | Lower, posterior portion |
| Epicondyles (medial and lateral) | Rough projections at both sides of distal end | Pubic bone (pubis) | Medial, anterior section |
| Capitulum | Rounded knob below lateral epicondyle; articulates with radius; sometimes called *radial* head of humerus | Acetabulum | Hip socket; formed by union of ilium, ischium, and pubis |
| | | Iliac crests | Upper, curving boundary of ilium |
| | | Iliac spines | |
| Trochlea | Projection with deep depression through center similar to shape of pulley; articulates with ulna |   Anterior superior | Prominent projection at anterior end of iliac crest; can be felt externally as "point" of hip |
| Olecranon fossa | Depression on posterior surface just above trochlea; receives olecranon process of ulna when lower arm extends |   Anterior inferior | Less prominent projection short distance below anterior superior spine |
| | |   Posterior superior | At posterior end of iliac crest |
| Coronoid fossa | Depression on anterior surface above trochlea; receives coronoid process of ulna in flexion of lower arm |   Posterior inferior | Just below posterior superior spine |
| | |   Greater sciatic notch | Large notch on posterior surface of ilium just below posterior inferior spine |
| **RADIUS** | Bone of thumb side of forearm |   Ischial tuberosity | Large, rough, quadrilateral process forming inferior part of ischium; in erect sitting position body rests on these tuberosities |
| **Head** | Disk-shaped process forming proximal end of radius; articulates with capitulum of humerus and with radial notch of ulna | | |
| | |   Ischial spine | Pointed projection just above tuberosity |
| Radial tuberosity | Roughened projection on ulnar side, short distance below head; biceps muscle inserts here |   Symphysis pubis | Cartilaginous, amphiarthrotic joint between pubic bones |

From Thibodeau GA, Patton KT: *Anatomy and physiology,* ed 3, St Louis, 1996, Mosby.

## Lower extremity bones and their markings

| Bones and markings | Description | Bones and markings | Description |
|---|---|---|---|
| **COXAL—cont'd** | | Epicondyles | Blunt projections from the sides of the condyles; one on the medial aspect and one on the lateral aspect |
| Superior ramus of pubis | Part of pubis lying between symphysis and acetabulum; forms upper part of obturator foramen | Adductor tubercle | Small projection just above medial condyle; marks termination of medial supracondylar ridge |
| Inferior ramus | Part extending down from symphysis; unites with ischium | Trochlea | Smooth depression between condyles on anterior surface; articulates with patella |
| Pubic arch | Angle formed by two inferior rami | | |
| Pubic crest | Upper margin of superior ramus | Intercondyloid fossa (notch) | Deep depression between condyles on posterior surface; cruciate ligaments that help bind femur to tibia lodge in this notch |
| Pubic tubercle | Rounded process at end of crest | | |
| Obturator foramen | Large hole in anterior surface of os coxa; formed by pubis and ischium; largest foramen in body | | |
| Pelvic brim (or inlet) | Boundary of aperture leading into true pelvis; formed by pubic crests, iliopectineal lines, and sacral promontory; size and shape of this inlet have obstetrical importance, since if any of its diameters too small, infant skull cannot enter true pelvis for natural birth | **PATELLA** | Kneecap; largest sesamoid bone of body; embedded in tendon of quadriceps femoris muscle |
| | | **TIBIA** | Shin bone |
| | | Condyles | Bulging prominences at proximal end of tibia; upper surfaces concave for articulation with femur |
| True pelvis (or pelvis minor) | Space below pelvic brim; true "basin" with bone and muscle walls and muscle floor; pelvic organs located in this space | Intercondylar eminence | Upward projection on articular surface between condyles |
| | | Crest | Sharp ridge on anterior surface |
| | | Tibial tuberosity | Projection in midline on anterior surface |
| False pelvis (or pelvis major) | Broad, shallow space above pelvic brim, or pelvic inlet; name "false pelvis" is misleading, since this space is actually part of abdominal cavity, not pelvic cavity | Medial malleolus | Rounded downward projection at distal end of tibia; forms prominence on medial surface of ankle |
| | | **FIBULA** | Long, slender bone of lateral side of lower leg |
| Pelvic outlet | Irregular circumference marking lower limits of true pelvis; bounded by tip of coccyx and two ischial tuberosities | Lateral malleolus | Rounded prominence at distal end of fibula; forms prominence on lateral surface of ankle |
| Pelvic girdle (or bony pelvis) | Complete bony ring; composed of two hip bones (ossa coxae), sacrum, and coccyx; forms firm base by which trunk rests on thighs and for attachment of lower extremities to axial skeleton | **TARSALS** | Bones that form heel and proximal or posterior half of foot |
| | | Calcaneus | Heel bone |
| | | Talus | Uppermost of tarsals; articulates with tibia and fibula; boxed in by medial and lateral malleoli |
| **FEMUR** | Thigh bone; largest, strongest bone of body | Longitudinal arches | Tarsals and metatarsals so arranged as to form arch from front to back of foot |
| Head | Rounded, upper end of bone; fits into acetabulum | Medial | Formed by calcaneus, talus, navicular, cuneiforms, and three medial metatarsals |
| Neck | Constricted portion just below head | | |
| Greater trochanter | Protuberance located inferiorly and laterally to head | Lateral | Formed by calcaneus, cuboid, and two lateral metatarsals |
| Lesser trochanter | Small protuberance located inferiorly and medially to greater trochanter | Transverse (or metatarsal) arch | Metatarsals and distal row of tarsals (cuneiforms and cuboid) so articulated as to form arch across foot; bones kept in two arched positions by means of powerful ligaments in sole of foot and by muscles and tendons |
| Intertrochanteric line | Line extending between greater and lesser trochanter | | |
| Linea aspera | Prominent ridge extending lengthwise along concave posterior surface | | |
| Supracondylar ridges | Two ridges formed by division of linea aspera at its lower end; medial supracondylar ridge extends inward to inner condyle, lateral ridge to outer condyle | **METATARSALS** | Long bones of feet |
| | | **PHALANGES** | Miniature long bones of toes; two in each great toe; three in other toes |
| Condyles | Large, rounded bulges at distal end of femur; one medial and one lateral | | |

From Thibodeau GA, Patton KT: *Anatomy and physiology,* ed 3, St Louis, 1996, Mosby.

## Synovial (diarthrotic) and two cartilagenous (amphiarthrotic) joints

| Name | Articulating bones | Type | Movements |
|------|-------------------|------|-----------|
| Atlantoepistropheal | Anterior arch of atlas rotates about dens of axis (epistropheus) | Synovial (pivot) | Pivoting or partial rotation of head |
| Vertebral | Between bodies of vertebrae | Cartilaginous (symphyses) | Slight movement between any two vertebrae but considerable motility for column as whole |
| Sternoclavicular | Between articular processes | Synovial (gliding) | Gliding |
| | Medial end of clavicle with manubrium of sternum | Synovial (gliding) | Gliding |
| Acromioclavicular | Distal end of clavicle with acromion of scapula | Synovial (gliding) | Gliding; elevation, depression, protraction, and retraction |
| Thoracic | Heads of ribs with bodies of vertebrae | Synovial (gliding) | Gliding |
| | Tubercles of ribs with transverse processes of vertebrae | Synovial (gliding) | Gliding |
| Shoulder | Head of humerus in glenoid cavity of scapula | Synovial (ball and socket) | Flexion, extension, abduction, adduction, rotation, and circumduction of upper arm |
| Elbow | Trochlea of humerus with semilunar notch of ulna; head of radius with capitulum of humerus | Synovial (hinge) | Flexion and extension |
| | Head of radius in radial notch of ulna | Synovial (pivot) | Supination and pronation of lower arm and hand; rotation of lower arm on upper extremity |
| Wrist | Scaphoid, lunate, and triquetral bones articulate with radius and articular disk | Synovial (condyloid) | Flexion, extension, abduction, and adduction of hand |
| Carpal | Between various carpals | Synovial (gliding) | Gliding |
| Hand | Proximal end of first metacarpal with trapezium | Synovial (saddle) | Flexion, extension, abduction, adduction, and circumduction of thumb and opposition to fingers |
| | Distal end of metacarpals with proximal end of phalanges | Synovial (hinge) | Flexion, extension, limited abduction, and adduction of fingers |
| | Between phalanges | Synovial (hinge) | Flexion and extension of finger sections |
| Sacroiliac | Between sacrum and two ilia | Synovial (gliding) | None or slight |
| Symphysis Pubis | Between two pubic bones | Cartilaginous (symphysis) | Slight, particularly during pregnancy and delivery |
| Hip | Head of femur in acetabulum of os coxae | Synovial (ball and socket) | Flexion, extension, abduction, adduction, rotation, and circumduction |
| Knee | Between distal end of femur and proximal end of tibia | Synovial (hinge) | Flexion and extension; slight rotation of tibia |
| Tibiofibular (proximal) | Head of fibula with lateral condyle of tibia | Synovial (gliding) | Gliding |
| Ankle | Distal ends of tibia and fibula with talus | Synovial (hinge) | Flexion (dosiflexion) and extension (plantar flexion) |
| Foot | Between tarsals | Synovial (gliding) | Gliding; inversion and eversion |
| | Between metatarsals and phalanges | Synovial (hinge) | Flexion, extension, slight abduction, and adduction |
| | Between phalanges | Synovial (hinge) | Flexion and extension |

From Thibodeau GA, Patton KT: *Anatomy and physiology,* ed 3, St Louis, 1996, Mosby.

**Muscular system**

## Muscles that move the head

| Muscle | Origin | Insertion | Function | Innervation |
|---|---|---|---|---|
| Sternocleidomastoid | Sternum<br>Clavicle | Temporal bone<br>(mastoid process) | Flexes head (prayer muscle)<br>One muscle alone, rotates head toward opposite side; spasm of this muscle alone or associated with trapezius called torticollis or wryneck | Accessory nerve |
| Semispinalis capitis | Vertebrae (transverse processes of upper six thoracic, articular processes of lower four cervical) | Occipital bone (between superior and inferior nuchal lines) | Extends head; bends it laterally | First five cervical nerves |
| Splenius capitis | Ligamentum nuchae<br>Vertebrae (spinous processes of upper three or four thoracic) | Temporal bone (mastoid process)<br>Occipital bone | Extends head<br>Bends and rotates head toward same side as contracting muscle | Second, third, and fourth cervical nerves |
| Longissimus capitis | Vertebrae (transverse processes of upper six thoracic, articular processes of lower four cervical) | Temporal bone (mastoid process) | Extends head<br>Bends and rotates head toward contracting side | Multiple innervation |

From Thibodeau GA, Patton KT: *Anatomy and physiology*, ed 4, St Louis, 2000, Mosby.

## Muscles of facial expression and of mastication

| Muscle | Origin | Insertion | Function | Innervation |
|---|---|---|---|---|
| **MUSCLES OF FACIAL EXPRESSION** | | | | |
| Epicranius (occipitofrontalis) | Occipital bone | Tissues of eyebrows | Raises eyebrows, wrinkles forehead horizontally | Cranial nerve VII |
| Corrugator supercilii | Frontal bone (superciliary ridge) | Skin of eyebrow | Wrinkles forehead vertically | Cranial nerve VII |
| Orbicularis oculi | Enriches eyelid | | Closes eye | Cranial nerve VII |
| Orbicularis oris | Encircles mouth | | Draws lips together | Cranial nerve VII |
| Zygomaticus major | Zygomatic bone | Angle of mouth | Laughing (elevates angle of mouth) | Cranial nerve VII |
| Buccinator | Maxillae | Skin of sides of mouth | Permits smiling<br>Blowing, as in playing a trumpet | Cranial nerve VII |
| **MUSCLES OF MASTICATION** | | | | |
| Masseter | Zygomatic arch | Mandible (external surface) | Closes jaw | Cranial nerve V |
| Temporal | Temporal bone | Mandible | Closes jaw | Cranial nerve V |
| Pterygoids (internal and external) | Undersurface of skull | Mandible (mesial surface) | Grate teeth | Cranial nerve V |

From Thibodeau GA, Patton KT: *Anatomy and physiology*, ed 4, St Louis, 2000, Mosby.

## Muscles acting on the shoulder girdle

| Muscle | Origin | Insertion | Function | Nerve supply |
|---|---|---|---|---|
| Trapezius | Occipital bone (protuberance) | Clavicle | Raises or lowers shoulders and shrugs them | Spinal accessory; second, third, and fourth cervical nerves |
| | Vertebrae (cervical and thoracic) | Scapula (spine and acromion) | Extends head when occiput acts as insertion | |
| Pectoralis minor | Ribs (second to fifth) | Scapula (coracoid) | Pulls shoulder down and forward | Medial and lateral anterior thoracic nerves |
| Serratus anterior | Ribs (upper eight or nine) | Scapula (anterior surface, vertebral border) | Pulls shoulder down and forward; abducts and rotates it upward | Long thoracic nerve |
| Levator scapulae | C1-C4 (transverse processes) | Scapula (superior angle) | Elevates and retracts scapula and abducts neck | Dorsal scapular nerve |
| Rhomboideus | | | | |
| Major | T1-T4 | Scapula (medial border) | Retracts, rotates, fixes scapula | Dorsal scapular nerve |
| Minor | C6-C7 | Scapula (medial border) | Retracts, rotates, elevates, and fixes scapula | Dorsal scapular nerve |

From Thibodeau GA, Patton KT: *Anatomy and physiology*, ed 4, St Louis, 2000, Mosby.

## Muscles that move the upper arm

| Muscle | Origin | Insertion | Function | Nerve supply |
|---|---|---|---|---|
| **AXIAL\*** | | | | |
| Pectoralis major | Clavicle (medial half)<br>Sternum<br>Costal cartilages of true ribs | Humerus (greater tubercle) | Flexes upper arm<br>Adducts upper arm anteriorly; draws it across chest | Medial and lateral anterior thoracic nerves |
| Latissimus dorsi | Vertebrae (spines of lower thoracic, lumbar, and sacral)<br>Ilium (crest)<br>Lumbodorsal fascia\* | Humerus (intertubercular groove) | Extends upper arm<br>Adducts upper arm posteriorly | Thoracodorsal nerve |
| **SCAPULAR\*** | | | | |
| Deltoid | Clavicle<br>Scapula (spine and acromion) | Humerus (lateral side about half-way down—deltoid tubercle) | Abducts upper arm<br>Assists in flexion and extension of upper arm | Axillary nerve |
| Coracobrachialis | Scapula (coracoid process) | Humerus (middle third, medial surface) | Adduction; assists in flexion and medial rotation of arm | Musculocutaneous nerve |
| Supraspinatus† | Scapula (supraspinous fossa) | Humerus (greater tubercle) | Assists in abducting arm | Suprascapular nerve |
| Teres minor† | Scapula (axillary border) | Humerus (greater tubercle) | Rotates arm outward | Axillary nerve |
| Teres major | Scapula (lower part, axillary border) | Humerus (upper part, anterior surface) | Assists in extension, adduction, and medial rotation of arm | Lower subscapular nerve |
| Infraspinatus† | Scapula (infraspinatus border) | Humerus (greater tubercle) | Rotates arm outward | Suprascapular nerve |
| Subscapularis† | Scapula (subscapular fossa) | Humerus (lesser tubercle) | Medial rotation | Suprascapular nerve |

From Thibodeau GA, Patton KT: *Anatomy and physiology,* ed 3, St Louis, 1996, Mosby.
\**Axial* muscles originate on the axial skeleton. *Scapular* muscles originate on the scapula.
†Muscles of the rotator cuff.

## Muscles that move the lower arm

| Muscle | Origin | Insertion | Function | Innervation |
|---|---|---|---|---|
| **FLEXORS** | | | | |
| Biceps brachii | Scapula (supraglenoid tuberosity) | Radius (tubercle at proximal end) | Flexes supinated forearm<br>Supinates forearm and hand | Musculocutaneous nerve |
| Brachialis | Humerus (distal half, anterior surface) | Ulna (front of coronoid process) | Flexes pronated forearm | Musculocutaneous nerve |
| Brachioradialis | Humerus (above lateral epicondyle) | Radius (styloid process) | Flexes semipronated or semisupinated forearm; supinates forearm and hand | Radial nerve |
| **EXTENSOR** | | | | |
| Triceps brachii | Scapula (infraglenoid tuberosity)<br>Humerus (posterior surface—lateral head above radial groove; medial head, below) | Ulna (olecranon process) | Extends lower arm | Radial nerve |
| **PRONATORS** | | | | |
| Pronator teres | Humerus (medial epicondyle)<br>Ulna (coronoid process) | Radius (middle third of lateral surface) | Pronates and flexes forearm | Median nerve |
| Pronator quadratus | Ulna (distal fourth, anterior surface) | Radius (distal fourth, anterior surface) | Pronates forearm | Median nerve |
| **SUPINATOR** | | | | |
| Supinator | Humerus (lateral epicondyle)<br>Ulna (proximal fifth) | Radius (proximal third) | Supinates forearm | Radial nerve |

From Thibodeau GA, Patton KT: *Anatomy and physiology,* ed 4, St Louis, 2000, Mosby.

## Muscles that move the wrist, hand, and fingers

| Muscle | Origin | Insertion | Function | Nerve supply |
|---|---|---|---|---|
| **EXTRINSIC** | | | | |
| Flexor carpi radialis | Humerus (medial epicondyle) | Second metacarpal (base of) | Flexes hand<br>Flexes forearm | Median nerve |
| Palmaris longus | Humerus (medial epicondyle) | Fascia of palm | Flexes hand | Median nerve |
| Flexor carpi ulnaris | Humerus (medial epicondyle)<br>Ulna (proximal two thirds) | Pisiform bone<br>Third, fourth, and fifth metacarpals | Flexes hand<br>Adducts hand | Ulnar nerve |
| Extensor carpi radialis longus | Humerus (ridge above lateral epicondyle) | Second metacarpal (base of) | Extends hand<br>Abducts hand (moves toward thumb side when hand supinated) | Radial nerve |
| Extensor carpi radialis brevis | Humerus (lateral epicondyle) | Second, third metacarpals (bases of) | Extends hand | Radial nerve |
| Extensor carpi ulnaris | Humerus (lateral epicondyle)<br>Ulna (proximal three fourths) | Fifth metacarpal (base of) | Extends hand<br>Adducts hand (moves toward little finger side when hand supinated) | Radial nerve |
| Flexor digitorum profundus | Ulna (anterior surface) | Distal phalanges (fingers 2 to 5) | Flexes distal interphalangeal joints | Median and ulnar nerves |
| Flexor digitorum superficialis | Humerus (medial epicondyle)<br>Radius<br>Ulna (coranoid process) | Tendons of fingers | Flexes fingers | Median nerve |
| Extensor digitorum | Humerus (lateral epicondyle) | Phalanges (fingers 2 to 5) | Extends fingers | Radial nerve |
| **INTRINSIC** | | | | |
| Opponents pollicis | Trapezium | Thumb metacarpal | Opposes thumb to fingers | Median nerve |
| Abductor pollicis brevis | Trapezium | Proximal phalanx of thumb | Abducts thumb | Median nerve |
| Adductor pollicis | Second and third metacarpals<br>Trapezoid<br>Capitate | Proximal phalanx of thumb | Adducts thumb | Ulnar nerve |
| Flexor pollicis brevis | Flexor retinaculum | Proximal phalanx of thumb | Flexes thumb | Median and ulnar nerves |
| Abductor digiti minimi | Pisiform | Proximal phalanx of fifth finger (base of) | Abducts fifth finger<br>Flexes fifth finger | Ulnar nerve |
| Flexor digiti minimi brevis | Hamate | Proximal and middle phalanx of fifth finger | Flexes fifth finger | Ulnar nerve |
| Opponens digiti minimi | Hamate<br>Flexor retinaculum | Fifth metacarpal | Opposes fifth finger slightly | Ulnar nerve |
| Interosseous (palmar and dorsal) | Metacarpals | Proximal phalanges | Adducts second, fourth, fifth fingers (palmar)<br>Abducts second, third, fourth fingers (dorsal) | Ulnar nerve |
| Lumbricales | Tendons of flexor digitorum profundus | Phalanges (2 to 5) | Flexes proximal phalanges (2 to 5)<br>Extends middle and distal phalanges (2 to 5) | Median nerve (phalanges 2 and 3)<br>Ulnar nerve (phalanges 4 and 5) |

From Thibodeau GA, Patton KT: *Anatomy and physiology,* ed 3, St Louis, 1996, Mosby.

## Muscles that move the trunk

| Muscle | Origin | Insertion | Function | Innervation |
|---|---|---|---|---|
| Sacrospinalis (erector spinae) | | | Extend spine; maintain erect posture of trunk<br>Acting singly, abduct and rotate trunk | Posterior rami of first cervical to fifth lumbar spinal nerves |
| Lateral portion<br>Iliocostalis lumborum | Iliac crest, sacrum (posterior surface), and lumbar vertebrae (spinous processes) | Ribs, lower six | | |

From Thibodeau GA, Patton KT: *Anatomy and physiology,* ed 4, St Louis, 2000, Mosby.

## Muscles that move the trunk—cont'd

| Muscle | Origin | Insertion | Function | Innervation |
|---|---|---|---|---|
| Iliocostalis dorsi | Ribs, lower six | Ribs, upper six | | |
| Iliocostalis cervicis | Ribs, upper six | Vertebrae, fourth to sixth cervical | | |
| **Medial portion** | | | | |
| Longissimus dorsi | Same as iliocostalis lumborum | Vertebrae, thoracic ribs | | |
| Longissimus cervicis | Vertebrae, upper six thoracic | Vertebrae, second to sixth cervical | | |
| Longissimus capitis | Vertebrae, upper six thoracic and last four cervical | Temporal bone, mastoid process | | |
| Quadratus lumborum (forms part of posterior abdominal wall) | Ilium (posterior part of crest) Vertebrae (lower three lumbar) | Ribs (twelfth) Vertebrae (transverse processes of first four lumbar) | Both muscles together extend spine One muscle alone abducts trunk toward side of contracting muscle | First three or four lumbar nerves |
| Iliopsoas | See muscles that move the thigh | | Flexes trunk | |

## Muscles of the thorax

| Muscle | Origin | Insertion | Function | Innervation |
|---|---|---|---|---|
| External intercostals | Rib (lower border; forward fibers) | Rib (upper border of rib below origin) | Elevate ribs | Intercostal nerves |
| Internal intercostals | Rib (inner surface, lower border; backward fibers) | Rib (upper border of rib below origin) | Depress ribs | Intercostal nerves |
| Diaphragm | Lower circumference of thorax (of rib cage) | Central tendon of diaphragm | Enlarges thorax, causing inspiration | Phrenic nerves |

From Thibodeau GA, Patton KT: *Anatomy and physiology,* ed 4, St Louis, 2000, Mosby.

## Muscles that move the abdominal wall

| Muscle | Origin | Insertion | Function | Innervation |
|---|---|---|---|---|
| External oblique | Ribs (lower eight) | Ossa coxae (iliac crest and pubis by way of inguinal ligament)* Linea alba† by way of an aponeurosis‡ | Compresses abdomen Rotates trunk laterally Important postural function of all abdominal muscles is to pull front of pelvis upward, thereby flattening lumbar curve of spine; when these muscles lose their tone, common figure faults of protruding abdomen and lordosis develop | Lower seven intercostal nerves and iliohypogastric nerves |
| Internal oblique | Ossa coxae (iliac crest and inguinal ligament) | Ribs (lower three) Pubic bone | Same as external oblique | Last three intercostal nerves; iliohypogastric and ilioinguinal nerves |
| Transversus abdominis | Lumbodorsal fascia Ribs (lower six) Ossa coxae (iliac crest, inguinal ligament) Lumbodorsal fascia | Linea alba Pubic bone Linea alba | Same as external oblique | Last five intercostal nerves; iliohypogastric and ilioinguinal nerves |
| Rectus abdominis | Ossa coxae (pubic bone and symphysis pubis) | Ribs (costal cartilage of fifth, sixth, and seventh ribs) Sternum (xiphoid process) | Same as external oblique; because abdominal muscles compress abdominal cavity, they aid in straining, defecation, forced expiration, and childbirth; abdominal muscles are antagonists of diaphragm, relaxing as it contracts and vice versa Flexes trunk | Last six intercostal nerves |

From Thibodeau GA, Patton KT: *Anatomy and physiology,* ed 4, St Louis, 2000, Mosby.

*Inguinal ligament (or Poupart's)—lower edge of aponeurosis of external oblique muscle, extending between the anterior superior iliac spine and the tubercle of the pubic bone. This edge is doubled under like a hem. The inguinal ligament forms the upper boundary of the femoral triangle, a large triangular area in the thigh; its other boundaries are the adductor longus muscle medially and the sartorius muscle laterally.

†Linea alba—literally, a white line; extends from xiphoid process to symphysis pubis; formed by fibers of aponeuroses of the right abdominal muscles interlacing with fibers of aponeuroses of the left abdominal muscles; comparable to a seam up the midline of the abdominal wall, anchoring its various layers. During pregnancy the linea alba becomes pigmented and is known as the linea nigra.

‡Aponeurosis—sheet of white fibrous tissue that attaches one muscle to another or attaches it to bone or other movable structures, for example, the right external oblique muscle attaches to the left external oblique muscle by means of an aponeurosis.

## Muscles of the pelvic floor

| Muscle | Origin | Insertion | Function | Nerve supply |
|---|---|---|---|---|
| Levator ani | Pubis and spine of ischium | Coccyx | Together with coccygeus muscles form floor of pelvic cavity and support pelvic organs | Pudendal nerve |
| Ischiocavernosus | Ischium | Penis or clitoris | Compress base of penis or clitoris | Perineal nerve |
| Bulbospongiosus | | | | |
|    Male | Bulb of penis | Perineum and bulb of penis | Constricts urethra and erects penis | Pudendal nerve |
|    Female | Perineum | Base of clitoris | Erects clitoris | Pudendal nerve |
| Deep transverse perinei | Ischium | Central tendon (median raphe) | Support pelvic floor | Pudendal nerve |
| Sphincter urethrae | Pubic ramus | Central tendon (median raphe) | Constrict urethra | Pudendal nerve |
| Sphincter externus anii | Coccyx | Central tendon (median raphe) | Close anal canal | Pudendal and S4 |

From Thibodeau GA, Patton KT: *Anatomy and physiology*, ed 3, St Louis, 1996, Mosby.

## Muscles that move the thigh

| Muscle | Origin | Insertion | Function | Innervation |
|---|---|---|---|---|
| Iliopsoas (iliacus and psoas major) | Ilium (iliac fossa) Vertebrae (bodies of twelfth thoracic to fifth lumbar) | Femur (lesser trochanter) | Flexes thigh Flexes trunk (when femur acts as origin) | Femoral and second to fourth lumbar nerves |
| Rectus femoris | Ilium (anterior, inferior spine) | Tibia (by way of patellar tendon) | Flexes thigh Extends lower leg | Femoral nerve |
| **GLUTEAL GROUP** | | | | |
|    Maximus | Ilium (crest and posterior surface) Sacrum and coccyx (posterior surface) Sacrotuberous ligament | Femur (gluteal tuberosity) Iliotibial tract* | Extends thigh— rotates outward | Inferior gluteal nerve |
|    Medius | Ilium (lateral surface) | Femur (greater trochanter) | Abducts thigh—rotates outward; stabilizes pelvis on femur | Superior gluteal nerve |
|    Minimus | Ilium (lateral surface) | Femur (greater trochanter) | Abducts thigh; stabilizes pelvis on femur Rotates high medially | Superior gluteal nerve |
| Tensor fasciae latae | Ilium (anterior part of crest) | Tibia (by way of iliotibial tract) | Abducts thigh Tightens iliotibial tract* | Superior gluteal nerve |
| Piriformis | Sacrum, greater sciatic foramen sacrotuberous ligament | Femur (medial aspect of greater trochanter) | Rotates thigh outward Abducts thigh Extends thigh | First or second sacral nerves |
| **ADDUCTOR GROUP** | | | | |
|    Brevis | Pubic bone | Femur (linea aspera) | Adducts thigh | Obturator nerve |
|    Longus | Pubic bone | Femur (linea aspera) | Adducts thigh | Obturator nerve |
|    Magnus | Pubic bone | Femur (linea aspera) | Adducts thigh | Obturator nerve |
|    Gracilis | Pubic bone (just below symphysis) | Tibia (medial surface behind sartorius) | Adducts thigh and flexes and adducts leg | Obturator nerve |

From Thibodeau GA, Patton KT: *Anatomy and physiology*, ed 4, St Louis, 2000, Mosby.
*The iliotibial tract is part of the fascia enveloping all the thigh muscles. It consists of a wide band of dense fibrous tissue attached to the iliac crest above and the lateral condyle of the tibia below. The upper part of the tract encloses the tensor fasciae latae muscle.

## Muscles that move the lower leg

| Muscle | Origin | Insertion | Function | Innervation |
|---|---|---|---|---|
| **QUADRICEPS FEMORIS GROUP** | | | | |
| Rectus femoris | Ilium (anterior, inferior spine) | Tibia (by way of patellar tendon) | Flexes thigh Extends leg | Femoral nerve |
| Vastus lateralis | Femur (linea aspera) | Tibia (by way of patellar tendon) | Extends leg | Femoral nerve |
| Vastus medialis | Femur | Tibia (by way of patellar tendon) | Extends leg | Femoral nerve |
| Vastus intermedius | Femur (anterior surface) | Tibia (by way of patellar tendon) | Extends leg | Femoral nerve |
| Sartorius | Coxal (anterior, superior iliac spines) | Tibia (medial surface of upper end of shaft) | Adducts and flexes leg Permits crossing of legs tailor fashion | Femoral nerve |
| **HAMSTRING GROUP** | | | | |
| Biceps femoris | Ischium (tuberosity) Femur (linea aspera) | Fibula (head of) Tibia (lateral condyle) | Flexes leg Extends thigh | Hamstring nerve (branch of sciatic nerve) Hamstring nerve |
| Semitendinosus | Ischium (tuberosity) | Tibia (proximal end, medial surface) | Extends thigh | Hamstring nerve |
| Semimembranosus | Ischium (tuberosity) | Tibia (medial condyle) | Extends thigh | Hamstring nerve |

From Thibodeau GA, Patton KT: *Anatomy and physiology,* ed 4, St Louis, 2000, Mosby.

## Muscles that move the foot

| Muscle | Origin | Insertion | Function | Nerve supply |
|---|---|---|---|---|
| **EXTRINSIC** | | | | |
| Tibialis anterior | Tibia (lateral condyle of upper body) | Tarsal (first cuneiform) Metatarsal (base of first) | Flexes foot Inverts food | Common and deep peroneal nerves |
| Gastrocnemius | Femur (condyles) | Tarsal (calcaneus by way of Achilles tendon) | Extends foot Flexes lower leg | Tibial nerve (branch of sciatic nerve) |
| Soleus | Tibia (underneath gastrocnemius) Fibula | Tarsal (calcaneus by way of Achilles tendon) | Extends foot (plantar flexion) | Tibial nerve |
| Peroneus longus | Tibia (lateral condyle) Fibula (head and shaft) | First cuneiform Base of first metatarsal | Extends foot (plantar flexion) Everts foot | Common peroneal nerve |
| Peroneus brevis | Fibula (lower two thirds of lateral surface of shaft) | Fifth metatarsal (tubercle, dorsal surface) | Everts foot Flexes foot | Superficial peroneal nerve |
| Peroneus tertius | Fibula (distal third) | Fourth and fifth metatarsals (bases of) | Flexes foot Everts foot | Deep peroneal nerve |
| Extensor digitorum longus | Tibia (lateral condyle) Fibular (anterior surface) | Second and third phalanges (four lateral toes) | Dorsiflexion of foot; extension of toes | Deep peroneal nerve |
| **INTRINSIC** | | | | |
| Lumbricales | Tendons of flexor digitorum longus | Phalanges (2 to 5) | Flex proximal phalanges Extend middle and distal phalanges | Lateral and medial plantar nerve |
| Flexor digiti minimi brevis | Fifth metatarsal | Proximal phalanx of fifth toe | Flexes fifth (small) toe | Lateral plantar nerve |
| Flexor hallucis brevis | Cuboid Medial and lateral cuneiform | Proximal phalanx of first (great) toe | Flexes first (great) toe | Medial and lateral plantar nerve |
| Flexor digitorum brevis | Calcaneous Plantar fascia | Middle phalanges of toes (2 to 5) | Flexes toes two through five | Medial plantar nerve |
| Abductor digiti minimi | Calcaneous | Proximal phalanx of fifth (small) toe | Abducts fifth (small) toe Flexes fifth toe | Lateral plantar nerve |
| Abductor hallucis | Calcaneous | First (great) toe | Abducts first (great) toe | Medial plantar nerve |

From Thibodeau GA, Patton KT: *Anatomy and physiology,* ed 3, St Louis, 1996, Mosby.

## 4-4   Circulatory system

### Blood cells

| Cell type | Description | Function | Life span |
|---|---|---|---|
| Erythrocyte | 7 μm in diameter; concave disk shape; entire cell stains pale pink; no nucleus | Transportation of respiratory gases ($O_2$ and $CO_2$) | 105 to 120 days |
| Neutrophil | 12-15 μm in diameter; spherical shape; multilobed nucleus; small, pink-purple staining cytoplasmic granules | Cellular defense—phagocytosis of small pathogenic microorganisms | Hours to 3 days |
| Basophil | 11-14 μm in diameter; spherical shape; generally two lobed nucleus; large purple staining cytoplasmic granules | Secretes heparin (anticoagulant) and histamine (important in inflammatory response) | Hours to 3 days |
| Eosinophil | 10-12 μm in diameter; spherical shape; generally two-lobed nucleus; large orange-red staining cytoplasmic granules | Cellular defense—phagocytosis of large pathogenic microorganisms such as protozoa and parasitic worms; releases antiinflammatory substances in allergic reactions | 10 to 12 days |
| Lymphocyte | 6-9 μm in diameter; spherical shape; round (single lobe) nucleus; small lymphocytes have scant cytoplasm | Humoral defense—secretes antibodies; involved in immune system response and regulation | Days to years |
| Monocyte | 12-17 μm in diameter; spherical shape; nucleus generally kidney-bean or "horse-shoe" shaped with convoluted surface; ample cytoplasm often "steel blue" in color | Capable of migrating out of the blood to enter tissue spaces as a *macrophage*—an aggressive phagocytic cell capable of ingesting bacteria, cellular debris, and cancerous cells | Months |
| Platelet | 2-5 μm in diameter; irregularly shaped fragments; cytoplasm contains very small pink staining granules | Releases clot activating substances and helps in formation of actual blood clot by forming platelet "plugs" | 7 to 10 days |

From Thibodeau GA, Patton KT: *Anatomy and physiology,* ed 4, St Louis, 2000, Mosby.

### Structure of blood vessels

| Arteries | Veins | Capillaries |
|---|---|---|
| **COATS** | | |
| Outer coat (tunica adventitia or externa) of white fibrous tissue; causes artery to stand open instead of collapsing when cut<br>Muscle coat (tunica media) of smooth muscle, elastic, and some white fibrous tissues; this coat permits constriction and dilation<br>Lining (tunica intima) of endothelium | Same three coats but thinner and fewer elastic fibers; veins collapse when cut; semilunar valves present at intervals | Only lining coat present; therefore walls only one cell thick |

**BLOOD SUPPLY**

Endothelial lining cells supplied by blood flowing through vessels; exchange of oxygen, etc., between cells of middle coat and blood by diffusion; outer coat supplied by tiny vessels known as vasa vasorum or "vessels of vessels"

**NERVE SUPPLY**

Smooth muscle cells of tunica media innervated by autonomic fibers

**ABNORMALITIES**

Atherosclerosis—hardening of walls of arteries (arteriosclerosis) characterized by lipid deposits in tunica intima
Aneurysm—saclike dilation of artery wall
Varicose veins—stretching of walls, particularly around semilunar valves
Phlebitis—inflammation of vein; "milk leg," phlebitis of femoral vein of women after childbirth

From Thibodeau GA, Patton KT: *Anatomy and physiology,* ed 4, St Louis, 2000, Mosby.

### Coronary arteries

| Right coronary artery | Left coronary artery |
|---|---|
| Divides into two main branches:<br>  Posterior descending artery—sends branches to both ventricles<br>  Marginal artery—sends branches to right ventricle and right atrium | Divides into two main branches:<br>  Anterior descending artery—sends branches to ventricles<br>  Circumflex artery—sends branches to left ventricle and left atrium |

From Thibodeau GA, Patton KT: *Anatomy and physiology,* ed 4, St Louis, 2000, Mosby.

# White blood cells (leukocytes)

| Class | Differential count* | |
| --- | --- | --- |
| | Normal range (%) | Typical normal (%) |
| **THOSE WITH GRANULAR CYTOPLASM AND IRREGULAR NUCLEI** | | |
| Neutrophils (neutral staining) | 65 to 75 | 65 |
| Eosinophils (acid staining) | 2 to 5 | 3 |
| Basophils (basic staining) | ½ to 1 | 1 |
| **THOSE WITH NONGRANULAR CYTOPLASM AND REGULAR NUCLEI** | | |
| Lymphocytes (large and small) | 20 to 25 | 25 |
| Monocytes | 3 to 8 | 6 |
| TOTAL | | 100 |

From Thibodeau GA, Patton KT: *Anatomy and physiology,* ed 4, St Louis, 2000, Mosby.
*In any differential count the sum of the percentages of the different kinds of leukocytes must, of course, total 100%.

# Major systemic arteries

| Artery* | Region supplied | Artery* | Region supplied |
| --- | --- | --- | --- |
| **ASCENDING AORTA** | | **ARCH OF AORTA—cont'd** | |
| Coronary arteries | Myocardium | **Left common carotid** | Head and neck |
| | | Left internal carotid† | Brain, eye, forehead, nose |
| **ARCH OF AORTA** | | | |
| **Brachiocephalic (innominate)** | Head and upper extremity | Left external carotid† | Thyroid, tongue, tonsils, ear, etc. |
| Right subclavian | Head, upper extremity | **DESCENDING THORACIC AORTA** | |
| Right vertebral† | Spinal cord, brain | **Visceral branches** | Thoracic viscera |
| Right axillary | Shoulder, chest, axillary region | Bronchial | Lungs, bronchi |
| (continuation of subclavian) | | Esophageal | Esophagus |
| Right brachial | Arm and hand | | |
| (continuation of axillary) | | **Parietal branches** | Thoracic walls |
| Right radial | Lower arm and hand (lateral) | Intercostal | Lateral thoracic walls (rib cage) |
| Right ulnar | Lower arm and hand (medial) | Superior phrenic | Superior surface of diaphragm |
| Superficial and deep palmar arches (formed by anastomosis of branches of radial and ulnar) | Hand and fingers | **DESCENDING ABDOMINAL AORTA** | |
| | | **Visceral branches** | Abdominal viscera |
| Digital | Fingers | Celiac artery (trunk) | Abdominal viscera |
| Right common carotid | Head and neck | Left gastric | Stomach, esophagus |
| Right internal carotid† | Brain, eye, forehead, nose | Common hepatic | Liver |
| | | Splenic | Spleen, pancreas, stomach |
| Right external carotid† | Thyroid, tongue, tonsils, ear, etc. | Superior mesenteric | Pancreas, small intestine, colon |
| | | Inferior mesenteric | Descending colon, rectum |
| **Left subclavian** | Head and upper extremity | Suprarenal | Adrenal (suprarenal) gland |
| Left vertebral† | Spinal cord, brain | Renal | Kidney |
| Left axillary (continuation of subclavian) | Shoulder, chest, axillary region | Ovarian | Ovary, uterine tube, ureter |
| Left brachial (continuation of axillary) | Arm and hand | Testicular | Testis, ureter |
| Left radial | Lower arm and hand (lateral) | **Parietal branches** | Walls of abdomen |
| Left ulnar | Lower arm and hand (medial) | Inferior phrenic | Inferior surface of diaphragm, adrenal gland |
| Superficial and deep palmar arches (formed by anastomosis of branches of radial and ulnar) | Hand and fingers | Lumbar | Lumbar vertebrae and muscles of back |
| Digital | Fingers | Median sacral | Lower vertebrae |

From Thibodeau GA, Patton KT: *Anatomy and physiology,* ed 3, St Louis, 1996, Mosby.
*Branches of each artery are indented below its name.

*Continued*

## Major systemic arteries—cont'd

| Artery* | Region supplied | Artery* | Region supplied |
|---|---|---|---|
| **DESCENDING ABDOMINAL AORTA—cont'd** | | **DESCENDING ABDOMINAL AORTA—cont'd** | |
| **Common iliac (formed by terminal branches of aorta)** | Pelvis, lower extremity | Internal iliac | Pelvis |
| | |   Visceral branches | Pelvic viscera |
| **External iliac** | Thigh, leg, foot |     Middle rectal | Rectum |
|   Femoral (continuation of external iliac) | Thigh, leg, foot |     Vaginal | Vagina, uterus |
| | |     Uterine | Uterus, vagina, uterine tube, ovary |
|     Popliteal (continuation of femoral) | Leg, foot | | |
|       Anterior tibial | Leg, foot | **Parietal branches** | Pelvic wall and external regions |
|       Posterior tibial | Leg, foot |   Lateral sacral | Sacrum |
|         Plantar arch (formed by anastomosis of branches of anterior and posterior tibial arteries) | Foot, toes |   Superior gluteal | Gluteal muscles |
| | |   Obturator | Pubic region, hip joint, groin |
|         Digital | Toes |   Internal pedundal | Rectum, external genitals, floor of pelvis |
| | |   Inferior gluteal | Lower gluteal region, coccyx, upper thigh |

From Thibodeau GA, Patton KT: *Anatomy and physiology,* ed 3, St Louis, 1996, Mosby.

## Major systemic veins

| Vein* | Region drained | Vein* | Region drained |
|---|---|---|---|
| **SUPERIOR VENA CAVA** | Head, neck, thorax, upper extremity | **SUPERIOR VENA CAVA—cont'd** | |
| | | **Cephalic—cont'd** | |
| Brachiocephalic (innominate) | Head, neck, upper extremity |   Basilic (direct tributary of axillary) | Medial and lower arm, hand |
| Internal jugular (continuation of sigmoid sinus) | Brain |     Median cubital (basilic) (formed by anastomosis of cephalic and basilic) | Arm, hand |
| **Lingual** | Tongue, mouth |     Deep and superficial palmar venous arches (formed by anastomosis of cephalic and basilic) | Hand |
| Superior thyroid | Thyroid, deep face | | |
| **Facial** | Superficial face |     Digital | Fingers |
| Sigmoid sinus (continuation of transverse sinus/direct tributary of internal jugular) | Brain, meninges, skull | Azygos (anastomoses with right ascending lumbar) | Right posterior wall of thorax and abdomen, esophagus, bronchi, pericardium, mediastinum |
|   Superior and inferior petrosal sinuses | Anterior brain, skull | | |
|   Cavernous sinus | Anterior brain, skull | Hemiazygos (anastomoses with left renal) | Left inferior posterior wall of thorax and abdomen, esophagus, mediastinum |
|     Ophthalmic veins | Eye, orbit | | |
|   Transverse sinus (direct tributary of sigmoid sinus) | Brain, meninges, skull | Accessory hemiazygos | Left superior posterior wall of thorax |
|     Occipital sinus | Inferior, central region of cranial cavity | **INFERIOR VENA CAVA** | Lower trunk and extremity |
|     Straight sinus | Central region of brain, meninges | **Phrenic** | Diaphragm |
|       Inferior sagittal sinus | Central region of brain, meninges | Hepatic portal system | Upper abdominal viscera |
| | |   Hepatic veins (continuations of liver venules and sinusoids and, ultimately, the hepatic portal vein) | Liver |
|       Superior sagittal (longitudinal) sinus | Superior region of cranial cavity | | |
| **External jugular** | Superficial, posterior head, neck |   Hepatic portal vein | Gastrointestinal organs, pancreas, spleen, gallbladder |
| Subclavian (continuation of axillary/direct tributary of brachiocephalic) | Axilla, lower extremity |     Cystic | Gallbladder |
| | |     Gastric | Stomach |
| Axillary (continuation of basilic/direct tributary of subclavian) | Axilla, lower extremity |     Splenic | Spleen |
| | |       Inferior mesenteric | Descending colon, rectum |
| **Cephalic** | Lateral and lower arm, hand |       Pancreatic | Pancreas |
| Brachial | Deep arm |     Superior mesenteric | Small intestine, most of colon |
|   Radial | Deep lateral forearm | | |
|   Ulnar | Deep medial forearm |       Gastroepiploic | Stomach |

From Thibodeau GA, Patton KT: *Anatomy and physiology,* ed 3, St Louis, 1996, Mosby.
*Tributaries of each vein are indented below its name.

## Major systemic veins—cont'd

| Vein* | Region drained | Vein* | Region drained |
|---|---|---|---|
| **INFERIOR VENA CAVA—cont'd** | | **INFERIOR VENA CAVA—cont'd** | |
| **Renal** | Kidneys | **Renal—cont'd** | |
| Suprarenal | Adrenal (suprarenal) gland | Popliteal | Leg, foot |
| Left ovarian | Left ovary | Posterior tibial | Deep posterior leg |
| Left testicular | Left testis | Medial and lateral plantar | Sole of foot |
| Left ascending lumbar (anastomoses with hemiazygos) | Left lumbar region | Fibular (peroneal) (continuation of anterior tibial) | Lateral and anterior leg, foot |
| Right ovarian | Right ovary | Anterior tibial | Anterior leg, foot |
| Right testicular | Right testis | Dorsal veins of foot | Anterior (dorsal) foot, toes |
| Right ascending lumbar (anastomoses with azygos) | Right lumbar region | Small (external, short) saphenous | Superficial posterior leg, lateral foot |
| Common iliac (continuation of external iliac; common iliacs unite to form inferior vena cava) | Lower extremity | Great (internal, long) saphenous | Superficial medial and anterior thigh, leg, foot |
| External iliac (continuation of femoral/direct tributary of common iliac) | Thigh, leg, foot | Dorsal veins of foot | Anterior (dorsal) foot, toes |
| Femoral (continuation of popliteal/direct tributary of external iliac) | Thigh, leg, foot | Dorsal venous arch | Anterior (dorsal) foot, toes |
| | | Digital | Toes |
| | | **Internal iliac** | Pelvic region |

From Thibodeau GA, Patton KT: *Anatomy and physiology,* ed 4, St Louis, 2000, Mosby.

## 4-5 | Endocrine system

### Names and locations of endocrine glands

| Name | Location | Name | Location |
|---|---|---|---|
| Hypothalamus | Cranial cavity (brain) | Adrenal glands | Abdominal cavity (retroperitoneal) |
| Pituitary glands (hypophysis cerebri) | Cranial cavity | Pancreatic islets | Abdominal cavity (pancreas) |
| Pineal gland (epiphysis) | Cranial cavity (brain) | Ovaries | Pelvic cavity |
| Thyroid gland | Neck | Testes (interstitial cells) | Scrotum |
| Parathyroid glands | Neck | Placenta | Pregnant uterus |
| Thymus | Mediastinum | | |

From Thibodeau GA, Patton KT: *Anatomy and physiology,* ed 4, St Louis, 2000, Mosby.

### Hormones

| Hormone | Source | Target | Principal action |
|---|---|---|---|
| **HYPOTHALAMUS** | | | |
| Growth hormone-releasing hormone (GRH) | Hypothalamus | Adenohypophysis (acidophils) | Stimulates secretion (release) of growth hormone |
| Growth hormone-inhibiting hormone (GIH), or somatostatin | Hypothalamus | Adenohypophysis (acidophils) | Inhibits secretion of growth hormone |
| Corticotropin-releasing hormone (CRH) | Hypothalamus | Adenohypophysis (basophils) | Stimulates release of adrenocorticotropic hormone (ACTH) |
| Thyrotropin-releasing hormone (TRH) | Hypothalamus | Adenohypophysis (basophils) | Stimulates release of thyroid-stimulating hormone (TSH) |
| Gonadotropin-releasing hormone (GNRH) | Hypothalamus | Adenohypophysis (basophils) | Stimulates release of gonadotropins (FSH and LH) |
| Prolactin-releasing hormone (PRH) | Hypothalamus | Adenohypophysis (acidophils) | Stimulates secretion of prolactin |
| Prolactin-inhibiting hormone (PIH) | Hypothalamus | Adenohypophysis (acidophils) | Inhibits secretion of prolactin |
| **PITUITARY GLAND** | | | |
| Growth hormone (GH) (stomatotropin [STH]) | Adenohypophysis (acidophils) | General | Promotes growth by stimulating protein anabolism and fat mobilization |
| Prolactin (PRL) (lactogenic hormone) | Adenohypophysis (acidophils) | Mammary glands (alveolar secretory cells) | Promotes milk secretion |

From Thibodeau GA, Patton KT: *Anatomy and physiology,* ed 4, St Louis, 2000, Mosby.

*Continued*

# Hormones—cont'd

| Hormone | Source | Target | Principal action |
|---|---|---|---|
| **PITUITARY GLAND—cont'd** | | | |
| Thyroid-stimulating hormone (TSH)* | Adenohypophysis (basophils) | Thyroid gland | Stimulates development and secretion in the thyroid gland |
| Adrenocorticotropic hormone (ACTH)* | Adenohypophysis (basophils) | Adrenal cortex | Promotes development and secretion in the adrenal cortex |
| Follicle-stimulating hormone (FSH)* | Adenohypophysis (basophils) | Gonads (primary sex organs) | Female: promotes development of ovarian follicle; stimulates estrogen secretion Male: promotes development of testis; stimulates sperm production |
| Luteinizing hormone (LH)* | Adenohypophysis (basophils) | Gonads and mammary glands | Female: triggers ovulation; promotes development of corpus luteum Male: stimulates production of testosterone |
| Melanocyte-stimulating hormone (MSH) | Adenohypophysis (basophils) | Skin (melanocytes); adrenal glands | Exact function uncertain; may stimulate production of melanin pigment in skin; may maintain adrenal sensitivity |
| Antidiuretic hormone (ADH) | Neurohypophysis | Kidney | Promotes water retention by kidney tubules |
| Oxytocin (OT) | Neurohypophysis | Uterus and mammary glands | Stimulates uterine contractions; stimulates ejection of milk into mammary ducts |
| **ADRENAL GLANDS** | | | |
| Aldosterone | Adrenal cortex (zona glomerulosa) | Kidney | Stimulates kidney tubules to conserve sodium, which, in turn, triggers the release of ADH and the resulting conservation of water by the kidney |
| Cortisol (hydrocortisone) | Adrenal cortex (zona fasciculata) | General | Influences metabolism of food molecules; in large amounts, it has an antiinflammatory effect |
| Adrenal androgens | Adrenal cortex (zona reticularis) | Sex organs, other effectors | Exact role uncertain, but may support sexual function |
| Adrenal estrogens | Adrenal cortex (zona reticularis) | Sex organs | Thought to be physiologically insignificant |
| Epinephrine (adrenaline) | Adrenal medulla | Sympathetic effectors | Enhances and prolongs the effects of the sympathetic division of the ANS |
| Norepinephrine | Adrenal medulla | Sympathetic effectors | Enhances and prolongs the effects of the sympathetic division of the ANS |
| **THYROID AND PARATHYROID GLANDS** | | | |
| Triiodothyronine ($T_3$) | Thyroid gland (follicular cells) | General | Increases rate of metabolism |
| Tetraiodothyronine ($T_4$), or thyroxine | Thyroid gland (follicular cells) | General | Increases rate of metabolism (usually converted to $T_3$ first) |
| Calcitonin (CT) | Thyroid gland (parafollicular cells) | Bone tissue | Increases calcium storage in bone, lowering blood $Ca^{++}$ levels |
| Parathyroid hormone (PTH) or parathormone | Parathyroid glands | Bone tissue and intestinal tract | Increases calcium removal from storage in bone and increases absorption of calcium by intestines, increasing blood $Ca^{++}$ levels |
| **PANCREATIC ISLETS** | | | |
| Glucagon | Pancreatic islets (alpha [$\alpha$] cells or A cells) | General | Promotes movement of glucose from storage and into the blood |
| Insulin | Pancreatic islets (beta [$\beta$] cells or B cells) | General | Promotes movement of glucose out of the blood and into cells |
| Somatostatin | Pancreatic islets (delta [$\delta$] cells or D cells) | Pancreatic cells and other effectors | Can have general effects in the body, but primary role seems to be regulation of secretion of other pancreatic hormones |
| Pancreatic polypeptide | Pancreatic islets (pancreatic polypeptide [PP] or F cells) | Intestinal cells and other effectors | Exact function uncertain, but seems to influence absorption in the digestive tract |

From Thibodeau GA, Patton KT: *Anatomy and physiology,* ed 4, St Louis, 2000, Mosby.
*Tropic hormones.

## 4-6   Nervous system

### Major ascending tracts of the spinal cord

| Name | Function | Location | Origin* | Termination† |
|---|---|---|---|---|
| Lateral spinothalamic | Pain, temperature, and crude touch opposite side | Lateral white columns | Posterior gray column opposite side | Thalamus |
| Ventral spinothalamic | Crude touch and pressure | Anterior white columns | Posterior gray column opposite side | Thalamus |
| Fasciculi gracilis and cuneatus | Discriminating touch and pressure sensations, including vibration, stereognosis, and two-point discrimination; also conscious kinesthesia | Posterior white columns | Spinal ganglia same side | Medulla |
| Spinocerebellar | Unconscious kinesthesia | Lateral white columns | Posterior gray column | Cerebellum |

From Thibodeau GA, Patton KT: *Anatomy and physiology,* ed 4, St Louis, 2000, Mosby.
*Location of cell bodies of neurons from which axons of tract arise.
†Structure in which axons of tract terminate.

### Major descending tracts of the spinal cord

| Name | Function | Location | Origin* | Termination† |
|---|---|---|---|---|
| Lateral corticospinal (or crossed pyramidal) | Voluntary movement, contraction of individual or small groups of muscles, particularly those moving hands, fingers, feet, and toes of opposite side | Lateral white columns | Motor areas cerebral cortex (mainly areas 4 and 6) opposite side from tract location in cord | Lateral or anterior gray columns |
| Ventral corticospinal (direct pyramidal) | Same as lateral corticospinal except mainly muscles of same side | Anterior white columns | Motor cortex but on same side as tract location in cord | Lateral or anterior gray columns |
| Lateral reticulospinal | Mainly facilitatory influence on motoneurons to skeletal muscles | Lateral white columns | Reticular formation, midbrain, pons, and medulla | Lateral or anterior gray columns |
| Medial reticulospinal | Mainly inhibitory influence on motoneurons to skeletal muscles | Anterior white columns | Reticular formation, medulla mainly | Lateral or anterior gray columns |
| Rubrospinal | Coordination of body movement and posture | Lateral white columns | Red nucleus (of midbrain) | Lateral or anterior gray columns |

From Thibodeau GA, Patton KT: *Anatomy and physiology,* ed 4, St Louis, 2000, Mosby.
*Location of cell bodies of neurons from which axons of tract arise.
†Structure in which axons of tract terminate.

## Spinal nerves and peripheral branches

| Spinal nerves | Plexuses formed from anterior rami | Spinal nerve branches from plexuses | Parts supplied |
|---|---|---|---|
| **CERVICAL** 1 2 3 4 | Cervical plexus | Lesser occipital Great auricular Cutaneous nerve of neck Supraclavicular nerves Branches to muscles | Sensory to back of head, front of neck, and upper part of shoulder; motor to numerous neck muscles |
| **CERVICAL** 5 6 7 8 | Brachial plexus | Phrenic nerve Suprascapular and dorsoscapular Thoracic nerves, medial and lateral branches Long thoracic nerve Thoracodorsal Subscapular Axillary (circumflex) Musculocutaneous Ulnar Median Radial Medial cutaneous | Diaphragm Superficial muscles* of scapula Pectoralis major and minor Serratus anterior Latissimus dorsi Subscapular and teres major muscles Deltoid and teres minor muscles and skin over deltoid Muscles of front of arm (biceps brachii, coracobrachialis, and brachialis) and skin on outer side of forearm Flexor carpi ulnaris and part of flexor digitorum profundus; some of muscles of hand; sensory to medial side of hand, little finger, and medial half of fourth finger Rest of muscles of front of forearm and hand; sensory to skin of palmar surface of thumb, index, and middle fingers Triceps muscle and muscles of back of forearm; sensory to skin of back of forearm and hand Sensory to inner surface of arm and forearm |
| **THORACIC (OR DORSAL)** 1 2 3 4 5 6 7 8 9 10 11 12 | No plexus formed; branches run directly to intercostal muscles and skin of thorax | | |
| **LUMBAR** 1 2 3 4 5 **SACRAL** 1 2 3 4 5 **COCCYGEAL** 1 | Lumbosacral plexus  Coccygeal plexus | Iliohypogastric     Sometimes fused Ilioinguinal Genitofemoral Lateral femoral cutaneous Femoral Obturator Tibial† (medial popliteal) Common peroneal (lateral popliteal) Nerves to hamstring muscles Gluteal nerves Posterior femoral cutaneous Pudendal nerve | Sensory to anterior abdominal wall Sensory to anterior abdominal wall and external genitalia; motor to muscles of abdominal wall Sensory to skin of external genitalia and inguinal region Sensory to outer side of thigh Motor to quadriceps, sartorius, and iliacus muscles; sensory to front of thigh and medial side of lower leg (saphenous nerve) Motor to adductor muscles of thigh Motor to muscles of calf of leg; sensory to skin of calf of leg and sole of foot Motor to evertors and dorsiflexors of foot; sensory to lateral surface of leg and dorsal surface of foot Motor to muscles of back of thigh Motor to buttock muscles and tensor fasciae latae Sensory to skin of buttocks, posterior surface of thigh, and leg Motor to perineal muscles; sensory to skin of perineum |

From Thibodeau GA, Patton KT: *Anatomy and physiology,* ed 4, St Louis, 2000, Mosby.
*Although nerves to muscles are considered motor, they do contain some sensory fibers that transmit proprioceptive impulses.
†Sensory fibers from the tibial and peroneal nerves unite to form the *medial cutaneous* (or *sural*) *nerve* that supplies the calf of the leg and the lateral surface of the foot. In the thigh the tibial and common peroneal nerves are usually enclosed in a single sheath to form the *sciatic nerve,* the largest nerve in the body with a width of approximately ¾ of an inch. About two thirds of the way down the posterior part of the thigh, it divides into its component parts. Branches of the sciatic nerve extend into the hamstring muscles.

## Comparison of structural features of the sympathetic and parasympathetic pathways

| Neurons | Sympathetic | Parasympathetic |
|---|---|---|
| **PREGANGLIONIC NEURONS** | | |
| Dendrites and cell bodies | In lateral gray columns of thoracic and first four lumbar segments of spinal cord | In nuclei of brainstem and in lateral gray columns of sacral segments of cord |
| Axons | In anterior roots of spinal nerves to spinal nerves (thoracic and first four lumbar), to and through white rami to terminate in sympathetic ganglia at various levels or to extend through sympathetic ganglia, to and through splanchnic nerves to terminate in collateral ganglia | From brainstem nuclei through cranial nerve III to ciliary ganglion<br>From nuclei in pons: through cranial nerve VII to sphenopalatine or submaxillary ganglion<br>From nuclei in medulla through cranial nerve IX to otic ganglion or through cranial nerves X and XI to cardiac and celiac ganglia, respectively |
| Distribution | Short fibers from CNS to ganglion | Long fibers from CNS to ganglion |
| Neurotransmitter | Acetylcholine | Acetylcholine |
| GANGLIA | Sympathetic chain ganglia (22 pairs); collateral ganglia (celiac, superior, and inferior mesenteric) | Terminal ganglia (in or near effector) |
| **POSTGANGLIONIC NEURONS** | | |
| Dendrites and cell bodies | In sympathetic and collateral ganglia | In parasympathetic ganglia (for example, ciliary, sphenopalatine, submaxillary, otic, cardiac, celiac) located in or near visceral effector organs |
| Receptors | Cholinergic (nicotinic) | Cholinergic (nicotinic) |
| Axons | In autonomic nerves and plexuses that innervate thoracic and abdominal viscera and blood vessels in these cavities<br>In gray rami to spinal nerves, to smooth muscle of skin blood vessels and hair follicles, and to sweat glands | In short nerves to various visceral effector organs |
| Distribution | Long fibers from ganglion to widespread effectors | Short fibers from ganglion to single effector |
| Neurotransmitter | Norepinephrine (many); acetylcholine (few) | Acetylcholine |

From Thibodeau GA, Patton KT: *Anatomy and physiology,* ed 4, St Louis, 2000, Mosby.

**Cranial nerves***

| Nerve† | Sensory fibers | | | Motor fibers | | | Function‡ |
|---|---|---|---|---|---|---|---|
| | Receptors | Cell bodies | Termination | Cell bodies | Termination | | |
| I Olfactory | *Nasal mucosa* | *Nasal mucosa* | Olfactory bulbs (new relay of neurons to olfactory cortex) | | | | *Sense of smell* |
| II Optic | *Retina* | *Retina* | Nucleus in thalamus (*lateral geniculate body*); some fibers terminate in superior colliculus of midbrain | | | | *Vision* |
| III Oculomotor | *External eye muscles except superior oblique and lateral rectus* | *Trigeminal ganglion* | Midbrain (*oculomotor nucleus*) | **Midbrain (oculomotor nucleus)** | External eye muscles except superior oblique and lateral rectus; autonomic fibers terminate in ciliary ganglion and then to ciliary and iris muscles | | **Eye movements, regulation of size of pupil, accommodation (for near vision)**, *proprioception (muscle sense)* |
| IV Trochlear | *Superior oblique (proprioceptive)* | *Trigeminal ganglion* | Midbrain | **Midbrain** | Superior oblique muscle of eye | | **Eye movements**, *proprioception* |
| V Trigeminal | *Skin and mucosa of head, teeth* | *Trigeminal ganglion* | Pons (*sensory nucleus*) | **Pons (motor nucleus)** | Muscles of mastication | | *Sensations of head and face*, **chewing movements**, *proprioception* |
| VI Abducens | *Lateral rectus (proprioceptive)* | *Trigeminal ganglion* | Pons | **Pons** | Lateral rectus muscle of eye | | **Abduction of eye**, *proprioception* |
| VII Facial | *Taste buds of anterior two thirds of tongue* | *Geniculate ganglion* | Medulla (*nucleus solitarius*) | **Pons** | Superficial muscles of face and scalp, autonomic fibers to salivary and lacrimal glands | | **Facial expressions, secretion of saliva and tears**, *taste* |

| Cranial nerve | Sensory receptors (location) | Sensory ganglion | Termination in CNS (sensory) | Origin in CNS (motor) | Motor termination | Functions |
|---|---|---|---|---|---|---|
| VIII Vestibulocochlear | | | | | | |
| 1 Vestibular branch | *Semicircular canals and vestibule (utricle and saccule)* | *Vestibular ganglion* | *Pons and medulla (vestibular nuclei)* | | | *Balance or equilibrium sense* |
| 2 Cochlear or auditory branch | *Organ of Corti in cochlear duct* | *Spiral ganglion* | *Pons and medulla (cochlear nuclei)* | | | *Hearing* |
| IX Glossopharyngeal | *Pharynx; taste buds and other receptors of posterior one third of tongue* | *Jugular and petrous ganglia* | *Medulla (nucleus solitarius)* | **Medulla (nucleus ambiguus)** | **Muscles of pharynx** | *Sensations of tongue,* **swallowing movements, secretion of saliva,** *aid in reflex control of blood pressure and respiration* |
| | *Carotid sinus and carotid body* | *Jugular and petrous ganglia* | *Medulla (respiratory and vasomotor centers)* | **Medulla at junction of pons (nucleous salivatorius)** | **Otic ganglion and then to parotid salivary gland** | |
| X Vagus | *Pharynx, larynx, carotid body, and thoracic and abdominal viscera* | *Jugular and nodose ganglia* | *Medulla (nucleus solitarius), pons (nucleus of fifth cranial nerve)* | **Medulla (dorsal motor nucleus)** | **Ganglia of vagal plexus and then to muscles of pharynx, larynx, and autonomic fibers to thoracic and abdominal viscera** | *Sensations* **and movements** *of organs supplied; for example,* **slows heart, increases peristalsis, and contracts muscles for voice production** |
| XI Accessory | *Trapezius and sternocleidomastoid (proprioceptive)* | *Upper; cervical ganglia* | *Spinal cord* | **Medulla (dorsal motor nucleus of vagus and nucleus ambiguus)** | **Muscles of thoracic and abdominal viscera (autonomic) and pharynx and larynx** | **Shoulder movements, turning movements of head, movements of viscera, voice production,** *proprioception* |
| | | | | **Anterior gray column of first five or six cervical segments of spinal cord** | **Trapezius and sternocleidomastoid muscle** | |
| XII Hypoglossal | *Tongue muscles (proprioceptive)* | *Trigeminal ganglion* | *Medulla (hypoglossal nucleus)* | **Medulla (hypoglossal nucleus)** | **Muscles of tongue and throat** | **Tongue movements,** *proprioception* |

From Thibodeau GA, Patton KT: *Anatomy and physiology,* ed 4, St Louis, 2000, Mosby.

*Italics indicate sensory fibers and functions. Boldface type indicates motor fibers and functions.

†The first letters of the rods in the following sentence are the first letters of the names of the cranial nerves. Many generations of anatomy students have used this sentence as an aid to memorizing these names. "On Old Olympus' Tiny Tops, A Friendly Viking Grew Vines And Hops." (There are several slightly differing versions of this mnemonic.)

‡An aid for remembering the general function of each cranial nerve is the following 12-word saying: "Some Say Marry Money, But My Brothers Say Bad Business, Marry Money." Words beginning with S indicate sensory function. Words beginning with M indicate motor function. Words beginning with B indicate both sensory and motor functions. For example, the first, second, and eighth cranial nerves perform sensory functions.

## Cranial nerves contrasted with spinal nerves

| | Cranial nerves | Spinal nerves |
|---|---|---|
| Origin | Base of brain | Spinal cord |
| Distribution | Mainly to head and neck | Skin, skeletal muscles, joints, blood vessels, sweat glands, and mucosa except of head and neck |
| Structure | Some composed of sensory fibers only; some of both motor axons and sensory dendrites; some motor fibers belong to somatic nervous system, some to autonomic | All of them composed of both sensory dendrites and motor axons; some of latter somatic, some autonomic |
| Function | Vision, hearing, sense of smell, sense of taste, eye movements | Sensations, movements, and sweat secretion |

From Thibodeau GA, Patton KT: *Anatomy and physiology,* ed 4, St Louis, 2000, Mosby.

## Autonomic functions

| Autonomic effector | Effect of sympathetic stimulation | Effect of parasympathetic stimulation |
|---|---|---|
| **CARDIAC MUSCLE** | Increase rate and strength of contraction (beta receptors) | Inhibit pacemaker; decrease rate and strength of contraction |
| **SMOOTH MUSCLE OF BLOOD VESSELS** | | |
| Skin blood vessels | Constriction (alpha receptors) | No effect |
| Skeletal muscle blood vessels | Dilation (beta receptors) | No effect |
| Coronary blood vessels | Constriction (alpha receptors) Dilation (beta receptors) | Dilation |
| Abdominal blood vessels | Constriction (alpha receptors) | No effect |
| Blood vessels of external genitalia | Constriction (alpha receptors) | Dilation of blood vessels causing erection |
| **SMOOTH MUSCLE OF HOLLOW ORGANS AND SPHINCTERS** | | |
| Bronchioles | Dilation (beta receptors) | Constriction |
| Digestive tract, except sphincters | Decreased peristalsis (beta receptors) | Increased peristalsis |
| Sphincters of digestive tract | Constriction (alpha receptors) | Relaxation |
| Urinary bladder | Relaxation (beta receptors) | Contraction |
| Urinary sphincters | Constriction (alpha receptors) | Relaxation |
| Reproductive ducts | Contraction (alpha receptors) | Relaxation |
| Eye | | |
|   Iris | Contraction of radial muscle; dilated pupil | Contraction of circular muscle; constricted pupil |
|   Ciliary | Relaxation; accommodates for far vision | Contraction; accommodates for near vision |
| Hairs (pilomotor muscles) | Contraction produces "goose pimples" (piloerection) (alpha receptors) | No effect |
| **GLANDS** | | |
| Sweat | Increased sweat | No effect |
| Lacrimal | No effect | Increased secretion of tears |
| Digestive (salivary, gastric, etc.) | Decreased secretion of saliva; not known for others | Increased secretion of saliva |
| Pancreas, including islets | Decreased secretion | Increased secretion of pancreatic juice and insulin |
| Liver | Stimulate glycogenolysis; increase blood sugar level | No effect |
| Adrenal medulla | Increased epinephrine secretion | No effect |

From Thibodeau GA, Patton KT: *Anatomy and physiology,* ed 4, St Louis, 2000, Mosby.

## 4-7 | Reproductive system

### Female reproductive system

| Organ | Location | Function |
|---|---|---|
| Ovary (2) | On each side of pelvic cavity; attached to posterior surface of broad ligament of the ovary, to ovarian tubes by fimbraie | Produces ova and female sex hormones |
| Fallopian tube (oviduct) (2) | Extends from upper angles of uterus to sides of pelvic cavity | Conveys ova toward uterus; site of fertilization; conveys fertilized ovum to uterus |
| Uterus | In pelvic cavity between bladder and rectum | Protects and sustains life of embryo during pregnancy |
| Vagina | Extends from uterus to vulva—about 7.5-10 cm (3-4 in.); placed anterior to rectum, posterior to bladder and urethra | Conveys uterine secretions to outside of body; receives erect penis during intercourse; transports fetus during birth process |
| Labia majora | Two folds that extend from mons pubis to within an inch of anus | Encloses and protects other external reproductive organs; maintains secretions |
| Labia minora | Two folds situated between labia majora | Forms margins of vestibule; protects openings of vagina and urethra |
| Clitoris | Small protuberance at apex of triangle formed by junction of labia minora | Glans is richly supplied with blood vessels and with endings associated with feelings of pleasure |
| Vestibule | Space between labia minora that includes vaginal and urethral openings | |
| Greater vestibular (Bartholin's) gland (2) | On each side of vagina | Secretes fluid that moistens and lubricates vestibule |
| Mammary gland (2) | Anterior to pectoralis muscles, extending from second to sixth ribs and from sternum into axilla | Lactation |

From Thibodeau GA, Patton KT: *Anatomy and physiology,* ed 4, St Louis, 2000, Mosby.

### Male reproductive system

| Organ | Location | Function |
|---|---|---|
| Testis (2)    Seminiferous tubules    Interstitial cells | Positioned obliquely in scrotum | Produce spermatozoa    Produce and secrete male sex hormones |
| Epididymis (2) | Superior and posterior to testis | Storage and maturation of spermatozoa; conveys spermatozoa to vas deferens |
| Vas deferens (2) | Extends from scrotum into abdominal cavity, passes over the top, then down posterior surface of bladder, and joins ampulla of seminal vesicle | Conveys spermatozoa from epididymis to ejaculatory duct |
| Seminal vesicle (2) | Posterior to bladder | Secretes alkaline fluid containing nutrients and prostaglandins; fluid helps neutralize acidic seminal fluid |
| Prostate gland | Immediately inferior to internal urethral sphincter | Secretes alkaline fluid that helps neutralize acidic seminal fluid and enhances motility of spermatozoa |
| Bulbourethral (Cowper's) gland (2) | On each side of membranous urethra | Secretes fluid that lubricates end of penis |
| Scrotum | External pouch at base of penis | Encloses and protects testes |
| Penis | Suspended from front and sides of pubic arch | Conveys urine and seminal fluid to outside of body; inserted into vagina during intercourse; glans penis is richly supplied with sensory nerve endings associated with feelings of pleasure during sexual stimulation |

From Thibodeau GA, Patton KT: *Anatomy and physiology,* ed 4, St Louis, 2000, Mosby.

## 4-8  Urinary system

| Organ | Location | Function |
|---|---|---|
| Kidney (2) | Posterior part of lumbar region, behind peritoneum; on each side of spinal column, extending from upper border of twelfth thoracic to third lumbar vertebra | Excretes metabolic wastes; regulates acid-base balance; regulates osmotic pressure, electrolyte pattern, and volume of extracellular fluids; regulates renin-angiotensin system; manufactures erythropoietin |
| Ureter (2) | Duct connecting kidney with bladder | Conveys urine to bladder, acting as conduit |
| Bladder | In pelvic cavity behind pubes<br>In male, in front of rectum<br>In female, in front of anterior wall of vagina and neck of uterus | Conveys urine to bladder, acting as conduit<br>Serves as reservoir for urine |
| Urethra | Membranous canal extending from bladder to urinary meatus<br>In male, begins at bladder, passes through prostate gland, goes between two sheets of tissue connecting pubic bones, and passes through urinary meatus of penis<br>In female, directly behind symphysis pubis and anterior to vagina | Drains urine from bladder during voiding<br><br>In male, also serves as passageway for semen during ejaculation |

From Thibodeau GA, Patton KT: *Anatomy and physiology,* ed 4, St Louis, 2000, Mosby.

# LANGUAGE TRANSLATION GUIDE

## Spanish-French-English equivalents of commonly used medical terms and phrases

| English | Spanish | French |
|---|---|---|
| **General phrases** | | |
| What is your name? | ¿Cómo se llama usted? (¿Cuál es su nombre?) | Comment vous appelez-vous? |
| Where do you work? | ¿Dónde trabaja? (Cuál es su profesión o trabajo?) (¿Qué hace usted?) | Où travaillez-vous? |
| You will need blood and urine tests. | Usted va a necesitar pruebas de sangre y de orina. | Vous avez besoin d'une analyse de sang et d'urine. |
| You will be admitted to a hospital. | Usted será ingresado al hospital. | Vous allez être admis à un hôpital. |
| May I help you? | ¿Puedo ayudarle? | Puis-je vous aider? |
| How are you feeling? Where does it hurt? | ¿Cómo se siente? ¿Dónde le duele? | Comment vous sentez-vous? Où avez-vous mal? |
| Do you feel better today? | ¿Se siente mejor hoy? | Vous sentez-vous mieux aujourd'hui? |
| Are you sleepy? | ¿Tiene usted sueño? | Avez-vous sommeil? |
| The doctor will examine you now. | El doctor le examinará ahora. | Le médecin va vous examiner maintenant. |
| You should remain in bed today. | Usted debe guardar cama hoy. | Vous devriez rester au lit aujourd'hui. |
| We want you to get up now. | Queremos que se levante ahora. | Nous voulons que vous vous leviez maintenant. |
| You may take a bath. | Puede bañarse. | Vous pouvez prendre un bain. |
| You may take a shower. | Puede tomar una ducha. | Vous pouvez prendre une douche. |
| Have you noticed any bleeding? | ¿Ha notado alguna hemorragia? | Avez-vous remarqué un saignement? |
| Do you still have any numbness? | ¿Todavía siente adormecimiento? | Ressentez-vous encore un engourdissement? |
| Do you have any drug allergies? | ¿Es usted alérgico(a) algún médicamento? | Souffrez-vous d'allergie à des médicaments? |
| I need to change your dressing. | Necesito cambiar su vendaje. | Je dois changer votre pansement. |
| What medications are you taking now? | ¿Qué médicamentos está tomando ahora? | Quels médicaments prenez-vous actuellement? |
| Do you take any medications? | ¿Toma usted algunas medicinas? | Prenez-vous des médicaments? |
| Do you have a history of | ¿Padece | Avez-vous déjà souffert de |
| a. heart disease? | a. del corazón? | a. maladie du coeur? |
| b. diabetes? | b. de diabetes? | b. diabète? |
| c. epilepsy? | c. de epilepsia? | c. épilepsie? |
| d. bronchitis? | d. de bronquitis? | d. bronchite? |
| e. emphysema? | e. de enfisema? | e. emphysème? |
| f. asthma? | f. de asma? | f. asthme? |
| Do you need a sleeping pill? | ¿Necesita una pastilla para dormir? | Avez-vous besoin d'un somnifère? |
| Do you need a laxative? | ¿Necesita un laxante/purgante? | Avez-vous besoin d'un laxatif? |
| Relax. Try to sleep. | Relájese. Trate de dormir. | Détendez-vous. Essayez de dormir. |
| Please turn on your side. | Favor de ponerse de lado. | Veuillez vous tourner sur le côté. |
| Do you have to urinate? | ¿Tiene que orinar? | Avez-vous besoin d'uriner? |
| Have you had any sickness from any medicine? | ¿Le ha caido mal alguna medicina? | Avez-vous déjà eu des réactions à un médicament? |
| Are you allergic to anything? Medicines, drugs, foods, insect bites? | ¿Es usted alergico(a) a algo? ¿Medicinas, drogas, alimentos, picaduras de insectos? | Êtes-vous allergique à quelque chose? Médicaments, drogues, aliments, piqûres d'insectes? |
| Do you use contact lenses, dentures? Do you have any loose teeth, removable bridges, or any prosthesis? | ¿Usa usted lentes de contacto, dentadura postiza? ¿Tiene dientes flojos, dientes postizos, o cualquier prostesis? | Utilisez-vous des verres de contact, des prothèses dentaires? Avez-vous des dents qui se déchaussent, des ponts amovibles ou une prothèse? |
| Press the button when you want a nurse. | Apriete el botón cuando quiera a una enfermera. | Appuyez sur le bouton pour appeler une infirmière. |

Spanish adapted from Lister S, Wilber CJ: *Medical Spanish: the instant survival guide,* London, 1983, Butterworth.
French translations provided by Catherine Moor, translator, Montreal, Quebec, Canada.

## Spanish-French-English equivalents of commonly used medical terms and phrases—cont'd

| English | Spanish | French |
|---|---|---|
| **Vocabulary** | | |
| *Anatomy* | | |
| abdomen | el abdomen | l'abdomen |
| ankle | el tobillo | le cheville |
| anus | el ano | l'anus |
| appendix | el apéndice | le appendice |
| arm | el brazo | le bras |
| back | la espalda | le dos |
| lower back | la cintura | le bas du dos |
| bladder | la vejiga | la vessie |
| blood | la sangre | le sang |
| body | el cuerpo | le corps |
| bone | el hueso | le os |
| bowels | los intestinos, las entrañas | les intestins |
| brain | el cerebro | le cerveau |
| breasts | el pecho, los senos | les seins |
| buttocks | las nalgas, las posaderas, las sentaderas | les fesses |
| calf | la pantorrilla, el chamorro | le mollet |
| chest | el pecho | la poitrine |
| coccyx | la cóccix | le coccyx |
| collarbone | la clavícula | la clavicule |
| ear (inner) | el oído | l'oreille (interne) |
| ear (outer) | la oreja | l'oreille (externe) |
| eardrum | el tímpano | le tympan |
| ears | las orejas | les oreilles |
| elbow | el codo | le coude |
| eye | el ojo | l'oeil |
| face | la cara | le visage |
| fallopian tube | el tubo falopio | la trompe de Fallope |
| finger | el dedo | le doigt |
| foot | el pie | le pied |
| genitals | los genitales | les parties génitales |
| hair (of the head) | el pelo, el cabello | le cheveu |
| hand | la mano | la main |
| head | la cabeza | la tête |
| heart | el corazón | le coeur |
| heart valve | la válvula del corazón | la valvule cardiaque |
| hip | la cadera | la hanche |
| hormone | la hormona | la hormone |
| intestines | los intestinos | les intestins |
| jaw | la quijada | la mâchoire |
| joint | la coyuntura, la articulación | l'articulation |
| kidney | el riñón | le rein |
| knee | la rodilla | le genou |
| leg | la pierna | la jambe |
| ligament | el ligamento | le ligament |
| lip | el labio | la lèvre |
| liver | el hígado | le foie |
| lung | el pulmón | le poumon |
| mouth | la boca | la bouche |
| muscle | el músculo | le muscle |
| neck | el cuello | le cou |
| nerve | el nervio | le nerf |
| nose | la naríz | le nez |
| ovary | el ovario | l'ovaire |
| pelvis | la cadera, la pelvis | le bassin |
| penis | el pene, el miembro | le pénis |
| pulse | el pulso | le pouls |
| pupil | la niña del ojo, la pupila | la pupille |
| rib | la costilla | la côte |
| saliva | la saliva | la salive |
| shoulder | el hombro | l'épaule |
| sinus | el seno | le sinus |
| skin | la piel | l'épiderme |
| skin (of the face) | el cutis | la peau (du visage) |

# Spanish-French-English equivalents of commonly used medical terms and phrases—cont'd

| English | Spanish | French |
|---|---|---|
| **Vocabulary—cont'd** | | |
| *Anatomy—cont'd* | | |
| skull | el cráneo | la crâne |
| spine | el espinazo, la columna vertebral | la colonne vertébrale |
| stomach | el estómago, la panza, la barriga | l'estomac |
| tendon | el tendón | le tendon |
| thigh | el muslo | la cuisse |
| toe | el dedo del pie | l'orteil |
| tongue | la lengua | la langue |
| tonsils | las angínas, las amígdalas | les amygdales |
| tooth, molar | el diente, la muela | la dent, molaire |
| trachea | la tráquea | la trachée |
| urine | la orina | l'urine |
| uterus | el útero, la matríz | l'utérus |
| vagina | la vagina | le vagin |
| vein | la vena | la veine |
| wrist | la muñeca | le poignet |
| **Common medical problems** | | |
| abortion | el aborto | l'avortement |
| abscess | el absceso | l'abcès |
| appendicitis | la apendicitis | l'appendicite |
| arthritis | la artritis | l'arthrite |
| asthma | el asma | l'asthme |
| backache | el dolor de espalda | la lombalgie |
| blindness | la ceguera | la cécité |
| bronchitis | la bronquitis | la bronchite |
| bruise | moretón, magulladura | la contusion |
| burn (1st, 2nd, or 3rd degree) | la quemadura (de primer, segundo o tercer grado) | la brûlure (premier, deuxième, ou troisième degré) |
| cancer | el cáncer | le cancer |
| chickenpox | la varicela | la varicelle |
| chills | los escalofrios | les frissons |
| cold | el catarro, el resfriado | le froid |
| constipation | la constipación | la constipation |
| convulsion | la convulsión | la convulsion |
| cough | la tos | la toux |
| cramps | los calambres | las crampes |
| cut | cortada, cortadura | la coupure |
| deafness | la sordera | la surdité |
| diabetes | la diabetes | le diabète |
| diarrhea | la diarrea | la diarrhée |
| dizziness | el vértigo, el mareo | les vertiges |
| epilepsy | la epilepsia | l'épilepsie |
| fainting spell | el desmayo | l'évanouissement |
| fatigue | la fatiga | la fatigue |
| fever | la fiebre | la fièvre |
| flu | la influenza, la gripe | la grippe |
| food poisoning | el envenamiento por comestibles | l'intoxication alimentaire |
| fracture | la fractura | la fracture |
| gall stone | el cálculo biliar | le calcul biliaire |
| gastric ulcer | la úlcera gástrica | l'ulcère gastrique |
| hallucination | la alucinación | la hallucination |
| handicap | el impedimento | le handicap |
| headache | el dolor de cabeza | le mal de tête |
| heart attack | el ataque al corazón | la crise cardiaque |
| heartbeat | el latido-el palpito | la pulsation cardiaque le battement de coeur |
| heart disease | la enfermedad del corazón | la maladie du coeur |
| heart murmur | el soplo del corazón | le souffle cardiaque |
| hemorrhage | la hemorragia | la hémorragie |
| hemorrhoids | la almorranas, hemorroides | las hémorroïdes |
| hernia | la hernia | la hernie |
| herpes | el herpes | la herpès |
| high blood pressure | la presión alta | la hypertension artérielle |
| hives | la urticaria | l'urticaire |

*Continued*

## Spanish-French-English equivalents of commonly used medical terms and phrases—cont'd

| English | Spanish | French |
|---|---|---|
| **Common medical problems—cont'd** | | |
| illness | la enfermedad | la maladie |
| immunization | la inmunización | l'immunisation |
| infection | la infección | l'infection |
| inflammation | la inflamación | l'inflammation |
| injury | la herida, el daño | la blessure |
| itch | la picazón-la comezón | la démangeaison |
| laryngitis | la laringitis | la laryngite |
| lice | los piojos | le poux |
| malaria | la malaria | la malaria |
| malignant | maligno(a) | la malin, maligne |
| malnutrition | la desnutrición | la malnutrition |
| measles | el sarampión | la rougeole |
| meningitis | la meningitis | la méningite |
| menopause | la menopausia | la ménopause |
| miscarriage | un malparto, un aborto, una pérdida | la fausse couche |
| mononucleosis | la mononucleosis infecciosa | la mononucléose |
| multiple sclerosis | la esclerosis múltiple | la sclérose en plaques |
| mumps | las paperas | les oreillons |
| muscular dystrophy | la distrofía muscular | la dystrophie musculaire |
| mute | mudo(a) | le muet (muette) |
| obese | obeso(a) | l'obèse |
| obstruction | la obstrucción | l'obstruction |
| overdose | la sobredosis | la surdose |
| overweight | el sobrepeso | l'embonpoint |
| pain | el dolor | la douleur |
| palsy, cerebral | la parálisis cerebral | l'infirmité motrice cérébrale |
| paralysis | la parálisis | la paralysie |
| Parkinson's disease | la enfermedad de Parkinson | la maladie de Parkinson |
| pneumonia | la pulmonía | la pneumonie |
| poison ivy/oak | la hiedra venenosa | la herbe à la puce le sumac de l'Ouest |
| polio | la poliomielitis | la poliomyélite, polio |
| rabies | la rabia | la rage |
| rash | la roncha, el salpullido, la erupción | l'éruption cutanée |
| redness | enrojecimiento o inflamación | la rougeur |
| relapse | la recaída | la rechute |
| scar | la cicatriz | la cicatrice |
| shock | el choque | l'état de choc |
| sore | la llaga | la lésion cutanée |
| spasm | el espasmo | le spasme |
| spider bite | la picadura de araña | la morsure d'araignée |
| sprain | la torcedura | l'entorse |
| stomachache | el dolor de estómago | le mal d'estomac |
| sunstroke | la insolación | le coup de soleil |
| swelling | la hinchazón | l'enflure |
| tetanus | el tétano(s) | le tétanos |
| tonsillitis | amigdalitis | l'amygdalite |
| toothache | el dolor de muela | le mal de dent |
| trauma | el trauma | le traumatisme |
| tuberculosis | la tuberculosis | la tuberculose |
| tumor | el tumor | la tumeur |
| unconsciousness | la insensibilidad | l'inconscience |
| venereal disease | la enfermedad venérea | la maladie vénérienne |
| virus | el virus | le virus |
| vomit | el vómito, los vómitos | le vomissement |
| weakness | la debilidad | la faiblesse |
| welt | roncha, verdugón | la marque de coup, zébrure |
| whiplash | concusión de la espina cervical, lastimado del cuello | le traumatisme cranio-cervical dit <<coup du lapin>> |
| **General hospital equipment and supplies** | | |
| bandage | la venda | le bandage |
| bathtub | la tina | la baignoire |
| bed | la cama | le lit |
| bedpan | la chata | le bassin hygiénique |
| blanket | cobija | la couverture |

## Spanish-French-English equivalents of commonly used medical terms and phrases—cont'd

| English | Spanish | French |
| --- | --- | --- |
| **General hospital equipment and supplies—cont'd** | | |
| call bell | el timbre | la sonnette d'appel |
| catheter | el cateter | le cathéter, la sonde |
| crutches | las muletas | las béquilles |
| operating table | la mesa de operaciones | la table d'opération |
| pillow | la almohada | l'oreiller |
| shower | la ducha | la douche |
| soap | el jabón | le savon |
| stethoscope | el estetoscopio | le stéthoscope |
| stretcher | la camilla | la civière |
| syringe | la jeringa | la seringue |
| thermometer | el termometro | le thermomètre |
| toilet | el excusado | la toilette |
| tongue depressor | el pisalengua | le abaisse-langue |
| toothbrush | el cepillo de dientes | la brosse à dents |
| walker | el apoyador para caminar, el andador | le cadre de marche, déambulateur |
| wheelchair | la silla de ruedas | le fauteuil roulant |
| **Medications and related supplies** | | |
| alcohol | alcohol | l'alcool |
| amphetamine | anfetamina | l'amphétamine |
| antibiotic | antibiótico | l'antibiotique |
| application | aplicación | l'application |
| artifical limb | el miembro artificial | la prothèse orthopédique |
| aspirin (for children) | aspirina (para niños) | l'aspirine (pour enfants) |
| Band-Aid | la curita | le Band-Aid |
| barbiturate | barbitúrico | le barbiturique |
| birth control pill | la píldora anticonceptiva | la pilule anticonceptionnelle |
| booster shot | la inyección secundaria | l'injection de rappel |
| brace | el braguero | l'appareil orthopédique |
| calcium | calcio | le calcium |
| capsule | cápsula | la capsule |
| cocaine | cocaína | la cocaïne |
| codeine | codeína | la codéine |
| cold pack | el emplasto frío | l'enveloppement froid |
| compress (hot) | la compresa (caliente) | la compresse (chaude) |
| condom | goma, condón | le condom |
| contact lens | lentes de contacto | le verre de contact |
| contraceptive pills | pastillas anticonceptivas | les pilules contraceptives |
| cotton | algodón | le coton |
| cough syrup | jarabe para la tos | le sirop pour la toux |
| diuretic | diurético | le diurétique |
| dose | dosis | la dose |
| douche | la ducha, lavado interno | la douche |
| dressing | vendaje | le pansement |
| dropper | el gotero | le compte-gouttes |
| drops | gotas | les gouttes |
| enema | enema | le lavement |
| gauze | gasa | la gaze |
| glucose | glucosa | la glucose |
| hearing aid | el aparato para la sordera | la prothèse auditive |
| heroin | heroína | la héroïne |
| ice | hielo | le glace |
| ice pack | la bolsa de hielo | le sac de glace |
| insulin | insulina | l'insuline |
| intrauterine device (IUD) | el dispositivio intrauterino | le dispositif intra-utérin (DIU) |
| laxative | laxante, purgante, purga | le laxatif |
| lotion | loción | la lotion |
| narcotic | narcótico | le narcotique |
| needle | aguja | l'aiguille |
| Novocain | novocaína | la Novocaïne |
| ointment | ungüento | l'onguent |
| pacemaker | el marcapaso | le stimulateur cardiaque |
| penicillin | penicilina | la pénicilline |
| pill | píldora, pastilla | la pilule |

*Continued*

## Spanish-French-English equivalents of commonly used medical terms and phrases—cont'd

| English | Spanish | French |
|---------|---------|--------|
| **Medications and related supplies—cont'd** | | |
| prosthesis | miembro artificial (prótesis) | la prothèse |
| sedative | sedante, calmante | le sédatif |
| sling | el cabestrillo | l'écharpe |
| smelling salts | sales aromáticas | les sels |
| splint | la tablilla | l'attelle |
| support | el apoyo | l'appui |
| suppository | supositorio | le suppositoire |
| syrup of ipecac | jarabe de ipecacuana | le sirop d'ipéca |
| vitamin | vitamina | la vitamine |
| **Medication instructions** | | |
| right | derecho(a) | droit |
| left | izquierdo(a) | gauche |
| tablespoonful | cucharada | la cuillerée à soupe |
| teaspoonful | cucharadita | la cuillerée à thé |
| one-half teaspoonful | media cucharadita | une demi-cuillerée à thé |
| BID | dos veces al día | deux fois par jour |
| TID | tres veces al día | trois fois par jour |
| QID | cuatro veces al día | quatre fois par jour |
| every hour | cada hora | toutes les heures |
| each day, daily | cada día, diariamente | tous les jours, quotidiennement |
| every other day | cada otro día (cada tercer día) | tous les deux jours |
| till gone | hasta terminar (acabar) | jusqu'à disparition des symptômes |
| Let it dissolve in your mouth. | Que se le disuelva en la boca. | Laissez dissoudre dans la bouche. |
| as needed for pain | cuando la necesite para el dolor | quand la douleur se fait sentir |
| symptoms | sintomas | les symptômes |
| insert | inserte | insérer, introduire |
| when you get up in the morning | al levantarse | au lever |
| apply | aplique | appliquer |
| one-half hour after meals | una hora antes de comidas | une demi-heure après les repas |
| now (stat) | ahora (ahora mismo) | maintenant (immédiatement) |
| before bedtime | antes de acostarse | avant le coucher |
| before you exercise | antes de hacer ejercicios | avant de faire de l'exercice |
| chew | mastique | mastiquer |
| mix | mezcle | mélanger |
| dissolved in | disuelto en | dissous dans |
| Shake well. | Agite bien. | Bien mélanger. |
| as directed | de acuerdo con las instrucciones | suivant avis médical |
| by mouth | por la boca | par voie orale |
| rub | frote | frotter |
| gargle | haga gargaras | se gargariser |
| soak | remoje, empape | faire tremper, imbiber |
| **Tests and procedures** | | |
| allergy test | prueba para alergias | le bilan allergologique |
| analysis | análisis | l'analyse |
| blood count | recuento (conteo) globular | la numération globulaire |
| blood transfusion | la transfusion de sangre | la transfusion sanguine |
| cardiogram | cardiograma | le cardiogramme |
| checkup, medical | reconocimiento (chequeo) médico | l'examen médical complet |
| culture (throat) | cultivo de la garganta | la culture de la gorge |
| electrocardiogram | electrocardiograma | l'électrocardiogramme |
| electroencephalogram | electroencefalograma | l'électroencéphalogramme |
| enema | la enema | le lavement |
| eye test | examen de la vista (de los ojos) | l'examen de la vue |
| injection | la inyección | l'injection |
| laboratory | laboratorio | le laboratoire |
| massage | el masaje | le message |
| pregnancy test | prueba de embarazo | le test de grossesse |
| specimen | muestra (espécimen) | l'échantillon |
| traction | la traccion | la traction |
| urinalysis | análisis de orina | l'analyse d'urine |
| vaccination | la vacuna | la vaccination |
| x-rays | radiografias (rayos equis) | la radiographie |

## Spanish-French-English equivalents of commonly used medical terms and phrases—cont'd

| English | Spanish | French |
|---------|---------|--------|

**Assessment**

*General*

| English | Spanish | French |
|---------|---------|--------|
| I am _____. | Soy _____. | Je suis _____. |
| I would like to examine you now. Please take off your clothes, except for your underwear (and bra), and put on this gown. | Quisiera examinarlo(a) ahora. Por favor, quítese la ropa menos la ropa interior (y el sostén), y póngase este camisón. | Je voudrais vous examiner maintenant. Veuillez enlever vos vêtements, sauf votre slip (et votre soutien-gorge), et enfilez cette blouse. |
| I am going to take your temperature now. Open your mouth. | Le voy a tomar la temperatura ahora. Abra la boca. | Maintenant, je vais prendre votre température. Ouvrez la bouche. |
| I am going to take your blood pressure now. | Le voy a tomar la presión ahora. | Maintenant, je vais prendre votre tension artérielle. |
| Your blood pressure is low. | Su presión es baja. | Votre tension artérielle est basse. |
| Your blood pressure is too high. | Su presión es demasiado alta. | Votre tension artérielle est trop élevée. |
| Here is a prescription to reduce your blood pressure. | Aquí tiene una receta para bajar la presión de sangre. | Voici une ordonnance pour réduire votre tension artérielle. |
| You must follow a diet to lose weight. | Debe seguir una dieta para perder peso. | Vous devez suivre un régime pour perdre du poids. |
| I am going to start an IV. | Le voy a empezar un suero. | Je vais vous faire une intraveineuse. |
| Bend your elbow. | Doble el codo. | Pliez le coude. |
| Make a fist. | Haga un puño. | Faites un poing. |
| I am going to give you an injection. | Le voy a poner una inyección. | Je vais vous faire une injection. |
| Breathe normally. | Respire normalmente. | Respirez normalement. |
| Cough. | Tosa. | Toussez. |
| Squeeze my hand. | Apriete mi mano. | Serrez ma main. |
| You have a slight fever. | Ud. tiene un poco de fiebre. | Vous avez un peu de fièvre. |
| Hold your leg up. | Levante la pierna. | Levez la jambe. |
| Stand up and walk. | Parese y camine. | Levez-vous et marchez. |
| Straighten your leg. | Enderece la pierna. | Tendez la jambe. |
| Bend your knee. | Doble la rodilla. | Pliez le genou. |
| Push/pull. | Empuje/jale. | Poussez/tirez. |
| Up/down. | Arriba/abajo. | Vers le haut/vers le bas. |
| In/out. | Adentro/afuera. | Dedans/dehors. |
| Slow/fast. | Despacio/aprisa. | Lentement/vite. |
| Rest. | Descanse. | Reposez-vous. |
| Kneel. | Arrodíllese. | Agenouillez-vous. |

*Ambulation history*

| English | Spanish | French |
|---------|---------|--------|
| Do you use equipment (canes, crutches, braces)? | ¿Usa equipo (bastones, muletals, abrazaderas)? | Utilisez-vous un appareil (canes, béquilles, appareils orthopédiques)? |
| Do you use a wheelchair? | ¿Usa usted una silla de ruedas? | Utilisez-vous un fauteuil roulant? |
| Do you drive a car? | ¿Maneja usted un carro? | Conduisez-vous une voiture? |
| Can you climb stairs? | ¿Puede usted subir las escaleras? | Pouvez-vous monter les escaliers? |

*Cardiology*

| English | Spanish | French |
|---------|---------|--------|
| Have you ever had chest pain? Where? | ¿Ha tenido alguna vez dolor de pecho? ¿Dónde? | Avez-vous déjà éprouvé une douleur thoracique? Où précisément? |
| Do you notice any irregularity of heart beat or any palpitations? | ¿Nota cualquier latido o palpitación irregular? | Les battements de votre coeur sont-ils irréguliers ou avez-vous des palpitations? |
| Do you get short of breath? When? | ¿Tiene falta de aire? Cuándo? | Vous arrive-t-il d'être essoufflé? À quel moment? |
| Do you take medicine for your heart? How often? | ¿Toma medicina para el corazón? ¿Con qué frecuencia? | Prenez-vous des médicaments pour le coeur? À quelle fréquence? |
| Do you know if you have high blood pressure? | ¿Sabe usted si tiene la presión alta? | Savez-vous si vous souffrez d'hypertension? |
| Is there a history of hypertension in your family? | ¿Hay historia de hipertensión en su familia? | Des membres de votre famille font-ils de l'hypertension? |
| You have had a heart attack. | Ha tenido un ataque al corazón. | Vous avez fait une crise cardiaque. |
| Be sure to tell us if you have chest pains or if you feel anything unusual. | Debe avisarnos si tiene dolores de pecho o si siente algo anormal. | Ne manquez pas de nous dire si vous ressentez des douleurs thoraciques ou quoi que ce soit d'anormal. |

*Diabetes*

| English | Spanish | French |
|---------|---------|--------|
| You have diabetes. | Usted tiene diabetes. | Vous faites du diabète. |
| Your doctor will regulate your dosage. | Su médico le indicará su dosis. | Votre médecin déterminera la posologie. |

*Continued*

## Spanish-French-English equivalents of commonly used medical terms and phrases—cont'd

| English | Spanish | French |
|---------|---------|--------|

### Assessment—cont'd
*Drug-related problems*

| English | Spanish | French |
|---------|---------|--------|
| What drugs do you use? | ¿Cuáles drogas usa usted? | Quelles drogues prenez-vous? |
|   heroin? |   ¿heroína? |   héroïne? |
|   cocaine? |   ¿cocaína? |   cocaïne? |
|   uppers? |   ¿estimulantes? |   amphétamines? |
|   downers? |   ¿abajos? |   tranquillisants? |
|   barbiturates? |   ¿diablitos o barbitúricos? |   barbituriques? |
|   speed? |   ¿blancas? |   excitants? |
| Where do you shoot the drugs? | ¿Dónde se pone usted las drogas? | À quel endroit vous injectez-vous les drogues? |
| Have you ever been through a detoxification program before? | ¿Ha participado alguna vez en un programa de desintoxicación? | Avez-vous déjà suivi un programme de désintoxication? |
| Have you ever overdosed on drugs? | ¿Alguna vez se ha sobredrogado? | Avez-vous déjà pris une dose excessive de drogues? |

*Ears, nose, and throat*

| English | Spanish | French |
|---------|---------|--------|
| Do you have any hearing problems? | ¿Tiene Ud. problemas de oir? | Avez-vous des troubles de l'audition? |
| Do you use a hearing aid? | ¿Usa Ud. un audífono? | Portez-vous une prothèse auditive? |
| Do your ears ring? | ¿Siente un tintineo o silbido en los oídos? | Avez-vous des bourdonnements d'oreilles? |
| Do you have allergies? | ¿Tiene alergias? | Avez-vour des allergies? |
| Do you have a cold? | ¿Tiene usted un resfriado/resfrío? | Avez-vous un rhume? |
| Do you have sore throats frequently? | ¿Le duele la garganta con frecuencia? | Avez-vous souvent mal à la gorge? |
| Have you ever had strep throat? | ¿Ha tenido alguna vez (infección de la garganta)? | Avez-vous déjà eu une angine à streptocoques? |
| I want to take a throat culture. Open your mouth. This will not hurt. | Quiero hacer un cultivo de la garganta. Abra la boca. Esto no le va a doler. | Je veux vous faire un prélèvement dans la gorge. Ouvrez la bouche. Cela ne fera pas mal. |

*Endocrinology*

| English | Spanish | French |
|---------|---------|--------|
| Have you ever had problems with your thyroid? | ¿Ha tenido alguna vez problemas con la tiroides? | Avez-vous déjà eu des problèmes de thyroïde? |
| Have you noted any significant weight gain or loss? What is your usual weight? | ¿Ha notado pérdida o aumento de peso? ¿Cuál es su peso usual? | Avez-vous engraissé ou maigri de façon significative? Quel est votre poids normal? |
| How is your appetite? | ¿Qué tal su apetito? | Avez-vous de l'appétit? |
| (Women) How old were you when your periods started? How many days between periods? Have you ever been pregnant? How many children do you have? | ¿Cuántos años tenía cuando tuvo la primera regla? ¿Cuántos días entre las reglas? ¿Ha estado embarazada? ¿Cuántos hijos tiene? | (Pour les femmes) À quel âg avez-vous eu vos premières menstruations? Combien de jours séparent vos règles? Avez-vous déjà été enceinte? Combien d'enfants avez-vous? |

*Gastrointestinal*

| English | Spanish | French |
|---------|---------|--------|
| What foods disagree with you? | ¿Qué alimentos le caen mal? | Quels aliments ne vous conviennent pas? |
| Do you get heartburn? | ¿Suele tener ardor en el pecho? | Avez-vous des brûlures d'estomac? |
| Do you have indigestion often? | ¿Tiene indigestión con frecuencia? | Avez-vous souvent une indigestion? |
| Are you going to vomit? | ¿Va a vomitar (arrojar)? | Êtes-vous sur le point de vomir? |
| Do you have blood in your vomit? | ¿Tiene usted vómitos con sangre? | Vos vomissures contiennent-elles des traces de sang? |

*Headaches/head*

| English | Spanish | French |
|---------|---------|--------|
| Do you have headaches? | ¿Tiene Ud. dolores de cabeza (jaquecas)? | Avez-vous des maux de tête? |
| Do you have migraines? | ¿Tiene Ud. migrañas (jaquecas)? | Avez-vous des migraines? |
| Where is the pain exactly? | ¿Dónde le duele, exactamente? | Où avez-vous mal exactement? |
| What causes the headaches? | ¿Qué la causa los dolores de cabeza? | Qu'est-ce qui occasionne les maux de tête? |
| Are there any changes in your vision? | ¿Hay algunos cambios en su vista? | Votre vue a-t-elle changé? |

*Neurology*

| English | Spanish | French |
|---------|---------|--------|
| Have you ever had a head injury? | ¿Ha tenido alguna vez daño a la cabeza? | Avez-vous déjà eu une blessure à la tête? |
| Have you ever had a sports injury?/motorcycle accident? | ¿Ha tenido alguna vez un daño deportivo?/(accidente en su motocicleta?) | Avez-vous déjà subi un accident de sport?/un accident de motocyclette? |
| Do you have convulsions? | ¿Tiene convulsiones? | Avez-vous des convulsions? |
| Do you see double? | ¿Ve usted doble? | Voyez-vous double? |
| Do you have tingling sensations? | ¿Tiene hormigueos? | Avez-vous des fourmillements? |

## Spanish-French-English equivalents of commonly used medical terms and phrases—cont'd

| English | Spanish | French |
|---|---|---|
| **Assessment—cont'd** | | |
| *Neurology—cont'd* | | |
| Do you have numbness in your hands, arms, or feet? | ¿Siente entumecidos las manos, los brazos, o los pies? | Éprouvez-vous une sensation d'engourdissement? |
| Have you ever lost consciousness? For how long? | ¿Perdió alguna vez el sentido? ¿Por cuánto tiempo? | Avez-vous déjà perdu connaissance? Pendant combien de temps? |
| How frequently does this happen? | ¿Con qué frecuencia ocurre esto? | À quelle fréquence cela se produit-il? |
| Is this hot or cold? | ¿Está frío o caliente esto? | Est-ce chaud ou froid? |
| Am I sticking you with the point or the head of the pin? | ¿Le estoy pinchando con la cabeza del alfiler? | Est-ce que je vous pique avec la pointe ou la tête de l'épingle? |
| *Obstetrics and gynecology* | | |
| How often do you get your periods? | ¿Cada cuándo le viene la regla? | À quel intervalle avez-vous vos règles? |
| When was your last menstrual period? | ¿Cuándo fue su última regla? | À quand remontent vos dernières menstruations? |
| When was your last Pap smear? | ¿Cuándo fue su última prueba de Papanicolado? | À quand remonte votre dernier frottis vaginal? |
| Would you like information on birth control methods? | ¿Quiere usted. información sobre los métodos del control de la natalidad? (los métodos anticonceptivos)? | Voulez-vous des renseignements sur les méthodes contraceptives? |
| Do you have an IUD in place? | ¿Le han puesto un aparato intrauterino? | Avez-vous un stérilet? |
| Has your bag of waters broken? When? | ¿Se le rompió la bolsa de agua(s)? ¿Cuándo? | Votre poche des eaux s'est-elle rompue? Quand? |
| When did your pains begin? | ¿Cuándo le comenzaron los dolores? | Quand les douleurs ont-elles commencé? |
| How many minutes apart are they now? | ¿Cuántos minutos pasan entre uno y otro dolor? | À quel intervalle se succèdent-elles? |
| Do you have a lot of pain? | ¿Tiene usted mucho dolor? | Souffrez-vous beaucoup? |
| Open your mouth and breathe. Do not push. | Abra la boca y respire por la boca. No empuje. | Ouvrez la bouche et respirez. Ne poussez pas. |
| Every time the pain comes, push. | Cuando le venga el dolor, empuje. | Chaque fois que vous avez mal, poussez. |
| It is not possible for your baby to be born vaginally; we are going to do a cesarean section. | No es posible que su bebé nazca por la vagina; pore so vamos a hacerle una cesárea. | Votre bébé ne peut pas naître par voie vaginale; nous allons devoir procéder à une césarienne. |
| *Ophthalmology* | | |
| Have you had pain in your eyes? | ¿Ha tenido dolor en los ojos? | Avez-vous parfois mal aux yeux? |
| Do you wear glasses? | ¿Usa usted anteojos/gafas/lentes/espejuelos? | Portez-vous des lunettes? |
| Were you exposed to anything that could have injured your eye? | ¿Fue expuesto a cualquier cosa que pudiera haberle dañado el ojo? | Avez-vous été exposé à quelque chose qui aurait pu vous blesser l'oeil? |
| Do your eyes water much? | ¿Le lagrimean mucho los ojos? | Vos yeux larmoient-ils beaucoup? |
| I am going to put drops in your eyes in order to examine them. This medicine may burn at first. | Le voy a poner gotas en los ojos para examinarlos. Esta medicina puede arderle al principio. | Je vais vous mettre des gouttes dans les yeux pour les examiner. Ce médicament peut causer une sensation de brûlure au début. |
| Please look into this apparatus. | Favor de mirar dentro de este aparato. | Veuillez regarder dans cet appareil. |
| *Orthopedics* | | |
| You have broken (a bone). | Usted se ha quebrado/roto (un hueso). | Vous vous êtes fracturé (un os). |
| You have dislocated (a joint). | Usted se ha dislocado (una coyuntura). | Vous vous êtes déboîté (une articulation). |
| You have pulled (a muscle). | Usted se ha distendido (un músculo). | Vous vous êtes claqué (un muscle). |
| You have sprained (a muscle)/(a ligament). | Usted se ha torcido (un músculo)/(un ligamento). | Vous vous êtes foulé (un muscle)/(un ligament). |
| You will need a cast. | Necesita un yeso. | Il va vous falloir un plâtre. |
| Do you feel pain when you stand? | ¿Siente dolor al pararse? | Avez-vous mal lorsque vous vous tenez debout? |
| Do you feel pain when you bend? | ¿Siente dolor al doblarse? | Avez-vous mal lorsque vous vous courbez? |
| We need to take some x-rays. | Necesitamos tomarle unos rayos X. | Nous devons prendre quelques radiographies. |
| You must wear a sling whenever you are out of bed. | Usted debe llevar un cabestrillo cuando no este en la cama. | Vous devez porter une écharpe chaque fois que vous quittez le lit. |
| *Pain* | | |
| What were you doing when the pain started? | ¿Qué hacía usted cuando le comenzó el dolor? | Qu'étiez-vous en train de faire lorsque la douleur a commencé? |
| Where is the pain? | ¿Dónde está el dolor? | Où avez-vous mal? |

*Continued*

## Spanish-French-English equivalents of commonly used medical terms and phrases—cont'd

| English | Spanish | French |
| --- | --- | --- |
| **Assessment—cont'd** | | |
| *Pain—cont'd* | | |
| How severe is the pain? Mild, moderate, sharp, or severe? | ¿Qué tan fuerte es el dolor? ¿Ligero, moderado, agudo, severo? | Quelle est l'intensité de la douleur? Est-elle légère, modérée, forte, ou intense? |
| Have you ever had this pain before? | ¿Ha tenido este dolor antes? ¿Ha sido siempre así?) | Avez-vous déjà ressenti cette douleur auparavant? |
| Does it hurt when I press here? How did the accident happen? | ¿Le duele cuando le aprieto aquí? ¿Cómo sucedió el accidente? | Avez-vous mal lorsque j'appuie ici? Comment l'accident s'est-il produit? |
| How did this happen? How long ago? | ¿Cómo sucedío esto? ¿Cuanto tiempo hace? | Comment cela est-il arrivé? Il y a combien de temps? |
| *Poison control (telephone information)* | | |
| What was swallowed? | ¿Qué se tragó? | Quel produit la victime a-t-elle avalé? |
| Please spell the name of the product for me. | ¿Favor de deletrear el nombre del producto? | Veuillez épeler le nom du produit. |
| How old is the person who swallowed this? | ¿Cuántos años tiene la persona que se tragó esto? | Quel est l'âge de la victime? |
| How much does the person weigh? | ¿Cuánto pesa? | Qual est le poids de la victime? |
| Is the person breathing all right? | ¿Está respirando bien? | La personne respire-t-elle bien? |
| Is the person complaining of any pain or other difficulty? | ¿Se queja de algún dolor, o de otra dificultad? | La victime se plaint-elle de douleur ou d'un autre trouble? |
| How long ago did the person swallow the product? | ¿Cuánto hace que esta persona se tragó el producto? | Depuis combien de temps la personne a-t-elle avalé le produit? |
| *Pulmonary/respiratory* | | |
| Do you smoke? How many packs a day? | ¿Fuma usted? ¿Cuántos paquentes al día? | Fumez-vous? Combien de paquets par jour? |
| How long have you been coughing? | ¿Desde cúando tiene tos? | Depuis combien de temps toussez-vous? |
| Does it hurt when you cough? | ¿Le duele cuando tose? | Avez-vous mal lorsque vous toussez? |
| Do you cough up phlegm? | ¿Al toser, escupe usted flema(s)? | Expulsez-vous des sécrétions lorsque vous toussez? |
| Do you cough up blood? | ¿Al toser, arroja usted sangre? | Crachez-vous du sang? |
| Do you wheeze? | ¿Le silba a usted el pecho? | Votre respiration est-elle sifflante? |
| Have you ever had asthma? | ¿Ha tenido asma alguna vez? | Avez-vous déjà fait de l'asthme? |
| Have you ever had | ¿Ha tenido alguna vez | Avez-vous déjà souffert des maladies suivantes: |
| tuberculosis? | tuberculosis? | tuberculose? |
| pneumonia? | pulmonía? | pneumonie? |
| emphysema? | enfisema? | emphysème? |
| bronchitis? | bronquitis? | bronchite? |
| Breathe deeply. | Aspire profundamente. (Respire profundo.) | Respirez à fond. |
| *Sexually transmitted diseases* | | |
| Do you have urethral discharge? | ¿Tiene descho de la uretra? | Avez-vous un écoulement urétral? |
| Do you have burning with urination? | ¿Tiene ardor al orinar? | Avez-vous des brûlures lorsque vous urinez? |
| Do you have a vaginal discharge? | ¿Tiene descho vaginales? | Avez-vous des pertes vaginales? |
| Do you have abdominal pain? | ¿Tiene dolor en el abdomen? | Souffrez-vous de douleurs abdominales? |
| When did you last have intercourse? | ¿Cuándo fue la última vez que tuvo relaciones sexuales? | À quand remontent vos dernières relations sexuelles? |
| *Unconscious patient* | | |
| What happened to him/her? | ¿Que le pasó? (Que le sucedío?) | Que lui est-il arrivé? |
| Has he vomited? | ¿Ha vomitado? | A-t-il vomi? |
| Is she pregnant? | ¿Está embarazada? | Est-elle enceinte? |
| **Patient instructions** | | |
| *General* | | |
| Roll over and sit up over the edge of the bed. | Voltéese y siéntese sobre el borde de la cama. | Retournez-vous et asseyez-vous au bord du lit. |
| Stand up slowly. Put weight only on your right/left foot. | Párese despacio. Ponga peso sólo en la pierna derecha/izquierda. | Levez-vous lentement. Appuyez-vous seulement sur votre pied droit/gauche. |
| Lift your head up. | Levante la cabeza. | Levez la tête. |
| Take a step to the side. | Dé un paso al lado. | Faites un pas de côté. |
| Turn to your left/right. | Doble a la izquierda/derecha. | Tournez à gauche/à droite. |

## Spanish-French-English equivalents of commonly used medical terms and phrases—cont'd

| English | Spanish | French |
| --- | --- | --- |
| **Patient instructions—cont'd** | | |
| *Drugs* | | |
| I want you to take your medicine. | Quiero que tome su medicina. | Je veux que vous preniez votre médicament. |
| Let it dissolve in your mouth. | Que se le disuelva en la boca. | Laissez-le se dissoudre dans la bouche. |
| Apply _____ to the affected part. | Aplique _____ en la parte afectada. | Appliquez _____ sur la partie atteinte. |
| Cool in the refrigerator. | Enfrie en el refrigerador. | Refroidissez au réfrigérateur. |
| Here is some medication for _____.Take _____ tablets every _____ hours as needed. | Aquí tiene la medicina para _____. Tome _____ tabletas cada _____ horas según la necesite. | Voici des médicaments pour _____. Prenez _____ comprimés toutes les _____ heures selon les besoins. |
| These pills are vitamins. | Estas pastillas son vitaminas. | Ces pilules contiennent des vitamines. |
| These pills are for pain. | Estas pastillas son para dolor. | Ce sont des pilules antidouleur. |
| Take _____ of these pills each day. | Tome _____ de estas pastillas cada día. | Prenez _____ pilules chaque jour. |
| Here is enough medicine for _____ days. | Aquí tiene suficiente medicina para _____ días. | Voici suffisamment de médicaments pour _____ jours. |
| Take one of these pills every _____ hours. | Tome una de estas pastillas cada _____ horas. | Prenez l'une de ces pilules toutes les _____ heures. |
| Take one pill daily for _____ days. | Tome una pastilla por _____ días. | Prenez une pilule par jour pendant _____ jours. |
| But no more than _____ a day maximum. | Pero no más de _____ en total cada día. | Mais pas plus de _____ par jour. |
| Fill the medicine dropper to this line and mix with a glass of water, juice, or milk. | Llene el gotero hasta esta linea y mezcle con un vaso de agua, jugo, o leche. | Remplissez le compte-gouttes jusqu'à ce trait et mélangez le contenu dans un verre d'eau, de jus ou de lait. |
| It is important for you to eat/drink liquids. | Es importante que usted coma/beba o tome líquidos. | Il est important que vous mangiez/buviez. |
| | | |
| *Preparation for surgery* | | |
| I'm going to shave you. | Le voy a rasurar. | Je vais vous raser. |
| The pill (this shot) will make you sleep. | La pastilla (Esta inyeccion) le hará dormir. | Cette pilule (cette injection) vous fera dormir. |
| The doctor wants you to stay in bed. | El médico quiere que se quede en cama. | Le médecin veut que vous restiez au lit. |
| | | |
| *Anesthesia* | | |
| You are not allowed water. | No debe tomar agua. | Vous ne pouvez pas boire d'eau. |
| Have you have anything to eat or drink since midnight? | ¿Ha comido o tomado algo desde la medianoche? | Avez-vous mangé ou bu quoi que ce soit depuis minuit? |
| You must have nothing to eat or drink after midnight. | No debe comer ni tomar nada después de la medianoche. | Vous ne devez rien manger ni boire après minuit. |
| Did someone take a sample of your blood? | ¿Le han domado una muestra de sangre? | Vous a-t-on fait une prise de sang? |
| | | |
| *Radiology* | | |
| I am going to take an x-ray of your _____. | Le voy a hacer una radiografia de la (del) _____. | Je vais faire une radiographie de votre _____. |
| Please lie on the table, face up/face down. | Por favor, acuéstese sobre la mesa, boca arriba/boca abajo. | Veuillez vous allonger sur la table, sur le dos/sur le ventre. |
| Turn on your left/right side. | Voltéese al lado izquierdo/al lado derecho. | Tournez-vous sur le côté gauche/droit. |
| Turn over. | Voltéese al otro lado. | Retournez-vous. |
| Swallow this mixture. | Trague esta mezcla. | Avalez ce mélange. |
| Stand here and place your chest against this plate. | Parese aquí y apoye el pecho contra esta placa. | Mettez-vous debout ici et placez la poitrine contre cette plaque. |
| Rest your chin here. | Apoye el mentón aquí. | Posez votre menton ici. |
| Take a deep breath. Hold it. Now breathe normally. | Aspire profundamente. Manténgalo. Ahora respire normalmente. | Inspirez à fond. Retenez votre respiration. Maintenant, vous pouvez respirer normalement. |

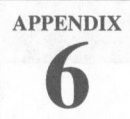

# AMERICAN SIGN LANGUAGE
# AND MANUAL COMMUNICATION

## Manual Alphabet

| A | B | C | D | E | F | G |
|---|---|---|---|---|---|---|
| H | I | J | K | L | M | N |
| O | P | Q | R | S | T | U |
| V | W | X | Y | Z | | |

## APPENDIX 7

# ASSESSMENT GUIDES

## 7-1 Adult health assessment

### HEALTH HISTORY
### Identifying information

Name, residence, telephone, age or date of birth, sex, race, ethnicity, religion, marital status/significant person/contact person, language, education, occupation, financial/insurance, source of information, advance directive

### Past history

- Statement about general health
- Other medical conditions and dates of onset or occurrence; health status in past year
- Surgeries and injuries and dates, known or suspected allergies (food, drugs, environmental allergens)
- Hospitalizations for injuries, surgery, or medical problems (condition, date, duration)
- Admittance to long-term care facility (reason, date, duration)
- Immunizations and dates
- Military history, travel and dates
- Childhood diseases and ages of occurrence
- Psychiatric illness and treatment
- Usual health care patterns and kind of practitioner used
- Use of rehabilitative and support personnel, past home care services
- Life-style patterns and personal habits in sleep, nutrition, fluid intake, urinary and bowel elimination, activity, sexual pattern, personal hygiene, others

### Present history

- Chief complaint or health concern (in client's words if possible)
- Onset and development of problem, where it took place, what was done
- Signs and symptoms, location, severity, duration, frequency, changes and effect on client, meaning of illness to client
- Factors that alleviate or aggravate symptoms
- Client's knowledge of disease, procedures, and planned therapy
- Client's adaptation to chronic disorder
- Laboratory and diagnostic tests and procedures performed and results
- Medications and treatments ordered since discharge
- Homebound status

### Family history

- Spouse, children, parents, siblings, including health status, ages, occupations, deaths and causes; pets in the home
- Roles and responsibilities of family members, relationship with family members, activities, response to stress or crisis
- Support systems within family, marital relationship
- History of abuse by family members or relatives
- Adaptation of family members to care of client in the home

### Psychosocial history

- General appearance
- Health goals and practices
- Alcohol, caffeine, and tobacco consumption: type, amount, frequency

From Jaffe MS, Skidmore-Roth L: *Home health nursing: assessment and care planning*, ed 3, St Louis, 1997, Mosby.

- Living arrangement (alone or with others and relations with them)
- Occupation and income, ability to pay for health care, insurance plan (Medicare, Medicaid, CHAMPUS, private insurance, workers' compensation)
- Education, degrees, profession if applicable
- Recreation and interests, social and other activities, hobbies, travel, retirement if applicable
- Friends, community involvement, clubs, organizations, or church activities
- Use of community agencies (Meals on Wheels, hospital or clinic, day care, transportation, home cleaning services, shopping services)
- English as a second language or no English spoken
- Review of a usual day's activities
- Emergency contact and telephone number

### Medications and treatments

- Prescribed and over-the-counter drugs: name, type, dose, frequency, route, length of use, side effects, desired effect, conditions being treated, drug form and how administered, contraindications, and risk for toxicity
- Oxygen and other inhalation medications or treatments
- General compliance with medication regimen
- Street or recreational drug use
- Aids to ensure safe, correct self-administration of medications
- Effect of client's age on absorption and excretion
- Treatment for adverse effects

### Review of systems

- Height, weight, vital signs, and temperature

### Pulmonary system

- Upper or lower respiratory disease or infections (acute or chronic)
- Dyspnea (at rest or exertional), pain in sinus, nose, throat, or chest; congestion or discharge from nose (rhinorrhea, epistaxis, snoring); hemoptysis; cough (productive or nonproductive, with sputum characteristics); hoarseness; olfactory perception; wheezing; abnormal breath sounds

### Cardiovascular system

- Heart disease (chronic, acute, congenital), vascular disease (hypertension, arterial or venous circulatory disorders)
- Chest, arm, throat, or jaw pain; leg pain or claudication; paresthesias; edema; varicosities or ulcer; dyspnea (exertion, nocturnal); palpitations; orthopnea; murmur; abnormal heart sounds

### Neurologic system

- Neuromuscular or neurosensory conditions; head or spinal trauma; seizure activity; vertigo or syncope; headache; tremors or spasms; paralysis; paresis; paresthesias; mentation changes (memory, orientation, level of consciousness); motor changes (gait, coordination); sensory perception changes (touch, taste, smell, vision, hearing); presbycusis; presbyopia; tinnitus; eye or ear pain or drainage; pruritus; photophobia; blurring; diplopia; floaters; use of glasses, contact lenses, hearing aid; sleep and rest pattern (rested, fatigue, muscle cramps); speech pattern (aphasia, slurred, alternate speech method)

## Gastrointestinal system

- Gastrointestinal, hepatic, biliary disorders; abdominal pain; nausea; vomiting; diarrhea; constipation; indigestion; heartburn; rectal bleeding; hematemesis; flatus; belching or eructation; jaundice; dysphagia (swallowing difficulty); chewing difficulty; anorexia; changes in appetite; presence and fit of dentures; caries; oral pain, bleeding, or lesions; halitosis; changes in gustatory perception; recent weight loss or gain; food intolerances, dislikes, and habits; special diet; 24-hour dietary intake review; bowel pattern review

## Endocrine system

- Glandular dysfunction (thyroid, pancreas, adrenal, pituitary), polyuria, polydypsia, changes in metabolic function, skin color and texture, hair, tolerance to heat and cold, Cushing's response to corticosteroid therapy

## Hematologic system

- Anemia, type and cause; weakness; pallor; night sweats; lymph node enlargement; skin hemorrhages; bruising; petechiae; bleeding from any site; previous transfusions (blood or blood products)

## Musculoskeletal system

- Bone or joint disease; fracture; pain or stiffness in joints and muscles; redness, swelling, or heat at joint sites; deformity; limited range of motion (ROM) and movement; fatigue; weakness; energy and endurance; ability to perform activities of daily living (ADL) (total, assisted), deficits and use of assistive devices; limb prosthesis; exercise or activity pattern review; rehabilitation services; reaction to disability; Katz index of ADL independence

## Renal/urinary system

- Upper or lower renal tract disorders, urinary pattern review, difficulty in urination (dysuria, dribbling, urgency, frequency, oliguria, nocturia, retention, incontinence), hematuria, calculi, dialysis, urinary tract infection, presence of catheter, 24-hour fluid intake and output, dialysis

## Integumentary system

- Skin color; eruptions; elasticity; turgor; texture; scarring; dryness or moisture; pruritis; alopecia; hair and nails characteristics and changes; corns; calluses; infection; pattern of daily skin, hair, nail care review

## Reproductive system

- Breast and male or female genital or organ disorders, sexually transmitted diseases, infection, lesions, discharges, bleeding, pain (testicular, pelvic, dyspareunia), infertility, impotence, pattern of sexual activity and changes, menstrual information (menarche, last period, abnormal bleeding or irregularities, menopause), pregnancies (live births, abortions, complications), penile implant

## Psychosocial/psychiatric/mental

- General appearance, depression, sadness, chronic anxiety or worry, dementia, delirium, mood swings, stressors, self-concept and self-esteem, delusions, combativeness, cognitive impairment (memory, attention span, orientation, judgment), intellectual function, disengagement or reclusiveness, thoughts of suicide; Mini-Mental State Exam, Short Portable Mental Status Questionnaire, Beck Depression Inventory, Yesavage Geriatric Depression Scale, OARS Social Resource Scale, Family APGAR

## 7-2   Pediatric assessment

### HEALTH HISTORY

Information in the health history is inclusive. It may be elicited from the caregiver or other family members or may be obtained from medical records. Modifications may be necessary to adapt to client and family needs and abilities.

### Identifying information

Date of interview, informant/complainant, source of referral
Name (of child), including nickname
First names of parents and last names, if different; their ages, occupations, educational levels
Others in household; their names, ages, relationships with client
Address
Home and work telephone numbers
Age, date of birth
Sex, race, religion, nationality, place of birth
Language ability (age appropriate), preference, need for translator
Community agencies used, telephone numbers
Support systems, telephone numbers

### Current illness

1. Chief complaint or reason for visit (in client's or caregiver's words)
2. Profile of illness, using PQRST mnemonic:
   P—prodromal, precipitating factors
   Q—qualitative, quantitative factors
   R—region, radiation
   S—severity (on a scale of 1 to 10)
   T—timings (date, onset, manner)
3. Progression of illness and effect of therapy

From Melson KA, Jaffe MS: *Pediatric and postpartum home health nursing: assessment and care planning,* St Louis, 1997, Mosby.

### History

1. Perinatal history
   a. Health of mother before, during pregnancy
      Maternal age, length of pregnancy, gravida and parity, extent of prenatal care
      Illnesses, medical conditions, exposure to communicable disease, complications relating to pregnancy, blood type
      Medications used and prescribed, exposure to toxins or chemicals
      Responses to pregnancy
   b. Duration, nature, severity of labor; use of sedatives, analgesics
      Type, date, location of delivery
      Procedures performed
      Complications
   c. Infant status, health at birth; Apgar score
      Weight, length, estimated gestational age
      Congenital anomalies, birth injuries
2. Developmental history
   Age, height, weight, dentition
   Performance of age-related developmental tasks, observed and recounted periods of delayed or accelerated growth, comparison with siblings, parental perceptions
   Grade expected and attained, quality of schoolwork
   Extracurricular activities, play
   Family/social relationships
3. Activity/performance history
   General disposition, personality, temperament
   Rituals, behaviors, responses to discipline or frustration
   Play and diversional activities, amount and type of exercise
   Eating patterns, food intake, alternative feeding management
   Sleep/nap patterns, duration, disturbances, aggravating and alleviating factors
   Urinary/bowel control, patterns, problems, remedies

Sexual maturity, activity, concerns

Drug use/abuse

4. Childhood diseases

Type, age, severity, complications, sequelae

5. Immunizations

Type, date, dosage, boosters, unusual reactions

Presence of written record

6. Medications

Over-the-counter, prescribed, borrowed; home remedies

Type, condition being treated, dose, frequency, duration, form, side effects; medication label, directions, pill count, as appropriate

Safe, accurate administration by observation, childproofing measures

7. Allergies

Hypersensitivity to foods, drugs, animals, insects, plants

Hay fever, asthma, allergic rhinitis, eczema, urticaria

8. Serious illness

Illness, injury, accidents: date, symptoms, family prevalence, course, pattern, recurrence, complications, sequelae

Dates and descriptions of hospitalizations, surgeries

Dates and results of special procedures, tests, screening panels

Presence of indwelling, central venous or peripheral catheters, tracheotomy; competence with use, maintenance

9. Family medical history

Age, sex, health status of family members

Genogram child's biologic maternal/paternal grandparents, parents, offspring, aunts, uncles, first cousins; indicate age, health status/problems, cause of death; include stillbirths, miscarriages, abortions

Familial illnesses, conditions, anomalies (e.g., cardiovascular disease, hypertension, cerebrovascular accidents, cancer, diabetes, any condition currently suspected or diagnosed in client)

Life-style choices (e.g., substance use/abuse, sedentary behaviors)

10. Psychosocial history

Family structure, roles and functions, cohesiveness

Family expectations, attitudes, outlook, bonding behaviors

Language spoken at home, communication patterns

Marital status, relationships, significant others

Educational levels, current and past employment, socioeconomic status, caregivers' work schedules

Home environment adequacy, safety

Ethnic, cultural, religious milieu

Lifestyle, health care beliefs; recreation, perceived stressors, health care concerns

Relationships with peers, employer, coworkers, schoolmates, community

Support systems, coping capacity of caregiver, resources

## REVIEW OF SYSTEMS

### General

General state of health, ability to perform age-dependent activities of daily living, unexplained weight change, fever, fatigue, constitutional symptoms, serious illness

### Pulmonary system

Shortness of breath (at rest, on exertion, positional), wheezing, stridor, frequent colds, infections, cough, hemoptysis, sputum production, date and results of last tuberculin skin testing and chest x-ray examination, use of ventilatory aids/devices

### Cardiovascular system

History of familial cardiac anomalies, congenital defects, heart murmurs, anemia, unexplained or disproportionate fatigue, activity intolerance, failure to gain weight, delayed growth/development, marked pallor, cyanosis, orthopnea or preference for squatting position, tachypnea, tachycardia, edema, dates and results of latest hematologic examination, electrocardiogram, echocardiogram

### Neurologic system

Maternal drug use, birth injury or anomaly, prematurity, trauma, delayed development, use of ototoxic drugs, tremors, spasms, seizures, ataxia, paresis, paresthesias, paralysis, any abnormal involuntary movement, difficulties with balance or coordination, difficulty swallowing, sensory defects or disturbances, delayed language development/speech problems, learning difficulties, altered level or loss of consciousness, memory loss, change in cognitive ability, behavior, affect

### Gastrointestinal system

Appetite, dietary intake, food intolerances, difficulty swallowing, weight change, anorexia, nausea, regurgitation, vomiting, pain, bowel control/habits, excessive eructation or flatulence, diarrhea, constipation, change in color/appearance of stools, infection, rectal pain/bleeding

### Endocrine system

Changes in weight, skin texture, hair distribution, pigmentation; weakness; fatigue; temperature intolerance; delayed/accelerated growth and development; polydipsia; polyphagia; polyuria; delayed/accelerated sexual maturation; personality changes; headache; visual disturbances

### Hematologic system

Local to generalized bleeding from any site (spontaneous or disproportionate to injury); petechiae; epistaxis; bruises; hyperbilirubinemia; anemias; fatigue; activity intolerance; weakness; pallor; exposure to/ingestion of chemicals, drugs, toxins; recent and past infections; chronic disease; transfusion history

### Musculoskeletal system

Strength, coordination, gait, ability to perform age-dependent activities of daily living, spinal curvature, back pain, movement limitations, fractures, deformities; muscle weakness, cramping, pain; joint stiffness, erythema, edema, pain; assistive/prosthetic devices

### Renal/urinary systems

Renal and nonrenal congenital anomalies, past infections, fever, trauma, exposure to nephrotoxic drugs or heavy metals, bladder control/habits, number of wet diapers, changes in color/odor of urine, force of stream, oliguria, polyuria, dysuria, hematuria, frequency, urgency, hesitancy, nocturia, enuresis, back or flank pain, anemia

### Reproductive system

Sexual maturity and activity; genital discharge; pruritus; lesions; rashes; breast pain, masses, discharge; measures to prevent pregnancy, sexually transmitted diseases

- Female: menarche, last menstrual period, menstrual pattern, date and results of last Papanicolaou smear, performance of breast self-examination
- Male: descended testicles, circumcision, scrotal swelling, lesions, masses, performance of testicular self-examination

### Integumentary system

Pruritus; jaundice; rashes; moles; birthmarks; congenital anomalies; scarring; petechiae; lesions; acne; ecchymoses; excessive oiliness or dryness; changes in amount/texture of hair; changes in appearance, configuration/color of nails; lice infestation; insect bites; exposure to drugs, plants, environmental toxins; recent travel

### Eye, ear, nose, and throat

- Eye: infection, discharge, excessive tearing, itching, photosensitivity, pain, edema of lids, yellowing of sclera, blurred or double vision, changes in vision, strabismus, use of corrective lenses, date and results of last eye examination
- Ear: infection, discharge, earache, tinnitus, change in hearing, vertigo, delayed speech development, date and results of latest auditory examination

- Nose: obstruction, stuffiness, discharge, sneezing, allergies, sinus pain, epistaxis, altered sense of smell
- Throat: difficulty chewing/swallowing, tongue soreness, sore throat, change in color/integrity of mucosa, hoarseness, voice aberrations, dentition, toothache, caries, gum swelling/bleeding, abscesses, pattern of dental hygiene, date and results of last dental examination

**Psychologic**

Facial expressiveness; body posture; grooming, personal hygiene; speech, language usage; mood; affect; tension; memory; cognitive function; performance of developmental tasks; activity patterns; coping abilities; relationship with family, peers, schoolmates, authority figures; school performance

## 7-3 | Geriatric functional and health assessment

### PURPOSE OF REFERRAL

What is the immediate problem for which the patient, family, or others need help? What event(s) led patient to seek help specifically at this time?

### HEALTH ASSESSMENT

1. Is patient under any unusual stress such as financial, home situation, transportation, health, family or personal relationships?
2. Which of the following best describes how patient feels?
   This is the best time of life.
   While some things are more difficult now, life is usually pleasant and acceptable.
   Just as happy now as when patient was younger.
   Life has become unpleasant and difficult to tolerate.
   Very unhappy with present situation.
3. Which of the following best describes patient's state of health?
   usually good.
   average health.
   below average.
   very poor.
4. Does patient have (or has patient had) any of the following symptoms? If yes, for how long?
   Frequent headaches
   Passing out or fainting
   Falling or stumbling
   Paralysis or leg or arm weakness
   Numbness or loss of feeling
   Tremor or shaking
   Forgetfulness
   Problem with memory
   Disorientation to time, person, or place
   Depression
   Agitation
   Hallucinations (hearing voices and/or seeing things)
   Suspiciousness of others
   Fearfulness
   Unusually high or low moods
   Difficulty sleeping
   Difficulty speaking
   Difficulty understanding what others say
   Difficulty swallowing
   Hoarseness or other change in voice
   Visual or eye problems (date of last visit to eye doctor)

   Hearing or ear trouble (date of last hearing examination)

   Dental problems, dental discomfort (date of last visit to dentist)

   Fever or sweats
   Swollen glands
   Lumps or sores
   Skin trouble
   Difficulty breathing
   Persistent cough
   Chest pain or tightness
   Irregular heartbeat
   Leg pain when walking
   High blood pressure
   Poor appetite

Change in weight
Frequent indigestion or stomach ache
Frequent nausea or vomiting
Change in bowel habits
Black bowel movements or rectal bleeding
Frequent diarrhea
Constipation
Urination at night
Painful urination
Difficulty starting or stopping urination
Difficulty holding urine or urine leakage
Sexual difficulties
Back or neck troubles
Joint pain or stiffness
Swelling of feet or ankles
Foot problems
Women only:
   Breast lumps or discharge
   Vaginal bleeding/discomfort
Men only:
   Discharge from penis
   Swelling/lump in testicle
   Ache in lower back or groin

5. Other problems:
   Sleeping problems
   Feeling lonely
   Change in sexual interest
   Feeling sad or depressed
   Change in sexual activity
   Thought of "ending it all"
   Feeling tense or anxious
   Change in appetite
6. Past medical history (approximate dates)
   Alcoholism
   Anemia
   Arthritis
   Asthma
   Bronchitis
   Cancer
   Cataracts
   Depression
   Diabetes
   Emotional problems
   Fractures
   Gallbladder problems
   Glaucoma
   Heart disease
   Hernia
   High blood pressure
   Jaundice
   Kidney disease
   Liver disease
   Lung disease
   Mental illness
   Nervous breakdown
   Prostate disease
   Phlebitis
   Pneumonia
   Seizures

Stomach ulcers
Stroke
Thyroid disease
Tuberculosis
Urinary tract infection
Venereal disease
Other

7. Hospitalizations (location, dates, reason)
8. Family health problems (for each, relationship to patient; if the patient has died, give age at time of death and cause of death)
Alcoholism
Cancer
Depression
Diabetes
Heart disease
High blood pressure
Kidney disease
Memory problems
Mental illness
Nervous breakdown
Speech or language disorder
Stroke
Other

9. Smoking history
Does patient now, or did patient ever, smoke cigarettes/cigar/ pipe, or chew tobacco?
How much?
For how long?
When did patient stop?

10. Does patient drink alcohol?
If no, why not?
If yes, how much?
How often? (less than 3 times a week, more than 3 times a week, daily)
Is alcohol a problem?

11. Prescription medicines (names, dosages, how often, how long taken)
12. Medicines taken in addition to prescription drugs (aspirin, antacids, cold pills/decongestants, hormones, laxatives, nerve pills, sleeping pills, vitamins/minerals, other)
13. Medication allergies
14. Are doing any of the following activities a problem for the patient? If yes, who helps?
Shopping for groceries
Preparing own meals
Eating
Doing housecleaning
Writing checks or paying bills
Taking medicines
Taking sponge or tub bath, or shower
Dressing
Using the telephone
Walking indoors
Walking outdoors
Going up or down stairs
Getting into or out of bed or chair
Getting off or on toilet

15. Does patient use any prosthetic devices or aids (glasses, hearing aids, cane, wheelchair, contact lenses, dentures, walker, other)?
16. Where does the patient live (apartment [nonpublic], home [owned], home [rented], foster home, public housing, subsidized housing, nursing home, other)?
17. With whom does patient live (alone, children, companion or friend, spouse or partner, another relative, other)?
18. With whom is patient in regular contact (spouse or partner, child or children, brother[s] or sister[s], other relative[s], friend[s], neighbor[s])?
19. Whom does patient call on for help?
20. How often in the past week has patient left home (e.g., going to church, meetings, or other activities)?

21. What interests and activities does patient most enjoy?
22. Which best describes patient's employment status
Never fully employed (outside the home)
Retired—when?
Presently working (full-time, part-time)
23. Patient's present or past occupations
24. Which of the following best describes patient's financial status?
Comfortably able to afford all necessities (food, clothing, and transportation)
Able to afford necessities with careful budgeting
Barely able to afford the basic needs
Unable to afford the necessities
25. What is patient's usual form of transportation?
Drives own car
Rides with a friend or relative
Takes a bus
Walks
Takes a cab
Doesn't go out of house or apartment
26. Which of the following services has patient used in the past 3 months? Who provided the service?
Personal care
Nursing services
Medical care (physicians)
Mental health services
Social services
Physical therapy
Occupational therapy
Hearing or speech testing or therapy
Sight center
Rehabilitation services
Nutritionist
Transportation
Day center
Meal program
Other
27. How many meals a day does patient eat?
28. How many snacks a day does patient eat?
29. How many cups of fluids per day does patient drink (including tea, coffee, water, juice, milk, soda pop, etc.)?
30. Concerns about diet or nutrition?

**MENTAL STATUS**

1. Appearance
2. Mood, affect (including check for depression, orientation)
3. Cognitive function (examples)
4. Communication

**SLEEPING**

1. Does patient sleep well?
2. Does patient feel well rested?
3. Ease of falling asleep
4. Nap pattern
5. Hours per night/times up during the night
6. Concerns of patient/family

**SENSES**

1. Sight
2. Hearing
3. Taste
4. Smell
5. Touch

**ACTIVITIES OF DAILY LIVING (for each, is patient independent or dependent?)**

1. Bathing
Initiation of bath
Type of bathing (tub, shower, sponge)
Bath preparation

Get in/out of tub
Ability to wash self
Hair washing
2. Dressing
Clothing selection
Putting on garments
Doing up buttons, etc.
Appropriateness of attire
Undressing
Laundry
3. Transfer
From bed to chair
From chair to standing
4. Toileting
Able to find bathroom
Able to use toilet appropriately
Hygiene
5. Bowel continence
Frequency and control
Constipation
6. Feeding
7. Telephone
Look up number
Dial
8. Medication
Preparation
Taking
9. Outside of home
Organization
Getting lost
10. Driving
11. Housework
Organization
Doing (List what able to do)
12. Food preparation
Planning
Shopping
Preparing
13. Finances
Banking
Paying bills
Balancing checkbook

## URINARY CONTINENCE

1. Does patient have "accidents"? (If "yes," when?)
2. Patient's knowledge of accidents
3. Frequency
4. Urgency
5. Can patient get to bathroom in time?
6. Does patient wet when coughing or sneezing or at other times?
7. Where is center of concern about wetting (patient, family, both)?
8. Other concerns

## MOBILITY

1. Walking ability (use of assistive devices)
2. Distance able to walk (and frequency)
3. Gait, posture
4. Stiffness (morning, after inactivity, evening, where?)
5. What does patient do to maximize mobility?
6. Hand dexterity and function
7. Problems with feet and shoes
8. Other concerns of patient/family

## NUTRITION

1. Number of meals per day
2. Number of glasses of fluid
3. Indigestion, nausea/vomiting, change in bowels
4. Dentition
5. Appetite
6. Weight stability
7. Concerns of family (need for referral to nutritionist)

## SAFETY

1. Is patient alone at any time?
2. Does patient get lost?
3. Kitchen safety
4. Household safety (rugs, cords, railings, stairs)
5. Other concerns

## CARE GIVER

1. Name of formal care giver, relationship
2. Informal care-giving system
3. Care giver's role/function
4. Impact of care giving on care giver/family
5. Assessment of stability/security provided in present care environment

---

| 7-4 | **Family assessment** |

## PHYSICAL HISTORY

- Chronic illness of family members
- Functional abilities or disabilities
- Energy levels of family members and how physical needs of its members are met
- Physical strength and ability to perform procedures
- Rigidity in functioning within family system
- Health practices
- Types of practitioners used
- Medications taken by family members

## PSYCHOSOCIAL HISTORY
### Emotional status/mental status

- Changes in family life and roles caused by client needs
- Family unable to meet emotional needs of its members
- Ability of family members to express feelings
- Ability of family to accomplish developmental tasks
- Ability to communicate clear message, solve problems, and make decisions

- Family attitude, overconcern toward illness or disability, relationship of client and family members
- Family patterns in use of coping mechanisms (denial, rationalization, projections, defensiveness) and ability to adapt
- Family organization (arguments, separations, divorces)
- Willingness to perform procedures and care for client
- Support of client by member most likely to become caregiver
- Family APGAR for family function

## PSYCHIATRIC DISORDERS

- General mental health of family
- Psychosomatic tendency
- Chronic anxiety in family members
- Depression in family members
- Behavior disorder of family member
- Presence of alcoholism, family violence, suicides, drug abuse

## CULTURAL INFLUENCES

- General values and ethnic identity of family
- Spiritual beliefs, religious affiliation
- Language barriers, English as a second language
- Beliefs regarding health care and health professionals

From Jaffe MS, Skidmore-Roth L: *Home health nursing: assessment and care planning*, ed 3, St Louis, 1997, Mosby.

## 7-5 Environmental assessment

### HOME EXTERIOR
- Primary entrance
- Steps or ramp available if needed
- Homebound or able to leave home safely

### HOME INTERIOR
- Condition and cleanliness, noise, waste disposal
- Space storage for extra equipment and supplies
- Counter space for preparation of supplies, cleaning of equipment
- Refrigeration for foods, medications, supplies
- Location of fuse or circuit breaker box
- Proper lighting, frayed or loose wiring or electrical connections, grounding of equipment
- Heating and air conditioning adequacy
- Woodstove or kerosene heater use and ability to fuel fire
- Ventilation, temperature control, drafts
- Laundry facilities for clothing, linens, supplies
- Doorways and if adequate to move through easily, to accommodate wheelchair, commode, and to allow for delivery of equipment
- Floors and pathways clear, dry, and not slippery; arrangement of furniture out of pathways but close enough to use for support when ambulating; small rugs and carpet edges out of pathways
- Stairway, number of stairs and height of stairs; room on first floor or need for client to be transported upstairs

From Jaffe MS, Skidmore-Roth L: *Home health nursing: assessment and care planning,* ed 3, St Louis, 1997, Mosby.

- Safety bars and holding aids for movement within environment
- Hot and cold running water or means to heat water, indoor plumbing versus drawn water
- Bathroom, commode within easy access
- Presence of allergens, dust, animals, plants, sprays, odors

### SAFETY FACTORS
- Client's feeling of safety in home
- Hospital bed, trapeze connection
- Side rails up or bed in low position if using hospital bed
- Call bell, water, tissues, wastebasket, telephone within reach
- Chair to assist to standing position
- Scales for weight in bathroom or near bed
- Proper body alignment and positioning if on bed rest
- Use of restraints, smoking and precautions taken
- Isolation or protective isolation procedures needed
- Nonslip mats in bath or shower
- Night-lights if out of bed at night to use bathroom or commode
- Safety aids for ADL to prevent falls, promote self-care; amount of assistance needed, proper fitting nonskid foot covering
- Proper hand-washing technique when required
- Proper administration of medications and use of aids to ensure accuracy
- Proper cleansing and disinfection of reusable supplies, removal and disposal of hazardous wastes
- Available emergency numbers to call

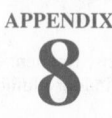

## APPENDIX 8

# NORMAL REFERENCE VALUES

### 8-1 Normal reference laboratory values

#### Reference intervals for hematology

| Test | Conventional units | SI units |
|---|---|---|
| Acid hemolysis (Ham test) | No hemolysis | No hemolysis |
| Alkaline phosphatase, leukocyte | Total score 14-100 | Total score 14-100 |
| Cell counts | | |
|   Erythrocytes | | |
|     Males | 4.6-6.2 million/mm³ | $4.6\text{-}6.2 \times 10^{12}/L$ |
|     Females | 4.2-5.4 million/mm³ | $4.2\text{-}5.4 \times 10^{12}/L$ |
|     Children (varies with age) | 4.5-5.1 million/mm³ | $4.5\text{-}5.1 \times 10^{12}/L$ |
| Leukocytes, total | 4500-11,000/mm³ | $4.5\text{-}11.0 \times 10^{9}/L$ |
| Leukocytes, differential counts* | | |
|   Myelocytes | 0% | 0/L |
|   Band neutrophils | 3%-5% | $150\text{-}400 \times 10^{6}/L$ |
|   Segmented neutrophils | 54%-62% | $3000\text{-}5800 \times 10^{6}/L$ |
|   Lymphocytes | 25%-33% | $1500\text{-}3000 \times 10^{6} L$ |
|   Monocytes | 3%-7% | $300\text{-}500 \times 10^{6}/L$ |
|   Eosinophils | 1%-3% | $50\text{-}250 \times 10^{6}/L$ |
|   Basophils | 0%-1% | $15\text{-}50 \times 10^{6}/L$ |
| Platelets | 150,000-400,000/mm³ | $150\text{-}400 \times 10^{9}/L$ |
| Reticulocytes | 25,000-75,000/mm³ (0.5%-1.5% of erythrocytes) | $25\text{-}75 \times 10^{9}/L$ |
| Coagulation tests | | |
|   Bleeding time (template) | 2.75-8.0 min | 2.75-8.0 min |
|   Coagulation time (glass tube) | 5-15 min | 5-15 min |
|   D-Dimer | <0.5 μg/mL | <0.5 mg/L |
|   Factor VIII and other coagulation factors | 50%-150% of normal | 0.5-1.5 of normal |
|   Fibrin split products (Thrombo-Wellco test) | <10 μg/mL | <10 mg/L |
|   Fibrinogen | 200-400 mg/dL | 2.0-4.0 g/L |
|   Partial thromboplastin time, activated (aPTT) | 20-35 s | 20-35 s |
|   Prothrombin time (PT) | 12.0-14.0 s | 12.0-14.0 s |
| Coombs' test | | |
|   Direct | Negative | Negative |
|   Indirect | Negative | Negative |
| Corpuscular values of erythrocytes | | |
|   Mean corpuscular hemoglobin (MCH) | 26-34 pg/cell | 26-34 pg/cell |
|   Mean corpuscular volume (MCV) | 80-96 μm³ | 80-96 fL |
|   Mean corpuscular hemoglobin concentration (MCHC) | 32-36 g/dL | 320-360 g/L |
| Haptoglobin | 20-165 mg/dL | 0.20-1.65 g/L |
| Hematocrit | | |
|   Males | 40-54 mL/dL | 0.40-0.54 |
|   Females | 37-47 mL/dL | 0.37-0.47 |
|   Newborns | 49-54 mL/dL | 0.49-0.54 |
|   Children (varies with age) | 35-49 mL/dL | 0.35-0.49 |
| Hemoglobin | | |
|   Males | 13.0-18.0 g/dL | 8.1-11.2 mmol/L |
|   Females | 12.0-16.0 g/dL | 7.4-9.9 mmol/L |
|   Newborns | 16.5-19.5 g/dL | 10.2-12.1 mmol/L |
|   Children (varies with age) | 11.2-16.5 g/dL | 7.0-10.2 mmol/L |
| Hemoglobin, fetal | <1.0% of total | <0.01 of total |
| Hemoglobin $A_{1c}$ | 3%-5% of total | 0.03-0.05 of total |
| Hemoglobin $A_2$ | 1.5%-3.0% of total | 0.015-0.03 of total |
| Hemoglobin, plasma | 0.0-5.0 mg/dL | 0.0-3.2 μmol/L |
| Methemoglobin | 30-130 mg/dL | 19-80 μmol/L |
| Sedimentation rate (ESR) | | |
|   Wintrobe: Males | 0-5 mm/h | 0-5 mm/h |
|        Females | 0-15 mm/h | 0-15 mm/h |
|   Westergren: Males | 0-15 mm/h | 0-15 mm/h |
|          Females | 0-20 mm/h | 0-20 mm/h |

From Rakel RE, ed.: *Conn's current therapy 2000*, Philadelphia, 2000, WB Saunders.
*Conventional units are percentages; SI units are absolute counts.

## Reference intervals* for clinical chemistry (blood, serum, and plasma)

| Analyte | Conventional units | SI units |
|---|---|---|
| Acetoacetate plus acetone | | |
|   Qualitative | Negative | Negative |
|   Quantitative | 0.3-2.0 mg/dL | 30-200 $\mu$mol/L |
| Acid phosphatase, serum (thymolphthalein monophosphate substrate) | 0.1-0.6 U/L | 0.1-0.6 U/L |
| ACTH (see Corticotropin) | | |
| Alanine aminotransferase (ALT) serum (SGPT) | 1-45 U/L | 1-45 U/L |
| Albumin, serum | 3.3-5.2 g/dL | 33-52 g/L |
| Aldolase, serum | 0.0-7.0 U/L | 0.0-7.0 U/L |
| Aldosterone, plasma | | |
|   Standing | 5-30 ng/dL | 140-830 pmol/L |
|   Recumbent | 3-10 ng/dL | 80-275 pmol/L |
| Alkaline phosphatase (ALP), serum | | |
|   Adult | 35-150 U/L | 35-150 U/L |
|   Adolescent | 100-500 U/L | 100-500 U/L |
|   Child | 100-350 U/L | 100-350 U/L |
| Ammonia nitrogen, plasma | 10-50 $\mu$mol/L | 10-50 $\mu$mol/L |
| Amylase, serum | 25-125 U/L | 25-125 U/L |
| Anion gap, serum, calculated | 8-16 mEq/L | 8-16 mmol/L |
| Ascorbic acid, blood | 0.4-1.5 mg/dL | 23-85 $\mu$mol/L |
| Aspartate aminotransferase (AST) serum (SGOT) | 1-36 U/L | 1-36 U/L |
| Base excess, arterial blood, calculated | 0 ± 2 mEq/L | 0 ± 2 mmol/L |
| Beta-carotene, serum | 60-260 $\mu$g/dL | 1.1-8.6 $\mu$mol/L |
| Bicarbonate | | |
|   Venous plasma | 23-29 mEq/L | 23-29 mmol/L |
|   Arterial blood | 21-27 mEq/L | 21-27 mmol/L |
| Bile acids, serum | 0.3-3.0 mg/dL | 0.8-7.6 $\mu$mol/L |
| Bilirubin, serum | | |
|   Conjugated | 0.1-0.4 mg/dL | 1.7-6.8 $\mu$mol/L |
|   Total | 0.3-1.1 mg/dL | 5.1-19.0 $\mu$mol/L |
| Calcium, serum | 8.4-10.6 mg/dL | 2.10-2.65 mmol/L |
| Calcium, ionized, serum | 4.25-5.25 mg/dL | 1.05-1.30 mmol/L |
| Carbon dioxide, total, serum or plasma | 24-31 mEq/L | 24-31 mmol/L |
| Carbon dioxide tension ($P_{CO_2}$), blood | 35-45 mm Hg | 35-45 mm Hg |
| Ceruloplasmin, serum | 23-44 mg/dL | 230-440 mg/L |
| Chloride, serum or plasma | 96-106 mEq/L | 96-106 mmol/L |
| Cholesterol, serum or ethylenediaminetetraacetic acid (EDTA) plasma | | |
|   Desirable range | <200 mg/dL | <5.20 mmol/L |
|   Low-density lipoprotein (LDL) cholesterol | 60-180 mg/dL | 1.55-4.65 mmol/L |
|   High-density lipoprotein (HDL) cholesterol | 30-80 mg/dL | 0.80-2.05 mmol/L |
| Copper | 70-140 $\mu$g/dL | 11-22 $\mu$mol/L |
| Corticotropin (ACTH), plasma, 8 AM | 10-80 pg/mL | 2-18 pmol/L |
| Cortisol, plasma | | |
|   8 AM | 6-23 $\mu$g/dL | 170-630 nmol/L |
|   4 PM | 3-15 $\mu$g/dL | 80-410 nmol/L |
|   10 PM | <50% of 8 AM value | <50% of 8 AM value |
| Creatine, serum | | |
|   Males | 0.2-0.5 mg/dL | 15-40 $\mu$mol/L |
|   Females | 0.3-0.9 mg/dL | 25-70 $\mu$mol/L |
| Creatine kinase (CK), serum | | |
|   Males | 55-170 U/L | 55-170 U/L |
|   Females | 30-135 U/L | 30-135 U/L |
| Creatine kinase MB isoenzyme, serum | <5% of total CK activity | <5% of total CK activity |
| | <5.0 ng/mL by immunoassay | <5.0 ng/mL by immunoassay |
| Creatinine, serum | 0.6-1.2 mg/dL | 50-110 $\mu$mol/L |
| Estradiol-17 beta, adult | | |
|   Males | 10-65 pg/mL | 35-240 pmol/L |
|   Females | | |
|     Follicular | 30-100 pg/mL | 110-370 pmol/L |
|     Ovulatory | 200-400 pg/mL | 730-1470 pmol/L |
|     Luteal | 50-140 pg/mL | 180-510 pmol/L |
| Ferritin, serum | 20-200 ng/mL | 20-200 $\mu$g/L |
| Fibrinogen, plasma | 200-400 mg/dL | 2.0-4.0 g/L |
| Folate, serum | 3-18 ng/mL | 6.8-41 nmol/L |
|   Erythrocytes | 145-540 ng/mL | 330-1220 nmol/L |

*Reference values may vary, depending on the method and sample source used.           *Continued*

## Reference intervals for clinical chemistry (blood, serum, and plasma)—cont'd

| Analyte | Conventional units | SI units |
|---|---|---|
| Follicle-stimulating hormone (FSH), plasma | | |
|   Males | 4-25 mU/mL | 4-25 U/L |
|   Females, premenopausal | 4-30 mU/mL | 4-30 U/L |
|   Females, postmenopausal | 40-250 mU/mL | 40-250 U/L |
| Gamma-glutamyltransferase (GGT), serum | 5-40 U/L | 5-40 U/L |
| Gastrin, fasting, serum | 0-100 pg/mL | 0-100 mg/L |
| Glucose, fasting, plasma or serum | 70-115 mg/dL | 3.9-6.4 nmol/L |
| Growth hormone (hGH), plasma, adult, fasting | 0-6 ng/mL | 0-6 $\mu$g/L |
| Haptoglobin, serum | 20-165 mg/dL | 0.20-1.65 gm/L |
| Immunoglobulins, serum (see table of Reference Intervals for Tests of Immunologic Function) | | |
| Iron, serum | 75-175 $\mu$g/dL | 13-31 $\mu$mol/L |
| Iron binding capacity, serum | | |
|   Total | 250-410 $\mu$g/dL | 45-73 $\mu$mol/L |
|   Saturation | 20-55% | 0.20-0.55 |
| Lactate | | |
|   Venous whole blood | 5.0-20.0 mg/dL | 0.6-2.2 mmol/L |
|   Arterial whole blood | 5.0-15.0 mg/dL | 0.6-1.7 mmol/L |
| Lactate dehydrogenase (LD), serum | 110-220 U/L | 110-220 U/L |
| Lipase, serum | 10-140 U/L | 10-140 U/L |
| Lutropin (LH), serum | | |
|   Males | 1-9 U/L | 1-9 U/L |
|   Females | | |
|   Follicular phase | 2-10 U/L | 2-10 U/L |
|     Midcycle peak | 15-65 U/L | 15-65 U/L |
|     Luteal phase | 1-12 U/L | 1-12 U/L |
|     Postmenopausal | 12-65 U/L | 12-65 U/L |
| Magnesium, serum | 1.3-2.1 mg/dL | 0.65-1.05 mmol/L |
| Osmolality | 275-295 mOsm/kg water | 275-295 mOsm/kg water |
| Oxygen, blood, arterial, room air | | |
| Partial pressure (PaO$_2$) | 80-100 mm Hg | 80-100 mm Hg |
|   Saturation (SaO$_2$) | 95-98% | 95%-98% |
| pH, arterial blood | 7.35-7.45 | 7.35-7.45 |
| Phosphate, inorganic, serum | | |
|   Adult | 3.0-4.5 mg/dL | 1.0-1.5 mmol/L |
|   Child | 4.0-7.0 mg/dL | 1.3-2.3 mmol/L |
| Potassium | | |
|   Serum | 3.5-5.0 mEq/L | 3.5-5.0 mmol/L |
|   Plasma | 3.5-4.5 mEq/L | 3.5-4.5 mmol/L |
| Porgesterone, serum, adult | | |
|   Males | 0.0-0.4 ng/mL | 0.0-1.3 mmol/L |
|   Females | | |
|     Follicular phase | 0.1-1.5 ng/mL | 0.3-4.8 mmol/L |
|     Luteal phase | 2.5-28.0 ng/mL | 8.0-89.0 mmol/L |
| Prolactin, serum | | |
|   Males | 1.0-15.0 ng/mL | 1.0-15.0 $\mu$g/L |
|   Females | 1.0-20.0 ng/mL | 1.0-20.0 $\mu$g/L |
| Protein, serum, electrophoresis | | |
|   Total | 6.0-8.0 g/dL | 60-80 g/L |
|   Albumin | 3.5-5.5 g/dL | 35-55 g/L |
|   Globulins | | |
|     Alpha$_1$ | 0.2-0.4 g/dL | 2.0-4.0 g/L |
|     Alpha$_2$ | 0.5-0.9 g/dL | 5.0-9.0 g/L |
|     Beta | 0.6-1.1 g/dL | 6.0-11.0 g/L |
|     Gamma | 0.7-1.7 g/dL | 7.0-17.0 g/L |
| Pyruvate, blood | 0.3-0.9 mg/dL | 0.03-0.10 mmol/L |
| Rheumatoid factor | 0.0-30.0 IU/mL | 0.0-30.0 kIU/L |
| Sodium, serum or plasma | 135-145 mEq/L | 135-145 mmol/L |
| Testosterone, plasma | | |
|   Males, adult | 300-1200 ng/dL | 10.4-41.6 nmol/L |
|   Females, adult | 20-75 ng/dL | 0.7-2.6 nmol/L |
|   Pregnant females | 40-200 ng/dL | 1.4-6.9 nmol/L |
| Thyroglobulin | 3-42 ng/mL | 3-42 $\mu$g/L |
| Thyrotropin (hTSH), serum | 0.4-4.8 $\mu$IU/mL | 0.4-4.8 mIU/L |
| Thyrotropin-releasing hormone (TRH) | 5-60 pg/mL | 5-60 mg/L |
| Thyroxine (FT$_4$), free, serum | 0.9-2.1 ng/dL | 12-27 pmol/L |
| Thyroxine (T$_4$), serum | 4.5-12.0 $\mu$g/dL | 58-154 nmol/L |

## Reference intervals for clinical chemistry (blood, serum, and plasma)—cont'd

| Analyte | Conventional units | SI units |
|---|---|---|
| Thyroxine-binding globulin (TBG) | 15.0-34.0 µg/mL | 15.0-34.0 mg/L |
| Transferrin | 250-430 mg/dL | 2.5-4.3 g/L |
| Triglycerides, serum, 12-h fast | 40-150 mg/dL | 0.4-1.5 g/L |
| Triiodothyronine ($T_3$), serum | 70-190 ng/dL | 1.1-2.9 nmol/L |
| Triiodothyronine uptake, resin ($T_3RU$) | 25%-38% | 0.25-0.38 |
| Urate | | |
|    Males | 2.5-8.0 mg/dL | 150-480 µmol/L |
|    Females | 2.2-7.0 mg/dL | 130-420 µmol/L |
| Urea, serum or plasma | 24-49 mg/dL | 4.0-8.2 nmol/L |
| Urea nitrogen, serum or plasma | 11-23 mg/dL | 8.0-16.4 nmol/L |
| Viscosity, serum | 1.4-1.8 × water | 1.4-1.8 × water |
| Vitamin A, serum | 20-80 µg/dL | 0.70-2.80 µmol/L |
| Vitamin $B_{12}$, serum | 180-900 pg/mL | 133-664 pmol/L |

## Reference intervals for therapeutic drug monitoring (serum)

| Analyte | Therapeutic range | Toxic concentrations | Proprietary name(s) |
|---|---|---|---|
| **Analgesics** | | | |
| Acetaminophen | 10-20 µg/mL | >250 µg/mL | Tylenol<br>Datril |
| Salicylate | 100-250 µg/mL | >300 µg/mL | Aspirin<br>Bufferin |
| **Antibiotics** | | | |
| Amikacin | 25-30 µg/mL | Peak >35 µg/mL<br>Trough >10 µg/mL | Amikin |
| Gentamicin | 5-10 µg/mL | Peak >10 µg/mL<br>Trough >2 µg/mL | Garamycin |
| Tobramycin | 5-10 µg/mL | Peak >10 µg/mL<br>Trough >2 µg/mL | Nebcin |
| Vancomycin | 5-35 µg/mL | Peak >40 µg/mL<br>Trough >10 µg/mL | Vancocin |
| **Anticonvulsants** | | | |
| Carbamazepine | 5-12 µg/mL | >15 µg/mL | Tegretol |
| Ethosuximide | 40-100 µg/mL | >150 µg/mL | Zarontin |
| Phenobarbital | 15-40 µg/mL | 40-100 ng/mL (varies widely) | Luminal |
| Phenytoin | 10-20 µg/mL | >20 µg/mL | Dilantin |
| Primidone | 5-12 µg/mL | >15 µg/mL | Mysoline |
| Valproic acid | 50-100 µg/mL | >100 µg/mL | Depakene |
| **Antineoplastics and immunosuppressives** | | | |
| Cyclosporine | 50-400 ng/mL | >400 ng/mL | Sandimmune |
| Methotrexate, high dose, 48-h | Variable | >1 µmol/L 48 h after dose | |
| Tacrolimus (FK-506), whole blood | 3-10 µg/L | >15 µg/L | Prograf |
| **Bronchodilators and respiratory stimulants** | | | |
| Caffeine | 3-15 ng/mL | >30 ng/mL | |
| Theophylline (aminophylline) | 10-20 µg/mL | >20 µg/mL | Elixophyllin<br>Quibron |
| **Cardiovascular drugs** | | | |
| Amiodarone<br>  (obtain specimen more than 8 h after last dose) | 1.0-2.0 µg/mL | >2.0 µg/mL | Cordarone |
| Digitoxin<br>  (obtain specimen 12-24 h after last dose) | 15-25 ng/mL | >35 ng/mL | Crystodigin |
| Digoxin<br>  (obtain specimen more than 6 h after last dose) | 0.8-2.0 ng/mL | >2.4 ng/mL | Lanoxin |
| Disopyramide | 2-5 µg/mL | >7 µg/mL | Norpace |
| Flecainide | 0.2-1.0 ng/mL | >1 ng/mL | Tambocor |
| Lidocaine | 1.5-5.0 µg/mL | >6 µg/mL | Xylocaine |
| Mexiletine | 0.7-2.0 ng/mL | >2 ng/mL | Mexitil |
| Procainamide | 4-10 µg/mL | >12 µg/mL | Pronestyl |
| Procainamide plus N-acetyl-p-aminophenol<br>  (NAPA) | 8-30 µg/mL | >30 µg/mL | |

*Continued*

## Reference intervals for therapeutic drug monitoring (serum)—cont'd

| Analyte | Therapeutic range | Toxic concentrations | Proprietary name(s) |
|---|---|---|---|
| **Cardiovascular drugs—cont'd** | | | |
| Propranolol | 50-100 ng/mL | Variable | Inderal |
| Quinidine | 2-5 $\mu$g/mL | >6 $\mu$g/mL | Cardioquin |
| | | | Quinaglute |
| Tocainide | 4-10 ng/mL | >10 ng/mL | Tonocard |
| **Psychopharmacologic drugs** | | | |
| Amitriptyline | 120-150 ng/mL | >500 ng/mL | Elavil |
| | | | Triavil |
| Bupropion | 25-100 ng/mL | Not applicable | Wellbutrin |
| Desipramine | 150-300 ng/mL | >500 ng/mL | Norpramin |
| Imipramine | 125-250 ng/mL | >400 ng/mL | Tofranil |
| Lithium | 0.6-1.5 mEq/L | >1.5 mEq/L | Lithobid |
| (obtain specimen 12 h after last dose) | | | |
| Nortriptyline | 50-150 ng/mL | >500 ng/mL | Aventyl |
| | | | Pamelor |

## Reference intervals* for clinical chemistry (urine)

| Analyte | Conventional units | SI units |
|---|---|---|
| Acetone and acetoacetate, qualitative | Negative | Negative |
| Albumin | | |
|    Qualitative | Negative | Negative |
|    Quantitative | 10-100 mg/24 h | 0.15-1.5 $\mu$mol/d |
| Aldosterone | 3-20 $\mu$g/24 h | 8.3-55 nmol/d |
| $\delta$-Aminolevulinic acid ($\delta$-ALA) | 1.3-7.0 mg/24 h | 10-53 $\mu$mol/d |
| Amylase | <17 U/h | <17 U/h |
| Amylase/creatinine clearance ratio | 0.01-0.04 | 0.01-0.04 |
| Bilirubin, qualitative | Negative | Negative |
| Calcium (regular diet) | <250 mg/24 h | <6.3 nmol/d |
| Catecholamines | | |
|    Epinephrine | <10 $\mu$g/24 h | <55 nmol/d |
|    Norepinephrine | <100 $\mu$g/24 h | <590 nmol/d |
|    Total free catecholamines | 4-126 $\mu$g/24 h | 24-745 nmol/d |
|    Total metanephrines | 0.1-1.6 mg/24 h | 0.5-8.1 $\mu$mol/d |
| Chloride (varies with intake) | 110-250 mEq/24 h | 110-250 mmol/d |
| Copper | 0-50 $\mu$g/24 h | 0.0-0.80 $\mu$mol/d |
| Cortisol, free | 10-100 $\mu$g/24 h | 27.6-276 nmol/d |
| Creatine | | |
|    Males | 0-40 mg/24 h | 0.0-0.30 mmol/d |
|    Females | 0-80 mg/24 h | 0.0-0.60 mmol/d |
| Creatinine | 15-25 mg/kg/24 h | 0.13-0.22 mmol/kg/d |
| Creatinine clearance (endogenous) | | |
|    Males | 110-150 mL/min/1.73 m$^2$ | 110-150 mL/min/1.73 m$^2$ |
|    Females | 105-132 mL/min/1.73 m$^2$ | 105-132 mL/min/1.73 m$^2$ |
| Cystine or cysteine | Negative | Negative |
| Dehydroepiandrosterone | | |
|    Males | 0.2-2.0 mg/24 h | 0.7-6.9 $\mu$mol/d |
|    Females | 0.2-1.8 mg/24 h | 0.7-6.2 $\mu$mol/d |
| Estrogens, total | | |
|    Males | 4-25 $\mu$g/24 h | 14-90 nmol/d |
|    Females | 5-100 $\mu$g/24 h | 18-360 nmol/d |
| Glucose (as reducing substance) | <250 mg/24 h | <250 mg/d |
| Hemoglobin and myoglobin, qualitative | Negative | Negative |
| Homogentisic acid, qualitative | Negative | Negative |
| 17-Ketogenic steroids | | |
|    Males | 5-23 mg/24 h | 17-80 $\mu$mol/d |
|    Females | 3-15 mg/24 h | 10-52 $\mu$mol/d |
| 17-Hydroxycorticosteroids | | |
|    Males | 3-9 mg/24 h | 8.3-25 $\mu$mol/d |
|    Females | 2-8 mg/24 h | 5.5-22 $\mu$mol/d |
| 5-Hydroxyindoleacetic acid | | |
|    Qualitative | Negative | Negative |
|    Quantitative | 2-6 mg/24 h | 10-31 $\mu$mol/d |

*Values may vary depending on the method used.

## Reference intervals for clinical chemistry (urine)—cont'd

| Analyte | Conventional units | SI units |
|---|---|---|
| 17-Ketosteroids | | |
|   Males | 8-22 mg/24 h | 28-76 μmol/d |
|   Females | 6-15 mg/24 h | 21-52 μmol/d |
| Magnesium | 6-10 mEq/24 h | 3-5 mmol/d |
| Metanephrines | 0.05-1.2 ng/mg creatinine | 0.03-0.70 mmol/mmol creatinine |
| Osmolality | 38-1400 mOsm/kg water | 38-1400 mOsm/kg water |
| pH | 4.6-8.0 | 4.6-8.0 |
| Phenylpyruvic acid, qualitative | Negative | Negative |
| Phosphate | 0.4-1.3 g/24 h | 13-42 mmol/d |
| Porphobilinogen | | |
|   Qualitative | Negative | Negative |
|   Quantitative | <2 mg/24 h | <9 μmol/d |
| Porphyrins | | |
|   Coproporphyrin | 50-250 μg/24 h | 77-380 nmol/d |
|   Uroporphyrin | 10-30 μg/24 h | 12-36 nmol/d |
| Potassium | 25-125 mEq/24 h | 25-125 mmol/d |
| Pregnanediol | | |
|   Males | 0.0-1.9 mg/24 h | 0.0-6.0 μmol/d |
|   Females | | |
|     Proliferative phase | 0.0-2.6 mg/24 h | 0.0-8.0 μmol/d |
|     Luteal phase | 2.6-10.6 mg/24 h | 8-33 μmol/d |
|     Postmenopausal | 0.2-1.0 mg/24 h | 0.6-3.1 μmol/d |
| Pregnanetriol | 0.0-2.5 mg/24 h | 0.0-7.4 μmol/d |
| Protein, total | | |
|   Qualitative | Negative | Negative |
|   Quantitative | 10-150 mg/24 h | 10-150 mg/d |
|   Protein/creatinine ratio | <0.2 | <0.2 |
| Sodium (regular diet) | 60-260 mEq/24 h | 60-260 mmol/d |
| Specific gravity | | |
|   Random specimen | 1.003-1.030 | 1.003-1.030 |
|   24-hour collection | 1.015-1.025 | 1.015-1.025 |
| Urate (regular diet) | 250-750 mg/24 h | 1.5-4.4 mmol/d |
| Urobilinogen | 0.5-4.0 mg/24 h | 0.6-6.8 μmol/d |
| Vanillylmandelic acid (VMA) | 1.0-8.0 mg/24 h | 5-40 μmol/d |

## Reference intervals for toxic substances

| Analyte | Conventional units | SI units |
|---|---|---|
| Arsenic, urine | <130 μg/24 h | <1.7 μmol/d |
| Bromides, serum, inorganic | <100 mg/dL | <10 mmol/L |
|   Toxic symptoms | 140-1000 mg/dL | 14-100 mmol/L |
| Carboxyhemoglobin, blood: | Saturation | |
|   Urban environment | <5% | <0.05 |
|   Smokers | <12% | <0.12 |
|   Symptoms | | |
|     Headache | >15% | >0.15 |
|     Nausea and vomiting | >25% | >0.25 |
|     Potentially lethal | >50% | >0.50 |
| Ethanol, blood | <0.05 mg/dL | <1.0 mmol/L |
| | <0.005% | |
|   Intoxication | >100 mg/dL | >22 mmol/L |
| | >0.1% | |
|   Marked intoxication | 300-400 mg/dL | 65-87 mmol/L |
| | 0.3%-0.4% | |
| Alcoholic stupor | 400-500 mg/dL | 87-109 mmol/L |
| | 0.4%-0.5% | |
| Coma | >500 mg/dL | |
| | >0.5% | >109 mmol/L |
| Lead, blood | | |
|   Adults | <25 μg/dL | <1.2 μmol/L |
|   Children | <15 μg/dL | <0.7 μmol/L |
| Lead, urine | <80 μg/24 h | <0.4 μmol/d |
| Mercury, urine | <30 μg/24 h | <150 nmol/d |

## Reference intervals for tests performed on cerebrospinal fluid (CSF)

| Test | Conventional units | SI units |
|------|--------------------|----------|
| Cells | <5/mm$^3$, all mononuclear | <5 × 10$^6$ L, all mononuclear |
| Protein electrophoresis | Albumin predominant | Albumin predominant |
| Glucose | 50-75 mg/dL (20 mg/dL less than in serum) | 2.8-4.2 mmol/L (1.1 mmol less than in serum) |
| IgG | | |
|   Children under 14 | <8% of total protein | <0.08 of total protein |
|   Adults | <14% of total protein | <0.14 of total protein |
| IgG index* $\left(\dfrac{\text{CSF/serum IgG ratio}}{\text{CSF/serum albumin ratio}}\right)$ | 0.3-0.6 | 0.3-0.6 |
| Oligoclonal banding on electrophoresis | Absent | Absent |
| Pressure, opening | 70-180 mm H$_2$O | 70-180 mm H$_2$O |
| Protein, total | 15-45 mg/dL | 150-450 mg/L |

## Reference intervals for tests of gastrointestinal function

| Test | Conventional units |
|------|--------------------|
| Bentiromide test | 6-h urinary arylamine excretion greater than 57% excludes pancreatic insufficiency |
| Beta-carotene, serum | 60-260 ng/dL |
| Fecal fat estimation | |
|   Qualitative | No fat globules seen by high-power microscope |
|   Quantitative | <6 g/24 h (>95% coefficient of fat absorption) |
| Gastric acid output | |
|   Basal | |
|     Males | 0.0-10.5 mmol/h |
|     Females | 0.0-5.6 mmol/h |
|   Maximum (after histamine or pentagastrin) | |
|   Males | 9.0-48.0 mmol/h |
|   Females | 6.0-31.0 mmol/h |
| Ratio: basal maximum | |
|   Males | 0.0-0.31 |
|   Females | 0.0-0.29 |
| Secretin test, pancreatic fluid | |
|   Volume | >1.8 mL/kg/h |
|   Bicarbonate | >80 mEq/L |
| D-Xylose absorption test, urine | >20% of ingested dose excreted in 5 h |

## Reference intervals for tests of immunologic function

| Test | Conventional units | SI units |
|------|--------------------|----------|
| **Complement, serum** | | |
|   C3 | 85-175 mg/dL | 0.85-1.75 gm/L |
|   C4 | 15-45 mg/dL | 150-450 mg/L |
|   Total hemolytic (CH$_{50}$) | 150-250 U/mL | 150-250 U/mL |
| **Immunoglobulins, serum, adult** | | |
|   IgG | 640-1350 mg/dL | 6.4-13.5 g/L |
|   IgA | 70-310 mg/dL | 0.70-3.1 g/L |
|   IgM | 90-350 mg/dL | 0.90-3.5 g/L |
|   IgD | 0.0-6.0 mg/dL | 0.0-60 mg/L |
|   IgE | 0.0-430 ng/dL | 0.0-430 $\mu$g/L |

## Lymphocyte Subsets, Whole Blood, Heparinized

| (Antigen(s) expressed) | Cell type | Percentage | Absolute cell count |
|---|---|---|---|
| CD3 | Total T cells | 56%-77% | 860-1880 |
| CD19 | Total B cells | 7%-17% | 140-370 |
| CD3 and CD4 | Helper-induced cells | 32%-54% | 550-1190 |
| CD3 and CD8 | Suppressor-cytotoxic cells | 24%-37% | 430-1060 |
| CD3 and DR | Activated T cells | 5%-14% | 70-310 |
| CD2 | E rosette T cells | 73%-87% | 1040-2160 |
| CD16 and CD56 | Natural killer (NK) cells | 8%-22% | 130-500 |
| Helper/suppressor ratio: 0.8-1.8 | | | |

## Reference values for semen analysis

| Test | Conventional units | SI units |
|---|---|---|
| Volume | 2-5 mL | 2-5 mL |
| Liquefaction | Complete in 15 min | Complete in 15 min |
| pH | 7.2-8.0 | 7.2-8.0 |
| Leukocytes | Occasional or absent | Occasional or absent |
| Spermatozoa | | |
|   Count | $60\text{-}150 \times 10^6$ mL | $60\text{-}150 \times 10^6$ mL |
|   Motility | >80% motile | >0.80 motile |
|   Morphology | 80%-90% normal forms | >0.80-0.90 normal forms |
| Fructose | >150 mg/dL | >8.33 mmol/L |

## 8-2   HERB-LABORATORY TEST INTERACTIONS

The table that follows lists known herb-laboratory test interactions. The reader should not assume that an herbal product not included here may not change given values. Research into herbal products is changing constantly, and new interactions are becoming known every day.

| Herb | Test affected | Results |
|---|---|---|
| Aloe | Serum potassium | ↓ test values with long-term aloe use |
| Angelica | Plasma partial thromboplastin time (PTT) | Possible ↑ PTT in clients taking warfarin concurrently |
| | Prothrombin time (PT) and plasma international normalized ratio (INR) | ↑ test values in clients taking warfarin concurrently |
| Astragalus | Semen specimen analysis | ↑ sperm motility in vitro |
| Cascara sagrada | Serum and 24-hour urine estrogens | ↑ or ↓ test values in serum and urine |
| Chaparral | Serum alanine aminotransferase (ALT, alanine transaminase, SGPT) | ↑ test values |
| | Serum aspartate aminotransferase (AST, aspartate transaminase, SGOT) | ↑ test values |
| | Serum bilirubin: total, direct (conjugated), and indirect (unconjugated) | Possible ↑ total bilirubin |
| | Urine bilirubin | + or ↑ test values |
| Chaste tree | Serum prolactin (human prolactin, HPRL) | ↓ test values |
| Chromium | Blood glucose | ↓ test values |
| Coffee | Diagnostic secretin stimulation for Zollinger-Ellison syndrome (secretion provocation test) | ↑ test values |
| | Serum 2-hour postprandial glucose | Falsely ↑ test values if caffeine is ingested during test |
| | Serum aspartate aminotransferase (AST, aspartate transaminase, SGOT) | ↓ test values in alcoholics |
| | Specimen infertility screen | Possible ↓ in number of motile spermatozoa with heavy coffee consumption |
| | Urine catecholamines | Falsely ↑ test values |
| Comfrey | Serum alanine aminotransferase (ALT, alanine transaminase, SGPT) | ↑ test values |
| | Serum aspartate aminotransferase (AST, aspartate transaminase, SGOT) | ↑ test values |
| | Serum bilirubin: total, direct (conjugated), and indirect (unconjugated) | Possible ↑ total bilirubin |
| | Urine bilirubin | + or ↑ bilirubin |
| Cranberry | Urine pH | ↓ pH |

*Continued*

| Herb | Test affected | Results |
|------|---------------|---------|
| Echinacea | Blood erythrocyte sedimentation rate (ESR, Zeta sedimentation) | Slightly ↑ ESR |
| | Blood gamma-glutamyltransferase | Possible hepatotoxicity if herb is taken for >8 weeks |
| | Peripheral blood differential leukocyte count (diff) | ↑ lymphocyte counts |
| | Serum alanine aminotransferase (ALT, alanine transaminase, SGPT) | ↑ test values |
| | Serum alkaline phosphatase | Possible hepatotoxicity if herb is taken for >8 weeks |
| | Serum alkaline phosphatase, heat stable | Possible hepatotoxicity if herb is taken for >8 weeks |
| | Serum aspartate aminotransferase (AST, aspartate transaminase, SGOT) | ↑ test values; possible hepatotoxicity if herb is taken for >8 weeks |
| | Serum immunoglobulin E (IgE) | ↑ test values |
| | Serum liver battery (profile) | Possible hepatotoxicity; risk ↑ when herb is taken with other hepatotoxic drugs |
| | Specimen semen analysis | High doses of herb interfere with sperm enzyme activity |
| Ephedra | Serum alanine aminotransferase (ALT, alanine transaminase, SGPT) | ↑ test values |
| | Serum aspartate aminotransferase (AST, aspartate transaminase, SGOT | ↑ test values |
| | Serum bilirubin: total, direct (conjugated), and indirect (unconjugated) | Possible ↑ total bilirubin |
| | Serum digoxin | Possible potentiation of cardiac glycoside effects |
| | Urine bilirubin | + or ↑ |
| Fenugreek | Blood cholesterol | ↓ total cholesterol |
| | Blood glucose | ↓ test values |
| Feverfew | Blood platelet aggregation; hypercoagulable state blood platelet aggregation | ↓ test values |
| | Duke's bleeding time | Possible inhibited platelet activity and ↑ bleeding |
| | Ivy's bleeding time | Possible inhibited platelet activity and ↑ bleeding |
| | Mielke's bleeding time | Possible inhibited platelet activity and ↑ bleeding |
| | Plasma partial thromboplastin time (PTT) | Possible ↑ PTT in clients taking warfarin concurrently |
| | Prothrombin time (PT) and plasma international normalized ratio (INR) | ↑ test values |
| Figwort | Blood glucose | ↓ test values |
| Garlic | Blood lipid profile | Possible ↓ test values |
| | Blood low-density lipoprotein (LDL) cholesterol | ↓ test values with aged garlic extract taken long-term |
| | Blood platelet aggregation; hypercoagulable state blood platelet aggregation | ↓ test values with aged garlic extract values with aged garlic extract taken long-term |
| | Blood triglycerides | ↓ test values with aged garlic extract taken long-term |
| | Diagnostic platelet adhesion test | ↓ test values with aged garlic extract taken long-term |
| | Duke's bleeding time | Possible inhibited platelet activity and ↑ bleeding |
| | Ivy's bleeding time | Possible inhibited platelet activity and ↑ bleeding |
| | Mielke's bleeding time | Possible inhibited platelet activity and ↑ bleeding |
| | Prothrombin time (PT) and plasma international normalized ratio (INR) | ↑ test values |
| | Serum immunoglobulin E (IgE) | ↑ test values |
| Ginger | Duke's bleeding time | Possible inhibited platelet activity and ↑ bleeding |
| | Ivy's bleeding time | Possible inhibited platelet activity and ↑ bleeding |
| | Mielke's bleeding time | Possible inhibited platelet activity and ↑ bleeding |
| | Plasma partial thromboplastin time (PTT) | Possible ↑ PTT in clients taking warfarin concurrently |
| | Prothrombin time (PT) and plasma international normalized ratio (INR) | ↑ test values |
| Ginkgo | Blood salicylate (aspirin, acetylsalicylic acid) | ↑ test values |
| | Diagnostic aspirin tolerance test (ASA tolerance test, bleeding time aspirin tolerance test) | Possible ↑ bleeding |
| | Duke's bleeding time | Possible inhibited platelet activity and ↑ bleeding |
| | Ivy's bleeding time | Possible inhibited platelet activity and ↑ bleeding |
| | Mielke's bleeding time | Possible inhibited platelet activity and ↑ bleeding |
| | Plasma partial thromboplastin time (PTT) | Possible ↑ PTT in clients taking warfarin concurrently |
| | Prothrombin time (PT) and plasma international normalized ratio (INR) | ↑ test values |

| Herb | Test affected | Results |
|------|--------------|---------|
| Ginseng | Blood glucose | ↑ test values |
| | Duke's bleeding time | Possible inhibited platelet activity and ↑ bleeding |
| | Ivy's bleeding time | Possible inhibited platelet activity and ↑ bleeding |
| | Mielke's bleeding time | Possible inhibited platelet activity and ↑ bleeding |
| | Plasma partial thromboplastin time (PTT) | Possible ↑ PTT in clients taking warfarin concurrently |
| | Prothrombin time (PT) and plasma international normalized ratio (INR) | ↑ test values |
| | Serum and 24-hour urine estrogens | Additive effects to estrogen |
| | Serum digoxin | Falsely ↑ results |
| Goldenseal | Calculated test (osmolar gap) blood osmolality | Possible ↑ osmolality |
| | Serum or urine plasma sodium | Relative ↑ in sodium values |
| | Serum osmolality | ↑ osmolality |
| Guar gum | Blood cholesterol | ↓ total cholesterol |
| | Blood glucose | ↓ test values |
| Gymnema | Blood cholesterol | ↓ total cholesterol |
| | Blood glucose | ↓ test values |
| Hawthorn | Serum digoxin | Falsely ↑ results |
| Lecithin | Blood lipid profile | ↓ cholesterol test values |
| Licorice | Blood anion gap | ↓ test values |
| | Qualitative urine myoglobin | Possible + test result |
| | Serum or urine plasma sodium | ↑ test values (hypernatremia) |
| | Serum myoglobin | Possible + test result |
| | Serum potassium | ↓ test values |
| | Serum prolactin (human prolactin, HPRL) | ↓ test values |
| Mayapple | Red blood cell (RBC) | ↓ test values |
| Mistletoe | Peripheral blood differential leukocyte count (diff) | ↑ lymphocyte counts |
| | Red blood cell (RBC) | ↓ test values |
| | Serum alanine aminotransferase (ALT, alanine transaminase, SGPT) | ↑ test values |
| | Serum aspartate aminotransferase (AST, aspartate transaminase, SGOT) | ↑ test values |
| | Serum bilirubin: total, direct (conjugated), and indirect (unconjugated) | Possible ↑ total bilirubin |
| | Urine bilirubin | + or ↑ test values |
| Mugwort | Serum bilirubin: total, direct (conjugated), and indirect (unconjugated) | Possible ↑ direct bilirubin |
| Pennyroyal | Red blood cell (RBC) | ↓ test values |
| | Serum alanine aminotransferase (ALT, alanine transaminase, SGPT) | ↑ test values |
| | Serum aspartate aminotransferase (AST, aspartate transaminase, SGOT) | ↑ test values |
| | Serum bilirubin: total, direct (conjugated), and indirect (unconjugated) | Possible ↑ total bilirubin |
| | Urine bilirubin | + or ↑ test values |
| Plantain | 24-hour urine quantitative 5-hydroxyindoleacetic acid (5-HIAA) | Falsely ↑ results if client ingests plantain within 5 days of test |
| | Serum digoxin | Falsely ↑ results |
| Poppy | Urine heroin | False + results if client ingested 5-15 g of poppy seeds 24 hours before sample was obtained |
| | Urine morphine | False + results possible with immunoassay method for up to 60 hours after ingestion of poppy seeds |
| Pycnogenol | Blood platelet aggregation; hypercoagulable state blood platelet aggregation | ↓ test values |
| Rauwolfia | Blood red blood cell (RBC) | ↓ test values |
| | Diagnostic basal nocturnal acid output gastric analysis | ↑ test values |
| | Serum gastrin | ↓ gastrin secretion in response to drug-stimulated increased gastric acidity |
| | Serum or urine plasma sodium | ↑ test values (hypernatremia) |
| Saw palmetto | Serum iron (Fe) | Possible ↓ test values |
| | Specimen semen analysis | Metabolic changes in sperm |
| Schisandra | Serum alanine aminotransferase (ALT, alanine transaminase, SGPT) | ↓ test values |
| | Serum aspartate aminotransferase (AST, aspartate transaminase, SGOT) | ↓ test values |
| Senna | 24-hour urine serum estriol | ↓ test values |
| Siberian ginseng | Serum androstenedione | ↑ test values |
| | Serum digoxin | Falsely ↑ results |

*Continued*

| Herb | Test affected | Results |
|---|---|---|
| Skullcap | Serum alanine aminotransferase (ALT, alanine transaminase, SGPT) | ↑ test values |
| | Serum aspartate aminotransferase (AST, aspartate transaminase, SGOT) | ↑ test values |
| | Serum bilirubin: total, direct (conjugated), and indirect (unconjugated) | Possible ↑ total bilirubin |
| | Urine bilirubin | + or ↑ |
| Soy | Blood high-density lipoprotein (HDL) cholesterol | ↓ LDL, triglycerides, and total cholesterol test values; ↑ HDL test values |
| | Blood lipid profile | Possible ↓ test values |
| | Blood low-density lipoprotein (LDL) cholesterol | ↓ test values |
| | Blood triglycerides | ↓ test values |
| Squill | Red blood cell (RBC) | ↓ test values |
| St. John's wort | Blood growth hormone (somatotropin, GH) | ↓ test values |
| | Blood theophylline (aminophylline) | ↓ test values |
| | Diagnostic Sims-Huhner test | ↓ sperm motility and viability |
| | Serum digoxin | ↓ digoxin peak and trough concentrations |
| | Serum iron (Fe) | Possible ↓ test values |
| | Serum prolactin (human prolactin, HPRL) | ↓ test values |
| | Specimen semen analysis | Mutagenic effects on sperm cells |
| Valerian | Serum alanine aminotransferase (ALT, alanine transaminase, SGPT) | ↑ test values |
| | Serum aspartate aminotransferase (AST, aspartate transaminase, SGOT) | ↑ test values |
| | Serum bilirubin: total, direct (conjugated), and indirect (unconjugated) | Possible ↑ total bilirubin |
| | Urine bilirubin | + or ↑ |

From Skidmore-Roth L: *Mosby's handbook of herbs and natural supplements,* ed 1, St Louis, 2001, Mosby.

## 8-3 Desirable weight for men and women of age 25 and over

| | | | Men (indoor clothing*) | | | | | |
|---|---|---|---|---|---|---|---|---|
| | | | Small frame | | Medium frame | | Large frame | |
| Feet | Inches | Cm | Pounds | Kilograms | Pounds | Kilograms | Pounds | Kilograms |
| 5 | 1 | 154.9 | 128-134 | 58.2-60.9 | 131-141 | 59.5-64.1 | 138-150 | 62.7-68.2 |
| 5 | 2 | 157.5 | 130-136 | 59.1-61.8 | 133-143 | 60.4-65.0 | 140-153 | 63.6-69.5 |
| 5 | 3 | 160.0 | 132-138 | 60.0-62.7 | 135-145 | 61.4-65.9 | 142-156 | 64.5-70.9 |
| 5 | 4 | 162.6 | 134-140 | 60.9-63.6 | 137-148 | 62.3-67.2 | 144-160 | 65.5-72.7 |
| 5 | 5 | 165.1 | 136-142 | 61.8-64.5 | 139-151 | 63.2-68.6 | 146-164 | 66.4-74.5 |
| 5 | 6 | 167.6 | 138-145 | 62.7-65.9 | 142-154 | 64.5-70.0 | 149-168 | 67.7-76.4 |
| 5 | 7 | 170.2 | 140-148 | 63.6-67.2 | 145-157 | 65.9-71.4 | 152-172 | 69.1-78.2 |
| 5 | 8 | 172.7 | 142-151 | 64.5-68.6 | 148-160 | 67.2-72.7 | 155-176 | 70.5-80.0 |
| 5 | 9 | 175.3 | 144-154 | 65.5-70.0 | 151-153 | 68.6-74.1 | 158-180 | 71.8-81.8 |
| 5 | 10 | 177.8 | 146-157 | 66.4-71.4 | 154-166 | 70.0-75.5 | 161-184 | 73.2-83.6 |
| 5 | 11 | 180.3 | 149-160 | 67.7-72.7 | 157-170 | 71.4-77.3 | 164-188 | 74.5-85.5 |
| 6 | 0 | 182.9 | 152-164 | 69.1-74.5 | 160-174 | 72.7-79.1 | 168-192 | 76.4-87.3 |
| 6 | 1 | 185.4 | 155-168 | 70.5-76.4 | 164-178 | 74.5-80.9 | 172-197 | 78.2-89.5 |
| 6 | 2 | 188.0 | 158-172 | 71.8-78.2 | 167-182 | 75.9-82.7 | 176-202 | 80.0-91.8 |
| 6 | 3 | 190.5 | 162-176 | 73.6-80.0 | 171-187 | 77.7-85.0 | 181-207 | 82.3-94.1 |

*Allow 5 pounds.

The weights presented are those associated with the lowest mortality. They are not necessarily the weights at which people are healthiest, perform their jobs optimally, or even look their best. Three weight ranges were determined for each sex on each size and attributed to a small, medium, or large frame. These tables correct the 1983 Metropolitan tables to height without shoe heels.

From Thompson JM: *Clinical outlines for health assessment,* St Louis, 1997, Mosby.

| | | | Women (indoor clothing*) | | | | | |
| | | | Small frame | | Medium frame | | Large frame | |
| Feet | Inches | Cm | Pounds | Kilograms | Pounds | Kilograms | Pounds | Kilograms |
|---|---|---|---|---|---|---|---|---|
| 4 | 9 | 144.8 | 102-111 | 46.4-50.0 | 109-121 | 49.5-55.0 | 118-131 | 53.6-59.5 |
| 4 | 10 | 147.3 | 103-113 | 46.8-51.4 | 111-123 | 50.0-55.9 | 120-134 | 54.5-60.9 |
| 4 | 11 | 149.9 | 104-115 | 47.3-52.3 | 113-126 | 51.4-57.2 | 122-137 | 55.5-62.3 |
| 5 | 0 | 152.4 | 106-118 | 48.2-53.6 | 115-129 | 52.3-58.6 | 125-140 | 56.8-63.6 |
| 5 | 1 | 154.9 | 108-121 | 49.1-55.0 | 118-132 | 53.6-60.0 | 128-143 | 58.2-65.0 |
| 5 | 2 | 157.5 | 111-124 | 50.5-56.4 | 121-135 | 55.0-61.4 | 131-147 | 59.5-66.8 |
| 5 | 3 | 160.0 | 114-127 | 51.8-57.7 | 124-138 | 56.4-62.7 | 134-151 | 60.9-68.6 |
| 5 | 4 | 162.6 | 117-130 | 53.2-59.0 | 127-141 | 57.7-64.1 | 137-155 | 62.3-70.5 |
| 5 | 5 | 165.1 | 120-133 | 54.5-60.5 | 130-144 | 59.0-65.5 | 140-159 | 63.6-72.3 |
| 5 | 6 | 167.6 | 123-136 | 55.9-61.8 | 133-147 | 60.5-66.8 | 143-163 | 65.0-74.1 |
| 5 | 7 | 170.2 | 126-139 | 57.3-63.2 | 136-150 | 61.8-68.2 | 146-167 | 66.4-75.9 |
| 5 | 8 | 172.7 | 129-142 | 58.6-64.5 | 139-153 | 63.2-69.5 | 149-170 | 67.7-77.3 |
| 5 | 9 | 175.3 | 132-145 | 60.0-65.9 | 142-156 | 64.6-70.9 | 152-173 | 69.1-78.6 |
| 5 | 10 | 177.8 | 135-148 | 61.4-67.3 | 145-159 | 65.9-72.3 | 155-176 | 70.5-80.0 |
| 5 | 11 | 180.3 | 138-151 | 62.7-73.6 | 148-162 | 67.3-73.6 | 158-179 | 71.8-81.4 |

*Allow 3 pounds.

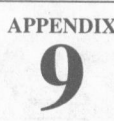

**APPENDIX 9**

# HEALTH PROMOTION

## 9-1 | Child preventive care timeline

### Clinical preventive services for normal-risk children

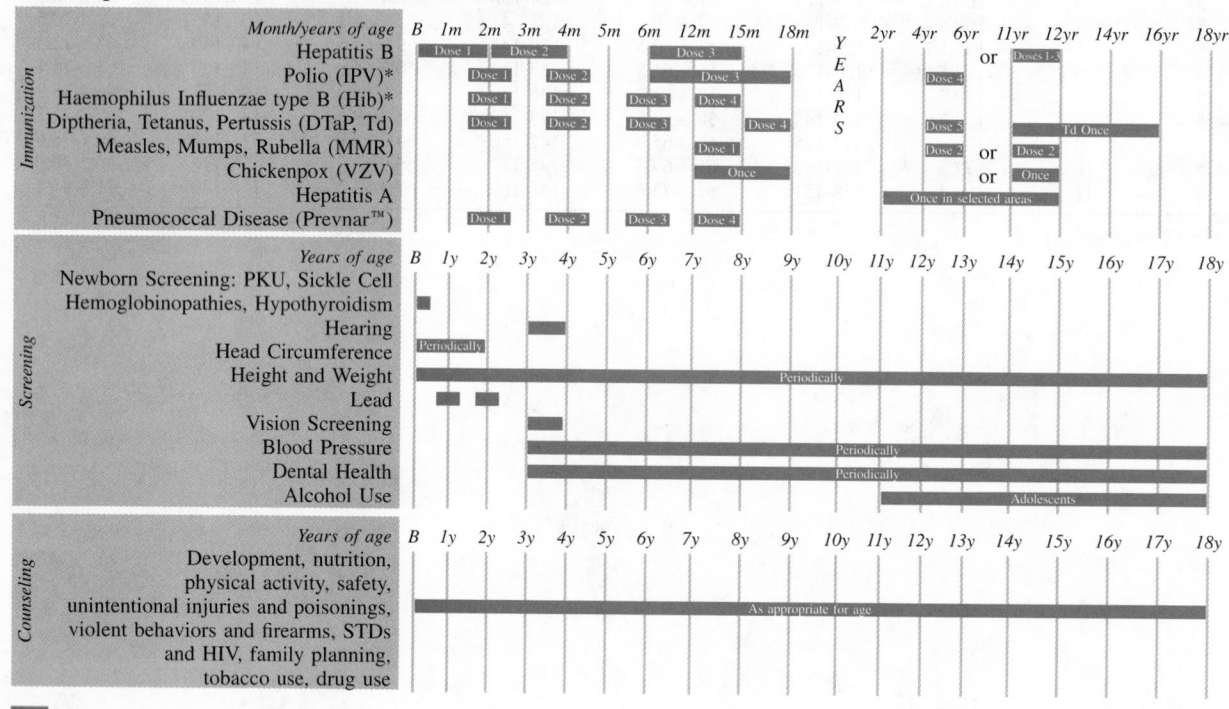

Recommended by most U.S. authorities

*Schedules may vary according to vaccine type.

From U.S. Department of Health and Human Services Public Health Service, 1998. The information on immunizations is based on recommendations issued by the Advisory Committee on Immunization Practices, the American Academy of Pediatrics, and the American Academy of Family Physicians.

# Recommended childhood immunization schedule, United States, January–December 2001*

| Age ▶<br>Vaccine ▼ | Birth | 1 mo | 2 mo | 4 mo | 6 mo | 12 mo | 15 mo | 18 mo | 24 mo | 4-6 yr | 11-12 yr | 14-18 yr |
|---|---|---|---|---|---|---|---|---|---|---|---|---|
| Hepatitis B[2] | | Hep B #1 | | | | | | | | | Hep B[2] | |
| | | | Hep B #2 | | | Hep B #3 | | | | | | |
| Diphtheria, tetanus, pertussis[3] | | | DTap | DTap | DTap | | DTaP[3] | | | DTap | Td | |
| H. influenzae type b[4] | | | Hib | Hib | Hib | Hib | | | | | | |
| Inactivated polio[5] | | | IPV | IPV | | IPV[5] | | | | IPV[5] | | |
| Pneumococcal conjugate[6] | | | PCV | PCV | PCV | PCV | | | | | | |
| Measles, mumps, rubella[7] | | | | | | MMR | | | | MMR[7] | MMR[7] | |
| Varicella[8] | | | | | | Var | | | | | Var[8] | |
| Hepatitis A[9] | | | | | | | | | Hep A—in selected areas[9] | | | |

Approved by the Advisory Committee on Immunization Practices (ACIP), the American Academy of Pediatrics (AAP), and the American Academy of Family Physicians (AAFP).

*Vaccines[1] are listed under routinely recommended ages. ⬚ Bars indicate range of recommended ages for immunization. Any dose not given at the recommended age should be given as a "catch-up" immunization at any subsequent visit when indicated and feasible. ⬭ Ovals indicate vaccines to be given if previously recommended doses were missed or given earlier than the recommended minimum age.

1. This schedule indicates the recommended ages for routine administration of currently licensed childhood vaccines, as of 11/1/00, for children through 18 years of age. Additional vaccines may be licensed and recommended during the year. Licensed combination vaccines may be used whenever any components of the combination are indicated and its other components are not contraindicated. Providers should consult the manufacturers' package inserts for detailed recommendations.
2. *Infants born to HBsAg-negative mothers* should receive the 1st dose of hepatitis B (Hep B) vaccine by age 2 months. The 2nd dose should be at least one month after the 1st dose. The 3rd dose should be administered at least 4 months after the 1st dose and at least 2 months after the 2nd dose, but not before 6 months of age for infants.
*Infants born to HBsAg-positive mothers* should receive hepatitis B vaccine and 0.5 mL hepatitis B immune globulin (HBIG) within 12 hours of birth at separate sites. The 2nd dose is recommended at 1-2 months of age and the 3rd dose at 6 months of age.
*Infants born to mothers whose HBsAg status is unknown* should receive hepatitis B vaccine within 12 hours of birth. Maternal blood should be drawn at the time of delivery to determine the mother's HBsAg status; if the HBsAg test is positive, the infant should receive HBIG as soon as possible (no later than 1 week of age).
*All children and adolescents* who have not been immunized against hepatitis B should begin the series during any visit. Special efforts should be made to immunize children who were born in or whose parents were born in areas of the world with moderate or high endemicity of hepatitis B virus infection.
3. The 4th dose of DTaP (diptheria and tetanus toxoids and acellular pertussis vaccine) may be administered as early as 12 months of age, provided 6 months have elapsed since the 3rd dose and the child is unlikely to return at age 15-18 months. Td (tetanus and diptheria toxoids) is recommended at 11-12 years of age if at least 5 years have elapsed since the last dose of DTP, DTaP or DT. Subsequent routing Td boosters are recommended every 10 years.
4. Three *Haemophilus influenzae* type b (Hib) conjugate vaccines are licensed for infant use. If PRP-OMP (PedvaxHIB® or ComVax® [Merck]) is administered at 2 and 4 months of age, a dose at 6 months is not required. Because clinical studies in infants have demonstrated that using some combination products may induce a lower immune response to the Hib vaccine component, DTaP/Hib combination products should not be used for primary immunization in infants at 2, 4 or 6 months of age, unless FDA-approved for these ages.
5. An all-IPV schedule is recommended for routine childhood polio vaccination in the United States. All children should receive four doses of IPV at 2 months, 4 months, 6-18 months, and 4-6 years of age. Oral polio vaccine (OPV) should be used only in selected circumstances. (See *MMWR* May 19, 2000/49(RR-5);1-22).
6. The heptavalent conjugate pneumococcal vaccine (PCV) is recommended for all children 2-23 months of age. It also is recommended for certain children 24-59 months of age. (See *MMWR* Oct. 6, 2000/49(RR-9);1-35).
7. The 2nd dose of measles, mumps, and rubella (MMR) vaccine is recommended routinely at 4-6 years of age but may be administered during any visit, provided at least 4 weeks have elapsed since receipt of the 1st dose and that both doses are administered beginning at or after 12 months of age. Those who have not previously received the second dose should complete the schedule by the 11-12 year old visit.
8. Varicella (Var) vaccine is recommended at any visit on or after the first birthday for susceptible children, i.e. those who lack a reliable history of chickenpox (as judged by a health care provider) and who have not been immunized. Susceptible persons 13 years of age or older should receive 2 doses, given at least 4 weeks apart.
9. Hepatitis A (Hep A) is shaded to indicate its recommended use in selected states and/or regions, and for certain high risk groups; consult your local public health authority. (See *MMWR* Oct. 1, 1999/48(RR-12);1-37).
**For additional information about the vaccines listed above, please visit the National Immunization Program Home Page at http://www.cdc.gov/nip/ or call the National Immunization Hotline at 800-232-2522 (English) or 800-232-0233 (Spanish).**

## Recommended immunization schedule for children not immunized in the first year of life in the United States

| Recommended time/age | Immunization(s)*† | Comments |
|---|---|---|
| **Younger than 7 years** | | |
| First visit | DTP, Hib, HBV,‡ MMR, OPV, VZV | If indicated, tuberculin testing may be done at same visit |
| | | If child is 5 years of age or older, Hib is not indicated |
| Interval after first visit: | | |
| 1 month | DTP, HBV | OPV may be given if accelerated poliomyelitis vaccination is necessary, such as for travelers to areas where polio is endemic |
| 2 months | DTP, Hib,‡ OPV | Second dose of Hib is indicated only in children whose first dose was received when younger than 15 months |
| ≥8 months | DTP or DTaP,§ HBV, OPV | OPV is not given if the third dose was given earlier |
| 4-6 years (at or before school entry) | DTP or DTaP,§ OPV | DTP or DTaP is not necessary if the fourth dose was given after the fourth birthday; OPV is not necessary if the third dose was given after the fourth birthday |
| 11-12 years | MMR | At entry to middle school or junior high school |
| 10 years later | Td | Repeat every 10 years throughout life |
| **7 years and older‖·**** | | |
| First visit | HBV,†† OPV, MMR, Td, VSV | After the 13th birthday, 2 doses of VZV are required 4 to 8 weeks apart |
| Interval after first visit: | | |
| 2 months | HBV,†† OPV, Td | OPV may also be given 1 month after the first visit if accelerated poliomyelitis vaccination is necessary |
| 8-14 months | HBV,†† OPV, Td | OPV is not given if the third dose was given earlier |
| 11-12 years | MMR | At entry to middle school or junior high |
| 10 years later | Td | Repeat every 10 years throughout life |

*If all needed vaccines cannot be administered simultaneously, priority should be given to protecting the child against those diseases that pose the greatest immediate risk. In the United States these diseases for children younger than 2 years usually are measles and *Haemophilus influenzae* type b infection; for children older than 7 years, they are measles, mumps, and rubella (MMR).

†DTP or DTaP, HBV, Hib, MMR, VZV, and OPV can be given simultaneously at separate sites if failure of the patient to return for future immunizations is a concern.

‡Any licensed Hib conjugate vaccine may be used.

§DTaP is not currently licensed for use in children younger than 15 months of age and is not recommended for primary immunization (i.e., first 3 doses) at any age.

‖If person is 18 years or older, routine poliovirus vaccination is not indicated in the United States.

**Minimal interval between doses of MMR is 1 month.

††Priority should be given to hepatitis B immunization of adolescents.

From American Academy of Pediatrics: *Report of the Committee on Infectious Diseases,* ed 23, Elk Grove Village, IL, 1994, The Academy. American Academy of Pediatrics, Committee on Infectious Diseases: Recommendations for the use of live attenuated varicella vaccine, *Pediatrics* 95(5):791-796, 1995.

# 9-2 | Adult preventive care time line

## Clinical preventive services for normal-risk adults

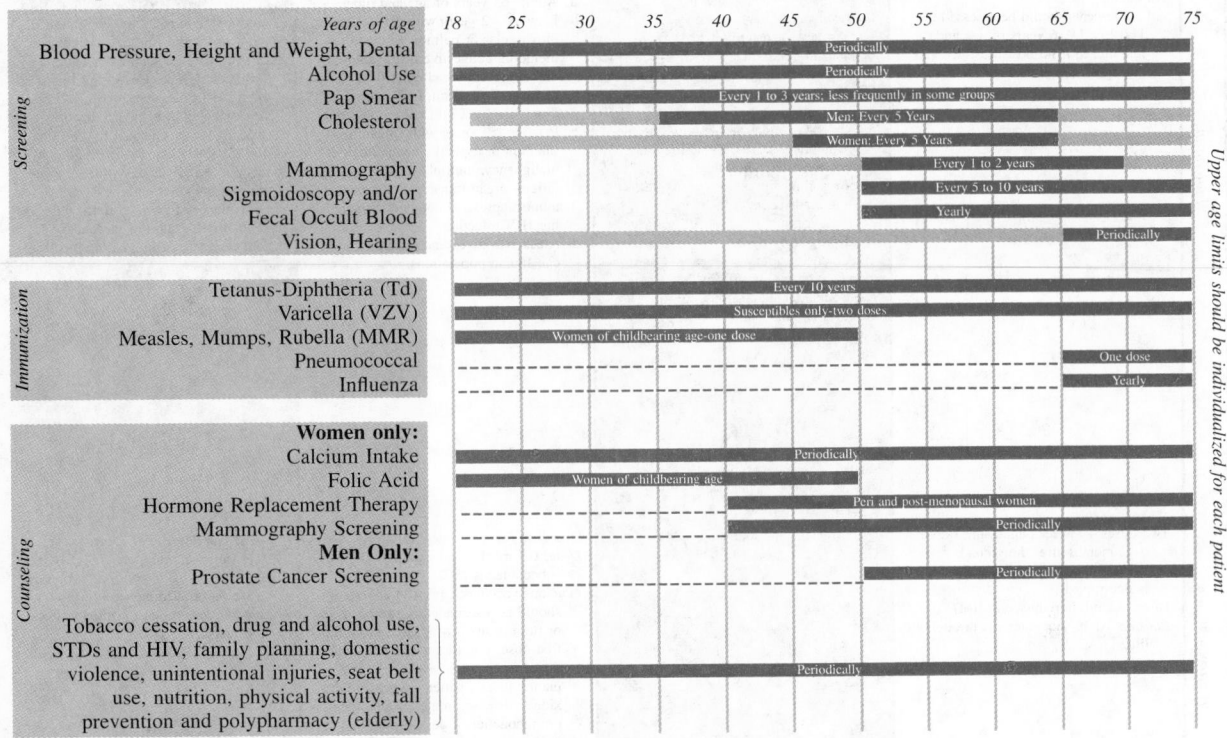

U.S. Department of Health and Human Services, Public Health Service, 1997.

■ Recommended by most U.S. authorities
■ Recommended by most U.S. authorities

# Summary of adolescent/adult immunization recommendations

| Agent | Tetanus & Diphtheria toxoids combined (Td) | Influenza vaccine | Pneumoccal polysaccharide vaccine (PPV) | Measles and mumps vaccines |
|---|---|---|---|---|
| **Indications** | All adults<br>All adolescents should be assessed at 11-12 or 14-16 years of age and immunized if no dose was received during the previous 5 years. | a. Adults 50 years of age and older.<br>b. Residents of nursing homes or other facilities for patients with chronic medical conditions.<br>c. Persons ≥6 mo. of age with chronic cardiovascular or pulmonary disorders, including asthma.<br>d. Persons ≥6 mo. of age with chronic metabolic diseases (including diabetes), renal dysfunction, hemoglobinopathies, immunosuppressive or immunodeficiency disorders.<br>e. Women in their 2nd or 3rd trimester of pregnancy during influenza season.<br>f. Persons 6 months-18 years of age receiving long-term aspirin therapy.<br>g. Groups, including household members and care givers, who can infect high risk persons. | a. Adults 65 years of age and older.<br>b. Persons ≥2 years with chronic cardiovascular or pulmonary disorders including congestive heart failure, diabetes mellitus, chronic liver disease, alcoholism, CSF leaks, cardiomyopathy, COPD or emphysema.<br>c. Persons ≥2 years with splenic dysfunction or asplenia, hematologic malignancy, multiple myeloma, renal failure, organ transplantation or immunosuppressive conditions, including HIV infection.<br>d. Alaskan Natives and certain American Indian populations. | a. Adults born after 1956 without written documentation of immunization on or after the first birthday.<br>b. Health care personnel born after 1956 who are at risk of exposure to patients with measles should have documentation of two doses of vaccine on or after the first birthday or of measles seropositivity.<br>c. HIV-infected persons without severe immunosuppression.<br>d. Travelers to foreign countries.<br>e. Persons entering post-secondary educational institutions (e.g., college). |
| **Primary schedule** | Two doses 4-8 weeks apart, third dose 6-12 months after the second.<br>No need to repeat doses if the schedule is interrupted.<br>*Dose:* 0.5 mL intramuscular (IM)<br>*Booster:* At 10-year intervals throughout life. | *Dose:* 0.5 mL intramuscular (IM)<br>Given annually, each fall. | One dose for most people*<br>*Dose:* 0.5 mL intramuscular (IM) or subcutaneous (SC)<br>*Persons vaccinated prior to age 65 should be vaccinated at age 65 if 5 or more years have passed since the first dose. For all persons with functional or anatomic asplenia, transplant patients, patients with chronic kidney disease, immunosuppressed or immunodeficient persons, and others at highest risk of fatal infection, a second dose should be given—at least 5 years after first dose. | At least one dose. (Two doses of *measles-containing vaccine* if in college, in health care profession or traveling to a foreign country with second dose at least 1 month after the first.)<br>*Dose:* 0.5 mL subcutaneous (SC) |
| **Contraindications** | Neurologic or severe hypersensitivity reaction to prior dose. | Anaphylactic allergy to eggs.<br>Acute febrile illness. | The safety of PPV during the first trimester of pregnancy has not been evaluated. The manufacturer's package insert should be reviewed for additional information. | a. Immunosuppressive therapy or immunodeficiency including HIV-infected persons with severe immunosuppression.<br>b. Anaphylactic allergy to neomycin.<br>c. Pregnancy.<br>d. Immune globulin preparation or blood/blood product received in preceding 3-11 months. |
| **Comments** | *Wound management:*<br>Patients with three or more previous tetanus toxoid doses:<br>a. give Td for clean, minor wounds only if more than 10 years since last dose;<br>b. for other wounds, give Td if over 5 years since last dose. Patients with less than 3 or unknown numbers of prior tetanus toxoid doses, give Td for clean, minor wounds and Td and TIG (Tetanus Immune Globulin) for other wounds. | Depending on season and destination, persons traveling to foreign countries should consider vaccination.<br>Any person ≥6 mo. of age who wishes to reduce the likelihood of becoming ill with influenza should be vaccinated.<br>Avoiding subsequent vaccination of persons known to have developed GBS within 6 weeks of a previous vaccination seems prudent; however, for most persons with a GBS history who are at high risk for severe complications, many experts believe the established benefits of vaccination justify yearly vaccination. | If elective splenectomy or immunosuppressive therapy is planned, give vaccine 2 weeks ahead, if possible.<br>When indicated, vaccine should be administered to patients with unknown vaccination status. All residents of nursing homes and other long-term care facilities should have their vaccination status assessed and documented. | Women should be asked if they are pregnant before receiving vaccine, and advised to avoid pregnancy for *30 days* after immunization. |

Adapted from the recommendations of the Advisory Committee on Immunization Practices (ACIP). Foreign travel and less commonly used vaccines such as typhoid, rabies, and meningococcal are not included, CDC, 1998.

| Rubella vaccine | Hepatitis B vaccine | Poliovirus vaccine: IPV—inactivated OPV—oral (Live) | Varicella vaccine | Hepatitis A vaccine |
|---|---|---|---|---|
| a. Persons (especially women) without written documentation of immunization on or after the first birthday or of seropositivity.<br>b. Health care personnel who are at risk of exposure to patients with rubella and who may have contact with pregnant patients should have at least one dose. | a. Persons with occupational risk of exposure to blood or blood-contaminated body fluids.<br>b. Clients and staff of institutions for the developmentally disabled.<br>c. Hemodialysis patients.<br>d. Recipients of clotting-factor concentrates.<br>e. Household contacts and sex partners of those chronically infected with HBV.<br>f. *Family members of adoptees from countries where HBV infection is endemic, if adoptees are HBsAg+.*<br>g. Certain international travelers.<br>h. Injecting drug users.<br>i. Men who have sex with men.<br>j. Heterosexual men and women with multiple sex partners or recent episode of a sexually transmitted disease.<br>k. Inmates of long-term correctional facilities.<br>l. All unvaccinated adolescents. | Routine vaccination of those ≥18 years of age residing in the U.S. is not necessary. Vaccination is recommended for the following high-risk adults:<br>a. Travelers to areas or countries where poliomyelitis is epidemic or endemic.<br>b. Members of communities or specific population groups with disease caused by wild polioviruses.<br>c. Laboratory workers who handle specimens that may contain polio-viruses.<br>d. Health care workers who have close contact with patients who may be excreting wild polioviruses.<br>e. Unvaccinated adults whose children will be receiving OPV. | Persons of any age without a reliable history of varicella disease or vaccination, or who are seronegative for varicella.<br>a. *Susceptible adolescents and adults living in households with children.*<br>b. All susceptible health care workers.<br>c. Susceptible family contacts of immunocompromised persons.<br>d. Susceptible persons in the following groups who are at high risk for exposure:<br>• persons who live or work in environments in which transmission of varicella is likely (e.g. teachers of young children, day care employees, residents and staff in institutional settings) or can occur (e.g., college students, inmates and staff of correctional institutions, military personnel)<br>• nonpregnant women of childbearing age<br>• international travelers | a. Persons traveling to or working in countries with high or intermediate endemicity of infection.<br>b. Men who have sex with men.<br>c. Injecting and non-injecting illegal drug users.<br>d. Persons who work with HAV-infected primates or with HAV in a research laboratory setting.<br>e. Persons with chronic liver disease.<br>f. Persons with clotting factor disorders.<br>g. Consider food handlers, where determined to be cost-effective by health authorities or employers. |
| One dose.<br>*Dose:* 0.5 mL subcutaneous (SC) | Three doses: second dose 1-2 months after the first, third dose 4-6 months after the first. No need to start series over if schedule interrupted. Can start series with one manufacturer's vaccine and finish with another.<br>*Dose (Adult):* intramuscular (IM)<br>Recombivax HB: 10:g/1.0 mL (green cap)<br>Engerix-B: 20:g/1.0mL (orange cap)<br>*Dose (Adolescents 11-19 years):* intramuscular (IM)<br>Recombivax HB: 5:g/0.5 mL (yellow cap)<br>Engerix-B: 10:g/0.5 mL (light blue cap)<br>*Booster:* None presently recommended. | Unimmunized adolescents/adults: IPV is recommended—two doses at 4-8 week intervals, third dose 6-12 months after second (can be as soon as 2 months).<br>*Dose:* 0.5 mL subcutaneous (SC) or intramuscular (IM).<br>Partially immunized adolescents/adults:<br>Complete primary series with IPV (IPV schedule shown above).<br>*OPV is no longer recommended for use in the United States.* | For persons <13 years of age, one dose.<br>For persons 13 years of age and older, two doses separated by 4-8 weeks. If >8 weeks elapse following the first dose, the second dose can be administered without restarting the schedule.<br>*Dose:* 0.5 mL subcutaneous (SC). | HAVRIX: Two doses, separated by 6-12 months.<br>Adults (19 years of age and older)—*Dose:* 1.0 mL intramuscular (IM);<br>Persons 2-18 years of age—*Dose:* 0.5 mL (IM).<br>VAQTA:<br>Adults (18 years of age and older): Two doses, separated by 6 months—*Dose:* 1.0 mL intramuscular (IM);<br>Persons 2-17 years of age: Two doses, separated by 6-18 months—*Dose:* 0.5 mL (IM) |
| Same as for measles and mumps vaccines. | Anaphylactic allergy to yeast. | *IPV:* Anaphylactic reaction following previous dose or to streptomycin, polymyxin B or neomycin. | a. Anaphylactic allergy to gelatin or neomycin.<br>b. Untreated, active TB.<br>c. Immunosuppressive therapy or immunodeficiency (including HIV infection).<br>d. Family history of congenital or hereditary immunodeficiency in first-degree relatives, unless the immune competence of the recipient has been clinically substantiated or verified by a laboratory.<br>e. Immune globulin preparation or blood/blood product received in preceding 5 months.<br>f. Pregnancy. | A history of hypersensitivity to alum or the preservative 2-phenoxyethanol |
| *Women should be asked if they are pregnant before receiving vaccine, and advised to avoid pregnancy for 3 months after immunization.* | a. Persons with serologic markers of prior or continuing hepatitis B virus infection do not need immunization.<br>b. For hemodialysis patients and other immunodeficient or immunosuppressed patients, vaccine dosage is doubled or special preparation is used.<br>c. Pregnant women should be sero-screened for HBsAg and, if positive, their infants should be given post-exposure prophylaxis beginning at birth.<br>d. Post-exposure prophylaxis: consult ACIP recommendations, or state or local immunization program. | In instances of potential exposure to wild poliovirus, adults who have had a primary series of OPV or IPV may be given 1 more dose of *IPV.*<br>Although no adverse effects have been documented, vaccination of pregnant women should be avoided. However, if immediate protection is required, pregnant women may be given IPV in accordance with the recommended schedule for adults. | Women should be asked if they are pregnant before receiving varicella vaccine, and advised to avoid pregnancy for one month following each dose of vaccine. | The safety of hepatitis A vaccine during pregnancy has not been determined, though the theoretical risk to the developing fetus is expected to be low. The risk of vaccination should be weighed against the risk of hepatitis A in women who may be at high risk of exposure to HAV. |

## 9-3   Canadian immunization guidelines

### Routine immunization schedule for infants and children

| Age at vaccination | DTaP[1] | Inactivated polio vaccine | Hib[2] | MMR | Td[3] | Hep B[4] (3 doses) |
|---|---|---|---|---|---|---|
| Birth | | | | | | |
| 2 months | X | X | X | | | Infancy |
| 4 months | X | X | X | | | |
| 6 months | X | (X)[5] | X | | | |
| 12 months | | | | X | | or |
| 18 months | X | X | X | (X)[6] or | | |
| 4-6 years | X | X | | (X)[6] | | |
| 14-16 years | | | | | X | preadolescence (9-13 yrs) |

DTaP, Diphtheria, tetanus, pertussis (acellular) vaccine: *Hib, Haemophilus influenzae* type b conjugate vaccine; *MMR,* measles, mumps and rubella vaccine; *Td,* tetanus and diphtheria toxoid, "adult type"; *Hep B,* hepatitis B vaccine.

### Routine immunization schedule for children <7 years of age not immunized in early infancy

| Timing | DtaP[1] | Inactivated polio vaccine | Hib | MMR | Td[3] | Hep B[4] (3 doses) |
|---|---|---|---|---|---|---|
| First visit | X | X | X | X[7] | | |
| 2 months later | X | X | (X)[8] | (X)[6] | | |
| 2 months later | X | (X)[5] | | | | Preadolescence |
| 6-12 months later | X | X | (X)[8] | | | |
| 4-6 years[9] | X | X | | | | (9-13 yrs) |
| 14-16 years | | | | | X | |

## Routine immunization schedule for children ≥7 years of age not immunized in early infancy

| Timing | Td[3] | Inactivated polio vaccine | MMR | Hep B[4] (3 doses) |
|---|---|---|---|---|
| First visit | X | X | X | |
| 2 months later | X | X | (X)[6] | Preadolescence |
| 6-12 months later | X | X | | (9-13 yrs) |
| 10 years later | X | | | |

1. DTaP (diptheria, tetanus, acellular or component pertussis) vaccine is the preferred vaccine for all doses in the vaccination series, including completion of the series in children who have received ≥1 dose of DPT (whole cell) vaccine.
2. Hib schedule shown is for PRP-T or HbOC vaccine. If PRP-OMP, give at 2, 4 and 12 months of age.
3. Td (tetanus and diphtheria toxoid), a combined adsorbed "adult type" preparation for use in persons ≥7 years of age, contains less diptheria toxoid than preparations given to younger children and is less likely to cause reactions in older persons.
4. Hepatitis B vaccine can be routinely given to infants or pre-adolescents, depending on the provincial/territorial policy; three doses at 0, 1 and 6 month intervals are preferred. The second dose should be administered at least 1 month after the first dose, and the third dose should be administered at least 4 months after the first dose, and at least 2 months after the second dose.
5. This dose is not needed routinely, but can be included for convenience.
6. A second dose of MMR is recommended, at least 1 month after the first dose given. For convenience, options include giving it with the next scheduled vaccination at 18 months of age or with school entry (4-6 years) vaccinations (depending on the provincial/territorial policy), or at any intervening age that is practicable.
7. Delay until subsequent visit if child is <12 months of age.
8. Recommended schedule and number of doses depend on the product used and the age of the child when vaccination is begun. Not required past age 5.
9. Omit these doses if the previous doses of DTaP and polio were given after the fourth birthday.

## Routine immunization of adults

| Vaccine or toxoid | Indication | Further doses |
|---|---|---|
| Diphtheria (adult preparation) | All adults | Every 10 years, preferably given with tetanus toxoid (Td) |
| Tetanus | All adults | Every 10 years, preferably given as Td |
| Influenza | Adults ≥65 years; adults <65 years at high risk of influenza-related complications | Every year using current vaccine formulation |
| Pneumococcal | Adults ≥65 years; conditions with increased risk of pneumococcal diseases | None usually |
| Measles | All adults born in 1970 or later who are susceptible to measles | Preferably given as MMR |
| Rubella | Susceptible women of childbearing age and health care workers | None |
| Mumps | Adults born in 1970 or later with no history of mumps | None |

## Routes of administration

| Vaccine | Preferred route of administration |
|---|---|
| BCG | Intradermal |
| Diphtheria toxoid (fluid) | Subcutaneous (SC)* |
| Diphtheria toxoid (adsorbed)† | Intramuscular (IM) |
| Hepatitis A | IM |
| Hepatitis B | IM |
| *Haemophilus influenzae* type b conjugate vaccine | IM |
| Influenza | IM; SC also permissible |
| Japanese encephalitis | SC |
| Meningococcal | SC |
| Measles | SC |
| MMR (measles, mumps, and rubella) | SC |
| MR (measles and rubella) | SC |
| Penta and Pentacel† | IM |
| Pertussis (monovalent acellular) | IM |
| Pertussis (monovalent whole cell) | SC |
| Plague | IM |
| Pneumococcal | IM, SC |
| Polio (IPV) | SC |
| Polio (OPV) | Oral |
| Rabies | IM |
| Rubella | SC |
| Tetanus toxoid (adsorbed)† | IM |
| Typhoid—oral | Oral |
| —Vi capsular | IM |
| Yellow fever | SC |

*The vaccines that are listed as SC only should not be given intramuscularly because of the lack of efficacy data for this route.
†Any vaccine combination containing adsorbed antigen *must* be administered intramuscularly because of the risk of subcutaneous nodule or sterile abscess if it is administered subcutaneously. Examples are Td (tetanus and diphtheria) and DaPT.

## Vaccination of individuals with immunodeficiency

| Vaccine | HIV/AIDS | Severe immuno-deficiency | Solid organ transplantation | BMT | Chronic disease age/alcoholism | Hyposplenia or asplenia |
|---|---|---|---|---|---|---|
| **Inactivated/component vaccines** | | | | | | |
| DPT (Td) | Routine use* | Routine use | Recommended† | Recommended | Routine use | Routine use |
| IPV | Routine use | Routine use | Recommended | Recommended | Routine use | Routine use |
| Hib | Routine use | Routine use | Recommended | Recommended | Routine use | Recommended (confirm response in children <10) |
| Influenza | Recommended | Recommended | Recommended | Recommended | Recommended | Recommended |
| Pneumococcal | Recommended | Recommended | Recommended | Recommended | Recommended | Recommended |
| Meningococcal | Use if indicated | Use if indicated | Use if indicated | Use if indicated | Use if indicated | Use if indicated |
| Hepatitis A | Recommended (gay men, IVDU) | Use if indicated | Use if indicated | Use if indicated | Recommended (chronic liver disease) | Use if indicated |
| Hepatitis B | Recommended (gay men, IVDU) | Routine use | Routine use | Routine use | Recommended (chronic liver or renal disease) | Routine use |
| *Live vaccines* | | | | | | |
| MMR | Routine use‡ (if no significant compromise) | Contraindicated | Consider at 24 mo (min. suppressive Rx) | Consider at 24 mo (no suppressive Rx, no GVHD) | Use if indicated | Use if indicated |
| OPV | Contraindicated (use IPV instead) | Contraindicated (use IPV instead) | Contraindicated (use IPV instead) | Contraindicated (use IPV instead) | If indicated use IPV | If indicated use IPV |
| Varicella | Use if indicated (asymptomatic disease) | Contraindicated | Consider at 24 mo (min. suppressive Rx) | Consider at 24 mo (no suppressive Rx, no GVHD) | Use if indicated | Use if indicated |
| Oral typhoid | Contraindicated (use IM vaccine instead) | Contraindicated (use IM vaccine instead) | Contraindicated (use IM vaccine instead) | Contraindicated (use IM vaccine instead) | If indicated use IM | If indicated use IM |
| BCG | Contraindicated | Contraindicated | Contraindicated | Contraindicated | Use if indicated | Use if indicated |
| Yellow fever | Contraindicated | Contraindicated | Consider at 24 mo (no suppressive Rx, no GVHD) | Consider at 24 mo (no suppressive Rx, no GVHD) | Use if indicated | Use if indicated |
| Oral cholera | Contraindicated | Contraindicated | Contraindicated | Contraindicated | Use if indicated | Use if indicated |

*Routine vaccination schedules should be followed with age-appropriate booster doses.

†Vaccination and/or revaccination recommended with or without verification of serologic response.

‡Most HIV-positive children can receive the first MMR vaccine without significant risk. Administration of the second MMR dose (particularly in adults) must be evaluated on a case-by-case basis.

## Contraindications and precautions to vaccinations

| Vaccine | True contraindications | Precautions* | Not contraindications |
|---------|------------------------|--------------|------------------------|
| All vaccines | Anaphylactic reaction to previous dose of vaccine<br>Anaphylactic reaction to a constituent of a vaccine | Moderate or severe illness with or without fever | Mild to moderate local reactions to previous injection of vaccine<br>Mild acute illness with or without fever<br>Current antimicrobial therapy<br>Convalescent phase of an acute illness<br>Prematurity<br>Recent exposure to infectious disease<br>Personal or family history of allergy |
| DPT | Anaphylactic reaction to previous dose of vaccine | Hypotonic-hyporesponsive state within 48 hr after prior dose of DPT | Fever ≥40.5° C after prior dose of DPT<br>Family history of sudden infant death syndrome<br>Convulsion within 48 hr of prior dose of DPT<br>Family history of convulsions<br>Persistent inconsolable crying lasting ≥3 hr within 48 hr after prior dose |
| IPV | Anaphylactic reaction to neomycin | — | — |
| MMR | Anaphylactic reaction to previous dose or to neomycin<br>Pregnancy<br>Immunodeficient state | Recent administration of G | Tuberculosis or positive TB skin test<br>Simultaneous TB skin testing<br>Current antimicrobial therapy<br>Infection with HIV<br>Egg allergy |
| Hib | | | History of Hib disease |
| Hepatitis B | | | Pregnancy |
| Influenza | Anaphylactic reaction to egg ingestion† | | Pregnancy |

*DPT,* diphtheria, pertussis and tetanus vaccine; *IPV,* inactivated poliovirus vaccine, MMR = measles, mumps, and rubella vaccine; *Hib, Haemophilus influenzae* type b conjugate vaccine.

*The events or conditions listed as precautions are not contraindications but should be carefully considered in determining the benefits and risks of administering a specific vaccine. If the benefits are believed to outweigh the risks (e.g., during an outbreak or foreign travel) the vaccine should be given.

†Persons with a history of anaphylaxis or systemic reactions after eating eggs should be vaccinated with influenza vaccine only with caution.

## 10-1   National Research Council Recommended Dietary Allowances,* Revised 1989

**Food and Nutrition Board, National Academy of Sciences**

| Category | Age (years) or condition | Weight[b] (kg) | Weight[b] (lb) | Height[a] (cm) | Height[a] (in) | Protein (g) | Fat-soluble vitamins Vitamin A (µg RE)[c] | Vitamin D (µg)[d] | Vitamin E (mg α-TE)[e] | Vitamin K (µg) |
|---|---|---|---|---|---|---|---|---|---|---|
| Infants | 0.0-0.5 | 6 | 13 | 60 | 24 | 13 | 375 | 7.5 | 3 | 5 |
| | 0.5-1.0 | 9 | 20 | 71 | 28 | 14 | 375 | 10 | 4 | 10 |
| Children | 1-3 | 13 | 29 | 90 | 35 | 16 | 400 | 10 | 6 | 15 |
| | 4-6 | 20 | 44 | 112 | 44 | 24 | 500 | 10 | 7 | 20 |
| | 7-10 | 28 | 62 | 132 | 52 | 28 | 700 | 10 | 7 | 30 |
| Males | 11-14 | 45 | 99 | 157 | 62 | 45 | 1,000 | 10 | 10 | 45 |
| | 15-18 | 66 | 145 | 176 | 69 | 59 | 1,000 | 10 | 10 | 65 |
| | 19-24 | 72 | 160 | 177 | 70 | 58 | 1,000 | 10 | 10 | 70 |
| | 25-50 | 79 | 174 | 176 | 70 | 63 | 1,000 | 5 | 10 | 80 |
| | 51+ | 77 | 170 | 173 | 68 | 63 | 1,000 | 5 | 10 | 80 |
| Females | 11-14 | 46 | 101 | 157 | 62 | 46 | 800 | 10 | 8 | 45 |
| | 15-18 | 55 | 120 | 163 | 64 | 44 | 800 | 10 | 8 | 55 |
| | 19-24 | 58 | 128 | 164 | 65 | 46 | 800 | 10 | 8 | 60 |
| | 25-50 | 63 | 138 | 163 | 64 | 50 | 800 | 5 | 8 | 65 |
| | 51+ | 65 | 143 | 160 | 63 | 50 | 800 | 5 | 8 | 65 |
| Pregnant | | | | | | 60 | 800 | 10 | 10 | 65 |
| Lactating | 1st 6 Months | | | | | 65 | 1,300 | 10 | 12 | 65 |
| | 2nd 6 Months | | | | | 62 | 1,200 | 10 | 11 | 65 |

[a]The allowances, expressed as average daily intakes over time, are intended to provide for individual variations among most normal persons as they live in the United States under usual environmental stresses. Diets should be based on a variety of common foods in order to provide other nutrients for which human requirements have been less well defined. See text for detailed discussion of allowances and of nutrients not tabulated.

[b]Weights and heights of Reference Adults are actual medians for the US population of the designated age, as reported by NHANES II. The use of these figures does not imply that the height-to-weight ratios are ideal.

NOTE: For more than 50 years, nutrition experts have produced a set of nutrient and energy standards known as the *Recommended Dietary Allowances (RDAs)*. A major revision is currently underway to replace the RDAs. The revised recommendations are called *Dietary Reference Intakes (DRIs)* and reflect the collaborative efforts of both the United States and Canada. Until 1997, the RDAs were the only standards available, and they will continue to serve health professionals until DRIs can be established for all nutrients. Current DRIs can be found in Appendix 10-3.

| Water-soluble vitamins | | | | | | | Minerals | | | | | | |
|---|---|---|---|---|---|---|---|---|---|---|---|---|---|
| Vita-min C (mg) | Thia-min (mg) | Ribo-flavin (mg) | Niacin (mg NE)$^f$ | Vita-min $B_4$ (mg) | Fo-late (μg) | Vita-min $B_{12}$ (μg) | Cal-cium (mg) | Phos-phorus (mg) | Mag-nesium (mg) | Iron (mg) | Zinc (mg) | Iodine (μg) | Sele-nium (μg) |
| 30 | 0.3 | 0.4 | 5 | 0.3 | 25 | 0.3 | 400 | 300 | 40 | 6 | 5 | 40 | 10 |
| 35 | 0.4 | 0.5 | 6 | 0.6 | 35 | 0.5 | 600 | 500 | 60 | 10 | 5 | 50 | 15 |
| 40 | 0.7 | 0.8 | 9 | 1.0 | 50 | 0.7 | 800 | 800 | 80 | 10 | 10 | 70 | 20 |
| 45 | 0.9 | 1.1 | 12 | 1.1 | 75 | 1.0 | 800 | 800 | 120 | 10 | 10 | 90 | 20 |
| 45 | 1.0 | 1.2 | 13 | 1.4 | 100 | 1.4 | 800 | 800 | 170 | 10 | 10 | 120 | 30 |
| 50 | 1.3 | 1.5 | 17 | 1.7 | 150 | 2.0 | 1,200 | 1,200 | 270 | 12 | 15 | 150 | 40 |
| 60 | 1.5 | 1.8 | 20 | 2.0 | 200 | 2.0 | 1,200 | 1,200 | 400 | 12 | 15 | 150 | 50 |
| 60 | 1.5 | 1.7 | 19 | 2.0 | 200 | 2.0 | 1,200 | 1,200 | 350 | 10 | 15 | 150 | 70 |
| 60 | 1.5 | 1.7 | 19 | 2.0 | 200 | 2.0 | 800 | 800 | 350 | 10 | 15 | 150 | 70 |
| 60 | 1.2 | 1.4 | 15 | 2.0 | 200 | 2.0 | 800 | 800 | 350 | 10 | 15 | 150 | 70 |
| 50 | 1.1 | 1.3 | 15 | 1.4 | 150 | 2.0 | 1,200 | 1,200 | 280 | 15 | 12 | 150 | 45 |
| 60 | 1.1 | 1.3 | 15 | 1.5 | 180 | 2.0 | 1,200 | 1,200 | 300 | 15 | 12 | 150 | 50 |
| 60 | 1.1 | 1.3 | 15 | 1.6 | 180 | 2.0 | 1,200 | 1,200 | 280 | 15 | 12 | 150 | 55 |
| 60 | 1.1 | 1.3 | 15 | 1.6 | 180 | 2.0 | 800 | 800 | 280 | 15 | 12 | 150 | 55 |
| 60 | 1.0 | 1.2 | 13 | 1.6 | 180 | 2.0 | 800 | 800 | 280 | 10 | 12 | 150 | 55 |
| 70 | 1.5 | 1.6 | 17 | 2.2 | 400 | 2.2 | 1,200 | 1,200 | 320 | 30 | 15 | 175 | 65 |
| 95 | 1.6 | 1.8 | 20 | 2.1 | 280 | 2.6 | 1,200 | 1,200 | 355 | 15 | 19 | 200 | 75 |
| 90 | 1.6 | 1.7 | 20 | 2.1 | 260 | 2.6 | 1,200 | 1,200 | 340 | 15 | 16 | 200 | 75 |

$^c$Retinol equivalents. 1 retinol equivalent = 1 μg retinol or 6 μg β-carotene.
$^d$As cholecalciferol. 10 μg cholecalciferol = 400 IU of vitamin D.
$^e$α-Tocopherol equivalents. 1 mg d-α tocopherol = 1 α-TE.
$^f$1 NE (niacin equivalent) is equal to 1 mg of niacin or 60 mg of dietary tryptophan.

**Estimated safe and adequate daily dietary intakes of selected vitamins and minerals**[a]

| Category | Age (years) | Vitamins | |
|---|---|---|---|
| | | Biotin (μg) | Pantothenic acid (mg) |
| Infants | 0-0.5 | 10 | 2 |
| | 0.5-1 | 15 | 3 |
| Children and adolescents | 1-3 | 20 | 3 |
| | 4-6 | 25 | 3-4 |
| | 7-10 | 30 | 4-5 |
| | 11+ | 30-100 | 4-7 |
| Adults | | 30-100 | 4-7 |

| Category | Age (years) | Trace elements[b] | | | | |
|---|---|---|---|---|---|---|
| | | Copper (mg) | Mangenese (mg) | Fluoride (mg) | Chromium (μg) | Molybdenum (μg) |
| Infants | 0-0.5 | 0.4-0.6 | 0.3-0.6 | 0.1-0.5 | 10-40 | 15-30 |
| | 0.5-1 | 0.6-0.7 | 0.6-1.0 | 0.2-1.0 | 20-60 | 20-40 |
| Children and adolescents | 1-3 | 0.7-1.0 | 1.0-1.5 | 0.5-1.5 | 20-80 | 25-50 |
| | 4-6 | 1.0-1.5 | 1.5-2.0 | 1.0-2.5 | 30-120 | 30-75 |
| | 7-10 | 1.0-2.0 | 2.0-3.0 | 1.5-2.5 | 50-200 | 50-150 |
| | 11+ | 1.5-2.5 | 2.0-5.0 | 1.5-2.5 | 50-200 | 75-250 |
| Adults | | 1.5-3.0 | 2.0-5.0 | 1.5-4.0 | 50-200 | 75-250 |

[a]Because there is less information on which to base allowances, these figures are not given in the main table of RDA and are provided here in the form of ranges of recommended intakes.

[b]Since the toxic levels for many trace elements may be only several times usual intakes, the upper levels for the trace elements given in this table should not be habitually exceeded.

## 10-2   Recommended nutrient intakes for Canadians, 1990

**Summary examples of recommended nutrient intake based on age and body weight expressed as daily rates**

| Age | Sex | Weight kg | Pro-tein g | Vit. A RE* | Vit. D μg | Vit. E mg | Vit. C mg | Folate μg | Vit. $B_{12}$ μg | Cal-cium mg | Phos-phorus mg | Mag-nesium mg | Iron mg | Iodine μg | Zinc mg |
|---|---|---|---|---|---|---|---|---|---|---|---|---|---|---|---|
| **Months** | | | | | | | | | | | | | | | |
| 0-4 | Both | 6.0 | 12 | 400 | 10 | 3 | 20 | 25 | 0.3 | 250† | 150 | 20 | 0.3§ | 30 | 2§ |
| 5-12 | Both | 9.0 | 12 | 400 | 10 | 3 | 20 | 40 | 0.4 | 400 | 200 | 32 | 7 | 40 | 3 |
| **Years** | | | | | | | | | | | | | | | |
| 1 | Both | 11 | 13 | 400 | 10 | 3 | 20 | 40 | 0.5 | 500 | 300 | 40 | 6 | 55 | 4 |
| 2-3 | Both | 14 | 16 | 400 | 5 | 4 | 20 | 50 | 0.6 | 550 | 350 | 50 | 6 | 65 | 4 |
| 4-6 | Both | 18 | 19 | 500 | 5 | 5 | 25 | 70 | 0.8 | 600 | 400 | 65 | 8 | 85 | 5 |
| 7-9 | M | 25 | 26 | 700 | 2.5 | 7 | 25 | 90 | 1.0 | 700 | 500 | 100 | 8 | 110 | 7 |
| | F | 25 | 26 | 700 | 2.5 | 6 | 25 | 90 | 1.0 | 700 | 500 | 100 | 8 | 95 | 7 |
| 10-12 | M | 34 | 34 | 800 | 2.5 | 8 | 25 | 120 | 1.0 | 900 | 700 | 130 | 8 | 125 | 9 |
| | F | 36 | 36 | 800 | 2.5 | 7 | 25 | 130 | 1.0 | 1100 | 800 | 135 | 8 | 110 | 9 |
| 13-15 | M | 50 | 49 | 900 | 2.5 | 9 | 30 | 175 | 1.0 | 1100 | 900 | 185 | 10 | 160 | 12 |
| | F | 48 | 46 | 800 | 2.5 | 7 | 30 | 170 | 1.0 | 1000 | 850 | 180 | 13 | 160 | 9 |
| 16-18 | M | 62 | 58 | 1000 | 2.5 | 10 | 40‖ | 220 | 1.0 | 900 | 1000 | 230 | 10 | 160 | 12 |
| | F | 53 | 47 | 800 | 2.5 | 7 | 30‖ | 190 | 1.0 | 700 | 850 | 200 | 12 | 160 | 9 |
| 19-24 | M | 71 | 61 | 1000 | 2.5 | 10 | 40‖ | 220 | 1.0 | 800 | 1000 | 240 | 9 | 160 | 12 |
| | F | 58 | 50 | 800 | 2.5 | 7 | 30‖ | 180 | 1.0 | 700 | 850 | 200 | 13 | 160 | 9 |
| 25-49 | M | 74 | 64 | 1000 | 2.5 | 9 | 40‖ | 230 | 1.0 | 800 | 1000 | 250 | 9 | 160 | 12 |
| | F | 59 | 51 | 800 | 2.5 | 6 | 30‖ | 185 | 1.0 | 700 | 850 | 200 | 13 | 160 | 9 |
| 50-74 | M | 73 | 63 | 1000 | 5 | 7 | 40‖ | 230 | 1.0 | 800 | 1000 | 250 | 9 | 160 | 12 |
| | F | 63 | 54 | 800 | 5 | 6 | 30‖ | 195 | 1.0 | 800 | 850 | 210 | 8 | 160 | 9 |
| 75+ | M | 69 | 59 | 1000 | 5 | 6 | 40‖ | 215 | 1.0 | 800 | 1000 | 230 | 9 | 160 | 12 |
| | F | 64 | 55 | 800 | 5 | 5 | 30‖ | 200 | 1.0 | 800 | 850 | 210 | 9 | 160 | 9 |

From *Recommended nutrient intakes for Canadians,* Health Canada, 1990. Reproduced with permission of the Minister of Public Works and Government Services Canada, 1997.

*Retinol Equivalents.

+Protein is assumed to be from breast milk and must be adjusted for infant formula.

†Infant formula with high phosphorus should contain 375 mg calcium.

§Breast milk is assumed to be the source of the mineral.

‖Smokers should increase vitamin C by 50%.

## Summary examples of recommended nutrient intake based on age and body weight expressed as daily rates—cont'd

| Age | Sex | Weight kg | Pro-tein g | Vit. A RE* | Vit. D μg | Vit. E mg | Vit. C mg | Folate μg | Vit. $B_{12}$ μg | Cal-cium mg | Phos-phorus mg | Mag-nesium mg | Iron mg | Iodine μg | Zinc mg |
|---|---|---|---|---|---|---|---|---|---|---|---|---|---|---|---|
| **Pregnancy (additional)** | | | | | | | | | | | | | | | |
| 1st Trimester | | 5 | 0 | 2.5 | 2 | 0 | 200 | 1.2 | 500 | 200 | 15 | 0 | 25 | 6 |
| 2nd Trimester | | 20 | 0 | 2.5 | 2 | 10 | 200 | 1.2 | 500 | 200 | 45 | 5 | 25 | 6 |
| 3rd Trimester | | 24 | 0 | 2.5 | 2 | 10 | 200 | 1.2 | 500 | 200 | 45 | 10 | 25 | 6 |
| Lactation (additional) | | 20 | 400 | 2.5 | 3 | 25 | 100 | 0.2 | 500 | 200 | 65 | 0 | 50 | 6 |

NOTE: While the above Recommended Nutrient Intake guidelines are the most up-to-date Canadian nutrition standards currently available, Health Canada and a number of U.S. government agencies are sponsoring the review of the scientific data concerning requirements and tolerable upper levels of nutrients and other food components. The review is intended to produce a series of Dietary Reference Intake (DRI) guidelines which will ultimately replace the current Canadian Recommended Nutrient Intakes. Currently DRIs can be found in Appendix 10-3.

## Summary of examples of recommended nutrients based on energy expressed as daily rates

| Age | Sex | Energy kcal | Thiamin mg | Riboflavin mg | Niacin Ne[+] | n-3 PUFA* g | n-6 PUFA g |
|---|---|---|---|---|---|---|---|
| **Months** | | | | | | | |
| 0-4 | Both | 600 | 0.3 | 0.3 | 4 | 0.5 | 3 |
| 5-12 | Both | 900 | 0.4 | 0.5 | 7 | 0.5 | 3 |
| **Years** | | | | | | | |
| 1 | Both | 1100 | 0.5 | 0.6 | 8 | 0.6 | 4 |
| 2-3 | Both | 1300 | 0.6 | 0.7 | 9 | 0.7 | 4 |
| 4-6 | Both | 1800 | 0.7 | 0.9 | 13 | 1.0 | 6 |
| 7-9 | M | 2200 | 0.9 | 1.1 | 16 | 1.2 | 7 |
| | F | 1900 | 0.8 | 1.0 | 14 | 1.0 | 6 |
| 10-12 | M | 2500 | 1.0 | 1.3 | 18 | 1.4 | 8 |
| | F | 2200 | 0.9 | 1.1 | 16 | 1.2 | 7 |
| 13-15 | M | 2800 | 1.1 | 1.4 | 20 | 1.5 | 9 |
| | F | 2200 | 0.9 | 1.1 | 16 | 1.2 | 7 |
| 16-18 | M | 3200 | 1.3 | 1.6 | 23 | 1.8 | 11 |
| | F | 2100 | 0.8 | 1.1 | 15 | 1.2 | 7 |
| 19-24 | M | 3000 | 1.2 | 1.5 | 22 | 1.6 | 10 |
| | F | 2100 | 0.8 | 1.1 | 15 | 1.2 | 7 |
| 25-49 | M | 2700 | 1.1 | 1.4 | 19 | 1.5 | 9 |
| | F | 1900 | 0.8 | 1.0 | 14 | 1.1 | 7 |
| 50-74 | M | 2300 | 0.9 | 1.2 | 16 | 1.3 | 8 |
| | F | 1800 | 0.8† | 1.0† | 14† | 1.1† | 7† |
| 75+ | M | 2000 | 0.8 | 1.0 | 14 | 1.1 | 7 |
| | F§ | 1700 | 0.8† | 1.0† | 14† | 1.1† | 7† |
| **Pregnancy (additional)** | | | | | | | |
| 1st Trimester | | 100 | 0.1 | 0.1 | 1 | 0.05 | 0.3 |
| 2nd Trimester | | 300 | 0.1 | 0.3 | 2 | 0.16 | 0.9 |
| 3rd Trimester | | 300 | 0.1 | 0.3 | 2 | 0.16 | 0.9 |
| Lactation (additional) | | 450 | 0.2 | 0.4 | 3 | 0.25 | 1.5 |

From *Recommended nutrient intakes for Canadians,* Health Canada, 1990. Reproduced with permission of the Minister of Public Works and Government Services Canada, 1997.

*PUFA, polyunsaturated fatty acids.

[+]Niacin equivalents.

†Level below which intake should not fall.

§Assumes moderate physical activity.

## 10-3 | Dietary reference intakes for the United States and Canada

**Food and nutrition board, institute of medicine, national academy of sciences dietary reference intakes: recommended intakes for individuals**

| Life stage group | Calcium (mg/d) | Phosphorus (mg/d) | Magnesium (mg/d) | Vitamin D (μg/d)[a,b] | Fluoride (μg/d) | Thiamin (mg/d) | Riboflavin (mg/d) | Niacin (mg/d)[c] | Vitamin B⁶ (mg/d) |
|---|---|---|---|---|---|---|---|---|---|
| **Infants** | | | | | | | | | |
| 0-6 mo | 210* | 100* | 30* | 5* | 0.01* | 0.2* | 0.3* | 2* | 0.1* |
| 7-12 mo | 270* | 275* | 75* | 5* | 0.5* | 0.3* | 0.4* | 4* | 0.3* |
| **Children** | | | | | | | | | |
| 1-3 y | 500* | **460** | **80** | 5* | 0.7* | **0.5** | **0.5** | **6** | **0.5** |
| 4-8 y | 800* | **500** | **130** | 5* | 1* | **0.6** | **0.6** | **8** | **0.6** |
| **Males** | | | | | | | | | |
| 9-13 y | 1,300* | **1,250** | **240** | 5* | 2* | **0.9** | **0.9** | **12** | **1.0** |
| 14-18 y | 1,300* | **1,250** | **410** | 5* | 3* | **1.2** | **1.3** | **16** | **1.3** |
| 19-30 y | 1,000* | **700** | **400** | 5* | 4* | **1.2** | **1.3** | **16** | **1.3** |
| 31-50 y | 1,000* | **700** | **420** | 5* | 4* | **1.2** | **1.3** | **16** | **1.3** |
| 51-70 y | 1,200* | **700** | **420** | 10* | 4* | **1.2** | **1.3** | **16** | **1.7** |
| >70 y | 1,200* | **700** | **420** | 15* | 4* | **1.2** | **1.3** | **16** | **1.7** |
| **Females** | | | | | | | | | |
| 9-13 y | 1,300* | **1,250** | **240** | 5* | 2* | **0.9** | **0.9** | **12** | **1.0** |
| 14-18 y | 1,300* | **1,250** | **360** | 5* | 3* | **1.0** | **1.0** | **14** | **1.2** |
| 19-30 y | 1,000* | **700** | **310** | 5* | 3* | **1.1** | **1.1** | **14** | **1.3** |
| 31-50 y | 1,000* | **700** | **320** | 5* | 3* | **1.1** | **1.1** | **14** | **1.3** |
| 51-70 y | 1,200* | **700** | **320** | 10* | 3* | **1.1** | **1.1** | **14** | **1.5** |
| >70 y | 1,200* | **700** | **320** | 15* | 3* | **1.1** | **1.1** | **14** | **1.5** |
| **Pregnancy** | | | | | | | | | |
| ≤18 y | 1,300* | **1,250** | **400** | 5* | 3* | **1.4** | **1.4** | **18** | **1.9** |
| 19-30 y | 1,000* | **700** | **350** | 5* | 3* | **1.4** | **1.4** | **18** | **1.9** |
| 31-50 y | 1,000* | **700** | **360** | 5* | 3* | **1.4** | **1.4** | **18** | **1.9** |
| **Lactation** | | | | | | | | | |
| ≤18 y | 1,300* | **1,250** | **350** | 5* | 3* | **1.4** | **1.6** | **17** | **2.0** |
| 19-30 y | 1,000* | **700** | **310** | 5* | 3* | **1.4** | **1.6** | **17** | **2.0** |
| 31-50 y | 1,000* | **700** | **320** | 5* | 3* | **1.4** | **1.6** | **17** | **2.0** |

From Food and Nutrition Board: *Dietary reference intakes for vitamin C, vitamin E, selenium, and carotenoids,* Washington, DC, 2000, National Academy Press.
NOTE: This table presents recommended dietary allowances (RDAs) in **bold type** and Adequate Intakes (AIs) in ordinary type followed by an asterisk (*). RDAs and AIs may both be used as goals for individual intake. RDAs are set to meet the needs of almost all (97% to 98%) individuals in a group. For healthy breastfed infants, the AI is the mean intake. The AI for other life-stage and gender groups is believed to cover needs of all individuals in the group, but lack of data or uncertainty in the data prevents being able to specify with confidence the percentage of individuals covered by this intake.
[a]As cholecalciferol. 1 pg cholecalciferol = 40 IU vitamin D.
[b]In the absence of adequate exposure to sunlight.
[c]As niacin equivalents (NE). 1 mg of niacin = 60 mg of tryptophan; 0-6 months = preformed niacin (not NE).

| Folate ($\mu$g/d)[d] | Vitamin $B_{12}$ ($\mu$g/d) | Pantothenic acid (mg/d) | Biotin ($\mu$g/d) | Choline[e] (mg/d) | Vitamin C (mg/d) | Vitamin E[f] (mg/d) | Selenium ($\mu$g/d) | Life stage group |
|---|---|---|---|---|---|---|---|---|
| | | | | | | | | **Infants** |
| 65* | 0.4* | 1.7* | 5* | 125* | 40* | 4* | 15* | 0-6 mo |
| 80* | 0.5* | 1.8* | 6* | 150* | 50* | 6* | 20* | 7-12 mo |
| | | | | | | | | **Children** |
| 150 | 0.9 | 2* | 8* | 200* | 15 | 6 | 20 | 1-3 y |
| 200 | 1.2 | 3* | 12* | 250* | 25 | 7 | 30 | 4-8 y |
| | | | | | | | | **Males** |
| 300 | 1.8 | 4* | 20* | 375* | 45 | 11 | 40 | 9-13 y |
| 400 | 2.4 | 5* | 25* | 550* | 75 | 15 | 55 | 14-18 y |
| 400 | 2.4 | 5* | 30* | 550* | 90 | 15 | 55 | 19-30 y |
| 400 | 2.4 | 5* | 30* | 550* | 90 | 15 | 55 | 31-50 y |
| 400 | 2.4[g] | 5* | 30* | 550* | 90 | 15 | 55 | 51-70 y |
| 400 | 2.4[g] | 5* | 30* | 550* | 90 | 15 | 55 | >70 y |
| | | | | | | | | **Females** |
| 300 | 1.8 | 4* | 20* | 375* | 45 | 11 | 40 | 9-13 y |
| 400[h] | 2.4 | 5* | 25* | 400* | 65 | 15 | 55 | 14-18 y |
| 400[h] | 2.4 | 5* | 30* | 425* | 75 | 15 | 55 | 19-30 y |
| 400[h] | 2.4 | 5* | 30* | 425* | 75 | 15 | 55 | 31-50 y |
| 400 | 2.4[g] | 5* | 30* | 425* | 75 | 15 | 55 | 51-70 y |
| 400 | 2.4[g] | 5* | 30* | 425* | 75 | 15 | 55 | >70 y |
| | | | | | | | | **Pregnancy** |
| 600[i] | 2.6 | 6* | 30* | 450* | 80 | 15 | 60 | ≤18 y |
| 600[i] | 2.6 | 6* | 30* | 450* | 85 | 15 | 60 | 19-30 y |
| 600[i] | 2.6 | 6* | 30* | 450* | 85 | 15 | 60 | 31-50 y |
| | | | | | | | | **Lactation** |
| 500 | 2.8 | 7* | 35* | 550* | 115 | 19 | 70 | ≤18 y |
| 500 | 2.8 | 7* | 35* | 550* | 120 | 19 | 70 | 19-30 y |
| 500 | 2.8 | 7* | 35* | 550* | 120 | 19 | 70 | 31-50 y |

[d]As dietary folate equivalents (DFE). 1 DFE = 1 $\mu$g food folate = 0.6 $\mu$g of folic acid from fortified food or as a supplement consumed with food = 0.5 $\mu$g of a supplement taken on an empty stomach.

[e]Although AIs have been set for choline, there are few data to assess whether a dietary supply of choline is needed at all stages of the life cycle, and it may be that the choline requirement can be met by endogenous synthesis at some of these stages.

[f]As $\alpha$-tocopherol, $\alpha$-Tocopherol includes RRR-$\alpha$-tocopherol, the only form of $\alpha$-tocopherol that occurs naturally in foods, and the 2R-stereoisomeric forms of $\alpha$-tocopherol (RRR-, RSR-, RRS-, and RSS-$\alpha$-tocopherol) that occur in fortified foods and supplements. It does not include the 2S-stereoisomeric forms of $\alpha$-tocopherol (SRR-, SSR-, SRS-, and SSS-$\alpha$-tocopherol), also found in fortified foods and supplements.

[g]Because 10% to 30% of older people may malabsorb food-bound $B_{12}$, it is advisable for those older than 50 years to meet their RDA mainly by consuming foods fortified with $B_{12}$ or a supplement containing $B_{12}$.

[h]In view of evidence linking folate intake with neural tube defects in the fetus, it is recommended that all women capable of becoming pregnant consume 400 $\mu$g from supplements or fortified foods in addition to intake of food folate from a varied diet.

[i]It is assumed that women will continue consuming 400 $\mu$g from supplements or fortified food until their pregnancy is confirmed and they enter prenatal care, which ordinarily occurs after the end of the periconceptional period—the critical time for formation of the neural tube.

## 10-4   Vitamins and minerals

### Summary of fat-soluble vitamins

| Vitamin | Physiologic functions | Results of deficiency | Requirement | Food sources |
|---|---|---|---|---|
| **Vitamin A**<br>Provitamin: beta-carotene<br>Vitamin: retinol | Production of rhodopsin and other light-receptor pigments<br>Formation and maintenance of epithelial tissue<br>Growth<br>Reproduction<br>Toxic in large amounts | Poor dark adaptation, night blindness, xerosis, xerophthalmia<br>Keratinization of epithelium<br>Growth failure<br>Reproductive failure | Adult male: 1000 μg or RE (5000 IU)<br>Adult female: 800 μg or RE (4000 IU)<br>Pregnancy: 1000 μg or RE (500 IU)<br>Lactation: 1200 μg or RE (6000 IU)<br>Children: 400 μg or RE (2000 IU) to 800 μg or RE (4000 IU) | Liver, cream, butter, whole milk, egg yolk<br>Green and yellow vegetables, yellow fruits<br>Fortified margarine |
| **Vitamin D**<br>Provitamins: ergosterol (plants); 7-dehydrocholesterol (skin)<br>Vitamins $D_2$ (ergocholecalciferol) and $D_3$ (cholecalciferol) | Calcitriol a major hormone regulator of bone mineral (calcium and phosphorus) metabolism<br>Calcium and phosphorus absorption<br>Toxic in large amounts | Faulty bone growth; rickets, osteomalacia | Adult: 5-10 μg cholecalciferol (200-400 IU)<br>Pregnancy and lactation: 10-12.5 μg (400-500 IU) depending on age<br>Children: 10 μg (400 IU) | Fortified milk<br>Fortifed margarine<br>Fish oils<br>Sunlight on skin |
| **Vitamin E**<br>Tocopherols | Antioxidant<br>Hemopoiesis<br>Related to action of selenium | Anemia in premature infants | Adult: 8-10 mg α-TE<br>Pregnancy and lactation: 10-11 mg α-TE<br>Children: 3-10 mg α-TE | Vegetable oils |
| **Vitamin K**<br>$K_1$ (phylloquinone)<br>$K_2$ (menaquinone)<br>Analog: $K_3$ (menadione) | Activates blood-clotting factors (for example, prothrombin) by alpha-carboxylating glutamic acid residues<br>Toxicity can be induced by water-soluble analogs | Hemorrhagic disease of the newborn<br>Defective blood clotting<br>Deficiency symptoms are produced by coumarin anticoagulants and antibiotic therapy | Adult: 70-140 μg<br>Children: 15-100 μg<br>Infants: 12-20 μg | Cheese, egg yolk, liver<br>Green leafy vegetables<br>Synthesized by intestinal bacteria |

From Williams SR: *Nutrition and diet therapy,* ed 8, St Louis, 1997, Mosby.

### Summary of vitamin C (ascorbic acid)

| Physiologic functions | Clinical applications | Requirement | Food sources |
|---|---|---|---|
| Antioxidant<br>Collagen biosynthesis<br>General metabolism<br>  Makes iron available for hemoglobin synthesis<br>  Influences conversion of folic acid to folinic acid<br>  Oxidation-reduction of the amino acids phenylalanine and tyrosine | Scurvy (deficiency)<br>Wound healing, tissue formation<br>Fevers and infection<br>Stress reactions<br>Growth | 60 mg | Fresh fruits, especially citrus<br>Vegetables such as tomatoes, cabbage, potatoes, chili peppers, and broccoli |

From Williams SR: *Nutrition and diet therapy,* ed 8, St Louis, 1997, Mosby.

## Summary of B-complex vitamins

| Vitamin | Coenzymes: physiologic function | Clinical applications | Requirement | Food sources |
|---|---|---|---|---|
| Thiamin | Carbohydrate metabolism<br>Thiamin pyrophosphate (TPP): oxidative decarboxylation | Beriberi (deficiency)<br>Neuropathy<br>Wernicke-Kosakoff syndrome (alcoholsim)<br>Depressed muscular and secretory symptoms | 0.5 mg/1000 kcal | Pork, beef, liver, whole or enriched grains, legumes |
| Riboflavin | General metabolism<br>Flavin adenine dinucleotide (FAD)<br>Flavin mononucleotide (FMN) | Cheilosis, glossitis, seborrheic dermatitis | 0.6 mg/1000 kcal | Milk, liver, enriched cereals |
| Niacin (nicotinic acid, nicotinamide) | General metabolism<br>Nicotinamine-adenine dinucleotide (NAD)<br>Nicotinamide-adenine dinucleotide phosphate (NADP) | Pellagra (deficiency)<br>Weakness, anorexia<br>Scaly dermatitis<br>Neuritis | 6.6 NE/1000 kcal | Meat, peanuts, enriched grains (protein foods containing tryptophan) |
| Vitamin $B_6$ (pyridoxine, pyridoxal, pyridoxamine) | General metabolism<br>Pyridoxal phosphate (PLP): transamination and decarboxylation | Reduced serum levels associated with pregnancy and use of oral contraceptives<br>Antagonized by isoniazid, penicillamine, and other drugs | 2 mg (men)<br>1.6 mg (women) | Wheat, corn, meat, liver |
| Pantothenic acid | General metabolism<br>CoA (coenzyme A): acetylation | Many roles through acyl-transfer reactions (for example, lipogenesis, amino acid activation, and formation of cholesterol, steroid hormones, heme) | 4 to 7 mg | Liver, egg, milk |
| Biotin | General metabolism<br>N-Carboxybiotinyl lysine: $CO_2$ transfer reactions | Deficiency induced by avidin (a protein in raw egg white) and by antibiotics<br>Synthesis of some fatty acids and amino acids | 30 to 100 μg | Egg yolk, liver<br>Synthesized by intestinal microorganisms |
| Folate (folic acid, folacin) | General metabolism<br>Single-carbon transfer reactions (for example, purine nucleotide, thymine, heme synthesis) | Megaloblastic anemia | 200 μg (men)<br>180 μg (women) | Liver, green leafy vegetables |
| Cobalamin | General metabolism<br>Methylcobalamin: methylation reaction (for example, synthesis of amino acids, heme) | Pernicious anemia induced by lack of intrinsic factor<br>Megaloblastic anemia<br>Methylmalonic aciduria<br>Homocystinuria<br>Peripheral neuropathy (strict vegetarian diet) | 2 μg | Liver, meat, milk, egg, cheese |

From Williams SR: *Nutrition and diet therapy,* ed 8, St Louis, 1997, Mosby

## Summary of major minerals (required intake over 100 mg/day)

| Mineral | Metabolism | Physiologic functions | Clinical applications | Requirements | Food sources |
|---|---|---|---|---|---|
| Calcium (CA) | Absorption according to body need; requires Ca-binding protein and regulated by vitamin D, parathyroid hormone, and calcitonin; absorption favored by protein, lactose, acidity<br>Excretion chiefly in feces: 70%-90% of amount ingested<br>Deposition-mobilization in bone tissue constant, regulated by vitamin D and parathyroid hormone | Constituent of bones and teeth<br>Participates in blood clotting, nerve transmission, muscle action, cell membrane permeability, enzyme activation | Tetany (decrease in serum Ca)<br>Rickets, osteomalacia<br>Osteoporosis<br>Resorptive hypercalciuria, renal calculuses<br>Hyperthyroidism and hypothyroidism | Adults: 800 mg<br>Pregnancy and lactation: 1200 mg<br>Infants: 400-600 mg<br>Children: 800-1200 mg | Milk, cheese<br>Green, leafy vegetables<br>Whole grains<br>Egg yolk<br>Legumes, nuts |
| Phosphorus (P) | Absorption with Ca aided by vitamin D and parathyroid hormone as for calcium; hundered by binding agents<br>Excretion chiefly by kidney according to serum level, regulated by parathyroid hormone<br>Deposition-mobilization in bone compartment constant | Constituent of bones and teeth, ATP, phosporylated intermediary metabolites<br>Participates in absorption of glucose and glycerol, transport of fatty acids, energy metabolism, and buffer system | Growth<br>Recovery from diabetic acidosis<br>Hypophosphatemia: bone disease, malabsorption syndromes, primary hyperparathyroidism<br>Hyperphosphatemia: renal insufficiency, hypothyroidism, tetany | Adults: 800 mg<br>Pregnancy and lactation: 1200 mg<br>Infants: 300-500 mg<br>Children: 800-1200 mg | Milk, cheese<br>Meat, egg yolk<br>Whole grains<br>Legumes, nuts |
| Magnesium (Mg) | Absorption according to intake load; hindered by excess fat, phosphate, calcium, protein<br>Excretion (regulated by kidney) | Constituent of bones and teeth<br>Coenzyme in general metabolism, smooth muscle action, neuromucular irritability<br>Cation in intracellular fluid | Low serum level following gastrointestinal losses<br>Tremor, spasm in deficiency induced by malnutrition, alcoholism | Adults: 280-350 mg<br>Pregnancy and lactation: 290-355 mg<br>Infants: 40-60 mg<br>Children: 80-170 mg | Milk, cheese<br>Meat, seafood<br>Whole grains<br>Legumes, nuts |
| Sodium (Na) | Readily absorbed<br>Excretion chiefly by kidney, controlled by aldosterone | Major cation in extracellular fluid, water balance, acid-base balance<br>Cell membrane permeability, absorption of glucose<br>Normal muscle irritability | Losses in gastrointestinal disorders, diarrhea<br>Fluid-electrolyte and acid-base balance problems<br>Muscle action | Adults: 500 mg<br>Infants: 120-200 mg<br>Children: 225-500 mg | Salt (NaCl)<br>Sodium compounds in baking and processing<br>Milk, cheese<br>Meat, eggs<br>Carrots, beets, spinach, celery |
| Potassium (K) | Readily absorbed<br>Secreted and resorbed in gastrointestinal circulation<br>Excretion chiefly by kidney, regulated by aldosterone | Major cation in intracellular fluid, water balance, acid-base balance<br>Normal muscle irritability<br>Glycogen formation<br>Protein synthesis | Losses in gastrointestinal disorders, diarrhea<br>Fluid-electrolyte, acid-base balance problems<br>Muscle action, especially heart action<br>Losses in tissue catabolism<br>Treatment of diabetic acidosis: rapid glycogen production reduces serum potassium level<br>Losses with diuretic therapy | Adults: 2000 mg<br>Infants: 500-700 mg<br>Children: 1000-2000 mg | Fruits<br>Vegetables<br>Legumes, nuts<br>Whole grains<br>Meat |

From Williams SR: *Nutrition and diet therapy* ed 8, St Louis, 1997, Mosby.

## Summary of major minerals (required intake over 100 mg/day)—cont'd

| Mineral | Metabolism | Physiologic functions | Clinical applications | Requirements | Food sources |
|---------|-----------|----------------------|----------------------|--------------|--------------|
| Chlorine (Cl) | Readily absorbed<br>Excretion controlled by kidney | Major anion in extra-cellular fluid, water balance, acid-base balance, chloride-bicarbonate shift<br>Gastric hydrochloride—digestion | Losses in gastrointestinal disorders, vomiting, diarrhea, tube drainage<br>Hypochloremic alkalosis | Adults: 750 mg<br>Infants: 180-300 mg<br>Children: 350-750 mg | Salt (NaCl) |
| Sulfur (S) | Elemental form absorbed as such; split from amino acid sources (methionine and cystine) in digestion and absorbed into portal circulation<br>Excreted by kidney in relation to protein intake and tissue catabolism | Essential constituent of protein structure<br>Enzyme activity and energy metabolism through free sulf-hydryl group (—SH)<br>Detoxification reactions | Cystine renal calculuses<br>Cystinuria | Diet adequate in protein contains adequate sulfur | Meat, eggs<br>Milk, cheese<br>Legumes, nuts |

## Summary of trace elements (required intake less than 100 mg/day)

| Mineral | Metabolism | Physiologic functions | Clinical applications | Requirements | Food sources |
|---------|-----------|----------------------|----------------------|--------------|--------------|
| Iron (Fe) | Absorption controls bioavailability; favored by body need, acidity, and reduction agents such as vitamins; hindered by binding agents, reduced gastric HCl, infection, gastrintestinal losses<br>Transported as transferrin, stored as ferritin or hemosiderin | Hemoglobin synthesis, oxygen transport<br>Cell oxidation, heme enzymes | Anemia (hypochromic, microcytic)<br>Excess: hemosiderosis, hemochromatosis<br>Growth and pregnancy needs | Adults:<br>men—10 mg,<br>women—15 mg<br>Pregnancy and lactation: 30 and 15 mg, respectively<br>Infants: 6-10 mg<br>Children: 10-12 mg | Liver, meats, eggs<br>Whole grains<br>Enriched breads and cereals<br>Dark green vegetables<br>Legumes, nuts<br>(Iron cookware) |
| Iodine (I) | Excreted in sloughed cells, bleeding<br>Absorbed as iodides, taken up by thyroid gland under control of thyroid-stimulating hormone<br>Excretion by kidney | Synthesis of thyroxin, which regulates cell metabolism, basal metabolic rate | Endemic colloid goiter, cretinism<br>Hypothyroidism and hyperthyroidism | Adults: 150 μg<br>Infants 40-50 μg<br>Children 70-150 μg | Iodized salt<br>Seafood |
| Zinc (Zn) | Absorbed with zinc-binding ligand from pancreas<br>Transported in blood by albumin; stored in many sites<br>Excretion largely intestinal | Essential coenzyme constituent; carbonic anhydrase, carboxypeptidase, lactic dehydrogenase | Growth: hypogonadism<br>Sensory impairment: taste and smell<br>Wound healing<br>Malabsorption disease | Adults:12-15 mg<br>Infants: 5 mg<br>Children: 10-15 mg | Widely distributed<br>Seafood, oysters<br>Liver, meat<br>Milk, cheese, eggs<br>Whole grains |
| Copper (Cu) | Absorbed with copper-binding protein metallothionein<br>Transported in blood by histidine and albumin<br>Stored in many tissues | Associated with iron in enzyme systems, hemoglobin synthesis<br>Metalloprotein enzyme constituent | Hypocupremia: nephrosis and malabsorption<br>Wilson's disease, excess copper storage<br>Menke's syndrome, kinky hair, discolored copper metabolism | Adults: 1.5-3 mg<br>Infants: 0.4-0.7 mg<br>Children: 0.7-2.5 mg | Widely distributed<br>Liver, meat<br>Seafood<br>Whole grains<br>Legumes, nuts<br>(Copper cookware) |

From Williams SR: *Nutrition and diet therapy,* ed 8, St Louis, 1997, Mosby.

Continued

## Summary of trace elements (required intake less than 100 mg/day)—cont'd

| Mineral | Metabolism | Physiologic functions | Clinical applications | Requirements | Food sources |
|---|---|---|---|---|---|
| Manganese (Mn) | Absorbed poorly<br>Excretion mainly by intestine | Enzyme component in general metabolism | Low serum levels in diabetes, protein-energy malnutrition<br>Inhalation toxicity | Adults: 2-5 mg<br>Infants: 0.3-1.0 mg<br>Children: 1-5 mg | Cereals, whole grains<br>Legumes, soybeans<br>Leafy vegetables |
| Chromium (Cr) | Absorbed in association with zinc<br>Excretion mainly by kidney | Associated with glucose metabolism; improves faulty glucose uptake by tissues; glucose tolerance factor | Potentiates action of insulin in persons with diabetes<br>Lowers serum cholesterol, LDL-cholesterol*<br>Increases HDL* | Adults: 50-200 $\mu$g<br>Infants: 10-60 $\mu$g<br>Children: 20-200 $\mu$g | Cereals<br>Whole grains<br>Brewer's yeast<br>Animal protein |
| Cobalt (Co) | Absorbed as component of food source, vitamin $B_{12}$<br>Elemental form shares transport with iron<br>Stored in liver | Constituent of vitamin $B_{12}$, functions with vitamin | Deficiency associated with deficiency of vitamin $B_{12}$ | Unknown; evidently minute | Vitamin $B_{12}$ source |
| Selenium (Se) | Absorption depends on solubility of compound form<br>Excreted mainly by kidney | Constituent of enzyme glutathione peroxidase<br>Synergistic antioxidant with vitamin E<br>Structural component of teeth | Marginal deficiency when soil content is low<br>Deficiency secondary to parenteral nutrition; malnutrition<br>Toxicity observed in livestock | Adults: 55-70 $\mu$g<br>Infants: 10-15 $\mu$g<br>Children: 20-50 $\mu$g | Varies with soil content<br>Seafood<br>Legumes<br>Whole grains<br>Low-fat meats and dairy products<br>Vegetables |
| Molybdenum (Mo) | Readily absorbed<br>Excreted rapidly by kidney<br>Small amount excreted in bile | Constituent of oxidase enzymes, xanthine oxidase | Deficiency unknown in humans | Adults: 75-250 $\mu$g<br>Infants: 15-30 $\mu$g<br>Children: 25-250 $\mu$g | Legumes<br>Whole grains<br>Milk<br>Organ meats<br>Leafy vegetables |
| Fluoride (F) | Absorption in small intestine; little known of bioavailability<br>Excreted by kidney—80% | Accumulates in bones and teeth, increasing hardness | Dental caries inhibited<br>Osteoporosis: may help control<br>Excess: dental fluorosis | Adults: 1.5-4 mg<br>Infants: 0.1-0.5 mg<br>Children: 0.5-2.5 mg | Fish<br>Fish products<br>Tea<br>Foods cooked in fluoridated water<br>Drinking water |

## 10-5 Daily dietary guide*

| Food group | Serving | Major contributions | Foods and serving sizes* |
|---|---|---|---|
| Milk, yogurt, and cheese | 2 (adult‖) <br> 3 (children, teens, young adults, and pregnant or lactating women) | Calcium <br> Riboflavin <br> Protein <br> Potassium <br> Zinc | 1 cup milk <br> 1½ oz cheese <br> 2 oz processed cheese <br> 1 cup yogurt <br> 2 cups cottage cheese <br> 1 cup custard/pudding <br> 1½ cups ice cream |
| Meat, poultry, fish, dry beans, eggs, and nuts | 2-3 | Protein <br> Niacin <br> Iron <br> Vitamin B-6 <br> Zinc <br> Thiamin <br> Vitamin B-12† | 2-3 oz cooked meat, poultry, fish <br> 1-1½ cups cooked dry beans <br> 4 T peanut butter <br> 2 eggs <br> ½-1 cup nuts |
| Fruits | 2-4 | Vitamin C <br> Fiber | ¼ cup dried fruit <br> ½ cup cooked fruit <br> ¾ cup juice <br> 1 whole piece of fruit <br> 1 melon wedge |
| Vegetables | 3-5 | Vitamin A <br> Vitamin C <br> Folate <br> Magnesium <br> Fiber | ½ cup raw or cooked vegetables <br> 1 cup raw leafy vegetables |
| Bread, cereals, rice, and pasta | 6-11 | Starch <br> Thiamin <br> Riboflavin§ <br> Iron <br> Niacin <br> Folate <br> Magnesium‡ <br> Fiber‡ <br> Zinc‡ | 1 slice of bread <br> 1 oz ready-to-eat cereal <br> ½-¾ cup cooked cereal, rice, or pasta |
| Fats, oils, and sweets | | Foods from this group should not replace any from the other groups. Amounts consumed should be determined by individual energy needs. | |

This is a practical way to turn the RDA into food choices. You can get all essential nutrients by eating a balanced variety of foods each day from the food groups listed here. Eat a variety of foods in each food group and adjust serving sizes appropriately to reach and maintain desirable weight.

---

*May be reduced for child servings.
†Only in animal food choices.
‡Whole grains especially.
§If enriched.
‖≥25 years of age.
Adapted from Williams SR: *Nutrition and diet therapy,* ed 8, St. Louis, 1997, Mosby.

# COMPLEMENTARY AND ALTERNATIVE MEDICINE

Complementary and alternative therapies increasingly are being used within the context of mainstream medicine. Various forms of complementary and alternative medicine (CAM) are practiced by health care professionals who offer therapies in relaxation, imagery, massage, and therapeutic touch to their patients.[1] It is important for health care professionals to know about CAM, to inquire about CAM therapies patients may be using, and to incorporate appropriate therapies into the plan of care of the patient.

The major categories of CAM are mind-body interventions, bioelectromagnetic applications, manual healing methods, pharmacologic and biologic treatments, diet and nutrition, other diagnostic and treatment methods, and alternative systems of medical practice. Under each of these major categories there are several CAM therapies, which are described throughout this appendix. It is important to remember that, in essence, the use of these therapies is not mutually exclusive with mainstream medicine, and in fact the patient may have a better outcome when a combination of therapies is used.[8]

## MIND-BODY INTERVENTIONS
### Art therapy

Art therapy involves the use of art media to lead an individual toward neutralization of conflict through sublimation or as a vehicle to moderate symbolic speech and move the individual toward verbalization of inner conflicts. Art therapy is often used when traditional forms of verbal psychotherapy have failed or have been rejected by an individual and when individuals have difficulty expressing feelings or use verbalization as a defense mechanism.[8]

American Art Therapy Association
1202 Allanson Rd.
Mundelein, IL 60060-3808
Phone: 888-290-0878
Phone: 847-949-6064
Fax: 847-566-4580

British Columbia Art Therapy Association
Suite 101
1001 West Broadway
Dept. 123
Vancouver, B.C.
Canada V6H 4E4
Phone: 604-878-6393

### Biofeedback

Biofeedback is a therapy in which sensors are placed on the body to measure muscle responses, heart rate, sweat responses, or neural activity. Information is provided by visual-auditory or body-muscle cell activation teaching to either increase or decrease physiologic activity to improve health problems (e.g., pain, anxiety, or high blood pressure).[10]

Association for Applied Psychophysiology and Biofeedback (AAPB)
10200 W. 44th Avenue, Suite 304
Wheat Ridge, CO 80033-2840
Phone: 303-422-8436
Fax: 303-422-8894

Biofeedback Certification Institute of America (BCIA)
10200 W. 44th Avenue, #310
Wheat Ridge, CO 80033
Phone: 303-420-2902
Fax: 303-422-8894

### Dance/movement therapy

Dance/movement therapy is a movement-based technique that aids in promoting feeling and awareness. The goal is to integrate body, mind, and self-esteem. This therapy uses different parts of the body, such as fingers, wrists, and arms, to respond to music.[10]

### Hypnotherapy

Selective attention is used in hypnotherapy to induce a specific altered state (trance) for memory retrieval, relaxation, or suggestion. This therapy is often used to alter habits (e.g., smoking, obesity), treat biologic mechanisms such as hypertension or cardiac arrhythmias, deal with the symptoms of a disease, alter an individual's reaction to disease, and affect an illness and its course through the body.[8]

### Interactive guided imagery

The focus of interactive guided imagery is on the target visual stimulus to produce a specific physiologic change that can promote healing. Imagery is effective in almost all of the major physiologic systems of the body, including respiration, heart rate, blood pressure, metabolic rates in cells, gastrointestinal mobility and secretion, sexual function, cortisol levels, blood lipids, and immune responsiveness.[8]

### Meditation

Meditation is an intentional self-regulation of posture, concentration, contemplation, and visualization to attenuate stress reactivity, affect neuroendocrine function, enhance a sense of control or self-efficacy, and prevent relapse for disorders such as chronic pain and anxiety.[8]

### Music therapy

The use of music, either in an active or in a passive mode, can be effective in helping individuals improve receptive communication, express or communicate feelings, reduce stress, enhance relaxation or pain management, improve perceptual-motor coordination, and improve socialization. Other types of vibratory sounds can be used, mainly to reduce stress, anxiety, and pain.[10]

American Music Therapy Association (AMTA)
8455 Colesville Road, Suite 1000
Silver Spring, MD 20910
Phone: 301-589-3300
Fax: 301-589-5175

Canadian Association for Music Therapy
Waterloo
Ontario, N2L 3C5
Canada
Phone: 800 996 CAMT
Fax: 519.884.8853

### Neurolinguistic programming

Neurolinguistic programming is the study of the structure of subjective experience, or how we make sense of our experiences and construct our mental world. The intent is to give individuals more choices in their own frames of reference. It can be used for various psychosomatic conditions, behavior-modification treatment, or stress management.[8]

### Poetry therapy

Poetry therapy is also called *bibliotherapy* and is the intentional use of poetry and other forms of literature for healing and personal growth. This therapy enables individuals to express what they may be unable to say in other ways and is used within individual, marital, and family psychotherapy formats.[8]

### Qi gong

Qi gong is a form of Chinese exercise-stimulation therapy that proposes to improve health by redirecting mental focus, breathing, coordination, and relaxation. The goal is to rebalance the body's own healing capacities by activating proposed electrical or energetic currents that flow along meridians located throughout the body. These meridians do not follow conventional nerve or muscle pathways. In Chinese medical training and practice, this therapy includes "external Qi," which is energy transmitted from one person to another for the purpose of healing. Qi Gong has been effective in the management of chronic illness (e.g., hypertension, asthma, allergies, chronic fatigue, fibromyalgia, diabetes, arthritis), wellness promotion, stress management, terminal illness as palliation, gastrointestinal conditions, musculoskeletal pains and sports injuries, tension headaches, colds and influenza, and tinnitus.[8,10]

National Qi Gong (Chi Kung) Association
P.O. Box 540
Ely, MN 55731
Phone: 218-365-6330
Fax: 218-365-6933

### Relaxation therapies

The relaxation therapies include lighter levels of altered states of consciousness through indirect or direct refocusing techniques, conscious breathing, and body awareness. These techniques are applicable for the stresses of everyday living, particularly stress disorders (e.g., anxiety and panic disorders), adjustment disorders, and addictions. Relaxation is also used for chronic illnesses of all kinds, including headache, irritable bowel syndrome, peptic ulcer disease, inflammatory bowel disease, hypertension, arrhythmias, coronary artery disease, and musculoskeletal pain/joint disorders.[8]

### Spiritual healing and prayer

Prayers are offered to a higher being or authority to reduce stress, promote healing, or arrest disease. Spiritual healing may be practiced by the individual patient, by groups, or by others with or without the patient's knowledge.[10]

### Tai chi

Tai chi is a technique that uses slow, purposeful, motor-physical movements of the body for the purpose of control to increase outer body mass strength and achieve a more balanced physiologic and psychologic state. Tai chi has positive effects on the respiratory, cardiovascular, and cerebral functions in both children and older adults, including reducing the incidence of falls in older people.[8,10]

### Yoga

Yoga involves the integration of posture and controlled breathing, relaxation, meditation, or a combination thereof. Hatha yoga involves physical exercise, breathing practices, and movement designed to have a salutary effect on posture, flexibility, and strength for the ultimate purpose of preparing the body to remain still for long periods of meditation. Raja yoga includes all of the other forms of yoga practice. The practitioner is instructed to follow moral directives, physical exercises, breathing exercises, meditation, devotion, and service to others to facilitate religious awakening. Yoga techniques have been effective in regulating heart rate, blood pressure, circulation, and digestion, as well as in healing chronic back pain, menstrual problems, carpal tunnel syndrome, and respiratory disease.

American Yoga Association
P.O. Box 19986
Sarasota, FL 34276
Phone: 941-927-4977
Fax: 941-921-9844

## BIOELECTROMAGNETIC APPLICATIONS
### Color therapy

With color therapy the wavelengths of the energy of light are used to assist the body in self-healing. This is often used as a complementary treatment for seasonal affective disorder, depression, and stress.[8]

### Diathermy

*Diathermy* refers to the use of high-frequency electrical currents as a form of physical therapy and in surgical procedures. The three forms of diathermy used by physical therapists are short-wave, ultrasound, and microwave.[10]

### Light therapy

Natural light or light of specified wavelengths is used to treat disease. This may include ultraviolet light, colored light, or low-intensity laser light. The eye is generally the initial entry point for the light because of its direct connection to the brain through the retinal hypothalamic pathway, which affects the autonomic nervous system and endocrine function. It has been used primarily for attention deficit disorders, cataracts, conjunctivitis, headaches, head trauma, hyperactivity, lazy eye, macular degeneration, migraine, night blindness, poor eyesight, stroke, and vision disorders. Secondarily, light therapy has been effective in treating eczema, fever, psoriasis, addictions, allergies, anxiety, autism, bronchitis, childbirth, glaucoma, insomnia, muscle spasm, premenstrual syndrome, stress, and strep throat. Light therapy complements many other treatments for these and other conditions.[8,10]

### Magnetic field therapy

Magnets are placed directly on the skin, stimulating living cells and increasing blood flow by ionic currents created from polarities on the magnets. Trigger points for magnets are acupuncture points where the action of the magnets serves to activate the tendinomuscular system to readily and widely transmit electrical stimuli. Magnets also increase tissue oxygen perfusion by decreasing vascular resistance, decreasing nerve cell firing, and stimulating various cellular structures (e.g., changes in calcium channels, sodium-potassium pump, RNA/DNA production, conversion of adenosine triphosphate to adenosine diphosphate, removal of oxygen and water from the cell, and stimulation of cyclic adenosine monophosphate). Common physiologic responses include vasodilation, analgesia, antiinflammatory action, spasmolytic activity, accelerated healing, and antiedema activity.[8,10]

### Neuroelectric therapy

Transcranial, cranial neuroelectric, or transcutaneous electric nerve stimulation (TENS) was initially used in the 1950s to treat insomnia. In a typical TENS session, surface electrodes are placed in the mastoid region (behind the ear) and, similar to electroacupuncture, are stimulated using a low-amperage, low-frequency alternating current. The action may stimulate endogenous neurotransmitters such as endorphins that produce symptomatic relief.[10]

## MANUAL HEALING METHODS
### Chiropractic

Chiropractic relies on adjustment of the spinal column to improve health or arrest disease through both stimulation and body manipulation. Treatment is achieved by applying controlled and directed forces to adjust the affected joint to alter, restore, and preserve musculoskeletal function and alleviate symptoms.[8] Doctors of chiropractic (DC) are licensed to perform this technique.

American Chiropractic Association (ACA)
1701 Clarendon Blvd
Arlington, VA 22209
Phone: 800-986-4636
Fax: 703-243-2593

Canadian Chiropractic Association
1396 Eglinton Avenue West
Toronto, Ontario
M6C 2E4
Canada
Phone: 416-781-5656
Phone: 800-668-2076
Fax: 416-781-7344

Chiropractors' Association of Australia (National) Limited
Suite 4
148 Station Street
Penrith NSW 2750
AUSTRALIA
PO Box 6246
South Penrith DC NSW 2750
Australia
Phone: 02-4731-8011
Fax: 02-4731-8088

Federation of Chiropractic Licensing Boards
901 54th Avenue, Suite 101
Greeley, CO 80634-4400
Phone: 970-356-3500
FAX: 970-356-3599

Foundation for Chiropractic Education and Research
P.O. Box 4689
Des Moines, IA 50306-4689
Phone: 800-622-6309

Idaho Association of Chiropractic Physicians
P.O. Box 1863
Boise, ID 83701
Phone: 208-377-4579
Fax: 208-377-3492

International Chiropractic Pediatric Association
5295 Highway 78, Suite #D362
Stone Mountain, GA 30087-3414
Phone: 770-982-9037
Fax: 770-736-1651

International Chiropractors Association
1110 N. Glebe Rd., Suite 1000
Arlington, VA 22201
Phone: 800-423-4690
Phone: 703-528-5000
Fax: 703-528-5023

International Federation of Sports Chiropractic
Chemin de la Joliette 5
CH-1006 Lausanne
Switzerland
Phone: 41 21 617-2933
Fax.: 41 21 617-3016

National Association for Chiropractic Medicine
15427 Baybrook Drive
Houston, TX 77062
Phone: 281-280-8262
Fax: 281-280-8262

Washington State Chiropractic Association
21400 Int'l Blvd. #207
SeaTac, WA 98198
Phone: 206-878-6055

## Osteopathic medicine

Osteopathic medicine is founded on basic principles of body unity, self-regulation, and the interrelationship of structure and function. Disease indicates a breakdown in the body's capacity for self-regulation. Osteopathic physicians, or Doctors of Osteopathy (DOs), use palpatory diagnosis and osteopathic manipulation to treat related somatic problems; however, they are complete and licensed physi-

cians who can practice in all areas of medicine and surgery, with the majority holding hospital staff privileges.[8]

American Association of Colleges of Osteopathic Medicine (AACOM)
5550 Friendship Blvd, Suite 310
Chevy Chase, MD 20815-7231
Phone: 301-968-4100

Australian Osteopathic Association
PO Box 242
Thornleigh NSW 2120
Australia
Phone: 61 2 9440 2511
Fax: 61 2 9440 9962

## Massage therapy

Massage therapy relies on soft tissue manipulation through stroking, kneading, friction, and vibration to improve health and provide comfort.

American Massage Therapy Association (AMTA)
820 Davis St.
Evanston, IL 60201
Phone: 847-864-0123
Fax: 847-864-1178

Associated Bodywork & Massage Professionals
1271 Sugarbush Drive
Evergreen, CO 80439-9766
Phone: 800-458-2267
Phone: 303-674-8478
Fax: 303-674-0859

National Association of Nurse Massage Therapists
2203 Woodridge Court
Grand Island, NE
68801 Phone: 800-262-4017

Nurse Touch & Massage Therapy Association International
1438 Shortcut, Suite E
Slidell, LA 70458
Phone: 504-893-8002
Fax: 504-892-3493

## Bodywork
*Alexander technique*

The Alexander technique is a bodywork technique in which rebalancing of "postural sets" (i.e., physical alignment) is taught by mentally focusing on the way correct alignments should look and feel and through verbal and tactile guidance by the practitioner.[8]

Alexander Technique International
1692 Massachusetts Ave, 3rd floor
Cambridge, MA 02138
Phone: 888-668-8996 (Canada and USA)
Phone: 617-497-2242
Fax: 617-497-2615

American Society for the Alexander Technique
P.O. Box 60008
Florence, MA 01062
Phone: 800-473-0620
Phone: 413-584-2359

Society of Teachers of the Alexander Technique
129 Camden Mews
London
NW1 9AH
UK
Phone: 44 020 7284 3338
Fax: 44 020 7482 5435

### Aston-patterning

Aston-Patterning is a bodywork technique to accommodate asymmetry and individual uniqueness of the human body to match human function to the environment. Appropriate alignment of the body provides the human structure with its most optimal support and adds the dynamic quality that facilitates motion. Alignment can be threatened by accidents, illnesses, or surgeries, and movement patterns are taught to include the asymmetric pattern rather than allowing a tension pattern to develop. This technique has been applied to fitness training and ergonomic and product design.[8]

### Bowen technique

The Bowen technique is a system of gentle but powerful soft tissue mobilizations using the thumbs and fingers over muscles, tendons, nerves, and fascia to restore the self-healing mechanism of the body. This technique has been used for conditions affecting the musculoskeletal system, including back, neck, hip, and shoulder pain.[8]

Bowen Research & Training Institute
P.O. Box 627
Palm Harbor, FL 34682
Phone: 727-937-9077
Fax: 727-942-9687

### Craniosacral therapy

Craniosacral therapy is a form of gentle manual manipulation used for diagnosis and for making corrections in a system made up of cerebrospinal fluid, cranial and dural membranes, cranial bones, and sacrum. This system is proposed to be dynamic with its own physiologic frequency. Through touch and pressure, tension is supposed to be reduced and cranial rhythms normalized, leading to improvement in health and disease.[8]

Craniosacral Therapy Association of the UK
Monomark House
27 Old Gloucester Street,
London WC1N 3XX
England
Phone: 07000 784 735

### FeldenKrais method

The FeldenKrais method is a bodywork technique in which its founder used the integration of physics, judo, and yoga. The practitioner directs sequences of movement using verbal or hands-on techniques or teaches a system of self-directed exercises to treat physical impairments through the learning of new movement patterns.[8]

### Hellerwork Structural integration

The Hellerwork structural integration is a bodywork technique that consists of deep pressure on soft tissues to improve alignment, movement reeducation to avoid unnecessary stress on the body structure, and dialogue with a practitioner to enhance the individual's awareness of how attitude affects structure and movement pattern.[8]

### Pilates method

Pilates method is a gentle but focused exercise-based system that tones, stretches, and strengthens the body in a nonimpact, balanced system of body-mind exercise and mobilizes the body to move with maximal efficiency and minimum effort. Classes include mat work and use of equipment designed to provide resistance against tensioned springs to isolate and develop specific muscle groups. This method can achieve an improvement of body alignment and breathing, increased body awareness, and efficient and graceful movement.

### Bonnie Prudden myotherapy

Bonnie Prudden Myotherapy is a method of applying manual pressure on muscles with the fingers, knuckles, and elbows to defuse trigger points and relax muscle spasm, improve circulation, and alleviate pain.[8]

### Polarity therapy

In polarity therapy there is a hands-on manipulation of bone, soft tissue, and energy points as well as vegetarian, nutritional, and attitudinal counseling. Specific stretching exercises using sound and movement remove energy blockages and restore the individual to balance and optimal health.[8]

American Polarity Therapy Association (APTA)
PO Box 19858
Boulder, CO 80308
Phone: 303-545-2080
Fax: 303-545-2161

### Reflexology

Reflexology is a bodywork technique that uses reflex points on the hands and feet. Pressure is applied at points that correspond to various body parts with the intention of eliminating blockages thought to produce pain or disease. The goal is to bring the body into balance.[10]

Association of Reflexologists
27 Old Gloucester Street
London
WC1N 3XX
England
Phone: 0870 5673320

### Reiki

Reiki is based on the Japanese word meaning "universal life force energy." The practitioner serves as a conduit for healing energy directed into the body or energy field of the recipient without physical contact with the body.[10]

### Rolfing structural integration

Rolfing is a bodywork technique that involves the myofascia. The body is realigned by using the hands to apply a deep pressure and friction that allows more efficient posture, movement, and the release of emotions from the body.[10]

### Rosen method

In the Rosen method, movement exercises are designed to move all of the joints in the body through their available range of motion and expand the chest to free up breathing capacity.[8]

### Therapeutic touch

Therapeutic touch is a body energy-field technique in which hands are passed over the body without actually touching to recreate and change proposed "energy imbalances" for restoring innate healing forces. Verbal interaction between patient and therapist helps to maximize effects.[10]

Healing Touch International
12477 W. Cedar Drive, Suite #202
Lakewood, CO 80228
Phone: 303-989-7982
Fax: 303-980-8683

### Trager approach

The Trager approach is a bodywork technique in which the practitioner enters a meditative state and guides the client through gentle, light, rhythmic nonintrusive movements. Mentastics, or movement education, exercises using self-healing movements are taught to clients.[8]

## PHARMACOLOGIC AND BIOLOGIC TREATMENTS
### Antineoplastons

Antineoplastons are naturally occurring peptides, amino acid derivatives, and carboxylic acids proposed to control neoplastic cell growth using the patient's own biochemical defense system, which works jointly with the immune system.[10]

## Chelation therapy

Chelation therapy involves the intravenous infusion of a chelating agent-synthetic amino acid ethylenediaminetetraacetic acid (EDTA)- of metal, toxins, lead, mercury, nickel, copper, cadmium, and plaque to treat certain diseases (e.g., cardiovascular). Ancillary treatments include the use of vitamins, changes in diet, and exercise.[10]

## Enzyme therapy

Enzyme therapy involves the use of enzymes to catalyze chemical reactions. Enzymes can accelerate the progress of inflammation necessary for healing, with some products useful in cases of trauma, acute and chronic inflammation, emboli, thrombosis, viral infections, and cancer. Proteolytic enzymes are used for wound debridement (i.e., collagenase, fibrinolysin; desoxyribonuclease ). Other enzymes are used to digest fibrin or blood clots, (i.e., streptokinase), and others are used as chemotherapeutic agents.[8]

## Flower essences

Derived from a flower, tree, bush, or water source, essences are used to address spiritual, mental, and emotional as well as physical problems.[8]

## Herbal medicine

Herbal medicine is the use of medicinal products containing as active ingredients exclusively plant material and/or vegetable drug preparations used to treat various health conditions. Herbal medicine (phytotherapy) is a major form of treatment for more than 70% of the world's population[6,8] (see Appendix 12).

American Botanical Council (ABC)
P.O. Box 144345
Austin, TX 78714-4345
Phone: 512-926-4900
Fax: 512-926-2345

American Herbal Pharmacopoeia
Box 5159
Santa Cruz, CA 95063
Phone: 831-461-6317
Fax: 831-475-6219

American Herbal Products Association (AHPA)
8484 Georgia Ave., Suite 370
Silver Spring, MD 20910
Phone: 301-588-1171
Fax: 301-588-1174

American Herbalists Guild
1931 Gaddis Road
Canton, GA 30115
Phone: 770-751-6021
Fax: 770-751-7472

The European Scientific Cooperative on Phytotherapy (ESCOP)
ESCOP Secretariat
Argyle House
Gandy Street, Exeter
Devon EX4 3LS
UK
Phone: 44 1392 424626
Fax: 44 1392 424864

Herb Research Foundation
1007 Pearl Street, Suite 200
Boulder, CO 80302
Phone: 303-449-2265
Fax: 303-449-7849

Herb Society of America
9019 Kirtland Chardon Rd
Kirtland, OH 44094
Ph: 440-256-0514
Fax: 440-256-0541

National Herbalist Association of Australia
Attn. The Secretary
P.O. Box 65
Kingsgrove, N.S.W. 2208
Australia
Phone: 61 2 5022938
Fax: 61 2 5543459

## Hyperthermia

Hyperthermia involves the use of various heating methods, such as electromagnetic therapy, to produce temperature elevations of a few degrees in cells and tissues, leading to a proposed antitumor effect. This is often used in conjunction with radiotherapy or chemotherapy for cancer treatment.[10]

## Immunoaugmentative therapy

Immunoaugmentative therapy, a cancer treatment, proposes that cancer cells can be arrested by the use of four different blood proteins. This approach is also proposed to restore the immune system and can be used as an adjunctive therapy.[10]

## Phytotherapy

Phytotherapy involves the use of plants for medicinal purposes (same as herbal medicine).[6]

# DIET AND NUTRITION
## Macronutrients

Proteins, fats, and carbohydrates are macronutrients. These nutrients can help to improve almost every acute and chronic disease.[8]

## Micronutrients

Vitamins and minerals are micronutrients. In the presence of inadequate nutrient intake, the provision of supplemental vitamins and minerals, as well as intake above the recommended daily allowance (RDA) of some nutrients (megavitamins), can reduce the risk of illness.[8]

## Oxidative stress

In oxidative stress the use of antioxidant intake in the diet may provide both preventive and therapeutic advantage and reduce the damaging effects of free radicals on cellular constituents.[8]

## Orthomolecular medicine

Orthomolecular medicine is a therapeutic approach that uses naturally occurring substances within the body, such as proteins, fat, and water, that promote restoration, balance, or both by using vitamins, minerals, or other forms of nutrition to subsequently treat disease, promote healing, or both.[10]

International Society for Orthomolecular Medicine
16 Florence Avenue
Toronto, Ontario
Canada M2N 1E9
Phone: 416-733-2117
Fax: 416-733-2352

## Nutritional oncology and integrative cancer care

The Bristol Cancer Help Center (BCHC) diet is a stringent diet of raw and partly and cooked vegetables with proteins from soy. It is claimed to enhance the quality of life and attitude toward illness in cancer patients.[10]

# OTHER DIAGNOSTIC AND TREATMENT METHODS
## Acupressure

In acupressure, manual pressure is applied at specific points on the body located along channels of energy. Shiatsu is a Japanese form of acupressure involving finger pressure at specific points on the body, mainly for the purpose of balancing energy in the body. The major focus is on prevention (i.e., keeping the body healthy), but this technique is also used to relieve common ailments and tensions, including sinus problems, shoulder and neck pain, back spasm, chronic fatigue, fibromyalgia, muscular tension, temporomandibular joint syndrome, and general aches and pains.[8]

**American Organization for Bodywork Therapies of Asia (AOBTA)**
1010 Haddonfield-Berlin Road
Suite 408
Voorhees, NJ 08043
Phone: 856-782-1616
Fax: 856-782-1653

## Acupuncture

Thin needles are inserted superficially on the skin at locations throughout the body. Points are located along meridians or channels of energy. Heat can also be applied by burning (moxibustion) or electric current (electroacupuncture). Healing is proposed by the restoration of a balance of energy flow called *Qi*. Another explanation suggests that the stimulation activates endorphin receptors. Acupuncture is highly effective in treating both acute and chronic pain associated with multiple causes. In addition, some common conditions are effectively treated; these include sinusitis, allergies, tinnitus, sore throats, high blood pressure, gastroesophageal reflex, hyperacidity and peptic ulcer disease, constipation, diarrhea, spastic colon, urinary incontinence, bladder and kidney infection, premenstrual syndrome (PMS), infertility, dysmenorrhea, memory problems, sensory disturbances, depression, anxiety, and other psychologic disorders.[8,10]

**Acupuncture and Oriental Medicine Alliance (Acupuncture Alliance)**
14637 Starr Road Southeast
Olalla, WA 98359
Phone: 253-851-6896
Fax: 253-851-6883

**Acupuncture Association of Chartered Physiotherapists (AACP) UK**
AACP Secretariat
Mere Complementary Practice
Castle Street
Mere
Wiltshire, BA12 6JE
UK
Phone: 01747 861151
Fax: 01747 861717

**Acupuncture Association of Washington**
PO Box 2271
Gig Harbor, WA 98335-4271
Phone: 253-851-4756

**Acupuncture Foundation of Canada (AFC)**
2131 Lawrence Avenue East, Suite 204
Scarborough, Ontario, M1R 5G4

**American Academy of Medical Acupuncture (AAMA)**
4929 Wiltshire Boulevard, Suite 428
Los Angeles, CA 90010
Phone: 323-937-5514

**American Academy of Veterinary Acupuncture (AAVA)**
Box 419
Hygiene, CO 80533-0419
Phone: 303-772-6726

**American Association of Acupuncture and Bioenergetic Medicine (AAABEM)**
2512 Manoa Road
Honolulu, HI 96822
Phone: 808-946-2069
Fax: 808-946-0378

**Association Europe Acupuncture**
167 Rue de la Convention
75015 Paris
France
Phone/Fax: 33 0 1 58 45 13 74

**Australian Acupuncture and Chinese Medicine Association Ltd.**
PO Box 5142
West End QLD 4101
Australia
Phone: 07 3846 5866
Fax: 07 3846 5276

**British Acupuncture Accreditation Board**
Suite D
206-208 Latimer Road
London W10 6RE
England
Phone/Fax: 0181 968 3469

**British Acupuncture Council**
63 Jeddo Road
London W12 9HQ
UK
Phone: +44 0 20 8735 0400
Fax: +44 0 20 8735 0404

**British Medical Acupuncture Society**
12 Marbury House
Higher Whitley
Warrington, Cheshire, WA4 4QW
UK
Phone: 01925 730727
Fax: 01925 730492

**Chinese Medicine and Acupuncture Association of Canada**
154 Wellington St.
London, Ontario
Canada N6B 2K8
Phone: 519-642-1970
Fax: 519-642-2932

**The Foundation for Traditional Chinese Medicine**
122A Acomb Road
York YO2 4EY
UK
Phone: 01904 785120 / 784828

**Illinois State Acupuncture Association**
1525 E. 53rd Street, Suite 705
Chicago, IL 60615
Phone: 773-363-0370
Fax: 773-955-9953

**International Council of Medical Acupuncture and Related Techniques**
American Division
800 Riverside Drive (8-1)
New York, NY 10032
Phone: 212-781-6262
Fax: 212-923-2279

**Maine Association of Acupuncture and Oriental Medicine**
PO Box 2131
South Portland, ME 04106

**National Certification Committee for Acupuncture and Oriental Medicine**
11 Canal Center Plaza, Suite 300
Alexandria, VA 22314
Phone: 703-548-9004
Fax: 703-548-9079

## Applied kinesiology

This form of treatment uses nutrition, physical manipulation, vitamins, diets, and exercise to restore and energize the body. Weak muscles are proposed to be a source of dysfunctional health.[8]

American Academy of Kinesiology and Physical Education
P.O. Box 5076
Champaign, IL 61820-2200
Phone: 800-747-4457
Phone: 217-351-5076
Fax: 217-351-2674

International College of Applied Kinesiology
6405 Metcalf Ave, Suite 503
Shawnee Mission, KS 66202-3929
Phone: 913-384-5336
Fax: 913-384-5112

## Aromatherapy

Aromatherapy is a form of herbal medicine that uses various oils from plants. Route of administration can be through absorption in the skin or inhalation. The action of antiviral and antibacterial agents is proposed to aid healing. The aromatic biochemical structures of certain herbs are thought to act in areas of the brain related to past experiences and emotions (e.g., limbic system).[10]

Aromatherapy Trade Council
PO Box 387
Ipswich IP2 9AN
UK
Phone/Fax: 01473 603 630

International Federation of Aromatherapists—Australia
PO Box 2210
Central Park, VIC 3145
Australia

International Federation of Aromatherapists—United Kingdom
182 Chiswick High Road
London W4 1PP
UK
Phone: 44 0 20 8742 2605/6

International Society of Professional Aromatherapists
82 Ashby Rd
Hinckley, Leics, LE10 1SN
UK
Phone: 01455 637987
Fax: 01455 890956

National Association for Holistic Aromatherapy
2000 2nd Avenue, Suite 206
Seattle, WA 98121
Phone: 206-256-0741
Fax: 206-770-5915

Register of Qualified Aromatherapists
P.O. Box 3431
Danbury, Chelmsford
Essex CM3 4UA
UK
Phone: 01245 227957
Fax: 01245 222152

## Biologic dentistry

Alternative or complementary dentistry may also be called *environmental, biocompatible,* or *holistic dentistry.* The concern is about the effect that dentistry may have on the overall health of an individual. The mouth is treated as a part of the human body, and dental care and dental health cannot be separated from the body and its influence on systemic health. When amalgams that contain mercury are replaced with nonmercury restoratives, the patient becomes "mercury-free."[8]

Holistic Dental Association
P.O. Box 5007
Durango, CO 81301
Fax: 970-259-1091

## Colon hydrotherapy

Colon hydrotherapy is an extended and more complete form of an enema as well as a safe and effective method of removing waste from the large intestine without using drugs. Colon hydrotherapy is used as a treatment for constipation or impaction, as a preparation for diagnostic studies of the large intestine (barium enema, sigmoidoscopy, or colonoscopy), and as a preparation for or after surgery. The procedure is also used for bowel training for paraplegics or quadriplegics, people with arthritis, and patients who have suspected autointoxication or intestinal toxemia.[8]

## Detoxification therapy

Cleansing of the body through nutritional action, centering on gastrointestinal function, characterizes detoxification therapy. It is used to assist in the transition from an unhealthy lifestyle to a healthier one by an improved selection of nutrients and elimination of some modern-day abuses, specifically, sugar, nicotine, alcohol, caffeine, and chemicals, often referred to *SNACCs.*[8]

## Environmental medicine

Environmental medicine involves a practice of medicine in which the major focus is on cause-and-effect relationships in health. Evaluations are made of factors such as eating and living habits and types of air breathed. Testing in the patient's own environment is performed to determine what precipitators are present that may be related to disease or other health problems. A treatment protocol is developed from this information.[10]

American Academy of Environmental Medicine
7701 East Kellogg, Suite 625
Wichita, KS 67207
Phone: 316-684-5500
Fax 316-684-5709

## Fasting

Fasting involves the elimination of foods with the addition of fluids such as mineral water, herbal and fruit teas, broth, and fruit juices for a limited period of time as a component of detoxification. This therapy requires the supervision of a health professional experienced in this form of therapy.[8]

## Juice therapy

In juice therapy, concentrated nutritional elixirs of fruit extracts and vegetables are used for nutritional maintenance, illness prevention, detoxification, and adjunctive treatment of allergies, digestive disorders, rheumatoid arthritis, skin diseases, and other conditions such as hypotension and hypertension, bronchitis, obesity, and insomnia.[8]

## Iridology

Iridology is the process of identifying certain problems or abnormalities occurring in the human body through indications shown in the iris of the eye, well before the appearance of clinical symptoms. This is also referred to as *iris diagnosis.*[8]

## Quartz crystal therapy

Quartz crystal therapy involves placement of a four- or six-sided quartz crystal over a chakra, or major energy station, of the body such as the brow, throat, heart, stomach, abdomen, base of the spine, or near the skull to act as a de-stressor and to support the immune system.[8]

## ALTERNATIVE SYSTEMS OF MEDICAL PRACTICE
### Professionalized health care systems
*Ayurveda*

Ayurveda is a major health-care system that emphasizes a preventive approach to health, focusing on an inner state of harmony and spiritual realization for self-healing. It includes special types of diets, herbs, and mineral parts and changes based on a system of constitutional categories in lifestyle. Enemas and purgation are used to cleanse the body of excess toxins. Ayurveda emphasizes lifestyle analysis and change as the most significant aspects of the healing process.[10]

Jiva Ayurvedic Research Institute
1144, Sector 19
Faridabad Harayana
India
Phone: 91 29 529 6174
Fax: 91 129 529 5547

*Homeopathy*

Homeopathy is a form of treatment in which substances (minerals, plant extracts, chemicals, or disease-producing germs), which in sufficient doses would produce a set of illness symptoms in healthy individuals, are given in microdoses to produce a "cure" of those same symptoms. The symptom is not thought to be part of the illness but rather part of a curative process. Homeopathy works by activating the self-healing capacity of the individual.[10]

American Institute of Homeopathy (AIH)
801 N. Fairfax St., Suite 306
Alexandria, VA 22314
Phone: 703-246-9501

British Homeopathic Association
15 Clerkenwell Close
London EC1R 0AA
England
Phone: 020 7566 7800
Fax: 020 7566 7815

European Committee for Homeopathy
Chaussée de Bruxelles 132, box 1
1190 Brussels
Belgium
Phone: 32-2-3453597
Fax: 32-2-3461826

Homeopathic Medical Association
6 Livingstone Rd
Gravesend. Kent
DA12 5DZ
UK
Phone: 01474 560336
Fax: 01474 327431

National Center for Homeopathy
801 N. Fairfax Street, Suite 306
Alexandria, VA 22314
Phone: 877-624-0613
Phone: 703-548-7790
Fax: 703-548-7792

North American Society of Homeopaths
1122 East Pike Street, #1122
Seattle, WA 98122
Phone: 206-720-7000
Fax: 206-329-5684

*Naturopathic medicine*

The basic philosophic premise of naturopathic medicine is that there is an inherent healing power in nature and in every human being.[9] This major health system includes practices that emphasize diet, nutrition, homeopathy, and various mind-body therapies. Emphasis is placed on self-healing and treatment through changes in lifestyle and the use of prevention techniques that promote health. Naturopathic doctors (NDs) are licensed in about one quarter of all states in the United States.[9,10]

American Association of Naturopathic Physicians (AANP)
8201 Greensboro Drive, Suite 300
McLean, VA 22102
Phone: 703-610-9037
Fax: 703-610-9005

American Naturopathic Medical Association (ANMA)
P.O. Box 96273
Las Vegas, NV 89193
Phone: 702-897-7053
Fax: 702-897-7140

American Naturopathic Medical Certification & Accreditation Board (ANCAB)
Phone: 702-897-4915

Canadian College of Naturopathic Medicine
Phone: 416-498-1255
Fax: 416-498-1576

Council on Naturopathic Medical Education
P.O. Box 11426
Eugene, OR 97440-3626
Phone: 541-484-6028

**Community-based health care systems**
*Oriental medical practices*

Oriental medical practices are ancient forms of medicine that focus on prevention and secondarily treat disease, with an emphasis on maintaining balance through the body by stimulating a constant, smooth-flowing Qi energy. Herbs, acupuncture, massage, diet, and exercise are also used.[8]

*Traditional Chinese herbal medicine*

Herbs are used to treat various health conditions, including chronic or acute pain, allergies, menopausal issues, arthritis, stress, fatigue, and digestive disorders. Herbs are also used to promote optimal well-being and prevent disease by strengthening resistance and the immune system.[8]

*Traditional medicine in Latin America*

Traditional Latin American medicine is an ethnomedical system representing many healing practices throughout Latin America. In Mexico it is known as curanderismo. This system of medicine combines various theoretical elements into a holistic approach to illness. The etiology of illness is framed in terms of imbalance, which can be between hot and cold in the body, between parts of the body, between patients and the social environment, or between patients and the spiritual realm. These illnesses can be treated by curanderismo and biomedicine, but only the curandero can treat supernatural ailments. This system has been used to treat susto (fear), believed to cause the soul to become dislodged from the body, resulting in illness; empacho, a gastrointestinal disorder believed to be caused by blockage in the stomach or intestine; and mal de ojo (evil eye), characterized by fever, irritability, headache, and weeping, generally affecting children.[8]

*Native American medicine*

Therapies used by many Native American Indian tribes include their own healing herbs and ceremonies that use components with a spiritual emphasis. This type of medicine is the opposite of science and focuses on the heart of spirit and the acknowledgment that the spirit, mind, and emotions all have interplay with the environment. An individual's connection to Nature and Mother Earth and communion with the spirit world is either in or out of harmony. The unique energies of the eight directions of the medicine wheel, as well as the sky, sun, moon, and earth, all play an integral part in Native American cosmology. Symptoms of illness are seen as connected with the spirit, and energy is then used as a catalyst to help patients come back into harmony.[8,10] There are several forms of therapy, which include the following: sweat lodge ceremony to heal; sacred pipe; sacred sage, sweet grass, cedar and other herbs wafted over the patient with the use of a feather; herbs used in a tea, eaten, used in a bath, or burned with the smoke inhaled; rattles to break up blocks of dead or jammed energy; and drums to align the person's spirit with the heartbeat of Mother Earth. All diseases have been treated with the use of Native American medicine, which does not preclude the use of additional mainstream medical therapies. This medicine is a safe modality when performed by the medicine person, who is an essential part of helping patients return to a state of harmony. It should not be attempted by individuals who do not have the education or training needed.[8]

Association of American Indian Physicians (AAIP)
    1225 Sovereign Row, Suite 103
    Oklahoma City, OK 73108 USA
    Phone: 405-946-7072
    Fax: 405-946-7651

*Shamanism*

Personal healing, transformation, and regeneration through access to a "higher power" forms the foundation of shamanic healing. Sickness, disease, and illness are indicators that the individual is out of balance and in disharmony within the essential nature. Success can be achieved if people are, first, willing to take responsibility for the creation of the disease and, second, open to nonphysical realities of life and willing to engage with their inner spirit and their higher selves. This type of healing has been effective for sexual dysfunction, chronic fatigue syndrome, mental health concerns, and obesity and other eating disorders.[8]

The Foundation for Shamanic Studies
    PO Box 1939
    Mill Valley, CA 94942
    Phone: 415-380-8282

## MISCELLANEOUS AND GENERAL RESOURCES

Advanced Nutrition
    3980 Virginia Beach Blvd., Suite 101
    Virginia Beach, VA 23452
    Phone: 800-527-6454
    Phone: 757-631-9363
    Fax: 757-631-9606

Alternative Medicine Foundation
    5411 W. Cedar Lane, Suite 205-A
    Bethesda, MD 20814
    Phone: 301-581-0116
    Fax: 301-581-0119

American Alternative Medicine Association (AAMA)
    708 Madelaine Drive
    Gilmer, TX 75644-3140
    Phone: 888-764-2237
    Phone: 903-843-6401

American Association for Therapeutic Humor (AATH)
    4534 W. Butler Drive
    Glendale, AZ 85302
    Phone: 623-934-6068
    Fax: 623-934-5902

American Holistic Health Association
    P.O. Box 17400
    Anaheim, CA 92817-7400
    Phone: 714-779-6152

American Holistic Medical Association
    6728 McLean Village Drive
    McLean, VA 22101-8729
    Fax: 703-556-8729

American Holistic Nurses Association
    P.O. Box 2130
    Flagstaff, AZ 86003-2130
    Phone: 800-278-2462

American Organization for Bodywork Therapies of Asia (AOBTA)
    1010 Haddonfield-Berlin Road, Suite 408
    Voorhees, NJ 08043
    Phone: 856-782-1616
    Fax: 856-782-1653

American Orthopsychiatric Association
    330 Seventh Ave, 18th Floor
    New York, NY 10001
    Phone: 212-564-5930
    Fax: 212-564-6180

American Physical Therapy Association (APTA)
    1111 N. Fairfax St.
    Alexandria, VA 22314-1488
    Phone: 703-684-2782
    Fax: 703-684-7343
    TDD: 703-683-6748

American Preventive Medical Association
    9912 Georgetown Pike
    Suite D-2
    P.O. Box 458
    Great Falls, VA 22066
    Phone: 800-230-APMA
    Phone: 703-759-0662
    Fax: 703-759-6711

American Society for Clinical Nutrition
    9650 Rockville Pike
    Bethesda, MD 20814-3998
    Phone: 301-530-7110
    Fax: 301-571-1863

American Society of Alternative Therapists
    P.O. Box 703
    Rockport, MA 01966
    Phone: 978-281-4400

Association for Integrative Health Care Practitioners
    201 Granby St.
    P.O. Box 3204
    Norfolk, VA 23514-3204
    Phone: 757-622-3400
    Fax: 757-622-1717

Association for Integrative Medicine
    Box 1
    Mont Clare, PA 19453
    Phone: 610-933-8145

Association of Natural Medicine
    19a Collingwood Road
    Witham
    Essex
    CM8 2DY
    UK
    Phone: 01376 502762

Association of Traditional Health Practitioners
    P.O. Box 346
    Elizabeth, South Australia 5112
    Australia
    Phone: 08 8284 2324
    Fax: 08 8254 8602

British Holistic Medical Association (BHMA)
    59 Lansdowne Place
    Hove
    East Sussex BN3 1FL
    UK
    Phone/Fax: 01273 725951

Canadian Orthopractic Manual Therapy Association (COMTA)
#207, 11520
100 Ave
Edmonton, AB
T5K 0J7
Canada
Phone: 780-482-7428
Fax: 780-488-2463

Canadian Physiotherapy Association
2345 Yonge Street
Suite 410
Toronto, Ontario M4P 2E5
Canada
Phone: 416-932-1888 or 1-800-387-8679
Fax: 416-932-9708

Center for Mind-Body Medicine
5225 Connecticut Ave. NW, Suite 414
Washington, DC 20015
Phone: 202-966-7338
Fax: 202-966-2589

Center for the Advancement of Health
2000 Florida Ave, N.W., Suite 210
Washington, DC 20009-1231
Phone: 202-387-2829
Fax: 202-387-2857

Chartered Society of Physiotherapy
14 Bedford Row
London WC1R 4ED
England
Phone: +44 0 20 7306 6666
Fax: +44 0 20 7306 6611

Complementary Alternative Medicine Association, Inc.
Phone: 404-284-7592

Dieticians of Canada
480 University Avenue, Suite 604
Toronto, Ontario, Canada M5G 1V2
Phone: 416-596-0857
Fax: 416-596-0603

Esalen Massage & Bodywork Association
Esalen Institute Highway One
Big Sur, CA 93920
Phone: 831-667-3018
Fax: 831-667-3048

Federation of Holistic Therapists
3rd Floor, Eastleigh House
Upper Market Street
Eastleigh, Hampshire SO50 9FD
UK

Foundation for the Advancement of Innovative Medicine
PO Box 7016
Albany, NY 12225-0016
Phone: 877-634-3246
Fax: 518-758-7967

Foundation for Innovation in Medicine
11 North Avenue East
Cranford, NJ 07016
Phone: 908-272-2967
Fax: 908-272-4583

Guild of Complementary Practitioners
Liddell House, Liddell Close
Finchampstead
Berkshire, RG40 4NS
UK
Phone: 0118 973 5757

Health Action Network Society
202-5262 Rumble Street
Burnaby, BC
Canada, V5J 2B6
Phone: 604-435-0512
Fax: 604-435-1561

International Breathwork Foundation
7 Silver Street
Buckfastleigh, Devon
TQ11 0BQ
UK
Phone: 44 0 1364 643 100

International Stress Management Association
United States Branch C/O Paul J. Rosch, M.D.
124 Park Ave.
Yonkers, NY 10703

National Association for Alternative Medicine
4433 Eagle Rock Blvd. #435
Los Angeles, CA 90041

National Association of Myofascial Trigger Point Therapists
251 Maitland Ave., Ste. 312
Altamonte Springs, FL 32701
Phone: 407-672-2344
Fax: 407-331-8825

National Center for Complementary and Alternative Medicine
P.O. Box 8218
Silver Spring, MD 20907-8218
Phone: 888-644-6226
Phone: 301-231-7537, ext. 5
TTY: 888-644-6226
Fax: 301-495-4957

Research Council for Complementary Medicine
Suite 5, 1 Harley Street
London W1G 9QD
UK

## REFERENCES

1. Caudell KA: Complementary and alternative therapies. In Lewis SM, Heitkemper MM, Dirksen SR, editors: *Medical-surgical nursing,* ed 5, St Louis, 2000, Mosby.
2. Eisenberg DM et al: Trends in alternative medicine use in the United States, 1990-1997: results of a follow-up national survey, *JAMA* 280(18):1569, 1998.
3. Lewis SM, Heitkemper MM, Dirksen SR, editors: *Medical-surgical nursing,* St Louis, 2000, Mosby.
4. Marriner A: *Nursing theorists and their work,* St Louis, 1986, Mosby.
5. Micozzi MS: *Fundamentals of complementary and alternative medicine,* New York, 1996, Churchill Livingstone.
6. Mills S, Bone K: *Principles and practice of phytotherapy,* London, 2000, Churchill Livingstone.
7. National Center for Complementary and Alternative Medicine, Washington DC, 2000, National Institutes of Health, http://nccam.nih.gov.nccam.
8. Novey DW: *Complementary/alternative medicine,* St Louis, 2000, Mosby.
9. Pizzorno JE, Murray MT: *Textbook of natural medicine,* ed 2, London, 1999, Churchill Livingstone.
10. Spencer JW, Jacobs, JJ: *Complementary/alternative medicine,* St Louis, 2000, Mosby.

# 12 HERBS AND NATURAL SUPPLEMENTS

## 12-1 Herbal glossary

**Arila**—A botanical term used to denote an accessory seed coating that may form a fleshy, cuplike structure around the immature seed (ovule), as in yew and nutmeg. The aril is often brightly colored and edible.

**Binomial**—The unique, two-part scientific name used to identify a plant. The first name is the genus; the second, the species. A designation of the variety may also follow to further differentiate the plant. Use of the binomial is the only reliable way to accurately specify a particular herb, since common names differ from region to region and a single common name may often denote several herbs that differ widely from one other.

**Concentration**—A means of expressing the amount of herb and solvent used in formulating an herbal preparation. For example, a tincture with a 1:5 concentration contains 1 part of the herb in grams to 5 parts of the solvent in milliliters. Concentration is not the same thing as potency (see below).

**Crude herb**—The raw plant, before it is processed or dried.

**Decoction**—A liquid preparation made by boiling plant parts (such as bark, roots, or rhizome) in water.

**Extract**—A concentrated form of the herb that is derived when the crude herb is mixed with water, alcohol, or another solvent and distilled or evaporated. Extracts may be either fluid or solid.

**Gall**—A lump or ball that forms most often on the stems, leaves, or roots of plants at the site of injuries caused by insects, fungi, bacteria, or other organisms. An example is the oak gall, which contains tannin.

**Herb**—A plant that is used for its medicinal purposes. (This differs from the biological definition of an herb as a plant with no woody above-ground parts.)

**Infusion**—A liquid preparation made by pouring water over plant parts (such as dried or fresh leaves, flowers, fruits, etc.) and allowing the mixture to steep. Boiling water is usually used, but cold water may also be used. Making a cup of herbal tea is an example.

**Minim**—A fluid measure constituting $\frac{1}{60}$ of a fluidrachm, which itself is about a teaspoonful ($\frac{1}{8}$ of a fluid ounce). A minim is about the equivalent of one drop of water.

**Nutraceutical**—A food that is used for its medicinal properties.

**Oil, essential**—The aromatic volatile oils extracted from various parts of the fresh herb. Essential oils are usually diluted before being used therapeutically.

**Oil, infused**—A mixture comprised of the herb's volatile oils and another oil. The so-called carrier oil is used to extract the herb's volatile oils by soaking plant parts in it for a specified time period.

**Pharmacognosy**—The study of chemicals taken from natural sources to be used as drugs or in the preparation of drugs. Sources may include plants, animals, or other life forms such as fungi, molds, and yeasts.

**Phytochemical**—The active chemical components, or constituents, present in a plant that account for its medicinal properties.

**Phytomedicine**—The use of plants, plant parts, and preparations made from them to prevent, treat, or cure various health conditions.

**Potency**—A measure of the strength of the active chemical components contained in an herb or herbal preparation. Standardized products ensure the consumer of receiving a dosage containing a consistent potency.

**Poultice**—Plant material (such as crushed fresh herbs) that has been wrapped in gauze or similar soft cloth, moistened, and applied topically.

**Powder**—The dried product of an extraction process in which the herb is first mixed with a solvent such as alcohol or water and is distilled; then the solvent is removed completely. The dry solid that remains either is already in powder form or may be ground into it.

**Rhizome**—An underground plant stem, growing more or less horizontally, that usually has roots on its underside and bears buds.

**Tincture**—A plant extract made by soaking herbs in a liquid (such as water, alcohol, vinegar, or glycerine) for a specified length of time, then straining and discarding the plant material. The remaining liquid is used therapeutically. Tinctures typically are made at a concentration of 1:5 to 1:10.

From Skidmore-Roth L: *Mosby's handbook of herbs & natural supplements*, St Louis, 2001, Mosby.

## 12-2 Common herbs and supplements

This table lists only a few of the most common herbs and supplements to provide a quick reference. For information on additional herbs, please see individual definitions. Information on herb–laboratory test interactions can be found in Appendix 8-2. Information on herb-drug interactions can be found in Appendix 12-3. For comprehensive information on many common and lesser-known herbs, consult *Mosby's Handbook of Herbs & Natural Supplements* by Linda Skidmore-Roth.

| Herb | Use | Contraindication |
|---|---|---|
| Agrimony | This herb is used for mild diarrhea, gastroenteritis, intestinal mucus secretion, inflammation of the mouth and throat, cuts and scrapes, and amenorrhea | Agrimony is not recommended in women during pregnancy and lactation, in children, or in those with known hypersensitivity to it or roses. |
| Alfalfa | This herb is used for poor appetite, hay fever and asthma, and high cholesterol. It may also be used as a nutrient source. | Alfalfa is not recommended in women during pregnancy and lactation, in children, or in those with known hypersensitivity. |

| Herb | Use | Contraindication |
|---|---|---|
| Aloe | Aloe vera gel is used externally for minor burns, skin irritations, minor wounds, frostbite, and radiation-caused injuries. Internally, it is used to heal intestinal inflammation and ulcers, and as a digestive aid to stimulate bile secretion. | *Topically:* hypersensitivity to this plant, garlic, onions, or tulips prohibits the use of aloe. Aloe also should not be used on deep wounds. *Internally:* the dried juice is contraindicated during pregnancy and lactation, in children younger than 12 years of age, and in those with kidney or cardiac disease or bowel obstruction. This product should not be used long-term. |
| Angelica | This herb is used for heartburn, indigestion, gas, colic, poor blood flow to the extremities, bronchitis, poor appetite, psoriasis, and vitiligo. It is also used as an antiseptic. | Angelica should not be used in women during pregnancy and lactation or in children; it should be used only with caution in people with diabetes or bleeding disorders. |
| Astragalus | This herb is used as an immune stimulant. It is also used for viral infections, HIV/AIDS, cancer, and vascular disorders. It can be used to improve circulation and to decrease blood pressure as well. It may show efficacy in treating myasthenia gravis. | Astragalus should not be used in women during pregnancy and lactation, in children, or in people with acute infections. |
| Bilberry | This herb is used for diabetic retinopathy, macular degeneration, glaucoma, cataract, capillary fragility, varicose veins, hemorrhoids, and mild diarrhea. | Bilberry should not be used in women during pregnancy and lactation or in children until more research is available. |
| Black cohosh | This herb is used to treat the symptoms of menopause (hot flashes and nervous conditions associated with menopause) and dysmenorrhea (menstrual cramps, pain, inflammation). | Black cohosh should not be used during pregnancy, since uterine stimulation can occur. It also should not be used in women during lactation or in children. |
| Black haw | This herb is used for dysmenorrhea, menstrual cramps and pain, menopausal metrorrhagia, hysteria, asthma, and heart palpitations. It is also used to lower blood pressure. | Black haw should be used with caution in people with kidney stones. |
| Blessed thistle | This herb is used for loss of appetite, indigestion, and intestinal gas. | Blessed thistle should not be used in women during pregnancy, in children, or in those with known hypersensitivity. |
| Blue cohosh | This herb is used to treat menopausal symptoms and uterine and ovarian pain and to improve the flow of menstrual blood. It is used as an antiinflammatory and antirheumatic as well. It is also a popular remedy in African-American ethnic medicine. | Blue cohosh should not be used in women during pregnancy, since the herb is a uterine stimulant. It is also contraindicated in women during lactation, in children, and in people with cardiac disease. |
| Borage | This herb is used as an antiinflammatory for premenstrual syndrome, rheumatoid arthritis, Raynaud's disease, and other inflammatory conditions. It is also used to treat atopic dermatitis, infant cradle cap, cystic fibrosis, high blood pressure, and diabetes. | Borage should not be used in women during pregnancy and lactation because of the possible presence of pyrrolizidine alkaloids. It is also contraindicated in children until more research is completed. |
| Burdock root | This herb is used for skin diseases, inflammation, rashes, colds and fever, cancer, gout, and arthritis. | Burdock is contraindicated in those who are hypersensitive to it. Burdock also should be used cautiously in people with diabetes or cardiac disorders. |
| Capsicum | This herb is used for muscle spasms, the pain of inflammation, neuromas, psoriasis, and dry mouth. It is also used as a food antioxidant and as a food seasoning. | Capsicum peppers are contraindicated in those with known hypersensitivity, in pregnant or lactating women, and in children until more research is available. It should not be used in open wounds or abrasions or near the eyes. Capsicum can cause extreme burns and blisters in its undiluted form. |
| Cascara | This herb is used for chronic constipation, hepatitis, and gallstones. | Cascara should not be used by those who are hypersensitive to it, by pregnant or lactating women, or by children until more research is available. Also, it is contraindicated in situations in which GI bleeding, obstruction, abdominal pain, nausea, vomiting, appendicitis, and Crohn's disease are present. |
| Cat's claw | This herb is used for cancer, herpes, HIV, rheumatoid arthritis, gastritis, gout, wounds, and gastric ulcers. | Cat's claw is contraindicated in women during pregnancy and lactation and in children younger than 3 years of age until more research is available. It also should not be used in people with muscular sclerosis, tuberculosis, AIDS, or hemophilia or in those who have had organ transplants. |

*Continued*

| Herb | Use | Contraindication |
|------|-----|------------------|
| Chamomile | This herb is used externally as an antiseptic and soothing agent for inflamed skin and minor wounds. Internally, it is used as an antispasmodic, gas-relieving, and antiinflammatory agent for the treatment of digestive problems; as a light sleep aid and sedative for adults and children; and as a possible anticancer agent. | Chamomile should not be used in women during pregnancy and lactation; it may be used in children. Cross-hypersensitivity may result from allergy to sunflowers, ragweed, or members of the aster family (e.g., Echinacea, feverfew, milk thistle). People with asthma should also avoid its use. |
| Chaparral | Use of this herb is not recommended because it is potentially toxic to the liver and kidneys. | Do not use chaparral in women during pregnancy and lactation or in children until more research is completed. People with liver or renal disease should also avoid the use of this herb. The American Herbal Product Association has recommended that companies not sell chaparral products until the hepatotoxicity question has been clarified. |
| Chicory | This herb is used as a coffee substitute, as a source of fructooligosaccharides, as a mild laxative for children, and as a treatment for gout, rheumatism, loss of appetite, and digestive distress. | Chicory is contraindicated in women during pregnancy and lactation. People who have cardiovascular disease or are hypersensitive to chicory or asteraceae/compositae herbs should also avoid its use, and people with gallstones should use under the supervision of a herbalist. |
| Comfrey | This herb is used for bruises, sprains, broken bones, acne, and boils. | The use of comfrey is not recommended in women during pregnancy and lactation, in children, and in those with are hypersensitive to it. Internal use may cause fatal hepatotoxicity. It should not be used for more than 6 weeks per year. It should not be used topically on broken skin. |
| Cranberry | This herb is used for urinary tract infections and in those with susceptibility to kidney stones. | Those with known hypersensitivity, oliguria, or anuria should not use cranberry. |
| Dong quai | This herb is used for the restoration of vitality in tired women; for a variety of gynecologic, menstrual, and menopausal symptoms; and for the treatment of cirrhosis of the liver. | Dong quai should not be used in women during pregnancy, in children, or in those with known hypersensitivity. In Chinese medicine, dong quai has been used during pregnancy, but its use must be monitored by an herbalist. It is contraindicated in people with bleeding disorders, excessive menstrual flow, or acute illness. |
| Echinacea | This herb is used for those with low immune status and for those with hard-to-heal superficial wounds. It is also used as a sun protectant. | Echinacea is not recommended in women during pregnancy and lactation or in children. It is also contraindicated in people who have autoimmune diseases such as lupus erythematosus, multiple sclerosis, HIV/AIDS, and collage disease and in people with tuberculosis or hypersensitivity to *Bellis* species or the Compositae family of herbs. Immunosuppression may occur after extended therapy with this herb. It should not be used for more than 8 weeks. |
| Elderberry | This herb may be useful for those with susceptibility to colds, influenza, and yeast infections; it is also used for nasal and chest congestion, earache associated with chronic congestion, and hay fever. | Elderberry is not recommended in women during pregnancy and lactation, in children, or in those with known hypersensitivity to it or similar plants. |
| Ephedra | This herb is used for seasonal and chronic asthma, nasal congestion, and cough. | Ephedra is contraindicated in those with known hypersensitivity to sympathomimetics, in women who are pregnant or lactating, in children younger than 12 years of age, and in people with narrow-angle glaucoma, seizure disorders, hyperthyroidism, diabetes mellitus, prostatic hypertrophy, arrhythmias, heart block, hypertension, psychosis, tachycardia, and angina pectoris. |
| Fenugreek | This herb is used for loss of appetite, skin inflammation, water retention, cancer, constipation, diarrhea, high cholesterol, high blood glucose levels, and calcium oxalate stones. | Fenugreek should not be used during pregnancy, since it can cause premature labor. It is also contraindicated in women during lactation, in children, and in those with known hypersensitivity. |
| Feverfew | This herb is used for migraines, cluster headaches, fever, psoriasis, and inflammation. | Feverfew should not be used in women during pregnancy and lactation, in children, or in those with known hypersensitivity. |

| Herb | Use | Contraindication |
|---|---|---|
| Flax | This herb is used for constipation and as a source of omega-3 fatty acids. | Flax is contraindicated in people with bowel obstruction and dehydration. It is also not recommended in women during pregnancy and lactation, in children, or in those with known hypersensitivity to this product. Flax should not be used as a poultice on open wounds. |
| Fo-ti | This herb is used for tiredness, constipation, and elevated cholesterol. | Fo-ti is contraindicated in women during pregnancy and lactation, in children, in those with known hypersensitivity, or in those with diarrhea. |
| Garlic | This herb is used for vascular disease, elevated levels of low-density lipoprotein or triglycerides, low levels of high-density lipoprotein, high blood pressure, poor circulation, risk of cancer, inflammatory disorders, childhood ear infection, and yeast infection. | Garlic should not be used in women during pregnancy, since it may stimulate labor, or during lactation, since it may cause colic in infants. It is also contraindicated in those with known hypersensitivity, stomach inflammation, gastritis, and hypothyroidism, since garlic may reduce iodine uptake. People who have had or who are about to have surgery should also avoid it, since clotting time may be increased. |
| Ginger | This herb is used for nausea, motion sickness, indigestion, and inflammation. | Ginger is not recommended in women during pregnancy (it is an abortifacient when taken in large amounts) or lactation, in children, or in those with known hypersensitivity. It should not be used in cholelithiasis unless directed by a physician. |
| Ginko | This herb is used for poor circulation, diabetes, vascular disease, cancer, inflammatory disorders, impotence, and degenerative nerve conditions. It is also used for age-related declines in cognition and memory. | Ginkgo is contraindicated in people with coagulation or platelet disorders or hemophilia, in children, and in those with known hypersensitivity. |
| Ginseng | This herb is used for physical and mental exhaustion, stress, viral infections, diabetes, sluggishness, fatigue, weak immunity, and convalescence. | Ginseng should not be used in women during pregnancy and lactation or in children. It is also contraindicated in those with known hypersensitivity, hypertension, and cardiac disorders. |
| Goldenseal | This herb is used for high blood pressure, poor appetite, infections, menstrual problems, minor sciatic pain, and muscle spasms. It is also used as an eye wash. | Goldenseal is contraindicated in women who are pregnant (it is a uterine stimulant). It also should not be used in people with known hypersensitivity or who have cardiovascular conditions such as heart block, arrhythmias, and hypertension. It should not be used locally for purulent ear discharge or a ruptured ear drum. |
| Gotu kola | This herb is used to treat chronic wounds and psoriasis. | Gotu kola should not be used in women during pregnancy and lactation or in children until more research is available. Those with known hypersensitivity to it or to members of the celery family should not use this product. |
| Grapeseed | This herb is used as an antioxidant, as a chronic disease preventative, and as an antiinflammatory. | Use of grapeseed should be avoided in women during pregnancy and lactation and in children until more research is available. |
| Green tea | This herb is used to prevent cancer and heart disease. It is also used for hypercholesterolemia; it is used as an antidiarrheal as well. | Green tea is contraindicated in those with known hypersensitivity and in those with kidney inflammation, GI ulcers, insomnia, cardiovascular disease, and increased intraocular pressure. |
| Guggul | This herb is used for high levels of low-density lipoprotein, elevated triglyceride levels, and weight loss. | Guggul is contraindicated during pregnancy, since it can cause uterine contractions. It also should not be used in women during lactation, in children, and in those with known hypersensitivity. |
| Gymnema | This herb is used to reduce high blood glucose levels. | Gymnema should not be used in women during pregnancy and lactation, in children, or in those with known hypersensitivity. |
| Hawthorn | This herb is used for poor circulation, chest pain, irregular heartbeat, high blood fats, and high blood pressure. | Hawthorn should not be used in women during pregnancy and lactation or in children. It is also contraindicated in those with known hypersensitivity to it or other members of the Rosaceae family. |
| Hops | This herb is used as a mild sedative, diuretic, and weak antibiotic. It is also used to improve appetite and to treat insomnia, hyperactivity, pain, fever, and jaundice. | Hops should not be used in people who are hypersensitive; who have breast, uterine, or cervical cancers; or who suffer from a depressive condition. |

*Continued*

| Herb | Use | Contraindication |
|------|-----|------------------|
| Horse chestnut | This herb is used for fever, fluid retention, frostbite, hemorrhoids, inflammation, lower extremity swelling, phlebitis, varicose veins, and wounds. | Horse chestnut is contraindicated in women during pregnancy and lactation and in children until more research has been completed. |
| Horsetail | This herb is used as a diuretic, a genitourinary astringent, and an antihemorrhagic. It is also used for Bell's palsy and for healing broken bones. | Horsetail should not be used in women during pregnancy and lactation or in children. It is also contraindicated in those with known hypersensitivity, edema, cardiac or renal disease, or nicotine sensitivity. It should not be used for prolonged periods. |
| Kava | This herb is used for nervous anxiety, restlessness, sleep disturbances, and stress. | Kava should not be used in women during pregnancy and lactation, in children younger than 12 years of age, or in those with known hypersensitivity, major depressive disorder, or Parkinson's disease. |
| Khat | This herb is used for obesity and gastric ulcers; it is also used as a stimulant. | Khat should not be used in women during pregnancy and lactation, in children, or in those with known hypersensitivity. People with renal, cardiac, or hepatic disease also should avoid its use. |
| Kudzu | This herb is used to reduce alcohol cravings and menopausal symptoms. | Kudzu should not be used in women during pregnancy and lactation, in children, or in those with known hypersensitivity. It should be used with caution by people who have heart disease. |
| Lemon balm | This herb is used for abdominal gas and cramping and for cold sores. | The use of lemon balm is not recommended in women during pregnancy and lactation, in children, or in those with known hypersensitivity. It should not be used in people with hypothyroidism. |
| Licorice | This herb is used for allergies, arthritis, asthma, constipation, esophagitis, gastritis, hepatitis, inflammatory conditions, peptic ulcers, poor adrenal function, and poor appetite. | Licorice should not be used in women during pregnancy and lactation, in children, or in those with known hypersensitivity. It is also contraindicated in people with liver disease, renal disease, hypokalemia, hypertension, arrhythmias, and congestive heart failure. |
| Maitake | This herb is used as an immunostimulant and as a treatment for diabetes, hypertension, high cholesterol, and obesity. | Maitake is not recommended in women during pregnancy and lactation, in children, or in those with known hypersensitivity until more information is available. |
| Melatonin | This supplement is used for jet lag, insomnia, and cancer protection; it is also used as an oral contraceptive. | Melatonin is not recommended in women during pregnancy and lactation, in children, or in those with known hypersensitivity. |
| Milk thistle | This herb is used to protect against alcoholic cirrhosis and hepatitis; it is also used as an antiinflammatory. | Milk thistle should not be used in women during pregnancy and lactation, in children, or in people with hypersensitivity it or to other plants in the Asteraceae family. |
| Monascus | This herb is used to help maintain acceptable cholesterol levels. | Monascus should not be used in women during pregnancy and lactation, in children, in those with known hypersensitivity to Monascus, or in those with hepatic disease such as cirrhosis or fatty liver. |
| Morinda | This herb is used for headache, arthritis, and digestive, heart, and liver conditions. | Morinda should not be used in women during pregnancy and lactation, in children, or in those with known hypersensitivity or hyperkalemia. |
| Nettle | This herb is used as a diuretic and as a treatment for hay fever. | Nettle should not be used in women during pregnancy and lactation, in children younger than 2 years of age, or in people with hypersensitivity. It should be used only with caution in children and the elderly. |
| Octacosanol | This herb is used for herpes, inflammation of the skin, and physical endurance. | Octacosanol should not be used in women during pregnancy and lactation or in children. |
| Passion flower | This herb is used as an antifungal and sedative and as a treatment for hypertension and group A hemolytic streptococcus. | Passion flower should not be used in women during pregnancy and lactation, in children, or in those with known hypersensitivity. |
| Pau d'arco | This herb is used for cancer, inflammation, and infection. | Pau d'arco should not be used in women during pregnancy and lactation, in children younger than 18 years of age, or in those with hemophilia, von Willebrand's disease, thrombocytopenia, or known hypersensitivity. |
| Pygeum | This herb is used for benign prostate hypertrophy; it is also used as an antiinflammatory. | Pygeum is not recommended in women during pregnancy and lactation, in children, or in those with known hypersensitivity. |

| Herb | Use | Contraindication |
|---|---|---|
| Raspberry leaves | This herb is used as a uterine tonic and as a treatment for dysmenorrhea, fever, and vomiting. | Raspberry should not be used medicinally in women during pregnancy and lactation and is contraindicated in those with known hypersensitivity. |
| Rose hips | This herb is used as a source of vitamin C and as a treatment for colds, fever, and mild infections. | Rose hips should not be used in women during pregnancy and lactation or in people with known hypersensitivity. |
| Saw palmetto | This herb is used to treat benign prostatic hypertrophy. | Saw palmetto should not be used during pregnancy and lactation, in children, or in those with known hypersensitivity. |
| Schisandra | This herb is used for GI disorders and for liver protection; it is also used as a tonic. | Schisandra should not be used in women during pregnancy and lactation, in children, or in those with known hypersensitivity. |
| Senna | This herb is used as a laxative. | Senna should not be used in women during pregnancy and lactation, in children younger than 12 years of age (unless prescribed by a physician), or in those with known hypersensitivity. Senna is also prohibited in those with intestinal obstruction, ulcerative colitis, GI bleeding, appendicitis, acute surgical abdomen, nausea, vomiting, and congestive heart failure. |
| Siberian ginseng | This herb is used to improve appetite, to improve circulation, and to treat memory loss, hypertension, insomnia, rheumatism, heart ailments, diabetes, and headache. | Siberian ginseng should not be used in women during pregnancy and lactation, in children, in those with known hypersensitivity to it or other ginsengs, or in those with hypertension. Siberian ginseng should not be used for more than 90 days without a rest period. |
| St. John's wort | This herb is used as an antidepressant and antiviral. | St. John's wort is not recommended in women during pregnancy and lactation, in children, or in those with known hypersensitivity. |
| Tea tree oil | This herb is used topically for infections and as an inhalant for respiratory disorders. | Tea tree oil should not be used in women during pregnancy and lactation or in those with known hypersensitivity. |
| Valerian | This herb is used as a sedative. | Valerian should not be used in women during pregnancy and lactation, in those with known hypersensitivity, or those with hepatic disease. It should be used only with caution in children, since research is lacking. |
| Yarrow | This herb is used to decrease bleeding, to improve circulation, and to treat GI disorders, hypertension, and thrombi. | Yarrow should not be used in women during pregnancy and lactation. It is also contraindicated in those with known hypersensitivity to it or other members of the Compositae family, such as *Chamomilla recutita, Tanacetum parthenium,* or *T. vulgare.* |
| Yerba maté | This herb is used as a diuretic and depurative. | Yerba maté should not be used in women during pregnancy and lactation, in children, or in those with anxiety disorders, hypertension, or known hypersensitivity. |
| Yohimbe | This herb is used to treat male organic impotence. | Yohimbe should not be used in women during pregnancy and lactation, in children, or in those with known hypersensitivity. Prolonged use is contraindicated, as is use in those with renal or hepatic disease, hypertension, angina pectoris, gastric or duodenal ulcers, bipolar disorder, anxiety disorder, schizophrenia, suicidal tendencies, and prostatitis. |

*AIDS,* Acquired immunodeficiency syndrome; *HIV,* human immunodeficiency virus.

## 12-3   Herb-drug interactions

| Herb | Drug | Interaction |
|------|------|-------------|
| Alfalfa | Diethylstilbestrol | Possible additive hormonal effect |
| | Warfarin | ↓ anticoagulant effect |
| Aloe | Acebutolol | Possible ↑ effect of acebutolol |
| | Adenosine | Possible ↑ effect of adenosine |
| | Amiodarone | Possible ↑ effect of amiodarone |
| | Amrinone | Possible ↑ action of amrinone |
| | Atropine | Possible ↑ action of atropine with chronic use or abuse of aloe |
| | Betamethasone | Potassium deficiency with chronic use or abuse of aloe |
| | Bretylium | ↑ action of bretylium with chronic use or abuse of aloe |
| | Chlorothiazide | Potassium deficiency with chronic use or abuse of aloe |
| | Chlorthalidone | Potassium deficiency with chronic use or abuse of aloe |
| | Cortisone | Potassium deficiency with chronic use or abuse of aloe |
| | Dexamethasone | Potassium deficiency with chronic use or abuse of aloe |
| | Digitoxin | ↑ action of digitoxin |
| | Digoxin | ↑ action of digoxin |
| | Disopyramide | ↑ action of disopyramide |
| | Esmolol | Potassium deficiency with chronic use or abuse of aloe |
| | Flecainide | Potassium deficiency with chronic use or abuse of aloe |
| | Fludrocortisone | Potassium deficiency with chronic use or abuse of aloe |
| | Hydrochlorothiazide | Potassium deficiency with chronic use or abuse of aloe |
| | Hydrocortisone | Potassium deficiency with chronic use or abuse of aloe |
| | Ibutilide | ↑ action of ibutilide |
| | Indapamide | Potassium deficiency with chronic use or abuse of aloe |
| | Lidocaine | ↑ action of lidocaine |
| | Methylprednisolone | Potassium deficiency with chronic use or abuse of aloe |
| | Metolazone | Potassium deficiency with chronic use or abuse of aloe |
| | Mexiletine | ↑ potassium loss; ↑ antidysrhythmic action |
| | Moricizine | ↑ potassium loss; ↑ antidysrhythmic action |
| | Phenytoin | ↑ potassium loss; ↑ antidysrhythmic action |
| | Prednisone | Potassium deficiency |
| | Prednisolone | Potassium deficiency |
| | Propafenone | Potassium deficiency; ↑ antidysrhythmic action |
| | Quinidine | Potassium deficiency; ↑ antidysrhythmic action |
| | Sotalol | Potassium deficiency; ↑ antidysrhythmic action |
| | Tocainide | Potassium deficiency; ↑ antidysrhythmic action |
| | Triamcinolone | ↑ potassium loss |
| Angelica | Doxazosin | ↑ effect of doxazosin |
| Broom | Glyburide | ↓ hypoglycemic effect |
| | Insulin | ↓ hypoglycemic effect |
| | Lithium | ↑ effects of lithium; ↑ toxicity |
| | Miglitol | ↓ hypoglycemic effect of miglitol |
| | Repaglinide | Possible ↓ hypoglycemic effect |
| Buchu | Glyburide | ↓ hypoglycemic effect |
| | Insulin | ↓ hypoglycemic effect |
| | Lithium | ↑ effects of lithium; ↑ toxicity |
| | Miglitol | ↓ hypoglycemic effect of miglitol |
| | Repaglinide | Possible ↓ hypoglycemic effect |
| Buckthorn | Acebutolol | Possible ↑ effect of acebutolol |
| | Adenosine | Possible ↑ effect of adenosine |
| | Amiodarone | Possible ↑ effect of amiodarone |
| | Amrinone | Possible ↑ action of amrinone |
| | Atropine | Possible ↑ action of atropine with chronic use or abuse of buckthorn |
| | Betamethasone | Potassium deficiency with chronic use or abuse of buckthorn |
| | Bretylium | ↑ action of bretylium with chronic use or abuse of buckthorn |
| | Chlorothiazide | Potassium deficiency with chronic use or abuse of buckthorn |
| | Chlorthalidone | Potassium deficiency with chronic use or abuse of buckthorn |
| | Cortisone | Potassium deficiency with chronic use or abuse of buckthorn |
| | Dexamethasone | Potassium deficiency with chronic use or abuse of buckthorn |
| | Digitoxin | ↑ action of digitoxin |
| | Digoxin | ↑ action of digoxin |
| | Disopyramide | ↑ action of disopyramide |
| | Esmolol | Potassium deficiency with chronic use or abuse of buckthorn |
| | Flecainide | Potassium deficiency with chronic use or abuse of buckthorn |
| | Fludrocortisone | Potassium deficiency with chronic use or abuse of buckthorn |

| Herb | Drug | Interaction |
|------|------|-------------|
| Buckthorn—cont'd | Hydrochlorothiazide | Potassium deficiency with chronic use or abuse of buckthorn |
| | Hydrocortisone | Potassium deficiency with chronic use or abuse of buckthorn |
| | Ibutilide | ↑ action of ibutilide |
| | Indapamide | Potassium deficiency with chronic use or abuse of buckthorn |
| | Lidocaine | ↑ action of lidocaine |
| | Methylprednisolone | Potassium deficiency with chronic use or abuse of buckthorn |
| | Metolazone | Potassium deficiency with chronic use or abuse of buckthorn |
| | Mexiletine | ↑ potassium loss; ↑ antidysrhythmic action |
| | Moricizine | ↑ potassium loss; ↑ antidysrhythmic action |
| | Phenytoin | ↑ potassium loss; ↑ antidysrhythmic action |
| | Prednisone | Potassium deficiency |
| | Prednisolone | Potassium deficiency |
| | Propafenone | Potassium deficiency; ↑ antidysrhythmic action |
| | Quinidine | Potassium deficiency; ↑ antidysrhythmic action |
| | Sotalol | Potassium deficiency; ↑ antidysrhythmic action |
| | Tocainide | Potassium deficiency; ↑ antidysrhythmic action |
| | Triamcinolone | ↑ potassium loss |
| Bugleweed | Levothyroxine | Do not use concurrently |
| | Liothyronine | Do not use concurrently with bugleweed |
| | Liotrix | Do not use concurrently with bugleweed |
| | Thyroid USP (desiccated) | Do not use concurrently with bugleweed |
| Capsicum peppers | Warfarin | ↑ risk of bleeding |
| Cascara sagrada | Acebutolol | Possible ↑ effect of acebutolol |
| | Adenosine | Possible ↑ effect of adenosine |
| | Amiodarone | Possible ↑ effect of amiodarone |
| | Amrinone | Possible ↑ action of amrinone |
| | Atropine | Possible ↑ action of atropine with chronic use or abuse of cascara |
| | Betamethasone | Potassium deficiency with chronic use or abuse of cascara |
| | Bretylium | ↑ action of bretylium with chronic use or abuse of cascara |
| | Chlorothiazide | Potassium deficiency with chronic use or abuse of cascara |
| | Chlorthalidone | Potassium deficiency with chronic use or abuse of cascara |
| | Cortisone | Potassium deficiency with chronic use or abuse of cascara |
| | Dexamethasone | Potassium deficiency with chronic use or abuse of cascara |
| | Digitoxin | ↑ action of digitoxin |
| | Digoxin | ↑ action of digoxin |
| | Disopyramide | ↑ action of disopyramide |
| | Esmolol | Potassium deficiency with chronic use or abuse of cascara |
| | Flecainide | Potassium deficiency with chronic use or abuse of cascara |
| | Fludrocortisone | Potassium deficiency with chronic use or abuse of cascara |
| | Hydrochlorothiazide | Potassium deficiency with chronic use or abuse of cascara |
| | Hydrocortisone | Potassium deficiency with chronic use or abuse of cascara |
| | Ibutilide | ↑ action of ibutilide |
| | Indapamide | Potassium deficiency with chronic use or abuse of cascara |
| | Lidocaine | ↑ action of lidocaine |
| | Methylprednisolone | Potassium deficiency with chronic use or abuse of cascara |
| | Metolazone | Potassium deficiency with chronic use or abuse of cascara |
| | Mexiletine | ↑ potassium loss; ↑ antidysrhythmic action |
| | Moricizine | ↑ potassium loss; ↑ antidysrhythmic action |
| | Phenytoin | ↑ potassium loss; ↑ antidysrhythmic action |
| | Prednisolone | Potassium deficiency |
| | Propafenone | Potassium deficiency; ↑ antidysrhythmic action |
| | Quinidine | Potassium deficiency; ↑ antidysrhythmic action |
| | Sotalol | Potassium deficiency; ↑ antidysrhythmic action |
| | Tocainide | Potassium deficiency; ↑ antidysrhythmic action |
| Cat's claw | Bepridil | ↑ antianginal effect of bepridil |
| Chaste tree | Bromocriptine | ↓ effect of bromocriptine |
| | Pramipexole | ↓ effect of pramipexole |
| | Ropinirole | ↓ action of ropinirole |
| | Selegiline | Possible ↓ action of selegiline |
| Chicory | Bepridil | ↑ antianginal effect of bepridil |
| Chromium | Glipizide | ↑ or ↓ hypoglycemic effect |
| | Glimepiride | ↑ or ↓ hypoglycemic effect |
| | Glyburide | ↑ or ↓ hypoglycemic effect |
| | Insulin | ↑ or ↓ hypoglycemic effect |
| | Miglitol | ↑ or ↓ hypoglycemic effect |
| | Repaglinide | Possible ↑ or ↓ hypoglycemic effect |

*Continued*

| Herb | Drug | Interaction |
|------|------|-------------|
| Dandelion | Glyburide | ↓ hypoglycemic effect |
|  | Insulin | ↓ hypoglycemic effect |
|  | Lithium | ↑ effects of lithium; ↑ toxicity |
|  | Miglitol | ↓ hypoglycemic effect of miglitol |
|  | Repaglinide | Possible ↓ hypoglycemic effect |
| Ephedra | Acebutolol | Dysrhythmias |
|  | Amrinone | Possible ↑ action of amrinone |
|  | Carboprost | Hypertension |
|  | Dexamethasone | Potassium deficiency with chronic use or abuse of ephedra |
|  | Digitoxin | Dysrhythmias |
|  | Digoxin | Dysrhythmias |
|  | Dinoprostone | Hypertension |
|  | Ephedrine | ↑ action of ephedrine |
|  | Epinephrine | ↑ action of epinephrine |
|  | Ergonovine | Hypertension |
|  | Metaproterenol | ↑ effect of metaproterenol |
|  | Oxtriphylline | ↑ action of ephedra and oxtriphylline |
|  | Oxytocin (injection) | Hypertension |
|  | Phenelzine | ↑ sympathomimetic action |
|  | Pirbuterol | ↑ action of ephedra and pirbuterol |
|  | Theophylline | Toxicity |
|  | Tranylcypromine | ↑ sympathomimetic action |
| Fenugreek | Glipizide | ↑ or ↓ hypoglycemic effect |
|  | Glimepiride | ↑ or ↓ hypoglycemic effect |
|  | Glyburide | ↑ or ↓ hypoglycemic effect |
|  | Insulin | ↑ or ↓ hypoglycemic effect |
|  | Miglitol | ↑ or ↓ hypoglycemic effect |
|  | Repaglinide | Possible ↑ or ↓ hypoglycemic effect |
| Feverfew | Warfarin | ↑ risk of bleeding |
| Garlic | Warfarin | ↑ risk of bleeding |
| Ginger | Warfarin | ↑ risk of bleeding |
| Ginkgo | Warfarin | ↑ risk of bleeding |
| Ginseng | Glipizide | ↑ or ↓ hypoglycemic effect |
|  | Glimepiride | ↑ or ↓ hypoglycemic effect |
|  | Glyburide | ↑ or ↓ hypoglycemic effect |
|  | Insulin | ↑ or ↓ hypoglycemic effect |
|  | Miglitol | ↑ or ↓ hypoglycemic effect |
|  | Phenelzine | Tension headaches, irritability, visual hallucinations |
|  | Repaglinide | Possible ↑ or ↓ hypoglycemic effect |
|  | Warfarin | ↓ anticoagulant effect |
| Gossypol | Amphotericin | ↑ risk of nephrotoxicity |
| Guarana | Adenosine | ↓ effect of adenosine |
| Hawthorn | Digitoxin | Cardiac toxicity |
|  | Digoxin | Cardiac toxicity |
| Horse chestnut | Aspirin | ↑ risk of bleeding |
|  | Choline salicylate | ↑ risk of bleeding |
| Juniper | Glyburide | ↓ hypoglycemic effect |
|  | Insulin | ↓ hypoglycemic effect |
|  | Lithium | ↑ effects of lithium; ↑ toxicity |
|  | Miglitol | ↓ hypoglycemic effect of miglitol |
|  | Repaglinide | Possible ↓ hypoglycemic effect |
| Kava | Alfentanil | ↑ CNS depression |
|  | Alprazolam | ↑ CNS depression; coma |
|  | Amitriptyline | ↑ CNS depression |
|  | Amoxapine | ↑ CNS depression |
|  | Amphetamine | Possible ↓ effect of amphetamine |
|  | Baclofen | Possible ↑ CNS depression |
|  | Brompheniramine | ↑ CNS depression |
|  | Buprenorphine | ↑ CNS depression |
|  | Bupropion | ↑ CNS depression |
|  | Buspirone | ↑ CNS depression |
|  | Butorphanol | ↑ CNS depression |
|  | Carbidopa-levodopa | ↑ Parkinson symptoms |
|  | Carisoprodol | Possible ↑ CNS depression |
|  | Cetirizine | ↑ CNS depression |
|  | Chloral hydrate | ↑ CNS depression |
|  | Chlordiazepoxide | ↑ CNS depression |

| Herb | Drug | Interaction |
|---|---|---|
| Kava—cont'd | Chlorpheniramine | ↑ CNS depression |
| | Chlorpromazine | ↑ CNS depression |
| | Chlorzoxazone | Possible ↑ CNS depression |
| | Clemastine | ↑ CNS depression |
| | Clomipramine | ↑ CNS depression |
| | Clonazepam | ↑ CNS depression |
| | Clorazepate | ↑ CNS depression |
| | Clozapine | ↑ CNS depression |
| | Codeine | ↑ CNS depression |
| | Cyclobenzaprine | ↑ CNS depression |
| | Cyproheptadine | ↑ CNS depression |
| | Diazepam | ↑ action of diazepam |
| | Doxepin | ↑ action of doxepin |
| | Droperidol | ↑ action of droperidol |
| | Estazolam | ↑ CNS depression |
| | Fentanyl | ↑ action of fentanyl |
| | Fluoxetine | ↑ action of fluoxetine |
| | Fluphenazine | Possible ↑ action of fluphenazine |
| | Flurazepam | ↑ action of flurazepam |
| | Fluvoxamine | ↑ effect of fluvoxamine |
| | Haloperidol | ↑ action of haloperidol |
| | Hydromorphone | ↑ action of hydromorphone |
| | Hydroxyzine | ↑ action of hydroxyzine |
| | Imipramine | ↑ action of imipramine |
| | Levodopa | ↑ Parkinson symptoms |
| | Levorphanol | ↑ action of levorphanol |
| | Lorazepam | ↑ action of lorazepam |
| | Loxapine | ↑ action of loxapine |
| | Remifentanil | ↑ CNS depression |
| | Risperidone | ↑ CNS depression |
| | Secobarbital | ↑ CNS depression |
| | Sufentanil | ↑ CNS depression |
| | Temazepam | ↑ CNS depression |
| | Thiopental | ↑ CNS depression |
| | Thioridazine | ↑ CNS depression |
| | Thiothixene | ↑ CNS depression |
| | Tramadol | ↑ CNS depression |
| | Trazodone | ↑ CNS depression |
| | Triazolam | ↑ CNS depression |
| | Trifluoperazine | ↑ CNS depression |
| | Triflupromazine | ↑ CNS depression |
| | Zolpidem | ↑ CNS depression |
| Kelpware | Aspirin | ↑ risk of bleeding |
| | Choline salicylate | ↑ risk of bleeding |
| Khat | Amoxicillin | Delayed or reduced absorption of amoxicillin; separate by 2 hr |
| | Ampicillin | Delayed or reduced absorption of ampicillin; separate by 2 hr |
| | Cloxacillin | Delayed or reduced absorption of cloxacillin; separate by 2 hr |
| | Dicloxacillin | Delayed or reduced absorption of dicloxacillin; separate by 2 hr |
| | Mezlocillin | Delayed or reduced absorption of mezlocillin; separate by 2 hr |
| | Nafcillin | Delayed or reduced absorption of nafcillin; separate by 2 hr |
| | Oxacillin | Delayed or reduced absorption of oxacillin; separate by 2 hr |
| | Penicillin | Delayed or reduced absorption of penicillin; separate by 2 hr |
| | Piperacillin | Delayed or reduced absorption of piperacillin; separate by 2 hr |
| | Ticarcillin | Delayed or reduced absorption of ticarcillin; separate by 2 hr |
| Licorice | Chlorothiazide | Potassium deficiency with chronic use or abuse of licorice |
| | Chlorthalidone | Potassium deficiency with chronic use or abuse of licorice |
| | Digitoxin | Digitoxin toxicity |
| | Digoxin | Digoxin toxicity |
| | Hydrochlorothiazide | Potassium deficiency with chronic use or abuse of licorice |
| | Indapamide | Potassium deficiency with chronic use or abuse of licorice |
| | Spironolactone | Hypokalemic alkalosis |
| Lily of the valley | Betamethasone | ↑ action and side effects of betamethasone |
| | Bisacodyl | ↑ action and side effects of bisacodyl |
| | Calcium products | ↑ action and side effects of calcium products |
| | Cascara products (OTC) | ↑ action and side effects of cascara product |

*Continued*

| Herb | Drug | Interaction |
|------|------|-------------|
| Oak | Sodium bicarbonate | ↓ action of sodium bicarbonate |
|  | Tromethamine | ↓ alkaline effect |
| Senna | Acebutolol | Possible ↑ effect of acebutolol |
|  | Adenosine | Possible ↑ effect of adenosine |
|  | Amiodarone | Possible ↑ effect of amiodarone |
|  | Amrinone | Possible ↑ action of amrinone |
|  | Atropine | Possible ↑ action of atropine with chronic use or abuse of senna |
|  | Betamethasone | Potassium deficiency with chronic use or abuse of senna |
|  | Bretylium | ↑ action of bretylium with chronic use or abuse of senna |
|  | Chlorothiazide | Potassium deficiency with chronic use or abuse of senna |
|  | Chlorthalidone | Potassium deficiency with chronic use or abuse of senna |
|  | Cortisone | Potassium deficiency with chronic use or abuse of senna |
|  | Dexamethasone | Potassium deficiency with chronic use or abuse of senna |
|  | Digitoxin | ↑ action of digitoxin |
|  | Digoxin | ↑ action of digoxin |
|  | Disopyramide | ↑ action of disopyramide |
|  | Esmolol | Potassium deficiency with chronic use or abuse of senna |
|  | Flecainide | Potassium deficiency with chronic use or abuse of senna |
|  | Fludrocortisone | Potassium deficiency with chronic use or abuse of senna |
|  | Hydrochlorothiazide | Potassium deficiency with chronic use or abuse of senna |
|  | Hydrocortisone | Potassium deficiency with chronic use or abuse of senna |
|  | Ibutilide | ↑ action of ibutilide |
|  | Indapamide | Potassium deficiency with chronic use or abuse of senna |
|  | Lidocaine | ↑ action of lidocaine |
|  | Methylprednisolone | Potassium deficiency with chronic use or abuse of senna |
|  | Metolazone | Potassium deficiency with chronic use or abuse of senna |
|  | Mexiletine | ↑ potassium loss; ↑ antidysrhythmic action |
|  | Moricizine | ↑ potassium loss; ↑ antidysrhythmic action |
|  | Phenytoin | ↑ potassium loss; ↑ antidysrhythmic action |
|  | Prednisone | Potassium deficiency |
|  | Prednisolone | Potassium deficiency |
|  | Propafenone | Potassium deficiency; ↑ antidysrhythmic action |
|  | Quinidine | Potassium deficiency; ↑ antidysrhythmic action |
|  | Sotalol | Potassium deficiency; ↑ antidysrhythmic action |
|  | Tocainide | Potassium deficiency; ↑ antidysrhythmic action |
|  | Triamcinolone | ↑ potassium loss |
| Siberian ginseng | Digitoxin | ↑ action of digitoxin |
|  | Digoxin | ↑ action of digoxin |
| Squill | Betamethasone | ↑ action and side effects of betamethasone |
|  | Bisacodyl | ↑ action and side effects of bisacodyl |
|  | Calcium products | ↑ action and side effects of calcium products |
|  | Cascara products (OTC) | ↑ action and side effects of cascara product |
| St. John's wort | Citalopram | Avoid concurrent use |
|  | Fluoxetine | Do not use concurrently |
|  | Fluvoxamine | ↑ effect of fluvoxamine, with possible fatal reaction; do not use concurrently |
|  | Oral contraceptives | ↓ effect of oral contraceptives |
|  | Sertraline | Potentiation of selective serotonin reuptake inhibitors; do not use concurrently |
| Yerba maté | Ciprofloxacin | Possible toxicity |
| Yew | Ketoconazole | ↓ action of ketoconazole |

From Skidmore-Roth L: *Mosby's handbook of herbs & natural supplements,* ed 1, St. Louis, 2001, Mosby.

# PHARMACOLOGY AND CLINICAL CALCULATIONS

## 13-1 | Formulas for drug calculations

**Surface area rule:**

$$\text{Child dose} = \frac{\text{Surface area (m}^2)}{1.73\text{m}^2} \times \text{Adult dose}$$

**Calculating strength of a solution:**

Solution strength:   Desired solution:

$$\frac{x}{100} = \frac{\text{Amount of drug desired}}{\text{Amount of finished solution}}$$

**Calculation of medication dosages:**

**Formula method:**

$$\frac{\text{Amount ordered}}{\text{Amount on hand}} \times \text{Vehicle} = \frac{\text{Number of tablets, capsules,}}{\text{or amount of liquid}}$$

Vehicle is the drug form or amount of liquid containing the dosage. Amounts used in calculation by formula must be in same system.

From Skidmore-Roth L: *Mosby's 1997 nursing drug reference,* St Louis, 1997, Mosby.

**Ratio—proportion method:**

1 tablet : tablet in mg on hand : : $x$ tablet order in mg
Know or have : : Want to know or order

Multiply means and extremes, divide both sides by known amount to get $X$. Amounts used in equation must be in same system.

**Dimensional analysis method:**

$$\text{Order in mg} \times \frac{\text{1 tablet or capsule}}{\text{What 1 tablet or capsule is in mg}}$$
$$= \text{Tablets or capsules to be given}$$

If amounts are in different systems:

$$\text{Order in mg} \times \frac{\text{1 tablet or capsule}}{\text{What 1 tablet or capsule is in g}} \times \frac{1}{1000\text{ mg}}$$
$$= \text{Tablets or capsules to be given}$$

## 13-2 | IV flow rate formulas

Use the following formulas to calculate IV flow rates.

$$\text{Flow rate (ml/hr)} = \frac{\text{Desired dose (mg/min)} \times 60 \text{ (min/hr)}}{\text{Drug concentration (mg/ml)}}$$

$$or = \frac{\text{Desired dose (}\mu\text{g/kg/min)} \times 60 \text{ (min/hr)} \times \text{wt } (kg)}{\text{Drug concentration (}\mu\text{g/ml)}}$$

$$or = \frac{\text{Drip rate (drops/min)} \times 60 \text{ (min/hr)}}{60 \text{ (drops/ml)}}$$

$$\text{Drip rate (drops/min)} = \frac{\text{Total volume to be infused (ml)} \times \text{drop factor (drops/ml)}}{\text{Total time for the infusion (min)}}$$

$$or = \frac{\text{Drops/ml}}{60 \text{ (min/hr)}} \times \frac{\text{Volume to be infused (ml/hr)}}{1}$$

From Thompson JM: *Quick reference for clinical nursing,* ed 2, St Louis, 1997, Mosby.

## 13-3 Common drug interactions*

| Drug category/representative drugs† | Interacting drug or substance | Effect |
|---|---|---|
| Antibiotics: macrolides (azithromycin, clarithromycin, dirithromycin, erythromycin) | Blood thinners (warfarin) | May enhance blood thinning effects |
| | Ergot alkaloids (ergotamine, methysergide) | Increased risk of toxicity |
| | HMG-CoA reductase inhibitors (lovastatin, pravastatin, simvastatin) | Toxic effects on muscle and severe muscle damage may occur |
| | Antiseizure drugs (carbamazepine) | May increase toxicity of carbamazepine |
| Antibiotics: penicillins (ampicillin, amoxicillin) | Birth control pills (norethindrone with ethinyl estradiol) | May interfere with birth control pills and result in unplanned pregnancy or menstrual problems |
| | Tetracyclines (doxycycline, tetracycline) | May interfere with effects of penicillins |
| | Blood thinners (warfarin) | May enhance blood thinning effects |
| Antibiotics: sulfonamides (trimethoprim/sulfamethoxazole, sulfamethizole) | Blood thinners (warfarin) | May increase blood-thinning effects |
| Antibiotics: tetracyclines (doxycycline, tetracycline) | Antacids (aluminum or magnesium containing) | Effects of tetracyclines may be reduced; separate by 3-4 hours |
| | Penicillins (ampicillin, amoxicillin) | May interfere with effects of penicillins |
| | Barbiturates (pentobarbital, phenobarbital, secobarbital) | May decrease effects of doxycycline; consider alternative tetracycline |
| Antidepressants: lithium | Sodium chloride (salt) | Low-salt diet or sudden changes in diet may cause lithium to build up |
| | Thiazide diuretics (hydrochlorothiazide) | May cause lithium toxicity |
| | Weight-loss agents (sibutramine) | May cause serious nervous system reactions |
| | Loop diuretics (furosemide) | May cause lithium toxicity |
| | ACE inhibitors (captopril, enalapril) | May cause lithium toxicity |
| Antidepressants: MAO inhibitors (isocarboxazid, phenelzine, tranylcypromine) | TCAs (amitriptyline, desipramine, doxepin, imipramine, nortriptyline) | Severe seizures and death may result; separate by at least 14 days |
| | SSRIs (citalopram, fluoxetine, fluvoxamine, paroxetine, sertraline) | Serious effects on nervous system, possibly life-threatening |
| | Sulfonylureas (glipizide, glyburide, tolbutamide) | May cause extremely low blood sugar |
| | Insulin | May cause extremely low blood sugar |
| | Dextromethorphan | May affect nervous system |
| | Tyramine-containing foods (avocados, bananas, beer, wine, caffeine, chocolate, cheese, liver, fava beans, fermented meats, canned figs, pickled herring, pineapple, raisins, sauerkraut, soy sauce, yeast extract, yogurt) | May cause severe and possibly fatal high blood pressure; warning signs are headache, vomiting, fever, and increased blood pressure |
| | Selective 5-HT$_1$ receptor agonists (naratriptan, rizatriptan, sumatriptan, zolmitriptan) | Increased risk of serious heart problems |
| | Painkillers: narcotic analgesics (codeine, meperidine) | May cause severe and possibly life-threatening reaction |
| | Weight-loss agents (sibutramine) | May cause serious nervous system reactions |
| Antidepressants: SSRIs (citalopram, fluoxetine, fluvoxamine, paroxetine, sertraline) | TCAs (amitriptyline, desipramine, doxepin, imipramine, nortriptyline) | Toxic effects may occur |
| | Blood thinners: warfarin | May increase or decrease effects of warfarin |
| | MAO inhibitors (isocarboxazid, phenelzine, tranylcypromine) | May cause serious effects on nervous system, possibly life-threatening |
| | Weight-loss agents (sibutramine) | May cause serious nervous system reactions |
| | Selective 5-HT$_1$ receptor agonists (naratriptan, rizatriptan, sumatriptan, zolmitriptan) | May cause serious nervous system reactions |
| Antidepressants: TCAs (amitriptyline, desipramine, doxepin, imipramine, nortriptyline) | Alcohol | May cause extreme drowsiness |
| | Antiseizure agents (carbamazepine) | Effects of antiseizure drug may be increased |
| | MAO inhibitors (isocarboxazid, phenelzine, tranylcypromine) | Severe seizures and death may result; separate by at least 14 days |
| | Narcotic analgesics (codeine, meperidine, oxycodone, propoxyphene) | May depress nervous system, slow breathing, and lower blood pressure |
| | SSRIs (citalopram, fluoxetine, fluvoxamine, paroxetine, sertraline) | Toxic effects may occur |

Updated by Jennifer L. McQuade, Pharm.D.

*ACE,* angiotensin-converting enzyme; *MAO,* monamine oxidase; *SSRI,* selective serotonin reuptake inhibitor; *TCA,* tricyclic antidepressant.

*This is a summary of common drug interactions and does not include all drugs and interactions. Some drugs may interact with other drugs or substances, and certain clinical situations may affect the likelihood of an interaction. Always consult detailed references and prescribing information before using or prescribing any medication.

†For herb-drug interactions, see Appendix 11-3.

| Drug category/representative drugs† | Interacting drug or substance | Effect |
|---|---|---|
| Antidiabetic agents: insulin | Beta-adrenergic blockers (pindolol, propranolol) | May mask symptoms of low blood sugar, especially with non-selective beta blockers |
| | Birth control pills (norethindrone with ethinyl estradiol) | May increase risk of high blood sugar |
| | MAO inhibitors (isocarboxazid, phenelzine, tranylcypromine) | May cause extremely low blood sugar |
| | Alcohol | May cause low blood sugar |
| Antidiabetic agents: sulfonylureas (glipizide, glyburide, tolbutamide) | Histamine $H_2$-antagonists (cimetidine, famotidine, nizatidine, ranitidine) | May cause low blood sugar |
| | Alcohol | May cause stomach upset, headaches, low blood sugar |
| | Beta-adrenergic blockers (metoprolol, propranolol) | May mask symptoms of low blood sugar; may increase or decrease blood sugar |
| | MAO inhibitors (isocarboxazid, phenelzine, tranylcypromine) | May cause extremely low blood sugar |
| | Salicylates (aspirin, aspirin-containing compounds) | May cause low blood sugar |
| Antihyperlipidemic agents: fibric acids (clofibrate, gemfibrozil) | HMG-CoA reductase inhibitors (lovastatin, pravastatin, simvastatin) | May have toxic effects on muscle and cause severe muscle damage |
| | Blood thinners (warfarin) | May increase blood-thinning effects and cause serious bleeding |
| Antihyperlipidemic agents: HMG-CoA reductase inhibitors (lovastatin, pravastatin, simvastatin) | Macrolides (azithromycin, clarithromycin, dirithromycin, erythromycin) | May have toxic effects on muscle and cause severe muscle damage |
| | Fibric acids (clofibrate, gemfibrozil) | May have toxic effects on muscle and cause severe muscle damage |
| Antiseizure agents (carbamazepine, phenytoin) | Alcohol | May cause drowsiness |
| | Birth control pills (norethindrone with ethinyl estradiol) | May interfere with birth control pills and result in unplanned pregnancy |
| | TCAs (amitriptyline, desipramine, doxepin, imipramine, nortriptyline) | May increase or decrease effects of antiseizure drug; may increase CNS effects; dosage may need adjusting |
| | Macrolides (azithromycin, clarithromycin, dirithromycin, erythromycin) | May increase toxicity of carbamazepine |
| Barbiturates (pentobarbital, phenobarbital, secobarbital) | Alcohol | May increase effects of drug, cause drowsiness, stop breathing, or cause blood pressure to drop too low |
| | Birth control pills (norethindrone with ethinyl estradiol) | May interfere with birth control pills and result in unplanned pregnancy |
| | Blood-thinners (warfarin) | May decrease blood-thinning effects |
| | Tetracyclines (doxycycline) | May decrease effects of doxycycline; consider alternative tetracycline |
| | Beta-adrenergic blockers (metoprolol, propranolol) | May decrease effects of beta-blockers |
| Benzodiazepines (alprazolam, chlordiazepoxide, clonazepam, diazepam) | Alcohol | Increased effects on central nervous system: drowsiness, confusion |
| | Narcotic analgesics (codeine, meperidine, oxycodone, propoxyphene) | May cause drowsiness and confusion |
| Birth control pills (norethindrone with ethinyl estradiol) | Antiseizure agents (carbamazepine, phenytoin) | May interfere with birth control pills and result in unplanned pregnancy; may decrease effects of antiseizure drugs |
| | Barbiturates (pentobarbital, phenobarbital, secobarbital) | May interfere with birth control pills and result in unplanned pregnancy |
| | Insulin | May increase risk of high blood sugar |
| | Penicillins (ampicillin, amoxicillin) | May interfere with birth control pills and result in unplanned pregnancy or menstrual problems |
| | Tobacco (smoking) | Increases chance of blood clots, stroke, and heart attack |
| Blood pressure drugs: ACE inhibitors (captopril, enalapril) | Potassium preparations | Increased potassium levels |
| | Digitalis glycosides (digoxin) | May increase digoxin levels |
| | Lithium | May cause lithium toxicity |

*Continued*

| Drug category/representative drugs† | Interacting drug or substance | Effect |
|---|---|---|
| Blood pressure drugs: beta-adrenergic blockers (propranolol, metoprolol) | Sulfonylureas (glipizide, glyburide, tolbutamide) | May mask symptoms of low blood sugar; may increase or decrease blood sugar |
| | Insulin | May mask symptoms of low blood sugar, especially with non-selective beta blockers |
| | Barbiturates (pentobarbital, phenobarbital, secobarbital) | May decrease effects of beta-blockers |
| | Digitalis glycosides (digoxin) | May cause extremely slow heartbeat, possibly heart block |
| | Calcium channel blockers (diltiazem, verapamil) | May increase effects on heart contractility |
| | Thiazide diuretics (hydrochlorothiazide) | May cause extremely low blood pressure |
| | Loop diuretics (furosemide) | May cause extremely low blood pressure |
| Blood pressure drugs: calcium channel blockers (diltiazem, verapamil) | Beta-adrenergic blockers (metoprolol, propranolol) | May increase effects on heart contractility |
| Blood pressure drugs: calcium channel blockers (diltiazem, verapamil) | Digitalis glycosides (digoxin) | May increase digoxin levels, increasing risk of toxicity |
| | Thiazide diuretics (hydrochlorothiazide) | May cause low blood pressure |
| | Loop diuretics (furosemide) | May cause low blood pressure |
| Blood pressure drugs: loop diuretics (furosemide) | Beta-adrenergic blockers (metoprolol, propranolol) | May cause extremely low blood pressure |
| | Digitalis glycosides (digoxin) | Can cause irregular heartbeat and extremely low blood pressure |
| | Lithium | May cause lithium toxicity |
| | Thiazide diuretics (hydrochlorothiazide) | May cause low blood pressure |
| Blood pressure drugs: thiazide diuretics (hydrochlorothiazide) | Beta-adrenergic blockers (metoprolol, propranolol) | May cause extremely low blood pressure |
| | Digitalis glycosides (digoxin) | Can cause irregular heartbeat and extremely low blood pressure |
| | Lithium | May cause lithium toxicity |
| | Loop diuretics (furosemide) | May cause low blood pressure |
| Blood thinners (heparin) | Blood thinners (warfarin) | May increase risk of bleeding |
| | Salicylates (aspirin, aspirin-containing compounds) | Increases risk of internal bleeding |
| | NSAIDs (etodolac, ibuprofen, naproxen, oxaprozin) | May cause internal bleeding or ulcers |
| Blood thinners (warfarin) | Acetaminophen, acetaminophen-containing combinations | High doses of acetaminophen may increase blood-thinning effects |
| | Barbiturates (pentobarbital, phenobarbital, secobarbital) | May decrease blood-thinning effects |
| | Blood thinners (heparin) | May increase risk of bleeding |
| | Penicillins (ampicillin, amoxicillin) | May enhance blood thinning effects |
| | Salicylates (aspirin, aspirin-containing compounds) | Increases risk of internal bleeding |
| | NSAIDs (etodolac, ibuprofen, naproxen, oxaprozin) | May cause internal bleeding or ulcers |
| | Sulfonamides (trimethoprim/sulfamethoxazole, sulfamethizole) | May increase blood-thinning effects |
| | Thyroid hormones (thyroid, levothyroxine) | May increase blood-thinning effects |
| | Vitamin K-containing foods and products | May decrease blood-thinning effects |
| | Macrolides (azithromycin, clarithromycin, dirithromycin, erythromycin) | May enhance blood thinning effects |
| | Fibric acids (clofibrate, gemfibrozil) | May increase blood-thinning effects and cause serious bleeding |
| Erectile dysfunction agents (sildenafil) | Nitrates (amyl nitrate, isosorbide dinitrate, isosorbide mononitrate, nitroglycerin) | Severe, possibly life-threatening drop in blood pressure |
| Heart drugs: digitalis glycosides (digoxin) | Beta-adrenergic blockers (propranolol, metoprolol) | May cause extremely slow heartbeat, possibly heart block |
| | Calcium channel blockers (diltiazem, verapamil) | May increase digoxin levels, increasing risk of toxicity |
| | Thiazide diuretics (hydrochlorothiazide) | Can cause irregular heartbeat and extremely low blood pressure |
| | Loop diuretics (furosemide) | Can cause irregular heartbeat and extremely low blood pressure |
| | ACE inhibitors (captopril, enalapril) | May increase digoxin levels |

Updated by Jennifer L. McQuade, Pharm.D.
*ACE,* angiotensin-converting enzyme; *MAO,* monamine oxidase; *SSRI,* selective serotonin reuptake inhibitor; *TCA,* tricyclic antidepressant.
†For herb-drug interactions, see Appendix 11-3.

| Drug category/representative drugs† | Interacting drug or substance | Effect |
|---|---|---|
| Heart drugs: nitrates (amyl nitrate, isosorbide dinitrate, isosorbide mononitrate, nitroglycerin) | Erectile dysfunction agents (Sildenafil) | Severe, possibly life-threatening drop in blood pressure |
| Histamine H2-antagonists (cimetidine, famotidine, nizatidine, ranitidine) | Sulfonylureas (glipizide, glyburide, tolbutamide) | Risk of low blood sugar |
| | Blood thinners (warfarin) | May increase effect of warfarin; possible bleeding risk, particularly with cimetidine |
| Migraine drugs: ergot alkaloids (ergotamine, methysergide) | Macrolides (azithromycin, clarithromycin, dirithromycin, erythromycin) | Increased risk of toxicity |
| | Selective 5-HT$_1$ receptor agonists (naratriptan, rizatriptan, sumatriptan, zolmitriptan) | Increased risk of serious heart problems |
| | Weight-loss agents (sibutramine) | May cause serious nervous system reactions |
| Migraine drugs: selective 5-HT$_1$ receptor agonists (naratriptan, rizatriptan, sumatriptan, zolmitriptan) | SSRIs (citalopram, fluoxetine, fluvoxamine, paroxetine, sertraline) | May cause serious nervous system reactions |
| | MAO inhibitors (isocarboxazid, phenelzine, tranylcypromine) | Increased risk of serious heart problems |
| | Ergot alkaloids (ergotamine, methysergide) | Increased risk of serious heart problems |
| | Weight-loss agents (sibutramine) | May cause serious nervous system reactions |
| Painkillers: acetaminophen, acetaminophen-containing combinations | Alcohol | May cause liver damage |
| | Blood thinners (warfarin, heparin) | High doses of acetaminophen may increase blood-thinning effects |
| Painkillers: narcotic analgesics (codeine, meperidine, oxycodone, propoxyphene) | Alcohol | May depress nervous system, slow breathing, and lower blood pressure |
| | MAO inhibitors (isocarboxazid, phenelzine, tranylcypromine) | May cause severe and possibly fatal reaction |
| | TCAs (amitriptyline, desipramine, doxepin, imipramine, nortriptyline) | May depress nervous system, slow breathing, and lower blood pressure |
| | Benzodiazepines (alprazolam, diazepam, chlordiazepoxide, clonazepam) | May cause drowsiness and confusion |
| | Weight-loss agents (sibutramine) | May cause serious nervous system reactions |
| Painkillers: NSAIDs (etodolac, ibuprofen, naproxen, oxaprozin) | Alcohol | May cause internal bleeding or ulcers |
| | Blood thinners (warfarin, heparin) | May cause internal bleeding or ulcers |
| | Salicylates (aspirin, aspirin-containing compounds) | May cause stomach upset without relieving pain; may cause internal bleeding or ulcers |
| Painkillers: salicylates (aspirin, aspirin-containing compounds) | Alcohol | May cause internal bleeding or ulcers |
| | Sulfonylureas (glipizide, glyburide, tolbutamide) | May cause low blood sugar |
| | Blood thinners (warfarin, heparin) | Increases risk of internal bleeding |
| | NSAIDs (etodolac, ibuprofen, naproxen, oxaprozin) | May cause stomach upset without relieving pain; may cause internal bleeding or ulcers |
| Thyroid hormones (thyroid, levothyroxine) | Blood thinners (warfarin) | May increase blood-thinning effects |
| Weight-loss agents (sibutramine) | Lithium | May cause serious nervous system reactions |
| | Ergot alkaloids (ergotamine, methysergide) | May cause serious nervous system reactions |
| | Selective 5-HT$_1$ receptor agonists (naratriptan, rizatriptan, sumatriptan, zolmitriptan) | May cause serious nervous system reactions |
| | Dextromethorphan | May cause serious nervous system reactions |
| | Lithium | May cause serious nervous system reactions |
| | MAO inhibitors (isocarboxazid, phenelzine, tranylcypromine) | May cause serious nervous system reactions |
| | SSRIs (citalopram, fluoxetine, fluvoxamine, paroxetine, sertraline) | May cause serious nervous system reactions |
| | Narcotic analgesics (codeine, meperidine, oxycodone, propoxyphene) | May cause serious nervous system reactions |

Updated by Jennifer L. McQuade, Pharm.D.
*ACE*, angiotensin-converting enzyme; *MAO*, monamine oxidase; *SSRI*, selective serotonin reuptake inhibitor; *TCA*, tricyclic antidepressant.
†For herb-drug interactions, see Appendix 11-3.

## 13-4 Top 200 brand name drugs by prescription

| Rank | Product | Total Rx retail units | Rank | Product | Total Rx retail units | Rank | Product | Total Rx retail units |
|---|---|---|---|---|---|---|---|---|
| 1. | Premarin Tablets | 41,755 | 64. | Monopril | 5,999 | 127. | BuSpar | 2,861 |
| 2. | Synthroid | 37,009 | 65. | Lescol | 5,698 | 128. | Elocon | 2,858 |
| 3. | Lipitor | 33,789 | 66. | Serevent | 5,657 | 129. | Levothroid | 2,844 |
| 4. | Prilosec | 28,033 | 67. | Xalatan | 5,614 | 130. | Humulin R | 2,836 |
| 5. | Norvasc | 24,093 | 68. | Flovent | 5,534 | 131. | Vicoprofen Non-Injection | 2,818 |
| 6. | Prozac | 23,598 | 69. | Celexa | 5,483 | 132. | Altace | 2,801 |
| 7. | Claritin | 23,062 | 70. | Propulsid | 5,441 | 133. | Endocet | 2,794 |
| 8. | Zithromax Z-Pak | 22,041 | 71. | Effexor XR | 5,387 | 134. | Mevacor | 2,732 |
| 9. | Zoloft | 21,189 | 72. | Nasonex | 5,218 | 135. | Ortho-Cept | 2,728 |
| 10. | Glucophage | 20,944 | 73. | Humulin 70/30 | 5,172 | 136. | Flomax | 2,618 |
| 11. | Prempro | 20,137 | 74. | Lotrisone | 5,126 | 137. | BuSpar Dividose | 2,615 |
| 12. | Paxil | 19,624 | 75. | Singulair | 4,933 | 138. | Alphagan | 2,611 |
| 13. | Zestril | 19,388 | 76. | Risperdal | 4,919 | 139. | Benzamycin | 2,603 |
| 14. | Augmentin | 19,321 | 77. | Lo/Ovral 28 | 4,674 | 140. | Tussionex | 2,541 |
| 15. | Lanoxin | 18,315 | 78. | Allegra-D | 4,547 | 141. | Nasacort AQ | 2,526 |
| 16. | Prevacid | 17,161 | 79. | Roxicet | 4,517 | 142. | Zantac | 2,486 |
| 17. | Zocor | 17,143 | 80. | Rezulin | 4,461 | 143. | Rhinocort | 2,477 |
| 18. | Celebrex | 15,922 | 81. | Ortho-Cyclen | 4,453 | 144. | Accolate | 2,477 |
| 19. | Vasotec | 14,265 | 82. | Vioxx | 4,447 | 145. | Estraderm | 2,470 |
| 20. | Levoxyl | 14,231 | 83. | Klor Con | 4,324 | 146. | Aricept | 2,465 |
| 21. | Cipro | 13,850 | 84. | Zyprexa | 4,268 | 147. | Cartia XT | 2,369 |
| 22. | Coumadin Tablets | 13,757 | 85. | Imitrex | 4,262 | 148. | Remeron | 2,351 |
| 23. | Amoxil | 13,595 | 86. | Atrovent Inhaler | 4,259 | 149. | Estrace Tablets | 2,321 |
| 24. | Ortho Tri-Cyclen | 13,077 | 87. | Desogen | 4,233 | 150. | Ultra Natalcare | 2,306 |
| 25. | Pravachol | 11,630 | 88. | Amaryl | 4,222 | 151. | Provera | 2,267 |
| 26. | Ambien | 11,604 | 89. | Adderall | 4,219 | 152. | Xanax | 2,265 |
| 27. | Biaxin | 11,217 | 90. | Serzone | 4,161 | 153. | Tri-Levlen | 2,262 |
| 28. | Ultram | 11,193 | 91. | Diovan | 4,132 | 154. | Premphase | 2,259 |
| 29. | Accupril | 10,580 | 92. | Hyzaar | 4,124 | 155. | Lasix Oral | 2,258 |
| 30. | Allegra | 10,578 | 93. | Necon 1/35 | 4,080 | 156. | Demadex | 2,218 |
| 31. | Zyrtec | 10,214 | 94. | Zestoretic | 4,080 | 157. | Estratest Tablets | 2,160 |
| 32. | Glucotrol XL | 10,174 | 95. | Vancenase AQ DS | 4,049 | 158. | Nizoral Topical | 2,156 |
| 33. | K-Dur 20 | 9,732 | 96. | Bactroban | 4,043 | 159. | Cleocin-T | 2,136 |
| 34. | Flonase | 9,661 | 97. | Plavix | 3,990 | 160. | Ritalin | 2,121 |
| 35. | Cardizem CD | 9,581 | 98. | Macrobid | 3,973 | 161. | Terazol 7 | 2,113 |
| 36. | Prinivil | 9,562 | 99. | Alesse-28 | 3,934 | 162. | Differin | 2,093 |
| 37. | Viagra | 9,422 | 100. | Ery-Tab | 3,847 | 163. | Skelaxin | 2,085 |
| 38. | Toprol XL | 9,228 | 101. | Daypro | 3,779 | 164. | Lac-Hydrin | 2,072 |
| 39. | Lotensin | 9,014 | 102. | Azmacort | 3,745 | 165. | Timoptic XE | 2,064 |
| 40. | Cardura | 8,750 | 103. | Evista | 3,662 | 166. | Vanceril | 2,062 |
| 41. | Procardia XL | 8,385 | 104. | Lotrel | 3,605 | 167. | Lamisil Oral | 2,037 |
| 42. | Fosamax | 8,121 | 105. | Combivent | 3,590 | 168. | Covera-HS | 2,008 |
| 43. | Wellbutrin SR | 7,911 | 106. | Imdur | 3,576 | 169. | Effexor | 2,007 |
| 44. | Humulin N | 7,865 | 107. | Detrol | 3,526 | 170. | Tegretol | 1,992 |
| 45. | Diflucan | 7,788 | 108. | Miacalcin Nasal | 3,292 | 171. | Patanol | 1,959 |
| 46. | Depakote | 7,608 | 109. | Avapro | 3,254 | 172. | Terazol 3 | 1,952 |
| 47. | Claritin D 12HR | 7,504 | 110. | Oxycontin | 3,226 | 173. | Zyrtec Syrup | 1,944 |
| 48. | Zithromax Suspension | 7,390 | 111. | Plendil | 3,216 | 174. | Lodine XL | 1,933 |
| 49. | Neurontin | 7,224 | 112. | Proventil HFA | 3,208 | 175. | Dyazide | 1,927 |
| 50. | Cozaar | 6,956 | 113. | Nitrostat | 3,173 | 176. | Accutane | 1,926 |
| 51. | Cefzil | 6,952 | 114. | Cycrin | 3,169 | 177. | Humalog | 1,904 |
| 52. | Adalat CC | 6,866 | 115. | Phenergan Suppository | 3,122 | 178. | Baycol | 1,903 |
| 53. | Pepcid | 6,842 | 116. | Tobradex | 3,105 | 179. | Nizoral Shampoo | 1,888 |
| 54. | Triphasil | 6,757 | 117. | Loestrin Fe 1/20 | 3,016 | 180. | One Touch Test Strip | 1,879 |
| 55. | Levaquin | 6,682 | 118. | Claritin RediTabs | 2,985 | 181. | Darvocet-N-100 | 1,870 |
| 56. | Relafen | 6,650 | 119. | Zithromax | 2,973 | 182. | Proscar | 1,858 |
| 57. | Dilantin Kapseals | 6,644 | 120. | Tiazac | 2,970 | 183. | MetroGel-Vaginal | 1,808 |
| 58. | Ortho-Novum 7/7/7 | 6,608 | 121. | Valtrex | 2,955 | 184. | Zovirax Topical | 1,788 |
| 59. | Hytrin | 6,414 | 122. | Loestrin Fe 1.5/30 | 2,942 | 185. | Premarin Vaginal | 1,767 |
| 60. | Claritin D 24HR | 6,309 | 123. | Climara | 2,937 | 186. | Ortho-Novum 1/35 | 1,763 |
| 61. | Veetids | 6,158 | 124. | Axid | 2,933 | 187. | Estrostep Fe | 1,747 |
| 62. | Ceftin | 6,018 | 125. | Arthrotec | 2,931 | 188. | Nasacort | 1,747 |
| 63. | Ziac | 6,017 | 126. | Sumycin | 2,889 | 189. | Estratab | 1,724 |

| Rank | Product | Total Rx retail units | Rank | Product | Total Rx retail units | Rank | Product | Total Rx retail units |
|------|---------|----------------------|------|---------|----------------------|------|---------|----------------------|
| 190. | K-Dur | 1,710 | 194. | Zyban | 1,664 | 198. | Micronor | 1,633 |
| 191. | Deltason | 1,710 | 195. | Diovan HCT | 1,640 | 199. | Zaroxolyn | 1,633 |
| 192. | Prinzide | 1,688 | 196. | Novolin 70/30 | 1,637 | 200. | Nitro-Dur | 1,629 |
| 193. | Biaxin Suspension | 1,670 | 197. | Retin-A | 1,634 | | | |

## 13-5 | Drug names that look alike and sound alike

| | | | | | |
|---|---|---|---|---|---|
| Accupril | Accutane | Bretylol | Brevital | CytoGm | Gamimune N |
| Acetazolamide | Acetohexamide | Brevibloc | Brevital | Cytosar (Cytara-bine) | Cytoxan |
| Achromycin | Actinomycin | Bumex | Buprenex | Cytosar | Cytovene |
| Achromycin | Aureomycin | Bumex | Permax | Cytotec | Cytoxan |
| Adderall | Inderal | Butabarbital | Butalbital | Danazol | Dantrium |
| Adenosine (Adeno-card) | Adenosine Phos-phate | Cafergot | Carafate | Darvon | Diovan |
| Adriamycin | Aredia | Calciferol | Calcitriol | Daunorubicin | Doxorubicin |
| Adriamycin | Idamycin | Calotan | Celtin | Daypro | Diupress |
| Albuterol | Atenolol | Capitrol | Captopril | DDAVP Nasal | DDAVP WI Rhinal Tube |
| Aldara | Alora | Carboplatin | Cisplatin | Decaderm | Decadron |
| Alkeran | Leukeran | Cardene SR | Cardizem SR | Decadron | Percodan |
| Alkeran | Myleran | Cardene | Cardizem | Demerol | Dilaudid |
| Allegra | Viagra | Cardizem CD | Cardizem SR | Demerol | Temaril |
| Allopurinol | Apresoline | Cardura | Coumadin | Denavir | Indinavir |
| Alprazolam | Lorazepam | Cardura | Ridaura | Depo-Estradiol | Depo-Testadiol |
| Altace | Alteplase | Cataflam | Catapres | Depo-Medrol | Solu-Medrol |
| Altace | Artane | Catapres | Catarase | DES | E.E.S. |
| Altenol | Atenolol | Cedax | Cidex | Desipramine | Imipramine |
| Altenuvax | Meruvax | Cefaclor | Cephalexin | Diabeta | Zebeta |
| Alupent | Atrovent | Cefazolin | Cefprozil | Dialose Plus (Docu-sate Potassium/ Casanthranol) | Dialose Plus (Docu-sate Sodium/ Phenolphtalein) |
| Amantadine | Ranitidine | Cefotaxime | Celtizoxime | | |
| Amantadine | Rimantadine | Cefprozil | Cefuroxime | Diamox | Dobutrex |
| Ambien | Amen | Ceftazidime | Ceftizoxime | Diamox | Trimox |
| Amicar | Amikin | Ceftin | Cefzil | Diazepam | Ditropan |
| Amiloride | Amiodipine | Cefuroxime | Cefotaxime | Dicyclomine | Diphenhydramine |
| Amiodarone | Amrinone (7/1/ 2000, changed to inamrinone) | Cefuroxime | Deferoxamine | Diflucan | Diprivan |
| | | Cefzil | Ketzol | Dilacor XR | Pilocar |
| Amitriptyline | Nortriptyline | Celebrex | Celexa | Dilone | Dyclone |
| Amoxapine | Amoxicillin | Celebrex | Cerebyx | Diphenatol | Diphenidol |
| Amoxapine | Amoxil | Celexa | Cerebyx | Dobutamine | Dopamine |
| Amoxicillin | Amoxil | Celexa | Zyprexa | Dolobid | Slobid |
| Amoxicillin | Atarax | Centoxin | Cyloxan | Doxcycline | Doxepin |
| Anfranil | Enalapril | Cephapirin | Cephradine | Doxil | Paxil |
| Ansaid | Asacol | Chlorpromazine | Chlorpropamide | Doxorubicin | Idarubicin |
| Antacid | Atacand | Chlorpromazine | Prochlorperazine | Drisdol | Drysol |
| Anusol | Anusol-HC | Chlor-Trimeton | Chlor-Trimeton (Non-drowsy) | Dyazide | Thiacide |
| Ara | C-Arasine | | | Dynacin | DynaCirc |
| Aredia | Meridia | Cisaprid | Cisplatine | Echogen | Epogen |
| Asacol | Os-Cal | Cisplatin | Cisplatinol | Edecrin | Eulexin |
| Asparaginase | Pegaspargasa | Clinoril | Clozaril | Edetate Calcium Disodium | Edetate Disodium |
| Avandia | Prandin | Clinoril | Oruvail | | |
| Aventyl | Bentyl | Clomiphene | Clomipramine | Elavil | Mellaril |
| Bactocil | Pathocil | Clomipramine | Norpramin (Desipramine) | Elavil | Oruvail |
| Banthine | Brethine | | | Eldepryl | Enalapril |
| Belladenal | Belladonna | Clonidine | Kionopin | Eludax | Eurax |
| Beloptic S | Betoptic 0.5% | Clonidine | Klonopin (Clonazepam) | Enalapril | Ramipril |
| Beloptic | Betagan | | | Enduron | Imuran |
| Benadryl | Benadryl Dye-Free | Codeine | Iodine | EquagesicO | EquiGesicO |
| Benadryl | Benylin | Codeine | Lodine | Erex | Urex |
| Benylin | Betalin | Cognex | Corgard | Eskalith | Estratest |
| Benylin | Ventolin | Compazine | Coumadin | Estraderm | Testoderm |
| Benzac W | Benzac W Wash | Cordarone | Inocor | Estratab | Estratest |
| Bepridil | Prepidil | Cortef | Lortab | Estratest | Estratest HS |
| Betagalen | Betagan | Cozaar | Zocor | Ethambutol | Ethmozine |
| Bicillin | V-Cillin | Cyclobenzaprine | Cyproheptadine | | |
| | | Cyclophosphamide | Cyclosporine | | |
| | | Cycloserine | Cyclosporine | | |

*Continued*

| | | | | | |
|---|---|---|---|---|---|
| Ethmozine | Erythrocin | Lanoxin | Xanax | Oprelvekin | Proleukin |
| Etidornate | Etretinate | Lasix | Lomotil | Organidin | Organidin NR |
| Etidronate | Etorridate | Lasix | Luvox | Orinase | Ornade |
| Eurax | Serax | L-Dopa (Levodopa) | Methyldopa | Paciltaxel | Paroxetine |
| Eurax | Urex | | | Paciltaxel | Paxil |
| E-vista | Evista | Lenoxin | Levoxine | Paraplatin | Platinol |
| Fam Pren Forte | Parafon Forte | Leucovorin | Leukeran | Parfodel | Pindolol |
| Feldene | Seldane | Leucovorin | Leukine | Pavulon | Peptavlon |
| Fentanyl | Sufenta | Leukeran | Myleran | Paxil | Taxol |
| Fentanyl | Sufentanil | Levbid | Lithobid | Pediapred | Pediaprofen |
| Flomax | Fosamax | Levobunolol | Levocabastine | Pediaprofen | Pediazole |
| Flomax | Volmax | Levoxine | Levsin | Pediaprofen | Prelone |
| Floricet | Florinal | Levoxyl | Luvox | Penicillamine | Penicillin |
| Flucytosine | Fluorouracil | Librax | Librium | Pentobarbital | Phenobarbital |
| Fludarabine | Flumadine | Lioresal | Lotensin | Perative | Periactin |
| Fludara | FUDR | Lithobid | Lithostat | Percodan | Percorten |
| Folic Acid | Folinic Acid | Lithobid | Lithotabs | Phenelzine | Phenylzin |
| Fortovase | Invirase | Loniten | Lotensin | Phenergan | Theragran |
| Furosemide | Torsemide | Lopid | Lorabid | Pindolol | Plendil |
| Gamulin Rh | MICRhoGAM | Lopurin | Lupron | Pitocin | Pitressin |
| Garamycin | Kanamycin | Lorabid | Lortab | Plendil | Prilosec |
| Gentamicin Ophthalamic Solution | Gentian Violet Solution | Lortab | Luride | Plendil | Prinivil |
| Gilipizide | Glyburide | Lotensin | Lovastalin | Pondimin | Prednisone |
| Glucophage | Glutofac | Lotrimin | Lotrisone | Posicor | Proscar |
| Glucotrol | Glyburide | Lotrimin | Otrivin | Potassium Phosphate | Sodium Phosphate |
| Granulex | Regranex | Loxitane | Soritane | Pravachol | Prevacid |
| Haldol | Stadol | Lupron | Nuprin | Pravachol | Propranolol |
| Haldrone | Halodrin | Magnesium Gluceptate | Magnesium Sulfate | PreCare | Precose |
| Halfprin | ½ Halfprin | Mapron (Meprobamate in Australia) | Mepron (Atovaquone in US) | Prednisolone | Prednisone |
| Haloperidol | Halotestin HC | Materna | Ibuprofen | Prednisone | Prilosec |
| Hemoccult | Seracult | Mazicon | Mivacron | Premarin | Primaxin |
| Heparin | Hespan | Medi-Gesic | Medigesic | Premarin | Provera |
| Hexadrol | Hexalol | Medrol ADT | Medrol Dosepak | Prilosec | Prinivil |
| Hycodan | Vicodin | Medroxyprogesterone | Methylprednisolone | Prilosec | Prozac |
| Hydrocodone | Hydrocortisone | Megace | Regian | Prinivil | Proventil |
| Hydromorphone | Meperidine | Meperidine Liquid | Morphine Liquid | Proctocort | Proctopream |
| Hydromorphone | Morphine | Methadone | Methylphenidate | Profen LA | Profen II |
| Hydroxyzine | Hyralazine | Methotrexate | Metolazone | Profen | Profen II |
| Hygroton | Regroton | Methylprednisolone | Prednisone | Prokine | Proleukin |
| Hytone | Vytone | Metoclopramide | Metolazone | Prolixin | Proloid |
| IMDUR | Inderal LA | Metoprolol | Misoprosiol | Promethazine | Promethazine with Codeine |
| IMDUR | K-Dur | Micro-K | Micronase | | |
| Imferon | Imuran | Minoxidil | Monopril | Propranolol | Propulsid |
| Imferon | Interferon | Monoket | Monopril | Proscar | Prosom |
| Imferon | Roferon-A | Mycelex | Myoflex | Proscar | Prozac |
| Imipenem | Omnipen | Mylanta Gas | Mylicon | Provera | Provir |
| Imovax | Imovax ID | Narcan | Norcuron | Psorcon | Psorion |
| Inderal | Isordil | Nasalcrom | Nasalide | Quinidine | Quinine |
| Inderal | Toradol | Navane | Norvasc | ReFresh (breath drops) | Refresh (lubricant eye drops) |
| Inhibace (Captopril in Israel) | Inhibace (Cilazapril in Switzerland & Japan) | Navelbine | Navoban | Renografin-60 | Reno-M-60 |
| | | Nelfinavir | Nevirapine | Reserpine | Risperdal (Risperidone) |
| Interferon 2 | Interleukin 2 | Neocare | Neocate | Retrovir | Ritonavir |
| Iodine | Lodine | Nicardipine | Nifedipine | Revex | ReVia |
| Isordil | Plendil | Nicobid | Nitro-Bid | Rifabutin | Rilampin |
| Isotretinoin | Tretinon | Nicoderm | Nitroderm | Ritalin | Ritodrine |
| Kaopectate | Kayexelate | Norflex | Noroxin (Norfloxacin) | Roxanol | Roxicet |
| K-Lor | Klor | | | Roxanol | Roxicodone Intensol |
| K-Phos Neutral | Neutra-Phos-K | Norpramin | Nortriptyline | | |
| Lactacare | Lacticare | Novclin 70/30 | Novolin 70/30 PenFill Prefilled | Salagen (Asprin, Buffered) name retired in 1993 | Salagen (Pilocarpine) name reissued in 1994 |
| Lamicel | Lamisil | | | | |
| Lamictal | Lomotil | Ocufen | Ocuflox (Ofloxacin) | Seldane D | Semprex D |
| Lamivudine | Lamotrigine | | | Serax | Xerac |
| Lanoxin | Lasix | Ocufen | Ocupress | Serentil | Sinequan |
| Lanoxin | Lenoxin | Ocu Mycin | Ocumycin | Seroquel | Serzone |
| Lanoxin | Levoxine | | | Soma | Soma Compound |
| Lanoxin | Lomotil | | | | |

| | | | | | |
|---|---|---|---|---|---|
| Sulfasalazine | Sulfixazole | Triad(Butalbital/ | Triad (Zinc Oxide/ | Vapesid | Versed |
| Sumatriptan | Zolmitriptan | Acetaminophen/ | Petrolatum/ | Verelan | Virilon |
| Symmetrel | Synthroida | Caffeine) | Mineral Oil) | Versed | Vistaril |
| Tedral | Teldrin | Triaminic | Triaminicin | Vexol | Vosol |
| Tegretol | Toradol | Trifluoperazine | Trihexyphenidyl | Viaracept | Viramune |
| Tenormin | Thiamine | Trimox | Tylox | Vinblastine | Vincristine |
| Terbinaline | Terfenadine | Tri-Norinyl | Triphasil | Vioxx | Zyvox |
| Tetracycline | Tetradcyl Sul- | Tronolane | Tronothane | Xanax | Zantac |
| | fate | Tussi-Organidin | Tussi-Organidin | Xeloda | Xenical |
| Thyrar | Thyrolar | | DM | Yocon | Zocor |
| Tiagabine | Tizanidine | Tylox | Wymox | Zantac | Zofran |
| Tiazac | Ziac | Tylox | Xanax | Zarontin | Zentron |
| Timoptic | Viroptic | Uridon | Vicodin | Zinacef | Zithromax |
| Tobradex | Tobrex | Urised | Urispas | Zocor | Zoloft |
| Toradol | Torecan | Valium | Versed | Zonalon | Zone A Forte |
| Toradol | Tramadol | Vancenase | Vanceril | Zosyn | Zotran |
| Trandate | Tridrate | Vantin | Ventolin | Zyprexa | Zyrtec |

## 13-6   Adverse drug effects during pregnancy*

| *Effect of drug* | *Drugs known to produce the effect in humans* |
|---|---|
| **First-trimester effects on embryonic development** | |
| Abortion | Acitretin, isotretinoin, misoprostol, quinine |
| Multiple anomalies involving craniofacial development | Acitretin, diazepam, dicumarol, ethanol, isotretinoin, methotrexate, para-methadione, phenytoin, quinine, thalidomide, trimethadione, warfarin |
| Neural tube defects | Valproate |
| Goiter | Iodide, methimazole, propylthiouracil |
| Abnormalities or reproductive organs | Androgens, diethylstilbestrol, estrogens, progestins |
| Inhibition of growth | Methotrexate, tetracycline, tobacco smoke |
| **Second- and third-trimester effects on fetal development** | |
| Abortion, mortality | Acitretin, captopril, heroin, isotretinoin, methotrexate, misoprostol, thalido-mide, tobacco smoke |
| Mental retardation | Dicumarol, ethanol, warfarin |
| Altered cardiovascular function | Anticholinergic drugs, propranolol, terbutaline |
| Hearing loss and loss of balance | Aminoglycoside antibiotics |
| Hyperbilirubinemia | Nitrofurantoin, sulfonamides |
| Hemolytic anemia | Nitrofurantoin |
| Goiter | Iodide, methimazole, propylthiouracil |
| Abnormalities of reproductive organs | Androgens, diethylstilbestrol, estrogens, progestins |
| Inhibition of growth | Captopril, dicumarol, ethanol, heroin, methotrexate, tetracycline, tobacco smoke, warfarin |
| Discoloration of teeth and reduced enamel | Tetracycline |
| **Labor, delivery, and perinatal period** | |
| Increased mortality | Tobacco smoking, cocaine abuse, warfarin |
| Altered cardiovascular function | Anticholinergic agents, caffeine, heroin, lidocaine, meperidine, propranolol, terbutaline |
| Gray-baby syndrome | Chloramphenicol |
| Respiratory depression | Diazepam, meperidine, morphine, phenobarbital, ethanol, tobacco smoking |
| Respiratory distress | Reserpine |
| Bleeding | Aspirin, dicumarol, indomethacin, warfarin |
| Hypoglycemia | Chlorpropamide, propranolol, tolbutamide |
| Hyperbilirubinemia | Nitrofurantoin, sulfonamides |
| Hemolytic anemia | Nitrofurantoin |
| Hyperirritability | Cocaine |

From Clark JBF, Queener SF, Karb VB: *Pharmacologic basis of nursing practice,* ed 5, St Louis, 1996, Mosby.
*This list does not include all drugs that affect fetal and neonatal function but is intended to give representative examples. The nurse should check sources of specific information about individual agents when drugs are administered to pregnant patients.

## 13-7    FDA pregnancy categories

| Category | Level of risk with drug exposure | Examples |
|:---:|---|---|
| A | Controlled studies in women fail to demonstrate risk in the first trimester (and there is no evidence of risk in later trimesters), and possibility of fetal harm appears remote. | Thyroid hormones |
| B | Animal reproduction studies have not demonstrated fetal risk, but there are no controlled studies in pregnant women. Animal reproduction studies have shown adverse effect (other than decreased fertility) that was not confirmed in controlled studies on women in first trimester. There is no evidence of risk in later trimesters. | Amoxicillin, buspirone, cimetidine, fluoxetine, hydrochlorothiazide, metronidazole, nizatidine, piperacillin |
| C | Studies in animals have revealed adverse effects on fetus, and there are no controlled studies in women. In some cases, studies in women and animals are not available. Drugs in this category should be given only if potential benefit justifies risk to fetus. | Alteplase, captopril, ciprofloxacin, codeine, enalapril, gentamicin, isoproterenol, lisinopril, morphine, reserpine, tubocurarine |
| D | There is positive evidence of human fetal risk, but the benefits for pregnant women may be acceptable despite the risk, as in life-threatening diseases for which safer drugs cannot be used or are ineffective. An appropriate statement must appear in the "warnings" section of the labeling of drugs in this category. | Amikacin, midazolam, netilmicin, tobramycin |
| X | Studies in animals or humans have demonstrated fetal abnormalities, there is evidence of fetal risk based on human experience, or both. The risk of using the drug in pregnant women clearly out-weighs any possible benefit. The drug is contraindicated in women who are or may become pregnant. An appropriate statement must appear in the "contraindications" section of the labeling of drugs in this category. | Isotretinoin, lovastatin, methotrexate |

From Clark JBF, Queener SF, Karb VB: *Pharmacologic basis of nursing practice,* ed 5, St Louis, 1996, Mosby.

# 14 INFECTION CONTROL

## 14-1 CDC isolation guidelines

The Centers for Disease Control and Prevention (CDC) has issued **new isolation guidelines** that contain two tiers of approach. The first and most important tier contains precautions designed to care for all clients in health care facilities regardless of their diagnosis or risk to have an infection. This new isolation is called **Standard Precautions** and uses the major features of Universal Precautions and body substance isolation. Standard Precautions apply to (1) blood, (2) all body fluids except sweat regardless of whether they contain blood, (3) non-intact skin, and (4) mucus membranes. Standard Precautions promote handwashing and use of gloves, masks, eye protection, or gowns when appropriate for patient contact.

The second tier condenses the old disease-specific and categories approach to isolation into three new transmission categories: Airborne Precautions, Droplet Precautions, and Contact Precautions. These are designed to interrupt transmission of infection from a known or probable source. These measures may be combined for diseases having more than one mode of transmission. For example, chickenpox is listed under Airborne and Contact Precautions. When used singularly or combined, these are to be used in addition to Standard Precautions.

**Airborne Precautions** are designed to reduce transmission of certain diseases such as tuberculosis, measles, or chickenpox or airborne droplet nuclei (5 microns or smaller). Microorganisms may be carried by air currents or dust particles and inhaled by a susceptible host. This requires the use of a private room with negative air flow and at least six air exchanges per hour, respiratory protection when entering rooms, and placement of surgical mask on client when out of room. Additional precautions may be necessary to prevent the transmission of tuberculosis.

**Droplet Precautions** are designed to reduce transmission of certain diseases such as rubella or pertussis known to be transmitted on large particle droplets (larger than 5 microns) inhaled by a susceptible host. In this type of Isolation, the client should be in a private room or cohorted with a client with the same microorganism.

## Standard precautions (Tier one)

- Standard precautions apply to blood, all body fluids, secretions, excretions (except sweat), non-intact skin, and mucous membranes.
- Hands are washed between patient contacts, after contact with blood, body fluids, secretions, and excretions and after contact with equipment or articles contaminated by them; and immediately after gloves are removed.
- Gloves are worn when touching blood, body fluids, secretions, excretions, non-intact skin, mucous membranes, or contaminated items. Gloves should be removed and hands washed between patient care.
- Masks, eye protection, or face shields are worn if patient care activities may generate splashes or sprays of blood or body fluid.
- Gowns are worn if soiling of clothing is likely from blood or body fluid. Wash hands after removing gown.
- Patient care equipment is properly cleaned and reprocessed and single use items are discarded.
- Contaminated linen is placed in leak-proof bag and handled as to prevent skin and mucous membrane exposure.
- All sharp instruments and needles are discarded in a puncture-resistant container. CDC recommends that needles be disposed of uncapped or use a mechanical device for recapping.
- A private room is unnecessary unless the patient's hygiene is unacceptable. Check with Infection Control Professional.

## Transmission categories (Tier two)

| Category | Disease | Barrier protection |
|---|---|---|
| Airborne precautions | Droplet nuclei smaller than 5 microns; measles; chickenpox (Varicella); disseminated varicella zoster; pulmonary or laryngeal TB* | Private room, negative airflow of at least six exchanges per hour, mask or respiratory protection device (see CDC TB Guidelines) |
| Droplet precautions | Droplets larger than 5 microns, diphtheria (pharyngeal); rubella; streptococcal pharyngitis, pneumonia, or scarlet fever in infants and young children; pertussis; mumps; mycoplasma pneumonia; meningococcal pneumonia or sepsis; pneumonic plague | Private room or cohort patients; mask |
| Contact precautions | Direct patient or environmental contact; colonization or infection with multidrug-resistant organism; respiratory syncytial virus; shigella and other enteric pathogens; major wound infections; herpes simplex; scabies; varicella zoster (disseminated) | Private room or cohort patients; gloves, gowns |

In addition to Standard Precautions, a mask should be worn when working within three feet of the client.

**Contact Precautions** are designed to reduce transmission of epidemiologically significant microorganisms from specific clients known or suspected to be infected or colonized. For example, multidrug-resistant organisms such as Methicillin-resistant Staphylococcus aureus (MRSA) or highly infectious microorganisms such as respiratory syncytial virus would be included in this category. Transmission occurs by direct contact with the client (skin-to-skin contact when performing patient care activities) or indirect contact (touching) of contaminated environmental surfaces. In this category, the client should be in a private room or cohorted with a client with a similar infection, and an emphasis is put on hand washing and the use of gloves and gowns.

The CDC further recommends the use of Standard Precautions for all immunocompromised clients. In addition, transmission-based precautions may be needed to reduce infection risks for these clients. Users of the Isolation Guidelines are referred to an additional CDC document to prevent nosocomial aspergillosis and Legionnaires' disease in immunocompromised clients.

Adapted from Garner JS and the Hospital Infection Control Practices Advisory Committee: *CDC Guideline for Isolation Precautions in Hospitals.* Am J Infect Control 24:26-52, 1996.

---

## 14-2   OSHA standard on occupational exposure to blood-borne pathogens

### INTRODUCTION

On December 6, 1991, the Occupational Safety and Health Administration (OSHA) issued its final standard on Occupational Exposure to Bloodborne Pathogens. In issuing this ruling, OSHA declared that healthcare workers face a significant health risk in the workplace if occupational exposure to bloodborne pathogens is a reasonable possibility. Although OSHA is concerned with the transmission of any bloodborne pathogen, the ruling is directed toward preventing or minimizing exposure to the Hepatitis B virus (HBV) and the Human Immunodeficiency Virus (HIV).

OSHA's ruling called "Occupational Exposure to Bloodborne Pathogens" and published in the Federal Register is a long-awaited response to a congressional mandate to create protection for healthcare workers against exposure to HBV and HIV. OSHA concluded that the danger of bloodborne pathogens could be minimized or eliminated by taking certain precautions in the workplace. These precautions include a combination of controls in engineering, general work practices, personal protective clothing and equipment, training of personnel, Hepatitis B vaccination of healthcare workers, and the use of warning signs and labels.

The OSHA standard mandates the Universal Precautions guidelines recommended by the CDC since August 1987. This is a system of infection control that is based on the assumption that medical history and examination cannot reliably identify all patients infected with HIV, HBV, or other potentially infectious diseases. Therefore, blood and body fluid precautions must be consistently used with ALL patients. In 1996, The Centers of Disease Control and Prevention published new recommendations for protection against bloodborne diseases and other pathogens (Appendix 14-1). The OSHA standard has not changed.

Surprisingly, however, OSHA far exceeded the CDC guidelines in both the scope of healthcare workers and employers covered under the standard, and the demands made in complying with the regulation. Most businessess were not prepared for addressing the scope of the new regulations. It is important to understand that the CDC guidelines presented in August 1987 and February 1996 are only recommendations, but a ruling from a powerful governmental agency like OSHA makes the practice of Universal Precautions a requirement, and an enforceable law.

OSHA identifies 24 sectors of industry and over 500,000 facilities that are subject to this ruling. Almost five million workers are employed in hospitals, nursing homes, medical and dental offices.

One of the surprises in the standard was OSHA's inclusion of almost a million workers employed in industry outside healthcare facilities. Among the businesses affected are linen and laundry services, waste removal services, funeral homes and mortuaries, veterinarian clinics, and medical equipment companies.

The standard applies to any workplace where any workers who, in the course of their duties, might come into contact with blood, body fluids, or other potentially infectious materials. The standard required all facilities to be in full compliance with the standard by July 6, 1992.

The standard covers employees in ALL health care facilities including hospitals, clinics, dentist and doctor offices, blood banks, plasma centers, occupational health clinics, nursing homes, hospices, emergency care centers, clinical laboratories, and institutions for the developmentally disabled. This includes part time, temporary, or probationary employees in both permanent and temporary worksites.

Healthcare facilities in 23 states and two territories that have state OSHA-approved plans are not covered by the federal standard. These states are: Alaska, Arizona, California, Connecticut, Hawaii, Indiana, Iowa, Kentucky, Maryland, Michigan, Minnesota, Nevada, New Mexico, New York, North Carolina, Oregon, Puerto Rico, South Carolina, Tennessee, Utah, Vermont, Virginia, the Virgin Islands, Washington, and Wyoming. In Connecticut and New York, the state plan covers only state and local government employees; all other employees are covered by the federal OSHA standard.

Because state standards must be "at least as effective" as the federal standard, healthcare facilities located in these states must assess their compliance with the federal standard as a starting point, and then review their individual state plan for any additional requirements.

### KEY PROVISIONS OF THE STANDARD

#### Purpose

The purpose of the standard is to limit occupational exposure to blood and other potentially infectious materials.

#### Scope

The ruling covers all employees who have the potential to come into contact with blood, body fluids, or other potentially infectious materials (OPIM).

#### Requirements

*Exposure control plan*

- Implementation of an Exposure Control Plan in which the employer must identify, in writing, workers who might be at risk for exposure to blood or other potentially infectious materials.

The employer's written plan must also explain how the facility will comply with the standard.

- The employer's plan must include:
- A determination by job task, procedure and/or job classification of how an employee might be exposed during the performance of the job. This must be done without regard to personal protective clothing and equipment. The list of procedures in which exposure may occur must be posted in the facility. The list of job classifications must include the names of employees who fill those positions.
- The method, including a schedule, of how the plan will be implemented. This must include details of personal protective equipment to be used, work practices in housekeeping, Hepati-

Adapted from Goodner B, Acello B: *The OSHA handbook,* ed 2, 1997, Skidmore-Roth Publishing.

tis B vaccinations, evaluation of exposure and required followup. Hazard communication and recordkeeping, detailed procedures for evaluating potentials of exposure in the workplace.

- A detailed plan for evaluating the circumstances if exposure occurs in the workplace. This plan should include first aid, evaluation by a healthcare professional, treatment, testing of source patient, follow up testing for the employee if indicated. A written report of the exposure incident must be provided to the employee within 15 days of the incident.
- The plan must be readily accessible to employees and available at all times to OSHA. All employees must know where the plan is kept in case of an OSHA inspection.

### Methods of compliance

- Implementation of Methods of Compliance, specifically, Universal Precautions, engineering and work practice controls.

Universal Precautions are now required. Every healthcare worker must take protective measures when in contact with any patient, and every patient must be approached as if the patient is HIV or HBV infected. This also includes emergency situations.

Examples of engineering controls include puncture-resistant containers for needles and other sharp instruments, proper packaging for specimens and infectious/hazardous waste products. Any device that is intended to remove or isolate bloodborne pathogens from the workplace is considered an engineering control.

Work practice controls are any practices that decrease the possibility of exposure to bloodborne pathogens by changing the way a task or procedure is performed. An example of work practice control is prohibiting recapping of needles by the two-handed method (changing to no recapping or recapping by one-handed method when necessary). Another example is the Hepatitis B vaccination requirement.

OSHA further requires that engineering and work practice controls be reviewed on a regular basis to ensure effective functioning. Other requirements that fall under general work practices and controls are:

- Proper and convenient handwashing facilities.
- To minimize needlesticks, needles and other sharps cannot be broken, and must be put in puncture-resistant containers that are labeled and color-coded. The containers must be leak-proof, top and bottom.
- Recapping of needles is strictly prohibited. If a medical procedure requires recapping, it must be done by the one-handed method or with the use of an instrument.
- Specimens (such as blood, body fluids, urine, tissue, biopsies) must be put in a leakage-proof container. Color-coding and labeling is required when a specimen is transported.
- Contaminated equipment must be decontaminated before servicing or shipping. If the equipment cannot be completely decontaminated, a label to that effect should be affixed.
- Any labels must include the red-orange biohazard symbol.
- The person or the business to whom the specimen is being sent must be notified and appropriately informed of the hazard before it is sent.
- Medical and nursing procedures must be performed in such a way as to prevent or decrease spraying, spilling or splashing of blood or body fluids.
- Eating, drinking, and smoking is prohibited in the work area where there is a potential for exposure.
- Housekeeping procedures for cleaning and decontamination must be developed for and by each department in the facility.

### Personal protective equipment

- Implementation of the use of personal protective equipment.

When a potential for occupational exposure exists, employers must provide, at no cost, and require employees to use appropriate personal protective equipment (PPE). Examples of PPE are gloves, gowns, lab coats, masks, mouthpieces, eye protection, and resuscitation bags. All items must be clean, in good repair, and replaced when necessary. Gloves are not necessarily required for routine phlebotomies in volunteer blood donation centers but must be made available to employees who want to glove. Gloves must be worn if the employee has nonintact skin on the hands.

PPE must be designed and made of the kind of material that will not allow potentially infectious material to penetrate through to the worker's clothes, skin, eye, mouth, or any part of the body with normal use.

The following requirements apply to PPE:

- The employer must make sure the employee uses the equipment correctly.
- PPE must be quickly accessible and always available in the correct and appropriate sizes.
- Special, nonallergenic equipment, such as gloves, must be provided for employees who have allergies.
- The employer must launder or dispose of the equipment at no charge to the employee.
- PPE must be placed in designated containers for cleaning or disposal.
- Gloves must be worn any time contact with blood or OPIM is anticipated. Disposal gloves are not to be reused. Other gloves may be reused after decontaminating as long as the glove is fully intact with no nicks or cuts.
- Gowns, masks and/or proper eye protection must be worn, depending upon the nature of exposure that is reasonably anticipated.

### Information and training

- Implementation of an information and training program for employees.

The employer is required to present information and training regarding occupational exposure to any employee immediately upon employment or upon assignment of any task or procedure in which the employee might be at risk for bloodborne exposure. This information and/or training must be repeated annually or as necessary when reassignments or modification of job descriptions occur, and training must be conducted by a person qualified to teach the subject matter.

All training sessions must include:

- An accessible copy of the regulatory text of the standard and explanation of what it means.
- A general explanation of the epidemiology, signs and symptoms of bloodborne diseases.
- An explanation of the modes of transmission of bloodborne pathogens.
- An explanation of the employer's exposure control plan along with a copy of the plan to each employee.
- An explanation of the appropriate methods for recognizing tasks/procedures that may involve exposure to blood or other potentially infectious material.
- An explanation of the use and limitations of methods that will prevent or reduce exposure, including appropriate engineering controls, work practices, and personal protective equipment.
- An explanation of why and how certain personal protective equipment is chosen and why employees are required to use it.
- Information and demonstration of the types, proper use, location, removal, handling, decontamination, and disposal of personal protective equipment.
- Information on Hepatitis B vaccine, including information on its efficacy, safety, method of administration, the benefits of vaccination, and that the vaccine and administration will be offered free of charge to the employee.
- Information on the correct procedure be taken if exposure to blood or other potentially infectious materials occurs. The name and title of the person to contact in an emergency must be included.
- Procedure on post-exposure evaluation and follow-up.
- An explanation of signs/labels and/or color coding used to identify hazards.
- An opportunity for interactive questions and answers with the person conducting the training.

*Hepatitis B vaccination*

- Implementation of Hepatitis B vaccinations to all employees. OSHA requires Hepatitis B series be made available to all employees who have reasonable or potential occupational exposure to blood or other potentially infectious materials within 10 working days of assignment. These vaccinations must be administered at no cost, at a reasonable time and place, under the supervision of licensed physician/licensed healthcare professional and according to the latest recommendations of the US Public Health Service (USPHS).

The following also applies to this requirement:

- If an employee does refuse the vaccination, the OSHA declination form must be signed.
- Prescreening can not be required as a condition of receiving the vaccine.
- Employees who decline to take the vaccination, may at any time reconsider and be given the vaccine free of cost.
- Should booster doses later be recommended by the USPHS, employees must be offered the injections at no cost.

*Post-exposure evaluation and follow-up:*

- Implementation of a plan for evaluation and follow-up if occupational exposure does occur.

OSHA places a great deal of emphasis on this part of its ruling. This requirement specifies procedures that must be made available to all employees who have had an exposure incident. The medical evaluation and follow-up must, at the very minimum, include the following:

- Initially, the employer must keep all information regarding the employee's exposure confidential.
- Document the circumstances of the exposure, identifying and testing the source individual.
- Laboratory tests must be conducted by an accredited laboratory at no cost to the employee.
- Test the exposed employee's blood if he/she consents.

If employee refuses HIV or HBV testing, be sure to document reasons given by the employee. If the employee consents to having blood drawn, but refuses testing for HIV, the blood can be preserved for 90 days. If the employee then elects, the blood can then be tested for HIV.

- Results of the source individual's blood testing must be made available to the employee as soon as those results are received.
- Postexposure prophylaxis, counseling and evaluation required by the employee must be provided by the facility.
- The employer must provide the employee with the physician's written evaluation within 15 days of the physician completing the evaluation.

The following information must be supplied to the physician who evaluates an employee involved in an exposure incident:

- A copy of the Bloodborne Pathogen Standard
- A description, in the employee's words, of how the exposure incident occurred.
- Documentation of the circumstances of the incident, including routes of entry.
- Any results that may be available on the source individual's blood testing or diagnosis.
- Any medical records that might be relevant to the treatment of the employee, including Hepatitis B vaccination status.

The physician's written evaluation must include only the following information. (Any other findings must be confidential and cannot be written in the report). The physician must state:

- Whether or not the Hepatitis B vaccine is indicated.
- Whether the employee has been informed of the results of the evaluation and testing.
- Whether further evaluation and treatment are required.

*Hazard communication*

- Implementation of a system of warning employees about potentially infectious materials by affixing the universal biohazard

symbol. This part of the standard requires warning labels, specifically the orange or orange-red biohazard symbol affixed to containers of regulated waste, refrigerators and freezers and other containers which are used to store or transport blood or other potentially infectious materials.

Other provisions regarding regulated infectious waste include:

- Red bags or containers may be used instead of labeling. When a facility uses Universal Precautions in its handling of all specimens, labeling is not required within the facility. Likewise, when all laundry is handled with Universal Precautions, the laundry need not be labeled.
- The biohazard label must be such that it cannot be easily removed from the site to which it is affixed.
- All regulated waste must be placed in containers and disposed of in a manner that is in keeping with state and local regulations as well as the federal requirements.
- Containers that are used for contaminated sharps must meet these criteria:
  - Must close automatically without any force necessary
  - Must be puncture resistant
  - Must be leak-resistant on sides, top and bottom
  - Must be labeled with the biohazard symbol or color-coded red
- Blood which has been tested and found free of HIV or HBV and released for clinical use, and regulated waste which has been decontaminated, need not be labeled. Signs must be used to identify restricted areas in HIV and HBV research laboratories and production facilities.

*Housekeeping and laundry*

- Implementation of requirements to maintain a clean and sanitary environment for employees

It is the employer's responsibility that the workplace be clean and sanitary. Specifically, the housekeeping requirements include:

- A written schedule for cleaning and decontamination must be posted.
- A method for decontamination must be listed on the schedule.
- Any surface or instrument must be cleaned immediately following any procedure or contamination with blood or OPIM with the appropriate disinfectant.
- Protective coverings used on equipment should be immediately replaced when necessary (such as after use) or at the end of the workday or shift.
- Any containers that are re-used must be decontaminated and inspected on a regular basis.
- Broken glass, especially glass that has a potential for contamination, cannot be picked up by hand, but must be cleaned with equipment or by some mechanical means.
- No storage container that would require an employee to reach into the container to retrieve a sharp is permitted.

The question about how laundry is to be handled has been an ongoing concern and one of the most confusing parts of the standard. Generally, these are considered to be the requirements:

- Laundry must be bagged at the location where it is used. It cannot be moved and later bagged.
- It cannot be sorted or rinsed in the same location where it is used. It must be moved to the laundry area for sorting or rinsing.
- Contaminated laundry must be placed in bags (or containers) that are either labeled or color-coded.
- If laundry is wet, it must be put in leak-proof bags.
- Any worker who has contact with laundry must wear gloves.
- Laundry may be done on site (at the facility) or can be sent to a laundry service.
- Any employee who does the laundry must be properly trained in bagging, handling, and disinfecting the laundry. Those training records must be kept on file.
- It is suggested that hot water and bleach be used.

*Recordkeeping*

- Implementation of accurate training records that must be kept for three years after the training

The recordkeeping system required by OSHA calls for medical records to be kept for each employee who is at risk for occupational exposure for the duration of employment plus 30 years. Other requirements include:

- The record must be confidential and must include name and Social Security number of the employee.
- Hepatitis B vaccination status, including dates of injections.
- The results of any evaluations following an exposure incident, medical testing and follow-up procedures. A copy of the physician's written opinion must be included.

In addition, training records must be maintained for three years and must include:

- Dates of training session.
- Contents and/or a summary of the training program.
- The trainer's name and qualifications.
- Names and job titles of all persons attending the sessions.

- Any of these training or medical records must be made available to the employee, anyone with written consent of the employee, and OSHA upon request of such documents.

*HIV and HBV research laboratories and production facilities*

- Implementation of special training and experience requirements for use in research laboratories and production facilities.
- Special standards for HIV and HBV research facilities are included in the standard, but are of such a highly-specialized nature that they are not covered here. These facilities must follow standard microbiological practices and specific additional practices intended to minimize exposures of employees working with concentrated viruses. These facilities must include required containment equipment and an autoclave for decontamination of regulated waste and must be constructed to limit risks and enable easy clean up. Additional training and experience requirements apply to workers in these facilities.

## 14-3   Immunizing agents and immunization schedules for health care workers (HCWs)*

| Generic name | Primary schedule and booster(s) | Indications | Major precautions and contraindications | Special considerations |
|---|---|---|---|---|
| **Immunizing agents strongly recommended for health care workers** | | | | |
| Hepatitis B (HB) recombinant vaccine | Two doses IM 4 weeks apart; third dose 5 months after second; booster doses not necessary. | *Preexposure:* HCWs at risk for exposure to blood or body fluids. *Postexposure:* See Table 3. | On the basis of limited data, no risk of adverse effects to developing fetuses is apparent. Pregnancy should *not* be considered a contraindication to vaccination of women. Previous anaphylactic reaction to common baker's yeast is a contraindication to vaccination. | The vaccine produces neither therapeutic nor adverse effects on HBV-infected persons. Prevaccination serologic screening is not indicated for persons being vaccinated because of occupational risk. HCWs who have contact with patients or blood should be tested 1-2 months after vaccination to determine serologic response. |
| Hepatitis B immune globulin (HBIG) | 0.06 mL/kg IM as soon as possible after exposure. A second dose of HBIG should be administered 1 month later if the HB vaccine series has not been started. | **Postexposure** prophylaxis: For persons exposed to blood or body fluids containing HBsAg and who are not immune to HBV infection—0.06 mL/kg IM as soon as possible (but no later than 7 days after exposure). | — | — |
| Influenza vaccine (inactivated whole-virus and split-virus vaccines) | Annual vaccination with current vaccine. Administered IM. | HCWs who have contact with patients at high risk for influenza or its complications; HCWs who work in chronic care facilities; HCWs with high-risk medical conditions or who are aged ≥65 years. | History of anaphylactic hypersensitivity to egg ingestion. | No evidence exists of risk to mother or fetus when the vaccine is administered to a pregnant woman with an underlying high-risk condition. Influenza vaccination is recommended during second and third trimesters of pregnancy because of increased risk for hospitalization. |

Centers for Disease Control and Prevention: Immunization of health-care workers: recommendations of the Advisory Committee on Immunization Practices (ACIP) and the Hospital Infection Control Practices Advisory Committee (HICPAC), *MMWR* 46(RR-18):4-9, 1997.

*IM,* Intramuscular; *HBV,* hepatitis B vaccine; *HBsAg,* hepatitis B surface antigen; *HIV,* human immunodeficiency virus; *MMR,* measles, mumps, rubella (vaccine); *TB,* tuberculosis; *IgA,* immunoglobulin A; *HAV,* hepatitis A virus.

*Persons who provide health care to patients or work in institutions that provide patient care (e.g., physicians, nurses, emergency medical personnel, dental professionals and students, medical and nursing students, laboratory technicians, hospital volunteers, and administrative and support staff in health-care institutions).

*Continued*

| Generic name | Primary schedule and booster(s) | Indications | Major precautions and contraindications | Special considerations |
|---|---|---|---|---|
| **Immunizing agents strongly recommended for health care workers—cont'd** | | | | |
| Measles live-virus vaccine | One dose SC; second dose at least 1 month later. | HCWs† born during or after 1957 who do not have documentation of having received 2 doses of live vaccine on or after the first birthday **or** a history of physician-diagnosed measles or serologic evidence of immunity. Vaccination should be considered for all HCWs who lack proof of immunity, including those born before 1957. | Pregnancy; immunocompromised persons,‡ including HIV-infected persons who have evidence of severe immunosuppression; anaphylaxis after gelatin ingestion or administration of neomycin; recent administration of immune globulin. | MMR is the vaccine of choice if recipients are likely to be susceptible to rubella and/or mumps as well as to measles. Persons vaccinated during 1963-1967 with a killed measles vaccine alone, killed vaccine followed by live vaccine, or with a vaccine of unknown type should be revaccinated with 2 doses of live measles virus vaccine. |
| Mumps live-virus vaccine | One dose SC; no booster. | HCWs† believed to be susceptible can be vaccinated. Adults born before 1957 can be considered immune. | Pregnancy; immunocompromised persons‡; history of anaphylactic reaction after gelatin ingestion or administration of neomycin. | MMR is the vaccine of choice if recipients are likely to be susceptible to measles and rubella as well as to mumps. |
| Rubella live-virus vaccine | One dose SC; no booster. | Indicated for HCWs,† both men and women, who do not have documentation of having received live vaccine on or after their first birthday **or** laboratory evidence of immunity. Adults born before 1957, **except women who can become pregnant,** can be considered immune. | Pregnancy; immunocompromised persons†; history of anaphylactic reaction after administration of neomycin. | The risk for rubella vaccine–associated malformations in the offspring of women pregnant when vaccinated or who become pregnant within 3 months after vaccination is negligible. Such women should be counseled regarding the theoretical basis of concern for the fetus. MMR is the vaccine of choice if recipients are likely to be susceptible to measles or mumps, as well as to rubella. |
| Varicella zoster live-virus vaccine | Two 0.5 mL doses SC 4-8 weeks apart if ≥13 years of age. | Indicated for HCWs† who do not have either a reliable history of varicella or serologic evidence of immunity. | Pregnancy, immunocompromised persons,§ history of anaphylactic reaction following receipt of neomycin or gelatin. Avoid salicylate use for 6 weeks after vaccination. | Vaccine is available from the manufacturer for certain patients with acute lymphocytic leukemia in remission. Because 71%-93% of persons without a history of varicella are immune, serologic testing before vaccination is likely to be cost-effective. |

Centers for Disease Control and Prevention: Immunization of health-care workers: recommendations of the Advisory Committee on Immunization Practices (ACIP) and the Hospital Infection Control Practices Advisory Committee (HICPAC), *MMWR* 46(RR-18):4-9, 1997.

†All HCWs (i.e., medical or nonmedical, paid or volunteer, full-time or part-time, student or non-student, with or without patient-care responsibilities) who work in health-care institutions (e.g., inpatient and outpatient, public and private) should be immune to measles, rubella, and varicella.

‡Persons immunocompromised because of immune deficiency diseases, HIV infection, leukemia, lymphoma or generalized malignancy or immunosuppressed as a result of therapy with corticosteroids, alkylating drugs, antimetabolites, or radiation.

§Persons immunocompromised because of immune deficiency diseases, HIV infection (who should primarily not receive BCG, POV, and yellow fever vaccines), leukemia, lymphoma or generalized malignancy or immunosuppressed as a result of therapy with corticosteroids, alkylating drugs, antimetabolites, or radiation.

| Generic name | Primary schedule and booster(s) | Indications | Major precautions and contraindications | Special considerations |
|---|---|---|---|---|
| **Immunizing agents strongly recommended for health care workers—cont'd** | | | | |
| Varicella-zoster immune globulin (VZIG) | Persons <50 kg: 125 μ/10 kg IM; persons ≥50 kg: 625 μ.‖ | Persons known or likely to be susceptible (particularly those at high risk for complications (e.g., pregnant women) who have close and prolonged exposure to a contact case or to an infectious hospital staff worker or patient. | — | Serologic testing may help in assessing whether to administer VZIG. If use of VZIG prevents varicella disease, patient should be vaccinated subsequently. |
| **BCG vaccination** | | | | |
| Bacille Calmette Guérin (BCG) Vaccine (tuberculosis) | One percutaneous dose of 0.3 mL; no booster dose recommended. | Should be considered only for HCWs in areas where multi-drug tuberculosis is prevalent, a strong likelihood of infection exists, and comprehensive infection control precautions have failed to prevent TB transmission to HCWs. | Should not be administered to immunocompromised persons,§ pregnant women. | In the United States, tuberculosis-control efforts are directed towards early identification, treatment of cases, and preventive therapy with isoniazid. |
| Immune globulin (hepatitis A) | *Postexposure:* One IM dose of 0.02 mL/kg administered ≤2 weeks after exposure. | Indicated for HCWs exposed to feces of infectious patients. | Contraindicated in persons with IgA deficiency; do not administer within 2 weeks after MMR vaccine, or 3 weeks after varicella vaccine. Delay administration of MMR vaccine for ≥3 months and varicella vaccine ≥5 months after administration of Ig. | Administer in large muscle mass (deltoid, gluteal). |
| Hepatitis A vaccine | Two doses of vaccine either 6-12 months apart (HAVRIX), or 6 months apart (VAQTA). | Not routinely indicated for HCWs in the United States. Persons who work with HAV-infected primates or with HAV in a research laboratory setting should be vaccinated. | History of anaphylactic hypersensitivity to alum or, for HAVRIX, the preservative 2-phenoxyethanol. The safety of the vaccine in pregnant women has not been determined; the risk associated with vaccination should be weighed against the risk for hepatitis A in women who may be at high risk for exposure to HAV. | — |
| Meningococcal polysaccharide vaccine (tetravalent A, C, W135, and Y) | One dose in volume and by route specified by manufacturer; need for boosters unknown. | Not routinely indicated for HCWs in the United States. | The safety of the vaccine in pregnant women has not been evaluated; it should not be administered during pregnancy unless the risk for infection is high. | — |

‖Some experts recommend 125 μ/10 kg regardless of total body weight.

*Continued*

| Generic name | Primary schedule and booster(s) | Indications | Major precautions and contraindications | Special considerations |
|---|---|---|---|---|
| **BCG vaccination—cont'd** | | | | |
| Typhoid vaccine, IM, SC, and oral | *IM vaccine:* One 0.5 mL dose, booster 0.5 mL every 2 years. *SC vaccine:* two 0.5 mL doses, ≥4 weeks apart, booster 0.5 mL SC or 0.1 ID every 3 years if exposure continues. *Oral vaccine:* Four doses on alternate days. The manufacturer recommends revaccination with the entire four-dose series every 5 years. | Workers in microbiology laboratories who frequently work with *Salmonella typhi.* | Severe local or systemic reaction to a previous dose. Ty21a (oral) vaccine should not be administered to immunocompromised persons† or to persons receiving antimicrobial agents. | Vaccination should not be considered an alternative to the use of proper procedures when handling specimens and cultures in the laboratory. |
| Vaccinia vaccine (smallpox) | One dose administered with a bifurcated needle; boosters administered every 10 years. | Laboratory workers who directly handle cultures with vaccinia, recombinant vaccinia viruses, or orthopox viruses that infect humans. | The vaccine is contraindicated in pregnancy, in persons with eczema or a history of eczema, and in immunocompromised persons† and their household contacts. | Vaccination may be considered for HCWs who have direct contact with contaminated dressings or other infectious material from volunteers in clinical studies involving recombinant vaccinia virus. |
| **Other vaccine-preventable diseases** | | | | |
| Tetanus and diphtheria (toxoids [Td]) | Two IM doses 4 weeks apart; third dose 6-12 months after second dose; booster every 10 years. | All adults. | Except in the first trimester, pregnancy is not a precaution. History of a neurologic reaction or immediate hypersensitivity reaction after a previous dose. History of severe local (Arthus-type) reaction after a previous dose. Such persons should not receive further routine or emergency doses of Td for 10 years. | Tetanus prophylaxis in wound management.¶ |
| Pneumococcal polysaccharide vaccine (23 valent). | One dose, 0.5 mL, IM or SC; revaccination recommended for those at highest risk ≥5 years after the first dose. | Adults who are at increased risk of pneumococcal disease and its complications because of underlying health conditions; older adults, especially those age ≥65 who are healthy. | The safety of vaccine in pregnant women has not been evaluated; it should not be administered during pregnancy unless the risk for infection is high. Previous recipients of any type of pneumococcal polysaccharide vaccine who are at highest risk for fatal infection or antibody loss may be revaccinated ≥5 years after the first dose. | — |

Centers for Disease Control and Prevention: Immunization of health-care workers: recommendations of the Advisory Committee on Immunization Practices (ACIP) and the Hospital Infection Control Practices Advisory Committee (HICPAC), *MMWR* 46(RR-18):4-9, 1997.
¶See CDC: Update on adult immunization: recommendations of the Advisory Committee on Immunization Practices (ACIP), *MMWR* 40(No. RR-12):1-94, 1991.

## 14-4   Work restrictions for health care workers (HCWs) exposed to or infected with certain vaccine-preventable diseases

| Disease/problem | Work restriction | Duration |
|---|---|---|
| **Diphtheria** | | |
|   Active | Exclude from duty. | Until antimicrobial therapy is completed **and** 2 nasopharyngeal cultures obtained ≥24 hours apart are negative. |
|   Postexposure | | |
|     (susceptible HCWs; previously vaccinated HCWs who have not had a Td booster dose within the previous 5 years) | Exclude from duty. | Same as active diphtheria |
|   Asymptomatic carriers | Exclude from duty. | Same as active diphtheria. |
| **Hepatitis A** | Restrict from patient contact and food handling. | 7 days after onset of jaundice. |
| **Hepatitis B:** HCWs with acute or chronic antigenemia | | |
| HCWs who do not perform exposure-prone invasive procedures | Standard precautions should always be observed. No restriction unless epidemiologically linked to transmission of infection. | Universal precautions should always be observed |
| HCWs who perform exposure-prone invasive procedures | These HCWs should not perform exposure-prone invasive procedures until they have sought counsel from an expert review panel that should review and recommend the procedures the worker can perform, taking into account the specific procedure as well as the skill and technique of the worker. | Until hepatitis B e antigen is negative. |
| **Upper respiratory infections** (persons at high risk for complications of influenza as defined by ACIP) | During particular seasons (e.g., during winter when influenza and/or RSV are prevalent), consider excluding personnel with acute febrile upper respiratory infections (including influenza) from care of high-risk patients. | Until acute symptoms resolve. |
| **Measles** | | |
|   Active | Exclude form duty. | 7 days after rash appears. |
|   Postexposure (susceptible personnel) | Exclude from duty. | 5th day after 1st exposure through 21st day after last exposure and/or 7 days after the rash appears. |
| **Mumps** | | |
|   Active | Exclude from duty. | 9 days after onset of parotitis. |
|   Postexposure (susceptible personnel) | Exclude from duty. | 12th day after 1st exposure through 26th day after last exposure **or** 9 days after onset of parotitis. |
| **Pertussis** | | |
|   Active | Exclude form duty. | Beginning of catarrhal stage through 3rd week after onset of paroxysms or until 5 days after start of effective antimicrobial therapy. |
|   Postexposure | | |
|     *Symptomatic personnel* | Exclude from duty. | 5 days after start of effective antimicrobial therapy. |
|     *Asymptomatic personnel* | No restriction, on antimicrobial prophylactic therapy. | |

Centers for Disease Control and Prevention: Immunization of health-care workers: recommendations of the Advisory Committee on Immunization Practices (ACIP) and the Hospital Infection Control Practices Advisory Committee (HICPAC), *MMWR* 46(RR-18):33-34, 1997.
Adapted from:
  CDC: Recommendations for preventing transmission of human immunodeficiency virus and hepatitis B virus to patients during exposure-prone invasive procedures, *MMWR* 40(RR-8):1-8, 1991.
  CDC: Guideline for isolation precautions in hospitals: recommendations of the Hospital Infection Control Practices Advisory Committee (HICPAC) and the National Center for Infectious Diseases, *Infect Control Hosp Epidemiol* 17:53-80, 1996.
  Williams WW: CDC guideline for infection control in hospital personnel, *Infect Control* 4(Suppl):326-349, 1983.
*Td,* Tetanus and diphtheria, *RSV,* respiratory syncytial virus; *VZIG,* varicella-zoster immune globulin.

| Disease/problem | Work restriction | Duration |
|---|---|---|
| **Rubella** | | |
| Active | Exclude from duty. | 5 days after the rash appears. |
| Postexposure (susceptible personnel) | Exclude from duty. | 7th day after 1st exposure through 21st day after last exposure and/or 5 days after rash appears. |
| **Varicella** | | |
| Active | Exclude from duty. | Until all lesions dry and crust. |
| Postexposure (susceptible personnel) | Exclude from duty. | 10th day after 1st exposure through 21st day (28th day if VZIG administered) after the last exposure; if varicella occurs, until all lesions dry and crust. |
| **Zoster** | | |
| (Localized in normal person) | Cover lesions; restrict from care of high-risk patients.* | Same as varicella. |
| Postexposure (susceptible personnel) | Restrict from patient contact. | |

*Patients who are susceptible to varicella and at increased risk for complications of varicella (i.e., neonates and immunocompromised persons of any age).

---

## 14-5 | Infectious diseases designated as notifiable at the national level: United States, 1997

Acquired immunodeficiency syndrome (AIDS)
Anthrax
Botulism
Brucellosis
Chancroid
*Chlamydia trachomatis*, genital infections
Cholera
Coccidioidomycosis
Cryptosporidiosis
Diphtheria
Encephalitis, California serogroup
Encephalitis, eastern equine
Encephalitis, St. Louis
Encephalitis, western equine
*Escherichia coli* O157:H7
Gonorrhea
*Haemophilus influenzae,* invasive disease
Hansen disease (Leprosy)
Hantavirus pulmonary syndrome
Hemolytic uremic syndrome, post-diarrheal
Hepatitis A
Hepatitis B
Hepatitis, C/Non A, Non B
HIV infection, pediatric
Legionellosis
Lyme disease

Malaria
Measles
Meningococcal disease
Mumps
Pertussis
Plague
Poliomyelitis, paralytic
Psittacosis
Rabies, animal
Rabies, human
Rocky Mountain spotted fever
Rubella
Rubella, congenital syndrome
Salmonellosis
Shigellosis
Streptococcal disease, invasive, Group A
*Streptococcus pneumoniae*, drug-resistant invasive disease
Streptococcal toxic-shock syndrome
Syphilis, congenital
Syphilis
Tetanus
Toxic-shock syndrome
Trichinosis
Tuberculosis
Typhoid fever
Yellow fever

### Infectious diseases and conditions that are not nationally notifiable but for which case definitions may be useful for surveillance*

Amebiasis
Aseptic meningitis
Bacterial meningitis, other
*Campylobacter* infection
*Cyclospora* infection
Dengue fever
Ehrlichiosis
Genital herpes (herpes simplex virus)
Genital warts
Giardiasis

Granuloma inguinale
Leptospirosis
Listeriosis
Lymphogranuloma venereum
Mucopurulent cervicitis
Nongonococcal urethritis
Pelvic inflammatory disease
Rheumatic fever
Tularemia
Varicella (chickenpox)

From Centers for Disease Control and Prevention: Case definitions for infectious conditions under public health surveillance, *MMWR* 46(No. RR-10), 1997.
*This list includes only the diseases and conditions that are not nationally notifiable for which case definitions are provided in the report; it is not a complete list of such diseases for which CDC and state and territorial health departments maintain surveillance systems.

# HEALTH ORGANIZATIONS AND RESOURCES

## 15-1 General resources

### ACQUIRED IMMUNODEFICIENCY SYNDROME (AIDS)

**AIDS Action**

1906 Sunderland Plc. NW
Washington, DC 20036
(202) 530-8030
FAX (202) 530-8031

**AIDS Information Hotline**

Based at the American Social Health
 Association
PO Box 13827
Research Triangle Park, NC 27709
(919) 361-8400
FAX (919) 361-8425
CDC National AIDS Hotline
 (800) 342-2437
CDC National AIDS Hotline Spanish
 Service (800) 344-7432
CDC National STD Hotline
 (800) 227-8922
CDC National AIDS Hotline TTY
 Service (800) 243-7889

**American Foundation for AIDS Research**

733 3rd Ave. 12th Floor
New York, NY 10017
(212) 682-7440
(800) 392-6327
(800) 342-2437
FAX (212) 682-9812

**HIV/AIDS Education Program**

431 18th St. NW
Washington, DC 20006
(202) 737-8300

**Division of HIV/AIDS Prevention**

A division of CDC's National Center for
 HIV, STD and TB Prevention
1600 Clifton Rd.
Atlanta, GA 30333
(404) 639-3311
(404) 639-3534
(800) 311-3435

**Elizabeth Glaser Pediatric AIDS Foundation**

Santa Monica (Headquarters)
2950 31st St. #125
Santa Monica, CA 90405
(310) 314-1459
FAX (310) 314-1469
e-mail: info@pedaids.org

**Elizabeth Glaser Pediatric AIDS Foundation**

*New York office*
41 Madison Ave. 29th Floor
New York, NY 10010
(212) 448-6654
e-mail: Ny@pedaids.org

*Washington, DC office*
805 15th St. NW, #500
Washington, DC 20005
(202) 371-0099
FAX (202) 371-2044
e-mail: Dc@pedaids.org

*General Information*
(888)-499-4673
e-mail (general): info@pedAIDS.org
e-mail (fundraising, donations):
development@pedAIDS.org
e-mail (research, grants):
research@pedAIDS.org

**Foundation for Children with AIDS**

1800 Columbus Ave.
Roxbury, MA 02119
(617) 442-7442
FAX (617) 442-1705

**Gay Men's Health Crisis**

The Tisch Building
119 W 24th St.
New York, NY 10011
(212) 807-6655
(800) 243-7692
FAX (212) 337-3656

**Lambda Legal Defense and Education Fund**

120 Wall St. Suite 1500
New York, NY 10005-3904
(212) 809-8585
FAX (212) 809-0055

**National Association of People With AIDS**

1413 K St. NW, 7th Floor
Washington, DC 20005
(202) 898-0414
FAX (202) 898-0435
e-mail: napwa@napwa.org

**National Hemophilia Foundation**

116 W 32nd Street, 11th Floor
New York, NY 10001
(212) 328-3700
(800) 424-2634
FAX (212) 328-3777
e-mail: info@hemophilia.org

**National Hospice and Palliative Care Organization**

1700 Diagonal Rd. Suite 300
Alexandria, VA 22314
(703) 243-5900
(800) 338-8619
(800) 658-8998
FAX (703) 525-5762
e-mail: info@nhpco.org

**National Pediatric & Family HIV Resource Center**

The François-Xavier Bagnoud Center
University of Medicine and Dentistry of
 New Jersey
30 Bergen St.-ADMC #4
Newark, NJ 07103
(973) 972-0410
(800) 362-0071
FAX (973) 972-0399

**National Resource and Consultation Center for AIDS and HIV Infection**

116 W 36th St. 11th Floor
New York, NY 10011
(888) 463-6643
FAX (212) 431-0906

**Project Inform**

205 13th St. #2001
San Francisco, CA 94103
(415) 558-8669
800-822-7422
FAX (415) 558-0684

**San Francisco AIDS Foundation**

995 Market St. #200
San Francisco, CA 94103
(415) 487-3000

### ADVOCACY

**American Civil Liberties Union**

125 Broad St. 18th Floor
New York, NY 10004-2400
(212) 549-2500
FAX (212) 549-2646

**Occupational Safety and Health Administration (OSHA)**

Public Affairs Office
US Department of Labor, Room N3637
200 Constitution Ave. NW
Washington, DC 20210
(202) 693-1999

## ALCOHOL AND DRUG ABUSE
**Al-Anon/Alateen Family Group Headquarters, Inc.**

1600 Corporate Landing Pkwy.
Virginia Beach, VA 23454-5617
(757) 563-1600
(800) 356-9996
FAX (212) 869-3757

**Alcohol Abuse Emergency 24-Hour Hotline**

107 Lincoln St.
Worcester, MA 01605-2499
(800) 345-3552

**Alcohol and Drug Problems Association of North America, Inc.**

307 N Main
St. Charles MO, 63301
(314) 589-6702
FAX (314) 940-2358

**Alcohol and Drug Helpline**

175 W 7200 S
Midvale, UT 84047
(800) 821-4357

**Alcoholics Anonymous World Services**

475 Riverside Dr.
New York, NY 10163
(212) 870-3400
FAX 212-870-3003

**American Council for Drug Education (ACDE)**

(800) 378-4435
e-mail: acde@phoenixhouse.org

**Center for Substance Abuse Treatment at SAMHSA**

5600 Fishers Ln.
Rockville, MD 20857
(301) 443-8956
email: info@samhsa.gov

**Cocaine Anonymous World Services**

3740 Overland Ave. Suite C
Los Angeles, CA 90034-6337
(310) 559-5833
FAX (310) 559-2554
e-mail: publicinfo@ca.org

**Drug Information Association, Inc.**

501 Office Center Dr. Suite 450
Fort Washington, PA 19034-3211
(215) 628-2288
FAX (215) 641-1229
e-mail: dia@diahome.org

**International Commission for Prevention of Alcoholism and Drug Dependency**

12501 Old Columbia Pike
Silver Springs, MD 20904
(301) 680-6719
FAX (301) 680-6090

**Mothers Against Drunk Driving (MADD)**

511 E John Carpenter Freeway, Suite 700
Irving, TX 75062
(972) 869-2206
(800) 438-6233
FAX (214) 869-2206

**National Association of Alcoholism and Drug Abuse Counselors (NAADAC)**

900 N Washington St. Suite 600
Alexandria, VA 22314-1535
(800) 548-0497
FAX (800) 377-1136
e-mail: naadac@naadac.org

**National Association of State Alcohol and Drug Abuse Directors, Inc.**

808 17th St. NW, Suite 410
Washington, DC 20006
(202) 293-0090
FAX (202) 293-1250
e-mail: dcoffice@nasadad.org

**National Association on Drug Abuse Problems, Inc.**

355 Lexington Ave.
New York, NY 10017
(212) 986-1170
FAX (212) 697-2939

**National Center On Addiction and Substance Abuse**

633 3rd Ave. 19th Floor
New York, NY 10017-6706
(212) 841-5200
FAX (212) 956-8020

**National Clearing House for Alcohol and Drug Information (PREVLINE)**

PO Box 2345
Rockville, MD 20852
(301) 468-2600
(800) 729-6686

**National Committee for the Prevention of Alcoholism and Drug Dependency**

12501 Old Columbia Pike
Silver Springs, MD 20904
(301) 680-6719
FAX (301) 680-6090

**National Council on Alcoholism and Drug Dependence, Inc.**

12 W 21st St.
New York, NY 10010
(212) 206-6770
(800) NCA-CALL
FAX (212) 645-1690
e-mail: national@ncadd.org

**National Institute on Alcohol Abuse and Alcoholism**

6000 Executive Blvd. Willco Building
Bethesda, Maryland 20892-7003
e-mail: niaaaweb-r@exchange.nih.gov

**National Institute on Drug Abuse**

6001 Executive Blvd. Room 5213
Bethesda, Maryland 20892-9651
(301) 443-1124
e-mail: Information@lists.nida.nih.gov

**Partnership for Drug-Free America**

405 Lexington Ave. Suite 1601
New York, NY 10174
(212) 922-1560
FAX (212) 922-1570

**Students Against Destructive Decisions (SADD)** (also Students Against Driving Drunk)

PO Box 800
Marlborough, MA 01752
(508) 481-3568
(800) 757-5777
FAX (508) 481-5759

## ALZHEIMER'S DISEASE
**Alzheimer's Association**

919 N Michigan Ave. Suite 1000
Chicago, IL 60611-1676
(312) 335-8700
(800) 272-3900
FAX (312)-335-1110

**Alzheimer's Disease Education and Referral**

a service of the National Institute on Aging
PO Box 8250
Silver Springs, MD 20907-8250
(800) 438-4380
e-mail: adear@alzheimers.org

**Alzheimer's Disease International**

45 / 46 Lower Marsh
London SE1 7RG
UK
44 20 7620 3011
FAX 44 20 7401 7351
e-mail info@alz.co.uk

## AMYOTROPHIC LATERAL SCLEROSIS
**Amyotrophic Lateral Sclerosis Association**

27001 Agoura Rd. Suite 150
Calabasas Hills, CA 91301-5104
(818) 880-9007
(800) 782-4747
FAX (818) 340-2060

## ARTHRITIS
**American Juvenile Arthritis Organization**

1330 W Peachtree St.
Atlanta, GA 30309
(404) 872-7100 ext. 6271
(800) 283-7800
FAX (404) 872-0457

**Arthritis Foundation**

1330 W Peachtree St.
Atlanta, GA 30309
(404) 872-7100
(800) 283-7800

**National Institute of Arthritis & Musculoskeletal & Skin Diseases**

1 AMS Cr.
Bethesda, MD 20892-3672
(301) 495-4484
(877) 226-4267
FAX (301) 718-6366

**Spondylitis Association of America**

14827 Ventura Blvd. Suite 222
Sherman Oaks, CA 91403
(800) 777-8189
(818) 981-1616
e-mail: info@spondylitis.org

**ASTHMA AND ALLERGIES**
**Asthma and Allergy Foundation of America**

1233 20th St. NW, Suite 402
Washington, DC 20036
(202) 466-7643
(800) 727-8462
FAX (202) 466-8940
e-mail: info@aafa.org

**National Institute of Allergy and Infectious Disease**

Office of Communications and Public
    Liaison
Building 31, Room 7A-50
31 Center Dr. MSC 2520
Bethesda, MD 20892-2520
(301) 496-5717
FAX (301) 402-0120

**National Jewish Medical and Research Center for Immunology and Respiratory Medicine**

1400 Jackson St.
Denver, CO 80206
(303) 388-4461
(800) 222-5864
FAX 303-398-1649

**BEREAVEMENT**
**American Association of Suicidology**

4201 Connecticut Ave. Suite 310
Washington, DC 20008
(202) 237-2280
FAX (202) 237-2282

**American Foundation for Suicide Prevention**

120 Wall St. 22nd Floor
New York, NY 10005
(888) 333-2377
(212) 363-3500
FAX (212) 363-6237
e-mail: inquiry@afsp.org

**Association for Death Education and Counseling**

342 N Main St.
West Hartford, CT 06117-2507
(860) 586-7503
FAX (860) 586-7550

**The Compassionate Friends, Inc.**

PO Box 3696
Oak Brook, IL 60522-3696
(630) 990-0010
(877) 969-0010
FAX (630) 990-0246

**Pregnancy and Infant Loss Center**

1421 E Wayzata Blvd. No 30
Wayzata, MN 55391
(612) 473-9372

**SHARE**

National SHARE Office
St Joseph's Health Center
300 1st Capitol Dr.
St. Charles, MO 63301-2893
(636) 947-6161
(800) 821-6819
FAX (636) 947-7486

**Widowed Persons Service, AARP**

601 E St. NW
Washington, DC 20049
(202) 434-2260
FAX (202) 434-6474

**BLINDNESS**
**American Council of the Blind**

1155 15th St NW, Suite 1004
Washington, DC 20005
(202) 467-5081
(800) 424-8666
FAX (202) 467-5085

**American Foundation for the Blind, Inc.**

11 Penn Plza. Suite 300
New York, NY 10001
(212) 502-7600
(800) 232-5463
FAX (212) 502-7777

**Association for Education and Rehabilitation of the Blind and Visually Impaired**

4600 Duke St. Suite 430
PO Box 22397
Alexandria, VA 22304
(703) 823-9690
FAX (703) 823-9695

**Association for Macular Diseases**

210 E 64th St. 8th Floor
New York, NY 10021
(212) 605-3719
FAX (212) 605-3795
e-mail: association@retinalresearch.org

**Blinded Veterans Association**

477 H St. NW
Washington, DC 20001-2694
(202)371-8880
e-mail: bva@bva.org

**Braille Institute**

(800) 272-4553
e-mail: info@BrailleInstitute.org

**Braille Revival League**

57 Grandview Ave.
Watertown, MA 02172
(617) 926-9198
(800) 424-8666

**Eye Care Foundation**

115 E 61st St.
New York City, NY 10021
(212) 832-7297
e-mail: contactus@eyecarefoundation.org

**The Glaucoma Foundation**

116 John St. Suite 1605
New York, NY 10038
(212) 285-0080
(800) 452-8266
e-mail: info@glaucoma-foundation.org

**Guide Dogs for the Blind**

PO Box 151200
San Rafael, CA 94915-1200
(415) 499-4000
(800) 295-4050
FAX (415)-499-4035

**Guide Dog Users, Inc.**

57 Grandview Ave.
Watertown, MA 02172
(617) 926-9198
(800) 424-8666

**Guiding Eyes for the Blind**

611 Granite Springs Rd.
Yorktown Heights, NY 10598
(914) 245-4024
(800) 942-0149

**National Alliance for Eye and Vision Research**

426 C St. NE
Washington, DC 20002
(202) 544-1880
FAX (202) 543-2565

**National Association for Visually Handicapped**

22 W 21st St. 6th Floor
New York, NY 10010
(212) 889-3141
FAX (212) 727-2931

**National Braille Association**

3 Townline Cr.
Rochester, NY 14623-2513
(716) 427-8620
FAX (716) 427-0263
e-mail: nbaoffice@compuserve.com

**National Eye Institute**

Information Officer
Building 31, Rm 6A32
Bethesda, MD 20205
(301) 496-5248

**National Federation of the Blind**

1800 Johnson St.
Baltimore, MD 21230
(410) 659-9314
e-mail: nfb@nfb.org

**National Library Service for the Blind and Physically Handicapped**

Library of Congress
1291 Taylor St. NW
Washington, DC 20542
(202) 707-9261
FAX (202) 707-0712

**Prevent Blindness America**

500 E Remington Rd.
Schaumburg, IL 60173
(708) 843-2020
(800) 331-2020
FAX (708) 843-8458

**Recording for the Blind and Dyslexic, Inc.**

20 Roszel Rd.
Princeton, NJ 08540
(609) 452-0606
(800) 803-7201
FAX (609) 987-8116

**CANCER**
**American Association for Cancer Education**

MD Anderson Cancer Center
Department of Epidemiology
1515 Holcombe Blvd.
Houston, TX 77030
(713) 792-6161
(800) 392-1611
FAX (713) 792-0807

**American Association for Cancer Research (AACR)**

Public Ledger Building, Suite 826
150 S Independence Mall W
Philadelphia, PA 19106-3483
(215) 440-9300
FAX (215) 440-9313

**American Brain Tumor Association**

2720 River Rd.
Des Plaines, IL 60018-4110
(847) 827-9910
(800) 886-2282
FAX (847) 827-9918
e-mail: info@abta.org

**American Cancer Society National Headquarters**

1599 Clifton Rd.
Atlanta, GA 30329
(404) 320-3333
(404) 329-7648
(800) 227-2345
FAX (404) 325-0230

**American Society of Clinical Oncology (ASCO)**

1900 Duke St. Suite 200
Alexandria, VA 22314
(703) 299-0150
FAX (703) 299-1044
e-mail: asco@asco.org

**Association of Community Cancer Centers (ACCC)**

1600 Nebel St. Suite 201
Rockville, MD 20852
(301) 984-9496
FAX (301) 770-1949

**Cancer Care, Inc.**

National Office
275 7th Ave.
New York, NY 10001
(212) 302-2400
(212) 221-3300
(800) 813-4673
FAX (212) 719-0263
e-mail: info@cancercare.org

**Cancer Federation, Inc.**

PO Box 1298
Banning, CA 92220
(800) 207-2873
FAX (909) 849-0156
e-mail: cancerfed@msn.com

**Cancer Hotline**

(800) 525-3777
(800) 638-6070
(800) 636-5700
(808) 524-1234

**CancerNet**

Building 31, Room 10A03
31 Center Dr. MSC 2580
Bethesda, MD 20892-2580
(800) 422-6237
TTY (800) 332-8615
FAX (800) 624-2511
FAX (301) 402-5874
e-mail: cancermail@cips.nci.nih.gov

**Leukemia & Lymphoma Society**

formerly the Leukemia Society of
    America
1311 Mamaroneck Ave.
White Plains, NY 10605
(800) 955-4572
FAX (212) 573-8925

**National Alliance of Breast Cancer Organizations**

9 E 37th St. 10th Floor
New York, NY 10016
(212) 889-0606
(888)-806-2226
FAX (212) 689-1213

**National Cancer Institute**

includes the Cancer Information Service
9000 Rockville Pike
NCI Building 31, Room 10A-18
Bethesda, MD 20892
(800) 422-6237
(800) 638-6070
(202) 636-5700
(808) 524-1234
FAX (301) 402-0555

**National Coalition for Cancer Research (NCCR)**

426 C St. NE
Washington, DC 20002
(202) 544-1880
FAX (202) 543-2565

**National Coalition for Cancer Survivorship (NCCS)**

1010 Wayne Ave. Suite 770
Silver Spring, MD 20910-5600
(301) 650-9127
(877) 622-7937
FAX (301) 565-9670

**National Hospice and Palliative Care Organization**

1700 Diagonal Rd. Suite 300
Alexandria, VA 22314
(703) 837-1500
(703) 243-5900
(800) 338-8619
(800) 658-8898
FAX (703) 525-5762
e-mail: info@nhpco.org

**Partnership for Caring Inc.**

incorporates Choice in Dying
325 E Oliver St.
Baltimore, MD 21202
(800) 989-9455

**Skin Cancer Foundation**

PO Box 561
New York, NY 10156
(212) 725-5176
(800) 754-6490
FAX (212) 725-5751
e-mail: info@skincancer.org

**Support for People with Oral and Head and Neck Cancer**

PO BOX 53
Locust Valley, NY 11560-0053
(800) 377-0928
FAX (516) 671-8794

**CEREBRAL PALSY**
**United Cerebral Palsy Association**

1660 L St. NW, Suite 700
Washington, DC 20036
(202)-776-0406
(800)-872-5827
FAX (202) 776-0414

**CHILD ABUSE**
**American Professional Society on the Abuse of Children**

National Office
940 NE 13th St.
CHO 3B-3406
Oklahoma City, OK 73104
(405) 271-8202
FAX (405) 271-2931
e-mail: jennifer-moslander@ouhsc.edu

**Child Abuse Listening and Mediation (CALM)**

1236 Chapala St.
PO Box 90754
Santa Barbara, CA 93190-0754
(805) 965-2376
FAX (805) 963-6707

**Child Help USA**

15757 N 78th St.
Scottsdale, AZ 85260
(480) 922-8212
(800) 422-4453
FAX (480) 922-7061

**Children's Defense Fund**

25 E St. NW
Washington, DC 20001
(202) 628-8787
(800) 233-1200
FAX (202) 662-3510

**National Clearinghouse on Child Abuse and Neglect Information**

330 C Street SW
Washington, DC 20447
(703) 385-7565
(800) 394-3366
FAX (703) 385-3206

**National Committee to Prevent Child Abuse**

200 S Michigan Ave. 17th Floor
Chicago, IL 60604
(312) 663-3520
FAX (312) 939-8962

**National Data Archive on Child Abuse and Neglect**

e-mail: NDACAN@cornell.edu

**Prevent Child Abuse America Fulfillment Center**

200 State Rd.
South Deerfield, MA 01373-0200
(800) 835-2671
FAX (800) 499-6464
e-mail PCAAmerica@channing-bete.com

**CHILDREN**
**American Sudden Infant Death Syndrome Institute**

2480 Windy Hill Rd.
Marietta, GA 30067
(770) 612-1030
(800) 232-7437

**Association for the Care of Children's Health**

19 Mantua Rd.
Mt. Royal, NJ 08061
(609) 224-1742
FAX (609) 423-3420
e-mail: amkent@tmg.smarthub.com

**Child Find of America, Inc.**

PO Box 277
New Paltz, NY 12561-0722
(845) 255-1848
FAX (845) 255-5706

**Children's Foundation**

725 15th St. NW, Suite 505
Washington, DC 20005-2109
(202) 347-3300
FAX (202) 347-3382
e-mail: info@childrensfoundation.net

**March of Dimes Birth Defects Foundation**

1275 Mamaroneck Ave.
White Plains, NY 10605
(914) 997-4526
(888) 663-4637
FAX (914) 997-4537

**Maternal and Child Health Bureau**

5600 Fishers Ln.
Rockville, MD 20857

**National Sudden Infant Death Syndrome Resource Center**

2070 Chain Bridge Rd. Suite 450
Vienna, VA 22182
(703) 821-8955
FAX (703) 821-2098
e-mail: sids@circsol.com

**National Tay-Sachs and Allied Diseases Association**

2001 Beacon St. #204
Boston, MA 02135
(617) 277-4463
(800) 906-8723
FAX (617) 277-0134

**National Youth Sports Safety Foundation, Inc.**

333 Longwood Ave. Suite 202
Boston, MA 02115
(617) 277-1171
FAX (617) 277-2278

**Starlight Children's Foundation**

5900 Wilshire Blvd. Suite 2530
Los Angeles, CA 90036
(323) 634-0080
FAX (323) 634-0090
e-mail: info@starlight.org

**Sudden Infant Death Syndrome Alliance**

1314 Bedford Ave. Suite 210
Baltimore, MD 21208
(410) 653-8226
(800) 221-SIDS
FAX (410) 653-8709

**Sudden Infant Death Syndrome Network, Inc.**

SIDS Network
PO Box 520
Ledyard, Connecticut 06339

**CYSTIC FIBROSIS**
**Cystic Fibrosis Foundation**

6931 Arlington Rd.
Bethesda, MD 20814
(301) 951-4422
(800) 344-4823
FAX (301) 951-6378

**DIABETES**
**American Association of Diabetes Educators**

100 W Monroe St. Suite 400
Chicago, IL 60603
(312) 424-2426
(800) 338-3633
FAX (312) 644-4411

**American Diabetes Association**

National Center
1701 N Beauregard St.
Alexandria, VA 22314
(703) 549-1500
(800) 342-2383
FAX (703) 836-7439

**Diabetes Action Research and Education Foundation**

426 C St. NE
Washington, DC 20002
e-mail: daref@diabetesaction.org

**International Diabetic Athletes Association**

1647B W Bethany Home Rd.
Phoenix, AZ 85015
(602) 433-2113
(800) 898-4322

**Juvenile Diabetes Foundation International**

120 Wall St.
New York, NY 10005-3904
(212) 889-7575
(800) 533-2873
FAX (212) 725-7259

**National Diabetes Information Clearinghouse**

1 Information Way
Bethesda, MD 20892-3560
(301) 654-3327
FAX (301) 907-8906

**DISABILITIES**
**Administration on Developmental Disabilities**

Commissioner
Administration for Children and Families
US Department of Health and Human
    Services
Mail Stop: HHH 300-F
370 L'Enfant Promenade SW
Washington, DC 20447
(202) 690-6590
e-mail: add@acf.dhhs.gov

## Alliance for Technology Access

2175 E Francisco Blvd. Suite L
San Rafael, CA 94901
(415) 455-4575
e-mail: ATAinfo@ATAccess.org

## Association for Children with Retarded Mental Development

345 Hudson St.
New York, NY 10014
(212) 741-0100
FAX (212) 627-8318

## The Association for Persons with Severe Handicaps (TASH)

29 W Susquehanna Ave. Suite 210
Baltimore, MD 21204
(410) 828-8274
FAX (410) 828-6706
TDD (410) 828-1306

## Association for Retarded Citizens (ARC)

1010 Wayne Ave. Suite 650
Silver Spring, MD 20910
(301) 565-3842
FAX (301) 565-5342

## Autism Society of America

7910 Woodmont Ave. Suite 300
Bethesda, MD 20814-3015
(800) 328-8476
(301) 657-0881
FAX (301)-657-0869

## Boy Scouts of America

Scouting for the Handicapped
1325 W Walnut Hill Ln.
PO Box 152079
Irving, TX 75015

## Department of Justice ADA Home Page

(800) 514-0301
TDD (800) 514-0383

## National Institute on Disability & Rehabilitation Research (NIDRR)

Switzer Building, Room 3132
Washington, DC 20202-2524
(202) 205-8241
FAX (202) 205-9252

## Council for Disability Rights

205 W Randolph, Suite 1650
Chicago, IL 60606
(312) 444-9484
TDD (312) 444-1967
FAX (312) 444-1977

## The Council for Exceptional Children

1110 N Glebe Rd. Suite 300
Arlington, VA 22201-5704
(888) 232-7733
(703) 620-3660
TTY (703) 264-9446
FAX (703) 264-9494

## Disability Resources, Inc.

Dept IN, 4 Glatter Ln.
Centereach, NY 11720-1032
FAX (631) 585-0290

## Disability Rights, Education, and Defense Funds

2212 6th St.
Berkeley, CA 94710
(510) 644-2555
FAX (510) 841-8645
TDD (800) 466-4232

## Federation for Children with Special Needs

1135 Tremont St. Suite 420
Boston, MA 02120
(617) 236-7210
(800) 331-0688
FAX (617) 572-2094
e-mail: fcsninfo@fcsn.org

## Independent Living for the Handicapped

1301 Belmont St. NW
Washington, DC 20009
(202) 797-9803
FAX (202) 483-5281
e-mail: ilhcph@erols.com

## Institute on Independent Living

Peterséns Väg 2
127 41 Stockholm-Skärholmen
Sweden

## International Council on Disability

25 E 21st St.
New York, NY 10010
(212) 420-1500
FAX (212) 505-0871

## International Council on Disability (ICOD)

Box 3488
Riyadh 11471
SAUDI ARABIA
966 1 488 2917
966 1 488 8260

## Learning Disabilities Association of America

4156 Library Rd.
Pittsburgh, PA 15234-1349
(412) 341-1515
(412) 341-8077
FAX (412) 344-0224

## Mental Disability Rights International (MDRI)

1156 15th St. NW, Suite 1001
Washington, DC 20005
(202) 296-0800
FAX (202) 728-3053
e mail: mdri@erols.com

## MOVE International

1300 17th St.
City Center
Bakersfield, CA 93301-4533
(800) 397-6683
e-mail: move-international@kern.org

## National Alliance for the Mentally Ill (NAMI)

Colonial Place Three
2107 Wilson Blvd. Suite 300
Arlington, VA 22201
(703) 524-7600
(800) 950-6264

## National Amputation Foundation

38-40 Church St.
Malverne, NY 11565
(516) 887-3600
FAX (516) 887-3667
e-mail: amps76@aol.com

## National Association of Developmental Disabilities Councils

1234 Massachusetts Ave. NW, Suite 103
Washington, DC 20005
(202) 347-1234
FAX (202) 347-4023

## National Center for Learning Disabilities

381 Park Ave. S, Suite 1401
New York, NY 10016
(212) 545-7510
(888) 575-7373
FAX (212) 545-9665

## National Center for the Dissemination of Disability Research

National Council on Disability
1331 F St. NW, Suite 1050
Washington, DC 20004-1107
(202) 272-2004
FAX (202) 272-2022
TTY (202) 272-2074

## National Council on Independent Living

1916 Wilson Blvd. Suite 209
Arlington, VA 22201
(703) 525-3406
TTY (703) 525-4153
FAX (703) 525-3409
e-mail: ncil@ncil.org

## National Information Center for Children and Youths with Disabilities

PO Box 1492
Washington, DC 20013
(202) 884-8200
(800) 695-0285
FAX (202) 884-8441

## National Organization on Disability

910 16th St. NW, Suite 600
Washington, DC 20006
(202) 293-5960
FAX (202) 293-7999

**National Parent Network on Disabilities (NPND)**

1130 17th St. NW, Suite 400
Washington, DC 20036
(202) 463-2299
FAX (202) 463-9405

**National Spinal Cord Injury Association**

6701 Democracy Blvd. Suite 300
Bethesda, MD 26817
(301) 588-6959
(800) 962-9629
FAX (301) 588-9414

**National Sports Center for the Disabled**

PO Box 1290
Winter Park, CO 80482
(970) 726-1540
(303) 316-1540
FAX (970) 726-4112
e-mail: info@nscd

**Rehabilitation International**

Secretary General
25 E 21st St.
New York, NY 10010
(212) 420-1500
FAX (212) 505-0871

**DOWN SYNDROME**
**National Association for Down Syndrome**

PO Box 4542
Oak Park, IL 60522-4542
(630) 325-9112

**National Down Syndrome Congress**

Lake Ridge 400 Office Park Building 5,
   Suite 100
Atlanta, GA 30328-1655
(800) 232-6372
(770) 604-9500
e-mail: NDSCcenter@aol.com

**National Down Syndrome Society**

666 Broadway
New York, NY 10012
(212) 460-9330
(800) 221-4602

**ELDERLY**
**Administration on Aging**

330 Independence Ave. SW
Washington, DC 20201
(202) 619-0724
(800) 677-1116
(202) 619-7501
(202) 401-4541
FAX (202) 260-1012

**American Academy of Physical Medicine and Rehabilitation**

One IBM Plaza, Suite 2500
Chicago, IL 60611-3604
(312) 464-9700
FAX (312) 464-0227
e-mail: info@aapmr.org

**American Association for Continuity of Care**

PO Box 7073
North Brunswick, NJ 08902
(800) 816-1575
FAX (301) 352-7086

**American Association for Geriatric Psychiatry**

7910 Woodmont Ave. Suite 1050
Bethesda, MD 20814
(301) 654-7850
FAX (301) 654-4137

**American Association of Homes and Services for the Aging** (note name change)

901 E St. NW, Suite 500
Washington, DC 20004
(202) 783-2242
FAX (202) 783-2255

**American Association for International Aging**

1900 L St. NW, Suite 512
Washington, DC 20036-5002
(202) 833-8893
FAX (202) 833-8762

**American Association of Public Health Dentistry (AAPHD)**

3760 SW Lyle Ct.
Portland, OR 97221
(503) 242-0712
FAX (503) 242-0721
e-mail: NATOFF@aol.com

**American Association of Retired Persons (AARP)**

601 E St. NW
Washington, DC 20049
(202) 434-2277
(800) 424-3410
FAX (202) 434-2320

**American Bar Association Commission on Legal Problems of the Elderly**

740 Fifteenth St. NW
Washington, DC 20005-1022
(202) 662-8690
(800) 285-2221
FAX (202) 662-8698
e-mail: abaelderly@abanet.org

**American Federation for Aging Research (AFAR)**

1414 Ave. of the Americas, 18th Floor
New York, NY 10019
(212) 752-2327
FAX (212) 832-2298
e-mail: amfedaging@aol.com

**American Geriatrics Society**

The Empire State Building
350 5th Ave. Suite 801
New York, NY 10118
(212) 308-1414
(800) 247-4779
FAX (212) 832-8646
e-mail: info@americangeriatrics.org

**American Psychological Association**

Division of Adult Development
750 1st St. NE
Washington, DC 20002-4242
(202) 336-5500
(800) 374-2721

**American Society on Aging**

833 Market St. Suite 511
San Francisco, CA 94103-1824
(415) 974-9600
FAX (415) 974-0300
info@asaging.org

**American Society for Geriatric Dentistry**

211 E Chicago Ave. Suite 948
Chicago, IL 60611
(312) 440-2661
FAX (312) 440-2824

**Association for Adult Development and Aging**

c/o American Counseling Association
5999 Stevenson Ave
Alexandria, VA 22304-3300
(703) 823-9800
(800) 347-6647
FAX (703) 823-0252

**Association for Gerontology in Higher Education**

1030 15th St. NW, Suite 240
Washington, DC 20005-1503
(202) 289-9806
FAX (202) 289-9824
e-mail: aghetemp@aghe.org

**Association of Humanistic Gerontology**

1711 Solano Ave.
Berkeley, CA 94707

**Beverly Foundation**

44 S Mentor Ave.
Pasadena, CA 91106
(626) 792-2292
FAX (626) 792-6117

**Catholic Charities USA**

1731 King St. Suite 200
Alexandria, VA 22314
(703) 549-1390
FAX (703) 549-1656

**Catholic Health Association of the United States**

4455 Woodson Rd.
St Louis, MO 63134-3797
(314) 427-2500
FAX (314) 427-0029

**Center for Social Gerontology**

2307 Shelby Ave.
Ann Arbor, MI 48103-3895
(734) 665-1126
FAX (734) 665-2071

**Children of Aging Parents**
¹609 Woodbourne Rd. Suite 302A
Levittown, PA 19057-1511
(215) 945-6900
(800) 227-7294
FAX (215) 945-8720

**City Meals on Wheels USA**
355 Lexington
New York, NY 10017
(212) 687-1234
FAX (212) 687-1296

**Consultant Dietitians in Healthcare Facilities**
A Practice Group of the American
   Dietetic Association
CD-HCF/ADA
216 W Saxon Blvd.
Chicago, IL 60606
(312) 899-0040
FAX (312) 899-1758

**Consumer Healthcare Products Association**
1150 Connecticut Ave. NW, 12th Floor
Washington, DC 20036-4193
(202) 429-9260
FAX (202) 223-6835

**Department of Veterans Affairs**
Veterans Health Administration
Nursing Strategic Healthcare Group
810 Vermont Ave. NW
Washington, DC 20420

**Design for Aging Center of the American**
Institute of Architects
1735 New York Ave. NW
Washington, DC 20006
(202) 626-7300
FAX (202) 626-7421

**Foundation for Hospice and Home Care**
519 C St. NE
Washington, DC 20002
(202) 547-7424
FAX (202) 546-8968

**Gerontological Nutritionists**
4103 44th St.
Sacramento, CA 95820

**Gerontological Society of America**
1030 15th St. NW, Suite 250
Washington DC 20005
(202) 842-1275
FAX (202) 842-1150
e-mail: webmaster@geron.org

**Gray Panthers**
733 15th St. NW, Suite 437
Washington, DC 20005
(202) 737-6637
(800) 280-5362
FAX (202) 737-1160
e-mail: info@graypanthers.org

**Health Promotion Institute**
c/o National Council on Aging
409 3rd St. SW
Washington, DC 20024
(202) 479-1200
FAX (202) 479-0735

**Hospice Association of America**
228 7th St. SE
Washington, DC 20003
(202) 546-4759
FAX (202) 547-9559

**House Select Committee on Aging**
House Office Building
Annex 1, Room 712
Washington, DC 20515

**Institute for Retired Professionals at New School of Social Research**
66 W 12th St.
New York, NY 10011
(212) 229-5683
FAX (212) 691-7172

**International Federation on Aging**
380 St. Antoine St. W, Suite 3200
Montreal, Quebec H2Y 3X7
(514) 287-9679
FAX (514) 987-1567

**International Senior Citizens Association, Inc.**
255 S Hill St. Suite 409
Los Angeles, CA 90012
(213) 625-5008
FAX (213) 625-7115

**International Senior Citizens' Association**
1102 S Crenshaw Blvd.
Los Angles, Ca 90019-3198

**Legal Services for the Elderly**
130 W 42nd St 17th Floor
New York, NY 10036
(212) 391-0120
FAX (212) 719-1939

**Meals on Wheels America**
280 Broadway, Suite 214
New York, NY 10007
(212) 964-5700
FAX (212) 442-3162

**Meals on Wheels Association of America**
1414 Prince St. Suite 202
Alexandria, VA 22314
(703) 548-5558
FAX (703) 548-8024

**Mental Disorders of the Aging**
Research Branch DCR
Room 11 C-03
5600 Fishers Ln.
Rockville, MD 20857

**National Aging Information Center**
330 Independence Ave. SW, Room 4656
Washington DC 20201
(202) 619-7501
FAX (202) 401-7620

**National Alliance of Senior Citizens**
1700 18th St. NW, Suite 401
Washington, DC 20009
(202) 986-0117
FAX (202) 986-2974

**National Asian-Pacific Center on Aging**
Melbourne Tower, Suite 914
1511 3rd Ave.
Seattle, WA 98101
(206) 624-1221
FAX (206) 624-1023

**National Association of Area Agencies on Aging**
927 15th St. NW, 6th Floor
Washington, DC 20005
(202) 296-8130
FAX (202)-296-8134

**National Association for Hispanic Elderly**
Asociacion Naciional Pro Personas
   Mayores
3325 Wilshire Blvd. Suite 800
Los Angeles, CA 90010
(213) 487-1922
FAX (213) 385-3014

**National Association for Home Care**
228 7th St. SE
Washington, DC 20003
(202) 547-7424
FAX (202) 547-3540

**National Association for Medical Equipment Services (NAMES)**
c/o American Association for Homecare
625 Slaters Ln. Suite 200
Alexandria, VA 22314-1171
(703) 836-6263
FAX (703) 836-6730

**National Association of Nutrition and Aging Services Programs (NANASP)**
1101 Vermont Ave. NW, Suite 1001
Washington, DC 20005
(202) 682-6899
FAX (202) 684-3984

**National Association of Spanish Speaking Elderly**
2025 I St. NW, Suite 219
Washington, DC 20006
(202) 293-9329

**National Association of State Units on Aging**
1225 I St. NW, Suite 725
Washington, DC 20005
(202) 898-2578
(800) 667-1116
FAX (202) 898-2583

**National Caucus and Center on Black Aged**

1424 K St. NW, Suite 500
Washington, DC 20005
(202) 637-8400
FAX (202) 347-0895

**National Council on Aging**

409 3rd St. SW
Washington, DC 20024
(202) 479-1200
FAX (202) 479-0735

**National Council of Senior Citizens**

8403 Colesville Rd. Suite 1200
Silver Spring, MD 20910-3314
(301) 578-8800
FAX (301) 578-8999

**National Hospice and Palliative Care Organization**

1700 Diagonal Rd. Suite 300
Alexandria, VA 22314
(703) 837-1500
(703) 243-5900
(800) 338-8619
(800) 658-8898
FAX (703) 525-5762
e-mail: info@nhpco.org

**National Indian Council on Aging**

10501 Montgomery Blvd. NE, Suite 210
Albuquerque, NM 87111-3846
(505) 292-2001
FAX (505) 888-3276

**National Institute on Age, Work, and Retirement**

c/o National Council on the Aging
409 3rd St. SW, Suite 200
Washington, DC 20024
(202) 479-1200
FAX (202) 479-0735

**National Rehabilitation Association**

633 S Washington St.
Alexandria, VA 22314
(703) 836-0850
FAX (703) 836-0848

**National Senior Citizens Law Center**

3435 Wilshire Blvd. Suite 2860
Los Angeles, CA 90010-1938
(213) 639-0930
FAX (213) 639-0934

**Older Women's League (OWL)**

666 11th St. NW, Suite 700
Washington, DC 20001
(202) 783-6686
(800) 825-3695

**Spanish Speaking Elderly Council (RAICES)**

30 3rd Ave. Room 617
Brooklyn, NY 11217
(718) 643-0232
FAX (718) 643-8257

**World Homecare and Hospice Organization**

228 7th St. SE
Washington, DC 20003
(202) 546-4756
FAX (202) 547-9312

## EPILEPSY
**American Epilepsy Society**

342 N Main St.
West Hartford, CT 06117
(860) 586-7505
FAX 860-586-7550

**Epilepsy Foundation of America**

4351 Garden City Dr. Suite 500
Landover, MD 20785
(301) 459-3700
(800) 332-1000
FAX (301) 577-2684

## FAMILY PLANNING/PREGNANCY
**American Society for Reproductive Medicine**

formerly American Fertility Society
1209 Montgomery Highway
Birmingham, AL 35216-2809
(205) 978-5000
FAX (205) 978-5005

**International Childbirth Education Association, Inc.**

PO Box 20048
Minneapolis, MN 55420
(952) 854-8660
FAX (952) 854-8772

**La Leche League International, Inc.**

1400 N Meacham
Schaumburg, IL 60173
(847) 519-7730
FAX (708) 519-0035

**Maternity Center Association**

281 Park Ave. S
New York, NY 10010
(212) 777-5000

**Planned Parenthood Federation of America, Inc.**

810 7th Ave.
New York, NY 10019
(212) 541-7800
(800) 230-7526
FAX 212-245-1845

## FOOD (see also Nutrition)
**Food and Drug Administration**

5600 Fishers Ln.
Rockville MD 20857-0001
(888) 463-6332

**Food and Nutrition Information Center**

National Agricultural Library Building,
    Room 304
10301 Baltimore Ave.
Beltsville, MD 20705
(301) 504-5719
FAX (301) 504-6409

## GASTROINTESTINAL DISORDERS
**American Society for Parenteral and Enteral Nutrition**

8630 Fenton St. Suite 412
Silver Spring, MD 20910
(301) 587-6315
(800) 727-4567
FAX (301) 587-2365

**Crohn's and Colitis Foundation of America**

386 Park Ave. S, 17th Floor
New York, NY 10016-8804
(212) 685-3440
(800) 932-2423
FAX (212) 779-4098

**National Association for Continence**

PO Box 8310
Spartanburg, SC 29305-8310
(864) 579-7900
(800) 252 3337
(864) 579-7902

**National Digestive Diseases Information Clearinghouse**

2 Information Way
Bethesda, MD 20892-3570
(301) 654-3810
FAX (301) 907-8906

**National Institute of Diabetes and Digestive and Kidney Diseases**

31 Center Dr. MSC 2560
Bethesda, MD 20892-2560

**United Ostomy Association**

19772 MacArthur Blvd. Suite 200
Irvine, CA 92612-2405
(949) 660-8624
(800) 826-0826
FAX (949) 660-9262

**Wound, Ostomy and Continence Nurse's Society (WOCN)**

2755 Bristol, Suite 110
Costa Mesa, CA 92626
(714) 476-0268
(800) 228-4238
FAX (714) 545-3643

## HEADACHE
**The American Council for Headache Education (ACHE)**

19 Mantua Rd.
Mt. Royal, NJ 08061
(856) 423-0258
FAX (856) 423-0082

**American Headache Society (AHS)**

19 Mantua Rd.
Mt. Royal, NJ 08061
(856) 423-0043
FAX (856) 423-0082
e-mail: ahshq@talley.com

**National Headache Foundation**
428 W St. James Place, 2nd Floor
Chicago, IL 60614-2750
(888) 643-5552
FAX (773) 525-7357

## HEALTH: GENERAL
**American Alliance for Health, Physical Education, Recreation and Dance**
1900 Association Dr.
Reston, VA 20191
(703) 476-3400
(800) 213-7193
FAX (703) 476-9527

**American Association for World Health**
1825 K St. NW, Suite 1208
Washington, DC 20006
(202) 466-5883
FAX (202) 466-5896

**American Health Care Association**
1201 L St. NW
Washington, DC 20005
(202) 842-4444
FAX (202) 842-3860

**American Health Foundation**
320 E 43rd St.
New York, NY 10017
(212) 953-1900
FAX (212) 687-2339

**American Red Cross National Headquarters**
431 18th St. NW
Washington, DC 20006
(202) 639-3520
FAX (202) 639-3141

**Health and Education Resources, Inc.**
4733 Bethesda Ave. Suite 700
Bethesda, MD 20814
(301) 656-3178
FAX (301) 656-3179

**National Association for Public Health Statistics & Information Systems**
NAPHSIS Headquarters
1220 19th St. NW, Suite 802
Washington, DC 20036
(202) 463-8851
FAX (202) 463-4870
e-mail: hq@naphsis.org

**National Center for Health Statistics**
Division of Data Services
Hyattsville, MD 20782-2003

**National Health Council, Inc.**
1730 M St. NW, Suite 500
Washington, DC 20036
(202) 785-3910
FAX (202) 785-5923

**National Institutes of Health**
9000 Rockville Pike
Bethesda, MD 20814
(301) 496-4000

**National Organization for Rare Disorders**
PO Box 8923
New Fairfield, CT 06812-8923
(203) 746-6518
(800) 999-6673
FAX (203) 746-6481

**National Wellness Institute**
PO Box 827
Stevens Point, WI 54481-2962
(715) 342-2969
FAX (715) 342-2979

**President's Council on Physical Fitness and Sports**
Hubert H. Humphrey Building Room 738H
200 Independence Ave, SW
Washington, DC 20201
(202) 690-9000
FAX (202) 690-5211

## HEALTH: MENTAL
**American Art Therapy Association**
1202 Allanson Rd.
Mundelein, IL 60060-3808
(888) 290-0878
(847) 949-6064
FAX (847) 566-4580
e-mail: arttherapy@ntr.net

**American Dance Therapy Association**
(410) 997-4040
FAX (410) 997-4048
e-mail: info@adta.org

**American Psychological Association**
750 1st St. NE
Washington, DC 20002-4242
(202) 336-5500

**National Mental Health Association**
1021 Prince St.
Alexandria, VA 22314-2971
(703) 684-7722
(800) 969-6642
FAX (703) 684-5968

**National Mental Health Consumer Self-Help Clearinghouse**
1211 Chestnut St.
Philadelphia, PA 19107
(215) 751-1800
(800) 668-4226
FAX (215) 735-0275

## HEARING AND SPEECH
**Alexander Graham Bell Association for the Deaf**
3417 Volta Place NW
Washington, DC 20007-2778
(202) 337-5220
TTY (202) 337-5221
FAX (202) 337-8314

**American Deafness and Rehabilitation Association**
PO Box 251554
Little Rock, AR 72225
(501) 868-8850
FAX (501) 868-8812

**Better Hearing Institute**
Box 1840
Washington, DC 20013
(703) 642-0580
(800) 327-9355
FAX (703) 750-9302

**Deafness Research Foundation**
*New York Office*
575 5th Ave. 11th Floor
New York, NY 10017
TDD (212) 599-0027
FAX (212) 599-0039

*Washington Office*
1050 17th St, NW, Suite 701
Washington, DC 20036
(202) 289-5850
FAX (202) 682-0356

**Laurent Clerc National Deaf Education Center**
Gallaudet University
800 Florida Ave. NE
Washington, DC 20002
(202) 651-5051
TTY (202) 651-5340
FAX (202) 651-5054

**National Association of the Deaf**
814 Thayer Ave.
Silver Spring, MD 20910-4500
(301) 587-1788
TTY (301) 587-1789
FAX (301) 587-1791
e-mail: NADinfo@nad.org

**National Center for Stuttering**
200 E 33rd St.
New York, NY 10016
(212) 532-1460
(800) 221-2483

**National Hispanic Council of the Deaf and Hard of Hearing**
c/o DEAF, Inc.
215 Brighton Ave.
Allston, MA 02134
(617) 254-4041

**National Institute on Deafness and Other Communication Disorders (NIDCD)**
31 Center Dr. MSC 2320
Bethesda, MD USA 20892-2320

**Self-Help for Hard of Hearing People**
7910 Woodmont Ave. Suite 1200
Bethesda, MD 20814
(301) 657-2248
FAX (301) 913-9413

**Telecommunications for the Deaf, Inc.**

8719 Colesville Rd. Suite 300
Silver Spring, MD 20910
(301) 589-3786
(301) 589-3006
FAX (301) 589-3797

## HEART
**American Heart Association**

7272 Greenville Ave.
Dallas, TX 75231-4596
(214) 373-6300
(800) 242-1793
FAX (214) 706-1341

**Cleveland Clinic Heart Center**

9500 Euclid Ave.
Mail Code EE3-37
Cleveland, OH 44195
(216) 444-3690
(800) 478-4255

**Citizens for Public Action on Blood Pressure and Cholesterol**

7200 Wisconsin Ave. Suite 1002
Bethesda, MD 20814
(301) 907-7790

**Mended Hearts, Inc.**

7272 Greenville Ave.
Dallas, TX 75231-4596
(214) 706-1442
FAX (214) 706-5231

**National Heart Lung and Blood Institute**

PO Box 30105
Bethesda, MD 20824-0105
(301) 251-1222
FAX (301) 251-1223

**National Marfan Foundation**

382 Main St.
Port Washington, New York 11050
(516) 883-8712
FAX (516) 883-8040
e-mail: staff@marfan.org

## HEMOCHROMATOSIS
**Hemochromatosis Foundation**

PO Box 8569
Albany, NY 12208
(518) 489-0972
FAX (518) 489-0027

## HEMOPHILIA
**Committee of Ten Thousand (COTT)**

236 Massachusetts Ave. NE, Suite 609
Washington, DC 20002
(800) 488-2688
(202) 543-0988
FAX (202) 543-6720
e-mail: cott-dc@rols.com

**National Hemophilia Foundation**

116 W 32nd St. 11th Floor
New York, NY 10001
(212) 328-3700
(800) 424-2634
FAX (212) 328-3777

## HOSPITAL CARE
**American Hospital Association**

*Headquarters*
1 North Franklin
Chicago, IL 60606-3421
(312) 422-3000

*Washington Office*
325 7th St. NW
Washington, DC 20004
(202) 638-1100

**Association for Professionals in Infection Control and Epidemiology, Inc.**

1275 K St. NW, Suite 1000
Washington, DC 20005-4006
(202) 789-1890
FAX (202) 789-1899
e-mail: APICinfo@apic.org

**Joint Commission on the Accreditation of Healthcare Organizations**

601 13th St. NW, Suite 1150N
Washington, DC 20005
(202) 783-6655
FAX (202) 783-6888

**National Association of Public Hospitals and Health Systems (NAPH)**

1301 Pennsylvania Ave. NW, Suite 950
Washington, DC 20004
(202) 585-0100

## HUNTINGTON'S DISEASE
**Huntington's Disease Society of America, Inc.**

140 W 22nd St. 6th Floor
New York, NY 10011-2420
(212) 242-1968
(800) 345-4372
FAX (212) 243-2443

## KIDNEY DISEASE
**National Institute of Diabetes and Digestive and Kidney Diseases**

31 Center Dr. MSC 2560
Bethesda, MD 20892-2560

**National Kidney Foundation**

30 E 33rd St. Suite 1100
New York, NY 10016
(212) 889-2210
(800) 622-9010
FAX (212) 689-9261

## LIVER DISEASE
**American Liver Foundation Home**

75 Maiden Ln. Suite 603
New York, NY 10038
(201) 256-2550
(800) 465-4837
(800) 223-0179
FAX (201) 256-3214
e-mail: webmail@liverfoundation.org

## MUSCULAR DYSTROPHY
**Muscular Dystrophy Association**

3300 East Sunrise Dr.
Tucson, AZ 85718
(800) 572-1717
FAX (602) 529-5356

## MYASTHENIA GRAVIS
**Myasthenia Gravis Foundation, Inc.**

5841 Cedar Lake Rd. Suite 204
Minneapolis, MN 55416
(952) 545-9438
(800) 541-5454
FAX (952) 545-6073

## NUTRITION (see also Food)
**American Dietetic Association**

*Headquarters*
216 W Jackson Blvd.
Chicago, IL 60606-6995
(312) 899-0040

*Washington, DC Office*
1120 Connecticut Ave. NW, Suite 480
Washington, DC 20036
(202) 775-8277

**Consumer Information Center**

(800) 688-9889
TTY (800) 326-2996
e-mail: catalog.pueblo@gsa.gov

**Council for Responsible Nutrition**

1875 Eye St. NW, Suite 400
Washington DC, 20006-5194
(202) 872-1488
FAX (202) 872-9594

**Food and Nutrition Service**

Room 421-A
US Department of Agriculture
Washington, DC 20250
(202) 447-7854

**National Dairy Council**

10255 W Higgins Rd. Suite 900
Rosemont, IL 60018-5616

## ORGAN DONORS
**The Living Bank**

PO Box 6725
Houston, TX 77265-6725
(713) 961-9431
(800) 528-2971
FAX (713) 961-0979

**United Network for Organ Sharing**

National Organ Procurement and
   Transplantation Network
1100 Boulders Pkwy. Suite 500
PO Box 13770
Richmond, VA 23225
(804) 330-8500
(888) 894-6301
FAX (804) 330-8517

## OSTEOPOROSIS
**National Osteoporosis Foundation**

1232 22nd St. NW
Washington, DC 20037-1292
(202) 223-2226
FAX (202)-223-2237

## PAIN

### American Academy of Orofacial Pain

AAOP Central Office
19 Mantua Rd.
Mount Royal, NJ 08061
(856) 423-3629
FAX (856) 423-3420

### American Academy of Pain Management

13947 Mono Way #A
Sonora CA 95370
(209) 533-9744
e-mail: aapm@aapainmanage.org

### American Academy of Pain Medicine

4700 W Lake
Glenview, IL 60025
(847) 375-4731
FAX (847) 375-6331
e-mail: aapm@amctec.com

### American Chronic Pain Association

PO Box 850
Rocklin, CA 95677
(916) 632-0922
FAX (916) 632-3208
e-mail: ACPA@pacbell.net

### American Fibromyalgia Syndrome Association (AFSA)

6380 E Tanque Verde, Suite D
Tucson, AZ 85715
(520) 733-1570

### American Pain Foundation

111 South Calvert St. Suite 2700
Baltimore, MD 21202
e-mail: webmaster@painfoundation.org

### American Pain Society

4700 W Lake Ave.
Glenview, IL 60025
(847) 375-4715
FAX (877) 734-8758
e-mail: info@ampainsoc.org

### Association for Applied Psychophysiology and Biofeedback

10200 W 44th Ave. Suite 304
Wheat Ridge, CO 80033-2840
(303) 422-8436
FAX (303) 422-8894

### International Association for the Study of Pain

IASP Secretariat
909 NE 43rd St. Suite 306
Seattle, WA 98105-6020
(206) 547-6409
FAX (206) 547-1703
e-mail: IASP@locke.hs.washington.edu

### Reflex Sympathetic Dystrophy Syndrome Association of America

PO Box 502
Milford, CT 06460
(203) 877-3790
e-mail: jwbroatch@aol.com

### TMJ Association, Ltd.

PO Box 26770
Milwaukee, WI 53226-0770
FAX (414) 259-8112
e-mail: info@tmj.org

## PARKINSON'S DISEASE

### American Parkinson Disease Association

1250 Hylan Blvd. Suite 4-B
Staten Island, NY 10305-1946
(718) 981-8001
(800) 223-2732
FAX (718) 981-4399

### The Michael J. Fox Foundation for Parkinson's Research

Grand Central Station
PO Box 4777
New York, NY 10163
(800) 708-7644

### National Parkinson Foundation Inc.

Bob Hope Parkinson Research Center
1501 NW 9th Ave.
Bob Hope Rd.
Miami, FL 33136-1494
(800) 327-4545
(800) 433-7022
(305) 547-6666
FAX (305) 243-4545

### Parkinson's Disease Foundation, Inc.

710 W 168th St.
New York, NY 10032-9982
(212) 923-4700
(800) 457-6676
FAX (212) 923-4778

## PEDICULOSIS

### National Pediculosis Association

PO Box 610189
Newton, MA 02161
(781) 449-6487
FAX (781) 449-8129
e-mail: npa@headlice.org

## PREGNANCY (See Family *Planning/Pregnancy*)

## REHABILITATION

### American Rehabilitation Counseling Association (ARCA)

5999 Stevenson Ave.
Alexandria, VA 22304-3300
(800) 545-2223
FAX (703) 823-0252

### CARF: The Rehabilitation Accreditation

Commission
4891 E Grant Rd.
Tucson, AZ 85712
TEL/TDD (520) 325-1044
FAX (520) 318-1129
e-mail: webmaster@carf.org

### National Foundation for Facial Reconstruction

317 E 34th St. Room 901
New York, NY 10016
(212) 263-6656
(800) 422-3223
FAX (212) 263-7534

### National Rehabilitation Information Center (NARIC)

1010 Wayne Ave. Suite 800
Silver Spring, MD 20910
(301) 562-2400
(800) 346-2742
FAX (301) 562-2401

### Rehabilitation International

25 E 21st St.
New York, NY 10010
(212) 420-1500
FAX (212) 505-0871

### Rehabilitation Services Administration

Department of Education
Office of Special Education and
   Rehabilitative Services
330 C St. SW
Washington, DC 20202
(202) 723-1282

## ROSACEA

### National Rosacea Society

800 S Northwest Highway, Suite 200
Barrington, IL 60010
(847) 382-8971
(888) 662-5874
FAX (847) 382-5567

## SAFETY

### Advocates for Highway and Auto Safety

750 First St. NE Suite 901
Washington, DC 20002
(202) 408-1711
FAX (202) 408-1699
e-mail: advocates@saferoads.org

### Medic Alert Foundation International

2323 Colorado Ave.
Turlock, CA 95382
(800) 432-5378
FAX (800) 863-3429

### National Highway Traffic Safety Administration

NTS-11, US Department of
   Transportation
400 7th St. SW
Washington, DC 20590
(202) 426-9294
(888) 327-4236
(202) 426-0123
FAX (202) 366-7882

### National Injury Information Clearinghouse

(301) 504-0424
FAX (301) 504-0025
e-mail: clearinghouse@cpsc.gov

**Poison Prevention Week Council**

PO Box 1543
Washington, DC 20013
(301) 504-0580 ext. 1184
FAX (301) 504-0399

## SCLERODERMA
**United Scleroderma Foundation**

12 Kent Way, Suite 101
Byfield, MA 01922
(800) 722-4673

## SEXUALLY TRANSMITTED DISEASES
**American Social Health Association**

PO Box 13827
Research Triangle Park, NC 27709
(919) 361-8400
FAX (919) 361-8425

**Sex Information and Education Council of the United States (SIECUS)**

130 W 42nd St. Suite 350
New York, NY 10036-7802
(212) 819-9770
FAX (212) 819-9776
e-mail: siecus@siecus.org

## SICKLE CELL ANEMIA
**Sickle Cell Anemia Research Foundation**

2625 3rd St.
Alexandria, LA 71302
(318)487-8019
FAX (318)487-9990
e-mail: alexscarf@aol.com

**Sickle Cell Disease Association of America (SCDAA)**

200 Corporate Pointe, Suite 495
Culver City, CA 90230-8727
(800) 421-8453
FAX (310) 215-3722

## SMOKING
**Action on Smoking and Health (ASH)**

2013 H St. NW
Washington, DC 20006
(202) 659-4310
FAX (202) 833-3921

**American Lung Association**

1740 Broadway
New York, NY 10019-4374
(212) 315-8700
(800) 586-4872
FAX (212) 265-5642

**Centers for Disease Control and Prevention**

National Center for Chronic Disease
    Prevention and Health Promotion
Office on Smoking and Health
Publications Catalog, Mail Stop K-50
4770 Buford Highway NE
Atlanta, GA 30341-3724
(770) 488-5705
TEL/FAX (800)-232-1311

**Coalition on Smoking or Health**

1150 Connecticut Ave. NW, Suite 820
Washington, DC 20036
(202) 452-1184
FAX (202) 452-1417

## SPINA BIFIDA
**Spina Bifida Association of America**

4590 MacArthur Blvd. NW, Suite 250
Washington, DC 20007-4220
(202) 944-3285
(800) 621-3141
FAX (202) 944-3295

## SPINAL CORD
**American Association of Spinal Cord Injury Psychologists and Social Workers**

75-20 Astoria Blvd.
Jackson Heights, NY 11370
(718) 803-3782

**American Spinal Injury Association (ASIA)**

2020 Peachtree Rd. NW
Atlanta, GA 30309-1402
(404) 355-9772
FAX (404) 355-1826

**Christopher Reeve Paralysis Foundation**

500 Morris Ave.
Springfield, NJ 07081
(800) 225-0292
FAX (973) 912-9433

**National Spinal Cord Injury Association**

8701 Georgia Ave. Suite 500
Silver Spring, MD 20910
(301) 588-6959
(800) 962-9629
FAX (301) 588-9414

**National Spinal Cord Injury Foundation**

369 Elliot St.
Newton Upper Falls, MA 02169
(800) 962-9629
(301) 588-6959
FAX (301) 588-9414

**Paralyzed Veterans of America**

801 18th St. NW
Washington, DC 20006-3517
(202) 872-1300
(800) 424-8200
FAX (202) 785-4452

**Spinal Cord Society**

19051 County Highway 1
Fergus Falls, MN 56537-7609
(218) 739-5252
(218) 739-5261
FAX (218) 739-5262

## SYSTEMIC LUPUS ERYTHEMATOSUS
**Lupus Foundation of America**

1330 Piccard Dr. Suite 200
Rockville, MD 20850-4303
(301) 670-9292
(800) 558-0121
FAX (301) 760-9486

## TUBEROUS SCLEROSIS
**Tuberous Sclerosis Alliance**

801 Roeder Rd. Suite 750
Silver Spring, MD 20910
(301) 562-9890
(800) 225-6872
FAX (301) 562-9870
e-mail: ntsa@ntsa.org

# Community resources: Canada

## ACQUIRED IMMUNODEFICIENCY SYNDROME (AIDS)
**Canadian Aboriginal AIDS Network**

251 rue Bank St. Suite 602
Ottawa, Ontario K2P 1X3
(613) 567-1817
FAX (613) 567-4652
e-mail: caan@storm.ca

**Canadian AIDS Hotlines and Service Organizations**

Canadian National AIDS Clearinghouse
(613) 725-3769
FAX (613) 725-9826

**Canadian AIDS Society**

309 Cooper St. 2nd Floor
Ottowa, Ontario K2T 0G5
(613) 230-3580
FAX (613) 563-4998

**Canadian HIV/AIDS Clearinghouse**

c/o Canadian Public Health Association
1565 Carling Ave. Suite 400
Ottawa, Ontario K1Z 8R1
(613) 725-3434
(877) 999-7740
FAX (613) 725-1205

## ADVOCACY
**Alliance for Children in Television**

60 St. Clair Ave. E, Suite 1002
Toronto, Ontario M4T 1N5
(514) 597-5417
FAX (416) 515-0467

**Canada Safety Council**

1020 Thomas Spratt Place
Ottawa, Ontario K1G 5L5
(613) 739-1535
FAX (613) 739-1566

**Canadian Association for Community Living**

Kinsman Building
York University Campus
4700 Keele St.
Toronto, Ontario M3J 1P3
(416) 661-9611
FAX (416) 661-5701
TTY (416) 661-2023
e-mail: info@cacl.ca

**Canadian Council on Social Development**

309 Cooper St. 5th Floor
Ottawa, Ontario K2P 0G5
(613) 236-8977
FAX (613) 236-2750

**Canadian Counselling Association**

116 Albert St. Suite 702
Ottawa, Ontario K1P 5G3
(613) 237-1099
FAX (613) 237-9786

**Consumers' Association of Canada**

National Office
Box 9300
307 Gilmore St.
Ottawa, Ontario K1G 3T9
(613) 238-2533
FAX (613) 563-2254
e-mail: info@consumer.ca

**Dying with Dignity**

55 Eglinton Ave. E, Suite 705
Toronto, Ontario M4P 1G8
(416) 486-3998
(800) 495-6156
FAX (416) 489-9010
e-mail: dwdca@web.net

**National Anti-Poverty Organization**

440-325 Dalhousie St.
Ottawa, Ontario K1N 7G2
(613) 789-0096
FAX (613) 789-0141
e-mail: napo@napo-onap.ca

**Non-Smokers' Rights Association**

720 Spadina Ave. Suite 221
Toronto, Ontario M5S 2T9
(416) 928-2900
FAX (416) 928-1860
e-mail: toronto@nsra-adnf.ca

**Patients' Rights Association**

170 Merton St.
Toronto, Ontario M4S 1A1
(416) 487-6287

**ALCOHOL AND DRUG ABUSE**
**Addiction Intervention Association**

PO Box 843, 400 Clyde Rd.
Cambridge, Ontario N1R 5X9
(519) 624-1911
FAX (519) 624-9972
e-mail: aia@aia.ca

**Al-Anon Family Groups (Canada)**

National Public Information
Capital Corporate Centre
9 Antares Dr. Suite 245
Nepean, Ontario K2E 7V5
(613) 723-8484
(800) 714-7498
FAX (613) 723-0151

**Alcohol and Drug Recovery Association of Ontario**

PO Box 843, 400 Clyde Rd.
Cambridge, Ontario N1R 5X9
(519) 624-8855
(800) 965-3307
FAX (519) 624-1383
e-mail: adrao@adrao.on.ca

**Alcoholics Anonymous**

234 Eglinton Ave. E, Suite 202
Toronto, Ontario M4P 1K5
(416) 487-5591
FAX (416) 487-5855

**Canadian Association for Children of Alcoholics**

164 Eglinton Ave. E, Suite 304
Toronto, Ontario M4P 1G4
(416) 813-5629
FAX (416) 813-5619

**Canadian Centre on Substance Abuse (CCSA)**

National Clearinghouse on Substance
  Abuse
75 Albert St. Suite 300
Ottawa, Ontario K1P 5E7
(613) 235-4048
FAX (613) 235-8101

**Canadian Foundation for Drug Policy**

70 MacDonald St.
Ottawa, Ontario K2P 1H6
(613) 236-1027
FAX (613) 238-2891

**Council on Drug Abuse**

16 Scarlett Rd.
Toronto, Ontario M6N 4K1
(416) 763-1491
FAX (416) 767-5343
e-mail: coda@ican.net

**MADD Canada**

6507C Mississauga Rd.
Mississauga, Ontario L5N 1A6
(905) 813-6233
(800) 665-6233
FAX (905) 813-8920

**Parent Resources Institute for Drug Education (PRIDE) Canada**

College of Pharmacy
University of Saskatchewan
Saskatoon, Saskatchewan S7N 0W0
(306) 975-3755
(800) 667-3747

**ALZHEIMER'S DISEASE**
**Alzheimer Society of Canada**

20 Eglinton Ave. W, Suite 1200
Toronto, Ontario M4R 1K8
(416) 488-8772
(800) 616-8816
FAX (416) 488-3778

**AMYOTROPHIC LATERAL SCLEROSIS**
**Amyotrophic Lateral Sclerosis Society of Canada**

265 Yorkland Blvd. Suite 300
Toronto, Ontario M2J 1S5
(416) 497-2267
(800) 267-4257
FAX (416) 497-1256
e-mail: alscanada@als.ca

**APLASTIC ANEMIA**
**Aplastic Anemia Association of Canada**

22 Aikenhead Rd.
Etobicoke, Ontario M9R 2Z3
(416) 235-0468
(888) 840-0039
FAX (416) 235-1756

**ARTHRITIS**
**Arthritis Society**

393 University Ave. Suite 1700
Toronto, Ontario M5G 1E6
(416) 979-7228
FAX (416) 979-8366

**ASTHMA AND ALLERGIES**
**Allergy Asthma Information Association**

Box 100
Toronto, Ontario M9W 5K9
(416) 679-9521
(800) 611-7011
FAX (416) 679-9524
e-mail: aaia.national@sympatico.ca

**Anaphylaxis Foundation of Canada**

2054-3080 Yonge St.
Toronto, Ontario M4N 3N1
(416) 438-1917
FAX (416) 431-3270
e-mail: foundation@anaphylaxis.org

**Asthma Society of Canada**

130 Bridgeland Ave. Suite 425
Toronto, Ontario M6A 1Z4
(416) 787-4050
FAX (800) 787-3880
FAX (416) 787-5807

**Canadian Society of Allergy and Clinical Immunology**

774 Echo Dr.
Ottawa, Ontario K1S 5N8
(613) 730-6272
(800) 668-3740 ext. 272
FAX (613) 730-1116
e-mail: csaci@rcpsc.edu

## BLINDNESS
### Canadian Council of the Blind
396 Cooper St. Suite 405
Ottawa, Ontario K2P 2H7
(613) 567-0311
FAX (613) 567-2728

### Canadian Guide Dogs For The Blind
PO Box 280
4120 Rideau Valley Dr. N
Manotick, Ontario K4M 1A3
(613) 692-7777
FAX (613) 692-0650

### Canadian National Institute for the Blind
1929 Bayview Ave.
Toronto, Ontario M4G 3E8
(416) 480-7569
FAX (416) 480-7699

### Canadian National Society of the Deaf-Blind
405-422 Willowdale Ave.
North York, Ontario M2N 5B1
FAX (604) 709-4206
e-mail: CNSDB@canada.com

### National Federation of the Blind
1455 Ellis St. Suite 107
Kelowna, British Columbia V1Y 2A3

## CANCER
### About Face International
123 Edward St. Suite 1003
Toronto, Ontario M5G 1E2
(800) 665-3223

### Breast Cancer Society of Canada
National Office 401 St. Clair St.
Point Edward, Ontario N7V 1P2
(800) 567-8767
e-mail: bcsc@bcsc.ca

### Canadian Association of Pharmacy in Oncology
Box 32
Don Mills Postal Station
Don Mills, Ontario M3C 2R6

### Canadian Breast Cancer Foundation
790 Bay St. Suite 1000
Toronto, Ontario M5G 1N8
(416) 596-6773
(800) 387-9816
FAX (416) 596-7857

### Canadian Cancer Society
10 Alcorn Ave. Suite 200
Toronto, Ontario M4V 3B1
(416) 961-7223
FAX (416) 961-4189

### National Cancer Institute of Canada
10 Alcorn Ave. Suite 200
Toronto, Ontario M4V 3B1
(416) 961-7223
FAX (416) 961-7327
e-mail: ncic@cancer.ca

## CHILD ABUSE
### Canadian Society for the Prevention of Cruelty to Children
356 1st St.
PO Box 700
Midland, Ontario L4R 4P4
(705) 526-5647
FAX (705) 526-0214

## CHILDREN
### Big Brothers & Sisters of Canada
3228 S Service Rd. Suite 113E
Burlington, Ontario L7N 3H8
(905) 639-0461
(800) 263-9133
FAX (905) 639-0214

### Boys and Girls Clubs of Canada
7100 Woodbine Ave. Suite 405
Markham, Ontario L3R 5G2
(905) 477-7272
FAX (905) 477-2056

### Canadian Child Care Federation
383 Parkdale Ave. Suite 201
Ottawa, Ontario K1Y 4R4
(800) 858-1412
(613) 729-5289
FAX (613) 729-3159

### Canadian Foundation for the Study of Infant Deaths
586 Eglinton Ave. E, Suite 308
Toronto, Ontario M4P 1P2
(416) 488-3260
(800)-363-7437
FAX (416) 488-3864
e-mail: sidsinfo@sidscanada.org

### Canadian Institute of Child Health
384 Bank St. Suite 300
Ottawa, Ontario K2P 1Y4
(613) 230-8838
FAX 613-230-6654

### Canadian Paediatric Society
100-2204 Walkley Rd.
Ottawa, Ontario K1G 4G8
(613) 526-9397
FAX (613) 526-3332

### SmartRisk Foundation
790 Bay St. Suite 401
Toronto, Ontario, M5G 1N8
(416) 977-7350
FAX (416) 596-2700

### Tracheo Esophageal Fistula Parent Network
c/o 42 Saskatoon Dr.
Etobicoke, Ontario M9P 2E9
(416) 249-8710

## CHRONIC FATIGUE SYNDROME
### National ME/FM Action Network
3836 Carling Ave.
Nepean Ontario K2K 2Y6
TEL/FAX (613)-829-6667
e-mail: ag922@freenet.carleton.ca

### Nightingale Research Foundation
Dedicated to the study and treatment of ME/CFS
121 Iona St.
Ottawa Ontario K1Y 3M1
FAX (613) 523-1958
e-mail: nightingale@nightingale.ca

## CYSTIC FIBROSIS
### Canadian Cystic Fibrosis Foundation
2221 Yonge St. Suite 601
Toronto, Ontario M4S 2B4
(416) 485-9149
(800) 378-2233
FAX (416) 485-0960

## DIABETES
### Canadian Diabetes Association
15 Toronto St. Suite 800
Toronto, Ontario M5C 2E3
(416) 363-3373
(800) 226-8464
FAX (416) 363-3393

### The Islet Foundation
61 Dalewood Rd.
Toronto, Ontario M4P 2N4
e-mail: a.t.gordon@attglobal.net

### Juvenile Diabetes Foundation Canada
7100 Woodbine Ave. Suite 311
Markham, Ontario L3R 5J2
(905) 994-8700
(877) 287-3533
FAX (905) 994-0800

## DISABILITIES
### Autism Society Ontario
1 Greensboro Dr. Suite 306
Toronto, Ontario M9W 1C8

### Autism Treatment Services of Canada
(403) 253-6961

### Canadian Coalition for the Prevention of Developmental Disabilities
c/o Canadian Institute of Child Health
384 Bank St. Suite 300
Ottawa, Ontario K2P 1Y4
(613) 230-8838

### Canadian Paraplegic Association
1101 Prince of Wales Dr. Suite 320
Ottawa, Ontario K2C 3W7
(613) 723-1033
FAX (613) 723-1060

### Canadian Rehabilitation Council for the Disabled
45 Sheppard Ave. E, Suite 801
Toronto, Ontario M2N 5W9
(416) 250-7490
FAX (416) 229-1371

### Council of Canadians with Disabilities
294 Portage Ave. Suite 926
Winnipeg, Manitoba R3C 0B9
(204) 947-0303
FAX (204) 942-4625

**DisAbled Women's Network (DAWN)**
123 Edward St. Suite 1112
Toronto, Ontario M5G 1E2

**The Easter Seals/March of Dimes National Council**
90 Eglinton Ave. E, Suite 511
Toronto, Ontario M4P 2Y3
(416) 932-8382
FAX (416) 932-9844
TTY (416) 932-8151
e-mail: national.council@esmodnc.org

**Learning Disabilities Association of Canada**
323 Chapel St. Suite 200
Ottawa, Ontario K1N 7Z2
(613) 238-5721
FAX (613) 235-5391

**Thalidomide Victims Association of Canada**
PO Box 9061, Sub 40
London, Ontario N6E 1V0
(519) 681-0357
FAX (519) 685-1518

**DOWN SYNDROME**
**Canadian Down Syndrome Society**
811-14 St. NW
Calgary, Alberta T2N 2A4
(403) 270-8500
(800) 883-5608
FAX (403) 270-8291
e-mail: dsinfo@cdss.ca

**ELDERLY**
**Canadian Association on Gerontology**
100-824 Meath St.
Ottawa, Ontario K1Z 6E8
(613) 728-9347
FAX (613) 728-8913

**Canadian Coalition on Medication Use and Seniors**
350 Sparks St. Suite 1005
Ottawa, Ontario K1R 7S8
(819) 770-3131

**EPILEPSY**
**Epilepsy Canada**
1470 Peel St. Suite 745
Montreal, Quebec H3A 1T1
(514) 845-7855
(800) 860-5499
FAX (514) 845-7866

**FAMILY PLANNING/PREGNANCY**
**Canadian Coalition on Depo Provera**
c/o Winnipeg Women's Health Clinic
419 Graham Ave. 3rd Floor
Winnipeg, Manitoba R3C 0M3
(204) 947-1517
FAX (204) 943-3844

**Canadian Mothercraft Society**
32 Heath St. W
Toronto, Ontario M4V 1T3
(416) 920-3515
FAX (416) 920-5983

**Canadian Pelvic Inflammatory Disease (PID)**
Society
PO Box 33804, Station D
Vancouver, British Columbia V6J 4L6
(604) 684-5704

**DES Action Canada**
5890 Monkland Ave. Suite 203
Montreal, Quebec H4A 1G2
(514) 482-3204
(800) 482-1337
FAX (514) 482-1445

**Endometriosis Association of Canada**
74 Plateau Crescent
Don Mills, Ontario M3C 1M8
(416) 651-2419
(800) 426-2363
FAX (416) 447-4384

**Infertility Awareness Association of Canada**
1 Nicholas St. Suite 406
Ottawa, Ontario K1N 7B7
(613) 244-7222
FAX (613) 244-8908

**La Leche League Canada**
PO Box 29
18C Industrial Dr.
Chesterville, Ontario K0C 1H0
(613) 448-1842
FAX (613) 448-1845

**Planned Parenthood Federation of Canada**
1 Nicholas St. Suite 430
Ottawa, Ontario K1N 7B7
(613) 241-4474
FAX (613) 241-7550

**FAMILY RESOURCES**
**Canadian Association for Community Care**
HomeSupport Canada
119 Rose Ave. Suite 104
Ottawa, Ontario K1Y 0N6
(613) 761-8609
FAX (613) 728-6101

**Canadian Association for Treatment and Study of the Family**
Department of Social Work
King's College
University of Western Ontario
266 Epworth Ave.
London, Ontario N6A 2M3
(519) 433-3491
(800) 265-4406
FAX (519) 433-8691

**Canadian Home Care Association**
17 York St. Suite 401
Ottawa, Ontario K1N 9J6
(613) 569-1585
FAX (613) 569-1604
e-mail: chca@cdnhomecare.on.ca

**College of Family Physicians of Canada**
2630 Skymark Ave.
Mississauga, Ontario L4W 5A4
(905) 629-0900
FAX (905)629-0893
e-mail: info@cfpc.ca

**Family Life Education Council**
12 Ave. SW, Suite 224
Calgary, Alberta T2R 0G9
(403) 262-3532
FAX (403) 265-6404

**Family Service Canada**
220 Laurier Ave. W, Suite 600
Ottawa, Ontario K1P 5Z9

**Family Therapy Program**
The University of Calgary Medical Clinic
3350 Hospital Dr. NW
Calgary, Alberta T2N 4N1
(403) 220-3300
FAX (403) 270-7446
e-mail: fraserm@ucalgary.ca

**One Parent Families Association of Canada**
National Head Office
1099 Kingston Rd. Suite 222
Pickering, Ontario L1V 1B5
(905) 831-7098
FAX (905) 831-2580
e-mail: Opfa222@aol.com

**Vanier Institute of the Family**
120 Holland Ave. Suite 300
Ottawa, Ontario K1Y 0X6
(613) 722-4007
FAX (613) 729-5249

**FOOD (see also Nutrition)**
**Canola Council of Canada**
400-167 Lombard Ave.
Winnipeg Manitoba R3B 0T6
(204) 982-2100
FAX (204) 942-1841

**GASTROINTESTINAL DISORDERS**
**Canadian Celiac Association, Hamilton Branch**
6519B Mississauga Rd.
Mississauga, Ontario L5N 1A6
(905) 567-7195
(800) 363-7296
FAX (905) 567-0710

**Crohn's and Colitis Foundation of Canada**
21 St. Clair Ave. E, Suite 301
Toronto, Ontario M4T 1L9
(416) 920-5035
(800) 387-1479
FAX (416) 929-0364

## HEADACHES
### Migraine Association of Canada
365 Bloor St. E, Suite 1912
Toronto, Ontario M4W 3L4
(416) 920-4916
(800) 663-3557
FAX (416) 920-3677

## HEALTH: GENERAL
### Alberta Centre for Well-Being
11759 Groat Rd. 3rd Floor
Edmonton, Alberta T5M 3K6
(780) 427-6949
(800) 661-4551
FAX (780) 455-2092

### Alberta Heart Health Project
3-18L 410 Agriculture Forestry Centre
University of Alberta
Edmonton, Alberta T6G 2P5
(780) 492-6502
FAX (780) 492-9130
e-mail: cynthias@ualberta.ca

### Atlantic Health Promotion Research Centre (AHPRC)
Room 5200, Dentistry Building
Dalhousie University
5981 University Ave.
Halifax, Nova Scotia B3H 3J5
(902) 494-2240
FAX (902) 494-3594
e-mail: AHPRC@DAL.CA

### British Columbia Consortium for Health
Promotion Research
University of British Columbia
Library Processing Centre
2206 E Mall, Room 324
Vancouver, British Columbia V6T 1Z3
(604) 822-2258
FAX (604) 822-9210

### Canadian Association for the Advancement of Women and Sport and Physical Activity
N202-801 King Edward Ave.
Ottawa, Ontario K1N 6N5
(613) 562-5667
FAX (613) 562-5668
e-mail: caaws@caaws.ca

### Canadian Association for Health, Physical Education, Recreation and Dance (CAHPERD)
403- 2197 Riverside Dr.
Ottawa, Ontario K1H 7X3
(613) 523-1348
(800) 663-8708
FAX (613) 523-1206
e-mail: info@cahperd.ca

### Canadian Consortium for Health Promotion Research
100 College St. Suite 207
Toronto, Ontario M5G 1L5
(416) 978-1100
FAX (416) 971-1365

### Canadian Association for School Health
2835 Country Woods Dr.
Surrey, British Columbia V4A 9P9
(604) 535-7664
FAX (604) 531-6454

### Canadian Association of Schools of Social Work
338 Parkdale Ave. Suite 206
Ottawa, Ontario K1Y 4R4
(613) 792-1953
FAX (613) 722-1956

### Canadian Association of Social Workers
383 Parkdale Ave. Suite 402
Ottawa, Ontario K1Y 4R4
(613) 729-6668
FAX (613) 729-9608
e-mail: casw@casw-acts.ca

### Canadian Consortium for Health Promotion Research
c/o Centre for Health Promotion,
   University of Toronto
100 College St. Suite 207
Toronto, Ontario M5G 1L5
(416) 946-3682
FAX (416) 971-1365

### Canadian Fitness and Lifestyle Research Institute
185 Somerset St. W, Suite 201
Ottawa, Ontario K2P 0J2
(613) 233-5528
FAX (613) 233-5536

### Canadian Health Services Research Foundation
11 Holland Ave. Suite 301
Ottawa, Ontario K1Y 4S1
(613) 728-2238
FAX (613) 728-3527
e-mail: webmaster@chsrf.ca

### Canadian Institute for Health Information
377 Dalhousie St. Suite 200
Ottawa, Ontario K1N 9N8
(613) 241-7860
FAX (613) 241-8120

### Canadian Institute of Public Health Inspectors
PO Box 5367, Station F
Ottawa, Ontario K2C 3J1
(888) 245-8180
FAX (613) 224-6055

### Canadian Institutes of Health Research (CIHR)
410 Laurier Ave. W, 9th Floor
Address Locator 4209A
Ottawa Ontario K1A 0W9
(613) 941-2672
FAX (613) 954-1800
e-mail: info@cihr.ca

### Canadian Intramural Recreation Association
740-B, rue Belfast Rd.
Ottawa, Ontario K1G 0Z5
(613) 244-1594
FAX (613) 244-4738
e-mail: cir@intramurals.ca

### Canadian Public Health Association
1565 Carling Ave. Suite 400
Ottawa, Ontario K1Z 8R1
(613) 725-3769
FAX (613) 725-9826

### Canadians for Health Research
PO Box 126
Westmount, Quebec H3Z 2T1
(514) 398-7478
FAX (514) 398-8631

### Canadian Society for International Health
1 Nicholas St. Suite 1105
Ottawa, Ontario K1N 7B7
(613) 241-5785
FAX (613) 241-3845

### Canadian Women's Health Network
419 Graham Ave. Suite 203
Winnipeg, Manitoba R3C 0M3
(204) 942-5500
(888) 818-9172
FAX (204) 989-2355
e-mail: cwhn@cwhn.ca
Clearinghouse: 1-888-818-9172

### Catholic Health Association of Canada
1247 Kilborn Place
Onawa, Ontario K1H 6K9
(613) 731-7148
FAX (613) 731-7797

### Center for Health Promotion
University of Toronto
The Banting Institute
100 College St. Room 207
Toronto, Ontario M5G 1L5
(416) 978-1809
FAX (416) 971-1365
e-mail:
   centre.healthpromotion@utoronto.ca

### Centre for Applied Health Research
University of Waterloo
200 University Ave. West, Room 3116
Waterloo, Ontario N2L 3G1
(519) 885-1211
FAX (519) 746-6776

### Centre for Health Promotion Studies
5-10 University Extension Centre
8303-112 St.
Edmonton, Alberta T6G 2T4
(780) 492-4039
FAX (780) 492-9579

**Consumer Health Association of Canada**

250 Sheppard Ave. E, Suite 205
Willowdale, Ontario M2N 6M9
(416) 222-6517
FAX (416) 225-1243

**Environmental Illness Society of Canada**

536 Dovercourt Ave.
Ottawa, Ontario K2A 0T9
(613) 728-9493
FAX (613)728-1757
e-mail: eisc@eisc.ca

**Health Canada**

Address Locator 0904A
Ottawa, Ontario K1A 0K9
(613) 957-2991
FAX (613) 941-5366

**McMaster Research Center for the Promotion of Women's Health**

McMaster University
1280 Main St. W, Room CNH-429
Hamilton, Ontario L8S 4L9
(905) 525-9140 ext. 23112
FAX (905) 524-2522

**Women's Health Interaction**

58 Arthur St.
Ottawa, Ontario K1R 7B9
(613) 563-4801
FAX (613) 594-4704

**HEALTH: DENTAL**
**Canadian Dental Association**

1815 Alta Vista Dr.
Ottawa, Ontario K1G 3Y6
(613) 523-1770
(613) 523-7736

**Canadian Dental Hygienists Association**

96 Centrepointe Dr.
Nepean, Ontario K2G 6B1
(613) 224-5515
FAX (613) 224-7283

**United Way of Canada**

404-56 Sparks Street
Ottawa, Ontario K1P 5A9
(613) 236-7041
FAX (613) 236-3087
e-mail info@unitedway.ca

**HEALTH: MENTAL**
**Canadian Mental Health Association National Office**

2160 Yonge St. 3rd Floor
Toronto, Ontario M4S 2Z3
(416) 484-7750
FAX (416) 484-4617
e-mail: cmhanat@interlog.com

**Canadian Psychiatric Association**

260-441 MacLaren St.
Ottawa, Ontario K2P-2H3
(613) 234-2815
FAX (613) 234-9857

**Canadian Psychiatric Research Foundation**

2 Carlton St. Suite 1007,
Toronto, Ontario M5B 1J3
(416) 351-7757
FAX (416) 351-7765
e-mail: admin@cprf.ca

**Canadian Psychological Association**

151 Slater St. Suite 205
Ottawa, Ontario K1P 5H3
(613) 237-2144
(888) 472-0657
FAX (613) 237-1674

**Schizophrenia Society of Canada**

75 The Donway W, Suite 814
Don Mills, Ontario M3C 2E9
(416) 445-8204
(800) 809-4673
FAX (416) 445-2270

**HEARING AND SPEECH**
**Acoustic Neuroma Association of Canada**

(780)428-3384
(800) 561-2622
e-mail: anac@compusmart.ab.ca

**Canadian Association of the Deaf**

251 Bank St. Suite 203
Ottawa, Ontario K2P 1×3
TEL/TTY (613) 565-2882
FAX (613) 565-1207

**Canadian Association of Speech-Language Pathologists and Audiologists**

130 Albert St. Suite 2006
Ottawa, Ontario K1P 5G4
(613) 567-9968
(800) 259-8519
FAX (613) 567-2859

**Canadian Cultural Society of the Deaf, Inc.**

CCSD Headquarters
11337-61 Ave. House 144
Edmonton, Alberta T6H 1M3
TTY 780-436-2599
FAX 780-430-9489
e-mail: ccsd@connect.ab.ca

**Canadian Deaf-Blind and Rubella Association**

34 Island View Dr. SS#1
Fredericton, New Brunswick E3C 1K3
(506) 452-1544
FAX (506) 451-8309
e-mail: albert@brunnet.net

**Canadian Hard of Hearing Association**

2435 Holly Ln. Suite 205
Ottawa, Ontario K1V 7P2
(613) 526-1584
(800) 263-8068
TTY (613) 526-2692
FAX (613) 526-4718

**Canadian Hearing Society**

271 Spadina Rd.
Toronto, Ontario M5R 2V3
(416) 964-9595
TTY (416) 964-0023
FAX (416) 928-2525

**HEART**
**Advanced Coronary Treatment Foundation of Canada**

379 Holland Ave. Suite 2
Ottawa, Ontario K1Y 0Y9
(613) 729-3455
FAX (613) 729-5837

**Canadian Cardiovascular Society**

222 rue Queen St. Suite 1403
Ottawa, Ontario K1P 5V9
(613) 569-3407
FAX (613) 569-6574
e-mail: ccsinfo@ccs.ca

**Canadian Marfan Association**

Centre Plaza Postal Outlet
PO Box 42257
128 Queen St. S
Mississauga, Ontario L5M 4Z0
(905) 826-3223
FAX (905) 826-2125
e-mail: info@marfan.ca

**Heart and Stroke Foundation of Canada**

222 Queen St. Suite 1402
Ottawa, Ontario K1P 5V9
(613) 569-4361
FAX (613) 569-3278

**HEMOCHROMATOSIS**
**Canadian Hemochromatosis Society**

272-7000 Minoru Blvd.
Richmond, British Columbia V6Y 3Z5
(877) 223-4766
(604) 279-7135
FAX (604) 279-7138
e-mail: (chcts@istar.ca)

**HEMOPHILIA**
**Canadian Hemophilia Society**

1450 City Councillors St. Suite 840
Montreal, Quebec H3A 2E6
(514) 848-0503
FAX (514) 848-9661

**HUNTINGTON'S DISEASE**
**Huntington Society of Canada**

151 Frederick St. Suite 400
Kitchener, Ontario N2H 2M2
(519) 749-7063
FAX (519) 749-8965

**KIDNEY DISEASE**
**Kidney Foundation of Canada**

5160 Decarie Blvd. Suite 780
Montreal, Quebec H3X 2H9
(514) 369-4806
FAX (514) 369-2472

## LIVER DISEASE
**Canadian Liver Foundation**

365 Bloor St. E, Suite 200
Toronto, Ontario M4W 3L4
(416) 964-1953
(800) 563-5483
FAX (416) 964-0024

## LUNGS
**Canadian Lung Association**

National Office
3 Raymond St. Suite 300
Ottawa, Ontario K1R 1A3
(613) 569-6411
FAX (613) 569-8860

## MUCOPOLYSACCHARIDE DISEASES
**Canadian Society for Mucopolysaccharide & Related Diseases, Inc.**

Instituts de recherche en santé du Canada
410, avenue Laurier ouest
Ottawa, Ontario K1A 0W9
(613) 957-8671
FAX (613) 954-1800
e-mail: srobertson@irsc.ca

## MULTIPLE SCLEROSIS
**Multiple Sclerosis Society of Canada**

250 Bloor St. E, Suite 1000
Toronto, Ontario M4W 3P9
(416) 922-6065
FAX (416) 922-7538

## MUSCULAR DYSTROPHY
**Muscular Dystrophy Association of Canada**

2345 Yonge St. Suite 900
Toronto, Ontario M4P 2E5
(416) 488-0030
FAX (416) 488-7523

## NUTRITION
**Anorexia Nervosa and Bulimia Association (ANAB)**

767 Bayridge Dr.
PO Box 20058
Kingston, Ontario K7P 1C0

**Dietitians of Canada**

480 University Ave. Suite 604
Toronto, Ontario M5G 1V2
(416) 596-0857
FAX (416) 596-0603

**National Eating Disorder Information Centre**

CW 1-211
200 Elizabeth St.
Toronto, Ontario M5G 2C4
(416) 340-4156
FAX (416) 340-4736
e-mail: nedic@uhn.on.ca

**National Institute of Nutrition**

265 Carling Ave. Suite 302
Ottawa, Ontario K1S 2E1
(613) 235-3355
FAX (613) 235-7032

**Organization for Nutrition Education**

Woodlawn Postal Outlet
PO Box 25
Guelph, Ontario N1H 8H6

## ORGAN DONORS
**Canadian Association of Transplantation**

College Park Post Office
777 Bay St.
PO Box 46060
Toronto, Ontario M5G 2P6

**Canadian Coalition on Organ Donor Awareness**

c/o Pharmaceutical Manufacturers' Association of Canada
1111 Prince of Wales Dr. Suite 302
Ottawa, Ontario K2C 3T2
(613) 727-1380
FAX (613) 724-1407

**Canadian Organ Replacement Register (CORR)**

(613) 241-7860 ext. 4140
FAX (613) 241-8120
e-mail: communications@cihi.ca

**Eye Bank of Canada**

1 Spadina Crescent
Toronto, Ontario
(416) 978-7355
e-mail: eye.bank@utoronto.ca

**Step By Step (Organ Transplant Association)**

509 St. Clair Ave. W
PO Box 73529
Toronto, Ontario M6C 1A1
(416) 658-3936
FAX (416) 658-7914
FAX (416) 964-0024

## ORTHOPEDICS
**Canadian Orthopaedic Association**

1440 St. Catherine St. W, Suite 421
Montreal, Quebec H3G 1R8
TEL/FAX (514) 874-9003

**Canadian Osteogenesis Imperfecta Society**

c/o 128 Thornhill Crescent
Chatham, Ontario N7L 4M3
(519) 436-0025
FAX (519) 627-0557

**Canadian Osteopathic Association**

575 Waterloo St.
London, Ontario N6B 2R2
(519) 439-5521
FAX (519) 439-2616

**Osteoporosis Society of Canada**

33 Laird Dr.
Toronto, Ontario M4G 3S9
(416) 696-2663
FAX (416) 696-2673

## PAIN
**Canadian Pain Society**

50 Driveway
Ottawa, Ontario K2P 1E2
(613) 234-0812
FAX (613)-234-9894
e-mail: jhoskins@cna-nurses.ca

**Canadian RSD (Reflex Sympathetic Dystrophy) Network**

107-60 Anderton Ave.
Courtenay, British Columbia V9N 2G8
TEL/FAX (250) 338-5835

**North American Chronic Pain Association of Canada**

150 Central Park Dr. Unit 105
Brampton, Ontario L6T 2T9
(905) 793-5230
(800) 616-7246
FAX (905) 793-8781

## PARKINSON'S DISEASE
**Parkinson Foundation of Canada**

4211 Yonge St. Suite 316
Toronto, Ontario M2P 2A9
(416) 227-9700
(800) 565-3000
FAX (416) 227-9600
e-mail: General.info@parkinson.ca

**PREGNANCY (see *Family Planning/Pregnancy*)**

## REHABILITATION
**Canadian Academy of Sport Medicine**

1010 Polytek St. Unit 14, Suite 100
Gloucester, Ontario K1J 9H9
(613) 748-5851
FAX (613) 748-5792
e-mail: jburke@casm-acms.org

**Canadian Art Therapy Association**

2400 Dundas St. W, Unit 6, Suite 601
Mississauga, Ontario L5K 2R8
(905) 469-9442

**Canadian Association of Occupational Therapists (CAOT)**

CTTC Building, Suite 3400
1125 Colonel By Dr.
Ottawa, Ontario K1S 5R1
(613) 523-2268
(800) 434-2268
FAX (613) 523-2552

**Canadian Association of Rehabilitation Professionals**

7030 Woodbine Ave. Suite 500
Markham, Ontario L3R 6G2
(888) 876-9992
(905) 940-9156
FAX (905) 940-8496

**Canadian Council on Rehabilitation and Work**

167 Lombard Ave. Suite 410
Winnipeg, Manitoba R3B 0T6
(204) 942-4862
TTY (204) 944-0341
FAX (204) 944-0753

## Canadian Injured Workers Alliance (CIWA)

PO Box 10098
Thunder Bay, Ontario P7B 6T6
(807) 345-3429
(877) 787-7010
FAX (807) 344-8683
TEL/FAX (807) 768-7240
e-mail: ciwa@norlink.net

## Canadian Physiotherapy Association

National Office
2345 Yonge St. Suite 410
Toronto, Ontario M4P 2E5
(416) 932-1888
(800) 387-8679
FAX (416) 932-9708
e-mail: information@physiotherapy.ca

## Canadian Society for Exercise Physiology

185 Somerset St. W, Suite 202
Ottawa, Ontario K2P 0J2
(613) 234-3755
(877) 651-3755
FAX (613) 234-3565
e-mail: info@csep.ca

## Institute for Work and Health

250 Bloor St. E, Suite 702
Toronto, Ontario M4W 1E6
(416) 927-2027 ext. 2131
FAX (416) 927-4167
e-mail: info@iwh.on.ca

## Sport Physiotherapy Canada

1010 Polytek, Unit 14, Suite 100
Gloucester, Ontario K1J 9J9
(613) 748-5794
FAX (613) 748-5792

## SAFETY
## Canadian Bike Helmet Coalition

c/o Canadian Institute of Child Health
885 Meadowlands Dr. E, Suite 512
Ottawa, Ontario K2C 3N2
(613) 230-8838
FAX (613) 224-4145

## Canadian Centre for Occupational Health and Safety

250 Main St. E
Hamilton, Ontario L8N 1H6
(800) 263-8466
(905) 572-4400
FAX (905) 572-4500

## Canadian Fire Safety Association (CFSA)

2175 Sheppard Ave. E, Suite 310
North York, Ontario M2J 1W8
(416) 492-9417
FAX (416) 491-1670
e-mail: cfsa@taylorenterprises.com

## The Canadian Network of Toxicology Centres

2nd Floor, Bovey Building, Gordon St.
University of Guelph
Guelph, Ontario N1G 2W1
(519) 837-3320
FAX (519) 837-3861
e-mail: dwarner@tox.uoguelph.ca

## Stay Alert . . . Stay Safe Organization

2190 Yonge St. 17th Floor
Toronto, Ontario M4P 2V8
(416) 480-8225
(800) 301-7277
FAX (416) 480-8556

## Traffic Injury Research Foundation of Canada

171 Nepean St. Suite 200
Ottawa, Ontario K2P 0B4
(613) 238-5235
FAX (613) 238-5292

## SERVICES
## Active Living Alliance for Canadians with a Disability

720 Belfast Rd. Suite 104
Ottawa, Ontario, K1G 0Z5
(613) 244-0052
(800) 771-0663
FAX (613) 244-4857

## Canada's Health Informatics Association (COACH)

2 Carlton St. Suite 1304
Toronto, Ontario M5B 1J3
(416) 979-5551
(888) 253-8554
FAX (416) 979-1144
e-mail: info@coachorg.com

## Canadian Advanced Medical Services International (CAMSI)

Executive Director
2170 Mt. Newton X Rd.
Saanichton, British Columbia V8M 2B2
(250)544-2554
FAX (250)544-2506

## Canadian Association for Community Care

1 Nicholas St. Suite 520
Ottawa, Ontario K1N 7B7
(613) 241-7510
FAX (613) 241-5923

## Canadian College of Health Service Executives

350 Sparks St. Suite 402
Ottawa, Ontario K1R 7S8
(613) 235-7218
(800) 363-9056
FAX (613) 235-5451
e-mail: cchse@cchse.org

## Canadian Healthcare Association

17 York St.
Ottawa, Ontario K1N 9J6
(613) 241-8005
FAX (613) 241-5055

## Canadian Healthcare Engineering Society

The Woolen Mill
4 Cataraqui St. Suite 310
Kingston, Ontario K7k 1Z7
(613) 531-2661
FAX (613) 531-0626
e-mail: info@ches.org

## Canadian Health Record Association

Canadian College of Health Record
    Administrators
1090 Don Mills Rd. Suite 501
Don Mills, Ontario M3C 3R6
(416) 447-4900
FAX (416) 447-4598
e-mail: chragen@attglobal.net

## Canadian Medic Alert Foundation

2005 Sheppard Ave. E, Suite 800
Toronto, Ontario M2J 5B4
(800) 668-1507
(800) 668-6381 French
FAX (416) 696-0156

## Canadian Parks and Recreation Association

CPRA National Office
404-2197 Riverside Dr.
Ottawa Ontario K1H 7X3
(613) 523-5315
FAX (613) 523-1182
e-mail: cpra@cpra.ca

## Canadian Pharmacists Association

1785 Alta Vista Dr.
Ottawa, Ontario K1G 3Y6
(800) 917-9489
(613) 523-7877
FAX (613)523-0445

## Canadian Red Cross Society

1800 Alta Vista Dr.
Ottawa, Ontario K1G 4J5
(613) 739-3000
FAX (613) 731-1411

## Canadian Society of Clinical Chemists

PO Box 1570
4 Cataraqui St. Suite 310
Kingston, Ontario K7L 5C8
(613) 531-8899
FAX (613) 531-0626
e-mail: cscc@adan.kingston.net

## Canadian Society of Hospital Pharmacists

1145 Hunt Club Rd. Suite 350
Ottawa, Ontario K1V 0Y3
(613) 736-9733
FAX (613) 736-5660
e-mail: www@cshp.ca

## Hope Air

Procter & Gamble Building
4711 Yonge St.
North York, Ontario, M2N 6K8
(416) 222-6335
FAX (416) 222-6930

**International Social Service Canada**
151 Slater St. Suite 714
Ottawa, Ontario K1P 5H3
(613) 236-6161
FAX (613) 233-7306

**Nonprescription Drug Manufacturers Association of Canada**
1111 Prince of Wales Dr. Suite 406
Ottawa, Ontario K2C 3T2
(613) 723-0777
FAX (613) 723-0779
e-mail: ndmac@ndmac.ca

**United Way of Canada**
56 Sparks St. Suite 404
Ottawa, Ontario K1P 5A9
(613) 236-7041
FAX (613) 236-3087

**YMCA Canada**
42 Charles St. E, 6th Floor
Toronto, Ontario M4Y 1T4
(416) 967-9622
FAX (416) 967-9618

**YWCA of Canada**
Canadian Headquarters
590 Jarvis St. 5th Floor
Toronto, Ontario M4Y 2J4
(416) 962-8881
FAX (416) 962-8084
e-mail: national@ywcacanada.ca

**SKIN**
**Canadian Dermatology Foundation**
450 Central Ave. Suite 308
London, Ontario N6B 2E8
(519) 432-3968

**Canadian Psoriasis Foundation**
824 Meath St.
Ottawa, Ontario K1Z 6E8
(613) 728-4000
(800) 265-0926
FAX (613) 728-8913
e-mail: cpf-fcp@psoriasis.ca

**Psoriasis Society of Canada**
PO Box 25015
HalifAX, Nova Scotia B3M 4H4
(902) 443-8680
FAX (902) 457-1664

**SLEEP DISORDERS**
**Canadian Sleep Society**
3080 Yonge St. Suite 5055
Toronto, Ontario M4N 3N1
(416) 483-6260
FAX (416) 483-7081

**Sleep/Wake Disorders Canada**
3089 Bathurst St. Suite 304
Toronto, Ontario M6A 2A4
(416) 787-5374
(800) 387-9253
FAX (416) 787-4431

**SMOKING**
**Canada's National Clearinghouse on Tobacco and Health**
170 Laurier Ave. W, Suite 1000
Ottawa, Ontario K1P 5V5
(800) 267-5234
(613) 567-3050
FAX (613) 567-2730
e-mail: info-services@cctc.ca

**Canadian Council for Tobacco Control**
170 Laurier Ave. W, Suite 1000
Ottawa, Ontario K1P 5V5
(613) 567-3050
FAX (613) 567-2730

**Canadian Lung Association**
National Office
3 Raymond St. Suite 300
Ottawa, Ontario K1S 5J1
(613) 747-6776
(613) 747-7430

**Physicians for a Smoke-Free Canada**
PO Box 4849, Station E
Ottawa, Ontario K1S 5J1
(613) 233-4878
FAX (613) 567-2730

**Smoking and Health Action Foundation**
120 Spadina Ave. Suite 22
Toronto, Ontario M5S 2T9
(416) 928-2900
FAX (416) 928-1860

**SPINA BIFIDA**
**Spina Bifida and Hydrocephalus Association of Canada**
167-167 Lombard Ave.
Winnipeg, Manitoba R3B 0T6
(204) 925-3650
(800) 565-9488
FAX (204) 925-3654
e-mail: spinab@mts.net

**SPINAL CORD**
**Canadian Chiropractic Association**
1396 Eglinton Ave. W
Toronto, Ontario M6C 2E4
(416) 781-5656
(800) 668-2076
FAX (416) 781-7344

**Canadian Spinal Research Organization**
120 Newkirk Rd. Unit 2
Richmond Hill, Ontario L4C 9S7
(905) 508-4000
(800) 361-4004
FAX (905) 508-4002
e-mail: csro@globalserve.net

**Spinal Cord Society Canada**
120 Newkirk Rd. Unit 32
Richmond Hill, Ontario L4C 9S7
(905) 508-4000
FAX (905) 508-4002

**STRESS**
**Canadian Institute of Stress**
Medcan Clinic Office
150 York St. Suite 1500
Toronto, Ontario M5H 3S5
(416) 236-4218

**SYSTEMIC LUPUS ERYTHEMATOSUS**
**Lupus Canada**
Box 64034
5512-4 St. NW
Calgary, Alberta T2K 6J1
(800) 661-1468
TEL/FAX (403) 274-5599
e-mail: info@lupuscanada.org

**THYROID**
**Thyroid Foundation of Canada**
PO Box/CP 1919 STN Main
Kingston, Ontario K7L 5J7
(613) 634-3426
FAX (613) 634-3483

**TOURETTE'S SYNDROME**
**Tourette Syndrome Foundation of Canada**
194 Jarvis St. Suite 206
Toronto, Ontario M5B 2B7
(800) 361-3120
(416) 861-8398
FAX (416) 861-2472

**TURNER'S SYNDROME**
**Turner's Syndrome Society**
7777 Keele St. 2nd Floor
Concord, Ontario L4K 1Y7
(905) 660-7766
(800) 465-6744
FAX 905-660-7450

## 15-2   Professional organizations

**NURSING ORGANIZATIONS**

**Air & Surface Transport Nurses Association**

Also known as the *National Flight Nurses Association*
9101 E Kenyon Ave. Suite 3000
Denver, CO 80237
(800) 897-6362
FAX (303) 770-1812

**Academy of Medical-Surgical Nurses**

AMSN National Office
E Holly Ave. Box 56
Pitman, NJ 08071-0056
(856) 256-2323
FAX (856) 589-7463
e-mail: amsn@ajj.com

**Alliance for Psychosocial Nursing (APN)**

6900 Grove Rd.
Thorofare, NJ 08094

**American Academy of Ambulatory Care Nursing**

E Holly Ave. Box 56
Pitman, NJ 08071-0056
(856) 256-2350
FAX (856) 589-7463

**American Academy of Nurse Practitioners**

PO Box 12846
Austin, TX 78711
(512) 442-4262
FAX (512) 442-6469

**American Academy of Nursing**

600 Maryland Ave. SW, Suite 100 W
Washington, DC 20024-2571

**American Assembly for Men in Nursing**

11 Cornell Rd.
Latham, NY 12110-1499
(518) 782-9400 Ext. 346
e-mail: aamn@aamn.org

**American Association of Colleges of Nursing**

1 Dupont Cr. NW, Suite 530
Washington, DC 20036
(202) 463-6930
FAX (202) 785-8320

**American Association of Critical Care Nurses**

101 Columbia
Aliso Viejo, CA 92656-1491
(949) 362-2000
(800) 899-2226
FAX (949) 362-2020
e-mail: info@aacn.org

**American Association of Diabetes Educators**

100 W Monroe St. Suite 400
Chicago, IL 60603-1901
(312) 424-2426
(800) 338-3633
FAX (312) 424-2427

**American Association for the History of Nursing, Inc.**

PO Box 175
Lanoka Harbor, NJ 08734
(609) 693-7250
FAX (609) 693-1037

**American Association of Legal Nurse Consultants**

4700 W Lake Ave.
Glenview, IL 60025-1485
(877) 402-2562
FAX (877) 734-8668
e-mail: info@aalnc.org

**American Association of Managed Care Nurses**

PO Box 4975
Glen Allen, VA 23058-4975
(804) 747-9698
FAX (804) 747-5316

**American Association of Neuroscience Nurses**

4700 W Lake Ave.
Glenview, IL 60025-1485
(847) 375-4733
(888) 557-2266
FAX (847) 375-6333
e-mail: info@aann.org

**American Association of Nurse Anesthetists**

222 S Prospect Ave.
Park Ridge, IL 60068-4001
(847) 692-7050
FAX (847) 692-6968

**American Association of Nurse Attorneys**

7794 Grow Dr.
Pensacola, FL 32514
(850) 474-3646
(877) 538-2262
FAX (850) 484-8762
e-mail: taana@puetzamc.com

**American Association of Occupational Health Nurses**

2920 Brandywine Rd. Suite 100
Atlanta, GA 30341
(770) 455-7757
FAX (770) 455-7271
e-mail: aaohn@aaohn.org

**American Association of Spinal Cord Injury Nurses**

75-20 Astoria Blvd.
Jackson Heights, NY 11370
(718) 803-3782
FAX (718) 803-0414

**American Board for Occupational Health Nurses**

201 E Ogden Rd. Suite 114
Hinsdale, IL 60521-3652
(630) 789-5799
FAX (630) 789-8901

**American College of Cardiovascular Nursing**

PO Box 3345
Riverview, FL 33568-3345
(813) 677-1116
FAX (813) 671-8912
e-mail: accn@accn.net

**American College of Nurse-Midwives**

818 Connecticut Ave. NW, Suite 900
Washington, DC 20006
(202) 728-9860
FAX (202) 728-9897

**American College of Nurse Practitioners**

503 Capitol Ct. NE, Suite 300
Washington, DC 20002
(202) 546-4825
FAX (202) 546-4797
e-mail: acnp@nurse.org

**American Holistic Nurses' Association**

PO Box 2130
Flagstaff, AZ 86003-2130
(800) 278-2462

**American Medical Informatics Association's Nursing Informatics Workgroup**

American Medical Informatics Association
4915 St. Elmo Ave. Suite 401
Bethesda, MD 20814
(301) 657-1291
FAX (301) 657-1296

**American Nephrology Nurses' Association**

E Holly Ave. Box 56
Pitman, NJ 08071-0056
(856) 256-2320
(888) 600-2662
FAX (856) 589-7463
e-mail: anna@ajj.com

**American Nurses Association**

600 Maryland Ave. SW, Suite 100 W
Washington, DC 20024-2571
(202) 651-7000
(800) 274-4262
FAX (202) 651-7001

**American Organization of Nurse Executives**

One N Franklin
Chicago, IL 60606
(312) 422-2800
FAX (312) 422-4503

**American Pediatric Surgical Nurses Association (APSNA)**

PO Box 200585
Boston, MA 02120
(203) 457-1275
e-mail: info@apsna.com

**American Psychiatric Nurses Association**

2025 M St. NW, Suite 800
Washington, DC 20036-3309
(202) 367-1133
FAX (202) 367-2133

**American Public Health Association, Public Health Nursing Section**

800 I St NW
Washington, DC 20001-3710
(202) 777-2742
FAX 202-777-2534

**American Radiological Nurses Association (ARNA)**

820 Jorie Blvd.
Oak Brook, IL 60523-2251
(630) 571-9072
FAX (630) 571-7837
e-mail: arna@rsna.org

**American Society of Ophthalmic Registered Nurses, Inc.**

PO Box 193030
San Francisco, CA 94119
(415) 561-8513
FAX (415) 561-8575

**American Society of Pain Management Nurses (ASPMN)**

7794 Grow Dr.
Pensacola, FL 32514
(888) 342-7766
FAX (850) 484-8762
e-mail: aspmn@puetzamc.com

**American Society for Parental and Enteral Nutrition, Nursing Practice Section**

8630 Fenton St. Suite 412
Silver Spring, MD 20910-3805
(301) 587-6315
(800) 727-4567
FAX (301) 587-2365

**American Society of PeriAnesthesia Nurses**

10 Melrose Ave. Suite 110
Cherry Hill, NJ 08003-3696
(877) 737-9696
FAX (856) 616-9601
e-mail: aspan@aspan.org

**American Society of Plastic & Reconstructive Surgical Nurses**

E Holly Ave. Box 56
Pitman, NJ 08071-0056
(856) 256-2340
FAX (856) 589-7463

**American Thoracic Society, ATS NUR Assembly**

c/o American Thoracic Society
1740 Broadway
New York, NY 10019
(212) 315-8700
FAX (212) 315-6498

**American Urological Association**

11512 Allecingie Pkwy.
Richmond, VA 23235
(804) 379-1306
FAX (804) 379-1386

**Arthritis Health Professionals Association, Nursing Section**

1800 Century Plc. Suite 250
Atlanta, GA 30345
(404) 633-3777
FAX (404) 633-1870

**Association of Camp Nurses (ACN)**

8504 Thorsonveien NE
Bemidji, MN 56601
(218) 586-2633
e-mail: acn@campnurse.org

**Association of Child and Adolescent Psychiatric Nurses (ACAPN)**

Part of the International Society of
  Psychiatric-Mental Health Nurses
1211 Locust St.
Philadelphia, PA 19107
(215) 545-2843
(800) 826-2950
FAX (215) 545-8107

**Association of Community Health Nursing Educators**

7794 Grow Dr.
Pensacola, FL 32514-7072
(850) 474-8821
FAX (850) 484-8762

**Association of Nurses in AIDS Care**

11250 Roger Bacon Dr. Suite 8
Reston, VA 20190-5202
(800) 260-6780
(703) 925-0081
FAX (703) 435-4390
e-mail: AIDSNURSES@aol.com

**Association of Nurses Endorsing Transplantation**

PO Box 541234
Merritt Island, FL 32954-1234
(407) 459-3777

**Association of PeriOperative Registered Nurses**

2170 S Parker Rd. Suite 300
Denver, CO 80231-5711
(303) 755-6300
(800) 755-2676
FAX (303) 750-3212

**Association of Pediatric Oncology Nurses**

4700 W Lake Ave.
Glenview, IL 60025-1485
(847) 375-4724
FAX (847) 375-6324
e-mail: info@apon.org

**Association for Practitioners in Infection Control & Epidemiology, Inc.**

1275 K St. NW, Suite 1000
Washington, DC 20005-4006
(202) 789-1890
FAX (202) 789-1899
e-mail: APICinfo@apic.org

**Association of Rehabilitation Nurses**

4700 W Lake Ave.
Glenview, IL 60025-1485
(847) 375-4710
(800) 229-7530
FAX (877) 734-9384
e-mail: info@rehabnurse.org

**Association of Women's Health Obstetrics, and Neonatal Nurses**

2000 L St. NW, Suite 740
Washington, DC 20036
(202) 662-1600
(800) 673-8499
FAX (202) 728-0575

**Baromedical Nurses Association**

PO Box 24113
Halethrope, MD 21227
(410) 789-5690

**Case Management Society of America**

8201 Cantrell Rd. Suite 230
Little Rock, AR 72227
(501) 225-2229
FAX (501) 221-9068
e-mail: cmsa@cmsa.org

**Center for The Study of The History of Nursing**

University of Pennsylvania School of
  Nursing
420 Guardian Dr.
307 Nursing Education Building
Philadelphia, PA 19104-6096
(215) 898-4502
e-mail: nhistory@nursing.upenn.edu

**Certification Board Perioperative Nursing**

2170 South Parker Rd. Suite 295
Denver, CO 80231
(888) 257-2667
FAX (303) 695-8464

**Chi Eta Phi Sorority, Inc.**
3029 13th St. NW
Washington, DC 20009
(202) 232-3858
FAX (202) 232-3460

**Commission of Graduates of Foreign Nursing Schools**
3600 Market St. Suite 400
Philadelphia, PA 19104-2651
(215) 222-8454
FAX (215) 662-0425
e-mail: info@cgfns.org

**Council of Nephrology Nurses and Technicians**
c/o National Kidney Foundation
30 East 33rd St. Suite 1100
New York, NY 10016
(800) 622-9010
(212) 889-2210
FAX (212) 689-9261
e-mail: info@kidney.org

**Dermatology Nurses Association**
E Holly Ave. Box 56
Pitman, NJ 08071-0056
(856) 256-2330
(800) 454-4362
FAX (856) 589-7463

**Developmental Disabilities Nurses Association (DDNA)**
PO Box 2749
Eugene, OR 97402
(800) 888-6733
FAX (541) 485-7372
e-mail: ddnahq@aol.com

**Division of Nurses, Bureau of Health Professionals**
9-35, Parklawn Building
5600 Fishers Ln.
Rockville, MD 20857
(301) 443-5786
FAX (301) 443-8586

**Drug and Alcohol Nursing Association**
660 Lonely Cottage Dr.
Upper Black Eddy, PA 18972-9313
(610) 847-5396
FAX (610) 847-5063

**Emergency Nurses Association**
915 Lee St.
Des Plaines, IL 60016-6569
(847) 698-9400
(800) 900-9659
FAX (847) 460-4001

**Federation of Nurses And Health Professionals (FNHP)**
A division of the American Federation of Teachers
555 New Jersey Ave. NW
Washington, DC 20001
(202) 879-4491
FAX (202) 879-4597

**Frontier Nursing Service**
132 FNS Dr.
Wendover, KY 41775

**The Helene Fuld Health Trust**
Jina Paik, Grants Manager
50 East 42nd St. 19th Floor
New York, NY 10017
(212) 681-1237
FAX (212) 681-1335

**Hospice & Palliative Nurses Association (HPNA)**
Penn Center W One, Suite 229
Pittsburgh, PA 15276
(412) 787-9301
FAX (412) 787-9305
e-mail: hpnahpna.org

**Infusion Nurses Society**
Fresh Pond Square
10 Fawcett St
Cambridge, MA 02138
(617) 441-3008
FAX (617) 441-3009

**Interagency Council on Information Resources for Nursing**
Attn: Mr. Frederick Pattison
ICIRN
10 W 16th Street, Apt. 1
New York, NY 10011

**International Association of Sickle Cell Nurses and Physician Assistants (IASCNAPA)**
c/o Deborah Boger
Wake Forrest University—Baptist
 Medical Center
Department of Pediatrics
Medical Center Blvd.
Winston-Salem, NC 27157-1081

**International Nurses Society on Addictions**
(formerly the National Nurses Society on
 Addictions)
1500 Sunday Dr. Suite 102
Raleigh, NC 27607
(919) 783-5871
FAX (919) 787-4916

**International Society of Nurses in Cancer Care**
ISNCC Secretariat
PO Box 297
Macclesfield, Cheshire SK11 7FZ
UK
44 162 566 9588
FAX 44 162 542 8128
e-mail: Secretariat@isncc.org

**International Society of Nurses in Genetics (ISONG)**
Executive Director
7 Haskins Road
Hanover, NH 03755
(603) 643-5706

**International Society of Psychiatric-Mental Health Nurses**
A division of which is the Association of
 Child and Adolescent Psychiatric
 Nurses (ACAPN)
1211 Locust St.
Philadelphia, PA 19107
(800) 826-2950
FAX (215) 545-8107
e-mail: ISPN@nursecominc.com

**Midwest Nursing Research Society**
4700 W Lake Ave.
Glenview, IL 60025
(847) 375-4711
FAX (847) 375-4777
e-mail: info@mnrs.org

**National Advisory Council On Nurse Education and Practice**
Elaine G. Cohen, MS, RN
NACNEP Executive Secretary
301-443-5786
e-mail: ecohen@hrsa.gov

**National Alliance of Nurse Practitioners**
325 Pennsylvania Ave. SE
L'Enfant Plaza SW
Washington, DC 20003-1100
(202) 675-6350

**National Association for Health Care Recruitment**
PO Box 5769
Akron, OH 44372
(330) 867-3088
FAX (330) 867-1630

**National Association of Clinical Nurse Specialists**
3969 Green Street
Harrisburg, PA 17110
(717) 234-6799
e-mail: info@nacns.org

**National Association of Directors of Nursing Administration/Long Term Care**
10999 Reed Hartman Highway #233
Cincinnati, OH 45242
(800) 222-0539
FAX (513) 791-3699
e-mail: info@nadona.org

**National Association of Geriatric Nursing Assistants**
214 West 5th St. Suite A
Joplin, MO 64801
(417) 623-6049
(800) 784-6049
FAX (417) 623-2230
e-mail: info@nagna.org

**National Association of Hispanic Nurses**
1501 Sixteenth St. NW
Washington, DC 20036
(202) 387-2477
FAX (202) 483-7183
e-mail: info@nahnhq.org

**National Association of Neonatal Nurses**

4700 W Lake Ave.
Glenview, IL 60025-1485
(800) 451-3795
FAX (888) 477-6266
e-mail: info@nann.org

**National Association of Nurse Massage Therapists**

2203 Woodridge Court
Grand Island NE 68801
(800) 262-4017

**National Association of Nurse Practitioners in Women's Health (NPWH)**

Formerly National Association of Nurse Practitioners in Reproductive Health
503 Capitol Ct. NE, Suite 300
Washington, D.C. 20002
(202) 543-9693
FAX (202) 543-9858
e-mail: info@npwh.org

**National Association of Orthopaedic Nurses**

E Holly Ave. Box 56
Pitman, NJ 08071-0056
(856) 256-2310
FAX (856) 589-7463
e-mail: naon@mail.ajj.com

**National Association of Pediatric Nurse Associates and Practitioners**

1101 Kings Highway N, Suite 206
Cherry Hill, NJ 08034-1912
(856) 667-1773
(877) 662-7627
FAX (856) 667-7187
e-mail: info@napnap.org

**National Association of School Nurses, Inc.**

*Eastern Office*
PO Box 1300
Scarborough, ME 04070-1300
(207) 883-2117
FAX (207) 883-2683

*Western Office*
111 Cantril St.
Castle Rock, CO 80104
(303) 663-2329
FAX (303) 663-0403
e-mail: nasn@nasn.org

**National Black Nurses Association, Inc.**

8630 Fenton St. Suite 330
Silver Spring, MD 20910-38
(301) 589-3200
FAX (301) 589-3223
e-mail: NBNA@erols.com

**National Conference of Gerontological Nurse Practitioners**

PO Box 232230
Centreville, VA 20120-2230
(703) 802-0088
FAX (703) 802-1436
e-mail: ncgnp@ncgnp.org

**National Council of State Boards of Nursing**

676 N St. Clair St. Suite 550
Chicago, IL 60611-2921
(312) 787-6555
FAX (312) 787-6898

**National Federation of Licensed Practical Nurses, Inc.**

893 US Highway 70 W, Suite 202
Garner, NC 27529
(919) 779-0046
(800) 948-2511
FAX (919) 779-5642

**National Federation of Specialty Nursing Organizations**

E Holly Ave. Box 56
Pitman, NJ 08071
(609) 256-2333
FAX (609) 589-7463
e-mail: nfsno@mail.ajj.com

**National Flight Nurses Association**

See Air & Surface Transport Nurses Association.

**National Gerontological Nursing Association**

7794 Grow Dr.
Pensacola, FL 32514
(850) 473-1174
(800) 723-0560
FAX (850) 484-8762
e-mail: ngna@puetzamc.com

**National Institute of Nursing Research**

31 Center Dr. Room 5B10
MSC 2178 Building 31B
Bethesda, MD 20892-2178
(301) 496-0207
FAX (301) 480-4969
e-mail: info@opae.ninr.nih.gov

**National League for Nursing**

61 Broadway, 33rd Floor
New York, NY 10006
(212) 363-5555
(800) 669-1656
FAX (212) 812-0393

**National Network of Career Nursing Assistants**

Director
3577 Easton Rd.
Norton, Ohio 44203
(330) 825 9342
FAX (330) 825 9378
e-mail: cnajeni@aol.com

**National Nurses Society on Addictions has changed to:**

International Nurses Society on Addictions

**National Nursing Staff Development**

7794 Grow Dr.
Pensacola, FL 32514
(800) 489-1995

**National Organization for Associate Degree Nursing**

11250 Roger Bacon Dr. Suite 8
Reston, VA 20190-5202
e-mail: noadn@noadn.org

**National Organization of Nurse Practitioner Faculties**

1522 K St. NW, #702
Washington, DC 20005
(202) 289-8044
FAX (202) 289-8046
e-mail: nonpf@nonpf.org

**National Student Nurses Association**

555 W 57th St.
New York, NY 10019
(212) 581-2211
FAX (212) 581-2368
e-mail: nsna@nsna.org

**North American Nursing Diagnosis Association (NANDA)**

1211 Locust St.
Philadelphia, PA 19107
(215) 545-8105
(800) 647-9002
FAX (215) 545-8107
e-mail: info@nanda.org

**Nurse Touch Massage Therapists Association**

1438 Shortcut, Suite E
Slidell, LA 70458
(504) 893-8002
FAX (504) 892-3493
e-mail: ntmta@aol.com

**Nurses Organization of Veterans Affairs**

1726 M Street, NW, Suite 1101
Washington, DC 20036
(202) 296-0888
FAX (202)-833-1577
e-mail: nova@vanurse.org

**Oncology Nursing Society**

501 Holiday Dr.
Pittsburgh, PA 15220-2749
(412) 921-7373
FAX (412) 921-6565
e-mail onsonline@ons.org

**Pediatric Endocrinology Nursing Society**

PO Box 2933
Gaithersburg, MD 20886-2933

## Philippine Nurses Association of America

151 Linda Vista Dr.
Daly City, CA 94014
(415) 468-7995
FAX (415) 468-7995

## Sigma Theta Tau International

550 W North St.
Indianapolis, IN 46202
(317) 634-8171
(317) 634-8188
(888) 634-7575

## Society for Education & Research in Psychiatric/Mental Health Nursing

1106 Little Magothy View Cape St Clair
Annapolis, MD 21401

## Society of Gastroenterology Nurses and Associates (SGNA)

401 N Michigan Ave.
Chicago, IL 60611-4267
(800) 245-7462
(312) 321-5165
FAX: (312) 527-6658

## Society of Otorhinolaryngology & Head-Neck Nurses, Inc.

116 Canal St. Suite A
New Smyrna Beach, FL 32168
(904) 428-1695
FAX (904) 423-7566

## Society of Pediatric Nurses

7794 Grow Dr.
Pensacola, FL 32514
(800) 723-2902
FAX (850) 484-8762

## Society for Peripheral Vascular Nursing

309 Winter St.
Norwood, MA 02062
(617) 762-3630
FAX (617) 762-5582

## Society of Urologic Nurses and Associates

E Holly Ave. Box 56
Pitman, NJ 08071-0056
(888) 827-7862
(856) 256-2335
FAX (856) 589-7463

## Society for Vascular Nursing

7794 Grow Dr.
Pensacola, FL 32414
(888) 536-4786
(850) 474-6963
FAX (850) 484-8762
e-mail: svn@puetzamc.com

## Southern Nursing Research Society

University of Alabama
College of Continuing Studies
Box 870388
Tuscaloosa, AL 35487-0388
(877) 314-7677
e-mail: info@snrs.org

## Transcultural Nursing Society

College of Nursing
University of Utah
25 S Dr.
Salt Lake City, UT 84112

## U.S. Public Health Service Nursing

Office of the Chief Nurse
5600 Fishers Ln. Room 18-40
Rockville, MD 20857
(301) 443-0577

## Wound Ostomy and Continence Nurses Society

1550 S Coast Highway, Suite #201
Laguna Beach, CA 92651
(888) 224-9626
FAX (949) 376-3456

## STATE NURSES ASSOCIATIONS

### Alabama

Alabama State Nurses' Association
360 N Hull St.
Montgomery, AL 36104-3658
(334) 262-8321
FAX (334) 262-8578
e-mail: alabamasna@mindspring.com

### Alaska

Alaska Nurses Association
237 E Third Ave.
Anchorage, AK 99501
(907) 274-0827
FAX (907) 272-0292
e-mail: aknurse@alaska.com

### Arizona

Arizona Nurses Association
1850 E Southern Ave. Suite 1
Tempe, AZ 85282-5832
(480) 831-0404
FAX (480) 839-4780
e-mail: lynazna@aol.com

### Arkansas

Arkansas Nurses Association
804 N University
Little Rock, AR 72205
(501) 664-5853
FAX (501) 664-5859

### California

American Nurses Association/California
801 Portola Dr. Suite 108
San Francisco, CA 94127-1234
(415) 664-3262
FAX (415) 664-3464

The California Nurses Association
2000 Franklin St.
Oakland, CA 94612
(510) 273-2200

California Coalition of Nurse
  Practitioners
2300 Bethards Dr. Suite K
Santa Rosa, CA 95405

### Colorado

Colorado Nurses Association
5453 E Evans Plc.
Denver, CO 80222-5295
(303) 757-7483
FAX (303) 757-2679
e-mail: CNA@Nurses-CO.ORG

### Connecticut

Connecticut Nurses' Association
377 Research Pkwy. Suite 2D
Meriden, CT, 06450-7160
(203) 238-1207
FAX (203) 238-3437
e-mail:
  ct_nurses_assoc@compuserve.com

### Delaware

Delaware Nurses Association
2644 Capitol Trail, Suite 330
Newark, DE 19711
(302) 368-2333
FAX (302) 366-1775
e-mail: delnurse@erols.com

### District of Columbia

District of Columbia Nurses Association,
  Inc.
5100 Wisconsin Ave. NW, Suite 306
Washington, D.C. 20016
(202) 244-2705
FAX (202) 362-8285
e-mail: dcnurses1@aol.com

### Florida

Florida Nurses Association
PO Box 536985
Orlando, FL 32853-6985
(407) 896-3261
FAX (407) 896-9042
e-mail: theFLNurse@aol.com

### Georgia

Georgia Nurses Association
1362 W Peachtree St. NE
Atlanta, GA 30309-2904
(404) 876-6624
(800) 324-0462
FAX (404) 876-4621
e-mail: gna@mindspring.com

### Guam

Guam Nurses Association
PO Box CG
Hagatna, Guam 96932
TEL/FAX (671) 477-6877
e-mail: guamnurs@ite.net

### Hawaii

Hawaii Nurses Association
677 Ala Moana Blvd. Suite 301
Honolulu, HI 96813
(808) 521-8361
FAX: (808) 524-2760

## Idaho

Idaho Nurses Association
200 N 4th St. Suite 200
Boise, Idaho 83702-6001
(208) 345-0500
FAX: (208) 385-0166
e-mail: idanurse@rmci.net

## Illinois

Illinois Nurses Association
105 W Adams, Suite 2101
Chicago, IL 60603
(312) 419-2900
FAX (312) 419-2920

## Illinois Nurses Association

107 W Cook, Suite E
Springfield, IL 62704
(217) 523-0783
FAX (217) 523-0838

## Indiana

Indiana State Nurses Association
Executive Director
2915 N High School Rd.
Indianapolis, IN 46224
(317) 299-4575
FAX (317) 297-3525
e-mail: isnarn@prodigy.net or
    erniekjr@aol.com

## Iowa

Iowa Nurses' Association
1501 42nd St. Suite 471
West Des Moines, IA 50266
(515) 225-0495
FAX (515) 225-2201
e-mail: iowanurses@aol.com

## Kansas

Kansas State Nurses Association
1208 SW Tyler
Topeka, KS 66612-1735
(785) 233-8638
FAX: (785) 233-5222
e-mail: troberts@echo.sound.net

## Kentucky

Kentucky Nurses Association
1400 S First St.
PO Box 2616
Louisville, KY 40201
(502) 637-2546
(800) 348-5411
FAX (502) 637-8236
e-mail: kentucky.nurses@prodigy.net

## Louisiana

Louisiana State Nurses Association
5700 Florida Blvd. Suite 720
Baton Rouge, LA 70806-4820
(225) 201-0993
FAX (225) 201-0971
e-mail: lsna@lsna.org

## Maine

Maine State Nurses Association
295 Water St.
PO Box 2240
Augusta, ME 04338-2240
(207) 622-1057
(800) 207-8611
FAX: (207) 623-4072
e-mail: mainenurse@aol.com

## Maryland

Maryland Nurses Association
849 International Dr. Suite 255
Linthicum, MD 21090
(410) 859-3000
FAX (410) 859-3001
e-mail:
    marylandnursesassociation@Erols.com

## Massachusetts

Massachusetts Nurses Association
340 Turnpike St.
Canton, MA 02021
(781) 821-4625
(800) 882-2056, ext. 726
FAX (781) 821-4445
e-mail: mna@mnarn.org

## Michigan

Michigan Nurses Association
2310 Jolly Oak Rd.
Okemos, MI 48864
(800) 832-2051
(517) 349-5640
FAX (517) 349-5818
e-mail: minurses@minurses.org

Michigan League for Nursing
33150 Schoolcraft Rd. Suite 201
Livonia, MI 48150-1646
(734) 427-1900
FAX (734) 427-0104
e-mail: mln@oeonline.com

## Minnesota

Minnesota Nurses Association
1625 Energy Park Dr.
St. Paul, MN 55108
(651) 646-4807
(800) 536-4662
FAX (651) 647-5301
e-mail: mnnurses@mnnurses.org

## Mississippi

Mississippi Nurses Association
31 Woodgreen Plc.
Madison, MS 39110
(601) 898-0670
FAX (601) 898-0190
e-mail: mna@netdoor.com

## Missouri

Missouri Nurses Association
1904 Bubba Ln.
PO Box 105228
Jefferson City, MO 65110
(888) 662-6662
(573) 636-4623
FAX (573) 636-9576

## Montana

Montana Nurses Association
104 Broadway, Suite 2-G
Helena, MT 59601
(406) 442 -6710
FAX (406) 442 -1841

## Nebraska

Nebraska Nurses Association
715 South 14th St.
Lincoln, NE 68508
(402) 475-3859
(800) 201-3625
FAX (402) 475-3961
e-mail: ne.nurses@prodigy.net

## Nevada

Nevada Nurses Association
PO Box 530399
Henderson, NV 89053-0399
(702) 260-7886
(888) 464-6622
FAX (702) 260-7052
e-mail: NvNurses@aol.com

## New Hampshire

New Hampshire Nurses Association
48 West St.
Concord, NH 03301-3595
(603) 225-3783
FAX (603) 228-6672
e-mail: nh_nurses@compuserve.com

## New Jersey

New Jersey State Nurses Association
1479 Pennington Rd.
Trenton, NJ 08618-2661
(609) 883-0175
FAX (609) 883-5343

## New Mexico

New Mexico Nurses Association
303 Washington SE
Albuquerque, NM 87108
or
PO Box 80300
Albuquerque, NM 87198
(505) 268-7744
FAX (505) 268-7711
e-mail: nmna@aol.com

## New York

New York State Nurses Association
11 Cornell Rd.
Latham, NY 12110
(518) 782-9400
e-mail: info@nysna.org

## North Carolina

North Carolina Nurses Association
103 Enterprise St.
PO Box 12025
Raleigh, NC 27605-2025
(919) 821-4250
(800) 626-2153
FAX: (919) 829-5807
e-mail: ncnurses@aol.com

## North Dakota

North Dakota Nurses Association
549 Airport Rd.
Bismarck, ND 58504-6107
(701) 223-1385
FAX (701) 223-0575
e-mail: ndna@prodigy.net

## Ohio

Ohio Nurses Association
4000 E. Main St.
Columbus, OH 43213-2983
(614) 237-5414
FAX (614) 237-6074

## Oklahoma

Oklahoma Nurses Association
6414 N. Santa Fe, Suite A
Oklahoma City, OK 73116
(405) 840-3476
(800) 580-3476
FAX (405) 840-3013
e-mail: audra@oknurses.com

## Oregon

Oregon Nurses Association
9600 SW Oak St. Suite 550
Portland OR 97223-6599
(503) 293-0011
FAX (503) 293-0013

## Pennsylvania

Pennsylvania State Nurses Association
PO Box 68525
Harrisburg, PA 17106
(717) 657-1222
(888) 707-7762
FAX (717) 657-3796

## Rhode Island

Rhode Island State Nurses Association
550 South Water St.
Corliss Landing
Providence, RI 02903-4344
(401) 421-9703
FAX (401) 421-6793

## South Carolina

South Carolina Nurses Association
1821 Gadsden St.
Columbia, SC 29201
(803) 252-4781
FAX (803) 779-3870
e-mail: info@scnurses.org

## South Dakota

South Dakota Nurses Association
818 East 41st St.
Sioux Falls, SD 57105
(605) 338-1401
FAX (605) 338-0516
e-mail: southdakota.nurses@prodigy.net

## Tennessee

Tennessee Nurses Association
545 Mainstream Dr. Suite 405
Nashville, TN 37228-1296
(615) 254-0350
FAX (615) 254-0303

## Texas

Texas Nurses Association
7600 Burnet Rd. Suite 440
Austin, TX 78757
(512) 452-0645
FAX (512) 452-0648
e-mail: tna@texasnurses.org

## Utah

Utah Nurses Association
3761 S 700 E, Suite 201
Salt Lake City, UT 84106
(801) 293-8351
FAX (801) 293-8458
e-mail: una@xmission.com

## Vermont

Vermont State Nurses Association
1 Main St. #26
Fifth Floor Champlain Mill
Winooski, VT 05404-2230
(802) 655-7123
FAX (802) 655-7187
e-mail:vtnurse@cwixmail.com

## Virgin Islands

Virgin Islands State Nurses Association
PO Box 583
Christiansted, St. Croix
U.S. Virgin Islands 00821-0583
(809) 773-1261
e-mail: vcgvina@viaccess.net

## Virginia

Virginia Nurses Association
7113 Three Chopt Rd.
Richmond, VA 23226
(804) 282-1808

## Washington

Washington State Nurses Association
575 Andover Park W, #101
Seattle, WA 98188
(206) 575-7979
FAX (206) 575-1908
e-mail: wsna@wsna.org

## West Virginia

West Virginia Nurses Association
119 Summers St.
Charleston, WV 25301
or
PO Box 1946
Charleston, WV 25327
(304) 342-1169
(800) 400-1226
FAX (304) 342-6973
e-mail: centraloffice@wvnurses.org

## Wisconsin

Wisconsin Nurses Association
6117 Monona Dr.
Madison WI 53716
(608) 221-0383
(800) 362-3959
FAX (608) 221-2788
e-mail: wna@execpc.com

## Wyoming

Wyoming Nurses Association
Majestic Building, Room 305
1603 Capitol Ave.
Cheyenne, WY 82001
(307) 635-3955
FAX (307) 635-2173
e-mail: wyonurse@aol.com or
bjmcdermot@aol.com

## CANADIAN NURSES ASSOCIATIONS

### Alberta

Alberta Association of Registered Nurses
11620 168th St.
Edmonton, Alberta T5M 4A6
(780) 451-0043
(800) 252-9392
FAX (780) 452-3276
aarn@nurses.ab.ca

United Nurses of Alberta
*Provincial Office*
#900, 10611-98 Ave.
Edmonton, Alberta T5K 2P7
(780) 425-1025
FAX (780) 426-2093
*Southern Alberta Regional Office*
#505, 700-6th Ave. SW
Calgary, Alberta T2P 0T8
(403) 237-2377
FAX (403) 263-2908
e-mail: nurses@una.ab.ca

### British Columbia

British Columbia Nurses Union
BC Nurses' Union
4060 Regent St.
Burnaby, British Columbia V5C 6P5
(604) 433-2268
FAX (604) 433-7945

College Of Registered Psychiatric Nurses
Of British Columbia
251 3041 Anson Ave.
Coquitlam, British Columbia V3B 2H6
(604) 944-4941
(800) 565-2505

Registered Nurses Association of British
Columbia (RNABC)
2855 Arbutus St.
Vancouver, British Columbia V6J 3Y8
(604) 736-7331
FAX (604) 738-2272

### Manitoba

Manitoba Association of R.N.
647 Broadway Ave.
Winnipeg, Manitoba R3C 0X2
(204) 774-3477
(800) 665-2027
FAX (204) 775-6052
e-mail: marn@marn.mb.ca

Manitoba Nurses Union
502-275 Broadway
Winnipeg, Manitoba R3C 4M6
(204) 942-1320
FAX (204) 942-0958

## New Brunswick

Nurses Association of New Brunswick
165 Regent St.
Fredericton, New Brunswick E3B 7B4
(506) 458-8731
(800) 442-4417
FAX (506) 459-2838

## Newfoundland

Association of Registered Nurses of
   Newfoundland and Labrador
55 Military Rd.
PO Box 6116
St. John's, Newfoundland A1C 5X8
(709) 753-6040
(800) 563-3200
FAX (709) 753-4940
e-mail: info@arnn.nf.ca

Newfoundland and Labrador Nurses'
   Union
PO Box 416
59A LeMarchant Rd.
St. John's, Newfoundland A1C 5J9
(709) 753-9961
(800) 563-5100
FAX (709) 753-1210
e-mail: nlnu@nlnu.nf.net

## Northwest Territories

Northwest Territories R.N. Association
PO Box 2757
Yellowknife, Northwest Territories X1A
   2R1
(867) 873-2745
FAX (867) 873-2336
e-mail: nwtrna@internorth.com

## Nova Scotia

Registered Nurses' Association of Nova
   Scotia
Suite 600, Barrington Tower
1894 Barrington Str.
HalifAX, Nova Scotia B3J 2A8
491-9744
FAX 491-9510

## Ontario

College of Nurses of Ontario
101 Davenport Rd.
Toronto, Ontario M5R 3P1
(416) 928-0900
(800) 387-5526
FAX (416) 928-6507
e-mail: cno@cnomail.org

Ontario Nurses' Association
*Toronto Office*
85 Grenville St. Suite 400
Toronto, Ontario M5S 3A2
(416) 964-8833 ext. 2272
(800) 387-5580 ext. 2272
FAX (416) 964-8864
e-mail: bevm@mail.ona.org
*London Office*
750 Baseline Rd. E, Suite 204
London, Ontario N6C 2R5
Telephone: (519) 438-2153 ext. 25
FAX: (519) 433-2050
e-mail: barbf@mail.ona.org

Registered Nurses Association of Ontario
   (RNAO)
438 University Ave. Suite 1600
Toronto, Ontario M5G 2K8
(416) 599-1925
(800) 268-7199
FAX (416) 599-1926
e-mail: info@rnao.org

## Prince Edward Island

Association of Nurses of Prince Edward
   Island
17 Pownal St.
Charlottetown, Prince Edward Island C1A
   3V7
(902) 368-3764
FAX (902) 628-1430

## Quebec

Ordre des infirmieres et infirmiers du
   Quebec
4200 Boul. Dorchester Ouest
Montreal, Quebec H3Z 1V4
(514) 935-2501
(800) 363-6048
FAX 514-935-1799
e-mail: inf@oiiq.org

## Saskatchewan

Saskatchewan R.N. Association (SRNA)
2066 Retallack St.
Regina, Saskatchewan S4T 7X5
(306) 757-4643
(800) 667-9945
FAX (306) 525-0849

## Yukon

Yukon R.N. Association
204-4133 4th Ave.
Whitehorse, Yukon Y1A 3T3
(867) 667-4062
FAX (867) 668-5123
e-mail: yrna@yukon.net

## CANADIAN SPECIALTY NURSING ASSOCIATIONS
### Aboriginal Nurses Association of Canada

12 Stirling Ave. 3rd Floor
Ottawa, Ontario K1Y 1P8

### Canadian Association of Critical Care Nurses (CACCN)

PO Box 25322
London, Ontario N6C 6B1
(519) 652-1989
FAX (519) 652-5545
e-mail: caccn@caccn.ca

### Canadian Association for Enterostomal Therapy

C.A.E.T. President
PO Box 48069
60 Dundas St.E
Mississauga, Ontario L5A 1W4

### Canadian Association of Nephrology Nurses and Technologists

Debbie Maure, Executive Director
336 Yonge St. Suite. 322
Barrie, Ontario L4N 4C8
(705) 720-2819,
FAX (705) 720-1451
e-mail: cannt@cannt.ca

### Canadian Association of Neuroscience Nurses

Bev Irwin, Membership Chairperson
#205 1818 West 6th Ave.
Vancouver, British Columbia V6J 1R6
e-mail: birwin@cw.bc.ca

### Canadian Association of Nurses in AIDS Care

Mario Savoie, Secretary
151, rue Champoux
Sainte-Mélanie, Quebec J0K 3A0
(450) 883-6955
FAX (450) 883-1078

### Canadian Council of Cardiovascular Nurses

222 Queen St. Suite 1402
Ottawa, Ontario K1P 5V9
(613) 569-4361
FAX (613) 569-3278

### Canadian Intravenous Nurses Association

18 Wynford Dr. Suite 516
North York, Ontario M3C 3S2
(416) 445-4516
FAX (416) 445-4513

### Canadian Nurses Protective Society

50 Driveway
Ottawa, Ontario K2P 1E2
(800) 267-3390
(613) 237-2092
FAX (613) 237-6300
e-mail: info@cnps.ca.

### Canadian Nurses Association

50 Driveway
Ottawa, Ontario K2P 1E2
(613) 237-2133
(800) 361-8404
FAX (613) 237-3520

### Canadian Nurses Foundation

50 Driveway
Ottawa, Ontario K2P 1E2
(613) 237-2133
FAX (613) 237-3520
e-mail cnf@cnursesfdn.ca

### Canadian Nursing Students' Association

325-350 Albert St.
Ottawa, Ontario K1R 1B1
(613) 563-1236
FAX (613) 563-7739

**Manitoba Operating Room Nurses Association (MORNA)**

Ray Larkins, Project/Systems Coordinator
St. Boniface General Hospital
235-3276
FAX 237-2587
e-mail: Rlarkins@sbgh.mb.ca

**Operating Room Nurses Association of Canada**

Marlene Hill, President
rfarley@cableregina.com

**Saskatchewan Operating Room Nurses Group**

Marla Ewen, President
SORNG
1702 20th St.
W Saskatoon, Saskatchewan S7M 0Z9

**Urology Nurses of Canada**

Sue Hammond, President
PO Box 731
Mount Pearl, Newfoundland A1N 2Y2

**Victorian Order of Nurses**

5 Blackburn Ave.
Ottawa, Ontario K1N 8A2
(613) 233-5694
FAX (613) 230-4376
e-mail: national@von.ca

**MEDICAL ORGANIZATIONS**
**American Academy of Addiction Psychiatry**

7301 Mission Rd. Suite 252
Prairie Village, KS 66208
(913) 262-6161
FAX (913) 262-4311
e-mail: info@aaap.org

**American Academy of Allergy, Asthma, and Immunology**

611 E Wells St.
Milwaukee, WI 53202
(414) 272-6071
(800) 822-2762
FAX (414) 272-6070

**American Academy of Child and Adolescent Psychiatry**

3615 Wisconsin Ave. NW
Washington, DC 20016-3007
(202) 966-7300
(800) 333-7636
FAX (202) 966-2891

**American Academy of Dermatology**

930 N Meacham Rd.
Schaumburg, IL 60173
(708) 330-0230
(888) 462-3376
FAX (708) 330-0050

**American Academy of Emergency Medicine (AAEM)**

611 East Wells St.
Milwaukee, WI 53202
(800) 884-2236
FAX (414) 276-3349
e-mail: info@aaem.org

**American Academy of Family Physicians**

11400 Tomahawk Creek Pky.
Leawood, KS 66211-2672
(913) 906-6000
(800) 274-2237
FAX (816) 822-0580
e-mail: fp@aafp.org

**American Academy of Neurology**

1080 Montreal Ave.
St. Paul, MN 55116
(651) 695-1940
(800) 879-1960
FAX (612) 623-3504

**American Academy of Ophthalmology**

655 Beach St.
San Francisco, CA 94109
(415) 561-8500
FAX (415) 561-8575
e-mail: comm@aao.org

**American Academy of Orthopedic Surgeons**

6300 N River Rd.
Rosemont, IL 60018-4262
(847) 823-7186
(800) 346-AAOS
FAX (847) 823-8125

**American Academy of Otolaryngology—Head and Neck Surgery, Inc.**

1 Prince St.
Alexandria, VA 22314-3357
(703) 836-4444
FAX (703) 683-5100

**American Academy of Pain Management**

13947 Mono Way, #A
Sonora, CA 95370
(209) 533-9744
FAX (847) 375-4777

**American Academy of Pain Medicine (AAPM)**

4700 W. Lake
Glenview, IL 60025
(847) 375-4731
FAX (847) 375-6331
e-mail: aapm@amctec.com

**American Academy of Pediatrics**

141 Northwest Point Blvd.
PO Box 927
Elk Grove Village, IL 60007-1098
(847) 434-4000
FAX (847) 434-8000
e-mail: kidsdocs@aap.org

**American Academy of Physical Medicine and Rehabilitation**

1 IBM Plz., 25th Floor
Chicago, IL 60611-3604
(312) 464-9700
FAX (312) 464-0227
e-mail: info@aapmr.org

**American Association of Clinical Endocrinologists**

1000 Riverside Ave. Suite 205
Jacksonville, FL 32204
(904) 353-7878
FAX (904) 353-8185
e-mail: info@aace.com

**American Association of Electrodiagnostic Medicine**

421 First Ave. SW, Suite 300
East Rochester, MN 55902
(507) 288-0100
FAX (507) 288-1225
e-mail: aaem@aaem.net

**American Association of Neurological Surgeons**

22 S Washington St.
Park Ridge, IL 60068-4287
(847) 692-9500
FAX (847) 692-2589
e-mail: info@aans.org

**American Board of Anesthesiology**

4101 Lake Boone Trail
The Summit, Suite 510
Raleigh, NC 27607-7506
(919) 881-2570
FAX (919) 881-2575

**American Board of Dermatology, Inc.**

Henry Ford Hospital
1 Ford Plc.
Detroit, MI 48202-3450
(313) 874-1088
FAX (313) 872-3221

**American Board of Emergency Medicine (ABEM)**

3000 Coolidge Rd.
East Lansing, MI 48823-6319
(517) 332-4800
FAX (517) 332-2234
e-mail: abem@abem.org

**American Board of Pain Medicine**

4700 W. Lake Ave.
Glenview, IL 60025
(847) 375-4726
FAX (847) 375-6326
e-mail: info@abpm.org

**American Board of Internal Medicine**

510 Walnut St., Suite 1700
Philadelphia, PA 19106-3699
(800) 441-2246
(215) 446-3500
FAX: (215) 446-3470

**American Board of Radiology**

5255 East Williams Cr., Suite 3200
Tucson, AZ 85711
(520) 790-2900
FAX (520) 790-3200
e-mail: info@theabr.org

**American College of Cardiology**

9111 Old Georgetown Rd.
Bethesda, MD 20814-1699
(301) 897-5400
(800) 253-4636
FAX (301) 897-9745
e-mail: resource@acc.org

**American College of Chest Physicians**

3300 Dundee Rd.
Northbrook, IL 60062
(708) 498-1400
(800) 343-ACCP
FAX (708) 498-5460
e-mail: accp@chestnet.org

**American College of Emergency Physicians**

1125 Executive Cr.
Irving, TX 75038-2522
(972) 550-0911
(800) 798-1822
FAX (972) 580-2816
e-mail: info@acep.org

**American College of Medical Genetics**

9650 Rockville Pike
Bethesda, MD 20814-3998
(301) 530-7127
FAX (301) 571-0677
e-mail acmg@faseb.org

**American College of Obstetricians and Gynecologists**

409 12th St. SW
PO Box 96920
Washington, DC 20090-6920
(202) 638-5577
FAX (202) 484-8107
e-mail: creog@acog.org

**American College of Occupational and Environmental Medicine**

1114 N. Arlington Heights Rd.
Arlington Heights, IL 60004
(847) 818-1800
FAX (847) 818-9266
e-mail: webmaster@ACOEM.org

**American College of Physician Executives**

4890 West Kennedy Blvd. Suite 200
Tampa, FL 33609
(800) 562-8088
(813) 287-2000
FAX (813) 287-8993
e-mail: webmaster@acpe.org

**American College of Physicians/ American Society of Internal Medicine**

Independence Mall W
6th St. at Race
Philadelphia, PA 19106-1572
(215) 351-2400
(800) 523-1546
FAX (215) 351-2448

**American College of Preventive Medicine**

1660 L St. Suite 206
Washington, DC 20036-5603
(202) 466-2044
FAX (202) 466-2662
e-mail: info@acpm.org

**American College of Radiology**

1891 Preston White Dr.
Reston, VA 20191
(703) 648-8900
(800) 227-5463
FAX (703) 648-9176

**American College of Rheumatology**

1800 Century Plc. Suite 250
Atlanta, GA 30345
(404) 633-3777
FAX (404) 633-1870
acr@rheumatology.org

**American College of Sports Medicine**

401 W. Michigan St.
Indianapolis, IN 46202-3233
(317) 637-9200
FAX: (317) 634-7817
e-mail: twest@acsm.org

**American College of Surgeons**

633 North St. Clair St.
Chicago, IL 60611-3211
(312) 202-5000
FAX (312) 202-5001
e-mail: postmaster@facs.org

**American Dermatological Association**

930 N. Meacham Rd.
Schaumburg, IL 60173-6016
(847) 330-9830
FAX (847) 330-1135
e-mail: info@amer-derm-assn.org

**American Gastroenterological Association**

7910 Woodmont Ave. 7th Floor
Bethesda, MD 20814
(301) 654-2055
FAX (301) 652-3890
e-mail: mgoslin@gastro.org

**American Geriatrics Society**

The Empire State Building
350 Fifth Ave. Suite 801
New York, NY 10118
(212) 308-1414
(800) 247-4779
FAX (212) 832-8646
e-mail: info@americangeriatrics.org

**American Institute of Ultrasound in Medicine**

14750 Sweitzer Ln. Suite 100
Laurel, MD 20707-5906
(301) 498-4100
(800) 638-5352
FAX (301) 498-4450
e-mail: prollins@aium.org

**American Medical Association**

515 N. State St.
Chicago, IL, 60610
(312) 464-5000

**American Medical Student Association**

1902 Association Dr.
Reston, VA 20191
(703) 620-6600
FAX (703) 620-5873
e-mail: amsa@www.amsa.org

**American Neurological Association**

5841 Cedar Lake Rd. Suite 204
Minneapolis, MN 55416-1491
(952) 545-6284
FAX (952) 545-6073
e-mail: lindawilkerson@msn.com

**American Orthopedic Foot and Ankle Society**

1216 Pine St. Suite 201
Seattle, WA 98101
(206) 223-1120
FAX (708) 223-1178
e-mail: aofas@aofas.org

**American Orthopsychiatric Association**

330 Seventh Ave. 18th Floor
New York, NY 10001
(212) 564-5930
FAX (212) 564-6180
e-mail: amerortho@aol.com

**American Psychiatric Association**

1400 K St. NW
Washington, DC 20005
(202) 682-6000
FAX (202) 682-6850
e-mail: apa@psych.org

**American Public Health Association**

800 I St. NW
Washington, DC 20001-3710
(202) 777-2742
FAX (202) 777-2534
e-mail: comments@apha.org

**American Roentgen Ray Society**

44211 Slatestone Ct.
Leesburg, VA 20176-5109
(703) 648-8992
(800) 438-2777
FAX (703) 729-4839
e-mail: webmaster@arrs.org

**American Society of Addiction Medicine (ASAM)**

4601 North Park Ave.
Arcade Suite 101
Chevy Chase, MD 20815
(301) 656-3920
FAX (301) 656-3815
e-mail: Email@asam.org

**American Society of Anesthesiologists**

520 N Northwest Hwy.
Park Ridge, IL 60068-2573
(708) 825-5586
FAX (708) 825-1692
e-mail: mail@asahq.org

## American Society of Cataract and Refractive Surgery

4000 Legato Rd. Suite 850
Fairfax, VA 22033
(703) 591-2220
(800) 451-1339
FAX (703) 591-0614
e-mail: ascrs@ascrs.org

## American Society of Clinical Oncology

1900 Duke St. Suite 200
Alexandria, VA 22314
(703) 299-0150
FAX (703) 299-1044
e-mail: asco@asco.org

## American Society of Colon and Rectal Surgeons (ASCRS)

85 W. Algonquin Rd. Suite 550
Arlington Heights, IL 60005
(847) 290-9184
FAX (847)290-9203
e-mail: ascrs@fascrs.org

## American Society for Dermatologic Surgery

930 N. Meacham Rd.
Schaumburg, IL 60173-6016
(847) 330-9830
FAX (708) 330-0050

## American Society of Dermatology, Inc.

2721 Capital Ave.
Sacramento, CA 95816-6004
(916) 446-5054
(561) 873-8335
FAX (916) 446-0500
e-mail: hautarzt@ix.netcom.com

## American Society of Hematology

1900 M Street NW, Suite 200
Washington, DC 20036
(202) 776-0544
FAX (202) 776-0545
e-mail: ash@hematology.org

## American Society of Internal Medicine

2011 Pennsylvania Ave. NW, Suite 800
Washington, DC 20006-1808
(202) 835-2746
FAX (202) 835-0443

## American Society of Neuroradiology

2210 Midwest Rd. Suite 207
Oak Brook, IL 60521
(708) 574-0220
FAX (708) 574-0661

## American Society of Plastic Surgeons

444 E Algonquin Rd.
Arlington Heights, IL 60005
(708) 228-9900
(888) 475-2784
FAX (708) 228-9131
e-mail: webmaster@plasticsurgery.org

## American Society of Regional Anesthesia and Pain Medicine

PO Box 11086
Richmond, VA 23230-1086
(804) 282-0010
FAX (804) 282-0090
e-mail: asra@societyhq.com

## American Society for Therapeutic Radiology and Oncology

12500 Fair Lakes Cr. Suite 375
Fairfax, VA 22033-3882
(703) 227-0187
(800) 962-7876
FAX (703) 502-7852
e-mail: webmaster@astro.org

## American Society of Transplantation

236 Route 38 W, Suite 100
Moorestown, NJ 08057
(856) 608-1104
FAX (856) 608-1103
e-mail: ast@ahint.com

## American Society of Transplant Surgeons

1020 North Fairfax St. Suite 200
Alexandria, VA 22314
(888) 990-2787

## American Thoracic Society

1740 Broadway
New York, NY 10019-4374
(212) 315-8700
FAX (212) 315-6498

## American Urological Association

1120 N Charles St
Baltimore, MD 21201
(410) 727-1100
FAX 410-223-4370
e-mail: aua@auanet.org

## Association of American Indian Physicians (AAIP)

1225 Sovereign Row, Suite 103
Oklahoma City, OK 73108
(405) 946-7072
FAX (405) 946-7651
e-mail: aaip@aaip.com

## Association of American Medical Colleges (AAMC)

2450 N St. NW
Washington, DC 20037-1126
(202) 828-0400
FAX (202) 828-1125

## Association of Emergency Physicians

127 Branchaw Blvd.
New Lenox, IL 60451
(800) 449-4237
FAX (815) 463-9230
e-mail: aep@interaccess.com

## College of American Pathologists

325 Waukegan Rd.
Northfield, IL 60093-2750
(847) 832-7000
(800) 323-4040
FAX (708) 446-8807

## Endocrine Society

4350 E West Highway, Suite 500
Bethesda, MD 20814-4410
(301) 941-0200
FAX (301) 941-0259
e-mail: endostaff@endo-society.org

## Radiological Society of North America

820 Jorie Blvd.
Oak Brook, IL 60523-2251
(630) 571-2670
FAX (630) 571-7837
e-mail: webmast2@rsna.org

## Society of American Gastrointestinal Endoscopic Surgeons

2716 Ocean Park Blvd. Suite 3000
Santa Monica, CA 90405
(310) 314-2404
FAX (310) 314-2585

## Society of Cardiovascular and Interventional Radiology

10201 Lee Hwy, Suite 500
Fairfax, VA 22030
(703) 691-1805
(800) 488-7284
FAX (703) 691-1855
e-mail: info@scvir.org

## Society of Critical Care Medicine

8101 E Kaiser Blvd. 3rd Floor
Anaheim Hills, CA 92808-2259
(714) 282-6000
(877) 291-7226
FAX (714) 282-6050
e-mail: info@sccm.org

## Society for Investigative Dermatology

Suite 340 820 W Superior Ave.
Cleveland, OH 44113-1800
(216) 579-9300
FAX (216) 579-9333
e-mail: sid@sidnet.org

## Society of Thoracic Surgeons

401 N Michigan Ave.
Chicago, IL 60611-4267
(312) 644-6610
FAX (312) 527-6635
e-mail: sts@sba.com

## DENTAL ORGANIZATIONS
### Academy of General Dentistry

211 East Chicago Ave.
Chicago, IL 60611
(312) 440-4300

### Academy of Orthotists & Prosthetists

526 King St. Suite 201
Alexandria, VA 22314
(703) 836-0788
FAX (703) 836-0737
e-mail: academy@oandp.com

**Academy for Sports Dentistry**
3705 Lincoln Trl.
Taylorville, IL 62568
(800) 273-1788
(217) 824-4990
e-mail: sportsdentistry@aol.com

**American Academy of Oral Medicine**
2910 Lightfoot Dr.
Baltimore, MD 21209-1452
(410) 602-8585
e-mail: info@aaom.com

**American Academy of Pediatric Dentistry**
211 E Chicago Ave. Suite 700
Chicago, IL 60611-2663
(312) 337-2169
FAX (312) 337-6329

**American Association of Dental Examiners**
211 E Chicago Ave. Suite 760
Chicago, IL 60611
(312) 440-7464
e-mail: info@aadexam.org

**American Association of Oral and Maxillofacial Surgeons**
9700 W Bryn Mawr
Rosemont, IL 60018-5701
(847) 678-6200
(800) 822-6637
FAX (847) 678-6286
e-mail: webadmin@aaoms.org

**American Association of Hospital Dentists**
211 E Chicago Ave. 5th Floor
Chicago, IL 60611
(312) 440-2661
(312) 440-2660
FAX (312) 440-2824

**American Association of Orthodontists**
401 North Lindbergh Blvd.
St Louis, MO 63141-7816
(314) 993-1700
FAX (314) 997-1745
e-mail: marketing@aaortho.org

**American Association of Public Health Dentistry**
3760 SW Lyle Ct.
Portland, OR 97221
(503) 242-0712
FAX (503) 242-0721
e-mail: natoff@aol.com

**American Board for Certification in Orthotics and Prosthetics, Inc.**
330 John Carlyle St. Suite 200
Alexandria, VA 22314.
(703) 836-7114
FAX (703) 836-0838

**American College of Dentists**
839-J Quince Orchard Blvd.
Gaithersburg, MD 20878-1614
(301) 977-3223
FAX (301) 977-3330
e-mail: info@facd.org

**American College of Oral and Maxillofacial Surgeons**
1100 NW Loop 410, Suite 420
San Antonio, TX 78213-2266
(800) 522-6676
(210) 344-5674
FAX (210) 344-9754
e-mail: info@acoms.org

**American College of Prosthodontists**
211 E Chicago Ave. Suite 1000
Chicago, IL 60611-2616
(312) 573-1260
FAX (312) 573-1257

**American Dental Association**
211 E Chicago Ave.
Chicago, IL 60611
(312) 440-2500
FAX (312) 440-2800

**American Orthotic and Prosthetic Association**
1650 King St. Suite 500
Alexandria, VA 22314
(703) 836-7116
FAX (703) 836-0838
e-mail: info@aopanet.org

**American Society of Dental Aesthetics**
635 Madison Ave.
New York, NY 10022
(212) 751-3263
(800) 454-2732
FAX (212) 755-3263

**American Society of Dentistry for Children**
211 E Chicago Ave. Suite 710
Chicago, IL 60611
(312) 943-1244
FAX (312) 943-5341
e-mail: asdckids@aol.com

**American Society for Geriatric Dentistry**
211 E Chicago Ave. Suite 948
Chicago, IL 60611
(312) 440-2661
FAX (312) 440-2824

**American Society of Maxillofacial Surgeons**
4900B South 31st St.
Arlington, VA 22206-1656
(703) 820-7400
FAX (703) 931-4520
e-mail: maxface@email.com

**The National Commission on Orthotic and Prosthetic Education**
330 John Carlyle St. Suite 200
Alexandria, VA 22314
(703) 836-7114
e-mail: info@ncope.org

**National Dental Association**
3517 16th Street NW
Washington DC 20010
(202) 588-1697
FAX (202) 588-1244
e-mail: admin@ndaonline.org

## ALLIED HEALTH ORGANIZATIONS
### CHIROPRACTIC
**American Chiropractic Association**
1701 Clarendon Blvd.
Arlington, VA 22209
(703) 276-8800
(800) 936-4636
FAX (703) 243-2593

**American College of Chiropractic Orthopedists**
1030 Broadway, Suite 101
El Centro, CA 92243
(619) 352-1452
FAX (619) 352-3966

**Council on Chiropractic Physiological Therapeutics**
Jan Sharp DC, DACRB
Sharp Chiropractic Center
7 Mystic Ln.
Malvern, PA 19355
e-mail: JSharpDC@aol.com

**Federation of Chiropractic Licensing Boards**
901 54th Ave. Suite 101
Greeley, CO 80634-4400
(970) 356-3500
FAX (970) 356-3599
e-mail: fclb@fclb.org

**Foundation for the Advancement of Chiropractic Education**
PO Box 1052
Levittown, PA 19058
e-mail: face@f-a-c-e.com

**Foundation for Chiropractic Education and Research**
PO Box 4689
Des Moines, IA 50306-4689
(800) 622-6309
FAX (515) 282-3347

**International Chiropractors Association**
1110 N Glebe Rd. Suite 1000
Arlington, VA 22201
(703) 528-5000
(800) 423-4690
FAX (703) 528-5023
e-mail: chiro@chiropractic.org

## DENTAL HYGIENE/DENTAL ASSISTING
**American Dental Assistants Association**

203 North LaSalle St. Suite 1320
Chicago, IL 60601-1225
(312) 541-1550
(800) 733-2322
FAX (312) 541-1496
e-mail: adaa1@aol.com

**American Dental Education Association**

1625 Massachusetts Ave. NW, Suite 600
Washington, DC 20036-2212
(202) 667-9433
FAX (202) 667-0642
e-mail: adea@adea.org

**American Dental Hygienists Association**

444 N Michigan Ave. Suite 3400
Chicago, IL 60611
(312) 440-8900
(800) 243-2342
FAX (312) 440-8929
e-mail: mail@adha.net

**Dental Assisting National Board**

676 N Saint Clair, Suite 1880
Chicago, IL 60611
(800) 367-3262
(312) 642-3368
FAX (312) 642-1475

## DIAGNOSTIC MEDICAL SONOGRAPHY
**American Institute of Ultrasound in Medicine**

14750 Sweitzer Ln. Suite 100
Laurel, MD 20707-5906
(301) 498-4100
(800) 638-5352
FAX (301) 498-4450

**American Registry of Diagnostic Medical Sonographers**

600 Jefferson Plz. Suite 360
Rockville, MD 20852-1150
(301) 738-8401
(800) 541-9754
FAX (301) 738-0312/0313

**Society of Diagnostic Medical Sonographers**

12770 Coit Rd. Suite 708
Dallas, TX 75251-1319
(972) 239-7367
(800) 229-9506
FAX (972) 239-7378

## MEDICAL ASSISTING
**American Association of Medical Assistants**

20 N Wacker Dr. Suite 1575
Chicago, IL 60606-2963
(312) 899-1500
FAX (312) 899-1259

**American Association for Medical Transcription**

3460 Oakdale Rd. Suite M
Modesto, CA 95355-9690
(209) 551-0883
(800) 982-2182
FAX (209) 551-9317

**American Registry of Medical Assistants**

69 Southwick Rd. Suite A
Westfield, MA 01085-4729
(413) 562-7336
(800) 527-2762

## MEDICAL TECHNOLOGY
**American Medical Technologists**

710 Higgins Rd.
Park Ridge, IL 60068-5765
(847) 823-5169
FAX 847-823-0458
e-mail amtmail@aol.com

**American Society for Clinical Laboratory Science**

7910 Woodmont Ave. Suite 530
Bethesda, MD 20814
(301) 657-2768
FAX (301) 657-2909

## NUCLEAR MEDICINE
**American College of Nuclear Medicine**

PO Box 175
Landisville, PA 17538
(717) 898-6006
FAX (717) 898-0713

**Nuclear Medicine Technology Certification Board**

2970 Clairmont Rd. Suite 935
Atlanta, GA 30329-4421
(404) 315-1739
FAX (404) 315-6502
e-mail: board@nmtcb.org

**Society of Nuclear Medicine**

1850 Samuel Morse Dr.
Reston, VA 20190
(703) 708-9000
FAX (703) 708-9015

## NUTRITION/DIETETICS
**American Dietetic Association(ADA)**

Headquarters
216 W Jackson Blvd.
Chicago, IL 60606
(312) 899-0040
FAX (312) 899-1979
*Washington, DC Office*
American Dietetic Association
1120 Connecticut Avenue NW, Suite 480
Washington, DC 20036
(202) 775-8277

**Association of Vegetarian Dieticians and Nutrition Educators**

3835 State Route 414
Burdett, NY 14818
(607) 546-7171
FAX (607) 546-4091

**Consultant Dieticians in Health Care Facilities**

A Dietetic Practice Group of the
American Dietetic Association
c/o American Dietetic Association
216 W Jackson Blvd. Suite 800
Chicago, IL 60606
(312) 899-0040
FAX (312) 899-1758

**Dietary Managers Association**

406 Surrey Woods Dr.
St. Charles, IL 60174
(800) 323-1908
FAX (630) 587-6308

## OCCUPATIONAL THERAPY
**American Occupational Therapy Foundation**

4720 Montgomery Ln.
PO Box 31220
Bethesda, MD 20824-1220
(301) 652-2682
FAX (301) 652-7711
e-mail: aotf@aotf.org

**National Board for Certification in Occupational Therapy, Inc. (NBCOT)**

800 S Frederick Ave. Suite 200
Gaithersburg, MD 20877-4150
(301) 990-7979
FAX (301) 869-8492

## OPTOMETRY AND OPTICIANRY
**American Academy of Optometry**

6110 Executive Blvd. Suite 506
Rockville, MD 20852
(301) 984-1441
FAX (301) 984-4737
e-mail: aaoptom@aol.com

**American Optometric Association**

243 N Lindbergh Blvd.
St Louis, MO 63141
(314) 991-4100
FAX (314) 991-4101

**American Optometric Student Association**

243 N Lindbergh Blvd.
St Louis, MO 63141
(314) 991-4100
FAX (314) 991-4101

**Association of Schools and Colleges of Optometry**

6110 Executive Blvd. Suite 510
Rockville, MD 20852
(301) 231-5944
FAX (301) 770-1828

**Joint Commission on Allied Health Personnel in Ophthalmology**

2025 Woodlane Dr.
St Paul, MN 55125-2995
(651) 731-2944
(888) 284-3937
FAX (651) 731-0410

**National Academy of Opticianry**

8401 Corporate Dr. #605
Landover, MD 20785
(301) 577-4828
(800) 229-4828
FAX (301) 577-3880

**National Association of Optometrists and Opticians**

PO Box 479
Marblehead, OH 43440
(419) 798-4071
FAX (419) 798-5548

**Opticians Association of America**

7023 Little RiverTurnpike, Suite 207
Annandale, VA 22003
(703) 916-8856
FAX (703) 916-7966
e-mail: oaa@oaa.org

## PHARMACY
**American Association of Colleges of Pharmacy**

1426 Prince St.
Alexandria, VA 22314
(703) 739-2330
FAX (703) 836-8982

**American Pharmaceutical Association**

2215 Constitution Ave. NW
Washington, DC 20037-2985
(202) 628-4410
FAX (202) 738-2351

**American Society of Consultant Pharmacists**

1321 Duke St.
Alexandria, VA 22314-3563
(703) 739-1300
(800) 355-2727
FAX (703) 739-132
e-mail: info@ascp.com

**American Society of Health-System Pharmacists**

7272 Wisconsin Ave.
Bethesda, MD 20814
(301) 657-3000
FAX (301) 652-8278

## PHYSICAL THERAPY
**American Physical Therapy Association**

1111 N Fairfax St.
Alexandria, VA 22314-1488
(703) 684-2782
(800) 999-2782
FAX (703) 684-7343

**Foundation for Physical Therapy**

1111 N Fairfax St. Suite 350
Alexandria, VA 22314-1488
(800) 875-1378
FAX (703) 706-8519
e-mail: foundation@apta.org

## PHYSICIAN ASSISTANT
**American Academy of Physician Assistants**

950 N Washington St.
Alexandria, VA 22314-1552
(703) 836-2272
FAX (703) 684-1924

**Association of Physician Assistant Programs**

950 N Washington St.
Alexandria, VA 22314
(703) 548-5538

**Association of Physician Assistants in Cardiovascular Surgery**

PO Box 4834
Englewood, CO 80155
(303) 221-5651
(877) 221-5651
FAX (303) 771-2550

**International Association of Sickle Cell Nurses and Physician Assistants (IASCNAPA)**

The Sickle Cell Information Center
PO Box 109
Grady Memorial Hospital
80 Butler Street SE
Atlanta, GA 30303
(404) 616-3572
FAX (404) 616-5998
e-mail: aplatt@emory.edu

**National Commission on Certification of Physician Assistants (NCCPA)**

157 Technology Pkwy. Suite 800
Norcross, GA 30092-2913
(770) 734-4500
FAX (770) 734-4535
e-mail: nccpa@nccpa.net

## PODIATRY
**American Academy of Podiatric Sports Medicine**

Rita Yates, Executive Director
4414 Ives St.
Rockville, MD 20853
(301) 962-1540
(800) 438-3355
FAX (301) 962-3850

**American Association of Podiatric Physicians and Surgeons**

1328 Southern Ave. SE, Suite 200
Washington, DC 20032
(202) 562-2777
FAX (202) 562-5351

**American College of Foot and Ankle Orthopedics & Medicine**

ACFAOM
3525 Ellicott Mills Dr. Suite N
Ellicott City, MD 21043
(800) 265-8263
FAX (410) 418-4805

**American College of Foot and Ankle Surgeons**

515 Busse Highway
Park Ridge, IL 60068
(847) 292-2237
(800) 421-2237
e-mail: mail@acfas.org

**American Podiatric Medical Association**

9312 Old Georgetown Rd.
Bethesda, MD 20814
(301) 571-9200
FAX (301) 530-2752

## RADIOLOGIC TECHNOLOGY
**American Registry of Radiologic Technologists**

1255 Northland Dr.
St. Paul, MN 55120-1155
(651) 687-0048

**American Society of Radiologic Technologists**

15000 Central Ave. SE
Albuquerque, MN 87123-3917
(505) 298-4500
(800) 444-2778
FAX (505) 298-5063

## RESPIRATORY CARE
**American Association for Respiratory Care**

11030 Ables Ln.
Dallas, TX 75229-4593
(972) 243-2272
FAX (972) 484-2720
e-mail: info@aarc.org

**Committee on Accreditation for Respiratory Care**

1248 Hardwood Rd.
Bedford, TX 76021-4244
(817) 283-2835
(800) 874-5615
FAX (817) 252-0773

**National Board for Respiratory Care**

8310 Nieman Rd.
Lenexa, KS 66214
(913) 599-4200
FAX (913) 541-0156

## SPEECH/LANGUAGE/HEARING
**American Academy of Audiology**

8300 Greensboro Dr. Suite 750
McLean, VA 22102
(800) AAA-2336
(703) 790-8466
FAX (703) 790-8631

**American Auditory Society**

512 East Canterbury Ln.
Phoenix, AZ 85022
(602) 789-0755
FAX (602) 942-1486
e-mail: Amaudsoc@aol.com

**American Speech-Language-Hearing Association**
10801 Rockville Pike
Rockville, MD 20852
(888) 321-2742
FAX (301) 897-7348
TTY (301) 571-0457

**Council on Professional Standards in Speech-Language Pathology and Audiology**
c/o American Speech-Language Hearing Association
10801 Rockville Pike
Rockville, MD 20852
(301) 897-5700
FAX (301) 571-0457

**National Student Speech Language Hearing Association**
Dawn D. Dickerson, Director of Operations
Holly Williams, Administrative Assistant
10801 Rockville Pike
Rockville, MD 20852
(800) 498-2071
e-mail: nsslha@asha.org

## 15-3   Poison control centers

**Alabama**
Poison Center
800-462-0800

**Alaska**
Anchorage Poison Control Center
800-478-3193
907-261-3193

**Arizona**
Arizona Poison and Drug Information Center
800-362-0101 (Arizona)
520-626-6016 (Tucson)

Samaritan Regional Poison Center
602-253-3334
800-362-0101

**Arkansas**
Arkansas Poison and Drug Information Center
800-376-4766
800-641-3805 (TDD)

**California**
California Poison Control System
800-876-4766

**Colorado**
Rocky Mountain Poison and Drug Center
800-332-3073 (outside Denver)
303-739-1123 (Denver)

**Connecticut**
Connecticut Poison Control Center
800-343-2722

**Delaware**
The Poison Control Center
800-722-7112
215-386-2100

**Florida**
Florida Poison Information Center
800-282-3171 (Jacksonville)
800-282-3171 (Miami)

**Georgia**
Georgia Poison Center
404-616-9000 (Metro Atlanta)
800-282-5846 (outside metro Atlanta)
404-616-9287 (TDD)

**Hawaii**
Hawaii Poison Center
808-941-4411

**Idaho**
Rocky Mountain Poison and Drug Center
800-860-0620

**Illinois**
Illinois Poison Center
800-942-5969
312-906-6185 (TDD)

**Indiana**
Indiana Poison Center
800-382-9097 (Indiana)
317-929-2323 (Indianapolis)
317-929-2336 (TDD)

**Iowa**
Iowa Statewide Poison Control Center
800-352-2222
712-277-2222

**Kansas**
Mid-America Poison Control Center
800-332-6633
913-588-6633
913-588-6639 (TDD)

**Kentucky**
Kentucky Regional Poison Center
502-589-8222

**Louisiana**
Louisiana Poison Control Center
800-256-9822

**Maine**
Maine Poison Control Center
800-442-6305
207-871-2950

**Maryland**
Maryland Poison Center
800-492-2414
410-706-7701
410-706-1858 (TDD)

**Massachusetts**
Massachusetts Poison Control System
617-232-2120 (Boston)
800-682-9211 (MA, RI only)
888-244-5313 (TDD)

**Michigan**
800-764-7661 (TDD available)

**Minnesota**
Minnesota Poison Control System
800-222-1222

Hennepin Regional Poison Center
800-764-7661 (MN, SD only)
612-347-3141
612-904-4691 (TDD)

**Missouri**
Cardinal Glennon Children's Hospital Regional
Poison Center
314-772-5200 (St. Louis)
800-366-8888 (outside St. Louis)

**Montana**
Rocky Mountain Poison and Drug Center
800-525-5042

**Nebraska**
The Poison Center
800-955-9119 (NE, WY only)
402-354-5555

**Nevada**
Rocky Mountain Poison and Drug Center
800-446-6179

Oregon Poison Center
503-494-8968

**New Hampshire**
New Hampshire Poison Information Center
800-562-8236
603-650-8000

**New Jersey**
New Jersey Poison Information and Education System
800-764-7661

**New Mexico**
New Mexico Poison and Drug Information Center
800-432-6866
505-272-2222

**New York**
800-336-6997
212-764-7667 (New York City)
212-689-9014 (TDD)

**North Carolina**
Carolinas Poison Center
800-848-6946
704-355-4000

## North Dakota

North Dakota Poison Information Center
800-732-2200 (ND, SD, MN only)
701-234-5575

## Ohio

Central Ohio Poison Center
800-762-0727 (Dayton only);
800-682-7625 (outside Dayton)
614-228-1323
614-228-2272 (TDD)

Cincinnati Drug and Poison Center and
Regional Poison Control System
800-872-5111
513-558-5111

Greater Cleveland Poison Control Center
888-231-4455
216-231-4455

## Oklahoma

Oklahoma Poison Control Center
800-764-766
1-405-271-5454

## Oregon

Oregon Poison Center
800-452-7165
503-494-8968

## Pennsylvania

Central Pennsylvania Poison Center
800-521-6110
412-681-6669 (Pittsburgh)

## Rhode Island

Massachusetts Poison Control System
617-232-2120 (Boston)
800-682-9211 (MA, RI only)
888-244-5313 (TDD)

## South Carolina

Palmetto Poison Center
800-922-1117
803-777-1117

## South Dakota

Hennepin Regional Poison Center
800-764-7661 (MN, SD only)
612-347-3141
612-904-4691 (TDD)

## Tennessee

Middle Tennessee Poison Center
615-936-2034 (Local)
800-288-9999

## Texas

Texas Poison Center Network
800-764-7661

## Utah

Utah Poison Control Center
800-456-7707

## Vermont

Vermont Poison Center
802-658-3456
877-658-3456

## Virginia

Blue Ridge Poison Center
800-451-1428
804-924-5543

National Capital Poison Center
202-625-3333
202-362-8563 (TDD)

Virginia Poison Center
800-552-6337
804-828-9123

## Washington

Washington Poison Center
206-526-2121 (Seattle)
800-732-6985 (outside Seattle)
206-517-2394 (TDD in Seattle)
800-572-0638 (TDD outside Seattle)

## Washington, DC

National Capital Poison Center
202-625-3333

## West Virginia

West Virginia Poison Center
800-642-3625

## Wisconsin

Wisconsin Poison System
800-815-8855
608-262-3702 (Madison)
414-266-2222 (Milwaukee)

## Wyoming

The Poison Center
800-955-9119 (NE, WY only)
402-354-5555

APPENDIX
**16**

# DIAGNOSIS-RELATED GROUPS

## 16-1  Major diagnostic categories

| Major diagnostic category | Group description | Major diagnostic category | Group description |
|---|---|---|---|
| 1 | Diseases and disorders of the nervous system | 14 | Pregnancy, childbirth, and the puerperium |
| 2 | Diseases and disorders of the eye | 15 | Newborns and other neonates with conditions originating in the perinatal period |
| 3 | Diseases and disorders of the ear, nose, mouth, and throat | 16 | Diseases and disorders of the blood and blood-forming organs and immunologic disorders |
| 4 | Diseases and disorders of the respiratory system | 17 | Myeloproliferative diseases and disorders and poorly differentiated neoplasms |
| 5 | Diseases and disorders of the circulatory system | | |
| 6 | Diseases and disorders of the digestive system | 18 | Infectious and parasitic diseases (systemic or unspecified sites) |
| 7 | Diseases and disorders of the hepatobiliary system and pancreas | 19 | Mental diseases and disorders |
| 8 | Diseases and disorders of the musculoskeletal system and connective tissue | 20 | Alcohol/drug use and alcohol/drug-induced organic mental disorders |
| 9 | Diseases and disorders of the skin, subcutaneous tissue, and breast | 21 | Injuries, poisonings, and toxic effects of drugs |
| 10 | Endocrine, nutritional, and metabolic diseases and disorders | 22 | Burns |
| 11 | Diseases and disorders of the kidney and urinary tract | 23 | Factors influencing health status and other contacts with health services |
| 12 | Diseases and disorders of the male reproductive system | 24 | Multiple significant trauma |
| 13 | Diseases and disorders of the female reproductive system | 25 | Human immunodeficiency virus infections |

## 16-2  List of diagnosis-related groups (DRGs)

| DRG | MDC | Type | DRG title |
|---|---|---|---|
| 1 | 01 | P | Craniotomy age >17 except for trauma |
| 2 | 01 | P | Craniotomy for trauma age >17 |
| 3 | 01 | P | *Craniotomy age 0-17 |
| 4 | 01 | P | Spinal procedures |
| 5 | 01 | P | Extracranial vascular procedures |
| 6 | 01 | P | Carpal tunnel release |
| 7 | 01 | P | Periph & cranial nerve & other nerv syst proc w CC |
| 8 | 01 | P | Periph & cranial nerve & other nerv syst proc w/o CC |
| 9 | 01 | M | Spinal disorders & injuries |
| 10 | 01 | M | Nervous system neoplasms w CC |
| 11 | 01 | M | Nervous system neoplasms w/o CC |
| 12 | 01 | M | Degenerative nervous system disorders |
| 13 | 01 | M | Multiple sclerosis & cerebellar ataxia |
| 14 | 01 | M | Specific cerebrovascular disorders except TIA |
| 15 | 01 | M | Transient ischemic attack & precerebral occlusions |
| 16 | 01 | M | Nonspecific cerebrovascular disorders w CC |
| 17 | 01 | M | Nonspecific cerebrovascular disorders w/o CC |
| 18 | 01 | M | Cranial & peripheral nerve disorders w CC |
| 19 | 01 | M | Cranial & peripheral nerve disorders w/o CC |
| 20 | 01 | M | Nervous system infection except viral meningitis |
| 21 | 01 | M | Viral meningitis |
| 22 | 01 | M | Hypertensive encephalopathy |
| 23 | 01 | M | Nontraumatic stupor & coma |

Excerpted from the *Federal Register* 65(148):47160-47169, Aug 1, 2000.
*P,* Surgical case; *M,* medical case; *CC,* comorbidity or complication.

| DRG | MDC | Type | DRG title |
|---|---|---|---|
| 24 | 01 | M | Seizure & headache age >17 w CC |
| 25 | 01 | M | Seizure & headache age >17 w/o CC |
| 26 | 01 | M | Seizure & headache age 0-17 |
| 27 | 01 | M | Traumatic stupor & coma, coma <1 hr |
| 28 | 01 | M | Traumatic stupor & coma, coma <1 hr age >17 w CC |
| 29 | 01 | M | Traumatic stupor & coma, coma <1 hr age ≤17 w/o CC |
| 30 | 01 | M | *Traumatic stupor & coma, coma <1 hr age 0-17 |
| 31 | 01 | M | Concussion age >17 w CC |
| 32 | 01 | M | Concussion age >17 w/o CC |
| 33 | 01 | M | *Concussion age 0-17 |
| 34 | 01 | M | Other disorders of nervous system w CC |
| 35 | 01 | M | Other disorders of nervous system w/o CC |
| 36 | 02 | P | Retinal procedures |
| 37 | 02 | P | Orbital procedures |
| 38 | 02 | P | Primary iris procedures |
| 39 | 02 | P | Lens procedures with or without vitrectomy |
| 40 | 02 | P | Extraocular procedures except orbit age >17 |
| 41 | 02 | P | *Extraocular procedures except orbit age 0-17 |
| 42 | 02 | P | Intraocular procedures except retina, iris & lens |
| 43 | 02 | M | Hyphema |
| 44 | 02 | M | Acute major eye infections |
| 45 | 02 | M | Neurological eye disorders |
| 46 | 02 | M | Other disorders of the eye age >17 w CC |
| 47 | 02 | M | Other disorders of the eye age >17 w/o CC |
| 48 | 02 | M | *Other disorders of the eye age 0-17 |
| 49 | 03 | P | Major head & neck procedures |
| 50 | 03 | P | Sialoadenectomy |
| 51 | 03 | P | Salivary gland procedures except sialoadenectomy |
| 52 | 03 | P | Cleft lip & palate repair |
| 53 | 03 | P | Sinus & mastoid procedures age >17 |
| 54 | 03 | P | *Sinus & mastoid procedures age 0-17 |
| 55 | 03 | P | Miscellaneous ear, nose, mouth & throat procedures |
| 56 | 03 | P | Rhinoplasty |
| 57 | 03 | P | T&A proc, except tonsillectomy &/or adenoidectomy only, age >17 |
| 58 | 03 | P | *T&A proc, except tonsillectomy &/or adenoidectomy only, age 0-17 |
| 59 | 03 | P | Tonsillectomy &/or adenoidectomy only, age >17 |
| 60 | 03 | P | *Tonsillectomy &/or adenoidectomy only, age 0-17 |
| 61 | 03 | P | Myringotomy w tube insertion age >17 |
| 62 | 03 | P | *Myringotomy w tube insertion age 0-17 |
| 63 | 03 | P | Other ear, nose, mouth & throat O.R. procedures |
| 64 | 03 | M | Ear, nose, mouth & throat malignancy |
| 65 | 03 | M | Dysequilibrium |
| 66 | 03 | M | Epistaxis |
| 67 | 03 | M | Epiglottitis |
| 68 | 03 | M | Otitis media & URI age >17 w CC |
| 69 | 03 | M | Otitis media & URI age >17 w/o CC |
| 70 | 03 | M | Otitis media & URI age 0-17 |
| 71 | 03 | M | Laryngotracheitis |
| 72 | 03 | M | Nasal trauma & deformity |
| 73 | 03 | M | Other ear, nose, mouth & throat diagnoses age >17 |
| 74 | 03 | M | *Other ear, nose, mouth & throat diagnoses age 0-17 |
| 75 | 04 | P | Major chest procedures |
| 76 | 04 | P | Other resp system O.R. procedures w CC |
| 77 | 04 | P | Other resp system O.R. procedures w/o CC |
| 78 | 04 | M | Pulmonary embolism |
| 79 | 04 | M | Respiratory infections & inflammations age >17 w CC |
| 80 | 04 | M | Respiratory infections & inflammations age >17 w/o CC |
| 81 | 04 | M | *Respiratory infections & inflammations age 0-17 |
| 82 | 04 | M | Respiratory neoplasms |
| 83 | 04 | M | Major chest trauma w CC |
| 84 | 04 | M | Major chest trauma w/o CC |
| 85 | 04 | M | Pleural effusion w CC |
| 86 | 04 | M | Pleural effusion w/o CC |
| 87 | 04 | M | Pulmonary edema & respiratory failure |
| 88 | 04 | M | Chronic obstructive pulmonary disease |
| 89 | 04 | M | Simple pneumonia & pleurisy age >17 w CC |
| 90 | 04 | M | Simple pneumonia & pleurisy age >17 w/o CC |

*Continued*

| DRG | MDC | Type | DRG title |
|-----|-----|------|-----------|
| 91 | 04 | M | Simple pneumonia & pleurisy age 0-17 |
| 92 | 04 | M | Interstitial lung disease w CC |
| 93 | 04 | M | Interstitial lung disease w/o CC |
| 94 | 04 | M | Pneumothorax w CC |
| 95 | 04 | M | Pneumothorax w/o CC |
| 96 | 04 | M | Bronchitis & asthma age >17 w CC |
| 97 | 04 | M | Bronchitis & asthma age >17 w/o CC |
| 98 | 04 | M | Bronchitis & asthma age 0-17 |
| 99 | 04 | M | Respiratory signs & symptoms w CC |
| 100 | 04 | M | Respiratory signs & symptoms w/o CC |
| 101 | 04 | M | Other respiratory system diagnoses w CC |
| 102 | 04 | M | Other respiratory system diagnoses w/o CC |
| 103 | PRE | P | Heart transplant |
| 104 | 05 | P | Cardiac valve & other major cardiothoracic proc w cardiac cath |
| 105 | 05 | P | Cardiac valve & other major cardiothoracic proc w/o cardiac cath |
| 106 | 05 | P | Coronary bypass w PTCA |
| 107 | 05 | P | Coronary bypass w cardiac cath |
| 108 | 05 | P | Other cardiothoracic procedures |
| 109 | 05 | P | Coronary bypass w/o PTCA or cardiac cath |
| 110 | 05 | P | Major cardiovascular procedures w CC |
| 111 | 05 | P | Major cardiovascular procedures w/o CC |
| 112 | 05 | P | Percutaneous cardiovascular procedures |
| 113 | 05 | P | Amputation for circ system disorders except upper limb & toe |
| 114 | 05 | P | Upper limb & toe amputation for circ system disorders |
| 115 | 05 | P | PRM card pacem impl w AMI, hrt fail or shk, or AICD lead or GNRTR PR |
| 116 | 05 | P | Oth perm card pacemak impl or PTCA w coronary artery stent implnt |
| 117 | 05 | P | Cardiac pacemaker revision except device replacement |
| 118 | 05 | P | Cardiac pacemaker device replacement |
| 119 | 05 | P | Vein ligation & stripping |
| 120 | 05 | P | Other circulatory system O.R. procedures |
| 121 | 05 | M | Circulatory disorders w AMI & major comp, discharged alive |
| 122 | 05 | M | Circulatory disorders w AMI w/o major comp, discharged alive |
| 123 | 05 | M | Circulatory disorders w AMI, expired |
| 124 | 05 | M | Circulatory disorders except AMI, w card cath & complex diag |
| 125 | 05 | M | Circulatory disorders except AMI, w card cath w/o complex diag |
| 126 | 05 | M | Acute & subacute endocarditis |
| 127 | 05 | M | Heart failure & shock |
| 128 | 05 | M | Deep vein thrombophlebitis |
| 129 | 05 | M | Cardiac arrest, unexplained |
| 130 | 05 | M | Peripheral vascular disorders w CC |
| 131 | 05 | M | Peripheral vascular disorders w/o CC |
| 132 | 05 | M | Atherosclerosis w CC |
| 133 | 05 | M | Atherosclerosis w/o CC |
| 134 | 05 | M | Hypertension |
| 135 | 05 | M | Cardiac congenital & valvular disorders age >17 w CC |
| 136 | 05 | M | Cardiac congenital & valvular disorders age >17 w/o CC |
| 137 | 05 | M | *Cardiac congenital & valvular disorders age 0-17 |
| 138 | 05 | M | Cardiac arrhythmia & conduction disorders w CC |
| 139 | 05 | M | Cardiac arrhythmia & conduction disorders w/o CC |
| 140 | 05 | M | Angina pectoris |
| 141 | 05 | M | Syncope & collapse w CC |
| 142 | 05 | M | Syncope & collapse w/o CC |
| 143 | 05 | M | Chest pain |
| 144 | 05 | M | Other circulatory system diagnoses w CC |
| 145 | 05 | M | Other circulatory system diagnoses w/o CC |
| 146 | 06 | P | Rectal resection w CC |
| 147 | 06 | P | Rectal resection w/o CC |
| 148 | 06 | P | Major small & large bowel procedures w CC |
| 149 | 06 | P | Major small & large bowel procedures w/o CC |
| 150 | 06 | P | Peritoneal adhesiolysis w CC |
| 151 | 06 | P | Peritoneal adhesiolysis w/o CC |
| 152 | 06 | P | Minor small & large bowel procedures w CC |
| 153 | 06 | P | Minor small & large bowel procedures w/o CC |
| 154 | 06 | P | Stomach, esophageal & duodenal procedures age >17 w CC |
| 155 | 06 | P | Stomach, esophageal & duodenal procedures age >17 w/o CC |
| 156 | 06 | P | *Stomach, esophageal & duodenal procedures age 0-17 |
| 157 | 06 | P | Anal & stomal procedures w CC |

**2051**

| DRG | MDC | Type | DRG title |
|-----|-----|------|-----------|
| 158 | 06 | P | Anal & stomal procedures w/o CC |
| 159 | 06 | P | Hernia procedures except inguinal & femoral age >17 w CC |
| 160 | 06 | P | Hernia procedures except inguinal & femoral age >17 w/o CC |
| 161 | 06 | P | Inguinal & femoral hernia procedures age >17 w CC |
| 162 | 06 | P | Inguinal & femoral hernia procedures age >17 w/o CC |
| 163 | 06 | P | Hernia procedures age 0-17 |
| 164 | 06 | P | Appendectomy w complicated principal diag w CC |
| 165 | 06 | P | Appendectomy w complicated principal diag w/o CC |
| 166 | 06 | P | Appendectomy w/o complicated principal diag w CC |
| 167 | 06 | P | Appendectomy w/o complicated principal diag w/o CC |
| 168 | 03 | P | Mouth procedures w CC |
| 169 | 03 | P | Mouth procedures w/o CC |
| 170 | 06 | P | Other digestive system O.R. procedures w CC |
| 171 | 06 | P | Other digestive system O.R. procedures w/o CC |
| 172 | 06 | M | Digestive malignancy w CC |
| 173 | 06 | M | Digestive malignancy w/o CC |
| 174 | 06 | M | G.I. hemorrhage w CC |
| 175 | 06 | M | G.I. hemorrhage w/o CC |
| 176 | 06 | M | Complicated peptic ulcer |
| 177 | 06 | M | Uncomplicated peptic ulcer w CC |
| 178 | 06 | M | Uncomplicated peptic ulcer w/o CC |
| 179 | 06 | M | Inflammatory bowel disease |
| 180 | 06 | M | G.I. obstruction w CC |
| 181 | 06 | M | G.I. obstruction w/o CC |
| 182 | 06 | M | Esophagitis, gastroent & misc digest disorders age >17 w CC |
| 183 | 06 | M | Esophagitis, gastroent & misc digest disorders age >17 w/o CC |
| 184 | 06 | M | Esophagitis, gastroent & misc digest disorders age 0-17 |
| 185 | 03 | M | Dental & oral dis except extractions & restorations, age >17 |
| 186 | 03 | M | *Dental & oral dis except extractions & restorations, age 0-17 |
| 187 | 03 | M | Dental extractions & restorations |
| 188 | 06 | M | Other digestive system diagnoses age >17 w CC |
| 189 | 06 | M | Other digestive system diagnoses age >17 w/o CC |
| 190 | 06 | M | Other digestive system diagnoses age 0-17 |
| 191 | 07 | P | Pancreas, liver & shunt procedures w CC |
| 192 | 07 | P | Pancreas, liver & shunt procedures w/o CC |
| 193 | 07 | P | Biliary tract proc except only cholecyst w or w/o C.D.E. w CC |
| 194 | 07 | P | Biliary tract proc except only cholecyst w or w/o C.D.E. w/o CC |
| 195 | 07 | P | Cholecystectomy w C.D.E. w CC |
| 196 | 07 | P | Cholecystectomy w C.D.E. w/o CC |
| 197 | 07 | P | Cholecystectomy except by laparoscope w/o C.D.E. w CC |
| 198 | 07 | P | Cholecystectomy except by laparoscope w/o C.D.E. w/o CC |
| 199 | 07 | P | Hepatobiliary diagnostic procedure for malignancy |
| 200 | 07 | P | Hepatobiliary diagnostic procedure for non-malignancy |
| 201 | 07 | P | Other hepatobiliary or pancreas O.R. procedures |
| 202 | 07 | M | Cirrhosis & alcoholic hepatitis |
| 203 | 07 | M | Malignancy of hepatobiliary system or pancreas |
| 204 | 07 | M | Disorders of pancreas except malignancy |
| 205 | 07 | M | Disorders of liver except malig, cirr, alc hepa w CC |
| 206 | 07 | M | Disorders of liver except malig, cirr, alc hepa w/o CC |
| 207 | 07 | M | Disorders of the biliary tract w CC |
| 208 | 07 | M | Disorders of the biliary tract w/o CC |
| 209 | 08 | P | Major joint & limb reattachment procedures of lower extremity |
| 210 | 08 | P | Hip & femur procedures except major joint age >17 w CC |
| 211 | 08 | P | Hip & femur procedures except major joint age >17 w/o CC |
| 212 | 08 | P | *Hip & femur procedures except major joint age 0-17 |
| 213 | 08 | P | Amputation for musculoskeletal system & conn tissue disorders |
| 214 | 08 | P | No longer valid |
| 215 | 08 | P | No longer valid |
| 216 | 08 | P | Biopsies of musculoskeletal system & connective tissue |
| 217 | 08 | P | Wnd debrid & skn grft except hand, for muscskelet & conn tiss dis |
| 218 | 08 | P | Lower extrem & humer proc except hip, foot, femur age >17 w CC |
| 219 | 08 | P | Lower extrem & humer proc except hip, foot, femur age >17 w/o CC |
| 220 | 08 | P | *Lower extrem & humer proc except hip, foot, femur age 0-17 |
| 221 | 08 | P | No longer valid |
| 222 | 08 | P | No longer valid |
| 223 | 08 | P | Major shoulder/elbow proc, or other upper extremity proc w CC |
| 224 | 08 | P | Shoulder, elbow or forearm proc, exc major joint proc, w/o CC |

*Continued*

| DRG | MDC | Type | DRG title |
|-----|-----|------|-----------|
| 225 | 08 | P | Foot procedures |
| 226 | 08 | P | Soft tissue procedures w CC |
| 227 | 08 | P | Soft tissue procedures w/o CC |
| 228 | 08 | P | Major thumb or joint proc, or oth hand or wrist proc w CC |
| 229 | 08 | P | Hand or wrist proc, except major joint proc, w/o CC |
| 230 | 08 | P | Local excision & removal of int fix devices of hip & femur |
| 231 | 08 | P | Local excision & removal of int fix devices except hip & femur |
| 232 | 08 | P | Arthroscopy |
| 233 | 08 | P | Other musculoskelet sys & conn tiss O.R. proc w CC |
| 234 | 08 | P | Other musculoskelet sys & conn tiss O.R. proc w/o CC |
| 235 | 08 | M | Fractures of femur |
| 236 | 08 | M | Fractures of hip & pelvis |
| 237 | 08 | M | Sprains, strains, & dislocations of hip, pelvis & thigh |
| 238 | 08 | M | Osteomyelitis |
| 239 | 08 | M | Pathological fractures & musculoskeletal & conn tiss malignancy |
| 240 | 08 | M | Connective tissue disorders w CC |
| 241 | 08 | M | Connective tissue disorders w/o CC |
| 242 | 08 | M | Septic arthritis |
| 243 | 08 | M | Medical back problems |
| 244 | 08 | M | Bone diseases & specific arthropathies w CC |
| 245 | 08 | M | Bone diseases & specific arthropathies w/o CC |
| 246 | 08 | M | Non-specific arthropathies |
| 247 | 08 | M | Signs & symptoms of musculoskeletal system & conn tissue |
| 248 | 08 | M | Tendonitis, myositis & bursitis |
| 249 | 08 | M | Aftercare, musculoskeletal system & connective tissue |
| 250 | 08 | M | Fx, sprn, strn & disl of forearm, hand, foot age >17 w CC |
| 251 | 08 | M | Fx, sprn, strn & disl of forearm, hand, foot age >17 w/o CC |
| 252 | 08 | M | *Fx, sprn, strn & disl of forearm, hand, foot age 0-17 |
| 253 | 08 | M | Fx, sprn, strn & disl of uparm, lowleg ex foot age >17 w CC |
| 254 | 08 | M | Fx, sprn, strn & disl of uparm, lowleg ex foot age >17 w/o CC |
| 255 | 08 | M | *Fx, sprn, strn & disl of uparm, lowleg ex foot age 0-17 |
| 256 | 08 | M | Other musculoskeletal system & connective tissue diagnoses |
| 257 | 09 | P | Total mastectomy for malignancy w CC |
| 258 | 09 | P | Total mastectomy for malignancy w/o CC |
| 259 | 09 | P | Subtotal mastectomy for malignancy w CC |
| 260 | 09 | P | Subtotal mastectomy for malignancy w/o CC |
| 261 | 09 | P | Breast proc for non-malignancy except biopsy & local excision |
| 262 | 09 | P | Breast biopsy & local excision for non-malignancy |
| 263 | 09 | P | Skin graft &/or debrid for skn ulcer or cellulitis w CC |
| 264 | 09 | P | Skin graft &/or debrid for skn ulcer or cellulitis w/o CC |
| 265 | 09 | P | Skin graft &/or debrid except for skin ulcer or cellulitis w CC |
| 266 | 09 | P | Skin graft &/or debrid except for skin ulcer or cellulitis w/o CC |
| 267 | 09 | P | Perianal & pilonidal procedures |
| 268 | 09 | P | Skin, subcutaneous tissue & breast plastic procedures |
| 269 | 09 | P | Other skin, subcut tiss & breast proc w CC |
| 270 | 09 | P | Other skin, subcut tiss & breast proc w/o CC |
| 271 | 09 | M | Skin ulcers |
| 272 | 09 | M | Major skin disorders w CC |
| 273 | 09 | M | Major skin disorders w/o CC |
| 274 | 09 | M | Malignant breast disorders w CC |
| 275 | 09 | M | Malignant breast disorders w/o CC |
| 276 | 09 | M | Non-malignant breast disorders |
| 277 | 09 | M | Cellulitis age >17 w CC |
| 278 | 09 | M | Cellulitis age >17 w/o CC |
| 279 | 09 | M | *Cellulitis age 0-17 |
| 280 | 09 | M | Trauma to the skin, subcut tiss & breast age >17 w CC |
| 281 | 09 | M | Trauma to the skin, subcut tiss & breast age >17 w/o CC |
| 282 | 09 | M | *Trauma to the skin, subcut tiss & breast age 0-17 |
| 283 | 09 | M | Minor skin disorders w CC |
| 284 | 09 | M | Minor skin disorders w/o CC |
| 285 | 10 | P | Amputat of lower limb for endocrine, nutrit, & metabol disorders |
| 286 | 10 | P | Adrenal & pituitary procedures |
| 287 | 10 | P | Skin grafts & wound debrid for endoc, nutrit & metab disorders |
| 288 | 10 | P | O.R. procedures for obesity |
| 289 | 10 | P | Parathyroid procedures |
| 290 | 10 | P | Thyroid procedures |
| 291 | 10 | P | Thyroglossal procedures |

| DRG | MDC | Type | DRG title |
|-----|-----|------|-----------|
| 292 | 10 | P | Other endocrine, nutrit & metab O.R. proc w CC |
| 293 | 10 | P | Other endocrine, nutrit & metab O.R. proc w/o CC |
| 294 | 10 | M | Diabetes age >35 |
| 295 | 10 | M | Diabetes age 0-35 |
| 296 | 10 | M | Nutritional & misc metabolic disorders age >17 w CC |
| 297 | 10 | M | Nutritional & misc metabolic disorders age >17 w/o CC |
| 298 | 10 | M | Nutritional & misc metabolic disorders age 0-17 |
| 299 | 10 | M | Inborn errors of metabolism |
| 300 | 10 | M | Endocrine disorders w CC |
| 301 | 10 | M | Endocrine disorders w/o CC |
| 302 | 11 | P | Kidney transplant |
| 303 | 11 | P | Kidney, ureter & major bladder procedures for neoplasm |
| 304 | 11 | P | Kidney, ureter & major bladder procedures for non-neopl w CC |
| 305 | 11 | P | Kidney, ureter & major bladder procedures for non-neopl w/o CC |
| 306 | 11 | P | Prostatectomy w CC |
| 307 | 11 | P | Prostatectomy w/o CC |
| 308 | 11 | P | Minor bladder procedures w CC |
| 309 | 11 | P | Minor bladder procedures w/o CC |
| 310 | 11 | P | Transurethral procedures w CC |
| 311 | 11 | P | Transurethral procedures w/o CC |
| 312 | 11 | P | Urethral procedures, age >17 w CC |
| 313 | 11 | P | Urethral procedures, age >17 w/o CC |
| 314 | 11 | P | *Urethral procedures, age 0-17 |
| 315 | 11 | P | Other kidney & urinary tract O.R. procedures |
| 316 | 11 | M | Renal failure |
| 317 | 11 | M | Admit for renal dialysis |
| 318 | 11 | M | Kidney & urinary tract neoplasms w CC |
| 319 | 11 | M | Kidney & urinary tract neoplasms w/o CC |
| 320 | 11 | M | Kidney & urinary tract infections age >17 w CC |
| 321 | 11 | M | Kidney & urinary tract infections age >17 w/o CC |
| 322 | 11 | M | Kidney & urinary tract infections age 0-17 |
| 323 | 11 | M | Urinary stones w CC, &/or ESW lithotripsy |
| 324 | 11 | M | Urinary stones w/o CC |
| 325 | 11 | M | Kidney & urinary tract signs & symptoms age >17 w CC |
| 326 | 11 | M | Kidney & urinary tract signs & symptoms age >17 w/o CC |
| 327 | 11 | M | *Kidney & urinary tract signs & symptoms age 0-17 |
| 328 | 11 | M | Urethral stricture age >17 w CC |
| 329 | 11 | M | Urethral stricture age >17 w/o CC |
| 330 | 11 | M | *Urethral stricture age 0-17 |
| 331 | 11 | M | Other kidney & urinary tract diagnoses age >17 w CC |
| 332 | 11 | M | Other kidney & urinary tract diagnoses age >17 w/o CC |
| 333 | 11 | M | Other kidney & urinary tract diagnoses age 0-17 |
| 334 | 12 | P | Major male pelvic procedures w CC |
| 335 | 12 | P | Major male pelvic procedures w/o CC |
| 336 | 12 | P | Transurethral prostatectomy w CC |
| 337 | 12 | P | Transurethral prostatectomy w/o CC |
| 338 | 12 | P | Testes procedures, for malignancy |
| 339 | 12 | P | Testes procedures, non-malignancy age >17 |
| 340 | 12 | P | *Testes procedures, non-malignancy age 0-17 |
| 341 | 12 | P | Penis procedures |
| 342 | 12 | P | Circumcision age >17 |
| 343 | 12 | P | *Circumcision age 0-17 |
| 344 | 12 | P | Other male reproductive system O.R. procedures for malignancy |
| 345 | 12 | P | Other male reproductive system O.R. proc except for malignancy |
| 346 | 12 | M | Malignancy, male reproductive system, w CC |
| 347 | 12 | M | Malignancy, male reproductive system, w/o CC |
| 348 | 12 | M | Benign prostatic hypertrophy w CC |
| 349 | 12 | M | Benign prostatic hypertrophy w/o CC |
| 350 | 12 | M | Inflammation of the male reproductive system |
| 351 | 12 | M | *Sterilization, male |
| 352 | 12 | M | Other male reproductive system diagnoses |
| 353 | 13 | P | Pelvic evisceration, radical hysterectomy & radical vulvectomy |
| 354 | 13 | P | Uterine, adnexa proc for non-ovarian/adnexal malig w CC |
| 355 | 13 | P | Uterine, adnexa proc for non-ovarian/adnexal malig w/o CC |
| 356 | 13 | P | Female reproductive system reconstructive procedures |
| 357 | 13 | P | Uterine & adnexa proc for ovarian or adnexal malignancy |
| 358 | 13 | P | Uterine & adnexa proc for non-malignancy w CC |

*Continued*

| DRG | MDC | Type | DRG title |
|-----|-----|------|-----------|
| 359 | 13 | P | Uterine & adnexa proc for non-malignancy w/o CC |
| 360 | 13 | P | Vagina, cervix & vulva procedures |
| 361 | 13 | P | Laparoscopy & incisional tubal interruption |
| 362 | 13 | P | *Endoscopic tubal interruption |
| 363 | 13 | P | D&C, conization & radio-implant, for malignancy |
| 364 | 13 | P | D&C, conization except for malignancy |
| 365 | 13 | P | Other female reproductive system O.R. procedures |
| 366 | 13 | M | Malignancy, female reproductive system w CC |
| 367 | 13 | M | Malignancy, female reproductive system w/o CC |
| 368 | 13 | M | Infections, female reproductive system |
| 369 | 13 | M | Menstrual & other female reproductive system disorders |
| 370 | 14 | P | Cesarean section w CC |
| 371 | 14 | P | Cesarean section w/o CC |
| 372 | 14 | M | Vaginal delivery w complicating diagnoses |
| 373 | 14 | M | Vaginal delivery w/o complicating diagnoses |
| 374 | 14 | P | Vaginal delivery w sterilization &/or D&C |
| 375 | 14 | P | *Vaginal delivery w O.R. proc except steril &/or D&C |
| 376 | 14 | M | Postpartum & post abortion diagnoses w/o O.R. procedure |
| 377 | 14 | P | Postpartum & post abortion diagnoses w O.R. procedure |
| 378 | 14 | M | Ectopic pregnancy |
| 379 | 14 | M | Threatened abortion |
| 380 | 14 | M | Abortion w/o D&C |
| 381 | 14 | P | Abortion w D&C, aspiration curettage or hysterotomy |
| 382 | 14 | M | False labor |
| 383 | 14 | M | Other antepartum diagnoses w medical complications |
| 384 | 14 | M | Other antepartum diagnoses w/o medical complications |
| 385 | 15 | M | *Neonates, died or transferred to another acute care facility |
| 386 | 15 | M | *Extreme immaturity or respiratory distress syndrome, neonate |
| 387 | 15 | M | *Prematurity w major problems |
| 388 | 15 | M | *Prematurity w/o major problems |
| 389 | 15 | M | *Full term neonate w major problems |
| 390 | 15 | M | Neonate w other significant problems |
| 391 | 15 | M | *Normal newborn |
| 392 | 16 | P | Splenectomy age >17 |
| 393 | 16 | P | *Splenectomy age 0-17 |
| 394 | 16 | P | Other O.R. procedures of the blood and blood forming organs |
| 395 | 16 | M | Red blood cell disorders age >17 |
| 396 | 16 | M | Red blood cell disorders age 0-17 |
| 397 | 16 | M | Coagulation disorders |
| 398 | 16 | M | Reticuloendothelial & immunity disorders w CC |
| 399 | 16 | M | Reticuloendothelial & immunity disorders w/o CC |
| 400 | 17 | P | Lymphoma & leukemia w major O.R. procedure |
| 401 | 17 | P | Lymphoma & non-acute leukemia w other O.R. proc w CC |
| 402 | 17 | P | Lymphoma & non-acute leukemia w other O.R. proc w/o CC |
| 403 | 17 | M | Lymphoma & non-acute leukemia w CC |
| 404 | 17 | M | Lymphoma & non-acute leukemia w/o CC |
| 405 | 17 | M | *Acute leukemia w/o major O.R. procedure age 0-17 |
| 406 | 17 | P | Myeloprolif disord or poorly diff neopl w maj O.R. proc w CC |
| 407 | 17 | P | Myeloprolif disord or poorly diff neopl w maj O.R. proc w/o CC |
| 408 | 17 | P | Myeloprolif disord or poorly diff neopl w other O.R. proc |
| 409 | 17 | M | Radiotherapy |
| 410 | 17 | M | Chemotherapy w/o acute leukemia as secondary diagnosis |
| 411 | 17 | M | History of malignancy w/o endoscopy |
| 412 | 17 | M | History of malignancy w endoscopy |
| 413 | 17 | M | Other myeloprolif dis or poorly diff neopl diag w CC |
| 414 | 17 | M | Other myeloprolif dis or poorly diff neopl diag w/o CC |
| 415 | 18 | P | O.R. procedure for infectious & parasitic diseases |
| 416 | 18 | M | Septicemia age >17 |
| 417 | 18 | M | Septicemia age 0-17 |
| 418 | 18 | M | Postoperative & post-traumatic infections |
| 419 | 18 | M | Fever of unknown origin age >17 w CC |
| 420 | 18 | M | Fever of unknown origin age >17 w/o CC |
| 421 | 18 | M | Viral illness age >17 |
| 422 | 18 | M | Viral illness & fever of unknown origin age 0-17 |
| 423 | 18 | M | Other infectious & parasitic diseases diagnoses |
| 424 | 19 | P | O.R. procedure w principal diagnoses of mental illness |
| 425 | 19 | M | Acute adjustment reaction & psychological dysfunction |

| DRG | MDC | Type | DRG title |
|-----|-----|------|-----------|
| 426 | 19 | M | Depressive neuroses |
| 427 | 19 | M | Neuroses except depressive |
| 428 | 19 | M | Disorders of personality & impulse control |
| 429 | 19 | M | Organic disturbances & mental retardation |
| 430 | 19 | M | Psychoses |
| 431 | 19 | M | Childhood mental disorders |
| 432 | 19 | M | Other mental disorder diagnoses |
| 433 | 20 | M | Alcohol/drug abuse or dependence, left AMA |
| 434 | 20 | M | Alc/drug abuse or depend, detox or oth sympt treat w CC |
| 435 | 20 | M | Alc/drug abuse or depend, detox or oth sympt treat w/o CC |
| 436 | 20 | M | Alc/drug dependence w rehabilitation therapy |
| 437 | 20 | M | Alc/drug dependence, combined rehab & detox therapy |
| 438 | 20 | | No longer valid |
| 439 | 21 | P | Skin grafts for injuries |
| 440 | 21 | P | Wound debridements for injuries |
| 441 | 21 | P | Hand procedures for injuries |
| 442 | 21 | P | Other O.R. procedures for injuries w CC |
| 443 | 21 | P | Other O.R. procedures for injuries w/o CC |
| 444 | 21 | M | Traumatic injury age >17 w CC |
| 445 | 21 | M | Traumatic injury age >17 w/o CC |
| 446 | 21 | M | *Traumatic injury age 0-17 |
| 447 | 21 | M | Allergic reactions age >17 |
| 448 | 21 | M | *Allergic reactions age 0-17 |
| 449 | 21 | M | Poisoning & toxic effects of drugs age >17 w CC |
| 450 | 21 | M | Poisoning & toxic effects of drugs age >17 w/o CC |
| 451 | 21 | M | *Poisoning & toxic effects of drugs age 0-17 |
| 452 | 21 | M | Complications of treatment w CC |
| 453 | 21 | M | Complications of treatment w/o CC |
| 454 | 21 | M | Other injury, poisoning & toxic effect diag w CC |
| 455 | 21 | M | Other injury, poisoning & toxic effect diag w/o CC |
| 456 | | | No longer valid |
| 457 | | | No longer valid |
| 458 | | | No longer valid |
| 459 | | | No longer valid |
| 460 | | | No longer valid |
| 461 | 23 | P | O.R. proc w diagnoses of other contact w health services |
| 462 | 23 | M | Rehabilitation |
| 463 | 23 | M | Signs & symptoms w CC |
| 464 | 23 | M | Signs & symptoms w/o CC |
| 465 | 23 | M | Aftercare w history of malignancy as secondary diagnosis |
| 466 | 23 | M | Aftercare w/o history of malignancy as secondary diagnosis |
| 467 | 23 | M | Other factors influencing health status |
| 468 | | M | Extensive O.R. procedure unrelated to principal diagnosis |
| 469 | | | **Principal diagnosis invalid as discharge diagnosis |
| 470 | | | **Ungroupable |
| 471 | 08 | P | Bilateral or multiple major joint procs of lower extremity |
| 472 | | | No longer valid |
| 473 | 17 | P | Acute leukemia w/o major O.R. procedure age >17 |
| 474 | | | No longer valid |
| 475 | 04 | M | Respiratory system diagnosis with ventilator support |
| 476 | | P | Prostatic O.R. procedure unrelated to principal diagnosis |
| 477 | | P | Non-extensive O.R. procedure unrelated to principal diagnosis |
| 478 | 05 | P | Other vascular procedures w CC |
| 479 | 05 | P | Other vascular procedures w/o CC |
| 480 | PRE | P | Liver transplant |
| 481 | PRE | P | Bone marrow transplant |
| 482 | PRE | P | Tracheostomy for face, mouth & neck diagnoses |
| 483 | PRE | P | Tracheostomy except for face, mouth & neck diagnoses |
| 484 | 24 | P | Craniotomy for multiple significant trauma |
| 485 | 24 | P | Limb reattachment, hip and femur proc for multiple significant tra |
| 486 | 24 | P | Other O.R. procedures for multiple significant trauma |
| 487 | 24 | M | Other multiple significant trauma |
| 488 | 25 | P | HIV w extensive O.R. procedure |
| 489 | 25 | M | HIV w major related condition |
| 490 | 25 | M | HIV w or w/o other related condition |
| 491 | 08 | P | Major joint & limb reattachment procedures of upper extremity |
| 492 | 17 | M | Chemotherapy w acute leukemia as secondary diagnosis |

*Continued*

| DRG | MDC | Type | DRG title |
|-----|-----|------|-----------|
| 493 | 07 | P | Laparoscopic cholecystectomy w/o C.D.E. w CC |
| 494 | 07 | P | Laparoscopic cholecystectomy w/o C.D.E. w/o CC |
| 495 | PRE | P | Lung transplant |
| 496 | 08 | P | Combined anterior/posterior spinal fusion |
| 497 | 08 | P | Spinal fusion w CC |
| 498 | 08 | P | Spinal fusion w/o CC |
| 499 | 08 | P | Back & neck procedures except spinal fusion w CC |
| 500 | 08 | P | Back & neck procedures except spinal fusion w/o CC |
| 501 | 08 | P | Knee procedures w PDX of infection w CC |
| 502 | 08 | P | Knee procedures w PDX of infection w/o CC |
| 503 | 08 | P | Knee procedures w/o PDX of infection |
| 504 | 22 | P | Extensive 3rd degree burns w skin graft |
| 505 | 22 | M | Extensive 3rd degree burns w/o skin graft |
| 506 | 22 | P | Full thickness burn w skin graft or inhal inj w CC or sig trauma |
| 507 | 22 | P | Full thickness burn w skin graft or inhal inj w/o CC or sig trauma |
| 508 | 22 | M | Full thickness burn w/o skin graft or inhal inj w CC or sig trauma |
| 509 | 22 | M | Full thickness burn w/o skin graft or inhal inj w/o CC or sig trauma |
| 510 | 22 | M | Non-extensive burns w CC or significant trauma |
| 511 | 22 | M | Non-extensive burns w/o CC or significant trauma |

# NURSING DIAGNOSES

For new and revised NANDA-approved definitions in 2003-2004, see Appendix 21.

## 17-1 NANDA-approved nursing diagnoses and definitions

### ACTIVITY INTOLERANCE

Insufficient physiological or psychological energy to endure or complete required or desired daily activities.

**Related factors**

Generalized weakness
Sedentary lifestyle
Imbalance between oxygen supply and demand
Bed rest or immobility

**Defining characteristics**

Verbal report of fatigue or weakness
Abnormal heart rate or blood pressure response to activity
Exertional discomfort or dyspnea
Electrocardiographic changes reflecting arrhythmias or ischemia

### ACTIVITY INTOLERANCE, RISK FOR

At risk of experiencing insufficient physiological or psychological energy to endure or complete required or desired daily activities.

**Risk factors**

History of previous intolerance
Deconditioned status
Presence of circulatory/respiratory problems
Inexperience with the activity

### ADAPTIVE CAPACITY, DECREASED INTRACRANIAL

Intracranial fluid dynamic mechanisms that normally compensate for increases in intracranial volumes are compromised, resulting in repeated disproportionate increases in intracranial pressure (ICP) in response to a variety of noxious and non-noxious stimuli.

**Defining characteristics**

Repeated increases in ICP > 10 mm Hg for more than 5 minutes following any of a variety of external stimuli.
Disproportionate increase in ICP following single environmental of nursing maneuver stimulus
Elevated P2 ICP waveform
Volume pressure response test variation (volume-pressure ratio >2, Pressure-volume index <10)
Baseline ICP ≥ 10 mm Hg
Wide amplitude ICP waveform

**Related factors**

Brain injuries
Sustained increase in ICP ≥ 10-15 mm Hg
Decreased cerebral perfusion pressure ≤ 50-60 mm Hg
Systemic hypotension with intracranial hypertension

### ADJUSTMENT, IMPAIRED

Inability to modify lifestyle/behavior in a manner consistent with a change in health status

**Defining characteristics**

Denial of health status change
Failure to achieve optimal sense of control
Failure to take actions that would prevent further health problems
Demonstration of non-acceptance of health status change

**Related factors**

Low state of optimism
Intense emotional state
Negative attitudes toward health behavior
Absence of intent to change behavior
Multiple stressors
Absence of social support for changed beliefs and practices
Disability or health status change requiring change in life style
Lack of motivation to change behaviors

### AIRWAY CLEARANCE, INEFFECTIVE

Inability to clear secretions or obstructions from the respiratory tract to maintain a clear airway

**Defining characteristics**

Dyspnea
Diminished breath sounds
Orthopnea
Adventitious breath sounds (rales, crackles, rhonchi, wheezes)
Cough, ineffective or absent
Sputum
Cyanosis
Difficulty vocalizing
Wide-eyed
Changes in respiratory rate and rhythm
Restlessness

**Related factors**
*Individual*

Smoking
Smoke inhalation
Second-hand smoke

*Obstructed airway*

Airway spasm
Retained secretions
Excessive mucus
Presence of artificial airway
Foreign body in airway
Secretions in the bronchi
Exudate in the alveoli

*Physiological*

Neuromuscular dysfunction
Hyperplasia of the bronchial walls
Chronic obstructive pulmonary disease
Infection
Asthma
Allergic airways

### ANXIETY

Vague uneasy feeling of discomfort or dread accompanied by an autonomic response (the source often non-specific or unknown to the individual); a feeling of apprehension caused by anticipation of danger. It is an alerting signal that warns of impending danger and enables the individual to take measures to deal with threat.

**Defining characteristics**
*Behavioral*

Diminished productivity
Scanning and vigilance
Poor eye contact
Restlessness
Glancing about
Extraneous movement (e.g., foot shuffling, hand/arm movements)
Expressed concerns due to change in life events
Insomnia
Fidgeting

*Affective*

Regretful
Irritability
Anguish
Scared
Jittery
Overexcited
Painful and persistent increased helplessness
Rattled
Uncertainty
Increased wariness
Focus on self
Feelings of inadequacy
Fearful
Distressed
Worried, apprehensive
Anxious

*Physiological*

Voice quivering
Trembling/hand tremors
Shakiness
Increased respiration (sympathetic)
Urinary urgency (parasympathetic)
Increased pulse (sympathetic)
Pupil dilation (sympathetic)
Increased reflexes (sympathetic)
Abdominal pain (parasympathetic)
Sleep disturbance (parasympathetic)
Tingling in extremities (parasympathetic)
Cardiovascular excitation (sympathetic)
Increased perspiration
Facial tension
Anorexia (sympathetic)
Heart pounding (parasympathetic)
Diarrhea (parasympathetic)
Urinary hesitancy (parasympathetic)
Fatigue (parasympathetic)
Dry mouth (sympathetic)
Weakness (sympathetic)
Decreased pulse pressure (parasympathetic)
Nausea (parasympathetic)
Urinary frequency (parasympathetic)
Faintness (parasympathetic)
Respiratory difficulties (sympathetic)
Increased blood pressure (sympathetic)

*Cognitive*

Blocking of thought
Confusion
Preoccupation
Forgetfulness
Rumination
Impaired attention
Decreased perceptual field
Fear of unspecified consequences
Tendency to blame others
Difficulty concentrating

Diminished ability to problem solve, learn
Awareness of physiological symptoms

**Related factors**

Exposure to toxins
Unconscious conflict about essential values/goals of life
Familial association/heredity
Unmet needs
Interpersonal transmission/contagion
Situational/maturational crises
Threat of death
Threat to self-concept
Stress
Substance abuse
Threat to or change in role status, health status, interaction patterns, role function, environment, economic status

**ASPIRATION, RISK FOR**

At risk for entry of gastric secretions, oropharyngeal secretions, or exogenous food or fluids into tracheobronchial passages.

**Risk factors**

Reduced level of consciousness
Depressed cough and gag reflexes
Presence of tracheotomy or endotracheal tube
Overinflated tracheotomy/endotracheal tube cuff
Inadequate tracheotomy/endotracheal tube cuff inflation
Gastrointestinal tubes
Bolus tube feedings/medication administration
Situations hindering elevation of upper body
Increased intragastric pressure
Increased gastric residual
Decreased gastrointestinal motility
Delayed gastric emptying
Impaired swallowing
Facial/oral/neck surgery or trauma
Wired jaws

**BODY TEMPERATURE, IMBALANCED, RISK FOR**

At risk for failure to maintain body temperature within normal range.

**Risk factors**

Extremes of age
Extremes of weight
Exposure to cold/cool or warm/hot environments
Dehydration
Inactivity or vigorous activity
Medications causing vasoconstriction/vasodilation, altered metabolic rate, sedation
Inappropriate clothing for environmental temperature
Illness or trauma affecting temperature regulation

**BODY IMAGE, DISTURBED**

Confusion in mental picture of one's physical self

**Defining characteristics**

Verbalization of feelings that reflect an altered view of one's body in appearance, structure, or function
Verbalization of perceptions that reflect an altered view of one's body in appearance, structure, or function
Nonverbal response to actual or perceived change in body structure and/or function
Behaviors of avoidance, monitoring, or acknowledgment of one's body

*Objective*

Missing body part
Trauma to nonfunctioning part
Not touching body part

Hiding or overexposing body part (intentional or unintentional)
Actual change in structure and/or function
Change in social involvement
Change in ability to estimate spatial relationship of body to environment
Extension of body boundary to incorporate environmental objects
Not looking at body part

*Subjective*

Refusal to verify actual change
Preoccupation with change or loss
Personalization of part or loss by name
Depersonalization of part or loss by impersonal pronouns
Extension of body boundary to incorporate environmental objects
Negative feelings about body (e.g., feelings of helplessness, hopelessness, or powerlessness)
Verbalization of change in lifestyle
Focus on past strength, function, or appearance
Fear of rejection or of reaction by others
Emphasis on remaining strengths
Heightened achievement

## Related factors

Psychosocial
Biophysical
Cognitive/perceptual
Cultural or spiritual
Developmental changes
Illness
Trauma or injury
Surgery
Illness treatment

## BREASTFEEDING, EFFECTIVE

Mother-infant dyad/family exhibits adequate proficiency and satisfaction with breastfeeding process

## Defining characteristics

Effective mother/infant communication patterns
Regular and sustained suckling/swallowing at the breast
Appropriate infant weight pattern for age
Infant content after feeding
Mother able to position infant at breast to promote a successful latch-on response
Signs and/or symptoms of oxytocin release
Adequate infant elimination patterns for age
Eagerness of infant to nurse
Maternal verbalization of satisfaction with the breastfeeding process

## Related factors

Infant gestational age >34 weeks
Support source
Normal infant oral structure
Maternal confidence
Basic breastfeeding knowledge
Normal breast structure

## BREASTFEEDING, INEFFECTIVE

Dissatisfaction of difficulty a mother, infant, or child experiences with the breastfeeding process

## Defining characteristics

Unsatisfactory breastfeeding process
Nonsustained suckling at the breast
Resisting latching on
Unresponsive to comfort measures
Persistence of sore nipples beyond first week of breastfeeding
Observable signs of inadequate infant intake
Insufficient emptying of each breast per feeding
Infant inability to attach on to maternal breast correctly

Infant arching and crying at the breast
Infant exhibiting fussiness and crying within the first hour after breastfeeding
Actual or perceived inadequate milk supply
No observable signs of oxytocin release
Insufficient opportunity for suckling at the breast

## Related factors

Nonsupportive partner/family
Previous breast surgery
Infant receiving supplemental feedings with artificial nipple
Prematurity
Previous history of breastfeeding failure
Poor infant sucking reflex
Maternal breast anomaly
Maternal anxiety or ambivalence
Interruption in breastfeeding
Infant anomaly
Knowledge deficit

## BREASTFEEDING, INTERRUPTED

Break in the continuity of the breastfeeding process as a result of inability or inadvisability to put baby to breast for feeding

## Defining characteristics

Infant receives no nourishment at the breast for some or all of feedings
Maternal desire to maintain and provide (or eventually provide) her breast for milk for her infant's nutritional needs
Lack of knowledge regarding expression and storage of breast milk
Separation of mother and infant

## Related factors

Contraindications to breastfeeding
Maternal employment
Maternal or infant illness
Need to abruptly wean infant
Prematurity

## BREATHING PATTERN, INEFFECTIVE

Inspiration and/or expiration that does not provide adequate ventilation

## Defining characteristics

Decreased inspiratory/expiratory pressure
Decreased minute ventilation
Use of accessory muscles to breathe
Nasal flaring
Dyspnea
Altered chest excursion
Shortness of breath
Assumption of 3-point position
Pursed lip breathing
Prolonged expiration phases
Increased anterior-posterior diameter
Respiratory rate/min: infants: <25 or 60; ages 1-4: <20 or <30; ages 5-14: <14 or 25; adults >14: <12 or >24
Depth of breathing: adult tidal volume: 500 ml at rest; infant tidal volume: 6-8 ml/Kg
Timing ratio
Orthopnea
Decreased vital capacity

## Related factors

Hyperventilation
Hypoventilation syndrome
Bony deformity
Pain
Chest wall deformity
Anxiety

Decreased energy/fatigue
Neuromuscular dysfunction
Musculoskeletal impairment
Perception/cognitive impairment
Obesity
Spinal cord injury
Body position
Neurological immaturity
Respiratory muscle fatigue

## CARDIAC OUTPUT, DECREASED

Inadequate blood pumped by the heart to meet metabolic demands of the body

### Defining characteristics
#### Altered heart rate/rhythm

Arrhythmias (tachycardia, bradycardia)
Palpitations
EKG changes

#### Altered preload

Jugular vein distention
Fatigue
Edema
Murmurs
Increased/decreased central venous pressure (CVP)
Increased/decreased pulmonary artery wedge pressure (PAWP)
Weight gain

#### Altered afterload

Cold/clammy skin
Shortness of breath/dyspnea
Oliguria
Prolonged capillary refill
Decreased peripheral pulses
Variations in blood pressure readings
Increased/decreased systemic vascular resistance (SVR)
Increased/decreased pulmonary vascular restaurants (PVR)
Skin color changes

#### Altered contractility

Crackles
Cough
Orthopnea/paroxysmal nocturnal dyspnea
Cardiac output <4 L/min
Cardiac index <2.5 L/min
Decreased ejection fraction, Stroke Volume Index (SVI), Left Ventricular Stroke Work Index (LVSWI)

#### Behavioral/emotional

Anxiety
Restlessness

### Related factors

Altered heart rate/rhythm

#### Altered stroke volume

Altered preload
Altered afterload
Altered contractility

## CAREGIVER ROLE STRAIN

Difficulty in performing caregiver role

### Defining characteristics
#### Caregiver activities

Difficulty performing/completing required tasks
Preoccupation with care routine
Apprehension about the future regarding care receiver's health and the caregiver's ability to provide care

Apprehension about care receiver's care if caregiver becomes ill or dies
Dysfunctional change in caregiving activities
Apprehension about possible institutionalization of care receiver

#### Caregiver health status
PHYSICAL

GI upset (e.g., mild stomach cramps, vomiting, diarrhea, recurrent gastric ulcer episodes)
Weight change
Rash
Hypertension
Cardiovascular disease
Diabetes
Fatigue
Headaches

EMOTIONAL

Impaired individual coping
Feeling depressed
Disturbed sleep
Anger
Stress
Somatization
Increased nervousness
Increased emotional lability
Impatience
Lack of time to meet personal needs
Frustration

SOCIOECONOMIC

Withdraws from social life
Changes in leisure activities
Low work productivity
Refuses career advancement

#### Caregiver-care receiver relationship

Grief/uncertainty regarding changed relationship with care receiver
Difficulty watching care receiver go through illness

#### Family processes

Family conflict
Concerns about family members

### Related factors
#### Care receiver health status

Illness severity
Illness chronicity
Increasing care needs/dependency
Unpredictability of illness course
Instability of care receiver's health
Problem behaviors
Psychological or cognitive problems
Addiction or codependency

#### Caregiving activities

Amount of activities
Complexities of activities
24-hour care responsibilities
Ongoing changes in activities
Discharge of family members to home with significant care needs
Years of caregiving
Unpredictability of care situation

#### Caregiver health status

Physical problems
Psychological or cognitive problems
Addiction or codependency
Marginal coping patterns

Unrealistic expectations of self
Inability to fulfill one's own or other's expectations

*Socioeconomic*

Isolation from others
Competing role commitments
Alienation from family, friends, and co-workers
Insufficient recreation

*Caregiver-care receiver relationship*

History of poor relationship
Presence of abuse or violence
Unrealistic expectations of caregiver by care receiver
Mental status of elder inhibiting conversation

*Family processes*

History of marginal family coping
History of family dysfunction

*Resources*

Inadequate physical environment for providing care (e.g., housing, temperature, safety)
Inadequate equipment for providing care
Inadequate transportation
Inadequate community resources (e.g., respite services, recreational resources)
Insufficient finances
Lack of support
Caregiver is not developmentally ready for caregiver role
Inexperienced with caregiving
Insufficient time
Lack of knowledge about or difficulty accessing community resources
Lack of caregiver privacy
Emotional strength
Physical energy
Assistance and support (formal and informal)

## CAREGIVER ROLE STRAIN, RISK FOR

Caregiver is vulnerable for felt difficulty in performing the family caregiver role

### Risk factors

Caregiver not developmentally ready for caregiver role (e.g., a young adult needing to provide care for middle aged)
Inadequate physical environment for providing care (e.g., housing, transportation, community services, equipment)
Unpredictable illness course or instability in the care receiver's health
Psychological or cognitive problems in care receiver
Presence of situational stressors that normally affect families (e.g., significant loss, disaster or crisis, economic vulnerability, major life events)
Presence of abuse or violence
Premature birth/congenital defect
Past history of poor relationship between caregiver and care receiver
Marginal family adaptation or dysfunction prior to caregiving situation
Marginal caregiver's coping patterns
Lack of respite and recreation for caregiver
Inexperience with caregiving
Caregiver is female
Addiction or codependency
Care receiver exhibits deviant, bizarre behavior
Caregiver's competing role commitments
Caregiver health impairment
Illness severity of the care receiver
Caregiver is spouse
Developmental delay or retardation of the care receiver or caregiver
Complexity/amount of caregiving tasks

Discharge of family member with significant home care needs
Duration of caregiving required
Family/caregiver isolation

## COMMUNICATION, IMPAIRED VERBAL

Decreased, delayed, or absent ability to receive, process, transmit, and use a system of symbols

### Defining characteristics

Willful refusal to speak
Disorientation in the three spheres of time, space, person
Inability to speak dominant language
Does not or cannot speak
Speaks or verbalizes with difficulty
Inappropriate verbalization
Difficulty forming words or sentences (e.g., aphonia, dyslalia, dysarthria)
Difficulty expressing thought verbally (e.g., aphasia, dysphasia, apraxia, dyslexia)
Stuttering
Slurring
Dyspnea
Absence of eye contact of difficulty in selective attending
Difficulty in comprehending and maintaining usual communication pattern
Partial or total visual deficit
Inability or difficulty in use of facial or body expressions

### Related factors

Decrease in circulation to brain
Cultural difference
Psychological barriers (e.g., psychosis, lack of stimuli)
Physical barriers (tracheostomy, intubation)
Anatomical defect (e.g., cleft palate, alteration of neuromuscular visual system, phonatory apparatus)
Brain tumor
Differences related to developmental age
Side effects of medication
Environmental barriers
Absence of significant others
Altered perceptions
Lack of information
Stress
Alteration of self-esteem or self-concept
Physiological conditions
Alterations of central nervous system
Weakening of the musculoskeletal system
Emotional conditions

## COMMUNITY COPING, INEFFECTIVE

A pattern of community activities for adaptation and problem solving that is unsatisfactory for meeting the demands or needs of the community

### Defining characteristics

Expressed community powerlessness
Deficits of community participation
Excessive community conflicts
Expressed vulnerability
High illness rates
Stressors perceived as excessive
Community does not meet its own expectations
Increased social problems (e.g., homicides, vandalism, arson, terrorism, robbery, infanticide, abuse, divorce, unemployment, poverty, militancy, mental illness)

### Related factors

Natural or man-made disasters
Ineffective or non-existent community systems (e.g., lack of emergency medical system, transportation system, or disaster planning systems)

Deficits in community social support services and resources
Inadequate resources for problem solving

## COMMUNITY COPING, READINESS FOR ENHANCED

Pattern of community activities for adaptation and problem solving that is satisfactory for meeting the demands or needs of the community but can be improved for management of current and future problems/stressors

### Defining characteristics

One or more characteristics that indicate effective coping:
Active planning by community for predicted stressors
Active problem solving by community when faced with issues
Agreement that community is responsible for stress management
Positive communication among community members
Positive communication between community/aggregates and larger community
Programs available for recreation and relaxation
Resources sufficient for managing stressors

### Related factors

Social supports available
Resources available for problem solving
Community has a sense of power to manage stressors

## CONFUSION, ACUTE

Abrupt onset of a cluster of global, transient changes and disturbances in attention, cognition, psychomotor activity level of consciousness, and/or sleep/wake cycle.

### Defining characteristics

Fluctuation in cognition
Fluctuation in sleep-wake cycle
Fluctuation in level of consciousness
Fluctuation in psychomotor activity
Increased agitation or restlessness
Misperceptions
Lack of motivation to initiate or follow through with goal-directed or purposeful behavior
Hallucinations

### Related factors

Over 60 years of age
Dementia
Alcohol abuse
Drug abuse
Delirium

## CONFUSION, CHRONIC

Irreversible, long-standing and/or progressive deterioration of intellect and personality characterized by decreased ability to interpret environmental stimuli, decreased capacity for intellectual thought processes and manifested by disturbances of memory, orientation, and behavior.

### Defining characteristics

Clinical evidence of organic impairment
Altered interpretation of or response to stimuli
Progressive or long-standing cognitive impairment
No change in level of consciousness
Impaired socialization
Impaired memory (short term, long term)
Altered personality

### Related factors

Alzheimer's disease
Korsakoff's psychosis
Multi-infarct dementia
Cerebrovascular accident
Head injury

## CONSTIPATION

Decrease in normal frequency of defecation accompanied by difficult or incomplete passage of stool and/or passage of excessively hard, dry stool

### Defining characteristics

Change in bowel pattern
Bright red blood with stool
Presence of soft paste-like stool in rectum
Distended abdomen
Bark or black or tarry stool
Increased abdominal pressure
Percussed abdominal dullness
Pain with defecation
Decreased volume of stool
Straining with defecation
Decreased frequency
Dry, hard, formed stool
Palpable rectal mass
Feeling of rectal fullness or pressure
Abdominal pain
Unable to pass stool
Anorexia
Headache
Change in abdominal growling (borborygmi)
Indigestion
Atypical presentations in older adults (e.g., change in mental status, urinary incontinence, unexplained falls, elevated body temperature)
Severe flatus
Generalized fatigue
Hypoactive or hyperactive bowel sounds
Palpable abdominal mass
Abdominal tenderness with or without palpable muscle resistance
Nausea and/or vomiting
Oozing liquid stool

### Related factors

*Functional*

Recent environment changes
Habitual denial/ignoring of urge to defecate
Insufficient physical activity
Irregular defecation habits
Inadequate toileting (e.g., timeliness, positioning for defecation, privacy)
Abdominal muscle weakness

*Psychological*

Depression
Emotional stress
Mental confusion

*Pharmacological*

Antilipemic agents
Laxative overdose
Calcium carbonate
Aluminum-containing antacids
Nonsteriodal anti-flammatory agents
Opiates
Anticholinergics
Diuretics
Iron salts
Phenothiazides
Sedatives
Sympathomimetics
Bismuth salts
Antidepressants
Calcium channel blockers

### Mechanical

Rectal abscess or ulcer
Pregnancy
Rectal anal fissures
Tumors
Megacolon (Hirschsprung's disease)
Electrolyte imbalance
Rectal prolapse
Prostate enlargement
Neurological impairment
Rectal anal stricture
Rectocele
Postsurgical obstruction
Hemorrhoids
Obesity

### Physiological

Poor eating habits
Decreased motility of gastrointestinal tract
Inadequate dentition or oral hygiene
Insufficient fiber intake
Insufficient fluid intake
Change in usual foods and eating patterns
Dehydration

## CONSTIPATION, PERCEIVED

Self-diagnosis of constipation and abuse of laxatives, enemas, and suppositories, to ensure a daily bowel movement.

### Defining characteristics

Expectation of a daily bowel movement with resulting overuse of
    laxatives, enemas, and suppositories
Expected passage of stool at same time every day

### Related factors

Cultural/family health beliefs
Faulty appraisal
Impaired thought processes

## COPING, DEFENSIVE

Reported projection of falsely positive self-evaluation based on a self-protective pattern that defends against underlying perceived threats to positive self-regard.

### Defining characteristics

Denial (of obvious problems, weaknesses)
Projection (of blame/responsibility)
Rationalization of failures
Defensiveness (hypersensitivity to criticism)
Grandiosity
Superior attitude toward others
Difficulty establishing/maintaining relationships
Hostile laughter or ridicule of others
Difficulty in reality testing of perceptions
Lack of follow-through or participation in treatment or therapy

### Related factors

To be developed

## CONSTIPATION, RISK FOR

At risk for a decrease in a person's normal frequency of defecation accompanied by difficult or incomplete passage of stool and/or passage of excessively hard, dry stool

### Risk factors

### Functional

Habitual denial/ignorance of urge to defecate
Recent environmental changes
Inadequate toileting (e.g., timeliness, positioning for defecation, privacy)

Irregular defecation habits
Insufficient physical activity
Abdominal muscle weakness

### Psychological

Emotional stress
Mental confusion
Depression

### Physiological

Insufficient fiber intake
Dehydration
Inadequate dentition or oral hygiene
Poor eating habits
Insufficient fluid intake
Change in usual foods and eating patterns
Decreased motility of gastrointestinal tract

### Pharmacological

Phenothiazides
Nonsteroidal anti-inflammatory agents
Sedatives
Aluminum-containing antacids
Laxative overuse
Iron salts
Anticholinergics
Antidepressants
Anticonvulsants
Antilipemic agents
Calcium channel blockers
Calcium carbonate
Diuretics
Sympathomimetics
Opiates
Bismuth salts

### Mechanical

Rectal abscess or ulcer
Pregnancy
Rectal anal stricture
Postsurgical obstruction
Rectal anal fissures
Megacolon (Hirschsprung's disease)
Electrolyte imbalance
Tumors
Prostate enlargement
Rectocele
Rectal prolapse
Neurological impairment
Hemorrhoids
Obesity

## COPING, FAMILY, READINESS FOR ENHANCED

Effective managing of adaptive tasks by family member involved with the patient's health challenge, who now is exhibiting desire and readiness for enhanced health and growth in regard to self and in relation to the patient

### Defining characteristics

Family members attempt to describe growth impact of crisis on their
    own values, priorities, goals, or relationships
Family member is moving in direction of health-promoting and enriching lifestyle that supports and monitors maturational processes, audits and negotiates treatment programs, and generally chooses experiences that optimize wellness
Individual expresses interest in making contact on a one-to-one basis or on a mutual-aid group basis with another person who has experienced a similar situation

## Related factors

Needs sufficiently gratified and adaptive tasks effectively addressed to enable goals of self-actualization to surface

## COPING, FAMILY, COMPROMISED

Usually supportive primary person (family member or close friend) provides insufficient, ineffective, or compromised support, comfort, assistance, or encouragement which may be needed by the client to manage or master adaptive tasks related to his or her health challenge

### Defining characteristics
#### Subjective

Client expresses or confirms a concern or complaint about significant other's response to his or her health problem

Significant person describes preoccupation with personal reaction (e.g., fear, anticipatory grief, guilt, anxiety to illness, disability, or to other situational or developmental crises)

Significant person describes or confirms an inadequate understanding or knowledge base that interferes with effective assistive or supportive behaviors

#### Objective

Significant person attempts assistive or supportive behaviors with less than satisfactory results

Significant person withdraws or enters into limited or temporary personal communication with the client at the time of need

Significant person displays protective behavior disproportionate (too little or too much) to the abilities or need for autonomy

### Related factors

Inadequate or incorrect information or understanding by a primary person

Temporary preoccupation by a significant person who is trying to manage emotional conflicts and personal suffering and is unable to perceive or act effectively in regard to needs

Temporary family disorganization and role changes

Other situational or developmental crises or situations the significant person may be facing

Little support provided by client, in turn, for primary person

Prolonged disease or disability progression that exhausts supportive capacity of significant people

## COPING, FAMILY, DISABLED

Behavior of significant person (family member or other primary person) that disables his or her own capacities and the capacity to effectively address tasks essential to either person's adaptation to the health challenge

### Defining characteristics

Neglectful care of the patient in regard to basic human needs and/or illness treatment

Distortion of reality regarding the health problem, including extreme denial about its existence or severity

Intolerance

Rejection

Abandonment

Desertion

Carrying on usual routines, disregarding client's needs

Psychosomaticism

Taking on illness signs of client

Decisions and actions by family that are detrimental to economic or social well-being

Agitation, depression, aggression, hostility

Impaired restructuring of a meaningful life for self

Impaired individualization, prolonged over concern for patient

Neglectful relationships with other family members

Client's development of helpless, inactive dependence

## Related factors

Significant person with chronically unexpressed feelings of guilt, anxiety, hostility, despair, etc.

Dissonant discrepant coping styles for dealing with adaptive tasks by the significant person and patient or among significant people

Highly ambivalent family relationships

Arbitrary handling of family's resistance to treatment, which tends to solidify defensiveness, as it fails to deal adequately with underlying anxiety

## COPING, INEFFECTIVE

Inability to form a valid appraisal of the stressors, inadequate choices of practiced responses, and/or inability to use available resources

### Defining characteristics

Lack of goal-directed behavior/resolution of problem including: inability to attend difficulty with organizing information

Sleep disturbance

Abuse of chemical agents

Decreased use of social support

Use of forms of coping that impede adaptive behavior

Poor concentration

Inadequate problem solving

Verbalization of inability to cope or inability to ask for help

Inability to meet basic needs

Destructive behavior toward self or others

Inability to meet role expectations

High illness rate

Change in usual communication patterns

Fatigue

Risk taking

### Related factors

Gender differences in coping strategies

Inadequate level of confidence in ability to cope

Uncertainty

Inadequate social support created by characteristics of relationships

Inadequate level of perception of control

Inadequate resources available

High degree of threat

Situational or maturational crises

Disturbance in pattern of tension release

Inadequate opportunity to prepare for stressor

Inability to conserve adaptive energies

Disturbance in pattern of appraisal of threat

## DEATH ANXIETY

The apprehension, worry, or fear related to death or dying

### Defining characteristics

Worrying about the impact of one's own death on significant others

Powerless over issues related to dying

Fear of loss of physical and/or mental abilities when dying

Anticipated pain related to dying

Deep sadness

Fear of the process of dying

Concerns of overworking the caregiver as terminal illness incapacitates self

Concern about meeting one's creator or feeling doubtful about the existence of a god or higher being

Total loss of control over any aspect of one's own death

Negative death images or unpleasant thoughts about any event related to death or dying

Fear of delayed demise

Fear of premature death because it prevents the accomplishment of important life goals

Worrying about being the cause of other's grief and suffering

Fear of leaving family alone after death

Fear of developing a terminal illness

Denial of one's own mortality or impending death

**Related factors**

To be developed

## DECISIONAL CONFLICT (SPECIFY)

Uncertainty about course of action to be taken when choice among competing actions involves risk, loss, or challenge to personal life values

**Defining characteristics**

Verbalizes uncertainty about choices
Verbalizes undesired consequences of alternative actions being considered
Vacillation between alternative choices
Delayed decision making
Verbalizes feelings of distress while attempting a decision
Self-focusing
Physical signs of distress or tension (e.g., increased heart rate, increased muscle tension, restlessness)
Questioning personal values and beliefs while attempting a decision

**Related factors**

Support system deficit
Perceived threat to value system
Lack of experience or interference with decision making
Multiple or divergent sources of information
Lack of relevant information
Unclear personal values/beliefs

## DENIAL, INEFFECTIVE

Conscious or unconscious attempt to disavow the knowledge or meaning of an event to reduce anxiety/fear to the detriment of health

**Related factors**

To be developed

**Defining characteristics**

Delays seeking or refuses medical attention to the detriment of health
Does not perceive personal relevance of symptoms or danger
Uses home remedies (self-treatment) to relieve symptoms
Does not admit fear of death or invalidism
Minimizes symptoms
Displaces source of symptoms to other organs
Unable to admit impact of disease on life pattern
Makes dismissive gestures or comments when speaking of distressing events
Displaces fear of impact of condition
Displays inappropriate affect

## DENTITION, IMPAIRED

Disruption in tooth development/eruption patterns or structural integrity of individual teeth

**Defining characteristics**

Excessive plaque
Crown or root caries
Halitosis
Tooth enamel discoloration
Toothache
Loose teeth
Excessive calculus
Incomplete eruption for age (may be primary or permanent teeth)
Malocclusion or tooth misalignment
Premature loss of primary teeth
Worn down or abraded teeth
Tooth fractures
Missing teeth or complete absence
Erosion of enamel
Asymmetrical facial expression

**Related factors**

Ineffective oral hygiene, sensitivity to heat or cold
Barriers to self-care
Access or economic barriers to professional care
Nutritional deficits
Dietary habits
Genetic predisposition
Selected prescription medications
Premature loss of primary teeth
Excessive intake of fluorides
Chronic vomiting
Chronic use of tobacco, coffee or tea, red wine
Lack of knowledge regarding dental health
Excessive use of abrasive cleaning agents
Bruxism

## DEVELOPMENT, DELAYED, RISK FOR

At risk for delay of 25% or more in one or more of the areas of social or self-regulatory behavior, or in cognitive, language, gross or fine motor skills

**Risk factors**
*Prenatal*

Maternal age <15 or >35 years
Substance abuse
Infections
Genetic or endocrine disorders
Unplanned or unwanted pregnancy
Lack of, late, or poor prenatal care
Inadequate nutrition
Illiteracy
Poverty

*Individual*

Prematurity
Seizures
Positive drug screening test
Brain damage (e.g., hemorrhage in postnatal period, shaken baby, abuse, accident)
Vision impairment
Hearing impairment or frequent otitis media
Chronic illness
Technology-dependent
Failure to thrive, inadequate nutrition
Foster or adopted child
Lead poisoning
Chemotherapy
Radiation therapy
Natural disaster
Behavior disorders
Substance abuse

*Environment*

Poverty
Violence

*Caregiver*

Abuse
Mental illness
Mental retardation or severe learning disability

## DIARRHEA

Passage of loose, unformed stools

**Defining characteristics**

Hyperactive bowel sounds
At least 3 loose liquid stools per day
Urgency
Abdominal pain
Cramping

**Related factors**

*Psychological*

High stress levels and anxiety

*Situational*

Alcohol abuse
Toxins
Laxative abuse
Radiation
Tube feedings
Adverse effects of medications
Contaminants
Travel

*Physiological*

Inflammation
Malabsorption
Infectious processes
Irritation
Parasites

## DISUSE SYNDROME, RISK FOR

At risk for deterioration of body systems as the result of pre-scribed or unavoidable inactivity

**Risk factors**

Paralysis
Mechanical immobilization
Prescribed immobilization
Severe pain
Altered level of consciousness

## DIVERSIONAL ACTIVITY, DEFICIENT

Decreased stimulation from (or interest or engagement in) recre-ational or leisure activities

**Defining characteristics**

Desire for something to do, to read, etc.
Usual hobbies cannot be undertaken in hospital

**Related factors**

Environmental lack of diversional activity as in long-term hospital-ization, frequent, lengthy treatments

## DYSREFLEXIA, AUTONOMIC

Life-threatening uninhibited sympathetic response of the nervous system attributable to a noxious stimulus after a spinal cord injury at T7 or above

**Defining characteristics**

Paroxysmal hypertension (sudden periodic elevated blood pressure where systolic pressure is over 140 mm Hg and diastolic pressure is above 90 mm Hg)
Bradycardia or tachycardia (pulse rate of less than 60 or over 100 beats per minute)
Diaphoresis (above injury)
Red splotches on skin (above injury)
Pallor (below injury)
Headache (diffuse pain in different portions of head and not confined to any nerve distribution area)
Chilling
Conjunctival congestion
Horner's syndrome (contraction of pupil, partial ptosis of eyelid, en-ophthalmos, and sometimes loss of sweating over affected side of face)
Paresthesia
Pilomotor reflex (gooseflesh formation when skin is cooled)
Blurred vision
Chest pain
Metallic taste in mouth
Nasal congestion

**Related factors**

Bladder distention
Bowel distention
Skin irritation
Lack of patient and caregiver knowledge

## DYSREFLEXIA, AUTONOMIC, RISK FOR

At risk for life-threatening, uninhibited response of the sympa-thetic nervous system, post spinal shock, in an individual with spinal cord injury or lesion at T6 or above (has been demonstrated in pa-tients with injuries at T7 and T8)

**Defining characteristics**

An injury/lesion at T6 or above AND at least one of the following noxious stimuli:

*Neurological stimuli*

Painful/irritating stimuli below level of injury

*Urological stimuli*

Bladder distension
Detrusor sphincter dyssynergia
Bladder spasm
Instrumentation or surgery
Epididymitis
Urethritis
Urinary tract infection
Calculi
Cystitis
Catheterization

*Gastrointestinal stimuli*

Bowel distension
Fecal impaction
Digital stimulation
Suppositories
Hemorrhoids
Difficult passage of feces
Constipation
Enemas
GI system pathology
Gastric ulcers
Esophageal reflux
Gallstones

*Reproductive stimuli*

Menstruation
Sexual intercourse
Pregnancy
Labor and delivery
Ovarian cyst
Ejaculation

*Musculo-skeletal-integumentary stimuli*

Cutaneous stimulation (e.g., pressure ulcer, ingrown toenail, dress-ings, burns, rash)
Pressure over bony prominences or genitalia
Heterotrophic bone
Spasm
Fractures
Range-of-motion exercises
Wounds
Sunburns

*Regulatory stimuli*

Temperature fluctuations
Extreme environmental temperatures

*Situational stimuli*

Positioning
Constrictive clothing (e.g., straps, stockings, shoes)

Drug reactions (e.g., decongestants, sympathomimetics, vasoconstrictors, narcotic withdrawal)

Surgical procedure

### Cardiac/Pulmonary Problems

Pulmonary emboli

Deep vein thrombosis

## ENERGY FIELD DISTURBED

Disruption of the flow of energy surrounding a person's being, which results in a disharmony of the body, mind, or spirit

### Defining characteristics

Temperature change (warmth or coolness)

Visual changes (image or color)

Disruption of the field (vacant/hold/spike/bulge)

Movement (wave/spike/tingling/dense/flowing)

Sounds (tone or words)

### Related factors

To be developed

## ENVIRONMENTAL INTERPRETATION SYNDROME, IMPAIRED

Consistent lack of orientation to person, place, time, or circumstances more than from 3 to 6 months, necessitating a protective environment

### Defining characteristics

Consistent disorientation in known and unknown environments

Chronic confusional states

Loss of occupation or social functioning from memory decline

Inability to follow simple directions or instructions

Inability to reason

Inability to concentrate

Slowness in responding to questions

### Related factors

Dementia (Alzheimer's disease, multi-infarct dementia, Pick's disease, AIDS dementia)

Parkinson's disease

Huntington's disease

Depression

Alcoholism

## FAILURE TO THRIVE, ADULT

Progressive functional deterioration of a physical and cognitive nature. The individual's ability to live with multisystem diseases, cope with ensuing problems, and manage his/her care are remarkably diminished.

### Defining characteristics

Anorexia: does not eat meals when offered

States does not have an appetite, not hungry, or "I don't want to eat"

Inadequate nutritional intake: eating less than body requirements

Consumption of minimal to no food at most meals (i.e., consumes <75% of normal requirements)

Weight loss (decreased from baseline weight): 5% unintentional weight loss in 1 month; 10% unintentional weight loss in 6 months

Physical decline (decline in bodily function): evidence of fatigue, dehydration, incontinence of bowel and bladder

Frequent exacerbations of chronic health problems (e.g., pneumonia, urinary tract infections)

Cognitive decline (decline in mental processing) as evidenced by: problems with responding appropriately to environmental stimuli; demonstrated difficulty in reasoning, decision making, judgement, memory, and concentration; decreased perception

Decreased social skills/social withdrawal: noticeable decrease from usual past behavior in attempts to form or participate in cooperative and interdependent relationships (e.g., decreased verbal communication with staff, family, friends)

Decreased participation in activities of daily living that the older person once enjoyed

Self-care deficit: no longer looks after or takes charge of physical cleanliness or appearance

Difficulty in performing simple self-care tasks

Neglect of home environment and/or financial responsibilities

Apathy as evidenced by lack of observable feeling or emotion in terms of normal activities of daily living and environment

Altered mood state: expresses feelings of sadness, being low in spirit

Expresses loss of interest in pleasurable outlets such as food, sex, work, family, friends, hobbies, or entertainment

Verbalizes desire for death

### Related factors

Depression

Apathy

Fatigue

## FALLS, RISK FOR

An increased susceptibility to falling that may cause physical harm

### Related factors

#### Adults

History of falls

Wheelchair use

Age 65 or over

Female (if elderly)

Lives alone

Lower limb prosthesis

Use of assistive devices (e.g., walker, cane)

#### Physiological

Presence of acute illness

Postoperative conditions

Visual difficulties

Hearing difficulties

Arthritis

Orthostatic hypotension

Sleeplessness

Faintness when turning or extending neck

Anemias

Vascular disease

Neoplasms (i.e., fatigue, limited mobility)

Urgency and/or incontinence

Diarrhea

Decreased lower extremity strength

Postprandial blood sugar changes

Foot problems

Impaired physical mobility

Impaired balance

Difficulty with gait

Proprioceptive deficits (e.g., unilateral neglect)

Neuropathy

#### Cognitive

Diminished mental status (e.g., confusion, delirium, dementia, impaired reality testing)

#### Medications

Antihypertensive agents

ACE inhibitors

Diuretics

Tricyclic antidepressants

Alcohol use

Antianxiety agents

Narcotics

Hypnotics or tranquilizers

#### Environment

Restraints

Weather conditions (e.g., wet floors/ice)

Throw/scatter rugs
Cluttered environment
Unfamiliar, dimly lit room
No antislip material in bath and/or shower

### Children <2 years of age

Male gender when <1 year of age
Lack of auto restraints
Lack of gate on stairs
Lack of window guard
Bed located near window
Unattended infant on bed/changing table/sofa
Lack of parental supervision

## FAMILY PROCESSES, ALCOHOLISM

Psychosocial, spiritual, and physiological functions of the family unit are chronically disorganized, leading to conflict, denial of problems, resistance to change, ineffective problem solving, and a series of self-perpetuating crises

### Defining characteristics
#### Feelings

Decreased self-esteem or sense of worthlessness
Anger or suppressed rage
Frustration
Powerlessness
Anxiety
Tension
Distress
Insecurity
Repressed emotions
Responsibility for alcoholic's behavior
Lingering resentment
Shame or embarrassment
Hurt
Unhappiness
Guilt
Emotional isolation and loneliness
Vulnerability
Mistrust
Hopelessness
Rejection
Being different from other people
Depression
Hostility
Fear
Emotional control by others
Confusion
Dissatisfaction
Loss
Misunderstood
Abandonment
Confused love and pity
Moodiness
Failure
Being unloved
Lack of identity

### Related factors

Abuse of alcohol
Family history of alcoholism, resistance to treatment
Inadequate coping skills
Genetic predisposition
Addictive personality
Lack of problem-solving skills
Biochemical influences

#### Roles and relationships

Deterioration in family relationships or disturbed family dynamics
Ineffective spouse communication or marital problems

Altered role function or disruption of family roles
Inconsistent parenting or low perception of parental support
Family denial
Intimacy dysfunction
Chronic family problems
Closed communication systems
Triangulating family relationships
Reduced ability of family members to relate to each other for mutual
growth and maturation
Lack of skills necessary for relationships
Lack of cohesiveness
Disrupted family rituals
Family unable to meet security needs of its members
Family does not demonstrate respect for individuality and autonomy
of its members
Pattern of rejection
Economic problems
Neglected obligations

#### Behaviors

Expression of anger inappropriately
Difficulty with intimate relationships
Loss of control of drinking
Impaired communication
Ineffective problem-solving skills
Enabling alcoholic to maintain drinking
Inability to meet emotional needs of its members
Manipulation
Dependency
Criticizing
Alcohol abuse
Broken promises
Rationalization or denial of problems
Refusal to get help or inability to accept and receive help appropriately
Blaming
Inadequate understanding or knowledge or alcoholism
Inability to meet spiritual needs of its members
Inability to express or accept wide range of feelings
Orientation toward tension relief rather than achievement of goals
Family special occasions are alcohol centered
Escalating conflict
Lying
Contradictory, paradoxical communication
Lack of dealing with conflict
Harsh self-judgment
Isolation
Nicotine addiction
Difficulty having fun
Self-blaming
Unresolved grief
Controlling communication and power struggles
Inability to adapt to change
Immaturity
Stress-related physical illnesses
Inability to deal with traumatic experiences constructively
Seeking approval and affirmation
Lack of reliability
Disturbances in academic performance in children
Disturbances in concentration
Chaos
Substance abuse other than alcohol
Failure to accomplish current or past developmental tasks or difficulty with life cycle transitions
Verbal abuse of spouse or parent
Agitation
Diminished physical contact

## FAMILY PROCESSES, INTERRUPTED

A change in family relationships and/or functioning

### Defining characteristics

Changes in power alliances
Changes in assigned tasks
Changes in effectiveness in completing assigned tasks
Changes in mutual support
Changes in availability for affective responsiveness and intimacy
Changes in patterns and rituals
Changes in participation in problem solving
Changes in participation in decision-making
Changes in communication patterns
Changes in availability for emotional support
Changes in satisfaction with family
Changes in stress-reduction behaviors
Changes in expressions of conflict with and/or isolation from community resources
Changes in somatic complaints
Changes in expressions of conflict within family

### Related factors

Power shift of family members
Family roles shift
Shift in health status of a family member
Developmental transition and/or crisis
Situation transition and/or crises
Informal or formal interaction with community
Modification in family social status
Modification in family finances

## FATIGUE

An overwhelming sustained sense of exhaustion and decreased capacity for physical and mental work at usual level

### Defining characteristics

Inability to restore energy even after sleep
Lack of energy or inability to maintain usual level or physical activity
Increase in rest requirements
Tired
Inability to maintain usual routines
Verbalization of an unremitting and overwhelming lack of energy
Lethargic or listless
Perceived need for additional energy to accomplish routine tasks
Increase in physical complaints
Compromised concentration
Disinterest in surroundings, introspection
Decreased performance
Compromised libido
Drowsy
Feelings of guilt for not keeping up with responsibilities

### Related factors
*Psychological*

Boring lifestyle
Stress
Anxiety
Depression

*Individual*

Humidity
Lights
Noise
Temperature

*Situational*

Negative life events
Occupation

*Physiological*

Sleep deprivation
Pregnancy
Poor physical condition
Disease states
Increased physical exertion
Malnutrition
Anemia

## FEAR

Response to perceived threat that is consciously recognized as a danger

### Defining characteristics

Report of: apprehension, increased tension, decreased self-assurance, excitement, being scared, jitteriness, dread, alarm, terror, panic

*Cognitive*

Identifies object of fear
Stimulus believed to be a threat
Diminished productivity, learning ability, problem-solving ability

*Behaviors*

Increased alertness
Avoidance or attack behaviors
Impulsiveness
Narrowed focus on "it" (i.e., the focus of the fear)

*Physiological*

Increased pulse
Anorexia
Nausea
Vomiting
Diarrhea
Muscle tightness
Fatigue
Increased respiratory rate and shortness of breath
Pallor
Increased perspiration
Increased systolic blood pressure
Pupil dilation
Dry mouth

### Related factors

Natural/innate origin (e.g., sudden noise, height, pain, loss of physical support)
Learned response (e.g., conditioning, modeling from or identification with others)
Separation from support system in potentially stressful situation (e.g., hospitalization, hospital procedures)
Unfamiliarity with environmental experience(s)
Language barrier
Sensory impairment
Innate releasers (neurotransmitters)
Phobic stimulus

## FLUID VOLUME, DEFICIENT

Decreased intravascular, interstitial and/or intracellular fluid. This refers to dehydration, water loss alone without change in sodium.

### Defining characteristics

Decreased urine output
Increased urine concentration
Sudden weight loss
Decreased venous filling
Increased hematocrit
Decreased skin/tongue turgor
Decreased BP
Dry skin/mucous membranes
Thirst

Increased pulse rate
Decreased pulse volume/pressure
Change in mental state
Increased body temperature
Weakness

### Related factors

Failure of regulatory mechanisms
Active fluid volume loss

## FLUID VOLUME, DEFICIENT, RISK FOR

At risk for experiencing vascular, cellular, or intracellular dehydration

### Risk factors

Extremes of age
Extremes of weight
Excessive losses through normal routes (e.g., diarrhea)
Loss of fluid through abnormal routes (e.g., indwelling tubes)
Deviations affecting access to, intake of, or absorption of fluids (e.g., physical immobility)
Factors influencing fluid needs (e.g., hypermetabolic states)
Knowledge deficiency related to fluid volume
Medications (e.g., diuretics)
Increased fluid output
Urinary frequency
Thirst
Altered intake

## FLUID VOLUME, EXCESS

Increased isotonic fluid retention

### Defining characteristics

Edema
Effusion
Anasarca
Weight gain
Shortness of breath
Intake greater than output
Abnormal breath sounds, rales (crackles)
Decreased hemoglobin and hematocrit
Increased central venous pressure‡
Jugular vein distention‡
Positive hepatojugular reflex
Clinical evidence lacking in fluid volume excess studies
Orthopnea
$S_3$ heart sound
Pulmonary congestion
Change in respiratory pattern
Change in mental status
Blood pressure changes
Pulmonary artery pressure changes
Oliguria
Specific gravity changes
Azotemia
Altered electrolytes, restlessness
Anxiety

### Related factors

Compromised regulatory mechanism
Excess fluid intake
Excess sodium intake

## FLUID VOLUME, IMBALANCED, RISK FOR

At risk for a decrease, increase, or rapid shift from one to the other of intravascular, interstitial, and/or intracellular fluid. This refers to the loss or excess or both of body fluids or replacement fluids.

### Risk factors

Scheduled for major invasive procedures
Other risk factors to be determined

## GAS EXCHANGE, IMPAIRED

Excess or deficit in oxygenation and/or carbon dioxide elimination at the alveolar-capillary membrane

### Defining characteristics

Visual disturbances
Decreased carbon dioxide
Tachycardia
Hypercapnia
Restlessness
Somnolence
Irritability
Hypoxia
Confusion
Dyspnea
Abnormal arterial blood gases
Cyanosis (in neonates only)
Abnormal skin color (pale, dusky)
Hypoxemia
Hypercarbia
Headache upon awakening
Abnormal rate, rhythm, depth of breathing
Diaphoresis
Abnormal arterial pH
Nasal flaring

### Related factors

Ventilation perfusion imbalance
Alveolar-capillary membrane changes

## GRIEVING, ANTICIPATORY

Intellectual and emotional responses and behaviors by which individuals (families, communities) work through the process of modifying self-concept based on the perception of potential loss

### Defining characteristics

Potential loss of significant object
Expression of distress at potential loss
Denial of potential loss
Denial of the significance of the loss
Guilt
Anger
Sorrow
Bargaining
Alteration in: eating habits, sleep patterns, dream patterns, activity level, libido
Altered communication patterns
Difficulty taking on new or different roles
Resolution of grief prior to the reality of loss

### Related factors

To be developed

## GRIEVING, DYSFUNCTIONAL

Extended, unsuccessful use of intellectual and emotional responses by which individuals (families, communities) attempt to work through the process of modifying self-concept based on the perception of loss

### Defining characteristics

Repetitive use of ineffectual behaviors associated with attempts to reinvest in relationships
Reliving of past experiences with little or no reduction (diminishment) of intensity of the grief
Prolonged interference with life functioning
Onset or exacerbation of somatic or psychomatic responses
Expression of distress at loss
Denial of loss
Expression of guilt
Expression of unresolved issues

Anger
Sadness
Crying
Difficulty in expressing loss
Alterations in: eating habits, sleep patterns, dream patterns, activity level, libido, concentration and/or pursuit of tasks
Idealization of lost object
Reliving of past experiences
Interference with life functioning
Developmental regression
Labile affect

### Related factors

Actual or perceived object loss (object loss is used in the broadest sense); objects may include: people, possessions, a job, status, home, ideals, parts and processes of the body.

## GROWTH AND DEVELOPMENT, DELAYED

Deviations from age-group norms

### Defining characteristics

Delay or difficulty in performing skills (motor, social, or expressive) typical of age-group
Altered physical growth
Inability to perform self-care or self-control activities appropriate for age
Flat affect
Listlessness, decreased responses

### Related factors

Inadequate caretaking: indifference, inconsistent responsiveness, multiple caretakers
Separation from significant others
Environmental and stimulation deficiencies
Effects of physical disability
Prescribed dependence

## GROWTH, DISPROPORTIONATE, RISK FOR

At risk for growth above the 97th percentile or below the 3rd percentile for age, crossing two percentile channels; disproportionate growth

### Risk factors
*Prenatal*

Congenital/genetic disorders
Maternal nutrition
Multiple gestation
Teratogen exposure
Substance use/abuse
Maternal infection

*Individual*

Infection
Prematurity
Malnutrition
Organic and inorganic factors
Caregiver and/or individual maladaptive feeding behaviors
Anorexia
Insatiable appetite
Chronic illness
Substance abuse

*Individual*

Deprivation
Teratogen
Lead poisoning
Poverty
Violence
Natural disasters

*Caregiver*

Abuse
Mental illness, mental retardation, severe learning disability

## HEALTH MAINTENANCE, INEFFECTIVE

Inability to identify, manage, and/or seek help to maintain health

### Defining characteristics

Demonstrated lack of knowledge regarding basic health practices
Demonstrated lack of adaptive behaviors to internal or external environmental changes
Reported or observed inability to take responsibility for meeting basic health practices in any or all functional pattern areas
History of lack of health-seeking behavior
Expressed interest in improving health behaviors
Reported or observed lack of equipment, financial, and/or other resources
Reported or observed impairment of personal support system

### Related factors

Lack of or significant alteration in communication skills (written, verbal, and/or gestural)
Lack of ability to make deliberate and thoughtful judgments
Perceptual or cognitive impairment
Complete or partial lack of gross and/or fine motor skills
Ineffective individual coping; dysfunctional grieving
Lack of material resources
Unachieved developmental tasks
Ineffective family coping; disabling spiritual distress

## HEALTH-SEEKING BEHAVIORS (SPECIFY)

Active seeking (by a person in stable health) ways to alter personal health habits and/or the environment in order to move toward optimal health. (*Stable health* is defined as age-appropriate illness prevention measures achieved; the patient reports good or excellent health, and signs and symptoms of disease, if present, are controlled.)

### Defining characteristics

Expressed or observed desire to seek higher level of wellness
Stated or observed unfamiliarity with wellness community resources
Demonstrated or observed lack of knowledge in health promotion behaviors
Expressed or observed desire for increased control of health practice
Expression of concern about effects of current environmental conditions on health status

### Related factors
To be developed

## HOME MAINTENANCE, IMPAIRED

Inability to independently maintain a safe growth-promoting immediate environment

### Defining characteristics
*Subjective*

Household members express difficulty in maintaining their home in a comfortable fashion
Household requests assistance with home maintenance
Household members describe outstanding debts or financial crises

*Objective*

Disorderly surroundings
Unwashed or unavailable cooking equipment, clothes, or linen
Accumulation of dirt, food wastes, or hygienic wastes
Offensive odors
Inappropriate household temperature
Overtaxed family members (e.g., exhausted, anxious family members)
Lack of necessary equipment or aids
Presence of vermin or rodents
Repeated hygienic disorders, infestations, or infections

**Related factors**

Disease or injury of individual or family member
Insufficient family organization or planning
Insufficient finances
Unfamiliarity with neighborhood resources
Impaired cognitive or emotional functioning
Lack of knowledge
Lack of role modeling
Inadequate support systems

## HOPELESSNESS

Subjective state in which an individual sees limited or no alternatives or personal choices available and is unable to mobilize energy on own behalf

**Defining characteristics**

Passivity, decreased verbalization
Decreased affect
Verbal cues (indicating despondency, "I can't," sighing)
Lack of initiative
Decreased response to stimuli
Turning away from speaker
Closing eyes
Shrugging in response to speaker
Decreased appetite; increased/decreased sleep
Lack of involvement in care; passively allowing care

**Related factors**

Prolonged activity restriction creating isolation
Failure or deteriorating physiological condition
Long-term stress
Abandonment
Loss of belief in transcendent values/God

## HYPERTHERMIA

Body temperature elevated above normal range

**Defining characteristics**

Increase in body temperature above normal range
Flushed skin
Warm to touch
Increased respiratory rate
Tachycardia
Seizures/convulsions

**Related factors**

Exposure to hot environment
Vigorous activity
Medications/anesthesia
Inappropriate clothing
Increased metabolic rate
Illness or trauma
Dehydration
Inability or decreased ability to perspire

## HYPOTHERMIA

Body temperature below normal range

**Defining characteristics**

Shivering (mild)
Cool skin
Pallor (moderate)
Slow capillary refill
Tachycardia
Cyanotic nail beds
Hypertension
Piloerection

**Related factors**

Exposure to cool or cold environment
Illness or trauma

Inability or decreased ability to shiver
Malnutrition
Inadequate clothing
Consumption of alcohol
Medications causing vasodilation
Evaporation from skin in cool environment
Decreased metabolic rate
Inactivity
Aging

## INCONTINENCE, BOWEL

Change in normal bowel habits characterized by involuntary passage of stool

**Defining characteristics**

Constant dribbling of soft stool
Fecal odor
Inability to delay defecation
Urgency
Self-report of inability to feel rectal fullness
Fecal staining of clothing and/or bedding
Recognizes rectal fullness but reports inability to expel formed stool
Inattention to urge to defecate
Inability to recognize urge to defecate
Red perianal skin

**Related factors**

Environmental factors (e.g., inaccessible bathroom)
Incomplete emptying of bowel
Rectal sphincter abnormality
Impaction
Dietary habits
Colorectal lesions
Stress
Lower motor nerve damage
Abnormally high abdominal or intestinal pressure
General decline in muscle tone
Loss of rectal sphincter control
Impaired cognition
Upper motor nerve damage
Chronic diarrhea
Self-care deficit—toileting
Impaired reservoir capacity
Medications
Immobility
Laxative abuse

## INCONTINENCE, FUNCTIONAL URINARY

Inability of usually continent person to reach toilet in time to avoid unintentional loss of urine

**Defining characteristics**

May only be incontinent in early morning
Senses need to void
Amount of time required to reach toilet exceeds length of time between sensing urge and uncontrolled voiding
Loss of urine before reaching toilet
Able to completely empty bladder

**Related factors**

Psychological factors
Impaired vision
Impaired cognition
Neuromuscular limitations
Altered environmental factors
Weakened supporting pelvic structures

## INCONTINENCE, REFLEX URINARY

Involuntary loss of urine at somewhat predictable intervals when a specific bladder volume is reached

**Defining characteristics**

No sensation of urge to void
Complete emptying with lesion above pontine micturition center
Incomplete emptying with lesion above sacral micturition center
No sensation of bladder fullness
Sensations associated with full bladder such as sweating, restlessness, and abdominal discomfort
Unable to cognitively inhibit or initiate voiding
No sensation of voiding
Predictable pattern of voiding
Sensation to urge without voluntary inhibition of bladder contraction

**Related factors**

Tissue damage from radiation cystitis, inflammatory bladder conditions, or radical pelvic surgery
Neurological impairment above level of sacral micturition center or pontine micturition center

## INCONTINENCE, STRESS, URINARY

Loss of less than 50 ml of urine occurring with increased abdominal pressure.

**Defining characteristics**

Reported or observed dribbling with increased abdominal pressure
Urinary urgency
Urinary frequency (more often than every 2 hours)

**Related factors**

Degenerative changes in pelvic muscles and structural supports associated with increased age
High intraabdominal pressure (e.g., obesity, gravid uterus)
Incompetent bladder outlet
Overdistention between voidings
Weak pelvic muscles and structural supports

## INCONTINENCE, TOTAL, URINARY

Continuous and unpredictable loss of urine

**Defining characteristics**

Constant flow of urine occurring at unpredictable times without distention or uninhibited bladder contractions/spasms
Unsuccessful incontinence refractory to treatments
Nocturia
Lack of perineal or bladder-filling awareness
Unawareness of incontinence

**Related factors**

Neuropathy preventing transmission of reflex indicating bladder fullness
Neurological dysfunction causing triggering of micturition at unpredictable times
Independent contraction of detrusor reflex due to surgery
Trauma or disease affecting spinal cord nerves
Anatomic (fistula)

## INCONTINENCE, URGE URINARY

Involuntary passage of urine occurring soon after a strong sense of urgency to void

**Defining characteristics**

Urinary urgency
Frequency (voiding more often than every 2 hours)
Bladder contracture/spasm
Nocturia (more than 2 times per night)
Voiding in small (less than 100 ml) or in large amounts (more than 550 ml)
Inability to reach toilet in time

**Related factors**

Decreased bladder capacity (e.g., history of pelvic inflammatory disease, abdominal surgeries, indwelling urinary catheter)

Irritation of bladder stretch receptors, causing spasm (e.g., bladder infection)
Alcohol
Caffeine
Increased fluids
Increased urine concentration
Overdistention of bladder

## INCONTINENCE, URGE URINARY, RISK FOR

Risk for involuntary loss of urine associated with a sudden, strong sensation or urinary urgency

**Risk factors**

Effects of medications, caffeine, alcohol
Detrusor hyperreflexia from cystitis, urethritis, tumors, renal calculi, central nervous system disorders above pontine micturition center
Detrusor muscle instability with impaired contractility
Involuntary sphincter relaxation
Ineffective toileting habits
Small bladder capacity

## INFANT BEHAVIOR, DISORGANIZED

Disintegrated physiological and neurobehavioral responses to the environment

**Defining characteristics**
*Regulatory problems*

Inability to inhibit
Irritability

*State-organization system*

Active-awake (fussy, worried gaze)
Diffuse/unclear sleep, state oscillation
Quiet-awake (staring, gaze aversion)
Irritable or panicky crying

*Attention-interaction system*

Abnormal response to sensory stimuli (e.g., difficult to soothe, inability to sustain alert status)

*Motor system*

Increased, decreased, or limp tone
Finger splay, fisting or hands to face
Hyperextension of arms and legs
Tremors, startles, twitches
Jittery, jerky, uncoordinated movement
Altered primitive reflexes

*Physiological*

Bradycardia, tachycardia, or arrhythmias
Pale, cyanotic, mottled, or flushed color
Bradypnea, tachypnea, apnea
"Time-out signals" (e.g., gaze, grasp, hiccough, cough, sneeze, sigh, slack jaw, open mouth, tongue thrust)
Oximeter desaturation
Feeding intolerances (aspiration or emesis)

**Related factors**
*Prenatal*

Congenital or genetic disorders
Teratogenic exposure

*Postnatal*

Malnutrition
Oral/motor problems
Pain
Feeding intolerance
Invasive/painful procedures
Prematurity

*Individual*

Malnutrition
Illness
Immature neurological system
Gestational age
Postconceptual age

*Individual*

Physical environment inappropriateness
Sensory inappropriateness
Sensory overstimulation
Sensory deprivation

*Caregiver*

Cue misreading
Cue knowledge deficit
Environmental stimulation contribution

## INFANT BEHAVIOR, DISORGANIZED, RISK FOR

Risk for alteration in integration and modulation of the physiological and behavioral systems of functioning (i.e., autonomic, motor, state, organizational, self-regulatory, and attentional-interactional systems)

**Risk factors**

Pain
Oral motor problems
Environmental overstimulation
Lack of containment or boundaries
Prematurity
Invasive or painful procedures

## INFANT BEHAVIOR, ORGANIZED, READINESS FOR ENHANCED

A pattern of modulation of the physiologic and behavioral systems of functioning of an infant (i.e., autonomic, motor, state, organizational, self-regulatory, and attentional-interactional systems) that is satisfactory but that can be improved, resulting in higher levels of integration in response to environmental stimuli

**Defining characteristics**

Stable physiologic measures
Definite sleep-wake states
Use of some self-regulatory behaviors
Response to visual or auditory stimuli

**Related factors**

Prematurity
Pain

## INFANT FEEDING PATTERN, INEFFECTIVE

Impaired ability to suck or coordinate the suck-swallow response

**Defining characteristics**

Inability to initiate or sustain an effective suck
Inability to coordinate sucking, swallowing, and breathing

**Related factors**

Prematurity
Neurological impairment/delay
Oral hypersensitivity
Prolonged NPO status
Anatomic abnormality

## INFECTION, RISK FOR

At increased risk for being invaded by pathogenic organisms.

**Risk factors**

Inadequate primary defenses (broken skin, traumatized tissue, decrease in ciliary action, stasis of body fluids, change in pH secretions, altered peristalsis)

Inadequate secondary defenses (e.g., decreased hemoglobin level, leukopenia, suppressed inflammatory response, immunosuppression)
Inadequate acquired immunity
Tissue destruction and increased environmental exposure
Chronic disease
Invasive procedures
Malnutrition
Pharmaceutical agents and trauma
Rupture of amniotic membranes
Insufficient knowledge to avoid exposure to pathogens

## INJURY, PERIOPERATIVE POSITIONING, RISK FOR

At risk for injury as a result of the environmental conditions found in the perioperative setting

**Risk factors**

Disorientation
Immobilization, muscle weakness
Sensory or perceptual disturbances resulting from anesthesia
Obesity
Emaciation
Edema

## INJURY, RISK FOR

At risk of injury as a result of environmental conditions interacting with the individual's adaptive and defensive resources.

**Risk factors**
*Internal*

Biochemical
  Regulatory function
    Sensory dysfunction
    Integrative dysfunction
    Effector dysfunction
  Tissue hypoxia
  Malnutrition
  Immune-autoimmune
  Abnormal blood profile
    Leukocytosis or leukopenia
    Altered clotting factors
    Thrombocytopenia
    Sickle cell
    Thalassemia
    Decreased hemoglobin level
Physical
  Broken skin
  Altered mobility
Developmental
  Age
    Physiological
    Psychosocial
Psychological
  Affective
  Orientation

*External*

Biological
  Immunization level of community
  Microorganism
Chemical
  Pollutants
  Poisons
  Drugs
    Pharmaceutical agents
    Alcohol
    Caffeine
    Nicotine
  Preservatives
  Cosmetics and dyes
  Nutrients (vitamins, food types)

Physical
  Design, structure, and arrangement of community, building, and/or
    equipment
  Mode of transport/transportation
  Nosocomial agents

*People or provider*
Nosocomial agents
Staffing patterns
Cognitive, affective, and psychomotor factors

## KNOWLEDGE DEFICIENT (SPECIFY)

Absence or deficiency of cognitive information related to specific
topic

### Defining characteristics

Verbalization of the problem
Inaccurate follow-through of instruction
Inaccurate performance of test
Inappropriate or exaggerated behaviors (e.g., hysterical, hostile, agi-
  tated, apathetic)

### Related factors

Lack of exposure
Lack of recall
Information misinterpretation
Cognitive limitation
Lack of interest in learning
Unfamiliarity with information resources

## LATEX ALLERGY RESPONSE

An allergic reaction to natural latex rubber products

### Defining characteristics
*Type I reactions*
Immediate

*Type IV reactions*
Eczema
Irritation
Reaction to additives causes discomfort (e.g., thiurams, carbamates)
Redness
Delayed onset (hours)

*Irritant reactions*
Erythema
Chapped or cracked skin
Blisters

### Related factors

No immune mechanism response

## LATEX ALLERGY RESPONSE, RISK FOR

At risk for allergic response to natural latex rubber products

### Risk factors

Multiple surgical procedures, especially from infancy (e.g., spina
  bifida)
Allergies to bananas, avocados, tropical fruits, kiwi, chestnuts
Professions with daily exposure to latex (e.g., medicine, nursing,
  dentistry)
Conditions needing continuous or intermittent catheterization
History of reactions to latex (e.g., balloons, condoms, gloves)
Allergies to poinsettia plants
History of allergies and asthma

## LONELINESS, RISK FOR

At risk of experiencing vague dysphoria.

### Risk factors
Affectional deprivation
Physical isolation
Cathectic deprivation
Social isolation

## MEMORY, IMPAIRED

Inability to remember or recall bits of information or behavioral
skills. Impaired memory may be attributed to pathophysiological or
situational causes that are either temporary or permanent.

### Defining characteristics

Inability to recall factual information
Inability to recall recent or past events
Inability to learn or retain new skills or information
Inability to determine if a behavior was performed
Observed or reported experiences of forgetting
Inability to perform a previously learned skill
Forgets to perform a behavior at a scheduled time

### Related factors

Acute or chronic hypoxia
Anemia
Decreased cardiac output
Fluid and electrolyte imbalance
Neurologic disturbances
Excessive environmental disturbances

## MOBILITY, IMPAIRED BED

Limitation of independent movement from one bed position to
another

### Defining characteristics

Impaired ability to: turn side to side; move from supine to siting or
  sitting to supine; "scoot" or reposition self in bed; move from supine to prone or prone to supine; move from supine to long sitting
  or long sitting to supine

## MOBILITY, IMPAIRED PHYSICAL

A limitation in independent, purposeful physical movement of the
body or of one or more extremities

### Defining characteristics

Postural instability during performance of routine Activities of Daily
  Living
Limited ability to perform gross motor skills
Limited ability to perform fine motor skills
Uncoordinated or jerky movements
Limited range of motion
Difficulty turning
Decreased reaction time
Movement-induced shortness of breath
Gait changes (e.g., decreased walk, speed, difficulty initiating gait,
  small steps, shuffles feet, exaggerated lateral postural sway)
Engages in substitutions for movement (e.g., increased attention to
  other's activity, controlling behavior, focus on pre-illness/disabil-
  ity activity)
Slowed movement
Movement-induced tremor

### Related factors

Medications
Prescribed movement restrictions
Discomfort
Lack of knowledge regarding value of physical activity
Body mass index about 75th age-appropriate percentile
Sensoriperceptual impairments
Neuromuscular impairment
Pain

Musculoskeletal impairment
Intolerance to activity/decreased strength and endurance
Depressive mood state or anxiety
Cognitive impairment
Decreased muscle strength, control and/or mass
Reluctance to initiate movement
Sedentary lifestyle or disuse or deconditioning
Selective or generalized malnutrition
Loss of integrity of bone structures
Developmental delay
Joint stiffness or contractures
Limited cardiovascular endurance
Altered cellular metabolism
Lack of physical or social environmental supports
Cultural beliefs regarding age appropriate activity

## MOBILITY, IMPAIRED WHEELCHAIR

Limitation of independent operation of wheelchair within environment (specify level of independence)

### Defining characteristics

Impaired ability to operate manual or power wheelchair on even or uneven surface
Impaired ability to operate manual or power wheelchair on an incline or decline
Impaired ability to operate wheelchair on curbs

## NAUSEA

An unpleasant, wave-like sensation in the back of the throat, epigastrium, or throughout the abdomen that may or may not lead to vomiting

### Defining characteristics

Usually precedes vomiting, but may be experienced after vomiting or when vomiting does not occur
Accompanied by pallor, cold and clammy skin, increased salivation, tachycardia, gastric stasis, and diarrhea
Accompanied by swallowing movements affected by skeletal muscles
Reports "nausea" or "sick to stomach"

### Related factors

Chemotherapy
Post-surgical anesthesia
Irritation to the gastrointestinal system
Stimulation of neuropharmacologic mechanisms

## NONCOMPLIANCE

Behavior of person and/or caregiver that fails to coincide with a health-promoting or therapeutic plan agreed on by the person (and/or family and/or community) and health-care professional. In the presence of an agreed-on, health-promoting or therapeutic plan, person's or caregiver's behavior is fully or partially nonadherent and may lead to clinically ineffective or partially ineffective outcomes.

### Defining characteristics

Behavior indicative of failure to adhere (by direct observation or by statements of patient or significant others)
Evidence of development of complications
Evidence of exacerbation of symptoms
Failure to keep appointments
Failure to progress
Objective tests (e.g., physiological measures, detection of physiologic markers)

### Related factors
*Healthcare plan*

Duration
Significant others
Cost

Intensity
Complexity

*Individual factors*

Personal and developmental abilities
Health beliefs, cultural influences, spiritual values
Individual's value system
Knowledge and skill relevant to the regimen behavior
Motivational forces

*Health system*

Satisfaction with care
Credibility of provider
Access and convenience of care
Financial flexibility of plan
Client-provider relationships
Provider reimbursement of teaching and follow-up
Provider continuity and regular follow-up
Individual health coverage
Communication and teaching skills of the provider

*Network*

Involvement of members in health plan
Social value regarding plan
Perceived beliefs of significant others

## NUTRITION, IMBALANCED: LESS THAN BODY REQUIREMENTS

Intake of nutrients insufficient to meet metabolic needs

### Defining characteristics

Loss of body weight with adequate food intake
Body weight 20% or more under ideal for height and frame
Reported inadequate food intake less than Recommended Daily Allowance
Weakness of muscles required for swallowing or mastication
Reported or evidence of lack of food
Lack of interest in food
Perceived inability to ingest food
Aversion to eating
Reported altered taste sensation
Satiety immediately after ingesting food
Abdominal pain with or without pathological conditions
Sore, inflamed buccal cavity

### Related factor[3]

Inability to ingest or digest food or absorb nutrients because of biological, psychological, or economic factors

## NUTRITION, IMBALANCED: MORE THAN BODY REQUIREMENTS

Intake of nutrients that exceeds metabolic needs

### Related factor

Excessive intake in relationship to metabolic need

### Defining characteristics

Weight 20% over ideal for height and frame
Triceps skinfold greater than 15 mm in men and 25 mm in women
Sedentary activity level
Reported or observed dysfunctional eating patterns (e.g., pairing food with other activities)
Concentrating food intake at end of day
Eating in response to external cues (e.g., time of day, social situation)
Eating in response to internal cues other than hunger (e.g., anxiety)

## NUTRITION, IMBALANCED, RISK FOR: MORE THAN BODY REQUIREMENTS

At risk for an intake of nutrients that exceeds metabolic needs.

## Risk factors

Hereditary predisposition

Excessive energy intake during late gestational life, early infancy, and adolescence

Frequent, closely spaced pregnancies

Dysfunctional psychological conditioning in relationship to food

Membership in lower socioeconomic group

Reported or observed obesity in one or both parents

Rapid transition across growth percentiles in infants or children

Reported use of solid food as major food source before 5 months of age

Observed use of food as reward or comfort measure

Reported or observed higher baseline weight at beginning of each pregnancy

Dysfunctional eating patterns

    Pairing food with other activities

    Concentrating food intake at end of day

    Eating in response to external cues (e.g., time of day, social situation)

    Eating in response to internal cues other than hunger (e.g., anxiety)

## ORAL MUCOUS MEMBRANE, IMPAIRED

Disruptions of the lips and soft tissue of the oral cavity

### Defining characteristics

Purulent drainage or exudates

Gingival recession, pockets deeper than 4 mm

Enlarged tonsils beyond what is developmentally appropriate

Smooth atrophic, sensitive tongue

Geographic tongue

Mucosal denudation

Presence of pathogens

Difficult speech

Self-report of bad taste

Gingival or mucosal pallor

Oral pain/discomfort

Xerostomia (dry mouth)

Vesicles, nodules, or papules

White patches/plaques, spongy patches or white curd-like exudate

Oral lesions or ulcers

Halitosis

Edema

Hyperemia

Desquamation

Coated tongue

Stomatitis

Self-report of difficulty eating or swallowing

Self-report of diminished or absent taste

Bleeding

Macroplasia

Gingival hyperplasia

Fissures, chelitis

Red or bluish masses (e.g., hemangiomas)

### Related factors

Chemotherapy

Chemical (e.g., alcohol, tobacco, acidic foods, regular use of inhalers)

Depression

Immunosuppression

Aging-related loss of connective, adipose, or bone tissue

Barriers to professional care

Cleft lip or palate

Medication side effects

Lack of or decreased salivation

Trauma (chemical, e.g., acidic foods, drugs, noxious agents, alcohol)

Pathological conditions—oral cavity (radiation to head or neck)

NPO for more than 24 hours

Mouth breathing

Malnutrition or vitamin deficiency

Dehydration

Infection

Ineffective oral hygiene

Mechanical (e.g., ill-fitting dentures, braces, tubes [endotracheal/nasogastric], surgery in oral cavity)

Decreased platelets

Immunocompromised

Impaired salivation

Radiation therapy

Barriers to oral self-care

Diminished hormone levels (women)

Stress

Loss of supportive structures

## PAIN, ACUTE

Unpleasant sensory and emotional experience arising from actual or potential tissue damage or described in terms of such damage (International Association for the Study of Pain); sudden or slow onset of any intensity from mild to severe with an anticipated or predictable end and a duration of less than 6 months

### Defining characteristics

Verbal or coded report

Observed evidence

Antalgic position

Protective behavior

Guarding behavior

Antalgic gestures

Facial mask

Sleep disturbance (eyes lack luster, "hecohe look," fixed or scattered movement, grimace)

### Related factors

Injuring agents

    Biological

    Chemical

    Physical

    Psychological

Self-focus; narrowed focus (altered time perception)

Impaired thought process

Reduced interaction with people and environment

Distraction behavior (pacing, seeking out other people and/or activities, repetitive activities)

Autonomic alteration in muscle tone (may span from listless to rigid)

Autonomic responses (diaphoresis, blood pressure, respiration, pulse change, pupillary dilatation)

Expressive behavior (restlessness, moaning, crying, vigilance, irritability, sighing)

Changes in appetite and eating

## PAIN, CHRONIC

Unpleasant sensory and emotional experience arising from actual or potential tissue damage or described in terms of such damage (International Association for the Study of Pain); sudden or slow onset of any intensity from mild to severe, constant or recurring without an anticipated or predictable end and a duration of greater than 6 months.

### Defining characteristics

Verbal or coded report or observed evidence of:

    Protective behavior

    Guarding behavior

    Facial mask

    Irritability

    Self focusing

    Restlessness

    Depression

Atrophy of involved muscle group

Changes in sleep pattern

Weight changes

Fatigue
Fear of reinjury
Reduced interaction with people
Altered ability to continue previous activities
Sympathetic mediated responses (temperature, cold, changes of body position, hypersensitivity)
Anorexia

### Related factor

Chronic physical/psychosocial disability

## PARENT/INFANT/CHILD ATTACHMENT, IMPAIRED, RISK FOR

Disruption of the interactive process between parent or significant other and infant that fosters the development of a protective and nurturing reciprocal relationship.

### Risk factors

Inability of parents to meet the personal needs
Anxiety associated with the parent role
Substance abuse
Premature infant
Ill infant or child who is unable to effectively initiate parental contact because of altered behavioral organization
Separation
Physical barriers
Lack of privacy

## PARENTAL ROLE CONFLICT

Parent experience of role confusion and conflict in response to a crisis.

### Defining characteristics

Parent(s) expresses concerns/feelings of inadequacy to provide for child's physical and emotional needs during hospitalization or in home
Demonstrated disruption in caretaking routines
Parent(s) expresses concerns about changes in parental role, family functioning, family communication, and/or family health
Expresses concern about perceived loss of control over decisions relating to child
Reluctant to participate in normal caretaking activities even with encouragement and support
Verbalizes/demonstrates feelings of guilt, anger, fear, anxiety, and/or frustrations about effect of child's illness on family process

### Related factors

Separation from child due to chronic illness
Intimidation with invasive or restrictive modalities (e.g., isolation, intubation)
Specialized care centers, policies
Home care of a child with special needs (e.g., apnea monitoring, postural drainage, hyperalimentation)
Change in marital status
Interruptions of family life due to home health-care regimen (treatments, caregivers, lack of respite)

## PARENTING, IMPAIRED

Inability of the primary caretaker to create an environment that promotes the optimum growth and development of the child

### Defining characteristics
#### Infant or child

Poor academic performance
Frequent illness
Runaway
Incidence of physical and psychological trauma or abuse
Frequent accidents
Lack of attachment
Failure to thrive

Behavioral disorders
Poor social competence
Lack of separation anxiety
Poor cognitive development

#### Parental

Inappropriate child care arrangements
Rejection or hostility to child
Statements of inability to meet child's needs
Inflexibility to meet needs of child, situation
Poor or inappropriate caretaking skills
High punitiveness
Inconsistent care
Child abuse
Inadequate child health maintenance
Unsafe home environment
Verbalization, cannot control child
Negative statements about child
Verbalization of role inadequacy frustration
Inappropriate visual, tactile, auditory stimulation
Inappropriate child care arrangements
Abandonment
Insecure or lack of attachment to infant
Inconsistent behavior management
Child neglect
Little cuddling
Maternal-child interaction deficit
Poor parent-child interaction

### Related factors
#### Social

Lack of access to resources
Social isolation
Lack of resources
Poor home environments
Lack of family cohesiveness
Inadequate child care arrangements
Lack of transportation
Unemployment or job problems
Role strain or overload
Marital conflict, declining satisfaction
Lack of value of parenthood
Change in family unit
Low socioeconomic class
Unplanned or unwanted pregnancy
Presence of stress (e.g., financial, legal, recent crisis, cultural move)
Lack of, or poor, parental role model
Single parents
Lack of social support networks
Father of child not involved
History of being abusive
History of being abused
Financial difficulties
Maladaptive coping strategies
Poverty
Poor problem-solving skills
Inability to put child's needs before own
Low self-esteem
Relocations
Legal difficulties

#### Knowledge

Lack of knowledge about child health maintenance
Lack of knowledge about parenting skills
Unrealistic expectation for self, infant, partner
Limited cognitive functioning
Lack of knowledge about child development
Inability to recognize and act on infant cues
Low educational levels or attainment
Poor communication skills

Lack of cognitive readiness for parenthood
Preference for physical punishment

*Physiological*

Physical illness

*Infant or child*

Premature birth
Illness
Prolonged separation from parent
Not gender desired
Attention deficit hyperactivity disorder
Difficult temperament
Separation from parent at birth
Lack of goodness of fit (temperament) with parental expectations
Unplanned or unwanted child
Handicapping condition or developmental delay
Multiple births
Altered perceptual abilities

*Psychological*

History of substance abuse or dependencies
Disability
Depression
Difficult labor and/or delivery
Young age, especially adolescent
History of mental illness
High number or closely spaced pregnancies
Sleep deprivation or disruption
Lack of, or late, prenatal care
Separation from infant/child
Multiple births

## PARENTING, IMPAIRED, RISK FOR

Risk for inability of the primary caretaker to create, maintain, or regain an environment that promotes the optimum growth and development of the child

### Risk factors
*Social*

Marital conflict, declining satisfaction
History of being abused
Poor problem solving skills
Role strain/overload
Social isolation
Legal difficulties
Lack of access to resources
Lack of value of parenthood
Relocation
Poverty
Poor home environment
Lack of family cohesiveness
Lack of or poor parental role model
Father of child not involved
History of being abusive
Financial difficulties
Low self-esteem
Unplanned or unwanted pregnancy
Inadequate child care arrangements
Maladaptive coping strategies
Lack of resources
Low socioeconomic class
Lack of transportation
Change in family unit
Unemployment or job problems
Single parent
Lack of social support network
Inability to put child's needs before own
Stress

*Knowledge*

Low educational level or attainment
Unrealistic expectations of child
Lack of knowledge about parenting skills
Poor communication skills
Preference for physical punishment
Inability to recognize and act on infant cues
Low cognitive functioning
Lack of knowledge about child health maintenance
Lack of knowledge about child development
Lack of cognitive readiness for parenthood

*Physiological*

Physical illness

*Infant or child*

Multiple births
Handicapping condition of developmental delay
Illness
Altered perceptual abilities
Lack of goodness of fit (temperament) with parental expectations
Unplanned or unwanted child
Premature birth
Not gender desired
Difficult temperament
Attention deficit hyperactivity disorder
Prolonged separation from parent
Separation form parent at birth

*Psychological*

Separation from infant/child
High number or closely spaced children
Disability
Sleep deprivation or disruption
Multiple births
Difficult labor and/or delivery
Young ages, especially adolescent
Depression
History of mental illness
Lack of, or late, prenatal care
History of substance abuse or dependence

## PERIPHERAL NEUROVASCULAR DYSFUNCTION, RISK FOR

At risk for disruption in circulation, sensation, or motion of an extremity

### Risk factors

Fractures
Mechanical compression (e.g., tourniquet, cast, brace, dressing, or restraint)
Orthopedic surgery
Trauma
Immobilization
Burns
Vascular obstruction

## PERSONAL IDENTITY, DISTURBED

Inability to distinguish between self and nonself

### Defining characteristic

To be developed

### Related factors

To be developed

## POISONING, RISK FOR

At accentuated risk of accidental exposure to or ingestion of drugs or dangerous products in doses sufficient to cause poisoning

**Risk factors**

*Internal*

Reduced vision
Verbalization of occupational setting without adequate safeguards
Lack of safety or drug education
Lack of proper precaution
Cognitive or emotional difficulties
Insufficient finances

*External*

Large supplies of drugs in house
Medicines stored in unlocked cabinets accessible to children or confused persons
Dangerous products placed or stored within reach of children or confused persons
Availability of illicit drugs potentially contaminated by poisonous additives
Flaking, peeling paint or plaster in presence of young children
Chemical contamination of food and water
Unprotected contact with heavy metals or chemicals
Paint, lacquer, etc., in poorly ventilated areas or without effective protection
Presence of poisonous vegetation
Presence of atmospheric pollutants

## POST-TRAUMA SYNDROME

A sustained maladaptive response to a traumatic, overwhelming event

**Defining characteristics**

Avoidance
Repression
Difficulty in concentrating
Grief
Intrusive thoughts
Neurosensory irritability
Palpitations
Enuresis (in children)
Anger and/or rage
Intrusive dreams
Nightmares
Aggression
Hypervigilant
Exaggerated startle response
Hopelessness
Altered mood states
Shame
Panic attacks
Alienation
Denial
Horror
Substance abuse
Depression
Anxiety
Guilt
Fear
Gastric irritability
Detachment
Psychogenic amnesia
Irritability
Numbing
Compulsive behavior
Flashbacks
Headaches

**Related factors**

Events outside the range of usual human experience
Physical and psychosocial abuse
Tragic occurrence involving multiple deaths

Sudden destruction of one's home or community
Epidemics
Being held prisoner of war or criminal victimization (torture)
Wars
Rape
Natural disasters and/or man-made disasters
Serious accidents
Witnessing mutilation, violent death, or other horrors
Serious threat or injury to self or loved ones
Industrial and motor vehicle accidents
Military combat

## POST-TRAUMA SYNDROME, RISK FOR

A risk for sustained maladaptive response to a traumatic, overwhelming event

**Risk factors**

Occupation (e.g., police, fire, rescue, corrections, emergency room staff, mental health)
Exaggerated sense of responsibility
Perception of event
Survivor's role in the event
Displacement from home
Inadequate social support
Non-supportive environment
Diminished ego strength
Duration of the event

## POWERLESSNESS

Perception that one's own action will not significantly affect an outcome; a perceived lack of control over a current situation or immediate happening

**Defining characteristics**

*Severe*

Verbal expressions of having no control or influence over situation
Verbal expressions of having no control or influence over outcome
Verbal expressions of having no control over self-care
Depression over physical deterioration that occurs despite patient compliance with regimens
Apathy

*Moderate*

Nonparticipation in care or decision making when opportunities are provided
Expressions of dissatisfaction and frustration over inability to perform previous tasks and/or activities
Does not monitor progress
Expression of doubt regarding role performance
Reluctance to express true feelings, fearing alienation from caregivers
Inability to seek information regarding care
Dependence on others that may result in irritability, resentment, anger, and guilt
Does not defend self-care practices when challenged

*Low*

Passivity
Expressions of uncertainty about fluctuating energy levels

**Related factors**

Health-care environment
Interpersonal interaction
Illness-related regimen
Lifestyle of helplessness

## POWERLESSNESS, RISK FOR

At risk for perceived lack of control over a situation and/or one's ability to significantly affect an outcome

## Risk factors

### Physiological

Chronic or acute illness (hospitalization, intubation, ventilator, suctioning)

Acute injury or progressive debilitating disease process (e.g., spinal cord injury, multiple sclerosis)

Aging (e.g., decreased physical strength, decreased mobility)

Dying

### Psychosocial

Lack of knowledge of illness or healthcare system

Lifestyle of dependency with inadequate coping patterns

Absence of integrality (e.g., essence of power)

Decreased self-esteem

Low or unstable body image

## PROTECTION, INEFFECTIVE

Decrease in the ability to guard the self from internal or external threats, such as illness or injury

### Defining characteristics

Deficient immunity

Impaired healing

Altered clotting

Maladaptive stress response

Neurosensory alterations

Chilling

Perspiring

Dyspnea

Cough

Itching

Restlessness

Insomnia

Fatigue

Anorexia

Weakness

Immobility

Disorientation

Pressure sores

### Related factors

Extremes of age

Inadequate nutrition

Alcohol abuse

Abnormal blood profiles (leukopenia, thrombocytopenia, anemia, coagulation)

Drug therapies (antineoplastic, corticosteroid, immune, anticoagulant, thrombolytic)

Treatments (surgery, radiation)

Diseases such as cancer and immune disorders

## RAPE-TRAUMA SYNDROME

Sustained maladaptive response to a forced, violent sexual penetration against the victim's will and consent

### Defining characteristics

Disorganization

Change in relationships

Confusion

Physical trauma (e.g., bruising, tissue irritation)

Suicide attempts

Denial

Guilt

Paranoia

Humiliation

Embarrassment

Aggression

Muscle tension and/or spasms

Mood swings

Dependence

Powerlessness

Nightmare and sleep disturbances

Sexual dysfunction

Revenge

Phobias

Loss of self-esteem

Inability to make decisions

Dissociative disorders

Self-blame

Hyperalertness

Vulnerability

Substance abuse

Depression

Helplessness

Anger

Anxiety

Agitation

Shame

Shock

Fear

### Related factors

Rape

## RAPE-TRAUMA SYNDROME: COMPOUND REACTION

Forced violent sexual penetration against the victim's will and consent. The trauma syndrome that develops from this attack or attempted attack includes an acute phase of disorganization of the victim's lifestyle and a long-term process of reorganization of lifestyle. This syndrome includes the following three sub-components: Rape-Trauma, Compound Reaction, and Silent Reaction.

### Defining characteristics

Change in lifestyle (e.g., changes in residence, dealing with repetitive nightmares and phobias, seeking family support, seeking social network support in long-term phase)

Emotional reaction (e.g., anger, embarrassment, fear of physical violence and death, humiliation, revenge, self-blame in acute phase)

Multiple physical symptoms (e.g., gastrointestinal irritability, genitourinary discomfort, muscle tension, sleep pattern disturbance in acute phase)

Reactivated symptoms of such previous conditions (i.e., physical illness, psychiatric illness in acute phase)

Reliance on alcohol/drugs (acute phase)

### Related factors

To be developed

## RAPE-TRAUMA SYNDROME: SILENT REACTION

Forced, violent sexual penetration against the victim's will and consent. The trauma syndrome that develops from this attack or attempted attack includes an acute phase or disorganization of the victim's lifestyle and a long-term process of reorganization of lifestyle.

### Related factors

To be developed.

### Defining characteristics

Abrupt changes in relationships with members of the opposite sex

Increase in nightmares

Increasing anxiety during interview (e.g., blocking of associations, long periods of silence, minor stuttering, physical distress)

Marked changes in sexual behavior

No verbalization of occurrence of the rape

Sudden onset of phobic reactions

## RELOCATION STRESS SYNDROME

Physiological and/or psychosocial disturbance following transfer from one environment to another

## Defining characteristics

Temporary or permanent move
Aloneness, alienation, loneliness
Depression
Anxiety (e.g., separation)
Sleep disturbance
Withdrawal
Anger
Loss of identity, self-worth, or self-esteem
Increased verbalization of needs, unwillingness to move, or concern over relocation
Increased physical symptoms/illness (e.g., gastrointestinal disturbance, weight change)
Dependency
Insecurity
Pessimism
Frustration
Worry
Fear

## Related factors

Unpredictability of experience
Isolation from family/friends
Past, concurrent, and recent losses
Feelings of powerlessness
Lack of adequate support system/group
Lack of predeparture counseling
Passive coping
Impaired psychosocial health
Language barrier
Decreased health status

## RELOCATION STRESS SYNDROME, RISK FOR

At risk for physiological and/or psychosocial disturbance following transfer from one environment to another

## Defining characteristics

Moderate to high degree of environmental change (e.g., physical, ethnic, cultural)
Temporary and/or permanent moves
Voluntary/involuntary move
Lack of adequate support system/group
Feelings of powerlessness
Moderate mental competence (e.g., alert enough to experience changes)
Unpredictability of experiences
Decreased psychosocial or physical health status
Lack of predeparture counseling
Passive coping
Past, current, recent losses

## ROLE PERFORMANCE, INEFFECTIVE

Patterns of behavior and self-expression do not match the environmental context, norms, and expectations

## Defining characteristics

Change in self-perception of role
Role denial
Inadequate external support for role enactment
Inadequate adaptation to change or transition
System conflict
Change in usual patterns of responsibility
Discrimination
Domestic violence
Harassment
Uncertainty
Altered role perceptions
Role strain
Inadequate self-management
Role ambivalence
Pessimistic
Inadequate role competency and skills
Inadequate knowledge
Inappropriate developmental expectations
Role conflict
Role confusion
Powerlessness
Inadequate coping
Anxiety or depression
Role overload
Change in other's perception of role
Change in capacity to resume role
Role dissatisfaction
Inadequate opportunities for role enactment

## Related factors
### Social

Inadequate or inappropriate linkage with the health care system
Job schedule demands
Young age, developmental level
Lack of rewards
Poverty
Family conflict
Inadequate support system
Inadequate role socialization (e.g., role model, expectations, responsibilities)
Low social economic status
Stress and conflict
Domestic violence
Lack of resources

### Knowledge

Inadequate role preparation (e.g., role transition, skill, rehearsal, validation)
Lack of knowledge about role
Role transition
Lack of opportunity for role rehearsal
Developmental transitions
Unrealistic role expectations
Education attainment level
Lack of or inadequate role model
Lack of knowledge about role skills

### Physiological

Inadequate/inappropriate linkage with health care system
Substance abuse
Mental illness
Body image alterations
Physical illness
Cognitive deficits
Health alterations (e.g., physical health, body image, self-esteem, mental health, psychosocial health, cognition, learning style, neurological health)
Depression
Low self-esteem
Pain
Fatigue

## SELF-CARE DEFICIT, BATHING/HYGIENE

Impaired ability to perform or complete bathing/hygiene activities for oneself

## Defining characteristics

Inability to get bath supplies
Inability to wash body or body parts
Inability to obtain or get to water source
Inability to regulate temperature or flow of bath water
Inability to get in and out of bathroom
Inability to dry body

**Risk factors**

Discomfort

**Related factors**

Decreased or lack of motivation
Weakness and tiredness
Severe anxiety
Inadequate to perceive body part or spatial relationship
Perceptual or cognitive impairment
Pain
Neuromuscular impairment
Musculoskeletal impairment
Environmental barriers

## SELF-CARE DEFICIT, DRESSING/GROOMING

An impaired ability to perform or complete dressing and grooming activities for oneself

**Defining characteristics**

Inability to choose clothing
Inability to use assistive devices
Inability to use zippers
Inability to remove clothes
Inability to put on socks
Inability to put on clothes on upper body
Impaired ability to put on or take off necessary items of clothing
Impaired ability to fasten clothing
Impaired ability to obtain or replace articles of clothing
Inability to maintain appearance at a satisfactory level
Inability to put on clothing on lower body
Inability to pick up clothing
Inability to put on shoes

**Related factors**

Decreased or lack or motivation
Pain
Severe anxiety
Perceptual or cognitive impairment
Neuromuscular impairment
Musculoskeletal impairment
Discomfort
Environmental barriers
Weakness or tiredness

## SELF-CARE DEFICIT, FEEDING

An impaired ability to perform or complete feeding activities

**Defining characteristics**

Inability to swallow food
Inability to prepare food for ingestion
Inability to handle utensils
Inability to chew food
Inability to use assistive device
Inability to get food onto utensil
Inability to open containers
Inability to manipulate food in mouth
Inability to ingest food safely
Inability to bring food from a receptacle to the mouth
Inability to complete a meal
Inability to ingest food in a socially acceptable manner
Inability to pick up cup or glass
Inability to ingest sufficient food

**Related factors**

Weakness or tiredness
Severe anxiety
Neuromuscular impairment
Discomfort
Environmental barriers
Decreased or lack of motivation
Musculoskeletal impairments

## SELF-CARE DEFICIT, TOILETING

An impaired ability to perform or complete own toileting activities

**Defining characteristics**

Inability to manipulate clothing
Unable to carry out proper toilet hygiene
Unable to sit on or rise from toilet or commode
Unable to get to toilet or commode
Unable to flush toilet or commode

**Related factors**

Environmental barriers
Weakness or tiredness
Decreased or lack of motivation
Severe anxiety
Impaired mobility status
Impaired transfer ability
Musculoskeletal impairment
Neuromuscular impairment
Pain
Perceptual or cognitive impairment

## SELF-ESTEEM, CHRONIC LOW

Long-standing negative self-evaluation/feelings about self or self-capabilities

**Defining characteristics**

Long-standing or chronic: self-negating verbalization
Expressions of shame/guilt
Evaluates self as unable to deal with events
Rationalizes away/rejects positive feedback and exaggerates negative feedback about self
Hesitant to try new things/situations
Frequent lack of success in work or other life events
Overly conforming, dependent on others' opinions
Lack of eye contact
Nonassertive/passive
Indecisive
Excessively seeks reassurance

**Related factors**

To be developed

## SELF-ESTEEM, SITUATIONAL LOW

Development of a negative perception of self-worth in response to a current situation (specify)

**Defining characteristics**

Verbally reports current situational challenge to self-worth
Self-negating verbalizations
Indecisive, nonassertive behavior
Evaluation of self as unable to deal with situation or events
Expressions of helplessness and uselessness

**Related factors**

Developmental changes (specify)
Disturbed body image
Functional impairment (specify)
Loss (specify)
Social role changes (specify)
Lack of recognition/rewards
Behavior inconsistent with values
Failures/rejections

## SELF-ESTEEM, SITUATIONAL LOW, RISK FOR

At risk for developing negative perception of self-worth in response to a current situation (specify)

## Risk factors

Developmental changes (specify)
Disturbed body image
Functional impairment (specify)
Loss (specify)
Social role changes (specify)
History of learned helplessness
History of abuse, neglect, or abandonment
Unrealistic self-expectations
Behavior inconsistent with values
Lack of recognition/rewards
Failures/rejections
Decreased power/control over environment
Physical illness (specify)

## SELF-MUTILATION

Deliberate self-injurious behavior causing tissue damage with the intent of causing nonfatal injury to attain relief of tension

### Defining characteristics

Cuts/scratches on body
Picking at wounds
Self-inflicted burns (e.g., eraser, cigarette)
Ingestion/inhalation of harmful substances/objects
Biting
Abrading
Severing
Insertion of object(s) into body orifice(s)
Hitting
Constricting a body part

### Related factors

Psychotic state (command hallucinations)
Inability to express tension verbally
Childhood sexual abuse
Violence between parental figures
Family divorce
Family alcoholism
Family history of self-destructive behaviors
Adolescence
Peers who self-mutilate
Isolation from peers
Perfectionism
Substance abuse
Eating disorders
Sexual identity crisis
Low or unstable self-esteem
Low or unstable body image
Labile behavior (mood swings)
History of inability to plan solutions or see long-term consequences
Use of manipulation to obtain nurturing relationship with others
Chaotic/disturbed interpersonal relationships
Emotionally disturbed; battered child
Feels threatened with actual or potential loss of significant relationship (e.g., loss of parent/parental relationship)
Experiences dissociation or depersonalization
Mounting tension that is intolerable
Impulsivity
Inadequate coping
Irresistible urge to cut/damage self
Needs quick reduction of stress
Childhood illness or surgery
Foster, group, or institutional care
Incarceration
Character disorder
Borderline personality disorder
Developmentally delayed or autistic individual
History of self-injurious behavior
Feelings of depression, rejection, self-hatred, separation anxiety, guilt, depersonalization

Poor parent-adolescent communication
Lack of family confidant

## SELF-MUTILATION, RISK FOR

At risk for deliberate self-injurious behavior causing tissue damage with the intent of causing nonfatal injury to attain relief of tension

### Risk factors

Psychotic state (command hallucinations)
Inability to express tension verbally
Childhood sexual abuse
Violence between parental figures
Family divorce
Family alcoholism
Family history of self-destructive behaviors
Adolescence
Peers who self-mutilate
Isolation from peers
Perfectionism
Substance abuse
Eating disorders
Sexual identity crisis
Low or unstable self-esteem
Low or unstable body image
History of inability to plan solutions or see long-term consequences
Use of manipulation to obtain nurturing relationship with others
Chaotic/disturbed personal relationships
Emotionally disturbed and/or battered children
Feels threatened with actual or potential loss of significant relationship
Loss of parent/parental relationships
Experiences dissociation or depersonalization
Experiences mounting tension that is intolerable
Impulsivity
Inadequate coping
Experiences irresistible urge to cut/damage self
Needs quick reduction of stress
Childhood illness or surgery
Foster, group, or institutional care
Incarceration
Character disorders
Borderline personality disorders
Loss of control over problem-solving situations
Developmentally delayed or autistic individuals
History of self-injurious behavior
Feelings of depression, rejection, self-hatred, separation anxiety, guilt, and depersonalization

## SENSORY PERCEPTION, DISTURBED (SPECIFY: VISUAL, AUDITORY, KINESTHETIC, GUSTATORY, TACTILE, OLFACTORY)

Change in the amount or patterning of incoming stimuli accompanied by a diminished, exaggerated, distorted, or impaired response to such stimuli

### Defining characteristics

Poor concentration
Auditory distortions
Change in usual response to stimuli
Restlessness
Reported or measured change in sensory acuity
Irritability
Disoriented in time, in place, or with people
Change in problem-solving abilities
Change in behavior pattern
Altered communication patterns
Hallucinations
Visual distortions

## Related factors

Altered sensory perception
Excessive environmental stimuli
Psychological stress
Altered sensory reception, transmission, and/or integration
Insufficient environmental stimuli
Biochemical imbalances for sensory distortion (e.g., illusions, hallucinations)
Electrolyte imbalance
Biochemical imbalance

## SEXUAL DYSFUNCTION

Change in sexual function that is viewed as unsatisfying, unrewarding, or inadequate

## Defining characteristics

Verbalization of problem
Alterations in achieving perceived sex role
Actual or perceived limitation imposed by disease and/or therapy
Conflicts involving values
Alterations in achieving sexual satisfaction
Inability to achieve desired satisfaction
Seeking of confirmation of desirability
Alteration in relationship with significant other
Change in interest in self and others

## Related factors

Biopsychosocial alteration of sexuality
 Ineffectual or absent role models
 Physical abuse
 Psychosocial abuse (e.g., harmful relationships)
 Vulnerability
 Misinformation or lack of knowledge
 Values conflict
 Lack of privacy
 Lack of significant other
 Altered body structure or function: pregnancy, recent childbirth, drugs, surgery, anomalies, disease process, trauma, radiation

## SEXUALITY PATTERNS, INEFFECTIVE

Expressions of concern regarding own sexuality

## Defining characteristics

Reported difficulties, limitations, or changes in sexual behaviors or activities

## Related factors

Knowledge/skill deficit about alternative responses to health-related transitions, altered body function or structure, illness, or medical treatment
Lack of privacy
Lack of significant other
Ineffective or absent role models
Conflicts with sexual orientation or variant preferences
Fear of pregnancy or of acquiring sexually transmitted disease
Impaired relationship with significant other

## SKIN INTEGRITY, IMPAIRED

Altered epidermis and/or dermis

## Defining characteristics

Disruption of skin surface
Destruction of skin layers
Invasion of body structures

## Related factors
### External

Hyperthermia or hypothermia
Chemical substance
Mechanical factors (e.g., shearing forces, pressure, restraint)

Radiation
Physical immobilization
Moisture
Medications
Extremes in age

### Internal

Altered nutritional state: obesity, emaciation
Altered metabolic state
Altered circulation
Altered sensation
Altered pigmentation
Skeletal prominence
Developmental factors
Immunological deficit
Alterations in turgor (change in elasticity)
Altered fluid status

## SKIN INTEGRITY, IMPAIRED, RISK FOR

At risk for skin being adversely altered

## Risk factors
### External

Hypothermia or hyperthermia
Chemical substance
Mechanical factors (e.g. shearing forces, pressure, restraint)
Radiation
Physical immobilization
Excretions and secretions
Humidity
Moisture
Extremes in age

### Internal

Medication
Altered nutritional state: obesity, emaciation
Altered metabolic state
Altered circulation
Altered sensation
Altered pigmentation
Skeletal prominence
Developmental factors
Alterations in skin turgor (change in elasticity)
Psychogenic
Immunological

## SLEEP DEPRIVATION

Prolonged periods of time without sleep (sustained natural, periodic suspension of relative consciousness)

## Defining characteristics

Daytime drowsiness
Decreased ability to function
Malaise
Tiredness
Lethargy
Restlessness
Irritability
Heightened sensitivity to pain
Listlessness
Apathy
Slowed reaction
Inability to concentrate
Perceptual disorders (e.g., disturbed body sensation, delusions, feeling afloat)
Hallucinations
Acute confusion
Transient paranoia
Agitated or combative
Anxious
Mild, fleeting nystagmus
Hand tremors

## Related factors

Prolonged physical discomfort
Prolonged psychological discomfort
Sustained inadequate sleep hygiene
Prolonged use of pharmacologic or dietary antisoporifics
Aging-related sleep stage shifts
Sustained circadian asynchrony
Inadequate daytime activity
Sustained environmental stimulation
Sustained unfamiliar or uncomfortable sleep environment
Non-sleep-inducing parenting practices
Sleep apnea
Periodic limb movement (e.g., restless leg syndrome, nocturnal myoclonus)
Sundowner's syndrome
Narcolepsy
Idiopathic central nervous system hypersomnolence
Sleep walking
Sleep terror
Sleep-related enuresis
Nightmares
Familial sleep paralysis
Sleep-related painful erections
Dementia

## SLEEP PATTERN, DISTURBED

Time limited disruption of sleep (natural, periodic suspension of consciousness) amount and quality

### Defining characteristics

Prolonged awakenings
Sleep maintenance insomnia
Self-induced impairment of normal pattern
Sleep onset greater than 30 minutes
Early morning insomnia
Awakening earlier or later than desired
Verbal complaints of difficulty falling asleep
Verbal complaints of not feeling well-rested
Increased proportion of Stage 1 sleep
Dissatisfaction with sleep
Less than age-normed total sleep time
Three or more nighttime awakenings
Decreased proportion of Stages 3 and 4 sleep (e.g., hyporesponsiveness, excess sleepiness, decreased motivation)
Decreased proportion of REM sleep (e.g., REM rebound, hyperactivity, emotional lability, agitation and impulsivity, atypical polysomnographic features)
Decreased ability to function

### Related factors
#### Psychological

Ruminative pre-sleep thoughts
Daytime activity pattern
Thinking about home
Body temperature
Temperament
Dietary
Childhood onset
Inadequate sleep hygiene
Sustained use of anti-sleep agents
Circadian asynchrony
Frequently changing sleep-wake schedule
Depression
Loneliness
Frequent travel across time zones
Daylight/darkness exposure
Grief
Anticipation
Shift work
Delayed or advanced sleep phase syndrome

Loss of sleep partner, life change
Preoccupation with trying to sleep
Periodic gender-related hormonal shifts
Biochemical agents
Fear
Separation from significant others
Social schedule inconsistent with chronotype
Aging-related sleep shifts
Anxiety
Medications
Fear of insomnia
Maladaptive conditioned wakefulness
Fatigue
Boredom

#### Individual

Noise
Unfamiliar sleep furnishings
Ambient temperature, humidity
Lighting
Other-generated awakening
Excessive stimulation
Physical restraint
Lack of sleep privacy/control
Nurse for therapeutics, monitoring, lab tests
Sleep partner
Noxious odors

#### Parental

Mother's sleep-wake pattern
Parent-infant interaction
Mother's emotional support

#### Physiological

Urinary urgency
Wet
Fever
Nausea
Stasis of secretions
Shortness of breath
Position
Gastroesophageal reflux

## SOCIAL INTERACTION, IMPAIRED

Insufficient or excessive quantity or ineffective quality of social exchange

### Defining characteristics

Verbalized or observed discomfort in social situations
Verbalized or observed inability to receive or communicate a satisfying sense of belonging, caring, interest, or shared history
Observed use of unsuccessful social interaction behaviors
Dysfunctional interaction with peers, family, and/or others
Family report of change in style or pattern of interaction

### Related factors

Knowledge/skill deficit about ways to enhance mutuality
Communication barriers
Self-concept disturbance
Absence of available significant others or peers
Limited physical mobility
Therapeutic isolation
Sociocultural dissonance
Environmental barriers
Altered thought processes

## SOCIAL ISOLATION

Aloneness experienced by an individual and perceived as imposed by others and as a negative or threatened state

**Defining characteristics**

*Objective*

Absence of supportive significant other(s)—family, friends, group

Sad, dull affect

Inappropriate or immature interests and activities for developmental age or stage

Uncommunicative, withdrawn; no eye contact

Preoccupation with own thoughts; repetitive, meaningless actions

Projects hostility in voice, behavior

Seeks to be alone or exists in subculture

Evidence of physical and/or mental handicap or altered state of wellness

Shows behavior unaccepted by dominant cultural group

*Subjective*

Expresses feeling of aloneness imposed by others

Expresses feelings of rejection

Experiences feelings of indifference of others

Expresses values acceptable to subculture but is unable to accept values of dominant culture

Inadequacy in or absence of significant purpose in life

Inability to meet expectations of others

Insecurity in public

Expresses interests inappropriate to developmental age or stage

**Related factors**

Factors contributing to the absence of satisfying personal relationships, such as the following:

Delay in accomplishing developmental tasks

Immature interests

Alterations in physical appearance

Alterations in mental status

Unaccepted social behavior

Unaccepted social values

Altered state of wellness

Inadequate personal resources

Inability to engage in satisfying personal relationships

**SORROW, CHRONIC**

A cyclical, recurring and potentially progressive pattern of pervasive sadness that is experience [by a client, parent or caregiver, or individual with chronic illness or disability] in response to continual loss, throughout the trajectory of an illness or disability

**Defining characteristics**

Feelings that vary in intensity, are periodic, may progress and intensify over time, and may interfere with the client's ability to reach his/her highest level of personal and social well-being

Client expresses periodic, recurrent feelings of sadness

Client expresses one or more of the following feelings: anger, being misunderstood, confusion, depression, disappointment, emptiness, fear, frustration, guilt/self-blame, helplessness, hopelessness, loneliness, low self-esteem, recurring loss, overwhelmed

**Related factors**

Death of a loved one

Person experiences chronic physical or mental illness or disability such as: mental retardation, multiple sclerosis, prematurity, spina bifida or other birth defects, chronic mental illness, infertility, cancer, Parkinson's disease

Person experiences one or more trigger events (e.g., crises in management of the illness, crises related to developmental stages and missed opportunities or milestones that bring comparisons with developmental, social, or personal norms)

Unending caregiving as a constant reminder of loss

**SPIRITUAL DISTRESS**

Disruption in the life principle that pervades a person's entire being and that integrates and transcends one's biological and psychosocial nature

**Defining characteristics**

Expresses concern with meaning of life and death and/or belief systems

Anger toward God (as defined by the person)

Questions meaning of suffering

Verbalizes inner conflict about beliefs

Verbalizes concern about relationship with deity

Questions meaning of own existence

Inability to choose or chooses not to participate in usual religious practices

Seeks spiritual assistance

Questions moral and ethical implications of therapeutic regimen

Displacement of anger toward religious representatives

Description of nightmares or sleep disturbances

Alteration in behavior or mood evidenced by anger, crying, withdrawal, preoccupation, anxiety, hostility, apathy, etc.

Regards illness as punishment

Does not experience that God is forgiving

Inability to accept self

Engages in self-blame

Denies responsibilities for problems

Description of somatic complaints

**Related factors**

Separation from religious and cultural ties

Challenged belief and value system (e.g., result of moral or ethical implications of therapy or result of intense suffering)

**SPIRITUAL DISTRESS, RISK FOR**

At risk for an altered sense of harmonious connectedness with all of life and the universe in which dimensions that transcend and empower the self may be disrupted

**Risk factors**

Energy-consuming anxiety

Low self-esteem

Mental illness

Physical illness

Blocks to self-love

Poor relationships

Physical or psychological stress

Substance abuse

Loss of loved one

Natural disasters

Situation losses

Maturational losses

Inability to forgive

**SPIRITUAL WELL-BEING, READINESS FOR ENHANCED**

Process of developing or unfolding of mystery through harmonious interconnectedness that springs from inner strengths

**Defining characteristics**

*Inner strengths*

A sense of awareness, self consciousness, sacred source, unifying force, inner core, and transcendence

*Unfolding mystery*

One's experience about life's purpose and meaning, mystery, uncertainty, and struggles

*Harmonious interconnectedness*

Relatedness, connectedness, harmony with self, others, higher power or God, and the environment

**SUFFOCATION, RISK FOR**

Accentuated risk of accidental suffocation (inadequate air available for inhalation)

## Risk factors
### Internal
Reduced olfactory sensation
Reduced motor abilities
Lack of safety education
Lack of safety precautions
Cognitive or emotional difficulties
Disease or injury process

### External
Pillow placed in infant's crib
Vehicle warming in closed garage
Children playing with plastic bags or inserting small objects into their mouths or noses
Discarded or unused refrigerators or freezers without doors removed
Children left unattended in bathtubs or pools
Household gas leaks
Smoking in bed
Use of fuel-burning heaters not vented to outside
Low-strung clothesline
Pacifier hung around infant's head
Eating large mouthfuls of food
Propped bottle placed in infant's crib

## SUICIDE, RISK FOR
At risk for self-inflicted, life-threatening injury

## Risk factors
### Behavioral
History of prior suicide attempt
Impulsiveness
Buying a gun
Stockpiling medicines
Making or changing a will
Giving away possessions
Sudden euphoric recovery from major depression
Marked changes in behavior, attitude, school performance

### Verbal
Threats to kill oneself
States desire to die/end it all

### Situational
Living alone
Retired
Relocation, institutionalization
Economic instability
Loss of autonomy/independence
Presence of gun in home
Adolescents living in nontraditional settings (e.g., juvenile detention center, prison, half-way house, group home)

### Psychological
Family history of suicide
Alcohol and substance use/abuse
Psychiatric illness/disorder (e.g., depression, schizophrenia, bipolar disorder)
Abuse in childhood
Guilt
Gay or lesbian youth

### Demographic
Age: elderly, young adult males, adolescents
Race: Caucasian, Native American
Gender: male
Divorced, widowed

### Physical
Physical illness
Terminal illness
Chronic pain

### Social
Loss of important relationship
Disrupted family life
Grief, bereavement
Poor support systems
Loneliness
Hopelessness
Helplessness
Social isolation
Legal or disciplinary problem
Cluster suicides

## SURGICAL RECOVERY, DELAYED
Extension of the number of postoperative days required to initiate and perform activities that maintain life, health, and well-being

### Defining characteristics
Evidence of interrupted healing of surgical area (e.g., red, indurated, draining, immobilized)
Loss of appetite with or without nausea
Difficulty in moving about
Requires help to complete self-care
Fatigue
Report of pain/discomfort
Postpones resumption of work/employment activities
Perception that more time is needed to recover

### Related factors
To be developed

## SWALLOWING, IMPAIRED
Abnormal functioning of the swallowing mechanism associated with deficits in oral, pharyngeal, or esophageal structure or function

### Defining characteristics
#### Pharyngeal phase impairment
Altered head positions
Inadequate laryngeal elevation
Food refusal
Unexplained fevers
Delayed swallow
Recurrent pulmonary infections
Gurgly voice quality
Nasal reflux
Choking, coughing, or gagging
Multiple swallows
Abnormality in pharyngeal phase by swallow study

#### Esophogeal phase impairment
Heartburn or epigastric pain
Acidic smelling breath
Unexplained irritability surrounding mealtime
Vomitous on pillow
Repetitive swallowing or ruminating
Regurgitation of gastric contents or wet burps
Bruxism
Nighttime coughing or awakening
Observed evidence of difficulty in swallowing (e.g., stasis of food in oral cavity, coughing/choking)
Hyperextension of head, arching during or after meals
Abnormality in esophageal phase by swallow study
Odynophagia
Food refusal or volume limiting
Complaints of "something stuck"

Hematemesis
Vomiting

### Oral phase impairment

Lack of tongue action to form bolus
Weak suck resulting in inefficient nippling
Incomplete lip closure
Food pushed out of mouth
Slow bolus formation
Food falls from mouth
Premature entry of bolus
Nasal reflux
Inability to clear oral cavity
Long meals with little consumption
Coughing, choking, gagging before a swallow
Abnormality in oral phase of swallow study
Piecemeal deglutition
Lack of chewing
Pooling in lateral sulci
Sialorrhea or drooling

### Related factors
### Congenital deficits

Upper airway anomalies
Failure to thrive or protein energy malnutrition
Conditions with significant hyptonia
Respiratory disorders
History of tube feeding
Behavioral feeding problems
Self injurious behavior
Neuromuscular impairment (e.g., decreased or absent gag reflex, decreased strength or excursion of muscles involved in mastication, perceptual impairment, facial paralysis)
Mechanical obstruction (e.g., edema, tracheostomy tube, tumor)
Congenital heart disease
Cranial nerve involvement

### Neurological problems

Upper airway anomalies
Laryngeal abnormalities
Achalasia
Gastroesophageal reflux disease
Acquired anatomic defects
Cerebral palsy
Internal traumas
Tracheal, laryngeal, esophageal defects
Traumatic head injury
Developmental delay
External traumas
Nasal or nasopharyngeal cavity defects
Oral cavity or oropharynx abnormalities
Premature infants

## THERAPEUTIC REGIMEN MANAGEMENT, COMMUNITY, INEFFECTIVE

Pattern of regulating and integrating into community processes programs for treatment of illness and the sequelae of illness that are unsatisfactory for meeting health-related goals.

### Defining characteristics

Deficits in persons and programs to be accountable for illness care of aggregates
Deficits in advocates for aggregates
Deficits in community activities for secondary and tertiary prevention
Illness symptoms above the norm expected for the number and type of population
Number of health care resources insufficient for the incidence or prevalence of illness(es)
Unavailable health care resources for illness care
Unexpected acceleration of illness

### Related factors

To be developed

## THERAPEUTIC REGIMEN MANAGEMENT FAMILIES, INEFFECTIVE

Pattern of regulating and integrating into family processes a program for treatment of illness and the sequelae of illness that is unsatisfactory for meeting specific health goals

### Defining characteristics

Inappropriate family activities for meeting the goals of a treatment or prevention program
Acceleration (expected or unexpected) of illness symptoms of a family member
Lack of attention to illness and its sequelae
Verbalized desire to manage the treatment of illness and prevention of the sequelae
Verbalized difficulty with regulation/integration of one or more effects or prevention of complications
Verbalizes that family did not take action to reduce risk factors for progression of illness and sequelae

### Related factors

Complexity of health care system
Complexity of therapeutic regimen
Decisional conflicts
Economic difficulties
Excessive demands made on individual or family
Family conflict

## THERAPEUTIC REGIMEN MANAGEMENT, EFFECTIVE

Pattern of regulating and integrating into daily living a program for treatment of illness and its sequelae that is satisfactory for meeting specific health goals

### Defining characteristics

Appropriate choices of daily activities for meeting the goals of a treatment or prevention program
Illness symptoms within a normal range of expectation
Verbalized desire to manage the treatment of illness and prevention of sequelae
Verbalized intent to reduce risk factors for progression of illness and sequelae

### Related factors

To be developed

## THERAPEUTIC REGIMEN MANAGEMENT, INEFFECTIVE

Pattern of regulating and integrating into daily living a program for treatment of illness and the sequelae of illness that is unsatisfactory for meeting specific health goals

### Defining characteristics

Choices of daily living ineffective for meeting the goals of a treatment or prevention program
Verbalizes that did not take action to reduce risk factors for progression of illness and sequelae
Verbalizes desire to manage the treatment of illness and prevention of sequelae
Verbalizes difficulty with regulation/integration of one or more prescribed regimens for prevention of complications and the treatment or illness or its effects
Verbalizes that did not take action to include treatment regimens in daily routines

### Related factors

Complexity of health care system
Complexity of therapeutic regimen
Decisional conflicts

Economic difficulties
Excessive demands made on individual or family
Family conflict
Family patterns of health care
Inadequate number and types of cues to action
Knowledge deficits
Mistrust of regimen and/or health care personnel
Perceived seriousness
Perceived susceptibility
Perceived barriers
Social support deficit
Powerlessness

## THERMOREGULATION, INEFFECTIVE

Temperature fluctuation between hypothermia and hyperthermia

### Defining characteristics

Fluctuations in body temperature above and below the normal range
Cool skin
Cyanotic nail beds
Flushed skin
Hypertension
Increased respiratory rate
Pallor (moderate)
Piloerection
Reduction in body temperature below normal range
Seizures/convulsions
Shivering (mild)
Slow capillary refill
Tachycardia
Warm to touch

### Related factors

Aging
Fluctuating environmental temperature
Immaturity
Trauma or illness

## THOUGHT PROCESSES, ALTERED

Disruption in cognitive operations or activities

### Defining characteristics

Inaccurate interpretation of environment
Cognitive dissonance
Distractibility
Memory deficit or problems
Egocentricity
Hypervigilance/hypovigilance
Inappropriate/nonreality-based thinking

### Related factors

To be developed

## TISSUE INTEGRITY, IMPAIRED

Damage to mucous membrane, corneal, integumentary, or subcutaneous tissues

### Defining characteristics

Damaged or destroyed tissue (e.g., cornea, mucous membrane, integumentary, subcutaneous)

### Related factors

Mechanical (e.g., pressure, shear, friction)
Radiation (including therapeutic radiation)
Nutritional deficit or excess
Thermal (temperature extremes)
Knowledge deficit
Irritants, chemical (including body excretions, secretions, medications)
Impaired physical mobility

Altered circulation
Fluid deficit or excess

## TISSUE PERFUSION, INEFFECTIVE (SPECIFY TYPE: RENAL, CEREBRAL, CARDIOPULMONARY, GASTROINTESTINAL, PERIPHERAL)

Decrease in oxygen resulting in the failure to nourish the tissues at the capillary level

### Defining characteristics
*Renal*

Altered blood pressure outside of acceptable parameters
Hematuria
Oliguria or anuria
Elevation in BUN/creatinine ratio

*Gastrointestinal*

Hypoactive or absent bowel sounds
Nausea
Abdominal distension
Abdominal pain or tenderness

*Peripheral*

Edema
Positive Homans' sign
Altered skin characteristics (hair, nails, moisture)
Weak or absent pulses
Skin discolorations
Skin temperature changes
Altered sensations
Claudication
Blood pressure changes in extremities
Bruits
Delayed healing
Diminished arterial pulsations
Skin color pale on elevations, color does not return on lowering the leg

*Cerebral*

Speech abnormalities
Changes in pupillary reactions
Extremity weakness or paralysis
Altered mental status
Difficulty in swallowing
Changes in motor response
Behavioral changes

*Cardiopulmonary*

Altered respiratory rate outside of acceptable parameters
Use of accessory muscles
Capillary refill >3 seconds
Abnormal arterial blood gases
Chest pain
Sense of "impending doom"
Bronchospasm
Dyspnea
Arrhythmias
Nasal flaring
Chest retraction

### Related factors

Hypovolemia
Hypervolemia
Interruption of flow, arterial
Exchange problems
Interruption of flow, venous
Mechanical reduction of venous and/or arterial blood flow
Hypoventilation
Impaired transport of the oxygen across alveolar and/or capillary membrane

Mismatch of ventilation with blood flow
Decreased hemoglobin concentration in blood
Enzyme poisoning
Altered affinity of hemoglobin for oxygen

## TRANSFER ABILITY, IMPAIRED

Limitation of independent movement between two nearby surfaces

### Defining characteristics

Impaired ability to transfer from bed to chair and chair to bed
Impaired ability to transfer on or off a toilet or commode
Impaired ability to transfer in and out of tub or shower
Impaired ability to transfer between uneven levels
Impaired ability to transfer from chair to car or car to chair
Impaired ability to transfer from chair to floor or floor to chair
Impaired ability to transfer from standing to floor or floor to standing

### Related factors

To be developed

## TRAUMA, RISK FOR

Accentuated risk of accidental tissue injury (e.g., wound, burn, fracture)

### Risk factors
*Internal*

Weakness
Poor vision
Balancing difficulties
Reduced temperature and/or tactile sensation
Reduced large—or small—muscle coordination
Reduced hand-eye coordination
Lack of safety education
Lack of safety precautions
Insufficient finances to purchase safety equipment or effect repairs
Cognitive or emotional difficulties
History of previous trauma

*External*

Slippery floors (e.g., wet or highly waxed)
Snow or ice on stairs, walkways
Unanchored rugs
Bathtub without hand grip or antislip equipment
Use of unsteady ladder or chairs
Entering unlighted rooms
Unsturdy or absent stair rails
Unanchored electric wires
Litter or liquid spills on floors or stairways
High beds
Children playing without gates at tops of stairs
Obstructed passageways
Unsafe window protection in homes with young children
Inappropriate call-for-aid mechanisms for bed-resting client
Pot handles facing toward front of stove
Bathing in very hot water (e.g., unsupervised bathing of young children)
Potential igniting of gas leaks
Delayed lighting of gas burner or oven
Experimenting with chemicals or gasoline
Unscreened fires or heaters
Wearing of plastic aprons or flowing clothing around open flame
Children playing with matches, candles, cigarettes
Inadequately stored combustibles or corrosives (e.g., matches, oily rags, lye)
Highly flammable children's toys or clothing
Overloaded fuse boxes
Contact with rapidly moving machinery, industrial belts, or pulleys
Sliding on coarse bed linen or struggling within bed restraints
Faulty electrical plugs, frayed wires, or defective appliances

Contact with acids or alkalis
Playing with fireworks or gunpowder
Contact with intense cold
Overexposure to sun, sun lamps, radiotherapy
Use of cracked dishware or glasses
Knives stored uncovered
Guns or ammunition stored unlocked
Large icicles hanging from roof
Exposure to dangerous machinery
Children playing with sharp-edged toys
High-crime neighborhood and vulnerable patient
Driving a mechanically unsafe vehicle
Driving after partaking of alcoholic beverages or drugs
Driving at excessive speeds
Driving without necessary visual aids
Children riding in front seat of car
Smoking in bed or near oxygen
Overloaded electrical outlets
Grease waste collected on stoves
Use of thin or worn pot holders or mitts
Unrestrained babies riding in car
Nonuse or misuse of seat restraints
Nonuse or misuse of necessary headgear for motorized cyclists or young children carried on adult bicycles
Unsafe road or road-crossing conditions
Play or work near vehicle pathways (e.g., driveways, lanes, railroad tracks)

## UNILATERAL NEGLECT

Lack of awareness and attention to one side of the body

### Defining characteristics

Consistent inattention to stimuli on affected side
Inadequate self-care
Positioning and/or safety precautions in regard to affected side
Does not look toward affected side
Leaves food on plate on affected side

### Related factors

Effects of disturbed perceptual abilities (e.g., hemianopsia)
One-sided blindness
Neurological illness or trauma

## URINARY ELIMINATION, IMPAIRED

Disturbance in urine elimination

### Defining characteristics

Dysuria
Frequency
Hesitancy
Incontinence
Nocturia
Retention
Urgency

### Related factors

Sensory motor impairment
Neuromuscular impairment
Mechanical trauma

## URINARY RETENTION

Incomplete emptying of the bladder.

### Defining characteristics

Bladder distention
Small, frequent voiding or absence of urine output
Sensation of bladder fullness
Dribbling
Residual urine
Dysuria
Overflow incontinence

## Related factors

High urethral pressure caused by weak detrusor
Inhibition of reflex arc
Strong sphincter
Blockage

## VENTILATION, IMPAIRED SPONTANEOUS

Decreased energy reserves results in an individual's inability to maintain breathing adequate to support life

## Defining characteristics

Dyspnea
Increased metabolic rate
Increased restlessness
Apprehension
Increased use of accessory muscles
Decreased tidal volume
Increased heart rate
Decreased $pO_2$ level
Increased $pCO_2$ level
Decreased cooperation
Decreased $SaO_2$ level

## Related factors

Metabolic factors
Respiratory muscle fatigue

## VENTILATORY WEANING RESPONSE, DYSFUNCTION (DVWR)

Inability to adjust to lowered levels of mechanical ventilator support, which interrupts and prolongs the weaning process

## Defining characteristics
## Mild DVWR

Responds to lowered levels of mechanical ventilator support with the following:
   Restlessness
   Slight increased respiratory rate from baseline
Responds to lowered levels of mechanical ventilator support with the following:
   Expressed feelings of increased need for oxygen; breathing discomfort; fatigue, warmth
   Queries about possible machine malfunction
   Increased concentration on breathing

## Moderate DVWR

Responds to lowered levels of mechanical ventilator support with the following:
   Slight increase from baseline blood pressure <20 mm Hg
   Slight increase from baseline heart rate <20 beats/minute
   Baseline increase in respiratory rate <5 breaths/minute
Hypervigilance to activities
Inability to respond to coaching
Inability to cooperate
Apprehension
Diaphoresis
Eye widening
Decreased air entry on auscultation
Color changes; pale; slight cyanosis
Slight respiratory accessory muscle use

## Severe DVWR

Responds to lowered levels of mechanical ventilator support with the following:
   Agitation
   Deterioration in arterial blood gas levels from current baseline
   Increase from baseline blood pressure >20 mm Hg
   Increase from baseline heart rate >20 beats/minute
   Respiratory rate increases significantly from baseline

Profuse diaphoresis
Full respiratory accessory muscle use
Shallow, gasping breaths
Paradoxical abdominal breathing
Discoordinated breathing with the ventilator
Decreased level of consciousness
Adventitious breath sounds, audible airway secretions
Cyanosis

## Related factors
### Physical

Ineffective airway clearance
Sleep pattern disturbance
Inadequate nutrition
Uncontrolled pain or discomfort

### Psychological

Knowledge deficit of the weaning process/patient role
Patient-perceived inefficacy about the ability to wean
Decreased motivation
Decreased self-esteem
Anxiety: moderate, severe
Fear
Hopelessness
Powerlessness
Insufficient trust in the nurse

### Situational

Uncontrolled episodic energy demands or problems
Inappropriate pacing of diminished ventilator support
Inadequate social support
Adverse environment (noisy, active environment; negative events in the room; low nurse-patient ratio; extended nurse absence from bedside; unfamiliar nursing staff)
History of ventilator dependence >1 week
History of multiple unsuccessful weaning attempts

## VIOLENCE, OTHER-DIRECTED, RISK FOR

At risk for behaviors in which an individual demonstrates that he/she can be physically, emotionally, and/or sexually harmful to others

## Risk factors

Body language: rigid posture, clenching of fists and jaw, hyperactivity, pacing, breathlessness, threatening stances
History of violence against others (e.g., hitting someone, kicking someone, spitting at someone, scratching someone, throwing objects at someone, biting someone, attempted rape, rape, sexual molestation, urinating/defecating on a person
History of threats of violence (e.g., verbal threats against property, verbal threats against person, social threats, cursing, threatening notes/letters, threatening gestures, sexual threats)
History of violent anti-social behavior (e.g., stealing, insistent borrowing, insistent demands for privileges, insistent interruption of meetings, refusal to eat, refusal to take medication, ignoring instructions)
History of violence, indirect (e.g., tearing off clothes, ripping objects off walls, writing on walls, urinating on floor, defecating on floor, stamping feet, temper tantrum, running in corridors, yelling, throwing objects, breaking a window, slamming doors, sexual advances)
Neurological impairment (e.g., positive EEG, CAT, MRI, neurological findings; head trauma; seizure disorders)
Cognitive impairment (e.g., learning disabilities, attention deficit disorder, decreased intellectual functioning)
History of childhood abuse
History of witnessing family violence
Cruelty to animals
Firesetting
Pre/perinatal complications/abnormalities

History of drug/alcohol abuse

Pathological intoxication

Psychotic symptomatology (e.g., auditory, visual, command hallucinations; paranoid delusions; loose, rambling, or illogical thought processes)

Motor vehicle offenses (e.g., frequent traffic violations, use of a motor vehicle to release anger)

Suicidal behavior

Impulsivity

Availability/possession of weapon(s)

## VIOLENCE, SELF-DIRECTED, RISK FOR

At risk for behaviors in which an individual demonstrates that he/she can be physically, emotionally and/or sexually harmful to self

### Risk factors

Age 15-19 or over 45

Marital status: single, widowed, divorced

Employment: unemployed, recent job loss/failure

Occupation: executive, administrator owner of business, professional, semiskilled worker

Interpersonal relationships: conflictual

Family background: chaotic or conflictual, history of suicide

Sexual orientation: bisexual (active), homosexual (inactive)

Physical health: hypochondriac, chronic or terminal illness

Mental health: severe depression, psychosis, severe personality disorder, alcoholism or drug abuse

Emotional status: hopelessness, despair, increased anxiety, panic, anger, hostility

History of multiple attempts

Suicidal ideation: frequent, intense prolonged

Suicidal plan: clear and specific

Lethality: method and availability of destructive means

Personal resources: poor achievement, poor insight, affect unavailable and poorly controlled

Social resources: poor rapport, socially isolated, unresponsive family

Verbal cues: talking about death, better off without me, asking questions about lethal dosages of drugs

Behavioral clues: writing forlorn love notes, directing angry messages at a significant other who has rejected the person, giving away personal items, taking out a large life insurance policy

Persons who engage in autoerotic sexual acts

## WALKING, IMPAIRED

Limitation of independent movement within the environment on foot

### Defining characteristics

Impaired ability to: climb stairs, walk required distances, walk on an incline or decline, walk on uneven surfaces, navigate curbs

### Related factors

To be developed

## WANDERING

Meandering, aimless, or repetitive locomotion that exposes the individual to harm; frequently incongruent with boundaries, limits, or obstacles

### Defining characteristics

Frequent or continuous movement from place to place, often revisiting the same destinations

Persistent locomotion in search of "missing" or unattainable people or places

Haphazard locomotion

Locomotion into unauthorized or private spaces

Locomotion resulting in unintended leaving of a premise

Long periods of locomotion without an apparent destination

Fretful locomotion or pacing

Inability to locate significant landmarks in a familiar setting

Locomotion that cannot be easily dissuaded or redirected

Following behind or shadowing a caregiver's locomotion

Trespassing

Hyperactivity

Scanning, seeking, or searching behaviors

Periods of locomotion interspersed with periods of nonlocomotion (e.g., sitting, standing, sleeping)

Getting lost

### Related factors

Cognitive impairment, specifically memory and recall deficits, disorientation, poor visuoconstructive (or visuospatial) ability, language (primarily expressive) defects

Cortical atrophy

Premorbid behavior (e.g., outgoing, sociable personality; premorbid dementia)

Separation from familiar people and places

Sedation

Emotional state, especially frustration, anxiety, boredom, or depression (agitation)

Over/understimulating social or physical environment

Physiological state or need (e.g., hunger/thirst, pain, urination, constipation)

Time of day

---

## 17-2    NANDA nomenclature conversion

| Taxonomy I nursing diagnosis | Taxonomy II nursing diagnosis | Taxonomy I nursing diagnosis | Taxonomy II nursing diagnosis |
|---|---|---|---|
| **Exchanging** | | **Exchanging—cont'd** | |
| Altered nutrition: More than body requirements | Imbalanced nutrition: More than body requirements | Constipation | Constipation |
| Altered nutrition: Less than body requirements | Imbalanced nutrition: Less than body requirements | Perceived constipation | Perceived constipation |
| | | Diarrhea | Diarrhea |
| Altered nutrition: Risk for more than body requirements | Risk for imbalanced nutrition: More than body requirements | Bowel incontinence | Bowel incontinence |
| | | Risk for constipation | Risk for constipation |
| Risk for infection | Risk for infection | Altered urinary elimination | Impaired urinary elimination |
| Risk for altered body temperature | Risk for imbalanced body temperature | Stress incontinence | Stress urinary incontinence |
| | | Reflex urinary incontinence | Reflex urinary incontinence |
| Hypothermia | Hypothermia | Urge incontinence | Urge urinary incontinence |
| Hyperthermia | Hyperthermia | Functional urinary incontinence | Functional urinary incontinence |
| Ineffective thermoregulation | Ineffective thermoregulation | Total incontinence | Total urinary incontinence |
| Dysreflexia | Autonomic dysreflexia | Risk for urinary urge incontinence | Risk for urge urinary incontinence |
| Risk for autonomic dysreflexia | Risk for autonomic dysreflexia | Urinary retention | Urinary retention |

| Taxonomy I nursing diagnosis | Taxonomy II nursing diagnosis | Taxonomy I nursing diagnosis | Taxonomy II nursing diagnosis |
|---|---|---|---|
| **Exchanging—cont'd** | | **Choosing—cont'd** | |
| Altered tissue perfusion (specify type: renal, cerebral, cardiopulmonary, gastrointestinal, peripheral) | Ineffective tissue perfusion (specify type: renal, cerebral, cardiopulmonary, gastrointestinal, peripheral) | Defensive coping | Defensive coping |
| | | Ineffective denial | Ineffective denial |
| | | Ineffective family coping: Disabling | Disabled family coping |
| Risk for fluid volume imbalance | Risk for imbalanced fluid volume | Ineffective family coping: Compromised | Compromised family coping |
| Fluid volume excess | Excess fluid volume | Family coping: Potential for growth | Readiness for enhanced family coping |
| Fluid volume deficit | Deficient fluid volume | Potential for enhanced community coping | Readiness for enhanced community coping |
| Risk for fluid volume deficit | Risk for deficient fluid volume | Ineffective community coping | Ineffective community coping |
| Decreased cardiac output | Decreased cardiac output | Ineffective management of therapeutic regimen: Individual | Ineffective therapeutic regimen management |
| Impaired gas exchange | Impaired gas exchange | | |
| Ineffective airway clearance | Ineffective airway clearance | Noncompliance (specify) | Noncompliance (specify) |
| Ineffective breathing pattern | Ineffective breathing pattern | Ineffective management of therapeutic regimen: Families | Ineffective family therapeutic regimen management |
| Inability to sustain spontaneous ventilation | Impaired spontaneous ventilation | | |
| Dysfunctional ventilatory weaning response | Dysfunctional ventilatory weaning response | Ineffective management of therapeutic regimen: Community | Ineffective community therapeutic regimen management |
| Risk for injury | Risk for injury | | |
| Risk for suffocation | Risk for suffocation | Effective management of therapeutic regimen: Individual | Effective therapeutic regimen management |
| Risk for poisoning | Risk for poisoning | | |
| Risk for trauma | Risk for trauma | Decisional conflict (specify) | Decisional conflict (specify) |
| Risk for aspiration | Risk for aspiration | Health-seeking behaviors (specify) | Health-seeking behaviors (specify) |
| Risk for disuse syndrome | Risk for disuse syndrome | | |
| Latex allergy response | Latex allergy response | **Moving** | |
| Risk for latex allergy response | Risk for latex allergy response | Impaired physical mobility | Impaired physical mobility |
| Altered protection | Ineffective protection | Risk for peripheral neurovascular dysfunction | Risk for peripheral neurovascular dysfunction |
| Impaired tissue integrity | Impaired tissue integrity | | |
| Altered oral mucous membrane | Impaired oral mucous membrane | Risk for perioperative-positioning injury | Risk for perioperative-positioning injury |
| Impaired skin integrity | Impaired skin integrity | | |
| Risk for impaired skin integrity | Risk for impaired skin integrity | Impaired walking | Impaired walking |
| Altered dentition | Impaired dentition | Impaired wheelchair mobility | Impaired wheelchair mobility |
| Decreased adaptive capacity: Intracranial | Decreased intracranial adaptive capacity | Impaired transfer ability | Impaired transfer ability |
| | | Impaired bed mobility | Impaired bed mobility |
| Energy field disturbance | Disturbed energy field | Activity intolerance | Activity intolerance |
| | | Fatigue | Fatigue |
| **Communicating** | | Risk for activity intolerance | Risk for activity intolerance |
| Impaired verbal communication | Impaired verbal communication | Sleep pattern disturbance | Disturbed sleep pattern |
| | | Sleep deprivation | Sleep deprivation |
| **Relating** | | Diversional activity deficit | Deficient diversional activity |
| Impaired social interaction | Impaired social interaction | Impaired home maintenance management | Impaired home maintenance |
| Social isolation | Social isolation | | |
| Risk for loneliness | Risk for loneliness | Altered health maintenance | Ineffective health maintenance |
| Altered role performance | Ineffective role performance | Delayed surgical recover | Delayed surgical recover |
| Altered parenting | Impaired parenting | Adult failure to thrive | Adult failure to thrive |
| Risk for altered parenting | Risk for impaired parenting | Feeding self-care deficit | Feeding self-care deficit |
| Risk for altered parent/infant/child attachment | Risk for impaired parent/infant/child attachment | Impaired swallowing | Impaired swallowing |
| | | Ineffective breastfeeding | Ineffective breastfeeding |
| Sexual dysfunction | Sexual dysfunction | Interrupted breastfeeding | Interrupted breastfeeding |
| Altered family processes | Interrupted family processes | Effective breastfeeding | Effective breastfeeding |
| Caregiver role strain | Caregiver role strain | Ineffective infant feeding pattern | Ineffective infant feeding pattern |
| Risk for caregiver role strain | Risk for caregiver role strain | | |
| Altered family processes: Alcoholism | Dysfunctional family processes: Alcoholism | Bathing/hygiene self-care deficit | Bathing/hygiene self-care deficit |
| | | Dressing/grooming self-care deficit | Dressing/grooming self-care deficit |
| Parental role conflict | Parental role conflict | | |
| Altered sexuality patterns | Ineffective sexuality patterns | Toileting self-care deficit | Toileting self-care deficit |
| | | Altered growth and development | Delayed growth and development |
| **Valuing** | | | |
| Spiritual distress (distress of the human spirit) | Spiritual distress | Risk for altered development | Risk for delayed development |
| | | Risk for altered growth | Risk for disproportionate growth |
| Risk for spiritual distress | Risk for spiritual distress | | |
| Potential for enhanced spiritual well-being | Readiness for enhanced spiritual well-being | Relocation stress syndrome | Relocation stress syndrome |
| | | Risk for disorganized infant behavior | Risk for disorganized infant behavior |
| **Choosing** | | | |
| Ineffective individual coping | Ineffective coping | | |
| Impaired adjustment | Impaired adjustment | | |

| Taxonomy I nursing diagnosis | Taxonomy II nursing diagnosis | Taxonomy I nursing diagnosis | Taxonomy II nursing diagnosis |
|---|---|---|---|
| **Moving—cont'd** | | **Feeling—cont'd** | |
| Disorganized infant behavior | Disorganized infant behavior | Dysfunctional grieving | Dysfunctional grieving |
| Potential for enhanced organized infant behavior | Readiness for enhanced organized infant behavior | Anticipatory grieving | Anticipatory grieving |
| | | Chronic sorrow | Chronic sorrow |
| **Perceiving** | | Risk for violence: Directed at others | Risk for other-directed violence |
| Body image disturbance | Disturbed body image | Risk for self-mutilation | Risk for self-mutilation |
| Chronic low self-esteem | Chronic low self-esteem | Risk for violence: Self-directed | Risk for self-directed violence |
| Situational low self-esteem | Situational low self-esteem | Post-trauma syndrome | Post-trauma syndrome |
| Personal identity disturbance | Disturbed personal identity | Rape-trauma syndrome | Rape-trauma syndrome |
| Sensory/perceptual alterations (specify: visual, auditory, kinesthetic, gustatory, tactile, olfactory) | Disturbed sensory perception (specify: visual, auditory, kinesthetic, gustatory, tactile, olfactory) | Rape-trauma syndrome: Compound reaction | Rape-trauma syndrome: Compound reaction |
| | | Rape-trauma syndrome: Silent reaction | Rape-trauma syndrome: Silent reaction |
| Unilateral neglect | Unilateral neglect | Risk for post-trauma syndrome | Risk for post-trauma syndrome |
| Hopelessness | Hopelessness | Anxiety | Anxiety |
| Powerlessness | Powerlessness | Death anxiety | Death anxiety |
| | | Fear | Fear |
| **Knowing** | | | |
| Knowledge deficit (specify) | Deficient knowledge (specify) | | **New to taxonomy II** |
| Impaired environmental-interpretation syndrome | Impaired interpretation syndrome | | Risk for falls |
| | | | Risk for powerlessness |
| Acute confusion | Acute confusion | | Risk for relocation stress syndrome |
| Chronic confusion | Chronic confusion | | |
| Altered thought processes | Disturbed thought processes | | Risk for situational low self-esteem |
| Impaired memory | Impaired memory | | |
| | | | Self-mutilation |
| **Feeling** | | | Risk for suicide |
| Pain | Acute pain | | Wandering |
| Chronic pain | Chronic pain | | |
| Nausea | Nausea | | |

## 17-3 Taxonomy II: domains, classes, diagnostic concepts, and diagnoses

### DOMAIN 1 HEALTH PROMOTION

The awareness of well-being or normality of function and the strategies used to maintain control of and enhance that well-being or normality of function

**Class 1 Health Awareness** Recognition of normal function and well-being

**Class 2 Health Management** Identifying, controlling, performing, and integrating activities to maintain health and well-being

| Diagnostic Concepts | Approved Diagnoses | |
|---|---|---|
| Therapeutic regimen management | 00082 | Effective therapeutic regimen management |
| | 00078 | Ineffective therapeutic regimen management |
| | 00080 | Ineffective family therapeutic regimen management |
| | 00081 | Ineffective community therapeutic regimen management |
| Health-seeking behaviors | 00084 | Health-seeking behaviors (specify) |
| Health maintenance | 00099 | Ineffective health maintenance |
| Home maintenance | 00098 | Impaired home maintenance |

### DOMAIN 2 NUTRITION

The activities of taking in, assimilating, and using nutrients for the purposes of tissue maintenance, tissue repair, and the production of energy

**Class 1 Ingestion** Taking food or nutrients into the body

| Diagnostic Concepts | Approved Diagnoses | |
|---|---|---|
| Infant feeding pattern | 00107 | Ineffective infant feeding pattern |
| Swallowing | 00103 | Impaired swallowing |
| Nutrition | 00002 | Imbalanced nutrition: Less than body requirements |
| Nutrition | 00001 | Imbalanced nutrition: More than body requirements |
| | 00003 | Risk for imbalanced nutrition: More than body requirements |

**Class 2 Digestion** The physical and chemical activities that convert foodstuffs into substances suitable for absorption and assimilation

**Class 3 Absorption** The act of taking up nutrients through body tissues

**Class 4 Metabolism** The chemical and physical processes occurring in living organisms and cells for the development and use of protoplasm, production of waste and energy, with the release of energy for all vital processes

**Class 5 Hydration** The taking in and absorption of fluids and electrolytes

| Diagnostic Concepts | Approved Diagnoses | |
|---|---|---|
| Fluid volume | 00027 | Deficient fluid volume |
| | 00028 | Risk for deficient fluid volume |
| | 00026 | Excess fluid volume |
| | 00025 | Risk for fluid volume imbalance |

### DOMAIN 3 ELIMINATION

Secretion and excretion of waste products from the body

**Class 1 Urinary System** The process of secretion and excretion of urine

| Diagnostic Concepts | Approved Diagnoses | |
|---|---|---|
| Urinary elimination | 00016 | Impaired urinary elimination |
| Urinary retention | 00023 | Urinary retention |
| Urinary incontinence | 00021 | Total urinary incontinence |
| | 00020 | Functional urinary incontinence |
| | 00017 | Stress urinary incontinence |
| | 00019 | Urge urinary incontinence |
| | 00018 | Reflex urinary incontinence |
| | 00022 | Risk for urge urinary incontinence |

**Class 2 Gastrointestinal System** Excretion and expulsion of waste products from the bowel

| Diagnostic Concepts | Approved Diagnoses | |
|---|---|---|
| Bowel incontinence | 00014 | Bowel incontinence |
| Diarrhea | 00013 | Diarrhea |
| Constipation | 00011 | Constipation |
| | 00015 | Risk for constipation |
| | 00012 | Perceived constipation |

**Class 3 Integumentary System** Process of secretion and excretion through the skin

**Class 4 Pulmonary System** Removal of byproducts of metabolic products, secretions, and foreign material from the lung or bronchi

| Diagnostic Concepts | Approved Diagnoses | |
|---|---|---|
| Gas exchange | 00030 | Impaired gas exchange |

# DOMAIN 4 ACTIVITY/REST

The production, conservation, expenditure, or balance of energy resources

**Class 1 Sleep/Rest** Slumber, repose, ease, or inactivity

| Diagnostic Concepts | Approved Diagnoses | |
|---|---|---|
| Sleep pattern | 00095 | Disturbed sleep pattern |
| | 00096 | Sleep deprivation |

**Class 2 Activity/Exercise** Moving parts of the body (mobility), doing work, or performing actions often (but not always) against resistance

| Diagnostic Concepts | Approved Diagnoses | |
|---|---|---|
| Disuse syndrome | 00040 | Risk for disuse syndrome |
| Mobility | 00085 | Impaired physical mobility |
| | 00091 | Impaired bed mobility |
| | 00089 | Impaired wheelchair mobility |
| Transfer ability | 00090 | Impaired transfer ability |
| Walking | 00088 | Impaired walking |
| Diversional activity | 00097 | Deficient diversional activity |
| Wandering | 00154 | Wandering |
| Self-care deficit | 00109 | Dressing/grooming deficit |
| | 00108 | Bathing/hygiene self-care deficit |
| | 00102 | Feeding self-care deficit |
| | 00110 | Toileting self-care deficit |
| Surgical recover | 00100 | Delayed surgical recovery |

**Class 3 Energy Balance** A dynamic state of harmony between intake and expenditure of resources

| Diagnostic Concepts | Approved Diagnoses | |
|---|---|---|
| Energy field | 00050 | Disturbed energy field |
| Fatigue | 00093 | Fatigue |

**Class 4 Cardiovascular/Pulmonary Responses** Cardiopulmonary mechanisms that support activity/rest

| Diagnostic Concepts | Approved Diagnoses | |
|---|---|---|
| Cardiac output | 00029 | Decreased cardiac output |
| Spontaneous ventilation | 00033 | Impaired spontaneous ventilation |
| Breathing patter | 00032 | Ineffective breathing pattern |
| Activity tolerance | 00092 | Activity intolerance |
| | 00094 | Risk for activity intolerance |
| Ventilatory weaning | 00034 | Dysfunctional ventilatory weaning response |
| Tissue perfusion | 00024 | Ineffective tissue perfusion (specify type: renal, cerebral, cardiopulmonary, gastrointestinal, peripheral) |

# DOMAIN 5 PERCEPTION/COGNITION

The human information processing system including attention, orientation, sensation, perception, cognition, and communication

**Class 1 Attention** Mental readiness to notice or observe

| Diagnostic Concepts | Approved Diagnoses | |
|---|---|---|
| Unilateral neglect | 00123 | Unilateral neglect |

**Class 2 Orientation** Awareness of time, place, and person

| Diagnostic Concepts | Approved Diagnoses | |
|---|---|---|
| Environmental interpretation | 00127 | Impaired environmental interpretation syndrome |

**Class 3 Sensation/Perception** Receiving information through the senses of touch, taste, smell, vision, hearing, and kinesthesia and the comprehension of sense data resulting in naming, associating, and/or pattern recognition

| Diagnostic Concepts | Approved Diagnoses | |
|---|---|---|
| Sensory perception | 00122 | Disturbed sensory perception (specify: visual, auditory, kinesthetic, gustatory, tactile, olfactory) |

**Class 4 Cognition** Use of memory, learning, thinking, problem solving, abstraction, judgment, insight, intellectual capacity, calculation, and language

| Diagnostic Concepts | Approved Diagnoses | |
|---|---|---|
| Knowledge | 00126 | Deficient knowledge (specify) |
| Confusion | 00128 | Acute confusion |
| | 00129 | Chronic confusion |
| Memory | 00131 | Impaired memory |
| Thought processes | 00130 | Disturbed thought processes |

**Class 5 Communication** Sending and receiving verbal and nonverbal information

| Diagnostic Concepts | Approved Diagnoses | |
|---|---|---|
| Verbal communication | 00051 | Impaired verbal communication |

# DOMAIN 6 SELF-PERCEPTION

Awareness about the self

**Class 1 Self-Concept** The perception(s) about the total self

| Diagnostic Concepts | Approved Diagnoses | |
|---|---|---|
| Identity | 00121 | Disturbed personal identity |
| | 00125 | Powerlessness |
| | 00152 | Risk for powerlessness |
| | 00124 | Hopelessness |
| Loneliness | 00054 | Risk for loneliness |

*Class 2 Self-esteem* Assessment of one's own worth, capability, significance, and success

| Diagnostic Concepts | Approved Diagnoses | |
|---|---|---|
| Self-esteem | 00119 | *Chronic low self-esteem* |
| | 00120 | *Situational low self-esteem* |
| | 00153 | *Risk for situational low self-esteem* |

*Class 3 Body Image* A mental image of one's own body

| Diagnostic Concepts | Approved Diagnoses | |
|---|---|---|
| Body image | 00118 | *Disturbed body image* |

## DOMAIN 7 ROLE RELATIONSHIPS

The positive and negative connections or associations between persons or groups of persons and the means by which those connections are demonstrated

*Class 1 Caregiving Roles* Socially expected behavior patterns by persons providing care who are not health care professionals

| Diagnostic Concepts | Approved Diagnoses | |
|---|---|---|
| Caregiver role strain | 00061 | *Caregiver role strain* |
| | 00062 | *Risk for caregiver role strain* |
| Parenting | 00056 | *Impaired parenting* |
| | 00057 | *Risk for impaired parenting* |

*Class 2 Family Relationships* Associations of people who are biologically related or related by choice

| Diagnostic Concepts | Approved Diagnoses | |
|---|---|---|
| Family processes | 00060 | *Interrupted family processes* |
| | 00063 | *Dysfunctional family processes: Alcoholism* |
| Attachment | 00058 | *Risk for impaired parent/infant/child attachment* |

*Class 3 Role Performance* Quality of functioning in socially expected behavior patterns

| Diagnostic Concepts | Approved Diagnoses | |
|---|---|---|
| Breastfeeding | 00106 | *Effective breastfeeding* |
| | 00104 | *Ineffective breastfeeding* |
| | 00105 | *Interrupted breastfeeding* |
| Role performance | 00055 | *Ineffective role performance* |
| | 00064 | *Parental role conflict* |
| Social interaction | 00052 | *Impaired social interaction* |

## DOMAIN 8 SEXUALITY

Sexual identity, sexual function, and reproduction

*Class 1 Sexual Identity* The state of being a specific person in regard to sexuality and/or gender

*Class 2 Sexual Function* The capacity or ability to participate in sexual activities

| Diagnostic Concepts | Approved Diagnoses | |
|---|---|---|
| Sexual function | 00059 | *Sexual dysfunction* |
| Sexual patterns | 00065 | *Ineffective sexuality patterns* |

*Class 3 Reproduction* Any process by which new individuals (people) are produced

## DOMAIN 9 COPING/STRESS TOLERANCE

Contending with life events/life processes

*Class 1 Post-Trauma Responses* Reactions occurring after physical or psychological trauma

| Diagnostic Concepts | Approved Diagnoses | |
|---|---|---|
| Relocation stress | 00114 | *Relocation stress syndrome* |
| Relocation stress | 00149 | *Risk for relocation stress syndrome* |
| Rape-trauma | 00142 | *Rape-trauma syndrome* |
| | 00144 | *Rape-trauma syndrome: Silent reaction* |
| | 00143 | *Rape-trauma syndrome: Compound reaction* |
| Post-trauma response | 00141 | *Post-trauma syndrome* |
| | 00145 | *Risk for post-trauma syndrome* |

*Class 2 Coping Responses* The process of managing environmental stress

| Diagnostic Concepts | Approved Diagnoses | |
|---|---|---|
| Fear | 00148 | *Fear* |
| Anxiety | 00146 | *Anxiety* |
| | 00147 | *Death anxiety* |
| Sorrow | 00137 | *Chronic sorrow* |
| Denial | 00072 | *Ineffective denial* |
| | 00136 | *Anticipatory grieving* |
| | 00135 | *Dysfunctional grieving* |
| Adjustment | 00070 | *Impaired adjustment* |
| Coping | 00069 | *Ineffective coping* |
| | 00073 | *Disabled family coping* |
| | 00074 | *Compromised family coping* |
| | 00071 | *Defensive coping* |
| | 00077 | *Ineffective community coping* |
| | 00075 | *Readiness for enhanced family coping* |
| | 00076 | *Readiness for enhanced community coping* |

*Class 3 Neurobehavioral Stress* Behavioral responses reflecting nerve and brain function

| Diagnostic Concepts | Approved Diagnoses | |
|---|---|---|
| Dysreflexia | 00009 | *Autonomic dysreflexia* |
| | 00010 | *Risk for autonomic dysreflexia* |
| Infant behavior | 00116 | *Disorganized infant behavior* |
| | 00115 | *Risk for disorganized infant behavior* |
| | 00117 | *Readiness for enhanced organized infant behavior* |
| Adaptive capacity | 00049 | *Decreased intracranial adaptive capacity* |

## DOMAIN 10 LIFE PRINCIPLES

Principles underlying conduct, thought and behavior about acts, customs, or institutions viewed as being true or having intrinsic worth

*Class 1 Values* The identification and ranking of preferred modes of conduct or end states

*Class 2 Beliefs* Opinions, expectations, or judgments about acts, customs, or institutions viewed as being true or having intrinsic worth

| Diagnostic Concepts | Approved Diagnoses | |
|---|---|---|
| Spiritual well-being | 00068 | *Readiness for enhanced spiritual well-being* |

*Class 3 Value/Belief/Action Congruence* The correspondence or balance achieved between values, beliefs, and actions

| Diagnostic Concepts | Approved Diagnoses | |
|---|---|---|
| Spiritual distress | 00066 | *Spiritual distress* |
| | 00067 | *Risk for spiritual distress* |
| Decisional conflict | 00083 | *Decisional conflict (specify)* |
| Noncompliance | 00079 | *Noncompliance (specify)* |

## DOMAIN 11 SAFETY/PROTECTION

Freedom from danger, physical injury or immune system damage, preservation from loss, and protection of safety and security

*Class 1 Infection* Host responses following pathogenic invasion

| Diagnostic Concepts | Approved Diagnoses |
|---|---|
| Infection | 00004   Risk for infection |

*Class 2 Physical Injury* Bodily harm or hurt

| Diagnostic Concepts | Approved Diagnoses |
|---|---|
| Oral mucous membrane | 00045   Impaired oral mucous membrane |
| Injury | 00035   Risk for injury |
| | 00087   Risk for perioperative positioning injury |
| | 00155   Risk for falls |
| Trauma | 00038   Risk for trauma |
| Skin integrity | 00046   Impaired skin integrity |
| | 00047   Risk for impaired skin integrity |
| Tissue integrity | 00044   Impaired tissue integrity |
| Dentition | 00048   Impaired dentition |
| Suffocation | 00036   Risk for suffocation |
| Aspiration | 00039   Risk for aspiration |
| Airway clearance | 00031   Ineffective airway clearance |
| Neurovascular function | 00086   Risk for peripheral neurovascular dysfunction |
| Protection | 00043   Ineffective protection |

*Class 3 Violence* The exertion of excessive force or power so as to cause injury or abuse

| Diagnostic Concepts | Approved Diagnoses |
|---|---|
| Self-mutilation | 00139   Risk for self-mutilation |
| | 00151   Self-mutilation |
| Violence | 00138   Risk for other-directed violence |
| | 00140   Risk for self-directed violence |
| | 00150   Risk for suicide |

*Class 4 Environmental Hazards* Sources of danger in the surroundings

| Diagnostic Concepts | Approved Diagnoses |
|---|---|
| Poisoning | 00037   Risk for poisoning |

*Class 5 Defensive Processes* The processes by which the self protects itself from the nonself

| Diagnostic Concepts | Approved Diagnoses |
|---|---|
| Latex allergy response | 00041   Latex allergy response |
| | 00042   Risk for latex allergy response |

*Class 6 Thermoregulation* The physiologic process of regulating heat and energy within the body for purposes of protecting the organism

| Diagnostic Concepts | Approved Diagnoses |
|---|---|
| Body temperature | 00005   Risk for imbalanced body temperature |
| Thermoregulation | 00008   Ineffective thermoregulation |
| | 00006   Hypothermia |
| | 00007   Hyperthermia |

## DOMAIN 12 COMFORT

Sense of mental, physical, or social well-being or ease

*Class 1 Physical Comfort* Sense of well-being or ease

| Diagnostic Concepts | Approved Diagnoses |
|---|---|
| Pain | 00132   Acute pain |
| | 00133   Chronic pain |
| Nausea | 00134   Nausea |

*Class 2 Environmental Comfort* Sense of well-being or ease in/with one's environment

*Class 3 Social Comfort* Sense of well-being or ease with one's social situations

| Diagnostic Concepts | Approved Diagnoses |
|---|---|
| Social isolation | 00053   Social isolation |

## DOMAIN 13 GROWTH/DEVELOPMENT

Age-appropriate increases in physical dimensions, organ systems, and/or attainment of developmental milestones

*Class 1 Growth* Increases in physical dimensions or maturity of organ systems

| Diagnostic Concepts | Approved Diagnoses |
|---|---|
| Growth | 00113   Risk for disproportionate growth |
| Failure to thrive | 00101   Adult failure to thrive |

*Class 2 Development* Attainment, lack of attainment, or loss of developmental milestones

| Diagnostic Concepts | Approved Diagnoses |
|---|---|
| Development | 00111   Delayed growth and development |
| | 00112   Risk for delayed development |

---

## 17-4   Nursing diagnoses relevant to diseases, disorders, and procedures

### ABDOMINAL SURGERY

Acute **Pain** related to surgical procedure

**Constipation** related to decreased activity, decreased fluid intake, anesthesia, narcotics

Imbalanced **nutrition**: less than body requirements related to high metabolic needs, decreased ability to digest food

Ineffective **health** maintenance related to deficit knowledge regarding self-care after surgery

Risk for ineffective **tissue** perfusion: peripheral related to immobility, abdominal surgery resulting in stasis of blood flow

Adapted from Ackley JB, Ladwig BG: *Nursing diagnosis handbook: a guide to planning care,* ed 5, St Louis, 2002, Mosby.

Risk for **infection** related to invasive procedure
See Surgery

### ACQUIRED IMMUNE DEFICIENCY SYNDROME

See AIDS

### ACTIVITY INTOLERANCE

**Activity** intolerance related to bedrest/immobility, generalized weakness, sedentary life-style, imbalance between oxygen supply/demand, pain

### ACTIVITY INTOLERANCE, POTENTIAL TO DEVELOP

Risk for **activity** intolerance related to deconditioned status, presence of circulatory/respiratory problems, inexperience with activity

## ACUTE BACK

Acute **Pain** related to injury to muscles, nerves
**Anxiety** related to situational crisis, back injury
**Constipation** related to decreased activity
Impaired physical **mobility** related to pain
Ineffective **coping** related to situational crisis, back injury
Ineffective **Health** Maintenance related to deficient knowledge regarding self-care with painful back

## ACUTE CONFUSION

Acute **confusion** related to being more than 60 years of age, dementia, alcohol abuse, drug abuse, delirium

## ADDICTION

See Alcoholism; Drug Abuse

## ADJUSTMENT DISORDER

**Anxiety** related to inability to cope with psychosocial stressor
Disturbed personal **identity** related to psychosocial stressor (specific to individual)
Impaired **adjustment** related to assault to self-esteem
Impaired **social** interaction related to absence of significant others or peers
Situational low **self-esteem** related to change in role function

## ADJUSTMENT IMPAIRMENT

Impaired **adjustment** related to disability requiring change in lifestyle, inadequate support systems, impaired cognition, sensory overload, assault to self-esteem, altered locus of control, incomplete grieving

## ADULT RESPIRATORY DISTRESS SYNDROME

See ARDS

## AFFECTIVE DISORDERS

Adult **failure** to thrive related to altered mood state
Chronic low **self-esteem** related to repeated unmet expectations
Chronic **sorrow** related to chronic mental illness
**Constipation** related to inactivity, decreased fluid intake
Disturbed **sleep** pattern related to inactivity
Dysfunctional **grieving** related to lack of previous resolution of former grieving response
**Fatigue** related to psychological demands
**Hopelessness** related to feeling of abandonment, long-term stress
Ineffective **coping** related to dysfunctional grieving
Ineffective **Health** Maintenance related to lack of ability to make good judgments regarding ways to obtain help
Risk for **loneliness** related to pattern of social isolation, feelings of low self-esteem
Risk for self-directed **violence** related to panic state
**Self-care** deficit: specify related to depression, cognitive impairment
**Sexual** dysfunction related to loss of sexual desire
**Social** isolation related to ineffective **coping**
See specific disorder: Depression; Manic Disorder, Bipolar I

## AIDS (ACQUIRED IMMUNE DEFICIENCY SYNDROME)

Anticipatory **grieving**: family/parental related to potential/impending death of loved one
Altered **sexuality** pattern related to possible transmission of disease
Anticipatory **grieving**: individual related to loss of physiopsychosocial well-being
Disturbed **body** image related to chronic contagious illness, cachexia
**Caregiver** role strain related to unpredictable illness course, presence of situation stressors
Chronic **pain** related to tissue inflammation and destruction
Chronic **sorrow** related to living with long-term chronic illness
Death **anxiety** related to fear of premature death
**Diarrhea** related to inflammatory bowel changes
Disturbed **energy** field related to chronic illness
**Fatigue** related to disease process, stress, poor nutritional intake

**Fear** related to powerlessness, threat to well-being
**Hopelessness** related to deteriorating physical condition
Imbalanced **nutrition**: less than body requirements related to decreased ability to eat and absorb nutrients secondary to anorexia, nausea, diarrhea
Ineffective **Health** Maintenance related to deficient knowledge regarding transmission of infection, lack of exposure to information, misinterpretation of information
Ineffective **protection** related to risk for infection secondary to inadequate immune system
Interrupted **family** processes related to distress about diagnosis of human immunodeficiency virus (HIV) infection
Risk for deficient **fluid** volume related to diarrhea, vomiting, fever, bleeding
Risk for **infection** related to inadequate immune system
Risk for **loneliness** related to social isolation
Risk for disturbed **thought** processes related to infection in brain
Risk for impaired **oral** mucous membranes related to immunological deficit
Risk for impaired **skin** integrity related to immunological deficit, diarrhea
Risk for **spiritual** distress related to physical illness
Situational low **self-esteem** related to crisis of chronic contagious illness
**Social** isolation related to self-concept disturbance, therapeutic isolation
**Spiritual** distress related to challenged beliefs or moral system
See AIDS in Child; Cancer; Pneumonia

## AIDS DEMENTIA

Impaired **environmental** interpretation syndrome related to viral invasion of nervous system
See Dementia

## AIRWAY OBSTRUCTION/SECRETIONS

Ineffective **airway** clearance related to decreased energy; fatigue; tracheobronchial infection, obstruction, secretions; perceptual/cognitive impairment; trauma; decreased force of cough because of aging

## ALCOHOL WITHDRAWAL

Acute **confusion** related to effects of alcohol withdrawal
**Anxiety** related to situational crisis, withdrawal
Chronic low **self-esteem** related to repeated unmet expectations
Disturbed **sensory** perception: visual, auditory, kinesthetic, tactile, olfactory related to neurochemical imbalance in brain
Disturbed **sleep** pattern related to effect of depressants, alcohol withdrawal, anxiety
Disturbed **thought** processes related to potential delirium tremors
Dysfunctional **family** processes: alcoholism related to abuse of alcohol
Imbalanced **nutrition**: less than body requirements related to poor dietary habits
Ineffective **coping** related to personal vulnerability
Ineffective **Health** Maintenance related to deficient knowledge regarding chronic illness or effects of alcohol consumption
Risk for deficient **fluid** volume related to excessive diaphoresis, agitation, decreased fluid intake
Risk for **violence** related to substance withdrawal

## ALCOHOLISM

Acute **confusion** related to alcohol abuse
**Anxiety** related to loss of control
Compromised/dysfunctional family **coping** related to codependency issues
**Coping**, defensive related to alcoholism
**Denial**, ineffective related to refusal to deny alcoholism
Disturbed **sleep** pattern related to irritability, nightmares, tremors
**Impaired** adjustment related to lack of motivation to change behaviors

Impaired **environmental** interpretation syndrome related to neurological effects of chronic alcohol intake

Impaired **home** maintenance related to memory deficits, fatigue

Impaired **memory** related to alcohol abuse

Ineffective **coping** related to use of alcohol to cope with life events

Imbalanced **nutrition**: less than body requirements related to anorexia

Ineffective **protection** related to malnutrition, sleep deprivation

Interrupted **family** process: alcoholism related to alcohol abuse

**Powerlessness** related to alcohol addiction

Risk for **injury** related to alteration in sensory/perceptual function

Risk for **loneliness** related to unacceptable social behavior

Risk for **violence** related to reactions to substances used, impulsive behavior, disorientation, impaired judgment

**Self-esteem** disturbance related to failure at life events

**Social** isolation related to unacceptable social behavior, values

## ALCOHOLISM, ALTERED FAMILY PROCESS

Altered **family** process, alcoholism related to abuse of alcohol, genetic predisposition, lack of problem-solving skills, inadequate coping skills, family history of alcoholism, resistance to treatment, biochemical influences, addictive personality

## ALLERGIES

Ineffective **Health** Maintenance related to deficient knowledge regarding allergies

Latex **allergy** related to hypersensitivity to natural rubber latex

Risk for latex **allergy** related to repeated exposure to products containing latex

## ALZHEIMER TYPE DEMENTIA

Adult **failure** to thrive related to difficulty in reasoning, judgment, memory, concentration

Disturbed **thought** processes related to chronic organic disorder

**Caregiver** role strain related to duration and extent of caregiving required

Chronic **confusion** related to Alzheimer's disease

Compromised family **coping** related to interrupted family processes

Disturbed **sleep** pattern related to neurological impairment, daytime naps

**Fear** related to loss of self

**Hopelessness** related to deteriorating condition

Impaired **environmental** interpretation syndrome related to Alzheimer's disease

Impaired **home** maintenance related to impaired cognitive function, inadequate support systems

Impaired **memory** related to neurological disturbance

Impaired physical **mobility** related to severe neurological dysfunction

Ineffective **Health** Maintenance related to deficient knowledge of caregiver regarding appropriate care

**Powerlessness** related to deteriorating condition

Risk for **injury** related to confusion

Risk for **loneliness** related to potential social isolation

Risk for other-directed **violence** related to frustration, fear, anger

**Self-care** deficit: specify related to psychological-physiological impairment

**Social** isolation related to fear of disclosure of memory loss

## AMPUTATION

Chronic **sorrow** related to grief associated with loss of body part

Disturbed **body** image related to negative effects of amputation, response from others

**Grieving** related to loss of body part, future life-style changes

Impaired physical **mobility** related to musculoskeletal impairment, limited movement

Impaired **skin** integrity related to poor healing, prosthesis rubbing

Ineffective **Health** Maintenance related to deficient knowledge of care of stump, rehabilitation

Ineffective **tissue** perfusion: peripheral related to impaired arterial circulation

**Pain** related to surgery, phantom limb sensation

Risk for deficient **fluid** volume: hemorrhage related to vulnerable surgical site

## ANAPHYLACTIC SHOCK

Impaired spontaneous **ventilation** related to acute airway obstruction

Ineffective **airway** clearance related to laryngeal edema, bronchospasm

Latex **allergy** response related to no immune mechanism response

See Shock

## ANEMIA

**Anxiety** related to cause of disease

Delayed **surgical** recovery related to decreased oxygen supply to body, increased cardiac workload

**Fatigue** related to decreased oxygen supply to the body, increased cardiac workload

Impaired **memory** related to anemia

Ineffective **Health** Maintenance related to deficient knowledge regarding nutritional and medical treatment of anemia

Ineffective **protection** related to bleeding disorder

Risk for **injury** related to alteration in peripheral sensory perception

## ANEMIA, SICKLE CELL

See Anemia; Sickle Cell Anemia/Crisis

## ANEURYSM, ABDOMINAL SURGERY

Risk for deficient **fluid** volume: hemorrhage related to potential abnormal blood loss

Risk for ineffective **tissue** perfusion: peripheral related to impaired arterial circulation

Risk for **infection** related to invasive procedure

See Abdominal Surgery

## ANEURYSM, CEREBRAL

See Craniectomy/Craniotomy; Subarachnoid Hemorrhage (if aneurysm has ruptured)

## ANGINA PECTORIS

**Activity** intolerance related to acute pain, dysrhythmias

Altered **sexuality** pattern related to disease process, medications, loss of libido

**Anxiety** related to situational crisis

Decreased **cardiac** output related to myocardial ischemia, medication effect, dysrhythmia

**Grieving** related to pain, life-style changes

Ineffective **coping** related to personal vulnerability to situational crisis of new diagnosis, deteriorating health

Ineffective **denial** related to deficient knowledge(delays seeking help when symptoms occur)

Ineffective **Health** Maintenance related to deficient knowledge of care of angina condition

**Pain** related to myocardial ischemia

## ANOREXIA

Deficient **fluid** volume related to inability to drink

Delayed **surgical** recovery related to inadequate nutritional intake

Imbalanced **nutrition**: less than body requirements related to loss of appetite, nausea, vomiting

## ANTISOCIAL PERSONALITY DISORDER

Defensive **coping** related to excessive use of projection

Disturbed **thought** processes related to internal turmoil and conflict (intrusive thinking)

**Hopelessness** related to abandonment

Impaired **social** interaction related to sociocultural conflict, chemical dependence, inability to form relationships

Ineffective **coping** related to frequently violating the norms and rules of society

Ineffective family **therapeutic** regimen management related to excessive demands on family

Risk for **loneliness** related to inability to interact appropriately with others

Risk for impaired **parenting** related to inability to function as parent or guardian, emotional instability

Risk for **self-mutilation** related to self-hatred, depersonalization

Risk for other directed **violence** related to history of violence

**Spiritual** distress related to separation from religious/cultural ties

## ANXIETY

**Anxiety** related to exposure to toxins, threat to or change in role status, unconscious conflict about essential goals and values of life, familial association/heredity, unmet needs, interpersonal transmission/contagion, situational/maturational crises, threat of death, threat to or change in health status, threat to or change in interaction patterns, threat to or change in role function, threat to self-concept, unconscious conflict regarding essential values/goals of life, threat to or change in environment, stress, threat to or change in economic status, substance abuse

## ANXIETY DISORDER

**Anxiety** related to unmet security and safety needs

Death **anxiety** related to fears of unknown, powerlessness

Decisional **conflict** related to low self-esteem, fear of making a mistake

Defensive **coping** related to overwhelming feelings of dread

Disabled family **coping** related to ritualistic behavior, actions

Disturbed **energy** field related to hopelessness, helplessness, fear

Disturbed **sleep** pattern related to psychological impairment, emotional instability

Disturbed **thought** processes related to anxiety

Ineffective **coping** related to inability to express feelings appropriately

Ineffective **denial** related to overwhelming feelings of hopelessness, fear, threat to self

**Powerlessness** related to life-style of helplessness

Risk for **spiritual** distress related to psychological distress

**Self-care** deficit related to ritualistic behavior, activities

**Sleep** deprivation related to prolonged psychological discomfort

## APPENDECTOMY

Deficient **fluid** volume related to fluid restriction, hypermetabolic state, nausea, vomiting

Ineffective **Health** Maintenance related to deficient knowledge regarding self-care following appendectomy

**Pain** related to surgical incision

Risk for **infection** related to perforation/rupture of appendix, surgical incision, peritonitis

See Surgery

## APPENDICITIS

Deficient **fluid** volume related to anorexia, nausea, vomiting

Delayed **surgical** recovery related to risk for infection

**Pain** related to inflammation

Risk for **infection** related to possible perforation of appendix

## ARDS (ADULT RESPIRATORY DISTRESS SYNDROME)

Death **anxiety** related to seriousness of physical disease

Delayed **surgical** recovery related to complications associated with respiratory difficulty

Impaired **gas** exchange related to damage to alveolar-capillary membrane, change in lung compliance

Impaired spontaneous **ventilation** related to damage to alveolar capillary membrane

Ineffective **airway** clearance related to excessive tracheobronchial secretions

See Ventilator Client

## ARRHYTHMIA

See Dysrhythmia

## ARTHRITIS

**Activity** intolerance related to chronic pain, fatigue, weakness

Chronic **pain** related to progression of joint deterioration

Chronic **sorrow** related to presence of chronic condition

Disturbed **body** image related to ineffective **coping** with joint abnormalities

Impaired physical **mobility** related to musculoskeletal impairment

Ineffective **Health** Maintenance related to deficient knowledge regarding care of arthritis

Risk for **spiritual** distress related to presence of chronic condition

**Self-care** deficit: specify related to pain, musculoskeletal impairment

See Rheumatoid Arthritis

## ARTHROPLASTY—TOTAL HIP REPLACEMENT

**Constipation** related to immobility

Impaired physical **mobility** related to decreased muscle strength, surgery

Impaired **walking** related to decrease muscle strength, surgery

**Pain** related to tissue trauma associated with surgery

Risk for **infection** related to invasive surgery, foreign object in body, anesthesia, immobility with stasis of respiratory secretions

Risk for **injury** related to interruption of arterial blood flow, dislocation of prosthesis

Risk for perioperative positioning **injury** related to immobilization, muscle weakness

Risk for **peripheral** neurovascular dysfunction related to orthopedic surgery

See Surgery

## ARTHROSCOPY

Ineffective **Health** Maintenance related to deficient knowledge regarding procedure, postoperative restrictions

## ASPIRATION, DANGER OF

Risk for **aspiration** related to reduced level of consciousness; depressed cough or gag reflexes; presence of tracheostomy or endotracheal tube; incomplete lower esophageal sphincter; presence of gastrointestinal tubes or tube feedings; medication administration; situations hindering elevation of upper body; increased intragastric pressure; increased gastric residual; decreased gastrointestinal motility; delayed gastric emptying; impaired swallowing; facial, oral, or neck surgery or trauma; wired jaws

## ASTHMA

**Activity** intolerance related to fatigue, energy shift to meet muscle needs for breathing to overcome airway obstruction

**Anxiety** related to inability to breathe effectively, fear of suffocation

Disturbed **body** image related to decreased participation in physical activities

Impaired **home** maintenance related to deficient knowledge regarding control of environmental triggers

Ineffective **airway** clearance related to tracheobronchial narrowing, excessive secretions

Ineffective **breathing** pattern related to anxiety

Ineffective **coping** related to personal vulnerability to situational crisis

Ineffective **Health** Maintenance related to deficient knowledge regarding physical triggers, medications, treatment of early warning signs

**Sleep** deprivation related to ineffective breathing pattern

## ATTENTION DEFICIT DISORDER

Disabled family **coping** related to significant person with chronically unexpressed feelings of guilt, anxiety, hostility, despair, etc.

Impaired **adjustment** related to intense emotional state

Risk for delayed **development** related to behavior disorders

Risk for impaired **parenting** related to lack of knowledge of factors contributing to child's behavior

Risk for **loneliness** related to social isolation

Risk for **spiritual** distress related to poor relationships

**Self-esteem** disturbance related to difficulty in participating in expected activities

**Social** isolation related to unacceptable social behavior

## AUTISM

Compromised family **coping** related to parental guilt over etiology of disease, inability to accept or adapt to child's condition, inability to help child and other family members seek treatment

Delayed **growth** and development related to inability to develop relations with other human beings, inability to identify own body as separate from those of other people, inability to integrate concept of self

Disturbed personal **identity** related to inability to distinguish between self and environment, inability to identify own body as separate from those of other people, inability to integrate concept of self

Disturbed **thought** processes related to inability to perceive self or others, cognitive dissonance, perceptual dysfunction

Impaired **social** interaction related to communication barriers, inability to relate to others

Impaired verbal **communication** related to speech and language delays

Risk for delayed **development** related to autism

Risk for **loneliness** related to health alterations, cognition

Risk for **self-mutilation** related to autistic state

Risk for **violence**: self- and other-directed related to frequent destructive rages toward self or others secondary to extreme response to changes in routine, fear of harmless things

See Mental Retardation

## AUTONOMIC DYSREFLEXIA

**Autonomic** dysreflexia related to bladder distention, bowel distention, noxious stimuli

Risk for **autonomic** dysreflexia related to bladder distention, bowel distention, noxious stimuli

## BACK PAIN

See Acute Back

## BATHING/HYGIENE PROBLEMS

Bathing/hygiene **self-care** deficit related to intolerance to activity, decreased strength and endurance, pain, discomfort, perceptual or cognitive impairment, neuromuscular impairment, musculoskeletal impairment, depression, severe anxiety

## BATTERED CHILD SYNDROME

**Anxiety**/fear related to threat of punishment for perceived wrongdoing

Chronic low **self-esteem** related to lack of positive feedback, excessive negative feedback

Chronic **sorrow** related to situational crises

Deficient **diversional** activity related to diminished/absent environmental or personal stimuli

Delayed **growth** and development: regression vs delayed related to diminished/absent environmental stimuli, inadequate caretaking, inconsistent responsiveness by caretaker

Disturbed **sleep** pattern related to hypervigilance, anxiety

Dysfunctional **family** process: alcoholism related to inadequate coping skills

Imbalanced **nutrition**: less than body requirements related to inadequate caretaking

Impaired **skin** integrity related to altered nutritional state, physical abuse

**Pain** related to physical injuries

**Post-trauma** syndrome related to physical abuse, incest, rape, molestation

Risk for delayed **development** related to shaken baby, abuse

Risk for disproportionate **growth** related to abuse

Risk for **poisoning** related to inadequate safeguards, lack of proper safety precautions, accessibility of illicit substances secondary to impaired home maintenance

Risk for **post-trauma** syndrome related to physical abuse, incest, rape, molestation

Risk for **self-mutilation** related to feelings of rejection, dysfunctional family

Risk for **suffocation**/aspiration related to propped bottle, unattended child

Risk for **trauma** related to inadequate precautions, cognitive or emotional difficulties

**Sleep** deprivation related to prolonged psychological discomfort

**Social** isolation: family imposed related to fear of disclosure of family dysfunction and abuse

## BED MOBILITY, IMPAIRED

Impaired bed **mobility** related to intolerance to activity, decreased strength and endurance, pain or discomfort, perceptual or cognitive impairment, neuromuscular impairment, musculoskeletal impairment, depression, severe anxiety

## BENIGN PROSTATIC HYPERTROPHY

See BPH; Prostatic Hypertrophy

## BIPOLAR DISORDER I (MOST RECENT EPISODE, DEPRESSED OR MANIC)

Chronic low **self-esteem** related to repeated unmet expectations

Disturbed **energy** field related to disharmony of mind, body, spirit

Dysfunctional **grieving** related to lack of previous resolution of former grieving response

**Fatigue** related to psychological demands

Impaired **adjustment** related to low state of optimism

Ineffective **coping** related to dysfunctional grieving

Ineffective **Health** Maintenance related to lack of ability to make good judgments regarding ways to obtain help

Risk for **loneliness** related to stress, conflict

Risk for **spiritual** distress related to mental illness

**Self-care** deficit: specify related to depression, cognitive impairment

**Social** isolation related to ineffective coping

See Depression; Manic Disorder, Bipolar I

## BODY IMAGE CHANGE

Disturbed **body** image related to psychosocial, biophysical, cognitive/perceptual, cultural, spiritual, developmental changes; illness; trauma or injury; surgery; illness treatment

## BODY TEMPERATURE, ALTERED

Risk for imbalanced **body** temperature related to extremes of age or weight, exposure to cold or hot environment, dehydration, change in activity, effects of medication, dysfunction of body temperature regulation center

## BORDERLINE PERSONALITY DISORDER

**Anxiety** related to perceived threat to self-concept

Disturbed **thought** process related to poor reality testing

Defensive **coping** related to difficulty with relationships, inability to accept blame for own behavior

Impaired **judgment** related to intense emotional state

Ineffective **coping** related to use of maladjusted defense mechanisms (e.g., projection, denial)

Ineffective family **therapeutic** regimen management related to manipulative behavior of client

**Powerlessness** related to life-style of helplessness

Risk for **caregiver** role strain related to inability of care receiver to accept criticism, care receiver taking advantage of others to meet own needs or having unreasonable expectations

Risk for **self-mutilation** related to ineffective **coping**, feelings of self-hatred

Risk for **spiritual** distress related to poor relationships associated with behaviors attributed to BPD

Risk for self-directed **violence** related to feelings of need to punish self, manipulative behavior

**Social** isolation related to immature interests

## BOWEL INCONTINENCE

**Bowel** incontinence related to decreased awareness of need to defecate, loss of sphincter control, fecal impaction

## BOWEL OBSTRUCTION

**Constipation** related to decreased motility, intestinal obstruction

Deficient **fluid** volume related to inadequate fluid volume intake, fluid loss in bowel

Imbalanced **nutrition**: less than body requirements related to nausea, vomiting

**Pain** related to pressure from distended abdomen

## BPH (BENIGN PROSTATIC HYPERTROPHY)

Disturbed **sleep** pattern related to nocturia

Ineffective **health** maintenance related to deficient knowledge regarding self-care with prostatic hypertrophy

Risk for **infection** related to urinary residual post voiding, bacterial invasion of bladder

Risk for urge urinary **incontinence** related to detrusor muscle instability with impaired contractility, involuntary sphincter relaxation

**Urinary** retention related to obstruction

## BRAIN INJURY

See Intracranial Pressure, Increased

## BRAIN SURGERY

See Craniectomy/Craniotomy

## BRAIN TUMOR

Anticipatory **grieving** related to potential loss of physiosocial-psychosocial well-being

Decreased **intracranial** adaptive capacity related to presence of brain tumor

Disturbed **sensory** perception: specify related to tumor growth compressing brain tissue

Disturbed **thought** processes related to altered circulation, destruction of brain tissue

**Fear** related to threat to well-being

**Pain** related to neurological injury

Risk for **injury** related to sensory-perceptual alterations, weakness

See Cancer; Chemotherapy; Condition; Craniectomy/Craniotomy

## BREAST CANCER

Chronic **sorrow** related to diagnosis of cancer, loss of body integrity

Death **anxiety** related to cancer diagnosis

**Fear** related to diagnosis of cancer

Ineffective **coping** related to treatment, prognosis

Risk for **spiritual** distress related to fear of diagnosis of cancer

**Sexual** dysfunction related to loss of body part, partner's reaction to loss

See Cancer; Chemotherapy; Mastectomy; Radiation

## BREAST-FEEDING, EFFECTIVE

Effective **breast-feeding** related to basic breast-feeding knowledge, normal breast structure, normal infant oral structure, infant gestational age >34 weeks, support sources, maternal confidence

## BREAST-FEEDING, INEFFECTIVE

Ineffective **breast-feeding** related to prematurity, infant anomaly, maternal breast anomaly, previous breast surgery, previous history of breast-feeding failure, infant receiving supplemental feedings with artificial nipple, poor infant sucking reflex, nonsupportive partner/family, **deficient knowledge**, interruption in breast-feeding, maternal anxiety or ambivalence

See Painful Breasts—Sore Nipples; Painful Breasts—Engorgement

## BREAST-FEEDING, INTERRUPTED

Interrupted **breast-feeding** related to maternal or infant illness, prematurity, maternal employment, contraindications to breast-feeding (e.g., drugs, true breast milk jaundice), need to abruptly wean infant

## BREATHING PATTERN ALTERATION

Ineffective **breathing** pattern related to neuromuscular impairment, pain, musculoskeletal impairment, perception/cognitive impairment, anxiety, decreased energy/fatigue

## BRONCHITIS

**Anxiety** related to potential chronic condition

**Health**-seeking behavior related to wish to stop smoking

Ineffective **airway** clearance related to excessive thickened mucus secretion

Ineffective **health** maintenance related to deficient knowledge regarding care of condition

## BURNS

Anticipatory **grieving** related to loss of bodily function, loss of future hopes and plans

**Anxiety**/fear related to pain from treatments, possible permanent disfigurement

Disturbed **body** image related to altered physical appearance

Delayed **surgical** recovery related to ineffective tissue perfusion

Deficient **diversional** activity related to long-term hospitalization

**Hypothermia** related to impaired skin integrity

Imbalanced **nutrition**: less than body requirements related to increased metabolic needs, anorexia, protein and fluid loss

Impaired **skin** integrity related to injury of skin

Ineffective **tissue** perfusion: peripheral related to circumferential burns, impaired arterial/venous circulation

Impaired physical **mobility** related to pain, musculoskeletal impairment, contracture formation

**Pain** related to injury, treatments

**Post-trauma** response related to life-threatening event

Risk for deficient **fluid** volume related to loss from skin surface, fluid shift

Risk for ineffective **airway** clearance related to potential tracheobronchial obstruction, edema

Risk for **infection** related to loss of intact skin, trauma, invasive sites

Risk for **peripheral** neurovascular dysfunction related to eschar formation with circumferential burn

Risk for **post-trauma** syndrome related to perception, duration of event that caused burns

## CANCER

**Activity** intolerance related to side effects of treatment, weakness from cancer

Anticipatory **grieving** related to potential loss of significant others, high risk for infertility

Chronic **pain** related to metastatic cancer

Chronic **sorrow** related to chronic illness of cancer

Compromised family **coping** related to prolonged disease or disability progression that exhausts supportive ability of significant others

**Constipation** related to side effects of medication, altered nutrition, decreased activity

Death **anxiety** related to unresolved issues regarding dying

Decisional **conflict** related to selection of treatment choices, continuation/discontinuation of treatment, "do not resuscitate" decision

Disturbed **body** image related to side effects of treatment, cachexia

Disturbed **sleep** pattern related to anxiety, pain

**Fear** related to serious threat to well-being

**Hopelessness** related to loss of control, terminal illness

Imbalanced **nutrition**: less than body requirements related to loss of appetite, difficulty swallowing, side effects of chemotherapy, obstruction by tumor

Impaired physical **mobility** related to weakness, neuromusculoskeletal impairment, pain

Impaired **skin** integrity related to immunological deficit, immobility

Impaired **oral** mucous membranes related to chemotherapy, oral pH changes, decreased/altered oral flora

Ineffective **denial** related to dysfunctional grieving process

Ineffective **health** maintenance related to deficient knowledge regarding prescribed treatment

Ineffective **protection** related to cancer suppressing immune system

Ineffective **role** performance related to change in physical capacity, inability to resume prior role

Ineffective **coping** related to personal vulnerability in situational crisis, terminal illness

Readiness for enhanced **spiritual** well-being related to desire for harmony with self, others, higher power/God when faced with serious illness

**Powerlessness** related to treatment, progression of disease

Risk for **disuse** syndrome related to severe pain, change in level of consciousness

Risk for impaired **home** maintenance related to lack of familiarity with community resources

Risk for **infection** related to inadequate immune system

Risk for **injury** related to bleeding secondary to bone marrow depression

Risk for **spiritual** distress related to physical illness of cancer

**Self-care** deficit: specify related to pain, intolerance to activity, decreased strength

**Social** isolation related to hospitalization, life-style changes

**Spiritual** distress related to test of spiritual beliefs

See Chemotherapy

## CARDIAC CATHETERIZATION

**Anxiety**/fear related to invasive procedure, uncertainty of outcome of procedure

Impaired **comfort** related to postprocedural restrictions, invasive procedure

Ineffective **health** maintenance related to deficient knowledge regarding procedure, postprocedural care, treatment and prevention of coronary artery disease

Risk for decreased **cardiac** output related to ventricular ischemia, dysrhythmias

Risk for ineffective **tissue** perfusion related to impaired arterial or venous circulation

Risk for **injury**: hematoma related to invasive procedure

Risk for **peripheral** neurovascular dysfunction related to vascular obstruction

## CARDIOGENIC SHOCK

Decreased **cardiac** output related to decreased myocardial contractility, dysrhythmia

See Shock

## CAREGIVER ROLE STRAIN

**Caregiver** role strain related to pathophysiological factors, developmental factors, psychosocial factors, situational factors

Risk for **caregiver** role strain related to pathophysiological factors, developmental factors, psychosocial factors, situational factors

## CAROTID ENDARTERECTOMY

**Fear** related to surgery in vital area

Ineffective **health** maintenance related to deficient knowledge regarding postoperative care

Risk for ineffective **airway** clearance related to hematoma compressing trachea

Risk for ineffective **tissue** perfusion: cerebral related to hemorrhage, clot formation

Risk for **injury** related to possible hematoma formation

## CARPAL TUNNEL SYNDROME

Impaired physical **mobility** related to neuromuscular impairment

**Pain** related to unrelieved pressure on median nerve

**Self-care** deficit; bathing/hygiene, dressing/grooming, feeding related to pain

## CASTS

Deficient **diversional** activity related to physical limitations from cast

Ineffective **health** maintenance related to deficient knowledge regarding cast care, personal care with cast

Impaired physical **mobility** related to limb immobilization

Impaired **walking** related to cast(s) on lower extremities, fracture of bones

Risk for impaired **skin** integrity related to unrelieved pressure on skin

Risk for **peripheral** neurovascular dysfunction related to mechanical compression from cast

**Self-care** deficit: bathing/hygiene, dressing/grooming, feeding related to presence of cast(s) on upper extremities

**Self-care** deficit: toileting related to presence of cast(s) on lower extremities

## CATARACT EXTRACTION

**Anxiety** related to threat of permanent vision loss, surgical procedure

Ineffective **health** maintenance related to deficient knowledge regarding postoperative restrictions

Risk for **injury** related to increased intraocular pressure, accommodation to new visual field

Disturbed **sensory** perception: vision related to edema from surgery

See Vision Impairment

## CATARACTS

Disturbed **sensory** perception: vision related to altered sensory input

See Vision Impairment

## CELLULITIS

Impaired **skin** integrity related to inflammatory process damaging skin

Ineffective **tissue** perfusion: peripheral related to edema

**Pain** related to inflammatory changes in tissues from infection

## CEREBRAL ANEURYSM

See Craniectomy/Craniotomy; Intracranial Pressure, Increased; Subarachnoid Hemorrhage

## CEREBROVASCULAR ACCIDENT

See CVA

## CHEMICAL DEPENDENCE

See Alcoholism; Drug Abuse

## CHEMOTHERAPY

Disturbed **body** image related to loss of weight, loss of hair

Death **anxiety** related to chemotherapy not accomplishing desired results

Delayed **surgical** recovery related to compromised immune system

**Fatigue** related to disease process, anemia, drug effects

Imbalanced **nutrition**: less than body requirements related to side effects of chemotherapy

Impaired **oral** mucous membranes related to effects of chemotherapy

Ineffective **health** maintenance related to deficient knowledge regarding action, side effects, way to integrate chemotherapy into life-style

Ineffective **protection** related to suppressed immune system, decreased platelets

**Nausea** related to effects of chemotherapy

Risk for deficient **fluid** volume related to vomiting, diarrhea

Risk for ineffective **tissue** perfusion related to anemia

Risk for **infection** related to immunosuppression

See Cancer

## CHF (CONGESTIVE HEART FAILURE)

**Activity** intolerance related to weakness, fatigue

**Constipation** related to activity intolerance

Decreased **cardiac** output related to impaired cardiac function

**Fatigue** related to disease process

**Fear** related to threat to one's own well-being

Excess **fluid** volume related to impaired excretion of sodium and water

Impaired **gas** exchange related to excessive fluid in interstitial space of lungs, alveoli

Ineffective **health** maintenance related to deficient knowledge regarding care of disease

**Powerlessness** related to illness related regimen

## CHILD ABUSE

See Battered Child Syndrome

## CHOLECYSTECTOMY

Imbalanced **nutrition**: less than body requirements related to high metabolic needs, decreased ability to digest fatty foods

Ineffective **health** maintenance related to deficient knowledge regarding postoperative care

**Pain** related to recent surgery

Risk for deficient **fluid** volume related to restricted intake, nausea, vomiting

Risk for ineffective **breathing** pattern related to proximity of incision to lungs resulting in pain with deep breathing

See Abdominal Surgery

## CHOLELITHIASIS

Imbalanced **nutrition**: less than body requirements related to anorexia, nausea, vomiting

Ineffective **health** maintenance related to deficient knowledge regarding care of disease

**Pain** related to obstruction of bile flow, inflammation in gallbladder

## CHRONIC OBSTRUCTIVE PULMONARY DISEASE

See COPD

## CHRONIC RENAL FAILURE

See Renal Failure

## CIRRHOSIS

Chronic low **self-esteem** related to chronic illness

Chronic **pain** related to liver enlargement

Chronic **sorrow** related to presence of chronic illness

**Diarrhea** related to dietary changes, medications

Disturbed **thought** processes related to chronic organic disorder with increased ammonia levels, substance abuse

**Fatigue** related to malnutrition

Imbalanced **nutrition**: less than body requirements related to loss of appetite, nausea, vomiting

Ineffective **health** maintenance related to deficient knowledge regarding correlation between life-style habits and disease process

Ineffective management of **therapeutic** regimen related to denial of severity of illness

Ineffective **protection** related to risk of impaired blood coagulation, bleeding from portal hypertension

**Nausea** related to irritation to gastrointestinal system

Risk for deficient **fluid** volume: hemorrhage related to abnormal bleeding from esophagus

Risk for **injury** related to substance intoxication, potential delirium tremens

Risk for impaired **oral** mucous membranes related to altered nutrition

Risk for impaired **skin** integrity related to altered nutritional state, altered metabolic state

## COLD, VIRAL

Impaired **comfort**: sore throat, aching, nasal discomfort related to viral infection

Ineffective **health** maintenance related to deficient knowledge regarding care of viral condition, prevention of further infections

## COLECTOMY

**Constipation** related to decreased activity, decreased fluid intake

Imbalanced **nutrition**: less than body requirements related to high metabolic needs, decreased ability to ingest/digest food

Ineffective **health** maintenance related to deficient knowledge regarding procedure, postoperative care

**Pain** related to recent surgery

Risk for **infection** related to invasive procedure

See Abdominal Surgery

## COLITIS

Deficient **fluid** volume related to frequent stools

**Diarrhea** related to inflammation in colon

**Pain** related to inflammation in colon

See Crohn's Disease; Inflammatory Bowel Syndrome; Ulcerative Colitis

## COLOSTOMY

Disturbed **body** image related to presence of stoma, daily care of fecal material

Ineffective **health** maintenance related to deficient knowledge regarding care of stoma, integrating colostomy care into life-style

Risk for altered **sexuality** pattern related to altered body image, self-concept

Risk for **constipation**/diarrhea related to inappropriate diet

Risk for impaired **skin** integrity related to irritation from bowel contents

Risk for **social** isolation related to anxiety about appearance of stoma and possible leakage

## COMA

Death **anxiety** (significant others) related to unknown outcome of coma state

Disturbed **thought** processes related to neurological changes

Ineffective family **therapeutic** regimen management related to complexity of therapeutic regimen

Interrupted family processes related to illness/disability of family member

Risk for **aspiration** related to impaired swallowing, loss of cough/gag reflex

Risk for **disuse** syndrome related to altered level of consciousness impairing mobility

Risk for impaired **skin** integrity related to immobility

Risk for impaired **oral** mucous membranes related to dry mouth

Risk for **injury** related to potential seizure activity

Risk for **spiritual** distress (significant others) related to loss of ability to relate to loved one, unknown outcome of coma

**Self-care** deficit: specify related to neuromuscular impairment

Total urinary **incontinence** related to neurological dysfunction

See cause of Coma

## COMMUNICABLE DISEASES, CHILDHOOD (MEASLES, MUMPS, RUBELLA, CHICKENPOX, SCABIES, LICE, IMPETIGO)

Deficient **diversional** activity related to imposed isolation from peers, disruption in usual play activities, fatigue, activity intolerance

Impaired **comfort** related to hyperthermia secondary to infectious disease process, pruritus secondary to skin rash or subdermal organisms

Ineffective **health** maintenance related to nonadherence to appropriate immunization schedules, lack of prevention of transmission of infection

**Pain** related to impaired skin integrity, edema

Risk for **infection**: transmission to others related to contagious organisms

See Meningitis/Encephalitis; Respiratory Infections, Acute Childhood; Reye's Syndrome

## COMMUNICATION PROBLEMS

Impaired verbal **communication** related to decrease in circulation to brain, brain tumor; physical barrier (e.g., tracheostomy, intubation); anatomical defect; impaired hearing; cleft palate; psychological barriers (e.g., psychosis, lack of stimuli); cultural difference; developmentally related or age-related factors; side effects of medication; environmental barriers; absence of significant others;

altered perceptions; lack of information; stress; alteration of self-esteem or self-concept; physiological conditions; alteration of central nervous system; weakening of musculoskeletal system; emotional conditions

## COMMUNITY COPING

Ineffective community **coping** related to natural or manmade disasters; ineffective or nonexistent community systems (e.g., lack of emergency medical, transportation, or disaster planning systems), deficits in community social support services and resources, inadequate resources for problem solving

Readiness for enhanced community **coping** related to community sense of power to manage stressors, social supports available, resources available for problem solving

## COMMUNITY MANAGEMENT OF THERAPEUTIC REGIMEN

Ineffective community **therapeutic** regimen management related to inadequate community resources

## COMPARTMENT SYNDROME

**Fear** related to possible loss of limb, damage to limb

Ineffective **tissue** perfusion: peripheral related to increased pressure within compartment

**Pain** related to pressure in compromised body part

## CONFUSION, ACUTE

Acute **confusion** related to over 60 years of age, alcohol abuse, delirium, dementia, drug abuse

## CONFUSION, CHRONIC

Chronic **confusion** related to Alzheimer's disease, Korsakoff's psychosis, multiinfarct dementia, cerebral vascular accident, head injury

## CONGESTIVE HEART FAILURE

See CHF

## CONJUNCTIVITIS

Disturbed **sensory** perception related to change in visual acuity resulting from inflammation

**Pain** related to inflammatory process

Risk for **injury** related to change in visual acuity

## CONSTIPATION

**Constipation** related to decreased fluid intake, decreased intake of foods containing bulk, inactivity, immobility, deficient knowledge of appropriate bowel routine, lack of privacy for defecation

## CONSTIPATION, PERCEIVED

Perceived **constipation** related to cultural or family health beliefs, faulty appraisal, impaired thought processes

## CONSTIPATION, RISK FOR

Risk for **constipation** related to functional factors impeding defecation, inappropriate diet, psychological factors, physical factors, medications

## CONVULSIONS

**Anxiety** related to concern over controlling convulsions

Impaired **memory** related to neurological disturbance

Ineffective **health** maintenance related to deficient knowledge regarding need for medication and care during seizure activity

Risk for **aspiration** related to impaired swallowing

Risk for delayed **development** related to seizures

Risk for **injury** related to seizure activity

Risk for disturbed **thought** processes related to seizure activity

See Seizure Disorders

## COPD (CHRONIC OBSTRUCTIVE PULMONARY DISEASE)

**Activity** intolerance related to imbalance between oxygen supply-demand

Altered **family** process related to role changes

**Anxiety** related to breathlessness, change in health status

Chronic low **self-esteem** related to chronic illness

Chronic **sorrow** related to presence of chronic illness

Death **anxiety** related to seriousness of medical condition, difficulty being able to "catch breath," feeling of suffocation

**Health**-seeking behavior related to wish to stop smoking

Imbalanced **nutrition**: less than body requirements related to decreased intake because of dyspnea, unpleasant taste in mouth left by medications

Impaired **gas** exchange related to ventilation-perfusion inequality

Impaired **social** interaction related to social isolation secondary to oxygen use, activity intolerance

Ineffective **airway** clearance related to bronchoconstriction, increased mucus, ineffective cough, infection

Ineffective **health** maintenance related to deficient knowledge regarding care of disease

**Noncompliance** related to reluctance to accept responsibility for changing detrimental health practices

**Powerlessness** related to progressive nature of disease

Risk for **infection** related to stasis of respiratory secretions

**Self-care** deficit: specify related to fatigue secondary to increased work of breathing

**Sleep** deprivation related to breathing difficulties when lying down

## COPING PROBLEMS

Defensive **coping** related to superior attitude toward others, difficulty establishing or maintaining relationships, hostile laughter or ridicule of others, difficulty in reality-testing perceptions, lack of follow-through or participation in treatment or therapy

Ineffective **coping** related to gender differences in coping strategies; inadequate level of confidence in ability to cope; uncertainty; inadequate social support created by characteristics of relationships; inadequate level of perception of control; inadequate resources available; high degree of threat; disturbance in pattern of tension release; inadequate opportunity to prepare for stressor; inability to conserve adaptive energies; disturbance in appraisal of threat

See Community Coping; Family Problems

## CRANIECTOMY/CRANIOTOMY

Adult **failure** to thrive related to altered cerebral tissue perfusion

Decreased **intracranial** adaptive capacity related to brain injury, intracranial hypertension

**Fear** related to threat to well-being

Impaired **memory** related to neurological surgery

Ineffective **tissue** perfusion: cerebral related to cerebral edema, decreased cerebral perfusion, increased intracranial pressure

**Pain** related to recent surgery, headache

Risk for disturbed **thought** processes related to neurophysiological changes

Risk for **injury** related to potential confusion

See Coma (if relevant)

## CROHN'S DISEASE

See Inflammatory Bowel Disease

## CROUP

See Respiratory Infections, Acute Childhood

## CVA (CEREBROVASCULAR ACCIDENT)

Adult **failure** to thrive related to neurophysiological changes

**Anxiety** related to situational crisis, change in physical or emotional condition

Ineffective **health** maintenance related to deficient knowledge regarding self-care following CVA

Interrupted **family** process related to illness, disability of family member

Caregiver role strain related to cognitive problems of care receiver, need for significant home care

Chronic confusion related to neurological changes

Constipation related to decreased activity

Disturbed body image related to chronic illness, paralysis

Disturbed sensory perception: visual, tactile, kinesthetic related to neurological deficit

Disturbed thought processes related to neurophysiological changes

Grieving related to loss of health

Impaired home maintenance related to neurological disease affecting ability to perform activities of daily living (ADLs)

Impaired memory related to neurological disturbances

Impaired physical mobility related to loss of balance and coordination

Impaired social interaction related to limited physical mobility, limited ability to communicate

Impaired swallowing related to neuromuscular dysfunction

Impaired transfer ability related to limited physical mobility

Impaired verbal communication related to pressure damage, decreased circulation to brain in speech center informational sources

Impaired walking related to loss of balance and coordination

Ineffective coping related to disability

Risk for aspiration related to impaired swallowing, loss of gag reflex

Risk for disuse syndrome related to paralysis

Risk for impaired skin integrity related to immobility

Reflex incontinence related to loss of feeling to void

Risk for injury related to disturbed sensory perception

Self-care deficit: specify related to decreased strength and endurance, paralysis

Total urinary incontinence related to neurological dysfunction

Unilateral neglect related to disturbed perception from neurological damage

## CYSTITIS
See UTI

## DECISIONS, DIFFICULTY MAKING

Decisional conflict related to support system deficit, perceived threat to value system; multiple or divergent sources of information, lack of relevant information, unclear personal values/beliefs

## DEEP VEIN THROMBOSIS
See DVT

## DEFENSIVE BEHAVIOR

Defensive coping related to nonacceptance of blame, denial of problems or weakness

Ineffective denial related to inability to face situation realistically

## DEHYDRATION

Deficient fluid volume related to active fluid volume loss

Impaired oral mucous membranes related to decreased salivation, fluid deficit

Ineffective health maintenance related to deficient knowledge regarding treatment and prevention of dehydration

See cause of Dehydration

## DELIRIUM

Acute confusion related to effects of medication, response to hospitalization, alcohol abuse, substance abuse, sensory deprivation or overload

## DELIRIUM TREMENS (DT)
See Alcohol Withdrawal

## DEMENTIA

Adult failure to thrive related to depression, apathy

Altered family process related to disability of family member

Chronic confusion related to neurological dysfunction

Chronic sorrow related to chronic mental illness

Disturbed sleep pattern related to neurological impairment, naps during the day

Imbalanced nutrition: less than body requirements related to psychological impairment

Impaired environmental interpretation syndrome related to dementia

Impaired home maintenance related to inadequate support system

Impaired physical mobility related to neuromuscular impairment

Risk for caregiver role strain related to number of care-giving tasks, duration of caregiving required

Risk for impaired skin integrity related to altered nutritional status, immobility

Risk for injury related to confusion, decreased muscle coordination

Self-care deficit: specify related to psychological or neuromuscular impairment

Total urinary incontinence related to neuromuscular impairment

## DENIAL OF HEALTH STATUS

Ineffective denial related to lack of perception about health status effects of illness

Ineffective management of therapeutic regimen related to denial of seriousness of health situation

## DENTAL CARIES

Impaired dentition related to ineffective oral hygiene, barriers to self-care, economic barriers to professional care, nutritional deficits, dietary habits

## DEPRESSION (MAJOR DEPRESSIVE DISORDER)

Adult failure to thrive related to depression

Chronic low self-esteem related to repeated unmet expectations

Chronic sorrow related to unresolved grief

Constipation related to inactivity, decreased fluid intake

Death anxiety related to feelings of lack of self-worth

Disturbed sleep pattern related to inactivity

Dysfunctional grieving related to lack of previous resolution of former grieving response

Disturbed energy field related to disharmony

Fatigue related to psychological demands

Hopelessness related to feeling of abandonment, long-term stress

Impaired environmental interpretation syndrome related to severe mental functional impairment

Ineffective coping related to dysfunctional grieving

Ineffective health maintenance related to lack of ability to make good judgments regarding ways to obtain help

Powerlessness related to pattern of helplessness

Risk for self-directed violence related to panic state

Self-care deficit: specify related to depression, cognitive impairment

Sexual dysfunction related to loss of sexual desire

Social isolation related to ineffective coping

## DERMATITIS

Anxiety related to situational crisis imposed by illness

Impaired comfort: pruritus related to inflammation of skin

Impaired skin integrity related to side effect of medication, allergic reaction

Ineffective health maintenance related to deficient knowledge regarding methods to decrease inflammation

## DEVELOPMENTAL CONCERNS
### Prenatal

Risk for delayed development related to maternal age

<15 or >35 years; substance abuse; infections; genetic or endocrine disorders; unplanned or unwanted pregnancy; lack of, late, poor prenatal care; inadequate nutrition; illiteracy; poverty

### Individual

Risk for delayed development related to prematurity; seizures; congenital or genetic disorders; positive drug screening test; brain damage (e.g., hemorrhage in postnatal period, shaken baby, abuse, accident); vision impairment; hearing impairment or frequent otitis media; chronic illness; technology dependence; failure to thrive, inadequate nutrition; foster or adopted child; lead poisoning; chemotherapy; radiation therapy; natural disaster; behavior disorders; substance abuse

### Environmental

Risk for delayed **development** related to poverty; violence

### Caregiver

Risk for delayed **development** related to abuse; mental illness; mental retardation or severe learning disability

## DIABETES MELLITUS

Adult **failure** to thrive related to undetected disease process
Disturbed **sensory** perception related to ineffective tissue perfusion
Imbalanced **nutrition**: less than body requirements related to inability to use glucose (type I diabetes)
Imbalanced **nutrition**: more than body requirements related to excessive intake of nutrients (type II diabetes)
Ineffective **health** maintenance related to deficient knowledge regarding care of diabetic condition
Ineffective management of **therapeutic** regimen related to complexity of therapeutic regimen
Ineffective **tissue** perfusion: peripheral related to impaired arterial circulation
**Noncompliance** related to restrictive life-style; changes in diet, medication, exercise
**Powerlessness** related to perceived lack of personal control
Risk for disturbed **thought** processes related to hypoglycemia, hyperglycemia
Risk for impaired **skin** integrity related to loss of pain perception in extremities
Risk for **infection** related to hyperglycemia, impaired healing, circulatory changes
Risk for **injury**: hypoglycemia or hyperglycemia related to failure to consume adequate calories, failure to take insulin
**Sexual** dysfunction related to neuropathy associated with disease

## DIARRHEA

**Diarrhea** related to infection, change in diet, gastrointestinal disorders, stress, medication effect, impaction

## DILATION AND CURETTAGE (D & C)

Ineffective **health** maintenance related to deficient knowledge regarding postoperative self-care
**Pain** related to uterine contractions
Risk for deficient **fluid** volume: hemorrhage related to excessive blood loss during or after procedure
Risk for ineffective **sexuality** patterns related to painful coitus, fear associated with surgery on genital area
Risk for **infection** related to surgical procedure

## DISSOCIATIVE DISORDER (NOT OTHERWISE SPECIFIED)

**Anxiety** related to psychosocial stress
Disturbance in **self-concept** related to childhood trauma, childhood abuse
Disturbed personal **identity** related to inability to distinguish self caused by multiple personality disorder, depersonalization, disturbance in memory
Disturbed **sensory** perception: kinesthetic related to underdeveloped ego
Disturbed **thought** processes related to repressed anxiety
Impaired **memory** related to altered state of consciousness
Ineffective **coping** related to personal vulnerability in crisis of accurate self-perception

## DISTURBED ENERGY FIELD

Disturbed **energy** field related to disruption in flow of energy as result of pain, depression, fatigue, anxiety, stress

## DISUSE SYNDROME, POTENTIAL TO DEVELOP

Risk for **disuse** syndrome related to paralysis, mechanical immobilization, prescribed immobilization, severe pain, altered level of consciousness

## DIVERSIONAL ACTIVITY, LACK OF

Deficient **diversional** activity related to environmental lack of **diversional** activity as in frequent hospitalizations, lengthy treatments

## DIVERTICULITIS

**Constipation** related to dietary deficiency of fiber and roughage
**Diarrhea** related to increased intestinal motility secondary to inflammation
Deficient **knowledge** related to diet needed to control disease, medication regimen
Imbalanced **nutrition**: less than body requirements related to loss of appetite
**Pain** related to inflammation of bowel
Risk for deficient **fluid** volume related to diarrhea

## DOWN SYNDROME

See Mental Retardation

## DRESS SELF (INABILITY TO)

Dressing/grooming **self-care** deficit related to intolerance to activity, decreased strength and endurance, pain, discomfort, perceptual or cognitive impairment, neuromuscular impairment, musculoskeletal impairment, depression, severe anxiety

## DRUG ABUSE

**Anxiety** related to threat to self-concept, lack of control of drug use
Disturbed **sensory** perception: specify related to substance intoxication
Disturbed **sleep** pattern related to effects of medications
Disturbed **thought** process related to mind-altering effects of drugs
Imbalanced **nutrition**: less than body requirements related to poor eating habits
**Impaired** adjustment related to failure to intend to change behavior
Impaired **social** interaction related to disturbed thought processes from drug abuse
Ineffective **coping** related to situational crisis
**Noncompliance** related to denial of illness
**Powerlessness** related to feeling unable to change patterns of abuse
Risk for **injury** related to hallucinations, drug effects
Risk for **violence** related to poor impulse control
**Sexual** dysfunction related to actions and side effects of drug abuse
**Sleep** deprivation related to prolonged psychological discomfort
**Spiritual** distress related to separation from religious, cultural ties

## DRUG WITHDRAWAL

Acute **confusion** related to effects of substance withdrawal
**Anxiety** related to physiological withdrawal
Disturbed **sensory** perception: specify related to substance intoxication
Disturbed **sleep** pattern related to effects of medications
Imbalanced **nutrition**: less than body requirements related to poor eating habits
Ineffective **coping** related to situational crisis, withdrawal
**Noncompliance** related to denial of illness
Risk for **injury** related to hallucinations
Risk for **violence** related to poor impulse control
See Drug Abuse

## DTS (DELIRIUM TREMENS)

See Alcohol Withdrawal

## DVT—DEEP VEIN THROMBOSIS

**Constipation** related to inactivity, bedrest
Delayed **surgical** recovery related to impaired physical mobility
Impaired physical **mobility** related to pain in extremity, forced bedrest

Ineffective **health** maintenance related to deficient knowledge regarding self-care needs, treatment regimen, outcome

Ineffective **tissue** perfusion: peripheral related to interruption of venous blood flow

**Pain** related to vascular inflammation, edema

See Anticoagulant Therapy

## DYING CLIENT

See Terminally Ill Adult

## DYSFUNCTIONAL GRIEVING

Dysfunctional **grieving** related to actual or perceived loss

## DYSFUNCTIONAL VENTILATORY WEANING

Dysfunctional **ventilatory** weaning response related to physical, psychological, situational factors

## DYSPHAGIA

Impaired **swallowing** related to neuromuscular impairment

Risk for **aspiration** related to loss of gag or cough reflex

## DYSRHYTHMIA

**Activity** intolerance related to decreased cardiac output

**Anxiety**/fear related to threat of death, change in health status

Decreased **cardiac** output related to altered electrical conduction

Ineffective **health** maintenance related to deficient knowledge regarding self-care with disease

Ineffective **tissue** perfusion: cerebral related to interruption of cerebral arterial flow secondary to decreased cardiac output

## DYSTHYMIC DISORDER

Altered **sexual** pattern related to loss of sexual desire

Chronic low **self-esteem** related to repeated unmet expectations

Disturbed **sleep** pattern related to anxious thoughts

Ineffective **coping** related to impaired social interaction

Ineffective **health** maintenance related to inability to make good judgments regarding ways to obtain help

**Social** isolation related to ineffective coping

See Depression

## EARACHE

Disturbed **sensory** perception: auditory related to altered sensory reception, transmission, integration

**Pain** related to trauma, edema

## ECZEMA

Disturbed **body** image related to change in appearance from inflamed skin

Ineffective **health** maintenance related to deficient knowledge regarding how to decrease inflammation and prevent further outbreaks

Impaired **skin** integrity related to side effect of medication, allergic reaction

**Pain**: pruritus related to inflammation of skin

## EMPHYSEMA

See COPD

## ENDOMETRIOSIS

Anticipatory **grieving** related to possible infertility

Ineffective **health** maintenance related to deficient knowledge about disease condition, medications, other treatments

**Nausea** related to prostaglandin effect

**Pain** related to onset of menses with distention of endometrial tissue

**Sexual** dysfunction related to painful coitus

## ENVIRONMENTAL INTERPRETATION PROBLEMS

Impaired **environmental** interpretation syndrome related to dementia, Parkinson's disease, Huntington's disease, depression, alcoholism

## EPIGLOTTITIS

See Respiratory Infections, Acute Childhood

## EPILEPSY

**Anxiety** related to threat to role functioning

Ineffective **health** maintenance related to deficient knowledge regarding seizures and seizure control

Impaired **memory** related to seizure activity

Ineffective **therapeutic** regimen managements related to deficient knowledge regarding seizure control

Risk for **aspiration** related to impaired swallowing, excessive secretions

Risk for delayed **development** related to seizure disorder

Risk for disturbed **thought** processes related to excessive, uncontrolled neurological stimuli

Risk for **injury** related to environmental factors during seizure

See Seizure Disorders

## EPISTAXIS

**Fear** related to large amount of blood loss

Risk for deficient **fluid** volume related to excessive fluid loss

## EYE SURGERY

**Anxiety** related to possible loss of vision

Disturbed **sensory** perception: visual related to surgical procedure

Ineffective **health** maintenance related to deficient knowledge regarding postoperative activity, medications, eye care

Risk for **injury** related to impaired vision

**Self-care** deficit related to impaired vision

## FAILURE TO THRIVE, ADULT

Adult **failure** to thrive related to depression, apathy, fatigue

## FALLS, RISK FOR

Risk for **falls** related to history of falls, physiological factors, cognitive impairment, medication effect, unsafe environment, young child or older adult

## FAMILY PROBLEMS

Compromised family **coping** related to inadequate or incorrect information or understanding by primary person; temporary preoccupation by significant person who is trying to manage emotional conflicts and personal suffering and is unable to perceive or act effectively in regard to client's needs; temporary family disorganization and role changes; other situational or developmental crises the significant person may be facing; little support provided by client for primary person; prolonged disease or disability progression that exhausts supportive capacity of significant people

Disabled family **coping** related to significant person with chronically unexpressed feelings such as guilt, anxiety, hostility, despair; dissonant discrepancy of coping styles for dealing with adaptive tasks by significant person and client or among significant people; highly ambivalent family relationships; arbitrary handling of family's resistance to treatment, which tends to solidify defensiveness as it fails to deal adequately with underlying anxiety

Interrupted **family** process related to situation transition and/or crises, developmental transition and/or crises

Readiness for enhanced family **coping** related to needs sufficiently gratified, adaptive tasks effectively addressed to enable goals of self-actualization to surface

## FATIGUE

**Fatigue** related to decreased or increased metabolic energy production, overwhelming psychological or emotional demands, increased energy requirements to perform ADLs, excessive social and/or role demands, states of discomfort, altered body chemistry

## FEAR

**Fear** related to identifiable physical or psychological threat to person

## FECAL INCONTINENCE

**Bowel** incontinence related to neurological impairment, gastrointestinal disorders, anorectal trauma

## FEMORAL POPLITEAL BYPASS

**Anxiety** related to threat to or change in health status

**Pain** related to surgical trauma, edema in surgical area

Risk for deficient **fluid** volume: hemorrhage related to abnormal blood loss

Risk for ineffective **tissue** perfusion: peripheral related to impaired arterial circulation

Risk for **infection** related to invasive procedure

Risk for peripheral **neurovascular** dysfunction related to vascular surgery, emboli

## FEVER

**Hyperthermia** related to infectious process, damage to hypothalamus, exposure to hot environment, medications, anesthesia, inability or decreased ability to perspire

Ineffective **thermoregulation** related to fluctuating environmental temperature, trauma, illness

## FLUID VOLUME DEFICIT

Deficient **fluid** volume related to active fluid loss, failure of regulatory mechanisms

## FLUID VOLUME EXCESS

Excess **fluid** volume related to compromised regulatory mechanism, excess sodium intake

## FLUID VOLUME IMBALANCE, RISK FOR

Delayed **surgical** recovery related to fluid volume imbalance

Risk for imbalanced **fluid** volume related to major invasive surgeries

## FRACTURE

Deficient **diversional** activity related to immobility

Impaired physical **mobility** related to limb immobilization

Impaired **walking** related to limb immobility

Ineffective **health** maintenance related to deficient knowledge regarding care of fracture

**Pain** related to muscle spasm, edema, trauma

Risk for impaired **skin** integrity related to immobility, presence of cast

Risk for ineffective **tissue** perfusion related to immobility, presence of cast

Risk for **peripheral** neurovascular impairment related to mechanical compression, treatment of fracture

## FUSION, LUMBAR

**Anxiety** related to fear of surgical procedure, possible recurring problems

Impaired physical **mobility** related to limitations from surgical procedure, presence of brace

Ineffective **health** maintenance related to deficient knowledge regarding postoperative mobility restrictions, body mechanics

**Pain** related to discomfort at bone donor site

Risk for **injury** related to improper body mechanics

Risk for perioperative positioning **injury** related to immobilization

## GALLSTONES

See Cholelithiasis

## GANGRENE

Delayed **surgical** recovery related to obstruction of arterial flow

**Fear** related to possible loss of extremity

Ineffective **tissue** perfusion: peripheral related to obstruction of arterial flow

## GAS EXCHANGE, IMPAIRED

Impaired **gas** exchange related to ventilation-perfusion imbalance

## GASTRIC ULCER

See Ulcer, Peptic

## GASTRITIS

Imbalanced **nutrition**: less than body requirements related to vomiting, inadequate intestinal absorption of nutrients, restricted dietary regimen

**Pain** related to inflammation of gastric mucosa

Risk for deficient **fluid** volume related to excessive loss from gastrointestinal tract secondary to vomiting, decreased intake

## GASTROENTERITIS

**Diarrhea** related to infectious process involving intestinal tract

Deficient **fluid** volume related to excessive loss from gastrointestinal tract secondary to diarrhea, vomiting

Imbalanced **nutrition**: less than body requirements related to vomiting, inadequate intestinal absorption of nutrients, restricted dietary intake

Ineffective **health** maintenance related to deficient knowledge regarding treatment of disease

**Nausea** related to irritation to gastrointestinal system

**Pain** related to increased peristalsis causing cramping

## GASTROESOPHAGEAL REFLUX

**Anxiety**/fear: parental related to possible need for surgical intervention (Nissen fundoplication, gastrostomy tube)

Deficient **fluid** volume related to persistent vomiting

Imbalanced **nutrition**: less than body requirements related to poor feeding, vomiting

Ineffective **airway** clearance related to reflux of gastric contents into esophagus and tracheal or bronchial tree

Ineffective **health** maintenance related to deficient knowledge regarding antireflux regimen (e.g., positioning, oral or enteral feeding techniques, medications), possible home apnea monitoring

**Pain** related to irritation of esophagus from gastric acids

Risk for **aspiration** related to entry of gastric contents in tracheal or bronchial tree

Risk for impaired **parenting** related to disruption in bonding secondary to irritable or inconsolable infant

## GI BLEED (GASTROINTESTINAL BLEEDING)

Deficient **fluid** volume related to gastrointestinal bleeding

**Fatigue** related to loss of circulating blood volume, decreased ability to transport oxygen

**Fear** related to threat to well-being, potential death

Imbalanced **nutrition**: less than body requirements related to nausea, vomiting

**Pain** related to irritated mucosa from acid secretion

Risk for ineffective **coping** related to personal vulnerability in crisis, bleeding, hospitalization

## GLAUCOMA

Disturbed **sensory** perception: visual related to increased intraocular pressure

See Vision Impairment

## GOUT

**Acute Pain** related to inflammation of affected joint

Impaired physical **mobility** related to musculoskeletal impairment

Ineffective **health** maintenance related to deficient knowledge regarding medications and home care

## GRAND MAL SEIZURE

See Seizure Disorders

## GRIEVING

Anticipatory **grieving** related to anticipated significant loss

Chronic **sorrow** related to unresolved grief

Dysfunctional **grieving** related to actual or perceived significant loss

**Grieving** related to actual significant loss; change in life status, style, or function

## GROOM SELF (INABILITY TO)

Dressing/grooming **self-care** deficit related to intolerance to activity, decreased strength and endurance pain, discomfort, perceptual or cognitive impairment, neuromuscular impairment, musculoskeletal impairment, depression, severe anxiety

## GROWTH AND DEVELOPMENT LAG

Delayed **growth** and development related to inadequate caretaking, indifference, inconsistent responsiveness, multiple caretakers, separation from significant others, environmental and stimulation deficiencies, effects of physical disability, prescribed dependence

## HEAD INJURY

Acute **confusion** related to brain injury
Disturbed **thought** processes related to pressure damage to brain
Disturbed **sensory** perception related to pressure damage to sensory centers in brain
Decreased **intracranial** adaptive capacity related to brain injury
Ineffective **breathing** patterns related to pressure damage to breathing center in brain stem
Ineffective **tissue** perfusion: cerebral related to effects of increased intracranial pressure
See Neurological Disorders

## HEADACHE

Acute **Pain**: headache related to lack of knowledge of pain control techniques or methods to prevent headaches
Disturbed **energy** field related to disharmony
Ineffective management of **therapeutic** regimen related to lack of knowledge, identification and elimination of aggravating factors

## HEALTH MAINTENANCE PROBLEMS

Ineffective **health** maintenance related to significant alteration in communication skills, lack of ability to make deliberate and thoughtful judgments, perceptual or cognitive impairment, ineffective coping, dysfunctional grieving, unachieved developmental tasks, ineffective family coping, disabling spiritual distress, lack of material resources

## HEALTH-SEEKING PERSON

**Health**-seeking behavior related to expressed desire for increased control of own personal health

## HEARING IMPAIRMENT

Disturbed **sensory** perception: auditory related to altered state of auditory system
Impaired verbal **communication** related to inability to hear own voice
**Social** isolation related to difficulty with communication

## HEART FAILURE

See CHF

## HEMIPLEGIA

See CVA

## HEMORRHAGE

**Fear** related to threat to well-being
Deficient **fluid** volume related to massive blood loss
See cause of Hemorrhage; Hypovolemic Shock

## HEMORRHOIDECTOMY

**Anxiety** related to embarrassment, need for privacy
**Constipation** related to fear of pain with defecation
Ineffective **health** maintenance related to deficient knowledge regarding pain relief, use of stool softeners, dietary changes
**Pain** related to surgical procedure
Risk for deficient **fluid** volume: hemorrhage related to inadequate clotting
**Urinary** retention related to pain, anesthetic effect

## HEMORRHOIDS

**Constipation** related to painful defecation, poor bowel habits
Impaired **Comfort**: pruritus related to inflammation of hemorrhoids
Ineffective **health** maintenance related to deficient knowledge regarding care of condition

## HEPATITIS

**Activity** intolerance related to weakness or fatigue secondary to infection
Acute **Pain** related to edema of liver, bile irritating skin
Deficient **diversional** activity related to isolation
**Fatigue** related to infectious process, altered body chemistry
Imbalanced **nutrition**: less than body requirements related to anorexia, impaired use of proteins and carbohydrates
Ineffective **health** maintenance related to deficient knowledge regarding disease process and home management
Risk for deficient **fluid** volume related to excessive loss of fluids via vomiting and diarrhea
**Social** isolation related to treatment-imposed isolation

## HERNIA

See Hiatus Hernia; Inguinal Hernia Repair

## HIATUS HERNIA

Imbalanced **nutrition**: less than body requirements related to pain after eating
Ineffective **health** maintenance related to deficient knowledge regarding care of disease
**Nausea** related to effects of gastric contents in esophagus
**Pain**: heartburn related to gastroesophageal reflux

## HIP FRACTURE

Acute **confusion** related to sensory overload, sensory deprivation, medication side effects
Acute **Pain** related to injury, surgical procedure
**Constipation** related to immobility, narcotics, anesthesia
**Fear** related to outcome of treatment, future mobility, present helplessness
Impaired physical **mobility** related to surgical incision, temporary absence of weight bearing
Impaired **transfer** ability related to immobilization of hip
Impaired **walking** related to temporary absence of weight bearing
**Powerlessness** related to health care environment
Risk for deficient **fluid** volume: hemorrhage related to postoperative complication, surgical blood loss
Risk for impaired **skin** integrity related to immobility
Risk for **infection** related to invasive procedure
Risk for **injury** related to dislodged prosthesis, unsteadiness when ambulating
Risk for perioperative positioning **injury** related to immobilization, muscle weakness, emaciation
**Self**-care deficit: specify related to musculoskeletal impairment

## HIV (HUMAN IMMUNODEFICIENCY VIRUS)

**Fear** related to possible death
Ineffective **protection** related to depressed immune system
See AIDS

## HOME MAINTENANCE PROBLEMS

Impaired **home** maintenance related to individual or family member disease or injury, insufficient family organization or planning, insufficient finances, unfamiliarity with neighborhood resources, impaired cognitive or emotional functioning, lack of knowledge, lack of role modeling, inadequate support systems

## HOPELESSNESS

**Hopelessness** related to prolonged activity restriction creating isolation, failing or deteriorating physiological condition, long-term stress, abandonment, lost belief in transcendent values or higher power/God

## HTN (HYPERTENSION)

Imbalanced **nutrition**: more than body requirements related to lack of knowledge of relationship between diet and disease process

Ineffective **health** maintenance related to deficient knowledge regarding treatment and control of disease process

**Noncompliance** related to side effects of treatments, lack of understanding regarding importance of controlling hypertension

## HUMAN IMMUNODEFICIENCY VIRUS

See AIDS; HIV

## HYGIENE, INABILITY TO PROVIDE OWN

Bathing/hygiene **self-care** deficit related to intolerance to activity, decreased strength and endurance, pain, discomfort, perceptual or cognitive impairment, neuromuscular impairment, musculoskeletal impairment, depression, severe anxiety

## HYPERTENSION

See HTN

## HYPERTHERMIA

**Hyperthermia** related to exposure to hot environment, vigorous activity, medications, anesthesia, inappropriate clothing, increased metabolic rate, illness, trauma, dehydration, inability or decreased ability to perspire

## HYPOTHERMIA

**Hypothermia** related to exposure to cold environment, illness, trauma, damage to hypothalamus, malnutrition, aging

## HYPOVOLEMIC SHOCK

See Shock

## HYSTERECTOMY

Acute **Pain** related to surgical injury

Anticipatory **grieving** related to change in body image, loss of reproductive status

**Constipation** related to opioids, anesthesia, bowel manipulation during surgery

Ineffective **coping** related to situational crisis of surgery

Ineffective **health** maintenance related to deficient knowledge regarding precautions and self-care following surgery

Risk for **constipation** related to narcotics, anesthesia, bowel manipulation during surgery

Risk for deficient **fluid** volume related to abnormal blood loss, hemorrhage

Risk for ineffective **tissue** perfusion related to thromboembolism

Risk for urge urinary **incontinence** related to edema in area, anesthesia, narcotics, pain

Risk for **urinary** retention related to edema in area, anesthesia, opioids, pain

**Sexual** dysfunction related to disturbance in self-concept

See Surgery

## IBS (IRRITABLE BOWEL SYNDROME)

**Chronic Pain** related to spasms, increased motility of bowel

**Constipation** related to low-residue diet, stress

**Diarrhea** related to increased motility of intestines associated with stress

Ineffective **health** maintenance related to deficient knowledge regarding self-care with IBS

Ineffective management of **therapeutic** regimen related to deficient knowledge, powerlessness

## IDENTITY DISTURBANCE

Disturbed personal **identity** related to situational crisis, psychological impairment, chronic illness, pain

## ILEUS

Acute **Pain** related to pressure, abdominal distention

**Constipation** related to decreased gastric motility

Deficient **fluid** volume related to loss of fluids from vomiting, fluids trapped in bowel

**Nausea** related to gastrointestinal irritation

## IMPACTION OF STOOL

**Constipation** related to decreased fluid intake, less than adequate amounts of fiber and bulk-forming foods in diet, immobility

## IMPOTENCE

**Self-esteem** disturbance related to physiological crisis, inability to practice usual sexual activity

**Sexual** dysfunction related to altered body function

## INCONTINENCE OF STOOL

**Bowel** incontinence related to decreased awareness of need to defecate, loss of sphincter control

Deficient knowledge related to lack of information on normal bowel elimination

## INCONTINENCE OF URINE

Functional **incontinence** related to altered environment; sensory, cognitive, or mobility deficits

Reflex **incontinence** related to neurological impairment

Risk for impaired **skin** integrity related to presence of urine

Risk for urge urinary **incontinence** related to effects of alcohol, caffeine, decreased bladder capacity, irritation of bladder stretch receptors causing spasm, increased urine concentration, overdistention of bladder

Stress urinary **incontinence** related to degenerative change in pelvic muscles and structural supports associated with increased age, high intraabdominal pressure (e.g., from obesity, gravid uterus), incompetent bladder outlet, overdistention between voidings, weak pelvic muscles and structural supports

Total urinary **incontinence** related to neuropathy preventing transmission of reflex indicating bladder fullness, neurological dysfunction causing triggering of micturition at unpredictable times, independent contraction of detrusor reflex due to surgery, trauma or disease affecting spinal cord nerves, anatomical fistula

Urge urinary **incontinence** related to decreased bladder capacity (i.e., history of pelvic inflammatory disease, abdominal surgeries, indwelling urinary catheter); irritation of bladder stretch receptors, causing spasm (e.g., bladder infection); alcohol; caffeine; increased fluids; increased urine concentration; overdistention of bladder

## INFANT BEHAVIOR

Disorganized **infant** behavior related to pain, oral/motor problems, feeding intolerance, environmental overstimulation, lack of containment/boundaries, prematurity, invasive/painful procedures

Readiness for enhanced organized Infant behavior related to prematurity, pain

## INFANT FEEDING PATTERN, INEFFECTIVE

Ineffective **infant** feeding pattern related to prematurity, neurological impairment or delay, oral hypersensitivity, prolonged NPO

## INFECTION

**Hyperthermia** related to increased metabolic rate

Ineffective **Protection** related to inadequate nutrition, abnormal blood profiles, drug therapies, treatments

## INFECTION, POTENTIAL FOR

Risk for **infection** related to inadequate primary defenses (e.g., broken skin, traumatized tissue, decrease in ciliary action, stasis of body fluids, change in pH secretions, altered peristalsis), inadequate secondary defenses (e.g., decreased hemoglobin, leukopenia suppressed inflammatory response), immunosuppression, inadequate acquired immunity, tissue destruction and increased environmental exposure, chronic disease, invasive procedures, malnutrition, pharmaceutical agents, trauma, rupture of amniotic membranes, insufficient knowledge to avoid exposure to pathogens

## INFLAMMATORY BOWEL DISEASE

Acute **Pain** related to abdominal cramping and anal irritation

Deficient **Fluid** volume related to frequent and loose stools

**Diarrhea** related to effects of inflammatory changes of the bowel

Imbalanced **Nutrition**: less than body requirements related to anorexia, decreased absorption of nutrients from gastrointestinal tract

Impaired **skin** integrity related to frequent stools, development of anal fissures

Ineffective **Coping** related to repeated episodes of diarrhea

**Social** isolation related to diarrhea

## INFLUENZA

Acute **Pain** related to inflammatory changes in joints

Deficient **Fluid** volume related to inadequate fluid intake

**Hyperthermia** related to infectious process

Ineffective **Health** maintenance related to Deficient Knowledge regarding self-care

Ineffective **Therapeutic** regimen management related to lack of knowledge regarding preventive immunizations

## INJURY

Risk for **falls** related to orthostatic hypertension, impaired physical mobility, diminished mental status

Risk for **injury** related to environmental conditions interacting with client's adaptive and defensive resources

## INSOMNIA

**Anxiety** related to actual or perceived loss of sleep

Disturbed **Sleep** pattern related to sensory alterations, internal factors, external factors

**Sleep** deprivation related to sustained inadequate sleep hygiene, prolonged use of pharmacological agents, aging-related sleep stage shifts

## INTRACRANIAL PRESSURE, INCREASED

Decreased **Intracranial** adaptive capacity related to sustained increase in intracranial pressure

See cause of Increased Intracranial Pressure

## IRRITABLE BOWEL SYNDROME

See IBS

## JOINT REPLACEMENT

Risk for **peripheral** neurovascular dysfunction related to orthopedic surgery

See Total Joint Replacement

## KIDNEY FAILURE

See Renal Failure

## KIDNEY STONE

Acute **Pain** related to obstruction from renal calculi

Deficient **Knowledge** related to fluid requirements and dietary restrictions

Impaired **urinary** elimination: urgency & frequency related to anatomical obstruction, irritation caused by stone

Risk for deficient **Fluid** volume related to nausea, vomiting

Risk for **infection** related to obstruction of urinary tract with stasis of urine

## KNOWLEDGE, DEFICIENT

Deficient **Knowledge** related to lack of exposure, lack of recall, information misinterpretation, cognitive limitation, lack of interest in learning, unfamiliarity with information resources

## LAMINECTOMY

Acute **Pain** related to localized inflammation and edema

**Anxiety** related to change in health status, surgical procedure

Deficient **Knowledge** related to appropriate postoperative and post-discharge activities

Impaired physical **mobility** related to neuromuscular impairment

Risk for impaired **tissue** perfusion related to edema, hemorrhage, or embolism

Risk for perioperative positioning **injury** related to prone position

Disturbed **Sensory** perception: tactile related to possible edema or nerve injury

**Urinary** retention related to competing sensory impulses, effects of narcotics/anesthesia

See Surgery

## LATEX ALLERGY

Latex **allergy** related to hypersensitivity to natural latex rubber

Risk for **latex** allergy response related to multiple surgical procedures, especially from infancy (e.g., spina bifida); allergies to bananas, avocados, tropical fruits, kiwi, chestnuts; professions with daily exposure to latex (e.g., medicine, nursing, dentistry); conditions needing continuous or intermittent catheterization; history of reactions to latex (e.g., balloons, condoms, gloves); allergies to poinsettia plants; history of allergies and asthma

## LEUKEMIA

Ineffective **Protection** related to abnormal blood profile

Risk for deficient **Fluid** volume related to nausea, vomiting, bleeding, side effects of treatment

Risk for **infection** related to ineffective immune system

See Cancer; Chemotherapy

## LONELINESS

Risk for **loneliness** related to lack of affection, physical isolation, cathectic deprivation, social isolation

## LOW BACK PAIN

See Acute Back

## MALNUTRITION

Imbalanced **Nutrition**: less than body requirements related to inability to ingest food, digest food, or absorb nutrients because of biological, psychological, or economic factors; institutionalization (i.e., lack of menu choices)

## MANIC DISORDER, BIPOLAR I

**Anxiety** related to change in role function

Deficient **Fluid** volume related to decreased intake

Disturbed **Thought** processes related to mania

Disturbed **Sleep** pattern related to constant anxious thoughts

Imbalanced **Nutrition**: less than body requirements related to lack of time and motivation to eat, constant movement

Impaired **Home** maintenance related to altered psychological state, inability to concentrate

Ineffective **Coping** related to situational crisis

Ineffective **denial** related to fear of inability to control behavior

Ineffective **Role** performance related to impaired social interactions

Interrupted **Family** processes related to family member's illness

Ineffective **Therapeutic** regimen management related to lack of social supports

Ineffective **Therapeutic** regimen management: families related to unpredictability of client, excessive demands on family, chronicity of condition

**Noncompliance** related to denial of illness

Risk for **caregiver** role strain related to unpredictability of condition, mood swings

Risk for **powerlessness** related to inability to control changes in mood

Risk for self-directed **violence** or other directed violence related to hallucinations, delusions

Risk for **suicide** related to bipolar disorder

**Sleep** deprivation related to hyperagitated state

## MASTECTOMY

Acute **Pain** related to surgical procedure

Disturbed **Body** image related to loss of sexually significant body part

Chronic **sorrow** related to Disturbed Body image, unknown long term health status

Death **anxiety** related to threat of mortality associated with breast cancer

Deficient **Knowledge** related to self-care activities

**Fear** related to change in body image, prognosis

**Nausea** related to chemotherapy

Risk for impaired physical **mobility** related to nerve or muscle damage, pin

Risk for **post-trauma** syndrome related to associated with loss of body part, surgical wounds.

Risk for **powerlessness** Related to fear of unknown outcome of procedure

**Sexual** dysfunction related to change in body image, fear of loss of feminism

See Cancer; Surgery

## MEMORY DEFICIT

Impaired **memory** related to acute or chronic hypoxia, anemia, decreased cardiac output, fluid and electrolyte imbalance, neurological disturbance, excessive environmental disturbances

## MENINGITIS/ENCEPHALITIS

Acute **Pain** related to neck (nuchal) rigidity, inflammation of meninges, headache, kinesthetic, Disturbed Sensory perception (i.e. pain felt when skin touched), fever, earache

Decreased **Intracranial** adaptive capacity related to sustained increase in intracranial pressure (10 to 15 mm Hg ICP)

Delayed **Growth** and development related to brain damage secondary to infectious process, increased intracranial pressure

Disturbed **Thought** processes related to inflammation of brain, fever

Excess **Fluid** volume related to increased intracranial pressure, syndrome of inappropriate secretion of antidiuretic hormone (SIADH)

Impaired **Comfort** related to central nervous system inflammation

Impaired **Comfort**: photophobia related to increased sensitivity to external stimuli secondary to central nervous system inflammation

Impaired **mobility** related to neuromuscular or central nervous system insult

Ineffective **airway** clearance related to seizure activity

Ineffective **Tissue** perfusion: cerebral related to inflamed cerebral tissues and meninges, increased intracranial pressure

Risk for **aspiration** related to seizure activity

Risk for **injury** related to seizure activity

Risk for **falls** related to neuromuscular dysfunction

Disturbed **sensory** perception: hearing related to CNS infection, ear infection

Disturbed **sensory** perception: kinesthetic related to CNS infection

Disturbed **sensory** perception: visual related to photophobia secondary to CNS infection

## MENOPAUSE

Effective **Therapeutic** regimen management related to verbalized desire to manage menopause

Ineffective **Sexuality** patterns related to altered body structure, lack of physiological lubrication, lack of knowledge of artificial lubrication

**Health**-seeking behavior related to menopause, therapies associated with change in hormonal levels

Impaired **memory** related to change in hormonal levels

Ineffective **thermoregulation** related to changes in hormonal levels

Readiness for enhanced **Spiritual** well-being related to desire for harmony of mind, body and spirit

Risk for Imbalanced **Nutrition**: more than body requirements related to change in metabolic rate caused by fluctuating hormone levels

Risk for **powerlessness** related to changes associated with menopause

Risk for situational low **self**-esteem related to developmental changes: menopause

Risk for urge urinary **Incontinence** related to changes in hormonal levels affecting bladder function

## MENTAL ILLNESS

Chronic **sorrow** related to presence of mental illness

Compromised family **Coping** related to lack of available support from client

Defensive **coping** related to psychological impairment, substance abuse

Disabled family **Coping** related to chronically unexpressed feelings of guilt, anxiety, hostility, or despair

Disturbed **Thought** processes related to head injury, mental disorder, personality disorder, organic mental disorder, substance abuse, severe interpersonal conflict, sleep deprivation, sensory deprivation or overload, impaired cerebral perfusion

Ineffective community **Therapeutic** regimen management: related to inadequate services to care for mentally ill clients, lack of information regarding how to access services

Ineffective **Coping** related to situational crisis, coping with mental illness

Ineffective **denial** related to refusal to acknowledge abuse problem, fear of the social stigma of disease

Ineffective **Therapeutic** regimen management: families related to chronicity of condition, unpredictability of client, unknown prognosis

Risk for **loneliness** related to social isolation

Risk for **powerlessness** related to life style of helplessness

## MENTAL RETARDATION

Chronic low **self**-esteem related to perceived differences

Delayed **Growth** and development related to cognitive or perceptual impairment, developmental delay

**Grieving** related to loss of perfect child; birth of child with congenital defect or subsequent head injury

Impaired **Home** maintenance related to insufficient support systems

Impaired **social** interaction related to developmental lag or delay, perceived differences

Impaired **swallowing** related to neuromuscular impairment

Impaired verbal **communication** related to developmental delay

Interrupted **Family** processes related to crisis of diagnosis and situational transition

Parental role **conflict** related to home care of child with special needs

Readiness for enhanced family **Coping** related to adaptation and acceptance of child's condition and needs

Risk for delayed **Development** related to cognitive or perceptual impairment

Risk for disproportionate **Growth** related to mental retardation

Risk for **self**-mutilation related to separation anxiety, depersonalization

**Self**-care deficit: bathing/hygiene, dressing/grooming, feeding, toileting related to perceptual or cognitive impairment

**Self** mutilation Related to inability to express tension verbally

See Child with Chronic Condition; Safety, Childhood

## MI (MYOCARDIAL INFARCTION)

Acute **Pain** related to myocardial tissue damage from inadequate blood supply

**Anxiety** related to threat of death, possible change in role status

**Constipation** related to decreased peristalsis from decreased physical activity, medication effect, change in diet

Death **anxiety** related to seriousness of medical condition

Decreased **cardiac** output related to ventricular damage, ischemia, dysrhythmias

**Fear** related to threat to well-being

Ineffective **Health** maintenance related to deficient knowledge regarding self-care and treatment

Ineffective **sexuality** patterns related to fear of chest pain, possibility of heart damage

Ineffective **denial** related to fear, deficient knowledge about heart disease

Ineffective family **coping** related to spouse or significant other's fear of partner loss

Interrupted **Family** processes related to crisis, role change

Risk for **powerlessness** Related to acute illness

Risk for **spiritual** distress Related to physical illness: MI

Situational low **self**-esteem related to crisis of MI

## MIGRAINE HEADACHE

Acute **Pain**: headache related to vasodilation of cerebral and extra-cerebral vessels

Disturbed **Energy** field related to Pain, disruption of normal flow of energy

Ineffective **Health** maintenance related to deficient knowledge regarding prevention and treatment of headaches

## MOBILITY, IMPAIRED PHYSICAL

Impaired physical **mobility** related to intolerance to activity, decreased strength and endurance, pain, discomfort, perceptual or cognitive impairment, neuromuscular impairment, musculoskeletal impairment, depression, severe anxiety

Risk for **falls** Related to impaired physical mobility

## MONONUCLEOSIS

**Activity** intolerance related to generalized weakness

Acute **Pain** related to enlargement of lymph nodes, irritation of oropharyngeal cavity

**Hyperthermia** related to infectious process

**Fatigue** related to disease state, stress

Impaired **swallowing** related to irritation of oropharyngeal cavity

Ineffective **Health** maintenance related to deficient knowledge concerning transmission and treatment of disease

Risk for **injury** related to possible rupture of spleen

## MUCOUS MEMBRANES, IMPAIRED ORAL

Impaired Oral mucous membrane related to pathological conditions-oral cavity (radiation to head or neck), dehydration, chemical trauma (e.g., acidic foods, drugs, noxious agents, alcohol), mechanical trauma (e.g., ill-fitting dentures, braces, endotracheal or nasogastric tubes, surgery in oral cavity), NPO for more than 24 hours, ineffective oral hygiene, mouth breathing, malnutrition, infection, lack of or decreased salivation, medication

## MULTIPLE SCLEROSIS (MS)

See Neurological Disorders

## MVA (MOTOR VEHICLE ACCIDENT)

See Fracture; Head Injury; Injury; Pneumothorax

## MYOCARDIAL INFARCTION

See MI

## NAUSEA

**Nausea** related to chemotherapy, postsurgical anesthesia, or irritation to the gastrointestinal system

## NEURITIS

**Activity** intolerance related to pain with movement

Acute **Pain** related to stimulation of affected nerve endings, inflammation of sensory

Ineffective **Health** maintenance related to deficient knowledge regarding self-care with neuritis

## NEUROGENIC BLADDER

Reflex **incontinence** related to neurological impairment

**Urinary** retention related to interruption in the lateral spinal tracts

## NEUROLOGICAL DISORDERS

Acute **confusion** related to dementia, alcohol abuse, drug abuse, delirium

Anticipatory **grieving** related to loss of usual body functioning

Imbalanced **Nutrition**: less than body requirements related to impaired swallowing, depression, difficulty feeding self

Impaired **Home** maintenance related to client's or family member's disease

Impaired **memory** related to neurological disturbance

Impaired physical **mobility** related to neuromuscular impairment

Impaired **swallowing** related to neuromuscular dysfunction

Ineffective **airway** clearance related to perceptual or cognitive impairment, decreased energy, fatigue

Ineffective **Coping** related to disability requiring change in life-style

Interrupted **Family** processes related to situational crisis, illness or disability of family member

**Powerlessness** related to progressive nature of disease

Risk for **disuse** syndrome related to physical immobility, neuromuscular dysfunction

Risk for impaired **skin** integrity related to altered sensation, altered mental status, paralysis

Risk for **injury** related to altered mobility, sensory dysfunction, cognitive impairment

**Self**-care deficit: specify related to neuromuscular dysfunction

**Sexual** dysfunction related to biopsychosocial alteration of sexuality

**Social** isolation related to altered state of wellness

## NEWBORN, NORMAL

Effective **breast**-feeding related to normal oral structure and gestational age greater than 34 weeks

Ineffective **Protection** related to immature immune system

Ineffective **thermoregulation** related to immaturity of neuroendocrine system

Readiness for enhanced organized **Infant** behavior related to appropriate environmental stimuli

Risk for **infection** related to open umbilical stump

Risk for **injury** related to immaturity, need for caretaking

## NONCOMPLIANCE

**Noncompliance** related to client value system, health beliefs, cultural influences, spiritual values, client-provider relationships, deficient knowledge

## NUTRITION, IMBALANCED

Imbalanced **Nutrition**: risk for more than body requirements related to obesity in parents, use of food as reward or comfort measure, dysfunctional eating pattern, eating in response to cues other than hunger

Imbalanced **Nutrition**: less than body requirements related to inability to ingest or digest food or absorb nutrients because of biological, psychological, economic factors

Imbalanced **Nutrition**: more than body requirements related to excessive intake in relation to metabolic need

## OBESITY

Disturbed **Body** image related to eating disorder, excess weight

Chronic low **self**-esteem related to Ineffective coping, overeating

Imbalanced **Nutrition**: more than body requirements related to caloric intake exceeding energy expenditure

## OBSESSIVE-COMPULSIVE DISORDER

**Anxiety** related to threat to self-concept, unmet needs

Decisional **conflict** related to inability to make a decision for fear of reprisal

Disabled family **Coping** related to family process being disrupted by client's ritualistic activities

Disturbed **Thought** processes related to persistent thoughts, ideas, impulses that seem irrelevant and will not relent

Ineffective **Coping** related to expression of feelings in an unacceptable way, ritualistic behavior

**Powerlessness** related to unrelenting repetitive thoughts to perform irrational activities

Risk for situational low **self**-esteem related to inability to control repetitive thoughts and actions

## OPEN REDUCTION OF FRACTURE WITH INTERNAL FIXATION (FEMUR)

**Anxiety** related to outcome of corrective procedure

Impaired physical **mobility** related to postoperative position, abduction of leg, avoidance of acute flexion

**Powerlessness** related to loss of control, unanticipated change in lifestyle

Risk for perioperative positioning **injury** related to immobilization

Risk for **peripheral** neurovascular dysfunction related to mechanical compression, orthopedic surgery, immobilization

See Surgery, Postoperative Care

## ORAL MUCOUS MEMBRANE, IMPAIRED

Impaired **oral** mucous membrane related to pathological conditions-oral cavity (radiation to head or neck), dehydration, chemical trauma (e.g., acidic foods, drugs, noxious agents, alcohol), mechanical trauma (e.g., ill-fitting dentures, braces, endotracheal and nasogastric tubes, surgery in oral cavity), NPO for more than 24 hours, ineffective oral hygiene, mouth breathing, malnutrition, infection, lack of or decreased salivation, medication

## OSTEOARTHRITIS

**Activity** intolerance related to pain after exercise or use of joint

Impaired **transfer** ability related to pain

Acute **Pain** related to movement

See Arthritis

## OSTEOMYELITIS

Acute **Pain** related to inflammation in affected extremity

Deficient **Diversional** activity related to prolonged immobilization, hospitalization

**Fear**: parental related to concern regarding possible growth plate damage secondary to infection, concern that infection may become chronic

**Hyperthermia** related to infectious process

Impaired physical **mobility** related to imposed immobility secondary to infected area

Ineffective **Health** maintenance related to continued immobility at home, possible extensive casts, continued antibiotics

Risk for **constipation** related to immobility

Risk for impaired **skin** integrity related to irritation from splint/cast

See Hospitalized Child

## OSTEOPOROSIS

Acute **Pain** related to fracture, muscle spasms

Deficient **Knowledge** related to diet, exercise, need to abstain from alcohol and nicotine

Effective **Therapeutic** regimen management: individual related to appropriate choices for diet and exercise to prevent and manage condition

Imbalanced **Nutrition**: less than body requirements related to inadequate intake of calcium and vitamin D

Impaired physical **mobility** related to pain, skeletal changes

Risk for **injury**: fracture related to lack of activity, risk of falling resulting from environmental hazards, neuromuscular disorders, diminished senses, cardiovascular responses, responses to drugs

Risk for **powerlessness** related to debilitating disease

## OTITIS MEDIA

Acute **Pain** related to inflammation, infectious process

Risk for delayed **Development** related to frequent otitis media

Risk for **infection** related to eustachian tube obstruction, traumatic eardrum perforation, infectious disease process

Disturbed **sensory** perception: auditory related to incomplete resolution of otitis media, presence of excess drainage in middle ear

## PACEMAKER

Acute **Pain** related to surgical procedure Anxiety related to change in health status, presence of pacemaker

Death **anxiety** related to worry over possible malfunction of pacemaker

Deficient **Knowledge** related to self-care program, when to seek medical attention

Risk for decreased **cardiac** output related to malfunction of pacemaker

Risk for **infection** related to invasive procedure, presence of foreign body (catheter and generator)

Risk for **powerlessness** related to presence of electronic devise to stimulate heart

## ACUTE PAIN

Acute **Pain** related to injury agents (biological, chemical, physical, psychological)

## PAIN, CHRONIC

Chronic **pain** related to chronic physical or psychosocial disability

## PANCREATITIS

Acute **Pain** related to irritation and edema of the inflamed pancreas

Chronic **sorrow** related to chronic illness

**Diarrhea** related to decrease in pancreatic secretions resulting in steatorrhea

Deficient **Fluid** volume related to vomiting, decreased fluid intake, fever, diaphoresis, fluid shifts

Imbalanced **Nutrition**: less than body requirements related to inadequate dietary intake, increased nutritional needs secondary to acute illness, increased metabolic needs caused by increased body temperature

Ineffective **breathing** pattern related to splinting from severe pain

Ineffective **denial** related to ineffective coping, alcohol use

Ineffective **Health** maintenance related to deficient knowledge concerning diet, alcohol use, medication

**Nausea** related to irritation of gastrointestinal system

## PANIC DISORDER

**Anxiety** related to situational crisis

Ineffective **Coping** related to personal vulnerability

**Post**-trauma syndrome related to previous catastrophic event

Risk for **loneliness** related to inability to socially interact because of fear of losing control

Risk for **Powerlessness** related to ineffective coping skills

Risk for **post**-trauma syndrome related to perception of the event, diminished ego strength

**Social** isolation related to fear of lack of control

## PARALYSIS

Acute **Pain** related to prolonged immobility

Chronic **sorrow** related to loss of physical mobility

**Constipation** related to effects of spinal cord disruption, diet inadequate in fiber

Disturbed **Body** image related to biophysical changes, loss of movement, immobility

**Disuse** syndrome related to paralysis

Impaired **Home** maintenance related to physical disability

Impaired physical **mobility** related to neuromuscular impairment

Impaired **transfer** ability related to paralysis

Ineffective **Health** maintenance related to deficient knowledge regarding self-care with paralysis

**Powerlessness** related to illness-related regimen

Reflex **incontinence** related to neurological impairment

Risk for impaired **skin** integrity related to altered circulation, altered sensation, immobility

Risk for **injury** related to altered mobility, sensory dysfunction

Risk for **falls** related to paralysis

Risk for **post**-trauma syndrome related to event causing paralysis

Risk for situational low **self**-esteem related to change in body image and function

**Self**-care deficit: specify related to neuromuscular impairment

**Sexual** dysfunction related to loss of sensation, biopsychosocial alteration

See Child with Chronic Condition; Hemiplegia; Hospitalized Child; Neurotube Defects; Spinal Cord Injury

## PARALYTIC ILEUS

See Ileus

## PARANOID PERSONALITY DISORDER

**Anxiety** related to uncontrollable intrusive, suspicious thoughts

Chronic low **self**-esteem related to inability to trust others

Impaired **adjustment** related to intense emotional state

Disturbed personal **Identity** related to difficulty in reality testing

Disturbed **Thought** processes related to psychological conflicts

Risk for **loneliness** related to social isolation

Risk for **post**-trauma syndrome related to exaggerated sense of responsibility

Risk for other directed **violence** related to being suspicious of others and others' actions

Risk for **suicide** related to psychiatric illness

Disturbed **sensory** perception: specify related to psychological dysfunction, suspicious thoughts

Social **isolation** related to inappropriate social skills

## PARENT ATTACHMENT

Risk for impaired parent/infant/child **Attachment** related to inability of parents to meet personal needs; anxiety associated with parental role; substance abuse; premature infant; ill infant/child who is unable to effectively initiate parental contact as a result of altered behavioral organization, separation, physical barriers, or lack of privacy

Risk for **spiritual** distress related to altered relationships

## PARENTAL ROLE CONFLICT

Chronic **sorrow** related to difficult parent-child relationship

Parental role **conflict** related to separation from child because of chronic illness, intimidation with invasive or restrictive modalities (e.g., isolation, intubation), specialized care center policies, home care of a child with special needs (e.g., apnea monitoring, postural drainage, hyperalimentation), change in marital status, interruptions of family life because of home care regimen (e.g., treatments, caregivers, lack of respite)

Risk for **spiritual** distress related to altered relationships

## PARENTING, IMPAIRED

Chronic **sorrow** related to difficult parent-child relationship

Impaired **Parenting** related to lack of available role model; ineffective role model; physical and psychosocial abuse of nurturing figure; lack of support between and from significant other(s); unmet social, emotional, or maturational needs of parenting figures; interruption in bonding process, (e.g., maternal, paternal, other); unrealistic expectations for self, infant, partner; physical illness; presence of stress (e.g., financial, legal, recent crisis, cultural move); lack of knowledge; limited cognitive functioning; lack of role identity; lack or inappropriate response of child to relationship; multiple pregnancies

Risk for **spiritual** distress related to altered relationships

## PARENTING, RISK FOR IMPAIRED

Risk for Impaired **Parenting** related to lack of available role model; ineffective role model; physical and psychosocial abuse of nurturing figure; lack of support between or from significant other(s); unmet social, emotional, or maturational needs of parenting figures; interruption in bonding process (e.g., maternal, paternal, other); unrealistic expectations for self, infant, partner; physical illness; presence of stress (e.g., financial, legal, recent crisis, cultural move); lack of knowledge; limited cognitive functioning; lack of role identity; lack of inappropriate response of child to relationship; multiple pregnancies

## PARKINSON'S DISEASE

Chronic **sorrow** related to loss of physical capacity

**Constipation** related to weakness of defecation muscles, lack of exercise, inadequate fluid intake, decreased autonomic nervous system activity

Imbalanced **Nutrition**: less than body requirements related to tremor, slowness in eating, difficulty in chewing and swallowing

Impaired verbal **communication** related to decreased speech volume, slowness of speech, impaired facial muscles

Risk for **injury** related to tremors, slow reactions, altered gait

See Neurological Disorders

## PELVIC INFLAMMATORY DISEASE

See PID

## PERICARDITIS

**Activity** intolerance related to reduced cardiac reserve, prescribed bedrest

Acute **Pain** related to biological injury, inflammation

Delayed **surgical** recovery related to complications associated with cardiac problems

Deficient **Knowledge** related to unfamiliarity with information sources

Ineffective **Tissue** perfusion: cardiopulmonary/peripheral related to risk for development of emboli

Risk for decreased **cardiac** output related to inflammation in pericardial sac, fluid accumulation compressing heart function

Risk for Imbalanced **Nutrition**: less than body requirements related to fever, hypermetabolic state associated with fever

Risk for decreased **cardiac** output related to inflammation in pericardial sac, fluid accumulation compressing heart function

## PERIOPERATIVE POSITIONING

Risk for perioperative positioning **injury** related to disorientation; immobilization; muscle weakness; sensory/perceptual disturbances resulting from anesthesia, obesity, emaciation, edema

## PERIPHERAL NEUROVASCULAR DYSFUNCTION, RISK FOR

Risk for **peripheral** neurovascular dysfunction related to fractures, mechanical compression, orthopedic surgery, trauma, immobilization, burns, vascular obstruction

## PERIPHERAL VASCULAR DISEASE

**Activity** intolerance related to imbalance between peripheral oxygen supply and demand

Chronic **pain**: intermittent claudication related to ischemia

Ineffective **Health** maintenance related to deficient Knowledge regarding self-care and treatment of disease

Ineffective **Tissue** perfusion: peripheral related to interruption of vascular flow

Risk for impaired **skin** integrity related to altered circulation or sensation

Risk for **falls** related to altered mobility

Risk for **injury** related to tissue hypoxia, altered mobility, altered sensation

Risk for **peripheral** neurovascular dysfunction related to possible vascular obstruction

## PERITONITIS

Acute **Pain** related to inflammation, stimulation of somatic nerves

**Constipation** related to decreased oral intake, decrease of peristalsis

Deficient **Fluid** volume related to retention of fluid in bowel with loss of circulating blood volume

Imbalanced **Nutrition**: less than body requirements related to nausea, vomiting

Ineffective **breathing** pattern related to pain, increased abdominal pressure

**Nausea** related to gastrointestinal irritation

## PERSONAL IDENTITY PROBLEMS

Disturbed personal **Identity** related to situational crisis, psychological impairment, chronic illness, pain

## PERSONALITY DISORDER

Chronic low **self**-esteem related to inability to set and achieve goals

Compromised family **Coping** related to inability of client to provide positive feedback to family, chronicity exhausting family

Decisional **conflict** related to low self-esteem, feelings that choices will always be wrong

Disturbed personal **Identity** related to lack of consistent positive self-image

Impaired **adjustment** related to ambivalent behavior toward others, testing of others' loyalty

Impaired **social** interaction related to knowledge or skill deficit regarding ways to interact effectively with others, self-concept disturbances

Risk for **loneliness** related to inability to interact appropriately with others

Risk for situational low **self**-esteem Related to history of learned **helplessness**

Risk for **self**-mutilation Related to disturbed interpersonal relationships, borderline personality disorders

**Spiritual** distress related to lack of identifiable values, lack of meaning to life

See Antisocial Personality Disorder; Borderline Personality Disorder

## PID (PELVIC INFLAMMATORY DISEASE)

Acute **Pain** related to biological injury; inflammation, edema, congestion of pelvic tissues

Ineffective **Health** maintenance related to deficient Knowledge regarding self-care, treatment of disease

Ineffective **Sexuality** patterns related to medically imposed abstinence from sexual activities until acute infection subsides, change in reproductive potential

Risk for **infection** related to insufficient knowledge to avoid exposure to pathogens; proper hygiene, nutrition, other health habits

Risk for urge urinary **Incontinence** related to inflammation, edema, congestion of pelvic tissues

## PNEUMONIA

**Activity** intolerance related to imbalance between oxygen supply and demand

Deficient **Knowledge** related to risk factors predisposing person to pneumonia, treatment

**Hyperthermia** related to dehydration, increased metabolic rate, illness

Impaired **Oral** mucous membrane related to dry mouth from mouth breathing, decreased fluid intake

Imbalanced **Nutrition**: less than body requirements related to loss of appetite

Impaired **gas** exchange related to decreased functional lung tissue

Ineffective **Health** maintenance related to deficient Knowledge regarding self-care and treatment of disease

Ineffective **airway** clearance related to inflammation and presence of secretions

Risk for deficient **Fluid** volume related to inadequate intake of fluids

See Respiratory Infections, Acute Childhood (for child)

## PNEUMOTHORAX

Acute **Pain** related to recent injury, coughing, deep breathing

**Fear** related to threat to own well-being, difficulty breathing

Impaired **gas** exchange related to ventilation-perfusion imbalance

Risk for **injury** related to possible complications associated with closed chest drainage system

## POISONING, RISK FOR
**Internal**

Risk for **poisoning** related to reduced vision, verbalization of occupational settings without adequate safeguards, lack of safety or drug education, lack of proper precaution, cognitive or emotional difficulties, insufficient finances

**External**

Risk for **poisoning** related to large supplies of drugs in house, medicine stored in unlocked cabinets accessible to children or confused persons, dangerous products placed or stored within the reach of children or confused persons, availability of illicit drugs potentially contaminated by poisonous additives, flaking or peeling paint or plaster in presence of young children, chemical contamination of food and water, unprotected contact with heavy metals or chemicals, paint or lacquer used in poorly ventilated areas or without effective protection, presence of poisonous vegetation, presence of atmospheric pollutants

## POSTOPERATIVE CARE

See Surgery, Postoperative

## POSTPARTUM, NORMAL CARE

Acute **Pain** related to episiotomy, lacerations, bruising, breast engorgement, headache, sore nipples, epidural or IV site, hemorrhoids

**Anxiety** related to change in role functioning, parenting

**Constipation** related to hormonal effects on smooth muscles, fear of straining with defecation, effects of anesthesia

Deficient **Knowledge**: infant care related to lack of preparation for parenting

Disturbed **Sleep** pattern related to care of infant

Effective **breast-feeding** related to basic breast-feeding knowledge, support of partner and health care provider

**Fatigue** related to childbirth, new responsibilities of parenting, body changes

**Health**-seeking behaviors related to postpartum recovery and adaptation

Impaired **skin** integrity related to episiotomy, lacerations

Ineffective **Role** performance related to new responsibilities of parenting

Impaired **Urinary** elimination related to effects of anesthesia, tissue trauma

Ineffective **breast**-feeding related to lack of knowledge, lack of support, lack of motivation

Readiness for enhanced family **Coping** related to adaptation to new family member

Risk for Impaired **Parenting** related to lack of role models, Deficient Knowledge

Risk for **constipation** related to hormonal effects on smooth muscles, fear of straining with defecation, effects of anesthesia

Risk for imbalanced **Fluid** volume related to shift in blood volume, edema

Risk for **infection** related to tissue trauma, blood loss

Risk for **post-trauma** syndrome related to trauma or violence associated with labor and birth process, medical/surgical interventions, history of sexual abuse

Risk for urge urinary **Incontinence** related to effects of anesthesia or tissue trauma

**Sexual** dysfunction related to fear of pain or pregnancy

## POST-TRAUMA SYNDROME

**Post**-trauma syndrome related to events outside the range of the usual human experience; physical and psychosocial abuse; tragic occurrence involving multiple deaths; sudden destruction of one's home or community; natural or produced disasters; wars; being held as a prisoner of war or criminal victimization (torture); epidemics; serious accidents; rape; assault; witnessing mutilation, violent death, or other horrors; serious threat or injury to self or loved one's; industrial and motor vehicle accidents; catastrophic illnesses or accidents; military combat

## POWERLESSNESS

**Powerlessness** related to Health care environment, illness-related regimen, interpersonal interaction, lifestyle of helplessness

Risk for **powerlessness** related to Chronic or acute illness, acute injury or progressive debilitative disease process, aging, dying, lack of knowledge of illness or healthcare style, lifestyle of dependency with inadequate coping patterns, absence of integrality, decrease self-esteem, low or unstable body image

## PREGNANCY-INDUCED HYPERTENSION/ PREECLAMPSIA

See PIH

## PREGNANCY—NORMAL

Deficient **Knowledge** related to primiparity

Disturbed **Body** image related to altered body function and appearance

Disturbed **Sleep** pattern related to sleep deprivation secondary to uncomfortable pregnant state

Imbalanced **Nutrition**: less than body requirements related to growing fetus, nausea

Imbalanced **Nutrition**: more than body requirements related to deficient knowledge regarding nutritional needs of pregnancy

Interrupted **Family** processes related to developmental transition of pregnancy

Readiness for enhanced family **Coping** related to satisfying partner relationship, attention to gratification of needs, effective adaptation to developmental tasks of pregnancy

**Fear** related to labor and delivery

**Health**-seeking behaviors related to desire to promote optimal fetal and maternal health

Ineffective **Coping** related to personal vulnerability, situational crisis

**Nausea** related to hormonal changes of pregnancy

**Sexual** dysfunction related to altered body function, self-concept, body image with pregnancy

See Discomforts of Pregnancy

## PREMATURE INFANT (CHILD)

Delayed **Growth** and development : developmental lag related to prematurity, environmental and stimulation deficiencies, multiple caretakers

Imbalanced **Nutrition**: less than body requirements related to delayed or understimulated rooting reflex, easy fatigue during feeding, diminished endurance

Disorganized **infant** behavior related to prematurity

Disturbed **Sleep** pattern related to noisy and noxious intensive care environment

Impaired **gas** exchange related to effects of cardiopulmonary insufficiency

Impaired **swallowing** related to decreased or absent gag reflex, fatigue

Ineffective **thermoregulation** related to large body surface/weight ratio, immaturity of thermal regulation, state of prematurity

Readiness for enhanced organized **Infant** behavior related to prematurity

Risk for delayed **Development** related to prematurity

Risk for disproportionate **Growth** related to prematurity

Risk for **infection** related to inadequate, immature, or undeveloped acquired immune response

Risk for **injury** related to prolonged mechanical ventilation, retrolental fibroplasia (RLF) secondary to 100% oxygen environment

Disturbed **sensory** perception related to noxious stimuli, noisy environment

## PREMATURE INFANT (PARENT)

Anticipatory **grieving** related to loss of perfect child possibly leading to dysfunctional grieving

Chronic **sorrow** related to threat of loss of a child, prolonged hospitalization

Compromised family **Coping** related to disrupted family roles and disorganization, prolonged condition exhausting supportive capacity of significant

Decisional **conflict** related to support system deficit, multiple sources of information

Dysfunctional **grieving** (prolonged) related to unresolved conflicts

Ineffective **breast**-feeding related to disrupted establishment of effective pattern secondary to prematurity or insufficient opportunities

Parental role **conflict** related to expressed concerns, expressed inability to care for child's physical, emotional, or developmental needs

Risk for impaired parent/infant/child **Attachment** related to separation, physical barriers, lack of privacy

Risk for **powerlessness** related to inability to control situation

Risk for **spiritual** distress related to challenged belief or value systems regarding moral or ethical implications of treatment plans

## PREOPERATIVE TEACHING

**Health**-seeking behaviors related to preoperative regimens, postoperative precautions, expectations of role of client during preoperative or postoperative time

See Surgery, Preoperative Care

## PRESSURE ULCER

Acute **Pain** related to tissue destruction, exposure of nerves

Imbalanced **Nutrition**: less than body requirements related to limited access to food, inability to absorb nutrients because of biological factors, anorexia

Impaired bed **mobility** related to intolerance to activity, pain, cognitive impairment, depression, severe anxiety

Impaired **skin** integrity: stage I or II pressure ulcer related to physical immobility, mechanical factors, altered circulation, skin irritants

Impaired **tissue** integrity: stage III or IV pressure ulcer related to altered circulation, impaired physical mobility

Risk for **infection** related to physical immobility, mechanical factors (shearing forces, pressure, restraint, altered circulation, skin irritants)

Total urinary **Incontinence** related to neurological dysfunction

## PROSTATECTOMY

See TURP

## PROSTATIC HYPERTROPHY

Disturbed **Sleep** pattern related to nocturia

Ineffective **Health** maintenance related to deficient knowledge regarding self-care and prevention of complications

Risk for **infection** related to urinary residual post voiding, bacterial invasion of bladder

Risk for urge urinary **Incontinence** related to small bladder capacity

**Urinary** retention related to obstruction

## PROTECTION, ALTERED

Ineffective **Protection** related to extremes of age, inadequate nutrition, alcohol abuse, abnormal blood profiles (leukopenia, thrombocytopenia, anemia, coagulation), drug therapies (antineoplastic, corticosteroid, immune, anticoagulant, thrombolytic), treatments (surgery, radiation), diseases (e.g., cancer, immune disorders)

## PRURITUS

Deficient **Knowledge** related to methods to treat and prevent itching

Impaired **Comfort**: pruritus related to inflammation in tissues

Risk for impaired **skin** integrity related to scratching from pruritus

## PSYCHOSIS

See **Schizophrenia**

## PULMONARY EMBOLISM

Acute **Pain** related to biological injury, lack of oxygen to cells

Deficient **Knowledge** related to activities to prevent embolism, self-care after diagnosis of embolism

Delayed **surgical** recovery related to complications associated with respiratory difficulty

**Fear** related to severe pain, possible death

Impaired **gas** exchange related to altered blood flow to alveoli secondary to lodged embolus

Ineffective **Tissue** perfusion: pulmonary related to interruption of pulmonary blood flow secondary to lodged embolus

Risk for altered **cardiac** output related to right ventricular failure secondary to obstructed pulmonary artery

See Anticoagulant Therapy

## PYELONEPHRITIS

Acute **Pain** related to inflammation and irritation of urinary tract

Disturbed **Sleep** pattern related to urinary frequency

Impaired **Comfort** related to chills and fever

Ineffective **Health** maintenance related to deficient knowledge regarding self-care, treatment of disease, prevention of further urinary tract infections

Impaired **Urinary** elimination related to irritation of urinary tract

Risk for urge urinary **Incontinence** related to irritation of urinary tract

## RAPE-TRAUMA SYNDROME

Chronic **sorrow** related to forced loss of virginity

**Rape**-trauma syndrome related to forced, violent sexual penetration against victim's will and consent

**Rape**-trauma syndrome: compound reaction related to forced and violent sexual penetration against victim's will and consent, activation of previous health disruptions (e.g., physical illness, psychiatric illness, substance abuse)

**Rape**-trauma syndrome: silent reaction related to forced and violent sexual penetration against victim's will and consent, demonstration of repression of incident

Risk for **post**-trauma syndrome related to trauma or violence associated with rape

Risk for **powerlessness** related to inability to control thoughts about incident

Risk for **spiritual** distress related to forced loss of virginity

## RASH

Impaired **Comfort**: pruritus related to inflammation in skin

Impaired **skin** integrity related to mechanical trauma

Risk for **infection** related to traumatized tissue, broken skin

Risk for latex **allergy** related to multiple surgical procedures, allergies to products associated with latex allergy, professions with daily associations with latex, history of reactions to latex

## REFLEX INCONTINENCE

Reflex **incontinence** related to neurological impairment

## RELOCATION STRESS SYNDROME

**Relocation** stress syndrome related to past, concurrent, and recent losses; losses involved with decision to move; feeling of powerlessness; lack of adequate support system; little or no preparation for the impending move; moderate to high degree of environmental change; history and types of previous transfers; impaired psychosocial health status; decreased physical health status; advanced age

Risk for Relocation stress syndrome related to see relocation stress syndrome

## RENAL FAILURE

**Activity** intolerance related to effects of anemia, congestive heart failure

Chronic **sorrow** related to chronic illness

Death **anxiety** related to unknown outcome of disease

Decreased **cardiac** output related to effects of congestive heart failure, elevated potassium levels interfering with conduction system

Excess **Fluid** volume related to decreased urine output, sodium retention, inappropriate fluid intake

**Fatigue** related to effects of chronic uremia and anemia

Impaired **Comfort**: pruritus related to effects of uremia

Imbalanced **Nutrition**: less than body requirements related to anorexia, nausea, vomiting, altered taste sensation, dietary restrictions

Impaired **Oral** mucous membrane related to irritation from nitrogenous waste products

Impaired **Urinary** elimination related to effects of disease, need for dialysis

Ineffective **Coping** related to depression secondary to chronic disease

Risk for Impaired **Oral** mucous membrane related to dehydration, effects of uremia

Risk for **infection** related to altered immune functioning

Risk for **injury** related to bone changes, neuropathy, muscle weakness

Risk for **noncompliance** related to complex medical therapy

Risk for **powerlessness** related to chronic illness

## RESPIRATORY INFECTIONS, ACUTE CHILDHOOD (CROUP, EPIGLOTTITIS, PERTUSSIS, PNEUMONIA, RESPIRATORY SYNCYTIAL VIRUS)

**Activity** intolerance related to generalized weakness, dyspnea, fatigue, poor oxygenation

**Anxiety**/fear related to oxygen deprivation, difficulty breathing

Deficient **Fluid** volume related to insensible losses (fever, diaphoresis), inadequate oral fluid intake

**Hyperthermia** related to infectious process

Imbalanced **Nutrition**: less than body requirements related to anorexia, fatigue, generalized weakness, poor sucking and breathing coordination, dyspnea

Impaired **gas** exchange related to insufficient oxygenation secondary to inflammation or edema of epiglottis, larynx, bronchial passages

Ineffective **airway** clearance related to excess tracheobronchial secretions

Ineffective **breathing** patterns related to inflamed bronchial passages, coughing

Risk for **aspiration** related to inability to coordinate breathing, coughing, sucking

Risk for **infection**: transmission to others related to virulent infectious organisms

Risk for **injury** (to pregnant others) related to exposure to aerosolized medications (e.g., ribavirin, pentamidine), resultant potential fetal toxicity

Risk for **suffocation** related to inflammation of larynx, epiglottis

## RHEUMATOID ARTHRITIS

Acute **Pain** related to swollen or inflamed joints, restricted movement, physical therapy

**Fatigue** related to chronic inflammatory disease

Impaired physical **mobility** related to pain, restricted joint movement

Risk for impaired **skin** integrity related to splints, adaptive devices

Risk for **injury** related to impaired physical mobility, splints, adaptive devices, increased bleeding potential secondary to antiinflammatory medications

Risk for situational low **self**-esteem related to disturbed in body image

**Self**-care deficits: feeding, bathing/hygiene, dressing/grooming, toileting related to restricted joint movement, pain

## ROLE PERFORMANCE, ALTERED

Ineffective **Role** performance related to inability to perform role as anticipated

## RSV (RESPIRATORY SYNCYTIAL VIRUS)

See Respiratory Infection, Acute Childhood

## SCHIZOPHRENIA

**Anxiety** related to unconscious conflict with reality

Chronic **sorrow** related to chronic mental illness

Deficient **Diversional** activity related to social isolation, possible regression

Disturbed **Sleep** pattern related to sensory alterations contributing to fear and anxiety

Disturbed **Thought** processes related to inaccurate interpretations of environment

**Fear** related to altered contact with reality

Imbalanced **Nutrition**: less than body requirements related to fear of eating, unaware of hunger, disinterest toward food

Impaired **Home** maintenance related to impaired cognitive or emotional functioning, insufficient finances, inadequate support systems

Impaired **social** interaction related to impaired communication patterns, self-concept disturbance, Disturbed Thought processes

Impaired verbal **communication** related to psychosis, disorientation, inaccurate perception, hallucinations, delusions

Ineffective **Coping** related to inadequate support systems, unrealistic perceptions, inadequate coping skills, Disturbed Thought processes , impaired communication

Ineffective **health** maintenance related to cognitive impairment, ineffective individual and family coping, lack of material resources

Ineffective **Therapeutic** regimen management: families related to chronicity and unpredictability of condition

Interrupted **Family** processes related to inability to express feelings, impaired communication

Risk for **caregiver** role strain related to bizarre behavior of client, chronicity of condition

Risk for **loneliness** related to inability to interact socially

Risk for **post**-trauma syndrome related to diminished ego strength

Risk for **powerlessness** related to intrusive, distorted thinking

Risk for self-directed other directed **violence** related to lack of trust, panic, hallucinations, delusional thinking

Risk for **suicide** related to psychiatric illness

**Self**-care deficit related to loss of contact with reality, impairment in perception

**Self**-esteem disturbance related to excessive use of defense mechanisms (e.g., projection, denial, rationalization)

**Sleep** deprivation related to intrusive thoughts, nightmares

**Social** isolation related to lack of trust, regression, delusional thinking, repressed fears

## SEIZURE DISORDERS

Ineffective **health** maintenance related to lack of knowledge regarding anticonvulsive therapy, fever reduction (febrile seizures)

Risk for delayed **development** and disproportionate growth related to effects of seizure disorder, parental overprotection

Risk for Disturbed **Thought** processes related to effects of anticonvulsant medications

Risk for **falls** related to possible seizure

Risk for ineffective **airway** clearance related to accumulation of secretions during seizure

Risk for **injury** related to uncontrolled movements during seizure, falls, drowsiness secondary to anticonvulsants

**Social** isolation related to unpredictability of seizures, community-imposed stigma

See Epilepsy

## SELF-CARE DEFICIT, BATHING/HYGIENE

Bathing/hygiene **Self**-care deficit related to intolerance to activity, decreased strength and endurance, pain, discomfort, perceptual or cognitive impairment, neuromuscular impairment, musculoskeletal impairment, depression, severe anxiety

## SELF-CARE DEFICIT, DRESSING/GROOMING

Dressing/grooming **Self-**care deficit related to intolerance to activity, decreased strength and endurance, pain, discomfort, perceptual or cognitive impairment, neuromuscular impairment, musculoskeletal impairment, depression, severe anxiety

## SELF-CARE DEFICIT, FEEDING

Feeding **Self-**care deficit: related to intolerance to activity, decreased strength and endurance, pain, discomfort, perceptual or cognitive impairment, neuromuscular impairment, musculoskeletal impairment, depression, severe anxiety

## SELF-CARE DEFICIT, TOILETING

Toileting **Self-**care deficit related to impaired transfer ability, impaired mobility status, intolerance to activity, decreased strength and endurance, pain, discomfort, perceptual or cognitive impairment, neuromuscular impairment, musculoskeletal impairment, depression, severe anxiety

## SELF-ESTEEM, CHRONIC LOW

Chronic low **self**-esteem related to long-standing negative self-evaluation

## SELF-ESTEEM, SITUATIONAL LOW

Situational low **self**-esteem related to developmental crisis, disturbed body image, functional impairment, loss, social role changes, lack of recognition/rewards, behavior inconsistent with values, failures, and rejections

## SELF-ESTEEM DISTURBANCE

**Self**-esteem disturbance related to inappropriate and learned negative feelings about self

## SELF-MUTILATION, RISK FOR

Risk for **self**-mutilation related to inability to cope with increased psychological or physiological tension in a healthy manner; feelings of depression, rejection, self-hatred, separation anxiety, guilt, and depersonalization; fluctuating emotions; command hallucinations; need for sensory stimuli; parental emotional deprivation; dysfunctional family

**Self** mutilation related to Psychotic state (command hallucinations) ; Inability to express tension verbally; Childhood sexual abuse; Violence between parental figures; Family divorce; Family alcoholism; Family history of self-destructive behaviors; Adolescence; Peers who self-mutilate; Isolation from peers; Perfectionism; Substance abuse; Eating disorders; Sexual identity crisis; Low or unstable self-esteem; Low or unstable body image; Labile behavior (mood swings); History of inability to plan solutions or see long-term consequences; Use of manipulation to obtain nurturing relationship with others; Chaotic/disturbed interpersonal relationships; Emotionally disturbed; battered child; Feels threatened with actual or potential loss of significant relationship (e.g., loss of parent/parental relationship); Experiences dissociation or depersonalization; Mounting tension that is intolerable; impulsivity; Inadequate coping; Irresistible urge to cut/damage self; Needs quick reduction of stress; Childhood illness or surgery; Foster, group, or institutional care; Incarceration; Character disorder; Borderline personality disorder; Developmentally delayed or autistic individual; History of self-injurious behavior; Feelings of depression, rejection, self-hatred, separation anxiety, guilt, depersonalization; Poor parent-adolescent communication; Lack of family confidant.

## SENSORY/PERCEPTUAL ALTERATIONS

Disturbed **sensory** perceptions: visual, auditory, kinesthetic, gustatory, tactile, olfactory related to altered, excessive, or insufficient environmental stimuli; altered sensory reception, transmission, and/or Integration; endogenous (electrolyte) or exogenous (e.g., drugs) chemical alterations; psychological stress

## SEPTICEMIA

Deficient **Fluid** volume related to vasodilation of peripheral vessels, leaking of capillaries

Imbalanced **Nutrition**: less than body requirements related to anorexia, generalized weakness

Ineffective **Tissue** perfusion related to decreased systemic vascular resistance

See Shock, Septic

## SEXUAL DYSFUNCTION

Chronic **sorrow** related to loss of ideal sexual experience, altered relationships

**Sexual** dysfunction related to biopsychosocial alteration of sexuality, ineffectual or absent role models, physical abuse or harmful relationships, vulnerability, conflicting values, lack of privacy, lack of significant others, altered body structure or function (pregnancy, recent childbirth, drug use, surgery, anomalies, disease process, trauma, radiation), misinformation or lack of knowledge

## SEXUALITY PATTERNS, INEFFECTIVE

Ineffective **Sexuality** patterns related to knowledge or skill deficit regarding alternative responses to health-related transitions, altered body function or structure, illness or medical problems, lack of privacy, lack of significant other, ineffective or absent role models, fear of pregnancy or acquiring a sexually transmitted disease, impaired relationship with a significant other

## SEXUALLY TRANSMITTED DISEASE

See STD

## SHINGLES

Acute **Pain** related to vesicular eruption along the nerves
Ineffective **Protection** related to abnormal blood profiles
Risk for **infection** related to tissue destruction
**Social** isolation related to altered state of wellness, contagiousness of disease
See Itching

## SHOCK

**Fear** related to serious threat to health status
Ineffective **Tissue** perfusion: cardiopulmonary, peripheral related to arterial/venous blood flow exchange problems
Risk for **injury** related to prolonged shock resulting in multiple organ failure, death
See Shock, Cardiogenic; Shock, Hypovolemic; Shock, Septic

## SHOCK, CARDIOGENIC

Decreased **cardiac** output related to decreased myocardial contractility, dysrhythmia
See Shock

## SHOCK, HYPOVOLEMIC

Deficient **Fluid** volume related to abnormal loss of fluid
See Shock

## SHOCK, SEPTIC

Deficient **Fluid** volume related to abnormal loss of fluid through capillaries, pooling of blood in peripheral circulation
Ineffective **Protection** related to inadequately functioning immune system
See Septicemia; Shock

## SICKLE CELL ANEMIA/CRISIS

**Activity** intolerance related to fatigue, effects of chronic anemia
Acute **Pain** related to viscous blood, tissue hypoxia
Deficient **Fluid** volume related to decreased intake, increased fluid requirements during sickle cell crisis, decreased ability of kidneys to concentrate urine
Impaired physical **mobility** related to pain, fatigue
Risk for Ineffective **Tissue** perfusion(renal, cerebral, cardiac, gastrointestinal, peripheral) related to effects of red cell sickling, infarction of tissues
Risk for **infection** related to alterations in splenic function

## SIDS

Anticipatory **grieving** related to potential loss of infant
**Anxiety**/fear: parental related to life-threatening event
Deficient **Knowledge**: potential for enhanced health maintenance related to knowledge or skill acquisition of CPR and home apnea monitoring
Disturbed **Sleep** pattern: parental/infant related to home apnea monitoring
Interrupted **Family** processes related to stress secondary to special care needs of infant with apnea
Risk for **powerlessness** related to unanticipated life-threatening event

## SKIN INTEGRITY, RISK FOR IMPAIRED

Risk for impaired **skin** integrity related to internal or external factors that are potentially harmful to skin

## SLEEP DEPRIVATION

**Sleep** deprivation related to Prolonged physical discomfort; Prolonged psychological discomfort; Sustained inadequate sleep hygiene; Prolonged use of pharmacologic or dietary antisoporifics; Aging-related sleep stage shifts; Sustained circadian asynchrony ; Inadequate daytime activity; Sustained environmental stimulation; Sustained unfamiliar or uncomfortable sleep environment; Non-sleep-inducing parenting practices; Sleep apnea; Periodic limb movement (e.g., restless leg syndrome, nocturnal myoclonus); Sundowner's syndrome; Narcolepsy; Idiopathic central nervous system hypersomnolence; Sleep walking; Sleep terror; Sleep-related enuresis; Nightmares; Familial sleep paralysis; Sleep-related painful erections; Dementia

## SLEEP PATTERN DISORDERS

**Sleep** pattern disorders related to sensory alterations, internal factors (illness, psychological stress), external factors (environmental changes, social cues)

## SOCIAL INTERACTION, IMPAIRED

**Social** interaction: impaired related to knowledge or skill deficit about ways to enhance mutuality, communication barriers, self-concept disturbance, absence of available significant others or peers, limited physical mobility, therapeutic isolation, sociocultural dissonance, environmental barriers, disturbed thought processes

## SOCIAL ISOLATION

**Social** isolation related to factors contributing to absence of satisfying personal relationships, such as delay in accomplishing developmental tasks, immature interests, alterations in physical appearance, alterations in mental status, unaccepted social behavior, unaccepted social values, altered state of wellness, inadequate personal resources, inability to engage in satisfying personal relationships, fear

## SOMATOFORM DISORDER

**Anxiety** related to unresolved conflicts being channeled into physical complaints or conditions
Chronic **pain** related to unexpressed anger, multiple physical disorders, depression
Ineffective **Coping** related to lack of insight into underlying conflicts

## SORROW

Chronic **sorrow** related to unresolved grief

## SPEECH DISORDERS

Impaired verbal **communication** related to anatomical defect, cleft palate, psychological barriers, decrease in circulation to brain

## SPINAL CORD INJURY

Chronic **sorrow** related to immobility, change in body function
**Constipation** related to immobility, loss of sensation
Deficient **Diversional** activity related to long-term hospitalization, frequent lengthy treatments
Disturbed **Body** image related to change in body function
Dysfunctional **grieving** related to loss of usual body function
**Fear** related to powerlessness over loss of body function
Impaired **home** maintenance related to change in health status, insufficient family planning or finances, Deficient Knowledge, inadequate support systems
Impaired physical **mobility** related to neuromuscular impairment
Ineffective **health** maintenance related to Deficient Knowledge regarding self-care with spinal cord injury
Reflex **incontinence** related to spinal cord lesion interfering with conduction of cerebral messages

Risk for **disuse** syndrome related to paralysis

Risk for **Autonomic** dysreflexia related to bladder or bowel distention, skin irritation, deficient knowledge of patient and caregiver

Risk for impaired **skin** integrity related to immobility, paralysis

Risk for ineffective **breathing** pattern related to neuromuscular impairment

Risk for **infection** related to chronic disease, stasis of body fluids

Risk for **loneliness** related to physical immobility

Risk for **powerlessness** related to loss of function

**Self-**care deficit related to neuromuscular impairment

**Sexual** dysfunction related to altered body function

**Urinary** retention related to inhibition of reflex arc

## SPIRITUAL DISTRESS

Risk for **spiritual** distress related to energy-consuming anxiety; low self-esteem; mental illness; physical illness; blocks to self-love; poor relationships; physical or psychological stress; substance abuse; loss of loved one; natural disasters; situation losses; maturational losses; inability to forgive

**Spiritual** distress related to separation from religious or cultural ties, challenged belief and value system resulting from moral or ethical implications of therapy or from intense suffering

## SPIRITUAL WELL-BEING

Readiness for enhanced **Spiritual** well-being related to desire for harmonious interconnectedness, desire to find purpose and meaning to life

## STD (SEXUALLY TRANSMITTED DISEASE)

Acute **Pain** related to biological or psychological injury

Ineffective **health** maintenance related to deficient knowledge regarding transmission, symptoms, and treatment of sexually transmitted disease

Ineffective **Sexuality** patterns related to illness, altered body function

**Fear** related to altered body function, risk for social isolation, fear of incurable illness

Risk for **infection**/spread of infection related to lack of knowledge concerning transmission of disease

**Social** isolation related to fear of contracting or spreading disease

## STOMATITIS

Impaired **Oral** mucous membrane related to pathological conditions of oral cavity

## STRESS URINARY INCONTINENCE

Stress urinary **Incontinence** related to degenerative change in pelvic muscles

## STROKE

See CVA

## SUBARACHNOID HEMORRHAGE

Acute **pain**: headache related to irritation of meninges from blood, increased intracranial pressure

Ineffective **Tissue** perfusion: cerebral related to bleeding from cerebral vessel

See Intracranial Pressure, Increased

## SUBSTANCE ABUSE

**Anxiety** related to loss of control

Compromised/dysfunctional family **coping** related to codependency issues

Defensive **coping** related to substance abuse

Disturbed **Sleep** pattern related to irritability, nightmares, tremors

Dysfunctional **Family** processes: alcohol related to inadequate coping skills

Imbalanced **Nutrition**: less than body requirements related to anorexia

Ineffective **Protection** related to malnutrition, sleep deprivation

Ineffective **denial** related to refusal to acknowledge substance abuse problem

Ineffective **Coping** related to use of substances to cope with life events

**Powerlessness** related to substance addiction

Risk for impaired **parent**/infant/child Attachment related to substance abuse

Risk for **injury** related to alteration in sensory perception

Risk for other or self directed **violence** related to reactions to substances used, impulsive behavior, disorientation, impaired judgment

Risk for **suicide** related to substance abuse

**Self-**esteem disturbance related to failure at life events

**Social** isolation related to unacceptable social behavior or values

## SUFFOCATION, RISK FOR
### Internal

Risk for **suffocation** related to reduced olfactory sensation, reduced motor abilities, lack of safety education, lack of safety precautions, cognitive or emotional difficulties, disease or injury process

### External

Risk for **suffocation** related to hazardous environment

## SUICIDE ATTEMPT

**Hopelessness** related to perceived or actual loss, substance abuse, low self-concept, inadequate support systems

Ineffective **Coping** related to anger, dysfunctional grieving

**Post-**trauma response related to history of traumatic events, abuse, rape, incest, war, torture

Readiness for enhanced **Spiritual** well-being related to desire for harmony and inner strength to help redefine purpose for life

Risk for **suicide** related to history of prior attempt, impulsiveness, buying a gun, stockpiling medicines, threats of killing self, family history of suicide, physical illness, hopelessness, social isolation

**Self-**esteem disturbance related to guilt, inability to trust, feelings of worthlessness or rejection

**Social** isolation related to inability to engage in satisfying personal relationships

**Spiritual** distress related to hopelessness, despair

## SURGERY, PERIOPERATIVE CARE

Risk for imbalanced **Fluid** volume related to surgery

Risk for perioperative positioning **injury** related to predisposing condition, prolonged surgery

## SURGERY, POSTOPERATIVE CARE

**Activity** intolerance related to pain, surgical procedure

Acute **Pain** related to inflammation or injury in surgical area

**Anxiety** related to change in health status, hospital environment

Deficient **Knowledge** related to postoperative expectations, life-style changes

Imbalanced **Nutrition**: less than body requirements related to anorexia, nausea, vomiting, decreased peristalsis

**Nausea** related to manipulation of gastrointestinal tract, post-surgical anesthesia

Risk for Ineffective **Tissue** perfusion: peripheral related to hypovolemia, circulatory stasis, obesity, prolonged immobility, decreased coughing, decreased deep breathing

Risk for **constipation** related to decreased activity, decreased food or fluid intake, anesthesia, pain medication

Risk for deficient **Fluid** volume related to hypermetabolic state, fluid loss during surgery, presence of indwelling tubes

Risk for ineffective **breathing** pattern related to pain, location of incision, effects of anesthesia/narcotics

Risk for **infection** related to invasive procedure, pain, anesthesia, location of incision, weakened cough due to aging

**Urinary** retention related to anesthesia, pain, fear, unfamiliar surroundings, client's position

## SURGERY, PREOPERATIVE CARE

**Anxiety** related to threat to or change in health status, situational crisis, fear of unknown

Deficient **Knowledge** related to preoperative procedures, postoperative expectations

Disturbed **Sleep** pattern related to anxiety about upcoming surgery

## SWALLOWING DIFFICULTIES

Impaired **swallowing** related to neuromuscular impairment (e.g., decreased or absent gag reflex, decreased strength or excursion of muscles involved in mastication), perceptual impairment, facial paralysis, mechanical obstruction (e.g., edema, tracheostomy tube, tumor), fatigue, limited awareness, reddened or irritated oropharyngeal cavity, improper feeding or positioning

## T & A (TONSILLECTOMY AND ADENOIDECTOMY)

Acute **Pain** related to surgical incision

Deficient **Knowledge**: potential for enhanced health maintenance related to insufficient knowledge regarding postoperative nutritional and rest requirements, signs and symptoms of complications, positioning

Impaired **Comfort** related to effects of anesthesia (nausea and vomiting)

Ineffective airway clearance related to hesitation or reluctance to cough secondary to pain

Risk for Imbalanced **Nutrition**: less than body requirements related to hesitation or reluctance to swallow

Risk for **aspiration**/suffocation related to postoperative drainage and impaired swallowing

Risk for deficient **Fluid** volume related to decreased intake secondary to painful swallowing, effects of anesthesia (nausea, vomiting), hemorrhage

## TBI (TRAUMATIC BRAIN INJURY)

Acute **confusion** related to brain injury

Chronic **sorrow** related to change in person's health status and functional ability

Decreased **Intracranial** adaptive capacity related to brain injury

Disturbed **Thought** processes related to pressure damage to brain

Interrupted **Family** processes related to traumatic injury to family member

Ineffective **Tissue** perfusion: cerebral related to effects of increased intracranial pressure

Ineffective **breathing** patterns related to pressure damage to breathing center in brain stem

Risk for **post**-trauma syndrome related to perception of event causing traumatic brain injury

Disturbed **sensory** perception: specify related to pressure damage to sensory centers in brain

## TEMPERATURE, DECREASED

**Hypothermia** related to exposure to cold environment

## TEMPERATURE, INCREASED

**Hyperthermia** related to dehydration, illness, trauma

## TEMPERATURE REGULATION, IMPAIRED

Ineffective **thermoregulation** related to trauma, illness

## TERMINALLY ILL ADULT

Anticipatory **grieving** related to loss of self or significant other

Compromised family **coping** related to inability to discuss impending death

Death **anxiety** related to unresolved issues relating to death and dying

Decisional **conflict** related to planning for advance directives

Disturbed **Energy** field related to impending disharmony of mind, body, spirit

Readiness for enhanced **Spiritual** well-being related to desire to achieve harmony of mind, body, spirit

Risk for **spiritual** distress related to impending death

**Spiritual** distress related to suffering before death

## THERAPEUTIC REGIMEN, EFFECTIVE MANAGEMENT

Effective **Therapeutic** regimen management related to adequate ability to manage needed health care

## THERAPEUTIC REGIMEN, INEFFECTIVE MANAGEMENT OF: FAMILIES

Ineffective family **Therapeutic** regimen management related to complexity of health care system, complexity of therapeutic regimen, decisional conflicts, economic difficulties, excessive demands on individual or family, family conflict

## THERAPEUTIC REGIMEN, INEFFECTIVE MANAGEMENT

Ineffective **Therapeutic** regimen management related to complexity of health care system; complexity of therapeutic regimen; decisional conflicts; economic difficulties; excessive demands made on individual or family; family conflict; family patterns of health care; inadequate number and types of cues to action; Deficient Knowledge; mistrust of regimen or health care personnel; perceived seriousness, susceptibility, barriers, or benefits; powerlessness; social support deficits

## THERAPEUTIC TOUCH

Disturbed **Energy** field related to low energy levels, disturbance in energy fields, pain, depression, fatigue

## THERMOREGULATION, INEFFECTIVE

Ineffective **thermoregulation** related to trauma, illness, immaturity, aging, fluctuating environmental temperature

## THOUGHT PROCESSES, DISTURBED

Disturbed **Thought** processes related to head injury, mental disorder, personality disorder, organic mental disorder, substance abuse, severe interpersonal conflict, sleep deprivation, sensory deprivation or overload, impaired cerebral perfusion

## THROMBOPHLEBITIS

See DVT

## TIA (TRANSIENT ISCHEMIC ATTACK)

Acute **confusion** related to hypoxia

**Health**-seeking behaviors related to obtaining knowledge regarding treatment, prevention of inadequate oxygenation

Ineffective **Tissue** perfusion: cerebral related to lack of adequate oxygen supply to brain

Risk for decreased **cardiac** output related to dysrhythmia contributing to inadequate oxygen supply to brain

Risk for **falls** related to hypoxia

Risk for **injury** related to possible syncope

## TISSUE DAMAGE—CORNEAL, INTEGUMENTARY, OR SUBCUTANEOUS

Impaired **tissue** integrity related to altered circulation, nutritional deficit or excess, fluid deficit or excess, Deficient Knowledge, impaired physical mobility, chemical irritants (including body excretions, secretions, medications), thermal irritants (temperature extremes), mechanical irritants (pressure, shear, friction), radiation irritants (including therapeutic radiation)

## TISSUE PERFUSION, DECREASED

Ineffective **Tissue** perfusion related to arterial or venous interruption of flow, exchange problems, hypovolemia, hypervolemia

## TONSILLECTOMY AND ADENOIDECTOMY

See T & A

## TOTAL URINARY INCONTINENCE

Total urinary **Incontinence** related to neuropathy, neurological dysfunction, compromised contraction of detrusor reflex, anatomical incontinence (fistula)

## TOTAL JOINT REPLACEMENT—TOTAL HIP/TOTAL KNEE

Acute **Pain** related to possible edema, physical injury, surgery

Deficient **Knowledge** related to self-care, treatment regimen, outcomes

Disturbed **Body** image related to large scar, presence of prosthesis

Impaired physical **mobility** related to musculoskeletal impairment, surgery, prosthesis

Risk for **infection** related to invasive procedure, anesthesia, immobility

Risk for **injury**: neurovascular related to altered peripheral tissue perfusion, altered mobility, prosthesis

## TRACTION AND CASTS

Acute **Pain** related to immobility, injury, or disease

**Constipation** related to immobility

Deficient **Diversional** activity related to immobility

Impaired physical **mobility** related to imposed restrictions on activity secondary to bone or joint disease injury

Impaired **transfer** ability related to presence of traction, casts

Risk for **disuse** syndrome related to mechanical immobilization

Risk for impaired **skin** integrity related to contact of traction or cast with skin

Risk for **peripheral** neurovascular dysfunction related to mechanical compression

**Self-care** deficit: feeding, dressing/grooming, bathing/hygiene, toileting related to degree of impaired physical mobility, body area affected by traction or cast

## TRANSFER ABILITY

Impaired **transfer** ability related to intolerant to activity, decreased strength and endurance, pain or discomfort, perceptual or cognitive impairment, neuromuscular impairment, musculoskeletal impairment, depression, severe anxiety

## TRANSIENT ISCHEMIC ATTACK

See TIA

## TRANSURETHRAL RESECTION OF THE PROSTATE

See TURP

## TRAUMA, RISK FOR
### Internal

Risk for **trauma** related to weakness, poor vision, balancing difficulties, reduced temperature and/or tactile sensation, reduced large or small muscle coordination, reduced hand-eye coordination, lack of safety education, lack of safety precautions, insufficient finances to purchase safety equipment or effect repairs, cognitive or emotional difficulties, history of previous trauma

### External

Risk for **trauma** related to unsafe environment, lack of supervision of child or elder adult

## TRAUMATIC BRAIN INJURY (TBI)

See TBI; Intracranial Pressure, Increased

## TURP (TRANSURETHRAL RESECTION OF THE PROSTATE)

Acute **Pain** related to incision, irritation from catheter, bladder spasms, kidney infection

Deficient **Knowledge** related to postoperative self-care, home maintenance management

Risk for deficient **Fluid** volume related to fluid loss, possible bleeding

Risk for **infection** related to invasive procedure, route for bacteria entry

Risk for **urinary** retention related to obstruction of urethra or catheter with clots

Risk for urge urinary **Incontinence** related to edema from surgical procedure

## ULCER, PEPTIC OR DUODENAL

Acute **Pain** related to irritated mucosa from acid secretion

**Fatigue** related to loss of blood, chronic illness

Ineffective **health** maintenance related to lack of knowledge regarding health practices to prevent ulcer formation

**Nausea** related to gastrointestinal irritation

See GI Bleed

## ULCERATIVE COLITIS

See Inflammatory Bowel Disease

## UNILATERAL NEGLECT OF ONE SIDE OF BODY

Unilateral **neglect** related to effects of disturbed perceptual abilities (e.g., hemianopsia), one-sided blindness, neurological illness or trauma

## URGENCY TO URINATE

Risk for urge urinary **Incontinence** related to effects of alcohol, caffeine, decreased bladder capacity, irritation of bladder stretch receptors causing spasm, increased urine concentration, overdistention of bladder

Urge urinary **Incontinence** related to decreased bladder capacity, irritation of bladder stretch receptors causing spasm, alcohol, caffeine, increased fluids, increased urine concentration, overdistention of bladder

## URINARY ELIMINATION, ALTERED

Impaired **Urinary** elimination related to anatomical obstruction, sensory motor impairment, urinary tract infection

## URINARY INCONTINENCE

See Incontinence of Urine

## URINARY RETENTION

**Urinary** retention related to high urethral pressure caused by weak detrusor, inhibition of reflex arc, strong sphincter, blockage

## UTI (URINARY TRACT INFECTION)

Acute **Pain**: dysuria related to inflammatory process in bladder

Impaired **urinary** elimination: frequency related to urinary tract infection

Ineffective **health** maintenance related to deficient knowledge regarding methods to treat and prevent UTIs

Risk for urge urinary **Incontinence** related to hyperreflexia from cystitis

## VAGINITIS

Acute **Pain**: pruritus related to inflamed tissues, edema

Ineffective **health** maintenance related to deficient knowledge regarding self-care with vaginitis

Ineffective **sexuality** patterns related to abstinence during acute stage, pain

Risk for **infection** related to spread of infection, risk of reinfection

## VARICOSE VEINS

Chronic **Pain** related to impaired circulation

Ineffective **health** maintenance related to deficient knowledge regarding health care practices, prevention, treatment regimen

Ineffective **Tissue** perfusion: peripheral related to venous stasis

Risk for impaired **skin** integrity related to altered peripheral tissue perfusion

## VENTILATION, INABILITY TO SUSTAIN SPONTANEOUS

Impaired spontaneous **Ventilation** related to metabolic factors, respiratory muscle fatigue

## VENTILATORY, DYSFUNCTIONAL WEANING RESPONSE (DVWR)

Dysfunctional **ventilatory** weaning response related to perceived inefficacy about the ability to wean, powerlessness, decreased motivation, adverse environment, inadequate social support, inadequate nutrition, sleep pattern disturbance, uncontrolled pain, ineffective airway clearance

## VIOLENT BEHAVIOR

Risk for other-directed **violence** related to body language, history of violence against others, history of violent antisocial behavior, history of violence, indirect, neurological impairment, cognitive impairment, history of childhood abuse, history of witnessing family violence, cruelty to animals, firesetting, pre/perinatal complications and abnormalities, history of drug/alcohol abuse, pathological intoxication, psychotic symptomatology, motor vehicle offenses, suicidal behavior, impusivity, availability/possession of weapon(s)

Risk for self-directed **violence** Related to suicidal ideation, suicidal plan, history of multiple suicide attempts, behavioral clues of suicide, verbal clues of suicide, emotional status, mental health, physical health, unemployment, age 15-19, age over 45, Marital status, occupation, conflictual interpersonal relationships, family background, sexual orientation, personal resources, social resources, engage in autoerotic sexual acts

## VISION IMPAIRMENT

Disturbed **sensory** perception related to altered sensory reception associated with impaired vision

**Fear** related to loss of sight

Risk for **injury** related to Disturbed sensory perception

**Self-care deficit**: specify related to perceptual impairment

**Social** isolation related to altered state of wellness, inability to see

## VOMITING

**Nausea** related to chemotherapy, post-surgical anesthesia, irritation to the gastrointestinal system, stimulation of neuropharmacologic mechanisms

Risk for deficient **Fluid** volume related to decreased intake, loss of fluids with vomiting

Risk for Imbalanced **Nutrition**: less than body requirements related to inability to ingest food

## WALKING IMPAIRMENT

Impaired **walking** related to intolerance to activity, decreased strength and endurance, pain or discomfort, perceptual or cognitive impairment, neuromuscular impairment, musculoskeletal impairment, depression, severe anxiety, lower extremity amputation

## WANDERING

**Wandering** related to Cognitive impairment, specifically memory and recall deficits, disorientation, poor visuoconstructive (or visuospatial) ability, language (primarily expressive) defects; Cortical atrophy; Premorbid behavior (e.g., outgoing, sociable personality; premorbid dementia); Separation from familiar people and places; Sedation; Emotional state, especially frustration, anxiety, boredom, or depression (agitation); Over/under stimulating social or physical environment; Physiological state or need (e.g., hunger related to thirst, pain, urination, constipation); Time of day

## WHEELCHAIR USE PROBLEMS

Impaired wheelchair **mobility** related to intolerance to activity, decreased strength and endurance, pain or discomfort, perceptual or cognitive impairment, neuromuscular impairment, musculoskeletal impairment, depression, severe anxiety, amputation

# NURSING INTERVENTIONS CLASSIFICATION

## 18-1 | Steps for implementing NIC in a clinical practice agency

### A. ESTABLISH ORGANIZATIONAL COMMITMENT TO NIC

- Identify the key person responsible for implementation (e.g., person in charge of nursing informatics).
- Create an implementation task force with representatives from key areas.
- Provide NIC materials to all members of the task force.
- Invite a member of the NIC project team to do a presentation to the staff nurses and to meet with the task force.
- Purchase copies of the NIC book.
- Circulate readings about NIC and The NIC/NOC Letter to units. Show the NIC video.
- Have members of the task force and other key individuals begin to use the NIC language in everyday discussion.
- Have key individuals from the task force sign onto the Center for Nursing Classification ListServ.

### B. PREPARE AN IMPLEMENTATION PLAN

- Write the specific goals to be accomplished with implementation.
- Do a force field analysis to determine driving and restraining forces.
- Determine if an in-house evaluation will be done and, if so, what is the nature of the evaluation effort.
- Identify which of NIC interventions are most appropriate for the agency/unit.
- Determine the extent to which NIC is to be implemented; for example, in standards, care planning, documentation, discharge summary, performance evaluation.
- Prioritize the implementation efforts.
- Choose 1-3 pilot units. Get members from these units involved in the planning.
- Develop a written timeline for implementation.

- Review current system and determine the logical sequence of actions to integrate.
- Create work groups of expert clinical users to review NIC interventions and activities, determine how these will be used in agency, and develop needed forms.
- Distribute the work of the expert clinicians to other users for evaluation and feedback before implementation.
- Encourage the development of a *NIC champion* on each of the units.
- Keep other key decision makers in agency informed.
- Determine the nature of the total nursing data set. Work to ensure that all units are collecting data on all variables in a uniform manner so that future research can be done.
- Make plans to ensure that all nursing data are retrievable.
- Identify learning needs of staff and plan ways to address these.

### C. CARRY OUT THE IMPLEMENTATION PLAN

- Develop the screens/forms for implementation. Review each NIC intervention and decide whether all parts (e.g., label, definition, activities, reference) are to be used.
- Provide training time for staff.
- Implement NIC on the pilot unit(s) and obtain regular feedback.
- Update content or create new computer functions as needed.
- Use focus groups to clarify issues and address concerns/questions.
- Use data on positive aspects of implementation in house-wide presentations.
- Implement NIC house-wide.
- Collect post implementation evaluation data and make changes as needed.
- Identify key markers to use for ongoing evaluation and continue to monitor and maintain the system.
- Provide feedback to the Center for Nursing Classification.

From McCloskey JC, Bulechek GM, eds: *Nursing interventions classification,* ed 3, St Louis, 2000, Mosby.

## 18-2 | NIC interventions

†Abuse protection support
†Abuse protection support: child
*Abuse protection support: domestic partner
†Abuse protection support: elder
Abuse protection support: religious
Acid-base management
Acid-base management: metabolic acidosis
Acid-base management: metabolic alkalosis
Acid-base management: respiratory acidosis
Acid-base management: respiratory alkalosis
Acid-base monitoring
Active listening
Activity therapy

Acupressure
Admission care
Airway insertion and stabilization
†Airway management
Airway suctioning
†Allergy management
Amnioinfusion
Amputation care
Analgesic administration
Analgesic administration: intraspinal
*Anaphylaxis management
Anesthesia administration
Anger control assistance
†Animal-assisted therapy
Anticipatory guidance
Anxiety reduction
Area restriction
Art therapy

Artificial airway management
Aspiration precautions
Assertiveness training
Attachment promotion
Autogenic training
Autotransfusion
†Bathing
Bed rest care
Bedside laboratory testing
†Behavior management
Behavior management: overactivity/inattention
Behavior management: self-harm
Behavior management: sexual
Behavior modification
Behavior modifications: social skills
Bibliotherapy
Biofeedback

*Interventions new to the third edition.
†Interventions revised for the third edition.

Birthing
Bladder irrigation
Bleeding precautions
Bleeding reduction
Bleeding reduction: antepartum uterus
Bleeding reduction: gastrointestinal
Bleeding reduction: nasal
Bleeding reduction: postpartum uterus
Bleeding reduction: wound
Blood products administration
†Body image enhancement
Body mechanics promotion
†Bottle feeding
Bowel incontinence care
Bowel incontinence care: encopresis
Bowel irrigation
†Bowel management
Bowel training
*Breast examination
†Breastfeeding assistance
Calming technique
†Cardiac care
†Cardiac care: acute
†Cardiac care: Rehabilitative
Cardiac precautions
Caregiver support
*Case management
Cast care: maintenance
Cast care: wet
Cerebral edema management
Cerebral perfusion promotion
Cesarean section care
Chemotherapy management
Chest physiotherapy
Childbirth preparation
*Circulatory care: arterial insufficiency
Circulatory care: mechanical assist device
*Circulatory care: venous insufficiency
Circulatory precautions
Code management
†Cognitive restructuring
Cognitive stimulation
*Communicable disease management
†Communication enhancement: hearing
   deficit
Communication enhancement: speech
   deficit
Communication enhancement: visual
   deficit
*Community disaster preparedness
*Community health development
Complex relationship building
*Conflict mediation
†Conscious sedation
†Constipation/impaction management
*Consultation
Contact lens care
Controlled substance checking
Coping enhancement
*Cost containment
Cough enhancement
†Counseling
Crisis intervention
Critical path development
†Culture brokerage
Cutaneous stimulation
Decision-making support
Delegation
Delirium management
Delusion management

Dementia management
*Developmental care
*Developmental enhancement: adolescent
†Developmental enhancement: child
†Diarrhea management
Diet staging
Discharge planning
Distraction
†Documentation
†Dressing
Dying care
Dysreflexia management
Dysrhythmia management
Ear care
Eating disorders management
Electrolyte management
Electrolyte management: hypercalcemia
Electrolyte management: hyperkalemia
Electrolyte management:
   hypermagnesemia
Electrolyte management: hypernatremia
Electrolyte management:
   hyperphosphatemia
Electrolyte management: hypocalcemia
Electrolyte management: hypokalemia
Electrolyte management:
   hypomagnesemia
Electrolyte management: hyponatremia
Electrolyte management:
   hypophosphatemia
Electrolyte monitoring
Electronic fetal monitoring: antepartum
Electronic fetal monitoring: intrapartum
Elopement precautions
Embolus care: peripheral
Embolus care: pulmonary
Embolus precautions
Emergency care
Emergency cart checking
Emotional support
Endotracheal extubation
Energy management
†Enteral tube feeding
†Environmental management
Environmental management: attachment
   process
Environmental management: comfort
†Environmental management: community
Environmental management: home
   preparation
†Environmental management: safety
Environmental management: violence
   prevention
Environmental management: worker
   safety
*Environmental risk protection
Examination assistance
†Exercise promotion
*Exercise promotion: strength training
Exercise promotion: stretching
†Exercise promotion: ambulation
Exercise promotion: balance
†Exercise promotion: joint mobility
†Exercise promotion: muscle control
†Eye care
†Fall prevention
Family integrity promotion
Family integrity promotion: childbearing
   family
†Family involvement promotion

Family mobilization
Family planning: contraception
Family planning: infertility
Family planning: unplanned pregnancy
Family process maintenance
Family support
Family therapy
Feeding
Fertility preservation
Fever treatment
*Financial resource assistance
Fire-setting precautions
First aid
*Fiscal resource management
Flatulence reduction
†Fluid management
Fluid/electrolyte management
Fluid monitoring
Fluid resuscitation
Foot care
*Forgiveness facilitation
Gastrointestinal intubation
Genetic counseling
Grief work facilitation
Grief work facilitation: perinatal death
Guilt work facilitation
Hair care
Hallucination management
Health care information exchange
†Health education
Health policy monitoring
Health screening
†Health system guidance
†Heat exposure treatment
Head/cold application
Hemodialysis therapy
Hemodynamic regulation
*Hemofiltration therapy
Hemorrhage control
High-risk pregnancy care
Home maintenance assistance
Hope instillation
Humor
Hyperglycemia management
Hypervolemia management
Hypnosis
†Hypoglycemia management
Hypothermia treatment
Hypovolemia management
†Immunization/vaccination management
Impulse control training
Incident reporting
†Incision site care
Infant care
Infection control
Infection control: intraoperative
Infection protection
Insurance authorization
Intracranial pressure (ICP) monitoring
Intrapartal care
Intrapartal care: high-risk delivery
Intravenous (IV) insertion
Intravenous (IV) therapy
†Invasive hemodynamic monitoring
Kangaroo care
Labor induction
Labor suppression
Laboratory data interpretation
†Lactation counseling
Lactation suppression

Laser precautions
Latex precautions
Learning facilitation
Learning readiness enhancement
Leech therapy
Limit setting
Malignant hyperthermia precautions
†Mechanical ventilation
Mechanical ventilatory weaning
Medication administration
*Medication administration: ear
Medication administration: enteral
*Medication administration: epidural
*Medication administration: eye
*Medication administration: inhalation
Medication administration: interpleural
*Medication administration: intradermal
*Medication administration: intramuscular (IM)
Medication administration: intraosseous
*Medication administration: intravenous (IV)
†Medication administration: oral
*Medication administration: rectal
*Medication administration: skin
*Medication administration: subcutaneous
*Medication administration: vaginal
†Medication administration: ventricular reservoir
†Medication management
Medication prescribing
†Meditation facilitation
Memory training
Milieu therapy
†Mood management
Multidisciplinary care conference
†Music therapy
†Mutual goal setting
Nail care
*Nausea management
Neurologic monitoring
†Newborn care
†Newborn monitoring
†Nonnutritive sucking
Normalization promotion
Nutrition management
Nutrition therapy
Nutritional counseling
Nutritional monitoring
Oral health maintenance
Oral health promotion
Oral health restoration
Order transcription
Organ procurement
†Ostomy care
†Oxygen therapy
Pain management
Parent education: adolescent
Parent education: childrearing family
*Parent education: infant
*Parenting promotion
Pass facilitation
Patient contracting
Patient-controlled analgesia (PCA) assistance
Patient rights protection
Per review
†Pelvic muscle exercise
Perineal care
Peripheral sensation management

Peripherally inserted central (PIC) catheter care
Peritoneal dialysis therapy
*Pessary management
Phlebotomy: arterial blood sample
Phlebotomy: blood unit acquisition
Phlebotomy: venous blood sample
†Phototherapy: neonate
Physical restraint
Physician support
Pneumatic tourniquet precautions
†Positioning
Positioning: intraoperative
Positioning: neurologic
Positioning: wheelchair
Postanesthesia care
Postmortem care
Postpartal care
Preceptor: employee
Preceptor: student
†Preconception counseling
Pregnancy termination care
Prenatal care
†Preoperative coordination
†Preparatory sensory information
†Presence
Pressure management
†Pressure ulcer care
†Pressure ulcer prevention
Product evaluation
*Program development
Progressive muscle relaxation
*Prompted voiding
Prosthesis care
*Pruritus management
Quality monitoring
Radiation therapy management
†Rape-trauma treatment
Reality orientation
Recreation therapy
Rectal prolapse management
Referral
*Religious addiction prevention
*Religious ritual enhancement
†Reminiscence therapy
Reproductive technology management
†Research data collection
*Resiliency promotion
Respiratory monitoring
Respite care
Resuscitation
Resuscitation: fetus
Resuscitation: neonate
Risk identification
Risk identification: childbearing family
*Risk identification: genetic
Role enhancement
Seclusion
Security enhancement
Seizure management
Seizure precautions
Self-awareness enhancement
Self-care assistance
Self-care assistance: bathing/hygiene
Self-care assistance: dressing/grooming
Self-care assistance: feeding
Self-care assistance: toileting
Self-esteem enhancement
Self-modification assistance
Self-responsibility facilitation

Sexual counseling
Shift report
Shock management
Shock management: cardiac
Shock management: vasogenic
Shock management: volume
Shock prevention
†Sibling support
Simple guided imagery
Simple massage
Simple relaxation therapy
†Skin care: topical treatments
Skin surveillance
Sleep enhancement
†Smoking cessation assistance
†Socialization enhancement
Specimen management
*Spiritual growth facilitation
Spiritual support
Splinting
*Sports-injury prevention: youth
*Staff development
Staff supervision
Subarachnoid hemorrhage precautions
Substance use prevention
Substance use treatment
†Substance use treatment: Alcohol withdrawal
Substance use treatment: Drug withdrawal
Substance use treatment: Overdose
†Suicide prevention
Supply management
Support group
Support system enhancement
Surgical assistance
Surgical precautions
†Surgical preparation
Surveillance
*Surveillance: community
Surveillance: late pregnancy
*Surveillance: remote electronic
Surveillance: safety
Sustenance support
Suturing
Swallowing therapy
†Teaching: disease process
†Teaching: group
Teaching: individual
*Teaching: infant nutrition
*Teaching: infant safety
Teaching: preoperative
Teaching: prescribed activity/exercise
Teaching: prescribed diet
Teaching: prescribed medication
†Teaching: procedure/treatment
Teaching: psychomotor skill
Teaching: safe sex
Teaching: sexuality
*Teaching: toddler nutrition
*Teaching: toddler safety
Technology management
†Telephone consultation
*Telephone follow-up
Temperature regulation
Temperature regulation: intraoperative
†Therapeutic play
†Therapeutic touch
Therapy group
Total parenteral nutrition (TPN) administration

Touch
Traction/immobilization care
Transcutaneous electrical nerve
  stimulation (TENS)
†Transport
†Triage: disaster
*Triage: emergency center
*Triage: telephone
Truth telling
Tube care
Tube care: chest
†Tube care: gastrointestinal
Tube care: umbilical line

†Tube care: urinary
Tube care: ventriculostomy/lumbar drain
Ultrasonography: limited obstetric
Unilateral neglect management
Urinary bladder training
Urinary catheterization
†Urinary catheterization: intermittent
†Urinary elimination management
Urinary habit training
Urinary incontinence care
Urinary incontinence care: enuresis
Urinary retention care
Values clarification

*Vehicle safety promotion
†Venous access devices (VAD)
  maintenance
†Ventilation assistance
†Visitation facilitation
Vital signs monitoring
*Vomiting management
Weight gain assistance
Weight management
Weight reduction assistance
†Wound care
Wound care: closed drainage
Wound irrigation

# APPENDIX 19
# NURSING OUTCOMES CLASSIFICATION

## 19-1 | Steps for implementing NOC in a clinical practice setting

### ESTABLISH ORGANIZATIONAL COMMITMENT
- Establish commitment of key personnel in the organization.
- Identify key person responsible for implementation (e.g., person in charge of nursing informatics).
- Create an implementation task force with representatives from key areas.
- Provide NOC book to all members of the task force and staff on the units where NOC will be implemented.
- Have key individuals sign onto the Center for Nursing Classification List Serve.

### PREPARE AN IMPLEMENTATION PLAN
- Write specific goals to be accomplished.
- Keep key personnel informed of progress throughout the planning and implementation stages.
- Do a force field analysis to determine driving and restraining forces.
- Prepare materials for an in-house evaluation.
- Choose 1 to 3 pilot units for implementation. Get members from these units involved in the planning.
- Develop a written timeline for implementation.
- Review current system and determine the sequence of actions to integrate NOC.
- Create work groups of expert clinical users to review NOC, indicators, and measures for use on the pilot units.
- Identify which of the NOC are most appropriate for the unit. This can be done by reviewing outcomes currently used on the unit and determining the NOC most appropriate for measuring the concept. The outcome and definition should not be changed.

- Review each NO and decide if indicators will be used and which are critical to document. Indicators can be made more specific if needed, e.g.. replacing IER or WNL with values. Indicators can be added if needed. The five point measurement scale should be retained, but the words used to anchor the scale can be made more specific if desired. If you add indicators or make changes in the wording of the scale, we would appreciate your sharing this with the research team.
- Distribute the work of the clinical experts to other users for evaluation.
- Determine the variables of the total nursing data set. Work to ensure that all units are collecting data on all variables in a uniform manner and that all nursing data are retrievable. Be sure the data set includes the Nursing Minimum Data Set variables.
- Identify the learning needs of staff and plan ways to address these.

### CARRY OUT THE IMPLEMENTATION PLAN
- Develop the screen/forms for implementation.
- Provide training time for staff.
- Implement NOC on the pilot units and obtain feedback. Use staff to clarify issues and concerns.
- Update content as needed.
- Use data from the pilot units in housewide presentations.
- Implement NOC housewide.
- Collect postimplementation evaluation data and make changes as needed. Identify key items to use for on-going evaluation and continue to monitor and maintain the system.
- Provide feedback to the Iowa Outcomes Research Team.

From Johnson M and Maas M, eds: *Nursing outcomes classification (NOC)*, St Louis, 1997, Mosby.

## 19-2 | NOC outcomes

| | | |
|---|---|---|
| Abuse cessation | Bone healing | Child development: 2 months |
| Abuse protection | Bowel continence | Child development: 4 months |
| Abuse recovery: emotional | Bowel elimination | Child development: 6 months |
| Abuse recovery: financial | Breastfeeding establishment: infant | Child development: 12 months |
| Abuse recovery: physical | Breastfeeding establishment: maternal | Child development: 2 years |
| Abuse recovery: sexual | Breastfeeding: maintenance | Child development: 3 years |
| †Abuse behavior self-control | Breastfeeding: weaning | Child development: 4 years |
| †Acceptance: health status | Cardiac pump effectiveness | Child development: 5 years |
| *Activity tolerance | Caregiver adaptation to patient | Child development: middle childhood |
| Adherence behavior | institutionalization | (6-11 years) |
| †Aggression control | Caregiver emotional health | Child development: adolescence |
| Ambulation: walking | Caregiver home care readiness | (12-17 years) |
| Ambulation: wheelchair | Caregiver lifestyle disruption | Circulation status |
| †Anxiety control | Caregiver-patient relationship | *Coagulation status |
| *Aspiration control | Caregiver performance: direct care | Cognitive ability |
| *Asthma control | Caregiver performance: indirect care | Cognitive orientation |
| Balance | Caregiver physical health | †Comfort level |
| *Blood glucose control | Caregiver stressors | Communication ability |
| Blood transfusion reaction control | Caregiver well-being | Communication: expressive ability |
| Body image | Caregiving endurance potential | †Communication: receptive ability |
| †Body positioning: self-initiated | Child adaptation to hospitalization | *Community competence |

From Johnson M, Maas M, Moorhead S: *Nursing Outcomes Classification (NOC)*, ed. 2, St. Louis, 2000, Mosby.
*Outcomes new to the second edition.
†Outcomes revised for the second edition.

*Community health status
*Community health: immunity
*Community risk control: chronic disease
*Community risk control: communicable disease
*Community risk control: lead exposure
Compliance behavior
Concentration
Coping
Decision making
*Depression control
*Depression level
*Dialysis access integrity
Dignified dying
†Distorted thought control
Electrolyte & acid/base balance
†Endurance
Energy conservation
*Family coping
*Family environment: internal
*Family functioning
*Family health status
*Family integrity
*Family normalization
*Family participation in professional care
†Fear control
*Fetal status: antepartum
*Fetal status: intrapartum
Fluid balance
Grief resolution
Growth
Health beliefs
Health beliefs: perceived ability to perform
Health beliefs: perceived control
Health beliefs: perceived resources
Health beliefs: perceived threat
Health orientation
Health promoting behavior
Health seeking behavior
*Hearing compensation behavior
Hope
Hydration
Identity
†Immobility consequences: physiological
Immobility consequences: psycho-cognitive
Immune hypersensitivity control
Immune status
†Immunization behavior
†Impulse control
Infection status
Information processing
Joint movement: active
Joint movement: passive
Knowledge: breastfeeding
Knowledge: child safety
*Knowledge: conception prevention
*Knowledge: diabetes management
Knowledge: diet
Knowledge: disease process
Knowledge: energy conservation
*Knowledge: fertility promotion
Knowledge: health behaviors
*Knowledge: health promotion
Knowledge: health resources
*Knowledge: illness care
*Knowledge: infant care
Knowledge: infection control
*Knowledge: labor & delivery

*Knowledge: maternal-child health
Knowledge: medication
Knowledge: personal safety
*Knowledge: postpartum
*Knowledge: preconception
*Knowledge: pregnancy
Knowledge: prescribed activity
*Knowledge: sexual functioning
Knowledge: substance use control
Knowledge: treatment procedure(s)
*Knowledge: treatment regimen
Leisure participation
Loneliness
*Maternal status: antepartum
*Maternal status: intrapartum
*Maternal status: postpartum
*Medication response
Memory
Mobility level
Mood equilibrium
Muscle function
Neglect recovery
Neurological status
Neurological status: autonomic
Neurological status: central motor control
Neurological status: consciousness
Neurological status: cranial sensory/motor function
Neurological status: spinal sensory/motor function
*Newborn adaptation
Nutritional status
Nutritional status: biochemical measures
Nutritional status: body mass
Nutritional status: energy
Nutritional status: food & fluid intake
Nutritional status: nutrient intake
Oral health
†Pain control
Pain: disruptive effects
Pain level
*Pain: psychological response
Parent–infant attachment
Parenting
Parenting: social safety
Participation: health care decisions
Physical aging status
*Physical fitness
Physical maturation: female
Physical maturation: male
Play participation
*Prenatal health behavior
*Preterm infant organization
Psychomotor energy
Psychosocial adjustment: life change
Quality of life
*Respiratory status: airway patency
†Respiratory status: gas exchange
Respiratory status: ventilation
Rest
Risk control
Risk control: alcohol use
*Risk control: cancer
*Risk control: cardiovascular health
Risk control: drug use
*Risk control: hearing impairment
Risk control: sexually transmitted diseases (STDs)
Risk control: tobacco use
Risk control: unintended pregnancy

*Risk control: visual impairment
Risk detection
Role performance
Safety behavior: fall prevention
Safety behavior: home physical environment
Safety behavior: personal
Safety status: falls occurrence
Safety status: physical injury
Self-care: activities of daily living (ADL)
Self-care: bathing
Self-care: dressing
Self-care: eating
Self-care: grooming
Self-care: hygiene
Self-care: instrumental activities of daily living (IADL)
Self-care: non-parenteral medication
Self-care: oral hygiene
Self-care: parenteral medication
Self-care: toileting
*Self-direction of care
Self-esteem
Self-mutilation restraint
*Sensory function: cutaneous
*Sensory function: hearing
*Sensory function: proprioception
*Sensory function: taste & smell
*Sensory function: vision
*Sexual functioning
*Sexual identity: acceptance
*Skeletal function
†Sleep
Social interaction skills
Social involvement
Social support
Spiritual well-being
Substance addiction consequences
*Suffering level
†Suicide self-restraint
*Swallowing status
*Swallowing status: esophageal phase
*Swallowing status: oral phase
*Swallowing status: pharyngeal phase
†Symptom control
Symptom severity
*Symptom severity: perimenopause
*Symptom severity: premenstrual syndrome (PMS)
*Systemic toxin clearance: dialysis
Thermoregulation
Thermoregulation: neonate
Tissue integrity: skin & mucous membranes
Tissue perfusion: abdominal organs
†Tissue perfusion: cardiac
Tissue perfusion: cerebral
Tissue perfusion: peripheral
Tissue perfusion: pulmonary
Transfer performance
Treatment behavior: illness or injury
Urinary continence
Urinary elimination
*Vision compensation behavior
Vital signs status
*Weight control
Well-being
Will to live
Wound healing: primary intention
Wound healing: secondary intention

# APPENDIX 20 | OMAHA CLASSIFICATION SYSTEM

## PROBLEM CLASSIFICATION SCHEME:

An orderly, nonexhaustive, mutually exclusive, client-focused taxonomy of domains, modifiers, problems, and signs/symptoms addressed by nurses and other professionals. The four domains represent priority areas of professional and client health-related concerns. Each of the 40 problems may be referenced as health promotion, potential, or deficit/impairment/actual as well as individual or family. Actual problems are described by a cluster of signs and symptoms. As an open system of language and codes, the Problem Classification Scheme is used as a comprehensive method for collecting, sorting, classifying, documenting, and analyzing client data.

## INTERVENTION SCHEME:

An organized framework designed to address specific client problems or nursing diagnoses and consisting of three levels of nursing actions or activities. Four broad categories of interventions are further delineated by targets or objects of nursing action and by client-specific information generated by the nurse or other professional. Because the Intervention Scheme is the basis for planning and intervening, it enables professionals to describe and communicate their practice including improving, maintaining, or restoring health and preventing illness. The Scheme is intended to be used in conjunction with the Problem Classification Scheme and the Problem Rating Scale for Outcomes.

## PROBLEM RATING SCALE FOR OUTCOMES:

A five-point, Likert-type scale for measuring the entire range of severity for the concepts of knowledge, behavior, and status. Each of the three subscales is a continuum providing an evaluation framework for examining problem-specific client ratings at regular or predictable times. Suggested times include admission, specific interim points, and dismissal. The ratings are a guide for the nurse or other professional as client care is planned and provided; the ratings offer a method to monitor client progress throughout the period of service. A comprehensive problem-solving model is created when the Problem Rating Scale for Outcomes is used with the other two schemes of the Omaha System.

## Domains and problems of the problem classification scheme

### DOMAIN I. ENVIRONMENTAL:

The material resources, physical surroundings, and substances both internal and external to the client, home, neighborhood, and broader community; appears at the first level of the Problem Classification Scheme.
01. Income
02. Sanitation
03. Residence
04. Neighborhood/workplace safety
05. Other

### DOMAIN II. PSYCHOSOCIAL:

Patterns of behavior, communication, relationships, and development; appears at the first level of the Problem Classification Scheme.
06. Communication with community resources
07. Social contact
08. Role change
09. Interpersonal relationship
10. Spirituality
11. Grief
12. Emotional stability
13. Human sexuality
14. Caretaking/parenting
15. Neglected child/adult
16. Abused child/adult
17. Growth and development
18. Other

### DOMAIN III. PHYSIOLOGICAL:

Functional status of processes that maintain life; appears at the first level of the Problem Classification Scheme.

19. Hearing
20. Vision
21. Speech and language
22. Dentition
23. Cognition
24. Pain
25. Consciousness
26. Integument
27. Neuromusculoskeletal function
28. Respiration
29. Circulation
30. Digestion-hydration
31. Bowel function
32. Genitourinary function
33. Antepartum/postpartum
34. Other

### DOMAIN IV. HEALTH RELATED BEHAVIORS:

Activities that maintain or promote wellness, promote recovery, or maximize rehabilitation potential; appears at the first level of the Problem Classification Scheme.
35. Nutrition
36. Sleep and rest patterns
37. Physical activity
38. Personal hygiene
39. Substance misuse
40. Family planning
41. Health care supervision
42. Prescribed medication regimen
43. Technical procedure
44. Other

# Intervention scheme

## I HEALTH TEACHING, GUIDANCE, AND COUNSELING

Health teaching, guidance, and counseling are nursing activities that range from giving information, anticipating client problems, encouraging client action and responsibility for self care and coping, to assisting with decision making and problem solving. The overlapping concepts occur on a continuum with the variation due to the client's self-direction capabilities.

## II TREATMENTS AND PROCEDURES

Treatments and procedures are technical nursing activities directed toward preventing signs and symptoms, identifying risk factors and early signs and symptoms, and decreasing or alleviating signs and symptoms.

## III CASE MANAGEMENT

Case management includes nursing activities of coordination, advocacy, and referral. These activities involve facilitating service delivery on behalf of the client, communicating with health and human service providers, promoting assertive client communication, and guiding the client toward use of appropriate community resources.

## IV SURVEILLANCE

Surveillance includes nursing activities of detection, measurement, critical analysis, and monitoring to indicate client status in relation to a given condition or phenomenon.

01. Anatomy/physiology
02. Behavior modification
03. Bladder care
04. Bonding
05. Bowel care
06. Bronchial hygiene
07. Cardiac care
08. Caretaking/parenting skills
09. Cast care
10. Communication
11. Coping skills
12. Day care/respite
13. Discipline
14. Dressing change/wound care
15. Durable medical equipment
16. Education
17. Employment
18. Environment
19. Exercises
20. Family planning
21. Feeding procedures
22. Finances
23. Food
24. Gait training
25. Growth/development
26. Homemaking
27. Housing
28. Interaction
29. Lab findings
30. Legal system
31. Medical/dental care
32. Medication action/side effects
33. Medication administration
34. Medication set-up
35. Mobility/transfers
36. Nursing care, supplementary
37. Nutrition
38. Nutritionist
39. Ostomy care
40. Other community resource
41. Personal care
42. Positioning
43. Rehabilitation
44. Relaxation/breathing techniques
45. Rest/sleep
46. Safety
47. Screening
48. Sickness/injury care
49. Signs/symptoms—mental/emotional
50. Signs/symptoms—physical
51. Skin care
52. Social work/counseling
53. Specimen collection
54. Spiritual care
55. Stimulation/nurturance
56. Stress management
57. Substance use
58. Supplies
59. Support group
60. Support system
61. Transportation
62. Wellness
63. Other

## Problem rating scale for outcomes

| Concept | 1 | 2 | 3 | 4 | 5 |
|---|---|---|---|---|---|
| **Knowledge:** the ability of the client to remember and interpret information | No knowledge | Minimal knowledge | Basic knowledge | Adequate knowledge | Superior knowledge |
| **Behavior:** the observable responses, actions, or activities of the client fitting the occasion or purpose | Not appropriate | Rarely appropriate | Inconsistently appropriate | Usually appropriate | Consistently appropriate |
| **Status:** the condition of the client in relation to objective and subjective defining characteristics | Extreme signs/symptoms | Severe signs/symptoms | Moderate signs/symptoms | Minimal signs/symptoms | No signs/symptoms |

# APPENDIX 21

# 2003-2004 NURSING DIAGNOSES SUPPLEMENT

## 21-1 New NANDA-approved nursing diagnoses and definitions

### COMMUNICATION, READINESS FOR ENHANCED

A pattern of exchanging information and ideas with others that is sufficient for meeting one's needs and life's goals and can be strengthened

**Defining Characteristics**

Expresses willingness to enhance communication
Able to speak or write a language
Forms words, phrases, and language
Expresses thoughts and feelings
Uses and interprets nonverbal cues appropriately
Expresses satisfaction with ability to share information and ideas with others

### COPING, READINESS FOR ENHANCED

A pattern of cognitive and behavioral efforts to manage demands that is sufficient for well-being and can be strengthened.

**Defining Characteristics**

Defines stressors as manageable
Seeks social support
Uses a broad range of problem-oriented and emotion-oriented strategies
Uses spiritual resources
Acknowledges power
Seeks knowledge of new strategies
Is aware of possible environmental changes

### FAMILY PROCESSES, READINESS FOR ENHANCED

A pattern of family functioning that is sufficient to support the well-being of family members and can be strengthened

**Defining Characteristics**

Expresses willingness to enhance family dynamics
Family functioning meets physical, social, and psychological needs of family members
Activities support the safety and growth of family members
Communication is adequate
Relationships are generally positive; interdependent with community; family task are accomplished
Family roles are flexible and appropriate for developmental stages
Respect for family members is evident
Family adapts to change
Boundaries of family members are maintained
Energy level of family supports activities of daily living
Family resilience is evident
Balance exists between autonomy and cohesiveness

### FLUID BALANCE, READINESS FOR ENHANCED

A pattern of equilibrium between fluid volume and chemical composition of body fluids that is sufficient for meeting physical needs and can be strengthened

**Defining Characteristics**

Expresses willingness to enhance fluid balance
Stable weight
Moist mucous membranes
Food and fluid intake adequate for daily needs
Straw-colored urine with specific gravity within normal limits
Good tissue turgor
No excessive thirst
Urine output appropriate for intake
No evidence of edema or dehydration

### KNOWLEDGE OF (specify), READINESS FOR ENHANCED

The presence or acquisition of cognitive information related to a specific topic is sufficient for meeting health-related goals and can be strengthened

**Defining Characteristics**

Expresses an interest in learning
Explains knowledge of the topic
Behaviors congruent with expressed knowledge
Describes previous experiences pertaining to the topic

### NUTRITION, READINESS FOR ENHANCED

A pattern of nutrient intake that is sufficient for meeting metabolic needs and can be strengthened

**Defining Characteristics**

Expresses willingness to enhance nutrition
Eats regularly
Consumes adequate food and fluid
Expresses knowledge of healthy food and fluid choices
Follows an appropriate standard for intake (e.g., the food pyramid or America Diabetic Association guidelines)
Safe preparation and storage for food and fluids
Attitude toward eating and drinking is congruent with health goals

### PARENTING, READINESS FOR ENHANCED

A pattern of providing an environment for children or other dependent person(s) that is sufficient to nurture growth and development and can be strengthened

**Defining Characteristics**

Expresses willingness to enhance parenting
Children or other dependent person(s) express satisfaction with home environment
Emotional and tacit support of children or dependent person(s) is evident; bonding or attachment evident
Physical and emotional needs of children/dependent person(s) are met
Realistic expectations of children/dependent person(s) exhibited

### SELF-CONCEPT, READINESS FOR ENHANCED

A pattern of perceptions or ideas about the self that is sufficient for well-being and can be strengthened

**Defining Characteristics**

Expresses willingness to enhance self-concept
Expresses satisfaction with thoughts about self, sense of worthiness, role performance, body image, and personal identity
Actions are congruent with expressed feelings and thoughts
Expresses confidence in abilities
Accepts strengths and limitations

## SLEEP, READINESS FOR ENHANCED

A pattern of natural, periodic suspension of consciousness that provides adequate rest, sustains a desired lifestyle, and can be strengthened

### Defining Characteristics

Expresses willingness to enhance sleep
Amount of sleep and REM sleep is congruent with developmental needs
Expresses a feeling of being rested after sleep
Follows sleep routines that promote sleep habits
Occasional or infrequent use of medications to induce sleep

## SUDDEN INFANT DEATH SYNDROME, RISK FOR

Presence of risk factors for sudden death of an infant under 1 year of age

### Risk Factors
*Modifiable*

Infants placed to sleep in the prone or side-lying position
Prenatal and/or postnatal infant smoke exposure
Infant overheating/overwrapping
Soft underlayment/loose articles in the sleep environment
Delayed or nonattendance of prenatal care

*Potentially Modifiable*

Low birth weight
Prematurity
Young maternal age

*Nonmodifiable*

Male gender
Ethnicity (e.g., African American, Native American race of mother)

Seasonality of SIDS deaths (higher in winter and fall months)
SIDS mortality peaks between infant age of 2-4 months

## THERAPEUTIC REGIMEN MANAGEMENT, READINESS FOR ENHANCED

A pattern of regulating and integrating into daily living a program(s) for treatment of illness and its sequelae that is sufficient for meeting health-related goals and can be strengthened

### Defining Characteristics

Expresses desire to manage the treatment of illness and prevention of sequelae
Choices of daily living are appropriate for meeting the goals of treatment or prevention
Expresses little to no difficulty with regulation/integration of one or more prescribed regimens for treatment of illness or prevention of complications
Describes reduction of risk factors for progression of illness and sequelae
No unexpected acceleration of illness symptoms

## URINARY ELIMINATION, READINESS FOR ENHANCED

A pattern of urinary functions that is sufficient for meeting eliminatory needs and can be strengthened

### Defining Characteristics

Expresses willingness to enhance urinary elimination
Urine is straw colored with no odor
Specific gravity is within normal limits
Amount of output is within normal limits for age and other factors
Positions self for emptying of bladder
Fluid intake is adequate for daily needs

## 21-2 | Revised NANDA-approved nursing diagnoses and definitions

### NAUSEA

A subjective unpleasant, wavelike sensation in the back of the throat, epigastrium, or abdomen that may lead to the urge or need to vomit

#### Defining Characteristics

Report of nausea ("sick to my stomach")
Increased salivation
Aversion toward food
Gagging sensation
Sour taste in mouth
Increased swallowing

#### Related Factors
*Treatment Related*

Gastric irritation: Pharmaceuticals (e.g., aspirin, nonsteroidal anti-inflammatory drugs, steroids, antibiotics), alcohol, iron, and blood
Gastric distention: Delayed gastric emptying caused by pharmacological interventions (e.g., narcotics administration, anesthesia agents)
Pharmaceuticals (e.g., analgesics, antiviral for HIV, aspirin, opioids, chemotherapeutic agents)
Toxins (e.g., radiotherapy)

*Biophysical*

Biochemical disorders (e.g., uremia, diabetic ketoacidosis, pregnancy)
Cardiac pain
Cancer of stomach or intra-abdominal tumors (e.g., pelvic or colorectal cancers)
Esophageal or pancreatic disease
Gastric distention due to delayed gastric emptying, pyloric intestinal obstruction, genitourinary and biliary distension, upper bowel sta-

sis, external compression of the stomach (liver, spleen, or other organ enlargement which slows the stomach functioning (squashed stomach syndrome), excess food intake
Gastric irritation due to pharyngeal and/or peritoneal inflammation
Liver or splenetic capsule stretch
Local tumors (e.g., acoustic neuroma, primary or secondary brain tumors, bone metastases at base of skull)
Motion sickness, Menière's disease, or labyrinthitis
Physical factors (e.g., increased intracranial pressure, meningitis)
Toxins (e.g., tumor-produced peptides, abnormal metabolites due to cancer)

*Situational*

Psychological factors (e.g., pain, fear, anxiety, noxious odors, taste, unpleasant visual stimulation)

### SPIRITUAL DISTRESS

Impaired ability to experience and integrate meaning and purpose in life through a person's connectedness with self, others, art, music, literature, nature, or a power greater than oneself

#### Defining Characteristics
*Connections to Self*

Expresses lack of:
Hope
Meaning and purpose in life
Peace/serenity
Acceptance
Love
Forgiveness of self
Courage
Anger

Guilt

Poor coping

### *Connections With Others*

Refuses interactions with spiritual leaders

Refuses interactions with friends, family

Verbalizes being separated from their support system

Expresses alienation

### *Connections With Art, Music, Literature, Nature*

Inability to express previous state of creativity (singing/listening to music/writing)

No interest in nature

No interest in reading spiritual literature

### *Connections With Power Greater Than Self*

Inability to pray

Inability to participate in religious activities

Expresses being abandoned by or having anger toward God

Inability to experience the transcendent

Requests to see a religious leader

Sudden changes in spiritual practices

Inability to be introspective/inward turning

Expresses being without hope, suffering

### **Related Factors**

Self-alienation

Loneliness/social alienation

Anxiety

Sociocultural deprivation

Death and dying of self or others

Pain

Life change

Chronic illness of self or others

## SPIRITUAL WELL-BEING, READINESS FOR ENHANCED

Ability to experience and integrate meaning and purpose in life through connectedness with self, others, art, music, literature, nature, or a power greater than oneself

### **Defining Characteristics**
### *Connections to Self*

Desire for enhanced: hope, meaning and purpose in life, peace/serenity, acceptance, surrender, love, forgiveness of self, satisfying philosophy of life, joy, courage

Heightened coping

Meditation

### *Connections With Others*

Provides service to others

Requests interactions with spiritual leaders

Requests forgiveness of others

Requests interactions with friends, family

### *Connections With Art, Music, Literature, Nature*

Displays creative energy (e.g., writing, poetry)

Sings/listens to music

Reads spiritual literature

Spends time outdoors

### *Connections With Power Greater Than Self*

Prays

Reports mystical experiences

Participates in religious activities

Expresses reverence, awe

# APPENDIX 22

# BIOTERRORISM AND EMERGING INFECTIONS

**bioterrorism** the calculated use, or threatened use, of biologic agents against civilian populations in order to attain political or ideological goals by intimidation or coercion.

**biotoxins** poisons produced by and derived from plants and animals. Biotoxins include abrin, from the jequirity bean or rosary pea *(Abrus precatorius)*; ricin, from castor beans; and strychnine, from *Strychnos nux vomica*. Biotoxins can be absorbed by ingesting or inhaling the toxin. Inhalation of ricin or abrin causes severe respiratory distress and ingestion of these agents causes nausea and vomiting; multisystem organ failure and death may occur. Strychnine attacks communication between the nerves and muscles and may lead to death from respiratory failure as the respiratory muscles tire. Treatment consists of removal of the toxin from the body and supportive care.

**blister agents/vesicants** chemicals that cause blistering of the skin or mucous membranes on contact. These agents include phosgene oxime, lewisite, distilled mustard, mustard gas, nitrogen mustard, sesqui mustard, and sulfur mustard. Exposure is mainly by inhalation or by contact with the skin or eyes. Inhalation causes shortness of breath, tachypnea, and hemoptysis, and death may result from the accumulation of fluid in the lungs; contact with the skin causes blistering and necrosis; and ocular contact causes swelling of the eyelids and corneal damage and can lead to blindness. Exposure to high doses affects the cardiovascular and nervous systems and may lead to cardiac arrest, convulsions, and coma. If these agents are ingested, nausea, vomiting, hematemesis, and diarrhea result. No antidote exists for most blister agents and treatment consists of removal of clothing, washing of the exposed areas, and supportive care. Lewisite can be neutralized by the application of British anti-Lewisite if it is done soon after exposure.

**blood agents** poisons that affect the body by being absorbed into the blood. Blood agents include arsine and cyanide. Exposure to both may occur by inhalation, and cyanide exposure may also occur by ingestion and absorption through the skin and eyes. Arsine causes hemolysis, resulting in generalized weakness, jaundice, delirium, and renal failure; high doses may result in death. There is no antidote and treatment is supportive. Cyanide prevents cells from using oxygen, leading to cell death, and poisoning especially affects the cardiovascular and nervous systems and can lead to heart and brain damage and death from respiratory failure. Treatment consists of the administration of an antidote and supportive care.

**Category A Diseases/Agents** bioterrorism diseases or agents that can be easily disseminated or transmitted from person to person, result in high mortality rates and have the potential for major public health impact, might cause public panic and social disruption, and require special action for public health preparedness.

**Category B Diseases/Agents** bioterrorism diseases or agents that are moderately easy to disseminate, result in moderate morbidity rates and low mortality rates, and require specific enhancements of CDC's diagnostic capacity and enhanced disease surveillance.

**Category C Diseases/Agents** emerging pathogens that could be engineered for mass dissemination in the future because of availability, ease of production and dissemination, and potential for high morbidity and mortality rates and major health impact.

**caustics (acids)** chemicals, such as hydrofluoric acid, that cause burns and corrosion of the skin, eyes, and mucous membranes on contact. Exposure may be by inhalation or ingestion. Treatment of exposure to these agents involves irrigation of exposed areas and neutralization of the substance.

**choking/lung/pulmonary agents** chemicals that cause severe irritation or swelling of the respiratory tract. Agents include ammonia, bromine, chlorine, osmium tetraoxide, phosgene, phosphine, and phosphorus. When inhaled, they cause damage to the lungs, either by their corrosive effects or by cytotoxicity, leading to respiratory distress and death from respiratory failure. Treatment consists of supportive care.

**dirty bomb** an explosive device that disperses radioactive material over a wide area, contaminating land, buildings, and people; its purpose is to cause fear and to make an area unusable for a long time.

**incapacitating agents** drugs that interfere with the inability to think clearly or cause unconsciousness or some other altered state of consciousness; their primary use is not to kill, although they can be lethal in high doses. They include aerosolized opioids and the anticholinergic BZ. Treatment of exposure to incapacitating agents is supportive.

**Laboratory Response Network (LRN)** a network of federal, state, and local laboratories, established in 1999 by the Centers for Disease Control and Prevention (CDC), whose purpose is to provide the laboratory infrastructure and capacity to respond to biological and chemical terrorism and other public health emergencies.

**long-acting anticoagulants** compounds that interfere with the blood's clotting ability. Exposure leads to uncontrollable bleeding, resulting in shock. Treatment is by administration of vitamin K.

**LRN** abbreviation for **Laboratory Response Network.**

**nerve agents** chemicals that interfere with the proper functioning of the nervous system; they are highly potent and very small amounts can have serious effects. Nerve agents include sarin, soman, tabun, and VX. Exposure is by inhalation or by skin or eye contact. Nerve agents can also be mixed with water and can be used to poison water supplies so that people can be exposed by drinking contaminated water or getting contaminated water on the skin. These agents act by inhibiting acetylcholinesterase, which allows the muscles to be stimulated constantly, and fatigue of the muscles used for breathing can cause death from respiratory failure. Treatment consists of removing the agent from the body and administration of an antidote (which must be done within minutes of exposure).

**ricin** a poison made from waste produced in processing castor beans. It can take the form of a powder, mist, or pellet, or can be dissolved in water or weak acid and can be used as a poison by ingestion, inhalation, or injection. As little as 500 micrograms can be a fatal dose. It cannot be spread by person-to-person contact. Poisoning is treated by minimizing exposure and by supportive care. There is no antidote.

**riot control agents/tear gas** agents normally used for crowd control; they include the compounds chloroacetophenone, chlorobenzylidenemalononitrile, chloropicrin, bromobenzylcyanide, and benzoxazepine. They are used as liquids or aerosols and exposure is by inhalation or by contact with the eyes or skin. They incapacitate by irritating the area of contact and cause irritation of the skin and mucous membranes and respiratory distress. High doses can cause blindness and death. Treatment is by removal of clothing and removing the agent from the skin and eyes; effects cease shortly after the agent is removed.

**toxic alcohols** poisonous alcohols that can damage the heart, kidneys, and nervous system. Ethylene glycol, commonly used in antifreeze, is a toxic alcohol. Severe poisoning is caused only by ingestion and is marked by progressive stages of central nervous system depression, acidosis, and renal failure. Treatment consists of administration of an antidote, hemodialysis, and supportive care.

**vomiting agents** chemicals that induce nausea and vomiting. Vomiting agents include adamsite, diphenylchlorarsine, and diphenylcyanoarsine. They are used as aerosols, and exposure is primarily by inhalation, also by ingestion and by skin and eye contact. They initially act like tear gas their effects progress to difficulty in breathing, nausea, and vomiting. Effects are self-limited, generally disappearing within two hours. Death may occur with exposure to high concentrations in confined spaces.

**weapons of mass destruction (WMD)** weapons, such as nuclear or chemical weapons, whose purpose is to kill large numbers of people indiscriminately.

**WMD** abbreviation for **weapons of mass destruction.**

# COMMONLY USED ABBREVIATIONS

NOTE: Abbreviations in common use can vary widely from place to place. Each institution's list of acceptable abbreviations is the best authority for its records.

ā — Before
abd — Abdominal/abdomen
ABG — Arterial blood gas
ABO — Three basic blood groups
ACLS — Advanced cardiac life support
ADD — Attention deficit disorder
ADH — Antidiuretic hormone
ADL — Activities of daily living
AF — Atrial fibrillation
AFB — Acid-fast bacillus
AICD — Automatic implantable cardiac defibrillator
AIDS — Acquired immunodeficiency syndrome
AK — Above the knee
ALS — Advanced life support; amyotrophic lateral sclerosis
ALT — Alanine aminotransferase
AM — Morning
ama — Against medical advice
AMI — Acute myocardial infarction
A-P; AP; A/P — Anterior-posterior
ASD — Atrial septal defect
ASHD — Arteriosclerotic heart disease
AST — Aspartate aminotransferase (formerly SGOT)
A-V; AV; A/V — Arteriovenous; atrioventricular
Ba — Barium
BBB — Blood-brain barrier
BCLS — Basic cardiac life support
BE — Barium enema
bid; b.i.d. — Twice a day (bis in die)
BK — Below the knee
BM — Bowel movement
BMR — Basal metabolic rate
BP — Blood pressure; buccopulpal
BPH — Benign prostatic hypertrophy
bpm — Beats per minute
BRP — Bathroom privileges
BSA — Body surface area
BSE — Breast self-examination
BUN — Blood urea nitrogen
Bx — Biopsy
c̄ — With
Ca — Calcium; cancer; carcinoma
CABG — Coronary artery bypass graft
CAD — Coronary artery disease
C&S — Culture and sensitivity
CAT — Computerized (axial) tomography scan
CBC; cbc — Complete blood count
CC — Chief complaint

CCU — Coronary care unit; critical care unit
CF — Cystic fibrosis
CHD — Congenital heart disease; coronary heart disease
CHF — Congestive heart failure
CHO — Carbohydrate
CK — Creatinine kinase
CMV — Cytomegalovirus
CNS — Central nervous system
c/o — Complaints of
CO — Carbon monoxide; cardiac output
CO2 — Carbon dioxide
COLD — Chronic obstructive lung disease
COPD — Chronic obstructive pulmonary disease
CP — Cerebral palsy; cleft palate
CPAP — Continuous positive airway pressure
CPK — Creatine phosphokinase
CPR — Cardiopulmonary resuscitation
CSF — Cerebrospinal fluid
CT — Computed tomography
CVA — Cerebrovascular accident; costovertebral angle
CVP — Central venous pressure
CXR — Chest x-ray
D & C — Dilation (dilatation) and curettage
dc; DC; D/C — Discontinue
DIC — Disseminated intravascular coagulation
diff — Differential blood count
DKA — Diabetic ketoacidosis
DM — Diabetes mellitus, diastolic murmur
DNA — Deoxyribonucleic acid
DNR — Do not resuscitate
DOA — Dead on arrival
DOB — Date of birth
DOE — Dyspnea on exertion
DPT — Diphtheria-pertussis-tetanus
DRG — Diagnosis-related group
DSM-IV — *Diagnostic and Statistical Manual of Mental Disorders*
DT — Delirium tremens
DTR — Deep tendon reflex
D5W — Dextrose 5% in water
Dx — Diagnosis
EBV — Epstein-Barr virus
ECF — Extended care facility; extracellular fluid
ECG — Electrocardiogram, electrocardiograph
ECHO — Echocardiography
ECT — Electroconvulsive therapy
ED — Emergency department; effective dose

EDD — Estimated date of delivery
EEG — Electroencephalogram, electroencephalograph
EENT — Eye, ear, nose, and throat
ELISA — Enzyme-linked immunosorbent assay
EMG — Electromyogram
EMS — Emergency medical service
EMT — Emergency medical technician
ENT — Ear, nose, and throat
ER — Emergency room (hospital); external resistance
ERV — Expiratory reserve volume
ESR — Erythrocyte sedimentation rate
ESRD — End-stage renal disease
FBS — Fasting blood sugar
Fe — Iron
FEV — Forced expiratory volume
FH, Fhx — Family history
FHR — Fetal heart rate
FTT — Failure to thrive
FUO — Fever of unknown origin
fx — Fracture
GB — Gallbladder
GC — Gonococcus or gonorrheal
GI — Gastrointestinal
Grav I, II, etc. — Pregnancy one, two, three, etc. (Gravida)
GSW — Gunshot wound
gtt — Drops (guttae)
GU — Genitourinary
Gyn — Gynecology
H & P — History and physical
HAV — Hepatitis A virus
Hb — Hemoglobin
HBV — Hepatitis B virus
HCG — Human chorionic gonadotropin
HCT — Hematocrit
HDL — High-density lipoprotein
HEENT — Head, eye, ear, nose, and throat
Hg — Mercury
HIV — Human immunodeficiency (AIDS) virus
h/o — History of
H2O2 — Hydrogen peroxide
HPI — History of present illness
HR — Heart rate
HSV — Herpes simplex virus
HT; HTN — Hypertension
hx; Hx — History
I & O — Intake and output
IBW — Ideal body weight
ICP — Intracranial pressure
ICU — Intensive care unit
IDDM — Insulin-dependent diabetes mellitus
Ig — Immunoglobulin
IM — Intramuscular